Surgery

SCIENTIFIC PRINCIPLES
AND PRACTICE

Surgery SECOND EDITION

SCIENTIFIC PRINCIPLES AND PRACTICE

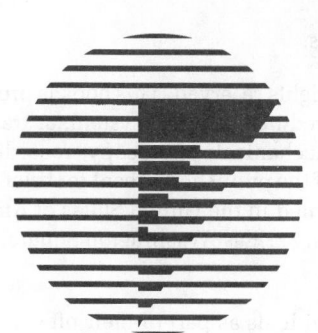

EDITOR-IN-CHIEF

Lazar J. Greenfield, MD
Frederick A. Coller Professor of Surgery
Chairman, Department of Surgery
University of Michigan Medical School
Surgeon-in-Chief
University of Michigan Hospitals
Ann Arbor, Michigan

ASSOCIATE EDITORS

Michael W. Mulholland, MD, PhD
Professor and Associate Chairman
Department of Surgery
University of Michigan Medical School
University of Michigan Hospitals
Ann Arbor, Michigan

Keith T. Oldham, MD
Professor of Surgery and Pediatrics
Duke University School of Medicine
Chief, Division of Pediatric Surgery
Duke University Medical Center
Durham, North Carolina

Gerald B. Zelenock, MD
Professor of Surgery
Section of Vascular Surgery
University of Michigan Medical School
University of Michigan Hospitals
Ann Arbor, Michigan

Keith D. Lillemoe, MD
Associate Professor of Surgery
Johns Hopkins University School of Medicine
Johns Hopkins Hospital
Baltimore, Maryland

With 183 contributors

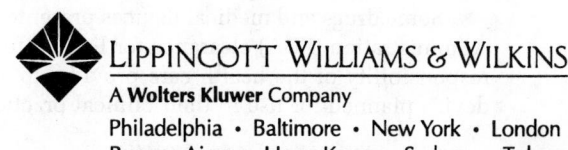

A **Wolters Kluwer** Company
Philadelphia · Baltimore · New York · London
Buenos Aires · Hong Kong · Sydney · Tokyo

Acquisitions Editor: Lisa McAllister
Associate Editor: Paula Callaghan
Associate Managing Editor: Grace R. Caputo
Production Manager: Caren Erlichman
Senior Production Coordinator: Kevin P. Johnson
Design Coordinator: Melissa Olson
Indexer: Alexandra Nickerson
Compositor: Tapsco, Inc.
Printer: Courier Book Company/Westford

Illustrations new to this edition were rendered by Holly R. Fischer, MFA.
Some radiographs in this book were electronically modified to enhance clarity.

Edition 2

Library of Congress Cataloging-in-Publication Data

Surgery: scientific principles and practice/edited by Lazar J. Greenfield . . . [et al.]
    with 183 contributors.—2nd ed.
        p. cm.
    Includes bibliographical references and index.
    ISBN 0-397-51481-6 (alk. paper)
    1. Surgery. 2. Medicine. I. Greenfield, Lazar J., 1934– .
    [DNLM: 1. Surgery. 2. Surgery, Operative. WO 100 S9617 1997]
    RD31.S922 1997
    617—dc20
    DNLM/DLC
    for Library of Congress   96-21918
                                                                     CIP

Care has been taken to confirm the accuracy of the information presented and to describe
generally accepted practices. However, the authors, editors, and publisher are not responsible for errors or omissions or for any consequences from application of the information in this book and make no warranty, express or implied, with respect to the
contents of the publication.

The authors, editors, and publisher have exerted every effort to ensure that drug
selection and dosage set forth in this text are in accordance with current recommendations and practice at the time of publication. However, in view of ongoing research,
changes in government regulations, and the constant flow of information relating to
drug therapy and drug reactions, the reader is urged to check the package insert for
each drug for any change in indications and dosage and for added warnings and precautions. This is particularly important when the recommended agent is a new or infrequently employed drug.

Some drugs and medical devices presented in this publication have Food and Drug
Administration (FDA) clearance for limited use in restricted research settings. It is the
responsibility of the health care provider to ascertain the FDA status of each drug or
device planned for use in their clinical practice.

9 8 7 6 5 4 3

Contributors

Dana K. Andersen, MD
Professor of Surgery
Chief, Section of Surgical Gastroenterology
Yale University School of Medicine
Chief, General Surgery Service
Yale–New Haven Hospital
New Haven, Connecticut

W. Scott Arnold, MD
Chief Resident in Surgery
University of Virginia Health Sciences Center
Charlottesville, Virginia

David A. August, MD
Associate Professor of Surgery
Cancer Institute of New Jersey
University of Medicine and Dentistry of New Jersey
Robert Wood Johnson Medical School
New Brunswick, New Jersey

William G. Austen, Jr., MD
Edward D. Churchill Professor of Surgery
Harvard Medical School
Surgeon-in-Chief
Massachusetts General Hospital
Boston, Massachusetts

Dennis F. Bandyk, MD, FACS
Professor of Surgery
Director, Vascular Surgery Division
University of South Florida College of Medicine
Tampa, Florida

Robert H. Bartlett, MD
Professor of Surgery
University of Michigan Medical School
University of Michigan Medical Center
Ann Arbor, Michigan

James M. Becker, MD
James Utley Professor and Chairman of Surgery
Boston University School of Medicine
Boston City Hospital
Surgeon-in-Chief
Boston University Medical Center Hospital
Boston, Massachusetts

Richard H. Bell, Jr., MD
Professor and Vice Chairman
Department of Surgery
University of Washington School of Medicine
Chief, Surgical Service
Department of Veterans Affairs Medical Center
Seattle, Washington

William D. Belville, MD
Associate Professor of Surgery
Section of Urology
University of Michigan Medical Center
Ann Arbor, Michigan

David A. Bloom, MD
Professor, Department of Surgery
University of Michigan Medical School
Chief, Pediatric Urology
C.S. Mott Children's Hospital
Ann Arbor, Michigan

C. Richard Boland, MD
Professor of Medicine
Chief, Division of Gastroenterology
University of California, San Diego, School of Medicine
UCSD Hospitals
Veterans Affairs Medical Center
La Jolla, California

Michael F. Boland, MD
Neurosurgeon
Neurosurgical Associates, Incorporated
St Louis, Missouri

Steven F. Bolling, MD
Associate Professor of Surgery
University of Michigan Medical School
Section of Thoracic Surgery
University of Michigan Hospitals
Ann Arbor, Michigan

R. Morton Bolman III, MD
Professor and Chief
Division of Cardiovascular and Thoracic Surgery
University of Minnesota Medical School—Minneapolis
Minneapolis, Minnesota

Edward L. Bove, MD
Professor of Surgery
University of Michigan Medical School
Chief, Pediatric Cardiovascular Surgery
C.S. Mott Children's Hospital
Ann Arbor, Michigan

Robert S. Bresalier, MD
Associate Professor of Medicine
University of Michigan Medical School
Ann Arbor, Michigan
Director, Gastrointestinal Oncology
Henry Ford Health Sciences Center
Detroit, Michigan

David C. Brewster, MD
Clinical Professor of Surgery
Harvard Medical School
Massachusetts General Hospital
Boston, Massachusetts

Jonathan S. Bromberg, MD, PhD
Associate Professor of Surgery and Microbiology
   and Immunology
Transplant Surgeon
University of Michigan Medical Center
Ann Arbor, Michigan

F. Charles Brunicardi, MD
Professor of Surgery
Chief, Section of General Surgery
Baylor University College of Medicine
Houston, Texas

David R. Byrd, MD
Assistant Professor of Surgery
Chief, Surgical Oncology
University of Washington School of Medicine
Seattle, Washington

Darrell A. Campbell, Jr., MD
Professor of Surgery
Head, Section of General Surgery
Associate Chairman for Hospital Affairs
University of Michigan Medical Center
Ann Arbor, Michigan

Howard R. Champion, FRCS, FACS
Professor of Surgery
Chief, Division of Surgery for Trauma
Uniformed Services University of the Health Sciences
Bethesda, Maryland

William F. Chandler, MD
Professor of Surgery
Section of Neurosurgery
University of Michigan Medical School
Ann Arbor, Michigan

Alfred E. Chang, MD
Professor of Surgery
University of Michigan Medical School
Chief, Division of Surgical Oncology
University of Michigan Medical Center
Ann Arbor, Michigan

Randall M. Chesnut, MD
Assistant Professor of Surgery in Residence
Department of Neurosurgery
University of California, San Francisco, School
   of Medicine
Chief, Neurosurgical Services
San Francisco General Hospital
San Francisco, California

Paul J. Chiao, PhD
Assistant Professor of Surgical Oncology and Tumor
   Biology
University of Texas M.D. Anderson Cancer Center
Houston, Texas

Kyung J. Cho, MD
Associate Professor of Radiology
University of Michigan Medical School
University of Michigan Hospital
Ann Arbor, Michigan

G. Patrick Clagett, Jr., MD
Chairman, Division of Vascular Surgery
University of Texas Southwestern Medical Center
Parkland Memorial Hospital
Zale-Lipshy University Hospital
Dallas Veterans Affairs Medical Center
Dallas, Texas

Alexander W. Clowes, MD
Professor of Surgery
University of Washington School of Medicine
Chief, Division of Vascular Surgery
University of Washington Medical Center
Seattle, Washington

Lisa M. Colletti, MD
Assistant Professor of Surgery
University of Michigan Medical School
University of Michigan Hospitals
Ann Arbor, Michigan

Robert L. Conter, MD
Associate Professor of Surgery
Pennsylvania State University College of Medicine
Milton S. Hershey Medical Center
Hershey, Pennsylvania

Arnold G. Coran, MD
Professor of Surgery
Head, Section of Pediatric Surgery
University of Michigan Medical School
Surgeon-in-Chief
C.S. Mott Children's Hospital
Ann Arbor, Michigan

Jack L. Cronenwett, MD
Professor of Surgery
Dartmouth Medical School
Chief, Section of Vascular Surgery
Dartmouth-Hitchcock Medical Center
Hanover, New Hampshire

Peter F. Crookes, MD
Assistant Professor of Surgery
University of Southern California School of Medicine
Attending Physician
Los Angeles County–University of Southern California
   Medical Center
University of Southern California University Hospital
North Comprehensive Cancer Center
Los Angeles, California

H. Gill Cryer, MD
Associate Professor of Surgery
University of California, Los Angeles, UCLA School
   of Medicine
Chief, Trauma and Emergency Surgery Service
UCLA Medical Center
Los Angeles, California

Louis G. D'Alecy, PhD
Professor of Physiology
Department of Physiology and Department of Surgery
University of Michigan Medical School
Ann Arbor, Michigan

James W. Davis, MD, FACS
Associate Clinical Professor of Surgery
University of California, San Francisco, School
  of Medicine
Chief of Trauma
Assistant Chief of Surgery
UCSF/Fresno Valley Medical Center
Fresno, California

Lillian G. Dawes, MD
Assistant Professor of Surgery
Northwestern University Medical Center
Chicago, Illinois

David C. Dawson, PhD
Professor and Associate Chair
Department of Physiology
University of Michigan Medical School
Ann Arbor, Michigan

Tom R. DeMeester, MD
Professor and Chairman
Department of Surgery
University of Southern California School of Medicine
Chief of Surgery
University of Southern California Hospital
Los Angeles, California

Verdi J. DiSesa, MD
Professor of Medicine and Cardiothoracic Surgery
Medical College of Pennsylvania and Hahnemann
  University School of Medicine
Medical College of Pennsylvania Hospital
Hahnemann University Hospital
Philadelphia, Pennsylvania

Gerard M. Doherty, MD
Assistant Professor of Surgery
Washington University School of Medicine
Barnes-Jewish Hospital
St Louis, Missouri

Lisa S. Dresner, MD
Assistant Professor of Surgery
State University of New York Health Science Center
  at Brooklyn
Director, Surgical Intensive Care Unit
Kings County Hospital Center
Brooklyn, New York

David L. Dunn, MD, PhD
Jay Phillips Professor and Head
Department of Surgery
University of Minnesota Medical School—Minneapolis
Minneapolis, Minnesota

Frederic E. Eckhauser, MD
Professor of Surgery
University of Michigan Medical School
Chief, Division of Gastrointestinal Surgery
University of Michigan Medical Center
Ann Arbor, Michigan

Lee M. Ellis, MD
Assistant Professor of Surgery and Cell Biology
University of Texas M.D. Anderson Cancer Center
Houston, Texas

Calvin B. Ernst, MD
Clinical Professor of Surgery
University of Michigan Medical School
Ann Arbor, Michigan
Head, Division of Vascular Surgery
Henry Ford Hospital
Detroit, Michigan

Steve Eubanks, MD
Assistant Professor of Surgery
Director, Surgical Endoscopy
Duke University Medical Center
Durham, North Carolina

Gary J. Faerber, MD
Assistant Professor of Surgery
Section of Urology
University of Michigan Medical Center
Ann Arbor, Michigan

F. Robert Fekety, MD
Professor Emeritus of Internal Medicine
Division of Infectious Diseases
University of Michigan Medical School
University of Michigan Hospitals
Ann Arbor, Michigan

Ronald M. Ferguson, MD, PhD
Professor and Chairman
Department of Surgery
Ohio State University College of Medicine
Chief, Division of Transplantation
Ohio State University Hospital
Columbus, Ohio

Mark F. Fillinger, MD
Assistant Professor of Surgery
Dartmouth Medical School
Dartmouth-Hitchcock Medical Center
Lebanon, New Hampshire

Neil A. Fine, MD
Assistant Professor of Surgery
Division of Plastic and Reconstructive Surgery
Northwestern University Medical School
Northwestern University Memorial Hospital
Chicago, Illinois

Heidi L. Frankel, MD
Assistant Professor of Surgery
Hospital of the University of Pennsylvania
Philadelphia, Pennsylvania
Department of Traumatology
Brandywine Hospital
Coatesville, Pennsylvania

Lawrence M. Gentilello, MD
Associate Professor of Surgery
University of Washington School of Medicine
Associate Director, Trauma Intensive Care Unit
Harborview Medical Center
Seattle, Washington

Dan I.N. Giurgiu, MD
Research Fellow in Surgery
Medical College of Pennsylvania and Hahnemann
   University School of Medicine
Philadelphia, Pennsylvania

Steven A. Goldstein, MD
Professor of Surgery
Director of Orthopaedic Research
Assistant Dean for Research and Graduate Studies
Professor of Mechanical Engineering and Applied
   Mechanics
College of Engineering
Research Scientist
Institute of Gerontology
University of Michigan
Ann Arbor, Michigan

Jerry Goldstone, MD
Professor of Surgery
University of California, San Francisco, School
   of Medicine
UCSF Medical Center
San Francisco Veterans Affairs Medical Center
San Francisco, California

Linda M. Graham, MD
Professor of Surgery
Case Western Reserve University School of Medicine
Chief, Division of Vascular Surgery
University Hospitals of Cleveland
Cleveland Veterans Affairs Medical Center
Cleveland, Ohio

Lazar J. Greenfield, MD
Frederick A. Coller Professor of Surgery
Chairman, Department of Surgery
University of Michigan Medical School
Surgeon-in-Chief
University of Michigan Hospitals
Ann Arbor, Michigan

Anita K. Gregory, MD
Chief Resident in General Surgery
St Luke's–Roosevelt Hospital Center
Columbia University College of Physicians and Surgeons
New York, New York

H. Barton Grossman, MD
Professor of Urology and Cell Biology
W.A. "Tex" and Deborah Moncrief, Jr., Chair in Urology
University of Texas M.D. Anderson Cancer Center
Houston, Texas

Karen S. Guice, MD
Professor of Surgery
Duke University Medical Center
Durham, North Carolina

John M. Ham, MD
Assistant Professor of Surgery
Medical College of Virginia
Virginia Commonwealth University
Richmond, Virginia

John B. Hanks, MD
C. Bruce Morton Professor of Surgery
Chief, Division of General Surgery
University of Virginia Health Sciences Center
Charlottesville, Virginia

E. John Harris, Jr., MD
Assistant Professor of Surgery
Division of Vascular Surgery
Stanford University School of Medicine
Stanford, California

Mark A. Healey, MD
Clinical Instructor in Surgery
Division of Trauma
University of California, San Diego, School of Medicine
UCSD Medical Center
San Diego, California

Mitchell L. Henry, MD
Associate Professor of Surgery
Ohio State University College of Medicine
Director, Clinical Transplantation
Ohio State University Medical Center
Columbus, Ohio

Anil P. Hingorani, MD
Resident
Columbia University College of Physicians and Surgeons
St Luke's–Roosevelt Hospital Center
New York, New York

Daniel B. Hinshaw, MD
Associate Professor of Surgery
University of Michigan Medical School
Chief of Surgery
Department of Veterans Affairs Medical Center
Ann Arbor, Michigan

Julian T. Hoff, MD
Professor of Surgery
University of Michigan Medical School
Head, Section of Neurosurgery
University of Michigan Medical Hospitals
Ann Arbor, Michigan

David B. Hoyt, MD, FACS
Professor of Surgery
University of California, San Diego, School of Medicine
Chief, Division of Trauma
Director, Surgical Intensive Care Unit
UCSD Medical Center
San Diego, California

Thomas S. Huber, MD, PhD
Assistant Professor of Surgery
University of Florida College of Medicine
Shands Teaching Hospital
Veterans Affairs Medical Center
Gainesville, Florida

W. Glenn Hurt, MD
Professor of Obstetrics and Gynecology
Virginia Commonwealth University
Medical College of Virginia
Richmond, Virginia

Mark D. Iannettoni, MD
Assistant Professor of Surgery
University of Michigan Medical School
University of Michigan Medical Center
Ann Arbor, Michigan

O. Wayne Isom, MD
Professor of Cardiothoracic Surgery
Cornell University Medical College
Cardiothoracic Surgeon-in-Chief
New York Hospital
New York, New York

Lloyd A. Jacobs, MD
Associate Professor of Surgery
University of Michigan Medical School
University of Michigan Hospitals
Ann Arbor, Michigan

Timothy M. Johnson, MD
Assistant Professor
University of Michigan Medical School
University of Michigan Medical Center
Ann Arbor, Michigan

Dennie V. Jones, Jr., MD
Assistant Professor of Medicine
University of Texas M.D. Anderson Cancer Center
Houston, Texas

Gregory J. Jurkovich, MD
Professor of Surgery
University of Washington School of Medicine
Chief of Trauma
Director, Emergency Surgical Services
Harborview Medical Center
Seattle, Washington

Kim U. Kahng, MD
Associate Professor of Surgery
Vice Chairman, Administrative Affairs
Medical College of Pennsylvania and Hahnemann
   University School of Medicine
Philadelphia, Pennsylvania

Larry R. Kaiser, MD
Associate Professor of Surgery
University of Pennsylvania School of Medicine
Director, Section of General Thoracic Surgery
University of Pennsylvania Medical Center
Philadelphia, Pennsylvania

Gordon L. Kauffman, Jr., MD
Professor of Surgery and Cellular and Molecular
   Physiology
Chief, Division of General Surgery
Milton S. Hershey Medical Center of the Pennsylvania
   State University
Hershey, Pennsylvania

James A. Knol, MD
Associate Professor of Surgery
University of Michigan Medical School
University of Michigan Hospitals
Ann Arbor, Michigan

M. Margaret Knudson, MD
Associate Professor of Surgery in Residence
University of California, San Francisco, School
   of Medicine
Director, Pediatric Trauma
San Francisco General Hospital
San Francisco, California

Walter A. Koltun, MD
Assistant Professor of Surgery
Pennsylvania State University College of Medicine
Milton S. Hershey Medical Center of the Pennsylvania
   State University
Hershey, Pennsylvania

John W. Konnak, MD
Professor of Surgery and Urology
University of Michigan Medical School
University of Michigan Hospitals
Ann Arbor, Michigan

William C. Krupski, MD
Professor of Surgery
Chief, Vascular Surgery Section
University of Colorado Health Sciences Center
Denver, Colorado

Steven L. Kunkel, MS, PhD
Professor of Pathology
University of Michigan Medical School
Ann Arbor, Michigan

Michael P. LaQuaglia, MD, FACS, FAAP
Associate Professor of Surgery
Cornell University Medical College
Chief, Pediatric Surgery
Memorial Sloan-Kettering Cancer Center
New York, New York

Baxter Larmon, PhD, MICP
Associate Professor of Medicine
Emergency Medicine Center
University of California, Los Angeles, UCLA School
   of Medicine
Los Angeles, California

Raymond W. Lee, MD
Fellow in Vascular Surgery
Oregon Health Sciences University
Portland, Oregon

L. Scott Levin, MD
Assistant Professor of Orthopaedic and Plastic Surgery
Acting Chairman, Division of Plastic, Reconstructive,
   Oral and Maxillofacial Surgery
Duke University Medical Center
Durham, North Carolina

Keith D. Lillemoe, MD
Associate Professor of Surgery
Johns Hopkins University School of Medicine
Johns Hopkins Hospital
Baltimore, Maryland

S. Martin Lindenauer, MD
Professor of Surgery and Health Services Management
School of Public Health
University of Michigan Medical School
Assistant Chief of Staff
Veterans Affairs Medical Center
Ann Arbor, Michigan

Carson D. Liu, MD
Clinical Instructor
UCLA Center for the Health Sciences
Los Angeles, California

Ricardo V. Lloyd, MD, PhD
Professor of Pathology
Mayo Clinic
Rochester, Minnesota

Michael R. Lucey, MD, FRCPI
Associate Professor of Medicine
University of Pennsylvania School of Medicine
Associate Chief, Division of Gastroenterology
Director, Division of Hepatology
Medical Director, Liver Transplant Program
Hospital of the University of Pennsylvania
Philadelphia, Pennsylvania

Flavian M. Lupinetti, MD
Associate Professor of Cardiovascular Surgery
University of Washington School of Medicine
Chief, Division of Cardiac Surgery
Children's Hospital and Medical Center
Seattle, Washington

Robert C. Mackersie, MD, FACS
Associate Professor of Surgery
University of California, San Francisco, School
   of Medicine
Director, Trauma and Surgical Critical Care
San Francisco General Hospital
San Francisco, California

Samuel M. Mahaffey, MD
Assistant Professor
Division of Pediatric Surgery
Department of Surgery
Duke University Medical Center
Durham, North Carolina

Ronald V. Maier, MD, FACS
Professor and Vice Chair
Department of Surgery
University of Washington School of Medicine
Surgeon-in-Chief
Harborview Medical Center
Seattle, Washington

Philippe A. Masser, MD
Staff Surgeon
Salem Memorial Hospital
Salem, Oregon

Larry S. Matthews, MD
Professor and Program Director
Section of Orthopaedic Surgery
University of Michigan Medical Center
Ann Arbor, Michigan

David W. McFadden, MD
Associate Professor and Chief
Division of General Surgery
University of California, Los Angeles, UCLA School
   of Medicine
Los Angeles, California
Chief, General Surgery
Sepulveda Veterans Affairs Medical Center
North Hills, California

David S. Medich, MD
Assistant Professor of Surgery
University of Pittsburgh School of Medicine
University of Pittsburgh Medical Center
Pittsburgh, Pennsylvania

Robert M. Merion, MD
Associate Professor of Surgery
Chief, Division of Transplantation
University of Michigan Medical School
Director, Kidney/Pancreas Transplantation Program
University of Michigan Medical Center
Ann Arbor, Michigan

Charles L. Mesh, MD
Vascular Surgery Associates of Cincinnati
Cincinnati, Ohio

Louis M. Messina, MD
Professor of Surgery
Chief, Division of Vascular Surgery
University of California, San Francisco, School
   of Medicine
San Francisco, California

Anthony A. Meyer, MD, PhD
Professor of Surgery
Chief, Division of General Surgery
University of North Carolina at Chapel Hill School
    of Medicine
Medical Director, Critical Care Services
Assistant Director, North Carolina Jaycee Burn Center
University of North Carolina Hospitals and Clinics
Chapel Hill, North Carolina

Thomas A. Miller, MD, FACS
C. Rollins Hanlon Professor and Chairman
Department of Surgery
St Louis University Medical School
Chief of Surgery
St Louis University Hospital
St Louis, Missouri

R. Scott Mitchell, MD
Associate Professor of Cardiovascular Surgery
Stanford University School of Medicine
Stanford, California

Ralph S. Mosca, MD
Assistant Professor of Surgery
C.S. Mott Children's Hospital
University of Michigan Medical Center
Ann Arbor, Michigan

Michael W. Mulholland, MD, PhD
Professor and Associate Chairman
Department of Surgery
University of Michigan Medical School
University of Michigan Hospitals
Ann Arbor, Michigan

Michel M. Murr, MD
Research Fellow in Gastrointestinal Surgery
Mayo Clinic and Foundation
Rochester, Minnesota

Thomas A. Mustoe, MD
Professor of Surgery
Chief, Division of Plastic Surgery
Northwestern University Medical School
Northwestern University Hospital
Chicago, Illinois

David L. Nahrwold, MD
Loyal and Edith Davis Professor and Chairman
Department of Surgery
Northwestern University Medical School
Surgeon-in-Chief
Northwestern Memorial Hospital
Chicago, Illinois

James P. Neifeld, MD
Professor of Surgery
Division of Surgical Oncology
Virginia Commonwealth University
Medical College of Virginia
Richmond, Virginia

H.H. Newsome, Jr., MD
Professor of Surgery
Virginia Commonwealth University
Medical College of Virginia
Medical College of Virginia Hospitals
Richmond, Virginia

Santhat Nivatvongs, MD, FACS
Professor of Surgery
Mayo Medical School
Consultant, Colon and Rectal Surgery
Mayo Clinic
Rochester, Minnesota

Patrick J. O'Hara, MD
Associate Professor of Surgery
Ohio State University College of Medicine
Department of Vascular Surgery
Cleveland Clinic Foundation
Cleveland, Ohio

Dana A. Ohl, MD
Associate Professor of Surgery
Section of Urology
University of Michigan Medical School
Ann Arbor, Michigan

Keith T. Oldham, MD
Professor of Surgery and Pediatrics
Duke University School of Medicine
Chief, Division of Pediatric Surgery
Duke University Medical Center
Durham, North Carolina

Geneva M. Omann, PhD
Associate Professor of Surgery and Biological Chemistry
University of Michigan Medical School
Research Chemist
Veterans Affairs Medical Center
Ann Arbor, Michigan

Lisa A. Orloff, MD
Assistant Professor of Surgery
Division of Otolaryngology
University of California, San Diego, School of Medicine
UCSD Medical Center
San Diego, California

Mark B. Orringer, MD
Professor of Surgery
Head, Section of Thoracic Surgery
University of Michigan Medical Center
Ann Arbor, Michigan

Mary F. Otterson, MD, MS
Associate Professor of Surgery and Physiology
Medical College of Wisconsin
Froedtert Memorial Lutheran Hospital
Milwaukee, Wisconsin

Theodore N. Pappas, MD
Professor of Surgery
Chief, Gastrointestinal Surgery
Duke University Medical Center
Durham, North Carolina

Neal R. Pellis, PhD
Associate Professor of Surgery and Immunology
University of Texas Graduate School of Biomedical
    Sciences
Adjunct Associate Professor of Immunology and Surgical
    Oncology
University of Texas M.D. Anderson Cancer Center
Program Manager, Biotechnology Program
NASA-Johnson Space Center
Houston, Texas

William S. Pierce, MD
Evan Pugh Professor of Surgery
Jane A. Fetter Professor of Surgery
Director of Surgical Research
Pennsylvania State University College of Medicine
Milton S. Hershey Medical Center
Hershey, Pennsylvania

John M. Porter, MD
Professor of Surgery
Head, Division of Vascular Surgery
Oregon Health Sciences University
Portland, Oregon

Bruce M. Potenza, MD, MPH
Instructor in Surgery
University of Massachusetts Medical Center
Worcester, Massachusetts

Jeffrey D. Punch, MD
Assistant Professor of Surgery
University of Michigan Medical School
University of Michigan Hospitals
Ann Arbor, Michigan

Steven E. Raper, MD
Associate Professor of Surgery
Institute for Human Gene Therapy
University of Pennsylvania School of Medicine
Philadelphia, Pennsylvania

Joseph H. Rapp, MD
Associate Professor of Surgery
University of California, San Francisco, School
    of Medicine
Chief, Vascular Surgery Service
San Francisco Veterans Affairs Medical Center
San Francisco, California

Daniel J. Reddy, MD
Clinical Associate Professor of Surgery
University of Michigan Medical School
Ann Arbor, Michigan
Vascular Surgeon
Henry Ford Hospital
Detroit, Michigan

Riley S. Rees, MD
Professor of Surgery and Plastic and Reconstructive
    Surgery
University of Michigan Medical School
Ann Arbor, Michigan

Linda M. Reilly, MD
Associate Professor of Surgery
University of California, San Francisco, School
    of Medicine
San Francisco Veteran's Affairs Medical Center
San Francisco, California

Michael L. Ritchey, MD
Associate Professor
University of Texas Health Science Center
Pediatric Urologist
Department of Pediatric Surgery
Hermann Children's Hospital
Texas Children's Hospital
Houston, Texas

Lawrence Rosenberg, MSc, MD, PhD, FRCSC, FACS
Associate Professor of Surgery
McGill University Faculty of Medicine
Associate Surgeon
Montreal General Hospital
Montreal, Quebec, Canada

Todd K. Rosengart, MD
Assistant Professor of Cardiothoracic Surgery
Cornell University Medical College
Assistant Attending Cardiothoracic Surgeon
New York Hospital
New York, New York

Joel J. Roslyn, MD
Professor and Chairman
Department of Surgery
Medical College of Pennsylvania and Hahnemann
    University School of Medicine
Philadelphia, Pennsylvania

Grace S. Rozycki, MD, FACS
Assistant Professor of Surgery
Emory University School of Medicine
Director of Trauma-Surgical Critical Care
Grady Memorial Hospital
Atlanta, Georgia

Valerie W. Rusch, MD
Professor of Surgery
Cornell University Medical College
Member and Attending Surgeon, Thoracic Service
Memorial Sloan-Kettering Cancer Center
New York, New York

Timothy W. Rutter, MBBS, FFARCS
Associate Professor of Anesthesiology
University of Michigan Medical School
Clinical Director and Associate Chair, Department
    of Anesthesiology
University of Michigan Hospitals
Ann Arbor, Michigan

John S. Sapirstein, MD
General Surgery Resident
Department of Surgery
University of Chicago Hospitals
Chicago, Illinois

Michael G. Sarr, MD
Professor of Surgery
Mayo Medical School
Chairman, Division of General and Gastroenterologic
   Surgery
Mayo Clinic and Mayo Foundation
Rochester, Minnesota

Felix H. Savoie, MD
Co-Director of Upper Extremity Service
Mississippi Sports Medicine and Orthopaedic Center
Jackson, Mississippi

Wolfgang H. Schraut, MD, PhD, FACS
Professor of Surgery
University of Pittsburgh School of Medicine
Chief, Gastrointestinal Surgery
Presbyterian University Hospital
Pittsburgh, Pennsylvania

Brian J. Sennett, MD
Clinical Instructor of Orthopaedic Surgery
Medical College of Pennsylvania and Hahnemann
   University School of Medicine
Associate Director, Joe Torg Center for Sports Medicine
Philadelphia, Pennsylvania

Steven R. Shackford, MD, FACS
Professor and Chairman
Department of Surgery
University of Vermont College of Medicine
Surgeon-in-Chief
Medical Center Hospital of Vermont
Burlington, Vermont

Alexander D. Shepard, MD
Clinical Associate Professor of Surgery
University of Michigan Medical School
Ann Arbor, Michigan
Senior Staff Surgeon
Medical Director, Vascular Laboratory
Henry Ford Hospital
Detroit, Michigan

Robert L. Sheridan, MD
Assistant Professor of Surgery
Harvard Medical School
Assistant Chief of Staff
Shriners Burns Institute
Boston, Massachusetts

Sara J. Shumway, MD
Professor of Surgery
University of Minnesota Medical School—Minneapolis
Surgical Director, Heart Transplantation
University of Minnesota Hospital and Clinics
Minneapolis, Minnesota

Richard Keith Simons, MB, BChir, FRCS, FRCS(C)
Assistant Professor of Surgery
Division of Trauma
University of California, San Diego, School of Medicine
UCSD Medical Center
San Diego, California

Michael J. Sise, MD
Associate Clinical Professor of Surgery
University of California, San Diego, School of Medicine
Chief, Division of Trauma
Mercy Hospital and Medical Center
San Diego, California

Vernon K. Sondak, MD
Associate Professor of Surgery
University of Michigan Medical School
Director, Sarcoma Program
University of Michigan Comprehensive Cancer Center
Ann Arbor, Michigan

David E. Soper, MD
Professor of Obstetrics and Gynecology
Director, Division of Benign Gynecology
Medical University of South Carolina College
   of Medicine
Charleston, South Carolina

Nathaniel J. Soper, MD
Associate Professor of Surgery
Washington University School of Medicine
Barnes Hospital
St Louis, Missouri

Wiley W. Souba, MD, ScD
Professor of Surgery
Harvard Medical School
Chief, Division of Surgical Oncology
Massachusetts General Hospital
Boston, Massachusetts

David I. Soybel, MD
Assistant Professor of Surgery
Harvard Medical School
Associate in Surgery
Brigham and Women's Hospital
Boston, Massachusetts

James C. Stanley, MD
Professor of Surgery
University of Michigan Medical Center
Head, Section of Vascular Surgery
University of Michigan Medical Center
Ann Arbor, Michigan

Thomas Ray Stevenson, MD
Professor of Surgery
Chief, Division of Plastic Surgery
University of California, Davis, School of Medicine
Sacramento, California

James R. Stewart, MD
Associate Professor of Surgery
Department of Cardiac and Thoracic Surgery
Vanderbilt University School of Medicine
Vanderbilt University Medical Center
Veterans Affairs Medical Center
Nashville, Tennessee

Robert M. Strieter, MD
Professor of Internal Medicine
Division of Pulmonary and Critical Care Medicine
University of Michigan Medical School
University of Michigan Medical Center
Ann Arbor, Michigan

Harvey J. Sugerman, MD
David M. Hume Professor of Surgery
Vice-Chairman, Department of Surgery
Virginia Commonwealth University
Medical College of Virginia
Richmond, Virginia

David S. Sumner, MD
Distinguished Professor of Surgery
Chief, Section of Peripheral Vascular Surgery
Southern Illinois University School of Medicine
Springfield, Illinois

Lloyd M. Taylor, Jr., MD
Professor of Surgery
Division of Vascular Surgery
Oregon Health Sciences University
Portland, Oregon

Gordon L. Telford, MD
Professor of Surgery
Medical College of Wisconsin
Froedtert Memorial Lutheran Hospital
Milwaukee, Wisconsin

Norman W. Thompson, MD
Henry King Ransom Professor of Surgery
University of Michigan Medical School
Chief, Division of Endocrine Surgery
University of Michigan Hospitals
Ann Arbor, Michigan

M. David Tilson, MD
Alisa Mellon Bruce Professor of Surgery
Columbia University College of Physicians and Surgeons
Professor of Surgery
St Luke's–Roosevelt Hospital Center
New York, New York

Ronald G. Tompkins, MD, ScD
Associate Professor of Surgery
Harvard Medical School
Visiting Surgeon
Massachusetts General Hospital
Boston, Massachusetts

Kevin K. Tremper, PhD, MD
Professor and Chair
Department of Anesthesiology
University of Michigan Medical School
University of Michigan Medical Center
Ann Arbor, Michigan

Jeremiah G. Turcotte, MD
Professor of Surgery
University of Michigan Medical School
Director, Organ Transplantation Center
University of Michigan Hospitals
Ann Arbor, Michigan

Richard H. Turnage, MD
Assistant Professor of Surgery
University of Texas Southwestern Medical School
Dallas Veterans Affairs Medical Center
Dallas, Texas

Richard Wait, MD, PhD
Professor and Chairman
Department of Surgery
State University of New York Health Sciences Center
  at Brooklyn
Brooklyn, New York

Thomas W. Wakefield, MD
Associate Professor of Surgery
University of Michigan Medical School
University of Michigan Medical Center
Veterans Affairs Medical Center
Ann Arbor, Michigan

Samuel A. Wells, Jr., MD
Bixby Professor of Surgery
Chairman, Department of Surgery
Washington University School of Medicine
Surgeon-in-Chief
Barnes-Jewish Hospital
St Louis, Missouri

John R. Wesley, MD
Clinical Professor of Surgery
University of California, Davis, School of Medicine
Chief, Pediatric Surgery
UCD Medical Center
Sacramento, California

Rodney A. White, MD
Professor of Surgery
University of California, Los Angeles, UCLA School
  of Medicine
Chief, Vascular Surgery
Associate Chairman, Department of Surgery
Harbor-UCLA Medical Center
Los Angeles, California

Glenn J.R. Whitman, MD
Professor of Surgery
Medical College of Pennsylvania and Hahnemann
  University Medical School
Chief, Section of Cardiothoracic Surgery
Medical College of Pennsylvania Hospital
Philadelphia, Pennsylvania

David M. Williams, MD
Associate Professor of Radiology
University of Michigan Medical Center
Ann Arbor, Michigan

John A. Williams, MD, PhD
Professor of Physiology and Internal Medicine
Chair, Department of Physiology
University of Michigan Medical School
Ann Arbor, Michigan

Robert J. Winchell, MD
Assistant Professor of Surgery
Division of Trauma
University of California, San Diego, School of Medicine
La Jolla, California

David H. Wisner, MD
Professor of Surgery
University of California, Davis, School of Medicine
Chief of Trauma Surgery
University of California, Davis, Medical Center
Sacramento, California

James S.T. Yao, MD, PhD
Magerstadt Professor of Surgery
Northwestern University Medical School
Chief, Division of Vascular Surgery
Vice Chair, Department of Surgery
Northwestern Memorial Hospital
Chicago, Illinois

Charles J. Yeo, MD
Associate Professor of Surgery and Oncology
Johns Hopkins University School of Medicine
Johns Hopkins Hospital
Baltmore, Maryland

Gerald B. Zelenock
Professor of Surgery
Section of Vascular Surgery
University of Michigan Medical School
University of Michigan Hospitals
Ann Arbor, Michigan

Preface

Our concept that the exciting new knowledge in the basic sciences was of vital importance to surgeons and needed to be presented in a readable and well-illustrated format was the impetus for the first edition of *Surgery: Scientific Principles and Practices*. The text has been well received by the surgical community, and many of the advances cited in the first edition have been rapidly and effectively integrated into surgical practice. The success of that concept has exceeded our expectations and provides an incremental stimulus to us to continue to refine and improve the approach. In the second edition, we have maintained our commitment to solicit the contributions of younger authors who are on the leading edge of their fields, and we have expanded our educational concept to include a more comprehensive review book with referenced questions, answers, and discussion. To facilitate the latter and broaden our editorial scope, we are delighted to welcome Keith Lillemoe of Johns Hopkins to our editorial group. He not only lowers our average age but adds a new perspective in general surgery. In fulfilling our objective to lay the scientific foundation for surgery, we have not neglected the practice component, adding new chapters by Steve Eubanks and Scott Levin to cover the ever-expanding fields of endosurgery and reconstructive plastic surgery, respectively. New chapters in applied science include human gene therapy by Steven Raper and the equally fascinating subject of cytokines by Lisa Colletti. Many chapters have been condensed and revised by their previous authors. In addition, 41 chapters have a total of 68 new authors who bring fresh insights to their subjects. Throughout, the consistency of illustrations and the highlighting that were so favorably received in the first edition were maintained.

As we progress through this final decade of the 20th century, there are many forces of change in medicine as a whole and surgery in particular. Hospitals are feeling enormous pressure. The operating room has shifted from a revenue producer to a cost center. More patients are undergoing procedures on an ambulatory basis. Some of the traditional physician–patient and teaching–training relationships have been strained. The relationships among and between physicians and with hospitals, delivery systems, and the medical bureaucracy are also in transition. Accountants and managers dedicated to reducing the costs of care are omnipresent but not omniscient. These functions must not interfere with the quality of care that has always been the hallmark of surgical practice. Our covenant with the patient must remain paramount. Physician leadership and management are needed. These important issues represent a challenge to improve our efficiency and broaden our perspective to ensure that managed care is not minimal care. An informed expert is a cost-effective decision maker.

The specialist is still in the best position to direct the evaluation and management of a clinical problem without the expensive and often irrelevant testing that so often characterizes the approach of the generalist. The widespread availability of noninvasive testing modalities and less-invasive diagnostic and therapeutic procedures, which are constantly undergoing revision and improvement, makes it difficult or impossible for anyone but a specialist to determine the safest and most effective strategy for a given patient. This places the obligation for current knowledge of surgical disorders directly on the surgeon, who must be able to incorporate new science and technology into his or her practice. It is this goal that we have established as our mission statement: To provide the scientific principles that serve as foundation for current and future surgical practice.

LAZAR J. GREENFIELD, MD
Editor-in-Chief

Preface to the First Edition

Our predecessors in surgery would be amazed at the scope and sophistication of the current practice of surgery. Yet, those who have witnessed this impressive expansion of clinical science are also acutely aware of the exponential growth of knowledge in the basic sciences. Surgical research has undergone a transformation from physiologic to cellular investigation, and we have now entered the era of molecular biology. These developments are changing the fundamental ways in which we think about injury and disease. The accelerated rate of scientific progress demands not only an expanded vocabulary but also a willingness to adopt new ideas and strategies and to readjust basic biologic concepts. Without this approach, future surgeons would be in danger of becoming surgical technicians and would fail their heritage as major contributors to medical progress.

These challenges prompted us to develop a new textbook of surgery that would balance scientific principles and clinical practice. The classic textbooks of past decades served their purpose well, emphasizing the rich heritage of clinical surgery. But new knowledge dictates new approaches to the integration of the basic sciences and clinical surgery. Therefore, *Surgery: Scientific Principles and Practice* begins with a major section devoted to basic topics such as cell biology, metabolism, inflammation, immunology, and wound healing. On this foundation we have added organ system chapters designed to include normal physiology and anatomy. Our commitment to clinical practice is demonstrated by the comprehensive list of topics, the emphasis on modern approaches to diagnosis and management, and descriptions of surgical techniques. We expect this book to be as useful to experienced practitioners as to students and residents in surgery.

In a departure from the customary approach, we have selected many younger authors who are scientifically sophisticated and currently active contributors to the field. Many are the authors of seminal papers in their disciplines and are joining a textbook of surgery for the first time. Their fresh and pragmatic approaches enhance both the substance and readability of the book.

Because surgery is a very visual craft, we have aspired to set a new standard for illustration by having one group of artists provide all the line drawings. This commitment, along with the color highlighting, ensures a uniformity of presentation for maximal teaching effectiveness and clinical usefulness.

The final and perhaps most important concept of *Surgery: Scientific Principles and Practice* is that we have tried to anticipate future developments. In choosing authors who are active investigators, we have endeavored to synthesize current concepts and to look ahead to the most promising areas for future progress. Armed with these concepts and the comprehensive state-of-the-art knowledge that this book provides, students and practitioners of surgery will be well prepared for the new challenges of the 21st century.

LAZAR J. GREENFIELD, MD
Editor-in-Chief

Acknowledgment

The editors are a remarkably synergistic group who have worked diligently to improve the second edition of *Surgery: Scientific Principles and Practice,* and we wish to express our thanks to the contributors, old and new, whose efforts made the work so gratifying. We were fortunate to have the opportunity to continue to work with our original editorial team of Lisa McAllister as Senior Editor for Medical Books, Paula Callaghan as Associate Editor, and Grace Caputo as Associate Managing Editor. Their stimulation and encouragement have been instrumental in sustaining the communication and procedural processes necessary for so large a project. We are also grateful to Holly Fischer for continuing to provide the distinctive artwork that contributes so much to the educational effectiveness of the work. Finally, we dedicate our efforts to those whose support and understanding makes it all worthwhile, our families.

Contents

PART ONE   SCIENTIFIC PRINCIPLES

CHAPTER 1   CELL STRUCTURE AND FUNCTION 3
John A. Williams and David C. Dawson

CHAPTER 2   NUTRITION AND METABOLISM 42
Wiley W. Souba and William G. Austen, Jr.

CHAPTER 3   WOUND HEALING 67
Neil A. Fine and Thomas A. Mustoe

CHAPTER 4   HEMOSTASIS 83
Thomas W. Wakefield

CHAPTER 5   CYTOKINES 108
Lisa M. Colletti, Steven L. Kunkel, and Robert M. Strieter

CHAPTER 6   INFLAMMATION 130
Geneva M. Omann and Daniel B. Hinshaw

CHAPTER 7   INFECTION 159
David L. Dunn

CHAPTER 8   SHOCK 182
Ronald V. Maier

CHAPTER 9   CRITICAL CARE 215
Robert H. Bartlett

CHAPTER 10 FLUIDS AND ELECTROLYTES AND ACID–BASE BALANCE 242
Richard Wait, Kim U. Kahng, and Lisa S. Dresner

CHAPTER 11 TRAUMA 267

            Introduction 267
            David B. Hoyt

            General Considerations 269
            Bruce M. Potenza and David B. Hoyt

            Trauma Systems 278
            David B. Hoyt

            Patient Care Phase: Prehospital and Resuscitation Care 279
            H. Gill Cryer and Baxter Larmon

            Patient Care Phase: Shock 285
            James W. Davis

            Definitive Care Phase: Head Injuries 291
            Randall M. Chesnut

            Definitive Care Phase: Maxillofacial Injuries 298
            Lisa A. Orloff

            Definitive Care Phase: Neck Injuries 309
            Gregory J. Jurkovich

Definitive Care Phase: Chest Injuries 317
Robert J. Winchell

Definitive Care Phase: Abdominal Injuries 331
David H. Wisner and David B. Hoyt

Definitive Care Phase: Retroperitoneal Injuries 353
Robert C. Mackersie

Definitive Care Phase: Vascular Injuries 361
Michael J. Sise and Steven R. Shackford

Definitive Care Phase: Orthopedic and Spinal Injuries 373
Mark A. Healey and Robert J. Winchell

Definitive Care Phase: Pediatric Trauma....................................... 377
M. Margaret Knudson

Definitive Care Phase: Geriatric Trauma....................................... 386
M. Margaret Knudson

Definitive Care Phase: Trauma in Pregnancy 390
Heidi L. Frankel, Grace S. Rozycki, and Howard R. Champion

Definitive Care Phase: Critical Care and Postinjury Management 395
Richard Keith Simons and David B. Hoyt

Envenomation and Environmental Injuries 402
Gregory J. Jurkovich and Lawrence M. Gentilello

CHAPTER 12   BURNS 422
Robert L. Sheridan and Ronald G. Tompkins

CHAPTER 13   ANESTHESIOLOGY AND PAIN MANAGEMENT 438
Timothy W. Rutter and Kevin K. Tremper

CHAPTER 14   TUMOR BIOLOGY.. 455
Lee M. Ellis, Dennie V. Jones, Jr., Paul J. Chiao, and Neal R. Pellis

CHAPTER 15   HUMAN GENE THERAPY.. 506
Steven E. Raper

CHAPTER 16   TRANSPLANTATION AND IMMUNOLOGY 527

Transplant Immunology 527
Jonathan S. Bromberg

Organ Preservation 556
Jeffrey D. Punch and Robert M. Merion

Renal Transplantation... 571
Mitchell L. Henry and Ronald M. Ferguson

Hepatic Transplantation 581
Darrell A. Campbell, Jr., John M. Ham, Jeremiah G. Turcotte, and Robert M. Merion

Cardiac Transplantation 599
Sara J. Shumway and R. Morton Bolman III

Pulmonary Transplantation.. 606
Larry R. Kaiser

Pancreatic and Islet Transplantation... 615
Lawrence Rosenberg

PART TWO   SURGICAL PRACTICE

SECTION A   HEAD AND NECK

CHAPTER 17   Head and Neck... 635
James P. Neifeld

SECTION B ESOPHAGUS

CHAPTER 18 ESOPHAGEAL ANATOMY AND PHYSIOLOGY,
            AND GASTROESOPHAGEAL REFLUX.. 653
            Peter F. Crookes and Tom R. DeMeester

CHAPTER 19 TUMORS, INJURIES, AND MISCELLANEOUS CONDITIONS
            OF THE ESOPHAGUS 694
            Mark B. Orringer

CHAPTER 20 ENDOSURGICAL PRINCIPLES.. 735
            Steve Eubanks

SECTION C STOMACH AND DUODENUM

CHAPTER 21 GASTRIC ANATOMY AND PHYSIOLOGY... 745
            Michael W. Mulholland

CHAPTER 22 DUODENAL ULCER.. 759
            Michael W. Mulholland

CHAPTER 23 STRESS ULCER AND GASTRIC ULCER.. 773
            Gordon L. Kauffman, Jr., and Robert L. Conter

CHAPTER 24 MORBID OBESITY 788
            Harvey J. Sugerman

CHAPTER 25 GASTRIC NEOPLASMS 795
            Michael W. Mulholland

SECTION D SMALL INTESTINE

CHAPTER 26 ANATOMY AND PHYSIOLOGY OF THE SMALL INTESTINE.................... 805
            Walter A. Koltun and Theodore N. Pappas

CHAPTER 27 ILEUS AND BOWEL OBSTRUCTION.. 817
            David I. Soybel

CHAPTER 28 CROHN'S DISEASE 831
            Wolfgang H. Schraut and David S. Medich

CHAPTER 29 SMALL INTESTINAL NEOPLASMS 844
            Michael G. Sarr and Michel M. Murr

SECTION E PANCREAS

CHAPTER 30 PANCREATIC ANATOMY AND PHYSIOLOGY..................................... 857
            Dana K. Andersen and F. Charles Brunicardi

CHAPTER 31 ACUTE PANCREATITIS 874
            Karen S. Guice

CHAPTER 32 CHRONIC PANCREATITIS 889
            Michael W. Mulholland

CHAPTER 33 NEOPLASMS OF THE EXOCRINE PANCREAS 901
            Richard H. Bell, Jr.

CHAPTER 34   NEOPLASMS OF THE ENDOCRINE PANCREAS 918
Charles J. Yeo

SECTION F   LIVER AND PORTAL VENOUS SYSTEM

CHAPTER 35   HEPATOBILIARY ANATOMY 931
David R. Byrd

CHAPTER 36   HEPATIC PHYSIOLOGY 943
Steven E. Raper

CHAPTER 37   HEPATIC INFECTION AND ACUTE HEPATIC FAILURE 958
Michael R. Lucey

CHAPTER 38   CIRRHOSIS AND PORTAL HYPERTENSION 972
Frederic E. Eckhauser, Steven E. Raper, and Jeremiah G. Turcotte

CHAPTER 39   HEPATIC NEOPLASMS 1008
John B. Hanks and W. Scott Arnold

SECTION G   GALLBLADDER AND BILIARY TRACT

CHAPTER 40   BILIARY ANATOMY AND PHYSIOLOGY 1023
Nathaniel J. Soper

CHAPTER 41   CALCULOUS BILIARY DISEASE 1033
Dan I.N. Giurgiu and Joel J. Roslyn

CHAPTER 42   BILIARY NEOPLASMS 1056
David L. Nahrwold and Lillian G. Dawes

CHAPTER 43   BILIARY STRICTURES AND SCLEROSING CHOLANGITIS 1067
Keith D. Lillemoe

SECTION H   COLON, RECTUM, AND ANUS

CHAPTER 44   COLONIC ANATOMY AND PHYSIOLOGY 1083
Thomas A. Miller

CHAPTER 45   ULCERATIVE COLITIS 1093
James M. Becker

CHAPTER 46   COLONIC POLYPS AND POLYPOSIS SYNDROMES 1109
C. Richard Boland and Robert S. Bresalier

CHAPTER 47   COLORECTAL CANCER 1128
Alfred E. Chang

CHAPTER 48   ANAL CANCER 1146
Santhat Nivatvongs

CHAPTER 49   DIVERTICULAR DISEASE 1151
Gordon L. Telford and Mary F. Otterson

CHAPTER 50   ACUTE GASTROINTESTINAL HEMORRHAGE 1158
Richard H. Turnage

CHAPTER 51 ANTIBIOTIC-ASSOCIATED COLITIS 1172
F. Robert Fekety

CHAPTER 52 ANORECTAL DISORDERS 1180
Santhat Nivatvongs

SECTION I HERNIA, MESENTERY, AND RETROPERITONEUM

CHAPTER 53 INGUINAL ANATOMY AND ABDOMINAL WALL HERNIAS 1207
James A. Knol and Frederic E. Eckhauser

CHAPTER 54 ACUTE ABDOMEN AND APPENDIX 1246
Carson D. Liu and David W. McFadden

CHAPTER 55 SPLEEN 1262
Anthony A. Meyer

SECTION J SURGICAL ENDOCRINOLOGY

CHAPTER 56 THYROID GLAND 1283
Norman W. Thompson

CHAPTER 57 PARATHYROID GLANDS 1308
Gerard M. Doherty and Samuel A. Wells, Jr.

CHAPTER 58 ADRENAL GLANDS 1331
H.H. Newsome, Jr.

CHAPTER 59 PITUITARY GLAND 1347
William F. Chandler and Ricardo V. Lloyd

CHAPTER 60 BREAST 1357
David A. August and Vernon K. Sondak

SECTION K THORAX

CHAPTER 61 LUNG NEOPLASMS 1417
Valerie W. Rusch

CHAPTER 62 CHEST WALL, PLEURA, MEDIASTINUM, AND NONNEOPLASTIC
LUNG DISEASE 1440
Mark D. Iannettoni and Mark B. Orringer

SECTION L CARDIOVASCULAR SYSTEM

CHAPTER 63 CONGENITAL HEART DISEASE AND CARDIAC TUMORS 1483
Ralph S. Mosca, Flavian M. Lupinetti, and Edward L. Bove

CHAPTER 64 VALVULAR HEART DISEASE 1503
O. Wayne Isom and Todd K. Rosengart

CHAPTER 65 ISCHEMIC HEART DISEASE 1534
Glenn J.R. Whitman and Verdi J. DiSesa

CHAPTER 66 MECHANICAL CIRCULATORY SUPPORT 1550
John S. Sapirstein and William S. Pierce

CHAPTER 67   CARDIAC ARRHYTHMIAS AND PERICARDIUM...................................1565
Steven F. Bolling and James R. Stewart

SECTION M   ARTERIAL SYSTEM

Basic Considerations in Vascular Disease

CHAPTER 68   ATHEROSCLEROSIS AND THE PATHOGENESIS
OF OCCLUSIVE DISEASE...1585
Alexander W. Clowes

CHAPTER 69   NONATHEROSCLEROTIC VASCULAR DISEASE..........................1596
Lloyd M. Taylor, Jr., Raymond W. Lee, E. John Harris, Jr., and John M. Porter

CHAPTER 70   OCCLUSIVE DISEASE: THROMBOSIS 1608
G. Patrick Clagett, Jr.

CHAPTER 71   PERIPHERAL ARTERIAL EMBOLISM 1621
Louis M. Messina

CHAPTER 72   ARTERIAL COMPRESSION SYNDROMES...1635
Lloyd A. Jacobs

CHAPTER 73   TISSUE ISCHEMIA 1643
Gerald B. Zelenock and Louis D'Alecy

CHAPTER 74   ARTERIAL HEMODYNAMICS...1656
Jack L. Cronenwett and Mark F. Fillinger

CHAPTER 75   VASCULAR DIAGNOSTICS 1668
David S. Sumner

CHAPTER 76   DIAGNOSTIC ANGIOGRAPHY..1678
David M. Williams and Kyung J. Cho

CHAPTER 77   NONOPERATIVE MANAGEMENT OF ATHEROSCLEROSIS.....................1710
Joseph H. Rapp, Linda M. Reilly, and William C. Krupski

CHAPTER 78   VASCULAR INFECTIONS 1720
Dennis F. Bandyk

CHAPTER 79   ENDOVASCULAR SURGICAL TECHNIQUES 1733
Rodney A. White

Occlusive Disease Involving Specific Vascular Territories

CHAPTER 80   CEREBROVASCULAR OCCLUSIVE DISEASE 1745
Louis M. Messina and Gerald B. Zelenock

CHAPTER 81   UPPER EXTREMITY OCCLUSIVE DISEASE 1758
James S.T. Yao

CHAPTER 82   VISCERAL OCCLUSIVE DISEASE..1764
Gerald B. Zelenock

CHAPTER 83   RENAL ARTERY OCCLUSIVE DISEASE 1780
James C. Stanley

CHAPTER 84   AORTOILIAC DISEASE..1796
David C. Brewster

CHAPTER 85   FEMOROPOPLITEAL AND INFRAPOPLITEAL OCCLUSIVE DISEASE...........1810
Lloyd M. Taylor, Jr., John M. Porter, and Philippe A. Masser

CHAPTER 86   LOWER EXTREMITY AMPUTATION 1823
Thomas S. Huber

Aneurysmal Disease

CHAPTER 87   PATHOGENESIS OF ANEURYSMS..1840
M. David Tilson, Anil P. Hingorani, and Anita K. Gregory

CHAPTER 88   EXTRACRANIAL CAROTID, INNOMINATE, SUBCLAVIAN,
AND AXILLARY ANEURYSMS...1849
Patrick J. O'Hara

CHAPTER 89   THORACIC AORTIC ANEURYSMS 1859
R. Scott Mitchell

CHAPTER 90   THORACOABDOMINAL AORTIC ANEURYSMS...................................1873
Daniel J. Reddy, Calvin B. Ernst, and Alexander D. Shepard

CHAPTER 91   ABDOMINAL AORTIC ANEURYSMS...1881
Jerry Goldstone

CHAPTER 92   SPLANCHNIC ARTERY ANEURYSMS 1893
James C. Stanley

CHAPTER 93   RENAL ARTERY ANEURYSMS..1901
James C. Stanley

CHAPTER 94   FEMORAL AND POPLITEAL ANEURYSMS......................................1909
Charles L. Mesh and Linda M. Graham

CHAPTER 95   VASCULAR MALFORMATION AND ARTERIOVENOUS FISTULA...............1916
S. Martin Lindenauer

SECTION N   VENOUS AND LYMPHATIC SYSTEMS

CHAPTER 96   VENOUS PHYSIOLOGY AND DISORDERS OF THE SUPERFICIAL
AND DEEP VEINS...1935
Thomas W. Wakefield and Lazar J. Greenfield

CHAPTER 97   VENOUS THROMBOSIS AND PULMONARY THROMBOEMBOLISM..........1944
Lazar J. Greenfield

CHAPTER 98   CHRONIC VENOUS INSUFFICIENCY 1958
Lazar J. Greenfield

CHAPTER 99   LYMPHATIC SYSTEM DISORDERS 1966
Lazar J. Greenfield

SECTION O   PEDIATRICS

CHAPTER 100   NEONATAL AND PEDIATRIC PHYSIOLOGY....................................1973
Samuel M. Mahaffey

CHAPTER 101   PEDIATRIC HEAD AND NECK 1994
John R. Wesley

CHAPTER 102   PEDIATRIC THORAX...2001
Chest Wall, Lung, and Mediastinum...2001
Arnold G. Coran
Congenital Abnormalities of the Diaphragm 2019
Keith T. Oldman

CHAPTER 103   PEDIATRIC ABDOMEN...2028
Abdominal Wall Defects 2028
John R. Wesley
Gastrointestinal Disorders 2034
Keith T. Oldham
Pediatric Liver...2078
Arnold G. Coran
Pediatric Biliary Tract..2083
Keith T. Oldham
Pediatric Pancreas..2094
Arnold G. Coran

CHAPTER 104   PEDIATRIC GENITOURINARY SYSTEM 2101
Urinary and Testicular Anomalies...2101
David A. Bloom and Michael L. Ritchey
Intersex, Vaginal, and Uterine Anomalies...................................2111
Arnold G. Coran

CHAPTER 105   CHILDHOOD TUMORS 2118
Michael P. LaQuaglia

SECTION P   MUSCULOSKELETAL SYSTEM

CHAPTER 106   ORTHOPEDIC SURGERY...2141
Larry S. Matthews and Steven A. Goldstein

CHAPTER 107   SURGERY OF THE HAND..2153
Brian J. Sennett and Felix H. Savoie

SECTION Q   NERVOUS SYSTEM

CHAPTER 108   CENTRAL NERVOUS SYSTEM 2165
Julian T. Hoff and Michael F. Boland

SECTION R   GENITOURINARY SYSTEM

CHAPTER 109   MALE ANATOMY AND PHYSIOLOGY.......................................2199
H. Barton Grossman, William D. Belville, Gary J. Faerber, John W. Konnak, and Dana A. Ohl

CHAPTER 110   FEMALE GENITAL SYSTEM 2216
W. Glenn Hurt and David E. Soper

SECTION S   SKIN AND SOFT TISSUE

CHAPTER 111   CUTANEOUS NEOPLASMS 2231
Alfred E. Chang, Timothy M. Johnson, and Riley S. Rees

CHAPTER 112   SARCOMAS OF BONE AND SOFT TISSUE 2246
Vernon K. Sondak

CHAPTER 113   AESTHETIC SURGERY 2269
Thomas Ray Stevenson

CHAPTER 114   RECONSTRUCTIVE PLASTIC SURGERY...2280
L. Scott Levin

INDEX 2291

ONE

SCIENTIFIC PRINCIPLES

SURGERY: SCIENTIFIC PRINCIPLES AND PRACTICE, Second Edition, edited by
Lazar J. Greenfield, Michael W. Mulholland, Keith T. Oldham, Gerald B. Zelenock,
and Keith D. Lillemoe. Lippincott–Raven Publishers, Philadelphia, © 1997.

CHAPTER 1

CELL STRUCTURE AND FUNCTION

JOHN A. WILLIAMS AND DAVID C. DAWSON

Clinical medicine is in the midst of a revolution. The explosive growth in basic biologic science during the past two decades has provided unprecedented insights into normal physiology and disease processes. The bases of human illness are understood increasingly in cellular and molecular terms, and novel approaches to treatment have resulted. The pace of scientific advancement is likely to accelerate. This new knowledge requires that future surgeons learn a new scientific vocabulary. All clinicians must understand the tenets of cellular and molecular biology to appreciate both the power and the limitations of these approaches.

CELL STRUCTURE

The human body, like all living organisms, is composed of cells. Individual cells express widely differing shapes and functions, but all possess common structural and functional elements that allow the cell to use energy, maintain homeostasis, grow, and divide.[1,2] Cells become differentiated for specific functions by expressing particular, spe-

cialized elements. For example, all cells possess membrane proteins that act as ion channels and participate in the maintenance of the intracellular ionic milieu, but in nerve cells, these ion channels have diversified and are highly voltage dependent, providing the basis for information transmission in the form of electrical impulses.

In many cases, proteins do not function as individual molecules but within larger structures specialized for specific functions. These structures, when visible by light and electron microscopy, are termed *organelles* (Fig. 1-1). In most cases, organelles compartmentalize the cell; they are surrounded by a biologic membrane based on a lipid bilayer that is structurally similar to the plasma membrane. This section reviews the structure of the major cell organelles as well as that of the cytoskeleton, a collection of structural proteins that form large, supramolecular aggregates.

Membranes and Organelles

Plasma Membrane

The plasma membrane defines the boundary of the cell and serves to contain and concentrate enzymes and the other macromolecular constituents.[3] The plasma membrane is composed of amphipathic molecules, mainly phospholipids and proteins that contain distinct regions that are either insoluble in water (hydrophobic) or soluble in water (hydrophilic). By orienting themselves so that their hydrophobic portions are in contact with each other, phospholipids can spontaneously form lipid bilayers, within which proteins and hydrophobic components such as cholesterol are embedded (Fig. 1-2). Individual lipid molecules are able to diffuse within the bilayer. Embedded proteins can also move, although their movement is slower

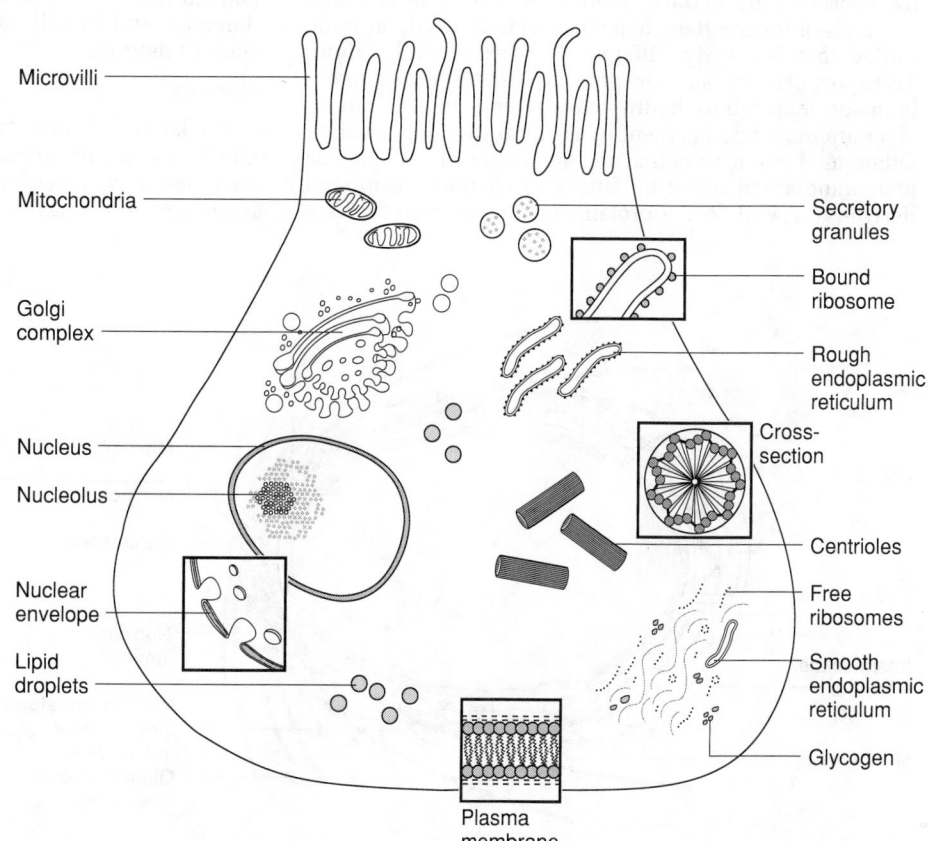

Figure 1-1. Schematic diagram of a typical epithelial cell, showing the common internal organelles.

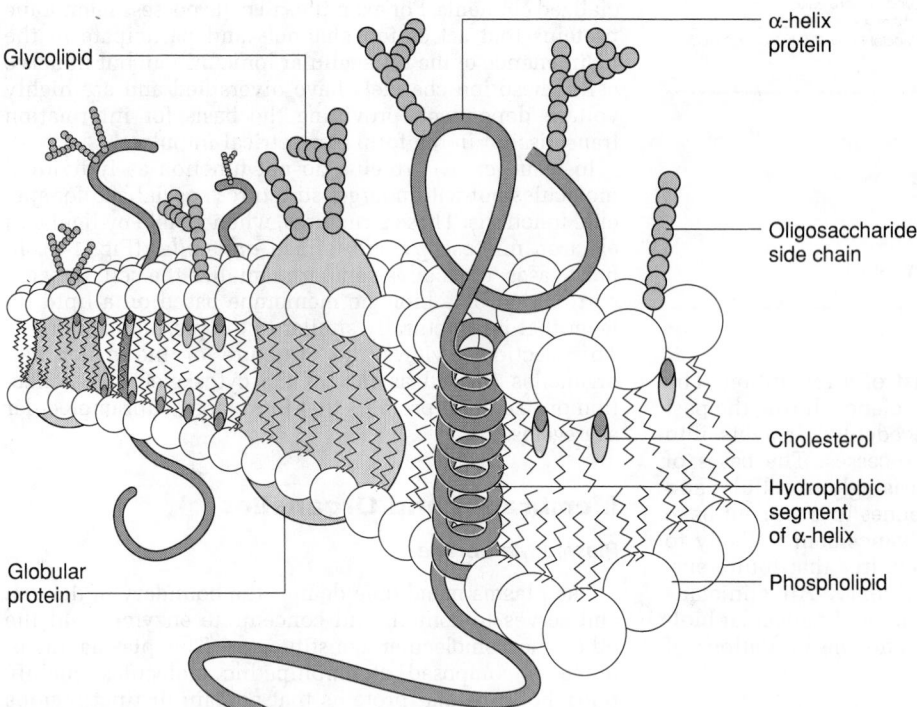

Figure 1-2. Structure of the cell membrane as a fluid mosaic consisting of a phospholipid bilayer that contains cholesterol and embedded proteins.

and often restricted by cytoskeletal attachment. The plasma membrane forms a continuous barrier between the aqueous extracellular and intracellular fluids. In addition to physically restraining macromolecules within the cell, the hydrophobic core of the lipid bilayer presents a barrier to small, charged molecules such as ions and adenosine triphosphate (ATP). This arrangement allows specialized transport proteins in the membrane, which act as regulated channels or transporters, to maintain an intracellular ionic milieu that is clearly different from extracellular fluid. Transport proteins and receptors are generally transmembrane proteins whose hydrophobic regions in the lipid bilayer are most often present in an α-helical configuration. Other membrane proteins on the inside of the plasma membrane are attached by fatty acid chains or isoprenyl derivatives, while some proteins on the external face are

linked to phosphatidylinositol (PI) situated in the outer leaflet of the bilayer. Most plasma membrane proteins extending externally bear carbohydrate moieties primarily as oligosaccharide chains, which contribute to the cell coat or glycocalyx. Finally, cells can restrict lipid and protein components to specific membrane domains. This is especially prominent in ion-transporting epithelial cells of gut and kidney, which have distinct apical and basolateral domains, and in cells with specialized secretory regions such as neurons.

Nucleus

The largest of the cellular organelles is the nucleus, usually 3 to 8 μm in diameter. The nucleus is defined by an envelope consisting of two membranes, the inner and outer nuclear membranes (Fig. 1-3). Just inside the inner nuclear

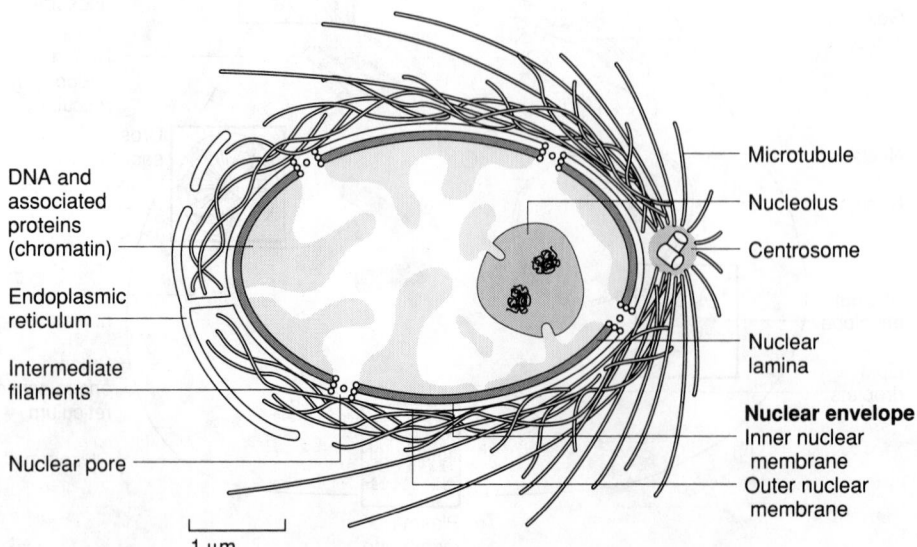

Figure 1-3. Detailed structure of the cell nucleus.

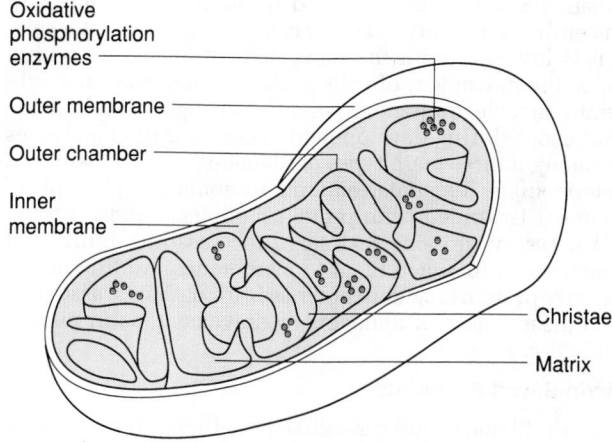

Oxidative
phosphorylation
enzymes

Outer membrane

Outer chamber

Inner
membrane

Christae

Matrix

Figure 1-4. Schematic structure of a typical mitochondrion.

membrane is a supporting meshwork of intermediate filaments, the nuclear lamina. The outer membrane is continuous with the rough endoplasmic reticulum (ER) and is studded with ribosomes. All of the chromosomal DNA is contained within the nucleus in association with a specialized class of acidic proteins, termed *histones.* Histones and DNA exist together as chromatin fibers. The contents of the nucleus communicate with the cytoplasm by means of openings in the nuclear envelope, called *nuclear pores.* These ringlike pores are composed of specialized proteins that function as channels to regulate the movement of material between nucleus and cytoplasm. The nucleus also contains a specialized region, the nucleolus, where ribosomes are assembled.

The remainder of the cell, external to the nucleus and contained by the plasma membrane, is termed *cytoplasm.* Cytoplasm is composed of a nonparticulate "soup," or cytosol, as well as a number of membranous organelles and the filamentous cytoskeleton.

Mitochondria

Mitochondria are sausage-shaped organelles, 0.2 to 0.5 μm in diameter and up to several micrometers in length. They are defined by a smooth outer membrane and an inner membrane characterized by infoldings, called *cristae,* which protrude into the central matrix (Fig. 1-4). Mitochondria are the major source of energy production in eukaryotic cells. The enzymes involved with electron transport and oxidative phosphorylation exist in an ordered array of small, stalked particles protruding inward from the inner membrane. Enzymes involved in the final oxidation of sugars and lipids are present in the matrix space, which also contains granules of mitochondrial DNA and a few ribosomes. Mitochondria contain the genetic codes for and synthesize some of their own proteins. They also divide by fission, consistent with the notion that mitochondria originated from captive or symbiotic bacteria. Both mitochondrial membranes have unique characteristics. The outer membrane contains porins, proteins forming large channels that render the membrane permeable to molecules of up to 10,000 daltons. The inner mitochondrial membrane is almost entirely protein, with the lowest lipid content of common biologic membranes. Oxidative phosphorylation at the inner membrane generates an electrochemical proton gradient, and the downhill movement of H^+ through adenosine triphosphatase (ATPase) molecules provides energy to synthesize ATP.

Endoplasmic Reticulum

The ER is a network of interconnected membranes forming closed vesicles, tubules, and saccules. The ER has a number of functions and is primarily involved in the synthesis of protein and lipids. The ER is divided into rough ER, which is studded with ribosomes and involved in the synthesis of exportable proteins (Fig. 1-5), and smooth ER, which lacks ribosomes and is involved in the synthesis of fatty acids and lipids (Fig. 1-6). Rough ER is especially prominent in cells such as pancreatic acinar cells and plasma cells that secrete large amounts of protein; its functional role in protein synthesis is discussed later. Smooth ER is especially prominent in cells producing lipid derivatives such as the adrenal cortex and in the hepatocyte. Smooth ER also contains enzymes that modify or detoxify endogenous metabolites and foreign molecules such as drugs and pesticides.

Golgi Complex

Adjacent to the rough ER and functionally involved in the sorting and packaging of secreted protein is the Golgi complex (see Figs. 1-1 and 1-5). Each complex consists of a series of flattened membrane sacs, or cisternae, surrounded by a number of vesicles. These vesicles are transport containers that shuttle proteins destined for secretion from the rough ER to the Golgi complex. During this process, secretory proteins are modified or processed, for example, by addition of sugar residues. The Golgi complex is also the compartment involved in directing secretory proteins into either lysosomes, small vesicles that rapidly move to the periphery of the cell and release their contents, or larger secretory granules where the contents condense and are stored to await a regulatory signal that initiates fusion with the plasma membrane and secretion (see section on intracellular synthesis, transport, and organization of macromolecules).

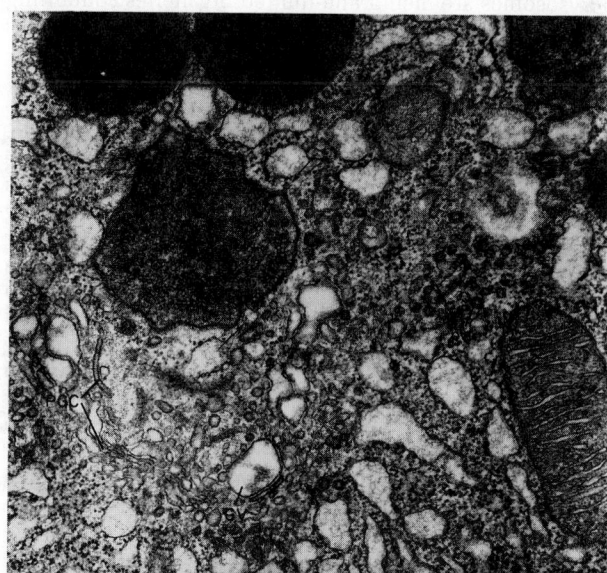

Figure 1-5. Electron photomicrograph of a portion of a pancreatic acinar cell showing endoplasmic reticulum, Golgi apparatus, and forming secretory granules. There is an abundance of small transport vesicles, which shuttle secretory proteins between the various membrane-limited organelles. CV, condensing vacuole; PGC, post-Golgi cisternae; PV, peripheral vesicles; GV, Golgi vacuole; t, transition element of the RER. (Courtesy of J. Jamieson, Yale University, New Haven, CT)

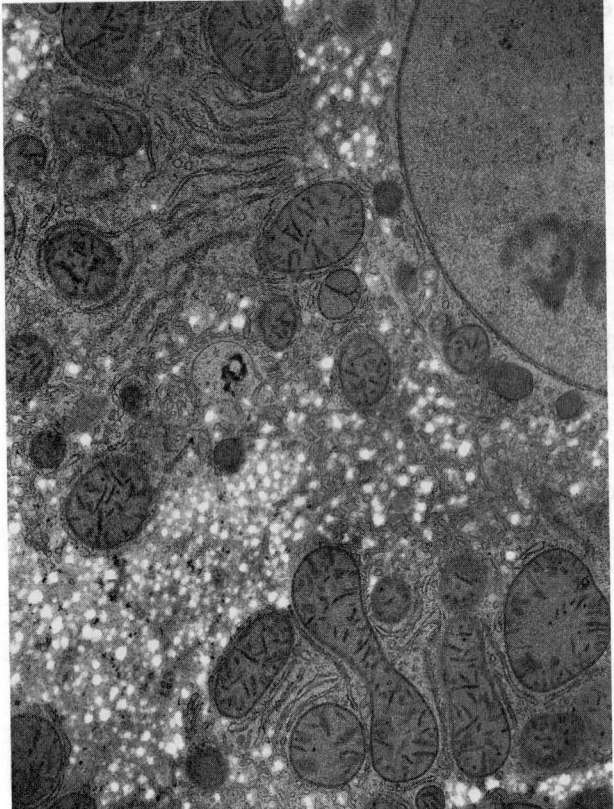

Figure 1-6. Electron photomicrograph of a portion of a hepatocyte, showing a nucleus, mitochondria, and smooth and rough endoplasmic reticulum. (Courtesy of A.K. Christensen, University of Michigan, Ann Arbor)

Lysosomes

Lysosomes are membrane-limited organelles containing acid hydrolytic enzymes that degrade polymers such as proteins, carbohydrates, and nucleic acids. Lysosomal enzymes all work best at an acid pH. The interior of the lysosome is maintained at pH of about 5.0 by an H^+-transporting ATPase located in the lysosomal membrane. This enzyme uses ATP hydrolysis to pump H^+ into the lysosomal lumen. Lysosomes are frequently classified as primary lysosomes, small, spherical structures containing only hydrolytic enzymes, or secondary lysosomes, larger and irregularly shaped, containing membranes or particles that are being digested. Secondary lysosomes result from the fusion of primary lysosomes with engulfed or abnormal organelles or with endocytotic vesicles that are bringing extracellular material into the cell for degradation. The cell is normally protected from lysosomal enzymes by their sequestration within a membrane-limited compartment. In addition, if the lysosome ruptures into the cytoplasmic compartment, the digestive enzymes become inactivated because cytoplasmic pH is maintained near 7.0. The lysosomal membrane is permeable to amino acids, monosaccharides, and other similarly sized molecules that are released after hydrolysis. These molecules can be reused by the cell.

Cytoskeleton

The cytoskeleton is a collection of filamentous protein structures that allows cells (1) to assume and maintain a variety of shapes, (2) to produce directed movement of

organelles within the cell, and (3) to effect movement of the entire cell relative to other cells.[4,5] Thus, the cytoskeleton is involved with the movement of organelles within cells, the movement of cells such as leukocytes on a substrate, muscle contraction, and the changes in cell shape that occur during development. These multiple activities depend on three main types of filaments—actin filaments, intermediate filaments, and microtubules. Each type of filament is formed from protein monomers and a variety of accessory proteins that serve to cross-link individual filaments or to attach them to membranes. Additional accessory proteins regulate polymerization, that is, assembly and disassembly of filaments or movement, as in muscle and cilia.

Actin-Based Filaments

Actin filaments are threadlike structures, about 8 nm in diameter, composed of a tight helix of actin monomers (Fig. 1-7). Actin filaments are polar structures with two different ends that are in equilibrium with free monomers. In muscle cells, most actin exists in stable filaments made from the globular subunits. In nonmuscle cells, about half of the actin is in the free monomer pool, and filaments can form by addition of subunits to the positive end. Disassembly occurs by deletion from the negative end. This equilibrium is also regulated by a number of actin-binding proteins, including thymosin and profilin. Polymerization is also regulated by cell surface receptors acting through heterotrimeric and small guanosine triphosphate (GTP)-binding proteins.

In skeletal muscle, actin forms a regular array of thin filaments, each with the positive end attached to a Z disk. The other major protein of skeletal muscle, myosin, contains two heavy chains, each of molecular weight 230,000, which together form two globular heads, a hinge region, and a coiled, rodlike tail (see Fig. 1-7). Also attached to each head are two distinct light chains of molecular weight about 20,000. In skeletal and cardiac muscle, 300 to 400 of these myosin dimers pack together by interaction between their rodlike tails to form a bipolar aggregate, called the *thick filament.* The protruding heads of the thick-filament myosin bundles interact with actin in an ATP-dependent manner to create movement by ratcheting the myosin head down the actin filament toward the positive end. This movement causes the thick and thin filaments to overlap and the muscle to shorten. Other proteins, including troponins and tropomyosin, are involved in the regulation of this interaction. One of the troponins (troponin C) binds Ca^{2+}, leading to activation of the myosin ATPase. In smooth muscle and nonmuscle cells, myosin is not as abundant or as well organized, but bipolar filaments of 15 to 20 myosin molecules exist and can interact with actin to produce movement. In this case, activation is controlled by Ca^{2+} interaction with the calcium-binding protein, calmodulin. Calmodulin activates the enzyme, myosin light-chain kinase, which phosphorylates one of the light chains of myosin and thus promotes the actin–myosin interaction.

Nonmuscle cells also contain a distinct, smaller form of myosin, termed *minimyosin* or *myosin I,* which does not form filaments. Rather, its smaller tail is attached to membranes or organelles, whereas its single head, which is similar to that of regular myosin, can interact with and move along an actin filament. When the actin is fixed, this can lead to organelle movement, as in cytoplasmic streaming.

Muscle-like bundles of actin and myosin can form transiently in nonmuscle cells and can be involved in specialized functions. An example of such a temporary cellular structure is the contractile ring that leads to the separation of the two daughter cells during cell division. The contractile ring con-

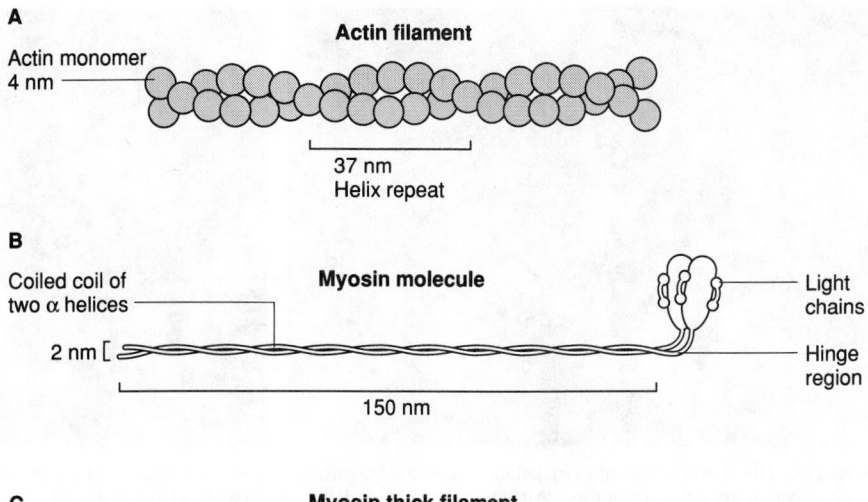

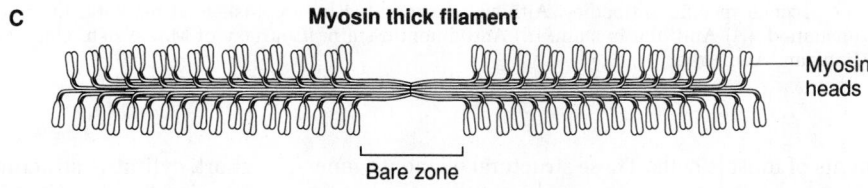

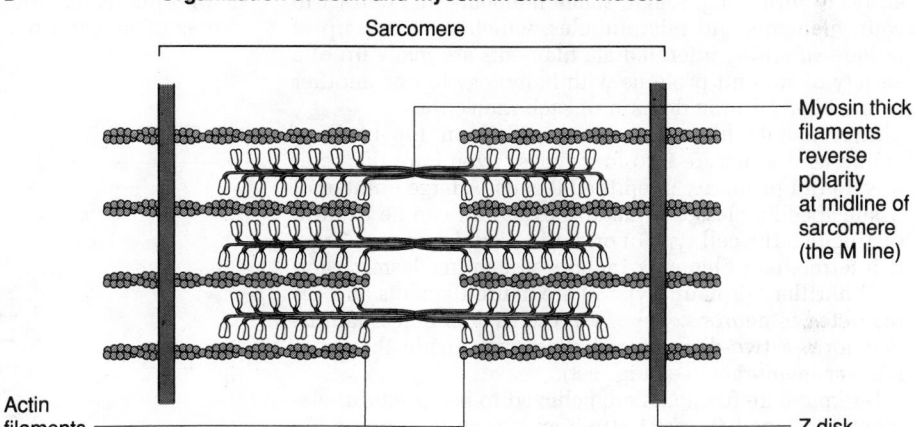

Figure 1-7. Structures of actin and myosin, their organization into filaments, and the organization of actin thin filaments and myosin thick filaments in striated muscle.

tains actin and myosin, and its formation constricts the middle of a cell. When cell division is complete, the ring disappears. Other, less transitory assemblies of actins and myosin are involved in the folding of epithelial cell sheets and in the maintenance of epithelial polarity. The latter is maintained by a belt of filaments running circumferentially around the apical end of the cell. The filaments attach to junctional complexes that connect adjacent cells.

Actin filaments are also involved in the maintenance of cell shape. An especially dense network of actin, sometimes termed the *cell web,* is present just beneath the plasma membrane. The cell web consists of a three-dimensional network of actin filaments stabilized by cross-linking proteins, one of the most abundant of which is filamen. Filamen exists as a dimer joined head-to-head with each tail possessing an actin-binding site. The loose actin network is also connected to the plasma membranes by other proteins, including spectrin and fodrin. Because the network must disassemble to allow secretion or endocytosis, it is not surprising that actin-severing proteins also exist. When activated by Ca^{2+}, one of these, gelsolin, severs and forms a cap on the new positive end of the actin fila-

ment, thereby leading to a local and usually transient disappearance of the network.

Another example of a specialized structure based on an actin-containing cytoskeleton are the microvilli found on many cells but especially on intestinal enterocytes. In the intestine, microvilli serve to increase absorptive surface area. The core of each microvillus contains a bundle of 20 to 30 parallel actin filaments attached at the tip by the positive end and extending down to anchor in a specialized cortex at the apical pole of the cell. The actin filaments are held together by several small actin-binding proteins, such as fimbrin. Fimbrin contains two actin-binding sites on a single polypeptide chain such that the actin filaments are tied into a compact bundle with regular spacing. The bundle is also connected to the overlying plasma membrane by lateral arms that contain a minimyosin-like molecule.

Intermediate Filaments

Intermediate filaments are a heterogeneous class of tough protein fibers named for their thickness (about 10 nm), which is intermediate between the thin and thick

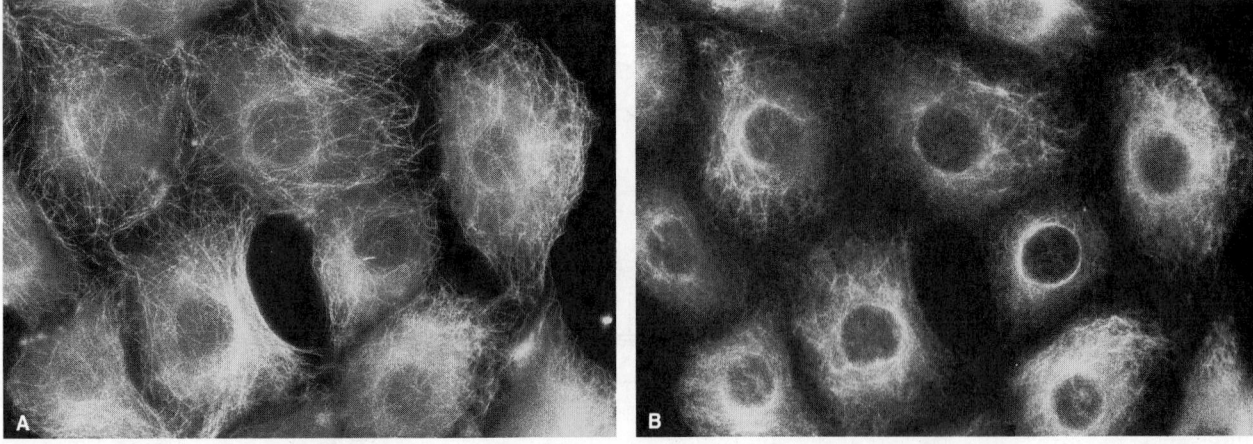

Figure 1-8. The distribution of cytoskeletal elements in pulmonary endothelial cells as detected by fluorescence-specific antibodies. Although surrounded by a cytoskeletal network, the nuclei are unstained. (*A*) Antitubulin stain. (*B*) Antivimentin stain. (Courtesy of M.J. Welsh, University of Michigan, Ann Arbor)

filaments of muscle cells. These structural elements generally form a basket around the nucleus and extend out to the cell periphery. Intermediate filaments are formed from fibrous proteins that associate side to side in overlapping arrays to form long, tough, stable filaments. In contrast to actin filaments and microtubules, which are made up of unique subunits, intermediate filaments are made up of a variety of subunit proteins with homology to one another in the fiber-forming domain of each molecule.

Intermediate filaments are classified on the basis of amino acid structure into four types. Type I are the keratins, found primarily in epithelial cells. A large number of tissue-specific classes of keratin exist and can be used to distinguish the cell type of origin for certain tumors. Type II intermediate filaments include vimentin, desmin, and glial fibrillary protein. Type III are neurofilaments and are restricted to neurons. Type IV proteins are nuclear lamins that form a two-dimensional sheet just inside the inner nuclear membrane (see Fig. 1-3).

Intermediate filaments are believed to be structural elements designed to resist stress and provide support. As such, they are often associated with other, more dynamic cytoskeletal elements such as microtubules (Fig. 1-8). In some cases, their assembly is controlled by phosphorylation. This is especially true for nuclear lamins, which are phosphorylated and disassemble during mitotic division as the nuclear envelope disappears.

Microtubules

Microtubules are found in all cells except erythrocytes. Structurally, they are hollow fibers 24 nm in diameter that vary in length from less than a micron to up to hundreds of microns. Their basic structure consists of 13 parallel rows, or protofilaments, each composed of globular subunits (Fig. 1-9). Chemically, microtubules contain two related major proteins, α- and β-tubulin, each with a molecular weight of about 50,000. In the cell, these subunits exist as an $\alpha\beta$ heterodimer, called *tubulin*. Tubulin dimers arranged $\alpha\beta-\alpha\beta-\alpha\beta$ make up the protofilament. As a result of this organization, microtubules are oriented with a positive and a negative end, and all structures that contain microtubules are polarized. Specialized cellular structures based on microtubules include cilia, neuronal axons, and the mitotic spindle.

Microtubules are frequently associated with a specialized organelle, the centriole (see Fig. 1-1). A centriole is a short, cylindric structure composed of nine groups of triplet microtubules. Centrioles usually exist in pairs oriented at right angles to each other. All cells contain at least one pair of centrioles near the nucleus, surrounded by a cloud of amorphous material, called the *microtubule-organizing center*. The centriole divides during DNA replication.

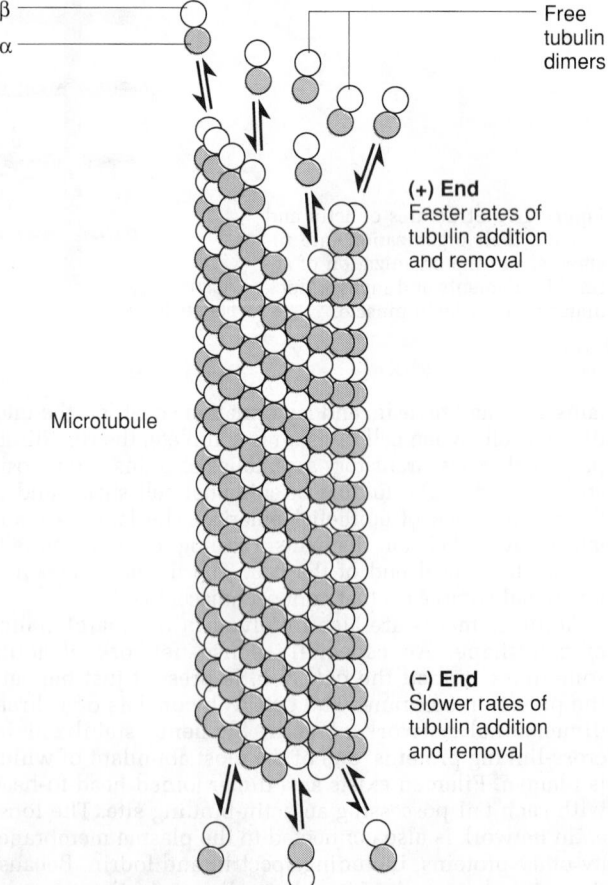

Figure 1-9. Diagram of a microtuble composed of longitudinal rows of tubulin dimers. The α- and β-tubulin dimers add to or dissociate from the two ends.

After forming the organizing center for each pole of the mitotic spindle, one centriole remains with each daughter cell. Because microtubules always have their negative pole associated with a centriole or microtubule-organizing center, and because growth occurs faster on the positive end, microtubules can be observed to grow out from the organizing center. Cilia are made up of an ordered array of microtubules, and each is attached to a modified centriole, termed the *basal body.*

Within the cell, microtubules exist in a dynamic state in which they are continually forming and dissociating as tubulin subunits add to or leave the ends. This dynamic equilibrium involves the conversion of GTP bound to tubulin to guanosine diphosphate (GDP). Each tubulin molecule possesses a binding site for colchicine, and binding of this drug prevents microtubule formation. Colchicine binding leads to the disappearance of formed microtubules and is the basis of the antimitotic action of this class of compounds. Other antimitotic agents that act on microtubules include vinblastine, which induces formation of paracrystalline aggregates of tubin, and paclitaxel (Taxol), which stabilizes formed microtubules, preventing their depolymerization. Microtubules also depolymerize at low temperatures. Although microtubules in dividing or motile cells such as leukocytes rapidly disappear in response to colchicine or low temperature, microtubules in organized parenchymal or epithelial cells disappear more slowly, and some microtubules, such as those in cilia, appear resistant. This difference, which is related to the function of the organelle (ie, whether it needs to be stable or dynamic) is due in large part to other associated proteins, termed *microtubule-associated proteins* (MAPs). The MAPs are responsible for holding microtubules together in permanent arrays, attaching them to other organelles, including membrane vesicles, and generating the force that is involved in microtubule-based movement. Many MAPs are high-molecular-weight proteins or complexes of proteins. One prominent lower-molecular-weight class is termed *tau protein;* it acts to facilitate microtubule polymerization.

The transport of organelles in cytoplasm is usually associated with microtubules. The most specialized case is axonal flow, whereby vesicles move at rates of 3 μm/s (250 mm/d) along the axon. When viewed in the electron microscope, a cross-bridge structure exists, connecting the moving particle to the microtubule. A motor protein, kinesin, has been isolated that mediates movement along microtubules in the negative-to-positive direction and is responsible for antegrade rapid axonal transport. Kinesin is composed of heavy-chain subunits, which bind tubulin and possess ATPase activity, and light chains, which attach to cellular organelles. When ATP is hydrolyzed, the kinesin moves along the microtubule, transporting the bound vesicle (Fig. 1-10). Other distinct proteins are believed to be involved in mediating transport in the opposite direction.

A specialized form of microtubule-based motility is the beating cilium. Each cilia has a basic structure of nine microtubule doublets surrounding a central microtubule pair. The entire structure, called an *axoneme,* also contains other linker proteins that hold the unit together and a specialized MAP protein, dynein, which makes contact with the adjacent microtubule doublet. Dynein is a large protein (400,000 daltons) with ATPase activity and, like kinesin, generates force on the adjacent microtubule in one direction. Because the microtubules are attached to one another, what would otherwise be a sliding motion is converted into a bending or whiplike motion. Cilia are especially prominent in the respiratory tract, where they generate movement of mucus out of the bronchial system.

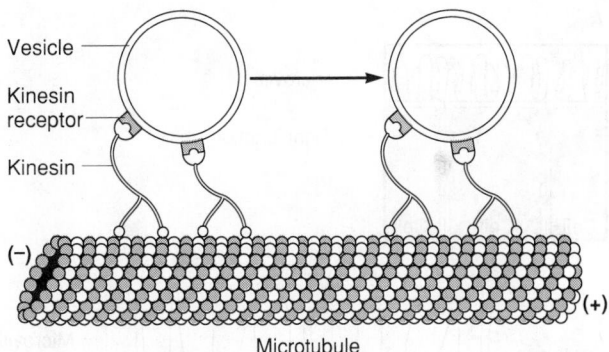

Figure 1-10. Model of kinesin-mediated transport of vesicles along a microtubule. The kinesin molecules move along the microtubule by interacting with tubulin in an ATP-requiring manner.

CELL–CELL INTERACTION

All cells must interact with their neighbors, and most are arranged in assemblies called tissues. The cells in a tissue are in contact with the extracellular matrix, which in cases such as connective tissue may surround the cells. In other cases, epithelial cells are directly attached to each other and the extracellular matrix is reduced to a thin layer, the basal lamina, which underlies the cellular sheet. Although cells such as neurons and endocrine cells influence other cells by specialized secretions, this section considers direct physical interactions mediated by molecules in the cell membrane and by the cytoskeleton.

Cell Junctions

Cell junctions were originally identified and classified by their structure as observed using the electron microscope. Functionally, cell junctions can be classified as occluding, anchoring, or communicating.[2] The major occluding junction is the tight junction or zonula occludens, which connects cells in epithelia and thereby allows epithelia to serve as selective permeability barriers. As discussed later, epithelia are almost always engaged in transcellular transport. Tight junctions make this possible both by preventing backflux between cells of transported molecules and by maintaining distinct apical and basal membrane proteins. Tight junctions are normally located near the apical pole of the cell and form a belt that completely encircles the cell (Fig. 1-11). In transmission electron microscopy, the junction appears as a series of focal contacts between the outer leaflets of adjacent plasma membrane. In freeze-fracture electron microscopy, the junction appears as an anastomosing network of sealing strands. Although all tight junctions are impermeable to macromolecules, the barrier to ions and water is related to the number of sealing strands. The strands are composed of long rows of transmembrane proteins, which have not been molecularly characterized.

Anchoring junctions connect the cytoskeleton of the cell to extracellular matrix or neighboring cells. Morphologically, these are adherens junctions or desmosomes. Adherens junctions occur in epithelia as a continuous adhesion belt, the zonula adherens, located just below the tight junction. Morphologically, this consists of a long stretch of continuous contact between cell membranes. The membranes are held together by a linker protein, E-cadherin, also called *uvomorulin*. E-cadherin is a single-pass transmembrane glycoprotein with four extracellular Ca^{2+}-binding domains and a terminal domain that binds to the same

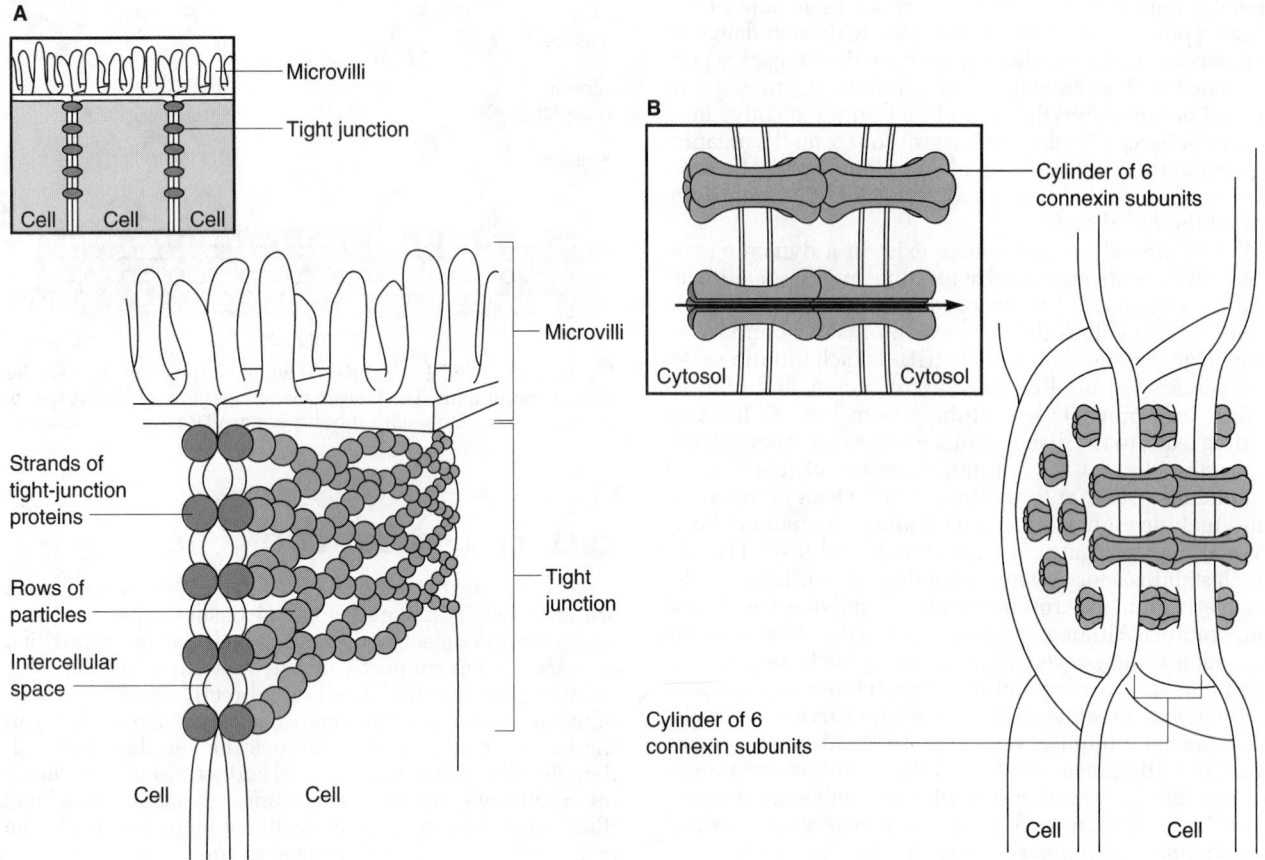

Figure 1-11. Schematic view of two intracellular junctions.

domain on another cadherin molecule. The properties of this molecule account for the Ca²⁺ dependence of cell adhesion. Within the cell, the adhesion belt is attached by the cytoplasmic end of cadherin molecules to contractile bundles of actin filaments by a set of intracellular linker proteins, including catenins, vinculin, and α-actinin. In nonepithelial cells, adherens junctions are localized as focal contacts or adhesion plaques where bundles of actin filaments terminate and serve primarily as attachment sites to the extracellular matrix. In addition to participating in anchoring junctions in adult cells, the cadherin family of cell-adhesion molecules, along with the structurally distinct CAM molecules (N-CAM, ICAM) and selectins, play important roles in morphogenesis and in the adhesion of leukocytes to endothelial cells during inflammation.

The other type of anchoring junction is the desmosome. Desmosomes are button-like points of attachment with a prominent intracellular plaque that weld together adjacent cells by serving as anchoring sites for intermediate filaments within the cell. The particular type of intermediate filament depends on the cell type being keratin in most epithelial cells and desmin in cardiac muscle cells. The transmembrane-linker proteins in desmosomes are cadherins that, as discussed earlier, bind each other by a Ca²⁺-dependent mechanism. Hemidesmosomes, or half-desmosomes, are morphologically similar to desmosomes but are chemically and functionally distinct and are considered in the next section, Cell–Matrix Adhesion.

The third functional type of cell junction is the gap junction, which is specialized for cell communication (see Fig. 1-11*B*). In conventional electron micrographs, it appears as a patch where adjacent membranes are separated by a uniform narrow gap of about 20 nm. This gap, however, is

spanned by protein molecules forming an array of channels through which ions and small molecules up to about 1000 daltons can pass. Thus, the junction mediates both electrical and chemical coupling. This is most dramatic in cardiac and smooth muscle but also plays an important role in embryogenesis. Gap junctions are formed from transmembrane proteins called *connexins*. A ring of six identical connexins, each of which spans the membrane four times, forms a *connexon,* with a central aqueous pore. The connexons protrude from the membrane and, when aligned with a connexon on an adjacent cell, both hold the two membranes at the characteristic distance and form a channel. These channels are not continuously open but regulated by Ca²⁺, intracellular pH, and protein phosphorylation.

Cell–Matrix Adhesion

Extracellular matrix is a meshwork of negatively charged polysaccharide glycosaminoglycan chains and protein fibers. The protein fibers are mainly structural, such as collagen and elastin, or adhesive, such as fibronectin and laminin. The principle protein molecules in the plasma membrane that serve as receptors for matrix molecules are the integrins.[6] Integrins are so named to indicate that they integrate the extracellular matrix and the cytoskeleton. Evidence is now emerging that integrins are functional as well as structural integrators and that they are involved in bidirectional signaling across the plasma membrane.

Integrins are noncovalently attached heterodimeric glycoproteins composed of α and β subunits. So far, 15 α and 8 β subunits have been identified. Different cell types express and synthesize different αβ complexes, with the combination of α and β determining the ligand specificity.

For example, $\alpha_5\beta_1$ is a fibronectin receptor, while $\alpha_6\beta_1$ is a laminin receptor; both are expressed on most cells. β_2 Chains, by contrast, are primarily expressed on white blood cells and mediate cell–cell interactions (eg, between white blood cells and vascular endothelium). A significant amount of redundancy occurs; most integrins bind several adhesive glycoproteins, and most adhesive glycoproteins bind to more than one protein.

Each integrin subunit spans the membrane once with a large extracellular domain and a small cytoplasmic domain. Divalent cation binding motifs are present in both subunits near the presumed ligand binding site. Most integrins are clustered into focal adhesion plaques and attach to actin through linker proteins, particularly talin and α-actinin. In fibroblasts, these focal adhesions colocalize with the termination of stress fibers. Other proteins in the adhesion plaque include a 125-kd tyrosine kinase termed *p125*^FAK (focal adhesion kinase). By virtue of this connection to the cytoskeleton, cells can orient the matrix macromolecules they secrete, and in turn, matrix macromolecules can organize the cytoskeleton. A special case is the integrin found in hemidesmosomes $\alpha_6\beta_4$, which connects intracellularly to intermediate filaments by distinct linker proteins. Whereas keratin filaments associated with desmosomes have lateral attachments to the desmosome, many filaments associated with hemidesmosomes end in the plaque.

Integrins are components of inside-out signal transduction. Various β_2-integrins on monocytes and neutrophils are stimulated (ie, show an increased binding affinity) in response to inflammatory mediators. Platelet activation induces its integrins to bind fibrinogen. In other cases, phosphorylation of a β_1-integrin during mitosis inhibits binding of fibronectin, allowing the cell to round up or detach. Integrins also mediate outside-in signaling. The binding of antibodies or glycoproteins to integrins can affect intracellular pH and Ca^{2+} as well as tyrosine phosphorylation and lead to cellular differentiation, activation, or proliferation. An integrin-associated protein appears to function as a Ca^{2+} channel. The protein p125^FAK can be activated by both integrins and peptide growth factors, although its role in cell function remains to be determined.

MEMBRANE TRANSPORT

The plasma membrane physically defines the boundaries of the cell and acts as a dynamic interface that mediates all interactions of the cell with the extracellular environment. The survival of the cell requires that cytosolic composition be maintained within narrow limits, despite the constant influx of nutrients and the simultaneous outflow of waste. This section focuses on the membrane transport mechanisms that enable the cell to maintain its unique composition despite the continual turnover of its contents.

A striking feature of living cells is the marked difference between the composition of the cytosol, the fluid within the cell, and the fluid of the extracellular milieu as illustrated in Figure 1-12. The most familiar example is the distribution of sodium (Na^+) and potassium (K^+). Cells are typically rich in K^+ and contain relatively little Na^+, despite the fact that they are constantly bathed by a fluid with precisely the opposite composition. Even more impressive is the distribution of ionized (as opposed to bound) Ca^{2+}. The extracellular concentration of this ion is typically of the order of 10^{-3} mol/L (1 mmol/L), whereas that of the cytosol is typically 10^{-7} mol/L (10^{-4} mmol/L), a 10,000-fold gradient. These and many other examples establish the fact that the cell and its environment are not in equilibrium. Such nonequilibrium ion distributions are all the more remarkable in light of the fact that the plasma

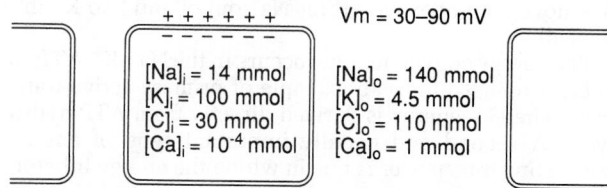

Figure 1-12. Intracellular ionic composition differs markedly from that of the surrounding extracellular fluid. Representative values for intracellular and extracellular ion concentrations are shown.

membrane is, to varying degrees, leaky to ions such as Na^+, K^+, and Ca^{2+}. The key to understanding the ability of the cell to maintain nonequilibrium cellular composition is found in two fundamental properties of the plasma membrane—selectivity and energy conversion.

Selectivity and Its Modulation

The plasma membrane is leaky to a variety of substances, but it exhibits an astounding ability to discriminate, or select, one substance over another. For example, the plasma membrane of many cells is 10 to 100 times more leaky to K^+ than Na^+. Even more spectacular is the selectivity for some organic compounds: D-glucose is often favored over the L-isomer by 1000-fold. The molecular basis for this selectivity lies in the properties of membrane-spanning proteins, which exhibit an enzyme-like specificity for particular molecules and can thus catalyze their selective transport across the plasma membrane. Much of the research in the field of membrane transport is devoted to identifying and characterizing the specific membrane proteins that constitute highly selective transport pathways.

The selectivity of biologic membranes can be altered drastically as a result of regulatory or signaling processes that occur within the cell. In nerve and muscle cells, for example, the resting membrane is 10- to 100-fold selective for K over Na, but in a matter of milliseconds, at the peak of an action potential, this selectivity can be completely reversed so that the membrane becomes 100-fold selective for Na over K. In the appropriate cell types, insulin can cause a 30-fold increase in the leakiness to glucose. This modulated selectivity is the basis for cellular signaling as well as regulatory processes that protect the integrity of individual cells and act as crucial elements in epithelial transport processes.

Energy-Converting Transport

The selectivity of the plasma membrane, although impressive, cannot account for the nonequilibrium composition of living cells. A cell can be maintained in a nonequilibrium state only by the continual expenditure of energy. The maintenance of steady-state, nonequilibrium cellular composition is possible because the plasma membrane is the site of energy converters, membrane proteins that function as biologic transport machines using the energy derived from metabolic processes to perform transport work. The archetype for the biologic transport machine is the Na^+-K^+-ATPase, a membrane protein that hydrolyzes cytosolic ATP and couples the resulting free energy to the transport of Na^+ and K^+. The catalytic cycle involves the binding of internal Na and external K in such a way that the hydrolysis of one molecule of ATP is associated with the movement of exactly three Na$^+$ out of and two K$^+$ into the cell.

The energy conversion that occurs in the Na$^+$-K$^+$-ATPase is often referred to as an example of primary active transport, whereby energy is derived directly from ATP hydrolysis. A second and equally important type of energy-converting transporter is one in which the energy inherent in a transmembrane ion gradient, usually that of Na$^+$, can be used to drive the transport of a second species (eg, protons, calcium, amino acids, or glucose). Such secondary active transport processes are extremely important to the cell because they allow energy that has been invested in the transmembrane Na gradient by the Na$^+$-K$^+$-ATPase to be used to perform various kinds of transport work (Fig. 1-13).

Cell composition is determined by the interaction of energy converters and selective leak pathways. This can be seen in Figure 1-14. Two cells are diagrammed, one a symmetric cell and the other a polarized cell, such as is found in an epithelial cell layer. Mechanisms for Na transport are diagrammed for both cells. In either case, a steady-state, intracellular Na concentration is achieved by a balance between the net inflow of Na and the net efflux of Na. In the case of the symmetric cell, Na is shown entering by a variety of mechanisms, Na channels, Na-dependent cotransport, and countertransport. Na leaves the cell through the Na$^+$-K$^+$-ATPase. The balance between these opposing processes determines the level of intracellular Na. Similarly, in the polarized cell net, transcellular Na transport is achieved by the serial arrangement of apical Na entry and basolateral Na exit, so that the level of intracellular Na is determined by the balance between these two processes. Despite similarities, these two cellular processes may differ significantly with regard to one important variable, the turnover rate. The symmetric cell is typically designed to maintain static gradients at a minimum rate of turnover; that is, leak rates are low, so pump rates are low. In contrast, the polarized cell is specialized for throughput. Entry and exit rates are elevated to produce significant transcellular Na transport that is important, for example, in the function of the airways, kidney, and gastrointestinal tract.

Membrane Composition: Implications for Selectivity and Energy Conversion

Plasma membranes are mosaic structures, consisting of a matrix of lipid in which are embedded the membrane proteins responsible for the specialized transport proper-

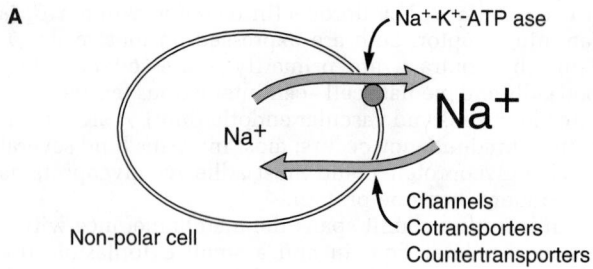

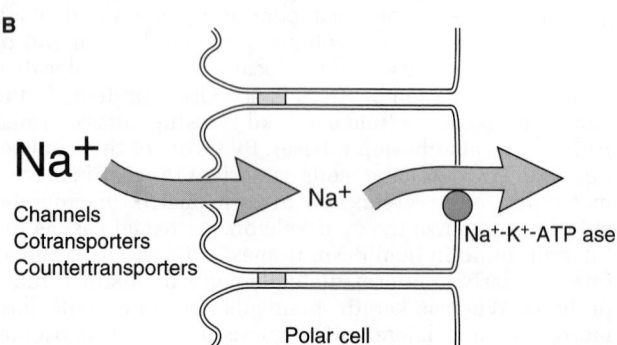

Figure 1-14. Cytosolic composition is maintained in a steady state by balancing pumps and leaks. Shown here are mechanisms that maintain low intracellular Na$^+$ concentration in two cells, one a symmetric cell (*A*) and the other a polar, epithelial cell (*B*). In the symmetric cell, Na$^+$ efflux by the pump is balanced by the sum of all the Na$^+$ leaks into the cell. In the polar cell, Na$^+$ influx at the apical (lumen-facing) side is balanced by active Na$^+$ efflux at the basolateral (blood-facing) side. The rates of Na$^+$ transport are typically much greater for the polar cell, which is designed to effect the net transcellular movement of Na$^+$ that is important for the function of the kidney and gastrointestinal tract.

ties of the cell interface (see Fig. 1-2). It is instructive to consider some of the general features of the lipid and protein regions of the plasma membrane, as an introduction to the molecular basis for membrane selectivity.

Lipid is a major component of the plasma membrane. Membrane phospholipids, being amphipathic molecules with polar and nonpolar ends, exhibit a strong tendency to organize into a stable, bimolecular layer (Fig. 1-15). The hydrocarbon layer formed by the fatty acid tails of phospholipids exhibits the transport properties that are expected for a layer of oil. Substances can penetrate this layer by a process of solubility–diffusion, that is, dissolving into the hydrocarbon and diffusing across. A model based on the simple notion of dissolving (partitioning) and diffusion predicts the transport properties of a lipid bilayer with amazing accuracy, and the tenet that plasma membranes are generally permeable to lipophilic molecules remains one of the most useful generalizations in cell biology.

The planar nature of the bimolecular lipid layer, combined with the physical properties of the fatty acid hydrocarbon tails of the phospholipids, has led to the concept of the plasma membrane as a "two-dimensional fluid." Experiments with labeled molecules indicate that individual phospholipids can move about relatively freely within the plane of each monolayer, but the polar head groups anchor the molecules so effectively in the aqueous phase that movement from one monolayer to another is relatively rare. Another reflection of the fluidity of the lipid bilayer is that some membrane proteins exhibit lateral mobility; that is, they can move about within the plane of the bilayer. The degree of fluidity exhibited by a lipid bilayer is af-

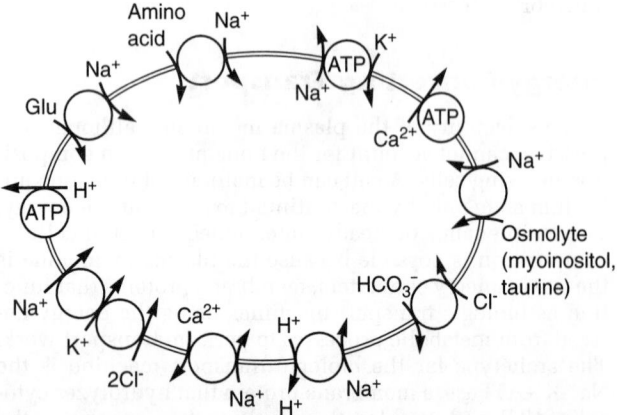

Figure 1-13. The plasma membrane contains a variety of energy-converting transporters, which function to maintain intracellular composition away from equilibrium.

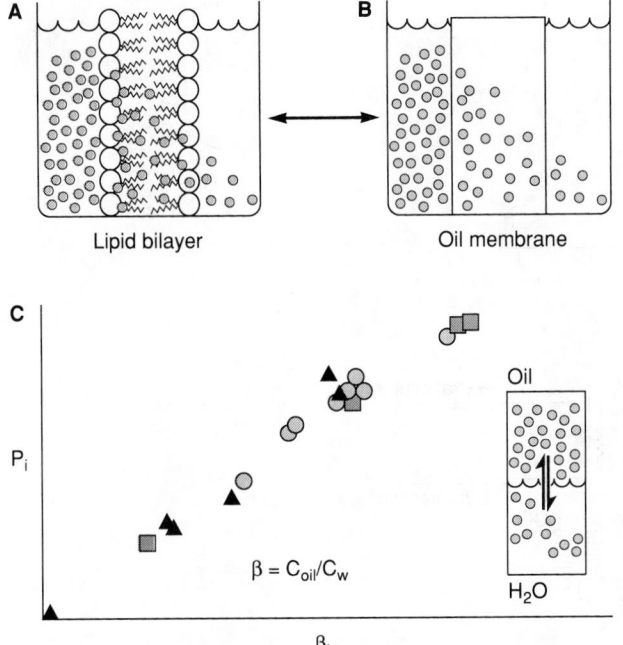

Figure 1-15. Lipophilic substances can cross a lipid bilayer by solubility diffusion. The lipid bilayer (*A*) can be approximated by a layer of oil (*B*), and the permeability of the oil membrane to various substances is expected to be proportional to β_i, the oil–water partition coefficient or solubility of the substance in oil (*C*). The inset in *C* illustrates the determination of β_i as an oil–water partition coefficient.

fected by the type of phospholipid (particularly the degree of unsaturation of the fatty acid side chains) and the cholesterol content. Cholesterol intercalates between phospholipids and decreases membrane fluidity.

Membrane Proteins: Specific Transport Pathways

The movement of substances like glucose and ions across the plasma membrane requires specialized permeation pathways, which are formed by membrane-spanning proteins. In the earlier literature, a variety of transmembrane transport processes were attributed to components referred to as "carriers." The word *carrier* naturally evokes a picture of a mobile membrane component that could bind the transported substance and shuttle it back and forth across the lipid bilayer. Some antibiotic molecules, such as valinomycin, facilitate transmembrane ion movement in precisely this way. There is little doubt, however, that the endogenous mediators of specific transmembrane transport processes are proteins that span the bilayer to provide a path from one side to the other, which is a hospitable environment for non–lipid-soluble (hydrophilic) moieties such as ions, sugars, and amino acids. These transport proteins can be divided into two broad categories: channels and carriers. In the former, the protein forms a pore that can open and close and provides a mechanism for passive flow of solutes or water across membranes. In the latter, the protein is likely to form a porelike structure, but translocation is coupled to specific conformational changes in the protein (see later).

The transport function of membrane-spanning proteins requires that they have a dual nature chemically—they must interact both with the hydrocarbon of the bilayer and

the transported substrate. Accordingly, such proteins are amphiphilic, with a hydrophobic portion that permits the protein to pass through the lipid layer and hydrophilic portions that are stable in the aqueous environments of the cytoplasm and the extracellular fluid. The functional, three-dimensional structure of such a protein may require that it cross the membrane as many as 10 or 12 times. Such proteins may consist of alternating hydrophilic and hydrophobic regions (Fig. 1-16). If the amino acid sequence is known, as a result of cloning the cDNA, it is possible to estimate the relative ability of various portions of the protein to interact with the bilayer. Stretches of amino acids that are highly hydrophobic (or hydropathic) are more likely to reside in the bilayer. A plot of the hydropathy index versus the position of the amino acids in the primary sequence (see Fig. 1-16) is used to identify regions of the protein that are likely to be associated with the membrane. This hydropathy plot provides a valuable first guess as to the number of membrane-spanning regions of the protein and points to possible large intracellular or extracellular domains. In the case of transport proteins, one expectation is that the membrane-spanning region is associated with the transport process per se, whereas large cytoplasmic or extracellular regions may be involved in regulatory functions, such as the binding of second messengers or hormones.

A membrane-spanning polypeptide chain generally adopts an α-helical conformation. This conformation is dictated by the fact that, in the absence of water, the polar peptide bonds tend to form hydrogen bonds with each other. The α-helical conformation maximizes the number of such bonds and generally forms in such a way as to also enable nonpolar amino acid side chains to interact with the lipid bilayer matrix. An important tertiary structure thought to be common to ion channel proteins is the juxtaposition of a number of membrane-spanning α helices, arranged like barrel staves, to form a central pore that is highly polar and thus a hospitable environment for ion conduction (see Fig. 1-16*B*).

Transport: Energetics and Mechanism

All transport mechanisms, regardless of their complexity, can be viewed as consisting of three steps: (1) the entry of the transported substance into the membrane on one side, (2) a translocation event that conveys the substance to the other side, and (3) the exit of the substance from the membrane and into the aqueous compartment. Understanding the mechanism for this process means comprehending the physical processes that govern each of these three steps. A complementary approach to understanding transport mechanisms is to inquire about the energetics of the transport process. Is the transporter a passive leak pathway, or does the transport event involve energy conversion?

The basis for energetic analysis of transport processes is the concept of equilibrium.[7,8] If the distribution of any substance, say glucose, Na, or K, is not at equilibrium, then flow of that substance is expected to be in a direction so as to restore equilibrium. If the distribution is maintained away from equilibrium, this means that some process is moving the substance "uphill," and such a process must involve energy conversion. For uncharged substances, the analysis is particularly simple. Consider, for example, the distribution of glucose across a cell membrane (Fig. 1-17). The equilibrium condition is [glucose]$_\text{in}$ = [glucose]$_\text{out}$. In this condition, there is no net flow of glucose through a simple glucose leak pathway. If [glucose]$_\text{in}$ is less than [glucose]$_\text{out}$, net passive glucose flow through a leak pathway is into the cell. If [glucose]$_\text{in}$ is greater than [glucose]$_\text{out}$,

A

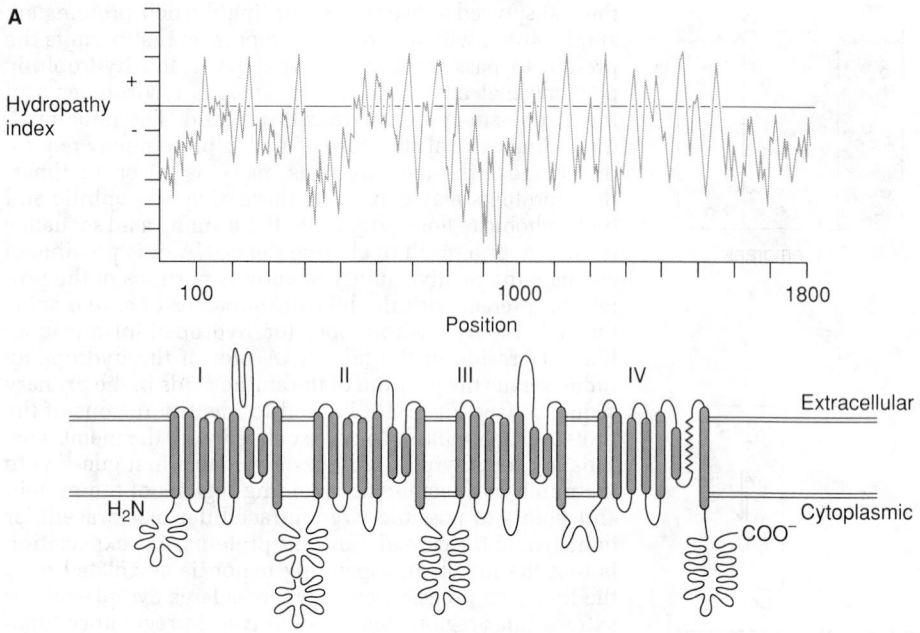

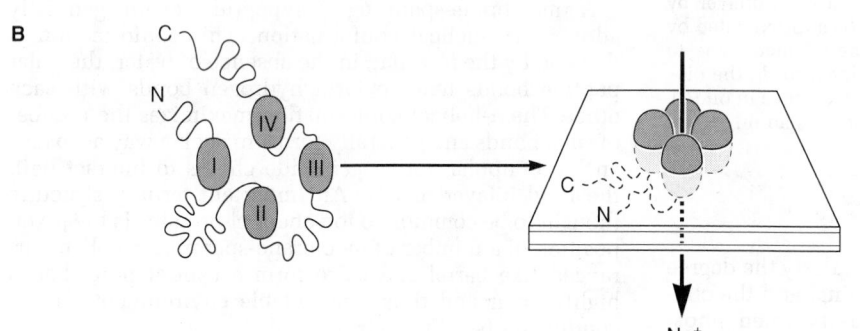

Figure 1-16. (*A*) The amino acid sequence of a sodium-channel protein derived from the cDNA can be analyzed by plotting the hydropathy index versus the position of the amino acid. (*B*) Regions predicted to be hydrophobic (+) are represented in the diagram as putative membrane-spanning domains. The four repeated motifs are shown as folding around a central pore to form an ion channel. (After Trimmer JS, Agnew WS. Molecular diversity of voltage-sensitive Na channels. Annu Rev Physiol 1989; 51:401)

glucose leaves the cell through such a transporter. Because this is a leak pathway (non–energy converting), glucose flow can only be "downhill," from a high glucose concentration to a low glucose concentration.

It is useful to analyze equilibrium for such a solute in terms of free energy, rather than concentration. To do this, we define the difference in chemical potential for glucose across the membrane, $\Delta\mu_{glu}$, as follows:

$$\Delta\mu_{glu} \text{ (in J/mol)} = RT \ln ([glucose]_i/[glucose]_o)$$
where:
R = the universal gas constant
T = the absolute temperature

In terms of free energy, the equilibrium condition is specified by $\Delta\mu_{glu} = 0$. If $\Delta\mu_{glu} \neq 0$, there is a driving force for net flow, and the flow occurs in a direction so as to restore equilibrium.

Ion flow through a channel can be driven by either an ion concentration gradient or an electrical potential difference (Fig. 1-18). To express both of these driving forces in the same units, the electrochemical potential difference, $\Delta\bar{\mu}_i$, can be defined. For K ions, $\Delta\bar{\mu}_K$ is given by the following equation:

$$\Delta\bar{\mu}_K = RT \ln ([K]_i/[K]_o) + zFV_m$$
where:
$[K]_i$ and $[K]_o$ = K concentrations
z = the valence

F = the Faraday
and V_m = the membrane potential

If $\Delta\bar{\mu}_K = 0$, the driving force for ion flow is zero, and the ion is distributed at equilibrium. If $\Delta\bar{\mu}_K \neq 0$, there is a driving force for ion flow. The total driving force, $\Delta\bar{\mu}_K$, is the sum of two parts—one due to the K concentration gradient [(RT ln ($[K]_i/[K]_o$)], and the other due to the electrical potential (zFV_m). The electrochemical potential difference can be regarded as a generalized potential function that encompasses driving forces due to both concentration gradients and electrical potential. $\Delta\bar{\mu}_K$ enables one to express the driving forces due to a concentration gradient and an electrical potential in the same units. This is perhaps most obvious as illustrated in Figure 1-18, in which all terms are expressed using electrical units (ie, millivolts), so that the driving force for K^+ flow can be written as follows:

$$\Delta\bar{\mu}_K/zF = V_m - E_K$$
where:
$E_K = RT/zF \ln ([K]_o/[K]_i)$, a measure of the driving force due to the potassium concentration gradient in electrical units

Driving Force for Water Flow

The energetics of water movement across cell membranes is simplified by the fact that water moves only passively owing to gradients of hydrostatic pressure or water

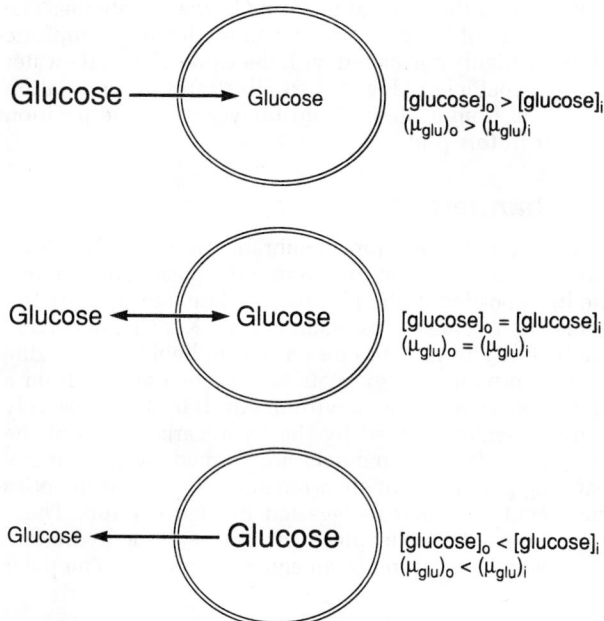

Figure 1-17. For a substance that moves by a non–energy-dependent transport mechanism, the direction of the net flow is determined by the passive driving force. In this example, the movement of glucose is determined by the orientation of the concentration gradient (the chemical potential gradient).

concentration. Hydrostatic pressure is an important driving force only for certain specialized cells—the capillary endothelium and the glomerulus of the kidney. For most of the cells in the body, the transmembrane hydrostatic pressure is zero (due to membrane elasticity), and water moves only in response to water concentration gradients.

Because the concentration of water is determined by the amount of dissolved solute, the difference in water concentration is typically expressed as a function of the difference in solute concentration or, as it is more commonly known, osmotic pressure difference (Fig. 1-19). Because there are no specialized, energy-converting transport mechanisms for water, water is distributed at equilibrium. Water distribution is determined entirely by solute distribution. If a cell gains solute, it swells by gaining water. If a cell loses solute, it shrinks due to the obligatory efflux of water.

Active Transport: Conservation of Energy

Transport processes can be conceptualized in terms of the relation between work available and work done, as suggested by Figure 1-20, which illustrates an example of a coupled transport process: Na^+–H^+ antiport or Na^+–H^+ exchange. From this perspective, the function of an Na^+–H^+ antiporter is to use the energy available in the transmembrane Na^+ gradient to drive protons out of the cell. This available energy has been invested in the Na^+ gradient by the action of the Na^+-K^+-ATPase. The work done moving protons is given by the electrochemical potential difference for protons multiplied by the number of protons (or moles of protons) moved per cycle. Similarly, the work *available* is given by the electrochemical potential difference for Na^+ times the mole number.

What would happen if we were to artificially *increase* ΔpH by acidifying the solution bathing the cell in Figure 1-20 so that ΔH^+ exceeds ΔNa^+? Like any chemical reaction, the antiporter would run backward. Protons would

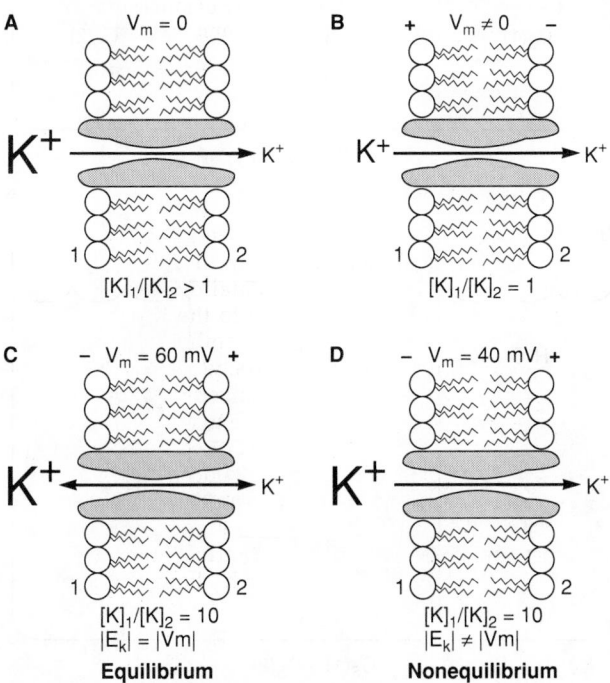

Figure 1-18. The direction of passive ion flow is determined by the *electrochemical potential gradient*. The total driving force is the sum of that due to the K concentration gradient (*A*) and that due to the electrical potential difference (*B*). If the driving force due to the concentration gradient is equal in magnitude and opposite in direction to the electrical potential (*C*), the total passive force is zero (ie, the ion is distributed at equilibrium). (*D*) A net driving force exists because there is an imbalance between E_k and V_m.

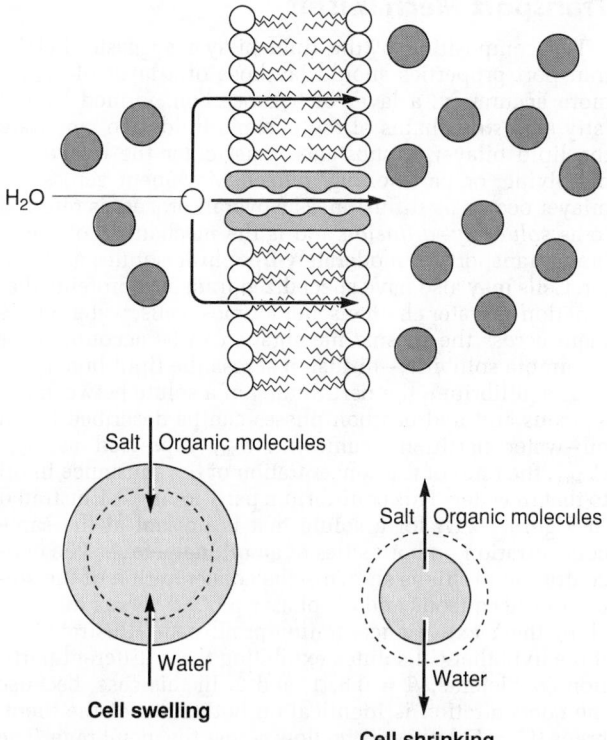

Figure 1-19. Water permeates the plasma membrane by means of *solubility–diffusion* through the lipid bilayer and, in some cells, through specialized water channels. Cell volume is normally determined by *solute* distribution because plasma membrane water permeability is high and cells tend to approach osmotic equilibrium.

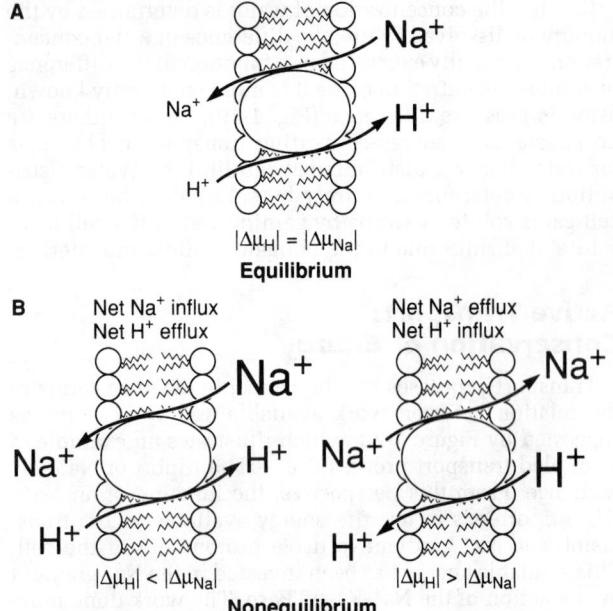

Figure 1-20. The $Na^+–H^+$ exchanger is an example of a *counter-transporter*, a mechanism by which energy invested in the Na gradient can be used to drive protons out of the cell. The direction of turnover of the exchange process is determined by the balance of the chemical potential gradients for Na and H.

enter the cell and drive Na^+ out. The energetics of any coupled transporter is an important experimental test for the coupling process.

Transport Mechanisms

The composition of the lipid bilayer suggests that its transport properties should be those of a layer of oil or, more accurately, a layer of hydrocarbon, formed by the fatty acid side chains of the phospholipids. To penetrate the lipid bilayer, a substance must enter the bilayer by dissolving, or partitioning, into it. Movement across the bilayer occurs by diffusion. The overall process is referred to as *solubility–diffusion* and is the mechanism of membrane transport for moderately lipophilic solutes and water. Cells may also have specialized transport proteins that function as water channels, but for most cells, water movement across the plasma membrane can be accounted for by simple solubility–diffusion across the lipid bilayer.

At equilibrium, the partitioning of a solute between the aqueous and hydrocarbon phases can be described by an oil–water partition coefficient, β_{oil}, expressed as C_{oil}/C_{water}, the ratio of the concentration of the substance in oil to that in water. This equilibrium partitioning is illustrated in Figure 1-21A for a solute that is present at the same concentration on both sides of an oil membrane. The concentration profile is shown—the concentration of the solute in the aqueous and oil phases plotted versus distance along the Y axis. Concentration profiles are illustrated for three hypothetical solutes exhibiting three different partition coefficients, $\beta = 0.5$, 1, and 2. In this case, because the concentration is identical on both sides of the membrane ($C_1 = C_2$), there is no flow across the membrane. The diffusion of lipophilic nonelectrolytes is a purely passive leak process; if there is no concentration gradient, there is no driving force for net flow. Figure 1-21B shows the concentration profiles in the presence of a concentration gradient ($C_1 > C_2$) illustrating the influence of the partition

coefficient on the amount of solute in the membrane. The permeability of lipid membranes to moderately lipophilic solutes is highly correlated with the value of the oil–water partition coefficient. Figure 1-22 illustrates the correlation using data from a planar lipid bilayer. Note the position of water in this plot.

Ion Channels

Ion channels are transmembrane proteins that form pores that can conduct ions across the plasma membrane. The lipid portion of the plasma membrane is virtually impermeable to small ions such as Na^+, K^+, Cl^-, and Ca^{2+}. The inability of ions to cross a hydrophobic layer is due to the enormous energy required to move an ion from a highly polar aqueous environment into the relatively nonpolar region formed by the hydrocarbon tails of the phospholipids. Ion channels are formed by membrane-spanning peptides that are arranged so that polar moieties line a central pore, as suggested in Figure 1-16B. These polar groups take the place of the water of hydration, which stabilizes an ion in an aqueous solution. The polar

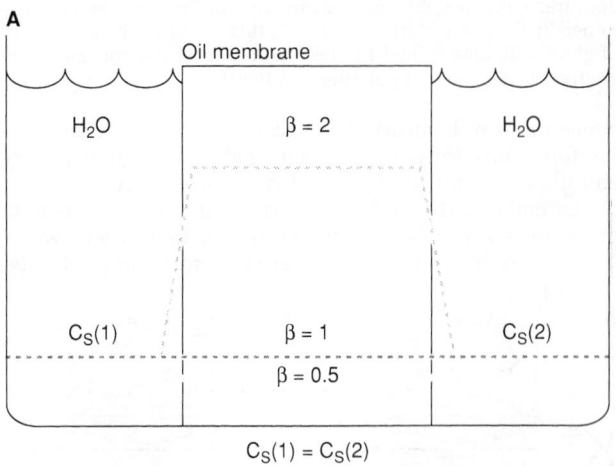

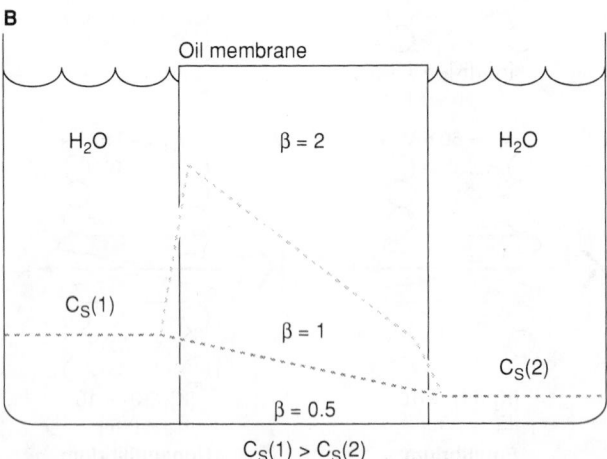

Figure 1-21. Moderately lipophilic solutes can cross the plasma membrane by solubility diffusion through the lipid bilayer, modeled here as an oil membrane. Three hypothetical solutes are depicted as having oil–water partition coefficients (β) of 0.5, 1, and 2. The concentration profiles in the absence (A) and in the presence (B) of a concentration gradient are shown. The dominant factor in the determination of permeability is the partition coefficient β_i.

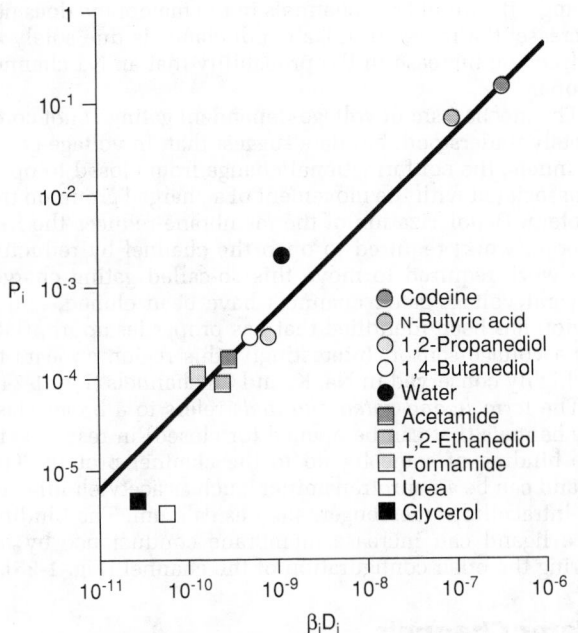

Figure 1-22. The permeability of a planar lipid bilayer to a series of lipophilic solutes is highly correlated with the product of the oil–water partition coefficient and the diffusion coefficient (ie, $\beta_i D_i$).

groups create, in essence, a water-like environment into which the ion can partition and move in the presence of an appropriate driving force.

The movement of an ion through a channel implies the movement of charge or current flow and hence is referred to as a *conductive process.* The physical interactions that underlie the conduction process determine both the rate at which ions can traverse the channel and the selectivity of the channel, the degree to which the channel discriminates between ions. The size of the single-channel conductance and the selectivity of the channel provide important criteria for distinguishing one channel from another on the basis of function. For example, most cells contain a variety of channels that are selective for specific ions (eg, Na^+, K^+, Cl^- Ca^{2+}, HCO_3^-). Selectivity provides a broad classification of channels. Most cells contain several subtypes of selective channels, which are often distinguished on the basis of the size of the single-channel conductance. It is likely that channels differentiated on the basis of function reflect the properties of distinctly different membrane proteins. The existence of channel diversity suggests that different channel proteins may play different roles in the life of the cell.

Gating of Ion Channels

Ion channels are permissive transport elements: ions flow through a channel only in the presence of an appropriate driving force. Records of the current flowing through single channels (Fig. 1-23) show clearly that even in the presence of a driving force, an ion channel does not conduct all of the time. Rather, the form of the single-channel current record suggests that the channel protein undergoes conformational changes between conducting (open) states and nonconducting (closed) states. These conformational changes are collectively referred to as *gating.* Gating of ion channels is crucial to the survival of cells and organisms because gating is the basis for the regulation of ion flow through membrane channels.

The simplest model for the gating process recognizes two states of the ion channel protein—closed (nonconducting) and open (conducting), which can be represented as a reversible chemical reaction:

$$\text{closed} \underset{\alpha}{\overset{\beta}{\rightleftharpoons}} \text{open}$$

The gating process can be envisioned as being the result of the incessant thermal vibration, or "twitching," of the protein. Every once in a while, one such thermal twitch has enough energy to precipitate a change in the conformation of the protein, a change from closed to open, for example. The rate coefficients, α and β, are a measure of the likelihood of these conformational changes. The relative values of α and E1 determine the fraction of time that the channel spends in one state or another, or more accurately, the probability of finding the channel in a particular state. For example, if $\alpha = \beta$, then, regardless of the individual values of α and E1, the channel conducts half the time. In general, the probability of finding the channel in the open state would be given by the following equation:

$$P_o = \beta/(\alpha + \beta)$$

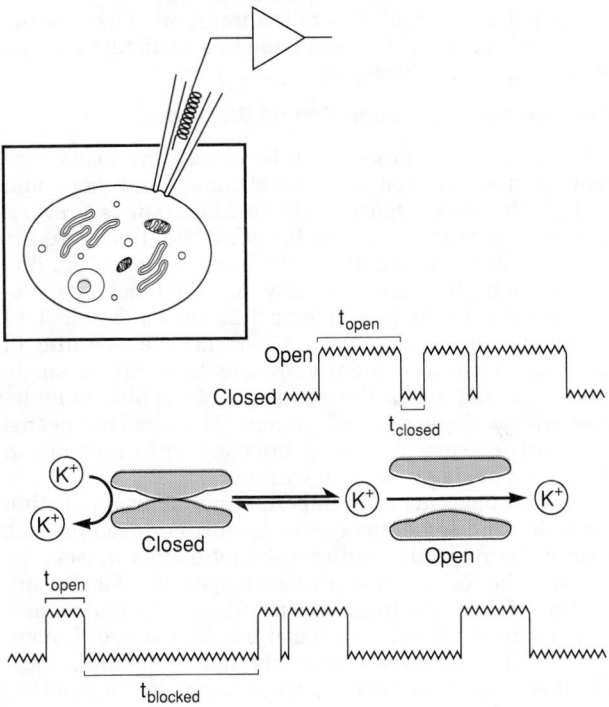

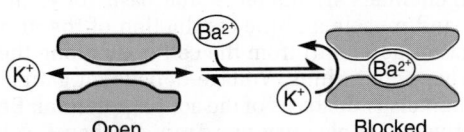

Figure 1-23. The patch–clamp method permits the recording of the currents that flow through a single open ion channel. The gating (opening and closing) of the channel is reflected in the changes in the single channel current between two values—zero and the open channel value. A channel blocker such as barium can induce long, nonconducting intervals because it binds in the channel and blocks ion flow.

Channel gating provides the molecular basis for exquisite regulation of the rate of ion flow across a membrane. For example, consider the rate of K flow through a population, or ensemble, of a particular type of K channel. The total conductance due to the population is given by g_K using the formula:

$$g_K = \gamma_K \langle N_K \rangle_o$$

where:

γ_K = conductance of a single K channel
$\langle N_K \rangle_o$ = average number of open channels

$\langle N_K \rangle_o$, however, is given by the formula

$$\langle N_K \rangle_o = N_K P_o$$

where:

N_K = *total* number of channels in the cell membrane (counting open *and* closed)
P_o = probability of finding any one channel in the open state

Combining, this relation is obtained:

$$g_K = \gamma_K N_K P_o$$

This important equation relates the macroscopic conductance, g_K, to the properties of individual channel proteins. Contained within the three parameters γ_K, N_K, and P_o is the basis for the regulation of ion transport. The conductance, or leakiness, of a membrane to a particular ion can be modulated by altering P_o, N_K, or γ_K.

Ion Channel Conduction Can Be Blocked

The conduction process can be blocked by ions or organic compounds that enter the channel, bind there, and occlude the pore. Typically, channel blockade is a reversible binding reaction, so that the efficacy of the blocker is determined by the affinity of the blocker for the binding site; this affinity determines how long the blocking molecule remains in the pore. Figure 1-23 shows the block of a K channel by the divalent ion, barium. The recording of the single channel current allows us to resolve a single blocking event, that is, the interaction of one blocker molecule with a single-channel protein. The blocking events are clearly discernible as long, nonconducting intervals in the record of single-channel current.

Channel blockade is an important mechanism of action for toxins and some therapeutic agents. For example, the deadly toxin of the puffer fish, tetrodotoxin, acts by blocking the Na^+ channels that are responsible for the conduction of the nerve impulse. The diuretic, amiloride, acts by blocking the Na channels that inhabit the apical membrane of the epithelial cells of the distal nephron. Local anesthetics such as lidocaine (Xylocaine) act by blocking ion channels.

Modulation of Ion Channel Gating

Two of the most important mechanisms that operate to gate ion channels are voltage and ligand binding. Voltage-gated ion channels are the molecular basis for excitability in nerve and muscle and the conduction of the nerve impulse (action potential) from the cell body along the axon to the synaptic terminus. Voltage-dependent gating of Na and K channels is the basis of the action potential. Because Na-selective channels open more rapidly than K-selective channels, the initial effect of a depolarizing stimulus is to increase an inward Na current and further depolarize V_m. Subsequently, K channels are opened by the depolarization, and the increased K conductance tends to repolarize V_m. It is important to realize that during an action potential, the Na conductance of the axon membrane can increase by 100-fold in less than 1 second. During this change, the number of channels in the membrane does not increase; the increase in Na conductance is due solely to a dramatic increase in the probability that an Na channel is open.

The mechanism of voltage-dependent gating is not completely understood, but data suggest that, in voltage-gated channels, the conformational change from closed to open is associated with the movement of a charged group on the protein. Depolarization of the membrane reduces the free energy (work) required to open the channel by reducing the work required to move this so-called gating charge. Several voltage-gated channels have been cloned, and a region has been identified that has properties appropriate for a voltage sensor. Interestingly, this region appears to be highly conserved in Na, K, and Ca channels (Fig. 1-24).

The term *ligand-gated channels* refers to a broad class of channels that can be opened (or closed) in response to the binding of some ligand to the channel protein. The ligand can be a neurotransmitter, such as acetylcholine, or an intracellular messenger, such as calcium. The binding of a ligand can increase membrane conductance by favoring the open configuration of the channel (Fig. 1-25).

Water Channels

The plasma membrane of most cells is highly permeable to water because water can cross the lipid bilayer at significant rates by means of solubility–diffusion. A few cells in the body are specialized so that they can exhibit a highly regulated water permeability. These cells include epithelial cells found in the distal tubule of the mammalian kidney. In such cells, the water permeability can be exquisitely regulated by antidiuretic hormone (ADH). ADH is a peptide hormone that binds to receptors located in the basolateral membranes of epithelial cells and, by means of a cAMP-dependent mechanism, leads to the insertion of water-conducting channels in the apical membrane. Regulated water permeability requires that two basic conditions be met: (1) there must be a regulatable pathway for water transport (ie, water channels); and (2) the background, or non–ADH-dependent water permeability of the membrane, must be relatively low. The apical membranes of ADH-sensitive epithelia are specialized in both of these ways. The resting water permeability (or hydraulic conductivity) of these membranes is relatively low, so that in the absence of ADH, even a substantial osmotic gradient produces little water flow. ADH can effect a dramatic increase in water permeability by inducing the insertion of water-conducting channels into the apical membrane of such cells. To be an effective instrument for the regulation of body fluid composition, these channels must be selective for water. If water channels exhibited significant ion permeability, for example, the ability of the kidney to regulate body fluid osmolality would be compromised by salt flows.

Carrier Proteins

Most transport proteins appear to function as carriers rather than as channels. Membrane carriers are a broad class of transmembrane proteins that include simple leaks as well as energy-converting mechanisms such as the ATPases, countertransporters, and cotransporters. For membrane carriers, the mechanism of translocation is probably more complicated than for an open channel. Although the details of the mechanisms are not well understood, important distinctions can be made between carrier-type and channel-type mechanisms on the basis of transport kinetics.

The most important difference between a channel mech-

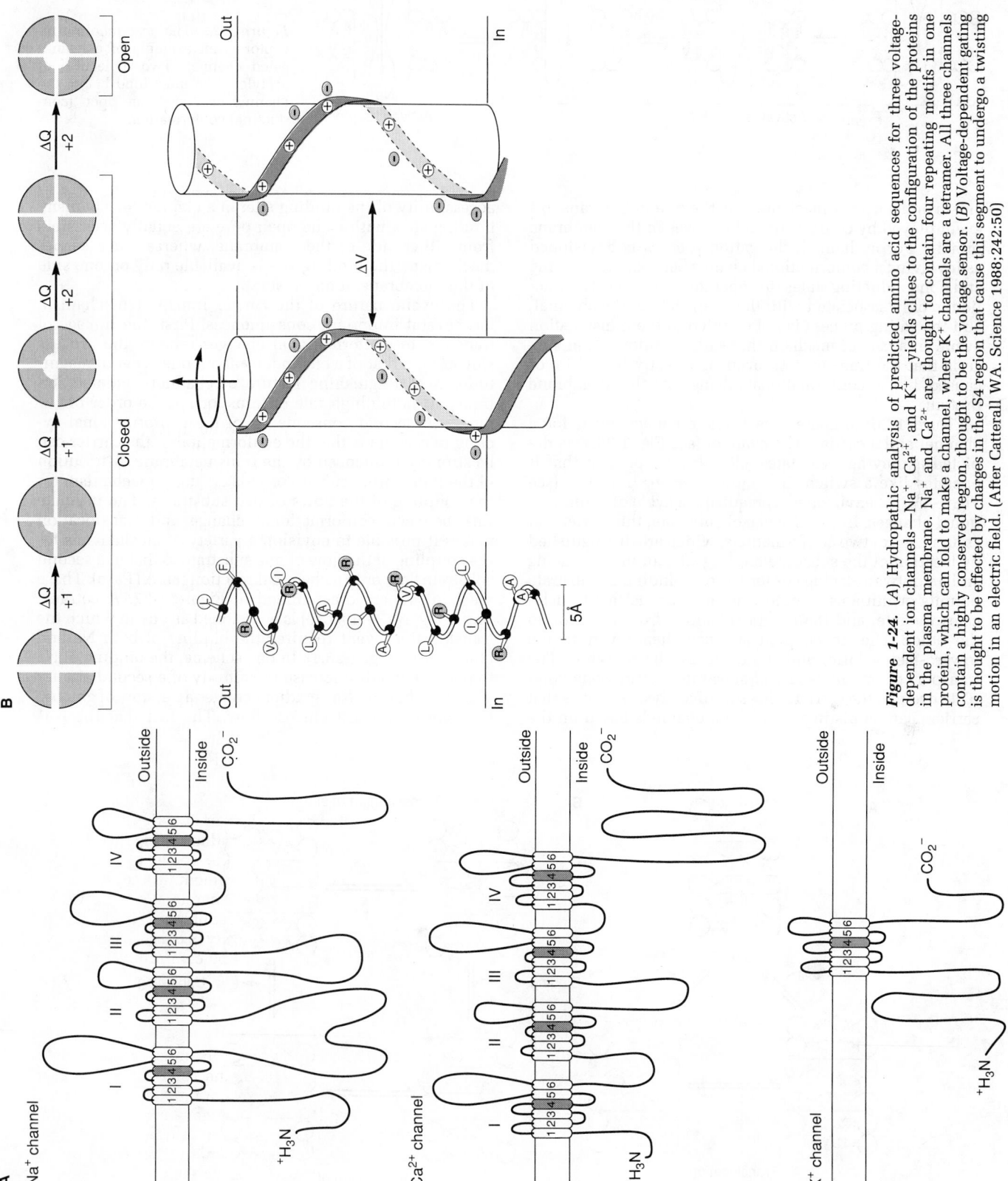

Figure 1-24. (*A*) Hydropathic analysis of predicted amino acid sequences for three voltage-dependent ion channels—Na^+, Ca^{2+}, and K^+—yields clues to the configuration of the proteins in the plasma membrane. Na^+ and Ca^{2+} are thought to contain four repeating motifs in one protein, which can fold to make a channel, where K^+ channels are a tetramer. All three channels contain a highly conserved region, thought to be the voltage sensor. (*B*) Voltage-dependent gating is thought to be effected by charges in the S4 region that cause this segment to undergo a twisting motion in an electric field. (After Catterall WA. Science 1988;242:50)

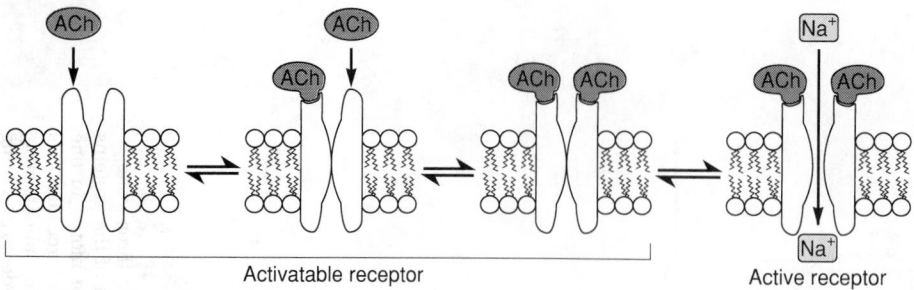

Figure 1-25. The acetylcholine receptor is an example of a ligand-gated channel. Two molecules of acetylcholine must bind before the channel can reach the open (conducting) conformation.

anism and a carrier mechanism is the role in the transport event played by conformational changes in the membrane protein. For a channel, the gating process is envisioned as involving a conformational change between conducting and nonconducting states that operates like a gate. Conduction is only associated with the open state of the channel, and the gating process is not coupled to the translocation event. In a carrier mechanism, available information suggests that the translocation event is directly linked to, or caused by, a conformational change in the membrane protein.

Figure 1-26 compares the transport mechanism for a channel and a carrier. The channel (see Fig. 1-26A) is depicted as having two states, closed and open, so that it operates like a switch. In contrast, carrier transport (see Fig. 1-26B) is envisioned as requiring a cycle of conformational changes. In the absence of substrate, the carrier can assume one of two conformations, which are distinguished by location of the substrate binding site, an inward-facing and an outward-facing conformation. Binding of substrate permits or initiates a conformational change that translocates the site, and the bound substrate, from one side to the other. The unoccupied site can then revert to the inward-facing form, and the cycle can be repeated. The transport of one molecule of substrate requires one complete cycle of the carrier. This sort of analysis suggests that carriers can be distinguished from channels based on the

accessibility of the binding site. In a channel mechanism, binding sites within the open pore are equally accessible from either side of the membrane, whereas in a carrier mechanism, the binding site is available only on one side of the membrane at any instant.

The cyclic nature of the carrier transport mechanism has several important consequences. First, the linkage of transport to conformational changes renders the process slower than that of a channel by about one order of magnitude. A distinguishing feature of channel-mediated ion transport is the high rate of transport, of the order of 10^6 ions/s. A second consequence of the conformational cycling in carriers is that the conformation of the carrier can be strongly influenced by the transmembrane distribution of the transported substrate. This creates a mechanism for the coupling of the flows of two substrates. The intimate link between conformational change and translocation makes it possible to envision a variety of mechanisms for the coupling of the flow of one substrate to that of a second substrate flow or to a chemical reaction (an ATPase). These mechanisms are diagrammed in Figure 1-27. A cotransporter (eg, Na^+–glucose) is envisioned as one in which the translocation event requires the binding of both Na and glucose (see Fig. 1-26A). In one scheme, the binding of Na to one site would increase the affinity of a second site for glucose. Thus, an Na^+ gradient creates a net flow of glucose by favoring inward glucose flow. The fact that the Na^+

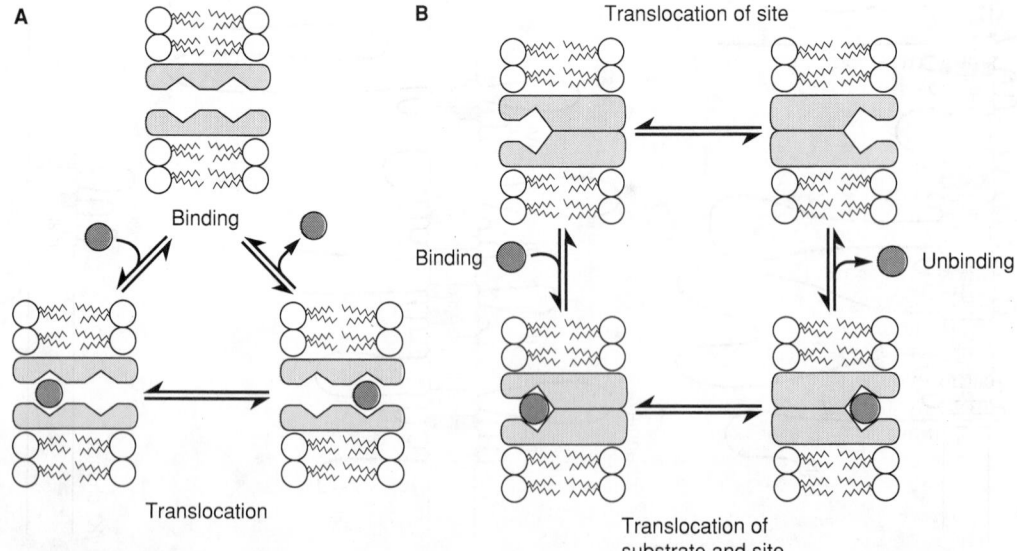

Figure 1-26. (A) Ion translocation through an open channel can be envisioned as involving a binding step, followed by translocation and unbinding of the ion. (B) In contrast, carrier-mediated flow involves binding followed by a conformational change that is coupled to the translocation of the substrate. In this model, the unbound site can translocate.

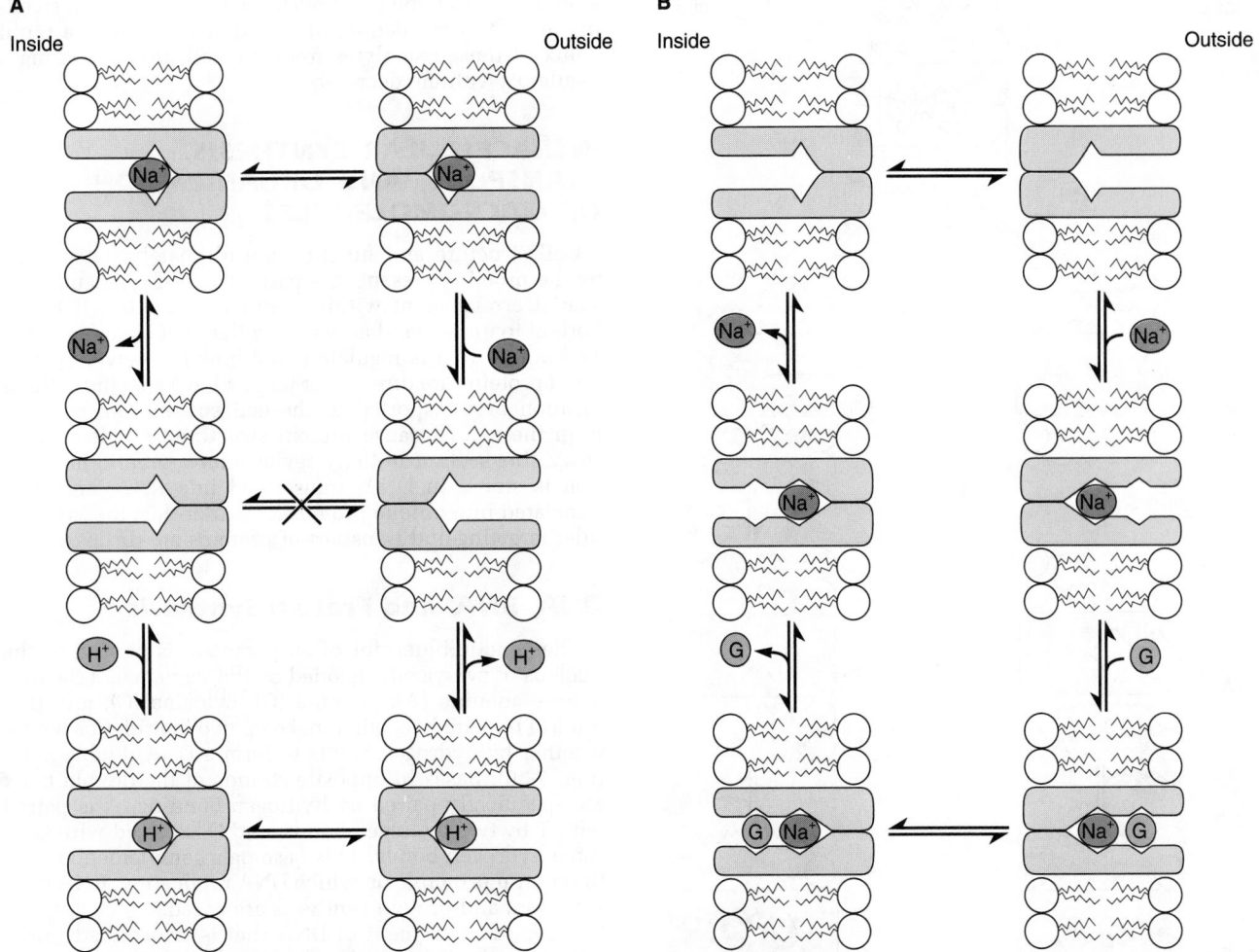

Figure 1-27. (A) An exchanger, or antiporter, is created by disallowing the translocation of the unbound site. For example, the catalytic cycle diagrammed here leads to the exchange of Na$^+$ for H$^+$ (ie, Na$^+$–H$^+$ antiport). (B) An obligatory cotransporter is created by permitting only two forms of the protein to undergo translatory conformational changes—the doubly bound and the unbound. Here, the binding of Na$^+$ facilitates the subsequent binding of glucose, leading to the Na$^+$-dependent cotransport of Na$^+$ and glucose.

binds with its charge means that the inside negative membrane potential represents another force, which drives the cycle so as to favor inward glucose flow.

If the conformational changes of the unbound site are disallowed, the resulting mechanism is an exchanger or antiporter because the only possible transport event is the obligatory exchange, or swapping, of one substrate molecule for another. This process is presumed to be the basis for the energy-converting countertransport that occurs, for example, in Na$^+$–H$^+$ exchange (see Fig. 1-26A). Here, the imposition of an Na$^+$ gradient can drive protons out of the cell. Because of the Na$^+$ gradient, Na$^+$ dominates the out-to-in portion of the cycle, whereas H$^+$ dominates the in-to-out portion of the cycle. There is evidence for an activation site on the cytoplasmic face of the Na$^+$–H$^+$ antiporter, which functions to turn on Na$^+$–H$^+$ exchange only when cytosolic pH falls below a certain set-point. It has been suggested that hormones and growth factors that influence Na$^+$–H$^+$ exchange do so in part by modulating the activating site.

The archetype for biologic pumps is the Na$^+$-K$^+$-ATPase. For this transporter, the biochemical events in the catalytic cycle have been examined in great detail, although the exact nature of the translocation events are still not well understood. Figure 1-28 illustrates how the inclusion of a phosphorylation event in the catalytic cycle could result in the coupling of the free energy of hydrolysis of ATP to the translocation of ions, in this case, the exchange of Na$^+$ for K$^+$ in the ratio of three Na$^+$ to two K$^+$. This unequal stoichiometry results in the transfer of net charge during the catalytic cycle, so that the normal pumping mode is associated with an outwardly directed membrane current.

Volume Regulation

One important function of the solute transport mechanisms that inhabit the plasma membrane is the maintenance and regulation of cell volume. Water distribution, as noted earlier, is determined in most cells entirely by solute distribution. Thus, the volume of a cell is determined by the same mechanisms that maintain the steady-state solute composition of the cell. Many, if not all, cells have the capacity to respond actively to a perturbation in cell volume; that is, they are capable of volume regulation. Volume regulatory responses are based on membrane transporters that enable the cell to undergo a net loss or a

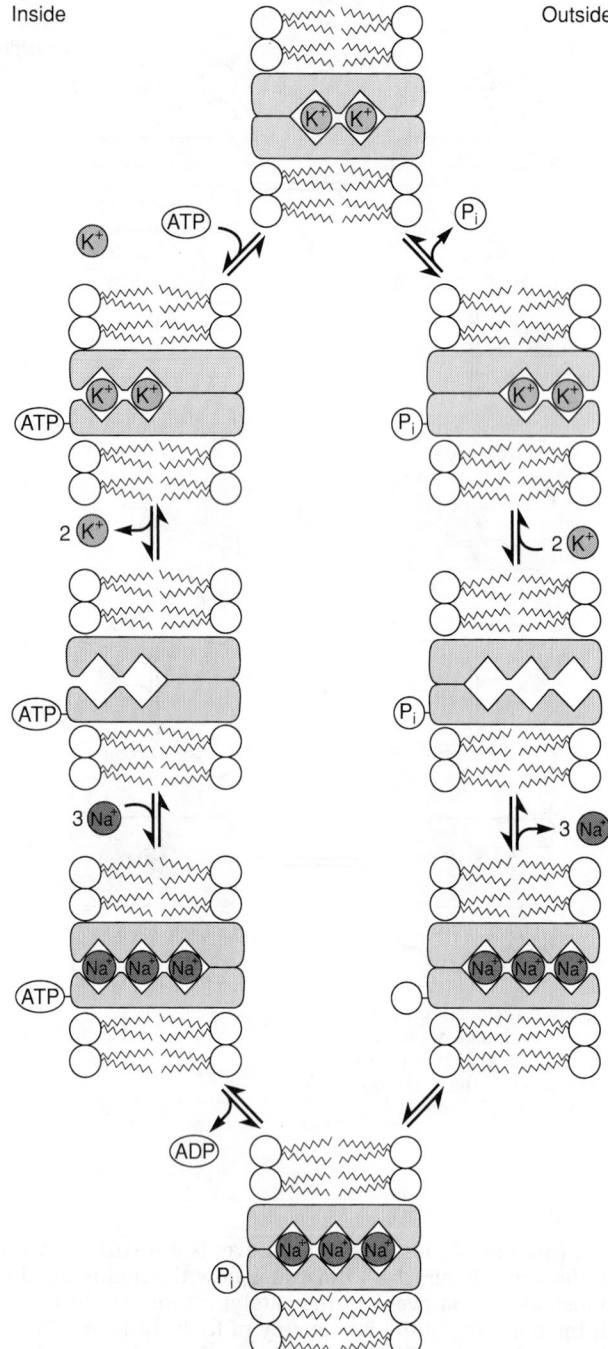

Inside   Outside

Figure 1-28. The Na⁺-K⁺-ATPase has a complicated catalytic cycle that involves not only the binding and unbinding of Na⁺ and K⁺ but also the binding of ATP, phosphorylation of the protein, and subsequent dephosphorylation, so that one ATP is hydrolyzed per transport cycle.

net gain of solute and hence lose or gain water. For example, if a cell is swollen by exposure to a hypotonic medium, the permeability of the cell membrane to K^+ and Cl^- is markedly increased, such that a net efflux of salt and water occurs, bringing about a regulatory volume decrease (Fig. 1-29). Similarly, shrinking a cell by exposing it to an impermeant solute activates mechanisms for solute entry, usually NaCl. Another type of volume regulatory mechanism involves the movements of organic solutes such as taurine or myoinositol. These solutes are accumulated by cells through Na-dependent cotransporters and can account for

a significant fraction of intracellular osmolality. Cell swelling leads to the opening of channels that mediate rapid efflux of these osmolytes from the cell, thus initiating a regulatory volume decrease.

INTRACELLULAR SYNTHESIS, TRANSPORT, AND ORGANIZATION OF MACROMOLECULES

Cell structure and function are ultimately determined by the proteins present in a particular cell type and their spatial arrangement within distinct organelles. It is important to understand how the synthesis of proteins is carried out, how it is regulated, and how the newly synthesized proteins are directed or targeted to a specific cellular location or transported to the cell surface and secreted from the cell. Because protein structure is coded for by DNA, this section initially reviews how genetic information is stored in DNA, transcribed into RNA, and then translated into unique proteins.[1,2,9] After this, the intracellular targeting and transport of proteins are discussed.

DNA, RNA, and Protein Synthesis

The genetic blueprint of an organism is carried in the nucleus of every cell, encoded by the sequence of the four bases—adenine (A), guanine (G), cytosine (C), and thymine (T)—which together make up two long chains bound together by hydrogen bonds to form a DNA double helix (Fig. 1-30). Bases in opposite strands of the double helix are specifically paired by hydrogen bonding. A is paired with T by two hydrogen bonds, and C is paired with G by three hydrogen bonds. This base-pair complementarity is the central principle on which DNA replication, RNA transcription, and protein synthesis are based.

A gene is a segment of DNA that is transcribed into a corresponding RNA molecule that either codes for a protein or forms a structural RNA molecule (Fig. 1-31). Genes are commonly between 10,000 and 100,000 base pairs in length and include, in addition to the coding sequence, flanking regions and intervening sequences, called *introns*. Introns are removed from the primary RNA transcript by a process called *splicing*. Each strand of DNA has polarity, and information is read from the 5′ to the 3′ direction, with the numbers referring to the free hydroxyl group on the deoxyribose moiety. The basic unit of information is the codon, a sequence of three bases or a triplet. The four nucleotide bases arranged as triplets lead to 64 possible codons. Sixty-one of these code for the 20 known amino acids, and 3 are termination signals called *stop codons*. The code is degenerate in that some amino acids are specified by up to 6 codons.

When cells divide, the two DNA chains that constitute the double helix separate, and each serves as a template for synthesis of a complementary strand directed by the enzyme DNA polymerase. One of the new double helices goes to each daughter cell, so that the amount and sequence of DNA in each new cell is the same as that of the parent cell. To direct the synthesis of protein, the DNA sequence has to be transcribed into three types of RNA—messenger RNA (mRNA), transfer RNA (tRNA), and ribosomal RNA (rRNA). RNA contains the nucleoside uridine (U) instead of thymidine and usually exists as a single-stranded, linear polymer. RNA synthesis is directed by an RNA polymerase enzyme that makes an RNA copy of DNA. Eukaryotic cells contain three types of RNA polymerase—termed I, II, and III—each of which catalyzes the formation of a different type of RNA. RNA polymerase II directs the formation of mRNA.

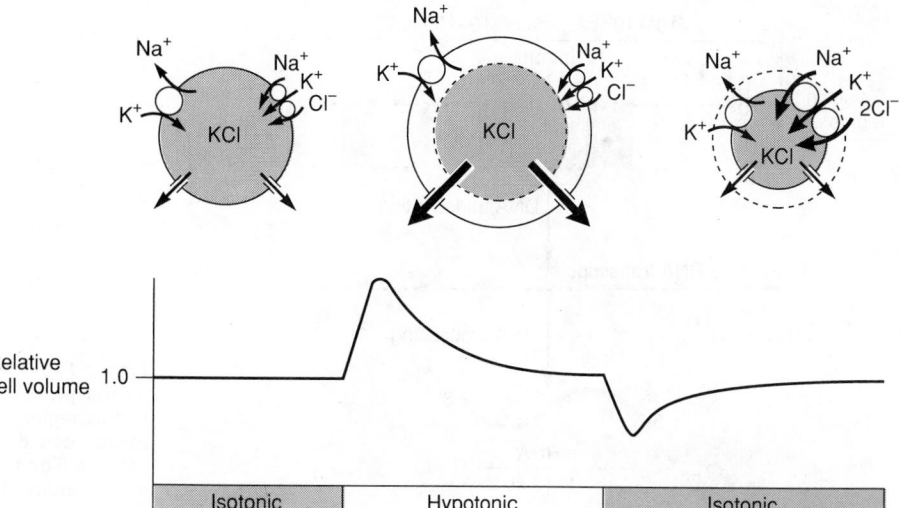

Figure 1-29. Many cells actively regulate their volume by turning on and off specific transport pathways. A hypotonic solution is shown here as causing cell swelling and activating channels for K$^+$ and Cl$^+$ so that salt leaves the cell, promoting shrinkage. A return to isotonic conditions leads to water efflux and cell shrinkage, which activates a coupled, Na$^+$-K$^+$-2Cl$^-$ entry process that results in a gain of salt and water and a return to normal volume.

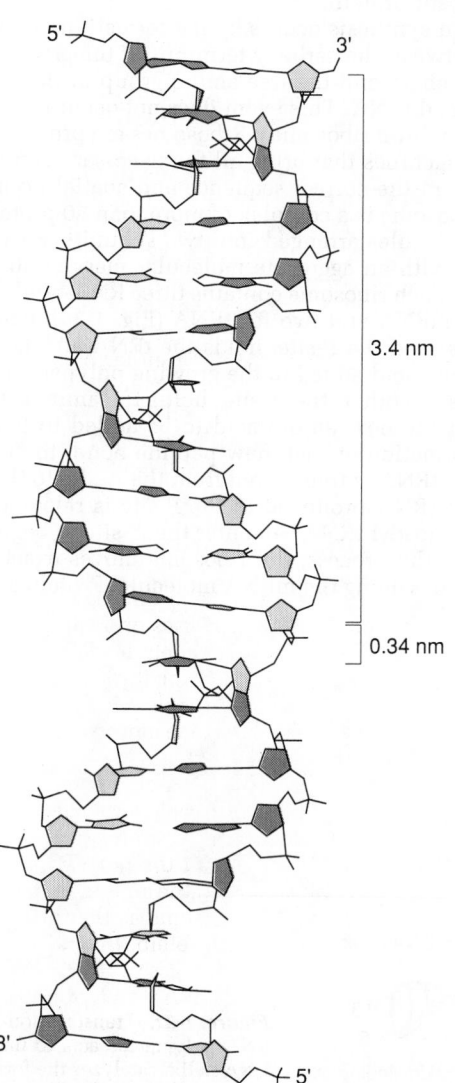

Figure 1-30. A section of a DNA double helix. The helix repeats every 3.4 nm and is composed of two DNA strands running in opposite directions. The opposite strands are shown as different colors; the bases project into the center and are held together by hydrogen bonds.

Transcription of a gene begins at an initiation site associated with a specific DNA sequence, called a *promotor region*. Recognition of this region by the polymerase is aided by specific proteins, called *transcription factors,* which bind to the DNA, and by *initiation factors,* which bind to the polymerase. Some transcription factors determine tissue specificity, whereas others, such as steroid hormone receptors, are regulatory and act in various cells to increase or decrease transcription rates of specific genes. After binding to DNA, the RNA polymerase opens up a short region of the double helix to expose the nucleotides. Once the two strands of DNA are separated, the strand containing the promoter acts as a template to which ribonucleoside triphosphates base pair by hydrogen bonds. Nucleotides are then joined together with elongation, proceeding in a 5′ to 3′ direction as the RNA polymerase moves stepwise along the DNA (Fig. 1-32). Behind the polymerase, the DNA double helix reforms, displacing the nascent RNA polymer. When a termination signal is reached, the polymerase releases both the template and the newly made RNA strand and is free to rebind to another promoter region. The average length of the RNA transcript is about 8000 nucleotides, although much longer molecules are common.

The initial products of RNA polymerase II are known as heterogeneous nuclear RNA because of their large size variation. These primary transcripts are then processed to form mRNA. Processing includes addition of a methylguanosine to the 5′ end as a cap, addition of a long sequence of adenosine bases to the 3′ end as a tail, and removal of a number of long nucleotide sequences. As mentioned earlier, these sequences, or introns, are present in the gene but not in mature RNA (see Fig. 1-31). The gene regions represented in mRNA are termed *exons,* for expressed regions. The joining of coding regions on either side of an intron sequence, or splicing, accounts for mature mRNA being much shorter than nuclear RNA. Moreover, alternative splicing can lead to the production of different mRNA molecules and, in some cases, different proteins from the same gene. mRNA is exported from the nucleus only after processing is complete. A typical mammalian cell can contain as few as 1 or 2 or up to 10,000 copies of each mRNA molecule at any one time. Although the number of copies is primarily a function of the rate of transcription (synthesis), mature mRNA is degraded in the cytoplasm, and the rate of degradation of each species also contributes to its relative

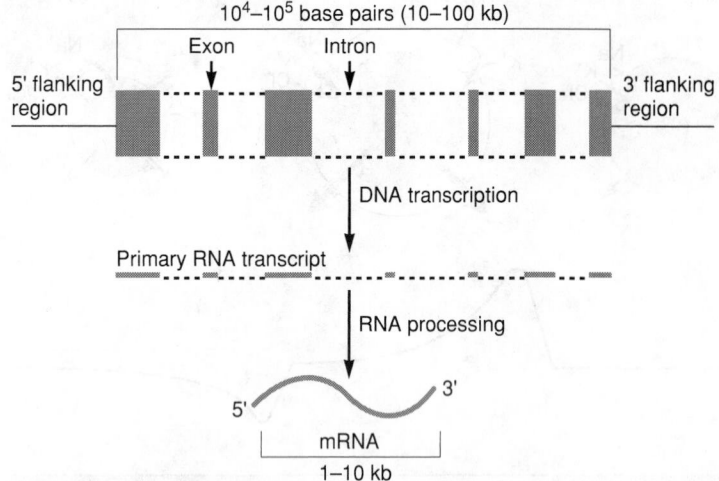

Figure 1-31. Structure of a typical gene, its primary RNA transcript, and the resulting mature mRNA. The entire coding region of the gene is initially transcribed, and the regions coded for introns are then spliced out during processing. The mature mRNA is then an RNA copy of the exon regions of the gene.

abundance. mRNA species that need to be rapidly regulated probably carry a sequence that tags them for more rapid destruction.

The synthesis of protein involves conversion from a four-letter nucleotide language to one of 20 chemically distinct amino acids. Accordingly, this process is referred to as *translation.* There is no mechanism for direct chemical recognition between specific nucleic acid bases and specific amino acids. Instead, an adapter molecule, tRNA, is used. tRNAs are small RNA molecules of 70 to 90 nucleotides, traditionally represented as a cloverleaf (Fig. 1-33). The loop on one end contains an anticodon nucleotide triplet that lines up with the complementary sequence of the mRNA, whereas the other end binds the amino acid specified by the mRNA codon. Each tRNA carries only one amino acid and must be recognized by a distinct enzyme, termed an *aminoacyl tRNA synthetase,* which catalyzes the covalent attachment of the carboxy end of the amino acid to the 3′ end of the tRNA in a process using ATP. Covalent attachment to the tRNA allows amino acids to be added to a growing protein in the sequence specified by the nucleic acid code. The attachment to tRNA also activates the amino acid by generating a high-energy intermediate. This energy is used to drive the reaction by which the amino acid is added to the nascent protein.

Protein synthesis occurs by the formation of a peptide bond between the carboxy terminus of the growing polypeptide chain and the free amino group of the activated amino acid tRNA. This event does not occur in free solution but within ribosomes. Ribosomes are protein synthesizing machines that bring all the necessary components together in the correct sequence and spatial orientation. Each ribosome is a complex of more than 80 proteins and RNA molecules arranged into two subunits, a small and a large, with an aggregate molecular mass of about four million. Each ribosome contains three RNA-binding sites, one for mRNA and two for tRNA (Fig. 1-34). One of the latter, termed the *P-site,* holds the tRNA attached to the last amino acid added to the growing polypeptide chain, whereas the other, the A-site, holds the aminoacyl tRNA carrying the next amino acid to be added to the chain. After formation of each new peptide bond, the resulting peptidyl tRNA is transferred from the A-site to the P-site. The free tRNA produced in the P-site is released, and a new aminoacyl tRNA can enter the A-site to begin a new cycle. In the process, the ribosome moves exactly three nucleotides along the mRNA molecule. Protein synthesis

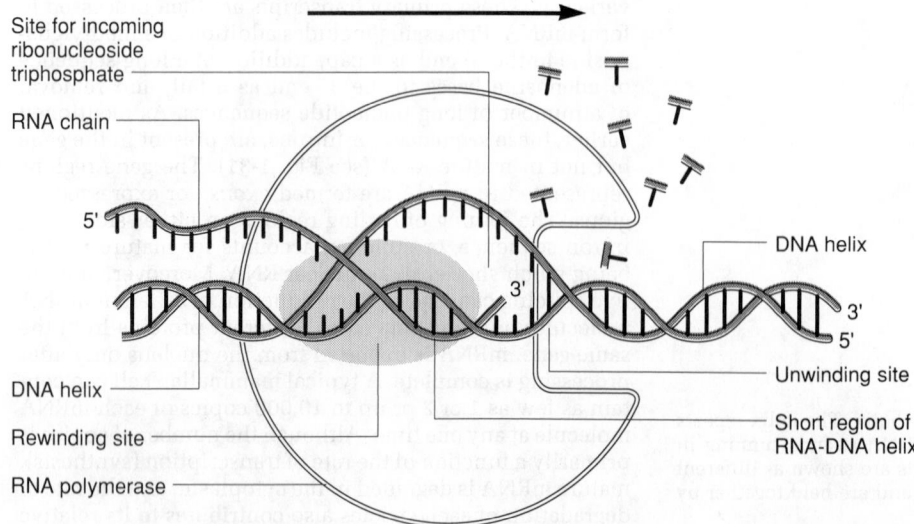

Figure 1-32. Transcription of DNA. RNA polymerase acts to unwind the DNA helix, catalyzes the formation of a transient RNA–DNA helix, and then releases the RNA as a single-strand copy while the DNA rewinds. In the process, the polymerase moves along the DNA from a start sequence to a stop sequence.

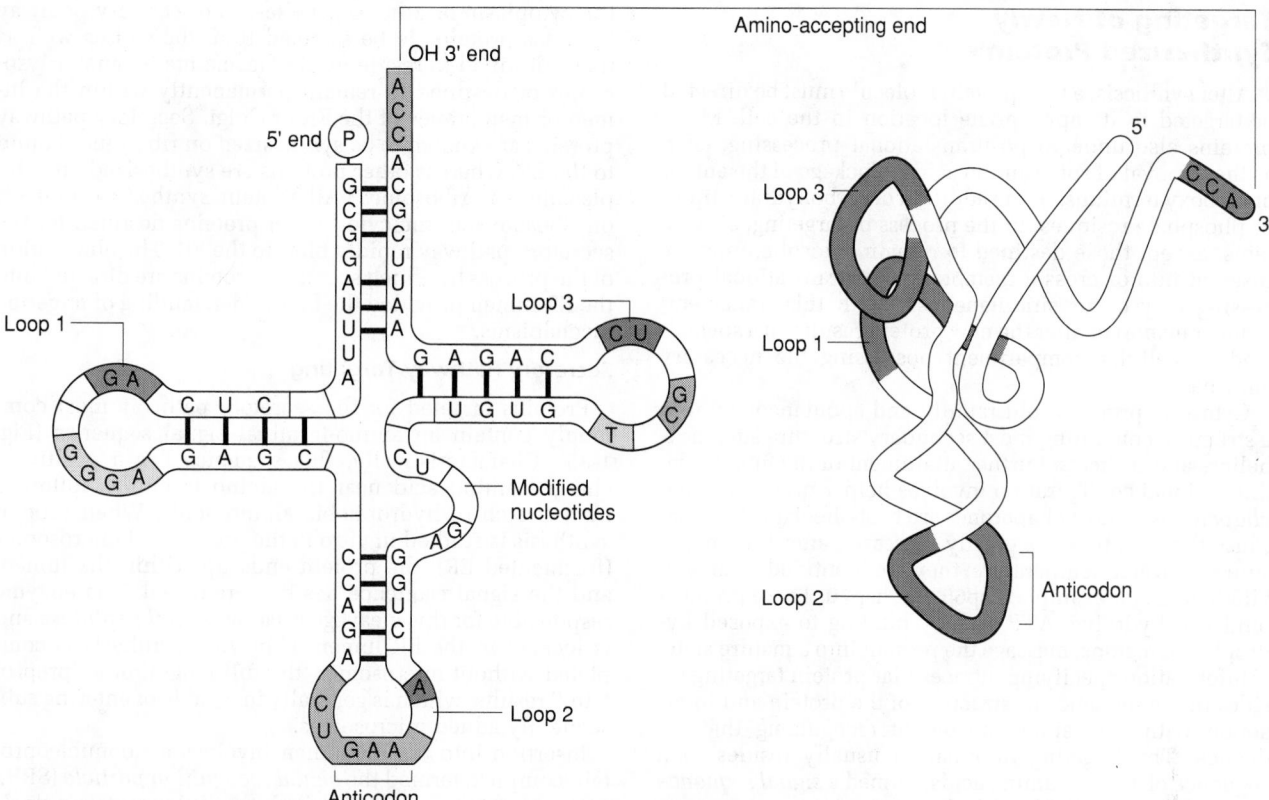

Figure 1-33. Structure of a transfer or tRNA molecule. The structure is shown as a stylized clover leaf (*left*) and as it is believed to exist in three dimensions (*right*). Note the opposite regions for binding an amino acid and the anticodon that forms a base pair with mRNA.

consumes a great deal of energy because four high-energy phosphate bonds must be split to make each peptide bond.

Protein synthesis requires identification of the appropriate starting and ending points on the mRNA. The synthesis of all eukaryotic proteins begins with a methionine coded for by an AUG triplet. Only one specific methionine

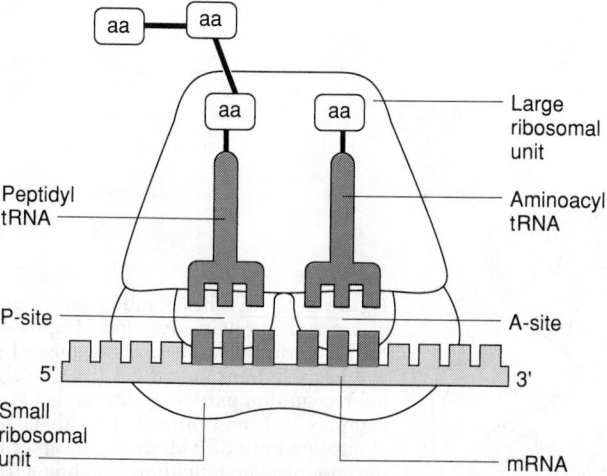

Figure 1-34. Schematic view of the elongation phase of protein synthesis on a ribosome. As the ribosome moves along the mRNA, incoming aminoacyl–tRNA complexes bind to the A-site on the ribosome, after which a new peptide bond is formed with the nascent polypeptide chain previously attached to the peptide tRNA. The ribosome then moves, ejecting the now-empty tRNA and opening the A-site for the next aminoacyl–tRNA complex.

tRNA can initiate synthesis. This initiator tRNA, charged with methionine, forms a complex with the small ribosomal subunit and a protein, eukaryotic initiation factor 2. This complex then binds to an mRNA, which is identified as such by its 5′ methylguanosine cap, and is then joined by other proteins (initiation factors). The small ribosomal subunit moves along the RNA until its initiating tRNA reaches the start site defined by the AUG sequence. At this time, some of the initiating factors dissociate, and a large ribosomal subunit joins the complex. Chain elongation can then occur by the binding of a free aminoacyl tRNA. Chain termination occurs when the ribosome reaches one of three different stop codons. Termination involves additional proteins, called *release factors,* which catalyze the addition of a water molecule rather than an amino acid to the carboxy terminus of the polypeptide chain. At this point, there is no longer attachment to a tRNA, and the completed polypeptide is released into the cytoplasm. The ribosome then dissociates into its two subunits and releases the mRNA.

The complete synthesis of a single protein takes 30 seconds to a few minutes, but multiple ribosomes can initiate translation and be moving down the mRNA molecule simultaneously, thus increasing the rate of protein synthesis. This complex of multiple ribosomes on an mRNA molecule is called a *polyribosome.* Protein synthesis can be blocked by a number of antibiotic molecules. Some, such as tetracyclines and streptomycin, selectively block prokaryotic protein synthesis and are therefore therapeutic agents for bacterial infections. Others, such as puromycin and cycloheximide, which act on eukaryotic protein synthesis, are useful as experimental tools. All of these inhibitors block specific steps in the complex sequence of initiation and elongation.

Targeting of Newly Synthesized Protein

After synthesis, a new protein molecule must be directed or targeted to its appropriate location in the cell. Many proteins also undergo posttranslational processing, such as the removal of some amino acids, blockage of the amino or carboxy terminus, or the addition of carbohydrate, lipid, or phosphate residues. In the process of targeting, all proteins, except those destined to remain cytosolic, must be inserted into or cross a membrane. Posttranslational processing may occur simultaneously with this transmembrane transport or after the new protein resides in a specialized subcellular compartment possessing the necessary enzymes.

Cytosolic proteins fold rapidly and spontaneously into a structure containing most secondary structure such as α helices and β sheets. Further attainment of the final three-dimensional configuration involves helper proteins called *chaperones*.[10] Most chaperones are heat-shock proteins because their synthesis is greatly increased after brief exposure to elevated temperature; they are identified by size in kilodaltons, for example, hsp60 and hsp70. These proteins bind and hydrolyze ATP and, by binding to exposed hydrophobic regions, massage the protein into a mature state.

Information specifying intracellular protein targeting resides in the sequence or structure of the protein and interaction with a receptor capable of recognizing that sequence. The targeting information usually resides in a sequence of 15 to 40 amino acids, termed a *signal sequence* or *signal peptide*.[11] The sole function of this sequence is to direct targeting, and the sequence is frequently removed after that function is complete. In other cases, targeting information resides in a signal patch of amino acid residues, which are adjacent after protein folding but are located at different regions in the primary sequence. The definition of signal areas on proteins is evolving, and only some of the better understood examples are presented.

After protein synthesis, the first "decision" in the targeting process is whether a newly synthesized protein is to enter the secretory pathway or remain in the cell in the cytoplasm or other organelles. The secretory pathway includes proteins to be secreted from the cell as well as those destined to reside in the plasma membrane or lysosomes or destined to remain permanently within the lumen or membranes of the ER or Golgi. Secretory pathway proteins are known to be synthesized on ribosomes bound to the ER, whereas other proteins are synthesized on cytoplasmic free ribosomes. All protein synthesis originates on ribosomes in the cytosol, but proteins destined for the secretory pathway rapidly bind to the ER. The elucidation of the process by which secretory proteins are directed into the ER lumen provided the first understanding of targeting mechanisms.

Secretory Pathway Targeting

Proteins targeted for the secretory pathway most commonly contain an amino-terminal signal sequence (Fig. 1-35). Characteristically, this sequence has a positively charged amino acid near the amino terminus, followed by a stretch of hydrophobic amino acids. When protein synthesis is studied in vitro in the presence of microsomes (fragmented ER), the protein ends up within the lumen, and the signal sequence has been removed. The enzyme responsible for this cleavage is called *signal peptidase* and is located in the ER lumen. If in vitro synthesis is completed without microsomes, the full length, or a "preprotein," results, which is generally incapable of entering subsequently added microsomes.

Insertion into the ER lumen involves a ribonucleoprotein complex, termed the *signal recognition particle* (SRP), and a receptor on the ER, called the *SRP receptor* or *docking protein*.[11] The SRP is a complex of six polypeptide chains and a 300-nucleotide RNA molecule that binds to the nascent signal peptide emerging from the ribosome after the synthesis of about 70 amino acids (see Fig. 1-35). After this interaction, translational arrest occurs until the ribosome SRP complex binds to an SRP receptor. The SRP receptor is an integral membrane protein of two polypeptide subunits exposed on the cytosolic surface of the ER membrane. At this point, translation resumes, the ribosome is passed on to bind to a ribosomal receptor protein,

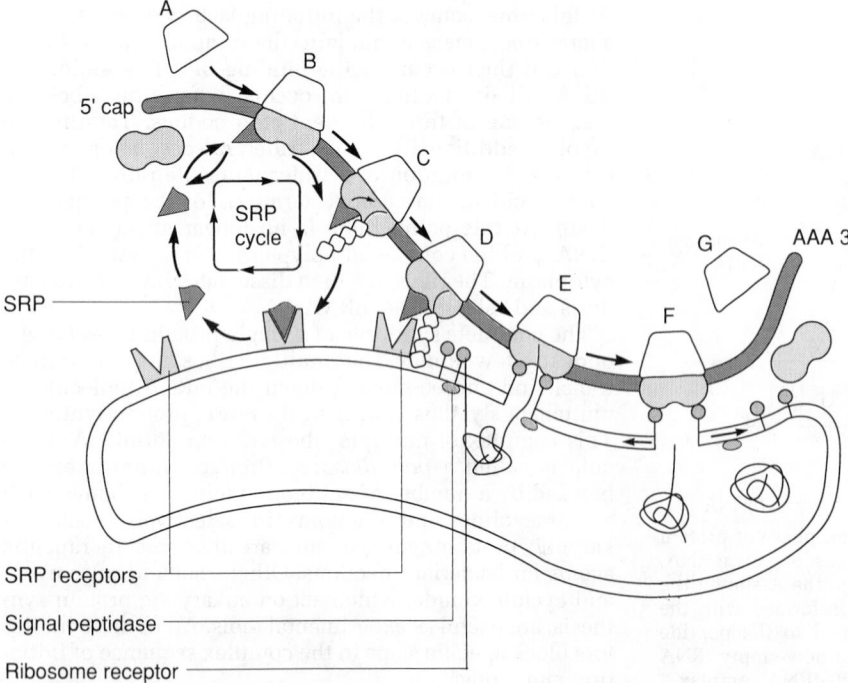

Figure 1-35. Synthesis and sequestration of secretory protein. Synthesis begins on the left as ribosomal subunits aggregate (A) and begin to translate mRNA (B). The signal-recognition particle (SRP) binds to the complex (C) and arrests peptide-chain elongation until SRP binds to a receptor in the endoplasmic reticulum membrane (D). The nascent polypeptide is then extruded into the lumen (E and F) with the aid of ribosome receptors, and SRP is released to recycle. The amino-terminal sequence may be cleaved by a signal peptidase. On chain termination, the ribosome dissociates (G), and its subunits can recycle.

and SRP dissociates. Next, the signal peptide binds to another ER membrane protein, the signal sequence receptor. This latter protein is believed to form part of a water-filled channel, through which the nascent secretory protein is extruded. In the most common case, the secretory protein is completely extruded into the lumen, the signal peptide is cleaved off, and the ribosome dissociates. Insertion of the nascent peptide through the membrane requires metabolic energy from ATP. Energy released by the spontaneous folding of the secretory protein in the ER lumen may also help to pull it across. Translocation and folding are also assisted by the intraluminal binding protein, BiP, which is related to hsp70 proteins.

Lysosomal proteins are similarly inserted into the ER and later sorted into their appropriate organelles. As is the case for many other secretory proteins, lysosomal enzymes are glycosylated on certain asparagine residues as protein synthesis is occurring. This process involves the transfer of a preformed oligosaccharide-containing glucose, mannose, and N-acetylglucosamine from a lipid-linked dolichol phosphate (Fig. 1-36). While still in the ER, the glucose is removed, exposing mannose. The oligosaccharide moiety is then further processed in the Golgi.

Proteins destined to reside in the plasma membrane or in the ER membrane (such as ribosome receptor) have to stop part way through their transmembrane passage (Fig. 1-37). This placement is directed by another amino acid sequence in the nascent protein, termed a *stop transfer* or *membrane anchor sequence*. In the simplest case, the amino terminus of the molecule is extruded through the membrane, the process stops at the anchor sequence, and synthesis of the carboxy terminus continues in the cytosol. An example of such a protein is the low-density lipoprotein (LDL) receptor. As the lumen of the ER corresponds topologically to the outside of the cell, after vesicular transport through the Golgi to the surface, the amino terminus of the LDL receptor ends up on the external surface of the plasma membrane. This portion of the molecule may be glycosylated within the ER and Golgi lumina, with the

result that the carbohydrate residues are located on the external surface of the plasma membrane. A more complex sequence of events occurs for proteins with an amino terminus that remains in the cytoplasm or for proteins that have multiple membrane-spanning regions. Both are thought to involve internal signal–anchor sequences. These internal sequences generally form α helices and are thought to insert into the bilayer as a hairpin loop (see Fig. 1-37). In the case of membrane proteins that span the bilayer multiple times, this process must be repeated with a separate insertion for each extracellular loop. Examples of such proteins are rhodopsin and heterotrimeric G-protein–coupled receptors that contain seven membrane-spanning segments.

Nuclear and Mitochondrial Targeting

Nuclear proteins, such as histones, DNA and RNA polymerases, and gene regulatory proteins, are synthesized on cytoplasmic free ribosomes and must then enter the nucleus through the nuclear pores. Studies with fluorescent-labeled proteins have shown free passage through these pores by polypeptides with a size cutoff point of about 60,000 daltons, consistent with a water-filled pore about 9 nm in diameter. This pore serves to keep cytoplasmic organelles and large proteins out of the nucleus, except those specifically targeted. Entry of large proteins into the nucleus is energy dependent and involves use of ATP. Nuclear targeting is specified by a short amino acid sequence rich in positively charged lysine and arginine residues and usually containing proline. The sequence can occur anywhere in the molecule and is not cleaved after entry. In contrast to secretory proteins, which are targeted only once, long-lived nuclear proteins may have to be targeted multiple times because the nuclear envelope breaks down and reforms during each mitosis, after which nuclear proteins must reaccumulate.

Mitochondria contain DNA and synthesize some proteins, but most mitochondrial proteins are imported from the cytoplasm (Fig. 1-38). Translocation of matrix proteins

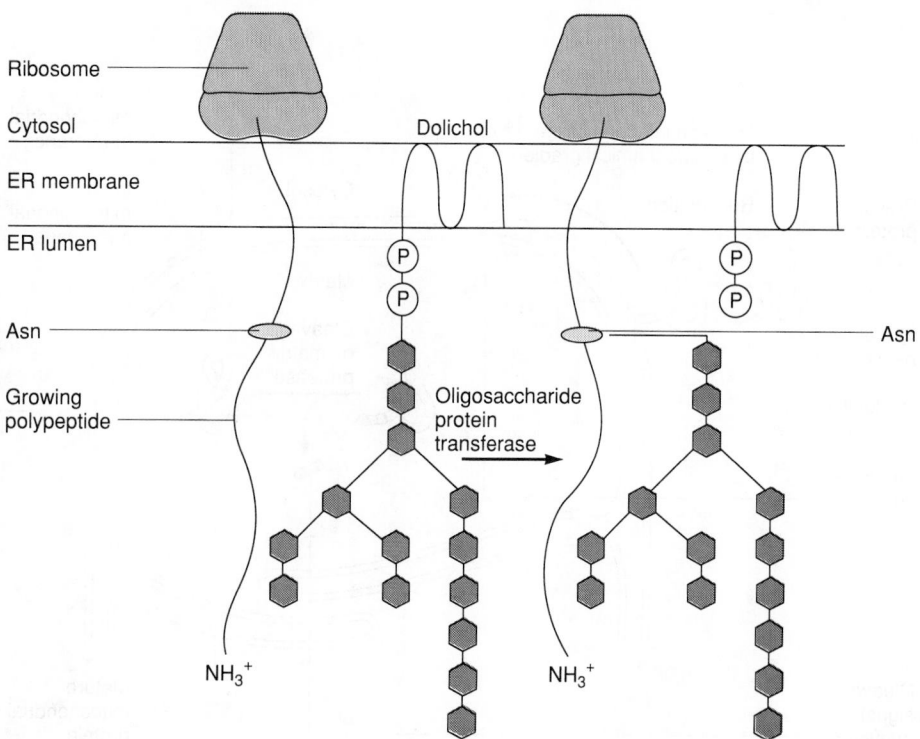

Figure 1-36. Biosynthesis of an asparagine-linked glycoprotein in the endoplasmic reticulum (ER) lumen. The sugar core is transferred as a preformed unit from a carrier lipid, dolichol phosphate, to the protein as it is being synthesized.

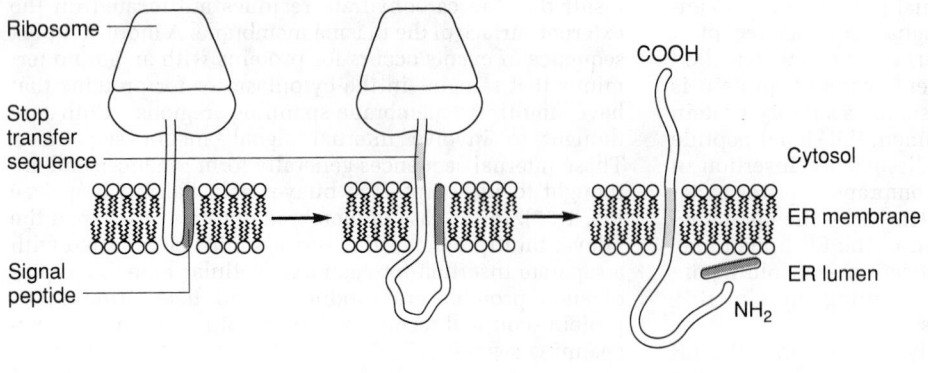

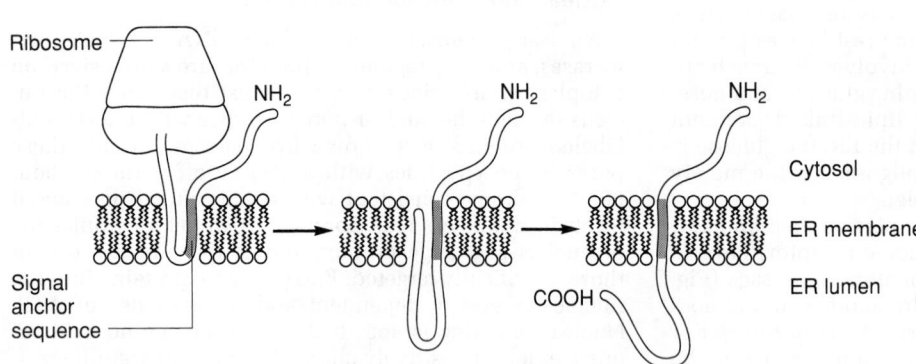

Figure 1-37. The topology of membrane proteins is the result of signals in the primary sequence. In this case, the two proteins end up with their opposite ends external. The occurrence of multiple signal anchor sequences can result in multiple transmembrane domains.

must occur across two membranes, the outer and inner mitochondrial membranes, and with the protein in an unfolded state. Cytosolic chaperone proteins of the hsp70 family bind the precursor protein as it is released from the ribosome and prevent it from folding spontaneously before it binds to a receptor protein on the mitochondria. Protein import is believed to occur at points of contact where the two membranes appear to be joined. Mitochondrial proteins have a signal sequence at their amino terminus. Mo-

lecular genetic studies have shown that the signal sequence can be as short as 12 amino acids, and, if engineered onto the amino terminus of a cytosolic protein, the sequence causes its insertion into the mitochondria. The signal sequence contains positively charged amino acids every third or fourth residue and form an amphipathic α helix, with all the positive residues on one side and relatively hydrophobic amino acids on the other. This amphipathic helix then inserts through the membrane,

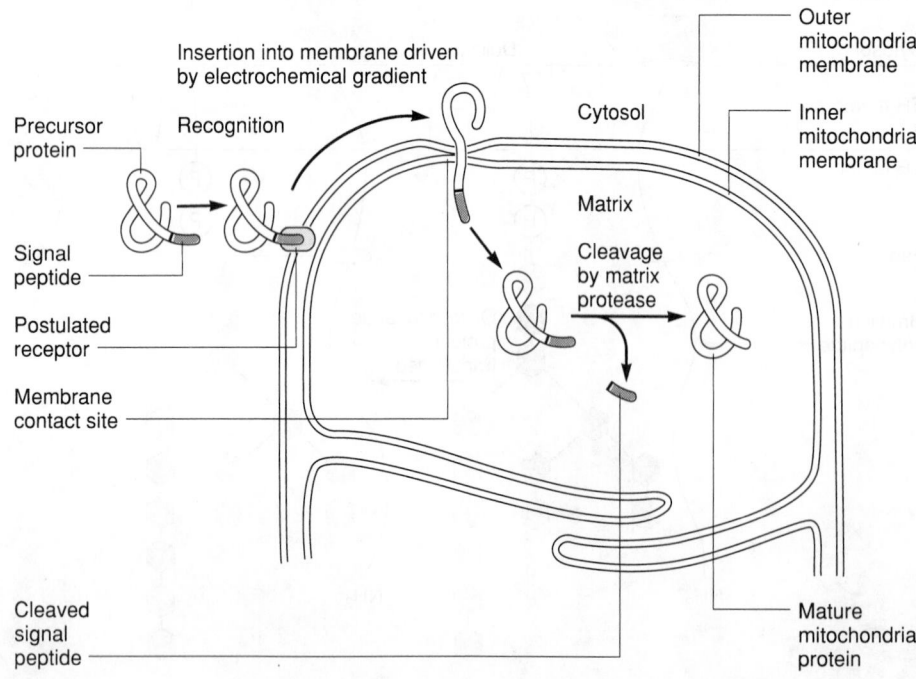

Figure 1-38. Insertion of newly synthesized protein into the mitochondrion is specified by a terminal signal peptide that interacts with a postulated receptor. These proteins are originally synthesized on free ribosomes and released into the cytoplasm, from which they insert into the mitochondrion.

probably in association with a receptor protein. The electrochemical proton gradient across the inner mitochondrial membrane provides energy for translocation across this membrane. Once within the mitochondrial matrix, the signal peptide is cleaved, and the protein folds to assume its mature configuration, which may also require assembly of multiple protein subunits.

Secretory Pathway

Once secretory proteins have been translocated across a lipid bilayer into the lumen of the ER, they must then pass through a number of compartments, including the Golgi, where they are further processed and sorted and end up in a secretory vesicle or lysosome[12,13] (Fig. 1-39). This passage involves movement by a distinct process, that of vesicular transport. In this mechanism, the proteins do not cross membranes but are transferred between the lumina of compartments. A small vesicle buds off from one compartment

such as ER and then fuses with another—in this case, the Golgi. In some cases, vesicular transport is a bulk movement of all luminal contents; in other cases, it is selective, with vesicular receptors binding only certain proteins in the luminal fluid.

The first vesicular transport event in the secretory pathway is movement of newly synthesized protein from ER to Golgi. The Golgi apparatus, which is made up of flattened saccules, can be subdivided into cis, medial, and trans elements, cis being adjacent to the ER. Vesicles about 50 nm in diameter bud off from smooth areas of ER, called *transitional elements,* by an ATP-requiring process and fuse with the *cis*-Golgi cisternae. These vesicles are coated; that is, they have a protein visible in electron micrographs that surrounds the vesicle. The coat is composed of coat proteins called *COPs;* these are distinct from the first identified coat protein, clathrin, and a low-molecular-weight GTP-binding (LMWG) protein, ARF, which is related to the protooncogene ras. LMWG proteins serve as molecular

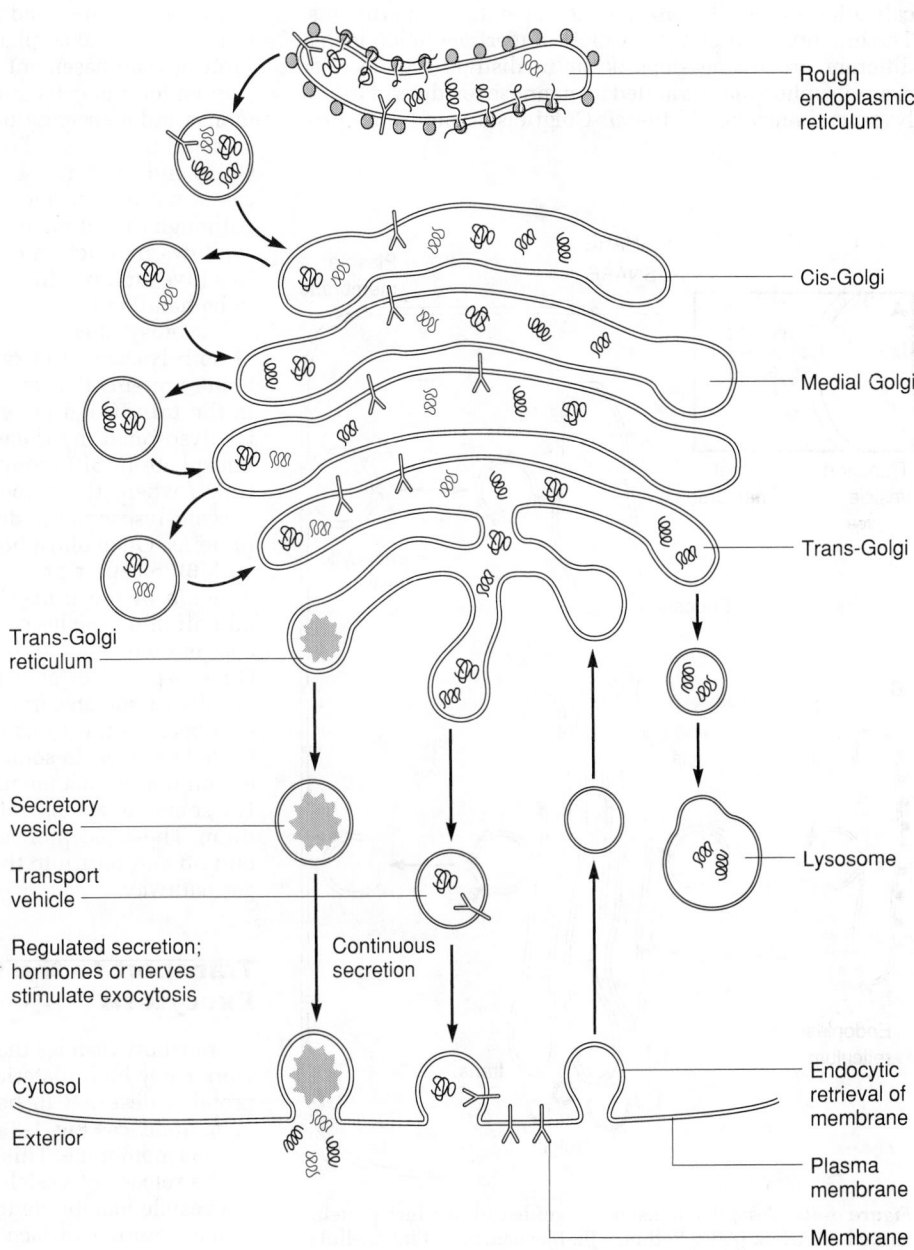

Figure 1-39. Intracellular transport and sorting of proteins destined for secretion, insertion into the plasma membrane, or targeting to the lysosome. After insertion into the endoplasmic reticulum lumen, movement from one compartment to another is by vesicular transport, which buds off one compartment and fuses with the next. Sorting signals intrinsic to the newly synthesized proteins specify the pathway to be taken.

Rough endoplasmic reticulum

Cis-Golgi

Medial Golgi

Trans-Golgi

Trans-Golgi reticulum

Secretory vesicle

Transport vehicle

Regulated secretion; hormones or nerves stimulate exocytosis

Continuous secretion

Cytosol

Exterior

Lysosome

Endocytic retrieval of membrane

Plasma membrane

Membrane protein

switches in that they are active when binding GTP and inactive when binding GDP. Coat assembly is initiated by ARF and GTP binding to a receptor that initiates COP binding, coat assembly, and budding. Transport vesicles also contain membrane-targeting proteins called *v-SNARES*. After GTP hydrolysis and uncoating, the v-SNARE binds to a docking protein in the target membrane termed the *t-SNARE* (Fig. 1-40), a process that also requires additional cytosolic proteins. A large family of LMWG proteins, the rab proteins, also appear to be involved in imposing specificity because different rab species are associated with different membrane compartments in the cell.

The transport event moves both content and membrane proteins. Proteins destined to reside in the ER lumen, such as protein disulfide isomerase, an enzyme that assists correct folding of nascent polypeptides, are not transported but are retained in the ER lumen by virtue of a signal sequence that presumably interacts with a receptor in the ER.

The Golgi apparatus is structurally and functionally divided. Each cisternae constitutes a functional compartment. This compartmentation is demonstrated by the localization of specific enzymes to separate compartments. The functional corollary of Golgi compartmentation is that different processing steps occur in distinct regions. For example, phosphate is added to mannose residues of future lysosomal enzymes in the *cis*-Golgi cisternae. In the pro-

cessing of secreted glycoproteins, the removal of mannose residues occurs in the medial cisternae, whereas the addition of sialic acid occurs in the trans cisternae. Such events have been used to develop test-tube models demonstrating vesicular transport from one Golgi compartment to another, which occurs similarly to transport from ER to Golgi. Coated vesicles bud from cisternal rims, uncoat, and then fuse selectively with the next compartment. Because all secretory proteins flow unidirectionally from *cis-* to medial to *trans*-Golgi compartments, vesicles must only be able to fuse with the next compartment. From the trans cisternae, secretory proteins move directly into a tubular network, called the *trans-Golgi network*. It is here that sorting takes place between secretory proteins and lysosomal enzymes.

The Golgi complex is especially prominent in exocrine cells, such as pancreatic and parotid acinar cells, and in endocrine cells, such as the islets of Langerhans or anterior pituitary. In goblet and other mucus-secreting cells, the Golgi is also prominent and is where proteoglycan synthesis takes place on the nascent protein core. This involves the addition of large glycosaminoglycan polymers to serine residues on the protein core. In a later step in the trans cisternae, sulfate is added. The same process, albeit to a lesser extent, takes place in many cell types that secrete proteoglycan basement membrane components.

In endocrine cells and neurons, many polypeptide hormones and neuropeptides are synthesized as larger precursors and then cleaved or processed beginning in the *trans*-Golgi and continuing in the secretory granule. In some cases, more than one biologically active peptide results. Although the rationale for this process is not always clear, it allows production of small peptides, such as enkephalins (five amino acids), that otherwise would be too small to be handled by the secretory pathway.

The biosynthesis of lysosomes[13] involves the production of both lysosomal enzymes and specific lysosomal membrane proteins that separate from other secretory proteins in the *trans*-Golgi network (Fig. 1-41). The sorting signal for lysosomal hydrolases is known to be mannose-6-phosphate (M6P) groups. Phosphate is added in the *cis*-Golgi, where the responsible enzymes must distinguish nascent lysosomal hydrolases from other secretory glycoproteins. Once phosphorylated, the M6P can interact with an M6P receptor protein to concentrate these enzymes in a region of the *trans*-Golgi network. These regions then bud off into vesicles coated with the protein clathrin. The coat is then shed, and the vesicle fuses with a lysosome. Once exposed to acid pH, the lysosomal acid hydrolase rapidly dissociates from the M6P receptor, which then cycles back to the *trans*-Golgi network, again by means of coated vesicles. In some cells, M6P receptors are also present on the plasma membrane, where they concentrate any lysosomal enzymes released into the extracellular medium. These receptors are concentrated in coated pits that bud off and return to the *trans*-Golgi network as a scavenger pathway.

Transport to the Cell Surface: Exocytosis

Transport vesicles that bud off from the *trans*-Golgi network carry both material to be secreted from the cell and proteins destined to become components of the plasma membrane (see Fig. 1-39). These vesicles can fuse with the plasma membrane. This process, termed *exocytosis*, results in the release of vesicle content and the incorporation of the vesicle membrane into the plasma membrane with the former internal surface of the vesicle now facing the outside of the cell.

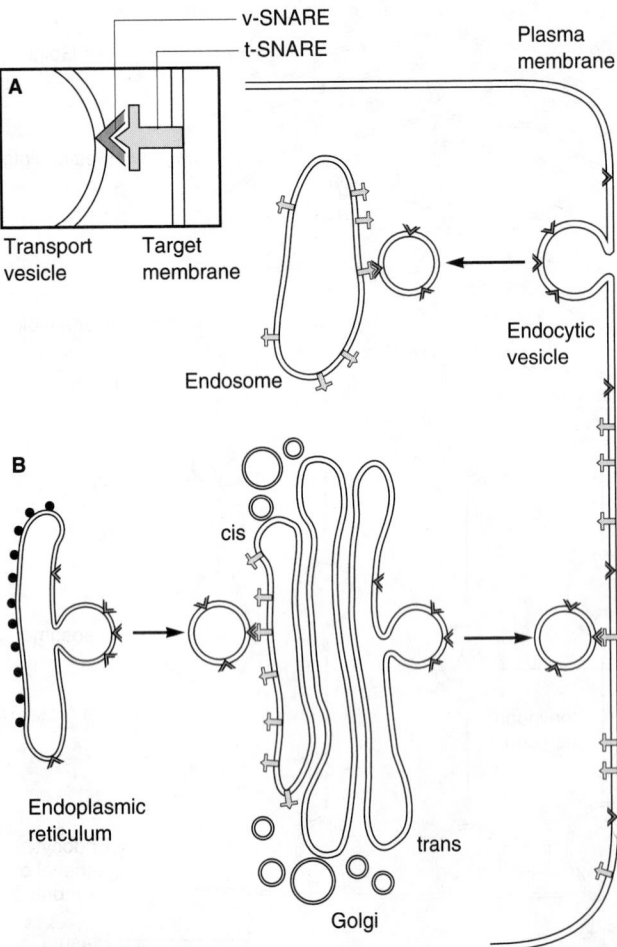

Figure 1-40. Vesicular transport is guided by distinct proteins termed *SNARES*. (After Rothman JE. Mechanisms of intracellular protein transport. Nature 1994;372:55)

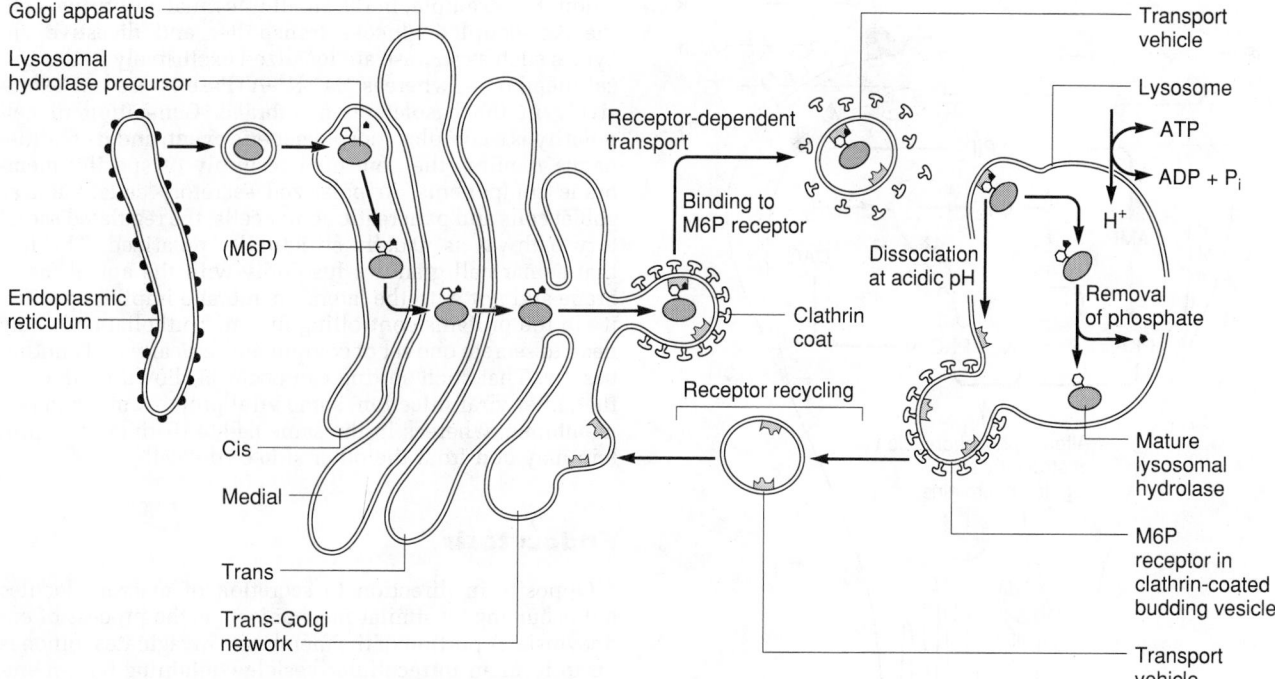

Figure 1-41. Biosynthesis of lysosomal proteins. Targeting is specified by phosphorylation of mannose and interaction with a mannose-6-phosphate receptor. The role of clatherin in the budding-off of transport vesicles is also illustrated.

Vesicular transport to the cell surface can be divided into two components—constitutive and regulated secretion.[14] Constitutive secretion involves small, coated vesicles that rapidly move to the plasma membrane and fuse. This mechanism, which occurs in all cells, is probably analogous to vesicular transport from ER to Golgi and that between Golgi cisternae. In the absence of a specific sorting mechanism, secretory and plasma membrane proteins take this route, which can be thought of as a default pathway. This pathway appears to transport basement membrane components that are secreted by all cells and also delivers membrane proteins such as Na^+-K^+-ATPase to the plasma membrane. Liver cells exhibit an active constitutive secretion of serum proteins, such as albumin and clotting factors.

Regulated secretion occurs in cells secreting digestive enzymes, hormones, and other regulatory molecules and neurotransmitters. In regulated secretion, the material to be secreted is sorted into a storage vesicle or granule; fusion with the plasma membrane and exocytosis then takes place in response to external stimulation.

In the case of digestive enzymes and protein and polypeptide hormones, there must be a signal sequence or patch on the molecules that directs it into the regulated pathway. When, for example, a pituitary cell is genetically engineered to synthesize trypsinogen or insulin, the foreign protein is packaged into secretory granules along with endogenous pituitary hormones. The production of secretory granules involves budding of clathrin-coated vesicles from the *trans*-Golgi network, which then fuse to form a large vesicle of dilute content. This vesicle, sometimes termed a *condensing vacuole,* concentrates secretory proteins and, in some cases, completes the processing of the secretory protein. In the case of insulin, its precursor, proinsulin, is cleaved to yield insulin and C peptide in the condensing vacuoles. In the process of condensation, secretory proteins may form complexes with ions such as

Ca^{2+} or Zn^{2+} and may even assume a crystalline array. This process is facilitated by other packaging or organizing proteins attached to the inner face of the granule membrane and by an H^+-ATPase in the granule membrane that acidifies the granule content. Most secretory granule membranes contain a relatively limited set of specialized proteins.

In the case of some neurons and mast cells, newly formed secretory granules do not contain secretory material but rather contain transporters and enzymes necessary for the uptake or synthesis of small molecules such as histamine and norepinephrine. These molecules are then condensed with counter-ions and proteins and are stored until regulated secretion is triggered.

Regulated secretion is triggered in most cases by a hormone or neurotransmitter (Fig. 1-42). The ensuing process is called *stimulus-secretion coupling.* In most cases, the coupling involves an increase in the cytoplasmic concentration of Ca^{2+}, but it may also involve generation of diacylglycerol or production of cAMP, which activate kinases or phosphatases. Evidence has accumulated invoking a role for small, GTP-binding proteins in this process, possibly analogous to their role in vesicular fusion in intracellular transport. In some secretory cells, such as mast cells and neurons that secrete within seconds, secretory vesicles or granules are prepositioned adjacent to the plasma membrane and may need only an increase in Ca^{2+} to fuse. In other cases, granules are dispersed in the cytoplasm and must be continually moved to the membrane over minutes or hours. Such a process, as occurs in pancreatic acinar cells after a meal, involves the cytoskeleton and particularly microtubules. The fusion event itself most likely involves protein–protein interactions between the outside of the granule membrane and the cytosolic face of the plasma membrane. This interaction generates a small fusion pore, which then widens by flow of membrane lipids. At this point, decondensation of secretory granule contents oc-

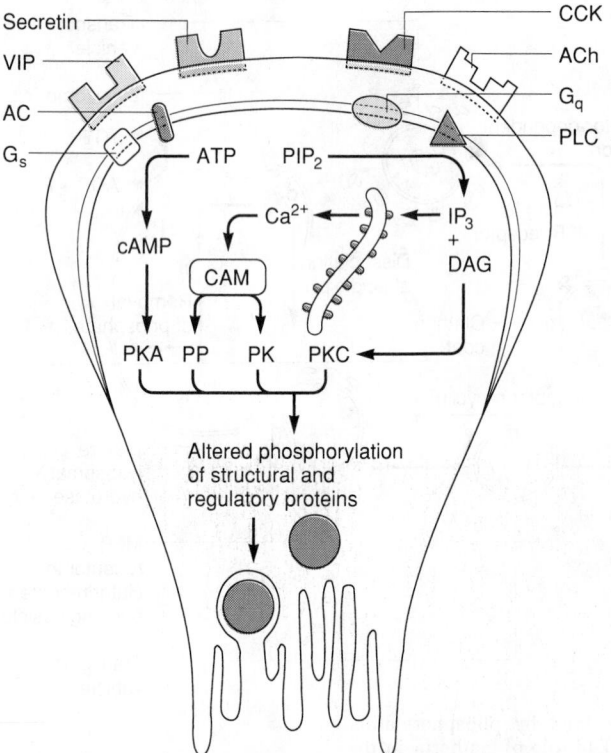

Figure 1-42. Scheme for control of regulated secretion for pancreatic acinar cells that secrete digestive enzymes. Vasoactive intestinal peptide (VIP) and secretin activate adenylate cyclase to promote AMP formation, whereas CCK and acetylcholine (ACh) activate phospholipase C (PLC), leading to production of inositol trisphosphate (IP_3) and diacylglycerol (DAG). IP_3 releases intracellular Ca^{2+}, which interacts with calmodulin (CAM). These second messengers (cAMP, Ca^{2+}, DAG) activate a battery of protein kinases (PK) and protein phosphotases (PP), which then induce secretion.

curs, facilitated by a flow of ions and water across the granule membrane.

The protein machinery involved in mediating docking and fusion is best known for synaptic vesicles and involves proteins functioning as v-SNARES and t-SNARES, which are believed to be synaptobrevin and syntaxin, respectively. Synaptic vesicle fusion is triggered directly by Ca^{2+} entering the cell through gated channels in the plasma membrane and binding to a Ca^{2+} sensor protein, probably synaptotagmin. The LMWG rab3a is also involved.

Because fusion of secretory granules with the plasma membrane greatly increases membrane surface area, there may be a transient increase in plasma membrane surface area. This increase is compensated for by an increase in endocytosis, by which coated vesicles bud from the plasma membrane and return to the *trans*-Golgi network. Endocytosis also serves a recycling function because components of the secretory granule membrane can be reused without requiring resynthesis.

Polarized Secretion in Epithelial Cells

Many cells are polarized with two distinct membrane domains. Polarization is especially prominent in epithelial cells, such as those that compose the renal tubule or the intestinal epithelium. Tight junctional complexes form a connecting belt around and between epithelial cells near their apical borders and allow apical and basolateral membranes to maintain distinct protein and even lipid compo-

sition. For example, in the small intestinal absorptive cell, the Na^+-coupled glucose transporter and digestive enzymes such as sucrase are localized exclusively in the apical membrane, whereas Na^+-K^+-ATPase is present exclusively in the basolateral membrane. Generation of cell polarity is a complex morphogenetic event, and its maintenance requires the continual resupply of specific membrane components. In polarized secretory cells, such as goblet cells and pancreatic acinar cells, the regulated secretory pathway is usually structurally polarized. The fact that acinar cell granules fuse only with the apical membrane and not with the lateral membrane implies specificity in the proteins controlling fusion. Epithelial cells may need to secrete one set of components apically and another basally. That such sorting can occur is shown by the fact that, after viral infection, some viral proteins move to one membrane, whereas in the same cell, a distinct viral protein may bud from the other side of the cell.

Endocytosis

Opposite in direction to secretion of macromolecules but occurring by similar mechanisms is the process of endocytosis. A portion of the membrane invaginates, pinches off to form an intracellular vesicle containing both membrane proteins and ingested material. As in the secretory pathway, the ingested macromolecules do not mix with the cytoplasm and are transferred within the cell by budding and fusion of vesicles. The process of endocytosis or pinocytosis, which involves the formation of small vesicles, is mechanistically distinct from phagocytosis, by which specialized cells take up larger particles, such as bacteria or erythrocytes (Fig. 1-43).

All cells continually take up portions of their cell membranes in the form of small endocytic or pinocytic vesicles. Pinocytosis, or "cell drinking," refers to the capture of surrounding fluid in the vesicle. The recovery of membrane molecules and any attached ligands is more importantly functionally. Endocytosis begins at a specialized region, the coated pit, which appears in electron micrographs as a depression of the membrane. The coated pit is further identified by a bristle-like coating on the cytoplasmic surface. This coating is composed of the protein clathrin, whose individual unit is a three-armed structure called a *triskelion*. Triskelions assemble into a basket-like lattice, and this assembly is believed to provide the force resulting in the invagination. The lifetime of a coated pit is short; the pit pinches off within minutes to form a coated vesicle. Specific LMWG proteins of the rab family are also involved in this process. Coated vesicles rapidly shed their coats, which can be reused at the membrane. The vesicle moves into the cell, guided by microtubules, to a perinuclear area near the *trans*-Golgi network. At this point, the vesicles fuse to form a larger structure, the endosome. Unless specifically removed, the contents of the endosome are passed on to lysosomes, where they are digested.

Many membrane receptor molecules have a cytoplasmic portion that allows them to localize in coated pits (Fig. 1-44). This may occur spontaneously, as with the LDL receptor, or after binding of ligand, as is the case for the epidermal growth factor (EGF) receptor. Concentration of receptors in coated pits allows their selective uptake, a process called *receptor-mediated endocytosis*. In the case of the LDL receptor, this is the major mechanism whereby cells take up cholesterol. A more specialized case is the asialoglycoprotein receptor, expressed only on hepatocytes, which take up plasma glycoproteins lacking terminal sialic acid residues. Other examples of receptor-mediated endocytosis are the uptake of transferrin with its

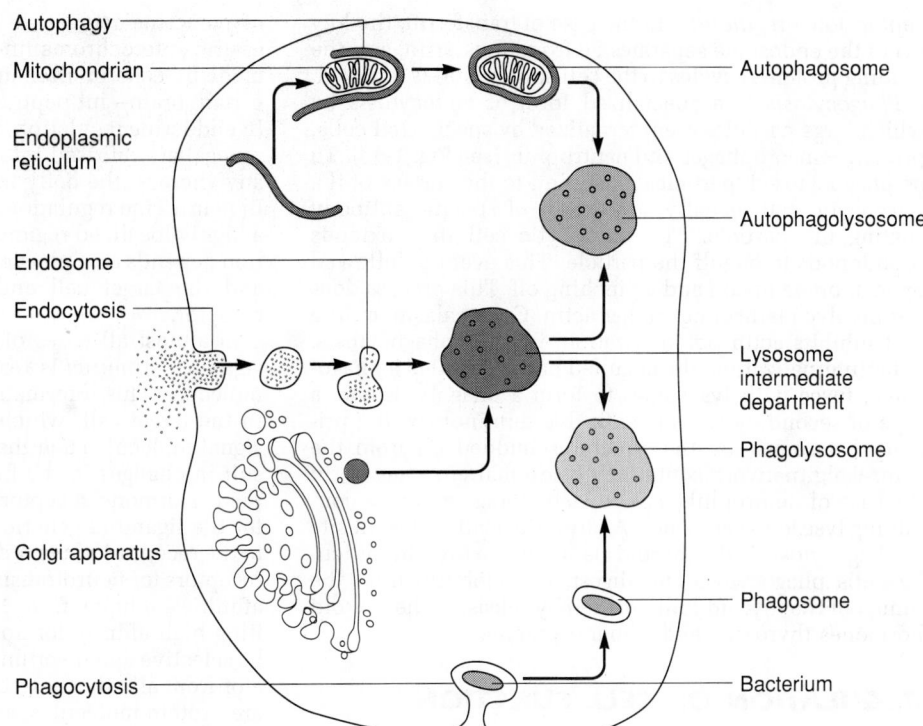

Figure 1-43. Formation of lysosomes by combination of transport vesicles from the Golgi-containing lysosomal enzymes with material that has been phagocytosed, endocytosed, or internalized by autophagy.

bound iron and the uptake by absorptive cells of the ileum of vitamin B_{12}.

Ligand–receptor complexes are sorted in the endosome. The contents of the endosome are maintained at an acidic pH of about 5.0 as a result of a specific vacuolar H^+-ATPase that transports H^+ into the endosomal lumen. Many ligand–receptor interactions are pH sensitive. The ligands dissociate in the endosome, after which the dissociated

ligand is transported to lysosomes and digested. The freed receptor is sorted and buds off as part of a transport vesicle that returns to the cell membrane, where the receptor can undergo another round of endocytosis. This sequence occurs for the LDL and asialoglycoprotein receptors. Some receptors, such as the EGF receptor, do not recycle but are degraded in the lysosome, resulting in a reduced number of cell surface receptors. This process is referred to as *re-*

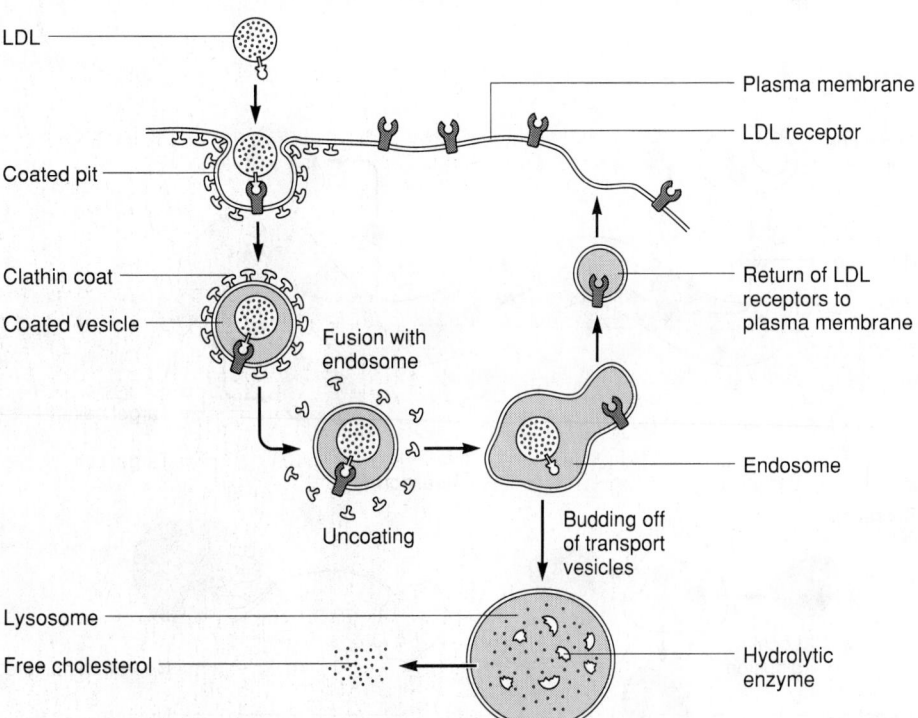

Figure 1-44. Receptor-mediated endocytosis of low-density lipoprotein (LDL), with resultant degradation of the endocytosed LDL and recycling of the receptor.

ceptor down-regulation. In the case of transferrin, the low pH of the endosome separates Fe from transferrin, and the binding protein recycles to the cell surface and is released.

Phagocytosis is a specialized form of endocytosis by which large particles are internalized by specialized cells, primarily macrophages and neutrophils (see Fig. 1-43). To be phagocytosed, particles must bind to the surface of the phagocytic cell, usually as a result of specific antibody coating the particle. The phagocytic cell then extends pseudopods to engulf the particle. This event is followed by membrane fusion and a pinching off. This process does not involve clathrin but rather actin. Cytochalasin, a drug that inhibits actin polymerization, inhibits phagocytosis. After internalization, the engulfed particle, called a phagosome, fuses with lysosomes to form a phagolysosome, a type of secondary lysosome. In this terminology, the primary lysosomes are the structures budded off from the *trans*-Golgi network containing lysosomal enzymes or, in the case of neutrophils, specialized storage granules containing lysosomal enzymes. A physiologically relevant site of phagocytosis is the thyroid gland, where thyroid follicular cells phagocytose and digest thyroglobulin from the lumen of the thyroid follicle, thereby releasing the thyroid hormones thyroxine and triiodothyronine.

REGULATION OF CELL FUNCTION

The growth, differentiation, and function of all cells are highly regulated events. Cell regulation can be thought of as the effector side of cell communication. Communication can occur in a number of ways, including direct physical contact or passage of small molecules from cell to cell through gap junction channels (see Fig. 1-11). Most commonly, cell regulation occurs by means of extracellular chemical messengers. Depending on how the extracellular messenger arrives, cell regulation can be classified as paracrine, endocrine, or neurocrine (Fig. 1-45). In paracrine regulation, a chemical messenger or mediator is produced and acts locally. This restricted domain of action is due to the limitations of diffusion and to the fact that the mediators are taken up or inactivated by target cells. Examples of paracrine regulators include histamine released from gastric enterochromaffin-like cells, prostaglandins that are made by cells in all mammalian tissues, nitric oxide, and certain brain–gut peptide regulators such as somatostatin. In endocrine regulation, the extracellular messengers (hormones) are released into the blood and act on target cells anywhere in the body that possess appropriate receptors. In neurocrine regulation, neurons secrete transmitters into a highly localized region, the synaptic cleft, so that regulation depends on a physical connection between the neuron and the target cell and on the presence of a specific receptor.

In almost all cases of cell regulation, the extracellular signal or stimulus is restricted to being an informational molecule. This information is received by a receptor on or in the target cell, which generally has an affinity for the signal molecule such that changes in its concentration result in changes in the fraction of receptors that are occupied. Hormone receptors generally have an affinity (K_d) for the ligand (a generic term for the molecule that binds to the receptor) of the order of 10^{-11} to 10^{-9} mol/L, whereas receptors for neurotransmitters more usually display lower affinities, ranging from 10^{-7} to 10^{-4} mol/L. Besides exhibiting high affinity for appropriate ligands, receptors must be selective and discriminate a specific extracellular mediator from all other extracellular molecules. Most receptors are protein molecules, existing either in the plasma membrane or intracellularly. Clearly, one important determinant of cell regulation is the nature of the specific complement of receptors and receptor subtypes expressed by a particular cell. Another major determinant of the cell response is its genetic programming. Thus, the same regulator may have different actions on different tissues. For example, adrenal corticosteroids such as cortisol cause cytolysis of lymphocytes but induce the synthesis of enzymes necessary for the production of glucose in the liver.

Most hormones, local mediators, and neurotransmitters are water soluble and cannot readily cross plasma membranes. They vary in size from small amines, such as histamine and norepinephrine, to medium-sized glycoproteins, such as follicle-stimulating hormone and thyroid-stimulat-

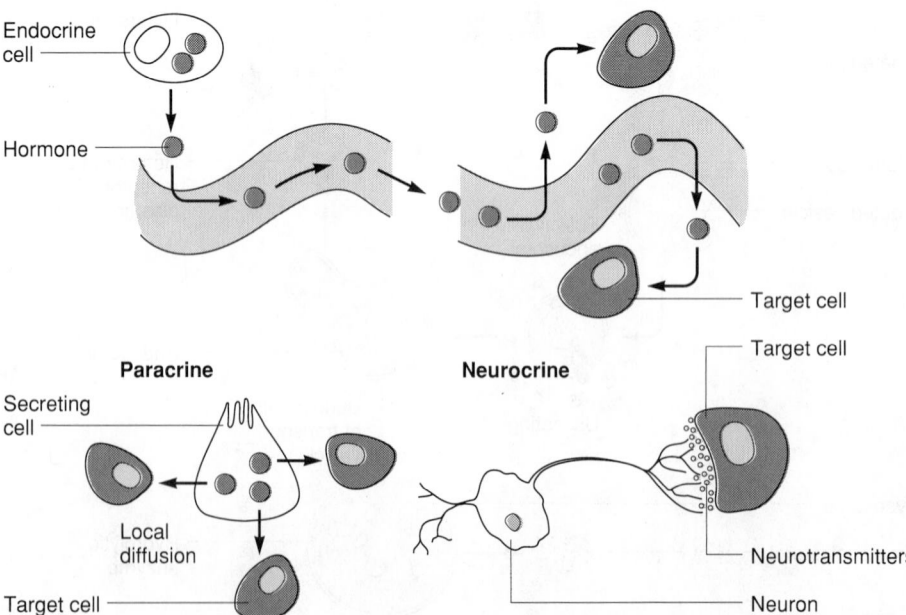

Figure 1-45. Endocrine, paracrine, and neurocrine modes of cell-to-cell communication.

ing hormone. Receptors for these mediators are localized on the cell membrane and transduce hormone binding into altered levels of intracellular messengers. The ligand itself, particularly polypeptide hormones, may enter the cell by receptor-mediated endocytosis, but intracellular actions of internalized peptides have not been convincingly documented. Another group of regulators, including steroid and thyroid hormones, are lipophilic. These molecules are generally carried in the plasma, bound to specific binding proteins. By virtue of their hydrophobic nature, they are able to penetrate readily the lipid portion of the cell membrane. Receptors for these hormones exist intracellularly in the cytoplasm or nucleus and generally act as regulators of gene expression. These hydrophobic signaling molecules exist in plasma bound to protein, so that the concentration of this class of regulators does not fluctuate rapidly in plasma, and their actions are generally slower in onset and more prolonged than those of the water-soluble class.

Intracellular Receptors and the Control of Gene Expression

The primary molecular structure of most intracellular receptors is known from molecular cloning. Receptors for steroid hormones, thyroid hormones, vitamin D, and retinoic acid are homologous and form a superfamily of receptors with similar structure and function. All have two properties in common: they bind DNA, and they also bind a particular ligand (hormone). The DNA-binding region in the center of the molecule is highly homologous within the superfamily. The carboxy-terminal end binds the ligand, and the amino terminus is a variable region believed to be active in regulating gene transcription (Fig. 1-46).

Most cells contain about 10,000 receptors for one or more steroid hormones or other similar receptors. Some types of steroid receptors, particularly for glucocorticoids, are located in the cytosol in the inactive state; others, in-

cluding thyroid hormone receptors, are located in the nucleus.[15] Once the ligand binds, the receptor undergoes a conformational change, termed *activation*. This allows cytoplasmic receptors to move into the nucleus and bind to DNA. Receptors already in the nucleus increase their affinity for DNA. In the case of glucocorticoid receptors and probably others of this class, the inactive receptor is associated with another protein, the heat-shock protein (molecular weight of 90,000). Heat-shock proteins block the DNA-binding domain of the receptor. Activation involves the dissociation of the inhibitor protein.

Activated steroid and thyroid receptors bind to specific regions of DNA and influence the synthesis of specific mRNA,[15,16] thereby regulating the production of proteins that mediate the cellular response to the hormone (Fig. 1-47). The specific region of DNA occupied by the receptor can be identified because the bound protein makes this region resistant to cleavage by nucleases. Electrophoretic analysis of a mixture of DNA fragments resulting from a nuclease digestion in the presence of bound receptor is called *DNA footprinting*. The receptor-binding DNA sequence (called a *response element*) consists of 8 to 10 base pairs. Response elements for glucocorticoids (termed *glucocorticoid response elements*) exhibit homology sufficient that the consensus sequence can be used to identify potential glucocorticoid-regulated genes. Deletion of these sequences abolishes glucocorticoid regulation, and their transfer to another gene confers regulation. Thyroid hormone receptors interact with a different sequence, termed a *thyroid hormone response element*. The interaction of these receptors with DNA is believed to involve a cysteine-rich region of the receptor that forms loops or fingers coordinated by Zn^{2+}. This so-called zinc finger structure is also present in other transcription factors that interact with DNA.

Only a small number of genes are immediately influenced by a particular steroid hormone (primary response). Synthesis of other steroid-regulated proteins occurs later.

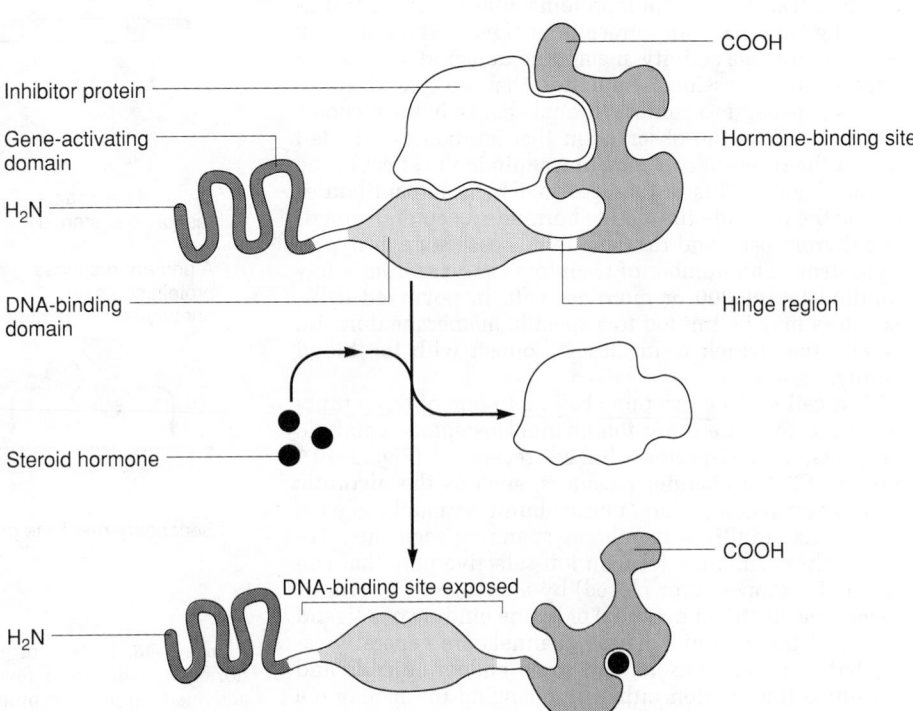

Figure 1-46. Schematic diagram of the domain structure of a steroid hormone receptor and its associated inhibitor protein. After steroid binding, the inhibitor dissociates, exposing the DNA-binding site.

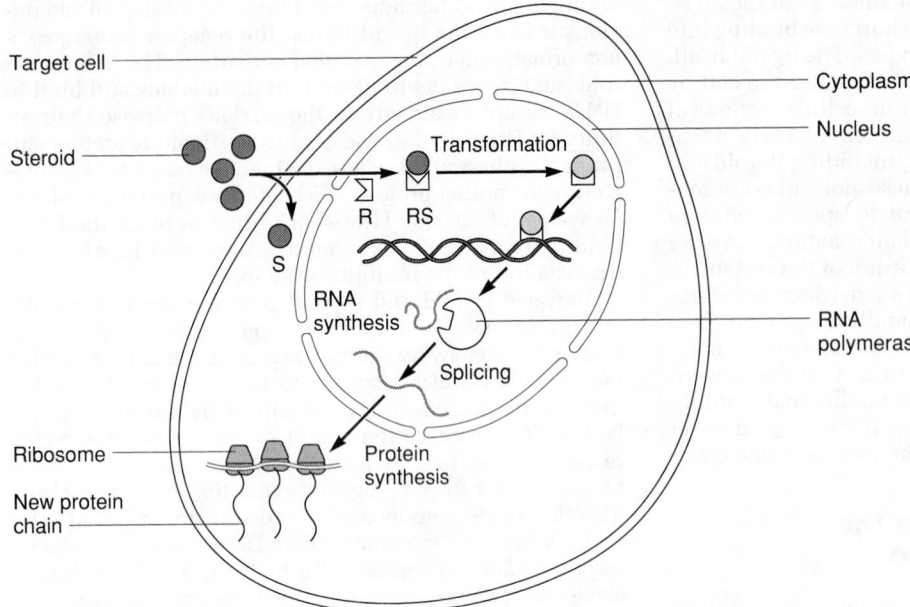

Figure 1-47. Schematic diagram of steroid hormone action. Steroids (S) enter the target cell and bind to a receptor (R), which is then transformed and binds to DNA in the nucleus, where it acts as a transcription factor to regulate the binding of RNA polymerase and the synthesis of new mRNA.

This observation has led to the concept that some of the primary gene products may in turn activate other genes responsible for the later or secondary response (Fig. 1-48). In addition to stimulating gene expression, steroid hormones may also inhibit transcription of genes. Furthermore, steroids do not induce the same gene in all cells. This latter observation indicates that the steroid receptor does not work alone but must interact with other transcription factors, some of which are cell-type specific.

Transduction by Cell Surface Receptors

All water-soluble regulatory molecules, including peptide and protein hormones and smaller neurotransmitters, bind to cell surface receptor proteins. Binding of the appropriate ligand evokes an intracellular signal, which usually regulates enzyme activity, membrane transport, or in some cases, gene expression. The notion that the role of the ligand is to generate a conformational change in the receptor is supported by the observation that antibodies directed against the receptor can sometimes mimic the effect of the normal ligand. This is the case in which autoantibodies against the thyroid-stimulating hormone receptor overactivate thyroid cells and result in the disease state of hyperthyroidism. The number of receptors can vary from a few hundred to 100,000 or more per cell. In polarized cells, receptors may be limited to a specific membrane domain, usually that which is in closest contact with the blood supply.

Most cell surface receptors belong to one of three functional classes. These are ion channel receptors, catalytic receptors, and G-protein–linked receptors (Fig. 1-49*A* through *C*). Ion channel receptors, such as the nicotinic cholinergic receptor, are multisubunit assemblies; each subunit has multiple membrane-spanning segments. Together, these subunits form an ion-selective pore that can be gated (ie, opened or closed) by a change in the transmembrane electrical potential or by the binding of a ligand to one of the subunits. These channels are generally restricted to nerve, muscle, and some endocrine cells and transduce information either by changing the membrane potential or by allowing entry of Ca^{2+}.

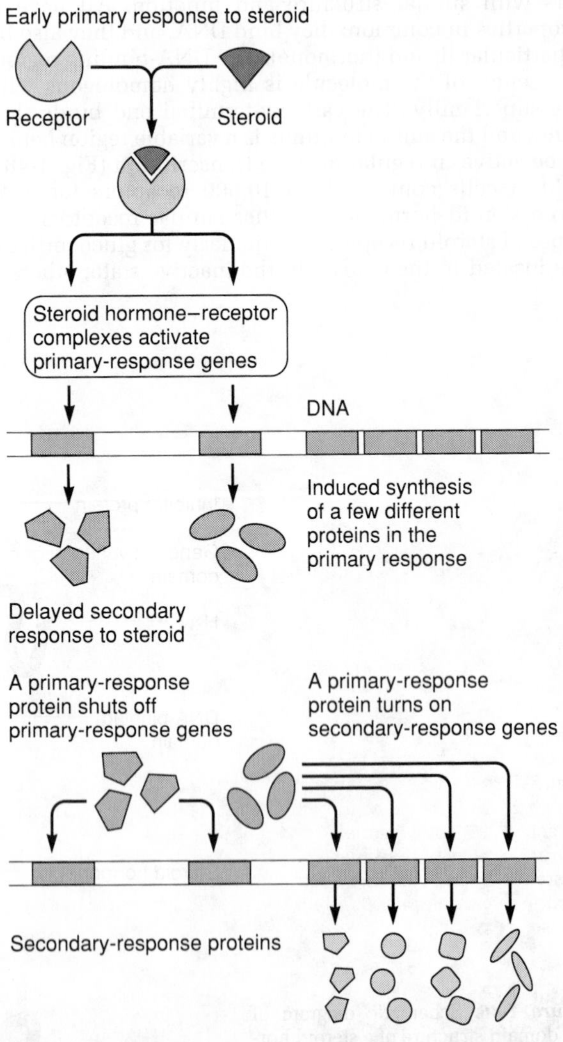

Early primary response to steroid

Receptor   Steroid

Steroid hormone–receptor complexes activate primary-response genes

DNA

Induced synthesis of a few different proteins in the primary response

Delayed secondary response to steroid

A primary-response protein shuts off primary-response genes

A primary-response protein turns on secondary-response genes

Secondary-response proteins

Figure 1-48. Pattern of gene expression in response to steroid hormone, whereby a few different primary-response genes are activated, and their products then regulate the expression of secondary-response genes.

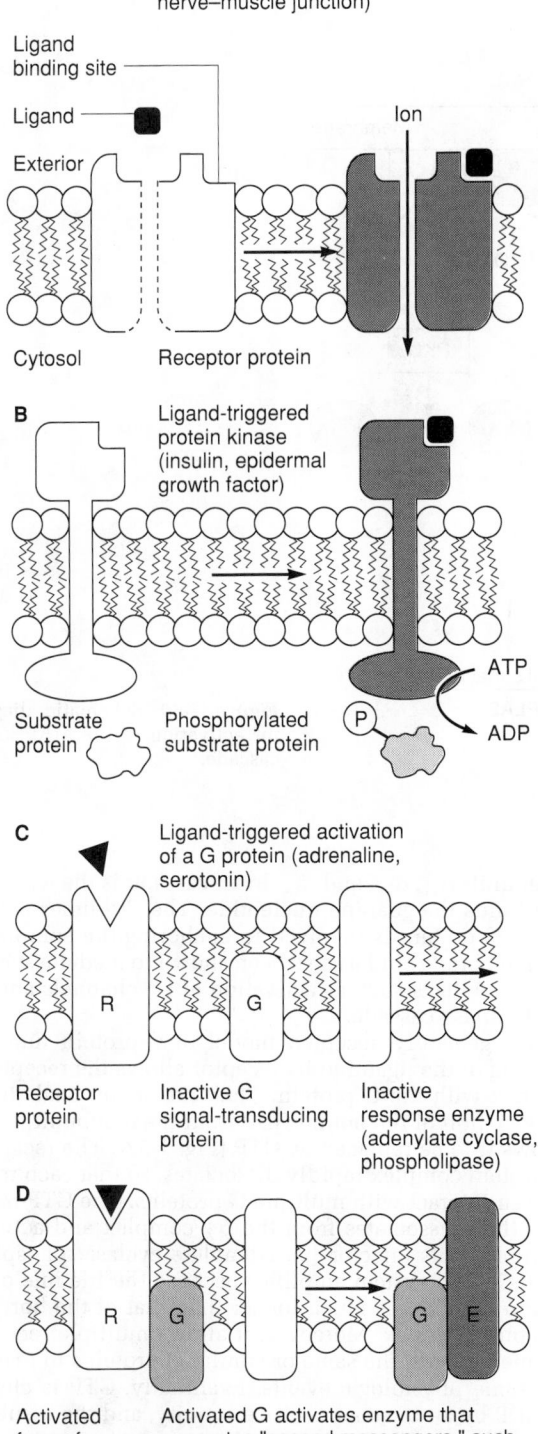

A Ligand-triggered ion channel (acetylcholine receptor at nerve–muscle junction)

Ligand binding site
Ligand
Exterior
Ion
Cytosol
Receptor protein

B Ligand-triggered protein kinase (insulin, epidermal growth factor)

Substrate protein
Phosphorylated substrate protein
ATP
ADP
P

C Ligand-triggered activation of a G protein (adrenaline, serotonin)

R
G
Receptor protein
Inactive G signal-transducing protein
Inactive response enzyme (adenylate cyclase, phospholipase)

D

R
G
G   E
Activated form of G protein
Activated G activates enzyme that generates "second messengers," such as cAMP or inositol 1,4,5-triphosphate

Figure 1-49. Types of cell-surface receptors. (*A*) Ligand-activated ion channel; binding results in a conformational change, opening or activating the channel. (*B*) Ligand-activated protein kinase; binding activates the kinase domain, which phosphorylates substrate proteins. (*C* and *D*) Ligand activation of a G protein, which then activates an enzyme that generates second, or intracellular, messengers.

Catalytic receptors are membrane proteins that possess enzymatic activity. They generally consist of three regions—an extracellular ligand-binding domain, a transmembrane-spanning region, and an intracellular catalytic domain. The best understood receptors of this class are tyrosine kinases,[17] which transfer phosphate from

ATP to tyrosine residues. Other catalytic receptors possess enzymatic activity as tyrosine phosphatases and as a form of guanylate cyclase, the enzyme synthesizing cyclic guanosine monophosphate (cGMP) from GTP. Receptors with tyrosine kinase activity include those for EGF, platelet-derived growth factor, and insulin. The insulin receptor contains four disulfide-linked chains, two of which span the membrane and are in proximity. The EGF receptor is a single chain but has been shown to dimerize in the membrane after binding EGF. Interaction between protein subunits may be involved in the signal transduction mechanism by which extracellular ligand binding alters the activity of an intracellular enzyme. In the case of the tyrosine kinase receptors, the kinase initially phosphorylates itself on tyrosine residues (autophosphorylation), a process that may involve the adjacent member of the dimer. Subsequently, the kinase may also phosphorylate tyrosine residues on cytoplasmic proteins such as the insulin-receptor substrate-1 (IRS-1). Multiple signaling pathways are initiated by the binding of intracellular proteins to the phosphotyrosine residues on the receptor or on IRS-1. These proteins include a GTPase-activating protein, phospholipase Cγ, a tyrosine phosphatase, and PI 3-kinase, all of which possess a highly conserved domain called SH2 for *src* homology, which was first found in the oncogene *src*. A pathway for activation of MAP kinase[18] (Fig. 1-50) involves the adaptor protein Grb2, which binds the activated receptor by an SH2 domain and then binds an effector, SOS (named after a gene in *Drosophila* sp), which promotes the release of GDP from ras, allowing it to bind GTP and thereby becoming active. Activated ras binds the protein kinase raf, causing it to translocate to the plasma membrane, where it is activated. The protein kinase raf initiates a kinase cascade by phosphorylating MAP kinase kinase (also called MEK), which phosphorylates and activates MAP kinase. MAP kinase is a key enzyme in initiating cell growth because it phosphorylates various transcription factors. Other receptors, such as those for growth hormone, erythropoietin, and interleukins, are not themselves tyrosine kinases; but when activated by a specific ligand, the cytoplasmic portion of the receptor binds a cytoplasmic tyrosine kinase of the janus family, which then autophosphorylates and activates similar mechanisms.

The largest family of cell surface receptors are the G-protein–linked receptors. These are homologous structurally in that they possess seven membrane-spanning hydrophobic domains, an extracellular amino terminus, three extracellular connecting loops, three intracellular connecting loops, and a carboxy tail (Fig. 1-51). They are also functionally homologous in that they all interact with guanine nucleotide–binding proteins (G proteins), which both activate the production of the intracellular message and influence the affinity of the receptor.

The transmembrane segments form a binding pocket for small molecules such as acetylcholine and catecholamines. The external segments are more important in the interaction with peptide hormones. The third cytoplasmic loop between the fifth and sixth transmembrane domains is the largest and most variable and is believed to interact with the appropriate G protein. Phosphorylation of serine, threonine, and tyrosine residues in the carboxy tail are important in desensitization, whereby continued occupancy of the receptors leads to the loss of the cell response.

G proteins are a family of proteins that bind and hydrolyze GTP.[19,20] Those in the plasma membrane were originally identified as a component in the activation of adenylate cyclase but are now known also to be involved in the inhibition of adenylate cyclase, the activation of phospholipases C and A₂, the regulation of Ca²⁺ and K⁺ channels, and the perception of light and odor. G proteins in-

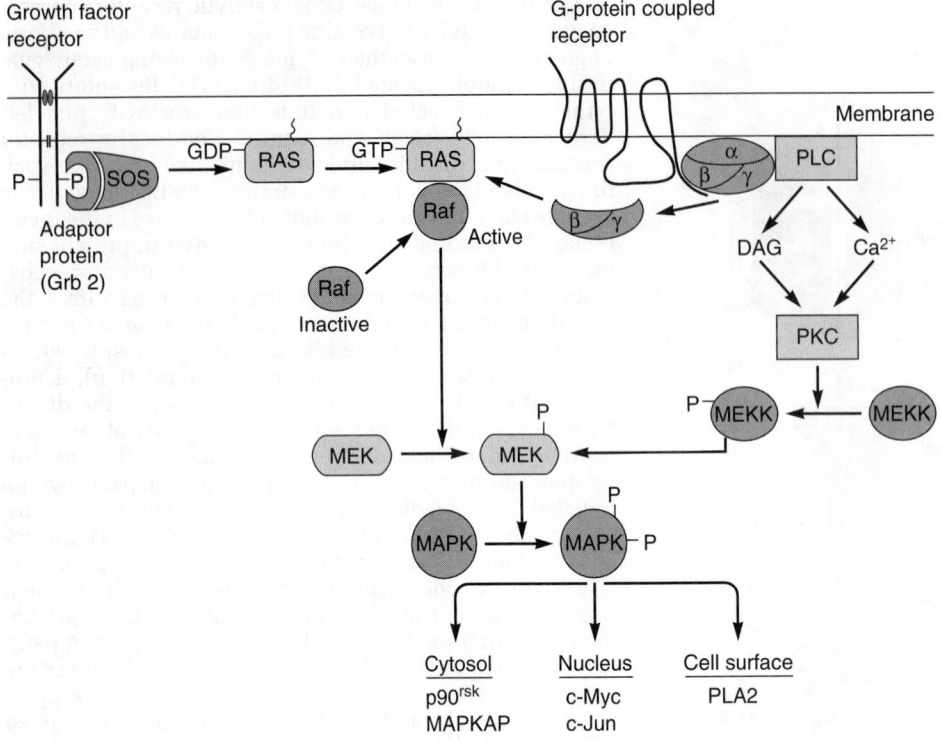

Figure 1-50. Schematic diagram for activation of the MAP kinase cascade.

volved in membrane signal transduction are heterotrimeric proteins with unique α subunits and common or extremely similar β and γ subunits.[20] The α subunits for the G-protein–stimulating adenylate cyclase (α_s) and for the G-protein–inhibiting adenylate cyclase (α_i) have been identified and have been shown to exist in multiple isoforms. Other homologous α subunits have been identified by purification and molecular cloning, which regulate other membrane effectors. One, termed α_o (the G protein is termed G_o), is especially abundant in brain and is believed to regulate ion channels. A G-protein–activating phospholipase C, termed G_q, and its α subunit, α_q, also exist, as do related

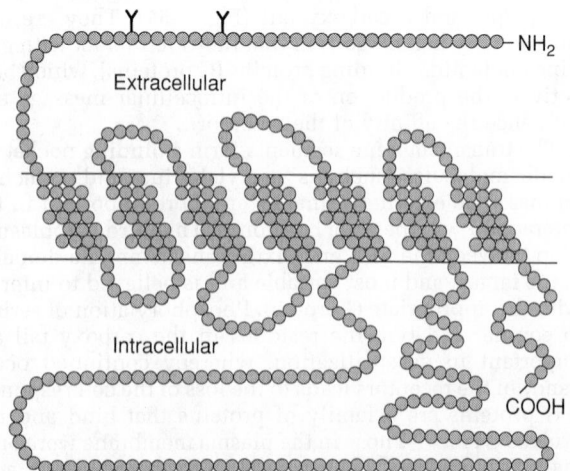

Figure 1-51. Schematic view of a G-protein–coupled receptor, showing the typical seven-transmembrane domain structure. Each sphere represents an amino acid. Y indicates N-linked sugar side chain.

α subunits α_{11}, α_{14}, and α_{15}. In all cases, it is the α subunit that binds the guanine nucleotide. The $\beta\gamma$ dimer portion of the G protein is involved in anchoring the complex to the membrane but has also been shown to mediate specific biologic effects such as activation of K^+ channels and the MAP kinase cascade.

In a generally accepted model of G-protein function, binding of the ligand to its receptor allows the receptor to interact with the G protein. This interaction leads to the dissociation of the bound GDP from the α subunit, which allows it to be replaced by GTP (Fig. 1-52). The receptor–G protein complex rapidly dissociates, so that each receptor can interact with multiple G proteins. The GTP-α subunit then dissociates from the $\beta\gamma$ complex and activates or inhibits its effector (ie, adenylate cyclase, phospholipase C). The system amplifies because the lifetime of the GTP-α complex is much longer than that of the hormone receptor complex. Moreover, it allows multiple receptors to interact with the same or similar G proteins to regulate the same physiologic events. Eventually, GTP is cleaved to GDP by an intrinsic GTPase activity, and the α subunit reassociates with $\beta\gamma$.

The final component in signal transduction by G–protein-linked cell surface receptors is the effector that generates the intracellular messenger. The two best understood effectors are adenylate cyclase, which converts ATP to cAMP, and the polyphosphoinositide-specific phospholipase C, which cleaves PI 4,5-bisphosphate, producing 1,4,5-inositol trisphosphate and 1,2-diacylglycerol (DAG). Adenylate cyclase has been cloned, and its primary structure is consistent with an integral membrane protein of molecular size of 150,000 with multiple membrane-spanning domains. The catalytic site is clearly intracellular. The PI-specific phospholipase C has also been purified and cloned and is known to exist in multiple forms (β, γ, and δ), which are expressed in different tissues. The importance of multiple forms and whether they

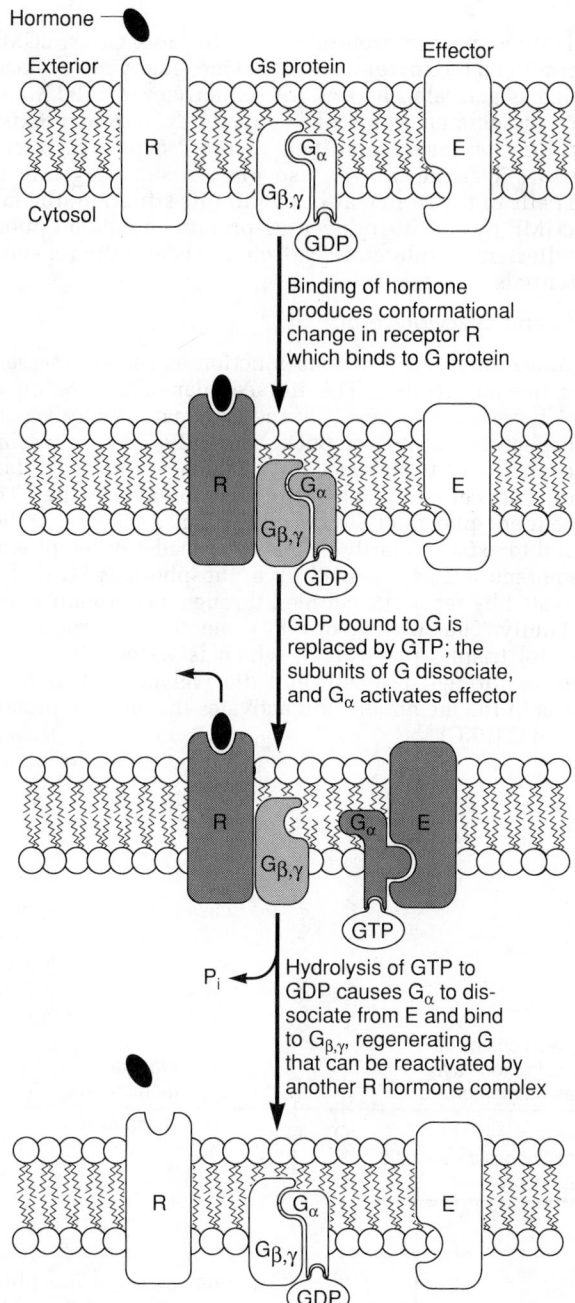

Figure 1-52. Activation of a membrane enzyme such as adenylate cyclase by the binding of hormone to its receptor. The G protein is here shown with its constituent α, β, and γ subunits. Blue units are in the activated state.

Labels in figure:
Hormone
Exterior — Gs protein — Effector
R — G_α — $G_{\beta,\gamma}$ — GDP — E
Cytosol

Binding of hormone produces conformational change in receptor R which binds to G protein

GDP bound to G is replaced by GTP; the subunits of G dissociate, and G_α activates effector

P_i Hydrolysis of GTP to GDP causes G_α to dissociate from E and bind to $G_{\beta,\gamma}$, regenerating G that can be reactivated by another R hormone complex

couple to the same or distinct G proteins remains to be established. The γ isoform, however, can be activated in a different manner, involving tyrosine phosphorylation by the EGF receptor.

Other specific effectors activated by G proteins may include phosphatidylcholine-specific phospholipases C and D, phospholipase A_2, Na^+–H^+ ion exchangers, and various ion channels. Regulation of ion channels is distinct mechanistically from that in which a ligand binds directly to a subunit of the channel. An example of G-protein regulation of ion channels occurs in the heart, where certain types of α_i activate K^+ in response to cholinergic receptor occupancy channels, thereby slowing the heart rate.

Intracellular Messengers

Cyclic Nucleotides

The prototypic intracellular messenger is cAMP. cAMP is produced by the plasma membrane. In liver cells, cAMP causes glycogenolysis by activation of the enzyme glycogen phosphorylase. To function as a mediator, the concentration of cAMP must change rapidly. In resting cells, cAMP exists at a concentration of 10^{-8} to 10^{-6} mol/L and is continually being degraded by a specific enzyme, cAMP phosphodiesterase. cAMP levels can increase 10-fold or more within seconds of receptor binding through activation of adenylate cyclase. The rise is reversed on cessation of stimulation by the phosphodiesterase. The cAMP response system can also be modulated in some cases by regulation of phosphodiesterase activity. The increase in cAMP can also be inhibited by regulators activating the inhibitory G protein (Fig. 1-53).

cAMP acts as an allosteric regulator, and most if not all of its actions are mediated by activation of cAMP-dependent protein kinase A (PKA), which catalyzes the phosphorylation of proteins. In its inactive form, PKA consists of two regulatory subunits that bind cAMP and two catalytic subunits (Fig. 1-54). cAMP binds to the regulatory subunit, causing it to release the active catalytic subunit. The active kinase then catalyzes the phosphorylation from ATP of serine and threonine residues of target proteins, thus effecting a change in their activity. For example, phosphorylation of phosphorylase kinase in liver and muscle activates glycogenolysis. Phosphorylation of hormone-sensitive lipase in fat cells activates lipolysis. A great many other structural and enzymatic proteins are known to be phosphorylated in response to various hormones, but the physiologic significance of the phosphorylation is not understood in most instances. In some cases, cAMP is known to activate gene expression. In eukaryotic cells, this is probably

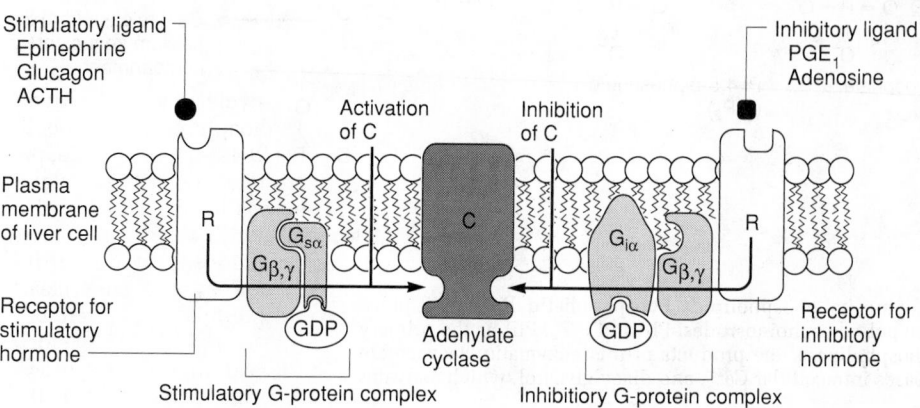

Labels in figure:
Stimulatory ligand — Epinephrine — Glucagon — ACTH
Inhibitory ligand — PGE$_1$ — Adenosine
Activation of C   Inhibition of C
Plasma membrane of liver cell
R — $G_{s\alpha}$ — $G_{\beta,\gamma}$ — GDP — C — $G_{i\alpha}$ — $G_{\beta,\gamma}$ — GDP — R
Receptor for stimulatory hormone
Adenylate cyclase
Receptor for inhibitory hormone
Stimulatory G-protein complex   Inhibitiory G-protein complex

Figure 1-53. Stimulatory and inhibitory regulation of adenylate cyclase (C) by different G proteins. The $\beta\gamma$ subunits are the same in both stimulatory and inhibitory G proteins, whereas the α subunits and receptors differ.

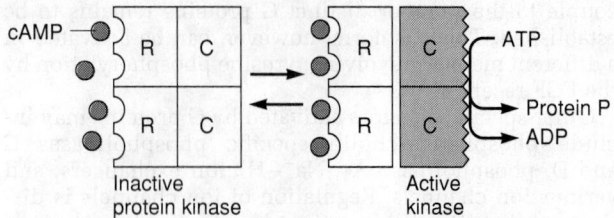

Figure 1-54. Activation of AMP-dependent protein kinase by cAMP. Binding of cAMP to the regulatory (R) subunits induces dissociation and activation of the catalytic (C) subunits. C is enzymatically active only when dissociated.

brought about by phosphorylation and activation by PKA of a DNA-binding transcription factor.

cAMP also inhibits the dephosphorylation by intracellular phosphatases of proteins phosphorylated by PKA. It does so by phosphorylating an inhibitor protein, which allows it to bind to and inhibit certain protein phosphatases.

cAMP is not the only cyclic nucleotide active as an intracellular messenger. Most animal cells also produce cGMP from GTP, and this cyclic nucleotide is known to activate a specific protein kinase. In most cases, cGMP is produced by a cytoplasmic enzyme, guanylate cyclase, which is activated by Ca^{2+} or oxidative radicals. Membrane-associated forms of guanylate cyclase also exist, and one has been identified as the receptor for atrial natriuretic factor. cGMP also plays a signaling role in rod cells of the retina, although in this situation, the fall in cGMP by a light-induced, G-protein–mediated phosphodiesterase influences Na^+ channels and the receptor potentials of these cells.

Ca^{2+} and Diacylglycerol

Intracellular calcium ions function as second messengers in many cells.[21] The intracellular concentration of Ca^{2+} increases as a result of the enzymatic hydrolysis of phosphatidylinositol bisphosphate (PIP$_2$) by a specific phospholipase C enzyme. PIP$_2$, which accounts for less than 1% of cellular phospholipid, is produced by the ATP-dependent phosphorylation of PI (Fig. 1-55) and is believed to exist primarily in the inner leaflet of the plasma membrane. PIP$_2$ is cleaved by a phospholipase C that is activated by receptors coupled through a G protein of the G_q family. The cleavage of PIP$_2$ generates two products— inositol trisphosphate (IP$_3$), which is water-soluble and diffuses through the cell, and diacylglycerol, which remains in the membrane and activates the enzyme protein kinase C (PKC).[22,23]

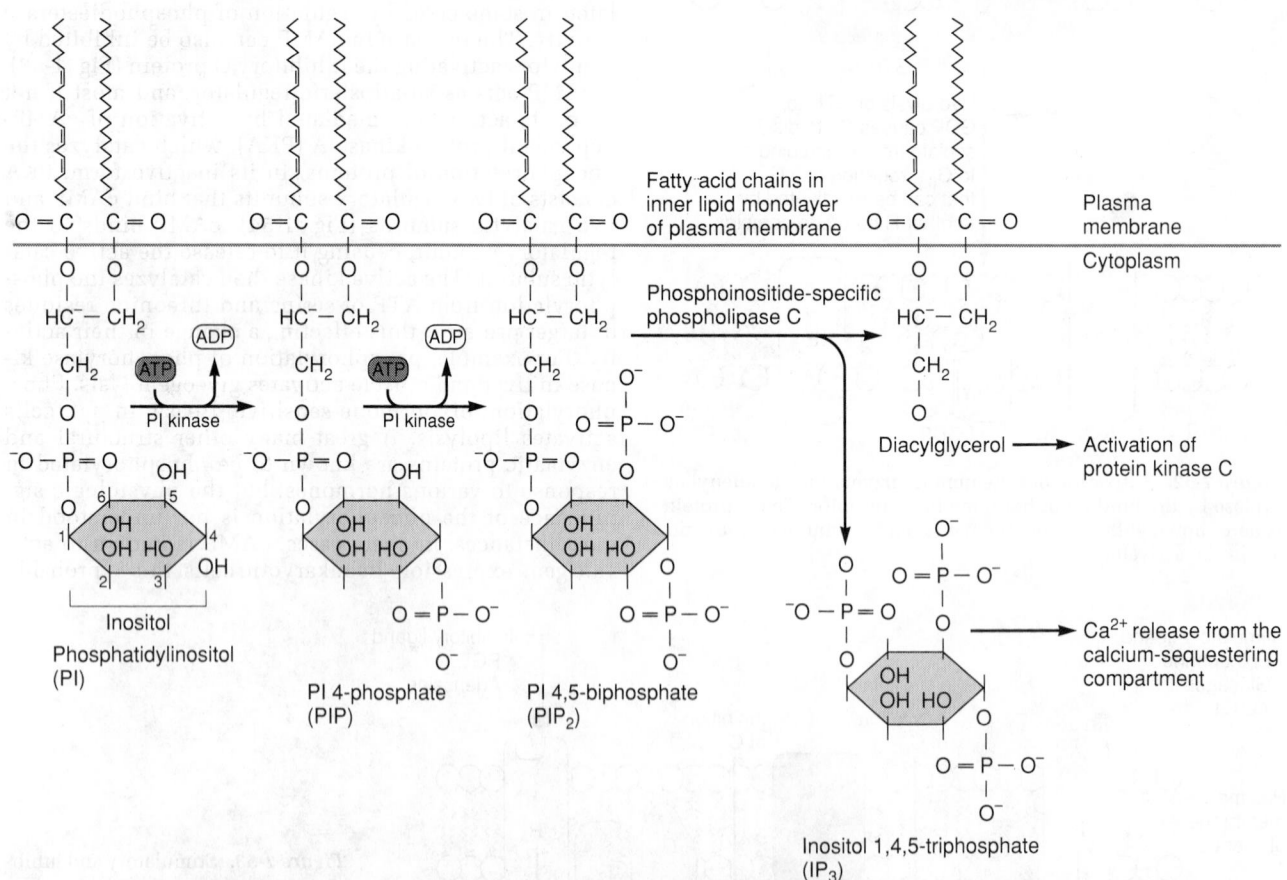

Figure 1-55. Synthesis and hydrolysis of inositol phospholipids. Phosphophatidylinositol is phosphorylated in the membrane to produce polyphosphoinositides, PIP and PIP$_2$. PIP$_2$ is the primary target for phosphoinositide-specific phospholipase; the products of this enzymatic cleavage are inositol trisphosphate (IP$_3$), which releases intracellular Ca^{2+}, and diacylglycerol, which activates protein kinase C.

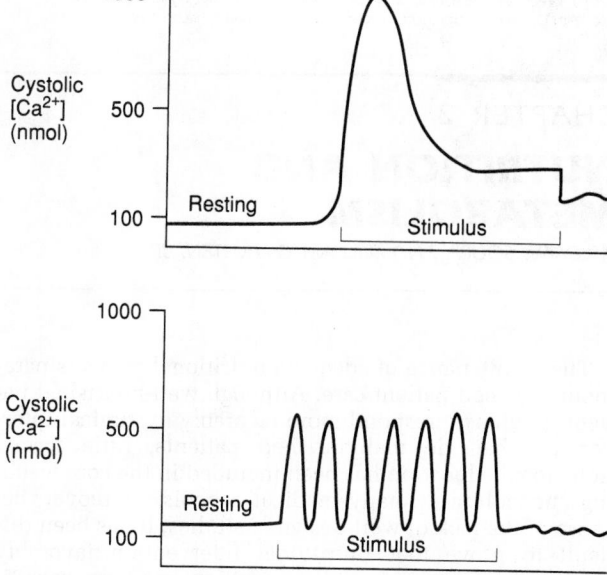

Figure 1-56. Patterns of Ca^{2+} signaling in hormone- and neuro-transmitter-regulated cells. (*Top*) A high concentration of stimulus induces a large amount of IP$_3$, which transiently increases Ca^{2+} to about 1 μmol by release of Ca^{2+} from intracellular stores, followed by a much lower sustained increase, which is due to Ca^{2+} influx across the cell membrane. (*Bottom*) Low concentrations of stimulant that induce small increases in IP$_3$ lead to transient release and reuptake of sequestered intracellular Ca^{2+}, leading to oscillations in intracellular free Ca^{2+}.

IP$_3$ in the cytoplasm binds to a receptor on the ER, which as a homotetramer forms a gated Ca^{2+} channel; its opening leads to the release of sequestered Ca^{2+}. Normally, cytoplasmic Ca^{2+} ([Ca^{2+}]$_i$) is maintained at a concentration of about 100 nmol/L by a system of pumps and leaks in the plasma membrane and by a Ca^{2+}-ATPase, which sequesters Ca^{2+} in intracellular organelles. By releasing sequestered Ca^{2+}, an increase in IP$_3$ can transiently increase [Ca^{2+}]$_i$ to as much as 1 μmol/L, although this level usually falls within a few minutes (Fig. 1-56). Continued maintenance of an elevated [Ca^{2+}]$_i$ requires additional Ca^{2+} influx from extracellular fluid, which may be controlled by a metabolite of IP$_3$ or by virtue of depletion of the intracellular stores. This latter mechanism, known as the *capacitative model,* implies an unknown mediator that regulates plasma membrane Ca^{2+} channels. After its production, IP$_3$ is rapidly hydrolyzed to IP$_2$ and IP by specific phosphatases or phosphorylated to 1,3,4,5-IP$_4$ and higher phosphate derivatives by IP$_3$ kinase.[23] 1,3,4,5-IP$_4$ is hydrolyzed to yield the inactive isomer, 1,3,4-IP$_3$.

When cells are stimulated by submaximal concentrations of agonist, Ca^{2+} is released and taken back up by intracellular stores, leading to repetitive [Ca^{2+}]$_i$ oscillations. In some larger cells, such as oocytes or neurons, an increase in [Ca^{2+}]$_i$ can be seen to propagate across the cell. This propagation, along with other evidence, has led to the concept of Ca^{2+}-induced Ca^{2+} release as being important after an initial triggering of Ca^{2+} release by IP$_3$.

Both Ca^{2+} and diacylglycerol exert many of their effects by altering protein phosphorylation. Most of the actions of Ca^{2+} are mediated by binding to proteins that can be thought of as intracellular Ca^{2+} receptors. The most common of these are troponin C in skeletal muscle and calmodulin, which is found in all animal and plant cells. Calmodulin binds four Ca^{2+} ions with an affinity of around 1 μmol/L. Calmodulin must bind at least four Ca^{2+} ions before it undergoes a conformational change and is able to activate enzymes. In some cases, calmodulin exists as a permanent regulatory subunit of a multisubunit enzyme, as is the case for phosphorylase kinase; in most cases, the calmodulin exists free, and after binding Ca^{2+} can interact with target proteins, which include cyclic nucleotide phosphodiesterase, some Ca^{2+} transport ATPases, and nitric oxide synthase (Fig. 1-57). A variety of Ca^{2+}-calmodulin–activated protein kinases exist, including myosin light-chain kinase, which is specific for myosin, and Ca^{2+}-calmodulin–regulated kinase II, which has a broad substrate specificity. These are all serine- and threonine-specific kinases. Ca^{2+}-calmodulin also activates a specific serine threonine phosphatase, calcineurin. This phosphatase has been shown to be essential for T-cell activation and is the target for immunosuppressants such as cyclosporine A.

The diacylglycerol that is produced by PIP$_2$ hydrolysis has as its primary function the activation of another kinase, PKC,[24] which also requires the presence of Ca^{2+} and acidic phospholipids. The action of diacylglycerol is to lower the K_m for Ca^{2+}, such that the enzyme can be activated even at resting [Ca^{2+}]$_i$ concentrations. An increase in [Ca^{2+}]$_i$ probably contributes to activation because Ca^{2+} also promotes binding of the cytoplasmic enzyme to membranes. When activated by DAG and Ca^{2+}, PKC transfers phosphates from ATP to serine and threonine residues on target proteins. PKC can also be activated by phorbol esters, tumor promoters that bind to PKC and are used experimentally to activate this pathway. DAG can be produced not only by PIP$_2$ hydrolysis but also by hydrolysis of other membrane phospholipids, particularly

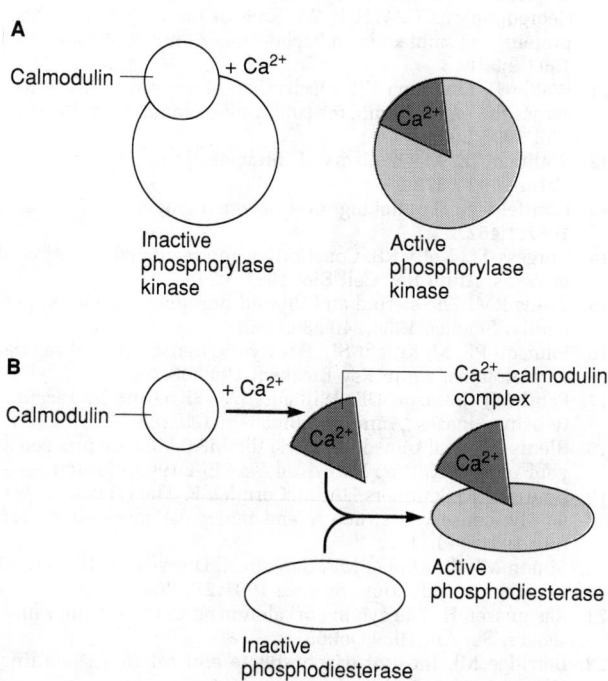

Figure 1-57. Ca^{2+} binding to the protein calmodulin alters its conformation and thereby activates enzymes. In the case of phosphorylase kinase, calmodulin is an integral subunit of the enzyme, whereas for other enzymes, such as phosphodiesterase, the activated calmodulin binds to the inactive enzyme, thereby activating it.

phosphatidyl choline, which may be cleaved by either a phospholipase C or phospholipase D enzyme. This means that DAG and Ca^{2+} signals, although initially coordinated, may diverge and that some extracellular signals can increase DAG without an increase in Ca^{2+}. It has also been discovered that PKC is actually a family of kinases and that some forms possess lipid binding but lack Ca^{2+}-binding domains.

PKC is believed to phosphorylate a number of important membrane molecules, including the Na^+–H^+ exchanger, ion channels, and certain receptors. Much of the evidence for this is based on the use of phorbol esters to activate PKC artificially. PKC is also able to activate the MAP kinase cascade. In some cases, the activation of PKC increases the transcription of specific genes, which are said to contain a phorbol ester response element. This probably involves activation of a DNA-binding transcription factor after a PKC-mediated phosphorylation.

REFERENCES

1. Darnell J, Lodish H, Baltimore D. Molecular cell biology, ed 2. New York, Scientific American Books/WH Freeman, 1990.
2. Aberts B, Bray D, Lewis J, Raff M, Roberts K, Watson JD. Molecular biology of the cell, ed 3. New York, Garland, 1994.
3. Bretscher MS. The molecules of the cell membrane. Sci Am 1985;253:100.
4. Schliwa M. The cytoskeleton. New York, Springer-Verlag, 1986.
5. Brady D. Cell movements. New York, Garland, 1992.
6. Hynes RO. Integrins: versatility, modulation and signalling in cell adhesion. Cell 1992;69:11.
7. Finkelstein A, Mauro A. Physical principles and formalisms of electrical excitability. In: Handbook of physiology: the nervous system I. Bethesda, MD, American Physiological Society, 1991:161.
8. Dawson D. Principles of membrane transport. In: Schultz SG, ed. Handbook of physiology: the gastrointestinal system. Bethesda, MD, American Physiological Society, 1991:1.
9. Stryer L. Biochemistry, ed 3. New York, WH Freeman, 1988.
10. Georgopoulous C, Welch WJ. Role of the major heat shock proteins as molecular chaperones. Annu Rev Cell Biol 1993;9:601.
11. Walter P, Lingoppa VR. Mechanism of protein translocation across the endoplasmic reticulum membrane. Annu Rev Cell Biol 1986;2:499.
12. Rothman JE. Mechanisms of intracellular protein transport. Nature 1994;372:55.
13. Kornfeld S. Trafficking of lysosomal enzymes. FASEB J 1987;1:462.
14. Burgess TL, Kelly RB. Constitutive and regulated secretion of proteins. Annu Rev Cell Biol 1987;3:243.
15. Evans RM. The steroid and thyroid hormone receptor superfamily. Science 1988;240:889.
16. Johnson PF, McKnight SL. Eukaryotic transcriptional regulatory proteins. Annu Rev Biochem 1989;58:799.
17. Fantl WJ, Johnson DE, Williams LT. Signaling by receptor tyrosine kinases. Annu Rev Biochem 1993;62:453.
18. Blenis J. Signal transduction via the MAP kinases: proceed at your own RSK. Proc Natl Acad Sci USA 1993;90:5889.
19. Bourne HR, Saunders DA, McCormick F. The GTPase superfamily: conserved structure and molecular mechanism. Nature 1991;349:117.
20. Simon MI, Strathman MP, Gautam N. Diversity of G proteins in signal transduction. Science 1991;252:802.
21. Rasmussen H. The cycling of calcium as an intracellular messenger. Sci Am 1989;Oct:66.
22. Berridge MJ. Inositol trisphosphate and calcium signalling. Nature 1993;361:315.
23. Majerus PW. Inositol phosphate biochemistry. Annu Rev Biochem 1992;61:225.
24. Nishizuka Y. Intracellular signaling by hydrolysis of phospholipids and activation of protein kinase C. Science 1992;258:607.

SURGERY: SCIENTIFIC PRINCIPLES AND PRACTICE, Second Edition, edited by Lazar J. Greenfield, Michael W. Mulholland, Keith T. Oldham, Gerald B. Zelenock, and Keith D. Lillemoe. Lippincott–Raven Publishers, Philadelphia, © 1997.

CHAPTER 2

NUTRITION AND METABOLISM
WILEY W. SOUBA AND WILLIAM G. AUSTEN, JR.

The maintenance of adequate nutritional status is paramount to good patient care. Although well-nourished patients obviously respond more favorably to surgical intervention than do malnourished patients, little formal nutritional education has been included in the core teaching curriculum at many medical schools. Moreover, because of the lack of well-designed studies, it has been difficult to prove that nutritional intervention favorably affects outcome. Historically, nutrition has been considered the province of physicians treating chronic medical diseases. Before the introduction of total parenteral nutrition (TPN), the surgeon was not involved in the care of debilitated malnourished individuals. It is now well established that malnutrition is common in hospitalized surgical patients and that the usual kinds of diets provided to patients may contain inadequate amounts or proportions of certain nutrients. Recent developments have increased our understanding of the relation between nutrition and metabolism, and it is increasingly clear that the optimal nutritional care for a given patient depends in large part on the primary diagnosis and underlying metabolic status. The mediators that regulate the body's metabolic and nutritional responses to injury, sepsis, and cancer have now been well described. Today, nearly all hospitalized patients can be fed safely and effectively. As a consequence, surgeons must be familiar both with the changes in body metabolism that occur during catabolic illnesses and with the indications for and delivery of perioperative nutritional support.

Although the disease process is usually the major cause of malnutrition, many patients lose additional weight during hospitalization because meals are withheld for diagnostic tests. Critically ill patients are frequently anorexic secondary to illness and confinement. These patients can now be fed; however, controlled trials in patients with normal body composition who undergo elective operations show that such nutritional support produces little improvement in outcome. Therefore, limited weight loss in selected hospitalized patients is acceptable because short-term undernutrition neither prolongs a life-limiting illness nor complicates convalescence after a major operation or other therapy. Other patients, such as those sustaining major injury or a life-threatening complication such as sepsis, require vigorous nutritional care. This chapter reviews the field of nutrition and metabolism as it relates to surgical patients.

BASIC NUTRITIONAL BIOCHEMISTRY
Body Composition

Total body mass is composed of an aqueous component and a nonaqueous component. The nonaqueous portion is made up of bone, tendons, and mineral mass as well as adipose tissue. The aqueous phase contains the body cell mass, which comprises skeletal muscle, intraabdominal

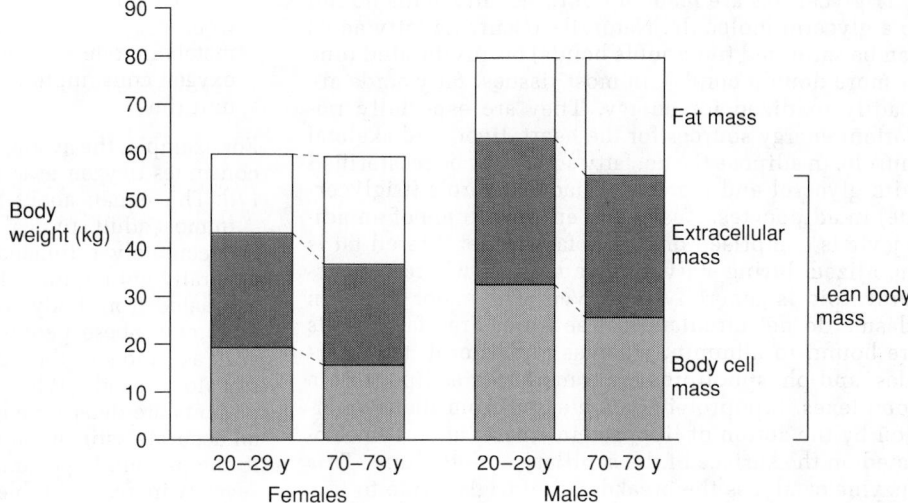

Figure 2-1. Body composition as a function of sex and age. (Data from Cohn SH, Vaartsky D, Yasumura S, et al. Compartmental body composition based on total-body nitrogen, potassium, and calcium. Am J Physiol 1980;239:E524.)

and intrathoracic organs, skin, and circulating blood cells. Also contributing to the aqueous portion is the interstitial fluid and the intravascular volume. Total body water (about 40 L) in an average-sized (70 kg) man makes up about 55% to 60% of total body mass. Of this 40 L, about 22.5 L are intracellular, 14 L are interstitial fluid, and 3 to 3.5 L are plasma volume. Body composition varies as a function of age and sex (Fig. 2-1) and is altered after injury or surgery. These changes are characterized by a loss of lean and fat body mass and expansion of the extracellular fluid compartment. Thus, the metabolically active body mass is diminished.

The body contains fuel reserves, which it can mobilize and use during times of starvation or stress (Table 2-1). By far, the greatest energy component is fat, which is calorically dense and provides about 9 kcal/g. Body protein constitutes the next largest mass of usable energy, but amino acids yield only about 4 kcal/g. Unlike fat reserves, body protein is not a stored form of energy but rather serves as a structural and functional component. Severe loss of body protein is associated with functional consequences. Following injury, proteolysis accelerates to generate amino acids to support gluconeogenesis and other key synthetic processes. In the long run, a chronic catabolic state can lead to erosion of body protein stores, which increases susceptibility to infection, impairs wound healing, and unfavorably affects outcome.

Energy Metabolism

From a simplistic mechanical standpoint, the human body is nothing more than an engine. It burns fuel to generate energy that is used to perform work. The human body does several kinds of work, including mechanical work (eg, locomotion, breathing), transport work (eg, carrier-mediated uptake of nutrients into cells), and synthetic work (biosynthesis of proteins and other complex molecules). Indeed, all of these kinds of work are essential for life. The energy used to do such tasks comes from the energy present in the chemical bonds of nutrients that are consumed. The human body has the capacity to oxidize several types of fuels, including glucose (carbohydrates), amino acids (proteins), fatty acids (lipids), ketone bodies, and alcohol. Thus, the human body converts energy stored in chemical bonds of nutrients into internal work (ie, enzymatic catalysis) and external work (ie, muscular contraction for locomotion). During starvation or after operative procedures when nutrition is not provided, the body oxidizes stored energy sources to generate work. In humans, this process is relatively inefficient, since about half of this potential energy is lost as heat. Some of the heat generated during this process is used to help maintain body temperature by means of carefully controlled regulatory mechanisms in the hypothalamus. Excess heat is released primarily through the skin through evaporation, radiation, convection, and conduction. In surgical patients, these central regulatory mechanisms are often "reset," leading to the development of fever, which under most circumstances is an appropriate response to injury and infection. A rise in body temperature, for example, results in increased enzymatic reactions, which are necessary to support the inflammatory process.

Amino acids, glucose, and fatty acids are the major energy sources the body uses to perform work. Amino acids are derived from endogenous or dietary proteins or are provided as crystalline L-amino acids when administered intravenously. Glucose either is produced when carbohydrates are broken down in the gut lumen or is generated in the liver from other sugars. Fatty acids are derived from the hydrolysis of triglycerides. Glucose provided in TPN solutions is in the form of dextrose, a hydrated glucose molecule that provides 3.4 kcal/g. One liter of D_5W contains 50 g of dextrose or 170 kcal. Therefore, the typical postoperative surgical patient who is given an intravenous glucose solution at 125 mL/h receives about 500 kcal/d. This is far less than the actual number of kilocalories needed to meet daily adult energy requirements. However, this amount of glucose is sufficient to stimulate pancreatic release of insulin, the primary anabolic hormone, which stimulates amino acid uptake and protein synthesis.

Table 2-1. FUEL RESERVES OF A HEALTHY (70-KG) ADULT MAN

Energy Source	kg	kcal Value
Fat	14	125,000
Protein		
Skeletal muscle	6	24,000
Other	6	24,000
Glycogen		
Muscle	0.15	600
Liver	0.075	300
Free glucose	0.02	80

Triglycerides are made up of three fatty acids bound to a glycerol molecule. Naturally occurring fatty acids can be saturated (no double bonds) or unsaturated (one or more double bonds). In most tissues, fatty acids are readily oxidized for energy. They are especially important energy sources for the heart, liver, and skeletal muscle. In adipose tissue, fatty acids may be reesterified with glycerol and stored as triacylglycerols (triglyceride) in adipocytes. Nearly the entire volume of an adipocyte is comprised of a large fat droplet. Stored fat is mobilized during starvation and stress, whereas structural lipid is generally preserved. The major lipids in plasma do not circulate in free form. Free fatty acids are bound to albumin, whereas cholesterol, triglycerides, and phospholipids are transported as lipoprotein complexes. Lipoproteins are cleared from the circulation by the action of lipoprotein lipase, an enzyme located on the surface of the capillary endothelium. This enzyme catalyzes the breakdown of triglyceride to free fatty acids and glycerol. The second lipase that regulates the supply of free fatty acids to tissues is hormone-sensitive lipase. It is present only in adipose tissue and catalyzes the breakdown of stored triglycerides into glycerol and fatty acids. The fatty acids produced are released into the bloodstream.

Hormone-sensitive lipase is rapidly activated by the counterregulatory hormones epinephrine, norepinephrine, and glucagon, which bind to a cell membrane receptor. Growth hormone and glucocorticoids also increase the activity of hormone-sensitive lipase, but this process takes time, since it involves de novo protein synthesis. Thus, during stress the activity of hormone-sensitive lipase increases, which mobilizes fat stores. Conversely, stress decreases the activity of lipoprotein lipase on endothelial cells, which, under certain circumstances, can impair the clearance of fat from the bloodstream of stressed catabolic patients. Nonetheless, fat is an important fuel source for critically ill patients; as a general rule, the amount of fat administered to patients receiving TPN should constitute about 15% to 30% of total nonprotein caloric needs.

Free fatty acids must be activated in the cytoplasm by condensation with coenzyme A (CoA) before they can be oxidized. The resulting fatty acyl-CoA molecules are transported into the mitochondria by a shuttle system in which L-carnitine acts as an acyl carrier. This process can be rate limiting during severe stress. Carnitine depletion has been shown to accompany critical illness, so supplementing TPN solutions with carnitine has been proposed to enhance the endogenous utilization of fats as fuel. Although this has not proved to be effective, it is an example of an attempt to improve the metabolic care of critically ill patients through nutrition.

A calorie is the amount of heat required to raise the temperature of 1 g of water from 14.5°C to 15.5°C at a pressure of one standard atmosphere. A kilocalorie is 1000 cal and is the unit of energy used in the United States to discuss body metabolism and nutrition. Basal energy requirements are measured with the subject at rest when no external work is being done; the energy is used mainly for transport work and synthetic work within cells. A small percentage (less than 5%) of this energy is spent on cardiac output and breathing in normal subjects. In contrast, the work of breathing in a person who has chronic obstructive lung disease or who is using a ventilator can account for 15% to 20% of caloric expenditure.

Caloric requirements (metabolic rate) are related to oxygen consumption by the formula:

$$\text{metabolic rate} = 4.83 \times \text{oxygen consumption}$$

where:
metabolic rate = kilocalories per unit time
oxygen consumption = liters consumed per unit time

For example, the average resting postabsorptive 70-kg man consumes oxygen at a rate of about 200 mL/min, or 288 L/d. This equals about 1450 kcal/d.

In most adult surgical patients, energy requirements can be accurately estimated, and complicated formulas are generally not required. Basal metabolic rate (BMR) can be estimated from body weight alone (Table 2-2) except in extremely obese people. Although metabolic rate varies with age and sex, these factors are not major determinants of caloric needs. When caloric requirements for surgical patients are determined, they provide the physician with an accurate estimate of how many kilocalories to provide to the patient. In general, energy needs increase as illness severity increases (Table 2-3). Interestingly, the caloric expenditure increases minimally after elective surgery. The largest increase in energy expenditure occurs in patients with severe multiple trauma or major thermal injury. Thus, an average-sized adult who sustains a major burn rarely requires more than 3500 kcal/d for maintenance.

Only the bond between carbon and hydrogen in carbohydrates, fats, and amino acids is significant as a source of usable energy in mammalian tissues. When the bond is broken by intracellular catalysis, energy is liberated and carbon dioxide and water are formed. The general formula for glucose oxidation is as follows:

$$C_6H_{12}O_6 + 6\ O_2 \rightarrow 6\ CO_2 + 6\ H_2O$$

The respiratory quotient (RQ) for this reaction is the ratio of 6 volumes of carbon dioxide to 6 volumes of oxygen, which equals 1.

For the oxidation of fats, more oxygen is required to oxidize the multiple carbon–carbon bonds; thus, the RQ is less than 1. The oxidation of triglyceride is as follows:

$$2\ C_{51}H_{98}O_6 + 145\ O_2 \rightarrow 102\ CO_2 + 98\ H_2O$$

The RQ for this reaction is 102 divided by 145, or 0.703.

The RQ for proteins is more difficult to calculate, since the composition of the various amino acids varies from protein to protein. On average, however, the RQ for protein is 0.8. The process of lipogenesis, in which fatty acids are synthesized from glucose, has an RQ much greater than 1. For a sample fat ($C_{55}H_{104}O_6$) containing a balanced mixture of fatty acids, the equation is as follows:

$$27\ C_6H_{12}O_6 + 6\ O_2 \rightarrow 2\ C_{55}H_{104}O_8 + 52\ CO_2 + 58\ H_2O$$

The RQ for this reaction is 52 divided by 6, which equals 8.67. The clinical significance of this reaction is that when very high carbohydrate loads are given, the patient's RQ may increase to 1.3 or even 1.4, indicating that a portion

Table 2-2. APPROXIMATE BASAL METABOLIC RATES IN ADULTS

Weight (kg)	Basal Metabolic Rate (kcal/d)
50	1300
60	1450
70	1600
80	1750
90	1900
100	2050

Table 2-3. CALORIC REQUIREMENTS FOR AN AVERAGE (70-KG) ADULT MAN

Disease Process	kcal/d
Basal	1450
Postoperative (uncomplicated)	1500–1700
Sepsis	2000–2400
Multiple trauma (ventilator)	2200–2600
Major burn	2500–3000

of the infused glucose is being converted to fat. In this process, considerable quantities of carbon dioxide are produced. Under normal circumstances, this extra carbon dioxide is removed from the body during breathing. On occasion, however, patients with pulmonary insufficiency develop carbon dioxide retention during high-glucose feedings, necessitating a decrease in glucose calories to prevent acid–base abnormalities.

Protein and Amino Acid Metabolism

About 15% of total body weight is made up of proteins, of which half are intracellular and half are extracellular. Extracellular proteins include those that circulate in the bloodstream (eg, albumin, transferrin, hemoglobin) and those that compose the intracellular matrix, such as collagen and other fibrous proteins. In humans and other mammals, dietary protein is the source of most amino acids. Intestinal absorption is the only physiologic pathway by which the body obtains exogenous amino acids, except through intravenous parenteral amino acid supply. Enterocytes are responsible for amino acid absorption and can transport amino acids across the brush border or basolat-

eral membrane. The active transport of amino acids into the cytoplasm of intestinal epithelial cells occurs by means of functionally and biochemically distinct amino acid transport systems defined by their amino acid selectivities and physicochemical properties. Each system presumably relates to an integral membrane-associated transporter protein that resides in the cell membrane and translocates the amino acid from the extracellular environment into the cytoplasm.

Many factors, including nutritional status, have been shown to specifically or nonspecifically alter amino acid transport activities. The first mechanism is reversible hyperplasia of the intestinal mucosa after a prolonged period of oral hyperalimentation, resulting in an increase in epithelial cells and in the absorptive surface area. This nonspecific hyperplasia can increase amino acid uptake by a factor of five. The second mechanism is a reversible several-fold increase of specific amino acid transport activities. Intestinal transport activity is also influenced by surgery, infection, and cancer. In conjunction with ileus, which precludes enteral nutrition altogether, specific changes in brush-border transport activity can also alter nutrition in surgical patients.

Digestion of ingested protein provides free amino acids that are absorbed by the small intestine and delivered to the body, where they can be incorporated into new proteins or other biosynthetic products. Excess amino acids are degraded, and their carbon skeletons are oxidized to produce energy or are incorporated into glycogen or free fatty acids. In addition to the metabolism of dietary amino acids, the existing proteins in the cell are continuously recycled, such that total protein turnover in the body is about 300 g/d (Fig. 2-2). Vertebrates cannot reuse nitrogen with 100% efficiency. Therefore, obligatory nitrogen losses occur, mainly in the urine. Most of the nitrogen lost in the urine is in the form of urea (85%) with lesser amounts as

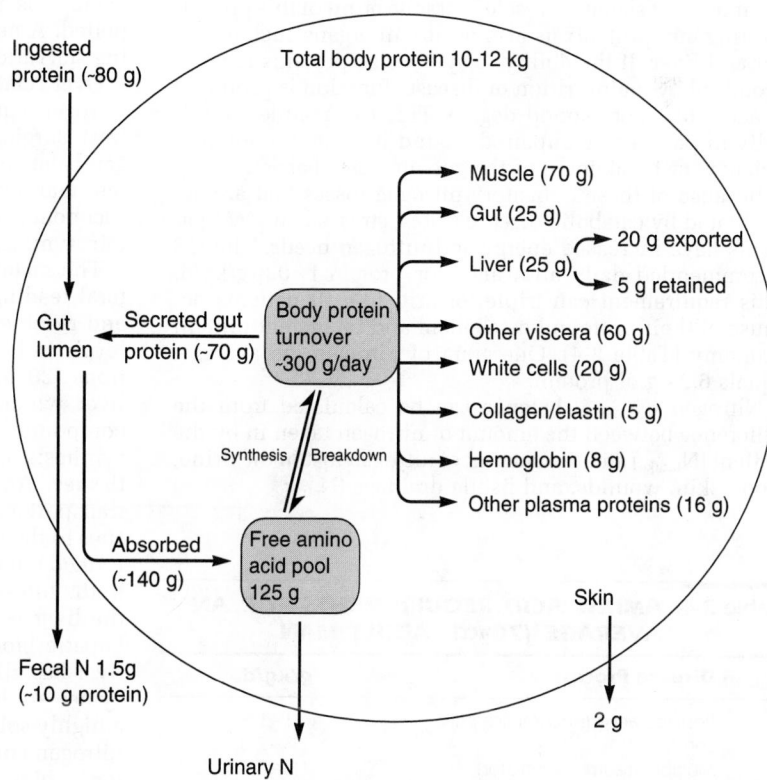

Figure 2-2. Whole body protein metabolism in a normal 70-kg man.

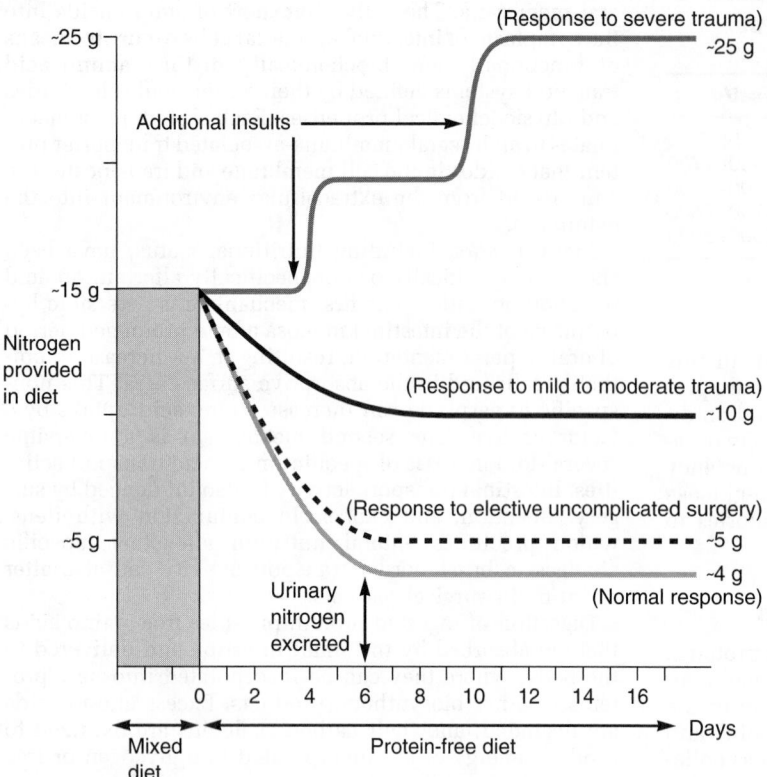

Figure 2-3. The response to starvation in normal, postoperative, and septic individuals. The normal person adapts to starvation by conserving body protein, which manifests as decreased nitrogen excretion in the urine. Septic patients do not adapt to starvation by using ketones for energy; therefore, urinary nitrogen losses are much greater.

creatine and ammonia. Urinary nitrogen losses diminish in patients who are fed a protein-free diet, but they never reach zero because the body cannot completely reuse nitrogen. In stressed patients, this ability to adapt to starvation is compromised such that proteolysis of body proteins continues at a substantial rate (Fig. 2-3). Although it is often assumed that skeletal muscle bears the brunt of this protein wasting, net proteolysis also occurs in organs such as the gut and liver. If the ability to synthesize proteins is compromised by malnutrition or disease, function is generally affected to a correspond degree. This can manifest clinically in patients as impaired wound healing, immunodeficiency, or breakdown of the gut–mucosal barrier.

Because of these obligatory nitrogen losses that are accentuated by catabolic disease states, stressed surgical patients have increased energy and nitrogen needs. The US recommended daily allowance for protein is 0.8 g/kg/d. This requirement can triple for critically ill patients because of their profound catabolism and inefficient protein economy (Table 2-4). One gram of nitrogen, on average, equals 6.25 g of protein.

Nitrogen ($N_{balance}$) balance can be calculated from the difference between the amount of nitrogen taken in by the patient (N_{intake}) and the amount of nitrogen lost in the urine, stool, skin, wounds, and fistula drainage (N_{out}):

$$N_{balance} = N_{intake} - N_{out}$$

When the nitrogen balance is positive, nitrogen intake exceeds the amount expelled. A positive nitrogen balance is usually associated, for example, with growth during childhood and anabolism after surgery. When the nitrogen balance is negative, intake is less than the amount expelled. A negative balance often occurs, for example, during starvation, injury, and severe infection.

Over relatively long periods, healthy adults maintain a nitrogen equilibrium (ie, zero nitrogen balance). In contrast, surgical patients are prone to develop negative nitrogen balances because of underlying disease. This most often manifests clinically as wasting of skeletal muscle secondary to rates of protein breakdown that exceed protein synthesis.

The metabolism of amino acids (from enteral or parenteral feedings) generates ammonia, one of the most toxic and reactive compounds in physiologic fluids. Ammonia levels in blood are generally kept at nontoxic concentrations (20 to 40 μmol/L). This is done primarily by the liver, which converts ammonia to urea, a nontoxic soluble compound. A large portion of the ammonia used for urea synthesis arises from nitrogen catabolism in extrahepatic tissues. Amino acids, primarily glutamine and alanine, transport ammonia in a nontoxic form from peripheral tissues to the visceral organs. In these organs, ammonia is reformed but is either excreted (kidneys) or detoxified (liver). In the intestinal tract, the large ammonia load delivered to the liver escapes the systemic circulation because of the hepatic biochemical pathways that detoxify it. Only the liver has all the enzymes of urea synthesis, and these enzymes are located only in periportal hepatocytes. Urea is a highly soluble (2 mol/L), nontoxic molecule with a high nitrogen content (47%). Little chemical energy is required for its biosynthesis. Normal humans that ingest a Western diet excrete about 30 g of urea daily. This can increase

Table 2-4. **AMINO ACID REQUIREMENTS FOR AN AVERAGE (70-KG) ADULT MAN**

Disease Process	g/kg/d
Postoperative (uncomplicated)	1–1.5
Sepsis	1.5–2.0
Multiple trauma (ventilator)	1.5–2.0
Major burn	2.0–3.0

to more than 60 g/d in catabolic surgical patients. Urea accounts for 85% of total urinary nitrogen, with the remaining 15% contributed by ammonia and creatinine.

The biosynthesis of urea involves four important steps: transamination, oxidative deamination, ammonia transport, and the reactions of the urea cycle. Transamination, catalyzed by enzymes called transaminases or aminotransferases, interconverts a pair of amino acids and a pair of keto acids. Transamination is generally a freely reversible process that permits transaminases to function both in amino acid catabolism and biosynthesis. The most important transamination reaction in the body is catalyzed by glutamate transaminase. This reversible reaction forms glutamate from α-ketoglutarate using a variety of amino acids as nitrogen donors. Hence, the amino acid groups of most amino acids ultimately are transferred to α-ketoglutarate by transamination with glutamate. This is important because glutamate is the only amino acid in mammalian tissues that undergoes oxidative deamination at an appreciable rate. Release of the nitrogen as ammonia is catalyzed by glutamate dehydrogenase, an enzyme with the highest activity in the liver. This enzyme plays an important role funneling nitrogen from glutamate to urea.

In the postabsorptive state (eg, after an overnight fast), the gut lumen is empty of ingested proteins. Therefore, absorption of luminal amino acids is relatively low. Circulating amino acid levels are maintained by the release of preformed amino acid pools and the breakdown of cellular proteins. Protein degradation generates amino acids that are exported directly and also provides amino acid precursors for synthesizing other amino acids that are subsequently released. In catabolic surgical patients, protein synthesis in skeletal muscle may be increased but protein breakdown is accelerated to a greater extent, such that net proteolysis and depletion of the amino acid pool are ob-

served (Fig. 2-4). This is manifested clinically as a loss of lean body mass and negative nitrogen balance.

Thermoregulation

Alterations in the body's central thermostat located in the hypothalamus are almost always observed in patients with systemic infection. Core temperature reflects the balance between heat production and heat loss, which can both be altered in surgical patients. Most of the heat produced in the postabsorptive basal state occurs in the brain and abdominal organs. An increase in heat production occurs following an infectious challenge as the result of revision of the hypothalamic setpoint, which is mediated by proinflammatory cytokines such as interleukin-1. This increase in body temperature is thought to be adaptive, since cellular reaction rates increase as a function of temperature. Metabolic rate increases about 10% for each 1°C increase in temperature.

Heat loss is regulated by adjustments in skin blood flow and perspiration. In cooler environments, heat dissipates from the skin. In warmer environments, heat loss occurs primarily through sweating. Burn patients exhibit an impaired ability to preserve body heat; therefore, warmer ambient temperatures in the intensive care unit and operating room are essential to maintain thermoneutrality in such patients. General anesthesia can reduce the capacity for shivering and lead to heat loss and mild hypothermia.

HOMEOSTATIC RESPONSES AND ADJUSTMENTS TO STRESS

Built into the body's defense mechanisms is a complex set of orchestrated responses that are initiated within moments of injury or insult. These responses are indelible,

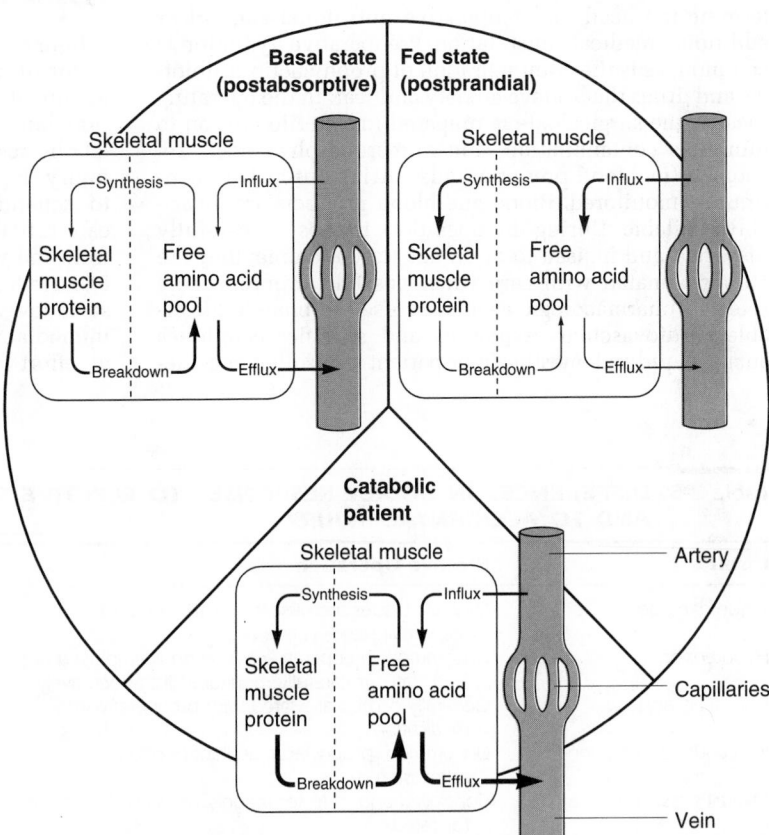

Figure 2-4. Relative rates of protein synthesis and breakdown in skeletal muscle in postabsorptive, postprandial, and catabolic states. After an overnight fast, muscle releases amino acids to help maintain circulating pool. Breakdown exceeds synthesis, although this may not be measurable using standard techniques. Following a meal, muscle amino uptake is greater than release, and protein synthesis is greater than catabolism. In catabolic surgical patients, protein synthesis may increase, but this rate is less than the rate of breakdown. In the absence of nutritional support, profound muscle wasting can occur.

essential for survival, and designed to maintain body homeostasis at a time when key physiologic processes are threatened. They are immediately set into motion by various components of the injury response, such as volume loss, tissue damage, fear, and pain. Subsequent factors that can reinitiate or perpetuate these responses include invasive infection and starvation. The events are generally related to the severity of injury; that is, the greater the insult, the more pronounced the specific response. Incorporated into the human genome are genes that encode the synthesis of key hormones and peptides that allow the body to respond to such insults with remarkable resilience. From an evolutionary standpoint, these biologic responses are the result of a process that favors survival of the fittest. From a teleologic standpoint, these responses are designed to benefit the organism, enhance recovery, and ensure a relatively speedy return to good health.

The response to trauma is similar whether the body is injured accidentally or in the carefully monitored confines of an operating room. The extent and magnitude of the stress response, however, are influenced by differences in the settings (Table 2-5). Accidental injury is unplanned and uncontrolled; tissues are torn, ripped, bruised, and contaminated. The associated volume loss can be substantial, leading to tissue underperfusion, which, if prolonged, can cause cellular deterioration and death in tissues that may not have been initially traumatized. Pain, excitement, and fear are generally heightened and uncontrolled. As a consequence, the magnitude of the physiologic responses to major accidental injury is considerable.

In contrast, the elective tissue trauma that is inflicted within the confines of an operating room is calculated, planned, and monitored. Although elective surgery causes pain, often interrupts food intake, and is generally associated with the removal of an organ or tissue, the perioperative treatment of elective surgical patients is often designed to attenuate such changes. Patients are seen before surgery by anesthesiologists and surgeons and are evaluated to determine the need for preoperative nutritional support or additional medical consultation. Preoperative hydration is common, as is the administration of prophylactic antibiotics and drugs that relieve anxiety and fear. In the operating theater, the surgical site is prepared in a sterile fashion to minimize contamination, and numerous physiologic responses (ie, blood pressure, pulse, urine output) are continually monitored. Blood and blood products are invariably available. During the operation, tissues are carefully dissected and incised to minimize tissue trauma; they are reapproximated with care when possible. Appropriately selected pharmacologic agents are used to block undesirable cardiovascular responses, and specific techniques such as epidural anesthesia or patient-controlled anesthe-

sia can be used to minimize postoperative pain. As a consequence, the physiologic responses to elective surgery are generally of a lesser magnitude than those seen with major accidental injury. Improvements in surgical and anesthetic care allow the performance of major elective operations with minimal morbidity and mortality.

SPECIFIC COMPONENTS OF THE STRESS RESPONSE

Volume Loss and Tissue Underperfusion

When the circulating blood volume is reduced, the body immediately compensates to maintain adequate organ perfusion. Detecting the fall in blood volume, pressure receptors in the aortic arch and carotid artery and volume (stretch) receptors in the wall of the left atrium signal the brain. Heart rate and stroke volume, the two determinants of cardiac output, increase. Afferent nerve signals are initiated and stimulate the release of both antidiuretic hormone (ADH) and aldosterone. Produced by the posterior pituitary gland in response to hypotonicity, ADH increases water reabsorption in the kidney. Aldosterone is produced by means of the renin–angiotensin system, which is activated when a fall in pulse pressure stimulates the juxtaglomerular apparatus in the kidney. Aldosterone increases renal sodium reabsorption, conserving intravascular water. These mechanisms are only partially effective, however, and in the absence of adequate resuscitation, severe hemorrhage often leads to a prolonged low-flow state. Under these circumstances, oxygen delivery is inadequate to meet tissue demands, and the cell is forced to switch to anaerobic metabolism, leading to lactic acidosis.

Tissue Damage

Injury of body tissues appears to be the most important factor in triggering the stress response. Hypovolemia and malnutrition can act synergistically with tissue destruction, but they do not initiate a hypermetabolic or hypercatabolic response unless they cause an infection or tissue injury. For example, prolonged underperfusion can lead to ischemia, cellular death, and the release of toxins that can initiate the stress response. Afferent neural pathways from the wound signal the hypothalamus that injury has occurred. A conscious patient generally senses tissue destruction as pain. Efferent pathways from the brain are immediately triggered and stimulate several responses in an effort to maintain homeostasis.

Table 2-5. DIFFERENCES IN BODILY RESPONSES TO ELECTIVE SURGERY AND TO ACCIDENTAL INJURY

Insult	Elective Operation	Accidental Injury (Trauma)
Tissue damage	Minimal; tissues are dissected with care and reapproximated	Can be substantial; tissues usually torn or ripped; débridement often necessary
Hypotension	Uncommon; preoperative hydration is employed and fluid status is carefully monitored intraoperatively	Fluid resuscitation often not immediate; blood loss can be substantial, leading to shock
Pain, fear, anxiety	Generally can be alleviated with preoperative medication	Generally present
Infectious complications	Uncommon; prophylactic antibiotics often administered	More common as the result of contamination, hypotension, and tissue devitalization
Overall stress response	Controlled and of lesser magnitude; starvation better tolerated	Uncontrolled; proportional to the magnitude of the injury; malnutrition poorly tolerated

Pain and Fear

Pain and fear are established components of the stress response. Both lead to excessive production of the catecholamines that prepare the body for the fight-or-flight response.

Lack of Nutrient Intake and the Consequences of Malnutrition

The metabolic response to injury and surgery increases energy expenditure. In many patients undergoing surgery, nutrient intake is inadequate for 1 to 5 days after the operation. If energy intake is less than expenditure, body fat stores are oxidized and lean body mass erodes, resulting in weight loss. Body glycogen stores are limited and become depleted in 24 to 36 hours. Consequently, glucose, which is required by the central nervous system and white blood cells, must be synthesized de novo. Amino acids, which are released principally by skeletal muscle, are the major gluconeogenic precursors. Most injured patients can tolerate a 15% loss of body weight without a significant increase in the risks of surgery. When weight loss exceeds this amount, the complications of undernutrition interact with the stress process and can impair the body's ability to respond appropriately to the injury and to complications such as infection.

The goal of nutritional support provided to the trauma patient is to match the energy and nitrogen expenditure that occurs after injury and to aid host defense. In contrast, the catabolic and hypermetabolic responses that occur after elective operations are not as significant because there is less tissue destruction and the neurohormonal–inflammatory response is less intense. Consequently, well-nourished patients undergoing major operations do not require nutritional support after surgery unless it is anticipated that food intake will be precluded for more than 7 days.

Invasive Infection

The major complication observed in surgical patients is infection. Most patients, particularly those in intensive care unit, are exposed to a variety of infectious agents in the hospital. The normal barrier defense mechanisms are disrupted by multiple indwelling catheters, nasotracheal and nasogastric tubes, and breakdown of skin and mucous membranes. Infection alone initiates catabolic responses that are similar but not identical to those described following injury in noninfected patients. Both processes cause fever, hyperventilation, tachycardia, accelerated gluconeogenesis, increased proteolysis, and lipolysis, with fat as the principal fuel. Inflammatory cells release various soluble mediators that aid host resistance and wound repair. Nutritional depletion can compromise the available host defense mechanisms and thereby increase the likelihood of invasive sepsis, multiple organ system failure, and death.

DETERMINANTS OF HOST RESPONSES TO SURGICAL STRESS

The pattern of physiologic changes elicited in response to surgical stress results from the specific interaction of a patient with the stressful stimulus. The host must be capable of transmitting and integrating injury signals, both neural and humoral, and of then mounting an appropriate response that requires the interaction of a number of organ systems. The nature, intensity, and duration of the stress are fundamental determinants of both the host mediators

activated and the physiologic changes observed. The responses that follow a minor elective operation are similar to those observed during a comparable period of fasting and bed rest. On the other hand, major thermal injury causes prolonged hypermetabolism and severely drains the body's energy and protein stores, resolving only with wound closure and resolution of the sepsis that may have developed. Thus, profound metabolic differences are seen between the body's response to simple starvation and to major stress (Table 2-6).

Body Composition

Body composition is a major determinant of the metabolic responses observed during surgical illness. Posttraumatic nitrogen excretion is directly related to the size of the body protein mass. The balance of nitrogen intake versus output serves as a marker of protein metabolism. The net loss of nitrogen from the body implies the net breakdown of the corresponding amount of protein. In women, skeletal muscle mass is about half that of age-matched men. Thus, nitrogen loses are most marked in muscular young men after injury and least marked in elderly, sedentary women.

Nutritional Status

Major elective surgery in patients with preexisting nutritional depletion is associated with diminished nitrogen losses compared with normally nourished patients, although endocrine responses are similar. A strong relationship between protein depletion and postoperative complications has been demonstrated in nonseptic, nonimmunocompromised patients who undergo elective major gastrointestinal surgery. Protein-depleted patients have significantly lower preoperative respiratory muscle strength and vital capacity, increased incidence of postoperative pneumonia, and longer postoperative hospital stays. Impaired wound healing and respiratory, hepatic, and muscle function in protein-depleted patients awaiting surgery have also been reported.

Age

Many of the changes in metabolic responses to surgical illness that occur with aging can be attributed to alterations in body composition and to long-standing patterns of physical activity. Although weight remains more or less stable, fat mass tends to increase with age, and muscle mass tends to decrease. The loss of strength that accompanies immobility, starvation, and acute surgical illness can have marked functional consequences. The capacity of muscle to serve as a substrate source can be limited during pro-

Table 2-6. **METABOLIC DIFFERENCES IN BODILY RESPONSES TO SIMPLE STARVATION AND TO INJURY**

Parameter	Simple Starvation	Severe Injury
Basal metabolic rate	–	++
Presence of mediators	–	+++
Major fuel oxidized	Fat	Mixed
Ketone body production	+++	±
Hepatic ureagenesis	+	+++
Negative nitrogen balance	+	+++
Gluconeogenesis	+	+++
Muscle proteolysis	+	+++
Hepatic protein synthesis	+	+++

longed illness in elderly patients, and muscle strength can rapidly become inadequate for respiratory and other vital muscle functions.

The changes in resting energy expenditure that occur with aging can be accounted for, in large part, by changes in body composition, specifically decreases in muscle mass. After the limited stress of elective operation, increases in energy expenditure are independent of age.

Endocrine responses to elective operation and to trauma appear to remain intact in older patients in terms of plasma cortisol levels and urinary excretion of adrenaline, noradrenaline, and 17-hydroxycorticosteroids.

The prevalence of cardiovascular and pulmonary diseases increases with age. Diminished arterial compliance, impaired vasoconstriction, altered autonomic function and sensitivity to catecholamines, and decreased baroreflex sensitivity can all impair the maintenance of cardiovascular homeostasis during acute surgical illness. Thus, the delivery of oxygen to the tissues can be impaired in the elderly at every step of the oxygen transport pathway and can be inadequate when oxygen demands increase. The physiology of aging, in general terms, is marked by a diminished sensitivity to perturbations of homeostasis and diminished effectiveness of the mechanisms to restore and maintain homeostasis.

Gender

Observed differences between the metabolic responses of men and women in general reflect differences in body composition. Lean body mass, expressed as a proportion of body weight, is lower in women than in men. This difference is thought to account for the generally lower net loss of nitrogen in women after major elective abdominal surgery.

MEDIATORS OF THE STRESS RESPONSE

The response to operative stress (elective injury) or accidental injury (trauma) has two components—a neurohormonal arm and an inflammatory arm. These pathways work together to determine the magnitude of the response. The principal counterregulatory hormones involved are the catecholamines, the corticosteroids, and glucagon. The inflammatory component of injury involves the local elaboration of cytokines and the systemic activation of humoral cascades involving complement, eicosanoids, and platelet-activating factor. These mediators promote wound healing by stimulating angiogenesis, white cell migration, and ingrowth of fibroblasts. During elective surgery, the local inflammatory response is confined to the wound, and significant amounts of these mediators do not gain access to the systemic circulation. Following accidental injury involving massive tissue destruction or prolonged hypotension leading to cell injury, excessive amounts of these substances can be produced locally, resulting in spillover into the systemic circulation. In addition, cells in other tissues, such as Kupffer cells in the liver, can be activated to produce these mediators. Such responses can lead to a systemic response in which these mediators cause detrimental effects, such as hypotension and remote organ dysfunction.

Counterregulatory Hormones

Following moderate to severe injury, a marked rise occurs in the elaboration of the counterregulatory hormones glucagon, glucocorticoids, and epinephrine. During the ebb phase of injury, the sympathoadrenal axis helps to maintain the pressure–flow relations necessary for an intact cardiovascular system. With the onset of hypermetabolism, characteristic of the flow phase, these and other hormones exert a variety of metabolic effects. Glucagon has potent glycogenolytic and gluconeogenic effects on the liver, signaling the hepatocytes to produce glucose from hepatic glycogen stores and gluconeogenic precursors. Cortisol mobilizes amino acids from skeletal muscle and increases hepatic gluconeogenesis. The catecholamines stimulate hepatic glycolysis and gluconeogenesis and increase lactate production from peripheral tissues (eg, skeletal muscle). Catecholamines also increase metabolic rate and stimulate lipolysis. The level of growth hormone is elevated, even in the presence of hyperglycemia, and thyroid hormone levels are reduced to low-normal concentrations. An infusion of counterregulatory hormones into normal patients reproduces many of the metabolic alterations that are characteristic of injury.[1]

Cytokines

Cytokines, which are produced both by endothelial cells at the site of injury and by diverse immune cells throughout the body, also occupy a pivotal position in the stress response.[2] Cytokines differ from classic endocrine hormones in that they are produced by a variety of cell types and have the capacity to exert their tissue effects locally by direct cell-to-cell communications (networking) in a paracrine or autocrine fashion. Cytokines can also stimulate the production of other cytokines, leading to important cascades that both amplify and diversify the effects of the proximal cytokine. Occasionally, when produced in excess, cytokines act as hormones and enter the systemic circulation in detectable levels. Under these circumstances, cytokines produce systemic responses by endocrine mechanisms.

The cytokines that appear to play the most important role in regulating the metabolic response to injury are tumor necrosis factor-α (TNF, cachectin), interleukin-1 (IL-1), interleukin-2 (IL-2), interleukin-6 (IL-6), and interferon-γ (IFN). These polypeptide signals—produced by an organism in response to tissue injury or necrosis, bacteremia, or endotoxemia—induce both adaptive responses (eg, stimulation of the acute-phase response) and adverse responses (eg, organ dysfunction; Fig. 2-5). Production of cytokines is likely to be greatest with the most severe injuries. Under these circumstances, locally produced cytokines can enter the systemic circulation. Detrimental responses, such as hypotension and organ dysfunction, can follow. Tissue injury and necrosis produced by high concentrations of TNF are mediated by effects on the microvasculature that produce intense inflammation, leading to ischemic and hemorrhagic necrosis.

TNF is considered to be the primary mediator of the systemic effects of endotoxin, producing anorexia, fever, tachypnea, and tachycardia at low doses and hypotension, organ failure, and death at higher doses. TNF is produced primarily by macrophages, but lymphocytes, Kupffer cells, and a number of other cell types have been identified as other sources of TNF. In healthy humans, plasma levels of TNF are quite low, generally ranging from 0 to 35 pg/mL. Concentrations in tissues are likely to be higher. In animal models, stimulation of TNF-producing cells with endotoxin induces both transcription and translation of the protein within minutes, with detection in serum after 20 minutes. In both humans and animals, TNF levels peak 1.5 to 2 hours after injection of endotoxin.

IL-1, like TNF, has a variety of proinflammatory activities. A single low in vivo dose of IL-1 causes fever, neutro-

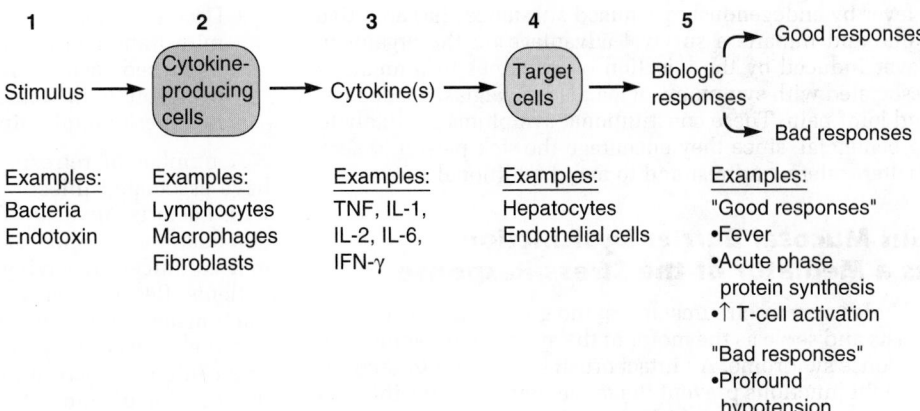

Figure 2-5. Cytokines can elicit both beneficial and deleterious responses.

philia, hypozincemia, increased hepatic acute-phase protein synthesis, decreased albumin synthesis, anorexia, sleep, and release of adrenocorticotropic hormone (ACTH), glucocorticoids, and insulin. At higher doses, IL-1 induces hypotension, leukopenia, tissue injury, and death in a manner characteristic of septic shock. IL-1 induces many of the same biologic effects as TNF, and the combined effect of these two cytokines is often greater than the effect of either alone.

IL-6 is recognized as the primary mediator of altered hepatic protein synthesis known as the acute-phase protein synthetic response. Glucocorticoid hormones augment the cytokine effects on acute-phase protein synthesis. Elevated levels of IL-6 are found in the circulation of patients with infections, traumatic injuries, and cancer. Interferons are a family of proteins originally noted for their ability to inhibit viral replication in infected cells.

IFN-γ is a type II interferon totally unrelated in structure and function to the type I interferons, which have antiviral properties. IFN-γ can up-regulate the number of TNF receptors on various cell types.

Cytokine Effects

If cytokines have detrimental effects, why do they exist? The genes that regulate cytokine biosynthesis are highly conserved, indicating that these peptides confer a survival benefit after injury. Although excess production can endanger the host, cytokines usually exert several beneficial effects, which appear to outweigh the detrimental effects seen in extreme pathophysiologic states.

Mobilization of Amino Acids and Stimulation of Acute-Phase Protein Synthesis. Cytokines act in concert with other mediators to promote mobilization of amino acids from skeletal muscle. This response provides key nutrients to support cellular metabolism at a time when the animal generally cannot acquire food because of the associated immobility and anorexia. IL-6 is now recognized as the cytokine primarily responsible for altering hepatic protein synthesis, recognized as the acute-phase response. The glucocorticoid hormones augment the response.

The primary metabolic component of the acute-phase response is a qualitative alteration in hepatic protein synthesis with a resulting alteration in plasma protein composition. Characteristically, the number of proteins that act as serum transport and binding molecules (eg, albumin, transferrin) decreases, and acute-phase proteins (eg, fibrinogen, C-reactive protein) increase. Acute-phase proteins are elaborated, in part, to reduce the systemic effects of tissue damage. Although the true physiologic role of

many of the acute-phase proteins remains unclear, many act as antiproteases, opsonins, or coagulation and wound-healing factors, and they probably inhibit the generalized tissue destruction associated with initiating local inflammation. For example, increases in fibrinogen enhance thrombus formation, whereas antiproteases reduce tissue damage resulting from proteases released by dead or dying cells. It has been hypothesized that C-reactive protein has a scavenger function. This acute-phase response confers a significant survival advantage after injury and infection.

Elevation in White Blood Cell Count. Leukocytosis is recognized clinically by an elevated circulating white blood cell count, with an increase in the proportion of immature cells. This phenomenon has been attributed, in part, to the release of neutrophils and their precursors into the circulation from the bone marrow. Both TNF and IL-1 increase the number and immaturity of circulating neutrophils through a direct action on the bone marrow. Locally produced TNF and IL-1 are also chemotactic for neutrophils.

Hypoferremia. Serum iron and zinc levels are reduced in septic patients, an event that is cytokine mediated. Decreased serum iron is probably important in protecting the host against various bacteria. The reduction of iron can inhibit the growth rate of microorganisms that have a strict requirement for iron as a growth factor. Both TNF and IL-1 mediate hypoferremia, hypozincemia, and other alterations in trace element metabolism.

Localization of the Wound and Inflammatory Site. Localizing or containing a tissue injury can be important to minimize systemic effects from the inflammation at the trauma site. This is accomplished by vasodilatation, migration of neutrophils and monocytes to the wound, initiation of the coagulation cascade, and proliferation of endothelial cells and fibroblasts in later stages of wound healing. These effects confine the insult as much as possible and activate defense mechanisms to minimize adverse systemic effects, such as cardiovascular collapse and subsequent organ failure. Cytokines are involved in all of these functions. The wound becomes an organ of cytokine production in which local metabolism is controlled in part by cytokines.

Fever and Subjective Discomfort. The systemic response to invading microorganisms and their toxins, fever is elicited by changes in the microenvironment of the anterior hypothalamus. These febrile responses are cytokine mediated. Fever has both beneficial and detrimental effects on the host, but it is generally believed that the generation of a fever by endogenously produced substances has adaptive value and imparts a survival advantage on the organism. Fever induced by the injection of cytokines in humans is associated with symptoms of malaise, myalgias, headaches, and joint pain. These constitutional symptoms are likely to be beneficial, since they encourage the sick person to seek shelter, safety, and rest and to avoid additional stresses.

Gut Mucosal Barrier Dysfunction as a Mediator of the Stress Response

Under certain circumstances, the gut can be a source of sepsis and serve as the motor of the systemic inflammatory response syndrome. An intact brush border and intercellular tight junctions prevent the movement of toxins into the intestinal lymphatics and circulation. These conditions can be altered in critically ill patients. Maintaining a gut mucosal barrier that effectively excludes luminal bacteria and toxins requires an intact epithelium and normal mucosal immune mechanisms.

Microbial translocation is the process by which microorganisms migrate across the mucosal barrier and invade the host. Translocation can be promoted in the following three general ways:

- Altered permeability of the intestinal mucosa (as caused by hemorrhagic shock, sepsis, distant injury, or administration of cell toxins)

- Decreased host defense (secondary to glucocorticoid administration, immunosuppression, or protein depletion)
- Increased bacteria in the intestine (caused by bacterial overgrowth, intestinal stasis, or the feeding of bacteria to experimental animals)

A number of retrospective and epidemiologic studies have associated infection in specific patient populations with bacterial invasion from the gut. These studies have demonstrated an increase in mucosal permeability in normal volunteers receiving endotoxin and in infected burn patients. Because many of the factors that facilitate bacterial translocation occur simultaneously in surgical patients and their effects may be additive or cumulative, patients in an intensive care unit can be extremely vulnerable to the invasion of enteric bacteria or to the absorption of their toxins. Such patients do not generally receive enteral feedings, and current parenteral therapy results in gut atrophy. The current methods for supporting critically ill patients neither facilitate repair of the intestinal mucosa nor maintain gut barrier function.

ELECTIVE OPERATIONS

Physiologic Responses to Surgery

The physiologic responses to surgical stress are multiple and complex (Fig. 2-6). One of the earliest consequences of surgery is an increase of circulating cortisol in response

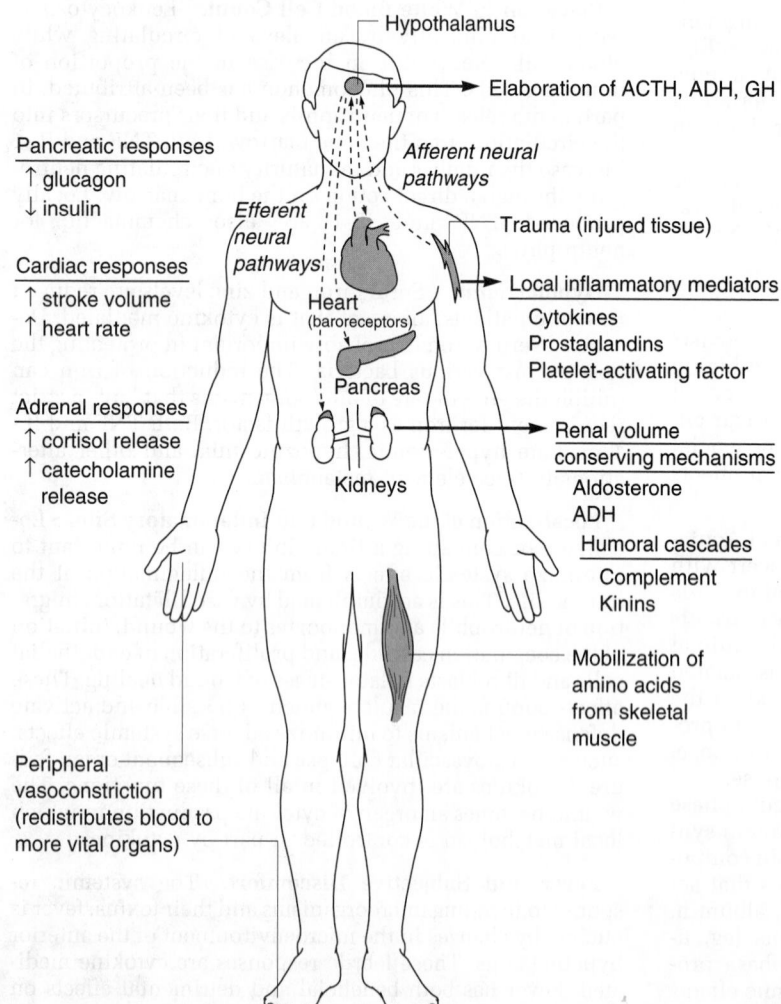

Figure 2-6. Homeostatic adjustments initiated after injury.

to a sudden outpouring of ACTH from the anterior pituitary gland. The rise in ACTH stimulates the adrenal cortex to elaborate cortisol, which remains elevated in plasma for 24 to 48 hours after operation. Cortisol has generalized effects on tissue catabolism and mobilizes amino acids from skeletal muscle to provide substrates for wound healing and to serve as precursors for the hepatic synthesis of acute-phase proteins or gluconeogenesis. When the adrenal cortex is activated, the adrenal medulla is stimulated through the sympathetic nervous system, with elaboration of epinephrine and norepinephrine. These circulating neurotransmitters play an important role in circulatory adjustment but can also elicit metabolic responses if the augmented secretion rate continues for a prolonged time.

The neuroendocrine responses to operation also modify the various mechanisms that regulate salt and water excretion. Alterations in serum osmolarity and tonicity of body fluids secondary to anesthesia and operative stress stimulate the secretion of aldosterone and ADH. Aldosterone is a potent stimulator of renal sodium retention, whereas ADH stimulates renal tubular water reabsorption. Thus, the ability to excrete a water load after elective surgery is restricted, and weight gain secondary to salt and water retention is typical. Edema occurs to a varying extent in all surgical wounds, and this accumulation is proportional to the extent of tissue dissection and local trauma. This "third-spaced" fluid eventually returns to the circulation as the wound edema subsides and diuresis commences 2 to 4 days after the operation.

The response of the endocrine pancreas also changes after elective operation. In general, insulin elaboration is diminished, and glucagon concentrations rise. This response may be related to increased sympathetic activity or to the rise in levels of circulating epinephrine, which suppresses insulin release. The rise in glucagon and the corresponding fall in insulin are a potent signal to accelerate hepatic glucose production. With other hormones (eg, epinephrine and glucocorticoids) gluconeogenesis is maintained.

The period of catabolism initiated by an operation, a combination of inadequate nutrition and alteration of the hormonal environment, is known as the adrenergic–corticoid phase. This phase generally lasts 1 to 3 days and is followed by the adrenergic-corticoid withdrawal phase, also lasting 1 to 3 days. This is followed by the onset of anabolism, which occurs at a variable time in the patient's convalescence. In general, in the absence of postoperative complications, this phase starts 3 to 6 days after an abdominal operation of the magnitude of a colectomy or gastrectomy, often concomitant with the commencement of oral feedings. The patient then enters a prolonged period of early anabolism, characterized by positive nitrogen balance and weight gain. Protein synthesis is increased as a result of sustained enteral feedings, and this change is related to the return of lean body mass and muscular strength.

Nutritional Support of Elective Surgical Patients

Most patients who undergo elective operations are adequately nourished. Unless the patient has suffered significant preoperative malnutrition, characterized by a weight loss exceeding 10% to 15%, or has a major intraoperative or postoperative complication, solutions containing 5% dextrose can be administered for 5 to 7 days before initiating enteral nutrition with no detrimental effect on outcome. Therefore, the increased cost of feedings and the potential complications associated with intravenous nutri-

tion cannot be justified. Jejunal feedings in the postoperative period can be useful for some patients, especially those undergoing extensive upper gastrointestinal surgery.

Nutritional Assessment

The two major objectives of nutritional assessment are to determine the patient's nutritional status and to determine energy, protein, and other nutrient requirements. A careful medical history and physical examination should consider associated diseases and any history of weight loss and should establish the diagnosis of cachexia, protein-energy malnutrition, or specific nutrient deficiencies. Measurements of skinfold thickness are helpful to determine fat mass, and a 24-hour urine collection with measurement of creatine allows determination of the creatinine-height index, a factor proportional to the size of muscle mass.

Immunologic status is used to evaluate nutritional status. Indicators of immunocompetence in the critically ill patient include total peripheral lymphocyte count, delayed hypersensitivity using a skin-test response to common antigens, and lymphocyte transformation. The depressed immune function often returns to normal with nutritional repletion, but altered immunologic responses are not specific for nutritional deficiencies and are observed in patients with advanced malignant disease or severe injuries. Serum albumin and transferrin are the most common serum proteins measured. They correlate well with body protein deficiency in isolated cases of malnutrition.

Determining Nutritional Requirements

A person's total energy requirements are based on the following factors: the BMR, the degree of stress imposed by the disease process, and the amount of energy expended with activity. Standard nomograms relate normal metabolic requirements to a person's age, sex, height, and weight. The principal determinants of nitrogen requirements in surgical patients are total energy intake, nitrogen intake, and the metabolic state of the patient. Malnourished patients with intact protein-conserving mechanisms can achieve nitrogen equilibrium when 7% to 8% of the total caloric needs are provided by protein. This translates into a calorie/nitrogen ratio of approximately 350:1. Hypermetabolic, catabolic patients, on the other hand, have a diminished protein economy and require much more protein.

Routes of Feeding

For patients who can eat and who have functional gastrointestinal tracts, adequate nutrition can best be provided by the regular hospital diet. The enteral route of feeding is always preferable, and a variety of enteral diets are available for patients with functional intestinal tracts who do not or cannot eat. In these patients, nasogastric or nasojejunal feedings may be indicated. For patients with diseased or nonfunctional gastrointestinal tracts, parenteral nutrition may be necessary. Peripheral venous feedings provide dilute nutrients in a large fluid volume and rely on fat emulsions as a principal calorie source. Central venous feedings consist of hypertonic glucose and amino acid solutions that are infused into the central circulation, generally through a catheter placed in the superior vena cava. Adequate calories can be administered in a small volume of fluid, but this method of feeding requires placement and care of a central venous catheter.

TRAUMA

General Overview and Time Course of the Injury Response

In the 1930s, Cuthbertson[3] described the time course for many of the posttraumatic responses, identifying two distinct periods. The early *ebb* or shock phase is usually brief (12 to 24 hours) and occurs immediately after injury. Blood pressure, cardiac output, body temperature, and oxygen consumption are reduced. These events are often associated with hemorrhage and result in hypoperfusion and lactic acidosis. With the restoration of blood volume, ebb-phase alterations give way to more accelerated responses. The *flow* phase is characterized by hypermetabolism, increased cardiac output, increased urinary nitrogen losses, altered glucose metabolism, and accelerated tissue catabolism. The flow-phase responses to accidental injury are similar to those seen after elective operation. The response to injury, however, is usually much more intense and extends over a long time.

Characteristics of the Flow Phase of the Injury Response

Hypermetabolism

Hypermetabolism is defined as an increase in BMR above what is considered normal for the patient's age, sex, and body size. BMR is usually determined by measuring the exchange of respiratory gases and by calculating heat production from oxygen consumption and carbon dioxide production. The degree of hypermetabolism (increased oxygen production) is generally related to the severity of the injury. Patients with long-bone fractures have a 15% to 25% increase in metabolic rate, whereas the metabolic needs of patients with multiple injuries increase by 50%. Patients with severe burn injury (over 50% of body surface area) have resting metabolic rates that can reach twice basal levels. These metabolic rates in trauma patients are contrasted with those in postoperative patients, who rarely experience BMR increases of more than 10% to 15% after operation.

Altered Glucose Metabolism

Hyperglycemia commonly occurs after an injury, and this elevation of fasting blood sugar levels generally parallels the severity of stress in the ebb phase. During the ebb phase, insulin levels are low and glucose production is only slightly elevated. Later, during the flow phase, insulin concentrations are normal or elevated, yet hyperglycemia persists. This phenomenon suggests an alteration in the relation between insulin sensitivity and glucose disposal. Hepatic glucose production increases and studies show that much of the new glucose generated by the liver arises from three-carbon precursors released from peripheral tissues.

Measurements of substrate exchange across injured and uninjured extremities of severely burned patients indicate that glucose is used in small amounts by uninjured extremities. In contrast, injured extremities extract large amounts of glucose. The wound converts most of the glucose to lactate, which is recycled to the liver in the Cori cycle. Additional studies have shown that uninjured volunteers (controls) can dispose of an exogenous glucose load much more readily than injured patients. Moreover, the quantity of insulin elaborated by the patients was greater than in control subjects. Nonetheless, these rising insulin concentrations failed to increase glucose clearance in these patients. Other studies have demonstrated a failure to suppress hepatic glucose production in trauma patients during glucose loading or insulin infusion. Either of these perturbations usually inhibits hepatic glucose production in normal patients. Thus, profound insulin resistance occurs in injured patients.

Alterations in Protein Metabolism

Extensive urinary nitrogen loss occurs after major injury. Like other responses, this loss is related to the extent of the trauma. It also depends, however, on the previous nutritional status as well as the age and sex of the patient because these factors in part determine the muscle mass. In unfed patients, protein breakdown rates exceed synthesis, and negative balance results. Providing exogenous calories and nitrogen increases synthesis, and, when adequate nutrients are provided, the two rates are matched and nitrogen balance is maintained.

Skeletal muscle is the major source of nitrogen lost in the urine after extensive injury. Although it is recognized that amino acids are released by muscle in greater quantities following injury, understanding that the composition of amino acid efflux does not reflect the composition of muscle protein is new. The release is skewed toward glutamine and alanine, each of which constitutes about one third of the total amino acids released by skeletal muscle. Glutamine is also extracted by the kidney, where it contributes ammonium groups for ammonia generation, a process that excretes acid loads. Glutamine is also taken up by the gastrointestinal tract and serves as an oxidative fuel. The gut enterocytes convert glutamine primarily to ammonia and alanine, and these two substances are released into the portal venous blood. This ammonia is then removed by the liver and is converted to urea. The alanine can also be removed by the liver and can serve as a gluconeogenic precursor. Following elective surgical stress, glutamine consumption by the bowel and the kidney accelerates, a reaction that appears to be regulated by the increased elaboration of the glucocorticoids. Although skeletal muscle releases alanine at an accelerated rate, the gastrointestinal tract and kidney also release increased amounts of alanine. Alanine is extracted by the liver and is used in the synthesis of glucose and acute-phase proteins. Hence, glutamine and alanine are important participants in the transfer of nitrogen from skeletal muscle to visceral organs. Their metabolic pathways, however, favor the production of urea and ammonia, which are both lost from the body.

Alterations in Fat Metabolism

To support hypermetabolism, increased gluconeogenesis, and interorgan substrate flux, stored triglyceride is mobilized and oxidized at an accelerated rate. Lipolysis is poorly attenuated after glucose administration. This phenomenon may be the result of continuous stimulation of the sympathetic nervous system. Although mobilization and use of free fatty acids increase in injured subjects, ketosis is blunted during brief starvation, and the accelerated protein catabolism remains unchecked. If unfed, severely injured patients rapidly deplete their fat and protein stores. Such malnutrition increases their susceptibility to added stresses of hemorrhage, operations, and infection and can contribute to organ system failure, sepsis, and death.

Nutritional Support of Injured Patients

Case Example

A 37-year-old nonobese man (2 m² body surface area) is admitted to the hospital with blunt abdominal trauma. He is resuscitated and has a positive diagnostic peritoneal lavage. At operation, a liver laceration is repaired, and it is observed that the patient has a large retroperitoneal hematoma that is not expanding. The patient is admitted to the trauma intensive care unit of the hospital, and a nasogastric tube is placed. During the next 24 hours, blood volume is restored, and the patient is given maintenance solutions with 5% dextrose and appropriate electrolytes at the rate of 125 mL/h. Because of a prolonged ileus, he is not fed, and TPN is begun on postoperative day 7. Twelve days after the accident, the patient starts taking clear liquids and is gradually advanced to a regular diet over the next 3 days. He is discharged from the hospital.

Nitrogen balance studies from hospital day 1 through day 7 reveal a cumulative nitrogen loss of 122 g. During this 7-day period, the patient had 0 nitrogen intake and about 500 glucose cal/day. When TPN was started, he had lost 9 lb, of which half was lean body mass, and half was fat. He gained his weight back over the next 4 weeks.

Consequences of Malnutrition

The metabolic response to injury results in an increased energy expenditure. If energy intake is less than expenditure, body fat stores are oxidated and lean body mass erodes, causing weight loss. When weight loss exceeds 10% to 15% of body weight, the complications of malnutrition interact with the disease process, increasing morbidity and mortality rates. Malnutrition to this extent after injury can impair the body's ability to respond appropriately to the injury and to inhibit responses to added stress, such as infection.

The major impact of nutritional support in the trauma patient is aid for the host defenses. These patients are exposed to a variety of infectious agents in the hospital, and their injuries and care requirements increase the risk of infection. The normal barrier defense mechanisms are disrupted by multiple indwelling catheters, nasotracheal and nasogastric tubes, and breakdown of skin and mucous membrane. Malnutrition can compromise the available host defense mechanism and thus increase the likelihood of invasive sepsis, multiple organ system failure, and death. Additional consequences include poor wound healing, decreased mobility and activity, the occurrence of pressure sores and decubitus ulcers, altered gastrointestinal function, and the occurrence of edema secondary to reduced colloid osmotic pressure.

Priorities of Care

Resuscitation, oxygenation, and arrest of hemorrhage are immediate priorities for survival. Wounds should then be repaired or stabilized as expeditiously as possible. Nutritional support is an essential part of the metabolic care of the critically ill trauma patient and should be instituted before significant weight loss occurs. Adequate nutrition supports normal responses that optimize wound healing and recovery.

Goals of Nutritional Support

The majority of injured persons are not malnourished at the time of injury, but the increased metabolic demands following injury quickly lead to a malnourished state if the patient is not nutritionally supported. On stabilization of the patient's condition and development of a care plan, nutritional support can be gradually initiated. The goal of nutritional support is to maintain body cell mass and limit weight loss to less than 10% of preinjury weight. The nutritional requirements of the trauma patient can be determined as follows:

1. Determine BMR (in kcal/d) for age, sex, and body surface area.

2. Determine the percentage of increase in metabolic rate due to the injury.
3. Multiply 25% × BMR to account for hospital activity (eg, walking, physical therapy, sitting, treatment).
4. The sum of the amounts calculated in steps 1 to 3 is an estimated daily caloric requirement for maintaining body weight.
5. Divide step 4 by 150 to determine nitrogen requirements (protein = 6.25 × nitrogen).
6. Administer about 70% of caloric requirement as glucose. Give remaining caloric requirement as fat. Reassess energy and nitrogen needs at least twice weekly.
7. If nutritional support appears inadequate because of progressive weight loss, consider directly measuring oxygen consumption or nitrogen balance.

SEPSIS

General Overview and Time Course of the Metabolic Response to Sepsis

The response patterns following a major infection are less predictable than those following elective operations and trauma. The invasion of the body by microorganisms initiates many host responses, including mobilization of phagocytes, an inflammatory response at the local site, fever, and tachycardia. Systemic events during the hyperdynamic phase of sepsis can be categorized into two general types of responses—those related to the host's immunologic defenses and those related to the body's general metabolic and circulatory adjustments to the infection. The changes in metabolism relate both to alterations in glucose, nitrogen, and fat metabolism and to redistribution of trace metals.

Systemic Metabolic Responses

Severe infection is characterized by fever, hypermetabolism, diminished protein economy, altered glucose dynamics, and accelerated lipolysis, much as in injury. Anorexia is commonly associated with systemic infection and contributes to the loss of body tissue. These effects are compounded in patients with sepsis by multiple organ system failure, which includes the gastrointestinal tract, liver, heart, and lungs.

Hypermetabolism. Oxygen consumption is usually elevated in patients with infections. The extent of this increase is related to the severity of infection, with peak elevations reaching 50% to 60% above normal. This response often occurs in the postoperative and postinjury periods secondary to severe pneumonia, intraabdominal infection, or wound invasion. If the patient's metabolic rate is already elevated to a maximal extent because of severe injury, no further increase will be observed. In patients with only slightly accelerated rates of oxygen consumption, infection causes a rise in metabolic rate that appears additive to the preexisting state. The metabolism increase is partly due to the increase in reaction rate associated with fever (Q_{10} effect). The metabolic rate increases 10% to 13% for each 1°C elevation in central temperature. On resolution of the infection, the metabolic rate returns to normal.

Altered Glucose Dynamics. The increased glucose production observed in infected patients appears to be additive to the augmented gluconeogenesis that occurs following injury. For example, uninfected burn patients have an accelerated glucose production rate about 50% above normal. With the onset of bacteremia in similar patient cases, hepatic glucose production increases to twice basal levels. Glucose dynamics following infection are complex, and profound hypoglycemia and diminished hepatic glucose production have also been described in both animals and humans. Studies in animals and humans also show that deterioration in glucogenesis is associated with more progressive stages of infection and may be related to alterations in splanchnic blood flow.

Alterations in Protein Metabolism. After an infection, accelerated proteolysis, increased nitrogen excretion, and prolonged negative nitrogen balance occur. The response pattern is similar to that described for injury. Amino acid efflux from skeletal muscle is accelerated in patients with sepsis, and this flux is matched by accelerated visceral amino acid uptake. In infected burn patients, splanchnic uptake of amino acids increases 50% above rates in uninfected burn patients with injuries of comparable size. These amino acids serve as glucose precursors and are used to synthesize acute-phase proteins. Studies in animals have demonstrated that an increase in hepatic amino acid uptake during systemic infection is caused by an increase in the activities of specific amino acid transporters that reside in the hepatocyte plasma membrane.

Severe infection is often associated with a hypercatabolic state that initiates marked changes in interorgan glutamine metabolism (Fig. 2-7). The cycle can begin with a breakdown in the gut mucosal barrier, which results in microbial translocation. Bacteria and their endotoxins stimulate macrophages to release cytokines, which activate the pituitary–adrenal axis. The release of cortisol stimulates glutamine synthesis and release by tissues such as the lungs and skeletal muscle. This supports the glutamine requirements of other tissues. The bulk of the glutamine

is taken up by the liver at the expense of the gut. It is unclear why organs such as the gut should subserve other tissues, but if the cycle persists, or if the patient cannot take oral feedings or remains glutamine deficient, a prolonged catabolic state develops.

Acidosis frequently occurs in patients with sepsis, and this stimulus serves as a signal for accelerated glutamine uptake by the kidney. Glutamine liberates an ammonia ion that combines with a hydrogen ion and is excreted in the urine, thus participating in acid–base homeostasis. Because the glutamine arises from skeletal muscle proteolysis, this complication of sepsis is yet another stimulus of heightened skeletal muscle breakdown.

Alterations in Fat Metabolism. Fat is a major fuel oxidized in infected patients, and the increased metabolism of lipids from peripheral fat stores is especially prominent during inadequate nutritional support. Lipolysis is most likely mediated by the heightened sympathetic activity that is a potent stimulus for fat mobilization and accelerated oxidation. Serum triglyceride levels reflect the balance between rates of triglyceride production by the liver and use and storage by peripheral tissues. Marked hypertriglyceridemia has been associated with gram-negative infection on occasion, but plasma triglyceride concentrations are usually normal or low, indicating enhanced clearance by other organs. Persons with infections cannot efficiently convert fatty acids to ketones in the liver, and hence do not adapt to starvation as do fasted, unstressed individuals. It has been suggested that the hypoketonemic state of infection may be a consequence of the hyperinsulinemia associated with catabolic states.

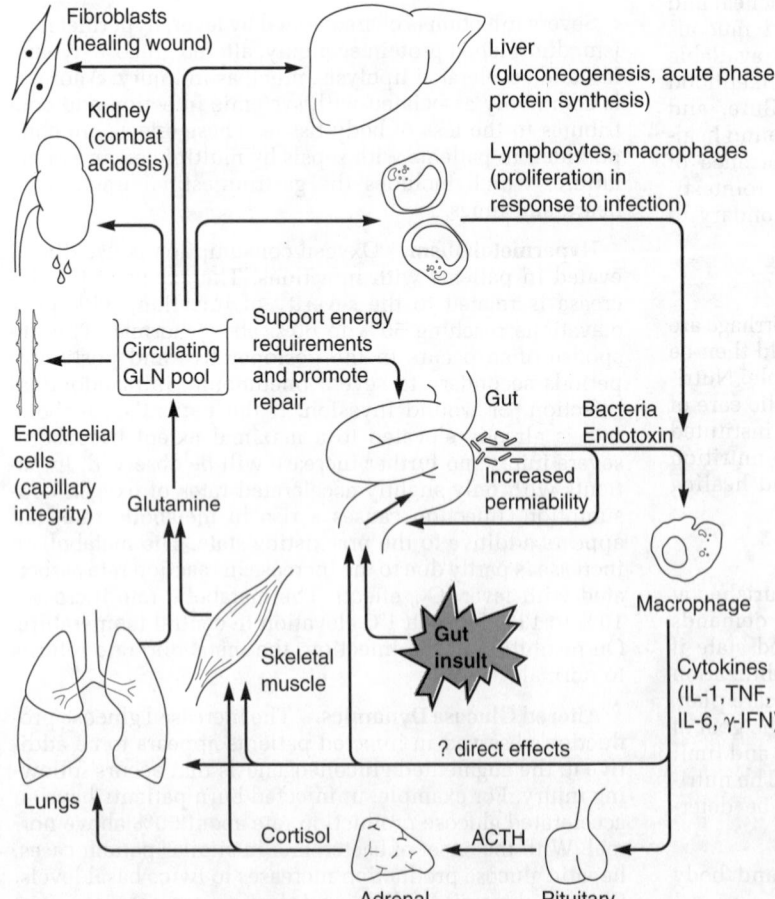

Figure 2-7. The interorgan glutamine (GLN) cycle can be initiated by any local or systemic catabolic insult that redirects the flow of glutamine and results in glutamine depletion. This patient developed a breakdown in the gut mucosal barrier, causing an increase in bowel permeability and bacterial translocation. Bacteria and endotoxins stimulate macrophages to release cytokines (TNF, IL-1, IL-6) that exert direct effects on glutamine metabolism in various organs and also stimulate release of the counterregulatory hormones. These mediators work together to mobilize glutamine stores from muscle and to stimulate glutamine production by the lungs. A central goal is to support the increased glutamine requirements in other tissues. It is unclear why organs such as the gut should subserve other tissues, but if the cycle persists, or if the patient is unable to take oral feedings or remains glutamine deficient, a prolonged catabolic state develops.

Changes in Trace Mineral Metabolism. Changes in the balance of magnesium, inorganic phosphate, zinc, and potassium generally follow alterations in nitrogen balance. Although the iron-binding capacity of transferrin is usually unchanged in early infection, iron disappears from the plasma, especially during severe pyrogenic infections. Similar alterations are observed with serum zinc levels. These decreases cannot be totally accounted for by losses of the minerals from the body. Rather, both iron and zinc accumulate in the liver, and this accumulation appears to be another host defense mechanism. The administration of iron to the infected host, especially early in the disease, is contraindicated because increased serum iron concentrations can impair resistance. Unlike iron and zinc, copper levels generally rise, and the increased plasma concentrations can be ascribed almost entirely to the increase in ceruloplasmin produced by the liver.

Nutritional Requirements and Special Feeding Problems

As with all patients, the primary objectives of nutritional assessment are to evaluate the patient's present nutritional status and to determine energy, protein, macronutrient, and micronutrient requirements. Weight gain and anabolism are generally difficult to achieve during the septic process, but they do occur once the disease process has abated. Total energy requirements can be calculated using the stress equation: mild to moderate infections increase energy requirements 20% to 30%, and severe infection increases caloric needs about 50% above basal levels.

The most severe complication of sepsis is the multiple organ dysfunction syndrome, which can result in death. The current treatment of systemic infection consists of (1) removal or drainage of the septic source; (2) use of appropriate antibiotics; (3) supportive therapy of specific organ failure, whether cardiac, pulmonary, hepatic, renal, or gastrointestinal; and (4) vigorous support of the host through nutritional means.

Respiratory Insufficiency

Common problems associated with systemic infection are inadequate oxygenation and elimination of carbon dioxide. Patients often require endotracheal intubation and vigorous ventilatory support. Most of the enteral and parenteral formulas used to provide nutritional support for critically ill patients contain large amounts of carbohydrate, which generate substantial quantities of carbon dioxide following oxidation. Such a large carbon dioxide load can worsen pulmonary function or delay weaning from the ventilator. If this becomes a problem, the carbohydrate load should be reduced to half of metabolic requirements and fat emulsion should be administered to provide the necessary additional calories.

Renal Failure

When renal failure becomes progressive, the early use of hemodialysis minimizes the effects of uremia on the metabolism of sepsis. Some authors have advocated that patients with acute and chronic renal failure receive a limited intake of nonessential amino acids in an attempt to lower urea production. Proteins of high biologic value, but in much smaller quantities (less than 0.5 g/kg/d) than usually given, are administered with adequate calories, usually in the form of glucose. When enteral feedings are not feasible, a central venous infusion of an essential amino acid solution and hypertonic dextrose provides calories and a small quantity of nitrogen to reduce protein catabolism while simultaneously controlling the rise in blood urea nitrogen. During dialysis, protein intake is liberalized, but the blood urea nitrogen is maintained below 100 mg/dL.

Gut Dysfunction

Sepsis causes marked changes in gastrointestinal function. The most common abnormality is ileus, which can result from intraabdominal disease or the effects of bacteria elsewhere. Breakdown of the gut mucosal barrier with translocation of luminal bacteria and their toxins can initiate a prolonged hypermetabolic state.

Hepatic Failure

Hepatic dysfunction is a common manifestation of septicemia. The degree of dysfunction varies and can appear early as a slight elevation of liver enzymes, or it can cause severe hyperbilirubinemia. Hepatic dysfunction generally resolves with treatment of the sepsis, but if the inflammation persists, adjustments in the feeding formula are necessary. The carbohydrate load is usually reduced to consist of no more than half of metabolic requirements, and the additional calories should be provided as fat emulsion. The patient should be observed for the presence of encephalopathy. If this complication occurs, the protein load should also be reduced.

Cardiac Dysfunction

The myocardial dysfunction that occurs in sepsis can be secondary to the elaboration of cytokines or to heart failure that is the result of pulmonary insufficiency. Malnourished patients with sepsis may be sensitive to volume overload, and use of a concentrated solution of hypertonic dextrose with amino acids may be indicated to maximize calories and to minimize the intravascular volume administered. In addition, 20% fat emulsion can be used as a source of additional energy.

NUTRITION AND METABOLISM IN CANCER PATIENTS

Cachexia is especially common in patients with advanced malignant disease, and it has been shown to have a negative effect on outcome. Malnutrition is associated with increased postoperative complications, including sepsis, ileus, and wound dehiscence, and it has been shown to have adverse effects on immune function and treatment tolerance. The rationale for providing nutritional support is an attempt to prevent or reverse host tissue wasting, broaden the spectrum of therapeutic options, improve the clinical course, and ultimately prolong patient survival.

The use of nutritional support in cancer patients, especially TPN, was initially heralded with enthusiasm. However, conflicting conclusions were drawn from numerous subsequent clinical studies. The discrepancies were due to poor study design and the use of different endpoints to assess efficacy. Consequently, enthusiasm has waned and a more conservative approach has governed patient selection. Nonetheless, nutritional support remains an important component of overall therapy for cancer patients.

Which Cancer Patients Should Receive Specialized Nutritional Support?

If the patient has a functional gastrointestinal tract and can consume adequate calories by mouth, a regular hospital diet should be provided, and no specialized nutritional support is necessary. In patients with head and neck cancers who have difficulty chewing or swallowing, a blenderized diet can be consumed orally or through a soft nasogastric tube inserted into the stomach through the nasal or oral route. If the cancer obstructs the nasopharyngeal route such that tube passage is contraindicated, placement of a feeding gastrostomy or jejunostomy (in the operating room) is almost always well tolerated. Because it is anticipated that head and neck cancer patients will continue to lose weight, this feeding strategy should be initiated early.

Preoperative nutritional support should be given only to patients who do not require an emergency operation and who have severe weight loss (more than 15% of preillness body weight) and a serum albumin level below 2.9 mg/dL. If the patient can tolerate preoperative tube feedings, this route is preferred as long as adequate calories and nitrogen can be delivered. For patients in whom this is not feasible (eg, a patient with profound weight loss from an obstructing carcinoma of the stomach), admission to the hospital for administration of preoperative TPN has been shown to decrease the rate of postoperative complications (Fig. 2-8). Preoperative nutrition (enteral or parenteral) should not be given for longer than 7 to 10 days. If it is anticipated that oral intake after surgery will be delayed for more than 7 days, placement of a jejunal feeding tube at the time of surgery should be strongly considered, especially if the patient was malnourished preoperatively.

In patients who develop gastrointestinal side effects from chemotherapy or radiotherapy (eg, mucositis, crampy pain, nausea, diarrhea), enteral feeding is often possible, although voluntary intake is likely to be diminished. These patients can tolerate 5 to 7 days of inadequate nutrition, especially if they were previously well nourished. If the side effects are severe, resulting in a longer period of gastrointestinal toxicity, the use of TPN should be considered. TPN has been shown to be a valuable component of the overall care of patients receiving bone marrow transplants.

Enteral Nutrition

Enteral nutrition is always the preferred method of feeding cancer patients if the gastrointestinal tract is functional. Infusing nutrients into the gastrointestinal tract (as opposed to intravenously) allows them to be processed and absorbed in a normal physiologic fashion. Use of the bowel lumen for nutrient delivery has several benefits. The trophic effects of enteral feeding on the small bowel mucosa have been well described. The integrity of the mucosal lining is maintained and can provide an effective barrier to intraluminal enteric organisms that might otherwise enter the systemic circulation. Atrophic changes can be seen in the intestinal epithelium after several days of bowel rest. This atrophy is not reversed by the available TPN solutions. Newer enteral diets contain pharmacologic amounts of gut-specific nutrients such as glutamine, a conditionally essential amino acid required for intestinal function.

Total Parenteral Nutrition

Numerous clinical trials have failed to yield a consensus about the efficacy of TPN in cancer patients. Several recent prospective studies, however, have helped to clarify both the indications for and contraindications to the use of TPN in surgical patients with cancer. The 1991 multicenter Veterans Affairs Cooperative trial demonstrated that preoperative TPN benefits surgical patients (many with cancer) who have severe preoperative malnutrition.[4] TPN was not effective in patients who were minimally or moderately malnourished. Brennan and colleagues[5] examined the use of routine postoperative TPN after major pancreatic resection. In patients randomly assigned to receive TPN starting on postoperative day 1, the investigators found a statistically significant increase in the incidence of intraabdominal abscesses, as well as a tendency toward an increased incidence of peritonitis and bowel obstruction. The control group received a standard peripheral infusion of dextrose, suggesting that the increase in complications was not caused by the absence of luminal nutrients but rather to some toxic effect of the TPN. The authors concluded that routine use of postoperative TPN is not indicated and may in fact have harmful side effects after pancreatic resection. Many surgeons would elect to place a feeding jejunostomy in such patients.

In contrast to the study of Brennan and associates, Fan and colleagues[6] examined perioperative TPN (starting 7 days before the planned procedure) in patients undergoing hepatectomy for hepatocellular carcinoma. They found that patients randomly assigned to receive perioperative TPN had a statistically significant reduction in infectious complications and a decreased diuretic requirement com-

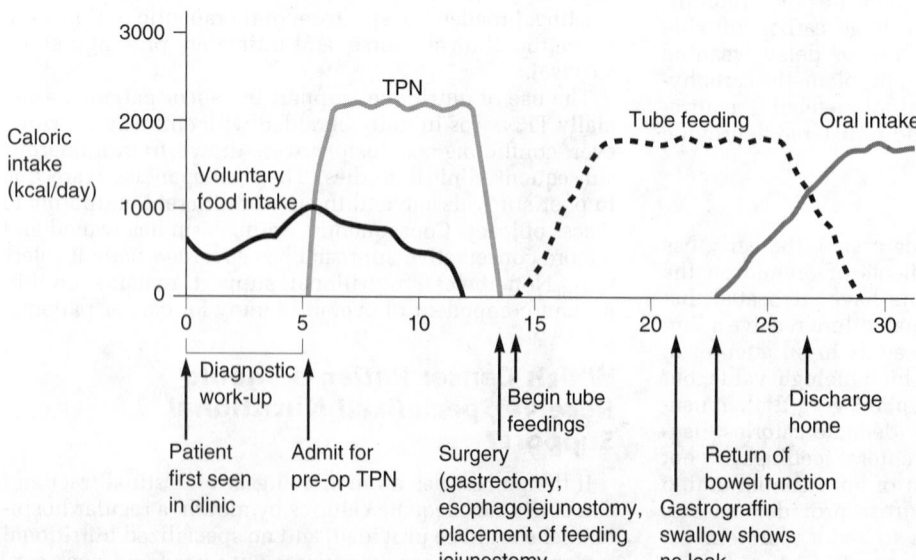

Figure 2-8. The use of total parenteral nutrition (TPN) in a cancer patient with an obstructing carcinoma of the stomach in whom preoperative enteral nutrition is contraindicated. The gastrointestinal tract should be used as soon as bowel function returns. Placement of a feeding jejunostomy at the time of operation may be useful.

pared with similar patients who did not receive TPN. The significance of this study is that it is one of only two reports that show a benefit to using routine perioperative TPN in patients not suffering from severe malnutrition. In addition, it establishes a select group of patients in whom routine perioperative TPN may be of benefit.

As a general rule, the most important factor to consider when making decisions about the use of TPN in patients with cancer is the response of the tumor to antineoplastic therapy. The guidelines listed here for the use of TPN in oncology patients will surely undergo future revision as more effective antitumor regimens become clinically available:

Relatively Short Hospital Stays (7 to 14 Days)

TPN Not Indicated

- In well-nourished or mildly malnourished patients undergoing chemotherapy, radiotherapy, or surgery. Such patients can usually consume some nutrition enterally and can tolerate short periods (up to 7 days) of inadequate intake
- In patients with rapidly progressive malignant disease who fail to respond to treatment. The condition of such patients is terminal, and they should not receive TPN.

TPN Indicated

- In severely malnourished patients or those with gastrointestinal or other toxicities that preclude adequate enteral intake for 7 days or longer. Evidence suggests that patients who are candidates for TPN under these circumstances should, when feasible, receive TPN before or in conjunction with the institution of therapy.

Lengthy Periods of In-Hospital TPN (More Than 2 Weeks) or Home TPN

TPN Not Indicated

- In patients with rapidly progressive tumor growth that is unresponsive to therapy. The condition of such patients is terminal.

TPN Indicated

- In patients for whom treatment-associated toxicities preclude the use of enteral nutrition and represent the primary impediment to the restoration of performance status. Such patients usually respond to antitumor therapy.
- In selected malnourished cancer patients in whom the natural history of the disease can be expected to permit a period of normal or near-normal performance status. Such patients should be receiving antitumor therapy with a reasonable anticipation of response, or the natural history of the untreated tumor should be such that a reasonable quality of life can be expected.

NUTRITION IN SURGICAL PATIENTS

Although the physiologic advantage of enteral nutrition is apparent, preoperative nutritional repletion by the enteral route has not been as extensively studied as preoperative TPN. Although its use can be associated with the development of nausea, diarrhea, and distention, enteral nutrition (through a feeding tube or as between-meal supplements) in malnourished patients is recommended if feasible. Candidates must have a functional gastrointestinal tract and must be able to receive adequate amounts of calories and nitrogen.

Total Parenteral Nutrition

Primary Therapy

Patients With Enterocutaneous Fistulas. Patients with gastrointestinal–cutaneous fistulas represent a classic indication for TPN. In such patients, oral intake of food almost invariably results in increased fistula output, which can lead to metabolic disturbances, dehydration, and death. Several comprehensive reviews have concluded that TPN clearly affects the treatment and course of disease in patients with gastrointestinal fistulas. The following conclusions can be drawn from studies evaluating the use of TPN in patients with enterocutaneous fistulas:

1. TPN increases the spontaneous closure rate of enterocutaneous fistulas but does not markedly decrease the mortality rate for patients with fistulas. (Improvements in mortality rates are mainly the result of improved surgical and metabolic care.)
2. If spontaneous closure of the fistula does not occur, patients are better prepared for operative intervention because of the nutritional support that they have received.
3. Certain fistulas (eg, radiated bowel) are associated with a higher failure rate of closure than others and should be treated more aggressively surgically after a defined period of nutritional support (unless closure occurs).

Patients With Short-Bowel Syndrome. Prospective randomized trials designed specifically to examine the impact of TPN on patients with short-bowel syndrome have not been initiated, mainly because such patients have no choice but to receive TPN. Most of these patients, who would have certainly died before the availability of TPN, now survive for long periods on home parenteral nutrition. In selected patients with residual small intestine (at least 18 inches), postresectional hyperplasia may develop with time, so they can tolerate enteral feedings. A recent study has demonstrated that the requirement for TPN could be decreased or even eliminated in patients with short-gut syndrome by providing a nutritional regimen consisting of supplemental glutamine, growth hormone, and a modified high- carbohydrate, low-fat diet.[7] The authors observed a marked improvement in the absorption of nutrients and a decrease in stool output with this combination therapy. In addition, TPN requirements were reduced by 50% as were the costs associated with care for these individuals. Discontinuing use of the growth hormone did not increase TPN needs in these patients once they had undergone successful gut rehabilitation.

Patients With Hepatic Failure. Individuals with liver disease are often malnourished because of alcohol abuse and diminished food intake. These individuals are protein depleted yet intolerant of protein because of their tendency to become encephalopathic with high nitrogen intake. Because of chronic liver damage and portalsystemic shunting, these patients experience derangements in circulating levels of amino acids. The ratio of plasma aromatic amino acids to branched-chain amino acids is increased, favoring the transport of aromatic amino acids across the blood–brain barrier. These amino acids are precursors of false neurotransmitters that contribute to lethargy and encephalopathy. Treating individuals who have liver failure with solutions rich in branched-chain amino acids and deficient in aromatic amino acids increases tolerance to the administered protein and clinically improves the encephalopathic state.

Patients With Major Thermal Injury. Aggressive nutritional support in patients with major burns appears to improve survival, particularly when increased amounts of dietary protein are provided.[8] Burned patients often require ventilatory support and suffer from ileus, which prevents use of the gastrointestinal tract for feeding. Even if the gastrointestinal tract is usable, such patients are often unable to eat enough because of frequent trips to the operating room combined with the anorexia of severe injury. Most burn authorities believe that aggressive nutritional support in patients with major thermal injury has improved their outcome.

Patients With Acute Renal Failure. TPN with amino acids of high biologic value may decrease the mortality rate of patients with acute renal failure.[9] Using solutions containing high-quality amino acids can improve nitrogen balance and diminish urea production. The concept is that providing only essential amino acids allows the body to maximally reuse nitrogen for synthesizing nonessential amino acids and thereby helps prevent rapid rises in blood urea nitrogen. This reduces the need for dialysis. There appears to be no advantage to using essential amino acid solution if the patient is already undergoing dialysis every other day. Therefore, a balanced standard amino acid formula is recommended.

Secondary Therapy

Prolonged Ileus After Operative Procedure. Occasional patients experience a prolonged ileus after an abdominal procedure, precluding the use of the intestinal tract as a route of feeding. This occurrence is generally unpredictable, and the cause of the ileus is often not demonstrated. If the patient is unable to eat by the seventh postoperative day, TPN should be started. The ileus can persist for several weeks. Although provision of TPN does not influence the disease process per se, it prevents further erosion of lean body mass.

Acute Radiotherapy and Chemotherapy Enteritis. Malnourished patients who undergo abdominal or pelvic radiotherapy or chemotherapy may develop mucositis and enterocolitis, which precludes using the gastrointestinal tract for prolonged periods. For these patients, TPN should be provided until the enteritis resolves and oral feeding can be resumed.

In the Perioperative Setting. In general, it is difficult to justify the use of perioperative nutrition (particularly parenteral feedings). The results of prospective randomized trials evaluating the efficacy of preoperative TPN conflict because of the variations in the nutritional status of patients studied, the differences in their disease types, the differences in the type and length of nutritional support administered, and the failure to accrue enough patients to avoid type II statistical errors. The following questions are important to consider: Does preoperative nutritional support decrease the morbidity and mortality associated with major operative procedures? How long should nutritional support be administered? What type of nutritional repletion should be administered?

One of the best studies evaluating the efficacy of preoperative TPN was published by the Veterans Affairs Total Parenteral Nutrition Cooperative Study Group.[4] More than 3500 patients requiring mainly elective abdominal surgery were included in this prospective randomized trial. They were initially screened for malnutrition using subjective criteria or by determining their Nutritional Risk Index score, which included objective criteria such as weight loss percentage and serum albumin level. The patients were further divided into one of four groups: well-nourished, borderline malnourished, moderately malnourished, or severely malnourished. Patients in each malnourished category were randomly assigned to receive at least 7 days of preoperative TPN or to proceed with surgery without it. Patients assigned to TPN therapy received 1000 kcal/d in excess of calculated caloric requirements. Lipid was provided daily. One criticism of this study was that patients were allowed to eat in addition to receiving parenteral feedings.

The analysis of the study data indicated no difference in short- or long-term complications between groups. Infectious complications, including pneumonia, abscess, and line sepsis, were statistically significantly higher in patients receiving TPN. Noninfectious complications (eg, impaired wound healing) were significantly lower only in those patients receiving TPN who were in the severely malnourished group (over 15% weight loss and serum albumin level below 2.9 mg/dL). This study strongly suggests that preoperative TPN should be provided only to severely malnourished patients who cannot be nourished by the enteral route. Contraindications to using preoperative TPN include problems requiring emergency operation and mild or moderate malnourishment. In these patients, TPN should be continued postoperatively only if the gastrointestinal tract cannot be used for tube feedings. Jejunostomy tubes should also be considered in patients undergoing major upper abdominal procedures when it is anticipated that they will not resume oral feedings for 7 to 10 days after surgery.

Composition of Formulas

Total parenteral nutrition solutions are administered through a central venous catheter that generally is inserted in the subclavian vein (Fig. 2-9). The composition of a standard TPN solution is shown in Table 2-7. Because of the hyperosmolarity of such solutions, they must be delivered into a high-flow system to prevent venous sclerosis. Patients receiving TPN should be monitored regularly by measuring blood sugar, serum electrolytes, and liver function. Elevations in serum glucose are common in surgical patients receiving TPN, especially if the patient is stressed and relatively glucose intolerant. Hyperglycemia can generally be controlled by adding insulin to the TPN formula or by decreasing the amount of glucose in the solution. Injured patients can maximally oxidize glucose at a rate of 5 to 6 mg/kg/min. For a 70-kg man, this equals 500 to 600 g/d. Glucose calories in excess of this amount are converted to fat or result in hyperglycemia and glycosuria. The amounts of various electrolytes provided to patients receiving TPN vary depending on factors such as previous nutritional and hydration status. Careful monitoring is critical because as new cell mass accrues, the intracellular ions potassium and phosphate can accumulate, leading to severe hypokalemia or hypophosphatemia. These electrolyte disturbances can develop rapidly and are much more life-threatening than hyponatremia. Requirements for vitamins (Table 2-8) and trace minerals (Table 2-9) must also be considered.

The use of lipids in TPN was developed to meet the requirement for linoleic acid and the full caloric needs in hypermetabolic patients, in light of the complications associated with infusing large amounts of dextrose. Intravenous fat emulsions are composed of soy or safflower oil (vegetable fat emulsions), which contain primarily long-chain triglycerides made up of fatty acids with 16- and 18-carbon chain lengths. Fat provides essential linoleic acid, inhibits lipogenesis from carbohydrates, and lowers the respiratory quotient, which can benefit patients with respiratory compromise. The high content of ω-6 polyunsaturated fatty acids, particularly linoleic acid, in these emulsions may be harmful, however. Linoleic acid is a precursor for the synthesis of various prostaglandins and

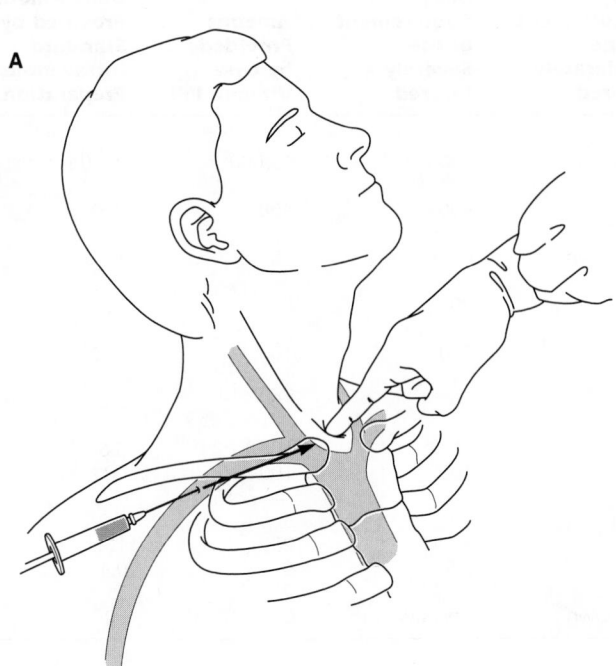
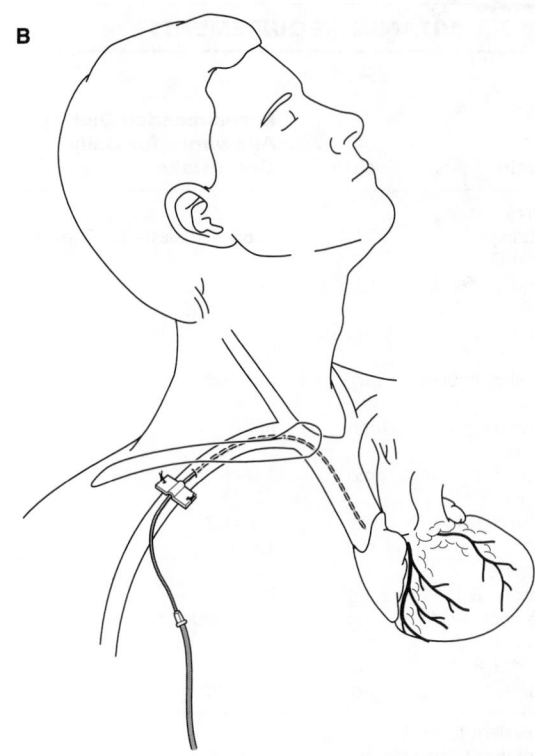

Figure 2-9. Technique for insertion of a subclavian catheter.

leukotrienes, which can suppress the immune system and cytokine activity. Standard intravenous fat emulsions can alter the cell membrane phospholipid composition of cells of the reticuloendothelial system, resulting in changes in membrane fluidity that impair clearance of bacteria and toxins. In addition, ω-6 polyunsaturated fatty acids can

alter the local production of cytokines, impairing chemotaxis. Newer nutritional methods of modifying the catabolic response to injury and infection use ω-3 fatty acids, which can decrease eicosanoid biosynthesis and thereby diminish the vasoconstriction, platelet aggregation, and immunosuppression that can occur when ω-6 derivatives are administered. Data suggest that ω-3 fatty acids may benefit critically ill patients.

Fat is an important fuel source for critically ill patients. Septic and injured patients seem to use endogenous fat preferentially as an energy source, which may be related to the effects of counterregulatory hormones on stimulating fat mobilization. These patients are relatively unresponsive to the administration of carbohydrates in that free fatty acid mobilization only is marginally decreased and free fatty acid oxidation is not suppressed as in pure starvation. Despite glucose infusion that exceeds energy expenditure, a hormonal milieu is maintained that favors fat mobilization and oxidation.

Potential Complications

Advances in technology, monitoring, and catheter care have greatly reduced the incidence of complications associated with TPN. The establishment of a nutrition support team (physician, dietician, nurse, and pharmacist) and the recognition that this team plays an important part in overall patient care has also been a key factor in reducing complications. The three types of TPN complications are mechanical, metabolic, and infectious (Table 2-10). The treatment of a patient who becomes septic while receiving TPN is shown in Figure 2-10.

Effects on the Gastrointestinal Tract

Most studies examining the effects of TPN on intestinal function and immunity have been performed on animals. These studies clearly demonstrate that TPN poses risks

Table 2-7. COMPOSITION OF A STANDARD CENTRAL VENOUS SOLUTION

VOLUME

10% amino acid solution	500 mL
50% dextrose solution	500 mL
Fat emulsion	—
Electrolytes + vitamins + minerals	~50 mL
Total volume	~1050 mL

COMPOSITION

Amino acids	50 g
Dextrose	250 g
Total potassium	50/6.25 = 8 g
Dextrose kcal	250 g × 3.4 kcal/g = 840 kcal
mOsm/L	~2000

Electrolytes Added to TPN Solutions	Usual Concentration (mEq/L)	Range of Concentrations (mEq/L)
Sodium	60	0–150
Potassium	40	0–80
Acetate	50	50–150
Chloride	50	0–150
Phosphate	15	0–30
Calcium*	4.5	0–20
Magnesium	5	5–15

* Generally added as calcium gluconate or calcium chloride. One ampule of calcium gluconate = 1 g of calcium = 4.5 mEq.

Table 2-8. VITAMIN REQUIREMENTS

Vitamin	Unit	Recommended Dietary Allowance for Daily Oral Intake	Daily Requirement of the Moderately Injured	Daily Requirement of the Severely Injured	Amount Provided by One Vitamin Pill	Daily Amount Provided by Standard Intravenous Preparations
Vitamin A (retinol)	IU	1760 (females)–3300 (males)	5000	5000	10,000	3300 (retinol)
Vitamin D (ergocalciferol)	IU	200	400	400	400	200
Vitamin E (tocopherol)	mg TE	8–10	Unknown	Unknown	15	10*
Vitamin K (phylloquinone)	µg	20–40†	20	20	0	0‡
Vitamin C (ascorbic acid)	mg	60	75	300	100	100
Thiamine (vitamin B_1)	mg	1.0–1.5	2	10	10	3.0
Riboflavin (vitamin B_2)	mg	1.2–1.7	2	10	10	3.6
Niacin	mg	13–19	20	100	100	40
Pyridoxine (vitamin B_6)	mg	2.0–2.2	2	40	5	4.0
Pantothenic acid	mg	4–7 (adults)†	18	40	20	15
Folic acid	mg	0.4	1.5	2.5	0	0.4
Vitamin B_{12}	µg	3.0	2	4	5	5
Biotin	µg	100–200†	Unknown	Unknown	0	60

* Equivalent to RDA.
† Estimated to be safe and adequate in dietary intakes.
‡ Must be supplemented in peripheral venous solutions.
(Rombeau JL, Rolandelli RH. Nutritional support. In: Wilmore DW, Brennan MF, Harken RH, et al, eds. Care of the surgical patient. II. Care in the ICU. New York, Scientific American Medicine, 1989:6)

related to intestinal disuse. A unique feature of TPN is that patients can remain on bowel rest for prolonged periods without concomitant malnutrition, thereby facilitating the study of intestinal disuse as an independent variable. In rats, TPN significantly disrupts the intestinal microflora and bacterial translocation from the gut lumen to the mesenteric lymph nodes. In addition, when stresses such as burn injury, chemotherapy, or radiotherapy are introduced in these models, animals receiving TPN have a much higher mortality rate. These studies suggest that, under certain circumstances, TPN can predispose patients to an increase in gut-derived infectious complications.[10]

In a provocative study in human volunteers,[11] those receiving TPN had an accentuated systemic response to endotoxin challenge compared with enterally fed volunteers. The results are consistent with an impairment in gut barrier function during parenteral feedings, which can promote the release of bacteria or cytokines and lead to pronounced systemic responses and possibly multiple organ failure.

Nutritional Support of the Gut in Critically Ill Patients

The intestinal tract has long been considered an inactive organ following operation or injury. Ileus is generally present, nasogastric decompression is often necessary, and the gut is usually unused in the immediate postoperative period. In the past, digestion and absorption were thought to be the only physiologic role of the gut. Disuse of the gastrointestinal tract, due to either starvation or TPN support, can lead to numerous physiologic derangements as well as to changes in gut microflora, impaired gut immune

Table 2-9. MINERAL AND TRACE ELEMENT REQUIREMENTS

Mineral	Recommended Dietary Allowance for Daily Oral Intake (mg)	Suggested Daily Intravenous Intake (mg)	Daily Amount Provided by a Commercially Available Mixture (mg)
Zinc	15	2.5–5.0*	5.0
Copper	2–3†	0.5–1.5	1.0
Manganese	2.5–5.0†	0.15–0.8	0.5
Chromium	0.05–0.2†	0.01–0.015	0.1
Iron	10 (males)–8 (females)	3	—

* Burn patients require an additional 2 mg.
† Estimated to be safe and adequate in dietary intakes.
(Rombeau JL, Rolandelli RH. Nutritional support. In: Wilmore DW, Brennan MF, Harken RH, et al. eds. Care of the surgical patient. II. Care in the ICU. New York, Scientific American Medicine, 1989:6)

Table 2-10. **COMPLICATIONS ASSOCIATED WITH THE USE OF TOTAL PARENTERAL NUTRITION (TPN)**

Complication	Cause	Treatment
MECHANICAL		
Pneumothorax	Puncture or laceration of lung pleura	Serial chest radiographs; chest tube if indicated
Subclavian artery injury	Penetration of subclavian artery during needlestick	Chest radiograph; serial monitoring of vital signs
Air embolism	Aspiration of air into the subclavian vein and right side of heart	Place patient in Trendelenberg and left lateral decubitus positions; aspirate air
Catheter embolization	Shearing off the tip when withdrawing catheter	Retrieve catheter transvenously under fluoroscopic guidance
Venous thrombosis	Clot formation in great vein secondary to catheter	Heparinization if clinically significant
Catheter malposition	Tip of catheter directed outside of superior vena cava or right atrium	Reposition under fluoroscopy
METABOLIC		
Hyperglycemia	Excessive glucose calories or glucose intolerance	Decrease glucose calories; administer insulin
Hypoglycemia	Sudden cessation of TPN	Bolus 50% glucose solution; monitor blood glucose
Carbon dioxide retention	Infusion of glucose calories in excess of energy needs	Decrease glucose calories and replace with fat
Hyperglycemic, hyperosmolar, nonketotic coma	Dehydration from excessive diuresis	Discontinue TPN immediately; give insulin; monitor glucose and electrolytes
Hyperchloremic metabolic acidosis	Excessive chloride administration	Give sodium and potassium as acetate salts
Azotemia	Excessive amino acid administration with inadequate calories	Decrease amino acids; increase glucose calories
Essential fatty acid deficiency	Inadequate essential fatty acid administration	Administer fat solution
Hypertriglyceridemia	Rapid fat infusion of decreased fat clearance	Slow rate of fat infusion
Hypophosphatemia, hypocalcemia, hypomagnesemia, hypokalemia	Inadequate administration of electrolyte in question	Increase administration
Bleeding	Vitamin K deficiency	Administer vitamin K
SEPTIC		
Line sepsis	Catheter tip infected	Remove catheter; antibiotics
Infection at skin site	Bacteria at site of catheter entry into skin	Remove catheter; local wound care

function, and disruption of the integrity of the mucosal barrier. Thus, maintaining gut function in the perioperative period can be essential to minimize septic complications and organ failure.

Treatment strategies to support the gut during critical illness should provide appropriate nutrition and maintenance of mucosal structure and function. Presumably, these efforts can assist the gut in its role as a metabolic processing station and barrier.

Enteral Feeding

Enteral feeding is probably the best method for maintaining mucosal structure and function. The trophic effects of luminal nutrition are key, and the benefits are well documented even when relatively small amounts of nutrients are provided.

Gut-Specific Nutrients

Both the composition of the diet and the route of delivery play important roles in maintaining gut structure and function. Several gut-specific nutrients have been studied, but glutamine has received the most attention. Glutamine has been classified as a nonessential or nutritionally dispensable amino acid. Because this implies that glutamine can be synthesized in adequate quantities from other amino acids and precursors, it has not been considered necessary to include glutamine in nutritional formulas. It has been eliminated from TPN solutions because of its relative instability and short shelf life compared with other amino acids. With few exceptions, glutamine is present in oral and enteral diets only at the relatively low levels characteristic

of most animal and plant proteins (about 7% of total amino acids).

Several recent studies have demonstrated that glutamine may be a conditionally essential amino acid during critical illness, particularly in supporting the metabolic requirements of the intestinal mucosa. In general, these studies demonstrate that dietary glutamine is not required during states of good health but appears to be beneficial when glutamine depletion is severe or when the intestinal mucosa is damaged by insults such as chemotherapy or radiotherapy. Adding glutamine to enteral diets reduces the incidence of gut translocation, but these improvements depend on the amount of supplemental glutamine and the type of insult studied. Glutamine-enriched TPN partially attenuates the villous atrophy that develops during use of parenteral nutrition. The use of intravenous glutamine in humans appears to be safe and effective, and it has been shown to diminish complications and reduce hospital stay.[12,13]

In contrast to glutamine, short-chain fatty acids are the primary energy source for colonocytes. In rats, diets rich in short-chain fatty acids have been shown to increase colonic DNA content and several mucosal morphometric parameters as well as to strengthen colonic anastomoses.

Growth Factors

Specific growth factors that promote intestinal mucosal growth appear to be involved in various physiologic processes, including growth, tissue repair, and regeneration. Among them is epidermal growth factor, a polypeptide secreted by submaxillary glands and by the Brunner glands

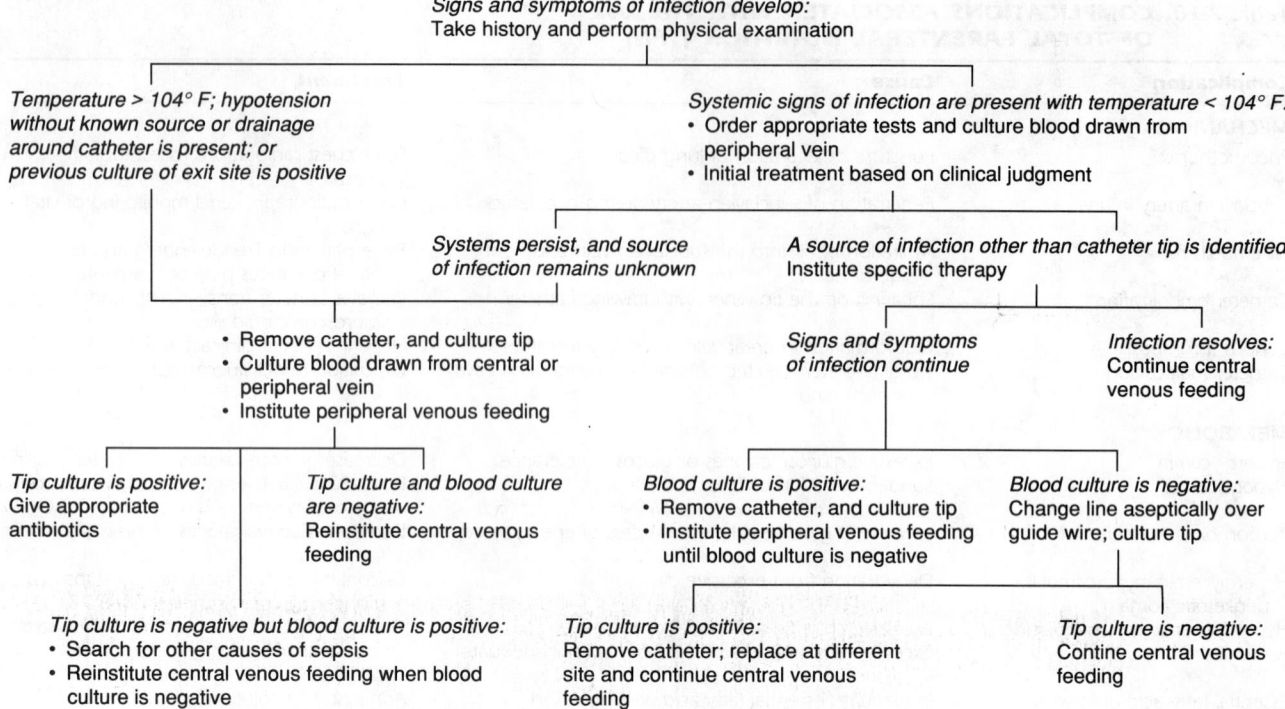

Figure 2-10. Treatment of a patient receiving total parenteral nutrition who becomes septic.

of the small intestine. The most widespread effect of epidermal growth factor on the gastrointestinal mucosa is the overall stimulation of DNA synthesis as evidenced by thymidine incorporation.

Other Methods of Modifying the Catabolic Response to Surgery and Critical Illness

Besides nutritional intervention, several other methods of modifying the physiologic and biochemical responses to an elective operation have been evaluated in an effort to reduce the magnitude of operative stress and to provide insight about mechanisms that negate these responses. The data suggest that regional anesthesia blocks afferent signals from the wound and interrupts sympathetic nervous efferent signals to the adrenal gland and possibly the liver. Sympathetic blockade reduces the apparent magnitude of the stress response. Other researchers have studied stress responses in sympathectomized animals by blocking the efferent limb of the neuroendocrine reflex response. Their data indicate that blockade of the central nervous system interrupts the afferent signals stimulated by operative procedures.

More recent studies have documented the safety and efficacy of long-term, postoperative exogenous recombinant growth hormone administration.[14] Growth hormone stimulates protein synthesis during hypocaloric feedings and increases sodium and potassium retention by the kidney. The potential synergistic effects of specialized nutrition combined with growth hormone require further study. Cyclooxygenase inhibitors, such as aspirin and ibuprofen, attenuate the symptoms and endocrine responses that occur during critical illness without altering cytokine elaboration. It is anticipated that researchers will eventually be able to selectively block the deleterious effects of excessive cytokines and preserve their benefits.

TECHNIQUES OF NUTRITIONAL SUPPORT

Transnasal (Nasogastric and Nasoduodenal) Feeding Catheters

Transnasal feeding catheters for intragastric feeding and for duodenal intubation are popular adjuncts for providing nutritional support by the enteral route. The stomach is easily accessed by passing a soft, flexible feeding tube. Intragastric feedings provide several advantages for the patient. The stomach has the capacity and reservoir for bolus feedings. Feeding into the stomach stimulates the biliary–pancreatic axis, which is probably trophic for the small bowel. Also, gastric secretions dilute the osmolarity of the feedings, reducing the risk of diarrhea. The major risk of intragastric feeding is regurgitation of gastric contents, which can result in aspiration into the tracheobronchial tree. This risk is highest in patients with altered mental sensorium or who are paralyzed.

Placing the feeding tube through the pylorus into the distal duodenum reduces the risk of regurgitating and aspirating the formulas. To place a transnasal intraduodenal feeding catheter, the patient should be sitting with the neck slightly flexed. This allows for the passage of a lubricated 8F polyurethane feeding catheter (with a stylet in place) through the patient's nose in a posterior and inferior direction, bringing the catheter to the level of the pharynx. The head should be brought back to a neutral position and the patient instructed to swallow while the feeding catheter is passed into the esophageal lumen. The catheter is then advanced 45 to 50 cm. The stylet is removed, and the position of the catheter is confirmed radiographically before feedings are begun. Tubes can be positioned fluoroscopically if necessary. Patients who frequently extubate the feeding catheter are candidates for a feeding tube bridle (Fig. 2-11). A variety of enteral formulas are commercially available.

a needle jejunostomy, which can be quickly performed at the end of the definitive operation. A 14- or 16-gauge needle is used to create a tunnel subserosally about 30 to 40 cm distal to the ligament of Treitz. The needle tip is introduced into the jejunal lumen. A feeding catheter is inserted through the needle and advanced 30 to 40 cm distally into the bowel lumen to the desired location; the needle is then withdrawn. The loop of jejunum is anchored to the parietal peritoneum with permanent sutures, and the catheter is secured to the skin with nylon sutures.

A feeding jejunostomy can also be performed using the Witzel technique. A loop of proximal jejunum 20 to 30 cm from the ligament of Treitz is delivered into the wound. A pursestring suture is placed on the antimesenteric border of the bowel, and an incision is made with electrocautery in the intestinal wall in the center of the pursestring suture. A red rubber catheter is inserted into the lumen of the jejunum and advanced distally. The pursestring suture is secured in place. A serosal tunnel is constructed with 3-0 silk sutures from the catheter's exit site, extending 5 to 6 cm proximally. The catheter is delivered through the abdominal wall through a separate stab incision. The adjacent loop of intestine is anchored with two 3-0 silk sutures. The catheter is secured to the skin with a monofilament nylon suture. Jejunal feeding catheters can be used for feedings immediately after the operation.

Peripheral Intravenous Feedings

Peripheral veins can be used for infusing glucose, amino acid solutions, and fat emulsions. These solutions must be nearly isotonic, however, to avoid peripheral vein sclerosis. Ten percent glucose solutions can be used to increase the efficacy of amino acid utilization. Fat emulsions can be administered simultaneously with glucose and amino acid solutions; they provide an efficient fuel source and are isotonic. The major disadvantage of these peripherally administered mixtures is limited caloric delivery to meet catabolic demands within tolerated fluid volumes. Indications for peripheral vein feeding include the following:

- As a supplement when enteral feedings can be only partially tolerated because of gastrointestinal dysfunction
- As a method of nutritional support when the gastrointestinal tract must be kept relatively empty for short periods during diagnostic workup
- As preliminary feedings before central venous catheter insertion in patients who require TPN

Technique of Central Venous Catheter Placement

The preferred method of access to the superior vena cava is by percutaneous cannulation of the subclavian vein (see Fig. 2-9). Alternate sites include the jugular approach, but when the catheter exits the neck region, it is more difficult to secure the dressing site and maintain sterility.

Central venous catheter placement should be performed by someone experienced in the technique. To reduce the risk of bleeding complications, patients with platelet counts below 50,000 mL should receive fresh platelets before catheter insertion. The procedure is performed using the aseptic technique; the surgeon should wear a hat, mask, gown, and gloves. The procedure can be done in the operating room or the patient's room if there is adequate lighting and assistance. An environment should be created to minimize patient anxiety, and informed consent must be obtained. The patient is placed in the Trendelenberg position, with both arms at the sides and the head turned away from the site of insertion. The chest is shaved, pre-

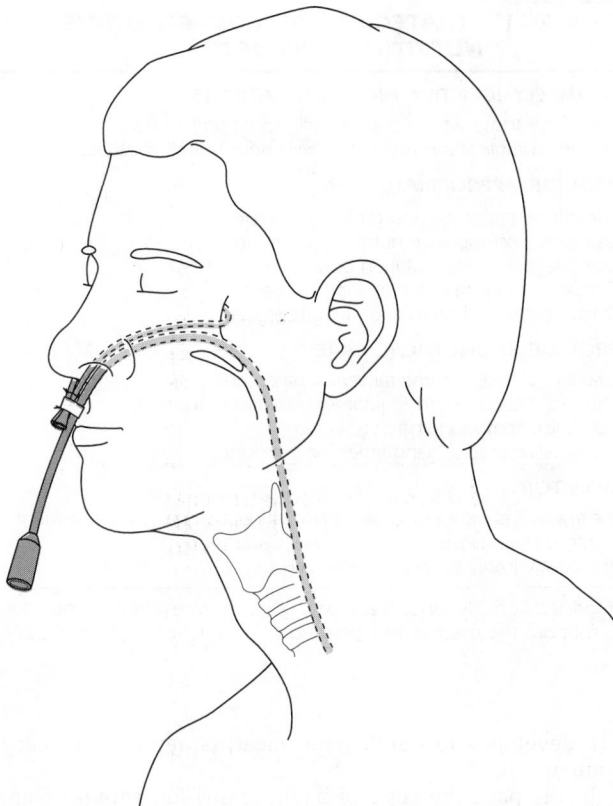

Figure 2-11. Use of a feeding tube bridle for patients who are prone to extubate the feeding catheter.

Technique for Gastrostomy Placement

A feeding gastrostomy should be considered for patients requiring long-term enteral nutrition and for those with esophagus obstructions or locally advanced head and neck cancers that preclude eating. A temporary Stamm gastrostomy is a popular method for access to the gastric lumen and can be performed at the time of any major abdominal procedure. A circular pursestring suture (3-0 silk) 1.5 cm in diameter is placed in the body of the anterior wall of the stomach. The ideal location is in the midportion of the stomach, closer to the greater curvature, in a relatively avascular site. A second circular pursestring suture is placed outside the first one. The feeding catheter is brought through the abdominal wall in the left upper quadrant. With electrocautery, a stab wound is made in the anterior portion of the stomach, directly in the center of the concentric pursestring sutures. The feeding catheter is introduced into the gastric lumen, and the inner concentric suture is secured in place. The second pursestring is secured, inverting the gastric mucosa completely. The stomach is drawn upward toward the anterior abdominal wall. Placing Lembert silk sutures in all four quadrants around the catheter secures the stomach to the anterior abdominal wall. The catheter is secured to the skin by placing sutures at the base of the catheter exit site. A percutaneous endoscopic gastrostomy to provide access for gastric feedings can be safely performed without either a laparotomy or general anesthesia.

Feeding Catheter Jejunostomy Placement and Witzel Jejunostomy

A feeding catheter jejunostomy should be considered after any major upper abdominal procedure if prolonged support with enteral nutrition is anticipated. The simplest method is

pared, and draped in a sterile fashion. Local anesthesia is infiltrated near the insertion site and the underlying tissues along the inferior border of the clavicle. The tip of the needle is inserted into the skin and subcutaneous tissues in the midclavian line; at the junction of the medial and middle thirds of the clavicle, it is directed posterior to the clavicle toward the suprasternal notch.

The needle is oriented parallel to the patient's bed and inserted beneath the clavicle with negative pressure applied to the syringe. The prompt inflow of blood into the syringe indicates entrance into the subclavian vein, and the needle is advanced a few millimeters to ensure the bevel is in the lumen of the vessel. The patient is instructed to perform a Valsalva maneuver to prevent an air embolism, the syringe is disconnected from the needle, and the flexible guide wire is passed through the needle lumen. The needle is then withdrawn over the guidewire. The passage of the wire through the needle should be met with minimal resistance, and the needle should be removed only after 15 cm of wire has been passed into the vessel. A small incision is made at the guide wire exit site, and a dilator is passed over the wire. The dilator is removed over the wire and is replaced by the catheter, which is fully advanced. The wire is withdrawn, and the catheter is flushed with sterile, heparinized saline. The catheter is then sutured into position, the insertion site cleaned, and a sterile dressing placed. Portable chest radiography is performed to confirm placement of the catheter and to rule out pneumothorax.

Complications from long-term central venous catheterization include venous thrombosis and catheter-related infections (see Table 2-10). Thrombosis of the central vessels is often overlooked. The clinical suspicion of subclavian vein or superior vena cava thrombosis is only about 3%, whereas studies that use phlebography or radionuclide venography indicate that the incidence is as high as 35%. Febrile episodes are not uncommon in cancer patients, particularly in those who aree neutropenic. If primary catheter sepsis is confirmed, the catheter must be removed immediately and the tip cultured.

NUTRITION SUPPORT AND HEALTH CARE REFORM

Health care reform is forcing hospitals to scrutinize expensive therapies such as nutrition support and the personnel involved in delivering them.[15] Nutrition support teams are now considered a cost center rather than a revenue center. The risk to the nutrition support team is that it will lose its independence, becoming a passive participant in the care of patients who require nutritional support. The risk to the patient is that cost issues may override those of quality care.

The evolution of an interdisciplinary nutrition support team approach was seen as a way to maximize efficiency and to improve patient care. The recent tendency has been to diminish the size of these units. At the same time, the challenge to nutrition support professionals is to coordinate efficient and early intervention and to document its efficacy and outcomes. In the absence of documented efficacy, many argue, there is no need for formal nutrition support or the team in charge of that service. Therefore, it becomes imperative that the team justify its importance to the hospital, pointing out that a formal nutrition support team provides quality control and polices the administration of nutritional support. To do this, the nutrition support team must do the following: (1) identify specific patient populations that will benefit from nutrition support, (2) establish clinical pathways (guidelines), and

Table 2-11. STRATEGIES FOR COST-EFFECTIVE NUTRITION SUPPORT

PROMPTLY IDENTIFY HIGH-RISK PATIENTS

Screen for those who would benefit from nutritional support
Prevent complications associated with poor nutritional status

PROVIDE APPROPRIATE CARE

Use critical pathways and clinical guidelines
Use early postoperative nutrition when indicated
Use total parenteral nutrition only when indicated
Transition to regular diet as soon as feasible
Document use of feeding on length of stay

PROVIDE ECONOMICAL CARE

Evaluate oral versus enteral versus parenteral
Shop for best prices for equipment, solutions, formulas
Centralize compounding
Standardize orders, hang times, and so forth

MONITOR

Incorporate patient outcomes and continuous quality improvement into daily practice
Proactively justify team costs and savings

(Modified from Nelson J. The impact of health care reform on nutrition support: the practitioner's perspective. Nutr Clin Prac 1995;5:22)

(3) develop and implement measurements of efficacy (outcomes).

In the past, the costs of paying nutrition support team members were more than offset by the reimbursements for the services provided, particularly for the delivery of TPN. In a capitated environment, hospitals find themselves in the peculiar situation where less is better. The danger of this approach as it relates to the nutritional support of hospitalized patients, particularly those with complicated problems and complex diseases, is that withholding nutritional support from certain patients can result in serious consequences. Aggressive early feeding may be the best approach if it reduces complications in the long run. Various methods to ensure that nutrition support is cost-effective have been suggested (Table 2-11).

REFERENCES

1. Bessey PQ, Watters JM, Aoki TT, et al. Combined hormonal infusion simulates the metabolic response to injury. Ann Surg 1984;200:264.
2. Fong Y, Lowry SF. Cytokines and the cellular response to injury and infection. In: Wilmore DW, Brennam MF, Harker AH, et al, eds. Care of the surgical patient. IV. Trauma. New York, Scientific American Medicine, 1992:1.
3. Cuthbertson DP. Observations of disturbance of metabolism produced by injury ot the limbs. Q J Med 1932;25:233.
4. Buzby GP, the Veterans Affairs Total Parenteral Nutrition Cooperative Study Group. Perioperative total parenteral nutrition in surgical patients. N Engl J Med 1991;325:525.
5. Brennan MF, Pisters PWT, Posner M, et al. A prospective randomized trial of total parenteral nutrition after major pancreatic resection for malignancy. Ann Surg 1994;220:436.
6. Fan ST, Lo CM, Lai ECS, et al. Perioperative nutritional support in patients undergoing hepatectomy for hepatocellular carcinoma. N Engl J Med 1994;331:1547.
7. Byrne TA, Persinger RL, Young LS, et al. A new treatment for patients with the short bowel syndrome: growth hormone, glutamine, and a modified diet. Ann Surg 1995;222:243.
8. Alexander JW, MacMillan BG, Stinnert JD, et al. Beneficial effects of aggressive protein feeding in severely burned children. Ann Surg 1980;192:505.
9. Abel RM, Beck CH, Abbott WM, Ryan JA, Barnett GO, Fischer JE: Improved survival from acute renal failure following treatment with intravenous essential L-amino acids and glucose:

results of a prospective, double-blind study. N Engl J Med 1973;288:695.

10. van der Hulst RRWJ, van Kreel BK, von Meyenfeldt MF, et al. Glutamine and the preservation of gut integrity. Lancet 1993;341:1363.

11. Fong Y, Marano MA, Barber A, et al. Total parenteral nutrition and bowel rest modify the metabolic response to endotoxin in humans. Ann Surg 1989;210:449.

12. Ziegler TR, Young LS, Benfell K, et al. Clinical and metabolic efficacy of glutamine-enriched parenteral nutrition following bone marrow transplantation: a double-blind randomized controlled trial. Ann Intern Med 1992;116:821.

13. Scheltinga MR, Young LS, Benfell K, et al. Glutamine-enriched intravenous feedings attenuate extracellular fluid expansion after standard stress. Ann Surg 1991;214:385.

14. Jiang ZM, He GZ, Zhang SY, et al. Low-dose growth hormone and hypocaloric nutrition attenuates the protein-catabolic response after major operation. Ann Surg 1989;210:514.

15. Nelson J. The impact of health care reform on nutrition support: the practitioner's perspective. Nutr Clin Pract 1995;5:22.

SURGERY: SCIENTIFIC PRINCIPLES AND PRACTICE, Second Edition, edited by Lazar J. Greenfield, Michael W. Mulholland, Keith T. Oldham, Gerald B. Zelenock, and Keith D. Lillemoe. Lippincott–Raven Publishers, Philadelphia, © 1997.

CHAPTER 3

WOUND HEALING

NEIL A. FINE AND THOMAS A. MUSTOE

Wound healing is a fundamental homeostatic process in response to injury. It involves the activation of basic cellular processes of inflammation, cell proliferation, and growth as well as regulation of these processes once repair is complete. An understanding of wound healing is fundamental to all of surgery and involves a broad range of cellular actions and interactions. For many years, it was a relatively inactive area for research, but increased understanding of the cellular and molecular events involving growth factors and cytokines, and the realistic prospects for pharmacologic manipulation, have focused a great deal of interest from a broad range of disciplines. Although much new knowledge has been gained, there remain many unanswered questions. This chapter outlines a basic set of concepts regarding wound healing, with emphasis on the clinical principles of basic surgical techniques and the care of open acute and chronic wounds.

NORMAL WOUND HEALING

Wound healing is the response to injury. Injury can be acute or chronic and involve multiple tissues, but wound healing is most clearly illustrated by examining the response to full-thickness injury (eg, a cut or an incision) to the epidermis and dermis. This injury sets in motion a sequence of interrelated reparative forces. Although the events overlap in time, it is helpful to consider the stages or phases of wound healing separately. This provides for clear conceptualization of the individual events. These events, however, do not occur independently, and the degree of temporal overlap is significant (Fig 3-1).

Every tissue in the body undergoes reparative processes after injury. Bone has the unique ability to heal without scar. Liver has the potential to regenerate parenchyma and is the only organ that has maintained that ability in the adult human. Although liver does regenerate, it often heals with scar (cirrhosis). With these exceptions, all other negative human tissues heal with scar. This chapter reviews the healing process of human skin with particular emphasis on surgical applications. Delineation of the individual mediators is still evolving, so the emphasis is on the underlying physiologic processes and the patterns of response.

Inflammatory Phase

The inflammatory phase of acute wound healing begins immediately after injury. The initial response to the disruption of blood vessels is bleeding. The homeostatic response to this is clot formation to stop hemorrhage. Platelet plug formation initiates the hemostatic process along with clotting factors activated by collagen and basement membrane proteins exposed by the injury. Fibrin, produced by the clotting cascade, binds the platelet plug and forms a matrix for the cellular responses that follows. After injury, transient vasoconstriction is mediated by catecholamines, thromboxane, and prostaglandin $F_{2\alpha}$ ($PGF_{2\alpha}$). Platelet degranulation provides the contents of α granules and dense granules, most notably platelet-derived growth factor (PDGF) and transforming growth factor β (TGF-β). These substances initiate chemotaxis and proliferation of inflammatory cells, beginning the inflammatory response that will ultimately heal the wound (Table 3-1). Transient vasoconstriction is necessary to decrease blood loss at the time of the initial wounding and also to allow clot formation. Vasoconstriction lasts for 5 to 10 minutes. Once a clot has been formed and active bleeding has stopped, vasodilation increases local blood flow to the wounded area, supplying cells and substrate necessary for further wound repair. The vascular endothelial cells also deform, increasing vascular permeability. The vasodilation and increased endothelial permeability are mediated by histamine, prostaglandin E_2 (PGE_2), and prostaglandin I_2 (prostacyclin; PGI_2) as well as vascular endothelial cell growth factor. These vasodilatory substances are released by injured endothelial cells and mast cells and enhance the egress of cells and substrate into the wounded tissue (Fig 3-2).

At this stage, the wound is full of debris from the initial injury. This material consists of a mixture of injured, devitalized tissue (fat, muscle, epithelium), clot (platelets, erythrocytes, fibrinogen), bacteria (from the skin surface and external environment), extravasated serum proteins (glycoproteins and mucopolysaccharides), and foreign material introduced at the time of injury (suture, dirt). During the next several days, the wound is cleared of bacteria, devitalized tissue, and foreign material by recited and activated phagocytic cells. Polymorphonuclear leukocytes (PMNs) begin to arrive immediately, attaining large numbers within 24 hours. The process of clearing the wound of debris usually takes several days, but the time varies depending on the amount of material to be cleared. The PMNs are followed temporarily by macrophages, which appear in wounds in significant numbers within 2 or 3 days. The macrophages are mononuclear phagocytic cells derived from circulating monocytes or resident tissue macrophages. They complete the process of removing all material not necessary for the ensuing steps of wound healing.

In the absence of significant bacterial contamination, macrophages promptly replace PMNs as the dominant cell type during the inflammatory phase. The role of the macro-

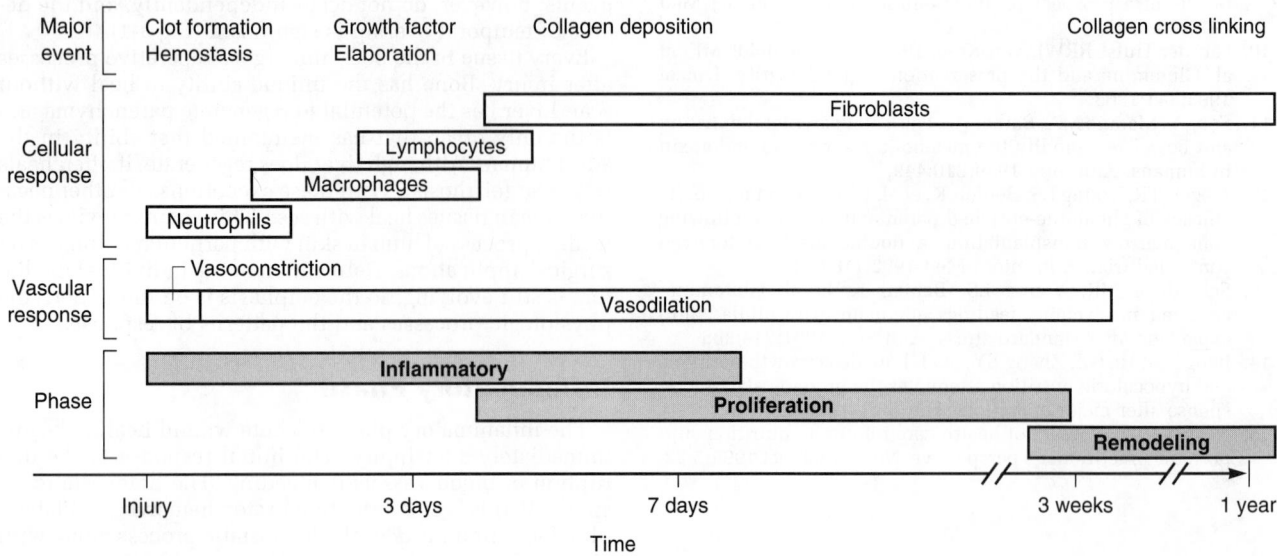

Figure 3-1. Time line of phases of wound healing with dominant cell types and major physiologic events.

phages is not limited to phagocytosis.[1] In addition, macrophages are the sources of more than 30 different growth factors and cytokines. These growth factors induce fibroblast proliferation, endothelial cell proliferation (angiogenesis), and extracellular matrix production, and they recruit and activate additional macrophages. The result is the induction of a wound healing amperification cycle as growth factors recruit macrophages and elicit additional growth factor release. Specific antibodies that destroy PMNs or block certain aspects of amplification function (such as adhesion) have shown that wounds heal normally in the absence of bacteria, but that healing is significantly impaired without functional macrophages. These studies confirm the dominant role of the macrophage in the inflammatory phase of wound healing.

Lymphocytes also appear in wounds in small numbers during the inflammatory phase. The role of lymphocytes in the wound healing process remains to be clarified, but they are thought to be related more to chronic inflammatory processes than to the initial response to wounding. Because recombinant growth factors are available in suffi-

cient quantities for clinical use, the prospect of using growth factors as pharmacologic agents to stimulate wound healing (and potentially modulate abnormal scarring) is the focus of research. No agent, however, has yet been approved for human use. Increased knowledge of the role of growth factors in wound healing has also provoked the evaluation of strategies using other pharmacologic agents to indirectly modulate growth factor levels in wounds.

Proliferative Phase

The proliferative phase begins with the formation of a provisional matrix of fibrin and fibronectin as part of initial clot formation. Initially, the provisional matrix is populated by macrophages; however, by day 3, fibroblasts appear in the fibronectin–fibrin framework and initiate collagen synthesis. Fibroblasts proliferate in response to growth factors to become the dominant cell type during this phase. Growth factors produced by macrophages simultaneously induce angiogenesis, which induces the ingrowth and proliferation of endothelial cells, forming new capillaries. This neovascularity is visible through the epithelium and gives the wound a pink or purple-red appearance. Capillary ingrowth provides the fibroblasts with oxygen and nutrients to sustain cell proliferation and support the production of the permanent wound matrix. This is composed of collagen and proteoglycans or ground substance and replaces the provisional fibronectin–fibrin matrix.

Collagen is the dominant structural molecule in the wound matrix and in the final scar. This is not surprising because collagen is the principal structural protein in skin, bone, and indeed all human tissue. Collagen is synthesized into an organized cable-like network in a multistep process with both intracellular and extracellular components (Fig. 3-3). The collagen molecule has abundant qualities of two unique amino acids, hydroxyproline and hydroxylysine. The hydroxylation process that forms these amino acids requires ascorbic acid (vitamin C) and is necessary for the subsequent stabilization and cross-linkage of collagen. Procollagen is formed within the fibroblasts as a long linear amino acid segment with regular repeats of hydroxypro-

---

Table 3-1. PLATELET GRANULES AND MEDIATORS OF PLATELET AGGREGATION

PLATELET GRANULES

α Granules: Contain Platelet-Specific Proteins

Platelet factor 4
β-Thromboglobulin
Platelet-derived growth factor
Transforming growth factor β

Dense Granules

Adenosine diphosphate
Serotonin
Calcium

MEDIATORS OF PLATELET AGGREGATION

Thromboxane A_2
Thrombin
Platelet factor 4

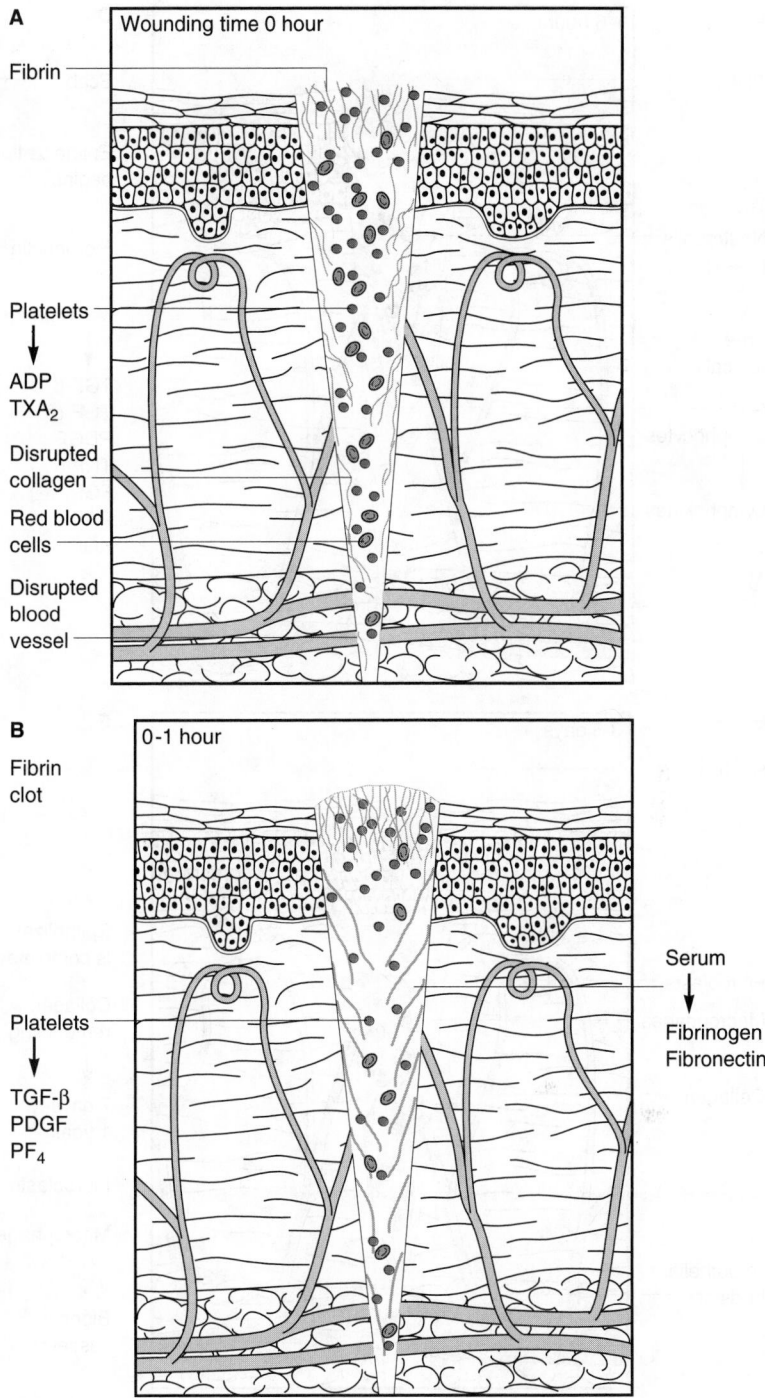

A Wounding time 0 hour

Fibrin

Platelets
↓
ADP
TXA₂

Disrupted collagen

Red blood cells

Disrupted blood vessel

B 0-1 hour

Fibrin clot

Platelets
↓
TGF-β
PDGF
PF₄

Serum
↓
Fibrinogen
Fibronectin

Figure 3-2. Schematic representation of wound healing processes. ADP, adenosine diphosphate; TXA₂, thromboxane A₂; TGF, transforming growth factor; PDGF, platelet-derived growth factor; PF₄, platelet factor 4; TNF-α, tumor necrosis factor α; FGF, fibroblast growth factor; PAF, platelet-activating factor; KGF, keratinocyte growth factor. *(continues)*

line every third amino acid and with terminal extension peptides. Procollagen molecules aggregate in the case of type 1 collagen (the most common) as three α chains to form a triple-helical complex (see Fig. 3-3*A*). The triple helix is maintained by intramolecular disulfide bonds between specific cystine residues. Procollagen is secreted in its triple-helical form; extracellular peptidases cleave the extension peptides at the amino and carboxy termini, leaving the central collagen molecule. Collagen cross-linking (see Fig. 3-3*B*) then occurs in the extracellular space as the collagen molecules aggregate into larger structures. Lysyl oxidase catalyzes the conversion of lysine and hydroxylysine into aldehyde forms. These aldehydes form intermo-

lecular bonds by undergoing spontaneous condensation. This produces stable, cross-linked collagen fibrils. These intramolecular and intermolecular bonds provide strength and stability. As the wound matures, fibrils cross-link to form large cables of collagen, providing increased tensile strength (see Fig 3-3*C*). The wound is now more appropriately considered a scar.

Although there are many types of collagen, type I predominates throughout the body. The principal collagen in scar is type I, with lesser amounts of type III collagen present. Other collagen types make important contributions to the basement membrane, cartilage, and other structures (Table 3-2).

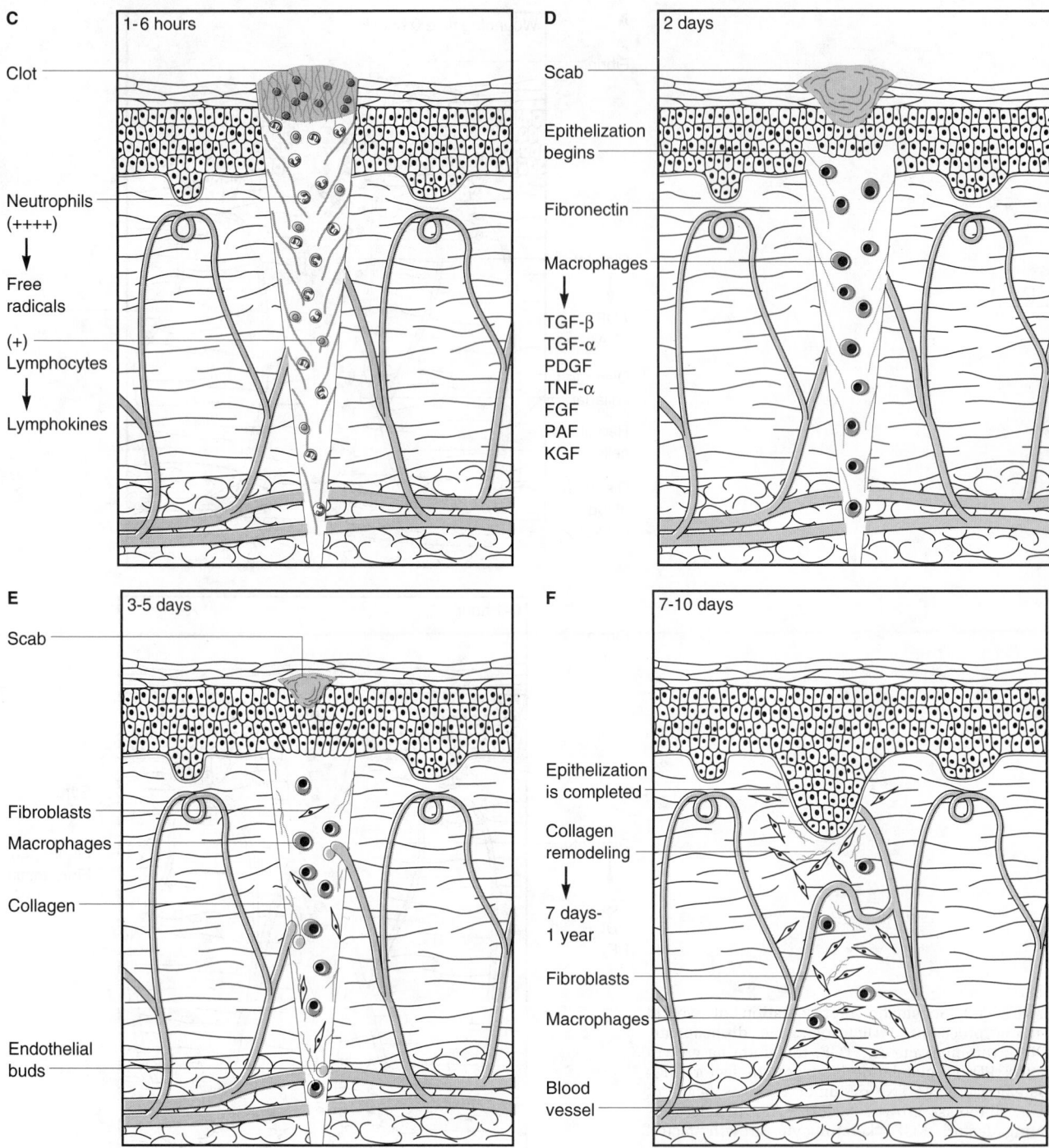

C 1-6 hours
Clot
Neutrophils (++++)
↓
Free radicals
(+)
Lymphocytes
↓
Lymphokines

D 2 days
Scab
Epithelization begins
Fibronectin
Macrophages
↓
TGF-β
TGF-α
PDGF
TNF-α
FGF
PAF
KGF

E 3-5 days
Scab
Fibroblasts
Macrophages
Collagen
Endothelial buds

F 7-10 days
Epithelization is completed
Collagen remodeling
↓
7 days-1 year
Fibroblasts
Macrophages
Blood vessel

Figure 3-2. *(Continued)*

Remodeling Phase

The transition from the proliferative phase to the remodeling phase is defined by reaching collagen equilibrium. Collagen accumulation within the wound reaches a maximum within 2 to 3 weeks after wounding. Although supranormal rates of synthesis and degradation continue throughout remodeling, there is no further change in total collagen content.[2] Tensile strength gradually increases as random collagen fibrils are replaced by organized fibrils with more intermolecular bonds. During the initial phase of wound healing, there is a relative abundance of type III collagen in the wound. With remodeling, the normal adult ratio of 4:1 (type I to type III) collagen is restored. Under normal wound healing conditions, the capillary density gradually diminishes, and the number of fibroblasts is reduced. The wound loses its pink or purple vascular color and becomes progressively pale. The collagen undergoes constant remodeling. New collagen is formed, and collagen degradation by specific collagenases is ongoing. Collagenase activity is balanced against new production of collagen to produce a steady state. As equilibrium is achieved, the collagen fibrils align themselves in a longitudinal arrangement as dictated by stress placed on the wound. Scars never achieve the degree of order achieved by collagen in normal skin or tendons, but they do increase in strength

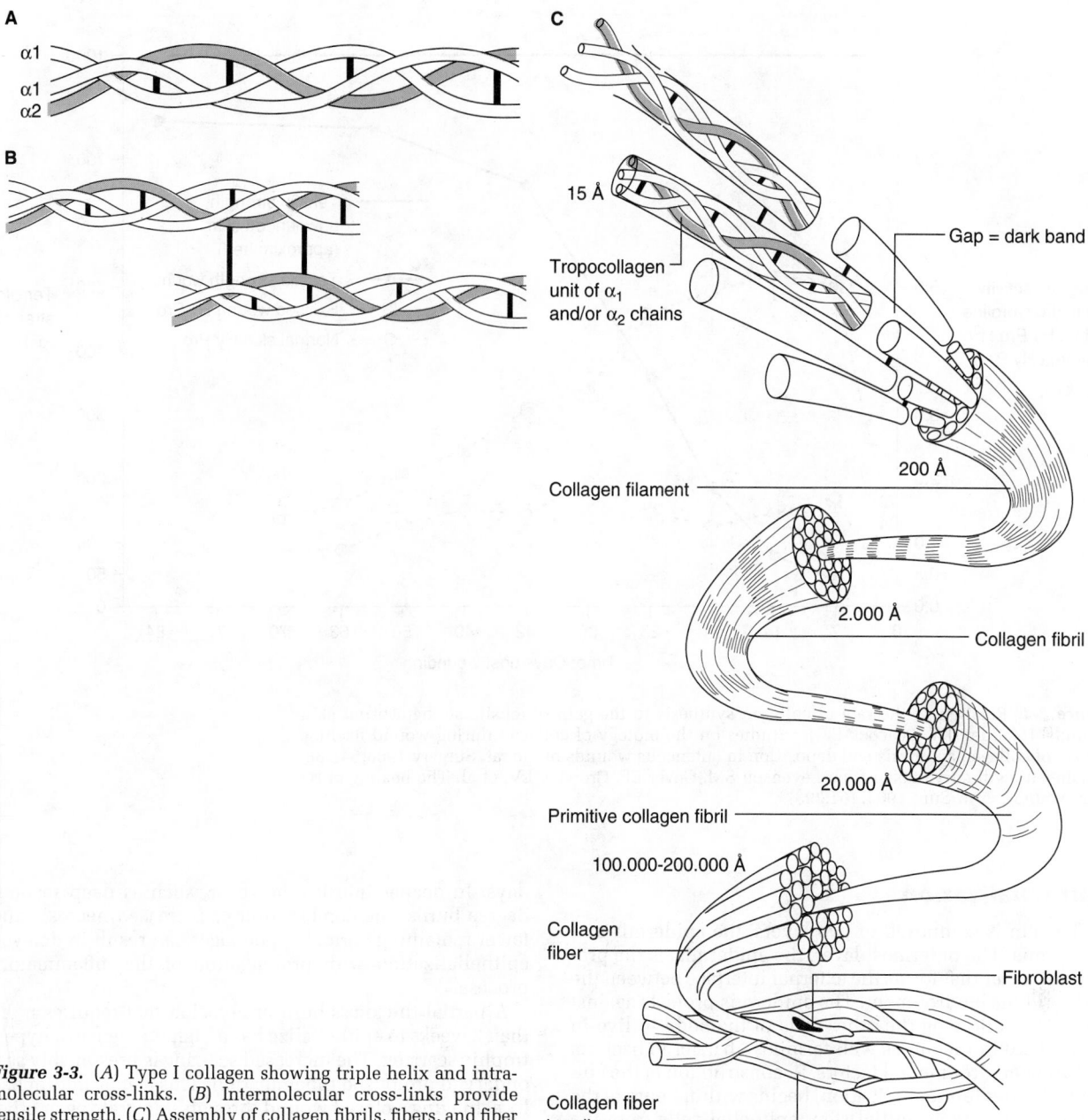

Figure 3-3. (*A*) Type I collagen showing triple helix and intramolecular cross-links. (*B*) Intermolecular cross-links provide tensile strength. (*C*) Assembly of collagen fibrils, fibers, and fiber bundles.

Table 3-2. COLLAGEN TYPES

Type	Property of Aggregate Unit	Tissue Distribution
I	Rigid fibrils	All connective tissue except cartilage
II	Rigid fibrils	Cartilage and vitreous
III	Elastic fibrils	Elastic tissue (eg, fetal skin, blood vessels, uterus)
IV	Sheet	Basement membrane
V	Fibril	Widespread
VI	Beaded filaments	Widespread
VII	Anchoring fibrils	Interface of basement membrane and underlying stroma
VIII	Sheet	Descemet membrane
IX	Fibril	Hyaline cartilage
X	Sheet	Hypertrophic cartilage
XI	Fibril	Hyaline cartilage
XII	Fibril	Similar to type I

for 6 months or longer, eventually reaching 70% of the strength of unwounded skin (Fig 3-4).

The other important component of the extracellular matrix is the ground substance or proteoglycans. These substances are composed of a protein backbone with long hydrophilic carbohydrate side chains. The hydrophilic nature of these molecules accounts for much of the water content of scar. In the early immature wound, there is a disproportionately large amount of proteoglycans (particularly hyaluronic acid). During the maturation phase, the proteoglycan content returns to a level that closely approximates that of normal skin.

Until recently, the extracellular matrix (predominantly collagen and proteoglycans) was thought to be inert. It is becoming increasingly clear, however, that extracellular matrix signals certain cells through cell attachment receptors (integrins) and serves as a reservoir for growth factors; no doubt other roles are still unknown. The role of proteoglycans as signaling molecules is just beginning to be understood.

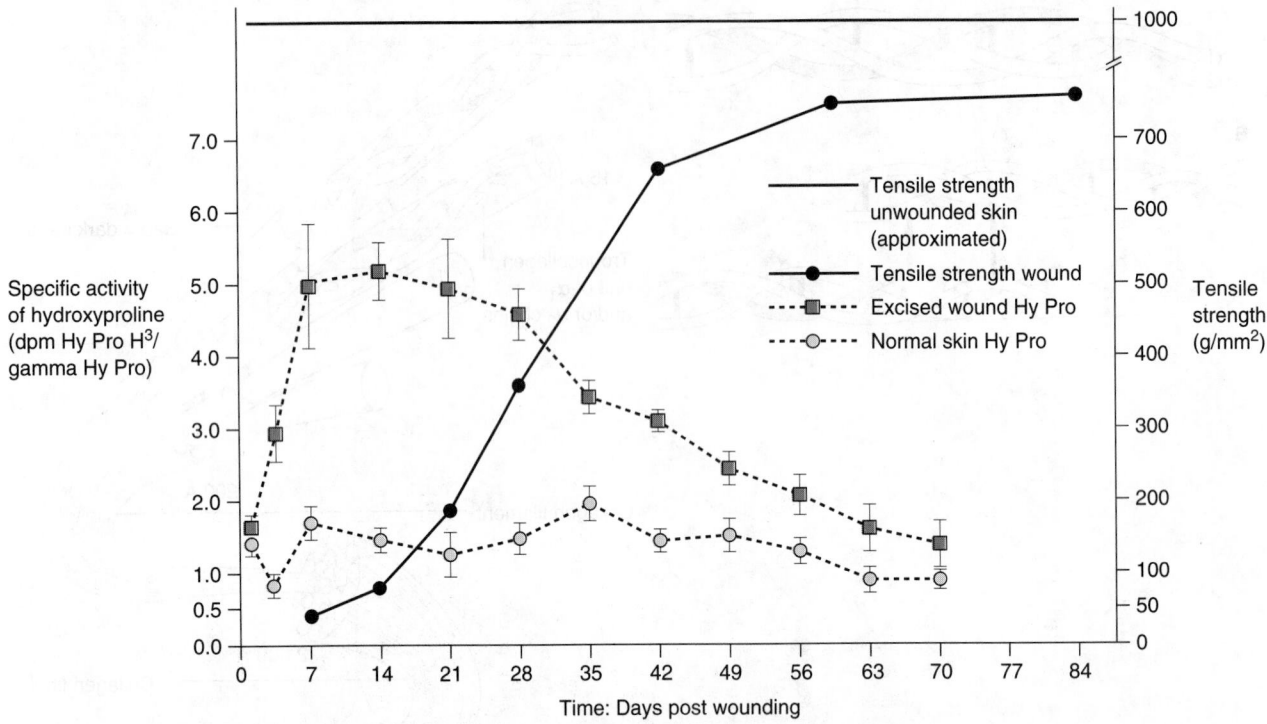

Figure 3-4. Relation of the rate of collagen synthesis to the gain of tensile strength of rat skin wounds. (Madden JW, Peacock EE Jr. Studies on the biology of collagen during wound healing. 1. Rate of collagen synthesis and deposition in cutaneous wounds of the rat. Surgery 1968;64:288. Tensile strength curve taken from Levenson SM, Gever EF, Crowley LV, et al. The healing of rat skin wounds. Ann Surg 1965;161:293)

Epithelialization

The skin is composed of two layers, the epidermis and the dermis. The outermost layer, the epidermis, is the protective barrier that forms the external interface between the body and the environment. The epidermis protects against water loss, allowing the other cells of the body to live in a liquid environment, as well forming a barrier to bacteria and other environmental factors. Reconstruction of the epithelial barrier (epithelialization) begins within hours of the initial injury. As an initial step, epithelial cells from the basal layer at the wound edge flatten and migrate across the wound, completing wound coverage within 24 to 18 hours in a coapted surgical wound. The cells along the margin are also dividing to reform the multilayered mature epithelium (see later). Epithelial cells exhibit contact inhibition; that is, they continue to migrate across an appropriate bed until a single continuous layer is formed. Epithelial cell migration occurs by a process in which the epithelial cells send out pseudopods, attaching to the underlying extracellular matrix by integrin receptors. Bacteria, large amounts of protein exudate from leaky capillaries, and necrotic tissue all compromise this process, delaying epithelialization. Delayed epithelialization results in a more profound and prolonged inflammatory process, thereby contributing to unsatisfactory or hypertrophic scarring.

In the case of open wounds, epithelialization results from migration of epithelial cells from remaining dermal appendages, sweat glands, and hair follicles, if the dermis is not destroyed (Fig 3-5). This is relatively rapid because the distance between hair follicles and sweat glands is short; epithelialization is usually complete within 7 to 10 days. In deeper injuries, however, such as deep second-degree burns, the combination of increased necrosis and fewer remaining dermal appendages can result in delayed epithelialization with prolongation of the inflammatory process.

A partial-thickness burn or abrasion that requires more than 2 weeks to epithelialize has a high incidence of hypertrophic scarring. The increased scarring is presumably secondary to prolonged inflammation. This can be minimized by achieving a closed wound through skin grafting or other techniques.

After the first layer of cells restores the epithelial barrier, additional layers develop, restoring the basilar-to-apical order. As the cells mature, they resume keratin formation. This regenerates the stratum corneum of the epidermis and completes the restorative process of epithelialization.

In full-thickness injury, the entire dermis is destroyed or removed. Epithelialization occurs only from the margins of the wound, at a maximal rate of 1 to 2 mm/d. In practice, adequate coverage of sizable wounds is rarely achieved. Thus, lower leg ulcers rarely heal faster than 1 cm/mo; that is, a 2-cm diameter ulcer typically takes 2 months to heal under ideal conditions. In an open wound, the rate of epithelialization is critically dependent on the vascularity and health of the underlying granulation tissue (neodermis) across which it migrates. Thus, although chronic wounds are manifested by a failure of epithelial migration, the cause is most often a problem in the underlying wound bed.

The epithelial cells alone provide little strength when not anchored to dermis. They are therefore prone to injury. The basal epidermal cells are attached to the underlying

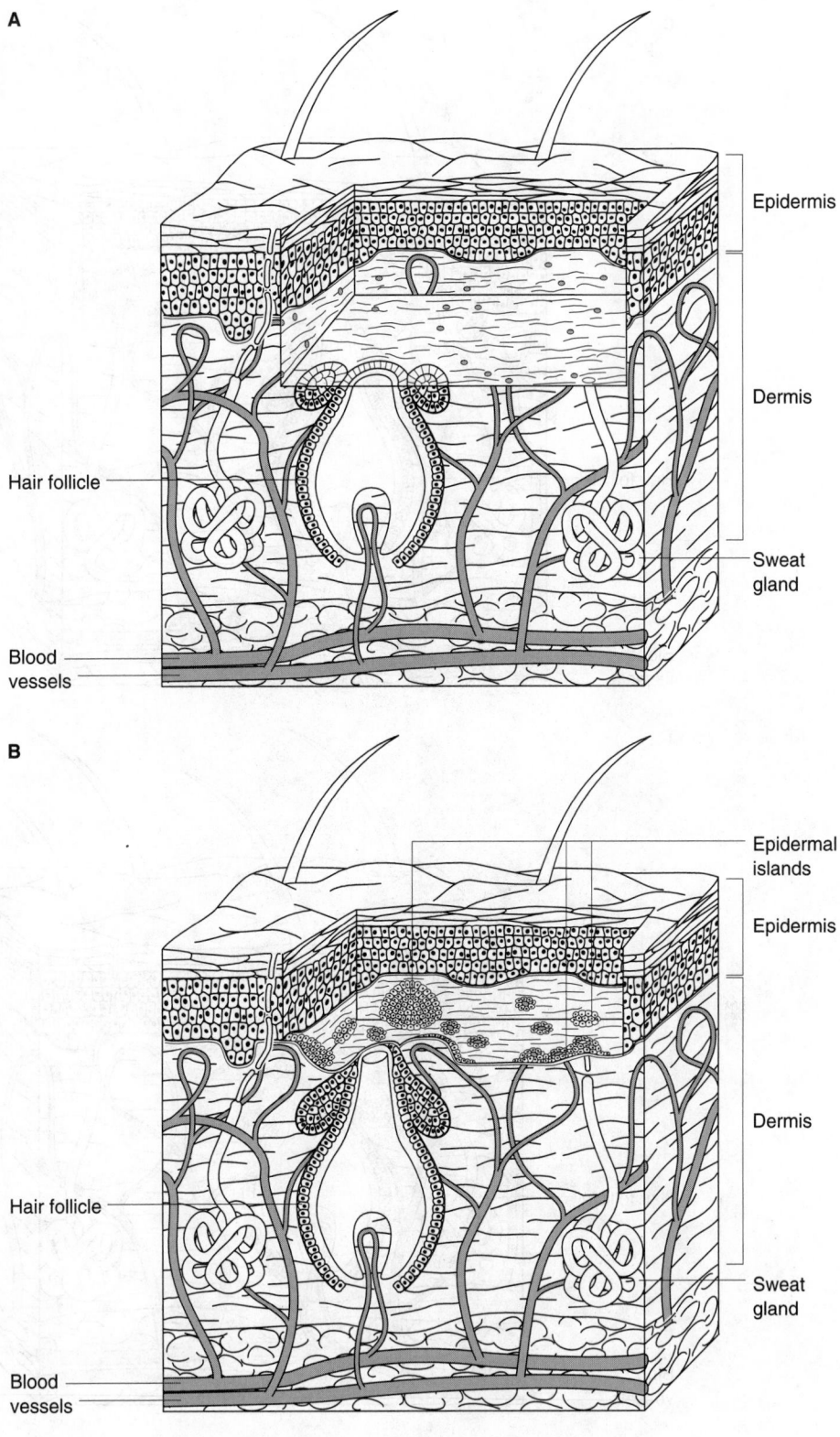

A

Epidermis

Dermis

Hair follicle

Sweat gland

Blood vessels

B

Epidermal islands

Epidermis

Dermis

Hair follicle

Sweat gland

Blood vessels

Figure 3-5. Reepithilialization of a partial-thickness wound. *(continues)*

dermis by hemidesmosomes. These structures attach to keratin filaments within the epithelial cells. The hemidesmosomes connect by a series of intermediate proteins to anchoring filaments, long proteins that intertwine with the collagen network of the dermis. Intact epithelium is resistant to sheer forces due to these strong dermal attachments. Without an adequate dermal base, however, epidermis provides unstable wound coverage and is characterized by chronic and recurrent breakdown.

Visible scarring occurs only when the injury extends deeper than the superficial dermis. Superficial abrasions and burns usually heal without scarring, but deeper abrasions and burns can scar significantly. Whenever the dermis is incised, a scar forms. The prominence of the scar is

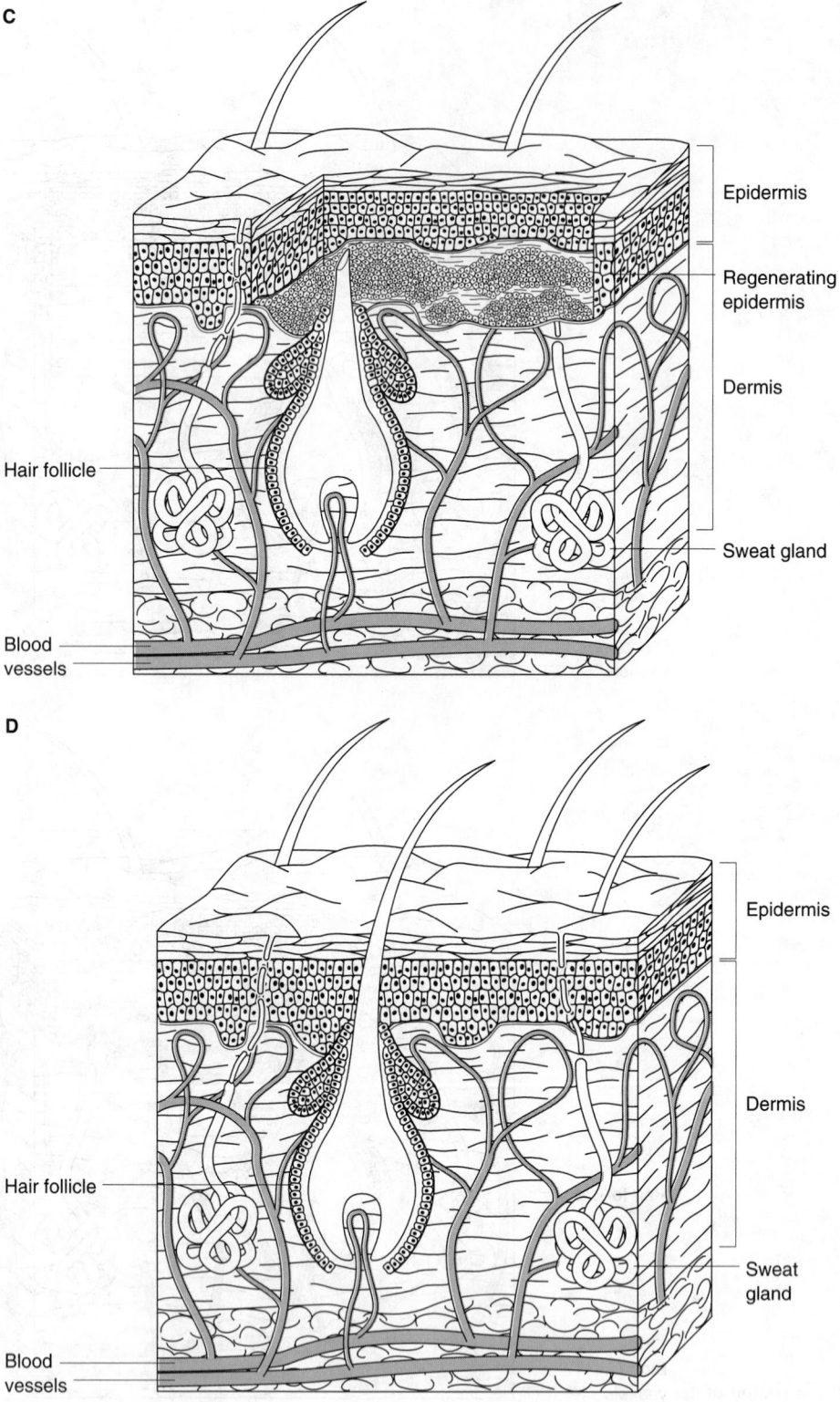

C

Epidermis

Regenerating
epidermis

Dermis

Hair follicle

Sweat gland

Blood
vessels

D

Epidermis

Dermis

Hair follicle

Sweat
gland

Blood
vessels

Figure 3-5. (Continued)

variable and can be minimized by location and closure
technique. If an incision is made, however, a scar is
inevitable.

Stretch marks are a unique type of scar. Stretch marks
occur when the collagen fibers in the dermis are stretched
to the point of disruption, but the epidermis is not disrupted. This results in scar formation in the dermis that is
visible through an intact, unscarred epidermis.

Clinical Implications

This review of normal wound healing has numerous
practical implications to the care of wound and surgical
incisions. Meticulous hemostasis reduces the inflammation and phagocytosis necessary to clear the wound of
blood. Atraumatic handling of tissue decreases the load of
necrotic or nonviable cells at the wound margin. This is

best achieved using fine forceps or skin hooks to retract and assist in coapting the dermis. Crush injury to the epidermis with forceps should be avoided. Deep sutures are best placed only into collagen-laden structures that can hold tension, that is, fascia and dermis. These tissues have the tensile strength to hold sutures under tension. Fat does not contain collagen and does not hold tension. Therefore, fatty tissue should not be sutured as a separate layer. Dead space obliteration and fluid evacuation are best achieved by suction drainage rather than by adding additional foreign material to the wound in the form of suture material. Therefore, in closing a laparotomy incision, even in a morbidly obese patient with a 2-inch panniculus, the closure should be limited to the abdominal fascia, the skin, and rarely the Scarpa fascia.

Under normal circumstances, epithelialization of an incision is complete within 24 to 48 hours, and there is no reason to protect the incision from water beyond this time period. Allowing the patient to wash or shower 1 or 2 days after surgery has significant psychologic benefit and gently débrides the incision and keeps it clean by rinsing away surface bacteria and debris. Blood and protein exudate are an excellent culture media for any skin surface bacteria. Showers reduce the chance of bacterial accumulation in surface crusts along the incision and on the sutures. This decreases inflammation and prevents breakdown of the fragile epithelial layer over the incision, improving the quality of the scar.

OPEN WOUNDS (ACUTE)

Open wounds, whether ulcers or open surgical incisions closing by secondary intention, heal with the same sequence of inflammation, matrix deposition, epithelialization, and scar maturation as previously described. However, there are some important differences. In the incisional wound, the healing process progresses through an orderly temporal sequence. In an open wound, the healing events are spatially separated. In the healing wound, a bed of granulation tissue forms over the exposed subcutaneous tissue. Granulation tissue is composed of new capillaries, proliferating fibroblasts, and an immature matrix of collagen, proteoglycans, substrate adhesion molecules (including fibronectin, laminin, and tenascin), and acute and chronic inflammatory cells. In addition, there are variable amounts of bacteria and protein exudate, depending on the ''health'' of the wound. At the advancing edge of epithelium, the process of acute inflammation is present. Behind the advancing edge, there is a proliferative area; and further behind, the scar is maturing and remodeling. An understanding of the biologic principles of wound healing has direct clinical implications in wound care, particularly in the case of chronic wounds (eg, pressure sores, lower leg ulcers, diabetic foot ulcers).

The most important clinical factor in the healing of surgical incisions is the gain in tensile strength of the wound. This was discussed previously and depends almost entirely on collagen deposition. The rate of collagen synthesis determines the initial wound strength; ultimate wound strength is determined by the degree of collagen organization and cross-linking. The healing of open wounds is defined primarily by epithelialization, and successful healing is related more to the maintenance of epithelial integrity than to the tensile strength of the scar. At the edge of a healing wound, the basal epithelial cells flatten out, lose their hemidesmosome attachments, and migrate over the wound base.

As discussed earlier, the rate of epithelialization in open wounds is limited by the rate of migration of the proliferating epithelial edge. Factors that regulate epithelial migration are an area of active research. There is clear evidence that the extracellular matrix (collagen, fibronectin, basement membrane proteins, glycosaminoglycans) is composed of structural elements that are not inert. They function as an essential substrate, with adhesion molecules regulating intercellular communication. The cellular occupants of the matrix express specific receptors that recognize amino acid sequences on the matrix proteins. This allows for cellular attachment at specific sites, cell locomotion, and intracellular signal transduction. Rapid epithelialization is therefore dependent on an optimal matrix, manufactured by the underlying granulation tissue, as well as on optimal delivery of nutrients and oxygen by an adequate blood supply.

Inflammatory cells in open wounds, especially the macrophages, release growth factors. Growth factors enhance migration and proliferation of fibroblasts and endothelial cells in wounds. In an open wound, however, this leads to the formation of granulation tissue, the cobblestone-like, pink surface of healthy new tissue. The ability of an open wound to form granulation tissue is governed by the blood supply to the tissue and the relative absence of devitalized tissue and bacteria.

Wound Contraction

Wound contraction is an important event that contrasts the healing of open wounds with closed incisions. When open wounds contract, the surrounding skin is pulled over the wound to reduce its size. This can occur much faster than epithelialization. In addition to increasing the speed of wound closure, another advantage is that the open wound is resurfaced by the normal sensate skin surrounding the wound. Most animals are loose skinned—meaning that the skin (epithelium, dermis, subcutaneous fat) is only loosely attached to the underlying muscle fascia. Some animal wounds heal almost entirely by contraction; for example, a 2-cm ulcer heals to a 3-mm point. Humans however, do not have this degree of skin mobility in most sites; the skin is tightly adherent and less elastic, especially in the lower leg. Therefore, although contraction may account for 90% of the reduction in wound size on the perineum, it accounts for at most 30% to 40% of the healing of a lower leg ulcer. This is one important reason why leg ulcers are so slow to heal. All healing wounds generate a strong contractile force.[3] When this contractile force is exerted across a joint, such as the neck, axilla, or elbow, it may result in a scar contracture. A scar contracture is a scar that limits the functional range of motion of a joint.

At the cellular level, the forces that drive wound contraction come from the fibroblasts. Fibroblasts, like muscle cells, contain actin microfilaments. When these filaments increase in number, the cells take on the morphologic appearance of myofibroblasts. Myofibroblasts are seen in increased numbers in contracting wounds, but their role is unclear. In addition, it is unknown whether the fibroblasts that attach to the collagen fibrils by means of integrin receptors move collagen fibers together using a locomotor action or whether the contraction comes from intrinsic cellular contraction.

Unless created and dressed under sterile conditions, all open wounds are contaminated by the bacterial flora on the surrounding skin and from the environment. Bacterial colonization of the wound is routine and is not deleterious to normal healing. Bacterial infection, however, is deleterious and can delay or prevent healing. Cellulitis or invasive bacterial infection of the surrounding tissues is relatively easy to diagnose with experience. This requires systemic antibiotic therapy. Distinguishing wound colonization from invasive infection, however, can be difficult. The burn wound experience has demonstrated that bacterial counts of more than 10^5 organisms per gram of tissue on quantitative analysis are associated with failure of surgical wound closure. This is an important technique, because clinical judgment is inadequate. The failure of wound closure in this circumstance is in part from bacterial and phagocytic proteases that prevent healing. In a similar fashion, if the bacterial count is above this threshold in the wound granulation tissue, the excessive proteases and endotoxins delay epithelialization.

Any nonepithelialized wound leaks plasma. With more inflammation, capillary permeability is further increased. Increased microvascular permeability results from endothelial cell injury or dysfunction. This is mediated by many components of the inflammatory cascade, including histamine, kinins, complement, PGE_2, PGI_2, and others. This exudate of serum proteins and inflammatory cells serves as a rich culture medium, which may continue the cycle of bacterial proliferation and leads to more exudate formation. The net result of this cycle is delayed or absent wound healing. In addition, the edema that results from capillary dysfunction increases the distance for diffusion from oxygen and nutrient sources to their metabolic targets.

Clinical Features

Basic principles of wound care are related to the mechanism elaborated earlier, although many varieties of wound care are practiced. Winter and Scales[4] first recorded that epithelialization is more rapid under moist conditions than dry conditions. Without dressings, a superficial wound, or one with minimal devitalized tissue, forms a scab or crust, meaning that the blood and serum coagulate, dry, and form a protective moisture barrier over the open wound (Fig 3-6). Epithelialization occurs with controlled clot proteolysis and migration of the epithelium under the clot. If the wound is kept moist with an occlusive dressing, however, and the exudate does not become infected, then epithelial migration is optimized. A skin graft donor site, for example, epithelializes several days faster under an occlusive dressing than a dry dressing. In addition, the pain of an open wound or skin graft donor site is dramatically reduced under an occlusive dressing.

Moist healing can be achieved by occlusive dressings, occlusive ointments or creams, or continually moistened dressings. The traditional wet to dry dressing, however, if truly left to dry, simply produces desiccation and necrosis of the surface layer of the wound, delaying epithelialization. Although wet to dry dressings can be effective for débridement of wound exudate, they are generally less desirable than a moist healing environment combined with effective cleaning of the wound (ie, water irrigation).

Role of Oxygen

Oxygen is necessary for normal metabolic cellular function, but in wounds with actively proliferating and metabolically stimulated cells, it is even more critical. Polymorphonuclear leukocytes require ambient PO_2 levels of 25 mmHg to produce superoxide radicals, which serve an essential role in bacterial killing. The enzyme system that generates superoxide and its derivative oxidant products functions optimally at PO_2 levels greater than 50 mmHg. Collagen synthesis is highly dependent on an adequate tissue oxygen tension, and the cells in a healing wound are metabolically active, creating a potentially competitive microenvironment in the wound. A fresh wound is ini-

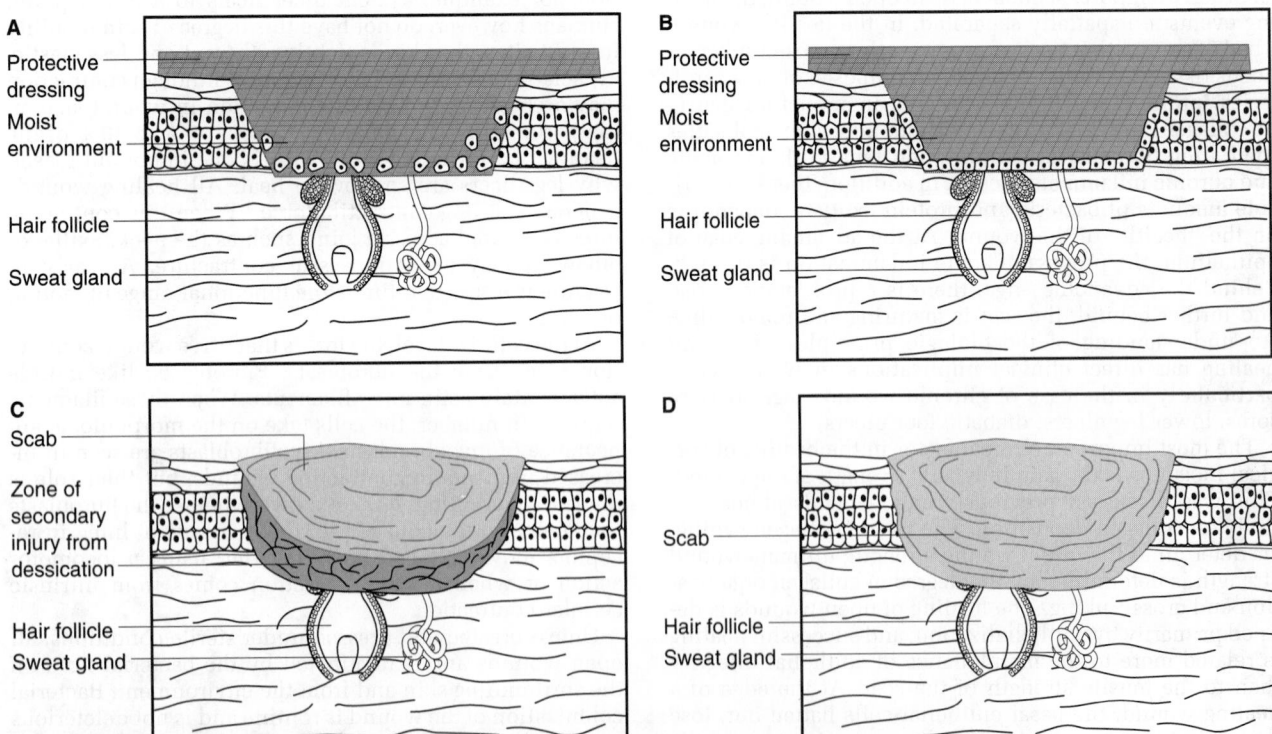

Figure 3-6. Rapid epithilialization occurs in a moist environment. Desiccation delays healing by causing tissue necrosis in the exposed wound. The scab ultimately forms a moisture barrier, and epithilialization occurs from the wound edge and any remaining dermal appendages (see Fig. 3-5).

tially avascular and is always hypoxic relative to the surrounding tissues. In the center of a new wound, the tissue PO_2 can drop to near zero. After angiogenesis and the delivery of oxygenated blood, the tissue PO_2 quickly rises. Generally, the tissue oxygen tension in a wound is lower than that of surrounding normal tissues. Atherosclerosis of major arteries, small vessel disease from other causes, impaired oxygen delivery, local scarring with fibrosis, and other events may reduce local tissue PO_2 levels from normal (about 40 mmHg) to less than 25 mmHg. If so, tissue hypoxia results in significantly impaired wound healing. In the postoperative patient, suboptimal skin perfusion due to even modest hypovolemia, smoking-related arteriopathy, or excess circulating epinephrine can result in a low tissue PO_2. Subcutaneous tissue oxygen levels have been correlated clinically with surgical complication rates. Supplemental oxygen, optimal fluid administration, pain control, and arterial reconstruction all have potential roles in the effort to enhance the tissue PO_2. Oxygen delivery to tissue determines the outcome; anemia alone is not specifically detrimental to wound healing.[5]

Role of Edema

In normal tissue, each cell is only a few cell diameters away from the nearest capillary, and receives nutrients and oxygen by diffusion. However, with inflammation, venous insufficiency, or any other causes of edema formation, the sequestered extracellular and extravascular fluid increases the diffusion distance for oxygen and results in a lower tissue PO_2. In the case of lower extremity venous insufficiency, the chronic protein leak from the capillaries results in pericapillary deposition. This "cuffing" is a further barrier to oxygen and nutrient diffusion, and possibly functions as a site of nonspecific binding of growth factors, making them less available to the wound environment. The importance of edema control is often underestimated. Even in extremities that are not noticeably swollen, elevation and other methods of edema control (elastic wraps, compression stockings, sequential compression machines) can be of substantial benefit. The most important therapeutic maneuver in the healing of leg ulcers associated with venous insufficiency is edema control with leg elevation, compression stockings or compressive dressings, and in severe cases, intermittent or sequential compression devices.

Role of Tissue Necrosis and Exudate

Open wounds often contain devitalized tissue as a result of injury, and possibly aggravated by infection or suboptimal tissue perfusion. If the amount of dead tissue is large, the impairment to healing is obvious, but it is often not fully appreciated that smaller amounts of necrotic tissue or fibrinous exudate also delay healing. In addition, any open wound constantly produces an exudate of serum proteins and dead inflammatory cells, which increases devitalized tissue if present. The net result is increased exudate, higher bacterial counts, edema, more proteases and other inflammatory mediators, and a deleterious effect on healing. Therefore, devitalized tissue, especially dermis requires surgical excision, although enzymatic débridement with collagenases may occasionally be acceptable. If necrotic dermis is left in place, the underlying subcutaneous tissue (fat), which is less vascular, eventually becomes infected. Small amounts of devitalized tissue and exudate can be débrided or removed with dressings, enzyme application, whirlpools, water irrigation or simple washing. However, the mechanical débriding action must be sufficient and frequent enough to remove the exudate and debris, producing a clean wound before healing is optimal. Because wounds are painful and the dressings or washing

insufficient, the exudate is often not removed adequately. This results in delayed healing.

CHRONIC WOUNDS

A practical definition of a chronic wound is one that has failed to heal within 3 months. Although there are a variety of underlying causes, most can be categorized as pressure sores, diabetic foot ulcers or leg ulcers. An important question is whether chronic wounds are intrinsically different than acute wounds. For instance, does local tissue senescence make healing a chronic wound impossible? Or, do chronic wounds have the inherent potential to heal, but a combination of factors lead to delayed healing? Research in the past few years has begun to address the question of what is different about the environment in a chronic wound.

Clinicians have long recognized that most chronic wounds do indeed have the potential to heal. Healing usually does not occur because of inadequate attention to the basic principles open wound care—adequate cleansing, débridement, edema control, avoidance and treatment of ischemia, and achievement of a moist wound healing environment. However, the wound environment in many chronic wounds does differ in important ways from acute wounds. Recent studies have examined wound fluid and biopsies collected from chronic wounds. These reveal significant increases in tissue levels in proteases and collagenases, which are capable of degrading matrix proteins and growth factors. Degradation of growth factors inhibits their crucial functions of proliferation and chemotaxis. When wound fluid from a chronic wound is compared with fluid from an acute surgical wound, there is indeed a decreased level of growth factors. It is not clear what influence bacteria have in this process, although the direct release of bacterial proteases and the indirect effect of protease release from phagocytic cells are both relevant. It is unknown whether growth factor levels are depressed because of proteolysis, primary inhibition of release, or secondary phenotypic changes in the cells of the chronic wound.

WOUND MANAGEMENT
Surgical Incisions

It takes at least three weeks for collagen to undergo sufficient remodeling and cross linking to attain moderate strength. Figure 3-4 shows that at 1 to 2 weeks, the time when most sutures are removed, a wound has a small fraction of its eventual strength and may therefore disrupt with even modest stresses. Therefore, deep sutures are placed in collagen containing structures to hold prolonged tension. Dermis, intestinal submucosa, muscular fascia, tendon, ligament, Scarpa fascia and blood vessel wall represent a partial list of tissues with high collagen content. These deep sutures are often absorbable. The most common absorbable material, polygalactic acid (Vicryl, Dexon) retains tensile strength for about 3 weeks. Sutures used for tendon and abdominal fascia are usually permanent or if absorbable should ideally retain their tensile strength for close to 6 weeks. After 6 weeks, wounded tissue has gained about 50% of its eventual strength. To prevent hernia formation, heavy lifting is avoided after major abdominal surgery for six weeks. Tendon repairs are splinted and activity restricted to avoid full tension for a similar period of time.

Open Wound Dressings

There are at least 150 dressing products commercially available at present. These include multiple topical antibiotics, irrigants and débriding agents. No treatment has been shown to improve healing beyond that of standard treatment, which adheres to the principles outlined earlier. There are many good alternative treatments, but to avoid confusion they should be judged according to the following criteria:

1. How effectively is the wound cleaned or débrided?
2. Is moist wound healing achieved?
3. Is edema minimized in the periwound tissue?
4. Are new pressure insults or wound soilage prevented?
5. Is tissue oxygenation (blood flow) adequate?

In some situations, reduction of tissue bacteria is also an important additional need although this is addressed by adequate cleaning and débridement most often. In the absence of large amounts of necrotic tissue, wound débridement does not need to be accomplished surgically. Proteinaceous exudate can be tenacious, however, and simple application of moist dressings may not be adequate to remove it. Water irrigation either in whirlpools or by water from a handheld shower spray or even from dental water cleaning devices can be gentle, and yet generate enough power to effectively débride.[6] Frequent moist dressing changes can accomplish this as well, and in some cases, occlusive absorptive dressings can generate enough tissue proteases to effectively degrade proteins that the absorptive dressings remove. This deceptively simple principle is the most frequently overlooked in wound care. The typical open surgical wound may be deep with interstices that packing or other absorptive dressings may not effectively reach. The deeper portions of the wound may then accumulate exudate and bacteria. This is one example where water irrigation may be particularly useful. Commonly used agents such as hydrogen peroxide are actually harmful to normal tissue, and are weak oxidants and thus do a poor job of débriding. These are to be avoided. Enzymatic débriding agents can be effective when properly used.

As discussed, a desiccated wound undergoes delayed healing. Most wounds require an absorptive dressing to remove exudate. This can be gauze, which is inexpensive and effective but which requires frequent dressing changes and is not occlusive so that an ointment or cream must be added. Skin graft donor sites do well with an occlusive polyurethane film dressing. Most of the newer dressing products have been designed to be more absorptive and achieve moist healing without infection from excess exudate. An emphasis has been to decrease the frequency of dressing changes. It must be emphasized that although factors such as convenience, patient acceptance and cost are good reasons for choosing a product, as long as moist healing is achieved, there is no evidence that one is better than another.

Edema is quite detrimental to wound healing and is often undertreated, in part because of difficulties in patient education. Edema can be a factor in virtually any ulcer of the lower extremity, although venous insufficiency is the most important. Because patients often have personal habits that are hard to modify, this can be a refractory problem. Patients often object to compression stockings, the most effective method for limiting edema. This leaves intermittent leg elevation, elastic wraps, and elevation of the foot of the bed as alternative measures. The critical factor is getting the patient to realize that leg swelling must be avoided, and so in the course of their day, each patient must modify behavior sufficiently to treat this problem.

Systemic Factors Affecting Wound Healing

Several important systemic factors or conditions influence wound healing. Interestingly, there are no known systemic conditions that lead to more rapid wound healing.

The discussion that follows relates to factors that may retard or inhibit wound healing.

Nutrition

Wound healing requires energy and is an anabolic process. Patients who are severely malnourished or who are actively catabolic demonstrate impaired healing. While there is no single measure of nutritional adequacy, the serum albumin level is the most readily available and clinically useful parameter. A serum albumin greater than 3.5 g/dL suggests adequate protein stores and positive nitrogen balance. However, albumin has a serum half life of nineteen days. Therefore, the serum albumin level does not drop early in a catabolic process and is slow to rise when protein stores are repleted and an anabolic state returns. Serum transferrin has a shorter half-life and, therefore, responds more promptly to nutritional fluctuations, but it is not part of a routine chemistry panel and has not gained widespread clinical usage. There is no consensus on nutritional parameters that accurately predict surgical complications. In considering closure of a chronic wound such as a pressure sore, the ability to form good granulation tissue is a clinical indication of acceptable wound healing potential. Certainly an albumin level of less than 3 mg/dL raises concern for potential wound healing problems. Most surgeons avoid trying to close chronic wounds surgically until nutritional levels are considered acceptable.

Vitamins play an important role in wound healing as well. Vitamin A is involved in the stimulation of fibroplasia, collagen cross linking, and epithelialization. In animal studies, vitamin A reverses the inhibitory effects of glucocorticoids on the inflammatory phase of wound healing.[7] While there is no conclusive evidence in humans, vitamin A may be useful clinically for steroid dependent patients who have problematic wounds, or who are undergoing an extensive surgical procedure. Vitamin A may be used either topically or systemically, but attention should be paid to the dosage and duration of therapy as vitamin A is fat soluble and has a well-defined toxicity state. An oral dose of 25,000 IU daily or topical application of 200,000 IU ointment three times a day should be sufficient.

Vitamin C is a necessary cofactor in the hydroxylation of lysine and proline in collagen synthesis and cross linkage. The deficiency state, scurvy, is rarely seen in the Western world today. The utility of vitamin C supplementation in patients who are taking a normal diet is not established.

Vitamin E is applied to wounds and incisions by many patients. The evidence to support this practice is entirely anecdotal. In fact, large doses of vitamin E have been found to inhibit wound healing.[8] However, massage and pressure have been shown to flatten and soften scars. It is possible that some of the perceived benefit by patients is due to these benefits obtained in the cause of application.

Essential fatty acids are required for all new cell synthesis. Essential fatty acid deficiency is first noted in areas of high cellular turnover, such as healing wounds, skin, and gastrointestinal mucosa. Early experience with total parenteral nutrition in which essential fatty acids were lacking showed that patients developed difficult wounds and dramatic skin changes. These were rapidly reversed with the addition of fat to the parenteral nutritional program.

Zinc and copper are also important cofactors for many enzyme systems that are important to wound healing. Deficiency states have been seen with parenteral nutrition but are rare and now readily recognized and treated with supplements.

Vitamin and mineral deficiency states clearly show the necessity of these agents for wound healing. However, these deficiency states are extremely rare in the absence of parenteral nutrition or other extreme dietary restrictions.

There is no evidence to support the concept that supranormal provision of these factors enhances wound healing in normal patients. Significant complications, especially with excessive fat soluble vitamin supplementation, are reported. However, malnutrition can be a significant problem in the elderly and debilitated patient. These patients require nutritional supplementation and should receive vitamin and mineral supplementation as part of their protein and caloric repletion.

Aging

There are important age-dependent aspects of wound healing. The elderly heal more slowly and with less scarring. There is gradual attenuation of the inflammatory response with age and decreased wound healing is one of the consequences. In vitro studies have documented an age dependent decrease in the proliferative potential of fibroblasts and epithelial cells. Clinically, these account for the formation of finer scars and improved cosmetic appearance in the elderly. Hypertrophic scars are rarely seen in the elderly. Sutures should be left in place longer to allow for the slower gain in tensile strength in the aged. This may be done without formation of suture marks as slower epithelialization occurs along the sutures. Although the aged usually heal surgical incisions without complications, the combination of age to other adverse factors can result in severe healing deficits and high surgical complication rates.

Pharmacologic Impairment to Wound Healing

Bone marrow suppression, a common consequence of chemotherapy, is detrimental to wound healing. Quantitative and qualitative lymphocyte and monocyte deficiency impairs cellular proliferation in the inflammatory phase of wound healing. Any chemotherapeutic agent that suppresses the bone marrow will impair healing. Fortunately, this is predictably reversible with cessation of chemotherapy. Glucocorticoids inhibit wound healing based on their antiinflammatory and immunosuppressive effects. The antiinflammatory effect of steroids is in part the result of inhibiting arachidonic acid metabolism by impairing macrophage migration and by altering neutrophil function. Glucocorticoids also inhibit synthesis of procollagen by fibroblasts, delaying wound contraction. Steroid dependent patients have a persistent decrease in wound tensile strength even after healing is complete. Patients who require chronic systemic steroids have attenuation of the dermis and it is therefore susceptible to injury. Even minor shearing forces may produce tearing of the skin and full thickness wounds due to the decreased tensile strength.

Ischemia

Adequate tissue oxygenation plays a critical role in wound healing.[9] It is needed for aerobic metabolism and also for proper neutrophil function, especially in bacterial killing. It is also a requirement for hydroxylation of proline and lysine to form stable collagen fibrils (Table 3-3).

Smoking. Smoking or nicotine patches inhibit oxygen delivery via sympathomimetic vasoconstriction. Also, smoking elevates carboxyhemoglobin levels in the blood. This shifts the oxygen delivery curve to the left due to the high affinity of carboxyhemoglobin for oxygen, resulting in less available oxygen in the wound. Animal studies demonstrate that even moderate decreases in tissue oxygen tension result in severe impairment of wound healing with substantially increased infection rates. Smoking has been shown to increase wound complication rates when skin flaps are elevated with marginal distal blood supply.

Table 3-3. FACTORS THAT CONTRIBUTE TO WOUND ISCHEMIA

Poor arterial inflow—atherosclerosis
Poor venous flow—venous stasis
Smoking
Radiation
Edema
Diabetes mellitus—accelerates atherosclerosis
Vasculitis
Fibrosis—chronic scarring
Pressure—pressure sores or decubitus ulcers

Radiation. Radiation injury leads to arteriolar fibrosis and impaired oxygen delivery. In addition, there is progressive obliteration of blood vessels in the radiated area over time. Radiation also causes intranuclear and cytoplasmic damage to fibroblasts, and this appears to limit their proliferative potential.

Edema. Edema impairs local oxygen delivery as outlined earlier. Also, edema is often associated with increased venous pressure. This post capillary obstruction decreases the perfusion pressure in the capillary bed, resulting in ischemia. Increased venous pressure also leads to protein extravasation and pericapillary cuffing. This acts as a diffusion barrier to oxygen, further impairing tissue oxygenation and wound healing.

Diabetes. Diabetes mellitus is often associated with decreased healing of open wounds and increased susceptibility to infection. Many factors contribute to poor healing in diabetic patients, and most of these reflect local wound ischemia. However, healing is not impaired in a normally perfused area in a well controlled diabetic patient. This subject is discussed in detail later.

Other Local Conditions

Peripheral arterial occlusive disease secondary to atherosclerosis can be a primary cause of impaired healing, and may also be a cofactor with other conditions discussed. Also, conditions such as vasculitis, prolonged pressure, lower leg venous insufficiency and tissue fibrosis affect wound healing through the mechanism of local tissue ischemia.

Chronic Wound Care

As noted, a chronic wound is commonly defined as an open wound that has failed to respond to standard care and remains open at three months. Typically, the wound size is static with an absence of a visible advancing epithelial edge. The etiology of a chronic wound is often multifactorial. One or more factors that impair wound healing, such as advanced age, ischemia, bacterial contamination, edema, and malnutrition or immunosuppression, are often present in patients with chronic wounds. A systematic approach is needed to identify these factors. Once all of the potentially applicable factors have been identified those amenable to treatment are reversed. While age is fixed, some impact can be made on most other factors. Wounds should be débrided and topical as well as systemic antibiotics given for bacterial infection. Arterial revascularization can increase oxygenation in the wound and elevation and compression dressings can decrease edema. Skin grafting or other surgical procedures are indicated as long as the underlying processes has been identified and is appropriately treated. The underlying causes of some chronic wounds cannot be corrected. Patients with diabetes or venous insufficiency are among these.

Specific chronic wounds are discussed in the sections that follow.

Pressure Sores

Pressure sores are sometimes mistakenly referred to as bed sores or decubitus ulcers. These sores are not always developed in bed or while lying flat in a decubitus position. All pressure sores, regardless of location, do involve prolonged pressure over a bony prominence. The ability of tissue to withstand pressure is defined by the duration of the pressure, the amount of pressure and related sheer forces. The most frequent locations of pressure sores are overlying the ischium, sacrum, and trochanter. The heel, knee, ankle, are less common locations.

The prolonged pressure produces ischemia in the tissue by occluding the microcirculation. This occurs when the tissue pressure exceeds the capillary filling pressure of 25 mmHg. Pressure on the tissue overlying the sacrum can reach 80 mmHg in a recumbent patient, so that tissue necrosis can occur within hours if not relieved by frequent changes in position.

Skin is more resistant to pressure than the underlying subcutaneous fat or muscle. This accounts for the common finding of a small skin ulceration overlying a large area of subcutaneous necrosis. Efforts to identify and control factors that contribute to impaired wound healing should be made. Nutrition is often a problem as is bacterial overgrowth. If the patient can avoid pressure on the involved area and other contributing factors are controlled, most pressure sores will heal. However, there is a higher incidence of recurrence if pressure sores are allowed to heal by secondary intention rather than by surgical closure. This is explained by the increased scarring that occurs in healing by secondary intention. This places a large amount of scar over a known pressure point. Because scars are never as strong as intact skin, they are more prone to breakdown than if intact skin has been placed over these pressure points by surgical closure.

Leg Ulcers

Leg ulcers are perhaps the most common type of chronic ulcer. The underlying disease process is most often local tissue ischemia. The underlying cause of this local tissue ischemia should be identified and appropriate treatment initiated.

About 90% of all leg ulcers in the United States are secondary to venous insufficiency (valvular incompetence). Venous ulcers lead to local tissue ischemia by increased venous pressure, which lowers the transcapillary perfusion pressure, and by leg edema. Initial treatment should be directed to cleansing and débriding the wound of proteinaceous exudate and limiting the edema and protein loss with compression dressings and elevation. A common treatment has been the Unna boot, a paste bandage that is absorptive, that limits edema to some extent, and that can be changed weekly, allowing the physician to totally control treatment with weekly visits. If this dressing is made compressive by adding an elastic wrap, it is highly effective in reducing edema, absorbing the exudate, and providing an occlusive wound environment. Its limitations are that it requires weekly visits and precludes normal showering or bathing. Compression garments or elastic wraps with frequent dressing changes, thorough cleaning, and an occlusive dressing can be equally effective. Surgical treatment of venous insufficiency is addressed elsewhere.

Additional causes of leg ulcers include arterial insufficiency and other vasculitis syndromes. These are treated best by correcting the underlying disease and local wound care. If the underlying problem cannot be treated, there is little hope of securing a stable, healed wound.

Diabetic Foot Ulcers

Diabetic foot ulcers are caused by pressure over bony prominences, usually the metatarsal heads, in the setting of neuropathy. However, there is no evidence to support the often cited concept that these ulcers may result from small vessel disease. This theory originated with a nonblinded study of the microvasculation in amputation specimens by Goldenberg in 1959. Subsequent blinded studies have failed to reveal any architectural differences in small blood vessels of diabetic amputation specimens. The ischemia in diabetic foot ulcers is most likely due to prolonged pressure on insensate toes and feet. This pressure ischemia is enhanced by the increase in blood viscosity related to nondeforming erythrocytes, which develop because of nonenzymatic glycosylation of cell membrane proteins. These rigid red blood cells plug capillary beds and decrease microvascular flow. In addition, the glycosylated hemoglobin has increased affinity for oxygen, thereby making less oxygen available to the tissues. Diabetic patients also have a predilection for infrapopliteal arterial occlusive disease and may therefore benefit from arterial reconstructive surgery. In addition, the requirements for successful treatment of diabetic ulcers include pressure relief with non−weight-bearing strategies and aggressive débridement of callus and marginally vascularized wound edges. Preventive measures with appropriate orthotic shoes are essential once healing is achieved.

Agents to Optimize Wound Healing

Dressings

Many types of dressings are commercially available, but none has been demonstrated to accelerate healing over standard care, despite marketing claims.

The ideal dressing should be simple, inexpensive, highly absorptive, and nonadherent. It should achieve moist healing and have antibacterial properties. Other factors to be considered are less frequent dressing changes, an all-in-one dressing that does not require tape or an overlay, and a gentle adhesive that is effective but not injurious to the skin when removed.[10]

The simplest dressing is gauze and tape—it is inexpensive, is absorptive, and when used with an antibacterial ointment, can achieve moist healing. The primary disadvantages are the necessity for frequent dressing changes and the potential for tape irritation and wound desiccation. Other products are classified into films, foams, hydrocolloids, hydrogels, and absorptive powders (Table 3-4). Films are semipermeable to water, generally made of polyurethane, and nonabsorptive. These are useful to achieve a moist wound healing environment over minimally exudative wounds, such as a split-thickness skin graft donor site.

Other dressing types have been designed to increase the absorptive capacity of the dressing. This requires fewer dressing changes and maintains an environment for moist healing.

The hydrocolloids deserve special mention because they have achieved widespread use. These contain hydrophilic materials, such as quar, karaya, gelatin, or carboxymethylcelluose, with an adhesive material and are covered by a semipermeable polyurethane film. The material adheres to the skin surrounding a wound, is highly absorptive, and achieves a moist healing environment. Adhesion is maintained until the absorptive capacity is exhausted, and then atraumatic removal is easily done. Similar materials have

Table 3-4. WOUND DRESSINGS

Classification	Composition	Indications	Functions	Examples
Films	Semiocclusive (semipermeable)— polyurethane or copolyester	Acute partial- or full-thickness wounds with minimal exudate Nondraining primarily closed wounds	Mimics skin performance Is water vapor permeable Is water and bacteria impermeable Is retention dressing for gel Is retention dressing for tubes Provides moist environment	Op-site Bioclusive Tegaderm Blisterfilm Visulin
Hydrocolloids	Contain hydrophilic colloidal particles (quar, karaya, gelatic, carboxymethl cellulose) in an adhesive mass (usually polysorbutylene)	Acute or chronic partial- or full-thickness wounds Stage I to IV decubitus ulcers	Absorbs fluid Débrides soft necrotic tissue by autolysis Protects wounds Provides good adhesiveness without adherence to wound Encourages granulation Promotes reepithelialization Protects wounds from trauma	Cutinova Hydro Duoderm Comfeel Restore Intrasite Ultec J&J ulcer dressing
Hydrogels	Contain 80%–99% water Cross-linked polymer such as polyethyleneoxide, polyvinyl pyrrolidone, or acrylamide	Acute or chronic partial-thickness wound with minimal exudate	Creates moist environment Usually requires secondary dressing Has low absorbancy Débrides minimally Decreases pain Does not adhere to wound	Vigilon Geliperm Elastogel Intrasite gel
Foams	Either hydrophilic or hydrophobic Nonocclusive Usually polyurethane or gel film–coated High absorbency	Acute or chronic partial-thickness wounds that are highly secreting and require mechanical débriding	Débrides Has high absorbancy Water vapor permeable	Cutinova Plus Lyofoam Allevyn
Impregnates	Fine mesh gauze impregnated with either moisturizing, antibacterial, or bactericidal compounds Nonadherent	Acute or chronic partial-thickness wounds with minimal to moderate exudate	Does not adhere to wound Promotes reepithelialization May contain antibacterial or bactericidal agents Requires secondary dressing	Aquaphor-Gauze Adaptic Biobrane Scarlet Red
Absorptive powders and pastes	Consist of starch, copolymers, or colloidal hydrophilic particles Can absorb up to 100 times their weight in fluid	Chronic full-thickness wounds with large amounts of exudate	Has high absorbancy Débrides necrotic and fibrous material from wound	Spand-Gel Geliperm Envisan paste Bard absorption dressing Duoderm granules Hydrogran Hollister Exudate Absorber

(Compiled by M.C. Crossland, RN, Wound Healing Center, Medical College of Virginia, Richmond)

been extensively used for peristomal care. These are best used for open wounds that have only moderate exudate.

The increased absorptive capacity of these products allows infrequent, minimally traumatic dressing changes. Increased absorptive capacity, ease of use, and achievement of moist healing are their principal advantages.

Antibiotics

The role of antibiotics in wound care is controversial. All open wounds are colonized with bacteria. Only when the surrounding tissue is invaded (cellulitis) are systemic antibiotics clearly indicated. Antibiotics may be useful in other situations, such as when the granulation tissue has

a high bacterial count, or in a case of reduced resistance to bacteria, such as in a diabetic foot ulcer, but these situations are not clearly defined. The routine use of systemic antibiotics for chronic wounds should be avoided to reduce the development of resistant bacterial strains within the wound.

Topical antibiotics are frequently used and can be useful. The ointment vehicle may help keep the wound moist, and the bacteria count in a wound may be lowered as a result. With most antibiotics, however, resistant organisms emerge quickly. The expense is substantial, and the benefits are not well demonstrated. Silver sulfadiazine, frequently used for burn care, is also useful for chronic wounds. Its broad spectrum of activity, the lack of relevant drug-resistant plasmids in bacterial, and its low cost make it a good choice.

Débriding Agents

Collagenases have been used to débride wounds for 20 years and can be a highly effective adjunct in the treatment of chronic wounds with necrotic tissue. These agents are used after surgical débridement to help clean a wound and to avoid a painful mechanical débridement. Collagenases that are combined with antibiotic powder have been proposed as a useful treatment for chronic wounds.

Pharmacologic Agents

No approved clinical agents accelerate normal healing. Growth factors found naturally in wounds have improved healing in both normal and complex animal wounds (Table 3-5). The growth factors with the most evidence for efficacy are PDGF, TGF-β, epidermal growth factor, and members of the fibroblast growth factor family; although insulin-like growth factor 1, IL-1, IL-2, granulocyte-macrophage colony-stimulating factor, and vascular endothelial cell growth factor have also shown improved rates of healing in animal models.[11,12] Clinical trials are in progress, and no agent has yet been approved by the Food and Drug Administration, although PDGF is in advanced trials. PDGF has shown efficacy in accelerating healing for patients with pressure sores, and in increasing the percentage of healing wounds in patients with diabetic ulcers. A limiting factor in these clinical trials has been the variability in patients, in terms of both systemic factors that impact healing and the number of variables in the wounds. The clinical studies are therefore difficult to perform and interpret.

Growth hormone deserves brief mention because it has been used successfully in some situations to reverse the catabolic impact of many severe injuries. Wound healing is a fundamentally anabolic event (creating new tissue), and in the setting of a severe burn, growth hormone administration significantly accelerates donor site healing, presumably because of its effects in minimizing catabolism.

EXCESSIVE SCARRING

Many factors are involved in the formation of an ideal scar. The most important of these are as follows:

- Accurate alignment of sharply incised tissue parallel to the natural lines of resting skin tension
- Closure of the wound without tension on the epidermis and without underlying dead space
- Primary healing without complications such as infection or dehiscence

The patient's genetic makeup and the location of the wound on the body are also important factors. The more negative the factors associated with a particular wound, the more likely it will form a scar that is less than ideal. From an evolutional viewpoint, wound healing has been programmed to be rapid and exuberant to minimize the problems of an open wound. As part of the aging process, the proliferative phase of wound healing becomes less exuberant, and although wound healing is slower, scars are improved.

The distinctions between an unsightly scar, a hypertrophic scar, and a true keloid can be confusing. An accurate diagnosis of most scars can be made by clinical observation and the history of the lesion.

Keloids

True keloids are uncommon and occur predominantly in dark-skinned people with a genetic predisposition for keloid formation.[13] In most cases, the gene appears to be transmitted in an autosomal dominant pattern. The primary difference between a keloid and a hypertrophic scar is that a keloid extends beyond the boundary of the original tissue injury. It behaves as a benign tumor and extends into or invades the normal surrounding tissue. This creates a scar that is larger than the original wound.

Histologically, keloids contain an overabundance of collagen. The absolute number of fibroblasts is not increased, but the production of collagen continually outpaces the activity of collagenase, resulting in a scar of ever-increasing dimensions. The cause of keloid formation is unknown. Immunoglobulin G levels are increased, which suggests possible autoimmune stimulation resulting in a chronic inflammatory response with continued collagen deposition.

The treatment of keloids is difficult: The cause is unknown, and the underlying disorder is not resolved by any specific therapy. Some improvement is usually seen with excision followed by intralesional steroid injection.[14] In unresponsive cases, excision followed by a short course of radiotherapy has been successful, but the resulting scar is unpredictable and potentially worse. Keloids typically develop several months after injury and rarely, if ever, subside. Although many therapies have been tried, with anecdotal reports of success, none is ideal.[15]

Table 3-5. SELECTED GROWTH FACTORS RELEVANT TO WOUND HEALING

Factor	Source	Target	Function
TGF-β	All cells	All cells	Fibrosis Proliferation
TGF-α	Platelets Keratinocytes Macrophages	Epithelial cells Fibroblasts Endothelial cells	Proliferation
PDGF	Platelets Macrophages Fibroblasts Endothelial cells Smooth muscle cells	Neutrophils Macrophages Fibroblasts Smooth muscle cells	Chemotaxis Proliferation Collagenase synthesis
FGF	Macrophages Fibroblasts Endothelial cells	Endothelial cells Epithelial cells Fibroblasts Chondroblasts	Proliferation Chemotaxis Angiogenesis
EGF	Platelets Macrophages Keratinocytes	Epithelial cells Endothelial cells Fibroblasts	Proliferation Chemotaxis
IGF-I/Sm-C	Fibroblasts	Fibroblasts Endothelial cells	Cell replication Collagen synthesis
IL-1	Macrophages	Fibroblasts Neutrophils	Proliferation Collagenase synthesis Chemotaxis

TFG-β, transforming growth factor β; TGF-α, transforming growth factor α; PDGF, platelet-derived growth factor; FGF, fibroblast growth factor; EGF, epidermal growth factor; IGF-I/Sm-C, insulin-like growth factor I/somatomedin C; IL-1, interleukin-1.

Hypertrophic Scars

Hypertrophic scars are histologically similar to keloids. They contain an overabundance of dermal collagen. Hypertrophic scars, however, respect the boundaries of the original injury and do not extend into normal unwounded tissue. They have less genetic predisposition, but hypertrophic scars also occur more frequently in Asians and blacks. They are often seen on the upper torso and across flexor surfaces. They usually develop within the first month after wounding and often subside gradually.

Improvement of hypertrophic scars may be obtained with pressure garments, topical silicone sheeting applications, or reexcision and closure.[16] Reexcision and closure should be considered if conditions of the closure can be improved. This is especially true for wounds that originally healed by secondary intention or were complicated by infection. Simple reexcision and closure is unlikely to improve a scar that was closed with proper alignment and that healed primarily without complications.[17]

Unsightly Scars

A wound that is closed under tension or without adequate or accurate alignment, or a wound that runs across the lines of natural skin tension, is often unsightly. Surgical excision and closure with attention directed to correcting the underlying cause of the unsightly scar usually results in improvement.

FETAL WOUND HEALING

Much interest and research have focused on the process of fetal wound healing. It has been demonstrated that humans and several other mammalian species undergo fetal skin healing with little or no scar if the injury occurs early enough during gestation.[18,19]

The physiologic mechanisms involved in scarless fetal healing are under active investigation. Adult wounds heal with a significant inflammatory response followed by abundant collagen deposition and remodeling into a mature scar. Numerous studies have shown that fetal wounds heal with little or no inflammation and no excess collagen formation. The fetal wound matrix is also higher in hyaluronic acid than the adult wound. This substance is seen only early in adult healing. Amniotic fluid is rich in hyaluronic acid and may provide the hyaluronic acid found in the fetal wound. Experiments that have exposed adult skin to amniotic fluid, however, demonstrate adult-type healing with scar formation.

Clearly, the fetal wound differs from the adult wound in several ways. The scarless healing appears multifactorial. Further research may identify factors (ie, growth factors) that can be applied to wounds to diminish scar formation. This has potentially important application in virtually all of surgery.

REFERENCES

1. Leibovich SJ, Ross R. The role of the macrophage in wound repair: a study with hydrocortisone and antimacrophage serum. Am J Pathol 1975;78:71.
2. Madden JW, Peacock EE. Studies on the biology of collagen during wound healing. I. Rate of collagen synthesis and deposition in cutaneous wounds of the rat. Surgery 1968;64:288.
3. Peacock EE Jr. Wound repair, ed 3. Philadelphia, WB Saunders, 1984.
4. Winter GD, Scales JT. Effect of air drying and dressings on the surface of a wound. Nature 1963;197:91.
5. Jonsson K, Jensen JA, Goodson WH, et al. Tissue oxygenation,

anemia, and perfusion in relation to wound healing in surgical patients. Ann Surg 1991;214:6.
6. Gross A, Cutright DE, Bhaskar SN. Effectiveness of pulsating water jet lavage in treatment of contaminated crushed wounds. Am J Surg 1972;124:373.
7. Seifter E, Rettura G, Padawer J, et al. Impaired wound healing in streptozotocin diabetes: prevention by supplemental vitamin A. Ann Surg 1981;194:42.
8. Ehrlich P, Tarver H, Hunt TK. Inhibitory effect of vitamin E on collagen synthesis and wound repair. Ann Surg 1972;175:235.
9. LaVan FB, Hunt TK. Oxygen and wound healing. Clin Plast Surg 1990;17:463.
10. Carver N, Leigh IM. Synthetic dressings. Int J Dermatol 1992;31:10.
11. Mustoe TA, Pierce GF, Thomason A, et al. Accelerated healing of incisional wounds in rats induced by transforming growth factor-β. Science 1987;237:1333.
12. Brown GL, Nanney LB, Griffen J, et al. Enhancement of wound healing by topical treatment with epidermal growth factor. N Engl J Med 1989;321:76.
13. Rockwell WB, Cohen IK, Enrlich HP. Keloids and hypertrophic scars: a comprehensive review. Plast Reconstr Surg 1989;84:827.
14. Griffith H. The treatment of keloids with triamcinolone acetonide. Plast Reconstr Surg 1966;38:202.
15. Lawrence WT. In search of the optimal treatment of keloids: report of a series and a review of the literature. Ann Plast Surg 1991;27:164.
16. Ahn ST, Monafo WW, Mustoe TA. Topical silicone gel: a new treatment for hypertrophic scars. Surgery 1989;106:781.
17. Khouri RK, Mustoe TA. Trends in the treatment of hypertrophic scars. Adv Plast Reconstr Surg 1991;8.
18. Mast BA, Diegelmann RF, Krummel TM, et al. Scarless wound healing in the mammalian fetus. Surg Gynecol Obstet 1992;174:441.
19. Siebert JW, Burd AR, McCarthy JG, et al. Fetal wound healing: a biochemical study of scarless healing. Plast Reconstr Surg 1990;85:503.

SURGERY: SCIENTIFIC PRINCIPLES AND PRACTICE, Second Edition, edited by Lazar J. Greenfield, Michael W. Mulholland, Keith T. Oldham, Gerald B. Zelenock, and Keith D. Lillemoe. Lippincott–Raven Publishers, Philadelphia, © 1997.

CHAPTER 4

HEMOSTASIS

THOMAS W. WAKEFIELD

BASIC CONSIDERATIONS

The coagulation mechanism is a dynamic interactive network that relies on the interaction between platelets and coagulation complexes for clot formation. Initiating agents for coagulation include collagen and tissue factor. Tissue factor, released from injured cells, activates the extrinsic pathway of coagulation. Disruption of the endothelium of blood vessels exposes underlying collagen to platelets, activating them. In the blood, tissue factor complexes with activated factor VII, activating factors IX and X to factors IXa and Xa (activated factors IX and X).[1] The enzyme responsible for the initial activation of factor VII is unknown. However, factors Xa and VIIa catalyze activation of factor VII, so there is amplification for the formation of factor VIIa.[2] At the same time, activated platelets spread in shape with their procoagulant phospholipid (platelet factor 3), becoming externalized. This allows for the coagulation proteins to assemble on the surfaces of platelets,

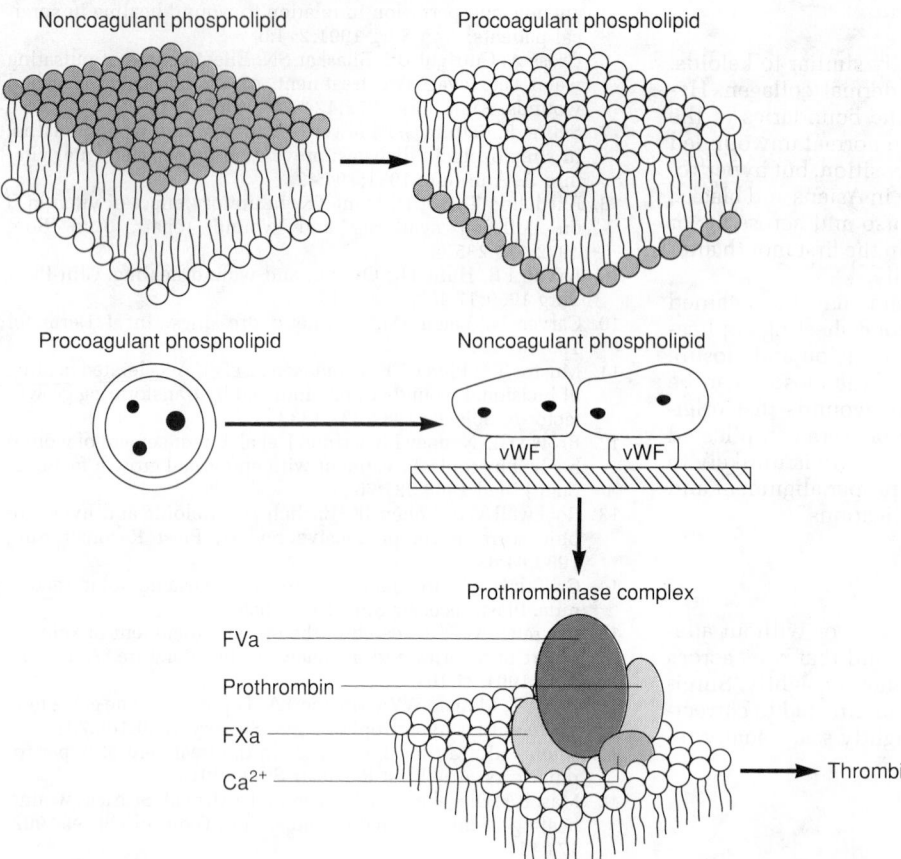

Noncoagulant phospholipid   Procoagulant phospholipid

Procoagulant phospholipid   Noncoagulant phospholipid

vWF   vWF

Prothrombinase complex

FVa

Prothrombin

FXa

Ca^{2+}

Thrombin

Figure 4-1. Formation of coagulation cascade assembly on the platelet phospholipid surface. (After Hassouna HI. Laboratory evaluation of hemostatic disorders. In: Penner JA, Hassouna HI, eds. Coagulation disorders II. Hematol Oncol Clin North Am 1993;7:1188)

accelerating the coagulation reactions[3] (Fig. 4-1). Platelet membranes contribute critical surfaces for coagulation complex assembly. Activated but not resting platelets express binding sites for coagulation factors. During platelet activation in vitro, microparticles are released that are rich in receptors for factors Va and VIIIa.[4,5] Von Willebrand factor (vWF) is responsible for platelet adhesion through binding to glycoprotein (Gp) Ib,[6] whereas fibrinogen forms bridges between activated platelets by binding to Gp IIb/IIIa on adjacent stimulated platelets.[7] Unstimulated platelets attach to immobilized fibrinogen by the same receptor.[8]

Once the platelet plug has formed, the stage is set for coagulation protein assembly. Activated factor X (Xa), activated factor V (Va), ionized calcium, and factor II (prothrombin) form on the platelet phospholipid surface to initiate the prothrombinase complex, which catalyzes the formation of thrombin faster than can be achieved with factor Xa alone[3] (Fig. 4-2). When the amount of tissue factor is limited, activation of factor IX rather than factor X is favored,[9,10] allowing for tissue factor activation in situations of low tissue factor concentration. The pathway so described up to this point corresponds to the classic extrinsic pathway of coagulation. Thrombin is central to all of coagulation and acts to cleave fibrinopeptide A (FPA) from the α chain of fibrinogen and fibrinopeptide B (FPB) from the β chain.[11] This leads to the release of fibrinopeptides and the formation of new fibrin monomers, which then cross-link, resulting in fibrin polymerization. Thrombin also activates factor XIII, which catalyzes the cross-linking of fibrin to make the clot firm,[12] activates platelets, and activates factors V and factors VIII, two nonenzymatic cofactors, to factors Va and VIIIa.[3] This is important because only factors Va and VIIIa are involved in coagulation. Fac-

tor XIIIa also cross-links other plasma proteins, such as fibronectin and α_2-antitrypsin, resulting in their incorporation into clot.[13]

The intrinsic pathway of blood coagulation requires activation of factor XI to XIa. This may occur by both the contact activation system through activation of factor XII, plasma prekallikrein, and high-molecular-weight kininogen, and more importantly through thrombin with negatively charged surfaces.[14] Factor XIa activates factor XI in an autocatalytic nature[14] and also catalyzes the conversion of factor IX to IXa.[15] Factor IXa, X, ionized calcium, and thrombin-activated factor VIII (VIIIa) then assemble on the platelet surface in a complex called the *Xase complex* to catalyze the activation of factor X to Xa[3] (see Fig. 4-2). Factor Xa then shunts into the prothrombinase complex for further amplification of thrombin formation. The importance of a mechanism of factor XI activation independent of the contact activation system is apparent because patients deficient in those factors of the contact activation system, including factor XI, bleed, whereas patients deficient in factor XII, prekallikrein, and high-molecular-weight kininogen do not usually bleed.[13]

NATURAL ANTICOAGULANT MECHANISMS

At the same time that thrombin forms, natural anticoagulant mechanisms oppose further thrombin formation. Just as thrombin generation is key to coagulation, antithrombin III is the most central anticoagulant protein. This glycoprotein of 70,000 MW binds to thrombin, preventing the removal of FPA and FPB from fibrinogen,[16] preventing the activation of factors V and VIII, and inhibiting the activa-

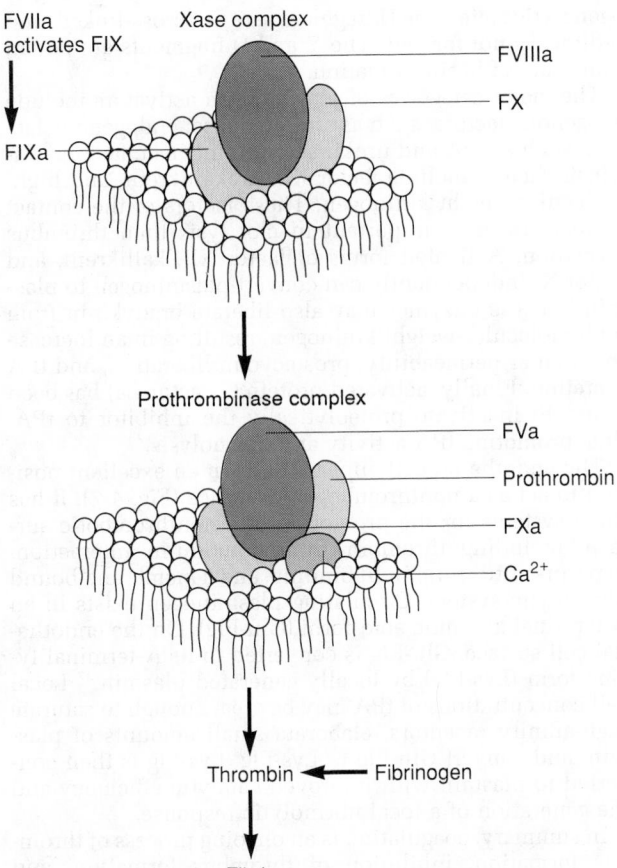

Figure 4-2. Formation of the Xase complex and prothrombinase complex with amplification of thrombin and fibrin formation (After Hassouna HI. Laboratory evaluation of hemostatic disorders. In: Penner JA, Hassouna HI, eds. Coagulation disorders II. Hematol Oncol Clin North Am 1993;7:1177)

tion and aggregation of platelets. In addition, antithrombin III inhibits factors IXa,[17] Xa, and XIa.[18] A second natural anticoagulant is activated protein C, which inactivates factors Va[19,20] and VIIIa,[21] thus reducing the Xase and prothrombinase complex acceleration of the rate of thrombin formation. In the circulation, protein C is activated to protein Ca on endothelial cell surfaces by thrombin complexed with one of its receptors, thrombomodulin[22–24] (Fig. 4-3), in a one to one complex,[25] highlighting another important role for thrombin. The formation of this thrombin–thrombomodulin complex accelerates the activation of protein C as compared with thrombin alone. Thrombin at the same time, by binding to thrombomodulin, loses its platelet-activating activity[26] as well as its enzymatic activity on fibrinogen and factor V.[27] Protein S is a cofactor for protein Ca[28] (Fig. 4-4). A third natural anticoagulant is heparin cofactor II.[29] Its concentration in plasma is estimated to be significantly less than antithrombin III, and its action is implicated primarily in the regulation of thrombin formation in extravascular tissues. Finally, thrombin is inactivated when it becomes incorporated into the clot.

The extrinsic pathway is short-lived owing to an inhibitor called the *lipoprotein-associated coagulation inhibitor*,[30] or *extrinsic pathway inhibitor*.[31] This protein inactivates the tissue factor–factor VIIa complex activation of factor X to Xa, but not of factor IX to IXa.[13] This inhibitor has also been termed *tissue factor pathway inhibitor*.

FIBRINOLYSIS

During the process of thrombus formation, there is a constant process of clot lysis, which prevents physiologic thrombus formation from leading to pathologic intravascular thrombosis. Plasminogen, tissue plasminogen activator (tPA), and α_2-antiplasmin (α_2-AP) become incorporated into the fibrin clot as it forms[3] (Fig. 4-5). In fact, thrombin (both α and γ) promotes tPA release from endothelial cells as well as the production of plasminogen activator inhibitor (PAI-1) from endothelial cells.[32,33] tPA converts plasminogen to plasmin, the main fibrinolytic enzyme. This is a serine protease whose main substrates include fibrin, fibrinogen, and other coagulation factors. Plasmin also interferes with platelet adhesion through vWF by proteolysis of Gp Ib.[34] Fibrin, when digested by plasmin, yields one molecule of fragment E and two molecules of fragment D. In physiologic clot formation, fragment D is released in dimeric form (D-dimer).[3] The D-dimer fragment is a marker

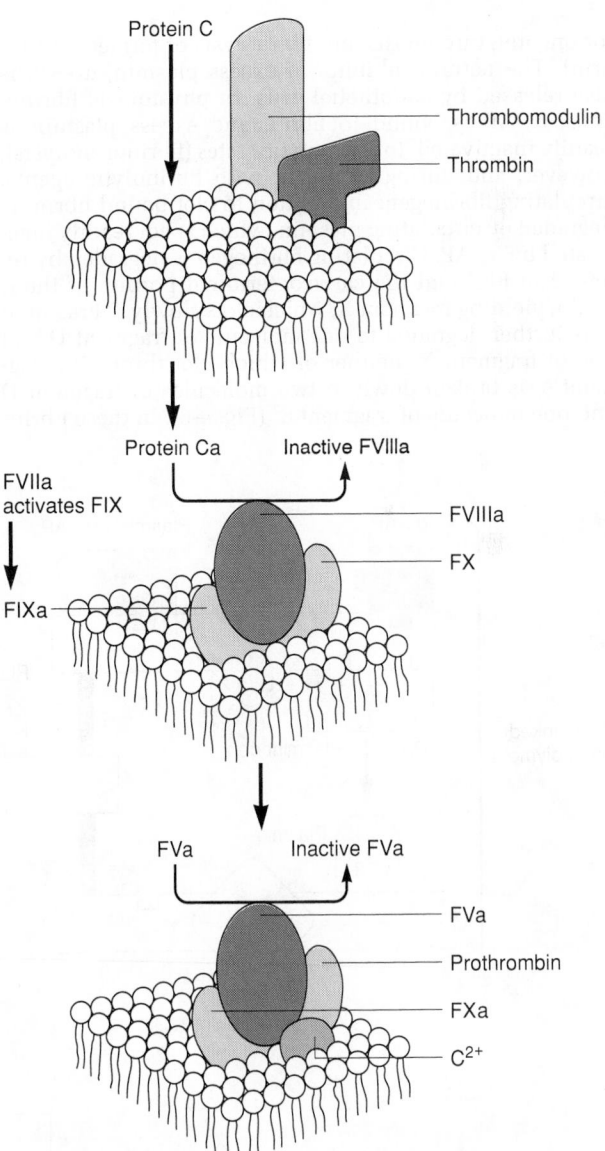

Figure 4-3. Activation of protein C by thrombin–thrombomodulin interaction. (After Hassouna HI. Laboratory evaluation of hemostatic disorders. In: Penner JA, Hassouna HI, eds. Coagulation disorders II. Hematol Oncol Clin North Am 1993;7:1175)

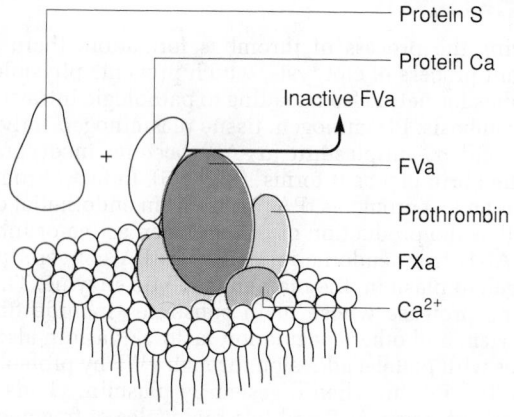

Figure 4-4. Actions of protein S. (After Hassouna HI. Laboratory evaluation of hemostatic disorders. In: Penner JA, Hassouna HI, eds. Coagulation disorders II. Hematol Oncol Clin North Am 1993;7:1176)

for ongoing thrombosis and fibrinolysis of formed clot (fibrin). The natural inhibitor of excess plasmin, α_2-AP, is also released by endothelial cells. In physiologic fibrinolysis, α_2-AP is bound to fibrin, and excess plasmin is readily inactivated. In fibrinolytic states (fibrinogenolysis), however, and during treatment with fibrinolytic agents, circulating fibrinogen, in addition to clot bound fibrin, is degraded by circulating plasmin, which is not readily inactivated by α_2-AP. Circulating fibrinogen is degraded by removal of FPB and the carboxy-terminal portion of the α chain, yielding fragment X, which clots slowly.[35] Fragment X is further degraded to one molecule of fragment D and one of fragment Y, neither of which clot thrombin; fragment Y is broken down to two molecules of fragment D and one molecule of fragment E[3] (Fig. 4-6). In these fibrin-ogenolytic states, the D fragments are not cross-linked, and D-dimer is not formed. The Y and D fragments are potent inhibitors of fibrin formation.

The major categories of plasminogen activators include exogenous factors, such as streptokinase; endogenous factors, such as tPA and urokinase; and intrinsic factors.[3] Intrinsic factors include factor XII, prekallikrein, and high-molecular-weight kininogen. These factors of the contact system are more important in clot lysis than thrombus formation. Activated forms of factor XII, kallikrein, and factor XI independently can convert plasminogen to plasmin.[36] These enzymes may also liberate bradykinin from high-molecular-weight kininogen, resulting in an increase in vascular permeability, prostacyclin liberation, and tPA secretion. Finally, activated protein C (factor Ca) has been found to inactivate proteolytically the inhibitor to tPA, thus promoting tPA activity and fibrinolysis.[25]

The endothelial cell appears to be in an excellent position to act as a nonthrombogenic surface (Fig. 4-7). It has three systems for the promotion of a nonthrombotic surface, including thrombin–thrombomodulin interaction, heparin–antithrombin III binding, and a membrane-bound fibrinolytic system. Circulating plasminogen exists in an N-terminal glutamic acid form (Glu-Plg). On the endothelial cell surface, Glu-Plg is converted to its N-terminal lysine form (Lys-Plg) by locally generated plasmin.[37] Local cell concentrations of tPA may be great enough to saturate high-affinity receptors, elaborate small amounts of plasmin, and convert Glu-Plg to Lys-Plg. Lys-Plg is then converted to plasmin with improved catalytic efficiency and the generation of a local fibrinolytic response.

In summary, coagulation is an ongoing process of thrombus formation, inhibition of thrombus formation, and thrombus dissolution. The central mediator is thrombin[3] (Fig. 4-8). Abnormalities in coagulation occur when one process, either thrombus formation, thrombus inhibition, or fibrinolysis, overcomes the others and dominates the delicate balance that is hemostasis.

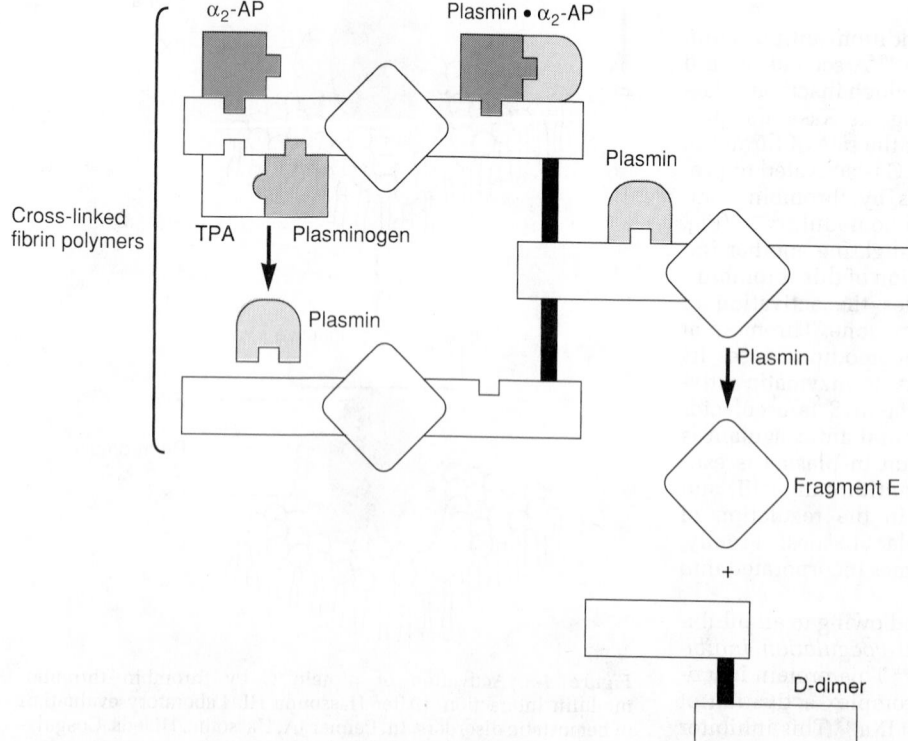

Figure 4-5. Incorporation of plasminogen, tissue plasminogen activator (TPA), and α_2-antiplasmin (α_2-AP) into the fibrin clot as it forms with production of D-dimer fragments. (After Hassouna HI. Laboratory evaluation of hemostatic disorders. In: Penner JA, Hassouna HI, eds. Coagulation disorders II. Hematol Oncol Clin North Am 1993;7:1186)

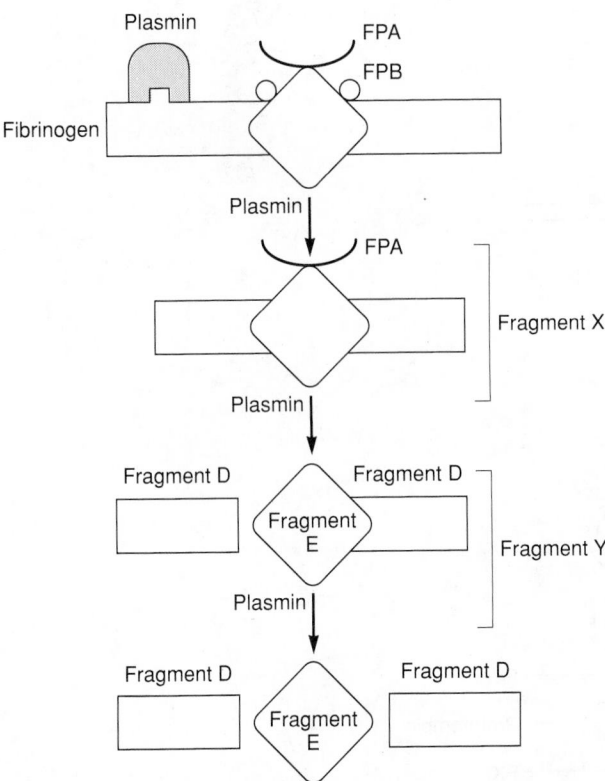

Figure 4-6. Process of fibrinogenolysis and formation of non–cross-linked fragments D. (After Hassouna HI. Laboratory evaluation of hemostatic disorders. In: Penner JA, Hassouna HI, eds. Coagulation disorders II. Hematol Oncol Clin North Am 1993;7:1193)

THROMBOSIS AND INFLAMMATION

Thrombosis and inflammation are closely linked. Tumor necrosis factor (TNF), a polypeptide cytokine of stimulated macrophages released in response to inflammation and sepsis, down-regulates thrombomodulin expression through endocytosis and degradation of thrombomodulin.[38] TNF increases the level of C4b-binding protein, decreasing the amount of free protein S available to function as a cofactor for protein C. Additionally, TNF induces tissue factor expression on the surface of endothelial cells. In a study of six normal human volunteers given TNF, factor X was activated to Xa early after administration, followed by prothrombin activation in a more gradual pattern of increase observed hours after maximal concentrations of factor Xa had been reached.[39] TNF also inhibits fibrinolysis by suppressing the release of tPA and inducing the expression of tPA inhibitor type I.[40-45] In vivo, TNF initially increases plasma plasminogen activator activity, followed by an even greater increase in PAI-1 antigen, leading to an overall inhibition of the fibrinolytic system.[46] Additionally, by down-regulating thrombomodulin, TNF decreases protein C production. Because protein C inhibits PAI, a decrease in protein C decreases the fibrinolytic potential of the blood. Along with its effects on coagulation, TNF facilitates inflammation. TNF and other cytokines stimulate adherence proteins on endothelial cells[47–50] for leukocytes and induce endothelial and vascular wall smooth muscle cell production of interleukin-8 (IL-8) gene expression and monocyte chemotactic protein 1 mRNA expression.[51] These cytokines activate neutrophils in vitro and stimulate neutrophil and monocyte movement in vivo. They are also in-

volved in the process of cytokine networking in which one cytokine activates other cytokines, producing a physiologic response. The association between TNF and activation of both the coagulation and inflammatory pathways has been firmly established.

A model for the possible interactions between thrombosis and inflammation has been proposed[52] (Fig. 4-9). In this model, vascular injury results in the margination of circulating platelets along the vessel wall, probably mediated by vWF binding to Gp Ib on the platelet surface. The platelets then activate and aggregate in an interaction mediated by fibrinogen, resulting in platelet plug formation. Blood clotting is stimulated by the expression of tissue factor, and the clotting complexes are propagated on the phospholipid surfaces of activated platelets, resulting in the formation of a fibrin clot. Circulating neutrophils and monocytes then interact with the platelets through P-selectin and with the endothelial cells through P-selectin and E-selectin, events that result in the stable interaction between leukocytes and platelets at the thrombus–wall interface. Neutrophils and monocytes participate in this local inflammatory response, and monocytes may specifically contribute to clot formation by further tissue factor expression on their surfaces. This has been suggested in a study involving fibrin formation under the influence of a monoclonal antibody to P-selectin in a primate arteriovenous fistula model.[53]

In the venous circulation, a series of steps linking thrombosis and inflammation has been suggested.[54] In step 1, thrombus formation involving platelets, neutrophils, and monocytes is initiated at venous confluences, saccules, and valve pockets. In step 2, adherent neutrophils and platelets become activated, releasing substances such as ADP (platelets) and neutrophil-activating peptide 2 (NAP-2; platelets and neutrophils), activating and attracting more platelets and neutrophils. Cathepsin G, secreted from activated neutrophils, converts β-thromboglobulin (secreted from platelets) into NAP-2 by proteolytic cleavage.[55] This NAP-2 stimulates more cathepsin G secretion, which in turn stimulates more platelet secretion,[56,57] providing more substrate for NAP-2 and causing feedback activation for the recruitment of more platelets and neutrophils. In step 3, coagulation is initiated and promoted on the phospholipid surface of the platelets. Finally, in step 4, new layers of neutrophils and platelets form on the surface of fibrin, activate, and begin another round of the clotting process. Leukocytes extravasate into the vein wall by a chemotactic gradient that develops in the wall in response to venous thrombosis. In a baboon model of deep venous thrombosis (DVT) induced by stasis, the presence of a venous catheter for a short time, and the administration of the thrombogenic reagents TNF and antibody to protein C, we have observed by enzyme-linked immunosorbent assay

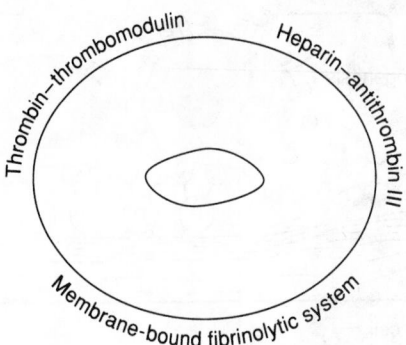

Figure 4-7. Vessel wall endothelial cell antithrombotic properties.

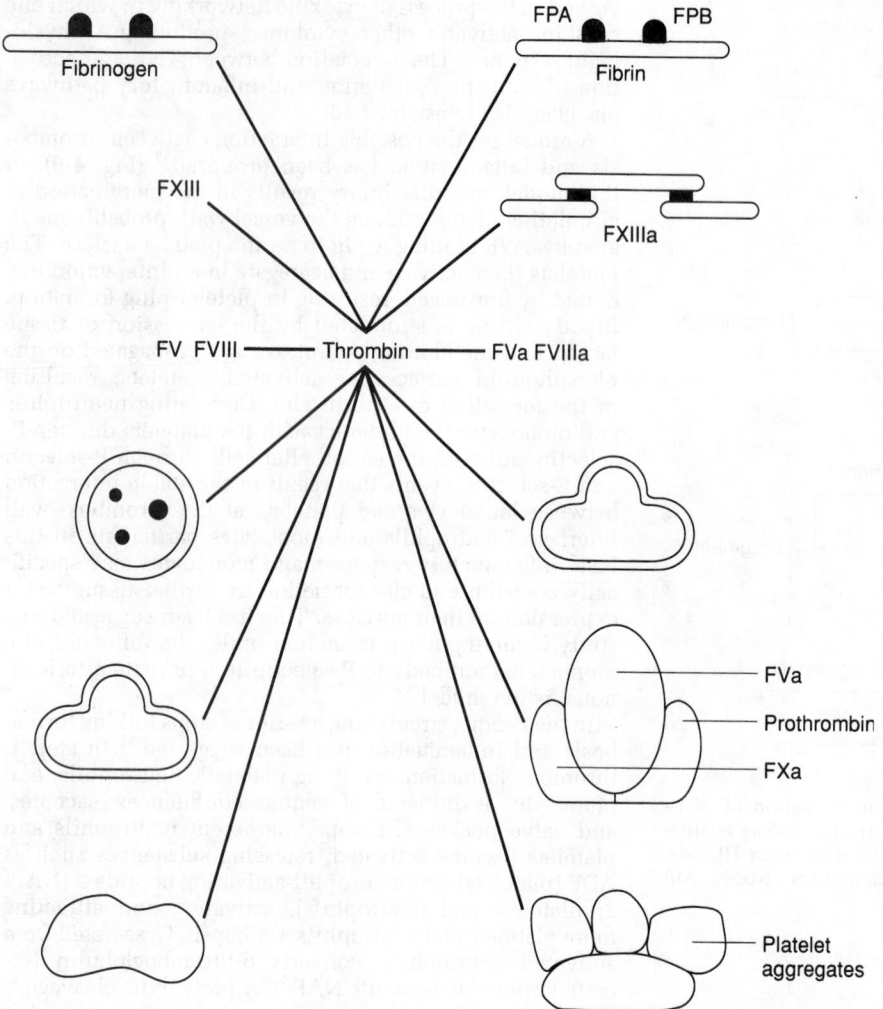

Figure 4-8. Thrombin as the central mediator of coagulation. (After Hassouna HI. Laboratory evaluation of hemostatic disorders. In: Penner JA, Hassouna HI, eds. Coagulation disorders II. Hematol Oncol Clin North Am 1993;7:1177)

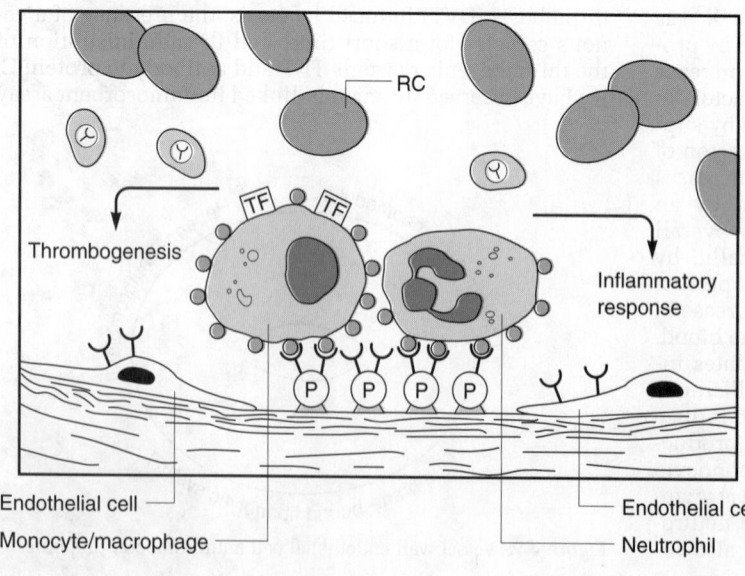

Figure 4-9. Cellular basis for blood coagulation, including platelets (P), neutrophils, monocytes, P-selectin (Y), and red blood cells (RC). (After Furie B, Furie BC. Molecular and cellular biology of blood coagulation. N Engl J Med 1992;326:803)

(ELISA) protein measurements and immunohistochemical tissue staining the presence of inflammatory cytokines in the vein wall directly beneath the luminal thrombus, including IL-8, IL-6, monocyte chemotactic protein 1, ENA-78, and MIP-1a.[58] We have similarly observed in a pure stasis model of inferior venal caval thrombosis in both primates and rats a similar occurrence in the vein wall with the early influx of neutrophils followed by the later extravasation of monocytes, macrophages, and lymphocytes in a typical inflammatory progression. This suggests that the sequence may lead to a complete inflammatory response in the vein wall. Further research to block the inflammatory response and the subsequent effect this interference may have on the detrimental interactions between the thrombus and the vein wall and valves may have significant implications for treatment of venous thrombosis. Approaches to interfere with the inflammatory response include blocking initial leukocyte adhesion, blocking leukocyte activation, or both.

PROCOAGULANT STATES

A number of conditions can lead to a procoagulant state, including heparin-associated thrombocytopenia, antithrombin III deficiency, protein C and S deficiencies, resistance to activated protein C, lupus anticoagulant and the presence of antiphospholipid antibodies, fibrinogen abnormalities, defective fibrinolytic activity, platelet abnormalities, disseminated intravascular coagulation (DIC), and other less common conditions, such as hyperhomocysteinemia and elevations in lipoprotein a.

Heparin-Associated Thrombocytopenia

Heparin-associated thrombocytopenia occurs in 0.6% to 30% of patients who receive heparin, although severe thrombocytopenia (platelet counts less than 100,000) is seen much less frequently.[59] It is caused by a plasma factor, most likely a heparin-dependent immunoglobulin G (IgG) platelet antibody, that causes platelet aggregation when exposed to heparin. The antibody may not be heparin specific, the main contributing mechanism being the degree of sulfonation of the heparin-like compound,[60] and the actual platelet aggregation is likely dependent on the Fc region of the antibody.[61] Activation of platelets in this setting can result in thrombocytopenia, thrombosis, and embolic episodes. Morbidity and mortality rates as high as 61% and 23%, respectively, have been reported.[62] Both bovine and porcine heparin have been associated with this syndrome, although bovine heparin appears to be more commonly associated. The syndrome usually begins 5 to 15 days after heparin administration, although it may begin earlier if the patient has been exposed to heparin in the past with preformed antibodies present. Arterial and venous thromboses have been reported and are likely to occur in diseased or traumatized vessels. Even small exposure as with heparin coating on pulmonary artery catheters has been reported to cause this problem. Low-molecular-weight heparins have also been associated with this syndrome, although isolated reports have suggested that these heparin fragments may occasionally be safely substituted for standard heparin in situations of heparin-associated thrombocytopenia.[63]

Heparin-associated thrombocytopenia should be suspected in a patient when thrombosis occurs while receiving heparin or when there is a fall in platelet count to less than 100,000/μL. The laboratory diagnosis is suggested by demonstrating 20% or higher platelet aggregation within 15 minutes or 6% or higher ^{14}C serotonin release within 45 minutes when heparin is added to donor platelets and the patient's own platelet-poor plasma, which has the antibody present. If the patient's platelet count is greater than 100,000/μL, the patient's own platelet-rich plasma may be used. If the platelet count is less than 100,000/μL, alternative platelet-rich plasma from another patient not treated with antiplatelet agents must be used. Other coagulation tests are usually normal in these patients. Treatment consists of cautious administration of protamine sulfate to reverse the heparin if active thrombosis has occurred or discontinuation of heparin, allowing its effects to wear off, followed by another anticoagulant, such as dextran sulfate or sodium warfarin (Coumadin). Aspirin has been used with limited success, but Iloprost, a prostacyclin analogue, has been found to be useful in treatment of these patients.[64] Iloprost, however, is no longer available for compassionate use due to its potential to cause severe vasodilation and hypotension. Other possible anticoagulants that have been suggested include ancrod, hirudin, low-molecular-weight heparins, and heparin-like compounds called heparinoids.

Antithrombin III Deficiency

Antithrombin III deficiency accounts for about 2% of venous thrombotic events. Arterial thrombosis, although much less common, has also been described with this deficiency. Antithrombin III deficiency was observed to be associated with arterial thrombosis in 1981, with four cases of thrombosis after reconstruction and two cases of spontaneous thrombosis.[65] Antithrombin III is a serine protease inhibitor of thrombin and factors Xa, IXa, and XIa. This α_2-globulin, present in normal plasma, has a half-life of 2.8 days. As heparin potentiates the anticoagulant effects of antithrombin III by changing its shape, a patient with antithrombin III deficiency usually presents with thrombosis on heparin or demonstrates an inability to become adequately anticoagulated despite heparin. This deficiency may be either congenital or acquired. Most cases become apparent early in life, and by 50 years of age, 85% of patients have suffered a thrombotic event, usually venous in origin. Homozygous patients usually die in infancy; heterozygous patients demonstrate a decreased plasma level, usually lower than 70%. Acquired deficits occur with inadequate production in liver disease, malignancy, nephrotic syndrome, DIC, malnutrition, or increased protein catabolism.[66] A temporal relation occurs between antithrombin III levels and protein metabolism. A second, less frequent condition exists in which a defective antithrombin III is made with normal levels quantitatively (progressive deficiency). There is also a third, less frequent condition in which there is an abnormal interaction between antithrombin III and heparin (antithrombin III heparin cofactor activity).[67] Thrombotic episodes are often related to events such as operations, childbirth, and infections; recurrent episodes are common. The diagnosis is made by measuring antithrombin III levels, preferably with the patient off anticoagulants. Both antigen and activity levels should be assessed. Heparin has been shown to decrease antithrombin III levels, whereas sodium warfarin tends to increase these levels. In addition, measuring the level during the acute thrombotic event may be misleading because antithrombin III may be low due to thrombotic consumption. Once the diagnosis is established, fresh-frozen plasma should be administered, beginning with 2 U every 8 hours and decreasing over 72 hours to 1 U every 12 hours, followed by sodium warfarin. Antithrombin III concentrates are available and may find use in situations when heparin administration is necessary for a short period, such as during operative procedures requiring anticoagulation and during management of DIC.[68]

Protein C and S Deficiencies

Protein C and S deficiencies are frequently described causes of the procoagulant state. Protein Ca inactivates factors Va and VIIIa of the Xase and prothrombinase complexes (Fig. 4-10). Protein C is activated to protein Ca 20,000 times faster than by thrombin alone through the interaction of thrombomodulin and thrombin on the endothelial cell surface.[69] Additionally, protein C inactivates the inhibitor to tPA, thus increasing the fibrinolytic activity of plasma. Protein S is a cofactor for protein C. Although most reports describe venous thrombosis, with deficiencies of protein C and S seen in as many as 4% or 5% of young patients with venous thrombotic disorders, arterial thrombosis has also been reported. In patients younger than 51 years of age requiring arterial revascularization, protein S deficiency was reported in 20%, and protein C deficiency was found in 15% of cases.[70] The half-life of proteins C and S is about 6 hours, and both deficiency states can be either congenital or acquired. In congenital conditions, patients homozygous for protein C deficiency usually die in infancy from unrestricted clotting of the microcirculation, called *purpura fulminans,* whereas heterozygous patients have protein C levels lower than 55% of normal. Levels between 55% and 65% are consistent with both heterozygous deficiency and the lower end of the distribution of normal values, so overlap does occur.[3] Both protein C antigen levels and activity should be measured, but only protein S antigen levels can be measured. Acquired deficiencies usually follow conditions that interfere with hepatic synthesis because these factors are produced in the liver along with the other vitamin K–dependent factors II, VII, IX, and X. The onset of episodes of thrombosis, especially venous, is typically between 15 and 30 years of age. The treatment for those with thrombotic events is lifelong anticoagulant therapy with sodium warfarin. Not all patients with these deficiencies experience episodes of thrombosis. Low levels of either protein C or protein S in patients without symptoms are not alone an indication for anticoagulation. In a large population of blood donors, 0.3% were found to have low protein C levels without any overt clinical thrombotic episodes, whereas many heterozygous family members of homozygous protein C–deficient infants are clinically unaffected.[25] It has also been reported that protein C deficiency may be associated with an abnormality in the protein C molecule, resulting in the generation of minimal enzymatic activity, as would be reflected in the protein C activity assay.

A dangerous paradox may occur during the administration of oral anticoagulants in patients with protein C deficiency. When oral anticoagulants are given, protein C levels decline more rapidly than most of the other vitamin K–dependent liver factors, which have half-lives of 5 to 7 days (II, IX, and X), thus rendering the patient receiving the sodium warfarin procoagulant for a short time. This may result in skin necrosis from clotting in the microcirculation.[71] To avoid this devastating complication, which leads to full-thickness necrosis of the skin and subcutaneous tissues on fatty areas of the body (but has been seen over all parts of the body, including the extremities), requires full heparin anticoagulation while beginning sodium warfarin until the vitamin K–dependent liver factors have all reached low levels, or using low doses of sodium warfarin initially.

Resistance to Activated Protein C

Resistance to activated protein C is reported in about 40% of patients who present with idiopathic venous thrombosis.[72] In this syndrome, the activated partial thromboplastin time (aPTT) is measured, with the addition of activated protein C and calcium chloride to the patient's

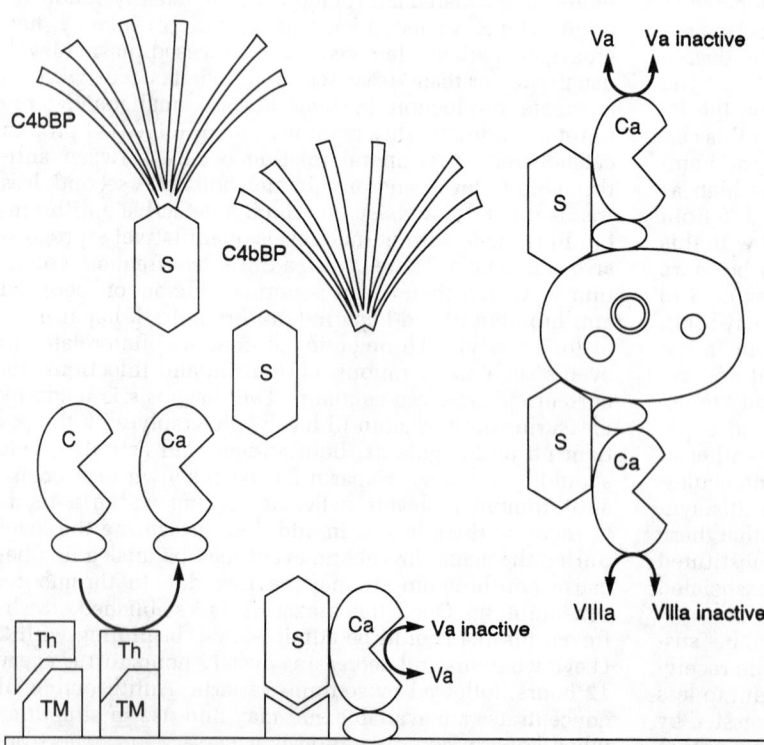

Figure 4-10. Role of proteins C and S. Th, thrombin; TM, thrombomodulin; C4bBP, C4b binding protein. (After Esmon CT. The regulation of natural anticoagulant pathways. Science 1987;235:1348)

serum, and the result is compared with the same test without the addition of activated protein C. It is thought that the defect in this syndrome is due to a selective decrease in the anticoagulant function of factor V, and formal genetic testing for this abnormal factor should be performed. Arterial and venous thrombosis has been reported with this syndrome and there has been tremendous interest in this syndrome, with more than 80 publications in the past 2 years.[73-76] Treatment options include anticoagulation at the time of thrombosis and long-term oral anticoagulation therapy thereafter, based on the patient's overall thrombotic risk profile.

Lupus Anticoagulant–Antiphospholipid Syndrome

The lupus anticoagulant–antiphospholipid syndrome involves one of a number of antiphospholipid antibodies that may cause a hypercoagulable state or be associated with liberated cellular phospholipid from thrombosis (such as cardiolipin) and act as a marker for ongoing coagulation.[77] The antiphospholipid syndrome (APS) consists of the presence of antiphospholipid antibody or the lupus anticoagulant along with any or all of the following: recurrent thromboses, recurrent fetal losses, thrombocytopenia, or livido reticularis. A prolonged aPTT not corrected by normal plasma in the face of other standard coagulation tests that are normal is considered indicative of this problem, as is the prolongation of another much less common test, the Russell viper venom time. Also, one can measure directly the antiphospholipid or anticardiolipin antibody. In fact, the abnormality in the aPTT is a laboratory artifact because phospholipid is added to the test, and the antiphospholipid antibody and lupus anticoagulant IgG or IgM immunoglobulins are specifically directed against anionic phospholipid. Thrombosis-promoting antibodies are most often IgG. In addition, the antiphospholipid antibody may cross-react with cardiolipin, the antigen used in blood screening for syphilis, producing a false-positive syphilis serology.

Imperfect concordance exists among the tests used to identify the abnormality responsible for APS. About 80% of patients with the lupus anticoagulant have a positive ELISA antiphospholipid antibody, but only 10% to 50% of patients with a positive ELISA antiphospholipid antibody have a lupus anticoagulant.[78] Patients with both tests positive appear to have a similar prognosis as those with either alone. Possible mechanisms for the procoagulant state associated with APS that have been proposed include inhibition of prostacyclin synthesis or release from endothelial cells, inhibition of protein C activation by the thrombin–thrombomodulin complex on endothelial cell surfaces, inhibition of plasminogen activator synthesis or plasminogen activator release from endothelial or other cells, and direct platelet activation. Although the lupus anticoagulant has been reported to exist in about 5% to 40% of patients with systemic lupus erythematosus (SLE), this condition can exist in patients without SLE, can be induced by medications, and can be seen in patients with cancer and certain infectious disorders. The lupus anticoagulant is a better predictor for thrombotic events, whereas a high-titer antiphospholipid antibody measured by ELISA (40 GPL units or more) is more sensitive for identifying female patients with pregnancies at risk for fetal loss. A low-titer ELISA test (5 to 40 GPL units) is a common, nonspecific finding of no real clinical significance.[78]

Thrombosis can involve both the venous and the arterial circulation, especially the peripheral vessels of the extremities, although aortic occlusion has been reported in association with the lupus anticoagulant. Antibodies to phospholipids and cardiolipin have also been demonstrated in the cerebral circulation of young stroke patients. Less common manifestations include livedo reticularis, pulmonary hypertension, vascular heart disease, labile hypertension, migraine headaches, chorea, Guillain-Barré syndrome, positive Coombs test, lesions of the multiple sclerosis type, digital gangrene, coronary thrombosis, epilepsy, repeated strokes, and subacute lupus erythematosus. At least one third of patients with the lupus anticoagulant have a history of one or more thrombotic events, with 70% of these in the venous circulation.[77] Concerning arterial thrombosis with this abnormality, 9 of 18 vascular reconstructions were associated with thrombosis in patients positive for antiphospholipid antibodies, versus only 2 of 33 nonvascular procedures in this same group of patients.[79] In another series of 158 patients with peripheral vascular disease (including 27 with abdominal aortic aneurysms, 1 with renovascular hypertension, 28 with cerebrovascular insufficiency, 31 with aortoiliac occlusive disease, and 71 with infrainguinal occlusive disease), 137 patients underwent peripheral vascular surgical reconstructions.[80] Fifteen patients were identified with procoagulant states, including 5 with protein C and S deficiencies and 5 with a lupus-like anticoagulant. Of patients undergoing 137 vascular procedures, 5 demonstrated thrombosis within 30 days, including 3 of 14 (21%) with either a lupus anticoagulant or heparin-associated thrombocytopenia, as opposed to only 2 of 123 (1.6%) with no procoagulant state identified ($P < .01$). A particular problem associated with this syndrome has been recurrent spontaneous abortions with both the lupus anticoagulant and antiphospholipid and anticardiolipin antibodies due to thrombosis of placental vessels. About 10% of women with two or more unexplained abortions are found to have a positive antiphospholipid antibody. Treatment for thrombosis associated with APS includes heparin followed by long-term sodium warfarin therapy. It is unfortunate that this entity has been misnamed as an anticoagulant, and it is important to realize that it is one of the entities associated with the procoagulant state.

Defective Fibrinolytic Activity

Defective fibrinolytic activity is another cause of the procoagulant state. Plasminogen is a normal plasma protein consisting of a single polypeptide chain of about 90,000 MW. It exists in 10 different forms. Abnormal plasminogen activity has been demonstrated in more than 30 cases of spontaneous arterial or venous thromboses and may affect 10% of the normal population, but it only becomes clinically evident once a thrombotic-prone event occurs.[81] Once this diagnosis is made, treatment is with long-term sodium warfarin therapy. Fibrinogen itself, as a marker of disease states, has been found more useful as an indicator for the development of atherosclerosis in a number of studies than as a marker for a hypercoagulable state,[82] although proposed mechanisms for a procoagulant state with dysfibrinogenemias have been suggested.[67]

Fibrinolytic activity of blood is derived from plasminogen activators produced in the endothelium of small blood vessels and continuously presented to the bloodstream. These include tPA in response to thrombin, histamine, and bradykinin, and the binding of thrombin to thrombomodulin on the endothelial cell surface, enhancing fibrinolysis by activating protein C (which inactivates the tPA inhibitor).[83] In addition factors of the contact system of coagulation are direct activators of plasminogen as indicated earlier. Defective fibrinolytic activity may be due to either decreased content of plasminogen activators, decreased release of the same, or an increase in the level of their inhibitors. In a study of 100 patients with recurrent DVT or pulmonary embolism and no other known underlying disease, 67 had normal tPA levels after a venous occlusion test, 22 had increased PAI in their serum, and 11 had low activator levels.[84] It has been observed that fibrinolytic activity of blood is reduced postoperatively for 7 to 10 days, owing to an altered relation between tPA and its inhibitor. Studies have demonstrated that pneumatic compression devices exhibit their antithrombotic effects systemically through prevention of this fibrinolytic shutdown. Adequate evidence appears to exist supporting a relation between impaired preoperative or postoperative fibrinolysis and venous thrombosis.[85] Arterial graft thrombosis has also been associated with plasminogen deficiency. Major inhibitors of the fibrinolytic system include α_2-AP and PAI. As secretion of endothelial cell–derived PAI is stimulated by thrombin, endotoxin, and IL-1, elevated levels of PAI have been found circulating during certain infections.[86] Also, TNF down-regulates the activity of protein C. Down-regulated protein C is less able to inactivate PAI, shifting the balance in the direction of thrombosis and linking the coagulation system with sepsis.

Abnormal Platelet Aggregation

Abnormal platelet aggregation has been seen in two clinical situations separate from heparin-associated abnormal platelet aggregation. The first is advanced malignancy, especially of the lung and uterus, and the second is in the occasional patient who undergoes carotid endarterectomy and then experiences thrombosis at the endarterectomy site due to platelet activation and aggregation. Hyperreactive platelets have also been associated with arterial graft thrombosis in patients undergoing peripheral vascular reconstructions.[70] However, platelet function may be more dependent on external factors, such as the circulating level of fibrinogen or the production of thrombin, rather than on an intrinsic feature of the platelets themselves. This suggests that antiplatelet agents alone are unlikely to eliminate a thrombogenic potential.[87]

Disseminated Intravascular Coagulation

Disseminated intravascular coagulation is the primary form of acute thrombosis. Causes of DIC include abruptio placenta, gram-positive and gram-negative sepsis, endotoxemia, malignant tumors, pelvic operations, certain snake bites, hematologic malignancies, and hepatic failure.[3] Coagulation is activated by the release into the circulation of tissue factor, which activates factor VII to VIIa, leading to massive thrombin production and fibrin generation. Fibrinolysis then becomes activated, leading to bleeding in the later stages of the syndrome due to the consumption of clotting factors, depletion of fibrinogen, and unchecked plasmin activity. Laboratory values in DIC reveal a decline in platelet count and fibrinogen level with a concomitant elevation in fibrin split products. A more chronic form of DIC has been reported, with the release of small amounts of tissue factor into the circulation in conditions such as tumors of the prostate, diabetes mellitus, use of factor IX concentrates, total hip replacement, and abdominal aortic aneurysm.[3] In a prospective study of 76 patients with extensive aortic aneurysms, 4% of patients (especially those with thoracoabdominal involvement) exhibited clinically overt DIC preoperatively.[88] In this more chronic form of DIC, fibrinogen tends to remain within the normal range, and the laboratory diagnosis depends more on the inhibitory capacity of plasma.

In summary, a number of conditions can lead to a procoagulant state. A procoagulant screen should include routine coagulation tests, such as the aPTT and platelet count; antithrombin III activity and antigen assay; protein C antigen and activity levels; protein S antigen level; mixing studies to identify a lupus anticoagulant (if indicated); an antiphospholipid antibody screen that includes anticardiolipin antibody; fibrinogen level; functional plasminogen assay; and platelet aggregation testing if possible. Although conditions exist that lead to these hypercoagulable states, only 10% to 15% of patients with venous thrombosis have one of the conditions listed here, the most frequent condition involving abnormalities in proteins C and S. The incidence increases with the concentration of patients at high risk in specialized coagulation centers[67] and may be even higher with the measurement of new parameters, such as resistance to protein C.[72–74] Thus, not every patient with a thrombotic event should be screened. However, patients with strong positive family histories, young patients with arterial and venous thromboses without obvious cause, and patients with multiple episodes of thrombosis without an underlying anatomic abnormality should be investigated and screened.

BLEEDING DISORDERS

Although the surgeon deals more often with procoagulant states than bleeding disorders, it is important to recognize these disorders when they occur.

Coagulation Factor Deficiency

Coagulation factor deficiency states are important causes of bleeding. Factor VIII and IX deficiency states are involved in hemophilia A and B and type I von Willebrand disease. Hemophilia A (Fig. 4-11) is inherited as a sex-linked recessive deficiency of factor VIII, with fewer cases secondary to spontaneous mutation. The incidence of this abnormality is about 1 in 10,000 births. Clinical findings range from bleeding into joints and muscles, epistaxis, hematuria, and bleeding after minor trauma to prolonged postoperative bleeding, retroperitoneal bleeding, and intramural bowel hemorrhage. Laboratory screening tests usually reveal a prolongation of aPTT, with other tests being normal. The minimum level of factor VIII required for hemostasis is 30%, and spontaneous bleeding is uncommon with factor VIII levels greater than 5% to 10% of normal.[89] Levels less than 2% constitute severe, 2% to 5% moderate, and greater than 5% mild deficiency.[90] Severe deficiency with levels less than 1% are at risk for spontaneous bleeding episodes. Although the half-life of factor VIII is 2.9 days in normal subjects, the half-life of factor VIII concentrates is only 9 to 18 hours.[3] Levels between 80% to 100% of normal should be attained for surgical bleeding or life-threatening hemorrhage. Acquired deficiency has been reported to occur with the development of antibodies to factor VIII after therapy. About 10% to 15% of patients with hemophilia A develop inhibitor antibodies, although the incidence of antibody formation may be much higher in previously untreated patients and in those with severe hemophilia A. A new recombinant factor VIII preparation has been developed and tested in children and infants. Despite the development of low levels of inhibitors in 20% of children at a mean 9 days after first administration, these inhibitors either disappeared or remained at low levels.[91] Because of the fact that this recombinant preparation is virus free, the benefits outweigh the risks of low levels of inhibitor development for the treatment of hemophilia A

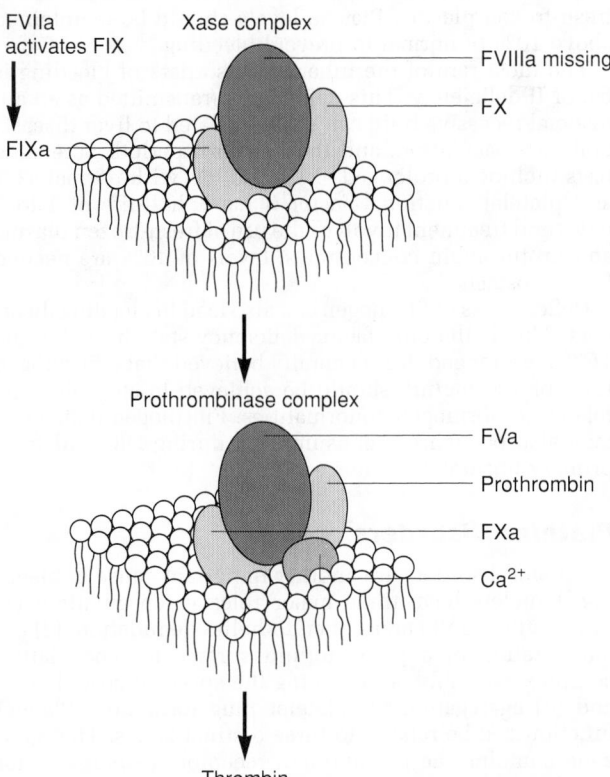

Complete assembly is incomplete

FVIIa activates FIX

Xase complex

FVIIIa missing

FX

FIXa

Prothrombinase complex

FVa

Prothrombin

FXa

Ca²⁺

Thrombin

Figure 4-11. Hemophilia A involves a deficiency of factor VIII. (After Hassouna HI. Laboratory evaluation of hemostatic disorders. In: Penner JA, Hassouna HI, eds. Coagulation disorders II. Hematol Oncol Clin North Am 1993;7:1187)

(especially in view of the fact that in 1992, almost 30% of the entire hemophilic population in the United States had reported acquired immunodeficiency syndrome [AIDS], and more than 22% had died of AIDS).[92] Factor IX deficiency (Christmas factor), known as hemophilia B (Fig. 4-12), is transmitted as an X-linked recessive trait. It may also be acquired due to enhanced factor IX clearance in states such as the nephrotic syndrome, abnormal protein production in vitamin K deficiency, and acquired specific inhibitors to factor IX in various autoimmune diseases, such as SLE. It is clinically indistinguishable from hemophilia A, and laboratory screening tests reveal a prolonged aPTT, with other tests normal, although a greater proportion of patients have only mild or moderate deficiency.[93] Severe deficiency (about 30% of cases) is defined as a level of activity less than 4% of normal, whereas moderate deficiency is reported with activity levels between 20% and 40%.[3] Treatment consists of plasma or factor IX concentrates and vitamin K. It has been recommended to achieve levels greater than 30% for hemostasis.[89]

Von Willebrand factor causes platelet adhesion to collagen, initiating platelet plug formation. It also forms a complex with factor VIII in the blood. Produced in endothelial cells and megakaryocytes (compared with the liver for factor VIII), it has a circulating half-life of 6 to 20 hours.[3] A number of different subtypes have been identified for its deficiency state (Fig. 4-13), and the syndrome is transmitted as both autosomal dominant (heterozygous) and autosomal recessive (homozygous). Variants that have been described include types I and III (quantitative decreases in normal-appearing vWF) and type II (qualitative abnor-

malities in structure and function of vWF).[94] vWF is most likely as common as hemophilia A, although the true incidence may surpass what is generally appreciated because many mild cases probably remain undiagnosed. The classic syndrome is caused by a reduction of factor VIII activity (although not as great as in hemophilia A) and vWF (vWF–factor VIII complex). Clinical manifestations include mild to moderate epistaxis, gingival bleeding, menorrhagia, rare joint or muscle bleeding, and subcutaneous bleeding.[3] Spontaneous bleeding is not as common as in hemophilia A. Screening laboratory tests include prolonged aPTT, with other coagulation tests normal; prolonged bleeding time; decreased level of factor VIII activity; decreased immunoreactive level of the vWF; and abnormal platelet aggregation response to ristocetin.[3] The most reliable source of vWF is cryoprecipitate, although many concentrates of factor VIII have vWF present and show promise. Desmopressin acetate (DDAVP) is available for the treatment of mild cases. Levels of 25% to 50% are needed for hemostasis.[89]

Other specific factor deficiencies are much less common and receive only a brief overview here. Factor XI (plasma thromboplastin antecedent), complexed to high-molecular-weight kininogen in the plasma, has a half-life of 40 to 80 hours.[3] Deficiency of this factor carries an autosomal recessive inheritance. Homozygous patients have levels up to 20% of normal, whereas heterozygous patients typically show levels between 30% and 65% of normal.[3] This syndrome is particularly frequent in certain ethnic groups, such as Ashkenazi Jews. Screening tests include a prolonged aPTT and whole blood clotting time, with other

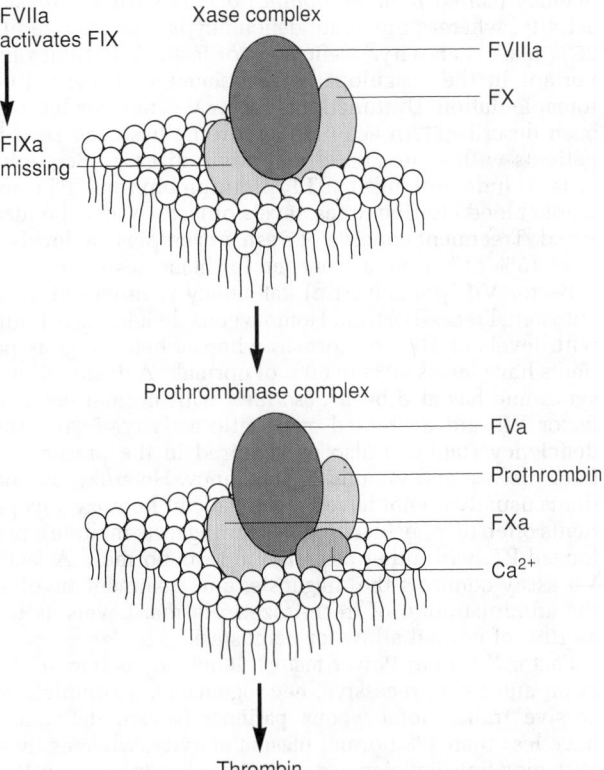

Complete assembly is incomplete

FVIIa activates FIX

Xase complex

FVIIIa

FX

FIXa missing

Prothrombinase complex

FVa

Prothrombin

FXa

Ca²⁺

Thrombin

Figure 4-12. Hemophilia B involves a deficiency of factor IX. (After Hassouna HI. Laboratory evaluation of hemostatic disorders. In: Penner JA, Hassouna HI, eds. Coagulation disorders II. Hematol Oncol Clin North Am 1993;7:1190)

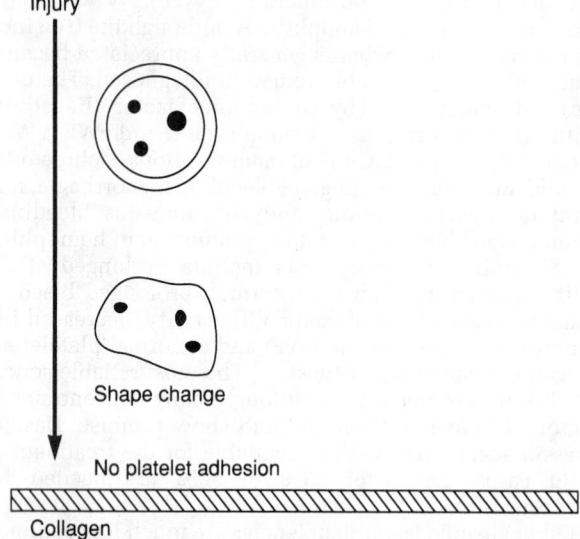

Injury

Shape change

No platelet adhesion

Collagen

Figure 4-13. von Willebrand disease involves an absence of platelet adhesion to collagen. (After Hassouna HI. Laboratory evaluation of hemostatic disorders. In: Penner JA, Hassouna HI, eds. Coagulation disorders II. Hematol Oncol Clin North Am 1993; 7:1187)

coagulation tests normal.[3] A factor XI assay is the definitive test for the diagnosis. Treatment includes administration of fresh-frozen plasma, and hemostasis requires at least 25% of normal factor XI activity.[89]

Factor V (proaccelerin) deficiency is rare. This liver-produced factor has a half-life of 12 to 36 hours, and its deficiency is inherited as autosomal recessive.[3] Severe deficiency (called *parahemophilia*) occurs with 1% plasma activity, whereas moderate deficiency is characterized by 25% plasma activity.[3] Deficiency of factor V becomes important in the coagulopathy associated with early liver transplantation. Dysfunctional factor V syndrome has also been described. An acquired syndrome has been seen in patients with acute and chronic liver disease.[3] Screening tests include prolonged aPTT, prothrombin time (PT), and whole blood clotting times; levels of factor V may be measured. Treatment consists of fresh-frozen plasma; levels at least 15% of normal are needed for hemostasis.[89]

Factor VII (proconvertin) deficiency is inherited as an autosomal recessive trait. Homozygous deficiency is found with levels of 10% of normal, whereas heterozygous patients have levels 40% to 60% of normal.[3] A dysfunctional syndrome has also been described with normal levels of factor VII and decreased enzymatic activity. Again, this deficiency state can also be acquired in the presence of liver disease and vitamin K deficiency. Heterozygous patients usually do not have symptoms, but homozygous patients often display bleeding. Screening tests include a prolonged PT, with other coagulation tests normal.[3] A factor VII assay confirms the diagnosis, and treatment involves the administration of fresh-frozen plasma. Levels as low as 10% of normal allow for hemostasis.[89]

Factor X (Stuart-Power factor) deficiency is transmitted as an autosomal recessive, heterogeneous, incomplete recessive trait.[3] Homozygous patients (severe deficiency) have less than 1% normal plasma activity, whereas those with moderate deficiency demonstrate levels between 10% and 20% of normal plasma activity.[3] Acquired deficiency states have been described. Screening tests include a prolonged aPTT, PT, and whole blood clotting time with a normal thrombin clotting time (TCT), and a specific factor

X assay exists.[3] Clinical findings include minor or more major bleeding episodes, and treatment involves the use of fresh-frozen plasma. Plasma levels should be maintained above 10% of normal to prevent bleeding.[89]

The most rare of the inherited disorders of bleeding is factor II deficiency. This deficiency, transmitted as an autosomal recessive trait, can also be related to liver disease, oral anticoagulation, and the newborn period. Screening tests include a prolonged aPTT and PT, with normal TCT and platelet function.[3] Factor II has a half-life of 2 to 5 days, and treatment involves the use of fresh-frozen plasma and prothrombin concentrates; levels of 40% are needed for hemostasis.[89]

Deficiencies of fibrinogen can also lead to bleeding disorders. This is the only factor deficiency state in which the TCT is prolonged. It is generally believed that a fibrinogen level of 100 mg/mL should be achieved to stop bleeding related to fibrinogen abnormalities. Fibrinogen deficiency may also occur from consumption during DIC and from primary fibrinolytic states.

Platelet Disorders

Platelet disorders are another important cause of bleeding. Platelets have three major roles in coagulation: (1) initial adhesion to areas of endothelial denudation; (2) externalization of a phospholipid surface for coagulation complex assembly, accelerating the speed of coagulation; and (3) aggregation for platelet plug formation. Platelet function can be related to three distinct zones. The outer zone contains the glycoprotein receptors responsible for platelet adhesion (Gp Ib) and platelet aggregation (Gp IIb/IIIa); receptors for fibrinogen, vWF, and fibronectin (Gp IIb/IIIa); and receptor for thrombospondin (Gp IIIb).[3] The second zone, the sol-gel zone, contains elements that allow platelet contraction; the third zone, the organelle zone, contains electron-dense bodies that store calcium serotonin, ADP, and ATP and the nondense α granules that store markers for platelet activation.[3] Bleeding associated with platelets includes mucosal bleeding, such as epistaxis, easy bruisability, petechiae, purpura, and menorrhagia.

Extracorporeal bypass circuits, such as cardiopulmonary bypass and extracorporeal membrane oxygenation circuits (ECMO), activate platelets regardless of the type of oxygenator employed and can produce bleeding. During cardiopulmonary bypass, after fibrinogen and IgG become absorbed onto the bypass circuit, platelets are immediately activated. These activated platelets change their shape, aggregate, and adhere to the fibrinogen surface through multiple interactions between the Gp IIb/IIIa receptor and the exposed binding sites on the carboxy terminus of the γ chain of fibrinogen and the Fc regions of IgG antibodies. Additionally, fibrinogen can induce both platelet activation and aggregation. Platelets release granule contents, such as platelet factor 4, β-thromboglobulin, serotonin, adenine nucleotides, and thromboxane, and their sensitivities to various platelet agonists decrease. Some adherent platelets break away and leave membrane fragments on the surface of the extracorporeal circuit. Platelet aggregates form; new, larger platelets arrive from the bone marrow; and a heterogeneous mixture of platelet fragments, degranulated platelets, resealed platelets with damaged membranes, reversibly activated, and new platelets occurs.[95] Thus, bleeding time increases are usually recorded. In addition, cardiopulmonary bypass activates factor XII and complement (the contact activation system), leading to neutrophil activation, release of lysosomal enzymes, generation of oxygen-free radicals, and the harmful "inflammatory" response seen with extracorporeal circuits along with the direct activation of the fibrinolytic system by plas-

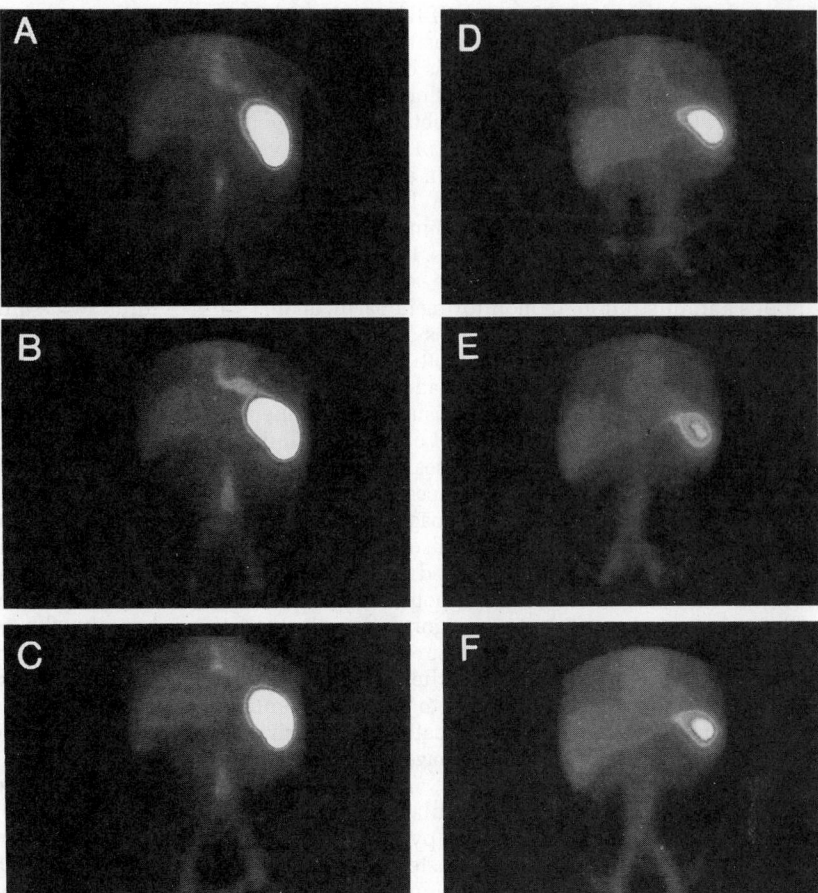

Figure 4-14. Human Dacron aortic graft platelet activity at 1 week (*A*), 3 months (*B*), and 6 months (*C*) versus absent human ePTFE aortic graft platelet activity at 1 week (*D*), 3 months (*E*), and 6 months (*F*). (Wakefield TW, Shulkin BL, Fellows EP, Petry NA, Spaulding SA, Stanley JC. Platelet reactivity in human aortic grafts: a prospective, randomized mid-term study of platelet adherence and release products in Dacron and ePTFE grafts. J Vasc Surg 1989;9:238)

min activation. Prosthetic vascular grafts likewise activate platelets, and platelet uptake on both Dacron (Fig. 4-14) and expanded polytetrafluoroethylene grafts has been found in a number of animal models and in patients for up to 6 months to 10 years after graft implantation.[96] This platelet uptake appears to be mostly a phenomenon of recruitment, with three different mechanisms: the release of ADP from activated platelets, the production of thromboxane from activated platelets, and the generation of thrombin.

Inherited defects of platelet receptors include defects of Gp IIb/IIIa (Glanzman thrombasthenia), characterized by impaired platelet binding to vWF, fibrinogen, and fibronectin. In patients with defects in Gp Ib (Bernard-Soulier syndrome), the absolute number of platelets is decreased, the platelets are larger, and platelet aggregation and adhesion are abnormal.[3] Acquired deficits occur in uremia, with both Gp Ib and Gp IIb/IIIa receptors defective, resulting in impaired adhesion and aggregation. Acquired deficits also occur in patients who previously received platelet transfusions and then develop immune-mediated platelet antibodies. Patients with Glanzman thrombasthenia also show abnormalities in the sol-gel zone, and their platelets lack the ability to contract and retract. A number of platelet disorders associated with abnormalities of the organelle zone have also been described.

Abnormalities in Fibrinolysis

Abnormalities in fibrinolysis may play a role in abnormal bleeding disorders. Genetic or acquired deficiencies in α_2-AP may be associated with bleeding, whereas deficiencies in factor XIII (fibrin-stabilizing factor) may lead to highly lysable clot. Treatment of α_2-AP deficiency is with epsilon aminocaproic acid or tranexamic acid. Homozygous patients with factor XIII deficiency with less than 1% of normal plasma activity often show bleeding from the umbilical cord at birth, bleeding after trauma or surgery, and delayed bleeding 24 to 36 hours later.[3] Intracranial bleeding has also been reported. Screening test results include a shortened euglobulin lysis time and the presence of clot solubility in 5M urea, 2% acetic acid, or 1% monochloroacetic acid.[3] A specific assay for factor XIII activity exists. Treatment consists of fresh-frozen plasma, cryoprecipitate, and factor XIII concentrates. Finally, a deficiency of PAI-1 has been described that may lead to bleeding.

PHARMACOLOGIC AND NONPHARMACOLOGIC INTERVENTIONS

Heparin

Heparin, discovered by Jay McLean in 1916, is a heterogeneous mixture of sulfated polysaccharide molecules of varying molecular weights. Heparin accelerates the reaction between thrombin and antithrombin III, accelerating the inhibition of thrombin and other serine proteases by antithrombin III. Heparin also directly binds and inhibits coagulation proteases and is important for the selective inhibitor of thrombin, heparin cofactor II. After bolus injection, heparin's half-life is about 90 to 120 minutes, although the half-life is dependent on the amount injected.

The more injected, the longer its half-life. Activated factor X and activated factor II are most sensitive to the heparin–antithrombin III complex. Heparin is cleared through the reticuloendothelial system and does not cross the placental barrier. Commercial heparin is obtained from pork or beef lung or intestine. Clinical use of heparin in venous thrombosis and pulmonary embolism and as a prophylactic agent has been established.[97] A lower frequency of bleeding complications has been found with continuous infusion rather than bolus injections. In addition, a lesser degree of thrombin accumulation has been found with continuous administration. In monitoring heparin, an aPTT of 1.5 times control or a TCT of 2 times control reflects adequate anticoagulation. Activated clotting times in a range of 150 to 200 seconds also suggest adequate anticoagulation. In many situations, direct measurements of heparin levels do not correlate with the level of anticoagulation as measured by aPTT. Heparin decreases platelet aggregability at the same time that it enhances the generation of thromboxane from platelets.[98] Noncoagulant high-molecular-weight heparin fragments may also potentiate platelet aggregation, and heparin-associated thrombocytopenia from an immune mechanism is a potential complication of heparin use. Any patient undergoing heparin therapy should have a platelet count measured every other day after the 4th day of therapy (or earlier if known to have been exposed to heparin in the past) to look for thrombocytopenia. The most common complication of heparin therapy is bleeding. The risk of hemorrhage is increased in the elderly, in postmenopausal women, and in patients with preexisting abnormalities of coagulation, thrombocytopenia, and uremia. Long-term therapy may be associated with alopecia and osteoporosis; osteoporosis has been found in patients receiving large doses of heparin for longer than 6 months.

Heparin use in venous thrombosis prophylaxis has received considerable attention. Low-dose heparin protects against venous thrombosis through three different mechanisms. First, antithrombin III activity, with its inhibition of factor Xa, is enhanced by trace amounts of heparin; second, there may be a decrease in thrombin availability, preventing its activation and its fibrin-stabilizing effect; and third, small doses of heparin may inhibit the second wave of platelet aggregation and the subsequent platelet release reaction. In a review of 27 clinical trials concerning the use of low-dose heparin for venous thromboembolism prophylaxis, the incidence of venous thrombosis in the nontreated patients averaged 25%, compared with only 7% in those receiving low-dose heparin.[99] Additionally, thrombi likely to produce major pulmonary embolism were decreased from 6% in the nontreated patients to 0.6% in the group treated with low-dose heparin. Low-dose heparin was found to decrease the incidence of massive pulmonary embolism seen at autopsy. Low-dose heparin does, however, carry an increased risk of wound hematoma, and only high-risk patients should be treated. The sodium and calcium salts of heparin appear to be equally effective for prophylaxis, and the incidence of wound hematoma is not related to the type of salt in the heparin preparation. In addition, there is only a slight advantage to giving 5000 units three times a day as compared with twice a day.

The use of low-dose heparin therapy has been endorsed for a number of applications by the National Institutes of Health Consensus Conference on venous thrombosis prophylaxis.[100] In a metaanalysis of 70 randomized trials in 16,000 patients comparing low-dose heparin with standard therapy for venous thrombosis prophylaxis, the odds of development of DVT with low-dose heparin decreased 67%±4%, whereas for pulmonary embolism (both fatal and nonfatal), the odds decreased 47%±10%.[101] For fatal pulmonary embolism, the odds reduction was even greater (64%±15%). No increase in mortality from other causes was found in patients treated with low-dose heparin. Importantly, these reductions were seen in urologic, elective orthopedic, and traumatic orthopedic procedures. This is somewhat at variance concerning urologic and orthopaedic patients in whom low-dose heparin is not thought to be efficacious, but it may reflect previous errors in interpretation of studies with small numbers of patients (type II errors). Bleeding complications were more frequent in the heparin-treated patients, with no difference between 5000 units twice a day and 5000 units three times a day. Low-dose heparin prophylaxis appears to be a good means of preventing venous thromboembolic events during many surgical procedures but should be confined to those patients known to be at high risk owing to the potential for increased bleeding complications. Other methods of pharmacologic prophylaxis are not reviewed here. Heparin plus other agents, such as dihydroergotamine, sodium warfarin, dextran, and aspirin, and mechanical measures have been evaluated and are reviewed in the National Institutes of Health Consensus Conference report.[100]

Due to the bleeding complications related to low-dose heparin, there is considerable interest in low-molecular-weight heparin for venous thrombosis prophylaxis. Standard heparin is a mixture of polysaccharide molecules that vary in size from 2 to 40 kd. The anticoagulant effect is primarily centered over the lower end of the molecular weight spectrum. Heparin effect requires a three-way complex among heparin, antithrombin III, and thrombin. A two-way complex between antithrombin III and thrombin, with heparin binding to antithrombin III but not thrombin (due to its small size in low-molecular form), allows for anti–factor Xa activity with less inhibition of thrombin. Theoretically, this should result in a decrease in systemic bleeding complications. In addition, with size below 5 to 8 kd, heparin cannot bind to both antithrombin III and platelets at the same time, thus decreasing the antiplatelet effect of the drug and potential bleeding complications. Although many types of low-molecular-weight heparin are available, they generally are eliminated from the bloodstream more slowly than unfractionated heparin, have a half-life about twice as long, and have a rate of disappearance from the bloodstream that is not dose dependent. In addition, their reversal by protamine sulfate is not complete as measured by anti–factor Xa levels.[102] In addition, low-molecular-weight heparins are readily absorbed from subcutaneous injection sites and do not cross the placental barrier. Although promising studies on the use of low-molecular-weight heparins in thromboembolism prophylaxis have been reported,[103] bleeding complications still have been reported and are not appreciably different than with standard heparin prophylaxis.[102] Clearly, more work with low-molecular-weight heparin is necessary not only for venous thrombosis prophylaxis but also for its routine use in other cardiovascular applications, such as during extracorporeal bypass.

Reversal of heparin anticoagulation with protamine sulfate is often associated with adverse hemodynamic and hematologic side effects, including hypotension, bradycardia, pulmonary artery hypertension or hypotension, declines in oxygen consumption, leukopenia, and thrombocytopenia.[104,105] Although the pulmonary changes have been observed in up to 3% to 4% of cases, hypotension is more frequent. In addition, deaths have been reported after the use of protamine, with noncardiogenic pulmonary edema and right heart failure accompanying the most severe reactions. In a survey sent to members of the Society for Vascular Surgery and the European Society for Vascular Surgery, the incidence of noteworthy protamine-related side effects was significant at 4% to 5%, as reported by about 650 surgeons. The most likely cause of the hypotension appears to involve the elaboration of a vasodilator factor, such as nitric oxide, as well as a direct depression of myocardial function, including the development of bradycardia.[106,107] Pulmonary artery hypertension, on the contrary, is thought to result from thromboxane release from nonplatelet sources in the pulmonary circulation.[108] Finally, thrombocytopenia and leukopenia are most likely the result of a direct effect of protamine on phospholipid membranes of these blood elements.[109] Additionally, immunologic reactions may also occur in patients with prior exposure to protamine, especially in diabetic patients taking NPH insulin that contains protamine (to allow for more prolonged absorption) or those previously exposed to protamine. Unfortunately, no other effective and safe agent for heparin neutralization exists, and in those situations when heparin must be reversed, such as at the completion of major aortic reconstructions and cardiopulmonary bypass, protamine must be given. Although it has been suggested that the rate of administration is the most crucial factor in protamine-related reactions, declines in hemodynamic parameters and oxygen consumption still occur with slow administration.[105] Work from our laboratory has demonstrated that total cationic charge appears to be an important determinant for both anticoagulation reversal efficacy and hemodynamic toxicity.[110] Effective and less toxic alternatives to protamine for the reversal of both standard unfractionated heparin and low-molecular-weight heparin anticoagulation should be possible in the future.

Warfarin

Oral anticoagulant therapy is recommended for chronic treatment of venous thromboembolism. Warfarin interferes with the vitamin K–dependent clotting factors II, VII, IX,

and X; protein C; and protein S. In the liver, these factors are γ-carboxylated in a reaction catalyzed by the reduced form of vitamin K. During this reaction, 10 to 12 glutamic acid residues are converted to γ-carboxyglutamic acid residues (Fig. 4-15). When these factors are released from the liver, they are secreted as active proteins.[3] The carboxyglutamic acid residues are responsible for these proteins binding to phospholipid membranes and the formation of the Xase and prothrombinase complexes on activated platelet surfaces. Warfarin prevents the reduction of vitamin K once it has functioned as a cofactor for the γ-carboxylation (Fig. 4-16). There are two classes of compounds possessing anticoagulant effects: 4-hydroxycoumarins (of which crystalline warfarin sodium [Coumadin], is the most common) and the 2-substituted 1,3-indanediones.[3] Bleeding complications are associated with the level of anticoagulation. The level of anticoagulation is monitored with the PT. At levels higher than a one-stage PT of 1.4 × control, there is nearly a five-fold increase in the frequency of bleeding complications.[111] Because of variations in the thromboplastins used for the prothrombin time determinations in various countries, a new international normalized ratio (INR) system, in which the sensitivity of thromboplastins can be standardized, has been developed.[112] Using this system, the proper range for treatment of venous thrombosis by warfarin is an INR of 2 to 3.

Major complications of sodium warfarin therapy include recurrent thrombosis, bleeding, and skin necrosis. It is recommended that warfarin be continued 4 to 6 months after an initial episode of DVT. Between 10 weeks and 4 months after DVT, the recurrent thrombosis rate is 8.3 episodes per 1000 patient months. Between 4 months and 3 years, this incidence falls to 4 episodes per 1000 patient months. At about 4 months, the risk of bleeding matches and exceeds the benefit from anticoagulant therapy. With recur-

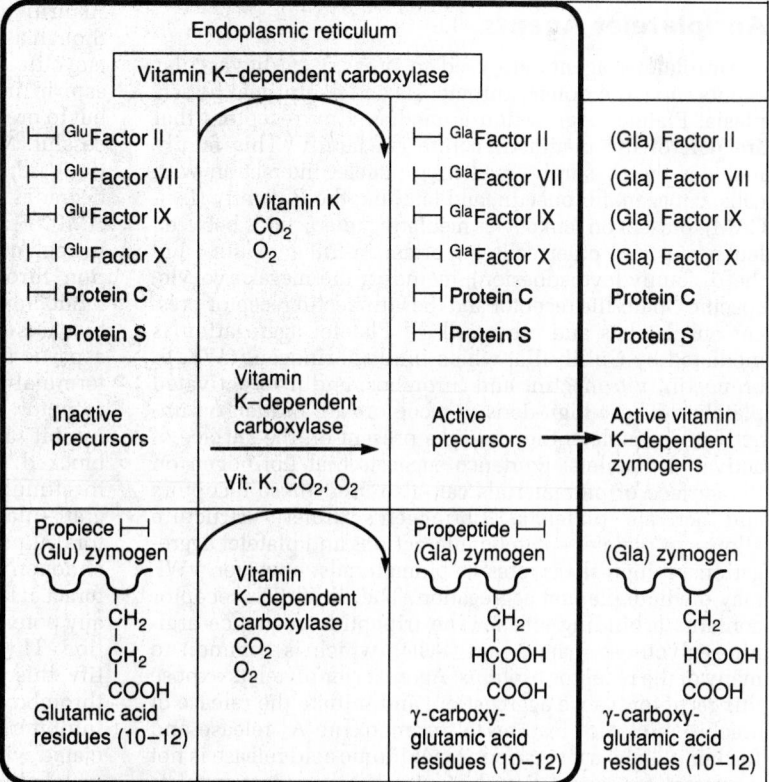

Figure 4-15. Conversion of glutamic acid residues to γ-carboxyglutamic acid residues by vitamin K–dependent carboxylase for factors II, VII, IX, and X; protein C; and protein S. (After Hassouna HI. Laboratory evaluation of hemostatic disorders. In: Penner JA, Hassouna HI, eds. Coagulation disorders II. Hematol Oncol Clin North Am 1993;7:1219)

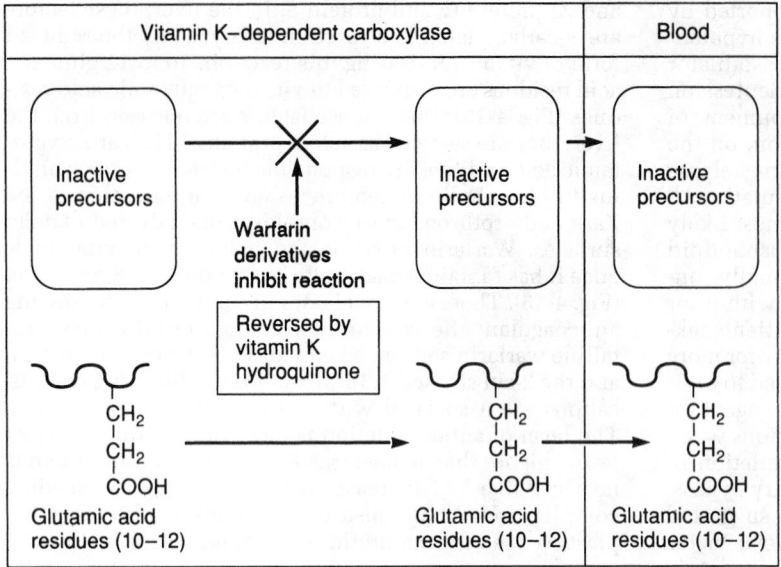

Figure 4-16. Secretion of inactive vitamin K–dependent precursor factors from the liver into the blood after warfarin administration. (After Hassouna HI. Laboratory evaluation of hemostatic disorders. In: Penner JA, Hassouna HI, eds. Coagulation disorders II. Hematol Oncol Clin North Am 1993;7:1220)

rent DVT, however, the thrombotic risk is greater, and sustained anticoagulation is appropriate. Repeat venous thrombosis has been found in up to 20% of patients with recurrent venous thrombosis who are treated with only a short, 6-month course of warfarin.[113] Patients at highest risk for bleeding on warfarin include the elderly, patients with gynecologic or urologic disorders, women after childbirth, and patients given large warfarin loading doses. A final important complication of warfarin is skin necrosis both in patients with and without protein C deficiency. This usually involves full-thickness skin sloughing over fatty areas such as the breasts and buttocks, and can also be seen in other anatomic distributions such as the extremities and digits.

Antiplatelet Agents

Antiplatelet agents are used to prevent cardiovascular events such as coronary thrombosis and neointimal hyperplasia. Platelet aggregation is mediated by receptors that are part of the mammalian integrin family. This family includes the β_1 family, mediating platelet interaction with cells, collagen, fibronectin, and laminin; the β_2 family (Leu-CAM), present on leukocytes mediating interactions between leukocytes and other cells important in inflammation; and the β_3 family (cytoadhesion), including the megakaryocyte-specific Gp IIb/IIIa receptor and the vitronectin receptor present on platelets and other cells.[114] Platelet aggregation is mediated by Gp IIb/IIIa, which binds fibrinogen, vWF, fibronectin, vitronectin, and thrombospondin to activated platelets. These high-density receptors are hidden on unactivated platelets; they become present on the surface of activated platelets. Evidence suggests that fibrinogen on the surface of biomaterials can also bind these receptors and activate platelets. Fibrinogen's dimeric structure allows for platelet–platelet interactions and platelet aggregation. At high shear rates on biomaterials, however, vWF may mediate platelet aggregation. The Gp IIb/IIIa receptor contains a binding site for the tripeptide sequence arginine–glycine–aspartic acid (RGD), which is common to many of the receptor proteins. Agonists for platelets expose this receptor, cause aggregation, and initiate the release of arachidonic acid, leading to thromboxane A_2 release and further platelet aggregation. Arachidonic acid release is not necessary for aggregation, however, because most agonists can directly expose Gp IIb/IIIa. In addition, initial platelet adhesion is a stimulus for platelet aggregation and receptor exposure.

Platelet aggregation can be inhibited by the following methods:

- Blocking cyclooxygenase, the first step converting arachidonic acid to thromboxane and prostacyclin
- Blocking thromboxane synthase, the enzyme leading to thromboxane A_2
- Blocking the thromboxane A_2 receptor
- Increasing intraplatelet levels of cyclic AMP or GMP, which inhibit the exposure of the platelet Gp IIb/IIIa receptor
- Directly blocking the platelet receptor Gp IIb/IIIa

Aspirin and indomethacin inhibit cyclooxygenase. Although aspirin inhibits thromboxane, it also inhibits prostacyclin. In clinical situations, the use of lower doses of aspirin in an attempt to inhibit thromboxane generation but to preserve prostacyclin generation has not proved successful. Methylxanthines, such as dipyridamole (Persantine), inhibit phosphodiesterase, the enzyme that normally degrades cyclic AMP, leading to a higher level of cyclic AMP. Endothelium-derived relaxing factor (nitric acid), nitroglycerin, and nitroprusside mediate platelet aggregation through modulation of cyclic GMP. Additionally, monoclonal antibodies to Gp IIb/IIIa or synthetic peptide blockers of this receptor containing the arginine-glycine-aspartic acid sequence or the fibrinogen γ-chain carboxy-terminal sequence directly inhibit the function of this receptor. Receptor blockage is the most specific way to inhibit aggregation; when the Gp IIb/IIIa receptor is blocked, even high concentrations of agonists are not able to stimulate platelets. In models of prosthetic vascular graft–platelet interactions, thromboxane synthase inhibitors appear less effective than aspirin, suggesting that endoperoxide intermediates are proaggregatory and can interact at the platelet thromboxane receptor, thus subverting any potential antiaggregatory effect of thromboxane reduction. Thromboxane receptor antagonists thus should rectify this situation and exhibit a synergistic effect with thromboxane synthase inhibitors. Thromboxane synthase inhibitors, not thromboxane receptor antagonists, are associated with a decreased urinary excretion of thromboxane metabolites and a marked increase in prostacyclin generation. Combined compounds with both thromboxane synthase inhibition and receptor antagonism have been developed with the intent of enhancing prostacyclin production from endoperoxide intermediates (antiaggregatory) while preventing these intermediates from combining with the thromboxane receptor and augmenting platelet aggregation. Ticlopidine, a relatively new antiplatelet agent, inhibits the exposure of the Gp IIb/IIIa receptor by unknown mechanisms. This agent, however, takes several days to become effective. Other agents with the possibility of inhibiting the generation of platelet thrombi include monoclonal antibodies to vWF, inhibitors of thrombin production such as activated protein C, and direct inhibitors of thrombin such as hirudin. Activated protein C has appeal because it may not increase the bleeding time, as do most other agents.

New Agents

New agents for anticoagulation include hirudin, aprotinin, desmopressin acetate, and ancrod. Hirudin, obtained from the saliva of leeches, is a single-chain polypeptide composed of 65 amino acids, with three disulfide bonds and 8000 to 9000 MW. It is highly specific for thrombin inhibition. Hirudin has a short half-life and is excreted unchanged in the urine. Hirudin has no natural inhibitors, compared with heparin, which has natural inhibitors platelet factor 4 and fibrin II—monomer. As an inhibitor of thrombin, hirudin prevents conversion of fibrinogen to fibrin; thrombin-catalyzed activation of factors V, VIII, and XIII; and importantly, thrombin-induced platelet aggregation. In addition to its small size and high potency for thrombin, hirudin has a dominant antiplatelet effect, even with platelet-rich thrombi. Hirudin has been found to be more effective than heparin in reducing platelet deposition and mural thrombus at similar aPTT levels.[115] Levels of aPTT of 2 to 3 × control (0.7 to 1 mg/kg hirudin) are effective in limiting arterial thrombosis and platelet deposition. Hirudin prevents thrombus growth at both high and low shear rates of blood flow and has even been found to stop thrombus growth in severe stenoses. However, the high incidence of bleeding complications from this drug may limit its clinical usefulness. The gene for hirudin was cloned in 1986, and a recombinant hirudin has been produced (hirulog). Hirulog is a polypeptide of 20 amino acids that has two domains: one that inhibits the active site of thrombin, and a second that prevents the binding of thrombin to fibrinogen.

One area of interest for all prosthetic surfaces, ranging from cardiopulmonary bypass and ECMO circuits to prosthetic vascular grafts, is the ability to *passivate* the surface, which means to lessen platelet—surface interactions in addition to leukocyte activation. Inhibition of platelet function during cardiopulmonary bypass has been accomplished using iloprost, but at the cost of hypotension owing to its vasodilatory properties.[116] A unique finding is that passivation lasts far beyond the time when the drug is present in the circulation. Other compounds that have been suggested for this purpose include a class of reversible platelet—fibrinogen receptor inhibitors, the RGD-containing peptides called *disintegrins* obtained from viper venom that inhibit receptors associated with platelet Gp IIb/IIIa receptor complexes.[117,118] In sheep, disintegrins limit thrombocytopenia, preserve platelet responsiveness to ADP, attenuate release of platelet factor IV, and decrease the Gp IIIa antigen associated with a 24-hour ECMO circuit surface.[118] Inhibitors of the contact activation portion of extracorporeal systems are less well described. Factor XII is activated by the cardiopulmonary bypass circuit. Corn trypsin inhibitor is a weak inhibitor of factor XII activa-

tion,[95] whereas aprotinin inhibits prekallikrein, kallikrein, and fibrinolysis, and preserves platelet function (perhaps by inhibiting the high deleterious levels of plasmin).[119] The inhibition of prekallikrein and kallikrein produces an anticoagulant state, whereas the inhibition of plasmin prevents fibrinolysis. Aprotinin has greater affinity for plasmin than kallikrein, and an anticoagulant effect is seen only at very high doses.[120] This agent has successfully reduced transfusion requirements and blood loss in open heart surgery.[121] Another agent that has been suggested to preserve platelet function is desmopressin acetate. Desmopressin acetate, a synthetic analogue of vasopressin, releases preformed vWF from storage sites (Weibel-Palade bodies) in endothelial cells.[122] vWF then stimulates the production of factor VIII coagulant protein, stabilizes its structure, and forms a circulating noncovalent complex with factor VIII. This vWF—factor VIII complex supports platelet adhesion and improves platelet—platelet interactions. The aPTT shortens and prothrombin consumption increases owing to the increase in factor VIII coagulant protein. Additionally, desmopressin elevates the plasma levels of larger vWF multimers, which are more effective than smaller vWF multimers. Finally, tPA secretion is stimulated by desmopressin. Desmopressin corrects the hemorrhage tendency in mild hemophilia A and von Willebrand disease, and has been found to reduce blood loss and the need for transfusion by 30% to 40% in complex cardiac operations. Additionally, qualitative platelet defects found in uremia and cirrhosis of the liver may be corrected transiently.[123] The platelet lesion caused by small doses of aspirin may also be corrected by desmopressin acetate. Despite the effectiveness of desmopressin acetate, it has not been shown to increase the risk of thrombosis.

Another anticoagulant that has been used in place of heparin is ancrod, a thrombin-like enzyme derived from the Malayan pit viper.[124] This enzyme produces a controlled decrease in fibrinogen levels by depleting FPA from fibrinogen but not FPB. The fibrin monomers that result stimulate the local production of tPA. Both of these actions lead to a state of anticoagulation. The amount of fibrinogen depletion must be carefully titrated to prevent bleeding.

Fibrinolytic Agents

Fibrinolytic agents are direct or indirect activators of plasminogen, the inactive proteolytic enzyme of plasma that binds to fibrin during the formation of thrombus. Fibrin-bound plasminogen is more susceptible to activation than is plasminogen free in plasma. Streptokinase isolated from group C β-hemolytic streptococci, and acylated plasminogen-streptokinase (APSAC) act through a streptokinase—plasmin complex; urokinase, single-chain urokinase-type plasminogen activator (SCU-PA), and recombinant tPA act directly on plasmin without an intermediate drug—plasmin complex[125](Fig. 4-17). tPA (originally isolated from a melanoma cell line and now produced through recombinant DNA technology) APSAC, and SCU-PA are termed *fibrin selective* because of their high ratio of activity for fibrin-bound plasminogen compared with circulating plasminogen.

Acylation of the streptokinase—plasminogen complex on the active serine moiety on the light chain stabilizes the catalytic serine site, making this complex inert to circulating plasminogen. Binding occurs by virtue of the heavy-chain lysine—plasminogen portions to fibrin; over time, the acetyl group leaves the complex, resulting in a fibrin-specific thrombolytic effect. Urokinase, a double-chain polypeptide, is formed by the cleavage of SCU-PA by plasmin single-chain urokinase (a proenzyme-like substance); this cleavage is fibrin specific and occurs through a mecha-

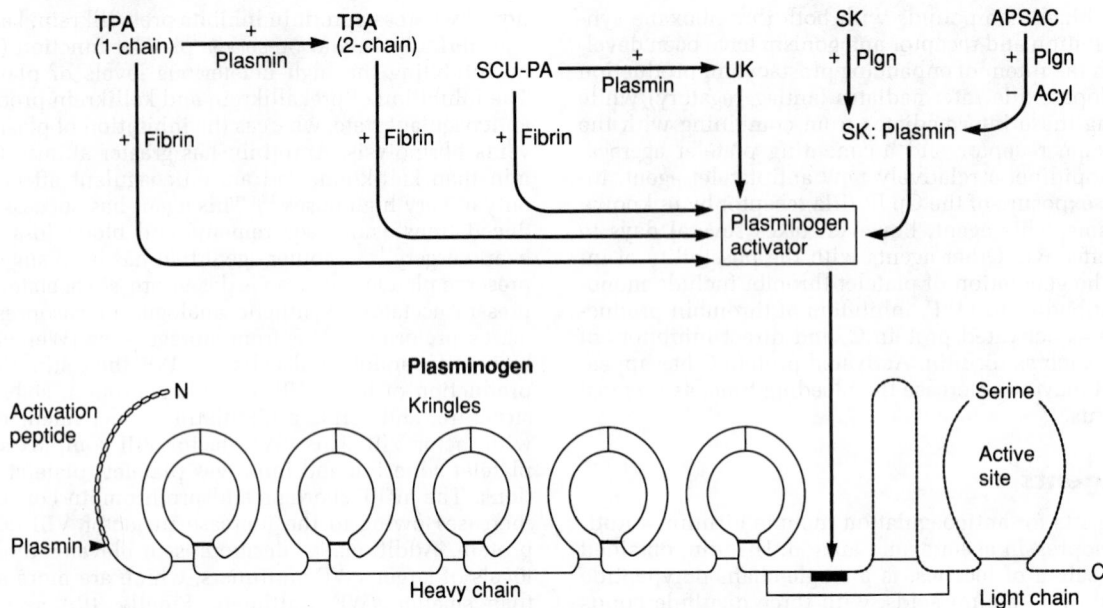

Figure 4-17. Sites of action of plasminogen activators on plasminogen. TPA, tissue plasminogen activator; SCU-PA, single-chain urokinase plasminogen activator; UK, urokinase; SK, streptokinase; Plgn, plasminogen; APSAC, acylated plasminogen–streptokinase. (After Marder VJ, Sherry S. Thrombolytic therapy: current status. N Engl J Med 1988;318:1513)

nism whereby SCU-PA activates plasminogen at the fibrin surface, converting it to plasmin. This activation is 10-fold more active at a fibrin surface than in circulating blood. Thus, only the fibrin-bound plasminogen is converted to plasmin for thrombolysis at the fibrin clot surface. tPA occurs in either a single or double polypeptide chain form. tPA has a fibrin-binding site and a catalytic site that are widely separated from each other. This separation allows tPA to be activated to its fibrin target, thus establishing its fibrin-specific nature. The level of the lytic state is greatest with streptokinase and APSAC, intermediate with urokinase, less with SCU-PA, and least with single-chain tPA[125] (Table 4-1). Half-lives also vary among different agents

from 5 minutes for single-chain recombinant tPA to 90 minutes for APSAC.[125] Streptokinase and APSAC, produced by group C β-hemolytic streptococci, are antigenic; urokinase and SCU-PA, produced from human fetal kidney cells in tissue culture, are nonantigenic. Because of its antigenicity, allergic reactions to streptokinase have been reported in 2% to 20% of cases. In addition, serum sickness has been reported with streptokinase.

Bleeding complications associated with fibrinolytic agents (reported in up to half of patients receiving systemic fibrinolytic agents for venous thrombosis) are related to the invasive procedures associated with drug therapy. Factors involved in bleeding include hypofibrinogenemia and fi-

Table 4-1. CHARACTERISTICS OF FIBRINOLYTIC AGENTS*

	SK	APSAC	UK	SCU-PA	rTPA 2-CHAIN	rTPA 1-CHAIN
Half-life (min)	23	90	16	7	8	5
Fibrin enhancement	1+	1+	2+	4+	4+	3+
Plasma proteolytic state	4+	4+	3+	2+	2+	1+
Duration of infusion	60 min	2–5 min	5–15 min	Several hours	Several hours	Several hours
Thrombus specificity (vs hemostatic plug)	0	0	0	0	0	0
Incidence of reperfusion (% within 3 h)	60–70	60–70	60–70	60–70	60–70	60–70
Speed of reperfusion (min)	45	45	45	45	45	45
Frequency of reocclusion (estimated %)	15	10	10	NA	20	20
Simultaneous administration of heparin	No	No	No	Yes	Yes	Yes
Bleeding complications	4+	4+	4+	4+	4+	4+
Allergic side effects	Yes	Yes	No	No	No	No
Antigenicity	Yes	Yes	No	NK	NK	NK
Expense	1+	2+	3+	4+	4+	4+

SK, streptokinase; APSAC, acylated plasminogen–streptokinase activator complex; UK, urokinase; SCU-PA, recombinant single-chain urokinase plasminogen activator; rTPA, recombinant tissue-type plasminogen activator; NA, data not available; NK, not known; 0, none; 4+, highest.
* The clinical data were derived mostly from reported experience with current intravenous dosages in the treatment of acute myocardial infarction.
(Marder VJ, Sherry S. Thrombolytic therapy: current status. N Engl J Med 1988;318:1514)

brin degradation products. The latter inhibit fibrin polymerization and, in combination with a decrease in the clotting factors V and VIII (from excess plasmin not neutralized by α_2-AP), inhibit the ability of blood to clot. Although coagulation tests in general do not correlate well with bleeding, a fibrinogen level of less than 100 mg/dL is associated with an increased risk and severity of bleeding. In addition, newly formed thrombi are easily lysed as they are formed. Platelets are both inhibited and stimulated by fibrinolytic agents. Because fibrinogen is a necessary cofactor for ADP-induced platelet aggregation, low fibrinogen levels aggravate a platelet defect. At the same time, plasminogen bound to platelets leads to impaired adhesion and a decrease in their ability to aggregate. Plasmin-induced cleavage of adhesive proteins, such as thrombospondin, fibronectin, and fibrin, also disrupt the bonds that hold platelet aggregates together. Additionally, plasmin formed on the endothelial cell surface impairs platelet adhesion to areas of vascular injury during therapy with fibrinolytic agents. Despite these mechanisms producing a decrease in the ability of the blood to clot during fibrinolytic therapy, it has been found that these agents promote reocclusion in up to 30% of cases early after thrombolysis through platelet activation, suggesting that platelet activation occurs early after lysis and that platelet inhibition occurs later.[114] Additionally, increased synthesis of endothelial cell PAI-1 has been demonstrated experimentally after treatment with tPA, another mechanism that could potentially contribute to early thrombotic reocclusion.[126]

Indications for thrombolytic therapy remain controversial. Clearly, in DVT, fibrinolytic agents allow for greater clot lysis than heparin and help preserve valve function to a greater degree, but at the risk of a higher rate of bleeding complications.[127] Thirteen studies of thrombolytic therapy for acute DVT have been compiled from the literature.[128] In these studies, patients were assessed with venography. Of those patients treated with anticoagulants, only 4% had complete lysis, and 14% revealed partial lysis. In contrast, 45% of patients treated with thrombolytic agents showed significant or complete clot lysis, and an additional 18% revealed partial lysis. Two studies evaluated the long-term success of thrombolytic therapy compared with anticoagulation for DVT. In 39 patients with follow-up of 1.6 to 5 years, 21% of patients treated with heparin had no evidence of postthrombotic symptoms, and 64% of patients treated with streptokinase did not have symptoms.[129,130] Similarly, significant functional benefit was reported 5 to 10 years after therapy in patients with significant clot lysis as measured by PPG times and foot volumetric studies, although PPG did not completely normalize in the lysis group. In addition, in a large prospective study in patients followed after DVT with either heparin or streptokinase, no major improvement in deep venous valvular competence was found with lytic agents at 2-year follow-up, and venous functional preservation appeared the same whether clot lysis was complete or incomplete.[131] About half of patients who present with their first episode of DVT and who begin lytic therapy within 72 hours of the onset of symptoms achieve significant dissolution of the thrombus. Only about 15% of patients who present acutely with lower extremity DVT, however, fit into this category because most patients who develop leg swelling or leg pain for the first time do not immediately seek medical attention.[132] The use of thrombolytic therapy for DVT remains controversial.

The main questions about the use of lytic therapy for DVT are which agent, what dose, and for how long? In a study comparing streptokinase to urokinase in DVT,[133] little cost difference was found after considering the longer infusion time and greater bleeding complications associated with streptokinase versus urokinase. Another study[134] compared tPA, 0.5 mg/kg twice over 4 hours or over 8 hours, with heparin versus placebo plus heparin for proximal venous thrombosis. Over 50% total clot lysis was found in 58% of a group of patients treated for 4 hours, 23% in a group treated for 8 hours, and only 7% complete clot lysis in the placebo-treated group. Follow-up of patients who achieved greater than 50% clot lysis revealed evidence of chronic venous insufficiency in only 25%, as compared with 56% of those with less than 50% clot lysis, a difference that was close to but not statistically significant ($P = .07$). This study suggests that further investigation into the use of the fibrin-specific agents for proximal DVT may be enlightening. Fibrinolytic therapy has been suggested for use in upper extremity effort venous thrombosis, catheter-induced venous thrombosis, Paget-Schroetter syndrome, and superior vena caval thrombosis. An interesting approach combining thrombolytic therapy and thoracic outlet decompression has been proposed.[135] Thrombolytic therapy is initiated locally with urokinase (250,000 IU bolus, then 1000 to 4000 IU/min) by a small catheter positioned from a basilic vein approach. After clot lysis, anticoagulation is continued for 3 months, with heparin followed by sodium warfarin to allow for thrombophlebitis (the inflammatory response in the vein that occurs due to the thrombus) to resolve. In about 3 months, thoracic outlet decompression is performed. Percutaneous transluminal angioplasty is not successful in the presence of an anatomic defect. Long-term results have been reported to be excellent and correlate well with the initial ability to clear the thrombus.

Thrombolytic therapy in pulmonary embolism has been extensively studied. Two carefully designed studies have evaluated the use of either urokinase or streptokinase. Although both agents rapidly lysed clot and improved pulmonary hemodynamics, there was no difference in patient mortality or recurrence rate of pulmonary embolism when compared with heparin alone.[136,137] Urokinase dissolved pulmonary arterial clot within 24 hours of treatment and, in certain instances, reversed shock. By 7 days, both the thrombolytic- and heparin-treated patients revealed equal improvement in pulmonary hemodynamics, and there was no difference in lung scan resolution. Additionally, no difference was seen between urokinase and streptokinase. Bleeding complications were more frequent in the thrombolysis-treated patients. Patients who received urokinase responded better if they were younger, if the embolus was less than 48 hours old, or if the embolus was of large magnitude. As a general guide, thrombolytic therapy for pulmonary embolism should be considered when there is angiographically documented lobar or greater pulmonary embolism causing acute pulmonary hypertension and shock; lesser degrees of pulmonary embolism should be treated with standard heparin anticoagulation.

Tissue plasminogen activator, 0.6 mg/kg over 2 minutes, plus heparin, versus placebo plus heparin for patients with pulmonary embolism has also been reported using lung scans at 24 hours and 7 days to document treatment efficacy.[134] No increase in bleeding complications was seen, and lysis was significantly improved at 24 hours in the tPA group (34.4%) versus the placebo group (12%; $P = .026$). Again, the advantage for tPA had disappeared by 7 days (59% lysis as compared with 56% lysis). The benefit for tPA thus would be expected only early in the small number of patients who die as a result of massive pulmonary embolism in the first hour after the embolus occurs.

Thrombolytic therapy for peripheral arterial applications is becoming more frequently used, especially when the agents are given intraarterially. The method of McNamara and Fischer[138] has gained the most recognition, involving passage of a guide wire through the thrombus and then infusion of a high dose of urokinase at 4000 IU/min for 1 to 2 hours, directly into the clot. If progress is made, further thrombolytic therapy is given at 1000 to 2000 IU/min for 6 to 12 hours or until complete clot lysis has occurred. Using this method, the mean infusion time was found to be 18 hours, and the incidence of bleeding was significantly lessened. McNamara and Fischer[138] compared these results to those of streptokinase from the literature and found a 13% incidence of severe bleeding with streptokinase versus only a 4% incidence with high-dose intraarterial urokinase therapy. McNamara and Bomberger[139] reported on their first 100 cases of selective intraarterial infusion of urokinase and found complete clot lysis in 77%, with native arterial occlusions responding better than arterial graft occlusions (71% versus 41% success) at 6-month follow-up. After thrombolytic therapy has reopened an occluded vessel or graft, however, radiologic or surgical correction of the lesion responsible for the thrombosis must be addressed for long-term success. A 1-year graft patency rate of 89% in those grafts in which an underlying lesion was successfully repaired, compared with 23% in grafts without a correctable lesion, has been reported.[140] At 2 years, this difference was even greater (79% compared with 10%). Complications associated with thrombolytic therapy for arterial thrombosis include bleeding, rethrombosis, embolization treated with further thrombolytic therapy, and sepsis from prolonged catheter placement. The most recent innovation in intraarterial thrombolytic therapy involves lacing the entire length of the thrombus with high-dose urokinase before continuous infusion and then using pulse-spray techniques. The application of tPA to peripheral vascular cases has been reported; and although promising results were described, 17% of patients still responded with a decrease in systemic fibrinogen levels to less than 100 mg/dL.[140a] In addition, three patients developed groin hematomas, and one developed a stroke soon after therapy had been completed. Although fibrin specific, tPA can still cause systemic thrombolytic effects.

The use of intraoperative thrombolytic therapy has been advocated for situations in which complete clot evacuation cannot be accomplished (as may be seen in up to 40% of patients undergoing balloon embolectomy with an embolectomy catheter for acute arterial occlusion), or when the distal vasculature is occluded and precludes appropriate inflow patency.[127] One method involves urokinase administration distal to an occluding clamp, infused at 250,000 IU combined with 1000 U of heparin in 250 mL saline, and allowed to remain for 30 minutes. If necessary, another 125,000 IU is infused for 30 minutes. Using this technique, 70% of limbs with critical ischemia at the completion of successful balloon embolectomy were spared amputation, with only one bleeding complication.[141] For patients with multivessel occlusions or for whom any degree of systemic fibrinolysis would be risky, a new high-dose isolated limb perfusion technique has been described. This technique involves anticoagulation, limb exsanguination with an Esmarch bandage, application of a proximal tourniquet, and direct arterial infusion of 1,000,000 IU or more of urokinase for 45 to 60 minutes, with direct drainage of the venous effluent below the tourniquet.

Although much work has been carried out on the use of thrombolytic agents in the sphere of acute myocardial infarction, this area is also evolving. Generally, the use of streptokinase reduces in-hospital mortality by 30%, although prospective comparisons between various thrombolytic agents has not been reported.[142] The clinical benefits associated with coronary thrombolysis most likely are determined by the rapidity of coronary artery reperfusion.

Platelet-mediated thrombotic events may be responsible for the 25% to 30% incidence of reocclusions associated with current protocols and agents. Heparin therapy added to tPA may improve the efficacy of this thrombolytic agent during coronary thrombolysis and helps to prevent reocclusion after thrombolysis is completed.

Contraindications to thrombolytic therapy, whether regional or systemic, are well defined and consist of active internal bleeding, recent surgery or trauma (generally within 10 days of infusion), recent cerebrovascular accident (within 2 months), or documented left heart thrombus (Table 4-2). Relative contraindications include recent surgery, gastrointestinal bleeding or trauma, severe hypertension, mitral valve disease, endocarditis, a history of a defect in hemostasis, and pregnancy.

Dextran

Dextran is a high-molecular-weight polysaccharide produced from sucrose by *Leuconostoc mesenteroides*. Fractionation and hydrolysis produce a product with an average molecular weight of either 40,000 (dextran-40; Rheomacrodex) or 70,000 (dextran-70). Dextran-40 has been studied in detail for its ability to augment patency of difficult lower extremity bypass grafts in the early postoperative period. Dextran-40 acts as a volume expander, causing hemodilution, decreasing blood viscosity, decreasing platelet adhesiveness, reducing factor VIII activity, and increasing the lysability of clot.[143] In addition, dextran has been found to coat endothelial cell surfaces, decreasing their electronegativity. Two 500-mL bottles on the day of bypass surgery followed by one on each of the succeeding 3 postoperative days at 75 mL/h increases bypass patency 1 day, 1 week, and 1 month postoperatively for femorotibial bypasses and all infrainguinal bypasses in which autologous vein was not able to be used. A number of other applications for dextran-40 have been suggested, including vascular trauma, endarterectomy, arterial and venous

---

Table 4-2. CONTRAINDICATIONS TO THROMBOLYTIC THERAPY

ABSOLUTE

Active internal bleeding
Recent (<2 mo) cerebrovascular accident
Intracranial pathology

RELATIVE

Major

Recent (<10 d) major surgery, obstetric delivery, or organ biopsy
Left heart thrombus
Active peptic ulcer or gastrointestinal abnormality
Recent major trauma
Uncontrolled hypertension

Minor

Minor surgery or trauma
Recent cardiopulmonary resuscitation
Atrial fibrillation with mitral valve disease
Bacterial endocarditis
Hemostatic defects (ie, renal or liver disease)
Diabetic hemorrhagic retinopathy
Pregnancy

CONTRAINDICATIONS FOR STREPTOKINASE

Known allergy
Recent streptococcal infection
Previous therapy within 6 mo

(Data from NIH Consensus Development Conference. Thrombolytic therapy in treatment. Ann Intern Med 1980;93:141)

thrombectomy, and venous reconstruction, and as a prophylactic agent for prevention of the development of venous thrombosis. None of these other indications has been substantiated by a clinical study, such as in the case of difficult lower extremity bypass procedures.

Mechanical Measures

Mechanical measures are used for the prevention of DVT during operative procedures or in patients who cannot be given pharmacologic prophylaxis. These measures include early ambulation, elastic stockings, electrical calf muscle stimulation, and external pneumatic compression, either with uniform-pressure stockings or graded-pressure stockings. In many well-controlled studies of venous prophylaxis, intermittent pneumatic compression has been found as effective as low-dose heparin therapy. In addition to augmentation of venous return with these devices, local and systemic fibrinolysis appears to be stimulated, even in areas remote from the application of the compression. The length of time that intermittent pneumatic compression should be used has not been adequately determined, but most data suggest that at least 5 days or longer in the face of prolonged immobilization may be optimal.

Vena caval interruption for venous thromboembolism is appropriate if traditional methods of anticoagulation fail or if the use of anticoagulant agents is contraindicated (see Chap. 97). Early results with direct vena cava ligation resulted in a high incidence of lower extremity venous complications and an unacceptably high rate of recurrent embolization. Thus, intraoperative caval compartmentalization and clip devices, followed by intravascular venous clot-trapping devices, were developed. These devices have resulted in a much lower incidence of venous stasis complications. The most effective device available is the Greenfield vena cava filter, a cone-shaped device. This cone shape allows for 85% of the length of the device to contain clot and still maintain flow around its periphery, allowing for natural fibrinolysis to take place. Indications for vena caval filtration include venous thrombosis or pulmonary embolism in patients with contraindications to anticoagulation, complications during anticoagulation, recurrent pulmonary embolisms in the face of adequate anticoagulation, chronic pulmonary embolism with associated pulmonary hypertension and cor pulmonale, and immediately after pulmonary embolectomy. Free-floating iliofemoral DVT may be associated with a 60% incidence of pulmonary embolism despite adequate anticoagulation[144]; free-floating inferior vena caval thrombi demonstrate a 27% incidence of pulmonary embolism despite adequate anticoagulation[145]; and bilateral free-floating femoral thrombi have a 43% incidence of pulmonary embolism despite anticoagulation[146]. These are all additional indications for filter placement. In 469 patients reported in the largest experience in the literature with the Greenfield filter, a contraindication to anticoagulation was the most frequent reason for filter insertion (38% of cases), followed by failure of anticoagulation (27% of cases).[147] Recurrent pulmonary embolism was reported in only 4% of patients during 12-year follow-up, the long-term inferior vena caval patency rate was 98% independent of anticoagulation, and venous ulceration was seen in only 3% of patients. No patient with suprarenal filter placement (32 cases) was found to have occluded inferior vena cava or renal veins during the follow-up period.

Percutaneous insertion versus direct surgical technique offers a number of advantages for the Greenfield filter, including decreased patient discomfort, decreased time of insertion, and decreased cost. Using a percutaneous approach, the incidence of venous thrombosis at the insertion site has been reported to be as high as 41%.[148] In response to this problem, a titanium Greenfield filter with modified hooks has been developed that reduces to a size of 12F in a 14F sheath. Testing of this filter in 186 patients revealed 97% successful placement and a recurrent pulmonary embolism rate of only 3%.[149] The venous thrombosis rate at the insertion site was only 8.7%

Surgical approaches for pulmonary thromboembolism are indicated in patients who have massive embolism with hypotension and who require massive doses of vasopressors (see Chap. 97). Open pulmonary embolectomy as practiced in the past is associated with a high morbidity and mortality. Today, open pulmonary embolectomy (or the placement on ECMO) is limited to patients who require cardiac massage manually for hypotension and patients who fail catheter pulmonary embolectomy. A catheter for the removal of pulmonary emboli has been developed. Catheter pulmonary embolectomy is performed by operative insertion under local anesthesia from either the jugular or common femoral vein. The cup catheter is inserted through a transverse venotomy, and the radiopaque catheter is then visualized under fluoroscopy as it is guided into the right side of the heart. The left main pulmonary artery is entered most easily. The cup is juxtaposed to the embolus, syringe suction is used to aspirate the clot into the cup, and the entire catheter and clot are withdrawn. Entry into the right pulmonary artery is performed by deflecting the cup in that direction as it reaches the superior edge of the cardiac shadow. Multiple retrievals may be necessary to remove enough thrombus to improve the pulmonary hemodynamics. In a series of 46 patients treated with this device, emboli were extracted in 76% of cases (35 of 46), and the 30-day survival was excellent at 70% (32 of 46).[150] Embolectomy was most successful for major pulmonary embolism and massive pulmonary embolism and least helpful for chronic pulmonary embolism. Successful embolectomy predicted long-term survival.

LABORATORY MONITORING OF COAGULATION AND ANTICOAGULATION

Tests of Platelet Function

Platelet tests include peripheral platelet counts, bleeding times, and platelet aggregation. Usually, a platelet count of 50,000/μL or more ensures adequate hemostasis, whereas counts less than 10,000/μL are dangerous and may lead to spontaneous bleeding. Thrombocytosis is considered a platelet count greater than 500,000/μL; in some cases (especially those involving myeloproliferative disorders), counts may be greater than 1,000,000/μL.[3] Bleeding time assays assess the ability of platelets to form hemostatic plugs and are usually shorter than 8 minutes. A bleeding time between 8 and 15 minutes most often reflects a low plasma level of vWF, the use of antiplatelet drugs, the presence of lupus-like antibodies, or a factor XI deficiency.[3] A bleeding time greater than 15 minutes is clearly prolonged and indicates severe platelet functional impairment, very low levels of vWF, or afibrinogenemia and severe factor V deficiency.[3] Platelet aggregation testing involves the use of a number of different agonists, such as ADP, collagen, epinephrine, arachidonic acid, calcium inophores, platelet-activating factor, thromboxane, and thrombin. Thrombin and collagen appear to be the primary in vivo stimuli, whereas thromboxane, ADP, serotonin, and platelet-activating factor appear to be amplifiers of aggregation after platelet secretion. Although a strong agonist, such as thrombin, can produce irreversible platelet aggregation independent of the arachidonic acid pathway, weak agonists, such as epinephrine, ADP, and collagen, require an intact cyclooxygenase pathway for the induction of irreversible platelet aggregation. Although a relatively straightforward technique, platelet aggregation is not available in most laboratories, probably because of the observer-dependent nature of the test. Characteristic curves for the various agonists have been reported, such as the presence of a second wave of aggregation for ADP at relatively low concentration (10^{-6} mol/L) versus only a single wave at higher levels (2×10^{-5} mol/L). The first wave is due to ADP, and the second wave arises from products released from the platelets on activation, such as thromboxane. Platelet aggregability has been studied in 685 male and 273 female patients in a prospective study of the role of hemostasis on the development of peripheral vascular occlusive disease.[87] Platelet aggregability was found to increase with age, was greater in white than in black patients (especially among men), and tended to decrease with higher levels of habitual alcohol intake. Platelet aggregability was less among smokers, especially among men, but it was increased in the presence of elevation in plasma fibrinogen levels. A variant of platelet aggregation testing has been proposed as the best diagnostic test for the presence of heparin-associated thrombocytopenia.[64]

Coagulation Tests

Coagulation tests include PT (intrinsic and extrinsic pathways and fibrinogen), PTT, and aPTT (contact and intrinsic pathway), TCT (fibrinogen conversion to fibrin), and activated clotting time (whole blood and platelets). The only abnormality that causes an isolated elevation in PT with all of the other tests normal is factor VII deficiency, the factor that is activated by tissue factor and then stimulates the generation of the extrinsic pathway of coagulation.[3] In addition, the PT is sensitive to small decreases in factor V levels. The PT is the most common manner of measuring the level of oral anticoagulant therapy. The aPTT identifies abnormalities of the contact and intrinsic phases of coagulation. The aPTT evolved from the PTT first described in 1953 and 1954. The PTT uses a phospholipid derived from either brain or lung tissue to mimic the function of the platelets in the scheme of coagulation. The aPTT incorporated the standardization of the activation of factor XII by agents such as cephaloplastin. Because the blood specimen, activator, and phospholipid must be incubated for a period of time, the blood specimen must be anticoagulated during the activation step; this is usually accomplished with sodium citrate. After incubation, the specimen is recalcified to begin the test. Conditions that cause a prolongation of aPTT include the presence of heparin; deficiencies in factors VIII, IX, and XII; and the presence of lupus-like anticoagulants.[3] Values of aPTT have variably been shown to correlate with heparin dosages and serum heparin levels. Heparin levels of 0.2 IU/mL or greater usually correlate with an aPTT of 1.5 times or greater. TCT is a measurement of the time it takes for exogenously added thrombin to turn plasma fibrinogen into fibrin clot. As such, it is extremely sensitive to levels of heparin and is an excellent means of measuring the level of heparin-induced anticoagulation. The beauty of the TCT is that it is not specific for any disease condition; thus, it may be used to differentiate factor deficiencies from the presence of heparin or to separate lupus anticoagulant from abnormalities in fibrinogen levels.[3] The ACT is a measurement of the ability of whole blood to clot, and as such is an available technique for monitoring heparin levels intraoperatively. The ACT responds in a linear fashion to increasing heparin dosage and correlates well with observed clinical anticoagulation (thrombus-free surface on cardio-

pulmonary bypass devices).[151] Adequate anticoagulation for extracorporeal circulation is defined as an ACT of 480 seconds or more, but most cardiovascular surgeons would agree that any value between 300 and 600 seconds is acceptable. For peripheral vascular applications, values of 250 seconds or greater are considered appropriate levels representative of full intraoperative anticoagulation. The ACT may be affected by hemodilution, cardioplegia solutions, hypothermia, platelet dysfunction, hypofibrinogenemia, and other coagulopathies as well as by certain medications and excess protamine administration.

Tests of Fibrinolysis

Tests of fibrinolysis are less well characterized. The euglobulin lysis test time is a crude but effective screening test for problems with fibrinolysis.[3] Patients with accelerated fibrinolysis are often found to have a deficiency of α_2-antiplasmin (of which the total amount normally is only half of the total plasmin that can be generated) or the fibrin clot–stabilizing factor XIII.[3] In addition, a deficiency of PAI may also lead to accelerated fibrinolysis. During normal clot formation and breakdown, the D-dimer fragment of fibrinogen is a marker for ongoing thrombosis and physiologic fibrinolysis, whereas for fibrinogenolysis, the two D fragments that are produced are not cross-linked into the D-dimer form.[3]

RISKS OF BLOOD TRANSFUSIONS

Risks of blood transfusions include immediate and delayed hemolytic reactions; nonhemolytic reactions; infectious disease transmission, including hepatitis, cytomegalovirus (CMV), and AIDS; and complications of massive transfusions. Immediate hemolytic reactions are usually caused by blood group ABO incompatibility, although they may also be caused by antigens of other blood group systems on the transfused red blood cells. The clinical manifestations depend on the antigen on the red-cell stroma and the antibody in the patient's serum, and include the production of bradykinin complement activation, release of vasoactive agents from platelets, and initiation of systemic clotting. Chills and fever, chest pain and lumbar pain, tachycardia and hypotension in the conscious patient, and often diffuse bleeding in the anesthetized unconscious patient constitute this syndrome. Death related to this syndrome is uncommon, unless associated with the transfusion of more than 100 mL of blood; it occurs from acute renal failure or hemorrhage due to DIC.[152] Delayed hemolytic reactions result from the amnestic response of preformed antibody to transfused red blood cells several days after the transfusion. In these reactions, clinical abnormalities are relatively mild and primarily consist of failure of the correction of anemia by transfusions or the presence of an unexpected positive direct antiglobulin test after transfusion. Although more severe reactions, such as hemoglobinuria, hemoglobinemia, and increased serum bilirubin, may be seen in some cases, acute renal failure occurs only rarely. Treatment is infrequently necessary.

Nonhemolytic reactions occur with the frequency of 1% to 2% of all transfusions and consist primarily of chills and fever during the transfusion or during the first 2 or 3 hours after the transfusion is complete.[153] The severity of this condition is variable, and management is symptomatic, including antipyretics. The mechanism of these reactions includes the presence of antibodies to white-cell antigens in the transfused blood, especially in the multitransfused or multiparous patient. These reactions can be prevented by the use of acetaminophen pretreatment, steroids, and leukocyte-free blood or by the use of filters that remove leukocytes from the transfused blood. Allergic reactions are also commonly associated with transfusions, with urticaria and pruritus seen in as many as 1% to 3% of all transfused patients.[154] Acute anaphylaxis occurs infrequently at a rate of about 1 per 150,000 components given.[155]

Infectious disease transmission is an important issue in clinical practice. The most common entities include viral hepatitis, CMV, and AIDS. Posttransfusion hepatitis in 90% of the cases consists of a non-A, non-B hepatitis, recently identified as hepatitis C. The incubation period is between 2 weeks and 1 year, with a median of 6 to 8 weeks.[152] Most patients are relatively symptom free, although the eventual development of chronic liver disease, cirrhosis, and hepatocellular carcinoma are the greatest concerns. All blood products except for immune serum globulin and albumin can carry and transmit this form of hepatitis. A screening assay for antibody marking previous exposure to hepatitis C became available in 1990. Surrogate tests available for this diagnosis include ALT and hepatitis B core antigen. Other forms of hepatitis are much less common, including hepatitis A, hepatitis B, and hepatitis D (associated with hepatitis B).

CMV exists in three forms: primary, reinfection, and reactivation. Primary exposure results in an IgM response to the virus, followed by an IgG antibody response. Reactivation is most commonly related to pregnancy, transplantation, and immunosuppression and is the most important cause of posttransfusion disease accompanying immunosuppression of patients. Fresh blood is used more frequently than stored blood, and although screening for CMV is said not to be feasible, two particularly susceptible groups whose blood should be screened include low-birthweight infants (less than 1500 g) and bone marrow transplant recipients.[152] AIDS is less frequently transmitted in blood than is hepatitis. Because heat treatment eliminates the risk of this viral transmission, products from pooled plasma that are heat treated are not at risk for human immunodeficiency virus type 1 transmission, such as albumin. In addition, public awareness has led to a number of programs, such as the routine screening of blood for antibody levels and the use of autologous blood transfusions during and after surgical procedures whenever possible. These programs have continued to lessen the risk of AIDS transmission from blood and blood products. Other infection-related complications are rare and include malaria, Chagas disease, human T-cell leukemia/lymphoma virus type 1, babesiosis, syphilis and other venereal diseases, and Epstein-Barr virus–related syndromes.

Massive transfusion complications relate to the rate and volume of blood transfused. The most common complication is dilutional thrombocytopenia.[156] Factor deficiency of the labile factors V and VIII rarely is of sufficient magnitude to result in problems with hemostasis. For hypocalcemia to occur with massive transfusion, 1 U of citrated blood must be administered every 5 minutes. Routine empiric calcium supplementation is unnecessary during most massive transfusion episodes.[152] Conversely, hypothermia is clearly a problem, especially when associated with massive transfusion during complex intraoperative procedures, such as thoracoabdominal aneurysm resection. The use of autotransfusion devices that can warm the blood has helped to solve this problem. Hyperkalemia is usually not a clinically significant problem during massive transfusions. Finally, although microaggregates present in blood may theoretically lead to lodgement in the pulmonary bed and contribute to respiratory distress, it is generally agreed that these aggregates are not a frequent cause of the adult respiratory distress syndrome.

In view of the many possible risks associated with blood transfusion, the use of autotransfusion devices is becoming increasingly more popular during surgical procedures. These devices allow the amount of nonautologous blood transfused to be minimized and decrease the overall risk of the various processes described. Their use is somewhat restricted during procedures requiring massive transfusion because of the limits of suctioning and the time needed to process the recovered blood (except for the power infuser–type units). In addition, great interest in autologous blood donation has been generated. Patients may donate as often as every 4 days for up to 14 days before their operative procedure,[152] and a hemoglobin as low as 11 g/dL is acceptable for proceeding with the operation. Directed relative donation programs, although popular with the public, have not been shown to enhance the safety of blood for the recipient[157] and carry the possible risk of coercion for the directed donation. Autologous programs are therefore of far greater potential widespread clinical use, along with new and improved autotransfusion devices.

REFERENCES

1. Zur M. Radcliffe RD, Oberdick J, et al. The dual role of factor VII in blood coagulation: initiation and inhibition of a proteolytic system by a zymogen. J Biol Chem 1982;257:5623.
2. Radcliffe R, Nemerson Y. Mechanism of activation of bovine factor VII: products of cleavage by factor Xa. J Biol Chem 1976;251:4749.
3. Hassouna HI. Laboratory evaluation of hemostatic disorders. In: Penner JA, Hassouna HI, eds. Coagulation disorders II. Hematol Oncol Clin North Am 1993;7:1161.
4. Sims PJ, Faioni EM, Wiedmer T, et al. Complement proteins C5b–9 cause release of membrane vesicles from the platelet surface that are enriched in the membrane receptor for coagulation factor Va and express prothrombinase activity. J Biol Chem 1988;263:18205.
5. Gilbert GE, Sims PJ, Wiedmer T, et al. Platelet-derived microparticles express high affinity receptors for factor VIII. J Biol Chem 1991;266:17261.
6. Hickey MJ, Williams SA, Roth GA. Human platelet glycoprotein IX: an adhesive prototype of leucine-rich glycoproteins with flank-center-flank structures. Proc Natl Acad Sci USA 1989;86:6773.
7. Bennett JS, Vilaire G, Cines DB. Identification of the fibrinogen receptor on human platelets by photoaffinity labeling. J Biol Chem 1982;257:8049.
8. Savage B, Ruggeri ZM. Selective recognition of adhesive sites in surface-bound fibrinogen by glycoprotein IIb/IIIa on non-activated platelets. J Biol Chem 1991;266:11277.
9. Osterud B, Rapaport SI. Activation of factor IX by the reaction product of tissue factor and factor VIII: additional pathway for initiating blood coagulation. Proc Natl Acad Sci USA 1977;74:5260.
10. Bauer KA, Kass BL, ten Care H, et al. Factor IX is activated in vivo by the tissue factor mechanism. Blood 1990;76:731.
11. Blomback B, Blomback M. The molecular structure of fibrinogen. Ann NY Acad Sci 1972;202:77.
12. Folk JE, Finlayson JS. The epsilon-(gamma-glutamyl) lysine crosslink and the catalytic role of transglutamines. Adv Protein Chem 1977;31:1.
13. Davie EW, Fujikawa K, Kisiel W. The coagulation cascade: initiation, maintenance, and regulation. Biochemistry 1991; 30:10363.
14. Naito K, Fujikawa K. Activation of human blood coagulation factor XII independent of factor XII: factor XI is activated by thrombin and factor XIa in the presence of negatively charged surfaces. J Biol Chem 1991;266:7353.
15. DiScipio RG, Kurachi K, Davie EW. Activation of human factor IX (Christmas factor). J Clin Invest 1978;61:1528.
16. Rosenberg RD, Damus PS. The purification and mechanism of action of human antithrombin-heparin cofactor. J Biol Chem 1973;248:6490.
17. Kurachi K, Fujikawa K, Schmer G, et al. Inhibition of bovine factor IXa and factor Xab by antithrombin III. Biochemistry 1976;15:373.

18. Kurachi K, Davie EW. Activation of human factor XI (plasma thrombo-plastin antecedent) by factor XIIa (activated Hageman factor). Biochemistry 1977;16:5831.

19. Kisiel W, Canfield WM, Ericsson LH, et al. Anticoagulant properties of bovine plasma protein C following activation by thrombin. Biochemistry 1977;16:5824.

20. Marlar RA, Kleiss AJ, Griffin JH. Mechanism of action of human activated protein C, a thrombin dependent anticoagulant enzyme. Blood 1982;59:1067.

21. Vehar GA, Davie EW. Preparation and properties of bovine factor VIII (antihemophilic factor). Biochemistry 1980; 19:401.

22. Esmon CT, Owen WG. Identification of an endothelial cell cofactor for thrombin-catalyzed activation of protein C. Proc Natl Acad Sci USA 1981;78:2249.

23. Owen WG, Esmon CT. Functional properties of an endothelial cell cofactor for thrombin-catalyzed activation of protein C. J Biol Chem 1981;256:5532.

24. Esmon NL, Owen WG, Esmon CT. Isolation of a membrane-bound cofactor for thrombin-catalyzed activation of protein C. J Biol Chem 1982;257:859.

25. Esmon CT. The regulation of natural anticoagulant pathways. Science 1987;235:1348.

26. Esmon NL, Carroll RC, Esmon CT. Thrombomodulin blocks the ability of thrombin to activate platelets. J Biol Chem 1983;258:12238.

27. Esmon CT, Esmon NL, Harris KW. Complex formation between thrombin and thrombomodulin inhibits both thrombin-catalyzed fibrin formation and factor V activation. J Biol Chem 1982;257:7944.

28. Walker FJ. Regulation of activated protein C by a new protein: a possible function for bovine protein S. J Biol Chem 1980;255:5521.

29. Tollefsen DM, Majerus PW, Blank MK. Heparin cofactor II: purification and properties of a heparin-dependent inhibitor of thrombin in human plasma. J Biol Chem 1982;257:2162.

30. Broze GJ, Girard TJ, Novotny WF. Regulation of coagulation by a multivalent Kunitz-type inhibitor. Biochemistry 1990; 29:7539.

31. Rapaport SI. Inhibition of factor VIIa/tissue factor-induced blood coagulation: with particular emphasis upon a factor Xa-dependent inhibitory mechanism. Blood 1989;73:359.

32. Gelehrter TD, Sznycer-Laszuk R. Thrombin induction of plasminogen activator inhibitor in cultured human endothelial cells. J Clin Invest 1986;77:165.

33. Dichek D, Quertermous T. Thrombin regulation of mRNA levels of tissue plasminogen activator and plasminogen activator inhibitor-1 in cultured human umbilical vein endothelial cells. Blood 1989;74:222.

34. Adelman B, Michelson AD, Loscalzo J, et al. Plasmin effect on platelet glycoprotein Ib–von Willebrand factor interactions. Blood 1985;65:32.

35. Schmaier AH. Disseminated intravascular coagulation: pathogenesis and management. J Intensive Care Med 1991; 6:209.

36. Coleman RW. Activation of plasminogen by human plasma kallikrein. Biochem Biophys Res Commun 1969;35:273.

37. Hajjar KA, Nachman RL. Endothelial cell–mediated conversion of Glu-plasminogen to Lys-plasminogen: further evidence for assembly of the fibrinolytic system on the endothelial cell surface. J Clin Invest 1988;82:1769.

38. Esmon NL, Esmon CT. Protein C and the endothelium. Sem Thromb Haemost 1988;14:210.

39. Van der Poll T, Buller HR, ten Cate H, et al. Activation of coagulation after administration of tumor necrosis factor to normal subjects. N Engl J Med 1990;322:1622.

40. Nawroth PP, Stern DM. Modulation of endothelial cell hemostatic properties by tumor necrosis factor. J Exp Med 1986;163:740.

41. Bevilacqua MP, Pober JS, Majeau GR, et al. Recombinant tumor necrosis factor induces procoagulant activity in cultured human vascular endothelium: characterization and comparison with the actions of interleukin-1. Proc Natl Acad Sci USA 1986;83:4533.

42. Conway EM, Bach R, Rosenberg RD, et al. Tumor necrosis factor enhances expression of tissue factor mRNA in endothelial cells. Thromb Res 1989;53:231.

43. Schleef RR, Bevilacqua MP, Sawdey M, et al. Cytokine activation of vascular endothelium: effects on tissue-type plasminogen activator and type I plasminogen inhibitor. J Biol Chem 1988;263:5797.

44. Van Hinsbergh VW, Kooistra T, van den Berg EA, et al. Tumor necrosis factor increases production of plasminogen activator inhibitor in human endothelial cells in vitro and rats in vivo. Blood 1988;72:1467.

45. Medina R, Schocher SH, Han JH. Interleukin-1, endotoxin, or tumor necrosis factor/cachectin enhance the level of plasminogen activator messenger RNA in bovine aortic endothelial cells. Thromb Res 1989;54:41.

46. Van der Poll T, Levi M, Buller HR, et al. Fibrinolytic response to tumor necrosis factor in healthy subjects. J Exp Med 1991;174:729.

47. Pohlman TH, Stanness KA, Beatty PG, et al. An endothelial cell surface factor(s) induced in vitro by lipopolysaccharide, interleukin-1, and tumor necrosis factor-alpha increases neutrophil adherence by CD18 dependent mechanism. J Immunol 1986;136:4548.

48. Schleimer RP, Rutledge BK. Cultured human endothelial cells acquire adhesiveness for neutrophils after stimulation with interleukin-1, endotoxin, and tumor-promoting phorbol diesters. J Immunol 1986;136:649.

49. Rothlein R, Dustin ML, Marlin SD, et al. A human intercellular adhesion molecule (ICAM-1) distinct from LFA-1. J Immunol 1986;137:1270.

50. Bevilacqua MP, Stengelin S, Gimbrone MA, et al. Endothelial leukocyte adhesion molecule 1: an inducible receptor for neutrophils related to complement regulatory proteins and lectins. Science 1989;243:1160.

51. Kunkel SL, Standiford T, Metinko AP, et al. Endothelial cell-derived novel chemotactic cytokines. In: Lefant C, ed. Lung vascular injury: molecular and cellular response. New York, Marcel Dekker, 1991.

52. Furie B, Furie BC. Molecular and cell biology of blood coagulation. N Engl J Med 1992;326:800.

53. Palabrica T, Lobb R, Furie BC. Leukocyte accumulation promoting fibrin deposition is mediated in vivo by P-selectin on adherent platelets. Nature 1992;359:848.

54. Stewart GJ. Neutrophils and deep venous thrombosis. Haemostasis 1993;23:127.

55. Holt JC, Yan Z, Lu W, et al. Isolation, characterization and immunological detection of neutrophil-activating peptide 2: a proteolytic degradation product of platelet basic protein. Proc Soc Exp Biol Med 1992;199:171.

56. Ferrer-Lopez P, Renesto P, Schattner M, et al. Activation of human platelets by C5a-stimulated neutrophils: a role for cathepsin G. Am J Physiol 1990;258:C1100.

57. Evangelista V, Rajtar G, de Gaetano G, et al. Platelet activation by fMLP-stimulated polymorphonuclear leukocytes: the activity of cathepsin G is not prevented by antiproteases. Blood 1991;77:2379.

58. Wakefield TW, Greenfield LJ, Rolfe MW, et al. Inflammatory and procoagulant mediator interactions in an experimental baboon model of venous thrombosis. Thromb Haemost 1993;69:164.

59. Ansell JE, Price JM, Shah S, et al. Heparin-induced thrombocytopenia: what is its real frequency? Chest 1985;88:878.

60. Greinacher A, Michels I, Mueller-Eckhardt. Heparin-associated thrombocytopenia: the antibody is not heparin specific. Thromb Haemost 1992;67:545.

61. Adelman B, Sobel M, Fujimura Y, et al. Heparin-associated thrombocytopenia: observations on the mechanism of platelet aggregation. J Lab Clin Med 1989;113:204.

62. Silver D, Kapsch DN, Tsoi EK. Heparin-induced thrombocytopenia, thrombosis and hemorrhage. Am Surg 1983;198: 301.

63. Robitaille D, Leclerc JR, Laberge R, et al. Cardiopulmonary bypass with a low-molecular weight fraction (enoxaparin) in a patient with a history of heparin-associated thrombocytopenia. J Thorac Cardiovasc Surg 1992;103:597.

64. Kappa JR, Fisher CA, Berkowitz HD, et al. Heparin-induced platelet activation in sixteen surgical patients: diagnosis and management. J Vasc Surg 1987;5:101.

65. Towne JB, Bernhard VM, Hussey C, et al. Antithrombin de-

ficiency: a cause of unexplained thrombosis in vascular surgery. Surgery 1981;89:735.

66. Flinn WR, McDaniel MD, Yao JST, et al. Antithrombin III deficiency as a reflection of dynamic protein metabolism in patients undergoing vascular reconstruction. J Vasc Surg 1984;1:888.

67. Eby CS. A review of the hypercoagulable state. In: Penner JA, Hassouna HI, eds. Coagulation disorders II. Hematol Oncol Clin North Am 1993:1121.

68. Menache D. Antithrombin III concentrates. In: Penner JA, Hassouna HI, eds. Coagulation disorders I. Hematol Oncol Clin North Am 1992:1115.

69. Clouse LH, Comp PC. The regulation of hemostasis: the protein C system. N Engl J Med 1986;314:1298.

70. Eldrup-Jorgensen J, Flanigan DP, Brace L, et al. Hypercoagulable states and lower limb ischemia in young adults. J Vasc Surg 1989;9:334.

71. Cole MS, Minifee PK, Wolma FJ. Coumadin necrosis: a review of the literature. Surgery 1988;103:271.

72. Svensson PJ, Dahlback B. Resistance to activated protein C as a basis for venous thrombosis. N Engl J Med 1994;330:517.

73. Koster T, Rosendaal FR, deRonde H, et al. Venous thrombosis due to poor anticoagulant response to activated protein C: Leiden thrombophilia study. Lancet 1993;342:1503.

74. Griffin JH, Evatt B, Wideman C, et al. Anticoagulant protein C pathway defective in majority of thrombophilic patients. Blood 1993;82:1989.

75. Bauer KA. Hypercoagulability: a new cofactor in the protein C anticoagulant pathway. (Editorial) N Engl J Med 1994; 330:566.

76. Dahlback B. Inherited resistance to activated protein C, a major cause of venous thrombosis, is due to a mutation in factor V gene. Haemostasis 1994;24:139.

77. Greenfield LJ. Lupus-like anticoagulants and thrombosis. J Vasc Surg 1988;7:818.

78. Lockshin MD. Antiphospholipid antibody syndrome. JAMA 1992;268:1451.

79. Ahn SS, Kalunian K, Rosove M, et al. Postoperative thrombotic complications in patients with the lupus anticoagulant: increased risk after vascular procedures. J Vasc Surg 1988;7:749.

80. Donaldson MC, Weinberg DS, Belkin M, et al. Screening for hypercoagulable states in vascular surgical practice: a preliminary study. J Vasc Surg 1990;11:825.

81. Towne JB, Bandyk DF, Hussey CV, et al. Abnormal plasminogen: a genetically determined cause of hypercoagulability. J Vasc Surg 1984;1:896.

82. Wu KW. Hypercoagulability in arterial thrombosis: new perspectives from epidemiologic studies. J Vasc Surg 1990; 12:208.

83. Rodgers GM. Hemostatic properties of normal and perturbed vascular cells. FASEB J 1988;2:116.

84. Nilsson IM, Ljungner H, Tengborn L. Two different mechanisms in patients with venous thrombosis and defective fibrinolysis: low concentrations of plasminogen activator or increased concentration of plasminogen activator inhibitor. Br Med J 1985;290:1453.

85. Prins MH, Hirsh J. A clinical review of the evidence supporting a relationship between impaired fibrinolytic activity and venous thromboembolism. Arch Intern Med 1991;151:1721.

86. Paramo JA, Perez JL, Serrano M, et al. Type 1 and 2 plasminogen activator inhibitor and tumor necrosis factor alpha in patients with sepsis. Thromb Haemost 1990;64:3.

87. Meade TW, Vickers MV, Thompson SG, et al. Epidemiological characteristics of platelet aggregability. Br Med J 1985; 290:428.

88. Fisher DF Jr, Yawn DH, Crawford ES. Preoperative disseminated intravascular coagulation associated with aortic aneurysms: a prospective study of 76 cases. Arch Surg 1983; 118:1252.

89. Collins JA. Blood transfusion and disorders of surgical bleeding. In: Sabiston DC, ed. Textbook of surgery, ed 14. Philadelphia, WB Saunders, 1991:85.

90. Lusher JM, Warrier I. Hemophilia A. In: Penner JA, Hassouna HI, eds. Coagulation disorders I. Hematol Oncol Clin North Am 1992:1021.

91. Lusher JM, Arkin S, Abildgaard CF, et al. Recombinant factor VIII for the treatment of previously untreated patients with hemophilia A: safety, efficacy and development of inhibitors. N Engl J Med 1993;328:453.

92. Telfer MC. Clinical spectrum of viral infections in hemophilic patients. In: Penner JA, Hassouna HI, eds. Coagulation disorders I. Hematol Oncol Clin North Am 1992:1047.

93. Larson PJ, High KA. Biology of inherited coagulopathies: factor IX. In: Penner JA, Hassouna HI, eds. Coagulation disorders I. Hematol Oncol Clin North Am 1992:999.

94. Ginsburg D. Biology of inherited coagulopathies: von Willebrand factor. In: Penner JA, Hassouna HI, eds. Coagulation disorders I. Hematol Oncol Clin North Am 1992:1011.

95. Edmunds LH. Blood contact activation during cardioplumonary bypass. J Vasc Surg 1990;12:213.

96. Wakefield TW, Shulkin BL, Fellows EP, et al. Platelet reactivity in human aortic grafts: a prospective randomized midterm study of platelet adherence and release products in Dacron and ePTFE grafts. J Vasc Surg 1989;9:234.

97. Hirsh J. Heparin. N Engl J Med 1991;324:1565.

98. Saba HI, Saba SR, Morelli GA. Effect of heparin on platelet aggregation. Am J Hematol 1984;17:295.

99. Kakkar VV. The current status of low-dose heparin in the prophylaxis of thrombophlebitis and pulmonary embolism. World J Surg 1978;2:3.

100. Prevention of venous thrombosis and pulmonary embolism: NIH consensus development. JAMA 1986;256:744.

101. Collins R, Scrigmeour A, Yusuf S, et al. Reduction in fatal pulmonary embolism and venous thrombosis by perioperative administration of subcutaneous heparin: overview of results of randomized trials in general, orthopedic, and urologic surgery. N Engl J Med 1988;318:1162.

102. Salzman EW. Low-molecular weight heparin: is small beautiful? (Editorial) N Engl J Med 1986;315:957.

103. Colwell CW, Spiro TE, Trowbridge AA, et al. Use of enoxaparin, a low-molecular weight heparin, and unfractionated heparin for the prevention of deep venous thrombosis after elective hip replacement. J Bone Joint Surg 1994;76A:3.

104. Horrow JC. Protamine: a review of its toxicity. Anesth Analg 1985;64:348.

105. Wakefield TW, Ucros I, Kresowik TF, et al. Decreased oxygen consumption as a toxic manifestation of protamine sulfate reversal of heparin anticoagulation. J Vasc Surg 1989;9:772.

106. Pearson PJ, Evora RR, Ayrancioglu K, et al. Protamine releases endothelium-derived relaxing factor from systemic arteries: a possible mechanism of hypotension during heparin neutralization. Circulation 1992;86:289.

107. Wakefield TW, Bies LE, Wrobleski SK, et al. Impaired myocardial function and oxygen utilization due to protamine sulfate in an isolated rabbit heart preparation. Ann Surg 1990;212:387.

108. Morel DR, Zapol WM, Thomas SJ, et al. C5a and thromboxane generation associated with pulmonary vaso- and bronchoconstriction during protamine reversal of heparin. Anesthesiology 1987;66:597.

109. Eika C. On the mechanism of platelet aggregation induced by heparin, protamine, and polybrene. Scand J Haematol 1972;9:248.

110. DeLucia A, Wakefield TW, Andrews PC, et al. Efficacy and toxicity of differently charged polycationic protamine-like peptides for heparin anticoagulation reversal. J Vasc Surg 1993;18:49.

111. Coon WW. Anticoagulant therapy. Am J Surg 1985;150:45.

112. Hirsh J. Oral anticoagulant drugs. N Engl J Med 1991; 324:1865.

113. Hull R, Carter C, Jay R, et al. The diagnosis of acute, recurrent, deep-vein thrombosis: a diagnostic challenge. Circulation 1983;67:901.

114. Coller BS. Platelets and thrombolytic therapy. N Engl J Med 1990;322:33.

115. Jang IK, Gold HK, Ziskind AA, et al. Prevention of platelet-rich arterial thrombosis by selective thrombin inhibition. Circulation 1990;81:219.

116. Addonzio VP Jr, Fisher CA, Jenkin BK, et al. Iloprost (ZK 36 374), a stable analogue of prostacyclin, preserves platelets during simulated extracorporeal circulation. J Thorac Cardiovasc Surg 1985;89:926.

117. Musial J, Niewiarowski S, Rucinski B, et al. Inhibition of

platelet adhesion to surfaces of extracorporeal circuits by disintegrins: RGD-containing peptides from viper venoms. Circulation 1990;82:261.

118. Shigeta O, Gluszko P, Downing SW, et al. Protection of platelets during long-term extracorporeal membrane oxygenation in sheep with a single dose of a disintegrin. Circulation 1992;86(Suppl II):398.

119. Mohr R, Goor DA, Lusky A, et al. Aprotinin prevents cardiopulmonary bypass-induced platelet dysfunction: a scanning electron microscope study. Circulation 1992;86(Suppl II):405.

120. Quereshi A, Lamont J, Burke P, et al. Aprotinin: the ideal anti-coagulant? Eur J Vasc Surg 1992;6:317.

121. Royston D, Bidstrup BP, Taylor KM, et al. Effect of aprotinin on need for blood transfusion after repeat open heart surgery. Lancet 1987;2:1289.

122. Salzman EW, Weinstein MJ, Reilly D, et al. Adventures in hemostasis: desmopressin in cardiac surgery. Arch Surg 1993;128:212.

123. Mannucci PM. Desmopressin: a nontransfusional form of treatment for congenital and acquired bleeding disorders. Blood 1988;72:1449.

124. Cole CW, Bormanis J, Luna GK, et al. Ancrod versus heparin for anticoagulation during vascular surgical procedures. J Vasc Surg 1993;17:288.

125. Marder VJ, Sherry S. Thrombolytic therapy: current status. N Engl J Med 1988;318:1512.

126. Fuji S, Sawa H, Saffitz JE, et al. Induction of endothelial cell expression of the plasminogen activator inhibitor type I gene by thrombosis in vivo. Circulation 1992;86:2000.

127. Quinones-Baldrich WJ. Principles of thrombolytic therapy. In: Rutherford RB, ed. Vascular surgery, ed 4. Philadelphia, WB Saunders, 1995;334.

128. Comerota AJ, Aldridge SC. Thrombolytic therapy for acute deep vein thrombosis. Semin Vasc Surg 1992;5:76.

129. Elliot MS, Immelman EJ, Jeffrey P, et al. A comparative randomized trial of heparin versus streptokinase in the treatment of acute proximal venous thrombosis: an interim report of a prospective trial. Br J Surg 1979;66:838.

130. Arnsen H, Hoiseth A, Ly B. Streptokinase or heparin in the treatment of deep vein thrombosis: follow-up results of a prospective study. Acta Med Scand 1982;211:65.

131. Kakkar VV, Lawrence D. Hemodynamic and clinical assessment after therapy for acute deep vein thrombosis: a prospective study. Am J Surg 1985;150:54.

132. Porter JM, Taylor LM. Current status of thrombolytic therapy. J Vasc Surg 1985;2:239.

133. Graor RA, Young JR, Risius B. Comparison of cost effectiveness of streptokinase and urokinase in the treatment of deep vein thrombosis. Ann Vasc Surg 1987;1:524.

134. Turpie AGG. Thrombolytic agents in venous thrombosis. J Vasc Surg 1990;12:196.

135. Machleder HI. Evaluation of a new treatment strategy for Paget-Schroetter syndrome: spontaneous thrombosis of the axillary-subclavian vein. J Vasc Surg 1993;17:305.

136. National Heart and Lung Institute Cooperative Study Group. Urokinase pulmonary embolism trial: phase 1 results. JAMA 1970;214:2163.

137. National Heart and Lung Institute Cooperative Study Group. Urokinase-streptokinase embolism trial: phase 2 results. JAMA 1974;229:1606.

138. McNamara TO, Fischer JR. Thrombolysis of peripheral arterial and graft occlusions: improved results using high-dose urokinase. AJR 1985;144:769.

139. McNamara TO, Bomberger RA. Factors affecting initial and 6 months patency rates after intraarterial thrombolysis with high-dose urokinase. Am J Surg 1986;152:709.

140. Gardiner GA, Sullivan KL. Catheter directed thrombolysis for the failed lower extremity bypass graft. Semin Vasc Surg 1992;5:99.

140a. Graor RA, Risius B, Young JR, et al. Peripheral artery and bypass graft thrombolysis with recombinant tissue-type plasminogen activator. J Vasc Surg 1986;3:115.

141. Comerota AJ, White JV. Intraoperative, intra-arterial thrombolytic therapy as an adjunct to revascularization in patients with residual and distal arterial thrombus. Semin Vasc Surg 1992;5:110.

142. Doorey AJ, Michelson EL, Topol EJ. Thrombolytic therapy for acute myocardial infarction: keeping the unfulfilled promises. JAMA 1992;268:3108.

143. Rutherford RB, Jones DN. The role of dextran-40 in preventing early graft thrombosis. In: Bergqvist D, Lindblad B, eds. Pharmacological intervention to increase patency after arterial reconstructions. Malmö, Sweden, ICM AB, 1989:44.

144. Norris CS, Greenfield LJ, Herrmann JB. Free-floating iliofemoral thrombus: a risk for pulmonary embolism. Arch Surg 1985;120:806.

145. Radomski JA, Jarrell BE, Carabasi RA, Yang SL, Koolpe H. Risk of pulmonary embolus with inferior vena cava thrombosis. Ann Surg 1987;53:97.

146. Berry RE, George JE, Shaver WA. Free-floating deep venous thrombosis: a retrospective analysis. Ann Surg 1990;211:719.

147. Greenfield LJ, Michna BA. Twelve-year clinical experience with the Greenfield vena caval filter. Surgery 1988;104:706.

148. Kantor A, Glanz S, Gordon DH, et al. Percutaneous insertion of the Kimray-Greenfield filter: incidence of femoral vein thrombosis. AJR 1987;149:1065.

149. Greenfield LJ, Cho KJ, Proctor M, et al. Results of a multicenter study of the the modified hook-titanium Greenfield filter. J Vasc Surg 1991;14:253.

150. Greenfield LJ, Proctor MC, Williams DM, et al. Long-term experience with transvenous catheter pulmonary embolectomy. J Vasc Surg 1993;18:450.

151. Stenbjerg S, Berg E, Albrechtsen OK. Heparin levels and activated clotting times (ACT) during open heart surgery. Scand J Haematol 1981;26:281.

152. Oberman HA. Complications of blood transfusion. In: Greenfield LJ, ed. Complications in surgery and trauma, ed 2. Philadelphia, JB Lippincott, 1990:183.

153. Barton JC. Nonhemolytic, noninfectious transfusion reactions. Semin Hematol 1981;18:95.

154. Menitove JE. Complications of blood transfusion. In: McClatchey KD, ed. Clinical laboratory medicine. Baltimore, Williams & Wilkins, 1993:1783.

155. Moore SB. Anaphylactic transfusion reactions: a concise review. Ir Med J 1985;78:54.

156. Moore SB. Management of transfusion in the massively bleeding patient. Hum Pathol 1983;14:267.

157. Umlas J. Transfusion-related acquired immunodeficiency syndrome and directed donations: would the national blood supply be safer with directed donations? Hum Pathol 1986;17:108.

SURGERY: SCIENTIFIC PRINCIPLES AND PRACTICE, Second Edition, edited by Lazar J. Greenfield, Michael W. Mulholland, Keith T. Oldham, Gerald B. Zelenock, and Keith D. Lillemoe. Lippincott–Raven Publishers, Philadelphia, © 1997.

CHAPTER 5

CYTOKINES

LISA M. COLLETTI, STEVEN L. KUNKEL, AND ROBERT M. STRIETER

Cytokines are soluble protein mediators that are secreted by one cell to influence another cell, tissue, or organ in either an autocrine, paracrine or endocrine fashion. In recent years, a multitude of soluble protein mediators with a wide range of biologic effects have been described. Cytokines play an important role in regulating the immune response and act in various ways on T cells, B cells, cells of the monocyte/macrophage lineage, neutrophils, fibroblasts, smooth muscle cells, and endothelial cells. The immunologic functions that are influenced by these polypeptides include the host response to both acute and chronic bacterial, viral, fungal, and parasitic infections, the development of sepsis, adult respiratory distress syndrome, multiple organ system failure (MOSF), allograft rejection, and autoimmune diseases. Cytokines also play important roles in tumor biology, in response to the tumor and in mediating tumor growth and metastasis. Cytokines are important molecules in regulating angiogenesis and cellular growth and differentiation. Although cytokines have a variety of actions and effects, this chapter focuses on their role in tissue injury, inflammation, and wound repair. Particular emphasis is placed on the classic early-response cytokines, tumor necrosis factor (TNF), interleukin-1 (IL-1), and interleukin-6 (IL-6), as well as the C-X-C chemokine family of molecules. The latter has important neutrophil, chemotactic, and angiogenic properties. Their angiogenic properties are important in wound repair and may also play an important role in tumor growth and metastasis.

Cytokine production at various tissue sites depends in part on the proximity of the site to an injurious stimulus. It has been suggested that cytokine concentrations increase concomitantly with the magnitude of injury. However, in

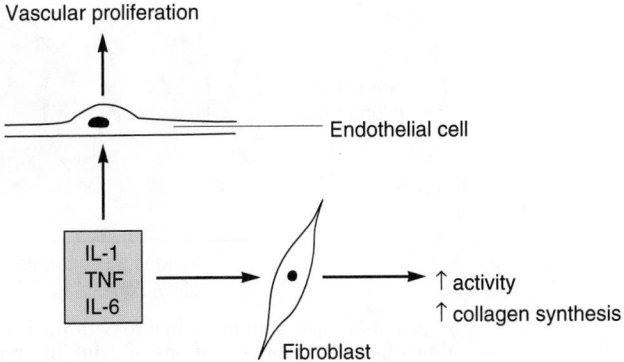

Figure 5-2. Effects of TNF, IL-1, and IL-6 on acute tissue injury and wound repair. Following injury, TNF, IL-1, and IL-6 regulate fibroblast activity and collagen synthesis, as well as vascular proliferation in the initiation of tissue repair.

both laboratory and clinical settings, it has been difficult to correlate plasma cytokine concentrations with the extent of tissue damage. The reason appears to be that cytokines typically function in an autocrine and paracrine fashion and are therefore designed to signal the presence of local, rather than systemic, inflammation. TNF and IL-1 are important early mediators of the inflammatory response and trigger a variety of host responses. These include an increase in neutrophil margination, activation of the antimicrobial activity of monocytes, macrophages, neutrophils, and eosinophils, induction of the acute-phase response, and increased skeletal muscle degradation to yield amino acids for gluconeogenesis[1-10] (Fig. 5-1). During wound repair, the same molecules play an important role in regulating vascular proliferation, fibroblast and osteoclast activity, and collagen synthesis[11-20] (Fig. 5-2). Although these activities constitute the normal physiologic response to injury and appear to be directed by relatively low, local concentrations of cytokines, excessive concentrations of these molecules can cause adverse effects[21-24] (Fig. 5-3). They include tachycardia, hypotension, pulmonary inflammation, edema, vascular congestion and hemorrhage, acute renal tubular necrosis and fibrinous renal thrombi, acute hepatic inflammation, and lactic acidosis, all of which can be associated with sepsis, systemic inflammation, and MOSF[21-24] (Table 5-1).

INFLAMMATION: THE INITIAL HOST RESPONSE TO INJURY OR INFECTION

Early-Response Cytokines

Polypeptide mediators, such as TNF and IL-1, are early-response cytokines and are actively involved in initiating the cascade of events that precipitate acute inflammation. They trigger other cytokines that are important in the inflammatory network and also appear to promote the adherence of inflammatory cells to the endothelium, thus enhancing the trafficking of immunologically active cells into an area of injury or infection. The actual physical interaction between the endothelium and neutrophils is a critical event in initiating the inflammatory response and is responsible for localizing inflammatory cells into an area of injury (Fig. 5-4). Adhesion molecules are grouped according to their protein structures, and three classes of molecules are important for leukocyte-endothelial interactions (Table 5-2)—the immunoglobin gene superfamily,

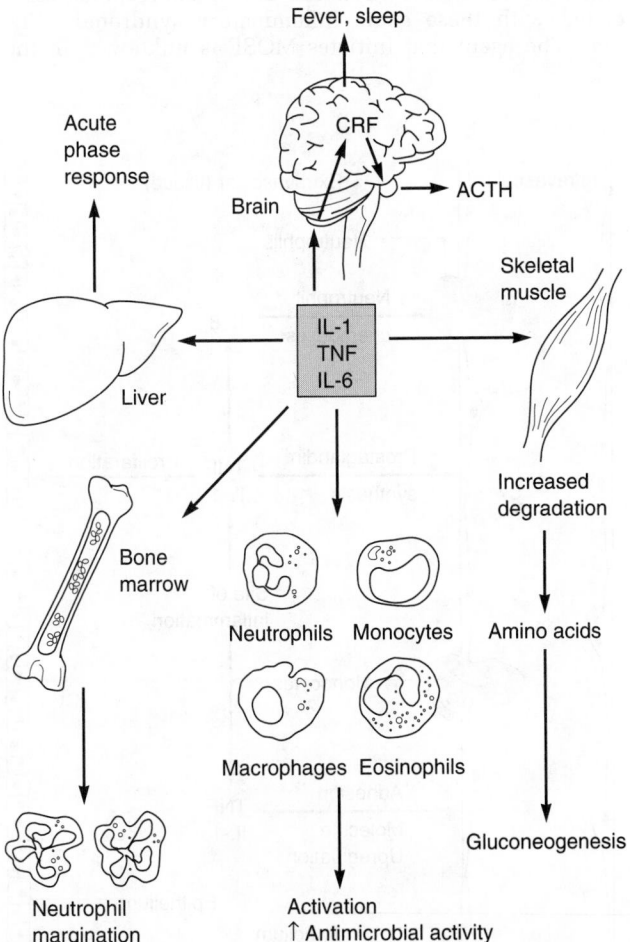

Figure 5-1. Early-response cytokines and the initiation of inflammation. TNF, IL-1, and IL-6 have a multitude of effects in the initiation of the inflammatory response, including the increased breakdown of skeletal muscle to yield amino acids for gluconeogenesis; the activation of monocytes, macrophages, neutrophils, and eosinophils, with an increase in neutrophil margination and an overall increase in leukocyte antimicrobial activity; and the induction of the acute-phase response. In the brain, these molecules cause changes that induce fever and sleep. In addition, they up-regulate corticotropin-releasing factor, which stimulates the production of ACTH.

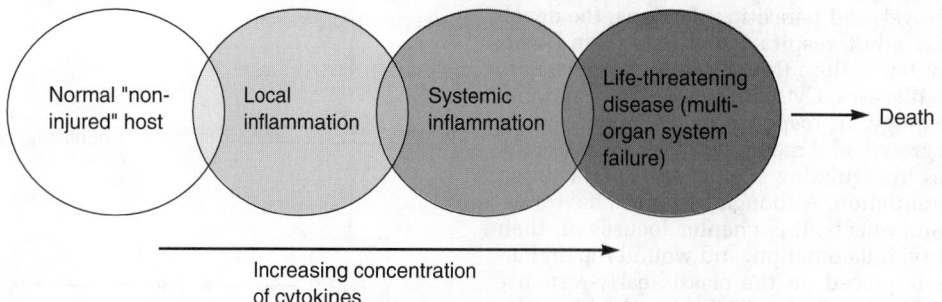

Figure 5-3. Spectrum of normal to pathologic effects of cytokines based on increasing concentrations. Low local concentrations of cytokines represent normal physiology and the normal initial response to injury or infection. Increasing concentrations of cytokines, resulting in systemic cytokine levels, result in severe physiologic derangements, often leading to multiple organ system failure and death of the host.

the selectins, and the integrins.[25] The major cytokine-induced adherence proteins that are expressed on the surface of endothelial cells include intercellular adhesion molecule-1 (ICAM), platelet-endothelial cell adhesion molecule (PECAM), vascular cell adhesion molecule (VCAM), all members of the immunoglobin gene superfamily, E-selectin, and P-selectin.[25-27] The major groups of cytokine-induced adherence proteins expressed on polymorphonuclear leukocytes (PMNs) include members of the integrin and selectin families.[25] The most important integrins expressed on the neutrophil cell surface that mediate neutrophil-endothelial adherence are the β_2 integrins. These include CD11a/CD18, CD11b/CD18, and CD11c/CD18.[28] The L-selectins and the very late after activation (VLA) antigens are also important leukocyte adhesion molecules.[28-29]

Tumor Necrosis Factor-α

Septic shock is a pathologic condition characterized by circulatory failure and collapse. It is typically associated with adult respiratory distress syndrome, MOSF, and death.[22-24] The interplay between monocytes, tissue macrophages, neutrophils, and endothelial cells appears to be particularly important in the pathophysiology of this process. At the cellular level, this syndrome is associated with hypermetabolism and an energy deficit, ultimately leading to cellular injury and death. The cascade of inflammatory events that ultimately culminates in MOSF is initiated by

trauma, microorganisms, microbial by-products, and cytokines.[22-24] Although MOSF can also occur in an aseptic state, particularly with multiple trauma or severe pancreatitis, there is always a cytokine-dependent response associated with these acute inflammatory syndromes (Fig. 5-5). The agent that initiates MOSF is unknown. In the

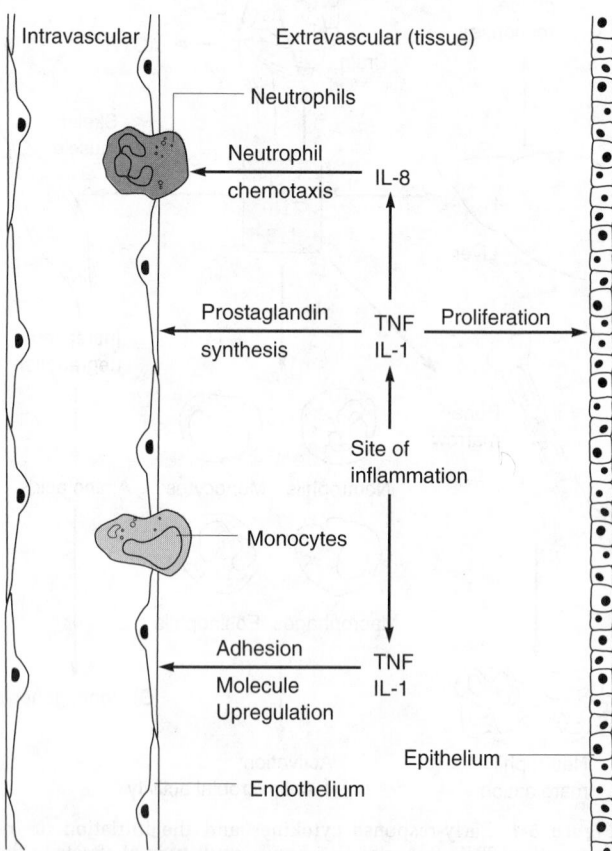

Figure 5-4. Initial interaction between leukocytes and the endothelium. TNF and IL-1 are important early mediators in the initial interaction between the endothelium and leukocytes. The early adherence of leukocytes to the endothelium is an important first step in the elicitation of leukocytes into an area of injury or inflammation, and TNF and IL-1 are critical mediators in this process, since they are capable of up-regulating endothelial and leukocyte adhesion molecules. TNF and IL-1 can also induce IL-8, a powerful neutrophil chemotactic agent.

Table 5-1. ADVERSE PHYSIOLOGIC EFFECTS SEEN WITH SYSTEMIC CYTOKINE LEVELS LEADING TO MULTIPLE ORGAN SYSTEM FAILURE

Organ System	Effect
Cardiovascular	Tachycardia
	Hypotension
Pulmonary	Inflammation
	Edema
	Vascular congestion
	Hemorrhage
Renal	Acute tubular necrosis
	Fibrinous renal thrombi
Hepatic	Acute hepatic inflammation
Musculoskeletal	Skeletal muscle breakdown
	Lactic acidosis

Table 5-2. MAJOR SUBFAMILIES OF ADHESION MOLECULES

Subfamily	Major Glycoprotein	Primary Distribution
IgG superfamily	ICAM-1	Endothelial cells, fibroblasts, epithelial cells, hematopoietic cells
	VCAM-1	Endothelial cells
	PECAM-1	Intercellular junction of endothelial cells, platelets
Selectins	L-selectin	All leukocytes
	E-selectin	Activated endothelial cells
	P-selectin	Platelets, Weibel-Palade bodies of endothelial cells
Integrins	β_1: VLA Antigens	T-lymphocytes (types 1-6)
	β_2: CD$_{11a}$, LFA-1	All leukocytes
	CD$_{11b}$, MAC-1	PMNs, monocytes
	CD$_{11c}$, gp150,95	PMNs, monocytes
	β_3: CD$_{11b}$, gp11b/111a	Platelets, endothelium

PMNs, polymorphonuclear leukocytes.

septic state, however, endotoxin triggers the expression of several cytokines, particularly TNF and IL-1, which can orchestrate the subsequent inflammatory response in a cascade fashion. If unchecked, this cascade can precipitate MOSF and eventual death. Interestingly, TNF has pleiotropic effects on many cellular functions. At local inflammation sites, this cytokine mediates the normal initiation, maintenance, and repair of tissue injury. In contrast, exaggerated systemic levels of TNF can cause MOSF and increase the host morbidity and mortality rate.[30–34] Cells of the monocyte–macrophage lineage are the principal cellular sources of TNF. However, TNF can also be expressed by glial cells in the brain, Kupffer cells in the liver, keratinocytes in the skin, mast cells, NK cells, T cells, and B cells.[35,36] A variety of exogenous and endogenous factors produced by bacteria, viruses, parasites, and tumors can induce cells to produce TNF; however, endotoxin is the most potent stimulus for TNF production and release.[35–38] The regulation of TNF gene expression is multi-

factorial, and several factors, such as interferon-gamma, can increase TNF production, while others, such as IL-4, IL-10, corticosteroids, and pentoxyfyllineor, decrease TNF production.[6,35,39]

Pathologic Changes Induced by Tumor Necrosis Factor

Tumor necrosis factor is clearly involved in the pathogenesis of septic shock. Administering recombinant TNF to experimental animals produces a clinical and pathologic syndrome, similar to that seen in septic shock and MOSF in humans.[21] When administered before the infusion of TNF or endotoxin, passive immunization with neutralizing antibodies against TNJ has been shown to prevent this syndrome in animals.[33,40] Several pathophysiologic alterations have been identified in animals treated with TNF. These include hemorrhage and ischemic necrosis of the gastrointestinal tract, hemorrhage and leukocyte infiltration into the lungs, acute tubular necrosis of the kidneys, metabolic acidosis, hypermetabolism, hypotension, and increased pituitary and stress hormone release.[21,38,41]

Mechanisms of Tumor Necrosis Factor–Induced Injury

Tumor necrosis factor has a marked procoagulant effect on endothelial cells, precipitating intravascular thrombosis[42,43] (Fig. 5-6 and Table 5-3). TNF causes endothelial cells to release factors with procoagulant activity factor, including tissue factor, platelet-activating factor, and von Willebrand factor, which all favor thrombosis.[42,43] TNF also down-regulates the expression of thrombomodulin, which has the potential to block the assembly of protein-C and protein-S complexes, further decreasing the anticoagulant properties of the endothelial cell surfaces.[44] Fibrinolysis is also influenced by TNF through modulation of the plasminogen-activator inhibitors and tissue-type plasminogen activator.[42,43,45] In addition, the antithrombotic properties of the vascular endothelium are profoundly altered by exposure to TNF. TNF enhances thrombin formation on the endothelial surface by inducing the synthesis of thromboplastin[46] and concomitantly suppressing thrombomodulin gene expression.[43,44] Further, TNF induces platelet-activating factor synthesis.[47] This phospholipid is a potent platelet and leukocyte activator, as well as a powerful vasoconstrictor.[47] Although most TNF-induced changes facilitate a hypercoagulable state, this cytokine can also stimulate endothelial synthesis of prostacyclin and urokinase-type plasminogen activator, thus facilitating antithrombotic tendencies (Fig. 5-7; see Table 5-3). Prostacyclin

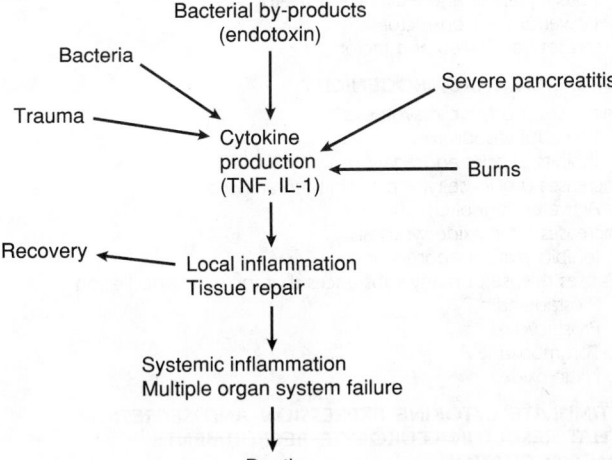

Figure 5-5. Multiple organ system failure (MOSF). A multitude of potential insults to the host can initiate the cascade of events that can ultimately culminate in MOSF and death. Trauma, burns, bacterial infection, or severe pancreatitis are all well-known initiating events precipitating MOSF. These events cause expression of TNF and IL-1, which initiate the inflammatory cascade. When the cascade proceeds in a controlled, well-orchestrated fashion, tissue repair and recovery of the host occurs. However, if this cascade continues in an exaggerated, uncontrolled fashion, with elevated systemic concentrations of a variety of inflammatory cytokines, MOSF ensues with potential death of the host.

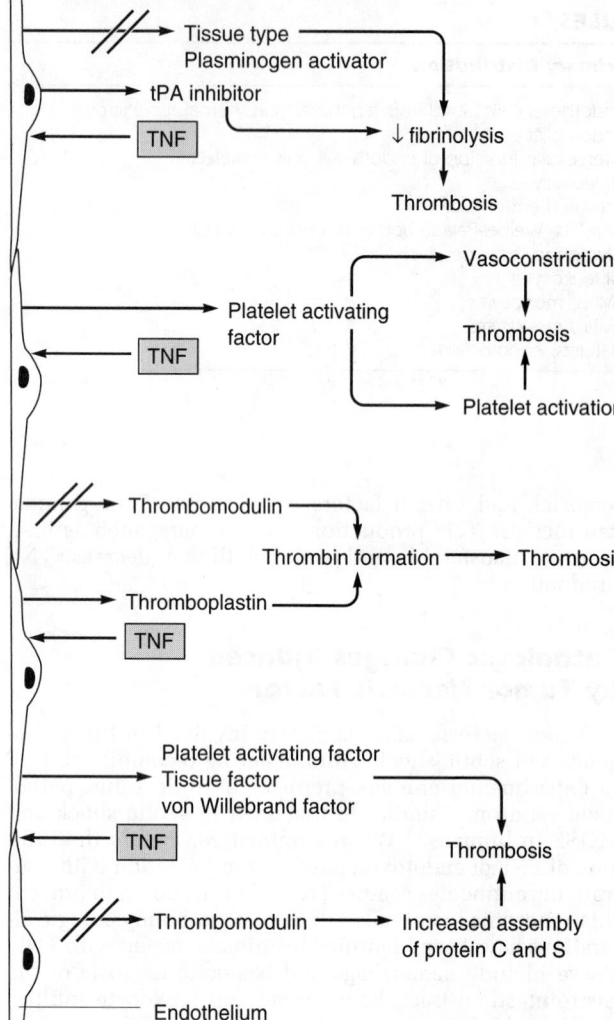

Figure 5-6. Actions of TNF favoring thrombosis. TNF has numerous procoagulant effects, favoring intravascular thrombosis. TNF causes endothelial cells to release a variety of factors with procoagulant properties including tissue factor, platelet-activating factor, von Willebrand factor, thromboplastin, and tissue-type plasminogen-activator inhibitor. It also inhibits the formation of tissue-type plasminogen activator and thrombomodulin. The inhibition of thrombomodulin increases coagulation through two mechanisms. A decrease in thrombomodulin allows both an increase in the assembly of protein C and S complexes, as well as increasing thrombin formation. In addition, both the decrease in thrombomodulin and the increase in thromboplastin further facilitate thrombin formation. Similarly, the decrease in tissue-type plasminogen activator and the increase in tissue-type plasminogen-activator inhibitor decrease overall fibrinolysis, again favoring thrombosis. The TNF-mediated increase in platelet-activating factor favors thrombosis through platelet activation and vasoconstriction.

inhibits platelet aggregation and is a potent vasodilator; urokinase-type plasminogen activator activates the fibrinolytic system.[48,49] This TNF-induced increase in prostacyclin facilitates vasodilation at sites of inflammation, as well as the hypotension associated with systemic cytokine release (ie, septic shock). Cyclooxygenase inhibitors prevent hypotension in this setting.[50,51] TNF also triggers the release of prostaglandin E_2, prostacyclin I_2, thromboxane A_2, and nitric oxide from endothelial cells, all of which have vasodilatory effects.[48-51] It is clear that this multitude of mediators can exert conflicting effects, and the net effect of TNF may de-

pend on the location and quantity in which it is produced and the vascular bed with which it interacts.

TNF also enhances endothelial procoagulant activity by inducing tissue factor, an important cofactor in the initiation of the extrinsic coagulation pathway, and by concurrently suppressing the anticoagulant protein-C pathway.[43] TNF also induces the production and release of IL-1 from endothelial cells.[52] IL-1 has procoagulant activities similar to those of TNF,[42-46] and these procoagulant activities are further increased by the induction of plasminogen-activator inhibitor by IL-1.[53] The overall effect of TNF clearly favors thrombosis, and this can be important in the pathogenesis of the hypercoagulable state associated with inflammatory and malignant disorders.

As discussed earlier, TNF alters cell surface molecule expression on neutrophils and endothelial cells, stimulat-

Table 5-3. PRIMARY EFFECTS OF TNF AND IL-1 ON THE VASCULAR ENDOTHELIUM

INCREASE LEUKOCYTE ADHESION BY INCREASING THE EXPRESSION OF ENDOTHELIAL ADHESION MOLECULES; FACILITATES EXTRAVASATION OF NEUTROPHILS

ICAM-1
PECAM-1
VCAM-1
E-selectin
P-selectin

INCREASE THROMBOGENICITY

Increases tissue factor
Decreases thrombomodulin
   Blocks assembly of protein C and S complexes
Increases synthesis of thromboplastin
   Increase in thromboplastin plus a decrease in thrombomodulin results in an increase in thrombin formation at the endothelial surface
Decreases fibrinolysis
   Increases tissue-type plasminogen activator inhibitor
   Decreases tissue-type plasminogen activator
Increases platelet-activating factor
   Potent platelet and leukocyte activator
   Powerful vasoconstrictor
Increases von Willebrand factor

DECREASE THROMBOGENICITY

Increases prostacyclin synthesis
   Powerful vasodilator
   Inhibits platelet aggregation
Increases urokinase-type plasminogen activator
   Activates fibrinolysis
Increases nitric oxide synthesis
   Inhibits platelet aggregation
Causes release of many substances that increase vasodilation
   Prostaglandin E_2
   Prostacyclin
   Thromboxane A_2
   Nitric oxide

STIMULATE CYTOKINE EXPRESSION AND SECRETION THAT RESULT IN LEUKOCYTE RECRUITMENT AND ACTIVATION

IL-1
IL-6
GM-CSF
G-CSF
IL-8
MCP-1

INCREASE PDGF

CAUSE MORPHOLOGIC CHANGE

STIMULATE ANGIOGENESIS

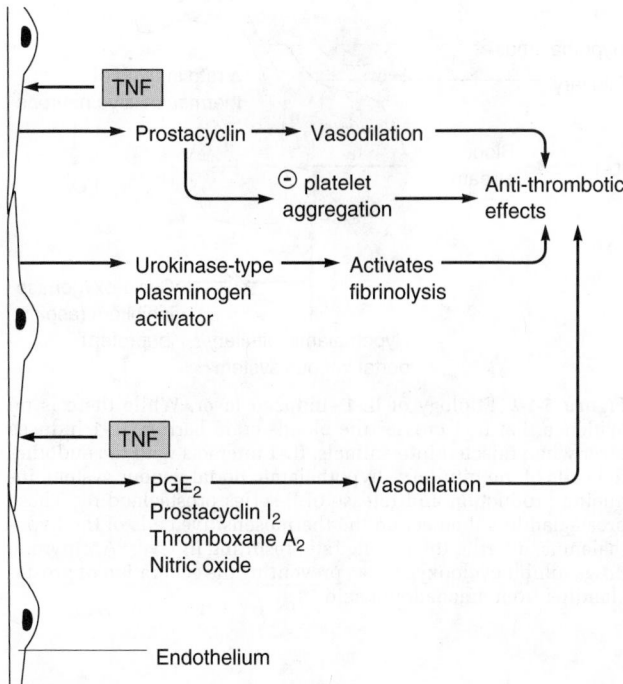

Figure 5-7. Anticoagulant effects of TNF. Although most TNF-induced effects on the endothelium favor thrombosis, this cytokine also has antithrombotic actions. These include an increase in endothelial synthesis of prostacyclin and urokinase-type plasminogen activator. Prostacyclin inhibits platelet aggregation and is a potent vasodilator. Urokinase-type plasminogen activator induces fibrinolysis. TNF also up-regulates endothelial production of PGE_2, prostacyclin I_2, thromboxane A_2, and nitric oxide, which are all powerful vasodilators.

ing endothelial-neutrophil adhesion and altering chemotaxis and procoagulant and antimicrobial neutrophil activity by up-regulating more distal inflammatory cytokines, particularly IL-8 and other chemokines.[54] TNF activates PMNs directly and indirectly through the release of more distal inflammatory cytokines. This induces the production and release of reactive oxygen metabolites and induces the production of additional cytokines[8,9] (Fig. 5-8). Neutrophil recruitment and activation is a key process in the development of MOSF, since the activated neutrophil appears to be one of the primary effector cells mediating the development of tissue injury in MOSF, regardless of the precipitating event.[22,23,28,55-57] Activated neutrophils release a variety of inflammatory mediators, including proteolytic enzymes, arachadonic acid metabolites, reactive oxygen species, and cytokines, which can all directly affect the microvasculature, leading to increased microvascular permeability, hemorrhage, and accentuated leukocyte migration into the affected tissues.[22,23,55-57]

Metabolic Effects of Tumor Necrosis Factor

In addition its important role in initiating the inflammatory response, TNF is also a potent regulator of cellular metabolism. Certain chronic infections, as well as malignancy, are associated with a condition termed *cachexia*, a syndrome involving weight loss, profound wasting, anorexia, and muscle weakness. TNF appears to mediate this syndrome.[58,59] Lipopolysaccharide (LPS), as well as other cytokines, activate a variety of inflammatory cells, most importantly macrophages, to produce TNF. This induction

is regulated both at the transcriptional and the posttranslational levels.[6,60] Both the chronic administration of TNF to rats and implantation of tumors secreting TNF in mice induce a syndrome of cachexia.[58,59] In vitro, higher TNF concentrations alter glucose metabolism in cultured myotubules by increasing glucose uptake and glycogen breakdown.[7] Purified TNF also suppresses lipoprotein lipase activity and stimulates lipolysis in cultured adipocytes.[61-63] Furthermore, TNF not only inhibits the differentiation process of preadipocytes but partially reverses differentiated adipocytes to a preadipocyte morphology and pattern of gene expression.[64] All of these cellular metabolic effects of TNF at least partially explain the chronic syndromes of anorexia, weight loss, and cachexia, which are associated with both chronic infection and malignancy.

Tumor Necrosis Factor Kinetics and Tolerance

The early release of TNF can clearly be shown during experimental endotoxemia, because systemic TNF levels are increased within 1 hour and then return to baseline

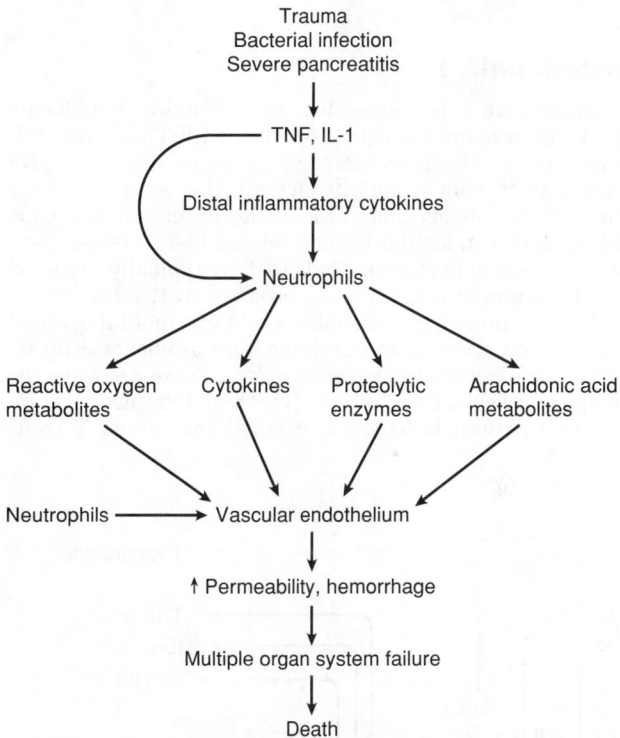

Figure 5-8. Cascade leading to multiple organ system failure. A variety of noxious events—including trauma, burns, infection, and pancreatitis—can trigger this cascade of events. TNF and IL-1 are important early mediators, initiating adherence of neutrophils to the vascular endothelium by up-regulating both leukocyte and endothelial adhesion molecules. TNF and IL-1 are also responsible for triggering the release of more distal inflammatory cytokines, which are important neutrophil chemotactic and activating agents. These activated neutrophils are recruited into the area of injury or infection where they elaborate reactive oxygen metabolites, other cytokines, proteolytic enzymes, and arachadonic acid metabolites, all of which injure the surrounding tissues and microvasculature, resulting in increased microvascular permeability, hemorrhage, and accentuated leukocyte migration into these tissues. Neutrophil recruitment and activation is one of the key events in this cascade, since the activated neutrophil appears to be one of the most important effector cells in mediating tissue injury in multiple organ system failure, regardless of the precipitating event.

within 3 hours of endotoxin administration.[37] Although TNF levels peak and return to baseline within a short time, systemic levels of this molecule can precipitate a vigorous inflammatory cascade, which continues despite the subsequent absence of detectable TNF.

In vivo treatment with a small, nonlethal dose of LPS results in the production and release of TNF. However, when the same animal is subsequently exposed to a greater (lethal) dose of LPS, TNF production is limited, and the animal tolerates the subsequent lethal dose of LPS.[39,60] Similarly, pretreatment with either TNF or IL-1 protects against the susceptibility to TNF cytotoxicity from subsequent TNF challenge.[15,65] TNF induces TNF production, and TNF-resistant cells constituitively express TNF mRNA and protein, which decreases TNF receptor levels.[66,68] It is difficult to completely explain the protective effect of TNF, IL-1, or LPS pretreatment simply by receptor down-regulation, because TNF and IL-1 are structurally unrelated and bind to different cell surface receptors.[69,70] It seems more likely that TNF-sensitive cells up-regulate the production of certain molecules, such as manganese superoxide dismutase and other antioxidants, in response to pretreatment with TNF, IL-1, or LPS and that these molecules are subsequently involved in protecting against TNF cytotoxicity.

Interleukin-1

Interleukin-1 is a complex, multifunctional molecule that shares many biologic properties with TNF.[71] In addition, IL-1 markedly potentiates the lethal effects of TNF when given concurrently.[71] Overall, IL-1 alone probably has weaker effects than TNF in the induction of shock. Many cells can synthesize and release IL-1 in response to a wide variety of stimuli. Cells that are typically involved in the immune response can produce IL-1, most importantly the monocyte/macrophage cell line, including blood monocytes, alveolar and peritoneal macrophages, Kupffer cells, and synovial macrophages.[1,2,72] These cells are the major sources of secreted IL-1 (Fig. 5-9). Lymphocytes, including natural killer cells, B cells, and helper T cells,

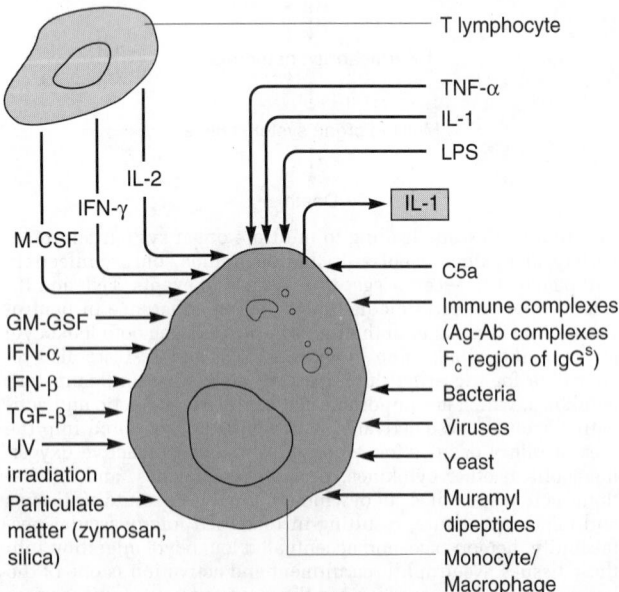

Figure 5-9. Stimuli for IL-1 production in cells of the monocyte/macrophage lineage. The macrophage is the most important cellular source of IL-1 in vivo.

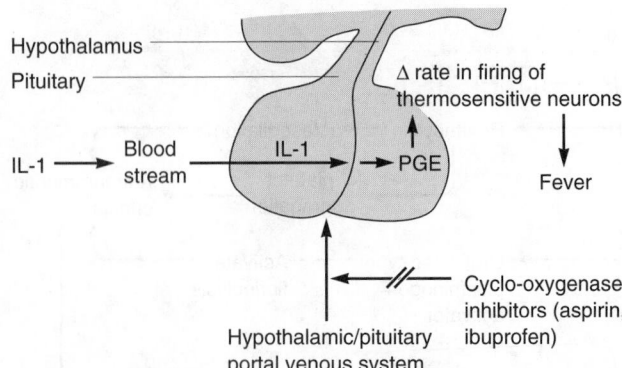

Figure 5-10. Etiology of IL-1–induced fever. While there is no evidence that IL-1 crosses the blood–brain barrier, IL-1 induces fever when injected into animals. IL-1 interacts with the endothelial cells of the pituitary–hypothalamic portal venous system, inducing production and release of E-series prostaglandins. These prostaglandins then act on the thermosensitive cells of the hypothalamus, altering their firing rate, resulting in fever. Antipyretic drugs inhibit cyclooxygenase, preventing the generation of prostaglandins from arachadonic acid.

are also sources of IL-1.[1,2,72] In addition, a variety of other "nonimmune" cells produce IL-1. In the central nervous system, astrocytes, microglia, and glioma cells produce IL-1 as do vascular smooth muscle cells and endothelial cells.[1,2,72] Neutrophils, fibroblasts, chondrocytes, epithelial cells, keratinocytes, Langerhans cells, and renal mesangial cells have also been shown to produce IL-1.[2–4] Interleukin-2 (IL-2), granulocyte macrophage colony stimulating factor (GM-CSF), transforming growth factor-β (TGF-β), TNF-α, all of the interferons, and IL-1 are all endogenous mediators that can induce IL-1 production.[1,2] Other endogenous stimuli for IL-1 production include antigen-antibody complexes, the Fc region of IgG, and C5a. Other nonspecific exogenous stimuli include silica particles and ultraviolet irradiation.[1,2] For macrophages to present antigen to T cells, macrophage-derived IL-1 participation and synthesis are required.[1,2] Exogenous products, such as endotoxins, peptidoglycans, muramyl dipeptide, virus particles, yeast particles, and zymosan, are also IL-1–stimulating agents.[1,2] In contrast to TNF, small doses of endotoxin or other cytokines have no tolerizing effect on subsequent IL-1 production.

Metabolic and Inflammatory Effects of Interleukin-1

The proinflammatory effects of IL-1 are well documented and include effects on fibroblasts, synovial cells, chondrocytes, endothelial cells, hepatocytes, and osteoclasts. A key feature of IL-1–induced actions is the stimulation of arachadonic acid metabolism and the secretion of a variety of inflammatory proteins, including other cytokines and proteases.[2,73] IL-1 stimulates the release of pituitary stress hormones, increases the synthesis of collagenases, resulting in the destruction of cartilage, and stimulates prostaglandin production.[73–76] IL-1 induces fever when injected into experimental animals.[73,77] There is no evidence that IL-1 crosses the blood–brain barrier, and it is likely that this pyrogenic action occurs by interacting with the endothelial cells of the hypothalamic-pituitary portal venous system, which generates prostaglandins of the E series[73,78] (Fig. 5-10). These prostaglandins then act on the hypothalamus to alter the firing rates of the thermo-

Table 5-4. MAJOR ACUTE-PHASE REACTANTS

Protein	Function
C-reactive protein	Opsonin
Serum amyloid A	Apolipoprotein
α_2-Macroglobulin	Antiproteinase
α_1 Acid glycoprotein	Transport
Fibrinogen	Coagulation
α_1-Proteinase inhibitor	Antiproteinase
α_1-Antichymotrypsin	Antiproteinase
Haptoglobin	Binds and removes hemoglobin
Hemopexin	Binds heme
Ceruloplasmin	Oxygen scavenger, transport
Complement C_3	Opsonin
Serum amyloid P	Unknown
Albumin	Unknown
Transferrin	Transport

sensitive neurons, resulting in fever.[73,78] Antipyretic drugs, such as aspirin, are effective because they inhibit the cyclooxygenase enzyme involved in converting arachadonic acid to prostaglandins. Fever is an evolutionarily conserved nonspecific reaction to infection and inflammation. While IL-1 can serve as an endogenous pyrogen, other cytokines can also induce an elevated body temperature.

An increase in the synthesis of hepatic acute-phase proteins and the associated decrease in albumin synthesis is another hallmark of inflammation. While IL-1 appears to play a role in inducing acute-phase proteins, IL-6 may be the cytokine responsible for directly stimulating hepatic acute-phase proteins.[3,79] Injections of either TNF or IL-1 induce IL-6 synthesis, which appears to be the most potent stimulus for hepatic acute-phase protein production.[3,79] IL-6 induces the production and release of C-reactive protein, serum amyloid, fibrinogen, alpha-1 antitrypsin, alpha-1 antichymotrypsin, and haptoglobin, with an associated reduction in albumin, transferrin, and fibronectin[3,79] (Tables 5-4 and 5-5).

Experimental evidence suggests that IL-1 has some interesting functions in physiologic homeostasis. For example, somnolence and anorexia are common manifestations of acute infection, and the central administration of IL-1 can induce slow-wave sleep in experimental animals.[80,81] IL-1 administration has an anorexigenic effect, inhibits lipoprotein lipase activity,[82,83] and mobilizes neutrophils from the bone marrow with a resultant neutrophilia.[84]

The effects of TNF and IL-1 overlap.[71] TNF can stimulate the production of IL-1, and the effects of the two cytokines together are far greater than the the the effects of either molecule alone[71] (Table 5-6). IL-1 is also produced in the sepsis syndrome in concert with TNF; however, the mechanism of IL-1–induced shock appears to be related to the release of other small mediator molecules, such as platelet-activating factor, prostaglandins, and nitric oxide, which all potentiate hypotension.[48,50] In animals, a single intravenous dose of IL-1 decreases the mean arterial pressure, lowers systemic vascular resistance, and induces leukopenia and thrombocytopenia.[50]

One of the most important properties of IL-1 involves its interaction with the vascular endothelium. These particular actions are again quite redundant, however, and overlap with those of TNF. The adherence of neutrophils, basophils, eosinophils, monocytes, and lymphocytes to the vascular endothelium involves the interaction between adhesion molecules on leukocytes (CD 11/CD 18 complex, L-selectin, and VLA-4 integrins) and the adhesion-receptor complex on the endothelial cell (ICAM-1, E-selectin, and VCAM-1).[4,5,25,27,29] By inducing the expression of ICAM-1,

E-selectin, and VCAM-1 on endothelial cells, IL-1 provides a key step in extravasating leukocytes to sites of local inflammation and injury. Other manifestations of IL-1–endothelial cell interactions include prostaglandin production, production of platelet-activating factor, and a variety of colony-stimulating factors.[4,46,47] These responses facilitate the mobilization and activation of appropriate leukocyte populations for specific localized immune responses. IL-1 also affects the vascular endothelium by shifting the balance toward thrombosis and a procoagulant state by down-regulating the fibrinolytic system and enhancing the activity of plasminogen-activator inhibitor and tissue-factor-like procoagulant, as well as thrombomodulin and the protein-C system.[42, 85-87] IL-1 shifts the fibrinolytic properties of the endothelium by increasing plasminogen-activator inhibitor-1 production while leaving unchanged or decreasing tissue-type plasminogen activator.[45,86,87] IL-1 enhances thrombin formation on the endothelial surface by inducing the synthesis of thromboplastin[46] and concomitantly suppressing thrombomodulin gene expression.[43,44] Furthermore, IL-1 induces platelet-activating factor synthesis.[47] This phospholipid is a potent platelet and leukocyte activator, as well as a powerful vasoconstrictor.[47]

Although most IL-1–induced changes facilitate a hypercoagulable state, this cytokine can also stimulate the endothelial synthesis of prostacyclin and urokinase-type plasminogen activator. This facilitates antithrombotic tendencies. Prostacyclin inhibits platelet aggregation and is a potent vasodilator, while urokinase-type plasminogen activator activates the fibrinolytic system.[48,49] This IL-1–induced increase in prostacyclin facilitates vasodilation at sites of inflammation, as well as the hypotension associated with systemic cytokine release (ie, septic shock). Cyclooxygenase inhibitors prevent hypotension in this setting.[50,51] It is clear that this multitude of mediators can exert conflicting effects, and the net effect of IL-1 can depend on its location and quantity, as well as the vascular bed with which it interacts.

Interleukin-6

Interleukin-6 also is important in host defense because it regulates the hepatic response to inflammation. IL-6 was initially termed *hepatocyte-stimulating factor* (HSF), and

Table 5-5. ACUTE-PHASE PROTEINS REGULATED BY CYTOKINES

INDUCED BY IL-6

C-reactive protein
α_2-macroglobulin
α_1 Acid glycoprotein
Fibrinogen
α_1-Proteinase inhibitor
α_1-Antichymotrypsin
Haptoglobin
Hemopexin
Ceruloplasmin
Complement C_3
Serum amyloid P
Serum amyloid A

INDUCED BY IL-1

C-reactive protein
α_1 Acid glycoprotein
Complement C3
Serum amyloid P
Serum amyloid A
Haptoglobin
Hemopexin

Table 5-6. SOME TISSUE SOURCES AND EFFECTS OF EARLY-RESPONSE CYTOKINES

	TNF	IL-1	IL-6
Source	Monocytes/macrophages, keratinocytes, Kupffer cells, fibroblasts, astrocytes, glial cells, mast cells, NK cells, T and B lymphocytes	Monocytes/macrophages, keratinocytes, Kupffer cells, fibroblasts, endothelial cells, astrocytes, microglial cells, epithelial cells, PMNs, vascular smooth-muscle cells, epithelial cells, NK cells, T and B lymphocytes	Monocytes/macrophages, keratinocytes, Kupffer cells, fibroblasts, endothelial cells, astrocytes, microglial cells, PMNs, T and B lymphocytes, epithelial cells
Induction of fever	++	+++	+
Induction of shock	+++	++	+/−
Stimulation of acute-phase response	+	++	+++
Endothelial cell activation	+++	++	+/−
Procoagulant activity	+++	++	+/−
Anorexia, weight loss	+++	++	+/−
Fibroblast proliferation	++	++	−

NK, natural killer; PMNs, polymorphonuclear leukocytes.

its most important function appears to be regulating the hepatic acute-phase response.[88–90] The hepatic acute-phase response is a series of homeostatic responses induced by injury or infection. Following the injurious or infectious stimulus, several physiologic changes develop within several hours. These changes typically reflect alterations in the set-point of a variety of physiologic parameters and include alterations in thermoregulation typically manifested by fever, nitrogen balance manifested by the development of a catabolic state, and changes in circulating levels of a group of particular proteins, classically termed *acute-phase proteins*. These physiologic changes allow the host to recover from the injury or infection. IL-6 is one of the primary stimuli for the production of these proteins by the liver.[91] Most of these proteins are glycoproteins, and they play various roles in the homeostatic response to injury and infection.[91,92] IL-6 expression is stimulated by a multitude of cytokines and growth factors, as well as by bacterial endotoxins.[93] In monocytes and macrophages, LPS is the most potent stimulus for IL-6 production; the most potent stimuli for fibroblast-derived IL-6 is IL-1 and TNF.[93–95] Platelet-derived growth factor (PDGF) and fibroblast growth factor (FGF) can also cause significant induction of IL-6 in fibroblasts.[93] Steroids inhibit IL-6 induction in cells of the monocyte–macrophage lineage.[13,96] Most if not all nucleated cells have the capacity

to express IL-6 in vitro. In vivo, the most prominent source of IL-6 appears to be LPS-stimulated monocytes or macrophages and IL-1- or TNF-stimulated stromal cells, particularly fibroblasts, epithelial cells, and endothelial cells[93,97,98] (Fig. 5-11). In vitro studies have shown that IL-6 can be expressed by central nervous system cells, particularly astrocytes, microglial cells, and folliculostellate cells.[99,100] Despite this in vitro data, it appears that only a few cell types in vivo secrete IL-6 in pathologic situations. Plasma levels of IL-6 rise rapidly following an in vivo challenge by LPS.[94,95,101] There appears to be a temporal lag between elevations in plasma TNF and subsequent elevations in plasma IL-6. Thus, it is likely that macrophage-derived IL-1 and TNF are responsible for producing IL-6.[101,102] These macrophage-derived, early-response cytokines can activate adjacent stromal cells, such as fibroblasts and endothelial cells, to release high levels of IL-6.[102] This cascade increases plasma levels of IL-6 and subsequently stimulates the hepatic acute-phase response.

Leukocyte–Endothelial Cell Interactions: The Role of Adhesion Molecules and Chemotactic Factors

Leukocyte extravasation is a crucial determinant of inflammatory and immunologic reactions. Endothelial cells and leukocytes interact closely in initiating the hemostatic, inflammatory, and immune responses to injury and infection. While cytokines are an important mechanism of communication between leukocytes and endothelial cells, the expression of a receptor and counter-receptor on the surface of these cells also permits physical interaction and subsequent communication between them. The binding of inflammatory cells to the endothelium is a key proximal event in initiating the inflammatory response that precedes chemotaxis. This event localizes inflammatory cells to an area of inflammation, infection, or injury. The endothelium is another important source of cytokines, which are then responsible for continuing to propagate the inflammatory response. Although this recruitment process is not unique to any particular organ, certain tissues, such as the lung, appear to be particularly susceptible to leukocyte recruitment and subsequent inflammatory injury. Leukocyte-endothelial adherence is unique in that it must both be strong enough to allow significant attachment of the

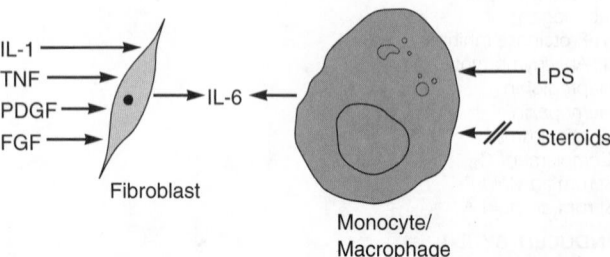

Figure 5-11. Stimuli for IL-6 production in fibroblasts and cells of the monocyte/macrophage lineage. In vivo, TNF and IL-1 are the most potent stimuli for fibroblast IL-6 production, while LPS is the most potent stimulus for monocyte/macrophage IL-6 production. Steroids inhibit monocyte/macrophage IL-6 production and release. PDGF and FGF are also capable of inducing fibroblast IL-6 production in vivo.

leukocyte to the endothelium and be controlled by one or more mechanisms that allow the adherence process to be transient and reversible. Once the adherence process occurs, a chemotactic signal triggers the inflammatory cells to transmigrate across the basement membrane into the interstitium.

Leukocytes and Endothelial Adhesion Molecules

Although many of the specific mechanisms that elicit neutrophils into tissues during acute inflammation are not fully known, the temporal events that initiate and propagate neutrophil recruitment likely include endothelial cell activation and expression of endothelial-derived neutrophil adhesion molecules, neutrophil activation and expression of neutrophil-derived adhesion molecules, neutrophil-endothelial cell adherence, and neutrophil transendothelial migration via established neutrophil chemotactic gradients.[28] The initial neutrophil-endothelial cell adhesion is a requisite event for successful neutrophil extravasation at sites of inflammation[28] (see Table 5-2).

Three major families of adhesion molecules are expressed on the surface of leukocytes and endothelial cells, and they are important for leukocyte-endothelial interactions.[25,28] These include the immunoglobin supergene family, the selectins, and the integrins. The immunoglobin supergene family includes ICAM-1, VCAM-1, and PECAM-1, which all can be expressed on endothelial cells and are important for leukocyte adherence.[25,28] E-selectin and P-selectin are members of the selectin family that are expressed on the surface of endothelial cells and are also important for leukocyte adherence.[25] L-selectin is also a member of the selectin family, and this molecule is expressed on the cell surface of all leukocytes.[25,28] It is particularly important for the early adherence of PMNs to the activated endothelium.

The family of integrins is further divided into 3 subfamilies: β_1, β_2, and β_3.[25] The β_1 subfamily includes the VLA antigens 1 through 6.[25] These molecules are primarily dis-

tributed on T lymphocytes. However, the interaction of monocyte-derived VLA-4 with VCAM-1 may be an important mechanism for monocyte adherence to the activated endothelium.[25,29] The β_2 subfamily includes CD11a, CD11b, CD11c, which represent lymphocyte function associated antigen (LFA-1), MAC-1, and gp150,95 (Fig. 5-12). CD11a, CD11b, and CD11c exist in a heterodimeric form, complexed to CD18. All of these molecules are expressed on the cell surface of a variety of leukocytes and are probably the most important subgroup of this family with respect to leukocyte-endothelial interactions.[25,28] Included in the β_3 subfamily are IIb and gpIIb/IIIa, which are expressed on platelets as well as the endothelium.[25]

The leukocyte β_2-integrin adhesion molecule family consists of a complex group of heterodimeric glycoproteins that are expressed only on the surface of leukocytes. The three members of the β_2-integrin family display a variable alpha and a constant beta chain with the cluster designations CD11a/CD18, CD11b/CD18, CD11c/CD18.[103-107] The CD11a/CD18 complex is expressed on all leukocytes; CD11b/CD18 is predominantly expressed on neutrophils and monocytes.[103-107] Neutrophils have a substantial pool of CD11b/CD18 in their secondary and tertiary granules, and when the neutrophil is activated, CD11b/CD18 rapidly translocates to the cell surface.[106-108] The ligand–receptor for neutrophil-derived CD11b/CD18 complex is the split product of complement (iC3b) and ICAM-1.[109]

ICAM-1 is a member of the immunoglobulin supergene family and is found on the surface of both immune and nonimmune cells.[107] Although originally described as the counter-receptor for CD11a/CD18 complex, ICAM-1 is also an important ligand/receptor for CD11b/CD18 complex expressed on neutrophils.[28] ICAM-1 is constituitively expressed on endothelial cells and is up-regulated in response to endotoxin, TNF, or IL-1.[106,107] Neutralizing monoclonal antibodies to either CD11b, CD18, or ICAM-1 in models of acute lung injury have been shown to attenuate neutrophil-dependent lung injury.[109-112] These findings suggest that neutrophil-derived β_2-integrins and endothe-

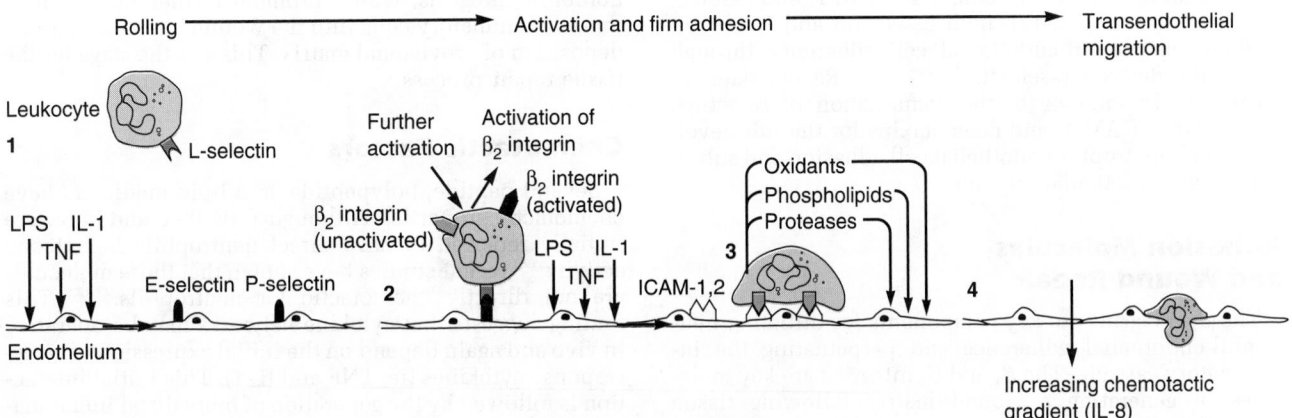

Figure 5-12. Neutrophil recruitment and activation into areas of inflammation. (1) Selectins mediate early loose adhesion or "rolling." This is a low-affinity adherence between constituitively expressed L-selectin on the neutrophil and E-selectin or P-selectin on the activated vascular endothelium. (2) This rolling slows the neutrophil enough to allow it to be activated, with expression and activation of β_2-integrins on the cell surface. Further activation of the endothelium by TNF, IL-1 or LPS leads to increased expression of ICAM-1 and ICAM-2, with subsequent firm adherence of the neutrophil to the endothelium. This is mediated through ICAM-β_2-integrin interactions. (3) The activated adherent neutrophil can then release proteases, oxidants, and phospholipids, resulting in endothelial cell injury and increased microvascular permeability. (4) Neutrophils then diapedese into the extravascular space via established chemotactic gradients. PECAM-1 may be important in transendothelial migration.

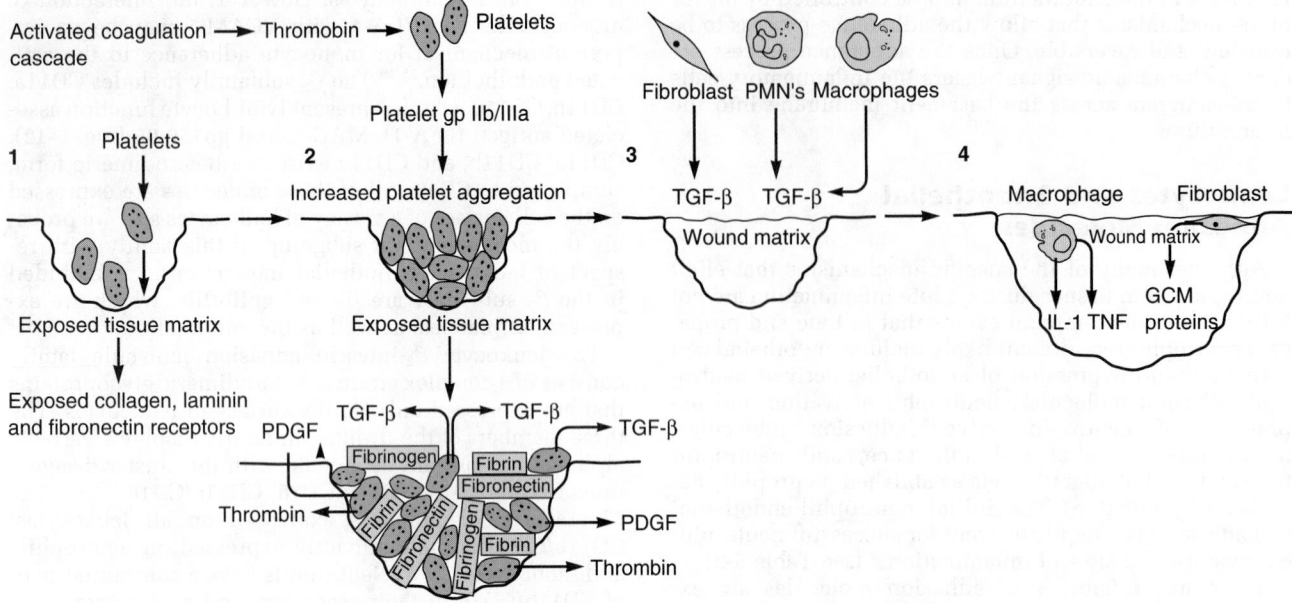

Figure 5-13. Establishment of a provisional wound matrix. (1) Platelets bind to exposed wound matrix via interaction of β_1 and β_3 integrins and collagen, laminin, and fibronectin receptors. (2) Following wounding, the coagulation cascade is activated, generating thrombin, which activates platelet gp IIb/IIIa and increases platelet aggregation. A provisional wound matrix is formed and is made up of platelets, fibrin, fibrinogen, and fibronectin. The activated platelets in the wound generate TGF-β, PDGF, and thrombin. (3) TGF-β is strongly chemotactic for neutrophils, macrophages, and fibroblasts, recruiting these cells into the provisional wound matrix, where they are also subsequently activated by TGF-β. (4) Increasing concentrations of TGF-β result in macrophage activation, producing increased amounts of TNF and IL-1. TGF-β also stimulates fibroblast production of extracellular matrix proteins. These reactions further enhance migration of macrophages and fibroblasts into the wound, facilitating tissue repair.

lial cell-derived ICAM-1 play a pivotal role in the pathogenesis of acute inflammation and lung injury.

Another group of molecules involved in neutrophil-endothelial adhesion are selectins.[108,113,114] These include L-selectin, which is constituitively expressed on leukocyte cell surfaces, E-selectin, which is induced on activated endothelial cells by endotoxin, TNF or IL-1, and P-selectin[25,113-118] (see Fig. 5-12). Both E-selectin and P-selectin facilitate neutrophil-endothelial cell adherence through neutrophil-derived L-selectin.[113,114,116,117] Recent data indicate the importance of the combination of selectins, β_2-integrins, ICAM-1, and chemotaxins for the full development of neutrophil-endothelial cell adhesion and subsequent transendothelial migration.[28]

Adhesion Molecules and Wound Repair

The β_2 integrins are key components for initiating neutrophil-endothelial adherence and perpetuating the inflammatory cascade. The β_1 and β_3 integrins are key molecules in generating a wound matrix following tissue injury.[25] Following tissue damage, platelets bind to the exposed matrix. This requires the interactions of the β_1 and β_3 integrins and the collagen, laminin, and fibronectin receptors (Fig. 5-13).[25] Activation of the coagulation cascade generates thrombin. This activates platelet gp IIb/IIIa, promoting further platelet aggregation.[25,26] A wound matrix is subsequently formed, containing platelets, fibrinogen, fibrin, and fibronectin. The activated platelets in the wound matrix elaborate TGF-β, PDGF, and thrombin.[16,25,26,118] TGF-β is strongly chemotactic for neutrophils, macrophages, and fibroblasts.[118,119] In addition, as these

inflammatory cells migrate into the wound, they encounter increasing concentrations of TGF-β, which subsequently activate these inflammatory cells. Macrophages increase their synthesis of TNF and IL-1, and fibroblasts increase their synthesis of extracellular matrix proteins.[118,119] These reactions stimulate the up-regulation of macrophage and fibroblast integrins, which promote further migration of these inflammatory cells into the wound site and increase deposition of provisional matrix. This sets the stage for the tissue repair process.

Chemotactic Factors

Several peptide, polypeptide, and lipid mediators have chemotactic properties. Although TNF, IL-1, and LPS were initially reported to have direct neutrophil chemotactic activity,[120] recent studies have shown that these molecules are not directly chemotactic for neutrophils.[22,121] This finding suggests that cytokine networks may be operative in vivo and again depend on the initial expression of early-response cytokines (ie, TNF and IL-1). This initial interaction is followed by the generation of more distal inflammatory mediators that directly influence neutrophil chemotaxis and activation.[54,122,123]

There is a particularly important group of novel chemotactic cytokines that share significant homology with the presence of four conserved cysteine amino acid residues.[123-126] These cytokines in their monomeric forms are all less than 10 kD, are characteristically basic heparin-binding proteins, have specific neutrophil chemotactic activity, and display four highly conserved cysteine amino acid residues, with the first two cysteines separated by one nonconserved amino acid residue. Because of their chemotactic properties and the presence of the C-X-C cysteine motif, these cytokines have been designated the C-X-C chemokine family. Interestingly, these chemokines are all clustered on human chromosome 4, and exhibit 20% to 50% homology at the amino acid level.[22,124,127–129] Since the mid-1980s, at least 12 different C-X-C chemokines have been identified. They include NH$_2$-terminal truncated forms of platelet basic protein (PBP; connective tissue activating protein-III, beta-thromboglobulin, and neutrophil-activating peptide-2), growth-related oncogene-α (GRO-α), growth-related oncogene-β (GRO-β), growth-related oncogene-γ (GRO-γ), IL-8, epithelial neutrophil-activating protein (ENA-78), granulocyte chemotactic protein-2 (GCP-2), platelet factor-4 (PF-4), γ-interferon–inducible protein (IP-10), and monokine induced by γ-interferon (MIG)[124,125,127–130] (Table 5-7). The NH$_2$-truncated forms of PBP are generated when PBP is released from platelet α-granules and undergoes proteolytic cleavage by monocyte-derived proteases.[123–125] GRO-α, GRO-β, and GRO-γ are closely related C-X-C chemokines,[124,125,127–131] with GRO-α originally described as a mitogen for human melanoma cells.[42,132] IL-8, ENA-78, and GCP-2 were all initially identified on by their ability to induce neutrophil activation and chemotaxis.[124,125,127–131] IL-8 is the most studied C-X-C chemokine family member and has been found to be produced by an array of both immune and nonimmune cells, including monocytes, alveolar macrophages, neutrophils, keratinocytes, mesangial cells, epithelial cells, hepatocytes, fibroblasts, and endothelial cells.[124,127,128,131] IL-8 is one of the most potent mediators of chemotaxis in this family of molecules.[54,122,123] Interestingly, the host-derived early-response cytokines, TNF and IL-1, are key molecules for inducing IL-8, which in turn plays an important role in inducing neutrophil recruitment and activation and in continuing the inflammatory response.[54,123] Similarly, in vitro studies have identified ENA-78 as a potent neutrophil chemotaxin that is produced by endothelial cells stimulated by either TNF or IL-1, neutrophils, monocytes, pulmonary epithelial cells, and pulmonary fibroblasts.[126] PF-4, the first member of the C-X-C chemokine family to be described, was originally identified by its ability to bind to heparin, inactivating heparin's anticoagulant function.[133] Both IP-10 and MIG are interferon-inducible C-X-C chemokines.[125,129,130,133,134] Although IP-10 induces all three interferons (IFN-α, IFN-β, and IFN-γ), MIG is unique in that it appears to be expressed only in the presence of IFN-γ.[129] IFN-γ also attenuates the expression of both IL-8 and ENA-8.[134] These concepts support the idea that both immune and nonimmune cells can produce neutrophil chemotactic cytokines and thus help to propagate the inflammatory response. They

also suggest that members of the C-X-C chemokine family demonstrate disparate regulation by IFN-γ.

Other Factors in Neutrophil Recruitment

Although chemotactic signals and adhesion molecules are generally considered to be the major determinants of leukocyte recruitment, changes in the rheologic properties of blood can also play a role in extravasating leukocytes. In addition, prostaglandins greatly amplify the activity of locally injected chemoattractants, such as IL-8.[135] Cytokine-induced prostaglandin production acts in concert with the expression of adhesion molecules and the production of chemotactic cytokines.

WOUND HEALING

Normal wound repair rapidly restores tissue integrity and function following various insults, such as trauma, burns, and infection. Healing involves a complex interplay between humoral, cellular, and extracellular matrix networks. Nevertheless, it occurs in a controlled, sequential manner that depends on the cells to communicate with one another (Fig. 5-14). While this communication often occurs by direct cell-to-cell contact through specific cellular adhesion molecules, cells can also signal one another through soluble mediators, such as cytokines. Chemokines have been previously discussed as chemotactic factors, but they also appear to have reparative activities. Recent findings support the importance of these molecules in angiogenesis, which is an important process in tissue repair and wound healing. As described earlier, these cytokines have been designated as the C-X-C family of chemokines because of their highly conserved four cysteine amino acids and their neutrophil chemotactic properties.

Following injury, the reparative process immediately begins with hemorrhage and extravasation of plasma into the wound (Fig. 5-15). This activates the intrinsic and extrinsic coagulation pathways, leading to fibrin deposition and establishment of a provisional matrix.[136] Platelet activation and degranulation also occur during coagulation, leading to the deposition of cytokines into the provisional matrix. These cytokines include TGF-α, TGF-β, PDGF, and neutrophil activating peptide-2, which is a proteolytic cleavage product of platelet basic protein.[119] These cytokines are either important growth factors or chemotaxins that elicit leukocytes, endothelial cells, fibroblasts, and keratinocytes, which are important in tissue repair.[119] Thus, coagulation and platelet activation provide the initial foundation for subsequent cellular recruitment.

Neutrophils are typically the first leukocytes to arrive at the wound, with their primary function to phagocytize debris. These cells can also produce cytokines that help to orchestrate the progression of wound repair. These cytokines include, but are not limited to, interferon-α (IFN-α), GM-CSF, TNF, IL-1, IL-1 receptor antagonist (IL-1ra), IL-6, IL-8, macrophage inflammatory protein-1-α (MIP-1-α), and TGF-β.[17,137,138] While neutrophils are important for initial host defense, the second wave of leukocytes consists of mononuclear cells, with the mononuclear phagocyte representing a pivotal leukocyte in the progression of wound repair. The mononuclear phagocyte can generate inflammatory mediators that are important in transforming the provisional matrix to more mature granulation tissue.[17,137–139]

The transition of wound repair from acute inflammation to granulation tissue is essential because granulation tissue consists of appropriate extracellular matrix constituents, fi-

Table 5-7. C-X-C CHEMOKINES

Name	Abbreviation
Connective tissue activating protein III β-Thromboglobulin	CTAP-III
Neutrophil-activating peptide-2	NAP-2
Growth-related oncogene-α	GRO-α
Growth-related oncogene-β	GRO-β
Growth-related oncogene-γ	GRO-γ
Interleukin-8	IL-8
Epithelial neutrophil-activating protein	ENA-78
Granulocyte chemotactic protein-2	GCP-2
Platelet factor-4	PF-4
γ-Interferon-inducible protein	IP-10
Monokine induced by γ-interferon	MIG

broblasts, endothelial cells, leukocytes, and mediators that form either the connective tissue foundation or stimulus for neovascularization. The process of angiogenesis is important because it sustains a continual supply of oxygen and nutrients to the cellular constituents of the wound and provides a substructure for the eventual reepithelialization of the wound surface (Table 5-8). Recent data suggest that the cytokines of the C-X-C chemokine family play an important role in the angiogenic process that occurs during wound healing. During the early phases of granulation tissue formation, the immature connective tissue resembles undifferentiated mesenchyme with persistent fibrin, an embryonic form of fibronectin, a predominance of collagen type I, fibronectin, and protease-dependent remodeling of the extracellular matrix[140] (see Fig. 5-14). The granulation tissue provides the foundation for reepithelialization of the wound surface. As basal keratinocytes migrate from the wound edge over the surface of the mature granulation tissue, keratinocytes at the wound margin begin to proliferate. This response is followed by epidermal regeneration and production of basement membrane extracellular constituents (ie, fibronectin, type IV and VII collagen, heparin sulfate proteoglycans and laminin) that provide the integrity of the epidermal to dermal structures.[119] The sequential yet overlapping interplay of coagulation, inflammation, and formation of granulation tissue provides the foundation for the subsequent reepithelialization that is necessary to restore tissue function under normal conditions of wound repair.

Cytokines and Angiogenesis

Angiogenesis is an important component of tissue repair and wound healing. The ingrowth of new blood vessels is critical for a continued supply of oxygen and nutrients to the regenerating tissues. One of the key features of the normal, physiologic process of angiogenesis is that it is a local, transient event under strict control. Strong evidence suggests that a biologic imbalance in the production of angiogenic and angiostatic factors contributes to the pathogenesis of several angiogenesis-dependent disorders. These disease states are typically associated with an overexpression of angiogenic activity, which may be associated with the maintenance and progression of a chronic disease state. Disorders associated with chronic inflammation, such as rheumatoid arthritis, scleroderma, psoriasis, atherosclerosis, and idiopathic pulmonary fibrosis are examples of nonmalignant diseases with chronic angiogenic activity.[141]

Persistent neovascularization in these disorders is a prerequisite for perpetuating fibroproliferation.[16,141] For example, in rheumatoid arthritis, the unrestrained proliferation of fibroblasts and neovascularization leads to the formation of persistent granulation tissue, whose degradative enzymes contribute to the profound destruction of joint spaces.[142] A subpopulation of macrophages isolated from rheumatoid synovium produce factors that are potentially angiogenic in vivo and chemotactic for capillary endothelial cells in vitro.[143,144]

The inability of macrophages to express appropriate angiogenic activity may also contribute to the pathogenesis of diseases that are associated with defective angiogenesis. Blood monocyte–derived macrophages from patients with scleroderma fail to generate the expected angiogenic activity when exposed to the agonist LPS,[145] suggesting that a defect in macrophage responsiveness to activating signals contributes to the attenuated neovascularization encountered in scleroderma.

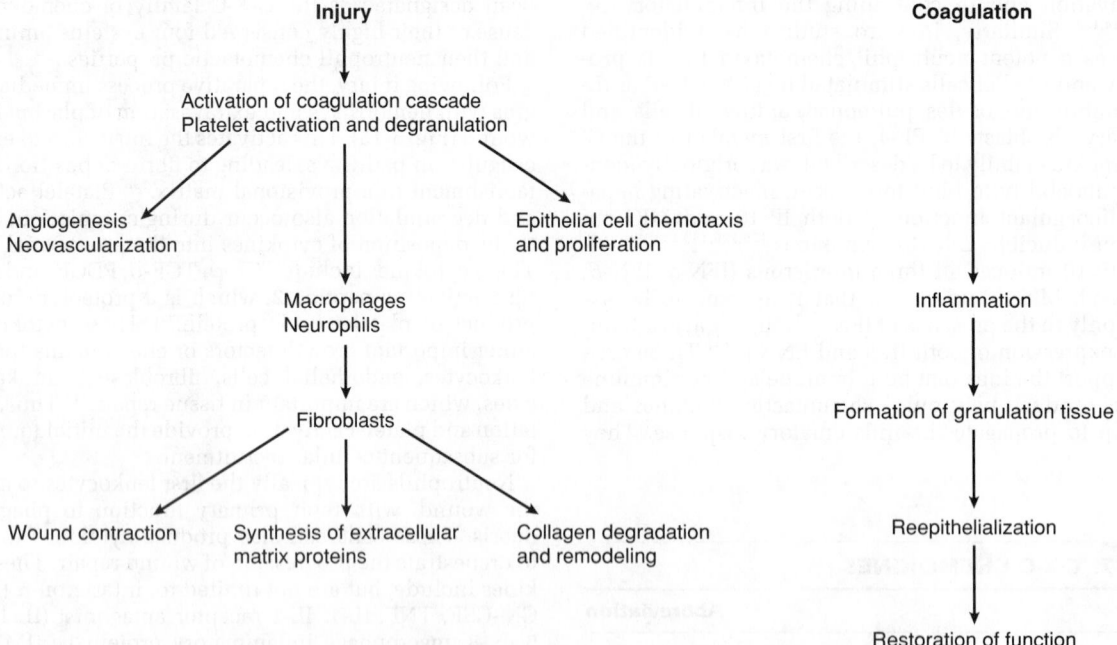

Figure 5-14. Wound healing and tissue repair. Injury initially results in platelet activation and degranulation, as well as activation of the coagulation cascade. The release of a variety of factors both from the activated platelets and through the coagulation cascade initiates the process of angiogenesis and neovascularization, activates neutrophils, monocytes, and macrophages, and recruits these cells into the area of injury. In addition, the process of epithelial cell chemotaxis and proliferation also begins. These processes represent acute inflammation. Macrophages and neutrophils and the cytokines and mediators that they elaborate are then important progressing from acute inflammation to active tissue repair with the formation of granulation tissue. Recruitment and activation of fibroblasts within the provisional wound matrix is the next key step in tissue repair. Fibroblasts increase their synthesis of extracellular matrix proteins, as well as elaborate proteases and collagenases which are important for tissue remodeling. This progresses to wound contraction, reepithelialization, and restoration of function.

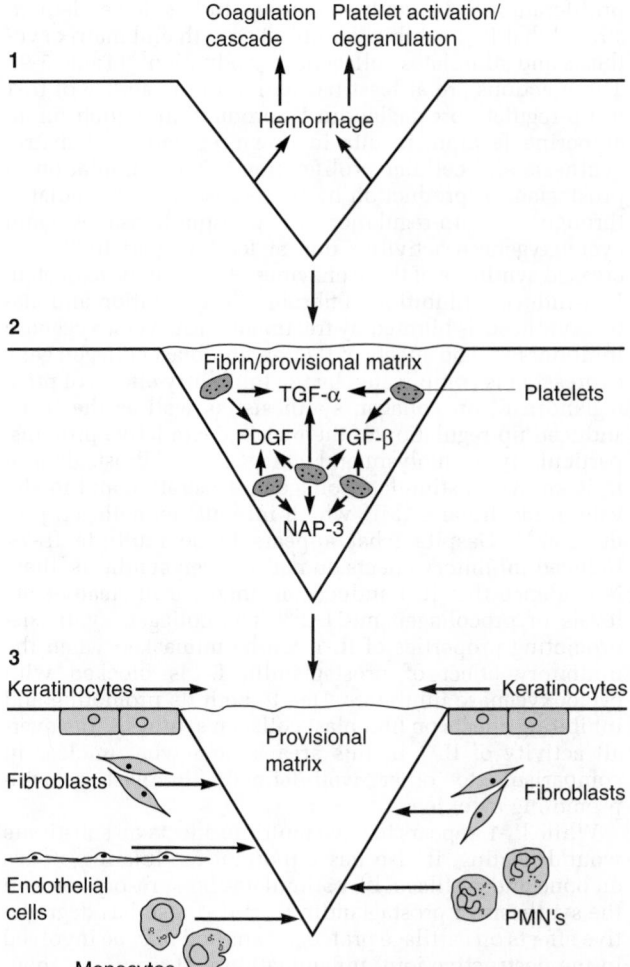

Figure 5-15. The wound matrix. (1) Following injury, hemorrhage occurs, with activation of coagulation and deposition of fibrin in the wound. (2) Concurrently, platelets are activated, resulting in degranulation, with the deposition of TGF-α, TGF-β, PDGF, and NAP-2 within the provisional wound matrix. (3) TGF-α, TGF-β, PDGF, and NAP-2 are important growth factors and chemotaxins for recruiting or activating fibroblasts, endothelial cells, monocytes, and neutrophils into the wound. Neutrophils are typically the first cells recruited into a site of injury, and produce a number of cytokines that are important for initiating wound repair. While neutrophils are important in initial host defense, the monocyte/macrophage is recruited into the wound after inflammation is established and is important in converting the provisional wound matrix into mature granulation tissue. Thus, coagulation and platelet degranulation are key processes for the subsequent cellular recruitment and activation necessary for wound healing.

Psoriasis is a well-known angiogenesis-dependent disorder, characterized by marked dermal neovascularization. Keratinocytes derived from psoriatic plaques are angiogenic compared to keratinocytes obtained from normal individuals. This appears to be at least partly due to an overproduction of the angiogenic cytokine, IL-8, and a deficiency in the production of the angiogenesis inhibitor, thrombospondin-1, with the net result being a proangiogenic environment.[146-149]

It is well established that angiogenesis is a tightly regulated process that is under complex positive and negative controls. It is also apparent that overexuberant angiogenesis is common with most chronic inflammatory disorders.

Angiogenesis and C-X-C Chemokines

While IL-8 is clearly a potent neutrophil chemotaxin and activator, findings strongly suggest that IL-8 is also a potent angiogenic factor.[143,150,151] In vitro, recombinant IL-8 mediates endothelial cell chemotaxis and proliferation. IL-8 also demonstrates potent angiogenic activity in an in vivo angiogenesis model using a corneal micropocket system in rabbits or rats. Endothelial cell chemotaxis occurs in response to recombinant IL-8 at a concentration of 1.25 nmol/L and is comparable to chemotaxis toward recombinant FGF at a concentration of 6 nmol/L.[143] Similar concentrations of IL-8 are angiogenic in the corneal micropocket model. Since monocytes and macrophages can represent a major source of angiogenic activity in wounds, chronic diseases, and solid tumors,[152] IL-8 may be an important angiogenic factor liberated by these cells in a variety of pathologic states, as well as during normal wound repair.

In contrast, another member of the C-X-C chemokine family, PF-4, has angiostatic properties.[153] In vivo, PF-4 was found to attenuate the growth of murine melanoma and human colon cancer, and this appeared to be related to its angiostatic properties.[154] This angiostatic activity was initially postulated to be secondary to the heparin binding domain in the carboxy terminus of the molecule.[153,154] This does not appear to be the case, however, since a recently produced PF-4 analog without the heparin binding domain was equipotent in vivo to native PF-4 in attenuating tumor growth.[155] The ELR motif (ie, the three amino acids that precede the first cysteine in the C-X-C chemokines) appears to be critically important in binding and activating neutrophils (Fig. 5-16). This particular motif is absent in certain members of the C-X-C chemokine family, notably PF-4, IP-10, and MIG. These particular molecules display a markedly reduced potency in mediating neutrophil chemotaxis.[28] When the ELR motif is introduced into these molecules, they gain significantly in their potency for neutrophil chemotaxis. Thus, this particular structural difference may also explain, at least in part, the disparate angiogenic activity between members of the C-X-C chemokine family.[28] This suggests that the C-X-C chemokines can function as either angiostatic or angiogenic factors, and the biologic balance that is maintained between these factors can govern overall angiogenic potential in a variety of physiologic and pathophysiologic states.

Cytokines and Fibroblasts

The replacement of normal functional organs by nonfunctional scars has long been associated with the exchange of differentiated parenchymal cells for fibroblasts and collagen. By virtue of their inability to express the differentiated and often highly specialized functions of the original parenchymal cells, these fibroblasts have been

Table 5-8. KERATINOCYTE-DERIVED CYTOKINES WITH ACTIVITY IN WOUND HEALING

Cytokine	Major Effect
TNF	Tissue remodeling
IL-1	Matrix deposition
	Tissue remodeling
IL-6	Inflammation
IL-8	Inflammation
TGF-β	Matrix deposition
TGF-α	Epithelialization
PDGF	Granulation tissue formation

viewed as passive structural cells and devoid of vital functions. Their unchecked proliferation inhibits the successful repair and regeneration of normal functional tissues. In the past, little attention was paid to the fibroblast's potentially active role in the inflammatory response. Because these cells are the primary source of the connective tissue found in fibrotic lesions, an increasing effort has been devoted to studying the mechanisms underlying the regulation of fibroblast growth, chemotaxis, and extracellular matrix synthesis and deposition. The fibroblast is appreciated as an important element in both normal and pathologic processes, particularly those surrounding tissue injury and repair. Because fibroblasts are present in virtually all tissues, cytokine production by these cells plays an important role in most if not all tissues. The fibroblast is involved in many functions, including regulation of tissue repair and fibrosis, hematopoiesis, bone metabolism, inflammation, and immune response.

Fibroblasts, Interleukin-1, and Tissue Remodeling

Interleukin-1 is important for normal wound repair, with tissue levels of IL-1 peaking along with TNF levels within the first day of wounding.[19] In vitro studies suggest that IL-1 is important for a variety of skin functions. Keratinocytes are known to synthesize IL-1 in response to injury, and IL-1 has been shown to stimulate fibroblast and keratinocyte growth as well as fibroblast collagen synthesis and keratinocyte chemotaxis[20] (Fig. 5-17). IL-1 also promotes increased transcription of the matrix degradative enzymes collagenase[76] and stromelysin.[156] Stromelysin is a potent tissue-degrading proteinase that is important in the tissue-remodeling processes associated with wound healing. The up-regulation of stromolysin may also be an important component of many pathologic processes, such as those involved in joint destruction in arthritis and tumor invasion. In addition, IL-1 induces macrophages to produce plasminogen-activator inhibitor, which is also important for tissue remodeling and repair[157] and also for fibroblast

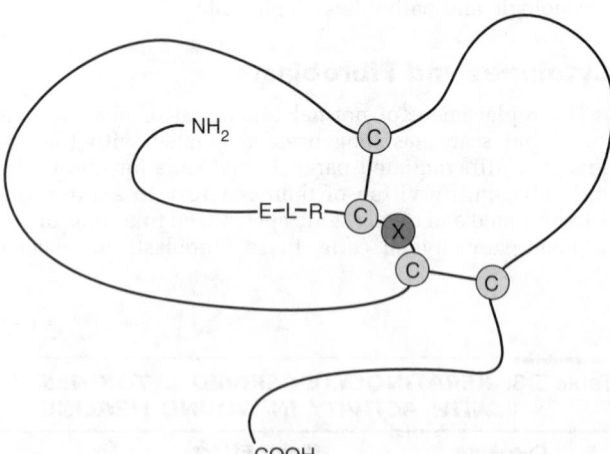

Figure 5-16. Schematic structure of C-X-C cytokines, demonstrating the 4 highly conserved cysteine amino acids. The first 2 cysteines are separated by 1 nonconserved amino acid. The ELR motif that precedes the first cysteine amino acid is also illustrated. The presence of the ELR motif appears to be important for neutrophil chemotactic activity and possibly also for angiogenic activity. PF-4, IP-10, and MIG lack the ELR motif and have a significantly reduced ability to induce neutrophil chemotaxis. This property is restored when the ELR motif is added to these molecules.

proliferation.[12] In contrast, other studies have demonstrated that IL-1 inhibits fibroblast growth and matrix synthesis and stimulates collagenase production[75] (Table 5-9). These actions are at least partly due to the ability of IL-1 to up-regulate prostaglandin E_2 production, which, in an autocrine fashion, results in down-regulation of matrix synthesis and cellular proliferation.[75] The stimulation of prostaglandin production by IL-1 appears to be mediated through the up-regulation of phospholipase A_2 and cyclooxygenase activities due at least in part to the increased synthesis of these enzymes. As would be expected, IL-1-induced inhibition of fibroblast proliferation and matrix synthesis is blunted by treatment with cyclooxygenase inhibitors.[158] The effects of IL-1 on fibroblast collagen gene expression is complicated by the inhibitory effects of prostaglandin E_2 on collagen synthesis, as well as the IL-1–induced up-regulation of the matrix degradative proteins, particularly stromolysin and collagenase.[159] Prostaglandin E_2 is known to stimulate collagenase secretion and to elevate intracellular cAMP, which inhibits net collagen production.[160] Despite what appears to be multiple IL-1–induced inhibitory effects on net collagen synthesis, there is evidence that IL-1 induces an increase in steady-state levels of procollagen mRNA.[161] The collagen synthesis-promoting properties of IL-1 can be unmasked when the inhibitory effect of prostaglandin E_2 is blocked with cyclooxygenase inhibitors. Due to both its promoting and inhibiting effects on fibroblast collagen synthesis, the overall activity of IL-1 in this area is somewhat unclear in comparison to other well-defined fibroblast growth-promoting cytokines.[162]

While IL-1 appears to have multiple effects on soft-tissue wound healing, it also has important modulating effects on bone and cartilage. IL-1 stimulates bone resorption and the synthesis of prostaglandin E_2.[11] IL-1 also has degradative effects on cartilage proteoglycans and may be involved in the destructive joint inflammation that occurs in rheumatoid arthritis.[11,74,75] In fact, the effects of IL-1 on fibroblasts were initially studied in arthritic joints.[74]

In addition to regulating fibroblast collagen synthesis, IL-1 also controls some aspects of fibroblast cytokine production. IL-1 participates in a positive feedback loop by stimulating additional fibroblast IL-1 production. In addition, IL-1 also induces fibroblast production of IL-6, IL-8, TNF, MCP-1, and several of the colony stimulating factors.[163] The fibroblast production of IL-1 is also induced by TNF and interferon-γ[164]; it is inhibited by steroids.[165] Although other cytokines can regulate fibroblast IL-1 production, the lack of significant secretion makes it unlikely that the fibroblast is an important in vivo source of IL-1. Many of the effects of IL-1 on the fibroblast are similar to those induced by TNF, and synergistic effects are seen when the two agents are used together.[163]

Fibroblasts, Tumor Necrosis Factor, Interleukin-6, and Wound Healing

As with other cytokines, the effects of TNF on the fibroblast are varied and difficult to separate in vivo from the influence of other cytokines, particularly IL-1. TNF appears to be important in the early inflammatory response to wounding and in orchestrating tissue repair. Studies suggest that TNF is important for normal wound repair, with tissue levels of TNF peaking within the first day of wounding.[19] Furthermore, TNF has potent angiogenic activity as demonstrated in an in vivo subcutaneous sponge-implant model.[166] Other studies suggest that abnormal levels of TNF or the continued presence of TNF in the wound inhibit healing, demonstrating that TNF inhibits the ingrowth of granulation tissue, retards the accumulation of collagen hydroxyproline, and down-regulates collagen synthesis.[167] Although TNF inhibits fibroblast collagen synthesis,[168] it also has potent mitogenic effects. The mitogenic response correlates well with an increased stimulation of tyrosine phosphorylation and is down-regulated by interferon-γ.[169] TNF has no chemotactic effect on fibroblasts and does not alter the fibroblast response to other chemoattractants. TNF does, however, stimulate the production of fibroblast prostaglandin E_2 and enhances transcription and translation of IL-6.[167] IL-6 may play a role in fibroblast extracellular matrix metabolism through its ability to enhance the production of tissue inhibitor of metalloproteinase.[170] More recent studies suggest that TNF acting locally may block wound healing by inhibiting the expression of the gene for type-I collagen.[18] TNF also stimulates cartilage resorption and the release of proteoglycans from cartilage by a limited proteolytic degradation, and it inhibits proteoglycan synthesis[14] (Fig. 5-18). These particular phenomena may be mediated and promoted by collagenase and prostaglandin E_2, because both are up-regulated

in fibroblasts and macrophages by TNF and are involved in the degradation of collagen matrix and stimulation of the intracellular proteases responsible for tissue remodeling.[140,167,168] TNF may also inhibit fracture healing in experimental animals. The decline in the rate of fracture repair appears to be related to TNF-induced inhibition of cartilage formation early in new bone synthesis. This is due to its inhibition of mesenchymal cell differentiation into chondroblasts.[171] All of these functions may be important in the normal process of wound healing and remodeling, as well as in the pathologic settings of degenerative joint diseases and altered wound healing.

Fibroblasts and Epithelial Growth Factor

The family of epithelial growth factor (EGF)-like molecules are characterized by high affinity binding to the EGF receptor, thus inducing mitogenesis in EGF-sensitive cells. EGF stimulation is associated with the activation of a phos-

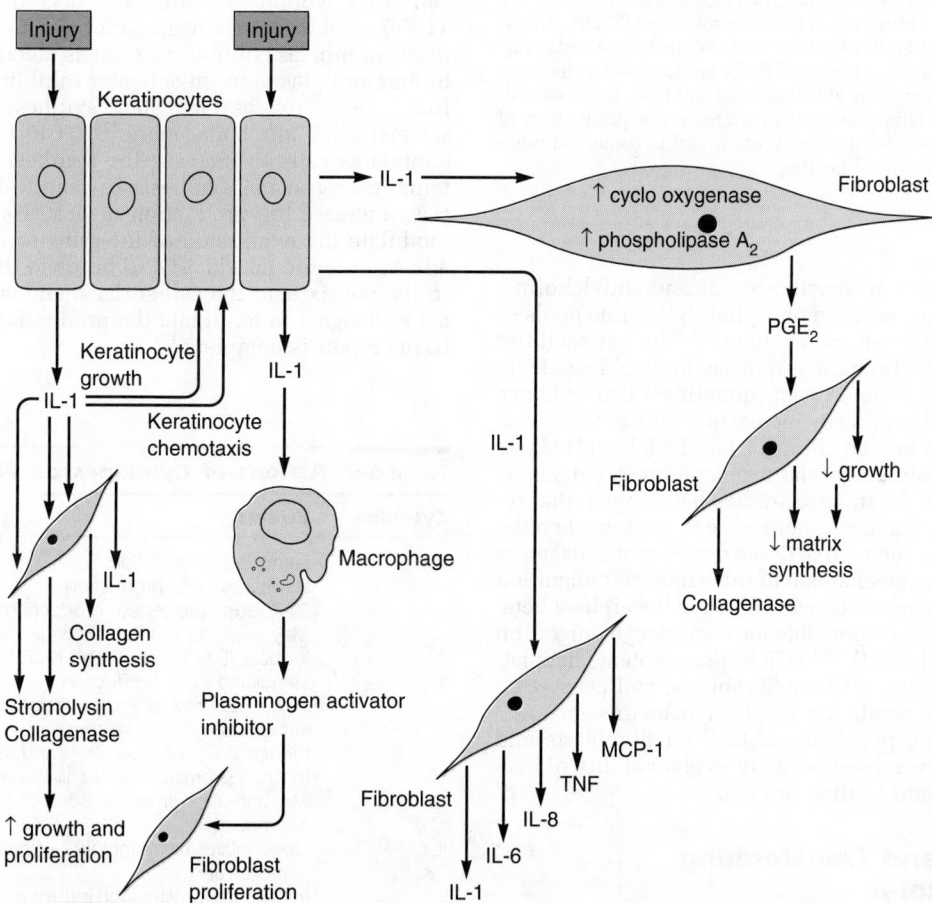

Figure 5-17. Actions of IL-1 on keratinocytes, macrophages, and fibroblasts in the context of wound healing. Keratinocytes produce IL-1 in response to injury. IL-1 then stimulates keratinocyte growth and chemotaxis. In addition, this keratinocyte-derived IL-1 has multiple effects on other cells, particularly fibroblasts and macrophages. IL-1 induces fibroblasts to produce many cytokines that are important for wound healing, including IL-1, IL-6, IL-8, TNF, and MCP-1. IL-1 also induces fibroblast growth and proliferation, collagen synthesis, and the synthesis of collagenase and stromolysin. Collagenase, and stromolysin are important in the process of tissue remodeling, which is a vital component of wound healing. In the macrophage, IL-1 induces the synthesis of plasminogen-activator inhibitor, which is important for tissue remodeling and also increases fibroblast proliferation. IL-1 also has some inhibitory actions on the fibroblast, which are mediated through the up-regulation of PGE_2. IL-1 increases cyclooxygenase and phospholipase A_2, increasing the synthesis of PGE_2. PGE_2 then functions in an autocrine fashion to decrease fibroblast growth and matrix synthesis and further increases collagenase production.

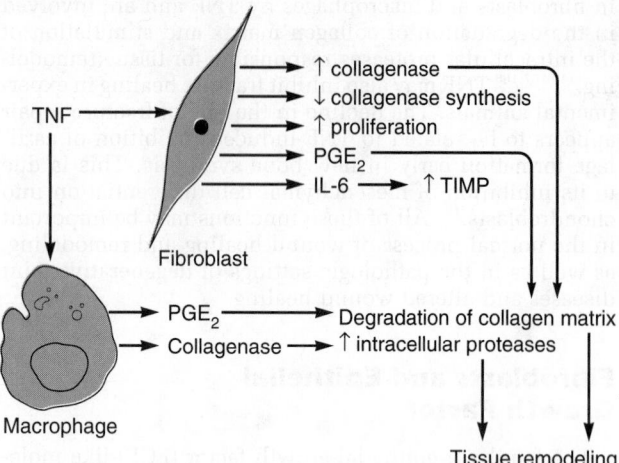

Figure 5-18. Effects of TNF on fibroblasts and macrophages in the context of wound healing. TNF has powerful mitogenic actions on the fibroblast, increasing proliferation. Conversely, it also inhibits collagen synthesis and increases collagenase production. TNF also increases fibroblast production of IL-6 and PGE$_2$. IL-6 appears to play a role in extracellular matrix metabolism by increasing production of tissue inhibitor of metalloproteinase (TIMP). In addition to increasing fibroblast production of collagenase and PGE$_2$, TNF also increases collagenase and PGE$_2$ production by the macrophage. Increased amounts of collagenase and PGE$_2$ facilitate collagen matrix degradation, as well as increase the production of intracellular proteases, which are all important in tissue remodeling, a key aspect of wound healing.

pholipase C, which is specific for phosphatidylcholine, reflecting cytokine-sensitive phosphatidylcholine pools or selective diacylglycerol metabolism.[159] The extracellular matrix influences fibroblast responses to cytokines. EGF, applied topically in microgram quantities, can enhance soft-tissue wound healing by increasing soft-tissue neovascularization.[172] In human clinical trials, EGF has also been shown to accelerate epidermal regeneration in cutaneous wounds.[172] Similarly, in vitro studies have shown that recombinant EGF enhances keratinocyte migration when the cells are grown on connective tissue matrices of collagen or fibronectin.[173] The mechanism of this enhanced migration may be related to increased expression of the alpha-2 beta-1 integrin, which is responsible for keratinocyte migration on collagen type I and IV.[173] EGF is also a potent chemoattractant for granulation tissue fibroblasts, and cells at all stages of wound repair are responsive to this factor.[174] These chemotactic properties of EGF for fibroblasts and keratinocytes may at least partially explain ability of EGF to accelerate wound healing in vivo.

Fibroblasts and Transforming Growth Factor-β

Transforming growth factor-β appears to be one of the key cytokines in controlling tissue repair. Furthermore, the sustained production of this cytokine has been implicated in the development of tissue fibrosis in various chronic disease states. Wound healing is a complex series of coordinated events. It begins with platelet-induced hemostasis, followed by an influx of inflammatory cells and fibroblasts, the deposition of extracellular matrix and neovascularization, and the proliferation of cells that reconstitute the injured tissue.[119] TGF-β plays a role in each of these events.[119] Platelets contain high concentrations of TGF-β and PDGF, which are released into the tissue at the site of

injury.[16] TGF-β is strongly chemotactic for neutrophils, T cells, monocytes, and fibroblasts.[16] As these inflammatory cells move into the site of injury, they are activated as they encounter increasing concentrations of TGF-β.[118] Monocytes begin to elaborate FGF, TNF, and IL-1, and fibroblasts increase their synthesis of extracellular matrix proteins.[119] TGF-β also induces both the infiltrating cells and resident cells to produce more TGF-β. This autoinduction amplifies its biologic effects at the site of injury and may contribute to the development of chronic fibrosis in various pathologic states.[175] At physiologic concentrations, TGF-β regulates PDGF production in smooth muscle cells and fibroblasts, FGF production in endothelial cells, and TNF and IL-1 production in monocytes.[175] TGF-β also modulates macrophage cytotoxicity by suppressing the production of superoxide and nitric oxide.[175]

The extracellular matrix is a dynamic superstructure of self-aggregating macromolecules, including fibronectin, collagens, and proteoglycans, to which cells attach by means of surface receptors called *integrins*.[119] TGF-β is a potent inducer of extracellular matrix production, stimulating the synthesis of collagen types I, II, V, fibronectin, and glycosaminoglycans.[176,177] The matrix surrounding the cells in a wound is continually degraded by proteases. TGF-β inhibits matrix degradation by increasing the synthesis of protease inhibitors, such as metalloproteinase inhibitor and plasminogen-activator inhibitor, and by inhibiting gene expression and synthesis of protease, stromelysin, and collagenase.[178] TGF-β simultaneously stimulates cells to increase the synthesis of matrix proteins, decrease the synthesis of matrix-degrading proteases, increase the production of protease inhibitors, and modulate the expression of integrins to increase cellular adhesion to the matrix. TGF-β binds to the proteoglycans in the matrix near the cell surface, and such binding can act as a signal to terminate the production of TGF-β after tissue repair is complete.[178]

Table 5-9. Actions of Cytokines on Fibroblasts

Cytokine	Effects
TNF	Stimulates proliferation
	Stimulates PGE$_2$ production
	Stimulates collagenase production
	May stimulate or inhibit collagen synthesis
	Induces IL-1, IL-6, IL-8, and MCP-1
IL-1	Stimulated PGE$_2$ production
	Stimulates growth and proliferation
	Stimulates collagen synthesis
	Induces IL-1, IL-6, IL-8, TNF, and MCP-1
	Induces stromelysin and collagenase
	May stimulate or inhibit extracellular matrix production
IL-6	Up-regulates tissue inhibitor of metalloproteinase production
	Inhibits the proliferation-inducing properties of TNF
PDGF	Potent chemotactic agent for fibroblasts
	Increases cellular proliferation
TGF-β	Induces TGF-β and PDGF
	Stimulates PGE$_2$ production
	Enhances collagen synthesis, deposition, and maturation
	Stimulates extracellular matrix production
	Inhibits matrix degradation by increasing synthesis of protease inhibitors
	May inhibit or promote cellular proliferation
EGF	Stimulates cellular proliferation and collagen synthesis
	Induces PDGF
	Potent chemotactic agent for fibroblasts

TGF-β can function as a mitogen or growth inhibitor for a wide variety of cell types, including selected mesenchymal-type cells. Whether TGF-β stimulates or inhibits proliferation depends on the presence of other growth factors, the concentration of TGF-β, and the cell density.[175] Thus, at low doses, TGF-β stimulates the proliferation of densely plated human marrow fibroblasts, but it is inhibitory at high concentrations.[179]

Fibrosis represents a pathologic excess of the normal process of tissue repair. The excessive or sustained production of TGF-β is a key molecular event in inducing tissue fibrosis, and this molecule may be an important mediator in a variety of disease states, including pulmonary fibrosis, liver cirrhosis, scleroderma, keloid formation and rheumatoid arthritis. The topical application of TGF-β accelerates wound healing.[180] In rats, topical or limited intravenous administration of TGF-β normalizes wound healing that is impaired by age or glucocorticoids.[181] In contrast, repeated injections of high-dose TGF-β induces serious systemic effects, including marked fibrosis of the kidneys and liver.[182] Recombinant TGF-β has been shown to accelerate soft-tissue wound healing in both normal and diabetic animals.[118,183] Normal healing was accelerated by 30% in wounds treated with recombinant TGF-β.[118] Further in vivo studies demonstrated that this cytokine enhances collagen synthesis, deposition, and maturation.[118] TGF-β also appears to enhance keratinocyte migration across a wound surface by increasing the expression of keratinocyte cell-surface integrins that facilitate the migratory component of reepithelialization.[184] Thus, the overall in vivo effects of TGF-β clearly favor its role as an important promoter of tissue repair, wound healing, and reepithelialization. These actions are clearly relevant for many potential clinical applications, including surgical wound healing in debilitated patients or those undergoing chemotherapy and treatment of diabetic, decubitus, varicose ulcerations, and burns.

Fibroblasts and Platelet-Derived Growth Factor

A heterodimeric protein comprised of A and B chains, PDGF is one of the most important mediators of the tissue repair process. This molecule was originally described as the most potent mitogen for cells of mesenchymal origins.[185–187] In addition, the homodimers of both the A and B chains are also potent growth factors, encoded by separate genes that are independently regulated and expressed.[186,187] PDGF is synthesized by megakaryocytes, fibroblasts, endothelial cells, macrophages, and smooth muscle cells. It is a potent mitogen for fibroblasts, smooth muscle cells, and endothelial cells.[188–190] This molecule is also a chemotactic and activating factor for neutrophils, smooth muscle cells, and fibroblasts.[190,191] PDGF is also a fibroblast chemoattractant, with the chemotactic response inversely related to the rate of cellular proliferation. PDGF has also been shown to accelerate the normal wound healing process by as much as 30%.[118] This is attibuted to a PDGF-dependent increase in early deposition of fibronectin and glycosaminoglycans, which accelerates the deposition of the provisional wound matrix.[118] There is a subsequent increase in collagen synthesis.[192] Topically applied PDGF accelerates the healing of surgical incisions in both normal and healing-impaired animals.[193,194] Enhanced wound-breaking strength was seen for as long as 49 days postwounding after a single topical application of PDGF at the time of wounding.[193,194] Other studies have shown that PDGF enhances the healing of dermal ulcers in both porcine and diabetic mouse models.[192–194] In one prospec-

tive randomized, double-blind study in humans, topically applied PDGF enhanced the healing of stage 3 and 4 decubitus ulcers.[195] It appears that during tissue injury and wound healing, PDGF stimulates a cascade of autocrine and paracrine activities. The accelerated healing responses that are seen in response to PDGF are associated with an enhanced influx and activation of macrophages, followed by the accumulation, activation, and proliferation of fibroblasts. Increases then occur in extracellular matrix deposition, particularly glycosaminoglycans and fibronectin, neovascularization, and acceleration of the reepithelialization process.[192]

Cytokines are important intercellular polypeptides that carry out a plethora of actions in various normal and pathologic states. The host response to infection, trauma, and acute surgical injury is mediated at least in part by the release of cytokines, particularly TNF, IL-1, and IL-6 in the early phase of the response. An orchestrated cytokine cascade is essential for maintaining normal immune func-

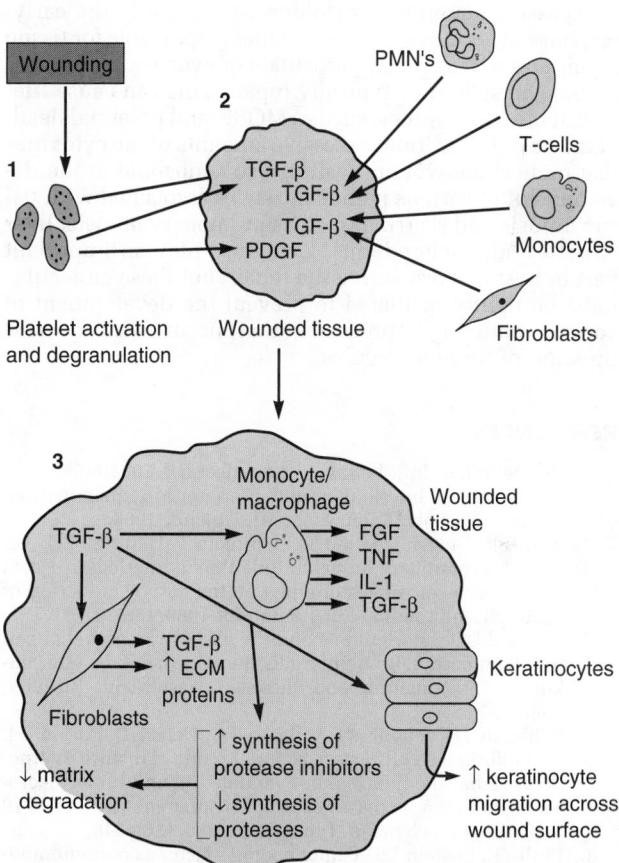

Figure 5-19. TGF-β in wound healing. TGF-β is one of the key cytokines in the orchestration of tissue repair. Immediately after wounding, platelets are activated and degranulated, releasing large amounts of TGF-β and PDGF into the wounded tissue. TGF-β is a powerful chemotactic agent for neutrophils, T-lymphocytes, monocytes, and macrophages, which are all recruited into the wound. As these cells encounter increasing concentrations of TGF-β, they become activated and release a variety of other factors that are important for perpetuating wound healing. Monocytes and macrophages release FGF, TNF, IL-1, and additional TGF-β. Fibroblasts also generate more TGF-β and increase their synthesis of extracellular matrix proteins. TGF-β inhibits matrix degradation by increasing the synthesis of extracellular matrix proteins, as well as increasing synthesis of protease inhibitors, and decreasing protease synthesis. TGF-β also increases keratinocyte migration across the wound surface, facilitating reepithalialization.

tion. Systemic levels of the early-response cytokines, TNF, IL-1 and IL-6, can profoundly affect many organ systems in the intact organism. Increased levels of these early-response cytokines, either systematically or locally, trigger a cascade of additional cytokines and mediators, which perpetuate the inflammatory response. In particular, alterations occur in the vascular endothelium and leukocytes that are critical for the migration of leukocytes into the area of injury. TNF, interleukins, and chemokines are particularly important molecules in this process. This integrated response results in an organized cascade of mediators and subsequent localization of cells to an area of injury or infection. This process then progresses to tissue repair to restore the organism to a functional, noninjured state. TGF-β and PDGF are particularly important mediators in wound repair. The up-regulation of macrophage and fibroblast integrins promotes further migration of these cells into the wound with increased deposition of provisional matrix. These cytokines are further responsible for recruiting and activating fibroblasts, in addition to increasing connective tissue deposition within the wound matrix to further facilitate tissue repair.

Excessive amounts of cytokines, particularly the early-response cytokines and the cytokines responsible for tissue repair and scarring, can perpetuate or even exacerbate the pathologic state they typically repair. This can cause life-threatening syndromes, such as MOSF, and potential death of the host. In addition, excessive amounts of the cytokines that orchestrate wound healing also contribute to the development of various pathologic states associated with tissue fibrosis and scarring, such as pulmonary fibrosis, liver cirrhosis, and scleroderma. Cytokines play an important part in host defense and tissue repair, but these molecules must be tightly regulated to prevent the development of various pathologic processes that occur with overexpression of these molecules.

REFERENCES

1. Dinarello CA. Interleukin 1. Rev Infect Dis 1984;6:51.
2. Oppenheim JJ. Interleukins and interferons in inflammation: current concepts. Kalamazoo, MI, Upjohn, 1986.
3. Andus T, Geiger T, Hiran T, Kishimoto T, Heinrich PC. Action of recombinant human interleukin 6, interleukin 1 beta and tumor necrosis factor alpha on the mRNA induction of acute phase proteins. Eur J Immunol 1988;18:739.
4. Haskard DO. Interleukin 1 and the vascular endothelial cell in inflammation. In: Bomford R, Henderson B, eds. Interleukin 1, inflammation and disease. Amsterdam, Elsevier, 1989:123.
5. Pohlman TH, Stanness KA, Beatty PG, Ochs HD, Harlan JM. An endothelial cell surface factor(s) induced in vitro by lipopolysaccharide, interleukin-1, endotoxin, and tumor necrosis factor alpha increases neutrophil adherence by a CDW18 dependent mechanism. J Immunol 1986;136:4548.
6. Philip R, Epstein LB. Tumor necrosis factor as immunomodulator and mediator of monocyte cytotoxicity induced by itself, gamma interferon and interleukin-1. Nature 1986; 323:86.
7. Lee MD, Zentella A, Pekala PH, Cerami A. Effect of endotoxin-induced monokines on glucose metabolism in the muscle cell line L6. Proc Natl Acad Sci USA 1987;84:2590.
8. Shalaby MR, Aggarwal BB, Rinderknecht E, Svedersky LP, Finkle BS, Palladino MA Jr. Activation of human polymorphonuclear neutrophil function by interferon gamma and tumor necrosis factor. J Immunol 1985;135:2069.
9. Klebanoff SJ, Vadas MA, Harlan JM, et al. Stimulation of neutrophils by tumor necrosis factor. J Immunol 1986; 136:4220.
10. Larrick JW, Kunkel SL. The role of tumor necrosis factor and interleukin-1 in the immunoinflammatory response. Pharm Res 1988;5:129.
11. Gowen M, Wood DD, Ihrie EJ, McGuire MKB, Russell GG. An interleukin-1 like factor stimulates bone resorption in vitro. Nature 1983;306:378.
12. Schmidt JA, Mizel SB, Cohen D, Green I. Interleukin 1: a potential regulator of fibroblast proliferation. J Immunol 1982;128:82.
13. Kohase M, Hendrickson-Destefano D, Sehgal PB, Vilcek J. Dexamethasone inhibits feedback regulation of the mitogenic activity of TNF, IL-1 and EGF in human fibroblasts. J Cell Physiol 1987;132:271.
14. Saklatvala J. Tumor necrosis factor alpha stimulates resorption and inhibits synthesis of proteoglycan in cartilage. Nature 1986;322:547.
15. Kirstein M, Baglioni C. Tumor necrosis factor induces synthesis of two proteins in human fibroblasts. J Biol Chem 1986;261:9565.
16. Clark RAF. Basics of cutaneous wound repair. J Dermatol Surg Oncol 1993;19:693.
17. Leibovich SJ, Weisman DM. Macrophages, wound repair and angiogenesis. Prog Clin Biol Res 1988;266:131.
18. Salomon GD, Kasid A, Cromack DT, et al. The local effects of cachectin/tumor necrosis factor on wound healing. Ann Surg 1991;214:175.
19. Fahey TJ 3d, Sherry B, Tracey KJ, et al. Cytokine production in a model of wound healing: the appearance of MIP-1, MIP-2, cachectin/TNF and IL-1. Cytokine 1990;2:92.
20. Sauder DN, Kilian PL, McLane JA, et al. Interleukin-1 enhances epidermal wound healing. Lymphokine Res 1990; 9:465.
21. Tracey KJ, Beutler B, Lowry SF, et al. Shock and tissue injury induced by recombinant human cachectin. Science 1986;234:470.
22. Strieter RM, Lynch III JP, Basha MA, Standiford TJ, Kasahara K, Kunkel SL. Host responses in mediating sepsis and the adult respiratory distress syndrome. Semin Respir Infect 1990;5:233.
23. Tracey KJ, Lowry SF, Cerami A. Cachectin/TNF-alpha in septic shock and septic adult respiratory distress syndrome. Am Rev Respir Dis 1988;138:1377.
24. Schlag G, Redl H, Hallstrom S. The cell in shock: the origin of multiple organ failure. Resuscitation 1991;21:137.
25. Benton LD, Khan M, Greco RS. Integrins, adhesion molecules surgical research. Surg Gynecol Obstet 1993;177:311.
26. Talbott GA, Sharar SR, Harlan JM, Winn RK. Leukocyte-endothelial interaction and organ injury: the role of adhesion molecules. New Horizons 1994;2:545.
27. Kumar AG, Dai XY, Kozak CA, Mims MP, Gotto AM, Ballantyne CM. Murine VCAM-1: molecular cloning, mapping, and analysis of a truncated form. J Immunol 1994;153:4088.
28. Strieter RM, Lukacs NW, Standiford TJ, Kunkel SL. Cytokines and lung inflammation. Thorax 1993;48:765.
29. Chuluyan HE, Issekutz AC. VLA-4 integrin can mediate CD11/CD18-independent transendothelial migration of human monocytes. J Clin Invest 1993;92:2768.
30. Waage A, Halstensen A, Espevik T. Association between tumor necrosis factor in serum and fatal outcome in patients with meningococcal disease. Lancet 1987;11:355.
31. Girardin E, Grau GE, Dayer JM, Roux-Lombard P, the J5 Study Group, Lambert PH. Tumor necrosis factor and interleukin-1 in the serum of children with severe infectious purpura. N Engl J Med 1988;319:397.
32. Marks JD, Marks CB, Luce JM, et al. Plasma tumor necrosis factor in patients with septic shock: mortality rate, incidence of adult respiratory distress syndrome. Am Rev Respir Dis 1990;141:94.
33. Tracey KJ, Fong Y, Hesse DG, et al. Anti-cachectin/TNF monoclonal antibodies prevent septic shock during lethal bacteremia. Nature 1987;330:662.
34. Shalaby MR, Halgunset J, Haugen OA, et al. Cytokine-associated tissue injury and lethality in mice: a comparative study. Clin Immunol Immunopathol 1991;61:69.
35. Kunkel SL, Remick DG, Strieter RM, Larrick JW. Mechanisms that regulate the production and effects of tumor necrosis factor-alpha. Crit Rev Immunol 1989;9:93.
36. Cerami A. Inflammatory cytokines. Clin Immunol Immunopathol 1992;62:S3.
37. Michie HR, Manogue KR, Spriggs DR, et al. Detection of

circulating tumor necrosis factor after endotoxin administration. N Engl J Med 1988;318:3972.

38. Bauss F, Droge W, Mannel DN. Tumor necrosis factor mediates endotoxic effects in mice. Infect Immun 1987;55:1622.

39. Waage A. Production and clearance of tumor necrosis factor in rats exposed to endotoxin and dexamethasone. Clin Immunol Immunopathol 1987;45:345.

40. Beutler B, Milsark IW, Cerami AC. Passive immunization against cachectin/tumor necrosis factor protects mice from lethal effects of endotoxin. Science 1985;229:869.

41. Remick DJ, Kunkel RG, Larrick JW, Kunkel SL. Acute in vivo effects of human recombinant tumor necrosis factor. Lab Invest 1987;56:583.

42. Bevilacqua MP, Pober JS, Majeau GR, Fiers W, Cotran RS, Gimbrone MA Jr. Recombinant tumor necrosis factor induces procoagulant activity in cultured human vascular endothelium: characterization and comparison with the actions of interleukin-1. Proc Natl Acad Sci USA 1986; 83:4533.

43. Nawroth PP, Stern DM. Modulation of endothelial cell hemostatic properties by tumor necrosis factor. J Exp Med 1986;163:740.

44. Conway EM, Rosemberg RD. Tumor necrosis factor suppresses transcription of the thrombomodulin gene in endothelial cells. Mol Cell Biol 1988;8:5588.

45. Emeis JJ, Kooistra T. Interleukin-1 and lipopolysaccharide induce an inhibitor of tissue type plasminogen activator in vivo and in cultured endothelial cells. J Exp Med 1986; 163:1260.

46. Bevilacqua MP, Pober JS, Majeau GR, Cotran RS, Gimbrone MA Jr. Interleukin 1 (IL-1) induces biosynthesis and cell surface expression of procoagulant activity in human vascular endothelial cells. J Exp Med 1984;160:618.

47. Bussolino F, Breviario F, Tetta C, Aglietta M, Mantovani A, Dejana E. Interleukin 1 stimulates platelet activating factor production in cultured human endothelial cells. J Clin Invest 1986;77:2027.

48. Rossi V, Brevario F, Ghessi P, Dejana E, Mantovani A. Prostacylin synthesis induced in vascular cells by interleukin-1. Science 1985;229:174.

49. van Hinsberg VWM, van der Berg EA, Fiers W, Dooijewaard G. Tumor necrosis factor induces the production of urokinase type plasminogen activator by human endothelial cells. Blood 1990;10:1991.

50. Okusawa S, Gelfand JA, Ikeijma T, Connolly RJ, Dinarello CA. Interleukin-1 induces a shock-like state in rabbits: synergism with tumor necrosis factor and the effect of cyclooxygenase inhibition. J Clin Invest 1988;81:1162.

51. Kettelhut IC, Fiers W, Goldberg AL. The toxic effects of tumor necrosis factor in vivo and their prevention by cyclooxygenase inhibitors. Proc Natl Acad Sci USA 1987;84:4273.

52. Libby P, Ordovas JM, Auger KR, Robbins AH, Birinyi LK, Dinarello CA. Endotoxin and tumor necrosis factor induce interleukin-1 gene expression in adult human vascular endothelial cells. Am J Pathol 1986;124:179.

53. Dejana E, Brevario F, Erroi A, et al. Modulation of endothelial cell function by different molecular species of interleukin-1. Blood 1987;69:695.

54. Strieter RM, Kunkel SL, Showell HJ, et al. Endothelial cell gene expression of a neutrophil chemotactic factor by TNF-alpha, LPS, and IL-1 beta. Science 1989;243:1467.

55. Flick MR, Perel A, Staub NC. Leukocytes are required for increased lung microvascular permeability after microembolization in sheep. Circ Res 1981;48:344.

56. Baird BR, Cheronis JC, Sandhaus RA, Berger EM, White CW, Repine JE. O_2 metabolites and neutrophil elastase synergistically cause edematous injury in isolated rat lungs. J Appl Physiol 1986;61:2224.

57. Weiss SJ, Regiani S. Neutrophils degrade subendothelial matrices in the presence of alpha-1-protease inhibitor: cooperative use of lysosmal proteases and oxygen metabolites. J Clin Invest 1984;73:1297.

58. Tracey KJ, Wei H, Manogue KR, et al. Cachectin/tumor necrosis factor induces cachexia, anemia and inflammation. J Exp Med 1988;167:1211.

59. Oliff A, Defeo-Jones D, Boyer M, et al. Tumors secreting human TNF/cachectin induce cachexia in mice. Cell 1987;50:555.

60. Beutler B, Tkacenko V, Milsark R, Krochin N, Cerami A. Control of cachectin (tumor necrosis factor) synthesis: mechanisms of endotoxin resistance. Science 1986;232:977.

61. Torti FM, Dieckmann B, Beutler B, Cerami A, Ringold GM. A macrophage factor inhibits adipocyte gene expression: an in vitro model of cachexia. Science 1985;229:867.

62. Semb H, Peterson J, Tavernier J, Olivecrona T. Multiple effects of tumor necrosis factor on lipoprotein lipase in vivo. J Biol Chem 1987;262:8390.

63. Kawakami M, Murase T, Ogawa H, et al. Human recombinant TNF suppresses lipoprotein lipase activity and stimulates lipolysis in 3T3-L1 cells. J Biochem 1987;101:331.

64. Torti FM, Torti SV, Larrick JW, Ringold GM. Modulation of adipocyte differentiation by tumor necrosis factor and transforming growth factor beta. J Cell Biol 1989;108:1105.

65. Hahn T, Toker L, Budilovsky S, Aderka D, Eshhar Z, Wallach D. Use of monoclonal antibodies to a human cytotoxin for its isolation and for examining the self-induction of resistance to this protein. Proc Natl Acad Sci USA 1985;82:3814.

66. Rubin BY, Anderson SL, Sullivan SA, Williamson BD, Carswell EA, Old LJ. Nonhematopoietic cells selected for resistance to tumor necrosis factor produce tumor necrosis factor. J Exp Med 1986;164:1350.

67. Spriggs D, Imamura K, Rodriguez C, Horiguchi J, Kufe DW. Induction of tumor necrosis factor expression and resistance in a human breast cancer cell line. Proc Natl Acad Sci USA 1987;84:6563.

68. Niitsu Y, Watanabe N, Neda H, et al. Induction of synthesis of tumor necrosis factor in human and murine cell lines by exogenous recombinant human tumor necrosis factor. Cancer Res 1988;48:5407.

69. Matsushima K, Akahoshi T, Yamada M, Furutani Y, Oppenheim JJ. Properties of a specific interleukin-1 (IL-1) receptor on human Epstein-Barr virus–transformed B lymphocytes: identity of the receptor for IL-1 alpha and IL-1 beta. J Immunol 1986;136:4496.

70. Holtman H, Wallach D. Down regulation of the receptors for tumor necrosis factor by interleukin 1 and 4b-phorbol-12 myristate-13-acetate. J Immunol 1987;139:1161.

71. Le J, Vilcek J. TNF and IL-1: cytokines with multiple overlapping biological activities. Lab Invest 1987;56:234.

72. Oppenheim JJ, Kovacx EJ, Mastsushima K, Durum SK. There is more than one interleukin 1. Immunol Today 1986;7:45.

73. Bernheim HA. Is prostaglandin E-2 involved in the pathogenesis of fever? Effects of interleukin-1 on the release of prostaglandins. Yale J Biol Med 1986;59:151.

74. Dayer JM, Russell RGG, Krane SM. Collagenase production by rheumatoid synovial cells: stimulation by a human lymphocyte factor. Science 1977;195:181.

75. Dayer JM, Bierard J, Chess L, Krane SM. Participation of monocyte/macrophages and lymphocytes in the production of a factor that stimulates collagenase and prostaglandin release by rheumatoid synovial cells. J Clin Invest 1979; 64:1386.

76. Postlethwaite AE, Lachman LB, Mainardi CL, Kang AH. Interleukin 1 stimulation of collagenase production by cultured fibroblasts. J Exp Med 1983;157:803.

77. Atkins E. Pathogenesis of fever. Physiol Rev 1960;40:580.

78. Stitt JT. Prostaglandin E as the neural mediator of the febrile response. Yale J Biol Med 1986;59:137.

79. Castell JV, Gofmez-Lechon MJ, David M. Interleukin 6 is the major regulator of acute phase protein synthesis in adult human hepatocytes. FEBS Lett 1989;242:237.

80. Krueger JM, Walter J, Dinarello CA, Wolff SM, Chedid L. Sleep promoting effects of endogenous pyrogen (interleukin 1). Am J Physiol 1984;246:R994.

81. Walter J, Davenne D, Shoham S, Dinarello CA, Krueger JM. Brain temperature changes coupled to sleep states persist during interleukin 1 enhanced sleep. Am J Physiol 1986; 250:R96.

82. McCarthy DO, Kluger MJ, Vander AJ. Suppression of food intake during infection: is interleukin 1 involved? Am J Clin Nutr 1985;42:1179.

83. Beutler BA, Cerami A. Recombinant interleukin 1 sup-

presses lipoprotein lipase activity in 3T3L1 cells. J Immunol 1985;135:3969.

84. Kampschmidt RF, Pulliam LA. The effect of human monocyte pyrogen on plasma iron, plasma zinc and blood neutrophils in rabbits and rats. Proc Soc Exp Biol Med 1978;158:32.

85. Nachman RL, Hajjar KA, Silverstein RL, Dinarello CA. Interleukin 1 induces endothelial cell synthesis of plasminogen activator inhibitor. J Exp Med 1986;163:1595.

86. Bevilacqua MP, Scheel RR, Gimbrone MA Jr, Loskutoff DJ. Regulation of the fibrinolytic system of cultured human endothelial cells by interleukin-1. J Clin Invest 1986;78:587.

87. Gramse M, Brevario F, Pintucci G, Millet I, Dejana E, Mussoni L. Enhancement by interleukin-1 (IL-1) of plasminogen activator inhibitor (PA-I) activity in cultured human endothelial cells. Biochem Biophys Res Commun 1986;139:720.

88. Ritchie DG, Fuller GM. Hepatocyte-stimulating factor: a monocyte-derived acute-phase regulatory protein. Ann NY Acad Sci 1983;408:490.

89. Koj A, Gauldie J, Regoeczi E, Saunder DN, Sweeney GD. The acute-phase response of cultured rat hepatocytes: system characterization and the effect of human cytokines. Biochem J 1984;224:505.

90. Gauldie J, Richards C, Harnish D, Lansdorp P, Baumann H. Interferon b$_2$/B-cell stimulatory factor type 2 shares identity with monocyte-derived hepatocyte-stimulating factor and regulates the major acute-phase protein response in liver cells. Proc Natl Acad Sci USA 1987;84:7251.

91. Gauldie J, Baumann H. Cytokines and acute phase protein expression. In: Kimball EH, ed. Cytokines in inflammation. Toronto, Telford Press, 1991:136.

92. Sehgal PB. Interleukin-6: a regulator of plasma protein gene expression in hepatic and non-hepatic tissues. Mol Biol Med 1990;7:113.

93. Van Snick J. Interleukin-6: an overview. Annu Rev Immunol 1990;8:253.

94. Fong Y, Moldawer LL, Marano M, et al. Endotoxemia elicits increased circulating b$_2$-IFN/IL-6 in man. J Immunol 1989;142:2321.

95. Hack CE, DeGroot ER, Felt-Bersma RJF, et al. Increased plasma levels of interleukin 6 in sepsis. Blood 1989;74:1704.

96. Baffet G, Braciak T, Fletcher RG, Gauldie J, Fey GH, Northeman W. Autocrine activity of IL-6 secreted by hepatocarcinoma cell lines. Mol Biol Med 1991;8:141.

97. Kato K, Yokio T, Takano N, et al. Detection by in situ hybridization and phenotypic characterization of cells expressing IL-6 mRNA in human stimulated blood. J Immunol 1990;144:1317.

98. Cicco NA, Lindeman A, Content J, et al. Inducible production of interleukin-6 by human polymorphonuclear neutrophils: role of granulocyte-macrophage colony-stimulating factor and tumor necrosis factor-alpha. Blood 1990;75:2049.

99. Frie K, Malipiero UV, Leist TP, Zinkernagel RM, Schwab ME, Fontana A. On the cellular source and function of interleukin 6 produced in the central nervous system in viral diseases. Eur J Immunol 1989;19:689.

100. Vankelecom H, Carmeliet P, Van Damme J, Billiau A, Denef C. Production of interleukin-6 by folliculostellate cells of the anterior pituitary gland in a histiotypic cell aggregate culture system. Neuroendocrinology 1989;49:102.

101. Brouckaert P, Spriggs DR, Demetri G, Kufe DW, Fiers W. Circulating interleukin-6 during a continuous infusion of tumor necrosis factor and interferon-gamma. J Exp Med 1989;169:2257.

102. Libert C, Brouckaert P, Shaw A, Fiers W. Induction of IL-6 by human and murine recombinant IL-1 in mice. Eur J Immunol 1990;20:691.

103. Kishimoto TK, Larson RS, Corbi AL, Dustin ML, Staunton DE, Springer TA. The leukocyte integrins: LFA-1, Mac-1, and p150,95. Adv Immunol 1989;46:149.

104. Hogg N. The leukocyte integrins. Immunol Today 1989;10:111.

105. Kishimoto TK, Larson RS, Corbi AL, Dustin ML, Staunton DE, Springer TA. Leukocyte integrins. In: Springer TA, Anderson DC, Rosenthal AS, Rothlein R, eds. Leukocyte adhesion molecules: structure, function, and regulation. New York, Springer-Verlag, 1990:7.

106. Arnout MA. Structure and function of the leukocyte adhesion molecules CD11/CD18. Blood 1990;75:1037.

107. Springer TA. Adhesion receptors of the immune system. Nature 1990;346:425.

108. Springer TA. The sensation and regulation of interactions with the extracellular environment: the cell biology of lymphocyte adhesion receptors. Annu Rev Cell Biol 1990;6:359.

109. Vedder NB, Winn RK, Rice CL, Chi EY, Arfors KE, Harlan JM. A monoclonal antibody to the adherence-promoting leukocyte glycoprotein CD18 reduces organ injury and improves survival from hemorrhagic shock and resuscitation in rabbits. J Clin Invest 1988;81:939.

110. Barton RW, Rothlein R, Ksiazek J, Kennedy C. Role of anti-adhesion monoclonal antibodies in rabbit lung inflammation. In: Springer TA, Anderson DC, Rosenthal AS, Rothlein R, eds. Leukocyte adhesion molecules: structure, function, and regulation. New York, Sringer-Verlag, 1990:149.

111. Mulligan MS, Varani J, Warren JS, et al. Roles of β2 integrins on rat neutrophils in complement and oxygen radical mediated acute inflammatory injury. J Immunol 1992;148:1847.

112. Mulligan MS, Warren JS, Smith CW, et al. Lung injury after deposition of IgA immune complexes: requirements for CD18 and L-arginine. J Immunol 1992;148:3086.

113. Lasky LA. Lectin cell adhesion molecules (LEC-CAMs): a new family of cell adhesion proteins involved with inflammation. J Cell Biochem 1991;45:139.

114. Stoolman LM. Selectins (LEC-CAMs): lectin-like receptors involved in lymphocyte recirculation and leukocyte recruitment. In: Fukuda, M, ed. Cell surface carbohydrates and cell development. Boca Raton, CRC, 1992:71.

115. Bevilacqua MP, Wheeler ME, Pober JS, et al. Endothelial-dependent mechanisms of leukocyte adhesion: regulation by interleukin-1 and tumor necrosis factor. In: Movat HZ, ed. Leukocyte emigration and its sequelae. Basel, Karger, 1987:79.

116. Stoolman LM. Adhesion molecules controlling lymphocyte migration. Cell 1989;56:907.

117. Picker LJ, Warnock RA, Burns A, Doerschuk CM, Berg EL, Butcher EC. The neutrophil selectin LECAM-1 presents carbohydrate ligands to the vascular selectins ELAM-1 and GMP-140. Cell 1991;66:921.

118. Pierce GF, Tarpley JE, Yanagihara D, Mustoe TA, Fox GM, Thomason A. Platelet-derived growth factor (BB homodimer), transforming growth factor-beta 1, and basic fibroblast growth factor in dermal wound healing: neovessel and matrix formation and cessation of repair. Am J Pathol 1992;140:1375.

119. Davidson JM. Wound repair. In: Gallin JI, Goldstein IM, Snyderman R, eds. Inflammation: basic principles and clinical correlates. New York, Raven, 1992:244.

120. Sauder DN, Mounessa NL, Katy SI, Dinarello CA, Gallin JI. Chemotactic cytokines: the role of leukocyte pyrogen and epidermal cell thymocyte-activating factor in neutrophil chemotaxis. J Immunol 1984;132:828.

121. Yoshimura T, Matsushima K, Oppenheim JJ, Leonard EJ. Neutrophil chemotactic factor produced by LPS-stimulated human blood mononuclear leukocytes: partial characterization and separation from interleukin-1. J Immunol 1987;139:788.

122. Strieter RM, Kunkel SL, Showell HR, et al. Monokine-induced neutrophil chemotactic factor gene expression in human fibroblasts. J Biol Chem 1989;264:10621.

123. Matushima K, Oppenheim JJ. Interleukin 8 and MCAF: novel inflammatory cytokine inducible by IL-1 and TNF. Cytokine 1989;1:2.

124. Baggiolini M, Walz A, Kunkel SL. Neutrophil-activating peptide-1/interleukin-8, a novel cytokine that activates neutrophils. J Clin Invest 1989;84:1045.

125. Walz A, Burgener R, Car B, Baggilini M, Kunkel SL, Strieter RM. Sturcture and neutrophil-activating properties of a novel inflammatory peptide (ENA-78) with homology to IL-8. J Exp Med 1991;174:1355.

126. Strieter RM, Kunkel SL, Burdick MD, Lincoln PM, Walz A. The detection of a novel neutrophil-activating peptide (ENA-78) using a sensitive ELISA. Immunol Invest 1992;21:589.

127. Baggioloini M, Dewald B, Walz A. Interleukin-8 and related chemotactic cytokines. In: Gallin JI, Goldstein IM, Sny-

derman R, eds. Inflammation: basic principles and clinical correlates. New York, Raven, 1992:69.

128. Miller MD, Krangel MS. Biology and biochemistry of the chemokines: a family of chemotactic and inflammatory cytokines. Crit Rev Immunol 1992;12:17.

129. Farber JM. HuMIG: a new member of the chemokine family of cytokines. Biochem Biophys Res Commun 1993;192:223.

130. Proost P, De Wold-Peeters C, Conings R, Opdenakker G, Billiau A, Van Damme J. Identification of a novel granulocyte chemotactic protein (GCP-1) from human tumor cells: in vitro and in vivo comparison with natural forms of GRO alpha, IP-10, and IL-8. J Immunol 1993;150:1000.

131. Oppenheim JJ, Zachariae OC, Mukaida N, Matsushima K. Properties of the novel proinflammatory supergene "intercrine" cytokine family. Annu Rev Immunol 1991;9:617.

132. Ansiowicz A, Zajchowski D, Stenman G, Sager R. Functional diversity of gro gene expression in human fibroblasts and mammary epithelial cells. Proc Natl Acad Sci USA 1988;85:9645.

133. Deutsch E, Kain W. Studies on platelet factor 4. In: Jonson SA, Monto RW, Rebuck JW, Horn RC, eds. Blood platelets. Boston, Little, Brown, 1961:337.

134. Kaplan G, Luster AD, Hancock G, Cohn Z. The expression of a gamma interferon-induced protein (IP-10) in delayed immune responses in human skin. J Exp Med 1987; 166:1098.

135. Rampart M, Van Damme J, Zonnekeyn L, Herman AG. Granulocyte chemotactic protein/interleukin-8 induces plasma leakage and neutrophil accumulation in rabbit skin. Am J Pathol 1989;135:21.

136. Clark RA, Lanigan JM, Dellapelle P, Manseau E, Dvorak HF, Colvin RB. Fibronectin and fibrin provide a provisional matrix for epidermal cell migration during wound re-epithelialization. J Invest Dermatol 1982;79:264.

137. Folkman J. Tumor angiogenesis. Adv Cancer Res 1985; 43:175.

138. Folkman J, Kagsbrun M. Angiogenic factors. Science 1987; 235:442.

139. Engerman RL, Pfaffenbach D, Davis MD. Cell turnover of capillaries. Lab Invest 1967;17:738.

140. Donoff RB, Mclennan JE, Grillo HC. Preparation and properties of collagenases from epithelium and mesenchyme of healing mammalian wounds. Biochem Biophys Acta 1971;227:639.

141. Zetter BR. Angiogenesis: state of the art. Chest 1988;93:159S.

142. Harris ED Jr. Recent insight into the pathogenesis of the proliferative lesion in rheumatoid arthritis. Arthritis Rheum 1976;19:68.

143. Koch AE, Polverini PJ, Leibovich SJ. Stimulation of neovascularization by human rheumatoid synovial tissue macrophages. Arthritis Rheum 1986;29:471.

144. Koch AE, Podlverini PJ, Kunkel SL, et al. Interleukin-8 (IL-8) as a macrophage-derived mediator of angiogenesis. Science 1992;258:1798.

145. Koch AE, Litvak MA, Burrows JC, Polverini PJ. Decreased monocyte-mediated angiogenesis in scleroderma. Clin Immunol Immunopathol 1992;64:153.

146. Rastinejad F, Polverini PJ, Bouck NP. Regulation of the activity of a new inhibitor of angiogenesis by a cancer suppressor gene. Cell 1989;56:345.

147. Good DJ, Polverini PJ, Rastinejad F, et al. A tumor suppressor-dependent inhibitor of angiogenesis is immunologically and functionally indistinguishable from a fragment of thrombospondin. Proc Natl Acad Sci USA 1990;87:6624.

148. Tolsma SS, Volpert OV, Good DJ, Frazier WA, Polverini PJ, Bouck NP. Peptides derived from two separate domains of the matrix protein thrombospondin-1 have antiangiogenic activity. J Cell Biol 1993;122:497.

149. DiPeitro LA, Polverini PJ. Angiogenic macrophages produce the angiogenic inhibitor thrombospondin 1. Am J Pathol 1993;143:678.

150. Strieter RM, Kunkel SL, Elner VM, et al. Interleukin-8: a corneal factor that induces neovascularization. Am J Pathol 1992;141:1279.

151. Hu DE, Hori Y, Fan TPD. Interleukin-8 stimulates angiogenesis in rats. Inflammation 1993;17:135.

152. Polverini PJ. Cytokines, vol 1. S. Basel, Karger, 1989:54.

153. Maione TE, Gray GS, Petro J, et al. Inhibition of angiogenesis by recombinant human platelet factor 4 and related peptides. Science 1990;247:77.

154. Sharpe RJ, Byers HR, Scott CF, Bauer SI, Maione TE. Growth inhibition of murine melanoma and human colon carcinoma by recombinant human platelet factor 4. J Natl Cancer Inst 1990;82:848.

155. Maione TE, Gray GS, Hunt AJ, Sharpe RJ. Inhibition of tumor growth in mice by an analog of platelet factor 4 that lacks affinity for heparin and retains potent angiogenic activity. Cancer Res 1991;51:2077.

156. Frisch SM, Ruley HE. Transcription from the stromolysin promoter is induced by interleukin 1 and repressed by dexamethasone. J Biol Chem 1987;262:16300.

157. Kuraoka S, Campeau JD, Rodgers KE, Nakamura RM, diZerega GS. Effects of interleukin-1 (IL-1) on postsurgical macrophage secretion of protease and protease inhibitor activities. J Surg Res 1992;52:71.

158. Mauvial A, Teyton L, Bhatnagar R, et al. Interleukin 1 alpha modulates collagen gene expression in cultured synovial cells. Biochem J 1988;252:247.

159. Bhatnagar R, Penfornis H, Mauvial A, Loyau G, Saklatvala J, Pujol J. Interleukin-1 inhibits the synthesis of collagen by fibroblasts. Biochem Int 1986;13:709.

160. Clark JG, Lostal KM, Marino BA. Modulation of collagen production following bleomycin-induced pulmonary fibrosis in hamsters: presence of a factor in lung that increases fibroblast prostaglandin E-2 and cAMP and suppresses fibroblast proliferation and collagen production. J Biol Chem 1982;257:8098.

161. Postlethwaite AE, Raghow R, Stricklin GP, Poppleton J, Seyer JM, Kang AH. Modulation of fibroblast functions by interleukin 1: increased steady state accumulation of type I procollagen messenger RNA's and the stimulation of other functions but not chemotaxis by human recombinant interleukin 1 alpha and beta. J Cell Biol 1988;106:311.

162. Bronson RE, Argenta JG, Bertolami C. Interleukin-1-induced changes in extracellular glycosaminoglycan composition of cutaneous scar-derived fibroblasts in culture. Collagen 1988;8:199.

163. Elias JA, Freundlich B, Kern JA, Rosenbloom J. Cytokine networks in the regulation of inflammation and fibrosis in the lung. Chest 1990;97:1439.

164. Johnson WJ, Breton J, Newman-Tarr T, Connor JR, Meunier PC, Dalton BJ. Interleukin-1 release by rat synovial cells is dependent on the sequential treatment with gamma interferon and lipopolysaccharide. Arthritis Rheum 1990;33:261.

165. Larsson EL. Cyclosporin A and dexamethasone suppress T cell response by selectively acting at distinct sites of the triggering process. J Immunol 1980;124:2828.

166. Mahadevan V, Hart IR, Lewis GP. Factors influencing blood supply in wound granuloma quantitated by a new in vivo technique. Cancer Res 1989;49:415.

167. Elias JA, Gustilo K, Baeder W, Freundlich B. Synergistic stimulation of fibroblast prostaglandin production by recombinant interleukin-1 and tumor necrosis factor. J Immunol 1987;138:3812.

168. Scharffetter K, Heckman M, Hatamochi A, et al. Synergistic effect of tumor necrosis factor alpha and interferon-gamma on collagen synthesis of human skin fibroblasts in vitro. Exp Cell Res 1989;181:409.

169. Kohno M, Nishizawa N, Tsujimoto M, Nomoto H. Mitogenic signaling pathway of tumor necrosis factor involves the rapid tyrosine phosphorylation of 41,000 and 43,000-Mr cytosol proteins. Biochem J 1990;267:91.

170. Sato T, Ito A, Mori Y. Interleukin 6 enhances the production of tissue inhibitor of metalloproteinases (TIMP) but not that of matrix metalloproteinases of human fibroblasts. Biochem Biophys Res Commun 1990;170:824.

171. Hashimoto J, Yoshikawa H, Takaoka K, et al. Inhibitory effects of tumor necrosis factor alpha on fracture healing in rats. Bone 1989;10:453.

172. Hom DB, Maisel RH. Angiogenic growth factors: their effects and potential in soft tissue wound healing. Ann Otol Rhinol Laryngol 1992;101:349.

173. Chen JD, Kim JP, Zhang K, et al. Epidermal growth factor (EGF) promotes human keratinocyte locomotion on collagen

by increasing the alpha 2 integrin subunit. Exp Cell Res 1993;209:216.

174. Buckley-Sturrock A, Woodward SC, Senior RM, Griffin GL, Klagsbrun M, Davidson JM. Differential stimulation of collagenase and chemotactic activity in fibroblasts derived from rat wound repair tissue and human skin by growth factors. J Cell Physiol 1989;138:70.

175. Barnard JA, Russette ML, Moses HL. The biology of transforming growth factor beta. Biochem Biophys Acta 1990; 1032:79.

176. Sporn MB, Roberts AB, Wakefield LM, de Crombrugghe B. Some recent advances in the chemistry and biology of transforming growth factor beta. J Cell Biol 1987;105:1039.

177. Ignotz RA, Massague J. Cell adhesion protein receptors as targets for transforming growth factor beta action. Cell 1987; 51:189.

178. Overall CM, Wrana JL, Sodek J. Transforming growth factor beta regulation of collagenase, 72-kDa progelatinase, TIMP, and PAI-1 expression in rat bone cell populations and human fibroblasts. Connect Tissue Res 1989;20:289.

179. Kimura A, Katoh O, Hyodo H, Kuramoto A. Transforming growth factor beta regulates growth as well as collagen and fibronectin synthesis of human marrow fibroblasts. Br J Haematol 1989;72:486.

180. Roberts AB, Joyce ME, Bolander ME, Sporn MB. Transforming growth factor-beta (TGF-β): a multifunctional effector of both hard and soft tissue regeneration. In: Westermark B, Betsholtz C, Hokfelt B, eds. Growth factors in health and disease: basic and clinical aspects. Amsterdam, Excerpta Medica, 1990:89.

181. Beck LS, DeGuzman L, Lee WP, Xu Y, Siegel MW, Amento EP. One systemic administration of transforming growth factor-β1 reverses age- or glucocorticoid-impaired wound healing. J Clin Invest 1993;92:2565.

182. Terrell TG, Working PK, Chow CP, Green JD. Pathology of recombinant human transforming growth factor-β1 in rats and rabbits. Int Rev Exp Pathol 1993;34:43.

183. Greenhalgh DG, Sprugel KH, Murray MJ, Ross R. PDGF and FGF stimulate wound healing in the genetically diabetic mouse. Am J Pathol 1990;136:1235.

184. Gailit J, Welch MP, Clark RA. TGF-β1 stimulates expression of keratinocyte integrins during re-epithelialization. J Invest Dermatol 1994;103:221.

185. Kohler N, Lipton A. Platelets as a source of fibroblast growth-promoting activity. Exp Cell Res 1974;87:297.

186. Deuel TF. Polypeptide growth factors: role in normal and abnormal cell growth. Annu Rev Cell Biol 1987;3:443.

187. Ross R. Platelet-derived growth factor. Lancet 1989;1:1179-1182.

188. Pierce GF, Mustoe TA, Altrock BA, Deuel TF, Thomason A. The role of platelet-derived growth factor in wound healing. J Cell Biochem 1991;45:319.

189. Deuel TF, Senior M, Huang JS, Griffin GL. Chemotaxis of monocytes and neutrophils to platelet-derived growth factor. J Clin Invest 1982;69:1046.

190. Paulsson Y, Hammacher A, Heldin CH, Westermark B. Possible positive autocrine feedback in the prereplicative phase of human fibroblasts. Nature 1987;328:715.

191. Libby P, Warner SJC, Salomon RN, Birinyi LK. Production of platelet-derived growth factor mitogen by smooth muscle cells from human atheroma. N Engl J Med 1988;318:1492.

192. Lynch SE, Colvin RB, Antoniades NH. Growth factors in wound healing. J Clin Invest 1989;84:640.

193. Greenhalgh DG, Sprugel KH, Murray MJ, Ross R. PDGF and FGF stimulate wound healing in the genetically diabetic mouse. Am J Pathol 1990;136:629.

194. Mustoe TA, Purdy J, Gramates P, Deuel TF, Thomason A, Pierce GF. Reversal of impaired wound healing in irradiated rats by platelet-derived growth factor BB: requirement for an active bone marrow. Am J Surg 1989;158:345.

195. Mustoe TA, Cutler NR, Allman RM, et al. A phase II study to evaluate recombinant platelet-derived growth factor-BB in the treatment of stage 3 and 4 pressure ulcers. Arch Surg 1994;150:213.

SURGERY: SCIENTIFIC PRINCIPLES AND PRACTICE, Second Edition, edited by Lazar J. Greenfield, Michael W. Mulholland, Keith T. Oldham, Gerald B. Zelenock, and Keith D. Lillemoe. Lippincott–Raven Publishers, Philadelphia, © 1997.

CHAPTER 6

INFLAMMATION

GENEVA M. OMANN AND DANIEL B. HINSHAW

Nature has endowed the human body with the ability to protect itself from invading organisms such as bacteria, which might otherwise view the body as a convenient source of nutrient broth. This ability is conferred by the immune system, a complex system of cellular and molecular elements that destroys these organisms. In addition, the immune system enables the body to eliminate dead tissue that has resulted from injury or from normal cell senescence and to combat transformed neoplastic tissue. The components of this complex system can be categorized as cellular and humoral. Humoral components are molecules circulating in the blood, including antibodies and the complement system, which together can cause lysis of foreign cells. Cellular components include phagocytic cells and antibody interactions with lymphocytes that result in cell-mediated lysis of foreign cells. These mechanisms presumably function continuously without presenting clinical symptoms.

Inflammation occurs when an invading organism is present in unusually large quantities or when tissue injury and cell death have occurred. This injury can occur by mechanical, chemical, or autoimmune processes. The classic symptoms of inflammation are swelling, redness, heat, pain, and altered function. Within minutes of the assault, mediators are released that cause dilation of the vasculature (resulting in redness) and increased vascular permeability. This leads to the accumulation of fluid (swelling) at the site of injury. Within 30 to 60 minutes, neutrophils marginate, extravasate, and accumulate at the site of injury, where they carry out nonspecific phagocytic functions and release oxidants and proteinases. Within 4 to 5 hours, mononuclear cells (monocytes and lymphocytes) begin to accumulate. Monocytes participate in nonspecific phagocytic activity, and lymphocytes orchestrate specific, antibody-dependent lysis of cells. Normally, these processes limit the site of injury, destroy the injurious agent, and remove necrotic tissue to clear the way for healing.

This chapter discusses the basic anatomy of the immune system and the cellular and biochemical components of inflammation, with a particular focus on acute inflammation. Details regarding the role of the immune system in infection, self-recognition (transplantation), and elimination of neoplastic tissue are discussed elsewhere.

OVERVIEW OF ANATOMY AND CELL DEVELOPMENT

The system of cells responsible for immunity is known as the *lymphoreticular system*.[1] These cellular elements are distributed throughout the body, some circulating in the blood, and others present in specialized organs (eg, spleen and lymph nodes) or as subunits within other organs (eg, Kupffer cells in the liver and Peyer patches in the ileum). Many of the lymphoid tissues are strategically located in tracts exposed to the external environment, such as the respiratory, gastrointestinal, and urogenital tracts. The cellular constituents of this system include lymphocytes, granulocytes, monocytes, macrophages, platelets, erythrocytes, and mast cells. In addition, endothelial cells that line the vasculature play an important part in immunity and inflammation. With the exception of endothelial cells, all these cells originate from pluripotent stem cells in the bone marrow (Fig. 6-1). Platelets, erythrocytes, monocytes, and granulocytes are released into the circulation after maturation in the bone marrow. Circulating monocytes migrate into tissues and develop into resident macrophages, such as Kupffer cells in the liver and glial cells of the nervous system. Pre–B lymphocytes and pre–T lymphocytes are released from the bone marrow, and further differentiation occurs in lymphoid organs and the thymus, respectively. Mast cells develop from precursors in the bone marrow that move into tissues, where they complete differentiation and continue to proliferate.

The peripheral lymphoid tissues consist of the thymus, where T-lymphocyte development occurs. In addition, lymph nodes, spleen, and lymph nodules serve as sites for the development of B lymphocytes, which become the antibody-producing cells in the body. Lymph nodules (eg, tonsils, Peyer patches, and the appendix) are dispersed in the submucosal tissues of the respiratory, urogenital, and intestinal tracts. Antibodies are produced and secreted by the salivary glands, respiratory tract, mammary glands, gastrointestinal tract, and urogenital tract. Because many of these sites represent cavities where microorganisms normally grow without the development of pathologic conditions, these systems have been strategically placed to respond to and guard against the external environment. The lymphoid tissues, especially the spleen, also contain phagocytic capabilities and serve as sites for the destruction of senescent circulating cells. In addition, the liver is rich in resident macrophages (Kupffer cells) and can serve to sequester and destroy senescent cells.

The development of inflammation at a site of tissue injury involves the following: (1) the release of chemoattractants that recruit cells to the site of injury and induce the release of proteinases, toxic oxidants, and cytotoxic cationic proteins; (2) the release of "priming" agents that enhance the ability of the cells to respond to the chemoattractants; and (3) the release of growth factors that increase the production of leukocytes. It is not uncommon for a mediator to induce two or three of these effects in different or the same cell types. For example, several growth factors also prime neutrophils for response to

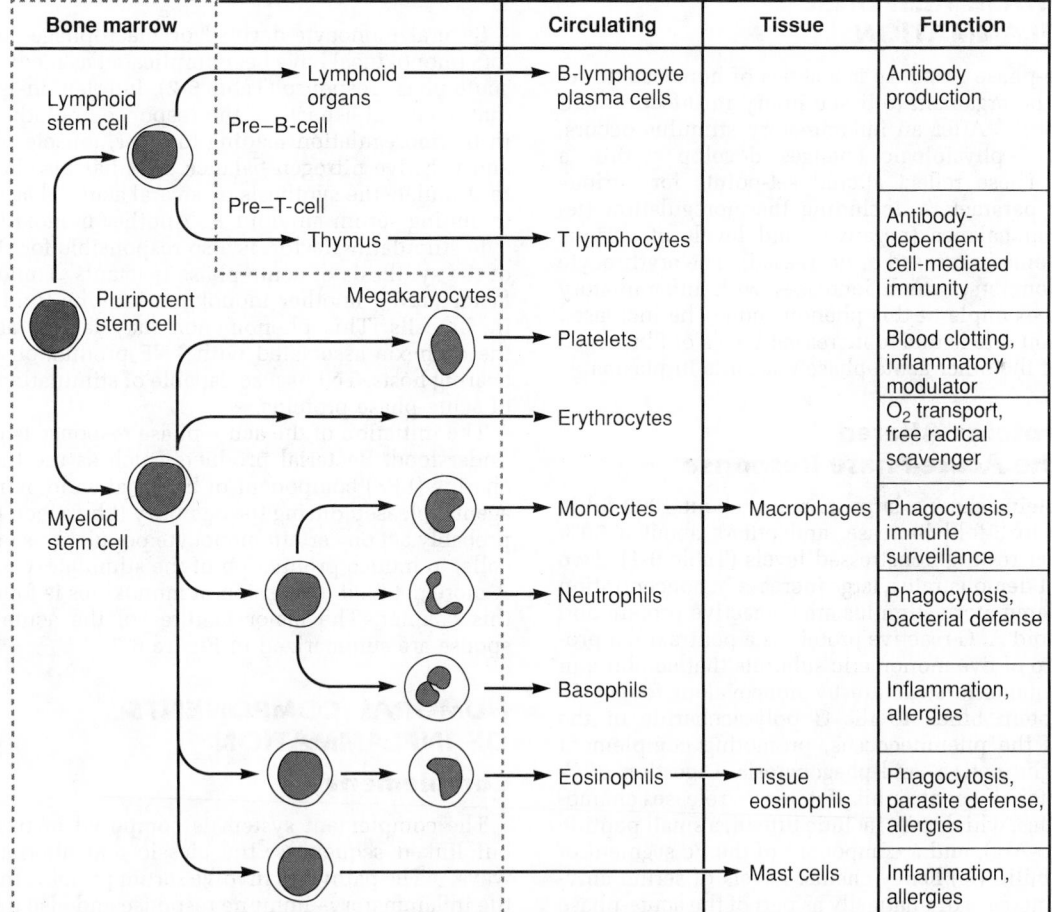

Figure 6-1. Cells of the hemopoietic cell system. Pluripotent stem cells in the bone marrow differentiate into lymphoid or myeloid stem cells. Lymphoid stem cells differentiate into pre–B cells or pre–T cells. In lymphoid organs, pre–B cells differentiate into B cells, which are released into the circulation. B cells further develop in the lymphoid organs into plasma cells, the antibody-producing cells of the immune system. Myeloid stem cells further differentiate in the bone marrow to produce mature cells. These mature cells are released into the circulation with the exception of mast cells, which are not found in the circulation. Circulating monocytes migrate into tissues, where they develop into macrophages.

Table 6-1. RESPONSES OF SOME HUMAN ACUTE-PHASE PROTEINS

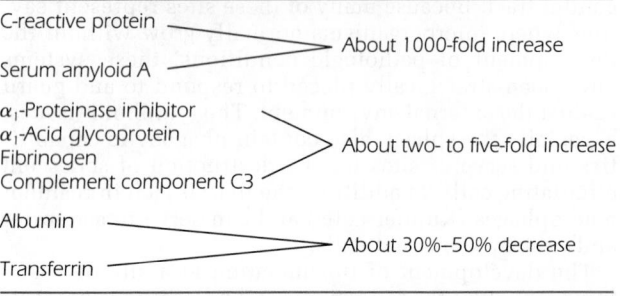

C-reactive protein
Serum amyloid A
    About 1000-fold increase

α_1-Proteinase inhibitor
α_1-Acid glycoprotein
Fibrinogen
Complement component C3
    About two- to five-fold increase

Albumin
Transferrin
    About 30%–50% decrease

stimulation by the bacterial cell wall product, *N*-formyl-peptide. The effect of the priming agents and growth factors is to amplify and augment the inflammatory response. Countering these events are inherent inhibitory pathways that serve to modulate leukocyte functions. Pathologic conditions apparently arise when the stimulatory and inhibitory pathways are not properly balanced.

ACUTE-PHASE RESPONSE AND INFLAMMATION

The acute-phase response is a series of homeostatic responses of the organism to tissue injury in infection and inflammation.[2-4] After an inflammatory stimulus occurs, a number of physiologic changes develop within a few hours. These reflect altered set-points for various physiologic parameters, including thermoregulation (fever), nitrogen balance (negative), and levels of various plasma proteins (increased or decreased). The erythrocyte sedimentation rate, which increases with inflammatory states, is an example of this phenomenon. The increased sedimentation rate is due to increased levels of fibrinogen and some of the other acute-phase reactants in plasma.

Serum Proteins Altered During the Acute-Phase Response

Some proteins show a large increase (about 1000-fold), some a 4- to 5-fold increase, and others about a 50% decrease over resting nonstressed levels (Table 6-1). Two proteins that demonstrate a large increase in concentration after an inflammatory stimulus are C-reactive protein and serum amyloid A. C-reactive protein is a pentraxin, a protein made up of five monomeric subunits that combine in a cyclic pentameric structure by noncovalent forces. C-reactive protein binds to the C polysaccharide of the cell wall of the pneumococcus, promoting complement fixation, agglutination, and phagocytosis. Digestion of C-reactive protein by neutrophil proteinases releases chemotactic peptides, which may include tuftsin, a small peptide (Thr-Lys-Pro-Arg), and a component of the Fc segment of immunoglobulin (Ig) heavy chains. Levels of serum amyloid A also increase dramatically as part of the acute-phase response, although the role in inflammation is unclear. Amyloid A is a major component of the deposits seen in secondary amyloidosis and thus may play a role in chronic inflammation.

A major inhibitor of neutrophil proteinases, especially elastase, is α_1-proteinase inhibitor (α_1-PI), which is synthesized not only by the liver but also by monocytes and macrophages. The elastase released from neutrophils acts

to regulate the synthesis of α_1-PI by monocytes, providing a way of modulating its destructive action at local sites of inflammation. Levels of α_1-PI increase 2-fold to 4-fold as part of the acute-phase response, and levels of α_1–acid glycoprotein rise 2-fold to 5-fold and can be induced by glucocorticoids. α_1–Acid glycoprotein may have a role as an inhibitor of platelet activation and as a possible modulator of T-lymphocyte function. The key coagulation protein, fibrinogen, increases 2-fold to 2.5-fold after an inflammatory stimulus. The elevation of fibrinogen persists for several weeks. Fibrinopeptides, by-products of fibrin formation, can increase chemotaxis of leukocytes and vascular permeability, in addition to their role in clot formation. The levels of two important complement components, C3 and properdin, also increase in the acute-phase response. Both are involved in bacterial opsonization (see later discussion), and their increase probably represents part of the attempt of the organism to anticipate this need.

Albumin is a negative acute-phase reactant. Levels of albumin drop after an inflammatory stimulus. This drop is usually 30% to 50% of the level before injury. The iron-binding protein transferrin undergoes a similar decrease. The reason for the decrease in production of these proteins in inflammation is poorly understood.

Mediators of the Acute-Phase Response

Several monocyte-derived or macrophage-derived factors (monokines) have been implicated as mediators of the acute-phase response (Table 6-2). Interleukin-1 (IL-1) mediates several aspects of the response, including changes in thermoregulation leading to fever, muscle proteolysis, and negative nitrogen balance. IL-1 has also been shown to stimulate the synthesis of several acute-phase reactants, including serum amyloid A. Another monokine, hepatocyte-stimulating factor, is also responsible for stimulation of the synthesis of acute-phase reactants. Tumor necrosis factor (TNF), another monokine, inhibits lipid synthesis in fat cells. This phenomenon may largely account for the cachexia associated with TNF production in cancer-bearing hosts. TNF is also capable of stimulating synthesis of acute-phase proteins.

The initiation of the acute-phase response is not clearly understood. Bacterial products, such as the lipopolysaccharide (LPS) component of bacterial endotoxin, or other agents released during tissue injury (fibrinogen fragments) probably act on certain monocyte populations (eg, Kupffer cells) to induce production of the stimulatory monokines. A more detailed discussion of monokines is found later in this chapter. The major features of the acute-phase response are summarized in Figure 6-2.

HUMORAL COMPONENTS OF INFLAMMATION
Complement

The complement system is composed of two different but linked sequences, the classic and alternative pathways.[5,6] The pathways involve serum proteins that amplify the inflammatory–immune response and also directly mediate tissue injury. The complement system represents the wedding of many classic immune responses to inflammation. Complement activation by either pathway has been associated with a cascade of events, some of which are mediated directly at a physiologic level by activated complement components (eg, the anaphylatoxins C3a and C5a) and also indirectly by activated leukocytes. Some of the direct physiologic effects of complement activation medi-

Table 6-2. CYTOKINES

Component	Sources*	Role in Inflammatory Response
Granulocyte-macrophage colony-stimulating factor	T lymphocytes, fibroblasts, endothelial cells	Increased production of granulocyte and mononuclear phagocytes; enhanced function of granulocytes and mononuclear phagocytes
Macrophage colony-stimulating factor	Lymphocytes (and others?)	Increased production of mononuclear phagocytes; enhanced function of mononuclear phagocytes
Granulocyte colony-stimulating factor	Lymphocytes?	Increased production of granulocytes; enhanced function of granulocytes
Platelet-derived growth factor	Platelets, macrophages	Leukocyte chemoattractant
Transforming growth factor β (TGF-β)	Platelets, lymphocytes, macrophages	Mononuclear phagocyte chemoattractant
Interleukin-1 (IL-1)†	Mononuclear phagocytes, fibroblasts, endothelial cells, keratinocytes, smooth muscle cells	Lymphocyte differentiation and activation; production of lymphokines; production of hepatic acute-phase proteins
IL-2	Lymphocytes	Lymphocyte differentiation; antiinflammatory effects on monocytes and macrophages; regulation of B-cell function and endothelial cell expression of adhesion molecules
IL-3	T lymphocytes	Early myeloid and lymphoid differentiation
IL-4	T lymphocytes	Lymphocyte proliferation and priming; enhanced myeloid differentaition (with other growth factors)
IL-5	Lymphocytes	B-cell activation; eosinophil differentiation
IL-6	Fibroblasts, mononuclear phagocytes, endothelial cells, T and B cells, mesangial cells, keratinocytes	Synergistic with IL-1 in lymphocyte proliferation, induction of hepatic acute-phase proteins
IL-7	Thymic stromal cells; bone marrow	Early B-cell precursor differentiation; induces lymphokine-activated killer cell activity; promotes tumor-specific, tumor-infiltrating lymphocytes
IL-8	Mononuclear phagocytes, endothelial cells, fibroblasts, epithelial cells	Neutrophil chemotactic factor
IL-9	T cells; peripheral blood mononuclear cells	Increases mast cell proliferation; increases IgE and IgG production by B cells; supports erythropoiesis
IL-10	T cells; macrophages; others	Inhibits monocyte and macrophage secretion of several interleukins; inhibits antigen-presenting capabilities of monocytes; increases IL-2 and IL-4 proliferative action on T cells
IL-11	Stromal cells	Stimulatory for lymphopoietic and myeloid and erythroid systems
IL-12	Monocytes	Growth factor for T cells and natural killer cells; promotes Th1 cell differentiation
IL-13	T cells	Antiinflammatory effects on monocytes and macrophages; regulation of B-cell function and endothelial cell expression of adhesion molecules
Tumor necrosis factor‡ (TNF)	Macrophage (TNF-α), lymphocytes (TNF-β)	Induction of hepatic acute proteins; enhances leukocyte function
Interferon-γ	T cells, macrophage?	B- and T-cell activation; enhances neutrophil and mononuclear phagocyte function

* These sources need to be activated to release these compounds. Activation can result from injury, autoimmune reactions, antigen challenge, or activation by cytokines.

† IL-1 and TNF share many biologic properties, but they are coded on separate genes, and TNF does not promote cell growth.

‡ TNF is composed of two components. TNF-β is derived from lymphocytes and is also known as *lymphocytoxin*. TNF-α is derived from macrophages. These two compounds both appear to bind to the same cell receptor and induce similar physiologic responses, although they share only a 30% sequence homology. Because TNF-α has been cloned, more work has been done with this compound.

ated by C3a and especially C5a include increased vascular permeability and contraction of smooth muscle. Indirectly, histamine release from mast cells mediated by C5a can also increase vascular permeability. The production of these anaphylaxis-like effects has led to the description of these complement components as *anaphylatoxins*. Complement activation also produces a large number of physiologic and pathologic effects by activating leukocytes. Some of the altered behavioral characteristics of leukocytes activated by C5a include enhanced adherence, chemotactic activity, release of proteinases (degranulation), and production of toxic metabolites of oxygen (oxidants). This complement-dependent activation of leukocytes is thought to play a key role in the generation of remote organ injury and dysfunc-

tion during inflammation. The adult respiratory distress syndrome that develops after a major burn is a good example of this phenomenon. Systemic complement activation as a result of a burn or other massive traumatic insult can lead to neutrophil activation by C5a and subsequent pulmonary sequestration of the activated, adherent neutrophils. The sequestered neutrophils then release a combination of toxic oxidants, proteinases, and cationic proteins that injure the alveolar capillary membrane. This leads to a diffuse, protein-rich capillary leak and causes the interstitial edema and alveolar flooding characteristic of the syndrome. Complement component C3, on the other hand, plays a key role in bacterial opsonization resulting in enhanced phagocytosis of invading microorganisms (see later

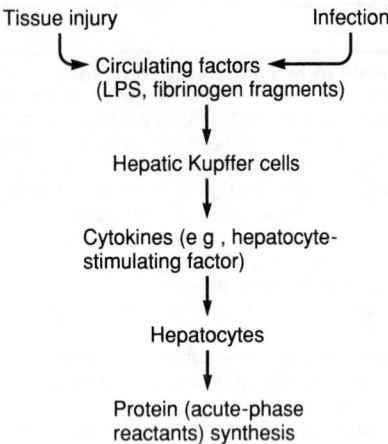

Figure 6-2. Acute-phase response. Certain soluble factors, such as the lipopolysaccharide (LPS) component of bacterial endotoxin or fibrinogen fragments, are released into the circulation after tissue injury or during infection. These factors stimulate Kupffer cells in the liver to secrete cytokines, which may in turn stimulate or inhibit the synthesis of certain proteins (acute-phase reactants) by hepatocytes.

discussion). Figure 6-3 summarizes the interrelations between the classic and alternative pathways of complement activation.

Classic Complement Pathway

Immune complexes are the typical activators of the classic pathway. Combinations of both IgM or IgG with antigen activate the first component of complement, C1. C1 is made up of three components, C1q, C1r, and C1s in the proportions $C1q(C1r)_2(C1s)_2$. The immune complex is bound by C1q, which causes indirect conformational changes in C1r. These changes lead to enzymatic activity and ultimately to cleavage of C1s, so that the active site of C1 then becomes located in the C1s subunit. Active C1 cleaves C4 to C4a and C4b and also cleaves C2 to yield C2a and C2b. C4b and C2a then complex tightly and form an enzyme, C3 convertase. C4b2a (C3 convertase) cleaves C3, releasing C3a and binding C3b to form C5 convertase (C4b2a3b), which leads to cleavage of C5 with release of C5a. C3a, C4a, and C5a act as anaphylatoxins, activating mast cells and basophils to release mediators that can induce local erythema and increased vascular permeability. C5a is also a potent stimulatory ligand and chemoattractant for granulocytes and monocytes. Neutrophils also have receptors for C3b and IgG, and they bind and phagocytose the antigen–antibody–complement complex. This stimulates release of specific and azurophilic granules by the neutrophil, further augmenting the local inflammatory injury. Some cells, such as erythrocytes, have membrane receptors for C5b that allow the formation of the membrane–attack complex (C5b-9) and lead to cell lysis. In the lysis sequence, membrane-bound C5b binds C6, C7, and C8. This complex binds C9, which induces circular polymerization of C9. The poly-C9 acts to create a hole in the cell membrane, which leads to cell death.

Alternative Complement Pathway

The alternative pathway differs from the classic pathway in that the first steps involving C1, C4, and C2 are bypassed. This pathway can be directly activated by agents other than antigen–antibody complexes (eg, complex polysaccharides like LPS and zymosan). Other serum pro-

tein factors (eg, factors B and D, which are discussed later) are involved in the activation sequence.

C3 has a thiol ester bond within its α chain—

$$(-S-\overset{\overset{\displaystyle O}{\displaystyle \|}}{C}-)$$

—which mediates covalent binding of C3 to carbohydrate (alcoholic) or amino side groups of surface molecules on bacteria or other target cells. A small portion of C3 in plasma exists in a hydrated form—

$$(-SH\ HO-\overset{\overset{\displaystyle O}{\displaystyle \|}}{C}-)$$

—and may complex in the presence of Mg^{2+} with factor B. This complex is then cleaved by factor D, yielding free Ba and $C3(H_2O)Bb$. $C3(H_2O)Bb$ can act on unhydrated C3 to produce C3a and C3b. The cascade usually continues only if C3b is bound to a surface (eg, bacterial cell walls) by means of the thiol ester. Surface-bound C3b again binds to factor B and becomes a substrate for factor D to yield C3bBb. When the protein properdin binds to the complex, its half-life is extended. The surface-bound C3bBb is a much more potent C3 convertase than the $C3(H_2O)Bb$. By cleaving an additional C3 and binding the released C3b, C3bBb is converted into the alternative pathway C5 convertase. The remaining steps (C5b-9) are identical to the classic pathway.

C3 and Opsonization of Bacteria

After C3 activation, the internal thiol ester of C3 can react nonspecifically with alcoholic or amino side groups of surface molecules of bacteria and other cells to form a tight covalent bond[7] (Fig. 6-4). This binding of C3b to target surfaces is resistant to changes in temperature, pH, and ionic strength. The covalently bound C3b is responsible for the opsonization of gram-positive and gram-negative bacteria as well as certain parasites. Phagocytic cells possess complement receptors on their surfaces, including receptors for C3b and its subfragments, that direct the phagocytosis of the opsonized target cells. Cell surfaces containing sialic acid residues (eg, sheep erythrocytes) tend to limit the binding of C3b, thus inhibiting progression of the alternative pathway as well as opsonization and phagocytosis of that cell type.

The alteration of the thiol ester in the C3b portion of C3 is in many respects responsible for the activity of C3b and subsequent activation of the alternative complement pathway. Ammonia (NH_3), for example, can attack the thiol-ester–producing amidated C3 and activate the alternative pathway, leading to membrane attack complex formation (C5b-9) and activation of a number of phagocytic cell functions, including toxic oxidant production. This phenomenon may have relevance to several in vivo disease states. In animal models of renal failure, elevated levels of renal vein NH_3 have been correlated with impaired renal function and the presence of complement components at the sites of renal injury. Also, erythrocytes often present at sites of inflammation may indirectly activate the alternative pathway by the formation of amidated C3 (see the section on erythrocytes later in this chapter).

Plasma proteins (eg, the complement inhibitor, C1 INH, C4b-binding protein) also act either to prevent complement activation (C1 INH) or to block progression of the pathway (C4b-binding protein). These proteins limit the extent of complement-mediated tissue injury during acute inflammation. In addition to C4b-binding protein, another plasma protein (factor H) and three membrane proteins (decay-accelerating factor, membrane cofactor protein, and

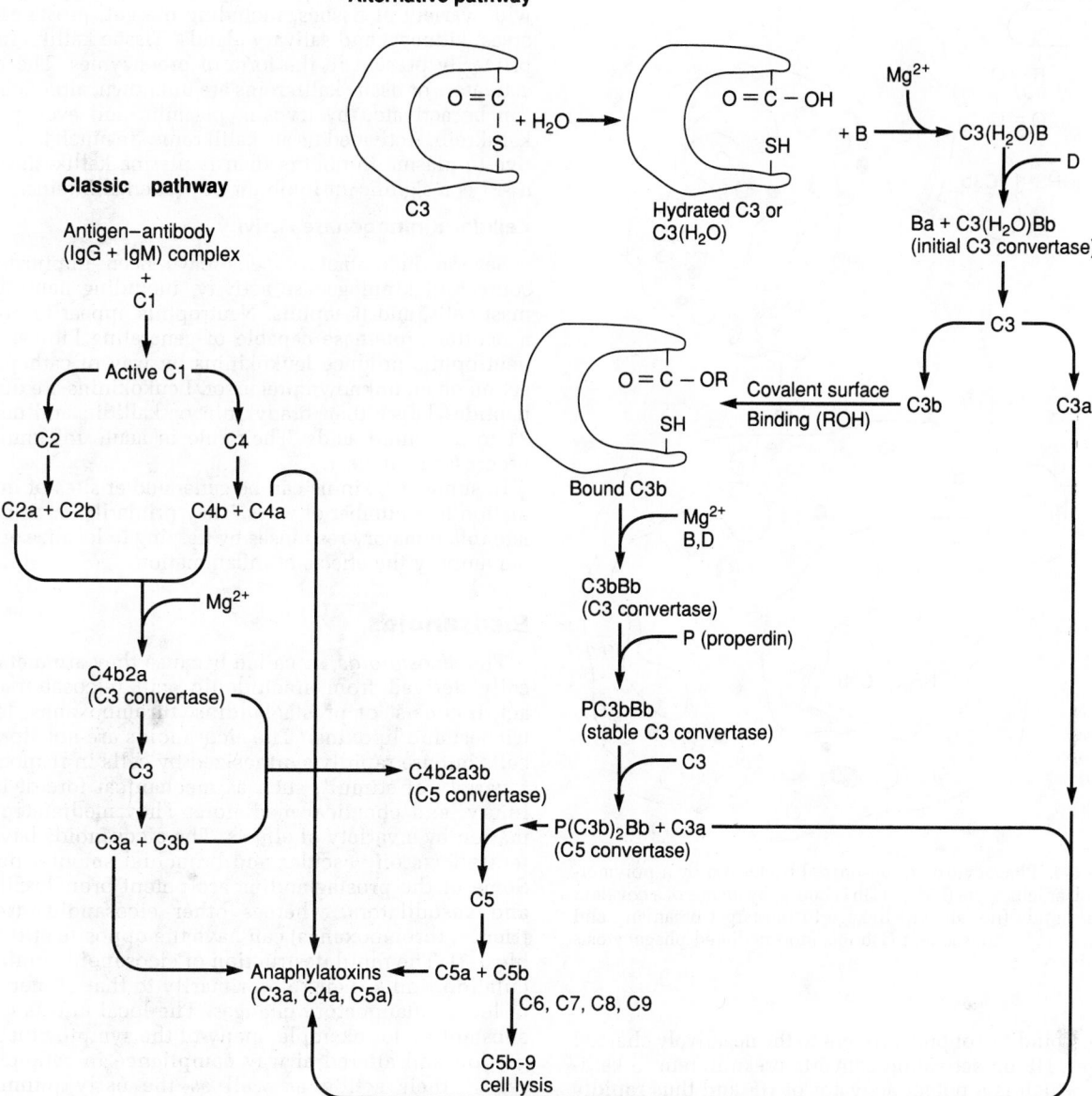

Figure 6-3. The classic and alternative pathways of complement activation.

complement receptor 1 [CR1]) also inhibit the activation of C3 and C5. It has been demonstrated that human recombinant CR1 that lacks the transmembrane and cytoplasmic domains—soluble CR1—can effectively block complement activation in serum. Soluble CR1 also inhibited complement-dependent tissue injury in a rat model of myocardial ischemia–reperfusion injury.

Kinins

Bradykinin and lysyl bradykinin are small vasoactive peptides generated during the acute inflammatory response.[8] They can cause increased vascular permeability, vasodilation, and pain. Much of the local pain at a wound site is attributable to these agents. Kinin formation is closely linked to the activation of the clotting cascade (see Chap. 4). Pain and local vascular congestion at a site of injury and hemorrhage not only notify the organism of the location of the injury but also serve to direct delivery of greater quantities of blood to the local area so that inflam-

matory cells can then respond to chemoattractants generated in the vicinity. Bradykinin, like the mast cell mediator histamine, acts primarily at the postcapillary venule to cause a reversible and usually short-lived capillary leak. Kinins, or inflammatory mediators, may be generated during inflammation by three different mechanisms: one involves plasma proteins, the second involves similar proteins in tissue, and the third involves cellular proteinases. The different pathways of kinin formation are summarized in Figure 6-5.

Production of Bradykinin in Plasma

Three plasma proteins are involved in the production of bradykinin: clotting factor XII (Hageman factor [HF]; see Chap. 4), prekallikrein, and high-molecular-weight kininogen. HF becomes activated on contact with a variety of negatively charged surfaces (eg, silicates, glass, heparin, dextran sulfate, and lipid A of endotoxin). Prekallikrein is largely bound to high-molecular-weight kininogen in plasma. High-molecular-weight kininogen acts to enhance

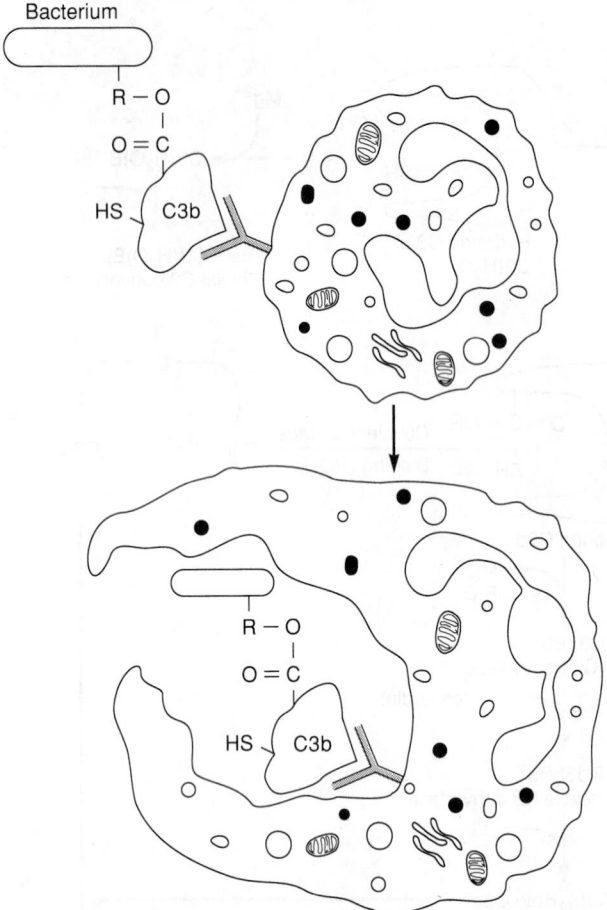

Bacterium

R—O

O=C

HS   C3b

R—O

O=C

HS   C3b

Figure 6-4. Phagocytosis of opsonized bacterium by a polymorphonuclear leukocyte (PMN). C3b is bound by means of a covalent ester or amide (not shown) linkage to the target organism, and opsonizes it for subsequent C3b receptor-mediated phagocytosis by the PMN.

contact (binding) of prekallikrein to the negatively charged surfaces. HF on activation converts prekallikrein to kallikrein, which is a potent activator of HF and thus rapidly expands and amplifies the response. The kallikrein also selectively cleaves high-molecular-weight kininogen, releasing the nine–amino acid peptide bradykinin. Control of HF activity occurs by way of further cleavage after activation. One cleavage product of activated HF, HFf, is still capable of activating prekallikrein, so that bradykinin formation may continue. Once HFf has lost its surface attachment, however, it is no longer capable of activating factor XI in the surface-dependent clotting cascade. The only major plasma inhibitor of activated HF is C1 INH. The main inhibitors of kallikrein in plasma are α_2-macroglobulin and C1 INH.

In addition to the functions discussed earlier, bradykinin is also an activator of phospholipase A_2, leading to the formation of arachidonic acid metabolites. It is also a potent constrictor of smooth muscle at many different sites. Bradykinin is metabolized sequentially to a partially active eight–amino acid peptide, Des-Arg bradykinin by carboxypeptidase N, and then to inactive five–amino acid and three–amino acid peptide fragments by angiotensin-converting enzyme.

Kinin Production in Tissue

Lysyl bradykinin (kallidin) is the product of cleavage of either high- or low-molecular-weight kininogen by tissue kallikreins. Tissue kallikreins are distinct proteins, differ-

ent from their plasma counterparts. They are present in a wide variety of tissues, including the gut, prostate, pancreas, kidneys, and salivary glands. Tissue kallikreins are primarily present in the form of proenzymes. The major activators of tissue kallikreins are unknown, although they can be activated by trypsin, plasmin, and even plasma kallikrein. Activated tissue kallikreins are much less sensitive to plasma inhibitors than is plasma kallikrein. Only α_1-PI is a significant inhibitor of tissue kallikreins.

Cellular Kininogenase Activity

Several inflammatory cells have been implicated as sources of kininogenase activity, including neutrophils, mast cells, and basophils. Neutrophils appear to possess a neutral proteinase capable of generating kinins. Also, neutrophils produce leukokinins by way of cathepsin D action on an unknown precursor. Leukokinins are distinct peptides larger than bradykinin or kallidin and contain 21 to 25 amino acids. Their role in acute inflammatory processes is unclear.

In summary, kinins can be generated at sites of inflammation in a number of ways. They primarily act to modulate inflammatory responses by helping to localize and often amplify the effects of inflammation.

Eicosanoids

The *eicosanoids*, so called because they are metabolically derived from arachidonic acid (eicosatetraenoic acid), consist of prostaglandins, thromboxanes, leukotrienes, and lipoxins.[9] The eicosanoids are not stored in cells but are rapidly synthesized by cells in response to a variety of stimuli, such as mechanical forces, tissue injury, and chemical mediators. They mediate inflammation by a variety of effects. The eicosanoids have potent effects on vascular and bronchial smooth muscle. Some of the prostaglandins are potent bronchodilators and vasodilators, whereas other eicosanoids (leukotrienes, thromboxanes) can have the opposite effect (Table 6-3). The rapid destruction of eicosanoids in the circulation limits their role primarily to that of mediators of local inflammatory changes. The local effects can be substantial; for example, many of the symptoms of congestion and altered airway compliance in asthma may reflect their action as well as the early pulmonary changes in adult respiratory distress syndrome. In addition to their role as vasodilators, the prostaglandins potentiate the increased vascular permeability induced by bradykinin. The leukotrienes LTC_4, LTD_4, and LTE_4 are vasoconstrictors responsible for the wheal and flare reaction in skin. By their alteration of blood flow, eicosanoids, like the kinins, play an important role in determining the local extent of an inflammatory process. They also help direct and accelerate the delivery of inflammatory cells to an injury site. LTB_4 is chemotactic for neutrophils, enhances neutrophil adherence to the endothelium, and enhances neutrophil oxidant release in response to other stimuli. Lipoxin A_4 and B_4 are potent vasoactive compounds.[10] In most tissues, lipoxin A_4 is a potent vasodilator, whereas lipoxin B_4 is a vasodilator in some tissues and a vasoconstrictor in other tissues. Lipoxin A_4 and B_4 also appear to be important immunoregulators. In vitro, lipoxin A_4 is a modest activator of neutrophil chemotaxis and oxidant production and is unable to stimulate cell aggregation; however, lipoxin A_4 inhibits other chemoattractants. It has been shown to inhibit LTB_4 and N-formyl-methionyl-leucyl-phenylalanine (FMLP)-induced responses, block LTC_4-induced contraction in guinea pig ileum and human pulmonary artery, trigger relaxation and reversal of the prostaglan-

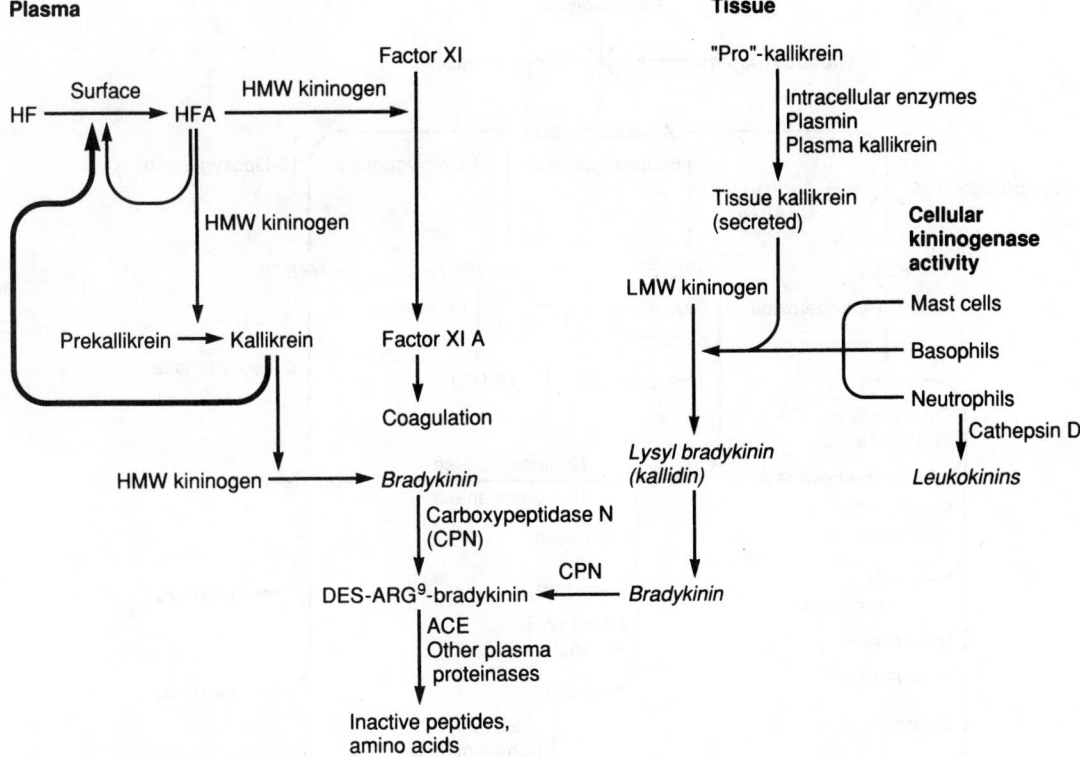

Figure 6-5. Three pathways of kinin formation. HF, Hageman factor; HFA, activated Hageman factor; HMW, high molecular weight; LMW, low molecular weight; ACE, angiotensin-converting enzyme. (After Proud D, Kaplan AP. Kinin formation: mechanisms and role in inflammatory disorders. Annu Rev Immunol 1988;6:49)

din $PGF_{2\alpha}$ and endothelin-induced contraction in human pulmonary artery, and antagonize the action of LTD_4 in rat renal cells. Because of these counterinflammatory functions, it has been hypothesized that the lipoxins are endogenously generated stop signals necessary for the inflammatory response to be self-limiting. Further studies are required to verify this hypothesis.

In general, the eicosanoids are rapidly metabolized or are so chemically unstable that they primarily exert their effects near the site of synthesis. Arachidonic acid does not exist in cells but is esterified to membrane phospholipids. Thus, the first step in the production of eicosanoids is phospholipase action, which liberates arachidonic acid. Depending on the cell type, the arachidonic

Table 6-3. SOME EFFECTS OF EICOSANOIDS IN INFLAMMATION

PROSTAGLANDINS

PGE_2, PGI_2	Bronchodilation
	Vasodilation
	Potentiate effect of other mediators (eg, histamine, bradykinin, C5a) that increase vascular permeability
	Block platelet aggregation
	Stimulate bone resorption by osteoclasts
PGD_2	Bronchoconstriction
	Vasodilation
	Potentiates effect of other mediators (eg, histamine, bradykinin) that increase vascular permeability
	Stimulates random movement (chemokinesis) of neutrophils and eosinophils

LEUKOTRIENES

LTC_4, LTD_4, LTE_4	Account for the slow-reacting substance of anaphylaxis
	Bronchoconstriction (more severe in distal airways than in proximal airways)
	Increased secretion of bronchial mucus
	Vasoconstriction and increased vascular permeability
	Produce wheal and flare reaction in skin
LTB_4	Induces chemotaxis (directed movement) and chemokinesis of neutrophils, eosinophils, and monocytes
	Promotes adhesion of leukocytes especially to endothelium
	Stimulates production of O_2^{-} and release of hydrolytic enzymes by neutrophils

LIPOXINS

LXA_4, LXB_4	Vasoactive
	Inhibit inflammatory response

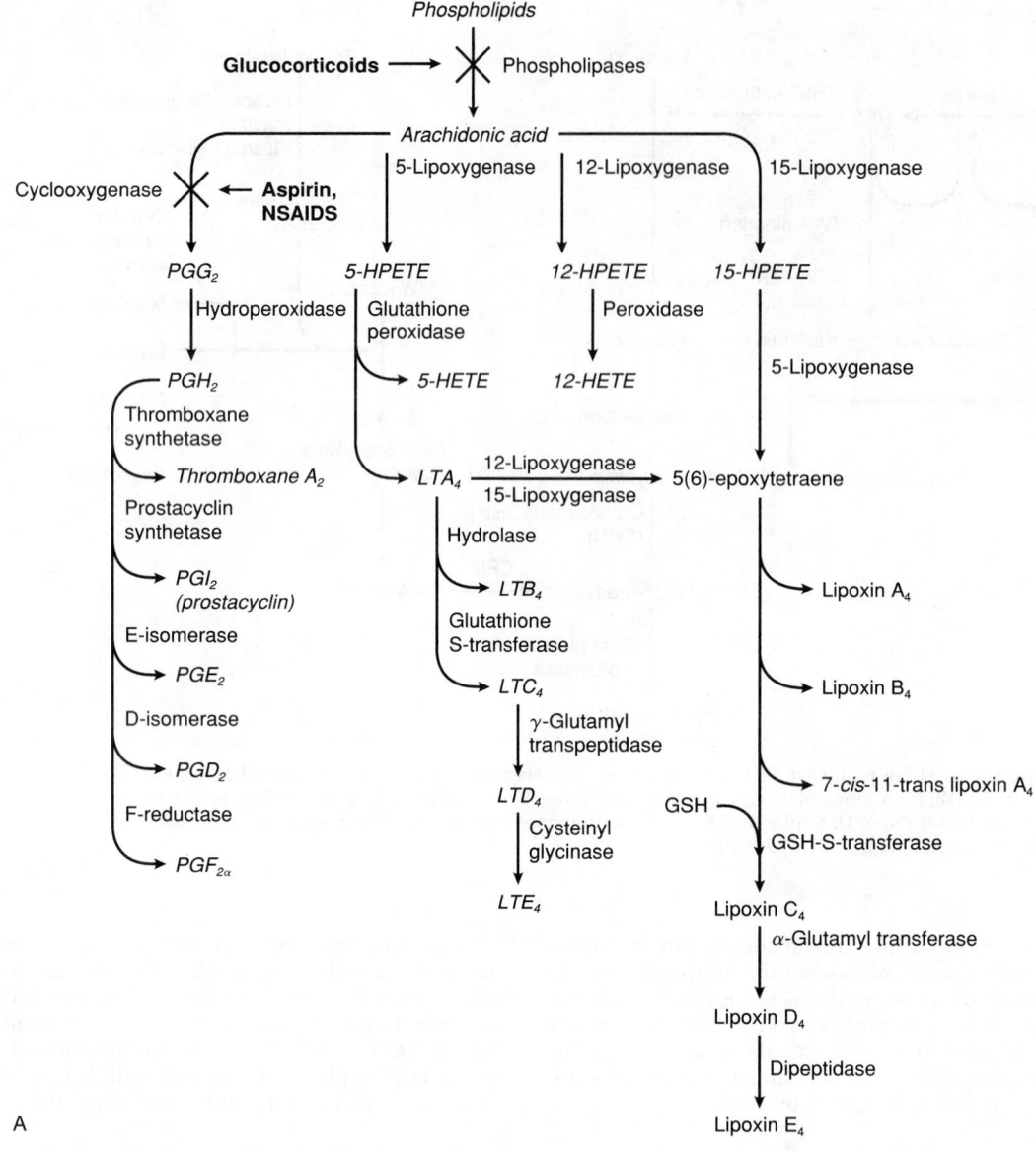

Figure 6-6. Pathways of eicosanoid production. Inflammatory mediators derived from arachidonic acid (*A*) and their structures (*B*). Sites of inhibition by antiinflammatory drugs are shown. NSAIDs, nonsteroidal antiinflammatory drugs (eg, ibuprofen). *(continues)*

acid may have several fates. Figure 6-6 outlines the pathways of arachidonic acid metabolism that lead to production of leukotrienes, lipoxins, thromboxane, and prostaglandins.

Cyclooxygenase Products

Cyclooxygenase catalyzes the first step in a series of reactions that converts arachidonic acid to prostaglandins or thromboxanes.[11] Cyclooxygenase converts arachidonic acid to PGG_2, which is subsequently reduced to PGH_2 by a peroxidase. PGH_2 is converted to prostaglandins and thromboxane by the action of specific enzymes. The specific eicosanoid produced varies from tissue to tissue depending on the activity of the specific enzyme in that tissue. Thus, the production of prostacyclin (PGI_2) in endothelial cells and thromboxane A_2 in platelets parallels the increased activities of prostacyclin synthetase and thromboxane synthetase, respectively, in these tissues. Countering the synthetic pathways are pro-

cesses for inactivation of these bioactive compounds. PGE_2, PGD_2, and PGF_2 are rapidly converted to inactive products by enzymatic pathways. Thromboxane A_2 and PGI_2 are chemically unstable and rapidly convert to the inactive compounds thromboxane B_2 and 6-keto-$PGF_{1\alpha}$.

Lipoxygenase Pathways

The enzyme 5-lipoxygenase catalyzes the first of a series of reactions that leads to the production of the leukotrienes. Arachidonic acid is converted by 5-lipoxygenase to 5-hydroperoxyeicosatetraenoic acid (5-HPETE). 5-HPETE is next converted to LTA_4 by a dehydrase. LTA_4 has two fates. It may be converted to LTC_4 by the addition of glutathione (GSH) by means of glutathione-S-transferase. Amino acids are then successively hydrolized from LTC_4 to give the dipeptide derivative LTD_4 and the single–amino acid derivative LTE_4. LTC_4, LTD_4, and LTE_4 are classified as the sulfidopeptide leukotrienes and constitute the slow-reactivity substance of anaphylaxis. Alternatively, LTA_4 can be

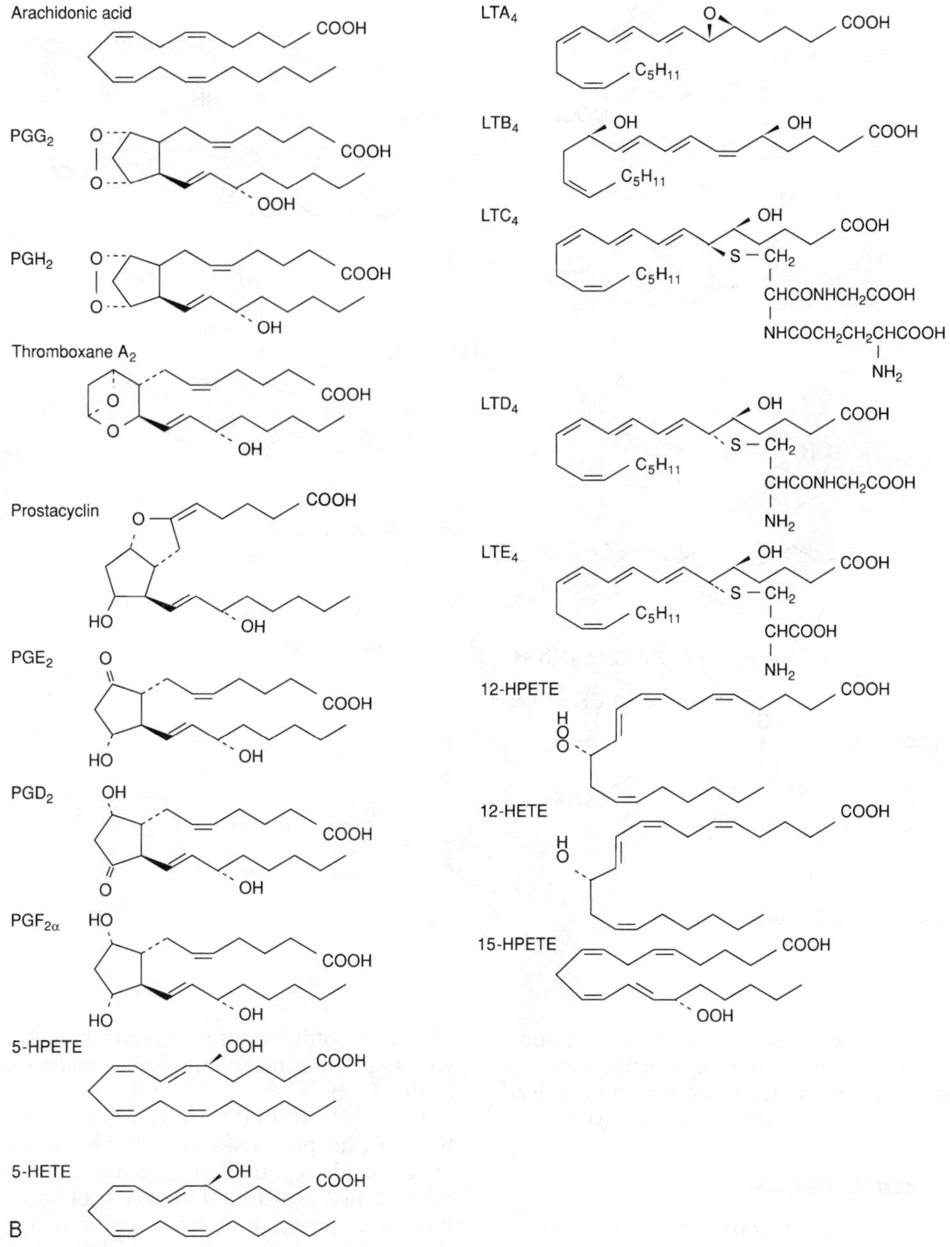

Arachidonic acid

PGG$_2$

PGH$_2$

Thromboxane A$_2$

Prostacyclin

PGE$_2$

PGD$_2$

PGF$_{2\alpha}$

5-HPETE

5-HETE

B

LTA$_4$

LTB$_4$

LTC$_4$

LTD$_4$

LTE$_4$

12-HPETE

12-HETE

15-HPETE

Figure 6-6. *(Continued)*

converted to LTB$_4$ by a hydrolase. Additional lipoxygenase activity results in the production of 12-HPETE and 12-hydroxyeicosatetraenoic acid (12-HETE; 12-lipoxygenase) and 15-HPETE (15-lipoxygenase). These compounds exhibit biologic activity, although they are not as potent as the cyclooxygenase products and leukotrienes. Lipoxin biosynthesis can occur by several routes, depending on the tissue.[10] A 5(6)-epoxytetraene intermediate can be formed by 5-lipoxygenase activity on 15-HPETE or by 12-lipoxygenase and 15-lipoxygenase activity on LTA$_4$. This intermediate is then converted to lipoxin A$_4$, lipoxin B$_4$, or lipoxin C$_4$. Lipoxin C$_4$ can be sequentially modified to form lipoxin D$_4$, then lipoxin E$_4$. Of these, lipoxin A$_4$ and B$_4$ appear to have the greatest (or at least most studied) biologic activities. Like the cyclooxygenase products, the lipoxygenase products are rapidly inactivated. For example, LTB$_4$ is enzymatically converted to 20-OH-LTB$_4$, then 20-COOH-LTB$_4$, each progressively less potent than LTB$_4$ in stimulating neutrophil chemotaxis.

The importance of these pathways in inflammation is accentuated by the fact that a large number of antiinflammatory drugs act to disrupt eicosanoid synthetic pathways (see Fig. 6-6). Corticosteroids inhibit inflammation at least in part by inhibiting the release of arachidonic acid from phospholipids. Nonsteroidal antiinflammatory drugs (NSAIDs) such as aspirin inhibit cyclooxygenase activity and block synthesis of prostaglandins and thromboxanes. In contrast to the other NSAIDs, aspirin inhibits cyclooxygenase in an irreversible manner. Because platelets are anucleated cells and cannot synthesize new cyclooxygenase, the effects of aspirin on platelet function can only be reversed by the arrival of new platelets that have not been exposed to aspirin. One of the potential negative effects of NSAID use is that inhibition of cyclooxygenase can shunt arachidonic acid through 5-lipoxygenase and result in the synthesis of higher levels of leukotrienes, thus minimizing any benefit achieved from reduction of other eicosanoid levels. Unfortunately, NSAIDs act systemically in a nonse-

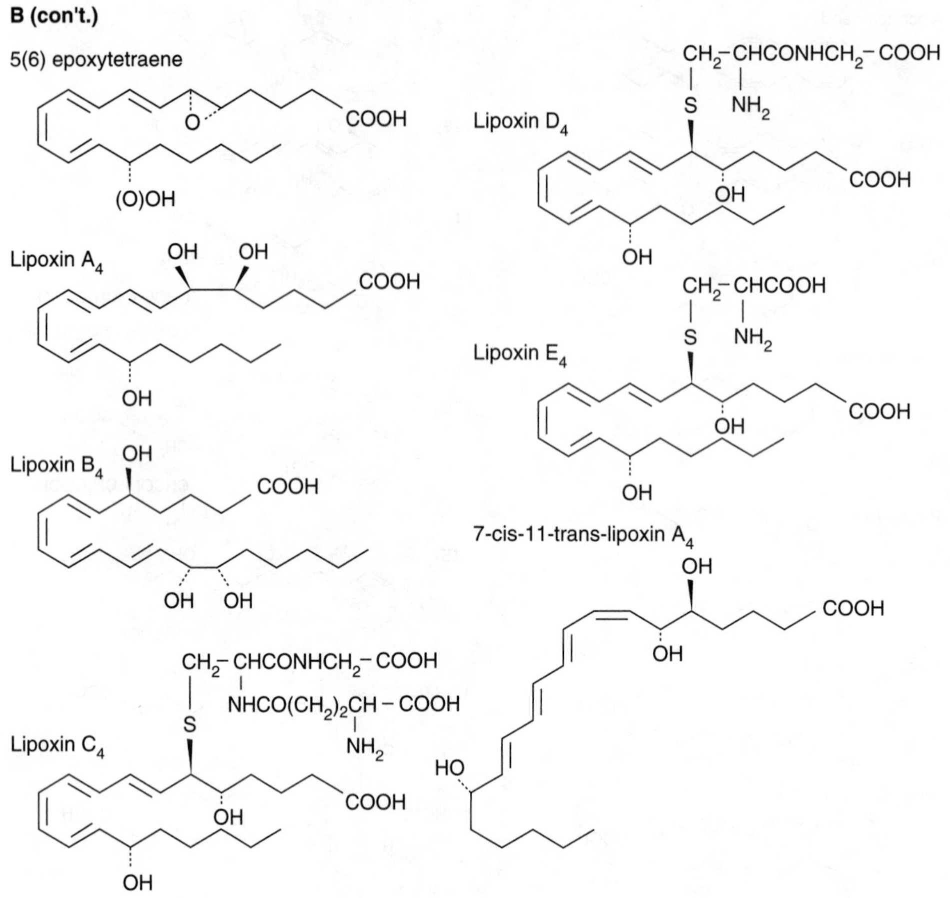

B (con't.)

5(6) epoxytetraene

Lipoxin A₄

Lipoxin B₄

Lipoxin C₄

Lipoxin D₄

Lipoxin E₄

7-cis-11-trans-lipoxin A₄

Figure 6-6. *(Continued)*

lective manner, so that prostaglandin synthesis at some locations where prostaglandins may be exerting cytoprotective effects (eg, stomach) is also inhibited and can lead to dangerous side effects (eg, mucosal ulceration).

Platelet-Activating Factor

Like the eicosanoids, platelet-activating factor (PAF) is not stored in cells but is rapidly produced during inflammation by activated leukocytes, mast cells, and vascular endothelium.[12] Pathophysiologic effects in vivo include bronchoconstriction, hypotension, and increased vascular permeability. In addition, PAF is chemotactic for leukocytes and enhances neutrophil oxidant production in response to other stimuli. Benveniste[13] originally reported that antigen stimulation of rabbit leukocytes, including IgE-sensitized basophils, caused the release of a soluble factor that induced platelet aggregation and secretion. They coined the name *platelet-activating factor* because of this functional activity. Subsequent studies identified the factor as a heterogeneous mixture of 1-0-alkyl-2-acetyl-*sn*-glycero-3-phosphocholine, with the alkyl moiety including saturated and unsaturated alkyl chains ranging from 14 to 22 carbons in length. Perhaps because of this molecular heterogeneity, the functional term has persisted, rather than a precise molecular term. PAF exerts a variety of biologic effects that are platelet independent.

The membrane phospholipid precursor of PAF is 1-0-alkyl-2-acyl-*sn*-glycero-3-phosphocholine (ether-PC), which is different from the more common membrane phosphatidyl-choline, which has acyl chains in both the 1 and 2 positions.

The neutrophil has uncommonly high levels of ether-PCs, with as much as half of the choline containing phospholipids in this form.

The synthesis of PAF (Fig. 6-7) is initiated by the activation of phospholipase A_2, which releases the fatty acyl chain to yield 1-0-alkyl-*sn*-glycerophosphocholine (lyso-PAF). The 2 position of the glycerol backbone is then acetylated by acetyl transferase, with acetyl CoA serving as the source of the acetyl group. This active PAF compound may be released from the cell, or it may be converted back to lyso-PC by acetylhydrolase. Cellular acyltransferases readily acylate the 2 position of lyso-PAF through fatty acyl CoA-dependent and CoA-independent mechanisms, converting it back to the precursor ether-PC. The mechanisms by which PAF production and release from cells are regulated are not clear. Calcium modulation of phospholipase A_2 appears to be crucial. In addition, acetyl transferase may be regulated through phosphorylation–dephosphorylation reactions.

A large percentage of the ether-PCs have arachidonic acid esterified at the 2 position. Thus, activation of phospholipase A_2 releases arachidonic acid in addition to lyso-PAF. Hence, PAF synthesis and eicosanoid production are coordinately regulated (Fig. 6-8). Although little is known about the mechanism of release of PAF from cells, a plasma acetylhydrolase has been characterized that is responsible for the inactivation of PAF released from cells.

PAF is synthesized on activation of a variety of inflammatory cells, including platelets, neutrophils, basophils, mast cells, mononuclear phagocytes, eosinophils, and vascular endothelium. PAF has been isolated from a number

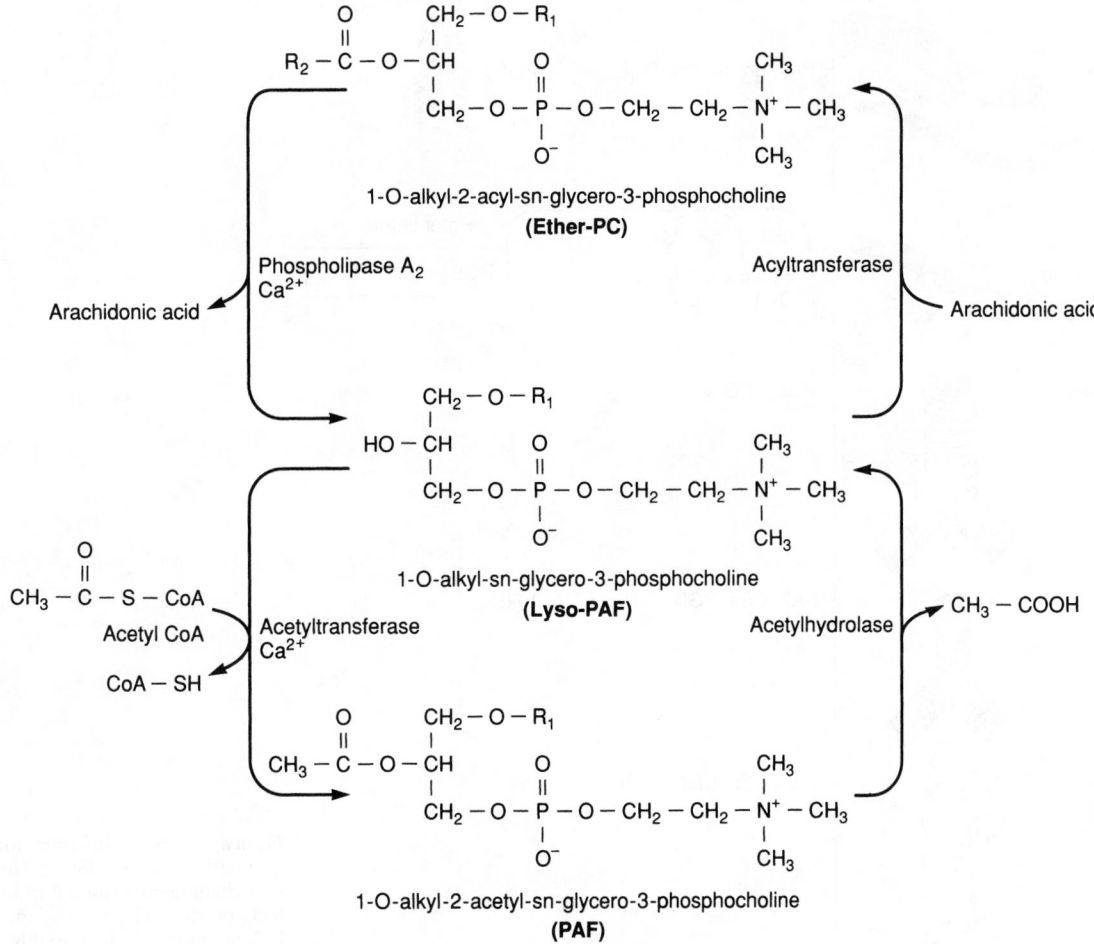

Figure 6-7. Pathways of platelet-activating factor (PAF) biosynthesis and breakdown.

of physiologically stressed tissues, including the brain, skin, lung, heart, liver, and kidney, although the cell of origin in these tissues is not known.

PAF is a stimulatory agonist for many of the inflammatory cells as well as for smooth muscle cells, renal mesangial cells, epithelial cells, and the vascular endothelium. PAF stimulates these cells to release other autocoids, additional modulators of cellular behavior. PAF is chemotactic for migratory inflammatory cells and promotes adherence of these cells to the vascular endothelium. It induces secretion and oxidant production by cells capable of those functions (mononuclear phagocytes, neutrophils, eosinophils). PAF also enhances the ability of neutrophils to respond to challenge with N-formylpeptides (bacterial peptides) and LTB_4. The ability of PAF to affect other cells is mediated

by a specific cell-surface receptor that rapidly induces intracellular enzymatic activity. There is considerable overlap and redundancy in the effects produced by the early humoral mediators of inflammation. Figure 6-9 depicts some of these interrelations and common effects produced by the different mediators.

Cytokines and Growth Factors

The cytokines consist of protein molecules that are released from inflammatory cells and induce activation of other cells[14,15] (see Table 6-2). Several of these proteins are frequently categorized as *growth factors* or *interleukins*. This is not exclusive terminology because many interleukins are growth factors. In general, these factors are not preformed in

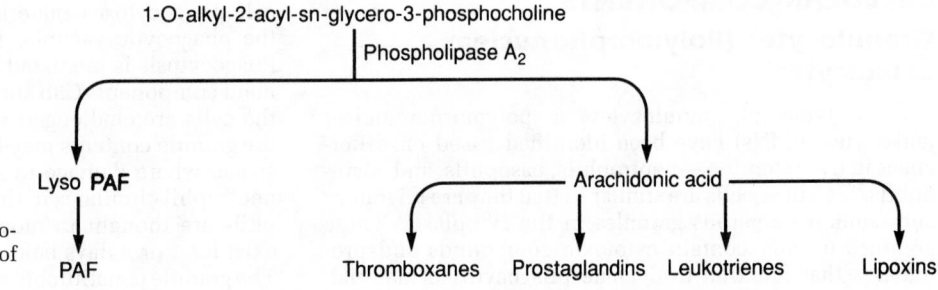

Figure 6-8. Phospholipase A_2 as a coordinate enzyme in the production of platelet-activating factor (PAF).

Function

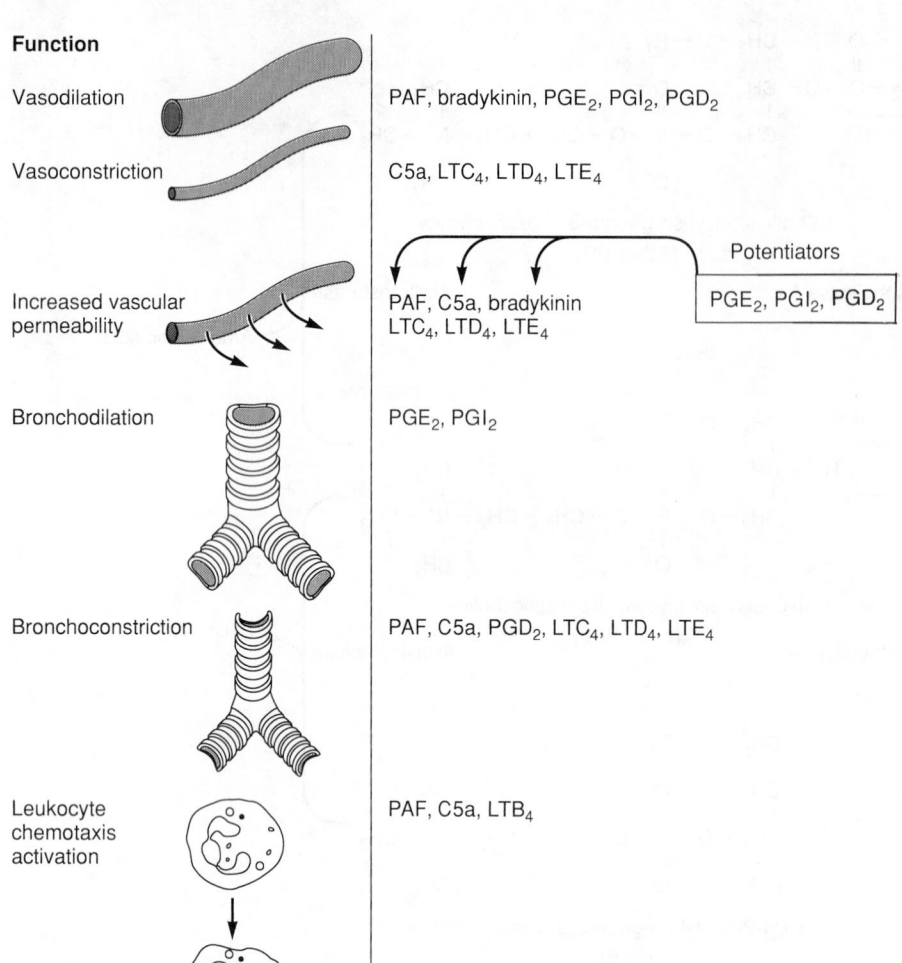

Vasodilation — PAF, bradykinin, PGE_2, PGI_2, PGD_2

Vasoconstriction — C5a, LTC_4, LTD_4, LTE_4

Potentiators

Increased vascular permeability — PAF, C5a, bradykinin LTC_4, LTD_4, LTE_4 | PGE_2, PGI_2, PGD_2

Bronchodilation — PGE_2, PGI_2

Bronchoconstriction — PAF, C5a, PGD_2, LTC_4, LTD_4, LTE_4

Leukocyte chemotaxis activation — PAF, C5a, LTB_4

Figure 6-9. Some inflammatory mediators with common effects. These examples demonstrate the redundancy of effects produced by various mediators in inflammation. It is possible that this feature of the inflammatory mediators leads to occasional overkill responses with pathologic results.

cells. Rather, activation of cells turns on expression of the genes encoding for these proteins. The effects of these proteins on other cells appear to be mediated predominantly through cell-surface receptors. The effects on cells represent two time scales. On an immediate time scale, cytokines may enhance activation of the existing leukocytes. Over longer time periods, cytokines may increase differentiation and production of more hemopoietic cells. Some cytokines do both. The sources and effects of several cytokines are summarized in Table 6-2, which is an introduction to the cytokines, not an exhaustive list. The involvement of cytokines in the acute-phase response was discussed earlier, and additional examples of how these proteins mediate inflammation appear in subsequent sections. Effects of growth factors on wound healing (eg, fibroblast recruitment and growth) are discussed in Chapter 3.

CELLULAR COMPONENTS

Granulocytes (Polymorphonuclear Leukocytes)

Three types of granulocytes or polymorphonuclear leukocytes (PMNs) have been identified based on differences in dye retention—neutrophils, basophils, and eosinophils.[16,17] These cells are similar in that they are migratory and contain numerous granules in the cytoplasm. These granules usually contain cytotoxic compounds and proteinases that function to degrade phagocytosed material,

and they function as mediators of inflammatory responses. Neutrophils represent 60% of the circulating leukocyte population, whereas basophils and eosinophils represent 0.1% to 0.5% and 1% to 3%, respectively. Because of their greater abundance, neutrophils have been the most studied. Thus, detailed discussions of neutrophil activation and function are presented here. Mechanisms of activation and regulation of basophil and eosinophil functions appear to be analogous.

Neutrophils

The neutrophil is a migratory, phagocytic cell that defends the host against bacteria and eliminates necrotic tissue. The neutrophil matures in the bone marrow and is released to the circulation as a fully differentiated cell. It is loaded with granules that contain a variety of proteinases, hydrolases, and antimicrobial agents (Table 6-4). The cell phagocytoses material, and the granules fuse with the phagocytic vacuoles to degrade the foreign material. Phagocytosis is mediated by surface receptors for complement components C3b and C3bi and by Fc receptors. When the cells are challenged with a large amount of material, the granule contents may be released into the extracellular space, where damage to surrounding tissues occurs. The neutrophil circulates in the blood for 7 to 10 hours. Neutrophils are thought to move into tissues, where they may exist for 1 or 2 days before being cleared from the system. The granule constituents are formed during differentiation,

Table 6-4. NEUTROPHIL GRANULE CONSTITUENTS

	Primary (Azurophilic)	Secondary (Specific)	Tertiary
Bactericidal enzymes	Myeloperoxidase	Lysozyme	
	Lysozyme		
Proteinases	Elastase	Collagenase	Gelatinase
	Cathepsin B		
	Cathepsin D		
	Cathepsin G		
	Proteinase 3		
Acid hydrolases	β-glycarophosphatase		
	β-glucuronidase		
	N-acetyl-β-glucuronidase		
	α-Mannosidase		
Bactericidal proteins	Defensins		
	Bactericidal permeability–increasing protein		
	Azurophil-derived bactericidal factors		
	Cationic proteins		
Cell-surface receptors		FMLP receptors	Laminin receptors
		C3bi receptors	C3bi receptors
Other		Lactoferrin	Alkaline
		Vitamin B_{12}–binding protein	phosphatase
		Histaminase	Cytochrome b
		Cytochrome b	
		Plasminogen activator	

(Data from Bainton DF. Phagocytic cells: developmental biology of neutrophils and eosinophils. In: Gallin JI, Goldstein IM, Snyderman R, eds. Inflammation: basic principles and clinical correlates. New York, Raven, 1988:265; and Smolen JE, Boxer LA. Functions of neutrophils. In: Williams WJ, Beutler E, Ersley AJ, Lichtman MA, eds. Hematology. New York, McGraw-Hill, 1990:780)

and replenishment of spent granules does not occur once the cells are in the circulation, nor do tissue neutrophils reenter the circulation. Hence, the neutrophil is a fully differentiated end cell that is poised to respond rapidly to stimuli but is rapidly spent in the process. Neutrophil function is replenished only by the formation of new neutrophils. In addition to their physiologic roles, neutrophils have been implicated as important mediators of inflammatory tissue injury in a wide range of conditions, including rheumatoid arthritis, gout, adult respiratory distress syndrome, other forms of organ failure in the multiple organ failure syndrome, and tissue injury after reperfusion of ischemic organs.

Neutrophils have an NADPH oxidase enzyme system on the plasma membrane, which can be activated to produce the toxic oxygen species superoxide anion ($O_2^{\bullet-}$). The oxidase is oriented in the plasma membrane, so that the oxidase present in the phagosomal membrane releases $O_2^{\bullet-}$ to the inside of the phagosome. Patients with chronic granulomatous disease have a defective NADPH oxidase system in their neutrophils, which is unable to generate $O_2^{\bullet-}$. Although their neutrophils are able to phagocytose bacteria, they are unable to kill the intracellular microbes, and chronic, unresolved infections result. Observations of these patients' neutrophils provided the definitive evidence for the essential role of neutrophil-derived oxidants in bacterial killing. NADPH oxidase in the plasma membrane is also capable of releasing $O_2^{\bullet-}$ into the extracellular space. Hence, neutrophils are thought to be a major source of injurious oxidants present at sites of inflammatory injury.

To counter the effects of neutrophil release of proteinases and oxidants, a variety of extracellular agents are present. These antiproteinases include plasma α_1-PI, α_2-macroglobulin, α_1-antichymotrypsin, and antileukoproteinases. In addition, superoxide dismutase is present in tissues and plasma to convert $O_2^{\bullet-}$ to hydrogen peroxide. The hydrogen peroxide is then removed by the action of catalase.

The neutrophil is a motile cell, as are many of the leukocytes. In vivo, neutrophils respond to injury by adhering to the vascular endothelium near the site of injury, extravasating, and migrating through tissues to the site of infection. In vitro, the cells migrate up a concentration gradient of chemoattractant. Studies indicate that there is both a temporal and spatial component to this mechanism. The cell can distinguish as little as 1% difference in the concentration of a chemoattractant[18] and is also sensitive to the rate of stimulus presentation.[19]

Signal Transduction in the Neutrophil. The ability of the neutrophil to respond to injury is partly due to its ability to respond to N-formylpeptides released by bacteria and to LPS, which is a component of the cell wall of gram-negative bacteria. In addition, the neutrophil responds to endogenously generated chemoattractants, LTB_4, PAF, complement component C5a, and IL-8 (also known as neutrophil-activating protein 1, or neutrophil chemotactic factor). The neutrophil's function is modulated by a variety of cytokines that are released during tissue injury (eg, TNF, IL-1, granulocyte-macrophage colony-stimulating factor [GM-CSF], and granulocyte colony-stimulating factor [G-CSF]; see Table 6-2). These stimuli can be categorized as chemotactic (N-formylpeptide, C5a, PAF, LTB_4, IL-8) or as priming agents that enhance chemotactic stimulation (TNF, GM-CSF, G-CSF, PAF). In addition, several physiologic compounds have been shown to inhibit chemoattractant-induced responses (PGE_1, adenosine triphosphate [ATP], epinephrine). Thus, the potential for regulation of neutrophil function is great.

Stimulation by Chemoattractants. The ability of the neutrophil to respond to assault is conferred by specific receptors on the membrane surface that bind an activator (ligand) and transmit signals inside the cell. The most studied ligand receptor system in the neutrophil is the N-formylpeptide receptor, which serves as a model for stimulation by other endogenous chemoattractants, such as LTB_4, PAF, C5a, and IL-8. All of these activators appear to initiate neutrophil responses by similar signal transduction pathways, although each has its own specific receptor, and subtle differences are evident.

Guanine Nucleotide–Binding Proteins in Signal Transduction. Heterotrimeric guanine nucleotide–binding proteins (G proteins) have been recognized as a widely distributed family of proteins involved in membrane signal transduction.[20,21] This protein is composed of an α, β, and γ subunit, and numerous isoforms of each have been found. Isoforms of the α subunit are the most abundant, with more than 20 known so far. There are at least 5 β and 10 γ isoforms. The size of the α subunits vary from about 39 to 52 kd. The β subunits are about 35 kd, and the γ subunits are about 5 to 10 kd. The G protein is located on the inside of the plasma membrane and transduces a signal of the ligand receptor–binding event on the outside of the plasma membrane to an effector on the inside of the plasma membrane. The G proteins function in a common cycle of events as follows.

The ligand binds to the receptor on the cell surface and transmits a signal to the G protein on the cytoplasmic side of the membrane. The G protein moves through an elaborate cycle of events that regulates the activation of effectors inside the cell (Fig. 6-10). In the unactivated state, the G_α subunit has guanosine diphosphate (GDP) bound at a guanine nucleotide–binding site and is associated with the $\beta-\gamma$ subunit. When ligand binds to the receptor, a

Table 6-5. cDNA CLONES OF G-PROTEIN α SUBUNITS

Subunit	Molecular Weight	Toxin	Effectors
G_s	45	Cholera	Adenylate cyclase
T_1	40	Pertussis, cholera	cGMP phosphodiesterase
T_2	40.5	Pertussis, cholera	cGMP phosphodiesterase
G_0	39	Pertussis	Unknown
G_{i-1}	41	Pertussis	Unknown
G_{i-2}	40	Pertussis	Phospholipase C
G_{i-3}	41	Pertussis	Unknown

(Data from Spiegel A, Carter A, Brann M, et al. Signal transduction by guanine nucleotides binding proteins. Recent Prog Horm Res 1988;44:337; and Casey PJ, Gilman AG. G protein involvement in receptor–effector coupling. J Biol Chem 1988;263:2577)

ternary complex of ligand–receptor–G protein is formed, causing the release of GDP from the G protein. This site is rapidly filled by guanosine triphosphate (GTP), which is at comparatively high concentrations in the cell. The binding of GTP to the site on the G protein causes the release of the ligand–receptor complex and the $\beta-\gamma$ complex from the G_α subunit. The G_α–GTP complex is activated and complexes with and activates the effector. The freed ligand–receptor complex may be available to complex with and activate another G-protein complex. Hence, amplification of the ligand receptor–binding event may occur. As long as the G_α–effector complex is associated, the effector is active. Thus, additional amplification occurs at this catalytic step. The G protein has an intrinsic GTPase activity that hydrolyzes the GTP and produces the G_α–GDP–effector complex. This complex is unstable, and a released G_α–GDP can complex again with the $\beta-\gamma$ subunit complex. It is then available to cycle again. Several types of G proteins have been identified based on functions and cDNA identification (Table 6-5).

In some systems, the $\beta-\gamma$ subunit, not the α subunit, has been implicated as the species responsible for activating the effector. In this case, amplification can still occur while the effector–$\beta-\gamma$ complex exists. Cycling of the G protein, however, is still dependent on the GTPase activity of the α subunit because it is thought that when G_α–GDP is generated, it complexes with the $\beta-\gamma$ subunit and thereby renders it inactive.

A second major class of G proteins are the small GTP-binding proteins. These proteins are about half the size of G_α. The group is represented by the Ras super family of proteins, which contains about 50 different proteins.[22] Whereas the heterotrimeric G proteins function in transmembrane signal transduction, the small GTP-binding proteins are important for regulating intracellular events. Like the heterotrimeric G proteins, the small GTP-binding proteins are also involved in a cycle of GDP–GTP exchange and hydrolysis that regulates their function (Fig. 6-11). The inactive state consists of the protein with GDP bound to its guanine nucleotide–binding site. Activation is induced by another protein, GDP-dissociation stimulator (GDS), which catalyzes the release of GDP, allowing GTP to bind at the open site. Inactivation occurs by autocatalytic hydrolysis of GTP to GDP. This autocatalytic activity can be modulated by GTPase activating proteins (GAPs). In addition, the small GTP-binding proteins can be inactivated and sequestered from regulation by GDS and GAP by complex formation with another protein, GDP-dissociation inhibitor (GDI).

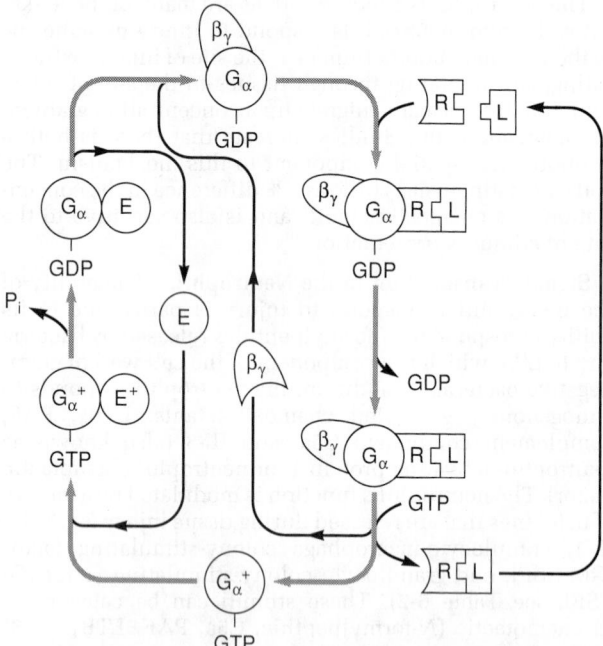

Figure 6-10. The G-protein cycle of activation. When a ligand (L) binds to its receptor (R) on the cell surface, this complex of LR activates a GTP-binding protein located on the cytoplasmic side of the cell membrane. Formation of the LR complex causes the release of GDP from the G protein. The vacant guanine nucleotide-binding site is rapidly filled by GTP from the cytosol, causing the release of the G protein from the LR complex and the dissociation of the Gα subunit from the β-γ subunit of the G protein. The GTP–Gα complex represents the activated G protein component that binds and activates an effector (E) in the cell. The catalytic activity of the effector continues until the bound GTP is hydrolyzed by the Gα subunit. The GDP–Gα complex rapidly dissociates from the effector (which is no longer active) and associates with a β-γ subunit and is ready for another cycle of activation. P_i, inorganic phosphate.

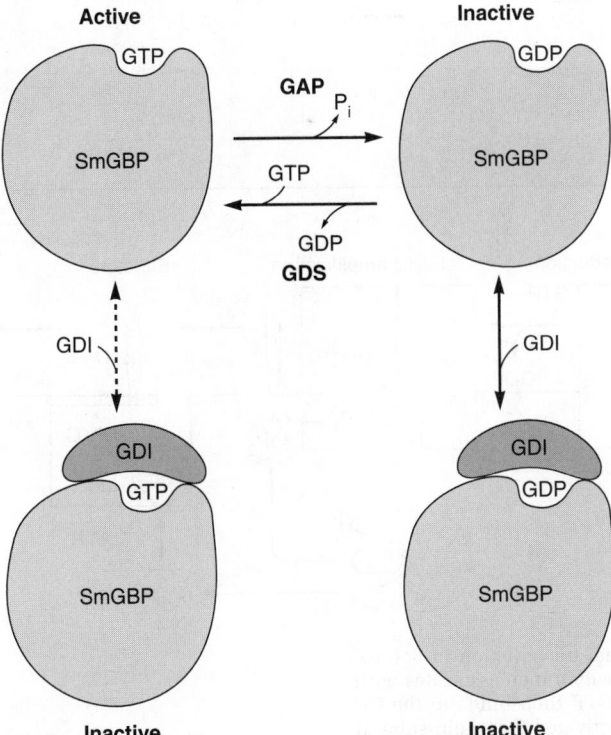

Active   Inactive

Figure 6-11. The GTPase cycle of small GTP-binding proteins (SmGBP). The inactive state consists of the protein with GDP bound to its guanine nucleotide-binding site. Activation is induced by another protein, GDP dissociation stimulator (GDS), which catalyzes the release of GDP, allowing GTP to bind at the open site. Inactivation occurs by autocatalytic hydrolysis of GTP to GDP. This autocatalytic activity can be modulated by GTPase-activating proteins (GAPs). In addition, the small GTP-binding protein can be inactivated and sequestered from regulation by GDS and GAP by complexation with another protein, GDP-dissociation inhibitor (GDI). GDI binds the GDP-bound form of SmGBP with higher affinity than the GTP-bound form.

G-Protein Coupling to Phospholipase C and Subsequent Events in Neutrophils.

The neutrophil G proteins, which transduce N-formylpeptide responses, are substrates for adenosine diphosphate (ADP) ribosylation by pertussis toxin. Immunologic identification has detected 40-kd and 41-kd pertussis toxin substrates that appear to be similar to $G_{i\alpha2}$ and $G_{i\alpha3}$, respectively.[23,24] The signal transduction pathway for N-formylpeptide–induced responses in the neutrophil are summarized in Figure 6-12. Substantial evidence implicates N-formylpeptide in activation of G proteins that mediate phospholipase C activation on ligand binding. This phospholipase C is specific for phosphatidylinositol 4,5-bisphosphate (PIP$_2$), which is cleaved to form inositol 1,4,5-trisphosphate (IP$_3$) and diacylglycerol (DAG). IP$_3$ causes the release of calcium from intracellular stores into the cytosol. Ca^{2+} and DAG cause activation of a Ca^{2+}, phospholipid-dependent protein kinase C, which also requires ATP. Phosphorylation events are thought to be important for activation of the NADPH oxidase system. Ca^{2+} is a central signal for degranulation.[25,26]

In addition to activation of phospholipase C, phospholipase A$_2$ and phospholipase D are activated.[27] Phospholipase A$_2$ cleaves arachidonate from the *sn*-2 position of glycerophospholipids. In the neutrophil, the most abundant sources of arachidonate are from phosphatidylethanolamine, phosphatidyl choline, and phosphatidylinositol. Not only is arachidonate the precursor for eicosanoid

synthesis, it has also been shown to stimulate NADPH oxidase in a cell-free assay system. Phospholipase D cleaves the polar head group from phospholipids to release phosphatidate. The phosphate group can be readily cleaved by phosphatidate phosphohydrolase to produce DAG. This DAG can then participate in sustaining protein kinase C activation. In addition, phosphatidate has been shown to be a potent activator of NADPH oxidase in a cell-free assay system. There is evidence that phospholipase A$_2$ and D are both directly activated by G proteins. It is also clear, however, that activation of both requires elevated Ca^{2+} and protein kinase C activation. Thus, activation of both phospholipase A$_2$ and D is dependent on phospholipase C activation. The proposed sequence of chemoattractant-induced phospholipase activation is summarized in Figure 6-13.

Activation of NADPH Oxidase.

The manner in which this activation cascade is coupled to responses is not well understood. Perhaps the best known system is that of NADPH oxidase, which generates superoxide in response to several chemoattractants.[22] The cytochrome b_{558} of the NADPH oxidase system is composed of two subunits, gp91 and p22, is membrane bound, and contains flavin and NADPH-binding sites. Also associated with the cytochrome b_{558} is the small GTP-binding protein Rap1A. On activation, three cytosolic proteins, p47-*phox*, p67-*phox*, and the small GTP-binding protein Rac2, translocate to the membrane and form a complex with the oxidase. These six components appear to constitute the activated NADPH oxidase in the cell. How this is coupled to the early events in signal transduction has not been completely resolved. Phosphorylation of p47-*phox* by protein kinase C, however, correlates with translocation and activation and appears to be one link. In addition, Rac2 in the cytosol exists as a complex with GDI. On activation, Rac2 and GDI dissociate, and this step appears to be essential for allowing exchange of GDP and GTP and translocation of Rac2 to the membrane. What, then, regulates dissociation of Rac2 and GDI? In vitro studies have shown that lipids such as arachidonate and phosphatidate stimulate the release of Rac2 from GDI. A model of NADPH activation is presented in Figure 6-14. Thus, lipid second messengers may regulate the activation of Rac2. Because the story is not complete, other factors and mechanisms may also be involved.

Alternative Signal Pathways.

Cytoskeletal changes appear to occur independent of increased Ca^{2+} levels and phospholipase C activation.[26,28] The rearrangement of the cytoskeleton depends on the same class of receptors and the pertussis toxin–sensitive G_i-protein. In addition, Ca^{2+}-independent oxidant production has been reported.[29,30] These pathways may be regulated by the activation of a phosphatidylinositol-specific kinase, which appears to be activated by chemoattractant activation. In particular, it has been shown that N-formylpeptide activation induces an increase of PIP$_3$, with activation kinetics that parallel oxidant production.[31] Thus, there appear to be additional pathways involved in neutrophil activation. This is an area of intense research.

Processing of the ligand–receptor complex that is freed from the G protein is an important mechanism (although not the only one) by which the cells adapt or desensitize to the stimulus.[25] The ligand–receptor complex appears to be modified to yield a complex that is no longer capable of transducing signals. This may occur by receptor phosphorylation or by interaction with molecules that block the G-protein–binding site. Ultimately, the ligand–receptor complex associates with the cytoskeleton and is internalized. Additional adaptation mechanisms appear to in-

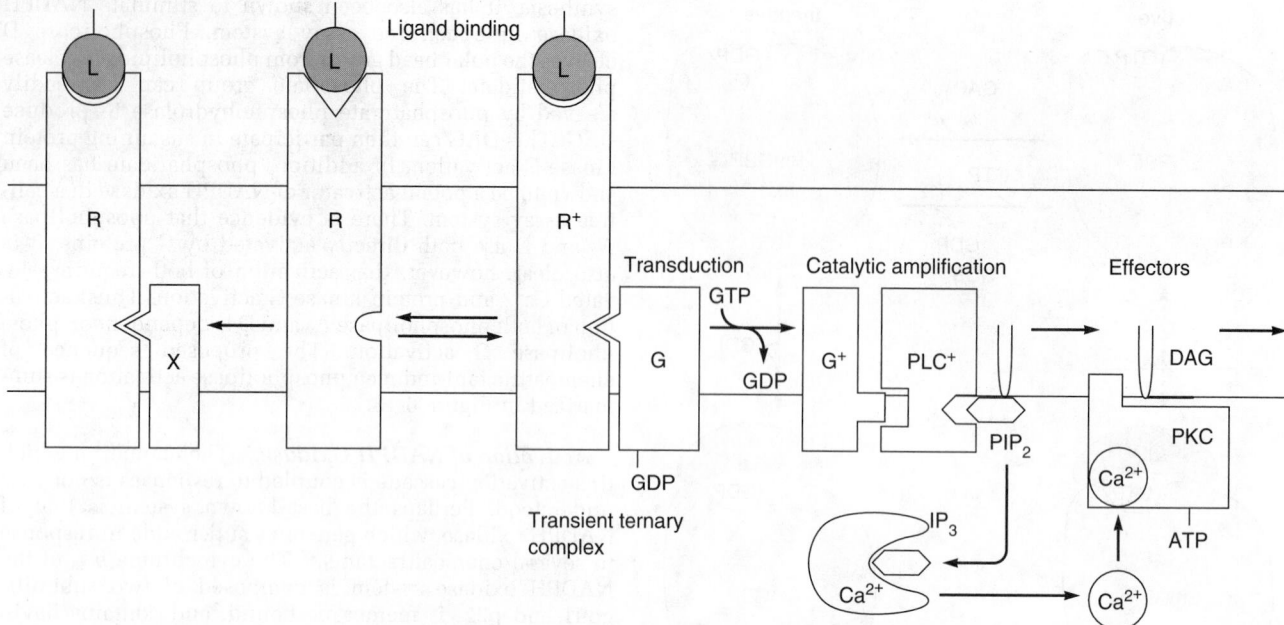

Figure 6-12. Early events of *N*-formylpeptide receptor–mediated signal transduction in neutrophils. *N*-formylpeptide (L) binds to the *N*-formylpeptide receptor (R), which then associates with a G protein and catalyzes the release of GDP from the Gα subunit. GTP then binds to the Gα subunit, releasing it and the $\beta\gamma$ subunit from the LR complex. This activated G protein subunit (G$^+$; either Gα-GTP or $\beta\gamma$) associates with phospholipase C and its substrate phosphatidyl inositol 4,5-bisphosphate (PIP$_2$) to catalyze the production of inositol 1,4,5-trisphosphate (IP$_3$) and diacylglycerol (DAG). IP$_3$ causes the release of Ca^{2+} from intracellular stores, and Ca^{2+} and DAG bind protein kinase C (PKC) to turn on protein phosphorylation. The LR complex that is released from the G protein may then be modified (x) in a manner that prevents the receptor from further association with the G protein, a step that results in desensitization of the cell to the *N*-formylpeptide. (After Sklar LA, Omann GM. Kinetics and amplification in neutrophil activation and adaptation. Cell Biol 1990;1:115)

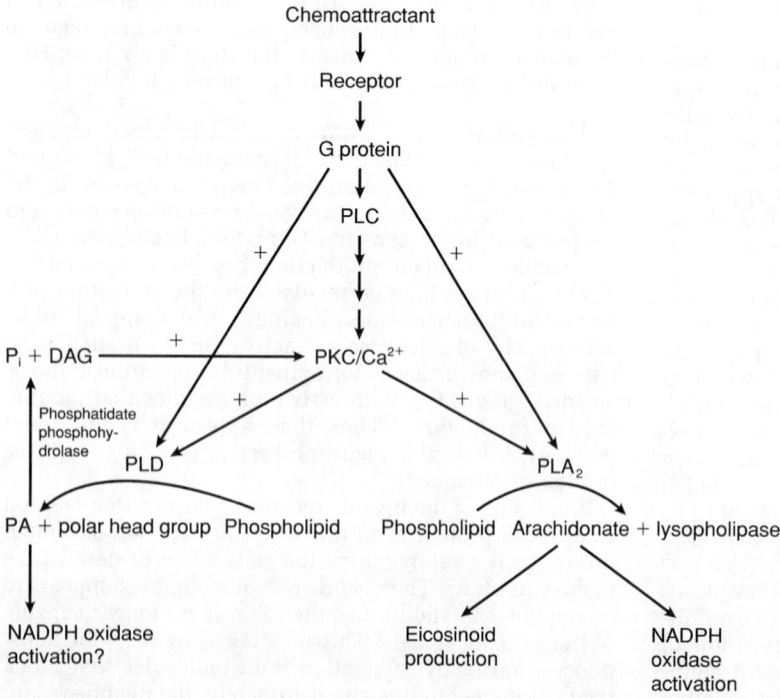

Figure 6-13. The role of phospholipases in neutrophil signal transduction. Ligand binding to its receptor activates G proteins, which activate phospholipase C (PLC). This in turn results in increased cytosolic Ca^{2+} and activation of protein kinase C (PKC) through the cascade of events summarized in Figure 6-12. Activated G proteins also activate phospholipases D and A$_2$ (PLD and PLA$_2$), but elevated Ca^{2+} levels and PKC activation are also required. Thus, PLC activation is required for activation of PLD and PLA$_2$. PLD produces phosphatidate (PA), which can be dephosphorylated to give diacylglycerol (DAG). PLA$_2$ cleaves arachidonate from the *sn*-2 position of glycerophospholipids, leaving a lysophospholipid. P$_i$, inorganic phosphate.

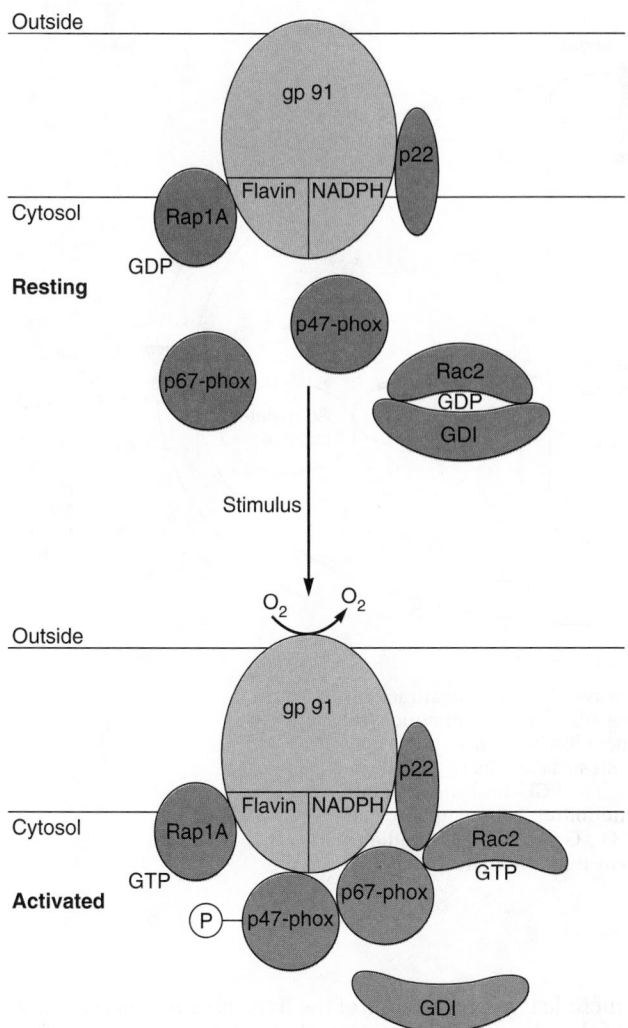

Outside

gp 91

p22

Flavin | NADPH

Cytosol

Rap1A

GDP

Resting

p47-phox

p67-phox

Rac2

GDI

GDP

Stimulus

O_2 O_2

Outside

gp 91

p22

Flavin | NADPH

Cytosol

Rap1A

Rac2

GTP

GTP

Activated

(P)   p47-phox

p67-phox

GDI

Figure 6-14. Activation of the NADPH oxidase in human neutrophils. In the resting neutrophil, the cytochrome subunits gp91 and p22 are tightly bound in the membrane, with Rap1A also bound to the gp91 subunit. p47-*phox,* p67-*phox,* and GDP dissociation inhibitor (GDI)–Rac2 complex are in the cytosol. On activation, GDI releases Rac2, and p47-*phox* becomes phosphorylated. This causes translocation of Rac2, p47-*phox,* and p67-*phox* to the membrane and complexation with the cytochrome components, thus completing the assembly of the active oxidase. Phosphorylation of p47-*phox* is mediated by protein kinase C, and dissociation of GDI–Rac2 may be mediated by lipid signal, such as arachidonate or phosphatidate. Other components may also be involved.

volve the decreased ability of the G protein to transduce signals.[32]

Inhibitory Pathways. Several compounds inhibit the ability of neutrophils to respond to *N*-formylpeptides. These include β-adrenergic agonists, such as epinephrine, PGE_1, and adenosine and related compounds.[33] There appear to be receptors for these ligands on the cell surface. These receptors increase cytosolic levels of cyclic adenosine monophosphate (cAMP) by activating adenylate cyclase by way of the stimulatory neutrophil G_s proteins. The mechanism by which these ligands modulate the chemotactic signal transduction pathways is not known, but it is likely due to cAMP-mediated phosphorylation of components of the chemoattractant signal pathway.

Priming of Neutrophil Function by Cytokines and Lipid Mediators. Several cytokines and lipid mediators cause neutrophils to respond more potently to activation by *N*-formylpeptides. Priming has been reported for LPS, PAF, LTB_4, TNF, and the growth factors GM-CSF and G-CSF. These growth factors play two important roles: they promote differentiation to produce new leukocytes, and they enhance the ability of the existing neutrophils to respond to chemotactic stimuli. Neutrophil priming generally occurs on a rapid time scale (within 1 hour) and does not appear to require protein synthesis. This suggests that priming may result from enhanced coupling of the signal transduction systems. In this regard, it has been shown that priming by LPS and GM-CSF causes an increase in *N*-formylpeptide receptors on neutrophils. There is not always a consistent correlation between receptor number and response, which suggests that other mechanisms also exist.

Many different factors act to regulate neutrophil behavior—some to enhance their activity, and others to diminish it. It is still unclear how much of a role the various priming agents (eg, LPS) play in producing a pathologic level of neutrophil activation. Figure 6-15 summarizes the balance of forces influencing neutrophil behavior during inflammation.

Eosinophils

Eosinophils constitute a small percentage (1% to 3%) of the leukocytes in the bloodstream. They also reside in tissues; for every circulating eosinophil, there are 100 tissue eosinophils. Unlike neutrophils, they appear to reside outside the circulation for several days and may later reenter the circulation. They exhibit phagocytic capabilities and contain granules with peroxisome-like proteins, lysophospholipase, and cytotoxic proteins specific to the eosinophil.[34,35] These proteins include major basic protein, eosinophil cationic protein, eosinophil-derived neurotoxin, and eosinophil peroxidase. Eosinophils are less effective as bactericidal agents than neutrophils but appear to play a major role in defense against parasites. They contain an NADPH oxidase system that is probably similar to that of the neutrophil. C5a, FMLP, and IL-5 are chemoattractants for this cell, and eosinophil function is enhanced by IL-3 and GM-CSF. Eosinophils are primary effectors in allergic reactions by virtue of IgE receptors (which are not found on neutrophils). Their role in tissue injury due to mechanical damage is not clear, although they may be important by virtue of their ability to affect the function of basophils and mast cells. Eosinophils contain histaminase, and the major basic protein has been shown to cause release of histamine from basophils and mast cells. In contrast, eosinophils may release prostaglandins that inhibit mast cell function by cAMP-dependent pathways. In addition, eosinophils produce LTC_4 and PAF, both of which increase vascular permeability.

Basophils

Basophils are fully differentiated cells released into the circulation from the bone marrow. Their granules contain histamine, proteoglycans, proteinases, acid hydrolases, eosinophil chemotactic factor, and a neutrophil chemotactic factor. Basophils contain the major, if not sole, source of histamine in the blood. Histamine is a vasoactive amine and the major mediator of the IgE-mediated immediate hypersensitivity response. Basophils also appear to be involved in defense against parasites. Besides the release of granule constituents, activation of basophils also results in the production of leukotrienes and PAF. Histamine release from basophils is induced by FMLP, C5a, and C3a as well as by IgE. C5a is also chemotactic for basophils. Thus, basophils may play a role in inflammation due to other types of injury (not IgE mediated).

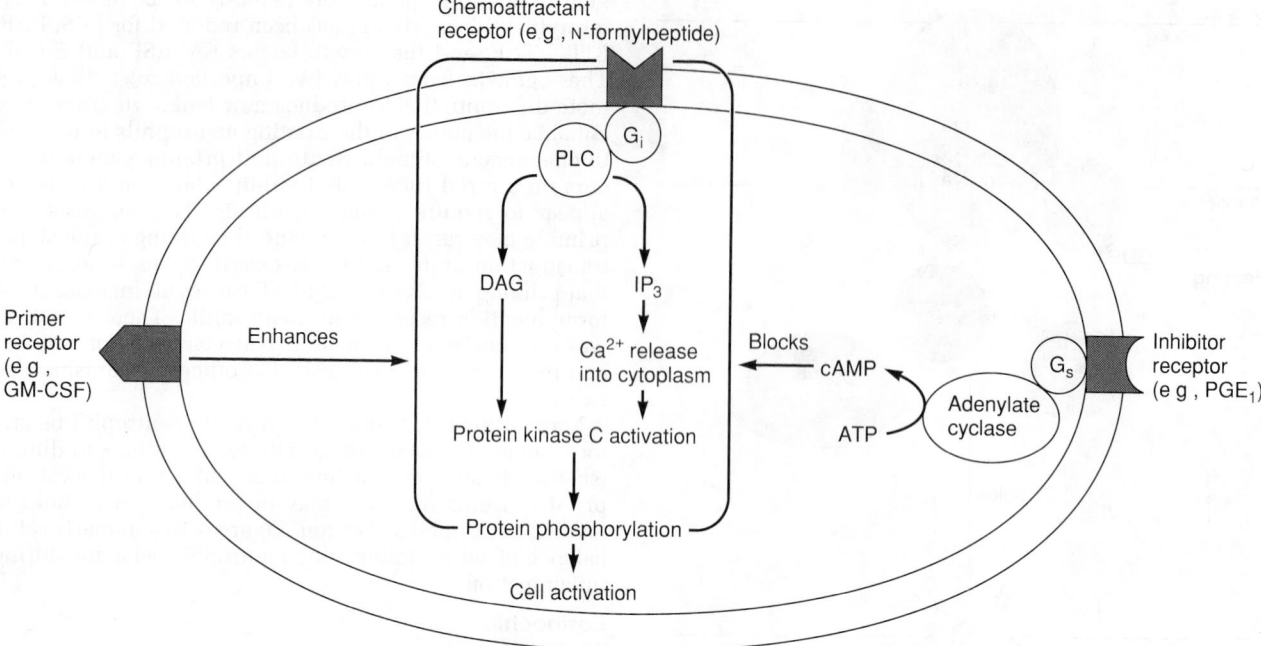

Figure 6-15. Modulation of neutrophil signal transduction pathways. The chemoattractant-mediated signal transduction pathway is enhanced by priming agents, such as granulocyte-macrophage colony-stimulating factor (GM-CSF). The mechanism is not clearly defined, but it may involve an enhanced expression of chemoattractant receptors on the cell surface. The chemoattractant-mediated signal transduction pathway is inhibited by agents such as PGE_1 and β-adrenergic agonists that cause G_s-mediated activation of adenylylcyclase. This inhibition is thought to occur by way of cyclic AMP (cAMP)-mediated phosphorylation events. G_i, G protein that mediates phospholipase C (PLC) activation by chemoattractants; G_S, G protein that stimulates adenylate cyclase; DAG, diacylglycerol; IP_3, inositol 1,4,5-trisphosphate.

Mast Cells

Mast cells are formed from bone marrow precursors that differentiate and proliferate in connective tissue. Numerous similarities exist between mast cells and basophils, although mast cells do not enter the circulation, and basophils do not significantly populate tissues. Mast cell granules contain histamine and proteoglycans. They represent the major source of histamine in most tissues except the stomach and central nervous system. They also function primarily in IgE-mediated immediate hypersensitivity reactions. Although they do not have FMLP receptors, C5a and C3a receptors are present and stimulate histamine release. It has become evident that mast cells release histamine when they are injured. For example, histamine release has been documented in models of rat thermal skin injury, hepatic ischemia–reperfusion injury, rat hepatic ischemia–reperfusion injury, and acute pancreatitis as well as in a human model of ischemia–reperfusion injury. It is hypothesized that histamine causes the activation of xanthine oxidase, which results in increased production of toxic oxygen radicals.[36,37]

Monocytes and Macrophages

The monocyte–macrophage system (collectively referred to as *mononuclear phagocytes*) consists of phagocytic cells scattered throughout the body. Monocytes are derived from precursors that mature in the bone marrow and are released into the circulation. Monocytes migrate into tissue, where they further differentiate into mature macrophages. There are various forms of macrophages, depending on the tissue in which they differentiate. These

include the Kupffer cells of the liver, alveolar macrophages of the lung, and brain microglial cells.

The mononuclear phagocytic cells play numerous effector and modulatory roles in immunity and inflammation (Fig. 6-16). The phagocytic function of macrophages is crucial to removal of senescent cells and cell debris. The release of lysosomal enzymes and oxidants (including the free radical nitric oxide, NO•; see later) during this process may contribute to inflammation. Mononuclear phagocytes are antigen-presenting cells that take up and process foreign proteins and make the processed epitopes available at the cell surface for recognition by and activation of T lymphocytes. These cells are migratory. During acute inflammation, monocytes respond to chemoattractants released during the inflammatory response (eg, PAF, C5a) and are recruited to the site of inflammation. Mononuclear phagocytes respond to inflammatory stimuli by releasing macrophage colony-stimulating factor, GM-CSF, IL-1, and TNF (in addition to a variety of growth factors). These factors induce fibroblasts and endothelial cells to produce cytokines as well. The growth factors ultimately increase the production of mononuclear phagocytes. In addition, several of these factors enhance the ability of effector cells (eg, neutrophils and mononuclear phagocytes) to respond to chemotactic stimuli released at the site of injury. Mononuclear phagocytes produce chemoattractants, such as neutrophil-activating peptide 1, PAF, and LTB_4, which serve to recruit additional leukocytes. Thus, the mononuclear phagocytes are important in initiating and augmenting the cycle of events that results in recruitment and activation of inflammatory cells at sites of inflammation.

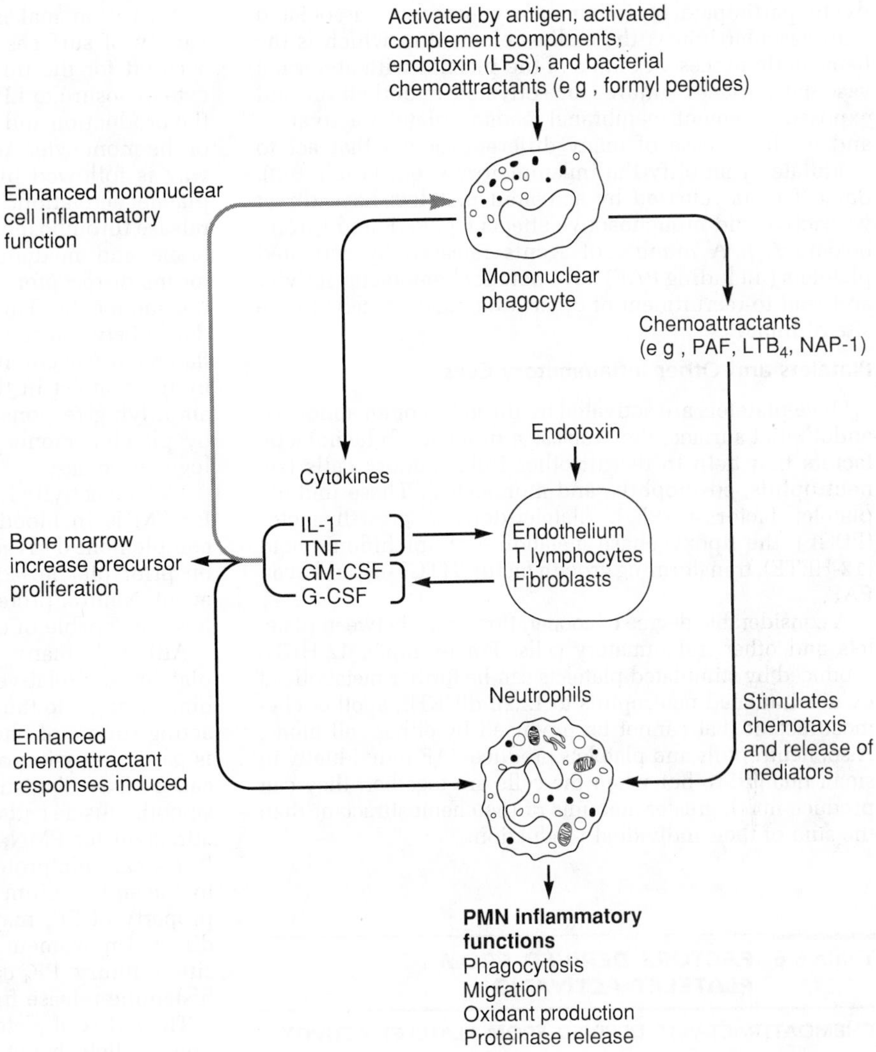

Figure 6-16. The central role of the mononuclear phagocyte in initiating and augmenting the inflammatory response. Activation of mononuclear phagocytes results in the release of neutrophil chemoattractants, growth factors, and interleukins, enhancing the ability of neutrophils to respond to the chemoattractants. In addition, these growth factors and interleukins can modulate the release of additional growth factors from the vascular endothelium, T lymphocytes, and fibroblasts. This function is also produced by endotoxin acting directly on these cells. The growth factors feed back to enhance mononuclear phagocyte function. On a longer time scale, they stimulate myeloid cell differentiation in the bone marrow. LPS, lipopolysaccharide; PAF, platelet-activating factor; NAP-1, neutrophil-activating protein 1; IL-1, interleukin-1; TNF, tumor necrosis factor; GM-CSF, granulocyte macrophage colony-stimulating factor; G-CSF, granulocyte colony-stimulating factor; PMN, polymorphonuclear leukocyte.

Lymphocytes

Lymphocyte responses in inflammation usually involve a much longer, slower time frame than those seen with other inflammatory effector cells (eg, neutrophils), which can manifest within seconds of exposure to a noxious stimulus. An example of this response is delayed hypersensitivity, in which protein antigens injected intradermally in a previously immunized host elicit a local response of induration and erythema that develops over many hours.

A detailed discussion of B- and T-lymphocyte biology is presented in Chapters 14 and 15. The primary role of lymphocytes in inflammation is to orchestrate chronic inflammatory processes. Presentation of processed antigen (eg, digested bacterial products) primarily by macrophages or other antigen-presenting cells to T lymphocytes sets the stage for chronic inflammation.[38] The stimulated T lymphocytes produce cytokines (see earlier discussion and Chap. 5), which further enhance the activity of the antigen-presenting cells. Cytokines also stimulate the differentiation and proliferation of B lymphocytes, and they have the ability to make antigen-specific antibodies. In addition, the stimulated T lymphocytes also can directly injure target cells at sites of inflammation by action of the lymphotoxin TNF-β (one of the cytokines) on cellular DNA.[39]

Platelets

Platelets are anucleated cells derived from megakaryocytes in the bone marrow.[40-42] Their central role in hemostasis is discussed in Chapter 4. This discussion focuses on their function as inflammatory cells, although their role in hemostasis often represents their initial involvement in an acute inflammatory process. Platelets possess a wide array of functions in inflammation, including the following:

- Synthesis and release of vasoactive eicosanoids
- Release of chemotactic factors
- Interaction with other inflammatory cells
- Interaction with endothelial cells
- Adherence to and coating of bacterial and tumor cells
- Increase of vascular permeability

Few of the factors released or the functions carried out by platelets during inflammation are unique to this cell type. Other inflammatory cells often have the same or similar capabilities. Indeed, some platelet functions (eg, adherence to and coating of bacteria or tumor cells) may reflect vestigial functions inherited from a primitive precursor inflammatory cell.

Because of its redundant functions in inflammation, the platelet serves primarily as an amplifier or modulator of the inflammatory response. Platelets are recruited primarily to participate in inflammatory processes associated with vascular injury, the earliest element of which is the hemostatic process. Contact of the platelet with abnormal vascular surfaces (injured or activated endothelium and exposed basement membrane) leads to platelet activation and to the release of many different factors that act to modulate or amplify the inflammatory event (Table 6-6). Some factors released by activated platelets have direct vasoactive and bronchoactive effects (eg, PAF and thromboxane A_2). A number of agents released by activated platelets (including PAF) have potent chemotactic activity and lead to recruitment of other inflammatory cells to the site of injury.

Platelets and Other Inflammatory Cells

Once platelets are activated by thrombin or an abnormal endothelial surface, they release a number of chemotactic factors that help to recruit other inflammatory cells (eg, neutrophils, eosinophils, and monocytes). These include platelet factor 4 (PF_4), platelet-derived growth factor (PDGF), the lipoxygenase metabolite of arachidonic acid (12-HETE), transforming growth factor β (TGF-β), and even PAF.

A considerable degree of cooperation exists between platelets and other inflammatory cells. For example, 12-HETE produced by stimulated platelets can be further metabolized by unstimulated neutrophils to 12,20-diHETE, another chemoattractant that cannot be produced by either cell alone. Also, neutrophils and platelets produce PAF individually in small quantities, but when the cells are together, they can produce much greater amounts of the chemoattractant than the sum of their individual production.

Table 6-6. FACTORS DERIVED FROM PLATELET ACTIVATION

CHEMOATTRACTANTS DERIVED FROM PLATELET ACTIVITY

C5a derived from complement cleavage by neutral proteinases released from activated platelets

Lipids
  12-Hydroxy eicosatetraenoic acid (12-HETE)
  Platelet-activating factor
α-Granule proteins
  Platelet-derived growth factor
  Platelet factor 4

GROWTH FACTORS PRODUCED BY PLATELETS

Transforming growth factors α and β
Fibroblast growth factor
Platelet-derived growth factor

ANTIMICROBIAL ACTIVITY FROM PLATELETS

Cationic bactericidal protein (β lysin)
IgE-mediated oxidant production by platelets directed at schistosomes

VASOACTIVE SUBSTANCES FROM PLATELETS

Vasodilators
  Prostaglandin E_2
  Prostaglandin I_2
Vasoconstrictors
  Prostaglandin $F_{2\alpha}$
  Serotonin
  Platelet-derived growth factor

AGENTS RELEASED BY PLATELETS AND THAT INCREASE VASCULAR PERMEABILITY

Serotonin
Platelet-activating factor
Prostaglandin E_2
Cationic proteins (eg, prostaglandin F_4)

Activation makes platelets adhere more strongly to a variety of surfaces. This phenomenon may in large part account for the thrombocytopenia seen in sepsis. Monocyte exposure to LPS from gram-negative bacteria leads to the production and exposure of tissue factor on the surface of the monocyte. Activation of the extrinsic clotting pathway is followed by thrombin formation and subsequent platelet activation. The thrombin-stimulated platelets then release thrombospondin, which binds to the platelet membrane and mediates platelet binding to monocytes by means of receptors for thrombospondin on the surface of the monocyte. This example illustrates the interdependence between the various cells involved in an acute inflammatory event. It also shows the central place occupied by the platelet in this process and how this type of self-amplifying response (generation of procoagulant activity by platelet–monocyte interaction) might lead to pathologic extremes.

Platelet activity is the primary source of chemoattractant for PMNs in blood and blood clots. Even much of the complement-derived chemotactic activity (C5a) depends on prior platelet activation during the initial hemostatic event. Neutral proteinases released from stimulated platelets are capable of cleaving C5.

Although many of the chemoattractants released by platelets are relatively evanescent, PDGF is stable and can bind strongly to the extracellular matrix, providing a long-acting source of chemoattractant. This property of PDGF is particularly important in relation to wound healing because PDGF also stimulates chemotaxis of fibroblasts and smooth muscle cells (see Chap. 3). Another platelet chemoattractant for PMN, PF_4, has some interesting properties. It is a cationic protein that on release is taken up rapidly by the endothelium and penetrates the vascular wall. This property of PF_4 may be responsible in large part for the directed movement of PMNs through the vessel wall to a site of injury. PF_4 can also act as a stimulatory ligand for histamine release from basophils.

The influx of platelets to sites of injury during inflammation parallels that of PMNs, with the typical peak accumulation occurring 1 to 3 hours after the beginning of injury. Almost every PMN response at the site of inflammation is modulated by the presence of platelets, including enhancement of PMN adherence to the endothelium, augmented release of leukocyte enzymes, increased production of leukocytic inflammatory mediators, and altered oxygen radical generation. Thus, platelets have the ability to augment or decrease PMN-mediated tissue injury. As an example of this relation, platelet lipoxygenase activity can be stimulated by high shear stress, such as might occur during cardiopulmonary bypass or across prosthetic cardiac valves. The precursor of 12-HETE, 12-HPETE, is then released from the stressed platelets, and it in turn can serve as a substrate for PMN synthesis of leukotrienes that induce PMN aggregation and chemotaxis.

Other Inflammatory Activity of Platelets

Bacteria can induce platelet aggregation with fibrin accumulation. Sometimes this phenomenon results in enhanced bacterial phagocytosis by PMNs, but it may also impair phagocytosis. Platelets also aggregate in some malignant diseases and may actually influence the pattern of metastasis of some tumors (enhancement of pulmonary metastases).

Platelets possess IgE receptors on their surfaces and participate to some extent in allergic phenomena. In schistosomiasis, sensitized platelets kill the parasites by the IgE-dependent generation of oxidants. This is further evidence for the pluripotent nature of platelets in their capacity to reproduce so many of the same functions of PMNs and

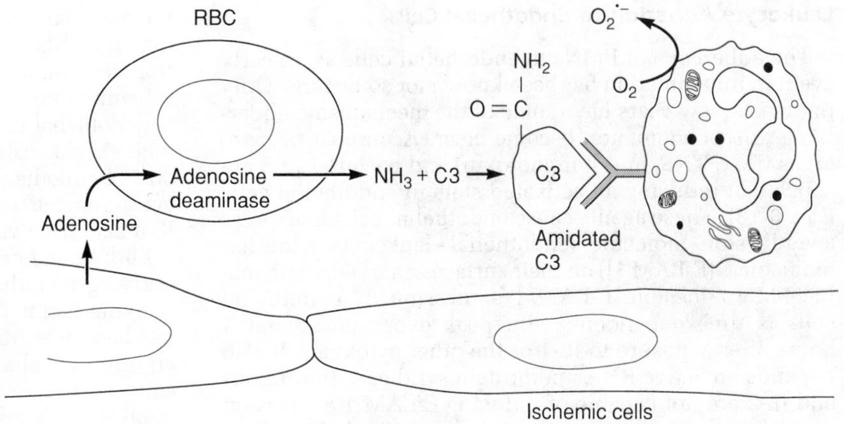

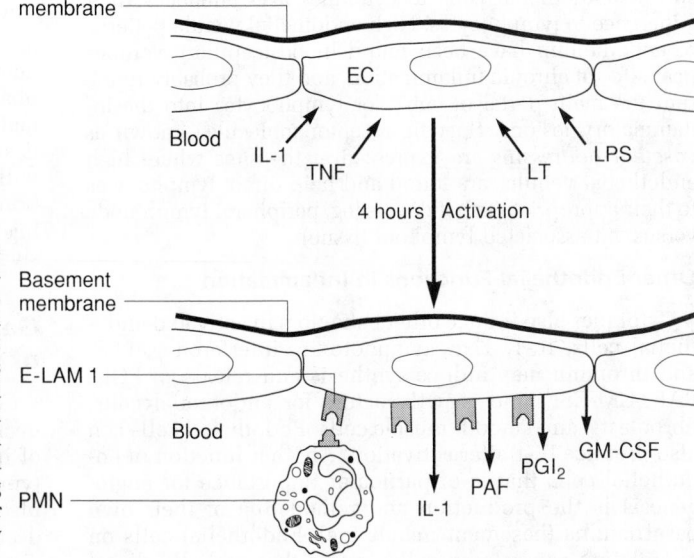

Figure 6-17. Erythrocytes in inflammation. Adenosine released from ischemic cells can be taken up by erythrocytes (RBCs) in the vicinity and deaminated by the RBC enzyme adenosine deaminase. The NH_3 released can then react with the third component of complement (C3) and amidate it. The amidated C3 can substitute for C3b in the alternative pathway of complement activation or bind to receptors on phagocytic cells, activating them.

monocytes. Also, platelet activation appears to occur in allergic asthma and may be a prerequisite for the accumulation of eosinophils in the lung that occurs 24 hours after exposure to an allergen. Platelets, by virtue of their early, crucial involvement in hemostasis, play an important if not central role in modulating the acute inflammatory response, especially at sites of traumatic tissue injury.

Erythrocytes

Although the primary function of the erythrocyte is oxygen transport, two features of red blood cell function may directly influence an acute inflammatory process. Erythrocytes have large quantities of the antioxidant enzymes, superoxide dismutase, and catalase. Erythrocytes may represent a large reservoir of antioxidant activity in whole blood. At sites of acute inflammation where oxidant generation occurs in the presence of hemorrhage, the presence of erythrocytes may help attenuate the deleterious effects of the oxidants on the surrounding tissue.

Another possible role for erythrocytes in the acute inflammatory response after ischemia–reperfusion injury involves adenosine deaminase, the erythrocyte enzyme (Fig. 6-17). Hostetter and Gordon[7] proposed that adenosine re-

leased from ischemic cells is taken up by erythrocytes at the site of ischemic injury. The adenosine is then deaminated by adenosine deaminase, and the NH_3 liberated by the process acts on the third component of complement, C3, to form amidated C3. Amidated C3 is capable of substituting for C3b in the complement activation sequence, thus activating the complement system. It also can bind to complement receptors on phagocytic cells to initiate release of inflammatory mediators, including superoxide anion. These observations provide a role for erythrocytes present at sites of injury where there is hemorrhage as initiators and amplifiers of the inflammatory response.

Vascular Endothelium

Only recently has the active role that the endothelium plays in the inflammatory process been appreciated.[43,44] This discussion focuses on changes in endothelial cells that are induced during the acute inflammatory event. A later section examines the biochemical changes associated with cellular (including endothelial) injury in inflammation. The roles of endothelial cells in wound healing (angiogenesis) and hemostasis are discussed in Chapters 3 and 4, respectively.

Figure 6-18. Endothelial cell (EC) activation and expression of endothelial–leukocyte adhesion molecule 1 (ELAM-1). In response to interleukin-1 (IL-1), tumor necrosis factor (TNF), lymphotoxin (LT), or the lipopolysaccharide of endotoxin (LPS), dramatic changes occur in the vascular endothelium. Four hours after exposure to these agents, endothelial cells express ELAM-1 on their surfaces, which leads to marked enhancement of neutrophil (PMN) adhesion to endothelial cells. Also as a part of the activation process, endothelial cells release IL-1, platelet-activating factor (PAF), PGI_2, and the cytokine granulocyte-macrophage colony-stimulating factor (GM-CSF). These changes in endothelial cell behavior play an important role in directing the traffic of inflammatory cells to a site of injury.

Leukocyte Adhesion to Endothelial Cells

The adherence of PMNs to endothelial cells as an early event in inflammation has been known for some time. Only in the past few years have some of the mechanisms underlying this phenomenon become clear. A number of cytokines (IL-1, TNF, and lymphotoxin) and bacterial LPS are capable of inducing an activated state in endothelial cells (Fig. 6-18). These agents cause endothelial cells to express an adhesion molecule (endothelial–leukocyte adhesion molecule 1 [E-LAM 1]) on their surfaces, markedly enhancing PMN adhesion. E-LAM 1 expression by endothelial cells is time dependent, with peak expression about 4 hours after exposure to IL-1 or the other cytokines. It also depends on active RNA and protein synthesis. Interferons and IL-2 are not capable of inducing E-LAM 1 expression by endothelial cells. The monoclonal antibody H18/7 reacts with E-LAM 1 effectively to block PMN–endothelial adhesion.

An important difference between E-LAM 1 and other adhesive proteins (eg, platelet glycoproteins IIb and IIIa; intercellular adhesion molecule 1, and HLA-DR) that may also be expressed on endothelial surfaces is that E-LAM 1 is *only* expressed *after* stimulation of the endothelial cells. The expression is usually of a transient nature in association with the pathologic process that initiates the production or release of the endothelial activators. The same cytokines (eg, IL-1, TNF, lymphotoxin) that induce expression of E-LAM 1 on endothelial cell surfaces also stimulate endothelial procoagulant activity. By initiation of the coagulation cascade, endothelial cells can indirectly act to stimulate platelets and then other leukocytes, increasing the adherence of inflammatory effector cells to endothelium. The expression of procoagulant activity and E-LAM 1 activity by endothelial cells may provide the crucial signals that direct phagocytic cell traffic out of the circulation into a site of injury.

High Endothelial Venules and Lymphocytes

The term *high endothelial venules* refers to specialized postcapillary venules that contain enlarged, cuboidal (high) endothelial cells. Lymphocytes bind to high endothelial venules in frozen tissue sections of lymphoid organs and other lymphoid tissues. High endothelial venules are thought to be central to the process of lymphocyte homing to lymph nodes and lymphoid tissues.[45,46] Ultrastructural analysis of high endothelial venules has demonstrated endothelial changes consistent with an activated metabolic state. Exposure of endothelial cells to cytokines also enhances their adherence to lymphocytes. High endothelial venule patterns of endothelium have been found in postcapillary venules near sites of chronic inflammation, and they probably represent the main portal of entry for lymphocytes into the inflammatory lesions. Specific receptor molecules known as *vascular addressins* are expressed at the sites where high endothelial venules are found and help direct lymphocytes to their appropriate target organs (eg, peripheral lymph node versus gut-associated lymphoid tissue).

Other Endothelial Functions in Inflammation

Cytokines also induce other behaviors in activated endothelial cells. IL-1, TNF, lymphotoxin, interferon-γ, LPS, and thrombin may induce synthesis and release of PGI_2, PAF, GM-CSF, and growth factors for endothelial cells, fibroblasts, and smooth muscle cells. Endothelial cells can also produce IL-1 after activation. Another function of endothelial cells that is of particular importance for angiogenesis is the production and remodeling of their own basal lamina (basement membrane). Endothelial cells on stimulation can release collagenases that partially digest the basal lamina and allow new vessel growth. This function may also enhance the egress of inflammatory cells from the circulation through the endothelium during acute inflammation.

Endothelial cells play a major role in regulating vascular tone. Angiotensin-converting enzyme is present on the surface of endothelial cells. In addition to its function of converting angiotensin I to the active vasoconstrictor angiotensin II, it also inactivates the potent inflammogen, bradykinin.

Endothelial cells also exert regulatory effects on the underlying smooth muscle by means of endothelium-derived relaxing factor (EDRF) and a peptide, endothelin. EDRF has been identified with NO•, a free radical generated by arginine metabolism. It exerts potent relaxant effects locally on the vessel wall. Endothelin is a 21–amino acid peptide with potent vasoconstrictive properties that appear to balance the effect of EDRF. Both agents play important physiologic roles in determining the distribution of blood flow, which can have significant effects on the magnitude of a local inflammatory response.

The enzyme nitric oxide synthase (NOS), which generates NO• from the terminal guanidinonitrogen of L-arginine, has three isoforms based on molecular weight and other characteristics.[47] Types I (brain) and III (endothelium) are constitutively expressed. Type II (macrophages) is the inducible form and plays an important role in mediating the pathologic host response to the LPS of endotoxin.

The main effect of constitutively generated, low levels of NO• is to activate cellular processes (eg, regulation of protein phosphorylation) through stimulation of the enzyme guanylyl cyclase to produce cGMP. Induction of type II NOS in macrophages after LPS exposure can lead to high levels of local NO• production throughout the vascular system, resulting in severe hypotension in endotoxin shock, apparently due to direct effects of NO• on vascular smooth muscle.

Under unusual circumstances, endothelial cells can exhibit macrophage-like properties in that they can act as antigen-presenting cells and also phagocytose particles. They may also be a significant source of oxidants in inflammatory reactions after ischemic insults. Endothelial cells are not passive participants in inflammatory processes; rather, they can direct and focus many aspects of an inflammatory event.

CELLULAR INJURY IN INFLAMMATION

A major effect of the inflammatory cascade is cellular injury and death. This may be beneficial, as in the neutrophil-mediated destruction of invading bacteria or phagocytic killing of tumor cells. It may be harmful if the main force of the inflammatory response is directed at host tissues. Tissue injury and organ dysfunction associated with inflammation after multiple trauma, major operations, or acute ischemic events account for an ever-increasing portion of the morbidity and mortality seen in intensive care units.

General Characteristics of Cell Injury and Death

Cell death usually results from one of two processes: (1) necrosis, a pathologic form of death that occurs as a result of injury; or (2) apoptosis.[48] Injury leading to necrosis is typically associated with cellular swelling and loss of plasma membrane integrity. Apoptosis is the form of cell death characterized by a morphologic pattern of nuclear fragmentation and condensation associated with cell shrinkage.

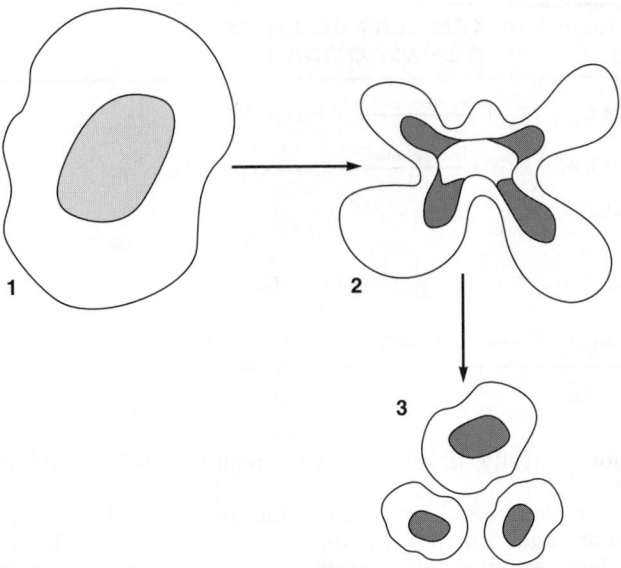

Figure 6-19. Schematic depiction of a cell (1) undergoing apoptosis. Chromatin condensation and DNA fragmentation (2) are followed rapidly by cellular shrinkage and blebbing, leading to the formation of multiple smaller apoptotic bodies (3). Colored portions of 2 and 3 represent condensed, fragmented chromatin.

This ultimately leads to fragmentation of the cell into many smaller, membrane-enclosed fragments (apoptotic bodies) that contain portions of the fragmented chromatin (Fig. 6-19). The apoptotic bodies retain intact plasma membranes for some time and are phagocytized in vivo by neighboring cells. Typically, apoptotic cell death is not accompanied by the inflammatory response seen with necrosis.

A wide variety of stimuli can induce the apoptotic process, including physiologic and pathologic stimuli (Table 6-7). Many of the pathologic agents that at low concentrations induce apoptosis in a given cell cause necrosis in the same cell at higher concentrations.

A fairly uniform sequence of events leads to necrotic cell death, and a wide variety of injurious agents may exert their toxic effects on cells through key pathways. Key elements in cellular function that have been identified as crucial to survival include the ATP synthetic pathways and maintenance of ion gradients across the plasma membrane.[49,50] Na^+ and K^+ normally have a reciprocal relation with their intracellular and extracellular concentrations (K^+ is high within cells and low in the plasma, whereas Na^+ is the reverse). This relation helps create the electrical potential difference that exists across the plasma membrane of viable cells. The intracellular (cytosolic) Ca^{2+} concentration is 10,000-fold less than that outside the cell. A number of cellular functions (eg, adherence) and intracellular enzyme systems require the presence of Ca^{2+}. Elevation of cytosolic Ca^{2+} levels more than 1 μmol/L above the normal range of about 100 to 200 nmol/L is associated with a number of important effects, including fragmentation and depolymerization of microtubules. This leads to morphologic changes, activation of phospholipase A_2, and degradation and destabilization of the phospholipid bilayer with the formation of lysophospholipids. Failure of ATP synthesis in injured cells not only limits energy available for biosynthetic and repair processes but also limits the function of the membrane ATPases responsible for maintaining the ion gradients. The combination of elevated cytosolic Ca^{2+} and depleted energy stores then work

together rapidly to collapse the transmembrane electrical potential and destroy membrane integrity. The result is cell death. Considerable controversy exists concerning the precise role of Ca^{2+} elevations in cell death. Some work supports a central role for Ca^{2+}, and other work suggests that it may represent an epiphenomenon.[49] Activation of a Ca^{2+}-dependent endonuclease by elevation of intranuclear Ca^{2+}, with the resultant fragmentation of DNA, has been postulated to play a critical role in apoptotic cell death.[51] This hypothesis may also help clarify the role that changes in intracellular Ca^{2+} homeostasis may play in cellular injury. With the accumulation of data from a number of laboratories using different models of cellular injury, it is clear that generalizations regarding cell death have limited usefulness, and mechanistic descriptions should be focused on a particular model and injurious agent.

An important concept that has been applied to cellular injury comes from extensive work with the response of cells to thermal stress.[52] Not only are there molecular lesions (eg, denatured proteins) produced within cells as a result of thermal stress or other forms of injury (eg, oxidant stress), but the cellular response to this stress involves a highly coordinated synthesis of a number of proteins of different molecular weight, the most prominent of which are a series of proteins of about 70 kd, which help to confer protection from a subsequent stress. Although the specific proteins induced vary with the particular stress (eg, heat shock versus oxidant exposure or hypoxia), there are sufficient common features to the responses that cross protection may be seen (Table 6-8). Some antioxidant proteins are induced as part of the stress response.[53] The precise

Table 6-7. STIMULI OF APOPTOSIS

PHYSIOLOGIC
Normal development
Removal of trophic factors
Steroid hormones
Spontaneous (some tumors)
Cytotoxic T lymphocytes
Tumor necrosis factor

PATHOLOGIC
Ischemia, oxidant stress
Ultraviolet and x-irradiation
Thermal stress (hyperthermia and hypothermia)
Anticancer agents
Agents that disrupt the cytoskeleton
Human immunodeficiency virus infection (lymphocytes)

Table 6-8. STRESS PROTEINS AND THEIR PRIMARY INDUCERS

Stress Proteins	Inducers
Heat-shock protein (HSP) groups HSP (110, 90, 70, 65 kd) Small HSPs (20–28 kd)	Thermal stress
Glucose-regulated proteins (GRPs) GRP (78, 96 kd)	Glucose starvation
Ubiquitin (8 kd)	Degraded proteins
Metallothioneins	Heavy metals (eg, Zn^{2+}, Ca^{2+}, Hg^{2+}, cd^{2+})
Oxidant-related stress proteins Superoxide dismutase (Mn-SOD; 90 kd)	Oxidant stress (also thermal stress)
Heme oxygenase (32 kd)	

role this response plays in modulating the acute features of oxidant injury is not clear.

Some stress proteins have the ability to bind ATP.[54] ATP has been noted to play a role in the association of stress proteins (particularly of the 70-kd series of proteins) with unfolded (denatured) or newly synthesized proteins.[55,56] Because dissociation of the stress proteins from unfolded proteins requires hydrolysis of ATP, it has been hypothesized that under ATP-depleted conditions, the stressed cell perceives a decrease in the level of free, unassociated stress protein, and this leads to initiation of the stress response. Thus, the energy status (ATP level) within a cell may play an important role in coordinating the cellular response to stress.

Oxidants and Cellular Injury

Humans live by oxygen-dependent cellular respiration, and yet oxygen, the necessary, central element of aerobic life, may also provide the means of death. Abundant evidence has implicated a number of reactive species of oxygen (oxidants) as sources of tissue injury in inflammation.[57,58] Normally, cellular respiration involves the four-electron reduction of oxygen to water. Reactive oxygen species represent intermediate stages in this process and under some circumstances may be released from a dysfunctional electron transport chain in the mitochondria to cause cellular injury. Most of the reactive O_2 species implicated in inflammatory tissue injury are probably generated by different mechanisms (Table 6-9). Some oxidants are free radicals. Free radicals are chemical species that have an unpaired electron, usually designated as •; for example, superoxide anion, a one-electron reduction product of oxygen, is designated as $O_2^{\bullet-}$. Oxidants that are free radicals have been implicated as the initiators of free radical chain reactions involving unsaturated fatty acids in the lipid bilayer of cell membranes. In much the same manner as the rancidification of fat, an initial attack of a fatty acid side chain by a free radical can lead to a self-propagating chain of reactions after formation of a lipid peroxide. This series of lipid oxidations theoretically can lead to disruption of the lipid bilayer with cell lysis. It is not entirely clear how often this mechanism of injury predominates as the source of lytic events because of the difficulties inherent in measuring the highly reactive free radicals and the products of their attack. It has been shown, however, that supplementation of endothelial cells in vitro with saturated and monounsaturated fatty acids, thereby decreasing the amount of polyunsaturated fatty acids within cellular membranes, markedly enhances cellular resistance to oxidant stress.[59] This observation may have real significance for designing the most beneficial type of lipid supplement

Table 6-9. OXIDANTS GENERATED IN INFLAMMATION

$$O_2 + 1e^- \xrightarrow[\text{oxidase}]{\text{NADPH}} O_2^{\bullet-} \qquad \text{Superoxide anion}$$

$$2H^+ + O_2^{\bullet-} + O_2^{\bullet-} \xrightarrow[\text{or superoxide dismutase}]{\text{spontaneous}} O_2 + H_2O_2 \qquad \text{Hydrogen peroxide}$$

$$H_2O_2 + Fe^{2+} \longrightarrow Fe^{3+} + OH^- + OH\bullet \qquad \text{Hydroxyl radical}$$

$$H_2O_2 + Cl^- + H^+ \xrightarrow{\text{myeloperoxidase}} H_2O + HOCl \qquad \text{Hypochlorous acid}$$

$$R'RNH + HOCl \longrightarrow H_2O + R'RNCl \qquad \text{Chloramines}$$

Table 6-10. CELLULAR DEFENSES AGAINST OXIDANTS

$$H_2O_2 + 2\ GSH \xrightarrow{\pm GSH\ peroxidase} 2\ H_2O + GSSG$$

$$ROOH + 2\ GSH \xrightarrow{GSH\ peroxidase} ROH + GSSG + H_2O$$

$$GSSG \xrightarrow[GSH\ reductase]{NADPH} 2\ GSH$$

$$O_2^{\bullet-} + O_2^{\bullet-} + 2H^+ \xrightarrow[\text{dismutase}]{\text{superoxide}} O_2 + H_2O_2$$

$$2H_2O_2 \xrightarrow{catalase} 2H_2O + O_2$$

for critically ill patients who require total parenteral nutrition.

Oxidants are also capable of attacking many other molecular targets, including amino acids in proteins and DNA. Many enzymes have cysteine or methionine residues (sulfur-containing amino acids) at their active sites. These amino acids are vulnerable to oxidative attack at the sulfur group, which may lead to inactivation and loss of potentially crucial function. Hydrogen peroxide (H_2O_2) can inactivate the glycolytic enzyme, glyceraldehyde 3-phosphate dehydrogenase (GAPDH) by oxidative attack on cysteine-149, which is located at its active site.[60] Inhibition of GAPDH blocks the generation of ATP from the catabolism of glucose through substrate-level phosphorylation in the distal glycolytic pathway as well as through mitochondrial respiration. As a result, ATP levels fall in injured cells after exposure to H_2O_2. Other biochemical events that occur in cells after oxidant exposure include the following: (1) rapid DNA strand breakage with activation of the nuclear enzyme poly (ADP-ribose) polymerase, (2) reduction of cellular NAD levels, (3) activation of the GSH redox cycle, (4) loss of intracellular Ca^{2+} regulation, and (5) profound changes in the organization of the cytoskeleton. Disruption of microfilaments (one of the main constituents of the cytoskeleton) appears to be directly related to the reduction in ATP levels after injury.[61]

Cells have evolved a variety of ways to deal with reactive oxygen species (Table 6-10). Some of the major elements in this system include the enzymes superoxide dismutase, catalase, GSH peroxidase, and GSH reductase. Catalase is probably the major means of H_2O_2 removal in most cells. Sensitivity to H_2O_2 is inversely related to cellular catalase activity. GSH, a three–amino acid peptide, has a number of functions within cells, but probably its most important role is to defend against oxidant attack. Although GSH can interact with H_2O_2 or other peroxides (eg, lipid peroxides) either directly or by way of the catalysis of GSH peroxidase, its major role in oxidant defense may be in protection and reduction of oxidizable sulfhydryl groups on proteins within the cell. During a massive oxidant attack, considerable-S-S-cross-linking of structural and functional proteins occurs, which may lead to cell death secondary to loss of important cytoskeletal functions. GSH-mediated reduction of these oxidized and cross-linked proteins may play a crucial role in the repair of oxidative damage in surviving cells.

Other oxidants are notable for their rapid reactivity, which alters the pattern of injury seen when they are the predominant oxidant. Hydroxyl radical (OH•) is so reactive it is difficult to measure. It is usually formed in the presence of reduced iron (Fe^{2+}; see Table 6-9) and may actually be the species responsible for initiating the DNA strand breakage seen in H_2O_2 injury.[62] Hypochlorous acid (HOCl), generated from H_2O_2 by the neutrophil enzyme myeloperoxidase, is also highly reactive and primarily targets the cell membrane, apparently killing cells by producing holes in the plasma membrane.[63] Peroxynitrite ($ONOO^-$), formed by the interaction of $NO^{\bullet}$ with $O_2^{\bullet-}$, has been implicated as a potential source of $NO^{\bullet}$-associated toxicity in inflammatory lung injury.[64] Other, less reactive, stable chlorinated oxidants (chloramines) are also thought to play a physiologic role in bacterial destruction by neutrophils.[65]

In addition to having potent toxic effects on cells, there is evidence that low levels of oxidants (eg, 30 to 100 μM H_2O_2) can act as important intracellular signals during inflammation.[66] Activation of cytokine gene expression in lymphocytes depends on release of the nuclear transcription factor NF-κB from an inhibitory subunit in the cytosol, IκB. This process can be induced by low levels of H_2O_2. Furthermore, when antioxidants are added to lymphocytes exposed to ligands that normally activate cytokine gene expression through NF-κB, the activation of NF-κB is blocked. These observations have provided strong evidence in support of the concept that nuclear transcription factors like NF-κB may depend on relatively subtle changes in the cellular redox potential for their activity.

Proteinases in Inflammation: Synergism With Oxidants

Phagocytic proteinases (especially neutrophil elastase) have been implicated as important mediators of tissue injury in inflammation.[65] The proteolytic activity that makes it possible for neutrophils to migrate between endothelial cells on their way out of blood vessels is apparently also capable of injuring endothelial cells. According to in vitro studies, elastase can cause cells to detach from surfaces, decrease the barrier function of cell monolayers, and even kill cells. The mechanism of proteolytic killing of cells is unclear, although a direct attack on integral membrane proteins, resulting in altered permeability of the plasma membrane, may account for the toxicity.

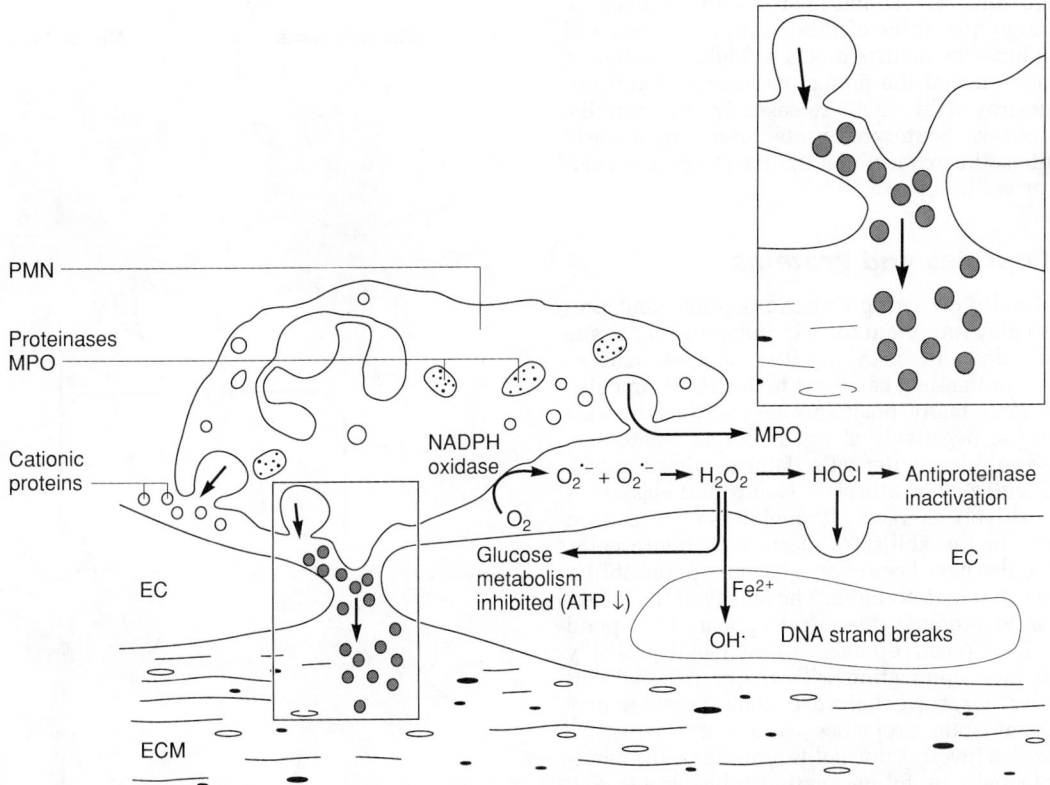

Figure 6-20. Phagocyte-derived mediators of inflammatory tissue injury. Polymorphonuclear leukocytes (PMNs) produce three major types of toxic agents involved in inflammatory tissue injury—oxidants, proteinases, and cationic proteins. An NADPH-oxidase enzyme system at the plasma membrane can produce $O_2^{\bullet-}$ by a one-electron reduction of O_2. Two of the $O_2^{\bullet-}$ molecules can react spontaneously or by the catalysis of superoxide dismutase to form H_2O_2. H_2O_2 can react with halide ions (Cl^-) in the presence of the neutrophil enzyme myeloperoxidase (MPO) to form hypochlorous acid (HOCl), or it can be reduced by Fe^{2+} in the target endothelial cell (EC) to the very reactive free radical species $OH^{\bullet}$. H_2O_2 is capable of damaging membrane lipids and some cellular enzymes (eg, glyceraldehyde 3-phosphate dehydrogenase, leading to inhibition of ATP synthesis). It can also disrupt intracellular Ca^{2+} homeostasis. The $OH^{\bullet}$ radical can produce DNA strand breaks in target cells, and HOCl appears to play an important role in oxidatively inactivating the plasma antiproteinases responsible for protecting the endothelium and extracellular matrix (ECM) from PMN-derived proteinases like elastase. Positively charged cationic proteins and peptides released by PMN are also thought to mediate damage to endothelial cells by virtue of their electrostatic effects on cellular membranes. (*Inset*) Controlled or limited release by degranulation of PMN proteinases at intercellular junctions may be involved in creating a path for PMN migration between endothelial cells and through the extracellular matrix to a site of inflammation outside of a blood vessel.

In the tissue destruction seen in acute inflammation, a close synergism has been proposed between neutrophil-derived oxidants and proteinases.[65] Of the 20 or more enzymes present in neutrophil granules, 3 are thought to have the greatest ability to cause tissue injury—serine proteinase elastase and two metalloproteinases, gelatinase and collagenase. These 3 enzymes can attack specific components of the extracellular matrix. The extracellular matrix, which is located underneath the endothelium and other epithelial surfaces as well as surrounding connective tissue cells, is made up of a complicated mixture of proteoglycans, glycoproteins, collagens, and elastin. The extracellular matrix plays a crucial function in regulating the morphology, pattern of growth and movement, and differentiation of the overlying cells. It may also be an important part of the normal capillary permeability barrier. Several effective plasma proteinase inhibitors oppose neutrophil-derived proteolytic activity, including α_1-PI, α_2-macroglobulin, and secretory leukoproteinase inhibitor. The most important inhibitor of neutrophil elastase is α_1-PI. The chlorinated oxidant HOCl can effectively inactivate α_1-PI by oxidation of a methionine residue. This oxidative inactivation makes the antiproteinase susceptible to proteolytic cleavage and irreversible inactivation.[67] Because plasma has large quantities of these antiproteinases and the HOCl produced by neutrophils is so highly reactive, it has been proposed that the protective barrier of antiproteinases is destroyed by HOCl released by neutrophils, which then allows neutrophil proteinases (particularly elastase) to attack the extracellular matrix and perhaps cellular targets as well.

Cationic Peptides and Proteins

Several naturally occurring cationic peptides and proteins may also play important roles in inflammatory tissue injury.[68] Molecules with many positive charges, such as polylysine and protamine, can exert toxic effects on cells. By virtue of their many positive charges, they interact strongly with the negatively charged plasma membrane. They may also be able to enter cells, damage mitochondria, and interfere with ATP synthesis.[69] Neutrophil elastase is also highly positively charged, although it is unclear what role this plays in the ability of elastase to injure cells. Cationic molecules have been shown to cause permeability changes in vascular endothelium. The ability of the different molecules to produce this effect appears to depend on the amount of positive charge present and probably represents an ionic interaction with the endothelial cell surface. Smaller phagocyte-derived cationic peptides may have natural antibiotic properties as potent bactericidal agents. This area of investigation holds promise for the development of potentially useful new antimicrobial agents. Figure 6-20 provides an overview of the various phagocyte-derived mediators of cellular injury and their roles in inflammatory tissue injury.

Other Mediators of Injury in Inflammation

In addition to the phagocyte-derived mediators of tissue injury described earlier, other factors are involved in inflammatory tissue injury. Some of these act independently of and others synergistically with the phagocyte-derived factors to kill cells. The complement system has already been described. It represents a system that can independently lyse cells by formation of the membrane attack complex (C5b-9) but that also can amplify tissue injury by recruitment and activation of neutrophils by C5a release.

TNF-α and TNF-β (lymphotoxin) released by cytolytic T lymphocytes may mediate cell killing by inducing DNA fragmentation in target cells.[39]

Ischemia, the loss of oxygen and substrate delivery to cells, represents a type of injury that is often discussed separately from inflammation. Where inflammation is present, however, it is highly likely that some element of ischemia is also present, and the reverse is true as well. Because the coagulation cascade is so intimately associated with inflammation, it would be almost impossible to imagine a major inflammatory event occurring without some associated vascular thrombosis and resultant ischemia. Also, at the time of restoration of blood flow to ischemic tissue (reperfusion), there is evidence that considerable inflammatory injury develops and is largely derived from oxidants generated in the reperfused tissue[70] (see Chap. 74). Evidence suggests that reperfused ischemic endothelium can generate $O_2^{\bullet-}$ during the conversion of hypoxanthine to xanthine and xanthine to uric acid by way of xanthine oxidase present in endothelial cells. During a period of ischemia, the enzyme xanthine dehydrogenase

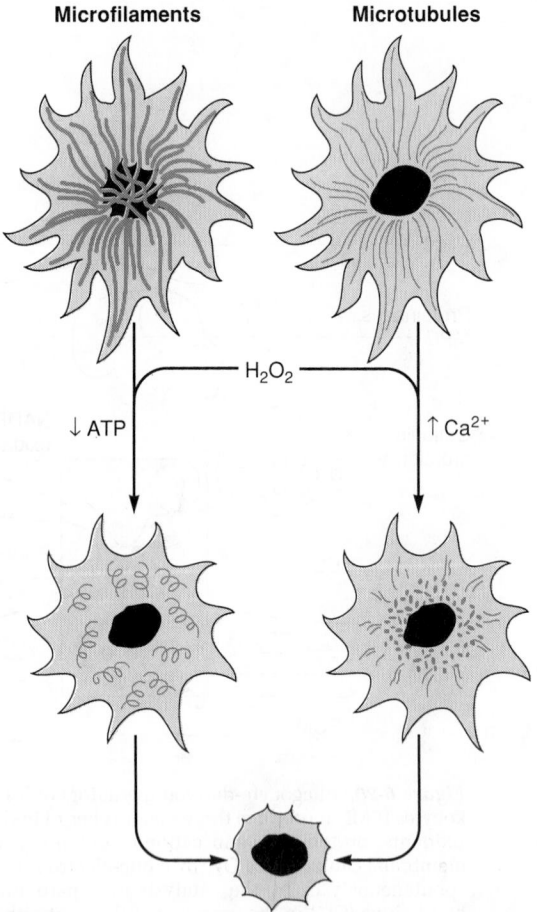

Figure 6-21. Interplay of metabolic factors and cytoskeletal structures that alters cellular morphology in oxidant injury. Diagram of metabolic changes and associated effects on cytoskeletal structures and cellular morphology induced by H_2O_2 injury to endothelial cells. Changes in microfilament (stress fiber) organization after H_2O_2-induced decline in ATP levels are shown on the left. Microtubule depolymerization occurring after H_2O_2-induced elevation of the intracellular Ca^{2+} concentration is depicted on the right. The combination of both events leads to cell rounding and loss of normal morphology. (After Hinshaw DB, Burger JM, Armstrong BC, Hyslop PA. Mechanism of endothelial cell shape change in oxidant injury. J Surg Res 1989;46:339).

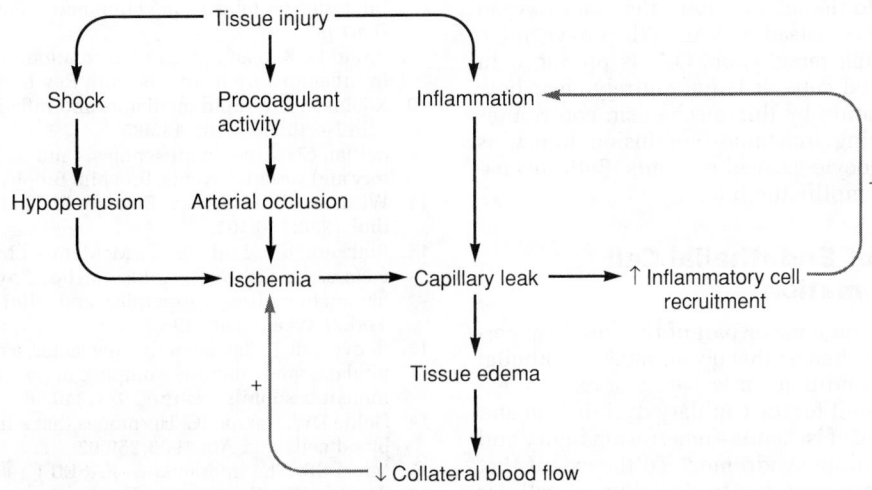

Figure 6-22. Cycle of organ dysfunction in inflammatory tissue injury. Tissue injury can lead to the expression of procoagulant (tissue factor) activity, followed by activation of the coagulation cascade and subsequent vascular occlusion. Ischemia may then develop, leading to capillary leak. Massive tissue injury with shock can produce global ischemic changes associated with hypoperfusion of multiple organs. Concomitant activation of inflammatory cascades (eg, complement activation, kinin formation, and generation and release of cytokines) can also lead to capillary leak secondary to the various mediators described in the text. The capillary leak in turn accentuates the inflammatory process by allowing greater accumulation of inflammatory cells at the site of the leak. Also, the associated tissue edema further exacerbates the hypoperfusion and ischemia by compromising collateral blood flow, establishing a vicious cycle.

Figure 6-23. Homeostasis of inflammatory mediators. Many relatively common clinical situations, such as exposure of blood to extracorporeal membranes (eg, dialysis, cardiopulmonary bypass), lead to activation of inflammatory pathways (eg, the alternative complement pathway). Activation of these pathways results in the generation of mediators (eg, anaphylatoxins) that produce a number of physiologic and cellular effects. Under most circumstances, all affected parameters normalize rapidly, with no persistent adverse effect on the organism. The actual determinants that convert typically transient phenomena into persistent responses leading to organ dysfunction and failure are still poorly understood. LPS, lipopolysaccharide.

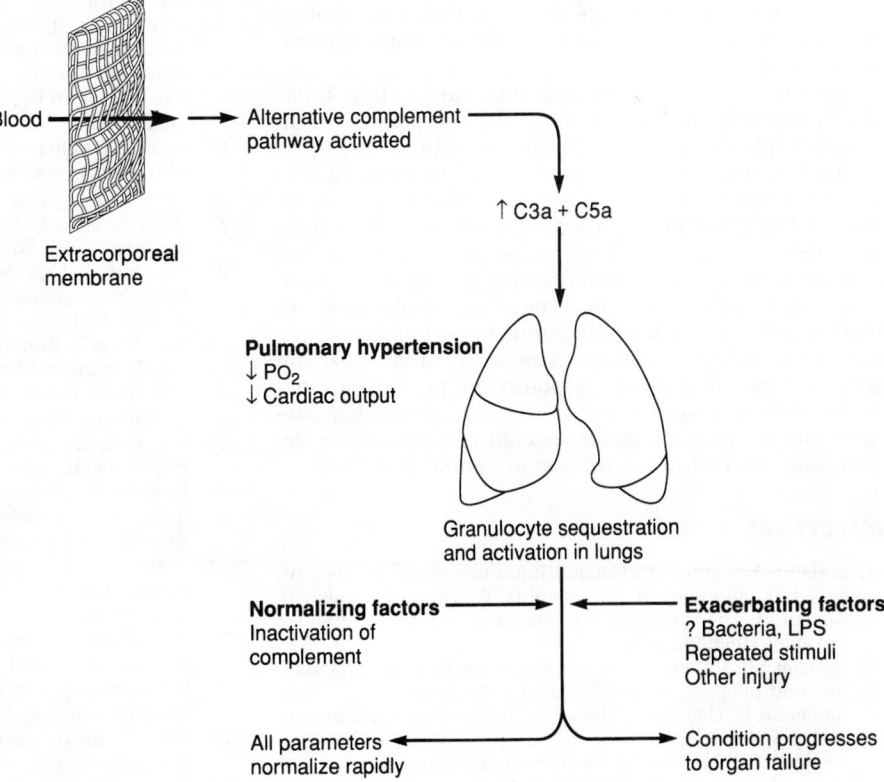

undergoes cleavage to the oxidase form that uses oxygen as an electron acceptor instead of NAD. When oxygen becomes available during reperfusion, $O_2^{\bullet-}$ is produced in the injured endothelial cells. It is not entirely clear how much oxidant generation by this mechanism contributes to tissue injury during ischemia–reperfusion injury as compared with phagocyte-derived oxidants. Both mechanisms may serve to amplify the injury.

Consequences of Endothelial Cell Injury in Inflammation

Endothelial cells form a major part of the capillary permeability barrier. The changes that occur in the endothelial cytoskeleton under conditions of ischemia or oxidant exposure probably account for the capillary dysfunction and leak seen in the setting of ischemia–reperfusion injury and the multiple organ failure syndrome.[50] To the extent that the cytoskeletal changes are due to depletion of cellular energy stores in ischemia, the changes may be reversible. Once the level of Ca^{2+} in the cytosol exceeds 1 μmol/L, the microtubule depolymerization that occurs in combination with the ATP-dependent disruption of microfilament architecture leads to a complete loss of normal endothelial morphology that is probably irreversible (Fig. 6-21).

Histamine is an inflammatory mediator that exerts a transient effect on postcapillary venular endothelium, producing local capillary leak and tissue edema. Its effect on the permeability of the endothelium is thought to be mediated by the transient changes it induces in endothelial morphology. Some breakdown products of fibrinogen may also alter the cytoskeleton of endothelial cells.

Whether the capillary leak is transient or of greater duration, the resultant edema can disrupt the normal pattern of function of most tissues involved. In the lung, such injury interferes with gas exchange. In the heart and other organs, the edema limits collateral blood flow, further reducing oxygen and substrate delivery, thus exacerbating the ischemic injury. Some of these concepts are summarized in Figure 6-22.

Figure 6-23 provides a schematic summary of the interplay between the humoral and cellular components of inflammation in one clinically relevant situation—exposure of blood elements to extracorporeal membranes (eg, hemodialysis, cardiopulmonary bypass).[71] Under most circumstances, the inflammatory cascade initiated by situations like these is aborted without tissue injury. It is unclear why the same apparent stimulus that evokes a minor inflammatory response in one person can create havoc in another and lead to the full gamut of pathologic events seen in multiple organ failure. The ability of the organism to control its inflammatory response and produce limited but effective responses to various external threats (eg, bacteria) may represent a major element responsible for determining survival in the process of natural selection.

REFERENCES

1. Bellanti A, Kadlec JV. General immunobiology. In: Ballanti JA, ed. Immunology III. Philadelphia, WB Saunders, 1985:16.
2. Kushner I. The acute phase response: an overview. Methods Enzymol 1988;163:373.
3. Dowton SB, Colten HR. Acute phase reactants in inflammation and infection. Semin Hematol 1988;25:84.
4. Baumann H, Gauldie J. The acute phase response. Immunol Today 1994;15:74.
5. Kaplan AP, Silverberg M. Mediators of inflammation: an overview. Methods Enzymol 1988;163:3.
6. Deitch, EA, Mancini, MC. Complement receptors in shock and transplantation. Arch Surg 1993;128:1222.
7. Hostetter MK, Gordon DL. Biochemistry of C3 and related thiolester proteins in infection and inflammation. Rev Infect Dis 1987;9:97.
8. Proud D, Kaplan AP. Kinin formation: mechanisms and role in inflammatory disorders. Ann Rev Immunol 1988;6:49.
9. Robinson DR. Lipid mediators and inflammation. Rheum Dis Clin North Am 1987;13:385.
10. Serhan CN. Lipoxin biosynthesis and its impact in inflammatory and vascular events. Biochim Biophys Acta. 1994;1212:1.
11. Williams KI, Higgs GA. Eicosanoids and inflammation. J Pathol 1988;156:101.
12. Pinckard RN, Ludwig JC, McManus LM. Platelet-activating factors. In: Gallin JI, Goldstein IM, Snyderman R, eds. Inflammation: basic principles and clinical correlates. New York, Raven, 1988:139.
13. Benveniste J. Platelet-activating factor, a new mediator of anaphylaxis and immune complex deposition from rabbit and human basophils. Nature 1974;249:581.
14. Golde DW, Gasson JC. Hormones that stimulate the growth of blood cells. Sci Am 1988;259:62.
15. Mizel SB. The interleukins. FASEB J 1989;3:2379.
16. Bainton DF. Phagocytic cells: developmental biology of neutrophils and eosinophils. In: Gallin JI, Goldstein IM, Snyderman R, eds. Inflammation: basic principles and clinical correlates. New York, Raven, 1988:265.
17. Smolen JE, Boxer LA. Functions of neutrophils. In: Williams WJ, Beutler E, Ersley AJ, Lichtman MA, eds. Hematology. New York, McGraw-Hill, 1990:780.
18. Zigmond SH. Mechanisms of sensing chemical gradients by polymorphonuclear leukocytes. Nature (Lond) 1974;249:450.
19. Omann GM, Sklar LA. Response of neutrophils to stimulus infusion: differential sensitivity of cytoskeletal activation and oxidant production. J Cell Biol 1988;107:951.
20. Freissmuth M, Casey PJ, Gilman AG. G-proteins control diverse pathways of transmembrane signaling. FASEB J 1989;3:2125.
21. Spiegel A, Carter A, Brann M, et al. Signal transduction by guanine nucleotide binding proteins. Recent Prog Horm Res 1988;44:337.
22. Bokoch GM, Knaus UG. The role of small GTP-binding proteins in leukocyte function. Curr Opin Immunol 1994;6:98.
23. Goldsmith P, Rossiter K, Carter A, et al. Identification of the GTP-binding protein encoded by G_{i3} complementary DNA. J Biol Chem 1988;263:6476.
24. Rotrosen D, Gallin JI, Spiegel AM, Malech HL. Subcellular localization of $G_{1\alpha}$ in human neutrophils. J Biol Chem 1988;263:10958.
25. Sklar LA, Omann GM. Kinetics and amplification in neutrophil activation and adaption. Cell Biol 1990;1:115.
26. Omann GM, Allen RA, Bokoch GM, Painter RG, Traynor AE, Sklar LA. Signal transduction and cytoskeletal activation in the neutrophil. Physiol Rev 1987;67:285.
27. Cockcroft S. G-protein-regulated phospholipase C, D, and A_2-mediated signalling in neutrophils. Biochim Biophys Acta 1992;1113:135.
28. Bengtsson T, Rundquist I, Stendahl O, Wymann MP, Andersson T. Increased breakdown of phosphatidylinositol 4,5-bisphosphate is not an initiating factor for actin assembly in human neutrophils. J Biol Chem 1988;263:17385.
29. Grinstein S, Furuya W. Receptor-mediated activation of electropermeabilized neutrophils. J Biol Chem 1988;263:1779.
30. Dewald B, Thelan M, Baggiolini M. Two transduction sequences are necessary for neutrophil activation by receptor agonists. J Biol Chem 1988;263:16179.
31. Traynor-Kaplan AE. Phosphoinositide metabolism during phagocytic cell activation. Curr Top Membrane Transpl 1990;35:303.
32. Wilde MW, Carlson KE, Manning DR, Zigmond SH. Chemoattractant-stimulated GTPase activity is decreased on membranes from polymorphonuclear leukocytes incubated in chemoattractant. J Biol Chem 1989;264:190.
33. Sklar L. Ligand-receptor dynamics and signal amplification in the neutrophil. Adv Immunol 1986;39:95.
34. Zucker-Franklin D. Eosinophils: morphology, production, biochemistry, and function. In: Williams WJ, Beutler E, Erslev AJ, Lichtman MA, eds. Hematology. New York, McGraw-Hill, 1990:780.

35. Gleich GJ, Adolphson CR. The eosinophilic leukocyte: structure and function. Adv Immunol 1986;39:177.

36. Friedl HP, Till GO, Trentz O, Ward PA. Roles of histamine, complement and xanthine oxidase in thermal injury of skin. Am J Pathol 1989;135:203.

37. Friedl HP, Smith DJ, Till GO, Thomson PD, Louis DS, Ward PA. Ischemia–reperfusion in humans: appearance of xanthine oxidase activity. Am J Pathol 1990;136:491.

38. Geppert TD, Lipsky PE. Antigen presentation at the inflammatory site. Crit Rev Immunol 1989;9:313.

39. Ruddle NH, Homer R. The role of lymphotoxin in inflammation. Prog Allergy 1988:162.

40. de Gaetano G, Cerletti C, Nanni-Costa MP, Poggi A. The blood platelet as an inflammatory cell. Eur Respir J 1989;6(Suppl):441.

41. Page CP. Platelets as inflammatory cells. Immunopharmacology 1989;17:51.

42. Weksler BB. Roles for human platelets in inflammation. Platelet membrane receptors: molecular biology, immunology, biochemistry, and pathology. New York, Alan R Liss, 1988:611.

43. Bevilacqua MP, Gimbrone MA Jr. Inducible endothelial functions in inflammation and coagulation. Semin Thromb Hemost 1987;13:425.

44. Fajardo LF. Special report: the complexity of endothelial cells. Am J Clin Pathol 1989;92:241.

45. Jutila MA, Berg EL, Kishimoto TK, et al. Inflammation-induced endothelial cell adhesion to lymphocytes, neutrophils, and monocytes. Transplantation 1989;48:727.

46. Cavender DE. Lymphocyte adhesion to endothelial cells in vitro: models for the study of normal lymphocyte recirculation and lymphocyte emigration into chronic inflammatory lesions. J Invest Dermatol 1989;93:88.

47. Schmidt HHHW, Lohmann SM, Walter, U. The nitric oxide and cGMP signal transduction system: regulation and mechanism of action. Biochim Biophys Acta 1993;1178:153.

48. Gerschenson LE, Rotello RJ. Apoptosis: a different type of cell death. FASEB J 1992;6:2450.

49. Bonventre JV, Malis CD, Cheung JU. Calcium. In: Zelenock G, D'Alecy L, Fantone J III, et al, eds. Clinical ischemic syndromes: mechanisms and consequences of tissue injury. St Louis, CV Mosby, 1990:227.

50. Hinshaw DB. The role of alterations in the endothelial cytoskeleton in ischemic injury. In: Zelenock G, D'Alecy L, Fantone J III, et al, eds. Clinical ischemic syndromes: mechanisms and consequences of tissue injury. St Louis, CV Mosby, 1990:243.

51. McConkey DJ, Hartzell P, Nicotera P, Orrenius S. Calcium-activated DNA fragmentation kills immature thymocytes. FASEB J 1989;3:1843.

52. DonatI YRA, Slosman DO, Polla BS. Oxidative injury and the heat shock response. Biochem Pharmacol 1990;40:2571.

53. Keyse SM, Tyrrell RM. Heme oxygenase is the major 32-kDa stress protein induced in human skin fibroblasts by UVA radiation, hydrogen peroxide, and sodium arsenite. Proc Natl Acad Sci USA 1989;86:99.

54. Welch WJ, Kang HS, Beckman RP, Mizzen LA. Response of mammalian cells to metabolic stress; changes in cell physiology and structure/function of stress proteins. Curr Top Microbiol Immunol 1991;167:31.

55. Beckmann RP, Lovett M, Welch WJ. Examining the function and regulation of hsp70 in cells subjected to metabolic stress. J Cell Biol 1992;117:1137.

56. Brown CR, Martin RL, Hansen WJ, Beckmann RP, Welch WJ. The constitutive and stress inducible forms of hsp70 exhibit functional similarities and interact with one another in an ATP-dependent fashion. J Cell Biol 1993;120:1101.

57. Dormandy TL. Free-radical pathology and medicine. J R Coll Physicians Lond 1989;23:221.

58. Halliwell B, Hoult JR, Blake DR. Oxidants, inflammation, and anti-inflammatory drugs. FASEB J 1988;2:2867.

59. Hart CM, Tolson JK, Black ER. Supplemental fatty acids alter lipid peroxidation and oxidant injury in endothelial cells. Am J Physiol 1991;(Lung Cell Mol Physiol 4):L481.

60. Hyslop PA, Hinshaw DB, Halsey WA Jr, et al. Mechanisms of oxidant-mediated cell injury: the glycolytic and mitochondrial pathways of ADP phosphorylation are major intracellular targets inactivated by hydrogen peroxide. J Biol Chem 1988;263:1665.

61. Hinshaw DB, Armstrong BC, Burger JM, Beals TF, Hyslop PA. ATP and microfilaments in cellular oxidant injury. Am J Pathol 1988;132:479.

62. Schraufstatter IU, Hyslop PA, Jackson JH, Cochrane CG. Oxidant-induced DNA damage of target cells. J Clin Invest 1988;82:1040.

63. Schraufstatter IU, Browne K, Harris A, et al. Mechanisms of hypochlorite injury of target cells. J Clin Invest 1990;85:554.

64. Mulligan MS, Hevel JM, Marletta MA, Ward PA. Tissue injury caused by deposition of immune complexes is L-arginine dependent. Proc Natl Acad Sci USA 1991;88:6338.

65. Weiss SJ. Tissue destruction by neutrophils. N Engl J Med 1989;320:365.

66. Schreck R, Rieber P, Baeuerle PA. Reactive oxygen intermediates as apparently widely used messengers in the activation of the NF-κB transcription factor and HIV-1. EMBO J 1991;10:2247.

67. Cochrane CG, Spragg R, Revak SD. Pathogenesis of the adult respiratory distress syndrome: evidence of oxidant activity in bronchoalveolar lavage fluid. J Clin Invest 1983;71:754.

68. Henson PM, Johnston RB Jr. Tissue injury in inflammation. J Clin Invest 1987;79:669.

69. Wakefield TW, Hinshaw DB, Burger JM, Burkel WE, Stanley JC. Protamine induces reductions of endothelial cell ATP. Surgery 1989;106:378.

70. McCord JM. Oxygen-derived radicals: a link between reperfusion injury and inflammation. Fed Proc 1987;46:2402.

71. Chenoweth DE. The properties of human C5a anaphylatoxin. Contrib Nephrol 1987;59:51.

SURGERY: SCIENTIFIC PRINCIPLES AND PRACTICE, Second Edition, edited by Lazar J. Greenfield, Michael W. Mulholland, Keith T. Oldham, Gerald B. Zelenock, and Keith D. Lillemoe. Lippincott–Raven Publishers, Philadelphia, © 1997.

CHAPTER 7

INFECTION

DAVID L. DUNN

Although we live in a constant state of invasion by microbial pathogens within the environment and within ourselves, the occurrence of infection is the exception rather than the rule. This is because potentially invasive microbes are held in check by a series of host defense barriers—physical, chemical, and immunologic—that act to maintain the integrity of the mammalian organism. When these barriers are breached or depressed, these omnipresent microorganisms can proliferate and produce infection. This is of importance to surgeons because host barriers are violated routinely in obtaining access to a particular portion of the body to perform the required procedure. Because this process predisposes patients to infection, surgeons have studied infectious disease entities and almost invariably have been the investigators who have determined how to reduce the incidence of infection in surgical patients.

Infection may develop in surgical patients as the result of many different types of bacterial, fungal, viral, and parasitic microorganisms. In an attempt to describe the interaction of host and invading microbe, many organisms have been categorized in relation to virulence and pathogenicity. Both are relative terms, reflecting a composite of microbial and host factors. Some organisms possess virulence factors that facilitate the development of severe infection in both the normal and the immunosuppressed host, whereas others that are nonpathogenic and rarely cause infection in a healthy person may produce infection and mortality in the immunocompromised patient. In general, virulence is exaggerated in the immunosuppressed host, and thus virtually any microorganism can become pathogenic in a patient who lacks intact host defenses.

HOST DEFENSES

Host defenses act to prevent microbes from causing infection and to contain and eradicate infection once it occurs. For many years, scientific doctrine has divided host defenses into humoral and cellular components. It has become increasingly clear, however, that host defenses are exceedingly complex and that additional stratification is necessary, primarily because of the intricate interactions that occur among various facets of host defense. Two points should be emphasized: (1) although individual host defenses act as a series of barriers to infection, many components of host defense also may act in tandem or synergistically to prevent and contain infection; and (2) many host defense components are capable of exerting deleterious effects on the host, such that an overexuberant host defense response may itself produce disease. Host defenses can be classified as barrier, microbial flora, humoral, cellular, and cytokine.

Barriers

The barrier defenses of the mammalian host are numerous and varied, but all serve to separate sterile body tissue from either the external environment or those portions of the body (eg, oropharynx, gut) that possess resident microbial flora (see later). Thus, the skin, mucous membranes, and epithelial layers of various organs of the body constitute effective physical barriers against microbial invasion. In certain portions of the body, these barriers have developed ancillary adaptations to increase the effectiveness of the barrier functions. For example, the skin of those areas of the body that are in direct contact with the environment (hands, feet) is particularly thick and durable. In addition, skin structures such as sebaceous glands secrete chemical compounds that serve to maintain a relatively low pH, providing effective bacterial stasis. Mucous secretion by specialized glands within the bronchi and gut provides a mucous layer that represents a physical and chemical barrier to microbial invasion. Within the respiratory tract, ciliary function serves to extrude microorganisms trapped within this mucous layer. In the alimentary tract, the very low pH within the stomach and gut peristalsis both serve to prevent microbial adherence and invasion. Although traumatic disruption of any of these barriers can immediately produce infection, disease states that affect barriers within a particular organ may also diminish protective function and lead to acute or chronic infections.

Microbial Flora

The terms commensal, resident, indigenous, and autochthonous have all been used to describe those microorganisms that reside in the human body and that continually come into contact with various aspects of host defenses. Many of these organisms are indeed symbionts, acting to promote host defense and health, while concomitantly benefiting from sequestration within the host milieu. The importance of this microflora should not be underestimated. Under normal circumstances, it is critical to the developing neonatal immune system and acts in concert with other host defenses to prevent the invasion of nonresident pathogens. Unfortunately, because of proximity and composition, the autochthonous microflora also can provide the initial inoculum that may lead to established infection once host barrier defenses are breached.[1]

The composition of the gut microflora is established in neonates after ingestion of microbes that are acquired during contamination from the birth canal and during initial feeding, and it remains relatively constant thereafter. Although this flora acts to promote development of the immune system, the specific interactions that produce this effect have not been elucidated fully. Studies performed with gnotobiotic animals have demonstrated that the absence of the gut microflora leads to poor development of gut-associated lymphoid tissue and absence of local responses to many antigens. Gnotobiotic rodents possess a huge, distended cecum and are susceptible to otherwise nonlethal bacterial inocula through a variety of routes of administration. Hepatic Kupffer cell numbers and responses are markedly diminished, as are a wide variety of systemic cellular and humoral immune responses.

The gut microflora also contributes to physical and chemical barriers at the mucous membrane level, in that many autochthonous microbes possess adhesion proteins by which they bind only to certain areas of the mucosal cell, or to specific types of other bacteria. This serves two purposes: (1) potential binding sites for pathogenic organisms are occupied (organisms that cannot adhere cannot cause infection, a phenomenon termed colonization resistance); and (2) a substantial physical mucobacterial layer is present. This layer is maintained despite the constant shedding of enterocytes, mucous cells, and bacteria through the high division rates of both bacterial and mammalian cells within this microenvironment.

The oropharynx contains both aerobic and anaerobic microorganisms, generally consisting of a variety of gram-positive aerobic and anaerobic organisms, lactobacilli, Branhamella, Bacteroides melaninogenicus and Bacteroides oralis, and other anaerobic forms. Microbial inhabitants of the oropharynx do not usually pass into the intestine because the stomach represents a significant barrier to invading microorganisms by virtue of its low pH, which kills most microbes unless very large numbers are present or the organisms are acid resistant (eg, Mycobacterium). This barrier function, coupled with the rapid transit time within the normal stomach and upper small intestine, probably explains why so few microbes (0 to 100 gram-positive facultative aerobes, lactobacilli, and Candida) are present in this portion of the gut. Passage of oropharyngeal microflora and ingested microbes into the small intestine can occur during meals, at which time the gastric pH is temporarily elevated, or in patients with diseases that cause alterations in gastric pH or motility.

The upper small intestine also contains few organisms, mainly gram-positive aerobes and lactobacilli. Conversely, the lower small intestine contains large numbers of aerobes and anaerobic forms, especially in patients in whom the ileocecal valve allows free backwash of cecal contents into the terminal ileum. Within the colon, a wide diversity and large number of facultative and strict anaerobic isolates are present. Only a relatively small number of aerobes (Enterococcus faecalis, Escherichia coli, and other Enterobacteriaceae) are present, these microbes being outnumbered 100 to 300 to 1 by anaerobes (Bacteroides fragilis, other Bacteroides species, Fusobacterium, and many others). Microbes are as much as 30% of the dry weight of feces, with as many as 10^{11} to

10^{12} organisms present per gram of feces. Thus, the number of bacteria in the colon approaches 10^{10} to 10^{12} per gram of feces for *Bacteroides* sp and is typically 10^8 to 10^{10} per gram of feces for *E coli*. Other microorganisms are present at variable, but often high, numbers.

Although both aerobic and anaerobic microorganisms may provide the initial inoculum should perforation of a viscus occur, the anaerobes appear to provide the greatest contribution to colonization resistance and thus prevent aerobic gram-negative bacilli from achieving numeric predominance and host invasion. Two points should be emphasized: (1) anaerobic organisms are found in great quantity and diversity at both ends of the gastrointestinal tract (oropharynx and colorectum), although the specific types of organisms differ between the two sites; and (2) an increase in both diversity and number of both total organisms and anaerobic isolates is noted as the gut microflora is progressively examined in an aboral direction, progressing from the stomach to the colon and rectum (Fig. 7-1).

Humoral Defenses

Stimulation of the immune system occurs after a variety of antigen-presenting cells (B lymphocytes, macrophages, dendritic cells, Langerhans cells) act to engulf, process, and present antigen to T lymphocytes of the helper lineage. These T lymphocytes, in turn, act to stimulate B lymphocytes to become mature plasmacytes (through secretion of cytokines such as interleukins 4 and 6 [IL-4 and IL-6]), dedicated to the production of antibody directed against this specific antigen. An *antigen* can be defined as any substance that stimulates the host immune response, that is, that the host immune system recognizes as foreign. Thus, an antigen may be an invading microorganism, an inert particle, or any type of chemical compound (eg, protein, lipid, saccharide, complex biomolecule) that triggers the host immune system. Although some antigens stimulate B lymphocytes directly to produce antibody (many polysaccharides), most antigens require the coordinated efforts of these various components of the immune system.[2]

Humoral defenses consist of antibody (immunoglobulin [Ig]) and complement (Fig. 7-2). All Ig classes (IgM, IgG, IgA, IgE, and IgD) and IgG subclasses (1 to 4 in humans) are composed of one type (M, G, A, E, D) of heavy (H) and one type (κ or γ) of light (L) protein chains that consist of several domains both structurally and functionally. Each Ig molecule contains one or more units that consist of two H- and two L-chains linked by disulfide bonds. The amino terminus of both H- and L-chains contains several hypervariable regions that fold in three dimensions to produce the antigen-binding site. The carboxy terminus of the H-chains contains regions that activate complement and bind Fc receptors, by which direct adherence to polymorphonuclear leukocytes (PMNs) and macrophages takes place after antigen binding occurs.

Initially, antibody of the IgM class is produced in response to an antigenic challenge. IgM is a pentameric molecule and thus possesses 10 binding sites per molecule. A second exposure to the same antigen, or a cross-reactive antigen, leads to the so-called second set response, in which antibody of the IgG class with two binding sites is produced more rapidly and in larger quantity compared with the initial IgM primary response. Evidence also indicates that antibody of increasing affinity is produced in response to the second antigenic challenge. Immunoglobulin of the IgA class is secreted by gut-associated lymphoid tissue and is combined with a secretory component protein to form a dimer termed *secretory IgA*. This antibody acts at a variety of epithelial sites to prevent microbial adherence and invasion. IgD and IgE exist in smaller amounts in the circulation and do not appear to play a major role as host defense components, the latter immunoglobulin class being associated with many hypersensitivity reactions and mast cell activation. Membrane-bound forms of

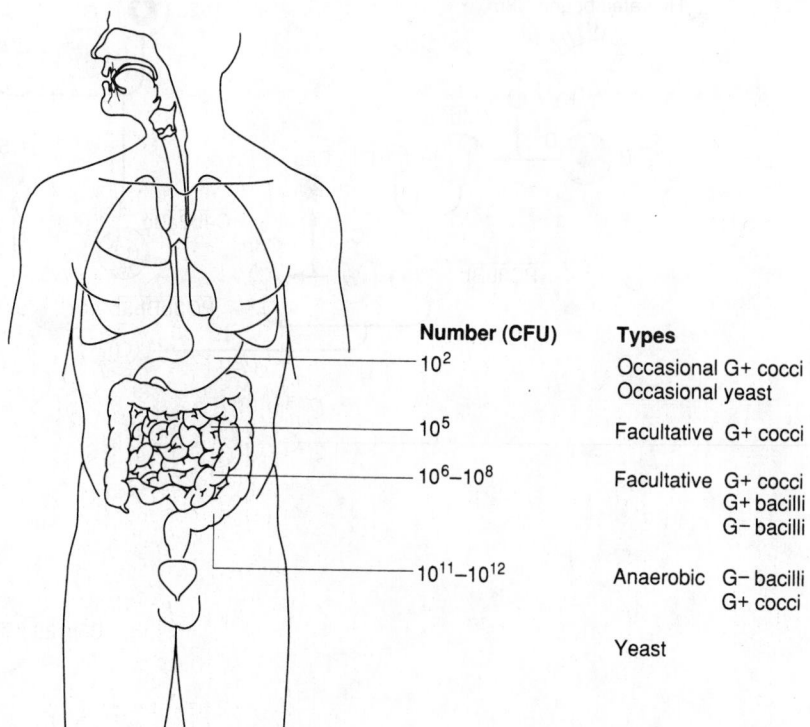

Figure 7-1. Autochthonous microflora of the gastrointestinal tract. Large numbers and different types of anaerobic bacteria are present in both the oropharynx and distal gut. The stomach is virtually sterile in normal individuals, but the number of microorganisms increases in an aboral direction. These organisms provide the initial inoculum of microorganisms when perforation of a viscus occurs. G+, gram-positive; G−, gram-negative.

Number (CFU)	Types
10^2	Occasional G+ cocci Occasional yeast
10^5	Facultative G+ cocci
10^6–10^8	Facultative G+ cocci G+ bacilli G− bacilli
10^{11}–10^{12}	Anaerobic G− bacilli G+ cocci
	Yeast

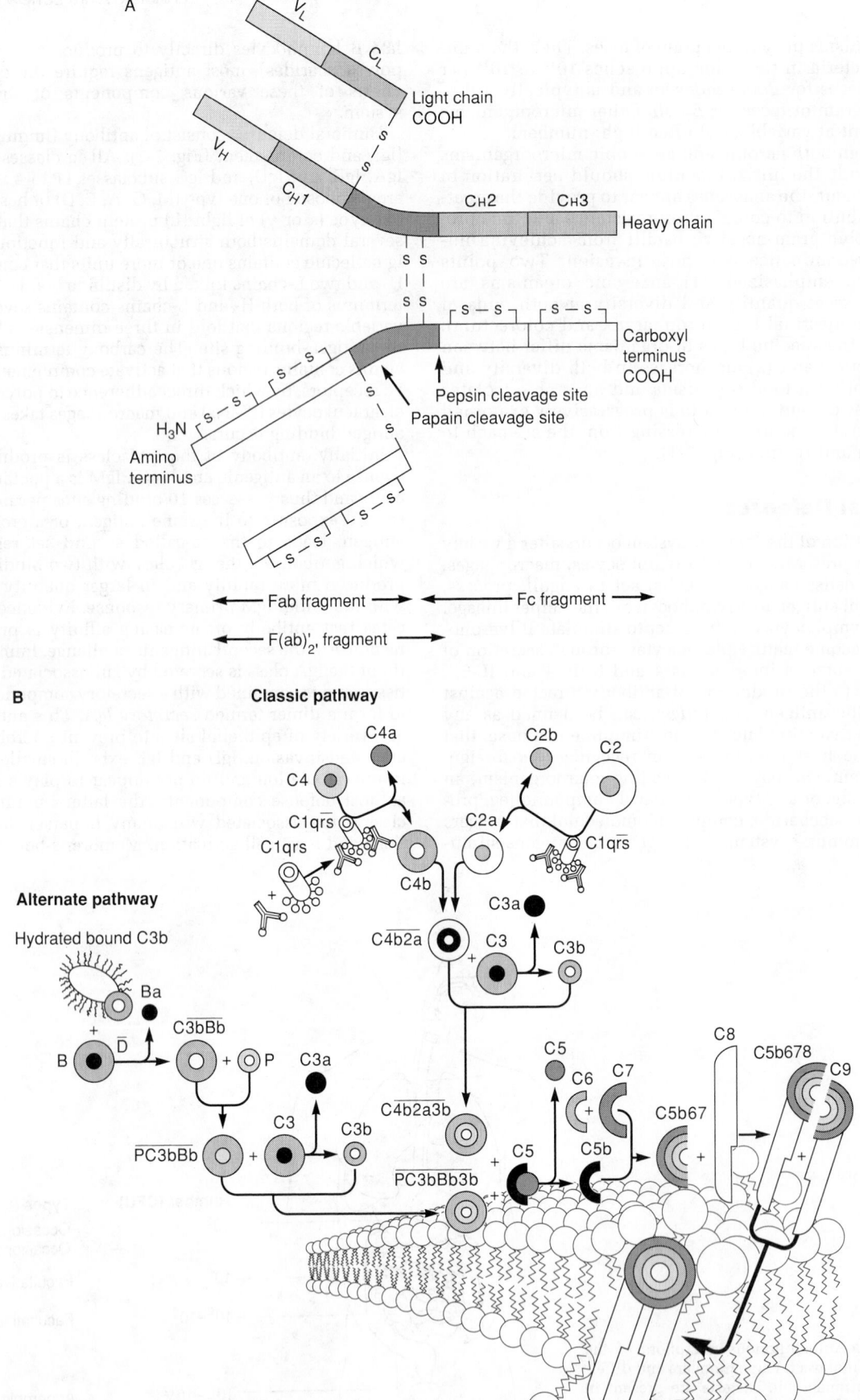

A

V_L
C_L
Light chain
COOH

V_H
C_{H1}
C_{H2}
C_{H3}
Heavy chain

Carboxyl terminus COOH

Pepsin cleavage site
Papain cleavage site

H_3N
Amino terminus

Fab fragment
Fc fragment
$F(ab)'_2$ fragment

B

Classic pathway

C4a
C4
C2b
C2
C1qr̄s̄
C2a
C1qrs
C4b
C1qr̄s̄
C3a
C4b2a
C3
C3b

Alternate pathway

Hydrated bound C3b
Ba
B
D̄
C3bB̄b̄
P
C3a
C4b2a3b
C5
C8
C5b678
C6
C7
C9
PC3bB̄b̄
C3
C3b
C5b67
PC3bB̄b̄3b
C5
C5b

C5b789

IgM and IgD serve as antigen receptors on B lymphocytes and are thus important in antigen recognition and subsequent T- and B-lymphocyte activation.

Ongoing antigenic stimulation enhances plasmacyte replication so that a clone of identical cells develops that secretes the same Ig. Each plasmacyte secretes Ig that is of only one class and only one specificity and that acts to bind a particular antigen. This binding process may serve to neutralize toxic compounds, but it also may produce enhanced phagocytosis by cellular components of the immune system. The Fc receptor portion of the heavy chain of some subclasses of IgG binds to a specific receptor present on many opsonophagocytic cells (PMNs and macrophages) and serves to markedly enhance phagocytosis. In addition, many but not all Igs activate complement after binding to antigen.

The complement system consists of a series of serum proteins that exist in a quiescent or very-low-level state of activation in the uninfected host. Complement activation can occur through either classic or alternate (properdin) pathways, both of which eventuate in deposition of terminal complement pathway components on the antigenic cell surface. Activation of the classic pathway of complement begins with C1qrs activation, usually after binding to IgG (IgG1, IgG2, and IgG3, not IgG4) or IgM that has bound antigen. After C1 binding, complement components C4, C2, and then C3 are sequentially activated through cleavage to subunit forms. Alternate pathway activation occurs in response to activation of alternate factors D and B by IgG4 binding to antigen or directly through contact with fungal and bacterial cell wall compounds, such as zymosan and gram-negative bacterial lipopolysaccharide (LPS; endotoxin). Either the C4b2a or the C3bBb complexes serve as C3 convertases to amplify conversion of C3 in each pathway, exponentially increasing the reaction's power. Subsequent activation steps include C5 cleavage and formation of the C5b-9 complex, which involves interaction of all the terminal portions of the complement cascade.

Several complement components represent important host defenses, acting to recruit or augment cellular host defenses or to inactivate invading microbes directly through lytic activity. The production of complement component fragments C3a and C5a during activation of this cascade serves to increase vascular permeability markedly, and C5a functions as a PMN and macrophage chemoattractant. This process leads to the recruitment of additional humoral and cellular defenses to a specific area of infection. In addition, C3b deposition on an antigenic surface serves to enhance opsonophagocytosis by means of receptors separate from those of the Fc class. Finally, C5b-9 complex deposition on membrane targets leads to lysis after the formation of gaps in the cell membrane and osmotic fluid shifts.

Although certain types of antibody are extremely effective activators of complement, many foreign substances activate either the classic or alternate pathways of complement. For example, many gram-negative microorganisms are able to activate one or both pathways of the complement system, whereas many yeast cell wall components directly activate the alternative complement pathway. The complement cascade most likely represents a relatively primitive host defense mechanism that is extremely effective in preventing infection, particularly when acting with other host defense components.

Excessive complement activation can produce deleterious effects in some instances. Complement activation causes enhanced PMN adhesion, margination, and release of lysosomal enzymes that can directly damage certain target tissues, such as the lung. This has been demonstrated to occur during hemodialysis, after hemofiltration membrane activation of complement. Some investigators hypothesize that this process also occurs during certain types of severe infection, such as gram-negative bacterial sepsis, although a consistent demonstration of this end-organ response phenomenon has not been established in either experimental models or the clinical setting, despite the evidence that complement activation occurs. Overall, antibody and complement act together to neutralize microbial toxins, lyse invading microbial organisms, or markedly enhance phagocytosis of those organisms that escape initial neutralization and lysis. Simultaneously, fragments of certain complement components act to recruit additional cellular components of host defenses and direct them toward the area of infection.

Cellular Defenses

A wide variety of cell types serve to provide host defense at several levels. As mentioned, macrophages can act as initial antigen-processing cells that serve to present antigen to helper T cells, thus initiating the immune response. Macrophages, however, are pluripotent cells that, in the process of engulfing and processing antigen, may become activated. Activated macrophages secrete a variety of cytokines, which are described later. Macrophages also act as phagocytic cells in the tissues and within the bloodstream and, because of their resident nature in many tissues, also represent the first line of host defenses in many areas of the body, even before activation. PMNs are present within the bloodstream, but only in small numbers within the tissue, and enter an area of infection through diapedesis after chemotactic stimuli are exuded by macrophages, bacterial breakdown products such as N-formylpeptides, and complement activation. This recruitment process generally takes several hours and clearly coincides with the critical time period during which the interplay between microbial proliferation and abrogation of infection by host defenses occurs. Unfortunately, it has become increasingly clear that activation of host defenses can also exert deleterious effects on the mammalian host. Secretion of lysosomal enzymes (cathepsin, elastase), free radicals (superoxide, hydroxyl), nitric oxide, and cytokines by macrophages and PMNs can directly injure nearby cells as well as tissues distant from the site of infection.

Cytokines

Macrophages, endothelial cells, lymphocytes, and other cells secrete a large number of different compounds, termed *cytokines,* that most probably evolved for the purpose of local intercellular and intracellular signaling. Lymphocytic cytokines have been termed *lymphokines,* and those secreted by macrophages are often referred to as *monokines.* Cytokines are generally low-molecular-weight polypeptides that exert a wide variety of biologic effects at both the local and systemic levels. The gene for many cytokines has been sequenced, isolated, and cloned; cellular receptors have been identified for many as well. Cytokines frequently are secreted after initial lymphocyte or macrophage activation and may act on

Figure 7-2. Humoral defenses consist of immunoglobulin (*A*) and complement (*B*). (*A*) All Ig classes and IgG subclasses are composed of one type (M, G, A, E, D) of heavy (H) and one type (κ or γ) of light (L) protein chains. The complement system consists of a series of serum proteins that may become activated through either a classic pathway or alternate (properdin) pathways, both of which eventuate in deposition of terminal complement pathway components on the antigenic cell surface.

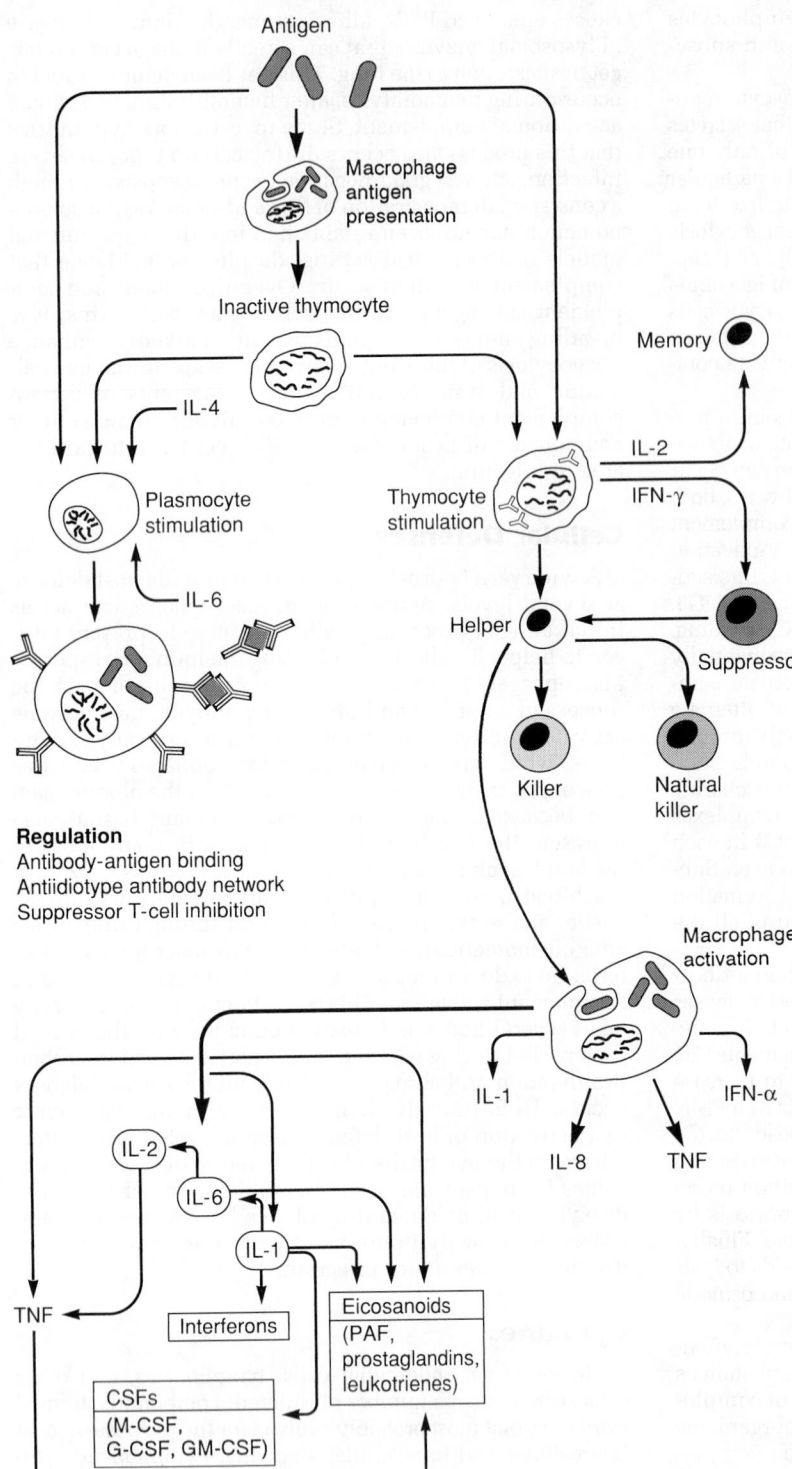

Figure 7-3. Inflammatory and immune response cytokine cascade. After initial antigen processing and presentation by macrophages and other cells, T lymphocytes act to stimulate B lymphocytes to become mature plasmacytes through secretion of cytokines such as IL-4 and IL-6, dedicated to the production of antibody directed against a specific antigen. Initial macrophage stimulation in response to bacterial products, interferon-γ (IFN-γ) release by T cells, and IL-1 release by macrophages themselves may be followed by macrophage tumor necrosis factor-α (TNF-α) production and subsequent secretion of IL-6 and other cytokines.

the secreting cell (autocrine activation) or on other cells within the same local environment (paracrine activation) to cause increased secretion of the same cytokine or other cytokines, respectively. For example, IL-2 is secreted by helper T lymphocytes and serves to increase the expression of IL-2 receptors, followed by additional IL-2 production by this same cell. Simultaneously, IL-2 secretion activates other cell types.

In all probability, a series of activation steps occur in which various cytokines serve to provide regulation of the cellular response. Thus, during initial macrophage stimulation in response to bacterial products, interferon-γ (IFN-γ) release by T cells and IL-1 release by macrophages may be followed by macrophage tumor necrosis factor (TNF) production; subsequently, secretion of IL-6 and other cytokines takes place (Fig. 7-3). Some cytokines are produced by several cell types, and most produce a wide array of effects. Interferons as a class consist of IFN-γ, IFN-α, and IFN-β. TNF-α and TNF-β are both produced by macrophages, whereas TNF-β is also produced by T cells.[3] In experimental model systems, IL-1 is capable of producing fever and hypotension, whereas TNF produces fever, hypotension, gut ischemia, and death. Previous administration of anti-TNF antibody ameliorates these effects. Administration of LPS to human volunteers has provided evidence that IL-1 and TNF are produced about 1.5 to 2 hours after LPS challenge, after which IL-6 and then IL-8 secretion occurs. Administration of TNF to human volunteers leads to many of the physiologic effects evidenced after LPS challenge (see later).

The duality of the effects of the cytokine component of host defenses, exerting both salutary and deleterious effects on the host, is becoming increasingly evident. For example, experimental models in which TNF or IL-1 is administered have provided evidence that this process actually leads to host defense enhancement and provides protection against a subsequent and otherwise lethal TNF or LPS challenge. Initial administration of high doses of TNF, however, produces lethality. Most likely, many cytokines act within the local host defense environment to provide feedback signals and regulate various components of the host defense microenvironment. Thus, cytokines may serve to regulate the set-point of host defenses on a continual basis. During overwhelming infection, the body's attempt to contain infection with humoral, cellular, and cytokine defenses after physical barriers are breached may limit infection in some cases. In extreme cases, however, it may limit infection while simultaneously allowing the egress of cytokines into the systemic circulation, with widespread triggering of host defenses throughout the body. This process most probably represents the explanation for the appearance of the septic state in patients in whom no active infection can be identified.

Host Defense Component Interactions

Several different components of the immune response are subsequently invoked after the primary initiation steps. A humoral response network exists in which plasmacyte stimulation is markedly enhanced by the presence of IL-4 and IL-6, which are derived from thymocytes and macrophages. Regulation of the humoral immune response network occurs at three different levels: (1) antibody–antigen binding, (2) antiidiotype antibody networks, and (3) inhibition through suppressor T-lymphocyte activation (see Fig. 7-3). The initial stages of the immune response are closely linked with the initiation of the host defense response. Invading microorganisms encounter preformed antibody and complement as well as PMNs and macrophages. These factors represent the first-line or resident host defenses and are able to prevent the development of infection in many cases. These first-line host defenses work closely together as second-line, or activation, host defenses become operative. For instance, antibody and complement act together through immunoglobulin Fc receptor interactions, C3b deposition, and the lytic effects of terminal complement factors C5b-9 to enhance bacteriolysis as well as phagocytosis of microorganisms. In addition, macrophage stimulation occurs so that enhanced cytokine release and further T-cell activation occurs (Fig. 7-4). T-cell activation is regulated by both positive and negative feedback systems. For instance, initial activation leads to IL-2 secretion, which induces the formation of additional IL-2 receptors on T cells that, in turn, causes further stimulation of helper T cells and the induction of memory T cells. Conversely, suppressor T cells are activated and serve to regulate the

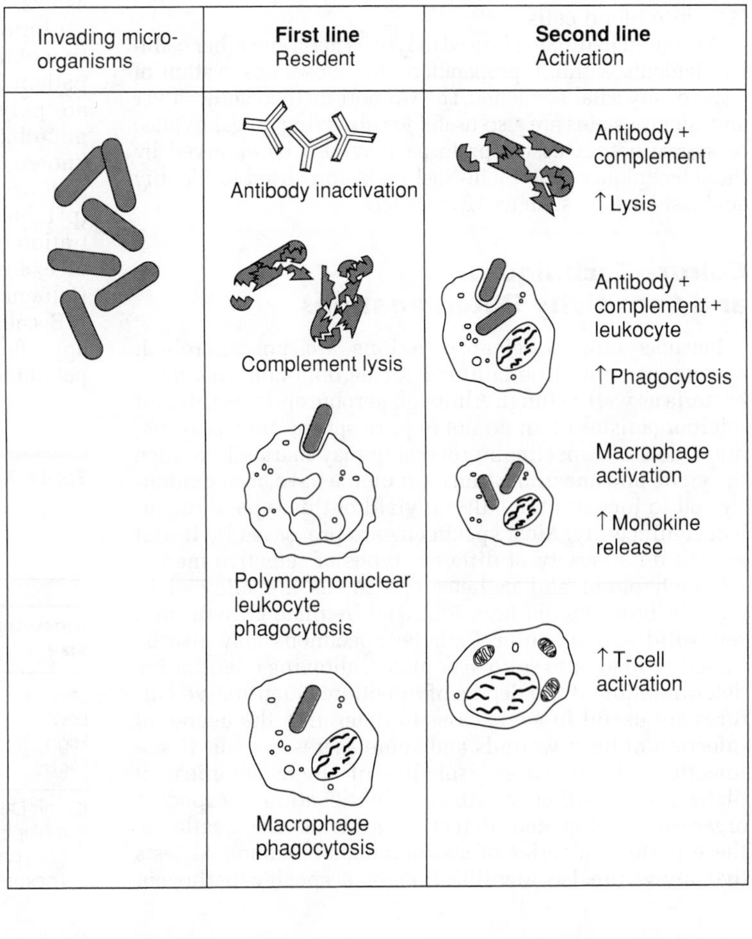

Figure 7-4. Interactions of various portions of mammalian host defenses. Antibody and complement act in concert to enhance bacteriolysis and phagocytosis, simultaneously recruiting additional humoral and cellular components to the site of infection. Macrophages act as pluripotent cells involved in first-line (resident) host defense, antigen presentation and T-cell activation, and subsequent activation and cytokine secretion.

cellular and humoral immune responses. Effector cells (killer T cells and natural killer cells) are also stimulated, and additional macrophage stimulation occurs through T-cell–mediated effects. The macrophage acts as a key cell in the initiation of the immune response as well as a first-line resident and as a second-line activated phagocytic and cytokine-secreting cell.

MICROBIOLOGIC DIAGNOSTIC TECHNIQUES

The surgeon must rely heavily on receiving appropriate information from the microbiology laboratory to prevent and treat perioperative infection. Simultaneously, expeditious preparation and transport of specimens and provision of salient clinical information allows the microbiologist to assist the surgeon in interpreting the cultural data.

Staining Techniques

Initially, a Gram stain can be rapidly performed on a specimen. This simple technique involves (1) fixation of the specimen with heat; (2) staining with a basic dye, such as crystal violet; (3) stain fixation with an iodine–potassium iodide solution; (4) washing with ethanol–acetone; and (5) counterstaining with safranin red. Gram-positive organisms do not decolorize and thus remain dark blue, whereas gram-negative microorganisms are decolorized during washing and exhibit retention of only the lighter red counterstain. Observation under high-power oil immersion light microscopy may indicate significant infection in a normally sterile body area, based on the presence of (1) more than two bacteria (gram-positive, gram-negative, or both) per 1000× magnification high-power field that is equivalent to 5×10^4 to 10^5 colony-forming units (CFU) per milliliter within the initial specimen; and (2) white blood cells.

Potassium hydroxide is used to lyse bacteria and other cellular elements within a preparation and allows observation of yeast or mycelial elements. The Gomori methenamine-silver and Giemsa stains are also useful for observing fungal hyphae or spores within tissue; protozoa may also be observed by these techniques. The Ziehl-Neelsen stain is used to identify acid-fast bacteria such as *Mycobacteria*.

Culture Techniques and Sensitivity Determinations

Because most surgical infections are polymicrobial, specimens should be cultured for aerobic and anaerobic bacteria as well as fungi. Although aerobic and aerotolerant microorganisms often do not require special transport media, a delay in specimen processing may markedly reduce the yield, and anaerobic transport media have been demonstrated to increase the cultural yield of this type of organism significantly. Most specimens are processed by initial growth on a variety of different types of selective media, although blood and catheter specimens are allowed to grow in broth media first, followed by plate growth on a semisolid agar medium. Catheter specimens may also be directly rolled onto solid agar plates, allowing quantitative determination of the degree of infection. Quantitative cultures are useful in some cases to determine the degree of infection of burn wounds and some aggressive soft tissue infections. In all cases, isolation of single colonies on plates allows further growth and identification of a specific organism. Automated detection systems are available; these perform a series of simultaneous biochemical tests that allow precise identification of a specific pathogen.

Automated techniques also allow determination of sensitivity patterns to a wide array of antimicrobial agents active against aerobes, anaerobes, fungi, and viruses. Most laboratories, however, routinely perform sensitivity analyses for solely aerobic isolates.

Initial cultural results may indicate solely that microorganisms are growing, but full characterization may require 2 or 3 days, sometimes longer. An initial report may tentatively indicate the number of different organisms, Gram stain characteristics, and simple biochemical characteristics, such as the presence or absence of lactose fermentation. In some cases, sensitivity reports may be available before complete identification of the organism. Once a specific microorganism is identified, a sample of about 10^5 CFU is inoculated during the log phase into Mueller-Hinton broth containing varying amounts of an antibiotic. After an 18- to 24-hour period, the tube or well that exhibits no visible growth is then noted, and the reciprocal of this dilution is termed the *minimal inhibitory concentration* (MIC). This value may be compared to either measured or known achievable serum levels for a particular antimicrobial agent. Determination of serum bactericidal levels may be of use in some cases and involves obtaining serum from a patient after antimicrobial agent administration. This antibiotic-containing serum is then used to determine inhibitory concentrations against a specific pathogen or series of pathogens. This test may be especially helpful in patients who are being treated with several antimicrobial agents and who are infected with several different pathogens. In general, antimicrobial agents that achieve in excess of a four- to eight-fold increase over the MIC during the peak serum level have been demonstrated to be efficacious in experimental animal models of infection as well as in clinical studies. This information may lead the clinician to at least consider a change in the antimicrobial agent regimen, although in some cases, this may be premature, especially if the patient is doing well.

Confounding factors that do not allow direct extrapolation of this microbiologic information to a specific surgical patient include evidence that (1) most surgical infections are polymicrobial in nature and may involve synergistic microbial interactions, (2) the initial inoculum size is not known and almost assuredly differs from the inoculum size used to determine the MIC, and (3) the host milieu (pH, blood supply) may affect both the activity and penetration of antimicrobial agents. Table 7-1 provides a series of examples in which variations in these factors might influence outcome during infection.[4]

Because the ultimate decision to alter antimicrobial therapy often resides with the initial response of the surgical patient to both the operation and empiric antimicrobial ther-

Table 7-1. DISPARATE HOST AND MICROBIAL FACTORS THAT CAN INFLUENCE ANTIMICROBIAL EFFICACY AND STILL EVENTUATE IN THE ERADICATION OF INFECTION

Inoculum Size	In Vitro Sensitivity	Antimicrobial Tissue Level
Low	Moderate	Adequate
Low	Exquisite	Low
High	Moderate	High
High	Exquisite	Adequate

(Dunn DL. The role of infection and use of antimicrobial agents during multiple system organ failure. In: Deitch EA, ed. Multiple organ failure: pathophysiology and basic concepts of therapy. New York, Theme, 1990:161)

apy, it is not unreasonable to ask why cultures should be obtained and how the information will be used. The answer revolves around two issues—the patient's response and the types and antimicrobial resistance patterns of the infecting organisms. For example, although many patients improve and do not require a change in antimicrobial agent regimen, those patients who exhibit evidence of persistent infection require an assiduous search for the reason. In some cases, the cause may be an undrained source of infection or the presence of necrotic tissue, both of which require surgical intervention; in other cases, an organism not normally within the spectrum of activity of the antimicrobial agents selected or resistant to the antimicrobial agents may be present. Thus, if an initial lack of response to therapy is coupled with evidence of microorganisms resistant to the antimicrobial agents initially chosen, the surgeon has the information available to alter the agents appropriately, by changing or adding other agents, once the microbiologic data become available. Incidentally, it is not infrequent that the availability of this information coincides with alterations in the clinical course of the patient.

Newer Detection Methods

Classically, the detection of microorganisms has taken place based on the clinical evidence of infection (eg, fever, leukocytosis) and cultural evidence of a specific organism. Increasing reliance is being placed on assays that do not employ cultural data. Specifically, the antibody and cytokine host response is being intensely examined, and extremely sensitive amplified assays that rely on antigen, antibody, or microbial DNA detection are being employed in the clinical setting. Routinely, antigen and antibody detection assays have employed hemagglutination, complement fixation, and radioimmunoassay techniques. In addition, enzyme-linked immunosorbent assay (ELISA), immunodot blot, Western immunotransblot, and immunofluorescence are being more frequently employed. Antigen-based assays such as the ELISA typically rely on the nonspecific binding of antigen within the well of a microtiter plate, after which a blocking agent is added to occupy unbound well sites. A specimen that may contain antibody that will bind to the antigen is added and allowed to react with antigen, and then a secondary labeled (eg, peroxidase) antibody is added that can be used for detection based on colorimetric changes after substrate and an indicator are added. This type of assay represents a rapid immunologic assay that can be used for both antigen and antibody detection for determination of antibody titer as well as screening for monoclonal antibody production of a certain specificity by a hybridoma cell line.

Transblot techniques also are being increasingly used in the clinical setting. In most cases, nucleic acid or protein is subjected to electrophoresis so that separation is achieved based on molecular weight. Sodium dodecyl sulfate polyacrylamide gel electrophoresis is commonly used. Immunoelectrophoretic transfer to nitrocellulose paper then takes place, and a probe may be employed to detect the presence of a certain antigen, antibody, or nucleic acid sequence. Direct blotting can take place using dot or slot blots, in which DNA or RNA digests are directly layered onto nitrocellulose, and the probe consists of a labeled cDNA sequence. Similarly, antigen or antibody can be directly blotted onto nitrocellulose, and the probe can consist of labeled antibody or antigen. Southern, Northern, and Western immunotransblot techniques are used to detect DNA, RNA, or proteins, respectively.

The polymerase chain reaction (PCR) is being used in some centers as a sensitive assay to detect small amounts of microbial DNA. In this assay, nucleic acid is extracted from the test sample, which may include the microbial nucleic acid in question. Amplification takes place in vitro through repeated nucleic acid denaturing and polymerization of complementary portions of nucleic acid, so that the gene copy number increases exponentially. The probe for this assay consists of a copy of a portion of the nucleic acid sequence of the microorganism. Because the probe itself can be copied and used in large quantity, and because the sample nucleic acid has been markedly amplified with regard to gene copy number, the test is extremely sensitive and can detect infection in its early stages.

These tests are being used in the clinical setting to detect a wide variety of infectious agents, including cytomegalovirus (CMV) and human immunodeficiency virus (HIV). Some preliminary observations also indicate that it may be possible to detect fungal pathogens such as *Candida* by using monoclonal antibodies directed against cell wall structures such as mannan, but this test has not found widespread clinical utility.

ANTIMICROBIAL AGENTS

Because the practicing surgeon is frequently called on to diagnose and treat infection, he or she is continually bombarded with persuasive arguments regarding the attributes and potential benefit of an increasingly large number and wide diversity of antimicrobial agents. For this reason, it has become increasingly difficult to choose those agents that are appropriate for a specific indication. Primarily, the surgeon must observe the clinical course of the patient and interpret the available microbiologic data in this context. In this regard, it must be remembered that (1) antimicrobial agents do not supplant but are adjunctive to surgical therapy (débridement of devitalized tissue and drainage of infected material), and (2) there is frequently no requirement to alter antimicrobial therapy in the face of clinical improvement, despite the data obtained from the cultural results. The rational use of antimicrobial agents in surgical patients involves (1) prophylaxis, (2) empiric therapy, and (3) directed therapy.

Classes of Antimicrobial Agents

Antibacterial agents can be categorized with regard to their structure, mechanism of action, and activity pattern against various types of bacterial pathogens. Penicillins (including several classes of extended-spectrum drugs, such as carboxypenicillins, ureidopenicillins, and penicillins plus β-lactamase inhibitors), cephalosporins, carbapenems, and monobactams possess a β-lactam ring of some type and act to bind to bacterial division plate proteins, thus inhibiting cell wall peptidoglycan synthesis and either causing or inducing autolytic bacteriolysis (Fig. 7-5). Because gram-positive and gram-negative bacteria possess different types of division plate proteins, many of these agents exhibit differential activity between these two types of microorganisms. For example, whereas first-generation cephalosporins bind avidly to gram-positive division plate proteins and poorly to those of most gram-negative bacteria, the converse is true for many third-generation cephalosporins, explaining their spectrum of activity.

Tetracyclines, chloramphenicol, and macrolides (eg, erythromycin) inhibit bacterial ribosomal activity and thus overall protein synthesis by a variety of different mechanisms. Aminoglycosides act to inhibit protein synthesis and also presumably act on a second target site, a supposition based on the fact that aminoglycosides are bacteriolytic and the other agents are bacteriostatic. Vancomycin inhibits assembly of peptidoglycan polymers, whereas quinolones bind to DNA helicase proteins and inhibit bacterial DNA synthesis. Sulfonamides inhibit paraaminobenzoic acid incorporation into dihydropteroic acid, thus reducing folic acid synthesis and thereby purine synthesis. Trimethoprim acts to inhibit dihydrofolate reductase, an enzyme also in the purine synthesis pathway, such that these two agents in combination act synergistically. Rifampin binds to bacterial RNA polymerase, acting to inhibit directly bacterial replication. Remember that each agent may possess significant clinical toxicity, which may be related to structure and mechanism of action, combined with the degree of differential activity between bacterial and mammalian enzyme systems. The general spectrum of activity of each antimicrobial agent class is shown in Figure 7-6.

Prophylaxis

Intravenous administration of an antimicrobial agent is clearly indicated for those patients undergoing clean-contaminated operations. Most information is derived from studies performed on patients undergoing either biliary or upper gastrointestinal surgery and receiving first-generation cephalosporin agents. The combined use of orally administered intraluminal antiaerobic and antianaerobic antimicrobial agents plus mechanical preparation of the bowel significantly reduces the superficial and deep wound infection rates after elective colonic resection (compared with mechanical bowel preparation alone or mechanical bowel preparation plus only an antiaerobic or an antianaerobic intraluminal antimicrobial agent). However, the addition of an intravenous antimicrobial agent has not been demonstrated to reduce further the rate of infection in a significant fashion. This is because the large number of patients required to demonstrate this effect has

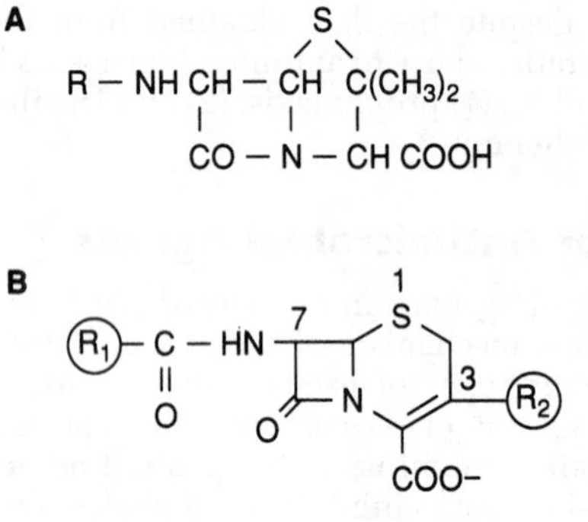

Figure 7-5. Structure of β-lactam antimicrobial agents. The ring structure of each of the four classes is slightly different, accounting for their different spectra of activity: (*A*) penicillin, (*B*) cephalosporin, (*C*) carbapenem, (*D*) monobactam. R, side chain.

precluded performance of a study designed to test this as an independent variable.[5]

Because of this finding, the use of an intravenous prophylactic antimicrobial agent with a spectrum of activity directed against the microflora in that region of the body has not been entirely substantiated, although conceptually it would make little sense to administer agents not directed against those organisms that form the initial inoculum. This complex issue remains unresolved largely because both superficial and deep wound infections occur as the result of *either or both* skin (superficial wound) flora (eg, *Staphylococcus aureus*) and body site (deep wound) flora. For this reason, administration of agents that possess activity directed against those expected pathogens is reasonable. The exact choice of agents is confusing, however, because some studies indicate that antistaphylococcal coverage is often adequate, whereas others indicate that additional coverage may be required. The beneficial results of antimicrobial prophylaxis in a given patient probably depend on the initial numbers and types of microbial pathogens within the skin and body site, the degree of contamination produced during the procedure, the activity of local and systemic host defenses, and the tissue level and activity of the antimicrobial agent against specific pathogens.

For instance, although administration of a first-generation cephalosporin is acceptable, second-generation cephalosporins or extended-spectrum penicillins with gram-positive and gram-negative activity and biliary tract excretion might be more suitable for patients undergoing extensive biliary tract procedures. Similarly, the use of agents with additional anaerobic activity for patients undergoing gastrointestinal procedures such as a small bowel resection for obstruction or colonic resection should be considered. Administration of broad-spectrum agents (eg, third-generation cephalosporins, carbapenems) for prophylaxis does not provide additional benefit in comparison to the above-mentioned types of agents and may foster the development of resistant organisms within a given institution or the development of superinfections within a given patient, particularly if administration of these agents is continued in the postoperative period.

Two additional points should be mentioned: (1) the added benefit of additional postoperative antimicrobial agent administration is unproved with regard to prophylaxis, and (2) some evidence also exists that for certain types of cases (eg, biliary tract surgery), the topical use of antimicrobial agents is equivalent to the administration of intravenous antimicrobial agents. This has not become dogma, although the concept that the combination of topical plus intravenous antimicrobial prophylaxis may further reduce the wound infection rate is intriguing.

Empiric Therapy

The surgeon must frequently decide whether to institute therapy with antimicrobial agents based on the clinical course of a given patient without the benefit of well-defined microbiologic data. The dilemma thus centers around an attempt to determine whether the patient has a source of infection and at what point the evidence provides enough support of this diagnosis, such that it would be imprudent to withhold antimicrobial therapy. Several tenets should be followed in this setting: (1) an assiduous search for a septic source should be undertaken and continued (cultures, radiographic procedures, and so forth), and (2) initial limits should be placed on the course of empiric therapy, and these should be continually reevaluated based on the clinical course of the patient. Care must also be taken to select antimicrobial agents based on known activity patterns in a given institution.

Controversial issues regarding the use of empiric antimicrobial therapy in this setting include the use of multiple-agent regimens in which each agent is specifically targeted against a specific class of pathogens, versus the use of more broad-spectrum agents (many second- and third-generation cephalosporins, carboxypenicillins, ureidopenicillins, penicillins plus β-lactamase inhibitors, carbapenems) that may suffer slightly from a lack of individual pathogen specificity but that overall are directed against several groups of pathogens. These broad-spectrum agents are being used more and more commonly as empiric therapy, particularly because they often avoid many of the toxic effects, such as nephrotoxicity, that are present with combined-modality regimens. Other broad-spectrum classes of agents remain virtually untested in surgical patients with severe sepsis (eg, amdinocillin, spectinomycin analogues such as trospectomycin, and newer quinolones). Careful selection among all of these agents is required, based on known spectra of activity.

Directed Therapy

In simple terms, directed antimicrobial therapy consists of the targeting of specific antibacterial agents against identified pathogens, once sensitivity reports are available. Cultural reports from patients with severe polymicrobial infections create confusion and often lead to administration of three or more antibacterial agents. Because there are no absolute rules, only general guidelines can be provided. Primarily, because experimental and clinical evidence supports the concept of aerobic–anaerobic synergy, therapy should be directed against both potential components of the infection if the body site is such that these microorganisms may be present. This issue is less well defined clinically regarding enterococcal infection, although several experimental studies indicate that this organism also can act with other components of the infection to enhance lethality. Secondarily, agents should be administered that exhibit specific activity against various components of the infection; an attempt should be made to select those agents that exhibit minimal toxicity while retaining suitable efficacy. This can often be achieved by administration of extended-spectrum penicillins or second- or third-generation cephalosporins in combination with other agents, or perhaps with carbapenem agents alone. Single-agent therapy has been demonstrated to be equivalent to an aminoglycoside plus an antianaerobic agent (clindamycin or metronidazole) for the treatment of peritoneal contamination due to gangrenous appendicitis, penetrating gastrointestinal injury, and established secondary bacterial peritonitis as long as the spectrum of activity includes aerobes and anaerobes. As mentioned, extended-spectrum agents should not be used for prophylaxis, nor when less expensive, more routine agents can be directed against a specific pathogen. They are often ideal for treatment of the patient with several pathogenic organisms or with a nosocomial

	Microorganism						
Antimicrobial agent	Gram-Positive			Gram-Negative		Anaerobic	
	Streptococci	Staphylococci	Enterococci	Enterics	Pseudomonas	Cocci	Bacteroides
Penicillins							
Penicillin G	3	1	1	0	0	2	1
Ampicillin	2	1	3	1	0	1	0
Carboxypenicillins	1	1	1	3	2	1	1
Ureidopenicillins	2	2	3	3	3	1	2
Ampicillin + β-lactamase inhibitor	2	2	3	2	1	2	2
Carboxypenicillins + β-lactamase inhibitor	2	2	2	3	2	2	3
Cephalosporins							
First generation	2	3	0	1	0	2	0
Second generation*	1	2	0	2	1	1	2
Third generation*	0	0	0	3	3	1	1
Monobactams	0	0	0	3	2	0	0
Carbapenems	3	3	0	3	3	2	3
Aminoglycosides	0	1	1	3	3	0	0
Vancomycin	3	3	3	0	0	3	0
Erythromycin	2	2	2	0	0	2	0
Quinolones*	2	1	1	3	2	1	0
Tetracyclines	2	1	1	1	0	1	2
Chloramphenicol	2	2	1	1	0	2	2
Clindamycin	2	1	2	0	0	2	3
Metronidazole	0	0	0	0	0	1	3
Trimethoprim-sulfamethoxazole	2	1	0	3	2	1	0

Figure 7-6. General spectrum of activity of commonly used antimicrobial agents. Higher numbers correspond to higher sensitivity of the organism to the antibiotic. *Specific agents vary markedly with respect to spectrum of activity.

infection due to a resistant organism that is within the spectrum of activity of a particular extended-spectrum agent and not other antimicrobials.

Clinical Manifestations of Infection

The interaction of invading microbes and host defenses produces the clinical manifestations of infection. In many cases, the classic local symptoms and signs of pain, swelling, and redness at the infected site and fever as part of the systemic response all occur, but their absence does not exclude infection, particularly in the immunocompromised host. Systemic leukocytosis with a preponderance of PMNs may be noted, and severe systemic infections may produce confusion, ileus, hypotension, and profound shock. Thus, any of these premonitory signs mandates a thorough diagnostic evaluation to establish or exclude the presence of significant infection.

Initially, a carefully directed review of the patient's previous history, operative procedures, and current physical status should be undertaken. Pertinent laboratory and physiologic monitoring data should also be carefully studied. Several diagnostic procedures should be performed to collect specimens to obtain concrete microbiologic information. Blood, urine, sputum, and any obviously infected site should be cultured for potential bacterial pathogens as well as fungi and viruses. Although a number of routine studies (eg, chest radiograph) should be performed, a concentrated effort should be directed toward the superficial and deep components of the surgical wound (see later) because this is the area in which most infections occur. For example, close examination of the wound may reveal a small amount of drainage, which prompts opening the wound to reveal a significant wound infection. Studies such as chest and sinus radiographs in a patient who has undergone prolonged intubation for the purpose of mechanical ventilation may identify diffuse pneumonitis, a discrete infiltrate, or sinusitis and can serve to direct further studies. Subsequent bronchoscopy or sinus aspiration can then be performed to obtain specific site cultures. Catheter sepsis, urinary tract infections, and systemic sepsis must also be considered. Of course, numerous disease entities not related to infection can cause fever in the immediate postoperative period (atelectasis, thrombophlebitis, pulmonary embolism, drug allergy), and these must also be weighed in the differential diagnosis.

Wound Infection

Many factors influence the occurrence of wound infections. Preoperative hair removal with instruments that cause abrasions, lack of antiseptic skin preparation, host immunosuppression, administration of antimicrobial agents after the wound is created, and the degree of bacterial contamination at the time of wounding are all important variables that enhance the rate of infection. Wound infection occurs when the inoculum of contaminating microorganisms is not contained by host defenses, proliferates, and produces established infection. Because of the accessibility of the wound, a great deal is known regarding the pathophysiology of this particular disease process. In fact, most concepts regarding how surgical infections develop and how they are prevented and treated, have evolved from seminal work done in this particular area.

Initial experimental studies demonstrated that a finite number of organisms in the initial inoculum to which the wound was exposed determined whether infection would result. Studies by Burke[6] and others led to the conclusion

that, for many organisms, this number was 10^5 CFU/g tissue. In an attempt to prevent infection, antimicrobial agents were administered before and at a series of time points after wounding and bacterial contamination of the wound. These studies unequivocally demonstrated that antimicrobial agents reduce infection to the greatest extent when administered before contamination and that the progressive loss of antimicrobial efficacy after contamination is directly related to growth of microbes within the tissues surrounding the wound and within the wound. Thus, a limited time period existed during which antimicrobial efficacy could be demonstrated. It has become increasingly clear that antimicrobial agents act in conjunction with resident and recruited host defenses to contain invading microbes, thus preventing established infection. Immunosuppression and inadequate antimicrobial tissue levels or use of antimicrobial agents to which an organism is resistant may foster the development of infection even when low inocula are present. Even the normal host with adequate levels of an appropriate antimicrobial agent may not be able to combat the development of infection if an extremely large bacterial inoculum is introduced.

Although the mentioned studies may seem mundane today, clinical practice at that time did not include administration of antimicrobial agents before creating an incision. Subsequently, a series of carefully controlled clinical studies were performed that established the tenet that antimicrobial agents must be administered before wounding during elective surgery to achieve both adequate tissue levels within the wound fluid and a reduction in the wound infection rate. Today, wounds are classified into three classes according to the likelihood of bacterial contamination: (1) clean (no viscus is entered; eg, herniorrhaphy); (2) clean-contaminated (minimal contamination; eg, elective colon resection with adequate mechanical and antimicrobial preparation of the bowel); and (3) contaminated (heavily contaminated surgery; eg, resection of unprepared, obstructed bowel with gross spillage of intestinal contents or stool, drainage of abscesses, débridement of traumatic neglected wounds). In addition, the surgical wound has been redefined to encompass both the superficial (extrafascial skin and subcutaneous tissue) and deep (body cavity) compartments. Antimicrobial agents generally should be administered for class 2 and 3, but patients undergoing clean surgery do not always require antimicrobial agents. Some studies, however, indicate that a reduction in the wound infection rate can also be achieved in clean cases by administration of prophylactic antimicrobial agents. In most cases, the wounds of patients undergoing contaminated surgery should be managed without initial closure. Healing can occur by delayed primary closure (5 to 7 days after the initial operation) or by secondary intention.

Intraabdominal Infection

The peritoneal cavity is a mesothelium-lined potential space that under normal circumstances contains only a small amount of serous, sterile fluid. Infection of this potential space can occur after the introduction of microorganisms during peritoneal dialysis or in patients with ascites in whom no viscus perforation has occurred (primary microbial peritonitis) or after perforation of a viscus with spillage of the autochthonous flora takes place (secondary microbial peritonitis). The change in microbial flora in patients with initial secondary bacterial peritonitis so that ongoing infection with normally low-virulence pathogens (eg, *Staphylococcus epidermidis, Candida albicans*) occurs has been termed *tertiary* or *persistent microbial peritonitis.* The introduction of microorganisms into the normally sterile peritoneal environment invokes several potent specialized host antimicrobial defense mechanisms—clearance, phagocytosis and killing, and sequestration[7] (Fig. 7-7).

Bacterial clearance, also termed *translymphatic absorption*, occurs through specialized structures found only on the peritoneal mesothelium on the underside of the diaphragm that act as conduits for both fluid and particulate matter. Stomata (10 to 16 μm) between mesothelial cells lead into lymphatic structures (lacunae), which subsequently drain into larger mediastinal lymphatic vessels.

These in turn pass material through the thoracic duct into the venous circulation. Particulates of all types, including bacteria, are rapidly cleared from the peritoneal cavity into the systemic circulation. Inoculation of bacteria into the peritoneum leads to bacteremia within minutes, and more than half of an inoculum of 2×10^8 killed radiolabeled *E coli* are cleared from the peritoneal cavity within 1 hour in experimental animal models.

Those microbes that are not cleared are rapidly engulfed by resident and recruited phagocytic cells. During the ini-

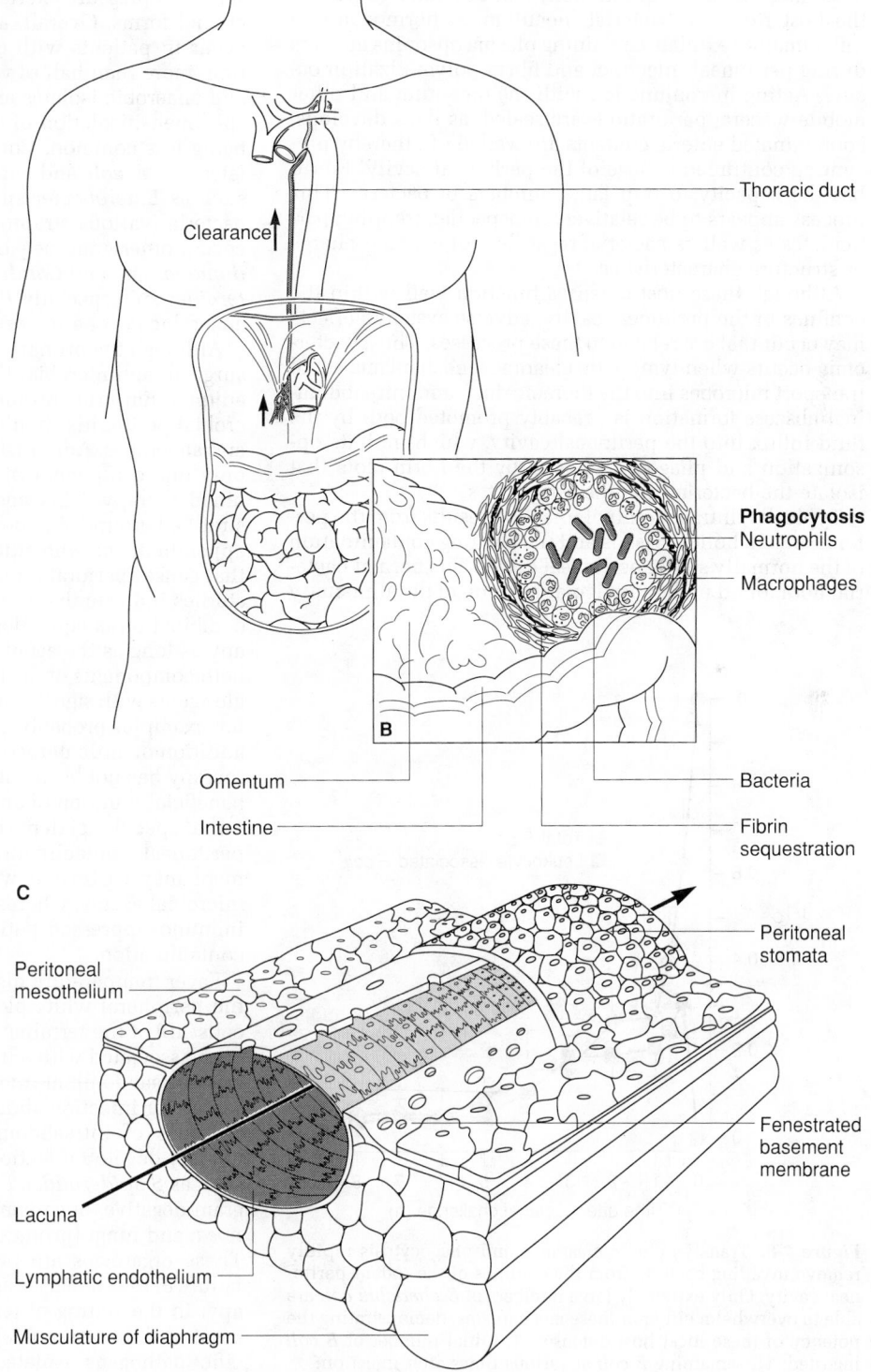

Figure 7-7. (*A*) Host defenses of the peritoneal cavity consist of sequestration and phagocytosis (*B*), followed by clearance. Clearance also occurs directly through translymphatic absorption (*C*), and resident macrophages engulf invading microorganisms. These two components represent the first line of peritoneal host defense, and recruitment of polymorphonuclear leukocytes after 3 to 4 hours and sequestration serve to further limit the development of infection.

tial stages of infection, resident macrophages act as the first line of peritoneal host defense in concert with clearance to diminish bacterial numbers. After the first several hours, there is an influx of PMNs into the peritoneal cavity. These cells act to engulf those invading microbes that have escaped other defense mechanisms. There are quantitative limitations to the capacity of each of these mechanisms to deal with contamination. In experimental animal models, only extremely large bacterial inocula (2×10^{10} E coli) are capable of saturating both clearance and phagocytosis mechanisms simultaneously (Fig. 7-8). The limits of these defenses in humans have not been established.

Those microorganisms that evade both clearance and phagocytosis are confronted by a final, primitive host defense mechanism (sequestration) that functions to protect the host from the bacterial inoculum. A fibrinogen-rich inflammatory exudate containing plasma opsonins appears during peritoneal infection, and fibrin polymerization occurs. Acting in conjunction with the omentum and other mobile viscera, perforations are sealed; as ileus develops, contaminated enteric contents are walled off, thereby preventing continued soilage of the peritoneal cavity. Fibrin has the capacity to trap large numbers of bacteria. This process appears to be relatively nonspecific, trapping particulates as well as bacteria, regardless of external charge or structure characteristics.

Although these host defenses function well within the confines of the peritoneal cavity, adverse systemic effects may occur that are related to these processes. Thus, bacteremia occurs when lymphatic clearance mechanisms act to transport microbes into the thoracic duct, and intraabdominal abscess formation is probably promoted both by the fluid influx into the peritoneal cavity, which inhibits opsonization and phagocytosis, and by the fibrin clots that isolate the bacteria from the phagocytes.

Typically, intraabdominal infection results from the perforation of a hollow viscus and the ensuing contamination of the normally sterile peritoneal cavity. The normal bacterial flora found in that particular location of the alimentary

tract thus determines the initial inoculum. In parallel with the overall quantity of microorganisms (both aerobes and anaerobes, but predominantly anaerobes), perforations of the lower small bowel and colon produce a higher frequency of infections that contain anaerobic microorganisms, and these patients develop a greater number of infectious complications and exhibit a higher mortality rate. In addition, certain predictable patterns of bacterial isolates are found, and the isolation of these organisms is independent of the site of perforation, indicating that a marked simplification of the numerous microbial forms present in the initial inoculum occurs. This simplification process may be related to synergistic interactions occurring among certain components of the initial inoculum as well as the selection pressure exerted by host defenses on certain microbial forms. Overall, an average of four or five isolates occur in patients with established intraabdominal infection, more than half of which are anaerobes. Both aerobic and anaerobic isolates are encountered in 80% to 90% of specimens, isolation of either aerobes or anaerobes alone being less common. Commonly encountered aerobic isolates are E coli and other gram-negative enteric bacilli, such as Enterobacter sp and Klebsiella sp, gram-positive bacteria (various streptococci, staphylococci, and enterococci), other gram-negative pathogens (Proteus and Pseudomonas sp), and Candida sp. Among the anaerobes, Bacteroides sp (especially B fragilis), Clostridium sp, and the anaerobic cocci are most consistently isolated.[8]

Although the primary treatment of a perforated viscus is surgical, antimicrobial therapy is an extremely important adjunct. Empiric antimicrobial therapy for secondary microbial peritonitis should be directed against both aerobes and anaerobes. Administration of an agent directed against only one component of the infection is inferior to combined therapy. This has been substantiated in carefully stratified groups of patients with perforated or gangrenous appendicitis or who suffer penetrating abdominal trauma that causes perforation of a viscus. As mentioned, several studies indicate that the results of using several agents in combination is equivalent to the use of single-agent therapy as long as the agents selected possess activity against both components of the infection. Selection of inferior single agents with significantly less activity against anaerobes, for example, probably produces deleterious results. The addition of antienterococcal or antifungal agents as initial therapy has not been substantiated. Determining the most beneficial duration of antimicrobial therapy in this setting for a specific patient is difficult. In general, minimal peritoneal contamination with adequate surgical treatment may be treated with a 3- to 5-day course of antimicrobial agents, whereas longer courses are indicated for immunosuppressed patients and patients with extensive contamination.

Fever (temperature higher than 37.6°C) and elevation of the peripheral white blood cell count (more than 10,000 cells/μL) at the termination of antimicrobial therapy have been associated with a high incidence of ongoing or recurrent intraabdominal infection. In this setting, an intensive search for infection should be instituted. During repeated episodes of intraabdominal soilage, patients more frequently develop infections caused by gram-positive cocci, such as S epidermidis, Enterococcus faecalis and faecium, gram-negative organisms such as Pseudomonas aeruginosa, and fungi (primarily C albicans and other species).[9] These organisms are probably selected out by both the failure of host defenses and initial antimicrobial agent therapy. In the setting of tertiary microbial peritonitis, treatment with antimicrobial agents directed against the specific pathogens isolated seems reasonable, although a

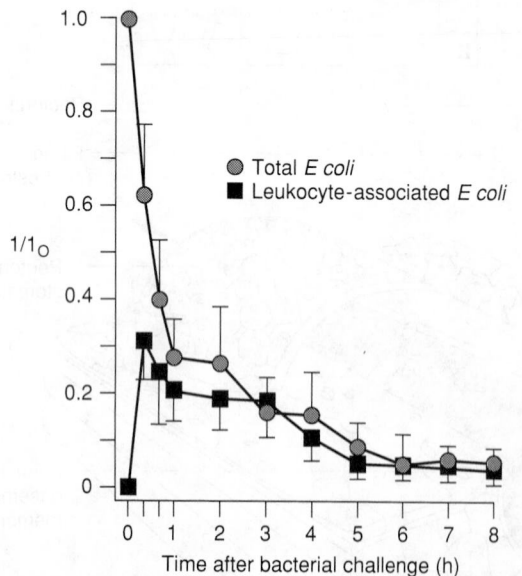

Figure 7-8. Translymphatic clearance and phagocytosis rapidly remove invading bacteria from the confines of the rodent peritoneal cavity. Only extremely large numbers of *Escherichia coli* are able to overwhelm either of these mechanisms, demonstrating the potency of these local host defenses. 1, initial number of *E coli* ingested; 1_o, remaining *E coli* at various times after injection.

salutary effect on patient mortality has been demonstrated with respect to only anticandidal therapy.

Evaluation of the patient with suspected intraabdominal infection should begin with physical examination and an initial flat plate and upright or decubitus roentgenogram of the abdomen. If no obvious viscus perforation is noted, and there is no obvious need for emergent laparotomy (ie, acute abdomen), an ultrasound or a computed tomographic (CT) scan of the abdomen should be performed to exclude the presence of biliary tract disease or an intraabdominal abscess. Intraabdominal fluid collections may be readily diagnosed (greater than 90% accuracy), safely sampled using a small needle, and drained by means of a percutaneously placed catheter should purulent material be aspirated, or if the initial Gram stain or potassium hydroxide preparation is positive. Cultures can be obtained at the time of percutaneous aspiration or laparotomy and can serve to direct therapy, perhaps through alterations in the initial empiric antimicrobial regimen. Should the patient who undergoes percutaneous drainage of an intraabdominal abscess deteriorate, laparotomy should be performed in almost all cases.

When the diagnostic evaluation proves unrevealing in the setting of suspected intraabdominal sepsis, minilaparotomy should be considered. The value of empiric laparotomy in this setting is controversial, and some authors have advocated performing this procedure only when clinical signs and symptoms or diagnostic studies indicate the presence of a potential intraabdominal source of infection, or in younger patients without a defined intraabdominal source of infection but with single organ failure.

Necrotizing Soft Tissue Infections

In 1924, Meleney described a lethal and rapidly progressive soft tissue infection due to a microaerophilic streptococcus (*S evolutus*) and *S aureus*.[10] Subsequent reports have established that necrotizing deep soft tissue infections may involve either the skeletal muscles, the deep muscular fascia, the superficial fascia, or a combination of all these areas. The nomenclature used to categorize severe deep soft tissue infections has become progressively more confusing because there have been many eponyms (eg, Meleney synergistic gangrene) applied to what is probably the same disease process occurring in different layers or sites. Thus, the disease process has been categorized according to the involved body site or tissue plane, the causative organism, the clinical course (clinical symptoms and signs, rapidity of progression), or any combination of these three. The most common entity seen by a surgeon is some form of necrotizing fasciitis, an uncommon infection of the deep and superficial fascia that is associated with a mortality rate as high as 40% in many series. This disease is probably best categorized by site, infecting organism, and extent of initial disease and rapidity of progression.

Although many underlying disease processes predispose patients to necrotizing fasciitis, three common factors are almost invariably present: (1) impairment of the immune system (eg, diabetes mellitus, malignancy, alcoholism); (2) compromise of the fascial blood supply; and (3) the presence of microorganisms that are able to proliferate within this area. Thus, patients who may be immunocompromised and who develop perineal or lower extremity decubitus ulcers, those who undergo closure of heavily contaminated wounds, and those who suffer heavy contamination in the process of traumatic wounding are predisposed to develop this type of infection. Infections of this type are usually polymicrobial in nature, with gram-positive organisms such as staphylococci and streptococci (aerobic and anaerobic), gram-negative enteric bacteria, and gram-

negative anaerobes being frequently identified. These polymicrobial cultural results indicate the occurrence of a synergistic process, perhaps in large part accounting for the severity of these infections. Some microorganisms, however, possess virulence factors that, in conjunction with an underlying host predisposition, allow this disease process to occur without dependence on other bacteria. Examples of this form of disease include necrotizing fasciitis due to *Clostridium, Pseudomonas*, and *Aeromonas* sp. In these patients, the process is often fulminant and is frequently associated with cellulitis, myositis, fasciitis, and bacteremia with an attendant high mortality, probably due to both the soft tissue infection and the bacteremia with concurrent bacterial exotoxin production. Although rare, tetanus and toxic shock syndrome (due to *Clostridium tetani* and certain toxin-producing strains of *S aureus*, respectively) may occur in or around the surgical wound. These unusual infections are associated with few if any of the classic signs of wound infection (eg, erythema, pain, fluctuation, drainage) and are frequently associated with signs of septic shock, organ failure, and high lethality.

Identification of a necrotizing soft tissue infection mandates immediate operative intervention with aggressive resection of all involved tissues and the empiric administration of antimicrobial agents active against gram-positive, gram-negative, and anaerobic bacteria. In most cases, this involves the use of several antimicrobial agents in combination. Because of the concern in all such cases for the presence of *Clostridium* infection, high doses of aqueous penicillin G are administered. Gram-positive organisms are treated with vancomycin or a semisynthetic penicillin, and gram-negative organisms are treated with an aminoglycoside or a monobactam. Anaerobic coverage is typically achieved by use of metronidazole or clindamycin. The use of extended-spectrum agents (eg, carbapenem, ticarcillinclavulinic acid, piperacillin-tazobactam) to treat gram-negative and anaerobic organisms may be acceptable, but it remains untested in this setting.

In most cases, there is a high index of suspicion that this type of disease process is based solely on clinical signs present within the soft tissues (eg, skin discoloration or necrosis; blebs; drainage of thin, watery, grayish, foul-smelling fluid; subcutaneous crepitus). Confirmatory evidence can be provided through local exploration of the wound (with direct observation and performance of a Gram stain) and radiologic studies (plain films, CT, or magnetic resonance imaging of the involved area), but performance of these studies should not preclude immediate operative intervention in a clearcut case or when the diagnosis is highly probable in a patient with evidence of clinical deterioration. Early recognition based on clinical signs, local site exploration, or CT scanning in selected patients, in conjunction with prompt, aggressive, and extensive débridement to remove all devitalized and infected tissue, broad-spectrum antibiotics, fluid resuscitation, hemodynamic monitoring, and nutritional support would appear to afford patients the best chance of survival. Often, such aggressive surgery is mutilating, requiring the removal of large amounts of body tissue and one or more extremities. The clearest guidelines to determine the limits of resection involve removal of clearly infected, necrotic tissue so that margins several centimeters into grossly normal, healthy tissue are achieved. Some authors advocate the use of frozen-section analysis to determine adequacy of excision, and this may be useful in some cases, particularly those in which the observer is unsure whether infected tissue remains at the margin of resection. Many surgeons débride well beyond the border of infection that is grossly visible at the time of surgery and rely on planned reexploration to a greater degree.

Continued areas of controversy include the efficacy of hyperbaric oxygen therapy, particularly in cases of clostridial gangrene, the need for performing a colostomy in patients with the perineal form of the disease (referred to as Fournier gangrene when this process involves the perineum and scrotum in males), and the continuing high mortality rate in patients with all forms of necrotizing fasciitis. Unfortunately, the rarity of the disease has made prospective, randomized data difficult to obtain, so that the literature remains without controlled trials demonstrating any additional benefits derived from hyperbaric oxygen therapy. This form of therapy may be a useful adjunct in some cases but is not available at every facility. Because the entire perineal region and buttocks are frequently involved in patients with perineal necrotizing fasciitis, performance of fecal stream diversion by means of colostomy often improves wound and patient care, although it has not invariably improved outcome. Interestingly, several authors have speculated that the mortality rate of necrotizing fasciitis has remained unchanged because improvements in treatment and critical care may have been offset by the occurrence of this disease process in an increasingly high-risk group of older or immunocompromised patients.

Gram-Negative Bacterial Sepsis, Shock, and Multiple-System Organ Failure

Gram-negative bacterial sepsis is a serious disease process that produces substantial morbidity and mortality in both normal and immunocompromised patients (10% to 20% and 30% lethality, respectively), despite therapeutic intervention with antimicrobial agents, aggressive hemodynamic monitoring, fluid resuscitation, and metabolic support. This disease process represents one of the most severe infections that can occur in the surgical patient. During the past several decades, nosocomial infections due to gram-negative pathogens have increased in frequency, several series reporting an average incidence of 3 to 13 cases of gram-negative bacteremia per 1000 hospital admissions. Many factors predispose patients to these infections:

- Underlying host disease processes such as malignancy, renal insufficiency, congestive heart failure, and diabetes mellitus
- Old age and disability
- Malnutrition
- Previous or concurrent antimicrobial therapy
- Major operations
- Respiratory or urinary manipulation or intubation
- Immunosuppression (acquired or inherited)

Fatality in most series has paralleled the presence and severity of the underlying host disease, polymicrobial bacteremia, shock, and lack of early appropriate antimicrobial therapy.

Although many different organisms cause this form of sepsis, *E coli* predominates in overall frequency. Also common are isolates of *Klebsiella*, *Enterobacter*, and *Serratia*; *Pseudomonas* bacteremia is somewhat less common. Sepsis due to *Proteus*, *Providencia*, *Acinetobacter*, *Aeromonas*, *Citrobacter*, *Achromobacter*, *Salmonella*, *Shigella*, *Bacteroides*, and numerous other organisms also has been reported. Some studies have demonstrated that non–*E coli* sepsis is more lethal than sepsis caused by *E coli*, and that *Pseudomonas* sepsis is associated with the highest lethality, but not all investigators have been able to substantiate this finding. In several series, 10% to 20% of patients had polymicrobial sepsis, and most investigators agree that polymicrobial sepsis is more lethal. This appears to be true even when patients are stratified regarding severity of underlying disease and appropriate or inappropriate antimicrobial therapy.

The manner in which gram-negative bacterial infection causes the initial physiologic host septic response (ie, fever, systemic acidosis, arterial hypoxemia, disordered substrate and oxygen usage, abnormal metabolism, hyperkalemia, hyperglycemia, decreased systemic vascular resistance, elevated cardiac output, and hypotension), the failure of organs separated spatially from the infected site, and eventual lethality has intrigued investigators for years. Although initially it seemed patent that blood-borne bacteria or bacterial toxins were responsible, it appears that more complex interactions probably take place. The triggering and amplification of numerous components of several host mediator systems play an important role, and increasing evidence indicates that organ failure and death may occur subsequent to such an overexuberant host response.

Activation of the complement and coagulation cascades occurs and has been associated with leukopenia due to PMN aggregation, macrophage stimulation, and thrombocytopenia. Release of cellular products such as superoxide radicals, lysosomal enzymes (eg, cathepsin, elastase), prostaglandins, and monokines appears to follow the initial activation steps. Bacteria, bacterial toxins, and host-mediated events alone cannot account for all the alterations that occur in host physiology, and thus some composite effect may be responsible. In particular, several groups of investigators have developed experimental models and have made clinical observations that make it clear that cellular mediators are released in response to a variety of stimuli, including bacterial products, and that excessive mediator secretion causes target organ damage and failure. Precise translation of this information to the clinical setting and demonstration of similar pathogenetic mechanisms have been difficult, and a unified sequence of events that eventuate in lethality has proved elusive.

Increasing evidence has implicated gram-negative bacterial LPS (endotoxin) as that portion of the gram-negative bacterial cell membrane responsible for many, if not all, of the toxic effects that occur during gram-negative bacterial sepsis. For this reason, LPS has been intensively examined from an immunologic, physiologic, and microbiologic standpoint. The biochemical structure of LPS has been determined for many species of gram-negative microorganisms, and generally consists of repeating O-antigen polysaccharide subunits linked to a polysaccharide core region that, in turn, is attached to membrane-bound lipid A (Fig. 7-9). The O-antigen polysaccharide subunits are unique for each organism, and thus largely are responsible for the wide serotypic diversity seen among strains of even a particular gram-negative bacterial species. The core region of LPS demonstrates a significant degree of structural conservation among genera of gram-negative bacteria and consists of a short series of saccharide residues. The innermost or deep portion of core LPS consists of three saccharide residues in most gram-negative bacteria and is the most highly conserved portion of this region. Lipid A is embedded within the outer membrane and consists of diglucosamine residues associated with nonhydroxylated fatty acids of 12- to 16-carbon atom chain length. Although relatively insoluble in aqueous solutions, injection of isolated lipid A produces toxicity in a variety of animal models, leading to the hypothesis that the hydrophilic O antigen solubilizes LPS in the mammalian host milieu, whereas lipid A interacts with lipid components of the host cell membrane.

The LPS molecule exerts diverse effects on the mamma-

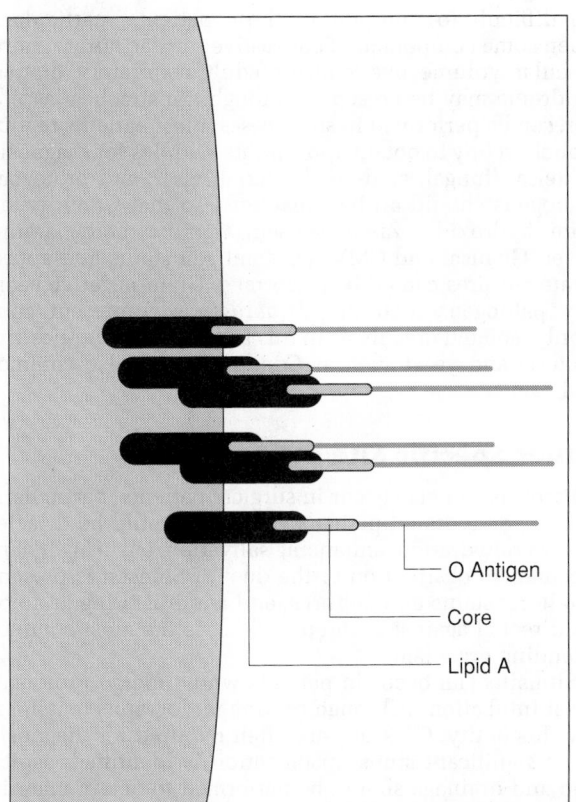

Figure 7-9. Structure of gram-negative bacterial lipopolysaccharide (LPS). LPS consists of three regions: (1) O antigen, a series of repeating polysaccharide units; (2) core LPS, a short series of biochemically and immunologically conserved saccharide residues; and (3) lipid A, which consists of diglucosamine residues associated with nonhydroxylated fatty acids embedded within the outer membrane and responsible for most toxicity.

lian host. Immunologic responses to LPS include nonspecific polyclonal B-cell proliferation, macrophage activation and cytokine secretion, tolerance to a subsequent LPS or bacterial challenge, and production of antibody directed against various portions of the LPS molecule after repeated challenge with either LPS or intact bacteria. Physiologic responses similar to those seen during gram-negative bacterial sepsis occur during LPS administration and include hypotension, hypoxemia, acidosis, bacterial translocation across the gut, complement and coagulation cascade activation, white blood cell and platelet margination, and death.

LPS exerts direct and indirect effects on host tissues to produce the septic response. Indirect (ie, mediated) effects result from LPS triggering of host macrophages. Activated macrophages secrete a wide array of cytokines that include TNF-α, IL-1α, IL-1β, IL-6, and IFN-α. Excessive secretion of monokines produces substantial systemic effects in the mammalian host. The most compelling evidence supporting this contention is the demonstration in experimental models and humans that administration of TNF by itself produces manifestations nearly identical (fever, leukopenia, hypotension, death) to the administration of LPS. Other evidence comes from study of endotoxin-resistant C3H/HeJ mice that do not produce TNF in response to endotoxin challenge. Although these animals are resistant to an otherwise lethal endotoxin challenge, a normal shock response is conferred by bone marrow transplantation from TNF-producing C3H/HeN mice. In addition, serum levels of TNF are elevated in patients with gram-negative

bacterial sepsis, and administration of LPS to humans and nonhuman primates is associated with elevations of TNF after 1.5 to 2 hours. In several animal models, anti-TNF antibody ameliorates lethal effects of either an LPS challenge or a TNF challenge.

TNF-α and IL-1β appear to be primary mediators within the local host milieu, exerting deleterious effects on the host only after large amounts are secreted and reach the systemic circulation. Macrophage IL-2 and IL-6 (and perhaps IL-8 in humans) appear to be secreted after TNF or IL-1 stimulation events occur, whereas IFN-α is secreted at low levels by macrophages during both the initial and subsequent activation and secretion stages. IFN-α may act to facilitate the continued activation of macrophages, recruitment of additional activated macrophages, and ongoing output of the mentioned cytokines. Serum IL-1β levels are increased in humans after exogenous endotoxin administration and are elevated after gram-negative bacterial challenge in nonhuman primates. Protective doses of anti-TNF antibody abrogates this increase in IL-1. IL-1 also has been shown to enhance survival in neutropenic mice after gram-negative bacterial challenge.

Similarly, IL-6 levels are elevated systemically and at the site of infection in animal and clinical studies. In humans, administration of LPS leads to increased serum levels of IL-6, and anti-TNF antibody abrogates the serum increase in IL-6 seen after gram-negative bacterial challenge in animal models. Although IL-6 administration does not itself lead to increased mortality, anti–IL-6 antibodies have been shown to improve survival after experimental gram-negative bacterial challenge. Several studies have also indicated that previous administration of low-dose LPS, TNF, or high-dose IL-2 may actually enhance survival during experimental gram-negative bacterial infection, indicating that the level of activation or ability of the host to respond to cytokine secretion may be of critical importance.

Thus, this portion of the host response that normally acts to contain and localize infection may injure the host during systemic infection, leading to the high mortality events of septic shock and multiple-system organ failure (MSOF). Isolated pulmonary failure (adult respiratory distress syndrome) is common after systemic sepsis, whereas gut, hepatic, and renal failure may occur subsequently. Many studies have clearly correlated mortality during MSOF with the number of organs failing.

The diagnosis of systemic sepsis is frequently suspected when the physiologic alterations occur after a known or suspected source of infection is identified, but the diagnosis is truly confirmed only after blood cultures become positive for a specific microorganism. Identification of the presence of gram-negative LPS is problematic at best because available assays, such as the limulus lysate test, are subject to a great deal of variation. Antibody detection tests for LPS, gram-positive, or fungal cell wall components have been examined experimentally and clinically, but most suffer from lack of specificity when biologic fluids are tested and are not routinely available. During the time in which a diagnosis is being established, clinical deterioration frequently occurs, and therapy must be instituted before the availability of confirmatory cultural data, based on a high index of suspicion that bacteremia may be present.

Many studies have demonstrated a salutary effect when appropriate treatment is begun early in the course of disease. Evidence also exists that empiric antimicrobial therapy directed against gram-negative aerobes may have a salutary effect in febrile, neutropenic patients with hematologic malignancies. Most of these studies indicate that two agents in combination may provide greater survival than the use of a single agent, and this information has been extended to therapy in nonneutropenic patients (a reasonable, put perhaps unwarranted, assumption). Other studies have demonstrated that gram-positive microorganisms are also important nosocomial pathogens, particularly in the former group of patients. Both gram-negative and gram-positive facultative aerobes play an important role in the development of nosocomial infections in the surgical intensive care unit, and anaerobic microorganisms are common components of intraabdominal and soft tissue infections. For that reason, empiric antimicrobial therapy is often directed against these two former types of pathogens, and against the latter type if a nonnosocomial source is concomitantly suspected.

Catheter and Prosthetic Device Infections

Prosthetic device and catheter infections are frequently the result of low-virulence organisms such as *S epidermidis*, although *S aureus* is also a frequent pathogen, and infection due to gram-negative bacteria and yeast can also occur. Gram-positive organisms are capable of adhering to synthetic polymers with great avidity and forming an exopolysaccharide slime layer that inhibits antimicrobial agent penetration. Treatment consists of device removal and antimicrobial agents directed against the infecting organism. Although this is a simple proposition with regard to percutaneously inserted catheters, many types of chronic indwelling catheters and devices require operative removal. A prolonged course of antibiotic therapy serves to eradicate infection in some cases but not in overtly bacteremic or fungemic patients. This latter approach may be indicated in patients who experience relatively few systemic manifestations due to the infection and who would be adversely affected by removal of the device (eg, loss of access for intravenous nutrition). Removal should never be delayed, nor should antimicrobial agents be withheld, in a patient who has obvious purulence in the region of the catheter and evidence of systemic sepsis.

Urinary Tract Infections

Urinary tract infections are often of concern, particularly in the hospitalized patient, because they represent the most common cause of gram-negative bacterial sepsis. The presence of more than 10^5 CFU/mL in a patient without a Foley catheter in place is diagnostic of infection, and 10^2 to 10^3 CFU/mL is considered significant in a patient who has been catheterized for a short time. Prostatitis should also be considered in this setting in the male patient and usually can be identified based on rectal examination findings, although transrectal ultrasonography may prove useful in selected cases. Because many antimicrobial agents concentrate to a high degree in the urine, it is often possible to eradicate a urinary tract infection quickly. Cultural and sensitivity reports should be obtained, and follow-up urine specimens should be sent to the laboratory to ensure the successful treatment of such infections. Gram-negative bacilli are frequent pathogens involved in these infections, but gram-positive organisms such as enterococci and even staphylococci are not uncommonly identified.

Nosocomial Pneumonia

Nosocomial pneumonia also represents a difficult diagnostic and therapeutic problem, frequently being suspected in the septic patient who requires prolonged intubation and mechanical ventilation. Chest radiographs often are difficult to interpret in these patients, particularly when some component of congestive cardiac failure, intravascular volume overload, or adult respiratory distress syndrome may be present. Although transtracheal aspiration can be performed in some cases, most patients require bronchoscopy to obtain appropriate samples for diagnosis. Bacterial, fungal, acid-fast bacterial, viral, and protozoan pathogens should all be considered so that Gram, potassium hydroxide, Ziehl-Neelsen, Gomori methenamine-silver, Giemsa, and CMV rapid antigen stains and appropriate cultures can all be performed. Gram-negative bacillary pathogens including *P aeruginosa* represent commonly isolated organisms in this setting, but gram-positive bacteria and yeast such as *Candida* sp are also common pathogens.

Other Specific Site Infections

Parotitis can also occur in surgical patients, particularly elderly, dehydrated patients. Therapy should be directed toward rehydration, enhancing salivation, ensuring that no mechanical obstruction of the duct of Stensen is present, obtaining stains and cultures, and administering antibiotics directed against *S aureus*, which is the most common offending organism.

Sinusitis can occur in patients who undergo prolonged nasal intubation. Although routine radiographs may identify this entity, CT scans are often required for diagnosis. Once significant sinus opacification is identified, aspiration and drainage should be performed to obtain material for stain and culture, but this procedure is also therapeutic.

Pseudomembranous colitis is caused by *Clostridium difficile* overgrowth and toxin secretion within the colon. It is associated with alterations in the colonic microflora that occur most frequently during antimicrobial agent administration but that also may take place during debilitating illness. Treatment consists of oral metronidazole or vancomycin, and it is prudent to discontinue or truncate the intravenous antimicrobial treatment course.

FUNGAL INFECTIONS

Infections due to fungal pathogens have become increasingly common, frequently occurring in patients undergoing prolonged hospitalization in the surgical intensive care unit and in immunocompromised patients. *Candida* sp (*C albicans*, *C tropicalis*, *C parapsilosis*, *C krusei*, and *C glabrata*) are the most frequent fungal pathogens isolated and are common elements of the host microflora. Prophylaxis with oral antifungal agents is warranted, especially during periods of maximal immunosuppression in transplant recipients, in patients with uncontrolled diabetes, or during some cases of prolonged antibacterial antimicrobial therapy.

In general, local, apparently noninvasive candidal infections involving the integument and mucous membranes are treated with oral decontamination and topical antifungal therapy using agents such as nystatin. Candidal urinary tract infections can be treated either with an oral antifungal agent or with topical amphotericin B as a continuous bladder irrigation. More difficult decisions concern the use of amphotericin B in patients who have fungal pathogens isolated from several sites. Several studies have demonstrated that patients with three positive sites, or with peritoneal or blood cultures positive for *Candida* sp, exhibit higher survival rates when amphotericin B therapy is instituted early in the course of infection. Thus, an obvious site of infection, such as pneumonitis with a positive fungal culture on bronchoscopy, positive fungal blood cultures, the presence of retinal changes compatible with candidal retinitis, or *Candida* sp present within the peritoneal cavity are generally considered indications for a limited course of amphotericin B therapy (300 to 500 mg). This issue remains controversial, and the role of combination therapy with 5-fluorocytosine or therapy with azole class drugs (eg, miconazole, ketoconazole, fluconazole, itraconazole) remains to be established.

Infection due to *Aspergillus niger*, *A fumigatus*, *A flavus*, and *A terreus* and other less common species can involve the lung, upper respiratory tract, oropharyngeal region, ear, sinuses, skin and soft tissue, and central nervous system. Preexisting pulmonary cavities with subsequent invasion by fungi and formation of an aspergilloma or fungus ball has been the classic description of this disease, but patients more commonly develop a diffuse pneumonia with patchy infiltrates on chest roentgenograms. Central nervous system involvement can also occur as an extremely insidious but lethal process, with the development of a fungal brain abscess. Therapy with systemic amphotericin B should be instituted based on even a presumptive diagnosis. Patients with severe infections probably should also receive 5-fluorocytosine and rifampin, although their added efficacy has not been unequivocally demonstrated. Deep fungal infections such as these require long-term systemic amphotericin B therapy with a total dose of between 2 and 3 g. The timing of surgical extirpative therapy has not been well defined. In general, however, fungal lesions that do not regress after 1 to 3 weeks of antifungal therapy may require excision, after which antifungal agent therapy is continued. Occasionally, the location of discrete areas of fungal infection in proximity to vital structures or progression while on initial therapy mandates early surgical intervention.

Cryptococcus neoformans is an encapsulated fungus that causes pulmonary, central nervous system, and disseminated cutaneous infection in immunosuppressed patients. Pulmonary disease can be insidious, producing mild fever, malaise, and a nonproductive cough. Central nervous system disease may present as malaise, fever, or headache either alone or in combination. Any patient with pulmonary cryptococcosis should undergo lumbar puncture. India ink preparations may demonstrate the organism in the cerebrospinal fluid, but tests for cerebrospinal fluid cryptococcal antigen and systemic antibody directed against this organism may also be helpful in establishing the diagnosis. Therapy consists of combined amphotericin B and 5-fluorocytosine. The total dose of amphotericin B that should be administered is between 1 and 1.5 g. Azole agents such as fluconazole also may be effective in the treatment of this disease.

Histoplasma capsulatum can cause both pulmonary and disseminated disease in transplant recipients. It can produce skin lesions that resemble erythema nodosum, and recognition of these lesions may be a key to the diagnosis. *Coccidioides immitis* can produce disease in healthy or immunosuppressed people who inhale the highly infective arthrospores in an endemic region. Treatment of either disease consists of the long-term administration of systemic amphotericin B. Phycomycoses due to *Mucor* and *Rhizopus* spp can produce locally destructive rhinocerebral or soft tissue infections that are difficult to eradicate. Central nervous system involvement is common and often fatal. Treatment consists of local aggressive surgical excision and long-term systemic amphotericin B.

Treatment of fungal infection consists of a clinical assessment to determine the severity of disease (superficial versus deep) as well as any laboratory information concerning the sensitivity patterns of the organism. As a general rule, superficial infections and those due to relatively low-virulence organisms (candidal esophagitis or sepsis) can be treated with 350 to 500 mg of systemic amphotericin B. Increasing evidence indicates that azole agents such as fluconazole may be efficacious in this setting, but until randomized, comparative trials are performed, this remains suppositional. More aggressive candidal infections and organisms with more invasive potential, such as *C neoformans*, require a more prolonged course of this agent and often the addition of a second agent, such as 5-fluorocytosine. Infections due to *Aspergillus* sp, *Mucor* sp, and other organisms require prolonged treatment (2 to 3 g total dose) with amphotericin B and 5-fluorocytosine; often, the addition of a third agent such as rifampin may be beneficial. The use of ketoconazole, and more potent azole class agents such as fluconazole and itraconazole, also may be considered in selected cases. These agents are less toxic but have not been demonstrated to be of equivalent efficacy to amphotericin B for the treatment of many organisms. Finally, patients receiving exogenous immunosuppressive agents should undergo a marked dosage reduction, and some agents should be discontinued until the infection is adequately controlled or is eradicated.

VIRAL INFECTIONS

Formerly, outside of the field of transplantation, the practicing surgeon was not frequently called on to treat viral disease. Solid organ transplant recipients are prone to develop viral infections by virtue of exogenous immunosuppression. Although this section emphasizes the nature of viral infections in transplant recipients, it is increasingly recognized that viral infections exert a significant impact on other groups of patients that the practicing surgeon may be called on to treat.

Herpesvirus Infections

The most common posttransplantation viral infections are those caused by herpes viruses (CMV, herpes simplex virus [HSV], Epstein-Barr virus [EBV], and varicella-zoster virus [VZV], and herpes virus type 6). All are most common during the periods of maximal host immunosuppression that occur immediately after transplantation and during treatment of allograft rejection. CMV is a common cause of fever after solid organ transplantation, and evidence of CMV infection occurs in about 30% of patients. Incidence factors associated with the occurrence of CMV infection include antirejection therapy, especially with antilymphocyte antibody preparations, increasing age, or cadaveric source. Patients who have no serologic evidence of CMV and who receive an organ from a CMV-seropositive donor are at highest risk for developing primary CMV infection and disease. Reactivation CMV infection can occur in CMV-seropositive recipients, and superinfection CMV disease (eg, the occurrence of both primary and reactivation disease due to distinct strains of CMV) has also been reported.

Manifestations of CMV infection range from asymptomatic evidence of infection based on a rise in anti-CMV titers or cultural evidence of viral shedding; to mild to moderate disease in which systemic signs and symptoms such as fever, leukopenia, malaise, lethargy, and myalgias occur; to severe disease manifestations in which the mentioned signs and symptoms are accompanied by profound hypotension, pulmonary failure, hepatitis, pancreatitis, massive gastrointestinal hemorrhage (upper or lower) due to virus-induced mucosal ulcerations, MSOF, and death. The most common presentation is that of a febrile, leukopenic patient with a cough, diffuse interstitial infiltrates on a chest radiograph, and hypoxia. A small subset of patients who have only gastrointestinal manifestations has also been recognized.

The diagnosis of CMV can be supported based on the mentioned symptoms and signs and can be confirmed by several tests. Serologic evidence is usually based on evidence of a greater than four-fold increase in anti-CMV antibody titer in two specimens obtained at separate times. Cultural evidence or the demonstration of typical CMV inclusion bodies from body fluid or a tissue specimen provide unequivocal evidence of CMV infection. Fluorescein-labeled anti-CMV monoclonal antibodies have been used in either direct or growth-augmented (shell vial) tests to provide a rapid diagnosis in less than 24 hours. Direct observation of the stained specimen by fluorescence microscopy is performed to detect the presence of CMV. Direct nucleic acid blotting and PCR analysis also have been used to detect the presence of CMV in body fluid samples with high specificity and sensitivity, although these tests are not routinely available.

Previously, the diagnosis of CMV relied heavily on serologic data, and cultural data were often not available for several days or several weeks. The earlier-mentioned tests allow the diagnosis of CMV to be made much more rapidly, and their development has coincided with the availability of effective anti-CMV therapy with agents such as ganciclovir. Thus, the surgical clinician is able to both diagnose and treat CMV in an effective fashion.

Although CMV disease continues to be associated with decreased patient and allograft survival, several studies indicate that a reduction in disease incidence is possible by use of either prophylactic administration of ganciclovir, acyclovir, anti-CMV immunoglobulin preparations, or a combination of these modalities. Treatment of CMV disease with ganciclovir, a drug that possesses substantially more in vitro activity against CMV than acyclovir, is efficacious, and preliminary data indicate that it may be possible to treat patients with mild CMV disease with ganciclovir and concurrently treat rejection as well. Foscarnet is another drug with considerable activity against CMV that has also been demonstrated to be efficacious in a limited number of patients, although this agent possesses neurotoxicity and nephrotoxicity.

HSV infection causes painful oropharyngeal ulcerations in most cases, although sporadic cases of disseminated disease (meningoencephalitis, hepatitis, pneumonitis) have been reported. Although HSV alone does not appear to affect patient or allograft survival adversely, combined HSV and CMV infections exert a deleterious effect on these parameters over and above the effect of CMV alone. EBV causes an occasional case of a mononucleosis-type syndrome but has also been clearly implicated in the pathogenesis of posttransplantation lymphomas. VZV infection can present as disseminated and occasionally life-threatening infection in nonimmune transplant recipients, or as painful herpes zoster in patients who had previously developed chicken pox. Primary HSV, EBV, and VZV infections are effectively treated with acyclovir. Evidence of initial life-threatening disease or of rapid disease progression mandates a concurrent reduction in immunosuppression, intravenous acyclovir, and hospitalization. VZV hyperimmune globulin may also provide benefit as prophylaxis for VZV-seronegative patients with clearcut VZV exposure or for treatment of severe cases in conjunction with acyclovir.[11]

Acquired Immunodeficiency Syndrome

A great deal of information has accumulated within the last several years with regard to cause and pathogenesis of acquired immunodeficiency syndrome (AIDS). This syndrome is caused by a human retrovirus (HIV-1) that infects T lymphocytes and causes severe immunosuppression. HIV-1 is a member of a family of lymphotrophic viruses, many of which appear to primarily affect other mammalian hosts, such as felines or primates. Infection is acquired through parenteral or sexual transmissions. Intravenous drug abuse, male homosexuality, and prostitution all represent high-risk types of behavior that predispose to HIV infection. People who live or travel in Haiti or sub-Saharan Africa, where the virus is endemic, also represent a potential high-risk group.

HIV detection typically consists of initial ELISA screening, but this test has a 1% to 3% false-positive rate. Although sensitive, the significant false-positive rate of this test mandates that all patients with positive ELISA tests be retested by the sensitive and specific Western immunotransblot analysis, in which viral capsid antigens are first subjected to electrophoresis, followed by immunoelectrophoretic transblotting onto nitrocellulose, where antibody directed against specific antigens can be detected. In particular, the HIV p24 antigen appears to be a sensitive indicator of HIV infection. Evidence indicates that initial infection with HIV is followed by a latent period that may last several months, after which viremia can be detected by cultural data, after which evidence of anti-HIV antibody is detectable.

Southern transblot detection and amplified PCR analysis are also available on an investigational basis at some institutions; both (particularly the latter) are extremely sensitive tests for detecting viral nucleic acid replication. These tests may become increasingly important in the diagnosis of HIV because many patients who are infected with HIV

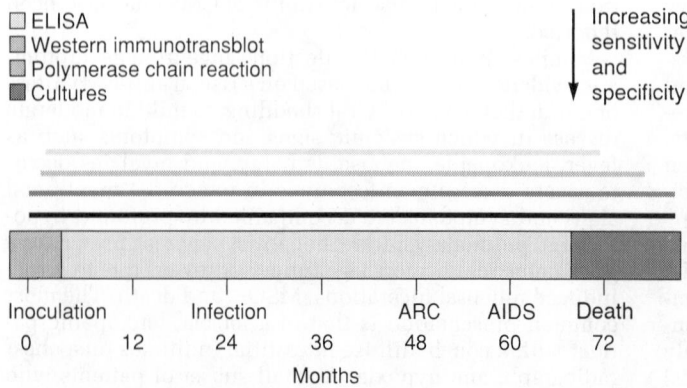

☐ ELISA
☐ Western immunotransblot
☐ Polymerase chain reaction
■ Cultures

Increasing sensitivity and specificity

Figure 7-10. Diagnostic tests used to identify the human immunodeficiency virus (HIV) and the general time courses during infection in which they may be positive. The enzyme-linked immunosorbent assay (ELISA) has a 0.1% false-positive rate, whereas the Western immunotransblot is more sensitive and specific. The polymerase chain reaction test is also used for HIV detection and may become increasingly important in the diagnosis of HIV because many patients who are infected with HIV may not exhibit an initial antibody response, so that the infection is undetected by either ELISA or Western immunotransblot analysis.

may not develop an initial antibody response, so that the infection is undetected by either ELISA or Western immunotransblot analysis (Fig. 7-10).

Several concerns about HIV disease transmission have arisen with regard to surgical patients. First, transfusion-associated HIV transmission has been documented; this has increased enthusiasm for limiting blood transfusions, for cell salvage and autotransfusion devices, and for autodonation of blood before elective operative procedures. Screening of all blood products before transfusion and exclusion of blood donors based on a history of high-risk activities have reduced the possibility of transfusion-associated AIDS to a low level. It is possible, however, to transfuse HIV-infected blood or blood products that are ELISA negative because a person may donate before developing an anti-HIV antibody response. Second, surgeons are concerned about the risk to themselves and other health care workers who are exposed to blood or body fluids from HIV-infected patients. Several cases of HIV transmission due to accidental punctures from hollow core needles used in patients with AIDS have been reported. Although HIV transmission appears to require a larger inoculum than hepatitis B virus, the disease is obviously potentially more lethal. Third, the concern about possible transmission of HIV from an HIV-infected surgeon to a patient has arisen. For that reason, the highly controversial issues of HIV screening of both patients and surgeons have been deliberated, although no resolution has emerged.

Many institutions have employed universal blood and body substance precautions, which entail treating all invasive procedures as having the potential to transmit disease such as HIV and hepatitis. HIV-infected patients may not be detected by routine antibody tests even though they are infective they reason, so stringent precautions to prevent disease transmission to health care workers should be applied to each and every case. Some surgeons believe that all patients should undergo preoperative HIV testing so that additional measures (eg, only one surgeon operating at a time with minimal assistance, use of Kevlar gloves) can be undertaken, and that the benefits of such a policy may outweigh the potential risk of being unable to maintain the anonymity of a patient identified as being infected with HIV or the occasional initial labeling of a patient as being HIV-positive who subsequently is found to be negative. The issue of HIV transmission from surgeon to patient is a difficult one and has yet to be unequivocally documented. Except when performing procedures in which the surgeon's blood intermingles with the patient's tissues because of a deep cut or needle stick, transmission seems a remote possibility, and the examples (orthopedic procedures, vaginal hysterectomy) of procedures during which this might occur do not really seem concordant with the manner in which these procedures can be performed to minimize this risk. These highly controversial issues continue to be deliberated but are unlikely to be resolved in the immediate future. The HIV-exposed person may consider use of prophylactic azidothymidine (AZT) or sequential serologic testing.

Patients who become infected with HIV are prone to a variety of infections and different types of malignancy. A spectrum exists in which patients progress from asymptomatic infection, to development of the AIDS-related complex of diseases, to AIDS itself. Common infections occurring in patients with AIDS are *Pneumocystis carinii* pneumonia, CMV pneumonitis, gastroenteritis, hepatitis, meningitis due to *C neoformans*, and pneumonia and disseminated infection due to atypical mycobacteria such as *Mycobacterium avium-intracellu-*

lare, M kansasii, and *M chelonei,* as well as gastrointestinal infections due to *Cryptosporidium* sp and *Campylobacter jejuni.* Predisposition to these infections is due in large part to the lymphotrophic nature of HIV, which markedly reduces the number of helper T cells as well as the absolute number of T cells.

Treatment of the AIDS-related complex and AIDS consists of aggressive antiinfective therapy, once a specific infection occurs, and use of AZT. AZT appears to prolong survival when administered early in the course of disease and is considered routine therapy. It is by no means clear that it is possible to eradicate this type of infection. Identification of CD3 antigen as the target molecule on the human T cell for HIV has led to proposals for drugs that mimic this receptor and prevent binding. This approach holds much promise, but prevention of disease transmission by education and by convincing people in high-risk groups to use condoms during sexual intercourse and to avoid sharing of needles may have the greatest impact on reducing the incidence of AIDS.

Hepatitis Viruses

Five distinct hepatitis viruses have been identified—hepatitis A, B, C (formerly non-A, non-B), D (δ), and E. Hepatitis A is usually spread through fecal—oral routes and only occasionally comes to the attention of the surgeon. Hepatitis B is transmitted through parenteral routes in most cases, although oral and sexual transmissions have been described. Infection can lead to either asymptomatic or symptomatic disease, depending on the extent of infection within the liver. Patients may have jaundice, lethargy, malaise, and evidence of acute hepatic transaminase elevations that persist for several weeks. During this stage, IgM antibody directed against surface and subsequently core antigens occurs, followed by the development of IgG antibody production.

Acute infection usually resolves without further sequelae, but 10% to 15% of patients subsequently experience chronic active or chronic persistent hepatitis with evidence of chronic antigenemia. Rarely, acute hepatitis progresses to fulminant hepatic failure, coma, and death. This type of infection and chronic active hepatitis appear to be more commonly associated with infection due to e antigen hepatitis B virus.

High-risk groups of patients (eg, hemodialysis, transplantation, hemophilia patients) and health care workers (eg, surgeons, dentists, hemodialysis unit personnel) should receive three vaccinations of the recombinant DNA hepatitis B vaccine if no previous exposure has been documented. Vaccination is not recommended in people who possess anti—hepatitis B antibody. Examination of post-vaccination antibody titers indicates that hemodialysis patients do not invariably respond to the initial vaccination series and so may require subsequent antibody level determination and booster vaccinations. Administration of anti—hepatitis B immunoglobulin and subsequent vaccination should occur in nonimmune patients after exposure to hepatitis B virus.

Hepatitis C can cause acute elevations in hepatic enzyme and chronic antigenemia, in much the same way as occurs with hepatitis B. Transmission occurs by blood products, and this virus is probably responsible for most cases of transfusion-related hepatitis. Identification is possible by an ELISA-based technique as well as more sophisticated recombinant immunoblot assays and PCR. Hepatitis D cannot in and of itself cause disease but acts as a secondary virus to hepatitis B. The disease caused by both together is more severe than hepatitis B alone.

PROTOZOAN AND PARASITIC PATHOGENS

Surgeons occasionally treat patients with disease caused by either protozoan or parasitic organisms, and this depends largely on geographic location because these types of infections are more common in semitropical and tropical habitats. Thus, occasional cases of amebic or echinococcal liver abscesses require operation, and rare cases are seen of bowel obstruction with or without free peritoneal perforation and widespread dissemination (due to various helminths) or of biliary tract disease (due to the oriental liver fluke Clonorchis sinensis). Solid organ transplant recipients and patients with AIDS can develop unusual infections caused by some more common protozoan pathogens, such as P carinii and Toxoplasma gondii.

P carinii causes cough, tachypnea, and mild fever; bilateral diffuse alveolar infiltrates and interstitial pneumonia are seen on the chest roentgenogram. The diagnosis must be rapidly established by bronchoscopy and in some cases open lung biopsy because of the high attendant mortality rate if untreated. Treatment consists of parenteral trimethoprim-sulfamethoxazole, trimethoprim-dapsone, or pentamidine, even if the diagnosis is presumptive. This disease rarely occurs in patients receiving trimethoprim-sulfamethoxazole prophylaxis. T gondii can cause a mononucleosis syndrome in healthy patients; in immunosuppressed patients, necrotizing encephalitis, myocarditis, pneumonitis, and death can occur. Toxoplasma-naive solid organ transplantation patients are more prone to infection if they receive organs from donors with evidence of previous Toxoplasma infection, and this disease is more common in cardiac allograft recipients. Treatment consists of administration of pyrimethamine and sulfadiazine.

NEW TREATMENT MODALITIES

Although the concept of host defense modulation is by no means new, increasing understanding of the host response has led to the accumulation of significant amounts of new information. The imperfect level of our understanding of the pathophysiology of infection makes difficult the prediction of the ultimate ramifications of even precisely targeted intervention. Thus, many antiinflammatory and antiinfective agents have been tested experimentally and clinically, with few concrete changes in clinical practice. For instance, although many experimental studies have provided evidence that administration of corticosteroids may reduce septic lethality, in most cases, the effect is maximized by corticosteroid treatment before the septic insult. Two clinical trials examining the effect of corticosteroid administration during septic shock reached the conclusion that administration of these agents did not reduce septic lethality and may adversely influence outcome in some patients. Other antiinflammatory agents have been tested experimentally but have also not clearly been found to be efficacious in the treatment of clinical sepsis.

Endogenous opioids (eg, β-endorphin) are released into the cerebral ventricles and systemic circulation in conjunction with endogenous adrenocorticotropic hormone, which promotes corticosteroid secretion during various types of stress and shock, including LPS administration. Many studies have demonstrated the salutary effects of opioid antagonist administration in animals subjected to shock for a variety of causes, including sepsis. Mortality has not been affected routinely when opioid antagonists are administered without other agents. Clinical studies have not uniformly indicated a successful treatment for septic shock. Other opioid antagonists, such as thyrotropin-releasing hormone, may prove to be more efficacious. Fibronectin has been administered to septic patients in an effort to enhance bacterial clearance, bacteriolysis, and host leukocyte phagocytosis. Despite several clinical trials, administration of cryoprecipitate that contains high levels of fibronectin has not been clearly demonstrated to be efficacious.

Gut Decontamination

The composition of the gut microflora is altered during hospitalization, antimicrobial agent administration, and various disease states. In most cases, the number of facultative aerobic isolates increases throughout the intestine, the number of anaerobic forms decreases, and thus the ability of anaerobic colonization resistance to prevent microbial adherence and invasion is presumably diminished. In addition to providing the initial inoculum when overt intestinal perforation occurs, the altered upper gastrointestinal microflora has been implicated in the development of nosocomial pneumonia, and the lower gastrointestinal microflora is implicated in the process of bacterial translocation.

Prolonged intubation for the purpose of mechanical ventilation is associated with initial or oropharyngeal and subsequent gastric colonization with facultative gram-negative aerobic organisms such as E coli, P aeruginosa, and Klebsiella pneumoniae. This phenomenon has also been associated with gram-negative respiratory infections caused by the identical organisms in a given patient. These same organisms may colonize and proliferate in the distal gastrointestinal tract despite so-called colonization resistance resulting from the presence of anaerobic organisms.

Bacterial translocation is a process in which bacteria are able to transgress the gut barrier and are engulfed by local macrophages that reside within mesenteric lymph nodes. Portal and systemic bacteremia and endotoxemia occur in some cases, depending on the severity of the insult. This process has been primarily documented in experimental models in two ways: (1) through so-called monoassociation of gnotobiotic or conventional antibiotic gut decontaminated animals with specific types of bacteria, and (2) by subjecting conventional animals to a variety of insults (eg, endotoxemia, thermal injury, intestinal ischemia). Although experimental and some clinical evidence supports the role of bacterial translocation during sepsis, exact cause and effect have not been clearly established. Of critical importance may be the influence of translocating bacteria and LPS on hepatic metabolism because hepatic macrophages (Kupffer cells) may be stimulated to produce cytokines such as TNF or IL-1 that act at the local and systemic levels to produce adverse effects on the host.

To reduce the quantity of aerobic gram-negative bacillary organisms present within the intestinal tract, several groups have studied the impact of selective gut decontamination. This technique involves the use of orally administered antimicrobial agents that achieve high intraluminal levels directed against gram-negative aerobes and yeast, leaving the host anaerobic intestinal microflora relatively undisrupted. Although a reduction or alteration in the microorganisms responsible for infectious episodes has been demonstrated in neutropenic patients with underlying hematologic malignancies and in intensive care unit patients, a clearcut impact on host mortality has not been clearly shown, particularly in the latter group.

Lipopolysaccharide Neutralization

Because LPS may be responsible for toxicity both directly and through host mediator systems, the ability of various agents to bind to this portion of the gram-negative bacterial outer membrane to reduce mortality has been intensively examined. Polymyxin B, a polypeptide antibiotic, binds stoichiometrically to the lipid A region of LPS but is extremely toxic when administered systemically. Administration of this drug may reduce lethality during experimental gram-negative bacteremia or endotoxemia, but toxicity has largely precluded clinical utility, although selective removal using extracorporeal hemofiltration may be possible.

Gram-negative bacterial infection or injection of LPS in experimental models results in the development of antibody primarily directed against O antigen, whereas little antibody directed against the core–lipid A region of LPS is produced. Anti–O-antigen antibody is serotype specific and is not cross-reactive. This same phenomenon appears to occur clinically. Because of the wide range of gram-negative bacterial serotypes that cause clinical infection, an intensive effort has been directed toward the identification of cross-reactive components of LPS against which antibody can be directed. A series of so-called rough mutants of both *Salmonella minnesota* and *E coli* 0111:B4 have been defined that consists of *S minnesota* Ra, Rb, Rc, Rd$_1$, Rd$_2$, and Re and *E coli* J5. These bacteria express progressively larger portions of the core region (inner or deep, intermediate, and outer) of LPS on their outer membranes as follows: *S minnesota* Re (deep, lipid A plus 3 sugars); Rd (intermediate, lipid A plus 5 sugars); Rc (intermediate, lipid A plus 6 sugars); *E coli* J5 (intermediate, lipid A plus 7 sugars); *S minnesota* Rb (outer, lipid A plus 10 sugars); and Ra (outer, lipid A plus 11 sugars). Rough mutants have also been defined for other gram-negative microorganisms, including other types of *E coli*, *Salmonella typhimurium*, and *P aeruginosa*. These organisms, or their derived outer membrane LPS, therefore represent suitable immunogens for the development of cross-reactive antibodies, and the deep core–lipid A region of LPS may represent the ideal candidate for a target antigen because (1) it is biochemically and immunologically highly conserved among a wide variety of gram-negative microorganisms, and (2) it represents the toxic moiety of LPS.

All of the initial studies performed in this field used polyclonal antibody derived from animal or human sources and indicated that type-specific (anti–O-antigen) antibody could provide potent non–cross-reactive protection during experimental gram-negative bacterial sepsis. These initial studies were hampered by the fact that monospecific antibody reagents were not available, and thus nonspecific effects could not be excluded. Subsequent studies using monoclonal antibodies have indicated that anti-LPS antibody can provide protection against either an LPS or a bacterial challenge. Although some authors have stated that only IgM antibodies enhance survival, others have provided evidence demonstrating that anti-LPS antibodies of similar but not identical specificity of either IgG or IgM classes provided similar protective capacity. Several groups have developed monoclonal antibodies directed against various portions of the core region of LPS as well as lipid A, and have demonstrated that administration of these cross-reactive anticore LPS reagents provides protective capacity during experimental endotoxemia and gram-negative bacteremia or peritonitis. In general, although anti–core LPS–lipid A monoclonal antibodies are more cross-reactive in vitro, these antibodies provide less potent protective capacity in vivo than anti–O-antigen reagents.[12]

That the presence of an anti–core LPS antibody titer occurs naturally and may be protective during clinical gram-negative bacterial infection has been demonstrated in several retrospective clinical studies. In addition, immunization of human volunteers with rough mutant organisms produces an antibody titer, and this serum or plasma is protective in experimental models of sepsis. Using polyclonal anti–*E coli* J5 human antibody preparations, several authors have demonstrated a reduction in mortality when

antiserum was administered to septic patients, although one group could not demonstrate protection when this antiserum was administered as single-dose prophylaxis to neutropenic patients to prevent septic complications. Several recent clinical trials have been performed using anti–core LPS–lipid A monoclonal antibody preparations. Although preliminary evidence indicated that a reduction in lethality can occur using either HA-1A or ES anti–lipid A IgM monoclonal antibody for the treatment of gram-negative bacterial sepsis, subsequent large, multicenter randomized trials provided no evidence of benefit. It remains unclear whether this was due to lack of anti-LPS activity of the reagents or inability to select out appropriate patients with gram-negative bacterial sepsis rather than infection due to other types of microbes. Both factors probably serve to explain the lack of efficacy of these antibody preparations. Trials are also underway to determine the effect of anti-TNF antibody preparations and TNF-binding protein during gram-negative bacterial sepsis, both of which abrogate TNF activity. Bacteriocidal permeability–increasing protein, an endogenous substance found in leukocyte granules that demonstrates anti-LPS activity, also is being tested in clinical trials.

Immunostimulants

Although many compounds have been studied experimentally, few have provided clinical efficacy in reducing the rate or severity of infection. Several compounds derived from mycobacterial or yeast cell wall extracts (muramyl dipeptide, zymosan, and glucan) probably act as direct macrophage stimulants, thereby directly enhancing the state of activation of host defenses. Levamisole, an antihelminthic agent, appears to stimulate PMNs directly and has been shown to possess limited clinical efficacy in a single trial. Thymopentin and several other synthetic compounds have undergone clinical testing. Thymopentin is a peptide that contains the active site of thymopoetin, a thymic hormone that acts to stimulate T-lymphocyte activity. Preliminary trials indicate that this agent ameliorates the host septic response after major operations and trauma, but conclusive evidence that a concurrent reduction in infection-related mortality occurs is not available. Other immune stimulatory agents, such as granulocyte-macrophage colony-stimulating factor and monophosphoryl lipid A, also are being studied.

REFERENCES

1. Dunn DL. Autochthonous microflora of the gastrointestinal tract. Perspect Colon Rectal Surg 1990;2:105.
2. Dunn DL, Meakins JL. Humoral immunity to infection and the complement system. In: Howard RJ, Simmons RL, eds. Surgical infectious diseases. Norwalk, CT, Appleton & Lange, 1988:175.
3. Durum SK, Oppenheim JJ. Macrophage-derived mediators: interleukin-1, tumor necrosis factor, interleukin-6, interferon, and related cytokines. In: Paul WE, ed. Fundamental immunology, ed 2. New York, Raven Press, 1989:639.
4. Dunn DL. The role of infection and use of antimicrobial agents during multiple system organ failure. In: Deitch EA, ed. Multiple organ failure: pathophysiology and basic concepts of therapy. New York, Thieme, 1990:150.
5. Bartlett JG, Condon RE, Gorbach SL, et al. Veterans Administration Cooperative Study on Bowel Preparation for Elective Colorectal Operations: impact of oral antibiotic regimen on colonic flora, wound irrigation cultures and bacteriology of septic complications. Ann Surg 1978;188:249.
6. Burke JF. Preventing bacterial infection by coordinating antibiotic and host activity: a time-dependent activity. South Med J 1977;1:24.
7. Dunn DL, Barke RA, Knight NB, et al. The role of resident

macrophages, peripheral neutrophils, and translymphatic absorption in bacterial clearance from the peritoneal cavity. Infect Immunol 1985;49:257.

8. Dunn DL, Simmons RL. The role of anaerobic bacteria in intraabdominal infections. Rev Infect Dis 1984;6:S139.

9. Rotstein OD, Pruett TL, Simmons RL. Microbiologic features and treatment of persistent peritonitis in patients in the intensive care unit. Can J Surg 1986;29:247.

10. Meleney FL. Hemolytic *Streptococcus* gangrene. Arch Surg 1924;9:317.

11. Dunn DL, Najarian JS. Infectious complications in transplant surgery. In: Shires GT, Davis J, eds. Principles and management of surgical infection. Philadelphia, JB Lippincott, 1990:425.

12. Dunn DL. Immunotherapeutic advances in the treatment of gram-negative bacterial sepsis. World J Surg 1987;11:233.

SURGERY: SCIENTIFIC PRINCIPLES AND PRACTICE, Second Edition, edited by Lazar J. Greenfield, Michael W. Mulholland, Keith T. Oldham, Gerald B. Zelenock, and Keith D. Lillemoe. Lippincott–Raven Publishers, Philadelphia, © 1997.

CHAPTER 8

SHOCK

RONALD V. MAIER

Shock can be described as a clinical syndrome arising from inadequate perfusion of tissues, often complicated by cellular metabolic dysfunction. Independent of the cause, hypoperfusion creates a disparity between the flow of nutrients to tissues and the metabolic needs of those tissues. The clinical manifestations of shock are the changes in end-organ function and sympathetic and neuroendocrine effects caused by inadequate perfusion and an insufficient cellular supply/demand ratio for oxygen. Because oxygen is the most labile vital substrate delivered by the circulation, inadequate oxygen delivery is implicated as a principal defect in shock, and timely restoration of perfusion and oxygen delivery often reverses the progression of shock.

Persistence or progression of shock can occur as a consequence of an ongoing perfusion defect, a cellular injury, or a combination of the two. After cellular injury, elaboration of inflammatory mediators can further compromise perfusion through the induction of functional and structural changes within the microvasculature. A vicious cycle then develops, whereby cellular injury further compromises perfusion, which again leads to cellular injury, producing more widespread derangements of cellular metabolism. During the recovery process, a period of diffuse immunoinflammatory mediator activation develops, termed the *systemic inflammatory response syndrome* (SIRS), and the multiple organ failure syndrome (MOFS) arises when these excessive systemic responses persist, become autonomous, and cannot be reversed.[1-3]

Fundamental in the treatment of shock is the timely restoration of perfusion. If the cause of shock is not immediately apparent, treatment, including volume resuscitation, is initiated empirically to prevent progression to an irreversible state while the underlying cause is defined. Ideally, control of the inciting pathologic process occurs simultaneously with interventions directed at optimizing cardiovascular dynamics and the institution of supportive care.[4-15]

CLASSIFICATION OF SHOCK

Classification schemes based on cause have been developed for the seemingly dissimilar processes leading to circulatory collapse and the shock state. The classic scheme proposed by Blalock in 1930[9] recognized hypovolemic, cardiogenic, neurogenic, and vasogenic shock as separate entities, but a somewhat more elaborate classification better serves the purposes of this discussion.

CLASSIFICATION OF SHOCK BASED ON CAUSE

- Hypovolemic
- Traumatic
- Cardiogenic
  - Intrinsic
  - Compressive
- Septic
  - Hyperdynamic
  - Hypodynamic
- Neurogenic
- Hypoadrenal

Strict adherence to a classification scheme can at times be troublesome, however, because clinical shock syndromes often involve a combination of processes, particularly those involving trauma and sepsis.

Hypovolemic Shock

Hypovolemic shock, the most common type, is the result of intravascular volume depletion through loss of red blood cell mass (hemorrhage) or plasma volume (extravascular fluid sequestration or gastrointestinal, urinary, and insensible losses). Microvascular hypoperfusion results from the combination of low intravascular blood volume, diminished cardiac output, and compensatory sympathetic peripheral vasoconstriction.

Traumatic Shock

Shock associated with trauma arises as a consequence of hypovolemia due to hemorrhage in conjunction with direct soft tissue injury and bone fractures. Hypovolemia caused by blood loss and fluid extravasation into injured tissues is compounded by activation of maladaptive inflammatory cascades initiated by the tissue injury. In contrast to pure hemorrhagic shock, subsequent organ injury and MOFS occur much more frequently after traumatic shock as a result of the overexpression of these immunoinflammatory cascades and initiation of SIRS. In fact, tissue injury alone significantly up-regulates multiple inflammatory mediator systems, priming the host for a potentially devastating response to a subsequent inflammatory challenge—the *second-hit phenomenon*. Traumatic shock requires a more demanding resuscitation, and there is a markedly greater propensity for postshock sequelae.

Cardiogenic Shock

Cardiogenic shock is the consequence of failure of the heart as an effective pump, resulting in inadequate cardiac output, tissue perfusion, and oxygen delivery. *Intrinsic* causes include myocardial infarction, cardiomyopathy, valvular heart disease, and rhythm disturbances. Right-sided heart failure can result from massive pulmonary embolism or other causes of pulmonary hypertension that limit systolic ejection. Inadequate left heart function leads to diminished peripheral perfusion and contributes to congestion of fluid in the pulmonary circulation. Adrenergic discharge in response to decreased perfusion induces peripheral vasoconstriction and tachycardia, producing physical findings similar to those noted in association with hypovolemic shock.

Compressive (or obstructive) cardiogenic shock is a discrete entity that results when extrinsic compression of the heart limits diastolic filling and thus systolic ejection and cardiac output. Blood or fluid within the poorly distensible pericardial sac may cause pericardial tamponade. Likewise, *any cause of increased intrathoracic pressure*—such as tension pneumothorax, herniation of abdominal viscera through a diaphragmatic hernia, and, in some instances, excessive positive-pressure ventilation—can cause compressive cardiogenic shock. The obstruction to cardiac filling is accompanied by jugular venous distention, clinical findings consistent with hypovolemia, increased sympathetic discharge, and diminished peripheral perfusion.

Septic Shock

In septic shock, hypotension and circulatory insufficiency develop as a consequence of infection and the systemic response to that infection. In its *hyperdynamic* form, septic shock is marked by diminished peripheral vascular resistance and generalized vasodilation causing relative hypovolemia. A compensatory increase in cardiac output occurs in an attempt to meet the metabolic needs of sepsis-induced cellular dysfunction. In contrast, *hypodynamic* septic shock occurs in situations of inadequate resuscitation or preterminal cardiovascular decompensation and is associated with vasoconstriction and a greatly increased mortality risk.

Inflammatory mediators associated with infection are the same as those seen in SIRS and contribute to cellular metabolic derangements and inability to use oxygen optimally as well the hemodynamic and endothelial abnormalities of sepsis. Complications develop as the circulatory system and metabolic machinery are unable to meet the energy demands of the tissues.

Neurogenic Shock

Sympathetic denervation through spinal cord injury, spinal anesthesia, or severe head injury produces generalized arteriolar *vasodilation* and *venodilation*. Peripheral vascular resistance is decreased, and vascular capacitance is increased. Shock occurs when the normal blood volume fails to fill the available intravascular space, and a severe relative hypovolemia exists. Despite hypotension, there is a noteworthy absence of sympathetic activity, as occurs in hypovolemic or cardiogenic shock. Both expansion of the circulating blood volume and correction of the inappropriate vasodilation are required to maintain cardiac output and perfusion pressure to supply metabolic needs.

Hypoadrenal Shock

The surgical patient with undiagnosed or unappreciated adrenal insufficiency may present with profound shock after stress due to loss of the homeostatic corticosteroid response. Hemodynamic instability may develop after an operative procedure or coincident with an unrelated illness. The profound circulatory collapse is often refractory to vigorous resuscitation with fluids and pressor agents. The response to exogenous corticosteroids is usually dramatic and potentially life-saving.

SYSTEM AND ORGAN RESPONSES TO SHOCK

The principal determinants of shock are microcirculatory hypoperfusion and cellular metabolic dysfunction. Restoration of perfusion at the cellular level is the common goal of resuscitation from all forms of shock. Correction of the inciting pathology, restoration of effective circulating blood volume, enhancement of cardiac function, or a combination of these measures addresses the perfusion deficit. Metabolic derangements must be identified and appropriate measures taken to address the underlying pathophysiology concurrent with the institution of appropriate support.

Microcirculation

The microcirculation is central to the pathophysiologic responses in shock. The normal transport of substances to tissue depends on microcirculatory flow, capillary surface area, capillary permeability, concentration gradients, diffusion through the interstitium, and cellular membrane exchange.

Primitive life forms were limited in size by the distances over which nutrients would diffuse. Developed circulatory systems allow the individual cells of a sizable being and complex structure to remain viable and function properly. Nutrients brought to the tissue capillary bed through the circulatory system diffuse through the interstitial space to a given cell. In shock, the failure of delivery (perfusion) at the level of the capillary bed results in metabolic failure at the cellular level.

The clinical parameters used to assess circulatory function in contemporary practice focus on systemic factors and are not particularly sensitive indicators of microcirculatory circumstances. A systolic blood pressure of 105 mmHg may be a normal finding in a healthy person or a worrisome finding in an person suffering a moderate degree of hemorrhagic shock. Tachycardia may be associated with increased tissue perfusion during exercise or with decreased tissue perfusion in hypovolemia. Urine output, level of mentation, and capillary refill can offer some additional guidance because these physical findings are related to the perfusion of the respective tissues; fluctuations of these parameters are not specific, however, to changes in perfusion. Invasive hemodynamic monitoring allows measurement of central venous pressure (CVP), pulmonary capillary wedge pressure (PCWP), and cardiac output and estimation of oxygen consumption. These measurements can provide a greater appreciation of systemic circulatory dynamics but do not precisely assess tissue capillary perfusion. Although the clinical approach measures central or systemic parameters, the focus is gradually shifting to organ-specific criteria as the appropriate assessment technology develops.

Microvascular Anatomy

The microcirculation includes arterioles, capillaries, and venules (Fig. 8-1). The arterioles are resistance vessels, having a high muscle content and a high wall thickness/channel diameter ratio. Arterioles divide into smaller metarterioles, which precede the capillary bed. The smooth muscle surrounding the metarterioles is much more sparse than that associated with larger arterioles. In many tissues, there is a spiral of smooth muscle, the precapillary sphincter, at the origin of the capillary bed. In most tissues, arteriolar smooth muscle is innervated by sympathetic nerves, which generally course with the arterial tree (Fig. 8-2). Capillaries join to form venules, which in turn empty into small veins. The small veins have smooth muscle within

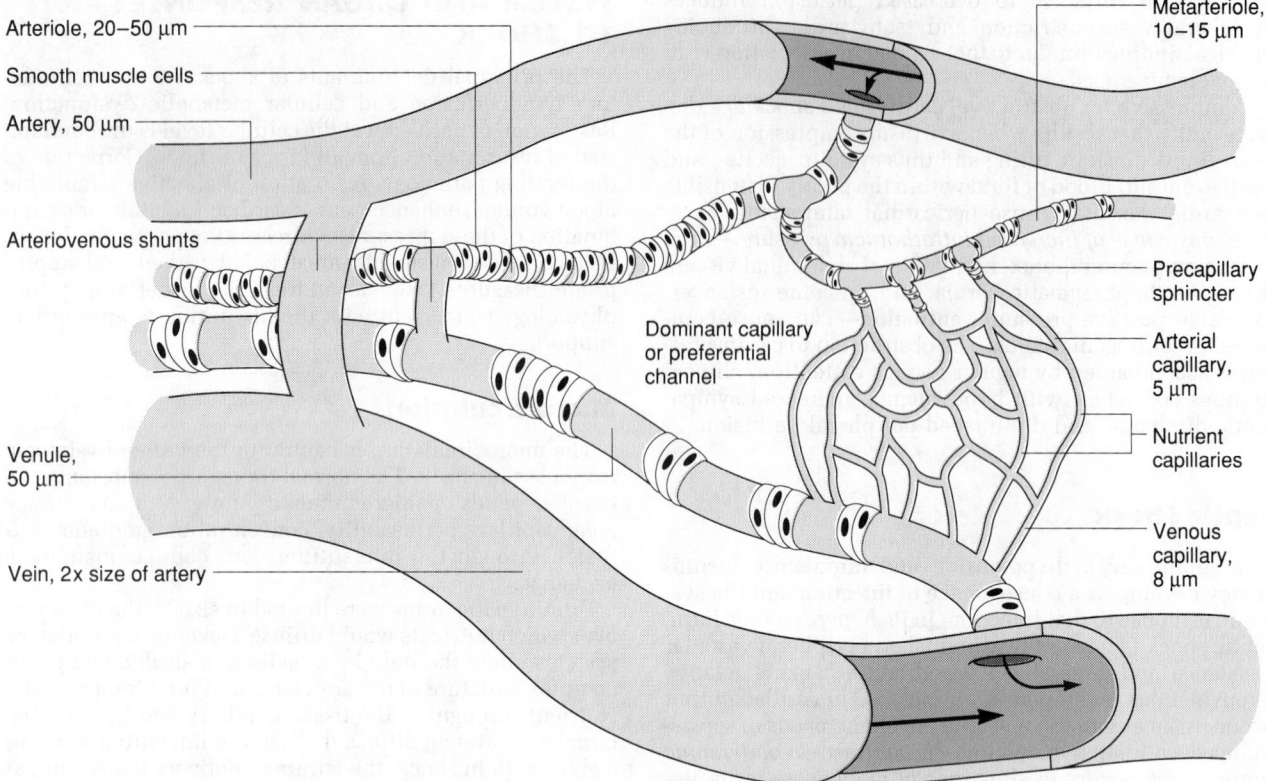

Figure 8-1. A typical zone of the microcirculation. Arteriolar smooth muscle regulates flow resistance and venous smooth muscle capacitance. The capillaries are single-cell layers of endothelium and contain no smooth muscle.

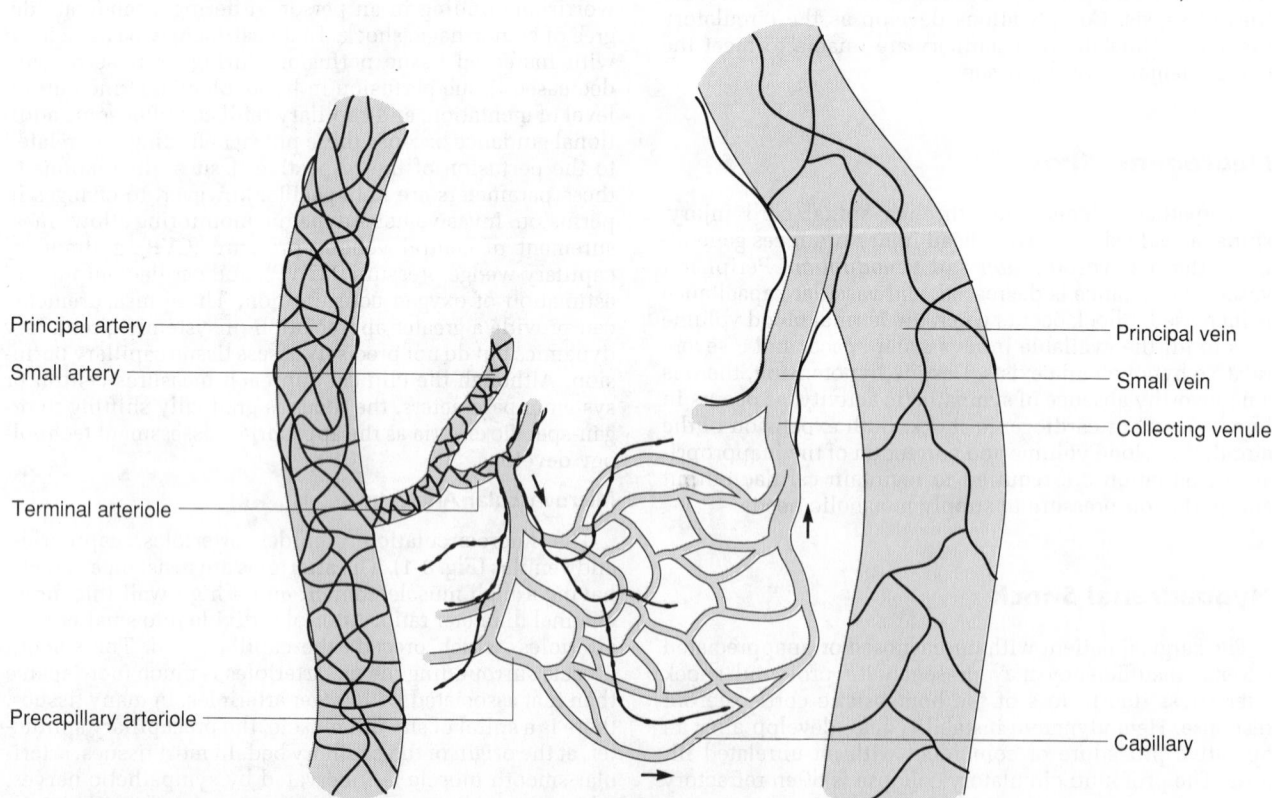

Figure 8-2. The innervation of a microcirculatory zone is diagrammatically presented. The precapillary arteriole and collecting venule are not innervated. Heavy lines indicate adrenergic nerves.

their walls, which again is innervated by the sympathetic nerves. Both the muscularity and the sympathetic innervation of the larger venules and small veins are less than in arteries of corresponding size but are still of considerable physiologic significance—especially in hypovolemic states[15-19] (see Figs. 8-1 and 8-2).

Capillaries consist of endothelial cells with a basal lamina and pericytes. Most capillaries have a continuous endothelium, making them relatively impermeable to larger molecules and cellular elements but freely permeable to water and solutes. A fenestrated endothelium is found in renal glomerular and peritubular capillaries, and discontinuous capillaries are present in the liver sinusoids and hematopoietic tissues. The pulmonary endothelium regulates the movement of plasma proteins similar to other microvascular beds to maintain an osmotic gradient to counteract hydrostatic forces. The ratio of functional large (20- to 22-nm radius) pores to small (5- to 7-nm radius) pores is 1:200, however, rather than up to 1:5000 found in other tissue beds. To compensate for this increased leak and to clear the proteins and fluid from the interstitium to maintain optimal gas exchange, an extensive lymphatic system that can increase flow 10 to 15 times normal exists.[20] Due to these differences, the lung is particularly sensitive to "flooding," early pulmonary dysfunction, and the acute respiratory distress syndrome (ARDS). These features are of particular importance during SIRS and other inflammatory-induced capillary injury. Finally, the inner lumen of the capillary may be as narrow as 4 μm. Red blood cells, which measure about 7 μm in diameter, and other similar-sized cellular elements of blood must be sufficiently deformable to pass through these channels[17] (Fig. 8-3).

Microvascular Physiology

Exchange of material between the vascular space and the cell of various tissues through the interstitial space is essential for organ viability and occurs at the capillary level. This exchange is accomplished through a number of mechanisms, including diffusion, filtration–absorption, and transcytosis. Blood flow through the microvasculature of a particular tissue is autoregulated to correspond with its metabolic needs. Similarly, when the metabolic needs are increased elsewhere in the body, blood flow to inactive (or less active) tissues can be significantly limited. This capacity to regulate the distribution of blood flow is essential because typically only 10% to 15% of the closed fluid system of the vasculature is perfused at any given moment. These normal homeostatic mechanisms play an integral role in the dynamics of shock states.[15-17,19,21]

The filtration of capillary fluid into the interstitium and its subsequent reabsorption into the postcapillary venule is governed by microvascular permeability in conjunction with the balance between hydrostatic and oncotic pressures. The relation of these forces to one another (and their net effects) is illustrated by what has been termed *Starling's law* of ultrafiltration:

$$\text{net filtration} = K_f[(P_c - P_i) + (\pi_i - \pi_c)]$$

where:
K_f = filtration coefficient
P_c = capillary hydrostatic pressure
P_i = interstitial hydrostatic pressure
π_i = interstitial oncotic pressure
π_c = capillary oncotic pressure

In normal circumstances, a net filtration from capillary to interstitium is effected by a relatively higher capillary hydrostatic pressure, whereas net reabsorption from the interstitium back into the postcapillary venule occurs as hydrostatic pressure falls and oncotic forces predominate. This dynamic process maintains a constant flux of fluid between the plasma and interstitium. Deviations from this dynamic equilibrium occur in shock, during which there may be dramatic reductions in capillary pressure, increases in permeability, alterations in endothelial cell function, and changes in venous pressure.

Although the mechanisms controlling blood flow to the capillary bed are complicated and vary among the different tissues, certain concepts are useful. *Poiseuille's law* describes the relation between flow of a fluid through a tube and the tube length and radius, the fluid viscosity, and the pressure gradient between ends of the tube.

$$Q = \frac{\Delta P \pi r^4}{8 \eta l}$$

where:
Q = *flow*
P = *pressure gradient*
r = *radius*
l = *length*
η = *viscosity*

The radius of the tube (or vessel) is the single most important variable because flow is proportional to the radius to the fourth power. Both the vessel radius and the pressure gradient are extremely dynamic. Vessel length and fluid viscosity may also have additional significant impact on flow dynamics. Strictly speaking, Poiseuille's law applies to Newtonian fluids flowing at a constant rate (ie, nonpulsatile flow) through straight, rigid tubes of uniform diameter, without branches or bifurcations. Poiseuille's law has additional limitations with respect to flow of blood in the microcirculation; in particular, rheologic changes due to deformability and aggregation of cellular elements have important effects. Despite such limitations, Poiseuille's law has attained universal acceptance as the best approximation of physical forces governing flow in the circulatory system.

Vasoconstrictive and vasodilatory influences directly impact local blood flow, as well as flow to other tissues through secondary effects on the systemic pressure. This secondary effect of peripheral vasoconstriction maintains the pressure gradient for central perfusion of the heart and the brain. Systemic blood flow meets most of its resistance at the arteriolar level. Although the individual capillary radius is significantly smaller, the vast numbers of capillaries (coursing in parallel) offer less total resistance.

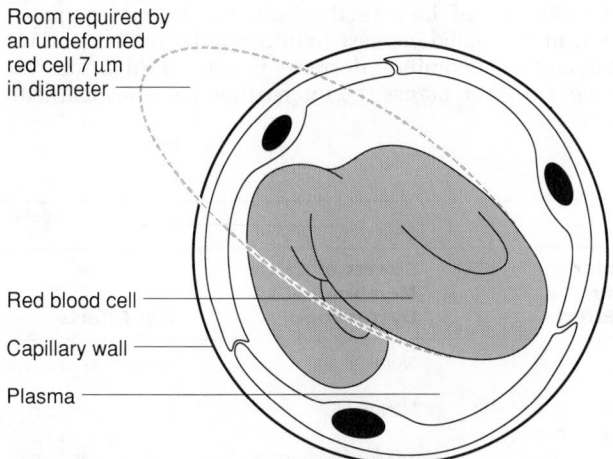

Room required by an undeformed red cell 7 μm in diameter

Red blood cell

Capillary wall

Plasma

Figure 8-3. The average capillary is 4 μm in diameter, and mean red-cell diameter is 7 μm. The red blood cell must be deformable to pass through the capillary.

A multiplicity of factors participate in the modulation of vasoconstriction and vasodilation in normal and shock states. The most apparent vasoconstrictive mechanism in hypovolemia is that involving the stimulation by norepinephrine of α-adrenergic receptors of vascular smooth muscle. Other known constrictive substances include angiotensin II, vasopressin, epinephrine, endothelin, and thromboxane A_2 (TXA_2). Vasodilatory effectors include epinephrine, prostacyclin (PGI_2), and local metabolic products, such as nitric oxide. There are a multitude of other vasoactive substances, including most notably the inflammatory cytokines produced by endothelium, macrophages, leukocytes, and other cells that express a proinflammatory phenotype in response to hypoperfusion and other inflammatory stimuli.

The vascular smooth muscle of arterioles has both α- and β-adrenergic receptors. The α-receptors located at the neuroeffector junction at the termination of the postganglionic sympathetic fibers are termed α_1. The β-receptors are also located on the vascular smooth muscle but are geographically separate from the sympathetic endings (noninnervated or extrajunctional receptors). α-Stimulation effects vasoconstriction, whereas β-stimulation effects vasodilation. The efferent sympathetic fibers innervating the precapillary resistance vessels and the venous capacitance vessels release norepinephrine on stimulation, which induces smooth muscle contraction and narrowing of the caliber of the vessels. These contractions are potent enough that blood flow to entire capillary beds can be arrested by adrenergic vasoconstriction. Arterioles can also close or collapse as the pressure within the resistance vessel diminishes. This occurs because blood vessels are distensible and require transmural pressure to overcome vessel wall tension and the pressure of the surrounding tissues (closing pressure). Blood flow to whole capillary beds can thus be arrested through the effects of adrenergic vasoconstriction (with or without hypotension).

The disruption of nutrient flow to tissues may be further compounded by secondary microvascular pathology. Stagnation or interruption of microvascular flow may result from increased viscosity, platelet aggregates and other debris, decreased deformability of cellular elements, increased adherence of activated leukocytes to endothelial cells expressing a proinflammatory phenotype, and compromise of the capillary channel by damaged, detached, and swollen endothelium. During shock, these changes may develop in association with tissue injury, ischemia, and the elaboration of inflammatory mediators.

Microvascular and Cellular Response

Moderate hypovolemia results in a relatively rapid spontaneous restitution of intravascular volume through expansion of the plasma space. This plasma reexpansion by erythrocyte-free fluid occurs within 1 hour as a result of alterations in pressure and osmolarity and produces an associated hemodilution.[22] Sympathetic discharge, associated arteriolar constriction, and induced metabolic changes in osmolarity initiate the compensatory events at the microcirculatory level. The ensuing fluid fluxes are governed by Starling forces.[23] Constriction of arterioles and precapillary sphincters occurs under the influence of sympathetic stimulation, circulating catecholamines, vasopressin, angiotensin II, and other mediators, and leads to diminished capillary hydrostatic pressure. The same factors limit the number of capillary beds perfused, limiting the surface area available for filtration. By virtue of diminished capillary hydrostatic pressure, with constant or increased intravascular oncotic pressure, there is rapid net reabsorption of fluid into the microcirculation.[22]

This initial pressure-related phase of restitution of blood volume in shock is overlapped by a second phase involving osmotically induced mobilization of intracellular fluid[23,24] (Table 8-1). Hyperglycemia and elevations of the soluble products of glycolysis, lipolysis, and proteolysis contribute to extracellular interstitial hyperosmolarity. The activity of glucose in this process is in part related to the relative impermeability of most cells to glucose. The osmotic gradient thus generated between the cells and interstitium leads to loss of intracellular volume and increases in interstitial volume and pressure. Increased interstitial pressure augments transcapillary reabsorption of fluid to enhance intravascular fluid volume. It also provides a driving force for mobilization of interstitial fluid and protein by the lymphatics, particularly in the lungs. If only red blood cells or red cells plus plasma are used for volume resuscitation, the red-cell mass and plasma volume are restored. The interstitial fluid deficit, however, persists.[12,13] To replete all fluid compartments, (intravascular, interstitial, and intracellular), volume resuscitation with blood *plus* electrolyte solution similar in composition to interstitial fluid (eg, lactated Ringer solution) is necessary. Resuscitation from hemorrhage with blood alone or with red cells plus plasma yields mortality rates comparable to those seen in untreated animals. Resuscitation with blood plus lactated Ringer solution significantly reduces mortality after hemorrhagic shock.[12,13]

The osmotic mechanisms contributing to the restitution of blood volume after moderate hemorrhage are not adequate in hemorrhage of greater magnitude. Plasma volume restitution is no greater with hemorrhage of 30% blood volume than with 10% blood volume hemorrhage. In larger hemorrhages (more than 25% blood volume), there is also deterioration of the normal cellular transmembrane potential, an associated increase in intracellular sodium and water, and a concomitant decrease in extracellular fluid volume. Diffusion across the interstitium becomes markedly

Table 8-1. FLUID SHIFT AFTER HEMORRHAGE

	Capillary Hydrostatic Effects (Starling Forces)	Extracellular Osmolarity-Induced Effects	Effects of Cell Membrane Dysfunction	Net Effects
Mild hemorrhage	↑	Minimal	None	Restitution of blood volume
Moderate hemorrhage	Transcapillary refill of intravascular space	Expansion of extracellular volume	Minimal	Partial restitution of blood volume
Severe hemorrhage	↓	None	Influx of sodium and fluid into cells	Intracellular fluid sequestration Minimal restitution of blood volume

impaired due to the increase in colloid density from fluid volume losses. The decrease in capillary surface area that occurs with vasoconstriction also decreases the ability to provide adequate nutrient transport to the tissues, further compromising cell membrane function and causing deterioration of intracellular energy stores, primarily adenosine triphosphate (ATP), in metabolically active cells. Tissue hypoxia results, anaerobic metabolites accumulate, and the cell cannot maintain the normal cell membrane potential. Accumulation of hydrogen ion, lactate, and other products of anaerobic metabolism overrides normal homeostatic vasomotor tone and contributes to maladaptive vasodilation, further augmenting hypotension and hypoperfusion. Extensive cellular swelling with intracellular fluid sequestration offsets the osmotically induced blood volume restitution seen with lesser hemorrhage.

The uptake of fluid by the failing cell is a major source of fluid sequestration after shock. Loss of cell membrane function is proportional to both the extent and duration of shock or degree of sepsis. The cause of the membrane failure is unclear but appears to be multifactorial. Loss of intracellular ATP energy stores during hypoperfusion or direct toxicity during sepsis may inhibit the membrane Na^+-K^+-ATPase pump. This is particularly true in metabolically active cells, such as hepatocytes.[25] Mitochondrial dysfunction is the most likely underlying cause for this loss in ATP due to uncoupling of oxidative phosphorylation during shock and sepsis.[26-29] In addition, direct inhibition or malfunction of the Na^+-K^+-ATPase pump may also cause cell membrane dysfunction and loss of active ion transport. Red blood cells from patients after shock have impaired function of the Na^+-K^+-ATPase pump.[30] Na^+-K^+-ATPase pump failure as a mechanism of membrane failure is supported by the ability of ouabain, a direct pump poison, to mimic shock-induced cell membrane dysfunction.[31] Also, a protein isolated from plasma of animals after hemorrhagic shock or sepsis has been demonstrated to induce cell membrane depolarization.[32-34] Thus, cell membrane dysfunction may represent a common pathophysiologic pathway among the various causes of shock.

Cellular dysfunction also appears to be related to abnormal intracellular calcium homeostasis. Intracellular calcium concentrations are normally controlled in a narrow range and are crucial for protease activity, contraction coupling, membrane stability, and coupling of electron and hydrogen ion transport during oxidative phosphorylation. Calcium is also a major second messenger for membrane signal transduction and inflammatory mediator production through the calcium–calmodulin pathway.[35] Abnormal accumulation of intracellular calcium has been noted after shock and sepsis and has been associated with many of the pathologic cellular abnormalities identified. Abnormal calcium homeostasis and increased intracellular levels of calcium both prime the inflammatory cell and enhance the inflammatory response, leading to the overproduction of potent mediators of SIRS and MOFS. A rapid influx of calcium occurs in many tissues after injury, including ischemia–reperfusion.[36,37] The continued loss of membrane integrity and accumulation of calcium can induce irreversible damage and cell death. Prevention of cellular and organ dysfunction and improved survival have been achieved in various shock states through use of calcium-channel blockers.[38,39]

Although the exact mechanisms of cell membrane dysfunction are unclear, the best and most consistent therapeutic intervention to reverse the abnormalities and prevent decompensation is rapid aggressive volume resuscitation. With adequate resuscitation, the changes in transmembrane potential and abnormalities of intracellular sodium concentration and water content can be reversed.[12-14]

If hypoperfusion persists, a paradoxical vasodilation occurs, which has been termed the *decompensated phase* of shock.[40,41] Decompensated shock has been associated with relaxation of the small precapillary arterioles in conjunction with a generalized loss of vasomotor tone in multiple vascular beds.[41,42] The exact cause of uncompensated shock is unclear, but it has a strong association with an increase in local factors, such as acidosis, which is known to be capable of overriding the homeostatic vasomotor responses.[43] Systemically, decompensated shock has been associated with increases in circulating lactate levels and increased products of glycolysis. In studies measuring membrane potential, there is a marked derangement, particularly in skeletal muscle, of membrane energy charge and membrane potential.[44] A narrow time frame separates the derangements found in severe shock that can be reversed with aggressive and timely resuscitation from the progressive decompensation and cellular injury that has become nonreversible and terminal.

Neuroendocrine Response

The neuroendocrine response to shock attempts to achieve restoration of effective blood volume, mobilization of metabolic substrates, and maintenance of central perfusion. Both peripheral and central afferent stimuli to the central nervous system are involved in inducing this response. Painful stimuli, relayed from viscera and peripheral tissue by autonomic and somatic afferent fibers, are recognized by the sensory cortex. En route, the hypothalamus is stimulated, inducing autonomic nervous activity and the central endocrine response. Hypovolemia, hypotension, or hypoxia appreciated by baroreceptors and chemoreceptors further contributes to this autonomic response.[45]

Hypotension, associated with a decrease in impulses from the aortic and carotid baroreceptors, *disinhibits* the vasomotor center. This disinhibition results in increased adrenergic output and decreased vagal activity. Sympathetic nerve endings release norepinephrine, inducing peripheral and splanchnic vasoconstriction, which is responsible for greater than 80% of systemic vascular resistance (SVR) and is the major contributor to maintenance of central organ perfusion pressure and venous return. Decreased vagal activity prompts an increased heart rate, increasing cardiac output.

Plasma levels of both epinephrine and norepinephrine are elevated with injury, and the degree of catecholamine elevation corresponds to the magnitude of injury.[46] In shock, the effects of endogenous epinephrine are largely metabolic. These effects include an increased metabolic rate, increased glycogenolysis and gluconeogenesis, and decreased insulin release by the pancreas.[45]

In addition to initiating autonomic nervous activity, the hypothalamus secretes releasing hormones, which induce the stress hormone release of the pituitary. As part of this response, adrenocorticotropic hormone (ACTH) secretion by the anterior pituitary is increased, stimulating cortisol secretion by the adrenal cortex. Other nonpituitary mechanisms enhance cortisol secretion,[47] and endorphins and encephalins are released by the central nervous system in the process. Cortisol affects cellular metabolism by alterations in substrate usage and protein synthesis. It contributes to decreased peripheral uptake of glucose and amino acids, enhanced lipolysis, and increased gluconeogenesis. Glucose intolerance or overt hyperglycemia can result.[48] At levels secreted during stress, cortisol exerts a significant degree of mineralocorticoid activity and concomitant fluid retention by the kidney. The importance of a cortisol response to stress is illustrated by the profound circulatory collapse that occurs in hypoadrenal patients not receiving corticosteroid supplementation in times of stress.

In conjunction with elevated plasma levels of cortisol and epinephrine, increased pancreatic secretion of glucagon, which accelerates hepatic gluconeogenesis, further aggravates the glucose intolerance that follows injury and sepsis.[45] Although cortisol, epinephrine, and glucagon individually lead to a mild degree of hyperglycemia, their action in concert is much more dramatic. This synergistic action accounts for much of the hyperglycemia associated with trauma and sepsis, which often occurs in the face of elevated plasma insulin levels.[49] It has been hypothesized that the hyperglycemia serves as an osmolar mechanism to contribute to reexpansion of blood volume during shock.

Insulin secretion in sepsis and shock is variable. Although levels are commonly elevated in association with hyperglycemia, in low output states, there may be depressed insulin secretion, perhaps the result of catecholamine inhibition of pancreatic β cells.[45]

The secretion of renin is increased in response to adrenergic discharge and decreased perfusion of the juxtaglomerular apparatus in the kidney. Renin allows formation of angiotensin I in the liver, which is then converted to angiotensin II in the lungs. Angiotensin II is an extremely effective vasoconstrictor that further augments sympathetic-mediated vasoconstriction. Other actions include stimulation of aldosterone release by the adrenal cortex and vasopressin release by the posterior pituitary. Aldosterone serves to maintain intravascular volume. Increased levels during shock induce tubular reabsorption of sodium, resulting in the excretion of a low-volume, concentrated, but relatively sodium-free urine. Aldosterone secretion is increased in response to ACTH stimulation of the adrenal and to circulating angiotensin II. Vasopressin (antidiuretic hormone; ADH), although usually secreted in response to increases in serum osmolarity,[50] is also elaborated in shock in response to volume loss. Decreased cardiac filling, appreciated by receptors in the ventricles, is the initiating event.[51,52] Vasopressin has a direct action on vascular smooth muscle (V_1 receptors), contributing to splanchnic and peripheral vasoconstriction. In the kidney, it acts on the distal tubules (V_2 receptors) to effect water reabsorption and hence conservation of volume.[53]

Cardiovascular Response

The neuroendocrine compensations of the individual in shock serve to maintain the immediate needs of the vital organs—the brain and heart. The metabolic rates of the heart and brain are high and their stores of energy substrates low. When the circulation is compromised, the continuous supply of nutrients and substances falls below demand levels. As a result, neither vital organ tolerates ischemia for more than brief periods. In conjunction with those mechanisms that sustain central blood pressure, autoregulation maintains coronary and cerebral perfusion despite significant degrees of shock.

Although peripheral vasoconstriction may maintain central pressure in shock, it occurs at the expense of other tissue beds, where supply is less than demand. Differential resistance to flow determines the degree to which each vascular bed is perfused. Physiologic compensations or therapeutic interventions that optimize effective circulating blood volume and restore peripheral perfusion are necessary to halt the progressive microcirculatory derangements of shock.

Cardiac Dynamics

Central in the general cardiovascular response to shock is the action of the heart. The principal determinants of cardiac function in the normal heart are the volume of blood available for the heart to pump (preload), the systolic contractile capability, and the diastolic filling of the ventricles. In hypovolemia, the two dynamic variables of cardiac function—ventricular filling and myocardial contractility—remain paramount and determine the stroke volume. The product of stroke volume and heart rate in turn determines the cardiac output. Increases in ventricular end-diastolic volume, reflecting venous return, cause ventricular distention. Ventricular distention in turn produces increased volume output with each stroke, the Frank-Starling mechanism (Fig. 8-4A). In the clinical setting using a pulmonary artery catheter, stroke volume can be seen to vary as a function of PCWP (see Fig. 8-4B and C).

Intravascular volume loss causes decreased ventricular end-diastolic distention and diminished stroke volume. Repletion of intravascular volume is accompanied by increased stroke volume. In the presence of reduced diastolic compliance, depletion of intravascular volumes causes a greater decrease in stroke volume; and repletion of intravascular volume restores stroke volume but at higher filling pressures. These changes move to corresponding points *along* the Starling curve (see Fig. 8-4D).

Contractile function can vary independent of volume status. Changes in contractile function *shift* the Starling curve up or down, producing increases or decreases in stroke volume for any given end-diastolic volume (see Fig. 8-4E). The inotropic state of the heart increases in the face of higher catecholamine levels (upward shift of the Starling curve). Contractile dysfunction (downward shift of the Starling curve) may follow myocardial infarction, septic insult, severe trauma, general anesthesia, prolonged shock, or acid–base derangements.

Venous System

A fundamental requirement for cardiovascular function is adequate cardiac filling, and cardiac output cannot exceed venous return. Interruption of venous return is of immediate consequence to pump function. Hypoperfusion has its initial impact on the filling of the venous system, and compensatory venous mechanisms are activated to maintain cardiac filling.[18]

The venous system contains nearly two thirds of the total circulating blood volume, including 20% to 30% within the splanchnic venous system. Most of this volume resides in the small veins, which constitute the bulk of venous capacitance. The venous system, especially that of the splanchnic circulation, is important in the physiologic compensation to hypoperfusion because it serves as a dynamic reservoir for an autoinfusion of blood volume involving both active and passive mechanisms.[18,54,55]

The volume of blood contained within a vessel is dependent on the compliance of the vessel and the transmural distention pressure. Compliance ($\Delta V/\Delta P$) is variable; it is greatest when vessels are partially collapsed and much lower when they are distended by high pressures. Decreases in transmural distention pressure are accompanied by passive recoil and flattening of the veins. This collapse passively mobilizes venous blood toward the heart. Further passive mobilization occurs through flow-related phenomena. Diminished cardiac output or arteriolar vasoconstriction results in decreased flow to tissues and the corresponding venous bed. This produces further passive recoil, collapse of the veins, and mobilization of venous blood, which may mimic active *venoconstriction*.

Venoconstriction, a consequence of α-adrenergic activity, is an additional but less significant mechanism by which venous return is optimized in shock. Small veins of skin, muscle, and the splanchnic viscera have sympathetic innervation and vascular smooth muscle with α-adrenergic receptors. The degree of sympathetic-mediated response

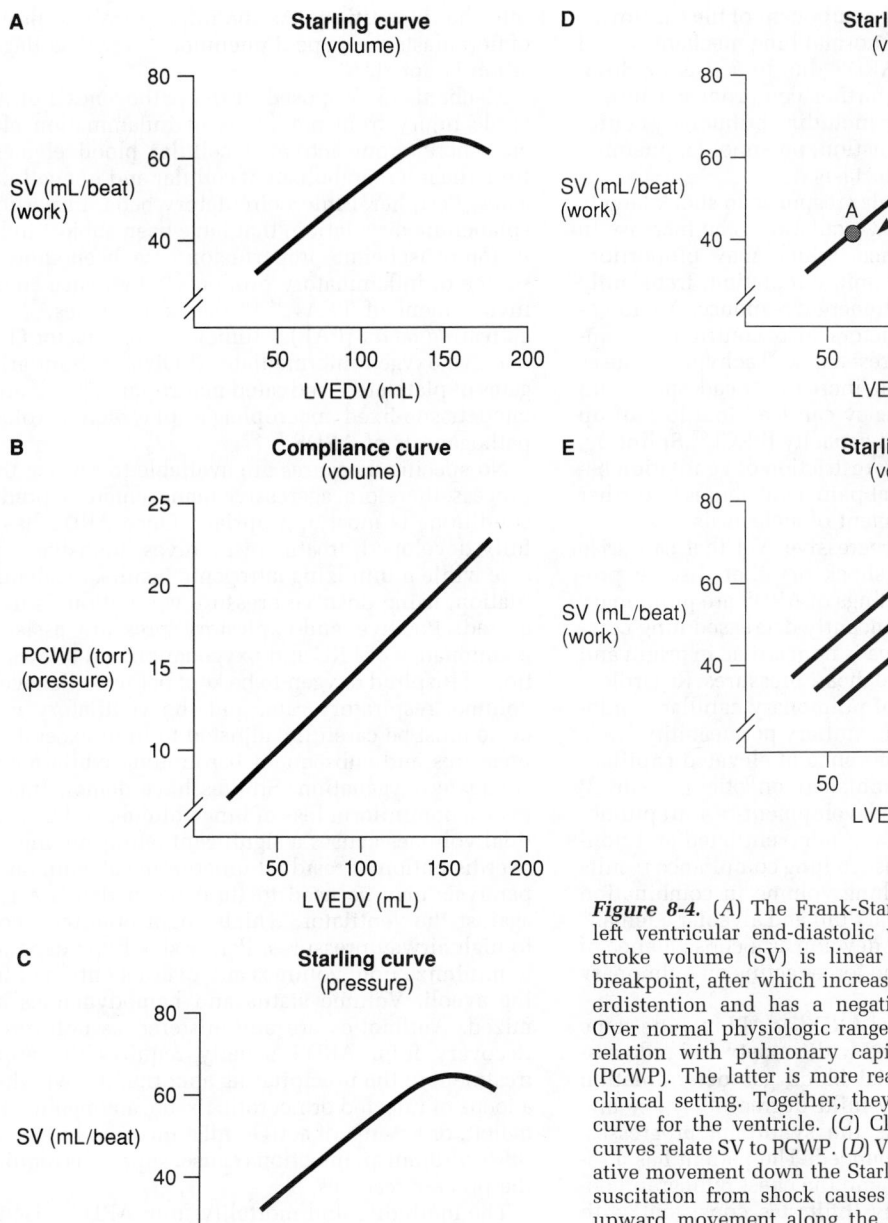

Figure 8-4. (*A*) The Frank-Starling relation between left ventricular end-diastolic volume (LVEDV) and stroke volume (SV) is linear and positive until a breakpoint, after which increasing LVEDV causes overdistention and has a negative effect on SV. (*B*) Over normal physiologic ranges, LVEDV has a linear relation with pulmonary capillary wedge pressure (PCWP). The latter is more readily measured in the clinical setting. Together, they define a compliance curve for the ventricle. (*C*) Clinically used Starling curves relate SV to PCWP. (*D*) Volume loss causes negative movement down the Starling curve, whereas resuscitation from shock causes an increased SV and upward movement along the curve. (*E*) Contractile function may vary independent of volume status. Upward shifts result in increased contractility (catecholamines and other inotropes), and downward shifts occur with myocardial infarction, sepsis, and acid–base derangements.

is unclear because it is difficult to measure independently active and passive changes. The splanchnic circulation makes major contributions to the maintenance of venous return; in healthy men subjected to 1-L hemorrhages, splanchnic blood volume decreases by about 500 mL. With this, there is little associated change in vital signs or in cardiac output.[18] It is likely that sympathetic venoconstriction is responsible for a portion of blood mobilized from the splanchnic venous circulation, but sympathetic-mediated venoconstriction in skin and skeletal muscle is probably not significant as a source of blood volume.

Peripheral Vascular Response

Selective vasoconstriction occurs in response to α-adrenergic receptor stimulation with the increased sympathetic activity in shock. The distribution of sympathetic fibers innervating arterioles and precapillary sphincters defines the

hierarchy of microcirculations. Blood flow to the skin is sacrificed early, followed by that to the kidneys and splanchnic viscera. Evidence also suggests that some degree of sympathetic-mediated arteriolar constriction occurs in skeletal muscle.[56] Arteriolar constriction increases SVR, maintaining arterial pressure in the face of a decreasing cardiac output.

Sympathetic stimulation does not cause significant vasoconstriction of either cerebral or coronary vessels. Normal blood flow is maintained in these circulations through complementary autoregulatory mechanisms as long as arterial pressure is above 70 mmHg.

Pulmonary Response

The pulmonary manifestations of shock are often related to pathology of extrathoracic origin as well as pathology intrinsic to the lungs. Contributing pathophysiologic processes include the pulmonary component of the cardiovascular response, disruption of normal lung mechanics, and acute lung injury (ALI) or ARDS due to sepsis or SIRS. Pulmonary function can be further compromised by pathologies intrinsic to the lung, including pulmonary contusion, aspiration, airway obstruction, pneumonia, pneumothorax, hemothorax, and atelectasis.

The acute pulmonary vascular response to shock largely parallels that of the systemic vasculature. The increase in pulmonary vascular resistance, which may proportionately exceed that of the systemic circulation, transiently accompanies the systemic adrenergic response. Angiotensin II and other vasoconstrictors also contribute to increased pulmonary vascular resistance. Tachypnea causes a decreased tidal volume but increased dead space and minute ventilation. Recumbency can lead to a loss of up to 20% of functional residual capacity (FRC).[57] Splinting, the voluntary and involuntary restriction of ventilation because of thoracic or abdominal pain, contributes to further loss of FRC and the development of atelectasis.

ARDS is a syndrome of progressive ALI that can arise as a direct consequence of shock or other disease processes. The characteristic findings of ARDS are pulmonary edema, hypoxemia, and significantly decreased lung compliance. The pulmonary edema is noncardiac in origin and occurs in the face of normal left heart pressures. Regardless of the specific mechanisms of pulmonary capillary endothelial injury, the increase in capillary permeability leads to pulmonary edema in the absence of elevated capillary hydrostatic presence or diminished oncotic pressure.[58] The hypoxemia results from development of intrapulmonary shunting and perfusion of underventilated and nonventilated alveoli. The decrease in lung compliance results from loss of surfactant and lung volume in combination with the presence of interstitial fluid and alveolar edema.[59] Pulmonary hypertension can develop as a consequence of vasoconstrictive mediators and forces acting on pulmonary arterioles.[60]

The early clinical findings of ARDS or ALI include some degree of tachypnea, associated with anxiety and mild respiratory distress. Early arterial blood gas determination may demonstrate a relatively mild degree of hypoxemia and respiratory alkalosis. As the syndrome progresses, hypoxia becomes more pronounced. The patient has a restrictive pattern of breathing, and the chest radiograph begins to show bilateral patchy infiltrates consistent with pulmonary edema. Chest radiograph findings may initially be relatively normal and often lag behind the development of symptoms of respiratory distress by 24 hours or longer. By this point, hypoxemia has almost invariably necessitated intubation and positive-pressure ventilation. Placement of a pulmonary artery catheter confirms the presence of normal left heart pressures (PCWP less than 18 mmHg) and the noncardiogenic nature of the edema. The fairly marked degree of intrapulmonary shunting is evident as a high alveolar–arterial gradient. Decreased compliance and loss of FRC necessitates the use of relatively high airway pressures to achieve normal tidal volumes, maintain FRC, and attain a reasonable arterial oxygen saturation.

Progressive histologic changes of ARDS become apparent in pulmonary capillaries, interstitium, and alveoli. Initially, interstitial edema develops with swelling of capillary endothelial cells and type I pneumocytes. The type I pneumocytes subsequently slough, and alveolar edema ensues. Functional surfactant is lost with a significant increase in alveolar opening pressure and decrease in alveolar surface tension. Decreased alveolar volume and development of alveolar edema and microatelectasis cause decreases in FRC. Capillary endothelial injury allows extravasation of plasma protein, fibrin, and red blood cells

into the interstitium. As the injury resolves, proliferation of fibroblasts and type II pneumocytes with collagen deposition is noted.[61,62]

Mechanisms proposed in the pathogenesis of ARDS include injury from mediators of inflammation elaborated elsewhere, from activated cellular blood elements, and from the microembolism of cellular and noncellular aggregates. Peripheral microcirculatory beds, in particular the splanchnic circulation, that have been subject to hypoperfusion or ischemia preperfusion have been shown to be a source of inflammatory products.[63] Evidence suggests the involvement of TXA_2,[64-66] the leukotrienes,[67,68] platelet-activating factor (PAF),[68] tumor necrosis factor (TNF), and reactive oxygen intermediates (ROIs).[60,69] Similarly, aggregates of platelets,[61] activated neutrophils,[60,70-72] and stimulated tissue-fixed macrophages play active roles in the pathogenesis of ARDS.[73-75]

No specific measures are available to reverse the ARDS process; therefore, aggressive management of predisposing conditions is most appropriate. Once ARDS has become fully developed, treatment involves intensive supportive care while minimizing iatrogenic insults. Mechanical ventilation, using positive-pressure ventilation, is usually required. Positive end-expiratory pressure assists in the maintenance of FRC and oxygenation and allows the fraction of inspired oxygen to be kept below toxic levels. Tidal volume, respiratory rate, and the ventilatory mode and cycle must be carefully adjusted to limit excessive airway pressures and subsequent barotrauma while maintaining adequate oxygenation. Studies have demonstrated ARDS to be a nonuniform loss of lung volume, and use of normal tidal volumes causes a significant iatrogenic injury due to overdistention of residual functioning alveoli. Sedation or paralysis may be used to limit the patient's active work against the ventilator, which might otherwise contribute to high airway pressures. Permissive hypercapnia is used to minimize tidal volumes and overdistention of functioning aveoli. Volume status and hemodynamics are optimized. Antibiotics are administered as cultures dictate. Recovery from ARDS usually requires the appropriate treatment of the precipitating abnormality, whether this is a focus of infected or necrotic tissue, an ongoing perfusion deficit, or an area of active inflammation. In the setting of SIRS, without an infectious cause, support is required until the process resolves.

The morbidity and mortality from ARDS arise not only from the consequences of respiratory failure but also from the underlying immunoinflammatory pathologic processes that caused it. Intercurrent infection, other complications of prolonged treatment in an intensive care unit, overly aggressive mechanical ventilation, and the development of MOFS also contribute. If the underlying process is controlled, perfusion deficits corrected, and appropriate supportive measures instituted, significant recovery of pulmonary function can occur over many days or weeks. In some cases, progressive pulmonary fibrosis complicates the healing process, resulting in permanent restriction of pulmonary function or progressive respiratory failure and death.[62]

Renal Response

Renal failure, as an acute complication of shock, has become less frequent because of the trend toward more aggressive resuscitation. Oliguric acute tubular necrosis (ATN) that develops after a period of hypovolemic shock is a foreseeable end-organ complication. The acquired renal insufficiency and renal failure in modern surgical intensive care units does not usually develop in such a straightforward manner. Shock, sepsis, and the administration of nephrotoxic agents, such as aminoglycosides and iodine dye, are major predisposing processes to the development of renal failure.[76] Renal failure is also a common component of MOFS, the major cause of late intensive care unit mortality.

When subjected to shock, the physiologic response of the kidney is to conserve salt and water. As a consequence of selective vasoconstriction, whole-organ blood flow to the kidneys and the other viscera is limited to preserve central arterial pressure. Within the kidney, sympathetic-mediated vasoconstriction increases resistance at the level of the afferent arteriole, as do angiotensin II and circulating catecholamines. Disruption of the thromboxane–PGI_2 balance from microvascular injury further contributes to vasoconstriction.[76] The increased preglomerular resistance accounts for a diminished glomerular filtration rate (GFR) as well as decreased renal blood flow.[77] Decreased filtration in conjunction with the effects of increased circulating levels of ADH (vasopressin) and aldosterone produce oliguria and azotemia. At diminished filtration rates, there is increased back-diffusion of filtered urea, causing elevation of blood urea nitrogen (BUN) out of proportion to that of the creatinine level, that is, prerenal azotemia. Appropriate resuscitation in the absence of other injury restores GFR and urine output.

Profound or prolonged decreases in renal cortical blood flow produce ischemia and subsequent reperfusion injury. The exact nature of the renal injury in this circumstance is not entirely clear. In animal models of ATN from toxic injury, there is histologic necrosis of tubular epithelium and obstruction of the tubules with debris. It has been postulated that the associated renal dysfunction is a consequence of tubular obstruction with back-leak of filtrate. Such structural abnormality may play a role in some forms of acute renal failure. It is apparent, however, that these mechanical abnormalities are not the only mechanisms involved. The disordered vasomotor influences causing vasoconstriction of the afferent and efferent arterioles can also account for the observed decreases in GFR and redistribution of renal blood flow.[77] Disruption of normal renal energetics and metabolism have also been implicated in animal models of acute renal failure. Hypoxia without hypoperfusion has been shown to cause decreases in GFR, urine output, tubular reabsorption of sodium, and renal oxygen consumption, which are partially reversed through restoration of oxygenation.[78] In hemorrhagic hypotension, renal ATP stores can be depleted, and this correlates with impairment of renal function.[79]

Metabolic Derangements in Sepsis and the Systemic Inflammatory Response Syndrome

A broad spectrum of metabolic abnormalities is apparent in sepsis and SIRS (Fig. 8-5). Disruption of the normal cycles of carbohydrate, lipid, protein, and oxygen metabolism occur as hypermetabolism develops. The early stages of sepsis and SIRS are marked by a shift in the use of energy substrates; and clinical deterioration in the late stages corresponds with the progressive inability to use glucose, fat, ketone bodies, and protein, accompanied by failure to use available oxygen.

Through the Cori cycle, lactate from the periphery is shuttled back to the liver, where it is used in the production of glucose. Because pyruvate is converted to alanine in the periphery, flux of alanine also contributes to hepatic gluconeogenesis. The glycolytic oxidation of glucose to pyruvate and its subsequent gluconeogenic regeneration from lactate represent an inefficient cycling of substrate.

There is no net energy production, but heat is released in significant quantities (Fig. 8-6).

Alterations in lipid metabolism cause a progressive rise in the serum triglyceride level as a result of a less efficient clearance of exogenous triglycerides coupled with increased hepatic lipogenesis. Glycerol turnover is also increased. In the early stages of sepsis, there is an increase in the circulating ketone bodies, β-hydroxybutyrate, and acetoacetate. The latter declines in the progressive stages of organ failure, leading to an elevated β-hydroxybutyrate/acetoacetate ratio.

Profound alterations in protein and amino acid metabolism develop with characteristic changes in amino acid levels, nitrogen balance, and skeletal muscle mass. Initially, levels of the branch chain amino acids (leucine, isoleucine, and valine) are reduced, whereas those of the aromatic amino acids (phenylalanine, tyrosine, and tryptophan) are elevated. There is an increase in the oxidative metabolism of protein to meet energy needs and a tremendous mobilization of nitrogen with net negative nitrogen balance. These changes are particularly prominent in the periphery and occur even in the face of amino acid loading. Marked urinary losses of nitrogen accompany muscle protein catabolism. The branch chain amino acids are preferentially used in the Kreb cycle, maintaining activity that otherwise would be lost from the diminished entry of carbohydrate- and fatty acid–generated acetylcoenzyme A. This results in reduced serum levels of leucine, isoleucine, and valine. The breakdown of skeletal muscle also liberates other amino acids that are metabolized in less efficient pathways, some of which contribute to gluconeogenesis. Profound consequences of this protein-based energy economy include marked ureagenesis, negative nitrogen balance, and often dramatic muscle wasting. The process is a state of autocannibalism, and the effects persist until the septic or inflammatory process is controlled and the cellular injury resolves.[80] This phase of postresuscitative hypermetabolism is not characterized by an energy deficit. Adequate energy appears to be available, but the carbon sources for its production are altered. Rather than being primarily glucose dependent, energy is derived from the oxidation of carbohydrate, fats, and amino acids.

Immunoinflammatory Responses

Inflammatory mediators play a significant role in the clinical manifestations and progression of shock and in the development of subsequent complications. These mediator systems function primarily as paracrine and autocrine agents in the local environment and are not usually detectable systemically. They are activated or produced by many different cell types throughout the body. Similar to hormones, inflammatory mediators evolved as part of the protective immunoinflammatory host response to potentially toxic conditions, such as devitalized tissues, or invasive agents, such as bacteria and viruses. The overexpression and systemic dissemination of these mediators produces the toxic autodestructive processes underlying SIRS and MOFS, with attendant high mortality. The relative importance of each mediator remains unclear because the pathologic processes defining the various types of shock involve a multitude of interrelated actions and reactions (see Chap. 6).

Many of the processes associated with shock participate in the initiation of this inflammatory response. Local tissue trauma with disruption of vascular integrity and the exposure of collagen activates the coagulation cascade, induces platelet aggregation, and disrupts endothelial cells. Activated platelets release TXA_2. Injured

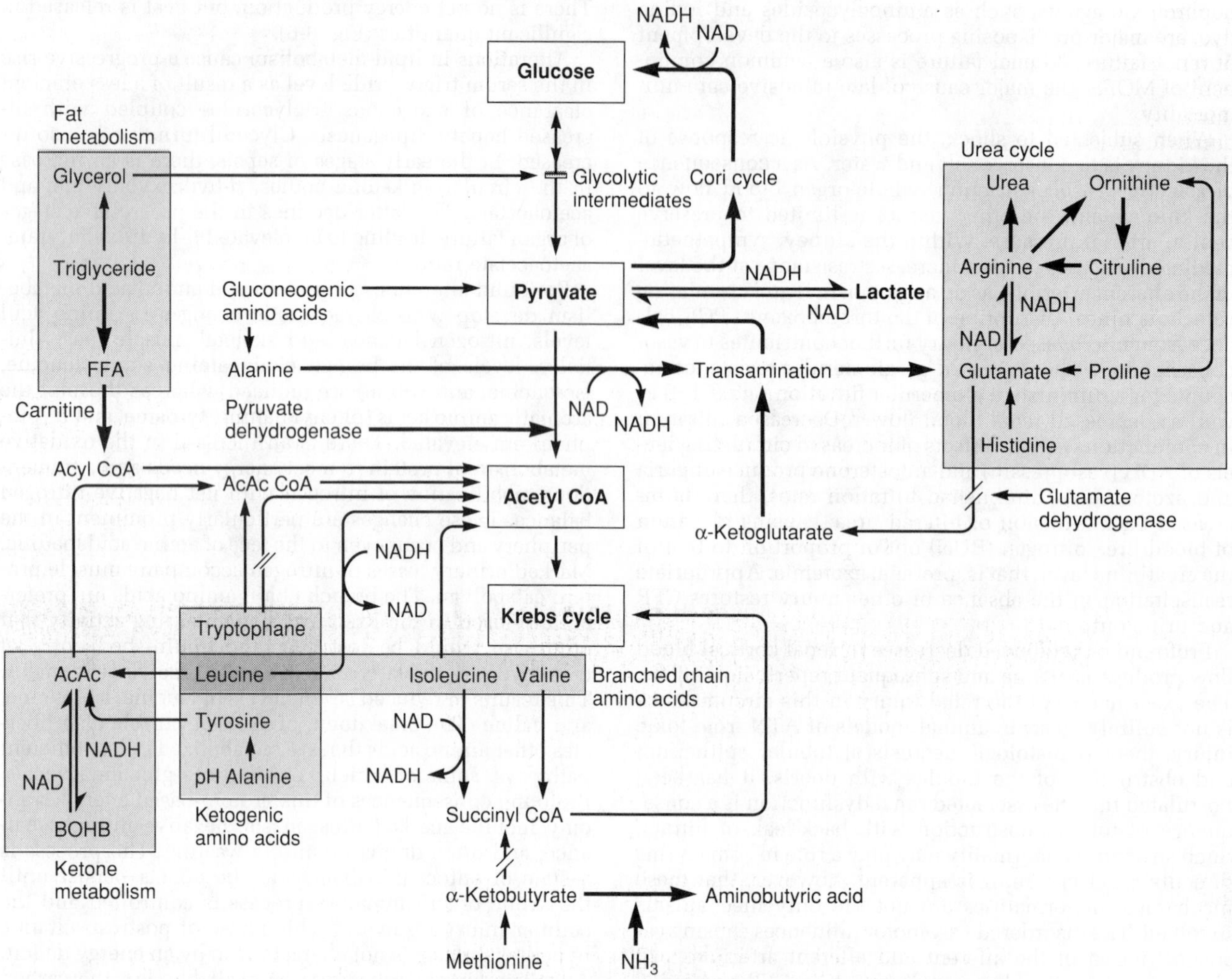

Figure 8-5. The metabolic response to injury affects carbohydrate, fat, and amino acid metabolism to maintain energy availability, protein synthesis, and cellular integrity. (After Stahl TJ, Cerra FB. Hemodynamic and metabolic responses. In: Howard RJ, Simmons RL, eds. Surgical infectious diseases, ed 2. Norwalk, CT, Appleton & Lange, 1988:209)

tissue activates factor XII (Hageman factor), which initiates a number of important reactions, including activation of complement and kinins. Tissue perfusion is compromised as a consequence of inadequate cardiac output, vasoconstrictive influences, and microvascular coagulation, which causes local ischemia and contributes to cellular metabolic dysfunction, cellular injury, and activa-

tion of additional inflammatory mediators. Damaged endothelial cells swell and, in combination with platelet and neutrophil aggregates and other debris, contribute to further obstruction of blood flow. Stasis and sludging develop, and the products of anaerobic metabolism accumulate. These inflammatory stimuli cause tissue-fixed macrophages to become extremely active metabolically

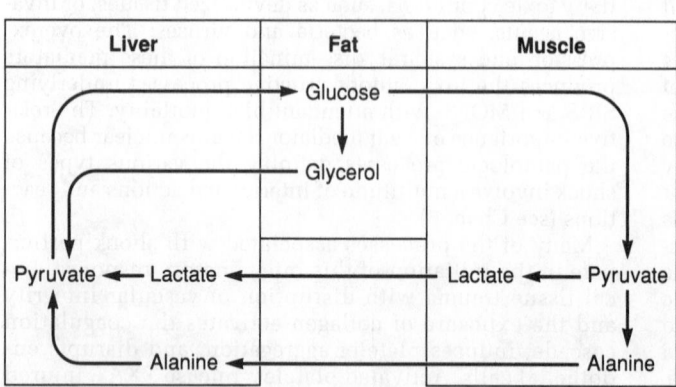

Figure 8-6. The lactate–glucose and alanine–glucose cycles are depicted. These cycles serve to transport carbon and nitrogen between peripheral and central tissue. The "center" of the cycles is the liver. Heat is a major by-product.

and fully capable of producing virtually all inflammatory mediators central to SIRS and MOFS.[3,81]

With resuscitation, restoration of oxygenated blood flow allows formation of potentially injurious ROIs. Reestablishment of flow also flushes inflammatory mediators and activated cellular elements from the hypoperfused vascular beds into the systemic circulation. In shock, ischemia of multiple tissues occurs; with resuscitation, a whole-body reperfusion injury may develop. Microvascular injury and increased capillary permeability lead to a diffuse leak of capillary fluid, development of generalized edema, organ dysfunction, further hemodynamic instability, and if severe or prolonged, subsequent development of MOFS.

Complement

The complement cascade is activated in shock and tissue injury through both the classic and alternative pathways.[82] Initiation of the intrinsic coagulation cascade and activation of factor XII induces the reactions of the classic pathway. Foreign material, dead tissue, antigen–antibody complexes, and bacterial products, in particular endotoxin or lipopolysaccharide from the outer cell membrane, stimulate the alternative pathway. Activation of either pathway results in the generation of the anaphylatoxins, C3a and C5a, soluble products with potent systemic hemodynamic effects.[83,84] C3a, a polypeptide, increases capillary permeability, causes smooth muscle contraction, and stimulates histamine release. C5a, a major chemotactic factor for neutrophils, stimulates degranulation of mast cells and increases vascular permeability, most markedly in the presence of the vasodilator prostaglandins PGE_1, PGE_2, and PGI_2. Small amounts of C5a not only attract neutrophils to foci of inflammation but also activate them, which induces diffuse endothelial injury and elaboration of secondary inflammatory mediators.[83] Direct complement fixation to altered tissues, such as endothelial cells expressing a proinflammatory phenotype, can progress through the C5-9 attack complex, causing cell membrane damage, permeability, and death.

Eicosanoids

Eicosanoids, which includes the prostaglandins and leukotrienes, are formed acutely from arachidonic acid released from membrane phospholipid by phospholipase A_2. Eicosanoids are not stored to any measurable level and are generated as needed from readily available arachidonic acid in response to various inflammatory phenomena. Platelets, white cells, and endothelial cells are a rich source of these compounds. Prostaglandins are formed by the cyclooxygenase pathway of arachidonic acid metabolism, and leukotrienes by the lipoxygenase pathway (Fig. 8-7). Elaboration of each specific metabolite depends on the local environment and enzyme pathway active in the cell of origin.[64,85] The prostaglandins, in particular TXA_2 and PGI_2, are not stored and are metabolized rapidly. As a result, their effects and those of all eicosanoids are largely exerted locally in paracrine and autocrine fashion.[86,87]

TXA_2 is the major arachidonic acid metabolite elaborated by platelets, but it is also produced by activated neutrophils and, in large amounts, by tissue-fixed macrophages. Prostaglandin G_2 (formed from arachidonic acid by cyclooxygenase) is converted to TXA_2 under the influence of thromboxane synthetase. TXA_2 induces intense vasoconstriction, platelet aggregation and degranulation, neutrophil margination in the microcirculation, and bronchoconstriction. It has a half-life of about 30 seconds and is quickly metabolized to the more stable but inactive thromboxane B_2. The exact role of TXA_2 in shock has not been fully defined. Thromboxane production has been shown to be induced by tissue ischemia.[88] The vasoconstriction and neutrophil margination induced by TXA_2 locally in response to inflammation limits perfusion of injured tissues, contributing to further extension of the injury.[89] Levels of thromboxane B_2 (the stable metabolite) have been shown to be elevated in patients with ARDS[65] as well as in models of ischemia-induced ATN.[76] TXA_2 also appears to be the major mediator responsible for the acute pulmonary hypertension seen after shock and resuscitation and with endotoxemia.

PGI_2, the major arachidonic acid metabolite formed by endothelial cells, serves as a check against the actions of TXA_2. PGI_2 is a vasodilator and a potent inhibitor of platelet aggregation. Elaboration of PGI_2 by normal endothelium prevents platelet adherence and aggregation from progressing beyond areas of vessel injury. It follows that endothelial injury upsets this TXA_2–PGI_2 balance. PGI_2 has a half-life of 2 to 3 minutes and is released into blood passing through the lung, producing significant systemic levels. Circulating PGI_2 may therefore reinforce the actions of PGI_2 that is produced locally.[90] PGI_2 is a potent vasodilator and markedly enhances microvascular flow and permeability induced during shock and resuscitation. The E-series prostaglandins, such as PGE_1 and PGE_2, exert actions similar to those of PGI_2, although with less potency. Together, these three prostaglandins function as antiinflammatory agents that down-regulate mediator production from inflammatory cells.[87,91] Although production of these antiinflammatory prostanoids provides homeostasis by maintaining a localized response and preventing systemic dissemination, overproduction and maintenance of high systemic levels of PGE_2 are a major cause of immunosuppression after trauma.[89,92] PGE_2 decreases interleukin-2 (IL-2) production, antibody induction, expression of major histocompatibility antigen type II (necessary for antigen presentation), and production of TNF by macrophages while inhibiting neutrophil migration.[87,92] The major source for PGE_2 production after shock or sepsis is the tissue-fixed macrophage.[87,93,94]

The leukotrienes are products of the lipoxygenase pathway arising from a variety of cell types, including macrophages, neutrophils, and vascular smooth muscle.[67,75]

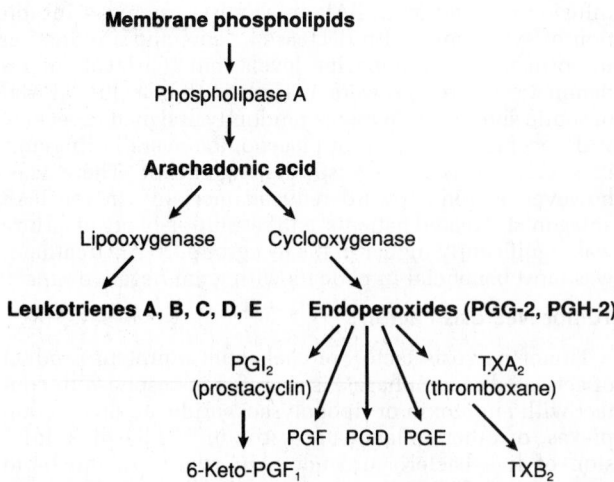

Figure 8-7. Membrane phospholipids containing polyunsaturated fatty acids of the omega-6 family are the parent elements in the cell membrane from which the vasoactive eicosanoids are derived. After their release, membrane enzymes facilitate the production and release of leukotrienes and prostaglandins. (After Stahl TJ, Cerra FB. Hemodynamic and metabolic responses. In: Howard RJ, Simmons RL, eds. Surgical infectious diseases, ed 2. Norwalk, CT, Appleton & Lange, 1988:209)

Their systemic effects are thought to play a major role in the cardiorespiratory derangements of anaphylaxis, and before being isolated and characterized, they were termed the *slow-reacting substance of anaphylaxis*. The leukotrienes produce similar cardiorespiratory derangements in shock. In animal models involving trauma, burns, and endotoxemia, leukotriene metabolites increase locally and systemically to levels greater than those required to induce pathophysiologic effects.[68,95] Leukotriene B4, C4, and D4 cause platelet aggregation, vasoconstriction, venoconstriction, and increases in postcapillary venular permeability. Decreases in cardiac output and lung compliance and increased pulmonary vascular resistance and bronchoconstriction are also noted. Leukotriene B4 is a potent chemoattractant and activator of neutrophils, similar to C5a. The recruitment, activation, and induction of neutrophil margination in the microcirculation may contribute to the early microvascular injury in ARDS and other tissue injuries. Leukotrienes may also produce an amplified formation of microthrombi in the lungs, leading to further ischemic injury. These microthrombi can lead to the release of multiple secondary mediators by activated platelets, neutrophils, and macrophages and to reperfusion injury on restoration of perfusion.[67,68] Inhibition of the lipoxygenase pathway in experimental shock blocked metabolic derangements and improved survival.[96]

Platelet-Activating Factor

Platelet-activating factor, a potent phospholipid mediator, is released by neutrophils, platelets, macrophages, and endothelial cells in response to ischemia, tissue injury, and sepsis.[97-99] Its effects include decreased cardiac function, increased pulmonary vascular resistance, bronchoconstriction, peripheral vasodilation, increased vascular permeability, priming of macrophages to subsequent stimuli, platelet and neutrophil aggregation, and enhanced neutrophil adherence to endothelium. The actions of PAF may be modulated and amplified by induction of secondary mediators. Elevated PAF levels with evidence of neutrophil priming have been found in models of endotoxemia, bacterial peritonitis, and trauma shock.[68,98,100] PAF produces clinical symptoms of stress after shock and contributes to the metabolic and counterregulatory hormone responses of endotoxemia. In human volunteers given an infusion of endotoxin, PAF antagonists produced inhibition of symptoms, with decreased rigors and a reduction in cortisol and epinephrine levels, but the levels of inflammatory cytokines were unaffected.[101] In a clinical trial of septic shock with patients randomly assigned to receive PAF receptor antagonist or placebo, the overall difference in survival was not statistically significant. There was, however, a trend toward reduced mortality in the PAF antagonist–treated patients, and resolution of organ failure was significantly higher in the test group.[102] The treatment was most beneficial in patients with gram-negative sepsis.

Tumor Necrosis Factor

Tumor necrosis factor, or cachectin, a protein product of activated macrophages, is secreted in response to contact with endotoxin or lipopolysaccharide, antibody complexes, or other inflammatory stimuli.[103] Likewise, infusion of live bacteria or endotoxin results in the rapid appearance of TNF in experimental models.[104] Elevation of serum levels of TNF have been reported shortly after experimental trauma and shock.[105-107] Documentation of elevated circulating levels of TNF in human shock is less clear.[108-111] This variability is thought to be due to the rapid clearance and uptake by membrane receptors and by soluble membrane receptors that are released from multiple cells after stress and injury. After hypoperfusion, the liver and gut appear to be major sources of TNF that is rapidly cleared but responsible for inducing hepatocyte changes after shock. The release of breakdown products and escape of bacteria and endotoxin through the damaged mucosal barrier of the gut after shock allow or induce activation of the tissue-fixed macrophages (Kupffer cells) of the liver. These macrophages then produce secondary inflammatory mediators, contributing to the postresuscitation clinical response and inflammatory mediator activation seen in SIRS.[112]

TNF is central to the inflammatory response, particularly in sepsis and after endotoxemia or bacteremia. TNF induces the secondary inflammatory responses through direct interaction with specific membrane receptors. This interaction causes neutrophils to undergo activation, a respiratory burst, and degranulation. It also causes T-cell activation and induction of the proinflammatory phenotype on endothelial cells. The latter results from expression of cell surface ligands that enhance neutrophil adherence, coagulation, endothelial injury, and increased vascular permeability.[103,113] TNF, either directly or through secondary mediators produced by the activated Kupffer cell, induces the hepatocyte acute-phase protein synthesis response. Hypotension, lactic acidosis, and respiratory failure are seen after infusion of TNF experimentally, as are other induced metabolic abnormalities, including hyperglycemia, hypertriglyceridemia, and a wasting diathesis (hence the original name, *cachectin*). TNF has been shown to contribute to the production and release of leukotrienes and PGE$_2$ by macrophages and endothelium.[103,114] It is likely that much of the tissue injury associated with TNF is a result of multiple secondary mediators of inflammation and other indirect effects of this potent molecule.

Systemic effects of TNF can also be modulated and down-regulated by the release of soluble TNF receptors. Interaction of TNF with soluble TNF receptors blocks binding and activation of target cells and tissues. Trauma and shock cause cells to release two forms of soluble TNF receptors, the 55-kd and 75-kd membrane receptors, which are elevated within 1 hour of injury and remain elevated for as long as 15 days.[108-110] In contrast to circulating levels of TNF, the circulating levels of soluble TNF receptors correlate well with the severity of tissue injury and shock, and higher levels correlate with an increased mortality and subsequent complications from SIRS. Soluble TNF receptors appear to be better markers of shock severity than TNF, which, due to rapid clearance, is rarely found elevated.[115]

Treatment with anti-TNF antibody in the experimental setting protects animals from the deleterious effects of lethal bacteremia and endotoxemia.[116] However, clinical trials in septic patients using infusions of monoclonal antibodies to the TNF molecule have shown no overall survival benefit. Experimentally, the evolutionary benefit of an appropriate response in TNF production and release is apparent because *complete* neutralization of TNF with passive immunity before infectious challenge increases mortality.

Interleukin-1

Interleukin-1 is a major inflammatory mediator produced by the tissue-fixed macrophage and circulating monocyte. Similar to TNF, IL-1 has been shown to have a crucial role in modulating and controlling the systemic inflammatory response. These effects are noted primarily after endotoxic and bacteremic insults, and documentation of IL-1 contributions to the inflammatory response after shock are less clear. Most clinical studies have been unable to document consistent elevation of IL-1b after shock. However, increased mRNA levels specific for IL-1 have been noted in pulmonary macrophages after shock in animal models.[117] It appears that IL-1, similar to TNF and other inflammatory cytokines, functions primarily in a paracrine and autocrine fashion with erratic and inconsistent release into the systemic circulation. Rapid receptor binding and the production and release of circulating natural antagonists to IL-1 also contribute to the variable systemic levels noted after shock. IL-1 receptor antagonist (IL-1ra) is produced by macrophages and other cells in response to IL-1, endotoxin, and other by-products of tissue injury and shock. IL-1ra levels correlate with severity of injury and also with increased risk of mortality and complication.[118] IL-1ra binds to IL-1 receptors on the cell membrane and blocks IL-1–induced cell activation. Similar to anti-TNF antibodies, the passive infusion of human recombinant IL-1ra has been shown to prevent death in animal models of endotoxemia and gram-negative bacteremia, but clinical trials in patients with sepsis and septic shock showed no overall improvement in survival, but there was a trend for lower mortality rates with treatment in septic shock.[119]

Interleukin-8

Interleukin-8 is produced predominantly by the macrophage–monocyte cell line, with additional production by endothelium with a proinflammatory phenotype and other interstitial cells. IL-8 is the most potent neutrophil chemokine and activates the neutrophil to undergo respiratory burst and degranulation. IL-8 up-regulates adhesion molecules on the neutrophil to enhance aggregation, which causes direct adhesion to the vascular endothelium, microvascular occlusion, and subsequent release of ROIs and destructive proteases. Elevated levels of IL-8 have been found in the bronchoalveolar lavage fluid from patients with ALI and ARDS. Induction of IL-8 with recruitment and activation of neutrophils after stress states appears central to the underlying pathophysiology of MOFS.[120,121]

Adhesion Molecules

Neutrophils are capable of extensive inflammatory tissue destruction and are strongly implicated in the pathogenesis of cell injury and organ dysfunction after shock, trauma, and sepsis. Margination of the neutrophil in the microcirculation is a ubiquitous pathologic finding in the various organs involved in MOFS. The ability of the neutrophil to induce damage requires activation and adherence to endothelial cells. Adherence is particularly prominent in the postcapillary venule and is accompanied by release of destructive ROIs and proteases. The adherence of the neutrophil requires enhanced expression of adhesion molecules on the surface of the endothelial cell and the neutrophil. Up-regulation of these adherence molecules is stimulated by C5a, IL-8, leukotriene B4, TNF, IL-1, and other inflammatory mediators inducing the proinflammatory phenotype on the endothelial cell surface and the activated neutrophil. Subsequent to induction, there is a rapid release of adhesion molecules from both the endothelial and neutrophil surfaces in an attempt to control and down-regulate the spread of the inflammatory process. Circulating adhesion molecules can be used as markers for the intensity of the inflammatory response and likelihood of organ injury. Circulating levels of soluble intercellular adhesion molecule 1 and E-selectin, major endothelial cell-surface adhesive molecules for neutrophils, correlate well with subsequent organ dysfunction and development of MOFS. High levels of E-selectin are also predictive of an increased mortality rate. The extent of endothelial cell activation after shock and injury appears important in the pathogenesis of MOFS. Therapeutic interventions to minimize the endothelial proinflammatory state and potentially prevent

neutrophil-induced tissue injury and organ dysfunction are the focus of investigations.[122,123]

Nitric Oxide

Nitric oxide influences both normal physiologic functions and abnormal maladaptive immunoinflammatory responses. Endothelium constitutively produces nitric oxide, which is a physiologic vasodilator maintaining normal vascular tone.[124,125] Inhibition of constitutive nitric oxide produces about a 30% increase in vascular resistance. Constitutive production is increased by flow stresses and vasomotor responses to tissue nutrient needs. Vasodilation is maintained by nitric oxide activation of guanylate cyclase in vascular smooth muscle cells.[126] Conditions that stimulate inflammatory mediator systems, such as prolonged hypoperfusion, ischemia–reperfusion, or sepsis stimulate an inducible isoform of nitric oxide synthase.[127] Induction of the nitric oxide synthase isoform is part of the host immunoinflammatory response and causes direct cytotoxicity, immune cell regulation, and inflammatory vasodilation. The nitric oxide isoform is thought to contribute significantly to the hyperdynamic cardiovascular response of sepsis and SIRS. It has also been postulated that induction of the nitric oxide synthase isoform by prolonged hypoperfusion is responsible both locally and, ultimately, systemically for reversal of the adaptive vasoconstrictive response to hypovolemia and the transition to a decompensated and maladaptive vasodilation. This transition is not well defined. It is hypothesized that after resuscitation from hypovolemic shock, the ability to generate nitric oxide is initially suppressed, and a beneficial increase in vascular tone is noted. Later, the constitutive and inducible forms of nitric oxide synthase reverse the vasoconstrictive responses to hypoperfusion, producing decompensation.

CLINICAL FEATURES AND TREATMENT

Although the causes of shock is vary, the common denominators are inadequate tissue perfusion and the imbalance between delivery of metabolic substrate and cellular metabolic needs. Early microvascular hypoperfusion is difficult to detect clinically and can occur in a variable pattern that depends on the underlying cause. The progression of shock leads to an increasing metabolic derangement with ultimate loss of homeostasis (decompensation) and inability to maintain mean arterial pressure, producing the organ dysfunction and hypotension recognized clinically. In the following sections, the clinical manifestations and treatment of the various forms of shock are described, recognizing the frequent multiplicity of responses and overlapping actions of the various causes of shock.

Monitors

Patients in shock not requiring emergent operation are usually cared for in the intensive care unit or other critical care setting. Careful and continuous assessment of physiologic status is essential. Blood pressure, pulse, and respiratory rate are monitored and the adequacy and effectiveness of resuscitation routinely determined by measuring urine output and mental status. More aggressive monitoring, including a variety of on-line invasive monitors and intermittent physiologic assessments, is common.

Use of the Pulmonary Artery Catheter

Invasive hemodynamic monitoring using the flow-directed pulmonary artery catheter (Swan-Ganz catheter) is essential in the optimal management of patients in shock

Table 8-2. NORMAL CARDIOVASCULAR PRESSURES

Pressures	Values (mm Hg)
Right atrium or central venous	0–6
Right ventricle	20–30/0–6
Pulmonary artery	20–30/6–12
Pulmonary artery mean	12–18
Pulmonary capillary wedge	6–12
Left atrium	4–12
Left ventricle	100–140/5–14
Arterial (systolic/diastolic)	100–140/60–80
Mean arterial	75–100

or those suffering postshock sequelae. The ability to predict accurately hemodynamic profiles of patients in shock without pulmonary artery catheterization is poor; incorrect predictions occur in more than one third of cases. The overall mortality rate is significantly lower in critically ill patients who have changes in therapy directed by pulmonary artery catheter data.[128]

The Swan-Ganz catheter, placed percutaneously, courses through the central venous circulation and the right heart to the pulmonary artery; both proximal (right atrial) and distal (pulmonary artery) ports provide data about cardiovascular dynamics. Right atrial and pulmonary artery pressures can be measured directly, and pulmonary artery wedge pressure serves as a reasonable approximation of left atrial pressure; cardiac output is readily determined by thermodilution technique. Systemic and pulmonary vascular resistance are calculated as the ratio of the respective pressures to cardiac output. Normal cardiovascular pressures and hemodynamic parameters are listed in Tables 8-2 and 8-3. Blood gas determinations on mixed venous blood from the distal (pulmonary artery) port of the catheter and from systemic arterial blood allow calculation of arterial and venous blood oxygen content. This information, in conjunction with the cardiac output, is sufficient to calculate oxygen consumption and oxygen delivery (Table 8-4). Characteristic hemodynamic patterns associated with the various forms of shock are shown in Table 8-5. An oximetric Swan-Ganz catheter offers additional advantages, and its use is described in Chapter 9.

The restoration of tissue perfusion and appropriate tissue oxygen delivery is best accomplished through hemodynamic manipulations based on pulmonary artery catheter measurements and oxygen transport calculations. The goal of resuscitation is to ensure delivery in a quantities sufficient to meet tissue demand. Although there is no prospective way of determining oxygen needs, there are two techniques for establishing whether oxygen delivery

is adequate. One method is to induce increases in oxygen delivery through increasing red-cell mass, improving arterial oxygen saturation, or augmenting cardiac output. Increases in oxygen delivery not accompanied by increases in oxygen consumption imply that oxygen availability is adequate and that oxygen consumption is flow independent. Increases in oxygen delivery that are accompanied by increases in oxygen consumption imply inadequacy of oxygen supply and that consumption is flow dependent. Similarly, elevated lactate levels that decrease with increased cardiac output and oxygen delivery imply that the lactate production is flow dependent and a consequence of anaerobic metabolism. A lactate/pyruvate ratio of greater than 20:1 is also consistent with anaerobic metabolism and therefore reflects inadequate flow. Resuscitation should thus be geared toward achieving a state in which oxygen consumption and lactate production are flow independent.

Gastric Tonometry

Techniques for evaluating the adequacy of resuscitation at the cell and tissue level are insensitive and, in large part, rely on surrogate markers. Evaluation of new technologies to measure oxygen delivery and tissue perfusion continues. One potential monitor of adequate tissue perfusion after resuscitation from shock is gastric intramucosal pH using gastric tonometry. Serial measurements of intramucosal gastric pH are based on hydrogen ion diffusion and equilibration with normal saline in the balloon-tipped gastric tonometer catheter. During resuscitation from shock, systemic hemodynamics and oxygen transport variables correlate poorly with gastric intramucosal pH. Inadequate visceral perfusion, however, as evidenced by persistent low intramucosal pH after resuscitation, is associated with subsequent organ dysfunction and death. Patients with low intramucosal pH whose defects are not corrected with seemingly adequate resuscitation to usual hemodynamic endpoints may need additional resuscitation. Correction of low intramural pH has not yet been correlated with an improvement in outcome, but persistence of a low intramucosal pH may identify patients unable to increase physiologic delivery of oxygen who are less likely to survive despite maximal resuscitative efforts.

Hypovolemic Shock

Any process that contributes to intravascular volume depletion can cause hypovolemic shock, including hemorrhage, extravascular fluid sequestration, gastrointestinal and urinary losses, or insensible loss. Hemorrhage is the form of volume loss that can be most readily quantified and reproduced. It historically has been vitally important

Table 8-3. NORMAL HEMODYNAMIC PARAMETERS

Parameter	Calculation	Normal Values
Cardiac output (CO)	SV × HR	4–8 L/min
Cardiac index (CI)	CO/BSA	2.5–4 L/min/m^2
Stroke volume (SV)	CO/HR × 1000	60–100 mL/beat
Systemic vascular resistance (SVR)	(MAP − RAP)/CO × 80	800–1400 dynes/s/cm^{-5}
Systemic vascular resistance index (SVRI)	SVR × BSA	1500–2400 dynes/s/cm^{-5}/m^2
Pulmonary vascular resistance (PVR)	(PAP$_m$ − PCWP)/CO × 80	100–150 dynes/s/cm^{15}
Pulmonary vascular resistance index (PVRI)	PVR × BSA	200–400 dynes/s/cm^{-5}/m^2
Left ventricular stroke work (LVSW)	SV/(MAP − PCWP) × 0.0136	60–80 g-m/beat
Left ventricular stroke work index (LVSWI)	LVSW/BSA	45–60 g-m/beat/m^2
Right ventricular stroke work (RVSW)	SV (PAP$_m$ − PAP) × 0.0136	10–15 g-m/beat
Right ventricular stroke work index (RVSWI)	RVSW/BSA	6–10 g-m/beat/m^2

Table 8-4. OXYGEN TRANSPORT CALCULATIONS

Parameters	Calculation	Normal Values
Oxygen-carrying capacity of Hgb		= 1.38 mL O_2/g Hgb
Plasma O_2 content		= Po_2 × 0.0031
Arterial O_2 content (Cao_2)	= Sao_2 (range, 0–1.00) × Hgb (g/dL) × 1.38 (mL/g)	20 vol%
Venous O_2 content (Cvo_2)	= Svo_2 × Hgb × 1.38	15.5 vol%
Arteriovenous O_2 difference (AV O_2 difference)	= Cao_2 − Cvo_2	3.5 vol%
	= (Sao_2 − Svo_2) × Hgb × 1.38	
Systemic oxygen delivery (Do_2)	= Cao_2 × CO (L/min) × 10 L/dL	800–1600 mL/min
	= Sao_2 × Hgb × 1.38 × CO × 10	
Systemic oxygen consumption (Vo_2)	= (AV)O_2 difference × CO × 10	150–400 mL/min
	= (Sao_2 − Svo_2) × Hgb × 1.38 × CO × 10	
Oxygen consumption index (Vo_2I)	= Vo_2/BSA	115–165 mL/m²/min

to patients and their physicians, and it is the best-studied form of shock. The signs and symptoms of the nonhemorrhagic forms of hypovolemic shock are the same as with hemorrhage, although they can be more insidious in onset.

The physiologic responses to hypovolemic shock are geared toward maintenance of central perfusion and the restoration of effective circulating blood volume. The compensatory mechanisms include an increase in sympathetic activity, hyperventilation, passive collapse of capacitance vessels, release of stress hormones, expansion of intravascular volume through resorption of interstitial fluid and mobilization of intracellular fluid, and conservation of fluids and electrolytes by the kidney. The clinical signs and symptoms encountered are recognized as the consequence of the intense adrenosympathetic response to diminishing blood volume (see Chap. 11).

Clinical stages of hemorrhagic shock have been based on the volume of blood lost. Mild volume loss can be tolerated with relatively few external signs, especially in the supine, resting patient (Table 8-6). Loss of 10% to 15% of the blood volume or class I hemorrhage (500 to 750 mL in a 70-kg patient) causes minimal change in the patient's clinical condition, with little or no alteration in blood pressure and heart rate. Adrenergic discharge can cause pallor, diaphoresis, and diminished capillary refill, and subcutaneous veins become less prominent as they passively collapse. With class II hemorrhage, consisting of a 20% to 30% decrease in blood volume (1000 to 1500 mL), the patient becomes anxious and mildly tachycardiac but is able to maintain a normal blood pressure. The skin changes are more prominent and are accompanied by oliguria. The oliguria is a function of the adrenergic-mediated renal arteriolar constriction as well as the production of circulating stress hormones—vasopressin and aldosterone. With blood volume loss of 30% to 40%, or class III hemorrhage (1500 to 2000 mL), the classic findings of hemorrhagic

shock appear. Initially, blood pressure may be relatively well maintained. Postural changes of heart rate and blood pressure are readily appreciated, and if hypovolemia is prolonged, the blood pressure is compromised and the patient extremely tachycardiac, oliguric, and agitated or confused. Severe blood loss, or class IV hemorrhage, with 40% or more blood volume loss (more than 2000 mL in a 70-kg patient), represents a severe physiologic insult. The hemodynamic instability results in progressive tachycardia and profound hypotension even while supine and resting. Mental status changes progress from restlessness and agitation to listlessness and obtundation, producing a moribund condition because blood flow to the brain is insufficient to maintain function.[54] Passage from an initially unrecognized class II stage to class IV can occur rapidly unless extreme attentiveness and caution are applied. Obtundation is an ominous clinical sign and requires aggressive volume resuscitation and emergent intervention. Decompensation of homeostatic mechanisms and inability to maintain systolic blood pressure above 90 mmHg after trauma-induced hypovolemia is associated with a mortality rate of more than 50%. Even severe hemorrhagic shock can be reversed, however, if there is rapid and adequate restoration of circulating blood volume and control of ongoing losses. If shock is prolonged, hypoperfusion of the various microvascular beds leads to cellular injury and the elaboration of inflammatory mediators, contributing to further hypoperfusion, organ dysfunction, and irreversible decompensation.

Diagnosis

Hypovolemic shock is readily diagnosed when there is an obvious source of volume loss and when overt signs of hemodynamic instability and increased adrenergic output are present. The diagnosis is more difficult when there is an occult source of volume loss. Under these circum-

Table 8-5. PHYSIOLOGIC CHARACTERISTICS OF THE VARIOUS FORMS OF SHOCK

Type of Shock	CVP and PCWP	Cardiac Output	Systemic Vascular Resistance	Venous O_2 Saturation
Hypovolemic	↓	↓	↑	↓
Cardiogenic	↑	↓	↑	↓
Septic				
Hyperdynamic	↓↑	↑	↓	↑
Hypodynamic	↓↑	↓	↑	↑↓
Traumatic	↓	↓↑	↑↓	↓
Neurogenic	↓	↓	↓	↓
Hypoadrenal	↓↑	↓	↑↓	↓

CVP, central venous pressure; PCWP, pulmonary capillary wedge pressure.

Table 8-6. PHYSICAL FINDINGS IN HEMORRHAGIC SHOCK*

Mild (<20% Blood Volume)	Moderate (20%–40% Blood Volume)	Severe (>40% Blood Volume)
Pallor	Pallor	Pallor
Cool extremities	Cool extremities	Cool extremities
Diminished capillary refill	Diminished capillary refill	Diminished capillary refill
Diaphoresis	Diaphoresis	Diaphoresis
Collapsed subcutaneous veins	Collapsed subcutaneous veins	Collapsed subcutaneous veins
	Tachycardia	Tachycardia
	Oliguria	Oliguria
	Postural hypotension	Hypotension
		Mental status changes

* Alcohol or drug intoxication may alter physical findings.

stances, physical findings may not be particularly well developed, and unreplaced gastrointestinal or urinary losses, excessive insensible loss, or intraabdominal fluid sequestration should be considered. Likewise, significant blood loss into the chest, abdomen, retroperitoneum, pelvis, and thigh may initially occur with relatively few specific findings. Plasma losses from tissue trauma or burns, free water deficit, or unreplaced insensible loss may also lead to hypovolemia.

Plasma losses cause hemoconcentration, and free water loss causes hemoconcentration and hypernatremia. Elevations of BUN and creatinine are consistent with hypovolemia but may occur in conjunction with other forms of shock. After acute hemorrhage, hemoglobin and hematocrit values do not change until compensatory fluid shifts have occurred or exogenous fluid is administered. Their values decrease once transcapillary refill, osmotic-induced shifts, or non–red cell volume resuscitation reexpands the blood volume.

It is imperative that the distinction be made between hypovolemic and cardiogenic forms of shock because appropriate therapy differs dramatically. The physical findings of jugular venous distention, rales, and the presence of an S_3 gallop in cardiogenic shock may assist in distinguishing the two. Both forms of shock, however, are associated with a diminished cardiac output and a compensatory sympathetic-mediated response.

Because physical findings can be confusing and multiple factors may be contributing to hemodynamic instability, more information may be needed to identify the degree of hypovolemia or the degree of cardiac dysfunction. Invasive monitoring using a pulmonary artery catheter provides this information. Diminished cardiac filling pressures (CVP and PCWP) and a low cardiac output responsive to volume resuscitation are found in situations of hypovolemia (see Table 8-5).

Treatment

Restoration of perfusion in hypovolemic shock requires reexpansion of the circulating blood volume in conjunction with necessary interventions to control ongoing volume loss. Vigorous volume resuscitation is paramount. Repletion of circulating volume reexpands capacitance vessels, restores venous return, and reestablishes ventricular filling. Contractile function, stroke volume, and cardiac output respond positively, consistent with Frank-Starling dynamics. Even after adequate resuscitation, diastolic

compliance may remain abnormal for some time, owing to increased myocardial interstitial fluid, and require relatively high filling pressures to maintain ventricular performance. In severe, prolonged hypovolemia, ventricular contractile function may become depressed and require inotropic support to maintain ventricular performance. In general, however, pharmacologic interventions directed toward increasing contractility in situations of inadequate preload are ineffective, further complicate metabolic derangements, and are not indicated until adequate volume resuscitation has been completed.

Measures designed to increase central blood pressure through increasing resistance to flow may maintain cerebral and coronary perfusion temporarily. These temporizing measures include use of the pneumatic antishock garment (PASG), use aortic cross-clamping, and infusion of α-adrenergic agents. Each of these, however, contributes to a further decrease in peripheral perfusion and may therefore contribute to the progression of shock to a potential irreversible stage. These measures cannot replace appropriate fluid resuscitation and control of volume loss as the essential components of resuscitation if metabolic and perfusion defects leading to organ failure are to be prevented.

In hypovolemia, as with other forms of shock, a principal consequence of hypoperfusion is the diminished transport of oxygen to tissues and the ineffective removal of toxic wastes. Successful resuscitation is accomplished through restitution of tissue oxygenation, and initial therapy is directed toward support of both respiratory and circulatory function. Immediate concerns therefore include establishment of an airway, ventilation, and intravenous access. Supplementary oxygen should be provided. If ventilatory function is in question, mechanical assistance should be instituted. Endotracheal intubation is desirable if the airway is tenuous because of obtundation or injury, or if ventilation is required for more than a brief period. The presence or possibility of cervical spine fracture or instability requires that measures be taken to attain airway control with as little manipulation of the neck as possible. In these circumstances, nasotracheal intubation, tracheostomy, or cricothyroidotomy may be life-saving.

Volume resuscitation is readily initiated through peripheral intravenous lines during the initial stages of evaluation. Rapid infusion of isotonic saline or a balanced salt solution is of diagnostic value and therapeutic benefit. Infusion of 2 to 3 L of crystalloid for 10 to 30 minutes restores an adequate blood pressure in most cases. Continued hemodynamic instability implies that shock has not been reversed or that there is ongoing blood or volume loss. Further volume resuscitation should therefore include simultaneous blood transfusion, either as fully crossmatched blood or, in dire circumstances, type-specific or O-negative packed cells (O-positive blood is acceptable for patients older than 50 years). In all patients resuscitated, measures should be taken to avoid hypothermia and its associated consequences.

Hypovolemic shock poorly responsive to volume resuscitation is suggestive of ongoing volume loss. It also raises the concern that other causes of instability, such as pericardial tamponade, tension pneumothorax, or ventricular dysfunction, are present. In the first two settings, prompt treatment is essential; although invasive monitoring is indicated, it should not delay treatment. Likewise, despite the desirability and utility of invasive monitoring, it should not delay the surgical control of ongoing blood loss.

Complications are less frequent after treatment of hemorrhagic shock than in situations of septic or traumatic shock. In the latter circumstances, the massive activation of inflammatory mediator response systems and consequences of their disseminated, indiscriminate cellular injury can be profound. Complications after simple hemorrhage are also more frequent if concomitant underlying arterial occlusive or comorbid end-organ disease is present.

Traumatic Shock

The major contributor to shock after trauma is hypovolemia, and acute hemorrhage is often the cause of early demise after injury. Even when hemorrhage ceases or is controlled, patients can continue to suffer loss of plasma volume into the interstitium of injured tissues and develop progressive hypovolemic shock. In addition, tissue injury evokes a broader pathophysiologic immunoinflammatory response and a potentially more devastating degree of shock than that produced by hypovolemia alone. Specific injuries can produce superimposed cardiogenic or neurogenic shock. Pericardial tamponade, or tension pneumothorax, can produce hemodynamically significant compression of the heart, and myocardial contusion can cause pump failure. Neurogenic shock can accompany spinal cord injury.

The degree to which direct tissue injury and an inflammatory response participate in the development and progression of traumatic shock distinguishes it from purely hypovolemic shock. Cellular injury, tissue devitalization, ischemia with subsequent reperfusion, bacterial contamination, and accumulations of blood or other body fluids contribute to the development of SIRS. It is the inflammatory, or toxic, response that evokes the dramatic functional and metabolic disturbances that follow. In many cases, the mediators involved in traumatic shock are the same or similar to those seen in sepsis. These inflammatory mediators amplify the original injury and contribute to the nondiscriminating injury of nontraumatized "by-stander" tissues.

Initial management of the seriously injured requires the assurance of an airway, breathing, and circulation; the latter requires appropriate volume resuscitation and control of ongoing losses. Control of hemorrhage is a major concern and demands priority over attention to other injuries. After resuscitation and control of volume losses, efforts necessary to minimize the potentially lethal postshock sequelae, including MOFS, are undertaken. These include restoration of perfusion to ischemic areas, stabilization of fractures, débridement of devitalized or contaminated tissues, and evacuation of hematomas.

Postresuscitation hypermetabolism driven by SIRS exists even in the absence of bacterial contamination or infection. This common process is thought to contribute to the development of organ dysfunction and MOFS.[3] It is not unusual to see a temperature of 38.8°C (102°F), tachycardia, and a widened pulse pressure, reflecting an elevated cardiac output. Other findings include transient increases in serum lactate, oxygen consumption, and amino acid clearance. Fluid sequestration and salt and water retention are common and contribute to weight gain. These effects of the local and systemic inflammatory response resolve and reverse as hemodynamic stability is maintained and repair processes ensue. Persistence of SIRS with progression to MOFS may be related to a persistent inflammatory focus, intercurrent infection, or an ongoing perfusion deficit.

Cardiogenic Shock

Intrinsic Cardiogenic Shock

Intrinsic cardiogenic shock results from failure of the heart as an effective pump. Such failure may be the result of myocyte, structural, or electrical abnormalities. Coronary artery disease is the most common cause of myocardial insufficiency, but contractile dysfunction may also arise as a consequence of cardiomyopathy, myocarditis, or metabolic abnormalities. Adequate output of oxygenated blood may be compromised by valvular or other cardiac structural abnormalities or with significant dysrhythmias. Right-sided heart failure may follow acute pulmonary embolism or the subacute chronic pulmonary hypertension that follows extensive microembolism. Chronic right-sided heart failure from pulmonary hypertension may also be seen with advanced chronic pulmonary disease. It can also arise as a result of direct injury or complicate ARDS and can lead to biventricular failure. Management of intrinsic cardiogenic shock can be focused more exclusively on the heart than is possible in other forms of shock.

Manifestations of cardiogenic shock develop as a consequence of failure of peripheral perfusion, the associated adrenergic response, and the inability of the heart to accommodate blood returning from the lungs and the periphery. In the absence of sepsis or tissue injury, however, there is not usually an associated increase in the metabolic needs of the peripheral tissues. As with hemorrhagic shock, the adrenergic response is initiated through baroreceptor and visceral afferent inputs to the medullary vasomotor center. Cardiac pain and hypoxia contribute to the adrenergic response, and if hypotension is profound, a central neurogenic response greatly increases sympathetic activity. Sympathetic-mediated constriction of the peripheral vasculature attempts to maintain central blood pressure and perfusion of cerebral and coronary circulations. The clinical findings of cardiogenic shock may thus be similar to those of hypovolemic shock because both involve induction of the adrenosympathetic response.

Diminished or ineffective contractile activity of the right or left side of the heart allows blood to accumulate in the respective venous circulations. Right-sided failure leads to accumulation of blood in the systemic veins and capacitance vessels. If this is severe or chronic, peripheral edema hepatomegaly and hepatojugular reflux may develop. In left-sided failure, the pulmonary vasculature initially accommodates blood accumulation by dilation of the capacious pulmonary veins. As the limits of capacity are reached, pressures within the vasculature increase. With normal pulmonary capillary permeability, pulmonary interstitial fluid flow overwhelms the capacity of pulmonary lymphatics, and edema develops at capillary pressures higher than 20 mmHg. Overt pulmonary alveolar edema develops at pressures of more than 24 mmHg. *Noncardiogenic* pulmonary edema develops in the face of left atrial pressures of 18 mmHg or less. Pulmonary edema impacts pulmonary function by limiting diffusion of oxygen by increasing the distances from alveoli to capillaries. In addition, interstitial and intraalveolar fluid causes a progressive decrease in lung compliance. As compliance falls, ventilatory work increases with accompanying atelectasis, thereby increasing the fraction of blood shunted past unventilated alveoli. Increases in cardiac interstitial fluid cause a significant decrease in diastolic compliance, a major feature of cardiogenic shock. In this setting, high ventricular filling pressures are necessary to ensure adequate cardiac output, but the elevated cardiac filling pressures make pulmonary edema a prominent clinical feature.

In making the diagnosis of cardiogenic shock, any history of cardiac disease is of diagnostic value. Associated physical findings include those of hemodynamic instability, peripheral vasoconstriction, and congestive fluid accumulation as well as findings specific to the underlying cardiac abnormality. Tachycardia, tachypnea, hypotension, and cool, pale, mottled, or cyanotic extremities in an agitated oliguric patient are typical. With severe or progressive shock, the level of consciousness may deteriorate from agitation to obtundation. The posture of a conscious patient in congestive heart failure is typically upright; subsequent collapse occurs once the hypotension of cardiogenic shock develops. Rales and an S_3 gallop rhythm may be appreciated. Jugular venous distention and peripheral edema are seen in right-sided or biventricular failure.

An electrocardiogram may provide evidence of preexisting cardiac disease as well as any acute changes. Chest radiographs may demonstrate abnormalities consistent with the specific underlying heart disease as well as the presence of pulmonary vascular congestion, pulmonary edema, pleural effusions, and cardiomegaly. Surface or transesophageal echocardiograms may demonstrate the presence of structural abnormalities or the functional impairment of cardiac contractility. Laboratory data are supportive and may offer critical information for optimal management. Cardiac enzymes may provide evidence of acute myocardial injury. Arterial blood gas determinations confirm the presence of hypoxia and assess the adequacy of ventilation and acid–base status. Urinary indices are consistent with prerenal azotemia (elevated urine osmolarity, decreased urinary sodium, and decreased fractional excretion of sodium).

In some cases, it is difficult to ascertain the precise role of cardiac dysfunction in the shock state. Pulmonary edema associated with an increased pulmonary capillary permeability may arise from noncardiac causes. Pulmonary disease and mechanical ventilation may obscure or otherwise alter the typical findings of cardiogenic failure. Occasionally, a sudden cardiac event may lead to a fall, a motor vehicle accident, or another type of trauma. The shock apparent in the emergency department may be mistakenly ascribed to traumatic rather than cardiac causes (or vice versa).

Invasive hemodynamic monitoring often establishes the specific nature of shock and allows appropriate treatments to be delivered in an effective and expedient manner. Hemodynamic findings consistent with cardiogenic shock include a low cardiac output (cardiac index less than 2.2 L/min/m^2) and high SVR, despite elevated cardiac filling pressures (PCWP usually 18 mmHg or greater). Tissues compensate for diminished oxygen delivery with an increased oxygen extraction; the mixed venous oxygen saturation is decreased and the arteriovenous oxygen difference increased. An increased plasma lactate concentration is commonly present, indicating a shift to anaerobic metabolism in major tissue beds.

Management of shock of cardiac origin involves the principles used in treating other forms of shock. Restoration of peripheral perfusion is accomplished through optimizing cardiovascular and respiratory dynamics. Initial measures include administration of supplemental oxygen, mechanical ventilation (as needed), and appropriate treatment of dysrhythmias. Cardiopulmonary resuscitation is instituted when indicated. When acute myocardial infarction is the cause of shock, coronary angiography and aggressive therapy with thrombolytic agents, balloon dilation, or surgery should be considered.

In any patient in shock, especially in those with compromised cardiac function, consideration should be given to the institution of mechanical ventilation. The work of breathing can be considerable, especially for the patient in a state of agitation or distress or with decreased compliance. Oxygen needs are decreased through intubation and mechanical ventilation. In this manner, the patient can be comfortably sedated with a secure airway; the work of breathing is undertaken by the ventilator, and gas exchange can be optimized. If there is a tenuous balance between myocardial oxygen needs and availability, the balance can thus be shifted in the patient's favor.

Hypotension precludes the use of morphine sulfate and nitrates, drugs typically used in simple congestive failure to alleviate cardiac pain and ameliorate pulmonary vascular congestion. Likewise, β-blockers are often ideal for the treatment of ischemic heart disease because they effectively decrease heart rate and the inotropic state of the heart, but their use in cardiogenic shock is usually contraindicated, and decisions to continue their use must be carefully planned and monitored.

Systematic manipulation of preload, afterload, and contractility using information provided by the pulmonary artery catheter allows optimization of tenuous cardiac dynamics. Because an adequate preload is a fundamental determinant of cardiac function, attention to cardiac filling pressures should be a primary concern. A PCWP of 15 to 20 mmHg should be the initial goal and is achieved by manipulations of intravascular volume or capacitance or by increasing contractile activity. During cardiogenic shock, wedge pressure is not typically lower than 15 to 18 mmHg. Because of inadequate homeostatic responses, however, filling pressures may not be optimal, and a relative intravascular hypovolemia may exist. If it does, volume expansion should be judiciously accomplished through infusion of crystalloid, colloid, or blood products. Packed cells offer both volume expansion and an increased oxygen-carrying capacity. The latter is vitally important in critically ill patients.

Alternatively, if excessively elevated, the PCWP may be returned to more optimal levels with infusion of moderate doses of inotropic agents. Dobutamine increases contractility without dramatic increases in heart rate, and associated increases in cardiac output may be accompanied by decreases in wedge pressure. Dopamine, which offers more α-adrenergic activity, may be a more appropriate inotrope in situations of persistent hypotension. Diuretics decrease cardiac filling pressures and help to clear excess water and salt. Morphine or nitrates produce venodilation, which may exacerbate hypotension, but these may be judiciously employed in conjunction with pressor agents. Preload is manipulated with the intention of finding an optimal point on the Starling curve. This can be ascertained only by repetitive measurements of filling pressures and simultaneous determination of cardiac output after each intervention. The optimal PCWP varies and may be significantly higher than 15 to 18 mmHg in patients with a poorly compliant or "stiff" left ventricle, as can be seen in ischemic cardiomyopathy or in septic myocardial dysfunction.

Afterload reduction can prompt increases in cardiac output through decreases in the resistance to flow. The use of nitroprusside or other dilators requires relative blood pressure stability and close hemodynamic monitoring. Infusion of afterload-reducing agents can be administered in conjunction with inotropic support. Dopamine may be ideal by providing afterload reduction through dopaminergic splanchnic receptors, causing vasodilation and a decrease in SVR.

After correction of preexisting or relative hypovolemia, the mainstay of treatment of cardiogenic shock is inotropic support. The β-adrenergic agonists, dopamine and dobutamine, in moderate doses offer positive inotropic support without excess α-adrenergic activity. Ultralow doses of α-agents, such as norepinephrine, are used occasionally as a means to stimulate contractile function selectively through the α-receptor. Increasing the inotropic state of the heart shifts the entire Starling curve upward, resulting in increased cardiac output for each level of cardiac filling. It is important to note that these increases are accompanied by increases in myocardial oxygen consumption and therefore can exacerbate myocardial ischemia. The overall increase in oxygen consumption may incorrectly imply a flow-dependent state of perfusion and inadequate resuscitation.[129]

Patients with cardiogenic shock and an inadequate response to volume expansion and drug therapy can be supported for significant periods using intraaortic balloon counterpulsation (IABC). This is achieved by placing the counterpulsation balloon catheter in the descending thoracic aorta using a peripheral arterial approach.[130] Inflation of the balloon during diastole augments diastolic pressure and improves coronary perfusion; deflation during systole then provides some degree of afterload reduction. After myocardial infarction, use of the IABC pump in patients with cardiogenic shock has been shown to provide significant hemodynamic support. Objective findings include immediate and significant increases in cardiac index, stroke volume, and diastolic pressure—stroke work index. In 12 to 24 hours, significant decreases in PCWP and SVR are noted, and improved maintenance of systemic pressure occurs.[131] IABC is generally used as a means of temporary support for the patient in cardiogenic shock, either with the hope of recovering myocardial function or while preparations are made for other intervention.[132] Additional measures to consider in cases of refractory cardiogenic shock include placement of ventricular assist devices, urgent myocardial revascularization, correction of other anatomic cardiac defects, or even urgent cardiac transplantation.[133]

Compressive Cardiogenic Shock

Shock from cardiac compression occurs when external pressure on the heart impairs ventricular filling. Because ventricular filling is a function of venous return and myocardial compliance, any process that places pressure on the heart can cause compressive cardiogenic shock. Included among these are pericardial tamponade, tension pneumothorax, mediastinal hematoma, and positive pressure from mechanical ventilation. With compression, the heart and surrounding structures become less compliant. Although initially responsive to increased filling pressures, eventually, even in the face of high venous pressure, there is inadequate ventricular filling. The lesser degree of myocardial stretch also causes diminished myocardial contraction and a decreased stroke volume and cardiac output, resulting in hypotension and shock. Cardiac compression is accompanied by the adrenergic response and characteristic clinical manifestations typical of other forms of shock. Diagnosis of compressive cardiogenic shock can therefore be difficult, especially in trauma. With trauma, shock most commonly arises as a consequence of hypovolemia; however, if it is associated with distended neck veins, measures must be taken to exclude cardiac compression as the cause. The greatest diagnostic challenge occurs when both conditions are present simultaneously.

The diagnosis of hypotension due to compressive cardiogenic shock is made largely on clinical findings and the chest radiograph. Physical findings of tension pneumothorax include ipsilateral decreased breath sounds, tracheal deviation away from the affected thorax, and jugular venous distention. Radiographic findings are those of a pneumothorax with signs of *increased intrathoracic volume* in the affected hemithorax, including tracheal and mediastinal deviation to the contralateral side, splaying of the ipsilateral ribs, and depression of the diaphragm. Absence of those findings in the presence of pneumothorax *does not exclude* tension pneumothorax because pressure may affect the various structures differentially. All such patients require urgent chest decompression. Release of air with tube thoracotomy restores normal cardiovascular dynamics. If chest tube placement cannot be immediately accomplished, tension may be relieved by placement of a 14-gauge needle over the third rib in the midclavicular line. Creation of an open pneumothorax by making a defect in an interspace appropriate for subsequent chest tube placement relieves the hemodynamic abnormality while materials for tube thoracostomy are gathered. Standard 32F to 36F chest tubes should be used because smaller catheters may not be adequate.

The classic clinical findings of pericardial tamponade include the Beck triad of hypotension, neck vein distention, and muffled heart sounds. Pulsus paradoxus may also be noted (this involves a decrease rather than the normal increase of systolic blood pressure with inspiration; values of more than 10 mmHg are significant). These findings may be obscured in a noisy emergency room environment, by positive-pressure ventilation, or by associated injuries. Tachycardia and peripheral vasoconstriction are always present but are nonspecific signs. Placement of a CVP catheter confirms the elevation in right-sided filling pressure. If a pulmonary artery catheter has been placed, findings consistent with tamponade (or other forms of cardiac compression) are a trend toward equalization of chamber pressures as hypotension progresses. In the patient at risk, echocardiography is an extremely sensitive and noninvasive approach to demonstrate pericardial fluid and need for operation. In most circumstances, use of blind pericardiocentesis is of limited diagnostic value because of the likelihood of a direct ventricular stick causing a false-positive diagnosis; it may also cause significant iatrogenic injury. Likewise, the inability to withdraw clotted pericardial blood that has not lysed limits this technique to acute and urgent situations. In truly desperate situations in which tamponade is a concern but not yet clearly diagnosed, a subxiphoid or intraoperative pericardial window establishes the diagnosis and relieves tamponade. True pericardiocentesis occurs in only about 30% of patients with tamponade due to acute injury.

A diaphragmatic hernia can cause cardiac compression and also presents with neck vein distention and decreased breath sounds on the affected side. Diagnosis may be difficult. A chest radiograph may establish the diagnosis, demonstrating abdominal viscera or a radiopaque nasogastric tube within the chest. Alternatively, it may demonstrate only what appears to be elevation (eventration) of the hemidiaphragm or a pleural effusion. Peritoneal lavage fluid exiting through a chest tube establishes the diagnosis, as does palpation of a defect or intrathoracic position of abdominal organs during chest tube placement.

After trauma, hypotension associated with distended neck veins or a wound in proximity to the heart should be considered to be compressive cardiogenic shock until proved otherwise. Chest tube placement (or bilateral chest tube placement) is appropriate treatment to resolve a potential tension pneumothorax. Pericardial tamponade must be relieved, and cardiac injuries require emergent sternotomy. Traumatic diaphragmatic defects require operative repair to avoid cardiac compression and other complications.

Septic Shock

The clinical findings in sepsis and septic shock represent the host response to infection.[84,134] Gram-positive and gram-negative bacteria, viruses, fungi, rickettsiae, and protozoa have all been reported to produce the clinical picture of septic shock, but the overall response is independent of the specific type of invading organism.[133,135] Septic shock develops as a consequence of the combination of metabolic and circulatory derangements accompanying systemic infection. It appears that the circulatory deficits are preceded by the metabolic abnormalities induced by infection. In fact, the circulatory changes in hyperdynamic sepsis appear to be an adaptive response to the underlying metabolic dysfunction and represent cardiovascular excess rather than low-output failure.

A broad spectrum of clinical findings are found with infection and sepsis. Local responses include redness (rubor), warmth (calor), pain (dolor), and swelling (tumor). More generalized findings in sepsis may include fever, tachypnea, tachycardia, or end-organ dysfunction. The term *septic shock* implies hemodynamic instability in association with these findings.

The hemodynamic changes in septic shock consist of two fairly characteristic patterns, termed *early* and *late* septic shock.[136,137] It is more accurate and useful to designate the septic response as *hyperdynamic* or *hypodynamic*. Hyperdynamic, or "warm," septic shock is marked by peripheral vasodilation, increased cardiac output, and warm extremities. The hypodynamic response of "cold" septic shock is accompanied by inadequate cardiac output, peripheral vasoconstriction, mottling, and cool extremities. A hypodynamic response results from inadequate effective circulating blood volume and depressed cardiac function, which promotes a tissue perfusion deficit. Hypoperfusion then enhances the elaboration of additional inflammatory mediators initiated by products of infection. The subsequent inflammatory response causes further microvascular compromise, progression of shock, and secondary organ dysfunction. The principal target areas affected by the pathophysiologic process are the heart, the vascular endothelium, and the metabolic machinery of the peripheral tissues.[84] Progression from hyperdynamic to hypodynamic sepsis is frequently a preterminal event signaling collapse of adaptive homeostatic mechanisms.

Hyperdynamic Response

Cardiac output is high and SVR low in hyperdynamic septic shock. Splanchnic vasoconstriction is pronounced, however, even in the absence of systemic hypotension and even though SVR is reduced. Venous capacitance is increased and results in diminished effectiveness of the circulating blood volume. The associated compromise of ventricular filling results in a cardiac output that, although normal or increased, may still not be adequate at the tissue level. The microcirculation is relatively underperfused, and the splanchnic viscera appear particularly vulnerable in this setting. Expansion of the circulating blood volume can occur through either transcapillary refill or fluid resuscitation. Because of ongoing inflammatory mediator-induced increases in capillary permeability and continued loss of intravascular volume, exogenous volume resuscitation must be provided to restore venous return and ventricular filling.[84] After optimal blood volume expansion, cardiac output may be tremendously, but *appropriately*, increased. Adequate volume resuscitation without appropriate increases in cardiac output may indicate the presence of underlying cardiac disease, sepsis-induced myocardial depression, or the end stages of progressive shock.

In septic shock, oxygen consumption depends not only on the *needs* of the tissues for oxygen but also, to a significant degree, on the *ability* of the tissues to use oxygen. This stands in contrast to other forms of shock. In septic shock, oxygen consumption may be increased, normal, or decreased, depending on the metabolic state of the tissue. Often, the total oxygen consumption is increased—but not proportionately to the degree that cardiac output is increased.[84,138] Oxygen extraction is diminished relative to cardiac output because of inefficient extraction and metabolic dysfunction, and this results in an abnormally high mixed venous oxygen saturation and correspondingly low

arteriovenous oxygen difference.[139] In this setting, the central mixed venous oxygen saturation is a less effective means of monitoring adequate peripheral perfusion.

In situations of regional infection, as in the septic hind limb,[138] demonstrable increases in blood flow to the affected area account for only a portion of the total increase in cardiac output. The region of sepsis, however, does seem to command a disproportionate share of the augmented cardiac output. In addition, splanchnic and hepatic blood flow can be increased, even in the absence of intraabdominal infection.

Despite tremendous increases in cardiac output, severely ill septic patients frequently develop progressive metabolic and mitochondrial derangements. This would indicate either that the increases in cardiac output are not adequate to meet metabolic needs or, more likely, that the metabolic derangements are not a function of inadequate blood flow but rather of direct toxicity due to infectious agents and their by-products or the massive systemic inflammatory response of sepsis. It appears that metabolic dysfunction, with or without hypoperfusion, drives the persistence of the hyperdynamic septic state.

Hypodynamic Response

The patient with a hypodynamic response to sepsis presents with hypotension as a consequence of diminished cardiac output. The patient is usually tachycardiac, tachypneic, febrile, and diaphoretic. The extremities are cool, mottled, and often cyanotic. Oliguria or overt renal failure and hypothermia may develop. The patient may be confused, obtunded, or comatose. The physical findings are similar to those seen with end-stage hemorrhagic shock, although they occur with a much lesser degree of intravascular volume depletion. A significant compromise of ventricular function associated with sepsis-induced metabolic derangements may cause a decreased cardiac output, even with normal or elevated filling pressures. The leukocyte count may initially be misleading because severe sepsis can lead to a consumptive neutropenia; however, the differential count almost always demonstrates a marked left shift, with many immature granulocytes. Elevations of serum lactate may be dramatic, with or without associated acidosis.

The hypodynamic cardiovascular response to sepsis is a critical condition that develops as a result of a number of interrelated factors, including inadequate volume resuscitation, underlying cardiac disease, or myocardial dysfunction associated with sepsis. The hypodynamic response is a state of gross decompensation; therefore, the morbidity and mortality are much greater than in patients who are able to mount a hyperdynamic response. Emergent therapeutic measures are necessary to restore more normal cardiovascular dynamics and to offer a greater chance of survival.

Myocardial Dysfunction

Hemodynamic instability in sepsis, initially a consequence of relative hypovolemia and vasodilatory influences, may progress as a consequence of concomitant myocardial dysfunction. The significance of myocardial depression in well-resuscitated patients with a hyperdynamic response is controversial.[140,141] Gated cardiac scans at times have demonstrated normal or supranormal ventricular function in these patients. In hypodynamic septic shock, significant degrees of myocardial dysfunction develop.[142,143]

Despite manifestation of a hyperdynamic response, some patients with septic shock have significant reductions in contractile function and ejection fraction, in association with ventricular dilation, apparently a consequence of increased static diastolic compliance.[142] In this setting, stroke volume and cardiac output are generally preserved. The dilation may be compensatory because the increased ventricular filling and stretch allow a normal stroke volume to be maintained even though contractility is impaired. Starling dynamics are maintained, but the Starling curve is shifted downward. This depression in myocardial function appears to be independent of volume status, SVR, and coronary perfusion pressure.[84,143] The cardiac dysfunction is reversible with resolution of ventricular dilation and return of contractile function once sepsis resolves.[142] The primary myocardial depressive substance appears to be a water-soluble protein of low molecular weight.[32–34,144] Serum from septic patients with depressed ejection fraction caused depressed contractility in an in vitro myocardial cell preparation,[144] and once sepsis resolved, the in vitro depressive activity was no longer evident.

Reduced dynamic diastolic compliance can also become a major feature of septic myocardiopathy. The ventricle becomes stiff during diastole, with resultant requirement for increases in filling pressures and propensity for hydrostatic pulmonary edema, relative tachycardia, and, sometimes, limited global function. Myocardial depression and diastolic dysfunction have been demonstrated in patients with both hyperdynamic and hypodynamic septic responses. Although *not* typically implicated as the sole cause of the hypodynamic response to sepsis, myocardial depression and diastolic dysfunction may be a significant contributing factor, particularly in preterminal stages. Persistent absolute or relative hypovolemia or underlying cardiac disease, however, is more commonly the cause of the hypodynamic response.

Treatment

Whether septic shock presents with a hyperdynamic or a hypodynamic response, the measures taken to reverse the shock are based on similar principles of management. These therapeutic principles are restoration of tissue perfusion and oxygen delivery to a degree sufficient to meet metabolic demands; correction or control of the source of sepsis; and supportive care to ensure the optimal environment for maintaining functional reserves, healing, and recovery (Fig. 8-8).

In sepsis, resuscitation and restoration of nutrient flow to tissues is often most appropriately accomplished before embarking on a significant operation for source control. This differs from situations of hemorrhage or cardiac compression, in which immediate intervention is accomplished concurrently with resuscitation. In septic shock, priorities are shifted toward alleviation of the perfusion deficit and restoration of oxygen transport, avoiding the dangerous combination of sepsis and microcirculatory hypoperfusion. It appears that the propagation of shock and the development of postshock organ dysfunction arise as a consequence of increased activation of inflammatory cells and elaboration of mediators in areas of hypoperfusion. Restoration of perfusion may break the cycle of shock, inflammation, and further shock. Interventions then can be taken to manage the sepsis in a stable patient, with diminished risk of further deterioration and postshock sequelae. Surgical manipulations of infected or necrotic tissues may liberate bacteria, their toxins, and inflammatory mediators. When such manipulations are undertaken in an underresuscitated patient, hemodynamic deterioration can be dramatic and difficult to reverse. Interventions directed at source control, such as the administration of antibiotics, can be provided safely and concurrently with resuscitation and should not be delayed.

The initial therapy of septic shock includes volume resuscitation; placement of invasive monitoring lines (ie, Swan-Ganz catheter, an arterial line, and Foley catheterization to quantify urine output); and administration of antibiotics appropriate to the clinical situation. Attention should be given to the patient's respiratory status, with support provided as indicated. Laboratory studies of immediate concern include arterial blood gas determinations, serum electrolytes, BUN, creatinine, lactate, and complete blood count with differential. Blood, sputum, urine, and other cultures are obtained as appropriate. If the source of sepsis is obvious but would require major operation for control, this is deferred until the patient has been resuscitated. If the source is not obvious, additional diagnostic studies are undertaken, including lumbar puncture and CT scanning. Unusual sites, such as the facial sinuses, can also be a source of sepsis.

The general venodilation and vasodilation seen in sepsis may limit effective venous return and ventricular end-diastolic volume even if the true circulating blood volume is not depleted. To restore an *effective* circulating blood volume, aggressive fluid resuscitation is needed, similar to the patient who is hypovolemic from hemorrhage. Optimal end-diastolic volume and pressure to support a dysfunctional myocardium may require an *increase* in circulating blood volume. Resuscitation to a PCWP of 15 mmHg is a reasonable initial goal. This may be accomplished with isotonic crystalloid, colloid, or blood products. Further interventions may still be required to achieve hemodynamic stability and flow-independent oxygen consumption. If the hemoglobin level is less than 12 to 13 g/dL, oxygen transport may be optimally restored with red-cell transfusion. If septic shock is accompanied by a hypodynamic response, augmentation of cardiac output may require inotropic support, vasodilators, or a combination of the two. Instability may preclude the use of vasodilators, in which case further support is accomplished solely through the use of inotropic agents.

If operative intervention is required for control of the septic process, it is ideally undertaken once the hemodynamic status has been optimized. Control of the septic focus in conjunction with restoration of perfusion offers the greatest opportunity to avoid persistent hypermetabolism and MOFS.

Neurogenic Shock

Neurogenic shock results from interruption of sympathetic vasomotor input and develops after spinal cord injury, spinal anesthesia, and severe head injury. Under normal conditions, baseline sympathetic activity establishes a degree of arteriolar and venous constriction. Ablation of this tone results in decreased SVR and a dramatic increase in venous capacitance, causing hypotension due to the relative hypovolemia. Arteriolar dilation not only lowers the SVR but also allows previously unopened vascular beds to be perfused, greatly expanding venous capacitance. Removal of sympathetic inputs to innervated portions of the venous system allows further venodilation. The increase in venous capacitance decreases venous return and ventricular filling, causing cardiac output and blood pressure to decrease.

In most cases, the patient has fairly obvious signs of neurologic injury or spinal anesthesia is planned. Hypotension and tachycardia may be present, but the extremities are warm and appear well perfused. With high cervical lesions, a relative bradycardia inappropriate for the degree of hypotension is present. CVP, PCWP, stroke volume, and SVR are all decreased; cardiac output is typically decreased. Blood pressure is usually responsive to postural changes.

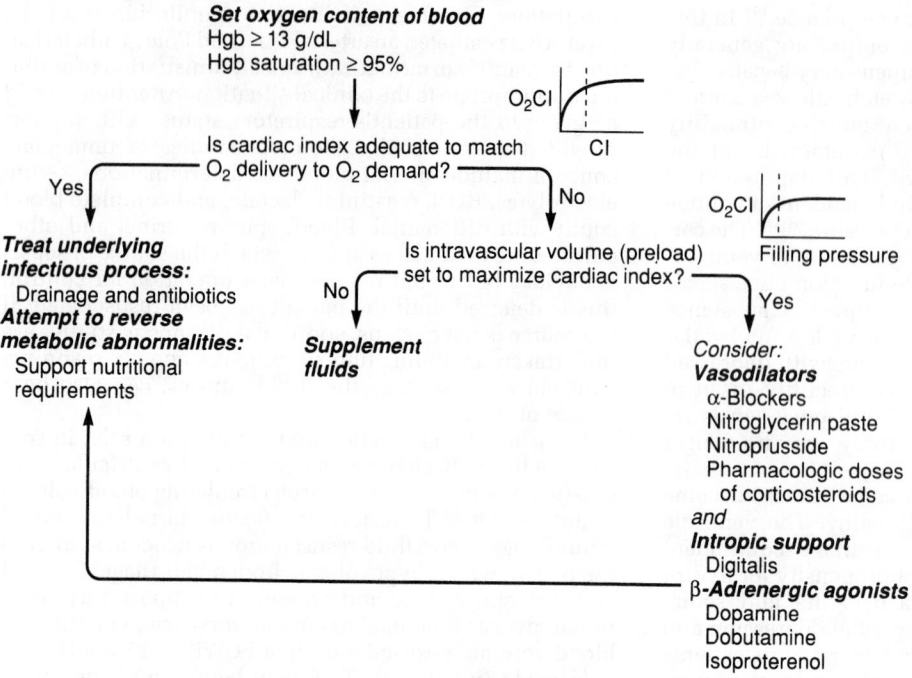

Figure 8-8. The basic algorithm for resuscitation. The goal is to match oxygen delivery with oxygen demand. The outcome variable is oxygen consumption; the managed variables are preload, afterload, and contractile function. (After Stahl TJ, Cerra FB. Hemodynamic and metabolic responses. In: Howard RJ, Simmons RL, eds. Surgical infectious diseases, ed 2. Norwalk, CT, Appleton & Lange, 1988:209)

Restoration of an effective, albeit expanded, intravascular volume may require extremely large volumes of resuscitation fluid to restore normal cardiac filling pressures. This restores cardiac output and, in most cases, reverses hypotension. Pharmacologic intervention with vasoactive agents may be necessary, however, and this is preferable to excessive volume resuscitation. Postshock sequelae are infrequent. Although there is significant hypotension with neurogenic shock, there is usually little if any hypoperfusion. Thus, activation of inflammatory cascades and subsequent organ injury rarely occurs. A major pitfall in the management of neurogenic shock arises when there is coexistent hemorrhage or ongoing volume loss that is not appreciated. This is not an unusual situation because cervical spine trauma causing paraplegia or severe head injury is frequently associated with multiple injuries. Thus, in trauma, the initial response to neurogenic shock is large volume resuscitation regardless of presumed cause. If hemodynamic instability persists after initial trauma resuscitation, the cause is probably not neurogenic, and occult blood loss or cardiogenic causes of shock should be explored. Severe brain injury causing acute loss of sympathetic tone is virtually nonsalvageable, and despite concerns regarding cerebral edema formation, volume administration is still appropriate initial therapy. After the acute phase, severe head injury may exacerbate hypovolemia through other mechanisms. Head injury and loss of ADH from the posterior pituitary can allow excessive urinary free water loss. Brain injury can also initiate or, more commonly, contribute to a generalized severe coagulopathy, leading to increased hemorrhage from multiple sites.

Hypoadrenal Shock

Shock of a dramatic nature that is poorly responsive to resuscitation can develop as a consequence of adrenal insufficiency. Clinically, this occurs most often when unknown or overlooked adrenal insufficiency complicates the course of another illness. Clinical deterioration, despite what would otherwise seem to be appropriate treatment,

is an important sign suggesting the diagnosis. In the United States, adrenal insufficiency most commonly arises as a consequence of the chronic therapeutic administration of high-dose exogenous corticosteroids, causing adrenal suppression. Other causes include idiopathic adrenal atrophy (Addison disease), tuberculosis, metastatic disease, bilateral hemorrhage, and amyloidosis. The stress of illness, operation, or trauma typically requires that the adrenal glands secrete cortisol in excess of that required in the nonstressed state (about three- to four-fold). Insufficiency not otherwise clinically apparent may manifest only after major physical stress.

Findings associated with adrenal insufficiency include weakness, fatigue, anorexia, abdominal pain, nausea, vomiting, and weight loss. In Addison disease, there may be hyperpigmentation of the skin and mucous membranes. Hyponatremia, hypochloremia, and hyperkalemia are consistent with decreased mineralocorticoid activity. Adrenal insufficiency may also present acutely as fever, hypotension, and an acute abdomen.

Surgical patients with significant adrenal insufficiency need not present with these findings. More typical is the development of refractory shock, frequently with hyperthermia, in the course of injury or illness. Hypotension can be dramatic despite massive volume resuscitation and pressor support. There may be no findings suggestive of the diagnosis other than the failure to respond to appropriate therapy. Anytime tht shock does not respond to appropriate therapeutic measures, the diagnosis should be reconsidered.

The diagnosis of adrenal insufficiency may be confirmed or excluded by means of an ACTH stimulation test. A significant measurable cortisol response should be elicited by ACTH administration. Confirming the diagnosis does not impede therapy, and dexamethasone may be given if exogenous corticosteroids are necessary during the time that the test is administered.

Successful therapy of an Addisonian crisis often requires significant cardiovascular support as well as stress doses of corticosteroids. Hydrocortisone, 100 mg every 6 to 8 hours, is given with a rapid taper to maintenance level.

Volume resuscitation and pressor support may be required for hours to days after therapy is initiated. Monitoring with a pulmonary artery catheter should be maintained until the hemodynamic instability resolves. Concurrently, the precipitating illness should be treated.

ADJUNCTIVE MEASURES IN THE THERAPY OF SHOCK

Inotropic Agents

Therapeutic adjustments of intravascular volume (preload) and SVR (afterload) form the basis of treatment strategies in all forms of shock. Optimal volume resuscitation should precede measures to augment the contractile function of the heart. Inotropic agents are used in shock when there is an inadequate cardiac output despite an adequate circulating blood volume.[145] Inotropic support is also indicated in situations of persistent shock and when, despite apparent hemodynamic stability, there remains evidence of a perfusion deficit (flow-dependent oxygen consumption, persistent elevation of serum lactate, or an elevated lactate/pyruvate ratio). Clinical evidence of end-organ dysfunction may also imply inadequate perfusion. Both catecholamine and noncatecholamine inotropic agents are used clinically, and the agents differ in their degree of α and β activity, chronotropic effects, and influence on myocardial oxygen consumption.

Dopamine

Dopamine is an endogenous sympathetic amine that is a biosynthetic precursor of epinephrine and functions as a central and peripheral neurotransmitter. At low doses (less than 2 to 3 μg/kg/min), stimulation of dopaminergic receptors produces renal arteriolar vasodilation with associated increases in renal blood flow, urine output, and sodium excretion. Because the splanchnic vasculature also contains dopaminergic receptors, low-dose dopamine may also enhance intestinal perfusion, reverse gut ischemia, and protect against mucosal barrier dysfunction. At moderate doses (5 μg/kg/min), stimulation of cardiac β-receptors produces increases in contractility and cardiac output with little effect on heart rate or blood pressure. With increasing doses (5 to 10 μg/kg/min), β-adrenergic effects still predominate, but further increases in cardiac output are accompanied by increases in heart rate and blood pressure. At higher doses (above 10 μg/kg/min), peripheral vasoconstriction from increasing α activity becomes more pronounced, prompting significant increases in vascular resistance and blood pressure. The relative degree of α, β, and dopaminergic activity evoked for a given dose varies among patients.

Dobutamine

Dobutamine is a synthetic catecholamine that has been used for its β-adrenergic effects and the absence of significant α activity. The predominant effect at infusion rates of 5 to 15 μg/kg/min is an increase in cardiac contractility with lesser increases in heart rate. Some reduction in peripheral vascular resistance may also occur. Improved cardiac function contributes to lowering ventricular filling and PCWP. When compared with dopamine, dobutamine produces less peripheral vasoconstriction and a diminished chronotropic response. Peripheral vasodilation may occur. As a consequence, dobutamine is ideally used in situations in which the therapeutic goal is augmentation of cardiac output without significant increase in blood pressure and potential mild afterload reduction.

Epinephrine

Epinephrine, the endogenous adrenal catecholamine, is released physiologically in response to stress. It has a broad spectrum of systemic actions, including significant cardiovascular effects. Pharmacologically, β-adrenergic responses predominate at lower rates of infusion (0.01 to 0.05 μg/kg/min). An increase in heart rate and contractility (β_1) in conjunction with peripheral vasodilation (β_2) produces a net increase in stroke volume and cardiac output, with a variable blood pressure response. At a higher rate of infusion, there is increasing α-mediated activity. SVR and blood pressure increase with incremental but variable change in cardiac output. Limitations of the use of epinephrine arise from its renal vasoconstrictive activity, its arrhythmogenic potential, and its substantial contribution to increasing myocardial oxygen demands. As a consequence of the presence of underlying cardiovascular disease, these limitations are of greater concern in adults than in children. In fact, epinephrine remains the inotrope of choice in the acute resuscitation of children.[146]

Norepinephrine

Norepinephrine, the sympathetic neurotransmitter, also exerts both α- and β-adrenergic effects; the β-adrenergic effects are evident at lower infusion rates, whereas the α-mediated effects are more prominent at higher doses. At lower rates of infusion, increases in heart rate and contractility are evident; with increasing α-mediated vasoconstriction, the increases in systemic resistance and blood pressure may blunt the initial chronotropic response through baroreceptor reflexes. Norepinephrine is used mainly in patients with hypotension that persists despite appropriate volume resuscitation and the use of other inotropic agents. Renal and mesenteric vasoconstrictive effects of norepinephrine complicate its use in shock, especially when support is needed for significant periods of time. Some evidence suggests that when low-dose dopamine is used in conjunction with norepinephrine, compromise of renal blood flow may be lessened.

Isoproterenol

Isoproterenol is a synthetic catecholamine with potent β-adrenergic effects. From a cardiovascular standpoint, both cardiac and peripheral effects are significant. Stimulation of cardiac β_1-receptors prompts an increase in contractility, heart rate, and conduction velocity. The chronotropic response, however, may predominate. These activities, in conjunction with peripheral vasodilation predominantly due to smooth muscle relaxation in skeletal muscle beds, from β_2-stimulation, generate significant increases in cardiac output and pulse pressure. With isoproterenol, myocardial oxygen demand is increased, and diastolic coronary filling is limited by tachycardia or diminished diastolic pressure. Tachyarrhythmias may also develop. Indications for the use of isoproterenol are limited because agents with fewer adverse effects have become available. It is still useful as a temporizing measure in patients with hemodynamically significant bradyarrhythmias while preparations are made for electrical pacing.

Amrinone

Amrinone, a noncatecholamine inotrope, has no adrenergic activity. Its actions result in part from phosphodiesterase inhibition as well as from alterations in cellular calcium fluxes. There are induced increases in cardiac contractility, stroke volume, heart rate, and cardiac output. Increased cyclic adenosine monophosphate concentration in vascular smooth muscle prompts vasodilation and therefore decreases systemic resistance. Blood pressure is usually unchanged at low rates of infusion. Higher rates of infusion or bolus treatment may evoke further potentially detrimental vasodilation, with less cardiac effect. In general, the increases in cardiac contractility in conjunction with a relative afterload reduction produce significant increases in cardiac output, often without increases in myocardial oxygen consumption. These considerations make amrinone attractive in the treatment of cardiogenic shock. Drawbacks to the use of amrinone are the variability of individual response, its relatively long half-life (3.6 hours), and the potential for significant hypotension.

Vasodilators

Vasodilators are used as a means to augment cardiac function through optimization of ventricular filling pressures (preload) and SVR (afterload), both of which reduce demands on the myocardium.[147]

The *failing ventricle* responds to afterload reduction with significant increases in stroke volume. The reason for this is that the compromised myocardium is working past the plateau and on the down slope of the Starling curve. Changes in ventricular filling therefore offer little compensation. It follows that increases in afterload in the compromised myocardium are accompanied by reductions in stroke volume and pressure. In these patients, afterload reduction with vasodilator agents may allow cardiac output to increase. As increases in cardiac output accompany the fall in SVR, the net decrease in blood pressure is limited.

Vasodilators vary in their relative effects on the arterial and venous systems. Venodilation, with associated increases in venous capacitance, lowers ventricular end-diastolic pressure. This decreases the pressure-related contributions to pulmonary edema. Such decreases in preload, when on the plateau of the Starling curve, do not limit cardiac output. With further decreases of left ventricular end-diastolic pressure, generally to below 15 mmHg, decreased cardiac output and instability can develop.

Nitroprusside

Nitroprusside is a balanced vasodilator that acts directly on arterial and venous smooth muscle. The subsequent relaxation is independent of adrenergic effects. Decreases in afterload prompt increases in cardiac output, and venodilation contributes to decreases in both pulmonary venous pressure and CVP. Nitroprusside is potent and has an immediate onset and a duration of action of 1 to 3 minutes. Administration is therefore by constant infusion with adjustments as indicated. Hypotension may develop, particularly in patients with inadequate preload. Although cardiac output is typically stable or improved with nitroprusside therapy, it may fall in patients with inadequate ventricular filling. In patients with compromised cardiac function, its use requires constant monitoring of arterial pressure and repeated hemodynamic measurements with a pulmonary artery catheter. As adjustments are made, hemodynamic effects are followed with serial measurements of systemic pressure, pulmonary artery pressures, PCWP, and cardiac output. Thiocyanate and cyanide toxicity may arise as a consequence of the presence of cyanide within the molecular structure of nitroprusside, especially when infusions of more than 3 μg/kg/min are continued for more than 72 hours. Monitoring of blood thiocyanate levels and surveillance for metabolic acidosis aid in avoiding toxicity.

Nitroglycerin

Nitroglycerin and related organic nitrates cause venodilation and some arterial vasodilation through direct action on vascular smooth muscle. In contrast to nitroprusside,

their effects are predominantly on the venous circulation. Their efficacy in the treatment of angina pectoris is based on mechanisms that both directly and indirectly affect the balance of myocardial oxygen supply and demand. Reduction of ventricular end-diastolic volume after venodilation allows decreased ventricular wall tension and decreased ventricular end-diastolic pressure with a corresponding decrease in myocardial oxygen demand. Reductions in end-diastolic pressure also allow improved subendocardial blood flow and myocardial oxygen delivery. These factors, in conjunction with a modest direct influence on coronary flow, restore a more favorable balance of myocardial supply and demand.

The use of nitroglycerin in cardiogenic and other forms of shock relies in part on these mechanisms. A primary concern when nitroglycerin is used in this manner is the avoidance of a compromise of cardiac function that can arise through undue reductions of preload. Serial hemodynamic measurements using a pulmonary artery catheter allow appropriate adjustments of preload as reductions in systemic resistance are achieved. The arterial vasodilatory effects of nitroglycerin, although less dramatic than those of nitroprusside, do allow afterload reduction.[148] A significant vasodilatory response is usually seen at an infusion rate of 1 to 2 μg/kg/min.

Captopril

Captopril is an oral angiotensin-converting enzyme inhibitor and provides some degree of afterload reduction, especially in patients who may have inappropriately high levels of angiotensin II. Captopril has an onset of action of 30 minutes, with peak effect at 1 to 3 hours.

Trendelenburg Position

Positioning of the patient has been thought to be an adjunct in the treatment of hypovolemic shock. Most recommendations are for the patient to be placed in the Trendelenburg position without flexion at the knees as originally described. The intent is to autotransfuse pooled blood from the capacitance or venous side to the central circulation, thus raising the central venous filling pressures and simultaneously increasing the arterial pressure by raising SVR. Although it is true that some forms of shock, particularly neurogenic shock, respond to the head-down position, the effect on cerebral perfusion has not been clearly defined. More importantly, placing the patient in Trendelenburg position increases the risk of aspiration of gastric contents and interferes with respiratory exchange due to abdominal contents putting increased upward pressure on the diaphragms. Investigations in normal volemic and hypovolemic patients also showed that the use of Trendelenburg position has an inconsistent effect on venous return and SVR. The purported beneficial effects can be easily obtained by elevating both legs while maintaining the trunk and the remainder of the patient in the supine position.[149,150]

Pneumatic Antishock Garment

The PASG has been widely used in the prehospital setting as a means of providing temporary support of the central hemodynamics of patients in shock. The PASG, or military antishock trousers, is an inflatable external compression device that can be wrapped around the legs and abdomen in the form of trousers. The three compartments (one abdominal and one for each lower extremity) can be inflated independently, which compresses vascular structures in the legs and abdomen.[151]

Increases in blood pressure seen with application of

PASG were in the past ascribed to the displacement of blood from capacitance vessels of the lower body toward the heart. Although the inflation pressures transmitted to the lower body do provide an increased driving pressure for venous return, they also produce narrowing of large veins, with increased resistance to flow. The net effect on venous structures is compression without significant increase in venous return.[47,152]

The inflated PASG also produces a significant increase in arterial resistance through mechanical compression of arteries encompassed by the suit.[153] Blood pressure increases as a consequence of the resistance to arterial flow in the lower body, resulting in an overall increase in SVR but no significant change in cardiac output.[154] The maintenance of central blood pressure at the expense of flow limitation to the lower body mimics to some degree the selective vasoconstriction seen in hypovolemic shock.

Use of PASG has been recommended in noncardiogenic forms of shock, when there is a systolic blood pressure of less than 80 mmHg, or in the presence of constitutional signs of shock, with a blood pressure of less than 100 mmHg. The most appropriate use of PASG, however, appears to be as a means to tamponade bleeding and augment hemostasis. Inflation of the suit provides splinting of complex fractures of the pelvis and lower extremities, similar to other air splints. The utility of PASG in arresting hemorrhage from pelvic fractures arises from a combination of fracture stabilization and tamponade.

Complications and the adverse effects of PASG arise from the effects of pressure applied to the viscera and body compartments. Increased intraabdominal pressure can cause limitation of ventilation and respiratory embarrassment. The PASG also compounds the hypotensive effects of cardiac compression from pericardial tamponade or tension pneumothorax, and severe cardiac compression may arise from use of PASG in patients with diaphragmatic rupture. In other circumstances, dangerous elevation of intracranial pressure may occur if there is associated head injury. Also, muscular compartment syndromes have developed after prolonged application as external pressure is transmitted to the musculature of the legs.

Use of PASG is contraindicated in compressive cardiogenic shock, and use of the abdominal compartment is contraindicated in pregnancy, esophageal variceal bleeding, diaphragmatic herniation, and evisceration. If PASG has been used, care must be taken as the garment is deflated. Sequential deflation of the compartments, beginning with the abdominal, should be undertaken. Ongoing volume resuscitation may be required because further instability can arise from the relatively sudden afterload reduction as well as from the consequences of reperfusion (hyperlactatemia, acidosis, and the elaboration of vasoactive mediators).

The appropriate use of PASG is not entirely clear. Military and initial civilian clinical studies suggested that it could be safely used to support temporarily the unstable trauma patient in the prehospital setting. A subsequent study of PASG in shock after trauma, however, demonstrated no specific advantage in improving survival, reducing morbidity, or decreasing costs.[155] In the urban environment, with in-field volume resuscitation and short transport times, use of PASG appears unwarranted. The use of PASG as a splint for pelvic and lower extremity fractures, however, does appear to have merit.

Hypothermia and Rewarming

A potential adverse consequence of massive volume resuscitation to reverse shock is hypothermia.[156] The use of refrigerated bank blood and room-temperature crystalloid solutions rapidly drops core temperatures if caution is not exercised to run all solutions through warming devices, such as the Level-One counter-current warmer. The consequences of hypothermia are numerous. During resuscitation, however, there are two critical issues. First, the detrimental impact of hypothermia on cardiac contractility can further impair cardiac output and oxygen delivery. Second, hypothermia directly impairs the enzymatic steps of the coagulation pathway, producing a significant coagulopathy. These effects can be prominent at temperatures below 35°C. Because coagulation assays are routinely performed after warming blood samples to 37°C, the clinical impact of the patient's hypothermia is often underestimated by routine testing. In fact, coagulation assays that appear normal at 37°C are significantly prolonged and clinically important when performed at the core body temperature of the hypothermic patient.[157] Rapid rewarming produces a significant decrease in the requirement for blood products and an improvement in cardiac function and survival in hypovolemic, hypothermic patients.[158,159] The most efficacious method for rewarming is extracorporeal counter-current warmers through femoral artery and vein cannulation. This process does not require a pump and rapidly rewarms from 30°C to 36°C in less than 30 minutes.

Caution must be expressed regarding the timing of the rewarming. Studies showing an improvement in outcome have all been performed after control of surgical bleeding and restoration of perfusion.[158,159] As is known from transplantation experiences, cooling of tissues during hypoperfusion significantly protects and enhances subsequent function. During resuscitation, ischemia–reperfusion injury occurs, in large part, from adherence of activated neutrophils. Reducing the core temperature reduces neutrophil activation and adherence and may protect against reperfusion injury. Normothermia during reperfusion optimizes neutrophil function, which allows massive microvascular injury, capillary leak, and interstitial edema, leading to compartment syndromes and other organ dysfunction. The focus on the abdominal compartment syndrome may in part be attributable to the maintenance of a normal core temperature during massive fluid resuscitation of severe hypovolemic states.[160] Further investigation is required to identify the ideal rate and sequence of rewarming. A relative hypothermic condition during hypoperfusion and resuscitation that avoids severe coagulopathy and cardiac depression and is subsequently followed by rapid restoration of normothermia may provide optimal protection against reperfusion injury and preservation of organ function.

Supranormal Resuscitation

Resuscitation to supranormal physiologic endpoints has been advocated for hypovolemic patients after noting improved survival among patients with higher values for cardiac index and oxygen delivery. The best survival occurred in patients that achieved hemodynamic parameters well above the standard values used as goals during resuscitation. Increased survival among those achieving greater than normal physiologic endpoints supports the concept that hypovolemic shock has induced an "oxygen debt" through deprivation of oxygen to the tissues. Resuscitation to supranormal endpoints and a hyperdynamic cardiovascular response is thought to replete this oxygen debt and prevent organ dysfunction. Cardiac index values greater than 4.5 L/min/m^2, oxygen delivery greater than 600 to 650 L/min/m^2, and an oxygen consumption of at least 170 L/min/m^2 are proposed as the endpoint parameters necessary to achieve enhanced survival and optimal organ function.[161–165] In these preliminary studies, however, patients in the aggressive resuscitation treatment arm rarely achieved supranormal endpoints and yet had significantly improved outcomes. In addition, patients undergoing standard resuscitation who spontaneously achieved supranormal values had the lowest mortality rates. Several large prospective trials have been unable to confirm the protective effect of trying to reach supranormal resuscitation endpoints, and there may be adverse effects.[165-170] Inotropes increase cardiac output and allow supranormal oxygen delivery, but use of these agents to increase oxygen delivery is accompanied by an increase in oxygen consumption, which is derived from an increase in cardiac work and metabolic rate. The increase in use more than offsets the increase in oxygen delivery.

The ability to reach supranormal hemodynamic levels spontaneously in response to the significant stress and metabolic derangements of severe shock may have prognostic value, but this approach appears not to improve survival, decrease organ dysfunction, nor shorten length of stay in the intensive care unit. In addition, it may be detrimental to outcome, particularly with excessive use of inotropes, because of their concomitant risk for cardiac morbidity. Supranormal oxygen delivery is not better than adequate oxygen delivery in patients who are fully resuscitated. There is potential danger in trying to drive poor responders beyond physiologic capabilities. Hypovolemic patients who have adequate volume replacement and sufficient reperfusion to reach normal hemodynamic levels do not benefit from the use of inotropes solely to reach supranormal target values.[129,169]

COMPLICATIONS OF SHOCK

Ischemia–Reperfusion Injury

Homeostatic responses to shock divert blood from nonvital tissue beds to preserve oxygen delivery to critical organs, such as the myocardium and brain. As a consequence, there is significant hypoperfusion and hypoxia in large vascular beds, such as the skin, subcutaneous tissue, skeletal muscle, and splanchnic bed. The patient who undergoes inadequate volume resuscitation may have unrecognized ongoing hypoperfusion of these tissues even though apparently normal cardiovascular dynamics have been restored. During these episodes of hypoperfusion, there is a direct ischemic insult, which varies dependent on the metabolic activity of the tissue. As resuscitation and restoration of microvascular perfusion occurs, a diffuse reperfusion injury develops.

During periods of hypovolemia and reduced microvascular flow, there is an increased transit time, sludging, and initiation of microvascular thrombosis, producing subclinical disseminated intravascular coagulopathy. Thrombin and other enzymes provide potent stimuli for induction of the proinflammatory phenotype of endothelial cells and activation inflammatory cells, such as macrophages and neutrophils. As the coagulolytic pathways are activated to restore perfusion, recurring cycles of ischemia, reperfusion, and capillary injury occur throughout the microvasculature of the hypoperfused tissues.

During the ischemia and hypoperfusion phase, degradation of ATP stores essential to maintain cell integrity and significant loss of diffusible intracellular adenine nucleotides occur. As ATP further degrades, there is an elevation in plasma and intracellular levels of hypoxanthine and xanthine, which on restoration of perfusion, reoxygenation, and catalyzation by xanthine oxidase, results in the formation of the superoxide radical.[171] Other ROIs, such as hydrogen peroxide and hydroxyl radical, are generated and lead to endothelial and parenchymal cell injury through membrane lipid peroxidation and inactivation of critical enzymes.[172] ROIs have also been shown to be involved in expression of the proinflammatory phenotype on endothelial cells and on macrophages, neutrophils, and other inflammatory cells.[173]

The proinflammatory phenotype of the endothelium includes increased procoagulant activity and expression of adhesion molecules on the membrane surface, including intercellular adhesion molecule 1 (ICAM-1) and the selectins E-selectin and P-selectin. Simultaneously, the activated neutrophil up-regulates the potent adhesive complex, CD-11/18. The subsequent adhesion of activated neutrophils to the endothelium leads to an explosive oxidative burst, producing additional ROIs, and to extensive release of proteolytic enzymes, leading to injury and disruption of the endothelial lining, extensive capillary leak, and massive interstitial edema.

Passive immunization of animals with monoclonal antibodies to either the neutrophil adhesive complex or to endothelial selectins dramatically lessens ischemia–reperfusion microvascular injury. Blood loss and ischemic tissue-flap models both demonstrate significant reductions in the volume of fluid required for resuscitation, lesser adherence of neutrophils during reperfusion, and diminished postresuscitation edema. Evidence of endothelial and parenchymal cell injury is reduced.

Abdominal Compartment Syndrome

Abdominal compartment syndrome is a highly morbid complication of reperfusion injury to the splanchnic viscera. The syndrome appears to be increasingly prominent due to aggressive resuscitation techniques that allow salvage of profoundly hypotensive and hypovolemic patients. In the past, such patients would have died. At present, after resuscitation, they experience extensive reperfusion injury with extensive capillary leak and massive interstitial edema. The loss of resuscitation fluid into the interstitium of the abdominal viscera produces effects similar to other compartment syndromes. The massive swelling of intraabdominal organs, in particular the intestines, compromises microvascular perfusion, impairs organ function, and significantly elevates intraabdominal pressures. The increased intraabdominal pressure elevates the diaphragm and, in combination with the simultaneous microvascular injury to the pulmonary vasculature, causes a marked impairment in gas exchange and significant compromise of ventilation. If adequate oxygenation and ventilation cannot be accomplished, decompressive celiotomy, leaving the abdomen open and covered with Silastic or other artificial covering, is required. With improved diaphragmatic excursion, a dramatic decrease in pulmonary ventilatory pressures and a marked improvement in oxygenation occur.

Immune Suppression

Resuscitation from shock has a significant impact on the subsequent immune response of the host. At least a portion of this effect may be due to blood transfusions. Their specific effect on the immune system has not been fully defined and has been debated for decades. In both the transplantation and oncology literature, however, an immunosuppressive effect of blood transfusion and a decreased host responsiveness are apparent. The quantity of blood transfused may simply be a marker for the severity of injury.

The immunosuppression after shock resuscitation is thought to contribute to the enhanced risk for nosocomial infections. Loss of major histocompatibility complex on antigen-presenting cells (monocytes), along with decreased production of IL-2 and altered lymphocyte function, persists for several weeks after major trauma and resuscitation.[107,174] A similar defect has been shown after major burn injury and hypovolemia. In experimental models, shock and resuscitation are followed by a prolonged period of altered lymphocyte function and an increased susceptibility to infection. Production of interferon-γ (IFN-γ), a major immunomodulator, is depressed after shock and gradually returns to normal as immunosuppression resolves.[175] Repletion of IFN-γ reverses shock-induced macrophage and lymphocyte immunosuppression in animal models.[175,176] A clinical trial of IFN-γ therapy after major trauma did not significantly reduce infectious complications but did improve sepsis-related mortality.[177]

A major cause of immunosuppression appears to be prolonged and excessive production of immunosuppressive agents, such as PGE_2 and IL-10, by the tissue-fixed macrophage.[178] Release of these antiinflammatory agents as endocrine, paracrine, and autocrine effectors to down-regulate and control the inflammatory response is appropriate, but prolonged and excessive production after severe shock states induces a maladaptive immunosuppressed condition.

Multiple Organ Failure Syndrome

Advances in resuscitation during the past three decades have made survival from previously fatal conditions common. Patients who survive experience complications not previously recognized, including ARDS and MOFS. ARDS can occur in relative isolation but is often a prelude to full-blown MOFS. The latter can develop after a variety of insults, including hemorrhage, sepsis, trauma, ischemia, and reperfusion. Alternatively, there may not be a well-identified precipitating cause, or combinations of processes may contribute to MOFS. Shock in combination with a significant inflammatory response (ie, SIRS) is a particularly high risk for MOFS development. In clinical practice, the process is usually multifactorial.

Shock and massive blood transfusion are major risk factors for the development of ARDS and MOFS. The transfusion of multiple units of banked blood leads to the filtration of microparticulates by the pulmonary microvasculature. These microparticles are not removed by blood filters, and they contribute to diffuse microvascular thrombosis and the resultant ischemia and reperfusion sequences underlying ARDS. Successful resuscitation from severe shock drives the excessive inflammatory response underlying MOFS and ARDS and induces an immunosuppressed state with subsequent risk for infectious complications.

The initial concern that shock lung was a consequence of excessive volume resuscitation gave way as the noncardiogenic nature of ARDS became apparent. It is now known that ARDS is part of SIRS, a nondiscriminating systemic injury response.[179,180] Strictly speaking, SIRS refers to signs and symptoms of systemic inflammation in the absence of infection. In actual clinical practice, the presence or absence of infection is not always obvious, and the clinical manifestations are the same. As a consequence of this diffuse autodestructive process, there is coincident or sequential failure of the lungs, kidneys, and liver, occurring simultaneously or sequentially after trauma, sepsis, or shock.[181] Instead of being the consequence of excessive resuscitation, SIRS and the resultant ARDS or MOFS are the consequence of prolonged hypoperfusion and subsequent activation of multiple inflammatory mediators. This process is similar to the way in which other, long recognized conditions, such as ischemic and necrotic tissue and primary or nosocomial infections,

can drive the inflammatory mediator systems. The various forms of shock tend to blend and become difficult to distinguish from one another, especially in the postresuscitation period. Despite seemingly appropriate resuscitation and correction of the process precipitating shock, gross metabolic and physiologic dysfunction may persist and progress.

The nature of MOFS is that of a diffuse cellular injury, developing *systemically* as a consequence of losing homeostatic control of *local* inflammation and microcirculatory hypoperfusion. Endothelial injury, platelet aggregation, and activation of macrophages and neutrophils occur, and the clotting, fibrinolytic, kinin, and complement cascades are activated along with release of potent inflammatory cytokines, such as granulocyte-macrophage colony-stimulating factor, TNF, IL-1, IL-6, IL-8, and PAF. All of these processes have been implicated in the systemic inflammatory response contributing to the diffuse organ injury of MOFS.[3] Reperfusion of areas of arrested or compromised microcirculatory flow contribute further to local and systemic inflammation through the generation of ROIs and the secondary activation of inflammatory cells and mediators. These products and cellular debris from locally injured tissue are released into the general circulation. Although they are recognized as having important roles in the progression of shock and the development of MOFS, the specific role that each plays has not been fully elucidated.

The effects of shock, resuscitation, and reperfusion and the subsequent development of MOFS appear to depend on changes in the splanchnic and pulmonary microcirculations. These vascular beds appear to be major sites of the activation and subsequent immunoinflammatory mediator production that underlies the diffuse systemic inflammatory response of SIRS. As splanchnic microcirculatory flow decreases in response to homeostatic vasoconstrictive responses during hypovolemia, excessive and prolonged hypoperfusion of the gut results in extensive microvascular injury and subsequent activation of endothelium, neutrophils, and macrophages. In addition, mucosal barrier disruption permits translocation of bacteria and bacterial toxins, such as endotoxins, to circulate and reach the large tissue-fixed macrophage population in the liver (Kupffer cells). Extensive activation of the Kupffer cells and release of inflammatory mediators, coupled with the ongoing release of activated neutrophils and by-products of activated gut macrophages, then cause injury to the pulmonary microcirculation and secondary induction of the alveolar macrophage and additional inflammatory mediator systems. These inflammatory mediators released from the pulmonary circulation induce the systemic inflammation seen in SIRS that underlies MOFS. The widespread activation of inflammatory mediator systems causes diffuse endothelial and parenchymal cell injury and ultimately organ dysfunction and failure.

Excessive and persistent macrophage activation plays a central role in SIRS and MOFS and is hypothesized to represent the penultimate step in a series of continuous immunoinflammatory stimulating events, including local hypoxia, exposure to bacteria and toxins, and mediator release from localized areas of inflammation.[181] Endotoxins (lipopolysaccharides) and other inflammatory stimuli provoke and activate the macrophage to release a number of potentially injurious central inflammatory mediators, including TNF, PAF, IL-1, IL-8, and IL-6. These secondary mediators modulate many of the detrimental effects seen in experimental conditions that mimic clinical sepsis, SIRS, and MOFS.[182] As hepatic macrophages or Kupffer cells remove bacteria, toxins, and other products of inflammation from the splanchnic circulation, they become activated, which leads to the release of multiple mediator substances that directly affect adjacent hepatocyte function. Using in vitro co-culture techniques, activated Kupffer cells induce alterations in hepatocyte protein synthesis rates, decreasing rates of albumin synthesis and increasing the production of acute-phase proteins. These cell–cell interactions appear bidirectional; the presence of hepatocytes enhances Kupffer cell production of IL-1, TNF, nitric oxide, and other mediators. Thus, the Kupffer cell—hepatocyte interaction modulates liver function. Tissue-fixed macrophage—parenchymal cell interactions in the lung, kidney, and other organs affected by SIRS lead to similar organ dysfunction and subsequent development of MOFS.[16]

When infection is the underlying process or a major contributing process, the diffuse inflammatory response develops independent of the specific type of microorganism. In noninfectious cases, the response also appears independent of the specific underlying cause. The excessive immunoinflammatory response may resolve relatively quickly, persist for long periods, or progress to multiple organ failure. Once initiated, the systemic response follows a predictable time course. After the initial insult and resuscitation, there is a 48- to 72-hour period of relative stability. During this time, the inflammatory response is initiated. Although the exact degree and the precise time of onset vary, this response typically peaks in 3 to 4 days and resolves within 9 to 14 days. Resolution generally requires that resuscitation and support have been adequate, that there is no significant ongoing perfusion deficit, that the inciting event has been eliminated, and that no second-hit intervening events (such as nosocomial infection) occur. If the inflammatory state or SIRS does not resolve, it is usually because a complication has occurred, an ongoing perfusion deficit remains, or the underlying source has not been controlled. Intercurrent infection, most commonly pulmonary, is the most common complication. If the cause of the persistent inflammatory state can be found and corrected, recovery may then occur. If the source cannot be controlled or further complications develop, a phase of persistent systemic inflammation is entered, from which multiple organ failure can develop. The persistent inflammatory phase is associated with a mortality rate of at least 25% to 40%. In general, patients who will recover show evidence of recovery within 2 weeks of injury. If SIRS persists for more than 7 to 10 days, organ failure and mortality rates rise, and dysfunction of virtually all organ systems develops.

Hemodynamic consequences of SIRS and the multiple inflammatory mediators include increased cardiac index, decreased SVR, hyperglycemia, hyperlactatemia, elevated oxygen consumption index, and elevated urine urea nitrogen excretion.

Pulmonary dysfunction typically arises early in the development of systemic inflammation; it may represent mild, localized ALI or be the prelude to fulminant ARDS. Decreased compliance in conjunction with increases in oxygen consumption and carbon dioxide production almost always cause respiratory distress and commonly necessitate mechanical ventilation. The lung injury and associated dysfunction may resolve during the initial 7 to 10 days or persist, depending on the ongoing pathologic processes.

Renal function tends to be maintained early in the course of SIRS unless the precipitating insult has prompted a sudden oliguric ATN. With persistent activation of inflammatory mediators, glomerular filtration rate falls, and the development of oliguric or polyuric renal failure marks the gradual transition from SIRS to MOFS. The renal dysfunction initially appears to be a prerenal azotemia, with low fractional excretion of sodium and modest elevations in the serum creatinine despite a normal or high cardiac output. Hemodynamic support, maintaining adequate levels of perfusion and flow-independent oxygen consumption, may offer maintenance or improvement of renal function. Despite optimal support, renal failure may progress.

Gastrointestinal abnormalities include ileus, stress ulceration, diarrhea, and mucosal atrophy. Breakdown of the mucosal barrier allows translocation of bacteria and endotoxin. Hepatic dysfunction is marked by a progressive rise in serum bilirubin levels after a latent period of several days. The hyperbilirubinemia is accompanied by mild elevations of serum alkaline phosphatase and hepatic transaminases. As clinical hepatic failure develops, these laboratory findings are accompanied by reduced hepatic protein synthesis and amino acid clearance, increased ureagenesis, and a falling hepatic redox potential despite exogenous nutritional support. Potentially treatable causes of hyperbilirubinemia, such as calculous or acalculous cholecystitis, hematoma, or abscess, are usually easily demonstrated with appropriate imaging studies and must be excluded. Functional deterioration of the nervous system is manifested by encephalopathy and peripheral neuropathies.

In the absence of a treatable underlying process, the mortality rate for MOFS is more than 90%.[183] Treatment of MOFS is directed at interrupting the evolving pathophysiologic processes and providing an optimal physiologic environment for healing and recovery. Fundamental concerns are control of the source of infection, inflammation, or instability; restoration of microcirculatory blood flow and oxygen transport; and institution of optimal supportive care. The presence of an inflammatory or infectious source and the persistence of an ongoing perfusion deficit are both primary causes of SIRS and the major reasons for transition to MOFS. Both prevention and therapy of MOFS therefore require source control and restoration of adequate perfusion. Control of hemorrhage, drainage of infection and large hematomas, débridement of devitalized and necrotic tissue, excision and grafting of burn wounds, fixation of fractures, and institution of appropriate antibiotics should be accomplished as early as possible.

Resuscitation efforts are directed toward restoration of adequate microcirculatory blood flow in all organ systems. Restoration of normal clinical parameters, such as blood pressure, pulse rate, urine output, and acid–base balance, does not ensure optimal resuscitation. The physiologic endpoints that most closely correspond to adequate microcirculatory flow are the levels of cardiac output and oxygen delivery at which oxygen consumption and lactate production remain independent of flow. The use of an oximetric pulmonary artery catheter to monitor adequate mixed venous oxygenation and other invasive monitoring should be used in patients who are at risk for developing MOFS as well as in those who develop the overt syndrome.

Advances in technology have made possible support of poorly functioning or failing organ systems. Mechanical assistance allows prolonged maintenance of adequate oxygenation and ventilation in all but the most extreme cases of pulmonary insufficiency. The various means of cardiac support are well defined and effective. The life-threatening consequences of renal failure can be avoided through hemodialysis and other measures for indefinite periods. Total parenteral nutrition (TPN) and enteral feeding can provide prolonged nutritional support in patients who otherwise would not be able to take in adequate calories. Although various therapies exist for some of the consequences of hepatic insufficiency, there is no specific means of prolonged support in the face of hepatic failure. The best means available to support the dysfunctional liver is the

Table 8-7. RELATIVE EFFECTS OF STARVATION AND HYPERMETABOLISM

Event	Starvation	Hypermetabolism
Energy expenditure	↓	++
Mediator activation	+	+++
Respiratory quotient	0.7	0.8–0.85
Fuel	Glucose/fat	Mixed
Gluconeogenesis	+	+++
Protein synthesis (relative to catabolism)	↓	↓↓
Catabolism	+	+++
Amino acid oxidation	±	+++
Ureagenesis	±	++
Ketonemia	+++	±
Rate of malnutrition	+	+++

+, increased; ±, increased or decreased.

provision of adequate nutrition and maintenance of optimal blood flow.

The importance of metabolic support in the patient with MOFS cannot be overemphasized. The malnutrition of MOFS is markedly different from that of starvation, and the nutritional requirements also differ (Table 8-7; see Chaps. 2 and 9). Although skeletal muscle catabolism proceeds despite amino acid infusion, the protein synthetic rate responds appropriately to optimal support. If optimal quantities of appropriately formulated amino acid solutions are given, protein synthetic rates can approach catabolic rates, and the goal of nitrogen balance is achieved. Formulas rich in branched-chain amino acids appear more efficient in promoting nitrogen retention and minimizing urea production. Excess glucose calories contribute to increased carbon dioxide production, fatty infiltration of the liver, and hyperosmolar complications. Using fat as a calorie source avoids these problems and provides essential fatty acids.

In the stressed patient, 1.5 to 2 g/kg/d of protein is required. The nonprotein calorie requirement is generally 25 to 35 kcal/kg/d, administered as 4 to 5 g/kg of glucose and 1 to 1.5 g/kg of fat. The ideal ratio of nonprotein kilocalories to grams of nitrogen administered is 100:1 or less. Whenever feasible, enteral feeding is preferred to TPN because evidence suggests that bacterial translocation from the gut can be limited through the use of enteral feedings. Enteral absorption and processing of nutrients appears superior to TPN and lessens overall complications. Delivery of nutrients beyond the pylorus lessens the risk of aspiration. Additionally, the cost of enteral nutrition is less than that of TPN.

General physical and emotional support gain greater importance as the length of hospitalization progresses. With the patient completely reliant on caretakers, attention must be given to positioning of the patient and equipment so that the breakdown of tissues does not occur. Pressure necrosis can cause decubitus ulcers, breakdown of nasal and auricular cartilages, and subglottic stenosis. Inattention to maintaining range of motion of extremities contributes to the development of contractures with associated disability. The time required for rehabilitation increases in proportion to the period of intensive care.

REFERENCES

1. American College of Chest Physicians/Society of Critical Care Medicine Consensus Conference Committee. Definitions for sepsis and organ failure and guidelines for the use of innovative therapies in sepsis. Crit Care Med 1992;20:864.
2. Bone RC, Fisher CJJ, et al. Sepsis syndrome: a valid clinical entity. Crit Care Med 1989;17:389.
3. Carrico CJ, Meakins JL, Marshall JC, Fry D, Maier RV. Multiple-organ-failure-syndrome. Arch Surg 1986;121:196.
4. Thal AP. Shock: a physiologic basis for treatment. Chicago, Year Book Medical Pub, 1971.
5. Simeone FA. Shock, trauma, and the surgeon. Ann Surg 1963;158:759.
6. Guthrie GJ. On gunshot wounds of the extremities. London, Longman, 1815.
7. Crile GW. An experimental research into surgical shock. Philadelphia, JB Lippincott, 1899.
8. Gesell R, Foote F, Copp ES. On the relation of blood volume to tissue nutrition (V). Am J Physiol 1922;63:32.
9. Blalock A. Experimental shock, the cause of the low blood pressure produced by muscle injury. Arch Surg 1930;20:959.
10. Wiggers CJ. The failure of transfusions in irreversible hemorrhagic shock. Am J Physiol 1945;144:91.
11. Reynolds M. Cardiovascular effects of large volumes of isotonic saline infused intravenously into dogs following severe hemorrhagic shock. Am J Physiol 1949;158:418.
12. Shires GT, Coln D, Carrico J, Lightfoot S. Fluid therapy in hemorrhagic shock. Arch Surg 1964;88:688.
13. Shires GT, Cunningham JN, Baker CRF, et al. Alterations in cellular membrane function during hemorrhagic shock in primates. Ann Surg 1972;176:288.
14. Shires GT, Williams J, Brown F. Acute changes in extracellular fluids associated with major surgical procedures. Ann Surg 1961;154:803.
15. Hardaway RM. Capillary perfusion in health and disease. New York, Futura, 1981:1.
16. West MA, Keller FA, Hyland B, et al. Kupffer cell modulation of hepatocellular function in multiple systems organ failure. J Leukocyte Biol 1984;36:436.
17. Simionescu N, Simionescu M. The cardiovascular system. In: Weiss L, ed. Cell and tissue biology: a textbook of histology. Baltimore, Urban & Schwarzenberg, 1988:353.
18. Rothe CF. Venous system: physiology of the capacitance vessels. In: Shepherd JT, ed. Handbook of physiology. Bethesda, American Physiological Society, 1983:397.
19. Guyton AC. Textbook of medical physiology, ed 7. Philadelphia, WB Saunders, 1986.
20. Taylor AE, Barnard JW, Barman SA, Adkins WK. Fluid balance. In: Crystal RG, West JB, eds. The lung: scientific foundations. New York, Raven Press, 1991:1147.
21. Rudolpho RR. Cardiovascular adrenoreceptors: physiology and critical care implications. In: Chernow B, ed. The pharmacologic approach to the critically ill patient. Baltimore, Williams & Wilkins, 1988:167.
22. Lister J, McNeill IF, Marshall VC, et al. Transcapillary refilling after hemorrhage in normal man. Ann Surg 1963;158:698.
23. Drucker WR, Cadwick CDJ, Gann DS. Transcapillary refill in hemorrhage and shock. Arch Surg 1981;116:1344.
24. Gann DS, Carlson DE, Byrnes GJ, et al. Role of solute in early restitution of blood volume after hemorrhage. Surgery 1983;94:439.
25. Peitzman AB, Corbett WA, Shires GT III, Illner H, Shires GT, Inamder R. Cellular function in liver and muscle during hemorrhagic shock in primates. Surg Gynecol Obstet 1985;161:419.
26. Chaudry IH. Cellular mechanisms in shock and ischemia and their correction. Am J Physiol 1983;245:R117.
27. Moreno-Sanchez R, Torres-Marquez MA. Control of oxidative phosphorylation in mitochondria, cells and tissues. Int J Biochem 1991;23:1163.
28. White IV, Mela L, Bacaizo LVJ, et al. Hepatic ultrastructure in endotoxemia, hemorrhage, and hypoxia: emphasis on mitochondrial changes. Surgery 1973;73:525.
29. Hirasawa H, Chaudry IH, Baue AE. Improved hepatic function and survival with adenosine triphosphate-magnesium chloride after hepatic ischemia. Surgery 1978;83:655.
30. Illner HP, Cunningham JNJ, Shires GT. Red blood cell sodium content and permeability changes in hemorrhagic shock. Am J Surg 1982;143:349.
31. Williams JA, Withrow CD, Woodbury DM. Effects of ouabain and diphenylhydantoin on transmembrane potentials, intra-

cellular electrolytes, and cell pH of rat muscle and liver in vivo. J Physiol (Lond) 1971;212:101.

32. Evans JA, Darlington DN, Gann DS. A circulating factor mediates cell depolarization in hemorrhagic shock. Ann Surg 1991;213:549.

33. Jones R, Carlson DE, Gann DS. A circulating shock protein that depolarizes cells in vitro depresses myocardial contractility and rate in isolated rat hearts. J Trauma 1994;37:752.

34. Eastridge BJ, Darlington DN, Evans JA, et al. A circulating shock protein depolarizes cells in hemorrhage and sepsis. Ann Surg 1994;219:298.

35. Mendez C, Garcia I, Maier RV. Oxidants augment endotoxin induced activation of alveolar macrophages. Shock 1996 (in press).

36. Smith A, Hayes G, Romaschin A, Walker P. The role of extracellular calcium in ischemia reperfusion injury in skeletal muscle. J Surg Res 1990;49:153.

37. Garcia JH, Anderson ML. Physiology of cerebral ischemia. Crit Rev Neurobiol 1989;4:303.

38. Wang P, Ba ZF, Dean RE, Chaudry IH. Diltiazem administration after crystalloid resuscitation restores active hepatocellular function and hepatic blood flow after severe hemorrhage shock. Surgery 1991;110:390.

39. Maitra SR, Krikhely M, Dulchavsky SA, et al. Beneficial effects of diltiazem in hemorrhagic shock. Circ Shock 1991;33:121.

40. Bond RF, Manley ES, Green HD. Cutaneous and skeletal muscle vascular responses to hemorrhage and irreversible shock. Am J Physiol 1967;212:488.

41. Garrison RN, Cryer HMI. Role of microcirculation to skeletal muscle during shock. Prog Clin Biol Res 1989;299:43.

42. Gustaffsson U, Wardell K, Nilsson GE, Lewis DH. Vasomotion in rat skeletal muscle induced by hemorrhage as recorded by laser-Doppler flowmetry. Microvasc Res 1991; 42:224.

43. Cryer HM, Kaebnick H, Harris PD, Flint LM. Effects of tissue acidosis on skeletal muscle microcirculatory responses to hemorrhagic shock in unanesthetized rats. J Surg Res 1985;39:59.

44. Amundson B, Jennische E, Haljamae H. Correlative analysis of microcirculatory and cellular metabolic events in skeletal muscle during hemorrhagic shock. Acta Physiol Scand 1980;108:147.

45. Clowes GHA Jr. Stresses, mediators, and responses of survival. In: Trauma, sepsis and shock: the physiological basis of therapy. New York, Marcel Dekker, 1988:1.

46. Davies CL, Newman RJ, Molyneux SG, Grahame-Smith DG. The relationship between plasma catecholamines and severity of injury in man. J Trauma 1984;24:99.

47. Holcroft JW, Link DP, Lanz BM, Green JF. Venous return and the pneumatic antishock garment in hypovolemic baboons. J Trauma 1984;24:928.

48. Baxter JD, Forsham PH. Tissues effects of glucocorticoids. Am J Med 1972;53:573.

49. Shamoon HM, Hendler R, Sherwin S. Synergistic interactions among anti-insulin hormones in the pathogenesis of stress hyperglycemia in humans. J Endocrinol Metab 1981;52:1235.

50. Goldsmith SR. Baro reflex control of vasopressin secretion in normal humans. In: Cowley AW, Laird JF, Ausiello D, eds. Vasopressin: cellular and integrative functions. New York, Raven Press, 1988:389.

51. Goetz, K.L. and B.C. Wang, Secretion of vasopressin during hemorrhagic: effects of receptors in the ventricles of the heart. In: Cowley AW, Laird JF, Ausiello D, eds. Vasopressin: cellular and integrative functions. New York, Raven Press, 1988:399.

52. Quillen EW, Reid IA, Keil LC. Cardiac and arterial baroreceptor influences on plasma vasopressin and drinking. In: Cowley AW, Laird JF, Ausiello D, eds. Vasopressin: cellular and integrative functions. New York, Raven Press, 1988:405.

53. Liard JF. Acute hemodynamic effects of anti-diuretic agones. In: Cowley AW, Laird JF, Ausiello D, eds. Vasopressin: cellular and integrative functions. New York, Raven Press, 1988:461.

54. Holcroft JW, Blaisdell FW. Shock: causes and management of circulatory collapse. In: Sabiston DC, ed. Textbook of surgery: the biological basis of modern surgical practice. Philadelphia, WB Saunders, 1986:38.

55. Holcroft JW. Shock. In: American College of Surgeons, ed. Care of the surgical patient. New York, Scientific American, 1988.

56. Garrison RN, Cryer HM. Role of the microcirculation to skeletal muscle during shock. In: Bond RF, Adams R, Chaudry I, eds. Perspectives in shock research: progress in clinical and biological research. New York, Alan R Liss, 1988:43.

57. Alexander F, Hechtman HB. Pulmonary and cardiovascular responses. In: Clowes GHA Jr, ed. Trauma, sepsis, and shock: the physiological basis of therapy. New York, Marcel Dekker, 1988:161.

58. Anderson RR, Holliday RL, Driedger AA, Lefcoe M, Reid B, Sibbald WJ. Documentation of pulmonary capillary permeability in the adult respiratory distress syndrome accompanying human sepsis. Am Rev Respir Dis 1979;119:869.

59. Brigham KL. Mechanisms of lung injury. Clin Chest Med 1982;3:9.

60. Sibbald WJ, Paterson NAM, Holliday RL, Anderson RA, Cobb TR, Duff JH. Pulmonary hypertension in sepsis. Chest 1978;73:583.

61. Tepliz C. The pathology and ultrastructure of cellular injury and inflammation in the progression and outcome of trauma, sepsis, and shock. In: Clowes GHA Jr, ed. Trauma, sepsis, and shock: the physiological basis of therapy. New York, Marcel Dekker, 1988:71.

62. Ashbaugh DG, Maier RV. Idiopathic pulmonary fibrosis in adult respiratory distress syndrome: diagnosis and treatment. Arch Surg 1985;120:530.

63. Maier RV, Hahnel GB. Potential for endotoxin-activated Kupffer cells to induce microvascular thrombosis. Arch Surg 1984;119:62.

64. Moncada S, Vane JR. Pharmacology and endogenous roles of prostaglandin endoperoxides, thromboxane A2 and prostacyclin. Pharmacol Rev 1979;30:293.

65. Deby-Duport A, Rodoux L, Mass M, et al. Release of thromboxane B2 during adult response distress syndrome and its inhibition by nonsteroidal anti-inflammatory substances in a man. Arch Int Pharmacodyn Ther 1982;259:317.

66. Slotman GJ, Burchard KW, D'Arezzo A, Gann DS. Ketoconazole prevents acute respiratory failure in critically ill surgical patients. J Trauma 1988;28:648.

67. Teupel GE, Strong JW, Wise WC, et al. The role of eicosanoids in mediating blood flow in endotoxin shock. In: Bond RF, Adams R, Chaudry I, eds. Perspectives in shock research: progress in clinical and biological research. New York, Alan R Liss, 1988:27.

68. Feuerstein G, Hallenbeck JM. Prostaglandins, leukotrienes, and platelet activating factor in shock. Annu Rev Pharmacol Toxicol 1987;27:301.

69. Taylor AE, Martin D, Parker JC. The effects of oxygen radicals on pulmonary edema formation. Surgery 1983;94:433.

70. Vedder NB, Winn RK, Rice CL, Harlan JM. Neutrophil-mediated vascular injury in shock and multiple organ failure. In: Passmore JC, Reichard SM, Reynolds DJ, et al, eds. Perspectives in shock research: metabolism, immunology, mediators, and models. New York, Alan R Liss, 1989:181.

71. Simons RK, Maier RV, Lennard ES. Neutrophil function in a rat model of endotoxin-induced lung injury. Arch Surg 1987;122:197.

72. Holman RG, Maier RV. Superoxide production by neutrophils in a model of adult respiratory distress syndrome. Arch Surg 1988;123:1491.

73. Maier RV, Hahnel GB. Is macrophage-induced macrothrombosis during endotoxemia dependent on prostaglandin synthesis? J Surg Res 1986;40:238.

74. Williams JG, Jurkovich GJ, Hahnel GB, Maier RV. Macrophage priming by interferon gamma: a selective process with potentially harmful effects. J Leukocyte Biol 1992;52:579.

75. Williams JG, Maier RV. Ketoconazole inhibits alveolar macrophage production of inflammatory mediators involved in acute lung injury (adult respiratory distress syndrome). Surgery 1992;112:270.

76. Lelcuk S, Alexander F, Kobzik G, et al. Prostacyclin and thromboxane A2 moderate postischemic renal failure. Surgery 1985;98:207.

77. Oken DE. Hemodynamic basis for human acute renal failure (vasomotor nephropathy). Am J Med 1984;176:702.

78. Galat JA, Robinson AV, Rhodes RS. Effect of hypoxia on renal flow. J Trauma 1988;28:955.

79. Ratcliffe RJ, Muonen CTW, Holloway PAH, Ledingham JGG, Redda GK. Acute renal failure in hemorrhagic hypotension: cellular energetics and renal function. Clin Nephrol 1980;13:73.

80. Cerra FB, Siegel JH, Coleman B, Border JR, McMenamy RH. Septic autocannibalism: a failure of exogenous nutritional support. Ann Surg 1980;192:570.

81. Maier RV. The angry macrophage and its impact on host response mechanisms. In: Faist E, Meakins J, Schildberg FW, eds. Host defense dysfunction in trauma, shock and sepsis. Heidelberg, Springer-Verlag, 1993:191.

82. Fosse E, Mollnes TE, Aasen AO, Trumpy JH, Stokke T. Complement activation following multiple injuries. Acta Chir Scand 1987;153:325.

83. Burke JF, Gelfand JA. Events in early inflammation. In: Howard RJ, Simmons RL, eds. Surgical infectious diseases. Norwalk, CT, Appleton & Lange, 1988:201.

84. Stahl TJ, Cerra FB. Hemodynamic and metabolic responses. In: Howard RJ, Simmons RL, eds. Surgical infectious diseases. Norwalk, CT, Appleton & Lange, 1988:209.

85. Reines HD, Cook JA. Arachidonic acid metabolites. In: Chernow B, ed. The pharmacologic approach to the critically ill patient. Baltimore, William & Wilkins, 1988:733.

86. Bachle YS. Synthesis and catabolism of cyclo-oxygenase products. Br Med Bull 1983;39:214.

87. Williams JG, Garcia I, Maier RV. Prostaglandin E2 mediates lipopolysaccharide-induced macrophage procoagulant activity by a cyclic adenosine monophosphate-dependent pathway. Surgery 1993;114:314.

88. Lelcuk S, Alexander F, Valeri CR. Ischemia stimulates thromboxane synthesis. Surg Forum 1984;35:76.

89. Patterson IS, Klausner JM, Goldman G, et al. Thromboxane mediates the ischemia-induced neutrophil oxidative burst. Surgery 1989;106:224.

90. Vane JR, Moncada S. Arachidonic metabolites in the cardiovascular system. In: Kovach AGB, Haumar J, Szabo H, eds. Cardiovascular physiology, microcirculation and capillary exchange. Elmsford, NY, Pergamon Press, 1981:37.

91. Williams JG, Garcia IA, Maier RV. Endothelial regulation of macrophage tumor necrosis factor production. Surg Forum 1992;43:94.

92. Faist E, Ertel W, Cohnert T, et al. Immunoprotective effects of cyclooxygenase inhibitors in patients with major surgical trauma. J Trauma 1990;30:8.

93. Ertel W, Mannion NH, Ayala A, et al. Eicosanoids regulate tumor necrosis factor synthesis after hemorrhage in vitro and in vivo. J Trauma 1991;31:609.

94. Ertel W, Morrison MH, Ayala A, et al. Chloroquine attenuates hemorrhagic shock-induced suppression of Kupffer cell antigen presentation and major histocompatibility complex class II antigen expression through blockade of tumor necrosis factor and prostaglandin release. Blood 1991;78:1781.

95. Denzlinger C, Rapp S, Hagmann W, et al. Leukotrienes as mediators in tissue trauma. Science 1985;230:330.

96. Bitterman H, Smith BA, Lefer AM. Beneficial actions of antagonism of peptide leukotrienes in hemorrhagic shock. Circ Shock 1988;24:159.

97. Snyder F. Chemical and biochemical aspects of platelet-activating factor: a novel class of acetylated ethel-linking choline phospholysates. Med Res Rev 1985;5:107.

98. Stahl GL, Craft DV, Lento PH. Detection of platelet-activating factor during traumatic shock. Circ Shock 1988;26:237.

99. Maier RV, Hahnel GB, Fletcher JR. Platelet-activating factor augments tumor necrosis factor and procoagulant activity. J Surg Res 1992;52:258.

100. Pitman JMI, Thurman GW, Anderson BO, et al. Platelet-activating factor may mediate neutrophil priming following clinical burns or blunt trauma. Surg Forum 1991;40:108.

101. Thompson WA, Coyle S, Van Zee K, et al. The metabolic effects of platelet-activating factor antagonism in endotoxemic man. Arch Surg 1994;129:72.

102. Dhainaut J, Tenaillon A, Le Tulzo Y, et al. Platelet-activating factor receptor antagonist BN 52021 in the treatment of severe sepsis: a randomized, double-blind, placebo-controlled, multicenter clinical trial. Crit Care Med 1994;22:1720.

103. Beutler BA. Orchestration of septic shock by cytokines: the role of cachectin (tumor necrosis factor). Prog Clin Biol Res 1989;286:219.

104. Hesse DG, Tracey KJ, Fong Y, et al. Cytokine appearance in human endotoxemia and primate bacteremia. Surg Gynecol Obstet 1988;166:147.

105. Ayala A, Wang P, Ba ZF, et al. Differential alterations in plasma II-6 and TNF levels after trauma and hemorrhage. Am J Physiol 1991;260:R167.

106. Chaudry IH, Ertel W, Ayala A. Alterations in inflammatory cytokine production following hemorrhage and resuscitation. In: Schlag G, Redle H, Traber DL, eds. Shock, sepsis and organ failure. Berlin, Springer-Verlag, 1993:73.

107. Svoboda P, Kantorova I, Ochmann J. Dynamics of interleukin 1, 2, and 6 and tumor necrosis factor alpha in multiple trauma patients. J Trauma 1994;36:336.

108. Schlag G, Redl H, Davies J, et al. Trauma and cytokines. In: Schlag G, Redle H, Traber DL, eds. Shock, sepsis and organ failure. Berlin, Springer-Verlag, 1993:128.

109. Schlag G, Redl H, Hallstrom S. The cell in shock: the origin of multiple organ failure. Resuscitation 1991;21:137.

110. Pretorius JP, Schlag G, Redl H, et al. The lung in shock as a result of hypovolemic traumatic shock in baboons. J Trauma 1987;27:1344.

111. Pullicino EA, Carli F, Poole S, et al. The relationship between the circulating concentrations of IL-6, TNF, and the acute phase response to elective surgery and accidental injury. Lymphokine Res 1990;9:231.

112. O'Neill PJ, Ayala A, Wang P, et al. Role of Kupffer cells in IL-6 release following trauma. Shock 1994;1:43.

113. Munro JM, Pober JS, Cotran RS, Tumor necrosis factor and interferon-gamma induce distinct patterns of endothelial activation and associated leukocyte accumulation in skin of papio anubis. Am J Pathol 1989;135:121.

114. Meyer JD, Yurt RW, Duhaney R, et al. Tumor necrosis factor—enhanced leukotriene B4 generation and chemotaxis in human neutrophils. Arch Surg 1988;123:1454.

115. Cinat ME, Waxman K, Granger GA, Pearce W, Annas C, Daughters K. Trauma causes sustained elevation of soluble tumor necrosis factor receptors. J Am Coll Surg 1994;179:529.

116. Tracey KJ, Fong Y, Hesse DG, Anti-cachectin/TNF monoclonal antibodies prevent septic shock during lethal bacteremia. Nature 1987;330:662.

117. Shenkar R, Coulson WF, Abraham E. Hemorrhage and resuscitation induce alterations in cytokine expression and the development of acute lung injury. Am J Respir Cell Mol Biol 1994;10:290.

118. Ertel W, Bonnacio M, Scholl F, et al. Release of anti-inflammatory mediator following mechanical trauma correlates with severity of injury and clinical outcome. Program of the American Association for the Surgery of Trauma, 1994:78.

119. Fisher CJ. Recombinant human interleukin 1 receptor antagonist in the treatment of patients with sepsis syndrome: results from a randomized, double-blind, placebo-controlled trial. JAMA 1994;271:1836.

120. Donnelly TJ, Meade P, Jagels M, et al. Cytokine, complement, and endotoxin profiles associated with the development of the adult respiratory distress syndrome after severe injury. Crit Care Med 1994;22:768.

121. Rot A. Endothelial cell binding of NAP-1/IL-8: role in neutrophil emigration. Immunol Today 1992;13:291.

122. Cowley HC, Heney D, Gearing AJH, Hemingway I, Webster NR. Increased circulating adhesion molecule concentrations in patients with the systemic inflammatory response syndrome: a prospective cohort study. Crit Care Med 1994;22:651.

123. Law MM, Cryer HG, Abraham E. Elevated levels of soluble ICAM-1 correlate with the development of multiple organ failure in severely injured trauma patients. J Trauma 1994;37:100.

124. Rees DD, Palmer RMJ, Moncada S. Role of endothelium-derived nitric oxide in the regulation of blood pressure. Proc Natl Acad Sci USA 1989;86:3375.

125. Aisaka K, Gross SS, Griffith OW, Levi R. Ng-methylarginine,

an inhibitor of endothelium-derived nitric oxide synthesis, is a potent pressor agent in the guinea pig: does nitric oxide regulate blood pressure in vivo? Biochem Biophys Res Commun 1989;160:881.

126. Ignarro LJ, Byrns RE, Buga GM, Wood KS, Chaudhuri G. Pharmacological evidence that endothelium-derived relaxing factor is nitric oxide: use of pyrogallol and superoxide-elicited vascular smooth muscle relaxation. J Pharmacol Exp Ther 1988;244:181.

127. Nussler AK, Billiar TR. Inflammation, immunoregulation, and inducible nitric oxide synthase. J Leukocyte Biol 1993;54:171.

128. Minoz O, Rauss A, Rekik N, Brun-Buisson C, Lemaire F, Brochard L. Pulmonary artery catheterization in critically ill patients: a prospective analysis of outcome changes associated with catheter-prompted changes in therapy. Crit Care Med 1994;22:573.

129. Hansen PD, Coffey SC, Lewis FRJ. The effects of adrenergic agents on oxygen delivery and oxygen consumption in normal dogs. J Trauma 1994;37:283.

130. Freed PS, Wasfre T, Zado B, Kentrowitz A. Intraaortic balloon pumping for prolonged circulatory support. Am J Cardiol 1988;61:554.

131. Eurich DA, Biddle TL, Kronenberg MW, Yu PN. The hemodynamic response to intra-aortic balloon counter-pulsation in patients with cardiogenic shock complicating acute myocardial infarction. Am Heart J 1977;93:274.

132. Bardet J, Mesquet C, Kahn JC, Gourgon R, Bourdarics JP. Clinical and hemodynamic results of intraaortic balloon counter-pulsation and surgery for cardiogenic shock. Am Heart J 1977;93:280.

133. Pennington DG. Emergency management of cardiogenic shock. Circulation 1989;79(Suppl 1):149.

134. Wiles J, Cerra FB, Border J. The systemic septic response: does the organism matter? Crit Care Med 1980;8:55.

135. Rackow EC. Clinical definition of sepsis and septic shock. In: Sibbald WJ, Sprung CL, eds. New horizons: perspectives on sepsis and septic shock. Fullerton, CA, Society of Critical Care Medicine, 1986:1.

136. Ayres SM. Sepsis and septic shock: a synthesis of ideas and proposals for the direction of future research. In: Sibbald WJ, Sprung CL, eds. New horizons: perspectives on sepsis and septic shock. Fullerton, CA, Society of Critical Care Medicine, 1986:375.

137. Clowes GHA Jr, Vucinic M, Weidner MG. Circulatory and metabolic alteration associated with survival or death in peritonitis: critical analysis of 25 cases. Ann Surg 1966; 163:866.

138. Duff JH, Groves AC, MacLean APH. Defective oxygen consumption in septic shock. Surg Gynecol Obstet 1969; 128:1051.

139. MacLean LD, Mulligan WG, MacLean APH, Duff JH. Patterns of septic shock in man: a detailed study of 56 patients. Ann Surg 1967;166:543.

140. Calvin JE, Driedger AA, Sibbald WJ. An assessment of myocardial function in human sepsis utilizing ECG gated cardiac scintigraphy. Chest 1981;80:579.

141. Parrillo JE. Cardiovascular dysfunction in human septic shock and endotoxemia. In: Passmore JC, Reichard SM, Reynolds DJ, et al, eds. Perspectives in shock research: metabolism, immunology, mediators, and models. New York, Alan R Liss, 1989:107.

142. Parker MM, Shelhauner JH, Bacharach SL, et al. Profound but reversible myocardial depression in patients with septic shock. Ann Intern Med 1984;100:483.

143. Ellrodt AG, Riedinger MS, Kimch A, et al. Left ventricular performance in septic shock: reversible segmental and global abnormalities. Am Heart J 1985;110:402.

144. Parrillo JE, Burch C, Shelhauner JH, Parker MM, Natanson C, Schuette W. A circulating myocardial depressant substance in humans with septic shock. J Clin Invest 1985; 76:1539.

145. Zantsky AL, Chernow B. Catecholamines and other inotropes. In: Chernow B, ed. The pharmacologic approach to the critically ill patient. Baltimore, Williams & Wilkins, 1988:346.

146. Chameides L, ed. Textbook of pediatric advanced life support. Dallas, American Heart Association, 1990:57.

147. Parrillo JE. Vasodilator therapy. In: Chernow B, ed. The pharmacologic approach to the critically ill patient. Baltimore, Williams & Wilkins, 1988:346.

148. Cerra FB, Hasset J, Siegel JH. Vasodilatory therapy in clinical sepsis with low output syndrome. J Surg Res 1978;25:180.

149. Sibbald WJ, Patterson N, Holliday R, et al. The Trendelenburg position: hemodynamic effects in hypotensive and normotensive patients. Crit Care Med 1979;7:218.

150. Guntheroth WG, Abel FL, Mullins GL. The effect of Trendelenburg's position on blood pressure and carotid flow. Surg Gynecol Obstet 1964;119:235.

151. Hands RD, Holcroft JW. Pneumatic antishock garment. In: Trunkey DD, Lewis FR, eds. Current therapy of trauma. Philadelphia, BC Decker, 1986:47.

152. Prizolo VE, Burchard KW, Singh AK, Moran JM, Gann DS. Trendelenburg versus PASG application: hemodynamic response in man. J Trauma 1986;26:718.

153. Palafox BA, Johnson MN, McEwen DK, et al. ICP changes following application of the MAST suit. J Trauma 1981; 21:55.

154. Geoffrey FA, Thal ER, Taylor WF, et al. Hemodynamic effects of military anti-shock trousers (MAST garment). J Trauma 1981;21:931.

155. Bickell WH, Pepe PE, Bailey ML, Wyatt CH, Maddox KL. Randomized trial of pneumatic antishock garments in the prehospital management of penetrating abdominal injuries. Ann Emerg Med 1987;16:653.

156. Luna GK, Maier RV, Pavlin EP, Anardi D, Copass MK, Oreskovich MR. Incidence and effect of hypothermia in seriously injured patients. J Trauma 1987;27:1014.

157. Gubler KG, Hassantash SA, Gentilello LM, Maier RV. The impact of hypothermia on dilutional coagulopathy. J Trauma 1994;36:847.

158. Gentilello LM, Cortes V, Moujaes S, et al. Continuous arteriovenous rewarming: experimental results and thermodynamic model simulation of treatment for hypothermia. J Trauma 1990;30:1436.

159. Gentilello LM, Cobean RA, Offner PJ, Soderberg RW, Jurkovich GJ. Continuous arteriovenous rewarming: rapid reversal of hypothermia in critically ill patients. J Trauma 1992; 32:316.

160. Schein M, Wittman DH, Aprahamian CC, Condon RE. The abdominal compartment syndrome: the physiological and clinical consequences of elevated intra-abdominal pressure. J Am Coll Surg 1995;180:745.

161. Shoemaker WC, Printen KJ, Amato JJ, Monson DO, Carey JS, O'Connor K. Hemodynamic patterns after acute anesthetized and unanesthetized trauma: evaluation of the consequence of changes in cardiac output and derived calculations. Arch Surg 1967;95:492.

162. Shoemaker WC, Appel PL, Waxman K, Schwartz S, Chang P. Clinical trial of survivors' cardiorespiratory patterns as therapeutic goals in critically ill postoperative patients. Crit Care Med 1982;10: 398.

163. Shoemaker WC, Montgomery ES, Kaplan E, Elwyn DH. Physiologic patterns in surviving and nonsurviving shock patients: use of sequential cardiorespiratory variables in defining criteria for therapeutic goals and early warning of death. Arch Surg 1973;106:630.

164. Bland RD, Shoemaker WC, Abraham E, Cobo JC. Hemodynamic and oxygen transport patterns in surviving and nonsurviving postoperative patients. Crit Care Med 1985;13:85.

165. Shoemaker WC, Appel PL, Kram HB, et al. Prospective trial of supranormal values of survivors as therapeutic goals in high risk surgical patients. Chest 1988;94:1176.

166. Boyd O, Grounds RM, Bennett ED. A randomized clinical trial of the effect of deliberate increase of oxygen delivery on mortality in high risk surgical patients. JAMA 1993; 270:2699.

167. Tuchschmidt J, Fried J, Astiz M, Rachow E. Elevation of cardiac output and oxygen delivery improves outcome in septic shock. Chest 1992;102:216.

168. Yu M, Levy MM, Smith P, Takiguchi SA, Miyasaki A, Meyers SA. Effect of maximizing oxygen delivery on morbidity and mortality rates in critically ill patients: a prospective, randomized, controlled study. Crit Care Med 1993;21:830.

169. Hayes MA, Timmins AC, Yau EHS, Palazzo M, Hinds CJ,

Watson D. Elevation of systemic oxygen delivery in the treatment of critically ill patients. N Engl J Med 1994;330:1717.

170. Gattinoni L, Brazzi L, Pelosi P, et al. A trial of goal-oriented hemodynamic therapy in critically ill patients. N Engl J Med 1995;333:1025.

171. Parks DA, Bulkely GB, Granger DN. Role of oxygen free radicals in shock, ischemia, and oxygen prevention. Surgery 1983;94:428.

172. McCord JM. The superoxide free radical: its biochemistry and pathophysiology. Surgery 1983;94:412.

173. Lo CJ, Garcia I, Cryer HG, Maier RV. Calcium and calmodulin regulate LPS-induced alveolar macrophage production of tumor necrosis factor and procoagulant activity. Arch Surg 1996;131:44.

174. Abraham E, Tanaka T, Change TH. Effects of hemorrhagic serum on IL-2 generation and utilization. Crit Care Med 1988;16:307.

175. Livingston DH, Malangoni MA. Interferon-gamma restores immune competence after hemorrhagic shock. J Surg Res 1988;45:37.

176. Ertel W, Morrison MH, Ayala A, Dean RE, Chaudry IH. Interferon-gamma attenuates hemorrhage-induced suppression of macrophages and splenocyte susceptibility to sepsis. Surgery 1992;111:177.

177. Dries DJ, Jurkovich GJ, Maier RV, et al. Effect of interferon gamma on infection-related death in patients with severe injuries. Arch Surg 1994;129:1031.

178. Faist E, Mewes A, Baker CC, et al. Prostaglandin E2 (PGE2) dependent suppression of IL-2 production in patients with major trauma. J Trauma 1987;27:837.

179. Bone RC. Toward an epidemiology and natural history of SIRS (systemic inflammatory response syndrome). JAMA 1992;268:3452.

180. Bone RC, Sibbald WJ, Sprung CL. The ACCP SCCM consensus conference on sepsis and organ failure. Chest 1992;101:1481.

181. Barton R, Cerra FB. The hypermetabolism multiple organ failure syndrome. Chest 1989;96:1153.

182. Ulevitch RJ, Wolfson N, Virca GD, et al. Macrophages regulate the host response to lipopolysaccharides. In: Passmore JC, Reichard SM, Reynolds DV, et al, eds. Perspectives in shock research: metabolism, immunology, mediators, and models. New York, Alan R Liss, 1989:193.

183. Fry DE, Pearlstein L, Fulton RL, et al. Multiple system organ failure: the role of uncontrolled infection. Arch Surg 1980;115:136.

SURGERY: SCIENTIFIC PRINCIPLES AND PRACTICE, Second Edition, edited by Lazar J. Greenfield, Michael W. Mulholland, Keith T. Oldham, Gerald B. Zelenock, and Keith D. Lillemoe. Lippincott–Raven Publishers, Philadelphia, © 1997.

CHAPTER 9

CRITICAL CARE

ROBERT H. BARTLETT

Although critical care has emerged as a distinct discipline, it involves nothing more or less than the care of our sickest patients. Intensive care units (ICUs) originated with the beginnings of cardiac surgery in the early 1960s. Cardiac surgical patients had new and special monitors—continuous electrocardiograms, intraarterial catheters, and central venous pressure catheters. It was often necessary to keep these patients on mechanical ventilators overnight and sometimes for 1 or 2 days. Monitors and devices made it possible to treat patients following the principles of cardiorespiratory physiology, theretofore only possible in the laboratory. As surgeons learned these techniques in cardiac surgery, they extended them to the care of other types

of surgical patients—vascular, trauma, and neurosurgical. Some of the recovery room nurses learned to manage ventilators, amplifiers, oscilloscopes, and the other gadgetry of the extended recovery room. Eventually, care of these patients became a full-time nursing responsibility. Nurses and machinery began to overflow the recovery room, and intensive care nursing units were established. Through the 1970s, critical care became a defined nursing specialty, with special training, certification, a society, and a journal. Every major hospital developed ICUs where these specialized nurses could practice. The concept spread among medical disciplines, from surgery to medicine to pediatrics to neonatology. By the 1980s, some physicians began to focus their practices on critically ill patients. Some internists and anesthesiologists limited their practices to critically ill patients of other primary physicians. "Reanimation" became a subspecialty of anesthesiology throughout Europe.

Surgeons have always been at the forefront of critical care as part of their routine practices. The concept of assigning preoperative or postoperative care to other colleagues runs counter to the training and responsibility of surgeons. Surgical intensive care nursing units, however, needed policies, administration, and supervision, and surgeons took on these jobs. Within the past decade, the discipline has been considered specialized enough to warrant fellowship training, examination, and certification by the American Board of Surgery in surgical critical care. Similar certification is offered by the boards of medicine, anesthesiology, and pediatrics.

Issues of administration and supervision aside, critical care remains simply the business of applied physiology and pharmacology in the treatment of the sickest patients. This chapter focuses on the basic principles and mechanics of that practice. Although principles of management and physiology are universal, the examples and numbers in this chapter relate to adult patients. This chapter assumes a thorough knowledge of basic physiology on the part of the reader.

The ICU affords the possibility to monitor a wide variety of physiologic variables continuously and to use that information to prevent and treat organ failure. Central to the intelligent use of this information is an understanding of homeostatic physiology: integrated cardiac, respiratory, and metabolic physiology (oxygen kinetics); respiratory physiology; body fluids and hemodynamics; nutrition and metabolism; and renal pathophysiology.

OXYGEN KINETICS: INTEGRATING HEMODYNAMIC, RESPIRATORY, AND METABOLIC PHYSIOLOGY

Oxygen Consumption

Oxygen consumed in this process of metabolism is expressed as the volume of oxygen per minute (Vo_2). Vo_2 is normally 100 to 120 mL/m^2/min, or 200 mL/min for a typical adult. Resting Vo_2 is a function of the metabolizing body cell mass, with fine-tuning control provided by the level of thyroid and catecholamine hormones and governed by a poorly understood metabolic controller in the hypothalamus. Vo_2 decreases under conditions of hypothermia, paralysis, and hypothyroidism. Vo_2 increases during exercise or other muscular activity, hyperthermia, profound hypothalamic injury, hyperthyroidism, catecholamines, and inflammatory mediators, particularly the interleukin cytokines. Under steady-state conditions, the amount of oxygen consumed in systemic metabolism is exactly equal to the amount of oxygen taken up in the pulmonary capillaries through the airway. This is true regardless of the status of pulmonary function

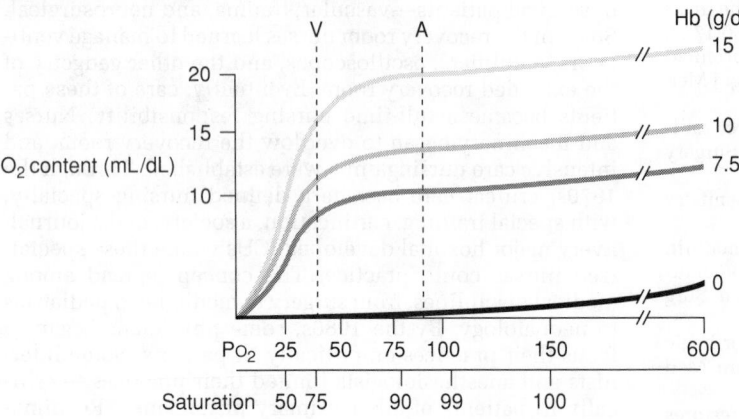

Figure 9-1. The relation of oxygen content, saturation, and PO_2. Typical normal arterial and venous blood levels are defined at various hemoglobin levels. (After Bartlett RH. University of Michigan surgical critical care review handbook. 1991)

or dysfunction, so VO_2 is measured across the lung with the assumption that this is exactly the amount consumed in systemic metabolism.

Oxygen Delivery

The amount of oxygen that is delivered to peripheral tissues is the product of the oxygen content in arterial blood and the cardiac output. Normally, the oxygen content of arterial blood (CaO_2) is about 20 mL/dL, and the normal cardiac index is 3.2 L/m^2/min, 5 L/min for a typical adult. Therefore, the normal systemic oxygen delivery (DO_2) is 20 mL/dL × 50 dL/min = 1000 mL/min. Although oxygen content is the most important measure of oxygen in blood, partial pressure of oxygen (PO_2) and oxyhemoglobin saturation are more commonly measured in the ICU; hence, it is necessary to convert these measurements. Each gram of hemoglobin can bind 1.36 mL of oxygen. If the hemoglobin of the blood is normal (15 g/dL) and the hemoglobin is 98% saturated, the amount of oxygen bound to hemoglobin is 19.9 mL/dL. In addition, a small amount of oxygen is physically dissolved in the water that makes up plasma and red blood cells. The solubility coefficient for oxygen is 0.0031 mL/mmHg/dL; therefore, the amount of oxygen dissolved in 1 dL of blood at PO_2 100 mmHg is 0.3 mL, making the oxygen content of normal arterial blood 19.9 + 0.3 = 20.2 mL/dL, conveniently rounded off to 20 mL/dL. Through the same arithmetic, the oxygen content of venous blood (CvO_2) is 16 mL/dL; hence, the normal arterial–venous difference is 4 mL O_2/dL. The relation between PO_2, saturation, and oxygen content for different concentrations of hemoglobin is shown in Figure 9-1. Notice that the arterial partial pressure of oxygen (PaO_2) and saturation are the same for normal arterial and venous

blood even though the oxygen content is severely decreased in anemia.

Autoregulation to Maintain Oxygen Delivery

The relations between VO_2 and DO_2 represent one of the most interesting autoregulation systems in hemostasis. First of all, if one of the three components of oxygen delivery is abnormal, endogenous mechanisms regulate the other two until normal oxygen delivery has been restored. In compensation for acute hypoxia or acute anemia, cardiac output increases, but only until normal oxygen delivery is reestablished. In chronic hypoxia, the red-cell mass increases until systemic oxygen delivery is normal at normal cardiac output. In chronic anemia, cardiac output increases and remains increased. When cardiac output is decreased, there is no mechanism to induce superoxygenation or polycythemia. In this situation, oxygen consumption generally continues at the normal rate of metabolism, and relatively more oxygen is extracted from the flowing blood, widening the arteriovenous oxygen difference ($AVDO_2$) difference. The various combinations of these compensatory mechanisms supply adequate oxygen for systemic metabolism through a wide range of variations in oxygen delivery. If oxygen delivery cannot be maintained at a level at least twice the oxygen consumption, an unstable state results, described later.

Autoregulation for Changing Oxygen Consumption

When a change in VO_2 occurs, a proportionate change in DO_2 occurs almost immediately, mediated completely by a change in cardiac output. For example, if a person

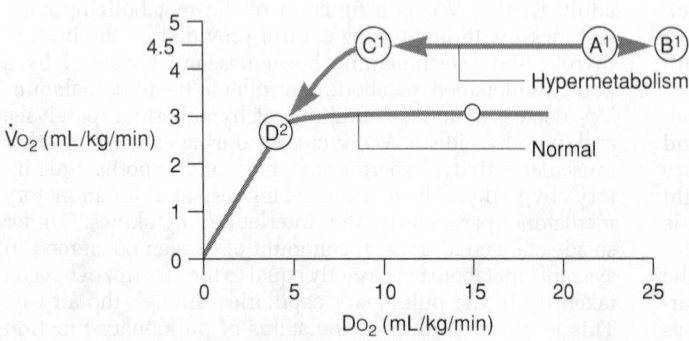

Figure 9-2. The relation of oxygen consumption when oxygen delivery is changed over a wide range. Examples are shown for normal metabolism and hypermetabolic status (A^1). (After Bartlett RH, Anderson HL. Multiorgan failure. In: Zelenock GB, et al, eds. Clinical ischemic syndromes: mechanisms and consequences of tissue injury. St Louis, CV Mosby, 1989:565)

goes from rest to mild exercise, V_{O_2} increases, followed promptly by an increase of cardiac output (A to A^1 in Fig. 9-2), reestablishing the ratio of delivery to consumption at about 5:1. The mechanism that mediates this change in cardiac output is not fully understood but is probably related to a chemoreceptor on the venous side of the circulation. This autoregulation occurs whether the change in V_{O_2} is up or down and whether it is caused by exercise, sepsis, catecholamines, or other mediators.

Autoregulation for Changing Oxygen Delivery

Conversely, a primary change in oxygen delivery is *not* followed by any change in oxygen consumption, nor would V_{O_2} be expected to change because systemic oxygen delivery is not included in the list of controllers of metabolism. If D_{O_2} fell below the level of V_{O_2}, however, V_{O_2} would become supply dependent. In theory, this situation would occur when the ratio of delivery to consumption was below 1:1. In actuality, this condition of supply dependency of V_{O_2} occurs when the D_{O_2} falls below twice V_{O_2}; that is, supply dependency occurs when the ratio of D_{O_2} to V_{O_2} is less than 2:1. This relation is shown in Figure 9-3, which demonstrates the biphasic nature of the V_{O_2} and D_{O_2} relation. When a state of supply dependency exists, anaerobic metabolism occurs, the patient experiences oxygen "debt," and hemodynamic instability eventually results. If the situation proceeds long enough, progressive organ failure occurs, and the patient can be said to be in a state of circulatory, ischemic, or hypoxic shock. The same relations exist when V_{O_2} is elevated during hypermetabolism (see Fig. 9-2). Supply dependency exists during hypermetabolism whenever the D_{O_2}/V_{O_2} ratio is less than 2:1, although during hypermetabolism, this occurs at a higher level of actual D_{O_2} than it does during normal metabolism. The primary goals of intensive care and management are to estimate or determine the V_{O_2} and D_{O_2}, maintain the patient near the normal ratio of 5:1, and, if oxygen delivery fails, intervene before the ratio reaches the critical low level of 2:1.

Venous Saturation Monitoring

The relation between D_{O_2} and V_{O_2} is reflected in the amount of oxygen in venous blood. Under normal conditions, D_{O_2} is 1000 mL/min and V_{O_2} is 200 mL/min. The amount of oxygen extracted is 20% of that delivered, and 80% of the oxygen is still present in venous blood returning to the heart. Usually, the arterial blood is fully saturated, and under normal circumstances, the saturation

of mixed venous blood ($S_{V_{O_2}}$) is 80%. (This measurement must be made in mixed venous blood because the relative extraction of organs served by the superior and inferior vena cava and coronary sinus are different.) If 80% $S_{V_{O_2}}$ corresponds to a 5:1 ratio, then 75% corresponds to 4:1, 60% to 3:1, 50% to 2:1, and so on. As long as the arterial blood is fully saturated, this observation holds true regardless of the absolute level of D_{O_2} or V_{O_2} (Fig. 9-4). If the arterial blood is less than fully saturated, the difference between arterial and venous saturation corresponds to the oxygen extraction, hence, the D_{O_2}/V_{O_2} ratio. For example, if the arterial blood were 80% saturated and the venous blood were 64% saturated, the ratio would be 5:1.

All of these interrelations were originally pointed out by Fick in 1870. Fick's axiom is that oxygen consumption through the airway is equal to that in peripheral tissues. His equation for calculating cardiac output is $CO = V_{O_2}$ divided by the AV_{O_2} difference, which can also be expressed as AV_{O_2} difference times cardiac output equals V_{O_2}.

In critically ill patients, V_{O_2} may be elevated or depressed, but slight to moderate elevation in V_{O_2} is the most common abnormality in critically ill patients. V_{O_2} is elevated in proportion to the amount of inflammation (either bacterial or sterile, as in burns and pancreatitis). A febrile patient with significant signs of septic toxicity typically has V_{O_2} that is 1.5 to 2 times normal. It is unusual for a critically ill patient to experience V_{O_2} greater than twice normal. This occurs only in situations of severe muscular exercise, such as seizures or tetanus. V_{O_2} is decreased in critically ill patients who are hypothermic.

During hypermetabolism, a change in V_{O_2} is followed promptly by a proportionate change in D_{O_2}; thus, it is normal for a hypermetabolic patient to have a high cardiac output and pulse rate, that is, to be hyperdynamic. Rarely, the hyperdynamic response exceeds the increase in V_{O_2}, reflected in a ratio higher than 5:1 and venous saturation greater than 80%. This situation can occur when a large arteriovenous fistula is present, either from direct vascular communication or through hyperperfusion of tissues such as occurs with portal hypertension with excessive perfusion of the splanchnic viscera. Some patients cannot mount an increased D_{O_2} in response to increased V_{O_2} because of any combination of hypoxia, anemia, and myocardial failure. If this occurs, then the D_{O_2}/V_{O_2} ratio is less than 5:1, AV_{O_2} difference widens, $S_{V_{O_2}}$ falls, the amount of oxygen extracted from each deciliter of blood increases, and the patient is using up the systemic oxygen reserves. This increased extraction is perfectly adequate compensation, however, and the patient remains stable as long as the ratio is greater than 2:1. When the various mechanisms

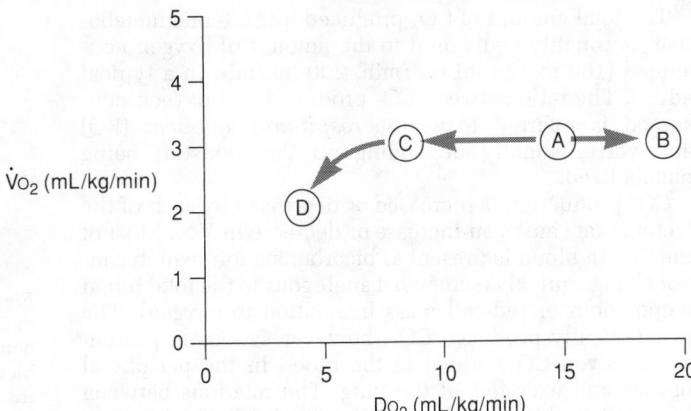

Figure 9-3. Normally (point A), systemic oxygen delivery is about 15 mL/kg/min and oxygen consumption 3 mL/kg/min. Consumption becomes supply dependent when delivery is very low (C to D). Delivery increases in response to increased metabolism (A to B). (After Bartlett RH, Anderson HL. Multiorgan failure. In: Zelenock GB, et al, eds. Clinical ischemic syndromes: mechanisms and consequences of tissue injury. St Louis, CV Mosby, 1989:565)

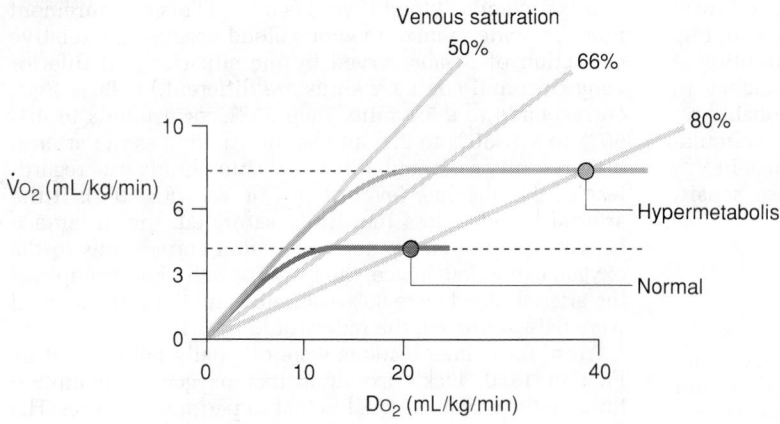

Figure 9-4. Mixed venous blood saturation over a wide range of oxygen delivery and consumption interrelations. Assuming that arterial blood is nearly saturated, venous saturation reflects the ratio between delivery and consumption. (After Bartlett RH. University of Michigan surgical critical care review handbook. 1991)

of delivery cannot maintain Do_2 at least twice Vo_2, supply dependency and shock occur.

A series of clinical studies have claimed that the biphasic relation is absent and that there is a continuous state of Vo_2 supply dependency in patients with acute respiratory distress syndrome or sepsis. These studies are marred by artifacts of clinical investigation and are not supported by laboratory studies in which all the variables can be evaluated. It appears, however, that the "knee" of the biphasic curve may be shifted to the right in sepsis, making the critical ratio closer to 3:1 than 2:1.

The shape of the oxyhemoglobin dissociation curve shown in Figure 9-1 changes in various conditions, moving to the right during acidosis, hypercarbia, and hyperthermia. Although these changes have physiologic importance (eg, facilitating systemic oxygen unloading during ischemia and acidosis), the effects on oxygen content and relation to Po_2 and saturation are relatively minor compared with the effects of hemoglobin on oxygen content.

RESPIRATORY PHYSIOLOGY AND PATHOPHYSIOLOGY

Carbon Dioxide Kinetics: Ventilation and Metabolism

As mentioned, oxygen uptake across the lung is related to ventilation–perfusion ($\dot{V}/\dot{Q}$) relations and alveolar Po_2. Carbon dioxide excretion, on the other hand, is related to the amount of ventilation. Because CO_2 is much more diffusible than oxygen, and because a small amount of hyperventilation excretes a large amount of CO_2, the limiting factors controlling oxygenation and CO_2 removal are different.

The total amount of CO_2 produced by systemic metabolism is roughly equivalent to the amount of oxygen consumed (100 to 120 mL/m²/min, 200 mL/min in a typical adult). The ratio between CO_2 produced and oxygen consumed is referred to as the *respiratory quotient* (RQ) and varies slightly depending on the foodstuff being metabolized.

CO_2 production is increased or decreased by each of the factors that causes an increase or decrease in Vo_2. Most of the CO_2 in blood is present as bicarbonate ion, which cannot change quickly (somewhat analogous to the total blood hemoglobin or red-cell mass in relation to oxygen). The metabolically produced CO_2, however, is mostly present as dissolved CO_2, added to the blood in the peripheral tissues and excreted in the lung. The relations between CO_2 content, bicarbonate, and dissolved CO_2 are shown in

Figure 9-5. Notice that the AVO_2 difference for CO_2 is 4 mL/dL, the same as that for oxygen. In a steady state, the amount of CO_2 excreted through the lung is exactly equal to the amount of CO_2 produced in peripheral tissues. Because the amount excreted is so easily influenced by minor changes in ventilation, however, the assurance of a steady state is particularly important when VCo_2 is measured at the airway. The amount of CO_2 excreted is a function of ventilation of perfused alveoli (ie, the alveolar ventilation per minute). The relation between alveolar ventilation and CO_2 excretion is shown in Figure 9-6.

Pathophysiology of Gas Exchange

The gas transfer in the lung and the causes of hypoxemia are demonstrated in Figure 9-7. Under normal conditions, red blood cells in the pulmonary capillaries become fully saturated, and oxygen dissolves in the plasma, resulting in blood Po_2 of 100 (after coming into equilibrium at the end of a resting expiration) and saturation of 100% (see alveolus A in Fig. 9-7). This equilibration may be disturbed by hypoventilation in relation to perfusion, or $\dot{V}/\dot{Q}$ mismatch; see alveolus B in Fig. 9-7), diffusion block caused

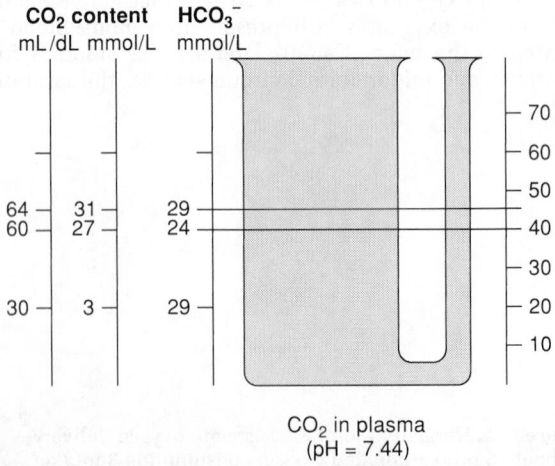

Figure 9-5. A beaker holding CO_2, representing the partitioning of CO_2 between the bicarbonate fraction and the dissolved or carbonic acid fraction in blood. Normal levels for arterial and venous blood are defined. (After Bartlett RH. Post-traumatic pulmonary insufficiency. In: Cooper P, Nyhus L, eds. Surgery annual, 1971. New York, Appleton-Century-Crofts, 1971)

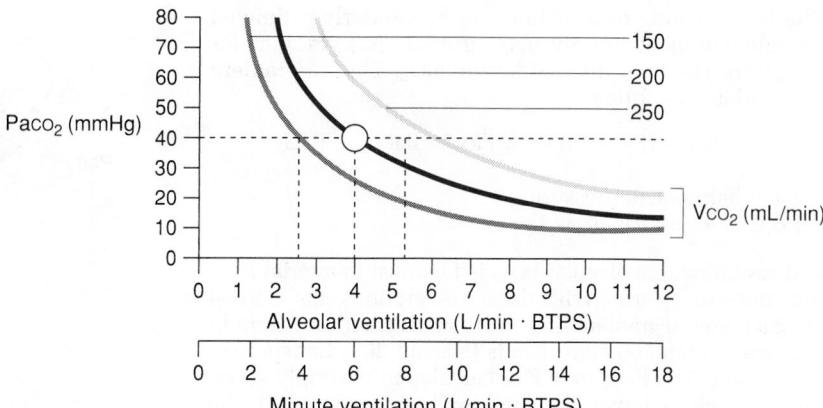

Figure 9-6. Alveolar ventilation required to excrete different levels of metabolically produced CO_2. (Adapted from Nunn JF. Applied respiratory physiology. London, Butterworth, 1969;2:9)

by interstitial fibrosis (see alveolus C in Fig. 9-7), or perfusion of nonventilated alveoli (simply the extreme of hypoventilation; see alveolus D in Fig. 9-7). Diffusion block and $\dot{V}/\dot{Q}$ mismatch can be almost completely overcome by breathing 100% oxygen; thus, hypoxemia during exposure to high alveolar PO_2 is caused by total $\dot{V}/\dot{Q}$ mismatch, called *transpulmonary shunting* or *venous admixture*. Under normal conditions, about 5% of the blood entering the left atrium has been shunted away from the pulmonary capillaries, either as a result of bronchial nutritive blood flow or through thebesian veins opening directly into the left side of the heart. This phenomenon, combined with the normal minor $\dot{V}/\dot{Q}$ mismatch associated with breathing at rest and positional effects on pulmonary blood flow, results in a normal arterial PO_2 of 90 to 100 mmHg and a normal arterial blood oxygen saturation (SaO_2) of 98%.

The extent to which various degrees of transpulmonary shunting affect arterial oxygenation is shown in Figure 9-8. The shunt fraction is actually calculated by assuming that the capillary oxygenation in those alveolar units that are functioning normally is fully saturated and oxygenated. In addition, it is assumed that blood passing through areas of transpulmonary shunt is identical to venous blood. With these assumptions, the fraction of blood passing through the shunt can be calculated as follows:

$$\frac{QS}{QT} = \frac{\begin{array}{c}\text{oxygen content of blood leaving the}\\\text{capillaries of normal alveoli}\\-\text{ oxygen content of arterial blood}\end{array}}{\begin{array}{c}\text{oxygen content of blood}\\\text{leaving normal alveoli}\\-\text{ oxygen content of venous blood}\end{array}}$$

Obviously, the effect of venous blood content on the shunt calculation is considerable; therefore, when oxygen delivery is decreased because of low cardiac output or low hemoglobin concentration, venous saturation falls, increasing the calculated shunt fraction. The shunt fraction can be calculated at any level of the fraction of inspired oxygen (FIO_2), but such a calculation includes components of diffusion block and $\dot{V}/\dot{Q}$ mismatch when FIO_2 is less than 1.

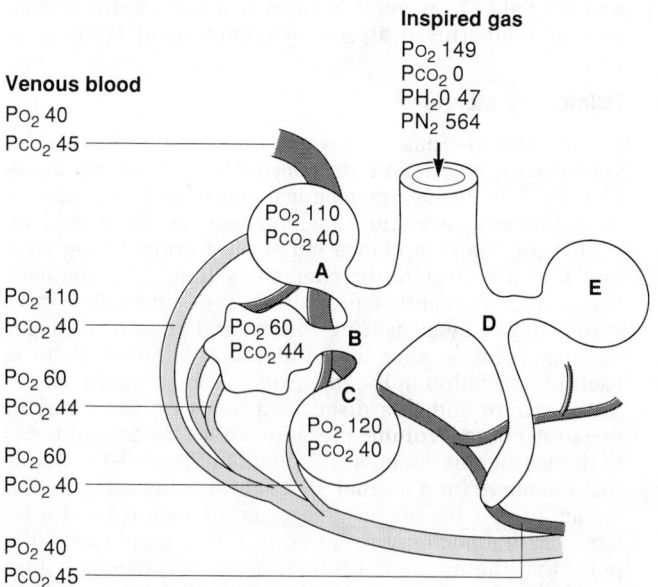

Inspired gas
PO_2 149
PCO_2 0
PH_2O 47
PN_2 564

Venous blood
PO_2 40
PCO_2 45

PO_2 110
PCO_2 40

PO_2 60
PCO_2 44

PO_2 60
PCO_2 40

PO_2 40
PCO_2 45

PO_2 110
PCO_2 40 — A

PO_2 60
PCO_2 44 — B

PO_2 120
PCO_2 40 — C

D   E

Figure 9-7. Variables affecting pulmonary gas exchange while breathing air. In alveolus A, distribution of blood flow and ventilation is equal and normal. The values in the alveolus and the exiting blood represent the end of a normal resting exhalation. Alveolus B represents hypoventilation. Alveolus C represents diffusion block. Alveolus D represents collapsed alveoli or transpulmonary shunt. Alveolus E is ventilated without blood flow. (After Bartlett RH. Posttraumatic pulmonary insufficiency. In: Cooper P, Nyhus L, eds. Surgery annual, 1971. New York, Appleton-Century-Crofts, 1971)

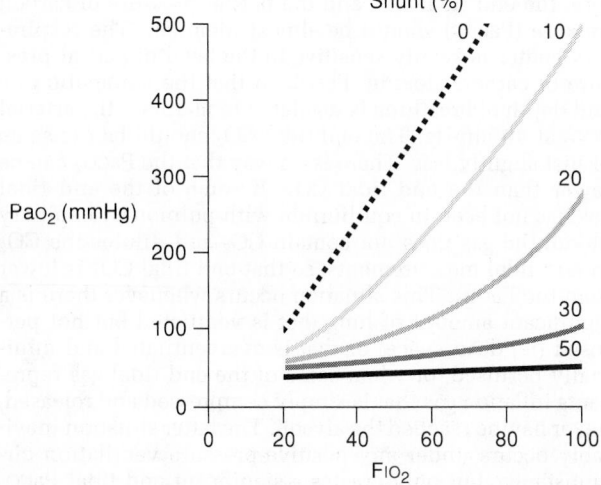

Figure 9-8. PaO_2 achieved at variable levels of FIO_2 at variable levels of shunt. These calculations assume normal hemoglobin and venous saturation of 75%. (After Bartlett RH. University of Michigan surgical critical care handbook. 1991)

The level of lung dysfunction can be similarly estimated by calculation of the alveolar–arterial (Aa) gradient for oxygen or the PaO_2 divided by the FIO_2. The Aa gradient is calculated as follows:

$$AaDO_2 = (P_B - P_{H_2O}) \times FIO_2 - PaCO_2 - PaO_2$$
where:
P_B = barometric pressure
P_{H_2O} = 47 mmHg at 37°C

and assuming that alveolar PCO_2 is identical to arterial PCO_2 (not necessarily true).With these assumptions, the normal alveolar arterial gradient is about 10 mmHg, and an Aa gradient greater than 500 corresponds to about 30% transpulmonary shunt. The PaO_2 over FIO_2 calculation is simply shorthand to characterize the Aa gradient without all the calculations. The normal value is 500, and a value of 100 corresponds to a 30% shunt. Finally, interruption of blood flow to alveoli has no effect on oxygenation, except by diverting blood flow to all the other areas of lung (see alveolus E in Fig. 9-7). If the remainder of the lung is basically normal, then occlusion of pulmonary arteries should have no effect on oxygenation. Patients with pulmonary embolism can become hypoxic, however, because (1) blood flow must increase through areas of $\dot{V}/\dot{Q}$ mismatch and shunting, (2) right atrial pressure increases to the point at which right-to-left shunting occurs through the foramen ovale, or (3) the residence time of red blood cells in pulmonary capillaries becomes so short that the time for oxygenation is inadequate. Of these causes, the latter can be largely corrected with supplemental oxygen, raising the gradient for oxygen diffusion in the pulmonary capillaries.

Carbon Dioxide Transfer in the Lung

The amount of CO_2 excretion is directly related to alveolar ventilation, as discussed earlier. Even if 70% to 80% of the alveoli are not inflated, hyperventilation of the remaining 25% can maintain normocarbia in arterial blood, whereas profound hypoxemia results from 70% to 80% shunt regardless of the level of FIO_2 or ventilation of remaining alveoli. These relations are shown in Figure 9-9, again illustrating that oxygenation is a function of matching blood flow to inflated alveoli, whereas CO_2 excretion is a function of ventilation or hyperventilation of alveoli with some blood flow. Normally, the end tidal CO_2 represents mixed alveolar gas that is in equilibrium with pulmonary capillary blood and hence with arterial blood. Therefore, the end tidal CO_2 and the partial pressure of carbon dioxide ($PaCO_2$) should be almost identical. The respiratory center is keenly sensitive to the level of partial pressure of carbon dioxide (PCO_2), so that the automatic rate and depth of breathing is regulated to maintain the arterial PCO_2 at 40 mmHg. The end tidal CO_2 should be the same or just slightly less. There is no way that the $PaCO_2$ can be lower than the end tidal CO_2. If some of the end tidal gas has not been in equilibrium with pulmonary capillary blood, the gas does not contain CO_2 and dilutes the CO_2 in end tidal measurements, so that end tidal CO_2 is lower than the $PaCO_2$. This situation occurs whenever there is a significant amount of lung that is ventilated but not perfused (ie, dead space) or that is overventilated and minimally perfused, or when some of the end tidal gas represents inflation gas that is simply compressed and released, never having reached the alveoli. The latter situation inevitably occurs under any positive-pressure ventilation circumstance, but only creates a significant end tidal $PaCO_2$ gradient when peak airway pressures are very high (more than 30 cm H_2O) and when the compression volume is a significant component of each exhaled breath. The end tidal CO_2 measurement, then, becomes a useful continuous

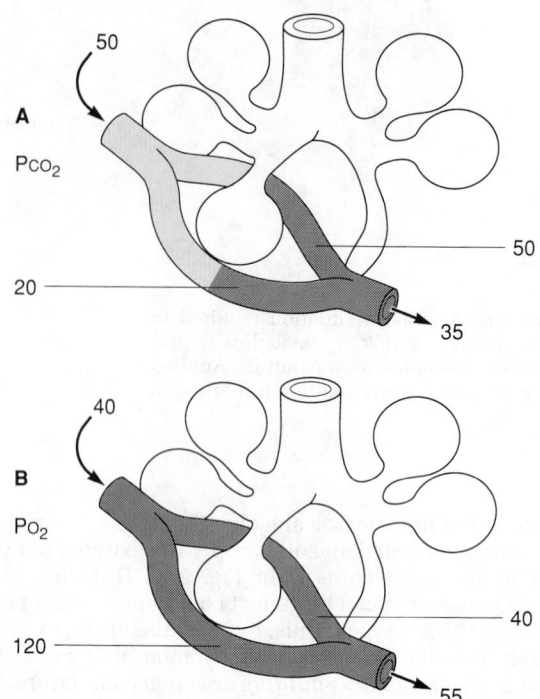

Figure 9-9. The effects of collapsed alveoli (transpulmonary shunt) on oxygen and CO_2 exchange in the lung. (*A*) CO_2 exchange is limited by ventilation or perfused lung. (*B*) Oxygen exchange is limited by blood oxygen uptake in ventilated lung. (After Bartlett RH. Pulmonary pathophysiology in surgical patients. Surg Clin North Am 1980;60:1323)

$PaCO_2$ monitor when the lung is nearly normal, as in ventilator weaning. In addition, the gradient between end tidal and arterial CO_2, when it is large, acts as an indirect measure of nonperfused alveoli or compression volume, or both.

Pulmonary Mechanics

The interrelations of gas volumes and pressures involved with ventilation are referred to as *pulmonary mechanics*. The use of a mechanical ventilator is an exercise in pulmonary mechanics, which may be illustrated by comparing the compliance curve for a normal lung with that for an atelectatic or edematous lung. The standard compliance or volume pressure curve shown in Figure 9-10 is drawn by measuring volume and pressure at stages of lung *deflation* after total inflation. (Although there is useful information in the *inflation* volume pressure curve, the literature and this discussion focus on the standard deflation curve.) Volume pressure curves for normal lungs in three different patients are shown in Figure 9-11. Notice that the curve for a normal 35-kg child is the same as that for an adult with major atelectasis. (It would be similar after pneumonectomy in an adult.) This emphasizes the point that the functional lung in acute respiratory failure is smaller, but not necessarily "stiffer." In the example shown in Figure 9-10, inflation of the normal lung with 500 mL requires 8 cm H_2O pressure, and moves the patient from point A to point B. When the pressure is released, exhalation occurs passively, and lung volume returns to point A. Periodic inflation to 25 or 30 cm H_2O would achieve near-total alveolar inflation without causing overdistention. Each exhaled breath includes gas that is compressed in the ventilator system and compressed in the air space of the lung during ventilation (appearing as addi-

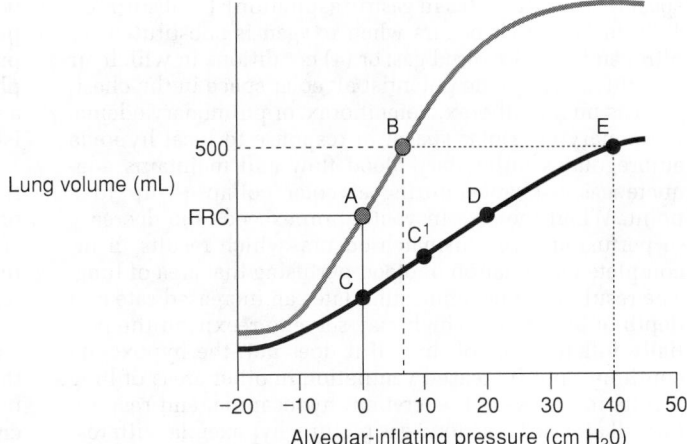

Figure 9-10. Volume pressure (compliance) curves representing a normal lung (points A and B) and an atelectatic or edematous lung (C through E). The functional reserve capacity is decreased (A to C), and more pressure is required for inflation (C to D to E). (After Bartlett RH. Use of mechanical ventilation. In: Holcroft J, ed. Care of the surgical patient. Part 1. Critical care. New York, Scientific American Medicine, 1989;2:9)

tional dead-space ventilation), but this compression volume is small, at the 8 cm H_2O required for normal tidal volume when compliance is normal.

In acute respiratory failure, the cause of decreased compliance is almost always associated with a decrease in the functional residual capacity (FRC; see Fig. 9-10). The decreased FRC represents the lost alveoli, which are either collapsed or filled with fluid but still perfused with blood. Because the lung is smaller, the compliance curve is shifted to the right, and much higher pressures are required to achieve the same level of inflation. To inflate the lung to point E, for example, a pressure of 40 cm H_2O would be necessary. One way of managing ventilation in this circumstance is to maintain positive end-expiratory pressure (PEEP) at 10 cm H_2O (see C^1 in Fig. 9-10) and ventilate to point D with tidal breathing. The PEEP is set at this level to maintain the inflation of alveoli that might close at lower end-expiratory pressures. The elevated peak inspiratory pressure is used to recruit closed alveoli. When that happens, the functional lung is bigger, and the entire compliance curve shifts back toward the left.

Several measurements must be taken to determine whether positive airway pressure is recruiting collapsed alveoli or simply distending normal alveoli (Fig. 9-12). As collapsed alveoli are reinflated, compliance improves, dead-space ventilation decreases, cardiac output is unaf-

fected, oxygenation improves at the same ventilator settings as shunt decreases, and the risk of air leak is minimal. These principles and measurements must be kept in mind during the treatment of the patient on a mechanical ventilator.

Lung damage can be caused by high airway pressure, so that overdistention as shown in Figure 9-12 is not merely inefficient, but actually detrimental. Because the most normal areas of lung have the best compliance, they are the most vulnerable to overdistention, contributing to the steady progression of lung dysfunction in patients ventilated at high peak pressure. Every effort should be made to keep the peak inspiratory pressure under 45 cm H_2O, preferably lower.

Pathophysiology of Respiratory Failure

Regardless of the specific cause, pulmonary dysfunction can be classified under two headings: (1) *alveolar collapse,* partial or complete (ie, decreased FRC); and (2) *pulmonary edema* caused by high hydrostatic pressure, increased capillary permeability, or both.

Alveolar Collapse

Decrease in FRC is caused by incomplete alveolar inflation related to (1) shallow breathing; (2) partial or complete airway occlusion, which can be generalized (as in broncho-

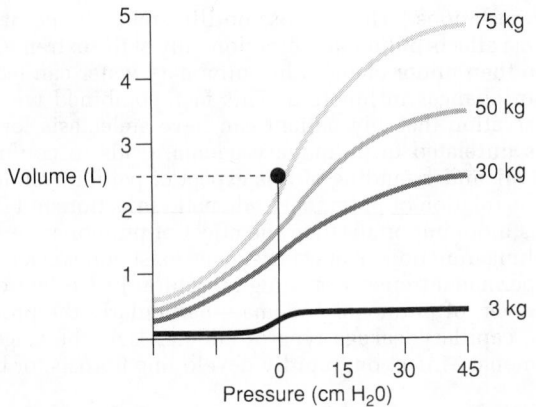

Figure 9-11. Lung volume and pressure in patients of different sizes (or lung volumes of different sizes in an adult patient). The decreased compliance in acute respiratory distress syndrome occurs because lung is smaller, not stiffer.

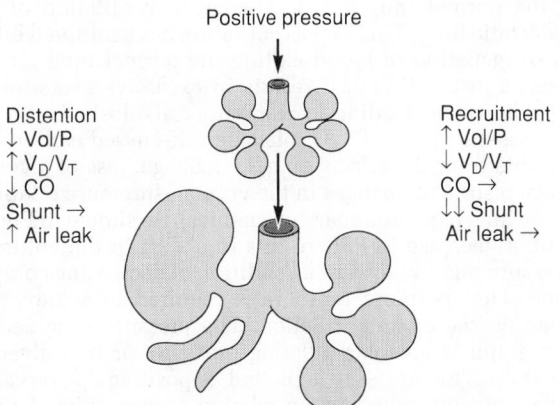

Figure 9-12. During mechanical ventilation, the gas volume might inflate alveoli equally (recruitment) or overdistend selected alveoli (distention). (After Bartlett RH. Pulmonary pathophysiology in surgical patients. Surg Clin North Am 1980;60:1323)

spasm) or localized (as in gastric aspiration); (3) absorption atelectasis, which occurs when oxygen is substituted for nitrogen in the inspired gas; or (4) conditions in which air or fluid is occupying potential alveolar space in the chest, such as pneumothorax, hemothorax, or pulmonary edema. Pulmonary arteriolar spasm in response to local hypoxia autoregulates pulmonary blood flow and maintains adequate gas exchange during alveolar collapse—up to a point. When the loss in ventilation exceeds the decrease in perfusion, $\dot{V}/\dot{Q}$ mismatch occurs, which results in incomplete oxygenation of blood perfusing that area of lung. The resultant hypoxemia stimulates an increased rate and depth of breathing, which may serve to reexpand the partially inflated area of lung. If it does not, the hypoxemia continues, but increased ventilation in other areas of lung results in excess CO_2 excretion, hypocapnia, and respiratory alkalosis. This blood gas picture, hypoxemia with respiratory alkalosis, is the most common abnormality of gas exchange in surgical patients and is the hallmark of $\dot{V}/\dot{Q}$ imbalance.

Oxygenation of blood in the poorly ventilated area of lung can be improved by the increasing concentration of oxygen in the inspired gas. As long as the airways are pinhole patent and the alveoli are inflated at all, the hypoxemia of $\dot{V}/\dot{Q}$ imbalance can be reversed by provision of supplemental oxygen. Of course, use of supplemental oxygen treats the symptom rather than the basic cause and may actually make the problems worse by adding to absorption atelectasis, depriving the poorly ventilated area of nitrogen to hold alveoli open. This may lead to total alveolar collapse. In that circumstance, blood perfusing the nonventilated area (transpulmonary shunt) mixes with blood from other areas of the lung, resulting in hypoxemia that does not improve significantly in response to administration of oxygen.

The reasons for this are shown in Figure 9-9. Blood perfusing the atelectatic lung mixes with blood perfusing the more normal lung, resulting in a decrease in oxygenation and an increase in blood CO_2. Increasing the inspired oxygen to 100% may result in a large increase in P_{O_2} in the blood exiting the normal lung. The major increase in P_{O_2}, however, is associated with a small increase in oxygen *content* because the oxygen that raises the P_{O_2} (eg, from 100 to 500) is the small amount dissolved in plasma. The oxygenation of the arterial blood is an average of the oxygen content of blood from the two areas of lung, not an average of the P_{O_2}. Therefore, systemic hypoxia persists regardless of the F_{IO_2}. When this hypoxemic hypercapnic blood reaches the respiratory center, the rate and depth of breathing are increased. This results in hyperventilation of the normal lung but no change in ventilation of the atelectatic lung. This hyperventilation has a minimal effect on oxygenation of blood exiting the normal lung for the reasons just outlined. It results in excessive excretion of CO_2, however, leading to respiratory alkalosis, just as in the lesser degrees of $\dot{V}/\dot{Q}$ mismatch discussed earlier.

Aside from the effects on gas exchange, loss of alveolar space results in changes in the volume–pressure relations in the lung (eg, pulmonary mechanics). As shown in Figure 9-10, a decrease in FRC results in a shift in the volume–pressure relation toward a condition of decreasing compliance. That is, more pressure is required to achieve the same degree of lung inflation. The pressure specified in this graph is alveolar inflating pressure, or transalveolar pressure. This pressure is plotted as positive if it serves to inflate alveoli, whether the relation to atmospheric pressure is positive (as in mechanical ventilation) or negative (as in spontaneous breathing). This method of expressing volume–pressure relations is a standard procedure and appears straightforward. It can become complex, however,

when a patient is breathing spontaneously while positive pressure is applied to the airway. Remember that negative pressure applied to the pleural space through the diaphragm and positive pressure applied to the airway with a ventilator are additive when volume–pressure characteristics are considered.

To measure compliance, the intrapleural pressure and the airway pressure must be measured exactly. In studies of pulmonary physiology, esophageal pressure is often substituted for intrapleural pressure. When the airway is intubated, airway pressure can be measured directly, and with some assumptions about pleural pressure, reasonable estimates of volume–pressure relations can be made. The compliance calculated using such pressures measured in the airway is referred to as *effective compliance*. The normal value is 100 mL/cm H_2O for adults, or 1 to 2 mL/kg/cm H_2O.

Pulmonary Edema

The causes of pulmonary edema are (1) increased hydrostatic pressure (left ventricular failure or gross fluid overload), (2) decreased plasma oncotic pressure (rarely a problem unless the concentration of plasma protein is very low), and (3) increased capillary permeability. When fluid begins to collect in the lung interstitium, it migrates to the loose areolar portions of the lung microanatomy that surround the small bronchioles and pulmonary arteries. Edema in these areas has the effect of narrowing bronchi and increasing resistance in the pulmonary vasculature. This decreases both ventilation and perfusion in the edematous area, but ventilation is often affected more than is blood flow, resulting in a decreased $\dot{V}/\dot{Q}$ ratio, with all of its attendant effects on gas exchange. As more fluid collects in the lung, it may compress alveoli, and eventually floods into the alveoli, further decreasing FRC and ultimately leading to transpulmonary shunting.

The interrelations between lung edema, atelectasis, and gas exchange in postoperative patients are often misunderstood. Significant changes in lung function do not occur until the level of interstitial water is grossly above normal, and at that point, $\dot{V}/\dot{Q}$ mismatch begins. With slightly more transcapillary filtrate, alveolar flooding and shunting occur. With these relations in mind, consider the effect of ventilator treatment: increased airway pressure tends to hold alveoli open, spread out the space available for water accumulation, and overcome the effects of small bronchial occlusion. These effects are observed during minimal edema, right up to the point at which the lung is filled with fluid. This is why positive airway pressure improves gas exchange in pulmonary edema. (Positive pressure does not affect the actual amount of edema in the lung, only its manifestations.) This discussion illustrates the point that edema affects pulmonary function only at the extreme, and even then minor changes in pulmonary water can lead to major changes in function. This fact, combined with the observation that any patient can have atelectasis for reasons unrelated to pulmonary edema, leads to confusion and misunderstanding of this aspect of pathophysiology.

The relation of pulmonary edema to infection and fibrosis is more important than the effect of pulmonary edema on lung function. Atelectasis may exist for weeks with no permanent effects on lung structure. Just a few days, however, of pulmonary edema—particularly the protein-rich, capillary-leakage type of edema—sets the stage for pulmonary infection, rapidly developing fibrosis, or both.

Management of Respiratory Failure

The University of Michigan algorithm for management of severe respiratory failure is shown in Figure 9-13. For purposes of this discussion, *severe respiratory failure* is

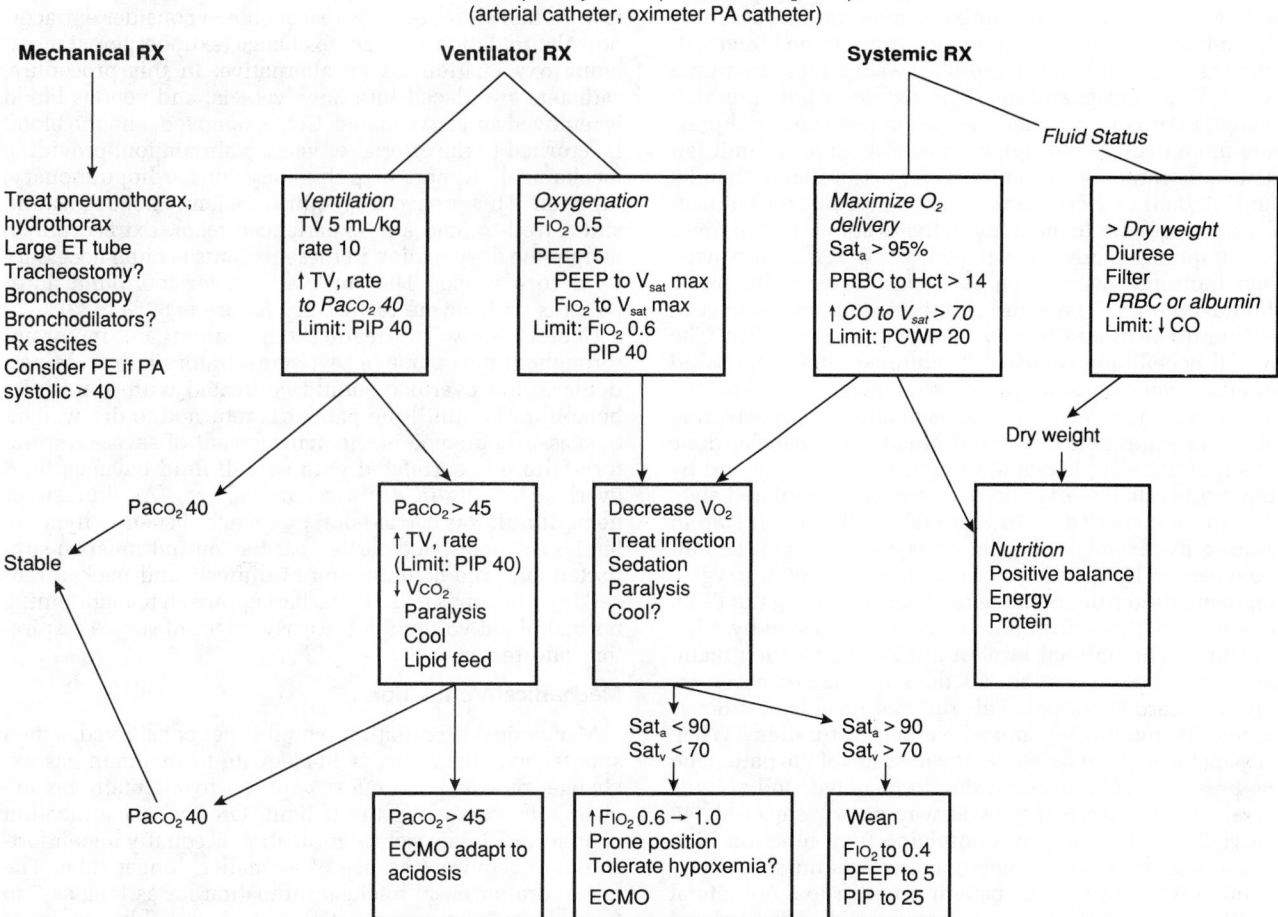

Figure 9-13. Respiratory failure algorithm. ET, endotracheal; PE, pulmonary embolism; PA, pulmonary artery; PEEP, positive end-expiratory pressure; ECMO, extracorporeal membrane oxygenation; PRBC, packed red blood cells; PCWP, pulmonary capillary wedge pressure. (After Bartlett RH. University of Michigan critical care handbook. 1991)

defined as the requirement for intubation, mechanical ventilation, and supplemental inspired oxygen. Although routine ventilator patients can be treated without a pulmonary artery catheter, that device provides essential information for the management of severe respiratory failure, and placement of a pulmonary artery catheter is assumed for purposes of this discussion. Whenever a pulmonary artery catheter is placed, we use a fiberoptic oximeter catheter (Oximetrix), which provides continuous measurement of mixed venous saturation. We do this because most of the important steps in management of severe respiratory failure are based on mixed venous saturation monitoring.

Although the cause of respiratory failure is usually in the lung interstitium and parenchyma, it is important not to overlook simple mechanical causes, such as pneumothorax, hydrothorax, plugged endotracheal tubes, occluded airways, or ascites. Bronchoscopy should be carried out if there is any question of aspiration or if there is any evidence of mucous plugging or impaction in the airways. Although ventilatory management with an indwelling endotracheal tube can be carried out for days or weeks, the incidence of bacterial pneumonia with chronic intubation, the gas flow resistance of endotracheal tubes, and the obligatory linkage of extubation with ventilator weaning all prompt us to recommend tracheostomy rather than chronic intubation for the treatment of patients with severe respiratory failure. Pulmonary embolism should be

considered as a cause of respiratory failure in any patient if the pulmonary artery systolic pressure is greater than 40 mmHg.

Optimizing systemic oxygen delivery in relation to oxygen requirement is the primary goal of management. Improving oxygenation of the blood by improving alveolar inflation is only one of the steps in optimizing oxygen delivery. Equally or more important are treating anemia and optimizing cardiac output. Most patients in the ICU are anemic, and oxygen delivery is maintained by a compensatory increase in cardiac output. This is an acceptable practice because most patients have adequate cardiac reserve to compensate anemia, and because of the potential infectious complications of blood transfusion. Patients with severe respiratory failure, however, are at risk of dying from decreased oxygen delivery (or related multiple organ failure), so that the risk of transfusion is minor compared with the risk of the primary problem. This is complicated by the fact that cardiac output may be compromised in these patients, either by the primary disease or by efforts to increase oxygenation by using airway pressure. Accordingly, oxygen delivery in these patients should be optimized first by maintaining a normal hematocrit. Second, cardiac output should be optimal (not necessarily maximal) to maintain delivery four to five times consumption. In general, this means avoiding situations that decrease cardiac output rather than actively trying to increase cardiac output. This includes keeping the airway pressure as low as possible to maximize venous return, avoiding abdominal distention, maintaining appropriate blood volume based on pulmonary capillary wedge pressure in the range of 15 mmHg, and maintaining blood pressure high enough to provide coronary perfusion (mean arterial pressure more than 50 mmHg), but not so high as to limit left ventricular function (mean arterial pressure more than 90 mmHg). If all of these steps are taken, cardiac output usually autoregulates to maintain delivery at four to five times consumption. If myocardial contractility is inadequate, then inotropic drugs such as dopamine or dobutamine should be used. These drugs, however, increase oxygen consumption in addition to increasing contractility. The overall benefit and titration of inotropes should be based on mixed venous saturation measurements.

Finally, oxygen delivery can be maintained by ensuring adequate saturation of arterial blood. This can be done by supplying supplemental oxygen to the airway and by improving inflation of collapsed or poorly ventilated alveoli. FIO_2 is increased to 50% or 60% as the initial step in treating hypoxemia. Alveolar collapse is treated, as outlined earlier, by cleaning airways, avoiding 100% oxygen, removing fluid from the lung or chest, and using the PEEP to hold open those alveoli that have been opened by other measures. The optimal level of PEEP is that which maintains arterial oxygenation but does not decrease venous return or cardiac output. This optimal level is best determined by monitoring mixed venous saturation. When varying the amounts of PEEP, the position of the patient on the pressure–volume curve should be noted, and volume should be decreased if peak airway pressure exceeds 40 cm H_2O. Another step in optimizing lung function is to take advantage of the gravitational effects on pulmonary blood flow by turning the patient prone or to a full lateral position to direct the blood flow to areas of optimal alveolar inflation. (This steps often result in the opening of closed posterior alveoli that had been compressed by the weight of fluid in the lung.)

At the same time that oxygen delivery is optimized, oxygen consumption should be decreased to normal, or even below normal if necessary. Treating infection, providing adequate sedation, and establishing muscular paralysis decrease oxygen consumption and decrease the need for oxygen delivery. The degree of sedation or paralysis, as with other steps and treatment, is based on mixed venous saturation. If oxygen delivery is still inadequate for metabolic needs despite these measures (ie, venous saturation is less than 60% to 70%), oxygen consumption can be further decreased by actively cooling the patient, realizing that cooling will result in coagulopathy and arrhythmia if the temperature is below 33°C.

Optimizing CO_2 removal is usually an easier step than optimizing oxygen delivery. Ventilator rate and tidal volume are adjusted to achieve normal arterial PCO_2, being careful to avoid peak airway pressure greater than 40 cm H_2O. If $PaCO_2$ exceeds 45 mmHg, the tidal volume, rate, or both are increased until PCO_2 is normal. CO_2 production can be minimized by sedation, paralysis, and treating infection. CO_2 production can be further decreased by avoiding heavy carbohydrate loads in the nutritional regimen and by cooling the patient. If $PaCO_2$ exceeds 45 mmHg despite these measures (and assuming tube or airway occlusion is ruled out), it is permissible to tolerate hypercarbia and achieve acid–base balance with bicarbonate or Tham buffer solution. This step is preferable to going to extremes of airway pressure, which further injures the lung. Some of the other details of mechanical ventilator management are discussed later.

If oxygen delivery or CO_2 excretion is inadequate despite all these measures, the likelihood of patient survival is low. In this situation, it is reasonable to consider extracorporeal circulation with gas exchange (extracorporeal membrane oxygenation) as an alternative. In this procedure, catheters are placed into large vessels, and venous blood is removed and oxygenated, CO_2 is removed, and the blood is returned to the arterial or venous circulation, providing mechanical support of pulmonary (or cardiopulmonary) function. This procedure requires systemic heparinization and a well-trained and experienced team. Extracorporeal membrane oxygenation in these patients is often necessary for 1 to 4 weeks. The survival rate for moribund adult patients with severe respiratory failure is 60% to 70%.

General steps in treating the patient are important throughout the course of severe respiratory failure. In particular, fluid overload should be treated with diuresis or hemofiltration until the patient is returned to dry weight. Successful outcome in the management of severe respiratory failure is correlated with overall fluid balance; fluid overload results in a lower survival rate. As diuresis or hemofiltration is carried out, the patient becomes hypovolemic. As mentioned earlier, cardiac output must be supported, and the combination of diuresis and packed red-cell transfusion is usually the best approach to maintaining normal blood volume in the early stages of severe respiratory failure.

Mechanical Ventilation

Mechanical ventilation should be considered when spontaneous breathing is inadequate to maintain gas exchange, or when the effort required to maintain gas exchange is exhausting the patient. Orotracheal intubation is preferred. Nasotracheal intubation is equally uncomfortable and requires the use of a smaller, longer tube. The use of oral or nasal tracheal intubation for as long as 2 to 3 weeks is common practice but is probably not wise. Aside from the obvious damage to the larynx and discomfort for the patient, the tube enters the sterile airway through the grossly contaminated pharynx. Despite the best attempts at oral hygiene, the posterior pharynx harbors a slurry of virulent organisms that inevitably track down along the endotracheal tube to colonize the airway, if not the alveoli. Tracheostomy is much more comfortable for the patient, offers much lower airway resistance, and, most importantly, avoids contamination of the lower airway. Having been through the phase of favoring chronic intubation, we now prefer early (in 1 to 2 days) tracheostomy for any patient with major respiratory failure.

The ventilator should be set on the assist-control mode at a low sensitivity. In this fashion, the patient breathes at a rate that regulates the $PaCO_2$ to normal, but each breath is mechanically assisted, providing maximal inflation. The volume of each breath is set by limiting the maximal pressure or maximal volume of each breath. Whichever method is used, the peak plateau pressure should generally not exceed 40 cm H_2O. If the patient is comatose or paralyzed, the assist mode cannot be used, and the rate is set in addition to the volume (controlled mechanical ventilation or intermittent mechanical ventilation). The use of the assist mode allows the patient to exercise respiratory muscles while getting the maximal benefit from the invasive endotracheal tube.

Adequate weaning indices are: inspiratory force greater than 20 cm H_2O, vital capacity twice the tidal volume, adequate gas exchange on assisted ventilation at FIO_2 of 0.3 and 5 cm H_2O of PEEP, and minute ventilation less than 10 L/min. Weaning from mechanical ventilation is best accomplished by going straight from the assist-control mode to spontaneous breathing with continuous gas flow (Fig. 9-14). Spontaneous breathing should be associated

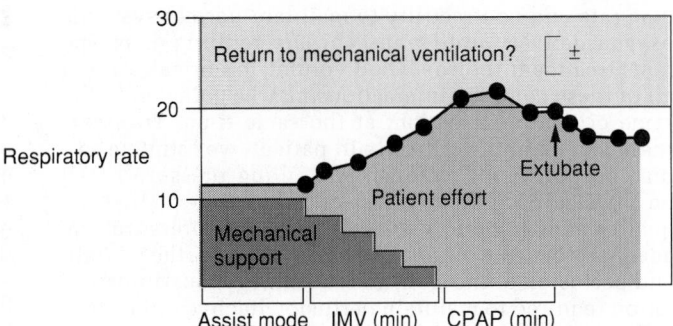

Figure 9-14. Weaning from mechanical ventilation. As mechanical support is decreased, patient effort must increase. If the respiratory rate is high and the tidal volume small, the patient is not ready for extubation. IMV, intermittent mechanical ventilation; CPAP, continuous positive airway pressure. (After Bartlett RH. Respiratory failure: life support systems. In: Bartlett RH, Whitehouse WM Jr, Turcotte JG, eds. Life support systems in intensive care. Chicago, Year Book, 1984:363)

with adequate gas exchange, adequate tidal volume, respiratory rate below 20 breaths/min, and pulse rate less than 120 beats/min. If the patient is hypermetabolic or is receiving excess carbohydrate as nutritional support, the minute ventilation is be elevated, even during assisted mechanical ventilation. If this is the case, the patient tires rapidly on spontaneous breathing, and the primary problem must be treated before attempting ventilator weaning.

Treatment of the Interstitial Space

Treatment of edema has two important goals: the first is to improve oxygenation if it is impaired, and the second is to minimize fibrosis and bacterial infection, which often accompany pulmonary edema caused by capillary injury. (Fibrosis and infection are unusual after hydrostatic edema.) The treatment of interstitial edema is to maintain the hydrostatic pressure as low as is compatible with adequate cardiac output and to raise the oncotic pressure selectively in the vascular space. These measures, combined with fluid restriction and diuresis, decrease the amount of pulmonary edema. Regulating the hydrostatic pressure and cardiac output requires the use of a pulmonary artery catheter and frequent determinations of cardiac output.

Because it is desirable to maintain the filling pressure of the left ventricle as low as possible while maintaining good cardiac output, inotropic drugs to improve left ventricular contractility are helpful. Isoproterenol or dopamine should be used, with serial cardiac output and filling pressure measurements. A Starling curve can be constructed and the optimal combination of filling pressure and inotropic drug determined.

Simple extracellular fluid (ECF) overload may contribute to interstitial edema in the lung. For example, in some centers, it is common practice to infuse 5 to 10 L of salt solution in addition to blood replacement for trauma patients. This is done as an attempt to replace presumed losses into the "third" extracellular space. (The plasma volume and the interstitial fluid are the normal interstitial spaces; the pathophysiologic third space is the transient edema in the area of operation or injury.) The third space expands as long as salt water is poured into the patient, and the difference between what is required and what is actually given is often measured in liters. The fact that most patients tolerate iatrogenic edema does not mean that this is a good practice. If sepsis occurs in an edematous patient, the increased capillary permeability can lead to pulmonary, myocardial, or brain dysfunction.

The first step in decreasing pulmonary edema is to decrease the pulmonary capillary hydrostatic pressure as low as is compatible with adequate cardiac output. This is done by diuresis and fluid restriction. As the patient falls behind in blood volume, signs of hypovolemia may appear. Blood volume is then replenished with a fluid that stays in the vascular space. Packed red blood cells are ideal for this

application. When the hematocrit is normal, concentrated salt-poor albumin should be used. This hyperoncotic fluid replenishes the blood volume by attracting interstitial fluid from throughout the body into the vascular space and supplementing diuresis. This technique is useful even in the septic patient, who may have increased capillary permeability and who may lose albumin from the vascular space at a rapid rate. Even when albumin "leaks out" at a rate three or four times normal, the short-term effects of expanding blood volume and decreasing edema appear. Experience with infusion of albumin solution into patients who are already hypervolemic has led to the mistaken impression that the use of concentrated albumin in the *hypo-*volemic patient may cause problems. On the contrary, it is an efficient way to reexpand blood volume. The use of concentrated globulins would be better yet, but such a preparation is not available. Although furosemide is usually used as the diuretic of choice, mannitol should be mentioned. This drug provides osmotic diuresis as well as a transient plasma hyperosmolarity, "pulling" fluid into the vascular space.

BLOOD VOLUME AND HEMODYNAMICS

Monitoring and management of systemic perfusion is one of the easier aspects of intensive care. In fact, an inordinate amount of attention is paid to blood pressure monitoring and management, sometimes to the exclusion of other, more important parameters, such as oxygen delivery or metabolic rate. This section reviews cardiac physiology and pathophysiology, cardiac function in relation to blood volume and filling pressure, and systemic vascular physiology in the management of hypotension and inadequate systemic perfusion.

Cardiac Function

Cardiac function is regulated by a complex set of baroreceptors and chemoreceptors, which continually adjust cardiac rate, strength of contractility, and ECF volume (by diuresis or antidiuresis), all acting to maintain systemic oxygen delivery at four to five times systemic oxygen consumption. Because normal oxygen consumption is 120 mL/m^2/min and normal arterial oxygen content is 20 mL/dL, normal cardiac output is autoregulated to a level of 3 L/m^2/min. If the rate of metabolism increases or decreases, chemoreceptors readjust the cardiac output proportionately. If arterial blood oxygen content falls because of anemia or hypoxemia, cardiac output increases until normal systemic oxygen delivery is reestablished. If cardiac output drops because of hypovolemia, increased catecholamine secretion results in increased cardiac rate and contractility to maintain normal systemic oxygen delivery until transcapillary refilling or exogenous treatment returns blood volume to normal. Any or all of these complex interactions may be going on in the same critically ill patient at the same time. To assess these factors in the critically ill patient, we estimate cardiac output, blood volume, and filling pressure based on physical examination. Specifically, we examine the quality and numeric values of the pulse pressure, the adequacy of urine output and brain function, the warmth and perfusion of the skin, and the endogenous autoregulation required to maintain perfusion (tachycardia, chest wall cardiac impulse). All of these findings give a reasonable estimation of cardiac output. Examination of the lungs for signs of vascular congestion and examination of the visible veins in the neck for estimation of venous pressure give some determination of filling pressure. Often, these physical findings are adequate to establish a diagnosis and institute management. If this level of monitoring is not satisfactory to solve clinical problems, direct measurement of filling pressure of the right heart (central venous pressure) or the left heart (pulmonary artery pressure) is required. Placement of a pulmonary artery catheter allows measurement of cardiac output by thermodilution and, more important, sampling of mixed venous blood for saturation measurements, which provides the ratio of systemic oxygen delivery to oxygen consumption.

From all these measurements, one can determine whether cardiac output is normal for the level of filling pressure of the left ventricle, or if contractility is decreased. In the latter case, cardiac output is lower than predicted for a given level of filling pressure. These relations are described in the familiar Frank-Starling curve (Fig. 9-15). If measurements indicate that the patient is in the normal range, then myocardial function can be assumed to be normal. If the patient is to the right of the normal range, then cardiac function is compromised because of valvular disease, extrinsic pressure such as paracardial tamponade, or (most commonly) a decrease in contractility.

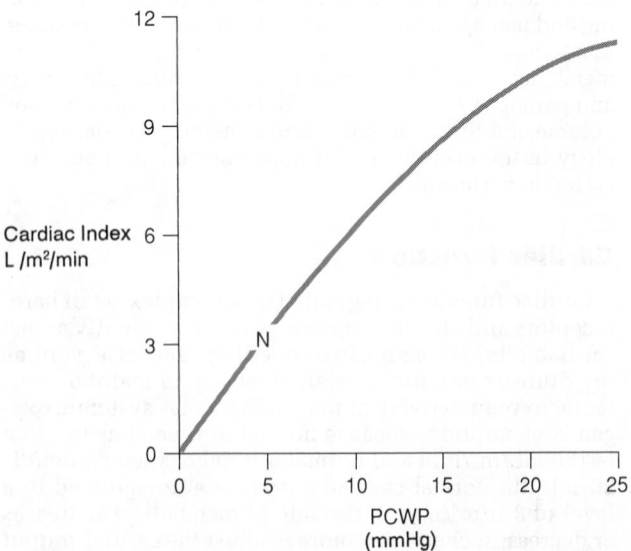

Figure 9-15. Left ventricular function curve (modified from the Frank-Starling curve). N is the normal resting status, and the curve represents normal cardiac output response to changes in filling pressure. PCWP, pulmonary capillary wedge pressure. (After Bartlett RH. University of Michigan critical care handbook. 1991)

Cardiac Function, Blood Volume, and Filling Pressure

The filling pressure described earlier and identified in Figure 9-15 reflects the relation between the cardiac function and the effective blood volume. If cardiac function and anatomy are normal, then blood volume, filling pressure, and cardiac function are related as shown in the normal area of the Starling curve. The intake and output of fluid and salt are autoregulated to maintain the filling pressure of the left ventricle at about 10 mmHg. ECF expansion (generalized edema) is usually associated with a normal blood volume. It is important to remember this fact when considering the critically ill patient with fluid overloaded. Gross expansion of the extracellular space with all the deleterious effects of tissue edema can and often does exist with perfectly normal blood volume. In other words, a pulmonary capillary wedge pressure of 5 to 10 mmHg does not rule out fluid overload as the cause of pulmonary or gastrointestinal dysfunction, for example. Even a minor decrease in ECF volume, however, leads to antidiuresis as soon as hypovolemia is reflected by decreased atrial filling pressures. Systemic blood pressure autoregulatory mechanisms increase cardiac output to compensate. In the case of bleeding, the change in blood volume is immediate and immediately reflected in these compensatory mechanisms. If the bleeding stops before a critical level of exsanguination occurs, the normal combination of hydrostatic and osmotic forces that control the flow of salt and water at the capillary level results in the net transfer of ECF back into the plasma volume (transcapillary refilling), which restores normal blood volume, albeit with hemodilution.

The fear of critically ill patients developing hypotension and ineffective perfusion, although it may be appropriate, usually results in infusion of intravenous salt and water in quantities that exceed losses. Consequently, most patients in the ICU have edema (worse in areas of injury or inflammation), anemia, dilutional hypoproteinemia, and compensatory increase in cardiac output. In response to anemia, these patients are tachycardic, even though blood volume is normal, filling pressures are normal, and total body ECF is excessive. All of these factors are reflected in the autoregulatory mechanisms designed to maintain systemic oxygen delivery four to five times consumption. If arterial saturation is close to 100%, then cardiac function is normal for that patient if the venous saturation is in the range of 75% to 80%.

Systemic and Regional Blood Flow

All of this discussion has addressed cardiac output as if blood flow were ideally distributed to each of the various organ systems. In fact, this is usually the case. Even in periods of high cardiac output and low cardiac output, the organs that require increased oxygen delivery (ie, blood flow) get the extra blood flow at the expense of other organs that need it less. This autoregulation is based primarily on the maintenance of total systemic vascular resistance as determined by arteriolar tone in all organs throughout the vascular system. Some organs, such as the heart and the brain, maintain constant blood flow over a wide range of inflow pressures. In other organs (such as the kidney), blood flow is more sensitive to arterial inflow pressure (or to state it more accurately, arteriolar resistance regulates organ blood flow in an active fashion). Management of regional or organ-specific blood flow is rarely possible or even considered in the treatment of critically ill patients. Notable exceptions are the use of vasopressin and glucagon to increase or decrease splanchnic blood flow, and the use of hypocarbic alkalosis to decrease cerebral blood flow.

Low doses of dopamine are said to improve selectively renal blood flow, although this phenomenon may be primarily the result of a generalized increase in cardiac output.

In the context of peripheral circulation, the calculation of resistance is a useful shorthand to describe the interrelations of cardiac output and systemic or pulmonary blood pressure, but it is no more than that. It is impossible to measure resistance. Resistance is simply a calculation in which blood pressure is divided by blood flow. The results should be expressed as Wood units, or millimeters of mercury per liter per minute per square meter. It is naive to apply other laws of fluid dynamic physics that are described for flow of newtonian fluids through rigid tubes, and it is ridiculous to convert resistance units to dyne per second per centimeter^{-5}, as if the resulting number will somehow be more accurate. (Multiplying Wood units times 79.9 to express resistance is common practice but has no rationale.) All cardiovascular measurements should be normalized to body weight or body surface area, and this is particularly true of resistance calculations. Cardiac index rather than cardiac output should always be used for resistance calculations to compare each patient to the theoretic norm. For example, imagine a 4-year-old with a blood pressure of 90 over 60 and a well-trained adult 300-pound athlete with a blood pressure of 110 over 80. Both have a normal cardiac index. The calculated systemic vascular resistance based on cardiac *index* is the same for both and is normal. The calculated systemic vascular resistance based on cardiac *output* would be pathologically high in the child and pathologically low in the athlete.

Management of Hypotension and Hypoperfusion

The University of Michigan algorithm for hemodynamics is shown in Figure 9-16. Despite the previous discussion, the first sign that brings hemodynamic problems to the physician's attention is often low blood pressure. If a patient who has low blood pressure or tachycardia, confusion, syncope, or narrow pulse pressure is identified as possibly having inadequate systemic oxygen delivery to meet metabolic needs (ie, shock), the first response is to make some assessment of venous pressure by physical examination. If the venous pressure is high, the problem is presumed to be related to the heart or some mechanical obstruction to blood flow. If venous pressure is low, the problem is presumed to be attributable to hypovolemia or systemic vasodilation. If the patient does not respond to initial simple management, more detailed monitoring is required in the form of a central venous pressure catheter or perhaps pulmonary artery catheter. If this level of monitoring provides a diagnosis, the physician can proceed to appropriate treatment. If signs of inadequate blood flow persist despite treatment based on venous pressure measurement, then transfer to the ICU and direct monitoring of pulmonary artery pressure, saturation, and cardiac output are required.

With pulmonary artery catheter monitoring in place, the physician can determine whether delivery is adequate to meet metabolic needs (ie, venous saturation is greater than 65% assuming that arterial saturation is more than 95%). If delivery is adequate, then no further acute treatment is needed. If delivery is not adequate, then an appropriate blood volume expander should be given until the wedge pressure is greater than 10 mmHg or the central venous pressure is greater than 5 mmHg. The appropriate blood volume expander may be blood, crystalloid, or plasma, depending on the presumed or proven fluid loss that led to hypovolemia.

If, despite adequate filling pressure, cardiac output is still decreased or venous saturation is less than 65%, then the cause is probably related to cardiac function, and appropriate treatment can be undertaken. If mechanical factors are ruled out and contractility is the limiting factor, then inotropic drugs are the appropriate treatment (Fig. 9-17). If cardiac output is high and hypotension persists, the cause may be related to systemic vasodilation (caused by sepsis, paralysis, or vasodilating drugs), or the problem may be metabolic in origin (hypoglycemia, hypocalcemia, or Addison disease). If blood pressure is normal or high and cardiac output is decreased despite adequate filling pressure, then the problem may be systemic hypertension or systemic hypertension combined with decreased contractility. Only in the latter circumstance is the use of systemic vasodilating drugs appropriate.

METABOLISM AND NUTRITION
Metabolic Requirements

The typical expenditures of energy and protein in normal subjects and critically ill patients are shown in Figure 9-18. Protein and energy requirements are continuous. These are met by endogenous sources during fasting or through exogenous treatment (nutrition). Energy expenditure is referred to as the *basal metabolic rate* or the *basal energy expenditure* (BEE). The BEE is properly expressed in joules, the standard unit of energy, but is more commonly and more practically expressed in calories. The BEE decreases with advancing age and varies with sex and body size. It is a function of cellular metabolism, hence of the body cell mass. The BEE is usually estimated from a chart combining age, sex, and body size.

Estimating and Measuring Energy Requirements

The actual metabolic rate of any given patient can be estimated by modifying the predicted basal rate according to the clinical condition. For example, the metabolic rate is decreased by 10% in a starving person and increased by 10% with minor activity. This further estimation of metabolic activity in the resting (as opposed to basal state) is referred to as the *resting energy expenditure*. Trauma, stress, sepsis, and surgical operations are all known to increase the metabolic rate. Several authors have proposed tables or formulas for estimating the metabolic rate depending on the degree of physiologic stress. This amount of energy is most conveniently expressed in calories per day. The metabolic rate is normalized to body surface area; however, the actively metabolizing tissue is the lean body cell mass. Consequently, reporting "per square meter" underestimates metabolism in a fat person and overestimates it in a lean person.

Although most of the studies on nutrition in critical illness have been based on estimated energy expenditure, actual measurement is much more accurate and is becoming an important aspect of critical care management. The most commonly used method of measurement is indirect calorimetry. In this method, the amount of oxygen absorbed across the lungs into the pulmonary blood is measured over a given period of time. Assuming the patient is at a metabolic steady state during this time, the amount of oxygen absorbed across the lungs is equal to the amount of oxygen consumed in metabolic processes. The energy released by oxidation of various food substrates is known from direct measurements, so that the metabolic rate measured in cubic centimeters of oxygen per minute can be converted to calories per hour or per day if the oxygenated

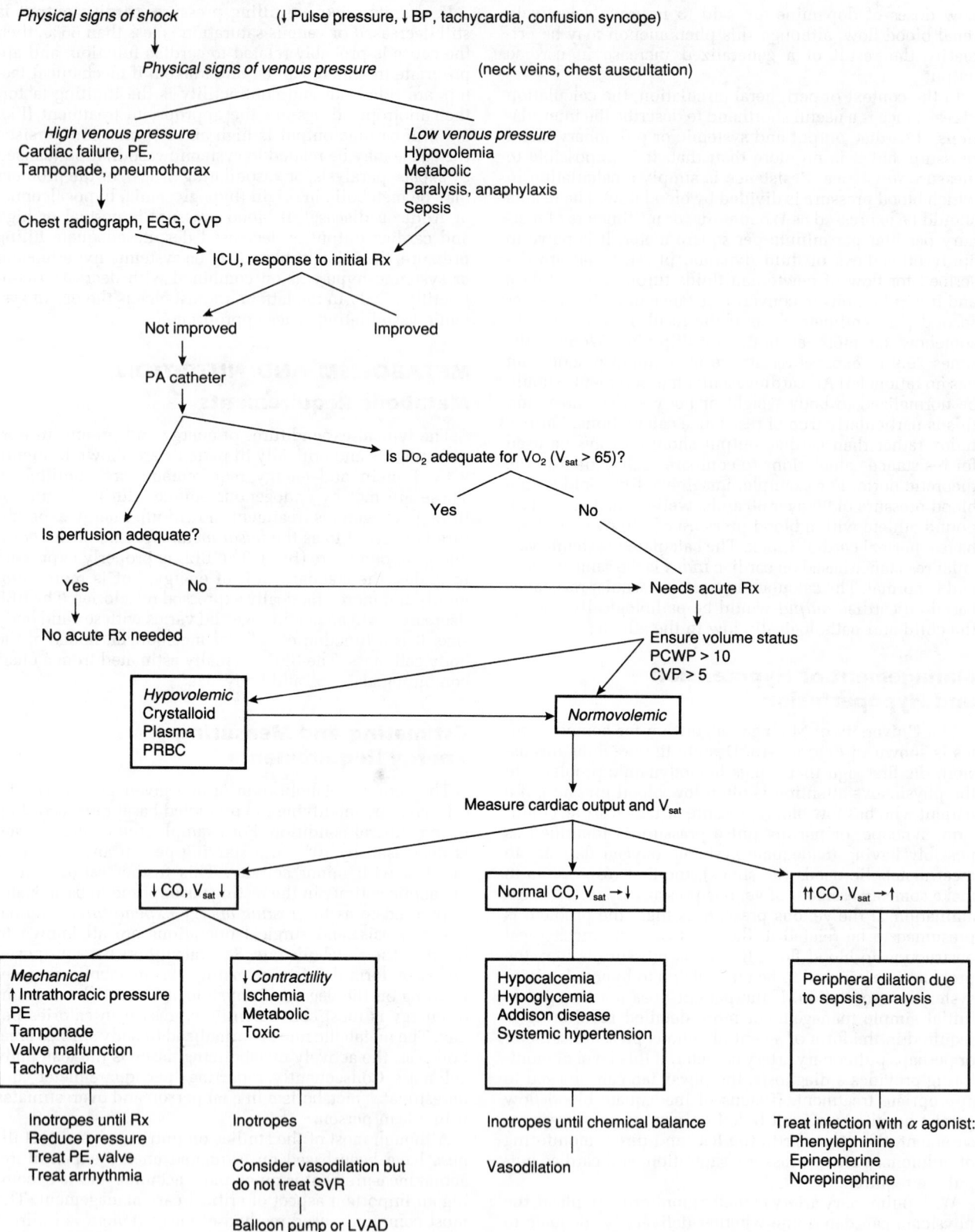

Figure 9-16. Hemodynamic algorithm. (After Bartlett RH. University of Michigan critical care handbook. 1991)

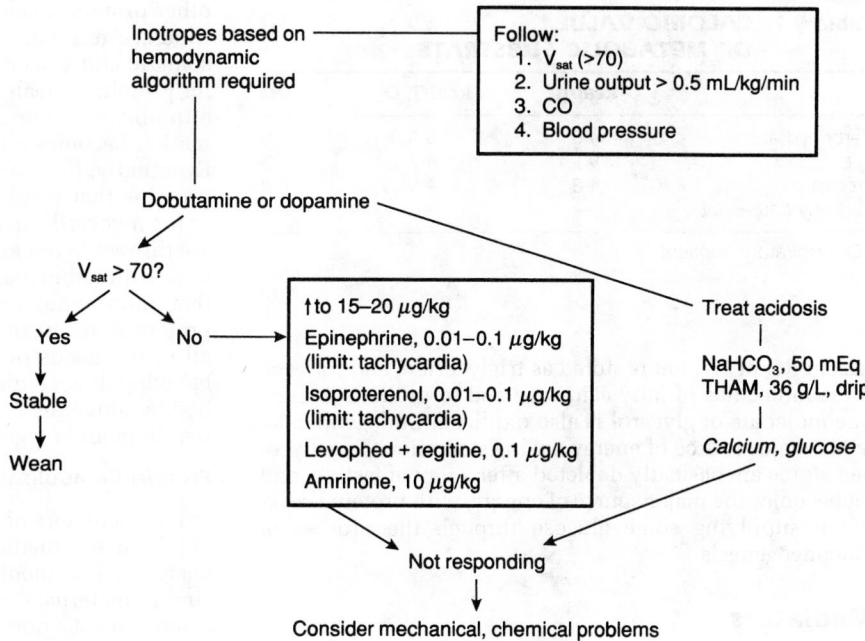

Figure 9-17. Commonly used inotropic drugs.

substrates are known. For practical purposes, a conversion factor of 5 kcal of energy per liter of oxygen consumed is a reasonable approximation. It overestimates the metabolic rate slightly, but it is a much more accurate approximation of the actual metabolic rate than a number derived from an arbitrary chart or table.

Energy Sources

The major sources of energy are carbohydrates (including ketones and alcohols) and fats. Protein can be oxidized through gluconeogenesis and is often a significant source of energy in critically ill patients. The goal of nutritional planning is to supply energy from nonprotein sources, allowing the use of endogenous and exogenous protein for anabolism rather than catabolism. In normal volunteers and surgical patients, protein breakdown is decreased by giving the subject exogenous fuel, be it glucose, fat, or xylitol. This is referred to as the *protein-sparing effect.*

Small amounts of glucose (400 cal/d) provide some degree of protein sparing, but full caloric support is required for maximal effect.

Carbohydrate is the major source of energy during normal, nonstarving existence. The brain, the red cells, and possibly other organs are obligate glucose users. They require glucose as the primary energy source under normal conditions. Other organs also use glucose preferentially as a source of energy. The brain and red blood cells can develop the capacity to use ketones as an energy source, a process called *starvation adaptation.* When fully oxidized, carbohydrate produces 4 cal of energy per gram of substrate, 5 cal of energy per liter of oxygen consumed, and one molecule of CO_2 for each molecule of oxygen consumed. The latter ratio is the RQ, which is 1 for carbohydrate (Table 9-1).

Fat is the most efficient source of energy. Fat produces 9 cal of energy per gram of substrate metabolized, produces 4.7 cal per liter of oxygen consumed in this oxidation, and

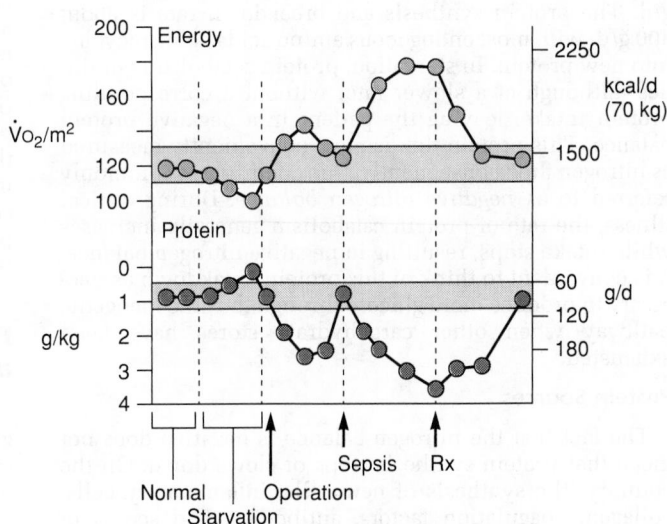

Figure 9-18. Energy and protein metabolism in normal, starving, operative, and septic states. (After Bartlett RH. Nutritional support. In: Dantzker DR, ed. Cardipulmonary critical care. Orlando, Grune & Stratton, 1986:263)

Table 9-1. CALORIC VALUE OF METABOLIC SUBSTRATES

	kcal/g	kcal/L O₂	RQ
Carbohydrate	4.0	5.0	1.0
Fat	9.5	4.7	0.7
Protein	4.8	4.5	0.8
Carbohydrate → fat	—	—	8.0

RQ, respiratory quotient.

has an RQ of 0.7. Fat is stored as triglyceride, and for each three molecules of fatty acid oxidized to produce energy, one molecule of glycerol is also oxidized. Endogenous fat is the major source of energy during starvation. The glycogen stores are basically depleted after a day of fasting, and fat becomes the major source of energy, with protein breakdown supplying some glucose through the process of gluconeogenesis.

Mediators

The mediators of the hypermetabolic state are incompletely understood. Elevated catecholamine levels have been identified in burn patients. Corticosteroids, glucagon, growth hormone, and thyroid hormone have all been implicated as mediators of the hypermetabolic state in various critical conditions. Interleukin-2 causes both hypermetabolism and protein catabolism. Certain amino acids may play a modulating role. Alanine, for example, has easy access into the gluconeogenic pathway, and it has been suggested that protein catabolism is dependent on the amount of alanine produced. Fischer and others have shown that infusing patients with branched-chain amino acids diminishes protein catabolism, and have proposed the use of solutions rich in branched-chain amino acids of patients in catabolic states. Whatever the mediator of the hypermetabolic state is, it appears best to treat the underlying cause while feeding metabolic fuel to the fire rather than attempting to reverse the hypermetabolic state per se.

Protein Metabolism

Estimating and Measuring Protein Requirements

In normal protein metabolism, there is a continuous excretion of nitrogen (mostly as urea) equivalent to about 50 g of protein each day, matched by protein intake of 50 g/d. The protein synthesis and breakdown rate is about 300 g/d, with most endogenous amino acids being recycled into new protein. In starvation, protein catabolism continues (although at a slower rate) without a corresponding protein intake, leaving the patient in a negative protein balance. This protein flux is most conveniently measured as nitrogen flux; consequently, this condition is commonly referred to as *negative nitrogen balance*. During critical illness, the rate of protein catabolism generally increases while intake stops, resulting in negative nitrogen balance. It is convenient to think of this protein breakdown as necessary to produce more glucose through the gluconeogenic pathway when other carbohydrate stores have been exhausted.

Protein Sources

The fact that the nitrogen balance is negative does not mean that protein synthesis stops or slows down. On the contrary, the synthesis of new cells, inflammatory cells, collagen, coagulation factors, antibodies, and scores of other proteins occurs at an accelerated rate during critical illness. Amino acids derived from muscle tissue or other somatic and visceral proteins become the building blocks for protein in healing tissue and host defenses. The site of a traumatic or surgical wound or an area of acute inflammation becomes a protein parasite on other body tissues. Eventually, this parasite may overwhelm the host because proteins that would otherwise strengthen the diaphragm or the myocardium or participate in host defense processes are thrown to the metabolic flames. A large part of the goal of nutritional management is to provide energy sources so that endogenous proteins are not required for energy (ie, protein sparing) and to supply exogenous proteins so that all of the needs of protein synthesis can be met without breaking down endogenous sources. Although oversimplified, a convenient number to remember for basal protein requirement is 1 g/kg/d or 40 g/m²/d.

Protein Catabolism Mediators

The mediators of protein catabolism appear to be different from the mediators of the metabolic rate. Although energy requirement and protein breakdown often follow similar patterns, there are patients who have major protein catabolism at a normal metabolic rate and patients who are hypermetabolic while conserving protein. Tumor necrosis factor is a specific mediator released from monocytes that stimulates endogenous protein breakdown. This follows clinical observations in which the degree of protein catabolism is generally related to the degree of inflammation and (presumed) neutrophil–monocyte activation.

Vitamins and Minerals

Vitamin stores are plentiful, and deficiency states develop slowly, so vitamin loss is not a concern during the early days of critical illness. A hypermetabolic patient catabolizes vitamins more rapidly than normal and can reach a deficiency state sooner. A patient who is severely malnourished before entry to the ICU may already have a vitamin deficiency. There is some evidence that high doses of vitamins A and C may be beneficial to patients with injuries. Because vitamins are inexpensive and safe, we deal with vitamins in the ICU the same way we do in the clinic—prescribe more than enough for the patient who is not eating. Commercial preparations for enteral or parenteral administration provide gross excesses but do not lead to overdose.

Trace metals must be managed more carefully than vitamins because deficiency can occur sooner and overdose can be deleterious. Calcium, phosphorous, magnesium, and sulfur are more than trace elements. They are lost continuously through the urine, stool, gastric juices, and other drainage. Although there are large body stores (particularly of calcium and phosphorous), deficiency can develop rapidly. Enteral and parenteral feeding must include these elements. Serum levels of calcium, phosphorus, and magnesium should be measured at regular intervals. Zinc, copper, chromium, selenium, and manganese must be supplied to patients who are supported with enteral or parenteral feeding for more than 2 weeks.

Endogenous Sources of Energy and Protein

In a normal 80-kg man, about 1000 cal are available as glycogen and other stored carbohydrates. About 140,000 cal are stored as fat. The body contains about 6 kg of protein, which could be consumed as an energy source or maintained to do work. Nutritional assessment is the process of measuring the amount of these energy and protein reserves.

Energy Reserves

The simplest measurement of nutritional status is body weight in relation to body height. Major changes in weight that are not caused by fluid shifts are related to changes in body fat. Energy reserves are generally estimates of body fat because the amount of carbohydrate held in reserve is negligible. The first approach to measuring energy reserve is an estimation of caloric balance. The daily resting energy expenditure is estimated as discussed earlier, and the daily energy intake is estimated from the caloric value of nutrients. The latter estimate is easy for critically ill patients because they usually receive nothing by mouth, with all calories supplied through parenteral or tube feeding routes. A 10,000-cal deficit in a critically ill patient is a severe, acute energy deficit, although this represents only 5 or 6 days of semistarvation. The problem associated with a 10,000-cal deficit is not the loss of a few pounds of fat but rather the associated protein catabolism that is commonly associated with this amount of energy deficit. Fat reserves can be estimated by measuring the thickness of the triceps skin fold or by examining changes in body weight, corrected for fluid balance. Measurement of arm circumference includes both fat and muscle mass. Any of these measurements of body fat is at best a gross approximation.

Protein Reserves

Because protein is the functional and structural chemical of the body, most nutritional assessment techniques are estimates of protein reserves. The creatinine–height index is basically a measurement of creatinine excreted (as a measure of muscle breakdown) normalized for body size. Because muscle is a major source of endogenous protein, muscle wasting is characteristic of the malnourished state. This can be detected by muscle strength and endurance testing. There are few standardized measures of muscle testing that are used as nutritional assessment. One such test is the maximal breathing capacity (also known as the *maximal voluntary ventilation*). In this test, the maximal amount of air that can be moved through rapid breathing over a period of 12 seconds is recorded. The values are expressed as ''percentage of predicted'' for a given age and sex and size (normal is 80% to 120%). In the absence of significant obstructive or restrictive disease, a low value usually indicates lack of muscular strength and endurance. Inspiratory force is another strength test that is easily and commonly done in the ICU. The normal range is 80 to 100 cm H_2O.

The actual nitrogen balance can be measured by measuring the amount of nitrogen excreted. This is most conveniently done by measuring the amount of urea excreted in the urine, assuming that urea constitutes 85% of the total nitrogen excretion. It is better to measure the total nitrogen in urine and other fluid losses because the percentage made up by urea can vary considerably. Knowing nitrogen excretion, the amount of protein catabolized can be estimated and compared with the amount of protein ingested by the patient. Indirect assessments of protein reserves are based on single measurement of body substances that are dependent on rapid protein synthesis for maintenance of normal levels. Conventional serum proteins, such as albumin and globulin, are not affected by malnutrition until it is severe. Proteins such as prealbumin and transferrin, which turn over more rapidly, are better indicators of protein status. Lymphocytes are rapidly destroyed, and protein is required for the formation of new cells. Consequently, the absolute lymphocyte count is a useful measure of the status of protein reserves. The lymphocyte count,

in our experience, is the best single static measurement characterizing nutritional status.

Protein is also required for synthesizing the cells and mediators involved in skin test reactivity. Although skin test reactivity is a manifestation of lymphocyte-mediated immunity, its usefulness in patient assessment is probably assessment of the inflammatory response rather than lymphocyte activity per se. Some chronically and acutely malnourished patients convert from reactive to anergic, and reactivity can be restored by nutritional repletion.

These methods of nutritional assessment are used to classify the nutritional status of patients at the time of injury, operation, or critical illness (Table 9-2). Patients who have both energy and protein depletion at the time of major physiologic stress have higher morbidity and mortality rates than patients with normal nutritional status. In an excellent study, Forse and Shizgal measured body cell mass (the gold standard measurement of nutrition) and found that the depleted state could not be reliably detected based on weight/height ratio, triceps skin fold, midarm circumference, albumin, total protein, hand strength, or creatinine/height ratio. Actual measurements of metabolic rate and nitrogen balance are the best methods of determining nutritional status in critically ill patients.

Energy Balance

Energy expenditure is most conveniently measured through the techniques of respirometry and indirect calorimetry. Respirometry is the process of measuring oxygen consumption and CO_2 production. Oxygen consumption can be measured by direct volumetric change in a closed-circuit rebreathing spirometer system with CO_2 absorber, by the volume and composition of exhaled gas and the composition and volume of inhaled gas, or by measuring the oxygen content of arterial and mixed venous blood and multiplying the $AVDO_2$ by the cardiac output. The latter method requires pulmonary artery catheterization and is complicated by potential errors in each step of the measurements, assumptions, and calculation. Mixed expired gas analysis is the easiest method for normal subjects but is not suitable for patients on supplemental oxygen or on mechanical ventilators because of minor variations in the inspired volume and oxygen concentration during the respiratory cycle. Direct volumetric spirometry is the best method for measuring oxygen consumption. This technique also lends itself well to simultaneous measurement of CO_2 production. With measurement of oxygen consumption and CO_2 production, the RQ can be calculated.

With the RQ, the relative amounts of carbohydrate and fat that are oxidized can be calculated. The RQ for protein is 0.8. By measuring urinary nitrogen, the amount of protein catabolized can be calculated, and the measured RQ can be corrected for the amount of O_2 and CO_2 involved in protein catabolism. For example, if the urinary nitrogen is 0.5 g/h, then protein was metabolized at a rate of 3 g/h, accounting for 3200 mL of O_2 consumed per hour and 2560 mL of CO_2 produced per hour. This nonprotein RQ is used to define the amount of fat or carbohydrate used as energy sources. Ketones have a low RQ (0.6), so ketone metabolism lowers the overall RQ. Conversely, the conversion of glucose to fat generates CO_2, so the RQ of that reaction is more than 1. Measurement of the RQ is helpful as an internal check on the accuracy of the calorimetry measurements and as a guideline to patient management. For example, if a patient has been receiving only 500 cal/d and has a metabolic rate of 2500 cal/d, one would expect that fat use would be maximum, and the RQ should be between 0.7 and 0.8. If such a patient is treated with parenteral nutrition using glucose as the major source of energy, the RQ should be 1 when the caloric replacement matches caloric losses. If the RQ exceeds 1, then some of the infused carbohydrate is being converted to fat, producing excess CO_2 that increases the need for breathing. Hypercaloric feeding with glucose can cause respiratory failure requiring mechanical ventilation, simply by increasing the load of CO_2. Energy balance is helpful because it serves to identify the high-risk patient. In our studies, acutely ill patients with caloric deficits greater than 10,000 cal had a much higher mortality rate than patients with positive caloric balances.

Nutrition Supplies

Energy and Protein

The goals of nutritional therapy in critical ill patients are to maintain a positive nitrogen balance and to avoid endogenous protein breakdown. Exogenous protein can be given through the gastrointestinal tract or parenterally. Parenteral administration is usually done in the form of amino acid solutions, although peptide solutions may be adequate for most conditions.

In the steady state, a 70-kg adult typically consumes 1800 cal and 60 g of protein each day, a ratio of 30 cal/g of protein or 187 cal/g nitrogen. This would be the appropriate amount of nutrients for a patient who is not nutritionally depleted and is not hypermetabolic—a patient on ventilator support for Guillain-Barré syndrome, for example. If the patient is nutritionally depleted but not hypermetabolic (eg, a patient with esophageal cancer being prepared for surgery), the maximal amount of protein that can be "loaded into" the active body cell mass should be given. The actual amount depends on the simultaneous caloric support because a greater degree of positive nitrogen balance can be achieved with a given nitrogen supply when a positive caloric balance is achieved at the same time. In such a patient, it would be appropriate to give 150 g of protein and 2500 cal daily (a ratio of 13 cal/g of protein or 85 cal/g of N). If the bulk of the calories are given as carbohydrate, some of this carbohydrate will be converted to fat, thus producing CO_2 and raising the minute ventilation requirement. A patient who is actively catabolizing protein because of depleted carbohydrate energy stores combined with a hypermetabolic state (eg, a major burn patient) requires an energy supply to match the hypermetabolic losses (eg, 3500 cal in a burn patient who is metabolizing 3000 cal/d). An exogenous supply of energy may slow down or turn off protein catabolism, but it may not, and it is common practice to provide gross excesses of protein to these patients. Such a patient would typically receive 3500 mL of a 4% protein formula, hence 140 g of protein with 3500 cal, or a ratio of 25 cal/g of protein (160 cal/g N).

Methods of Supplying Nutrition

Feeding by mouth is the most efficient way of providing energy and protein and is feasible in many critically ill patients. The possibility of oral feeding is one of several reasons why tracheostomy is preferable to endotracheal intubation for long-term management of patients with acute respiratory failure.

Enteral Feeding.   If the patient cannot or will not take food by mouth, liquid food should be administered directly into the stomach or intestine through a feeding tube.

Enteral feeding can be accomplished by a tube passed directly into the jejunum at surgery or into the duodenum or jejunum at surgery, or by a tube passed into the stomach through the nose or mouth. Soft, small-bore feeding catheters with weighted tips are commercially available, but small bore nasogastric tubes can serve just as well. It is generally possible to accomplish tube feeding with gastric infusion. Patients with gastric ileus, such as patients who have just had abdominal operations, can be fed in the jejunum during the period of gastric atony. Formulas for tube feeding range from milk to commercial preparations. These commercial preparations general have 1 to 2 cal/mL and include 3% to 7% protein. Most of the calories are supplied as glucose or sucrose, so that the solutions have a high osmolarity. Cramps or diarrhea can result when these high-osmolarity solutions are placed into the stomach or intestine. Diarrhea is the major complication with most tube feeding formulations, and it can usually be controlled by adding pectin to the feedings. A large amount of pectin may be required. Diarrhea can also be minimized by the use of starch or fat as an energy source in tube feedings. This can be supplied as part of the commercial preparation or added in the form of medium-chain triglycerides or other oils. The best results are usually achieved by supplying about half of the calories as carbohydrate and half as fat. Although some formulations are advertised as low residue, almost all of the liquid feeding formulas are completely absorbed in the small intestine. Typical formulas are shown in Table 9-3.

Table 9-2. ASSESSMENT OF ENERGY AND PROTEIN STORES

	Excess	Normal	Depletion Mild (kcal)	Depletion Severe (kcal)
Energy reserves				
Cumulative caloric balance	+	0	−5000	−10,000
Triceps skinfold	−	Per table	−5%	−40%
Arm circumference	−	Per table	−5%	−30%
Weight change	−	Variable		−20%
Protein reserves				
Creatinine/height index		Per table	−5%	−30%
Lymphocyte count	>2000	1800/μL	1600	500
Cumulative nitrogen balance	+	0	−30 g	−300 g
Albumin	>3	3 g/dL	2.5	1.5
Total protein	>8	6 g/dL	5.5	4.0
Muscle strength				
Inspiratory force	>100	100 cm H_2O	50	20
Maximal volume ventilation	>120	100% Predicted	60	30
Skin test reactivity		Reactive	Anergic	

Table 9-3. COMPONENTS OF COMMONLY USED ENTERAL FEEDING FORMULAS

Name	Nonprotein Calories			Protein (g)	Osmolarity (mOsm/kg)
	Total	Fat	Carbohydrate		
Milk	565	369	196	33	277
Eggnog	881	297	584	58	480
Isocal	924	396	528	34	300
Ensure	909	333	576	37	450
Vivonex	913	9	904	21	550
Vivonex HN	845	9	844	43	810
Magnacal	1720	720	1000	70	590

Feedings should be given by continuous infusion into the stomach rather than large boluses. It is rarely necessary to give more than 100 mL/h. When possible, the patient should be situated in a sitting position to prevent regurgitation along the tube. Gastric residuals should be checked if the patient feels uncomfortable or appears distended, but it is not necessary to check the residual more than once a day under most circumstances. With continuous tube feeding, a residual of 200 to 300 mL is normal.

It is better to start with a small amount of full-strength formula rather than a large amount of diluted formula. The amount (rather than the concentration) should be gradually increased until the desired volume is reached. Tube feedings can be supplemented by oral intake. Hypernatremia can result if the tube feeding is rich in sodium. This should be managed by the use of low-salt solutions or by the administration of free water. A serious problem with tube feeding is complete cessation of feedings by the nursing staff because of diarrhea or high gastric residual. If the tube feeding needs to be curtailed for any reason, it should be reinstituted the next hour at a smaller volume and gradually increased until the prescribed caloric load is reached.

Parenteral Feeding. Commercial preparations for parenteral feeding are limited to glucose (5% to 45%) and fat (10% to 20%) as energy sources and amino acid or peptide solutions (2% to 10%) as protein sources. Both parenteral and tube feedings are planned so that total energy requirements can be met through fat, carbohydrate, or both. Any protein administered should be available for anabolic processes. Parenteral feeding with carbohydrate is limited by the sclerotic effect of hyperosmolar solutions on veins. Effective parenteral feeding with carbohydrate alone requires solutions of at least 1 cal/mL (25% sugar). This type of solution must be given into an area of rapid blood flow, generally the superior vena cava. Complications still occur, which are discussed later in this chapter. Fat is a more efficient energy source and can be given through peripheral veins in concentrations of either 10% or 20%. The total daily energy requirement can be given as fat, or a major portion can be given as fat with the rest as carbohydrate.

Both fat and carbohydrate are equally effective sources of energy. The fat has the advantage of peripheral administration, the carbohydrate has the advantage of about 10% less expense. The ratio between fat and carbohydrate energy sources and the ratio between total energy sources and grams of protein vary depending on the clinical state. For example, a patient with cardiac failure may require a solution that is low in volume, low in sodium, but high in calories and protein. A patient with multiple intestinal fistulas may require large volumes, allowing less calories and grams of protein per milliliter. Because of the potential problems with central venous cannulation, the administration of 10% glucose, amino acid solutions, and fat through peripheral veins has become popular. Two liters of 10% glucose supply 800 cal, and 500 mL of 20% lipid supply 1000 cal. The total is ample for most patients who are not hypermetabolic.

Any hospital that routinely cares for critically ill patients should have a standardized approach to parenteral nutrition, including vascular access, catheter management, solution preparation, stock solutions, and protocols for the management of risks and complications. The standard solution for total parenteral nutrition is made by mixing equal amounts of 50% glucose and 9% amino acids. This solution contains the equivalent of 1 carbohydrate calorie per milliliter at a ratio of 25 cal/g of protein. The osmolarity of this solution is 1800 mOsm/L, and it must be given into an area of rapidly flowing blood. Insertion and care of the catheter must follow sterile technique. The standard solution can be modified for individual patients by raising or lowering the concentration of glucose and amino acids and by varying the electrolyte and trace metal composition. Vitamins and trace minerals are added to the solution at regular intervals, following the general principle of providing more than basal requirements, as discussed earlier. The standard solution is supplemented with intravenous fat to provide at least 100 g of fat emulsion each week to preclude fatty acid deficiency. We favor giving 25% to 50% of the calories each day as fat emulsion. Fat emulsion is usually given through a peripheral vein, although it can be given

Table 9-4. COMPONENTS OF COMMONLY USED PARENTERAL FEEDING FORMULAS*

	Glucose		Amino Acid (g)	mOsm	Calories: Gram of Nitrogen
	Grams	Calories			
Peripheral vein	100	400	25	880	85:1
Plus 500 mL 10% fat	100	900	25	880	222:1
Standard central	250	1000	45	1750	140:1
Concentrated cardiac	350	1400	45	2250	200:1

* Values per liter of solution.

through a central catheter at the same time as the hypertonic glucose solution. Typical formulas are shown in Table 9-4.

The most common complication of total parenteral nutrition is infection on or around the intravascular catheter. Of course, infection can occur with any indwelling vascular catheter, but it is more likely in the presence of hypertonic glucose and protein solutions. If catheter infection is suspected, the catheter must be removed and a new catheter placed. The second most common complication is hyperglycemia, which is treated with insulin, and by using fat rather than glucose as the primary calorie source. Other complications are largely those of hyperglycemia, that is, hyperosmolar coma, osmotic diuresis, and localized thrombosis. These complications can be caused by running the solution too rapidly. This is prevented by always using a rate-limiting pump when administering hypertonic solutions. The presence of systemic infection is an indication for nutritional support, not a contraindication to placing a central catheter. Other complications are related to disease states and specific amino acids. Aromatic amino acids are neurotransmitter precursors. Symptoms of central nervous system disturbances (confusion, seizures, coma) occur in total parenteral nutrition patients, particularly those with liver dysfunction. These symptoms often cease when amino acid infusion is stopped. A solution low in aromatic amino acids has been proposed for liver failure patients.

Application of Metabolic Economics to the Critically Ill Patient

Nutritional Status Assessment

Whenever possible, patients who are identified as malnourished through the nutritional assessment process listed previously should be returned to normal nutritional status before a major elective operation. Other than this circumstance, however, patients who require hospitalization because of critical illness cannot be nutritionally prepared ahead of time. Each patient admitted to the ICU should be evaluated for nutritional status. Patients who show evidence of malnutrition should be started on a feeding regimen soon after admission (Fig. 19-19).

During the period of critical illness, nutritional and metabolic status should be assessed daily. Although estimation from tables or graphs varies considerably from the actual protein and caloric requirements, estimation is better than nothing. Correlation of daily fluid balance with daily weight is an essential step in evaluating nutritional status during critical illness. Along with daily estimation or measurement of caloric balance, periodic measurement of acute-phase, protein-dependent reactants such as lymphocytes is also helpful. Many patients reach the state of hypoproteinemia in the critical care unit; however, this should never happen if appropriate attention is given to protein and calorie status. The University of Michigan algorithm for management of nutrition in critical illness is shown in Figure 9-20. In our studies, patients who were in a positive caloric balance at the time of ICU discharge had a higher survival rate than patients in a negative balance. In particular, patients with a 10,000-cal cumulative deficit at the time of discharge from the ICU had a high mortality rate.

Energy requirements should be measured, specifically in respiratory failure patients, because overfeeding with carbohydrate results in excess CO_2 production through the conversion of carbohydrate to fat. This positive RQ can require continuation of mechanical ventilation when a patient would otherwise be ready for weaning from the ventilator.

A patient with systemic infection (sepsis) has an elevated metabolic rate and an elevated protein catabolic rate. This patient requires an energy and protein supply to meet these needs. The fact that the patient has a systemic infection should not deter the physician from placing a central venous catheter or whatever access is required for enteral or parenteral feeding.

ACUTE RENAL FAILURE

Acute renal failure (ARF), by definition, is an abrupt decrease in kidney function that results in accumulation of nitrogenous solutes. Urine output in ARF may be oliguric (urine output less than 400 mL/d) or nonoliguric (urine output is normal or increased while solute clearance is markedly decreased; Table 9-5). The mortality of ARF in the surgical ICU is high (50% to 90%) because ARF is usually just one component of severe multiorgan failure. Mortality from nonoliguric ARF is significantly less than from oliguric, although many patients progress to oliguria and its poor outcome. Regardless of urine output, the sequelae of ARF result from retention of metabolic wastes and are indicated by a progressive rise in blood urea nitrogen (BUN) and serum creatinine concentrations. Hypervolemia and electrolyte imbalances further complicate management of oliguric ARF.

The pathogenesis of ARF is commonly classified as being prerenal, postrenal, or intrinsic parenchymal disease. This discussion is limited to parenchymal disease.

Parenchymal abnormalities include acute tubular necrosis (ATN), pigment nephropathy (due to circulating myoglobin and hemoglobin), and nephrotoxic agents (various drugs and contrast material). Other causes of parenchymal renal disease, such as acute glomerular nephritis and vasculitis, are not typically responsible for ARF in the surgical patient and are not discussed in this chapter.

Acute Tubular Necrosis

Acute tubular necrosis results from ischemia to the renal parenchyma and is the most common pathologic finding of ARF. Under conditions of diminishing renal blood flow, perfusion of the kidneys is first maintained by vasomotor responses, which dilate the afferent arteriole and constrict the efferent arteriole. As continued hypotension is de-

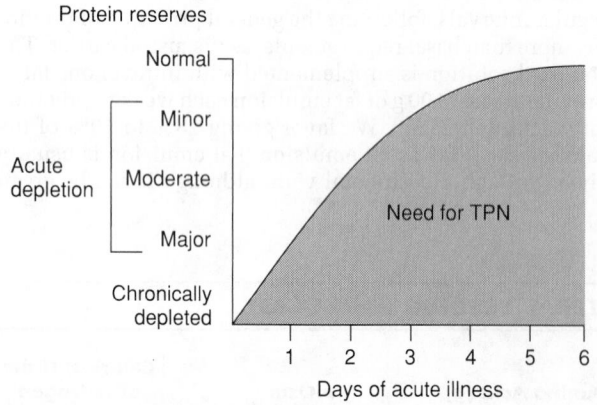

Protein reserves

Figure 9-19. General guidelines for determining when to institute parenteral nutrition after acute illness or operation. Patients at risk for multiple organ failure should be started on total parenteral nutrition (TPN) within 48 hours. (After Bartlett RH. Nutritional support. In: Dantzker DR, ed. Cardiopulmonary critical care. Orlando, Grune & Stratton, 1986:263)

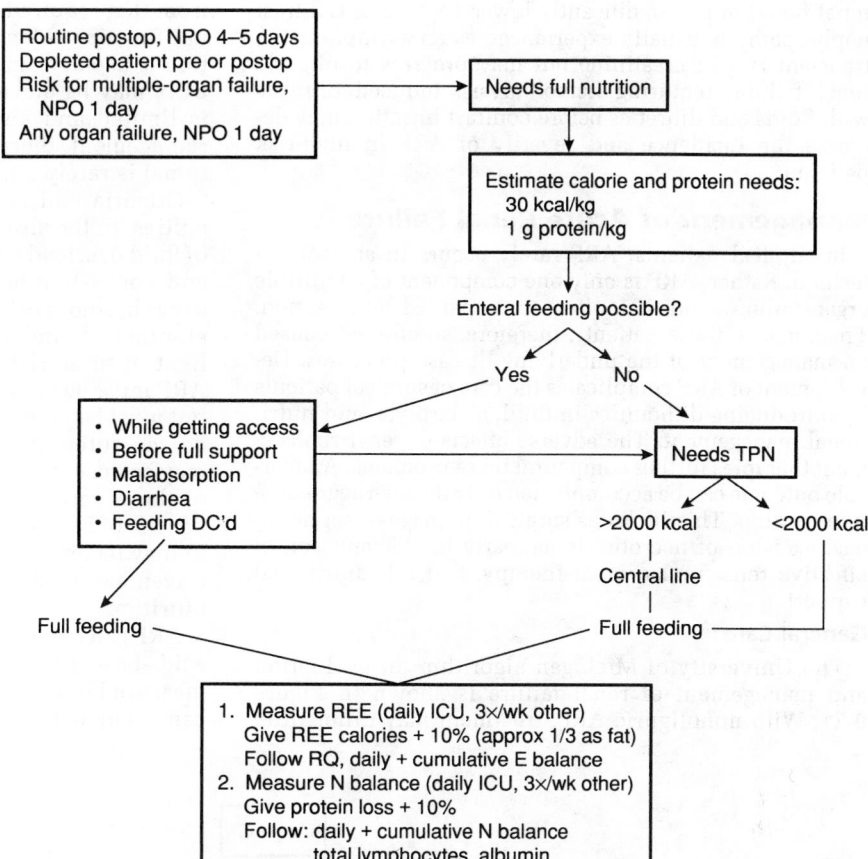

Figure 9-20. Nutritional management algorithm. TPN, total parenteral nutrition; REE, resting energy expenditure; RQ, respiratory quotient. (After Bartlett RH. University of Michigan critical care handbook. 1991)

tected by the juxtaglomerular apparatus, the renin–angiotensin system is activated in concert with sympathetic release of other vasoactive hormones. These substances produce vasoconstriction of the afferent arteriole and further exacerbate cortical hypoperfusion. Casts of cellular debris obstruct the lumen, and cellular edema occurs. As tubular cells necrose and slough off, glomerular ultrafiltrate leaks back across the proximal tubular membrane into the interstitium, causing edema. ATN is a spectrum of cortical ischemic injury ranging from polyuria with tubular dysfunction to temporary anuria to renal cortical necrosis with chronic anuria.

Pigment Nephropathy

Pigment nephropathy is a common cause of ARF and may occur after trauma, burn, operation, or hemodynamic catastrophe. With ischemia or blunt injury to large muscle masses, myoglobin is released to the circulation. In the kidney, it is filtered from blood and reabsorbed by the tubule. Although myoglobin is not a direct nephrotoxin, in the presence of aciduria, myoglobin is converted to ferrihemate, which is toxic to renal cells. Rhabdomyolysis should be suspected in patients with burns, trauma, seizures, alcohol or drug intoxication, prolonged ischemia to muscle groups, and extended coma. Diagnosis can be made with elevated creatine phosphokinase and a urine microscopy study that shows prominent heme pigment without red blood cells in the urine sediment. Hyperkalemia and elevated serum creatinine are also consistent with injury to muscle masses. Prevention of myoglobin-induced ARF may include the use of diuretics and alkalization of urine.

Nephrotoxic Agents

Drug-induced ARF is responsible for about 5% of all cases of ARF. Its pathophysiology differs according to the offending agent. Through normal reabsorption and secretion, the kidney is exposed to high concentrations of drugs and solutes, which may be toxic. This problem is compounded by hypovolemia, which causes increased reabsorption of water and solutes and exposes the lumen to even higher concentrations of toxins. Although the damage to tubular function can be significant, much drug-induced ARF remains nonoliguric because of sparing of glomerular function.

Radiographic contrast dye has been documented to cause ARF. The incidence of contrast nephropathy is about 1% to 10% and may be predicted according to a number of risk factors. These include contrast load, age, preexisting renal insufficiency, and diabetes, although some of these factors are disputed. The incidence in patients with normal

Table 9-5. **STANDARD MEASUREMENTS IN THE DIAGNOSIS OF RENAL FAILURE**

Test	Prerenal	Parenchymal
Urine osmolarity (mOsm)	>500	250–350
U/P osmolality	>1.5	<1.1
U/P creatinine	>20	<10
Urine sodium	<20	>40
FE_{Na}	<1%	>3%

FE_{NA}, fraction of excreted sodium; U/P, urine-to-plasma ratio.

renal function is a significantly lower 1% to 2%. Contrast nephropathy is usually experienced as an asymptomatic, transient rise in creatinine but may progress to oliguric renal failure, requiring hemodialysis. Induced diuresis with fluids and diuretics before contrast injection may decrease the incidence and severity of ARF in high-risk patients.

Management of Acute Renal Failure

In surgical patients, ARF rarely occurs in an isolated fashion. Rather, ARF is only one component of a multiple organ failure syndrome often accompanied by infection. Treatment of these patients, therefore, should be focused on management of the underlying disease processes. Development of ARF complicates the care of surgical patients by introducing difficulties in fluid, electrolyte, and nutritional management. The adverse effects of renal replacement therapies further compound these problems. A favorable outcome can be accomplished only through aggressive intervention. This includes surgical drainage of septic focus, excision of necrotic tissue, early implementation of effective renal replacement therapy, and full nutritional support.

General Care

The University of Michigan algorithm for evaluation and management of renal failure is shown in Figure 9-21. With nonoliguric ARF, treatment may differ little from that required for identical patients with normal renal function. Management of fluids, solutes, and nutrition is usually unaffected by nonoliguric ARF, although BUN may be elevated. The extent of renal dysfunction is limited and almost always reversible. Use of renal replacement therapies (and their inherent complications) is rarely necessary.

Oliguria and anuria pose several management difficulties. In the absence of normal urine output, problems of fluid overload can lead to anasarca, pulmonary edema, and congestive heart failure. The pharmacokinetics of drugs becomes difficult to predict as a result of decreased elimination and increased volume of distribution. In light of these risks, the volume status of patients with ARF must be carefully monitored. Fluid intake and output must be precisely tabulated, and body weight should be measured daily. Pulmonary artery catheterization may be necessary to monitor more closely the fluid status of these patients. Treatment options for hypervolemia consist of fluid restriction or fluid removal with artificial kidney techniques. Fluid restriction, however, limits intravenous medications and may preclude adequate nutrition.

ARF can create severe derangements in electrolyte and acid–base physiology. Serum electrolytes should be measured daily. Of all the electrolyte abnormalities that can occur with ARF, hyperkalemia is the most serious.

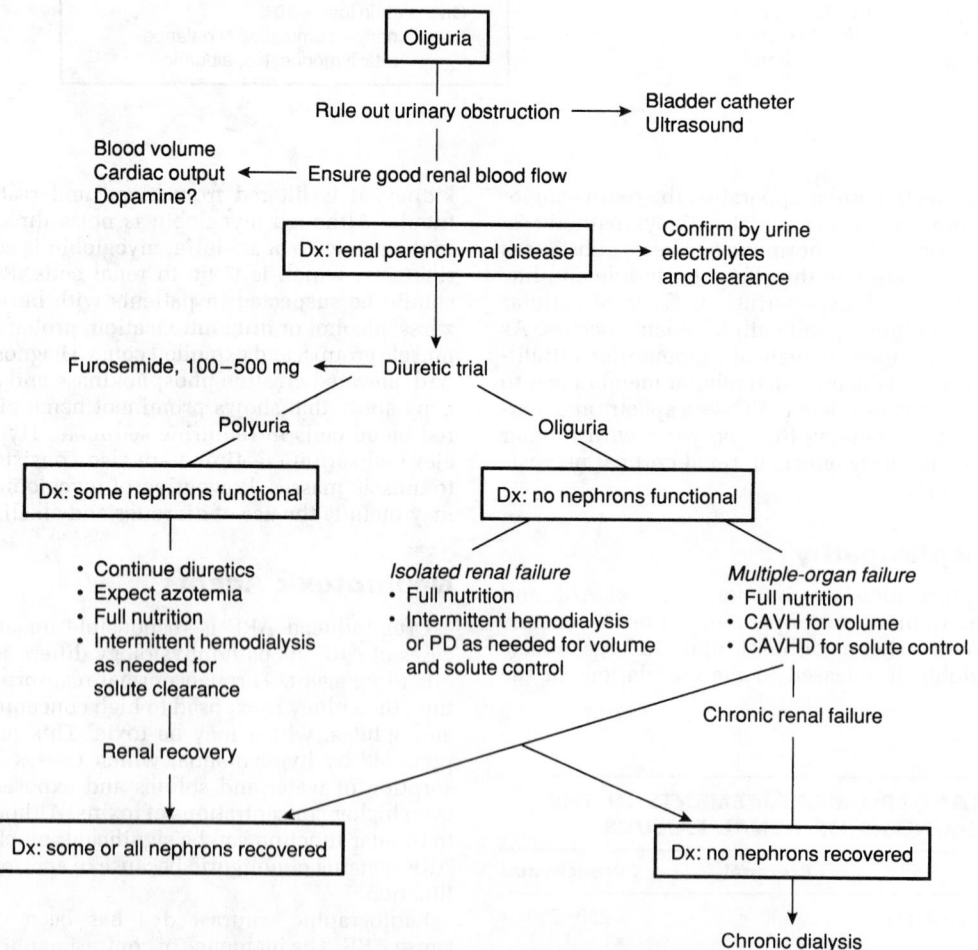

Figure 9-21. Acute renal failure management algorithm. PD, peritoneal dialysis; CAVH, continuous arteriovenous hemofiltration; CAVHD, continuous arteriovenous hemodialysis. (After Mault JR, Bartlett RH. Acute renal failure. In: Greenfield LJ, ed. Complications in surgery and trauma, ed 2. Philadelphia, JB Lippincott, 1989:149)

Under the conditions of hypercatabolism and tissue necrosis that characterize these patients, large amounts of potassium may be generated and may accumulate during a short period of time. Acute hyperkalemia decreases cardiac excitability, which may ultimately result in asystole. Removal of potassium must be accomplished with renal replacement therapy or ion-exchange resins. Other electrolyte abnormalities, such as hyponatremia, hyperphosphatemia, hypocalcemia, and metabolic acidosis, are common with ARF and must be monitored closely. Treatment consists of appropriate additions or restrictions of intravenous solutions and effective use of the artificial kidney.

Platelet dysfunction and coagulopathy are often associated with ARF. A reproducible platelet defect can be demonstrated experimentally with a BUN of 100 mg/dL.

Anemia also accompanies ARF in surgical patients. In addition to blood loss due to hemorrhage or operation, erythropoietin production has been shown to decrease in direct proportion to decreasing renal function.

Nutrition

The goal of nutritional support in ARF is to provide optimal amounts of calorie and protein substrates to minimize autocatabolism and allow tissue anabolism, wound healing, and sustained immune function. In any discussion of nutrition and renal failure, it is necessary to point out the distinction between acute and chronic renal failure. In chronic renal failure, patients are generally healthy and have energy requirements that differ little from those without chronic renal failure. Protein intake is required only for metabolic turnover and is restricted to minimize production of urea generation and other products of protein metabolism.

By contrast, the metabolic requirements of a patient with ARF are those of a critically ill hospitalized patient. Actual measurement of resting energy expenditure has shown that caloric requirements of multiple organ failure patients with ARF are often 50% above those of normal, healthy subjects. Measured protein requirements may be increased to as much as 2.5 g/kg to provide to anabolic wound healing and sustained immune function. For these patients, protein restriction is counterproductive and potentially detrimental. Urea generation is best minimized by providing enough energy substrates (carbohydrates and lipids) to prevent cannibalization of endogenous protein as an energy source. Investigations emphasizing energy and protein balance have demonstrated improvement of outcome from ARF.

Positive energy balance may also make management of uremia and hyperkalemia less difficult. When a patient receives fewer calories than those expended, the difference must be made up from endogenous stores. In a well-nourished person, carbohydrate stores rarely exceed 2500 kilocalories. After this has been depleted, lipid and protein stores are mobilized. In the diseased state, endogenous protein has been shown to be preferentially catabolized as an energy substrate in the absence of readily available glucose. With catabolism of protein, urea is generated. In addition, catabolic wasting of tissues and cells liberates excess potassium. Maintenance of positive energy balance with glucose and lipids should reduce protein catabolism, urea generation, and hyperkalemia.

Although protein restriction may be advocated in chronic renal failure, protein requirements in ARF are usually elevated. Abel and colleagues were among the first to suggest improved survival with addition of amino acids to intravenous nutrition. Others have confirmed these findings. The two important concerns regarding protein supplementation in ARF are what type and how much to administer. The rate of protein catabolism reported in various studies ranges from 70 to 200 g/d. In light of this wide range of protein catabolism, actual measurement of protein balance is desirable. In the oliguric patient, the protein catabolic rate of a patient can be reasonably approximated through calculation of the urea generation rate. In this calculation, changes in BUN and fluid balance are recorded for a 24-hour period. Nitrogen content is also determined from collections of dialysate or ultrafiltrate, nasogastric suction, wound drains, and so on, obtained over the same time interval. Assuming that urea produced by protein catabolism is not reused and that it is contained within the extracellular space, the urea generation rate can be calculated. With this information, daily protein balance can be monitored. Maintenance of positive protein balance is the goal, although this may be difficult to achieve. Most investigators have supplemented protein at a rate of 0.5 to 1 g/kg/d, and the effects of providing larger amounts have yet to be studied.

Much effort has been dedicated to determining the optimum proteins and amino acids to administer to ARF patients. Some contend that a solution of only essential amino acids should be given, whereas others have shown benefit with the use of mixed (essential and nonessential) amino acids. In addition, solutions containing a high ratio of branched-chain amino acids may enhance positive nitrogen balance.

Renal Replacement Therapy

Indications for use of renal replacement therapy include fluid overload (pulmonary edema, congestive heart failure), hyperkalemia, metabolic acidosis, uremic encephalopathy, coagulopathy, and acute poisoning. Three modalities of renal replacement therapy are available for treatment of ARF: hemodialysis, peritoneal dialysis, and continuous arteriovenous hemofiltration (CAVH). The features of each of these therapies are contrasted in Table 9-6 and described next.

Hemodialysis. In the contemporary form of hemodialysis, blood is circulated through a porous hollow-fiber membrane that is permeable to solutes of less than 2000 daltons. An isotonic solution surrounds the membrane that provides a concentration gradient for the selective removal of solutes, such as potassium, urea, and creatinine, while maintaining plasma concentrations of sodium, chloride, and bicarbonate. A roller pump is used to maintain an extracorporeal blood flow of about 300 mL/min through an arteriovenous shunt or a double-lumen venovenous access. The transmembrane pressure gradient created by the pump effects the desired amount of fluid removal. Full systemic anticoagulation is required for this procedure, although less heparin may be used on patients with a baseline coagulopathy. Hemodialysis is typically performed every other day for a 3- to 4-hour period but is required more frequently in catabolic patients with high urea generation rates. Solute and volume removal are considered very efficient with hemodialysis relative to the other methods of renal replacement. This property is reflected in the clearance of water-soluble drugs such as aminoglycosides, cephalosporins, and penicillins. Plasma concentrations may be decreased by as much as 50% per treatment; accordingly, these drugs should be administered on a post-treatment schedule with closer monitoring of serum concentrations. Hemodialysis is also the method of choice for rapid removal of life-threatening toxins and poisons.

Although the incidence of complications from hemodialysis is insignificant in the treatment of patients with chronic renal failure, frequent and often profound complications may occur with its use in critically ill patients with

Table 9-6. COMPARISON OF RENAL REPLACEMENT THERAPIES

	Hemodialysis	**Peritoneal Dialysis**	**CAVH/CAVHD**
Description	Rapid, intermittent	Slow, intermittent	Slow, continuous
Access	Arteriovenous or venovenous	Abdominal catheter	Arteriovenous
Anticoagulation	Required	None required	Required
Solute removal	Excellent	Excellent	Good with standard CAVH; excellent with CAVHD
Fluid removal	Good to excellent	Good	Excellent
Hemodynamic instability	Significant	None	None
Risks of procedure	Hypotension/hypoxemia, dysequilibrium syndrome	Infection or peritonitis; intraabdominal adhesions; respiratory distress	Dehydration; hemorrhage; electrolyte imbalance
Overall appraisal	Useful for urgent removal of solutes or poisons	Contraindicated with abdominal operation	Allows great flexibility with fluid and electrolyte balance
	Hemodynamic instability limits use in intensive care patients	Useful in burn patients and poor vascular access	Solute removal enhanced with CAVHD

CAVH, continuous arteriovenous hemofiltration; CAVHD, continuous arteriovenous hemodialysis.

ARF. In the acute setting, hemodialysis has been shown to cause hypotension, hypoxemia, and hemolysis and to precipitate cardiac arrhythmia. These events limit the application of dialysis in patients in unstable conditions.

Peritoneal Dialysis. Peritoneal dialysis is performed by infusion of several liters of a sterile electrolyte solution with hypertonic glucose into the abdominal space. Using the peritoneal membrane as a selective barrier, the dialysate solution creates an osmotic pressure gradient that extracts ECF and solutes out of the mesenteric circulation and into the peritoneal cavity, which is then drained after an equilibration period of 1 to 2 hours. Extracellular volume removal usually ranges from 0.5 to 1 L/h, although greater fluid and solute clearance can be accomplished by using larger volumes of dialysate and performing exchange cycles more frequently. Use of automated delivery systems makes this a relatively simple procedure with respect to nursing time and training.

Peritoneal dialysis has several advantages over other methods of renal substitution. This technique does not require vascular access or systemic anticoagulation, making it useful in patients with peripheral vascular disease or risk of hemorrhage. In addition, the slow rate of equilibration and fluid extraction with peritoneal dialysis minimizes the problems of disequilibrium and hemodynamic compromise experienced with conventional hemodialysis.

Peritoneal dialysis has many risks and complications, particularly in surgical patients. The most frequent and significant of these complications is catheter infection and peritonitis. Rigid peritoneal catheters inserted percutaneously in the acute setting become predictably colonized after 48 to 72 hours. Subcutaneously placed Silastic catheters are associated with a lower incidence of peritonitis (1.6 episodes per patient-year) and should be implanted with prolonged use of peritoneal dialysis. Other access-related complications include visceral injury at the time of catheter placement and formation of intraabdominal adhesions. In light of these risks, peritoneal dialysis is generally the last-choice method of renal replacement after abdominal operation or trauma.

Other complications of peritoneal dialysis include hyperglycemia secondary to the hypertonic glucose of the dialysate and respiratory distress due to reduced diaphragmatic compliance from increased intraabdominal pressure. Finally, repeated lavage of the peritoneal cavity causes protein loss of 10 g/d or greater and may exacerbate malnutrition in patients with catabolic ARF.

Continuous Arteriovenous Hemofiltration. CAVH was conceived by Kramer and colleagues in 1977 and is specifically intended for treatment of ARF. CAVH is an extracorporeal ultrafiltration technique that removes ECF across a synthetic membrane by means of the hydrostatic pressure gradient created between indwelling arterial and venous catheters. With a systolic blood pressure of 80 mmHg or greater, blood flows through the porous hollow-fiber capillary membrane at a rate of 50 to 150 mL/min, driving plasma water and solutes of up to 10,000 daltons out of the hemofilter at 500 to 700 mL/h. A replacement solution formulated to resemble ECF without toxic solutes is simultaneously infused into the venous access of the circuit at a rate to achieve a desired hourly fluid balance. This exchange transfusion of 12 to 17 L/d of ECF provides clearance of about 10 to 14 g/d of urea (assuming a BUN concentration of 80 mg/dL). Arteriovenous access is accomplished by percutaneous cannulation of the femoral artery and vein with a low incidence of complications. Although full systemic anticoagulation is not necessary for CAVH, heparinization of the extracorporeal circuit is required, usually at a rate of 500 U/h. CAVH is run continuously for as many days as renal replacement is required. Hemofilter performance (as monitored by the ultrafiltration rate) decreases over time, requiring replacement with a new hemofilter about every 2 days. Continuous hemofiltration can also be accomplished by venous drainage with a pump, with return to the venous system.

Experience with CAVH has demonstrated little or no incidence of hemodynamic instability with treatment of unstable critically ill ARF patients. The stable nature of this therapy is attributed to its slow and continuous fluid and solute removal and to the fact that the membrane (polysulfone) does not induce complement activation when in contact with blood.

With ultrafiltration rates averaging 10 to 12 L/d, CAVH also allows great flexibility with volume management and eliminates the need for fluid restriction in patients with oliguric ARF. Fluid balance and serum electrolyte concentrations can be titrated to any value in a matter of hours by manipulating the composition and rate of the replacement solution. CAVH facilitates the ability to provide optimum amounts of nutrition to ARF patients.

Solute clearance with CAVH is limited by the ultrafiltration and replacement fluid exchange rate. In patients with a high urea generation rate, solute removal with CAVH may be inadequate, and variations of the technique may be used to enhance clearance. The most promising of these variations is continuous arteriovenous hemodialysis (CAVHD), which uses the same filter and circuit as CAVH but additionally employs the use of a dialysate bath to increase solute clearing abilities equal to that achievable with standard hemodialysis. In CAVHD, ultrafiltration is diminished to about 150 mL/h, requiring little replacement fluid and thus simplifying the procedure. With either CAVH or CAVHD, complications of dehydration, electrolyte imbalance, and hemorrhage can occur. Accurate tabulation of fluid balance and frequent measurements of serum electrolytes and coagulation indices are necessary.

Guidelines for Renal Replacement Therapy in Acute Renal Failure. The current recommendations for renal replacement therapy in ARF are as follows:

1. Volume (intravenous fluids, total parenteral nutrition, and so on) should be supplemented as needed for the patient, independent of method of renal replacement.
2. Renal replacement therapy should be instituted early in the course of ARF, before hypervolemia, azotemia, or hyperkalemia occurs.
3. For severely ill patients with ARF, CAVH is the renal replacement therapy of choice.
4. If solute clearance is insufficient with CAVH, conversion to CAVHD or supplementation with standard hemodialysis should be done.
5. Peritoneal dialysis may be used when vascular access is unavailable or when risk of hemorrhage is prohibitive.
6. Hemodynamically stable patients with isolated ARF should be treated with intermittent hemodialysis or peritoneal dialysis.

Prognosis

Survival of patients with ARF is a function of the successful treatment of the primary disease from which the renal failure was derived. The anephric patient supported with renal replacement therapy survives until disease of some other organ system supervenes. In a study of patients with "pure" ATN after renal transplantation, Mentzer and colleagues described the mortality rate of ischemic ATN without other organ failure as 6%. By contrast, the mortality rate of multiple organ failure complicated by ARF ranges from 50% to 90%.

In patients who survive the acute phase of illness, recovery of renal function after ARF is dependent on the type and extent of injury to the renal parenchyma. Renal replacement therapy may be required for several weeks until urine output and solute excretion return to acceptable levels. If renal function has not returned after 6 weeks, recovery is unlikely, and provisions should be made for long-term renal substitution therapy.

MULTIPLE ORGAN FAILURE

For this discussion, multiple organ failure is defined as dysfunction of two or more of the six vital organ systems: cardiovascular, respiratory, nervous system, renal, liver, and host defenses. Failure of other organs (eg, skin, coagulation, digestive system) may occur, but these are of secondary importance compared with the major organ systems. A definition of organ system failure is included in Table 9-7.

One of the important contributions from the NIH-sponsored adult extracorporeal membrane oxygenation study was the identification of multiple organ failure as a syndrome and definition of the mortality risk. The 713 patients in that study were selected because they had respiratory

Table 9-7. CRITERIA FOR ORGAN FAILURE*

Cardiovascular	Cardiac index <2.5 L/m²/min with left atrial pressure >10 mmHg
	Inotropic or vasopressor drugs required to maintain adequate perfusion
Respiratory	Alveoloarterial O_2 gradient >300 mmHg
Nervous	Glasgow coma score <10
Renal	Creatinine >3 mg/dL
Liver	Bilirubin >5 mg/dL
Host defenses	Positive blood culture
	Invasive tissue infection
	Anergic to common antigens

* Arbitrary definitions of the University of Michigan Surgical Intensive Care Unit.

failure, and the mortality rate of respiratory failure alone was 40% in patients aged 12 to 65 years. With two organ systems failing, the mortality rate rose to 55%; it was 75% with three organs failing, and 90% with four or more organ systems failing. In a study of isolated acute postoperative renal failure with no other organ systems failing, the mortality rate was 6%. The mortality rate with multiple organ failure including renal failure was 70% to 90%. The failure of the host defense system, defined as locally invasive infection or systemic sepsis, is both a cause and a result of other organ system failure and carries a high mortality risk.

The specific mechanism of organ injury with ischemia is the subject of many other chapters in this book. Understanding the mechanism is of major importance because it may be possible to prevent or delay tissue injury by pharmacologic or mechanical means during periods of ischemia. There is major interest in pharmacologic prevention of tissue injury associated with ischemia using enzyme inhibitors, oxygen radical "scavengers," and other agents discussed in detail in other chapters in this book. The most effective short-term protectant during ischemia is hypothermia. Cooling of organs during the ischemic period of transplantation and cardiac operations has been standard practice for decades. Hypothermia offers protection from ischemic injury for minutes to hours. We rarely take advantage of this phenomenon in the ICU, but the use of moderate hypothermia (with paralysis and anesthesia to avoid shivering) is worthy of investigation as a short-term means of preventing tissue injury. In fact, this is a normal protective mechanism. Any patient in profound circulatory shock rapidly becomes hypothermic.

If a single organ sustains major ischemic injury, then perfusion is reestablished, and other organs may progress through the early phases of tissue injury identified earlier. Specifically, after prolonged ischemia and reperfusion of a leg, for example, generalized capillary leakage is commonly seen. The organs that malfunction when edematous are most obviously affected (the lung, brain, heart, and gut). Tissue edema, however, can be found in kidney, muscle, skin, and all other organs. This suggests that chemical or cellular mediators from the ischemic reperfused tissue are acting to increase capillary permeability throughout the body. The fact that permeability is increased in systemic organs as well as the lungs suggests that the mediator is not microemboli, which would be trapped in pulmonary capillaries, but rather humoral or cellular. A wide variety of mediators have been implicated as the cause of increased capillary permeability, including lysosomal enzymes, by-products of coagulation and fibrinolysis, platelets and the products of platelet activation, white cells and the products of white-cell activation, arachidonic acid metabolites, complement activation, leukocytic cytokines, and superoxide radicals. In addition to these general factors, tissue-specific agents may cause systemic toxicity, such as myoglobin after ischemia to muscle, or bacterial endotoxin after ischemia to gut. The actual mechanism of systemic capillary injury after local ischemia probably includes many or all of these mediators, suggesting that a single pharmacologic approach to prevention is naive.

Clinically, the multiple organ failure patient progresses through well-defined phases. Identification of these phases may help shed some light on the mechanisms of tissue injury with systemic ischemia. After an episode of shock and resuscitation, the phases of multiple organ failure can be described as follows:

Phase I: Generalized increased capillary permeability resulting in edema, weight gain, intravenous volume requirement, and increased protein concentration in urine and lymph. Although the pulmonary microvasculature has been the most thoroughly studied, it is apparent that the lung is the most obvious end organ in a generalized permeability defect.

Phase II: A hypermetabolic state, with increased V_{O_2}; and a compensatory increase in oxygen delivery characterized by tachycardia and high cardiac output. This condition after systemic ischemia and reperfusion is similar to hypermetabolism after endotoxemia, localized sterile inflammation, and infusion of stress hormones, suggesting a common mechanism.

Phase III: Organ malfunction due to localized edema (particularly in the lung and heart) and cellular injury, particularly in the kidney, liver, brain, and host defense system. Hemorrhagic shock predisposes to bacterial translocation and endotoxin absorption from the intestine. The theory that gut bacteria are the cause of systemic hypermetabolism and capillary leakage in shock is an old one that is receiving renewed attention.

Phase IV: In the absence of systemic sepsis, organs may recover to normalcy, or they may be irreversibly damaged, leading to the need for chronic support (eg, of the kidney). If the organ failure phases lead to systemic infection or irreversible tissue damage in the lung or brain, then death of the entire organ is likely.

The management of multiple organ failure is the business of intensive care, only briefly summarized here. The important principles are to avoid further episodes of local or systemic ischemia and to keep the brain viable by pharmacologic or mechanical support of the failing organs until organ recovery occurs.

Respiratory failure is treated by mechanical assistance for lung inflation and ventilation and by decreasing lung edema as much as possible. Airway intubation is usually required, using inflation (PEEP and CPAP) to achieve and sustain alveolar inflation for the purpose of systemic oxygenation, and using mechanical ventilation for the purpose of CO_2 removal. Peak airway pressures greater than 40 cm H_2O are damaging to the lung, and much of the progressive respiratory failure seen in the past decade in ICUs may be iatrogenic barotrauma. There is now good evidence that forced diuresis with negative fluid balance is associated with improved survival in acute respiratory failure.

Cardiac failure is treated with inotropic drugs and with mechanical devices (usually the intraaortic balloon pump) if inotropes are ineffective. Although inotropic drugs are usually titrated to achieve a desired arterial blood pressure, it is more sensible to titrate inotropes to achieve a normal D_{O_2}/V_{O_2} ratio. Pulmonary artery pressure and mixed venous saturation monitoring are essential for intelligent treatment of patients with severe respiratory or cardiac failure.

Adequate nutrition is important for recovery from multi-ple organ failure. Usually the gut is malfunctioning early in this syndrome (ileus), and it is necessary to provide nutrients intravenously. Sugar and fat are given to meet the measured requirements, based on V_{O_2} measurement and the arithmetic of indirect calorimetry. Protein is given to match protein losses, usually in the range of 1 to 2 g/kg/d. Our data indicates that results are improved if nutritional support is begun in critically ill patients within 24 hours of admission into the ICU.

Renal failure is treated by mechanical substitution of renal function. Although hemodialysis and peritoneal dialysis can serve this purpose, each has significant drawbacks in the critically ill, multiple organ failure patient. CAVH and CAVHD are the methods of choice for renal replacement therapy and have totally replaced intermittent dialysis for critically ill patients in our hospital. An important change in the management of renal failure in the last few years emphasizes the need for full nutritional support in these patients (rather than protein and fluid restriction, as had been practiced in the past).

Hepatic failure often occurs as part of this syndrome, and there is no specific treatment. The effects of hepatic failure (coagulopathy, hypoproteinemia, ascites, ammonia intoxication) are treated symptomatically.

Host defense failure (locally invasive or systemic infection) is treated by local drainage, excision, or both whenever possible, with the addition of systemic antibiotics. Despite an incredible proliferation of synthetic antibiotics, sepsis is the final common pathway in most of these patients.

BIBLIOGRAPHY

General

Pre and Post Op Care Committee of the American College of Surgeons, eds. Critical care, vol 1. Care of the surgical patient. New York, Scientific American, 1988.

Bartlett RH. Michigan critical care handbook and critical care physiology. Boston, Little, Brown, 1995.

Oxygen Kinetics

Bartlett RH. A critical carol: being an essay on anemia, suffocation, starvation, and other forms of intensive care, after the manner of Dickens. Chest 1984;85:687.

Cain SM. Oxygen delivery and uptake in dogs during anemic and hypoxic hypoxia. J Appl Physiol 1977;42:228.

Cilley RE, Scharenberg AM, Bongiorno PF, Bartlett RH. Low oxygen delivery produced by anemia, hypoxia and low cardiac output. J Surg Res 1991;51:425.

Fleming A, Bishop M, Shoemaker W, et al. Prospective trial of supranormal values as goals of resuscitation in severe trauma. Arch Surg 1992;127:1175.

Hirschl RB, Heiss KF, Cilley RE, Hultquist KA, Housner J, Bartlett RH. Oxygen kinetics in experimental sepsis. Surgery 1992;112:37.

Russel JA, Phang PT. Oxygen delivery/consumption controversy: approaches to management of critically ill. Am J Respir Crit Care Med 1994;149:533.

Shoemaker W, Appel PL, Kram HB. Hemodynamic and oxygen transport responses in survivors and nonsurvivors of high-risk surgery. Crit Care Med 1993;21:977.

Tremper KK, Barker SJ. Pulse oximetry. Anesthesiology 1989;70:98.

Tuchschmidt J, Fried J, Astiz M, Rackow E. Elevation of cardiac output and oxygen delivery improves outcome in septic shock. Chest 1992;102:216.

White KM. Completing the hemodynamic picture: S_{VO_2}. Heart Lung 1985;14:272.

Hemodynamics

Camm AJ, Garratt CJ. Adenosine and super ventricular tachycardia. N Engl J Med 1991;325:1261.

Fick A. On the measurement of the blood quantity in the ventricles of the heart. Proceedings of the Physiological, Medical Society of Wurzburg, July 9, 1870.

Hansen PD, Coffey SC, Lewis FR. The effects of adrenergic agents on oxygen delivery and oxygen consumption in normal dogs. J Trauma 1994;37:283.

Ognibene FP, Parker MM, Natanson C, et al. Depressed left ventricular performance: response to volume infusion in patients with sepsis and septic shock. Chest 1988;93:903.

Sarnoff SJ. Myocardial contractility as described by ventricular function curves: observations on Starling's law of the heart. Physiol Rev 1955;35:107.

Starling EH. The Linacre lecture on the law of the heart. Given at Cambridge, 1915. London, Longmans, Green, 1918.

Swan HJC, Ganz W, Forrester JS, et al. Catheterization of the heart in man with the use of a flow directed balloon tipped catheter. N Engl J Med 1970;283:447.

Vincent JL, Preiser JC. Inotropic agents. New Horizons 1993;1:137.

Respiration

Arensman R, Cornish JD, eds. Extracorporeal life support. Cambridge, MA, Blackwell, 1993.

Artigas A, Carlet J, LeGall JR, et al. Clinical presentation, prognostic factors and outcome of ARDS in the European collaborative study, 1985-1987: a preliminary report. In: Zapol W, Lamare F, eds. Adult respiratory distress syndrome. New York, Marcel Decker, 1991.

Bartlett RH. Use of mechanical ventilation. In: Holcroft J, ed. Care of the surgical patient, vol 1: critical care. New York, Scientific American Medicine, 1993.

Bartlett RH, Morris AH, Fairley HB, et al. A prospective study of acute hypoxic respiratory failure. Chest 1986;589:684.

Bernard GR, Artigas A, Brigham KL, et al. The American–European consensus conference on ARDS: definitions, mechanisms, relative outcomes, and clinical trial coordination. Am J Respir Crit Care Med 1994;149:818.

Gattinoni L, Bombino M, Pelosi P, et al. Lung structure and function in different stages of severe adult respiratory distress syndrome. JAMA 1994;271:1772.

Gattinoni L, D'Andrea L, Pelosi P, Vitale G, Pesenti A, Fumagali R. Regional effects and mechanism of positive end-expiratory pressure in early adult respiratory distress syndrome. JAMA 1993;269:2122.

Hechtman HB, Weisel RD, Vito L, et al. The independence of pulmonary shunting and pulmonary edema. Surgery 1973; 74:300.

Hickling KG, Walsh J, Henderson S, Jackson R. Low mortality rate in ARDS using low volume, pressure-limited ventilation with permissive hypercapnia: a prospective study. Crit Care Med 1994;22:1568.

Kolobow TA, Moretti MP, Fumagali R. Severe impairment of lung function induced by high peak airway pressure during mechanical ventilation: an experimental study. Am Rev Respir Dis 1987;135:312.

Pelosi P, D'Andrea L, Vitale G, Pesenti A, Gattinoni L. Vertical gradient of regional lung inflation in adult respiratory distress syndrome. Am J Respir Crit Care Med 1994;149:8.

Shanley CJ, Bartlett RH. The management of acute respiratory failure. Curr Opin General Surg 1994:7.

Simmons RS, Berdine GG, Seidenfeld JJ, et al. Fluid balance in the adult respiratory distress syndrome. Am Rev Respir Dis 1989;135:924.

Vasilyev S, Schaap RN, Mortensen JD. Hospital survival rates of patients with acute respiratory failure in the modern respiratory intensive care unit: an international, multi-center, prospective survey. Chest 1995;107:1083.

Nutrition and Metabolism

Bartlett RH, Dechert RE, Mault J, Ferguson S, Kaiser AM, Erlandson EE. Measurement of metabolism in multiple organ failure. Surgery 1982;92:771.

Bessey PQ. Metabolic response to critical illness. In: Wilmore DW, Brennan MF, Harken AF, Holcroft JW, Meakins JL, eds. Care of the surgical patient: critical care. New York, Scientific American Medicine, 1988.

Cahill G. Starvation in man. N Engl J Med 1970;282:668.

Christou NV, MacLean APH, Meakins JL. Host defense in blunt trauma interrelationships of kinetics of anergy and depressed neutrophil function: nutritional status in sepsis. J Trauma 1980;28:833.

Cook DJ, Laine LA, Guyatt GH, et al. Nosocomial pneumonia and the role of gastric pH: a meta analysis. Chest 1991;100:7.

Dudrick SJ, Wilmore DW, Vars HM, Rhoades JE. Can intravenous feeding as a sole means of nutrition support growth in the child and restore weight loss in an adult? An affirmative answer. Ann Surg 1969;169:974.

Kresowik TF, Dechert RE, Mault JR, Arnoldi DK, Whitehouse WM Jr, Bartlett RH. Does nutritional support affect survival in critically ill patients? Surg Forum 1984;35:108.

Moore FA, Moore EE, Kudsk KA, et al. Clinical benefits of an immune-enhancing diet for early postinjury enteral feeding. J Trauma 1994;37:607.

Shizgal HM, Milne CA, Spanier AH. The effect of nitrogen- sparing, intravenously administered fluids on postoperative body composition. Surgery 1979;85:496.

Tryba M. Sucoalfate vs antacids or H2 antagonists for stress ulcer prophylaxis: a meta analysis on efficacy and pneumonia rate. Crit Care Med 1991;19:942.

Renal Failure

Abel RM, Beck CH, Abbot WM, et al. Improved survival from acute renal failure after treatment with intravenous essential L-amino acids and glucose: results of a prospective double-blind study. N Engl J Med 1973;208:695.

Bartlett RH, Bosch J, Geronemus R, Paganini E, Ronco C, Swartz R. Continuous arteriovenous hemofiltration for acute renal failure: workshop summary. Trans ASAIO 1988;34:67.

Bartlett RH, Mault JR, Dechert RE, Palmer J, Swartz RD, Port FK. Continuous arteriovenous hemofiltration: improved survival in surgical acute renal failure? Surgery 1986;100:400.

Geronemus R, Schneider N. Continuous arteriovenous hemodialysis: a new modality for treatment of acute renal failure. Trans Am Soc Artif Intern Organs 1984;30:610.

Kolff WJ, Berk HTJ. Artificial kidney: dialyzer with great area. Acta Med Scand 1944;117:121.

Mault JR, Bartlett RH, Dechert RE, Clark SF, Swartz RD. Starvation: a major contributor to mortality in acute renal failure? Trans Am Soc Artif Intern Organs 1983;29:390.

Mault JR, Dechert RE, Lees P, Swartz RD, Port FK, Bartlett RH. Continuous arteriovenous filtration: an effective treatment for surgical acute renal failure. Surgery 1987;101:478.

Mentzer SJ, Fryd DS, Kjellstrand CM. Why do patients with post-surgical acute tubular necrosis die? Arch Surg 1985;120:907.

Teschan PE, Post RS, Smith LJ, et al. Post-traumatic renal insufficiency in military casualties. Am J Med 1955;18:172.

Fluids and Electrolytes

Brimioulle S, Berre J, Dufaye P, et al. Hydrochloric acid infusion for treatment of metabolic alkalosis associated with respiratory acidosis. Crit Care Med 1989;17:232.

Davenport HW, ed. The ABC of acid-base chemistry, ed 4. Chicago: University of Chicago Press, 1958.

Demling RH, Manohar M, Will JA, et al. The effect of plasma oncotic pressure on the pulmonary micro-circulation after hemorrhagic shock. Surgery 1979;86:323.

Huckabee WE. Abnormal resting lactate. I. Significance in hospital patients. Am J Med 1961;30:838.

Lyons LY, Owns JH, Moore FD. Posttraumatic alkalosis: incidence and pathophysiology of alkalosis in surgery. Surgery 1966; 60:93.

Moore FD. Determination of total body water and solids with isotopes. Science 1946;104:157.

Virgilio RW, Rice CL, Smith DE, et al. Crystalloid vs colloid resuscitation: is one better? Surgery 1979;85:129.

Central Nervous System

Arbit E, Krol G. Coma, seizures and brain death. In: Wilmore DW, Brennan MF, Harken AF, Holcroft JW, Meakins JL, eds. Care of the surgical patient. New York, Scientific American Medicine, 1988.

Griffin D, Fairman N, Coursin D, et al. Acute myopathy during treatment of status asthmaticus with corticosteroids and steroidal muscle relaxant. Chest 1992;102:510.

Kaufman HH, Bretaudiere JP, Rowlands BJ, et al. General metabolism in head injury. J Neurosurg 1987;20:254.

Marion DW. The Glasgow coma scale score: contemporary application. Intensive Care World 1994;11:101.

McGillicuddy JE. Cerebral protection: pathophysiology and treatment of increased intracranial pressure. Chest 1985;87:85.

Teasdale G, Jennett B. Assessment of coma and impaired consciousness. Lancet 1974;2:81.

Watling SM, Dasta JF. Prolonged paralysis in intensive care unit patients after the use of neuromuscular blocking agents: a review of the literature. Crit Care Med 1994;22:884.

Host Defenses

Abraham E. Sepsis: cellular and physiologic mechanisms. New Horizons 1993:1.

Baker JW, Deitch EA, Berg RD, Specian RD. Hemorrhagic shock induces bacterial translocation from the gut. J Trauma 1988;28:896.

Bernard GR, Loose JM, Sprung CL, et al. Hydrocorticosteroids in patients with the adult respiratory distress syndrome. N Engl J Med 1987;317:1565.

Christou NV, MacLean APH, Meakins JL. Host defense in blunt trauma: interrelationships of kinetics of anergy and depressed neutrophil function, nutritional status, and sepsis. J Trauma 1980;20:833.

Clagett P. Hemostasis in surgical patients. In: Miller TA, Rolands BJ, ed. Physiologic basis of modern surgical care. St Louis, CV Mosby, 1988.

Lacroix J, Infante-Rivard C, Jenicek M, Gauthier M. Prophylaxis of upper gastrointestinal bleeding in intensive care units: a meta-analysis. Crit Care Med 1989;17:862.

Pugin J, Aukenthler R, Lew D. Oropharyngeal decontamination decreases incidence of ventilator associated pneumonia: a randomized placebo control double blind clinical trial. JAMA 1991;265:2704.

Rock CS, Lowry SF. Tumor necrosis factor. J Surg Res 1991; 51:434.

Staab DB, Sorensen VJ, Fath JJ, et al. Coagulation defects resulting from ambient temperature-induced hypothermia. J Trauma 1994;36:634.

Weiss SJ. Tissue destruction by neutrophils. N Engl J Med 1989;320:365.

SURGERY: SCIENTIFIC PRINCIPLES AND PRACTICE, Second Edition, edited by Lazar J. Greenfield, Michael W. Mulholland, Keith T. Oldham, Gerald B. Zelenock, and Keith D. Lillemoe. Lippincott–Raven Publishers, Philadelphia, © 1997.

CHAPTER 10

FLUIDS AND ELECTROLYTES AND ACID–BASE BALANCE

RICHARD B. WAIT, KIM U. KAHNG, AND LISA S. DRESNER

A complete understanding of fluid and electrolyte balance is essential for surgeons and for those caring for surgical and other critically ill patients. Only with a thorough knowledge of normal physiologic control mechanisms can one hope to understand the complex pathophysiology of abnormal or disease states. Similarly, an understanding of the techniques used to evaluate and monitor patients must precede any attempt at treatment. This chapter reviews normal fluid and electrolyte physiology as well as acid–base physiology. In addition, the physiologic changes in fluids and electrolytes that commonly take place in response to disease, injury, and surgical therapy are discussed.

The study of body fluids began centuries ago, but our understanding of the complex interactions of the water and electrolyte and nonelectrolyte components that constitute the body fluids has increased substantially in recent decades. With these advances have come more sophisticated studies of the mechanisms regulating the exchange of fluids and electrolytes. To understand how the body's internal milieu is regulated, the basic concepts of fluid compartments, osmosis, and oncotic pressure must be addressed.

TOTAL BODY WATER AND THE FLUID COMPARTMENTS

The total volume of water within the body is termed *total body water* (TBW). The relation between TBW and body weight is relatively constant for any given person and depends on the amount of fat present within the body. Because fat contains little water, TBW as a percentage of body weight decreases with increasing body fat. Using isotopic water dilution techniques (deuterium or tritium), the estimated average TBW in men is 60% of body weight, whereas in women, who typically have more adipose tissue, the estimated average TBW is 50% of body weight.[1] The percentage of body weight accounted for by water also varies with age. In infants, water makes up about 80% of body weight. This value decreases to about 65% by 1 year of age. Throughout adult life, a gradual decrease occurs in TBW content because the amount of fat within the body usually increases with age. Estimates of TBW should be adjusted for very thin or obese patients. In obese patients, estimates of TBW should be decreased by 10% to 20%, whereas in lean patients, estimates should be increased by about 10%.

TBW is distributed within intracellular and extracellular compartments (Table 10-1). Intracellular fluid (ICF) makes up about two thirds of the TBW, or about 40% of body weight. ICF cannot be measured directly but is calculated as the difference between the TBW and the measured extracellular water. Although localized within cells, the ICF is readily exchangeable with the water in the extracellular compartment.

Extracellular fluid (ECF) volume can be measured directly. Methods for these measurements are much less reliable than those used to measure TBW because no substance used for the measurement of extracellular water distributes itself solely into the extracellular compartment. Use of inulin as a measure of extracellular volume yields results that range from 30% to 33% of TBW, or about 20% of body weight (see Table 10-1). The ECF compartment may be further subdivided into the intravascular and interstitial spaces. The intravascular space, which accounts for 25% of the ECF, contains the plasma volume, which is about 8% of the TBW or 5% of body weight. The interstitial water volume can be calculated as the difference between the total ECF and the intravascular fluid; it constitutes about 25% of TBW, or 15% of body weight. The interstitial

Table 10-1. BODY FLUID COMPARTMENTS

Total Body Water	Body Weight (%)	Total Body Water (%)
Total	60	100
Intracellular	40	67
Extracellular	20	33
Intravascular	5	8
Interstitial	15	25

space extends from the blood vessels to the cells themselves and includes the complex ground substance making up the acellular matrix of tissue. Although the water within this space is thought to be freely exchangeable with intravascular, lymphatic, and intracellular water, this water exists in two phases. The free phase contains water that is generally freely exchangeable and in a constant state of flux. The bound or gel phase is composed of water that is closely associated with glycosaminoglycans, mucopolysaccharides, and other matrix components. This water is much less freely exchangeable. An additional ECF compartment, the transcellular compartment, consists of water that is poorly exchangeable under normal circumstances. This fluid is separated from other compartments by both endothelial and epithelial barriers. Included in this category are cerebrospinal fluid, synovial fluid, water within cartilage and bone, fluids of the eye, and the lubricating fluids of the serous membranes. Together, these fluids constitute about 4% of TBW.

Thus, TBW is contained in intracellular, intravascular, and interstitial compartments. These three compartments are in dynamic equilibrium, and alterations in one ultimately lead to compensatory changes in the others.

COMPOSITION OF BODY FLUIDS

Sodium and potassium are the dominant cations within the body. Sodium is primarily restricted to the ECF and potassium to the ICF. Sodium content in the average adult is about 60 mEq/kg. About 25% of this sodium is nonexchangeable because it is confined to bone. Of the exchangeable fraction, about 85% is in the ECF. Small amounts of potassium, calcium, and magnesium make up the remainder of the cations present in the ECF (Table 10-2).

These extracellular cations are electrochemically balanced, primarily by chloride anions as well as by bicarbonate, phosphate, and sulfate ions. Within the plasma, anionic proteins also contribute to ion balance. The interstitial fluid, an ultrafiltrate of plasma, contains little protein. As a result of the Donnan equilibrium, the content of both cations and anions in interstitial fluid is slightly higher than within plasma (see Table 10-2). The Donnan equilibrium describes the unique relation between solutions of permeable and impermeable complex anions when these anions are unevenly distributed across a semiperme-

able membrane. This special type of equilibrium exists between the ICF and ECF because of the high concentration of protein and nondiffusible phosphates within the cell. Interstitial fluid, in contrast, contains little protein. The Donnan equilibrium exists across the capillary endothelial membrane because the concentration of protein is higher on the blood side of the capillary than on the interstitial fluid side. Because of the presence of complex anions, the concentrations of diffusible ions is not necessarily equal across these membranes. As mentioned, potassium is the dominant cation of the ICF. Total body potassium is normally about 42 mEq/kg, and most of this potassium is intracellular and freely exchangeable. Magnesium and sodium ions also contribute to the cationic component of the ICF. These cations are balanced by phosphate and sulfate anions and by bicarbonate and intracellular proteins.

Concentration of Body Fluids

Despite the difference in composition between the ECF and ICF, the overall concentration of water in these fluids is identical. When concentration differences of water occur, they are only transient because water freely equilibrates between compartments. The concentration of water within the fluid compartments depends on the osmotic activity generated by the ion species contained in each compartment.

Osmotic Activity of Body Fluids

Body fluids are aqueous solutions composed primarily of water and contained in the different compartments of the body. For the purpose of simplicity, we consider the fluid compartments to be static, although there is a continuous flux of both water and electrolytes among these compartments. The movement of water depends on a number of physical principles, the most important of which is osmosis. According to the principles of osmosis, if two solutions are separated by a semipermeable membrane (ie, a membrane that is permeable to water but impermeable to electrolytes and nonelectrolyte particles), water moves across the membrane to equalize the concentration of osmotically active particles. In so doing, osmotic equilibrium is achieved.

The osmotic activity across a semipermeable membrane is determined by the concentration of the solutes on each side of the membrane. Traditionally, electrolyte concentrations are expressed as milliequivalents per liter (mEq/L). The concentration of nonelectrolytes is usually expressed in milligrams per deciliter (mg/dL) or grams per deciliter (g/dL). The concentration of multivalent ions such as calcium and magnesium may be expressed as either mEq/L or mg/dL. The movement of water across a semipermeable membrane is based primarily on the number of particles rather than on the molar concentration of the solution, so this measurement is made by dividing the molar concentration of the substance by the number of particles into which it can freely dissociate in water. The unit of measurement for these particles is the osmole (osm) or milliosmole (mOsm). Therefore, when 1 mol of NaCl dissociates in water to Na^+ and Cl^-, it produces 2 osm, whereas 1 mol of a nondissociating molecule, such as glucose, produces 1 osm (1000 mOsm). Osmolarity, measured in mOsm/L, or osmolality, measured in mOsm/kg water, defines the osmotic activity of the particles in solution. Osmolality is measured by freezing-point depression techniques; however, the measured osmolality of a solution may not equal the calculated osmolality if the ions do not totally dissociate. This occurs more frequently as ionic solutions increase in concentration. The osmotic coefficient of a solution de-

Table 10-2. ELECTROLYTE CONCENTRATIONS OF INTRACELLULAR AND EXTRACELLULAR FLUID COMPARTMENTS

	Extracellular Fluid (mEq/L)		Intracellular Fluid
	Plasma	Interstitial Fluid	
CATIONS			
Na^+	140	146	12
K^+	4	4	150
Ca^{2+}	5	3	10^{-7}
Mg^{2+}	2	1	7
ANIONS			
Cl^-	103	114	3
HCO_3^-	24	27	10
SO_4^{2-}	1	1	—
HPO_4^{3-}	2	2	116
Protein	16	5	40
Organic anions	5	5	—

scribes the amount of dissociation of the ions in solution, and it can be calculated by dividing the observed (measured) osmolality by the calculated value:

osmotic coefficient

$$= \frac{\text{observed (measured) osmolality}}{\text{calculated osmolality}} \quad (1)$$

Because cells are bounded by a semipermeable membrane, adding free water to the fluid surrounding a cell causes water to move across the cell membrane to equalize the osmolality differential between the intracellular and extracellular compartments. On a larger scale, adding free water to the ECF of the body causes an immediate expansion of the extracellular space, followed by a redistribution of water into the intracellular compartment (Fig. 10-1A). Similarly, loss of free water from the extracellular space (contraction of the extracellular compartment) ultimately leads to a shift of water from the intracellular to the extracellular space (see Fig. 10-1B). These osmotic forces are not trivial. An osmotic gradient of just 1 mOsm generates a pressure equivalent to 19.3 mmHg. Thus, changes in the osmotic activity of the ECF determine in part the volume of water in the intracellular space. Osmolality defines the concentration of a solution in fluid, and tonicity refers to the effect of a fluid on cell volume.

In contrast to impermeant solutes that are excluded from the intracellular space, such as sodium, permeant solutes such as urea can freely cross cell membranes. Although urea contributes to the osmolality of a solution, it has no effect on the tonicity because it distributes equally across membranes, and as such does not contribute to the osmoles that effect cell volume. Urea is an ineffective osmole. Although hypoosmolar states (dilutional states) are always accompanied by hypotonicity, hyperosmolar states are not always associated with hypertonicity, for example, in the patient with a markedly elevated blood urea nitrogen (BUN) level. Glucose contributes effective osmoles to the ECF, whereas insulin increases the transport of glucose across cell membranes, rendering these osmoles ineffective. In the hyperglycemic diabetic patient, therefore, the elevated glucose level contributes to the hyperosmolality and hypertonicity of the ECF. In response, water shifts from the intracellular space to the extracellular space, causing expansion of the ECF and a decrease in the concentration of plasma sodium. For every 100 mg/dL elevation in blood glucose, measured serum sodium falls 1.5 mEq/L. When insulin is administered, glucose moves into the cells and no longer contributes to the hypertonic state. Water shifts back into the cells, correcting the apparent hyponatremia.

Plasma osmolality (P_{osm}) is an excellent measure of total body osmolality because osmolality differentials between fluid compartments are only transient, with fluid shifts maintaining isosmotic conditions. Because sodium is the predominant extracellular cation, estimates of P_{osm} can be made by simply doubling the serum sodium concentration (serum [Na^+]):

$$P_{osm}(\text{mOsm/L}) = 2 \times \text{serum}[Na^+] \quad (2)$$

Because glucose and BUN may make significant contributions to P_{osm} in certain disease states, this formula is modified for glucose and for BUN:

$$P_{osm}(\text{mOsm/L}) = 2 \times \text{serum}[Na^+] + \frac{\text{glucose}}{18} + \frac{\text{BUN}}{2.8} \quad (3)$$

A number of errors are inherent in this simple calculation, although most of these errors offset each other; thus, the formula has proved to be fairly accurate in most clinical settings. If there is a discrepancy of greater than 15 mOsm/L between the calculated P_{osm} and that measured by osmometry in the clinical laboratory, an osmolal gap exists. This gap may be the result of the presence of osmotically active particles, such as mannitol, ethanol, or ethylene glycol, or of a reduced fraction of plasma water secondary to myeloma proteins or hypertriglyceridemia.

Colloid Oncotic Pressure (Colloid Osmotic Pressure)

Plasma proteins are confined primarily to the intravascular space and contribute to the osmotic pressure developed between the plasma and the interstitial fluid. Normal plasma protein levels of 7 g/dL contribute about 0.8 mOsm/L. The van't Hoff equation can be used to convert osmolality to osmotic pressure:

$$\pi = CRT \quad (4)$$

where:
π = osmotic pressure
C = osmolal solute concentration
R = gas constant
T = absolute temperature

At body temperature, each milliosmole develops a 19.3-mmHg pressure gradient; thus, normal plasma protein concentrations generate a colloid oncotic pressure of 15.4 mmHg (19.3 mmHg × 0.8 mOsm/L). When measured directly, plasma oncotic pressure equals about 24 mmHg. The difference between the calculated and measured pressures is due to the shift in solute particles caused by the pressure of protein anions on one side of a semipermeable membrane (within the intravascular space). This redistribution is explained by the Donnan equilibrium, described previously.

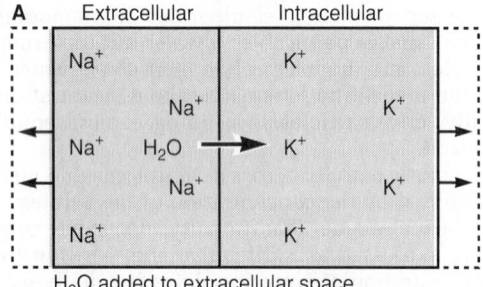

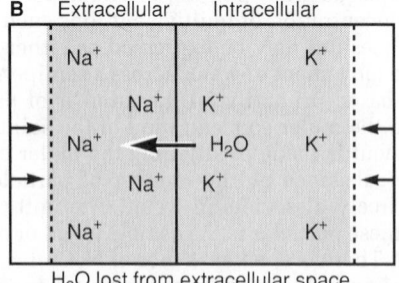

Figure 10-1. (A) The equilibration of water from the extracellular to the intracellular space after the addition of free water to the extracellular fluid compartment. Osmolality transiently decreases within the extracellular compartment, causing water to move across the cell membranes into the intracellular space. (B) Similar shifts after free water loss from the extracellular compartment. Water moves from the intracellular space to the extracellular space in response to the osmal gradient that is established.

Osmoregulation

The body is capable of fine regulation of solute and water concentrations, so that osmolality remains fairly constant at an average of 289 mOsm/kg H_2O. In response to small changes in cell volume, osmoreceptor cells in the paraventricular and supraoptic nuclei of the hypothalamus send signals to the neuronal centers that control the two primary regulators of water balance, thirst and antidiuretic hormone (ADH, arginine vasopressin) secretion. In the presence of excess free water, ECF osmolality falls. As the osmolality approaches 280 mOsm/kg H_2O, thirst is inhibited, and ADH levels decline.[2] In the absence of ADH, the permeability of the renal collecting tubules to water is decreased, and the urine becomes maximally dilute, with urine osmolality (U_{osm}) approaching 100 mOsm/kg H_2O (Fig. 10-2). This causes an increase in free water excretion, and the P_{osm} begins to rise. With water depletion, thirst is stimulated, and ADH secretion is increased as P_{osm} approaches 295 mOsm/kg H_2O. As ADH levels rise into the 5 pg/mL range, the renal collecting tubules become maximally permeable to water. Water is reabsorbed from the collecting ducts in response to the concentration gradient developed in the renal medullary interstitium. Thus, the final concentration of urine depends on both the permeability of the collecting ducts (controlled by ADH secretion) and the concentration of the medullary interstitium. Maximal U_{osm} may approach 1200 mOsm/kg H_2O. The net effect is to decrease dramatically free water excretion and to return P_{osm} toward normal. The high sensitivity of the osmoreceptors, combined with the high gain achieved through the ADH feedback system, ensures that even small changes in P_{osm} result in marked alterations in urine concentration. This relation can be expressed as follows:

$$\text{urine osmolality} = 95 \times \text{plasma osmolality} \qquad (5)$$

A 1-mOsm change in P_{osm}, therefore, results in a 95-fold change in U_{osm}.

In addition to the signals from the hypothalamic osmoreceptors, neural input from baroreceptor regions of the medulla as well as angiotensin II can influence ADH secretion and thirst. Consequently, changes in either osmolality or hemodynamics influence water balance. The response of ADH secretion to changes in pressure is exponential, so that relatively small changes in pressure have little effect, but large decreases in pressure can cause dramatic increases in ADH secretion. In general, changes in osmolality have a much greater effect on ADH secretion than do hemodynamic changes. The changes in ADH secretion elicited by changes in P_{osm} can be profoundly affected by large changes in blood pressure (Fig. 10-3).

Sodium Concentration and Water Balance

Changes in TBW content are reflected by changes in the extracellular solute concentration. Because sodium is the primary extracellular cation and potassium is the predominant intracellular cation, the serum $[Na^+]$ approximates the sum of the exchangeable total body sodium (Na_e^+) and exchangeable total body potassium (K_e^+) divided by TBW:

$$\text{serum}[Na^+] = \frac{Na_e^+ + K_e^+}{TBW} \qquad (6)$$

Because total body solute content ($Na_e^+ + K_e^+$) remains relatively stable over time, changes in TBW content result in inversely proportional changes in serum Na^+ (Fig. 10-4). Thus, abnormalities in serum sodium are an indication of abnormal TBW content.

Effective Circulating Volume

Effective circulating volume is a term used to describe that portion of the extracellular volume that perfuses the organs of the body and affects the baroreceptors. The effective circulating volume normally corresponds to the intravascular volume, but in certain disease states, the two can be substantially different. An example of this is the patient with congestive heart failure in whom the intravascular volume is actually high, while the effective circulating volume is low because of cardiac failure. Similarly, patients with arteriovenous fistulas, either surgically created or re-

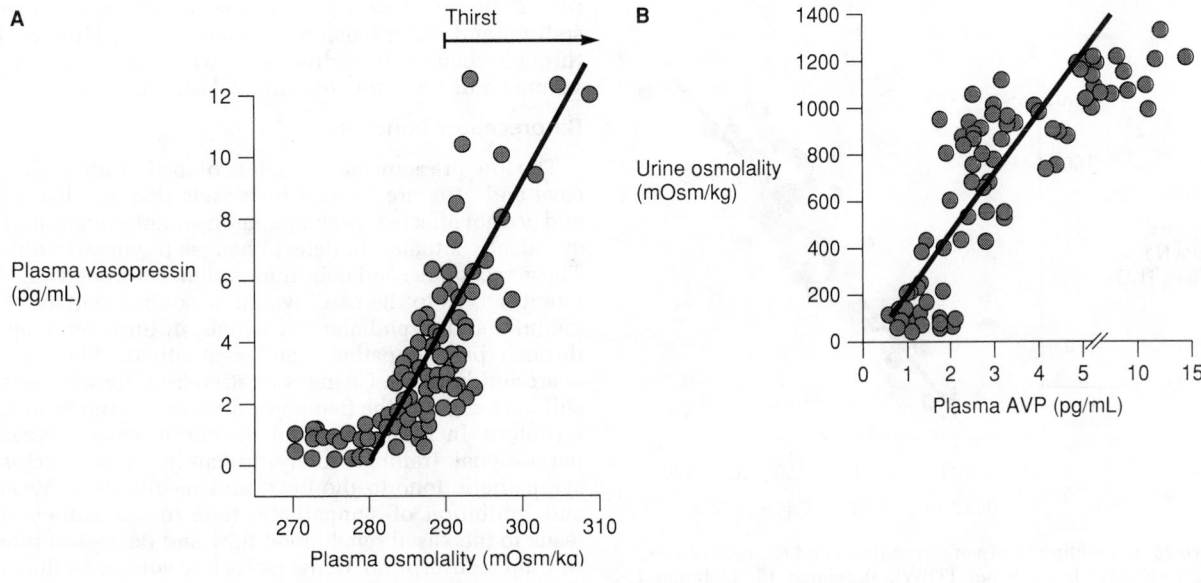

Figure 10-2. The relation of plasma ADH (arginine vasopressin or AVP) secretion to plasma (*A*) and urine (*B*) osmolality in healthy adults in varying states of water balance. (Robertson GL, Berl T. Water metabolism. In: Brenner BM, Rector FC Jr, eds. The kidney. Philadelphia, WB Saunders, 1986:392)

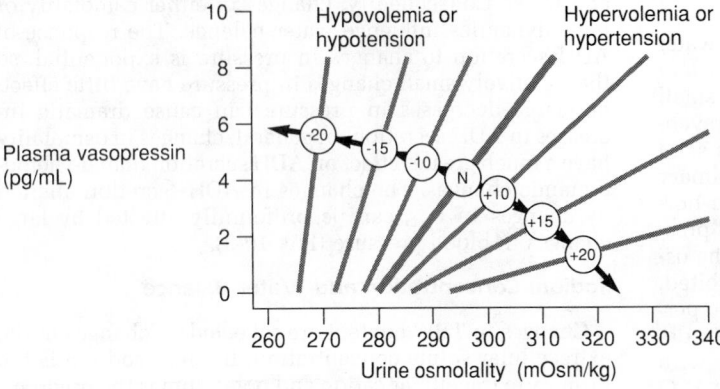

Figure 10-3. Effect of acute changes in blood volume or pressure on the osmoregulation of ADH (vasopressin). The heavy oblique line in the center represents the relation between plasma ADH and osmolality under normovolemic, normotensive conditions. The lines to the left and right show the shift in the relation when blood volume or blood pressure is acutely decreased or increased by the percentage indicated within the circles. (Robertson GL. Physiology of ADH secretion. Kidney Int 1987; 32[Suppl 21]:520)

sulting from trauma or aneurysms, have a deficit in effective circulating volume.

The effective circulating volume is usually in a state of equilibrium with the remainder of the extracellular volume, so that changes in the total extracellular volume are reflected by changes in the effective circulating volume. This relation can be drastically altered in certain disease states, many of which are familiar to the surgeon. Abnormal shifts of fluid from the intravascular space into the tissues is often termed *third-space* fluid loss. Examples of disorders that cause this third-space loss of fluid include bowel obstruction, which causes edema of the bowel wall and transudation of fluid into the bowel lumen, pancreatitis, which causes retroperitoneal fluid extravasation, and *sepsis syndrome*, with resulting capillary leak. Although this fluid remains in the extracellular compartment, it is poorly exchangeable while the disease process persists. In these situations, total ECF remains constant or increases, and interstitial water is increased at the expense of intravascular volume.

Volume Control

Changes in volume are detected both by osmoreceptors, which detect changes in P_{osm}, and baroreceptors, which are sensitive to changes in pressure. The osmoreceptors

are responsible for the day-to-day fine-tuning of volume, whereas the baroreceptors contribute relatively little to the control of fluid balance under normal conditions.[3] As mentioned earlier, large changes in circulating volume can modify the osmoregulation of ADH secretion. These changes must be on the order of a 10% to 20% loss of blood volume. In addition to having baroreceptors that control volume by means of sympathetic and parasympathetic connections, the atria appear to be endocrine organs capable of directly responding to volume changes with the elaboration of atrial natriuretic peptide (ANP).

Baroreceptor Modulation of Volume Control

Changes in the effective circulating volume are sensed by the volume receptors of the intrathoracic capacitance vessels and atria, the pressure receptors of the aortic arch and carotid arteries, the intrarenal baroreceptors, and, to a lesser extent, the hepatic and cerebrospinal volume receptors. These *stretch receptors* are sensitive to changes in pressure and also to changes in circulating volume that are manifested by changes in pressure. The responses of these receptors to altered circulating volume are neural, by way of the sympathetic and parasympathetic fibers, and hormonal. The primary hormonal mediators include the renin–angiotensin system, aldosterone, ANP, dopamine, and the renal prostaglandins. The end result of this complex system of receptors and messengers is a change in sodium and water balance mediated by the kidneys. It is through changes in sodium and water reabsorption that volume and pressure are ultimately normalized.

Baroreceptor Function

The low-pressure baroreceptors of the intrathoracic vena cava and atria are located in vessels that are distensible and are not affected by sympathetic stimulation; thus, they are ideally situated to detect changes in venous volume.[4] These receptors send continuous signals through vagal afferent nerves to the cardiovascular control centers of the medulla and hypothalamus, which, in turn, send signals through parasympathetic and sympathetic fibers to the heart and kidneys. Changes in stretch of these vessels result in changes in the frequency of signal output from these receptors. Increases in atrial distention cause decreased nerve-signal traffic, which ultimately causes increased sympathetic tone to the heart and results in tachycardia and inhibition of sympathetic tone to the kidney. This leads to increased renal blood flow and decreased tubular sodium reabsorption. Conversely, low volume in the intrathoracic vessels results in increased sympathetic tone to the kidneys, decreased renal blood flow, and increased sodium reabsorption.

The kidneys are richly innervated with sympathetic fi-

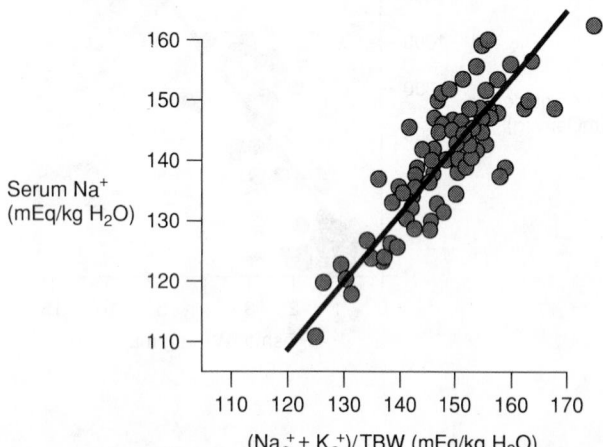

Figure 10-4. Relation between serum [Na^+] and the ratio of (Na_e^+ + K_e^+) to total body water (TBW). (Edelman IS, Liebman J, O'Meara MP, Birkenfeld LW. Interrelationships between serum sodium concentration, serum osmolarity and total exchangeable sodium, total exchangeable potassium and total body water. J Clin Invest 1958;37:1236)

bers whose terminals are located throughout the vascular tree, especially on afferent and efferent arterioles. In addition, the tubules are directly innervated by sympathetic nerves. The kidneys receive little parasympathetic innervation. Experimental evidence clearly indicates that renal sympathetic nerve stimulation results in decreased renal blood flow and increased tubular sodium reabsorption. The effects of renal sympathetic nerve activity on sodium reabsorption are probably mediated both by direct innervation of the renal tubule and by β-adrenergic stimulation of renin production. The renal sympathetic nervous system may not be crucial to the fine regulation of sodium balance under normal physiologic conditions because experiments in conscious, unstressed animals reveal minimal effects of renal denervation on either blood flow or sodium reabsorption. The effects of renal denervation become much more marked in the presence of anesthesia or hypotension, suggesting that sympathetic effects on renal function may be important during periods of stress.

Arterial baroreceptors are located in the aortic arch and carotid arteries. They respond to changes in heart rate, arterial pressure, and the rate of rise in the arterial pressure. Although a major role as a fine-tuning mechanism of volume control is unlikely, arterial baroreceptors are important during periods in which there are extremes in the changes in arterial pressure characteristics, as occur during hemorrhage. In addition, there are arterial baroreceptors in the afferent arterioles of the kidneys. Increases in transmural pressure cause suppression of renin release, and decreases in transmural pressure stimulate renin release.

Hormonal Mediators of Volume Control

Renin–Angiotensin System.   The key to much of the volume and pressure control exerted by the kidneys is the release of renin from the juxtaglomerular cells of the afferent arterioles. Renin is a 40-kd proteolytic enzyme that is released in response to changes in arterial pressure, changes in sodium delivery to the macula densa of the distal convoluted tubule, increases in β-adrenergic activity, and increases in cellular cAMP. The latter may be stimulated by prostaglandins, histamine, glucagon, and other hormonal influences. Renin cleaves the decapeptide angiotensin I from circulating angiotensinogen and α_2-globulin produced by the liver. Angiotensinogen is abundant, so this reaction is enzyme dependent rather than substrate dependent. Angiotensin I is further cleaved to the octapeptide angiotensin II by angiotensin-converting enzyme, which is produced by vascular endothelial cells. One pass through the pulmonary microvasculature converts most angiotensin I to angiotensin II. Until the discovery of endothelin, angiotensin was thought to be the most potent vasoconstrictor produced within the body. Angiotensin II acts both locally and systemically to increase vascular tone. In addition, it stimulates catecholamine release from the adrenal medulla, increases sympathetic tone by acting centrally, and stimulates catecholamine release from sympathetic nerve terminals. Angiotensin II also affects sodium reabsorption by decreasing renal plasma flow and the glomerular filtration coefficient. This results in altered glomerular–tubular feedback, the mechanism by which changes in distal tubular NaCl delivery alter glomerular blood flow. Finally, angiotensin II increases sodium reabsorption by direct tubular action as well as by stimulation of aldosterone release from the adrenal cortex. The multiplicity of actions of angiotensin are depicted in Figure 10-5. Angiotensin II can be further cleaved by aminopeptidase A to form angiotensin III. This hormone has actions similar to its precursor. Its half-life is short, and its physiologic significance has yet to be fully determined.

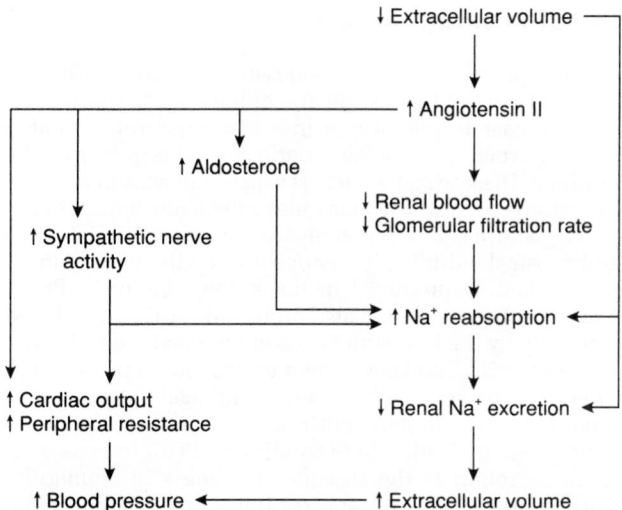

Figure 10-5. Multiple effects of increased angiotensin II release in response to the stimulus of decreased extracellular volume.

Aldosterone.   Aldosterone is a mineralocorticoid produced within the zona glomerulosa of the adrenal cortex. This hormone exerts a major influence over sodium balance by increasing renal tubular reabsorption of sodium. Aldosterone acts directly on the distal tubular segments, predominantly on the collecting tubules. By increasing protein production within these tubular cells, aldosterone induces an influx of sodium, which causes an increase in cellular Na^+-K^+-ATPase activity. The net result is increased sodium reabsorption and increased potassium excretion. Although the primary regulator of aldosterone secretion is angiotensin II, aldosterone release is also stimulated by increased potassium levels, ACTH, and prostaglandins.

ATRIAL AND RENAL NATRIURETIC PEPTIDES

The role of cardiac atria and renal tubules in sodium and volume control has only recently been recognized. ANP is synthesized and released by atrial myocytes in response to atrial wall distention. For each 1-mmHg increase in right atrial pressure, plasma ANP levels increase by about 30 pg/mL.[5] There is evidence that ANP has a direct inhibitory effect on renal sodium reabsorption, which is probably maximal at the level of the medullary collecting tubules. Although pharmacologic doses of ANP can cause changes in both renal blood flow and glomerular filtration rate, physiologic levels do not appear to have any major effect on these parameters. Other active fragments of the ANP prohormone have been found to have natriuretic activity. The best described is urodilatin, also known as *renal natriuretic* peptide. Urodilatin is a peptide with ANP-like activity that was first isolated from human urine. It is synthesized and luminally secreted by cortical-collecting tubule cells. Like ANP, it is released in the kidney tubules in response to atrial distention and saline loading. It is at least twice as potent as ANP, acting in the distal nephron to cause a rise in intracellular cGMP, leading to sodium, chloride, and water diuresis. Urodilatin and other peptides may play an important role in controlling intravascular volume and water and electrolyte secretion.[6]

Renal Prostaglandins

Renal prostaglandins are eicosanoids produced by the action of cyclooxygenase on arachidonic acid. These autocoids appear to play a role in volume control, although under normal physiologic conditions, this role may be minimal. Disease states such as sepsis and jaundice, or the induction of anesthesia, may make the contribution of the prostaglandins more pronounced. Prostaglandin E_2 (PGE_2) and prostaglandin I_2 (PGI_2) appear to be the predominant prostaglandins produced in the kidney, although $PGF_{1\alpha}$ and thromboxane A_2 are also produced. PGE_2 is produced primarily by the interstitial cells of the renal medulla. The release of PGE_2 has been shown to depend on increases in interstitial pressure, which can be induced by changes in renal perfusion, ureteral obstruction, or alterations in oncotic pressure. Under these conditions, PGE_2 increases sodium excretion in the absence of changes in glomerular filtration rate. PGE_2 antagonizes the action of vasopressin (ADH) and inhibits ADH-induced sodium reabsorption along the medullary collecting duct and thick ascending limb. PGI_2 is produced by the glomeruli and endothelial cells of the kidney and is present in the greatest concentrations in the renal cortex. PGI_2 is a vasodilator, and its effects on renal vascular resistance increase both renal blood flow and glomerular filtration rate. PGI_2 production is augmented by increases in angiotensin, catecholamines, and sympathetic tone, and may act to counterbalance their vasoconstricting effects. Although under normal physiologic conditions, inhibition of prostaglandin production has little effect on renal function, administration of nonsteroidal antiinflammatory agents, which inhibit cyclooxygenase, to patients with conditions known to cause renal dysfunction (eg, cirrhosis) can precipitate renal failure, presumably because of loss of the protective effects of the renal prostaglandins.[7]

Endothelins

Endothelins are peptide vasoconstrictors that are also involved in volume and pressure regulation. Endothelin is produced and released by endothelial and other cells acting in a paracrine fashion on adjacent smooth muscle cells. In addition, endothelin stimulates the release of other vasoactive mediators, particularly endogenous vasodilators, which act to limit its intense vasoconstrictor effect. In addition to increasing peripheral resistance, endothelin infusion has a direct inotropic effect on the myocardium, increasing cardiac output. Endothelin infusion increases the systemic release of ANP, nitric oxide, and PGI_2 (prostacyclin). In addition, endothelin inhibits the release of renin by the juxtaglomerular apparatus and activates angiotensin-converting enzyme. Endothelin also modulates the biosynthesis of aldosterone. Endothelin has complex effects on sodium and water balance, which adds to its actions by modulating release of other hormones. Endothelin inhibits water reabsorption while simultaneously inhibiting vasopressin-mediated water reabsorption. In animal experiments, endothelin decreases sodium excretion by lowering the filtered load of sodium and increasing circulating aldosterone. In other experiments, at much lower concentrations, endothelin-1 causes a dose-dependent natriuresis and diuresis. Endothelin appears to have complex interactions with other regulators of renal perfusion and handling of water and electrolytes, which has stimulated research to evaluate the contribution of endothelin to the pathophysiology of various renal diseases.[8]

Nitric Oxide

Nitric oxide is a gaseous free radical produced by nitric oxide synthases that are found in a wide variety of mammalian cells. Nitric oxide is synthesized by nitric oxide synthase from L-arginine, and its formation is blocked by a variety of L-arginine analogues, such as L-NG-monomethyl-arginine (L-NMMA). With a half-life of 3 to 5 seconds, nitric oxide is rapidly neutralized by hemoglobin, methylene blue, and superoxide anions.

Nitric oxide has many biologic functions. It is an endothelial-derived vasodilator that is an important physiologic regulator of vessel tone and tissue blood flow. In addition to its flow-regulating properties, nitric oxide also inhibits platelet aggregation and adhesion and participates in host defenses. Specifically, macrophages, after exposure to cytokines, produce nitric oxide, which has proved to be cytotoxic to tumor cells and bacteria. This induced macrophage nitric oxide production contributes to the vasodilation and low systemic vascular resistance that is characteristic of sepsis. In the gastrointestinal system, nitric oxide functions as a neurotransmitter, participating in the relaxation of the lower esophageal sphincter, sphincter of Oddi, stomach, small intestine, and anus. Nitric oxide is produced by the gastric mucosa, where, as a vasodilator, it protects mucosal blood flow.[9]

Nitric oxide participates in the regulation of renal hemodynamics and renal handling of water and electrolytes. Its production occurs throughout the kidney in smooth muscle cells, mesangial cells, tubules, and endothelial cells. Nitric oxide and PGI_2 each independently cause renal vasodilation in response to a variety of stimuli. Nitric oxide is important in the regulation of medullary (vasa recta) blood flow. Pressure-dependent sodium excretion is ablated with inhibitors like L-NMMA and restored with L-arginine. Nitric oxide also contributes to tubuloglomerular feedback, which modulates the delivery and reabsorption of sodium and chloride in the renal tubules. Nitric oxide synthase in macula densa cells is activated by tubular solute reabsorption to release nitric oxide as a vasodilating component of the tubuloglomerular feedback response. Nitric oxide also participates in regulating renin release by the juxtaglomerular apparatus. Finally, nitric oxide produced in the proximal tubule may mediate the affects of angiotensin on tubular reabsorption.[10]

NORMAL WATER AND ELECTROLYTE EXCHANGE

Under normal circumstances, the body's homeostatic mechanisms are capable of controlling the volume and composition of the fluid compartments at a remarkably constant level, so that a stable internal milieu is maintained. Surgical patients, however, are particularly prone to fluid and electrolyte abnormalities, not only because of disease but also because the necessities of surgical care may sidestep some of these homeostatic mechanisms. Although it is important to recognize and correct the abnormalities brought about by disease, trauma, and stress, it is equally important to know how to maintain normal fluid and electrolyte balance and thus avoid iatrogenic abnormalities.

Normal Water Exchange

Water losses are both sensible (able to be measured) and insensible. Sensible losses include losses through urine, stool, and sweat. Table 10-3 summarizes the normal sensible and insensible losses encountered in a 24-hour period. The volumes of these losses may vary considerably. Uri-

Table 10-3. WATER LOSSES IN A 60- TO 80-kg MAN

	Average Daily Volume (mL)	Minimal Daily Volume (mL)
Sensible losses		
Urinary	800–1500	300
Intestinal	0–250	0
Sweat	0	0
Insensible losses		
Lungs and skin	600–900	600–900

(Adapted from Shires GT, Canizaro PC. Fluid and electrolyte management of the surgical patient. In: Sabiston DC, ed. Textbook of surgery. Philadelphia, WB Saunders, 1986:77)

nary loss usually varies in proportion to intake plus other losses. The minimal amount of water needed to excrete normal metabolic waste products is about 300 mL/d.

Water loss in stool is usually small, on the order of 150 mL/d, but may increase markedly in disease conditions. The gastrointestinal tract has a net secretory action down to the level of the jejunum, and the reabsorptive capacity of the remainder of the small and large intestines keeps water loss by this route to a minimum. Bowel obstruction, severe diarrhea, and enterocolic fistulas are examples of conditions that may increase gastrointestinal losses of water and electrolytes.

Sweat does not usually account for much of the daily water loss. Sweating is an active process involving the secretion of a hypotonic mixture of electrolytes and water, and it should be differentiated from the insensible water loss of evaporation from the skin.

Insensible water loss is the evaporatory loss of water from both the skin and the respiratory tract (see Table 10-3). Evaporatory skin losses depend on the body surface area, the temperature of the patient, and the relative humidity of the environment. Evaporation through the skin functions as a mechanism for heat loss and is proportional to calories expended. About 30 mL of water is lost for every 100 kcal expended. Respiratory exchange depends on the ambient temperature and the relative humidity as well as on the rate of air exchange. Respiratory water loss is also energy dependent; thus, at normal respiratory rates, 13 mL of water is lost for every 100 kcal expended. Overall, normal insensible water losses average about 8 to 12 mL/kg/d. Insensible water loss increases 10% for each degree of body temperature above 37.2°C (99°F). In addition, patients with tracheostomies who breathe unhumidified air lose additional free water. Conversely, patients who are on respirators or who breathe air that is 100% humidified, have no respiratory losses and may gain free water.

A person normally consumes about 2000 mL/d of water, although this quantity is highly variable. About one third of this amount comes from water bound to food, and the remainder originates from free water intake. In addition, water may be gained when carbohydrates and proteins, which are kept in solution by water within the cell, are metabolized. Although this gain is usually minimal, catabolic states may increase the amount of oxidative free water gain to about 500 mL/d. To maintain proper fluid volumes, intake and excretion are well balanced through thirst mechanisms and the changes in renal excretion described earlier.

Normal Salt Exchange

In industrialized nations, daily salt intake averages 100 to 250 mEq/d Na$^+$, or 6 to 15 g/d NaCl. This amount of intake is normally balanced by losses through sweat, stool,

and urine. Renal sodium excretion is the mechanism by which fine control of sodium balance can be exerted. In cases of hyponatremia, the kidney can conserve sodium with urinary losses of less than 1 mEq/d. Conversely, urinary excretion can be maximized to rates up to 5000 mEq/d if necessary to achieve sodium balance. The normal sodium requirement is in the range of 1 to 2 mEq/kg/d.

Potassium balance in the body is also finely controlled. Because most potassium remains in the intracellular compartment, potassium homeostasis is maintained by a balance between intake and gastrointestinal and renal losses, and a balance between extracellular and intracellular potassium. In a normal diet, about 40 to 120 mEq of potassium is ingested daily. Of this potassium, 10% to 15% is excreted in the feces, and the remainder is excreted in the urine. Normal daily potassium requirements are about 0.5 to 1 mEq/kg/d. Abnormal renal function markedly changes this figure; consequently, potassium intake must be minimized in patients with renal failure.

FLUID AND ELECTROLYTE THERAPY

Parenteral Solutions

A number of electrolyte solutions are available for parenteral administration. Selection of the appropriate fluid is determined by assessment of the patient's maintenance fluid requirements, existing fluid deficits, and ongoing fluid losses. Table 10-4 lists the commonly available electrolyte solutions and the electrolyte composition of each. Although use of these solutions is convenient, there are occasions when a particular solution does not accurately replace the electrolyte components of the losses or deficits, and more than one type of solution may be indicated. Ions such as potassium, magnesium, or calcium may be necessary and can be added to parenteral solutions to suit the patient's requirements.

Lactated Ringer solution is a physiologic solution containing many of the electrolytes found in plasma. This solution is commonly used to replace losses of fluid with the ionic composition of plasma, such as edema fluid and small bowel losses. It is ideal for the replacement of existing fluid deficits when the serum electrolyte concentrations are normal. The disadvantage of this solution is the relatively low sodium content (130 mEq/L) as compared with plasma. Normal renal function usually ensures that the extra free water in this solution (150 mL/L) is excreted. Hyponatremia can occur with extended use of lactated Ringer solution, or with use in patients who have impaired renal function, especially dilutional abnormalities such as those secondary to increased ADH secretion. Because lac-

Table 10-4. ELECTROLYTE CONTENT OF COMMONLY USED INTRAVENOUS ELECTROLYTE SOLUTIONS

| Solution | Electrolyte (mEq/L) | | | | | |
	Na$^+$	K$^+$	Ca^{2+}	Mg^{2+}	Cl$^-$	HCO$_3$
0.9% NaCl (normal saline)	154	—	—	—	154	—
0.45% NaCl	77	—	—	—	77	—
0.33% NaCl	56	—	—	—	56	—
0.2% NaCl	34	—	—	—	34	—
Lactated Ringer solution	130	4	4	—	109	28
3.0% NaCl	513	—	—	—	513	—
5.0% NaCl	855	—	—	—	855	—

tate anions are readily metabolized to bicarbonate, the lactate ions in lactated Ringer solution rarely contribute to acidosis if tissue perfusion has been maintained or restored.

Isotonic saline (0.9% or normal saline) contains 154 mEq of both sodium and chloride. Although this solution can be useful in patients with hyponatremia or hypochloremia, the excess of both sodium and chloride can lead to electrolyte and acid–base disturbances. Infusion of large volumes of 0.9% saline can lead to total body sodium overload and hyperchloremia. The added chloride load can result in a hyperchloremic metabolic acidosis or can aggravate preexisting acidosis. In addition, the pH of this solution and of the related solutions (0.45%, 0.33%, and 0.2% saline) is 4.0 to 5.0.

The less-concentrated saline solutions are used to replace ongoing fluid losses, such as nasogastric tube losses, and are also used in maintenance fluid therapy. The solution is determined by the calculated requirements. The 0.45%, 0.33%, and 0.2% saline solutions are hypoosmotic and thus have excess free water. In addition, 0.33% and 0.2% saline solutions are hypotonic with respect to plasma and can result in red blood cell lysis if rapidly infused. For this reason, 5% dextrose (50 g of dextrose per liter) is added to these solutions to increase the tonicity. In addition, when metabolized, 5% dextrose represents 200 kcal for each liter of solution.

Hypertonic saline solutions (3% NaCl and 5% NaCl) are usually reserved for replacement of sodium deficits in patients with symptomatic hyponatremia or those at high risk for developing symptoms. Calculations for replacement of sodium deficits are addressed later in this chapter. Hypertonic saline solutions have been used in the early resuscitation of hypovolemic trauma and burn patients. These solutions appear to increase intravascular volume in these patients more quickly than lactated Ringer solution, and the total resuscitation volume requirement may be decreased. Patients resuscitated with hypertonic solutions require close monitoring of serum electrolytes to prevent hypernatremia and hyperosmolar coma. Although these experimental findings are of interest, the efficacy of hypertonic saline resuscitation has yet to be determined.

Plasma expanders are also commonly used in surgical patients. Some of these solutions and their contents are given in Table 10-5. These solutions are usually reserved for special clinical situations and are not used routinely in fluid management. Plasma protein solutions, such as 5% and 25% albumin, act initially by increasing plasma oncotic pressures. Exogenously administered protein is retained in the intravascular space, and interstitial water may move into the intravascular space. Abnormalities in microvascular permeability, such as those found in the pulmonary circulation in the adult respiratory distress syndrome, in regional circulatory beds in burns or infections, and in the systemic circulation in sepsis, can result in the extravasation of these proteins into the interstitial space. This, in turn, can lead to increased rather than decreased interstitial edema formation. About half of all exogenously administered albumin eventually ends up in the extravascular space. In addition, the half-life of exogenously administered albumin is about 11 days, considerably shorter than endogenously produced protein. Hydroxyethyl starch (hetastarch), and dextran are synthetic plasma expanders. They have longer or similar half-lives to albumen and are less expensive. The usefulness of oxygen-carrying synthetic plasma expanders, including stroma-free hemoglobin and perfluoro chemical compound–containing solutions, is under intense investigation. In the future, these solution may prove beneficial in selected clinical settings.

Goals of Fluid and Electrolyte Therapy

The goals of fluid therapy are the normalization of hemodynamic parameters and normalization of body fluid electrolyte concentrations. These are accomplished by the correction of preexisting volume and electrolyte abnormalities, administration of fluids to replace normal daily losses (maintenance fluid therapy), and replacement of additional ongoing fluid losses as they occur. Replacement of fluids is crucial for patients in situations such as trauma, operative manipulation, and postoperative fluid shifts, in which fluid losses can lead to major abnormalities in fluid balance.

Correction of Existing Volume Abnormalities

Volume Deficit

Volume deficits can be either acute or chronic. Chronic volume deficits may manifest as decreased skin turgor, weight loss, sunken eyes, hypothermia, oliguria, orthostatic hypotension, and tachycardia. In addition, serum BUN and creatinine may be elevated, with a high BUN/creatinine ratio (above 15:1), and the hematocrit may be elevated as well. Assuming no change in red-cell mass, the hematocrit can be expected to increase 6 to 8 points for each liter deficit in intravascular volume. In this situation, urine concentration is usually high, and urine sodium excretion is low (less than 20 mEq/L Na$^+$). Plasma sodium is not an indicator of intravascular volume, and if the fluid losses have been isotonic, plasma sodium concentration remains normal.

Acute volume losses are usually manifested by changes in vital signs without concomitant tissue changes. If organ perfusion is compromised, urine output may also be low. Oliguria and hypovolemia may be caused by intrinsic renal dysfunction. Attempts to quantify volume deficits are generally of little value. All deficits should be immediately addressed. Volume resuscitation should be continued until hemodynamic parameters are normalized. The volume of fluid required for resuscitation is the best estimate of what the volume deficit has been.

Table 10-5. PLASMA EXPANDERS

Solution	Concentration (%)
HUMAN ALBUMIN	
Albutein 5% (Alpha Therapeutic)	5
Albutein 25% (Alpha Therapeutic)	25
Albuminar-5 (Armour)	5
Albuminar-25 (Armour)	25
Buminate 5% (Hyland)	5
Buminate 25% (Hyland)	25
PLASMA PROTEIN FRACTIONS: ALBUMIN 4.4%	
Plasmanate (Cutter)	
Plasmatein (Alpha Therapeutic)	
Plasma-Plex (Armour)	
Proteinate (Hyland)	
DEXTRANS AND STARCH	
Dextran 40 (Rheomacrodex)	10
Dextran 70 (Macrodex)	6
Hetastarch (Hespan)	6

(Adapted from Carroll HJ, Oh MS. Water, electrolyte and acid–base metabolism. Philadelphia, JB Lippincott, 1989:82)

Fluid resuscitation for hypovolemia is initiated with an isotonic solution such as lactated Ringer solution. Urine flow in critically ill patients is monitored with an indwelling Foley catheter. In general, urine output of greater than 0.5 mL/kg/h is also desirable. After fluid resuscitation has been initiated, a thorough history and physical examination may help to determine the origins of the volume deficits, and the underlying causes can be appropriately addressed. Central venous pressure may be monitored with a central venous catheter or pulmonary artery catheter. Invasive monitoring with central venous catheter or pulmonary artery catheter should be considered in elderly patients or patients with cardiac disease. Placement of these catheters should occur concurrently with ongoing resuscitation and is used to guide fluid resuscitation as well as the need for inotropes or pressors in critically ill patients. The goal of initial therapy is the normalization of heart rate, blood pressure, and tissue perfusion.

Volume Excess

Surgical patients usually do not present with volume excesses, although it is not uncommon for patients to manifest volume excess during the course of their hospitalization. Large volumes of fluid can be sequestered in extravascular spaces (third-space losses) as a consequence of surgery, trauma, and disease processes. With the resolution of pathologic conditions and normalization of microvascular permeability, these fluid losses stop and eventually reverse. Thus, the sequestered fluid is autotransfused at variable rates. This may lead to volume overload if appropriate adjustments in fluid management are not made. In addition, postoperative patients and traumatized patients may be unable to excrete normal fluid loads secondary to increased ADH secretion. Frequent manifestations of volume overload are weight gain, elevated central venous pressure, pulmonary edema, peripheral edema, and an S3 gallop. Intravascular volume excess is best treated by appropriate volume restriction and by judicial use of loop diuretics if acute symptoms become evident.

Maintenance Fluid Therapy

Maintenance fluid replacement is aimed at replacing fluids normally lost during the course of a day. Calculation of maintenance fluid replacement does not include replacement of either preexisting deficits or ongoing additional losses. Maintenance fluid replacement should begin after the reestablishment of normal hemodynamic status with appropriate resuscitation fluids.

Basal requirements for water and electrolytes are determined by sensible and insensible losses. Insensible water loss averages about 8 to 12 mL/kg/d and increases 10% for every degree of body temperature above 37.2°C (99°F). For example, a 70-kg man without a fever has a daily insensible water loss of about 840 mL. In addition, urinary and stool losses must be added to this figure. A useful formula for calculating maintenance water requirements is provided in Table 10-6. This formula adjusts for differences in body weight and for changes in body water content. A smaller (or younger) person who has a high percentage of TBW in relation to body weight requires a greater amount of maintenance fluid per kilogram than a larger (or older) person. For example, a 10-kg child requires 100 mL H_2O/kg/d or 1000 mL/H_2O/d. A 70-kg man requires 1000 mL/d for the first 10 kg (100 mL/kg × 10 kg), plus 500 mL/d for the second 10 kg (20 mL/kg × 10 kg), plus 1000 mL/d for the last 50 kg (20 mL/kg × 50 kg). Thus, the total daily water requirement for a 70-kg man is about 2500 mL/d. Because hypervolemia is poorly tolerated in older patients and in patients with cardiac disease, the requirement per

Table 10-6. CALCULATION OF MAINTENANCE FLUID REQUIREMENTS

Body Weight	Fluid Requirement*	
For 0–10 kg	Give 100 mL/kg/d	A
For the next 10–20 kg	Given an additional 50 mL/kg/d	B
For weight > 20 kg†	Give 20 mL/kg/d	C

* Maintenance fluid requirements = sum of A + B + C.
† For elderly patients or patients with cardiac disease, this amount should be reduced to 15 mL/kg/d.

kilogram over 20 kg is decreased to 15 mL/kg/d in these patients. Thus, the volume calculated for a 50-kg octogenarian is 1950 mL/d (1000 mL + 500 mL + 450 mL). These calculations are only estimates, and each patient must be observed closely for signs of volume depletion or volume overload.

Sodium requirements in patients are variable, and excess sodium administration is usually balanced by increased urinary sodium excretion. As a general estimate, 1 to 2 mEq/kg/d of sodium is required for maintenance therapy. Potassium requirements are about half that of sodium; thus, 0.5 to 1 mEq/kg/d is the normal calculated potassium requirement. If sodium is replaced at the rate of 2 mEq/kg/d and potassium is replaced at the rate of 1 mEq/kg/d, then a 70-kg patient requires 2500 mL of water with 140 mEq of sodium and 70 mEq of potassium added to the solution. One liter of parenteral solution would therefore contain 56 mEq of sodium and 28 mEq of potassium. Of the available crystalloid solutions, 0.33% saline solution (56 mEq/L Na^+) is the solution that best fits this patient's daily requirements for maintenance therapy. Potassium chloride can be added to each liter of solution (20 to 30 mEq/L), but this is best done after clinical assessment of the patient's electrolyte, acid–base, and renal functional status. Normal maintenance therapy requires the administration of sodium and potassium. Replacement of calcium, phosphate, or magnesium is generally not necessary in patients requiring short-term therapy. In critically ill patients, however, critical deficits of these electrolytes may occur and must be replaced. In patients requiring long-term fluid replacement, addition of these electrolytes, as well as trace elements, vitamins, protein, and calories, is essential. For this reason, parenteral nutrition solutions should be started as soon as possible in all patients not expected to resume full enteral nutrition, or with fluid replacement expected for more than 1 week.

Replacement of Ongoing Fluid Losses

Surgical patients are likely to have extraordinary fluid losses at some point during their hospitalization, especially if they have undergone operative procedures. Once volume deficits have been replaced and maintenance fluids have been calculated and given, the overall fluid balance of the patient can be maintained by replacement of any fluid losses over and above those considered to be maintenance. Although intraoperative and postoperative losses as well as third-space fluid losses must be estimated, ongoing losses from nasogastric tubes, ileostomies, fistulas, and so forth can be easily measured and quantitated. In addition, the electrolyte contents of these fluids can often be predicted (Table 10-7), and the exact electrolyte content of the fluids can frequently be measured and replaced with precision. Ongoing losses should be detailed on a flow chart that documents the intake and output of all fluids. Patients needing emergent operation require adequate

Table 10-7. ELECTROLYTE CONCENTRATIONS IN GASTROINTESTINAL SECRETIONS

Secretion	Electrolyte (mEq/L)					Rate (mL/d)
	Na$^+$	K$^+$	Cl$^-$	HCO$_3^-$	H$^+$	
Salivary	50	20	40	30	—	100–1000
Gastric						
Basal	100	10	140	—	30	1000
Stimulated	30	10	140	—	100	4200
Bile	140	5	100	60	—	500–1000
Pancreatic	140	5	75	100	—	1000
Duodenum	140	5	80	—	—	100–2000
Ileum	140	5	70	50	—	100–2000
Colon	60	70	15	30	—	—

fluid resuscitation before being taken to the operating room, except in the circumstance of uncontrolled hemorrhage, for which operative intervention is the only means of stabilizing the volume loss. Operative and postoperative fluid management must be carefully controlled and monitored to ensure an optimal patient outcome.

Intraoperative Fluid Therapy

Anesthesia interrupts normal baroreceptor reflexes, so that the patient with volume depletion, which was compensated preoperatively by increased vascular resistance and heart rate, may become acutely hypotensive on induction of anesthesia. For this reason, adequate resuscitation before surgery is mandatory. During operative procedures, fluid losses result from blood loss, third-space sequestration from trauma or manipulation of tissues, and evaporative losses from the wound itself. Blood loss is grossly estimated during surgery, and estimates by the surgeon are usually considerably lower than those measures made by isotopic techniques. Although most patients can tolerate an unreplaced blood loss of at least 500 mL, losses above this level may require replacement during the operation. The shifts of fluid from the intravascular space to the extravascular space that occur in response to third-space volume losses from operative manipulation, tissue trauma, and evaporation cannot be measured but should be anticipated. Replacement with isotonic solutions, such as lactated Ringer solution, is given at a rate of 500 to 1000 mL/h during the operation. Close intraoperative monitoring of blood pressure and urine output aids the surgeon and anesthesiologist in avoiding periods of hypotension secondary to volume depletion. Central venous pressure is monitored in those patients undergoing more complex procedures. In critically ill patients or patients at high risk for developing cardiac or fluid balance abnormalities during surgery, cardiac output and pulmonary artery wedge pressures are used to gauge the adequacy of fluid resuscitation. Elderly patients and high-risk patients may also benefit from preoperative placement of a pulmonary artery catheter to optimize preoperative, operative, and postoperative cardiac function and fluid resuscitation.

Postoperative Fluid Therapy and Monitoring

Fluid therapy during the postoperative period should be tailored to each patient and depends on the adequacy of the patient's volume status at the completion of the operative procedure as well as on the ongoing fluid losses. Maintenance fluid therapy should be supplemented by replacement of the additional fluids needed to replace the ongoing third-space losses as well as losses from various tubes and drains. In general, isotonic solutions should be used for volume resuscitation during the early postoperative period. It is best not to give potassium supplements during this period unless they are specifically required as indicated by serum electrolyte measurements.

Monitoring fluid status during the postoperative period is best accomplished by careful monitoring of vital signs, urinary output, and central venous pressure if necessary. Urine output is maintained at a level greater than 0.5 mL/kg/h. Urine specific gravity is usually measured more easily than U_{osm} and serves as an indicator of both volume status and renal ability to concentrate and dilute the urine. Urine specific gravity of greater than 1.010 to 1.012 indicates that the urine is being concentrated (as compared with plasma), and a urine specific gravity of less than 1.010 indicates that dilute urine is being produced. Volume depletion or cardiac failure is usually accompanied by concentrated urine at low flow rates. Urine specific gravity in the range of plasma (1.010 to 1.012) may indicate adequate hydration or the inability of the kidneys to dilute or concentrate the urine. Renal failure in the postoperative period may be accompanied by either low urine volumes (oliguric renal failure, less than 500 mL/d) or normal or high urine volumes (nonoliguric or high-output renal failure). In patients at high risk for developing renal failure during the postoperative period, urine collections should be obtained for measurement of urine electrolytes as well as creatinine clearance. This group of patients includes those with preexisting renal disease, those who were hypotensive before or during surgery, and those receiving nephrotoxic drugs.

An accurate and direct method of monitoring a patient's fluid status is to measure central pressures. This may be performed with some accuracy using a central venous catheter placed in the superior vena cava. Central venous pressures of 5 to 12 mmHg or 6 to 15 cm H_2O are considered normal. Pressures above this range usually indicate volume overload or cardiac failure, whereas pressures below this range indicate intravascular volume depletion. Serial monitoring of central venous pressure is a valuable indicator of both volume status and adequacy of fluid management.

Because central venous pressure is affected by venomotor tone and cardiac performance as well as by circulating volume, measurements may not accurately define the causes of abnormalities in effective circulating volume, especially in conditions in which central venous pressures are high. Insertion of a pulmonary artery catheter enables much more accurate determinations of both volume status and cardiovascular performance. Pulmonary artery pressure, pulmonary artery wedge pressure, and thermodilution measurement of cardiac output can be easily accomplished using the Swan-Ganz catheter. In addition, venous saturation in the pulmonary artery, which may reflect global adequacy of oxygen delivery, can be continuously measured. Critically ill patients can be closely monitored using serial measurements of wedge pressure and cardiac output, achieving more precise control of fluid management.

Both short-term and long-term fluid management are facilitated by daily measurement of body weight and fluid intake and output, which are carefully recorded on the patient's chart. Insensible fluid losses are estimated and added to the total outputs. Balancing daily intake and output with appropriate fluid management is essential. Normally, hospitalized patients with no caloric intake lose weight at a rate dependent on the catabolic state. Weight gain usually indicates increases in TBW rather than in protein or fat content.

CONCENTRATION CHANGES IN BODY FLUIDS

Volume excess or deficits are often isotonic but may be accompanied by changes in extracellular sodium concentration and osmolality. Normal sodium homeostasis has been discussed in previous sections. The mechanisms controlling normal osmoregulation may be affected by the same processes responsible for the changes in volume. Volume depletion is most commonly encountered in surgical and trauma patients. These patients usually present with isotonic dehydration (Fig. 10-6*A*). In this condition, the volume lost is isotonic with plasma. Examples of isotonic volume deficits include blood loss, third-space losses, and gastrointestinal losses. Volume depletion may also be accompanied by hypoosmolar conditions (hypotonic dehydration; see Fig. 10-6*B*), which is often iatrogenic and the result of incomplete volume resuscitation with hypotonic solutions. Dehydration associated with hyperosmolar states (hypertonic dehydration; see Fig. 10-6*C*) is infrequent and usually indicates impaired consciousness and thirst mechanisms, or a patient's inability to drink or obtain water. As mentioned previously, volume excesses often occur some time after hospitalization rather than at presentation. The most frequent concentration defect associated with volume excess is hyponatremia.

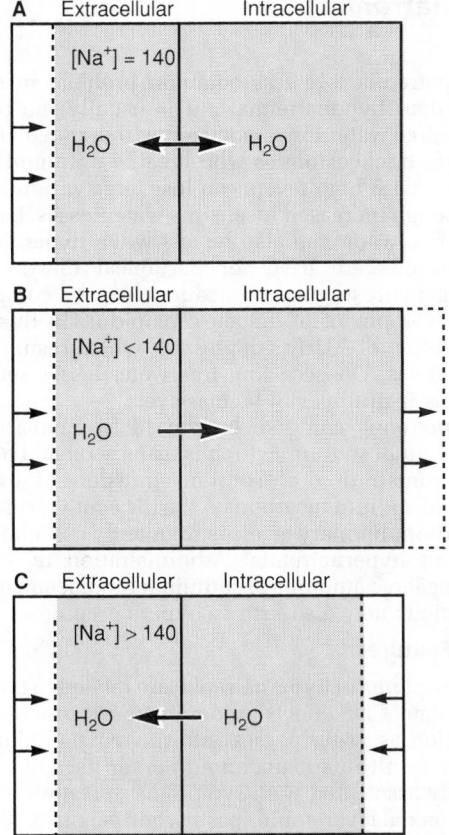

Figure 10-6. (*A*) Isotonic dehydration. Extracellular fluid is lost, but sodium concentration and osmolality remain unchanged. There is no change in intracellular volume. (*B*) Hypotonic dehydration caused by an extracellular fluid deficit with hyponatremia. Water moves into the intracellular space, causing further extracellular depletion and intracellular fluid (ICF) expansion. (*C*) Hypertonic dehydration caused by loss of extracellular free water resulting in hypernatremia. Water from the ICF shifts to the extracellular space, resulting in contraction of both ICF and extracellular fluid compartments.

Hyponatremia

Causes

The most common cause of hyponatremia is an excess of free water rather than a deficit in total body sodium. Hyponatremia in this situation is associated with a low P_{osm}. Hyponatremia is frequently seen in the postoperative or posttrauma period because increased ADH secretion acts on the collecting tubules of the kidney to increase free water reabsorption. Volume expansion due to increased free water reabsorption may stimulate natriuresis, which may exacerbate the problem. Hyponatremia per se results in increased sodium reabsorption, and both volume expansion and hyponatremia diminish the effects of ADH on the collecting tubules. Thus, hyponatremia is usually self-limiting, with serum [Na$^+$] rarely falling below 130 mEq/L unless aggravated by exogenous free water administration. Postinjury or postoperative elevations in ADH secretion are transient, but there are numerous other causes of the syndrome of inappropriate secretion of ADH (SIADH). Tumors of the lung, pancreas, duodenum, bladder, and prostate may secrete ADH. Virtually any pulmonary disease may result in elevation of ADH levels. Brain tumors, cerebral vascular accidents, and other central nervous system (CNS) disorders may also result in varying degrees of SIADH.

Hyponatremia is also associated with low effective circulating volume. This most commonly occurs in edematous states or cirrhosis with ascites, but it can also result from dehydration with concomitant volume replacement with hypotonic solutions. Because of the low intravascular volume, renal plasma flow and glomerular filtration rate are low, resulting in increased sodium reabsorption by the kidneys. This renal compensation may not be sufficient to correct the abnormality.

Although hyponatremia most often results from excess free water, it can occur in the presence of excess solute. In this situation, TBW content is either normal or diminished, and P_{osm} is increased. The hyperosmolality shifts water from the intracellular to the extracellular space, resulting in hyponatremia. The most common example of this hyperosmolar–hyponatremic state is untreated hyperglycemia. Excess solute may also be due to the exogenous administration or ingestion of mannitol, ethanol, methanol, or ethylene glycol. In addition to shifts in water, cellular exchange of potassium for sodium as a compensatory mechanism for potassium loss may result in hyponatremia. In both hyperosmolar and hypokalemic conditions, total body sodium remains normal.

Finally, hyperproteinemia and hyperlipidemia can cause falsely low sodium values. This has been termed *pseudohyponatremia*. This is an abnormality in laboratory measurement of sodium and is not accompanied by any symptoms attributable to hyponatremia.

Clinical Features

The development of symptoms depends on both the level of hyponatremia and the rapidity with which serum [Na$^+$] falls. Chronic hyponatremia is often asymptomatic until the serum [Na$^+$] level falls below 110 to 120 mEq/L. An acute drop in serum [Na$^+$] to 120 to 130 mEq/L may result in a variety of symptoms. The clinical manifestations of hyponatremia are primarily related to the CNS and are the result of cellular water intoxication, although gastrointestinal and musculoskeletal symptoms are also common. Weakness, fatigue, muscle cramps, mental confusion, anorexia, nausea, and vomiting occur frequently. Headaches, confusion, and delirium may herald frank seizure activity and coma. Permanent CNS damage can occur if hyponatremia is left untreated, but overzealous treatment may also lead to CNS injury. Rapid infusion of hypertonic saline may result in central pontine myelinolysis and the quadriplegia, dysarthria, and dysphasia of "locked-in" syndrome. Because of the dangers inherent in rapid treatment, the underlying causes and the risks to the patient with hyponatremia must be carefully considered before deciding on the appropriate therapy.

Diagnosis

Differentiating the causes of hyponatremia may be difficult. Once hyperosmolar hyponatremia (caused by hyperglycemia, mannitol administration, or radiologic contrast medium) has been excluded, and pseudohyponatremia has been eliminated from the differential diagnosis, one must determine whether the effective circulating volume is low (hyponatremic dehydration) or normal. Hyponatremic dehydration may be caused by renal or extrarenal sodium losses. Renal sodium losses are usually the result of diuretic use, chronic renal failure, adrenal insufficiency, or a defect in aldosterone secretion. The hallmark of these disorders is a urine sodium level above 20 mEq/L in the face of hyponatremia. Extrarenal sodium loss may be secondary to vomiting, diarrhea, or fluid loss through nasogastric tubes, fistulas, or drains. The dehydration resulting from these conditions causes increased renal sodium reabsorption and urine sodium levels below 20 mEq/L. Normal or high effective circulating volume in combination with hyponatremia is almost always caused by SIADH or by increased sensitivity of the renal collecting tubules to the action of normal levels of ADH.

Treatment

Treatment of hyponatremia depends on the severity of the symptoms, the chronicity with which the condition develops, and the hydrational status of the patient. Hypovolemic patients often benefit primarily from rehydration because their symptoms are frequently caused by dehydration rather than hyponatremia. Isotonic saline or lactated Ringer solution can often be used in these patients to normalize volume. Because rapid normalization of volume may lead to hypernatremia, serial monitoring of serum [Na$^+$] is performed during judicious volume replacement. Most surgical patients with hyponatremia are euvolemic or hypervolemic. Patients without symptoms in this category are best treated by free water restriction because free water overload is the usual cause of the condition.

Patients who have significant symptoms require aggressive treatment tempered by the duration of the hyponatremia. Because the risk of central pontine myelinolysis is greatest in patients who have been hyponatremic for longer than 48 hours, 5% or 3% saline solution is given relatively slowly to increase serum [Na$^+$] at a rate not exceeding 0.5 mEq/L/h. The amount of sodium needed to increase the serum [Na$^+$] to a desired level can be calculated as follows:

Na$^+$ required (in mEq)

$$= (\text{desired }[Na^+]_s - \text{actual }[Na^+]_s) \times TBW \quad (7)$$
where:
[Na$^+$]$_s$ = serum sodium concentration

For example, a 70-kg patient has been hyponatremic for more than 48 hours and has a serum sodium level of 120 mEq. To avoid central pontine myelinolysis, correction of serum [Na$^+$] during the first 24 hours is limited to 0.5 mEq/L/h × 24 = 12 mEq/L. Using formula 7,

$$Na^+ \text{ required} = (132 - 120) \times TBW$$

Because TBW is 60% of body weight,

$$Na^+ \text{ required} = (132 - 120) \times (0.6[70])$$
$$= 12 \times 42$$
$$= 504 \text{ mEq}$$

Because 5% saline contains 850 mEq/L of sodium,

$$504 \text{ mEq} \times \frac{1 \text{ L}}{850 \text{ mEq}} = 0.593 \text{ L 5% saline}$$

Administration of this fluid would supply 593 mL of water and expand the TBW by this amount, so that the increase in serum [Na$^+$] is slightly less than calculated. A high degree of accuracy is rarely needed in the formulation of treatment. Frequent serum electrolytes should be obtained, and increasing symptoms may necessitate more rapid therapy despite the inherent risks.

For acute hyponatremia (less than 48 hours), more rapid treatment may be used. Symptomatic acute hyponatremia may be treated with hypertonic saline to correct serum [Na$^+$] at a rate of 1 to 2 mEq/L/h. Hyperacute hyponatremia, which may result from inadvertent infusion of large volumes of water or from dialysis accidents, can be treated to increase serum [Na$^+$] at rates of 5 mEq/L/h. The treatment goal in any of these settings is to achieve a serum sodium level above 125 mEq/L or to achieve resolution of symptoms. It is unnecessary to increase serum sodium levels rapidly to normal values. Prophylactic anticonvulsant therapy may also be beneficial.

Hypernatremia
Causes

Hypernatremia is a less common problem in surgical patients than hyponatremia and is usually the result of excessive free water loss associated with hypovolemia. Patients with tracheostomies who breathe unhumidified air or patients with high fevers can lose large volumes of free water through increased insensible water losses. Large volumes of free water can also be lost when hypertonic glucose solutions are used for peritoneal dialysis. Head trauma or neurosurgical procedures may be complicated by the development of diabetes insipidus. In this condition, secretion of ADH is depressed, which results in free water diuresis. On occasion, free water losses secondary to diabetes insipidus can be massive.

Hypernatremia can also be caused by increased total body content of sodium, which is usually related to exogenous administration of sodium. Infusion of excessive amounts of sodium bicarbonate during acute resuscitation from cardiopulmonary arrest is frequently associated with subsequent hypernatremia. Administration of solutions containing large amounts of sodium for replacement of free water deficits may also lead to hypernatremia.

Clinical Features

The symptoms of hypernatremia are related to the hyperosmolar state. CNS effects predominate because of cellular dehydration as water passes into the extracellular space. This may result in subarachnoid hemorrhage but is more commonly associated with symptoms of restlessness, irritability, ataxia, fever, tonic spasms, and seizures. Moderate degrees of hypernatremia are tolerated well, and symptoms rarely develop unless serum [Na$^+$] levels exceed 160 mEq/L or serum osmolality exceeds 320 to 330 mOsm/kg. The development of symptoms also depends on the rapidity with which the hypernatremia develops.

Treatment

Once hypernatremia becomes symptomatic, it is associated with significant morbidity and mortality. Prompt treatment of hypernatremia is essential. Rapid correction of hypernatremia is associated with a significant risk of cerebral edema and herniation. In chronic hypernatremia, the cells within the brain gradually adapt by increasing intracellular osmotic solute content, thereby regaining cellular volume. These cellular changes are not readily reversed. A sudden decrease in extracellular sodium concentration, and therefore osmolality, results in cell swelling. Because chronic hypernatremia is relatively well tolerated, there are few advantages to correcting the free water deficit rapidly. Free water is administered to correct serum $[Na^+]$ at a rate not exceeding 0.7 mEq/L/h. The amount of water required to correct a hypernatremic state depends on the free water deficit, the insensible free water losses, and the urinary free water excretion rate. The water requirement to replace the free water deficit can be calculated using the following formula:

water requirement

$$= (actual\ [Na^+]_s/desired\ [Na^+]_s - 1) \times TBW \quad (8)$$

Because

desired change in $[Na^+]_s$ = actual $[Na^+]_s$ − desired $[Na^+]_s$

It follows that

$$\frac{desired\ change\ in\ [Na^+]_s}{desired\ [Na^+]_s} = \frac{actual\ [Na^+]_s}{desired\ [Na^+]_s - 1}$$

Substituting into formula 8,

water requirement

$$= \frac{desired\ change\ in\ [Na^+]_s}{desired\ [Na^+]_s} \times TBW \quad (9)$$

For example, a 70-kg patient with a TBW of 42 L (TBW 60% of body weight) has a serum sodium of 170 mEq/L. The maximum desired change in serum sodium over 1 day would be about 16 mEq (0.7 mEq/L/h). Substituting into formula 9,

$$water\ requirement = \frac{16}{154} \times 42$$

$$= 4.3\ L$$

The desired level of serum sodium would not be achieved unless insensible losses (about 8 mL/kg/d) and urinary free water losses were also replaced. Urinary losses of free water can be determined by calculating free water clearance:

$$C_{H_2O} = V - C_{osm} = V - \frac{(U_{osm} \times V)}{P_{osm}} \quad (10)$$

where:
C_{H_2O} = free water clearance
C_{osm} = osmolar clearance rate
V = urine flow rate
U_{osm} and P_{osm} = urine and plasma osmolalities

The U_{osm} and P_{osm} can be estimated by the total sodium and potassium concentrations. Therefore,

$$C_{H_2O} = V - [(U_{Na} + U_K) \times V]/[Na^+]_s \quad (11)$$

where:
U_{Na} and U_K = urinary sodium and potassium concentrations

A positive number signifies net free water loss and adds to the water requirement, whereas a negative number indicates free water absorption and is substracted from the water requirement. Thus, the total water requirement to achieve the desired decrease in serum $[Na^+]$ is the sum of the calculated water deficit plus the calculated insensible water loss plus the urinary free water clearance.

COMPOSITIONAL CHANGES

Potassium

Potassium is the major intracellular cation and is the major determinant of intracellular osmolality. Normally, intracellular potassium concentration is about 150 mEq/L, whereas extracellular potassium levels range from 3.5 to 5 mEq/L. Because of the large difference between intracellular and extracellular potassium concentrations, a transmembrane potential is generated. Alterations in the potassium concentration gradient have profound effects on transmembrane potential and consequently on cellular function. This is especially true for cardiac, skeletal, and smooth muscle. The membrane potential (E_m) developed in cells is described by the Nernst equation:

$$E_m = -\log 60\ [K_I]/[K_E] \quad (12)$$

where:
$[K_I]$ and $[K_E]$ = intracellular and extracellular potassium concentrations, respectively

Normally, the membrane potential of cells is about −90 mV as produced by a $[K_I]/[K_E]$ ratio of 30:1. Intracellular potassium levels are relatively stable, but extracellular potassium levels are often altered in pathologic situations. Overall potassium balance is determined by potassium intake and by renal and extrarenal excretion.

Extracellular potassium concentration is primarily determined by renal excretion. About 90% of ingested potassium is excreted in the urine. Most potassium filtered by the glomerulus is reabsorbed in the proximal tubule, so that net excretion of potassium is determined by the amount of potassium secreted by the distal tubule and collecting duct of the nephron. In these nephron segments, movement of potassium into the tubular lumen is determined by the difference between intracellular and luminal fluid potassium concentrations, the permeability of the luminal cell membranes to potassium, and the electrical potential gradient across the luminal cell membrane. Potassium secretion is stimulated by increased urine flow in the distal nephron segments, increased sodium delivery to these segments, high plasma potassium concentrations, and alkalosis. In addition, humoral factors, including aldosterone, vasopressin, and β-adrenergic agonists, stimulate renal excretion of potassium. Because of the central role of the kidneys in potassium excretion, renal failure (either acute or chronic) can easily lead to hyperkalemia.

Sweat accounts for a small amount of daily potassium excretion. Nonrenal excretion of potassium is primarily fecal, and 5 to 10 mEq/d is excreted in the feces. This amount may be greatly increased in hyperkalemic states or in renal failure.

Extracellular potassium levels can be greatly influenced by the acute flux of potassium into or out of the cells. Insulin causes potassium to move into the cell, inducing a change in membrane potential and stimulating glycolysis. Alkalosis causes potassium to shift into cells in exchange for H^+. Conversely, acidemia induces the cellular exchange of intracellular K^+ for extracellular H^+. A redistribution of potassium into the ECF can also occur in hyperosmolar conditions because the movement of water into the extracellular compartment causes "solvent drag" and may increase the flux of potassium in response to its concentration gradient.

Hyperkalemia

Causes. Hyperkalemia rarely develops from excessive potassium intake in the absence of renal insufficiency because the capacity for renal potassium excretion is large. In the surgical patient, diminished renal function is perhaps the most common problem leading to hyperkalemia. Both chronic and acute renal failure result in a defect in potassium excretion. Nonoliguric renal failure, a form of renal failure common in critically ill patients, may lead to potassium intoxication despite apparently adequate urine formation. Serum potassium levels may increase by 0.3 to 0.5 mEq/L/d in noncatabolic patients with acute renal failure, but this level can increase to 0.7 mEq/L/d or more in catabolic patients or those with other sources of potassium intake. In patients with chronic renal disease, colonic potassium excretion is increased, as is the amount of potassium excreted per functional nephron, thereby normalizing potassium balance. Insulin therapy may lead to hypokalemia if potassium supplementation is not given. Infusion of cationic amino acid solutions, such as arginine and lysine, can be associated with hyperkalemia because these amino acids are taken up by cells in exchange for potassium. In addition, hyperkalemia has been reported to occur with administration of β-blocking agents.

Cellular disruption with release of potassium may result in hyperkalemia. Crush injuries can cause massive release of potassium. Reperfusion of ischemic limbs can also lead to substantial elevations in potassium. Potassium released from lysed erythrocytes in large hematomas or after massive blood transfusion can lead to hyperkalemia, particularly in patients with impaired renal function. Similarly, potassium release from tumor lysis may result in increased serum potassium. Hyperkalemia can also be associated with the depolarizing muscle relaxants (eg, succinylcholine). Although unusual, hyperkalemia can also result from absorption of potassium after the use of solutions containing high potassium levels, such as cardioplegia solutions or organ preservation solutions (Collin or University of Wisconsin solutions).

Finally, a spuriously elevated serum potassium level due to hemolysis caused by application of a tourniquet and fist-squeezing is not uncommon. Hyperkalemia accompanying thrombocytosis and leukocytosis may also be a cause of spuriously elevated potassium determinations.

Clinical Features. The clinical manifestations of hyperkalemia are primarily related to membrane depolarization caused by a decrease in the $[K_I]/[K_E]$ ratio. The most life-threatening manifestations are related to the cardiac effects of membrane depolarization. Mild hyperkalemia results in peaked T waves on the electrocardiogram (ECG) and can cause paresthesia and weakness. More severe forms of hyperkalemia cause flattened P waves, prolongation of the QRS complex, and deep S waves on ECG. Ventricular fibrillation and cardiac arrest can result. Neuromuscular manifestations of severe hyperkalemia include weakness progressing to flaccid paralysis.

Treatment. The treatment of hyperkalemia is dictated by the serum level and by ECG changes or symptoms. Severe hyperkalemia with ECG abnormalities requires urgent treatment. The effects of hyperkalemia on membrane potentials can be reduced by increasing calcium levels. Rapid infusion of 10% to 20% calcium gluconate may be lifesaving. The effects are transient and usually last about 30 minutes. Administration of sodium bicarbonate is another temporary measure. The increase in serum sodium antagonizes the effects of hyperkalemia on the membrane potential, whereas the increase in extracellular pH shifts potassium into the cells. Movement of potassium into the intracellular compartment can also be achieved by giving 25 to 50 g of glucose (50 to 100 mL of 50% glucose solution) with 10 to 20 units of regular insulin.

Definitive therapy of hyperkalemia requires increasing potassium excretion. This may be accomplished by the administration of K^+–Na^+ exchange resins such as sodium polystyrene sulfonate (Kayexalate). The usual oral dose is 40 g dissolved in 20 to 100 mL of sorbitol. Each gram removes about 1 mEq of potassium. Kayexalate can also be given as a retention enema in a dose of 50 to 100 grams in 200 mL of water. Retention of the enema may be facilitated by inflating the balloon of a Foley catheter in the rectum. Each gram removes about 0.5 mEq of potassium. Peritoneal dialysis or hemodialysis is indicated for severe hyperkalemia and for patients with renal failure.

Hypokalemia

Causes. Hypokalemia can be caused by total body potassium depletion secondary to decreased potassium intake, increased extrarenal potassium losses, or increased renal potassium losses. Normally, hypokalemia is not secondary to diminished potassium intake, although intravenous fluid replacement with potassium-free solutions for prolonged periods can result in hypokalemia, especially in patients with increased potassium losses from the gastrointestinal tract.

Decreased serum potassium levels may also be caused by redistribution of potassium into the intracellular space. Acute increases in blood pH secondary to bicarbonate administration during resuscitation can cause acute hypokalemia, as can administration of insulin to hyperglycemic diabetics.

Causes of hypokalemia include the following:

- Shift of potassium to the intracellular space
  Acute alkalosis
  Administration of glucose and insulin
  Catecholamines
- Increased gastrointestinal loss
  Diarrhea
  Mucus-secreting colon tumors (villous adenoma)
- Excessive renal loss
  Metabolic alkalosis
  Magnesium deficiency
  Hyperaldosteronism (adrenal adenoma or hyperplasia)

Clinical Features. Symptoms of hypokalemia, like those of hyperkalemia, are manifestations of disturbances in the $[K_I]/[K_E]$ ratio with resultant alterations in membrane potentials. As potassium levels fall below 2.5 mEq/L, muscle weakness is common. Severe hypokalemia can cause paralysis involving the muscles of respiration. Intestinal peristalsis can be impaired and result in intestinal ileus. Cardiac muscle abnormalities are reflected by the predisposition to digitalis intoxication, the development of cardiac arrhythmia, including ventricular fibrillation, and sensitization to epinephrine-induced arrhythmia. ECG abnormalities include flattened T waves, depressed ST segments, prominent U waves, and prolongation of the QT interval. Renal changes include decreased renal blood flow and glomerular filtration rate. These effects may be relatively minor, and they may be accompanied by polyuria, polydipsia, metabolic alkalosis, and sodium retention. Decreased peripheral vascular resistance with ensuing hypotension may be due to a decrease in vascular sensitivity to angiotensin II.

Treatment. The primary treatment of hypokalemia is potassium replacement, although the patient's acid–base balance should be considered before initiating therapy. The route and rate of potassium replacement depends on the presence and severity of symptoms. A reduction in serum potassium of 1 mEq/L represents a total body potassium deficiency of about 100 to 200 mEq. Potassium should be administered intravenously if the symptoms are severe, if the serum concentration is below 2 mEq/L, or if the patient is unable to take oral potassium. Intravenous potassium can be administered at a rate of about 10 mEq/h, and the concentration of potassium should be 40 mEq/L or less. If less fluid is desired, up to 20 mEq in 100 mL of intravenous solution can be given, although no more than 40 mEq should be administered per hour. Potassium should be given orally if possible. Oral formulations include potassium salts such as potassium chloride, potassium phosphate, and potassium bicarbonate.

Calcium

Calcium is a divalent cation found in abundance in the human body. About 99% of total body calcium is located in bone in the form of hydroxyapatite crystals. Although the bulk of this calcium is not readily exchangeable, the calcium on the surface of bones can be exchanged and serves as the major store of calcium for maintenance of calcium balance. Calcium homeostasis depends on exchange of calcium between bone and ECF, renal excretion, and intestinal absorption. These three processes are controlled to a great extent by parathyroid hormone (PTH).

The total plasma calcium concentration is about 10 mg/dL. In ECF, calcium exists in three forms: ionized calcium, nonionized calcium, and protein-bound calcium. Ionized calcium, which makes up about 45% of total calcium, is responsible for most physiologic actions of calcium in the body, and its level is tightly controlled by regulatory mechanisms. Normal serum concentration of ionized calcium is about 4.5 mg/dL. Because laboratory measurement of the ionized form is more difficult than measurement of total calcium, many laboratories report only total calcium values. Some nonionized calcium is complexed with nonprotein anions, including phosphate and citrate, and does not easily dissociate. These molecular forms make up only 15% of the total calcium present in plasma. About 40% of extracellular nonionized calcium is bound to proteins. Most is bound to albumin, with the remainder bound to αa- and β-globulins. In contrast to non–protein-bound calcium (ionized and nonionized), protein-bound calcium is not ultrafiltratable.

Changes in either plasma protein levels or pH can alter the proportion of calcium in the ionized state. The protein binding of calcium is pH dependent because of competition by H^+ for protein binding sites. Prompt correction of changes in ionized calcium by various homeostatic mechanisms usually prevents symptoms from occurring, but rapid changes in pH can result in symptoms. The change in ionized calcium can be predicted if the changes in pH and protein concentrations are known. A 0.1 change in pH changes protein-bound calcium by 0.17 mg/dL in the same direction as the pH change. Thus, acidosis decreases protein-bound calcium levels and increases ionized calcium levels. Similarly, a change in albumin concentration of 1 g/dL changes protein-bound calcium by 0.8 mg/dL in the same direction. Because little of the calcium is bound to globulins, changes in globulin concentration of 1 g/dL change protein-bound calcium by only 0.16 mg/dL.

Despite a 10,000-fold concentration gradient with the ECF, the intracellular calcium concentration is normally maintained at extremely low levels, 10^{-7} mol/L. This is accomplished by active transport of calcium out of the cell and by sequestration of calcium within mitochondria and the endoplasmic reticulum. Calcium influx occurs through calcium channels, and cytosolic calcium is often bound to specific calcium-binding proteins such as calmodulin. These control mechanisms are key to the central role of calcium as a second messenger in multiple physiologic cellular functions such as neurovascular transmission, muscle contraction, and enzyme regulation.

Calcium Homeostasis

Calcium homeostasis is maintained through a balance of bone exchange, renal excretion, and intestinal absorption. All of these functions are controlled to a great degree by PTH. Of these three homeostatic mechanisms, calcium exchange with bone is the most important. Although the mechanisms are not clearly understood, it appears that decreased levels of ionized calcium lead to increases in PTH and increases in 1,25-dihydroxyvitamin D_3, both of which stimulate bone absorption by increasing osteoclastic activity. Increased levels of ionized calcium results in decreased PTH and 1,25-dihydroxyvitamin D_3, which decreases bone absorption. In addition, an elevated ionized calcium concentration results in increased calcitonin and 24,25-dihydroxyvitamin D, which increases osteoblastic activity.

Intestinal absorption of calcium depends primarily on 1,25-dihydroxyvitamin D_3, which stimulates calcium absorption from all parts of the small intestine. Renal excretion of calcium is regulated by PTH and vitamin D, which increase distal tubular reabsorption of calcium, and by calcitonin, which inhibits calcium reabsorption. Both metabolic and respiratory alkalosis can increase calcium excretion, but acidosis has the opposite effect. The basics of the regulation of calcium homeostasis are depicted in Figure 10-7.

Hypercalcemia

Causes. The most common cause of hypercalcemia is primary hyperparathyroidism, which occurs as a result of a parathyroid adenoma in about 80% of cases. Chief cell hyperplasia accounts for an additional 15% of cases. Secondary hyperparathyroidism, in which elevation of PTH secretion occurs because of a deficiency in vitamin D metabolism, occurs in patients with chronic renal failure but does not usually increase serum calcium. Tertiary hyperparathyroidism is the development of autonomously functioning parathyroid adenomas as a result of chronic parathyroid stimulation. Because parathyroid function does not always return to normal after correction of the underlying cause of hyperparathyroidism, hypercalcemia may persist for long periods, for example, after renal transplantation despite the fact that renal function has returned toward normal. In addition to these conditions, hypercalcemia secondary to thiazide diuretics or lithium therapy has been reported.

Hypercalcemia can be caused by malignant disease, by either metastases to bone or autonomous tumor secretion of hormone-like substances that alter calcium homeostasis. Bony involvement resulting in hypercalcemia is often due to multiple myeloma, lymphoma, or metastatic breast carcinoma. Interleukin-1, colony-stimulating factor, and tumor necrosis factor have been implicated as local mediators of the osteolytic activity associated with tumor metastases. Tumors that elaborate humoral factors resulting in hypercalcemia are primarily squamous cell carcinomas of the head and neck, esophagus, lung, kidney, and genitourinary tract. Secretion of PTH-like peptides, prostaglandins, transforming growth factor, and vitamin D metabolites has been reported. Humorally mediated hypercalcemia may also occur with metastatic breast carcinoma.

Clinical Features. The clinical manifestations of hypercalcemia depend on both the severity and duration of the abnormality. Neuromuscular effects may be the earliest manifestations and include muscle fatigue, weakness, personality disorders, psychoses, confusion, and coma. Cardiovascular effects are less prominent, with hypertension being the most frequent problem encountered. ECG changes include shortening of the Q-T interval. Gastroin-

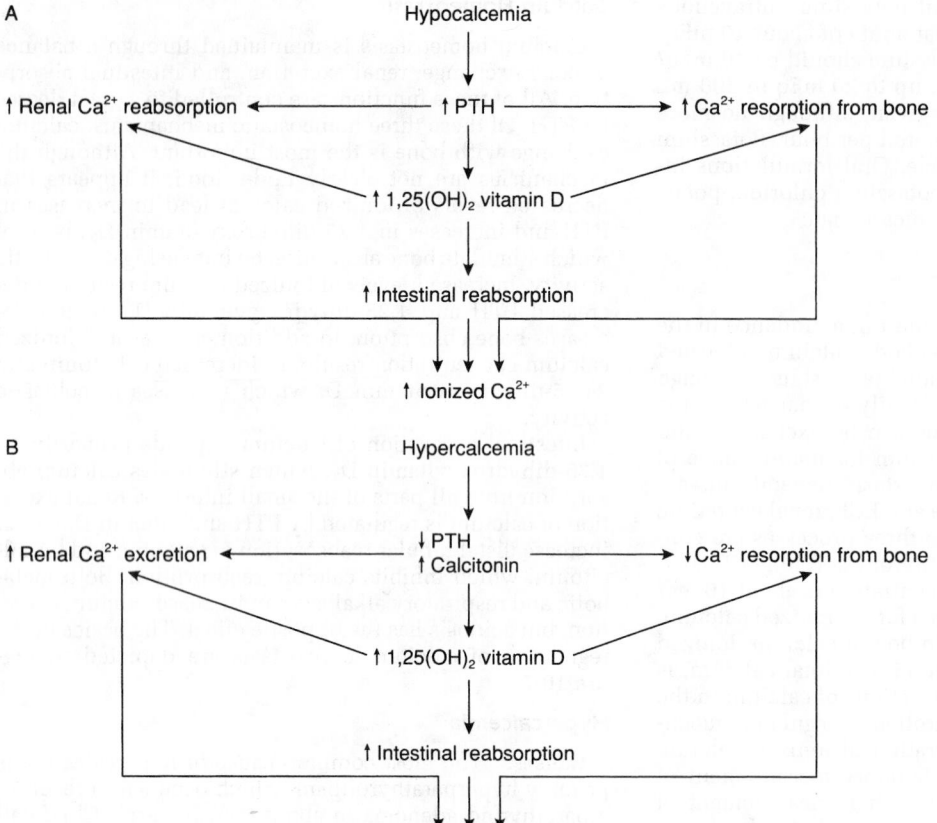

Figure 10-7. Effects of hypocalcemia (*A*) and hypercalcemia (*B*) on the mediators of calcium homeostasis. PTH, parathyroid hormone.

testinal side effects, such as nausea, vomiting, and abdominal pain, are not uncommon. Pancreatitis and increased gastric acid secretion with ulcer formation have also been reported.

The renal side effects of chronic hypercalcemia are numerous and can be severe. The combination of increased renal calcium excretion and decreased intestinal calcium reabsorption in response to hypercalcemia results in a new state of equilibrium at a higher serum concentration of calcium. A decrease in glomerular filtration rate, which may be a direct effect of hypercalcemia or secondary to dehydration from vomiting, can exacerbate the hypercalcemia by increasing calcium reabsorption by the kidney. In addition, nephrocalcinosis can occur, ultimately leading to chronic renal failure. Nephrolithiasis, interstitial nephropathy, renal tubular acidosis (RTA), and nephrogenic diabetes insipidus may also accompany prolonged hypercalcemia.

Treatment. Elevation of total serum calcium concentrations to greater than 14 mg/dL requires prompt treatment to prevent the many serious and potentially lethal complications. This is even more urgent for hypercalcemia associated with hyperphosphatemia because of the risk of metastatic calcification. Immediate measures are directed toward maximizing renal excretion of calcium. Because these patients are often dehydrated, 0.9% or 0.45% saline solution with 20 to 30 mEq/L of potassium is administered intravenously. Hydration should proceed at rates of 200 to 300 mL/h to promote diuresis. Furosemide may be given to further enhance calcium excretion, but adequate hydration must precede diuretic therapy.

Long-term treatment depends on the underlying cause of the hypercalcemia. Primary hyperparathyroidism is usually readily treated by resection of the parathyroid abnormality (adenoma or hyperplasia). Definitive treatment of secondary or tertiary hyperparathyroidism may be either subtotal parathyroidectomy or total parathyroidectomy with autonomous parathyroid transplantation. Hypercalcemia secondary to tumor secretion of hormonal mediators may be controlled by extirpation of the tumor. In the presence of metastatic bone disease, inhibition of bone resorption with mithramycin or calcitonin may yield good results. In addition, hypercalcemia due to metastatic breast carcinoma or hematologic malignancies may respond to steroid therapy. Patients with renal failure benefit from dialysis using a low-calcium dialysate.

Hypocalcemia

Causes. Hypocalcemia secondary to hypoparathyroidism can complicate thyroid or parathyroid surgery by either inadvertent total parathyroidectomy or loss of parathyroid function due to devascularization. This has been reported to occur in as many as 2% to 3% of total thyroidectomies, although this figure appears to be declining. After resection of a parathyroid adenoma, hypocalcemia can occur because of atrophy of the remaining glands. Calcium replacement therapy may be required until the remaining glands become totally functional.

Hypocalcemia can also be a complication of acute pancreatitis, soft tissue injury, and pancreatic and small bowel fistulas. Longstanding vitamin D deficiency secondary to malnutrition, malabsorption, or lack of sun exposure can lead to hypocalcemia. Renal failure can lead to a deficiency in 1,25-dihydroxyvitamin D_3 and result in diminished intestinal absorption of calcium. Severe magnesium deficiency can also lead to hypocalcemia because of suppression of PTH levels.

Clinical Features. Serum calcium levels below 8 mg/dL may be associated with symptoms and signs that are primarily manifestations of neuromuscular abnormalities. These include muscle cramps, perioral tingling, paresthesia, laryngeal stridor, tetany, seizures, and psychotic behavior. Classic signs of hypocalcemia include hyperactive deep tendon reflexes, Chvostek sign, and Trousseau sign. ECG changes include a prolonged QT interval caused by prolongation of the ST segment.

Treatment. Asymptomatic hypocalcemia, which may be secondary to low protein or albumin levels with normal ionized calcium levels, need not be treated. Symptomatic hypocalcemia is best treated with intravenous infusion of calcium in the form of calcium gluconate or calcium chloride. Calcium chloride dissociates primarily to the ionized form and is therefore more efficacious in raising ionized calcium levels. Calcium should be administered at a rate not exceeding 50 mg/min (2.5 mEq/min). Prolonged calcium replacement is given orally in the form of calcium lactate, calcium citrate, or calcium carbonate. Vitamin D_3, also known as calcitriol, increases the rate of intestinal absorption and decreases the oral calcium dose requirement.

Magnesium

Total body content of magnesium in the average adult is 2000 mEq, half of which is confined to bone. Most of the remaining magnesium is distributed in the intracellular space. Less than 1% of total body magnesium is located in the extracellular space at concentrations of 1.4 to 2 mEq/L (or 1.7 to 2.3 mg/dL). Sixty percent of this magnesium exists in the ionized form, 25% is in the protein-bound state, and the remainder is complexed with nonprotein anionic species.

Magnesium consumed in the diet is primarily absorbed by the small intestine. The amount absorbed depends on the intake, which averages 25 mEq/d. Magnesium absorption may also be influenced by the levels of 1,25-dihydroxyvitamin D_3. Bone stores constitute the other major source of available magnesium, although regulation of magnesium exchange with bone is poorly understood.

Magnesium is primarily excreted by the kidneys. About 40% of the filtered magnesium is reabsorbed in the proximal tubule, predominantly in the ascending limb of Henle. Thus, loop diuretics cause a marked increase in magnesium excretion. Magnesium excretion is also increased by hypermagnesemia, hypercalcemia, metabolic acidosis, and phosphate depletion. Conversely, magnesium excretion is decreased by metabolic alkalosis.

Hypermagnesemia

Causes. Renal failure is the primary cause of hypermagnesemia. Because of the ability of the kidneys to excrete large magnesium loads, hypermagnesemia rarely occurs if renal function remains normal. In patients with chronic or acute renal failure, administration of magnesium-containing antacids or laxatives is often the cause of magnesium excesses. Hypermagnesemia may also be due to the release of magnesium from injured tissues; thus, severe burns, crush injuries, and other causes of rhabdomyolysis may lead to high magnesium levels. Severe metabolic acidosis, extracellular volume depletion, and renal insufficiency with creatinine clearances below 30 mL/min may also cause hypermagnesemia.

Clinical Features. Neuromuscular function is depressed by hypermagnesemia because of the inhibition of synaptic acetylcholine release. Loss of deep tendon reflexes can occur with magnesium levels above 8 mg/dL. Paralysis and eventually coma can develop if levels exceed 12 to 18 mg/dL. Acute hypermagnesemia may be manifested by hypotension or even cardiac arrest if levels exceed 18 mg/dL.

Treatment. Hypermagnesemia is rare. Because it is usually associated with renal failure, withholding magnesium-containing drugs in these patients usually prevents the development of magnesium excesses. Calcium antagonizes the effects of magnesium, so that infusion of 5 to 10 mEq of calcium by slow intravenous injection may serve as adequate emergency treatment. Volume expansion, correction of acid–base disturbances, administration of loop diuretics, and hemodialysis may also be used to decrease magnesium levels.

Hypomagnesemia

Causes. Because the kidneys are able to conserve magnesium well in states of magnesium depletion, hypomagnesemia rarely occurs from poor intake alone. The combination of low intake and increased gastrointestinal loss can lead to hypomagnesemia. Malabsorptive states, especially steatorrhea, can result in significant losses of magnesium. Other causes of hypomagnesemia include prolonged periods of intravenous fluid replacement without magnesium replacement and chronic use of loop diuretics. Drugs, such as cyclosporine, aminoglycosides, cisplatin, and insulin, can also produce magnesium depletion. Burns, acute pancreatitis, treatment of diabetic ketoacidosis, and the diuretic phase of acute renal failure have been associated with the development of hypomagnesemia.

Clinical Features. Magnesium plays an integral role as a cofactor in many enzyme systems and also affects neuromuscular function. Deficiencies in magnesium may present symptoms and signs similar to hypocalcemia. Muscle fasciculations and weakness, tetany, carpopedal spasm, nausea, vomiting, and personality changes may occur. Electrolyte disturbances may also be caused by hypomagnesemia. Hypocalcemia caused by impaired PTH secretion and PTH resistance may develop. Hypokalemia caused by renal potassium wasting may also occur.

Treatment. Magnesium may be administered orally in mild cases of hypomagnesemia, but large oral doses frequently lead to diarrhea. Correction of major deficits is therefore managed by intravenous administration of magnesium sulfate at a dose of 50 to 100 mEq/d. Treatment of patients who have severe symptoms with up to 3 g of magnesium sulfate may be accomplished by bolus intravenous injection followed by an infusion of 1 to 2 mEq/kg/d.

ACID–BASE BALANCE
Definitions

An acid is defined as a chemical that can donate a hydrogen ion (H^+), for example, HCl and H_2CO_3, and a base is a chemical that can accept an H^+, for example, OH^- and HCO_3^-). Ampholytes are both acids and bases; an example is $H_2PO_4^-$, which can donate a H^+ to become HPO_4^{-2} but can also accept H^+ to become H_3PO_4. Because HCl is a strong acid that almost completely dissociates, Cl^- is not considered a base. Bases are commonly anions, but neutral substances can also function as bases (eg, ammonia and creatinine). Some chemicals do not fit the classic definition of an acid, although they retain acidic properties when dissociated in water. For example, when $CaCl_2$ is dissolved in water, the Ca^{2+} accepts OH^- to form $Ca(OH)_2$. Because $[H^+] \times [OH^-]$ in water remains constant at 10^{-14}, the consumption of OH^- by Ca^{2+} results in increased dissociation of water. Consequently, the concentration of hydrogen ions increases, and $CaCl_2$ dissolved in water is an acidic solution.

The concentration of hydrogen ions ($[H^+]$) determines the acidity of a solution. The pH is the negative logarithm of $[H^+]$ expressed in moles per liter (mol/L). The concentration of H^+ in biologic systems is in the range of nanomoles (10^{-9} mol) per liter (nmol/L). When

$$[H^+] = 40 \text{ nmol/L} = 4 \times 10^{-10} \text{ mol/L}$$

then

$$pH = -\log [H^+] = -(-7.4) = 7.4$$

When

$$[H^+] = 80 \text{ nmol/L} = 8 \times 10^{-10} \text{ mol/L}$$

then

$$pH = -\log [H^+] = -(-7.1) = 7.1$$

The degree to which an acid dissociates determines its strength. If an acid, HA, dissociates to H^+ and A^-, then

$$[H^+] \times [A^-]/[HA] = K \qquad (13)$$

where:
K = dissociation constant

The greater the value of K, the greater the ability to dissociate, and therefore the greater the strength of the acid. Because most acids have a K value considerably below 1.0,

$$pK = -\log K \qquad (14)$$

Rearranging,

$$[H^+] = K \times [HA]/[A^-]$$

$$-\log [H^+] = -\log K \times -\log [HA]/[A^-] \qquad (15)$$

$$pH = pK \times \log [A^-]/[HA]$$

This is the derivation for the Henderson-Hasselbalch equation.

Buffer Systems

Buffers are chemicals in solution that tend to minimize changes in pH that would otherwise occur after the addition of acid or alkali. If a strong acid is added to the salt of a weak acid and a strong base, the reaction produces another salt and a weak acid:

$$HCl + NaHCO_3 \rightarrow NaCl + H_2CO_3$$

Thus, the decrease in pH that would have occurred in the absence of $NaHCO_3$ is minimized. Conversely, if a strong base is added to a weak acid, the base is neutralized:

$$NaOH + H_2CO_3 \rightarrow NaHCO_3 + H_2O$$

The elevation in pH after the addition of NaOH is prevented.

Thus, one type of buffer is a mixture of a weak acid and its salt, which forms an amount of weak acid or base equivalent to the amount of strong acid or base added to the system. The presence of such buffer systems in the body is key to minimizing changes in pH secondary to the daily production of the 70 mEq of acid generated from dietary precursors. There is a relatively narrow range of pH for optimal function of the chemical reactions necessary for cell function.

The principal intracellular buffers are organic phosphates, bicarbonate, and peptides. In addition, hemoglobin functions as a significant buffer in red blood cells. The major extracellular buffer is bicarbonate. An approximation of the total body buffer capacity is 15 mEq/kg. More than half of the total body alkaline buffer content is located outside the ECF and may in large part reside in bone.[11]

The buffer pair carbonic acid–bicarbonate (H_2CO_3/HCO_3^-) is the focus of the ensuing discussion because it is the primary buffer system of the body and the components of this buffer system are easily measured. Because all body buffer systems are in equilibrium, the state of the H_2CO_3/HCO_3^- system essentially reflects the state of all the body buffers.

From a chemical point of view, the ideal buffer should have a pK that approximates the pH to be preserved. The H_2CO_3/HCO_3^- buffer system has a pK of only 6.1, but this buffer system is efficient because of the presence of large amounts of bicarbonate, the conversion of its acid H_2CO_3 to CO_2 that is rapidly excreted through the lungs, and an inexhaustible supply of CO_2, although at low concentrations.

The H_2CO_3/HCO_3^- buffer system is defined by the Henderson-Hasselbalch equation. This equation (equation 15), when applied to the H_2CO_3/HCO_3^- buffer system, yields the following:

$$pH = pK + \log [HCO_3^-]/[H_2CO_3] \qquad (16)$$

In the clinical use of this equation, $[H_2CO_3]$ is replaced by $[CO_2]$ because measurement of the low concentrations of $[H_2CO_3]$ present in body fluids is difficult, whereas $[CO_2]$, which is in equilibrium with $[H_2CO_3]$ in a fixed ratio, can be readily measured. Making this substitution, the equation becomes

$$pH = pK + \log [HCO_3^-]/[CO_2] \qquad (17)$$

Because the pK for this buffer system is 6.1,

$$pH = 6.1 + \log [HCO_3^-]/[CO_2] \qquad (18)$$

Using normal values for $[HCO_3]$ (24 mEq/L) and $[CO_2]$ (1.2 mmol/L),

$$pH = 6.1 + \log 24/1.2$$

$$= 6.1 + \log 20 = 7.4$$

A pH of 7.4 is maintained as long as the ratio of $[HCO_3^-]$ to $[CO_2]$ remains 20:1. The amount of $[CO_2]$ in solution is estimated from P_{CO_2} and its solubility coefficient (0.03 in plasma). Making these substitutions,

$$pH = 6.1 + \log [HCO_3^-]/(P_{CO_2} \times 0.03) \qquad (19)$$

Anion Gap

The anion gap is defined as follows:

$$\text{anion gap} = [Na^+] - ([Cl^-] + [HCO_3^-]) \qquad (20)$$

Normally, the difference between the serum $[Na^+]$ and the sum of the chloride and bicarbonate anion concentrations is a reflection of the sum of the serum proteins, sulfate anions, inorganic phosphates, and organic acids present in low concentrations. The anion gap is usually 12 ± 2 mEq/L. Variances from the normal may be caused by a change in unmeasured anions or cations. Calculation of the anion gap may help define both simple and mixed forms of acid–base disturbances. Acidosis associated with a high anion gap is generally secondary to increases in endogenously produced acids (eg, lactic or ketoacidosis), decreases in renal excretion of acids (eg, renal failure), or ingestion of toxins.

ACID–BASE DISTURBANCES

The four primary acid–base disturbances are related to changes in either $[HCO_3^-]$ or P_{CO_2}, which reflect equation 19, relating pH to the $[HCO_3^-]/P_{CO_2}$ ratio. Metabolic acidosis is a decrease in pH as a result of a primary decrease in $[HCO_3^-]$, whereas metabolic alkalosis is an increase in pH caused by a primary increase in $[HCO_3^-]$. Respiratory acidosis is a decrease in pH secondary to a primary increase in PCO_2. Likewise, respiratory alkalosis is an increase in pH because of a primary decrease in PCO_2. In each of these disorders, compensatory changes occur to minimize changes in the relative ratio of $[HCO_3^-]$ to PCO_2 and thereby blunt the effect on pH (Table 10-8).

Metabolic Acidosis

Three mechanisms result in a decrease in extracellular bicarbonate concentration and metabolic acidosis:

1. Dilutional acidosis. Rapid infusion of an alkali-free solution results in dilution of the bicarbonate concentration.
2. Cellular retention of K^+ in exchange for Na^+ and H^+. Buffering of the H^+ may result in a transient decrease in extracellular bicarbonate concentration.
3. Decreased body bicarbonate content. This occurs when net loss of bicarbonate exceeds bicarbonate generation.

The first two mechanisms are relatively infrequent and generally produce only mild, self-limiting metabolic acidosis. Most clinically significant metabolic acidosis is related to net loss of bicarbonate, which occurs when consumption due to either loss or titration is greater than bicarbonate generation. Under normal circumstances of ingestion of the average amount of protein in the American diet, about 70 mEq of acid is generated daily. The major source of acid production is sulfuric acid from the metabolism of sulfur-containing amino acids. In addition, normal physiologic processes result in the generation of organic acids, the titration of which consumes bicarbonate. Although the resulting organic anions are further metabolized with regeneration of bicarbonate, urinary excretion of some organic anions occurs and results in net loss of bicarbonate.

These sources of acid gain are partially offset by net gastrointestinal absorption of metabolizable anions, such as citrate, which are metabolized to yield bicarbonate. The remainder of the excess acid is balanced by renal excretion of acid with simultaneous generation of bicarbonate. A decrease in body bicarbonate content may therefore be the result of a primary increase in net acid generation, termed *extrarenal acidosis,* or a primary reduction in renal acid excretion, termed *renal acidosis.*

In extrarenal acidosis, the normal compensatory mechanism is increased renal excretion of acid, usually as ammonia, with generation of bicarbonate. This mechanism is sensitive to decreases in bicarbonate concentration and has the capacity to generate large amounts of bicarbonate.

In contrast, renal acidosis is not as readily compensated because the renal abnormality is the primary mechanism. The level to which serum bicarbonate concentration decreases depends on several factors, including the magnitude of the disparity in acid production and acid excretion as well as its duration. In general, the development of renal acidosis is slow but progressive, whereas the development of extrarenal acidosis is rapid but usually self-limiting. Despite persistent net loss of bicarbonate, extracellular bicarbonate concentration may stabilize at a subnormal level rather than continue to decrease. This may be due to bone buffering, which has the capacity to buffer as much as 28 to 37 mEq/d of acid.

Mechanisms Resulting in Decreased Body Bicarbonate Content

Increased Production of Organic Acids. Increased protein intake and tissue catabolism resulting in greater metabolism of sulfur-containing amino acids can lead to generation of increased amounts of sulfuric acid. With normal kidney function, any decline in serum bicarbonate concentration stimulates renal acid excretion, which can compensate nearly completely for the increase in acid production.

Administration of Exogenous Acid. Ingestion of a sufficient quantity of exogenous acid can exceed renal compensatory capacity and result in metabolic acidosis. Examples of acids that may be ingested include ammonium chloride, calcium chloride, nitric acid, sulfuric acid, and hydrochloric acid.

Nonrenal Loss of Bicarbonate. Diarrhea, intestinal or pancreatic fistulas, and burns can cause metabolic acidosis secondary to loss of bicarbonate. In addition, ureterosigmoidostomy and ureteroileostomy result in loss of bicarbonate because of reabsorption of NH_4Cl from the urine. The potential for fistulas to result in metabolic acidosis depends on the concentration of bicarbonate in the fluid and the rate of external drainage. Thus, metabolic acidosis is less common with biliary fistulas than pancreatic fistulas because bicarbonate concentration in bile is generally less than 50 to 60 mEq/L, and the amount of drainage tends to be modest. In pancreatic fistulas, bicarbonate concentration in pancreatic juice approaches 150 mEq/L, and the drainage can be profuse.

Organic Acidosis. The two most common types of organic acidosis are ketoacidosis and lactic acidosis. The abnormality primarily responsible for ketoacidosis is deficiency of insulin, whether primary, as in diabetic ketoacidosis, or secondary to hypoglycemia. Normally, free fatty acids generated from breakdown of triglycerides in adipose tissue are either used as an energy source by various organs such as muscle, or carried to the liver, where they are reesterified to triglycerides and incorporated into very-low-density lipoprotein, or further metabolized. Ketoacids are produced by mitochondrial metabolism of free fatty acids to acetyl-CoA with subsequent formation of acetoacetate and β-hydroxybutyrate (redox forms of the same compound). Under normal conditions, a small amount of ketoacids is produced. During prolonged starvation, production of ketoacids increases to modest levels, providing an important source of energy to nonhepatic tissues, particularly the brain. In ketoacidosis, the ketoacid production is excessive because of insulin deficiency, which drives ketoacid production by increasing free fatty acid release from adipose tissue, increasing transport of free fatty acids into hepatic mitochondria, promoting conversion of acetyl-CoA to ketoacids, and impairing extrahepatic use of ketoacids.[12] In diabetic ketoacidosis, insulin deficiency also contributes to hyperglycemia by decreasing the metabolism of glucose by extrahepatic tissues and increasing hepatic production of glucose. The resulting osmotic glucose diuresis causes increased renal excretion of sodium and water. Additional losses of sodium and potas-

Table 10-8. HCO_3^- AND PCO_2 DERANGEMENTS IN PRIMARY AND SECONDARY ACID–BASE DISTURBANCES

Disorder	Primary			Secondary	
	pH	HCO_3^-	PCO_2	HCO_3^-	PCO_2
Metabolic acidosis	↓	↓			↓
Metabolic alkalosis	↑	↑			↑
Respiratory acidosis	↓		↑	↑	
Respiratory alkalosis	↑		↓	↓	

sium occur as the result of renal excretion of the excess ketoacid anions. Potassium excretion is further enhanced by hyperaldosteronism as the result of the increased delivery of sodium to the distal tubule that occurs in association with the osmotic diuresis. Despite total body potassium depletion, serum potassium concentration is often increased in diabetic ketoacidosis secondary to metabolic acidosis, renal insufficiency, insulin deficiency, and hyperosmolality. These pathophysiologic changes result in the typical clinical presentation, which includes dehydration, polyuria, polydipsia, hyperglycemia, hyperventilation, and metabolic acidosis with an increased anion gap (normochloremic). Spontaneous decarboxylation of acetoacetate to acetone occurs with excretion of acetone through the lungs, resulting in the characteristic odor described in diabetic ketoacidosis. Patients may be lucid, although some degree of mental obtundation is common, and coma may occur.

In hyperosmolar, hyperglycemic, and nonketotic coma, moderate acidosis may be observed. The mechanism of the acidosis is not clear. In contrast to the moderate hyperglycemia, averaging 600 mg/dL, seen in diabetic ketoacidosis, the marked hyperglycemia, averaging 1200 mg/dL, that occurs in hyperosmolar nonketotic hyperglycemia is not associated with ketoacidosis.

Lactic acidosis can be divided into type A, caused by tissue hypoxia, and type B, caused by other mechanisms. Hypoxia, the most common cause of lactic acidosis, impairs the mitochondrial oxidation of NADH to NAD that is necessary for glycolysis. Under these conditions, NADH is oxidized by the reduction of pyruvate, the end product of glucose metabolism in the Embden-Meyerhof pathway, to lactic acid. Thus, generation of lactic acid is the final step of anaerobic glycolysis. Lactic acid is normally produced by muscle, blood elements, intestine, and skin, and is used by the liver and kidney. Normal serum lactate concentration is below 2 mEq/L. Lactic acidosis secondary to hypoxia is usually due to increased production of lactate as well as decreased use, and serum lactate concentration is greater than 6 mEq/L.

The most common cause of type B lactic acidosis is ethanol intoxication. Lactic acidosis is caused by increased generation of NADH by the metabolism of alcohol, which interferes with hepatic gluconeogenesis and, therefore, lactate use.

In lactic acidosis, the L-isomer is usually elevated because of the specificity of mammalian lactate dehydrogenase. Various bacteria found in colonic flora are capable of generating large amounts of D-lactic acid. D-Lactic acidosis has been reported in humans only in the presence of short-gut syndrome because the small bowel normally absorbs the dietary substrate for bacterial D-lactic acid production. In addition, the colon must be selectively colonized by bacteria that possess D-lactate dehydrogenase (D-LDH). Typically, the patient has short-gut syndrome, and the acidosis is preceded by food ingestion and is accompanied by characteristic neurologic findings, including mental confusion, slurred speech, staggering gait, and nystagmus. These neurologic manifestations are secondary to bacterial neurotoxins. The acidosis is accompanied by an increased anion gap, but L-lactate and ketone levels are normal. Treatment includes oral antibiotics, recolonization of the colon with non–D-lactate dehydrogenase–forming bacteria, and a low-carbohydrate diet.

Metabolic Acidosis Caused by Drugs and Toxins. Acetylsalicylic acid (aspirin) is rapidly metabolized to salicylic acid, which is eventually further metabolized and excreted by the kidney. Ingestion of more than 4 to 6 g/d results in excretion of unmetabolized salicylic acid. Salicy-

late intoxication causes a respiratory alkalosis secondary to direct stimulation of the respiratory center as well as a metabolic acidosis with an increased anion gap. In addition, acidosis increases the toxicity of salicylate by increasing the concentration of the nonionized form, which results in higher intracellular concentrations. Manifestations of salicylate overdose include tinnitus, asterixis, noncardiogenic pulmonary edema, hypotension, vascular collapse, vomiting, seizures, and coma. Blood levels of salicylate correlate poorly with the severity of the clinical presentation because of the variability in time between ingestion and hospitalization. Treatment is usually required when more than 10 g have been ingested. It includes alkalinization of the urine to prevent reabsorption of salicylate and hemodialysis in patients with severe neurologic symptoms.

Ethylene glycol, the principal component of antifreeze, is converted by alcohol dehydrogenase to glycoaldehyde, then to glycolic acid with production of one NADH at each step. The acidosis produced by ingestion of ethylene glycol is secondary to accumulation of glycolic acid, although lactate also accumulates because of the production of NADH. Bicarbonate is not regenerated when the glycolate is further metabolized, so exogenous alkali is required to replace what was titrated. In addition, 3% to 10% of ethylene glycol is converted to oxalic acid, which may result in hypocalcemia and contribute to acute renal failure. Three stages of toxicity are described. CNS dysfunction characterizes the first stage. This is followed by cardiopulmonary failure and finally by oliguric acute renal failure. Treatment includes the administration of ethanol, which has greater affinity for alcohol dehydrogenase and delays the metabolism of ethylene glycol to its toxic metabolites. Treatment also includes hemodialysis or peritoneal dialysis to remove ethylene glycol and glycolate.

Metabolism of methanol by alcohol dehydrogenase results in the formation of formaldehyde and formic acid, both of which are severely toxic. The acidosis is associated with an increase in anion gap secondary to the accumulation of formate. The clinical presentation includes blurred vision or blindness associated with the funduscopic findings of hyperemic discs and retinal edema, malaise, headache, abdominal pain, vomiting, convulsions, and coma. Treatment includes ethanol infusion to delay the metabolism of methanol by alcohol dehydrogenase, hemodialysis, bicarbonate administration, and intravenous folate to enhance metabolism of formate.

Renal Acidosis: Decreased Net Acid Excretion

The impaired ability of the kidney to excrete acid and hence generate bicarbonate may be secondary to a decrease in the number of functioning nephrons and is termed *uremic acidosis* or *renal tubular acidosis*. Uremic acidosis, which can occur in both acute and chronic renal failure, is primarily caused by a reduction in ammonia excretion secondary to a reduction in the number of functioning proximal tubular cells. In addition, decreased proximal tubular bicarbonate reabsorption contributes to the development of acidosis. Although the onset of uremic acidosis may be related to declining renal function, its appearance can also be influenced by diet-dependent protein and organic anion ingestion, use of diuretic therapy that stimulates acid excretion, and the extent of tubular versus glomerular injury.

RTA can be classified as distal (classic, type I) or proximal (type II), depending on the primary site of the renal tubular defect leading to acidosis. Distal RTA is characterized by a defect in urinary acidification. It is associated with either hypokalemia or hyperkalemia, depending on the underlying pathophysiologic mechanisms. Proposed mechanisms of distal RTA with hypokalemia include reduced H^+ pump activity and increased tubular permeability with backleak of secreted H^+ into the tubular cell. In RTA with hyperkalemia, the mechanism is decreased luminal negativity secondary to impaired sodium reabsorption. The major defect in proximal RTA is proximal tubular dysfunction resulting in diminished reabsorption of filtered bicarbonate. Urinary excretion greater than 15% of the filtered load of bicarbonate at normal serum bicarbonate levels is pathognomonic for proximal RTA. Other indicators of proximal tubular dysfunction include glycosuria, aminoaciduria, uricosuria, and phosphaturia.

Clinical Features of Acute Metabolic Acidosis

The major cardiovascular effects of acute metabolic acidosis are peripheral arteriolar dilation, decreased cardiac contractility, and central venous constriction. These can lead to cardiovascular collapse and pulmonary edema. Catecholamine secretion is stimulated by metabolic acidosis, and in mild cases (pH over 7.1), heart rate may be increased. In more severe metabolic acidosis (pH below 7.1), the direct effects of acidosis override the catecholamine effects and result in bradycardia and decreased contractility. These depressive effects are magnified by β-blockers. In addition to these cardiovascular effects, metabolic acidosis can affect oxygen delivery by shifting the oxygen–hemoglobin dissociation curve to the right. In more prolonged metabolic acidosis, this may be partially offset by decreased production of 2,3-diphosphoglycerate in red blood cells because of a slower rate of glycolysis. Metabolic acidosis can also cause gastric distention, abdominal pain, nausea, and vomiting.

Compensatory Mechanisms

Renal Compensation. The kidney is extremely sensitive to changes in serum bicarbonate concentration and responds by increasing net acid excretion primarily by increasing ammonia excretion. Maximal renal compensation requires 2 to 4 days. In addition, the maximal amount of ammonia excreted during acidosis depends on factors that include the rate of glutamine delivery, effects on glomerular filtration rate by associated conditions such as dehydration, and the type of anion that accompanies the acid because renal acid secretion is stimulated to varying degrees by different anions. Although renal compensation is effective in achieving normal net acid excretion with extrarenal causes of metabolic acid, variable results are seen with renal acidosis. Compensation at times is complete for proximal RTA, whereas compensation is generally incomplete for distal RTA.

Respiratory Compensation. Delay in achieving maximal renal response to an increased acid load causes blood pH to decline, which stimulates hyperventilation. Although effective in promptly raising blood pH, ventilatory compensation is only partial, and full respiratory compensation requires 12 to 24 hours. The mechanism behind this delay remains unclear. The magnitude of the decrease in P_{CO_2} in response to a given degree of metabolic acidosis can be used to determine whether the metabolic acidosis is complicated by coexisting respiratory acidosis or respiratory alkalosis. Although a number of sophisticated mathematic models relating P_{CO_2} to serum bicarbonate, serum hydrogen ion, and pH have been described, the following is a simple equation that is readily applicable to the clinical situation[12]:

$$dP_{CO_2} = 1.2 \times d[HCO_3^-] \pm 2.0 \qquad (21)$$

where:
dP_{CO_2} = expected decrease in P_{CO_2} given the

measured decrease in serum bicarbonate concentration

For example, if serum bicarbonate is 18, $d[HCO_3^-]$ is 6 (24 − 18). The expected dP_{CO_2} is 7.2 ± 2, or P_{CO_2} = 32.8 (40 − 7.2) ± 2 mmHg. This equation is applicable in mild to moderate metabolic acidosis because pulmonary edema complicating severe metabolic acidosis interferes with maximal ventilatory compensation.

Treatment

Acute Metabolic Acidosis. The major principle of treatment for mild to moderate acute metabolic acidosis is correction of the underlying cause. In surgical and trauma patients, metabolic acidosis is often the result of hypoxia secondary to inadequate tissue perfusion and subsequent lactic acidosis. Volume and blood resuscitation alone may be enough to correct the acidosis. Attempts to correct acidosis with exogenous bicarbonate without correction of inadequate tissue perfusion are usually unsuccessful. Likewise, attempts to treat hypotension in volume-depleted patients with vasopressor agents increase tissue hypoxia and acidosis and may exacerbate the problem. The immediate goals are volume replenishment and correction of acidosis, and the long-term goal is to identify and treat definitively the underlying disease process.

The use of bicarbonate for the treatment of lactic acidosis is controversial. In several studies, the use of bicarbonate in patients with lactic acidosis has not improved clinical parameters or outcome. In addition, bicarbonate administration does not change the clinical course or outcome of patients with diabetic ketoacidosis. The use of bicarbonate is best reserved for patients with other, not easily reversible causes of metabolic acidosis to prevent cardiovascular collapse and is generally not used until the pH falls to 7.1 to 7.2. Because older patients and those with cardiovascular disease have decreased tolerance for acidosis, bicarbonate may be given before pH has fallen to such low levels. The amount of bicarbonate required to increase its serum concentration to any given level cannot be calculated. The goal is to increase pH to 7.2 to 7.3 by administering one or two ampules of bicarbonate (44.5 to 50 mEq/amp) initially, basing the need for additional bicarbonate on repeated arterial blood gas results. Rapid correction to achieve normal serum bicarbonate concentration may be harmful because organic anions are precursors of bicarbonate, and their eventual metabolism combined with administered bicarbonate may result in metabolic alkalosis. This may be further complicated by persistent hyperventilation in the face of rapidly normalized serum bicarbonate concentration resulting in the superimposition of a respiratory alkalosis. In addition, rapid correction of serum bicarbonate concentration may not allow reversal of 2,3-diphosphoglycerate depletion in red blood cells. The resulting shift of the oxygen–hemoglobin dissociation curve to the left may result in tissue hypoxia.

Chronic Acidosis. Most cases of distal RTA require treatment with daily doses of alkali to correct acidosis and prevent nephrocalcinosis and nephrolithiasis. Patients with distal RTA and hypokalemia require potassium supplementation as well. In proximal RTA in adults, mild cases do not require specific therapy. Severe cases [HCO_3^-] below 18) are treated with thiazide diuretics and a low-salt diet to achieve a modest degree of volume depletion, which reduces the requirement for bicarbonate supplementation. Children are particularly susceptible to the growth-retarding effects of even mild acidosis, and the threshold for treatment should be low.

Diabetic Ketoacidosis. The correction of both acidosis and hyperglycemia are best achieved by the administration of insulin. Metabolism of the anions of the ketoacids begins promptly with insulin therapy and results in the generation of bicarbonate. In addition, insulin inhibits ketone formation and gluconeogenesis and stimulates peripheral use of ketones and glucose. A general recommendation is to administer a loading dose of 20 IU of regular insulin intravenously, followed by a continuous intravenous infusion of 5 to 10 IU/h. Infusion of small amounts of insulin (1 to 3 IU/h) should be continued until acidosis clears. Volume resuscitation is also required; the average amount is 4 or 5 L in the first 24 hours. Alternating liters of normal and half-normal saline is recommended, despite increased extracellular osmolality, to minimize the risk of cerebral edema. Potassium replacement is essential, even in the face of normal or high serum potassium, because hypokalemia develops as acidosis and hyperglycemia are corrected. Unrecognized hypokalemia is a major cause of death from diabetic ketoacidosis.

Hyperosmolar Nonketotic Acidosis.   The key to successful treatment is to seek, recognize, and treat any underlying cause for the hyperosmolar nonketotic hyperglycemia, such as gram-negative sepsis. Hyperglycemia is corrected by the administration of insulin as described previously. Volume depletion can be more severe than that seen with diabetic ketoacidosis. Potassium supplementation must be given as well.

Metabolic Alkalosis

Causes

Sustained metabolic alkalosis occurs only if extracellular bicarbonate concentration is increased and renal excretion of excess bicarbonate is inhibited. Alone, neither is sufficient to result in metabolic alkalosis. Extracellular bicarbonate concentration is increased by numerous mechanisms. Loss of HCl is a leading cause of metabolic alkalosis in surgical patients. The most common example of this cause of metabolic alkalosis is loss of pure gastric secretion due to vomiting or nasogastric drainage in the face of gastric outlet obstruction. The gastric secretion of HCl generates equal amounts of bicarbonate in the blood. External loss of gastric acid results in a net gain in bicarbonate, which causes metabolic alkalosis. Although the kidney can excrete excess bicarbonate, this must be accompanied by excretion of sodium. Renal excretion of sodium is limited in the face of the volume depletion, which also occurs with external losses of gastric secretion. As volume depletion progresses, sodium is conserved in exchange for hydrogen. Thus, in metabolic alkalosis secondary to gastric outlet obstruction, the urine initially is alkalotic but becomes paradoxically acidotic in prolonged or uncorrected cases.

Increased extracellular bicarbonate concentration can occur with administration of either bicarbonate or precursors of bicarbonate, such as lactate, citrate, or calcium carbonate, or as a result of increased renal production of bicarbonate. Conditions in which acid excretion exceeds endogenous acid production and in which the renal threshold for bicarbonate reabsorption is increased can result in metabolic alkalosis. Such conditions include moderate potassium depletion, excess mineralocorticoids, and high P_{CO_2}.

Hypokalemia and cellular exchange of potassium for hydrogen can also lead to metabolic alkalosis. Hypokalemia results in enhanced proximal tubular bicarbonate reabsorption and distal tubular acid excretion. When potassium leaves the cell, it is exchanged for either sodium or hydrogen to maintain electrical neutrality. Loss of potassium from the body then results in a net gain in bicarbonate in the ECF.

Maintenance of elevated extracellular bicarbonate concentration can occur by a number of mechanisms. Volume contraction leads to decreases in renal blood flow and glomerular filtration rate that reduce the filtered load of bicarbonate. This, in addition to decreased proximal tubular reabsorption of bicarbonate, maintains high extracellular concentrations of bicarbonate. High P_{CO_2} causes an increase in renal threshold for bicarbonate secondary to decreased intracellular pH of the renal tubular cell. The net result is increased bicarbonate reabsorption.

Hypercalcemia and low PTH levels both result in increased proximal tubular reabsorption of bicarbonate, which may be enhanced by a decrease in glomerular filtration rate. Renal failure also leads to an inability of the kidney to excrete excess bicarbonate. Diuretics can cause or exacerbate metabolic alkalosis by both causing rapid contraction of intravascular volume and increasing renal excretion of acid. Chloride deficiency is another common factor that maintains an alkalotic state. In some instances of metabolic alkalosis, urinary excretion of chloride is markedly reduced. Reversal of metabolic alkalosis in these cases can be readily achieved by administration of chloride-containing solutions. Although chloride deficiency per se can result in an increased renal threshold for bicarbonate and in increased renal reabsorption of bicarbonate, this apparent association may also be related to volume contraction. Metabolic alkalosis can be divided into chloride-responsive and chloride-resistant types.

Respiratory Compensation

The major compensatory mechanism in metabolic alkalosis is respiratory because the presence of the metabolic alkalosis implicates renal dysfunction in either generating or failing to excrete increased amounts of bicarbonate. Hypoventilation is limited by the development of hypoxemia, which stimulates ventilation, and P_{CO_2} rarely exceeds 60 mmHg (Table 10-9). Among the four major types of acid–base disorders, this compensatory mechanism is the least effective. For a given degree of metabolic alkalosis, the following equation can be used to predict the compensatory increase in P_{CO_2}:

$$dP_{CO_2} = 0.7 \times d[HCO_3^-] \pm 5 \qquad (22)$$

where:
dP_{CO_2} = expected increase in P_{CO_2} given the measured increase in serum bicarbonate concentration

Clinical Features

Clinical signs of metabolic alkalosis may not be prominent because the condition usually develops relatively slowly. If acute, CNS manifestations of confusion, obtun-

---

Table 10-9. CALCULATIONS FOR ESTIMATING THE COMPENSATORY RESPONSES TO PRIMARY ACID–BASE DISTURBANCES

Type of Disorder	Degree of Compensation	Time Required
Metabolic acidosis	$dP_{CO_2} = d[HCO_3^-] \times 1.2 \pm 2$	12–24 h
Metabolic alkalosis	$dP_{CO_2} = d[HCO_3^-] \times 0.7 \pm 5$	12–24 h
Acute respiratory acidosis	$d[HCO_3^-] = dP_{CO_2} \times 0.07 \pm 1.5$	Minutes
Chronic respiratory acidosis	$d[HCO_3^-] = dP_{CO_2} \times 0.4 \pm 3$	3–5 d
Acute respiratory alkalosis	$d[HCO_3^-] = dP_{CO_2} \times 0.2 \pm 2.5$	Minutes
Chronic respiratory alkalosis	$d[HCO_3^-] = dP_{CO_2} \times 0.5 \pm 2.5$	2–3 d

dation, stupor, and coma may be present as well as tetany and neuromuscular irritability.

Treatment

Correction of the underlying cause is the mainstay of treatment in this disorder. In general, correction of potassium depletion and volume depletion corrects the metabolic alkalosis. Renal excretion of bicarbonate cannot occur in the face of persistent volume depletion. Volume depletion should be corrected with chloride-containing solutions. In patients without intravascular volume deficits, renal excretion of bicarbonate can be enhanced by administration of the carbonic acid anhydrase inhibitor diuretic acetazolamide. If renal excretion of bicarbonate cannot be increased because of underlying renal insufficiency, or if the metabolic alkalosis is severe, acid may be administered to titrate directly the excess extracellular bicarbonate. Acids that can be used include ammonium chloride, arginine hydrochloride, lysine hydrochloride, or dilute hydrochloric acid (0.1 N). Partial correction of the alkalosis is the initial goal. A general guide is that 2.2 mEq/kg decreases serum bicarbonate by about 5 mEq/L. In the face of renal failure, dialysis may be necessary to remove excess bicarbonate.

Respiratory Alkalosis

A primary decrease in P_{CO_2} resulting in increased extracellular pH is referred to as *respiratory alkalosis.* Hyperventilation and the ensuing fall in P_{CO_2} may be secondary to hypoxia, reflex stimulation from decreased pulmonary compliance, drugs, mechanical ventilation, and other causes.

Hypoxia stimulates ventilation through peripheral chemoreceptors in the carotid and aortic body. Decrease in arterial P_{O_2}, rather than in oxygen content, is the main stimulus. Acute drops in arterial P_{O_2} result in sustained hyperventilation only when the P_{O_2} decreases below 60 mmHg. Although hyperventilation occurs with even slight degrees of hypoxia, the resulting increase in brain pH suppresses the stimulus for hyperventilation unless severe hypoxia is present. In contrast, chronic hypoxia results in hyperventilation even with mildly decreased P_{O_2} because brain pH is lowered by metabolic compensation. The two most common causes of hypoxia resulting in respiratory alkalosis are pulmonary disease and exposure to high altitudes.

Compensatory Mechanisms

Tissue buffering is the initial response to a decrease in P_{CO_2}. Red blood cells provide one third of the buffering. Consumption of bicarbonate results from cellular liberation of H^+. Although immediate, the magnitude of tissue buffering is slight and can be predicted by the following formula:

$$d[HCO_3^-] = dP_{CO_2} \times 0.2 \pm 2.5 \qquad (23)$$

Renal compensation is achieved, not by increasing excretion of bicarbonate, but by decreasing net acid excretion, primarily through reductions in ammonia excretion and increases in organic anion excretion. These organic anions are excreted as sodium and potassium salts. As a result, potassium excretion is increased, resulting in hypokalemia. Complete renal compensation requires 2 or 3 days.

Clinical Features

Chronic respiratory alkalosis is generally asymptomatic because compensatory mechanisms are successful in maintaining pH close to normal. Acute respiratory alkalosis may cause sensations of breathlessness, dizziness, and

nervousness and can result in circumoral and extremity paresthesias, altered levels of consciousness, and tetany. These signs are related to decreased cerebral blood flow secondary to decreased P_{CO_2}, and decreased ionized calcium concentration secondary to the increased blood pH.

Treatment

The underlying stimulus for the hyperventilation should be addressed. The cause of hypoxemia should be determined and corrected. In acute symptomatic respiratory alkalosis, rebreathing or breathing 5% CO_2 temporarily relieves the symptoms. If the condition is secondary to mechanical ventilation, adjustment of tidal volume or respiratory rate should result in resolution of the respiratory alkalosis.

Respiratory Acidosis

Respiratory acidosis, the decrease in extracellular pH from a primary increase in P_{CO_2}, is due to inadequate ventilation. Although pulmonary disease commonly causes hypoxemia, respiratory acidosis is far less common because diffusion of O_2 is more readily impaired than diffusion of CO_2. The main causes of hypoventilation include depression of the respiratory center, impaired respiratory excursion of the thorax, airway obstruction, and chronic obstructive pulmonary disease. In addition, inappropriate ventilatory settings in the mechanically ventilated patient may result in respiratory acidosis.

Compensatory Mechanisms

Increased P_{CO_2} results in increased H_2CO_3, which dissociates into H^+ and HCO_3^-. Cellular exchange of Na^+ and K^+ for H^+ allows the reaction to continue in this direction with increased extracellular bicarbonate. This tissue buffering is accomplished within minutes. Persistently elevated P_{CO_2} also stimulates increased renal acid excretion, primarily the chloride salt of ammonia, and results in increased renal generation of HCO_3^-. Full renal compensation occurs over 3 to 5 days. The following formula describes chronic respiratory acidosis:

$$d[HCO_3^-] = dP_{CO_2} \times 0.4 \pm 3 \qquad (24)$$

Clinical Features

The magnitude of clinical manifestations depends on the chronicity and rate of development of respiratory acidosis. Acute changes in P_{CO_2} result in acute cerebral acidosis, which may cause drowsiness, restlessness, and the development of a flapping tremor, or, if more severe, stupor or coma. The response of the cerebral vasculature to acidosis is dilation. The consequent increase in cerebral blood flow may result in increased intracranial blood pressure, headache, and papilledema. Systemic acidosis results in peripheral vasodilation, depressed cardiac contractility, and insensitivity to catecholamines.

Treatment

Treatment should be directed to the underlying cause of the hypoventilation. Endotracheal intubation to achieve adequate ventilation is key to the treatment of acute respiratory acidosis of any cause. The treatment of chronic, compensated respiratory acidosis may be complicated by the accompanying hypoxemia. In chronic hypercapnia, the central chemoreceptors may be insensitive, and the accompanying hypoxemia may supply the main respiratory drive through stimulation of peripheral chemoreceptors. In such patients, complete correction of the hypoxemia may further suppress respiration and worsen the respiratory acidosis. In addition, P_{CO_2} should not be normalized rapidly.

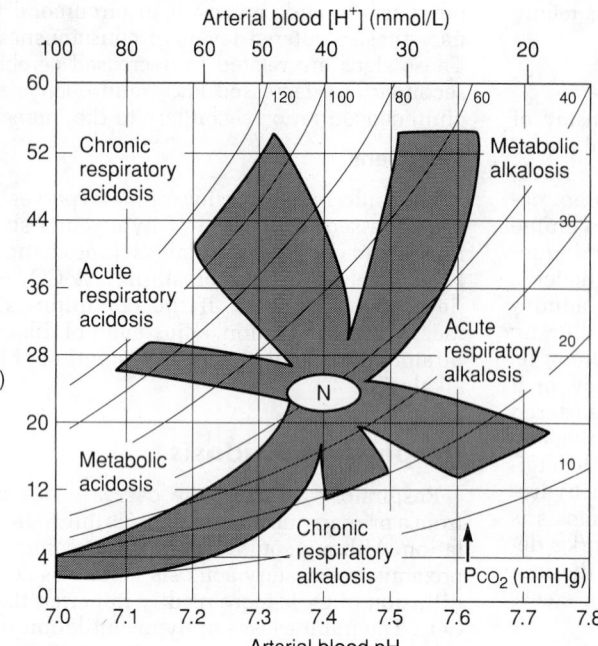

Figure 10-8. Acid–base nomogram. Shown are the 95% confidence limits of the normal respiratory and metabolic compensations for primary acid–base disturbances. (Cogan MG, Rector FC Jr. Acid–base disturbances. In: Brenner BM, Rector FC Jr, eds. The kidney. Philadelphia, WB Saunders, 1986;473)

Reequilibration of cerebral bicarbonate concentration lags behind systemic changes. Thus, even if P_{CO_2} is normal, cellular and cerebral metabolic alkalosis may develop.

Mixed Acid–Base Disorders

Combinations of two or more of the four primary acid–base disorders may occur and should be suspected when blood pH approaches normal despite abnormal P_{CO_2} and $[HCO_3^-]$, or when compensatory changes appear to be either excessive or inadequate (Fig. 10-8). The combination of respiratory acidosis and respiratory alkalosis is impossible, but any other combination is possible. Familiarity with the acid–base disorders associated with various clinical situations and the expectation of mixed abnormalities allows appropriate interpretation of arterial blood gases and serum electrolyte determinations. A summary of the calculations for estimating the compensatory responses and timing of these responses is presented in Table 10-9.[13]

REFERENCES

1. Edelman IS, Leibman J. Anatomy of body water and electrolytes. Am J Med 1959;27:256.
2. Robertson GL. Physiopathology of ADH secretion. In: Tolis G, Labrie F, Martin JB, et al, eds. Clinical neuroendocrinology: a pathophysiological approach. New York, Raven Press, 1979:247.
3. Briggs JP, Sawaya BE, Schnerman J. Disorders of salt balance. In: Kokko JP, Tannen RL, eds. Fluid and electrolytes. Philadelphia, WB Saunders, 1990:70.
4. Gauer OH, Henry JP. Neurohumoral control of plasma volume. In: Guyton AC, Cowley AW, eds. Cardiovascular physiology. II. International review of physiology, vol 9. Baltimore, University Park Press, 1976:145.
5. Salazar, FJ, Granger, JP, Joyce, MLM, et al. Effects of hypertonic saline infusion and water drinking on atrial peptides. Am J Physiol 1986;251:R1091.
6. Goetz KL. Renal natriuretic peptide (urodilatin?) and atriopeptin: evolving concepts. Am J Physiol 1991;261:F921.
7. Wait RB, Kahng KU. Renal failure complicating obstructive jaundice. Am J Surg 1989;157:256.
8. Reuzzi G, Benigni A. Endothelins in the control of cardiovascular and renal function. Nature 1993:342;589.
9. Rodeberg DA, Chaet MS, Bass RC, Arkovitz MS, Garcia VF. Nitric oxide: an overview, Am J Surg 1995;170;292.
10. Bachman S, Mundel P. Nitric oxide and the kidney: synthesis, localization and function. Am J Kid Dis 1994:24;112.
11. Lemann JJR, Lennon EJ. Role of diet, gastrointestinal tract, and bone in acid–base homeostasis. Kidney Int 1972;1:275.
12. Foster DW, McGarry JD. The metabolic derangements and treatment of diabetic ketoacidosis. N Engl J Med 1983; 309:159.
13. Carroll HJ, Oh MS. Water, electrolyte and acid–base metabolism. Philadelphia, JB Lippincott, 1989:206.

SURGERY: SCIENTIFIC PRINCIPLES AND PRACTICE, Second Edition, edited by Lazar J. Greenfield, Michael W. Mulholland, Keith T. Oldham, Gerald B. Zelenock, and Keith D. Lillemoe. Lippincott–Raven Publishers, Philadelphia, © 1997.

CHAPTER 11

TRAUMA

DAVID B. HOYT, BRUCE M. POTENZA, H. GILL CRYER, BAXTER LARMON, JAMES W. DAVIS, RANDALL M. CHESNUT, LISA A. ORLOFF, GREGORY J. JURKOVICH, ROBERT J. WINCHELL, DAVID H. WISNER, ROBERT C. MACKERSIE, MICHAEL J. SISE, STEVEN R. SHACKFORD, MARK A. HEALEY, M. MARGARET KNUDSON, HEIDI L. FRANKEL, GRACE S. ROZYCKI, HOWARD R. CHAMPION, RICHARD K. SIMONS, AND LARRY M. GENTILELLO

Introduction

DAVID B. HOYT

The beginnings of surgery can be linked closely with trauma care and casualty management during war. Today, trauma is a principal public health problem in every country, regardless of the level of socioeconomic development. In the United States, trauma is the leading cause of death among people between 1 and 44 years of age. The 150,000 annual deaths in the United States caused by trauma are more than three times the number of combat casualties that occurred during the entire Vietnam conflict. About 57 million people were accidentally injured in 1985 in the United States; this represents an annual injury incidence of about one in four people and accounts for one third of all hospital admissions. Individual loss, pain, suffering, incapacitation, and disability are difficult to quantify. Although injuries occur to people of all ages and both genders, young men are most often affected. Because many severe injuries result in long-term disability, consideration of the lifetime cost of injury should take into account acute and chronic care as well as the cost of lost economic productivity. Recent calculations have estimated the total cost of injury in the United States to be about $180 billion per year.[1]

MORTALITY PEAKS AFTER TRAUMATIC INJURY

Trauma-related deaths tend to occur at three traditionally recognized times after injury (Fig. 11-1). About half of all trauma-related deaths occur within seconds or minutes of injury and are related to lacerations of the aorta, heart, brain stem, brain, and spinal cord. Few of these patients can be saved by health care systems, regardless of efficacy. These injuries are best addressed by prevention strategies, either devices that prevent injury or laws that limit certain behavior patterns.[2]

The second mortality peak occurs within hours of injury and accounts for about 30% of deaths, half of which are caused by hemorrhage and half by injuries to the central nervous system (CNS).[3] Because many of these deaths can be averted by early treatment during the "golden hour" after injury, important reductions in second-peak mortality have resulted from the development of rapid transport and trauma treatment systems. Overall trauma mortality rates have been reduced from approximately 30% to between 2% and 9% where well-organized trauma care systems exist.[4,5] Only about 25% of the US population is served by such systems. Further development of trauma care systems, assisted by legislation, organized care protocols, and expansion of these systems to rural areas, will undoubtedly result in further reductions in mortality during this period.

The third mortality peak includes deaths that occur from 1 day after injury to weeks later. This late mortality usually is attributed to infection and multiple organ failure.[6] Ten to 20% of trauma-related deaths occur during this period. The development of efficient trauma care systems, however, has changed the epidemiology of these deaths. Refractory intracranial hypertension during the first week after severe head injury now accounts for a significant number of these deaths. The incidence of sepsis and multiple organ failure has diminished as a result of aggressive and better early resuscitation and care. Sepsis and multiple organ failure now account for about 5% of overall mortality and only 30% of late mortality where organized trauma care systems exist. Finally, fatal pulmonary embolism accounts for a significant number of these late deaths.[7]

Efforts to reduce the morbidity and mortality of trauma

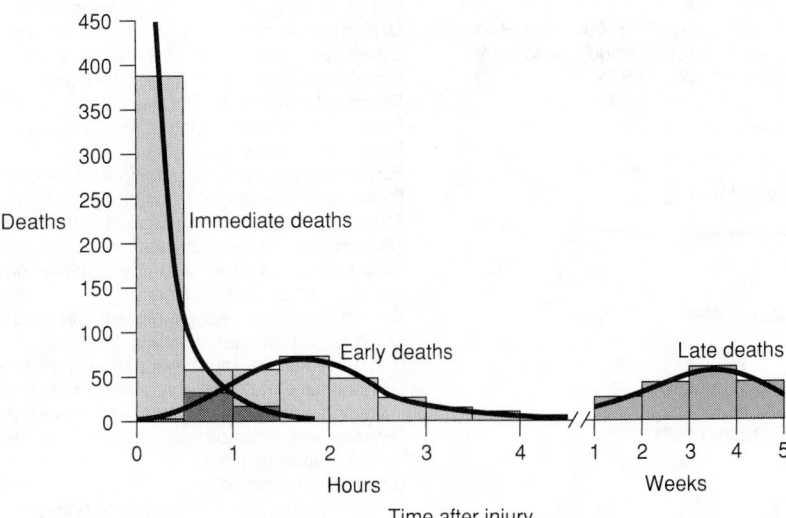

Figure 11-1. Three periods of peak mortality after injury.

must include specific programs for each of the three different mortality peaks. Early deaths can best be reduced by accident prevention programs or legislated protective devices. Focus on the regional planning and development of trauma care systems impacts the number of avoidable deaths during the second mortality peak. Finally, late deaths can be diminished as research generates better understanding of the processes related to sepsis, multiple organ failure, and CNS injury.[8]

HISTORICAL DEVELOPMENT OF TRAUMA CARE

The approach to modern trauma has evolved from the care of wounds and casualty management during war. Advances in rapid transport, volume resuscitation, wound management (both débridement and infection control), blood banking, enteric injury management, vascular surgery, surgical critical care, and early nutritional management have all grown out of military experience. Salient historical events are shown in Table 11-1. Although by no means complete, this table provides examples of the many significant contributions derived from the large military experience with multiple injuries.

Civilian progress has generally followed the evolution of military systems with regard to trauma care. In 1922, the importance of orthopedic trauma was first recognized in the United States with the establishment of the Committee on the Treatment of Fractures. This evolved into the Committee on Trauma of the American College of Surgeons in 1949. Increased awareness of traffic injuries and fatalities occurred during the 1950s and 1960s, among both surgeons and the general public. The first specific trauma unit was opened in 1961 at the University of Maryland, and the concept of the "golden hour" was established. In 1966, the National Academy of Sciences and the National Research Council published *Accidental Death and Disability: The Neglected Disease of Modern Society*, an important white paper that increased public awareness and led to a federal agenda for the general improvement of trauma care. Coupled with leadership from key academic centers and often by surgeons with recent military experience, the spread of advanced trauma systems began. The Maryland Institute of Emergency Medicine became the first completely organized, statewide, regionalized system in 1973. Prehospital provider programs were formalized, emergency medical technicians and other paramedical personnel were identified, and training programs were established. In 1973, the Emergency Medical Service Act became law, providing specific endorsement and financial assistance for the development of comprehensive emergency medical service systems. In addition to federal efforts, state and local legislatures began to organize strategies for caring for injured patients that employed prehospital care systems to deliver patients to major hospitals at which appropriate care could be given. Despite these efforts, organized trauma care is still underdeveloped in 60% to 70% of the United States.[9]

Two other factors influenced the rapid development of regionalized systems of trauma care in the late 1970s. First, major teaching hospitals in large cities had become regional trauma centers by default because of their experience and involvement in the trauma care of indigent patients. With strong academic leadership, these centers were able to develop regionalization of systems of trauma care by example. Of at least equal importance, a task force of the American College of Surgeons Committee on Trauma published, in 1976, a standard for evaluation of care entitled *Optimal Hospital Resources for the Care of the Seriously Injured*. The current and most comprehensive version of this report was published in 1993.[10] It establishes criteria for prehospital and trauma care personnel and establishes the importance of ongoing quality assessment. It also defines the elements of a trauma system. In addition, in 1980 the American College of Surgeons Committee on Trauma developed the Advanced Trauma Life Support course, which has contributed to uniformity of initial care and the development of a common language for all care providers.[11]

Table 11-1. SIGNIFICANT HISTORICAL DEVELOPMENTS RELATED TO TRAUMA CARE

Period or Person	Contribution
Greek medicine	Wound care and fracture management
Roman Empire	Realization that laudable pus was undesirable
	Healing by second intention
16th-century Paré	Use of dressing and ligature in wound management
French and Indian War, John Hunter	Differentiation between primary and secondary wound healing
Early 1800s Dominique, Jean Larrey	Developed the principle of the ambulance and the concept of triage
Crimean War, 1853–1856	Demonstrated value of nursing care (Florence Nightingale)
Samuel Gross, 1862	Described shock as the root unhinging of the machinery of life
Civil War	Rediscovery of importance of field ambulance, nonsuppurative wound care
	Initial use of antiseptics
	Further development of nursing care by Clara Barton, American Red Cross Founder
World War I	Principle of débridement and delayed closure for wounds more than 8 hours old
	Established primary closure for wounds less than 8 hours old only
	Field ambulance mechanized with automobile availability
	Recognition that shock was due to blood or fluid loss and use of seawater to replace blood volume
	Introduction of Dakin solution
World War II	Débridement and delayed closure practiced
	Diverting colostomies standard care
	Blood transfusion, rapid evacuation, specialized surgical units close to the front
Korean conflict	Development of MASH units, use of helicopters, development of vascular surgery, field research leading to better understanding of posttraumatic renal failure
Vietnam conflict	Development of an airbase regional emergency medical system with transport from injury to intervention in 1 hour
	Better fluid resuscitation
	Understanding of adult respiratory distress syndrome

In summary, the current awareness of trauma is the result of many historical factors, both military and civilian in origin. The prevalence and economic impact of trauma and the commitment required to provide optimal care make it a significant challenge for the surgeon.

General Considerations

BRUCE M. POTENZA AND DAVID B. HOYT

EPIDEMIOLOGY

In the United States, about 2.5 million people are hospitalized annually as a result of accidental injury, and more than 114 million physician contacts are generated for the outpatient management of injuries.[12] Although injury affects all age groups, it is epidemic among the younger members of society. In the United States, injury is the leading cause of death among persons younger than 44 years of age, and 70% of hospital admissions for injury are in this age group. Moreover, among those aged 15 to 24 years, 78% of all deaths are caused by injury.[12] Even in very young children, the 1- to 4-year-old age group, injury accounts for almost half the total number of deaths.

Although morbidity and mortality figures are important, another important cost of the injury toll for society is measured in years of productive life lost (YPLL). This figure reflects the potential productivity that is lost as a result of premature death and is calculated by subtracting the age of the patient at death from 70. Because injury is so prevalent among the young, traumatic deaths result in a high number of YPLL, more so than deaths from cancer or chronic disease, which are concentrated in the elderly population. In fact, the total number of YPLL as a result of injury is about 40% higher than the YPLL for the second and third leading causes of premature death—cancer and heart disease—combined. For each traumatic death there are, on average, 36 YPLL, compared with 16 for cancer and 12 for heart disease.[12]

Young men constitute the highest risk group, not because of physiologic distinctions but because of their propensity to engage in high-risk activities. The leading causes of injury are motor vehicle accidents, falls, firearms, cutting or piercing instruments, and burns. Fatalities after injury are mainly caused by motor vehicle accidents (32%), gunshot wounds (22%), and falls (9%).

Closer examination of these figures reveals some important differences among the various ethnic groups in the United States. The three leading causes of traumatic death for persons younger than 35 years of age are the same in all groups: motor vehicle accidents, homicide, and suicide. Their relative importance differs, however. In the African-American population, the leading cause of death in this age group is homicide (32 deaths per 100,000 persons per year); in all other groups, it is motor vehicle accidents. The mortality rate from motor vehicle accidents is about 42 per 100,000 among Native Americans, 20 per 100,000 among the white population, 11 per 100,000 in the Asian population.[12] Those who plan injury research and prevention projects must take into account the characteristics of the specific target populations.

BIOMECHANICS OF INJURY

All traumatic injury occurs as a result of deformation of tissues beyond a threshold that results in structural damage. Understanding the biomechanics of specific injuries is important in guiding initial evaluation. In general, injury is categorized as either penetrating or nonpenetrating (blunt) trauma. With blunt trauma, the injury is produced as the tissues are compressed or as deceleration occurs. In penetrating trauma, the injury is produced by crushing and separation of tissues along the path of the penetrating object.

Energy Transfer

The severity of any injury is directly proportional to the amount of kinetic energy transferred to the tissues and the properties of those tissues that accept and dissipate the energy. Kinetic energy (KE) is a function of the mass (M) of an object and its velocity (V):

$$KE = \frac{M \times V^2}{2}$$

Changes in velocity alter the magnitude of kinetic energy much more dramatically than changes in mass. This fact becomes critical, for example, for assessment of high- and low-velocity gunshot wounds. Likewise, a small child and a large adult, although significantly different in size and weight, are subjected to similar levels of energy transfer in a high-speed vehicular collision, the primary determinant being velocity rather than mass.

Cavitation

Cavitation occurs as tissue impacted by a moving body recoils from the point of impact, away from the object. An example of cavitation after blunt trauma is the temporary deformation of the tissues caused by a lap belt or steering wheel in a motor vehicle accident. The resulting transient tissue cavity may be caused by rapid acceleration or deceleration. Extreme strain occurs at points of anatomic fixation during the formation of these temporary cavities. Forces can be produced both along the longitudinal axis (tensile or compression strain) and across the longitudinal axis (shear strain) and can result in deformity, tearing, and tissue failure or fracture.

With penetrating trauma, transient cavitation is caused by the transfer of kinetic energy from the projectile and, in addition, a permanent cavity is produced by tissue displacement.

The tolerance of biologic tissue for traumatic injury is directly proportional to the elasticity of the organ—that is, its ability to return to its original shape and position. This characteristic is directly affected by the rate of loading, or the rate at which strain is applied. More rapid application of force increases the likelihood of exceeding the tolerance of the tissue. Tissue injury occurs when a low strain or shear force is applied at a high rate of loading.

BIOMECHANICS OF BLUNT TRAUMA

Blunt trauma produces two types of force during impact. Changes in speed (acceleration or deceleration) create shear strain, and deformity changes (stretch or compression) create tensile strain. Analyses of injuries associated with changes in speed have facilitated the understanding of specific injuries to the head, thorax, and abdomen. For example, shear stress to the head secondary to deceleration leads to stretching of the brain stem, and injury to the spinal cord occurs from shear stress at points of attachment. Contrecoup brain injuries include stretch forces placed on bridging veins, which can lead to hemorrhage and subdural hematoma. Understanding of how these injuries occur allows us to predict injury patterns for specific types of trauma.

Shear Strain Injuries

Differential acceleration in the thorax makes the aorta the most common site of shear injuries, the most frequent point of injury being the ligamentum arteriosum. Here, the descending aorta is tightly fixed to the thoracic spine, whereas it is relatively mobile more proximally. Shear stress in this area allows the proximal aorta to move in relation to the fixed distal aorta and, therefore, to tear. Abdominal injuries can result as a consequence of acceleration of the viscera at a rate out of proportion to movement of the points of attachment. The kidneys, small intestine, large intestine, and spleen are all vulnerable to this type of shear injury. Similarly, with deceleration, the liver may continue to travel relative to the ligamentum teres, generating shear forces that transect or lacerate the hepatic parenchyma. Rapid deceleration can place sudden flexion and extension forces on the cervical spine, which can cause cervical fractures, subluxation, or ligamentous injury.

Tensile Strain Injuries

Tensile strain creates injury by the direct compression of tissue. For the head, tensile strain results in fractures of the skull, which in turn can cause intracranial bleeding or contusions of the underlying brain. In the thorax, external chest compression can lead to cardiac contusion, pulmonary contusion, pneumothorax, and fractured ribs or a flail chest. In the abdomen, organs compressed between a frontal impact and the vertebral column may be injured. The pancreas, liver, spleen, and occasionally the kidneys are vulnerable to this type of injury. In addition, direct compression of the abdomen can increase intraabdominal pressure, rupturing the diaphragm. External compression of the pelvis is associated with bladder rupture and other pelvic injuries.

Motor Vehicle Collisions

Patterns of injury are recognized for several specific types of motor vehicle collisions: (1) head-on or frontal impact, (2) rear impact, (3) lateral or side impact, (4) rotational impact, and (5) rollover. Each causes a different kind of damage, and the presumption is usually that any or all of these forces may have been involved. Some estimate of injury pattern is possible by analysis of damage to the vehicle, however, and a description of vehicular damage can be useful for broad categorization of patients. In general, a vehicle's occupant receives a kinetic energy transfer similar to that of the vehicle itself. As an automobile collides with an object, passengers collide with the interior of the automobile, and the internal organs collide with the body wall or are sheared from anatomic attachment.

Injury research and better automotive design have greatly improved the outcome for occupants if the safety features of the vehicle are in use at the time of the accident. Active safety restraint systems include shoulder and lap seat belts and door locks; passive restraint systems include front and rear energy-absorbing collapsible chassis, and improved lateral wall design. All of these features are designed to minimize the transfer of the energy of the collision to the occupants.

Frontal and Rear Impact

With frontal impact, the vehicle stops abruptly, and unrestrained front-seat occupants move in one of two predictable pathways: down and under the dashboard or up and over the steering wheel. With the former movement, the knees strike the dashboard, and the upper legs absorb the primary energy transfer. Dislocated knees, fractured femurs, and posterior fracture dislocations of the hips are the expected injuries.

After the knees impact, the upper body flexes forward, moving up and over the steering wheel. The chest or abdomen impacts the steering wheel, and the head impacts the windshield. The head stops the forward momentum of the torso, and kinetic energy is absorbed by the cervical spine (Fig. 11-2). Predictable injury patterns resulting from the up-and-over component of a frontal impact:

1. The anterior chest wall compresses the steering wheel so that fractured ribs, flail chest, pulmonary contusion, and myocardial contusion result.
2. Compression injuries occur to hollow abdominal viscera and solid organs and can result in visceral organ perforation, mesenteric or solid organ hemorrhage, or parenchymal injury.
3. After the anterior chest stops, intrathoracic organs continue to move, resulting in shear injuries such as lacerations of the aorta or liver.
4. Shear injuries to the kidneys and other solid viscera may also occur.
5. Injury to the brain can occur from direct compression, with scalp lacerations, skull fractures, and cerebral contusions, or from deceleration and shear stress, which cause diffuse axonal injury and cerebral contusion or subdural hematoma.
6. Acute neck flexion, hyperextension, or both, can occur, causing cervical spine injury.

Rear impact collisions occur when stationary or slow-moving vehicles are struck from behind. The amount of kinetic energy generated depends on the difference between the velocities of the two vehicles, rather than their sum, as with forward collisions. After a rear impact, the vehicle and its occupants accelerate forward, during which time cervical spine hyperextension with injury can occur. If the vehicle slows to a stop spontaneously, often the occupants are not severely injured. If the car strikes another object, the occupants are thrown forward, with injury potentials similar to those seen with a frontal impact. Rear impact collisions therefore can cause two types of injury: those caused by the primary rear impact and those resulting from the secondary frontal impact.

Lateral Impact, Rotational Impact, and Rollover

Two patterns of injury result from lateral impact, depending on whether energy is transferred to the vehicle directly or imparts motion to the vehicle. If the target vehicle remains in place or there is significant passenger compartment intrusion, typical injuries include lateral crushing compression injuries to the torso, pelvis, and spine. Energy delivered to the chest with lateral compression can cause a flail chest, pulmonary contusion, and ruptured liver or spleen. Depending on the location of the occupant's arm, humeral and clavicular fractures may occur. The pelvis and femur are often impacted by the door, forcing the femoral head medially and causing an acetabular fracture. Head injuries range from simple lacerations to cerebral contusions with intracranial hemorrhage.

If the vehicle does not move away from the point of lateral impact, an occupant who is restrained remains fixed in place and is more vulnerable to the intruding vehicle. More commonly, the vehicle is moved by the force of the impact, and passenger restraints markedly reduce injury. In this case, the occupant begins lateral motion with the car and is pulled away from the impact point by the restraint. As the torso is pushed laterally, the head stays

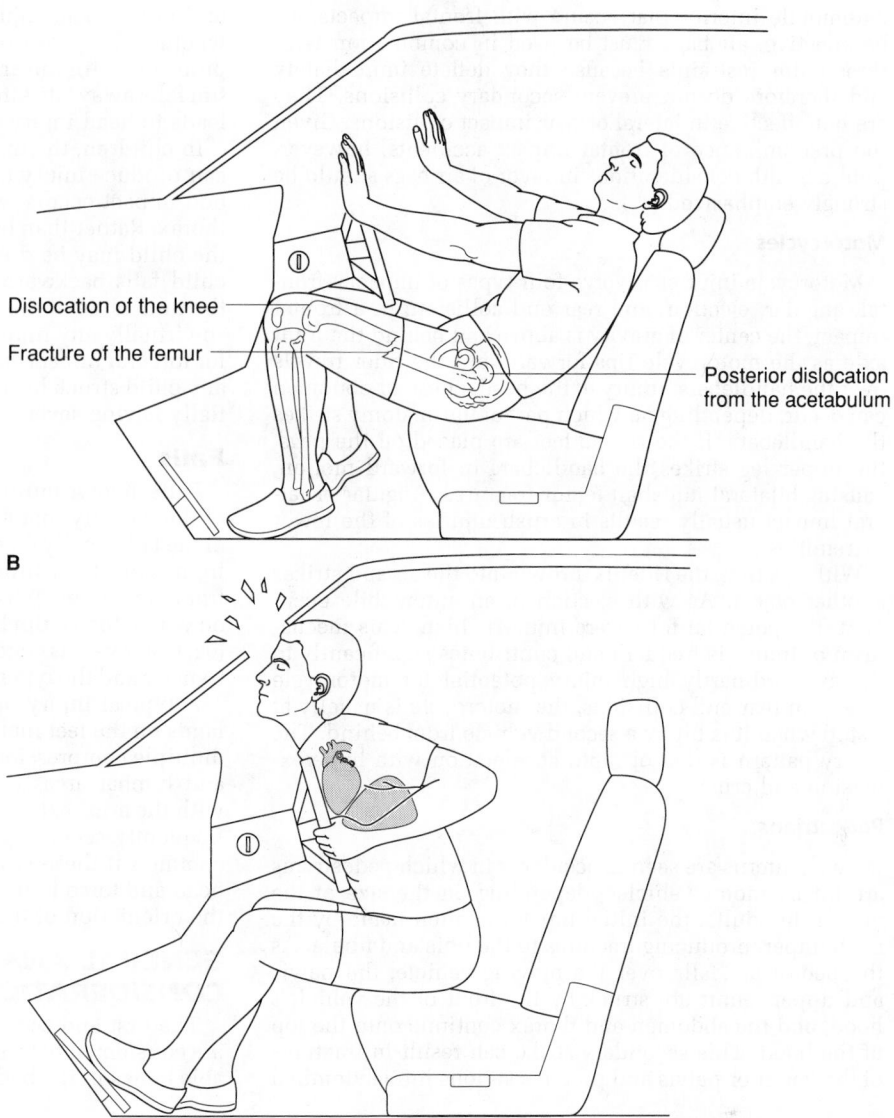

Dislocation of the knee

Fracture of the femur

Posterior dislocation from the acetabulum

B

Figure 11-2. Down-and-under (*A*) and up-and-over (*B*) mechanisms of injury after frontal deceleration impact.

in its original position. This produces lateral flexion and rotation of the cervical spine, and fractures of the spine are common with lateral collisions. Passengers sustaining lateral impact may also have injuries resulting from secondary collisions with other passengers.

Rotational impact injuries occur if the car strikes a moving vehicle laterally. The moving vehicle rotates around the point of impact, resulting in combinations of the injuries seen in head-on and lateral impacts. Many different injuries are possible.

During rollover accidents, the automobile may be hit many times from many different angles; as a result, an occupant can have virtually any type of injury, and all potential injury mechanisms should be considered. Rollover accidents with passenger ejection are associated with a profound increase in fatality rates, in part because the second impact can cause injuries that compound or exceed those resulting from the initial impact. Rollover accidents with passenger ejection are considered to have the greatest injury potential.

Restraint Device Injury

Theoretically, three-point passenger restraints allow the kinetic energy transferred by the impact to be absorbed by the bony pelvis and chest. If they are improperly posi-

tioned, however, lap belts can rise above the pelvis, delivering the compression force to the soft tissues of the abdominal cavity or retroperitoneum. The number of injuries related to restraint devices is increasing, probably because of the broader general use of these systems. Although there is no question of the overall efficacy of these devices, specific related injuries must still be recognized by the clinician.

Common injuries if lap belts are incorrectly strapped above the anterior iliac crest include compression injuries of the intraabdominal organs (liver, pancreas, spleen, small bowel, large bowel), increased intraabdominal pressure and diaphragmatic rupture, and anterior compression of the lumbar spine. Diagonal shoulder straps should be worn in combination with lap belts to prevent forward motion of the trunk. Diagonal shoulder straps should not be worn alone because this practice is associated with chest and neck injuries if the pelvis is not secured by the lap belt. Injuries associated with shoulder straps include clavicle and rib fractures and carotid artery injuries. Lap belt injuries include hollow organ perforation, mesenteric bleeding, and more severe solid organ injuries as well as thoracolumbar fractures.

Air bags have enormous potential for injury prevention because they prevent the initial collision of passenger and automobile interior that occurs with frontal impacts. To be effective, air bags must be used in combination with three-point restraints because they deflate immediately and therefore do not prevent secondary collisions. They are not effective in lateral or rear impact collisions. Given the predominance of frontal impact accidents, however, public health considerations in favor of air bags should be strongly emphasized.

Motorcycles

Motorcycle injuries involve four types of impacts: frontal, angular, ejection, and rear end collision. In a frontal impact, the center of gravity is above and behind the front axle as the motorcycle tips forward and the rider travels over the handlebars. Injury to the head, chest, or abdomen can occur, depending on which part of the anatomy strikes the handlebars. If the rider's feet are placed on the pegs, the upper leg strikes the handlebars in forward motion, causing bilateral midshaft femur fractures. Angular or lateral impact usually results in crush injuries of the lower extremities.

With ejection, the rider is thrown into the air and strikes another object. As with ejection of an automobile occupant, the potential for severe injury is high. This mechanism of injury is frequent and contributes significantly to the extraordinarily high injury potential for motorcycle riders. In rear end collisions, the motorcycle is usually at a stop when it is hit by a second vehicle from behind. The injury pattern is that of rapid acceleration with hyperextension and crush.

Pedestrians

Two patterns are seen in accidents in which pedestrians are hit by motor vehicles, depending on the size of the victim. In adults, the initial impact is often made by the car bumper, producing fractures to the tibia and fibula. As the pedestrian falls over the moving vehicle, the pelvis and upper femur are struck by the front of the vehicle's hood, and the abdomen and thorax continue onto the top of the hood. This secondary strike can result in fractures of the femur or pelvis and produce serious intraabdominal

or intrathoracic injury. Injury to the head depends on whether the pedestrian's head strikes the car hood or is protected with the arms. A third impact occurs as the victim falls away, striking the ground. This impact commonly leads to head injury as well.

In children, the initial impact is predictably higher and can produce injury to the pelvis or upper femur. The second impact occurs when the front of the hood strikes the thorax. Rather than being thrown onto the top of the hood, the child may be dragged underneath the vehicle. As the child falls backward, multiple impacts with the ground, the underside of the vehicle, and the wheels are possible, so virtually any injury can occur. Because of the potential for forceful impact and the direct blow to the middle torso, any child struck by a vehicle must be considered as potentially having severe injuries.

Falls

Falls involve multiple impacts. Energy transfer is a result of the velocity that develops during the fall, so the height of the fall usually determines the magnitude of injury. Falls from more than three times the height of the victim, or from more than 20 feet, are considered severe. The surface on which the victim lands and its degree of compressibility (eg, water versus concrete) also have an effect on the energy transfer and the types of shear and tensile strain that occur.

A typical injury pattern after falls in which the victim lands on the feet includes bilateral calcaneal fractures and multiple compression fractures of the spine in the thoracic and lumbar areas (Fig. 11-3). If the victim falls forward with the arms extended, bilateral Colles wrist fractures are frequently seen. Hip dislocation and pelvic fractures are common if these structures are impacted, and significant head and torso injuries are always possible, depending on the orientation of the victim at the time of impact.

GENERAL ANATOMIC CONSIDERATIONS IN BLUNT INJURY

The first and second ribs, sternum, scapula, and femur are considered to be some of the strongest and least vulnerable bones in the body. Therefore, fractures of these bones

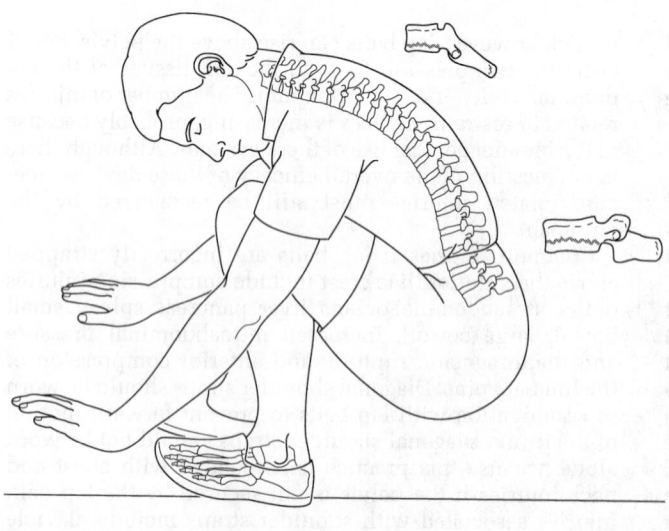

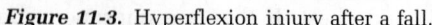

Figure 11-3. Hyperflexion injury after a fall.

are indicators of severe trauma. Significant association exists between first and second rib fractures and injuries to the head, chest, and abdomen. Similarly, fractures to the sternum, though unusual, have a relatively high frequency of associated myocardial contusion. Fractures to the scapula indicate significant thoracic trauma. The presence of a femur fracture in a frontal impact injury should raise suspicion of acetabular fractures or dislocation of the knee. An inventory of specific orthopedic injuries and their common associated findings is provided in Table 11-2. These associations should be considered routinely during initial evaluation of persons sustaining major blunt trauma.

The anatomic orientation of certain structures also leads to predictable injury patterns. For example, the right ventricle is the most anterior portion of the heart and therefore is the most commonly contused area. The association of the spleen with ribs on the left and the liver with ribs on the right, as well as the marked mobility of these two organs, leads to an obvious association when the overlying ribs are injured. If major pelvic fractures are encountered, urethral tears and bladder perforation should be suspected.

BIOMECHANICS OF PENETRATING INJURIES

Penetrating trauma involves the transfer of energy to a relatively small tissue area. The velocity of a gunshot wound is exceedingly high compared with any type of blunt trauma. The kinetic energy of a bullet disrupts and fragments cells and tissues, moving them away from the path of the bullet. The actual size of the frontal area of impact is determined by three factors: profile, tumble (spin and yaw), and fragmentation.

The profile, or frontal area, of a knife, screwdriver, or smooth bullet is that of a pointed missile. If the missile is crushed or deformed as a result of impact, the frontal area changes shape and disperses the impact over a wider tissue area, producing greater energy exchange and therefore greater injury. A knife or jacketed bullet does not deform significantly during impact, but a hollow-point bullet flattens, spreads, and fragments on impact, enlarging the area of injury.

Tumble results if the center of gravity of a bullet is eccentric, usually because it is located nearer the base than the

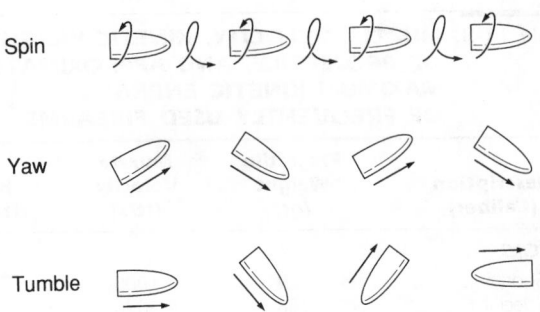

Figure 11-4. Specific aspects of bullet movement that affect tissue injury.

apex of the bullet. Spin and axial movement (yaw) are bullet movements that occur after a gun is fired (Fig. 11-4). At impact, spin and yaw continue to carry the base of the bullet forward, resulting in end-over-end motion, or tumble. This increases the area of energy exchange and results in greater tissue damage. Gunshot wounds are an example of fragmentation injury. The frontal impact damage can be estimated by classifying the instrument of penetrating injury according to energy capacity.

Low-Energy Stab Wounds

Low-energy missiles include knives and other objects that produce damage only by their sharp cutting edges. Cavitation is minimal, and injury can be predicted simply by tracing the pathway of the weapon within the body. Knowledge of the type of weapon and the sex of the attacker is sometimes helpful. Men tend to stab with the blade on the thumb side of the hand in an upward thrust; women tend to stab downward, holding the blade to the outside of the hand. The attacker may stab and move the knife or other weapon inside the body, which can lead to more injury than that deduced from the appearance of the cutaneous wound. Judgment of the potential scope of injury by examination of the entrance wound alone is not reliable.

Low- and Medium-Velocity Gunshot Wounds

Low-velocity gunshot wounds are defined as those with an initial muzzle velocity of less than 1200 ft/s. Medium-velocity projectiles have muzzle velocities between 1200 and 2000 ft/s. Most handguns and some rifles are low- or medium-energy weapons. Table 11-3 provides a comparison of bullets and initial muzzle velocity for firearms that are frequently associated with penetrating trauma in civilians. The primary point of classification is that these weapons not only damage the tissue directly in the path of the missile but also produce cavitation injury to tissues in close proximity to the impact. The size of the cavitation injury is directly proportional to the velocity of the bullet. With low- and medium-velocity gunshot wounds, this cavity is usually three to six times the area of the bullet's frontal surface. The amount of tumble, fragmentation, and profile change also influence the extent of injury.

High-Energy Weapons

High-velocity projectiles are those with a muzzle velocity of more than 2000 ft/s. The essential difference in these weapons is that their projectiles produce a much larger cavity or pressure cone than low- and medium-velocity

Table 11-2. PATTERNS OF INJURY TO THE HEAD, NECK, TRUNK, AND EXTREMITIES ASSOCIATED WITH ORTHOPEDIC INJURIES

Diagnosed Injury	Associated Injury
Fracture—temporal, parietal bone	Epidural hematoma
Maxillofacial fracture	Cervical spine fracture
Sternal fracture	Cardiac contusion
First and second rib fracture	Descending thoracic aorta, intraabdominal bleeding
Fractured scapula	Pulmonary contusion
Fractured ribs 8–12, right	Lacerated liver
Fractured ribs 8–12, left	Lacerated spleen
Fractured pelvis	Ruptured bladder, urethral transection
Fractured humerus	Radial nerve injury
Supracondylar humerus	Brachial artery injury
Distal radius fracture	Median nerve compression
Supracondylar femur fracture	Thrombosis popliteal artery
Anterior dislocation shoulder	Axillary nerve injury
Posterior dislocation of hip	Sciatic nerve injury
Posterior dislocation of knee	Popliteal artery thrombosis

Table 11-3. MUZZLE VELOCITY, KINETIC WEIGHT OF PROJECTILE, AND APPROXIMATE MAXIMUM KINETIC ENERGY OF FREQUENTLY USED FIREARMS

Description (Caliber)	Projectile Weight (gr)	Muzzle Velocity (ft/s)	KE (ft/lb)
PISTOLS			
.22 Short	29	1000	72
.38 Special	158	870	263
9-mm Luger	125	1150	440
.45	250	860	410
.357 Magnum	158	1430	695
.44 Magnum	240	1470	1150
RIFLES			
.22 Long	40	1150	150
.56-mm M-16	55	3200	1248
.30-30 Winchester	170	2200	1830

missiles. The temporary cavity extends well beyond the actual bullet tract, producing a wider injury. The vacuum created by the cavitation pulls clothing, bacteria, and other debris from the surrounding areas into the wound, creating the additional risk of contamination. The proliferation of semiautomatic weapons in society has also resulted in an increase in the number of wounds a victim may experience. Instead of a single gunshot wound, the surgeon may be facing with multiple wounds in multiple body locations.

GENERAL ANATOMIC CONSIDERATIONS FOR PENETRATING INJURIES

Evaluation of entrance and exit wounds is essential to assess the number of projectiles, their courses, and which organs are at risk of injury. Entrance wounds for bullets typically cause tattooing, burning, and abrasion as a result of the spin. Depending on the range, there may be direct burning of skin. Weapons fired within 5 to 8 cm of the skin cause burns. Tattooing occurs if the muzzle is within 30 cm of the skin at the time of firing. The range from which a gun is fired is also significant in that the air resistance that slows bullet velocity and reduces kinetic energy is directly proportional to the distance traveled.

After a missile penetrates tissue, the energy is distributed predictably within a closed space and, depending on the organs impacted and the types of tissue traversed, certain injuries can be anticipated. For example, a bullet penetrating the skull may have insufficient residual energy to traverse and exit the opposite side of the skull. It may instead follow the curvature of the interior of the skull, generating a more severe brain injury than would result from a simple linear passage.

In the thorax, lung parenchyma has low mass and therefore sustains less damage from penetrating injury than any other thoracic tissue. Similarly, blood vessels that are not fixed may be pushed aside without significant damage. Large fixed vessels, however, such as the aorta and vena cava, are particularly susceptible to fatal injury. If bones are penetrated, fragments can become secondary missiles that can lacerate the surrounding tissues. Low-velocity bullets may not follow a straight path but rather ricochet through the body cavity, injuring other organs. Muscles may expand out of the path of a missile, but this can result

in stretching and hemorrhage. Injury to adjacent blood vessels can result in intimal damage with subsequent thrombosis even if most of the vessel remains intact.

Penetrating injuries should also be evaluated with regard to topography. For example, penetrating wounds of the neck are commonly associated with injury to the jugular vein, trachea, and carotid artery. Injuries to the trachea are commonly associated with damage to the esophagus, and injuries to the carotid artery are frequently associated with injuries to the internal jugular vein. Penetrating wounds to the thorax raise the possibilities of injury to the heart, lung, and diaphragm. The anterior location of the right ventricle makes it particularly vulnerable to penetrating trauma. All penetrating wounds below the nipple line or inframammary groove must be considered for potential intraabdominal injury (Fig. 11-5). Similarly, wounds that cross the midline, so-called axial traverse wounds, are important to recognize. In the thorax, every mediastinal structure is at risk from such wounds, and in the abdomen, the possibility of major vascular injury, particularly to the aorta and vena cava, must be considered. Associated abdominal injuries often include the liver and spleen as well as the diaphragm, lung, or stomach. Duodenal and pancreatic injuries are commonly seen with injuries to the liver, inferior vena cava, stomach, and colon. Examples of injuries associated with specific vascular trauma include the following:

- Superior mesenteric artery or superior mesenteric vein injury with pancreas and liver
- Renal artery injury with liver, kidney, and colon
- Inferior vena cava injury with liver, small bowel, colon, pancreas, and duodenum
- Portal vein injury with inferior vena cava, liver, pancreas, and duodenum
- Axillary artery injury with brachial plexus trauma

SCORING SYSTEMS AND INJURY ASSESSMENT

Many systems have been developed to compare trauma injuries and trauma patients among institutions. Some provide considerable help, although none is perfect. The impetus for injury severity scoring systems is provided by the need to identify and classify severely injured patients in the prehospital phase, to predict mortality, to assess results, and to improve communication.

One simple way to classify trauma patients is to place them into three groups according to severity of injury: (1) those patients with injuries that are rapidly fatal, (2) those with injuries that are potentially fatal, and (3) those with injuries that are not fatal. The first group includes patients who have exsanguinating injuries, massive head injuries, cervical spinal cord transection, or major airway disruption; such injuries produce death in less than 10 minutes. Five percent of traumatic injuries and half of all deaths fall within this category. The third group accounts for 80% of trauma patients and includes those whose injuries are minor or confined to soft tissue and those who have isolated extremity fractures. This group does not have major injury, and urgent treatment is not essential. These patients survive without significant disability, even if prolonged delays occur before definitive therapy. The real impact of improved prehospital care and organized trauma care systems is on the second category of patients (about 15% of the total) those who can be saved if effective medical care is provided quickly. It is for this group that scoring systems have been developed.

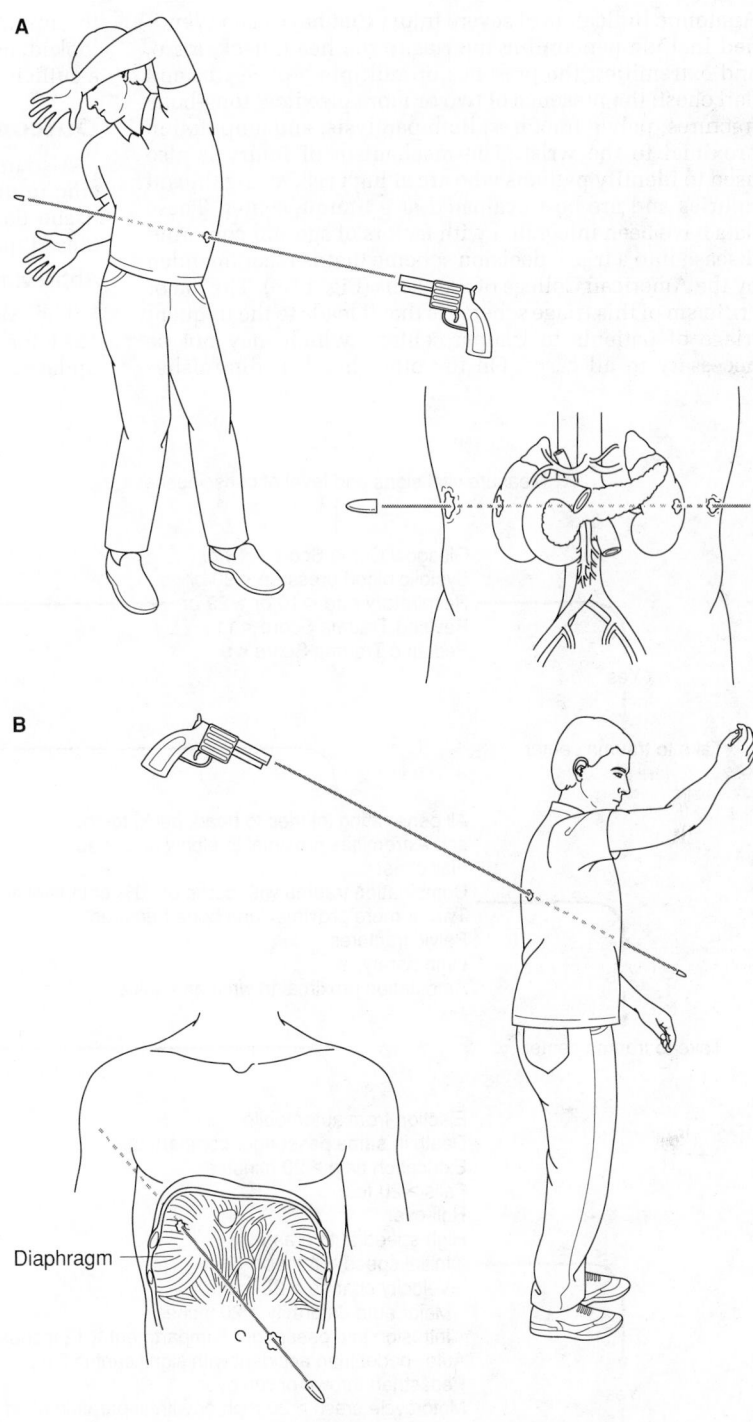

Figure 11-5. Axial traverse (*A*) and transdiaphragmatic (*B*) wounding mechanisms with associated injury potential for combined thoracic and abdominal injuries.

Revised Trauma Score and Triage

The trauma score developed by Champion and Sacco[13] in 1981 has been the most widely applied as well as the most useful scoring system for the initial evaluation of trauma victims. It mathematically combines the physiologic parameters of blood pressure, respiratory rate, and head injury (as assessed by the Glasgow Coma Score, described later) to assess injury severity and to predict which patients need the most timely and sophisticated medical care. Table 11-4 shows the components of the Revised Trauma Score (RTS).

In addition to physiologic scores, specific anatomic aspects of injury are correlated with high injury potential.

Table 11-4. REVISED TRAUMA SCORE COMPONENTS

Glasgow Coma Scale	Systolic Blood Pressure (mmHg)	Respiratory Rate (breaths/min)	Coded Value
13–15	>89	10–29	4
9–12	76–89	>29	3
6–8	50–75	6–9	2
4–5	1–49	1–5	1
3	0	0	0

Anatomic indicators of severe injury that have been identified include penetrating injuries to the head, neck, torso, and extremities; the presence of multiple broken ribs and flail chest; the presence of two or more proximal long-bone fractures; pelvic fractures; limb paralysis; and amputation proximal to the wrist. The mechanism of injury is also used to identify patients who are at high risk for significant injuries and are best evaluated at a trauma center. These data have been integrated with factors of age and comorbid disease into a triage decision scheme that is recommended by the American College of Surgeons (Fig. 11-6). The major criticism of this triage scheme is that it leads to the frequent triage of patients to trauma centers, which may not be necessary in all cases. On the other hand, it diminishes the number of patients with severe injury who are overlooked, and some overclassification is the inherent cost of a sufficiently sensitive scoring system.

Outcome Assessment

Also important are the needs to accurately compare specific injuries and to develop a scale for rating severity of tissue damage. Outcome analysis is a major objective of these types of scoring systems.[14]

Abbreviated Injury Scale

The Abbreviated Injury Scale (AIS) was developed in 1971 for use in blunt trauma. It has subsequently been updated and, as of the 1990 revision, includes descriptors

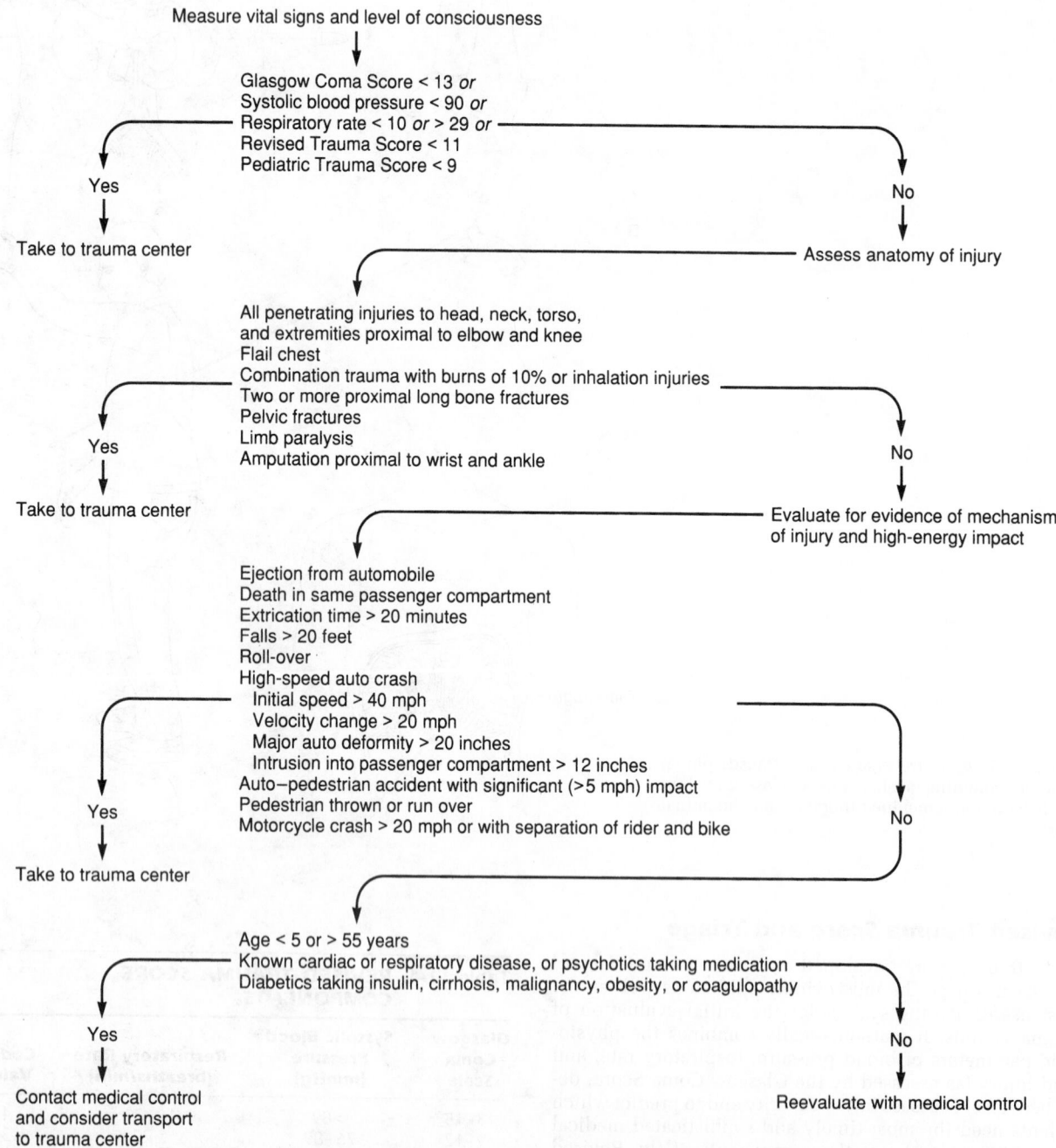

When in doubt take to a trauma center

Figure 11-6. Field triage decision scheme as recommended by the American College of Surgeons.

for penetrating trauma.[15] It is a specific anatomic index; the severity of nonfatal injuries is determined in six different body areas on a scale of 0 to 5, where 0 indicates no injury and 5 indicates critical injury. AIS codes 6 through 9 are uniformly fatal injuries and have therefore been eliminated. Table 11-5 shows an example of the AIS for abdominal injuries. The shortcoming of the AIS is that it evaluates only the most severe injury within a specified anatomic compartment and fails to account for multiple serious injuries within an individual compartment, thereby underscoring the true severity of injury.

Injury Severity Score

In 1974, Baker developed the Injury Severity Score (ISS), which is calculated by assigning AIS values to each injury in six body areas: (1) head and neck, (2) face, (3) chest, (4) abdomen and pelvic contents, (5) extremities and pelvis, and (6) general and cutaneous. To derive the ISS, the scores for the three most severely injured areas are squared and added.

The result is that substantial quadratic correlation between injury severity based on ISS and death can be developed. The ISS is extremely helpful and has been widely used. However, it does not adjust for patient age and comorbid risk factors such as chronic disease. In addition, the severity of head injury is disproportionately underscored in that combinations of injuries in other areas can result in a higher ISS score than a fatal head injury. Despite these drawbacks, the ISS is an excellent tool for the study of groups of patients with multiple injuries from blunt trauma, and it allows comparison of outcomes and quality assurance. Most recent reports of injured patients include descriptions of injury severity as measured by ISS.

TRISS

The TRISS methodology[16] is of great importance because it attempts to combine the trauma score, or physiologic component, and the ISS, or anatomic component. It also incorporates the patient's age. The equation for the TRISS is as follows:

$$P_s = \frac{1}{(1 + e^{-b})}$$

where:

P_s = probability of survival
$b = b_0 + b_1 (RTS) + b_2 (ISS) + b_3 (\text{patient age})$

(The coefficients b_0, b_1, b_2, and b_3 are derived from a regression analysis applied to data from thousands of patients analyzed in the Major Trauma Outcome Study.)

The TRISS method yields a specific probability of survival. Adjustments are made for age and type of injury sustained (blunt or penetrating). The methodology allows patient groups to be compared. Individuals with an unexpected outcome can be specifically identified. The American College of Surgeons Committee on Trauma continues to recommend that the TRISS methodology be used with a trauma registry to maintain a quality assurance program until an alternative is developed.

TRISS can be used for quality assurance evaluations both within and between institutions. Typically, a cutoff point (eg, $P_s = 50\%$) is chosen, and records of the deaths of patients who had a probability of survival greater than that number are submitted for peer review. TRISS can also be used to examine cases in which the survivors exceeded the chosen value. TRISS can also be used to compare a set of trauma outcomes from one institution to those from another institution. To achieve this goal, a Z factor is calculated: the Z factor is equal to the number of observed deaths minus the expected number of deaths, divided by a population variation factor specific to the institution. A positive Z statistic indicates more survivors than expected, and a negative Z statistic indicates fewer than the expected number of survivors. One other factor that is added to the comparison is a W statistic. This statistic attempts to compare the average increase or decrease in the number of survivors per 100 patients with the normal population. In theory, then, comparisons between institutions can be made.[17]

Other potentially relevant scoring systems are in various stages of development and validation. These include evaluation of specific mechanisms of injury, comparison of penetrating and blunt injuries, and provision of patient outcome indices in the intensive care unit. A specific Organ Injury Scaling system has been developed in an attempt to standardize the description of major parenchymal injuries. Another system, A Scoring Characterization of Trauma (ASCOT), uses descriptors of anatomic injury, patient physiology, age, and type of injury.[18] Like TRISS, the ASCOT system uses logistic modeling and multivariate analysis to calculate a probability of survival. Large groups of patients have been analyzed and compared with the reference patients in the Major Trauma Outcome Study using the ASCOT system. The results for probability of survival are equal to and in some instances surpass those calculated by the TRISS methodology. Long-term use of ASCOT has yet to be evaluated.

Finally, to simplify the coding of trauma scores, a method that uses discharge diagnoses based on the *International Classification of Diseases* (9th edition) is undergoing testing.[19,20] In this system, the first and second discharge diagnoses as well as the first operative code and the injury E code are used to calculate a Mortality Risk Ratio, which can be used in quality assurance. Again, the validity and applicability of this system for intrainstitutional and interinstitutional quality assurance remains to be documented.

Trauma is a major national health care problem that affects one of four US citizens annually. The cost of trauma injury and treatment in the United States is about $180 billion per year if loss of future productivity is considered. The causes of traumatic death vary considerably, depending on demographics. Urban and politically unstable areas typically have a higher incidence of penetrating trauma, whereas rural and stable communities have a predominance of blunt injuries, usually vehicular accidents. Nevertheless, causes of death after injury are remarkably similar. CNS injury accounts for about half of all fatalities, hemorrhage for 35%, and sepsis, multiple organ failure, and pulmonary embolism for about 15%. With the introduction of trauma care systems during the last two decades, the incidence of preventable death has dropped from about 25% to less than 5%. This is the result of improvements in care for acute head injuries and control of hemorrhage. In addition, the incidence of late death attrib-

Table 11-5. ABBREVIATED INJURY SCALE SCORING SYSTEM FOR ABDOMINAL INJURIES

Score	Injury Examples
1	Abdominal wall abrasion
2	Liver, stomach, colon, mesentery contusion
3	Minor liver or spleen laceration
	Bowel laceration without perforation
4	Major liver or spleen laceration
	Bowel laceration with perforation
5	Major liver or spleen laceration with tissue loss
	Bowel laceration with tissue loss

utable to sepsis and multiple organ failure has diminished, possibly as a result of better and early resuscitation.

The responsibility of the surgeon for trauma encompasses the early recognition of injury, the resuscitation, and then the definitive care of the patient. As we improve the operative and intensive care rendered to trauma patients, we are beginning to reach the flat portion of the outcome curve.[3,17] The area of injury prevention, however, is still open to substantial improvement. To reduce the morbidity and mortality from trauma, surgeons must take a more active role in the prevention of trauma at the community level.

Trauma Systems

DAVID B. HOYT

The development of civilian regional trauma systems has provided the single most significant improvement in the care of injured patients in the last two decades. Despite this, comprehensive systems are developed in less than 30% of the United States.[9] The necessary elements of a trauma system have been defined. These include four primary patient needs: access to care, prehospital care, hospital care, and rehabilitation. In addition, five issues require social and political solutions to supplement medical efforts: prevention, disaster medical planning, patient education, research, and rational financial planning. Recent federal legislation (The Trauma Care Systems Planning and Development Act) authorizes planning, implementation, and development of statewide trauma care systems.[21]

COMPONENTS OF A TRAUMA CARE SYSTEM

Access

A first step in providing broad access to trauma care is to establish adequate emergency communication systems. Although many urban centers have capitalized on modern electronic technology to establish emergency systems, most rural communities in the United States have not. This type of access includes emergency-only telephone numbers (eg, 911), emergency telephones located along major freeways, and a host of individualized radio and telephone networks. Access also requires that all potential users know how to enter the system. Public safety and information programs and school educational programs are used to inform health care providers and the public about emergency medical access.

Prehospital Care

Prehospital care encompasses many components. The primary focus is on education of paramedical personnel to provide initial resuscitation, triage, and treatment of injured patients. The development of coordinated response systems for ground ambulances, fixed-wing aircraft, and helicopters is an essential part of a modern trauma system. Effective prehospital care requires coordination between various public safety agencies and hospitals to maximize efficiency, minimize duplication of services, and provide care at a reasonable cost.

Hospital Care

Hospital care of the injured patient requires commitments from specific facilities to provide administrative support, medical staff, nursing staff, and other support personnel. The unpredictable nature of trauma care may generate demands for diagnostic services, operating rooms, laboratory services, and critical care beds that may disrupt other programs within a hospital. Ultimately, the responsibility for a decision to commit to becoming a trauma center rests with the board of trustees and the medical staff of a hospital. This decision must be made within a complex social, financial, and ethical framework that is beyond the scope of this review.

Rehabilitation

Rehabilitation, the long-term component of trauma patient care, is as important as prehospital and hospital care, although it is traditionally underdeveloped. Only 1 of 10 trauma patients in the United States has access to adequate rehabilitation programs. The long-term functional recovery of patients after injury is also poorly understood.[22] It makes little sense to develop sophisticated prehospital and hospital care systems, only to have patients obtain posttraumatic rehabilitation in inadequate facilities.

Other Essential Components

Effective trauma programs must focus on injury prevention. As noted, more than half of deaths occur within minutes of injury. Identification of risk factors and high-risk groups, development of strategies to alter personal behavior through education or legislation, and other preventive efforts are the only rational approach to reduce these types of injuries. Education is the second component of a trauma system, with the goal being both public and professional understanding of the available regional resources and how to access them. Disaster planning for a region is another responsibility of a trauma system, and emergency services within a community must be coordinated prospectively. Finally, a societal commitment to support effective research and to fund the financial operations of trauma systems is necessary. Most of the industrialized world has begun to approach this complex problem. Fitting trauma care systems into the changing managed health care environment remains a challenge.

PRIMARY ROLE OF SURGEONS IN A TRAUMA SYSTEM

The key individual participants in the development of a system of trauma care are the general surgeons. Surgeons have political responsibilities that include interaction with local police, fire, and emergency medical service authorities; interaction with the individual hospitals; and interaction with any other institutions that participate in the system of care. Planning with the recognized verification authorities at a state or local level is necessary. Implied is a fiscal responsibility to optimize the use of resources and to maintain cost containment so that the system can be successful.

Surgeons should be involved in needs assessment for both ground and air prehospital care services and should assume an active role in the training of emergency medical technicians and paramedical personnel. This includes responsibility for prehospital management protocols and for direct input to field personnel for treatment of injured patients before hospital admission. The final responsibility in the prehospital arena is to monitor and analyze prehospital care outcome and correct deficiencies as they occur.

During the resuscitation phase, surgeons should maintain a vital involvement in initial management of injured patients. Advanced trauma life support (ATLS) protocols have been established and provide a basis for initial care. Many models have worked well; in some, surgeons resuscitate patients initially, and in others, surgeons work together with emergency physicians and other members of the resuscitation team.

It is essential for the surgeon to maintain active involvement in initial resuscitation and to prioritize and orchestrate the sequence of evaluation and management of complex injuries. The greatest source of preventable death and morbidity occurs during the initial phase of care and is related to the need for rapid operative intervention. The central role of surgeons in this capacity is obvious. Establishment of protocols for evaluation of life-threatening injuries becomes the responsibility of the surgeon so that operative care can be provided in a timely fashion. Modern trauma care requires the ability to move rapidly, to prioritize multiple injuries, and to accomplish several tasks simultaneously. No training other than that of the general surgeon allows a single person to function effectively in such a capacity.

Postinjury care is ongoing and does not end after operation. Critical care, including mechanical ventilatory support, hemodynamic support, and management of renal, hepatic, and gastrointestinal dysfunction, are important postoperative surgical requirements that contribute to preventable death.[23] In addition, nutritional support in the treatment of multiple organ failure is an important domain of the general surgeon.

The quality of surgical leadership is of fundamental importance in the development of trauma systems. Successful trauma systems cannot develop without the commitment of the surgical department and the surgeons themselves within a hospital or community.

TRAUMA SYSTEM DEVELOPMENT

Trauma system development involves the redistribution of patients and of medical and economic resources. It therefore requires public and legislative support and community-wide education. The first step in the development of such a system is to determine the need. In general, this has been done in communities by a quality assurance program that reviews the outcome of trauma cases in that region. This review has traditionally been focused on trauma deaths and their potential preventability. It is at least as important, however, to demonstrate whether there is potential for preventing permanent disability. The involvement of local physicians in such an audit usually leads to unambiguous conclusions, and, with increased public awareness, the need for change becomes a community issue. The role of the surgeon is critical in both leadership and commitment to establishing a better standard of care.

The second phase of the review is to establish legal authority for the development of a system. This usually requires legislation at a state or local level that provides public agency authority. Recent federal and state legislative efforts continue to define this relationship.[21] The designated agency then works with trauma surgeons to develop criteria for the trauma system, to design facilities to care for the patients, and to establish a registry for tracking all injured patients and for maintaining a quality improvement program. A prehospital communications and transport system must be developed, along with a training program and specific qualifications for trauma care personnel

for every phase of hospital care, including resuscitation, surgery, critical care, and rehabilitation.

With criteria established, the process is democratized. The authoritative body requests proposals from major hospitals and appropriate local health care professionals. These proposals demonstrate the commitment of hospital and medical staff and their ability to comply with established standards. The standard criteria were developed by the American College of Surgeons Committee on Trauma and appear in their 1993 report entitled *Resources for the Optimal Care of the Injured Patient*.[10] External peer review is usually employed to critique proposals and to verify a specific hospital's capabilities. The purpose of peer review is not to certify a hospital within a region but to verify that the hospital and medical personnel can in fact deliver the appropriate level of care. The verification process can be accomplished through the American College of Surgeons Committee on Trauma or by inviting outside reviewers who are expert in the field of trauma.

After verification, formal designation is carried out by the authoritative body established at the outset. Designation is contractual and generally binding on prehospital providers. The designation process sets standards of care for the trauma system that can be monitored on an ongoing basis and implies a specific commitment from the providers.

The final component of program development involves design of the mechanisms for ongoing monitoring of needs assessment and quality assurance for the system. The trauma registry allows accurate documentation of epidemiologic data and monitoring of standards of care.[24] Clinical indicator cases in which care is questioned are selected for review, and care is improved over time. The use of the Injury Severity Score and the TRISS methodology previously discussed allows for the identification of patients who die and for analysis of the predicted mortality. This methodology also allows for unanticipated deaths to be automatically reviewed.

In summary, the development of a trauma system within a geographic area (city, county, or state) provides for access to trauma care and rapid transport of major trauma victims to specific hospitals within that region. The development of trauma systems has resulted in a significant reduction in patient mortality within the first hours after injury. These specific hospitals, called trauma centers, have concentrated resources and expertise to treat severely injured patients effectively, both immediately and throughout their care. Experience gained from the development of trauma systems has demonstrated the importance of the commitment required from surgeons to meet the specific problems encountered in the process.

Patient Care Phase: Prehospital and Resuscitation Care

H. GILL CRYER AND BAXTER LARMON

Care of the injured patient begins in the prehospital setting with a tightly integrated multidisciplinary emergency medical system. The goals of this system are to provide immediate access to lifesaving medical care. This usually entails the use of a first-response team, such as the fire department, with the capability of providing basic trauma life support (BTLS) within minutes of an accident. Next, a rapid transport team capable of providing advanced life support moves the injured patient to a trauma center, where a multidisciplinary team meets the patient to continue resuscitation, identify injuries, and provide expeditious therapy, with the aim of completing all of these processes within 1 hour (the so-called golden hour). The goals of a prehospital care system are to initiate emergency care of immediately life-threatening injuries and to transport the injured patient as expeditiously and safely as possible to a trauma center. The goals of the resuscitation phase are to identify and initiate therapy for immediately life-threatening and potentially life-threatening problems and to move the patient safely and rapidly to the treatment phase.

PREHOSPITAL CARE

Personnel

The initial goal of any emergency medical services system is to provide a rapid response of personnel trained in BTLS skills to the scene of the injured patient. The initial responsibility of the emergency medical services personnel is rapidly to assess the patient's airway, breathing, and circulation (ABCs) and evidence of obvious external hemorrhage. BTLS skills include extrication, spinal protection, immobilization, splinting, and control of external hemorrhage. Patients with medical problems such as myocardial infarction often require restoration of cardiac function and stabilization before transport. However, the injured patient is at risk for progressive deterioration from continued bleeding and requires rapid transport to a trauma center, with performance of stabilizing procedures en route rather than at the scene.[25] If delays in transport occur, as in complicated extrication procedures, then securing of the airway, placement of intravenous lines, and administration of intravenous fluid takes place in the field. Otherwise, these procedures are usually best performed en route to a trauma center. For these reasons, a second response team that includes emergency medical technicians–paramedics with advanced trauma life support (ATLS) training and a transport vehicle that contains ATLS equipment such as endotracheal tubes, intravenous fluids, and suctioning devices, is mobilized. Activation of this team occurs after communication between the first-response team and a base station with medical input from the trauma center.

The controversy between rapid transport ("scoop and run") and field stabilization philosophies continues to appear in the literature. The choice of procedure for the individual patient often requires complex judgments. Decisions made by experienced on-scene emergency medical technicians communicating with the trauma center that will receive the patient provide the best patient outcome.[25,26] The procedures performed and the time invested depend on factors such as hemodynamic stability, level of consciousness, complexity of extrication, distance from the receiving trauma center, and experience of the personnel at the scene and in the transport vehicle. Standardized training programs for emergency medical technicians–paramedics, such as prehospital ATLS and BTLS, taught in the trauma centers that work closely with the emergency medical technicians, provide the best background for making these complex decisions.[27]

Assessment and Management Priorities

Airway Assessment

Because the most immediately life-threatening problem to the injured patient is loss of airway patency, this is the first priority of the first-response team on arrival at the injury site. Patients who are awake, alert, and talking obviously have a patent airway, but patients who are unconscious or have evidence of respiratory insufficiency require immediate attention. Typical BTLS skills, such as suctioning, the placement of oropharyngeal airways, and the use of bag–mask devices, are usually sufficient to at least temporarily restore oxygenation at the injury scene. On the other hand, approximately 10% of patients require endotracheal intubation,[28] and up to 20% of patients would benefit from field intubation. Endotracheal intubation is the best procedure for airway control for patients who are in shock, have abnormal breathing patterns, or are unable to protect their airway because they are unconscious. Endotracheal intubation is a skill that requires proper training and regular use of the technique. In addition, ongoing quality assurance and reeducation are needed to maintain skills over time.

Training of paramedical personnel almost always includes endotracheal intubation, but the indications for intubation vary. Most trauma systems underutilize prehospital endotracheal intubation. Endotracheal intubation is far superior to bag-valve-mask systems because it provides larger tidal volumes and less risk of aspiration.[28] Unconscious or obtunded patients with absent or diminished gag reflexes have a high risk of aspiration of gastric contents. Positive-pressure ventilatory assistance by bag-valve-mask increases gastric distention and the risk of aspiration. Indications for endotracheal intubation in the field should include respiratory distress, hypovolemic shock, unconsciousness, significant head injury, and severe chest injury. Reported rates of successful intubation by paramedical personnel vary between 90% and 98%, and complications are rare.[29] More liberal indications for endotracheal intubation include all patients in major injury cases with unstable vital signs or altered mental status. On the other hand, there are problems with intubation at prehospital sites. Patients with head injuries may have cervical spine injuries, so in-line mobilization techniques are necessary to ensure intubation without further injury to the cervical spinal cord. Patients often clench their teeth, in which case either nasotracheal intubation or the use of paralytic agents such as succinylcholine may be necessary for successful intubation. Nasotracheal intubation is an effective technique if practiced frequently, but most paramedical personnel lack training in this technique. The use of paralytic agents in the field is currently under investigation. Some systems allow their use under direct supervision and with permission from a physician at the receiving facility or base station who is in direct communication with the field personnel.[29] Prehospital personnel should not use paralytic agents without physician control.

Breathing

After establishment of a patent and controlled airway, the next priority is to ensure that air exchange is taking place. Immediately life-threatening injuries that preclude air exchange include tension pneumothorax, massive open chest wounds, sucking chest wounds, and tracheal disruption. There are no maneuvers likely to correct tracheal disruption in the field. Both open chest wounds and sucking chest wounds respond to endotracheal intubation and positive-pressure ventilation. Tension pneumothorax occasionally requires field decompression. Field techniques to deal with tension pneumothorax include needle thoracostomy and chest tube thoracostomy.

Some trauma systems allow paramedical personnel to place chest tubes in the field or en route under medical control.[30] Chest tube placement is probably not necessary in urban trauma systems with short response times but can be of value in rural areas, where transport times can exceed

1 hour. For the most part, problems with breathing in the injured patient are best handled by endotracheal intubation and rapid transport to a trauma center. If endotracheal intubation is not successful, the laryngeal mask[31] offers advantages over the esophageal obturator airway, which is still used in many trauma systems. Occasionally, cricothyroidotomy may be the only way to establish an airway. Reasonable results have been obtained in the prehospital setting,[32,33] but few trauma systems have trained paramedical personnel for field cricothyroidotomy.

Circulation

The most common cause of death during the first hour after injury is hemorrhage. Therefore, after establishment of a patent airway and adequate air exchange, the next priority is support of the circulation. Direct pressure controls obvious external hemorrhage. The placement of one or two large-bore intravenous lines in the upper extremities en route to the trauma center facilitates resuscitation. However, placement of lines must not delay transport unless the patient is undergoing a complex extrication or is more than 30 minutes from a trauma center.[27] The standard of care in the prehospital setting for hypotensive patients has been volume replacement and application of the pneumatic antishock garment (PASG). However, recent data raise questions about both therapies.

In a large, prospective, randomized study, Mattox and colleagues[34] found that, in an urban setting with predominately penetrating trauma, the PASG offers no survival advantage and actually increases mortality if it is used in patients with thoracic injuries. On the other hand, there was a suggestion of benefit for patients who had a field blood pressure lower than 50 mmHg. Cayten and colleagues[35] also found that patients with a field blood pressure lower than 50 mmHg had increased survival with PASG use. Taken together, these studies suggest that PASG use is beneficial if the field blood pressure is less than 50 mmHg. It is also possible that the PASG is of value in other settings, particularly those involving lengthy transport times, or in patients with blunt trauma. These situations have not been adequately studied in prospective clinical trials.

The controversy between the scoop and run philosophy and the field resuscitation philosophy in seriously injured patients has more or less been resolved by common sense.[25] Patients who are a short distance from a trauma center should not undergo field placement of intravenous lines. Instead, they should be expeditiously transported to the trauma center with attempts made during transport to obtain intravenous access. This facilitates initiation of resuscitation on arrival at the trauma center. On the other hand, patients who are a long distance from a trauma center or who require long extrication times benefit from the placement of intravenous lines and administration of intravenous fluids. However, a new controversy has arisen regarding the use of intravenous fluids in the prehospital setting for injured patients.

Recent experimental and clinical evidence raises the possibility that internal hemorrhage from major vascular injuries should not be treated with intravenous fluid infusion until the bleeding can be controlled in the operating room.[36] In the hypotensive state, such major vascular injuries have a chance to clot and temporarily stop hemorrhage. But if intravenous volume restores normal blood pressure, the clot can dislodge and the rate of bleeding can significantly increase. This can lead to loss of both oxygen-carrying capacity and clotting factors and, ultimately, to exsanguination. If this theory is correct, it would be particularly relevant to the use of such agents as hypertonic saline. Hypertonic saline restores intravascular volume and blood pressure to almost normal levels very rapidly, albeit transiently. A prospective, randomized trial of normal saline versus hypertonic saline administration[37] demonstrated a significant improvement in survival when the data were compared with MTOS data for patients who had a probability of survival of 25% or lower, patients who had nontamponaded injuries, and patients who had an entry Glasgow Coma Scale (GCS) score of 8 or less. There was no evidence that nontamponaded bleeding was exacerbated by the use of hypertonic saline, despite the fact that blood pressure and intravascular volume increased. This study included patients in an urban trauma setting in which the median time from injury to arrival at the trauma center was 54 minutes. The median time from the beginning of infusion to arrival at the trauma center was 15 minutes. These data were confirmed by similar results obtained in a multiinstitution trial[38] in urban trauma systems. In this setting, it appears that the most severely injured patients can benefit from the use of hypertonic saline resuscitation. It is not known whether similar results would be obtained in settings with longer prehospital times.

RESUSCITATION PHASE

Adoption of the trauma center concept has increased dramatically over the last decade and produced documented improvement in survival of multiply injured patients in numerous reports. Trauma centers are hospitals committed to the total care of the trauma patient 24 hours a day. Multidisciplinary trauma teams consist of emergency physicians, general and orthopedic surgeons and neurosurgeons, critical care nurses, and diagnostic technicians. After notification of a major injury from the scene, the trauma team assembles in a specially equipped resuscitation room and waits for the patient to arrive. Care is immediately transferred from the prehospital team to the trauma team, and the trauma team rapidly initiates the resuscitation phase without a delay or lapse. Seriously injured patients should bypass hospitals without these resources and be taken to the nearest trauma center.

On the other hand, many patients have relatively minor injuries that do not require mobilization of this expensive team and resources. Therefore, an important function of a trauma system is to allow communication between prehospital personnel and the trauma center to identify those patients who can benefit from trauma hospital and trauma team care. In addition to communication between the prehospital care team and the trauma team, a written report briefly describing the mechanism and extent of injury, vital signs, and significant treatment started by the prehospital personnel should be provided. These details identify high-risk patients to alert the trauma center team to look for injury patterns of high probability and to guide further workup. Assessment and treatment then follow a logical sequence based on nationally standardized protocols through the ATLS format.

Team Composition

The trauma team consists of members from different disciplines, each of whom sees the patient from a particular point of view. By necessity, the team must have a single captain whose responsibility it is to organize and prioritize treatment efforts while the team is performing the primary and secondary survey to identify and treat life-threatening conditions. In a well-orchestrated team, the team leader integrates and coordinates several tasks simultaneously. In most level I and II trauma centers, the team captain is a general surgeon trained in trauma care. In the ideal situation, the trauma surgeon should be present when the patient arrives. This is true in every level I and level II trauma center. However, this may not be practical in many areas where the incidence of trauma is too low to justify the expense of an in-house trauma surgeon 24 hours a day, 365 days a year. In many rural and nonacademic level III trauma centers, the initial team captain is an emergency physician, with a general surgeon assuming the role when he or she arrives. Academic institutions with both emergency medicine and surgical residency programs have the obligation of training both specialties to assume the role of trauma team leadership.

Although responsibilities vary between institutions, anyone involved in the resuscitation of trauma patients must master several procedures: all types of airway management, including cricothyroidotomy; establishment of vascular access through both percutaneous and open approaches; decompression of the pleural space using needle or tube thoracostomy; and decompression of the pericardial space by pericardiocentesis, subxiphoid window, or emergency thoracotomy.

Primary Survey: Initial Assessment

The multidisciplinary trauma team receives the patient from the transport team in a specially equipped resuscitation room. The team's first priority is to simultaneously assess the airway, blood pressure, and level of consciousness of the patient. This examination begins with observation of the patient's ability to talk and breathe as well as palpation of the wrist for a pulse. Although in reality the primary survey is performed in a simultaneous fashion, for descriptive purposes it is broken down here into its individual components and their appropriate priorities.

The first priority is reassessment of the airway. Airway obstruction often responds to simple maneuvers such as suctioning, the chin lift, jaw thrust, or placement of an oropharyngeal airway. Protection of the cervical spine with in-line immobilization is imperative during these maneuvers. Persistence of respiratory insufficiency requires endotracheal intubation. Unsuccessful intubation necessitates cricothyroidotomy. Occasionally, the anatomy does not allow cricothyroidotomy, as can occur with laryngeal fracture. In these cases, a formal tracheotomy must be performed. After an airway is established, a physician auscultates the chest to confirm air exchange and obtains a chest radiograph to ensure proper tube position.

The next priority is to ensure adequate ventilatory exchange by rapid auscultation of both lung fields and assessment for mechanical factors that may interfere with breathing. These include compression of the lung from hemothorax, pneumothorax, or visceral herniation; loss of chest wall stability from flail chest; lung damage from pulmonary contusion; and airway obstruction from aspiration. A dramatic presentation with cyanosis, intense respiratory effort without air movement, distended neck veins, and lack of breath sounds on chest auscultation indicates that a tension pneumothorax is present. Clinical diagnosis of tension pneumothorax requires immediate needle thoracostomy followed by chest tube thoracostomy. Sucking chest wounds should be sealed with an occlusive dressing secured on three sides to function as a flap valve. Most other problems become evident on the initial chest radiograph and are relieved by chest tube insertion, suctioning, or repositioning of the endotracheal tube. The optimal position for chest tube insertion is the midaxillary line at the fifth or sixth interspace, avoiding the axilla, the large muscles of the back and chest, and the breast. Insertion of a finger into the chest before chest tube placement ensures entry into the pleural space and provides the opportunity to digitally search for defects in the diaphragm.

After establishment of an airway, ventilation, and appropriate pleural drainage, the next priority is an assessment of the patient's circulatory status. This includes estimation of blood volume and cardiac function. Blood pressure, pulse, skin perfusion and capillary refill, mental status, presence of breath sounds, and neck vein distention are all useful clinical indicators of hemodynamic status. The first issue is to establish whether the patient is in hypovolemic shock and, if so, the magnitude of this shock. The initial survey evaluates blood pressure, pulse, and skin perfusion. Circulatory collapse in the injured patient is almost always caused by hypovolemia secondary to hemorrhage. Occasionally, concurrent heart disease, spinal cord injury, and massive soft tissue swelling or cardiac tamponade also contribute. The mainstay of treatment for hypotension in the injured patient is volume resuscitation with crystalloid solution and packed red blood cells (RBCs). A lack of response to intravenous infusion of 2 L of lactated Ringer solution indicates significant, ongoing hemorrhage and necessitates immediate blood transfusion.

Effective resuscitation from hemorrhagic shock requires both restoration of intravascular volume and control of hemorrhage. Most hypotensive patients are compensating maximally on arrival in the emergency department (ED) and many have ongoing hemorrhage. The less responsive a patient is to initial volume resuscitation, the more urgent is the need for hemorrhage control. One need not wait for a response to resuscitation before taking the patient to the operating room. Another situation that requires vigilance is the cool, pale patient with relatively normal vital signs. These patients are compensating maximally and have a normal blood pressure because of intensive peripheral vasoconstriction. However, this compensatory mechanism is of only limited duration, and such patients require immediate rapid volume transfusion, blood transfusion, and operative control of bleeding. A similar trap exists for patients with the mangled extremity syndrome or multiple open fractures. Patients may have lost significant blood volume at the injury scene. Before resuscitation, there may be relatively little hemorrhage from the open wounds. However, the patient may exsanguinate after initiation of intravenous fluids that increase blood pressure and cause vasodilation of previously vasoconstricted extremities. These patients also require immediate volume resuscitation and operative control of their wounds.

The final priority in the primary survey is a brief neurologic evaluation using components of the GCS (Table 11-6). The GCS is scored by assessing eye opening, verbal responses, and motor responses. In addition, pupillary size and reactivity and the presence of other lateralizing signs are assessed. Mental status may improve in response to volume resuscitation; however, a patient with a GCS score of 8 or less is assumed to have a significant brain injury. In this case, aggressive brain resuscitation, including hyperventilation, restoration of circulating volume, and the provision of adequate oxygenation, are important considerations.

ED resuscitative thoracotomy is an aggressive, desperate attempt to save a dying patient. The dramatic return to full consciousness of a clinically dead patient after release of a pericardial tamponade from a stab wound to the heart provides complete justification for ED thoracotomy to those who have witnessed it. However, the widespread use of the technique in all patients arriving without vital signs has resulted in an extremely low survival rate at a very high cost. At first glance, the cost of an unsuccessful ED thoracotomy would seem to be nothing more than the cost of sterilizing the instruments and the physician's time.

Table 11-6. GLASGOW COMA SCALE

EYE OPENING

Spontaneous	___ 4
To voice	___ 3
To pain	___ 2
None	___ 1

VERBAL RESPONSE

Oriented	___ 5
Confused	___ 4
Inappropriate words	___ 3
Incomprehensible words	___ 2
None	___ 1

MOTOR RESPONSE

Obeys command	___ 6
Purposeful movement (pain)	___ 5
Withdraw (pain)	___ 4
Flexion (pain)	___ 3
Extension (pain)	___ 2
None	___ 1

TOTAL SCORE (1 + 2 + 3) ___

Many times, however, vital signs are temporarily restored, and the patient dies in the operating room or in the intensive care unit after massive blood transfusion and the use of considerable resources. Even worse from the resource management perspective is the rare patient who survives in a permanent vegetative state. The cost of the care for these patients must be included in any cost/benefit analysis.

Boyd and colleagues[39] performed a metaanalysis on 24 reports concerning the outcome of ED thoracotomy. They found that the overall survival rate after ED thoracotomy was 11% (264 of 2294 patients). There were no survivors among patients with no signs of life at the trauma scene. Signs of life were defined as supraventricular electrical activity, pupillary reaction, and agonal respirations. In addition, there were no neurologically intact survivors among blunt trauma patients who were without signs of life on arrival in the ED. Considering these findings, the researchers proposed an algorithm that would indicate ED thoracotomy for penetrating trauma only if the patient had signs of life at the scene and had lost signs of life less than 5 minutes before arrival in the ED. Blunt trauma patients would be allowed ED thoracotomy only if the patient had signs of life on arrival in the ED. For patients who meet these criteria and lose cardiac function, airway placement and fluid resuscitation are initiated simultaneously with, or are immediately followed by, left anterior thoracotomy, pericardiotomy, and internal cardiac massage.

Secondary Survey

The secondary survey is directed at specific identification of suspected and unsuspected injuries. It consists of a thorough physical examination that includes observation and palpation of the entire body for evidence and characterization of injury. However, the priorities of the secondary survey depend on the results of the primary survey and the patient's response to initial resuscitative efforts. The secondary survey for a patient in hemorrhagic shock unresponsive to initial resuscitative efforts during the primary survey consists only of rapid identification of the bleeding site and rapid transport to the operating room for definitive control of hemorrhage. At the other end of the spectrum, a completely stable patient with relatively mi-

nor injuries undergoes a complete physical examination with confirmatory laboratory and radiographic tests before initiation of the treatment phase. The secondary survey can be interrupted at any time if a patient's status deteriorates. Many aspects of the secondary survey, such as physical examination, radiographic examination, and blood drawing for laboratory tests and crossmatching of blood, are performed simultaneously. For the purposes of description, the secondary survey is broken down into its individual components.

Head and Face

The head-to-toe examination usually begins with palpation of the skull and the head to identify hematomas, lacerations, and fractures. Scalp lacerations can cause significant blood loss and should be closed with a full-thickness running suture to provide hemostasis. Potential ocular injuries are assessed by testing visual acuity, pupillary function, and ocular range of motion. A fundoscopic examination is important to identify increased intracranial pressure, vitriol hemorrhage, or retinal detachment. The findings of ecchymosis over the mastoid process, hemotympanum, otorrhea, rhinorrhea, and periorbital ecchymosis often indicate basilar skull fracture. Thorough palpation of the facial bones identifies step-offs or instability associated with facial fractures. Reassessment of the airway and a careful bimanual examination of the oral cavity identify loose teeth as well as mandibular and maxillary fractures. Bleeding from nasal fractures may require posterior and anterior packing for hemostasis.

Neck

Examination of the cervical region is conducted while axial immobilization of the cervical spine is maintained. The cervical collar is removed, and the neck is examined for tracheal deviation, subcutaneous emphysema, hematomas, or distended jugular veins. The posterior cervical spine is palpated to elicit tenderness or other signs of obvious fractures. Cranial nerve function should be determined and recorded. Evidence of laryngeal fracture includes subcutaneous emphysema, tenderness or distortion of the thyroid and cricoid cartilage, and voice change. The presence of a fractured larynx is a relative contraindication to endotracheal intubation because of the possibility of extending the injury or creating a false passage leading to loss of the airway. Patients with suspected laryngeal fractures should immediately be taken to the operating room for formal tracheotomy. Carotid pulses are assessed, and bruits or expanding hematomas that may be suggestive of carotid artery injury are identified.

Penetrating injuries should not be probed, cannulated, or explored past the platysma, because uncontrollable hemorrhage may ensue if a clot is dislodged from a major vascular injury. Wounds that have penetrated the platysma are evaluated either by formal operative exploration of the neck or by some combination of angiography, triple endoscopy (pharyngoscopy, laryngoscopy, and esophagoscopy), radiographic contrast study, computed tomography (CT) scan, and observation. If a water-soluble contrast swallow does not show a pharyngeal or esophageal leak, a subsequent barium swallow is indicated. Injuries encompassing the area from the cricoid cartilage to the angle of the mandible are usually explored. Angiography is mandatory for injuries between the cricoid cartilage and the clavicle and for injuries between the angle of the mandible and the base of the skull. Radiographic evaluation of the cervical spine should include anteroposterior, lateral, and odontoid views. CT scanning is often used to further evaluate suspicious bony injuries, and careful flexion and extension films may be necessary to rule out potentially unstable ligamentous injuries of the cervical spine.

Chest

The chest wall is inspected for evidence of instability (flail chest) and for lacerations, including sucking chest wounds, abrasions, and contusions. Auscultation is performed to identify hemothorax or pneumothorax, and palpation is used to elicit tenderness that may be associated with rib fractures. As has been mentioned, tension pneumothorax can be identified by cyanosis, tracheal deviation, distended neck veins, lack of breath sounds, and inability to move air. Tension pneumothorax causing cardiopulmonary collapse is a clinical diagnosis that requires immediate treatment by needle thoracostomy followed by chest tube insertion.

Virtually all other life-threatening and potentially life-threatening chest injuries are diagnosed or suspected on chest radiography. Hemothorax is identified by opacification of a hemithorax and is treated by chest tube thoracostomy. Most pulmonary parenchymal bleeding stops with reexpansion of the lung and evacuation of the pleural space. However, thoracotomy is indicated if the initial blood loss exceeds 1500 mL or if the rate of ongoing blood loss exceeds 200 to 300 mL/hour in an adult. Blood evacuated from the pleural space can be autotransfused with appropriate chest tube drainage systems. Pneumothorax is usually treated by chest tube thoracostomy. Occasionally, small, stable pneumothoraces can be treated successfully by needle aspiration or close observation.

Pulmonary contusion is identified by radiographic findings of an irregular interstitial pattern or frank consolidation in the lung parenchyma. The clinical manifestations of pulmonary contusion vary from mild dyspnea to overt pulmonary failure with development of adult respiratory distress syndrome. The magnitude of the injury is rarely appreciated during the initial evaluation, and it is important to follow up with serial blood gas determinations and a repeat chest radiographs at 6 hours.

All patients with chest trauma should have an electrocardiographic evaluation and continuous monitoring during the first hour in the ED. Patients with electrocardiographic changes during the initial hour may have myocardial contusions and should be monitored for at least 24 hours. If there is any sign of myocardial failure, the patient should undergo echocardiography. Most myocardial contusions are self-limited and require only careful monitoring and treatment of significant dysrhythmias during the first 24 to 48 hours. Rarely, patients have all of the manifestations of overt myocardial failure and require full support, including aortic balloon pump.

Patients with rapid deceleration blunt injuries to the chest may sustain a transection of the thoracic aorta. The chest radiograph should be evaluated for widening of the mediastinum (more than 8 cm on a 40-inch anteroposterior chest radiograph), apical capping of the lung with blood, tracheal displacement, depression of the left main-stem bronchus, loss of the aortic window, deviation of the nasogastric tube, and loss of the parispinous stripe. Each of these findings suggests the presence of a mediastinal hematoma, which is often associated with a transection of the aorta. Additional radiographic findings that indicate a substantial force to the mediastinum include fractures of the sternum, first or second ribs, or scapula. Patients with a significant mechanism of injury and suspicion of mediastinal hematoma on chest radiography should undergo arch aortography to rule out transection of the aorta. Recent use of spiral dynamic CT scanning and transesophageal echocardiography[40] are encouraging, and these techniques also have a place in the identification of aortic injury in patients with severe blunt chest trauma.

Evidence of a ruptured diaphragm on chest radiograph includes the presence of the nasogastric tube or bowel above the normal plane of the diaphragm. If the patient has a diagnosis of ruptured diaphragm and respiratory distress, consideration should be given to careful placement of a chest tube. Placement of the chest tube to water seal instead of suction decreases intrathoracic pressure and prevents further herniation. These patients should undergo expeditious exploratory laparotomy to repair the defect.

Major bronchial injuries typically present with massive subcutaneous mediastinal emphysema and pneumothorax. Chest tube placement results in a vigorous air leak.

Management of penetrating injuries to the chest depends on the trajectory of the missile. Wounds confined to one lung or pleural cavity are usually treated by chest tube placement alone, with reexpansion of the lung. If the missile trajectory may have traversed the mediastinum, further evaluation is necessary, potentially including bronchoscopy, esophagoscopy, and aortography. Echocardiography is used to rule out pericardial blood and heart injury. False-negative studies have occurred when blood in the pericardium decompresses into the pleural space. However, echocardiography may be a sufficient screening tool if there are no clinical signs or symptoms and no hemothorax.

Abdomen

The abdominal examination should attempt to determine whether there is a significant injury requiring surgical intervention. Although physical examination is often accurate and reliable, it can be misleading in 20% to 30% of patients.[41] This is particularly true in patients who are obtunded from head injury, alcohol, drug use, or shock. If patients are hemodynamically unstable, it is important to rapidly determine whether free intraperitoneal hemorrhage is responsible for the hypotension. Diagnostic peritoneal lavage (DPL) accomplishes this goal rapidly and safely and is extremely reliable in the hemodynamically unstable patient.

DPL is considered grossly positive if more than 10 mL of blood is aspirated after catheter insertion. If less than 10 mL of blood or no blood is aspirated, 1 L of normal saline solution is infused into the peritoneum and then drained. A sample of the drained fluid is sent to the laboratory for RBC count; DPL is considered microscopically positive if the RBC count is higher than 100,000/mL. If the goal is to find the source of hemorrhage in a hypotensive patient, a grossly positive DPL pinpoints the abdomen as at least one source, and the patient should undergo immediate laparotomy. On the other hand, a microscopically positive DPL indicates intraabdominal injury that will eventually require laparotomy, but the major source of hemorrhage causing the hypotension may be elsewhere (chest or pelvis).[42]

In the hemodynamically stable patient, the lack of specificity of the DPL often leads to nontherapeutic and therefore unnecessary laparotomies. For this reason, CT has become routine for the evaluation of the abdomen in hemodynamically stable patients. Sequential CT scans may be necessary. Injuries that often have subtle findings during the first several hours after injury but may be found on a delayed CT scan include duodenal rupture, pancreatic transection, and blunt rupture of the intestine. Laboratory evaluations that may be helpful include liver enzyme levels and, to a lesser extent, serum amylase levels. The use of ultrasound is popular in some institutions, replacing DPL for the diagnosis of free intraperitoneal fluid.

The workup for patients with penetrating abdominal injuries depends on the missile. Gunshot wounds to the abdomen are an indication for exploratory laparotomy, because 90% to 95% of these patients have intraabdominal injuries. The occasionally encountered patient with a tangential subcutaneous wound can be evaluated by laparoscopy[43] to determine whether peritoneal penetration injury has occurred. Stab wounds to the abdomen are often evaluated initially by local exploration of the wound. If the wound traverses the anterior fascia, then the patient can be evaluated by DPL or laparoscopy and should undergo exploratory laparotomy if the results are positive. Stab wounds to the flank and back are best evaluated by CT and serial observation.[44] CT findings that mandate exploratory laparotomy include retroperitoneal hematoma, free air, extravasation of contrast material, and free intraperitoneal fluid.

Pelvis

After evaluation of the abdomen, the pelvis is assessed by physical examination. The bones of the pelvis are palpated gently to elicit tenderness that could indicate fracture. The genitalia should be inspected for scrotal hematoma or blood at the urethral meatus, which indicates probable urethral transection. A bimanual pelvic examination in women identifies evidence of vaginal laceration, indicating an open pelvic fracture. A rectal examination is performed to identify blood indicative of bowel injury and, occasionally, a mobile prostate, which indicates urethral transection. Evidence of a free-floating prostate, blood at the urethra, or scrotal hematoma should prompt a retrograde urethrogram before placement of a bladder catheter is attempted. All patients sustaining blunt trauma should undergo plain radiography of the pelvis to diagnose potential pelvic fracture. If a pelvic fracture is present, the patient should be assessed for retroperitoneal pelvic bleeding.

If the patient is hemodynamically unstable, the pelvic fracture must be considered a potential source of hemorrhage. This is important because pelvic fracture bleeding is retroperitoneal and rarely controllable at exploratory laparotomy. Potential pelvic fracture bleeding should be evaluated and treated by early angiography. If the patient is hemodynamically stable, the pelvic fracture should be evaluated further with additional plain radiographs and CT scans.

Extremities

Finally, the extremities are evaluated for open wounds with potential sources of hemorrhage or occult open fractures. Evaluation of pulses may indicate vascular injury. Palpation and passive range of motion tests diagnose potential long-bone fractures, dislocations, and ligamentous injuries. Dislocations require prompt reduction, especially if there is any evidence of neurovascular compromise. Penetrating wounds to the extremities necessitate evaluation for potential vascular injury by palpation of pulses, auscultation for bruits, and recognition of expanding hematomas. Proximity wounds can be evaluated by duplex ultrasound scanning or arteriography.

The ideal trauma system consists of a prehospital care team that quickly and safely transports an injured patient to a trauma center, where a multidisciplinary trauma team immediately begins resuscitation of the patient. Treatment of immediately life-threatening injuries begins during transport and continues after arrival at the trauma center. Rapid initial evaluation, followed by a more detailed secondary survey, allows identification of injuries while therapy is simultaneously begun. The management priorities are to identify and treat airway obstruction, hemorrhage, epidural or subdural hematoma, retroperitoneal or medias-

tinal hematoma, peripheral vascular injury, nonbleeding visceral injury, and long-bone fracture, in that order. The secondary survey is interrupted as necessary to treat life-threatening and limb-threatening injuries as they are identified according to this priority list. If interruption occurs, the secondary survey is completed at a later time.

Patient Care Phase: Shock
JAMES W. DAVIS

Shock can result from a variety of insults, including hypovolemic, septic, cardiac, or neurologic compromise. It is a condition caused by blood flow that is insufficient to meet the metabolic demands of organs and tissues. This section describes the hemorrhagic and hypovolemic causes of shock; other causes of shock are covered elsewhere.

PATHOPHYSIOLOGY

Hemorrhage initiates both rapid and slower, more sustained compensatory responses. Rapid responses, which occur within 1 minute of injury, are primarily increased adrenergic output, reflex tachycardia, and vasoconstriction. More sustained responses include resorption of fluid into the intravascular space and renal conservation of water and electrolytes.

Rapid Response

The body responds to maintain homeostasis almost immediately after the onset of hemorrhage. Decreased activation of the arterial baroreceptors, through a decrease in blood pressure or, even more subtly, through a decrease in pulse pressure, causes an increased sympathetic discharge, which results in reflex tachycardia and vasoconstriction.

Increased adrenergic output with increased secretion of catecholamines also leads to vasoconstriction, increased heart rate, and increased myocardial contractility. Constriction of the systemic capacitance of small veins and venules shifts blood back to the central venous circulation, increasing right-sided cardiac filling pressures. Left-sided filling and pressure are augmented by pulmonary vasoconstriction. Concomitantly, vasoconstriction occurs in the skin, kidneys, and viscera, effectively shunting blood to those tissues with locally dominant blood flow regulatory mechanisms (ie, heart and brain). Adrenergically mediated vasoconstriction increases cardiac filling and causes increased contractility and reflex tachycardia, all of which combine to increase stroke volume and cardiac output.

Sustained Response

Sustained compensatory responses include the release of vasoactive hormones and fluid shifts from the interstitium and the intracellular space. Decreased renal blood flow and increased adrenergic activity lead to the secretion of renin from the juxtaglomerular complex. Renin stimulates the release of adrenocorticotropic hormone (ACTH) and also stimulates the formation and release of angiotensin I by the liver. Circulating angiotensin I is converted in the lungs to angiotensin II, which is probably the most potent known vasoconstrictor. The increased concentrations of angiotensin and ACTH also increase aldosterone secretion. Aldosterone acts to increase resorption of sodium (Na^+) in the renal tubules. The release of vasopressin is increased because of reduced stimulation from the arterial baroreceptors, and this hormone causes increased resorption of water from the renal ultrafiltrate. After hemorrhage, vasopressin is sufficiently elevated to also function as a vasoconstrictor.

Adrenergically mediated vasoconstriction affects arterioles, precapillary and postcapillary sphincters, and small veins and venules. The decrease in intravascular hydrostatic pressure distal to the precapillary sphincter leads to resorption of interstitial fluid (water, Na^+, and chloride [Cl^-]) into the vascular space and thereby functions to restore circulating volume. This is known as *transcapillary refill.*

The increased release of the stress hormones (epinephrine, ACTH, cortisol, and glucagon), coupled with relative insulin resistance after shock, leads to high extracellular concentrations of glucose. In addition to glucose, products of anaerobic metabolism (ie, lactate) from hypoperfused cells accumulate in the extracellular compartment, inducing hyperosmolarity. This extracellular hyperosmolarity draws water from the intracellular space, increasing interstitial osmotic pressure, which in turn drives water, Na^+, and Cl^- across the capillary endothelium into the vascular space.[45]

Loss of Compensation

If the shock state continues, the postcapillary sphincter remains in spasm, but the arteriolar and precapillary sphincters cannot maintain the tension, and they become relaxed. As the sphincters relax, the capillary hydrostatic pressure increases, and Na^+, Cl^-, and water are moved into the interstitium by Starling forces, leading to further depletion of intravascular volume.

Cellular membrane function is also impaired in hemorrhagic shock. The normal, negative membrane potential approaches neutrality, leading to increased permeability and interstitial concentration of potassium (K^+). This is caused at least in part by a decrease in the normal function of the adenosine triphosphate–dependent Na^+-K^+ membrane pump that is induced by cellular hypoxia. The loss of the membrane potential difference and the Na^+-K^+ pump also leads to an intracellular influx of fluid, with concomitant cellular swelling. Some experimental evidence indicates that the decrease in membrane potential may be partly mediated by endorphins and that the decrease is partially reversible with naloxone.

EVALUATION OF SHOCK

Shock is easily recognized by even the most inexperienced caregiver after the compensatory mechanisms have been overcome by the severity of the injury. It is more difficult to recognize the patient in compensated shock, who presents with vital signs that are almost normal. It is critically important to the patient's ultimate outcome that recognition and treatment of shock occur before decompensation. The clinical assessment must be guided by the knowledge that the severity of the symptoms and signs of shock varies from patient to patient and also in relation to the volume of blood lost. The patient is evaluated based on clinical appearance, hemodynamic measurements, and biochemical analysis.

The initial vasoconstriction described earlier causes the skin to be cool, with poor capillary refill. Patients in shock hyperventilate to compensate for metabolic acidosis. As the shock state progresses, mental status changes also occur; decreased cerebral perfusion pressure and increased catecholamine stimulation of the reticular activating formation may lead to anxiety and restlessness. With increasing blood loss, stupor or coma may result.

The hemodynamic assessment should include evaluation of the rate and character of the pulse, the blood pressure, and, in some cases, the central venous pressure (CVP) and pulmonary artery pressure. Tachycardia is a normal response to volume loss but also to pain, anxiety, and fear, all of which are commonly present in the trauma patient. Assessment of the pulse (full and strong or weak and thready) may be helpful in determining the proper diagnosis. Because of the body's ability to compensate for hypovolemia, changes in blood pressure do not occur reliably until 20% to 30% of blood volume has been lost. In patients for whom there is no concern of spinal injuries, postural vital signs can be assessed. A drop of more than 10 mmHg in the systolic blood pressure or an increase of 20 beats per minute in the heart rate with upright posture are suggestive of volume loss. In addition, the pulse pressure usually narrows, even in compensated shock, because of the effects of vasoconstriction on the diastolic blood pressure. In patients with multisystem injuries or significant premorbid medical conditions, more invasive cardiovascular monitoring may be necessary. The CVP reflects the efficiency of the cardiac pump, the adequacy of the blood volume, and the state of the venous tone. Changes in CVP in response to treatment or from continuing hemorrhage are more revealing than a solitary measurement.

An indirect but extremely valuable measure of perfusion and volume status is urine output. A urinary catheter should be inserted in every trauma patient evaluated for shock. Hourly urine output should be 0.5 to 1 mL/kg for adult patients, at least 1 mL/kg for most pediatric patients, and 1 to 2 mL/kg for patients younger than 2 years of age.

Biochemical analysis of shock is based on the shift from aerobic to anaerobic metabolism in underperfused tissues. Increased lactate production is associated with tissue hypoperfusion.[46] Broder and Weil[47] reported increased lactate levels in patients with shock, and Vitek and Cowley[48] determined the median lethal dose associated with increased serum lactate to be 7.3 mEq/L. A decrease in serum lactate levels occurs in hypovolemic patients after resuscitation.[49] The time required to normalize serum lactate levels through resuscitation is an important prognostic factor for survival.[50]

Another biochemical marker of shock and resuscitation is the base deficit. This is defined as the amount of a fixed base (or acid) that must be added to an aliquot of blood to restore the pH to 7.40. The base deficit can be obtained as part of the arterial blood gas analysis and is reflective of metabolic acidosis, oxygen debt, and of the changes in lactate[51] (Fig. 11-7). The base deficit is a useful guide to the fluid volume required for resuscitation, and changes in the base deficit with volume infusion can be used to judge the efficacy of resuscitation.[52] The biochemical changes associated with the hypoperfusion of shock (ie, increased lactate concentration and base deficit) occur even with compensation. Because of the potential difficulties in diagnosing compensated shock, an arterial blood gas analysis including base deficit should be obtained for every major trauma patient, and any patient with a base deficit of 6 mEq/L or less should be considered to be in shock until proved otherwise.

CLASSIFICATION OF HEMORRHAGE

The signs and symptoms of shock vary with both the severity and duration of blood loss. A review of the Advanced Trauma Life Support (ATLS) classification system of the American College of Surgeons is useful to compre-

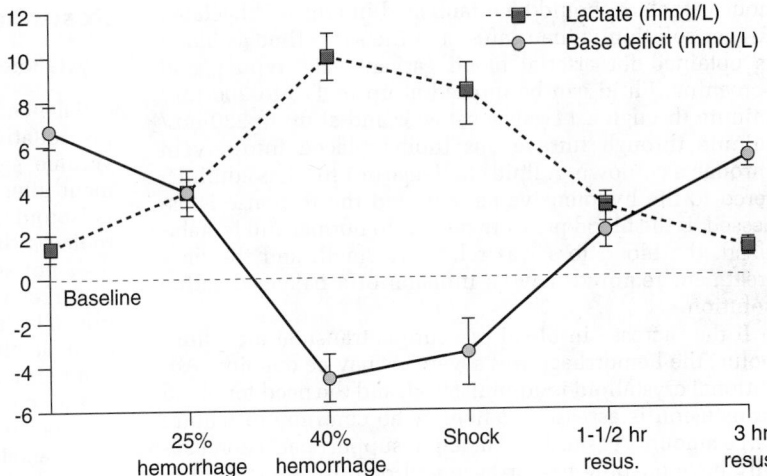

Figure 11-7. Correlation of serum lactate with base deficit after shock. Vertical axis is in milliequivalents per liter.

hend the manifestations and physiologic changes associated with hemorrhagic shock in adults[53] (Table 11-7). Blood volume is estimated at 7% of ideal body weight, or about 4900 mL in a 70-kg patient.

Class I: Mild hemorrhage, up to 15% of total blood volume. This condition is exemplified by voluntary blood donation. In the supine position, there are no measurable changes in heart or respiratory rates, blood pressure, or pulse pressure. Capillary refill is normal. This degree of hemorrhage requires little or no treatment, and blood volume is restored within 24 hours by transcapillary refill and the other compensatory methods.

Class II: Loss of 15% to 30% of blood volume (800 to 1500 mL). Clinical symptoms include tachycardia and tachypnea. The systolic blood pressure may be only slightly decreased, especially in the supine position, but the pulse pressure is narrowed (because of the diastolic increase from adrenergic discharge). Urine output is reduced only slightly (20 to 30 mL/hour). Mental status changes (eg, anxiety) are frequently present. Capillary refill is usually delayed. Patients with class II hemorrhage can usually be resuscitated with crystalloid solutions, but some may require blood transfusion.

Class III: Loss of 30% to 40% of blood volume (up to 2000 mL). Patients with class III hemorrhage present with inadequate perfusion that is obvious; marked tachycardia and tachypnea; cool, clammy extremities

with significantly delayed capillary refill; hypotension; and significant changes in mental status (eg, confusion, combativeness). Class III hemorrhage represents the smallest volume of blood loss that consistently produces a decrease in systolic blood pressure. The resuscitation of these patients frequently requires blood transfusion in addition to administration of crystalloids.

Class IV: Loss of more than 40% of blood volume (more than 2000 mL), representing life-threatening hemorrhage. Symptoms include marked tachycardia, a significantly depressed systolic blood pressure, and narrowed pulse pressure or unobtainable diastolic pressure. The mental status is depressed (eg, lethargy, stupor), and the skin is cold and pale. Urine output is negligible. These patients require immediate transfusion for resuscitation and frequently require immediate surgical intervention.

TREATMENT OF HEMORRHAGIC SHOCK

The treatment of hemorrhagic shock requires control and arrest of hemorrhage as well as restitution of the circulating blood volume. The search for the source of hemorrhage should occur simultaneously with the institution of volume infusion.

A minimum of two large-bore (14- to 16-gauge) intrave-

Table 11-7. CLASSIFICATION OF SHOCK IN ADULTS: ESTIMATED FLUID AND BLOOD REQUIREMENTS,* BASED ON PATIENT'S INITIAL PRESENTATION

	Class I	Class II	Class III	Class IV
Blood loss (mL)	≤750	750–1500	1500–2000	≥2000
Blood loss (% BV)	≤15	15–30	30–40	≥40
Pulse rate	<100	>100	>120	>140
Blood pressure	Normal	Normal	↓	↓
Pulse pressure	Normal or ↑	↓	↓	↓
Capillary refill	Normal	Positive	Positive	Positive
Respiratory rate	14–20	20–30	30–40	>35
Urine (mL/h)	≥30	20–30	5–15	Negligible
Mental status	Slightly anxious	Mildly anxious	Anxious/confused	Confused/lethargic
Fluid replacement (3:1 rule)	Crystalloid	Crystalloid	Crystalloid + blood	Crystalloid + blood

BV, blood volume.
* For a 70-kg man.

nous catheters should be established in adults.[53] Lactated Ringer solution is then infused at the same time as blood is obtained for arterial blood gas analysis, typing, and screening. Fluid can be infused at up to 175 to 200 mL/minute through a 14-gauge catheter and at up to 220 mL/minute through intravenous tubing placed into a vein through a cutdown. A fluid challenge of 1 to 2 L is administered to the hypotensive patient, and the response is assessed. If the blood pressure returns to normal and is stabilized, the blood loss was relatively small, and the only treatment required may be infusion of a balanced saline solution.

If the increase in blood pressure is transient after fluid bolus, the hemorrhage was severe or may be ongoing. Additional crystalloid is administered, and the need for blood transfusion is assessed. Patients who continue to require large amounts of fluid and blood to support perfusion usually have ongoing hemorrhage and require surgical intervention. No response or a minimal response to apparently adequate infusions of crystalloid solution and blood indicates exsanguinating hemorrhage and the need for urgent surgery.

Some controversy has developed over how much resuscitation should be attempted before definitive control of hemorrhage. Animal studies have demonstrated increased blood loss and increased mortality after infusion of isotonic and hypertonic solutions in models with uncontrolled hemorrhage.[54] In a similar study of uncontrolled hemorrhage, improved survival and decreased hemorrhage was achieved by infusion of only enough fluid to maintain a mean arterial pressure of 40 mm Hg (instead of 80 mm Hg).[55] It seems logical that restoration of normal blood volume would lead to increased hemorrhage if the sites of bleeding were not controlled. However, this approach to resuscitation (ie, withholding of intravenous fluids) in patients at high risk for ongoing hemorrhage, such as those with penetrating truncal trauma, remains unproved and controversial.[56]

The same clinical indicators used to evaluate shock are used to evaluate the patient's response to resuscitative efforts. The commonly considered endpoints of resuscitation include a normal blood pressure, decreased heart rate, adequate urine output, and normal CVP. The same compensatory mechanisms that can allow shock to go unrecognized, however, can also lead to underresuscitation. This is particularly true of blood pressure. CVP depends on intravascular volume and the state of venous tone. Assessment of the adequacy of volume replacement by CVP can be improved by observing the changes in CVP after rapid administration of small volumes (250 mL) of Ringer solution. A CVP that does not change after administration of a bolus may indicate that normovolemia is still not restored.

Metabolic parameters should also be used to assess the endpoints of resuscitation. With adequate restoration of volume, the metabolic acidosis should resolve, and the base deficit and serum lactate level should normalize. A base deficit that persists despite an apparently adequate volume of resuscitation necessitates a diligent search for ongoing hemorrhage.

Monitoring changes in cellular perfusion by measurement of tissue oxygen tension (tissue PO_2) has significant appeal as an endpoint of resuscitation. The measurement of tissue PO_2 during inspired oxygen challenges is both sensitive and specific in determining flow-dependent oxygen consumption.[57] Although this technology has significant potential, it is not widely available at present, and the confounding variables of vasoconstriction from hypothermia and catecholamine release have not been resolved.

Resuscitative Fluids

Crystalloids

Balanced salt solutions are the most commonly used resuscitative fluids, and their use to restore extracellular volume significantly decreases the transfusion requirement after hemorrhagic shock. Lactated Ringer solution is isotonic, readily available, and inexpensive. It rapidly replaces the depleted interstitial fluid compartment and does not aggravate any preexisting electrolyte abnormalities. Previous investigations have shown that administration of lactated Ringer solution does not lead to aggravation of the lactic acidosis that is present in shock.[49] As volume and perfusion are restored, lactate is mobilized and metabolized to bicarbonate in the liver. Mild metabolic alkalosis may occur 1 or 2 days after large-volume resuscitations with lactated Ringer solution. Normal saline solution is also effective for resuscitation of hypovolemic patients. Previous concerns about inducing hypernatremic, hyperchloremic metabolic acidosis with massive resuscitation volumes have not been borne out by further investigation with normal saline and the hypertonic saline solutions. Resuscitation with crystalloid solutions requires a volume administration ratio of 3:1 to 4:1 over volume lost.

Colloids

Although colloids do not replete the interstitial space, they have a volume-expanding effect somewhat greater than the amount infused. Colloids have the theoretic advantages of increasing the colloid oncotic pressure and of requiring smaller volumes for resuscitation than crystalloids do.[58] Colloids commonly used for volume expansion in hypovolemia include albumin, dextran 70, dextran 40, and hydroxyethyl starch.

Albumin solutions have been used during resuscitation to increase colloid oncotic pressure and, hypothetically, to protect the lung from interstitial edema; however, there is a relatively rapid flux of albumin across the pulmonary capillary membranes and relatively rapid clearance through the pulmonary lymphatics. In addition, it has been estimated that albumin passage from the intravascular to the extravascular space occurs at a rate of up to 500 mL/h.

Dextran 70 and dextran 40 are polysaccharides with molecular weights of 70,000 and 40,000, respectively. Dextran 40 (10%) is hyperoncotic and initially exerts a volume-expanding effect that is almost twice the volume infused. However, because of its lower molecular weight, it is more rapidly excreted than the other colloids. The gain in intravascular volume is roughly equal to the amount of dextran 40 infused within the first 3 or 4 hours of administration. Dextran 40 is more commonly used in cases of peripheral vascular disease and hyperviscosity syndromes. Dextran 70 is provided as a 6% solution and does not exert the hyperoncotic effect produced by dextran 40. The volume expansion is somewhat greater than the amount infused, but because of its larger molecular size, its volume-expanding effect may be maintained for 24 to 48 hours. The dextran preparations also cause decreased platelet adhesiveness and decreased factor VIII activity. They carry an incidence of allergic reaction of up to 5%, and of anaphylaxis of 0.6%.[58] In addition, because of the rheologic properties of dextran, blood incompatibility can be simulated, making identification of compatible blood more difficult.

Hydroxyethyl starch (hetastarch, Hespan) is an amylopectin. It exerts a volume-expanding effect similar to that of dextran 70. The duration of expansion is about 36 hours. Hetastarch is reported to have side effects similar to those of dextran, but to a lesser degree. The incidence of anaphylaxis is 0.006%. A new hydroxyethyl starch, pentastarch, has a lower molecular weight and fewer hydroxyethyl groups. Pentastarch has a shorter duration of action (2.5 hours) than hetastarch and has been reported to have less effect than other colloids on coagulation in burn resuscitation and in postoperative cardiac surgery patients.[59,60]

The controversy regarding use of crystalloids versus colloids in resuscitation has not been resolved. Both types of solutions can restore circulating volume. The effects of the solutions on pulmonary function are at issue and are summarized as follows: (1) The use of crystalloid solutions decreases plasma oncotic pressure, thereby leading to lung edema at lower microvascular pressures; and (2) colloids given in the face of pulmonary injury (contusion) can extravasate, promoting edema because of the reduced plasma interstitial oncotic gradient. Several studies have indicated an advantage to crystalloids in resuscitation. It has been demonstrated that saline and dextran are cleared from the alveolar space more rapidly than either starch or plasma.[61] In addition, a metaanalysis of colloid versus crystalloid resuscitation after hemorrhagic shock demonstrated a higher mortality rate among the colloid-resuscitated patients, partly because of pulmonary complications.[62]

Blood

Most patients with class I or II hemorrhage can be resuscitated with balanced salt solutions only. Patients who lose more than 25% to 30% of total blood volume need blood for resuscitation. Blood administered within 24 hours of its collection is probably ideal for resuscitation of trauma patients. The availability of whole blood, however, has progressively decreased with the increasing separation of donated blood into components such as packed red blood cells (RBCs), plasma, and platelets. There remains some controversy about whether fresh whole blood therapy is superior to component therapy in the treatment of hemorrhage and resuscitation-induced coagulopathy. The failure of component therapy to resolve nonsurgical bleeding in some trauma patients has led to recommendations that whole blood be used more often,[63] but there is no scientific evidence to indicate that whole blood has additional benefits.

The decision about the composition of blood to be transfused is determined in part by the urgency of the situation. Blood that has been fully typed and crossmatched carries the least risk of transfusion reactions, but it also takes the most time to obtain (usually 45 minutes or longer). Other transfusion options include the use of type O, Rh-negative or type-specific blood (Table 11-8).

Type O, Rh-Negative Blood

Type O, Rh-negative (universal donor) blood is immediately available without a crossmatch. Because type O blood contains no AB cellular antigens, administration of packed RBCs is relatively safe for patients of any blood type, with little risk of hemolytic reaction. The administration of more than 4 units of type O, Rh-negative blood to a non-O blood type patient, however, can theoretically result in an admixture of blood type. Rarely, administration of a high-titered anti-A or anti-B unit of type O blood to a non-O blood type patient results in a positive direct Coombs test or, even more rarely, a hemolytic reaction.

A pretransfusion blood specimen should be sent to the blood bank on admission of the patient, and type-specific blood should be transfused as soon as it is available. Previous concerns that administration of type O blood to patients with non-O blood types would lead to hemolytic reactions after the transfusion is changed to appropriate type-specific blood are probably unwarranted.

Type-Specific Blood

Type-specific blood is available from most blood banks within 5 to 10 minutes of receipt of the blood specimen, while the patient is being resuscitated with balanced salt solutions. Although not crossmatched, this blood can be administered safely, as demonstrated in both military[64] and civilian[65] experiences. The rapid availability and safety of type-specific blood makes it the blood of choice for resuscitation in trauma.

Autotransfusion

Autotransfusion involves collection of the shed blood and its reinfusion through a filter back into the patient. Autotransfusion can be as simple as aspiration of the blood into a citrate-containing collection chamber, followed by reinfusion through a 40-μm filter. A more elaborate system, the Haemonetics autotransfuser, centrifuges the collected blood and delivers washed, packed RBCs for reinfusion. The advantages of autotransfusion include transfusion with warm, compatible blood without delays and with no risk of transmission of hepatitis, human immunodeficiency virus, or other blood-borne pathogens.

Autotransfused blood can produce disseminated intravascular coagulation and activation of fibrinolysis. In addition, collection of blood from the peritoneal cavity after hollow viscous injury, even with cell washing, can lead to bacterial contamination of the autotransfused blood.[66] Successful autotransfusion of contaminated blood has been demonstrated,[67] but blood obtained from enteric-contaminated cavities should probably not be used until its safety is better determined. Inadequate scavenging of shed blood has been a problem because suction power is limited to 30 to 60 mmHg to avoid hemolysis. It appears, however, that this level could be increased to 100 mmHg with little effect on hemolysis and some improvement in blood scavenging.[68] Despite that improvement, investigators have found that the autotransfuser was used in only 22% of the trauma patients for whom it was prepared. The precise role of autotransfusion in trauma is not well defined, but, with increasing concerns about homologous blood transfusion, its use is likely to increase.

Experimental Resuscitation Fluids

Hypertonic Saline

Hypertonic saline solutions have been used in resuscitation of patients after burn shock, elective vascular surgery, and trauma. The exact mechanisms of hypertonic resuscitation have not been elucidated, but the expansion of plasma volume is caused by an osmotically induced shift of intracellular fluid into the intravascular compartment. In addition to expanding volume, hypertonic saline solutions have been shown to increase left ventricular performance,[69] decrease peripheral resistance from arteriolar di-

Table 11-8. TRANSFUSION OPTIONS: COMPARISON OF BLOOD AVAILABILITY

	Typing	Antibody Screen	Cross-match	Time
Type O negative	No	No	No	Immediately
Type specific	Yes	No	No	5 min
Type and screen	Yes	Yes	No	10 min
Type and crossmatch	Yes	Yes	Yes	45 min

lation,[70] and redistribute cardiac output to the kidneys and viscera.[70,71]

The optimal osmolarity of hypertonic saline solutions for resuscitation from hypovolemia has not been determined. Solutions in the range of 3600 to 4800 mOsm are associated with frequent seizure activity. Investigations with 2400-mOsm saline solutions administered in boluses of 4 mL/kg[72] have shown that this concentration rapidly restores blood pressure to baseline levels after hemorrhagic loss of 40% to 50% of blood volume. However, the response to bolus administration was not sustained. The addition of colloid to the hypertonic saline solution led to sustained increases in arterial pressure, cardiac output, and measured plasma volumes, with the colloid acting to hold the water drawn into the intravascular space by the hypertonic saline solution. Other reports[73] have described more effective volume replacement with smaller-volume infusions of 500-mOsm solutions than with lactated Ringer solution and suggest a mortality advantage in head-injured patients.[74]

Studies of hypertonic saline resuscitation in models of uncontrolled hemorrhage,[75] have demonstrated increased hemorrhage and increased mortality after administration of hypertonic saline solutions, compared with resuscitation with normal saline solution. The increased hemorrhage is thought to be caused in part by the peripheral vasodilatation produced by administration of hypertonic saline solutions. The optimal concentrations of saline and optimal combinations of components for these solutions have not been determined.

Stroma-Free Hemoglobin

After removal from an erythrocyte, hemoglobin retains its oxygen-carrying capacity. Hemoglobin solutions prepared from lysis of RBCs have been shown to be effective oxygen-carrying resuscitative fluids in animal models.[76] The side effects from the use of hemolyzed blood (eg, renal dysfunction, coagulopathy) are caused by stromal elements of the erythrocyte. Removal of these stromal elements by lysis decreases the incidence of such problems. Other problems with stroma-free hemoglobin as a blood substitute include a short half-life and a marked affinity for the oxygen molecule, becoming half-saturated at a P_{O_2} of 14 mmHg instead of the normal 27 mmHg.

An increased intravascular residence time of 140 minutes and a half-saturation pressure of 24 mmHg have been demonstrated in vivo with pyridoxylation of stroma-free hemoglobin.[76] Stroma-free hemoglobin can be given in concentrations of up to 7 g/dL without exceeding normal plasma oncotic pressure. The potential for significant fluid overload exists with the administration of large volumes of this substance.[77] Clinical trials are now underway.

Encapsulated Hemoglobin

Another blood substitute has been developed by using high-pressure extrusion and homogenization to produce liposomes with hemoglobin molecules in the center. These synthetic erythrocytes have more than half the oxygen-carrying capacity of RBCs and can be augmented to an affinity almost identical to that of whole blood by coencapsulation of pyridoxal-5-phosphate. The circulation half-life with various cofactors can be as long as 16 to 20 hours. Liposome-encapsulated hemoglobin has additional advantages in that it has no blood type, is virus-free, and can be manufactured in large volumes. Methods have been developed for rapid production of liters of liposome-encapsulated hemoglobin solution with a hemoglobin content of 16 g/dL.[78] Disaccharides can be incorporated into the liposomes; they stabilize the compound so that it can be frozen and dehydrated for long-term storage.

In rat studies, the injection of liposome-encapsulated hemoglobin caused a decrease in platelets to 40% of baseline and an increase in plasma levels of thromboxane B_2.[79] The primary sites of removal of liposome-encapsulated hemoglobin molecules are the liver and the reticuloendothelial system. The effects of liposome-encapsulated hemoglobin on the immune system, as well as the long-term side effects and toxicity, are unknown.

Liposome-encapsulated hemoglobin remains a promising area of investigation for artificial blood and RBC substitution. Liposome-encapsulated hemoglobin can also be combined with hypertonic saline; experimental data show improved blood pressure and survival and reduced acidosis versus with this combination, compared with lactated Ringer solution or hypertonic saline alone.[80] Further investigations of the possible side effects of liposome-encapsulated hemoglobin compounds on the immune system are needed before the true potential of this blood substitute can be assessed.

Perfluorocarbons

Perfluorocarbons are large, branched or cyclic aliphatic compounds in which carbon–hydrogen bonds have been replaced with carbon–fluorine bonds. These compounds have the ability to dissolve and carry oxygen. The most common of these substances is Fluosol DA 20%, a combination of perfluorocarbon compounds with stabilizing emulsifiers, hetastarch, and a buffered salt solution.[81] In experimental trials with canine and rat models, Fluosol DA 20% was effective in restoring plasma volume, oxygen delivery, and oxygen consumption.[82–84] Fluosol DA 20% is effective in volume restitution, with improved oxygen delivery and oxygen-carrying capacity in elective neurosurgery patients and in patients undergoing gastrectomy.[85]

Perfluorocarbon infusion, however, has been shown to depress platelet counts, plasma immune globulin levels, immunoglobulin G, and fibrinogen.[84] Other investigations have reported depressed immune function after perfluorocarbon resuscitation from hemorrhage, as demonstrated by decreased ability to respond to pneumococcal infection[86] and decreased survival rate after a standard intraabdominal polymicrobial infection.[87] Perfluorocarbons are expensive, and although they are capable of increasing oxygen delivery, the associated immune system depression is a marked disadvantage for the use of these substances in the resuscitation of trauma patients. Newer formulations offer potential for the future.

COMPLICATIONS OF SHOCK

Hemorrhagic shock can lead to a cascade of related complications, each requiring its own intervention if the clinician is to achieve the goal of resuscitating the patient from the shock state. The most commonly encountered of these complications are metabolic acidosis, hypothermia, and coagulopathy.

Metabolic Acidosis

The acidosis of hemorrhagic shock results from tissue hypoperfusion, anaerobic metabolism, and lactate accumulation. The treatment for acidosis from shock is restoration of adequate tissue perfusion. Acidosis can lead to cardiac compromise, however, and some therapeutic drugs (eg, lidocaine) are inactive if the pH is less than 7.2. Severe acidosis therefore should be treated with judicious administration of bicarbonate, with frequent monitoring of the pH and base deficit by arterial blood gases, to achieve a pH of 7.2 or higher. Overadministration of bicarbonate should be avoided because it shifts the oxyhemoglobin dissociation curve to the left, resulting in greater oxygen affinity for the hemoglobin molecule and less oxygen release into the tissues.

Hypothermia

Hypothermia (core temperature below 35°C) is common after severe injury. Heat loss is increased in the trauma patient. In addition to immobilization, both prehospital and postadmission exposure can lead to conductive, convective, and evaporative heat loss. The administration of room-temperature intravenous fluids and of cold, stored blood also contributes to hypothermia.

As the core temperature decreases, the rate of oxygen consumption also decreases, to about 50% at 28°C. The decrease in oxygen consumption is accompanied by increased production of acid metabolites. A leftward shift in the oxyhemoglobin dissociation curve also occurs with hypothermia but is partially compensated by the acidosis. Central nervous system effects progress from confusion and loss of manual dexterity to obtusion and frank coma as the core temperature decreases from 35° to 26.5°C. The heart rate decreases to about half of baseline at 28°C, with concomitant decrease in cardiac output. All cardiac electrical conduction intervals are prolonged, consistent with the changes in heart rate, and both atrioventricular dissociation and refractory ventricular fibrillation occur at 28°C. Other physiologic effects include ileus and pancreatitis (from cold enzyme activation) at temperatures lower than 35°C.

Compensatory responses to hypothermia include increased excretion of catecholamines, with potential doubling of the basal metabolic rate, and increased production of thyroid hormones, with potential increases in the basal metabolic rate to five times baseline. Shivering can increase heat production as well, but it represents a significant energy expenditure. Compensatory responses to hypothermia are lost at temperatures below 30° or 31°C, and a state of complete poikilothermy is reached.

The treatment for hypothermia is rewarming. The core temperature (rectal or bladder) should be obtained on admission of the trauma patient. Patients whose core temperatures are 33° to 35°C can be treated with passive rewarming, warm blankets, and hot packs. Patients with core temperatures lower than 33°C require active rewarming. If the patient is unconscious, airway control should first be obtained. Because severe hypothermia causes vasoconstriction, noninvasive blood pressure measurements may not be feasible or accurate, and an arterial line should be placed for monitoring and blood gas sampling. The inspired gas through the ventilator should be heated to 43° or 44°C and fully saturated with water vapor to increase heat conductance into the capillary beds of the lung.

The intravenous fluids should also be warmed. Commercially available rapid infusion systems with heating elements are useful for this purpose. In patients in extremis, extracorporeal pump systems can be used for both circulatory support and rewarming. Other warming methods include nasogastric or peritoneal lavage with saline solution warmed to 40°C.

Coagulopathy

Coagulopathy is a frequent problem in the trauma patient who has received large volumes of crystalloid solution and blood for resuscitation. Although this problem is incompletely understood, it is clear that posttraumatic coagulation defects are multifactorial. The presence of shock, the fluid volume required for resuscitation, the presence of hypothermia, and preexisting diseases (eg, liver,

renal, or congenital coagulation disorders) all influence the likelihood and severity of coagulopathy.

The major factor in coagulopathy has been postulated to be the dilutional thrombocytopenia that occurs after massive volume resuscitation. Although bleeding times can be prolonged with platelet counts less than 100,000 cells/mL, platelet counts of 50,000 cells/mL or greater are usually adequate for surgical hemostasis. Dilutional thrombocytopenia becomes more likely with infusions of more than one blood volume. Each unit of platelets administered increases the platelet count by 10,000 to 15,000 cells/mL. Control of surgically remediable hemorrhage is prudent before platelet transfusion to prevent the loss of the transfused platelets into the surgical field.

Dilution of other coagulation factors also plays a role in development of coagulopathy. Factors V and VIII are the most labile in banked blood, but levels of less than 10% of normal for factors VII, X, XI, XII, and XIII are associated with abnormalities in hemostasis, as demonstrated by prolonged partial thromboplastin time and prothrombin time. Fresh frozen plasma can be administered as a source of all the soluble coagulation factors. The administration of cryoprecipitate may be necessary as a concentrated source of factor VIII and fibrinogen, particularly if adequate hemostasis is not obtained with the use of fresh frozen plasma.

Definitive Care Phase: Head Injuries
RANDALL M. CHESNUT

EPIDEMIOLOGY

Brain injury is the most common cause of death in trauma victims, accounting for about half of deaths at the accident site. The injuries are usually a result of blunt trauma, and motor vehicle accidents are the most frequent cause. Of particular significance are motorcycle accidents involving unhelmeted passengers, which produce severe injuries. Up to two thirds of all motor vehicle accident victims sustain some head injury. Complications from closed head injuries are the single largest cause of morbidity and mortality in patients who reach the hospital alive. Of patients who require long-term rehabilitation, head trauma is usually the primary injury. These data are generally applicable to children as well as adults. Although the mechanisms vary, head injuries are the major cause of morbidity and mortality in childhood trauma victims, accounting for an annual mortality rate of 1 per 1000 in this age group.

PATHOPHYSIOLOGY

Traumatic injury to the brain involves a primary brain injury that occurs at impact and leads to disruption of brain substance and blood vessels. In addition, secondary brain injury may result from hypoxia, hypotension, the effects of increased intracranial pressure (ICP), and altered cellular biochemical processes.

Primary Injury

Energy transfer to the head causes direct disruption of neurons, glial cells, and microvasculature localized at the area of impact. As the brain accelerates within the skull, it is also vulnerable to impact with the opposite inner table, and contrecoup injury to the opposite underlying brain is relatively common. Diffuse axonal injury from brain distortion can lead to damage and disruption of deep brain structures. The brain is also subject to torsion injury resulting from rotation around the fixed brain stem. This type of injury can damage the reticular activating system, leading to unconsciousness. Intracranial hemorrhage results from disruption of bridging subdural veins and bleeding from cortical tissue damage (subdural hematoma), direct laceration of epidural arteries from impact fractures (epidural hematoma), or intraparenchymal bleeding (intracerebral contusion and hematoma). Bleeding and brain laceration from penetrating injuries are caused by direct energy transfer. Whether direct impact causes contusion, subdural hematoma, epidural hematoma, or diffuse axonal injury, little can be done therapeutically to change the magnitude or location of the primary injury after it has occurred.

Secondary Injury

Secondary brain injuries result from events occurring after the primary insult, as a result of either the direct consequences of a process initiated by the primary injury or deleterious outside influences. The occurrence and magnitude of secondary insults are often the determining factors in outcome from brain injury. Because secondary insults, in contrast to primary injuries, are amenable to medical management, they are the focus toward which the medical treatment of brain injury is directed.

Primary tissue injury initiates a variety of biochemical processes, including free radical–mediated lipid peroxidation, excitotoxic superactivation of glutamate–aspartate neurotransmitter systems, alterations in membrane receptor and ionic channel characteristics, and other effects. These processes can proceed for significant periods of time after primary injury and often are self-sustaining. Numerous clinical trials have investigated treatment of brain trauma patients with various pharmacologic agents to determine means by which these processes can be attenuated or reversed.

The primary external secondary injury processes occurring after brain injury are hypotension and hypoxia. Hypotension is the primary treatable determinant of severe head injury. A single episode of systolic blood pressure less than 90 mmHg, if it occurs during the period from injury through resuscitation, doubles the mortality and significantly increases the morbidity of any given brain injury in adults.[88] Furthermore, an early hypotensive episode strongly increases the probability of later intracranial hypertension. Rapid and complete restoration of blood pressure is therefore the most important goal in the resuscitation of brain-injured patients. It is also for this reason that the somewhat unconventional suggestion of using pressors as temporizing agents during volume resuscitation has been made.[88]

Hypoxia (apnea or cyanosis in the field or an arterial partial pressure of oxygen lower than 60 mmHg) is also an independent predictor of poor outcome. The frequency and magnitude of hypoxia have been notably decreased by modern airway management techniques, particularly by early endotracheal intubation and assisted ventilation.

Intracranial Pressure

ICP results from the aggregate volumes of brain, cerebrospinal fluid (CSF), and blood within the fixed intracranial compartment. Mild or slow expansion of one or two of these compartments can be buffered by compensatory decreases in the CSF or blood compartments (into the spinal subarachnoid space or the venous sinuses, respectively). If this buffering capacity is exceeded, the compliance of the brain is compromised, and small additional increases in intracranial volume produce marked elevations in ICP.

Intracranial hypertension causes harm by two somewhat separate mechanisms—herniation and ischemia. Herniation occurs when a pressure gradient exists across an incomplete barrier such as the tentorium or the falx cerebri. It is deleterious because of the tissue damage that results when herniation occurs. Transtentorial herniation, the most common form, is manifested by anisocoria, motor posturing, autonomic disturbances, and death. The possibility of herniation is the major determinant of the absolute threshold of ICP management, which is usually accepted as 20 to 25 mmHg, although this range has not been well determined empirically.

The second aspect of intracranial hypertension that is deleterious is elevated resistance to cerebral blood flow (CBF), which can cause or exacerbate ischemia. This resistance can be roughly approximated by cerebral perfusion pressure (CPP), which is defined as the difference between arterial blood pressure and ICP:

$$CPP = \text{mean arterial pressure} - ICP$$

Under normal circumstances, cerebral pressure autoregulation maintains stable CBF over a wide range of CPP (about 50 to 150 mmHg) (Fig. 11-8). After injury to the brain, this autoregulation is usually disrupted. The disruption can be complete, resulting in a pressure-passive system (*straight dashed line B* in Fig. 11-8). More frequently, the disruption is incomplete, characterized by a normal sigmoid shape but with abnormal elevation of the lower breakpoint above the normal value of 50 mmHg (*sigmoid dashed line*). The consequence of this disruption is that a CPP that is satisfactory for uninjured patients may be insufficient in patients with head trauma (range of hypoperfusion). In a pressure-passive system, cerebral blood volume (CBV) increases in proportion to CPP. In such an instance, the goal is to keep the CPP just above the level of cerebral ischemia. In the situation of incomplete disruption, the goal is to keep CPP within the range of autoregulation, because this not only avoids ischemia but also can decrease ICP if autoregulatory vasoconstriction in response to increased CPP decreases intracranial blood volume.

Confounding this situation is the recent information that CBF can be significantly depressed during the early postinjury period.[88a] Therefore, it is particularly critical that CPP be supported assiduously from the first point of patient contact. Because hyperventilation causes vasoconstriction, thereby decreasing CBF, the use of hyperventilation during this early period is somewhat more hazardous than after the first 24 to 48 hours.

In any instance, the goal is to maintain a CPP that meets the metabolic demands of the cells. Because metabolic information is often not readily available at the bedside, we must accept a reasonable estimate of an acceptable CPP, which for adult patients is usually thought to be 70 mmHg. If monitoring of jugular venous saturation and cerebral oxygen extraction are available, they can be useful in guiding CPP management in a more specific fashion.

Treatment of hypertension is rarely indicated in head-injured patients. There is no evidence that hypertension promotes continued intracranial hemorrhage, and hypertension related to brain injury usually resolves after the intracranial hypertension is controlled. If profound hypertension requires treatment, short-acting, selective β-blockers should be used. Vasodilators such as sodium nitroprusside should be avoided because they increase CBV.

Metabolic autoregulation is the other and somewhat

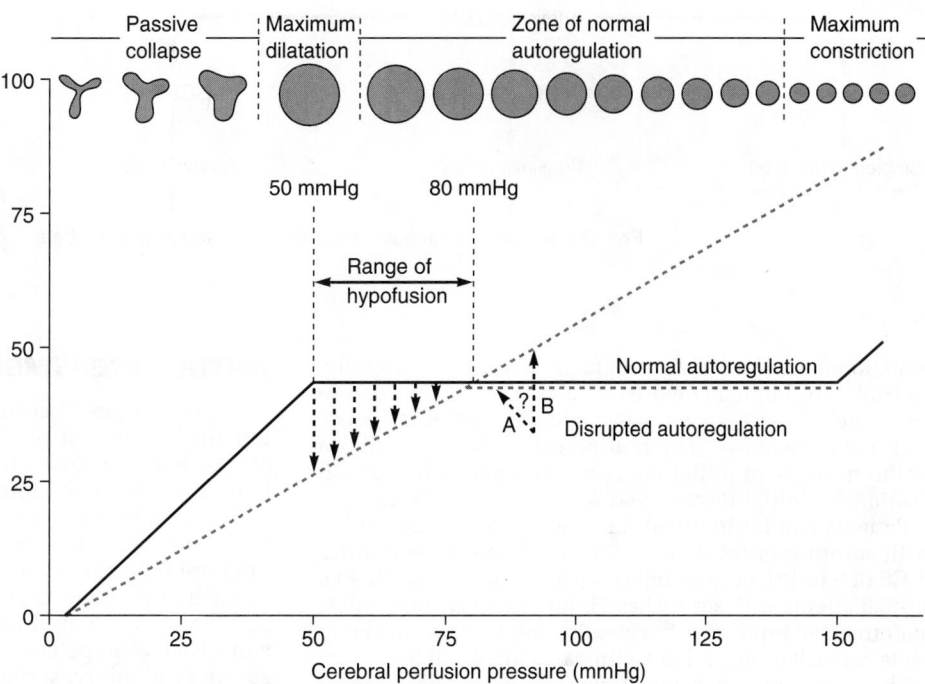

Passive collapse   Maximum dilatation   Zone of normal autoregulation   Maximum constriction

50 mmHg   80 mmHg

Range of hypofusion

Normal autoregulation

Disrupted autoregulation

A   ?   B

Cerebral perfusion pressure (mmHg)

Figure 11-8. Cerebral pressure autoregulation. The normal relation is indicated by the solid line with autoregulatory breakpoints at 50 and 150 mmHg. Two disrupted states are also diagrammed. Complete loss of autoregulation (*line B*) results in a pressure-passive system wherein cerebral blood flow (depicted on vertical axis in milliliters per 100 grams per minute) and cerebral blood volume increase linearly with cerebral perfusion pressure. With the more common case of incomplete disruption, a right shift in the lower breakpoint occurs. A shift in this relation to the right by 30 mmHg would represent the partially disrupted state. The circles at the top of the figure represent the diameters of the resistance vessels in the normal situation. The areas of the circles represent the cerebral blood volume.

more fundamental type of intrinsic CBF control. Vasoconstriction is nonlinearly proportional to pH and, therefore, is subject to manipulation of the arterial partial pressure of carbon dioxide ($PaCO_2$). As a result, hyperventilation-induced alkalosis produces vasoconstriction, resulting in a decrease of both CBF and CBV. Although the latter is beneficial in controlling ICP, the former is potentially deleterious and mandates caution when using hyperventilation.

Metabolic autoregulation is more robust than pressure autoregulation with respect to trauma. Also, metabolic autoregulation is the most fundamental physiologic safeguard against ischemia. Therefore, hyperventilation must be used with caution if ischemia is suspected.

Cerebral Edema and Osmolar Therapy (Mannitol)

Cerebral edema during the early postinjury period is generally cytotoxic (intracellular). Later, vasogenic (extracellular) edema may play a role in brain swelling. Although cerebral edema therefore results from two different mechanisms (cellular membrane dysfunction and breakdown of the blood–brain barrier, respectively), present treatment is limited to the administration of osmotic agents, most commonly mannitol. Mannitol increases the osmotic gradient, drawing fluid from the interstitial compartment into plasma and thereby reducing brain volume. In regions where the blood–brain barrier has been disrupted, however, mannitol is minimally effective and can actually leak into tissues.[89] Fortunately, the area of blood–brain barrier breakdown is usually much smaller than the area of edema that it creates, and mannitol is usually quite effective in lowering ICP.

Mannitol can produce significant diuresis. The resulting hypovolemia can cause hypotension, not only producing secondary insult to the brain but also causing intracranial hypertension because of autoregulatory vasodilatation. Therefore, mannitol should be avoided under conditions of hypovolemia, and fluid losses should be diligently re-

placed. Because small doses of mannitol (0.25 g/kg) are equally efficacious as large doses (1 g/kg) in lowering ICP, the smaller doses should be used.

CLINICAL ASSESSMENT

The objectives during early clinical assessment of the head-injured trauma patient are multiple and must be accomplished simultaneously. The establishment of adequate oxygenation, ventilation, and circulatory stability and the evaluation of the extent of brain injury must parallel avoidance of ICP elevation. Systemic hypotension is not often the result of a head injury; rather, one must initially presume that hypotension in a trauma patient is the result of hypovolemia. It is a significant error to withhold volume resuscitation in a misdirected effort to control cerebral edema. During initial assessment, mental status changes cannot be presumed to be the result of drugs or alcohol, although routine toxicology screening is appropriate. Any change in mental status or in the neurologic examination in general, or any evidence of herniation (eg, anisocoria), suggests an expanding intracranial mass lesion. Under such circumstances, therapeutic ICP reduction becomes the first priority, and emergency imaging or surgical decompression must be accomplished immediately.

Noxious stimuli such as placement of a urinary catheter, nasogastric tube, or vascular cannula, can precipitate ICP peaks during resuscitation. These procedures should therefore be done quickly and efficiently, preferably after sedation.

With regard to the brain injury, several critical assessments are necessary and should be recorded precisely because temporal change is at least as important as any single observation. The three key parameters are level of consciousness, pupillary reflexes and size, and the motor examination.

Glasgow Coma Scale

The single most important assessment for a head-injured patient is to evaluate the level of consciousness. In this regard, the Glasgow Coma Scale (GCS) has become an in-

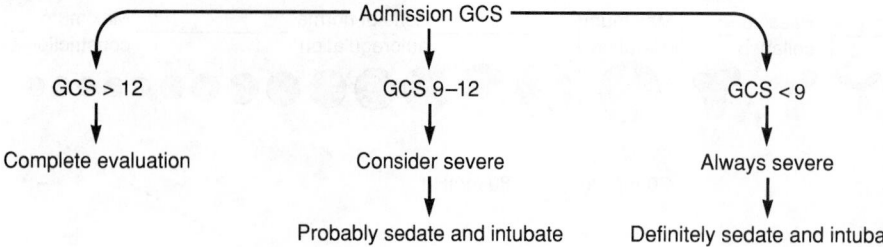

Figure 11-9. Glasgow Coma Scale (GCS) triage guide for initial evaluation of head injury.

ternational standard of measurement that is easily, rapidly, and reliably implemented (see Table 11-6). GCS components include assessment of eye opening, verbal response, and motor response. The routine use of GCS provides a useful measure of initial injury severity and allows stratification for initial therapy and for outcome analysis.

Patients can be stratified for triage purposes into those with severe injuries (GCS of 8 or less), moderate injuries (GCS of 9 to 12), or mild injuries (GCS greater than 12; Fig. 11-9). Patients with severe head injuries require immediate endotracheal intubation, mechanical ventilation, and complete resuscitation, and any clinical evidence of intracranial hypertension (eg, signs of herniation) mandates maximal therapy to decrease ICP. Many significant injuries carry GCS scores between 9 and 12. Although this is defined as the moderate injury group, all of these patients require maximal brain resuscitation until a definitive diagnosis can be made. A patient with a GCS of 12 or more tends to be confused but responsive to verbal stimulation. These patients need serial neurologic evaluations; this is the group that can "talk and die" because of missed or delayed intracranial pathology. In general, however, attention to other major injuries can take priority to cerebral imaging or management.

Pupils

Pupillary asymmetry, dilation, or loss of light reflex in an unconscious patient usually reflects herniation caused by mass effect from intracranial hemorrhage ipsilateral to the dilated pupil. The probability of an intracranial mass lesion can be roughly approximated given the degree of anisocoria (greater than 1 mm, greater than 3 mm), the mechanism of injury (motor vehicle accident or not), and the age of the patient[90] (Fig. 11-10). Occasionally, pupillary signs indicate direct injury to the second or third cranial nerve or trauma to the globe, but this is rare with blunt injuries. An unequal and nonreactive pupil is the cardinal sign that herniation is occurring and rapid lowering of ICP is essential. An ovoid pupil is also ominous and is associated with injuries that result in herniation in about 15% to 20% of patients.

Motor Examination

The motor system is examined for asymmetry, abnormal posturing, and lack of movement. Hemiparesis, paraparesis, or quadraparesis suggests a cervical or thoracolumbar spine fracture with spinal cord injury. Hemiparesis secondary to brain-stem herniation may occur either ipsilateral or contralateral to the side of the dilated pupil. Hemiparesis can also result from significant brain contusion. In the unconscious patient, a painful stimulus should be used to evaluate motor function. All four extremities should be examined and the results noted; only the response of the best limb is reflected in the GCS score.

INITIAL TREATMENT

Although there is currently no means to quantify it before the insertion of an ICP monitoring device, early intracranial hypertension can certainly exert a detrimental influence on outcome. However, all treatment modalities for intracranial hypertension have serious potential complications, and many of them (eg, use of diuretics) can directly interfere with resuscitation procedures. Because of its efficacy in improving the likelihood of survival after trauma and the acknowledged negative influence of secondary insults, such as hypotension and hypoxia, on outcome from severe head injury, systemic resuscitation provides a vital infrastructure on which treatment of intracranial hypertension must be based. In the absence of obvious evidence of raised ICP, any presumptive treatment must be consistent with optimal systemic resuscitation. Alternatively, signs of transtentorial herniation should be interpreted as definitive evidence of intracranial hypertension and must prompt rapid and definitive treatment specifically focused toward lowering ICP. In such circumstances, the balance of cerebral and general, systemic priorities must be reassessed.

The composition and volume of the intravenous fluids used to resuscitate patients with head injuries should be selected with the purpose of restoring intravascular blood volume. Usually, isotonic crystalloid solution in the form of lactated Ringer solution is chosen. Hypertonic saline solutions may have a role because they restore circulating blood volume, in part by inducing a fluid shift from the

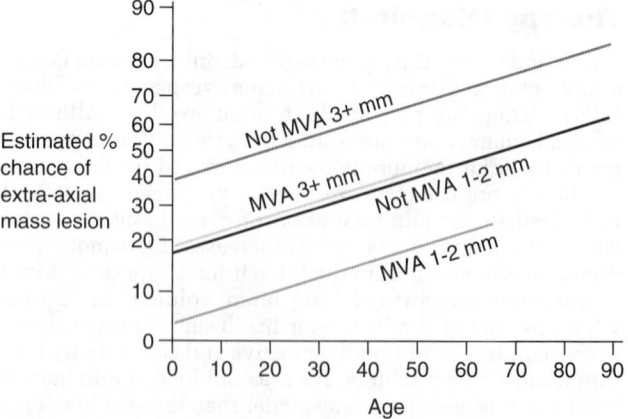

Figure 11-10. Estimated probability of an extraaxial intracranial mass lesion larger than 25 cc as a function of degree of anisocoria (in millimeters), age, and mechanism of injury. Mechanism of injury was defined as motor vehicle accident (MVA) or other mechanism (Not MVA). (Chesnut RM, Gautille TA, Blunt BA, et al. The localizing value of pupillary size asymmetry in severe head injury: relation to lesion type and location. Neurosurgery 1994;34:1)

intracellular compartment, and this can decrease ICP.[91] The endpoint of resuscitation does not depend on the presence or absence of a head injury. Blood volume should be normal, with an appropriate blood pressure and CVP, adequate urine output and peripheral perfusion, and progressive improvement of any base deficit. The systolic blood pressure should never be allowed to drop below 90 mmHg. In the absence of an ICP monitor, a mean blood pressure of 90 to 100 mmHg should be maintained. After ICP monitoring is available, a minimal CPP of 70 mmHg should be the goal.

Resuscitation in the Absence of Clinical Signs of Herniation

Elevation of the head of the bed (reverse Trendelenburg position in the absence of clearance of the axial skeleton) usually lowers the CPP in the absence of adequate volume resuscitation.[92] Because this can elevate the ICP per se, it is not advised until complete resuscitation has been accomplished. The confusion and agitation often attendant to head injury but can drive intracranial hypertension and render sedation desirable. Although patients with suspected head injury should usually be sedated, pharmacologic relaxation has the notable effects of limiting the neurologic examination to the pupils and the initial computed tomographic (CT) scan taken on arrival at the hospital. Therefore, its use in the absence of evidence of herniation should be limited to situations in which sedation alone is not sufficient to optimize safe and efficient patient transport and resuscitation. If it is used, short-acting agents are strongly preferred. The prophylactic administration of mannitol is not recommended because of its volume-depleting diuretic effect. In addition, although it is desirable to approximate the lower end of the normal range of $PaCO_2$ during transport of a patient with suspected brain injury, the risk of exacerbation of early ischemia by vigorous hyperventilation outweighs its questionable benefit for patients without evidence of herniation. Therefore, ventilatory parameters consistent with optimal oxygenation and normal ventilation are recommended. The tidal volume should be set at 15 mL/kg and the initial rate at about 10 respirations per minute. These settings should be adjusted to accomplish a $PaCO_2$ of 33 to 35 mmHg when arterial gas values are available.

Resuscitation in the Presence of Clinical Signs of Herniation

If there is evidence of transtentorial herniation (or progressive neurologic deterioration not attributable to extracranial explanations), aggressive treatment of suspected intracranial hypertension is indicated. Hyperventilation is easily accomplished by increasing the ventilatory rate, and it does not depend on or interfere with successful volume resuscitation. However, hyperventilation should be used with caution, because any resultant increase in mean intrathoracic pressure can interfere with cardiac preload, particularly in the setting of hypovolemia.

Because hypotension can produce both neurologic deterioration and intracranial hypertension, the use of mannitol is not desirable unless adequate volume resuscitation has been accomplished. If resuscitation is adequate, mannitol should be administered by bolus infusion. Under such circumstances, the neurologic injury must be managed with the utmost haste.

Radiographic Priorities

Neurosurgical evaluation and assessment is initiated as soon as the potential for significant head injury is realized. Prompt radiographic evaluation is essential, and CT is the imaging modality of choice for almost all acute neurologic conditions. Patients with mild head injuries usually can be observed with sequential examinations, and radiographic evaluation may be unnecessary unless the results determine whether or not the patient can be discharged from the hospital. Any evidence of neurologic deterioration or a situation in which the neurologic examination cannot be followed (eg, the need for general anesthesia) mandates CT scan or intraoperative ICP monitoring.

In general, indications for neurologic imaging (usually CT) include the following:

- Suspected skull penetration by a foreign body
- Discharge of CSF, blood, or both from the nose
- Hemotympanum or discharge of blood or CSF from the ear
- Protracted unconsciousness
- Altered state of consciousness at the time of examination
- Focal neurologic signs or symptoms
- Any situation precluding proper surveillance
- Head injury plus additional trauma
- Possible head injury in the presence of additional pathologic findings, such as stroke
- Head injury with alcohol intoxication

Patients with moderate or severe injuries require prompt neurosurgical consultation and rapid radiographic evaluation with CT. Hemodynamically stable patients with significant neurologic deterioration should go immediately for CT scanning. In hemodynamically unstable patients who require immediate surgical intervention to sustain intravascular volume, exploratory thoracotomy or laparotomy must take precedence, and measurement of ICP or air ventriculography can be performed concurrently to diagnose significant intracranial mass lesions.

The cervical spine should be cleared radiographically or immobilized and protected in every patient with a severe head injury. Although only 13% of patients with severe head injuries have spinal injuries, the potentially devastating consequences of an overlooked spine injury demand constant vigilance.

Plain Skull Radiographs

With the routine availability of CT, plain skull radiography has been criticized. Several authors have concluded that the presence of a fracture on a skull radiograph rarely influences treatment, does not reflect the severity of injury or predict outcome, and has seldom been a legal concern. On the other hand, the likelihood of a surgical intracranial hematoma is strongly correlated with the presence or absence of a skull fracture and the normalcy of the neurologic examination.[93] The utility of skull films in head injury remains controversial.

In general, any patient meeting one of the aforementioned criteria should undergo CT imaging. Skull radiographs should be reserved for the patient with a mild head injury who has a normal neurologic examination and for whom the results of the skull radiographic study will alter the care plan (eg, allow discharge from the hospital without a CT or determine the necessity for CT). If a CT is unavailable, a lateral displacement of the calcified pineal gland of greater than 2 mm on a skull radiograph suggests mass effect. However, if there is suspicion of intracranial pathology, more definitive diagnostic maneuvers are indicated.

Linear skull fractures appear as two radiolucent lines with sharp, well demarcated edges, typically coursing from the point of impact on the calvarium toward the base of the skull (Fig. 11-11). Depressed skull fractures are easily seen on plain frontal and lateral skull films. The mecha-

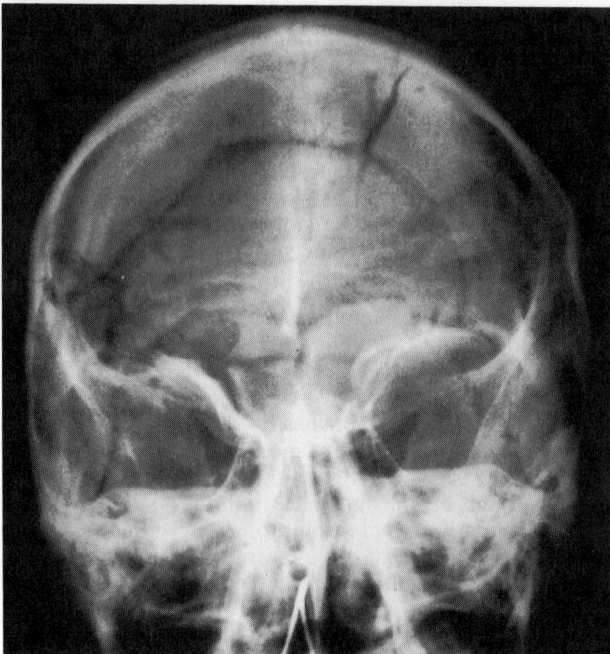

Figure 11-11. Large coronal bioccipital skull fracture.

nism of injury is usually a direct blow to the skull by a blunt object. Closed depressed skull fractures that are comminuted and those with a fragmented outer margin displaced beneath the inner table have usually been treated surgically, although there is growing evidence that many of these injuries can be treated nonoperatively if there is no neurologic dysfunction or CT evidence of underlying tissue injury. Open fractures are also usually treated surgically, but, again, there is growing evidence that fresh, noncomminuted fractures without neurologic deficit, CSF or brain extrusion, gross contamination, or underlying tissue injury can be closed and treated with prophylactic antibiotics.

Basilar skull fractures are usually diagnosed on clinical evidence because they are poorly visualized on plain films. Only about 20% of patients with clinical evidence of basilar skull fractures have discernible injury on plain skull radiographs. These clinical signs include otorrhea or rhinorrhea, subcutaneous ecchymoses overlying the mastoid region (Battle sign), bilateral periorbital ecchymoses (raccoon eyes), or hematotympanum. A basilar skull fracture can involve the paranasal sinuses, piriform sinus, petrous bone, sphenoid sinus, or sella turcica. Injury to adjacent structures, such as the seventh or eighth cranial nerve, brain stem, and carotid or basilar artery, are not uncommon. These fractures are usually visualized on CT scans, although special protocols may be required. In the acute situation, no specific therapy is indicated. A blood leak should not be tamponaded unless bleeding is brisk, and antibiotics should not be administered for the purpose of prophylaxis of meningitis.

Computed Tomography

The CT finding that correlates most significantly with intracranial hypertension is compression or obliteration of the basilar cisterns (Fig. 11-12). Not only does this finding portend a stormy ICP course, but the primary predictor of outcome in patients with this CT scan picture is the peak level of intracranial hypertension that occurs during the first 72 hours.[94,95] If cisternal compression is paired with a midline shift of more than 5 mm, the prognosis is even

more ominous. ICP monitoring should immediately be initiated in any patient with cisternal compression, and the intracranial hypertension should be vigorously treated. Such patients, particularly those with minimal evidence of contusions, die primarily from secondary insults; the implication is that they are potentially salvageable.

Acute epidural hematomas correlate well with skull fractures. The most common association is a linear, nondisplaced fracture in the temporoparietal region, crossing the middle meningeal artery. The classic clinical course involves a lucid interval after a brief loss of consciousness with subsequent neurologic deterioration. However, such a course occurs in less than half of patients with epidural hematoma cases, so clinical suspicion must remain high. The typical appearance on CT is a high- or mixed-density convex extraaxial hematoma with smooth borders (Fig. 11-13).

Acute subdural hematomas occur over the convexity of the brain. The hematoma can evolve as a result of rupture of bridging cortical veins or bleeding from the underlying parenchymal injury, which is common. It is this subjacent tissue damage that usually determines the neurologic outcome of patients not succumbing to intracranial hypertension. On CT, a subdural hematoma appears as an extraaxial, high- or mixed-density crescentic mass that spreads out over the hemisphere, following the cortical irregularities. The midline shift can be out of proportion to the size of the hematoma because of the contributing mass effect from a significant underlying brain contusion or brain swelling (Fig. 11-14).

Intracerebral hemorrhage and cerebral contusion are

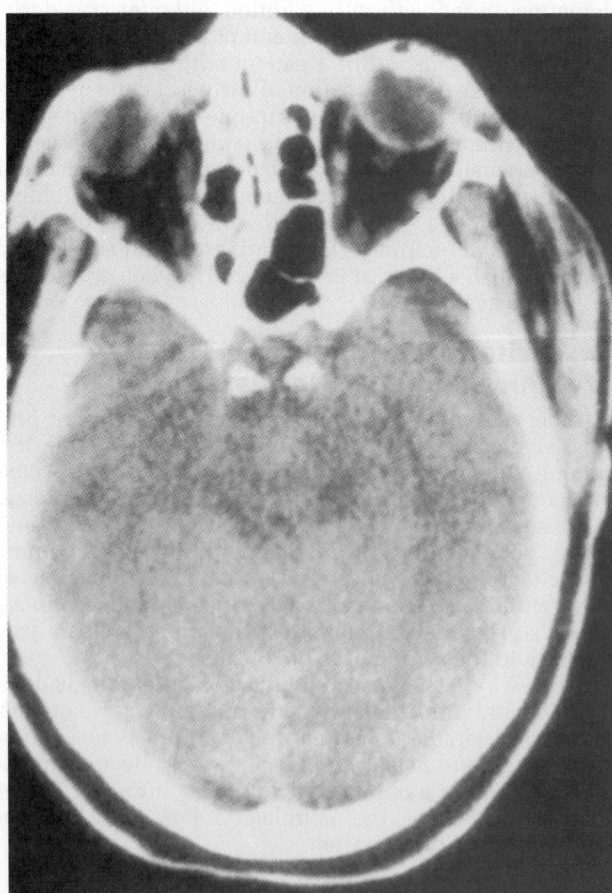

Figure 11-12. A CT scan that is highly predictive of intracranial hypertension. The basilar cisterns are obliterated, and the sulci are flattened.

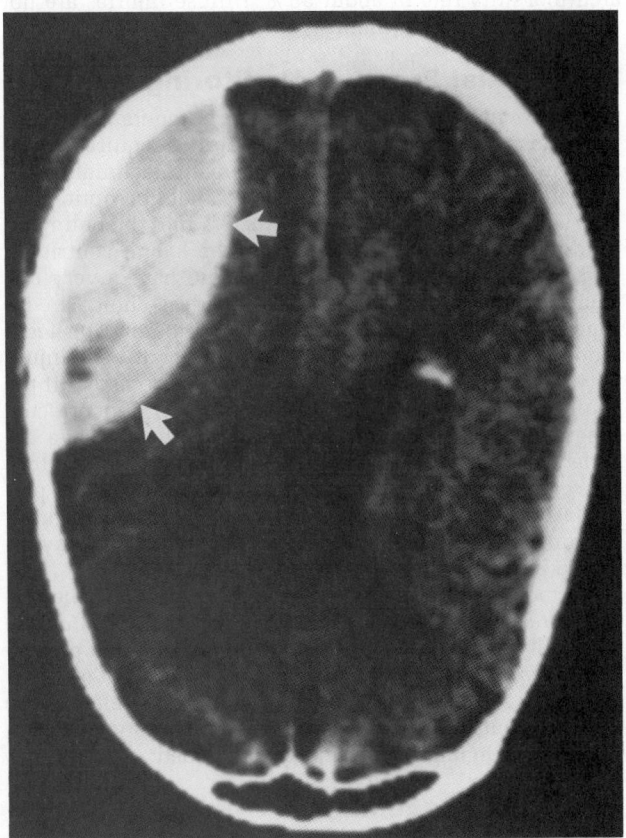

Figure 11-13. Typical CT scan appearance of mixed-density, lens-shaped, acute epidural hematoma with mass effect.

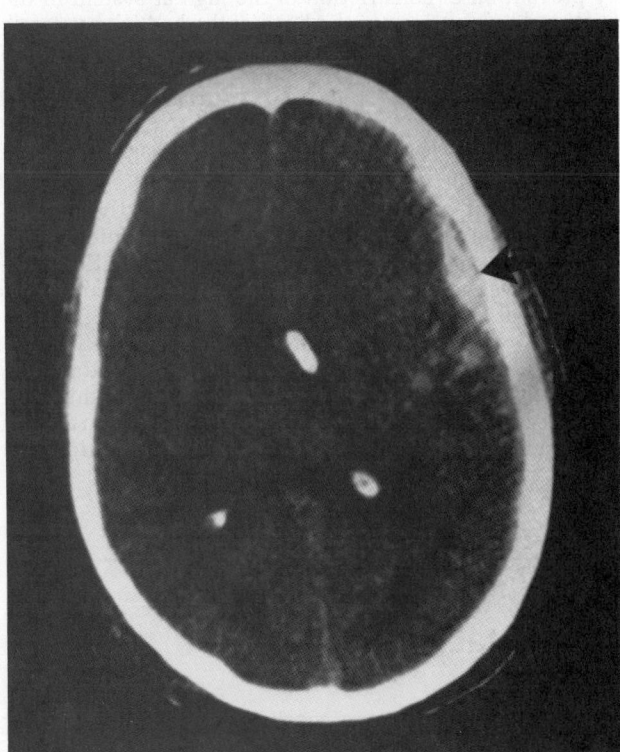

Figure 11-14. Usual CT scan appearance of a crescent-shaped, high-density blood collection conforming to the contour of the cerebral hemisphere in a subdural hematoma.

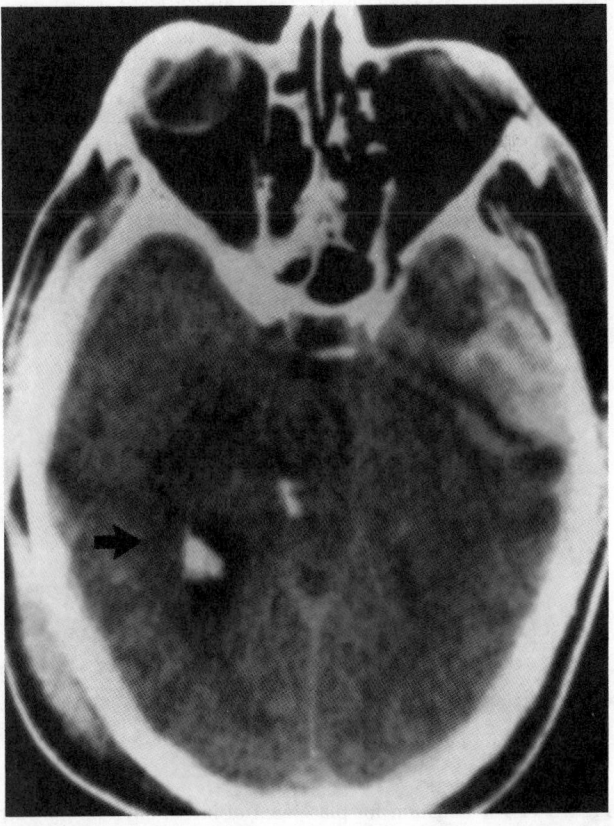

Figure 11-15. Contusion and associated intracerebral hematoma in the frontotemporal area.

common after trauma and are readily visualized on CT scans. Brain contusion appears as a focal, heterogeneous density with hemorrhage interspersed with injured tissue (Fig. 11-15). Intracerebral hematomas are usually more homogenous in their high-density appearance. These lesions tend to expand over time as the result of some continued hemorrhage and the development of edema. It is important to closely observe and monitor the ICP of patients with intracerebral hematomas, because significant and hazardous mass effect may evolve, requiring surgical extirpation.

The typical CT appearance of subarachnoid hemorrhage is a layer of blood over the cerebral cortex, layering over the tentorium, and, commonly, filling of the basal cisterns. Cerebral edema appears as areas of decreased density, which can be either focal or diffuse. Posttraumatic edema usually takes hours to days to develop unless it is compounded by hypoxia or hypotension. The swollen brain commonly seen in the setting of trauma may be caused by edema or by increased CBV (unclotted, intravascular blood has a low density). Diffuse axonal injury, typical of acute acceleration–deceleration injury, appears on CT scan as small areas of focal hemorrhage and cerebral swelling. Finally, gunshot wounds or other penetrating injuries can be evaluated with CT to allow accurate preoperative assessment of the anatomic injury for prognostic and therapeutic planning purposes.

DEFINITIVE MANAGEMENT
Surgical Decompression and Outcome

The objective of management for acute subdural or epidural hematomas is emergent surgical decompression. The timing of decompression is critical; a delay of more than

4 hours is associated with a poor outcome.[96] The possibility of a mass lesion must be entertained in any patient who develops evidence of herniation. Under optimal circumstances, this herniation can be reversed medically (with hyperventilation and mannitol), allowing emergency CT imaging, which demonstrates the location and size of any intracranial mass lesions and also identifies those patients who are herniating because of diffuse, nonsurgical processes.

If CT is not immediately available or herniation is refractory to medical management, emergency trephination is a useful and life-saving option. The first burr hole is placed in the ipsilateral temporal region, and the dura is opened if an epidural hematoma is not in evidence (Fig. 11-16). If this exploration is negative, the second hole is placed in the opposite temporal region. If this procedure is unrewarding, serial trephines are performed in the region of the parietal boss and the frontal convexity, first on the ipsilateral side and then contralaterally. A burr hole exploration is not considered to be negative until six holes have been drilled. A positive trephine is turned into a craniotomy, and the hematoma is thoroughly evacuated.

Epidural hematomas are frequently of arterial origin and have a tendency to expand. Prognosis varies directly with level of consciousness at time of surgery, with mortality rates that range from 0% for patients conscious throughout, to 27% with the classic lucid interval, to more than 50% if the patient never regains consciousness. Given these data, epidural hematomas should almost uniformly undergo immediate surgical evacuation. Such an approach has resulted in an overall mortality rate of about 9%.[97]

Subdural hematomas are more common, particularly in trauma not involving motor vehicles. For subdural hematomas, the prognosis is less optimistic, with mortality rates of about 50%. To a great extent, this is related to the often significant injury to the underlying brain. Cerebral contusions and intracerebral hematomas are treated operatively only if mass effect results in intracranial hypertension or signs of herniation. Diffuse brain injury has a mortality rate that is directly related to the significance of the associated intracranial hypertension. The mortality rate for patients with diffuse injury with open basilar cisterns is about 13%, whereas compression or absence of cisterns has an associated mortality rate of about 38%. Diffuse injuries are not amenable to surgical therapy.

Intracranial Pressure Monitoring

All patients with severe brain injuries and a significant percentage of those with moderate injuries require continuous monitoring of ICP. Although many techniques are available, the most common involve small fiberoptic pressure sensors placed several millimeters into the brain and fluid-coupled catheters placed into the lateral ventricles. The fiberoptic catheters are reliable and have a very low complication rate, making them an ideal choice in instances in which a minimum-risk ICP monitoring technique is desired (eg, in a patient with moderate head injury who needs general anesthesia). They are also useful if the ventricles are too small to cannulate or if an uncorrected coagulopathy exists. Ventriculostomy catheters have the added capability of allowing CSF drainage for ICP control. However, the complication rate is significantly higher, particularly for infection and hemorrhage. In any case, an appropriate monitoring technology is available for any instance in which ICP monitoring is desired.

ICP monitoring not only provides early warning of herniation but also, by allowing calculation of CPP, opens up the possibility of more precise optimization of CBF and prevention of secondary ischemic brain injury. Because all methods of lowering ICP have potentially harmful side effects, use of such agents to treat suspected intracranial hypertension without ICP monitoring is not recommended.

Medical Management

Aggressive restoration of intravascular volume, maintenance of adequate CPP, and avoidance of hypoxia are the mainstays of medical treatment for intracranial hypertension. In addition, it is necessary to control pain, response to noxious stimuli, seizures, and hypermetabolism. Egress of blood from the intracranial space should be facilitated by prevention of constriction of the jugular system in the neck and by elevation of the head of the bed in euvolemic patients. In addition, attention should be paid to intrathoracic pressures, particularly if the use of positive end-expiratory pressure or continuous positive airway pressure is being considered. Finally, meticulous general critical care is essential, because the rather protracted ICU stay and the necessity for intubation, mechanical ventilation, and other artificial support systems significantly increase the risk of nosocomial and iatrogenic complications.

CSF drainage, hyperventilation, mannitol, and barbiturates are the mainstays of therapy to control documented intracranial hypertension. However, each has significant potential complications that can obviate its beneficial effects and, therefore, caution and vigilance must attend the use of any of these treatments. Nevertheless, minimization of the secondary injuries that are often attendant on altered intracranial dynamics can offer profound contributions the patient's recovery from severe head injury.

Definitive Care Phase: Maxillofacial Injuries

LISA A. ORLOFF

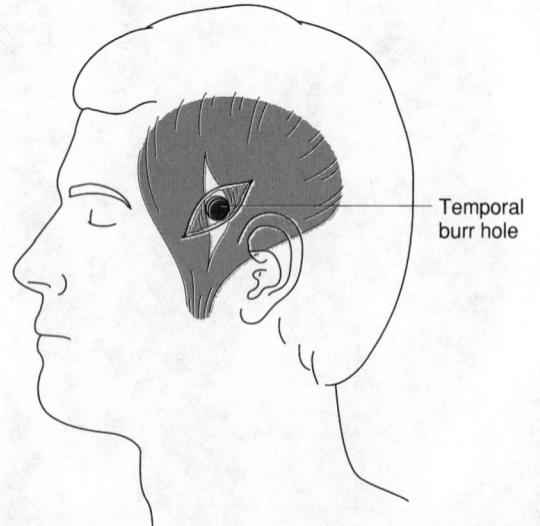

Figure 11-16. Location for placement of initial exploratory burr hole in the temporal region for emergency diagnosis and decompression.

Temporal burr hole

The major causes of maxillofacial trauma are motor vehicle accidents, direct assault, industrial injuries, sports-related injuries, and low- and high-velocity gunshot injuries. Maxillofacial injuries are present in one third of seriously injured patients with multisystem trauma,[98] and such injuries can be life-threatening. Airway compromise and hemorrhage are immediate concerns in patients with maxillofacial trauma; associated brain and cervical spine injuries must be sought and recognized, and appropriate timing of treatment must be coordinated with care of trunk and extremity injuries. An awareness of maxillofacial anatomy and dynamics is essential in order to effect survival from acute injuries and to restore normal form and function.

ANATOMY

Maxillofacial trauma constitutes most extracranial head injuries. Facial skeletal fractures and soft tissue damage in the frontal, orbital, nasal, zygomatic, maxillary, and mandibular regions are included. Ocular trauma, a specific form of maxillofacial injury that is the province of the ophthalmologic surgeon, is not discussed here.

The frontal bone, which houses the frontal sinuses, is particularly strong because of its arched configuration and its thick, hard bone. Up to 2200 lb of force is necessary to fracture the frontal sinus; this force is two to three times greater than that required to fracture other facial bones.[99] The frontal sinus is fully developed by about 19 years of age, but its size and degree of pneumatization are variable. The thick anterior wall makes up the central inferior portion of the forehead. The inferior wall or floor of the sinus is the roof of the orbit. The thin posterior wall abuts the frontal lobe of the brain. The frontonasal duct communicates with the nasal cavity.

The nasoethmoid complex, located at the junction of the frontal, nasal, lacrimal, and ethmoid bones and sinuses, is susceptible to compression and collapse during blunt facial trauma. The medial canthal tendons and the nasolacrimal drainage system are also vulnerable. Injury to these structures can result in telecanthus (widening of the intercanthal distance) and lacrimal dysfunction. Cerebrospinal fluid (CSF) rhinorrhea and anosmia secondary to cribriform plate or ethmoidal roof disruption with olfactory tract damage should be suspected.

The orbit is comprised of seven bones: frontal, zygoma, maxilla, lacrimal, ethmoid, sphenoid, and palatine. The four walls of the orbit form a pyramid, with its base anteriorly at the level of the eyelids and its apex posteriorly at the optic foramen. The lateral and superior walls are strong and are not easily fractured. On the other hand, the orbital floor (or roof of the maxillary sinus) and medial wall (mostly lamina papyracea) are thin and easily fractured. The orbital rims themselves are sturdy and protect the globe. Bony fragments of the orbit can impinge on the optic nerve or on the ophthalmic and retinal arteries and veins, especially at the orbital apex. Extraocular muscles, especially the inferior rectus, can become entrapped between bone fragments, limiting ocular movement.

The nasal bones are the most commonly fractured bones in the body. If injury to the nose is not detected and corrected, nasal obstruction and deformity can result. Traumatic epistaxis or nose bleeding can occur with blunt midface trauma with or without fracture of the nose. The thin, paired nasal bones project like a tent on the frontal process of the maxilla. The internal nasal septum provides tenuous support and is frequently injured.

The blood supply to the nose derives from the internal and external carotid arteries. The external carotid gives off the maxillary artery, whose sphenopalatine and descending pharyngeal branches supply the nose and ethmoid and maxillary sinuses, and the facial artery, whose superior labial branch supplies the anterior inferior nasal cavity.

The internal carotid artery gives off the ophthalmic artery, which in turn sends anterior and posterior ethmoidal arteries to the nose. The most common sites of epistaxis are along the anterior septum (the Kiesselbach or Little area) and behind the middle turbinate. However, any midface fractures and associated mucosal lacerations can present with epistaxis.

The zygoma is divided into the zygomatic arch and the malar bone. The zygoma articulates with the frontal, maxillary, temporal, and sphenoid bones. Predictable fracture patterns result from specific forces on the zygoma. Posterolateral blows cause zygomatic arch fractures. More anterior blows to the zygoma cause tripod (or trimalar) fractures, so called because of the three main fracture sites: the frontozygomatic suture line, the maxilla along the infraorbital rim, and the zygomatic arch.

The maxilla serves as a shock absorber for the skull and the cranial cavity. It is connected to the skull by the palatine bone, the zygoma, and the nasal processes. Consistent fracture patterns from blows to the maxilla, first classified by LeFort in 1901,[100] occur within and along the maxilla at its junction with the weaker and aerated bone of the paranasal sinuses and nasal cavity. Significant force is required to produce such fractures, and they are most often the result of motor vehicle accidents. With increased survival from automobile accidents, mainly as a result of increased seat belt use, has come an increased frequency of maxillofacial or LeFort fractures, perhaps because the upper torso and face are not completely restrained. The classic LeFort fractures are defined as follows (Fig. 11-17):

LeFort I: The fracture line runs along the floor of the maxillary sinus and posteriorly along the maxillary tubercle and into the pterygoid plates. A midpalatal split fracture, running anteroposteriorly, may be present.

LeFort II: Also called a pyramidal fracture, the apex of the fracture runs across the nasofrontal suture line; the fracture lines then run down the lamina papyracea of the ethmoid bone, across the orbital floor, and around the zygoma to the pterygoid plates.

LeFort III: Also known as craniofacial dysjunction, this fracture runs through all buttresses connecting the maxilla to the skull. Separation occurs across the root of the nose near the cribriform plate, across the frontoethmoidal suture and superior orbit to the region of the frontozygomatic suture, across the temporal fossa to the pterygomaxillary space, and usually across the

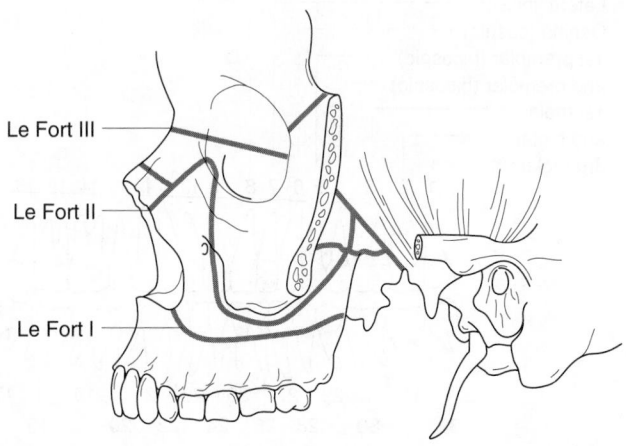

Figure 11-17. Le Fort classification system of maxillofacial fractures.

base of the pterygoid plates. The cribriform plate, ethmoidal arteries, optic nerve, and internal maxillary artery are all vulnerable in such fractures. The patient has a characteristic "mule" face, but initially this may not be obvious because of facial edema.

In practice, LeFort fractures are frequently asymmetric, mixed, or impure. For instance, there may be a "hemi-LeFort II" fracture, or a mixed LeFort I fracture on one side and a LeFort II fracture on the other side of the face.

The mandible is the second most frequently fractured facial bone, after the nasal bones. The configuration of an open arch, the position on the face, and the tendency to atrophy with age and the edentulous state make the mandible especially vulnerable to trauma. The most common cause of mandible fractures is interpersonal violence, especially among men. Mandible fractures are uncommon in children and are usually caused by child abuse or falls. Motor vehicle accidents account for most of the remaining mandible fractures. Sports injuries (even boxing) account for only 2% of mandible fractures.[101] The sites of fracture, in decreasing order of frequency, are the body, angle, condylar neck, symphysis and parasymphysis, ramus, and alveolar ridge. Multiple fractures occur in 53% of cases.[102] Although discussion of dental injuries is beyond the scope of this chapter, knowledge of dental anatomy is essential in the management of mandible injuries. The universal numbering system of permanent dentition (Fig. 11-18) and the Angle classification of occlusion (Fig. 11-19) facilitate description of injuries, planning of repair, and prediction of outcome.

Soft tissue injuries of the face are encountered even more often than facial fractures. Such injuries can be devastating, both functionally and cosmetically. Surgical management of soft tissue injuries requires attention to details of superficial anatomy in addition to awareness of subcutaneous structures.

The facial nerve is the most important underlying structure at risk, because blunt or penetrating trauma to the facial nerve trunk or branches can cause complete or partial ipsilateral facial paralysis. The most common cause of facial nerve injury is fracture of the temporal bone,[103] but injury can occur anywhere from the intracranial to the external facial course of the nerve. After exiting the stylomastoid foramen, the facial nerve trunk enters the parotid gland and divides into temporal, zygomatic, buccal, mar-

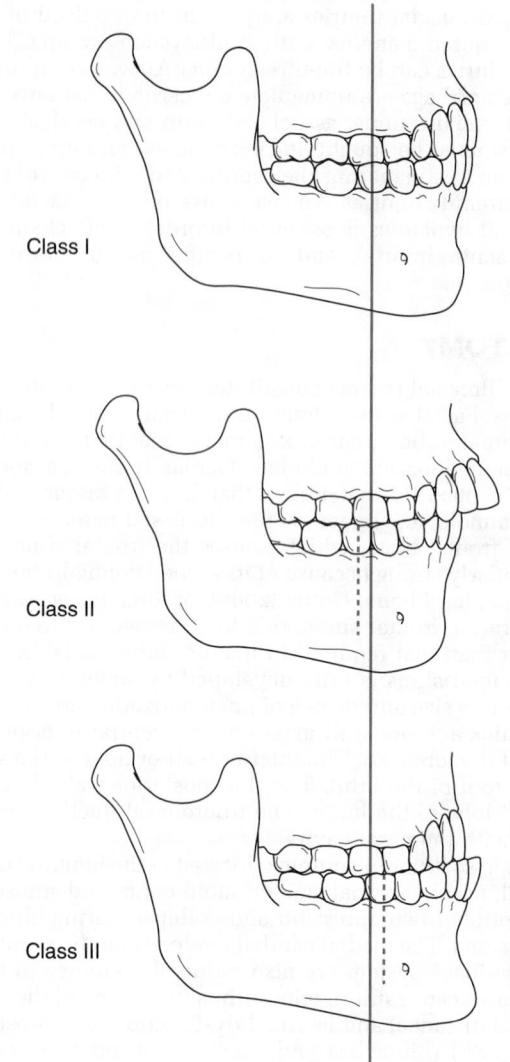

Figure 11-19. Angle classification of occlusion.

ginal mandibular, and cervical branches. Injuries to the middle branches distal to the parotid rarely result in significant deficit, but the temporal and marginal mandibular branches have the least cross-innervation with other branches, so they are vulnerable throughout their course.

In general, nonpenetrating trauma to the extracranial facial nerve is managed conservatively by expectant observation. Penetrating injuries are best repaired at the time of wound débridement and closure. If primary neurorrhaphy is not feasible, interposition grafts (usually from the greater auricular nerve or sural nerve) may be necessary.

EARLY CONSIDERATIONS

Initial priority in the patient with maxillofacial trauma, as in any trauma victim, must be directed at performing an efficient and orderly physical examination and stabilizing life-threatening problems. Because the airway is in the midst of the maxillofacial region, confirming and securing airway support may immediately lead to identification of maxillofacial injuries. Facial skeletal instability, soft tissue edema, and hemorrhage can hinder airway access. Teeth and blood may be aspirated, contributing to respiratory

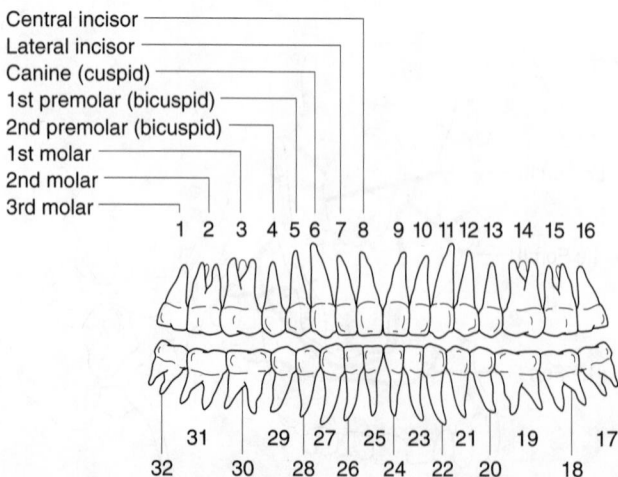

Figure 11-18. Universal numbering system of permanent dentition.

distress. If a patient cannot be safely intubated by either the orotracheal or the nasotracheal route, a tracheotomy or cricothyrotomy may be necessary. Although initial airway control should be obtained by the simplest and most direct route, management of midface and mandibular injuries may necessitate subsequent tracheotomy in the definitive phase of management.

Two to 4% of patients with maxillofacial injuries have concomitant cervical spine fractures.[104] Throughout the initial resuscitation and until proven otherwise, the patient with maxillofacial injuries should be treated as if the cervical spine is unstable. Any airway access maneuvers must be performed with attention toward maintaining in-line traction on the cervical spine.

Bleeding from facial injuries, especially in conjunction with blood loss from additional injuries, can be life-threatening and warrants immediate attention. Direct pressure can be applied to external sites of bleeding, but intranasal and pharyngeal hemorrhage are usually best treated initially by packing. However, packing of nasoethmoid or cribriform plate fractures can lead to direct intracranial injury. In this situation, a combined craniofacial approach to fracture reduction, dural repair, and control of epistaxis and rhinorrhea may be required.

Most nosebleeds come from anterior intranasal vessels. These can be controlled with anterior nasal packs consisting of 0.5- or 1-inch wide gauze impregnated with antibiotic ointment. In the conscious patient, the nasal mucosa is vasoconstricted and anesthetized topically with oxymetazoline (Neo-Synephrine) and tetracaine (Pontocaine) or 4% cocaine. Gauze is then layered into the nose, starting inferiorly along the floor and packing superiorly. The tail of gauze is brought out anteriorly to facilitate pack removal in 3 to 5 days. Various prefabricated nasal packs are often available in emergency departments.

Posterior nasal bleeding requires posterior packing for control. A no. 16 or 18 Foley catheter can be inserted through the nose into the nasopharynx; the balloon is then inflated with 10 to 15 mL of saline solution, and the catheter is pulled anteriorly against the vomer and sphenoid rostrum in the posterior naris. An anterior pack is then inserted to abut the Foley balloon. The catheter is secured anteriorly with a clamp, dental roll, or piece of plastic tubing, taking care to avoid pressure on the nasal ala or columella. The packs are removed in 3 to 5 days. Whenever a posterior pack is in place, the patient must be monitored for potential airway obstruction and hypoxemia.

Epistaxis that fails to respond to nasal packing requires more invasive management. Surgical ligation of the anterior and posterior ethmoidal arteries may be sufficient to control anterior bleeding. These vessels are approached through a standard external ethmoid incision between the medial canthus and the nasal root. If bleeding persists, a more posterior source should be suspected, and the internal maxillary artery is then ligated as well. This vessel is usually exposed through a transantral approach. The maxillary sinus is opened through a Caldwell-Luc (gingivobuccal sulcus) incision, and the posterior wall of the sinus is then opened to reach the pterygomaxillary space. In some cases of severely comminuted midface fractures, this approach is not feasible, and an intraoral approach is preferred.

An alternative but less specific means of controlling posterior epistaxis is by ligation of the external carotid artery. Because this vessel is somewhat removed from the actual site of bleeding, there is frequently collateral blood flow into the maxillary artery system distal to the point of ligation. Nevertheless, the external carotid artery can easily be accessed through the neck, even under local anesthesia. It is essential to identify at least two branches of the exter-

nal carotid artery before ligating it, in order to avoid accidental ligation of the internal carotid artery. Care must be taken to avoid injury to the vagus nerve, superior laryngeal nerve, hypoglossal nerve, sympathetic chain, and marginal mandibular nerve.

Patients with epistaxis and maxillofacial fractures who can be taken to surgery immediately and given a general anesthetic may have their bleeding controlled most effectively by fracture reduction. Early fracture treatment can obviate the need for formal nasal packing or vessel ligation.

Finally, a more recently developed technique is that of selective arterial catheterization and embolization for control of epistaxis. The bleeding sites are identified angiographically and then occluded with embolization materials (such as polyvinyl alcohol foam, polymerizing fluids, or even microballoons). This procedure is performed by interventional radiologists at specialized centers.[105]

Pharyngeal bleeding can occur as a result of mucosal laceration or penetrating injury to the internal carotid artery. Initial management after airway stabilization consists of packing the throat with layers of gauze wrap. The end of the gauze roll should be brought out through the mouth to facilitate pack retrieval after more definitive management is implemented.

EVALUATION

Physical Examination

After the airway has been secured and life-threatening hemorrhage controlled, the secondary survey can be performed. An efficient but systematic physical examination of the entire body should be carried out. The maxillofacial examination is part of the evaluation of the head and neck, including the neurologic system.

The scalp and face should be inspected for any lacerations or bruises. All loose soft tissue and bone fragments should be saved.

The eyes are checked for pupil size and reactivity to light and accommodation. Pupil asymmetry can indicate an elevation of intracranial pressure but may also be a sign of trauma to the globe. Extraocular movements are tested, and diplopia and unequal pupillary levels are assessed. Limitation suggests orbital injury with entrapment of periorbital tissues (Fig. 11-20). Visual acuity is evaluated (eg, by tests of light perception, ability to count fingers, ability to read print). Proptosis and enophthalmos suggest hemorrhage within and fracture of the orbital walls, respectively. Periorbital swelling frequently accompanies fracture of the zygoma or maxilla (Fig. 11-21) Subconjunctival hemorrhage suggests a fractured zygoma or direct trauma to the globe (Fig. 11-22). Pooling and leakage of tears may indicate disruption of the lacrimal system.

The nose is inspected for deformity, pain, mobility, septal hematoma, and obstruction. Bleeding should be managed immediately, as previously discussed. Leakage of CSF suggests a cribriform plate or ethmoidal roof fracture and, if present, should warn against insertion of any nasal tubes or packing. Any watery nasal discharge should be tested on filter paper: CSF will form a ring around blood or mucus. Intercanthal distance is measured; if it is more than 3.5 cm, a nasoethmoid fracture should be suspected.

The ears are examined for bleeding, CSF leakage, tympanic membrane perforation, and hemotympanum. Lacerations of the external auditory canal usually indicate the presence of a mandible fracture.

The facial soft tissues are examined for sensory and motor deficits. Peripheral or central injury to cranial nerves V and VII must be sought in relation to other injuries. Subcutaneous emphysema in the middle and upper face

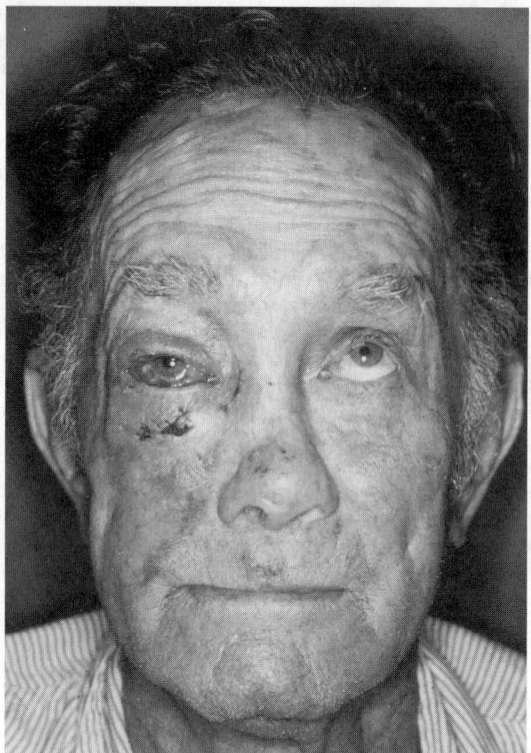

Figure 11-20. Orbital blowout fracture with entrapment of inferior rectus muscle and limitation of upward gaze on the patient's right side.

suggests paranasal sinus fracture, and in the lower face and neck it implies injury to the larynx, trachea, or lungs. Venous engorgement of the face suggests trauma to the major vessels of the neck or thorax. Leakage of clear or pink fluid from a facial wound may be a sign of parotid duct or gland injury.

The face as a whole is examined for asymmetry and deformity. Elongation with bilateral swelling suggests bilateral maxillary fracture. Step-off defects, tenderness, and ecchymoses around the orbit suggest maxilla and zygoma fractures. The midface is palpated for mobility. Bimanual palpation (with one hand grasping the maxilla and palate intraorally while the other hand stabilizes the forehead) may reveal palate, cheek, or nose mobility, indicating a LeFort I, II, or III fracture of the maxilla. Eye injuries occur in 60% of patients with midfacial trauma, and blindness is a particular risk in LeFort III fractures.[102] Therefore, any patient with suspected fractures should have a formal ophthalmologic examination.

The mandible is palpated externally from one temporomandibular joint to the other. Tenderness, step-off defects, and crepitus are external signs of fracture. Intraoral hematoma (especially involving the sublingual and gingival mucosa), lacerations, bleeding, loose or broken teeth, mobile jaw segments, and malocclusion are internal signs of mandible fracture (Fig. 11-23).

Radiographic Examination

In the conscious and cooperative patient with maxillofacial trauma, plain facial films and panoramic mandible radiographs can be performed initially to assess bony injury (Fig. 11-24). The cervical spine must be confirmed as uninjured before any manipulation of the head is done. Plain films are entirely adequate for isolated zygoma and orbit fractures. More detailed and definitive radiographic assessment is obtained with computed tomography (CT).

CT is part of the standard management of the head-injured patient, and sections through the facial skeleton can be obtained simultaneously, providing information on the extent of facial fractures in addition to the status of the brain. Axial and coronal sections are complementary; only axial views can be obtained in patients with cervical spine injury, although coronal reconstructions can be made. The coronal CT scan images (obtained with the patient's head hanging with the neck extended) are especially helpful in delineating the cribriform plate and ethmoid roof region, the orbital rims, and the overall vertical facial height (Fig. 11-25).

DEFINITIVE CARE

Timing of Repair

Most maxillofacial injuries do not require immediate definitive repair. Although soft tissue injuries usually are best treated as early as possible for optimum healing with minimum infection, treatment of facial fractures can be delayed while attention is directed toward more life-threatening injuries. Fracture reduction is difficult to perform and results are difficult to assess early after injury because of edema. If surgery can be performed within 3 to 6 hours of trauma and is planned for treatment of brain injury acutely, maxillofacial repair can be carried out simultaneously or serially. Otherwise, it is preferable to wait for edema to subside and to perform elective repair at 4 to 7 days after injury. After 2 weeks, fracture reduction become increasingly difficult as fibrosis develops. For mandible fractures, definitive repair should be performed within 24

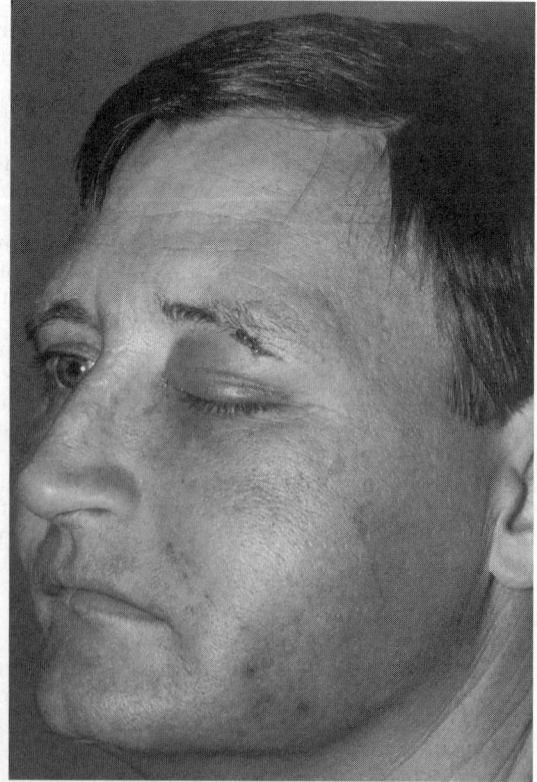

Figure 11-21. Patient with zygoma fracture with cheek and periorbital swelling.

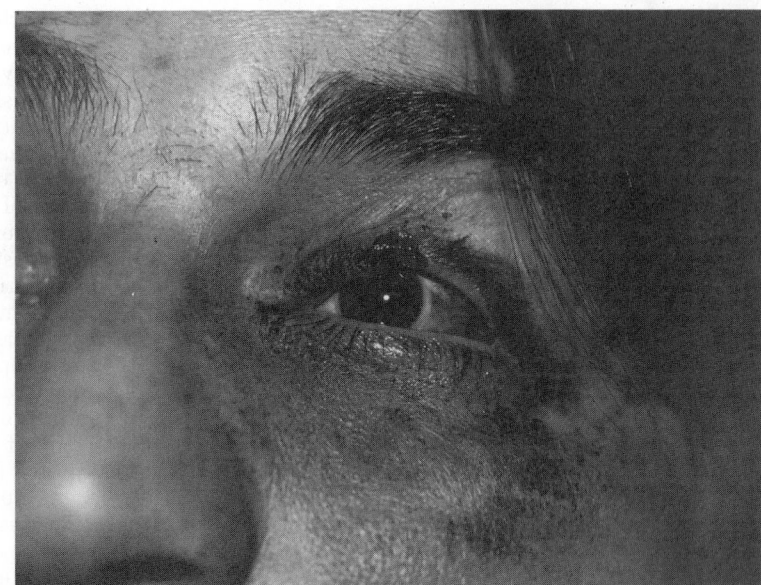

Figure 11-22. Subconjunctival hemorrhage is associated with direct ocular trauma or zygoma fracture.

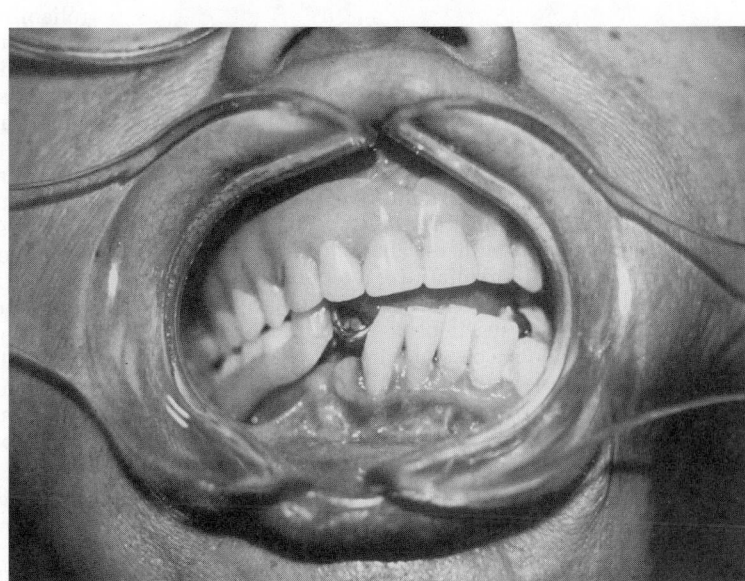

Figure 11-23. Malocclusion, even of dentures, is a sign of mandible fracture.

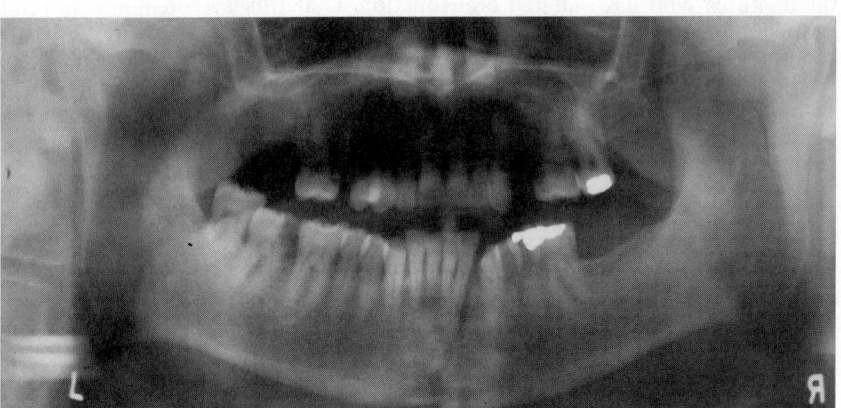

Figure 11-24. Panoramic radiograph showing fracture of the mandibular symphysis.

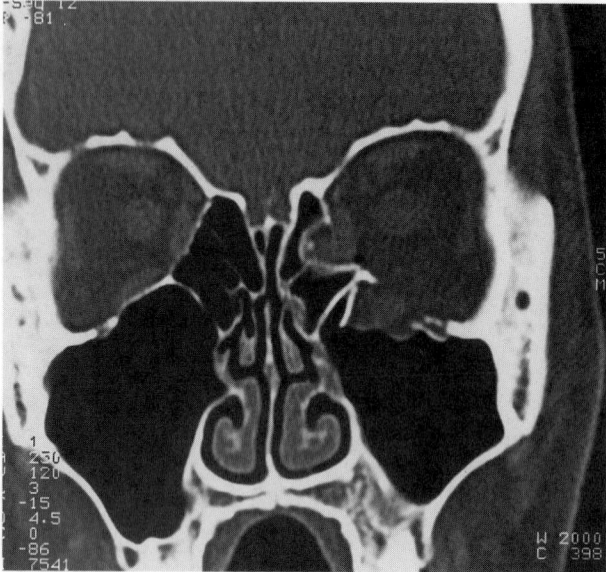

Figure 11-25. Coronal CT scan showing orbital floor fracture.

hours to minimize fracture contamination and risk of osteomyelitis, as well as to alleviate pain.

Infection Prophylaxis

Contaminated wounds usually should be treated with prophylactic antibiotics until definitive treatment has been delivered. Coverage against *Staphylococcus* and *Streptococcus* species usually suffices. The rich vascularity of the facial soft tissues helps to minimize infection and optimize wound healing. Even animal bites, a particularly common cause of facial soft tissue injuries in children, can be repaired primarily and successfully treated with antibiotics, unlike animal bites elsewhere on the body.

Facial fractures involving the paranasal sinuses usually cause bleeding into the sinuses, which, if stagnant, may lead to sinusitis. Nasal packing for epistaxis control should always be accompanied by antibiotic therapy to avoid inducing sinusitis or toxic shock syndrome.

Open reduction and fixation of facial fractures with alloplastic hardware carries a risk of prosthetic implant contamination and infection; therefore, perioperative antibiotic use is appropriate.

In addition to antibiotic therapy, oral hygiene is extremely important in patients with maxillary or mandibular fractures who have altered oral function. Oral rinses with saline and dilute hydrogen peroxide or commercial mouthwash are effective.

The use of antibiotic prophylaxis in the presence of CSF fistulas is controversial. Antibiotics in this setting have not been shown to reduce the incidence of meningitis, and they can encourage the growth of resistant organisms.[106]

Management of Soft Tissue Injuries

The outcome of soft tissue injuries can be greatly influenced by the surgeon. Although secondary reconstruction and scar revision are frequently necessary, the primary wound management should incorporate the principles of wound healing and aesthetic soft tissue surgery.

Wound cleansing is an extremely important preliminary step. Foreign bodies, gross debris, and bacterial contamination should be scrubbed and then rinsed from the wound.

Application of antiseptic solutions such as chlorhexidine gluconate, hexachlorophene, or povidone-iodine is followed by copious irrigation with sterile saline solution. Tissues should be kept moist with saline until they are actually closed.

Adequate anesthesia is essential to ensure patient comfort and cooperation. Even with general anesthesia, infiltration of local anesthetic can help with vasoconstriction during surgery and with pain relief postoperatively. Common anesthetic solutions include 1% or 2% lidocaine with epinephrine 1:100,000, mixed with the longer-acting 0.5% bupivacaine. Doses up to 300 mg lidocaine or 120 mg bupivacaine are generally safe for the average adult; the addition of epinephrine counteracts the vasodilatory effect of lidocaine and prolongs its duration of action. Local infiltration and regional nerve blocks are usually sufficient for repair of facial wounds, but general anesthesia is often required for repair of significant facial injuries in children, large wounds in adults, and lacrimal and facial nerve lacerations, as well as for prolonged cases and for multiply injured patients with concurrent repair of other sites.

The surgical instruments needed may not be available in the emergency department, and the surgeon should specifically request or bring a set of facial plastic surgery instruments. Choice of suture material depends on the location and dimensions of the wounds and the age and reliability of the patient. Absorbable suture is usually used for closure of subcutaneous layers. Chromic catgut is absorbed in tissues by macrophage activity and retains its tensile strength for 7 to 10 days. A fast-absorbing catgut can be used for skin closure in cases in which it is preferable not to have to remove skin sutures (eg, in young children or noncompliant patients). The longer-acting absorbable sutures derived from polyglycolic acid maintain their tensile strength for 30 to 45 days. They are absorbed by acid hydrolysis with less associated inflammatory reaction than chromic catgut. These are the preferred sutures for closure of wounds with considerable tension or inflammation. Nonabsorbable monofilament suture is the preferred material for skin closure because it incites very little tissue reaction and can be used for running intradermal or epidermal suturing.

Hemostasis is achieved with direct pressure, cautery, or ligation of identified vessels. Before wound closure, tissue should be assessed for damage and loss. Abraded skin heals with an abnormal texture and color; if small amounts of tissue are abraded or crushed, they should be excised. Larger areas should be allowed to heal acutely and undergo scar revision later. Jagged wound edges should be reapproximated without being trimmed; their closure often resembles running W-plasties or geometric broken line closures, which are preferable to linear scars. Avulsion wounds and defects with tissue loss should be closed. If the loss is small, the local tissue can be undermined and advanced to close the wound primarily. Larger defects can be closed with local skin flaps, skin grafts, or regional flaps. If in doubt, the surgeon can close the wound with a skin graft and perform a revision later under more elective conditions.

Avulsed tissue that has been saved can be cleaned and reimplanted. Avulsed ears are best reattached with microvascular repair of nutrient arteries and veins. Simple suturing of the ear itself is less successful but can be enhanced by multiple cutaneous incisions on both sides of the ear and by treatment of the patient with hyperbaric oxygen for 2 weeks. Avulsed cheek or lip defects are better treated by rearranging surrounding tissue to achieve closure.

Skin closure consists of deep stitches to approximate the dermis and remove tension from the wound edge, followed by skin approximation. Deep stitches of absorbable suture are placed with knots buried and wound edges everted. Cutaneous stitches should also be placed so as to evert the approximated wound edges; interrupted vertical mattress sutures, simple interrupted stitches, a running subcuticular suture, a simple running stitch, or a running locking stitch can be used.

Drains should be used for large wounds with oozing or with high potential for infection. A small rubber drain usually suffices. Antibiotic ointment or an occlusive dressing should be applied. Skin sutures are removed from the face after 4 or 5 days. Sutures left in longer are likely to cause permanent marks where epithelium grows down the suture track.

Facial scars, like those elsewhere on the body, mature over months and years. Even aesthetically unacceptable scars improve with maturation. Nevertheless, any scar that is larger than 2 cm, is wider that 2 mm, distorts normal anatomy, or does not lie in a favorable skin tension line can be improved by scar revision. Revision should be performed no sooner than 6 months after initial injury, and preferably about 1 year later.

Facial nerve lacerations are best repaired primarily at the time of soft tissue repair (Fig. 11-26). If primary repair is not feasible because of other life-threatening injuries, the severed nerve endings should be tagged with metal microvascular clips or nonabsorbable suture, if possible. The optimal technique of neurorrhaphy is debatable, but epineural, perineural, and interfascicular repair are all effective. The most important variables are the atraumatic handling of the nerve, the use of microsuture (eg, 8-0 to 10-0 monofilament nylon) in end-to-end anastomosis, and the absence of tension. If tension is present or a segment of facial nerve is missing, an interposition graft should be inserted. The greater auricular nerve in the neck and the sural nerve from the leg are the most common donor nerves.

Duct injuries (mainly the lacrimal ducts and the parotid ducts) should be repaired primarily. The duct is cannulated with fine silicone tubing and then, if possible, sutured over the cannula. The parotid duct can be marsupialized into the oral cavity, and the lacrimal duct can be diverted into the nasal cavity by dacryocystorhinostomy if primary repair fails. Medial and lateral canthal tendon injuries should be repaired with permanent suture that is passed through periosteum or even bone.

Management of Bony Injuries

Facial fractures are treated by closed or open reduction, with or without wire or rigid fixation. Nondisplaced fractures, such as those involving the nasal bones, zygoma, and maxilla, may require no treatment at all. On the other hand, displaced fractures require not only reduction and stabilization but also treatment of associated injuries to the facial soft tissues and intracranial structures.

Treatment of frontal sinus fractures is a function of fracture complexity (Fig. 11-27). Nondisplaced anterior wall fractures can be left alone. Displaced anterior wall fractures should be opened and repaired to avoid later mucocele formation and a residual depressed area over the fracture site. The frontal sinus mucosa adjacent to the fracture line is removed, and the anterior wall fragments are reduced and stabilized with either stainless steel wire (no. 26 or 28 gauge) or microplates and screws.

Posterior wall fractures should be explored, preferably using an osteoplastic flap[107] or craniotomy approach. Any dural defects are repaired first. The sinus mucosa is then either removed from all fracture lines or stripped from the sinus completely and replaced by autologous fat packing within the sinus. The frontonasal duct is also obliterated with a fat or muscle plug. The bony fragments are then reduced and stabilized. If posterior wall fractures are severely comminuted or bone is missing, the frontal sinus is best cranialized by removing the entire posterior wall and the sinus mucosa while preserving the anterior wall. The cranialization procedure[108] eliminates the sinus altogether and makes room for edematous brain to expand. The normal forehead contour is preserved, and the frontal lobes of the brain are still protected by bone.

Nasoethmoid fractures (Fig. 11-28) are rarely amenable to closed reduction because of the frequent disruption of the medial canthal tendons and nasolacrimal system. Open reduction is often performed with the help of an ophthalmologic surgeon. The bone fragments of the nasal, lacrimal, and ethmoid bones are restored to their correct anatomic positions and stabilized with stainless steel wires or microplates. The medial canthal tendons are realigned and stabilized with transnasal wires. Lacrimal injuries are repaired with a dacryocystorhinostomy, with the use of silicone catheters to reestablish routes for tear flow.

Orbital floor blow-out fractures are best exposed through a subciliary or transconjunctival lower eyelid incision. Herniated orbital contents, such as inferior rectus and inferior oblique muscles and orbital fat, are replaced within the periosteum of the orbit. Exposure of the fracture extent should be made with great caution, especially to avoid injury to the infraorbital nerve, the optic nerve, and the globe itself. The fractured orbital floor should be reduced if possible, or reconstituted with an implant if support is inadequate. Implants of silicone sheeting (0.04 inch [0.1 cm] thick), Gelfilm, autogenous bone and cartilage, or titanium mesh have all been used successfully.

Medial blow-out fractures should also be explored to reduce herniated fat and muscle and to assess the lacrimal system and ethmoid vessels. Implants are usually not necessary, but larger defects can be reconstituted with the same implant materials used for inferior wall blow-out fractures.

Superior and lateral orbital blow-out fractures are quite

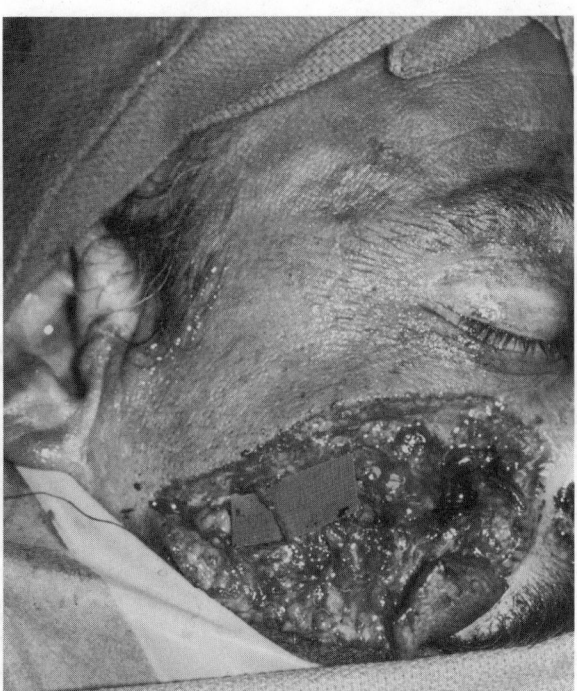

Figure 11-26. Repaired facial nerve after injury to face.

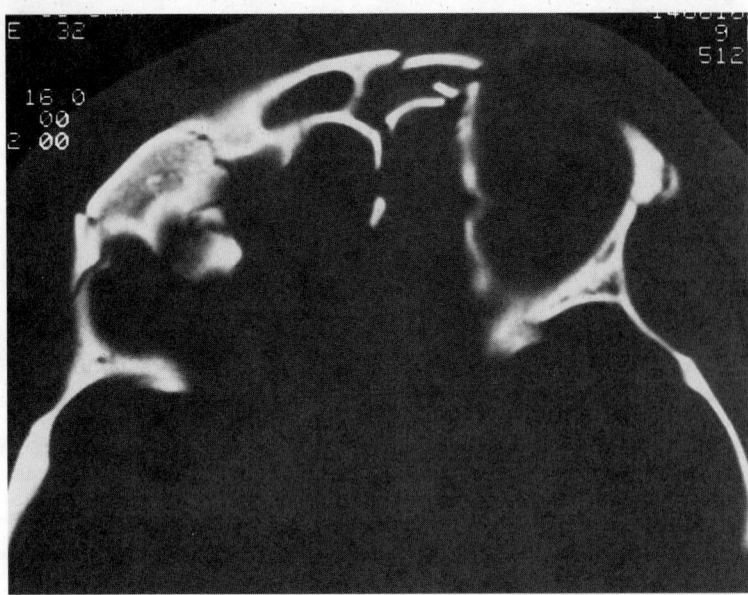

Figure 11-27. Axial CT scan showing displaced anterior and posterior table frontal sinus fracture.

rare. Orbital contents should be reduced, associated frontal sinus injuries addressed, and the fractures stabilized.

Orbital apex fractures (Fig. 11-29) are perhaps the most serious type of orbital fractures. The approach for exploration and decompression depends on the fracture site. Options include a lateral orbitotomy, an extended external sphenoethmoidectomy, a frontal craniotomy, or an endoscopic intranasal approach. The surgeon must be familiar with the entire three-dimensional anatomy of the orbit and its surrounding structures to achieve safe decompression of the optic nerve and the ophthalmic neurovascular bundle.

Reduction of nasal fractures often must await resolution of local swelling. Isolated nasal fractures identified within hours of their onset can be reduced early; otherwise, closed reduction is best carried out within 5 to 10 days. Most nasal fractures can be managed with closed techniques. Open reduction is used for early correction of nasal fractures that cannot be reduced adequately in a closed fashion and for correction of previously existing nasal deformity or malunion. Unsuccessful attempts at closed reduction and open wounds of skin and mucosa are indications for open reduction. Only surgeons experienced in rhinoplasty should perform open repair.

Topical intranasal anesthesia with regional local anesthetic blocks to the nasal dorsum, anterior maxilla, base of the septum, infraorbital nerve, greater palatine nerve, and superior alveolar nerve enable closed reduction of nasal fractures in the emergency department or clinic setting. General anesthesia may be necessary, but it should still be supplemented with topical and local anesthetics to enhance visualization and reduce bleeding. Depressed and displaced fractures are reduced with the use of an intranasal elevator and manual pressure or with special forceps. The septum can also be realigned with the use of these

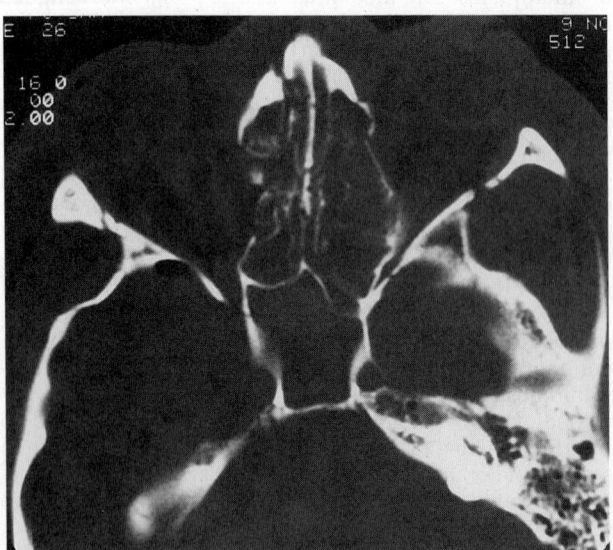

Figure 11-28. Complex nasoethmoid fracture.

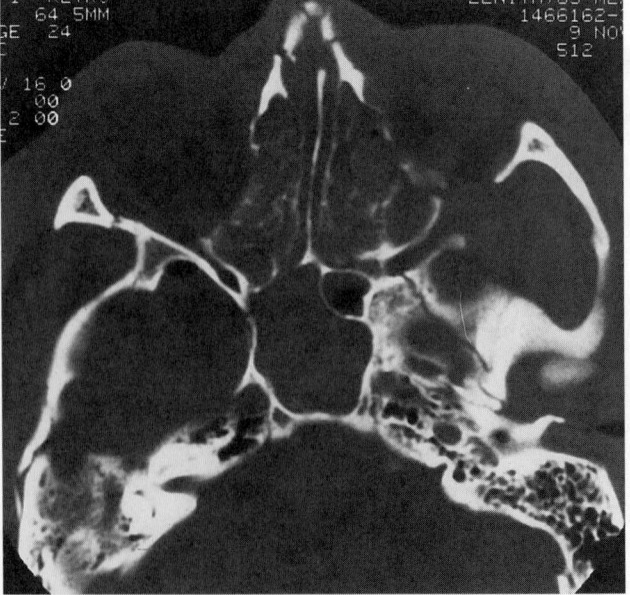

Figure 11-29. Left orbital apex fracture with optic nerve compression in same patient as Figure 11-28.

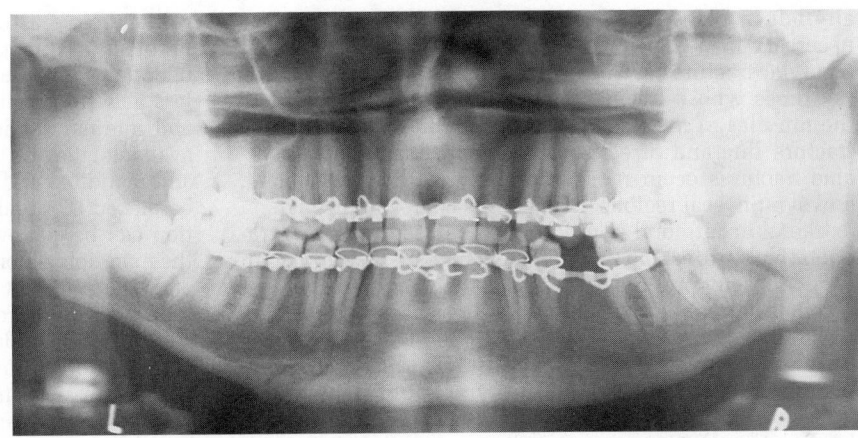

Figure 11-30. Intermaxillary fixation with arch bars and wires.

instruments. Internal packing and external splinting help to stabilize the reduction.

Most isolated zygomatic arch fractures cause purely cosmetic deformities. Reduction can be performed through a Gillies (temporal scalp), lateral brow, or intraoral incision. Fixation is usually unnecessary. Zygomatic arch fractures are particularly difficult to treat secondarily if they heal in a displaced position.

Malar complex and tripod fractures usually require reduction and fixation at a minimum of two points to maintain stability. The lateral brow and subciliary lower lid incisions yield access to zygomaticofrontal and inferior orbital rim fractures. The malar complex can be reduced and then wired or plated to these locations.

Maxillary fractures are some of the most challenging facial fractures to manage. The main goal is reestablishment of adequate dental occlusion, and secondary goals are reunion of the bony fractures and cosmetic facial restoration. The mainstay of treatment is open reduction and internal fixation of the maxillary fragments. Intermaxillary fixation (IMF), also known as maxillomandibular fixation, usually plays a role in the realignment and stabilization of the occlusion. IMF traditionally is achieved by wiring arch bars to the maxillary and mandibular teeth (Fig. 11-30) and then binding the arch bars and maxillae to one another with wires or rubber bands. A newer and safer method for achieving IMF is the four-screw technique, whereby self-tapping 2.7-mm bone screws are placed into the maxilla and mandible bilaterally, and wires are secured between the screws above and below[109] (Fig. 11-31).

Most LeFort I fractures are adequately reduced and stabilized by IMF with or without circumzygomatic and orbital rim suspension wires. LeFort II fractures are handled similarly. Miniplates or microplates are also used to stabilize individual maxillary fractures. Associated nasoethmoid and orbital fractures are managed concomitantly, as previously described. LeFort III fractures often require suspension wiring to the stable frontal bone. External fixation devices must be considered for severely comminuted maxillary fractures. Alveolar and palatal fractures associated with any LeFort-type injury are best managed with intraoral acrylic splints that are wired into place.

The general approach to proper midface reduction and stabilization is to establish the mandible as a solid base and to rebuild the facial skeleton vertically after centric occlusion has been restored. The upper midface is secured to the cranial base, and midfacial height is preserved. If mandible fractures are also present, these should be reduced first, if possible.

Successful management of mandible fractures requires not only restoration of premorbid occlusion but also complete immobilization of the fragments during healing. Infections must be prevented to avoid malunion or nonunion and osteomyelitis. In general, teeth in the line of fractures can and should be preserved, because they actually improve the likelihood of successful mandible fracture repair.[110] Exceptions include teeth that are grossly mobile within the bony mandible fragment, those with root fractures or periapical radiolucency, those with extensive caries, and those that interfere with fracture reduction.

IMF is the fundamental therapy for maxillary and mandibular arch fractures, as previously described. IMF is usu-

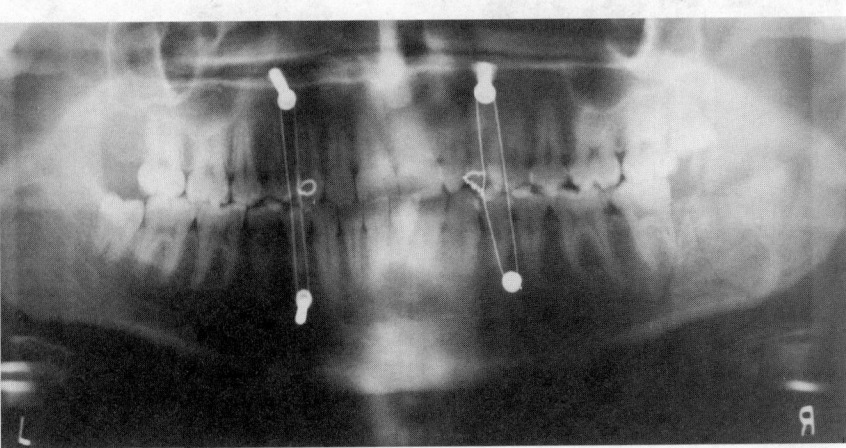

Figure 11-31. Intermaxillary fixation with the four-screw technique.

ally left in place for 4 to 6 weeks, although less time is necessary in pediatric patients and in patients with subcondylar fractures. Displaced and "unfavorable" fractures (ie, those whose fragments are distracted by the pull of the muscles of mastication) require open exposure of the fracture line and direct reduction and fixation. Unfavorable fractures occur most commonly in the angle, body, and symphyseal regions. Exposure is achieved through an extraoral or intraoral approach. IMF is used at least intraoperatively to establish proper occlusion. Fixation with wires does not provide rigid fixation, whereas miniplate or reconstruction plate osteosynthesis does have this primary advantage. Unless rigid fixation is obtained, IMF should be maintained for 4 to 6 weeks postoperatively. Dynamic compression plates have the ability to apply compressive forces to the fracture site that facilitate the primary bone healing process. Lag screws and even plates that use hollow screws that encourage osseointegration are also useful (Fig. 11-32).

Mandible fractures in edentulous patients pose special problems. Although occlusion is no longer a primary issue of concern, edentulous mandibles are typically atrophic and less able to accept hardware. Occasionally, open reduction and internal fixation is possible. Otherwise, if dentures are available, they can be wired circumferentially to the maxilla and mandible and then placed in IMF. Gunning splints can be placed intraorally to bridge the fracture, or external fixation can be achieved with percutaneous pins inserted into the mandible on either side of the fracture and connected by an acrylic bar that maintains reduction and immobilization. Elderly patients require immobilization for 6 to 10 weeks because of their slower rate of healing.

Nonunion is more likely to occur with mandible fractures than with fractures of other facial bones. Débridement, rewiring, and restabilization may not be adequate; bone grafts and external fixation are usually required. Hyperbaric oxygen therapy can be helpful in preparation for bone grafting.

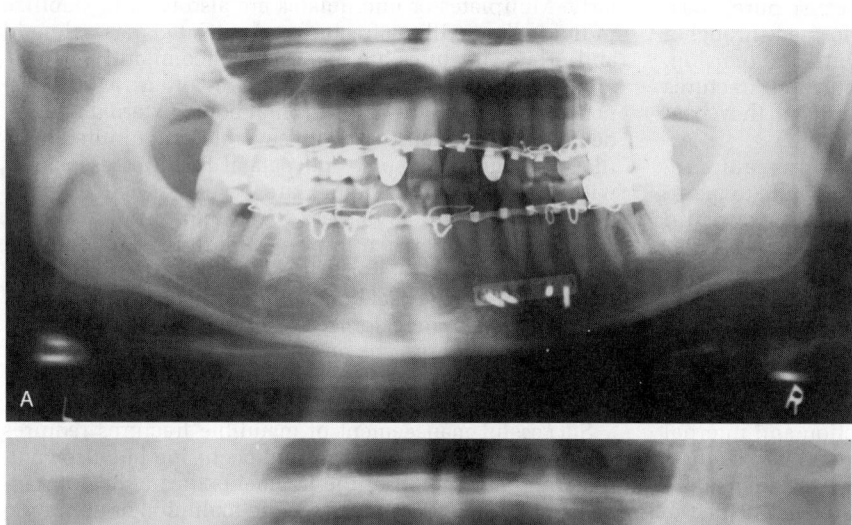

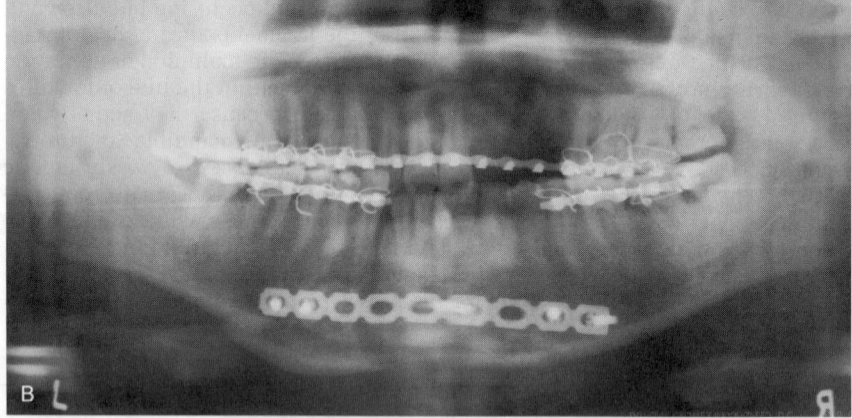

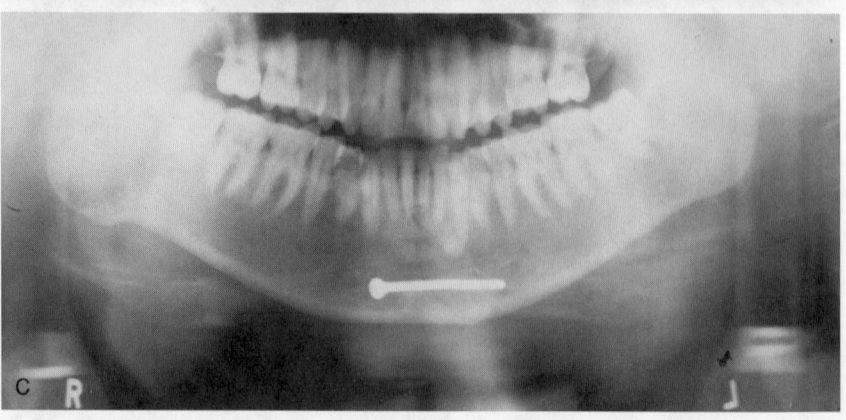

Figure 11-32. (*A*) Intermaxillary fixation (IMF) with rigid miniplate fixation. (*B*) IMF with rigid fixation using a mandibular reconstruction plate. (*C*) Lag-screw fixation of symphyseal fracture.

Definitive Care Phase: Neck Injuries

GREGORY J. JURKOVICH

The vital structures of the neck are concentrated in a small anatomic area, generally unprotected by bone or dense muscular covering. Yet, because of its relatively small size, only 5% to 10% of traumatic injuries involve the neck. Although infrequent in occurrence, neck injuries often require prompt surgical management. Disruption of the airway or carotid circulation is an immediate life-threatening problem, and esophageal or peripheral nerve injury can cause chronic morbidity. Penetrating injuries are most common and most severe, with fatality rates ranging from 1% to 2% for stab wounds, from 5% to 12% for gunshot wounds, and up to 50% for rifle or shotgun blasts.[111-113] Up to 50% of these deaths are preventable with appropriate early care. Significant blunt neck trauma is less common but can be particularly difficult to manage because it often involves the airway. Carotid or vertebral artery injury can also occur as a consequence of acute cervical spine hyperextension, even in the absence of bony injury. The initial diagnosis of these injuries can be difficult, yet the consequences of missing an injury are severe.

As a general guideline, all patients with penetrating neck wounds that traverse the platysma muscle should be admitted to the hospital for evaluation, observation, and treatment. Likewise, all patients with blunt traumatic injuries of the neck should be admitted. This section of the text focuses on the preferred and available diagnostic and treatment options for patients with blunt or penetrating neck trauma.

ANATOMY

The neck is classically divided into a number of anatomic triangles (Fig. 11-33). The two large anterior and posterior triangles are particularly important in neck trauma. Wounds to the posterior triangle rarely involve the esophagus, airway, or major vascular structures, although if the blow is directed inferiorly, intrathoracic injury can occur. In contrast, penetrating wounds that enter through either the sternocleidomastoid muscle or the anterior triangle carry a high likelihood of vascular, airway, or esophageal injury (Fig. 11-34).

The anterior neck is further divided into three zones defined by horizontal planes (Fig. 11-35). Zone I represents the base of the neck and is variably defined as extending from the sternal notch to the top of the clavicles or to the cricoid cartilage. Injuries here carry the highest mortality rate because of the risk of major vascular and intrathoracic injury. Zone II is the central and largest portion of the neck. It extends from the top of zone I to the angle of the mandible. Zone II injuries are most common but carry a lower mortality rate than either zone I or III injuries, because injury is usually apparent and exposure of vital structures is readily accomplished. Zone III is that part of the neck above the angle of mandible. The risk of injury to the distal carotid artery, salivary glands, and pharynx is greatest in this zone. Exposure in this region can be particularly difficult.

The other major anatomic landmark in the neck is the platysma muscle. This thin, broad muscle lies just beneath the skin and covers the entire anterior triangle and anteroinferior aspect of the posterior triangle. Wounds that fail to penetrate the platysma are considered superficial and do not warrant extensive evaluation. Wounds that penetrate the platysma must be considered a serious surgical problem that mandates hospital admission and further evaluation.

INITIAL MANAGEMENT

The same priorities for initial care of the multiply injured patient apply to the management of isolated neck trauma. Airway control remains the primary tenet of initial trauma care, and it takes precedence over all other aspects of the evaluation and resuscitation. If injury involves the airway itself or surrounding structures, this management task takes on special significance. Rapid inspection for air movement, crepitus, hoarseness, and subcutaneous em-

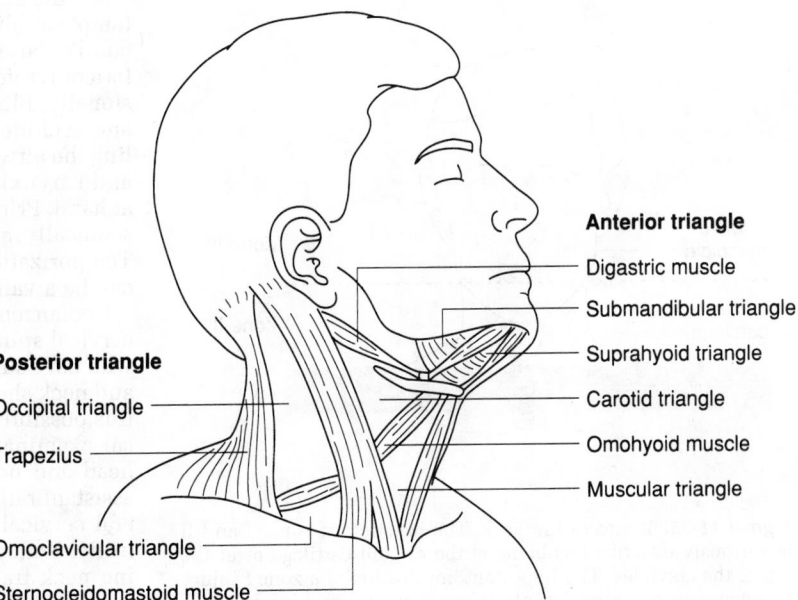

Figure 11-33. Anatomic triangles of the neck. The posterior triangle is composed of the smaller occipital and omoclavicular triangles. The anterior triangle has as smaller divisions the carotid, muscular, submandibular, and suprahyoid triangles.

Posterior triangle
Occipital triangle
Trapezius
Omoclavicular triangle
Sternocleidomastoid muscle

Anterior triangle
Digastric muscle
Submandibular triangle
Suprahyoid triangle
Carotid triangle
Omohyoid muscle
Muscular triangle

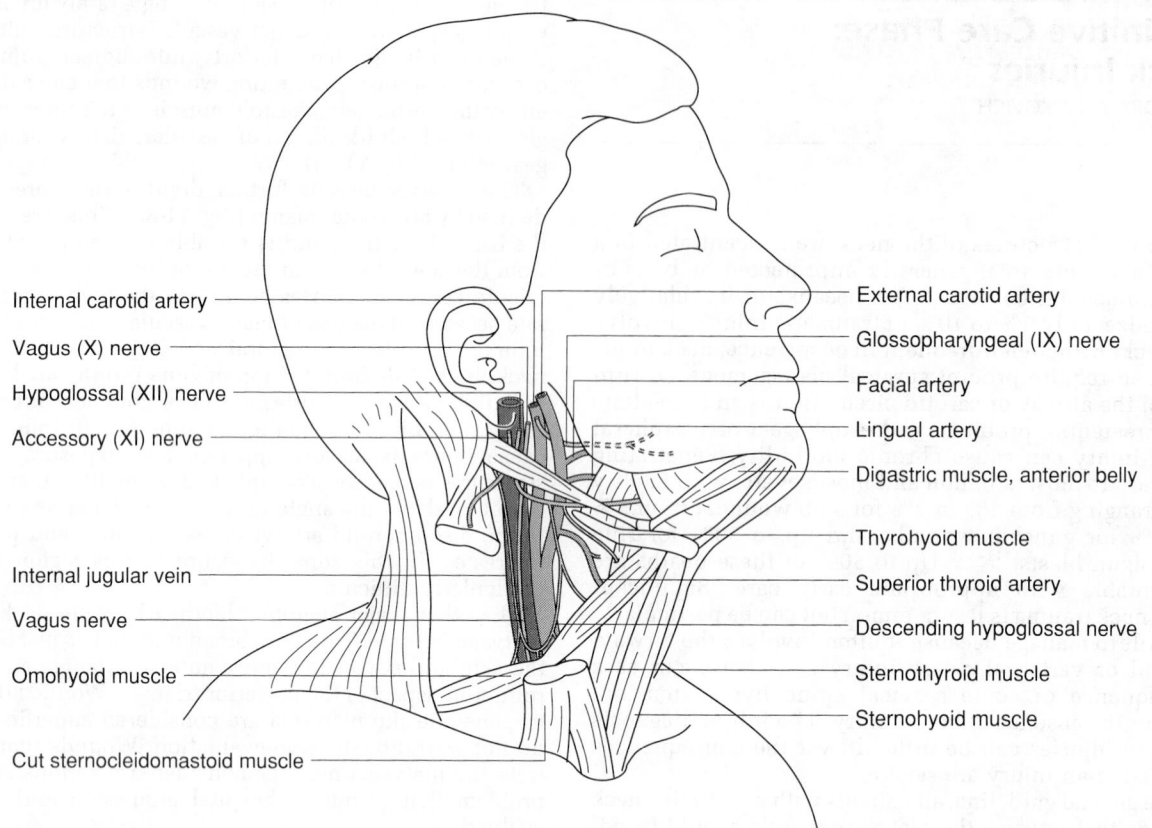

Internal carotid artery

Vagus (X) nerve

Hypoglossal (XII) nerve

Accessory (XI) nerve

Internal jugular vein

Vagus nerve

Omohyoid muscle

Cut sternocleidomastoid muscle

External carotid artery

Glossopharyngeal (IX) nerve

Facial artery

Lingual artery

Digastric muscle, anterior belly

Thyrohyoid muscle

Superior thyroid artery

Descending hypoglossal nerve

Sternothyroid muscle

Sternohyoid muscle

Figure 11-34. Proximity of cranial nerves to the carotid arteries of the neck. Trauma resulting in cranial nerve deficits in this region is often associated with vascular injury.

physema is the first step. Supplemental oxygen should always be administered, and adequate lighting and suction are essential. If spontaneous ventilation appears adequate, close observation and pulse oximetry monitoring are suggested, because acute decompensation can occur with little warning. If spontaneous respirations are inadequate, if blood or other material obstructs the airway, or if progressive cervical swelling from hemorrhage threatens to oc-

clude the airway, emergency intubation is necessary. Procrastination converts a simple intubation into a difficult and bloody emergency tracheostomy. Direct visualization of the vocal cords and oral endotracheal intubation are usually preferred. If cervical spine injury has not been excluded, hyperextension of the neck must be avoided. Two-man intubation with in-line cervical traction is an alternative to nasotracheal intubation.

Massive pharyngeal or neck hematoma can totally occlude the airway, making direct intubation impossible. Attempts at blind nasotracheal intubation cause further mucosal or laryngeal injury, and an emergency surgical airway (cricothyroidotomy or tracheostomy) is required. Occasionally, blunt laryngeal trauma is so severe as to disrupt and occlude the airway. The preferred method of controlling the airway in this setting is controversial (see Trachea and Larynx), but provisions for a surgical airway must be at hand. Primary tracheostomy or a single attempt at endoscopically assisted endotracheal intubation are options. Temporization with transtracheal needle-jet insufflation can be a valuable adjunct in these settings.

Concurrent with airway control is awareness of potential cervical spine injury, particularly in unconscious patients who have sustained blunt head and neck trauma. The head and neck should be supported in the neutral position until this possibility is excluded radiographically and by physical examination. In the emergency room, support of the head and neck is best accomplished by a strong, steady assistant rather than by collars, sandbags, or tape. The lateral cervical spine film is an essential component of the initial evaluation of patients with either blunt or penetrating neck trauma, both to assess the bony cervical spine and to evaluate soft tissues for edema or misplaced air.

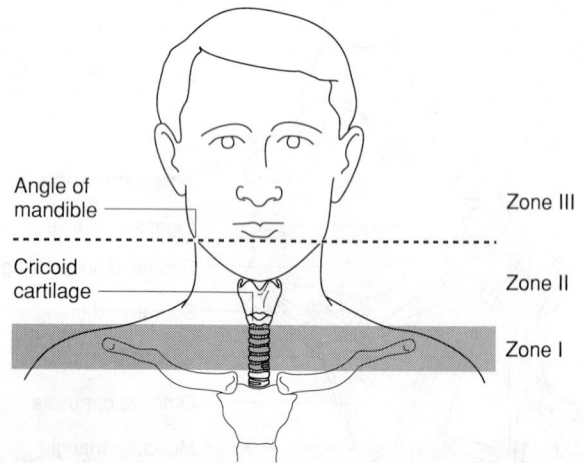

Angle of mandible

Zone III

Cricoid cartilage

Zone II

Zone I

Figure 11-35. Zones of the neck. The junction of zones I and II is variously described as being at the cricoid cartilage or at the top of the clavicles. The important implication of a zone I injury is the greater potential for intrathoracic great vessel injury.

Table 11-9. CLINICAL SIGNS OF SIGNIFICANT INJURY IN PENETRATING NECK TRAUMA

VASCULAR
Shock
Active bleeding
Large or expanding hematoma
Pulse deficit

DIGESTIVE TRACT
Hemoptysis
Dysphagia or odynophagia
Hematemesis
Subcutaneous emphysema

AIRWAY
Dyspnea
Stridor
Hoarseness
Dysphonia or voice change
Subcutaneous emphysema

NEUROLOGIC
Focal or lateralized neurologic deficit

The initial management continues to follow the ABC guidelines of trauma care advocated by the Advanced Trauma Life Support course of the American College of Surgeons, with particular attention directed at adequacy of ventilation, treatment of shock, and baseline neurologic examination. Patients with blunt neck trauma often have concomitant thoracic injuries, and penetrating neck wounds may follow a caudal trajectory, injuring lung or intrathoracic great vessels, particularly if the entrance is in zone I.[114] Rapid physical examination of the thorax is therefore part of the initial evaluation of neck trauma patients and should include inspection, palpation, and auscultation. Pneumothorax must be treated rapidly by needle decompression or tube thoracostomy, or both, and treatment should not necessarily be delayed for radiographic confirmation. Major neck hemorrhage is treated with direct pressure. Blind clamping of vessels is discouraged to avoid inadvertent injury to nerve or esophagus. Adequate peripheral intravenous access is required in all patients with neck trauma and usually requires at least two peripheral intravenous catheters lines of 16 gauge or larger. Blood is drawn for typing and crossmatching and routine laboratory evaluations, and fluid resuscitation is initiated based on the degree of shock and anticipated hemorrhage. A rapid yet thorough neurologic examination is also part of the initial management, with particular attention to the patient's level of consciousness and the status of cranial and brachial plexus nerves. Changes in the results of neurologic examination are key indicators of ongoing injury.

After the initial resuscitation, a complete physical examination is performed to detect associated injuries and to better define the extent of neck trauma. Close visual inspection of the neck alerts the physician to the possibility of underlying injuries and the mechanism of injury. For example, an oblique 4- to 6-cm bruise on the neck of a restrained passenger in a motor vehicle accident should alert the physician to the possibility of blunt cervical vascular trauma from a seat belt injury. Neck wounds should not be probed for fear of dislodging a clot and reinstituting hemorrhage. The neck should be palpated with attention to normal anatomic landmarks and areas of tenderness. Crepitus or subcutaneous emphysema indicates injury to the trachea, esophagus, or lung until proven otherwise. Never assume that a penetrating skin wound itself is responsible for subcutaneous air. If the patient is able to talk, the presence of hoarseness, dysphagia, or dysphonia should be determined. Hemoptysis and hematemesis are also signs of tracheal or esophageal injury. Table 11-9 lists the clinical signs of significant injury that usually mandate neck exploration to exclude or treat vascular, airway, esophageal, or nerve injuries.

All patients with blunt or penetrating neck trauma should have a chest radiograph to rule out thoracic trauma. Stable patients should have soft tissue neck films to look for retropharyngeal hematoma, tracheal narrowing or deviation, retained missile fragments and pathways, and subcutaneous or retropharyngeal air. Computed tomography (CT) of the neck is particularly helpful in blunt trauma to evaluate laryngeal structures. Patients who have sustained blunt neck trauma and whose neurologic examination is inconsistent with findings on head CT should undergo four-vessel cerebral angiography.

SELECTIVE VERSUS MANDATORY EXPLORATION

The relative indications for immediate, mandatory neck exploration versus selective, nonoperative management aided by invasive diagnostic studies remain controversial and subject to the experiences and preferences of individual surgeons and trauma centers. Two distinct schools of thought exist on this subject, one advocating mandatory surgical exploration of all wounds that penetrate the platysma[112,115,116] and one favoring a more selective approach.[117-121] More than two decades of literature reviews have concluded that either approach is acceptable, and the results are similar, although the more recent reports have favored some type of selective management policy.[118,121-124] The most recent comprehensive review of selective versus mandatory operative management again documents similar rates for injury incidence, overall mortality, and delayed complications, as well as similar hospital costs[125] (Table 11-10).

Perhaps more significant than this controversy are the areas of uniform agreement. All patients with clinical signs of significant injury require prompt exploration. All other patients with wounds that penetrate the platysma should at least be admitted to the hospital and observed. The disagreement concerns whether patients without positive clinical findings should routinely undergo surgical neck exploration, undergo extensive diagnostic evaluation, or simply be observed.[125,126]

Table 11-10. MANDATORY OPERATION COMPARED WITH SELECTIVE MANAGEMENT OF PENETRATING NECK TRAUMA*

	Mandatory	Selective
PATIENTS		
Number of series	11	24
Number of patients	1653	2540
OUTCOME		
Mortality rate	5.85%	3.75%
(range)	(0.3%–11.0%)	(0%–9.8%)
Cases explored	1492 (90.2%)	1596 (62.8%)
Positive explorations	803 (53.8%)	1117 (70.0%)
Cases observed	161 (9.8%)	944 (37.2%)
Delayed exploration	3 (1.9%)	20 (2.1%)
SYSTEM INJURED		
Arterial injuries	213 (12.9%)	303 (11.9%)
Venous injuries	310 (18.8%)	459 (18.0%)
Esophagus or pharynx	163 (9.9%)	191 (7.5%)
Larynx or trachea	150 (9.1%)	181 (7.1%)

(Modified from Asensio J, Valenziano C, Falcone R, Grosh J. Management of penetrating neck injuries: the controversy surrounding zone III injuries. Surg Clin North Am 1991;71:267)

Advocates of a mandatory exploration policy cite the low morbidity and negligible mortality rate after negative neck exploration as justification for the high rate of negative findings (40% to 60%). The disastrous complications of missed injuries further support this stance. A 67% mortality rate is reported after delayed operations for neck vascular injuries, and a 44% mortality rate for delayed operations for esophageal injuries.[113] A 1986 literature review reported an overall mortality rate of 16.7% for patients initially observed after penetrating neck trauma who subsequently required surgical exploration.[126] In addition, a few reports have documented major structural injury in a small percentage of patients who undergo exploration despite a clinically silent physical examination; in one report, 5.5% of patients with wounds that appeared innocuous but were nevertheless explored had significant injuries.[116] Transcervical gunshot injuries represent a special category of neck wounds, with one report documenting the high likelihood of injuries to cervical structures (83%) and supporting aggressive surgical exploration in all cases.[127]

Supporters of a more selective approach berate the high incidence of negative explorations, the cost of a surgical exploration, and the fact that some injuries are missed in spite of a surgical exploration. They also argue that the original data supporting mandatory neck exploration is based on World War II and Vietnam War experience with large-caliber, high-velocity projectiles, unlike the typical knife or hand gun injury observed in civilian trauma. The wide availability and diagnostic accuracy of angiography, endoscopy, and esophagography further support a selective management plan. Merion and colleagues,[119] as part of a review of the cost of managing penetrating neck trauma, analyzed 27 reported series in which the clinical courses of more than 4000 patients with penetrating neck trauma were documented. Fifty-two percent of patients treated by surgeons advocating selective exploration underwent immediate operation, compared with almost 90% of patients treated by those advocating mandatory exploration. Reexamination of these series revealed that mortality rate was no different in the two groups, and only 2.4% of initially observed patients required subsequent operation.[126]

At Harborview Medical Center in Seattle, all patients with neck wounds who are in hypovolemic shock or who have evolving stroke are immediately explored for vascular control. Most of those with neck wounds that penetrate the platysma in zone II undergo exploration, as do all patients with clinical signs of tracheal, esophageal, or major vascular injury. Preoperative angiography is usually not required for zone II injuries because of the relative ease of exposure and control of critical vascular structures. The track of the offending agent is followed throughout its course to exclude any possible vascular, tracheal, esophageal, or neurologic injury. Endoscopy is usually performed intraoperatively if pharyngeal, esophageal, or tracheal injury is suspected but cannot readily be identified.

Zone I and III penetrating injuries are selectively managed, based on clinical presentation and the results of diagnostic studies. Hemodynamically unstable patients undergo immediate exploration, with operative incision based on the most likely source of vascular injury. Zone I injuries are managed like mediastinal traversing wounds.[127,128] Angiography is performed in hemodynamically stable patients with penetrating wounds to zone I to identify potential injuries to the thoracic outlet vessels or to better plan the operative approach. Cinefluoroesophagography, first with water-soluble contrast material and then with barium, is performed after angiography for zone I injuries. Endoscopy is considered a complementary procedure to the esophagography, and should follow if there is any question of an abnormality. Angiography

is also performed for zone III injuries, because of the possible inaccessibility of internal carotid artery lesions or to demonstrate a need for systemic anticoagulation. In addition, most of the vascular lesions identified at the base of the skull are best managed by interventional angiography techniques. Esophageal studies are not done for zone III injuries.

If a nonoperative approach is selected for the asymptomatic patient, arteriography, esophagography, esophagoscopy, or a combination of these procedures is performed for all penetrating neck wounds.[129] Other experienced trauma surgeons argue that no diagnostic studies are required in the completely asymptomatic patient with a zone II or III injury.[118] Because a number of clinical reviews demonstrate that a mandatory exploration policy and a more selective diagnostic approach provide similar patient outcomes, each institution or surgeon should adopt a management plan most consistent with local resources and experience.

OPERATIVE EXPLORATION

Twenty-five to 50% of patients with penetrating neck trauma (depending on mechanism) present with obvious signs of injury requiring prompt operation. An additional 10% to 20% of patients without clinical signs of injury are discovered to have significant vascular, esophageal, or airway injury on further diagnostic testing. A physician treating patients with neck trauma must be capable of performing a complete neck exploration and repair of vascular and aerodigestive injuries. Neck exploration should be performed in the operating room under general endotracheal anesthesia. In the hemodynamically stable patient with a patent airway, intubation can be deferred until laryngoscopy and bronchoscopy have been performed. A nasogastric tube is usually passed to ensure an empty stomach. Preparation and draping of the patient before induction of anesthesia allows control of hemorrhage if the patient starts to gag at the time of placement of the endotracheal tube. The chest is also auscultated before surgery, and a chest radiograph is routinely performed, because penetrating injuries may follow a downward path with pleural penetration. A pneumothorax may not develop until positive-pressure ventilation is applied, and it may initially present as unexplained hypotension during anesthesia.

The incision is planned to allow full exposure of the tract of the injury (Fig. 11-36). The oblique incision along the anterior border of the sternocleidomastoid muscle is preferred for unilateral and high (zone III) injuries, whereas the transverse collar incision is preferable for bilateral or neck-traversing wounds. Extension of either neck incision into a median sternotomy affords excellent exposure of the thoracic great vessels. Proximal and distal control of the major vessels must also be considered in the length and position of the incision, and the patient is always surgically prepared for a possible median sternotomy. The tract of the injury is followed to its depth, systematically examining each structure in or near the tract.

MANAGEMENT OF SPECIFIC INJURIES
Blood Vessels

Blood vessels are the most commonly injured structures in the neck. Major arterial injuries occur in 18% of penetrating neck wounds, and major venous injuries in 26%.[126] Blunt vascular injury accounts for perhaps only 3% of all carotid injuries, but the initial diagnosis can be difficult and must be suspected if the mechanism of injury involves a direct blow to or compression of the neck, basilar skull

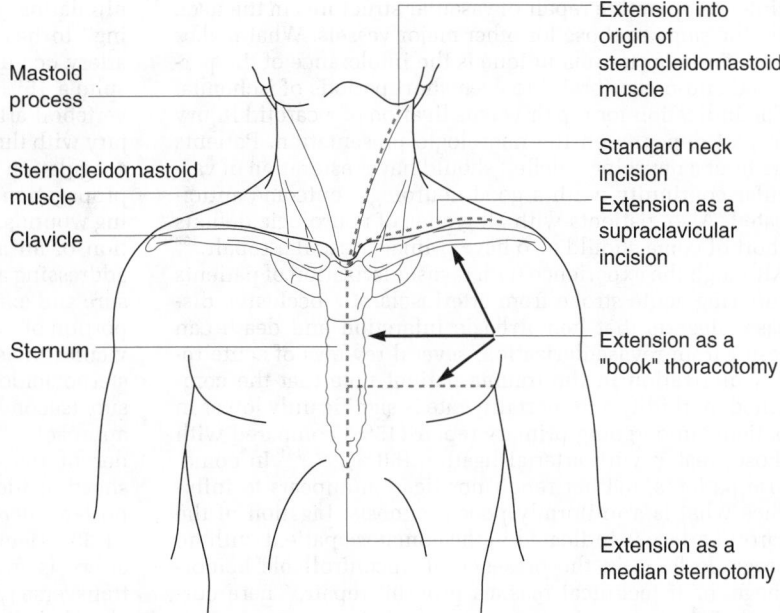

Figure 11-36. Neck exploration incisions. Extension of oblique or collar incision into a median sternotomy affords excellent exposure of the great vessels.

fracture, hyperextension and rotation, or blunt intraoral trauma.[130] Physical findings that should alert the clinical to blunt carotid injury include expanding hematoma, audible bruit, pulsatile neck mass, palpable thrill, Horner syndrome, or any neurologic symptom not explained by intracranial or other injuries.

Carotid Artery

In a recent multicenter review, 60 blunt carotid injuries were recognized in 49 patients over 6 years in 11 level I trauma centers.[131] Motor vehicle accidents were the most common injury mechanism (72%), followed by impingement between two solid objects (10%), falls and assaults (10%), and clothesline-type neck injuries (8%). Combinations of blunt carotid injury with head, facial, and cervical spine injuries occurred in 49%, 35%, and 18% of patients, respectively. The initial neurologic examination was normal in 49% of the patients, highlighting the point that, although its recognition is often delayed, blunt carotid trauma must be suspected in patients who develop focal neurologic signs or symptoms after a latent interval.[132] Twenty-nine percent of patients developed significant neurologic deficits more than 12 hours after admission. CT is usually the first diagnostic priority, because concomitant head injury is present in most of these patients. If the findings on head CT are not consistent with the clinical presentation, however, four-vessel cranial arteriography is indicated. Duplex ultrasound has been suggested as a screening tool.[133] In the multicenter study, duplex ultrasound demonstrated 86% (12 of 14) of the arterial injuries but was unable to discern dissection of the internal carotid artery at the base of the skull in two patients; proximal flow characteristics were also normal in both of these patients.[131]

The mortality rate remains high with blunt carotid injury, ranging from 20% to 40%, with permanent neurologic impairment in 40% to 80% of survivors.[131,134,135] Table 11-11 stratifies outcome by type of blunt carotid arterial injury; of note are the reasonably good outcome that can be anticipated for an uncomplicated arterial dissection and the uniformly poor outcome from complete arterial disruption. Treatment is highly variable and depends on the

vascular lesion as well as concomitant injuries. If it is anatomically feasible, pseudoaneurysms are probably best managed by resection. Small pseudoaneurysms in anatomically inaccessible sites can best be managed by systemic anticoagulation. Larger inaccessible pseudoaneurysms are a difficult management challenge; they may require balloon occlusion, ligation, or extracranial–intracranial bypass.[131,136,137] The best treatment of arterial dissection is likewise unresolved, although it would appear that systemic anticoagulation, if it is possible, is indicated to prevent propagation, embolization, or thrombosis. Resection is not required in most patients with arterial dissection. The outcome of an arterial injury with complete vascular thrombosis depends more on the neurologic status than on any treatment regime. Nonsurgical management seems appropriate for most of these patients.[135] The rare and fortunate patient with complete carotid thrombosis without neurologic deficits can best be treated with anticoagulation to prevent further or contralateral damage.[134]

Patients with penetrating carotid artery injury most commonly present with exsanguinating hemorrhage. The prin-

Table 11-11. **OUTCOME STRATIFIED BY TYPE OF BLUNT CAROTID ARTERIAL INJURY**

	Patients	Mortality	Patients With Good Neurologic Outcome
Arterial dissection*	25	2 (8%)	16 (64%)
Arterial thrombosis	20	8 (40%)	6 (30%)
Pseudoaneurysm*	11	1 (9%)	7 (64%)
Disruption	7	7 (100%)	0 (0%)
Carotid–cavernous fistula	3	0 (0%)	3 (100%)

* Pseudoaneurysm with concomitant arterial dissection occurred in six instances.

(Richardson J, Simpson C, Miller F. Management of transmediastinal gunshot wounds. Surgery 1981;90:671)

ciples of operative repair of vascular structures in the neck are the same as those for other major vessels. What makes neck vascular trauma unique is the intolerance of the perfused end-organ (brain) to even short periods of ischemia. The indication for repair versus ligation of a carotid injury in part depends on the neurologic presentation. Patients without a neurologic deficit should have restoration of vascular continuity, with a good neurologic outcome anticipated. Also, patients with all grades of neurologic deficits short of coma should also have primary vascular repair.[138] Although the experience with revascularization of patients suffering acute stroke from arteriosclerotic occlusive disease suggests that hemorrhagic infarction and death can result from revascularization, several reviews of acute revascularization in the trauma patient note that the combined morbidity and mortality rate is significantly lower in patients undergoing primary repair (15%) compared with those treated with arterial ligation (50%).[139–141] In comatose patients, neither repair nor ligation appears to influence what is a uniformly poor prognosis. Ligation of the carotid artery is indicated in the comatose patient with no prograde flow, in the presence of uncontrollable hemorrhage, or if technical reasons prohibit repair. There currently is little experience or evidence to favor extracranial-intracranial bypass in the patient requiring carotid artery ligation for trauma, although it has been used selectively in patients requiring selective carotid occlusion.[137,142]

Vertebral Artery

Traumatic injury to the vertebral artery, once only rarely diagnosed, is now more commonly identified, certainly because of the liberal application of neck angiography after both penetrating and blunt neck injuries. Blunt vertebral artery injuries occur more commonly than blunt carotid injuries, probably because of the close association of bony and ligamentous structures. Mechanisms reported to cause vertebral artery injury are remarkably diverse, including hyperextension and rotation, direct blows, chiropractic ma-

nipulation, yoga exercises, volleyball, and even "head banging" to heavy metal rock music.[143,144] Unilateral vertebral artery occlusion seldom results in a neurologic deficit, despite a 15% incidence of congenital unilateral hypoplastic vertebral arteries.[145] Treatment of blunt vertebral artery injury with thrombosis usually is nonoperative: systemic anticoagulation (if possible) is recommended to avoid further propagation of existing thrombus. More often with penetrating wounds, acute hemorrhage, pseudoaneurysm, or formation of an arteriovenous fistula are reasons for surgically addressing a known vertebral artery injury. Operative exposure and exploration can be difficult. The extraosseous first portion of the vertebral artery can be exposed by a supraclavicular incision with transection of the sternal head of the sternocleidomastoid muscle (Fig. 11-37). More distal exposure (second or third portion) is best obtained by an anterior approach.[146,147] An incision is made along the anterior border of the sternocleidomastoid muscle, and the carotid sheath is identified and retracted either anterosuperiorly or posteroinferiorly to expose the prevertebral space (Fig. 11-38). Hemoclips are blindly applied where the vertebral artery is free of the osseous vertebral canal between the transverse processes, behind the longus cervicis (colli) muscle. High ligation of the vertebral artery at the C1-2 level (fourth portion) is a satisfactory method of obtaining distal control without unroofing the bony canal of the vertebral artery.[145] Percutaneous embolization both distal and proximal to the site of arterial injury simplifies the management, but it requires a skilled and experienced interventional angiographer to cross the site of injury without causing further, uncorrectable damage. Contralateral vertebral angiography is recommended to accurately determine the extent of injury or the adequacy of embolization.

Trachea and Larynx

Blunt laryngeal trauma typically results from an anterior impact force (eg, dashboard, steering wheel) that drives the larynx posteriorly against the rigid cervical spine. The

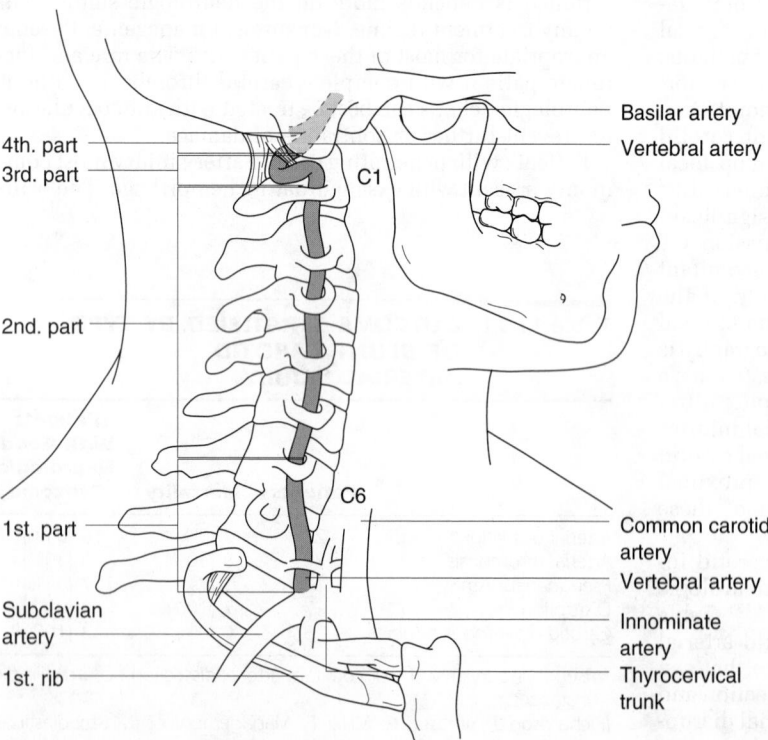

Figure 11-37. Normal anatomy of the vertebral artery, showing its division into four parts.

A

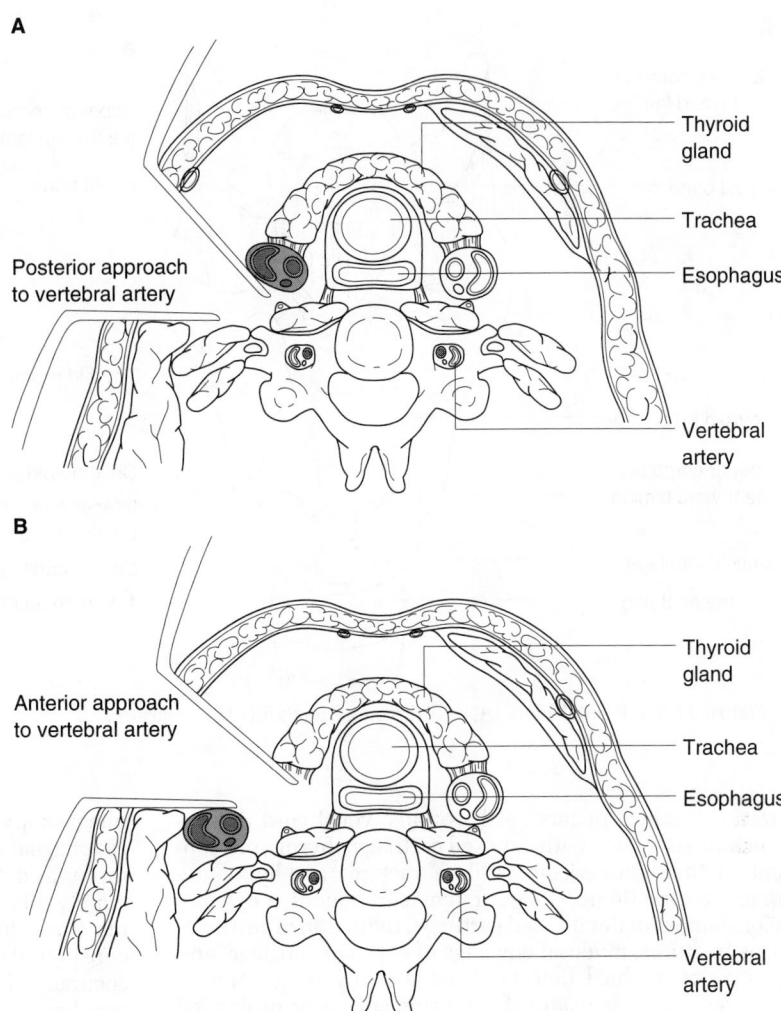

Posterior approach
to vertebral artery

Thyroid
gland

Trachea

Esophagus

Vertebral
artery

B

Anterior approach
to vertebral artery

Thyroid
gland

Trachea

Esophagus

Vertebral
artery

Figure 11-38. Operative approach to the vertebral artery. (*A*) Carotid artery and sheath retracted anteriorly. (*B*) Carotid artery and sheath retracted posteriorly.

impact can produce a simple or comminuted fracture of laryngeal cartilage, disruption of the mucosa of the endolarynx, or perforation and tears of the hypopharynx. Figure 11-39 depicts the critical laryngeal anatomy and the most common blunt injury pattern. These injuries are frequently occult and are often initially overlooked as attention is directed to injuries of the head, face, and thorax. Delayed recognition of blunt laryngeal trauma is the single greatest contributor to mortality, followed by aspiration of blood, missed esophageal injury, and overlooked concomitant intraabdominal injury. Subtle clinical signs and symptoms of laryngeal injury cannot be ignored. One report identifies hoarseness as the most common symptom, followed by shortness of breath, inability to tolerate the supine position, pain, dysphagia, and aphonia. Tenderness was identified as the most common clinical sign, followed by subcutaneous emphysema, neck contusion, tracheal deviation and hemoptysis.[148] Liberal use of fiberoptic endoscopy and neck CT aids in the diagnosis.[149]

Unlike blunt laryngeal trauma, penetrating injuries to the trachea and larynx are usually readily apparent and dramatic in their clinical presentation. Subcutaneous emphysema (occasionally massive), pain, hoarseness, and respiratory distress are hallmarks of tracheal injury. However, rapid endotracheal intubation by field paramedics can mask a high tracheal injury. Concomitant esophageal, vascular, and thoracic injuries are frequent. A 20-year review of 106 tracheobronchial injuries documented a 22% incidence of concomitant esophageal injuries, a 16% incidence of major vessel injury, and a 40% incidence of hemopneumothorax.[150]

As with any trauma victim, the first treatment priority for those with laryngotracheal injuries is to secure an adequate airway. With a laryngeal injury, this usually straightforward task can be extremely challenging. If an emergency airway is required, direct endotracheal intubation can be attempted initially if the laryngeal structures are well visualized and the endotracheal tube is passed over a flexible endoscope. However, this risks further damage to the trachea even in the most experienced hands. Equipment and preparation for emergency tracheostomy should always be at hand, and tracheostomy is usually recommended if an emergency airway is required, even though it also carries some risk of further injury.[151] Pulse oximetry monitoring is essential, and care must be taken to prevent episodes of hypoxia while alternative airway access techniques are attempted. Transtracheal needle-jet insufflation can temporize a critical situation and allow a more controlled tracheostomy.

Operative repair is usually not required for patients with simple laryngeal edema, hematomas without mucosal disruption, small lacerations of the endolarynx not involving the anterior commissure or the free margin of the vocal fold, and small lacerations of the supraglottic larynx that do not disrupt the integrity of this site.[151] Indications for primary open repair of the larynx include virtually all pen-

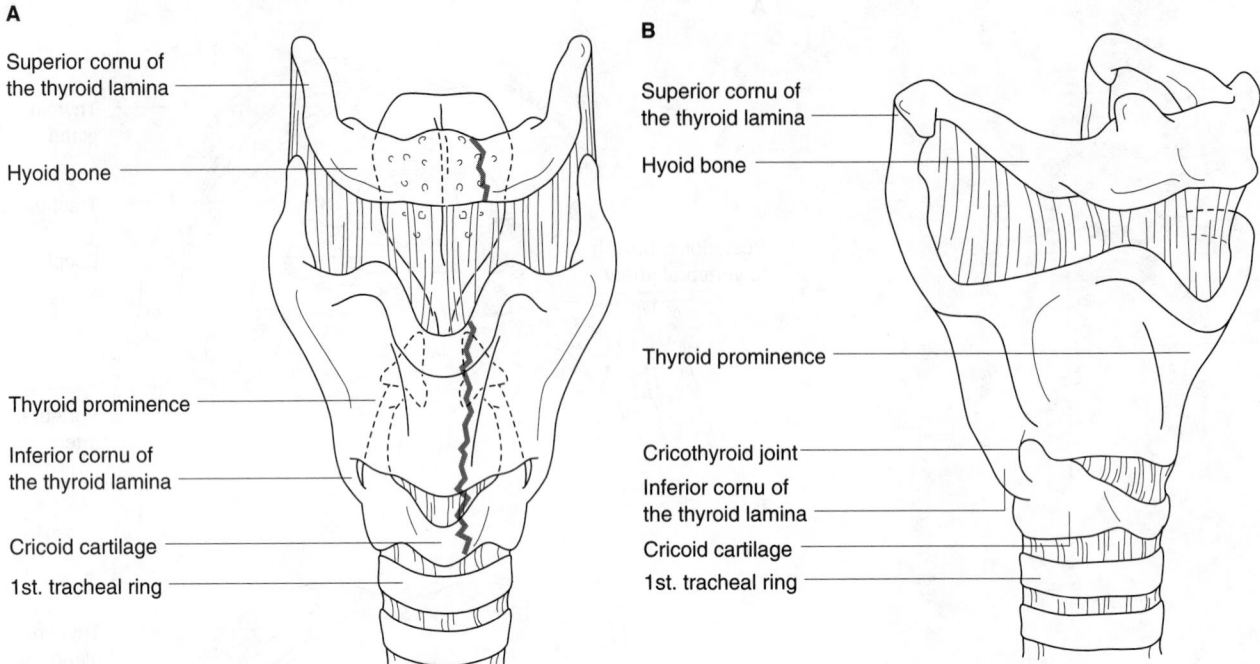

Figure 11-39. Frontal view (*A*) and three-quarters view (*B*) of larynx.

etrating tracheal or laryngeal wounds, vocal cord disruption, mucosal tears with exposed cartilage, thyrohyoid separation, thyroid or cricoid cartilage fractures, and hypopharyngeal perforations. The basic tenets of operative care are débridement of devitalized cartilage, reduction of cartilaginous fractures, mucosal coverage of exposed cartilage, and closure of tracheal defects. Tracheostomy is not always required, but it is useful if extensive edema or prolonged airway compression is anticipated. Controversial areas in the surgical care of laryngotracheal trauma patients include the timing of operation, the role of laryngeal stints, the use of steroids, indications for skin grafting, and the techniques of operative exposure of the larynx.[152]

Pharynx and Esophagus

Esophageal injuries occur in only 5% of patients with penetrating neck wounds, but the diagnosis of an esophageal injury can be difficult. The clinical signs of esophageal injury, such as hematemesis, odynophagia, neck pain, crepitus, and air in the soft tissues on chest and neck radiographs, are often absent or obscured by concomitant laryngotracheal injury.[153] In one review of 77 patients with penetrating esophageal injuries, 45 had cervical esophageal wounds.[154] Overall, physical findings were diagnostic in only 26% of patients. Furthermore, the morbidity of a missed esophageal injury is catastrophic. One review of penetrating neck wounds contained 109 cases of esophageal injuries; the mortality rate was 2% if operation was immediately performed but increased to 44% if operation was delayed because of an initially missed injury and to 100% if no operation was performed.[113] This information is widely used as support for a mandatory neck exploration policy. However, other authors have documented a small but significant incidence of missed esophageal injury even after neck exploration. In one report, cervical esophageal injury was initially missed at neck exploration in three patients, and all three died.[154] As a result, an aggressive effort at excluding esophageal injury is warranted, and some authors recommend routine esophagography or eso-

phagoscopy, or both, to aid in the diagnosis of isolated esophageal injuries. However, the sensitivity of esophagography in detecting esophageal injury varies from approximately 50% to 90%, and the sensitivity of endoscopy varies from 29% to 100%.[126] These modalities should be considered complementary; when combined, they have an accuracy of almost 100%.[155] The choice of rigid or flexible esophagoscopy is controversial and probably reflects individual preferences.

Careful evaluation of the entire tract of the offending penetrating agent or region of blunt hematoma is required to document esophageal integrity. This can be technically challenging and time consuming, but it is a crucial component of the neck exploration. Concomitant intraoperative endoscopy, esophageal air insufflation, or even vital dye instillation can be helpful in excluding injury. Because almost all reported deaths from cervical esophageal injuries are the result of a delayed or missed diagnosis, a particularly high level of suspicion is warranted. If it is injured, the esophagus should be meticulously débrided and repaired primarily, in two layers, with absorbable and nonabsorbable suture. Single-layer closure may be adequate.[156] All such wounds should be drained to avoid infection or development of a salivary fistula, which occurs in 9% to 18% of these patients.[153,156] Esophagography before drain removal is also recommended, because about half of postrepair fistulas are initially clinically silent. Muscle should always be placed between the trachea and esophagus in a combined repair. If there is massive loss of tissue, as with a shotgun blast, it may be necessary to perform a cutaneous esophagostomy for feeding purposes and a cutaneous pharyngostomy for salivary drainage. A secondary reconstructive procedure is then required after the initial healing is complete. Most surgeons advocate primary repair of all esophageal injuries, if it can be accomplished early. Delays of longer than 12 hours significantly increase the risk of repair dehiscence, wound abscess, and death. Neck esophageal injuries diagnosed more than 24 to 48 hours after injury are best managed initially by diversion and drainage.

Nerves

The preoperative determination of level of consciousness and lateralizing gross motor or sensory deficits is required in all patients; a more detailed neurologic examination of the brachial plexus, deep cervical plexus, phrenic nerve, and cranial nerves should be performed in all but the most unstable patients. A hypoglossal or spinal accessory nerve injury is particularly easy to miss unless a preoperative neurologic examination is performed. The vagus nerve can be evaluated by examination of the vocal cords. Primary débridement and repair of all severed or lacerated "named" nerves is preferred, with the use of fine interrupted nonabsorbable suture on the perineurium. Repair of a *single* recurrent nerve injury is controversial. An avulsed recurrent laryngeal nerve (blunt laryngotracheal disruption) should be implanted into the posterior cricoarytenoid muscle.[157] If a motor nerve deficit is apparent, an expendable sensory nerve such as the great auricular can be interposed as a nerve graft to allow anastomosis without tension. If the patient's condition precludes primary repair, the nerve ends should be marked with silver clips or nonabsorbable colored suture. Secondary repair 3 weeks after injury is advised.

Definitive Care Phase: Chest Injuries

ROBERT J. WINCHELL

Chest injuries are common after trauma and are frequently severe. About half of all accident fatalities include some element of chest injury, and about one fourth of these deaths can be directly attributed to thoracic injuries. Blunt injuries to the chest, such as from motor vehicle crashes or falls, are more common than those from penetrating trauma, except in some urban areas, where penetrating injuries predominate. Most penetrating injuries are stab wounds, but the incidence of injuries from gunshot wounds is increasing.

Most chest injuries can be treated with relatively simple methods, such as tube thoracostomy, appropriate analgesic management, and good pulmonary toilet.[158] However, delay in diagnosis and treatment of severe chest injuries (eg, tension pneumothorax, rib fractures with pulmonary contusion, aortic transection) is a common cause of preventable death after trauma. An organized structure for understanding chest injuries and their pathophysiology is necessary to avoid delays that may lead to morbidity and mortality.

ANATOMIC CONSIDERATIONS

For purposes of injury classification, the thorax can be divided into four anatomic zones: (1) the chest wall, (2) the pleural space, (3) the pulmonary parenchyma, and (4) mediastinal structures. Injuries to the chest wall include injuries to the bony thorax and shoulder girdle, as well as soft tissue injuries. Pleural space injuries include the various types of pneumothorax and hemothorax, in which the potential space between the visceral and parietal pleurae is occupied by either blood or air. Pulmonary parenchymal injuries include pulmonary contusion, laceration, hematoma, and pneumatocele. Mediastinal injuries are divided into aerodigestive tract and vascular injuries. The aerodigestive injuries include tracheal and bronchial disruptions, traumatic asphyxia, and esophageal injuries. Mediastinal vascular injuries include injuries to the heart, aorta, and great vessels.

EVALUATION

The initial evaluation and treatment of the patient with chest injuries is the same as for any trauma victim. An effective airway is secured, adequacy of breathing is ensured, and circulation is assessed and supported with control of external hemorrhage and establishment of large-bore peripheral venous access. Therapy for potentially serious problems should be initiated immediately.

Whenever possible, a careful history relevant to the chest should be obtained. The history should include details of the mechanism of injury. The speed at impact and the degree of frontal deceleration are important factors in motor vehicle crashes. Aortic transection is associated with severe deceleration injury. Patients not using restraint systems are likely to contact the steering wheel or the dashboard of the car. This places them at an increased risk for chest injuries, such as rib fractures, flail chest, and myocardial contusion, as well as tracheal or laryngeal injuries.

In patients who suffer penetrating trauma, the characteristics of the wounding instrument are important, but accurate information is often not available. External wounds can be misleading. All information from the patient should be carefully considered, even if the complaints are distant from the perceived trajectory of the injury. Patients with complaints of hoarse voice, dyspnea, local throat pain, and dysphasia should be carefully evaluated for injuries to the larynx and the cervical portion of the esophagus. Complaints of dyspnea or pressure in the chest with or without chest wall pain may be indicative of pneumothorax or hemothorax.

The patient's past medical history is also important. A history of pulmonary disease, heart disease, or prior thoracic surgery can alter interpretation of diagnostic studies and impact therapeutic decisions. In addition, a history of medications, allergies, smoking, and the recent ingestion of drugs and alcohol should be obtained.

The physical examination begins with complete exposure of the chest and inspection for signs of contusions, lacerations, or wounds. These visible signs may give clues to the mechanism of injury. The breathing pattern, its effectiveness in ventilation, and any abnormal motion of the chest wall should be observed. Chest wall splinting and shallow respiration may be noted in patients with rib fractures. Asymmetric chest wall expansion with hyperinflation is suggestive of tension pneumothorax. Paradoxical motion of a segment of chest wall is diagnostic of flail chest.

The presence of wounds should be noted, both anteriorly and posteriorly, and marked with radiopaque clips for radiographic reference. In general, these wounds should not be probed. Little if any valuable information is obtained from probing chest wounds, and the maneuver can turn a minor laceration injury into a pneumothorax, requiring a chest tube and longer hospitalization. The location of penetrating injuries, and the likely trajectory of missiles, should modulate the physician's search for mediastinal and pulmonary parenchymal injuries. Penetrating injuries below the nipple line must be presumed to involve the abdominal cavity as well.

The examination of the chest continues with auscultation. The breath sounds should be compared bilaterally for quality and symmetry. Absence of breath sounds on one side is highly suggestive of hemothorax or pneumothorax. Asymmetric hypoventilation may be secondary to splinting from rib fractures, pulmonary contusion, hemothorax or pneumothorax, or main-stem intubation. The presence of rales and rhonchi should alert the clinician to possible intercurrent problems, such as pneumonia or cardiogenic shock from a myocardial infarction.

Gentle but firm palpation of the chest wall demonstrates areas of point tenderness that may be associated with fractures of the ribs, sternum, or clavicles. Areas of referred pain or tenderness should be noted, such as sternal compression causing lateral rib pain in the case of lateral rib fractures. Shoulder pain may be associated with the diaphragmatic irritation of splenic injury (Kerr sign). The presence of crepitus over the manubrium or in the neck may be an early sign of tracheobronchial injury. Crepitus over the chest wall may be caused by rib fractures or by air in the subcutaneous tissues from a pneumothorax.

Percussion of the chest can also provide valuable information. Hyperresonance should raise suspicion of pneumothorax. This finding is most dramatic with tension pneumothorax, and it may be the most reliable physical finding. Dullness to percussion is suggestive of hemothorax.

ADJUNCTIVE DIAGNOSTIC MODALITIES

The chest radiograph is by far the most important diagnostic study, and it should be obtained early in all patients with significant chest trauma. Standard posteroanterior and lateral chest films provide the most accurate information and should be obtained whenever possible. Because of urgency, concerns about unstable spinal or pelvic injuries, and conflicting priorities, this is rarely possible in the trauma patient. For these patients, 100-cm supine anteroposterior chest radiographs are obtained.

Most thoracic injuries can be diagnosed simply from the plain films, making evaluation of chest films a vital skill for the trauma surgeon. A systematic approach to reading chest radiographs is important to ensure that all available information is considered. All chest films should be evaluated for abnormalities of the bony thorax, the soft tissues of the mediastinum, the diaphragm, the pleural space, and the pulmonary parenchyma.

In addition to rib fractures, injuries to the clavicle, scapula, and thoracic spine should be apparent on direct examination of the chest film. A lateral chest film may be necessary to make the diagnosis of sternal fracture, and specific oblique views may increase the diagnostic yield for rib fractures, although both are frequently clinical rather than radiographic diagnoses. Presence of significant bony injuries is indicative of major energy transfer to the chest and should raise suspicion of underlying injuries.

Evaluation of the mediastinum is performed next, looking not only for abnormal widening of the superior mediastinum but also for more subtle changes in mediastinal contour. Abnormalities of the aortic contour should raise the suspicion of vascular injury. The presence of air in the mediastinum is suggestive of injury to the esophagus or tracheobronchial tree. The diaphragmatic contours should be sharp and located in normal anatomic position. Poor visualization of a hemidiaphragm may result from traumatic rupture of the diaphragm or from hemothorax. A depressed hemidiaphragm associated with hyperexpansion of the hemithorax suggests tension pneumothorax.

Haziness over one hemithorax on supine chest radiograph can indicate a hemothorax. Conversely, lucency of one hemithorax should raise suspicion of pneumothorax. Pneumothorax is often confirmed by identification of lung

parenchyma collapsed away from the chest wall, but this finding is not always present, especially in patients on positive-pressure ventilation. The radiograph should also be carefully evaluated for lucency in the region of the diaphragm and deepening of the costophrenic sulcus, which are indicative of subpulmonic pneumothorax. The diagnostic accuracy for a suspected pneumothorax may be increased by upright inhalation and exhalation radiographic views.

In patients with potential esophageal injuries, contrast studies should be obtained. The use of a water-soluble contrast agent instead of barium in esophageal evaluation is controversial. The water-soluble medium causes less reaction in the mediastinum if there is an esophageal injury, but it can cause significant pneumonitis if there is a tracheoesophageal fistula. Barium contrast studies give superior mucosal detail in esophageal injuries. It is prudent to begin with water-soluble contrast and proceed with a larger volume of barium for better mucosal detail if no extravasation occurs. In patients who are conscious and alert, the oral contrast should be swallowed under fluoroscopic visualization. In unconscious adult patients, a nasogastric tube is placed just below the pharynx and a 30- to 50-mL bolus of contrast material is injected with enough pressure to gently distend the esophagus while obtaining a plain radiograph.

Angiography is the best study to rule out major injury to the great vessels in the chest, and angiography remains mandatory in most patients at risk for aortic disruption who have an abnormal chest radiograph. There has been considerable interest in the use of other modalities to make the diagnosis of aortic injury, primarily computed tomography (CT) and transesophageal echocardiography. CT scan of the chest appears to have a higher rate of missed injury than angiography for assessment of the aorta and should not be relied on in patients with abnormal chest films. CT scan of the chest may be of value to assess the mediastinum and aortic arch in patients with a normal chest film, where the concern for aortic injury is based on mechanism of injury alone. Findings of mediastinal hematoma would warrant angiography. Transesophageal echocardiography is a promising modality for the evaluation of the aortic arch that has been used successfully in some centers. It is a potential alternative for patients who cannot be transported to the angiography suite because of hemodynamic instability or immediate need for other surgery.

Angiography should be obtained whenever the diagnosis of occult vascular injury within the thoracic cavity is considered. Accurate knowledge of the anatomy of an injury may be essential to planning the correct surgical approach. Patients with penetrating injuries to the thoracic inlet, wounds that cross the midline, or penetrating injuries with trajectories that suggest vascular involvement should undergo angiography if they are hemodynamically stable. Such injuries may present with subtle angiographic findings, and biplanar views are mandatory. Patients with occult vascular injury are at risk to develop massive bleeding after angiography, and they must be monitored with great care throughout the procedure.

Thoracoscopy is emerging as a potential diagnostic tool for the evaluation of chest trauma. It provides good visualization of mediastinal structures as well as the pleural cavity. The procedure currently requires general anesthesia and intubation with a double-lumen endotracheal tube to facilitate complete examination, which may limit its usefulness as a screening tool. The ultimate role of thoracoscopy is still to be defined.

TREATMENT

General Considerations

Most injuries to the chest can successfully be managed without surgical intervention. The routine use of tube thoracostomy for treatment of hemothorax and pneumothorax is a cornerstone of therapy. Thoracotomy is most often needed for the control of massive bleeding or of bleeding that persists despite tube thoracostomy. About 80% to 85% of patients with hemorrhage within the chest can be treated by tube thoracostomy alone.

Partial or complete collapse of the lung associated with pneumothorax or hemothorax allows small tears or lacerations in the pulmonary parenchyma to continue to bleed. The insertion of a chest tube with subsequent evacuation of the air, blood, and clot allows for reexpansion of the lung and restoration of the normal negative intrathoracic pressure. The reexpanded parenchyma is then apposed against the relatively nondeformable chest wall, leading to tamponade of the low-pressure bleeding. For larger and deeper lacerations, still with relatively low-pressure bleeding from the pulmonary circulation, bleeding can be controlled by the reinflated parenchyma and by the edema in the injured tissue. Persistent bleeding is most commonly a result of injuries to major proximal branches of the pulmonary circulation or to systemic arteries, including the intercostal and internal mammary arteries.

The key to successful closed drainage is complete evacuation of blood and clot with full reexpansion of the lung. Patients with ongoing bleeding can form significant clot and are at risk to occlude the thoracostomy tube. Therefore, it is vital to use a relatively large tube in patients with hemothorax and to monitor the tube to ensure its continued patency. In most adults, a 36F chest tube is a reasonable choice.

Insertion of a chest tube should be performed as a sterile procedure. After appropriate skin preparation with povidone-iodine solution, local anesthetic is injected, and the chest tube is placed through a skin incision in the fifth or sixth intercostal space, slightly anterior to the midaxillary line. This relatively cephalad location for the chest tube is chosen to ensure intrathoracic placement of the tube and to avoid injury due to a potentially elevated or ruptured hemidiaphragm. The tube is directed posteriorly to facilitate evacuation of blood from the thorax when the patient is supine. A finger should be inserted through the incision into the thorax before placement of the thoracostomy tube. This digital exploration allows the physician to confirm the thoracic location, assess for the presence of pleural adhesions, feel for viscera (suggesting a ruptured diaphragm), and, possibly, palpate injuries in the diaphragm and pericardium before inserting the chest tube. After insertion, the thoracostomy tube should be placed to closed suction drainage until the air leak is resolved and the output is less than 2 mL/kg in a 24-hour period (or about 150 mL/day).

The use of prophylactic antibiotics is common with tube thoracostomy; however, the risk of empyema under appropriate sterile technique is minimal, and prophylactic antibiotics are probably unnecessary.

Indications for Surgery

Chest Wall Injuries

Most chest wall injuries do not require surgical repair; however, these patients frequently have associated abdominal, orthopedic, or other injuries that do require operative management.[159] The open pneumothorax, or sucking chest wound, requires operative débridement and closure. Ster-

nal fractures with significant posterior displacement also require operative repair.

Injuries Manifesting in the Pleural Space

Thoracotomy is indicated for control of ongoing hemorrhage. Pleural space injuries that require operative repair include massive hemothorax, ongoing bleeding, and clotted or caked hemothorax.

Parenchymal Injuries

The cause of massive hemothorax requiring surgery occasionally is ongoing hemorrhage from parenchymal lung injuries. Deep parenchymal injuries can produce severe hemoptysis that necessitates thoracotomy. In addition, operative repair is required for injuries to the trachea or major bronchi if there are large, continuing air leaks that cannot be controlled by insertion of chest tubes.

Mediastinal Injuries

Mediastinal injuries that require surgery include blunt or penetrating cardiac trauma with associated exsanguination, cardiac tamponade, or great vessel injury. Injuries to the thoracic esophagus require thoracotomy and repair.

Other Injuries

Thoracotomy can be of value in resuscitation of trauma patients with hypovolemia unresponsive to massive volume infusion. Resuscitative thoracotomy may also be indicated in patients with cardiac arrest after penetrating trauma but rarely after blunt trauma.

General Conduct of Surgery

The choice of position and surgical approach is dictated by the nature of the patient's thoracic injuries, the certainty of diagnosis, and the potential for associated injuries involving other body sites. The standard posterolateral thoracotomy (Fig. 11-40) provides optimal exposure to the contents of a particular hemithorax, but the lateral position of the patient makes access to the other side of the chest or the abdomen difficult if not impossible. Therefore, although posterolateral thoracotomy provides the best access, it can be used only in patients who have injuries isolated to a given hemithorax. Whether this is so can usually be determined in patients with clearly defined injury and in those who have been under observation for a period of time before thoracotomy.

In most patients undergoing emergency thoracotomy for

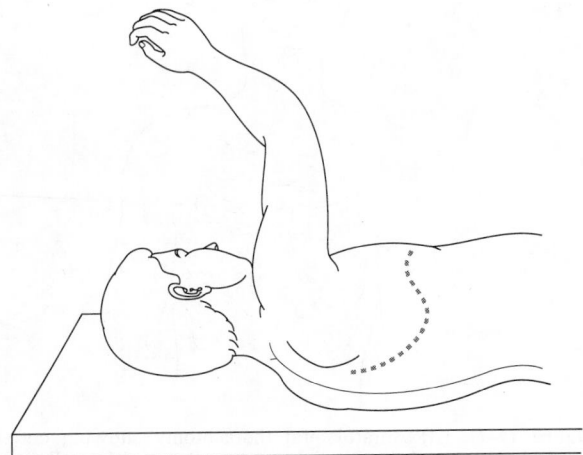

Figure 11-40. Posterolateral thoracotomy incision.

chest trauma, an anterolateral approach must be used, with the patient supine, to allow for access to the abdomen and contralateral chest cavity. Exposure through an anterolateral thoracotomy is considerably more difficult but is adequate with proper technique. The ipsilateral side of the body should be elevated to facilitate posterior exposure. The posterior aspect of the incision must extend as far as possible, at least to the border of the latissimus dorsi, and particular care must be taken to follow the curvature of the underlying rib. The mobility of the ribs is limited in the anterolateral approach, and it may be necessary to divide the costal cartilage at the sternum to gain sufficient access. The medial portion of the incision should curve superiorly to facilitate this maneuver (Fig. 11-41*A*).

The anterolateral thoracotomy incision can be carried transversely across the sternum into the opposite hemithorax to allow exposure to the heart, mediastinum, and structures in the opposite pleural cavity. The sternum can be divided with a sternal saw, a Lebsche knife, or heavy scissors. This bilateral, or clamshell, thoracotomy provides excellent exposure to the heart, mediastinum, and bilateral pulmonary hila (see Fig. 11-41*B*). It is necessary to divide both internal mammary arteries in making this incision, and they must be carefully ligated with suture at the time of closure to prevent recurrent bleeding.

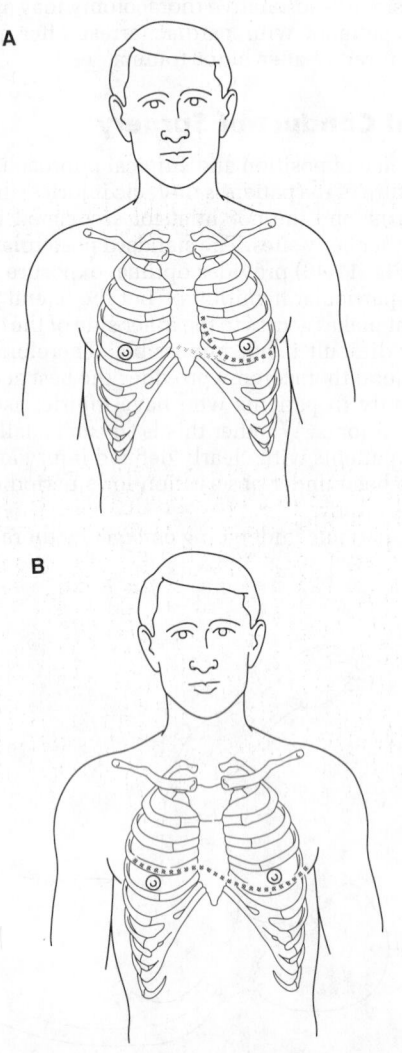

Figure 11-41. (*A*) Anterolateral thoracotomy showing correct (*dark*) and too-transverse (*light*) incisions. (*B*) A clamshell, or bilateral thoracotomy, incision.

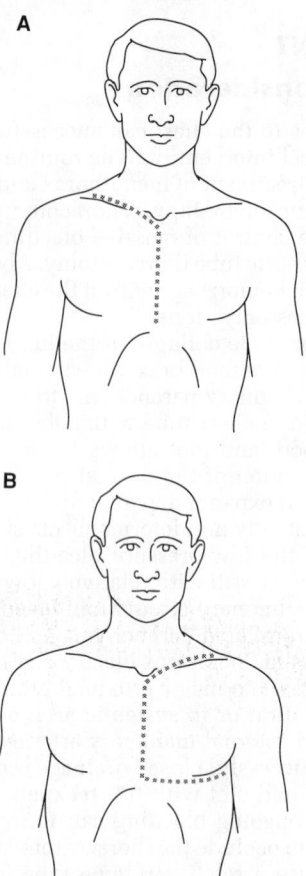

Figure 11-42. Median sternotomy with clavicular extension (*A*) and trapdoor incision (*B*) for exposure of the intrathoracic great vessels.

The median sternotomy incision provides excellent exposure to the heart and the great vessels in the anterior mediastinum, but it provides difficult exposure for repair of injuries of the lungs, descending aorta, chest wall, diaphragm, or esophagus. Therefore, like the posterolateral thoracotomy, it can be used only if the patient's injuries can be determined with relative certainty. This is not often the case, and most penetrating injuries to the heart are best approached through a left anterolateral thoracotomy, with extension across the sternum transversely if necessary.

The median sternotomy can be extended into the neck or over the clavicle for exposure of the aortic arch and innominate vessels (Fig. 11-42*A*); this may provide the best access to vascular injuries at the thoracic inlet. The median sternotomy combined with the clavicular extension and left anterolateral thoracotomy, the so-called trapdoor incision, can be used for exposure to the entire left thoracic inlet (see Fig. 11-42*B*). Such an incision may be the only way to approach proximal injuries in this difficult area. This exposure should be used only if it is absolutely necessary for control of hemorrhage, because it can lead to brachial plexus traction and disabling long-term sequelae. Care must also be taken to avoid injury to the phrenic nerve on the anterior border of scalenus anterior muscle.

Specific Injuries

Injuries to the Thoracic Cage

Rib Fractures.   Rib fractures are the most common injury associated with blunt chest trauma. They can occur directly at the site of force or laterally as a result of significant anteroposterior compression of the chest. The location and area of rib fracture may be indicative of associated injuries. The first rib is protected by the shoulder girdle and clavicle, so fractures of the first rib indicate a significant amount of energy transferred to the torso. First rib fractures have been associated with severe chest and abdominal injuries and with aortic injuries. Posterior rib fractures are also associated with significant energy transfer to the thorax. Fractures of the lower ribs may be associated with intraabdominal injury. A 20% incidence of splenic injury is associated with fractures of ribs 9, 10, and 11 on the left side.[160] There is similar association of right lower rib fractures and hepatic parenchymal injuries.

The diagnosis of rib fracture is primarily clinical, and fractures often cannot be seen on routine radiographs. Rib tenderness, either directly or on anteroposterior compression, crepitus over the possible area of fracture, and decreased breath sounds on the side of injury are all suggestive of rib fracture or injury. Specific rib detail films increase the diagnostic yield of chest radiographs, but radiologic confirmation of the diagnosis is not essential (Fig. 11-43). However, chest radiographs may demonstrate associated injuries, such as pneumothorax, pulmonary contusion, or hemothorax.

The treatment of rib fractures is directed primarily at control of their adverse effect on ventilation. Because of the pain associated with chest wall injury, poor inspiratory effort, splinting, and an ineffective cough commonly result. If these are not prevented or appropriately treated, atelectasis and pneumonia ensue. Elderly patients, especially those with preexisting pulmonary disease, are particularly prone to these complications. An assessment of the patient's ventilatory compromise from pain can be made by bedside pulmonary function tests, with primary attention to the forced vital capacity and tidal volume. A forced vital capacity of less than 10 mL/kg or a tidal volume of less than 5 to 7 mL/kg is indicative of significant respiratory compromise.

Adequate pain relief and pulmonary toilet are the primary therapeutic goals. Good analgesia and careful pulmonary care can markedly improve the patient's ventilatory

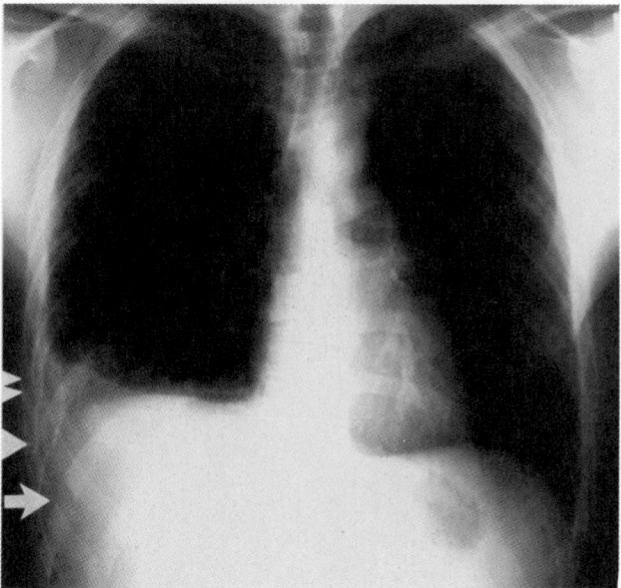

Figure 11-43. Chest radiograph showing multiple rib fractures (ribs 7 to 10). The costophrenic angle is blunted, representing a 400-mL hemothorax.

function. The use of intercostal nerve blocks is effective but has largely been supplanted by newer techniques such as patient-controlled analgesia, continuous opioid infusion, and epidural analgesia. Careful use of parenteral opioids, either on a routine basis or through patient-controlled analgesia, suffices in most cases. Epidural techniques are of particular value in elderly patients and in those with underlying pulmonary disease, in whom parenteral opioid use may be limited by respiratory side effects. One study showed that use of epidural opioid produces improvement in pulmonary function superior to that obtained from continuous intravenous administration of narcotic.[161] Ventilatory function should be measured both before and after analgesic treatment is begun, and the narcotic dose should be titrated for ventilatory response. The practice of taping fractured ribs is not only ineffective but counterproductive because it can increase the pain from the rib fractures and may further restrict an already compromised ventilatory ability.

Although epidural and continuous intravenous analgesia appear to be the most effective methods for pain control from rib fractures, not all patients with fractured ribs require hospitalization. Patients who are generally healthy with no underlying medical problems, and who demonstrate good ventilatory function with oral analgesics, may be treated on an outpatient basis with careful follow-up. Patients with a history of smoking, chronic obstructive pulmonary disease, or other pulmonary problems who sustain rib fractures are at increased risk for complications. These patients usually benefit from hospital admission to ensure adequate analgesia and to monitor pulmonary function.

Sternal Fractures.   Sternal fractures are frequently associated with a significant blow to the anterior chest. The incidence of sternal fractures historically is low, occurring in about 5% of patients with severe chest injuries. Sternal fracture has been reported to occur in unrestrained motor vehicle accident victims who impact the steering wheel. The mortality rate associated with sternal fractures in older series has been as high as 25% to 30%, mainly because of other injuries to the chest, such as aortic transection, cardiac contusion, tamponade, or tracheobronchial rupture. More recent studies have suggested a change in the pattern and severity of injuries associated with sternal fracture.[162] Widespread improvements in automobile safety, including collapsible steering columns, interior padding, and passive restraints, have probably contributed to this change. Isolated sternal fracture may result from shoulder belt use, and it does not necessitate hospital admission in the stable patient.

Sternal fractures are usually transverse but can be longitudinal, especially if they are associated with sternal flail chest. Posterior displacement of the fractured sternum can impinge on the heart. The diagnosis of sternal fracture is made by palpation of the sternum if an obvious step-off is present. A lateral chest radiograph reveals sternal fractures and the degree of posterior displacement (Fig. 11-44). The treatment of sternal fracture is primarily adequate pain relief and pulmonary toilet, as for rib fractures. If severe displacement is present, operative reduction with fixation of the fracture may be required. In addition, the possibility of other serious injuries associated with sternal fracture should be considered.

Flail Chest.   A flail chest occurs when consecutive ribs are fractured in more than one place, creating a free-floating segment of the chest wall. The free-floating segment can involve the sternum, with separation of the costochondral junction on either side (Fig. 11-45). Flail chest occurs in up to 20% of patients with severe blunt chest injuries.

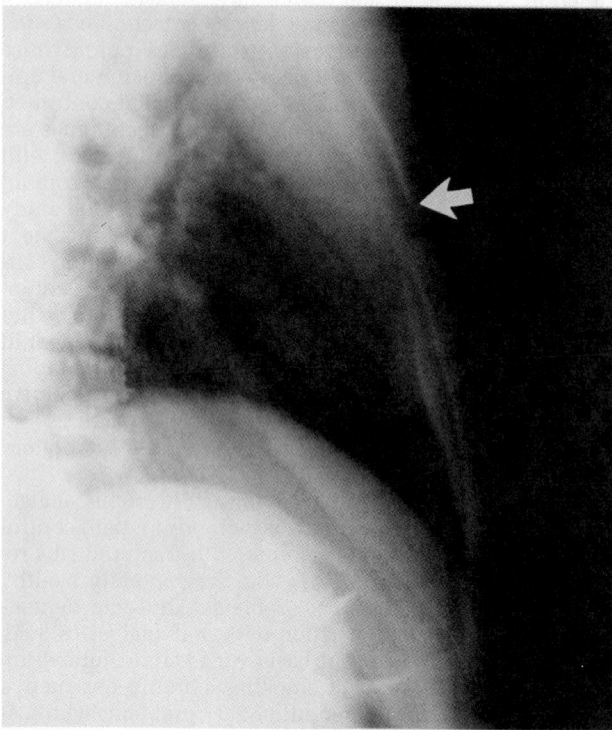

Figure 11-44. Posterior displacement of a sternal fracture (*arrow*), as demonstrated on a lateral chest radiograph.

The creation of the free-floating segment may result in paradoxical chest wall motion with respiration. The intact chest wall expands during inspiration, but the negative intrathoracic pressure generated causes the flail segment to move inappropriately inward. Historically, it was believed that this paradoxical motion was the cause of the severe ventilatory insufficiency associated with flail chest, and therapeutic efforts were focused on stabilization of the flail segment.[163-165] Stabilization was attempted with dressings, sandbags, surgical fracture fixation, even towel clips through the chest wall into the rib, attached to the frame of the bed. Mortality rates with these modes of treatment were between 30% and 40%.[166]

Gradually, understanding of the pathophysiology of the flail chest has evolved. The ventilatory impairment is not caused simply by the paradoxical motion of the chest wall but rather by the underlying pulmonary parenchymal injury in combination with the hypoventilation and splinting that result from the pain of multiple contiguous rib fractures. The weak and ineffective ventilatory effort frequently leads to progressive atelectasis and pneumonia. Improved understanding of the pathophysiology of flail chest also has altered the therapeutic focus, with dramatic improvements in survival. The current approach to the patient with flail chest stresses ventilatory support, as determined by the degree of pulmonary parenchymal injury, and good analgesia to prevent the cycle of pain, splinting, and hypoventilation. Using such methods, the mortality rate for flail chest has decreased to 2% in nonventilated patients and 19% in patients requiring mechanical ventilation.

The patient's ventilatory status is assessed at the time of initial presentation. Mechanical problems contributing to respiratory compromise, such as airway obstruction, pneumothorax, or hemothorax, should be treated rapidly. Patients with a flail chest who present with respiratory distress and hypoxemia require immediate endotracheal intubation and mechanical ventilation. If the patient's ventilatory function is initially adequate, aggressive measures to ensure analgesia are undertaken. Epidural techniques are often required, and they should be considered early. The patient is carefully monitored, because the pulmonary injuries commonly progress over the first several hours. Mechanical ventilation should be initiated at the first early signs of impending ventilatory failure, not after the patient is in an advanced state of respiratory compromise.

Vigorous chest physiotherapy and pulmonary toilet are an integral part of the treatment protocol. Usually, the amount of pain experienced by the patient decreases within 72 hours, and the amount of analgesia required is concomitantly less. These patients are continued on aggressive chest physiotherapy and pulmonary toilet under careful observation until their pain is well controlled, their tidal volume is adequate, and their cough has improved. They can then be weaned gradually from systemic to oral analgesia.

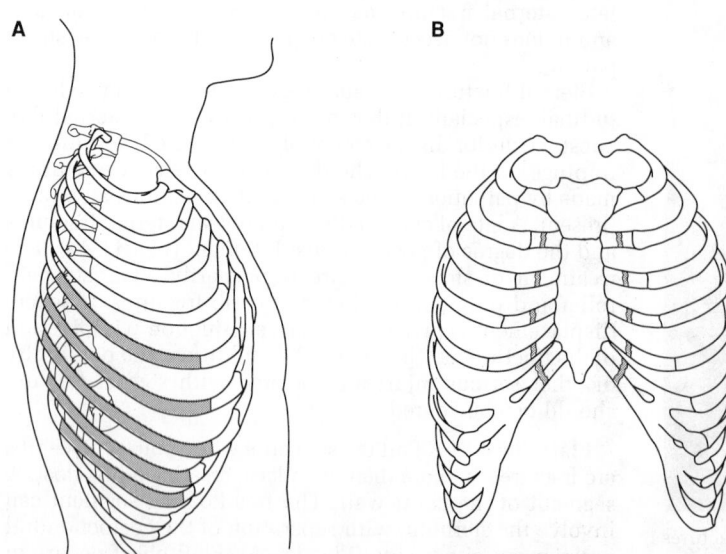

Figure 11-45. Right lateral flail chest (*A*) and sternal flail chest (*B*).

Open Pneumothorax. The open pneumothorax, or sucking chest wound, is an uncommon injury that produces a large chest wall defect and is usually caused by impalement, high-speed motor vehicle accident, or shotgun blast. These injuries can also occur from large lacerations in the chest wall after an assault. The defect in the chest wall allows equilibration of intrathoracic and ambient pressures, leading to collapse of the lung. If the defect is large enough, air flows through the chest wall defect rather than through the trachea and into the lungs with each inspiratory effort. This can result in rapid and profound ventilatory compromise, an immediately life-threatening situation. The diagnosis of a sucking chest wound can be made on simple inspection of the chest wall and hearing the flow of air through the wound. The defect should be occluded with an impermeable dressing, such as petrolatum gauze, essentially converting the situation to a closed pneumothorax. Tube thoracostomy is then performed to reexpand the lung. The chest wall defect usually requires operative débridement and formal chest wall closure. In most cases, closure can usually be accomplished primarily, although large soft tissue defects may require tissue transfer techniques.

Pleural Space Injuries

Simple Pneumothorax. Pneumothorax, defined as air in the potential space between the visceral and parietal pleurae, is a common occurrence. It ordinarily results from a ruptured alveolus or from small lacerations in the pulmonary parenchyma and is frequently associated with rib fractures. Pneumothorax also can result from lacerations through the chest wall (eg, stab or gunshot wounds) and from iatrogenic injuries (eg, misguided efforts at placement of a central venous catheter). The diagnosis of pneumothorax is suggested on physical examination by decreased ipsilateral breath sounds; decreased expansion of the affected hemithorax, with hyperresonance to percussion; crepitus; or subcutaneous emphysema. The chest radiograph is usually diagnostic (Fig. 11-46). In patients on positive-pressure ventilation, the radiologic diagnosis can be somewhat more difficult, and the diaphragmatic contour should carefully be evaluated for evidence of subpulmonic air, the deep sulcus sign.

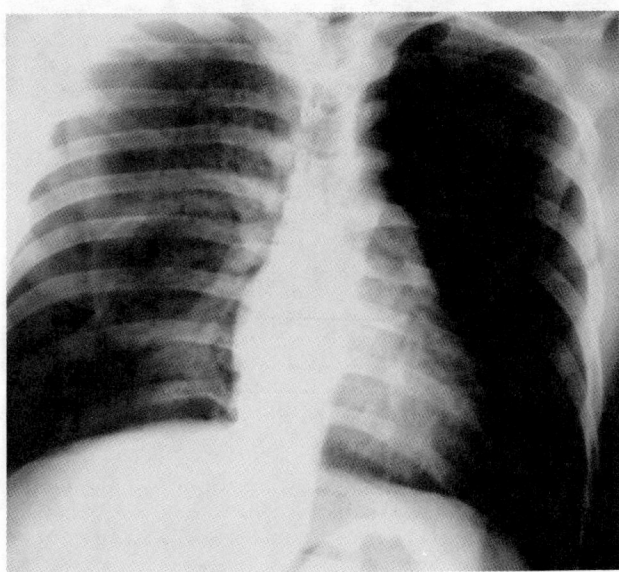

Figure 11-46. Right-sided simple pneumothorax with no significant mediastinal shift (arrow indicates lung margin).

In patients with penetrating trauma to the chest but no pneumothorax apparent on supine chest film, upright posteroanterior and inhalation-exhalation views may improve the diagnostic yield. Patients who manifest no evidence of pneumothorax on upright chest radiograph after 6 hours of observation may be discharged safely.[167]

Traumatic pneumothorax is treated by placement of a tube thoracostomy, as previously described. A large (36F) chest tube should be inserted to evacuate the air and any blood and blood clots that may be present. Patients with subcutaneous emphysema who are to undergo general anesthesia with positive-pressure ventilation should be considered for prophylactic tube thoracostomy to prevent the potentially lethal complication of tension pneumothorax. A chest radiograph should be obtained after insertion of the chest tube to confirm that proper tube position and reexpansion of the lung have occurred.

Patients with small, asymptomatic pneumothoraces not requiring general endotracheal anesthesia or positive-pressure ventilation may be observed carefully without placement of a tube thoracostomy. If the air leak between the parietal and visceral pleurae has sealed, the air in the pleural cavity will be reabsorbed, with subsequent complete expansion of the lung. Serial chest films should be obtained to ensure that the pneumothorax is progressively decreasing and that the lung is not collapsed. Very small pneumothoraces, particularly those from spontaneous bleb rupture or iatrogenic injury, can be drained effectively with smaller thoracostomy tubes, causing less patient discomfort and shortening hospital stay.

Tension Pneumothorax. A tension pneumothorax occurs if the pressure of accumulated air in the pleural space exceeds the ambient pressure, resulting in a net positive intrathoracic pressure. Although tension pneumothorax can occur in patients who are breathing spontaneously, it is most commonly associated with positive-pressure ventilation. Positive-pressure ventilation increases the air leak into the ipsilateral pleural space and can convert a simple pneumothorax to a tension pneumothorax. Mediastinal shift leads to decreased venous return to the heart and compression of the opposite functional lung. Tension pneumothorax often causes severe respiratory distress and hemodynamic compromise.

Patients with tension pneumothorax can have tachypnea, dyspnea, absent breath sounds on the affected side, and hyperresonance to percussion. As the situation progresses, central cyanosis, tracheal deviation, jugular venous distention, and arterial hypotension occur. Chest radiograph may reveal a collapsed lung, a depressed ipsilateral hemidiaphragm, widened intercostal spaces, and a mediastinal shift away from the hemithorax with positive intrathoracic pressure (Fig. 11-47).

Immediate decompression of the affected hemithorax is required in patients with respiratory and hemodynamic compromise from tension pneumothorax. Decompression is most rapidly accomplished by needle thoracostomy, which involves placing a large-bore (14- or 16-gauge) needle through the chest wall to relieve the positive intrathoracic pressure. Historically, the second intercostal space in the midclavicular line was suggested as the site for this procedure, but the anatomic landmarks are rather difficult, and the potential for mediastinal vascular injuries is significant. It is recommended that the needle thoracostomy be done in the fifth or sixth intercostal space at the midaxillary line, in the same position as the tube thoracostomy. The body wall is thinnest at this site, and the anatomy is much less complex. Placement of a tube thoracostomy after needle decompression constitutes definitive therapy.

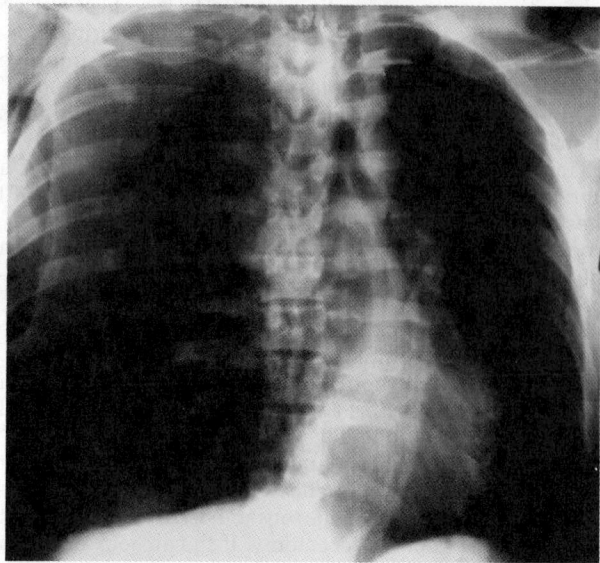

Figure 11-47. Right-sided tension pneumothorax with tracheobronchial and mediastinal shifts.

Hemothorax. A hemothorax is the accumulation of blood in the pleural space, and it occurs in 50% to 75% of patients with severe blunt or penetrating chest trauma. The amount of bleeding is often minimal with small lung lacerations or puncture wounds. Massive bleeding can occur from injuries to larger branches of pulmonary arteries and veins, major rents in the pulmonary parenchyma, or lacerations of systemic arteries. Patients may be relatively asymptomatic or in frank hypovolemic shock at the time of presentation. Patients may complain of dyspnea or shortness of breath. Physical examination may reveal decreased breath sounds and dullness to percussion of the injured side. Supine chest films usually show haziness of the affected lung field or, with massive hemothorax, complete opacification (Fig. 11-48).

The treatment of hemothorax begins with tube thoracostomy to evacuate the blood and reexpand the lung. The pressure of the pulmonary parenchymal circulation is relatively low, and reexpansion of the lung compresses the areas of injury against the interior of the relatively rigid chest wall. This acts to tamponade low-pressure bleeding. In addition, the pulmonary parenchyma has a high concentration of tissue thromboplastin, which probably contributes to hemostasis and sealing of air leaks. Simple tube thoracostomy is adequate treatment for up to 85% of patients with hemothorax.

Massive hemothorax (ie, larger than 1000 to 1500 mL) may require thoracotomy. Efforts should be made to evacuate all of the blood from the chest and to reexpand the lung, which leads to tamponade of the injured lung parenchyma. If reexpansion fails or if the patient continues to bleed rapidly, thoracotomy is required for control of bleeding. Persistent bleeding, at a rate greater than 200 mL/hour for 4 hours, or greater than 100 mL/hour for 8 hours, is also an indication for thoracotomy in adults. If the patient manifests any hemodynamic instability during this period, urgent thoracotomy is mandatory.

Caked or Clotted Hemothorax. In some patients with hemothorax, a clot remains around the lung despite the presence of an adequate, large-bore tube thoracostomy. This clot keeps the lung from completely reexpanding and can cause pulmonary entrapment or an eventual fibrothorax (Fig. 11-49). The incidence of infected, clotted, or caked hemothorax after tube thoracostomy is 5% to 15% in major trauma patients. Although some volume of a hemothorax is spontaneously absorbed over time, a large hemothorax will not resolve without mechanical drainage. The magnitude of the residual hemothorax that would necessitate thoracotomy has never been clearly defined (Fig. 11-50).

Surgical therapy for a clotted hemothorax consists of evacuation of retained clot and decortication of the lung. If done relatively early, before the clot has become organized,

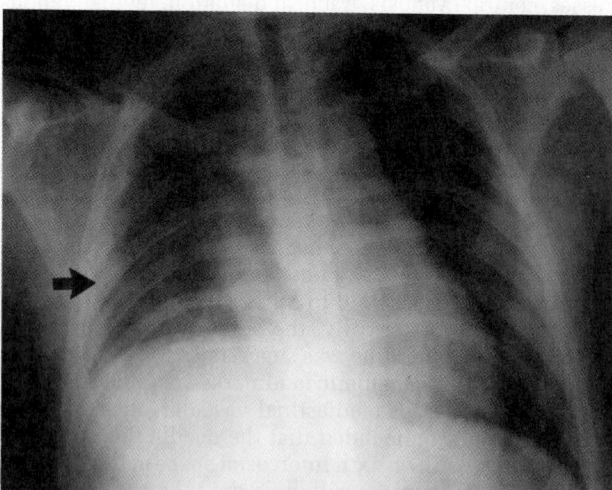

Figure 11-48. Right-sided hemothorax with diffuse unilateral haziness and pleural-based density (*arrow*), indicating intrapleural blood.

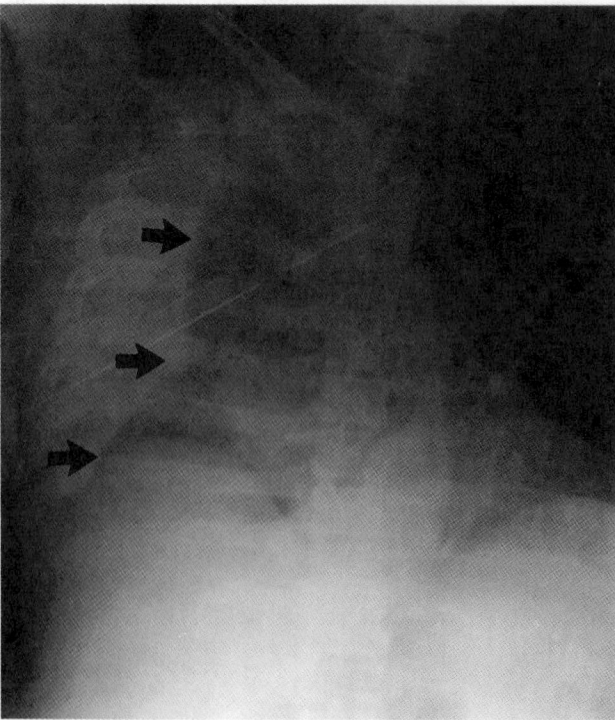

Figure 11-49. Large accumulation of intrapleural blood or clotted hemothorax with compression of right lung (*arrows*).

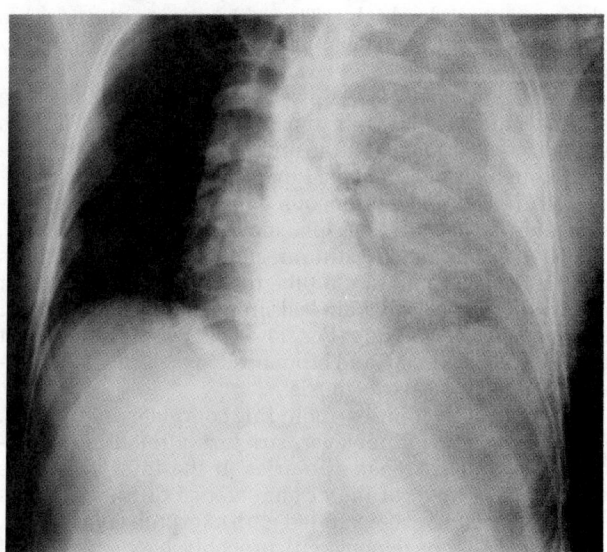

Figure 11-50. Hemothorax and associated massive left pulmonary contusion after blunt chest trauma.

evacuation often can be accomplished through a limited thoracotomy. This is usually well tolerated, with full re-expansion of the lung and discharge from the hospital within a week. After the first 7 to 10 days, removal of clot is likely to require full thoracotomy and decortication, which is a significantly larger operation. Thoracoscopy can offer a promising alternative to thoracotomy for the early evacuation of clot, and successful experience with thoracoscopic decortication has been reported.[168,169]

Parenchymal Injuries

Pulmonary Contusion. Pulmonary contusion occurs in up to 70% of patients with severe blunt chest trauma. It is associated with rib fractures, flail chest, and sternal fractures. Pulmonary contusion involves extensive interstitial hemorrhage within the parenchyma, with alveolar collapse and extravasation of blood and plasma into the alveoli. As a result, patients develop a ventilation–perfusion mismatch, which leads to arterial hypoxemia. Under these circumstances, the hypoxemia is usually refractory to increases in inspired oxygen concentration. In addition, pulmonary compliance decreases, and work of breathing increases. These effects tend to worsen over the first several hours after injury and can combine to produce severe respiratory failure. The diagnosis of pulmonary contusion should be considered in patients with rib fractures and flail chest or with any other severe blunt chest trauma. Such patients must be observed carefully for evidence of progressive ventilatory failure.

Physical examination may reveal contusions over the involved chest as well as the rib injuries previously described. The patient who is unable to meet the demands of increased work of breathing may present with significant respiratory distress. The classic radiographic appearance is that of a poorly defined infiltrate consistent with both alveolar and interstitial edema. These findings on the chest radiograph are present within 1 hour of injury in 70% of patients. The remainder, however, have a delay of 4 to 6 hours before the contusion becomes visible on the chest film. Hypoxemia and significant alveolar-arterial gradient may be evident on arterial blood gas examination.

Treatment of patients with pulmonary contusion is primarily supportive. Patients who can maintain satisfactory arterial blood gases (ie, partial pressure of oxygen greater than 60 mmHg with inspired oxygen concentration of 50%) and adequate ventilatory mechanics (ie, a respiratory rate of less than 24 breaths per minute, a tidal volume of more than 5 to 7 mL/kg, and a forced vital capacity of more than 10 mL/kg) may not require intubation. These patients should be carefully monitored, and care should be taken to provide adequate analgesia for rib fractures.

Patients who cannot sustain adequate respiratory function require mechanical ventilation. Gas exchange can be improved in most cases by use of a moderate level of continuous positive airway pressure. Careful optimization of intravascular volume status and cardiac performance is often required in more severely injured patients, and placement of a pulmonary artery catheter should be considered. The therapeutic goals are to maintain adequate peripheral oxygen delivery with airway pressure and inspired oxygen concentration at the lowest possible levels.

Depending on their size and severity, pulmonary contusions may start to resolve within 48 to 72 hours of injury, but 2 to 3 weeks may be required for complete resolution.

Pulmonary Laceration. Pulmonary lacerations result from mechanisms similar to those causing contusion but require more significant force for blunt trauma. They can also result from bony laceration of the lung after rib fractures, but they are more common with penetrating injuries to the chest. Patients with pulmonary lacerations may have complaints similar to those of patients with pulmonary contusion, but they also frequently have hemoptysis. Chest radiography often reveals an area of pulmonary contusion and hemothorax.

The hemorrhage from pulmonary lacerations is usually from the low-pressure pulmonary system and can be treated with tube thoracostomy and reexpansion of the lung. If the air leak from the tube thoracostomy is large and the lung is not completely reexpanded, the placement of a second tube may be necessary. Bronchoscopy should be performed in patients with large air leaks or hemoptysis, to rule out a bronchial injury.

Patients who have a pulmonary laceration and require positive-pressure ventilation are at risk for development of significant bronchopleural fistulas. If the air leak is very large, conventional modes of volume ventilation may not provide adequate alveolar ventilation. Strategies to improve alveolar ventilation include pressure-limited ventilatory modes, higher-frequency low-volume ventilation, and, in rare circumstances, independent lung ventilation. Bronchoscopic procedures to occlude the distal airway leading to the fistula have also been reported.[170,171] In most circumstances, the air leak eventually closes, especially if the patient can be weaned from positive-pressure ventilation. If a significant leak persists, if the lung fails to expand, or if hemorrhage from the pulmonary laceration continues at a significant rate, thoracotomy may be necessary.

Pulmonary Hematoma. Pulmonary hematoma occurs when bleeding from a laceration is contained within the surrounding parenchyma. The mechanisms of injury and presenting complaints are similar to those for contusion, but hemoptysis is more likely with intraparenchymal hematoma. On chest radiograph, the margins of a pulmonary hematoma are more clearly defined and spherical, in contrast to the diffuse, ill-defined borders of a contusion (Fig. 11-51). The degree of ventilatory compromise is usually less severe than in patients with pulmonary contusion.

Conservative treatment with good pulmonary toilet and chest physiotherapy is the rule, and these lesions usually resolve without therapy within 2 to 3 weeks. During this time, the patient may have intermittent low-grade fever; however, if the fever remains high or increases, the possibility of an infected pulmonary hematoma should be enter-

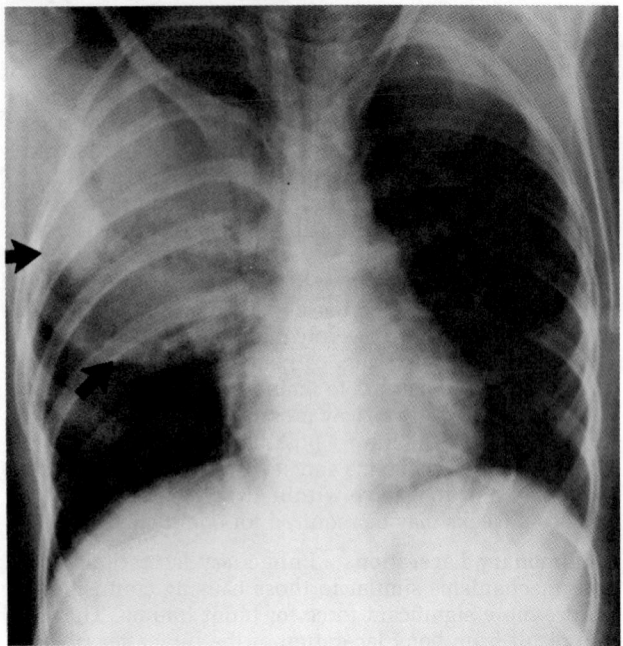

Figure 11-51. Right-sided pulmonary hematoma with well-defined spherical margins (*arrows*), in contrast to the ill-defined borders of a contusion.

tained. Bronchoscopy should be performed to rule out a retained foreign body or clot within the airway. Antibiotics should be started, and vigorous chest physiotherapy should be initiated. A CT scan of the chest may reveal an air–fluid level within the hematoma. Percutaneous placement of a drainage catheter can be effective in resolving infected pulmonary hematomas. If this is unsuccessful, surgical resection may be needed.

Pneumatocele. A traumatic pulmonary pneumatocele occurs if there has been sufficient force to rupture a small airway without causing major hemorrhage, forming an air-filled pulmonary cavity. Pneumatocele is usually well tolerated, but the patient may complain of mild chest pain, dyspnea, or hemoptysis. A chest radiograph reveals a spherical, air-filled cavity that may show a fluid level on upright chest film (Fig. 11-52). Preexisting disease, such as pulmonary abscess, tuberculosis, or other cavitary lesion in the lung, should be ruled out. A CT scan of the chest is helpful in establishing the diagnosis. Because infections occur in fewer than 10% of patients with these injuries, prophylactic antibiotics are not indicated. Conservative management with good pulmonary toilet and observation is the treatment of choice. Resolution of these lesions is slow, taking up to 4 months.

Mediastinal Injuries

Tracheobronchial Injuries. Tracheobronchial injuries from blunt trauma are relatively uncommon, occurring in fewer than 1% of patients with severe trauma. These injuries can result from blunt trauma (eg, high-speed motor vehicle accidents) or from crushing injuries. If significant anteroposterior compressive force is applied to the chest, it causes rapid lateral deformation of the thoracic cavity and results in traction injury of the trachea or main-stem bronchi, usually within 2 cm of the carina. Penetrating injuries to the tracheobronchial tree are most common in the cervical area but can occur anywhere. Clothesline-type injuries can occur in bicyclists, motorcyclists, or drivers of

other recreational vehicles. These blunt injuries can cause transection of the cervical trachea, resulting in airway obstruction.

Most patients with severe airway injuries die at the scene of the accident as a result of airway obstruction. Patients who survive to reach the hospital may complain of dyspnea, cough, or hemoptysis. Physical examination may reveal stridor, and subcutaneous emphysema is almost always found. Chest radiographs may reveal pneumothorax, extensive pneumomediastinum, and air in the soft tissues of the neck. Placement of a tube thoracostomy may result in a continued massive air leak from the chest tube with no expansion of the lung (Fig. 11-53). If so, a second chest tube should be placed, and bronchoscopy should be undertaken to confirm the diagnosis.

Most bronchial injuries, including complete disruptions, heal spontaneously; however, stricture formation is common with more extensive injuries. If the injury involves less than one third of the circumference of the bronchus and the lung can be reexpanded with chest tube placement, conservative management will probably be successful. If the injury involves more than one third to one half of the circumference of the airway, early surgical repair is indicated to prevent late stricture.[172] Persistent large air leak and inability to reexpand the lung may also necessitate surgical repair of bronchial injuries.

A right posterolateral thoracotomy gives excellent exposure to the thoracic trachea and right main-stem bronchus. Proximal left main-stem bronchial injuries can also be reached through this incision. Complete transection of the left main-stem bronchus requires left posterolateral thoracotomy, especially if the transection is more than 1 cm distal from the carina. Primary repair is the goal in most cases, although severe injuries may require sleeve resection of the bronchus or even lung resection. The repair should establish a mucosal closure with an absorbable suture material to decrease the incidence of suture-line granuloma formation or anastomotic stenosis.

Tracheal transection in the low cervical area may be associated with retraction of the tracheal stump into the

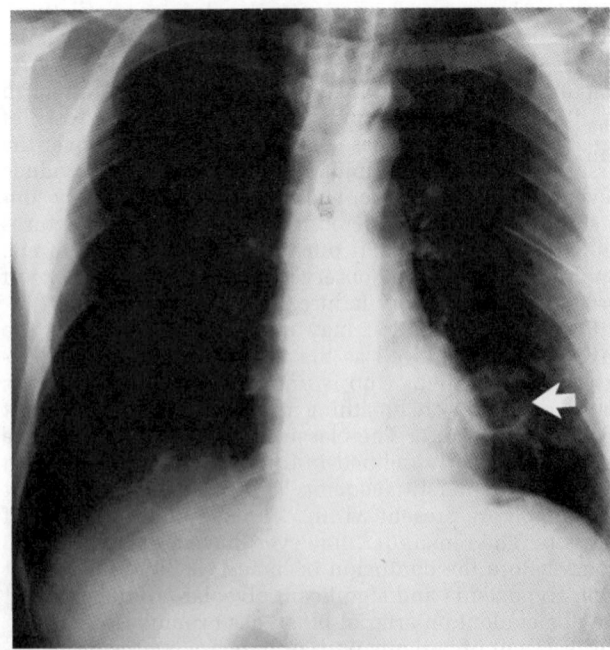

Figure 11-52. Left-sided pneumatocele with spherical air-filled cavity (*arrow*).

Patients with blunt aortic injuries frequently have associated injuries, with head trauma, fractures, and major visceral lacerations being most common. Specific symptoms include severe chest or back pain. The physical examination may reveal fractures of the clavicles, sternum, or ribs. Upper extremity hypertension and asymmetry of pulses in the upper and lower extremities (pseudocoarctation) may be diagnostic. This presentation occurs if the ends of the transected aorta are not in perfect alignment. A careful neurologic evaluation is important, because patients may develop paraplegia or paraparesis from loss of blood flow through the intercostal arteries that supply the spinal cord. The diagnosis of blunt injury of the thoracic aorta depends on a thorough search for it, which should be triggered initially by an appropriate mechanism of injury (ie, deceleration). A chest radiograph is a useful screening procedure. Numerous findings on chest film have been associated with thoracic aortic injury. These include the presence of a widened mediastinum (greater than 8 cm at the aortic knob in adults); obliteration of the aortopulmonary window and an indistinct aortic knob; deviation of the trachea, nasogastric tube, or endotracheal tube to the right; depression of the left main-stem bronchus more than 140 degrees with concomitant elevation of the right main-stem bronchus; and the presence of an apical cap (Fig. 11-54). Aortic injury is also associated with fractures of the first or second rib and with scapula fractures. The finding of abnormal architecture of the mediastinum or aortic knob contour is probably the most reliable early finding on chest film and demands further work-up. An anteroposterior chest film taken with the patient in the supine position tends to magnify the size of the mediastinum to some extent. It is often helpful to obtain an upright chest film, if it is not contraindicated.

Abnormal findings on the chest film, or suspicion of the injury, must be aggressively investigated. Because of the high morbidity of missed injuries, angiography is the diagnostic study of choice in patients at significant risk. It is important to obtain full arch aortography, four-vessel run-off, and a full aortogram to avoid missing injuries at the aortic root, the diaphragmatic hiatus, or the origins of the great vessels. CT scan of the chest has been proposed as a

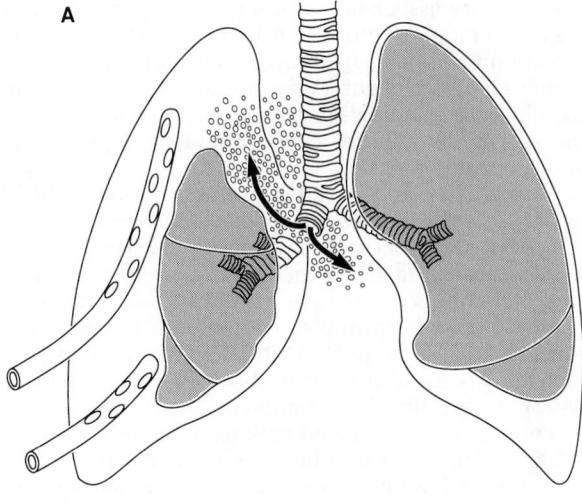
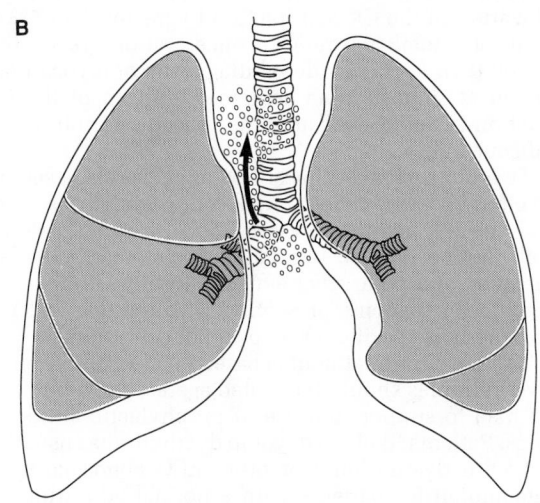

Figure 11-53. Ruptured bronchus demonstrating pneumothorax with intrapleural rupture (*A*) and pneumomediastinum with extrapleural rupture (*B*).

mediastinum. Preparations should therefore be made for extension of the incision into the median sternotomy if necessary. The repair of cervicotracheal injuries is discussed in greater detail in the section on neck trauma.

Aortic Injuries. Injuries to the aorta from penetrating trauma can occur anywhere along its course. Blunt injuries of the thoracic aorta occur in as many as 20% of fatalities in motor vehicle accidents. About half of these patients die at the scene; of the 50% who survive the initial injury, approximately half die within the first 24 hours and 90% within 10 weeks without surgical treatment.

Blunt aortic disruption is associated with the mechanism of abrupt deceleration. Shear forces act on the vessel at points of anatomic fixation, resulting in transection of the vessel. In patients who survive, the hemorrhage is contained by the adventitia and tissues of the mediastinum, forming a pseudoaneurysm. The most common sites are the proximal aortic arch near the aortic valve; just distal to the origin of the left subclavian artery origin at the ligamentum arteriosum; and at the diaphragmatic hiatus. Patients with ascending aortic tears have a high mortality rate and rarely reach the hospital alive. Most patients who present alive have injuries at the level of the ligamentum arteriosum. Injuries at the diaphragm occur infrequently.

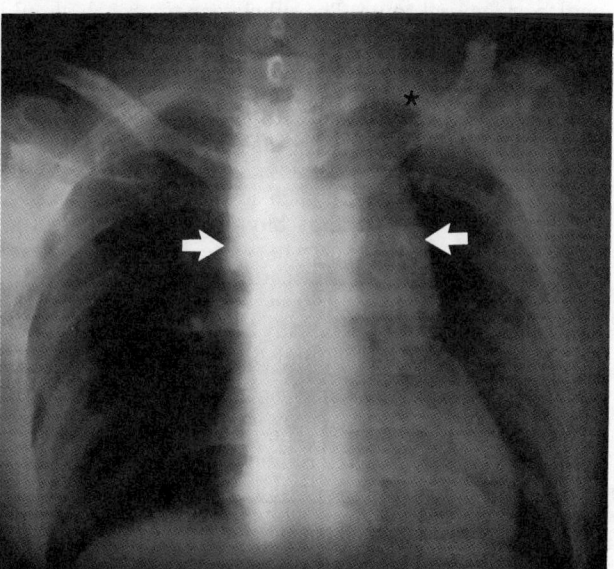

Figure 11-54. Chest radiograph demonstrating wide mediastinum (*arrows*), a left pleural cap (*asterisk*), and obliteration of the aortic notch, all consistent with an aortic transection.

diagnostic alternative, but studies continue to demonstrate a missed injury rate higher than for angiography. CT scan of the chest is not an optimal study for diagnosis of aortic injury because of its axial nature; at best, it provides circumstantial evidence of such injury.[173,174] It has been suggested that CT may be a useful screening procedure before angiography in relatively low-risk patients who have a normal chest film. Transesophageal echocardiography is a promising modality for the diagnosis of aortic injury, especially in patients who cannot be transported to the angiography suite. Early experience has shown transesophageal echocardiography to be a highly sensitive method, with few missed injuries in experienced hands.[175]

Injuries of the aorta require surgical repair. Injuries of the ascending aorta often require full cardiopulmonary bypass for repair, and median sternotomy provides the best exposure. The repair of aortic injuries at or below the level of the ligamentum arteriosum is accomplished through a left posterolateral thoracotomy. Relatively simple injures can be repaired primarily. In young patients, it is often prudent to use pledgetted sutures for the repair. The thoracic aorta has relatively limited mobility, and intercostal vessels should not be sacrificed to facilitate primary repair. More extensive injuries require placement of a prosthetic graft.

The technique of aortic repair has been the subject of some controversy, primarily because of the risk of spinal cord ischemia with cross-clamping of the thoracic aorta. One review[176] showed no difference in the rate of paraplegia (8%) with or without placement of a heparin-bonded shunt to maintain distal flow during repair. The use of complete cardiopulmonary bypass with full heparinization has been shown to increase the mortality rate in patients who have other cerebral and vascular injuries, and it is probably contraindicated in blunt trauma. Most surgeons favor cross-clamping of the aorta with expeditious repair of the injury.

Rapid surgical repair is vital to the survival of these patients. If the pseudoaneurysm ruptures before definitive repair, the mortality rate is extremely high. The preoperative treatment of patients with aortic disruption involves careful control of blood pressure and avoidance of hypertension. An intraarterial catheter should be placed for direct arterial pressure monitoring, and a central venous or pulmonary artery catheter should be placed by an internal jugular or femoral route. The subclavian approach should be avoided because of the danger of entering the mediastinal hematoma. Pharmacologic control of blood pressure is indicated to avoid possible rupture before surgical repair. The use of sodium nitroprusside should be avoided in patients with head injuries because the vasodilatory effect of this drug can cause an increase in intracranial pressure. A short-acting β-antagonist such as esmolol or labetalol is probably the best choice if blood pressure control is needed. These agents are easy to titrate, and they decrease both blood pressure and myocardial contractility, which should result is lower shear stress in the arterial wall. Trimethaphan camsylate (Arfonad) has also been proposed for blood pressure control and offers many of the same advantages.

Myocardial Contusion. The incidence of myocardial contusion is difficult to determine because there is no consensus with regard to its definition and diagnostic criteria. It has been suggested that as many as 75% of patients with major blunt chest injury sustain myocardial contusion, although the incidence of clinically significant findings or complications is clearly much less. Clinically significant arrythmias or pump failure probably occur in fewer than 5% of patients admitted to a trauma center. The mechanisms of injury associated with myocardial contusion include deceleration or crush injuries to the anterior thorax. There are no classic signs or symptoms, although the patient may complain of chest pain and sometimes of palpitations. Physical examination may reveal bruising and tenderness over the anterior chest. Findings of pericardial rubs or murmurs are rare.

The sensitivity and specificity of diagnostic tests for myocardial contusion cannot be determined because there are no universally accepted diagnostic criteria. Findings on electrocardiogram (ECG) that have been associated with myocardial contusion include ST-T wave alterations, supraventricular and ventricular dysrhythmia, and sinus and atrioventricular nodal dysfunction. Right and left bundle-branch blocks have also been observed. None of these, however, is specific. For example, the ST-T wave alterations may also be associated with pain, anxiety, hypoxia, and hypovolemia, all of which are common after severe trauma. Determination of creatine kinase (CK) isoenzymes, specifically the myocardial band (MB) fraction, has also been used to aid in the diagnosis of myocardial contusion. Elevation of the CK-MB fraction to greater than 5% of the total, or a total plasma CK concentration greater than 50 to 100 IU/mL, is considered diagnostic of myocardial contusion at some trauma centers. Elevation of the CK-MB fraction is neither sensitive nor specific for clinically significant injury.

Two-dimensional echocardiography has also been used in an effort to diagnose myocardial contusion. This is a sensitive and specific method to assess global cardiac performance, wall motion defects, intramural hematomas, valvular dysfunction, and pericardial effusion. Positive findings are uncommon in patients presenting with trauma, and none of these tests is specific for myocardial contusion.[177]

The need for treatment is based on clinical presentation. Dysrhythmias should be treated aggressively, but there are no data to support the use of prophylactic antidysrhythmics. Patients likely to develop dysrhythmias usually present with dysrhythmia or other ECG abnormalities. It is uncommon for patients with a normal admitting ECG to develop significant dysrhythmia. Patients with suspected myocardial contusion and clinical evidence of poor myocardial performance should undergo cardiac echocardiography. Patients at risk for myocardial contusion who require surgery for other problems should be carefully monitored, but emergency surgery can be accomplished without significant additional morbidity or mortality. Myocardial pump failure is rare, and its treatment is not specifically altered in the posttraumatic patient should it occur.

Some controversy has surrounded the asymptomatic patient. A typical scenario involves the patient with some chest wall pain after a motor vehicle accident but without dysrhythmia. Stable patients with no evidence of dysrhythmia or other injury that would mandate hospitalization can be monitored for as little as 8 hours and discharged safely.[178]

Cardiac Tamponade. Injuries to the heart resulting in cardiac tamponade can occur from either blunt or penetrating trauma, although penetrating injuries are much more common. The incidence of pericardial tamponade from blunt mechanisms is difficult to assess. Blunt cardiac injuries with tamponade can result from motor vehicle accidents, crush injuries, falls, construction injuries, and explosions. According to autopsy series, about 10% of motor vehicle accident fatalities show evidence of some cardiac damage, and 5% of deaths are from cardiac injuries, but patients presenting alive with tamponade from blunt injury are rare.

Pericardial tamponade occurs after blunt trauma from rupture of a chamber of the heart. This occurs with a severe blow to the chest at the moment when the heart is at end-diastole and maximally distended with blood. The part of the heart most likely to rupture in this scenario is the portion with the thinnest, least muscular wall, usually the right atrial appendage. Rupture of other chambers and disruption of the inferior vena cava from the right atrium can also occur, but these lesions are usually associated with death at the scene. A small atrial injury may allow the patient to survive to be transported to a hospital.

Penetrating trauma is the usual cause of pericardial tamponade, and the outcome is directly related to the character of the weapon. High-velocity, large-caliber weapons or shotguns are predictably lethal. Large stab wounds with free chamber perforation larger than 2 cm are also frequently fatal. Smaller stab wounds and iatrogenic cardiac injuries from central venous catheterization or percutaneous transcoronary angioplasty are more likely to have a good outcome.[179]

The diagnosis of pericardial tamponade should be considered in any patient with penetrating chest trauma, particularly to the central portion of the chest. Tamponade should also be considered in patients with severe blunt chest trauma who remain hypotensive and have no evidence of external blood loss or hemorrhage into the thorax, abdomen, or pelvis. The classic Beck triad, consisting of muffled heart sounds, decreased pulse pressure, and jugular venous distention, occurs in a minority of patients. If the patient is hypovolemic, jugular venous distention may not develop until late in the presentation. Chest radiography may reveal a pneumothorax or hemothorax or be entirely normal. The pericardium is not acutely distensible, and an enlarged cardiac silhouette is not usually seen in acute tamponade.

Placement of a central venous catheter to measure central venous pressure (CVP) has been advocated as a diagnostic test in the hemodynamically stable patient. A very high central venous pressure (more than 20 to 25 cm H_2O) is probably diagnostic, although elevations of this magnitude are usually associated with visible venous distention. Moderately elevated pressures, in the range of 14 to 16 cm of water, require further evaluation. Measurements of central venous pressure are neither sensitive nor specific for the diagnosis of pericardial tamponade, and they are dependent on the patient's volume status and level of agitation. Such tests may be of value, but they must be interpreted with extreme care. Two-dimensional echocardiography is highly sensitive for the presence of pericardial fluid and wall motion abnormalities. If available in a timely fashion, echocardiography is a good diagnostic study to rule out tamponade in the stable patient. Under most circumstances, there is little role for diagnostic pericardiocentesis.

In hemodynamically stable patients with high likelihood of cardiac tamponade, the preferred approach is to perform a subxiphoid pericardial window incision with the patient under general anesthesia (Fig. 11-55). An extraperitoneal approach is made through a midline incision, or a transperitoneal approach is used at the time of concurrent laparotomy. The xiphoid is retracted superiorly or resected, and an incision is made through the diaphragm into the pericardium. This test is highly accurate for the presence of blood in the pericardial sac, and it allows for decompression of the tamponade. Decompression of tamponade through a subxiphoid window may result in significant hemorrhage that cannot be well controlled. Necessary preparations for immediate median sternotomy must be made before a window incision is performed, in the event a cardiac injury is found.

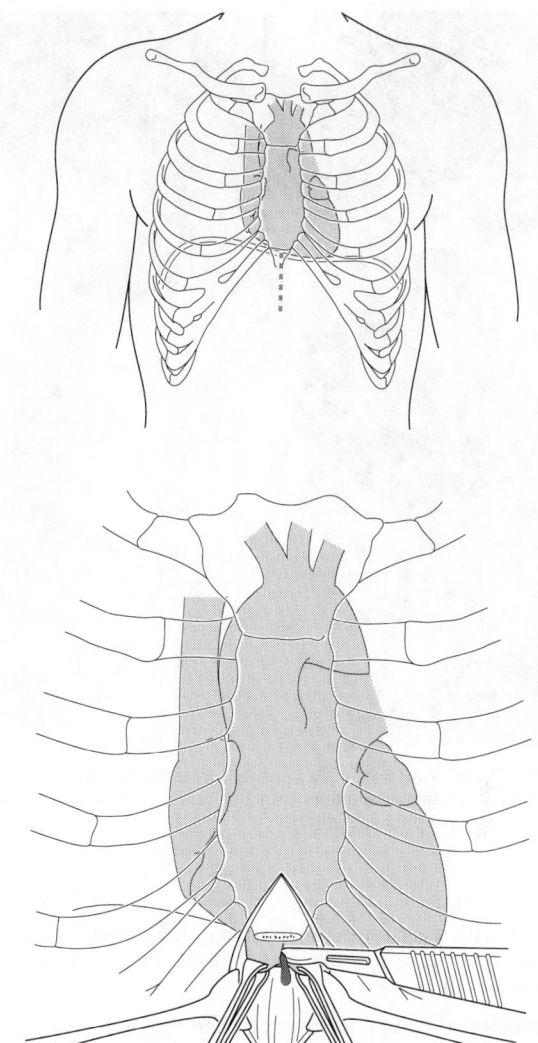

Figure 11-55. Subxiphoid window incision to definitively rule out pericardial tamponade.

Patients with profound hemodynamic instability and a penetrating wound in the left chest or parasternal region should undergo immediate left anterolateral thoracotomy with a wide, longitudinal opening of the pericardium. Cardiac lacerations should be digitally controlled until adequate blood volume is restored and the patient is relatively stable. The use of staples has also been advocated to rapidly but temporarily close cardiac lacerations for immediate hemostasis. Small lacerations in the beating heart can then be repaired using nonabsorbable sutures placed through Teflon pledgets. Larger lacerations may require cardiopulmonary bypass for adequate decompression and repair. The left thoracotomy incision can be carried transversely across the sternum into the right chest to facilitate exposure of the entire heart and great vessels.

Reported survival rates for small injuries to a single chamber are between 60% and 87%, although patients who arrive moribund do poorly regardless of care. The postpericardiotomy syndrome occurs commonly after repair of traumatic cardiac injury. It can occur in mild form in up to half of patients. The more severe form includes pericarditis with fever, malaise, and a friction rub. Pericarditis is usually treated with nonsteroidal antiinflammatory agents. Symptomatic pericardial effusions should be

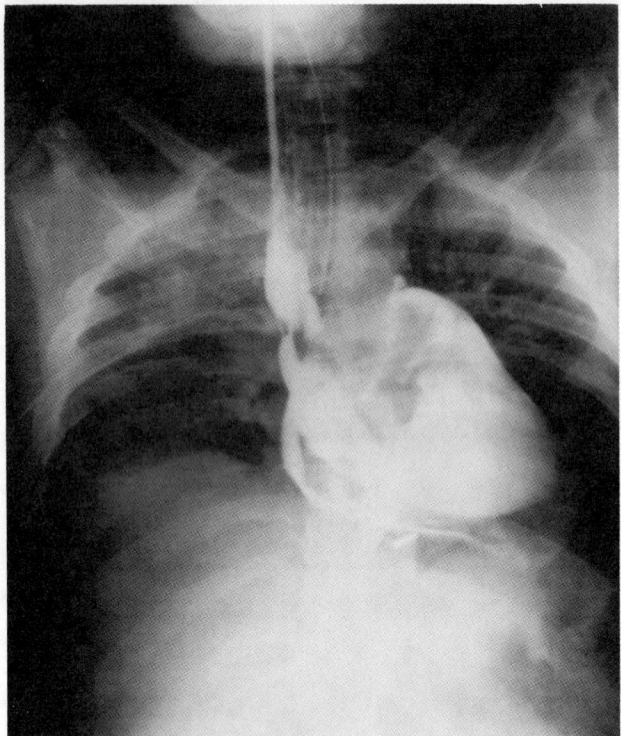

Figure 11-56. Water-soluble contrast esophagogram demonstrating leak from the esophagus into the pericardial sac consistent with a distal esophageal injury.

distend the esophagus. If the initial study is negative, a barium study is then performed.

Esophagoscopy is also of value in the diagnostic workup. Adequate examination requires rigid esophagoscopy under general anesthesia. Flexible endoscopy is not as effective at distention of the esophagus, and it has a high rate of missed injury. Visualization of an esophageal laceration is diagnostic, but a negative esophagoscopy must be accompanied by a contrast study of the esophagus to achieve sufficient diagnostic certainty. Esophagoscopy should be used to follow up suspicious or technically imperfect contrast studies and as a security measure in patients with a high likelihood of esophageal injury. If an esophageal injury is identified, immediate exploration is undertaken.

The surgical approach is dictated by the location of the injury. Cervical esophageal lesions can usually be approached through a collar incision, repaired primarily, and drained widely. This topic is covered more fully in the section on neck injuries. Most injuries of the proximal thoracic esophagus can be approached through a right posterolateral thoracotomy. Injuries near the diaphragmatic hiatus may be more accessible through a left posterolateral thoracotomy. If the diagnosis is made rapidly, most lacerations of the esophagus can be repaired primarily and the mediastinum drained widely. Reinforcement of the repair with a pleural flap or other tissue is recommended (Fig. 11-57). If an adequate pleural flap cannot be obtained, an intercostal muscle pedicle flap can be used to buttress the esophageal repair in a similar fashion. Esophageal injuries at the diaphragmatic hiatus may be repaired primarily and

treated with percutaneous drainage. Recurrent symptomatic pericardial effusions may require complete anterior pericardiectomy.

Esophageal Injury.   Injury to the thoracic esophagus from external force or compression is a rare event and occurs in fewer than 0.01% of patients who sustain multiple blunt injuries.[180] If it does occur, the site of blunt rupture is most often in the distal third of the esophagus, just above the gastroesophageal junction. This injury probably results from an abrupt increase in intraabdominal pressure while the glottis is closed during impact. The resultant rapid rise in pressure causes rupture at the weakest point of the esophagus, similar to that seen in Boerhaave syndrome. Penetrating trauma to the thoracic esophagus is also uncommon and is usually associated with injuries to the adjacent structures. Symptoms include chest pain and dysphagia, and a Hamman crunch may be noted on auscultation of the mediastinum. A nasogastric tube should be carefully passed for gastric decompression and may return blood. Late findings with missed esophageal rupture include subcutaneous emphysema, fever, and shock. The chest film may reveal air in the retroesophageal space, pneumomediastinum, pneumothorax, or left pleural effusion, but it may also be normal.

Esophagography should be performed in every patient with suspected esophageal injury. This is best begun with water-soluble contrast rather than barium because of the problems associated with barium contamination of the mediastinum (Fig. 11-56). Patients who are conscious and alert can swallow the contrast material under fluoroscopy. In unconscious and intubated patients, a nasogastric tube is carefully placed into the proximal esophagus, and 30 to 50 mL of water-soluble contrast medium is injected with pressure to

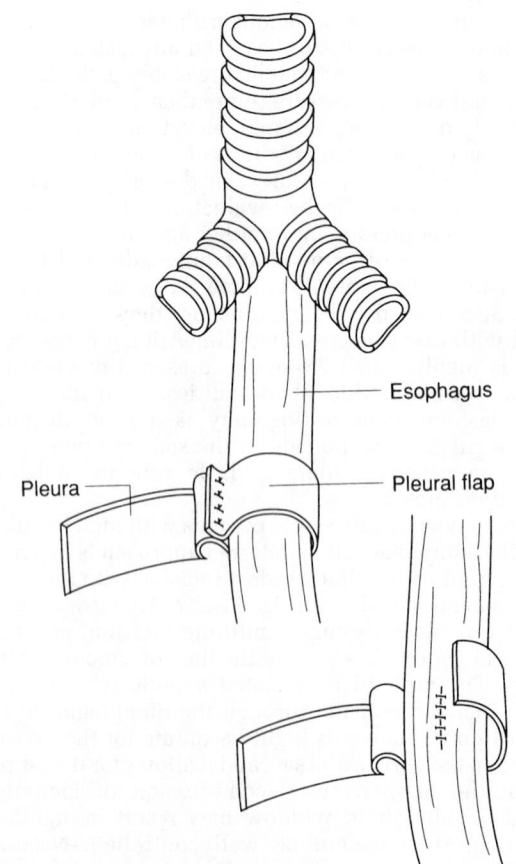

Figure 11-57. Pleural patch reinforcement of primary closure of the esophagus after penetrating injury.

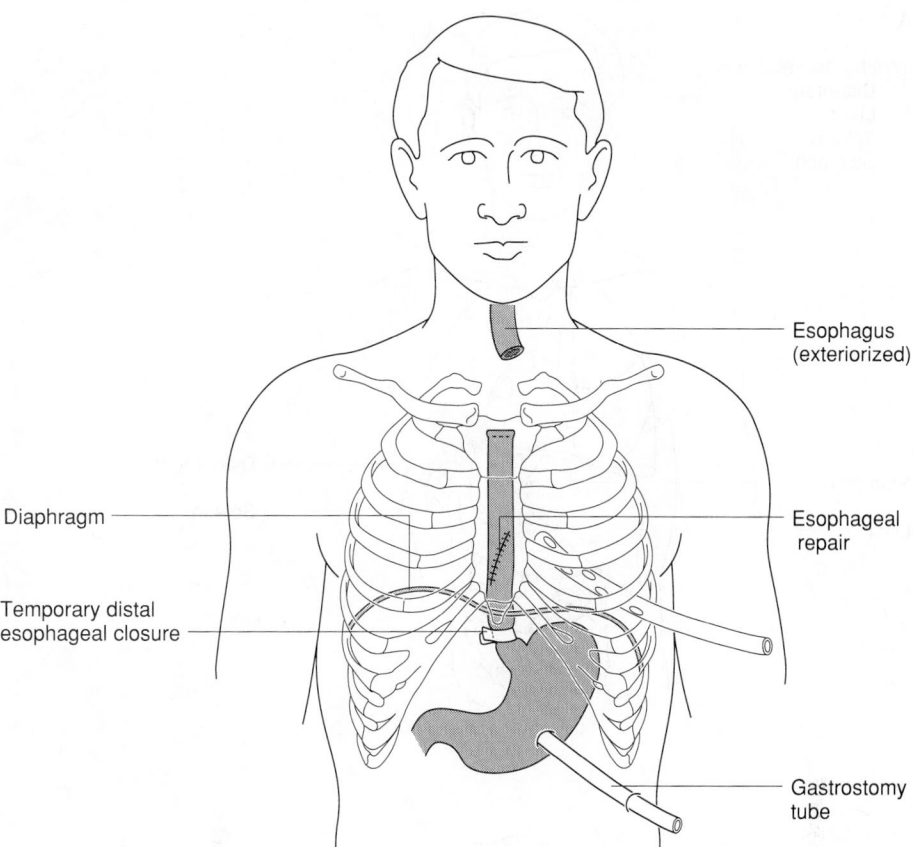

Figure 11-58. Esophageal exclusion including transection and proximal esophagostomy with temporary closure of the distal esophagus to prevent reflux and ongoing leak.

Labels in figure: Esophagus (exteriorized); Esophageal repair; Gastrostomy tube; Diaphragm; Temporary distal esophageal closure

reinforced with a circumferential (Nissen) or partial (Thal) fundoplication.

If the diagnosis of esophageal injury has been delayed, primary repair is probably not feasible because of established mediastinitis. In cases of severe mediastinal contamination, esophageal exclusion with wide mediastinal drainage, cervical esophagostomy, and temporary closure of the gastroesophageal junction with suture or band ligation is recommended. A proximal gastrostomy is performed for decompression, and a feeding jejunostomy is performed for nutritional support (Fig. 11-58). Later reconstruction is required and may be complex[181] (see Chap. 19).

Definitive Care Phase: Abdominal Injuries

DAVID H. WISNER AND DAVID B. HOYT

Most civilian abdominal injuries are caused by blunt trauma secondary to high-speed automobile accidents, although penetrating injuries are common in urban environments. The failure to successfully manage abdominal injuries accounts for most of the preventable deaths that follow multiple trauma. Failure to recognize occult abdominal hemorrhage and to control bleeding from intraabdominal organs leads to significant morbidity, and such injuries account for about 10% of the traumatic deaths that occur annually in the United States.

ANATOMIC CONSIDERATIONS

The abdomen is defined by the diaphragm at its superior aspect and by the infragluteal fold at its caudal aspect; it includes the entire circumference of the torso. Abdominal injury is often accompanied by trauma to other sites, such as the central nervous system, the chest, and the musculoskeletal system. To simplify the initial trauma evaluation, the abdomen can be divided into four areas: (1) intrathoracic abdomen, (2) true abdomen, (3) pelvic abdomen, and (4) retroperitoneal abdomen (Fig. 11-59). With the exception of the true abdomen, all of these areas are difficult to assess by physical examination alone.

The intrathoracic abdomen is the portion of the upper abdomen that lies beneath the rib cage (see Fig. 11-59A). Bony and cartilaginous structures make this area essentially inaccessible to palpation. Its contents include the diaphragm, liver, spleen, and stomach. Each of these organs can be injured when blunt or penetrating impact is delivered to the rib cage. Diagnostic peritoneal lavage (DPL) is useful in evaluating this anatomic area.

The pelvic abdomen is defined by the bony pelvis (see Fig. 11-59B). Its contents include the rectum, bladder, urethra, small intestine, and, in females, the uterus, fallopian tubes, and ovaries. Trauma to the pelvis, particularly pelvic fractures, can damage the organs within, and penetrating injuries of the buttocks can injure any or all of the pelvic organs. Injury to these structures may be extraperitoneal and therefore difficult to diagnose. For this reason, suspected injuries may require adjunctive procedures,

A

Intrathoracic abdomen
    Diaphragm
    Liver
    Spleen
    Stomach

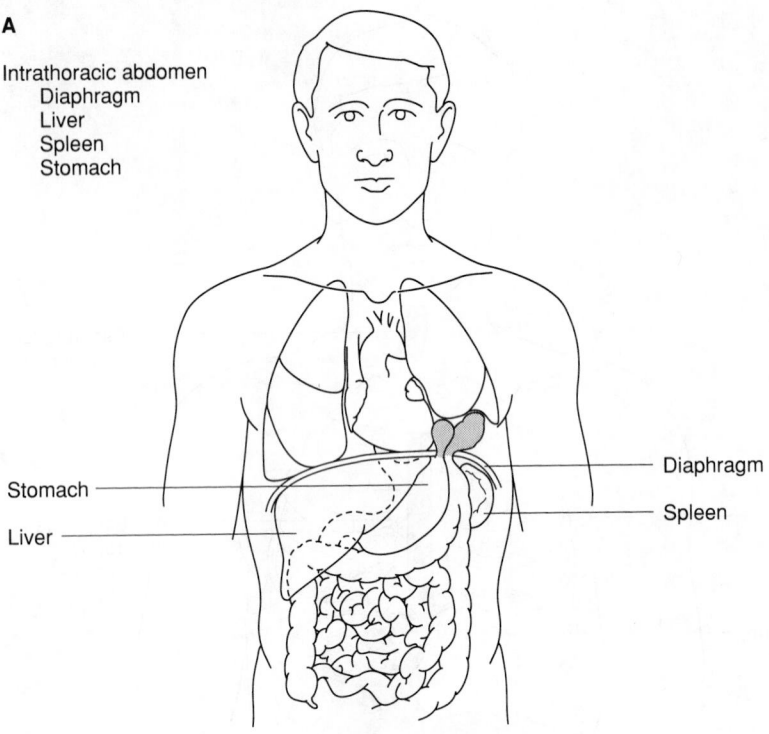

Stomach

Liver

Diaphragm

Spleen

B

Pelvic abdomen
    Urinary bladder
    Urethra
    Rectum
    Small intestine
  In addition
    Uterus, fallopian tubes,
    ovaries (female)

Bladder

Urethra

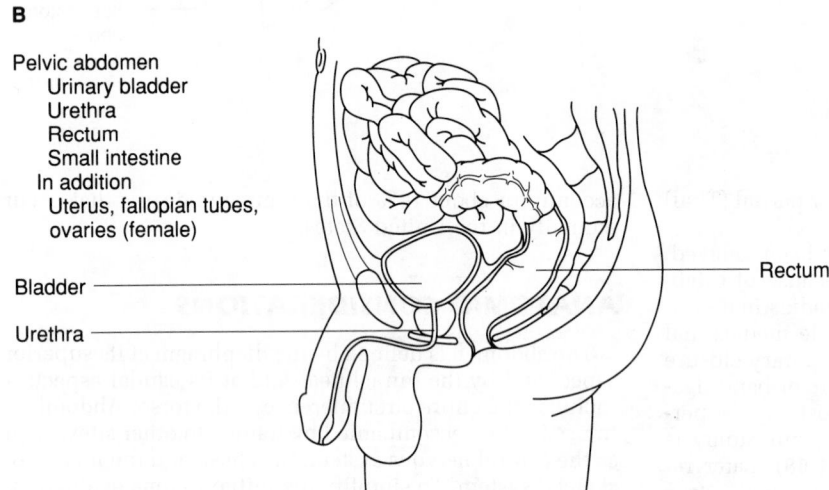

Rectum

C

Retroperitoneal abdomen
    Kidneys
    Ureters
    Pancreas
    Great vessels
    Duodenum (2nd
    and 3rd parts)

Duodenum

Inferior vena cava

Right kidney

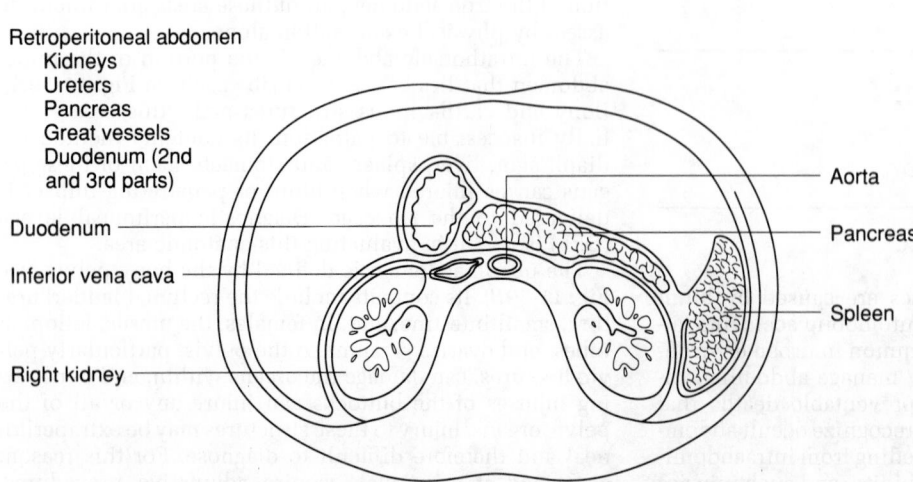

Aorta

Pancreas

Spleen

Figure 11-59. Four traditional anatomic divisions of the abdomen. (*A*) Intrathoracic abdomen. Contents of this area are subdiaphragmatic but cephalad to the costal margin. With respiration, the diaphragm is presumed to ascend to the level of the nipples (fourth intercostal space anteriorly). A ruptured left hemidiaphragm is illustrated with herniation of the stomach and distal transverse colon into the left hemithorax. (*B*) Similarly, the contents of the pelvic abdomen are within the bony pelvis. (*C*) The structures in the retroperitoneal abdomen. The true (intraperitoneal) abdomen contains the remainder of the viscera, and the inventory of its contents is dynamic, depending on body position and respiration (not shown).

such as bladder catheterization, urethrocystography, and sigmoidoscopy, for diagnosis.

The retroperitoneal abdomen contains the kidneys, ureters, pancreas, second and third portions of the duodenum, great vessels, aorta, and vena cava (see Fig. 11-59C). Injury to these structures can also occur secondary to penetrating or blunt trauma. The kidneys can be damaged by injury to the lower ribs posteriorly, and any of these structures can be damaged by crushing injuries to the front or side of the torso. Again, injury to these structures may result in few physical findings, and physical examination and DPL are of little use. Evaluation of the retroperitoneal abdomen requires use of radiographic imaging procedures, including computed tomography (CT), angiography, ultrasound, and intravenous pyelography.

The true abdomen contains the small and large intestines, the bladder when distended, and the uterus when gravid. Perforation of these organs is usually manifested by pain from peritonitis and is associated with significant abdominal physical findings. DPL is a useful adjunct if injury is suspected, and a plain abdominal film can be helpful if free air is present.

PENETRATING INJURY

Handguns are the most common cause of serious penetrating injury to the abdomen. Significant intraabdominal injury occurs in about 80% of patients who sustain abdominal gunshot wounds, but in only 20% to 30% of patients with stab wounds. The frequency of organ injury after penetrating abdominal trauma is shown in Table 11-12.

Injuries to both thoracic and abdominal cavities occur in 25% of patients with penetrating wounds of the abdomen. Patients with penetrating wounds of the thorax may also have significant intraabdominal injury because the bullet can readily traverse the diaphragm. Patients with gunshot wounds to the abdomen and lower chest should routinely undergo laparotomy, because the probability of significant intraabdominal injury is high. Whether selective management or mandatory laparotomy is the best method for treating stab wounds is a controversy discussed later. The difference in injury potential between the two is a function of the higher kinetic energy associated with a gunshot wound.

BLUNT TRAUMA

Automobile accidents are the cause of at least 60% of all traumatic injuries. Table 11-13 shows the frequency with which specific organs are injured by blunt abdominal

Table 11-12. FREQUENCY OF ORGAN INJURY IN PENETRATING ABDOMINAL TRAUMA

Organ	Occurrence (%)
Liver	37
Small bowel	26
Stomach	19
Colon	17
Major vascular	13
Retroperitoneal	10
Mesentery and omentum	10
Spleen	7
Diaphragm	5
Kidney	4
Pancreas	4
Duodenum	2
Biliary system	1
Other	1

Table 11-13. FREQUENCY OF ORGAN INJURY IN BLUNT ABDOMINAL TRAUMA IN ADULTS

Organ	Occurrence (%)
Liver	30
Spleen	25
Retroperitoneal hematoma	13
Kidney	7
Urinary bladder	6
Intestine	5
Mesentery	5
Pancreas	3
Diaphragm	2
Urethra	2
Vascular	2

trauma. Some series list the liver rather than the spleen as the most commonly injured intraabdominal organ; this difference probably reflects the means of diagnosis. Small liver injuries are often detected in patients who undergo CT scan of the abdomen, whereas splenic injuries in adults are more likely to be clinically significant and to require surgical intervention.

Solid organs are most frequently injured from blunt trauma. The sudden application of pressure to the abdomen is more likely to rupture a solid organ than a hollow viscus, and this accounts for the greater incidence of solid organ injury. The more elastic tissues of young people tolerate trauma better than those of older people, and this accounts in part for the differences in injuries between children and adults with blunt abdominal trauma.

PREHOSPITAL CARE

Little can be done outside of a hospital for patients with abdominal injuries. For penetrating wounds, sterile dressings should be applied, and the patient should be carefully monitored. Foreign bodies embedded in the trunk should not be removed because major bleeding can follow. Evisceration is best left undisturbed except for application of a moist sterile dressing and protection of the patient from further injury. General principles of stabilization and evaluation should be followed, including ensuring an adequately functioning airway, inserting intravenous lines (preferably in the upper extremity), beginning fluid resuscitation, and providing rapid transport to a trauma facility. The prehospital application of the pneumatic antishock garment (PASG) for severe intraabdominal hemorrhage is controversial, but it probably provides some additional time to resuscitate and transport the patient to the operating room.

HOSPITAL RESUSCITATION AND DIAGNOSIS

Diagnosis and treatment should proceed concurrently after established protocols, many of which have already been reviewed. A functioning airway must be established, particularly in the comatose patient, before evaluation of the abdomen. If necessary, an endotracheal tube is placed and assisted ventilation begun. Upper extremity, large-bore intravenous catheters are initiated, and resuscitation is begun with lactated Ringer solution. The protocol for initial management has been described. An early rapid assessment of the abdomen is performed.

History

Penetrating injuries present little diagnostic challenge other than the question of whether to explore the abdomen operatively. An attempt should be made to establish details of the trauma event and the weapon used. The blunt trauma assessment can be aided considerably by an accurate history. If the patient was involved in an automobile accident in which the steering wheel was struck or a seat belt was worn, specific thoracic and epigastric abdominal trauma should be suspected. If the patient was restrained, it can be helpful to determine whether the restraint was a two-point lap belt or a three-point shoulder belt. The patient who sustains rib fractures involving the lower left chest has a 20% chance of associated splenic injury; the patient with rib fractures on the right has a 10% chance of liver injury. A compression fracture of the lumbosacral region carries a 20% risk of significant renal parenchymal injury. A relevant history, combined with a directed physical examination, guides the initial assessment of patients with abdominal trauma.

Physical Examination

The objective of the physical examination in abdominal trauma is to rapidly identify the patient who needs laparotomy. Precise definition of specific organ injury is unnecessary because immediate operative indications are usually applicable to any specific organ. These fundamentally consist of significant hemorrhage or perforation of a hollow viscus. Unfortunately, the specificity and sensitivity of physical examination are not adequate to make these determinations. Associated injuries often cause tenderness and spasm in the abdominal wall and make diagnosis difficult. Lower rib fractures, pelvic fractures, or abdominal wall contusions can mimic the signs of peritonitis.

In patients with gunshot wounds, no presumptions should be made about entrance and exit wounds. Their determination is difficult in the emergency department, and unfounded presumptions can lead to inaccurate estimations about the number of times a patient was shot and the course of the bullets. If time permits, radiographs should be obtained to determine the location of any bullets or bullet fragments that remain in the patient. Presumptions about entrance and exit wounds can also lead to subsequent legal difficulties.

Because the primary manifestation of blunt solid organ injury is hemorrhage, the patient should be monitored closely during the initial assessment, and continuing or refractory shock is presumed to result from continuing or massive hemorrhage. In this instance, the PASG should be applied, and further evaluation should be conducted in the operating room. A hemodynamically stable patient can undergo complete evaluation, including physical examination, DPL, and adjunctive radiographic and laboratory studies.

The patient should be examined from head to toe for signs of blunt trauma and for penetrating wounds. Small abrasions or areas of ecchymosis suggest significant local intraabdominal injury. Penetrating wounds should be marked with radiopaque clips to allow radiographic delineation of the injury tract. The abdominal wall and back should be carefully inspected, and posterior ecchymosis should raise the possibility of retroperitoneal injury. The absence of bowel sounds is consistent with an ileus, but it is a nonspecific finding and, in the context of a busy emergency department, it is insensitive for discriminating between patients who do and do not need laparotomy.

The patient's respiratory pattern should be evaluated. Halting, labored breathing may be caused by diaphragmatic irritation or may accompany significant upper abdominal injury. Inspiratory left shoulder pain correlates with irritation of the left hemidiaphragm from bleeding, which is often the result of a splenic laceration.

Palpation can reveal localized tenderness, spasm, or rigidity of the abdominal wall. These findings and the finding of rebound tenderness are consistent with peritonitis and perforation of hollow viscera. Exploratory laparotomy is required for this presumed diagnosis. Suprapubic tenderness and pelvic lateral wall tenderness, which can indicate a pelvic fracture, are assessed in the conscious patient. Inspection of the perineum and urethral meatus for blood is routine to look for signs of pelvic fracture.

As assessment continues, a urinary catheter is placed, and a urine sample is sent for analysis for microscopic hematuria. If there is suspicion of injury to the lower urinary tract, the bladder, or the urethra because of an associated pelvic fracture, retrograde urethrography is performed before catheterization. Rectal examination is performed, and sphincter tone is evaluated. The integrity of the rectal wall and the position and mobility of the prostate are evaluated. The stool should be tested for the presence of gross or occult blood. A nasogastric tube is passed, and gastric contents are aspirated and tested for blood.

The physical findings for injuries to these different structures are often a function of the time interval between injury and examination. Hollow viscus perforations usually require several hours before peritonitis becomes apparent. Colon or gastric perforations produce peritonitis more rapidly, small bowel perforations less so. Because of the wide spectrum of injury, frequent reevaluation becomes an essential strategy in the treatment of patients with blunt abdominal trauma.

Laboratory Studies

Blood studies of value in the initial evaluation of a patient with abdominal trauma include the hematocrit, serum amylase, and plasma transaminase levels. Leukocyte counts, serum creatinine, glucose, and serum electrolyte determinations are often obtained for reference but ordinarily have little value in the early management period.

The diagnosis of massive hemorrhage is usually obvious from hemodynamic parameters, and the hematocrit merely confirms the diagnosis. Iatrogenic dilutional anemia is common and, in the presence of hemodynamic stability, is well tolerated. Urinalysis confirms the presence of microscopic hematuria. For blunt trauma, radiographic evaluation of the kidneys and bladder should be initiated if the patient has gross hematuria, or microscopic hematuria and shock (systolic blood pressure below 90 mmHg), at any point during the prehospital or emergency department course.[182] The serum amylase is insensitive and nonspecific as a marker for major pancreatic or enteric injury. Injuries to the head and face commonly cause increased plasma amylase concentrations. Persistent or symptomatic hyperamylasemia, however, should raise the concern of significant intraabdominal injury and is an indication for aggressive radiographic or surgical investigation. Pancreatic or duodenal injury is best assessed with the use of intraluminal gastrointestinal and intravenous contrast media with dynamic CT scan.

Radiographic Evaluation

Radiologic studies of potential value in the evaluation of abdominal trauma include abdominal plain films, retrograde urethrography and cystography, excretory urography, CT scans, radionuclide scans, ultrasound, and angiography. All injuries from penetrating trauma should be evaluated with a plain radiograph with the use of radio-dense markers on the wound sites to allow evaluation of the missile trajectory. With blunt trauma, an anteroposterior film of the pelvis can delineate pelvic fractures not detectable on physical examination. The initial pelvic film or chest radiograph can also demonstrate fractures of the thoracic or lumbar spine. The presence of a transverse fracture of the vertebral bodies, or Chance fracture, should increase the search for serious blunt intestinal injury. In addition, free intraperitoneal air, trapped retroperitoneal air from duodenal perforation, or loss of the psoas shadow from retroperitoneal bleeding all may be seen. The overall value of plain abdominal films after blunt trauma is limited.

Of greater value are CT scan, ultrasound, angiography, and radionuclide scan. CT has real value in the accurate assessment of solid organ injuries, particularly liver, kidney, and spleen, and contrast-enhanced CT has great accuracy in the delineation of intraabdominal bleeding. The accuracy of CT scan in evaluation of hollow viscus injury is limited, but this is not an obstacle because this limitation is well known. CT is specific in the evaluation of retroperitoneal injuries and is the single most useful and informative diagnostic study for patients with abdominal trauma. Ultrasound for the evaluation of abdominal trauma has been used for a number of years in Europe and has recently gained increased acceptance in the United States.[183,184] There is a learning curve for the use of ultrasonography in the emergency department, but in the hands of experienced personnel it is effective in determining the presence or absence of intraperitoneal blood. Ultrasound has proved better for evaluation of blunt trauma than for penetrating trauma. Further evaluation will establish its ultimate utility. Radionuclide scan has limited value in the early treatment of a trauma patient and is best used for serial observation during nonoperative management of solid organ injuries, such as subcapsular hematoma of the liver or splenic hematomas. Angiography is reserved for specific situations, such as suspected aortic or renal arterial injuries, and is not considered an initial screening investigation.

Laparoscopy has also been used for both diagnosis and therapy in trauma patients.[43,185,186] Published experience is relatively limited, but laparoscopy appears to have a role in the initial evaluation of penetrating trauma patients in whom it is unclear whether the peritoneum has been penetrated. Laparoscopy has also been used with some success to diagnose diaphragmatic injury in patients with penetrating injury to the lower chest. It has been less reliable in the diagnosis and management of hollow viscus injury after penetrating abdominal trauma. For patients with blunt trauma, the role of laparoscopy is still undetermined, and it is unclear whether it will offer a significant advantage over other diagnostic modalities.

Abdominal Paracentesis and Peritoneal Lavage

DPL is a standard technique to detect significant intraabdominal hemorrhage after blunt trauma. Its applicability after low-velocity gunshot or stab wounds is less clear, and it has no place in the evaluation of high-velocity gunshot wounds. Abdominal paracentesis can be used in place of DPL if the suspicion of intraabdominal hemorrhage is high and time is critical. A negative result on abdominal paracentesis is of no definitive diagnostic significance, however, and it is usually preferable to perform formal DPL if there is a need to establish whether a hemoperitoneum is present. DPL, like a paracentesis, is of greatest value in

patients whose physical findings do not clearly establish whether intraperitoneal injury is present.

The specific indications for DPL in blunt trauma include the following:

- Unconscious patient with question of potential abdominal injury
- Patient with a high-energy injury, suspected intraabdominal injury, and equivocal physical findings
- Patient with multiple injuries and unexplained shock
- Patient with major noncontiguous or thoracoabdominal injuries
- Patient with spinal cord injury
- Intoxicated patient in whom abdominal injury is suspected
- Patient who has a suspected intraabdominal injury with equivocal diagnostic findings and who will be undergoing prolonged general anesthesia for another injury, making continued reevaluation impossible.

Relative contraindications include patients with previous abdominal operations, pregnancy, morbid obesity, obvious peritonitis, and exsanguinating hemorrhage. If the patient is hemodynamically stable, CT scan is prudent and, if the patient is unstable, immediate exploratory laparotomy is called for. Children have somewhat different indications, and this is discussed separately.

DPL is not useful for patients with abdominal gunshot wounds, all of whom require immediate laparotomy.[187] If local exploration of a stab wound suggests penetration of the anterior fascia and peritoneum, DPL can help distinguish those with significant and insignificant injuries. It is most sensitive in the diagnosis of hemoperitoneum, but significant hemoperitoneum does not necessarily accompany hollow viscus lacerations.

In blunt trauma, DPL is considered positive if 10 mL of grossly bloody aspirate is obtained before instillation of lavage fluid, or if the siphoned lavage fluid has more than 100,000 red blood cells (RBCs) per milliliter. Evaluation of lavage fluid in stab wounds should be based on a different protocol. In general, more than 1000 RBCs/mL is considered a positive DPL result, and laparotomy should follow.

DPL and CT scan are both satisfactory tests for the diagnosis of visceral injury after blunt abdominal trauma.[188,189] DPL has distinct advantages, including higher sensitivity, lower cost, immediate interpretation, and rapidity (Table 11-14). The major disadvantages are a 1% to 3% risk of iatrogenic intraperitoneal injury and the high sensitivity of the test. The high sensitivity can lead to nontherapeutic laparotomies (ie, when there are no injuries requiring repair). False-positive DPL results are relatively common if an infraumbilical approach is used in a patient with a pelvic fracture. A pelvic radiograph should be obtained before DPL if a pelvic fracture is suspected, so that the

Table 11-14. COMPARISON OF DIAGNOSTIC PERITONEAL LAVAGE (DPL) AND COMPUTED TOMOGRAPHY (CT) IN THE DIAGNOSIS OF VISCERAL INJURY AFTER BLUNT ABDOMINAL TRAUMA

	DPL	CT
False-negative	<1%	5%–20%
False-positive	5%–12%	5%
Time to complete	5 min	55 min
Cost	$125	$900

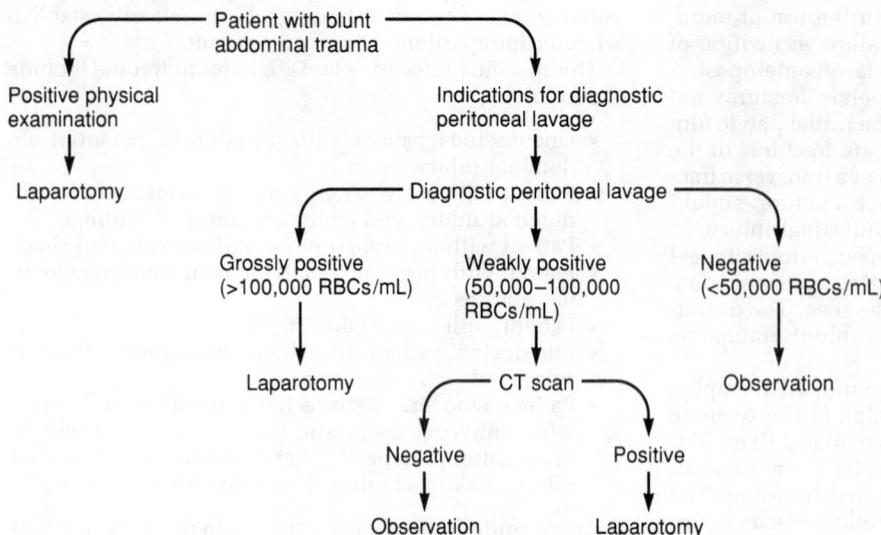

Figure 11-60. Diagnostic algorithm for blunt abdominal trauma.

incision is placed cephalad to the umbilicus. This avoids a false-positive result from traversing of a pelvic hematoma that has dissected into the anterior infraumbilical abdominal wall. Finally, an important related issue is whether every patient with hemoperitoneum from abdominal trauma requires laparotomy.

Before DPL, the bladder should be emptied by drainage with a catheter. The abdomen is prepared with povidone-iodine solution and draped with sterile towels. The lower abdominal midline is infiltrated by lidocaine with epinephrine, and a 3-cm incision is carried down to the linea alba. This is opened, and a peritoneal dialysis catheter is placed through the peritoneum under direct vision. After peritoneal entry, the catheter is directed at a 45-degree angle into the pelvis and aspirated. If the aspirate returns 5 to 10 mL of nonclotting blood, the study is considered positive and is terminated. If little or no blood is aspirated, 1000 mL of normal saline or lactated Ringer solution (or 10 mL/kg in a child) is rapidly infused into the peritoneal cavity. After the infusion is complete, the empty intravenous bottle is placed on the floor, allowing the intraperitoneal fluid to be siphoned into the bottle for analysis.

The general approaches to the diagnosis of blunt and penetrating trauma are outlined in Figures 11-60 and 11-61.

Indications for Surgery

It is the unique job of the general surgeon directing a trauma team to integrate the various specialties involved in the care of the multiply-injured patient. In this regard, judgments about specialized procedures for problems that are not life-threatening need to be made with an overall view of the patient's physiologic status. This requires both important managerial skills and technical skills. With specific regard to abdominal injuries, indications for laparotomy include signs of peritonitis, unexplained shock, evisceration, uncontrolled hemorrhage, clinical deterioration during observation, and, in general, a DPL consistent with hemoperitoneum.

In preparation for laparotomy, certain issues must be considered to protect the patient against hypotension during the early stages of surgical exploration. Vascular access must be secure. Femoral venous lines and large-bore catheters placed by saphenous cutdown at the ankle are options for the rapid infusion of large volumes of fluid. If the patient has lost a large amount of blood, central venous catheterization should be done prospectively. Arterial cannulas should be placed to allow perioperative blood pressure monitoring and sequential blood gas determinations.

Broad-spectrum antibiotics are given as soon as the decision to perform a laparotomy is made. The postoperative

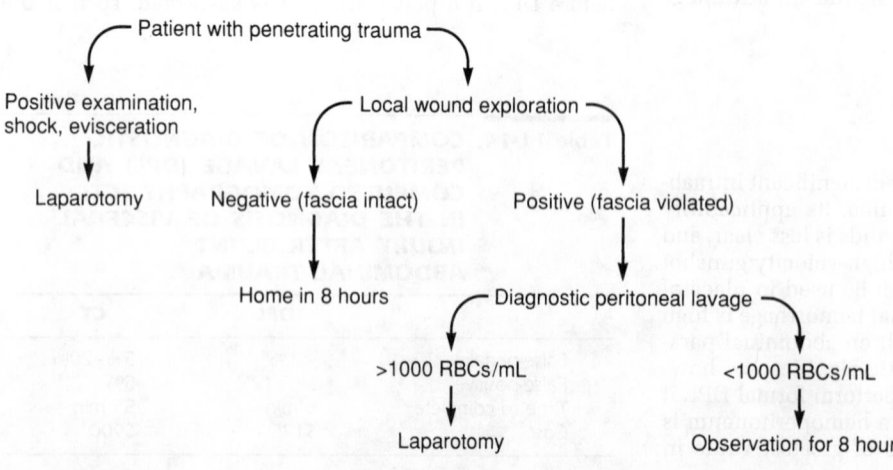

Figure 11-61. Diagnostic algorithm for low-velocity penetrating abdominal trauma.

use of antibiotics is dictated by the operative findings. The spectrum of coverage should include anaerobic and aerobic organisms. Several large studies have compared the efficacy of a second-generation cephalosporin (cefoxitin) compared with clindamycin plus an aminoglycoside (gentamicin or tobramycin) in abdominal trauma. Cefoxitin as a single agent is as effective as any combined treatment. The ideal length of coverage is uncertain. In general, if patients have gross enteric contamination with established peritonitis, treatment should last 5 to 7 days. Patients with minimal contamination can be treated with prophylaxis for 24 hours or less.

Tetanus prophylaxis should be administered, particularly with transenteric gunshot wounds. If fully immunized as a child, a patient is adequately treated with a booster immunization. If adequate childhood immunization is absent, unlikely, or unknown, then passive immunization should be provided with hyperimmune globulin (Hyper-Tet).

Operative Approach

The initial operative approach for abdominal trauma is straightforward. A midline incision is preferred, and there are few reasons to deviate from this choice. In addition, the patient should be routinely prepared from the sternal notch to the middle thigh to allow harvesting of the saphenous vein for any vascular injury encountered. This also allows extension into a median sternotomy in the event that more proximal control of the vena cava or aorta is needed.

After the abdomen is opened, obvious blood and clot is sequentially removed, first from the lower abdomen and then from the upper abdomen, by packing of all four quadrants of the abdomen. If the peritoneal cavity is full of blood, the location of clot is often a clue to the site of bleeding. Any area that is found to be the source of hemorrhage can be repacked. Inflow occlusion can be accomplished, if needed, by clamping of the aorta at the diaphragmatic hiatus. Obvious hollow viscus wounds should be rapidly sutured. This initial closure does not need to be definitive and is done primarily to minimize contamination during the course of the operation. Retroperitoneal hematomas may be the source of exsanguinating hemorrhage if rupture into the free peritoneal cavity has occurred. If not, these can be left for investigation at a later time, depending on the location. Hematomas of the pelvis that are associated with pelvic fractures should not be disturbed. Stable hematomas in the perinephric space lateral to the midline are also best left undisturbed. Central hematomas that can involve injury to the major vascular structures, pancreas, or duodenum are noted and explored after control of injuries within the peritoneal cavity.

After hemorrhage has been controlled by packing and ongoing contamination has been stopped, time is taken to allow resuscitation of the patient's circulating blood volume. Warming is also appropriate at this time if massive blood loss has occurred. Sustained periods of hypotension should be avoided at all costs, and this usually can be accomplished with packing. After the intraabdominal injuries have been repaired, a complete and thorough exploratory laparotomy is performed methodically to investigate the entire contents of the abdomen.

SPECIFIC INJURIES

Diaphragm

Injuries to the diaphragm occur in about 4% of patients with blunt abdominal or thoracic trauma; these injuries involve the left hemidiaphragm in 90% of patients. All diaphragmatic injuries must be repaired to avoid the long-term potential for herniation, incarceration, and strangulation of abdominal viscera. The diagnosis of diaphragm injury should be suspected if respiratory distress and radiologic evidence of pleural effusion are not relieved by tube thoracostomy or if an upright radiograph demonstrates obvious visceral herniation into the thorax (Fig. 11-62). Chest radiograph findings in patients with blunt diaphragmatic rupture are sometimes subtle and may appear only as a blurring of the costophrenic angle or the line of the hemidiaphragm.

Epigastric and low-thoracic penetrating injuries should be presumed to have traversed the diaphragm. During exploratory laparotomy, the entire diaphragmatic surface should be exposed and directly visualized. Linear lacerations can be repaired with a simple running suture or interrupted horizontal mattress sutures, whereas larger lacerations and tissue deficits occasionally require repair with prosthetic material. Frequently, the left side of the medial portion of the defect is directly adjacent to the pericardium, and care must be taken to avoid iatrogenic injury to the pericardium or heart. Exploration of acute traumatic diaphragmatic rupture is usually accomplished through the abdomen because of the high potential for associated intraperitoneal injury. Defects discovered at a later date can be addressed satisfactorily by a transthoracic approach, which facilitates lysis of adhesions. The principal complication of diaphragmatic rupture is visceral incarceration and possible strangulation associated with an unrecognized injury. After surgical repair, specific problems are rare.

Spleen

The spleen is the intraabdominal organ most frequently injured in blunt trauma. Splenic injury is often accompanied by rib fractures on the left because the spleen lies in

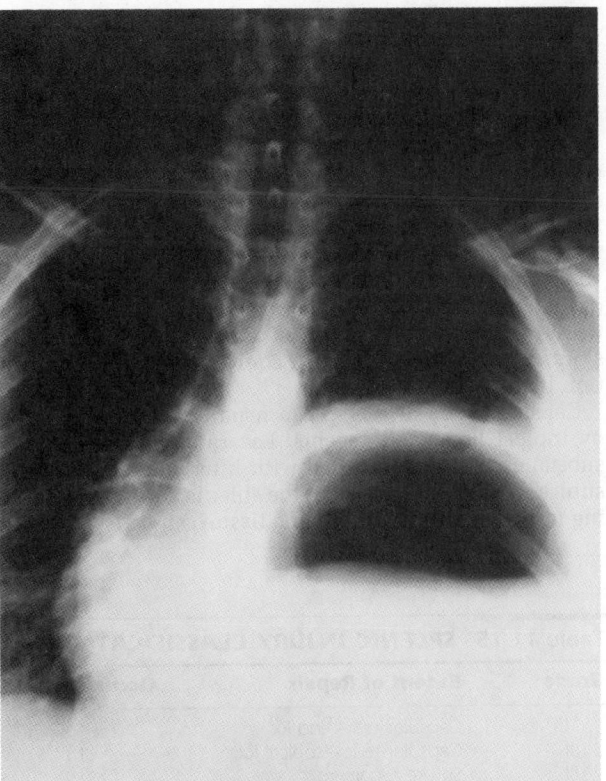

Figure 11-62. Chest radiograph showing gastric bubble in the left chest consistent with a rupture of the left hemidiaphragm.

the left upper quadrant of the abdomen just to the left and slightly posterior to the stomach. Blunt injury is usually the result of compression of the spleen between the anterior body wall and the posterior thorax. The history is helpful if the patient can describe a specific fall or direct blow to the left chest, flank, or abdomen. For penetrating trauma, a wound entry or exit in this area should raise the suspicion of splenic injury. The clinical signs may be few and subtle; a high level of suspicion must be maintained simply on the basis of mechanism of injury. Clinical evidence of splenic injury includes signs of blood loss, left upper quadrant abdominal pain or tenderness, and pain referred to the left shoulder.

In general, laboratory studies are of limited help. Leukocytosis and decreased hematocrit are present, but neither is specific for splenic injury. Plain abdominal films may show enlargement of the splenic shadow and medial displacement of the stomach. Radionuclide scan and CT scan reveal significant splenic injury, the CT scan being both more sensitive and more specific. DPL confirms a hemoperitoneum, if present, with splenic injury.

The management of splenic trauma has been the subject of major reexamination in the past 15 years. Historically, splenic injury was routinely treated with splenectomy. With increased appreciation of the danger of postsplenectomy sepsis (incidence, 0.5% to 5%; mortality rate, 50%), splenic salvage procedures and the nonoperative management of splenic injuries have become well accepted, although not uniformly endorsed. This is particularly true in children (discussed later). An individualized and possibly nonoperative approach in adults allows salvage of a substantial number of spleens in hemodynamically stable patients, but no compelling evidence indicates that this approach is clearly superior. Potential disadvantages include prolonged hospitalization and possibly more exposure to transfused blood, but the principal risk for the nonoperative approach is that significant associated intraperitoneal injuries may be missed. This remains a controversial area. The spectrum of splenic injury varies from a simple laceration or contusion without capsular disruption to total fragmentation. The classification of splenic injury may be relevant to the discussion of operative versus nonoperative therapy (Table 11-15).

The spleen is evaluated for hemorrhage during the course of laparotomy. If hemorrhage is noted, a decision must be made regarding splenic salvage. This assessment requires complete mobilization of the spleen from its attachments (see Pancreas), and care must be taken to prevent further injury. After the spleen is mobilized, the tail of the pancreas is released from the posterior retroperitoneum, and the spleen is delivered into the abdominal incision. Ongoing bleeding can be controlled during mobilization by manual compression.

Capsular tears of the spleen usually can be controlled by topical hemostatic agents. Lacerations of the splenic substance can be controlled with interlocking absorbable sutures. Major lacerations of the splenic substance involving less than half of the splenic tissue can be treated with

segmental splenic resection. Splenic salvage should not be attempted if the patient has protracted hypotension or other severe injuries or if undue delays are encountered in the attempt to repair the spleen. With penetrating injury, damage to adjacent structures, such as the stomach, pancreas, colon, and diaphragm, must be anticipated and investigated. The nonoperative management of splenic trauma in adults is most attractive if the patient is hemodynamically stable and has no other signs of abdominal injury. Nonoperative management is successful in such circumstances about 90% of the time in adults, and even more often in children. A noninvasive test, such as a CT scan, should be performed, and the patient should be observed clinically with repeat scans as indicated.

Complications after splenectomy include early transient thrombocytosis, which usually resolves spontaneously within 2 or 3 months. Anticoagulation is neither necessary nor helpful. Delayed hemorrhage, pancreatitis, and subphrenic abscess also may occur. Subphrenic abscess is primarily related to associated hollow viscus injuries and is uncommon after blunt trauma. Drainage of the subphrenic space should not be done; it is associated with an increased rather than decreased incidence of abscess.

Postsplenectomy Sepsis

Fatal pneumococcal septicemia after splenectomy was first noted 40 years ago in children. This postsplenectomy sepsis syndrome is caused by failure to clear one of several encapsulated bacteria in the absence of the spleen. The incidence varies from 0.5% to as much as 12% or 15%, depending on age and the underlying disease. The incidence is inversely related to age and is higher with underlying hematologic disorders such as lymphoma or thalassemia. The incidence of life-threatening sepsis in adult trauma patients is low, but it is higher than in the normal population. The overall clinical significance is not easily defined. Concern about the possibility of postsplenectomy sepsis should not obscure the fact that the initial priority is to arrest hemorrhage and deal with the patient's immediately life-threatening injuries.

Certainly in children and possibly in adults, efforts at splenic salvage are appropriate. If splenectomy is performed, postoperative follow-up is essential. Immunization with the polyvalent pneumococcal vaccine is required, and booster immunization should be done every 3 years. In addition, prophylactic antibiotics, usually oral penicillin, should be given any time the patient is undergoing instrumentation, such as during dental repair or surgery, and should probably be given prophylactically as well. Such patients should be advised of their increased potential for postsplenectomy sepsis and should carry an identification card to alert health care workers of this possibility if they have an infection. All infections should be considered emergencies and treated aggressively with intravenous antibiotics in the hospital.

Liver

The liver is the largest organ in the abdominal cavity and is commonly damaged in blunt and penetrating abdominal trauma as well as in thoracoabdominal injuries. Some series have found that the incidence of liver injuries exceeds that of injuries to the spleen. Regardless, the two together account for about 75% of all blunt intraabdominal injuries. Trauma sufficient to lacerate the liver is often associated with injuries to other organs. Spontaneous hemostatic mechanisms are sufficiently effective that about 85% of patients with liver injuries are not actively bleeding at the time of laparotomy, and these injuries are predictably well tolerated. At laparotomy, most liver injuries require no

---

Table 11-15. SPLENIC INJURY CLASSIFICATION

Grade	Extent of Repair	Occurrence (%)
I	Capsular tear—no Rx	6
II	Capsular tear—topical Rx	15
III	Suture repair	19
IV	Partial splenectomy	11
V	Splenectomy	49

specific therapy, and drainage is usually unnecessary. Those injuries that do require definitive surgical care present a complex and life-threatening series of problems.

Patients with significant liver injuries usually have a history of major blunt energy transfer to the right thorax or upper abdomen. Physical findings may be minimal because early bleeding may not cause peritoneal irritation or abdominal distention. Any patient with unexplained hypotension after blunt abdominal trauma must be considered at risk for a severe liver injury. Likewise, major liver injury should be suspected if a patient has a history of shock at the scene after blunt trauma. DPL is most helpful in establishing the diagnosis of hemoperitoneum, and if lavage results are positive, laparotomy is appropriate. In hemodynamically stable patients and in those with a contraindication to DPL, CT scan is precise in evaluating subcapsular hematomas, lacerations, and other hepatic parenchymal injuries. The possibility of injuries to other organs should lead to laparotomy in the event of a positive CT scan.

Injuries vary from simple capsular tears and nonbleeding lacerations, to complex fractures with lobar destruction and extensive parenchymal disruption, to bile duct disruption, to hepatic artery and venous injuries. The type of injury dictates the character of the surgical therapy required. The principles of liver injury management are the same regardless of the severity of injury. They involve control of bleeding, removal of devitalized tissue, and establishment of adequate drainage.

Simple lacerations that have stopped bleeding at the time of surgery do not require drainage unless they are deep into the parenchyma, in which case they have a high probability of postoperative biliary leakage. Subcapsular hematomas can be simply evacuated or left intact if there is no associated parenchymal injury. Lacerations that con-

tinue to bleed despite attempts at local control require exploration of the liver wound. The depths of the liver wound are explored, and specific vessels and biliary radicals are individually ligated.

In the event that bleeding continues despite segmental ligation of parenchymal vessels, the structures of the porta hepatis should be compressed as a diagnostic maneuver (Pringle maneuver; Fig. 11-63) If the bleeding stops as a result of this maneuver, it is presumed to originate from the portal veins or the hepatic artery. If the bleeding continues, it is presumed to arise principally from the hepatic veins or inferior vena cava, although this distinction is seldom clearcut in the operating room. The portal triad can also be intermittently occluded with this maneuver to allow improved visualization during placement of sutures as parenchymal vessels are ligated. If selective parenchymal ligation fails, ligation of the hepatic artery is an alternative if the trial Pringle occlusion has had a salutary effect. This can occasionally produce dramatic hemostasis without subsequent liver failure. The vessel is usually occluded as close to the liver injury as possible, and after initial efforts at hemostasis have failed.

An alternative for deep lacerations with persistent bleeding is resectional débridement of the involved segment of the liver. This is accomplished by the finger fracture technique, removing devitalized liver or an appropriate portion of the liver up to and including formal lobectomy. This is required in about 5% to 8% of all patients with liver injuries. Subsegmental resection may be adequate; if segmentectomy or lobectomy is required, a knowledge of the anatomy is imperative so as not to compromise inflow or outflow of the remaining segments. This decision should be made early in the exploration, the blood bank notified, adequate help procured, and exposure obtained. Exposure is best accomplished by complete division of the capsular

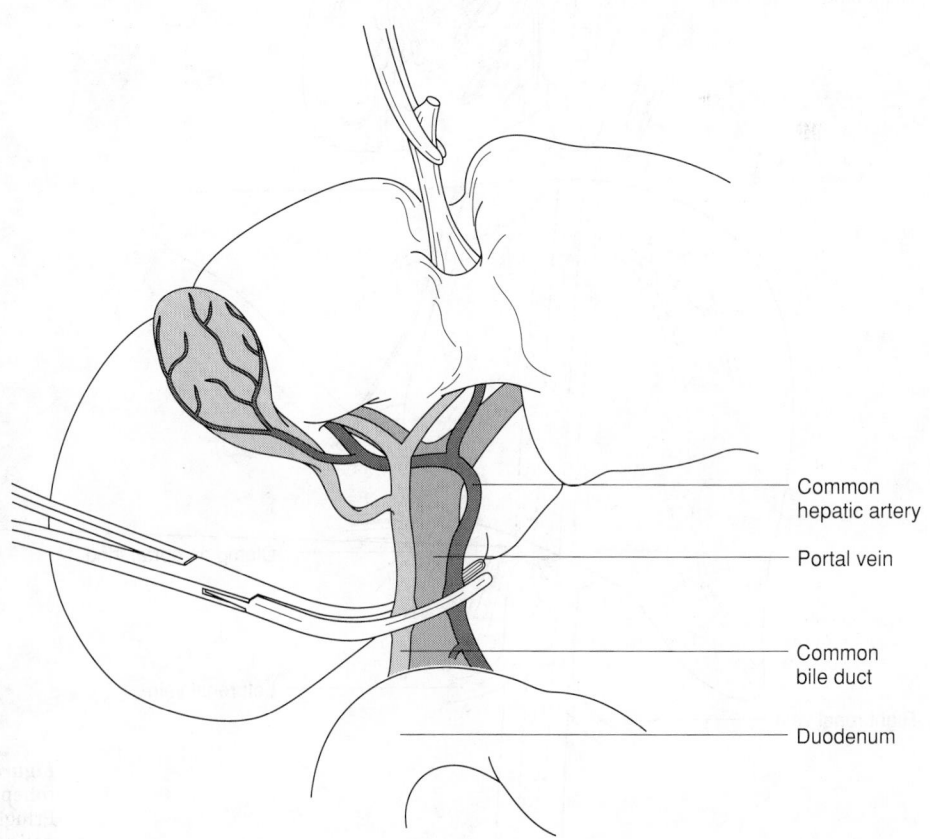

Figure 11-63. Pringle maneuver compression of the portal triad structures with a noncrushing vascular clamp for hepatic inflow control.

Common hepatic artery

Portal vein

Common bile duct

Duodenum

attachments of the liver. Parenchymal débridement and division is done after formal dissection of the porta hepatis. This is an alternative associated with operative mortality rates usually in the range of 10%.

In the event that parenchymal or hepatic vein bleeding cannot be controlled and the patient remains difficult to resuscitate, is hypothermic, and has a coagulopathy from massive transfusion, packing of the injury and further resuscitation after the abdomen is closed is appropriate. Subsequent operative removal of the packs 24 to 72 hours later can be accompanied by resection and suture ligation in a stable, resuscitated patient. After hemostasis has been achieved, the area should be drained. Either sump drainage or wide open drainage can be used. Packing has been enthusiastically advocated in the last 5 to 10 years, and good results suggest that it should be considered early in the treatment of this group of complex patients.

Inability to control bleeding by any of the previously described techniques suggests significant retrohepatic vena cava bleeding or bleeding from the hepatic veins. If bleeding is unilobar, débridement and resection may be sufficient. With bilobar involvement or uncontrollable hemorrhage from a single lobe, early consideration should

be given to the placement of an intracaval shunt or complete vascular isolation[190] (Fig. 11-64). To accomplish this, the midline laparotomy incision is extended into the chest, either by a right anterior thoracotomy or, preferably, by a median sternotomy. Infrahepatic (cephalad to the renal veins) and suprahepatic (usually intrapericardial) control of the vena cava is obtained. A shunt or other large conduit is then inserted through a right atrial pursestring into the vena cava, and vascular occlusion around the conduit at these sites is obtained. The resultant vascular isolation is always imperfect but may allow better visualization of hepatic vein and vena cava lacerations for direct suture ligation or repair. Total venous occlusion may be equally effective and serves the same general purpose. The risk of hypotension is significant with either approach. With the former, significant blood loss is inevitable during a trial cannulation. With the latter, diminished venous return to the right atrium is always a result. This is such an unusual injury that personal preference dictates the approach.

The major complications after liver injury include hemorrhage, respiratory insufficiency, coagulopathy, hypoglycemia, biliary fistula or other bile duct injury, hemobilia, and subdiaphragmatic or intraparenchymal abscess forma-

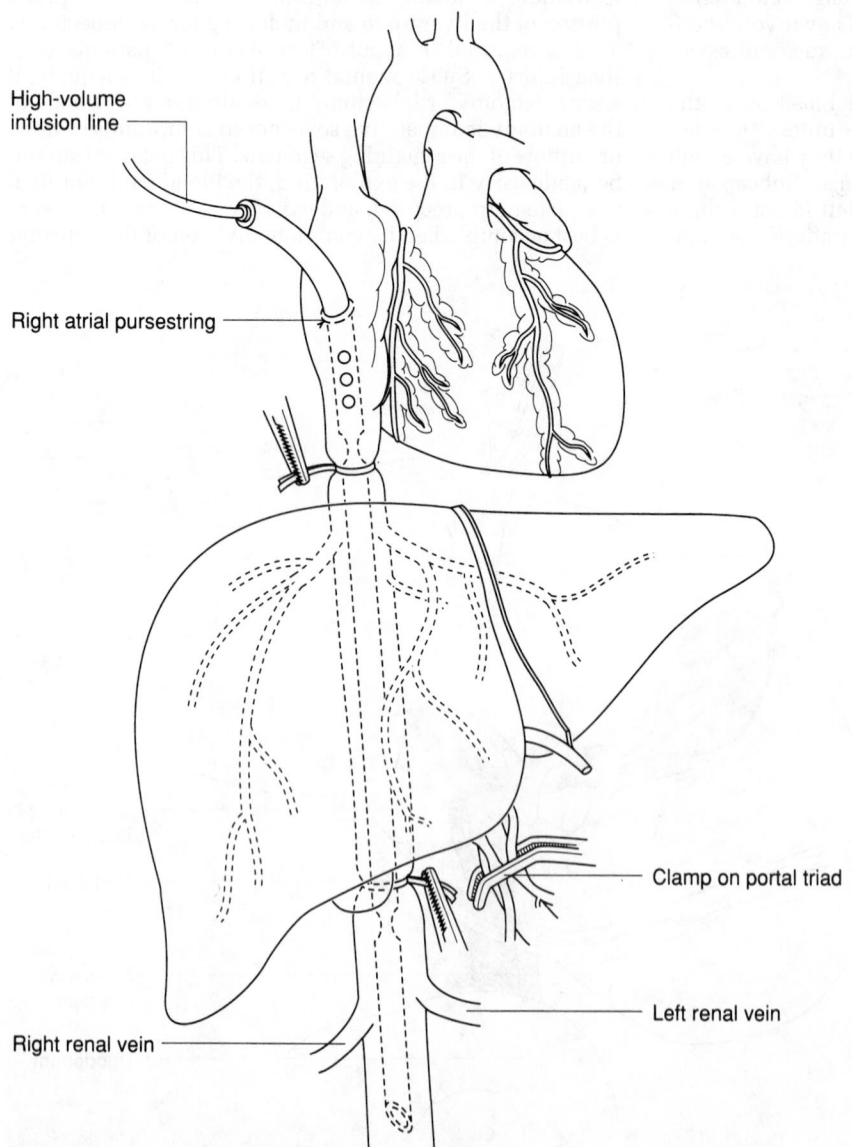

High-volume infusion line

Right atrial pursestring

Clamp on portal triad

Left renal vein

Right renal vein

Figure 11-64. Intracaval shunt used for retrohepatic venous injuries, combined with a Pringle maneuver for isolation of the retrohepatic vena cava for operative repair.

tion. The coagulopathy after liver resection is usually the result of hypothermia and inadequate replacement of blood components. Patients undergoing major hepatic resection after trauma need continuous glucose infusion, often 10% dextrose, during the early postoperative period. Hypoalbuminemia is not common and does not usually require albumin administration. It should be treated simply with aggressive nutritional support unless hemodynamic consequences arise. Hyperbilirubinemia is transient and usually peaks in 2 to 3 weeks after major resection; it usually does not exceed 10 mg/dL. Intrahepatic and subphrenic abscesses can develop, particularly if significant débridement has been necessary. These are diagnosed by clinical evidence of sepsis combined with ultrasound or CT scan. Biliary fistulas usually close spontaneously, and major extrahepatic ductal injuries are rare. A T-tube placed in an otherwise normal common bile duct is inappropriate unless the extrahepatic biliary tree is injured. Hemobilia is a rare complication presenting with intrahepatic bleeding into the bile ducts and is best diagnosed with angiography or endoscopy. Angiographic embolization is the treatment of choice.

Stomach

The stomach is vulnerable to penetrating injuries of the upper abdomen and lower chest. The upper abdominal viscera underlie the lower ribs to a level as high as the fourth intercostal space. The stomach is injured in 5% to 10% of patients with penetrating abdominal trauma. The location of external wounds should lead to the initial suspicion of gastric injury. As with injuries to other intraabdominal viscera, physical examination of the abdomen often points to the presence of injury. It is difficult to differentiate between gastric injuries and injuries to other intraabdominal viscera based on palpation of the abdomen alone, but a physical examination that is positive for peritoneal signs mandates expeditious abdominal exploration. Precise preoperative characterization of injuries is not necessary. Hematemesis or blood found on aspiration of the stomach with a nasogastric tube are other findings suggestive of gastric injury. Although many patients with blood in the stomach after penetrating abdominal trauma have a gastric injury, the absence of these signs does not rule out such an injury.

Abdominal exploration is begun by a standard upper midline incision. Adequate diagnosis requires mobilization and visualization of the entire stomach. Most of the anterior surface of the stomach can be adequately visualized without extensive mobilization. Visualization is facilitated if the edge of the greater curve of the stomach is grasped, either with the fingers or with several Babcock clamps, and the stomach is pulled down into the operative field. For greater traction, the Babcock clamps can be used to grasp the nasogastric tube through the stomach wall. If the clamps are placed far apart, this maneuver can also be used to spread out the stomach so that the entire surface can be seen. It is also helpful to place a nasogastric tube and empty the stomach with suction.

Exposure of the anterior surface of the gastroesophageal junction can be difficult if the flare of the costal margin is narrow or if the left lobe of the liver is in the way. Improved exposure is accomplished with extension of the midline incision as high as possible by creating a paraxiphoid extension. The left hepatic lobe is retracted to the right after division of the left triangular ligament, as would be done for exposure of the gastroesophageal junction for performance of a vagotomy or antireflux procedure. Finally, mobilization of the gastroesophageal junction, encirclement with a tape or drain, and caudal traction into the operative

field allow for improved visualization and the performance of any necessary repairs.

The posterior wall of the stomach should be examined for the presence of injuries. This is especially true if there is an injury on the anterior surface. The posterior stomach is exposed by opening the gastrocolic ligament. This can be done bluntly if the hole is made to the left of the midline about halfway between the stomach and the transverse colon in a relatively avascular area. The lesser sac is entered, and the posterior wall of the stomach can then be seen (Fig. 11-65).

As with exposure of the anterior surface, the greater curve of the stomach should be grasped. By lifting of the greater curve superiorly and out into the wound, the posterior wall of the stomach can be displayed and visualized. If necessary, the attachments of the gastrohepatic and gastrocolic ligaments to the lesser and greater curvature, respectively, should be cleared to rule out an underlying injury. The excellent blood supply of the stomach allows this to be done with minimal risk of devascularization.

Injuries to the stomach are usually easy to repair. Most can be repaired primarily in two layers, with an inner running layer of 3-0 or 4-0 absorbable sutures followed by an outer layer of 3-0 or 4-0 permanent Lembert sutures. Because of the ample blood supply and large lumen of the stomach in all areas except the gastroesophageal junction and pylorus, there is minimal concern for excessive inversion and luminal compromise. Good blood supply also leads to excellent healing in most cases. On rare occasions, especially after shotgun wounds, large injuries of the stomach may require resection. Injuries to the pylorus are rare. If they do occur, they should be closed with a Heineke-Mikulicz pyloroplasty if possible; a concomitant vagotomy is not necessary.

Because of the stomach's position high in the abdomen, injuries to the stomach are frequently associated with lacerations of the diaphragm. This is especially true for gunshot wounds. During spontaneous ventilation, there is negative pressure in the pleural cavity and positive pressure in the abdomen. The resultant pressure gradient causes movement of gastric fluid and particulate matter from the abdomen into the chest if both the stomach and diaphragm have been injured. The degree to which movement of such debris into the chest has occurred can be deceptive in the operating room because most of the movement occurs before the institution of positive-pressure ventilation and laparotomy. Small holes in the hemidiaphragm may appear innocuous when in fact significant pleural contamination has occurred.

Even small amounts of contamination with gastric contents can result in the development of an empyema. It is difficult to drain particulate matter with a chest tube, especially if there is associated clotted blood. In the presence of combined injuries to the stomach and diaphragm, therefore, the pleural cavity should be lavaged before closure of the diaphragmatic hole. The diaphragmatic laceration should be enlarged enough to allow lavage from the abdomen. The course of the phrenic nerve in the diaphragm should be borne in mind, and enlargement of the diaphragmatic laceration should be done either radially or as peripherally as possible (Fig. 11-66).

Occasionally, adequate lavage of the pleural cavity using an abdominal approach is difficult. This occurs if the amount of pleural contamination is massive or if enlargement of the diaphragmatic laceration cannot be done without risk of denervation of the diaphragm. In such instances, the abdomen should be closed and a limited anterolateral thoracotomy should be performed for removal of contaminating particulate debris and saline lavage fluid. Although this seemingly drastic strategy rarely proves necessary, it

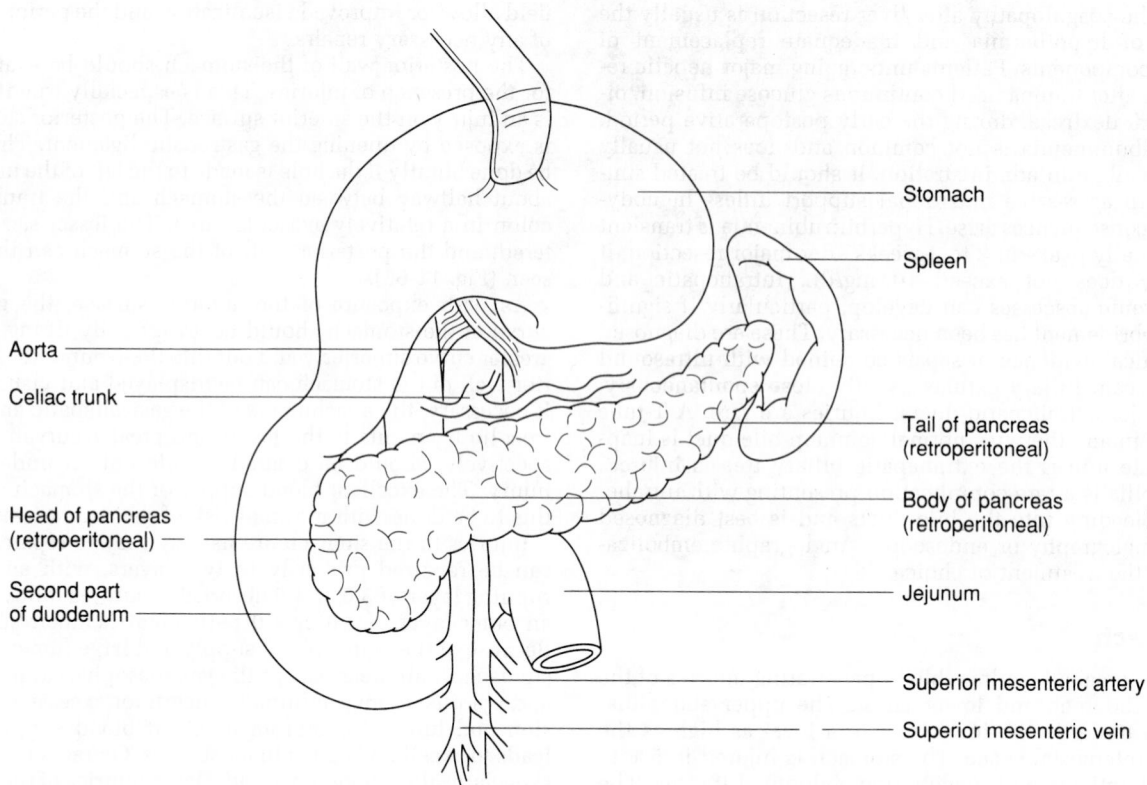

Stomach

Spleen

Aorta

Celiac trunk

Tail of pancreas
(retroperitoneal)

Body of pancreas
(retroperitoneal)

Head of pancreas
(retroperitoneal)

Second part
of duodenum

Jejunum

Superior mesenteric artery

Superior mesenteric vein

Figure 11-65. Posterior stomach exposure. The posterior wall of the stomach is exposed by entering the lesser sac through the gastrocolic ligament. This allows access to the body and tail of the pancreas.

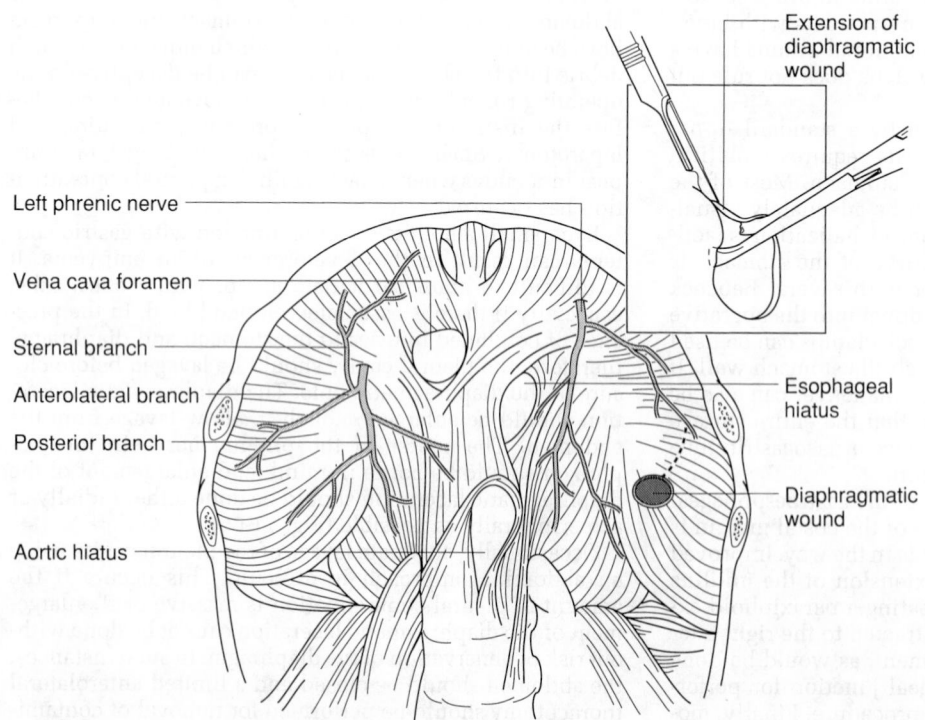

Extension of
diaphragmatic
wound

Left phrenic nerve

Vena cava foramen

Sternal branch

Anterolateral branch

Posterior branch

Esophageal
hiatus

Diaphragmatic
wound

Aortic hiatus

Figure 11-66. Phrenic nerve distribution of the diaphragm. Enlarging diaphragmatic wounds to carry out pleural lavage should be done with this innervation in mind. Either radial incision (as shown) or circumferential incisions should be used.

significantly reduces the risk of empyema development. A newer approach to this problem is the use of thoracoscopy to lavage the hemithorax. Experience with thoracoscopy in this setting is minimal to date, but it can be an attractive alternative to thoracotomy.

Blunt injuries to the stomach are rarer than penetrating injuries and account for only 1% of blunt hollow viscus injuries. The stomach is large, distensible, and mobile. A great deal of force is necessary to cause a blowout of the gastric wall. As a consequence, the mortality rate from associated injuries is high in patients with blunt stomach injuries. Blowout injuries of the stomach also tend to be large. The stomach may be more likely to be injured from blunt trauma if it is full at the time of the injury, and blunt trauma injuries are therefore often associated with significant intraperitoneal contamination. Associated injuries usually make the need for abdominal exploration obvious. Principles of operative exposure and repair are the same as for penetrating injuries.

Duodenum

Penetrating Injuries

Because of the retroperitoneal location of the duodenum in close proximity to a number of other viscera and major vascular structures, isolated penetrating injuries to the duodenum are rare. The need for abdominal exploration is usually dictated by associated injuries, and the diagnosis of duodenal injury is usually made in the operating room. Associated injuries lead to a mortality rate of 15% to 20% in patients with duodenal injury. The duodenum is also susceptible to complications of repair.[191]

In the rare instances in which isolated penetrating injury to the duodenum occurs, the most reliable means of making the diagnosis is with serial abdominal examinations. Although theoretically appealing as a means of diagnosis, the use of serum amylase concentrations in the diagnosis of penetrating duodenal injury is neither sensitive nor specific. The sensitivity of DPL in the diagnosis of penetrating duodenal injury is also poor because of the retroperitoneal location of the duodenum.

As with the stomach, diagnosis of duodenal injuries in the operating room depends on adequate exposure. The lateral and posterior portions of the duodenum cannot be visualized without mobilization. This mobilization is done by incising the lateral peritoneal reflection of the duodenum and mobilizing the duodenum from right to left with a combination of blunt and sharp dissection (Fig. 11-67). This technique is known as the Kocher maneuver, and it can be carried well across the midline to the level of the abdominal aorta, providing exposure of the underlying vena cava and aorta.

Entry into the lesser sac by way of the gastrocolic ligament provides exposure of the posterior aspect of the proximal part of the first portion of the duodenum and the medial aspect of the second portion. Exposure of the third and fourth portions of the duodenum, if necessary, is carried out by incising the ligament of Treitz and mobilizing the right colon from right to left so that the right colon and small intestine can be elevated. This is sometimes referred to as the Cattell maneuver (Fig. 11-68). With this combination of maneuvers, the entire duodenum can be mobilized and exposed for identification and thorough evaluation of any injury. It is critical to identify all injuries at the time of the initial abdominal exploration, because overlooked injuries are associated with a significant increase in subsequent morbidity.

Grading systems have been devised to characterize duodenal injuries. Although useful for research purposes, the specifics of the grading systems are less important than several simple aspects of the duodenal injury: (1) the anatomic relation to the ampulla of Vater, (2) the character of the injury (ie, a simple laceration versus destruction of the duodenal wall), (3) the involved circumference of the duodenum, and (4) associated injuries to the biliary tract, pancreas, or major vascular structures.

Most penetrating injuries to the duodenum are simple lacerations that can be repaired primarily. Such repairs should be done in two layers, with an inner absorbable layer of 3-0 or 4-0 running sutures followed by an outer layer of 3-0 or 4-0 permanent Lembert sutures. The closure should be oriented transversely if possible to avoid luminal compromise, but transverse orientation is not as critical in the duodenum as it is in the rest of the small intestine. Excessive inversion should be avoided. The biliary tract does not require drainage in such cases unless there is a primary biliary tract injury, and the duodenum does not require tube decompression, although both of these maneuvers have been advocated in the past. The periduodenal area should be drained with either closed suction drainage or passive rubber drains.

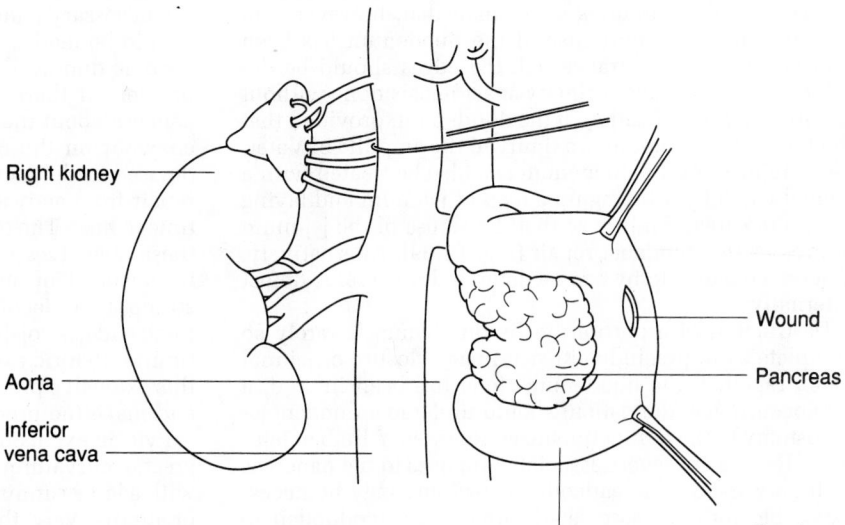

Figure 11-67. Duodenal mobilization. The Kocher maneuver is performed by mobilizing the duodenum from right to left. This exposes the underlying inferior vena cava and aorta and allows for visualization of the lateral and posterior aspects of the second portion of the duodenum.

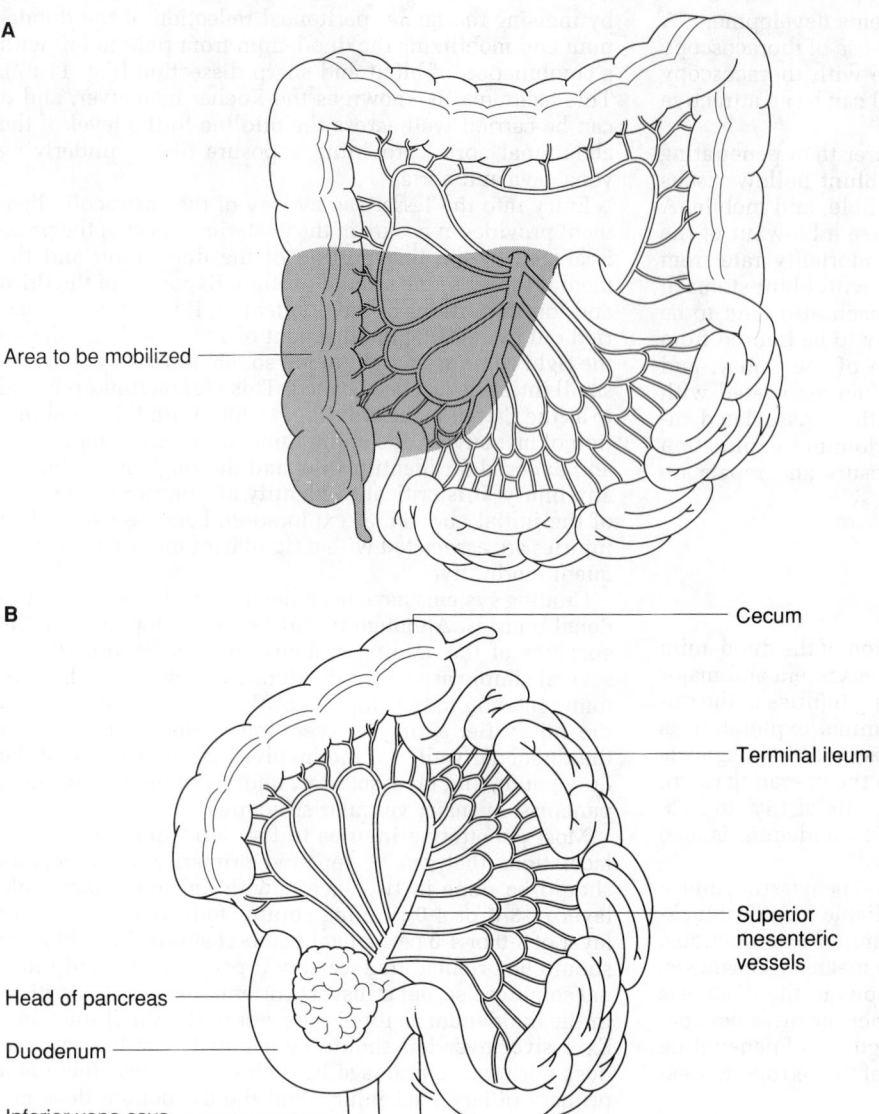

A

Area to be mobilized

B

Cecum

Terminal ileum

Superior mesenteric vessels

Head of pancreas

Duodenum

Inferior vena cava

Aorta

Figure 11-68. Right retroperitoneal exposure. (*A*) The third and fourth portions of the duodenum are exposed by mobilizing the right colon and small intestine from right to left. (*B*) The right colon and small intestine can then be lifted up, providing exposure of the duodenum from below. It is important to carefully replace the small intestine in the abdominal cavity at the conclusion of the operation. Iatrogenic volvulus of the mobilized bowel is possible if such care is not taken.

Large injuries to the duodenum are more difficult to repair. Injuries that encompass as much as 40% or 50% of the duodenal wall can be successfully closed primarily. Primary repair of injuries larger than that, however, can lead to luminal compromise. If the duodenum has been transected or almost transected, the edges should be débrided and a two-layer primary anastomosis done without tension after mobilization of the duodenum, provided that the transection is not in proximity to the ampulla of Vater. Large injuries of the duodenum can also be treated with a jejunal patch by bringing up a loop of jejunum and laying it onto the area of injury so that the serosa of the jejunum buttresses the duodenal repair (Fig. 11-69). Alternatively, a duodenojejunostomy can be done to drain a large defect internally.

Destruction of a portion of the duodenum is rarely so complete as to preclude either primary closure or jejunal patch repair. If the duodenum alone has been injured, a rare occurrence, the patient should undergo a duodenojejunostomy to the defunctionalized Roux-en-Y limb of jejunum. If there are severe associated injuries to the pancreas or biliary tract, pancreaticoduodenectomy may be necessary. The morbidity associated with pancreaticoduodenectomy is substantial, and this operation is indicated only if

the extent of injury is so great that the necessary resection has in essence been done by the injury. If débridement of devitalized tissue results in a pancreaticoduodenectomy, the necessary pancreatic, gastric, and biliary anastomoses should be made.

Some duodenal repairs are tenuous. This is a particular problem if there is associated pancreatic injury, raising concern about the digestive action of activated pancreatic enzymes on the repair. Pyloric exclusion is a technique devised to defunctionalize the duodenum and protect the repair from activated pancreatic enzymes until it has had time to heal. The original procedure devised to accomplish these objectives was called pyloric diverticulization, and it consisted of antrectomy, oversewing of the duodenal stump, tube decompression of the duodenum and biliary tract, and gastrojejunostomy to restore gastrointestinal continuity. Pyloric exclusion was devised as an alternative to this extensive procedure in order to shorten operating time and make the procedure reversible.

Pyloric exclusion is started with a gastrotomy along the greater curvature of the stomach. The pylorus is closed with a large running suture placed through the gastrotomy; or alternatively, the pylorus is stapled closed. Gastrointestinal continuity is then restored by a gastrojejunostomy

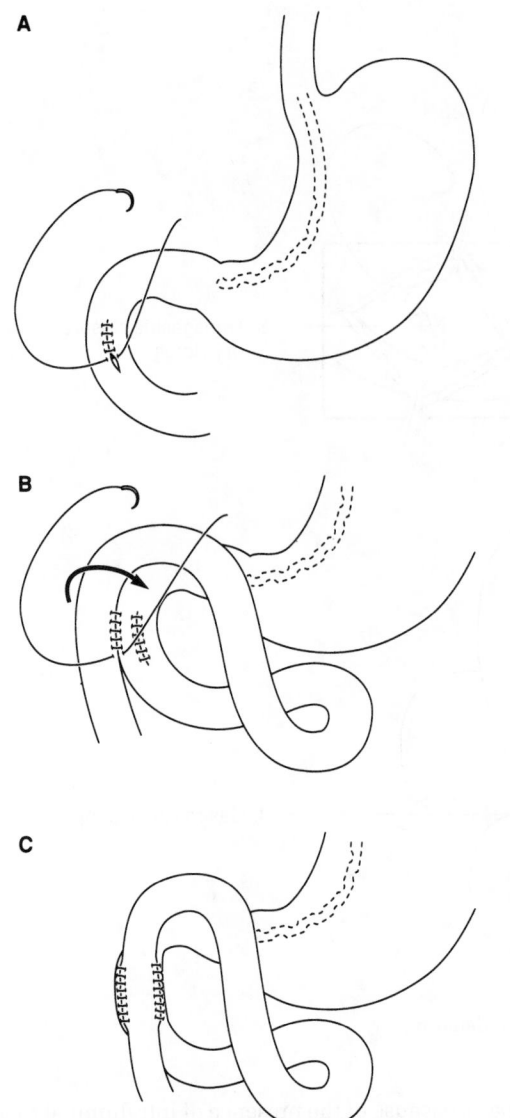

Figure 11-69. A jejunoileal patch can be used to reinforce repairs of the duodenum. (*A*) The duodenum is first repaired. (*B*) The retrocolic loop of jejunum is brought up to the area of repair. (*C*) The serosa is sewn over the repair.

(Fig. 11-70). Tube decompression of the duodenum should be performed in severe duodenal injuries, but the biliary tract does not require decompression unless there has been an associated biliary tract injury. As with all duodenal injuries, the periduodenal area should be externally drained to ensure that a postoperative leak becomes a controlled fistula.

If patients who undergo pyloric exclusion are studied a number of weeks after the exclusion procedure with upper gastrointestinal contrast series, most are found to have normal reconstituted gastrointestinal continuity. The closure of the pylorus breaks down, and the normal gastrointestinal route is reestablished. This occurs regardless of whether the pylorus was closed with absorbable or nonabsorbable suture. As the pylorus reopens, the gastrojejunostomy may gradually close of its own accord. It is for this reason that pyloric exclusion, although an inherently ulcerogenic procedure, does not require a concomitant vagotomy.

Blunt Injuries

Blunt injuries to the duodenum are both less common and more difficult to diagnose than penetrating injuries. They can occur in isolation or with pancreatic injury. These are instances in which the need for immediate abdominal exploration is not obvious. Because the duodenum is located in the retroperitoneum, findings on physical examination of the abdomen may be subtle unless there are associated intraabdominal injuries. Nonetheless, the physical examination is still one of the best methods for determining the presence of a duodenal injury. This is true even if the admission examination is indeterminate, emphasizing the need for serial abdominal examinations.

In theory, perforations of the duodenum should be associated with leak of amylase and other digestive enzymes, and it has been suggested that determination of the serum amylase concentration may be helpful in the diagnosis of blunt duodenal injuries. However, the test lacks sensitivity. The duodenum is retroperitoneal, the concentration of amylase in the fluid that leaks is variable, and amylase concentrations often take hours to days to increase after injury. Although serial determinations of serum amylase are better than a single, isolated determination on admission, sensitivity is still poor, and necessary delays are inherent in serial determinations.

Plain abdominal radiographs have been advocated for the diagnosis of blunt duodenal injuries. The characteristic finding is that of extraluminal retroperitoneal air in the area of the duodenum. If present, this finding on plain film is often indicative of duodenal injury and should prompt operative exploration. Because many blunt injuries to the duodenum do not demonstrate this finding, however, it is not a reliable way to rule out injury.

Upper gastrointestinal series and CT scans of the abdomen are more sensitive than plain abdominal radiographs for the presence of duodenal contusion or perforation after blunt trauma. Performance of these tests requires a stable patient without any other obvious indications for abdominal exploration. Upper gastrointestinal series are less expensive to perform than CT scans, are widely available, and may have slightly increased sensitivity for subtle injuries of the duodenum. An advantage of CT, on the other hand, is that the rest of the retroperitoneum and peritoneal viscera are also visualized. With either study, extravasation of contrast material from the duodenum constitutes an indication for surgical intervention and repair.

Operative exposure and repair of the duodenum after blunt trauma is the same as for penetrating injuries. Crush injuries are more common after blunt trauma and occasionally require extensive resection, but the injuries can be treated by simple techniques of repair if they are diagnosed in a timely fashion.

Intramural hematoma of the duodenum is a rare injury specific to patients with blunt trauma.[192] It is most common in children with isolated localized force to the upper abdomen, possibly because of the relatively flexible and pliable musculature of the child's abdominal wall. Intramural hematomas occur when the duodenum is crushed and there is bleeding in the submucosal or subserosal layers of the duodenum. The duodenum is not perforated. Such hematomas can lead to obstruction of the lumen. If the diagnosis is not made at the time of the initial injury, the obstruction usually takes several days to develop, presumably because of increased accumulation of intramural water as the hemoglobin in the hematoma begins to break down and osmotic forces increase absorption of water. This mechanism is similar to that proposed to explain the increase in size of subdural hematomas with time.

If exploration takes place shortly after injury, intramural

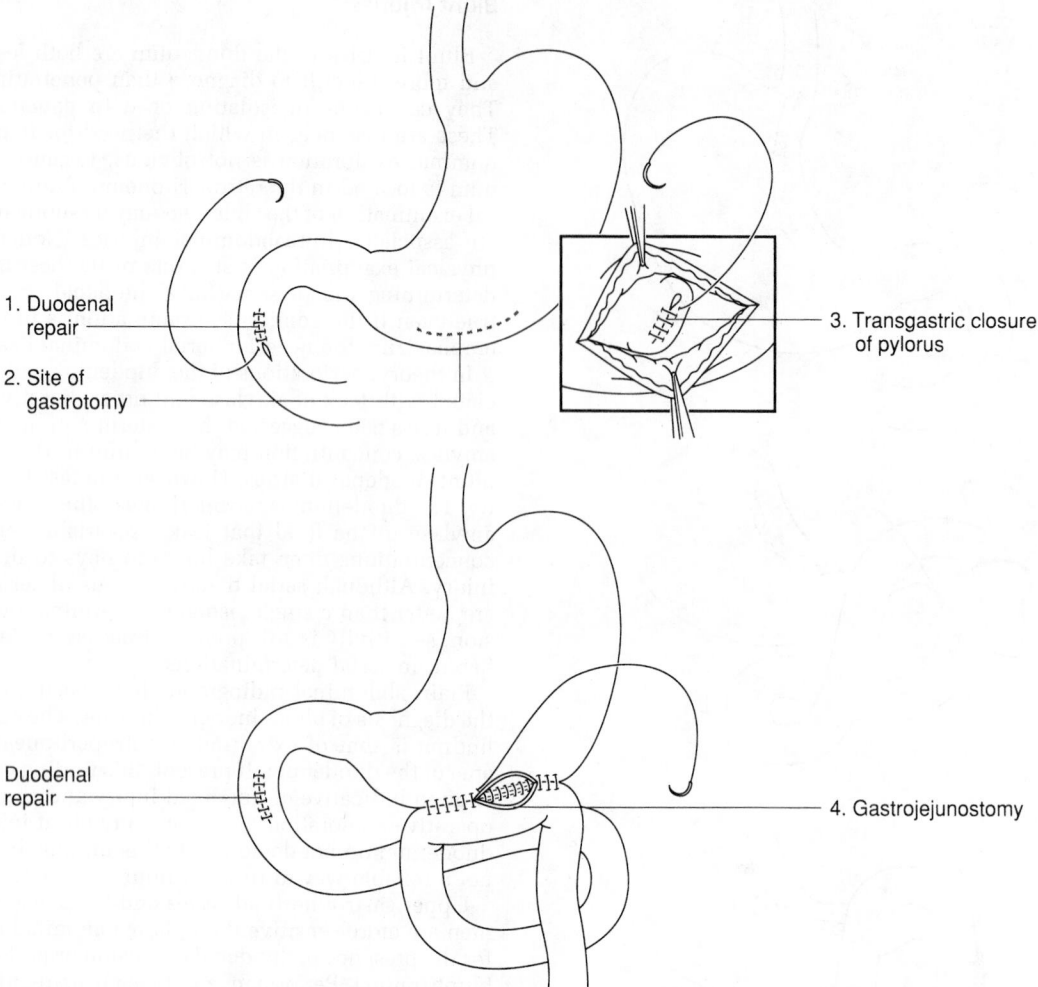

1. Duodenal repair

2. Site of gastrotomy

3. Transgastric closure of pylorus

Duodenal repair

4. Gastrojejunostomy

Figure 11-70. Technique of pyloric exclusion for complex duodenal injury.

hematomas of the duodenum are seen as periduodenal hematomas through the abdominal incision. At the time of initial operative evaluation, all hematomas in the area of the duodenum should be explored to rule out the possibility of perforation. Such exploration includes a Kocher maneuver and mobilization of the duodenum, which in most instances successfully drains subserosal hematomas. Submucosal hematomas may require drainage with deeper, separate incisions. If surgery does not occur shortly after injury, obstructive symptoms become manifest after a number of days. An upper gastrointestinal series or CT scan should be performed to demonstrate obstruction. The obstruction is usually in the second portion of the duodenum and, in the classic picture, demonstrates a coiled-spring appearance.

Some debate surrounds the treatment of intramural hematomas of the duodenum if the diagnosis is delayed, but the weight of opinion argues for initial nonoperative treatment. This strategy is usually successful because the hematoma gradually resolves and the obstructive symptoms subside without long-term residual sequelae. If obstructive symptoms persist beyond 10 to 14 days from the time of diagnosis, abdominal exploration should be undertaken to rule out the presence of a duodenal perforation or injury to the head of the pancreas that may be an alternative cause of duodenal obstruction.

Complications

Both penetrating and blunt injuries of the duodenum can lead to complications associated with leak of the duodenal repair. The duodenum is particularly susceptible to leak of repairs because of the presence of intraluminal digestive enzymes. Adequate drainage of the periduodenal area ensures that such leaks are controlled and do not result in an intraabdominal abscess. Placement of a decompressive duodenal tube to protect duodenal repairs is controversial but, in theory, lessens the incidence of failed repairs. If a duodenal repair breaks down and the duodenum is adequately drained, a duodenal fistula results. In the absence of distal obstruction, foreign body, or persistent infection (the chances of which are minimized by adequate drainage), many of these controlled fistulas ultimately close. They may be slow to resolve, and a wait of several months is advised to allow them to resolve spontaneously. Trials of total parenteral nutrition may increase the rate of spontaneous closure. If a fistula fails to close after an appropriate waiting period, further surgical intervention is warranted. It consists of reexploration of the abdomen and construction of a duodenojejunostomy as a form of internal drainage. The duodenojejunostomy should be constructed with the use of a defunctionalized Roux-en-Y limb of jejunum.

Pancreas

Penetrating Injuries

Penetrating injuries to the pancreas are usually diagnosed in the operating room.[193] Like the duodenum, the pancreas is located in the retroperitoneum, surrounded by a number of other viscera and major vascular structures. As a result, an isolated injury to the pancreas is unusual, and patients with penetrating pancreatic trauma usually have obvious indications for abdominal exploration. Major vascular injuries are seen in 40% to 50% of patients with penetrating pancreatic injuries, in 50% of those with injuries to the liver, and in 25% of those with injuries to the duodenum. Preoperative serum amylase concentrations are not helpful; they are elevated in only about 30% of patients with penetrating pancreatic injuries.

On abdominal exploration, signs of pancreatic injury include a projectile path that passes in proximity to the pancreas, a central hematoma in the upper abdomen, and injuries to the duodenum, vena cava, suprarenal aorta, or mesenteric vessels. In all these instances, the pancreas should be thoroughly explored.

The anterior surface of the pancreas is visualized by entry into the lesser sac of the peritoneal cavity. This is done in the same fashion as outlined previously for exposure of the posterior aspect of the stomach, with division of the gastrocolic ligament in a relatively avascular area to the left of the midline. A thin layer of peritoneum overlies the anterior surface of the pancreas at this point, and complete visualization of the surface sometimes requires incision of this layer.

The tail of the pancreas can be more fully visualized, especially in its posterior aspect, by mobilization of the spleen and the tail of the pancreas as a unit. This is accomplished by incision of any lateral attachments of the spleen to the abdominal wall and mobilization of the spleen with blunt dissection laterally to medially by development of the plane between the anterior surface of the left kidney and the posterior aspect of the spleen. This brings the spleen into the abdominal wound and elevates the posterior aspect of the pancreatic tail for inspection (Fig. 11-71).

The posterior aspect of the body of the pancreas is visualized by development of the avascular area at the inferior margin of the body and tail of the pancreas with a combination of sharp and blunt dissection. The pancreas can then be mobilized inferiorly to superiorly. This maneuver is also important for mobilization of the pancreas in preparation for distal pancreatic resection.

The posterior aspect of the head of the pancreas can be exposed by an extensive Kocher maneuver. In combination with entry into the lesser sac, this also allows for bimanual palpation of the pancreatic head, with one hand placed on the anterior surface of the pancreas through the hole in the lesser sac and the other hand placed behind the pancreas in the plane developed by the Kocher maneuver.

In the evaluation of penetrating pancreatic injuries, the key to operative management is the determination of whether a ductal injury is present. Transduodenal intraoperative pancreatography has been recommended, but the use of this technique in the identification of ductal injuries is controversial. The advantage of this maneuver is that it allows for more definitive determination of the type of operative intervention that should be undertaken. The major disadvantage is that it necessitates entry into the duodenum when there is no associated duodenal injury, which turns simple pancreatic injuries into combined pancreaticoduodenal injuries, with an attendant increase in potential postoperative morbidity. A further argument against intraoperative pancreatography is that most injuries to the pancreas can be adequately evaluated and decisions made about appropriate operative treatment without radiographic examination of ductal anatomy. In certain circumstances, the use of intraoperative endoscopic retrograde cholangiopancreatography (ERCP) eliminates this problem.

The operative management of penetrating pancreatic injuries is somewhat controversial. Injuries can be classified according to both location and severity. With respect to location, injuries can be subdivided into those of the head, body, and tail of the pancreas. With respect to severity, classification systems have been devised that not only have comparative and research applications but also can be used in the determination of the best treatment. Class I injuries are simple contusions of the pancreas; class II injuries are lacerations of the parenchyma in the body or tail of the pancreas; class III injuries are those with severe disruption of the head or body; and class IV injuries are those in which there is an associated injury to the duodenum.

It is usually agreed that class I injuries should be observed or simply drained externally. The optimal type of drainage is a matter of some debate, and a variety of different drainage methods have been espoused. For many years, passive rubber drains were routinely used. Several reports published in the 1970s and early 1980s sought to demonstrate the superiority of sump drainage for pancreatic injuries, although other reports published since that time have not demonstrated superiority for any particular form of drainage. A recent report on a randomized series of patients seemed to demonstrate an advantage of closed suction drainage over sump drainage, but the data were inconclusive. The type of drain used after pancreatic injury is probably not important as long as adequate drainage is effected. This can be accomplished with passive, sump, or closed suction systems.

If drains are used, they should be left in place for at least 5 to 7 days to ensure that a drain tract develops. Pancreatic fistulas can develop on a delayed basis 3 to 7 days after injury, and if the drains are removed before that time, drain-

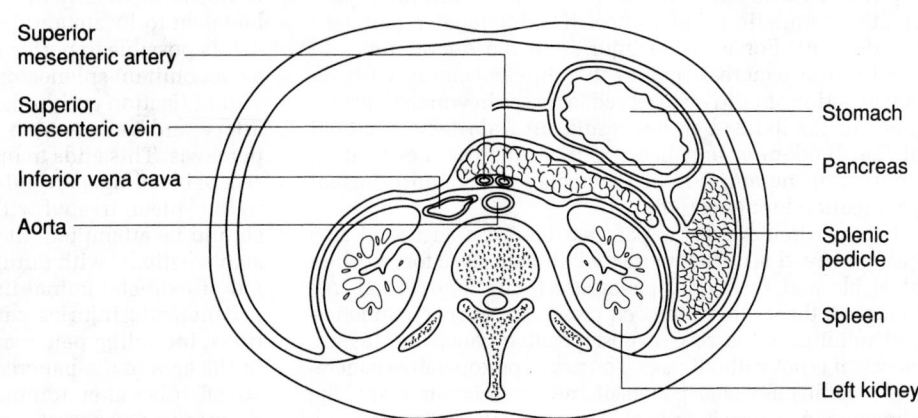

Figure 11-71. Left retroperitoneal exposure. The spleen and tail of the pancreas can be mobilized as a unit by developing a plane just anterior to the left kidney using a combination of sharp and blunt dissection. This allows visualization of the spleen and the posterior aspect of the tail of the pancreas and also simplifies the removal if splenectomy is to be done in conjunction with a distal pancreatectomy.

Superior mesenteric artery
Superior mesenteric vein
Inferior vena cava
Aorta
Stomach
Pancreas
Splenic pedicle
Spleen
Left kidney

age may be inadequate. The morbidity rate for patients with undrained pancreatic secretions is much greater than that for those with drained pancreatic secretions.

The timing of drain removal should be based on both the amount and character of the pancreatic drainage. Drain outputs in excess of 150 to 200 mL/d are suggestive of pancreatic fistulas. Determinations of drain amylase concentration are moderately helpful, but amylase concentrations in the drainage are of little benefit if patients are tested within a few days of injury, because even high levels (in excess of 50,000 IU/L) do not correlate with the development of a pancreatic fistula or other complications. Determinations done at 7 days after injury correlate with the presence of a pancreatic fistula or other pancreatic complication only if the level is higher than 100,000 IU/L. The negative predictive value of a concentration below 100,000 IU/L is poor, however, and does not rule out the presence or subsequent development of a pancreatic complication.

The treatment of class II injuries depends on the presence or absence of a ductal injury, a determination that can be difficult to make. The argument for intraoperative pancreatography is made for class II injuries. The presence of a ductal injury in the head of the pancreas does not usually make a difference with respect to treatment, because most of these injuries should be drained regardless. On the other hand, if a ductal injury is present in the body or tail of the pancreas, the appropriate treatment is resection of the distal pancreas, whereas if no ductal injury is present, simple drainage is adequate. Although this reasoning is clear, the difficulty lies in determining whether injuries to the body or tail of the pancreas do in fact include ductal injury. Intraoperative pancreatography is helpful, regardless of the technique employed, to make this determination.

Class III injuries of the body or tail of the pancreas, as mentioned previously, should be treated with a distal pancreatectomy. Distal resection can include up to 80% of the gland if necessary. Subsequent endocrine or exocrine insufficiency is rare if the pancreas is normal. Class III injuries of the head of the pancreas should be drained. Resection of these injuries requires internal drainage, near-total pancreatectomy, or pancreaticoduodenectomy, procedures that are associated with a high rate of morbidity and mortality. If the patient develops a pancreatic fistula, the fistula can be controlled by the drains. If the fistula does not resolve with time, the pancreas can be drained internally at a later date.

Class IV injuries of the pancreas involve injuries to the duodenum as well as the pancreas.[194] If the injuries to the duodenum and pancreas are simple, the duodenum can be repaired primarily, and the pancreas can be drained, or a distal resection can be carried out if the pancreatic injury is in the body or tail. For more complicated, combined injuries, pyloric exclusion can be done to minimize pancreatic stimulation and protect the duodenal repair (see Duodenum). For massive injuries to the duodenum and head of the pancreas, pancreaticoduodenectomy with reconstruction should be reserved for cases in which débridement of devitalized tissue results in a de facto removal of the duodenum and head of the pancreas. Penetrating injuries to the ampulla of Vater may also require formal pancreaticoduodenectomy.

Internal drainage of the pancreas has been suggested as a means of treating ductal injuries without the need for resection of viable and functional pancreatic tissue (Fig. 11-72). Although in theory this approach preserves pancreatic function and minimizes the risk of postoperative pancreatic insufficiency, it is not without risks. The risk of postoperative pancreatic insufficiency after pancreatic resection is minimal if the remaining pancreas is normal. The pancreaticojejunal anasto-

mosis is prone to break down and leak, especially if suboptimal conditions of associated injury and hemodynamic instability exist. The construction of a Roux-en-Y jejunal limb requires the opening of the intestine and the creation of a small bowel anastomosis. If the intestine has not been injured, this procedure increases the amount of contamination associated with the injury and also increases the likelihood of postoperative morbidity. For these reasons, most major trauma centers rarely carry out internal drainage procedures in the early postinjury period, relying instead on either resection or drainage. Internal drainage is usually reserved for cases in which persistent pancreatic fistulas or pseudocysts develop late.[195]

Distal pancreatectomy for traumatic injuries should be performed only after the pancreas has been thoroughly mobilized and exposed. In some cases, the pancreas has already been transected, and the site of resection has therefore already been determined for the surgeon. If this is not the case, the pancreas should be transected just proximal to the site of known or presumed ductal injury. If associated splenectomy is planned, elaborate dissection is unnecessary. The splenic artery can be identified near the superior margin of the pancreas and ligated. The splenic vein can also be individually ligated at this point. Commonly, the splenic vein lies behind the body and tail of the pancreas, and its isolation requires more dissection. As an alternative to extensive dissection to isolate the splenic vein behind the pancreas, the vein can be transected along with the pancreatic parenchyma. Individual ligation of the splenic vein stump can be done after the distal pancreas and spleen have been removed. It is helpful to first mobilize the spleen and tail of the pancreas.

The pancreas should be mobilized at the site of transection and can be encircled with a rubber drain. Mobilization and encirclement are best done by an approach to the pancreas along its inferior margin and mobilization inferiorly to superiorly. The pancreas can be divided either distal to a bowel clamp or with a stapler. There are some indications that a sutured closure is less likely to break down and lead to fistula formation than a stapled closure. If a bowel clamp is used, the pancreatic stump should be oversewn with a running suture. Typically, nonabsorbable suture has been recommended for this purpose, but the type of suture used is probably not of major consequence with respect to the subsequent development of complications. It is also recommended that an individual figure-of-eight suture be placed in the cut end of the pancreatic duct. This proves exceedingly difficult in patients with normal pancreatic ductal systems because the duct is small and not easily identified in the cut edge of the pancreatic stump. A pancreatic duct that can be seen easily may indicate preexisting proximal ductal obstruction. In this case, the duct should be individually ligated. If the cut end of the duct is not immediately apparent, time and effort should not be taken to locate and individually ligate it.

It is possible to perform a distal pancreatectomy without a concomitant splenectomy. Splenic salvage involves individual ligation and division of the branches of the splenic artery and vein, which supply the body and tail of the pancreas. This adds to operative time and can increase the risk of bleeding, particularly if there is an associated injury to the spleen treated with splenorrhaphy. Splenic salvage should be attempted, therefore, only in hemodynamically stable patients with minimal or no associated intraabdominal or extraabdominal injuries.

Pancreatic injuries can lead to a number of complications, including pancreatic fistulas, pseudocysts, bleeding in the area of the pancreatic bed, and pancreatitis. Pancreatic fistulas after trauma are characterized by persistent drainage of pancreatic enzymes and secretions from the

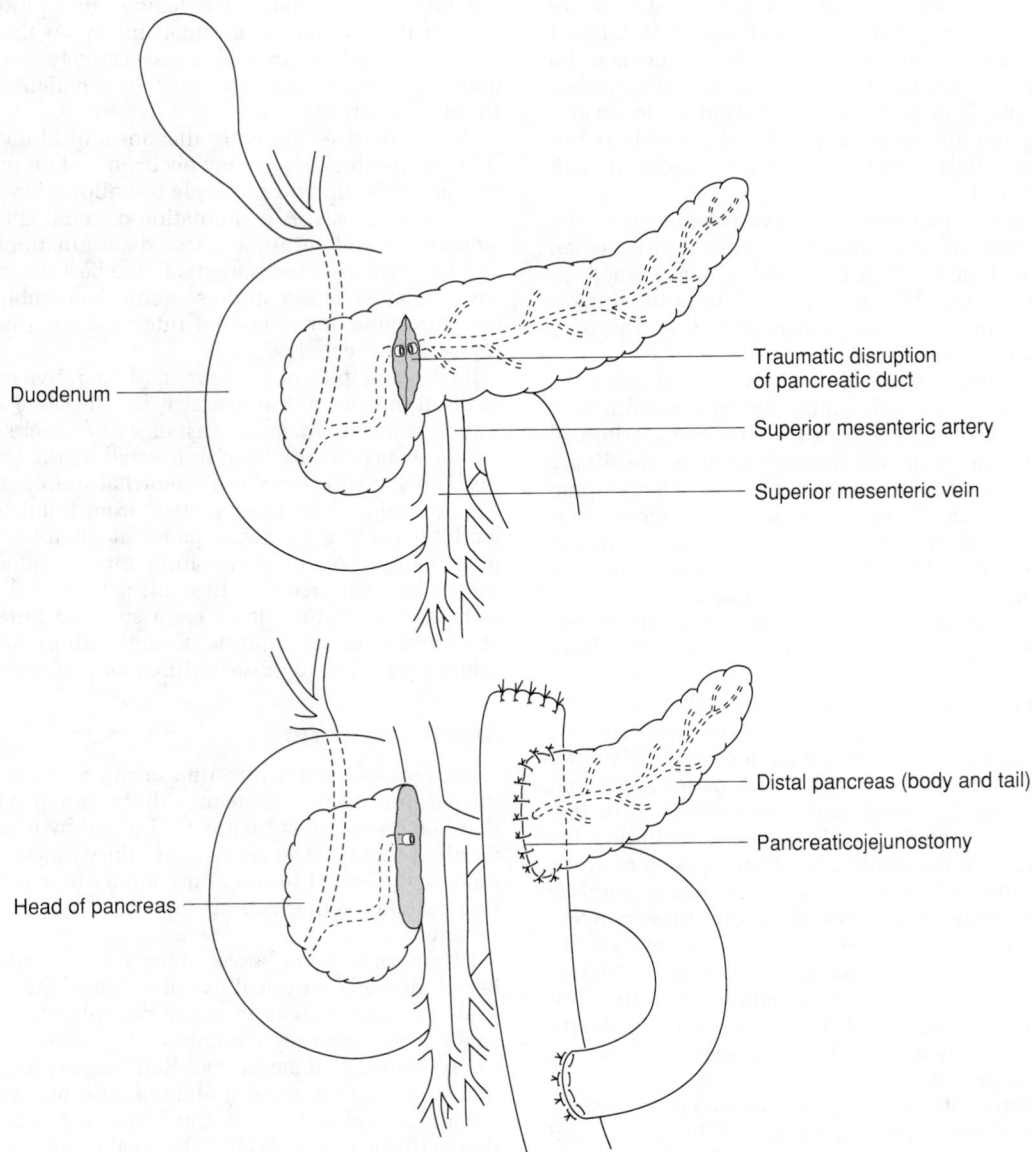

Duodenum

Traumatic disruption
of pancreatic duct

Superior mesenteric artery

Superior mesenteric vein

Distal pancreas (body and tail)

Pancreaticojejunostomy

Head of pancreas

Figure 11-72. Internal drainage of a pancreatic injury involving the ductal system. Illustrated is internal drainage with the creation of a Roux-en-Y jejunoileal limb and construction of a pancreaticojejunal anastomosis.

pancreatic injury for a number of weeks after injury. Most of these fistulas close spontaneously, especially if there is no proximal obstruction of the pancreatic ductal system. A trial of total parenteral nutrition may improve the rate and incidence of spontaneous closure. Somatostatin has not been used extensively in patients with posttraumatic pancreatic fistulas, but fistulas that develop after elective pancreatic surgery seem to close more quickly if somatostatin is given.[196,197] In recalcitrant posttraumatic fistulas, a trial of somatostatin should be given. In the rare instances in which fistulas fail to close spontaneously, surgical intervention may be required. The involved pancreas is resected, if possible; otherwise, procedures are performed to create internal drainage into the stomach or a defunctionalized limb of jejunum.

Pseudocysts that develop after pancreatic trauma often resolve on their own or with percutaneous aspiration. If, after 4 to 6 weeks of observation with serial ultrasound or CT scanning, the pseudocyst does not show signs of resolution, it should be drained internally with a defunctionalized limb of jejunum.

Bleeding in the area of the pancreatic bed is usually an early complication that is caused by inadequate drainage with resultant autodigestion of the pancreas and surrounding tissue. Bleeding can be avoided by identifying all injuries at the time of exploration and ensuring adequate drainage. If massive bleeding does occur, it should be dealt with through operative intervention.

Pancreatitis, another complication of pancreatic injury, is also related to inadequate drainage of pancreatic secretions. Treatment consists of provision of adequate drainage and supportive care. If the pancreatitis is localized to the distal pancreas and a trial of conservative management fails, distal pancreatectomy should be considered.

Blunt Injuries

The major difference between penetrating and blunt injuries of the pancreas concerns diagnosis. Penetrating injuries are usually discovered on abdominal exploration for associated injuries, but blunt injuries may occur in isolation, and the preoperative diagnosis can be difficult. Blunt pancreatic injuries are relatively rare, which increases the difficulty of diagnosis. In one series of pancreatic injuries, delays in diagnosis of blunt injuries ranged up to several days. Making the diagnosis as quickly as possible is important because delays in diagnosis are associated with increased morbidity.

The body of the pancreas lies directly anterior to the vertebral column and is vulnerable to crush injuries when the anterior abdominal wall is forceably compressed, as can occur from a seat belt or a sharp blow to the epigastrium. In such instances, the pancreas may be the only intraabdominal organ injured.

A number of different means are available to make the diagnosis of blunt pancreatic injury. Physical examination of the abdomen is useful, but because of the retroperitoneal location of the pancreas, the results can be misleadingly benign until a number of hours after injury. This emphasizes the importance of serial examinations. In most cases, the abdomen becomes progressively more tender to palpation during the first 24 to 48 hours after injury, and the need for abdominal exploration becomes more obvious. The physical examination of the abdomen is much less reliable in young children and in patients with head injuries.

The serum amylase concentration is elevated on admission in about 70% of patients with blunt pancreatic injury. However, elevated serum amylase has a poor positive predictive value and also occurs in many patients without pancreatic injury. The amylase concentration can be elevated because of trauma to other organs, including the salivary glands and the ovaries. In addition, the remaining 30% of patients with normal admission serum amylase concentrations must be considered. Serum lipase concentrations and serial determinations of serum amylase are occasionally helpful in monitoring the courses of patients with normal or only mildly elevated admission values, but reliance on these methods of diagnosis results in delays in diagnosis, and a percentage of diagnoses are missed for a considerable period.

DPL is of little help in the early diagnosis of pancreatic injury unless there have been associated intraperitoneal injuries. The retroperitoneal location of the pancreas results in minimal findings in the lavage fluid, and obtaining amylase concentrations in the lavage fluid is not helpful.

CT scan of the abdomen allows for visualization of the retroperitoneum, including the pancreas. In the case of isolated injury to the pancreas, the sensitivity of the CT scan is at its lowest shortly after injury. Although it may be a good test for the diagnosis of pancreatic injury after a number of hours have passed, immediate CT of the abdomen will miss some pancreatic injuries, particularly if expert interpretation is not available.

Finally, ERCP is a means of diagnosing pancreatic injury. ERCP is an attractive diagnostic method because it is less invasive than abdominal exploration and also provides information about the status of the ductal system, but there are several practical disadvantages of the technique. Most of the studies that have reported successful use of ERCP have involved stable patients studied hours to days after injury and sent to a referral center specifically because of suspicion of a pancreatic injury. These patients are a selected group, quite different from patients who are freshly injured. ERCP is not universally available and, even in large centers, is often unavailable at the odd hours necessary for early diagnosis in acutely injured patients. Many endoscopists are fearful of inducing an exacerbation of pancreatitis in patients with mild pancreatic injuries lacking ductal involvement. The logic of using ERCP dictates that, in the absence of a ductal injury on the study, the patient should be treated conservatively; worsening of traumatic pancreatitis in some of these patients is an undesirable side effect.

To summarize, the early diagnosis of blunt pancreatic injuries, particularly if they occur in isolation, can be extremely difficult, and no single test allows for an easy and reliable diagnosis. A combination of serial abdominal examinations and serum amylase determinations, CT scan, and ERCP in selected patients is the best diagnostic strategy available. These studies should be combined, with a low threshold for operative intervention if a pancreatic injury is suspected.

Basic principles of exposure and operative management of blunt injuries of the pancreas are the same as for penetrating injuries. In many instances of severe injury, the pancreas has already been transected by the trauma, making the pancreatic resection somewhat simpler to carry out. Isolated injuries of the pancreas from blunt trauma also lend themselves to distal pancreatectomy with splenic preservation. As in penetrating injury, splenic salvage should be attempted only in stable patients without associated splenic rupture or severe associated intraabdominal or extraabdominal injuries. Complications of pancreatic injury are similar to those outlined for penetrating injuries.

Small Intestine

Because the small intestine occupies more volume in the peritoneal cavity than any other organ, it is the intraabdominal viscus most frequently injured by penetrating abdominal trauma. The severity of injury ranges from trivial rents in the bowel serosa or mesentery to massive perforation or devascularization injuries requiring extensive resection.

Diagnosis of small bowel injury can be made by a number of methods. Physical examination of the abdomen reveals peritoneal signs in many patients with penetrating small bowel injuries. Patients with gunshot wounds routinely undergo laparotomy. Routine exploration of all other penetrating anterior abdominal injuries that violate the abdominal wall fascia can be carried out. An alternative to this is to use serial abdominal examinations, hematocrits, and leukocyte counts. If the patient develops increasing signs of intraperitoneal injury, abdominal exploration is performed. In stable patients with penetrating injuries to the anterior abdomen, a third approach is DPL. A variety of criteria for positivity in patients who undergo DPL for blunt trauma have been proposed, ranging from 1000 RBCs/mL of lavage fluid as a threshold for positivity up to the conventional 100,000 RBCs/mL used in blunt trauma patients. Use of the more stringent criteria naturally decreases the rate of false-negative results for small penetrating injuries to the small intestine and other subtle intraperitoneal injuries, but it does so at the cost of an increased rate of false-positive results.

Regardless of the approach taken for the preoperative diagnosis of penetrating injuries of the small intestine, the operative approach should be the same. The abdomen should be explored through a standard upper midline incision, and initial attention should be directed toward bleeding from associated injuries or from the small bowel mesentery. Bleeding from the mesentery can usually be controlled easily with suture ligation or with a rapid running closure of the mesenteric rent. This closure does not need to constitute definitive repair, but it temporarily controls bleeding until definitive treatment is delineated.

After bleeding has been controlled, steps to prevent ongoing leakage of intestinal contents from the injured small bowel should be taken. This is done by rapid examination of the small intestine and by either application of Babcock or Allis clamps or a temporizing running single-layer closure of injured areas. After initial control of the leak, the intestine should be examined more carefully. Definitive repair or resection should not be done until the entire length of the intestine has been carefully examined, because a thorough knowledge of the extent of injury is necessary for a logical and rational approach to management. It makes no sense, for example, to repair a segment of small intestine only to determine after further exploration that injuries to adjacent segments of the bowel dictate resection of the entire segment.

The entire length of the small intestine should be carefully examined, starting at the ligament of Treitz and moving sequentially, proximally to distally, at each successive loop. This should be done in a systematic manner and should include inspection of the small bowel mesentery by fanning out of the mesentery with examination of each new loop. If there is a suspicious area along the mesenteric border of the intestine, the mesentery should be cleared away to allow for adequate visualization. The small intestine has a good blood supply and easily tolerates this maneuver. Any blood or other debris found on the serosa of the bowel should be wiped away. Sometimes, such debris overlies an otherwise unsuspected area of injury.

In theory, the number of holes found in the small intestine should add up to an even number because there should be an identical number of entrance and exit wounds. This rule is sometimes violated in practice, however, because the intestine is extensively coiled in the peritoneal cavity and tangential wounds of the bowel are common. Rather than focusing on the number of holes in the bowel, attention should be directed to a close inspection of the entire length of the intestine. After all areas of injury have been identified, a decision about repair or resection is made. Areas of massive destruction of the bowel or the mesentery, with associated ischemia, should be treated with resection. If, after débridement, over 40% to 50% of a portion of the wall of the small intestine is missing, that segment should also be resected.

Knife wounds to the small intestine are usually easy to manage and rarely require extensive débridement or resection. On rare occasions, a large rent in the small bowel mesentery results in enough devascularization to require resection of a segment of intestine. Gunshot wounds require more débridement. However, because the small bowel is filled largely with air and is pliable and mobile, it is resistant to the effects of a bullet. Débridement of gunshot wounds does not need to be done beyond obviously devitalized areas, regardless of the type of gun used and the velocity of the bullet.

Minor mesenteric lacerations should be treated with suture ligation of bleeding points and closure of the rent. Major lacerations with devascularization should be treated with resection and primary anastomosis. Small bowel anastomoses, if properly done and after adequate débridement of devitalized tissue, have an excellent rate of healing even with severe associated injuries, shock, and peritonitis.

Shotgun wounds to the abdomen from close range are often associated with massive tissue destruction and should be treated in a manner similar to that described previously. At medium or long range, they sometimes result in a diffuse pattern of shot injury, creating multiple small perforations of the small intestine. In such instances, the general principles outlined previously should be followed and obvious areas of injury repaired. It is sometimes impossible to ensure closure of all the numerous areas of perforation. In such cases, obvious areas of injury should be closed; smaller areas of perforation often do not require surgical closure because they rarely leak and are of minimal consequence.

On rare occasions, injuries to the small intestine occur in patients who are hemodynamically unstable as a result of associated injuries. In such instances, the small intestine can be treated most expeditiously by application of the gastrointestinal anastomosis stapler as necessary to remove the injured areas of bowel. If a second operation is planned because of associated injuries, definitive anastomosis can be deferred and the stapled ends of the intestine simply returned to the abdomen until the second procedure is performed.

Blunt injuries to the small intestine are much less common than penetrating injuries. As with other blunt intraabdominal injuries, they are more difficult to diagnose because the need for urgent intraabdominal intervention is not always obvious. Blunt perforations and devascularizations of the small intestine often occur in isolation, either as the only injury or as the only intraabdominal injury present. This makes early diagnosis even more difficult.[198]

Seat belts have been implicated in the pathogenesis of blunt injuries of the small intestine. The intestine is compressed between the seat belt and the vertebral column and can be distended to the point of rupture or torn violently on its mesentery, resulting in either perforation or devascularization. Because of the severe degree of force necessary to produce a blunt intestinal injury, there is a frequent association with transverse fractures of a lumbar vertebral body (Chance fracture).

Diagnosis is made primarily by physical examination of the abdomen. Abdominal examination is usually positive shortly after injury, but initial findings in some cases can be subtle, resulting in delays in diagnosis. If head injury or intoxication makes physical examination of the abdomen unreliable, DPL should be performed. The false-negative rate of DPL for this injury is 5%. CT, particularly if done early after injury, is not reliable in ruling out blunt intestinal injury.[199,200] The injury itself may not be obvious, and small amounts of intraperitoneal fluid from the injury may not be detectable.

Blunt injuries to the small intestine are most common in either the proximal jejunum or the distal ileum, probably because the intestine is fixed at these two points and more vulnerable to compression and stretch injuries. Multiple injuries to the small intestine from blunt trauma occur in about 25% of cases. Second or even third areas of injury should be carefully sought if a blunt intestinal injury is discovered on abdominal exploration.

After the suspicion of blunt intestinal or other intraabdominal injury has been raised and the decision to explore the abdomen has been made, the basic principles of abdominal exploration and operative management of blunt small bowel injuries are the same as for penetrating injuries. Because of the nature of the mechanism of injury, the perforations are usually amenable to primary repair. Mesenteric rents that cause devascularization and require resection are relatively more common after blunt injury than after penetrating injury.

Colon and Rectum

Most injuries to the colon and rectum are the result of penetrating or perforating trauma. Blunt trauma accounts for only about 5% of colonic injuries. Rectal injuries can occur in association with pelvic fractures, and the possibility of rectal injury must be considered in any patient with a significant pelvic fracture, in addition to evaluation of other pelvic viscera such as the bladder, distal ureters, uterus, and vagina.

Signs and symptoms of peritonitis result from injury to the colon and rectum but are not specific. Injury to the extraperitoneal rectum is particularly difficult to recognize because peritonitis does not result. Conventional laboratory studies are not usually helpful, but plain radiographs may show free air in the peritoneal cavity. DPL may be of value if intraperitoneal colonic injury is present, yielding lavage fluid with blood, bacteria, or fecal material. If the injury is confined to the extraperitoneal colon and rectum, however, DPL is of no value. Extraperitoneal colonic or rectal injury is extremely difficult to diagnose. The possibility of rectal injury must be considered in any patient with penetrating trauma to the lower abdomen or buttocks. Digital examination is essential. The presence of blood on examination is strong evidence for colon or rectal injury, and proctoscopic and sigmoidoscopic examinations should be performed. Water-soluble contrast studies may also be useful, but direct bowel examination usually is preferable. About 95% of colon injuries are caused by gunshot, shotgun, or stab wounds, and whenever the possibility of colonic injury is entertained, broad-spectrum intravenous prophylactic antibiotics should be started immediately. The number of doses continued postoperatively is determined by the degree of colon injury, but it is prudent to treat most patients for 7 to 10 days, as for established peritonitis.

The central issue in the operative management of colonic injuries is the controversy between primary repair of low-risk colonic injuries and repair or resection with exteriorization.[201] Primary repair may be selected after additional risk factors have been excluded. Complications increase with primary repair in the presence of preoperative hypotension, intraperitoneal hemorrhage exceeding 1 L, more than two additional injured organs (hepatic, pancreatic, and splenic injuries have the highest morbidity), significant fecal spillage, or an elapsed time since injury of more than 6 hours. Many patients with low-risk penetrating colon injuries can be treated with primary closure in the absence of these risk factors. High-risk colon injuries or those associated with severe injuries, as indicated previously, should be treated with resection and colostomy. This is a relatively conservative approach, and recent series indicate that primary repair may be safe even in the presence of some of the circumstances listed.[202,203] At present, however, a conservative approach is recommended.

A compromise between colostomy and primary repair has been advocated, with exteriorization of the repaired segment. The success of this technique varies, and it probably has little benefit over exteriorization alone. Postoperative complications include abscess formation, anastomotic leak, peristomal hernia, and the morbidity and mortality associated with colostomy closure.

The morbidity and mortality from rectal injuries is primarily a result of inadequate initial therapy and the complications associated with delayed sepsis. Rectal injury must be suspected if there is any penetrating injury or if there is a sacral fracture that produces a pelvic ring disruption. Sigmoidoscopic examination is essential.

The principles of operative management include the following:

- Placement of the patient in the lithotomy position to provide simultaneous exposure of both the perineum and abdomen
- Wide débridement of all dead and devitalized tissue
- A totally defunctioning colostomy (simple loop colostomy may be inadequate)
- Rectal wall closure if possible
- Retrorectal drainage in selected severe injuries with

coccygectomy if necessary to attain adequate rectal drainage
- Distal rectal stump washout
- Broad-spectrum intravenous antibiotics, nutritional support, and serial débridement

Complete rectal destruction is a rare injury for which primary abdominoperineal resection with packing may be necessary. If done, the packing should be removed operatively in about 48 hours. Complications of rectal injuries include pelvic abscesses, urinary or rectal fistulas, rectal incontinence and stricture, urinary incontinence, and loss of sexual function.

Retroperitoneal Hematoma

The management of retroperitoneal hematomas found at laparotomy in patients with multisystem trauma has been a source of controversy for years. The optimal management of retroperitoneal hematoma depends on a number of factors, including its cause, its location, and the presence of associated injuries.

The retroperitoneum can be divided into anatomic zones for purposes of decision making (Fig. 11-73). Central retroperitoneal hematomas (zone 1) are associated with pancreaticoduodenal injuries or major abdominal vascular injury. Flank or perinephric hematomas (zone 2) may be associated with injuries to the genitourinary tract or, in the case of penetrating trauma, with injuries to the colon. Zone 3 injuries, which are confined to or originate from the pelvis, are most often associated with pelvic fractures.

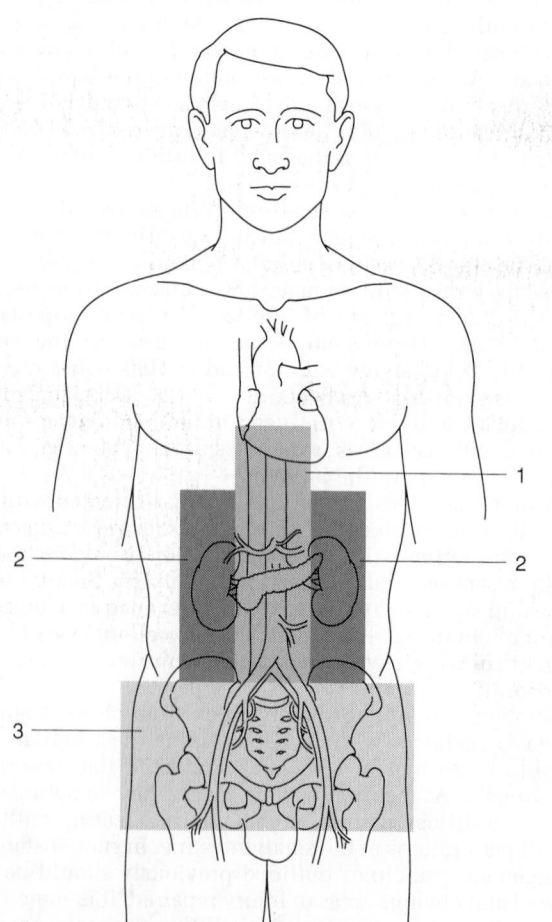

Figure 11-73. Zones of the retroperitoneum.

Retroperitoneal hematomas in zone 1, regardless of cause or size, are formally explored with inspection of each of the relevant structures. This is required because of the high incidence of associated major vascular, pancreatic, or duodenal injuries and the high morbidity and mortality if these are overlooked.

Zone 2 hematomas caused by penetrating injuries should routinely be explored. Whether proximal control of the renal pedicle should be obtained before exploration of a perinephric hematoma is controversial.[204-206] If there is severe ongoing hemorrhage, time should not be taken to obtain proximal control, and the kidney should be mobilized directly. If time and the degree of hemorrhage permit, however, it is probably safest to obtain vascular control before mobilization of the kidney. Zone 2 hematomas caused by blunt trauma can be left alone if they are not expanding and the intravenous urogram is normal.

Zone 3 retroperitoneal hematomas in patients with penetrating injuries are usually explored to exclude major vascular injuries. Local bleeding encountered at exploration under these circumstances is usually easy to control, and the associated injuries can be identified. Patients with zone 3 hematomas secondary to blunt trauma usually have associated pelvic fractures. Exploration of the hematoma can be hazardous and is usually avoided. There is often extensive injury to the rich presacral venous and arterial circulation. Incision of the peritoneum releases the tamponade, and dissection within the hematoma can produce catastrophic bleeding. Discrete bleeding points can rarely be identified. Exploration of these hematomas is associated with an increased requirement for transfusion and a higher mortality rate.

Definitive Care Phase: Retroperitoneal Injuries

ROBERT C. MACKERSIE

The process of identifying and controlling sources of major hemorrhage after injury is of primary importance early in the resuscitation of multiply-injured patients. This should be undertaken as a logical, stepwise process that includes evaluation of external, thoracic, abdominal, retroperitoneal, and fracture sites of hemorrhage. The initial diagnoses of fracture site hemorrhage and external hemorrhage can usually be made on the basis of the physical examination. The diagnoses of thoracic and abdominal hemorrhage are reliably made using chest radiography and diagnostic peritoneal lavage (DPL), as discussed earlier in this chapter. The diagnosis of retroperitoneal hemorrhage, however, cannot be made reliably with these methods and requires a separate set of screening and diagnostic studies. Two of the most common causes of major hemorrhage in the retroperitoneum after blunt trauma are pelvic fractures and injuries to the kidney. With appropriate screening and evaluation performed early in the resuscitation, timely therapeutic intervention can be instituted, resulting in decreased morbidity and mortality.

PELVIC FRACTURES

Most pelvic fractures occur as a result of blunt trauma with high energy transfer, such as occurs in motor vehicle accidents, motorcycle accidents, or falls. The spectrum of pelvic fracture injuries ranges from minor, isolated, nondisplaced fractures of the pubic rami to severe injuries with multiple fractures that can be rapidly lethal. The proximity of adjacent organs results in a high incidence of associated genitourinary and abdominal injuries. The potential complications of pelvic fracture injury may be underestimated in the face of other, more obvious injuries. Radiographic screening, early control of associated hemorrhage, and diagnosis and treatment of other injuries are essential to minimize morbidity and mortality.

Unlike most long-bone fractures, only about 25% of pelvic fractures are apparent on the basis of physical examination. The practice of forced bimanual manipulation of the iliac crests to elicit pelvic instability is to be condemned because it is neither sensitive nor specific diagnostically and it is painful at best in a patient with a pelvic fracture. Screening radiographs of the pelvis should be obtained on all patients with major blunt injuries or hypotension from any blunt mechanism.

A number of classification schemes have been proposed for pelvic fractures.[207-209] One of the simpler schemes is shown in Figure 11-74. Pelvic fractures are divided into fractures that are comminuted and unstable (type 1); fractures involving two separate breaks in the pelvic ring, which are also unstable (type 2); and stable fractures involving either single breaks in the ring or fractures of the pubic rami or iliac crest (type 3).[210]

Grouping pelvic fractures into those involving primarily the anterior arch and those involving primarily the posterior arch has also been proposed. This method is useful in that anterior arch fractures are most commonly associated with injury to the urethra in males or to the bladder, whereas posterior arch fractures are more commonly associated with major hemorrhage. Although a general relation exists between the number of breaks in the pelvic ring and the blood transfusion requirement, the precision with which the pelvic radiograph alone can predict massive transfusions is limited. This is particularly true of complex, crush-type injuries.

Hemorrhage resulting from injury to the sacral venous plexus, laceration of multiple arterial branches of the hypogastric vessels, or fractured cancellous bone presents a formidable challenge to the trauma surgeon. Massive hemorrhage is the principal cause of early death in patients with pelvic fracture, and survival depends principally on rapid identification and control. The presence of hemorrhage from associated intraperitoneal injuries should be considered first (Fig. 11-75). The presence of a major pelvic fracture, independent of other injuries, increases the probability of a significant intraabdominal injury by about 10%. For this reason, DPL is indicated for most patients with pelvic fractures. A supraumbilical lavage is preferable under these circumstances because of the possibility of catheter penetration of a large retroperitoneal hematoma dissecting into the preperitoneal space. If DPL is performed soon after injury using proper position and technique, the incidence of false-positive results caused by pelvic fracture hemorrhage has been reported to be as low as 1%.[211] DPL performed incorrectly in the infraumbilical site with a major pelvic fracture can yield an incidence of false-positive results as high as 45% (Fig. 11-76).

Grossly positive findings on DPL should prompt an expeditious exploratory laparotomy, because more than 90% of these patients have significant intraabdominal injuries. Patients with major pelvic fractures whose DPL results are positive only by cell count criteria have a lower incidence of major intraabdominal injuries, and that primary control of pelvic fracture hemorrhage may be considered first in these patients.[42]

At laparotomy, after a thorough abdominal exploration

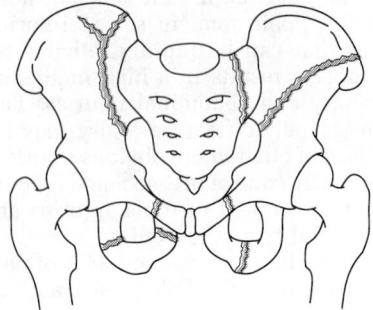

Type I: Unstable (crush)
Mortality: 20%–30%
Blood loss: >10 units
Complications: 60%–75%

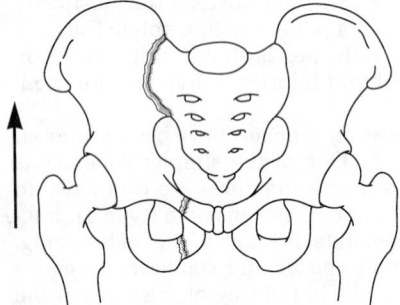

Type II: Unstable
Mortality: 8%–12%
Blood loss: 2–10 units
Complications: 30%–50%

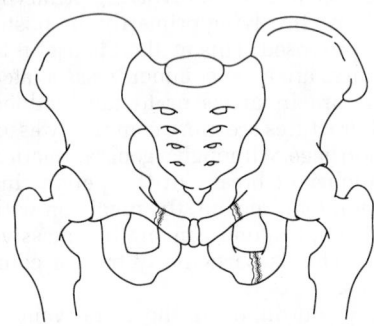

Type III: Stable
Mortality: <5%
Blood loss: 1–4 units
Complications: 10%–20%

Figure 11-74. Classification of pelvic fractures with relative stability, mortality rates, and blood loss indicated.

has been performed and injuries repaired, the size of the pelvic hematoma can be assessed. Exploration of retroperitoneal pelvic fracture hematomas is contraindicated under almost all circumstances. Pelvic fracture hemorrhage can rarely be controlled surgically, and decompression of the hematoma can further exacerbate bleeding. Ligation of the internal iliac arteries is ineffective in controlling bleeding because of the rich collateral blood supply and frequency of venous bleeding. On rare occasions, actual disruption of the iliac vessels requires operative control. For rapidly expanding pelvic hematomas, placement of laparotomy packs in the pelvis to aid tamponade can provide effective temporary control. The inferior extent of the laparotomy incision in patients with large pelvic fracture hematomas should be limited in order to facilitate wound closure and improve tamponade if packing is required. Rapid closure of the abdominal wound under these circumstances should be followed immediately by pelvic angiography and embolization of active arterial bleeding.

In patients with negative DPL results and evidence of major ongoing hemorrhage, three modalities are available to help reduce pelvic fracture blood loss: application of external counterpressure for venous tamponade, arteriography and embolization of arterial pelvic bleeding sites, and placement of an external pelvic fixator.[212]

The early identification of patients requiring specific pelvic fracture hemorrhage control is essential in reducing transfusion requirements and morbidity and mortality.

The combination of type and location of fractures, hemodynamic status on admission, and fluid and blood requirements in the first 30 to 60 minutes of resuscitation is usually sufficient to identify these patients. As a general rule, patients requiring six or more units of blood during the first 6 hours after injury may benefit from some form of specific hemorrhage control.

The application of external counterpressure (ie, the pneumatic antishock garment [PASG]) has been shown in several series to be effective in lowering transfusion requirements, presumably by producing tamponade of venous hemorrhage. Although the PASG can be used as the definitive method of hemorrhage control, its efficacy in controlling arterial hemorrhage or in reducing subsequent sacral plexus hemorrhage after removal is unclear. In addition, the prolonged use of external counterpressure has been associated with skin necrosis and lower-extremity compartment syndrome. For these reasons, the use of the PASG is limited to the resuscitation phase for immediate control of massive hemorrhage.

Definitive control of major arterial pelvic fracture bleeding is best accomplished by pelvic arteriography. Internal iliac arteriography with selective embolization of bleeding branches is associated with minimal morbidity and results in complete control of arterial bleeding in more than 85% of patients.[213,214]

In selected patients with unstable fractures involving the sacrum or pubic diastasis injuries, the application of pelvic

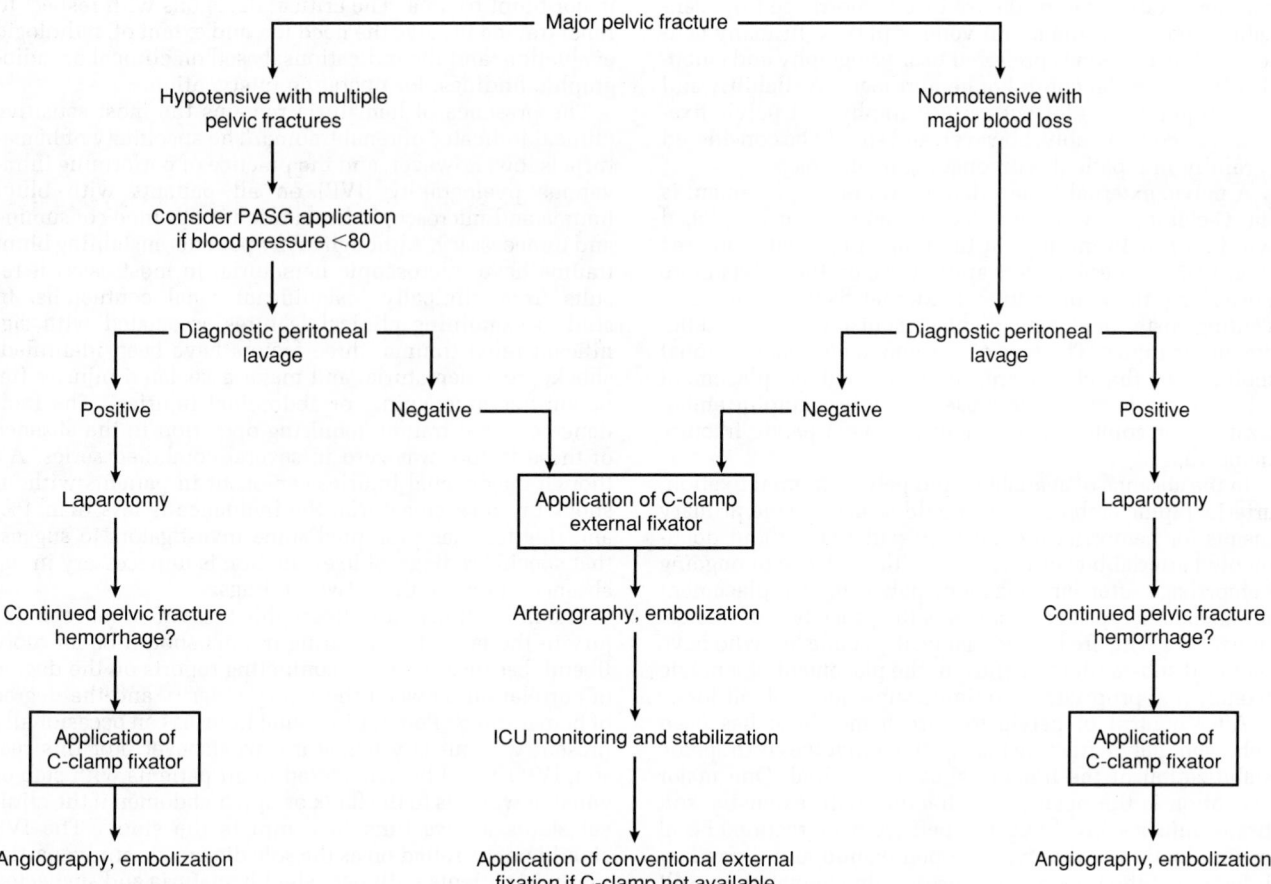

Figure 11-75. Algorithm for the initial management of abdominal and pelvic hemorrhage. External pelvic fixation should precede arteriography only if it is immediately available. PASG, pneumatic antishock garment.

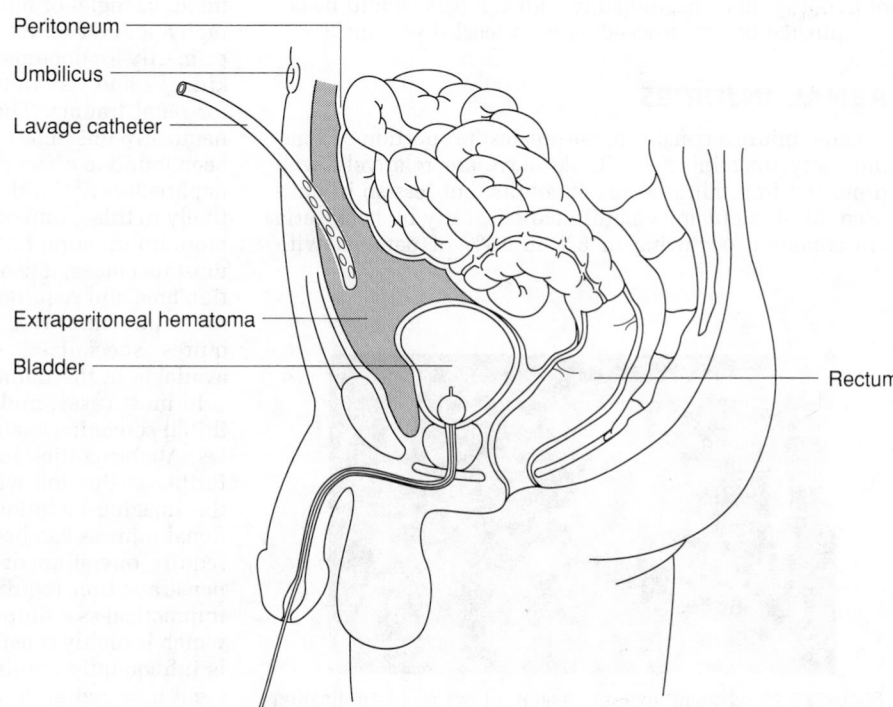

Figure 11-76. Peritoneal lavage performed through the infraumbilical site with pelvic fracture can be complicated by placement of the catheter into the extraperitoneal hematoma. Supraumbilical lavage is therefore indicated in the presence of a pelvic fracture.

external fixation can further reduce hemorrhage from cancellous bone and the sacral venous plexus. In many centers, pelvic fixation is preferred to arteriography and embolization for initial control of hemorrhage. Availability and time requirements for both arteriography and pelvic fixation vary considerably, however, and should be considered carefully in a patient with ongoing hemorrhage.

A pelvic external fixator that allows rapid placement is the C-clamp, or vice-type, fixator, which can be placed within 10 to 15 minutes in the trauma resuscitation area (Fig. 11-77). These fixators apply force on the pelvis more posteriorly than conventional external fixators, thus preventing posterior element displacement and associated ligamentous injury. The ease of placement and the rotational mobility of the clamp arm allow immediate placement without interference with subsequent arteriographic embolization for combined treatment of severe pelvic fracture hemorrhage.

In the absence of available rapid pelvic external fixation, arteriographic embolization should be used as the primary means for hemorrhage control. In patients without documented arterial bleeding sites or with evidence of ongoing hemorrhage after embolization, pelvic fixator placement for amenable types of fractures is the procedure of choice. In patients who are hemodynamically stable but who have required substantial transfusion, the placement of a pelvic fixator, if appropriate, also limits subsequent blood loss.

After control of pelvic fracture hemorrhage has been achieved, pelvic fracture management involves orthopedic stabilization of the fracture sites, if required. One major exception is the open pelvic fracture with extensive soft tissue injuries involving the perineum or rectum. Fecal contamination of this type of open wound and secondary infection of the fracture and surrounding hematoma result in a high incidence of sepsis and mortality in inadequately treated patients. Complete proximal fecal division produced by a divided colostomy or end-colostomy and Hartmann pouch has been shown to reduce the mortality rate by approximately 50% in patients with these injuries. The performance of a diverting colostomy should not be undertaken as a first priority, however. Control of hemorrhage, treatment of other life-threatening injuries, and correction of hypothermia, coagulopathy, and acidosis should be accomplished before proceeding with fecal diversion.

RENAL INJURIES

Renal injuries constitute the greatest proportion of genitourinary tract injuries. The kidneys are relatively well protected from blunt injury in adults, but less so in children. Mild contusions manifested clinically by hematuria are common, occurring in 6% to 15% of patients with major blunt trauma. The critical decisions with respect to renal trauma involve the need for, and extent of, radiologic evaluation, and the indications, based on clinical or radiographic findings, for operative intervention.

The presence of hematuria remains the most sensitive clinical indicator of renal trauma. The specificity of hematuria is low, however, and the practice of performing intravenous pyelography (IVP) on all patients with blunt trauma and microscopic hematuria is both time-consuming and unnecessary. Although many patients sustaining blunt trauma have microscopic hematuria, in most cases it results from clinically insignificant renal contusions. In studies examining clinical features associated with significant renal trauma, three factors have been identified: shock, gross hematuria, and major associated injuries (ie, pelvic fractures, spinal or abdominal injuries). The incidence of renal trauma requiring operation in the absence of these factors was zero in several combined series. Although major renal injuries can occur in patients without shock or gross hematuria, the incidence is less than 1%, and this fact has prompted some investigators to suggest that specific radiographic evaluation is unnecessary in the absence of one of these two findings.

The indications for radiographic assessment of renal injury in the face of penetrating trauma should be far more liberal, because there are conflicting reports on the degree of correlation between the injury severity and the degree of hematuria.[215] Penetrating renal injuries can occasionally present without any hematuria whatsoever. For this reason, IVP should be considered in all patients with stab or gunshot wounds to the flank or upper abdomen if the clinical status allows time to complete the study. The IVP should not be relied on as the sole diagnostic study, particularly in patients with persistent hematuria and suspected penetrating renal injury. In one report, the incidence of false-negative IVP studies was 75% for penetrating injuries.[216] Most of these false-negative studies were associated with smaller cortical lacerations not involving the collecting system. Computed tomography (CT) scanning should be used to stage any injury treated nonoperatively, and follow-up CT scans are usually indicated.

Radiographic options for the diagnosis of renal trauma include single- or multiple-film IVP, formal nephrotomography, and CT scan. Single-film ("one-shot") IVP is useful primarily for documenting the presence of two functioning kidneys and has limited use as a screening examination for renal trauma. The use of single-film IVP in hemodynamically unstable patients requiring laparotomy has not been found to affect the intraoperative decision to perform nephrectomy,[217] and the procedure should not be used routinely in this group of patients. Multiple-film IVP provides more information on the ureters and collecting system. In most instances, it can be performed easily in the resuscitation area and requires minimal time and effort. Nephrotomography improves diagnostic accuracy of IVP but requires specialized equipment that frequently is not available in the trauma resuscitation area.

In most cases, multiple-film IVP serves as an adequate initial screening examination, particularly for blunt injuries. Abnormalities suggesting renal injury should prompt further evaluation with CT scan. CT scan has emerged as the imaging technique of choice for most renal trauma. Renal injuries can be staged with respect to those likely to require operation or to develop complications. The expense and time required for the CT scan, however, makes it impractical as a simple screening modality. Arteriography, which is highly sensitive and specific for vascular injuries, is infrequently required, because renal CT provides sufficient information to allow exploration and repair of renal vascular injuries.

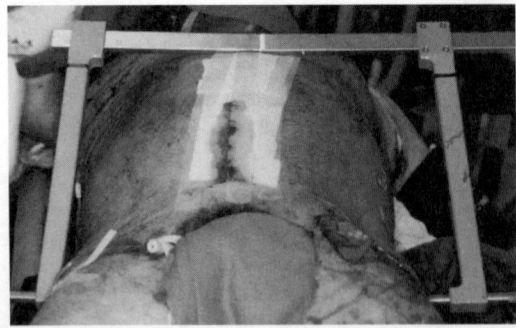

Figure 11-77. C-clamp external fixator allows rapid application of posterior fixation.

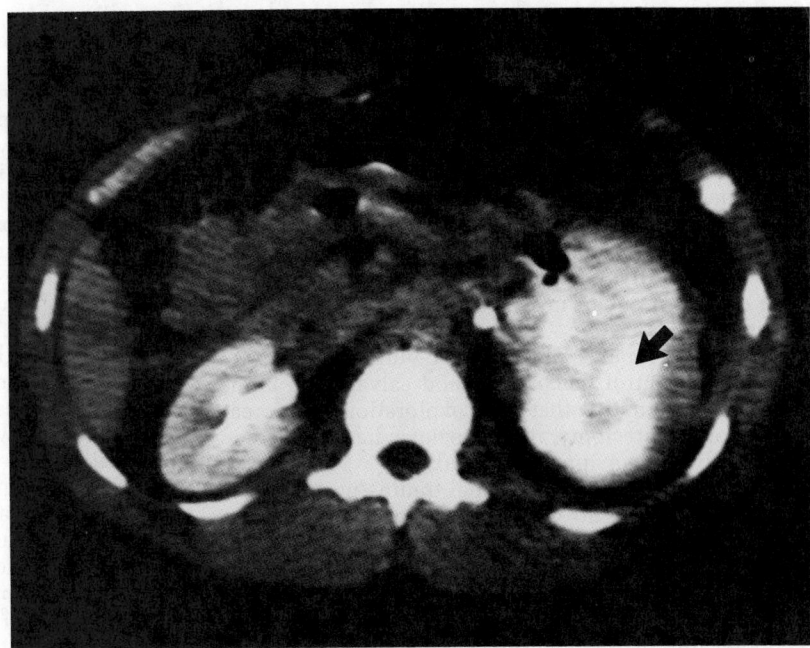

Figure 11-78. Ruptured kidney (*arrow*) requiring operation for intractable pain and continued hemorrhage.

The decision to perform renal exploration as an independent procedure should be based on both radiographic and clinical evaluation. CT allows more precise assessment of the degree of perinephric hemorrhage and the degree of collecting system disruption than operative inspection[218] (Figs. 11-78 and 11-79). Most blunt renal injuries diagnosed with preoperative CT are contusions and minor lacerations, and can be treated nonoperatively with close monitoring and follow-up CT. Renal parenchymal injuries and even minor lacerations of the collecting system caused by blunt trauma usually heal without complications. Patients with clinical evidence of ongoing hemorrhage, larger or expanding perinephric hematomas, major collecting system disruptions, or persistent hemorrhage into the collecting system usually benefit from early operation.

Penetrating injuries, particularly gunshot wounds, routinely require exploratory laparotomy because of the high incidence of associated intraabdominal injuries and the likelihood of complex renal injury. The overall incidence of renal injuries in penetrating torso trauma is 6% to 8%. Stab wounds occasionally produce only minor isolated renal lacerations, without hilar or collecting system involvement, and minimal hematomas. Selected patients have been successfully treated nonoperatively with close clinical examination and follow-up.

A number of major renal injuries are diagnosed at the time of initial laparotomy, often in hemodynamically unstable patients. Most commonly, a perinephric hematoma is encountered in association with blunt hepatic or splenic injuries. Indications for renal exploration at laparotomy

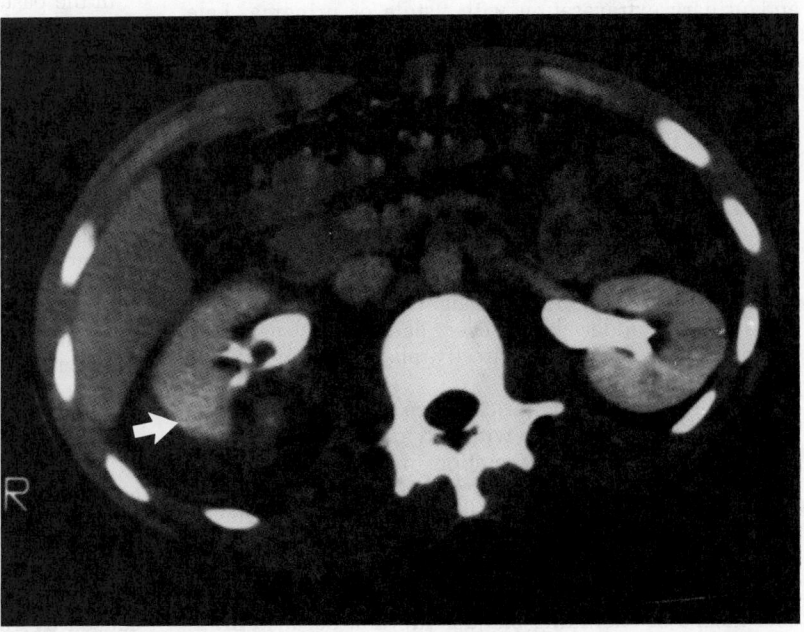

Figure 11-79. Ruptured kidney (*arrow*) treated nonoperatively.

after blunt trauma include an expanding or pulsatile perinephric hematoma and suspected renal vascular injury. In patients with blunt injuries, it is preferable to defer exploration of nonexpanding, nonpulsatile perinephric hematomas until treatment of intraabdominal and other associated life-threatening injuries is completed. Postoperative CT scanning can be used for formal staging of these injuries. In many instances, injuries can be better defined and treated nonoperatively. Perinephric hematomas found during laparotomy for penetrating trauma should usually be explored carefully. Continued or recurrent hemorrhage is more often a problem in penetrating than in blunt renal injuries.

The goal of renal exploration for blunt or penetrating injury is to control hemorrhage and salvage the kidney. Contrary to the notion that renal exploration often creates a need for nephrectomy, recent reviews have reported an overall salvage rate approaching 90%.[219]

The operative approach to renal trauma usually should include proximal control of both the renal artery and renal vein. After control of the renal hilum is obtained, the kidney can be explored by mobilization of either the right or left colon centrally and dissection through the Gerota fascia, with elevation of the kidney from the retroperitoneum. Although initial proximal renal vascular control can potentially result in a lower overall nephrectomy rate, it may not be appropriate in patients who are hemodynamically compromised as a result of their renal injury. Under these circumstances, rapid mobilization of the kidney with digital control of the hilum is necessary to stem what can be exsanguinating hemorrhage. Many of these patients ultimately require nephrectomy.

The specific operative approach is dependent on the injury. The general objectives are to control hemorrhage, repair any injury to the collecting system, and revascularize or remove nonperfused renal tissue. Options include simple suture repair of lacerations with or without pedicle flap coverage, partial nephrectomy with oversewing of vessels and repair of the collecting system, and total nephrectomy. Although some enthusiasm exists for revascularization of arterial injuries involving intimal tears and complete occlusion of the renal artery, this is rarely successful in patients with blunt trauma. To be successful, repair should be performed within 6 to 8 hours of injury.

Postoperative complications from renal trauma include recurrent or ongoing hemorrhage, arteriovenous fistula, and urinary extravasation with fistula or urinoma. Late hypertension may also occur in a small number of patients as a result of either central renal vascular injuries or severely injured kidneys treated nonoperatively. The outcome of complications from renal trauma depends on the extent and timeliness of postinjury evaluation.

BLADDER INJURIES

Injury to the urinary bladder, with its relatively protected position, is often associated with other serious injuries. Diagnostic methods are straightforward and effective and should be undertaken in every patient with suspected bladder injury. Outcome is directly related to early diagnosis and treatment.

Most blunt bladder injuries (more than 95% in some series) occur in association with pelvic fractures. The most common mechanism is laceration of the extraperitoneal bladder. Severe deceleration can also result in a bursting rupture at the dome of the bladder. Penetrating injuries to the bladder may occur in isolation but are more commonly associated with other intraabdominal injuries. The absence of peritoneal signs on physical examination is not a reliable means of excluding bladder rupture, because intra-

peritoneal rupture occurs less frequently, and urine, if present in the peritoneum, produces little inflammatory reaction. The diagnostic method of choice for suspected rupture of the urinary bladder is a static cystogram followed by a postvoid film. Cystography should be performed in any patient with visible blood in the urine in association with a pelvic fracture. Static cystography can be conducted easily in the trauma resuscitation area and involves the placement of a urinary catheter and the instillation of contrast medium. Large bladder perforations or dome ruptures are often visualized with smaller amounts of contrast, and the initial film should be taken using only 100 to 150 mL of contrast. If the initial film is negative, full distention of the bladder with 300 to 400 mL is required to reliably exclude injury, because small perforations, particularly those caused by penetrating injury, may not be apparent otherwise. Although most bladder ruptures are readily apparent after these studies, small retroperitoneal perforations may be missed because small amounts of extravasation can be concealed by the contrast medium within the bladder itself. For this reason, it is essential to empty the bladder completely and to obtain an additional post-void film. The diagnosis of urinary bladder rupture on the basis of CT scan is made occasionally as an incidental or serendipitous finding, but CT should not be relied on to exclude ruptured urinary bladder because of the frequency of false-negative findings.

Urethral injury in men is frequently associated with bladder rupture, and all male patients should be carefully examined for the presence of scrotal or urethral hematoma, free-floating prostate, or blood at the meatus. Retrograde urethrography should be performed before placement of urinary catheters in these patients.

Bladder ruptures are classified into those that rupture freely into the peritoneal cavity (Fig. 11-80) and those with extravasation limited to the retroperitoneum (Fig. 11-81). Intraperitoneal bladder ruptures, often involving burst injuries of the dome, are characteristically large injuries, and they require early operative repair. Occasionally, this form of bladder rupture is discovered at the time of laparotomy for other, immediately life-threatening problems. Bladder repair is accomplished by a layered closure using absorbable sutures. Although many urologists prefer to place a suprapubic cystostomy tube at the time of bladder repair, patients can also be managed with simple urethral catheter drainage alone.

In the past, extraperitoneal bladder ruptures were treated primarily by operative repair. It has since become evident that most extraperitoneal bladder injuries can be treated nonoperatively by urethral catheter drainage alone.[220] This method obviates bladder exploration with manipulation of the extraperitoneal hematoma. The early and late complications after nonoperative management of extraperitoneal bladder injuries are minimal. Follow-up cystography, performed after about 10 days, demonstrates healing of the bladder injury in approximately 85% of patients.[221] Occasionally, a patient requires prolonged catheter drainage, and consideration should be given to performing a suprapubic cystostomy under these circumstances. With this management regimen, even large extraperitoneal bladder injuries heal without the need for operative repair.

Most complications of bladder rupture involve delay or error in diagnosis. Contamination of the large pelvic hematoma with infected urine is reported rarely. Patients with extraperitoneal bladder rupture usually should be given antibiotics for the duration of urinary catheter placement.

URETERAL INJURIES

Ureteral injuries occur less frequently than injuries to either the bladder or the kidney. They are most often caused by gunshot wounds and stab wounds but in rare

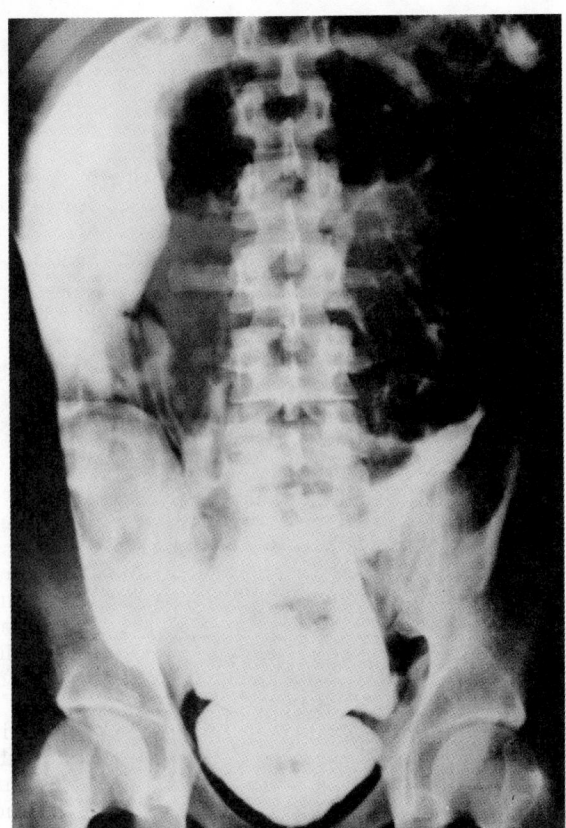

Figure 11-80. Intraperitoneal rupture of the bladder as demonstrated on cystogram.

cases are secondary to blunt external trauma. Because isolated ureteral injuries can present without even microscopic hematuria, a vigorous search for ureteral injury is required for any patient with penetrating trauma.

The diagnosis of a ureteral injury after trauma can usually be made on the basis of an IVP showing either a cutoff in ureteral drainage or contrast extravasation. About 15% of ureteral injuries are not evident initially on IVP,

and retrograde ureterography is necessary to confirm the diagnosis.

The luxury of preoperative IVP is frequently not available in patients with life-threatening intraabdominal injuries who require immediate laparotomy. Ureteral injuries under these circumstances must be excluded at the time of surgery. In most cases, exploration of the bullet or stab wound tract is sufficient to exclude or confirm ureteral injury. With massive retroperitoneal hematomas or the presence of multiple penetrating injuries, direct inspection of the entire ureter is not feasible, and extensive dissection should be avoided because of the danger of devascularization. Under these circumstances, an intraoperative IVP can be performed. An alternative is intraoperative chromopyelography using intravenous methylene blue to color the urine and better delineate any extravasation.

Treatment of ureteral injuries is best performed at the time of initial exploration. Specific treatment primarily depends on the location and extent of injury. In most cases with penetrating trauma, short segments of ureter are involved, and there is little if any loss of length. Under these circumstances, primary ureteroureterostomy with stenting or reimplantation of the distal ureter into the bladder is the preferred technique (Fig. 11-82A). For ureteral injuries involving long segment loss, such as those that occur with shotgun injuries, the problem is more complex. Lower ureteral injuries can be repaired by reimplantation of the distal ureter into the bladder, combined with either a psoas hitch (see Fig. 11-82B) or a bladder pedicle (Boari) flap (see Fig. 11-82C) to reduce tension. Transureteroureterostomy is an option for both lower and middle ureteral injuries (see Fig. 11-82D). For long segment loss in the upper ureter, autotransplantation of the kidney to the iliac fossa has been described, as has small bowel interposition.

Missed ureteral injuries can present as urinoma, characterized by nausea, vomiting, fever, and lower quadrant pain. Urinary fistulas with drainage through either a surgical wound or the original penetrating injury can also occur. Screening for these missed ureteral injuries is best done with IVP, ultrasound, or CT scanning to look for urinomas. A definitive diagnosis is best obtained by retrograde ureterography.

URETHRAL INJURIES

The occurrence of urethral injuries after trauma is limited almost entirely to the male population because of the length and exposure of the membranous urethra[222] (Fig.

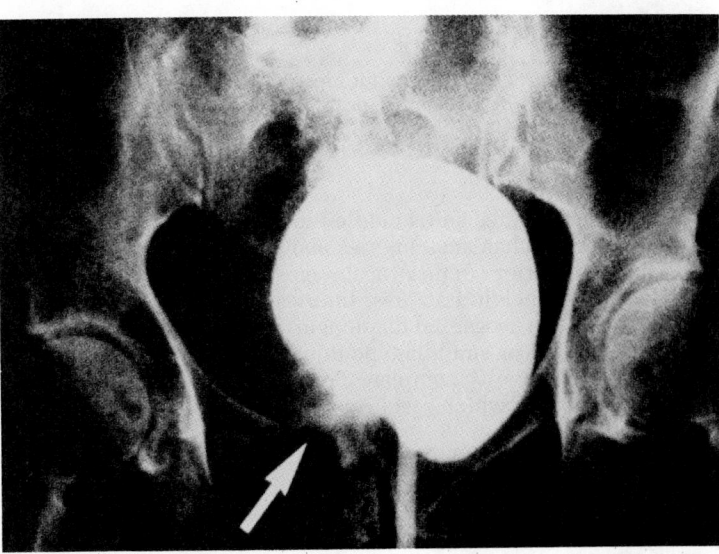

Figure 11-81. Cystogram demonstrating contained retroperitoneal bladder rupture.

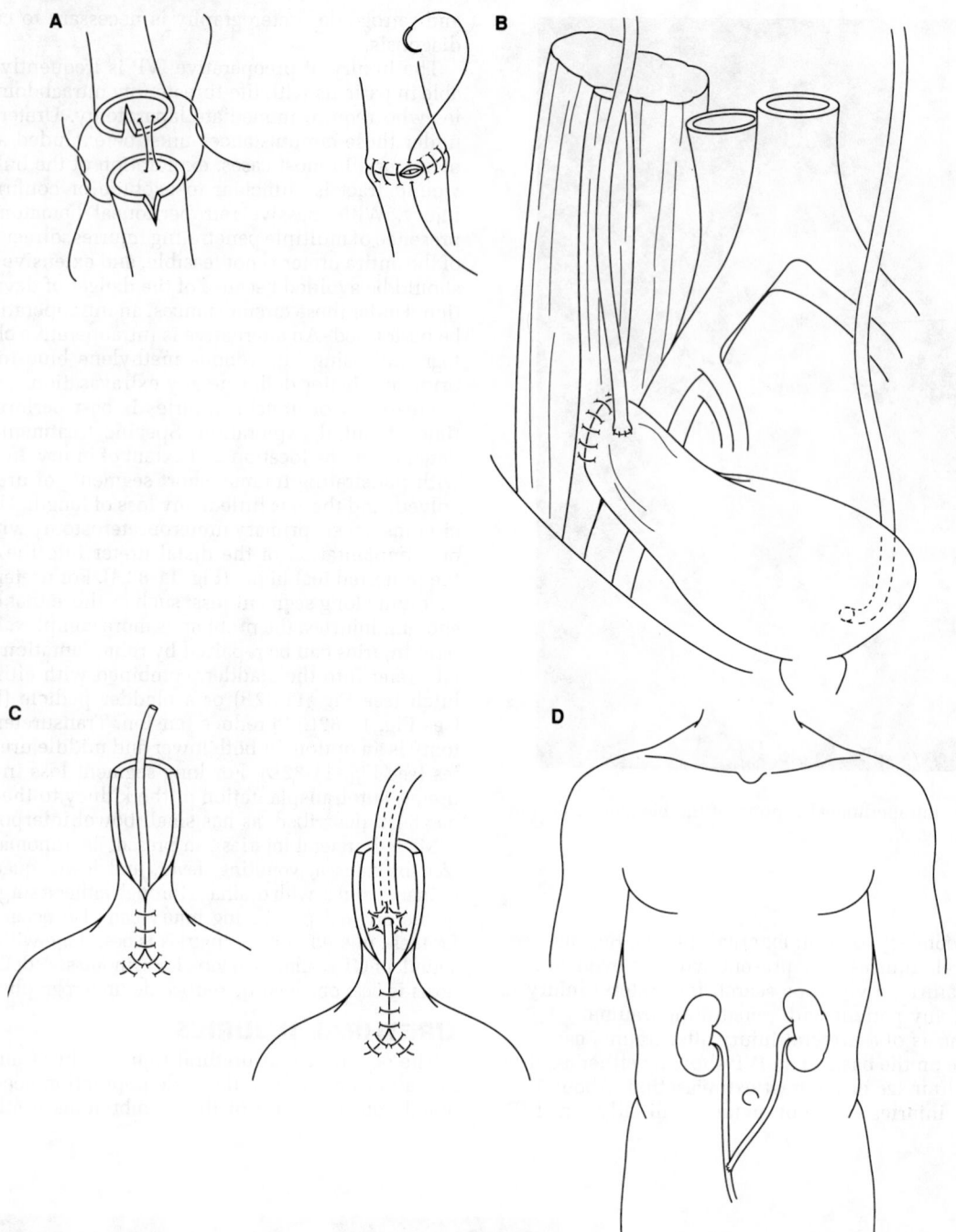

Figure 11-82. Options for repair of the ureter: primary ureteroureterostomy (*A*), psoas hitch (*B*), bladder (Boari) flap (*C*), or transureteroureterostomy (*D*).

11-83). Pelvic fractures and straddle-type injuries are the most common mechanisms. Injuries above the urogenital diaphragm (posterior urethra) occur most commonly in association with pelvic fractures. Injuries to the anterior urethra (below the urogenital diaphragm) occur usually as the result of a fall or straddle-type injury. Most posterior urethral injuries involve complete disruption, as opposed to anterior injuries, which result in partial tears in about half of patients.

A urethral tear should be suspected in any male patient with pelvic fracture. These patients should be examined carefully for signs of urethral injury, including scrotal or perineal hematomas, blood at the urethral meatus, or ante-

rior displacement of the prostate gland on rectal examination. The presence of any of these clinical findings constitutes a contraindication to immediate placement of a urethral catheter. A retrograde urethrogram should be obtained in these cases by the placement of a small balloon catheter in the fossa navicularis and gravity infusion of 10 to 15 mL of contrast material. This is a rapid, simple, and reliable means of diagnosing urethral injuries (Fig. 11-84). Contrast material should never be injected under pressure for this examination.

Urethral injuries, particularly partial tears that are not associated with prostate displacement, can occur in the absence of any clinical findings. Urinary catheters should

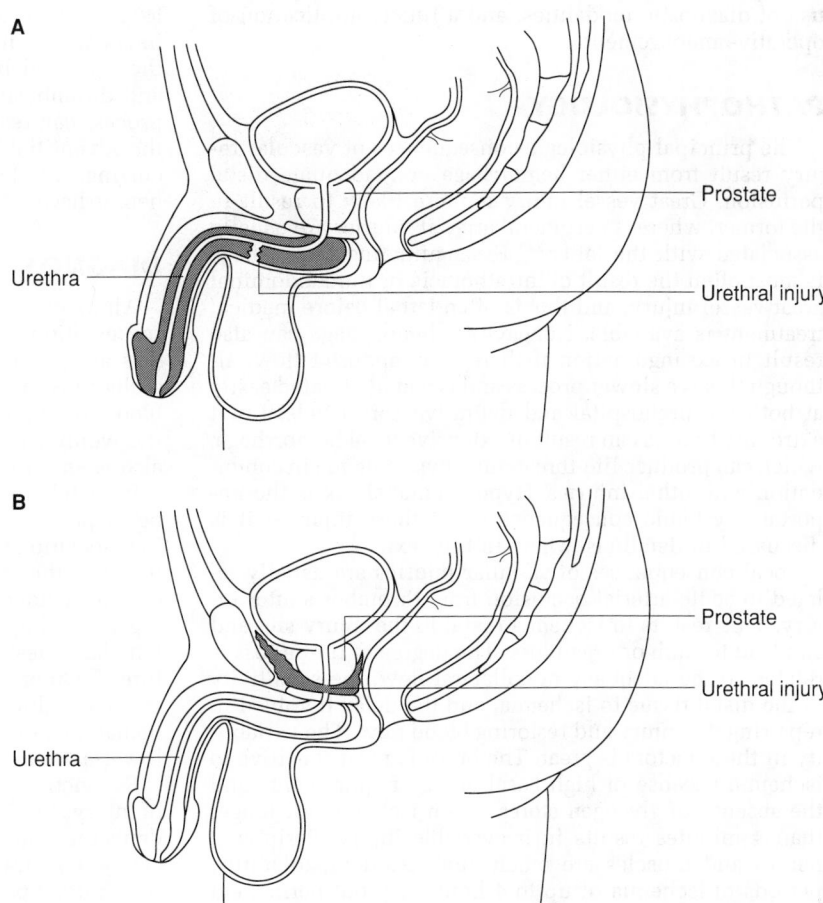

Figure 11-83. (*A*) Anterior tear of the urethra with the Buck fascia intact. (*B*) Posterior tear with prostate displacement.

be placed with great care in any patient with a pelvic fracture, and any difficulty in catheter placement should be an indication for a retrograde urethrogram.

Initial management of urethral tears consists of suprapubic cystostomy for urinary drainage. Because of the increased incidence of impotence and urinary stricture, immediate repair or reconstruction of the injured urethra usually is not attempted. Formal reconstruction of urethral tears can be undertaken after several months and usually involves a perineal urethroplasty. Impotence, which occurs in about 20% of late repairs, is the major complication, and its severity is related to the degree of initial injury.

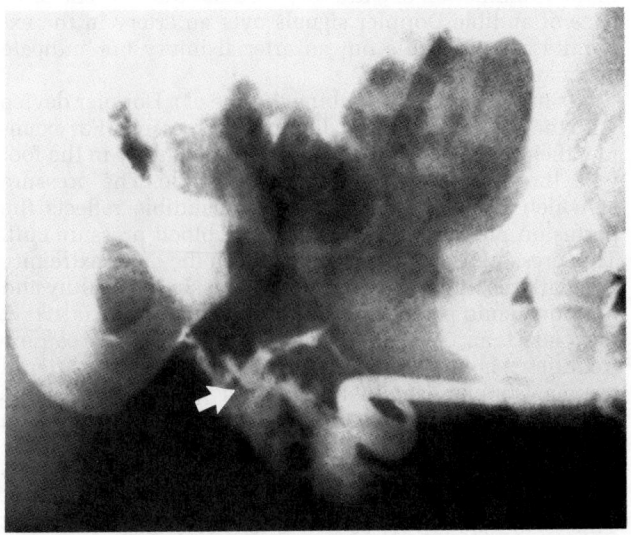

Figure 11-84. Retrograde urethrogram showing tear of the membranous urethra (posterior) with contrast extravasation (*arrow*).

Definitive Care Phase: Vascular Injuries

MICHAEL J. SISE AND STEVEN R. SHACKFORD

Vascular injuries have become increasingly common because of the epidemic of urban violence and the widespread application of invasive diagnostic and therapeutic techniques that use vascular access. The development of regional trauma systems with rapid transport has also contributed to the increased incidence of vascular injuries by delivering patients with previously fatal injuries to the trauma center in a timely fashion. Injuries range from isolated penetrating extremity trauma with minimal signs to major vessel injury with blunt-mechanism, multiple-system trauma. Early diagnosis and successful management require a thorough examination, a thorough search based on mechanism and location of injury, an efficient use of diagnostic modalities, and a timely application of operative management.

PATHOPHYSIOLOGY

The principal physiologic consequences of vascular injury result from either hemorrhage or inadequate distal perfusion. Great vessel injury is more likely to result in the former, whereas peripheral arterial injuries are usually associated with the latter.[223] Exsanguinating hemorrhage is most often the result of intrathoracic or intraabdominal great vessel injury, and this is often lethal before medical treatment is available. Noncavitary hemorrhage can also result in exsanguination if there is unopposed flow, although this is a slower process and is usually treated easily at both the prehospital and definitive care levels. Blunt extremity trauma can result in extensive local hemorrhage, which can produce life-threatening hypovolemia in combination with other injuries. Hypovolemic shock is the important systemic consequence of all these injuries; it is discussed in detail elsewhere in this text.

Local consequences of vascular injuries are usually related to acute arterial occlusion from thrombosis after injury. This results in ischemia distal to the injury site and can lead to limb or organ loss. The degree of tissue loss is related to the adequacy of collateral flow, the sensitivity of the distal tissue to ischemia, and the delay involved in repairing the injury and restoring blood flow. The variability in these factors is great. The brain is most sensitive to ischemia because of high basal energy requirements and the absence of glycogen stores. Brain ischemia for longer than 4 minutes results in irreversible injury. Peripheral nerves and muscles are much more resilient, tolerating periods of ischemia of up to 4 hours without permanent injury. An important principle of vascular repairs, however, is that outcome is time-dependent, necessitating an aggressive approach and a high priority.

The mechanism of injury from acute arterial ischemia includes both the initial anoxic phase, when blood flow has ceased, and a reperfusion phase, after blood flow has been restored. The events associated with the restoration of arterial blood flow after complete ischemia extend the magnitude and severity of the original insult in skeletal muscle and peripheral nerves. Reperfusion injury includes the production of toxic metabolites and an inflammatory response that causes significant endothelial damage.[224,225]

If the severity of ischemia is significant enough to cause skeletal muscle necrosis, rhabdomyolysis with the release of potassium and myoglobin into the systemic circulation follows. Acute acidosis, hyperkalemia, and myoglobin-induced renal failure can occur. Beyond the immediate threat of limb loss, the systemic effects of extremity ischemia with muscle necrosis can ultimately prove fatal.

The type of vascular injury is related to both the mechanism of trauma and the location of the target vessel. Simple lacerations are the most common penetrating injuries to both arteries and veins. Incomplete lacerations often cause more hemorrhage than complete transections because of the inability of a partially transected vessel to undergo retraction, vasoconstriction, and thrombosis as it would if completely transected. Complex associated soft tissue injuries also exacerbate local hemorrhage. Intimal flap occlusion, arterial contusion with thrombosis, and arteriovenous fistulas are all common outcomes of acute penetrating vascular injury. Chronic problems include pseudoaneurysm formation, thrombosis, and distal embolization.

Blunt trauma usually is caused by the deceleration injuries associated with motor vehicle accidents or falls from heights, and it commonly results in complete or partial disruption of the vessel wall. As the arterial wall is deformed, the elastic adventitia and muscular layers remain intact while the intima fractures. Blood dissects beneath the fractured intima, causing protrusion into the lumen and thrombosis. In the aorta and its major branches, this process can result in an acute pseudoaneurysm with only the adventitial layer remaining intact; delayed rupture, occurring minutes to days later, can cause exsanguinating hemorrhage.

DIAGNOSIS

Although vascular trauma may be apparent on initial presentation, it is frequently occult. Assessments of blood loss are predictably emotional and inaccurate; however, a clear history of arterial bleeding (pulsatile, oxygenated blood) or major venous bleeding (dark blood flowing from the wound) is noteworthy. The presence of hypotension also is an important observation.

Intraabdominal or intrathoracic vascular injury should be suspected if penetrating trauma to the torso is present in association with hypovolemic shock. Blunt great vessel injury in the chest should be suspected whenever there is external evidence of major thoracic trauma, such as a steering wheel imprint on the anterior chest, sternal fracture, left flail chest, thoracic spine fracture, or first rib fracture.[226] Other signs associated with intrathoracic vascular trauma include a widened mediastinum, thoracic outlet hematoma, upper-extremity hypotension, and diminished lower-extremity pulse.

For victims of blunt trauma, the mechanism and force of injury should be carefully reviewed. Motor vehicle accidents that cause fatalities are often associated with significant energy transfer. A history of altered mental status or intermittent paralysis also should alert the examiner to the possibility of aortic or arch vessel disruption.

The physical examination specific to the evaluation of vascular injuries should follow the initial assessment previously detailed. The course of a penetrating injury should be estimated both visually and radiographically, using plain films with radiopaque markers for entrance and exit site location. Patients with blunt injuries require a complete evaluation with emphasis on examination of the pulses. This can be difficult in a hypovolemic and hypotensive patient with multiple fractures and splints. After adequate fluid resuscitation has been completed, peripheral pulses should be palpable. Segmental arterial pressure determination by Doppler technique is a valuable adjunct in the examination of extremity vascular trauma. The presence of audible Doppler signals over an artery in the extremity does not rule out an arterial injury nor indicate adequate perfusion.

It is most helpful to combine the use of a Doppler device with the determinations of distal blood pressure. For example, the probe is placed over the selected artery in the foot with the blood pressure cuff at the ankle. The pressure at which Doppler signals become inaudible reflects the perfusion pressure at the level of the blood pressure cuff. This pressure is compared with that in the other extremity and with the upper-extremity pressures. In the healthy and normovolemic person, the ankle–brachial index is 1:1. A ratio less than 0.9, or a 20-mmHg difference between extremities, should arouse suspicion of significant arterial trauma. Doppler examination has not been widely used to screen for significant venous injuries and is of unproven value.

Duplex scanning in extremity vascular trauma is a valuable adjunct in the rapid evaluation of trauma patients. This technique is very sensitive for detecting vascular injury and can be used as a valuable screening technique in patients who do not have classic signs of vascular trauma.[227] This technique is particularly accurate in detecting thrombosis, pseudoaneurysm, intimal flap, and arteriovenous fistula. Although it is currently used on a limited basis, this technique can find broad application in the evaluation of trauma patients.

Complete proximal occlusion or arterial disruption results in distal ischemia, which in the extremities produces the classic findings of pain, pallor, pulse deficit, paresthesia, and diminished perfusion (Table 11-16). Partial occlusions produce lesser signs and symptoms and are therefore more likely to be missed.

The selective use of arteriography is fundamental to the evaluation of patients with suspected vascular trauma. In general, the purposes of arteriography are to rule out the presence of occult vascular injury in patients with a suggestive history or physical examination and to establish the anatomy and location of an injury, so as to direct appropriate surgical exposure. Arteriography is not necessary if there is unequivocal evidence of arterial injury and if the operative approach is easily established. For example, a patient with a posterior knee dislocation and popliteal artery occlusion does not need arteriography before operation. In this instance, arteriography is probably unnecessary and certainly time consuming. In contrast, a hemodynamically stable patient with a penetrating neck wound at the thoracic inlet cannot be efficiently managed without arteriography of the aortic arch and great vessels. It is essential to individualize the use of arteriography in vascular trauma.

The indications for arteriography include a history of moderate hemorrhage at the penetrating injury site, injury in proximity to major arterial structures, diminished pulses, and peripheral nerve injury in the distribution of a nerve that is in proximity to a major vessel. Proximity as the sole indication for arteriography, in the absence of a diminished ankle–brachial ratio or other signs of major injury, has proved to be an unreliable indicator of the need for arteriography.[228] In the absence of the classic signs of major vascular injury, patients with penetrating wounds in proximity to major vessels can be observed closely without arteriography.

Formal arteriography using the Seldinger technique is preferred in stable patients. In unstable patients with other major injuries and suspected occult extremity arterial trauma, arteriography can be performed in the emergency department or on the operating table. In these cases, rapid bolus injection of sufficient contrast material without inflow occlusion is most likely to produce adequate visualization of extremity vessels.

Arteriography for vascular trauma must be performed with attention to several essential details:

1. Entrance and exit wounds should be marked with radiopaque markers.

2. The contrast agent should be injected well above the suspected site of injury.
3. Biplanar views of at least 15 cm of artery above and below the site of injury should be obtained.
4. Early and late views should be taken to rule out the presence of early venous filling from an arteriovenous fistula or late filling of a pseudoaneurysm.
5. Any abnormality should be attributed to vessel injury unless there is unequivocal evidence of underlying chronic vascular disease in the contralateral noninjured extremity.

The appropriate use of arteriography can significantly reduce the rate of unnecessary explorations for suspected vascular trauma. If routine surgical exploration is performed whenever vascular injury is suspected, a negative exploration rate of about 60% or more can be expected. Selective use of arteriography reduces the negative exploration rate to about 35%. With experience, arteriography is an extremely reliable method of excluding vascular trauma. In this context, the sensitivity is 97% to 100%, and the specificity is 90% to 98%, with overall accuracy between 92% and 98%.[228] Arteriography has an associated minor complication rate of 2% to 4% and a major complication rate of 0.6%.

NONOPERATIVE MANAGEMENT

The aggressive application of arteriography for suspected occult vascular trauma results in the detection of clinically insignificant lesions that can be treated nonoperatively. These include intimal irregularity, focal spasm with minimal narrowing, and small pseudoaneurysms. Although these lesions have been aggressively managed with operative therapy in the past, considerable evidence suggests that nonoperative therapy of some asymptomatic lesions is safe and effective. Ongoing surveillance for subsequent occlusion or hemorrhage is mandatory, however. Duplex scanning offers an accurate, noninvasive method to follow these lesions in the extremities. Operative therapy is indicated for thrombosis, for chronic symptoms of occlusive disease, and for failure of small pseudoaneurysms to undergo thrombosis. Nonoperative therapy may also be indicated for clinically insignificant lesions in patients with multiple injuries for whom vascular repair would present a prohibitive risk.

OPERATIVE MANAGEMENT

The initial step in the management of all vascular injuries is the adequate restoration of circulating blood volume. External bleeding should be controlled by direct pressure. Blind clamp placement is to be condemned. Tourniquets also are to be avoided unless there is extensive soft tissue loss with extensive hemorrhage. If the use of a tourniquet is unavoidable, a pneumatic cuff of the type used for distal-extremity orthopedic procedures is preferred. Tourniquets occlude collaterals, making distal ischemia significantly worse. If applied improperly, they allow arterial inflow, occlude venous outflow, and increase bleeding.

The operative management of vascular injuries must be orchestrated with the overall care of the patient's other injuries. Although life-threatening abdominal or thoracic injuries take priority over limb-threatening arterial injuries, every attempt should be made to begin simultaneous vascular repair by an additional team of surgeons while the abdominal or chest injury is being treated.

The goal of operative management of vascular injuries is the rapid control of hemorrhage and the restoration of perfusion, with salvage of the extremity or organ in jeop-

Table 11-16. PHYSICAL FINDINGS ASSOCIATED WITH EXTREMITY VASCULAR INJURY

Classic Signs	Signs of Occult Injury
Pulsatile bleeding	History of significant hemorrhage
Thrill or bruit	Proximity wounds
Pain	Peripheral nerve deficit
Pulselessness	Diminished pulse
Pallor	Fracture dislocation (knee, elbow)
Paresthesias	Unexplained shock
Paralysis	
Poikliothemia	

ardy. Intravenous broad-spectrum antibiotics should be administered as preparations for surgery are being made. In isolated-extremity vascular injury with arterial occlusion, systemic heparin should also be administered to avoid the propagation of thrombus in vessels distal to the occlusion. In multiply-injured patients, especially those with central nervous system trauma, heparin is inappropriate. Tetanus prophylaxis should be included, as in the treatment of any penetrating wound. A wide sterile operative field should be prepared to allow for adequate exposure of vessels with both proximal and distal control. A lower extremity should always be prepared as a potential site for saphenous vein harvest. In patients with lower-extremity injury, the contralateral limb should be made ready for vein harvest. For patients with suspected neck or abdominal sites of vascular trauma, the chest should be prepared to allow access to the aorta and its branches.

The early involvement of an orthopedic surgeon is an essential part of the surgical management of extremity vascular trauma associated with skeletal injury. The surgical procedure should be a combined effort. In general, the vascular repair is performed first, followed by stabilization of the skeletal injury, but the vascular surgeon's role does not end after perfusion is restored. Careful surveillance to ensure that orthopedic appliances do not obstruct the arterial repair and reexamination to confirm patency before wound closure are essential to successful limb salvage. A similar approach should be taken to vascular injuries associated with large soft tissue defects. The early involvement of a surgeon experienced with plastic and reconstructive surgery is essential to the successful management of these wounds.

A few patients have extensive soft tissue loss in an extremity associated with neurologic deficit, extensive fractures, and vascular injuries, with limbs that appear mangled. Usually, there is little hope for functional recovery, and careful consideration should be given to primary amputation. An objective scoring system has been developed to aid with this difficult problem[229] (Table 11-17). A score of 7 or greater has been found to predict eventual amputation in 100% of patients. This decision must be made in consultation with orthopedic and reconstructive surgical colleagues and should take into account the patient's overall status. In cases of extensive skeletal damage and severe hemorrhage, primary amputation can be life-saving. The decision to take this course is complex and difficult.

Vascular reconstruction for trauma should be performed with attention to proper technique. The use of fine monofilament sutures on the appropriately sized needles, vascular instruments, and loupe magnification are all appropriate. It is in the best interest of the patient that surgeons unfamiliar with techniques of vascular reconstruction obtain assistance from experienced colleagues.

The initial step in the surgical management of vascular injuries is to obtain proximal and distal control of the injured vessel. This is most easily accomplished through uninjured areas adjacent to the injury, using incisions normally employed for elective exposure of these vessels. Direct approach through the site of injury is fraught with the hazards of severe hemorrhage and iatrogenic trauma to the vessel itself or to adjacent nerves. Balloon-tipped catheters can be valuable in obtaining proximal and distal control if they are inserted carefully through the site of injury and inflated. Subsequent dissection then establishes proximal and distal control.

After control has been established, careful thrombectomy of the proximal and distal arteries is carried out until there is no evidence of thrombus. Heparinized saline, 10 IU/mL, is then flushed proximally and distally into the lumen of the artery. The technique for arterial repair should not be selected until the entire extent of the injury is known and the injured vessel has been débrided. The injured arterial segment is inevitably longer than appreciated at first inspection. End-to-end anastomosis can be used in the repair of many larger arteries if there is sufficient length to perform the repair without undue tension. Although 2 cm has frequently been cited, there is no definitive length of artery for safe resection and primary repair.

In the repair of more extensive arterial injuries, reversed saphenous vein from an uninjured lower extremity is the first choice for interposition graft. Although Gore-Tex grafts have been used with success at many centers, saphenous vein remains the usual choice for interposition grafting.[230] Care must be taken to avoid either kinking from a redundant graft or stenosis from undue tension. A spatulated anastomosis should be performed between artery and graft to avoid stenosis. Intraoperative completion angiography is mandatory to determine the adequacy of repair, confirm patency, and visualize the distal arterial runoff.

The repair of concomitant venous injuries is controversial. The priority of venous repair in combined arterial and venous injuries has not been firmly established. Proximal extremity veins and the great veins are repaired whenever technically possible to avoid the sequela of venous occlusion. Techniques of repair vary from simple suture closure to saphenous vein patch or graft interposition. Venous repair should not be attempted in a hemodynamically unstable patient; rather, ligation should be performed to expedite the operation.

The use of intraluminal shunts provides a valuable adjunct for patients in need of complex arterial reconstructive procedures.[231] Standard shunts used in elective carotid operation function well in the early restoration of arterial and venous flow if extensive grafting or limb reimplantation is required. Limb ischemia time is significantly reduced when shunts are used properly. Interposition grafting can be performed by placing the interposition graft over the shunt. Shunts effectively restore flow to injured extremities in patients who are too unstable to undergo completion of peripheral arterial repair. Shunts have been

---

Table 11-17. COMPONENTS OF THE MANGLED EXTREMITY SEVERITY SCORE

	Points
SKELETAL OR SOFT TISSUE INJURY	
Low energy: stabs, simple fractures, low-velocity gunshot wounds	1
Medium energy: open or multiple fractures, dislocations	2
High energy: close-range shotgun wounds, high-velocity gunshot wounds, crush injuries	3
Very high energy: high-energy plus gross contamination, major soft tissue loss	4
LIMB ISCHEMIA	
Pulses reduced or absent, perfusion normal	1
Pulseless, with paresthesia, delayed capillary refill	2
Cool, paralyzed, insensate, numb	3
(All ischemia scores are doubled if ischemia time >6 h)	
SHOCK	
Systolic blood pressure always >90 mmHg	0
Transient hypotension	1
Persistent hypotension	2
AGE	
<30 y	0
30–50 y	1
>50 y	2

left in place for extended periods with ultimate salvage of the extremity.[231]

Extraanatomic bypass plays a limited but important role in arterial trauma. Penetrating abdominal trauma with aortic or iliac artery disruption associated with extensive bowel injury and contamination by enteric contents can make in situ arterial repair highly susceptible to infection and disruption. In this situation, arterial ligation and extraanatomic bypass through the axillofemoral or femorofemoral route may be the only acceptable means to restore distal perfusion. The long-term patency rate of such grafts is inferior to in situ reconstruction, but these grafts do provide an excellent means to maintain perfusion and avoid life-threatening complications. Patients must be observed closely for graft occlusion and the need for subsequent reconstructive procedures.

The development of an extremity compartment syndrome is a devastating complication after arterial trauma. The syndrome is uncommon in the thigh and forearm but is frequently seen in the calf. The most sensitive sign of compartment syndrome is pain on passive stretch of the involved muscle. Although many devices are available to measure compartment pressures in the calf, many trauma surgeons are aggressive in the application of four-compartment fasciotomy whenever there is extensive soft tissue

injury or skeletal trauma in the lower leg combined with vascular trauma or the history of prolonged ischemia (Fig. 11-85). In any patient with lower-extremity trauma who exhibits signs of pain or distal ischemia, the compartment pressure should be measured and fasciotomy performed as needed. An untreated or unrecognized compartment syndrome produces nerve and muscle damage and prevents good functional recovery despite the patency of the vascular repair. Factors that suggest the need for fasciotomy are as follows:

- Prolonged period (6 hours or more) between injury and restoration of perfusion
- Associated crush injury
- Preoperative calf swelling
- Combined arterial and venous injuries
- Extensive venous ligation
- Postoperative signs or disproportionate muscle pain, pain on passive stretch, or tender and firm muscles
- Elevated compartment pressures

Proper wound management is essential to successful limb salvage after vascular trauma in the extremities. Aggressive wound débridement and pulse irrigation with copious amounts of antibiotic solution should be performed routinely. Coverage of the vascular repair with viable mus-

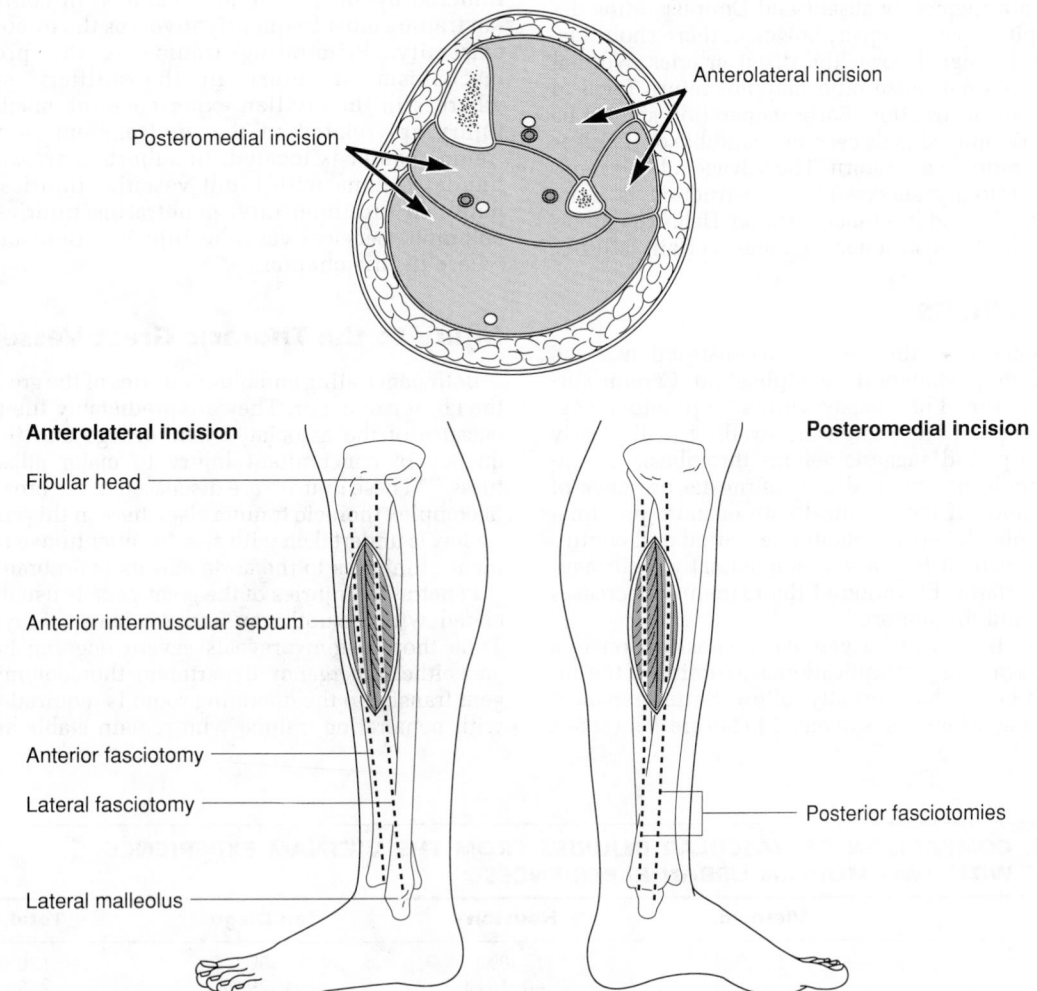

Figure 11-85. Surgical approach for four compartment fasciotomies through incisions on the medial and lateral aspects of the calf.

cle or fascia and subcutaneous tissue is essential to prevent desiccation and infection. The assistance of a plastic and reconstructive surgeon is essential in the management of injuries that involve extensive tissue loss. Flap rotation and, in the case of extreme tissue loss, myocutaneous free flap transfer may be required. Delayed primary skin closure should also be considered in all injuries except those involving minimal trauma and surgical dissection.

The use of low-molecular-weight dextran can prevent early thrombosis and improve microvascular circulation in patients with prolonged ischemia. Dextran 40 mL/h for 24 hours does not cause significant bleeding complications and can improve patency rates of arterial reconstructions, especially in small arteries. The routine use of a postoperative heparin infusion, however, significantly increases the incidence of wound hematoma. Heparin should be reserved for patients with documented thrombotic complications, including deep venous thrombosis and definable hypercoagulable states. Vasodilators are of limited value in the perioperative management of vascular injuries.

Postoperative monitoring for early failure of the vascular reconstruction is essential to ensure limb salvage. Monitoring in the intensive care unit with frequent peripheral vascular examination should be employed. The immediate challenges after operation are restoration of adequate intravascular volume and rewarming of the patient. Evaluation of distal circulation is difficult until the patient is normovolemic and normothermic. In the early postoperative period, pulses are frequently absent and Doppler ratios decreased, despite a patent repair; however, there should be audible Doppler signals over the distal arteries. Normal pulses and a normal pulse ratio may not return for 6 to 8 hours after reconstruction. Early reoperation should be performed if Doppler signals become inaudible or if pulses and a normal ratio do not return. The salvage rate for reoperation after initially successful reconstruction is more than 90% if performed in a timely fashion. Delay in reoperation dooms the reconstruction to almost certain failure.

COMPLICATIONS

Early thrombosis of the vascular reconstruction is the most immediate postoperative complication. Careful surveillance, as outlined previously, allows for prompt recognition and reoperation. Significant swelling in the early postoperative period suggests venous thrombosis. A duplex scan should be obtained to confirm the presence of venous thrombus. If the popliteal vein or more proximal veins are involved, heparin should be started and continued until the patient has been therapeutically anticoagulated with warfarin. Elevation of the extremity decreases the swelling and discomfort.

Infection in the area of a vascular reconstruction is a potentially devastating complication. Disruption of the suture line and hemorrhage usually follow. Suture repair of the disrupted anastomosis is doomed to failure. The safest

course is ligation in an area of the artery not involved in the infection, combined with extraanatomic bypass in uninvolved tissue to restore the distal perfusion.

Late complications include stenosis or occlusion of the arterial repair, aneurysmal changes in vein grafts, and the postthrombotic syndrome after venous thrombosis or ligation. All patients who require surgical treatment of vascular trauma should be monitored regularly on a long-term basis because of the potential for late complications. Early detection allows for timely treatment and a reduction in morbidity.

MANAGEMENT OF SPECIFIC VASCULAR INJURIES

Most patients presenting to trauma centers with vascular trauma have injuries of the extremities. Vascular injuries of the head, neck, chest, and abdomen are often immediately fatal. In contrast to the military experience, in which many of the wounds are from high-velocity missiles, civilian penetrating injuries tend to result from low-velocity weapons. As a result, more patients with torso and head and neck injuries survive to reach the trauma center. Table 11-18 compares the civilian experience to military experience with regard to the distribution of vascular injuries. Most military vascular injuries occur in the lower extremity and are inflicted by antipersonnel weapons. In contrast, civilian trauma most frequently involves the torso and upper extremity. Penetrating trauma is the predominant mechanism of injury in the military experience, whereas in the civilian experience the mechanisms of injury are related to the environment in which the trauma center is located. In suburban areas, motor vehicular trauma with blunt vascular injuries predominates. In the inner city, penetrating injuries are more common. Cervical vascular injuries are discussed elsewhere in this chapter.

Injury to the Thoracic Great Vessels

Both penetrating and blunt injuries of the great vessels in the chest can occur. They are predictably life-threatening because of the associated hemorrhage and the high frequency of concomitant injury to major adjacent structures.[226] These injuries are discussed in the broader context of complex thoracic trauma elsewhere in this chapter. This review is undertaken with specific attention to the management of injuries to the aorta and its main branches.

Penetrating injuries of the great vessels usually are associated with hemothorax and evidence of hypovolemia. Tube thoracostomy reveals severe ongoing hemorrhage, and either emergency department thoracotomy or an urgent transfer to the operating room is required. In patients with penetrating trauma who remain stable and who do

Table 11-18. COMPARISON OF VASCULAR INJURIES FROM THE VIETNAM EXPERIENCE WITH TWO MODERN URBAN EXPERIENCES

Site	Vietnam	Houston	San Diego	Total
Neck	50 (5%)	17 (8%)	53 (8%)	120 (6%)
Chest	11 (1%)	40 (18%)	194 (29%)	245 (13%)
Abdomen	29 (3%)	41 (18%)	154 (23%)	197 (11%)
Upper extremity	342 (34%)	64 (29%)	102 (16%)	508 (28%)
Lower extremity	568 (57%)	59 (27%)	161 (24%)	788 (42%)
TOTAL	1000	221	664	1858

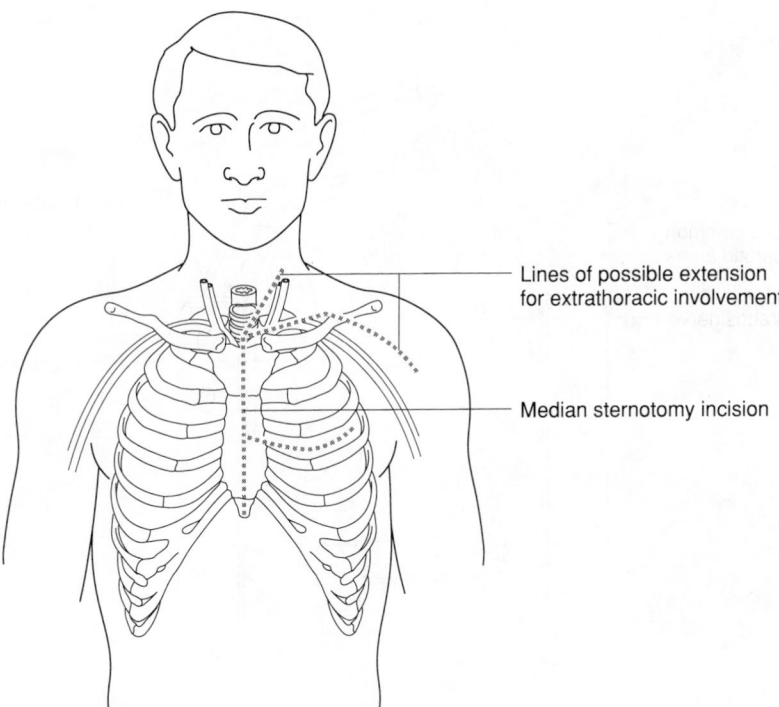

Figure 11-86. The proximal great vessels are best approached through a median sternotomy. Extrathoracic vascular exposure can be obtained by extending the incision along the course of the vessels.

not have significant ongoing hemorrhage after tube thoracostomy, there are a number of signs that suggest the need for arteriography to rule out great vessel injury. These include missile emboli to peripheral vessels, the presence of missiles or missile trajectories in proximity to great vessels, and a mediastinal hematoma on chest radiograph. Confirmation of the diagnosis is obtained at angiography, if possible, but the magnitude of hemorrhage may well preclude any maneuver other than immediate thoracotomy.

Penetrating wounds to the ascending aorta, innominate artery, and right subclavian artery are best approached by a median sternotomy. Extrathoracic extensions may be necessary to obtain proximal and distal vascular control (Fig. 11-86). The approach to a penetrating wound of the innominate vein and left common carotid artery is shown in Figures 11-87 through 11-89. In general, venous ligation is well tolerated, and arterial repair is performed. Left subclavian and descending thoracic aortic injuries require a left thoracotomy for exposure. If an emergency department thoracotomy is required, exposure of all but the apex of the mediastinum can be obtained by carrying the incision across the sternum into the right chest (see Fig. 11-41). Almost all survivable blunt great vessel injuries result in

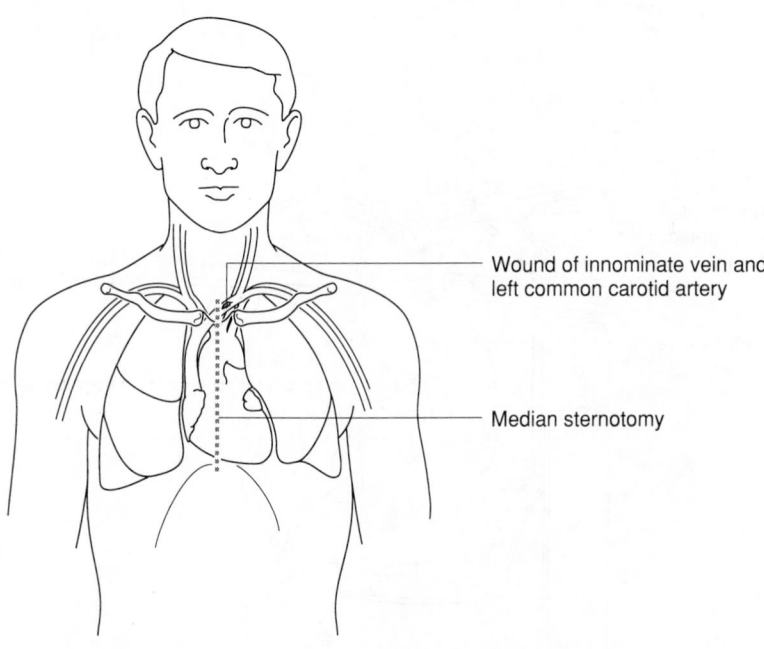

Figure 11-87. A penetrating wound to the innominate vein and left common carotid artery is best approached through a median sternotomy.

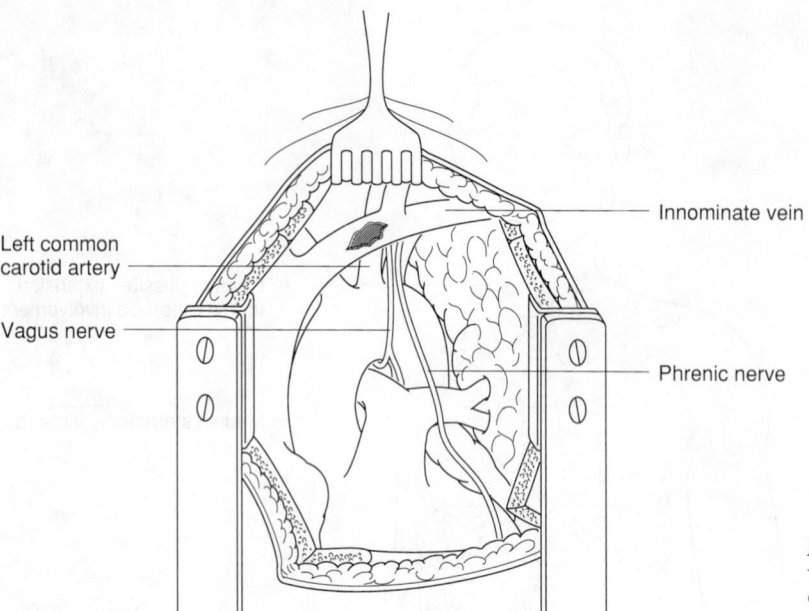

Figure 11-88. Proximal and distal control of both venous and arterial injuries must be obtained without injury to the adjacent structures, such as the phrenic, vagus, or recurrent laryngeal nerves.

acute pseudoaneurysms of the aortic isthmus or the proximal arch vessels (Figs. 11-90 through 11-92). The aortic isthmus (the area of the descending aorta between the ligamentum arteriosum and the origin of the left subclavian artery) is susceptible to shear injury in deceleration accidents. These typically involve transection of the intima and media with containment of hemorrhage by the elastic adventitia. The mortality rate from delayed rupture of this lesion approaches 50% in the first 24 hours if left untreated.

Surgical management of aortic injuries consists of direct suture repair or synthetic graft interposition. If possible, cardiopulmonary bypass capability should be available in the event that aortic occlusion proves necessary for repair. For patients who arrive at a trauma center without severe hypotension, the results of surgical therapy are encourag-

ing. Paraplegia is an important complication because the anterior spinal artery originates from branches of the thoracic intercostal arteries. Crossclamping of the aorta in the chest for arterial repair results in paraplegia in about 8% of these patients despite modern techniques to maximize distal perfusion. The best approach includes avoidance of hypovolemia and rapid vascular repair.

Abdominal Vascular Injury

The diagnosis of major intraabdominal vascular injury is most often made at celiotomy. The common exception to this is blunt disruption of the renal artery with thrombosis, which is typically detected on arteriography after nonvisualization of the involved kidney. Rarely, blunt aortic or iliac artery disruption is suspected from diminished or

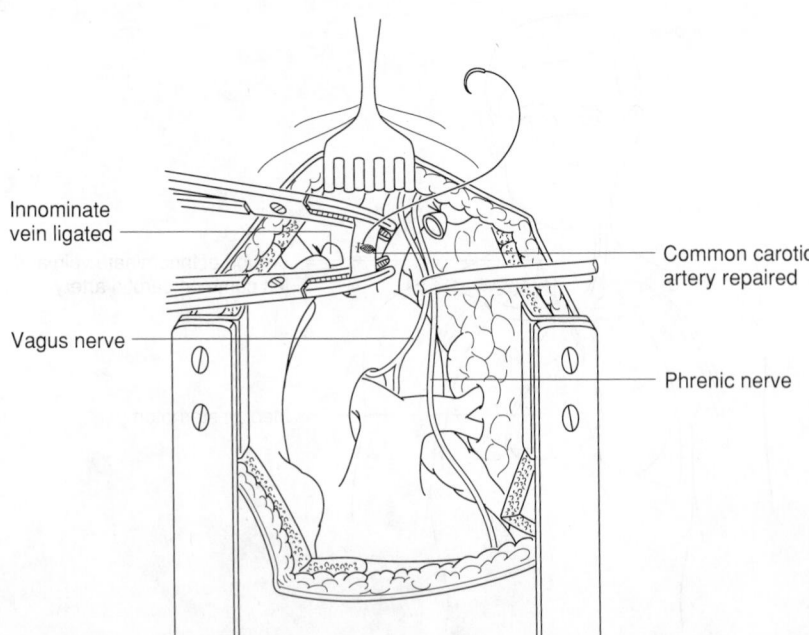

Figure 11-89. Combined arterial and venous injuries often are best treated with ligation of the vein, whereas isolated venous injuries may be safely repaired. Common carotid arterial repair is shown.

The infrarenal aorta and its bifurcation are best approached by mobilization of the small intestine to the right upper quadrant and opening of the retroperitoneum in the midline or lateral to either the ascending or descending colon (Fig. 11-94). The superior and inferior mesenteric arteries, the left renal hilum, and the left iliac artery can be exposed by reflection of the spleen and entire left colon for entry into the retroperitoneum (Fig. 11-95). Similarly, the vena cava, right renal hilum, and right iliac artery can be exposed by a Kocher maneuver combined with mobilization of the right colon (Fig. 11-96). The portal area is best exposed by the combination of a Kocher maneuver and mobilization of the hepatic flexure of the colon from the underlying duodenum and head of the pancreas.

Arterial and venous repair in the abdomen employ the same general principles of vascular technique used elsewhere. Primary suture repair, patch angioplasty, and saphenous vein interposition are used selectively to restore adequate flow. The use of synthetic graft material should be avoided if there is associated bowel or pancreatic injury. All mesenteric arterial repairs should include a careful inspection of the intestine for evidence of ischemia. Completion angiography after abdominal vascular repair is difficult and suboptimal. Therefore, documentation of patency of the repair is best achieved using Doppler ultrasound or, possibly, intraoperative duplex scanning.

Injuries to the vena cava or the portal vein present significant management challenges because of the insidious nature of ongoing blood loss, the difficulty of obtaining

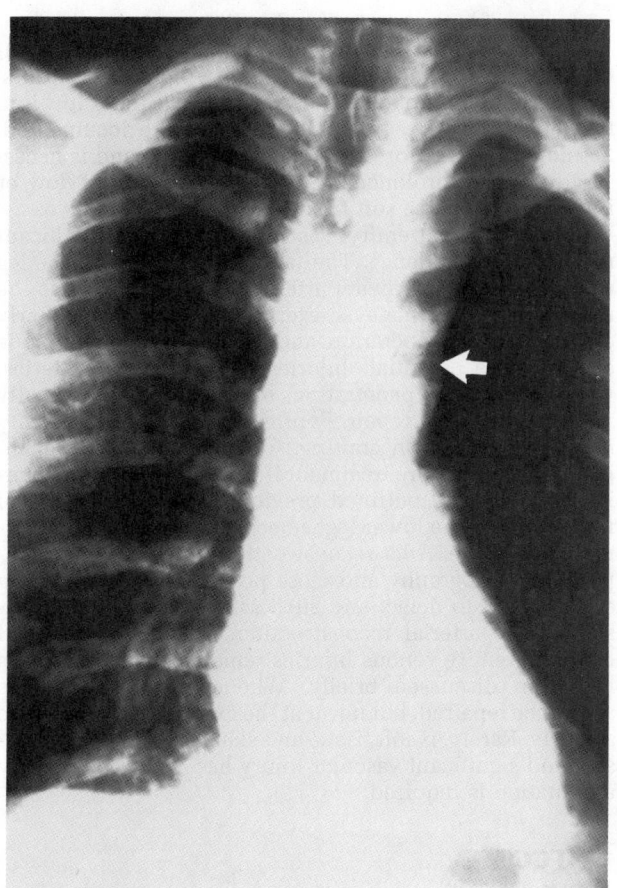

Figure 11-90. Portable chest radiograph demonstrating an indistinct aortic knob (*arrow*) and left apical pleural cap in a 21-year-old man who sustained a significant deceleration injury to the chest.

absent distal pulses, and the injury is documented by arteriography.

The initial management of patients with abdominal vascular trauma is dictated by the severity of hemorrhage from the site of injury. In the agonal patient, emergency department thoracotomy and aortic occlusion above the diaphragm must be performed to control hemorrhage during transport to the operating room. Rapid fluid resuscitation and expeditious celiotomy are required in all patients with abdominal vascular injury.

The priorities in the management of abdominal vascular trauma are similar to those employed in other areas. If active bleeding is encountered at celiotomy, it is controlled by direct pressure. If contained retroperitoneal hemorrhage is encountered, proximal and distal vascular control is obtained before the hematoma is opened. Associated bowel injury should be closed expeditiously to avoid ongoing contamination from enteric contents. The most common finding at celiotomy in patients with blunt abdominal trauma is either retroperitoneal or intramesenteric hematoma. Less commonly, intestinal ischemia may be present as a result of thrombosis or avulsion of mesenteric vessels.

Exposure of the great vessels of the posterior abdomen is essential in the management of significant abdominal vascular trauma. If active hemorrhage is encountered, precise identification of the source of bleeding can be difficult. If it is necessary, exposure of the aorta at the diaphragmatic hiatus for clamp placement is best performed by entering the lesser sac and longitudinally splitting the crural fibers (Fig. 11-93).

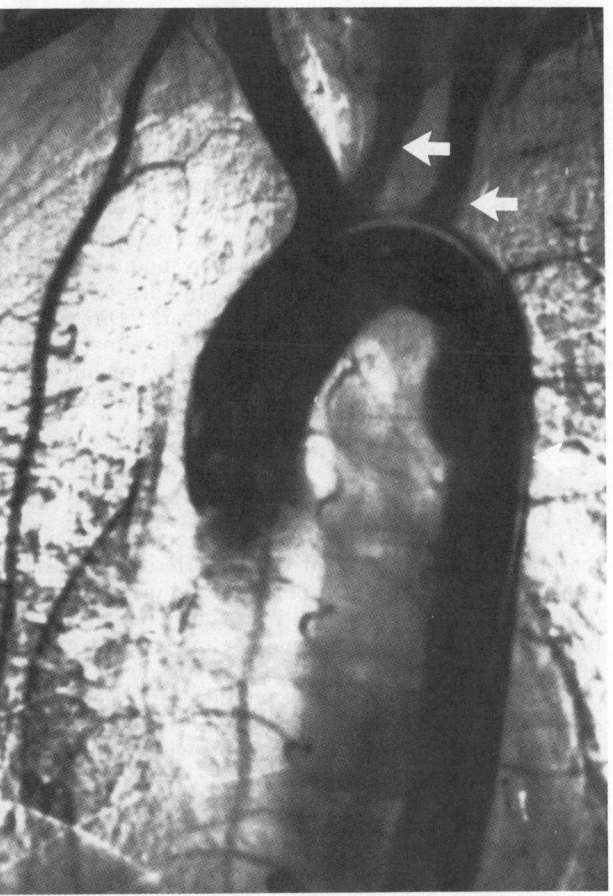

Figure 11-91. Thoracic aortogram revealing traumatic pseudoaneurysm of the aortic isthmus, the left common carotid artery, and the left subclavian artery (*arrows*) in the same patient shown in Figure 11-90.

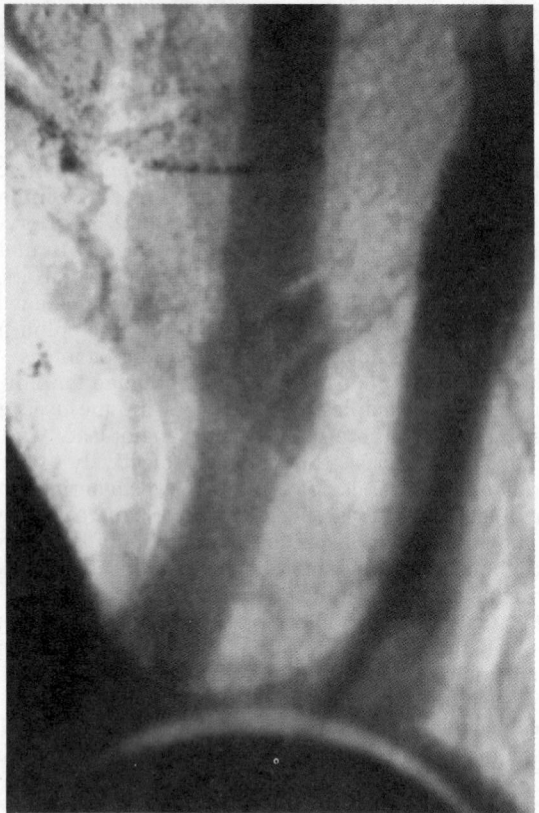

Figure 11-92. Enlarged view of the carotid and subclavian injury in the same patient shown in Figure 11-90.

proximal and distal control, and the high risk of subsequent thrombosis. Ligation of these vessels should be performed only as a desperate measure in unstable patients. Massive lower-extremity edema accompanies ligation of the infrarenal vena cava, and ligation above the renal veins is uniformly fatal. Portal venous ligation should be avoided if at all possible. The portal vein provides 80% of the oxygen and nutrient blood flow to the liver.[232] Direct suture and patch angioplasty are the most effective means to repair injuries of the great veins. Mesenteric venous injury can be managed by ligation without significant complications.

Extremity Vascular Trauma

The most common sites of extremity arterial trauma are the brachial and superficial femoral arteries. Penetrating injuries are more common than blunt injuries. If they do occur, blunt injuries are usually associated with major fractures or dislocations. Supracondylar humeral fractures and posterior dislocations of the knee are associated with significant risks of brachial and popliteal artery injury, respectively (Figs. 11-97 and 11-98). Concomitant peripheral nerve injuries occur in 60% of patients with vascular injuries in the extremities.

The extensive collateral circulation and the smaller muscle mass in the arm make acute arterial occlusion in the arm less likely to cause limb-threatening ischemia than in the leg. The priorities of prompt diagnosis and timely restoration of perfusion, however, remain applicable to upper-extremity arterial trauma. A potentially limb-threatening situation is caused by injury to the brachial artery proximal to the origin of the profunda brachii artery or by occlusion of both the ulnar and radial arteries in the forearm; prompt arterial repair should be undertaken. In contrast, if isolated radial or ulnar artery occlusion occurs, reconstruction is not required, provided adequate flow into the hand through the remaining vessel can be documented. Fasciotomy in the forearm is rarely required and is necessary only after prolonged delays in restoration of flow or if there is extensive soft tissue injury.

In the lower extremity, vascular trauma is a significant management challenge. The large muscle mass of the leg and the lack of significant arterial collaterals increase the risk of limb loss whenever arterial occlusion occurs. Early diagnosis, timely operation, and proper vascular technique are therefore essential. Injuries to the femoral arteries, whether blunt or penetrating, often can be successfully managed by direct repair. Popliteal artery injuries usually require interposition grafting.[230] Isolated tibial vessel injury does not require treatment if one of the other leg arteries is patent. As outlined previously, the liberal use of fasciotomy in the lower leg is necessary to avoid compartment syndrome. After reconstruction, intraoperative completion arteriography and close postoperative monitoring are essential to detect and successfully treat early occlusion of the arterial reconstruction. The management of lower extremity venous injuries remains controversial, as has been discussed briefly. Whenever possible, veins should be repaired, but never at the expense of physiologic stability. Rarely, if soft tissue and skeletal injury are extensive and significant vascular injury has occurred, primary amputation is required.

OUTCOME

The results of properly diagnosed and expeditiously treated vascular trauma are encouraging. The mortality rate after isolated peripheral vascular trauma is low, with no mortalities reported in many series. The mortality rate for suprarenal aortic injuries remains about 50% to 70%. In-

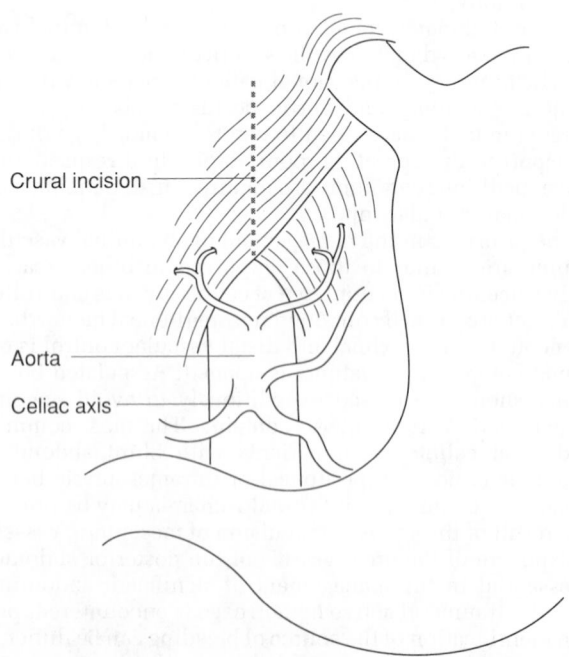

Figure 11-93. Supraceliac aortic exposure for proximal control is best obtained through the lesser sac by splitting the crural fibers of the diaphragm directly over the aorta.

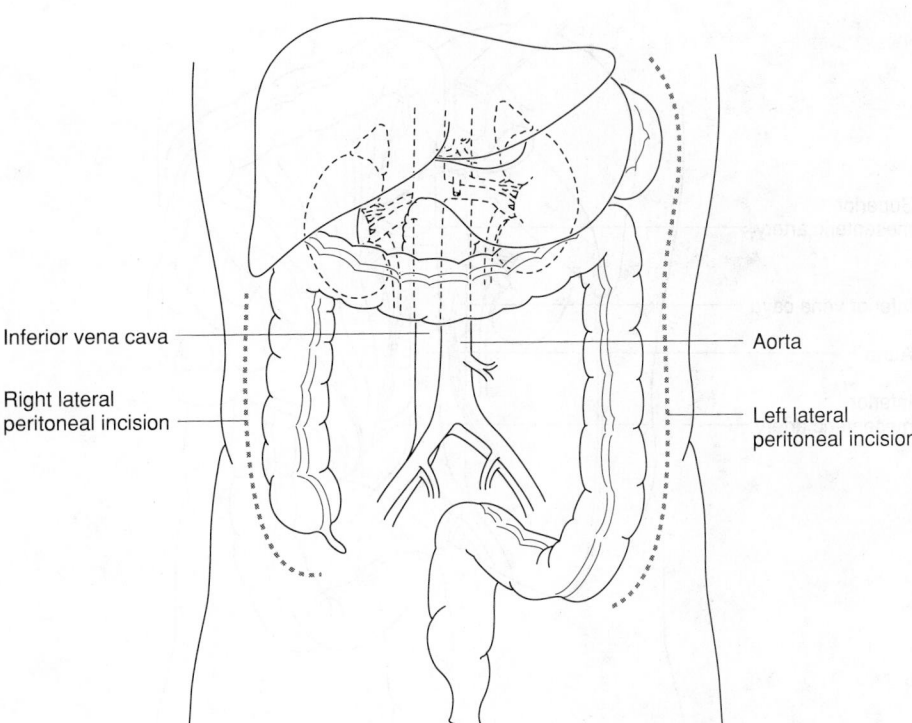

Figure 11-94. Lines of incision for entrance into the retroperitoneum on the left and right sides of the abdomen.

Inferior vena cava

Right lateral peritoneal incision

Aorta

Left lateral peritoneal incision

frarenal aortic injuries have mortality rates of 20% to 40%. The amputation rate after peripheral vascular trauma continues to decrease, with several series reporting amputation rates of less than 2%. The recent improvement in limb salvage is a result of a combination of factors, most of which decrease the warm ischemia time. Early amputa-

tion, if necessary, appears to be related to prolonged ischemia but is clearly multifactorial. Late amputation is done primarily for disability or infection.

Almost all vascular repairs can achieve at least temporary technical success as determined by immediate postoperative patency. Technical success, however, implies nei-

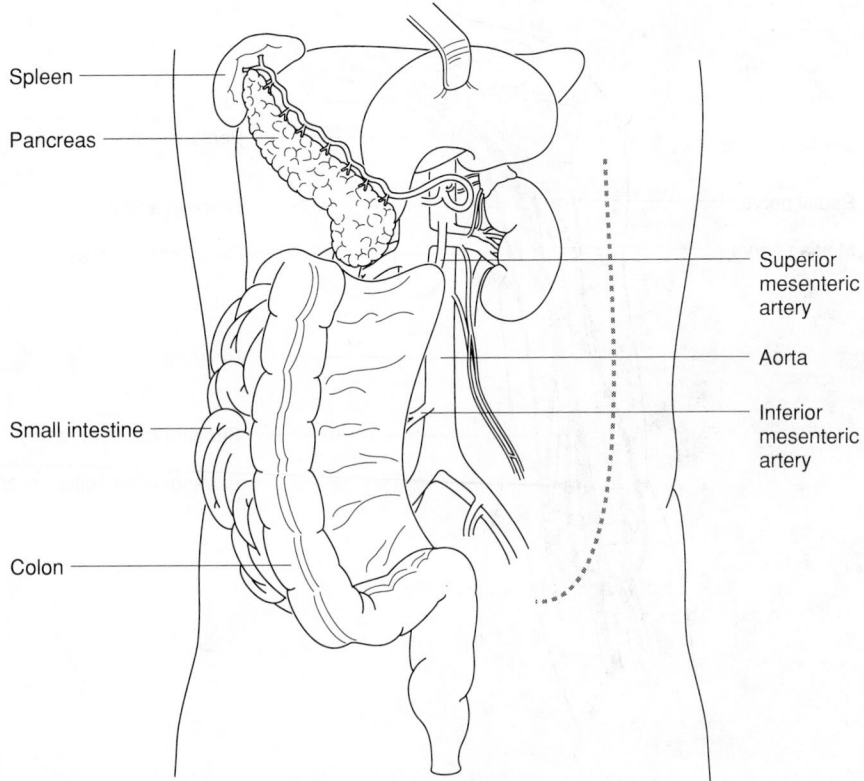

Spleen

Pancreas

Small intestine

Colon

Superior mesenteric artery

Aorta

Inferior mesenteric artery

Figure 11-95. Exposure of the aorta, its branches, and the left kidney is best obtained by an approach through the left side of the retroperitoneum.

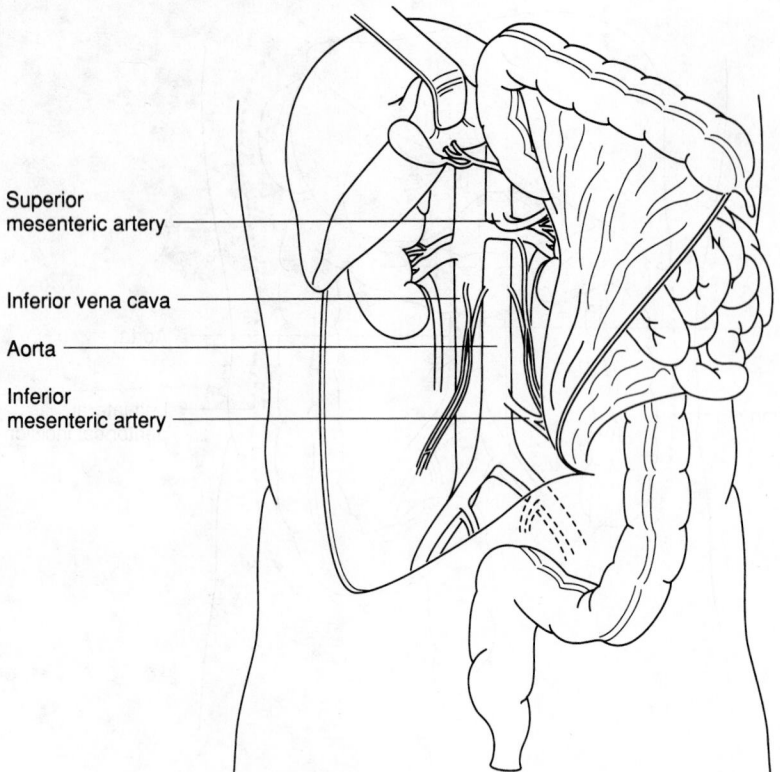

Superior mesenteric artery

Inferior vena cava

Aorta

Inferior mesenteric artery

Figure 11-96. The vena cava, right kidney, and portal area are best exposed by an approach through the right side of the peritoneum.

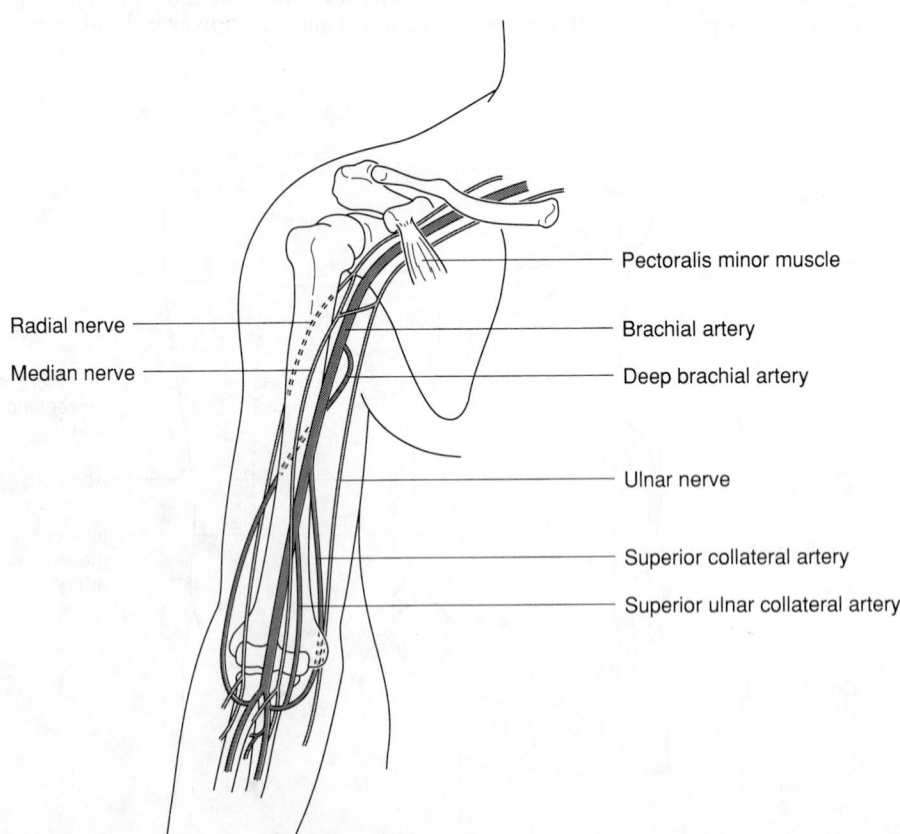

Radial nerve

Median nerve

Pectoralis minor muscle

Brachial artery

Deep brachial artery

Ulnar nerve

Superior collateral artery

Superior ulnar collateral artery

Figure 11-97. The proximity of the distal brachial artery to the humerus leads to a predisposition to arterial injury with supracondylar fractures.

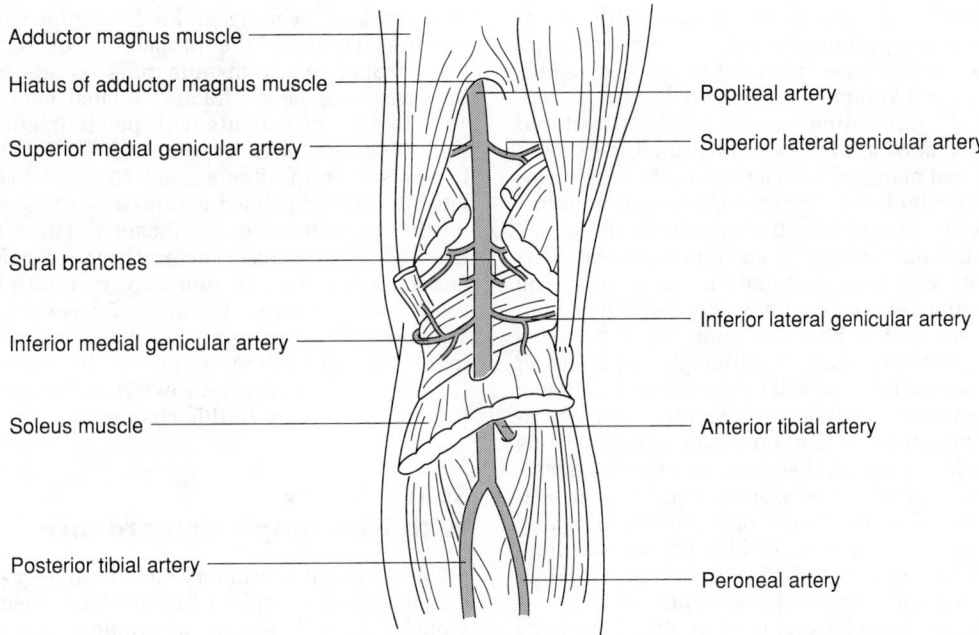

Figure 11-98. The popliteal artery is bound above and below the knee joint by the muscles of the thigh and calf and is immobile. Posterior knee dislocation frequently results in injury to the popliteal artery.

ther limb salvage nor satisfactory functional outcome. Although most series report low early rates of amputation, there is little information on return of function, incidence of late amputation, or incidence of long-term morbidity.

Definitive Care Phase: Orthopedic and Spinal Injuries

MARK A. HEALEY AND ROBERT J. WINCHELL

Significant orthopedic injuries occur in over 70% of multiply injured patients, more than twice as often as significant intrathoracic or intraabdominal injuries.[233] It is essential that the general surgeon involved in the care of multiply injured patients have a sound understanding of basic orthopedic principles. A patient's orthopedic problems rarely are a direct threat to life in the initial care phase, but untreated orthopedic injuries are a major contributing factor to in-hospital morbidity and are one of the principal determinants of later functional recovery.

ORTHOPEDIC INJURIES CONSIDERED IN THE PRIMARY SURVEY

The initial resuscitation of the multiply injured patient is always directed toward the identification and treatment of immediately life-threatening injuries involving the airway, ventilation, and circulation. Generally, major injuries to the head, thorax, and abdomen take precedence, but injuries to the axial spine and pelvis and multiple long-bone fractures can have a significant effect on hemodynamic stability and the ability to assess other injuries.

Fractures of the axial spine, especially in the high cervi-

cal spine, can cause varying degrees of respiratory compromise, ranging from the loss of abdominal muscles, intercostal muscles, and cervical accessory muscles to complete apnea if the cord level is above the phrenic outflow tract (C-3 to C-5). Patients with ventilatory failure from acute cord injury typically present with a paradoxical breathing pattern in which the abdomen protrudes on inhalation, creating a seesaw appearance. This is caused by paralysis of the abdominal musculature and is seen with injuries as low as T-10 to T-11. The loss of abdominal tone can cause marked ventilatory dysfunction, which is compounded by loss of the use of intercostal and accessory muscles and by loss of diaphragm function as the level ascends. Early endotracheal intubation and mechanical ventilation must be considered, even in patients who appear compensated on initial evaluation. There is a strong tendency for such patients to tire and to develop respiratory failure a few hours after the injury. With or without intubation, they are at high risk for development of early pulmonary complications related to atelectasis and inability to clear secretions.

In addition to ventilatory compromise, high axial spinal lesions can cause significant hypotension, confusing the initial evaluation of the patient. Most central nervous system (CNS) control of arteriolar tone is mediated through the sympathetic nervous system. The sympathetic nerves arise from contributions from the ventral roots of the thoracic spinal segments, but the system is controlled by descending pathways from the medulla. In high thoracic and cervical spinal cord injuries, these controlling pathways may be interrupted, with subsequent loss of vasomotor tone. The lack of sympathetic drive to the sinoatrial node results in a predominance of vagal stimulation and bradycardia. The combination produces the classic picture of spinal shock, hypotension, and relative bradycardia. In contrast to hypovolemic shock, the extremities of patients with high axial spinal lesions are warm and well perfused because the injury ablates sympathetically mediated vasoconstriction.

In the initial evaluation of hypotensive trauma patients,

hemorrhage must be presumed. The patient with spinal shock should be managed initially with volume expansion until diagnostic studies have ruled out sources of significant hemorrhage and volume deficits have been replaced. After the patient's circulating volume has been restored and no further hemorrhage has been identified, persistent hypotension is best managed with a pure α-adrenergic agonist, such as phenylephrine. Appropriate central monitoring lines should be placed to optimize volume status.

Fracture-related hemorrhage is an important consideration in patients who have sustained blunt trauma. The amount of bleeding from open fractures in the field is often unknown. The amount of bleeding from closed fractures is frequently underestimated.[234] Although hypotension should prompt a search for intraabdominal or intrathoracic bleeding, noncavitary bleeding from fractures and lacerations frequently contributes to hypotension and may be its sole cause.[235] It is important, therefore, to make an assessment of bleeding caused by orthopedic injuries. A closed femoral fracture, whether simple or complex, typically causes loss of one to two units of blood.[236] Closed tibia fractures usually result in loss of one unit or less. Although multiple fractures can produce shock, hypotension is unusual with a single closed femoral shaft or other long-bone fracture, and an additional bleeding source is likely in patients with these conditions who are hypovolemic.[237] Hemorrhage related to pelvic fractures requires special consideration and is discussed elsewhere.

Pain from multiple orthopedic injuries can also complicate the assessment of potential injuries at other locations. Physical examination of the chest, abdomen, and cervical spine frequently relies on the patient's ability to report pain on palpation. Pelvic fractures or rib fractures may produce pain during abdominal palpation. Alternatively, the intense competitive pain from long-bone fractures can extinguish the patient's response to visceral pain or to pain in the cervical region. Therefore, in multiple-trauma patients, especially those with significant long-bone fractures, there must be a strong emphasis on objective evaluation of all potential injuries. This equates to a liberal policy on obtaining radiographs and frequent use of diagnostic peritoneal lavage, computed tomography (CT), or ultrasound to objectively screen for intraabdominal injuries.

TRUE ORTHOPEDIC EMERGENCIES

Most orthopedic injuries do not require care on a truly urgent basis. The fixation of skeletal injuries can usually be safely deferred until the patient is stable from all other injuries. Certain circumstances, however, dictate immediate therapy to preserve life and functional recovery.

Pelvic Fracture

Pelvic fractures require special consideration in the trauma patient. High-energy impacts, such as those sustained in motor vehicle, pedestrian, and motorcycle accidents and falls from height, result in transfer of significant force to the torso. The surgeon must be alert to several immediate concerns in this subset of patients with pelvic fracture. First is the significant incidence of serious associated injuries, especially to the CNS and abdominal viscera, that contributes significantly to the 5% to 20% overall mortality rate that accompanies pelvic fracture in this setting. Of equal importance is hemorrhage related to the fracture itself. Even with closed pelvic fractures, bleeding is poorly tamponaded and can cause hemodynamic instability. Anterior pelvic ring fractures typically bleed 1 to 2 units each. Fractures of the posterior pelvic elements, especially vertical disruptions of the sacroiliac joint, can pro-

duce massive bleeding, and radiographic evidence of such fractures confirms the probability of significant blood loss.[208] Statistics from numerous reports underscore the importance of pelvic fracture-related hemorrhage. About 15% to 19% of patients with pelvic fractures from blunt trauma present with hypotension.[209,238,239] Mortality rates in this subgroup often exceed 40%.[235,239] Hemorrhage related to isolated pelvic fracture causes 12% to 41% of these deaths and contributes significantly to the remaining fatalities.[208,209,238] This makes hemorrhage the major preventable factor contributing to mortality in multiply injured patients with pelvic fracture. Successful management schemes require an aggressive multidisciplinary approach involving application of pneumatic antishock garment (PASG), angiography, and external fixation, as described in detail elsewhere in this chapter.

Spinal Injury With Neurologic Compromise

The potential ventilatory and circulatory problems associated with acute spinal injuries have been outlined previously. After these critical problems are controlled, the further approach to patients with spinal cord injuries is driven primarily by the stability of the patient's neurologic condition. The nature of the injury and the presence or absence of compromise of the spinal canal are also important in determining initial therapy. Patients with incomplete injuries and over 50% compromise of the spinal canal are potential candidates for emergency surgical decompression.

In all of these patients, the spine should be strictly immobilized. Early axial traction with a halo apparatus or Gardner-Wells tongs should be instituted for unstable cervical injuries. Careful neurologic assessment is then performed, and the level of sensory and motor function is determined. Patients with complete injuries, especially in the cervical spine, should be observed for 48 to 96 hours before surgical stabilization because of the risk of further compromise of the injured cord. Those with incomplete injury who improve are usually observed carefully with serial examinations. Patients with significant cord compromise and an examination that shows worsening should be considered for decompressive surgery. Patients with an examination that shows neurologic stability and incomplete injury represent a difficult management decision, and care must be individualized.

Clinical trials have demonstrated two treatments that improve neurologic outcome in patients with spinal cord injury. In one trial, the Second National Acute Spinal Cord Injury Study, patients who received high doses of methylprednisolone sodium succinate within 8 hours of injury had improved neurologic recovery.[240,241] Based on this evidence, patients with spinal cord injury should be treated with an initial bolus of 30 mg/kg of methylprednisolone, followed by the infusion of 5.4 mg/kg/h for 23 hours. Steroid treatment that begins more than 8 hours after injury results in worse recovery than placebo treatment[241] and is not recommended. In the second trial, intravenous administration of the monosialic ganglioside GM$_1$ to patients 48 to 72 hours after spinal cord injury and after low-dose treatment with methylprednisolone improved motor recovery.[242] More recent work with animals does not support a role for combined high-dose steroid and GM$_1$ therapy.[243] The ultimate role of these and other pharmacologic manipulations is still uncertain.

Patients with either complete or incomplete injuries should have definitive spinal stabilization at the earliest practical time. Evidence from many centers shows benefits in prevention of early complications as well as significant acceleration of rehabilitation in patients undergoing early stabilization. The precise method of stabilization must be tailored to the individual patient and injury.

Open Fracture

The association of a soft tissue injury with a fracture greatly increases the risk of infection and subsequent problems with osteomyelitis, nonunion, and late disability. The Gustilo classification, defined initially for fractures of the tibia, is a useful system for aiding in management decisions (Table 11-19).

All open fractures require thorough irrigation and débridement of devitalized tissue, which should be accomplished within 8 hours of injury. This is best performed in the operating room. Patients should receive broad-spectrum parenteral antibiotics, usually a cephalosporin, with the addition of an aminoglycoside for grade III fractures.

Early stabilization of bony injuries is also of paramount importance in the care of open fractures, although local soft tissue injuries can limit the options available for skeletal fixation. External fixation is the best option for tibial and femoral injuries with large soft tissue components, but internal fixation is safe and offers significant advantages in certain cases.

Fractures caused by gunshot wounds can be managed like other open fractures. With low-velocity gunshot fractures, superficial débridement of the external wound sites with immediate internal fixation of the fracture is well tolerated and has a very low infection rate. High-velocity wounds are less common and require careful open débridement and individualized treatment. Patients with fractures not requiring stabilization can be treated on an outpatient basis after débridement of the external wound sites. Admission for a course of antibiotics is not required.[244] Regardless of the mechanism of injury or the treatment method chosen, patients with early rather than late fixation of open fractures fare better in both the short term and the long term.

Dislocations With Potential for Neurovascular Compromise

Joint dislocations manifest as pain and deformity and may or may not be associated with fractures. Their immediate importance relates to associated neurovascular injuries. These injuries can be overlooked easily in the multiple-trauma patient unless each joint and pulse is systematically evaluated. In general, any dislocation causing symptoms of local neurovascular compromise must be reduced immediately. Postreduction radiographs should be obtained to rule out associated fractures. With most dislocations, vascular injuries are unlikely; they occur in only 1% to 2% of cases.[245] The dislocated knee is an important exception: associated popliteal artery injury is present in approximately one third of cases and is accompanied by a high frequency of limb loss if undetected or unrepaired. This problem is discussed in detail elsewhere in this chapter. Angiography should be considered in any patient with severe ligamentous disruption or multiple fractures around the knee, and for any dislocation with signs of vascular injury or for which the pulse was absent before reduction. Dislocations at the hip, shoulder, and elbow also have potential for neurovascular compromise, and reduction should take place as soon as possible, but angiography is usually not required.

Avascular necrosis of the femoral head is a disabling problem associated with acute dislocations of the hip. The blood supply to the femoral head is tenuous, and dislocation interferes with the primary supply by the central artery. In addition, the tension on the joint capsule can greatly impede collateral flow. It is therefore imperative to reduce hip dislocations as soon as possible.

Reduction of dislocations, particularly those involving large joints, may require considerable force to overcome muscular spasm and reestablish anatomic relations. Although reduction often relieves the pain dramatically, the actual process can be difficult for both patient and surgeon. Dislocations at smaller joints are commonly reduced with analgesia alone, but dislocations at major joints, especially the hip and knee, often are best reduced under general anesthesia, during which profound muscle relaxation and absence of pain provide optimal conditions for good anatomic reduction with minimal patient discomfort.

COMPARTMENT SYNDROME

If bleeding or edema occurs inside a closed fascial compartment, the pressures within that compartment may become sufficiently high to impair blood flow and lower oxygen tension, resulting in impaired cellular metabolism and, eventually, cell death. This syndrome occurs commonly after crush injury to an extremity with or without fractures and also after a period of ischemia followed by reperfusion. The ischemia reperfusion mechanism typically occurs with vascular injuries or, less frequently, after use of the PASG or after prolonged elevation of the legs during surgical procedures. Compartment syndrome may be present during the initial assessment, or it may not appear until the postoperative or postresuscitative period. If there has been prolonged elevation of the limb on a fracture table or prolonged use of the PASG, this complication can occur on the uninjured side. It must be diagnosed and treated early to avoid loss of a functional limb. In the patient with multiple injuries, this equates to a thorough search for and objective measurement of compartment pressures. The clinical presentation and treatment of this syndrome is described elsewhere in this chapter. In addition to occurring with blunt trauma and vascular injuries, compartment syndrome also occurs with gunshot wounds and can involve compartments in the foot.

SYSTEMIC IMPACT OF ORTHOPEDIC INJURIES

Although rarely lethal in their own right, orthopedic injuries often are the source of major morbidity and mortality in trauma patients. The immobility imposed by unsta-

Table 11-19. CLASSIFICATION OF OPEN FRACTURES

Type I	Wound generally less than 1 cm long; low-energy mechanism without significant crushing or contamination
Type II	Wound generally more than 1 cm long; high-energy mechanism and moderate soft tissue damage
Type III	Wound generally more than 10 cm long; high-energy mechanism, extensive soft tissue damage; fracture often highly comminuted; automatically includes high-velocity gunshot wounds, displaced segmental fractures, extensive crush injuries, concomitant vascular injuries, and extensive contamination of soft tissues
Type IIIA	Limited periosteal stripping; no major soft tissue defects; complex reconstruction not usually required
Type IIIB	Extensive periosteal stripping; major soft tissue loss; complex reconstruction required
Type IIIC	Type IIIA or IIIB injury associated with major vascular injury

ble extremity or spine fractures places the patient at greatly increased risk. Pulmonary complications are perhaps the most common cause of morbidity and mortality in the intensive care unit (ICU). Several studies have shown a dramatic decrease in the incidence of all types of pulmonary complications with early skeletal stabilization of long-bone and spinal fractures[246,247] and pelvic fractures.[248] A potential exception to this general rule is discussed below. Early mobilization and aggressive pulmonary care are vital in the care of the multiply injured patient and must be given priority.

Perhaps the most catastrophic of postinjury complications is pulmonary embolism; it is one of the leading causes of preventable death in young patients who survive their initial injuries. All patients with orthopedic injury, particularly those with fractures of the lower extremities or pelvis, are at high risk for deep venous thrombosis and subsequent pulmonary embolism, and a recent study suggests that patients with spinal cord injuries are at even greater risk. This randomized study[249] examined the incidence of deep venous thrombosis in trauma patients and found that prophylaxis with sequential compression devices or low-dose heparin reduced the incidence from 8.8% to 2.9%. Among patients with spinal cord injury, prophylaxis decreased the incidence from 27% to 10%. Prophylactic measures are therefore helpful but imperfect, and a subset of patients have deep venous thrombosis despite maximal therapy. Aggressive prophylaxis and surveillance are required in the multiple-trauma patient, and all patients require prophylaxis with pneumatic compression hose and, if possible, with subcutaneous heparin. In the same prospective study, it was possible to initiate low-dose heparin therapy within 24 hours of injury in 37% of cases and within 48 hours in 75%. Trauma patients who are paralyzed, or who are immobilized by head injury, spine injury, or multiple orthopedic injuries, should be considered for placement of a Greenfield filter.[250] Early stabilization of fractures to allow mobilization of the patient is the single most effective preventive therapy.

The fat embolism syndrome is manifested by the classic triad of acute respiratory failure, altered mental status, and petechiae of the head, torso, and sclera; it is frequently associated with long-bone and pelvic fractures. Less fulminant presentations, without petechiae and with lesser degrees of pulmonary dysfunction, are more common.[251] Attention has turned away from theories of simple embolization of fat to the pulmonary vasculature. Recent work suggests an interaction of platelets, the coagulation cascade, and fat that results in intravascular coagulation and leukocyte activation. This is followed by inflammation, endothelial damage, increased capillary permeability, and decreased functional surfactant levels in the lung. These changes produce hypoxemia and pulmonary edema, which may progress to the adult respiratory distress syndrome. Most of these patients manifest a CNS depression that is out of proportion to the degree of hypoxemia. At present, the only therapy for fat embolism syndrome is supportive care.[252] Therefore, prevention is critical and numerous studies indicate that early fracture fixation decreases the incidence of this and other pulmonary complications. However, in a recent study,[253] a subset of patients with femoral fractures and coexisting lung contusion was found to have a higher incidence of adult respiratory distress syndrome if the fracture was repaired early than if it was repaired late. Avoidance of reaming of the femoral canal can prevent this effect on outcome.[254] Further analysis of this subgroup of patients is required to define the optimal management scheme.

Patients who have spinal fractures with associated cord injuries are vulnerable to myriad immediate and delayed complications. Although these complications are not unique to patients with spinal cord injuries, their clinical presentation in such patients may be dramatically altered, leading to serious delays in diagnosis. Extra surveillance and prophylactic measures for gastrointestinal, genitourinary, and integumentary complications are warranted.

OTHER ISSUES IN ORTHOPEDIC TRAUMA

General Principles of Fracture Fixation of the Extremities

During the initial phases of treatment, adequate reduction and immobilization are sufficient to manage most extremity fractures. Definitive management ranges from simple anatomic reduction and casting to complex open reduction and internal fixation. The choice of treatment involves a number of variables and is aimed at optimizing functional recovery.

Fractures of the lower extremity can be categorized roughly by anatomic site, and there is a strong tendency toward early rigid fixation to facilitate mobilization. Fractures of the hip, including the proximal femur, almost always require rigid fixation to maintain anatomic relations and hip function. Although midshaft femur fractures can be treated adequately with balanced skeletal traction and bed rest, most of these fractures are managed by intramedullary rods, allowing rapid ambulation. Simple fractures of the lower leg are well managed with casting alone and crutch ambulation. Complex fractures usually require internal fixation to obtain adequate anatomic realignment. In addition, the tendency should be toward rigid fixation in multiply injured patients to allow early mobilization. Fractures of the ankle almost always require open reduction and internal fixation to achieve adequate functional recovery.

Upper-extremity fractures often can be managed with closed techniques. Fractures of the proximal and middle humerus rarely require rigid fixation because accurate anatomic reduction is not critical. Fractures in the region of the elbow are more likely to require internal fixation to preserve elbow function. In the lower arm, fractures involving only one bone (ulna or radius) are most commonly managed by casting. Complex fractures involving both bones almost always require internal rigid fixation to preserve rotational function of the forearm. Similarly, fractures around the wrist commonly require rigid fixation to maintain reduction. Fractures of the small bones of the hand often require rigid fixation because accurate anatomic reconstruction is vital to function.

Rigid fixation can be achieved by a wide variety of methods, including intramedullary instrumentation; various plates, wires, and screws; and external fixators. Completely implantable instrumentation is preferred, but in open fractures, especially those with soft tissue loss, inability to achieve soft tissue coverage and risk of infection often necessitate the use of external techniques. In addition, external fixators are usually more rapidly applied, obviating the need for long operations with significant blood loss in critically ill, multiply injured patients.

Mangled Extremities

The badly damaged extremity with significant skeletal, soft tissue, and neurovascular injury presents a difficult management problem. Complex open fractures with degloving, traumatic amputation, and associated nerve and vessel injuries may be technically repairable, but the salvage of a painful and functionally useless limb serves little purpose. Reconstructive efforts often require multiple operations and may continue for several years. By comparison, young patients suffering primary amputation usually return to productive life within a year of injury. The decision to proceed with primary amputation of a mangled extremity can be exceedingly difficult, but it is of vital importance.[229] Although such decisions mandate a multidisciplinary approach, it is the responsibility of the general trauma surgeon to consider the impact of attempts at limb salvage on the overall resuscitation of the patient.

Strategy and Timing

An important advance in the management of the trauma patient has been the recognition that early treatment of orthopedic injuries (ie, within 24 hours) is associated with decreased hospital stay, shortened ICU stay, and diminished morbidity and mortality. Early fixation of orthopedic injuries must be incorporated as part of the overall resuscitation of the patient and must be individualized. Previously accepted contraindications to early orthopedic surgery, such as extensive burns[255] or head injury,[256] are being challenged, but contraindications still exist.[257] These include hemodynamic instability, respiratory failure, significant hypothermia, or coagulopathy in cases in which prolonged or additional surgery or blood loss would jeopardize the patient's survival or meaningful neurologic recovery. If these problems are encountered, surgery should not be postponed arbitrarily. Rather, aggressive correction of the abnormality should be undertaken with frequent reappraisal of the patient's suitability for early orthopedic repair.

Early orthopedic intervention must be efficient and expert. Long operations by inexperienced personnel that involve excessive blood loss not only negate the benefits of early intervention but can cause increased morbidity and mortality. There are occasions where patient instability compromises the care of orthopedic injuries. This may mean that the washout of open fractures or fasciotomy must be performed in the ICU or, more rarely, that the life of the patient must be preserved at the expense of the viability of the injured limb. Because such patients often require the expertise of multiple subspecialties, the general trauma surgeon must be familiar with the diagnostic and therapeutic options and use this knowledge to coordinate the optimal care of these challenging patients.

Definitive Care Phase: Pediatric Trauma

M. MARGARET KNUDSON

If a disease were killing our children in the proportions that accidents are, people would be outraged and demand that this killer be stopped.

C. Everett Koop, MD, ScD

Injury is the most important threat to the lives of American children and the leading cause of death in children older than 1 year of age. Trauma is responsible for more pediatric deaths than all other diseases combined. Each year in the United States, almost 13 million children aged 0 to 14 years old require emergency treatment for injuries, 360,000 are hospitalized, and 20,000 die of accidental illness or injury. In addition, an estimated 100,000 children are permanently handicapped as the result of trauma. According to the National Safety Council, the annual fiscal cost of injuries to children is more than $15 billion. These direct monetary costs are minor in comparison with the tremendous toll that a premature death or disability has on a family and on society as a whole. In the last decade, there has been considerable improvement in the care of the adult trauma patient as a result of the development of highly organized trauma systems. Progress for pediatric trauma patients has been slower. Because there are fewer critically injured children than adults, regional cooperation is necessary to develop and sustain trauma centers with personnel trained in the special needs of children. A thorough understanding of the patterns of injury and knowledge of the physiologic, anatomic, and psychological characteristics unique to pediatric trauma patients are necessary to ensure the best outcome.

MECHANISMS OF INJURY

The leading cause of pediatric injury and death in the United States is blunt trauma. The major mechanisms that result in blunt injuries are motor vehicle accidents (involving children as passengers, pedestrians, or cyclists) and falls (Fig. 11-99). Falls are more prevalent in infants and

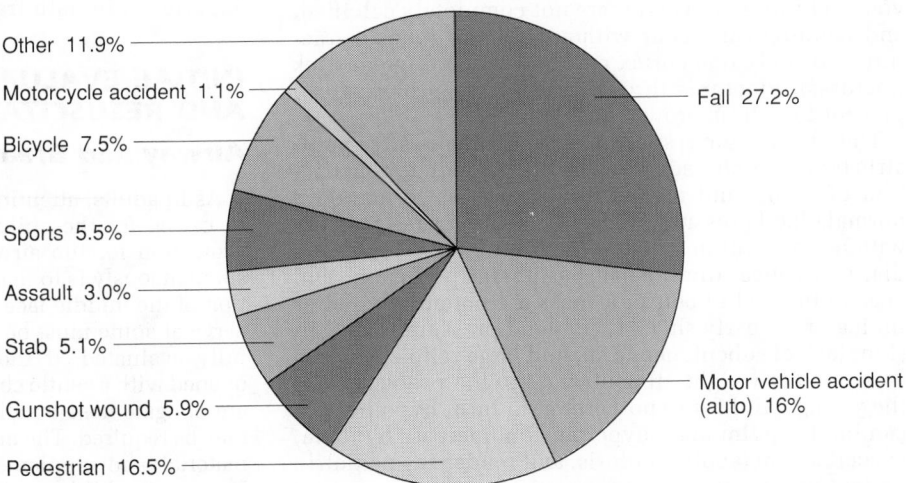

Figure 11-99. Mechanisms of injury in pediatric trauma in the United States. (Data from the National Pediatric Trauma Registry, phase II, 1990)

Other 11.9%
Motorcycle accident 1.1%
Bicycle 7.5%
Sports 5.5%
Assault 3.0%
Stab 5.1%
Gunshot wound 5.9%
Pedestrian 16.5%
Fall 27.2%
Motor vehicle accident (auto) 16%

toddlers and are a leading cause of death in urban areas. Children of school age are more likely to be struck by cars while walking or riding a bicycle. About 70% of cyclists injured or killed each year are under 15 years of age. Pediatric pedestrian injuries and deaths are also more common in urban areas. In adolescent years, high-speed motor vehicle crashes and penetrating trauma are the predominate mechanisms of injury. These different mechanisms of injury result in different injury patterns. Head injuries are frequently seen in children who have fallen or have been assaulted. Major thoracic and abdominal injuries are often the result of penetrating trauma or motor vehicle crashes. Lower-extremity fractures are common after pedestrian accidents. The highest mortality rates are associated with penetrating wounds, child abuse, and drowning, but motor vehicle accidents cause the greatest number of deaths.

The number of children and adolescents killed or injured by firearms has reached epidemic proportions, especially in urban areas. In the United States, an estimated 20,000 children and young adults are injured each year with firearms, and 4500 die. These gunshot wounds occur most frequently in the home, where the assailant is known to the child and the wounding instrument is readily available and unsecured. Handguns are the most common wounding instrument in urban areas, whereas rifle and shotgun wounds are more frequent in rural settings. Children who die from shootings most often have severe head and neck injuries, followed by thoracic and abdominal injuries.[258,259]

ANATOMIC AND PHYSIOLOGIC CONSIDERATIONS

Physical appearance is the most obvious difference between adults and children. The smaller size of pediatric patients results in an increased likelihood of multiple system trauma because the force of impact is dissipated over a relatively smaller area (Fig. 11-100). The higher frequency of head injuries in children is partially explained by the proportionately greater size of the head, the thin skull, and the weaker supporting cervical musculature. In infants with unfused cranial sutures and open fontanels, intracranial hemorrhage can be profuse and can result in shock. The mediastinum is mobile in childhood, and intrapleural pressure increases that are caused by a hemothorax or pneumothorax result in mediastinal shift and obstruction of venous return more readily in children than in adults. The protuberant abdomen of the child receives little protection from either the thoracic cage or the pelvis, accounting for the high incidence of intraabdominal injuries. In young children, the bones are not completely calcified, and bending can occur without fracture (buckle fractures), or only one cortex may be involved (greenstick fractures). Fractures through immature epiphyses can present long-term growth problems.

The physiologic response to hypovolemia after pediatric trauma is characterized by the immediate constriction of small- and medium-sized arteries to maintain normal blood pressure. Decompensation usually occurs with a blood volume deficit of 20% to 25%. Tachycardia, tachypnea, diminished peripheral perfusion, and change in level of consciousness are potentially better indicators of early shock than blood pressure. The thin skin, lack of subcutaneous fat, and large ratio of surface area to body weight all contribute to the propensity of the young child for hypothermia. In turn, hypothermia can induce pulmonary hypertension, increase hypoxia, exacerbate metabolic acidosis, and render the pediatric patient unresponsive to resuscitation.

TRIAGE AND PREHOSPITAL CARE

Optimal care of the severely injured pediatric trauma patient begins with early prehospital intervention and rapid transport of the child to the appropriate facility. The appropriate facility may not be the nearest hospital, but it should be the nearest center with the personnel and equipment needed to properly care for the injured child. Depending on the stability of the patient, it may be appropriate initially to evaluate and resuscitate the injured child in a general hospital while arranging prompt transfer to a specialized pediatric trauma center. A highly integrated system that includes emergency medical services and various levels of trauma centers, such as is present in the state of Maryland, should be the goal of every state.

The prehospital care of the injured child should be limited to assessment and securing of the airway and stabilization of the spine and obvious fractures. During short transport times, intravenous (IV) access is not necessary, and repeated attempts to establish IV access can delay definitive treatment. For longer transport times (more than 20 minutes), intraosseous infusions may be the most appropriate access, especially for children in shock. Numerous studies have demonstrated that properly trained prehospital personnel can rapidly establish intraosseous access with minimal complications. However, in large areas of the United States, emergency vehicles are not equipped with appropriately sized airways or with intravenous and intraosseus equipment for children. It should be a goal of all who care for sick and injured children to assure that pediatric emergency equipment is carried on all fire trucks and ambulances in their area.

Emergency medical personnel must also make triage decisions and transport children to appropriate facilities. Children with minor injuries are best cared for in the emergency department of their local hospital, close to their family and pediatrician. Children with potentially life-threatening injuries require evaluation in either an adult trauma center with pediatric capabilities or a specialized pediatric trauma center. Both the Revised Trauma Score and the Pediatric Trauma Score have been shown to function well in identifying children in need of trauma center care (Table 11-20). In addition to the physiologic data used in trauma scoring, the mechanism of injury also must be considered. No triage scheme is perfect, and even seemingly stable children with apparently minor injuries but a history of high-risk accident should be fully evaluated and resuscitated by a pediatric trauma team led by a surgeon with experience in both trauma and pediatric care.

INITIAL EVALUATION AND RESUSCITATION
Airway and Breathing

As in adults, attention to the airway is the first concern in caring for the child with multiple injuries. The best protection for the airway in the child who is breathing spontaneously is to maintain a superior and anterior position of the middle face (sniffing position). In addition, the cervical spine must be immobilized until the neck can be fully evaluated. If the airway is inadequate, it can be opened with a gentle chin lift or jaw thrust. Because infants are obligate nose-breathers, clearing of the nasal passages may be required. The mouth is cleared of blood and foreign material, and supplemental oxygen is applied in all cases. In a young child, respiratory compromise can result from

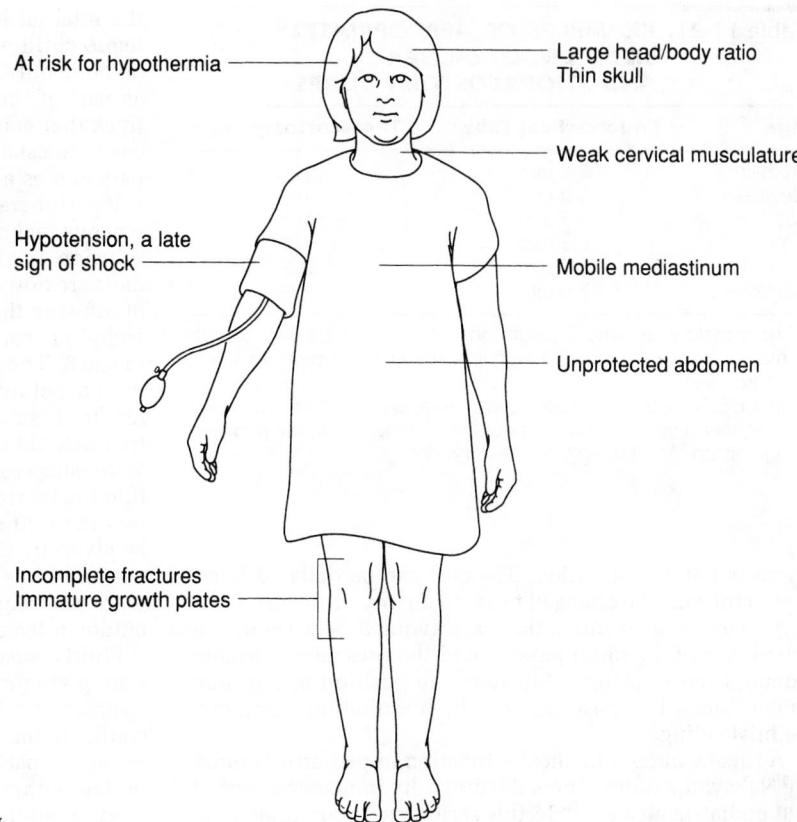

At risk for hypothermia

Hypotension, a late
sign of shock

Incomplete fractures
Immature growth plates

Large head/body ratio
Thin skull

Weak cervical musculature

Mobile mediastinum

Unprotected abdomen

Figure 11-100. Pediatric anatomy and physiology.

gastric dilatation or from compression of the diaphragm by intraabdominal blood or air. The use of nasogastric or orogastric tubes is therefore necessary in pediatric trauma patients.

Should intubation be required for oxygenation, ventilation, or airway protection, the anatomic differences in pediatric patients must be appreciated. The larynx in a small child is more anterior and caudad than in the adult. The trachea is soft and short, measuring only 5 cm in length in infants and 7 cm in 2-year-olds. Failure to appreciate these differences results in bronchial intubation or possible perforation. The proper size of the endotracheal tube can be approximated by choosing a tube with a diameter equal to that of the child's naris or fifth digit (Table 11-21). In the elective setting, if the child has an empty stomach, uncuffed endotracheal tubes are usually recommended to avoid airway edema and subglottic stenosis. However, in the trauma setting, a cuffed tube may be appropriate if

Table 11-20. TRAUMA SCORING SYSTEMS

Revised Trauma Score*

Glasgow Coma Scale Score	Systolic Blood Pressure (mmHg)	Respiratory Rate	Coded Value
13–15	>89	10–29	4
9–12	76–89	>29	3
6–8	50–75	6–9	2
4–5	1–49	1–5	1
3	0	0	0

Pediatric Trauma Score†

Size (kg)	Airway	Blood Pressure (mmHg)	CNS	Open Wound	Skeletal Wound	Score
>20	Normal	>90	Awake	None	None	+2
10–20	Maintained	50–90	Obtunded	Minor	Closed	+1
<10	Required	<50	Coma	Major	Multiple	−1

* An RTS of 11 or less predicts increased mortality and can be used as a triage index. (Boyd CR, Tolson MA, Cope WS. Evaluating trauma care: the TRISS method. J Trauma 1987;27:370).
† A PTS of 8 or less is associated with increased mortality.
(Tepas JJ, Ramenofsky ML, Mollit DL, Gaus BM, DiScala C. The Pediatric Trauma Score as a predictor of injury severity. J Pediatr Surg 1987;22:14)

Table 11-21. EXAMPLES OF APPROPRIATELY SIZED ENDOTRACHEAL AND THORACOSTOMY TUBES*

Age	Endotracheal Tube	Thoracostomy Tube
Premature	2.5 mm	12F
Newborn	3.0 mm	14F
Toddler	4.5 mm	20F
6 Y	5.5 mm	24F
10 Y	6.5 mm	28F
Adolescent	7.0 mm	32F

* The Broselow Pediatric Resuscitation Tape can also be used to estimate weight based on the height of the child, in order to select appropriate drug doses.
(Lubitz DS, Seidel JS, Chameides L, et al. A rapid method for estimating weight and resuscitation drug dosages from length in the pediatric age group. Ann Emerg Med 1988; 17:576)

there is risk of aspiration. The cuff can be deflated later, or the tube can be changed to avoid airway problems. Usually, nasotracheal intubations are avoided because of the small size of the nasal passage and the presence of friable adenoid tissue. After intubation, the position of the tube is confirmed by chest radiograph; auscultation alone can be misleading.

A review of endotracheal intubation in pediatric trauma by Nakayama underscores the difficulty in management of the pediatric airway.[260] In this series, early complications of airway management in children included right mainstem intubation, massive barotrauma, failure of adequate preoxygenation, esophageal intubation, and extubation during transport. Late complications that were recognized included vocal cord paresis and subglottic stenosis. Some of these airway complications resulted in the death of the child at the scene of the injury. The authors of this study emphasized the need for both special training and continued reeducation for life support specialists who deal with children.

Rarely, an endotracheal tube cannot be placed or is contraindicated because of massive facial trauma. In these situations, an emergency airway should be established by placing a 12- to 16-gauge angiocatheter through the cricothyroid membrane into the trachea and instituting jet insufflation. A formal cricothyroidotomy or tracheostomy can then be performed under controlled circumstances, with anesthesia and proper lighting and instruments.

Circulation

The recognition and treatment of hypovolemic shock in children allows little margin for error. Even seemingly minor blood loss can have major physiologic consequences in children, because the initial blood volume is relatively small. The estimated blood volume in young children is 80 mL/kg (or 8% of total body weight). Therefore, a healthy, 10-kg toddler has a blood volume of only about 800 mL. As mentioned, hypotension is a late sign of shock, and the trauma team must be attentive to other signs of diminished perfusion, such as tachycardia, tachypnea, decreased capillary filling, and disorientation (Table 11-22).

Volume resuscitation begins with establishment and maintenance of venous access. Initially, percutaneous placement of two peripheral IV catheters (20-gauge or larger) should be attempted. Favored sites in pediatric patients include the greater saphenous vein at the ankle, the cephalic vein in the antecubital fossa, and the external jugular vein. Percutaneous central line placement through the internal jugular or subclavian vein in small, hypovolemic children is fraught with complications and should be done only by an experienced clinician and not usually as part of the initial resuscitation. Percutaneous femoral lines that gain access to the inferior vena cava are much easier to establish, provided that the femoral pulse can be palpated as a reference.

If peripheral lines cannot be placed rapidly by the percutaneous technique and the child is in shock, intraosseous infusion is appropriate. Specially designed intraosseous nails are now available that allow for a safe and rapid route of infusion through the marrow cavity of a long bone. This technique can be applied in infants and small children up to age 6. The preferred site is the anterior tibial plateau, 2 to 3 cm below the tibial tuberosity. Alternatively, the distal femur, 3 cm above the external condyle, can be used. Extremities that are injured or fractured should not be used. With successful establishment of intraosseous infusion into the marrow cavity, the circulation time to the heart is less than 20 seconds. Crystalloids, blood, and drugs can be given by this route with minimal complications. After the child has been stabilized, time can be spent securing more permanent venous access by either percutaneous or cutdown techniques.

Fluid resuscitation is initiated with lactated Ringer solution, giving an initial bolus of 20 mL/kg if the patient is hypotensive. If the patient remains hypotensive, a second, similar bolus can be given, but if there is again no sustained response, packed red blood cells should be transfused (10 mL/kg; either type O, Rh-negative, or type-specific), and consideration should be given to surgical therapy to control hemorrhage. Ninety-five percent of pediatric patients with blunt trauma are hemodynamically stable with this initial approach, and further diagnostic studies can then be undertaken. For the child in shock, the administration of sodium bicarbonate usually is not necessary, because acidosis is best reversed by restoration of perfusion and correction of hypoventilation. In the child who is resistant to resuscitation and has a serum pH below 7.2, sodium bicarbonate can be administered while fluid resuscitation is continued. The estimated dose is calculated from the following formula:

$$NaHCO_3 = body\ weight \times 0.3 \times base\ deficit$$

Half the calculated dose can be given as an IV bolus, and the remainder is given at a rate of 3 to 5 mEq/min. Throughout the resuscitation, hypothermia must be avoided. This is done by warming all blood and crystalloid solutions and by using overhead radiant heaters and blankets. In intubated patients, the inspired oxygen should also be warmed. The urine output is monitored continuously as a guide to volume replacement. Adequate renal perfusion is indicated by an output of 1 to 2 mL/kg/h.

Emergency department resuscitative thoracotomy is attempted in children who arrive in cardiac arrest after penetrating chest injury. The role of resuscitative thoracotomy after blunt trauma is less clear, but the outcome in children appears similar to that in adults, with less then a 2% sal-

Table 11-22. NORMAL VITAL SIGNS BY AGE

	Pulse	Systolic Blood Pressure (mmHg)	Respiratory Rate
Infant (<1 y)	160	80	40
Preschool (<5 y)	140	90	30
Adolescent (>10 y)	120	100	20

vage rate overall. Therefore, emergency department thoracotomy is reserved for children who arrive at the hospital in cardiac arrest after penetrating trauma if there were signs of life at the scene, or after blunt trauma if the arrest was witnessed and the child does not have major head injuries.

PEDIATRIC TRAUMA PROTOCOL

After securing the airway and initiating fluid resuscitation, the trauma surgeon performs a rapid but thorough physical examination in search of injuries (Fig. 11-101). Findings from the examination, including neurologic findings and serial vital signs, are carefully documented. As IV lines are placed, blood is drawn for laboratory studies, including complete blood count, levels of serum electrolytes, blood urea nitrogen, creatinine, and amylase, and blood typing and crossmatching. The smallest acceptable blood collection tubes should be used, because repeated blood drawing in small children contributes to the need for blood replacement. Blood pressure and oxygen saturation, as measured by pulse oximetry, are monitored continuously, as is the urine output. Cervical spine, chest, and pelvic radiographs are routinely obtained in the trauma

room. Throughout this critical period, the special psychologic needs of the child must be considered. The frightened child is emotionally labile and may regress to infantile behavior. A calm and reassuring approach with attempted explanations of procedures gains the most cooperation and can help avert long-term psychological problems resulting from the accident.

MANAGEMENT OF SPECIFIC INJURIES
Thoracic Trauma

The prevalence of thoracic injury among children hospitalized after blunt or penetrating trauma ranges from 0.1% to 30%. The presence of thoracic trauma has increasingly been recognized as an indicator of increased mortality. The mortality rate from thoracic injuries in children ranges from 7% to 14% overall, but it increases to 25% in children younger than 5 years of age. The compliant thoracic cage of a child allows the kinetic energy to be transmitted to the underlying intrathoracic structures, often without obvious injury to the external chest wall. As a result, rib fractures are less common in children than adults, occurring only

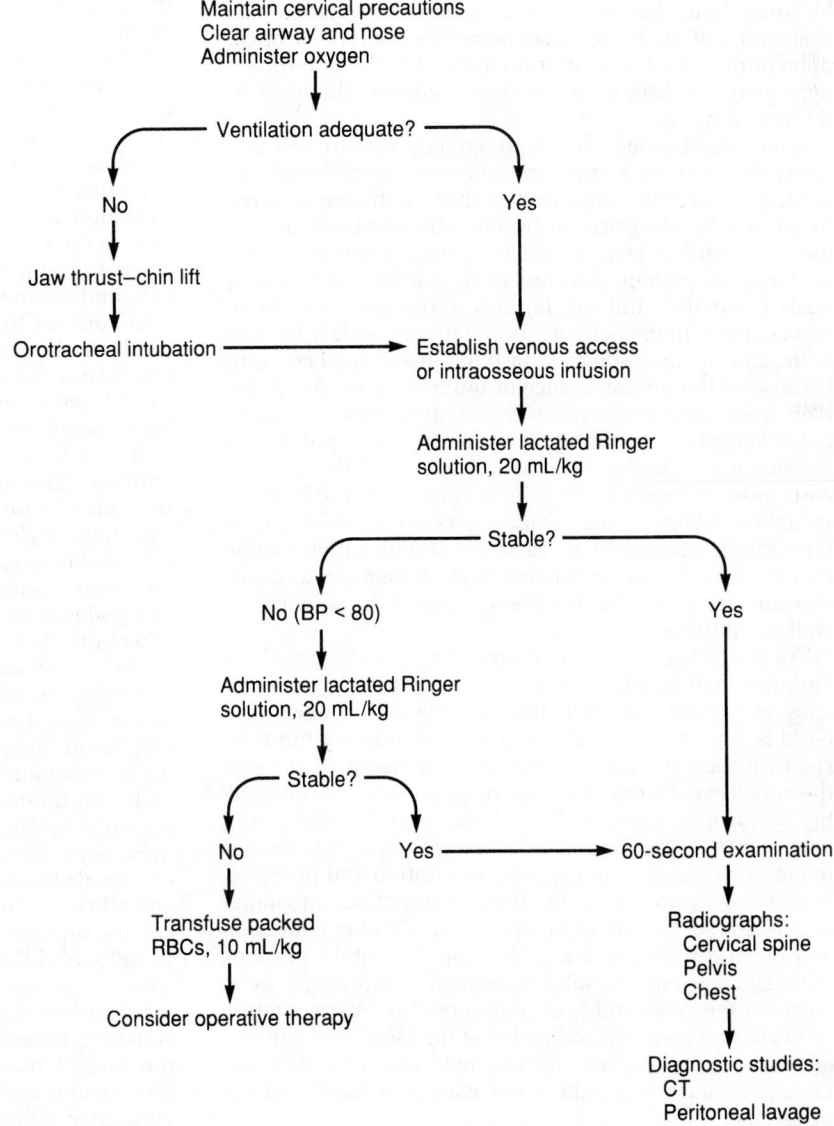

Figure 11-101. Pediatric resuscitation algorithm.

in about 50% of children with major thoracic injury. If rib fractures are diagnosed in children, they are a marker of severe trauma and are associated with an increased mortality rate. The combination of rib fractures and head injury is a particularly lethal situation.

The most common thoracic injury in children is pulmonary contusion. The recognition of pulmonary contusion may be delayed because the lung fields often appear normal on the initial chest radiograph. Therefore, children with evidence of chest trauma require careful monitoring of oxygen saturation levels for the first 24 to 48 hours. Computed tomography (CT) scan of the chest is also an excellent method of detecting pulmonary pathology that presents in a delayed fashion. The need for ventilatory support after blunt thoracic trauma in the pediatric population is relatively uncommon and, if required, it is usually of short duration.

A tension pneumothorax can cause severe hypotension in a child as a result of a rapid shift in the mobile mediastinum that obstructs venous return to the heart. About 25% of all traumatic pneumothoraces in children are under tension. These injuries must be recognized early and treated by chest decompression with a properly sized tube thoracostomy (see Table 11-21). A hemothorax can result in hypotensive shock as a result of a relatively large amount of blood loss, and this blood loss must be monitored by tube thoracostomy. Reexpansion of the lung decreases bleeding from the low-pressure pulmonary system, and evacuation of the hemothorax decreases the risk for development of a residual clot or infection. On the other hand, persistent bleeding from the chest indicates the need for thoracotomy.

Bronchial injuries and diaphragmatic rupture are relatively rare but very important concerns in children sustaining major crush injuries. Cardiac contusion is rarely diagnosed by electrocardiographic abnormalities in children, but cardiac arrhythmias may suggest this diagnosis. In the stable patient, the clinical significance of this diagnosis is usually minimal. Injuries to the great vessels are less common in the pediatric population, possibly because of the lack of atherosclerotic vascular disease and certainly because of the predominance of blunt injuries. Blunt thoracic vascular injuries most frequently involve the aorta, but other sites, including the vena cava and pulmonary vessels, are reported. Traumatic rupture of the thoracic aorta most commonly occurs in children involved in motor vehicle accidents, either as passengers or pedestrians. Even if promptly recognized, it is associated with a high mortality rate. An association between first rib fractures and subclavian artery injuries has been reported in pediatric as well as adult series.

Traumatic asphyxia is an injury seen more frequently in children than in adults. This syndrome results when the chest is compressed while the glottis is closed, as when a child is run over by a vehicle. The extraordinary but transient increase in thoracic pressure is transmitted through the vena cava. Children appear to be particularly vulnerable because of the compliant thorax and the absence of valves in the superior and inferior vena cava. This venous hypertension results in capillary disruption and petechial hemorrhage into the brain, skin, conjunctiva, and other organs above the site of compression. Cardiac contusion and hepatic injury may also develop. The child presents with facial cyanosis, subconjunctival hemorrhage, petechiae on the chest and head, and, possibly, disorientation or seizures. Treatment is directed at the associated injuries and complications; the term "traumatic asphyxia" is a misnomer, because asphyxia is not usually a feature of the syndrome.

Abdominal Trauma

Twenty-five percent of children who sustain multiple trauma have serious intraabdominal injuries. Detection of these injuries by physical examination is often difficult and requires a gentle examiner and a cooperative, communicative child. Children who are hemodynamically unstable after obvious blunt abdominal trauma should undergo emergency laparotomy. Similarly, those who are victims of gunshot wounds to the abdomen deserve immediate operative exploration, because over 90% of them have injuries requiring repair. Stable patients and victims of stabbings are candidates for further diagnostic studies, including diagnostic peritoneal lavage (DPL) or abdominal CT or ultrasound.

DPL is a rapid and sensitive test for the presence of intraabdominal hemorrhage. The technique has been previously described in this chapter. In general, DPL has a limited role in the care of pediatric patients because it provides confirmation of a finding (ie, hemoperitoneum) that does not mandate operation. It is rational only if the clinical situation requires laparotomy after a positive finding. Recently, ultrasound has also been used in pediatric blunt trauma patients to detect abdominal fluid.

CT scan of the abdomen is the preferred diagnostic approach for hemodynamically stable children with blunt abdominal trauma. Standard abdominal CT scan for traumatic injury requires the use of both oral and IV contrast agents. In some cases, a rectal contrast agent is also useful. CT scan not only detects blood in the abdomen but also identifies which organs are injured. Serial CT scans can be used to monitor the rate of bleeding as well as organ healing in patients selected for nonoperative management. CT also has the advantage of imaging the retroperitoneal structures that are not evaluated by DPL. No child who is hemodynamically unstable or whose airway is at risk should be sent to the CT scanner. A complete scan usually requires 30 to 45 minutes to perform. The relative indications for DPL and abdominal CT scan are listed in Table 11-23.

In contrast to adults, 95% of pediatric trauma patients are hemodynamically stable on admission and are thus candidates for evaluation by CT scan, which delineates solid visceral injuries with both a high sensitivity and a high specificity. Missed hollow viscus injury, the major failing of CT scan, is more of a problem in adults than in children. The incidence of this type of injury in children with blunt trauma is about 1% to 2%, whereas it is about five times higher in the adult population. This difference is probably a result of the different mechanisms involved; for example, children tend to be automobile passengers and pedestrians rather than drivers who impact a steering wheel during a motor vehicle accident.

The spleen and the liver are injured with about equal frequency in children sustaining blunt trauma, and together these two target organs account for about 75% of childhood abdominal injuries. The historical preference for splenectomy for splenic injury was first challenged in pediatric trauma patients in the late 1960s. The risks of postsplenectomy sepsis were recognized and found to be inversely related to age. Experience at almost every major children's trauma center in the world supports the safety and efficacy of nonoperative management of children with splenic ruptures. Most series report splenic salvage in 90% to 100% of children. Although therapy must be individualized, the general guidelines are that operation is not indicated unless there is refractory hypotension or a transfusion requirement in excess of 50% of blood volume within the first 24 hours. In reality, few patients approach this level, and transfusion practices are such that only 10% to 20% of children with isolated splenic injuries require

Table 11-23. EVALUATION OF THE ABDOMEN IN CHILDREN

Indications for Peritoneal Lavage	Indications for Abdominal CT
Unstable patient with no obvious abdominal injury	Stable patient after multiple trauma
Patient requiring *immediate* operation for associated injuries (eg, neurosurgical)	Patient requiring *emergent* operation for associated injuries (eg, orthopedic)
Unconscious patient or unreliable physical examination	Unconscious patient or unreliable physical examination
Patient with anterior abdominal stab wound without other indications for surgery	Patient with posterior abdominal stab wound without other indications for surgery
Patient with unexplained blood loss	Patient with unexplained blood loss
Patient with free fluid seen on CT scan that has no obvious source	Patient with hematuria or suspected pancreatic or liver injury

blood transfusion at all. It has been suggested that the child's spleen is more capable of contracting to limit hemorrhage after injury, although the physiologic reason for this ability is not known.

Nonoperative therapy requires that the child be continuously monitored for the first 48 hours and be examined serially by a surgeon for evidence of ongoing bleeding or the presence of other abdominal injuries requiring surgical intervention. A staffed operating room, a well-equipped blood bank, and an anesthesiologist also must be readily available. Children usually are hospitalized until the abdominal pain and ileus resolve, which typically takes 5 to 7 days. After discharge, contact sports should be avoided for 2 months after injury or until the CT scan demonstrates a healed spleen, which typically requires 4 to 6 weeks. Late complications are unusual.

Should nonoperative therapy fail or laparotomy be required for another purpose, the spleen often can be repaired surgically by various hemostatic topical agents, suture techniques, partial splenectomy, or reestablishment of the capsule with absorbable mesh. However, given the success of nonoperative therapy, experience with surgical salvage techniques has diminished in recent years.

The management of liver injuries in pediatric patients has also changed since the advent of routine abdominal CT scan for blunt trauma. Several reports describe successful nonoperative treatment of liver injuries detected radiologically in children. The degree of liver injury and the amount of free intraperitoneal blood are less important in determining the outcome with this method of management than is the stability of the child. This approach is applicable to most children, with a success rate of 90% and transfusion requirements similar to those for children with ruptured spleens. However, some children with liver injuries require operative intervention, and the need for surgery is more likely in the presence of severe multisystem injuries, lobar disruption of the liver exceeding 25%, and the need for transfusion within 2 hours of admission. Among children treated without operative intervention, delayed hepatic hemorrhage, sepsis, and hemobilia are potential complications, but the incidence of each is low. It appears that the liver stops bleeding spontaneously in most cases and, like the spleen, heals over time (Figs. 11-102 and 11-103). This is true of complex as well as simple injuries, so long as major vascular trauma is not involved.

Acute gastric dilatation is common in children and may mimic visceral injury. A nasogastric tube should be placed in all patients who have sustained serious trauma, to avoid aspiration of gastric contents and to allow for a more reliable physical examination. Rupture of the stomach is an injury that occurs in children, often after a blow to the abdomen with bicycle handlebars or after the child is hit by a car. Intramural duodenal hematomas may also occur after these types of events. This injury results from disruption of the submucosal vessels, which leads to formation

of submucosal hematoma with obstruction of the duodenal lumen. The hematoma usually resolves spontaneously, and the initial treatment for children with this injury is bowel rest and parenteral nutrition. Occasionally, operative therapy is required, particularly if there is no improvement after 2 to 3 weeks. Injuries to the small bowel are not infrequent in children and can result from seemingly insignificant trauma, but the incidence of actual perforation is low. Tears or hematomas of the bowel mesentery occur because the mesenteric attachments in a child are not as dense as in an adult and allow for increased visceral movement. An important association has been established among use of seat belts, flexion–distraction vertebral fractures (Chance fractures), and bowel injuries in children. The recognition of injuries to the small intestine can be difficult, because peritoneal signs may be delayed and CT scan is inaccurate. Subtle signs of intestinal injury on CT scan include the presence of unexplained fluid in the pelvis and an apparent thickening of the involved wall of the intestine. However, frequent abdominal examinations and a thorough search are the most reliable tools for the detection of intestinal injuries in children.

Pancreatic injuries can follow a blow to the upper abdomen and can be lethal if unrecognized and untreated. Pancreatic injuries are rare, but a notable pattern is that of seemingly minor but direct epigastric trauma leading to major injury. Infants and toddlers appear to be unable to protect themselves; in particular, this is one important pattern of child abuse. Posttraumatic pancreatitis is a poten-

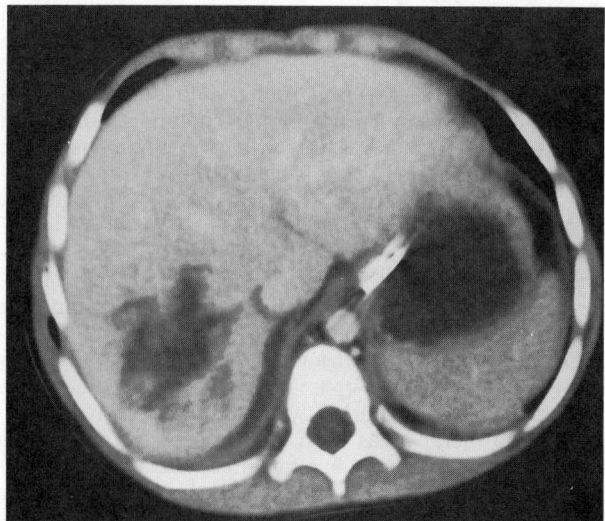

Figure 11-102. Abdominal CT scan of a 3-year-old child demonstrating a stellate laceration of the posterior right lobe of the liver after an auto–pedestrian accident.

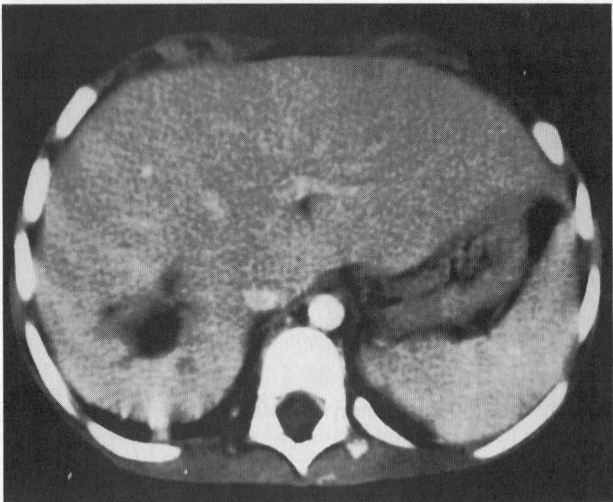

Figure 11-103. Follow-up CT scan 10 days after trauma demonstrating healing after nonoperative treatment for patient shown in Figure 11-102.

tially serious complication after blunt abdominal trauma and should be considered in a child who is slow to recover.

Central Nervous System Injuries

Head injuries are the leading cause of death and disability after pediatric trauma, and they result primarily from motor vehicle accidents or from falls. Although the morbidity and mortality associated with head injury relate in part to the nature of the primary injury, a process controlled only by prevention, secondary insults also significantly affect outcome. These secondary insults, which include hypoxia, hypotension, and intracranial hypertension, can be at least partially controlled by specific interventions. Severe brain injury in children is frequently associated with initial apnea or hypoventilation, or both. Hypoxia, particularily if it is accompanied by hypotension, adds insult to the already injured brain. Rapid establishment of a secure airway prevents hypoxia and allows for hyperventilation, which can assist in the control of cerebral hypertension. Recovery from head trauma is also affected by prompt surgical intervention for mass lesions such as epidural or subdural hematomas. Although they are less common in children than in adults, such injuries are readily detected by CT scan of the head.

Pediatric patients are more prone to development of intracranial hypertension after injury than are adults. Brain swelling with intracranial hypertension threatens about half of children with severe head injuries, and uncontrolled cerebral hypertension carries a poor prognosis. Control of intracranial hypertension includes elevation of the head, sedation and analgesia, hyperventilation, maintenance of normal vascular volume, and treatment of hyperthermia and seizures. Placement of a device to monitor intracranial pressure, such as the Camino fiberoptic catheter, should be considered for children in coma. Osmotic agents are also useful for treatment of brain edema, but they must be used cautiously in the hypotensive child. Barbiturate therapy has been used successfully by some pediatric neurosurgeons but remains controversial. Children with severe head injury clearly benefit from early institution of enteral nutrition and engagement of the services of a rehabilitation team. In general, the recovery is more rapid and the prognosis is better in children with serious head injuries than in adults.

Pediatric spinal cord injury is rare, with only 5% of all spinal injuries occurring in children. Radiologic evaluation of the cervical spine in pediatric patients is particularly difficult owing to some normal anatomic variations. For example, 40% of normal young children show a pseudosubluxation with anterior displacement of C-2 on C-3. Increased distance between the dens and the anterior arch of C-1 also can be observed in children. Skeletal growth centers can be misinterpreted as fractures of the spine. Spinal cord injury without radiographic abnormality is more commonly seen in children than in adults because vertebral fracture is not a prerequisite for spinal cord injury. A recent review of the outcome of pediatric cervical spine injuries demonstrated that younger children sustained more severe injuries than did older children. The incidence of paralysis after cervical spine fractures in children is about 25%. The increased mortality rate in younger children is explained by the frequent association between cervical spine injuries and severe closed head trauma.

Genitourinary Injuries

The kidneys are less protected in children than in adults and are more vulnerable to blunt traumatic injury. In addition, unsuspected congenital abnormalities are more likely to lead to posttraumatic hematuria in children. Hematuria is the hallmark of renal injury and is best evaluated with abdominal CT scan with IV contrast. Hematuria is also an excellent marker of other abdominal injuries, such as liver and spleen injuries, both of which are readily detected by CT scan. Over 80% of renal injuries are simple contusions or lacerations that can be managed nonoperatively. In a small percentage of cases, early operative intervention for the repair of major lacerations or vascular injuries is warranted in an attempt to salvage the injured kidney and to control hemorrhage. Rupture of the bladder usually is associated with pelvic fractures and can be confirmed with a cystogram. Urethral injuries can also result from pelvic fractures and should be suspected if the child is unable to void or if there is difficulty in passing a urinary catheter. Impalement injuries to the perineum can also injure the urethra. As in adults, urethral injuries are best treated initially with bladder drainage (possibly suprapubic) and delayed repair.

Pelvic Fractures and Extremity Trauma

Trauma to the growing extremity of a child can cause a bend without actual fracture of the bone. If the epiphysis of a long bone is involved, there may be long-term consequences in terms of growth and development. On the other hand, many fracture deformities in young children correct themselves spontaneously, a process termed *remodeling*. The blood loss associated with bony injuries, especially in the pelvis, is proportionately greater in the child than in the adult, and this must be considered during the resuscitation phase. Supracondylar fractures at the elbow are relatively common in children and should always raise the concern of an accompanying vascular injury. All injured extremities must be monitored carefully with frequent neurovascular examinations for possible development of a compartment syndrome.

Children with pelvic fractures are at risk for life-threatening hemorrhage as well as associated abdominal injuries. Patients at significant risk for hemorrhage are those with bilateral anterior and posterior fractures. The presence of multiple pelvic fractures also predicts the presence of associated genitourinary and abdominal injuries. Another marker for associated abdominal injury occurring with pelvic fracture is the addition of any other bony fracture. Pelvic fractures in children rarely occur in isolation, and associated injuries to the head, abdomen, chest, and extremities must be suspected.

Vascular injuries may accompany both blunt and penetrating extremity trauma. Fractures that are associated with the potential for vascular injuries are those about the knee and the elbow. Gunshot wounds to the extremities also threaten vessels in proximity to their path. Vascular injuries usually present with "hard signs" such as loss of pulses, pain, paralysis, or expanding hematomas. Occasionally, only "soft signs" or no signs of injury are apparent on the initial examination. Duplex arterial examination is an excellent, noninvasive study that is capable of detecting these occult and potentially limb-threatening vascular injuries.

INTENSIVE CARE CONSIDERATIONS

Although a complete description of pediatric intensive care is beyond the scope of this chapter, a few specific points essential for the care of the pediatric trauma patient should be mentioned. For all children, assurance of adequate oxygenation and ventilation is vital. In some cases, the monitoring of end-tidal carbon dioxide level and pulse oximetry may be adequate, but frequently, indwelling arterial lines are essential for optimal management of the unstable child. Ventilators should be adjusted to maintain oxygenation at the lowest possible fractional inspired oxygen and at the lowest possible peak airway pressures. Addition of small amounts of end-expiratory positive pressure may be helpful. Nosocomial infections are a constant threat in the environment of the intensive care unit (ICU), but antibiotics should be used only to treat specifically identified infections and cultured organisms. Prolonged use of prophylactic antibiotics only leads to superinfections with resistant organisms, as does the use of steroids. In general, steroids are reserved for the treatment of spinal cord injury (high doses for a very short time) and, occasionally, for airway edema that prevents extubation.

The nutritional needs of the injured child must also be addressed early in the ICU setting (within 24 to 48 hours of admission). The enteral route of administration is preferred, because there is now good evidence that the gut is an essential organ in resisting infection. The resting energy requirement for a typical 5-year-old child is 45 kcal/kg/24 h, and this increases to 90 kcal/kg/24 h in the face of major illness. Protein requirements are in the range of 1 to 2 g/kg/24 h. If the gut cannot be used to deliver the entire caloric requirement, it is still beneficial to give some nutrition by a nasoduodenal or jejunostomy tube, supplemented by IV central alimentation.

Rehabilitation from injury should be initiated in the ICU. Speech, physical, and occupational therapists are integral members of the pediatric intensive care team. Significant behavioral disturbance after nonneurologic trauma has been documented in 35% of young patients.[261] These dysfunctions include phobias, major scholastic difficulties, rage attacks, and episodic depressions. The child's reaction to trauma may be one of dependency, withdrawal, or guilt. Important therapies directed at resolving these issues in children include play and art therapy, which can be instituted in the ICU setting as soon as the child can participate. Involvement of the family is also essential, because severe injuries result in significant psychologic morbidity for both the child and the family.

CHILD ABUSE

All physicians caring for injured children have an ethical and legal responsibility to recognize and report the possibility of child abuse. This is a major public health issue in the United States. Most children who die or sustain serious injury from child abuse have been injured previously and frequently. These deaths and injuries are potentially preventable if the abusive behavior is detected early. The initial hint of abuse may be a discrepancy between the history offered and the apparent degree of injury. In addition, the history may be inconsistent among the adults involved. Frequently, the child has been taken to several different emergency departments to avoid raising suspicion. Physical signs of child abuse include perioral injuries, retinal hemorrhages, multiple subdural hematomas without a fresh skull fracture, genital or perianal injuries, burns in unusual areas (including burns caused by cigarettes), and radiographic evidence of multiple old or healed fractures.

If abuse is suspected, hospital admission is mandatory, and a formal report is required by law in most states. Medical therapy is of course provided, but a principal objective is to initiate the legal and social protection process.

QUALITY ASSURANCE

The quality of pediatric trauma care must be evaluated continuously by all those involved in this important specialty. Fundamental to any quality assessment is the evaluation of unexpected outcomes. The TRISS methodology, which uses the Injury Severity Score and the Revised Trauma Score to predict outcome, has been applied successfully to evaluate pediatric trauma care. Not only can TRISS analysis be used to identify cases for institutional review, but it is also useful for comparing results among trauma centers or with national norms. More in-depth quality assurance is conducted with the use of audit filters.[262] These audit filters can be used to generate valuable quality assurance reviews of patients with complications, delayed major surgeries, delayed diagnoses, or unexpected returns to the operating room.

Ideally, all seriously injured pediatric trauma patients would be cared for in a designated pediatric trauma center. However, with the existing constraints of geography and medical expertise, most pediatric patients are cared for by general surgeons in general hospitals. An integrated, regionalized pediatric trauma system would assure that all injured children receive the level of care appropriate for their needs. Without doubt, a pediatric surgeon or trauma surgeon must be intimately involved in all levels of trauma care, from prehospital care to prevention.

PREVENTION

The future of pediatric trauma care rests with the prevention of injuries. Most childhood deaths resulting from trauma are preventable. Epidemiologic studies have confirmed that more than two thirds of pediatric deaths after trauma occur before the child reaches the hospital; the only solution to these deaths is prevention.

Methods aimed at reducing childhood injury are described as active or passive. Active intervention requires a behavior change to be effective, such as securing a child in a safety seat. On the other hand, passive intervention requires little action from the individual. The most effective injury prevention programs incorporate the four Es[263]:

Engineering of products and environments
Enactment of legislation to promote safety

Education of children, caregivers, health care professionals, and legislators
Evaluation of the efficacy of specific interventions

Examples of successful pediatric injury prevention strategies include use of bicycle helmets, mandatory fencing of swimming pools, use of smoke detectors, lowering of hot water setpoints in homes, and use of window guards. The National Safe Kids Campaign is a comprehensive injury prevention campaign that provides educational material to the media and to local coalitions to help in the development of prevention programs and supportive legislation. Control of the current epidemic of violence requires complex programs integrating gun control legislation, conflict resolution techniques, and drug abuse prevention. It is through such programs that we can begin to combat the single greatest health problem that affects children today.

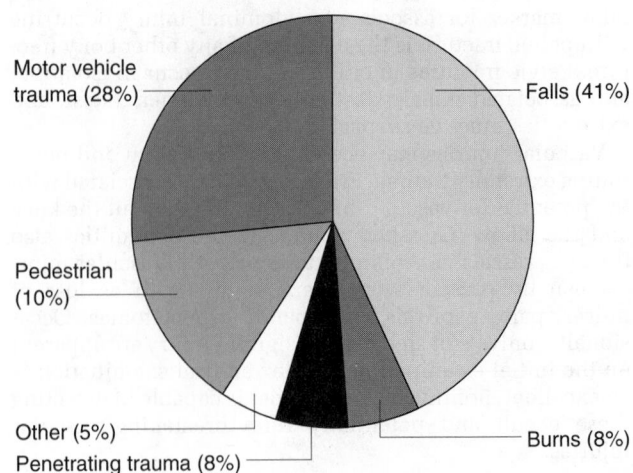

Figure 11-104. Causes of death among the elderly.

Definitive Care Phase: Geriatric Trauma

M. MARGARET KNUDSON

The population of the United States is aging. In 1980, 26.5 million Americans were older than 65 years of age. By the year 2050, this number is expected to double, and 20% of the population will be in the geriatric age group. Along with an increasing life expectancy, this group enjoys a healthier life-style, allowing them to be more active but also more prone to injury. Thus, geriatric trauma is becoming an important health care problem.

Although elderly persons are less likely to be injured than young people, their injuries are more likely to have fatal outcomes. Trauma is now the fifth leading cause of death in those aged 65 and older. Although elderly persons constitute only 11% of the US population, 25% of all trauma deaths occur in this group. Older trauma patients who survive their initial injuries are more likely to suffer complications and permanent functional dependency. Geriatric trauma patients also stay in the hospital an average of twice as long as younger patients with similar injuries, and they consume one third of all the health care resources expended on trauma care.[264]

A favorable outcome after trauma in an elderly person is best ensured by an aggressive approach toward resuscitation and diagnosis of injuries, avoidance of complications, and attention to the patient's preexisting medical conditions.

MECHANISMS OF INJURY

Falls

Falls are the leading cause of accidental death and disability among elderly persons; about 9500 elderly people die each year as the result of a fall (Fig. 11-104). Although most falls among geriatric patients are not fatal, a significant number result in injuries that are severe enough to require hospitalization. Most of these injuries are orthopedic in nature, but, according to one recent review, falls are also responsible for most head injuries in the elderly.

An extensive review of the causes of falls in the elderly population has been published.[264a] Risk factors for falls include chronic diseases and disabilities and visual, hearing, and vestibular impairments. Abnormalities in balance

and gait also contribute to the risk of falling, as do diseases that affect the bones, muscles, and joints. Orthostatic hypotension—a drop in systolic blood pressure of 20 mmHg or more with standing—is common in elderly persons and can result in falls. Syncope is another important cause of serious falls; it can be precipitated by decreases in cerebral blood flow or by a variety of metabolic problems, such as hypoxia or hypoglycemia. Falling may be the first presentation of an acute disease such as pneumonia. Alcohol and prescription drugs, particularly sedatives, antihypertensives, diuretics, and hypoglycemic agents, can also increase the tendency to fall.

Environmental hazards represent a largely preventable cause of falls in the elderly. Poor lighting, stairways without handrails, improper footwear, and obstacles on floors are factors that increase the risk of falling in the home. The physician caring for an elderly patient who has suffered a fall assumes the responsibility for evaluating the cause of the fall in addition to treating the injuries sustained.

Motor Vehicle Crashes

Trauma from motor vehicle crashes is the second leading cause of accidental death in the geriatric population, resulting in more than 4000 deaths each year. Although older people drive fewer miles, they have the seond highest accident rate of any age group, behind those younger than 25 years. In addition, the number of elderly drivers involved in fatal crashes is disproportionately high. For example, the risk of death at age 70 is three times higher than at age 20 after similar motor vehicular crashes. In contrast to younger drivers, elderly drivers are more likely to be involved in two-vehicle crashes than in single-vehicle crashes, and these accidents typically occur during the day, in good weather, and close to home. Alcohol and excessive speed are less likely to be causative factors, but visual impairment, poor judgment, and underlying medical conditions can contribute to the high incidence of motor vehicle crashes involving older drivers.

Pedestrian Injuries

The National Safety Council reports that 2000 elderly pedestrians are killed each year.[264b] Elderly pedestrians are struck more frequently than any other age group, including children.[265] Diminished visual acuity (especially at night), hearing impairment, and slowed gait are factors contributing to the increased risk of pedestrian fatalities in the elderly population. Senile mental and physical changes may delay the responses necessary to avoid injury from moving vehicles. The mortality rate is increased for all levels of injury to elderly pedestrians.[265] Like children, injured elderly pedestrians frequently suffer severe, and often fatal, closed head trauma.

Burns

Burns are responsible for about 8% of accidental deaths among elderly persons. Older people tend to suffer larger and deeper burns than younger people and are more likely to die from comparable injuries. Most of these burn injuries occur in the place of residence. Scalds are the most common burns suffered by elderly persons, but fatal burns also commonly involve alcohol, smoking in bed, or being trapped in a burning building. Elderly people can have more difficulty separating themselves from a burning object or environment because of physical and neurologic impairments. Burns involving over 50% to 70% of the total body surface area are almost uniformly fatal in patients older than 65 years of age. The presence of an inhalation injury adds to the mortality rate for any level of burn. In addition, approximately half of all elderly burn survivors are less independent after discharge than before the injury, and many require placement in care facilities outside the home.

ANATOMIC AND PHYSIOLOGIC CHARACTERISTIC OF AGING

A summary of the major physiologic changes of aging is provided in Table 11-24.

Cardiovascular System

The primary effects of aging on the cardiovascular system include increased stiffness and decreased distensibility of the myocardium and arterial system. The aged heart is characterized by decreases in strength of contraction, cardiac output, stroke volume, and heart rate in response to exercise and hypertension. There is also a diminished sensitivity to catecholamine stimulation. Dysrhythmia, including premature ventricular contractions and supraventricular beats, is more common in elderly persons. In addition to the aging process, acquired heart disease resulting from ischemia and atherosclerosis impacts the ability of

the heart to respond to stress. For these reasons, cardiac dysrhythmia, heart failure, and even sudden death may follow major trauma.[266]

Respiratory System

The alterations of pulmonary function with age include decreases in vital capacity, forced expiratory volume, diffusing capacity, and arterial oxygen tension. Functional residual capacity and residual volume both increase, and arterial carbon dioxide tension remains the same. The anteroposterior diameter of the chest increases, and the intervertebral disc space size decreases, often resulting in the barrel-chest deformity and diminished diaphragmatic excursion. Disordered patterns of breathing, such as Cheyne-Stokes respiration and sleep apnea, are observed more commonly in the elderly population. Older patients are more prone than younger patients to develop pneumonia, which can seriously complicate their care in the post-trauma setting.

Renal System

Age-related changes in the kidney include reduced glomerular filtration rate and diminished excretory capacity. The serum creatinine level is a less sensitive indicator of renal function in elderly patients, who normally have less lean body mass. The calculated creatinine clearance is a better guide to the dosage of drugs that are cleared by the kidney.

Osteoporosis

Increased bone resorption is the primary mechanism of the osteoporotic changes in bone that occur with aging. Other factors that contribute to osteoporosis in the older population include decreased levels of sex hormones; deficiencies of calcium, protein, and vitamin D; and lack of exercise. Osteoporotic changes in bone can explain the tendency toward fractures with seemingly minor trauma, and they are a factor in the occurrence of multiple, severe fractures after major trauma.

Nutrition and Metabolism

Preexisting protein-calorie malnutrition is common in elderly persons. Although there is a general reduction in the metabolic rate and caloric requirement with aging, the need for protein, minerals, and vitamins does not change significantly. After severe trauma, nutritional support necessarily includes correction of underlying deficiencies as well as provision of adequate protein and calories to meet the needs of a stressed patient. Early attention to nutrition may help to avoid such complications as infection, respiratory compromise, and poor wound healing.

Immune System

Changes in the immune system that occur with age have been collectively referred to as immune senescence. The number of suppressor T lymphocytes is diminished in the elderly, whereas the number of helper T cells increases, causing impairment of T-cell–mediated immunity. There also tend to be deficiencies in humoral immunity and immunoglobulin production among elderly patients. The results of these immunologic changes are an increased susceptibility to infection and a higher incidence of multiple organ failure after trauma.

Table 11-24. ANATOMIC AND PHYSIOLOGIC CHANGES OF AGING

Organ System	Changes
Cardiovascular	Decreased cardiac output
	Diminished compliance
	Decreased response to catecholamines
	Arrhythmias
Respiratory	Decreased oxygen tension
	Decreased compliance
	Decreased vital capacity
	Increased residual capacity
Renal	Decreased glomerular filtration
	Diminished concentrating ability
Nutritional	Decreased body mass
	Protein, calorie, vitamin deficiencies
Immunologic	Decreased cellular immunity
	Decreased humoral immunity

INITIAL EVALUATION AND RESUSCITATION

Basic prehospital triage decisions do not differ significantly for older patients. Impaired physiologic variables, as measured by the trauma score at the scene of the injury, predict the need for trauma center management. Elderly patients who are stable but have obvious head or thoracoabdominal injuries should be evaluated at a trauma center. In addition, it is important to consider the mechanism of injury when making triage decisions, because an older patient is more likely to sustain a significant injury from a particular mechanism than a younger person is.

The initial resuscitation of the elderly injured patient follows the basic principles of trauma care, with certain special considerations based on the expected physiologic alterations outlined previously. The general principles of securing the airway and assessing the adequacy of breathing remain the same. Early recognition of hypoxia and prompt intervention may prevent the consequences of decreased oxygen delivery to the brain, heart, and kidney. Elderly patients with impaired neurologic function are likely to aspirate, and airway protection should be considered in these patients. Arterial blood gases are obtained initially, and oxygen saturation monitored serially with pulse oximetry. Two large-bore intravenous catheters are inserted, and blood is drawn for laboratory studies and for typing and crossmatching.

In evaluating the circulatory system, it must be remembered that elderly patients probably are accustomed to higher than normal blood pressures. Although a systolic pressure of 100 mmHg is not alarming in a 25-year-old, in a 75-year-old it can represent hypotensive shock if the normal pressure is 150 mmHg systolic. As in children, there is little room for error in these fragile patients, and fluid resuscitation therapy must be precise. Aggressive monitoring benefits elderly injured patients.[267,268] Some have suggested that geriatric trauma patients with an Injury Severity Score greater than 9, evidence of shock or hypoperfusion, or a history of intercurrent disease should be considered for monitoring with pulmonary artery and intraarterial catheters during the initial resuscitation.[265] Injured patients with a measured pulmonary capillary wedge pressure of less than 15 can continue to receive volume replacement as needed, but those with a pulmonary capillary wedge pressure greater than 15 can benefit from inotropic support. Continued monitoring of oxygen transport variables, mixed venous oxygen saturation, and lactate level is suggested. Although there are limitations to these techniques, this type of approach can result in decreases in both mortality rate and complications.

Lactated Ringer solution remains the resuscitation fluid of choice in the elderly patient. However, the initial experience with hypertonic solutions has been very favorable. Hypertonic fluids can produce elevated blood pressures and improved cardiac performance with much smaller volumes than isotonic solutions. Their benefits may be substantial in elderly patients with limited cardiac reserve.

After the initial resuscitation efforts and the primary survey, it is important to obtain a detailed account of the events surrounding the trauma. A heart attack or stroke may have preceded a fall or motor vehicle crash. A thorough medical history should also be sought, with emphasis on the medications taken. β-Blocking agents are commonly used for hypertension in this age group, and they may prevent the tachycardia normally seen with hypovolemia. Hypoglycemic drugs can precipitate coma, mimicking head injury. Chronic diuretic therapy can lead to intravascular volume and electrolyte deficiencies, contributing to the development of shock after trauma.

Routine radiographs obtained in the trauma resuscitation room should include chest, spinal, and pelvic films. Degenerative changes in the cervical spine, which include narrowing of the spinal canal and development of osteophytes, increase the likelihood of spinal cord injury after trauma. Hyperextension injuries are common in older people who fall. The sclerotic changes and the osteophytes present on the bones of these patients make plain radiographs difficult to interpret. Computed tomography (CT) scan may be required to delineate spinal fractures.

Cerebral atrophy accompanies aging. In addition, the cerebral vasculature is fragile, particularly the veins. The combination of these factors makes elderly patients more prone to develop subdural hematomas, which may initially be subtle. Therefore, CT scanning of the head should be used liberally in elderly patients.

The abdomen must be suspected of harboring occult injuries in all victims of multiple trauma. Diagnostic peritoneal lavage and abdominal CT scanning are excellent methods of detecting abdominal trauma that is not evident on physical examination and can help to avoid the consequences of delayed diagnosis. Abdominal ultrasound is another excellent method for detecting blood in the peritoneum. These examinations are noninvasive and can be performed quickly at the bedside during the resuscitation phase.

MANAGEMENT OF SPECIFIC INJURIES

Thoracic Injuries

The combination of a less elastic chest wall and osteoporosis of the bones results in a high incidence of rib fractures in elderly persons sustaining trauma. Accompanying pneumothorax and hemothorax must be suspected as well. Early management of multiple rib fractures with epidural catheters for pain control is recommended and potentially can prevent the development of pneumonia and the need for mechanical ventilatory support in these patients. Atherosclerotic changes in the aorta make elderly persons more prone to suffer thoracic aortic disruption after deceleration injuries. Diagnostic aortography should be considered based on an appropriate history even in the presence of a normal-appearing mediastinum, especially if there are other signs of severe chest trauma. Recent data suggest that even with prompt recognition and treatment of thoracic aortic tears, these injuries are associated with an extremely poor prognosis in geriatric patients.[268a] Myocardial contusion should be suspected if arrythmia develops during electrocardiographic monitoring. If injury to the heart is suspected after blunt trauma, echocardiography demonstrates abnormal wall motion and the presence of pericardial fluid.

In a comparison of old and young trauma patients, a higher percentage of older patients presented without vital signs after severe blunt trauma to the chest.[268b] The elderly group had an overall higher mortality rate, especially if they had sustained additional extrathoracic injuries. In one series,[268c] 48 patients older than 60 years of age suffered blunt chest trauma, and 85% were able to manage without mechanical ventilation. Of these patients, 89% survived, and 81% returned to independent living. It appears that with proper initial management of chest trauma, avoidance of complications, and attention to pain control, pulmonary toilet, and nutritional support, a favorable outcome after thoracic injuries in elderly patients can be expected.

Abdominal Trauma

Occult intraabdominal injuries must be sought diligently in elderly trauma patients. Although these patients fare relatively well during abdominal operative therapy, they have little tolerance for the shock or sepsis that may follow unidentified injuries. As in younger patients, the liver and spleen are most likely to be injured after blunt trauma. One report suggests a relatively higher incidence of biliary tract injuries in people older than 60 years. If hematuria is present, the kidneys and bladder must be investigated by abdominal CT with intravenous contrast and cystography.

If operative therapy is required for either blunt or penetrating trauma, certain principles should guide management. The fluid requirements during major surgery must be carefully guided by the monitoring of central pressures. Intraarterial pressure monitoring is also required. Elderly persons have a tendency to develop hypothermia. It should be remembered that the cold patient quickly develops lactic acidosis and coagulopathy, which may not readily be reversible. Prevention of hypothermia with specially designed warming blankets and fluid infusers should be the goal.

Head Trauma

The general principles of management of closed head trauma, including early detection and treatment of intracranial hemorrhage and avoidance of secondary brain injury from hypoxia and hypovolemia, apply in geriatric patients as well as in younger patients. Subdural hematomas are three times more common in older people, and they may manifest as a subtle, gradual neurologic decline. Twenty percent of very old patients who present after trauma with an initial Glasgow Coma Scale (GCS) score of 13 or higher have intracranial hematomas, and 12% of these elderly patients with an initial GCS of 13 or higher die.[269] Most of these head injuries result from falls in the home. Studies of elderly patients with head injuries have documented prolonged length of hospital stay among those who survive. Even relatively minor head trauma can result in a loss of independent living for elderly patients.

Pennings and coworkers recently studied a group of 90 consecutive patients aged 60 years or older who had sustained severe blunt brain injury.[270] This group was compared with 79 randomly selected patients aged 20 to 40 years who also with severe head trauma. Although there were no significant differences between older and younger patients with respect to admission GCS score, Revised Trauma Score, Injury Severity Score, Abbreviated Injury Scale score, resuscitation, neurosurgical interventions, or nutritional support, 79% of the former died, compared with 36% of the latter. Of the 9 elderly patients who survived to leave the hospital, 6 were in a persistently vegetative state, and 2 were severely disabled at the time of transfer to nursing homes. Total charges per favorable outcome for the young patients were $154,155, compared with $1,550,971 for the older group. Clearly, present efforts should be directed toward the prevention of these devastating injuries in geriatric patients.

Intensive Care Considerations

The need for early invasive monitoring in elderly patients after multiple blunt trauma has been described (see Resuscitation). The mortality rate correlates with the development of sepsis and cardiac complications.[264,267] It is possible that aggressive intensive care monitoring can lead to improved outcome by decreasing complications in seriously injured elderly patients.

In addition to close monitoring for cardiopulmonary dysfunction, other important considerations in the intensive care unit (ICU) setting include early mobilization to improve pulmonary and musculoskeletal functions and provision of early and adequate nutritional support. Monitoring for changes in sputum cultures in intubated patients allows for early detection and treatment of hospital-acquired pneumonia. Acute renal failure may follow a period of shock in the elderly trauma patient. Other factors that contribute to renal injury are the administration of nephrotoxic drugs (eg, aminoglycosides, diuretics) and the presence of free hemoglobin or myoglobin in the plasma. Early recognition of renal failure in the nonoliguric stage, with elimination of all offending agents, offers the best outcome.

Sepsis and multiple-organ failure cause most late deaths after trauma in elderly patients. The urinary tract is a common source of septicemia in older patients. Pulmonary and intraabdominal sources are also possible. Acalculous cholecystitis can follow any type of trauma and should be suspected in a septic patient with abdominal pain, particularly if the bilirubin level is elevated. Infections from indwelling intravenous or intraarterial catheters can also occur in the ICU and, if suspected, require removal and culturing of the catheter.

Geriatric trauma patients are also at increased risk for development of thromboembolic complications after. Older patients at very high risk for development of deep venous thrombosis (DVT) and subsequent pulmonary embolism include those with hip and pelvic fractures requiring prolonged immobilization, those with neurologic trauma, and those with a prior history of DVT or pulmonary embolism. Institution of prophylactic methods, such as mechanical sequential leg compression devices or low-dose anticoagulants, should be considered in all elderly trauma patients after all bleeding injuries have been controlled. Most episodes of DVT are clinically silent, and monitoring of these high-risk patients with serial duplex venous ultrasound examinations allows prompt diagnosis and treatment of this life-threatening complication. Similarly, patients with unexplained hypoxia should be considered for ventilation–perfusion scans or for pulmonary angiography to detect pulmonary emboli.

Moral and ethical considerations have assumed an increasingly important role in the care of elderly patients in the ICU. Although aggressive care is indicated in most situations, decisions regarding operative and intensive care therapy necessarily involve the participation of the patient (if possible) and the family. Increasing numbers of elderly patients have expressed their wishes in terms of a living will. In the competent patient, autonomy must be protected. In other cases, the family may have a clear idea of the patient's attitude toward the quality of life and the use of life-support measures after a catastrophic injury.

PREDICTING OUTCOME AFTER GERIATRIC TRAUMA

Although aggressive care can benefit the elderly trauma patient, surgical and ICU care are both costly and in limited supply. Clearly, these resources should be reserved for the patients most likely to benefit from them. Many studies have sought to determine the predictors of outcome after trauma in the older population. Table 11-25 lists the factors that are correlated with poor outcome. In one large, multicenter study of 852 geriatric patients (aged 65 or older) with blunt trauma, the Injury Severity Score was found to be the variable that correlated most significantly with mortality.[271] Mortality rates were higher for men than for women at all ages and at all levels of injury severity. In addition, the geriatric population was found to be inhomogeneous. That is, mortality rates were significantly higher for patients aged 75 years and older, compared with those between 65 and 75 years of age. Admission variables that were associated with the highest relative risks of death were a Trauma Score lower than 7; hypotension (systolic blood pressure lower than 90 mmHg); hypoventilation (respiratory rate of less than 10 breaths per minute); or a GCS score equal to 3. These variables may be used not only to predict a poor outcome but also to help make decisions about the triage of elderly patients to trauma centers or the allocation of ICU beds. Mortality rate is only one outcome variable, however. The factors that influence the functional outcome of elderly patients who survive must also be identified.

INJURY PREVENTION

Prevention efforts in the elderly population should begin with a thorough assessment of the home environment. The greatest impact is afforded by measures to prevent falls. In addition to ensuring that the home is free of mechanical hazards, attention must be directed toward the medications that these patients are taking. Frequently, the geriatric patient is prescribed a wide variety of medications, some of which may interact to produce gait instability or orthostatic hypotension.

Pedestrian safety should be another major area of attention for injury prevention activists. Identification of particularly dangerous intersections by mapping of the frequency of pedestrian events allows for modification of crosswalks to provide improved visibility, longer crossing times, and other improvements.

Persons with visual or hearing deficits, dementia, or musculoskeletal disorders, and those taking certain kinds of medications, may be particularly dangerous drivers.[265] Both the American Association of Retired Persons and the National Retired Teachers Association encourage older adults to update their driving skills through educational courses. Allowing elderly people to renew their drivers licenses only after they pass driving, hearing, and visual tests helps to keep unfit drivers off the road. The cost of such injury prevention programs is minimal compared with the cost of caring for an elderly trauma patient in the ICU for weeks. At this time, both the prevention and acute care aspects of geriatric trauma are still in their infancy, awaiting advances by those challenged by this special population.

Definitive Care Phase: Trauma in Pregnancy

HEIDI L. FRANKEL, GRACE S. ROZYCKI, AND HOWARD R. CHAMPION

The maternal mortality rate in the United States has declined markedly during the past 50 years as a result of improved antenatal and obstetric care and a major reduction in the rate of septic abortions.[272] In contrast, the number of deaths caused by injury during pregnancy is on the rise, and trauma has emerged as the single greatest threat to both the gravid and nongravid woman. Trauma complicates 6% to 7% of all pregnancies and is the most frequent nonobstetric cause of death in the gravid patient. An active life-style during pregnancy, with gravid females driving

Table 11-25. FACTORS CORRELATED WITH POOR OUTCOME AFTER GERIATRIC TRAUMA

Increased age
Male gender
Hypotension
Hypoventilation
Low Glasgow Coma Scale score
Increased Injury Severity score
Decreased Trauma or Revised Trauma score
Presence of preexisting conditions
Development of cardiovascular complications
Development of septic complications

motor vehicles up to term, places these women at increased risk for blunt injury. In addition, penetrating trauma is now responsible for up to 20% of injuries requiring hospital admission of pregnant patients.[272]

Fetal death occurs in less than 1% of cases of trivial trauma, in 27% of minor trauma, and in 61% of major trauma, but in up to 80% if there is maternal shock.[273] The three to four times greater incidence of fetal death than maternal death implies that maternal survival alone is insufficient to ensure fetal well being. Although most trauma (52%) occurs in the third trimester, fetal demise is also related to birth weight and age of gestation. Fifty percent of fetuses die after trauma at 26 weeks gestational age, as do 90% of fetuses weight less than 750 g, compared with 40% of those weighing 750 to 1000 g.[274]

All trauma surgeons, emergency physicians, and obstetricians must understand the anatomic and physiologic characteristics unique to pregnancy as well as the principles of resuscitation and treatment after trauma in order to guarantee the best possible outcome for both the injured mother and her fetus.

ANATOMY AND PHYSIOLOGY UNIQUE TO THE GRAVID PATIENT

Anatomic and physiologic changes of pregnancy can alter injury response, necessitating a modified approach to resuscitation and therapy (Table 11-26). Knowledge of these changes must guide the evaluation and resuscitation of the pregnant trauma patient.[275]

Hemodynamic Changes

As pregnancy progresses, cardiac output increases up to 150% above normal until the 24th week and then plateaus. This increase in cardiac output is produced by a modest rise in heart rate and a greater elevation of stroke volume, changes that occur as a result of an expanded blood volume and the direct inotropic effect of estrogen.[276] This hypervolemic state is protective for the mother because fewer red blood cells are lost during hemorrhage (and delivery) and oxygen-carrying capacity therefore is minimally affected.[277] The increase in plasma volume, which is proportionally greater than the enlarged erythrocyte volume, results in the anemia of pregnancy. At term, the plasma volume continues to expand, but the red cell mass begins to increase, resulting in a near-normal hematocrit. This physiologic hypervolemia masks volume loss and may give the clinician an unfounded sense of security about thepatient's hemody-

Table 11-26. PHYSIOLOGIC ALTERATIONS IN PREGNANCY

System	Change	Implication
Cardiovascular	Cardiac output increased by 150%	Delayed signs of shock
	Plasma volume increased by 50%	
	Peripheral vascular resistance decreased	
	Vena cava compression	Supine hypotension syndrome
Respiratory	Residual lung volume decreased	Decreased buffering capacity
	Decreased Po_2	
	Chronic respiratory alkalosis	
Gastrointestinal	Decreased GI motility	Increased propensity toward aspiration
	Decreased GE sphincter competency	
	Intraabdominal organ displacement	Clinical examination unreliable
Genitourinary	Enlarged ovarian venous plexuses	Physiologic hydronephrosis and urinary stasis
	Dilitation of renal system	
Laboratory values	Increased WBC count	Difficulty interpreting clinical picture regarding hemorrhage
	Decreased hematocrit	
	Increased fibrinogen and factors VII, VIII, X, XII	Hypercoaguable state

namic stability. Almost 35% of maternal blood volume may be lost before signs of shock manifest.[278]

If the pregnant patient is in the supine position, the inferior vena cava is partially obstructed by the gravid uterus, which decreases venous blood return to the heart, lowers cardiac output, and causes supine hypotension. The enlarged uterus also compresses the abdominal aorta, reducing blood flow to the fetus through diminished uterine arterial flow. Turning the pregnant patient onto her left side restores circulation and increases cardiac output by 30%.[279]

Overall, cardiac work is increased because of the volume load and estrogen effect, despite the decrease in systemic vascular resistance mediated by prostaglandin, progestin, intracellular calcium, and endothelial-derived factors.[280] Early in pregnancy, the blood pressure, especially the diastolic component, decreases, but then it slowly returns to normal by term. Mean normal values for the first trimester are 105 systolic and 60 diastolic; for the second trimester, 102 and 55, and for the third trimester, 108 and 67. Significant elevations from these levels may indicate pregnancy-induced hypertension.[281]

Finally, as the diaphragm becomes progressively more elevated because of the enlarging uterus, the heart is displaced to the left and upward, resulting in a lateral shift of the cardiac apex (and a corresponding left axis deviation on electrocardiogram, with Q waves in lead III and aVF). Further, each pregnant woman has some degree of benign pericardial effusion. These changes result in an enlarged cardiac silhouette and increased pulmonary vascular markings on the chest radiograph.[282]

Pulmonary Changes

As the uterus enlarges, diaphragmatic displacement results in decreased residual lung volume, ventilatory reserve, and resting arterial oxygen tension. A chronic respiratory alkalosis results, more from increased tidal volume than from physiologic hyperventilation, results.[283] Progesterone stimulates the respiratory center to increase the depth of each breath without an increase in respiratory rate, but the flow rates remain unchanged. A progressive rise in cyclic adenosine monophosphate and higher levels of both free and bound cortisol may account for this flow rate maintenance in pregnancy. Pulmonary artery pressures remain normal, but pulmonary vascular resistance decreases to accommodate the incremental changes in blood volume and cardiac output.[276,283]

Gastrointestinal Changes

As pregnancy progresses, the enlarged uterus stretches the abdominal wall and compresses the viscera. This results in a diminished response to peritoneal irritation and altered or referred pain perception, making the clinical examination unreliable. An increased propensity toward aspiration occurs because of compression of the intraabdominal organs, which decreases gastrointestinal motility, and because of the relaxant effect of progesterone and estrogen on smooth muscle, which diminishes esophageal sphincter competency. Finally, gastrin is produced by the placenta and lowers gastric pH during pregnancy.

Renal System

Throughout pregnancy, the renal system enlarges to meet the demands of increased blood volume. The renal pelvis and ureter dilate early in the first trimester, resulting in a mild hydronephrosis. Urinary stasis in the collecting system predisposes pregnant women to pyelonephritis. In the first trimester, the renal blood flow and the glomerular filtration rate increase by 150%; consequently, the levels of creatinine and blood urea nitrogen decrease. This effect precedes significant increases in cardiac output or blood volume. The clinical significance is that normal or slightly elevated levels of creatinine or blood urea nitrogen may signify renal dysfunction. Because of hormonal and osmoreceptor alterations, the normal serum sodium concentration for a pregnant woman is about 132 mEq/L. Increased clearance of uric acid occurs in the first and second trimester, but reabsorption becomes normal later. An elevated serum uric acid level in the first or second trimester may portend toxemia even in the normotensive gravid female.

Musculoskeletal System

The relaxation of the interosseous ligaments during pregnancy causes increased mobility of the sacroiliac and sacrococcygeal joints and widening of the symphysis pubis. These changes, coupled with an enlarged uterus, disrupt the maternal center of gravity and increase the risk for falls.

Laboratory Values

The peripheral blood leukocyte count increases to about 12,000 cells/mL and may be as high as 25,000 cells/mL during labor. The platelet count may appear falsely low because of a dilutional effect. Fibrinogen, prothrombin, factors VII, VIII, X, and XII, and fibrin split products are increased, causing a hypercoagulable state with the attendant risks.

INITIAL ASSESSMENT AND MANAGEMENT

Priorities for resuscitation of the injured pregnant patient are the same as for any other trauma patient. Patient care, however, is altered to accommodate the unique anatomic and physiologic characteristics of the gravid woman.[284]

The best therapy for the unborn child is expedient maternal resuscitation. An adequate airway with supplemental oxygenation is essential to prevent fetal hypoxemia. The release of maternal catecholamines causes uteroplacental vasoconstriction, compromising fetal circulation. Because fetal blood functions on a different oxyhemoglobin dissociation curve, small positive increments in oxygen concentration improve oxygen content and physiologic reserve for the fetus, even if maternal arterial oxygen content does not change appreciably. Maternal hemorrhagic shock, with its resultant release of catecholamines, causes uterine artery vasoconstriction, reducing uterine perfusion and compromising fetal viability. Hence, vigorous crystalloid resuscitation is encouraged, even for patients who appear normotensive. In late pregnancy, compromised cardiac output and blood pressure secondary to vena cava compression occur when the patient is in a supine position. Placement of the patient in the left lateral decubitus or right hip-flexed position relieves this vascular compromise. The insertion of a nasogastric tube is prudent considering the pregnant patient's increased propensity toward vomiting and aspiration. Urinary volume per hour should be monitored to provide some indication of perfusion status. The pneumatic antishock garment can be used to stabilize fractures or control hemorrhage. However, the abdominal component should not be inflated, to avoid further diminution of venous return and direct fetal trauma.

History and Physical Examination

The secondary survey consists of a thorough history (including obstetric history), physical examination, and fetal monitoring.[285] Maternal prenatal history is crucial and may alter management decisions if medical problems such as preeclampsia, diabetes, essential hypertension, or congenital heart disease are present. Obstetric history includes the date of the last menstrual period, the expected date of confinement, the perception of fetal movement, and the status of this and previous pregnancies. Gestational age (ie, fetal maturity) can be estimated from the fundal height, as measured by palpation. (Fundal height at the umbilicus represents about 20 weeks' gestation.) These factors contribute to the decision regarding feasibility of delivery, if it is necessary. For example, a 26-week-old fetus is considered viable if given neonatal intensive care support.[285] Pelvic and rectal examinations are performed, with special attention to vaginal discharge (amniotic fluid or blood), effacement, dilatation, and fetal station.[286] Fetomaternal hemorrhage occurs in 6% of all pregnancies, but in 20% after trauma.

Although 0.01 mL of fetal blood (1 to 3 fetal cells per 500,000 maternal red blood cells) will sensitize 70% of Rh-negative patients, the remainder require up to 40 mL, or one third of fetal blood volume. The Kleihauer-Betke test detects fetal cells in the maternal circulation, indicating fetomaternal hemorrhage. Because this test can deter-

mine the risk of isosensitization in Rh-negative gravid females, it is recommended for injured Rh-negative pregnant patients in the second or third trimester to detect impending fetal exsanguination. If positive, the Kleihauer-Betke test should be repeated 24 hours later to identify ongoing fetomaternal hemorrhage. Treatment consists of an initial dose of Rh immune globulin of 300 μg with an additional 300 μg administered for every 30 mL of fetomaternal transfusion estimated by this test.

Fetal Assessment and Monitoring

Fetal evaluation consists of uterine assessment, fundal height measurement, and recording of heart tones, heart rate, and movement. A heart rate of 100 beats/min or less is considered bradycardia. Uterine tenderness and contraction may be related to abruptio placentae, which can occur in the absence of vaginal bleeding. Auscultation for a complete minute determines regularity (acceleration and deceleration) of the fetal heartbeat. However, continuous fetal monitoring is the best predictor of a healthy or distressed fetus.[287] There is still no consensus on the indications for fetal monitoring in trauma patients. A guideline for patients with major injuries, including shock, is to provide continuous fetal monitoring for 48 hours after stabilization. For those patients with minor injuries or insignificant trauma, monitoring for 24 hours is indicated.

Fetal heart rate and uterine activity can be monitored by either external (indirect) or internal (direct) methods. The external method is noninvasive and has wider clinical application. Internal monitoring requires insertion of an intrauterine catheter and application of a fetal scalp electrode. The normal fetal heart rate ranges between 120 and 160 beats/min. Abnormalities in variability may signal hypoxia or dysrhythmia in the fetus. Early decelerations of fetal heart rate, which conform closely to uterine contractions, are vagally mediated and not of significance. Similarly, variable decelerations, secondary to transient umbilical cord compression, are harmless. The presence of late decelerations of fetal heart rate after uterine contractions is thought to be related to uteroplacental insufficiency, an oxytocin effect, and may warrant routine tocographic monitoring after injury.

Ultrasonography is a valuable adjunct in determining fetal viability. It detects the changes of pregnancy 3 to 4 weeks after ovulation and is therefore useful in the gestational period, especially because it involves no radiation exposure. During the first trimester, an endovaginal ultrasound probe provides close approximation of the transducer to the uterus through cervical tissue. This method does not require bladder catheterization and filling and thus allows for a rapid examination. The real-time unit demonstrates fetal cardiac movement and the B-mode determines fetal size and placental location. Abruptio placentae is identified as a retroplacental lucency (blood clot) or an echogenic structure within amniotic fluid.

Diagnostic Modalities

After patient stabilization, diagnostic modalities are used to define the extent and type of injury for the mother and unborn child. Initially, laboratory studies are obtained. If blood is urgently needed, type O, Rh-negative blood is chosen. Evaluation of the abdomen may be performed by diagnostic peritoneal lavage, computed tomography (CT) scan, or ultrasound.[288] There is an increasing role for ultrasound in the diagnosis of hemoperitoneum secondary to blunt abdominal trauma. Studies are being conducted that compare the accuracy of ultrasound with the standard diagnostic modalities for abdominal evalua-

Table 11-27. REPRESENTATIVE ENTRANCE EXPOSURES AND FETAL DOSES FOR FREQUENTLY PERFORMED RADIOGRAPHIC EXAMINATIONS WITH A 200 SPEED IMAGE RECEPTOR

Examination	Entrance Exposure (mrad)	Fetal Dose (mrad)
Skull (lateral)	70	0
Cervical spine (AP)	110	0
Shoulder	90	0
Chest (PA)	10	0
Thoracic spine (AP)	180	1
Lumbosacral spine (AP)*	250	80
Intravenous pyelogram*	210	60
Hip*	220	50
Wrist or foot	5	0

AP, anteroposterior; PA, posteroanterior.
* Gonadal shields should be used if possible.
(Bushong SC. Radiologic science for technologists: physics, biology, and protection. St Louis, CV Mosby, 1988:550)

tion, peritoneal lavage, and CT scan. Diagnostic peritoneal lavage may be performed in the pregnant patient, but the open (supraumbilical) technique is recommended. Reliance on ultrasound to evaluate both the mother and the fetus, a technique with a 70% to 100% sensitivity and specificity in the diagnosis of blunt abdominal trauma, can obviate the need to perform a CT scan or lavage and can provide valuable information on fetal motion, tone, location, and placement.

Liberal but judicious use of radiographic studies is advised for evaluation of the pregnant trauma patient. A diagnostic modality deemed necessary should not be withheld for fear of potential hazard to the fetus. Factors contributing to the sequelae of prenatal exposure to ionizing radiation are the stage of development, the exposure time, the dose delivered, and the dose absorbed. The absorbed radiation dose varies according to many factors, including instrument model, desired image quality, and distance from the radioactive source. The developmental stages are the preimplantation phase (0 to 8 days after conception), major organogenesis (9 to 60 days), and the fetal period (61 to 270 days).

No estimates have been made of radiation risk during the first few days of human development. The roentgen (R) is the unit of exposure, and the centigray (cGy) or rad is the unit of absorbed dose. Exposure and absorbed fetal doses for radiographic tests are presented in Table 11-27. Because the natural prevalence of congenital anomalies is about 6%, any effects of such tests are undetectable at low radiologic doses. There is no medical justification for terminating pregnancy in women exposed to 5 cGy or less.[289] A 0.1% increase in the rate spontaneous abortion during the first 2 weeks of development follows a dose of 10 cGy, and there is a 1% increase in congenital abnormalities at the same dose.[290] Combined studies, such as CT scan of the abdomen with oral and intravenous contrast, obviate the need for multiple studies such as an intravenous pyelogram. Prudent judgment and foresight by the physician should ensure that specific radiographic studies are ordered and accurately performed to avoid repetition.

MANAGEMENT
Blunt Trauma

Motor vehicle accidents remain the chief cause of maternal blunt trauma. As pregnancy progresses, the uterus becomes more vulnerable, rising out of the protective bony pelvis, and absorbs most of the impact of blunt abdominal trauma. Pelvic fractures in the gravid patient cause extensive retroperitoneal hemorrhage as a result of engorged pelvic veins. These factors often result in direct fetal injury, usually skull fracture or intracerebral hemorrhage. Pregnancy is thought by some to increase the risk of splenic rupture after blunt trauma, although others do not support this claim.[291,292] Tension pneumothorax may be more dramatic in pregnancy because of decreased lung volumes.

Uterine rupture from blunt trauma occurs most often at the site of prior Caesarean section or at the posterior fundus. It can present with massive hemorrhage or more insidiously with minimal vaginal bleeding if rupture occurs at the fundus, far from the uterine vessels. Repair can be either primary in two layers or with a polytetrafluoroethylene (Gore-Tex) patch. There are cases of maternal survival reported when laparotomy was delayed up to 24 days.[275] Avulsion of the uterus has been reported, with associated bladder rupture being a common finding.

Abruptio placentae is the second most common cause of fetal death; it carries a 30% to 70% rate of fetal death and 1% maternal mortality rate. Over 50% separation invariably results in fetal demise.[293] Abruptio placentae can occur in the absence of obvious abdominal injury, because maternal shock is a far greater stimulus for abruption than are the mechanical forces of trauma disrupting the placenta.[286] Abruptio placentae is more common in the presence of hypertension, diabetes mellitus, advanced age, multiparity, and maternal use of tobacco or cocaine. Abruptio placentae presents with vaginal bleeding (in 80% of cases), abdominal pain, disseminated intravascular coagulation due to thromboplastin release, and inexplicable maternal hypovolemia. It invariably occurs within 48 hours after trauma, and pregnant patients who are at risk should be monitored accordingly.

Burns

Fewer than 0.1% of pregnant patients suffer severe burns. The successful approach to the management of the burn victim relies on maintaining a normal intravascular volume and avoiding hypoxia. In these patients, inadequate initial resuscitation is responsible for loss of the pregnancy. Burn patients are at a high risk for β-agonist tocolytic complications because of their high-output state, extensive fluid requirements, and capillary permeability problems. Magnesium sulfate has a vasodilator effect and therefore may not be the treatment of choice for these patients. Table 11-28 delineates the estimates of body surface area burned and associated mortality rates.

Operative Management

General anesthesia is preferred for the gravid patient with multisystem injury. The risks of anesthesia are related to the physiologic changes that accompany pregnancy. For

Table 11-28. CRUDE MORTALITY RATES AFTER MATERNAL BURN INJURIES

Body Surface Injured (%)	Maternal Mortality Rate (%)	Fetal Mortality Rate (%)
<40	3	22
50	25	53
>80	100	100

(Creasy RK, Resnick R. Maternal–fetal medicine: principles and practice, ed 2. Philadelphia, WB Saunders, 1989:871)

example, because aspiration is more likely, rapid-sequence induction is the method of choice. The effects of anesthetics are related to the stage of fetal development and the dose given. Because premature labor has been shown to be associated with surgery and with various anesthetic regimens, intraoperative fetal monitoring is imperative. If anesthesia is administered, adequate volume status, maintenance of normotension, and supplemental oxygenation must be considered. One study reported increased fetal demise after laparotomy, more so if the operation was performed in the first trimester or in the presence of peritonitis.[294] However, other authors downplay the effects of general anesthesia and surgery on fetal outcome.[295] In a multicenter study of pregnant, injured patients, fetal death occurred in 35% of cases in which the women underwent general anesthesia and surgery, compared with 11% of cases in which general anesthesia was not used. However, the mean ISS in the surgery group was 18.0, compared with 5.5 in the nonsurgery group.

If laparotomy is necessary, a standard vertical midline incision is employed. Adequate visualization is mandatory, and the pregnant uterus should not interfere with abdominal exploration or repair of an injury. Vaginal delivery is almost always encouraged. Even early in the postoperative period, vaginal delivery is still preferred and is not harmful to the mother or the neonate. Cesarean section prolongs the operative time and increases blood loss by about 1 L. During celiotomy for trauma, indications for cesarean section are as follows:

- Maternal shock, pregnancy near term
- Threat to life from exsanguination (injury or disseminated intravascular coagulation)
- Mechanical limitation for maternal repair
- Risk of fetal distress exceeding risk of prematurity
- Unstable thoracolumbar spinal injury

Successful outcome of a postmortem cesarean section depends on the duration of the gestation and the time interval between maternal death and delivery. Under optimal conditions, at 26 to 28 weeks' gestation, estimated fetal survival is about 50%. Therefore, postmortem cesarean section is justified if the estimated gestational age is about 26 to 28 weeks. Time since maternal death must be considered, however. If the time interval between maternal death and delivery is less than 5 minutes, the fetal prognosis is considered excellent. If the time interval since maternal death is prolonged to about 20 minutes, fetal prognosis is poor. Uncertainty of maternal death time is not a contraindication for this procedure.[273]

Medications

When administrating medications to the gravid patient, potential risk versus therapeutic benefit must be considered. Prophylactic tetanus immunization should be given appropriately, with anti-D globulin for patients who are Rh-negative and at risk for isoimmunization. Prophylactic antibiotics are administered as indicated; tetracycline and most sulpha drugs are avoided.

Critical Care Management

Critical care management of the traumatized pregnant patient covers a wide range of topics. The basic principles of hemodynamic monitoring, adequate ventilatory support, nutrition, and careful assessment of volume status apply here but are covered in detail in other chapters. A knowledge of the disease processes that can arise in the pregnant patient within the first 24 hours after injury completes the clinical scope and allows the physician to render quality critical care to the traumatized patient and unborn child.

Toxemia of Pregnancy or Preeclampsia (Pregnancy-Induced Hypertension)

Any traumatized pregnant patient presenting with seizures or in a coma should be presumed to have eclampsia, which complicates up to 0.29% of all deliveries. In the severe state, this process is manifested by hypertension, pulmonary edema, proteinuria, and seizure activity. The pathophysiology is vasospasm, which affects hepatic, renal, cerebral, and placental blood flow. Despite the presence of pulmonary edema, intravascular volume depletion is often present, and a fluid challenge may be appropriate. Rapid control of the hypertension is achieved with sodium nitroprusside, but thiocyanate levels should be monitored carefully in patients who require prolonged administration of the drug. Elevated maternal oxygen consumption compromises the uterine vascular bed, resulting in fetal distress. A smoother reduction in blood pressure and in myocardial oxygen consumption is accomplished by achieving volume expansion before vasodilation. Inotropic support, in combination with a vasodilator agent, maximizes oxygen delivery and affects afterload reduction. Magnesium sulfate causes a slight hypotensive effect but does not decrease afterload. Considering the compromised renal function, addition of low-dose dopamine improves renal blood flow. These hemodynamic parameters are guidelines for optimizing maternal hemodynamics, uteroplacental perfusion, and, ultimately, fetal well-being.

Thromboembolism

Pregnant patients are at increased risk of thromboembolism from all three components of the Virchow triad: stasis, intimal damage, and hypercoagulability. Increased venous capacitance, caval compression, and weight gain promote stasis. Labor and trauma cause intimal damage, and hypercoagulability results from elevated levels of fibrinogen and intrinsic coagulation factors. Advanced age and multiparity further increase the risk. No method of prophylaxis has been demonstrated to be both safe and universally effective in preventing thromboembolism, either in the patient with multiple injuries or in the pregnant patient.

Amniotic Fluid Embolism

Amniotic fluid embolism is characterized by hypotension, hypoxemia, and coagulopathy. The diagnosis is often difficult, and an 80% mortality rate has been reported. Amniotic fluid debris enters the maternal venous circulation, causing sudden dyspnea and hypotension. A mixed metabolic acidosis and respiratory alkalosis ensue. The chest radiograph shows the characteristic pulmonary edema or acute respiratory disease pattern. Hemodynamically, the patient has left ventricular failure—decreased left ventricular stroke work index, elevated pulmonary capillary wedge pressure, and a low systemic vascular resistance. About 30% of these patients experience disseminated intravascular coagulation. Although most cases of amniotic fluid embolism occur during labor, it has been reported to occur after abdominal trauma and abruptio placentae. This diagnosis is clinical, and the treatment is based on supportive care (ie, oxygenation, maximization of hemodynamic parameters, and correction of coagulopathy).

Hemorrhage

Although the basic principles of volume resuscitation apply to the gravid patient, definitive therapy, such as removal of retained products of conception, must be accomplished before hemorrhage control is achieved. Simultaneously, the coagulation disorder is corrected with the use of cryoprecipitate, fresh frozen plasma, platelets, blood, and other blood products. Proper treatment of shock is also necessary to prevent the long-term sequelae of pituitary necrosis (Sheehan syndrome) that results from the increased demand for blood flow.

Minor Trauma

The pregnant patient with minor injury should be observed for several hours. Patients with insignificant trauma do not require admission unless specific signs and symptoms are present, such as vaginal bleeding, abdominal cramps, or leakage of amniotic fluid. In one series,[295] only 1 of 11 patients developed symptoms after minor trauma, and pregnancy outcome was successful. Occult abruptio placentae has been reported after motor vehicle accidents in which the patient displayed only subtle signs and symptoms. Because placental separation can occur with rapid deceleration, a three-point restraint system appropriately applied is recommended. The mechanism of injury may provide invaluable information regarding potential injuries in even a healthy-appearing patient. At a minimum, a prompt and thorough assessment, fetal monitoring for 24 hours, and a thorough search for injuries are necessary for evaluating the pregnant patient with minor trauma.

SUMMARY

The pregnant trauma victim presents a unique challenge to the resuscitating physician. Two patients are being treated, and a high degree of expertise is needed to treat both. Initially, evaluation should involve the cooperative efforts of the emergency physician, trauma surgeon, obstetrician, and obstetric nurse. If the pregnancy is near term or delivery is anticipated, the pediatrician should also be consulted. The pregnancy should not distract the surgeon from initiating basic resuscitation. Equally important, the injury should not confound the obstetrician. The expertise of the obstetric nurse is useful in coordinating the overall care plan of the mother and her unborn child. Expedient, accurate resuscitation of the mother takes priority, because the best chance for fetal survival is maternal survival.

Definitive Care Phase: Critical Care and Postinjury Management

RICHARD K. SIMONS AND DAVID B. HOYT

Improvements in transport systems and resuscitation techniques and a more unified approach to operative management of many injuries have reduced early trauma mortality and shifted the burden of support to the postinjury and postoperative arena. Trauma patients represent a unique group among the population of intensive care unit (ICU) patients by virtue of their age (approximate mean, 33 years) and their general lack of chronic underlying disease. For these reasons, the prospects for functional recovery are good but depend on sophisticated and skillful critical care and postinjury management. This care, which frequently is complex and involves multiple systems, demands a level of expertise best provided by established trauma centers led by practiced trauma surgeons. Uncoordinated care rendered independently by multiple surgical subspecialists or nonsurgical ICU personnel is likely to be fragmented and may serve the patient poorly. This section reviews those critical care issues that are pertinent or unique to the patient with major trauma.

LOCAL EFFECTS OF TISSUE INJURY

Traumatic injury involves the transfer of kinetic energy to tissue, resulting in the primary possibilities of tissue damage and disruption, with loss of function, local hemorrhage, contamination, and embolization of air, tissue, or particulate matter. These effects occur immediately but can be exacerbated by inappropriate or poorly timed postinjury management. Secondary effects of tissue injury, which can occur from minutes to days later, include further hemorrhage, edema, immunosuppression, inflammation, infection, and ischemia. These secondary effects are major determinants of whether severe systemic complications develop and are an important focus of early postinjury critical care.

FACTORS RELATED TO POSTINJURY COMPLICATIONS
Shock, Ischemia, and Reperfusion Injury

Tissue ischemia after trauma can be either local or global. The related derangements in cellular metabolism and changes in ion transport across cell membranes have been a major focus of shock research for many years. Data suggest that an important component of posttraumatic tissue injury occurs after resuscitation and reperfusion with reoxygenation. Oxygen free radicals (eg, hydroxyl radical, superoxide anion), generated from tissue-derived xanthine oxidase and phagocyte-derived NADPH (nicotinamide-adenine dinucleotide phosphate, reduced form) oxidase systems, are thought to be important mediators. Reperfusion injury may be responsible for such diverse events as compartment syndromes and ongoing fluid sequestration after resuscitation. A more detailed discussion of these processes can be found in Chapter 73.

Therapeutic strategies aimed at ameliorating reperfusion injury remain experimental at this time. They include the use of xanthine oxidase inhibitors, inhibitors of neutrophil adherence, exogenous antioxidants, and other modalities such as cytokine blockade (see Chap. 5). Several of these approaches have shown promise in animal studies, but they have yet to enter the clinical arena.

Alterations in the Immune and Inflammatory Response

Major perturbations in the immune system occur in trauma patients and contribute to late septic mortality. The changes in the immune system are significant and global, affecting both humoral and cellular components of the system[296] (Table 11-29). Macrophage receptor expression and subsequent antigen presentation are impaired, and there is a shift toward an immunosuppressive phenotype. Similar defects appear in lymphocyte function, including shifts in T-cell populations with decreased CD3 and CD4 subpopulations, depression of B-cell and immunoglobulin produc-

Table 11-29. ALTERATIONS IN IMMUNOLOGIC RESPONSE AFTER MAJOR TRAUMA

	Inflammatory or Immune Component	Postinjury Change
Humoral factors	Fibronectin	Decreased
	Complement	Increased
	Immunoglobulin	Decreased (burns)
Cellular factors	Neutrophils	Decreased chemotaxis
		Decreased bactericidal activity (burns)
		Increased adherence
		Increased nonspecific proteolytic activity
	Macrophages	Decreased antigen processing
		Impaired T-cell interaction
		Increased in inhibitory macrophages
	Lymphocytes	Change in helper/suppressor ratio
		Decreased mitogen response
Cytokines and prostanoids	PGE$_2$	Increased
	IL-1	Decreased
	IL-6	Increased
	Tumor necrosis factor	Increased

tion, and loss of antigen recall. Many neutrophil antimicrobial functions are suppressed after trauma, including chemotaxis, phagocytosis, respiratory burst, and intracellular killing.

There are also significant changes in humoral mediators after trauma, with increased levels of proinflammatory cytokines, including tumor necrosis factor, interleukin-1, and interleukin-6, and decreased levels of interleukin-2, interleukin-3, and interferon-γ. Immunosuppressive complement activation products and other immunosuppressive peptides are present in the serum of trauma patients; serum fibronectin and opsonic activity are decreased.

The overall effect of these global changes in immune competence after trauma is a profound immunosuppression. The clinical results include septic complications, the systemic inflammatory response syndrome, and multiple-organ dysfunction.

The mechanisms by which this immunosuppression develops after trauma include the direct effects of tissue injury itself, the release of multiple immunosuppressive mediators, and the immunosuppressive effects of the neuroendocrine response to trauma. In addition, the gastrointestinal tract can play an important, perhaps central, role in the development of posttraumatic immunosuppression. Shock, trauma, endotoxemia, and starvation have all been shown to have a negative impact on the functional integrity of the intestine, resulting in translocation of bacteria or endotoxin to the portal circulation or to the mesenteric lymph nodes.[297] In addition, activation of gut-associated immune cells can lead to systemic release of gut-derived cytokines. The net result of this process appears to be a generalized, cytokine-mediated immunosuppression, although its clinical relevance remains to be fully demonstrated.

Immunomodulation

The importance of these immunosuppressive effects is becoming more apparent as our ability to modify this response improves. Early definitive care of wounds, restora-

tion of gastrointestinal tract function and integrity, selected immunologic stimulation using biologic response modifiers or specific metabolic or nutritional immunostimulants, and selective immunologic blockade of certain aspects of the immune response are all potential strategies to reduce the immune consequences of trauma. Many of these potential interventions remain experimental, although some are now moving into clinical critical care, including the following[296]:

- Rapid and complete resuscitation with restoration of organ dysfunction using global and regional indicators
- Early establishment of enteral nutrition with high-calorie, high-protein products and possible use of specific nutritional supplements with immunostimulatory activity
- Aggressive wound débridement
- Drainage of any septic focus, along with the use of appropriate antibiotics
- Restoration of normal epithelial barriers and, in particular, preservation of gastrointestinal tract integrity

Provider-Related Complications

Careful analysis and classification of complications after traumatic injury shows that most complications are directly related to the patient's injuries, although many can be termed provider related.[17,298,299] These complications include errors in diagnosis that result in delays of treatment, technical errors, and errors of judgment. If injuries are missed or their severity is unrecognized during the initial evaluation of a trauma patient, the burden of subsequent diagnosis is placed on the critical care phase of trauma management. Missed injuries and unexpected physiologic deterioration after recognized injuries should be anticipated, and frequent monitoring of vital signs and follow-up physical examinations are a required part of the treatment of multiply injured patients. Sudden neurologic deterioration can signify worsening of an intracerebral bleed, and deteriorating vital signs can signify ongoing hemorrhage from an apparently trivial splenic injury or pelvic fracture. A full secondary survey, performed on the second hospital day, frequently picks up new, minor injuries not appreciated by the patient or physician at the time of admission, particularly minor orthopedic injuries.

In addition to these early errors, 23% of provider-related complications in one report occurred during the critical care phase of trauma care and were associated with a disproportionate percentage of preventable deaths.[300] These data are particularly interesting because they come from hospitals participating in a well-established trauma system. Critical care errors included management errors, monitoring errors, errors in electrolyte management or drug administration, and technical and procedural errors. Collectively, these studies demonstrate the importance of continued vigilance in identifying and correcting provider-related complications, particularly recurrent process errors, in order to minimize preventable mortality and morbidity. Such quality control should be an essential component of any trauma care system.

COMPLICATIONS IN MAJOR ORGAN SYSTEMS

Pulmonary Complications

Pulmonary complications account for one third of disease-related complications after trauma. Age greater than 55 years, shock at time of admission, and severe head injury are significant risk factors for the development of serious pulmonary complications, including pneumonia, atelectasis, pulmonary embolus, and the adult respiratory distress syndrome.[301] Pulmonary complications can be divided into airway difficulties, mechanical problems, infectious events, and embolic occurrences.

The general indications for endotracheal intubation and mechanical ventilation in the trauma patient include the need for (1) a secure airway, (2) decrease in the work of breathing, for patients with acutely increased ventilatory work loads or decreased ventilatory capacity, (3) maintenance of arterial oxygen tension by increasing functional residual capacity and the partial pressure of oxygen in the alveoli, and (4) induced hyperventilation for treatment of intracranial hypertension. The most common clinical scenario for intubation and mechanical ventilation involves patients with neurologic injuries. Common indications for posttraumatic mechanical ventilation are shown in Table 11-30.

The presence of thoracoabdominal injuries, the degree of shock, and the patient's age and underlying diseases also play a role in the decisions regarding intubation and mechanical ventilation. The rapidly changing physiologic status of many trauma patients often requires that intubation be performed in anticipation of particular events. Under these circumstances, physiologic trends, including those that occur over short periods, are often an appropriate indication for intubation and mechanical ventilation. In the trauma setting, it is always prudent to err on the side of aggressive airway and ventilatory control.

Patients who develop high peak airway pressures as a result of severe thoracic injury, pulmonary edema, or acute respiratory distress are at greatly increased risk for the development of mechanical complications. Prolonged in-

Table 11-30. COMMON INDICATIONS FOR MECHANICAL VENTILATION WITH SPECIFIC INJURIES

AIRWAY COMPROMISE
Massive facial fractures
Arterial injury in neck
Aspiration (blood, debris)
Severe head injury

INADEQUATE VENTILATION
Cervical spine injury (high)
Shock
Ruptured diaphragm
Crushed chest or flail chest

INADEQUATE OXYGENATION
Pulmonary contusion or flail chest
Massive aspiration
Shock
Air or fat embolus

NEED FOR HYPOCAPNEIC VASOCONSTRICTION
Increased intracranial pressure
Glasgow Coma Scale score ≤8
Best motor response is posturing or flaccidity

tubation dramatically increases the risk of both infectious and mechanical complications (Table 11-31).

Many mechanical complications of the endotracheal tube can be avoided by close monitoring of tube position. Proximal displacement of the endotracheal tube can occur suddenly (usually by an iatrogenic mechanism) or gradually, usually in association with increased peak airway

Table 11-31. COMPLICATIONS OF MECHANICAL VENTILATION

Complication	Cause	Common Conditions
MECHANICAL		
Tube displacement	High airway pressure	ARDS or infection
	Iatrogenic	Any
Cuff leak	Tube displacement	Any
	Balloon perforation	Any
	Tracheal malacia or dilation	Prolonged ETT intubation
Balloon herniation	Overinflation, obstruction of ETT tip	Any
Main-stem intubation	Iatrogenic	Any
ETT stenosis or kink	Secretions or malposition	Any
Spontaneous pneumothorax	Parenchymal degeneration	ARDS
	High airway pressure	
Bronchopleural fistula	Barotrauma or lung laceration	Infection or ARDS
Nasal erosion	Iatrogenic	Any
Tracheoinominate fistula	Pressure necrosis	Tracheostomy—high pressure
Tracheoesophageal fistula		High pressure plus nasogastric tube
Vocal cord granulomas	Pressure necrosis	Prolonged ETT intubation
Aretynoid stenosis	Pressure necrosis	Prolonged ETT intubation
Tracheal stenosis	Pressure necrosis	Tracheostomy
Depressed cardiac output	Impaired venous return	High PEEP or PIP
Increased intracranial pressure	Impaired venous return	High PEEP or PIP
METABOLIC		
Hypoxia	Pulmonary edema, V/Q mismatch	Pneumonia, ARDS, PE
Hypercapnea	V/Q mismatch	ARDS
INFECTIOUS OR INFLAMMATORY		
Tracheobronchitis	Oropharyngeal colonization	Prolonged ETT intubation
Pneumonia	Gastric and oropharyngeal colonization	Prolonged ETT intubation
ARDS	Variable	Severe injury
Empyema	Iatrogenic pneumonia or gastrointestinal contamination	Variable
Pleural effusion	Reactive or fluid overload	Variable

ETT, endotracheal tube; ARDS, acute respiratory distress syndrome; PE, pulmonary embolus; PEEP, positive end-expiratory pressure; PIP, peak inspiratory pressure.

pressures. An endotracheal cuff leak is often the first clinical manifestation of proximal balloon displacement and mandates careful determination of tube position. The blind instillation of more air into the endotracheal tube cuff can result in its expulsion proximal to the vocal cords and can precipitate loss of the airway.

Endotracheal tube obstruction can result from mucous plugs, kinking, balloon herniation over the distal orifice, or gradual accumulation of proteinaceous debris. Failure to pass a suction catheter easily should prompt close examination of tube position and balloon volume. Bronchoscopy occasionally is required to confirm endotracheal tube position and patency.

Modern endotracheal tubes with high-volume, low-pressure cuffs have greatly reduced the incidence of laryngeal and subglottic injuries previously associated with prolonged endotracheal intubation. Patients who require prolonged intubation or have laryngeal injuries are candidates for tracheostomy, although the exact timing of this procedure remains a controversial issue. Certainly, patients with profound and persistent neurologic deficits, patients with significant airway injury or edema, and patients with severe respiratory failure requiring mechanical ventilation for more than 2 to 3 weeks are all candidates, and early tracheostomy can help reduce the incidence of iatrogenic airway injuries. Tracheostomy can be performed by standard surgical techniques or percutaneously at the bedside.

Mechanical ventilation in patients with normal lungs requires positive airway pressures, which rarely cause mechanical problems. Many trauma patients, however, develop lung abnormalities that require high-pressure ventilation because of diminished compliance. Peak and mean airway pressures must be monitored and ventilator settings adjusted to minimize the risk of barotrauma. Smaller tidal volumes, decreased flow rates, or pressure-controlled modes of ventilation may be required (see Chap. 9).

Bronchopleural fistulas may occur after penetrating injury to the chest. Most air leaks are uncomplicated, and they usually close spontaneously within 2 to 5 days. Positive-pressure ventilation, particularly in patients with more severe lung injury or disease and diminished lung compliance, potentiates tidal volume loss from a larger bronchopleural fistula. A reduction in tidal volume with an appropriate increase in ventilatory rate usually reduces the volume loss to tolerable levels. Occasionally, more complex ventilatory patterns are required to reduce airway pressures, such as time-cycle, pressure-controlled ventilation or high-frequency, independent lung ventilation.

Pneumonia and empyema comprise most posttraumatic thoracic infections. Penetrating trauma that results in pleural contamination sufficient to cause an empyema occurs infrequently. The more common causes are severe chest wall injuries or gastrointestinal contamination through a diaphragmatic defect. Staphylococcus aureus is the causative organism in most posttraumatic empyema unless there has been contamination from the intestinal tract. Iatrogenic contamination and failure or delay in adequately evacuating a hemothorax appear to be contributing factors. The prophylactic use of antibiotics, although possibly of benefit, should not be considered a substitute for aseptic technique, proper chest tube positioning, complete evacuation of a hemothorax or pneumothorax, or complete reexpansion of the lung.

Pneumonia is one of the most prevalent and troublesome infections after trauma. Most postinjury pneumonias occur in patients who require prolonged endotracheal intubation and mechanical ventilation. In patients with severe head injuries who require prolonged muscular paralysis, the incidence of pneumonia approaches 80% to 90%. Causative factors include reduced cough, impaired mucociliary clearance, immunosuppression, aspiration, and oropharyngeal and gastric bacterial colonization (Table 11-32).

Posttraumatic nosocomial pneumonia characteristically is caused by gram-negative enteric organisms such as Escherichia coli, Klebsiella pneumoniae, and Pseudomonas aeruginosa. These organisms are typically found in the gastrointestinal tract and frequently colonize the normally sterile upper gastrointestinal tract and oropharynx in critically ill patients admitted to the ICU. Contamination of the upper respiratory tract by microaspiration of these oropharyngeal or gastric organisms has been implicated in the pathogenesis of nosocomial pneumonia, and therapeutic strategies have evolved to minimize this process. These include prophylaxis of stress ulceration with the use of cytoprotective agents that preserve gastric acidity rather than with acid-neutralizing strategies, with the aim of reducing gastric colonization and subsequent inoculation of the respiratory tract. In addition, the use of topical antimicrobial agents in the oropharynx and stomach has been advocated on the theory that decontamination of these sites through reduction in the numbers of pathogenic gram-negative organisms is of benefit. The data comparing different stress ulceration prophylaxis strategies with regard to the incidence of nosocomial pneumonia have yet to demonstrate any consistent benefit of sucralfate over acid-neutralizing strategies.[302,303] The data on selective decontamination of the digestive tract suggest a decreased incidence of nosocomial pneumonia in patients given topical antibiotics, but this has yet to be translated into decreased length of stay in the ICU or improved survival.[304,305]

The diagnosis of pulmonary infection in trauma patients with prolonged endotracheal intubation is complicated by the certain presence of colonization and by the usual presence of concurrent noninfectious problems (eg, atelectasis, pulmonary edema, acute respiratory distress). The use of conventional findings on sputum Gram stain and radiographic findings is a problem. Clinical reports suggest that quantitative cultures of central respiratory secretions may also be inaccurate.[306,307] Bronchoscopy with either protected catheter brush sampling or bronchoalveolar lavage promises a higher degree of diagnostic accuracy in patients with recurrent or resistant respiratory infections.[308,309]

The development of nosocomial pneumonia necessitates appropriate and adequate antibiotic therapy. Treatment is often empiric, at least initially, and choice of antibiotic depends on Gram stain identification of predominant or-

Table 11-32. POTENTIAL FACTORS PREDISPOSING TO THE DEVELOPMENT OF POSTINJURY PNEUMONIA

Aspiration at the time of injury (blood, gastric contents)
Muscular paralysis (head injury)
Enforced immobilization (elevated head of bed, head injuries)
Orthopedic injuries (soft tissue emboli, immobilization)
Sinus infection (bacterial reservoir)
Infected pneumatocele (bacterial reservoir)
Endotracheal intubation (conduit for microaspiration)
Nasogastric intubation (wick for gastric contents)
Neutralization of gastric pH (bacterial overgrowth with aspiration)
Pulmonary contusion or laceration
Oropharyngeal colonization (increased bacterial adherence)
Tracheobronchial bacterial colonization (decreased mucociliary clearance)
Postinjury immunosuppression
Pain and reduced ventilatory capacity

ganisms and the knowledge of prevailing antibiotic sensitivities or organisms specific to the unit or hospital. After the organism and specific antibiotic sensitivities are identified, then treatment can be modified accordingly for the purposes of simplicity, consistency, and cost-effectiveness. Both empiric and specific antibiotic use for nosocomial pneumonia should be standardized by formal protocols and revised on a regular basis in light of unit or institutional changes in prevailing organisms or sensitivities.

Deep venous thrombosis and its lethal counterpart, pulmonary embolus, are not infrequent complications after traumatic injury. Deaths from pulmonary embolus contribute significantly to delayed mortality after trauma. Patients at high risk for this complication should be prospectively identified and adequately treated prospectively with a combination of mechanical calf compression stockings and low-dose anticoagulation. If this is not possible, then placement of a prophylactic inferior vena caval filter should be considered. Patients with multiple long-bone fractures, pelvic fractures, spinal cord injuries, or severe head injuries should be considered at high risk; because pulmonary embolus is a frequently unheralded but lethal complication, prophylaxis should initiated at the earliest opportunity.[310]

Relief of thoracic pain after blunt chest injury is an important but often neglected adjunct to the maintenance of good pulmonary toilet. Patients with multiple rib fractures derive substantial benefit from adequate analgesia. To this end, patient-controlled narcotic analgesia or the lumbar or thoracic epidural administration of opiate analgesics or local anesthetics can be helpful in appropriately selected trauma patients.[161] Adequacy of analgesia can be determined by intermittent assessment of objective parameters such as maximal inspiratory force and vital capacity.

Most trauma patients require mechanical ventilation for only short-term management, and guidelines for ventilator weaning and extubation are similar to those for other surgical patients. Increases in ventilatory work associated with massive volume resuscitation and chest wall or pulmonary edema usually resolve within the first 48 to 72 hours after trauma and rarely require formal weaning in the absence of additional lung disease. Patients requiring prolonged mechanical ventilation frequently require a formal program of stepwise reduction in ventilator support. This weaning process is discussed in detail in Chapter 9.

Cardiovascular Complications

Because most trauma patients are young and in good health, the frequency of major cardiovascular complications after injury is usually low. Complications occur most often in three major groups: elderly patients, particularly those with preexisting coronary artery or myocardial disease; patients who have sustained direct myocardial injury; and patients who develop sepsis or multiple-organ failure later in their hospital course.

Preinjury myocardial disease, particularly coronary artery disease, is clearly associated with decreased survival after major injury.[311] Indications for hemodynamic monitoring in high-risk or elderly patients after major trauma should be adjusted appropriately. Patients sustaining major thoracoabdominal or orthopedic injuries are usually monitored with central venous pressure and arterial lines. In addition, a flow-directed pulmonary artery catheter should be placed in patients with evidence of inadequate myocardial function, a history of coronary artery or heart disease, or impairment of gas exchange.

Survivors of penetrating cardiac injuries usually have an uncomplicated postoperative course. Lacerations involving the conduction system or a coronary artery are exceptions. Blunt cardiac injury does not often lead to clinical complications. Rhythm disturbances usually are transient and easily treated, and they occur within the first several hours after injury.[178] The recovery time for the occasional patient who exhibits cardiac insufficiency after myocardial contusion is usually shorter (48 to 72 hours) than for the patient with myocardial infarction, probably because of a lack of underlying coronary artery disease. Inotropic support is considered safe if required. Patients with evidence of significant cardiac injury should also be screened for pericardial effusion or tamponade, papillary muscle defects, and ventricular wall contractility with the use of echocardiography.

Cardiac failure unrelated to direct injury may occur after global ischemia and profound hemorrhagic shock or in the presence of sepsis. A variety of small polypeptides that are myocardial depressant factors have been isolated in experimental models of hemorrhagic and endotoxic shock. These appear to exert their effects by a negative inotropic action, but their relevance is uncertain. Care of these patients is simply supportive.

Central Nervous System Complications

The principal challenge in the management of head injury resides in postinjury critical care and involves management of increased intracranial pressure (ICP) as well as multisystem dysfunction. Failure to control ICP and maintain cerebral perfusion pressure is the most common and serious complication after severe head injury.[312] These issues were discussed in detail in a previous section of this chapter. Monitoring of the ICP and clinical course must be accompanied by the liberal use of sequential computed tomography (CT) scanning. Changes in clinical course should be considered absolute indications for restudy. This is the only practical method for the prompt identification of patients who develop surgically correctable mass lesions during the initial care phase of treatment.

ICP monitors include intraventricular catheters, subarachnoid or subdural bolts, and intraparenchymal or extradural fiberoptic sensors. Complications associated with these catheters are predictable and include hemorrhage and infection. Camino catheters are reliable monitors of ICP pressure and have a lower incidence of infection but do not allow drainage of cerebrospinal fluid for treatment.

A unique set of issues arises in patients with lethal head injuries who are identified as potential organ donors. The combined use of CT, clinical examination, and ICP monitoring usually allows prompt identification of these patients. The expansion of transplantation programs has increased the need for donor organs, and the effort to solicit donation is now a legal requirement in most of the United States. Physiologic support must be continued until the wishes of the patient or family regarding organ donation can be ascertained. Centrally mediated hypotension, pulmonary edema, massive diuresis from diabetes insipidus, hypothermia, and coagulopathy are all predictable problems that require aggressive support until either death or organ donation. The burden of this support is best minimized by prompt solicitation and expeditious organ donation.

Abdominal Complications

Missed injuries and postoperative intraabdominal infections are the most important abdominal complications after trauma. Missed injuries after diagnostic peritoneal lavage occur in about 0.5% to 3% of patients. These usually consist of diaphragmatic or retroperitoneal injuries of the duodenum, pancreas, colon, or genitourinary tract. Similarly, bowel and pancreatic injuries are difficult to identify with CT and ultrasound and may be missed. A high level of suspicion must be maintained, with frequent clinical examination of patients at risk for occult abdominal trauma. The onset of new abdominal signs mandates further workup or exploration.

Fever, leukocytosis, tachycardia, paralytic ileus, increased fluid requirements, and failure to wean from mechanical ventilation all represent warning signs of the development of intraabdominal infection. Infection usually results from either missed injury or a postoperative event in the trauma setting. CT is the most useful diagnostic tool in this clinical setting because it yields considerable information with regard to organ injury and the presence of intraabdominal abscesses or fluid collections. Ultrasonography may be useful as well. Its major advantages are portability and low cost, but it is less sensitive, less specific, and may well be more operator dependent in an ICU environment. Localized fluid collections, suggestive of intraabdominal abscesses, can be managed by surgical or interventional radiologic drainage procedures.

No method of noninvasive imaging is completely accurate, and none should be relied on to definitively exclude intraabdominal injury or infection in the face of contrary clinical data. Bowel perforations, mesenteric or segmental ischemia, and diaphragmatic injuries may be impossible to diagnose reliably by CT. Diagnostic peritoneal lavage for the evaluation of acute abdominal problems has been advocated. Although not routine, it may be a useful adjunct if suspicion of abdominal injury exists but the patient has an inconclusive initial diagnostic evaluation. Laparotomy as a diagnostic test for unexplained sepsis has a low yield in critically ill trauma patients and should not be used routinely. It is the rare patient with progressive sepsis but no identifiable source who benefits from laparotomy.

Intraabdominal compartment syndrome is becoming increasingly recognized in the postoperative period after laparotomy for intraabdominal injuries. Extensive retroperitoneal hematoma, bowel edema, and the need for intraabdominal packing all place the patient at risk for development of this syndrome. The trauma surgeon should be aware of this possibility not only at the time of abdominal wall closure but also in the postoperative period, when increasingly tense abdominal distention, increasing airway pressures, difficulty in ventilating, and finally, decreasing urine output in the face of normal vascular filling pressures should strongly suggest the diagnosis. Elevated intraabdominal pressures can be confirmed by transducing the bladder or stomach after instillation of saline solution, with pressures higher than 20 cm of water providing the confirmatory evidence. Patients with abdominal compartment syndrome must be returned to the operating room for expeditious reexploration and prosthetic closure. As packs are removed, hematomas and edema resolve, prosthetic material can gradually be imbricated, and abdominal contents eventually can be reduced below the level of the fascia by careful application of external packs. After this has been achieved, final definitive closure of fascia should be possible.

Hemorrhage or performation caused by stress ulceration of the gastric mucosa has been described after trauma. The incidence of this complication has greatly diminished in recent years, in temporal relation to the introduction of routine prophylactic pharmacotherapy aimed at either reducing gastric pH or providing gastric mucosal cytoprotection. Other factors are earlier and more aggressive use of intragastric tube feedings and the development of resusci-

tation endpoints that more clearly signal restoration of adequate organ perfusion. However, certain patients still appear to be at high risk for development of stress ulceration. Among these are patients who have septic complications, organ dysfunction, severe multisystem injury (Injury Severity Score greater than 20), spinal cord injury with neurologic deficit, or significant burn injury. These patients should be aggressively treated and monitored for evidence of gastrointestinal bleeding.[313] Omeprazole can be useful in patients who develop bleeding and may be preferable to surgical options except in the exsanguinating patient.

A small number of patients develop acute surgical problems unrelated to direct injury. Acalculous cholecystitis, acute appendicitis, acute diverticulitis, and perforated duodenal ulcer are among these complications. Diminished pain responses in patients with head or spinal cord injuries and the frequent need for endotracheal intubation and ventilatory support complicate accurate diagnosis. With the exception of acalculous cholecystitis, which can be evaluated by ultrasound and biliary scintigraphy, the diagnosis of nontraumatic intraabdominal infection after trauma is frequently delayed. The principal strategy for overcoming this problem is to educate those who provide care to remain alert to the possibilities.

Infection

Intraabdominal Infection

Posttraumatic intraabdominal infection is almost always the result of contamination from the gastrointestinal tract. Penetrating trauma accounts for most of these infections. Intestinal injuries accompany 40% to 50% of gunshot wounds and 15% to 30% of stab wounds and usual produce significant intraabdominal contamination. Because of its higher bacterial counts, isolated injuries of the colon are associated with a higher incidence of infectious complications than are isolated gastric, duodenal, or small bowel injuries. The precise incidence of intraabdominal or incisional wound infection after colonic injuries depends on factors present at the time of injury (eg, blood loss, degree of contamination, other associated injuries) and on whether the wound is closed or left open. The latter is often the safer situation.

The use of perioperative antibiotics for trauma has been investigated extensively. Most studies compared singleagent, second- or third-generation cephalosporins with combinations of antibiotics that are effective against anaerobic and coliform bacteria. Single-agent cephalosporins are at least as effective as multiagent regimens in retarding intraabdominal abscesses or wound infections resulting from a variety of contaminated traumatic wounds. Singleagent cephalosporins continue to be the first choice of prophylactic and perioperative antibiotics in the treatment of most abdominal traumas. The optimal duration of administration of postinjury antibiotics has not been determined, but a number of studies suggest that there is no advantage in administering these agents for more than 2 days.

Wound Infection

The incidence of incisional wound infection depends on the method of wound treatment and the degree of contamination. One study of wound infections in trauma patients found incidences of 3.2%, 8.1%, and 24.6% for clean, clean contaminated, and contaminated wounds, respectively.[314] The liberal use of delayed primary closure or secondary closure in heavily contaminated wounds (eg, colonic injuries) substantially reduces the incidence of wound infection in that group.

Wounds heavily contaminated at the time of injury require extensive débridement and washout. Shotgun wounds, degloving injuries, and crush injuries are at higher risk. The degree and source of contamination are critical; it may be appropriate to return patients to the operating room daily for débridement and washout of major wounds. Almost all contaminated wounds, assuming adequate nutritional repletion, respond to this regimen of repeated débridement and conscientious dressing care. Failure to respond initially should prompt a thorough investigation, including quantitative wound cultures and examination for invasive fungal infection. Patients with progressive tissue destruction in the absence of identifiable pathogens may benefit from an empiric course of an antifungal agent such as amphotericin B. Delays in recognition of invasive fungal infections under these circumstances are frequently lethal.

Large, degloving injuries or areas of extensive skin loss usually require thorough débridement and, eventually, skin grafting. Attempts at creative closures of large contaminated or devascularized flaps over drains are usually futile and increase the risk of serious infection and sepsis. Fresh cadaver autografts can provide an ideal interim dressing over débrided wounds and reduce the incidence of secondary infection, pain, and fluid loss.

Catheter Infection

Central venous pulmonary artery and arterial catheters continue to be a major source of nosocomial infections. Infection rates for central venous catheters vary depending on catheter type (single-lumen or multilumen), insertion site, duration of use, type of use, dressing type, and the patient's underlying condition. The placement of catheters during initial resuscitation may be less than optimal with respect to aseptic technique. In general, emergency lines are best removed within 24 hours; failure to do so has been associated with an increased risk of infection. Cutdown catheters are particularly prone to infection and usually should not be used any longer than is absolutely necessary.

The two principal sources of catheter infections are catheter hub colonization with internal migration of bacteria and external catheter contamination with migration of skin wound bacteria. The incidence of infection at each of these sites varies and is probably a function of placement technique and the frequency of catheter hub manipulation. Long duration of catheter use and septic condition of the patient are additional risk factors for catheter infections.

Multilumen catheters have been associated with an increased incidence of contamination and infection compared with single-lumen catheters. The reasons have not been precisely determined but are probably related to the increased frequency of catheter manipulation and the infusion of multiple agents.

Studies using a silver-impregnated antimicrobial subcutaneous cuff attached to a central venous catheter or an antibiotic-impregnated catheter have reported a decreased incidence of associated line infections.[315,316] Such devices offer the potential advantages of reduced infections and the less frequent need for line changes. However, the antimicrobial advantages of the cuffs are eliminated if catheters are changed over guide wires through the cuffs. The use of these devices in trauma patients and their efficacy has yet to be determined.

In general, the treatment of the complication of catheter sepsis is removal, with replacement at an alternative site if the line is necessary. Systemic antibiotic therapy may not be needed, but if it is given, the duration of treatment should be brief.

Sinusitis

Sinus infections are of importance both as primary infections and as a potential reservoir for secondary pulmonary infections. Sinusitis is most commonly associated with obstruction caused by indwelling nasotracheal or nasogastric tubes. Surveillance sinus films should be obtained routinely as part of the fever evaluation in patients with nasal tubes. Tube removal or alternative placement, sinus aspiration or drainage, and antibiotics usually provide adequate therapy.

Orthopedic and Soft Tissue Complications

Major orthopedic injuries to the pelvis, thoracolumbar spine, or long bones occur in one fourth of blunt trauma patients. Related morbidity and mortality usually result from hemorrhage, immobilization, or sepsis. Primary failure of fracture healing is relatively uncommon. Hemorrhage is the major source of mortality and has been discussed. Pelvic fractures are clearly the most problematic. Less dramatic but far more common are the pulmonary and septic complications related to prolonged immobilization and enforced bed rest. As has been discussed, early fixation of these injuries is associated with lower morbidity rates.[247]

Open fractures, particularly those associated with significant loss of soft tissue, are often heavily contaminated and prone to local infection, necrosis, and progressive tissue loss. Long-term disability, including amputation, can result. Aggressive and frequent operative débridement, dressing changes, and systemic antibiotics maximize the probability of a good outcome.

Potential development of compartment syndrome exists in any patient with prolonged ischemia, particularly if it is coupled with associated soft tissue trauma. Reperfusion edema can take several hours to develop, and continuous or frequent monitoring of compartment pressure should be performed for high-risk patients. Prophylactic fasciotomy, performed at the time of initial surgery, is often indicated for prolonged ischemia (longer than 4 to 6 hours) and for severe crush injuries. Monitoring of urine for the presence of myoglobin and monitoring of serum creatine kinase enzyme levels can be useful in detecting any progressive or ongoing rhabdomyolysis. Evidence of progressive muscle necrosis should prompt a complete inspection of the involved muscle groups, usually in the operating room.

Renal Failure

Despite the frequency of profound hypovolemic shock that occurs after major trauma, the incidence of renal failure in these patients is declining. A 1991 multicenter study of 72,757 trauma patients found an incidence of only 0.11% for renal failure requiring dialysis.[317] The combined effects of rapid transportation and appropriate fluid resuscitation are responsible for this remarkably low incidence. Inadequate renal perfusion caused by a variety of shock states remains the primary cause of renal dysfunction.[318] Hypovolemic shock can be produced by ongoing hemorrhage, inadequate fluid resuscitation, or excessive diuresis combined with volume restriction (eg, in head-injured patients). Causes of inadequate renal perfusion not related to hypovolemia include cardiogenic problems such as myocardial contusion, tamponade, and infarction. Occasionally, hypotension secondary to sympathectomy associated with high cervical spinal cord injuries is seen.

Direct renal injury in the posttraumatic patient is most commonly associated with prolonged shock or ischemia and is termed acute tubular necrosis. Pharmacologic agents, such as aminoglycosides, amphotericin B, and radiographic agents used for contrast studies, are all associated with primary nephrotoxicity. Compartment syndromes and crush injuries producing rhabdomyolysis can also precipitate renal failure on the basis of renal tubular precipitation of pigment compounds. Preexisting renal disease contributes to all of these insults.

The outcome for patients who develop posttraumatic renal failure is determined principally by their underlying disease, the cause of the renal failure, and any associated injuries. Previous reports have suggested that the mortality rate from oliguric renal failure is substantially greater (70% to 80%) than from nonoliguric renal failure (20% to 30%). Supportive treatment for posttraumatic renal failure includes correction of the underlying cause, nutritional support, and dialysis. Most centers rely on hemodialysis performed by means of percutaneously placed venous access lines. These methods are more suitable for acute, short-term hemodialysis, and they avoid the complications of infection and thrombosis associated with surgically placed arteriovenous shunts. Peritoneal dialysis is often impractical because of associated abdominal and pelvic injuries, but it can be done if necessary. The use of continuous arteriovenous hemodialysis or venovenous hemodialysis has recently been applied to patients with posttraumatic renal failure.[319] Advantages include ease of use, absence of systemic anticoagulation, and avoidance of the rapid fluid and electrolyte shifts that occur with intermittent dialysis. Studies are now evaluating this technique in comparison with conventional dialysis.

Envenomation and Environmental Injuries

GREGORY J. JURKOVICH AND LAWRENCE M. GENTILELLO

ENVENOMATION INJURIES
Snakes

More than 375 species of venomous snakes can be found worldwide, and they are responsible for about 300,000 bites and 30,000 deaths each year. In the United States, it is estimated that 45,000 snakebites occur annually, with 14 to 20 deaths.[320-322] However, in 1991, only 3805 snakebites were reported to the American Association of Poison Control Centers, and 1039 of these were from snakes usually considered to be nonpoisonous.[323] Occasionally, a bite by a garter snake (*Thamnophis* sp) can be confused early with the bite of a poisonous snake of the Crotalidae family.

Progressive local effects (eg, edema, erythema) are produced by the toxic salivary secretions of the snake's parotid-like Duverney glands if the victim's skin has been broken.[324] However, systemic signs fail to develop, and the local signs resolve spontaneously within a few days.

The five main families of poisonous snakes are the Colubridae, Elapidae, Hydrophidae, Viperidae, and Crotalidae. The Colubridae family consists primarily of the boomslang and the bird snake, which are found mainly in Africa. The Elapidae family includes the cobras, the coral snakes, and the adders, which are found throughout Asia, Africa, the Americas, and Australia. The Hydrophidae family consists of the sea snakes, which are found throughout the Pacific and along the west coast of South America. The Viperidae family consists of old world vipers, which are found throughout Africa, Europe, and the Middle East. The Crotalidae are the true pit vipers and are found worldwide. The native venomous snakes of North America are members of the phylum Chordata, class Reptilia, order Squamata, suborder Serpentes, and of the families Crotalidae and Elapidae (Table 11-33).

Rattlesnakes are members of the family Crotalidae, genus *Crotalus* or *Sistrurus*. Water moccasins (or cottonmouths) and copperheads are also members of the Crotalidae family, but of the genus *Agkistrodon*. The coral snakes are the major representatives of the Elapidae family and belong to the genera *Micrurus* and *Micruroides*. Other well-known members of the Elapidae family not indigenous to North America are the cobras and mambas. The distribution of venomous snakes in the United States is extensive, with at least one native species found in every state except Maine, Alaska, and Hawaii. Rattlesnakes are particularly widely distributed, and the water moccasin is found across the southeastern United States, in the Mississippi Valley, and in Illinois and Indiana. The copperhead's range is primarily from central Massachusetts to northern Florida and west to Illinois and Texas.

The Crotalidae, or pit vipers, have a number of characteristics that differentiate them from harmless snakes (Fig. 11-105). Their unique and characteristic thermoreceptor "pit" is an infrared sensor located between the nostril and the eye that helps the snake localize its prey. Pit vipers also have a vertical, elliptically shaped pupil, a triangular-shaped head, and retractable fangs. Venomous snakes have a single row of plates distal to the anal plate on their ventral surface, whereas harmless snakes have a double row of caudal plates.

Coloration is so variable as to be almost useless as a distinguishing characteristic. An exception is the coloration of the Elapidae coral snake, which can be identified by the simple rhyme, "Red on yellow, kill a fellow; red on black, venom lack." This refers to the fact that a coral snake has circular bands of colors with red adjacent to yellow, whereas the nonvenomous but similar-looking king snake has red on black bands that do not completely encircle it.

Table 11-33. SNAKES OF THE FAMILY CROTALIDAE

Genus	Common Name	Characteristics	Range
Agkistrodon	Water moccasin and copperhead	No rattles; large plates on crown	North America, southeastern Europe, and Asia
Bothrops	New World pit vipers	No rattles; small scales on crown; large scales ventral tail	Mexico to South America
Crotalus	Rattlesnakes	Rattles; small scales on crown	North, Central, and South America
Lachesis	Bushmaster	No rattles; small scales on crown; small scales ventral tail	Central and South America
Sistrurus	Massasaugas and pygmy rattlesnakes	Rattles; large plates on crown	North America
Trimeresurus	Asiatic pit vipers	No rattles; small scales on crown	Asia

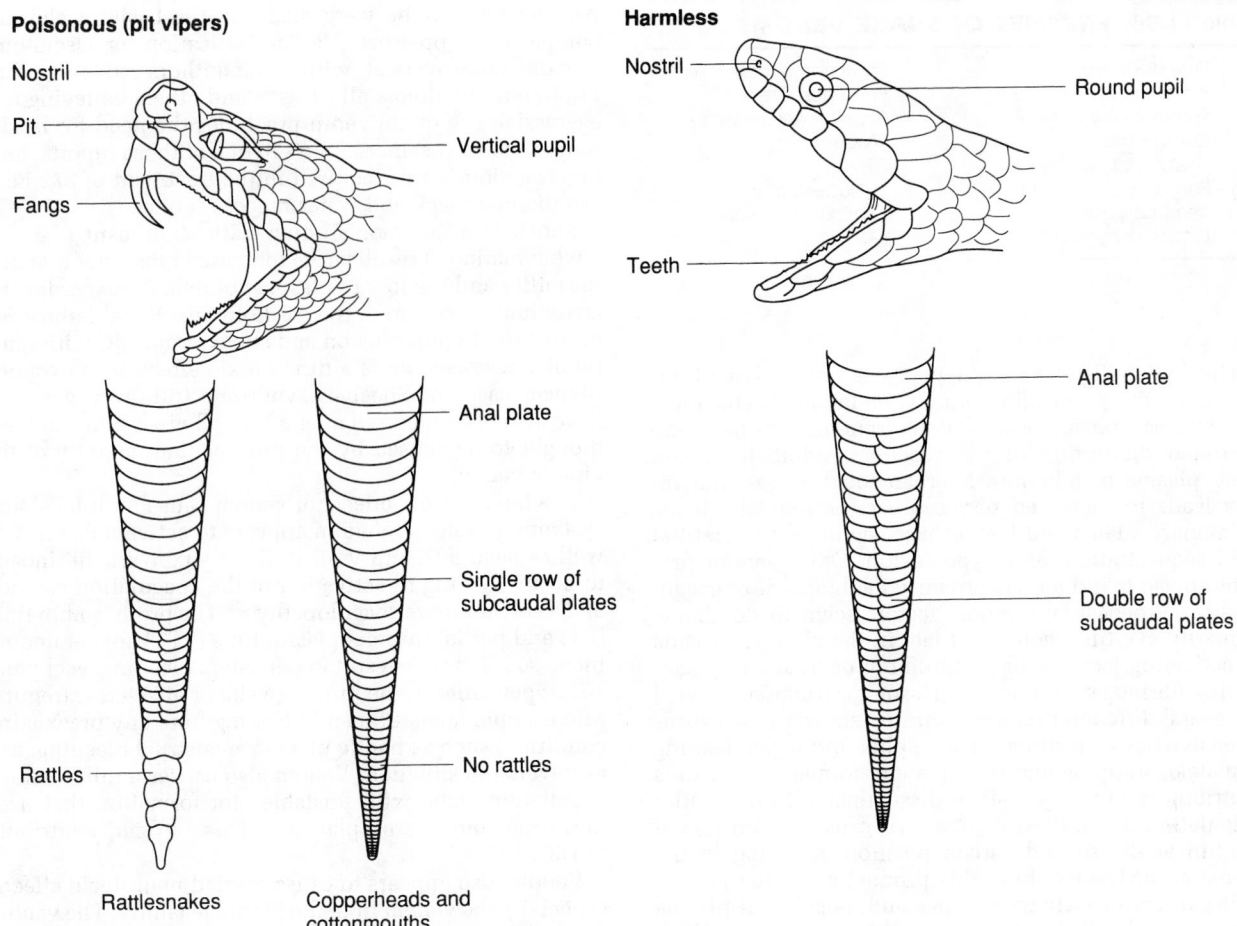

Figure 11-105. Characteristics of snakes that differentiate poisonous pit vipers from harmless snakes.

It has also been noted that the Eastern coral snake has a completely black nose, whereas the king snake usually does not.

Most snakebites occur in the United States in the Sunbelt region between April and October, with the peak occurring in the summer months of July and August. Snakes appear to be more aggressive before and after hibernation. The victims of snakebites are typically men between 18 and 50 years of age, and up to 60% of bites occur during deliberate handling of snakes.[325] In one report,[325] the ingestion of alcohol was associated with 56.5% of snakebites incurred while intentionally handling or knowingly not avoiding a snake. Other reports suggest that about 30% of all snakebite victims are intoxicated.[326]

Not every poisonous snakebite results in envenomation, and even the presence of fang marks does not necessarily correlate with envenomation. Venom is produced in large glands located on the dorsal sides of the head, corresponding to the parotid glands, that give the head its characteristic triangular shape. During the bite, the venom is forced through the hollow fangs by the palatine muscles and extruded out the orifices, which are located just proximal to the tip. Small thicknesses of clothing or foot gear can significantly diminish the depth of penetration and limit the amount of envenomation.

The severity of envenomation is related to the amount of venom injected, the concentration of the venom, and the size of the snake. Direct intravenous envenomation is unusual but particularly severe.[327] Snakebites that exhibit a distance between the fangs greater than 15 mm are representative of a large snake and suggest a potentially more significant envenomation. Hibernation also seems to play a role in severity. After hibernation, snakes are relatively dehydrated because they have been in a prolonged fasting state, and they produce a more potent, concentrated venom. Even if fang marks are present, 10% to 25% of bites have no significant envenomation. With each strike, the snake can discharge between 25% and 75% of its venom, so successive or repetitive strikes tend to diminish the amount of venom available. It has also been observed that snakes that are angered or fearful can discharge greater amounts of venom.

Venom

The function of venom is to kill or immobilize prey and to aid in digestion. Venom consists of a complex array of proteins and enzymes that are usually characterized as neurotoxins, hemotoxins, and cardiotoxins. More than 26 different proteins and nonenzymatic peptides have been isolated from various venoms.[322] The Crotalidae venom consists of about 90% water, 5 to 15 enzymes, 3 to 12 nonenzymatic proteins and peptides, and at least 6 other unidentified substances. A partial list of these enzymes is shown in Table 11-34 and includes several proteolytic enzymes, phospholipase, nucleotidase, acetylcholinesterase, and amino acid oxidase.

Table 11-34. ENZYMES OF SNAKE VENOMS

Proteolytic enzymes	Phosphomonoesterase
Arginine ester hydrolase	Phosphodiesterase
Thrombin-like enzyme	Acetylcholinesterase
Collagenase	RNase
Hyaluronidase	DNase
Phospholipase A$_2$ (A)	5'-Nucleotidase
Phospholipase C	L-Amino acid oxidase
Lactate dehydrogenase	

The low-molecular-weight peptides and polypeptides appear to act by damaging vascular endothelial cells. Electron microscopic analysis of tissue from humans has demonstrated disruption of the vascular endothelium and other plasma membranes. Microangiopathic vascular injury leads to increased permeability, peripheral edema, pulmonary edema and hemorrhage, significant interstitial fluid sequestration, and hypotension. Other venom proteins appear to induce a neuromuscular blockade or coagulopathy. Procoagulant venom factors seem to dominate, primarily exerting their effect late in the clotting cascade by activating factor X or prothrombin or by directly converting fibrinogen to fibrin.[328] Tissue destruction is aided by several different proteins. L-Amino-acid oxidase causes extensive tissue destruction and splits fibrinogen, leading to platelet trapping and unstable clot formation and thus contributing to the genesis of disseminated intravascular coagulation (DIC). Phospholipase A$_2$ causes hydrolysis of lecithin at the second carbon position, resulting in the formation of lysolecithin. This product alters the permeability of erythrocyte membranes and muscle cell plasma membranes, leading to hemolysis and tissue edema. Hyaluronidase induces the lysis of ground substance and thereby aids in the distribution of the venom throughout body tissues.

The Elapidae snakes also have specific neurotoxins and cardiotoxins, which have a more direct effect on the neuroactivity of the prey. Coral snake venom exhibits a direct blocking action on the acetylcholine receptor sites, which do not appear to be responsive to neostigmine. This causes ptosis, dysphagia, and slurred speech and can lead to seizures, coma, and death within 8 to 72 hours.

Signs and Symptoms

The important signs and symptoms of snakebites include both local and systemic effects. Immediate pain, edema, and erythema at the site of the bite are typical. Local signs and symptoms progressing at a rate of more than 30 cm/h, along with microscopic hematuria and bleeding from the puncture sites, indicate significant envenomation.[329]

Myonecrosis at or near the bite site is caused by both the direct toxic effects of the venom and the added ischemia of edema and increased compartment pressures. The development of a frank compartment syndrome after a snakebite of the extremity is an unusual occurrence. Studies using purified venom injected into the anterolateral leg compartment of mongrel dogs determined that only intramuscular injection leads to an increase in compartmental pressure.[330] Because most snakebites do not penetrate through the superficial fascia, compartment syndromes are unusual, and the principal cause of myonecrosis is probably direct toxicity of the venom rather than ischemia from elevated compartment pressure. Nonetheless, in one report of 36 rattlesnake bites, three definitive diagnoses of com-

partment syndrome were made on the basis of elevated compartment pressures.[331] The indication for fasciotomy remains controversial, with some authors recommending fasciotomy in almost all cases[332] and others believing that aggressive use of antivenin precludes the need for fasciotomy in most instances.[333–336] In one of those reports, only one fasciotomy was required in the treatment of 272 Eastern diamondback and water moccasin bites.[336]

Shock is a common finding with significant systemic envenomation. It results from increased microvascular permeability and the loss of plasma volume. Bradycardia and arrhythmia result from the cardiotoxins. Renal failure can occur from hypoperfusion and shock, from DIC with renal tubular necrosis, or as a direct toxic effect of the venom. Sixteen cases of Sheehan syndrome (pituitary necrosis) have also been reported after a Russell viper bite and were thought to be caused by the procoagulant activity of the viper's venom.[337]

The hematologic effects of venom cause both local and systemic problems. Venom appears to activate factor X as well as factors IX and V, or it directly converts fibrinogen to fibrin, leading to activation of the coagulation cascade and a consumptive coagulopathy.[328] The prothrombin time (PT) and partial thromboplastin time (PTT) are commonly increased. This can result in persistent bleeding, ecchymosis, or petechiae at the puncture site or affected extremity. Microscopic hematuria and bleeding from any preexisting condition, such as peptic ulcer or menstrual bleeding, can aggravate the situation. Venom also causes a mild defibrinogenation state, with unstable clot formation that uses fibrinogen but spares platelets. This too can contribute to DIC.

Venom also appears to cause myriad neurologic effects, especially the venom from the Elapidae family. The venom of coral snakes, cobras, and sea snakes contains an acetylcholinesterase receptor antagonist that causes ptosis, slurred speech, and impaired swallowing leading to hypersalivation. This venom also has central nervous system activity that results in progressive weakness, paresthesia, and eventually, respiratory muscle failure and respiratory arrest. Patients may develop seizures and psychotic behavior that can lead to coma or death in 8 to 72 hours. The toxins responsible include neurotoxin A, which appears to act on the central nervous system, and neurotoxin B, which acts at the myoneural junction.

Clinical Evaluation

Initial laboratory testing should include serum electrolytes, complete blood count with platelet count, PT, PTT, fibrinogen level, and urinalysis.[320] Frequent clinical examinations should focus on neurologic, hematologic, and hemodynamic profiles. Special immunodiagnostic studies have been developed to help identify the species of snake, but these tests are not yet clinically applicable in the United States.[338] Radioimmunoassay is extremely sensitive, with some venoms being detected at levels of 0.4 g/L. The limiting aspects of this assay are its expense and the fact that it can take 24 hours to produce a definitive result. The enzyme-linked immunosorbent assay has been widely used and is sensitive to 5 g/L of venom. This assay can be run on serum, urine, blister fluid, or aspiration fluid. This test is helpful in attempting to determine the specific snake in order to direct monovalent antivenin therapy. In the United States, however, there is only one Crotalidae antivenin and only one coral snake antivenin; therefore, this more detailed identification is usually unnecessary.[339]

Treatment

Initial first aid begins with immobilization and splinting of the infected part at the level of the heart or at a slightly dependent position, much as a fracture of the extremity would be treated. The utility of incision and suction at the puncture site has been debated for years. In dogs, up to half of the venom can be removed if incision and suction are begun within 3 minutes of the bite,[340] but these results have not been verified in humans. Russell has indicated that if immediate incision and suction is started and continued for 1 hour, at best 11% of the venom may be removed.[322,341] Most authorities do not recommend incision and suction therapy.[342]

The use of a proximal tourniquet should also be discouraged because it can lead to venous congestion and increased ischemia without demonstrated benefit. Firm but nonocclusive wrapping of the extremity, however, is a useful first aid measure, since it appears to delay dissemination of the venom. Cryotherapy (ice pack) is universally discouraged because it increases tissue ischemia. The effects of cryotherapy and steroids were studied in envenomated mongrel dogs, and no added benefit could be demonstrated by their use as adjuvants to antivenin alone.[343]

Tetanus prophylaxis and the prevention of secondary infections are important objectives of snakebite treatment. The gram-negative organisms *Aerobacter, Proteus*, and *Pseudomonas* are particularly common causes of bacterial infection, and appropriate systemic antibiotics are given routinely. Cholinergic agonists may be of benefit after an Elapidae bite, because this venom has a significant effect on acetylcholine receptors. Calcium gluconate can also be of benefit after an Elapidae bite to control the onset of seizures. Some snake venoms have been shown to contain metallopeptides, and for this reason, ethyletediaminetetraacetic acid (EDTA) has been tried experimentally in animals as a chelator to inactivate these proteins. The use of EDTA is to be discouraged, however, because it appears to hasten death in laboratory animals for unknown reasons.[337] Systemic steroids have no effect in the initial treatment of snakebites, but they play a significant role in treatment of the serum sickness that often follows antivenin therapy.[333]

Although there is debate concerning the efficacy and utility of antivenin therapy,[344] antivenin remains the mainstay of treatment of significant envenomation throughout the world.[345] More than 100 antivenin products are available worldwide, but there are only two in the United States. The Crotalidae antivenin by Wyeth is a polyvalent, hyperimmune equine serum that is produced by horse envenomation with the Eastern diamondback, Western diamondback, tropical rattlesnake, and fer-de-lance. The other available antivenin is the Eastern coral snake antivenin, also manufactured by Wyeth.

Before administration of antivenin, the patient must be tested for sensitivity to equine serum. Intradermal testing with 0.2 mL of 1:10 or 1:100 serum dilution should be performed in all patients, with a positive test being a wheal or erythema within the first 15 to 30 minutes. Similarly, two drops in the conjunctiva with 1:1000 dilution serum may be positive with the production of itching and erythema in the conjunctiva. These sensitivity tests have a false-positive rate of about 50% and a false-negative rate of 8% to 10%. Anaphylaxis is reported in 3% to 54% of patients treated with antivenin. This latter event is a type I immunoglobulin E–mediated anaphylactic reaction to the horse serum, which results in mast cell degranulation.

The occurrence of anaphylaxis during or after administration of antivenin mandates immediate cessation of therapy and countermeasures, including antihistamines (diphenhydramine HCl [Benadryl]), epinephrine infusion, or corticosteroids. The adequacy of the airway and volume status must be ensured. The risk of continuing antivenin must be weighed against the potential fatal nature of severe envenomation. The Wyeth antivenin product brochure describes a lengthy desensitization schedule. Concomitant administration of intravenous antihistamine and epinephrine in small, titrated microdrip doses to prevent the most severe manifestations of systemic anaphylaxis has been described in an allergic patient in whom antivenin therapy was deemed essential. This technique requires close physician observation because there are risks from both anaphylaxis and the treatment itself.[339]

The other major complication of antivenin therapy is serum sickness. Serum sickness occurs in about 50% to 75% of all patients treated with antivenin. It is a type III hypersensitivity reaction in which soluble antigen–antibody complexes are deposited diffusely in the presence of antigen excess. In 26 patients who were treated with a total of 507 vials of Crotalidae antivenin, there was an immediate hypersensitivity reaction in 23%, and serum sickness occurred in 50%.[333] Eighty-three percent of patients who received more than eight vials of antivenin experienced serum sickness, compared with 38% of those who received fewer than eight vials. The serum sickness symptoms of urticaria, itching, nephritis, and arthralgia can occur any time up to 3 weeks after antivenin therapy. The exact number of vials of antivenin required to induce serum sickness is not known, but it appears that increasing amounts of antivenin lead to a higher incidence of serum sickness, with almost universal occurrence after the administration of 7 to 10 vials of antivenin. The treatment for serum sickness is systemic corticosteroids in decreasing doses over a 7- to 14-day period.

Pit viper bites are graded by the following scale[333,346,347]:

Grade 0—visible bite but no envenomation
Grade I—minimal pain and edema of less than 25 cm
Grade II—moderate pain, edema of 25 to 40 cm, systemic weakness, and emesis
Grade III—severe pain, edema of 40 to 50 cm, petechiae, and systemic vertigo
Grade IV—lethal envenomation with widespread edema, shock, seizures, coma, and renal failure

The estimated initial amount of Crotalidae antivenin needed should correlate with the presenting clinical grade of envenomation. The package insert for Wyeth Crotalidae Antivenin Polyvalent suggests the following dosing estimations:

Grade 0—none
Grade I—none
Grade II—2 to 4 vials
Grade III—5 to 9 vials
Grade IV—More than 10 vials

Each vial is diluted in 10 mL of normal saline solution and given intravenously over a 15- to 20-minute period. Antivenin therapy is continued until the entire estimated dose is administered or until progression of symptoms has stopped. Repeated dosing may be necessary. Children and small adults appear particularly susceptible to envenomation and may require a larger dose than initially anticipated.

Although early surgical excision of the bite wound has been advocated by some, most authorities regard antivenin as the primary therapy and reserve surgery for the occasional compartment syndrome or for débridement of necrotic tissue at the site of the bite several days after envenomation. Unless deep intramuscular envenomation has occurred and antivenin therapy has been delayed, fasciotomy is rarely required. Because the musculature and deep compartments of the hand are relatively superficial, however, intramuscular penetration can occur at these sites. Myonecrosis and interstitial edema can cause enough compartmental hypertension in these upper-extremity sites to make linear finger fasciotomy and digital release helpful. Fasciotomy can help reduce the ischemic tissue damage caused by increased pressure, but it does not alleviate the myonecrosis caused by the direct toxic effect of the venom.[330,348] Noninvasive arterial studies may help select patients who require special surgical intervention for ischemia.[349]

VENOMOUS LIZARDS

Two species of venomous lizards exist, *Heloderma suspectum* and *Heloderma horridum*. *H suspectum*, or Gila monster, is found in the southwestern United States, and *H horridum*, or Mexican beaded lizard, is found in central and southern Mexico.[350] Physicians may, however, encounter a bite victim anywhere in the world, because these colorful animals are common in zoos and are often kept illegally as pets. Nonetheless, human envenomation is very unusual, with only 13 case reports of Gila monster envenomation in the medical literature since 1956, most from captive animals[351].

Gila monsters can be up to 55 cm long. They characteristically have slow, lingering movements, but they also have surprisingly quick reflexes and incredibly powerful jaws. Although they are usually docile, reports in the medical literature suggest that they can strike without warning or provocation. The mechanism of envenomation is fairly inefficient. The lizard has eight pairs of inferior labial glands, located on either side of the lower jaw, that secrete venom into the floor of the mouth. By capillary action alone, the venom travels out of the glands and into grooves of the posteriorly curved lower canines (teeth 4 through 7, counting from the central incisor). Only about 60% of bites have significant envenomation, because prolonged chewing is required to adequately disperse the venom into the prey. Dislodging of the animal from its prey, however, is difficult because of its extremely powerful jaws. It may be necessary to cut the powerful masseter muscles to pry open the lizard's mouth. More ill-advised techniques, such as grabbing the tail or igniting the lizard (flame under the lower jaw), have also been attempted. The teeth of the Gila monster are poorly anchored, and they are periodically shed. Wounds must be thoroughly explored for the teeth; radiographs of the soft tissue often fail to demonstrate these foreign bodies.[351]

Generally, Gila monster bites have local effects, with direct tissue destruction and capillary membrane injury by serotonin, amine oxidases, phospholipase A, hyaluronidase, and a variety of proteases. Pain is the most common clinical symptom; it usually subsides within 8 to 10 hours, although it can persist for several days. Generalized weakness, dizziness, perspiration, and anxiety are other common symptoms. Hypotension is a common clinical finding with envenomation, and it usually responds to fluid resuscitation alone. There has been one reported case of significant systemic hypotension and myocardial infarction in a 23-year-old after a Gila monster bite.[352] Other common signs include erythema, edema, and even lymphangitis, probably from pathogens injected at the time of the bite; injection of sterile venom produces none of these clinical signs. Severe nausea and vomiting may also be seen. Laboratory abnormalities are rare. The treatment of Gila monster bites consists largely of local wound care and systemic support of the patient (eg, fluids, pain relief, antibiotics, antiemetics). No antivenin is available. Tetanus immunization should be current. A period of observation after the bite to assess the potential for systemic toxicity is warranted.

SPIDERS

More than six genera of spiders in the United States can inflict painful bites, but the most widely known and the ones of medical significance are the *Loxosceles reclusa* (brown recluse spider) and the *Latrodectus mactans* (black widow spider).

The brown recluse spider is so named because it lives in dark, dry places, emerging only at night. It does not spin a web but catches prey by pursuit. It is small (0.5 to 1 cm wide) and is recognizable by the characteristic violin-shaped mark on its cephalothorax (Fig. 11-106). Viewed under a microscope, it has three pairs of eyes rather than two pairs, as most spiders have. In the United States, the brown recluse spider resides primarily in the South and Midwest. Like most biting spiders, they bite humans only if trapped or crushed against the skin. Brown recluse spider bites cause dermonecrosis with edema, ischemia, and cyanosis occurring within 12 hours of the bite, followed occasionally by extensive purpura or hemorrhage surrounding the ischemic halo of the bite site. Within 2 to 4 days, the site develops a characteristic crateriform ulcer, with induration and eschar formation.[353] The eschar may conceal a progressive, undermining necrosis, which can persist for 6 to 8 weeks. These wounds are most severe in the fatty parts of the body, such as the thighs and buttocks, perhaps because of the relatively poor blood supply to these tissues. There may also be a particular dermonecrotic factor in brown recluse venom. Sphingomyelinase D is

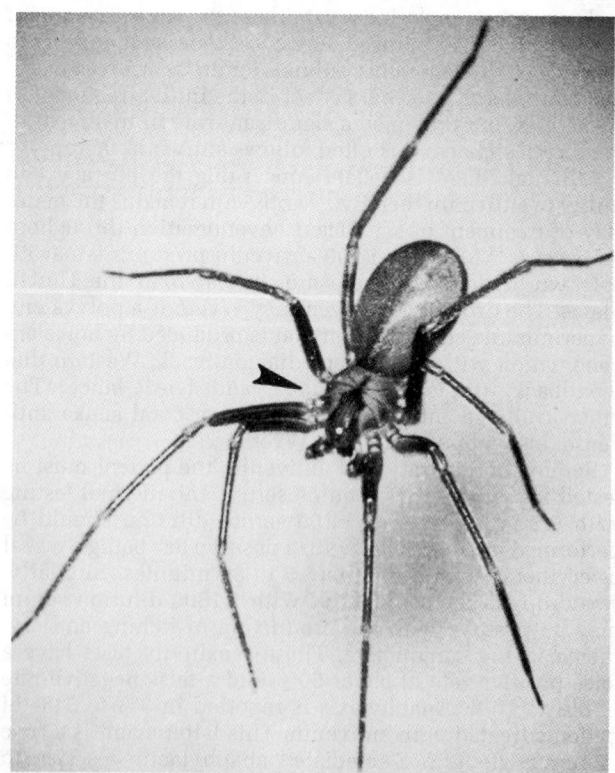

Figure 11-106. *Loxosceles reclusa*, or brown recluse spider. A dark stripe is visible on the dorsal surface of the cephalothorax, which is in the shape of a violin. (Rees R, Campbell D, Rieger E, King LE. The diagnosis and treatment of brown recluse spider bites. Ann Emerg Med 1987;16:945)

present in the venom and appears to interact with the sphingomyelin of the red cell membrane, and perhaps with capillary endothelial cell membranes, causing cell destruction.[354] Histologically, the site of the bite is said to resemble a cutaneous Arthus reaction, with the mechanism involving interactions between complement, neutrophils, and the clotting system.[355] Recent investigations suggest that the necrosis is completely dependent on the victim's neutrophils, yet these neutrophils are not activated by the venom. The *Loxosceles* venom appears to be a novel, yet potent, endothelial cell agonist that stimulates the release of interleukin-8 and granulocyte-macrophage colony-stimulating factor and expression of E-selectin.[356]

Treatment of brown recluse spider bites includes analgesics, antitetanus therapy, avoidance of early surgical débridement, and oral dapsone. Dapsone may work as a neutrophil inhibitor, and it appears to be effective in reducing the size of the skin lesion and limiting the need for surgical débridement.[357] The most common dose is 50 to 100 mg (0.7 mg/kg) twice daily for 3 days to 2 weeks, although it is not approved for this use by the Food and Drug Administration. One controlled trial of dapsone, in guinea pigs injected with spider venom, demonstrated a reduction in lesion induration and necrosis area 72 hours after envenomation.[358] Electric shock therapy had no benefit in that trial. Hyperbaric oxygen treatment of envenomation in rabbits also failed to demonstrate any effect on lesion healing time or superficial appearance, although hyperbaric treatments decreased the amount of necrosis visible histologically on day 24 after envenomation.[359] Local injections of lidocaine or phentolamine and systemic steroids and antihistamines have been widely used in the past but to no demonstrable benefit. Systemic corticosteroids probably have a role only in the rare case of systemic loxoscelism, which produces minimal skin changes but massive hemolysis.[353]

Black widow spiders are found throughout the United States, except for Alaska. Although both the male and the female possess potent venom, the male is smaller in size, and its bite cannot penetrate the skin. The mature female has a black body, about 6 mm in diameter, with a characteristic, red hourglass mark on the ventral aspect of the thorax (Fig. 11-107). This mark is not always present and may consist of only two red dots. The black widow prefers a dry, protected, dimly lit area with access to flies and other insects, such as the outdoor privy. During the period in which the female *L mactans* is guarding an egg sac, she is particularly aggressive and reportedly attacks the male if he disturbs the web, hence earning the common name, black widow.[360]

Black widow toxin contains a systemic neurotoxin, the primary effect of which is chest pain and abdominal pain. The abdominal pain may mimic an abdominal crisis, with marked cramping and a rigid abdomen. The neurologic signs of hyperreflexia, paresthesia, and cutaneous hyperesthesia help distinguish this from a true intraabdominal catastrophe. Profuse sweating, hypertension, and tachycardia are also common.[361] The primary treatment is supportive care and administration of narcotics and muscle relaxants (methocarbamol or benzodiazepam) for pain control, although antivenin therapy also provides effective pain relief in patients with severe envenomations.[362] Antivenin is a horse serum–derived immunoglobulin therapy that is usually suggested for use in children younger than 6 years of age, the very infirm, and patients with severe reaction. The usual dose is one ampule in 50 mL of normal saline solution. Calcium gluconate, 10 mL of a 10% solution given intravenously over a 15- to 20-minute period, has usually been considered to be first-line treatment of severe envenomation, although one report disputes its efficacy at pain relief.[362] Most black widow spider bite symptoms resolve within 1 day, but recurrent symptoms can persist for 2 to 3 days. Antivenin has been reported to be effective up to 30 hours after a bite.[363] The reported mortality rate is 2% to 6%, usually as a result of severe acute or delayed hypersensitivity reactions with paralysis, hemolysis, renal failure, and coma.

HYMENOPTERA

More than 100,000 species of Hymenoptera make up the well-known families of bees, wasps, and hornets and also include the fire ant, a nonwinged Hymenoptera present in the Southeastern United States.[364] More envenomations and more deaths (about 40 annually) in the United States are caused by Hymenoptera stings than by snakebites. The venom of most Hymenoptera species is as toxic as the rattlesnake's venom, the difference being the volume administered. The venom is primarily a hemolysin and neurotoxin, known for triggering anaphylactic reactions. It is estimated that about 0.4% of the population are at risk for anaphylaxis from Hymenoptera stings.[365] Most sting reactions are mild, involving only dermal manifestations such as hives and edema. The clinical effects are related to both the local toxic effects and the anaphylactic systemic effects. The local toxic effects include significant pain, swelling, and pruritus. If a significant amount of toxin is injected, the patient may develop signs of nausea, emesis, and muscle spasms.

Most deaths from Hymenoptera stings are a result of severe anaphylactic reaction, which can occur at any age but are relatively more common in adults. In this reaction, a preformed immunoglobulin E antibody activates mast cells, leading to degranulation with massive histamine release and prompting laryngeal and pulmonary edema, vasodilation, and vascular collapse. The treatment for Hymenoptera bites and stings is to remove the stinger, treat the local wound with ice and possibly an enzymatic meat tenderizer, and treat the anaphylactic reactions aggressively with antihistamines (diphenylhydramine HCl, 50 to 100 mg intramuscularly or intravenously) or epinephrine (1:1000 dilution, 0.3 to 0.5 mL intramuscularly or subcutaneously). Patients also require supplemental oxygen and intravenous fluids.

After sting anaphylaxis, approximately 50% of patients remain allergic to subsequent stings; this is in part determined by the severity of the initial anaphylactic symptoms. Children with benign dermal reactions only are un-

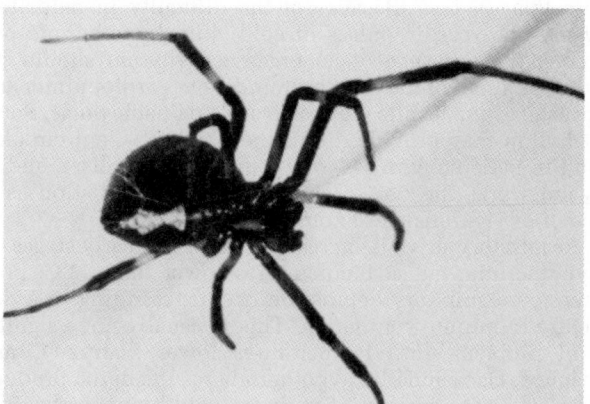

Figure 11-107. *Latrodectus mactans,* or black widow spider. It has a shiny black globular body with the red hourglass mark on the abdomen.

likely to have recurrent reactions. Patients with more severe reactions are at risk for repeat anaphylaxis. Patients with a history of insect sting anaphylaxis and positive venom skin tests should have epinephrine available and are candidates for venom immunotherapy, which provides almost 100% protection against reactions to subsequent stings. Such desensitization can take longer than 3 years.[365]

Two species of imported fire ants now infest large areas of the Gulf Coast states.[366] The most aggressive species, *Solenopsis invicta*, has adapted well to environmental conditions in the southern states, where it has become a considerable agricultural pest and a significant public health problem. Sting reactions typically include a dermal wheal and flare reaction, followed by sterile pustules at sting sites. Occasionally, large, local dermal reactions and pyoderma, or even life-threatening anaphylaxis, can occur. Four venom allergens have been isolated and characterized. Clinical studies are now in progress to compare the safety and efficacy of fire ant venom with whole-body extract for diagnosis and treatment of fire ant allergy.[364]

SCORPIONS

More than 650 types of scorpions can be found worldwide. In the United States, most are not lethal, and the sting results primarily in local effects. In parts of Brazil, Mexico, North Africa, India, and Israel, however, the scorpion sting can be lethal. The venom toxicity depends greatly on species, season, and the age of the scorpion. In a fatal response, the venom induces a sympathetic storm, resulting in hypertension, tachycardia, and high-output cardiac failure.[367] Serum biochemistry reveals increased potassium and glucose, decreased sodium, and markedly elevated catecholamine levels. The treatment is specific antivenin therapy and systemic support directed at controlling hypertension and acute pulmonary edema. The outcome in the United States is usually excellent, with complete resolution of local effects, but in some parts of Brazil, the mortality rates for a scorpion bite have been reported to be as high as 12% in adults and 60% in children.[368] In India, of 34 children admitted to hospital after scorpion sting, 14 had hypertension, 9 had acute pulmonary edema, 5 had myocardial failure, and 4 died.[367] In another study from Israel, respiratory distress was the main feature in 17 of 54 children with scorpion stings, but only 3 required mechanical ventilation. Two patients died, but both had failed to receive antivenom.[369]

HYPOTHERMIA

Because humans are homeotherms, we attempt to maintain a constant body temperature despite changes in environmental temperature. Humans have a remarkable capacity to dissipate heat at the cost of evaporating body water; however, our tropical evolutionary heritage has provided us with far less ability to cope with cold conditions. As a result, hypothermia can occur in a variety of clinical settings, and from a number of causes (Table 11-35).

To allow for the normal diurnal temperature variation of 1° to 2°C, hypothermia is considered to be present in humans if the core temperature drops below 35°C. Hypothermia is usually classified by temperature zone as mild (32° to 35°C), moderate (28° to 32°C), or severe (less than 28°C).[370,371] Primary accidental hypothermia is defined as a decrease in core temperature that occurs as a result of overwhelming environmental cold stress. It most often occurs as a result of recreational misadventures that lead to cold water immersion or prolonged environmental exposure. Secondary accidental hypothermia occurs as a result of abnormalities in thermoregulation and is often seen in

Table 11-35. CLINICAL DEFINITIONS OF HYPOTHERMIA AND EXAMPLES OF SETTINGS IN WHICH THEY OCCUR

Type	Settings
Accidental	Recreational environmental exposure, cold water immersion
Therapeutic	Treatment of Reye syndrome, cardiopulmonary bypass, organ preservation
Drug induced	Alcohol, anesthetics, barbiturates, phenothiazines, morphine, others
CNS dysfunction	Transection of spinal cord, hypopituitarism, cerebrovascular accidents
Hypothalamic dysfunction	Wernicke encephalopathy, anorexia nervosa, head trauma, pinealoma, other tumors
Metabolic	Hypoglycemia, hypothyroidism, hypoadrenalism, malnutrition
Dermal dysfunction	Burns, erythrodermas
Traumatic	Occurs after any major injury

(Adapted from Jurkovich GJ. Hypothermia in the trauma patient. Adv Trauma 1989;4:111)

neonates or in elderly persons, in patients with metabolic abnormalities (eg, hypothyroidism), and in association with alcohol intoxication, drug use, or anesthesia.

The physiologic response to hypothermia is one of transitional changes, with few exact temperature-dependent responses (Fig. 11-108). Broadly speaking, the transition from a "safe zone" of hypothermia (in which physiologic adaptations to heat loss are working) to a "danger zone" of hypothermia (in which shivering is abolished, metabolism decreases, and heat loss is passively accepted) occurs between 33° and 30°C. The initial effects of hypothermia mimic intense sympathetic stimulation, with tremulousness, profound vasoconstriction, tremendous increases in oxygen consumption, and acceleration of heart rate and minute ventilation.[372]

The cardiovascular response includes tachycardia, followed by progressive bradycardia, which starts at about 34°C and results in a 50% heart rate decrease at 28°C. The conduction system is particularly sensitive to hypothermia: the PR, then the QRS, and finally the QT interval become progressively prolonged.[373] At core temperatures lower than 32°C, a variety of atrial and then ventricular dysrhythmias occur. Asystole occurs at core temperatures less than 25°C.[374] Because of the difficulty in palpating weak, bradycardic pulses in cold, stiff, hypothermic patients, the presence of an organized rhythm should be taken as a sign of life that contraindicates cardiopulmonary resuscitation, despite the absence of a palpable pulse. Such a rhythm may provide diminished but sufficient circulation in patients with severely reduced metabolism, and it is not worth the risk of converting it to fibrillation as a result of vigorous chest compressions.

Respiratory drive is increased during the early stages of hypothermia, but at temperatures lower than 33°C, progressive respiratory depression occurs, resulting in a decrease in minute ventilation. This is usually not a significant problem until temperatures lower than 29°C are reached. Occasionally, hypothermia results in the production of a large amount of mucous (cold bronchorrhea).[375] Because ciliary action and the cough reflex are also depressed, this effect predisposes to atelectasis and aspiration. Noncardiogenic pulmonary edema is also occasion-

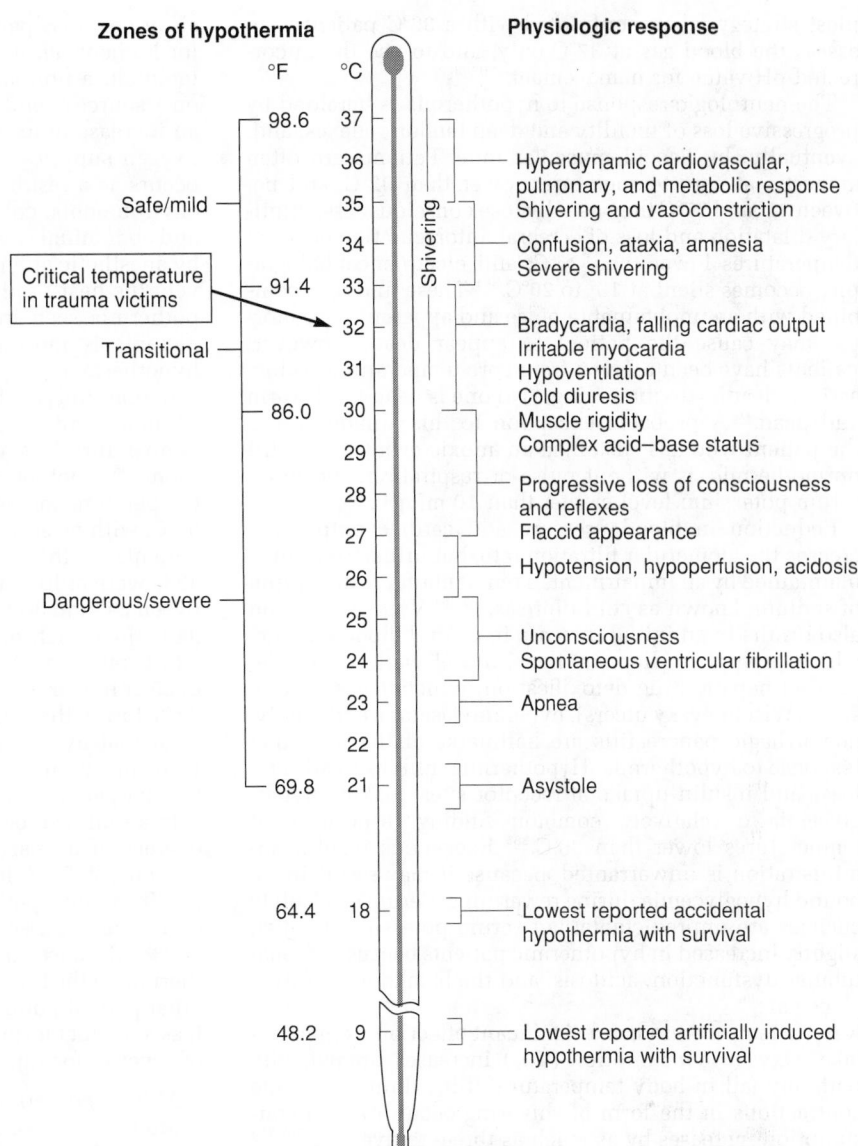

Zones of hypothermia

Physiologic response

°F   °C

— 98.6   37

— 36

Safe/mild —   35 — Hyperdynamic cardiovascular, pulmonary, and metabolic response
Shivering and vasoconstriction

— 34 — Confusion, ataxia, amnesia
Severe shivering

— 91.4   33

Transitional —   32 — Bradycardia, falling cardiac output
Irritable myocardia

— 31 — Hypoventilation
Cold diuresis

— 86.0   30 — Muscle rigidity

— 29 — Complex acid–base status

— 28 — Progressive loss of consciousness
and reflexes

— 27 — Flaccid appearance

— 26 — Hypotension, hypoperfusion, acidosis

Dangerous/severe —   25

— 24 — Unconsciousness
Spontaneous ventricular fibrillation

— 23 — Apnea

— 22

— 69.8   21 — Asystole

64.4   18 — Lowest reported accidental
hypothermia with survival

48.2   9 — Lowest reported artificially induced
hypothermia with survival

Critical temperature in trauma victims (label pointing to 32°C)

Shivering (bracket spanning ~37–32°C)

Figure 11-108. Zones of hypothermia and corresponding physiologic response. Because of wide biologic variability, physiologic changes rarely occur at the exact temperatures given. (Jurkovich GJ. Hypothermia in the trauma patient. Adv Trauma 1989;4:111)

ally reported, especially in elderly patients, and especially after prolonged periods of hypothermia.[376]

Perhaps the greatest controversy regarding the pulmonary effects of hypothermia concerns the need to correct blood gases to the patient's hypothermic body temperature. Arterial blood gas samples are always warmed to 37°C before measurement. A nomogram is then used to estimate the blood gas values at the patient's actual body temperature. With each 1°C temperature reduction, the partial pressure of carbon dioxide (PCO_2) decreases by 4.4%, and the partial pressure of oxygen (PO_2) decreases by 7.2%. Thus, a blood gas measurement at 37°C with a PCO_2 of 40 and a PO_2 of 70 in a 32°C patient is reported as having a PCO_2 of 32 and a PO_2 of 48 after temperature correction.

The decrease in partial pressure is related to the increased solubility of gases in cold fluids and is not a result of a change in carbon dioxide content, oxygen content, or serum bicarbonate level. Clinicians often assume that the normal PCO_2 and PO_2 at 37°C are the values that should be attained at all temperatures. However, if normothermic endpoints for PCO_2 were attained in a hypothermic patient they would represent an increase in total body stores of carbon dioxide, which would manifest as a rising PCO_2

and a falling pH during rewarming. Likewise, attempts to increase a PO_2 that reflects normal oxygen content at a lower temperature are also inappropriate. A far simpler strategy is to assess the blood gases at 37°C without temperature correction. Values that are normal and acceptable when reported at 37°C correspond to normal values and contents when corrected for hypothermic temperatures.

Temperature correction of blood gases for pH management is also unnecessary. A pH of 7.40 at 37°C would be temperature-corrected to 7.47 in a 32°C patient. At 37°C, the acid–base balance of water is neutral (pH=pOH) at a pH of 6.8, and the body functions optimally when its pH is offset by 0.6 pH units above the neutral point of water (ie, has a relatively alkaline pH of 7.40). The pH of water rises with cooling, causing the pH of blood to rise by 0.015 pH units per degree Celsius, without a change in bicarbonate content.[377,378] Maintaining a 30°C patient at a pH of 7.40 instead of 7.47 fails to maintain the normal pH offset above the neutral point of water (relative alkalinity) and results in an acidotic cellular and chemical environment that has a multiplicity of effects on enzyme systems. Because blood with a pH of 7.40 assessed at 37°C is reported as having a pH of 7.47 when temperature is corrected to 32°C, the simplest strategy when confronted with a 32°C patient is to assess the blood gas at 37°C only, and to use the uncorrected pH value for management.[379,380]

The neurologic response to hypothermia is heralded by progressive loss of lucidity and deep tendon reflexes, and, eventually, by flaccid muscular tone. Patients are often amnestic at core temperatures lower than 32°C, and between 31° and 27°C they usually lose consciousness. Pupillary dilatation and loss of cerebral autoregulation occur at temperatures lower than 26°C, and electroencephalography becomes silent at 19° to 20°C.[381] These findings, combined with an unobtainable pulse and apparent rigor mortis, may cause the patient to appear dead. However, patients have been revived from core temperatures as low as 17°C, leading to the saying, "No one is dead until warm and dead." A probable exception to this admonition is the patient who has sustained an anoxic event while still normothermic, is without pulse or respiration, and has a serum potassium level greater than 10 mEq/L.[382]

Reduction in blood pressure and cardiac output decreases the glomerular filtration rate, but urinary output is maintained by an impairment in renal tubular reabsorption of sodium, known as cold diuresis.[383,384] Vasoconstriction also results in an initial increase in central blood volume, which prompts a diuresis. Ileus, bowel wall edema, depressed hepatic drug detoxification, punctate gastric erosions (Wischnevsky ulcers), hyperamylasemia, and, rarely, hemorrhagic pancreatitis are hallmarks of the intestinal response to hypothermia. Hypothermia inhibits insulin release and insulin uptake at receptor sites, making hyperglycemia a relatively common finding, especially at temperatures lower than 30°C.[385] Exogenous insulin administration is unwarranted, because it may result in rebound hypoglycemia during rewarming. Serum electrolyte changes are unpredictable, but serum potassium is often slightly increased in hypothermic patients because of renal tubular dysfunction, acidosis, and the breakdown of liver glycogen.[386]

Body temperature has a significant effect on oxygen uptake. Oxygen consumption ($\dot{V}o_2$) increases dramatically with any fall in body temperature. If involuntary muscle contractions in the form of shivering occur, oxygen consumption increases by as much as three- to five-fold.[387,388] Shivering is inefficient because it produces heat near the surface of the body, causing most of it to be lost to the environment, with less than 45% being retained by the patient.[387]

The thermoregulatory drive is such a powerful one that it takes precedence over many other homeostatic functions. The consequent increase in oxygen use can result in anaerobic metabolism, acidosis, and significant cardiopulmonary stress.[389] One study noted a 35% increase in consumption of oxygen and a 65% increase in production of carbon dioxide in postsurgical patients after resolution of anesthesia, when the thermostatic drive reappeared.[390] In another study, a core temperature decrease of as little as 0.3°C in postoperative patients was associated with a 7% increase in $\dot{V}o_2$, and temperature reductions between 0.3° and 1.2°C were associated with a 92% increase in $\dot{V}o_2$, with proportional increases in minute ventilation.[391] Further details of the responses of specific organ systems to hypothermia are beyond the scope of this section, but the interested reader is referred to several excellent in-depth monographs.[371,392–395]

Hypothermia in Trauma Patients

Mild hypothermia is very common after traumatic injury. If ambient temperature falls below the thermoneutral temperature (ie, the temperature at which no thermogene-

sis or heat dissipation is necessary), which is 28°C (82.5°F) for humans, an increase in heat production is required to maintain a normal body temperature. Combustion is the only source of endogenous heat production, and it requires an increase in oxygen use. However, after shock or injury oxygen supplies are often limited, and further heat loss occurs as a result of cold emergency and operating room environments, cold fluid resuscitation, and open thoracic and abdominal cavities. This problem is further aggravated by anesthetic and neuromuscular blocking agents that prevent the heat-producing shivering response. Thus, the hypothermia seen in surgical patients or critically injured patients is most often a form of secondary accidental hypothermia.

In one study, 57% of trauma patients admitted to a level I trauma center were hypothermic at some time, and the temperature loss was most significant in the emergency room.[396] Another study reported that the average initial temperature for 94 intubated major trauma victims was 35°C, with no seasonal variation.[397] Sixty-six percent of all patients in this study were hypothermic on admission: 43% were mildly hypothermic, with core temperatures between 34° and 36°C, and 23% had temperatures lower than 34°C. Jurkovich and colleagues reported that 42% of 71 adult trauma victims with an Injury Severity Score (ISS) of 25 or higher reached a core temperature lower than 34°C, 23% lower than 33°C, and 13% lower than 32°C.[398] It is clear that hypothermia is a common occurrence after severe injury, and that any degree of hypothermia in the trauma patient can be detrimental.

In a multicenter review, the mortality rate for moderate degrees of primary accidental hypothermia (28° to 32°C) was only 21%.[399] In contrast, moderate levels of hypothermia in surgical patients, particularly those who are victims of trauma, are associated with a mortality rate approaching 100%. Because the mortality rate associated with hypothermia in the trauma victim is so high in comparison with other patient populations, some have proposed classifying it as a distinct form of hypothermia.[400] The following zones of severity for injury hypothermia have been proposed:

Mild hypothermia–36° to 34°C (96.8° to 93.2°F)
Moderate hypothermia—34° to 32°C (93.2° to 89.6°F)
Severe hypothermia—less than 32°C (less than 89.6°F)

Core hypothermia appears to occur only in victims of relatively severe trauma. Little and Stoner, reporting on a heterogeneous group of 82 trauma patients, observed that hypothermia occurred only in those patients with an ISS greater than 12.[401] Skin temperature fell from 32° to 31.7°C, whereas core temperature fell from 37.3°C to 36.5°C. Hypothermia did not occur in less severely injured patients, and shivering, which could have been expected, was noted in only one of the hypothermic patients. Mild degrees of injury have been associated with small elevations in core body temperature, particularly if the shivering response mechanism has not been ablated.[393,402]

Hypothermia should be considered an ominous sign in the trauma patient, an indicator of severe physiologic injury and a predictor of poor outcome; even mild hypothermia can be an ominous sign. Two reports have noted that regardless of the index temperature defining the degree of hypothermia, the mortality rate among hypothermic trauma patients is consistently greater than among those who remain warm.[398,403] Both the mortality rate and the incidence of hypothermia increase with higher ISS, massive fluid resuscitation, and the presence of shock. After controlling for each of these variables, the mortality rate of the hypothermic patient is still greater than that of the warm trauma patient. No patient whose core body temperature fell below 32°C in these studies survived. Steinemann and colleagues confirmed that early posttraumatic hypothermia correlated with hemorrhagic shock, although they did not demonstrate hypothermia as an independent variable of mortality if the patients were stratified by TRISS methodology.[404] However, hypothermia is known to affect the physiologic variables that determine TRISS calculations; this influence would result in an overestimation of the severity of injury in cold patients.

The apparent detrimental effect of hypothermia in the human trauma victim is in contrast to a large body of animal experimental evidence suggesting that hypothermia has a protective role in shock. This rather extensive body of literature is reviewed elsewhere[393], but in general animals subjected to combined hypothermia and shock (eg, hemorrhage, burn, blunt trauma) usually survive longer than similarly injured but actively warmed animals. Blalock and Mason were among the first in modern times to recognize the ability of hypothermia to prolong survival times after shock, but they emphasized that the overall survival rate was unchanged.[405] However, increased survival rates and times were shown recently in a rat hypothermia model after hemorrhagic shock.[406] More recently, the protective effects of hypothermia in preventing ischemia-reperfusion injury have been described in both an intestinal and muscle ischemia model.[407,408]

The role of hypothermia in patients with shock remains unclear. The physiologic consequence of severe trauma is a drop in core body temperature; it remains unclear, however, whether this is a protective response against shock or the result of diminished heat production due to failing metabolism. The frequent presence of lactic acid accumulation in cold, seriously injured patients supports the latter hypothesis. Clinical studies indicate that even mild hypothermia in the trauma patient is predictive of a poor outcome. Hypothermia does diminish metabolic demands and oxygen consumption in anesthetized patients, but the price appears to be malfunction of enzymes and physiologic systems necessary to recover from injury.

Perhaps the systems most affected in patients sustaining major trauma are those involved in clotting. Reports of coagulation abnormalities in patients with apparently normal clotting factor levels surfaced shortly after the introduction of hypothermic cardioplegia for cardiac surgery.[409,410] Although hemodilution with volume expanders that are deficient in clotting factors and platelets is thought to be the primary cause of nonsurgical bleeding, attempts to determine the cause of coagulopathy have recently focused on the affects of hypothermia on platelet and clotting factor function.

Levels of hypothermia commonly encountered in clinical practice have been found to have a significant effect on platelet function. Cold platelets undergo morphologic changes that affect adherence, including loss of shape, cytoplasmic swelling, and dissolution of cytoplasmic microtubules necessary for normal motility. These changes often render cold, transfused platelets inactive.[411] Platelet activation is also associated with activation of cell-membrane phospholipases; these enzymes hydrolyze phospholipids to arachidonic acid, a precursor to prostaglandin endoperoxides and thromboxane A_2, a potent vasoconstrictor that is necessary for normal platelet aggregation.[412] Valeri and associates induced systemic hypothermia to 32°C in baboons but kept one forearm warm by using heating lamps and a warming blanket.[413] Simultaneous bleeding time measurements in the warm and cold arms were 2.4 and 5.8 minutes, respectively. This effect, which was reversible with rewarming, appeared to be mediated by cold-induced slowing of the enzymatic reaction rate of thromboxane synthetase, which resulted in decreased production of thromboxane A_2.

As with blood gases, clinical tests of coagulation are temperature-standardized to 37°C. Fibrometers contain a thermal block that heats the plasma and reagents to 37°C before initiating the assay. Tests of coagulation therefore reflect clotting factor deficiencies but are corrected for any potential effect of hypothermia on clotting factor function. In a detailed study of the kinetic effects of hypothermia on clotting factor function, clotting tests (PT, PTT, and thrombin time) were performed on reference human plasma containing normal clotting factor levels at temperatures ranging from 25° to 37°C. The results showed a significant slowing of all coagulation tests at temperatures lower than 35°C, in proportion to the degree of hypothermia.[414] The prolongation of clot formation occurred at clinically relevant levels of hypothermia and was equivalent to that seen in normothermic patients with significant clotting factor depletion. For example, assays conducted at 35°, 33°, and 31°C prolonged the PTT to the same extent as would occur in a euthermic patient with reductions in factor IX levels to 66%, 32%, and 7% of normal, respectively.

Clotting factor supplementation is not the answer to a hypothermia-induced coagulopathy: rewarming is. However, in many seriously injured patients, clotting factor depletion exists in conjunction with hypothermia. It was recently demonstrated[415] that a potentiating effect of hypothermia on coagulation dysfunction occurs in plasma with deficient clotting factor levels, although there does not appear to be synergy between the two conditions. Hypothermic, coagulopathic trauma patients still benefit from coagulation profile testing. If prolongation of PT and PTT are evident in plasma warmed to 37°C, clotting factor replacement is indicated; if PT and PTT are almost normal, rewarming alone reverses the clinically apparent coagulopathy.

Treatment

Rewarming techniques are usually classified as passive external rewarming, active external rewarming, or active core rewarming.[371,416] Passive external rewarming simply implies allowing spontaneous rewarming to occur with the patient removed from a hypothermic environment; it is usually used only for the mildly hypothermic patient. Active external rewarming techniques include surrounding the patient with warm blankets or heating pads, use of infrared heating lamps, and immersion in warm water. Active core rewarming techniques include heated peritoneal or thoracic lavage; heated gastric, bladder, or colonic lavage; use of heated and water-saturated inhaled air; and extracorporeal circulatory rewarming.

The advantages and disadvantages of each technique are regularly debated, particularly regarding the role of external versus core rewarming. The rate of heat transfer to the hypothermic patient is greatest with active core rewarming, particularly extracorporeal circulation rewarming. This may be a critical factor in surgical patients, who need rapid restoration of clotting and cardiac function is necessary.

The technique of rewarming the hypothermic victim by extracorporeal circulation has been described by numerous authors in the past two decades, primarily on the basis of a small number of personal experiences.[417,418] The technique has limited applicability in surgical patients, but it has appeal in cases of primary accidental hypothermia, in which maintenance of circulation, correction of hypoxia, and replenishment of intravascular volume may play a role as large as correction of the temperature change itself. Improvements in heparin-bonded circuitry and the use of atraumatic centrifugal pumps may eventually remove the restriction that systemic anticoagulation places on extra-corporeal bypass.

A newly described active core rewarming technique has been termed continuous arteriovenous rewarming.[419] This technique makes use of the patient's own blood pressure to drive an extracorporeal circuit through a small, efficient countercurrent heat exchange device. Heparin-bonded short tubing lengths, the relative anticoagulated state of most hypothermic trauma victims, and its relative ease of use may make this device widely applicable in rewarming of severely hypothermic patients with intact circulations.

The use of body cavity lavage with warm solutions is a simple, less invasive method of accomplishing active core rewarming. However, rewarming rates with body cavity lavage vary greatly according to initial core temperature, dialysate temperature, infusion rate, and dwell time. Several studies support the notion that active core rewarming by peritoneal lavage is preferable to active external rewarming.[371,420] One group recently examined three techniques for rewarming hypothermic and cardiac-arrested dogs, concluding that both peritoneal lavage (55°C dialysate) and partial extracorporeal circulation were faster than active external rewarming with a heating blanket.[371] A frequently stated disadvantage of external rewarming is that the peripheral tissues are rewarmed in advance of the core, resulting in peripheral vasodilation. In the presence of inadequate volume resuscitation, this can result in vascular collapse (rewarming shock) and a subsequent fall in central temperature (afterdrop) as the cold peripheral blood returns to the core. It is debatable whether this is the mechanism of the core afterdrop, however, because a core afterdrop has been noted to occur in animal models even during complete circulatory arrest. Volume contraction caused by vasoconstriction, cold diuresis, and cellular swelling coupled with inadequate fluid resuscitation may be a more appropriate explanation for circulatory collapse during rewarming.

The thermodynamic principles of heat transfer to the hypothermic patient are reviewed in greater detail elsewhere, but a sense of rewarming rates and quantity of heat transferred by various techniques is instructional.[416,421,422] Ventilation of a patient with a core temperature of 32°C with water-saturated air at 41°C results in a maximum heat transfer rate of 9 kcal/h. For comparison, basal metabolic heat generation produces about 70 kcal/h, and shivering produces up to 250 kcal/h. Given the specific heat of the body (0.083 kcal/kg per degree Celsius), 58 kcal is required to raise the temperature of a 70-kg patient by 1°C. More than 6 hours would therefore be required to warm a 32°C patient using humidified inspired air at 41°C.

Heat transfer rates with body cavity lavage can be similarly calculated, based on the specific heat of water (1 kcal/kg per degree Celsius). If 1 L water at 44°C is infused into a body cavity and dwells long enough to exit at 40°C, 4 kcal of heat has been transferred to the patient. More than 14 L of fluid is needed to increase the patient's core temperature by 1°C. However, warming becomes less efficient as the patient rewarms, and a longer dwell time is required to reduce the temperature of the infusate to 40°C.

Warming by cardiopulmonary bypass or continuous arteriovenous rewarming is the most efficient method of core heating. With flow rates of 15 to 30 L/h, it is possible to deliver 120 to 240 kcal/h if the reinfused blood is heated to 40°C, a rate of heat transfer more than 10 times that of the other methods. In any case, the urgency with which rewarming must be accomplished depends on how adversely the hypothermia is affecting the patient. With the exception of extracorporeal circulatory methods, most rewarming techniques serve primarily to prevent loss of endogenously generated heat and are ineffective in circumstances in which rapid rewarming is indicated. Early attention to the mechanisms of heat loss is necessary to prevent the metabolic and hemorrhagic complications associated with hypothermia in surgical patients.

COLD INJURY AND FROSTBITE

Cold injuries limited to digits, extremities, or exposed surfaces are caused either by direct tissue freezing (frostbite) or by more chronic exposure to an environment just above freezing (chilblain or pernio; trench foot). Cold injury has been a major cause of morbidity during war experiences. It resulted in more than 7 million lost soldier fighting days by Allied forces in World War II and was reportedly the most common major injury sustained by British soldiers in the Falkland Islands expedition.[423]

Chilblain and pernio are descriptive terms for a form of local cold injury characterized by pruritic, red-purple papules, macules, plaques, or nodules on the skin. The lesions are often associated with edema or blistering and are caused by a chronic vasculitis of the dermis.[424] This pathology appears to be provoked by repeated exposure to cold, but not freezing, temperatures. This injury typically occurs on the face, the anterior surface of the tibia, or the dorsum of the hands and feet, areas poorly protected or chronically exposed to the environment. With continued exposure, ulcerative or hemorrhagic lesions may appear and progress to scarring, fibrosis, and atrophy. Treatment consists of sheltering the patient, elevating the affected part on sheepskin, and allowing gradual rewarming at room temperature. Rubbing and massage are contraindicated because they can cause further damage and secondary infection.

Trench foot or cold-immersion foot (or hand) describes a nonfreezing injury of the hands or feet, typically seen in sailors, fishermen, or soldiers, that is caused by chronic exposure to wet conditions and temperatures just above freezing.[425] It appears to involve an alternating arterial vasospasm and vasodilatation, with the affected tissue first cold and anesthetic and then hyperemic after 24 to 48 hours of exposure. With the hyperemia comes an intense, painful burning and dysesthesia, and tissue damage is characterized by edema, blistering, redness, ecchymosis, and ulceration. Complications of local infection or cellulitis, lymphangitis, and gangrene may occur. A posthyperemic phase occurs 2 to 6 weeks later and is characterized by tissue cyanosis with increased sensitivity to cold. Treatment is best started during or before the reactive hyperemia state and consists of immediate removal of the extremity from the cold, wet environment and exposure of the feet (or hands) to warm, dry air. Elevation to minimize edema, protection of pressure spots, and local and systemic measures to combat infection are indicated. Massage, soaking of the feet, and rapid rewarming are not indicated. Demyelination of nerves, muscle atrophy, fallen arches, and osteoporosis may all present long-term complications, and some patients develop a tendency toward marked vasospasm during subsequent exposure to cold.[426]

Frostnip is the mildest form of cold injury. It is characterized by initial pain and pallor, with subsequent numbness of the affected body part. Skiers and other winter outdoor enthusiasts are most likely to suffer this cold injury to the nose, ears, or tips of digits. The injury is reversible, and warming of the cold tissue results in return of sensation and function with no tissue loss.

Frostbite is a more severe and more common form of cold injury that essentially consists of local freezing of tissues. Frostbite is traditionally classified into four grades of injury severity:

First degree—tissue freezing with hyperemia and edema, but without blistering
Second degree—tissue freezing with hyperemia, edema, and characteristic large, clear blisters
Third degree—tissue freezing with death of subcutaneous tissues and skin, resulting in hemorrhagic vesicles that are usually smaller than second-degree blisters
Fourth degree—tissue necrosis, gangrene, and eventual full-thickness tissue loss

The affected body part almost always appears hard, cold, white, and anesthetic initially, regardless of the depth of injury. Because the appearance of the lesion changes frequently during the course of treatment, and because the initial treatment regimen is applicable for all degrees of insult,[427] some authorities suggest discarding this classification as a prognostic impossibility, and simply classify frostbite as either superficial or deep.[428]

Weather conditions, altitude, degree of protective clothing, duration of exposure, and degree of tissue wetness are all contributing external factors to the development of frostbite injury. Because sensory nerve activity is abolished at a skin temperature of 7° to 9°C, the disappearance of pain is an early warning sign of cold injury. Acclimation to cold may be protective, whereas a previous history of frostbite probably predisposes to another cold tissue injury. Smoking and a history of arterial disease also are contributing factors. In urban environments, over 50% of frostbite injuries are alcohol related, and a significant portion of these patients (16%) have an underlying psychiatric illness.[429]

Evidence suggests that frostbite injury has two components—the initial freeze injury and a reperfusion injury that occurs during rewarming. The initial response to tissue cooling is vasoconstriction and arteriovenous shunting, intermittently relieved (every 5 to 7 minutes) by vasodilation, the so-called hunting response.[430] With prolonged exposure, this response fails, and the temperature of the freezing tissue approximates ambient temperature until −2°C. At that point, extracellular ice crystals form, and as they enlarge, the osmotic pressure of the interstitium increases, resulting in movement of intracellular water into the interstitium. Cells begin to shrink and become hyperosmolar, with disruption of cellular enzyme function. If freezing is rapid, intracellular ice crystals form, resulting in immediate cell death. Intravascularly, disruption of endothelial cells and sludging of red cells result in cessation of circulation.

During rewarming, red cell, platelet, and leukocyte aggregation are known to occur and to cause patchy thrombosis of the microcirculation. These accumulated blood elements are thought to release, among other products, the toxic oxygen free radicals and the arachidonic acid metabolites $PGF_{2\alpha}$ and thromboxane A_2, which further aggravate vasoconstriction and platelet and leukocyte aggregation.[431] However, the exact mechanism of tissue destruction and death after freeze injury remains poorly defined. Animal studies suggest that vascular injury in the form of endothelial cell damage and subsequent interstitial edema, but not vessel thrombosis, predominates as the initial event in rewarming injury.[432] A substantial component of severe cold injury may be neutrophil mediated, as suggested by the observation that a monoclonal antibody to neutrophil-endothelial and neutrophil-neutrophil adherence can markedly ameliorate the pathology of a severe cold injury.[433] In this rabbit model, animals treated with the anti-CD11/CD18 adhesion molecule after cold injury (30 minutes at −15°C) but before rewarming (in a 39°C water bath) had significantly less tissue loss and edema. The implication of these observations is that much of the injury of severe frostbite occurs during rewarming or reperfusion. Clinical applications of these experimental observations remain untested.

Treatment

Prehospital or field care of the victim of cold injury should focus on removal of the patient from the hostile environment and protection of the injured body part from further damage. Rubbing or exercising of the affected tissue does not augment blood flow and risks further cold injury or mechanical trauma. Because repeated bouts of freezing and thawing worsen the injury, it is preferable to immediately seek definitive shelter and care for the patient with frostbite of the hands or feet rather than to rewarm the tissue in the field and risk refreezing. Although the initial symptoms may be mild and overlooked by the patient, severe pain, burning, edema, and even necrosis and gangrene may appear with rewarming. With severe injury, there is a progressive decrease in range of motion, and edema becomes prominent. The injury can progress to numbness and, eventually, to loss of all sensation in the affected tissue.

The emergency room treatment of a frostbite victim should first focus on the basic ABCs of trauma resuscitation, and systemic hypothermia should be identified and corrected. Most patients are dehydrated, and resuscitation with warm fluids is an important part of early treatment. Fractures often lead to frostbite in mountaineers, and although manipulation may be required to treat vascular compromise, open reduction is hazardous, and application of traction should be delayed until after postthawing edema has been assessed.

Gradual, spontaneous rewarming is inadequate, especially for deeper injuries, and delayed thawing or rubbing of the injured part in ice or snow often results in marked tissue loss.[434] Rapid rewarming is achieved by immersing the tissue in a large water bath of 40° to 42°C (104° to 108 °F). The water should feel warm, but not hot, to the normal hand. The bath should be large enough to prevent rapid loss of heat, and the water temperature should be maintained. Dry heat is not advocated because it is difficult to regulate and because the use of excessive heat can be disastrous. The rewarming process should take about 30 to 45 minutes for digits; the affected area appears flush after rewarming is complete and good circulation has been reestablished. Narcotics are required, because the rewarming process can be quite painful.

The skin is gently but meticulously cleaned and air dried, and the affected area is elevated to minimize edema. A tetanus toxoid booster is administered as indicated by the immunization history. Sterile cotton is placed between the toes or fingers to prevent skin maceration, and extreme care is taken to prevent infection and to avoid even the slightest abrasion. The affected tissue is protected by a tent or cradle, and pressure spots are prevented. In one review, infection developed in 13% of urban frostbite victims, but one half of these infections were present at time of admission.[429] Most clinicians reserve antibiotics for specific infections.[435]

After rewarming, the treatment goals are to prevent further injury while awaiting demarcation of irreversible tissue destruction. All patients should be hospitalized, and affected tissue should be gently cleansed once or twice a day in warm (38°C) whirlpool baths. Some clinicians add an antiseptic such as chlorhexidine or an iodophor to the bath.[435] Based on the findings of arachidonic acid metabolites in the blisters of frostbite victims, some authors have advocated the use of topical aloe vera (a thromboxane inhibitor) and systemic ibuprofen or aspirin. Heggers and colleagues described a nonrandomized trial in which 56 patients who were treated with these agents plus prophylactic penicillin had less tissue loss, a lower amputation rate, and shorter hospital stays than 98 patients treated with warm saline solution, silver sulfadiazine (Silvadene), or mafenide acetate (Sulfamylon) dressings.[431] Uninfected blebs should be left intact, because they provide a sterile biologic dressing for 7 to 10 days and protect underlying epithelialization. After resolution of edema, digits should be exercised during the whirlpool bath and physical therapy should be begun. Tobacco, nicotine, and other vasoconstrictive agents must be withheld. Weight bearing is prohibited until complete resolution of edema.

Numerous adjuvants have been suggested and tried in an effort to restore blood supply to frostbitten areas. The intense vasoconstrictive effect of cold injury has focused attention on increased sympathetic tone. Sympathetic blockade and even surgical sympathectomy has been advocated as early therapy, under the theory that it would reduce the vasospasm that precipitates thrombosis in the affected tissue.[436] This method of treatment has produced inconsistent results in experimental studies and is difficult to evaluate clinically. Although it can mollify the chronic pain, hyperhidrosis, and vasospasm of cold injuries, it may increase vascular shunting. In one series, physicians noted a more proximal demarcation of injury in sympathectomized limbs than in nonsympathectomized ones, despite apparently equal bilateral injury.[434]

Experience with intraarterial vasodilating drugs such as reserpine and tolazoline has also been unrewarding. Bouwman and colleagues demonstrated in a controlled clinical study that immediate (mean, 3 hours) ipsilateral intraarterial infusion of reserpine coupled with early (mean, 3 days) ipsilateral operative sympathectomy failed to alter the natural history of acute frostbite injury when compared with the contralateral limb.[437] Heparin, thrombolytic agents, and hyperbaric oxygen have also failed to demonstrated any substantial treatment benefit, whereas low-molecular-weight dextran alleviated postthawing circulatory obstruction as late as 2 hours after thawing and markedly reduced tissue loss in rabbit feet.[438,439]

The difficulty in determining the depth of tissue destruction in cold injury has led to a conservative approach to the care of frostbite injuries.[440,441] As a general rule, amputation and surgical débridement are delayed for 2 to 3 months unless infection with sepsis intervenes. The natural history of a full-thickness frostbite injury is the gradual demarcation of the injured area with dry gangrene or mummification clearly delineating nonviable tissue. Often the permanent tissue loss is much less than originally suspected. In an Alaska series, only 10.5% of patients required amputation, and it usually involved only phalanges or portions of phalanges.[442] The need for emergency surgery is unusual, but vigilance should be maintained during the rewarming phase for the development of a compartment syndrome requiring fasciotomy. Open amputations are indicated in patients with persistent infection and sepsis that is refractory to débridement and antibiotics. Mills and colleagues[434] convincingly demonstrated that of all the factors in the treatment of frostbite that can influence outcome, premature surgical intervention by any means, in any amount, was by far the greatest contributor to a poor result.

The use of technetium-99m methylene diphosphonate bone scanning has shown some promise in the early detection of eventual bone and soft tissue viability.[443] Preliminary data on small numbers of patients suggest that triple-phase scanning (1 minute, 2 hours, 7 hours) performed 48 hours after admission accurately predicts the eventual level of bone and soft tissue viability.

Frostbitten tissues seldom recover completely. Some degree of cold insensitivity invariably remains. Hyperhidrosis (in up to 72% of patients), neuropathy, decreased nail and hair growth, and a persistent Raynaud phenomenon in the affected part are frequent sequelae to cold injury.[438] The affected tissue remains at risk for reinjury and should be carefully protected during any cold exposure. As mentioned previously, chilblains (or chronic pernio) is a specific form of a dermopathy secondary to cold-induced skin vasculitis. Treatment with antiadrenergics (prazosin hydrochloride, 1 to 2 mg/d) or calcium-channel blockers (nifedipine, 30 to 60 mg/d) and careful protection from further exposure is often helpful.[424,444] However, few therapies afford significant relief to the chronic symptoms after tissue freeze injury, although β- and α-adrenergic blocking agents, calcium-channel blockers, topical and systemic steroids, and a host of home remedies have been tried, all with occasional individual success.

REFERENCES

1. Rice DP, MacKenzie EJ, et al, eds. Cost of injury in the United States: a report to Congress. Atlanta, Centers for Disease Control, 1989.
2. Kraus JF, Peek C, McArthur DL, Williams A. The effect of the 1992 California motorcycle helmet use law on motorcycle crash fatalities and injuries. JAMA 1994;272:1506.
3. Hoyt DB, Bulger EM, Knudson MM, et al. Death in the operating room: an analysis of a multi-center experience. J Trauma 1994;37:426.
4. Lowe DK, Gately HL, Goss JR, et al. Patterns of death, complication and error in management of motor vehicle accident victims: implications for a regional system of trauma care. J Trauma 1983;23:503.
5. Shackford SR, Hollingsworth-Fridlund P, Cooper G, et al. The effect of regionalization upon the quality of trauma care assessed by concurrent audit before and after institution of a trauma system: a preliminary report. J Trauma 1986;26:812.
6. Baker CC, Oppenheiner L, Stephens B, et al. Epidemiology of trauma deaths. Am J Surg 1980;140:144.
7. Shackford SR, Mackersie RC, Hollingsworth-Fridlund P, Hollbrook TL, Wolf PL, Hoyt DB. The epidemiology and pathology of traumatic death: a population-based analysis. Arch Surg 1993;128:571.
8. Grossblatt N, ed. Injury in America: a continuing public health problem. Washington, DC, National Academy Press, 1985.
9. National Highway Traffic Safety Administration. EMS system development: results of the statewide EMS assessment program. (Interim report) Washington, DC, US Department of Transportation, March 1994.
10. American College of Surgeons Committee on Trauma. Resources for optimal care of the injured patient: 1993. Chicago, American College of Surgeons, 1993.
11. American College of Surgeons Committee on Trauma. Advanced trauma life support course: instructor manual. Chicago, American College of Surgeons, 1994.
12. Baker S. The injury fact book. New York, Oxford University Press, 1992.
13. Champion HR, Fallen WF, Golocovsk M. The trauma score. Crit Care Med 1981;9:672.
14. Champion HR, Gainer PS, Yackee E. A progress report on the trauma score in predicting a fatal outcome. J Trauma 1986;26:927.
15. The abbreviated injury scale (AIS), rev. ed. Des Plaines, IL, American Association for Automotive Medicine, 1990.
16. Boyd CR, Tolson MA, Copes WS. Evaluating trauma care: the TRISS method. J Trauma 1987;27:370.
17. Hoyt DB, Hollingsworth-Fridlund P, Winchell RJ, et al. An analysis of recurrent process errors leading to provider-related complications on an organized trauma service: directions for care improvement. J Trauma 1994;36:377.
18. Wisner DH. History and current status of trauma scoring systems. Arch Surg 1990;127:115.

19. Rutledge R. Injury severity scoring in trauma patients. Adv Trauma Crit Care 1993;8:117.

20. Rutledge R. Injury severity grading in trauma patients: a simplified technique based upon ICD-9 coding. J Trauma 1993;35:497.

21. Model trauma care system plan. Washington, DC, US Department of Health and Human Services, September 30, 1992.

22. Holbrook TL, Hoyt DB, Anderson JP, Hollingsworth-Fridlund P, Shackford SR. Functional limitation after major trauma: a more sensitive assessment using the quality of well-being scale. The trauma recovery pilot project. J Trauma 1994;36:74.

23. Davis JW, Hoyt DB, McArdle MS, Mackersie RC, Shackford SR, Eastman AB. The significance of critical care errors in causing preventable death in trauma patients in a trauma system. J Trauma 1991;31:813.

24. Davis JW, Hoyt DB, McArdle MS, et al. An analysis of errors causing morbifity and mortality in a trauma system: a guide for quality improvement. J Trauma 1992;32:660.

25. Pepe PE, Maio RF. Evolving challenges in pre-hospital trauma services: current issues in suggested evaluation tools. Prehosp Diaster Med 1993;8;S25.

26. Sampalis JS, Lavoie A, Williams JI. Impact of on-site care, pre-hospital time, and level of in-hospital care on survival in severely injured patients. J Trauma 1993;34:252.

27. Cayten CG, Murphy JG, Stahl WN. Basic life support versus advanced life support for injured patients with an injury severity score of 10 or more. J Trauma 1993;35:460.

28. Pepe PE, Copass MK, Joyce TH. Pre-hospital endotracheal intubation: rationale for training emergency medical personnel. Ann Emerg Med 1985;14:1085.

29. Vilke GM, Hoyt DB, Epperson M, et al. Intubation techniques in the helicopter. J Emerg Med 1994;12:217.

30. York D, Dudek L, Larson R, et al. A comparison study of chest tube thoracostomy: air medical crew and in-hospital trauma service. Air Med J 1993;12:227.

31. Greene MK, Roden R, Hinchley G. The laryngeal mask airway: two cases of pre-hospital trauma care. Anesthesia 1992;47:688.

32. Salvino CK, Dries D, Gamelli R, et al. Emergency cricothyroidotomy in trauma victims. J Trauma 1993;34:503.

33. Xeropotamos NS, Coats T, Wilson AW. Pre-hospital surgical airway management: one year's experience from the Helicopter Emergency Medical Service. Injury 1993;24:222. (11 patients, 4 of whom survived)

34. Mattox KL, Bickel LW, Pepe PE, et al. Prospective MAST study in 911 patients. J Trauma 1989;29:1104.

35. Cayten CG, Berendt BM, Byrne DW, et al. A study of pneumatic anti-shock garments in severely hypotensive patients. J Trauma 1993;34:728.

36. Bickwell WH, Wall MJ, Pepe PE, et al. Immediate versus delayed fluid resuscitation for hypotensive patients with penetrating torso injuries. N Engl J Med 1994;331:1105.

37. Vassar MJ, Perry CA, Holcroft JW. Pre-hospital resuscitation of hypotensive trauma patients with 7.5% NaCl versus 7.5% NaCl with added dextran: a controlled trial. J Trauma 1993;34:622.

38. Vassar MJ, Fischer RP, O'Brien PE, et al. A multi center trial for resuscitation of injured patients with 7.5% sodium chloride: the effect of added dextran. The multicenter group for the study of hypertonic saline in trauma patients. Arch Surg 1993;128:1003.

39. Boyd MV, Vanek VW, Bourguet CC. Emergency room resuscitation thoracotomy: when is it indicated? J Trauma 1992;33:714.

40. Buckmaster MS, Kearney PA, Johnson SB. Further experience with transesophageal echocardiography in the evaluation of thoracic aortic injury. J Trauma 1994;30:989.

41. Miller FB, Cryer HM, Chilikuris S, et al. Negative findings on laparotomy for trauma. South Med J 1989;82:1231.

42. Evers BM, Cryer HM, Miller FB. Pelvic fracture hemorrhage: priorities in management. Arch Surg 1989;124:422.

43. Fabian TC, Croce MA, Stewart RM, et al. A prospective analysis of diagnostic laparoscopy in trauma. Ann Surg 1993;217:557.

44. Meyer DM, Thal ER, Weigelt JA. The role of abdominal CT in the evaluation of stab wounds to the back. J Trauma 1989;29:1226.

45. Gann DS, Carlson DE, Byrnes GJ, et al. Impaired restitution of blood volume after large hemorrhage. J Trauma 1981;12:598.

46. Huckabee WE. Relationships of pyruvate and lactate during anaerobic metabolism. II. Exercise and formation of O_2 debt. J Clin Invest 1958;37:255.

47. Broder G, Weil MH. Excess lactate: an index of reversibility of shock in human patients. Science 1964;143:1457.

48. Vitek V, Cowley RA. Blood lactate in the prognosis of various forms of shock. Ann Surg 1971;173:308.

49. Canizarro PC, Prager MD, Shires GT. The infusion of Ringer's lactate solution during shock. Am J Surg 1971;122:494.

50. Abramson DA, Scalea TM, Hitchcock R, et al. Lactate clearance and survival following injury. J Trauma 1993;35:584.

51. Davis JW. The relationship of base deficit to lactate in porcine hemorrhagic shock and resuscitation. J Trauma 1994;36:168.

52. Davis JW, Shackford SR, Mackersie RC, et al. Base deficit as a guide to volume resuscitation. J Trauma 1988;28:1464.

53. American College of Surgeons Committee on Trauma. Advanced trauma life support: shock. Chicago, American College of Surgeons, 1988:59.

54. Krausz MM, Bar-Ziv M, Rabinovici R, et al. "Scoop and run" or stabilize hemorrhagic shock with normal saline or small-volume hypertonic saline? J Trauma 1992;33:6.

55. Kowalenko T, Stern S, Dronen S, et al. Improved outcome with hypotensive resuscitation of uncontrolled hemorrhagic shock in a swine model. J Trauma 1992;33:349.

56. Martin RR, Bickell WH, Pepe PE, et al. Prospective evaluation of preoperative fluid resuscitation in hypotensive patients with penetrating truncal injury: a preliminary report. J Trauma 1992;33:354.

57. Waxman K, Annas C, Daughters K, et al. A method to determine the adequacy of resuscitation using tissue oxygen monitoring. J Trauma 1994;36:852.

58. Ross AD, Angaran DM. Colloids vs. crystalloids: a continuing controversy. Drug Intell Clin Pharmacol 1984;18:202.

59. Waxman K, Holness R, Tominaga G, et al. Hemodynamic and oxygen transport effects of pentastarch in burn resuscitation. Ann Surg 1989;209:341.

60. London MJ, Ho JS, Triedman JK, et al. A randomized clinical trial of 10% pentastarch (low molecular weight hydroxy ethel starch) vs. 5% albumin for plasma volume expansion after cardiac operations. J Thorac Cardiovasc Surg 1989;97:785.

61. Mackersie RC, Durelle J. Differential clearance of colloid and crystalloid solutions from the lung. J Trauma 1993;35:448.

62. Moss GS, Rice CL, Sehgal LR, et al. Management of traumatic and hemorrhagic shock. Anesth Rev 1990;17:25.

63. Gervin AS. Transfusion, autotransfusion, and blood substitutes. In: Mattox KL, Moore EE, Feliciano DV, eds. Trauma. Norwalk, CT, Appleton & Lange, 1988:161.

64. Whelan TJ, Burkhalter WE, Gomez A. Management of war wounds. In: Welch CE, ed. Advances in surgery, vol 3. Chicago, Year Book Medical Publishers, 1968:251.

65. Gervin AS, Fisher RP. Resuscitation of trauma patients with type-specific, uncrossmatched whole blood. J Trauma 1984;24:327.

66. Boudreaux JP, Bornside GH, Cohn I. Emergency autotransfusion: partial cleansing of bacteria-laden blood. J Trauma 1983;23:31.

67. Glover JL, Smith R, Yaw PB, et al. Autotransfusion of blood contaminated by intestinal contents. JACEP 1978;7:142.

68. Jurkovich GJ, Moore EE, Medina G. Autotransfusion in trauma: a pragmatic analysis. Am J Surg 1984;148:782.

69. Widenthal K, Mierzwial DS, Mitchell JH. Acute effects of increased serum osmolality on left ventricular performance. Am J Physiol 1969;216:898.

70. Kramer GC, Walsh JC. Future trends in emergency fluid resuscitation. In: Tuma RF, White JV, Messmer K, eds. The role of hemodilution in optimal patient care. Munich, Zuckschwerdt-Verlag, 1989:89.

71. Roche T, Silva M Jr, Negraes GA, et al. Hypertonic resuscitation from severe hemorrhagic shock: patterns of regional circulation. Circ Shock 1986;19:165.

72. Smith GJ, Kramer GC, Perron P, et al. A comparison of sev-

SURGERY: SCIENTIFIC PRINCIPLES AND PRACTICE

416

eral hypertonic solutions for resuscitation of bled sheep. J Surg Res 1985;39:517.

73. Shackford SR, Fortlage DA, Peters RM, et al. Serum osmolar and electrolyte changes associated with large infusions of hypertonic sodium lactate for intravascular volume expansion of patients undergoing aortic reconstruction. Surg Gynecol Obstet 1987;164:127.

74. Holcroft JW, Vassar MJ, O'Brien PE, et al. Hypertonic/hyperoncotic resuscitation of trauma victims undergoing helicopter transport: a multicenter trial. Arch Surg 1993;128:1003.

75. Gross D, Landau EH, Klin B, et al. Quantitative measurement of bleeding following hypertonic saline therapy in "uncontrolled" hemorrhagic shock. J Trauma 1989;29:79.

76. Greenburg AG, Hayashi R, Siefert I, et al. Intravascular persistence and oxygen delivery of pyridoxalated stroma-free hemoglobin during gradations of hypotension. Surgery 1979;86:13.

77. Moss GS, Gould SA, Sehgal LR, et al. Hemoglobin solution: from tetramer to polymer. Surgery 1984;95:249.

78. Farmer MC, Rudolph AS, Vandegriff KD, et al. Liposome encapsulated hemoglobin: oxygen binding properties and respiratory function. Biomater Artif Cells Artif Organs 1988; 16:289.

79. Rabinovici R, Rudolph AS, Feuerstein G. Characterization of hemodynamic, hematologic and biochemical responses to administration of liposome-encapsulated hemoglobin in the conscious, freely moving rat. Circ Shock 1989;29:115.

80. Rabinovici R, Rudolph AS, Vernick J, et al. A new salutary resuscitative fluid: liposome encapsulated hemoglobin/hypertonic saline solution. J Trauma 1993;35:121.

81. Messmer K. Blood substitutes in shock therapy. In: Shires GT, ed. Shock and related problems: clinical surgery international, vol 9. New York, Churchill Livingstone, 1984.

82. Tremper KK, Friedman AE, Levine EM, et al. The preoperative treatment of severely anemic patient with a perfluorochemical oxygen-transport fluid: Fluosol-DA. N Engl J Med 1982;307:277.

83. Elliot LA, Ledgerwood AM, Lucas CE, et al. Role of Fluosol-DA 20% in prehospital resuscitation. Crit Care Med 1989; 17:166.

84. McCoy LE, Elliot LA, Lucas CE, et al. Regenerative responses to exchange transfusion. Biomater Artif Cells Artif Organs 1988;16:575.

85. Nishimura N, Sugi T, Hiranuma N, et al. Changes of lung water and cardiovascular parameters during neurosurgical procedures associated with various types of infusion. Resuscitation 1983;10:227.

86. Hodges GR, Worley SE, Kemner JM, et al. Effect of exchange transfusion with an oxygen-carrying resuscitation fluid on the efficacy of penicillin therapy of pneumococcal infection in rats. Antimicrob Agents Chemother 1984;26:903.

87. Hoyt DB, Greenburg AG, Worley SE, et al. Resuscitation with Fluosol DA 20%: tolerance to sepsis. J Trauma 1986;26:713.

88. Chesnut RM, Marshall LF, Klauber MR, et al. The role of secondary brain injury in determining outcome from severe head injury. J Trauma 1993;34:216.

88a. Bouma GJ, Muizelaar JP, Stringer WA, et al. Ultra-early evaluation of regional cerebral blood flow in severely head-injured patients using xenon-enhanced computerized tomography. J Neurosurg 1992;77:360.

89. Kaufmann AM, Cardoso ER. Aggravation of vasogenic cerebral edema by multiple-dose mannitol. J Neurosurg 1992; 77:584.

90. Chesnut RM, Gautille TA, Blunt BA, Klauber MR, Marshall LR. The localizing value of pupillary size asymmetry in severe head injury: relation to lesion type and location. Neurosurgery 1994;34:1.

91. Todd MM, Tommasino C, Moore S. Cerebral effects of isovolemic hemodilution with a hypertonic saline solution. J Neurosurg 1985;63:944.

92. Rosner MJ, Coley IB. Cerebral perfusion pressure, intracranial pressure, and head elevation. J Neurosurg 1986;65:636.

93. Mendelow AD, Teasdale G, Jennett B, Bryden J, Hessett C, Murray G. Risks of intracranial haematoma in head injured adults. Br Med J 1983;287:1173.

94. Marmarou A, Anderson RL, Ward JD, et al. Impact of ICP instability and hypotension on outcome in patients with severe head trauma. J Neurosurg 1991;75(Suppl):S159.

95. Marshall LF, Bowers-Marshall S, Klauber MR, et al. A new classification of head injury based on computerized tomography. J Neurosurg 1991;75(Suppl):S14.

96. Seelig JM, Becker DP, Miller JD, Greenberg RP, Ward JD, Choi SC. Traumatic acute subdural hematoma: major mortality reduction in comatose patients treated within four hours. N Engl J Med 1981;304:1511.

97. Marshall LF, Gautille T, Klauber MR, et al. The outcome of severe head injury. J Neurosurg 1991;75(Suppl):S28.

98. Hayter JP, Ward, AJ, Smith EJ. Maxillofacial trauma in severely injured patients. Br J Oral Maxillofac Surg 29:370,1991.

99. Nahum, AM. The biomechanics of maxillofacial trauma. Clin Plast Surg 1975;2:59.

100. LeFort R. Etude experimentale sur les fractures de la machoire siperieuve. Riv Chir Paris 1901;23:208.

101. Stanley RB. Pathogenesis and evaluation of mandible fractures. In: Mathog RH, ed. Maxillofacial trauma. Baltimore, Williams & Wilkins, l984.

102. Holt GR. Maxillofacial trauma. In: Cummings CW, ed. Otolaryngology: head and neck surgery. St Louis, CV Mosby, l986.

103. Coker NJ. Management of traumatic injuries to the facial nerve. Otolaryngol Clin North Am 1991;24:2l5.

104. Haug RH. Cervical spine fractures and maxillofacial trauma. J Oral Maxillofac Surg 1991;49:727.

105. Valavanis A. Interventional neuroradiology for head and neck surgery. In: Cummings CW, ed. Otolaryngology: head and neck surgery, update II. St Louis, CV Mosby, l990.

106. Marentette LJ, Valentino J. Traumatic anterior fossa cerebrospinal fluid fistulae and craniofacial considerations. Otolaryngol Clin North Am 1991;24:152.

107. Goodale RL, Montgomery WW. Anterior osteoplastic frontal sinus operation. Ann Otol Rhinol Laryngol 1961;70:860.

108. Nadell J, Cline DG. Primary reconstruction of depressed frontal skull fractures including those involving the sinus, orbit and cribriform plate. J Neurosurg 1974;41:200.

109. Busch RF, Prunes F. Intermaxillary fixation with intraoral cortical bone screws. Laryngoscope 1991;101:1336.

110. Dierks EJ. Management of associated dental injuries in maxillofacial trauma. Otolaryngol Clin North Am 1991;24:177.

111. Ordog G. Penetrating neck trauma. J Trauma 1987;27:543.

112. Saletta J, Lowe R, Lim L, et al. Penetrating neck trauma. J Trauma 1976;16:579.

113. Sankaran S, Walt A. Penetrating wounds of the neck: principles and some controversies. Surg Clin North Am 1977; 57:139.

114. Flint L, Snyder W, Perry M, Shires G. Management of major vascular injuries in the base of the neck: an 11-year experience with 146 cases. Arch Surg 1973;106:407.

115. Bishara R, Pasch A, Douglas D, et al. The necessity of mandatory exploration of penetrating zone II neck injuries. Surgery 1986;100:655.

116. Jones R, Terrell J, Salyer K. Penetrating wounds of the neck: an analysis of 274 cases. J Trauma 1967;7:228.

117. Jurkovich G, Zingarelli W, Wallace J, Curreri P. Penetrating neck trauma: diagnostic studies in the asymptomatic patient. J Trauma 1985;25:819.

118. Mansour MA, Moore EE, Moore FA, Whitehill TA. Validating the selective management of penetrating neck wounds. Am J Surg 1991;162:517.

119. Merion RM, Harness JK, Ramsburgh SR. Selective management of penetrating neck trauma: cost implications. Arch Surg 1981;116:691.

120. Adolfo A, Kaledzi Y, Parsa M, Freeman H. Penetrating neck wounds: mandatory versus selective exploration. Ann Surg 1985;202:563.

121. Demetriades D, Charalambides D, Lakhoo M. Physical examination and selective conservative management in patients with penetrating injuries of the neck. Br J Surg 1993;80:1534.

122. Roden D, Pomerantz R. Penetrating injuries to the neck: a safe, selective approach to management. Am Surg 1993; 59:750.

123. Gerst PH, Sharma S, Sharma P. Selective management of penetrating neck trauma. Am Surg 1990;56:553.

124. Beitsch P, Weigelt JA, Flynn E, Easley S. Physical examina-

tion and arteriography in patients with penetrating zone II neck wounds. Arch Surg 1994;129:577.

125. Asensio J, Valenziano C, Falcone R, Grosh J. Management of penetrating neck injuries: the controversy surrounding zone II injuries. Surg Clin North Am 1991;71:267.

126. Carducci B, Lowe R, Dalsey W. Penetrating neck trauma: consensus and controversies. Ann Emerg Med 1986;15:208.

127. Hirshberg A, Wall MJ, Johnston RH Jr, et al. Transcervical gunshot injuries. Am J Surg 1994;167:309.

128. Richardson J, Simpson C, Miller F. Management of transmediastinal gunshot wounds. Surgery 1981;90:671.

129. Sclafani SJ, Cavaliere G, Atweh N, et al. The role of angiography in penetrating neck trauma. J Trauma 1991;31:557.

130. Welling R, Saul T, Tew J, et al. Management of blunt injury to the internal carotid artery. J Trauma 1987;27:1221.

131. Cogbill TH, Moore EE, Meissner M, et al. The spectrum of blunt injury to the carotid artery: a multicenter perspective. J Trauma 1994;37:473.

132. Pretre R, Reverdin A, Kalonji T, Faidutti B. Blunt carotid artery injury: difficult therapeutic approaches for an underrecognized entity. Surgery 1994;115:375.

133. Davis J, Holbrook T, Hoyt D, et al. Blunt carotid artery dissection: incidence, associated injuries, screening, and treatment. J Trauma 1990;30:1514.

134. Martin WSG-GS. Pediatric penetrating head and neck trauma. Laryngoscope 1990;100:1288.

135. Fakhry S, Jacques PF, Proctor H. Cervical vessel injury after blunt trauma. J Vasc Surg 1988;8:501.

136. Sundt T, Pearson B, Piepgras D, et al. Surgical management of aneurysms of the distal extracranial internal carotid artery. J Neurosurg 1986;64:169.

137. Gewertz B, Samson D, Ditmore QM, Bone G. Management of penetrating injuries of the internal carotid artery at the base of the skull utilizing extracranial-intracranial bypass. J Trauma 1980;20:365.

138. Brown MF, Graham JM, Feliciano DV, et al. Carotid artery injuries. Am J Surg 1982;144:748.

139. Weaver F, Yellin A, Wagner W, et al. The role of arterial reconstruction in penetrating carotid injuries. Arch Surg 1988;123:1106.

140. Unger S, Tucker W, Mrdeza M, et al. Carotid arterial trauma. Surgery 1980;87:477.

141. Liekweg W, Greenfield L. Management of penetrating carotid arterial trauma. Ann Surg 1978;188:587.

142. Vazquez Anon V, Aymard A, Gobin YP, et al. Balloon occlusion of the internal carotid artery in 40 cases of giant intracavernous aneurysm: technical aspects, cerebral monitoring, and results. Neuroradiology 1992;34:245.

143. DeBehnke DJ, Brady W. Vertebral artery dissection due to minor neck trauma. J Emerg Med 1994;12:27.

144. Egnor MR, Page LK, David C. Vertebral artery aneurysm: a unique hazard of head banging by heavy metal rockers. (Case report) Pediatr Neurosurg 1991;17:135.

145. Golueke P, Scalfani S, Phillips T, et al. Vertebral artery injury: diagnosis and management. J Trauma 1987;27:856.

146. Hatzitheofilou C, Strahlendorf C, Kakoyiannis S, et al. Penetrating external injuries of the oesophagus and pharynx. Br J Surg 1993;80:1147.

147. Meier D, Brink B, Fry W. Vertebral artery trauma: acute recognition and treatment. Arch Surg 1981;116:236.

148. Myers E, Iko B. The management of acute laryngeal trauma. J Trauma 1987;27:448.

149. Fuhrman G, Stieg F, Buerk C. Blunt laryngeal trauma: classification and management protocol. J Trauma 1990;30:87.

150. Kelly J, Webb W, Moulder P, et al. Management of airway trauma. I. Tracheobronchial injuries. Ann Thorac Surg 1985;40:551.

151. Schaefer SD. The acute management of external laryngeal trauma: a 27-year experience. Arch Otolaryngol Head Neck Surg 1992;118:598.

152. Gussack G, Jurkovich G. Treatment dilemmas in laryngotracheal trauma. J Trauma 1988;28:1439.

153. Glatterer M, Toon R, Ellestad C, et al. Management of blunt and penetrating external esophageal trauma. J Trauma 1985;25:784.

154. Defore W, Mattox K, Hansen H, et al. Surgical management of penetrating injuries of the esophagus. Am J Surg 1977;134:734.

155. Weigelt J, Thal E, Snyder W, et al. Diagnosis of penetrating cervical esophageal injuries. Am J Surg 1987;154:619.

156. Winter RP, Weigelt JA. Cervical esophageal trauma: incidence and cause of esophageal fistulas. Arch Surg 1990;125:849.

157. Snow J. Diagnosis and therapy for acute laryngeal and tracheal trauma. Otolaryngol Clin North Am 1984;17:101.

158. Shackford SR: Blunt chest trauma: the intensivist's perspective. J Intensive Care Med 1986;1:125.

159. Mattox KL: Thoracic injury requiring surgery. World J Surg 1983;7:49.

160. Trunkey DD: Spleen. In: Blaisdell FW, Trunkey DD, eds. Trauma management. New York, Thieme-Stratton, 1982.

161. Mackersie RC, Karagianes T, Hoyt DB, Davis JW. Prospective evaluation of epidural and intravenous opiates for pain control and restoration of ventilatory function following multiple rib fractures. J Trauma 31:443, 1991.

162. Roy-Shapira A, Levi I, Khoda J. Sternal fractures: A red flag or a red herring? J Trauma 1994;37:59.

163. Maloney JV, Schmotzer KJ, Raschke E. Paradoxical respiration and penduluft. J Thorac Cardiovasc Surg 1961;41:219.

164. Sarnoff SJ, Gaensler EA, Maloney JV. Electrophrenic respiration: the effectiveness of contralateral ventilation during activity of one phrenic nerve. J Thorac Cardiovasc Surg 1950;19:929.

165. Duff JH, Goldstein M, Maclean APH, et al. Flail chest: a clinical review and physiologic study. J Trauma 1968;8:63.

166. Thomas AN, Blaisdell FW, Lewis FR, Scholbohm RM. Operative stabilization for flail chest after blunt trauma. J Thorac Cardiovasc Surg 1978;75:793.

167. Weigelt J, Aurbakken CM, Meir D, Thal E. Management of asymptomatic patients following stab wounds to the chest. J Trauma 1982;22:291.

168. Mancini M, Smith LM, Nein A, et al. Early evacuation of clotted blood in hemothorax using thoracoscopy: case reports. J Trauma 1993;34:144.

169. Obrien J, Cohen M, Solit R, et al. Thoracoscopic drainage and decortication as definitive treatment for empyema thoracis following penetrating chest trauma. J Trauma 1994;36:536.

170. Ponn RB, D'Agostino RS, Stern H, Westcott JL. Treatment of peripheral bronchopleural fistulas with endobronchial occlusion coils. Ann Thorac Surg 1993;56:1343.

171. York EL, Lewall DB, Hirji M, Gelfand ET, Modry DL. Endoscopic diagnosis and treatment of postoperative bronchopleural fistula. Chest 1990;97:1390.

172. Jones WS, Mavroudis C, Richardson JD, et al. Management of tracheobronchial disruption resulting from blunt trauma. Surgery 1984;95:319.

173. Mirvis SE, Kostrubiak I, Whitely NO, et al. Role of CT in excluding major arterial injury after blunt thoracic trauma. AJR Am J Roentgenol 1987;149:601.

174. Miller FB, Richardson JD, Thomas HA, et al. Role of CT in diagnosis of major arterial injury after blunt thoracic trauma. Surgery 1989;106:596.

175. Kearney PA, Smith W, Johnson SB, et al. Use of transesophageal echocardiography in the evaluation of traumatic aortic injury. J Trauma 1993;34:696.

176. Mattox KL, Holtzman M, Pickard LR, et al. Clamp/repair: a safe technique for the treatment of blunt injury to the descending thoracic aorta. Ann Thorac Surg 1985;40:456.

177. Karalis DG, Victor MF, Davis GA, et al. The role of echocardiography in blunt chest trauma: a transthoracic and transesophageal echocardiographic study. J Trauma 1994;36:53.

178. Foil MB, Mackersie RC, Furst SR, et al. The asymptomatic patient with suspected myocardial contusion: is hospital admission really necessary? Am J Surg 1990;160:638.

179. Moreno C, Moore EE, Majure JA, et al. Pericardial tamponade: a critical determinant for survival following penetrating cardiac wounds. J Trauma 1986;26:821.

180. Kemmerer WT, Eckert WG, Gathright JB, et al. Patterns of thoracic injuries in fatal traffic accidents. J Trauma 1961;1:595.

181. Urschel HC Jr, Razzuk MA, Wood RE, et al. Improved management of esophageal perforation: exclusion and diversion in continuity. Ann Surg 1974;175:587.

182. Mee SL, McAninch JW, Robinson AL, et al. Radiographic assessment of renal trauma: a 10-year prospective study of patient selection. J Urol 1989;141:1095.

183. Hoffman R, Nerlich M, Muggia-Sullam M, et al. Blunt abdominal trauma in cases of multiple trauma evaluated by ultrasonography: a prospective analysis of 291 patients. J Trauma 1992;32:452.

184. Rozycki GS, Ochsner MG, Jaffin JH, et al. Prospective evaluation of surgeon's use of ultrasound in the evaluation of trauma patients. J Trauma 1993;34:516.

185. Ivatury RR, Simon RJ, Stahl WM. A critical evaluation of laparoscopy in penetrating abdominal trauma. J Trauma 1993;34:822.

186. Salvino CK, Esposito TJ, Marshall WJ, et al. The role of diagnostic laparoscopy in the management of trauma patients: a preliminary assessment. J Trauma 1993;34:506.

187. Moore E, Moore J, Van Duzer-Moore S. Mandatory laparotomy for gunshot wounds penetrating the abdomen. Am J Surg 1980;140:847.

188. Meyer DM, Thal ER, Weigelt JA. Evaluation of computed tomography and diagnostic peritoneal lavage in blunt abdominal trauma. J Trauma 1989;29:1168.

189. Federle MP, Crass RA, Jeffrey RB, et al. Computed tomography in blunt abdominal trauma. Arch Surg 1982;117:645.

190. Schrock T, Blaisdell FW, Mathewson C. Management of blunt trauma to the liver and hepatic veins. Arch Surg 1968;96:698.

191. Levison MA, Peterson SR, Sheldon GF, et al. Duodenal trauma: experience of a trauma center. J Trauma 1984;24:475.

192. Jones WR, Hardin WJ, Davis JT, et al. Intramural hematoma of the duodenum: a review of the literature and case report. Ann Surg 1971;173:534.

193. Wisner DH, Wold RL, Frey CF. Diagnosis and treatment of pancreatic injuries: an analysis of management principles. Arch Surg 1990;125:1109.

194. Feliciano DV, Martin TD, Cruse PA, et al. Management of combined pancreatoduodenal injuries. Ann Surg 1987;205:673.

195. Lucas CE. Diagnosis and treatment of pancreatic and duodenal injury. Surg Clin North Am 1977;57:49.

196. Schroder ST, Kivilaakso E, Kalima T, et al. Treatment of pancreatic fistulas with somatostatin and total parenteral nutrition. Scand J Gastroenterol 1989;24:859.

197. Williams ST, Woltering EA, O'Dorisio TM, et al. Effect of octreotide on pancreatic exocrine function. Am J Surg 1989;157:459.

198. Wisner DH, Chun Y, Blaisdell FW. Blunt intestinal injury: keys to diagnosis and management. Arch Surg 1990;125:1319.

199. Marx J, Moore EE, Jorden RC, et al. Limitations of computed tomography in the evaluation of acute abdominal trauma: a prospective comparison with diagnostic peritoneal lavage. J Trauma 1985;25:933.

200. Sherck JP, Oakes DD. Intestinal injuries missed by computed tomography. J Trauma 1990;30:1.

201. Stone HH, Fabian TC. Management of perforating colon trauma. Ann Surg 1979;190:430.

202. Chappuis CW, Frey DJ, Dietzen CD, et al. Management of penetrating colon injuries. Ann Surg 1991;213:492.

203. Levison MA, Thomas DD, Wiencek RG, et al. Management of the injured colon: evolving practice at an urban trauma center. J Trauma 1990;30:247.

204. Atala A, Miller FB, Richardson JD, et al. Preliminary vascular control for renal trauma. Surg Gynecol Obstet 1991;172:386.

205. Carroll PR, McAninch JW, Wong A, et al. Outcome after temporary vascular occlusion for the management of renal trauma. J Urol 1994;151:1171.

206. Corriere JN, McAndrew JD, Benson GS. Intraoperative decision-making in renal trauma surgery. J Trauma 1991;31:1390.

207. Looser KG, Crombie HD Jr. Pelvic fractures: an anatomic guide to severity of injury: review of 100 cases. Am J Surg 1976;132:638.

208. Cryer HM, Miller FB, Evers BM, et al. Pelvic fracture classification: correlation with hemorrhage. J Trauma 1988;28:973.

209. Burgess AR, Eastridge BJ, Young JWR, et al. Pelvic ring disruptions: effective classification system and treatment protocols. J Trauma 1990;30:848.

210. Trunkey DD, Chapman MW, Lin RC Jr, Dunphy JE. Management of pelvic fractures in blunt trauma injury. J Trauma 1974;14:912.

211. Mendez C, Gubler KD, Maier RV. Diagnostic accuracy of peritoneal lavage in patients with pelvic fractures. Arch Surg 1994;129:477.

212. Flint L, Babikian G, Anders M, Rodriguez J, Steinberg S. Definitive control of mortality from severe pelvic fracture. Ann Surg 1990;211:703.

213. Panetta T, Sclafani SJ, Goldstein AS, Phillips TF, Shaftan GW. Percutaneous transcatheter embolization for massive bleeding from pelvic fractures. J Trauma 1985;25:1021.

214. Ben Menachem Y, Coldwell DM, Young JW, Burgess AR. Hemorrhage associated with pelvic fractures: causes, diagnosis, and emergent management. AJR 1991;157:1005.

215. Nicolaisen GS, McAninch JW, Marshall GA, et al. Renal trauma: reevaluation of the indications for radiologic assessment. J Urol 1985;133:183.

216. Bergen CT, Chan FN, Bodzin JH. Intravenous pyelogram results in association with renal pathology and therapy in trauma patients. J Trauma 1987;27:515.

217. Stevenson J, Battistella FD. The "one-shot" intravenous pyelogram: is it indicated in unstable trauma patients before celiotomy? J Trauma 1994;36:828.

218. Carroll PR, McAninch JW. Staging of renal trauma. Urol Clin North Am 1989;16:193.

219. McAninch JW, Carroll PR, Klosterman PW, Dixon CM, Greenblatt MN. Renal reconstruction after injury. J Urol 1991;145:932.

220. Cass AS, Luxenberg M. Management of extraperitoneal ruptures of bladder caused by external trauma. Urology 1989;3:179.

221. Corriere JN Jr, Sandler CM. Management of the ruptured bladder: seven years' experience with 111 cases. J Trauma 1986;26:830.

222. Cass AS. Urethral injury in the multiple-injury patient. J Trauma 1984;24:901.

223. Shackford SR, Rich NM. Peripheral vascular injury. In: Mattox KL, Moore EE, Feliciano DV, eds. Trauma, ed 2. Norwalk, CT, Appleton & Lange, 1991.

224. Coimbra RA, Anderson RJ, Dikdan G, Teehan EP, Hernandez-Maldonado JJ, Hobson RW. Leukocyte activation in ischemia-reperfusion injury of skeletal muscle. J Surg Res 1991;51:13.

225. Jerome SN, Smith CW, Korthuis RJ. CD 18−dependent adherence reactions play an important role in the development of the no-reflow phenomenon. Am J Physiol 1993;264:H479.

226. Mattox KL, O'Gorman RB. Injury to the thoracic great vessels. In: Moore EE, Mattox KL, Feliciano DV, eds. Trauma. Norwalk, CT, Appleton & Lange, 1988:385.

227. Knudson MM, Lewis FR, Atkinson K, Newhaus A. The role of duplex ultrasound arterial imaging in patients with penetrating extremity trauma. Arch Surg 1993;128:1033.

228. Snyder WH, Thal ER, Bridges RA, et al. The validity of normal arteriography in penetrating trauma. Arch Surg 1978;113:424.

229. Johansen K, Davies M, Howie T, et al. Objective criteria accurately predicting amputation following lower extremity trauma. J Trauma 1990;30:568.

230. Feliciano DV, Mattox KL, Graham JM, et al. Five year experience with PTFE grafts in vascular wounds. J Trauma 1985;25:75.

231. Johansen K, Bandyk D, Thiele B, Hansen ST. Use of temporary intraluminal shunts: resolution of a management dilemma in complex vascular injuries. J Trauma 1982;22:395.

232. Graham JM, Mattox KL, Beall AC. Portal venous injuries. J Trauma 1978;128:843.

233. Court-Brown CM. Care of accident victims. Br Med J 1989;298:115.

234. Perry JF, McClellan RJ. Autopsy findings in 127 patients following fatal traffic accidents. Surg Gynecol Obstet 1964;119:586.

235. Pedowitz RA, Shackford SR. Non-cavitary hemorrhage pro-

ducing shock in trauma patients: incidence and severity. J Trauma 1989;29:219.

236. Lieurance R, Benjamin JB, Rappaport WD. Blood loss and transfusion in patients with isolated femur fractures. J Orthop Trauma 1992;6:175.

237. Ostrum RF, Verghese GB, Santer TJ. The lack of association between femoral shaft fractures and hypotensive shock. J Orthop Trauma 1993;7:338.

238. Mucha P Jr, Farnell MB. Analysis of pelvic fracture management. J Trauma 1984;24:379.

239. Riemer BL, Butterfield SL, Diamond DL, et al: Acute mortality associated with injuries to the pelvic ring: the role of early patient mobilization and external fixation. J Trauma 1993;35:671.

240. Bracken MB, Shepard MJ, Collins WF, et al. A randomized controlled trial of methylprednisolone or naloxone in the treatment of acute spinal cord injury. N Engl J Med 1990;322:1405.

241. Bracken MB, Shepard MJ, Collins WF, et al. Methylprednisolone or naloxone treatment after acute spinal cord injury: 1-year follow-up data. Results of the second National Acute Spinal Cord Injury Study. J Neurosurg 1992;76:23.

242. Geisler FH, Dorsey FC, Coleman WP. Recovery of motor function after spinal-cord injury: a randomized, placebo-controlled trial with GM-1 ganglioside. N Engl J Med 1991;324:1829.

243. Constantini S, Young W. The effects of methylprednisolone and the ganglioside GM1 on acute spinal cord injury in rats. J Neurosurg 1994;80:97.

244. Dickey RL, Brett CB, Kearns RJ, Tullos HS. Efficacy of antibiotics in low-velocity gunshot fractures. J Othop Trauma 1989;3:6.

245. Bunt TJ, Malone JM, Moody M, Davidson J, Karpman R. Frequency of vascular injury with blunt trauma-induced extremity injury. Am J Surg 1990;160:226.

246. Lozman J, Deno DC, Feustel PJ, et al. Pulmonary and cardiovascular consequences of immediate fixation or conservative management of long-bone fractures. Arch Surg 1986;121:992.

247. Seibel R, LaDuca J, Hassett JM, et al. Blunt multiple trauma (ISS 36), femur traction, and the pulmonary failure-septic state. Ann Surg 1985;202:283.

248. Latenser BA, Gentilello LM, Tarver AA, et al. Improved outcome with early fixation of skeletally unstable pelvic fractures. J Trauma 1991;31:28.

249. Dennis JW, Menawat S, Von Thron J, et al. Efficacy of deep venous thrombosis prophylaxis in trauma patients and identification of high-risk groups. J Trauma 1993;35:132.

250. Rogers FB, Shackford SR, Wilson J, et al. Prophylactic vena cava filter insertion in severely injured trauma patients: indications and preliminary results. J Trauma 1993;35:637.

251. Fabian, TC, Hoots AV, Stanford DS, et al. Fat embolism syndrome: prospective evaluation in 92 fracture patients. Crit Care Med 1990;18:42.

252. Demarest GB, Jabczenski F. Orthopedic complications. In: Mattox KL, ed. Complications of trauma. New York, Churchill Livingstone, 1994:567.

253. Pape H-C, Auf'm'Kolk M, Paffrath T, et al. Primary intramedullary femur fixation in multiple trauma patients with associated lung contusion: a cause of posttraumatic ARDS? J Trauma 1993;34:540.

254. Pape H-C, Regel G, Dwenger A, et al. Influences of different methods of intramedullary femoral nailing on lung function in patients with multiple trauma. J Trauma 1993;35:709.

255. Dossett AB, Hunt JL, Purdue GF, Schlegel JD. Early orthopedic intervention in burn patients with major fractures. J Trauma 1991;31:888.

256. Hofman PAM, Goris RJA. Timing of osteosynthesis of major fractures in patients with severe brain injury. J Trauma 1991;31:261.

257. Phillips TF, Contreras DM. Current concepts review: timing of operative treatment of fractures in patients who have multiple fractures. J Bone Joint Surg Am 1990;72:784.

258. Allshouse MJ, Rouse T, Eichelberger MR. Childhood injury: a current perspective. Pediatr Emerg Care 1993;9:159.

259. Eichelberger MR, ed. Pediatric trauma: prevention, acute care, rehabilitation. Chicago, Mosby–Year Book, 1993.

260. Nakayama DK, Gardner MJ, Rowe MI. Emergency endotracheal intubation in pediatric trauma. Ann Surg 1990;211:218.

261. Wesson DE, Scorpio RJ, Spence LJ, et al. The physical, psychological and socioeconomic costs of pediatric trauma. J Trauma 1992;33:252.

262. Nakayama DK, Gardner MJ, Waggoner T. Audit filters in quality assurance in pediatric trauma care. J Pediatr Surg 1993;28:19.

263. Stylianos S, Eichelberger MR. Pediatric trauma: prevention strategies. Pediatr Clin North Am 1993;40:1359.

264. DeMaria EJ: Evaluation and treatment of the elderly trauma victim. Clin Geriatr Med 1993;9:461.

264a.Tineti ME, Speechley M. Prevention of falls among the elderly. N Engl J Med 1989;320:1055.

264b.Champion HR, Copes WS, Buyer D, et al. Major trauma in geriatric patients. Am J Public Health 1989;79:1278.

265. Santora TA, Schinco MA, Trooskin SZ. Management of trauma in the elderly patients. Surg Clin North Am 1994;74:163.

266. Adkins RB, Scott HW, eds. Surgical care for the elderly. Baltimore, Williams & Wilkins, 1988.

267. Scalea TM, Simon HM, Duncan AO, et al. Geriatric blunt multiple trauma: improved survival with early invasive monitoring. J Trauma 1990;30:129.

268. DeMaria EJ, Kenney PR, Merriam MA, et al. Aggressive trauma care benefits the elderly. J Trauma 1987;27:1200.

268a.Camp PC, Rogers FB, Shackford SR, et al. Blunt traumatic thoracic aortic lacerations in the elderly: an analysis of outcome. J Trauma 1994;37:418.

268b.Shorr RM, Rodriquez A, Indeck MC, et al. Blunt chest trauma in the elderly. J Trauma 1989;29:234.

268c.Allen JE, Schwab CW. Blunt chest trauma in the elderly. Am Surgeon 1985;51:697.

269. Bybee DE. Toleration of head injury by the elderly. Neurosurgery 1987;20:954.

270. Pennings JL, Bachulis BL, Simons CR, et al. Survival after severe brain injury in the aged. Arch Surg 1993;128:787.

271. Knudson MM, Lieberman J, Morris JA, et al. Mortality factors in the geriatric blunt trauma patients. Arch Surg 1994;129:448.

272. Gould SF, Delaney JJ. Obstetrical and gynecological injuries. In: Zuidema CA, Rutherford RB, Ballinger WF, eds. Management of trauma, ed 4. Philadelphia, WB Saunders, 1985:505.

273. Rothenberger P, Quattelbaum FW, Perry JF Jr. Blunt maternal trauma: a review of 103 cases. J Trauma 1978;18:173.

274. Kissinger DP, Rozycki GS, Morris JA, et al. Trauma in pregnancy: predicting pregnancy outcome. Arch Surg 1991;126:1079.

275. Maull KI, Rozycki GS, Pedigo RE, et al. Female reproductive system trauma. In: Mattox KL, Moore EE, Feliciano DV, eds. Trauma. Norwalk, CT: Appleton & Lange, 1988:553.

276. Gonik B. Intensive care monitoring of the critically ill pregnant patient. In: Creasy RK, Resnick R, eds. Maternal-fetal medicine: principles and practice, ed 2. Philadelphia, WB Saunders, 1989:845.

277. Smith CV, Phelan JP. Trauma in pregnancy. In: Clark SL, Cotton DB, Hankins GPJ, Phalen JP, eds. Critical care obstetrics, ed 2. Boston, Blackwell, 1991:498.

278. Brinkman CR III, Morfio M, Assili NS. Circulation shock in pregnant sheep. Am J Obstet Gynecol 1974;118:77.

279. Bieniarz J, Branda LA, Maqueda E, et al. Aortocaval compression by the uterus in late pregnancy. Am J Obstet Gynecol 1968;102:1106.

280. Greiss FC, Anderson SG. Effect of ovarian hormones on the uterine vascular bed. Am J Obstet Gynecol 1970;107:829.

281. Clark SL, Cotton DB, Lee W, et al. Central hemodynamic assessment of normal term pregnancy. Am J Obstet Gynecol 1989;161:1439.

282. Lee W, Cotton DB. Cardiorespiratory changes during pregnancy. In: Clark SL, Cotton DB, Hankins GDU, Phelon JP, eds. Crit care obstetrics, ed 2. Boston, Blackwell, 1991:2.

283. Hume RF, Killam AP. Maternal physiology. In: Scott JR, Ki-Saia J, Hammon DB, Spellacy WN, eds. Obstetrics and gynecology. Philadelphia, JB Lippincott, 1990:93.

284. Bremer C. Trauma in pregnancy. Emerg Nurs 1986;21:708.

285. Higgins SD. Perinatal protocol: trauma in pregnancy. J Perinatol 1988;8:288.

286. Neufeld JDG, Moore EE, Marx JA, Rosen. Trauma in pregnancy. Emerg Med Clin North Am 1987;5:623.

287. Depp R. Clinical evaluation of fetal status. In: Scott JR, DiSaia PJ, Hammond CB, Spellacy WN, eds. Danforth's obstetrics and gynecology. Philadelphia, JB Lippincott 1990:293.

288. Reed KJ. Ultrasound in obstetrics. In: Scott JR, DiSaia PJ, Hammond CB, Spellacy WN, eds. Danforth's obstetrics and gynecology. Philadelphia, JB Lippincott, 1990:293.

289. Brent RJ. The effect of embryonic and fetal exposure to x-ray, microwaves, and ultrasound: counseling the pregnant and nonpregnant patient about these risks. Semin Oncol 1989;16:347.

290. Bushong SC. Radiologic science for technologists. Washington, DC, CV Mosby, 1983:550.

291. Sparkman RS. Rupture of the spleen in pregnancy. Am J Obstet Gynecol 1958;76:587.

292. Griswold R, Collier H. Blunt abdominal trauma. Int Abstr Surg 1961;112:309.

293. Higgins SD, Garite TB. Late abruptioplacental in trauma patients: implication for monitoring. Obstet Gynecol 1984; 63:105.

294. Sounders P, Milton PJ. Laparotomy during pregnancy: an assessment of diagnostic accuracy and fetal wastage. Br Med J 1973;3:165.

295. Pearlman MD, Tinthalli JE, Lornez RP. A prospective controlled study of outcome after trauma during pregnancy. Am J Obstet Gynecol 1990;162:1502.

296. Simons RK, Hoyt DB. Immunomodulation. Adv Trauma Crit Care 1994;9:135.

297. Deitch EA. The role of intestinal barrier failure and bacterial translocation in the development of systemic infection and multiple organ failure. Arch Surg 1990;125:403.

298. Cales RH, Trunkey DD. Preventable trauma deaths: a review of trauma care systems development. JAMA 1985;254:1059.

299. Hoyt DB, Hollingsworth-Fridlund P, Fortlage D, Davis JW, Mackersie RC. An evaluation of provider-related and disease-related morbidity in a level 1 university trauma service: directions for quality improvement. J Trauma 1992; 33:586.

300. Davis JW, Hoyt DB, Mackersie RC, Schackford SR, McArdle M. The significance of critical care errors in causing preventable deaths in trauma patients in a trauma system. J Trauma 1991;31:813.

301. Hoyt DB, Simons RK, Winchell RJ, et al. A risk analysis of pulmonary complications following major trauma. J Trauma 1993;35:524.

302. Driks MR, Craven DE, Celli BR, et al. Nosocomial pneumonia in intubated patients given sucralfate as compared with antacids or histamine type 2 blockers: the role of gastric colonization. N Engl J Med 1987;317:1376.

303. Simms HH, DeMaria E, McDonald L, Peterson D, Robinson A, Burchard KW. Role of gastric colonization in the development of pneumonia in critically ill trauma patients: results of a prospective randomized trial. J Trauma 1991;31:531.

304. Stoutenbeek CP, van Saene HK, Miranda DR, Zandstra DF, Langrehr D. The effect of oropharyngeal decontamination using topical nonabsorbable antibiotics on the incidence of nosocomial respiratory tract infections in multiple trauma patients. J Trauma 1987;27:357.

305. Johanson WG Jr, Seidenfeld JJ, de los Santos R, Coalson JJ, Gomez P. Prevention of nosocomial pneumonia using topical and parenteral antimicrobial agents. Am Rev Respir Dis 1988;137:265.

306. Johanson WG Jr, Pierce AK, Sanford JP, Thomas GD. Nosocomial respiratory infections with gram-negative bacilli: the significance of colonization of the respiratory tract. Ann Intern Med 1972;77:701.

307. Berger R, Arango L. Etiologic diagnosis of bacterial nosocomial pneumonia in seriously ill patients. Crit Care Med 1985;13:833.

308. Villers D, Derriennic M, Raffi F, et al. Reliability of the bronchoscopic-protected catheter brush in intubated and ventilated patients. Chest 1985;88:527.

309. Kahn FW, Jones JM. Diagnosis in bacterial respiratory infection by bronchoalveolar lavage. J Infect Dis 1987;155:862.

310. Winchell RJ, Hoyt DB, Walsh J, Simons RK, Eastman AB. Risk factors associated with pulmonary embolism despite routine prophylaxis: implications for improved protection. J Trauma 1994;37:600.

311. Morris JA Jr, MacKenzie EJ, Edelstein SL. The effect of preexisting conditions on mortality in trauma patients. JAMA 1990;263:1942.

312. Rosner MJ. Pathophysiology and management of increased intracranial pressure. In: Andrews BT, ed. Neurosurgical intensive care. New York, McGraw-Hill, 1993:57.

313. Simons RK, Hoyt DB, Winchell RJ, Holbrook T. A risk analysis of stress ulceration following trauma. J Trauma 1994; 36:165.

314. Weigelt JA. Risk of wound infections in trauma patients. Am J Surg 1985;150:782.

315. Maki DG, Cobb L, Garman JK, Shapiro JM, Ringer M, Helgerson RB. An attachable silver-impregnated cuff for prevention of infection with central venous catheters: a prospective randomized multicenter trial. Am J Med 1988;85:307.

316. Flowers RH III, Schwenzer KJ, Kopel RF, Fisch MJ, Tucker SI, Farr BM. Efficacy of the attachable subcutaneous cuff for the prevention of intravascular catheter-related infection: a randomized, controlled trial. JAMA 1989;261:878.

317. Morris JA, Much P, Ross S, et al. Acute posttraumatic renal failure: a multicenter perspective. J Trauma 1991;31:1584.

318. Stene JK. Renal failure in the trauma patient. Crit Care Clin 1990;6:111.

319. McDonald BR, Mehta RL, Ward DM. Decreased mortality in patients with acute renal failure undergoing continuous arteriovenous hemodialysis in the intensive care unit. Contrib Nephrol 1991;93:51.

320. Minton S. Poisonous snakes: part 1 and 2. Clin Med 1978; 85:13.

321. Parrish H. Incidence of treated snakebites in the United States. Public Health Rep 1966;81:269.

322. Russell F. Medical problems of snakebite: epidemiology. In: Snake venom poisoning. Great Neck, NY, Scholium International, 1983:250.

323. Litovitz T, Holm K, Bailey K, et al. Annual report of the American Association of Poison Control Centers national data collection system. Am J Emerg Med 1992;10:454.

324. Gomez H, Davis M, Phillips S, et al. Human envenomation from a wandering garter snake. Ann Emerg Med 1994; 23:1119.

325. Curry S, Horning D, Brady P, et al. The legitimacy of rattlesnake bites in central Arizona. Ann Emerg Med 1989;18:658.

326. Wingert W, Chan L. Rattlesnake bites in southern California and rationale for recommended treatment. West J Med 1988;148:37.

327. Davidson T. Intravenous rattlesnake envenomation. West J Med 1988;148:37.

328. Hutton RA, Warrell DA. Action of snake venom components on the haemostatic system. Blood Rev 1993;7:176.

329. Arnold R. Treatment of venomous snakebites in the Western hemisphere. Mil Med 1984;149:361.

330. Garfin S. Rattlesnake bites and surgical decompression: results using a laboratory model. Toxicon 1984;22:177.

331. Downey D, Omer G, Moneim M. New Mexical rattlesnake bites: demographic review and guidelines for treatment. J Trauma 1991;31:1380.

332. Glass T. Early débridement in pit viper bites. JAMA 1976; 235:2513.

333. Jurkovich GJ, Luterman A, McCullar K, et al. Complications of Crotalidae antivenin therapy. J Trauma 1988;28:1032.

334. Russell F, Carlson R, Wainschel J, et al. Snake venom poisoning in the United States: experiences with 550 cases. JAMA 1975;233:341.

335. Stewart R, Page C, Schwesinger W, et al. Antivenin and fasciotomy/debridement in the treatment of the severe rattlesnake bite. Am J Surg 1989;158:543.

336. White RR, Weber RA. Discussion of poisonous snakebite in central Texas: possible indicators for antivenin treatment. Ann Surg 1991;213:466.

337. Nelson B. Snake envenomation: incidence, clinical presentation, and management. Medical Toxicology 1989;4:17.

338. Minton S. Present tests for detection of snake venom: clinical applications. Ann Emerg Med 1987;16:932.

339. Wingert W, Wainschel J. Diagnosis and management of envenomation of poisonous snakes. South Med J 1975;68:1015.

340. McCullough N, Gennaro J. Evaluation of venomous snake bite in southern United States. J Fla Med Assoc 1963;40:959.

341. Kunkel D. Bites of venomous reptiles. Emerg Med Clin North Am 1984;2:563.

342. Treatment of snakebite in the United States. Med Lett Drugs Ther 1982;24:87.

343. Clark R. Cryotherapy and corticosteroids in the treatment of rattlesnake bite. Mil Med 1971;136:42.

344. Lindsey D. Controversy in snake bite: time for a controlled appraisal. J Trauma 1985;25:462.

345. Christopher DG, Rodning CB. Crotalidae envenomation. South Med J 1986;79:159.

346. McCullough N, Gennaro J Jr. Treatment of venomous snake bites in the United States. Clin Toxicol 1970;3:483.

347. Wood J, Hoback W, Green T. Treatment of snake venom poisoning with ACTH and cortisone. Va Med 1955;82:130.

348. Garfin SR, Castilonia RR, Mubarak SJ, et al. The effect of antivenin on intramuscular pressure elevations induced by rattlesnake venom. Toxicon 1985;23:677.

349. Curry S, Kraner J, Kunkel D, et al. Noninvasive vascular studies in management of rattlesnake envenomations to extremities. Ann Emerg Med 1985;14:1081.

350. Russell F. Gila monster. In: Russell F, ed. Snake venom poisoning. Great Neck, NY, Scholium International, 1983:395.

351. Hooker KR, Caravati EM. Gila monster envenomation. Ann Emerg Med 1994;24:731.

352. Preston C. Hypotension, myocardial infarction, and coagulopathy following Gila monster bite. J Emerg Med 1989;7:37.

353. Wilson DC, King LE Jr. Spiders and spider bites. Dermatol Clin 1990;8:277.

354. Wasserman G. Wound care of spider and snake envenomations. Ann Emerg Med 1988;17:1331.

355. Futrell JM. Loxoscelism. Am J Med Sci 1992;304:261.

356. Patel KD, Modur V, Zimmerman GA, et al. The necrotic venom of the brown recluse spider induces dysregulated endothelial cell-dependent neutrophil activation: differential induction of GM-CSF, IL-8, and E-selectin expression. J Clin Invest 1994;94:631.

357. DeLozier J, Reaves L, King L, et al. Brown recluse spider bites of the upper extremity. South Med J 1988;81:181.

358. Barrett SM, Romine-Jenkins M, Fisher DE. Dapsone or electric shock therapy of brown recluse spider envenomation? Ann Emerg Med 1994;24:21.

359. Strain GM, Snider TG, Tedford BL, et al. Hyperbaric oxygen effects on brown recluse spider (*Loxosceles reclusa*) envenomation in rabbits. Toxicon 1991;29:989.

360. Pennell T, Babu S, Meredith J. The management of snake and spider bites in the southeastern United States. Am Surg 1987;53:198.

361. Muller GJ. Black and brown widow spider bites in South Africa: a series of 45 cases. S Afr Med J 1993;83:399.

362. Clark RF, Wethern-Kestner S, Vance MV, et al. Clinical presentation and treatment of black widow spider envenomation: a review of 163 cases. Ann Emerg Med 1992;21:782.

363. Suntorntham S, Roberts J, Nilsen G. Dramatic clinical response to the delayed administration of black widow spider antivenin. (Letter) Ann Emerg Med 1994;24:1198.

364. Freeman TM. Imported fire ants: the ants from hell! Allergy Proc 1994;15:11.

365. Reisman RE. Stinging insect allergy. Med Clin North Am 1992;76:883.

366. Stafford CT. Fire ant allergy. Allergy Proc 1992;13:11.

367. Bawaskar HS, Bawaskar PH. Cardiovascular manifestations of severe scorpion sting in India (review of 34 children). Ann Trop Paediatr 1991;11:381.

368. Yarom R. Scorpion venom: a tutorial review of its effects in man and experimental animals. Clin Toxicol 1970;3:561.

369. Dudin AA, Rambaud-Cousson A, Thalji A, et al. Scorpion sting in children in the Jerusalem area: a review of 54 cases. Ann Trop Paediatr 1991;11:217.

370. Report of Committee on Accidental Hypothermia. Royal College of Physicians, 1966.

371. Moss J. Accidental severe hypothermia. Surg Gynecol Obstet 1986;162:501.

372. Brantigan C, Patton B. Clinical hypothermia, accidental hypothermia and frostbite. In: Goldsmith H, ed. Lewis practice of surgery. New York, Harper & Row, 1978.

373. Trevino A, Razi B, Beller B. The characteristic electrocardiogram of accidental hypothermia. Arch Intern Med 1971;127:470.

374. Ferguson N. Urban hypothermia. Anaesthesia 1985;40:651.

375. Cohen D, Cline J, Lepinski S, et al. Resuscitation of the hypothermic patient. Am J Emerg Med 1988;6:475.

376. Ledingham I, Mone J. Treatment of accidental hypothermia: a prospective clinical study. Br Med J 1980;1:1102.

377. Rahn H, Reeves R, Howell B. Hydrogen ion regulation, temperature, and evolution. Am Rev Respir Dis 1975;112:165.

378. Ream A, Reitz B, Silverberg G. Temperature correction of PaCO$_2$ and pH in estimating acid-base status: an example of emperor's new clothes? Anesthesiology 1982;56:41.

379. White F. A comparative physiologic approach to hypothermia. J Thorac Cardiovasc Surg 1982;82:821.

380. Hansen J, Sue D. Should blood gas measurements be corrected for the patient's temperature? (Letter) N Engl J Med 1980;303:341.

381. Orlowski J, Erenberg G, Lueders H, et al. Hypothermia and barbiturate coma for refractory status epilepticus. Crit Care Med 1984;12:367.

382. Schaller M, Fischer A, Perret C. Hyperkalemia: a prognostic factor during acute severe hypothermia. JAMA 1990;264:1842.

383. Moyer J, Morris GJ, DeBakey M. Effect on renal hymodynamics and excretion of water and electrolytes in dog and man. Ann Surg 1957;145:26.

384. Anderson M, Nielsen K. Renal function under experimental hypothermia in rabbits. Acta Med Scand 1955;151:191.

385. Curry D, Curry K. Hypothermia and insulin secretion. Endocrinology 1970;87:750.

386. Axelrod D, Bass D. Electrolytes and acid base balance in hypothermia. Am J Physiol 1956;186:31.

387. Iampietro P, Vaughan J, Goldman R, et al. Heat production from shivering. J Appl Physiol 1960;15:632.

388. Pozos R, Wittmers L. The nature and treatment of hypothermia. Minneapolis, University of Minnesota Press, 1983.

389. Flacke J, Flacke W. Frequent, insidious and often serious. Semin Anesth 1983;2:183.

390. Zwischenberger J, Kirsh M, Dechert R, et al. Supression of shivering decreases oxygen consumption and improves hemodynamic stability during postoperative rewarming. Ann Thorac Surg 1987;43:428.

391. Roe C, Goldberg M, Blair C, et al. The influence of body temperature on early postoperative oxygen consumption. Surgery 1966;60:85.

392. Gentilello L. Practical approaches to hypothermia. Adv Trauma Crit Care 1994;9:39.

393. Jurkovich G. Hypothermia in the trauma patient. Adv Trauma Crit Care 1989;4:111.

394. Paton B. Accidental hypothermia. Pharmacol Ther 1983;22:331.

395. Reuler J. Hypothermia: pathophysiology, clinical settings, and management. Ann Intern Med 1978;89:519.

396. Gregory JS, Flancbaum L, Townsend MC, et al. Incidence and timing of hypothermia in trauma patients undergoing operations. J Trauma 1991;31:795.

397. Luna G, Maier R, Pavlin E, et al. Incidence and effect of hypothermia in seriously injured patients. J Trauma 1987;27:1014.

398. Jurkovich G, Greiser W, Luterman A, et al. Hypothermia in trauma victims: an ominous predictor of survival. J Trauma 1987;27:1019.

399. Danzl D, Pozos R, Auerbach P, et al. Multicenter hypothermia surgery. Ann Emerg Med 1987;16:1042.

400. Gentilello L, Jurkovich G. Hypothermia in the penetrating trauma victim. In: Ivatury R, Cayten G, eds. Textbook of penetrating trauma. Baltimore, Williams & Wilkins, 1996:995.

401. Little R, Stoner H. Body temperature after accidental injury. Br J Surg 1981;68:221.

402. Hardy J, Randini I. Some physiologic aspects of surgical trauma. Am Surg 1952;136:345.

403. Psarras P, Ivatury R, Rohman M, et al. Hypothermia in trauma: incidence and prognostic significance. Longboat

Key, FL, Eastern Association for the Surgery of Trauma, 1988.

404. Steinemann S, Shackford S, Davis J. Implications of admission hypothermia in trauma patients. J Truama 1990;30:200.

405. Blalock A, Mason M. A comparison of the effects of heat and those of cold in the prevention and treatment of shock. Arch Surg 1945;42:1054.

406. Sori A, El-Assuooty A, Rush B, et al. The effect of temperature on survival in hemorrhagic shock. Am Surg 1987; 53:706.

407. Jurkovich G, Pitt R, Curreri P, et al. Hypothermia prevents increased capillary permeability following ischemia-reperfusion injury. J Surg Res 1988;44:514.

408. Wright J, Kerr J, Valeri C, et al. Regional hypothermia protects against ischemia-reperfusion injury in isolated canine gracilis muscle. J Trauma 1988;28:1027.

409. Bachmann F, McKenna, Cole E, et al. The hemostatic mechanism after open heart surgery. I. Studies on plasma coagulation factors and fibrinolysis in 512 patients after extracorporeal circulation. J Thorac Cardiovasc Surg 1975;79:76.

410. Harker L, Malpass T, Branson H, et al. Mechanism of abnormal bleeding in patients undergoing cardiopulmonary bypass: acquired transient platelet dysfunction associated with selective α-granule release. Blood 1980;56:824.

411. Kattlove H, Alexander B. The effect of cold on platelets. I. Cold-induced platelet aggregation. Blood 1971;38:39.

412. Patt A, McCroskey B, Moore E. Hypothermia-induced coagulopathies in trauma. Surg Clin North Am 1988;68:775.

413. Valeri C, Feingold H, Cassidy G, et al. Hypothermia induced reversible platelet dysfunction. Ann Surg 1987;205:175.

414. Reed R, Bracey A, Hudson J, et al. Hypothermia and blood coagulation: dissociation between enzyme activity and clotting factor levels. Circ Shock 1990;32:141.

415. Gubler K, Gentilello L, Hassantash S, et al. The impact of hypothermia on dilutional coagulopathy. J Trauma 1994; 36:847.

416. Gentilello L, Jurkovich G, Moujaes S. Hypothermia and injury: thermodynamic principles of prevention and treatment. In: Levine B, ed. Perspectives in surgery. St Louis, Quality Medical Publishers, 1991.

417. Fruehan A. Accidental hypothermia. Arch Intern Med 1960;105:218.

418. Kugelberg J, Schuller H, Berg B. Treatment of accidental hypothermia. Scand J Thorac Cardiovasc Surg 1967;1:142.

419. Gentilello L, Cortes V, Moujaes S, et al. Continuous arteriovenous rewarming: experimental results and thermodynamic model simulation of treatment for hypothermia. J Trauma 1990;30:1436.

420. Patton J, Doolittle W. Core rewarming by peritoneal dialysis following induced hypothermia in the dog. J Appl Physiol 1972;33:800.

421. Myers R, Britten J, Cowley R. Hypothermia: quantitative aspects of therapy. JACEP 1979;8:523.

422. Gentilello L, Moujaes S. Treatment of hypothermia in trauma victims: thermodynamic considerations. J Intens Care Med 1995;10:5.

423. Britt LD, Dascombe WH, Rodriguez A. New horizons in management of hypothermia and frostbite injury. Surg Clin North Am 1991;71:345.

424. Jacob J, Weisman M, Rosenblatt S, et al. Chronic pernio: a historical perspective of cold-induced vascular disease. Arch Intern Med 1986;146:1589.

425. Auerbach P. Disorders due to physical and environmental agents. In: Mills J, Ho MT, Salber PR, Trunkey DD, eds. Current emergency diagnosis and treatment. Los Altos, CA, Lange Medical Publications, 1985.

426. Francis T, Golden FSC. Non-freezing cold injury: the pathogenesis. J R Nav Med Serv 1985;71:3.

427. Lloyd E. Hypothermia and cold stress. Aspen 1986:84.

428. Mills WJ, Jr. Frostbite: a discussion of the problem and a review of the Alaskan experience (1973 classic article). Alaska Med 1993;35:28.

429. Urschel JD. Frostbite: predisposing factors and predictors of poor outcome. J Trauma 1990;30:340.

430. Dana H, Rex I, Samitz M. The hunting reaction. Arch Dermatol 1969;99:441.

431. Heggers J, Robson M, Weingarten M, et al. Experimental and clinical observations on frostbite. Ann Emerg Med 1987; 16:1056.

432. Bourne M, Piepkorn M, Clayton F, et al. Analysis of microvascular changes in frostbite injury. J Surg Res 1986;40:26.

433. Vedder NB, Winn RK, Rice CL, et al. Inhibition of leukocyte adherence by anti-CD 18 monoclonal antibody attenuates reperfusion injury in the rabbit ear. Proc Natl Acad Sci USA 1990;87:2643.

434. Mills WJ Jr, Whaley R. Frostbite: experience with rapid rewarming and ultrasonic therapy. Part I and II. (1960 classic article) Alaska Med 1993;35:6.

435. Treatment of frostbite. Med Lett Drugs Ther 1980;22:112.

436. Rakower S, Shahgoli S, Wong SL. Doppler ultrasound and digital plethysmography to determine the need for sympathetic blockade after frostbite. J Trauma 1978;18:713.

437. Bouwman D, Morrison S, Lucas C, et al. Early sympathetic blockade for frostbite: is it of value? J Trauma 1980;20:744.

438. Purdue G, Hunt J. Cold injury: a collective review. J Burn Care Rehabil 1986;7:331.

439. Mundth E. Frostbite symposium. In: Viereck E, ed. Arctic Aero Med Lab. Ft Wainwright Laboratory, Alaska, 1964.

440. Mills W Jr. Comment and recapitulation. Alaska Med 1993;35:69.

441. Edlich R, Chang D, Birk K, et al. Cold injuries. Compr Ther 1989;15:13.

442. Mills WJ Jr. Summary of treatment of the cold injured patient: frostbite. (1983 classic article) Alaska Med 1993;35:61.

443. Mehta RC, Wilson MA. Frostbite injury: prediction of tissue viability with triple-phase bone scanning. Radiology 1989;170:511.

444. Rustin M, Newton J, Smith N, et al. The treatment of chilblains with nifedipine: the results of a pilot study, a double-blind placebo-controlled randomized study and a long-term open trial. Br J Dermatol 1989;120:267.

SURGERY: SCIENTIFIC PRINCIPLES AND PRACTICE, Second Edition, edited by Lazar J. Greenfield, Michael W. Mulholland, Keith T. Oldham, Gerald B. Zelenock, and Keith D. Lillemoe. Lippincott–Raven Publishers, Philadelphia, © 1997.

CHAPTER 12

BURNS

ROBERT L. SHERIDAN AND RONALD G. TOMPKINS

Management of burn patients is a multifaceted challenge, requiring surgical, critical care, rehabilitative, and psychosocial skills. The prognosis of such patients has improved dramatically in the past two decades, with most not only surviving but enjoying excellent functional and cosmetic outcomes. This chapter reviews the clinical management of serious burns and relates progress in this management to the growing understanding of the pathophysiology of burn injury.

MANAGEMENT PHILOSOPHY

The management philosophy provides a systematic approach to patients that includes the following:

- Individualized resuscitation of virtually all patients regardless of injury severity (the exception being elderly patients with massive injuries for whom survival is highly unlikely and in whom the quality of survival is likely to be inconsistent with their own desires as expressed by health care proxy or close family members)
- Early excision and biologic closure of deep wounds
- Continuous rehabilitation

- Judicious use of broad spectrum antibiotics with early detection and specific treatment of septic foci
- Intensive patient and family psychosocial support
- Long-term follow-up with ongoing rehabilitative and reconstructive support

The acute hospitalization is organized into four phases: (1) initial evaluation and resuscitation, (2) initial wound excision and biologic closure, (3) definitive wound closure, and (4) intensification of the continuous rehabilitation effort. With this approach, regardless of injury size, quality survival can be expected for most burn patients who present without anoxic brain injury.

EPIDEMIOLOGY

Some 2 million Americans require medical attention each year for burn injuries. Children 6 months to 2 years of age[1] and elderly persons[2] are at particular risk of sustaining burns in domestic cooking and bathing accidents. Young adults are more often injured in the workplace. Structural fires spare no age group. As in motor vehicle trauma, alcohol use frequently contributes to these injuries. Although the life-threatening nature of large injuries is often emphasized, the potentially devastating impact of poorly managed smaller burns should not be neglected (Color Fig. 12-1). Extensive efforts have been made to diminish the incidence of pediatric burn injury through public education, but the effect is variable. For example, legislation that mandates lower temperatures for water heaters has been successful, leading to a decreased incidence of hot water injuries in children.[3] Inconsistent application of these laws remains a problem. About 15% of pediatric burn injuries are attributed to abuse or neglect, and an awareness of this important issue facilitates the prevention of repeated injuries.

NATURAL HISTORY

Teleologically, the skin envelope played a crucial role in allowing aquatic sea animals to adapt to the land environment. Our survival as individuals continues to depend on the vapor and bacterial barriers provided by normal skin. The epidermal layer provides these two essential functions, and the dermis provides flexibility and strength (Fig. 12-1). In addition, dermal appendages prevent desiccation of the skin by producing oils, and the reactive dermal microvasculature is responsible for heat dissipation and conservation, allowing humans to adapt to changes in environmental temperature. These important functions are compromised or lost when substantial areas of the skin are burned. An understanding of the natural history of any disease process facilitates an understanding of the success of intervention. This natural history is examined here at the level of the local tissue and the whole organism.

Local Response to Burn Injury

The local response to thermal injury is principally related to destruction and thrombosis of vessels in the dermis. Of particular interest are the microvascular reactions in the surrounding dermis, where progressive vasoconstriction and thrombosis are seen to a degree that varies in accordance with the severity of the primary injury.[4] In animal models, the secondary injury that follows these microvascular changes is truncated by cyclooxygenase inhibitors,[5] lazaroids,[6] and fibrinogen depletion.[7] These observations suggest possible future therapeutic interventions to minimize secondary injury.

Systemic Response to Burn Injury

The systemic response to cutaneous thermal injury is driven by the loss of the skin's barrier functions. This results in accelerated fluid losses, decreased host resistance to infection, release of mediators from the injured tissue with microvascular and end-organ dysfunction, and bacterial overgrowth within the eschar, resulting in systemic infection. Edema in tissue immediately surrounding the burn occurs secondary to local release of vasoactive mediators, such as prostaglandins, thromboxane A_2, and reactive oxygen radicals. When burn size exceeds 20% or 30% of the body surface, clinically significant interstitial edema is seen in distant soft tissues secondary to a combination of mediators generated in the wound and hypoproteinemia. Distant microvascular injury may interfere with the function of organ systems not directly injured by the burning process,[8] thus explaining the frequent occurrence of pulmonary and other end-organ dysfunction in patients with large burns.[9] Although exciting work is underway that may

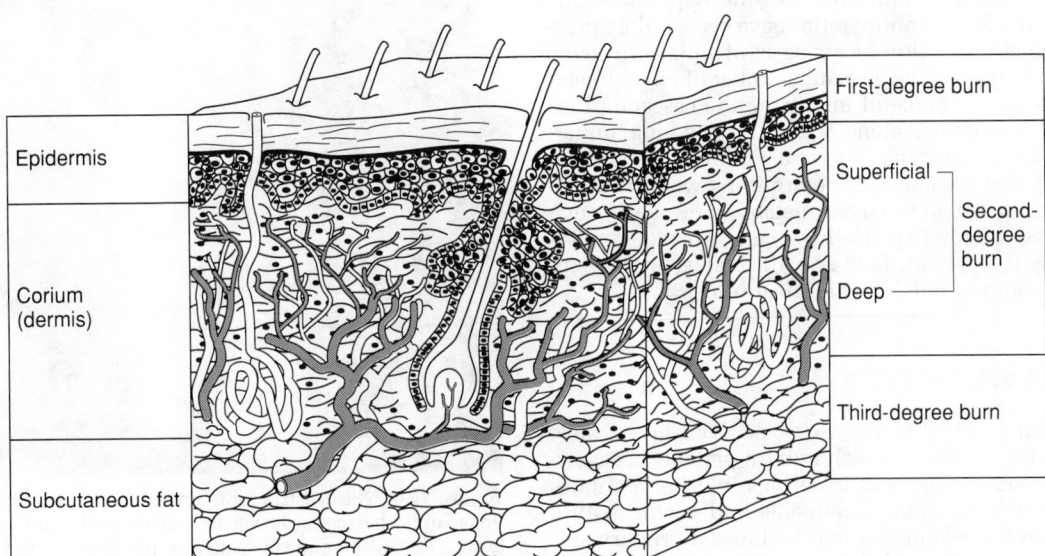

Figure 12-1. Schematic depiction of skin.

ultimately lead to clinically useful modifications of these mediator effects,[10] our understanding of these processes is as yet inadequate to allow intelligent intervention.

A burn wound is initially clean but is rapidly colonized by endogenous bacteria. As these bacteria multiply in the avascular eschar over succeeding days, proteases liquefy the eschar, which then separates, leaving a bed of granulation tissue or healing burn, depending on the depth of the original injury. If wounds are small, less than 20% of the total body surface (TBSA), this local infectious challenge is usually well tolerated. When injuries are larger, however, systemic infection frequently results, explaining the rare survival of patients with burns in excess of 40% of the TBSA when the wound is managed in this expectant fashion.[11]

The physiologic challenge of a burn in excess of 20% of the TBSA frequently results in an initial decrease in cardiac output and metabolic rate. Subsequently, a hypermetabolic response is seen, with a near doubling of cardiac output and resting energy expenditure over the next 24 to 48 hours in those who are successfully resuscitated. The magnitude of this response peaks with injuries of 60% or more of the TBSA when the metabolic rate is more than double resting values. Enhanced gluconeogenesis, relative insulin resistance, and increased protein catabolism associated with this response have major clinical implications for the support of burn patients. The etiology of the hypermetabolic response is not entirely understood but is assumed to involve a combination of the following and perhaps other factors:

- Change in hypothalamic function with coincident increases in glucagon, cortisol, and catecholamine secretion[12]
- Deficient gastrointestinal barrier function with translocation of bacteria and their by-products[13]
- Bacterial contamination of the burn wound with systemic release of similar products from this source[14,15]
- Some element of enhanced heat loss through evaporation of fluid across the eschar[16]

The hypermetabolic response probably has survival value because it is conserved so broadly over numerous species. An important element of successful treatment of patients who have sustained large injuries is to support this response through the provision of adequate quantity and quality of substrate.

Although limited modifications of the hypermetabolic response in the form of antipyretics have been widely practiced, elimination of this response is of unknown value and may be harmful. The growing number of recombinant protein products capable of impacting the cascade of inflammatory mediators, along with our fledgling understanding to the process, has lead to a plethora of laboratory and clinical projects aimed at determining whether seemingly adverse facets of the hypermetabolic response, such as the excessive protein catabolism, can be obviated without harming the patient. Data are still inadequate to support such therapies outside of clinical trials.

INITIAL EVALUATION

Meaningful survival can be expected even in the most severe injuries, so the approach to burn patients is aggressive. An organized approach to serious injuries facilitates the achievement of optimal outcome and begins with a systematic initial evaluation that includes a primary survey, effective vascular and airway access, and a systematic secondary survey.

Systematic Initial Evaluation

Many burn patients sustain concurrent injuries, and the initial evaluation should therefore be approached as for any victim of multiple trauma. After the airway is evaluated and secured while the cervical spine is controlled, breathing mechanics are assessed, a rough estimate is made of the circulating blood volume, the level of consciousness is documented, and the patient is completely exposed. This should be done in a warm environment to avoid hypothermia. Secure airway and vascular access is crucial and should be obtained early during the evaluation. A badly burned face precludes tape in securing the endotracheal tube; an umbilical tie harness should be used instead (Color Fig. 12-2). Secure venous access is best obtained centrally, although two peripheral intravenous lines are a reasonable option. In hypovolemic children, intraosseous resuscitation can be lifesaving (Color Fig. 12-3), but it should be promptly replaced with venous cannulae as soon as practical. All patients should have a nasogastric tube placed, particularly if they are to be transported by air, because a gas-filled stomach can lead to emesis and aspiration (Fig. 12-2). A bladder catheter facilitates smooth fluid resuscitation. Continuous temperature monitoring with rectal or esophageal probes and arterial access is helpful in selected patients.

The burn-specific secondary survey (Table 12-1) includes a complete history, vital signs, a detailed physical

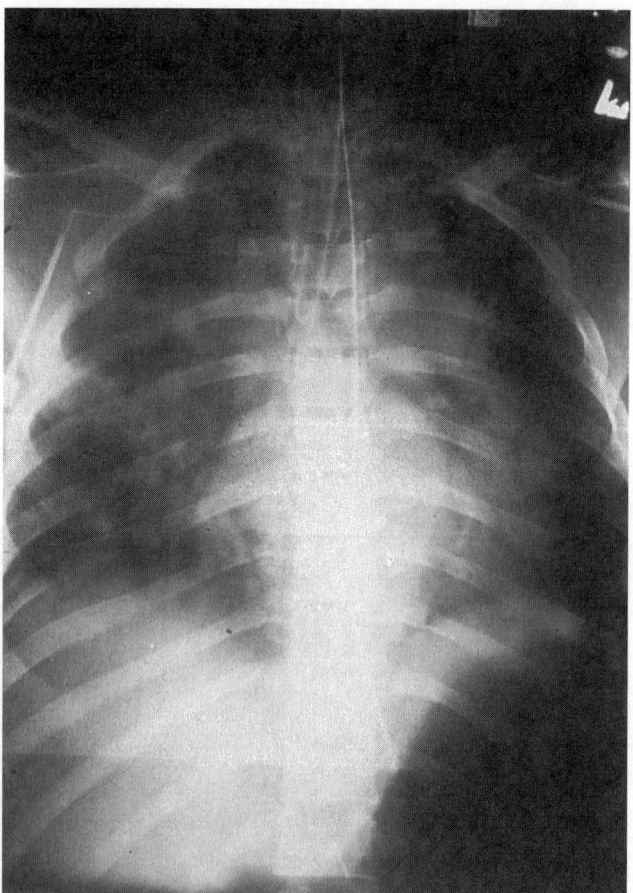

Figure 12-2. Nasogastric tube function, as well as physical presence, must be regularly verified to minimize the possibility of gastric distention and subsequent aspiration during burn resuscitation. Both of these potential problems are shown in this radiograph of a burn patient.

Table 12-1. IMPORTANT ASPECTS OF THE BURN-SPECIFIC SECONDARY SURVEY

HISTORY

Closed-space exposure
Extrication time
Delay in seeking attention
Fluid given during transport
Previous illnesses and injuries

HEAD, EYES, EARS, NOSE, AND THROAT

The globes should be examined and corneal epithelium stained with fluorescein before adnexal swelling makes examination difficult. Adnexal swelling provides excellent coverage and protection during the first days after injury. Tarsorrhaphy is virtually never indicated acutely.
Corneal epithelial loss can be overt, giving a clouded appearance to the cornea, but it is more often subtle, requiring fluorescein staining for documentation. Topical ophthalmic antibiotics constitute optimal initial treatment.
Signs of airway involvement include perioral and intraoral burns or carbonaceous material and progressive hoarseness.
Hot liquid can be aspirated with a facial scald injury and result in acute airway compromise requiring urgent intubation.
Endotracheal tube security is crucial and is best maintained with an umbilical tape harness, rather than adhesive tape, on the burned face.

NECK

The radiographic evaluation is driven by the mechanism of injury.
Neck escharotomies are rarely needed to facilitate venous drainage of the head.

CARDIAC

Cardiac rhythm should be monitored for 24 to 72 hours in electrical injury.
Elderly patients may experience transient atrial fibrillation if modestly overresuscitated.
Significant arrhythmias are unusual if intravascular volume and oxygenation are adequately supported.
History of myocardial infarction increases the risk of new infarct with the stress of burn injury, and appropriate monitoring is necessary.

PULMONARY

Inflating pressures should be kept below 40 cm H_2O by the performance of chest escharotomies when needed.
Severe inhalation injury may lead to slough of endobronchial mucosa and thick endobronchial secretions. Sudden endotracheal tube occlusions may occur.

VASCULAR

Burned extremities should be vigilantly monitored by serial examinations. Indications for escharotomy include decreasing temperature, increasing consistency, slowed capillary refill and diminished Doppler flow in the digital vessels. One should not wait until flow in named vessels is compromised to decompress the extremity.
Fasciotomy is indicated after electrical or deep thermal injury when distal flow is compromised. Compartment pressure measurement can be helpful, but clinical examination is an indication for decompression regardless of compartment pressure readings.

ABDOMEN

Nasogastric tubes should be placed and their function verified, particularly before air transport in unpressurized helicopters.
An inappropriate resuscitative volume requirement may be a sign of an occult intraabdominal injury.
Torso escharotomies may be required to facilitate ventilation of deep circumferential abdominal wall burns.
Immediate stress ulcer prophylaxis with histamine-receptor blockers and antacids is indicated with serious burns.

GENITOURINARY

Bladder catheterization is appropriate in all who require fluid resuscitation and urine output monitoring.
The foreskin should be reduced over the bladder catheter after insertion, since progressive swelling may otherwise result in paraphimosis.

NEUROLOGIC

Early neurologic evaluation is important, since the sensorium is altered by medication or hemodynamic instability during the hours after injury. CT scanning is appropriate if possible for head trauma.
Patients who require neuromuscular blockade for transport should also receive adequate sedation and analgesia.

EXTREMITIES

Extremities with circumferential thermal burns or electrical injury should be promptly decompressed by escharotomy or fasciotomy when clinical examination reveals diminished distal perfusion. Limbs at risk should be dressed so they can be frequently examined.
The need for escharotomy usually becomes evident during the early resuscitation. Most escharotomies can be delayed until transport has been effected if this is less than 6 hours.
Burned extremities should be elevated and splinted in a position of function.

WOUNDS

Wounds are often underestimated in depth and overestimated in size on initial examination.
Size, depth, and the presence of circumferential components are important issues.

LABORATORY TESTS

Arterial blood gas analysis is important when airway compromise or inhalation injury is present.
Normal carboxyhemoglobin concentration on admission does not eliminate the possibility of a significant exposure as the half-life of carboxyhemoglobin is 30 to 40 minutes in those effectively ventilated with 100% oxygen.
Baseline hemoglobin and electrolytes can be helpful later during resuscitation.
Urinalysis for occult blood should be performed with deep thermal or electrical injuries.

RADIOGRAPHIC EVALUATIONS

Radiographic evaluation is driven by the mechanism of injury and the need to document placement of supportive cannulae.

(continued)

Table 12-1. IMPORTANT ASPECTS OF THE BURN-SPECIFIC SECONDARY SURVEY (Continued)

ELECTRICAL BURNS

Cardiac rhythm should be monitored in high (greater than 1000 volts) or intermediate (greater than 220 volts) voltage exposures for 24 to 72 hours.

Low and intermediate voltage exposures can cause locally destructive injuries but uncommonly result in systemic sequelae.

After high-voltage exposures, delayed neurologic and ocular sequelae can occur, so a carefully documented admission examination is important.

Injured extremities should be serially evaluated for intracompartmental edema and promptly decompressed when necessary.

Bladder catheters are required for high-voltage exposure to assess the possibility of pigmenturia. This is treated adequately with volume loading in most patients.

CHEMICAL BURNS

Wounds should be irrigated with tapwater for at least 30 minutes. The globe is irrigated with isotonic crystalloid solution. Blepharospasm may require ocular anesthetic administration.

Exposure to hydrofluoric acid may be complicated by life-threatening hypocalcemia, particularly exposures to concentrated or anhydrous solutions. Close monitoring and supplementation of serum calcium is necessary. Subeschar injection of 10% calcium gluconate solution is appropriate after exposure to highly concentrated or anhydrous solutions.

TAR BURNS

Tar should be initially cooled with tapwater irrigation, then removed with a lipophillic solvent.

---

examination, and laboratory and radiographic studies appropriate for the mechanism of injury. The history, particularly details about the mechanism of injury, is important and is ideally obtained from witnesses, rescue personnel, and family members. The mechanism of injury often determines the need for special studies, such as computed tomography (CT) of the head and abdomen or radiography of the cervical spine. Other important historical points include medical and surgical history, time of the last meal, tetanus status, medications and allergies, water temperature in hot liquid injuries, and extrication time in closed-space injuries. Vital signs are determined during the secondary survey, and age-specific norms should be known (Table 12-2). A complete physical examination should proceed in an organized fashion; the presence of the burn should not distract the examiner from performing a complete assessment.

The patient's neurologic status should be carefully documented early in the evaluation, because many patients become progressively obtunded secondary to the administration of analgesics and sedatives and as the result of intravascular volume depletion. If injury mechanism is consistent with a head injury, CT should be performed.

Trauma to the head, face, and neck is determined by inspection and palpation. The corneal epithelium and globes should be examined before the development of adnexal edema, which makes examination more difficult. Major corneal epithelial burns are obvious by the resulting opaque appearance of the cornea. More subtle defects are apparent after staining with topical fluorescein. Upper airway injuries are suspected in the presence of a hoarse voice, burns of the lips or tongue, singed facial hair and nasal vibrissae, or carbonaceous sputum. Hot liquid aspiration may complicate facial scald burns in small children and should be suspected in if there is blistering in or around the mouth. If upper airway compromise is imminent, endotracheal intubation is mandatory, particularly before the initiation of long transports. Verification of endotracheal tube security is an important part of the head and neck examination.

The torso should be assessed for compliance, and if ventilation is restricted by overlying circumferential eschar, torso escharotomies should be performed promptly with coagulating electrocautery to minimize blood loss. Incisions are typically made axially along the flanks and are connected by one or more horizontal incisions (Fig. 12-3). The abdomen should be assessed for tenderness or distention. If the mechanism of injury suggests an abdominal injury, CT or peritoneal lavage is appropriate, particularly in the presence of an inappropriately high resuscitative volume requirement. Gastric distention is particularly common in distressed children, and nasogastric decompression is routinely recommended during the initial evaluation and transport. Proper nasogastric tube function should be verified regularly. All burned patients should receive immediate stress ulcer prophylaxis with intraluminal antacids and intravenous histamine-receptor blockers, since the incidence of stress ulceration is unacceptably high if this precaution is not taken. The presence of genital burns should be noted. If the patient is not circumcised, the foreskin should be reduced after placement of the bladder catheter to avoid paraphimosis secondary to progressive edema.

Regular assessment and documentation of peripheral perfusion is crucial during the first days after injury. Blood flow can be compromised by constricting circumferential eschar as subeschar tissues become progressively edematous or by progressive intracompartmental edema in patients with electrical or deep thermal burns. Both are detected by the development of a progressive increase in the extremity's consistency and a decrease in its distal temperature. Pulsatile Doppler signals in the lower pressure distal vasculature, such as the palmar arch and digital vessels, should be documented hourly; their loss is consistent with

Table 12-2. Age-Specific Resuscitation Endpoints

Evaluation	Target
Sensorium	Comfortable, arousable
Urine output	
Infants	1–2 mL/kg/h
Children	0.5–1 mL/kg/h
All others	0.5 mL/kg/h
Base deficit	<2 mEq/dL
Systolic blood pressure	
Infants	60–70 mmHg
Children	70–90 + (twice age in years) mmHg
Adolescents and adults	90–120 mmHg

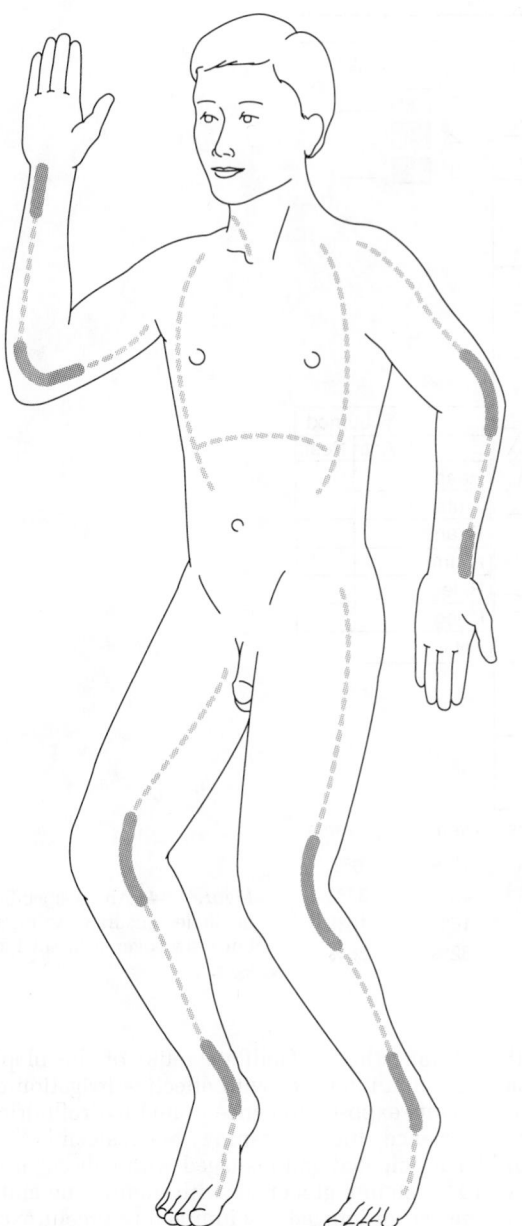

Figure 12-3. Preferred sites of escharotomy. Connecting lateral axial incisions across the midline facilitates ventilation with low inflating pressures. Extremity escharotomies are performed using medial and lateral axial incisions.

increasing tissue pressure if intravascular volume is adequate. Constricting circumferential eschar can be opened at the bedside using coagulating electrocautery. This is most commonly done using medial and lateral axial incisions with the patient lightly sedated. It is important to maintain hemostasis during the procedure and to verify that distal blood flow has been enhanced. Hand escharotomies are not often required once the proximal upper extremity has been adequately decompressed. If decompression of the arm to the level of the metacarpophalangeal joints has not resulted in adequate digital blood flow, axial digital incisions are made between the extensor tendons and the neurovascular bundles. Ideally, a single incision on the radial aspect of the thumb and the ulnar aspect of the digits suffices. The incisions on the central digits of the hand can be extended proximally between the extensors.

Weakness of intracompartmental muscle groups or pain with their passive stretch supports the suspicion of elevated intracompartmental pressures, although such signs can be obscured in many burn patients. It can be exceptionally difficult to diagnose an evolving compartment syndrome in acutely burned patients, and one should decompress such extremities based on clinical suspicion.[17] Compartment pressure measurements can be a useful adjunct in equivocal situations, but clinical judgment suffices in most cases. If missed, compartment syndromes lead to intracompartmental sepsis or functional deficits later in the patient's course.

Evaluation of the wound is deferred until higher priority evaluations are complete. Important to the initial evaluation are an assessment of the wound depth, size, and circumferential components. Early burn depth estimates are accurate in very deep or very superficial wounds. Many burns, however, particularly scald injuries, are of indeterminate depth on initial examination. Significant effort has been applied to develop technical aids that accurately gauge burn wound depth during the initial evaluation,[18] but none of these aids has had clinical success. Fortunately, an accurate determination of depth is not necessary to proceed with initial wound management or fluid resuscitation. In contrast, an accurate assessment of burn size can be made early and is important to initial management, since resuscitative fluid administration is determined primarily by overall burn size. Burn size in children is best estimated with an age-specific chart (Fig. 12-4), because the body's proportions change with growth. The major anthropometric change involves the head and legs. The infant head represents 18% and the legs 14% of the TBSA. In older adolescents and adults, the head represents 9% and the legs 18% of the TBSA. It is important to identify circumferential components of the wound, since these areas need to be closely monitored for compromise of peripheral perfusion in extremity or neck burns and ventilation in torso injuries. It is worthwhile to calculate both burned and unburned areas. Since the sum must equal 100%, mistaken estimates of burn wound size can be avoided easily.

Relatively few laboratory studies are essential during the initial evaluation. Patients with a history of exposure to noxious fumes should have the arterial PaO_2, $PaCO_2$, pH, and carboxyhemoglobin percentage determined. Since the half-life of carboxyhemoglobin is 30 to 45 minutes when patients are ventilated with high concentrations of oxygen, however, a normal carboxyhemoglobin of less than 5% does not preclude significant exposure when patients have been appropriately ventilated during transport. Patients with electrical or deep thermal injuries often require blood products during the initial resuscitation; a blood bank specimen should be sent routinely in such patients. Routine hematology and chemistry profiles are of limited usefulness initially, but a baseline should be established. Urinalysis for occult blood is helpful in patients with electrical or deep thermal burns if gross pigmenturia has been cleared with crystalloid administration. Radiographic evaluation during the initial evaluation is determined largely by the mechanism of injury and the need to evaluate placement of resuscitative cannulae.

The initial evaluation of patients with electrical, chemical, tar, or abuse-related injuries is generally the same as for patients with thermal injuries; a few unique aspects require emphasis, however. Burn units are often called on to manage nonburn diagnoses that require complex wound and critical care resources, such as purpura fulminans, toxic epidermal necrolysis, staphylococcal scalded skin syndrome, or major soft tissue avulsions. Such patients benefit from the unique combination of critical care and surgical resources available in burn units.[19] Special aspects of evaluation of patients with

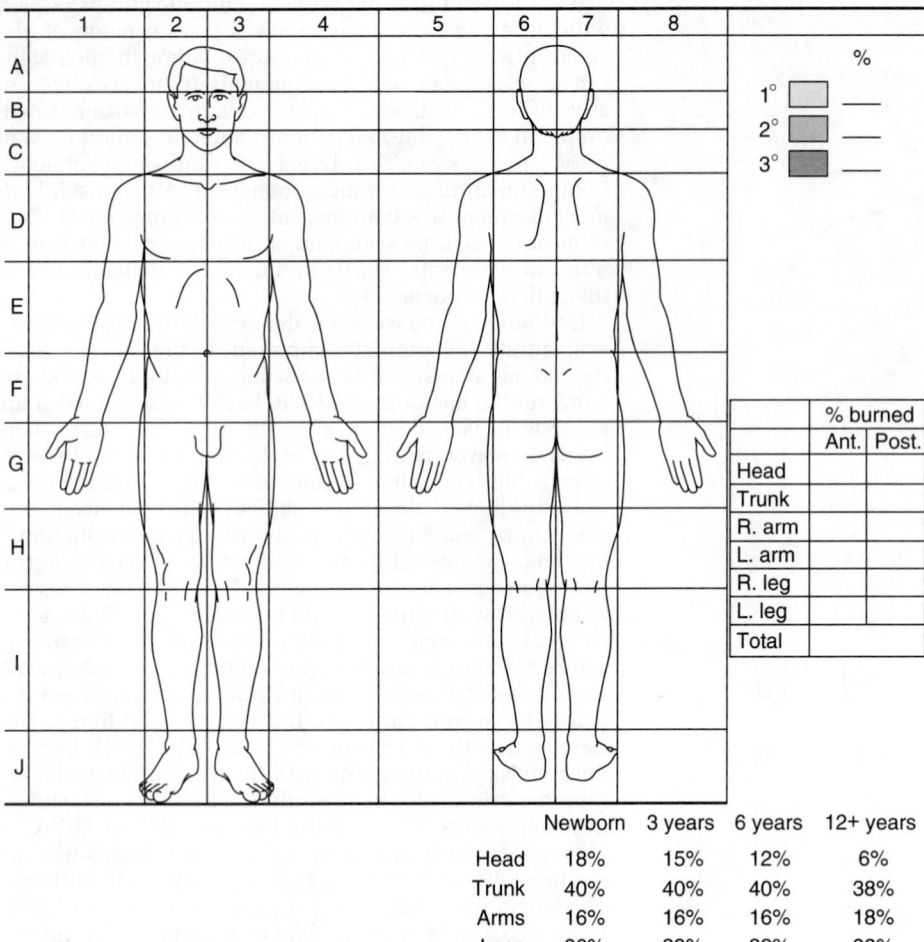

	Newborn	3 years	6 years	12+ years
Head	18%	15%	12%	6%
Trunk	40%	40%	40%	38%
Arms	16%	16%	16%	18%
Legs	26%	29%	32%	38%

Figure 12-4. An age-specific chart facilitates accurate estimation of burn size over a broad range of ages.

purpura fulminans, toxic epidermal necrolysis, and staphylococcal scalded skin syndrome are presented in Table 12-3 and Color Figure 12-4.

Electrical Injuries

Although lesser voltages can cause locally destructive injuries without systemic sequelae (Color Fig. 12-5), high voltage (more than 1000 volts) can cause a combination of deep tissue injury secondary to the passage of current, locally destructive entrance and exit wounds, deep wounds where current arches across flexed joints, flame burns secondary to clothing ignition, flash burns, axial spine fractures secondary to tetanic contraction of paravertebral muscles, and other injuries related to the fall or blast that so commonly accompanies high-voltage injury. Patients with burns caused by exposure to high-voltage electricity require a complete trauma evaluation, cardiac monitoring, bladder catheterization to evaluate the urine for pigment, serial monitoring of compartments at risk for pressure elevation, and spine immobilization pending radiographic examination of the axial spine. Compartment pressure elevation, secondary to edema of injured muscle, can result in additional ischemic injury if compartments are not promptly released (Color Fig. 12-6).

Chemical Injuries

Patients who suffer chemical burns (Color Fig. 12-7) are first treated with at least 30 minutes of copious tapwater irrigation. Ocular injuries are irrigated with saline. Topical

ophthalmic anesthetics facilitate relief of the blepharospasm that often interferes with effective irrigation of the globe. Patients exposed to concentrated hydrofluoric acid may experience life-threatening hypocalcemia.[20] This should be anticipated and managed with subeschar injection of 10% calcium gluconate with monitoring and support of the serum ionized calcium before urgent excision of selected extensive wounds. The more common limited exposures to dilute hydrofluoric acid are managed with irrigation and topical calcium gluconate gel.

Tar Injuries

Tar is often heated to more than 300°F, and contact commonly causes a deep burn. Adherent tar is initially cooled by tapwater irrigation to limit the progression of the injury and is later removed with a lipophilic solvent (Color Fig. 12-8). After initial irrigation, chemical, and tar burns are managed surgically as indicated by depth, which is frequently underestimated on initial examination.

Injuries of Abuse

All burned children should be evaluated for abuse or neglect. It is an ethical and legal mandate that suspicious injuries be filed with the appropriate local agency.[21] Table 12-4 lists important historical points and characteristics of the burn wound that can indicate the burn was caused by abuse, and Color Figure 12-9 is an example of this type of injury. All such children should be admitted to the hospi-

---

Table 12-3. **KEY ASPECTS OF THE DIAGNOSIS OF PURPURA FULMINANS, TOXIC EPIDERMAL NECROLYSIS, AND STAPHYLOCOCCAL SCALDED SKIN SYNDROME**

PURPURA FULMINANS

It is typically a complication of meningococcal sepsis.
It is likely a consequence of transient protein C deficiency; therefore, fresh frozen plasma should be considered as a resuscitative colloid.
It is frequently accompanied by organ failure.
Treatment involves management of organ failures and excision and grafting of wounds.

TOXIC EPIDERMAL NECROLYSIS (TENS)

A variant of erythema multiforme major, TENS is an epidermal slough at the dermal–epidermal junction.
The degree of mucous membrane and conjunctival involvement varies, and when severe is usually called Stevens-Johnson syndrome.
Differentiation from SSSS can be difficult on clinical grounds, and in such cases, skin biopsy is diagnostic. Treatment involves prevention of wound desiccation and superinfection with topical antimicrobials and xenografting of confluent areas of slough while awaiting healing. Ophthalmologic evaluation is important to prevent synechiae. Those with severe oropharyngeal involvement may require intubation for airway protection and enteral tube feeding for nutritional support.

STAPHYLOCOCCAL SCALDED SKIN SYNDROME (SSSS)

SSSS is a reaction to a staphylococcal toxin that causes a separation at the granular layer of the epidermis. This superficial wound generally heals quickly if superinfection and desiccation are prevented.
Involvement of the mucous membrane and conjunctiva is not seen, which is a helpful diagnostic point for separating SSSS from TENS.
A detailed search for a focus of staphylococcal infection is warranted, while empiric antistaphylococcic antibiotics are administered.

---

tal regardless of burn size. Radiographic screening of the head and long bones should be considered to further document possible abuse.

FLUID RESUSCITATION

The large number of fluid resuscitation formulas in common use is a tribute to the fact that no one formula accurately predicts fluid requirements in every patient. No formula can replace a physician at the bedside repeatedly evaluating the patient's physiologic response throughout the resuscitative period. Common controversies in fluid resuscitation relate to the role of colloid, the differences between children and adults, and the influence of inhalation injury and delayed resuscitation on fluid requirements. A reasonable consensus is represented by the Modified Brooke formula (Table 12-5), which serves as the basis for this discussion. Regardless of the formula chosen to initiate resuscitation, subsequent fluid administration is best guided by regular reassessment of resuscitation endpoints rather than by a formulaic prediction.

Vasoactive mediators released from injured tissue result in a diffuse capillary leak seen shortly after a major

---

Table 12-4. **IMPORTANT POINTS OF HISTORY AND PHYSICAL EXAMINATION THAT SUGGEST ABUSE OR NEGLECT**

HISTORY

Delayed presentation for medical care
Conflicting histories
Previous injuries

SUSPICIOUS BURN PATTERNS

Sharply demarcated margins
Uniform depth
Absence of splash marks
Stocking or glove patterns
Flexor sparing
Porcelain contact sparing
Dorsal location of contact injury of the hands
Very deep localized contact injury

---

burn injury. This loss of microvascular integrity results in the extravasation of crystalloid and colloid solutions for the first 18 to 24 hours after burn injury. This pathophysiology explains the enormous volume requirement in these patients and is the reason that most resuscitative formulas withhold colloid until 24 hours after injury. Despite controlled data to support this common clinical practice,[22] controversy over this point remains. Children commonly require intravenous fluid in excess of that predicted by several formulas.[23,24] A urine output of 1 to 2 mL/kg/h is one important resuscitation endpoint in children. Infants and very young children have renal concentrating abilities that are not completely mature. In toddlers and older children, however, whose concentrating abilities are adult, targeting a urine flow of 0.5 to 1 mL/kg/h results in lower overall fluid requirements that are closer to those of an adult. Patients with inhalation injury have overall volume requirements greater than are predicted by standard formulas,[25] possibly because of to the release of vasoactive mediators from injured pulmonary parenchyma.

During the first 24 hours, lactated Ringer solution, 2 to 4 mL/kg/% burn/24 h, is the primary resuscitative fluid. Because hypoglycemia can develop in children who weigh less than 10 kg if glucose is not administered, lactated Ringer solution or half normal saline with 5% dextrose at a maintenance rate (4 mL/kg/h) is given along with a reduced amount of the former (3 mL/kg/% burn/ 24 h). Dextrose-containing fluid should not be given as the primary resuscitative fluid, because hyperglycemia and osmotic diuresis may result. Half of the calculated 24-hour total should be administered during the first 8 hours after injury. These calculations should be based on the time of injury, not on the time that vascular access is achieved. During this first 24-hour period, the resuscitative infusion of lactated Ringer solution should be adjusted up or down in 10% increments every hour based on age-specific resuscitation endpoints, such as urine output, sensorium, base deficit, cardiac filling pressures, pulse, and blood pressure (see Table 12-2). The importance of an hourly bedside evaluation during this period cannot be overemphasized.

It is important to recognize a failing resuscitation as early as possible because this facilitates salvage of these patients. At any point during a resuscitation, the estimated total fluid administration can be calculated based on the known administered volume and the current rate of infusion. This figure is divided by the patient's weight and burn size, resulting in a numeral that describes the number of milliliters of fluid per kilogram of body weight per percentage of burn that the patient is targeted to receive during the first 24 hours. A failing resuscitation is one in which the patient is likely to receive 6 or more mL/kg/% burn during the first 24 hours after injury. Larger resuscitation fluid volumes are commonly required by patients for whom resuscitation is delayed, who have suffered inhalation injury, or who have extensive and deep burns. These patients often benefit from the early infusion of low-dose dopamine, 3 to 5 μg/kg/h, and placement of a pulmonary artery catheter, or the early administration of colloid (Table 12-5).

Patients with gross pigmenturia are at risk for myoglobin-induced acute tubular necrosis (Color Fig. 12-10). This situation is most common in patients who have sustained high-voltage electrical injury or deep thermal burns. In these patients, pigment must be cleared from the urine promptly. This is ideally accomplished with crystalloid loading, maintaining a brisk urine output of 2 mL/kg/h or more. Also helpful is alkalinization of the urine. This is best accomplished by administration of 0.12 to 0.5 mEq/kg/h of sodium bicarbonate intravenously as a part of the resuscitative fluid, with careful observation of the serum pH. Occasionally, osmotic diuresis using mannitol is required; however, the administration of osmotic diuretics obscures the urine output as a measure of intravascular volume status. Therefore, a pulmonary artery or central venous catheter should be placed when mannitol must be used so that cardiac filling pressures can be used to judge the adequacy of fluid administration.

Beginning 24 hours after injury, colloid administration is appropriate, as the diffuse microvascular injury abates and endothelial cell integrity returns. At this time, colloid will remain largely within the intravascular compartment. Colloid, generally 5% albumin in lactated Ringer solution, is infused at a dose based on burn size (see Table 12-5).

Table 12-5. MODIFIED BROOKE FORMULA

FIRST 24 HOURS

Adults and Children >10 kg

Lactated Ringer solution: 2–4 mL/kg/% burn/24 h
  (first half in first 8 h)
Colloid: none

Children <10 kg

Lactated Ringer solution: 2–3 mL/kg/% burn/24 h
  (first half in first 8 h)
Lactated Ringer solution with 5% dextrose: 4 mL/kg/h
Colloid: none

SECOND 24 HOURS

All Patients

Crystalloid: to maintain urine output. If silver nitrate is used, sodium
  leeching will mandate continued isotonic crystalloid. If a
  nonaqueous topical solution is used, free water requirement is
  significant. Serum sodium should be monitored closely.
  Nutritional support should begin, ideally by the enteral route.
Colloid (5% albumin in lactated Ringer solution)
  0%–30% burn: none
  30%–50% burn: 0.3 mL/kg/% burn/24 h
  50%–70% burn: 0.4 mL/kg/% burn/24 h
  >70% burn: 0.5 mL/kg/% burn/24 h

During this second 24-hour period, crystalloid requirements markedly diminish and transeschar free water loss dominates the electrolyte picture unless an aqueous topical antimicrobial such as 0.5% silver nitrate solution is used. In the former situation, free water administration is required; in the latter case, transeschar leeching of sodium (about 350 mEq/m²/24 h) mandates continued administration of isotonic crystalloid. Major morbidity is associated with aberrations of serum sodium concentrations at this time, so diligent electrolyte monitoring is important. Nutritional support, ideally enterally, should commence during the first 48 hours after injury.

INITIAL WOUND EXCISION AND BIOLOGIC CLOSURE

Early removal of extensive areas of devitalized tissue with immediate biologic closure of resulting wounds is the core surgical objective during the first postburn week. This policy of early excision is now widely practiced in the United States. It is accomplished as excision of the entire wound coincident with fluid resuscitation[26] or, more commonly, by staged excision of all deep partial- and full-thickness components of the wound during the first 3 to 7 days after injury.[27] Wounds of the face, palms, soles, and genitals generally are not excised early. The emphasis on early excision is based on several documented and perceived advantages over the traditional approach of allowing eschar to liquefy until separation occurs, leaving a bed of granulation tissue that is subsequently autografted. Documented advantages include an improved survival rate in patients with injuries involving more than 30% to 40% of the body surface,[28,29] truncated hospital stays,[30] lower costs, and fewer painful dressing changes. Although not proved, it appears that a decrease in the duration and intensity of the hypermetabolic response, improved immunologic function, and less hypertrophic scarring may result from early excision.

Estimation of Burn Depth

In practical terms, only deep partial- or full-thickness burns undergo early excision. Such an approach assumes an ability to accurately determine burn depth during the initial examination. Although numerous technical aids, such as laser Doppler flow meters, intravenous fluorescein, burn wound biopsy, thermography, light reflectance, and fluorescence of intravenous dyes, have been proposed,[18] none has yet equaled in accuracy or practicality the eye of an experienced examiner. The differentiation of superficial burns that will heal within 3 weeks with topical antimicrobial treatment from deeper injuries that will require excision can generally be made on clinical examination during the first days after injury. Certain patients have a component of their wound for which it is difficult to judge depth on initial examination. If overall wound size is not large (ie, less than 15% of TBSA), such indeterminate-depth wounds can be treated with topical antimicrobials initially until the portion that requires grafting becomes evident. This situation is common in patients with small injuries caused by hot liquid. In this case, it is prudent to apply topical antimicrobials for 5 to 7 days and to limit excision and grafting to full-thickness and deep dermal wounds.

Topical Antimicrobials

Topical antimicrobials play an important supportive role to excision and grafting because they delay the process of wound colonization and infection. Three topical agents are in common use in the United States today (Table 12-6). Silver sulfadiazine is perhaps the most common because it has a broad spectrum of activity, is painless and simple to apply, and has no metabolic or electrolyte implications. Mafenide acetate is an important element of the topical formulary because it alone reliably penetrates eschar. The major disadvantages are that it is a carbonic anhydrase inhibitor that causes a moderate metabolic acidosis and that is painful on application. It is typically applied to eschar at risk for infection and to all deep burns of the external ear. The latter practice has markedly diminished the incidence of auricular chondritis. Silver nitrate is applied to heavy gauze dressings every 2 hours as an aqueous 0.5% solution. Although it penetrates eschar poorly and can leech large quantities of sodium and potassium from the wounds, its broad antibacterial and antifungal activity, as well as its flexible use on burn wounds, donor sites, and fresh grafts, makes it a valuable topical agent.

Techniques of Excision

A common argument against early burn wound excision is the prodigious blood loss associated with these procedures. Modern blood-conserving practices and the selection of earlier timing for excision of wounds have diminished this concern, however. Tangential wound excisions of the torso, neck, and head are performed after subeschar injection of dilute epinephrine solutions. Tangential wound excisions of the extremities are done after exsanguination and inflation of a pneumatic tourniquet. Although substantial experience is required to differentiate marginal areas of wound, tissue viability is readily accessed by color and texture, rather than the presence of diffuse bleeding. The principle is simply to excise nonviable tissue and to conserve that which is viable. Instruments used to tangentially excise burned tissue include hand-operated, compressed gas–powered, and electric dermatomes. When required, excisions to the underlying fascia are performed with coagulating electrocautery, further diminishing blood loss. Although such procedures have traditionally been limited to 2 hours or 20% of TBSA, far larger procedures can be done safely if blood-conserving practices are rigorously followed and patients are kept warm by maintaining operating room temperatures above 90° or 100°F.

Temporary Wound Closure Alternatives

Once necrotic eschar is excised to a bed of viable tissue, immediate biologic closure is mandatory. Ideally, immediate autografting is performed. When donor sites are insufficient for this purpose, a temporary biologic cover must be chosen while donor sites heal. Such covers should prevent desiccation and provide a vapor and bacterial barrier over the excised wound. Fresh or cryopreserved human allograft is most appropriate for this purpose. It is placed in a meshed but unexpanded fashion exactly as autograft would be placed. When placed on a viable wound bed, it vascularizes and provide physiologic wound closure until rejected 2 to 4 weeks later; at this time or before it is replaced with reharvested autograft. Other temporary covers in common use are porcine xenograft, both fresh and reconstituted, and the synthetic bilaminate Biobrane, which has a porous nylon inner layer and a semipermeable outer layer. Only human allograft will vascularize, however, and it therefore remains the optimal temporary wound closure material. Although application of biologic covers to wounds with residual eschar is dangerous and should not be practiced, a second common use for biologic dressings is to cover selected clean superficial wounds as they epithelialize. This minimizes the pain associated with an open partial-thickness burn. Allograft, screened for malignant and infectious diseases, is a precious resource and is not commonly used as a biologic dressing in these circumstances. Rather, reconstituted porcine xenograft is preferred.

DEFINITIVE WOUND CLOSURE

During the phase of definitive wound closure, allograft is replaced with reharvested autograft, and burns of certain specialized areas are addressed. This phase generally begins 1 week after injury and lasts for several weeks thereafter, depending on the extent of burn and the availability of suitable donor sites. Prompt definitive wound closure in patients with large injuries remains an elusive goal despite encouraging early experience with two proposed permanent skin substitutes, artificial skin and cultured epidermal sheets (see later). At present, even in patients with extensive injuries, reharvested autograft provides the most practical and durable definitive wound closure material.

Burns of the Face, Ocular Adnexae, and Ears

Because of the thickness and deep appendages of the skin of the central face, relatively deep burns in these areas frequently heal. This is fortunate, because it is difficult to achieve a favorable result with primary excision and grafting of the central face. Unless burns in these areas are of extraordinary depth, they are commonly treated with topical antimicrobial agents for 2 weeks. Areas that remain unhealed are excised and closed with thick sheet autograft. The face can be considered to consist of cosmetic units (Fig. 12-5), and it is ideal if full-thickness facial burns can be autografted in cosmetic units if this does not require sacrifice of significant areas of healed burn or unburned skin.[31]

Burns of the ocular adnexae are common and potentially difficult management problems. During the first week after injury, lid edema generally ensures that the underlying globe is adequately protected and lubricated. As wound contracture occurs, exposure and desiccation of the globe can ensue (Color Fig. 12-11), with resulting keratitis and corneal ulceration. If this is unresponsive to ocular lubrication, prompt surgical release of the lid is mandatory. Tarsorrhaphy is an ineffective alternative, since the forces of wound contraction routinely disrupt the tarsorrhaphy and damage the underlying tarsal plate.

Burns of the external ear are treated with twice daily

Table 12-6. **THREE COMMON TOPICAL MEDICATIONS USED IN THE UNITED STATES**

Agent	Characteristics
Silver sulfadiazine	Painless on application
	Fair to poor eschar penetration
	No metabolic side effects
	Broad antibacterial spectrum
Mafenide acetate	Painful on application
	Excellent eschar penetration
	Carbonic anhydrase inhibitor
	Broad-spectrum antibacterial
0.5% Silver nitrate	Painless on application
	Poor eschar penetration
	Leeches electrolytes
	Broad-spectrum antibacterial and antifungal

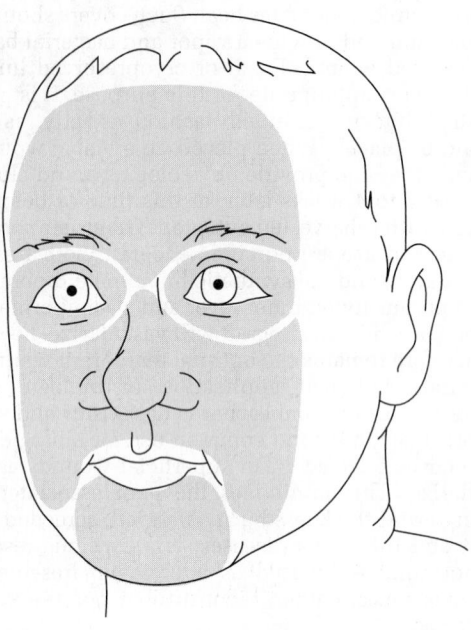

Figure 12-5. The cosmetic units of the face. It is ideal to autograft the face in cosmetic units if this does not require the sacrifice of significant areas of healed burn or unburned skin.

cleansing and application of mafenide acetate. It is essential to avoid pressure on the burned auricle from objects such as pillows. Simple devices such as foam ear protectors are effective preventive measures. Deep burns of the external ear are commonly complicated by acute suppurative chondritis if topical mafenide acetate is not applied. This complication is recognized by progressive auricular edema, erythema, and pain; it requires that the infected cartilage be immediately débrided to avoid complete loss of the cartilaginous support of the auricle.

Burns of the Hands and Feet

The increasing survival rates of patients with large burns have brought into greater focus the importance of the quality of life after such injuries. A crucial element of postinjury quality of life is hand function. Optimal functional outcome of hand burns is facilitated by an organized, multidisciplinary approach to the injuries.

The initial evaluation of the burned hand should begin with screening for other trauma. A complete hand examination is necessary, with particular attention being paid to perfusion by evaluation of capillary refill, temperature, consistency, and Doppler signals in the palmar arch, digital vessels, and distal pulp. It is not enough to simply demonstrate that there is blood flow in the radial or ulnar arteries. If the hands are cool and firm with distal circulation impaired, prompt escharotomies of the proximal upper extremity and hand are performed as previously described. When one is dealing with high voltage electrical injury or deep thermal burns, the need for urgent fasciotomy is indicated by progressive firmness of the compartments of the hand and forearm, or progressive neurologic impairment or pain. In equivocal cases, it is most prudent to proceed to decompression promptly, rather than to wait until ischemia has advanced.

Subsequent management of the burned hand is dictated by the depth of the injury. Superficial burns are managed with elevation, topical antimicrobials, and full passive range of motion twice daily for each joint. Splinting the hand in a functional position, with the metacarpophalangeal joints at 70 to 90 degrees, the interphalangeal joints in extension, the thumb in neutral position with the first web space open, and the wrist in 20 to 30 degrees of extension is indicated if there is significant edema. Healing can be expected within 2 to 3 weeks if injuries are superficial. Deep partial- and full-thickness injuries are best managed with excision and sheet grafting as soon as practical (Color Fig. 12-12). Hands are immobilized in a functional position for 7 days after surgery before passive and active therapy is resumed. Fourth-degree hand burns, which involve the underlying extensor mechanism, joint capsules, or bone are significantly more difficult problems and are managed by staged sheet autografting. They also often benefit from temporary axial Kirschner wire fixation of open and unstable interphalangeal or metacarpophalangeal joints. Patients with smaller overall burn sizes in association with fourth-degree hand burns are often well served by débridement and groin or abdominal flap coverage. When hand burns are addressed in an organized fashion that stresses continuous hand therapy, most patients with deep partial- and full-thickness burns have normal or near-normal long-term function.[32] Even patients with fourth-degree injuries, although rarely enjoying normal function, can expect to be able to function independently in activities of daily living.

The palmar skin is remarkably thick, so only about 20% of palmar burns require resurfacing. Therefore, a conservative approach facilitates preservation of the specialized attachment of the palmar skin to the underlying fascia. Full-thickness injuries are grafted with full-thickness or thick split-thickness sheet grafts and splinted in extension to maintain the palm in an open position.

Burns of the feet are managed in a similar fashion. Prompt excision and grafting of deep dermal and full-thickness injuries of the dorsum of the foot generally result in normal function. Fourth-degree injuries, although more difficult management problems, are entirely consistent with a normal functional result. Burns of the plantar surface of the feet are grafted with full- or thick split-thickness sheet grafts if they fail to heal within 3 weeks.

Genital Burns

On initial presentation, it is important to ensure that the burned foreskin is reduced into a normal position, since progressive edema may result in paraphimosis. Bladder catheter drainage is not required to limit contamination of perineal wounds with urine. Bladder catheters should be used only to facilitate resuscitation and should be promptly removed when genital edema is resolved and close monitoring of the urine output is no longer required. Likewise, diversion of the intestinal tract is not required in the management of perineal burns. On occasion, contraction of the deeply burned and desiccated foreskin may render the placement of bladder catheters in the acute setting impossible. In these cases, dorsal or ventral incisions through the contracted foreskin permit catheter placement. When a deeply burned foreskin is being débrided, any viable remnant should be preserved, because such tissue may be useful in later reconstruction.

Although there is some enthusiasm for early excision of deep genital burns, these limited surface area injuries can be managed with topical therapy for 2 to 3 weeks unless the wounds are remarkably deep. Unhealed injuries are

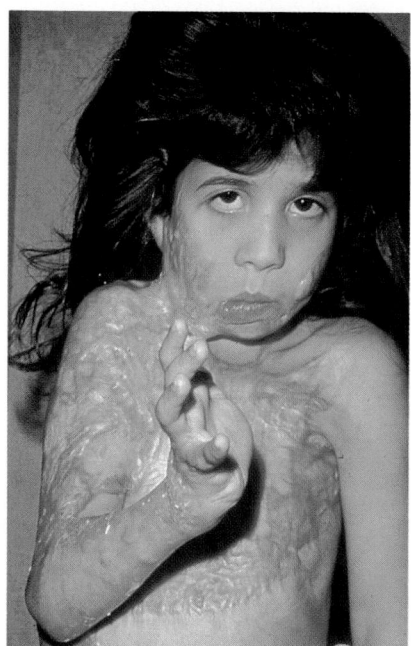

Color Figure 12-1. Suboptimal management of small burns can have major adverse functional and cosmetic implications.

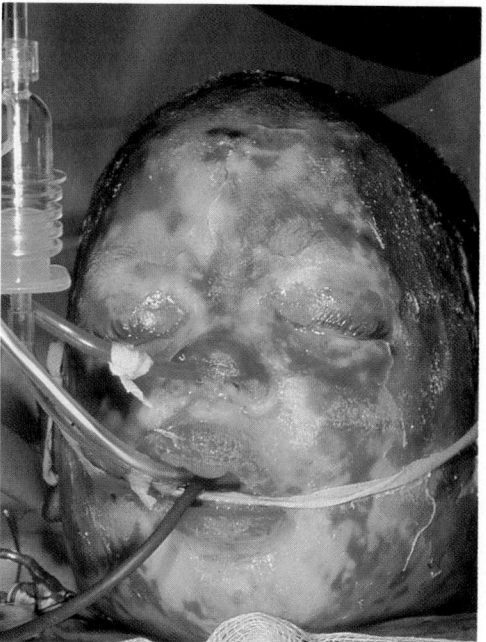

Color Figure 12-2. Endotracheal tube security is of the utmost importance during the first few postburn days, because airway edema can result in significant difficulty when one is attempting to reinsert displaced endotracheal tubes. Secure airway control is facilitated by the use of umbilical ties, rather than adhesive tape, to anchor endotracheal tubes.

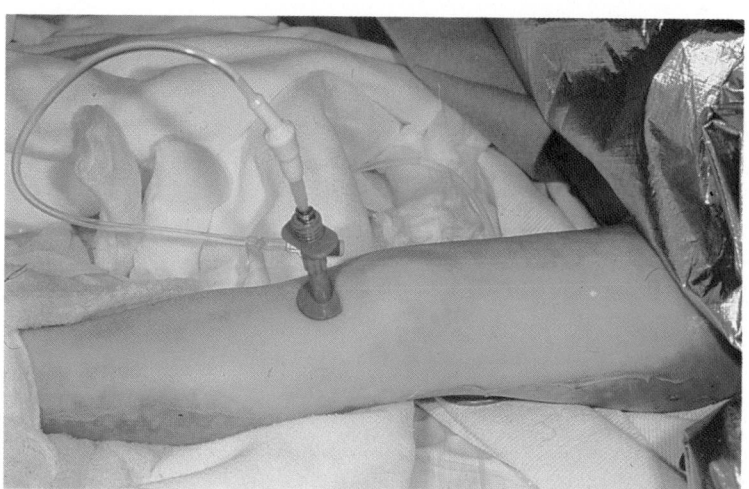

Color Figure 12-3. Intraosseous infusion can be life-saving in children in whom vascular access cannot be promptly achieved.

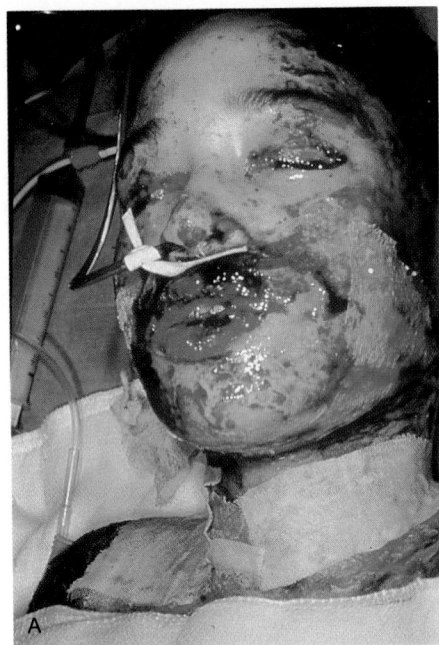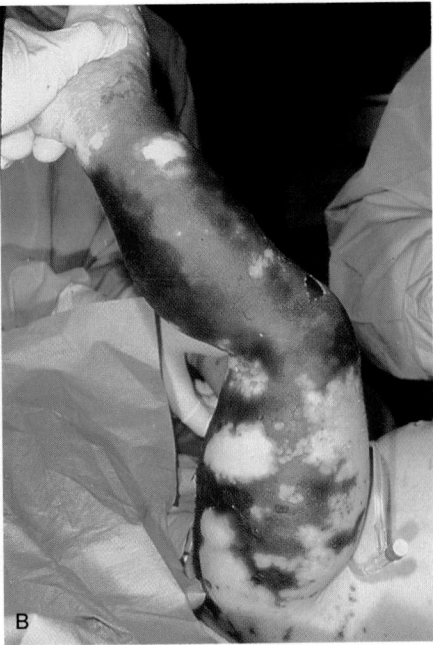

Color Figure 12-4. (*A*) Toxic epidermal necrolysis is a severe variant of erythema multiform. When there is major mucous membrane involvement, as in this patient, it is described as Stevens-Johnson syndrome. (*B*) Purpura fulminans describes a syndrome in which extensive soft tissue necrosis results from transient protein C or protein S deficiency complicating meningococcal sepsis.

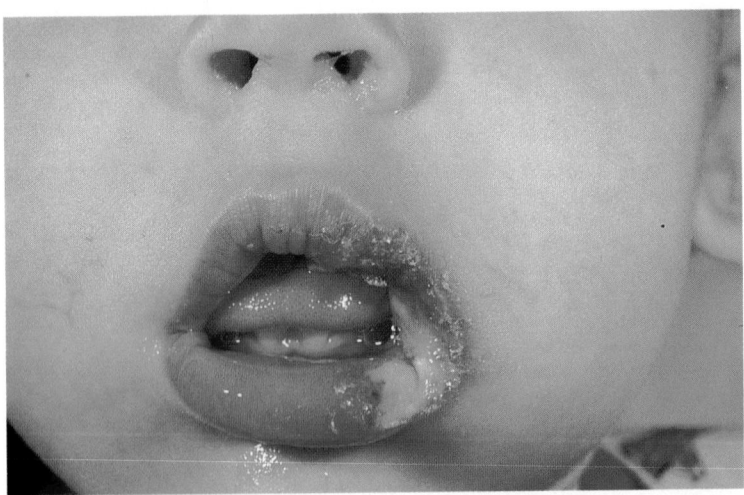

Color Figure 12-5. Low- and intermediate-voltage injuries can be locally destructive, as in this child who suffered a 110-volt commissure burn to the mouth by biting the cord of an electrical appliance. These injuries are rarely associated with serious systemic sequelae.

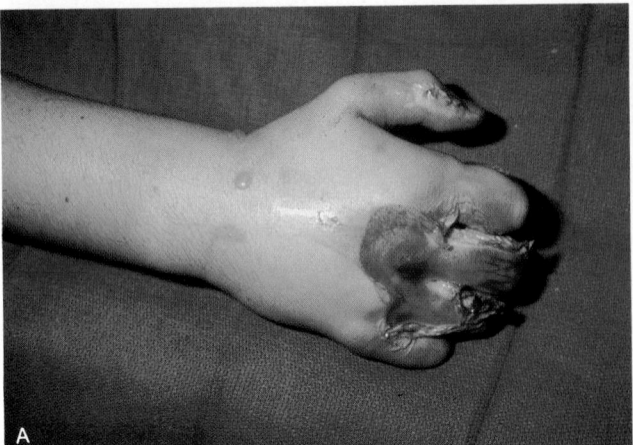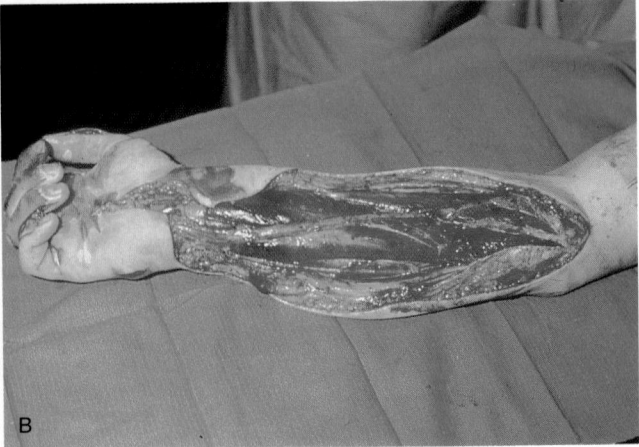

Color Figure 12-6. (*A*) This patient made contact with a 20,000-volt power line, resulting in a locally destructive entrance wound and occult muscle injury in the proximal extremity, leading to a compartment syndrome. (*B*) Prompt fasciotomy of the forearm and hand prevented the development of an additional ischemic injury secondary to high intracompartmental pressures.

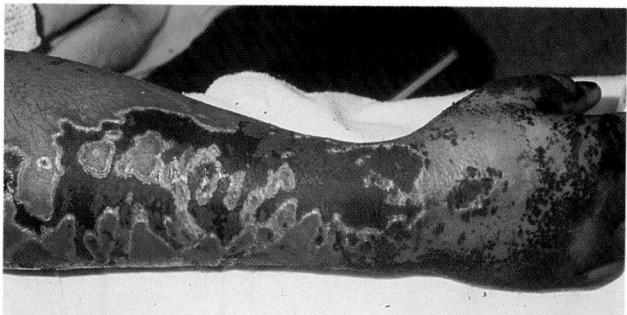

Color Figure 12-7. Chemical burns are often deeper than they appear on initial examination, as in this patient who suffered a sulfuric acid splash injury. Copious irrigation remains the mainstay of initial therapy.

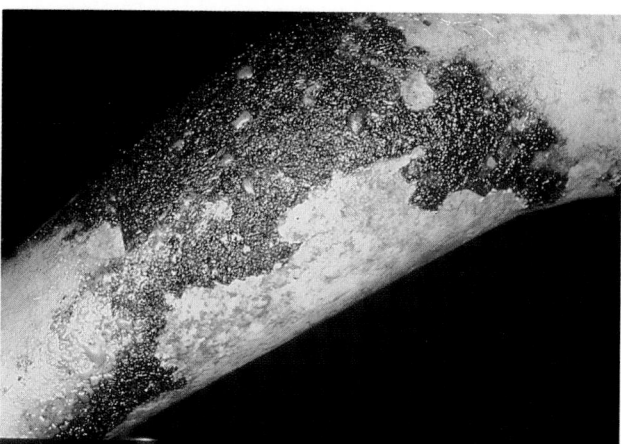

Color Figure 12-8. Tar burns are managed with initial cooling irrigation followed by later tar removal. In this patient, residual tar is being removed after softening in a lipophyllic solvent. Such burns are usually deep and generally require resurfacing.

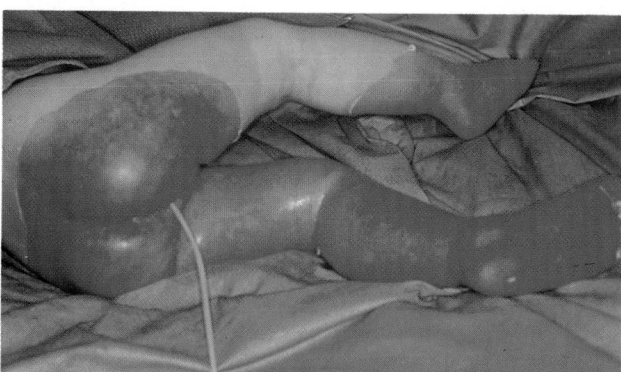

Color Figure 12-9. This child's wound is consistent with an intentional immersion in scalding water, demonstrating both flexor sparing and sharply defined margins around a deep burn of uniform depth.

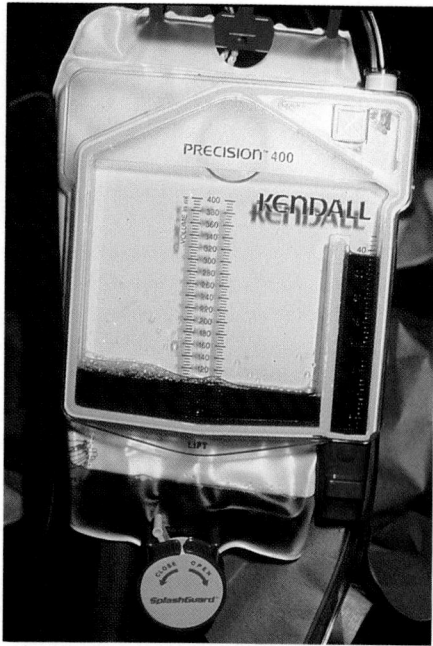

Color Figure 12-10. Heavily pigmented urine must be cleared of hemochromogens to avoid acute tubular necrosis.

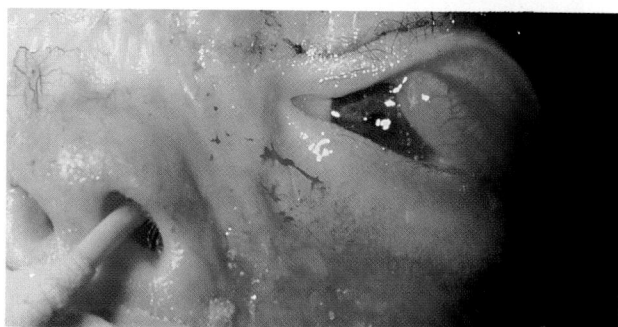

Color Figure 12-11. Contracture of burned ocular adnexae results in exposure and desiccation of the globe. When ocular lubrication is inadequate, lid release is mandatory.

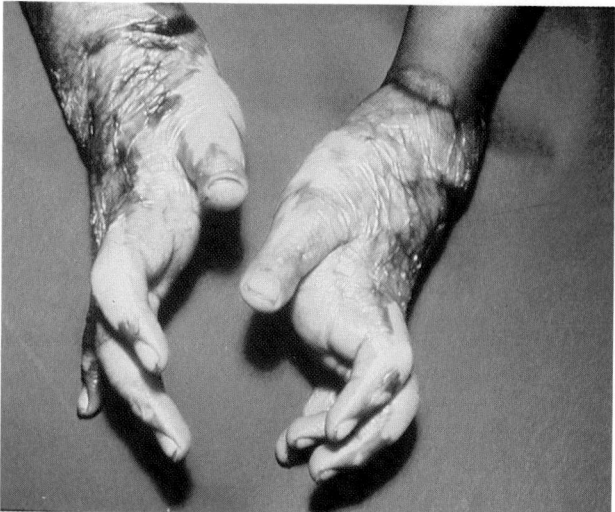

Color Figure 12-12. Spontaneous healing of deep dermal hand burns can result in a poor functional result.

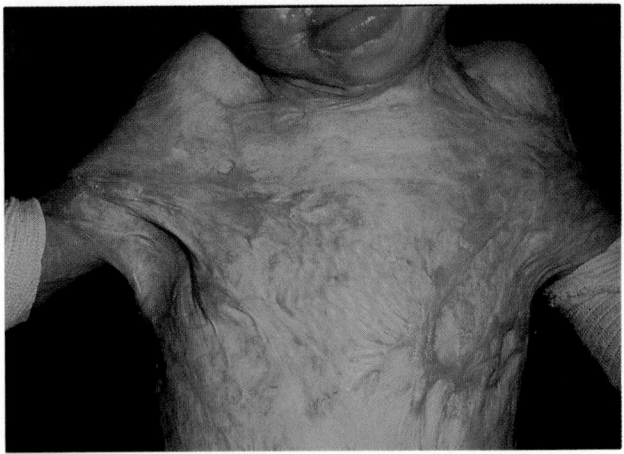

Color Figure 12-13. Hypertrophic scar formation has major adverse functional and cosmetic implications.

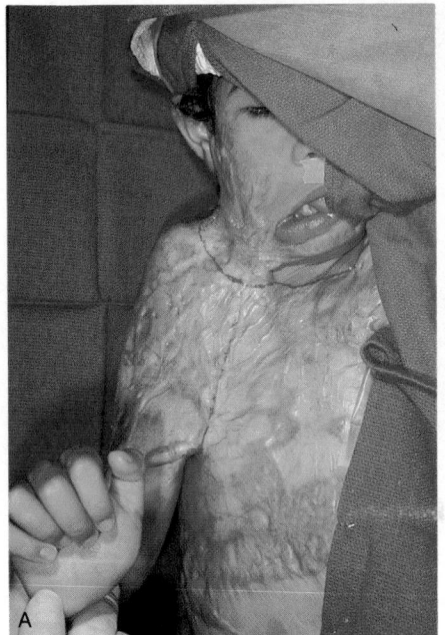

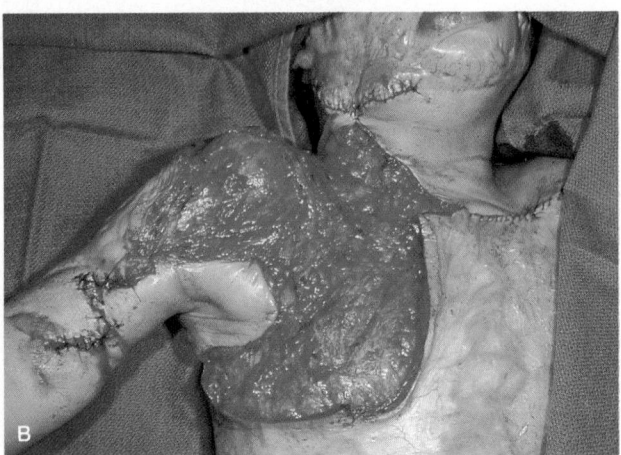

Color Figure 12-14. Prompt release and autografting is indicated when hypertrophic scar formation threatens to limit function.

débrided and grafted with sheet autograft at this time, with generally excellent cosmetic and functional results.

SELECTED CRITICAL CARE ISSUES

The enhanced survival of patients with large burns has been facilitated by increasing sophistication of the critical care techniques used to support an aggressive surgical approach to wounds, to manage failing organ systems, and to support the hypermetabolic response to injury. This section reviews some of the important points relevant to the management of inhalation injury and respiratory failure, techniques of arterial and venous access, nutritional support of the hypermetabolic response and the recognition and management of multiorgan failure.

Inhalation Injury and Respiratory Failure

The pathophysiology of inhalation injury is complex and varies with the aerosolized toxins particular to the circumstances of individual injuries.[33] However, these injuries routinely demonstrate the following:

- Upper airway obstruction secondary to progressive edema
- Reactive bronchospasm from aerosolized irritants
- Small airway occlusion initially from edema and subsequently from sloughed endobronchial debris and loss of the ciliary clearance mechanism
- Microatelectasis from loss of surfactant and alveolar edema
- Interstitial and alveolar edema secondary to loss of capillary integrity

The physiologic consequences of these aberrations are upper and lower airway obstruction, increased airway resistance, decreased compliance, an increase in the dead space/tidal volume ratio, and intrapulmonary shunting.

Determination of the severity of inhalation injury is surprisingly difficult because the components of the smoke to which a patient has been exposed are generally unknown. Since current treatment is exclusively supportive, diagnosis provides only prognostic information. Suggestive points in the patient's history include entrapment within a closed space or prolonged extrication time. Physical signs that support the diagnosis include singed nasal vibrissae and facial hair, burns of the central face, intraoral burns, carbonaceous debris in the oropharynx, and diffuse wheezing. Bronchoscopy frequently reveals carbonaceous endobronchial debris and mucosal pallor, erythema, or ulceration. Xenon scanning may reveal delayed or asymmetric clearance of the radiotracer secondary to small airway obstruction. Unfortunately, findings at the time of initial evaluation frequently do not correlate with the subsequent clinical course.

The earliest consequence of inhalation injury is upper airway edema, which is commonly seen during the first 6 to 24 hours after injury. It is more prominent in small children and patients with large surface area injuries who experience more significant aberrations of capillary integrity and therefore more soft tissue edema. Upper airway obstruction is best managed with prompt endotracheal intubation and elevation of the head maintained for 48 to 72 hours. In equivocal cases, diagnostic bronchoscopy is performed and patients with significant upper airway edema are intubated using the bronchoscope as a stylet. Endotracheal tubes are removed when facial edema has largely resolved and there is an audible air leak around the tubes at 30 cm H_2O of inflation with the cuff deflated.

Although severe steam inhalation can result in direct heat injury to the distal tracheobronchial tree, more distal airway injuries are usually caused by aerosolized toxins rather than thermal energy, the upper airway being a highly effective heak sink. The physiologic consequences of small airway injury are obstruction and intrapulmonary shunting with progressive respiratory failure. Small airway occlusion secondary to sloughed endobronchial debris and the loss of the ciliary clearance mechanism result in a high rate (20% and 50%) of pneumonia.[34] Successful treatment of patients with inhalation injury requires aggressive pulmonary toilet aided by frequent chest physiotherapy and bronchoscopic suctioning and lavage. Positive-pressure ventilation facilitates the treatment of patients with large shunts or compliance sufficiently poor to result in an excessive work of breathing. Positive end-expiratory pressure helps to optimize functional residual capacity, minimizing intrapulmonary shunt and enhancing compliance. Although moderate inflating pressures help to expand recruitable segments, peak inspiratory pressures in excess of 40 cm H_2O in adults should be avoided because they are associated with both overt barotrauma and more subtle overpressure injuries to the pulmonary microvasculature and alveoli. The combined effects of barotrauma and oxygen exacerbate respiratory failure.[35] High inflating pressures are also ineffective in recruiting additional respiratory units, because the compliance decrements are not homogeneous and high pressures simply overdistend more compliant segments. When ventilating patients with poor compliance, one approach is to use low-volume ventilation and to tolerate moderate hypercapnia and respiratory acidosis to facilitate control of inflating pressures (Table 12-7). This is associated with a low incidence of barotrauma and a high rate of survival.

Carbon Monoxide and Cyanide Exposure

Both carbon monoxide and cyanide are commonly inhaled by victims of closed-space fires. Carbon monoxide is a colorless and odorless gas with a high affinity for hemoglobin. Patients with significant amounts of carboxyhemoglobin suffer from a marked reduction in their ability to deliver oxygen to peripheral tissues despite a normal arterial partial pressure of oxygen. The 2.5-hour half-life of carboxyhemoglobin is reduced by a factor of five by ventilation with 100% oxygen. Fire victims who are well ventilated with high concentrations of oxygen by emergency response personnel from the time of extrication commonly have normal carboxyhemoglobin values (below 5%) on initial evaluation despite significant exposures to carbon

---

Table 12-7. CONVENTIONAL VOLUME VENTILATION PROTOCOL

Pressure-controlled ventilation is used in children under 8 kg; others are ventilated with volume-controlled machines.
Initial tidal volumes are set between 12 and 15 mL/kg.
Peak inspiratory pressure is monitored hourly.
If peak inspiratory pressure exceeds 40 cm H_2O:
   Mechanical problems, such as a need for torso escharotomy, are evaluated.
   Adequate sedation is ensured, the goal being a patient who is sedated but arousable.
   Tidal volumes are decreased in 10% to 20% increments.
   Respiratory rates are increased as long as auto-PEEP does not occur.
   Supranormal levels of $Paco_2$ are tolerated as long as pH > 7.2.

monoxide at the time of injury. Carboxyhemoglobin is not sensed by standard transmission pulse oximetry, so a normal saturation on such a monitor does not preclude the possibility of significant carboxyhemoglobinemia. In conjunction with a severe carbon monoxide exposure, patients frequently also suffer an hypoxic cerebral insult and on occasion experience late neurologic sequelae. Hyperbaric oxygen can reduce the half-life of carboxyhemoglobin more rapidly than 100% oxygen and may possibly reduce further the incidence of late neurologic sequelae. This later contention is debated, however, and the obvious danger associated with the loss of patient access during treatment in a monoplace hyperbaric chamber must temper the use of this modality in unstable patients undergoing resuscitation.[36]

Hydrogen cyanide, which is commonly present in the smoke of structural fires, interferes with oxidative metabolism at the cellular level and causes lactic acidosis. With proper ventilation and fluid resuscitation, the cyanide-induced acidosis corrects rapidly in most patients, and specific treatment with sodium thiosulfate in not generally required.[37]

Vascular Access Techniques

The successful management of large burns, particularly in the presence of respiratory or other organ failures, depends critically on reliable venous and arterial access, despite the high rates of catheter sepsis traditionally associated with these patients. Peripheral access is often impractical in burn patients and is associated with unacceptable rates of suppurative thrombophlebitis. For these reasons, central venous access is routine except in patients with small injuries who require venous access for only a few days.

Arterial access, when required, can be safely maintained through the percutaneous radial, pedal, or femoral route. The importance of proper technique cannot be overemphasized if complications are to be avoided. The risk of central nervous system emboli associated with axillary arterial lines and the difficulty maintaining catheters in the radial position for prolonged periods have led to a preference for the femoral position in children.[38] Patients intubated for airway protection only, who have no significant intrapulmonary shunt or dead space abnormalities, can be well treated with a transmission oximetry probe and central venous blood gasses.

Because most catheter infections arise from the central venous line tract rather than the hub, strict line care, including a nonocclusive insertion site cleansing every 4 hours, minimizes the risk of both arterial and central venous catheter sepsis. Catheters should be changed at least weekly and are inserted through unburned tissue whenever possible. Using this approach, central venous and arterial catheter sepsis rates are not significantly higher than in unburned critically ill patients.[38,39]

Nutritional Support

The hypermetabolic response to burn injury is intense until wound closure is complete. This physiologic response is considered by some to be detrimental to the patient. This assumption must be accepted with caution, however, since this response to injury has been retained by numerous species for millions of years and presumably plays a role in recovery from injury. Conventional wisdom indicates that bacteria and their products that translocate from an incompetent gut barrier, the burn wound itself, and infectious foci are the forces driving the hypermetabolic and inflammatory responses. Accurate nutritional

therapy for this response is crucial to achieving a favorable outcome.

Accurate support is essential because overfeeding is associated with hepatic steatosis, hepatic dysfunction, and increased carbon dioxide production exacerbating respiratory insufficiency. Underfeeding results in inanition and poor wound healing. These factors have led to a plethora of formulas by which nutritional support has been administered to burn patients. Patients treated with prompt wound excision and biologic closure have a reduced energy expenditure compared with historic controls,[40] and multiple studies have revealed that standard formulas are poorly predictive of actual energy requirements in individual burn patients. For these reasons, indirect calorimetry is commonly used to guide nutritional support of critically burned individuals. Total energy expenditure can be roughly estimated by using expired gas indirect calorimetry to determine a resting energy expenditure and then multiplying the resting energy expenditure by a factor of growth hormone 1.3 to 1.7.

Protein loads of 2.5 to 3 g/kg/d are recommended to support the requirements of seriously burned individuals. Reports have proposed that use of recombinant human growth hormone can accelerate donor site healing and produce an earlier positive nitrogen balance. Prompt donor site healing and reliable positive nitrogen balance can be achieved without this expensive therapy, however. Additionally, the long-term effects of pharmacologic doses of growth hormone remain undetermined, so the routine use of recombinant human growth hormone in burn patients should be approached with caution.

Multiple Organ Failure and Other Complications of Thermal Injury

It has been said that treatment of patients with large burns requires identification and management of a series of complications while the wound is progressively closed. Successful clinicians interpret any subtle deterioration as a manifestation of an occult complication, usually septic, until it is proved otherwise. Common complications of thermal injury are presented in Table 12-8.

Multisystem organ failure is the leading cause of late death in burn patients.[41] The etiology of the multisystem organ failure syndrome involves complex cellular and subcellular biology that is only now beginning to be unraveled by investigators with use of increasing numbers of recombinant products and receptor-blocking antibodies. Our fragmentary understanding of this biology makes it clear that we must use caution when considering therapeutic use of these products outside the laboratory. It is widely assumed that the hypermetabolic response is driven by several inciting events, including repeated infections, translocation of bacteria and their products from an incompetent gut barrier, and the burn wound itself, and that these underlying processes cause multiorgan failure through similar mediator cascades after an overly exuberant response.[13]

A deteriorating burn patient commonly has early evidence of multiple organ dysfunction in a predictable cascade: increasing obtundation is followed by progressive intrapulmonary shunting with hypoxia, ileus, nonoliguric renal failure, rising cholestasis, and thrombocytopenia. The most common initiating event is one of the many infections to which burn patients are prone. Certainly, wound sepsis is an obvious potential source. This should be infrequently seen now, however, since deep wounds are promptly removed before the onset of infection. The clinical team should search thoroughly for an occult infectious focus when multiorgan dysfunction first becomes evident

Table 12-8. COMMON COMPLICATIONS AFTER BURN INJURY

NEUROLOGIC

Transient delirium occurs in up to 30% of patients and generally resolves with supportive therapy. Evaluation is for anoxia, metabolic disturbance and structural lesions.

Seizures most commonly result from hyponatremia or abrupt benzodiazepine withdrawal.

Peripheral nerve injuries occur from direct thermal injury, compression from compartment syndrome or overlying nonelastic eschar, major metabolic disturbances, or improper splinting techniques.

Delayed peripheral nerve and spinal cord deficits develop weeks or months after high-voltage injury secondary to small vessel injury and demyelinization.

RENAL

Early acute renal failure follows inadequate perfusion during resuscitation or myoglobinuria.

Late renal failure complicates sepsis and multiple organ failure or the use of nephrotoxic agents.

ADRENAL

Acute adrenal insufficiency secondary to adrenal hemorrhage presents with hypotension, fever, hyponatremia, and hyperkalemia.

CARDIOVASCULAR

Endocarditis and suppurative thrombophlebitis typically present with fever and bacteremia without signs of local infection.

Hypertension occurs in up to 20% of children and is best managed with β-adrenergic blockers.

Venous thromboembolic complications are infrequent in patients with large burns.

Iatrogenic catheter insertion complications are minimized by meticulous technique.

PULMONARY

Pneumonia may occur with or without inhalation injury and is treated with pulmonary toilet and antibiotics.

Early respiratory failure may occur secondary to inhalation of noxious chemicals. Later respiratory failure may occur secondary to sepsis or pneumonia.

HEMATOLOGIC

Neutropenia and thrombocytopenia, as well as disseminated intravascular coagulation, are common indicators of impending sepsis.

Systemic immunologic deficits contribute to a high rate of infectious complications.

OTOLOGIC

Auricular chondritis secondary to bacterial infection results in rapid loss of viable cartilage. It is preventable by the routine use of topical mafenide acetate on all burned ears.

Sinusitis and otitis media can be caused by transnasal instrumentation and are treated by relocation of tubes, antibiotics, and judicious surgical drainage.

Complications of endotracheal intubation include nasal alar and septal necrosis, vocal cord erosions and ulcerations, tracheal stenosis and tracheoesophageal and tracheoinnominate artery fistulae. Complications are minimized by compulsive attention to tube position, avoidance of oversized tubes, and attention to cuff pressures.

ENTERIC

Hepatic dysfunction, secondary to transient hepatic blood flow deficits and manifested as hepatocellular enzyme (AST, ALT) elevations, is extremely common. Late hepatic failure begins with elevations of cholestatic enzymes and may progress through coagulopathy and hepatic failure. It is associated with sepsis and multiple organ failure.

Pancreatitis is generally coincident with splanchnic flow deficits early and sepsis induced organ failures later.

Acalculous cholecystitis can present as sepsis without localized symptoms or signs. Radiographic evaluation can be followed by bedside percutaneous cholecystostomy in unstable patients.

Gastroduodenal ulceration, secondary to splanchnic flow deficits that degrade mucosal defenses, is common and potentially life threatening if routine histamine-receptor blockers and antacids are not administered.

Intestinal ischemia is possible if it is secondary to inadequate resuscitation and splanchnic flow deficits.

OPHTHALMIC

Ectropion, from progressive contraction of burned ocular adnexae, results in exposure of the globe. This requires acute eyelid release. Tarsorrhaphy is rarely helpful, more often resulting in injury to the tarsal plate as contraction forces pull out tarsorrhaphy sutures.

Corneal ulceration can progress to full-thickness corneal destruction if secondary infection occurs. This is prevented by careful globe lubrication with topical antibiotics and possibly acute lid release for ectropion.

Symblepharon, or scarring of the lid to the denuded conjunctiva, occurs following chemical burns or corneal epithelial defects complicating toxic epidermal necrolysis. It is prevented by daily examination and adhesion disruption with a fine glass rod.

GENITOURINARY

Urinary tract infections are minimized by maintaining bladder catheters only when required. Neither bladder catheterization nor colonic diversion is required for management of perineal and genital burns.

Candidal cystitis occurs with bladder catheters and broad-spectrum antibiotics. Catheter change and amphotericin B irrigation for 5 days is generally therapeutic. If infections are recurrent, the upper tracts should be screened ultrasonographically.

(continued)

Table 12-8. COMMON COMPLICATIONS AFTER BURN INJURY (Continued)

MUSCULOSKELETAL

Burned exposed bone is generally débrided with a drill until viable cortical bone is reached. This is allowed to granulate and is autografted. Patients whose overall condition and wounds are appropriate are treated with local or distant flaps.

Fractured and burned extremities are best immobilized with external fixators while overlying burns are grafted. Burn patients with coincident fractures in unburned extremities benefit from prompt internal fixation.

Heterotopic ossification develops weeks after injury and is seen most commonly around deeply burned major joints such as the triceps tendon. It presents with pain and decreased range of motion. Most patients respond to physical therapy, but some require excision of heterotopic bone to achieve full function.

SOFT TISSUE

Hypertrophic scar formation is a major cause of long-term functional and cosmetic deformities. It is heralded by a secondary increase in neovascularity 9 to 13 weeks after epithelialization. Management options include grafting of deep dermal and full-thickness wounds, compression garments, judicious steroid injections, topical silicone products, and scar release and resurfacing procedures.

---

because addressing such processes promptly can prevent the full development of the syndrome. When an underlying infectious focus can be identified and addressed, organ function improves. If not, failures progress with a predictably fatal outcome. The occult infections that should be considered in such situations (see Table 12-8) include nosocomial sinusitis, which is particularly common in those with nasotracheal tubes; intravascular infections, such as endocarditis and suppurative thrombophlebitis, which typically present with fever and bacteremia without localized signs of infection; pneumonia or empyema; intraabdominal infections, such as acute cholecystitis and intestinal infarction; osteomyelitis; and infected intravascular devices.

REHABILITATION AND RECONSTRUCTION

With survival after large burns becoming more the rule than the exception, more attention has been focused on the quality rather than the simple fact of survival. Maximizing physical and psychosocial functional recovery is the key to optimizing the overall quality of life after serious burn injury.

Physical function is best optimized by the continuous involvement of dedicated burn occupational and physical therapists beginning during the acute resuscitation. At this time, their involvement may be limited to antideformity positioning and splinting of the hands and extremities with twice-daily full range-of-motion exercises of all joints. In more stable patients, and in those with large injuries nearing wound closure, therapy sessions may take many hours each day and involve strengthening, ambulation, active and passive range of motion, development of adaptive skills with modified utensils, performance of activities of daily living, and, in older adolescents and adults, development of work-related skills. These important activities are continued after discharge.

Psychosocial adaptation after severe burns can be difficult, particularly if serious injury involves the hands or face. Preburn psychiatric pathology or family dysfunction may further complicate recovery. The coordinated involvement of psychiatric, psychologic, and social work staff facilitates maximum psychologic recovery and social reintegration. These staff should be actively involved with the patient, family, and local outpatient support services throughout the hospitalization. Planning for discharge and arrangements and funding for needed outpatient services begin at the time of admission. The expectation for every burn patient should be a return to family and mainstream community life.

Hypertrophic Scarring and Reconstructive Surgery

Hypertrophic scar formation is a major source of long-term morbidity after burns (Color Fig. 12-13). All healed and grafted burns become hypervascular shortly after successful epithelialization. Wounds destined to become hypertrophic go through a second surge of neovascularization at 9 to 13 weeks.[42] Additional collagen is formed and contraction occurs during the next 4 to 6 months, at which time the hypervascular tissue involutes, becoming less erythematous and raised over the subsequent 8 to 12 months. Despite the importance of hypertrophic scar formation, our basic understanding of the process remains poor.[43] This lack of understanding is exacerbated by the absence of an animal model of scar hypertrophy.

Wounds that are associated most commonly with hypertrophy are deep dermal burns that heal in 3 or more weeks and full-thickness wounds that heal by contraction and epithelial spread from wound edges. Wounds across flexor surfaces and across the anterior neck and submental area, where there is much tension across the healed wounds, are also subject to scar hypertrophy with increased frequency. Any wound has the potential to become hypertrophic, however, and it is often difficult to predict accurately the probability that any individual patient will suffer from hypertrophic scar formation.

The ability to influence the development of hypertrophic scars is limited. Current tools include compression garments, topical silicone sheets, steroid injections, and release or excision and autografting. Compression garments are individually measured and worn beginning within 2 weeks of grafting or wound epithelialization. They are not advised for use on the head of a child less than 1 year old, since they can mold the calvarium. Topical silicone has been advocated by some for hypertrophic scar treatment, although the mechanism of action is not clear and the use of topical silicone sheeting is accompanied by frequent skin irritation and rashes. Judicious intradermal steroid injection has been of value in the management of limited areas of hypertrophic scarring, usually in cosmetically important areas of small size. Intradermal steroid injections can be painful, and the dose must be limited to avoid systemic effects. Patients with recalcitrant areas of hypertrophic scarring often are best served by release or excision. Resultant wounds are covered with sheet autograft or flaps. Tissue expanders can be of great value, particularly in the closure of defects of hair-bearing scalp. When function is not limited, it is ideal to wait 2 years for full scar maturation before one embarks on reconstructive procedures. When function is threatened, however, prompt surgery is indicated (Color Fig. 12-14). Patients with large burn wounds commonly require a series of reconstructive procedures during the first few years after injury to attain the best possible cosmetic and functional results.

FUTURE OF BURN MANAGEMENT

Several exciting potential adjuncts to current burn care are the topic of frequent discussion. They are, however, simply supportive and cannot replace excellent clinical care. Indeed, for any such adjunct to be at all effective, it must be used in the setting of optimal clinical care. These potential adjuncts fall into five broad groups: those intended to support or modify the hypermetabolic response, growth factors, innovations in wound management, new critical care technology, and permanent skin substitutes.

Recent work has shown that, although the factors driving the hypermetabolic response may vary from patient to patient, a common web of mediators effects the response. The adverse aspects of the hypermetabolic response are best obviated by minimizing release of inflammatory mediators from the wound by prompt excision and biologic closure. Support of gastrointestinal barrier function is ensured through establishment of adequate splanchnic blood flow by normalizing hemodynamics and providing enteral nutritional support as soon as possible after injury. Early detection and elimination of infectious foci are fundamental also. These measures are likely to be more effective than attempts to modify the complex cascade of mediators that affect the hypermetabolic response. Support, rather than major modification, of the hypermetabolic response seems most appropriate at present, since our understanding of the basic biology is quite fragmentary. Ongoing work with blocking antibodies and recombinant mediators in animal models and humans promises to enhance our understanding of the hypermetabolic response to injury and to facilitate treatment of such patients.

Use of topical epidermal growth factor or systemic human growth hormone has been associated with shortened donor site healing times in burn patients. The differences between control and treated patients have been limited, however, and any potential benefit should be weighed against the financial and as yet undefined long-term physiologic costs of these therapies. Ongoing animal and clinical work with transforming growth factors, platelet-derived growth factors, fibroblast growth factors, and colony-stimulating factors promises to enhance our understanding of the biology of wound healing and may lead to improvements in clinical care in the future.

The ability to accurately determine the depth of wounds on initial presentation has the potential to shorten hospital stays by eliminating the period of observation that is commonly used to facilitate accurate predictions of wound healing in patients with small burns of indeterminate depth. Although several such technical adjuncts, such as laser Doppler flow meters and high-resolution ultrasound, have been developed,[18] none has proved of practical clinical utility. The ability of low-power lasers to cause intravenously administered indocyanine green dye to fluoresce is under evaluation and may prove valuable. Bloodless wound débridement using a scanning carbon dioxide laser has been effective in a porcine model and holds potential promise as a means to decrease the blood loss associated with wound excision. Débriding enzymes have previously been associated with injury to normal tissue, bleeding, pain, infection, and inadequate débridement. New formulations of these enzymes that are inactivated by circulating proteases are under development. They are designed to liquefy necrotic tissue without injuring healthy tissue. If efficacious, these substances may also facilitate both wound depth evaluation and blood-conserving removal of eschar.

Critical care technologies under development that may affect burn care include newer modes of ventilation that stress avoidance of high inflating pressures and techniques of extracorporeal support. Nitric oxide, delivered into the ventilator circuit, has been shown to decrease intrapulmonary shunting by increasing pulmonary blood flow to well-ventilated lung segments and to decrease pulmonary vascular resistance in patients with respiratory failure.[44] Definitive wound closure using materials other than autograft is the goal of several ongoing research projects and, if realized, will have an enormous impact on the acute and reconstructive management of burn patients. Substitutes being developed include epidermal analogues, dermal analogues, and composite substitutes. Of the epidermal analogues, sheets of cultured autologous epithelium are in clinical use. Although expensive and associated with low engraftment rates and extreme graft fragility, this technology is of value in the treatment of patients with massive injuries, in whom less than 5% to 10% of the body surface is available for donor harvest.[45] Patients with smaller injuries are better served by a split-thickness autograft. If cultured epidermis becomes fully integrated with a functional dermal analogue, its value may increase substantially. Dermal substitutes, designed to be combined with ultrathin autograft or cultured epithelium, are best represented by a synthetic bilaminate artificial skin,[46] which was tested successfully in a large multicenter trial. Although currently unavailable for general clinical use, this artificial skin has been associated with gratifying long-term cosmetic and functional results and may play a role in the eventual solution to the problem of definitive wound closure in patients with massive burns. Other dermal substitutes under development include allogenic fibroblast-containing materials and cryopreserved human dermis. Experience with these substitutes is limited, and their general use cannot yet be recommended.

Enormous strides have been made in burn patient management during the past two decades. Although burn injuries remain a tremendous challenge to the patient, family, and burn unit team, the prognosis for those suffering such injuries continues to improve. Ongoing progress in the evolution of our ability to modify the hypermetabolic response, fully understand the potential roles of growth factors, develop more effective ways to evaluate and excise wounds, mature critical care technologies, and develop durable permanent skin substitutes will further enhance our patients' quality of survival.

REFERENCES

1. Simon PA, Baron RC. Age as a risk factor for burn injury requiring hospitalization during early childhood. Arch Pediatr Adolesc Med 1994;148:394.
2. Lindblad BE, Terkelsen CJ, Christensen H. Epidemiology of domestic burns related to products. Burns 1990;16:89.
3. Erdmann TC, Feldman KW, Rivara FP, et al. Tap water burn prevention: the effect of legislation. Pediatrics 1991;88:572.
4. Aggarwal SJ, Diller KR, Blake GK, et al. Burn-induced alterations in vasoactive function of the peripheral cutaneous microcirculation. J Burn Care Rehabil 1994;15:1.
5. Ehrlich HP. Promotion of vascular patency in dermal burns with ibuprofen. Am J Med 1984;77:107.
6. Choi M, Ehrlich HP. U75412E, a lazaroid, prevents progressive burn ischemia in a rat burn model. Am J Pathol 1993;142:519.
7. Ehrlich HP, McGrane WL, Rajaratnam JB. Ancrod prevents vascular occlusion in thermally injured rats. J Trauma 1987;27:420.
8. Katz A, Ryan P, LaLonde C, et al. Topical ibuprofen decreases

thromboxane release from the endotoxin-stimulated burn wound. J Trauma 1986;26:157.

9. Demling R, Picard L, Campbell C, et al. Relationship of burn-induced lung lipid peroxidation on the degree of injury after smoke inhalation and a body burn. Crit Care Med 1993;21:1935.

10. LaLonde C, Knox J, Daryani R, et al. Topical flurbiprofen decreases burn wound–induced hypermetabolism and systemic lipid peroxidation. Surgery 1991;109:645.

11. Gupta M, Gupta OK, Yaduvanshi RK, et al. Burn epidemiology: the Pink City scene. Burns 1993;19:47.

12. Youn YK, LaLonde C, Demling R. The role of mediators in the response to thermal injury. World J Surg 1992;16:30.

13. Deitch EA. Multiple organ failure. Adv Surg 1993;26:333.

14. Sasaki TM, Welch GW, Herndon DN, et al. Burn wound manipulation-induced bacteremia. J Trauma 1979;19:46.

15. Demling RH, LaLonde C, Liu YP, et al. The lung inflammatory response to thermal injury: relationship between physiologic and histologic changes. Surgery 1989;106:52.

16. Wilmore DW, Mason AD Jr, Johnson DW, et al. Effect of ambient temperature on heat production and heat loss in burn patients. J Appl Physiol 1975;38:593.

17. Sheridan RL, Tompkins RG, McManus WF, et al. Intracompartmental sepsis in burn patients. J Trauma 1994;36:301.

18. Heimbach D, Engrav L, Grube B, et al. Burn depth: a review. World J Surg 1992;16:10.

19. Sheridan RL, Gagnon SW, Tompkins RG. The burn unit as a resource for the management of acute nonburn conditions in children. J Burn Care Rehabil 1995;16:62.

20. Sheridan RL, Ryan CM, Quinby WC, et al. Emergency management of major hydrofluoric acid exposures. Burns 1995;21:62.

21. Montrey JS, Barcia PJ. Nonaccidental burns in child abuse. South Med J 1985;78:1324.

22. Goodwin CW, Dorethy J, Lam V, et al. Randomized trial of efficacy of crystalloid and colloid resuscitation on hemodynamic response and lung water following thermal injury. Ann Surg 1983;197:520.

23. Merrell SW, Saffle JR, Sullivan JJ, et al. Fluid resuscitation in thermally injured children. Am J Surg 1986;152:664.

24. Graves TA, Cioffi WG, McManus WF, et al. Fluid resuscitation of infants and children with massive thermal injury. J Trauma 1988;28:1656.

25. Navar PD, Saffle JR, Warden GD. Effect of inhalation injury on fluid resuscitation requirements after thermal injury. Am J Surg 1985;150:716.

26. Desai MH, Herndon DN, Broemeling L, et al. Early burn wound excision significantly reduces blood loss. Ann Surg 1990;211:753.

27. Sheridan RL, Tompkins RG, Burke JF. Management of burn wounds with prompt excision and immediate closure. J Intens Care Med 1994;9:6.

28. Herndon DN, Gore D, Cole M, et al. Determinants of mortality in pediatric patients with greater than 70% full-thickness total body surface area thermal injury treated by early total excision and grafting. J Trauma 1987;27:208.

29. Merrell SW, Saffle JR, Sullivan JJ, et al. Increased survival after major thermal injury: a nine year review. Am J Surg 1987;154:623.

30. Herndon DN, Barrow RE, Rutan RL, et al. A comparison of conservative versus early excision: therapies in severely burned patients. Ann Surg 1989;209:547.

31. Gonzalez-Ulloa M. Restoration of the face covering by means of selected skin in regional aesthetic units. Br J Plast Surg 1956;9:212.

32. Sheridan RL, Hurley J, Smith MA, et al. The acutely burned hand: management and outcome based on a ten year experience with 1,047 burned hands. J Trauma 1995;38:406.

33. Heimbach DM, Waeckerle JF. Inhalation injuries. Ann Emerg Med 1988;17:1316.

34. Rue LW III, Cioffi WG, Mason AD, et al. Improved survival of burned patients with inhalation injury. Arch Surg 1993;128:772.

35. Slutsky AS. Mechanical ventilation: American College of Chest Physicians' Consensus Conference. Chest 1993; 104:1833.

36. Grube BJ, Marvin JA, Heimbach DM. Therapeutic hyperbaric

37. Barillo DJ, Goode R, Esch V. Cyanide poisoning in victims of fire: analysis of 364 cases and review of the literature. J Burn Care Rehabil 1994;15:46.

38. Sheridan RL, Weber JM, Tompkins RG. Femoral arterial catheterization in pediatric burn patients. Burns 1994;20:45.

39. Sheridan RL, Weber JM, Peterson HF, et al. Central venous catheter sepsis with weekly catheter change in pediatric burn patients: an analysis of 221 catheters. Burns 1995;21:127.

40. Carlson DE, Cioffi WG Jr, Mason AD Jr, et al. Resting energy expenditure in patients with thermal injuries. Surg Gynecol Obstet 1992;174:270.

41. Saffle JR, Sullivan JJ, Tuohig GM, et al. Multiple organ failure in patients with thermal injury. Crit Care Med 1993;21:1673.

42. Kischer CW. The microvessels is hypertrophic scars, keloids and related lesions. J Submicrosc Cytol Pathol 1992;24:281.

43. Rockwell WB, Cohen IK, Ehrlich HP. Keloids and hypertrophic scars: a comprehensive review. Plast Reconstr Surg 1989;84:827.

44. Zapol WM, Falke KJ, Hurford WE, et al. Inhaling nitric oxide: a selective pulmonary vasodilator and bronchodilator. Chest 1994;105:87S.

45. Sheridan RL, Tompkins RG. Cultured autologous epithelium in patients with burns of 90% or more of the body surface. J Trauma 1995;38:48.

46. Heimbach D, Luterman A, Burke J, et al. Artificial dermis for major burns: a multi-center randomized clinical trial. Ann Surg 1988;208:313.

SURGERY: SCIENTIFIC PRINCIPLES AND PRACTICE, Second Edition, edited by Lazar J. Greenfield, Michael W. Mulholland, Keith T. Oldham, Gerald B. Zelenock, and Keith D. Lillemoe. Lippincott–Raven Publishers, Philadelphia, © 1997.

CHAPTER 13

ANESTHESIOLOGY AND PAIN MANAGEMENT

TIMOTHY W. RUTTER AND KEVIN K. TREMPER

Anesthesia is a combination of amnesia, analgesia, and muscle relaxation. This state can be achieved by inhaling various vapors that produce each of these conditions in proportion to the concentration achieved in the central nervous system. Anesthesia can also be achieved by using one of three pharmacologic agents that are each targeted to produce a specific effect. These are the amnesics, analgesics, and neuromuscular blocking agents. As the concentration of inhalation anesthetics increases, cardiovascular and respiratory function is progressively depressed. Because of the surgical procedure's requirements or the patient's preexisting cardiac disease, the concentration of inhalation agent that is required to produce sufficient muscle relaxation may be a relative overdose with respect to its effect on the cardiovascular system. For this reason, modern anesthetics usually require titration of these agents to optimize conditions for the surgery while maintaining cardiovascular stability.

The goals of modern anesthesia are (1) to achieve this state quickly and safely by choosing the appropriate techniques and agents for the patient's medical condition; (2) to maintain this state throughout the surgical procedure while compensating for the effects of varying degrees of painful stimuli and blood and fluid loss; and (3) to reverse the muscle relaxation and amnesia, bringing the patient back to physiologic control while maintaining sufficient analgesia to minimize postoperative pain. This process is accomplished with a high degree of safety 30 to 40 million times a year in the United States, in spite of the serious potential complications of technical or judgment errors. The high degree of success of both surgical and anesthetic outcomes is due to the efforts of thousands of surgeons and anesthesiologists who have advanced the art and science of their fields.[1] Although modern techniques and analgesics have made it possible to nearly eliminate all perioperative pain, judgmental feelings about patients who complain of pain still remain. Pain is not only unpleasant; it has significant adverse physiologic effects, and physicians should encourage patients to alert health care personnel when pain is felt.

ANESTHETIC AGENTS AND THEIR PHYSIOLOGIC EFFECTS

Inhalation Agents

Anesthetics are generalized depressants of consciousness, pain, cardiopulmonary function, motor function, and recall. The potent inhalation agents (eg, halothane, ethrane, isoflurane) produce these effects in a dose-dependent fashion with about 1% inhaled concentration. The measurement used to compare the potency of inhalation agents is the percentage of minimum alveolar concentration that prevents movement on painful stimulation (incision) in half of the subjects. There is significant patient-to-patient variability even when patients possess a similar degree of health. Compounding this variability are the effects of age, weight, preexisting heart disease, liver disease, and other medications other than the anesthetics. Table 13-1 lists the commonly used inhalation agents and their minimum alveolar concentrations and side effects. In general, all agents depress blood pressure by myocardial depression and vasodilation. There is a generalized depression of cerebral function and cerebral metabolic rate of oxygen consumption, although cerebral blood flow may increase because of vascular dilatation and a loss of autoregulation. Renal blood flow and glomerular filtration rate are reduced by 20% to 50%. Blood flow to the skin increases and cutaneous autoregulation is reduced, impairing the body's ability to conserve heat. The combination of these effects, the cold environment of the operating

room, and open body cavities make the patient extremely vulnerable to hypothermia.

Muscle Relaxants

To prevent movement and to facilitate the surgical exposure, neuromuscular blocking agents are generally used. These drugs are competitive or noncompetitive inhibitors of the neurotransmitter acetylcholine at the neuromuscular junction. The only noncompetitive inhibitor used clinically is succinylcholine. This drug rapidly binds to the neuromuscular junction and produces depolarization, clinically obvious as fine muscle fasciculations occurring about 60 seconds after injection. Succinylcholine cannot be reversed, but its effects are short-acting because it is quickly hydrolyzed in the plasma by cholinesterase. Because of rapid onset, succinylcholine is frequently used to facilitate endotracheal intubation when it must be accomplished quickly.

All other clinically useful muscle relaxants are termed *competitive inhibitors* and do not cause depolarization when they attach at the neuromuscular junction. Because these agents compete with acetylcholine, the block produced is in direct proportion to the concentration of the agent relative to the concentration of acetylcholine. If the concentration ratio is low enough, competitive relaxants can be reversed if the concentration of acetylcholine is artificially elevated. Acetylcholine concentration can be increased by giving a drug that blocks its metabolism, an anticholinesterase (neostigmine). The neuromuscular blocking agent is still present, but motor function returns if the acetylcholine concentration is high enough to outcompete the blocking agent. There is a ceiling to which anticholinesterase drugs can elevate acetylcholine; therefore, high levels of nondepolarizing relaxants cannot be reversed. Reversing neuromuscular relaxants is not analogous to using naloxone to reverse the effects of opioids. The reversal agent neostigmine does not compete or combine with the relaxant.

Unfortunately, there are systemic consequences to increasing the plasma concentration of acetylcholine. Acetylcholine is the predominant neurotransmitter in the preganglionic sympathetic and parasympathetic nervous systems and in the postganglionic parasympathetic nervous system. For this reason, an anticholinergic drug (atro-

---

Table 13-1. COMMON INHALATION AGENTS: MINIMUM ALVEOLAR CONCENTRATIONS AND EFFECTS

Agent	Minimum Alveolar Concentration (%)	Strengths	Weaknesses
Nitrous oxide	105	Analgesia Rapid uptake and elimination Little cardiac or respiratory depression	Sympathetic stimulation Expansion of closed air spaces Interference with vitamin B_{12} metabolism Limitation of FiO_2
Halothane	0.75	Low cost Effectiveness in low concentrations Little airway irritability Uterine relaxation	Less chemical stability Slow uptake and elimination Biodegradability Hepatic necrosis Cardiac depression and arrhythmias
Enflurane	1.68	Good muscle relaxation Stable cardiac rate and rhythm	Pungent odor Seizure activity on electroencephalography
Isoflurane	1.15	Good muscle relaxation Stable cardiac rate and rhythm Usability in neurosurgery	Pungent odor High cost

(Adapted from Miller FL, Marshall BE. The inhaled anesthetics. In: Longnecker DE, Murphy FL, eds. Introduction to anesthesia, ed 8. Philadelphia, WB Saunders, 1992:77)

Table 13-2. COMMON NEUROMUSCULAR BLOCKING DRUGS AND REVERSAL AGENTS

Muscle Relaxant	Intubating Dose (mg/kg)	Infusion Dose (µg/kg/min)	Strengths	Weaknesses
DEPOLARIZING				
Succinylcholine	1.0	100*	Fastest onset (30 to 60 s) Short duration† (5 min)	Associated with malignant hyperthermia, dysrhythmias, bradycardia, and hyperkalemia, especially in patients with burns or neurologic injury
NONDEPOLARIZING				
Long Acting (>1 h)				
Pancuronium	0.1	0.3	No histamine release	Tachycardia Slow onset Long duration
Pipecuronium	0.08	—	Similar to pancuronium, no cardiovascular effects	—
Doxacurium	0.07	—	Similar to pancuronium, minimal cardiovascular effects	—
Intermediate Acting (≈1 h)				
Atracurium	0.5	10	Spontaneous breakdown in plasma	Histamine release
Vecuronium	0.1	1	No cardiovascular effects	—
Rocuronium	0.8	10	Fast onset, no cardiovascular effects	—
Short Acting (10 min)				
Mivacurium	0.2	10	Fast onset, short duration	Histamine release

* This should not be used for longer than 1 hour.
† Duration is dramatically increased in patients with abnormal plasma pseudocholinesterase.

pine or glycopyrrolate) must be given with the anticholinesterase to prevent the undesirable effects of a generalized acetylcholine overdose. The common neuromuscular blocking drugs, their doses, durations, and side effects are listed in Table 13-2; common regimens of reversal agents are given in Table 13-3.

Nondepolarizing relaxants are frequently used in critically ill patients who are difficult to manage otherwise, for example, head-injured patients who require hyperventilation or patients with adult respiratory distress syndrome who require complex modes of ventilation. It is imperative that these drugs be given in conjunction with analgesics and amnesic agents. Neuromuscular blocking agents have no analgesic or amnesic properties and only prevent motion of voluntary muscles. Patients can be totally aware and in pain, but unable to communicate. When prolonged muscle relaxation is required, it is best to administer the relaxant by continuous infusion and then monitor the effect with a nerve stimulator. For these settings, relaxants should be administered only to achieve the degree of relaxation necessary and in a dose that allows reversal at any time. Table 13-2 includes the recommended ranges of infusion rates. In recent years, there have been reports of patients who have prolonged residual motor weakness after the muscle relaxant is cleared.[2] These problems have been primarily noted with the drug pancuronium bromide (Pa-

Table 13-3. DRUGS FOR ANTAGONIZING NONDEPOLARIZING NEUROMUSCULAR BLOCKADE*

Dose	Time to Peak Effect (min)	Dose	Use With
ANTICHOLINESTERASES			
Edrophonium	1–2	0.5–1.0 mg/kg	—
Neostigmine	3–5	0.04–0.07 mg/kg	—
Pyridostigmine	10–12	0.2–0.3 mg/kg	—
ANTICHOLINERGICS			
Glycopyrrolate	—	0.008 mg/kg (0.5–0.6 mg/70 kg)	Neostigmine Pyridostigmine
Atropine	—	0.007–0.02 mg/kg (0.05–1.5 mg/70 kg)	Edrophonium Neostigmine

* For reliable results in reversing the effects of nondepolarizing muscle relaxants, administration of anticholinesterases is delayed until spontaneous recovery permits three of four responses to a train-of-four stimulus. For patients with more profound blockade, larger amounts of anticholinesterases may be required, but doses of neostigmine higher than 0.14 mg/kg are unlikely to produce additional improvement.

(Adapted from Watling SM, Dasta JF. Prolonged paralysis in intensive care unit patients after the use of neuromuscular blocking agents: a review of the literature. Crit Care Med 1994;22:884)

vulon), especially when the patients are also being treated with steroids. It is therefore recommended that pancuronium bromide not be used for longer than 2 days.

All muscles in the body are not equally sensitive to muscle relaxants. The diaphragm is most resistant to neuromuscular blockade, while the neck and pharyngeal muscles that support the airway are most sensitive. It is possible for an intubated patient to spontaneously ventilate and even to produce a large negative inspiratory effort, and yet develop complete airway obstruction when extubated because of the effects of residual muscle relaxant on the upper airway muscles. The definitive clinical test for complete reversal of neuromuscular blockage is the patient's ability to sustain a head lift from the bed for 5 seconds.

Narcotics and Other Intravenous Analgesics

Narcotics and synthetic analogues belong to the class of drugs called *opioids.* The most commonly used drugs in this family are morphine, meperidine, and codeine. Since the mid–1980s, a series of synthetic narcotics have been developed with fentanyl as the prototype. More recently developed synthetics (sufentanil and alfentanil) are more potent and of shorter duration (Table 13-4). Narcotics produce profound analgesia and respiratory depression. They have no amnesic properties, no direct myocardial depressive effects, and no muscle-relaxant properties. Narcotics can produce significant hemodynamic effects indirectly by releasing histamine or blunting the patient's sympathetic vascular tone because of analgesic properties. The latter effect depends on the degree of sympathetic tone that is present. Acutely injured patients may be hypovolemic and in pain, with high sympathetic tone and peripheral vascular resistance. Patients in this condition can experience dramatic drops in systemic blood pressure with minimal doses of opioids. For this reason, it is important to titrate narcotics in small incremental doses. Because of the lack of direct myocardial depression and the absence of histamine release with the synthetic opioids, they are frequently used as the primary anesthetic in combination with an amnesic agent and a muscle relaxant in patients with significant myocardial dysfunction.

When opioids are titrated intravenously, patients first become apneic because of the respiratory depressive effect (shifting the CO_2 response curve), but they still breathe on command. As the dose increases, patients become apneic and unresponsive. An unusual side effect of high-dose intravenous opioids is chest-wall muscle rigidity, which can make it extremely difficult to ventilate a patient without the assistance of a muscle relaxant.

Opioids are primarily analgesic and not amnesic. Patients can be totally aware and have substantial recall of conversations in spite of appearing completely anesthetized. All opioids can be reversed with naloxone. The duration of action of naloxone can be shorter than that of the narcotic, and patients must be observed carefully after they have been treated with naloxone. Naloxone reversal of opioids can be dangerous because the agent acutely reverses not only the analgesic effects of the opioid, but also analgesic effects of native endorphins. Naloxone treatment has been associated with acute pulmonary edema and myocardial ischemia and should not be used electively to reverse the effects of a narcotic. It is appropriately used in an emergency situation when the airway is not controlled and the patient is not ventilating because of a narcotic overdose.

Propofol

Propofol is a lipid-soluble substituted isopropyl phenol that produces a rapid induction of anesthesia in 30 seconds followed by awakening in 4 to 8 minutes. Intravenous propofol can effectively produce total anesthesia, including amnesia, analgesia, and some degree of muscle relaxation. This agent is unique because it is rapidly cleared through hepatic metabolism to inactive metabolites in a way that the patient becomes alert very quickly after cessation of infusion. Propofol causes a lower incidence of nausea and vomiting when compared to opioid or inhalation anesthetics. It has important roles in intensive care units when used as a continuous infusion sedative at dosages of 25 to 50 mg/kg/min. When the infusion is discontinued, the patient becomes alert within minutes. Propofol can produce significant hypotension when intravenous induction doses are administered. It also produces significant pain on injection. Pain can be diminished or eliminated by pretreatment with intravenous lidocaine, 0.5 mg/kg. Propofol is insoluble in aqueous solution and therefore comes dissolved in a lipid emulsion.

Ketamine

Ketamine is a phencyclidine derivative that produces anesthesia characterized by dissociation between the thalamus and limbic systems. Induction of anesthesia is achieved within 60 seconds after intravenous injection of 1 to 2 mg/kg or within 2 to 4 minutes of intramuscular injection of 5 to 10 mg/kg. Patients appear to be in a cataleptic state in which their eyes remain open with a slow nystagmic gaze. The drug produces intense amnesia and analgesia, but has been associated with unpleasant visual and auditory hallucinations that can progress to delirium. The incidence of these problems can be significantly reduced if benzodiazepines are also administered with the

Table 13-4. ANALGESICS

	Potency	Sedation Dose	Duration	Infusion Dose
OPIOIDS				
Morphine	1	0.02–0.1 mg/kg IV	2–7 h	—
Meperidine	0.1	0.2–1 mg/kg IV	2–4 h	—
Fentanyl	100	0.5–1 μg/kg IV	30–60 min	—
Sufentanil	1000	Not recommended		—
Alfentanil	25	10–20 μg/kg IV	10–15 min	—
OTHER ANALGESICS AND ANESTHETICS				
Propofol		0.5–1 mg/kg IV		25–50 μg/kg/min
Ketamine		0.5–1 mg/kg IV		15–80 μg/kg/min

Table 13-5. ANXIOLYTICS AND AMNESICS (BENZODIAZEPINES)

Name	Dose	Duration (h)	Strengths	Weaknesses
Midazolam (Versed)	0.05 (infusion dose 0.25 µg/kg/min)	0.5	Water soluble Short duration Good for sedation for short procedures	Acute respiratory depression
Diazepam (Valium)	0.1	1	Intermediate duration	Irritation on IV injection Phlebitis Acute respiratory depression after IV overdose
Lorazepam (Ativan)	0.02–0.08	6–8	Long duration	—
BENZODIAZEPINE REVERSAL				
Flumazenil (Romazicon)	4–20 µg/kg (0.2 mg repeated every 2 to 10 min until reversal is achieved) Maximum dose 1 mg	45 to 90 min	—	May produce seizures, panic, arrhythmias

drug. At low doses, patients continue to spontaneously ventilate but cannot be expected to protect the airway should vomiting occur. At higher doses, ketamine acts as a respiratory depressant and produces complete apnea. Ketamine also has direct and indirect sympathetic nervous system stimulatory effects, which can be useful in hypovolemic patients. These effects are diminished or absent in patients who are catecholamine depleted. The sympathetic stimulatory effect increases myocardial oxygen consumption and intracranial pressure, and ketamine is relatively contraindicated in patients with ischemic heart disease or space-occupying intracerebral lesions. Ketamine is frequently used as anintravenousanalgesic during débridement procedures, at doses listed in Table 13-4.

Amnesics and Anxiolytics

Benzodiazepines are the primary class of agents used as amnesics and anxiolytics. The prototype drug, diazepam, has been more recently replaced by its water-soluble analogue of shorter duration, midazolam. Lorazepam also belongs in this family of agents, but because it has a very long duration of action, it is not routinely used intraoperatively. Lorazepam has intensive care unit applications (Table 13-5). Benzodiazepines produce anxiolysis and some degree of amnesia, but have no analgesic properties. Intraoperatively, midazolam is always used in conjunction with an opioid or inhalation agent. Midazolam can be used in combination with the short-acting opioid, fentanyl, to produce conscious sedation for minor procedures. Benzodiazepines can produce apnea and have synergistic effects with narcotics. Very small doses of midazolam and fentanyl can quickly produce an unconscious apneic patient. As with all anesthetics, benzodiazepines used as intravenous agents for sedation should be given in small incremental doses to achieve the desired effect. A reversal agent is also available for benzodiazepines (flumazenil). The recommended dosages of these drugs and the reversal agents appear in Table 13-5.

Local Anesthetics

Local anesthetics constitute a class of drugs that temporarily block nerve conduction by binding to neuronal sodium channels. As the concentration of the local anesthetic increases around the nerve, autonomic transmission will be blocked first, followed by sensory transmission, and then motor nerve transmission. These drugs can be in-

jected locally into tissue to produce a field block, around peripheral nerves to produce a specific dermatome block, or into the spinal or epidural space to produce a major conduction block.

Adverse consequences associated with the use of local anesthetics fall into three categories—acute central nervous system toxicity due to excessive plasma concentration, hemodynamic and respiratory consequences due to excessive conduction block of the sympathetic or motor nerves, and allergic reactions. Whenever a local anesthetic is injected, there can be inadvertent intravascular injection or an overdose of the drug because of rapid uptake from the tissues. All can produce seizures. Complications can be minimized by withdrawing before injection to avoid an intravascular injection and limiting dosages to the safe range (Table 13-6).

When local anesthetics are administered for a spinal or epidural block, they produce a progressive blockade of the sympathetic nervous system, which produces systemic vasodilation. Sympathetic nerves travel along the thoracolumbar region with the first four thoracic branches, including the cardiac sympathetic accelerators. A sympathetic blockade of this entire region produces profound systemic vasodilatation and bradycardia. This condition is referred

Table 13-6. LOCAL ANESTHETICS

	Maximum Single Dose (mg)	Duration (h)	Comments
AMIDES			
Lidocaine	500	1*	Fast onset Exaggerated cardiotoxicity with IV injection
Bupivacaine	200	4–12*	Slow onset Long duration
ESTERS†			
2-Chloroprocaine	1000	0.5–1*	Fast onset Lowest toxicity
Tetracaine	80	0.5–1	Slow onset

* Addition of 100 µg of epinephrine (0.1 mL of 1:1000) lowers the toxicity and increases the duration of the local anesthetic.
† Metabolism to para-aminobenzoic acid may cause allergic reactions.

to as *total sympathectomy*, and the hypotension that ensues is usually below the minimal cerebral perfusion pressure required to maintain consciousness. Affected patients are bradycardic, hypotensive, unconscious, and usually apneic. This disastrous situation is easily remedied if treated quickly with a vasopressor (phenylephrine or ephedrine) and atropine. If not treated promptly, the situation proceeds to cardiac arrest. Because the level of sympathetic block is two to six dermatomal levels higher than the sensory block, it is often difficult to obtain a high spinal sensory level without approaching a total sympathectomy.

Local anesthetics are chemically divided into two groups, esters and amides. The esters (2-chloroprocaine and tetracaine) produce metabolites that are related to *p*-aminobenzoic acid and have been associated with allergic reactions. Amides (lidocaine and bupivacaine) are rarely associated with allergic reactions.

These classes of drugs can be used in combination to produce an anesthetic state with minimal adverse physiologic consequences. Patients with serious preexisting medical problems undergoing very stimulating and traumatic procedures require not only a continuous titration of the level of these drugs but also concomitant use of cardiovascular drugs to improve myocardial function and to adjust systemic resistance. As procedures and patients' diseases become more complex and severe, need for continuous comprehensive physiologic data increases. Consequently, along with the development of shorter-acting, more targeted pharmacologic agents, the sophistication of electronic monitoring equipment has progressively increased.

RISKS ASSOCIATED WITH ANESTHESIA

Because the anesthetic agents effectively obtund or completely block nearly all physiologic protective mechanisms, there is an associated risk even without a surgical procedure. Fortunately, with the advent of newer agents and monitoring techniques, it is estimated that the mortality rate due to anesthesia alone has decreased from about 1 in 10,000 patients in the 1950s to as low as 1 in 100,000 or less for healthy patients today.[3] Although a 1 in 100,000 risk of death or serious neurologic impairment may appear small, when dire consequences occur in a young patient undergoing a purely elective procedure, the consequences are devastating for everyone involved. When patients are placed in a condition in which they cannot breathe, there is always the possibility of a technical or judgmental error resulting in hypoxia and brain damage or death. It has been estimated that between 50% and 75% of anesthetic-related deaths are due to human error and are preventable. Because the consequences of an anesthetic mishap are usually severe, the emotional and financial costs are high.

The most common problems associated with adverse outcomes are related to the airway and include inadequate ventilation, unrecognized esophageal intubation, unrecognized extubation, and unrecognized disconnection from the ventilator. The incidence of these problems has been significantly reduced by including capnometry and pulse oximetry in addition to other noninvasive monitors, although a cause-and-effect relation has been difficult to prove. Efforts to improve outcome can be approached at three levels: (1) reduction of the incidence of rare but catastrophic anesthetic-related problems; (2) improvement of the care and experience of every patient undergoing anesthesia and surgery; and (3) improvement of the preparation and management of patients with preexisting medical conditions who have higher morbidity and mortality rates. The first goal has been addressed in part with improved

monitoring techniques and anesthesia training. Others have been advanced by the addition of comprehensive pain management, as discussed later in this chapter. Issues of preexisting medical disease and how they affect the anesthetic plan are also briefly discussed later in this chapter.

Cardiovascular Diseases

Hypertension

Hypertension is the most common preexisting medical disease in patients presenting for surgery. Hypertensive patients should be treated medically to render them normotensive before elective surgery. These medications should be continued throughout the perioperative period. The incidence of hypotension and myocardial ischemia intraoperatively is higher in untreated hypertensive patients than in adequately treated hypertensive patients if the preoperative diastolic pressure is 110 mmHg or higher.[4] Inadequately treated hypertensive patients undergoing carotid endarteriectomies have an increased incidence of neurologic deficits, and those with a history of prior myocardial infarctions have an increased incidence of reinfarction. Patients commonly have an elevated blood pressure on admission to the hospital. Hypertensive patients can have exaggerated responses to painful stimuli and have a higher incidence of perioperative ischemia.

Coronary Artery Disease

Much of the anesthetic preoperative evaluation is directed toward detecting the presence and determining the degree of ischemic heart disease. Coronary artery disease is present in about 25% of patients who undergo surgery each year.[4] It is the leading cause of death in the United States and continues to be a major cause of postoperative morbidity and mortality. The goal of the preoperative cardiac evaluation is to identify patients who are at increased risk of perioperative cardiac morbidity. Although perioperative cardiac events are the leading cause of death following anesthesia and surgery, it has been difficult to define patient characteristics that accurately predict a high risk of adverse outcome.[5] Preoperative congestive heart failure (CHF) is clearly a significant risk factor, as is recent myocardial infarction or unstable angina. Diabetes melitis, atherosclerotic vascular disease, and hypertension also appear to confer risk, although less than CHF or unstable angina. Perioperative risk in patients with valvular heart disease varies with the severity of the disease as represented by CHF, pulmonary hypertension, and dysrhythmias. Dysrhythmias are also a concern in the presence of coronary artery disease. Age and stable angina remain controversial as predictors of perioperative risk, with equal numbers of supporting and refuting studies. Previous coronary artery bypass grafting appears to confer protection against perioperative cardiac events. Because of the incidence of silent ischemia, especially in patients with diabetes melitis, patients in high-risk groups (ie, men over age 40, women over age 50) should be evaluated with preoperative electrocardiography (ECG). In patients without significant pulmonary disease, the ability to climb two flights of stairs without stopping or experiencing symptoms of angina or shortness of breath is considered a good practical test of cardiac reserve. Unfortunately, many patients with ischemic heart disease have concomitant pulmonary disease or other medical problems that limit their activity. The resting 12-lead ECG remains the most cost-effective screening test for ischemic heart disease. ECG may be normal in patients with extensive ischemic heart disease and does not detect the presence of prior subendocardial myocardial infarction. For patients in high-risk groups, further stress evaluations may be required.

A history of myocardial infarction is important information. Large retrospective studies have found that the incidence of reinfarction is related to the time elapsed since the previous myocardial infarction.[5-7] The incidence of reinfarction appears to stabilize at about 6% after 6 months. The highest rate of reinfarction occurs in the 0- to 3-month period. Mortality from reinfarction, for patients undergoing noncardiac surgery, has been reported to be between 20% to 50% and usually occurs within the first 48 hours after surgery. Invasive hemodynamic monitoring with a pulmonary artery catheter and aggressive pharmacologic intervention has been shown to reduce reinfarction rates (Table 13-7). The incidence of reinfarction is also increased in patients undergoing intrathoracic or intraabdominal procedures lasting longer than 3 hours.[5] The site of surgery and anesthetic technique have not been shown to change the incidence of reinfarction if the procedure is shorter than 3 hours.[5] Patients with known three-vessel or left main coronary artery disease are at increased risk, whereas those who have undergone prior coronary artery bypass grafting are at a substantially decreased risk of reinfarction. Although prophylactic therapy with beta blockers, calcium-channel agents, and nitrates have not been proven beneficial, withdrawal of these agents has been associated with perioperative ischemia, myocardial infarction, and death.[5]

All patients in high-risk groups or with a history of ischemic heart disease must be evaluated and properly treated before elective surgery. All elective surgery should be delayed for 6 months after myocardial infarction. If this is not feasible, invasive monitoring should be considered in the perioperative period and intensive postoperative observation should continue for at least 48 hours.

Congestive Heart Failure

Congestive heart failure has been described as the single most important factor predicting postoperative cardiac morbidity[8] (Table 13-8). All elective surgical procedures should be deferred until congestive failure is treated. If surgery cannot be deferred, aggressive perioperative management is warranted with a goal of optimizing cardiac output. In contrast to isolated ischemic heart disease, CHF is more easily diagnosed by history, physical examination, and basic preoperative laboratory workup, including ECG and chest radiography. Because patients with left, right, or both left and right ventricular dysfunction are less tolerant of the fluid shifts associated with surgery and the myocardial depression associated with the anesthetic, they constitute the highest-risk group for postoperative cardiac complications.

Table 13-7. RISK OF MYOCARDIAL REINFARCTION AFTER SURGERY WITH AGGRESSIVE HEMODYNAMIC MONITORING AND INTERVENTIONS AND POSTOPERATIVE ICU ADMISSION

Age of Previous Infarction (mo)	Reinfarction Rate (%)
7–12	1.0
3–6	2.3
0–3	5.8

(Rao TKL, Jacobs KH, El Etr AA. Reinfarction following anesthesia in patients with myocardial infarction. Anesthesiology 1983;59:499)

Table 13-8. CLINICAL FACTORS INDEPENDENTLY RELATED TO PERIOPERATIVE CARDIAC COMPLICATIONS

Criteria	Points
S_3 gallop or jugular venous distention on preoperative physical examination	11
Transmural or subendocardial myocardial infarction in the previous 6 mo	10
Premature ventricular beats, more than 5 beats/min documented at any time	7
Rhythm other than sinus or presence of premature atrial contractions on last preoperative ECG	5
Age over 70 y	4
Emergency operations	3
Intrathoracic, intraperitoneal, or aortic site of surgery	3
Evidence for important valvular aortic stenosis	3
Poor general medical condition*	3

Total Points	Risks of Cardiac Complication (%)	Risk of Death (%)
0–5	0.7	0.2
6–12	5	2
13–25	11	2
≥26	22	5

* As evidenced by electrolyte abnormalities, renal insufficiency, abnormal blood gases, abnormal liver status, or any condition that has caused the patient to become chronically bedridden.
(Goldman L, Caldera DC, Nussbaum SR, et al. Multifactoral index of cardiac risk in noncardiac surgical procedures. N Engl J Med 1977;297,845)

Pulmonary Disease

Pulmonary disease is divided into acute and chronic restrictive and obstructive disease. Restrictive disease is defined by processes that reduce lung volumes, and obstructive disease is characterized by reduced flow rates on pulmonary function tests. Restrictive diseases are further subdivided into intrinsic and extrinsic forms. Intrinsic disease includes adult respiratory distress syndrome, and extrinsic disease is usually due to external restriction of lung volume by chest wall deformities or the patient's excessive weight. Although restrictive diseases can produce significant pulmonary dysfunction, less anesthetic preparation is necessary for these patients. A more sophisticated ventilator is needed in the perioperative period.

Obstructive diseases are present in patients with FEV_1/FPC ratios of less than 50%. Obstructive pulmonary disease can be either chronic or acute (asthma). In either case, the reversible component of obstruction should be reversed before elective surgery. Patients are maintained on bronchodilator medications, and those with chronic secretions are appropriately hydrated and receive therapy to mobilize secretions. In patients with reactive airway disease, the endotracheal tube can induce severe bronchiospasm. Even in patients who are well- treated preoperatively, reactive bronchospasm can complicate anesthetic induction and the emergence from anesthesia. The principal method used to prevent or diminish this "foreign body"–induced bronchospasm is intubation of the patient at a deep level of anesthesia when reflexes are blunted. The classic way to manage a patient with severe asthma is to induce with an agent that produces bronchodilation and to ventilate the patient with an inhalation agent until the patient is deeply anesthetized before laryngoscopy and intubation. The patient should be extubated while spontaneously ventilating, but with the inhalation agent still in effect. The patient is brought back to consciousness while ventilating by mask. Unfortunately, this technique may not be feasible in patients who have a full stomach because of the risk of aspiration or who are difficult to intubate or ventilate.

For elective surgery, patients should not be wheezing, and chronic patients should have no signs of bacterial infection, such as purulent sputum. Chest physiotherapy combined with hydration helps to remove secretions from the airways. The preoperative use of intermittent positive pressure breathing has not been shown to decrease the incidence of postoperative pulmonary complications.

Regional anesthetics can be useful in these patients for peripheral surgery or for procedures that require an anesthetic sensory level below T6. As the sensory and motor levels rise to T6 and above, patients lose significant accessory motor function that can decrease expiratory reserve volume and the ability to cough and clear secretions. Because of tenuous pulmonary status and the high incidence of postoperative pulmonary complications, pulmonary patients should be extubated with caution only when they meet adequate extubation criteria relative to preoperative test data. Changes in pulmonary mechanics and frequency of postoperative pulmonary complications are greatest after upper abdominal surgery. Both vital capacity and functional residual capacity are reduced, reaching lowest levels in the first 24 hours postoperatively. In the high-risk groups, therapy should be directed toward restoring functional residual capacity to preoperative levels. Such therapy improves compliance and gas exchange. Because of the potential adverse effects of systemic narcotics on respiratory drive, the use of epidural narcotics and local anesthetics for postoperative pain control is very popular. These techniques allow the patients to be extubated earlier and, in patients with intrathoracic and upper abdominal surgery, help restore pulmonary function toward preoperative values.[9]

Obesity

Obesity causes a host of problems on both sides of the surgical drapes. Obesity is defined as being 20% over ideal body weight. Ideal body weight can be easily estimated as height (cm) − 100 = ideal body weight (kg). The pathophysiologic changes associated with morbid obesity (twice the ideal body weight) affect the respiratory, cardiovascular, and gastrointestinal systems. Patients have an external restrictive disease that reduces functional residual capacity and worsens with the supine position. Breathing effort increases and ventilation becomes diaphragmatic and position dependent. Obese patients frequently desaturate at night and have a high incidence of sleep apnea. Because of increased blood volume and frequent desaturations, obese patients can develop pulmonary hypertension and right-sided heart failure. Obese individuals have a high incidence of coronary artery disease. Because of size alone, they have increased cardiovascular demands with limited cardiac reserve and exercise tolerance. Obese patients have a high incidence of hiatal hernia and gastroesophageal reflux, increasing the risk for aspiration on induction and emergence from anesthesia. Because of fatty liver infiltration and fat deposits elsewhere, these patients may experience prolonged effects of anesthetics and other analgesics. Issues as mundane as venous access can cause significant problems in this patient group.

The primary concern of the anesthesiologist is gaining adequate control of the airway. The combined problems of aspiration risk, rapid desaturation caused by reduced functional residual capacity and increased oxygen demand, as well as technical difficulties associated with intubation due to anatomic fat deposits, make intubation a high-risk procedure. If problems occur, there can be sig-

nificant technical difficulties in obtaining a rapid cricothyrotomy. For these reasons, a nasal or oral awake intubation can be useful. All patients should receive prophylactic administration of H_2-receptor antagonists and metachlopromide to decrease the volume of gastric contents. If intubations are to be done after induction of anesthesia, they should be performed in a rapid sequence using cycroid pressure. To prevent aspiration on emergence, obese patients should be extubated when fully awake, preferably in the sitting position. Regional anesthetics can be very useful when peripheral procedures are planned. Unfortunately, morbidly obese patients can develop pulmonary failure just by laying flat, making it difficult to use epidural or spinal anesthetics for abdominal procedures. Epidural analgesics for postoperative pain management allow earlier extubation and ambulation of these patients.[9]

Overall hospital mortality rate increases when several chronic diseases are present. Investigators have found that renal failure and CHF are associated with the highest increases in hospital mortality rates, especially in the elderly undergoing emergency procedures[10] (Table 13-9).

PREOPERATIVE EVALUATION

The three goals of the preoperative evaluation are: (1) to develop an anesthetic plan that considers the patient's medical condition, the requirements of the surgical procedure, and the patient's preferences; (2) to ensure that the patient's chronic disease is under appropriate medical therapy before an elective procedure; and (3) to gain rapport with and the confidence of the patient, answer any questions, and allay fears.

Optimally, to complete this task, an anesthesiologist would meet every patient before the planned surgical procedure to review the medical history, complete a physical examination, discuss the options and associated anesthetic risks, and develop an anesthetic plan. The anesthesiologist prefers to have a comprehensive evaluation of the medical status by the patient's family practitioner or internist, including the results of pertinent laboratory studies. In the past, this was accomplished when the anesthesiologist visited the patient in the hospital the night before surgery.

Table 13-9. HOSPITAL MORTALITY RATES IN RELATION TO AGE, PREOPERATIVE DISEASE, AND SURGERY

Preoperative Disease and Surgery	Age (y)		
	<50*	50–69*	>70*
Chronic heart failure	0.1%/0.5%	0.4%/2%	0.8%/4%
Renal failure	0.2%/1%	0.9%/2%	2%/9%
Abdominal surgery	0.3%/2%	1%/6%	3%/12%
Chronic heart failure and renal failure	0.7%/3%	3%/13%	6%/24%
Chronic heart failure and abdominal surgery	0.9%/4%	4%/17%	7%/30%
Renal failure and abdominal surgery	2%/8%	2%/32%	16%/50%
Chronic heart failure, renal failure, and abdominal surgery	6%/26%	22%/60%	37%/76%

* Figures are for elective surgery (first number) and emergency surgery (second number).
(Pedersen T, Eliasen K, Henriksen E. A prospective study of mortality associated with anesthesia and surgery: risk indicators of mortality in hospitals. Acta Anaesthesiol Scand 1990;34:176)

Currently, it is rare to have patients admitted the night before surgery even before the most comprehensive and complex surgical procedures. The evaluation must still be accomplished, but it must be done on an ambulatory basis, which creates associated logistical problems.

A patient's medical condition should be optimized before an elective surgical procedure. This optimization is best performed by the primary care physician, with medical specialty consultation if necessary. If the procedure is deemed a surgical emergency, the anesthesiologist is responsibile for assessing the patient quickly, developing the appropriate anesthetic plan, and proceeding to the operating room as soon as possible. In an emergency situation, the anesthesiologist is not obligated to seek medical consultation to evaluate chronic medical problems because time is essential. The following questions must be answered when evaluating a patient undergoing an elective surgical procedure. What must be included in the preoperative evaluation? Second, who is involved in this process? When and where are all the steps in this process to be conducted? How should all the information be coordinated so that it is available to the appropriate personnel at the appropriate time?

The following steps must be completed before moving the patient into the operating room:

1. A history and physical examination
2. Appropriate laboratory studies and medical consultations
3. An anesthesiologist preoperative evaluation with assignment of an American Society of Anesthesiologists (ASA) physical status
4. Discussion with the patient of the options and risks
5. Development of an anesthetic plan

The history and physical examination have repeatedly been shown to be the most valuable parts of the preoperative assessment. It is primarily the surgeon's responsibility to obtain a history that includes current medical conditions, current medication, and previous surgical and anesthetic history. Questions that are of unique interest to the anesthesiologist are those that involve previous anesthetic problems experienced by the patient or blood relatives and the patient's exercise tolerance. This evaluation not only determines the laboratory tests that may be required but also allows for the assignment of ASA physical status (Table 13-10). The classification serves as a general measure of the patient's state of well being, taking into account all problems the patient brings to the operating room, including systemic disturbances caused by the surgical illness. Although studies of anesthetic mortality show a correlation with the physical status classification, this categorization does not describe the risk directly. The risk of any operation is determined not only by patient-related factors, but also by procedure-specific ones. For patients with complex medical problems, it is frequently helpful to supplement the surgical history and physical examination with a recent assessment by the patient's primary physician.

The value of preoperative laboratory studies has undergone substantial reevaluation since the mid–1980s. In the past, a surgical procedure was an opportunity to obtain a battery of baseline laboratory tests, even for ASA PS-I patients. The current thinking is that a laboratory test should not be ordered unless a change in the surgical or anesthetic plan is anticipated. The only preoperative screening test required at the University of Michigan, for instance, is an ECG within a year of the planned surgical procedure for men older than 40 and women older than 50 years of age. Pregnancy tests should be obtained only for women who state that they could be pregnant. For procedures with significant anticipated blood loss, a type and

Table 13-10. PHYSICAL STATUS CLASSIFICATION OF THE AMERICAN SOCIETY OF ANESTHESIOLOGISTS

Physical Status Classification	Description
PS-1	A normal healthy patient
PS-2	A patient with mild systemic disease that results in no functional limitation *Examples:* Hypertension, diabetes mellitus, chronic bronchitis, morbid obesity, extremes of age
PS-3	A patient with severe systemic disease that results in functional limitation *Examples:* Poorly controlled hypertension, diabetes mellitus with vascular complications, angina pectoris, prior myocardial infarction, pulmonary disease that limits activity
PS-4	A patient with severe systemic disease that is a constant threat to life *Examples:* Congestive heart failure, unstable angina pectoris, advanced pulmonary, renal, or hepatic dysfunction
PS-5	A moribund patient who is not expected to survive without the operation *Examples:* Ruptured abdominal aneurysm, pulmonary embolus, head injury with increased intracranial pressure
PS-6	A declared brain-dead patient whose organs are being removed for donor purposes
Emergency operation (E)	Any patient in whom an emergency operation is required *Example:* An otherwise healthy 30-year old woman who requires dilation and curettage for moderate but persistent vaginal fleeding (PS-1E)

cross match is ordered, and a preoperative hematocrit is also required. All other tests should have an indication based on history and physical examination. A current strategy for selecting tests indicated by patient history is presented in Table 13-11. Electronic patient questionnaires have also been developed, allowing the patient to select his or her own preoperative tests.

Discussions of the options of anesthetic techniques and anesthetic risks are best performed by the anesthesiologist who will provide the anesthetic. If the surgeon prefers a specific anesthetic technique, this is best communicated directly to the anesthesiologist rather than recommended to the patient. The development of the anesthetic plan must be determined by the anesthesiologist.

The history and physical examination and laboratory studies should be performed by the surgeon as soon as the surgical procedure is scheduled. The results of the laboratory studies must be evaluated well in advance of the day of surgery so that positive findings can be attended to in a timely manner. For healthy patients (ASA PS-I and PS-II), the preoperative anesthetic assessment can be conducted by the anesthesiologist on the day of the procedure. If the patients have complex medical problems (ASA PS-III or greater) or have significant concerns they want to discuss with an anesthesiologist, they should be evaluated before the day of surgery. Because of the logistical prob-

Table 13-11. SIMPLIFIED STRATEGY FOR PREOPERATIVE TESTING*

Preoperative Condition	Hgb Male	Hgb Female	WBC	PT/PTT	PTL/BT	Electrolytes	Creatinine/BUN	Blood Glucose	SGOT/Alk PTase	X-ray	ECG	Pregnancy Test	T/S
Procedure with blood loss	O	O	—	—	—	—	—	—	—	—	—	—	O
Procedure without blood loss	—	—	—	—	—	—	—	—	—	—	—	—	—
Neonates													
<40 d old	—	O	—	—	—	—	—	—	—	?	M	—	—
40–49 d old	—	O	—	—	—	—	—	—	—	?	O	—	—
50–64 d old	O	O	—	—	—	—	—	—	—	O	O	—	—
≥65–74 d old	O	O	—	—	—	—	—	—	—	O	O	—	—
≥75 d old	O	O	—	—	—	—	—	—	—	O	O	—	—
Cardiovascular disease	O	O	—	—	—	—	O	—	—	—	O	—	—
Pulmonary disease	O	—	—	—	—	—	O	—	—	O	O	—	—
Malignancy	—	—	L	L	—	—	O	—	—	O	—	—	—
Radiotherapy	—	—	—	—	—	—	—	—	—	O	—	—	—
Hepatic disease	—	—	—	O	—	—	—	O	O	—	—	—	—
Exposure to hepatitis	O	O	—	O	—	—	—	O	O	—	—	—	—
Renal disease	—	—	—	—	—	O	O	—	—	—	—	—	—
Bleeding disorder	—	—	—	O	O	—	—	—	—	—	—	—	—
Diabetes	O	O	—	—	—	O	O	O	—	—	—	—	—
Smoking	—	—	—	—	—	—	—	—	—	O	—	—	—
Possible pregnancy	—	O	—	—	—	—	—	—	—	—	—	O	—
Drug use	O	—	—	—	—	—	—	—	—	—	—	—	—
Diuretics	—	—	—	—	—	O	O	—	—	—	—	—	—
Digoxin	—	—	—	—	—	O	O	—	—	—	O	—	—
Steroids	O	O	O	O	—	O	—	O	—	—	—	—	—
Anticoagulants	—	—	—	—	—	—	—	—	—	—	—	—	—
CNS disease	—	—	O	—	—	O	O	O	—	—	O	—	—

* Not all diseases are included in this table. The physician's own judgment is needed regarding patients with diseases not listed.

?, perhaps obtain; L, obtain for leukemias only; O, obtain; M, obtain for men only; HGB, hemoglobin; WBC, white blood cell count; PT, prothrombin time; PTT, partial thromboplastin time; PLT, platelet count; BT, bleeding time; BUN, blood urea nitrogen; SGOT, serum glutamic-oxaloacetic transaminase; Alk PTase, alkaline phosphatase; ECG, electrocardiogram; T/S, blood typing and screening for unexpected antibodies; CNS, central nervous system.

lems of scheduling, most institutions have developed pre-operative anesthesia clinics where this process can take place. When specialty medical consultation is considered, the following questions should be answered. Does this patient have ischemic heart disease that requires further medical management or workup? What is the degree of functional improvement of the organ system in question? Is medical treatment of these problems optimized? If not, what needs to be done and how long will it take?

An obvious problem that concerns anesthesiologists is the potential of a difficult intubation. Even if a patient has no medical problem, the possibility of a difficult airway warrants that the patient be seen preoperatively and evaluated. These patients can always be approached by an awake fiberoptic technique, but this takes planning and can cause a significant delay if there is no prior warning. Although there is no absolute standard to predict a difficult intubation, a simple four-step examination helps to determine the likelihood. First, the patient should have a normal mouth opening. Second, the patient should have normal neck flexion and extension. Third, the physician should be able to fit three finger widths under the patient's chin between the thyroid cartilage and the mentum. Finally, when the patient opens the mouth and is asked to stick out the tongue, the airway can be classified depending on whether the uvulae can be completely seen (class 1), only partly seen (class 2), or not seen, with only the hard and soft palate visible (class 3). This classification roughly predicts progressive difficulty in intubating due to difficulty in visualizing the larynx.[11]

MONITORING THE SURGICAL PATIENT

One of the more obvious changes in anesthesia care has been the routine use of an array of electronic monitoring devices to provide continuous surveillance of physiologic status. Because the art and science of anesthesiology involves titrating pharmacologic agents to produce desired physiologic effects, there must be a measured parameter to which drug dosages are titrated. Depending on the severity of preexisting disease and the extent and duration of the surgical procedure, invasive techniques can be used to provide comprehensive continuous data to guide the titration of fluid therapy and cardiovascular agents.

Monitors of Oxygenation

Pulse oximetry has been called the most significant advance in patient monitoring to date. This device continuously, noninvasively and inexpensively provides arterial hemoglobin saturation (SaO_2) and peripheral pulse by measuring light absorption in a manner similar to a laboratory co-oximeter. A co-oximeter shines light through a cuvette filled with a blood sample. Each hemoglobin species absorbs light in direct proportion to its concentration (Beer-Lambert law). A co-oximeter requires one wavelength of light for each hemoglobin species to be measured, that is one wavelength for oxyhemoglobin and one for reduced hemoglobin. To measure other hemoglobins, such as carboxyhemoglobin or methemoglobin, the device requires four wavelengths of light.

The pulse oximeter uses two wavelengths of light, one red and one infrared, that shine through a tissue bed, usually a finger. Opposite the light sources is a photodiode that measures the transmitted light intensity. A large proportion of the light absorbed as it passes through the tissues is not associated with arterial blood, but with other components of the tissue, such as skin, muscle, bone, and venous blood. Therefore, the device analyzes only the pulsatile component of absorption and assumes that anything that pulses within the tissue bed is arterial blood, hence the name *pulse oximeter*. Actually, the pulse oximeter measures the ratio of the pulsatile component of red light absorbed to the pulsatile component of the infrared light absorbed. This ratio changes with SaO_2. The exact relation between this ratio and SaO_2 has been empirically determined from volunteer studies and is programmed into the electronics of the oximeter. If any artifacts occur in a pulsatile nature, they may be erroneously integrated into the equation, causing erroneous SaO_2 estimates.

Several things should be remembered when using the pulse oximeter. First, the device measures SaO_2 and not arterial oxygen tension (PaO_2). The PaO_2 must drop below 80 mmHg before any significant change in SaO_2 occur. As the PaO_2 drops below 60 mmHg, the SaO_2 rapidly falls as the inflection point of the sigmoidal oxyhemoglobin dissociation curve is approached. As a rough rule of thumb, as SaO_2 drops below 90%, the PaO_2 can be estimated by subtracting 30 points from the SaO_2. For example, a SaO_2 of 85% corresponds to a PaO_2 of 55 mmHg. Second, the pulse oximeter measures saturation (mL oxygen/dL blood) and not arterial content or CaO_2. Although the dissolved oxygen is ignored because of its small contribution, the oxygen content is directly proportional to the SaO_2 and the hemoglobin concentration. Since the hemoglobin concentration is is about one third of the hematocrit, the following equation can be used to estimate CaO_2:

$$CaO_2 = 0.45 \text{ Hct} \times SaO_2$$

or, if SaO_2 is 100%:

$$CaO_2 \approx \tfrac{1}{2} \text{ Hct}$$

The oxygen-carrying capacity of blood can be quickly assessed by spinning a hematocrit and measuring the arterial saturation with a pulse oximeter.

Because the pulse oximeter uses only two wavelengths of light, it cannot detect the presence of carboxyhemoglobin (carbon monoxide poisoning) or methemoglobin. Because the absorption characteristics of carboxyhemoglobin are similar to those of oxyhemoglobin, the pulse oximeter will register approximately the sum of both these gases. A pulse-oximeter reading of 100% saturation for a patient with smoke inhalation injury may actually indicate severe carbon monoxide poisoning. The only method of determining carbon monoxide poisoning is to send an arterial blood sample for laboratory co-oximeter measurement of carboxyhemoglobin. The only clinically accepted device for invasive monitoring of oxygen saturation is the pulmonary arterial oximeter catheter (see Chap. 9).

Despite the potential drawbacks, the pulse oximeter has been shown to be impressively accurate in a wide variety of patients with a tremendous variation in pulse amplitude.[12]

Ventilation Monitors

By definition, a patient is appropriately ventilated when arterial carbon dioxide tension ($PaCO_2$) is 40 mmHg. Measuring the respiratory rate can only document the presence of ventilation, not its adequacy. Capnography, or end-tidal CO_2 monitoring, is the visual display of the CO_2 concentration at the airway. To understand the utility of capnography, one must understand dead-space components and how they affect CO_2 removal from the body.[13] Dead space (DS) is defined as the portion of the tidal volume (V_T) that does not participate in gas exchange.

$$V_T = DS + V_A$$

The alveolar volume (V_A) is the volume of the inspired gas that reaches well-perfused alveoli. The remainder of the V_T, which equals the DS, can be divided into three subcomponents—apparatus dead space (DS_{ap}), anatomic dead space (DS_{an}), and alveolar dead space (DS_{al}).

$$DS = DS_{ap} + DS_{an} + DS_{al}$$

At the end of inspiration, the respiratory apparatus (eg, endotracheal tube) is filled with inspired gas that should not contain CO_2. Similarly, all the anatomic airways (trachea, bronchi, and all conducting airways down to the alveoli) should be filled with inspired gas and should therefore contain no CO_2. In this model, there are two types of alveoli, those which that well-perfused, alveolar gas and those that are not perfused, DS_{al} gas. At the end of inspiration, the DS_{al} gas, since it is not perfused, does not pick up CO_2 and again contains inspired gas and no CO_2. The alveolar gas should completely equilibrate with the arterial blood and contain CO_2 at the same tension as the arterial blood, ideally Pa_{CO_2} should equal 40 mmHg. As the patient expires, the CO_2 detected at the patient's mouth first reflects the DS_{ap} gas having no CO_2, followed by the DS_{an} gas, again with no CO_2, and finally the alveolar gases, containing both dead space and well-perfused alveolar gas. When mixed alveolar gas reaches the airway, it produces a rapid rise in the CO_2 concentration to a level somewhere

Table 13-12. STANDARDS FOR POSTANESTHESIA CARE*

	Standards	Criteria to Be Fulfilled
Standard I†	All patients who have received general, regional, or monitored anesthesia care shall receive appropriate postanesthesia management.	1. A PACU or an area that provides equivalent postanesthesia care shall be available to receive patients after anesthesia care. All patients who receive anesthesia care shall be admitted to the PACU or its equivalent *except* by specific order of the anesthesiologist responsible for the patient's care. 2. The medical aspects of care in the PACU shall be governed by policies and procedures that have been reviewed and approved by the department of anesthesiology. 3. The design, equipment, and staffing of the PACU shall meet requirements of the facility's accrediting and licensing bodies.
Standard III	A patient transported to the PACU shall be accompanied by a member of the anesthesia care team who is knowledgeable about the patient's condition. The patient shall be continually evaluated and treated during transport with monitoring and support appropriate to the patient's condition.	
Standard III	On arrival in the PACU, the patient shall be reevaluated and a verbal report provided to the responsible PACU nurse by the member of the anesthesia care team who accompanies the patient.	1. The patient's status on arrival in the PACU shall be documented. 2. Information concerning the preoperative condition and the surgical/anesthetic course shall be transmitted to the PACU nurse. 3. The member of the anesthesia care team shall remain in the PACU until the PCAU nurse accepts responsibility for the nursing care of the patient.
Standard IV	The patient's condition shall be evaluated continually in the PACU.	1. The patient shall be observed and monitored by the methods appropriate to the patient's medical condition. Particular attention shall be given to monitoring oxygenation, ventilation, circulation, and temperature. During recovery from all anesthetics, a quantitative method of assessing oxygenation such as pulse oximetry shall be employed in the initial phase of recovery. This is not intended for application during the recovery of the obstetric patient in whom regional anesthesia was used for labor and vaginal delivery. 2. An accurate written report of the PCAU period shall be maintained. Use of an appropriate PACU scoring system is encouraged for each patient on admission, at appropriate intervals prior to discharge, and at the time of discharge. 3. General medical supervision and coordination of patient care in the PACU should be the responsibility of an anesthesiologist. 4. There shall be a policy to ensure the availability in the facility of a physician capable of managing complications and providing cardiopulmonary resuscitation for patients in the PACU.
Standard V	A physician is responsible for discharging the patient from the PACU.	1. When discharge criteria are used, they must be approved by the department of anesthesiology and the medical staff. They may vary depending on whether the patient is discharged to a hospital room, to the ICU, to a short stay unit, or home. 2. In the absence of the physician responsible for the discharge, the PACU nurse shall determine that the patient meets the discharge criteria. The name of the physician accepting responsibility for discharge shall be noted on the record.

* Based on ASA's Standards for Postanesthesia Care. A copy of the full text can be obtained from ASA, 520 N. Northwest Highway, Park Ridge, IL 60068-2573.
† For nursing care issues, refer to Standards of Postanasthesia Nursing Practice, published by the American Society of Postanesthesia Nurses.

Table 13-13. POSTANESTHESIA RECOVERY SCORE*

Parameter	Score
ACTIVITY	
Voluntary movement of all limbs to command	2
Voluntary movement of 2 extremities to command	1
Unable to move	0
RESPIRATION	
Breathes deeply and coughs	2
Dyspnea, hypoventilation	1
Apneic	0
CIRCULATION	
Blood pressure equals 80% of preanesthetic level	2
Blood pressure equals 50%–80% of preanesthetic level	1
Blood pressure equals <50% of preanesthetic level	0
CONSCIOUSNESS	
Fully awake	2
Arousable	1
Unresponsive	0
COLOR	
Pink	2
Pale, blotchy	1
Cyanotic	0

* Patients should score at least 7 before discharge from the postanesthesia care unit.

between the concentration in the alveolar gas (40 mmHg) and the DS_{al} (0 mmHg), depending on each component's proportion of volume. For example, if half of the alveoli are DS_{al} and $Paco_2$ equals 40 mmHg, then the plateau value of the capnogram should be 20 mmHg, implying that half of the alveoli are not being perfused. With inspiration, the CO_2 value again drops to 0 until another expiration, and a square wave appears again as the alveolar gas is detected at the mouth. With each breath, there should be a square wave, whose a height approaches the $Paco_2$ value as the amount of the DS_{al} gas approaches 0.

In a healthy young adult, there is no significant DS_{al} gas, and the end tidal CO_2 value equals the $Paco_2$. Therefore, the difference between these values indicates the proportion of DS_{al} in the patient. The presence of a capnogram itself implies there is metabolism (the production of CO_2), circulation (blood flow to the lungs), and ventilation (respiratory rate and an intact ventilator circuit).

Providing this information on a breath-to-breath basis, the continuous capnogram is extremely useful in many critical situations. It can be used as a surveillance monitor of both the respiratory circuit and the cardiovascular system. Any acute decrease in cardiac output will decrease blood flow to the lungs and increase the DS_{al}, causing an acute drop in end tidal CO_2. For this reason, the device was originally used during neurosurgical procedures in the sitting position to detect the presence of air emboli. This principle also allows the detection of pulmonary emboli or any acute drop in cardiac output. In fact, the only acute catastrophic cardiopulmonary problem that will not be detected by the capnometer is arterial desaturation. Therefore, the combination of the capnometer and the pulse oximeter creates a dynamic duo for beat-to-beat and breath-to-breath surveillance of metabolism, circulation, ventilation, and oxygenation.

Circulation Monitors

Hemodynamic stability can be monitored by a variety of methods, the most basic of which is systemic arterial blood pressure. Intermittent, noninvasive measure of systemic

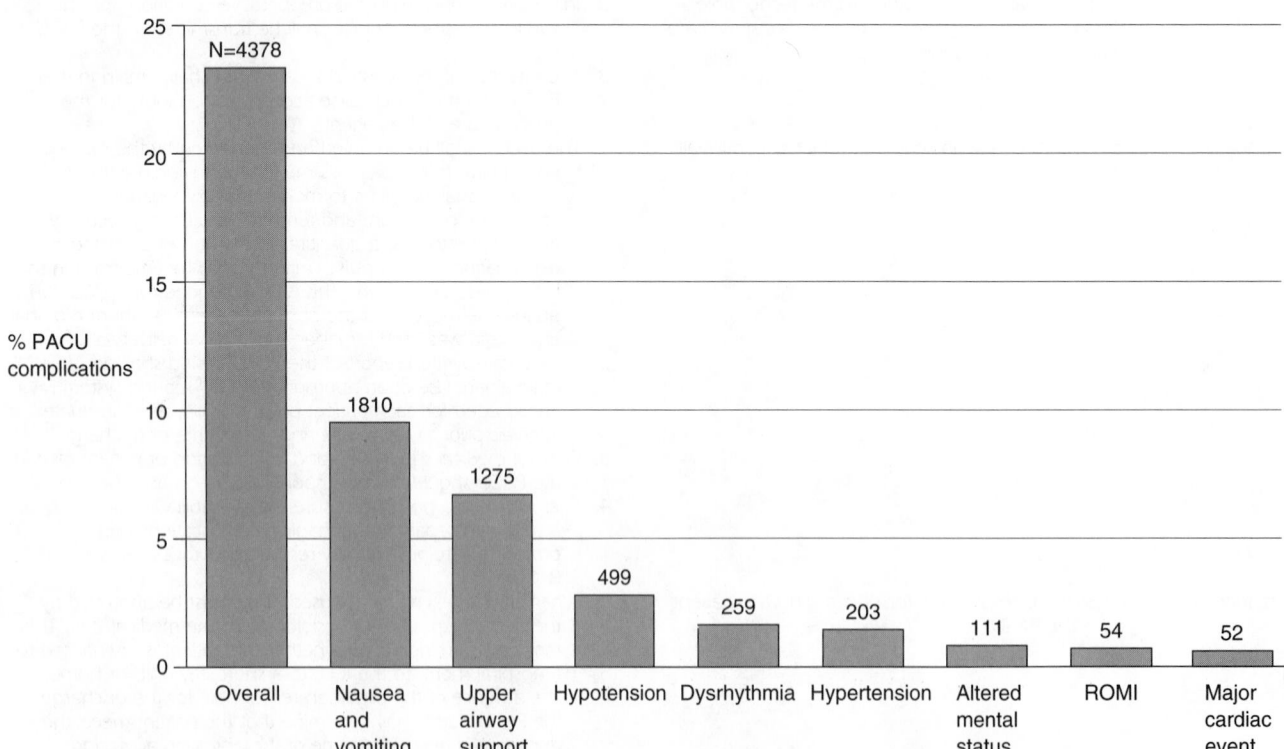

Figure 13-1. Major postanesthesia care unit complications by percentage of occurrence and number of patients experiencing each complication. Nausea and vomiting were the most frequently observed complications. ROMI, rule out myocardial infarction. (After Hines R, Barash PG, Watrous G, et al. Complications occurring in the postanesthesia care unit: a survery. Anesth Analg 1992;74:505)

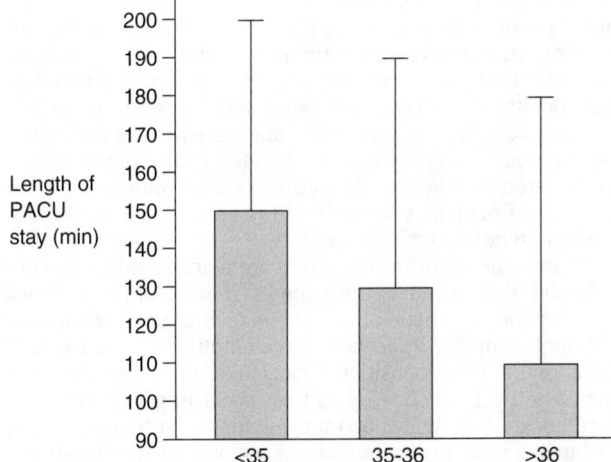

Figure 13-2. Patient body temperature at admission also affects the development of postanesthesia care unit (PACU) complications. The duration of PACU stay as a function of temperature at admission is shown. Stay was significantly reduced in patients whose temperature at admission was 36°C or higher ($P < .01$). (After Hines R, Barash PG, Watrous G, et al. Complications occurring in the postanesthesia care unit: a survey. Anesth Analg 1992;74:506)

blood pressure with an oscillometric blood pressure cuff is the standard in the operating room, and its accuracy equals that of clinical measurements by auscultation. Circulation monitors can be cycled as quickly as once per minute, but when used for an extended duration, they should be cycled no more than once every 3 to 5 minutes. When tighter control is required in patients with significant hypertension, serious heart disease, or those who may suffer acute blood loss, invasive arterial monitoring is used. Although pressure measurements provided by inva-

sive techniques are different from those of noninvasive techniques, they usually coincide closely. A continuous invasive arterial tracing can also be used to assess the adequacy of fluid resuscitation by following the systolic pressure variation with positive-pressure ventilation. A variation greater than 10 mmHg in the systolic pressure between peak inspiration and end expiration implies inadequate preload and the need for more aggressive fluid resuscitation.[14] In patients without left ventricular dysfunction, who are undergoing extended surgical procedures with significant fluid shifts and potential blood loss, central venous pressure monitoring is frequently used, with pulmonary arterial catheter monitoring reserved for more critically ill patients and those with significant left ventricular dysfunction. The adequacy of circulation can be objectively documented by thermodilution cardiac output measurements and mixed venous oxygen saturation monitoring. Transesophageal echocardiography is now commonly used to assess cardiac function. This technique is easily used in the anesthetized, intubated patient and can quickly assess systolic and diastolic function as well as valvular dysfunction.

COMMON PROBLEMS IN THE POSTOPERATIVE PERIOD

Postanesthesia care units are required in any setting where surgical procedures are conducted. The increased scope of surgery and the invasive technology used to monitor sicker patients has increased the service at and training required to operate these facilities. In 1994, the ASA revised the 1988 Standards for Postanesthesia Care (Table 13-12).

The scoring systems used to assess the postoperative patient direct attention to the primary areas of concern. The postanesthesia recovery score is an attempt to evaluate postanesthesia patient status[15] (Table 13-13). This basic information should be incorporated in a record that provides clear documentation of postoperative events. Documentation

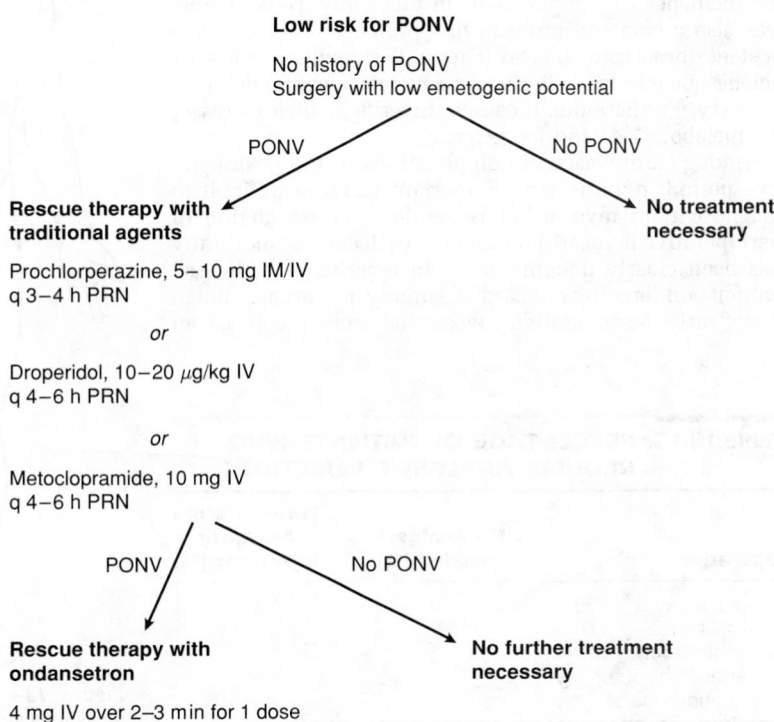

Figure 13-3. Algorithm for preventing and treating postoperative nausea and vomiting (PONV) in adults.

Table 13-14. DIFFERENTIAL DIAGNOSIS OF DELAYED EMERGENCE

NEUROLOGIC INJURY

Ischemia
Mass lesions
Seizure disorders

METABOLIC ABNORMALITIES

Hypoglycemia
Diabetic ketoacidosis
Nonketotic hyperosmolar hyperglycemic coma
Hepatic dysfunction
Electrolyte disturbances
Renal dysfunction
Thyroid dysfunction
Adrenocortical dysfunction
Cardiorespiratory failure
Hypothermia
Malignant hyperthermia

DRUG EFFECTS

Inhalational anesthetics
Opioids
Barbiturates
Benzodiazepines
Ketamine
Antichlorinergics
Muscle relaxants

should also include details of postoperative outpatient care, with a note indicating postoperative telephone contact made to elucidate problems. Problems should receive appropriate follow-up, and written postoperative discharge instructions should be provided for the patient.

Investigators have reported that 24% of patients experience a postanesthesia care unit complication. Nausea, vomiting, and the need for airway support constitute 70% of these complications[16] (Fig. 13-1). The need to maintain airway support was by far the most common respiratory complication. The duration of the procedure as well as ASA classification and type of procedure had a significant bearing on the incidence of complications in this study. Hypothermia was also a common problem that prolonged postoperative postanesthesia care unit stay (Fig. 13-2). Hypothermia has the deleterious effects of altering drug metabolism and delaying recovery. Furthermore, it causes shivering, which increases the metabolic demand for oxygen.

Among cardiovascular complications in the postoperative period, none is more important or more difficult to diagnose than myocardial ischemia. The association of perioperative myocardial ischemia with cardiac morbidity has been clearly documented.[17] In a series of high- risk patients undergoing noncardiac surgery, researchers noted that "early postoperative myocardial ischemia [was] an important correlate of adverse cardiac outcomes."[17] Diagnosis is complicated by the fact that only 10% to 30% of patients suffering documented myocardial infarction have pain and that postoperative ECG T-wave changes are often nonspecific.[18] Instead, one must seek secondary indications of ongoing ischemia or "angina equivalents," such as hypotension, arrhythmias, elevated filling pressures, or postoperative oliguria. Arrhythmias are common and are significant primarily because of the association with myocardial ischemia or hypoxemia.

Nausea and vomiting are rarely unifactoral and cause considerable discomfort to the patient. There is little evidence to favor one anesthetic or anesthetic technique over another, although propofol appears to have an antiemetic effect. Nitrous oxide, often considered causative, does not appear to increase the incidence of nausea, according to well-documented studies. It is not unusual for an antiemetic agent to be included preoperatively or as part of the anesthetic technique, especially in patients with a positive history or those deemed to be at risk, such as menstruating young women undergoing laparoscopy. Standard usage includes phenothiazines, butyrophenones, metoclopramide, and scopolamine. Recently, the Food and Drug Administration approved the use of the serotonin antagonist Odansetron, which was shown in several studies to be superior to other agents.[19] An algorithm for the treatment of postoperative nausea and vomiting is illustrated in Figure 13-3.

The most common cause of delayed emergence is the residual effects of anesthesia. A differential diagnosis of delayed anesthetic emergence is presented in Table 13-14. There should be little confusion about the implication of muscle relaxants because physical indications of ventilatory distress, combined with the readings of the blockade monitor, should clearly indicate the role of these drugs.

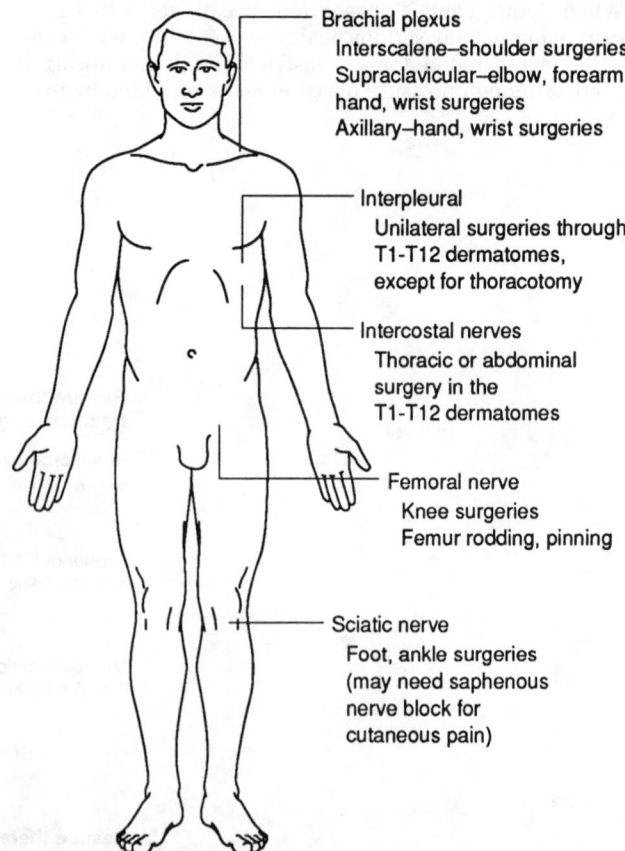

Figure 13-4. Surgical procedures in which peripheral nerve blockade can provide postoperative pain relief.

Table 13-15. PERCENTAGE OF PATIENTS WHO REQUIRE ANALGESIC INJECTIONS

Operation	No Analgesic Needed (%)	Three or More Analgesic Injections (%)
Minor chest wall	82	0
Inguinal hernia	52	0
Appendicectomy	25	10
Lower abdominal surgery	18	40
Upper abdominal surgery	10	45–65

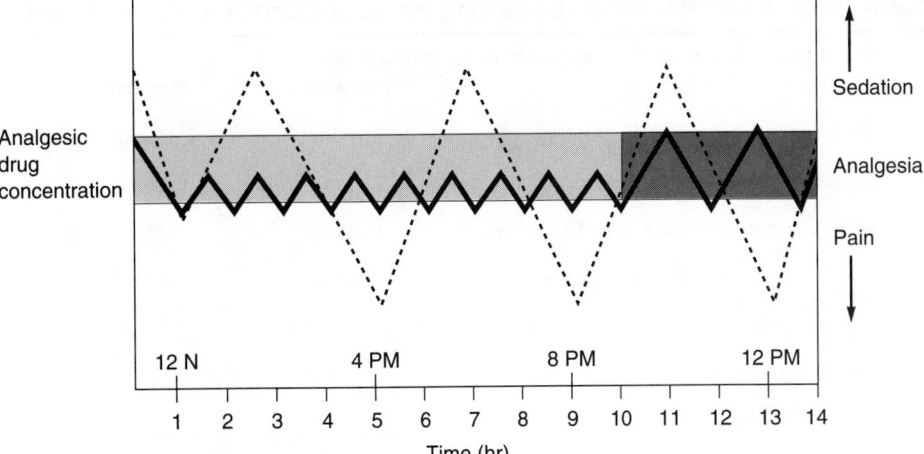

Figure 13-5. Theoretical relation between dosing interval, analgesic drug concentration, and clinical effects when comparing a patient-controlled analgesia system (*solid line*) to conventional intramuscular therapy (*dashed line*). (After White PF. Patient-controlled analgesia: a new approach to the management of postoperative pain. Semin Anesth 1985;4:261)

POSTOPERATIVE ACUTE PAIN MANAGEMENT

Postoperative pain is an inevitable consequence of surgery. Its severity is site dependent (Table 13-15), but the magnitude of the pain experienced by individual patients after similar surgical procedures is influenced by a multitude of factors. Variation in patient experience has been clearly demonstrated by several authors and is reflected in deficiencies in postoperative pain control.[20] The recognition of this clinical problem has prompted interest in underlying pain mechanisms and in innovative ways to alleviate postoperative suffering.

In 1965, the crucial role of nociceptive C fiber feedback behavior and its modulation by cells in the substantia gelatinosa of the dorsal horn was recognized.[21] Repetitive stimulation of these fibers by cellular mediators, such as kinins and catecholamines, promotes neural excitation, prolongs repetitive firing, and lowers the threshold to further excitation. As a result, C fibers do not show fatigue, and the stage is set for continuous pain. Counterirritation of large afferent activity has been shown empirically to have beneficial effects. The gate-control theory provides an explanation for the inhibition of C fiber–mediated pain. Serotonergic and enkephalinergic descending inhibitory pathways modulate activity in the dorsal horn before information is relayed to the somatosensory cortex through the spinothalamic tract. The common observation that pain is worse at night, when less sensory information is processed, and that it decreases with daytime activity is an example of how this complex neural system functions. Transcutaneous nerve stimulation is a technical attempt to use this principle.

Superficial somatic pain is well localized and has a protective function. Superficial somatic pain is readily treated by common analgesic techniques. Deep somatic pain may not be well localized, may have some protective function, as in joint immobilization, and is fairly responsive to a variety of analgesics. Visceral pain, served almost entirely by C fiber activity, is poorly localized, often referred, and difficult to treat. In major operations, all modes can be activated, compounding the clinical challenge of providing adequate pain management. These clinical observations direct the focus of postoperative pain management to the treatment of somatic pain by attacking the nociceptor and the subsequent transmission of the painful impulse by the nerve fiber. The use of nonsteroidal antiinflammatory drugs with or without the injection of local anesthetics into the wound is very effective. If done preemptively at the time of surgery, this approach can significantly benefit the patient's postoperative experience.[22] Examples of nerve blocks for various procedures are shown in Figure 13-4.

Including potent opioids in the treatment of deep pain, both somatic and visceral, has been routine. However, the responses to standard regimens have been notoriously unreliable, from inadequate pain relief to narcosis, with complications at both ends of the scale. It was not until the 1980s that variations in response were linked to variable serum concentrations of analgesic drugs. Interpatient variation in serum levels to any standard dose can be 5-fold, and interpatient therapeutic concentrations can vary on a similar scale. When factored together, there is the potential for a 25-fold variation in patient response to a standard drug prescription. Each patient has an individual therapeutic window (Fig. 13-5). The clinical implications are enormous.

Where appropriate, opioids can be reversed using titrated doses of naloxone. Flumazenil can be used for reversal of benzodiazepines.

Table 13-16. PROBLEMS THAT CAN OCCUR DURING PATIENT-CONTROLLED ANALGESIA (PCA) THERAPY

OPERATOR ERRORS

Misprogramming PCA device
Failure to clamp or unclamp tubing
Improperly loading syringe or cartridge
Inability to respond to safety alarms
Misplacing PCA pump key

PATIENT ERRORS

Failure to understand PCA therapy
Misunderstanding PCA pump device
Intentional analgesic abuse

MECHANICAL ERRORS

Failure to deliver on demand
Defective one-way valve at Y-connector
Faulty alarm system
Device malfunctions

Table 13-17. EXAMPLE OF ORDERS FOR PATIENT-CONTROLLED ANALGESIA (PCA)

1. Patient is to be initiated on PCA with standard monitoring protocol.
2. Drug selection →

	Morphine	Meperidine	Dilaudid	
	1 mg/mL	10 mg/mL	0.2 mg/mL	_____ mg/mL
3. Loading → Initial dose (start PRN for pain)	2–4 mg	20–40 mg	0.2–0.4 mg	_____ mg
Incremental dose, q 5–10 min PRN	1–2 mg	10–20 mg	0.1–0.2 mg	_____ mg
Maximum total loading dose	10 mg	100 mg	1 mg	_____ mg
Other:	_____ mg	_____ mg	_____ mg	_____ mg
4. Pump setting → PCA dose	_____ mg	_____ mg	_____ mg	_____ mg
Lockout interval	_____ min	_____ min	_____ min	_____ min
4-Hour limit	_____ mg	_____ mg	_____ mg	_____ mg

(University of Michigan Hospitals form RP-2044330/982, Rev. 7/93, Acute Pain Service, Patient Controlled Analgesia Standard Orders)

In 1968, investigators demonstrated the virtue of small intravenous doses given on demand.[23] As a result, the patient experienced greater pain relief, yet used the same or less total narcotic. Although there was significant patient variation, the demand from any individual patient, though cyclic, was constant. Patient-controlled analgesia (PCA) and the technologic and administrative systems to provide it have developed to a point of some sophistication, requiring servicing and a support structure with its own set of problems (Table 13-16). PCA administration requires a receptive environment, education of all personnel, and adequate patient instruction. PCA has received widespread acceptance by patients, nursing staff, and physicians because it provides more prompt and painless analgesia that more closely matches the patient's need over time. PCA is as safe as conventional intramuscular medication. Morphine and meperidine are commonly used drugs, and an example of orders is shown in Table 13-17.

Transdermal narcotic delivery is receiving attention and may become available for postoperative pain. The method is both practical and inexpensive and aims to maintain continuous delivery and constant blood levels. Fentanyl has been the drug of choice and has been well received by patients. The method appears to be safe, but there is a significant lag time between application and the attainment of therapeutic blood levels.

The discovery of endorphins in the 1970s and recognition of their importance in modulating pain at spinal sites lead to the supposition that it would be possible to selectively apply opioids directly to receptors. This led to the development of epidural opiate analgesia, in which opioids are applied directly to the receptors at spinal sites. The goal of epidural opiate analgesia is to obtain maximal analgesia while minimizing systemic side effects. For severe acute postoperative pain caused by major surgery, epidural opiate analgesia has proved to be a superior modality for pain control. In high-risk cases, there is evidence that it has an overall beneficial effect on morbidity.[9] The effective use of this sophisticated modality requires education and the establishment of protocols with rigorous attention to detail. The potential for respiratory depression demands adherence to monitoring standards. Morphine and fentanyl, often in combination with a dilute local anesthetic solution, are most often prescribed. A typical order form with monitored parameters is shown in Table 13-18.

A comprehensive postoperative pain management service demands resources and must use the physical and pharmacologic modalities available, while recognizing the significant subjective component of any individual's pain problem. The ability to recognize the impact of acute pain or an underlying chronic pain disorder requires that experience be brought to bear on difficult problems. The active involvement of nursing staff and surgeons is essential for the patient to achieve maximal benefit. It is incumbent on the pain management service to render efficient, continuous, and cost-effective care.

Table 13-18. OPIOID PROTOCOLS IN EPIDURAL OPIATE ANALGESIA

	Morphine*	Fentanyl†
Length of Onset	Longer (30–60 min)	Shorter (15–30 min)
Duration	Longer (6–24 h for single bolus)	Shorter (1–2 h for single bolus)
Cephalad Spread and Side Effects	More prone	Less prone
Indication	Favored for lumbar administration after abdominal surgery	Favored for thoracic administration after chest surgery
Dose	Typically 3–5 mg q 6–8 h	Typically 50–75 µg/h (±dilute bupivacaine)

* Hydrophilic: slow in, slow out.
† Lipophilic: fast in, fast out.

REFERENCES

1. Calverly RK. Anesthesia as a specialty: past, present, and future. In: Barash PG, Cullen BF, Stoelting RK, eds. Clinical anesthesia. Philadelphia, JB Lippincott, 1992.
2. Watling SM, Dasta JF. Prolonged paralysis in intensive care unit patients after the use of neuromuscular blocking agents: a review of the literature. Crit Care Med 1994;22:884.
3. Miller RD. Anesthesia, ed 3. New York, Churchill Livingstone, 1990.
4. Stoelting RK, Dierdorf SF. Anesthesia and co-existing disease, ed 3. New York, Churchill Livingstone, 1993.
5. Mangano DT. Perioperative cardiac morbidity. Anesthesiology 1990;72:153

6. Rao T, Jacobs K, El Etr A. Reinfarction following anesthesia in patients with myocardial infarction. Anesthesiology 1983;59:499.

7. Tarhan S, Moffitt EA. Myocardial infarction after general anesthesia. JAMA 1972;220:1451.

8. Goldman L, Caldera DC, Nussbaum SR, et al. Multi-factorial index of cardiac risk in noncardiac surgical procedures. N Engl J Med 1977;297:845.

9. Yaeger M, Glass D, Neff R, Brink-Johnsed T: Epidural anesthesia and analgesia in high risk surgical patients. Anesthesiology 1987;66:729.

10. Pedersen T, Eliasen K, Henriksen E. A prospective study of mortality associated with anaesthesia and surgery: risk indicators of mortality in hospitals. Acta Anaesthesiol Scand 1990;34:176.

11. Mallampati SR, Gatt SP, Guigino LD, et al. A clinical sign to predict difficult tracheal intubation: a prospective study. Can J Anaesth 1985;32:429.

12. Wahr JA, Tremper KK. Pulse oximetry. In: Blitt CD, Hines RL, eds. Monitoring in anesthesia and critical care medicine, ed 3. New York, Churchill Livingstone, 1994;385.

13. Nunn JF. Respiratory dead space and distribution of inspired gases. In: Applied respiratory physiology, ed 2. London, Butterworths, 1977;213.

14. Coriat P, Vrillon M, Perel A, et al. A comparison of systolic pressure variations and echo cardiographic estimates of end diastolic left ventricular size in patients after aortic surgery. Anesth Analg 1994;78:46.

15. Bonner S. Admission and discharge criteria. In: Post anesthesia care. Connecticut, Prentice Hall International, 1990.

16. Hines R, Barash PG, Waltons G, et al. Complications occurring in the postanesthesia care units: a survey. Anesth Analg 1992;74:503.

17. Mangao DT, Browner WS, Hollenberg M. Association of perioperative myocardial ischemia with cardiac morbidity and mortality in men undergoing noncardiac surgery. N Engl J Med 1990;323:1781.

18. Breslow MJ, Miller CF, Parker SD. Changes in T-wave morphology following anesthesia and surgery: a common recovery-room phenomenon. Anesthesiology 1986;64:398.

19. Alou E, Himmelseher S. Odansetron in the treatment of post-operative vomiting. Anesth Analg 1992;75:561.

20. Marks RM, Sacher EJ. Undertreatment of medical inpatients with narcotic analgesics. Ann Intern Med 1973;78:173.

21. Melzack R, Wall P. Pain mechanisms: a new theory. Science 1965;150:97.

22. Tverskoy M, Cozacov C, Ayache M. Post-operative pain after inguinal herniorrhaphy with different types of anesthesia. Anesth Analg 1990;70:29.

23. Sechzer PH. Studies in pain with the analgesic demand system. Anesth Analg 1971;50:1.

SURGERY: SCIENTIFIC PRINCIPLES AND PRACTICE, Second Edition, edited by Lazar J. Greenfield, Michael W. Mulholland, Keith T. Oldham, Gerald B. Zelenock, and Keith D. Lillemoe. Lippincott–Raven Publishers, Philadelphia, © 1997.

CHAPTER 14

TUMOR BIOLOGY

LEE M. ELLIS, DENNIE V. JONES, JR., PAUL J. CHIAO, AND NEAL R. PELLIS

Cancer affects both young and old, people of all ethnic and racial origins, and people from every socioeconomic stratum. Treatment up to and including the latter half of this century has employed surgery and, more recently, radiotherapy, chemotherapy, and immunotherapy. Technologic advances propel investigations toward an understanding of the causes and consequences of malignant changes at the tissue, cellular, genomic, and molecular levels.[1] This new knowledge is beginning to translate into clinical successes.

In an era of clinical specialization and subspecialization, it is apparent that cancer management requires a multimodality approach and understanding. The surgeon, medical oncologist, radiation oncologist, radiologist, and pathologist have become clinical partners. A second partnership is developing between the laboratory investigator and clinician, and reports of flow cytometry (FCM), receptor analysis, and serum tumor markers routinely appear on patients' medical records. Clinicians recognize that laboratory advances more rapidly are adapted to clinical medicine. Participation in multimodality patient care conferences requires at least a working knowledge of each specialty's perspective, tools, and limitations. An introduction to emerging laboratory technologies and clinical specialties must begin early in medical training. Otherwise, many clinicians may be relegated to a spectator role in the treatment of cancer.

EPIDEMIOLOGY

The distribution of cancer throughout populations is caused by many factors. Genetic predispositions may be reflected in complex racial or ethnic characterizations, or they may be as simple as hair and skin color. Although geographic influences include environmental factors, such as incident sunlight or domestic confinement, there are also dietary considerations determined by the available food resources. With worldwide advancement in travel, cultural exchange, migration, and communication, the geographic boundaries to various forms of cancer become less well defined. In this chapter, the distributive aspects of major forms of neoplasia are discussed and their respective risk factors reviewed.

Geographic Patterns

Although a genetic predisposition exists for some cancers, most available information favors environmental variation as the major contributor to the disparate geographic incidence of different cancer types. Examples from both extremes of the frequency spectrum for specific cancer sites are shown in Table 14-1. In many cases, the high incidence of a specific cancer in a particular region or country is linked to a specific causative agent. The chewing of a betel nut, tobacco, and lime mixture in regions of India has resulted in a high incidence of oropharyngeal tumors. The high incidence of gastric carcinoma in Japan is linked to a diet of smoked and highly salted foods and food contaminated with aflatoxin. The high incidence of hepatitis B infections in parts of Africa and China is thought responsible for the high incidence of hepatocellular carcinoma in these regions. Geographic differences in several other common solid tumors are less clearly explained. Breast and colon carcinomas are common in North America but rare in Africa and Asia (Fig. 14-1). Carcinomas of the stomach, esophagus, and cervix are more common in developed countries. Attempts have been made to create international and regional cancer maps to identify epidemiologic patterns of specific cancers (Fig. 14-2).

Cancer Statistics

The incidence of cancer is rising in nearly all populations. Estimates of overall cancer incidence by site and sex in the United States have been reported by the National Cancer Institute's Surveillance, Epidemiology and End Results program (Fig. 14-3). In men, lung, prostate, and colo-

Table 14-1. INTERNATIONAL VARIATION IN CANCER INCIDENCE

Cancer	Area of High Incidence	Rate	Area of Low Incidence	Rate
Melanoma	Australia	30.9	Japan	0.2
Lip	Canada	15.1	Japan	0.1
Nasopharynx	Hong Kong	30.0	United Kingdom	0.3
Prostate	United States	91.2	China	1.3
Liver	China	34.4	Canada	0.7
Penis	Brazil	8.3	Israel	0.2
Oral cavity	France	13.5	India	0.4
Cervix uteri (F)	Brazil	83.2	Israel	3.0
Esophagus	France	29.9	Romania	1.1
Stomach	Japan	82.0	Kuwait	3.7
Thyroid	Hawaii	8.8	Poland	0.4
Multiple myeloma	United States	8.8	Philippines	0.4
Kidney	Canada	15.0	India	0.7
Corpus uteri (F)	United States	25.7	India	1.2
Lung	United States	110.0	India	5.8
Colon	United States	34.1	India	1.8
Testis	Switzerland	10.0	China	0.6
Bladder	Switzerland	27.8	India	1.7
Lymphosarcoma	Switzerland	9.2	Japan	0.8
Pancreas	United States	16.4	India	1.5
Hodgkin disease	Canada	4.8	Japan	0.5
Brain	New Zealand	9.7	India	1.1
Larynx	Brazil	17.8	Japan	2.1
Ovary (F)	New Zealand	25.8	Kuwait	3.3
Rectum	Israel	22.6	Kuwait	3.0
Breast (F)	Hawaii	93.9	Israel	14.1
Leukemia	Canada	11.6	India	2.2

(Adapted from Fraumeni JF Jr, Hoover RN, Devesa SS, Kinlen LJ. Epidemiology of cancer. In: DeVita VT, Hellman S, Rosenberg SA, eds. Cancer: principles and practice of oncology, ed 3. Philadelphia, JB Lippincott, 1989:202)

rectal carcinomas have the highest incidence. Breast carcinoma accounts for 29% of all cancer in women, followed by colorectal, lung, and uterine carcinomas. Marked variations in cancer incidence at different sites occur within ethnic and racial subpopulations in the United States (Table 14-2). Environmental factors are at least partially responsible because within a few decades, migrant populations develop cancer risks nearly identical to the indigenous population (Fig. 14-4).

From 1973 to 1987, there was a 15% increase in incidence for all cancer sites (Fig. 14-5). Cutaneous melanoma showed the greatest increase at 83%, and non-Hodgkin lymphoma and prostate carcinoma followed with increases of about 50%. The reasons for these increases are unknown. Only a few cancers declined in incidence over the same interval. Carcinoma of the cervix showed the greatest reduction at 36%, followed by endometrial carcinoma and gastric carcinoma. The reduction in carcinoma of the cervix is likely due to the early detection and treatment of cervical dysplasia resulting from the widespread use of routine cervical cytologic screening.

Cancer remains the second most common cause of mortality in the United States after heart disease, accounting for 22% of all deaths. Analysis of age-adjusted mortality from cancer at selected sites for men and women from 1930 to 1986 (Fig. 14-6) demonstrates some remarkable trends. For both sexes, the dramatic increases in the death rate observed for lung carcinoma are attributed to increases in cigarette smoking. The decline in mortality from gastric cancer in both sexes is likely due to a true decrease in

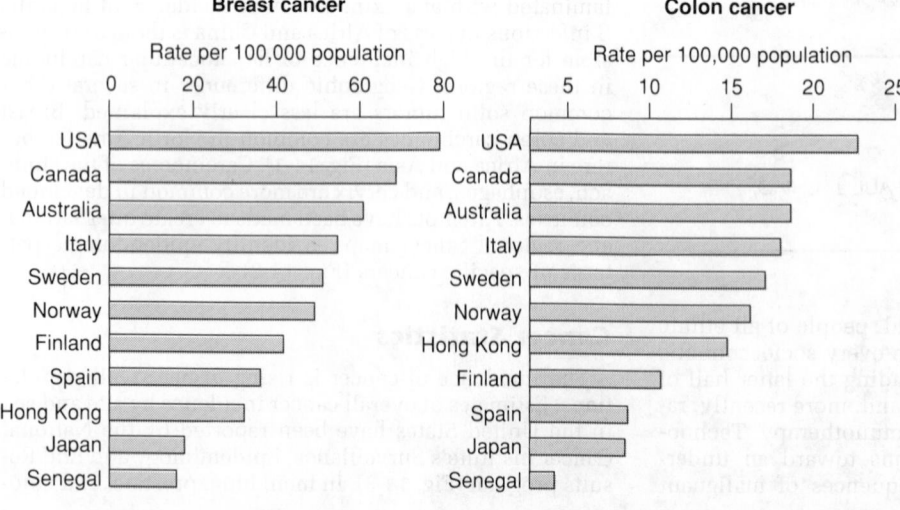

Figure 14-1. International variations in breast cancer and colon cancer incidence rates. (After Waterhouse J, Muir C, Shanmugarathnam K, Powell J. Cancer incidence in five continents. Lyons, France, IARC Scientific Pub, 1982)

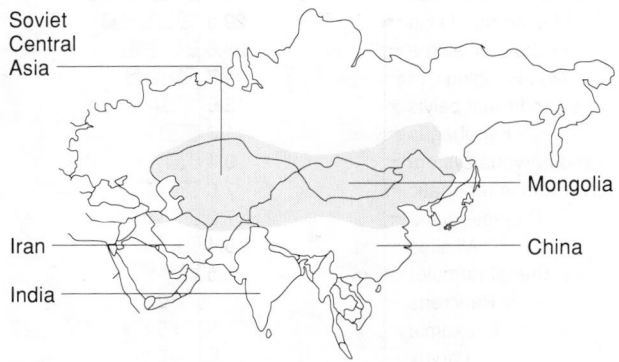

Figure 14-2. The esophageal cancer belt extends from the Caspian Sea across Soviet Central Asia. (After Kmet J, Mahboudi E. Esophageal cancer in the Caspian littoral of Iran: initial studies. Science 1972;175:846)

incidence because routine endoscopic screening has not gained acceptance in the United States, and therapeutic intervention has had little impact on survival. The top five causes of cancer mortality by age group in 1986 are shown in Figure 14-7. From 1973 to 1987, overall cancer mortality increased 13% in people aged 65 years and older, with an increase for all ages of 5.4%.

Mortality is dramatically affected for the few cancers highly sensitive to chemotherapy. From 1973 to 1987, cancer mortality from testicular carcinoma and Hodgkin disease has been reduced by 60% and 50%, respectively (see Fig. 14-5).

Cancer continues to be a major cause of loss of life and productivity worldwide. An emphasis on education, regular health evaluations, and screening for premalignant lesions or early malignancies in geographic regions with a high cancer incidence may result in a global reduction in cancer mortality. The goals of investigations in tumor biology include attempts to identify cancer causation, markers for early detection, mechanisms of cellular transformation and tumor cell growth regulation, alterations of host–tumor immune interactions, and novel and complementary therapeutic strategies.

Table 14-2. AVERAGE ANNUAL AGE-ADJUSTED INCIDENCE RATES PER 100,000 US MALES FOR SELECTED CANCER SITES BY RACIAL AND ETHNIC GROUP, 1975–1985

Cancer	Whites	Blacks	Hispanics	Native Americans
All sites	404	490	266	185
Lip	4	0	3	0
Nasopharynx	1	1	1	1
Other oral cavity and pharynx	12	21	5	2
Esophagus	5	18	3	2
Stomach	12	21	21	26
Colon	40	41	18	8
Rectum	20	15	12	5
Liver	3	5	4	5
Gallbladder	1	1	2	9
Other biliary	2	1	2	3
Pancreas	11	17	12	9
Larynx	9	12	4	1
Lung and bronchus	82	120	32	14
Melanoma of skin	10	1	2	2
Prostate	77	123	72	46
Testis	4	1	3	2
Bladder	30	15	11	4
Kidney	10	10	9	9
Brain and other nervous system	7	4	5	3
Thyroid	2	1	3	2
Hodgkin disease	4	3	3	1
Non-Hodgkin lymphoma	13	9	7	5
Multiple myeloma	5	10	3	3
Leukemia	14	11	8	6
All others	28	31	22	19

(Adapted from Fraumeni JF Jr, Hoover RN, Devesa SS, Kinlen LJ. Epidemiology of cancer. In: DeVita VT, Hellman S, Rosenberg SA, eds. Cancer: principles and practice of oncology, ed 3. Philadelphia, JB Lippincott, 1989:210)

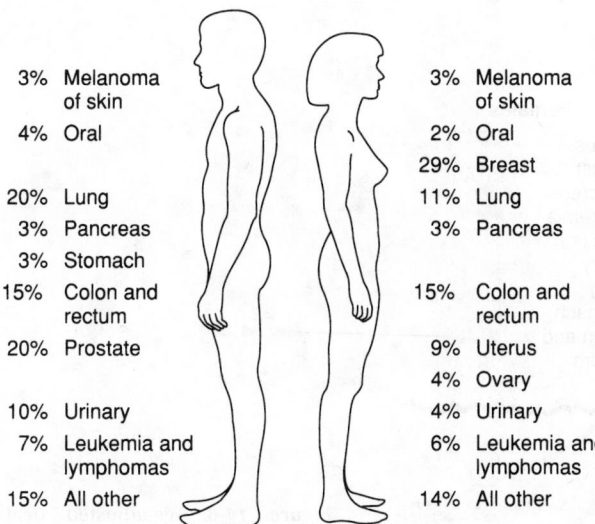

3%	Melanoma of skin	3%	Melanoma of skin
4%	Oral	2%	Oral
		29%	Breast
20%	Lung	11%	Lung
3%	Pancreas	3%	Pancreas
3%	Stomach		
15%	Colon and rectum	15%	Colon and rectum
20%	Prostate	9%	Uterus
		4%	Ovary
10%	Urinary	4%	Urinary
7%	Leukemia and lymphomas	6%	Leukemia and lymphomas
15%	All other	14%	All other

Figure 14-3. Estimated cancer incidence by site and sex, 1990. (After Silverberg E, Boring CC, Squires TS. Cancer statistics, 1990. CA 1991;40:9)

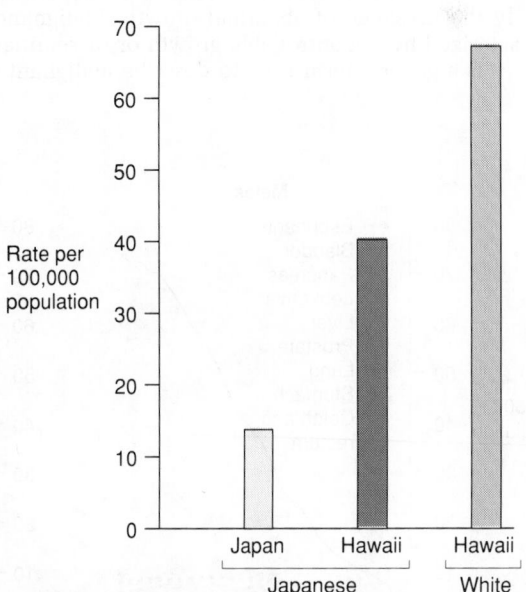

Figure 14-4. Breast cancer incidence in Japanese women born in Japan, Japanese women born in Hawaii, and white women born in Hawaii. (After Reddy BS, Cohen LA, McCoy GD, Hill P, Weisburger JH, Wynder EL. Nutrition and its relationship to cancer. Adv Cancer Res 1980;32:237)

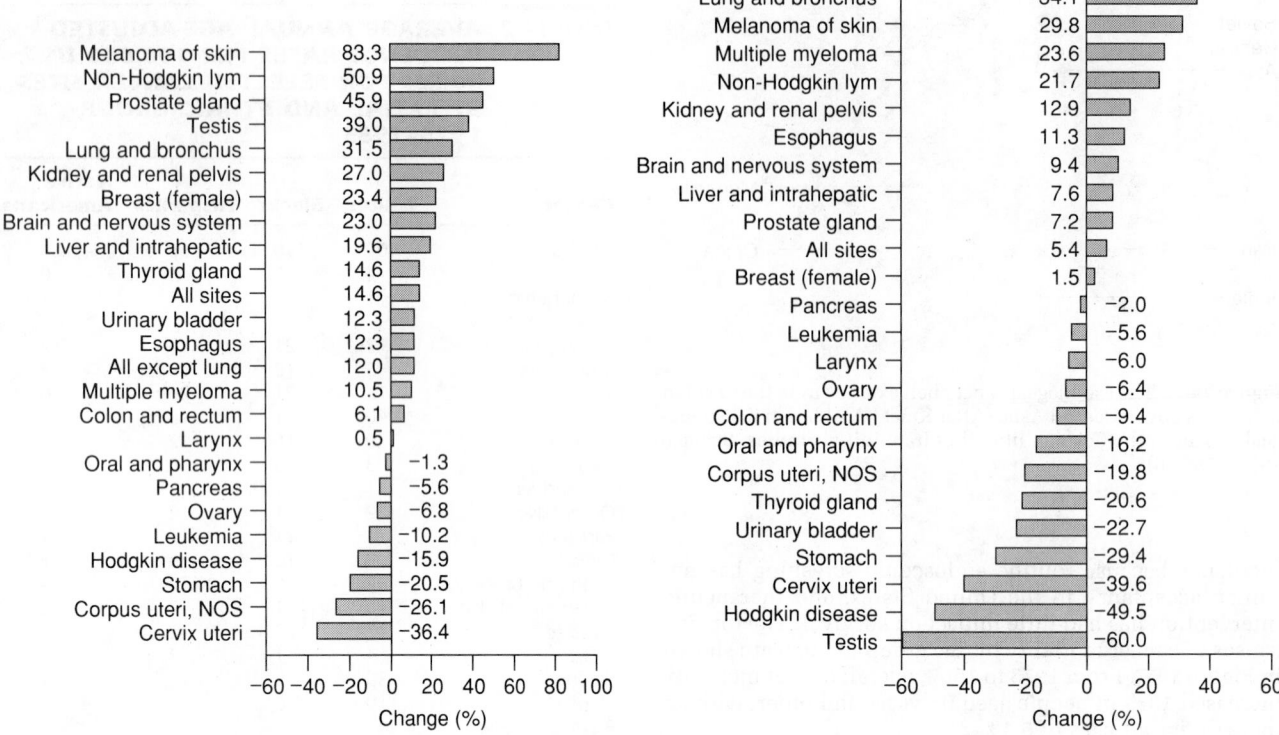

Figure 14-5. Changing patterns of cancer incidence (*left*) and mortality (*right*) in the United States in all races and both sexes, 1973 to 1987. (After Newman ME. New cancer statistics show losses, gains. J Natl Cancer Inst 1990;82:1238)

SPECTRUM OF NEOPLASIA

Neoplasia may be simply defined as new growth. Proliferation of neoplastic cells is more rapid than in most normal tissue and fails to respond to the cessation of a growth stimulus or to endogenous proliferation inhibitors. Neoplastic growth frequently results in an abnormal swelling or tumor, and the terms *neoplasm* and *tumor* are frequently used interchangeably. The designation of *benign* or *malignant* refers to the clinical behavior of a neoplasm, not merely the presence of abnormal growth. Malignancy is characterized by uncontrollable growth or dissemination. *Cancer* is a general term used to describe malignant neo-

plasia with implications of a tendency to local recurrence and dissemination.

Hyperplasia is an increase in cell number demonstrable in both normal and neoplastic tissues. High basal growth rates are normal for bone marrow, intestinal crypt epithelium, and skin. In response to injury, an increase in growth rate over baseline is a normal response in wound healing. Liver regeneration after hepatic injury or hepatectomy results in both a dramatic hyperplastic response with an increase in cell number and a hypertrophic response with an increase in cell size. Hyperplastic polyps in colonic mucosa are frequently seen, but a relation to subsequent malignancy has been difficult to establish. In breast ductal

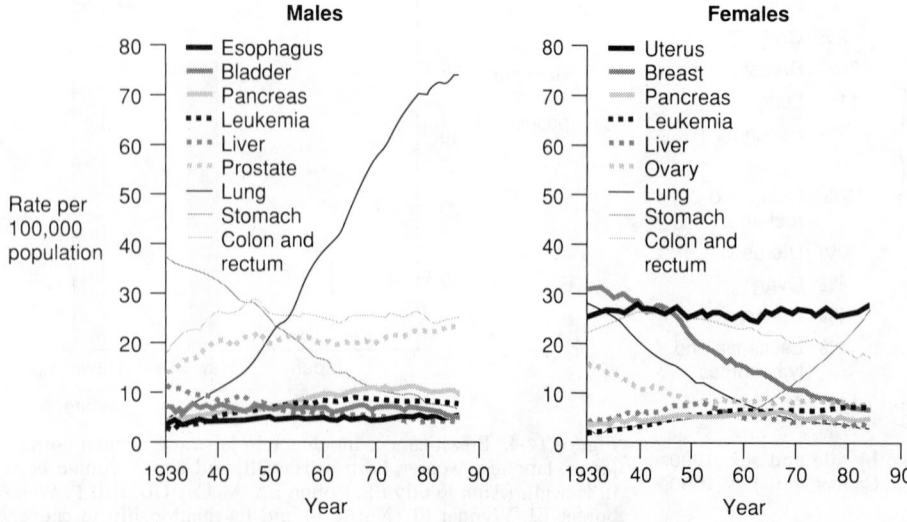

Figure 14-6. Age-adjusted death rates for cancer in the United States, 1930 to 1986. (After Silverberg E, Boring CC, Squires TS. Cancer statistics, 1990. CA 1991;40:9)

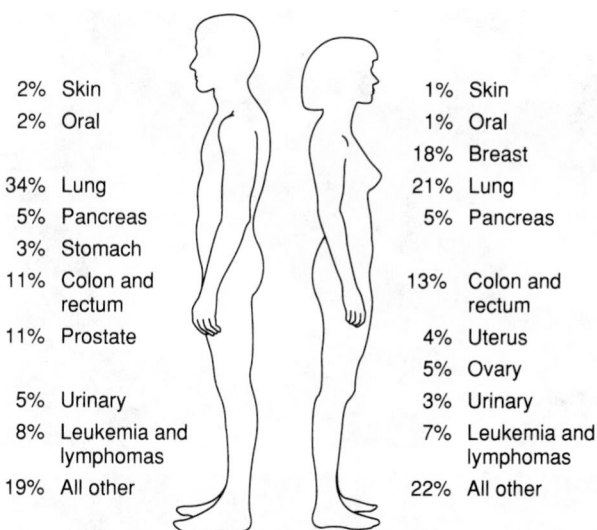

2%	Skin	1%	Skin
2%	Oral	1%	Oral
		18%	Breast
34%	Lung	21%	Lung
5%	Pancreas	5%	Pancreas
3%	Stomach		
11%	Colon and rectum	13%	Colon and rectum
11%	Prostate	4%	Uterus
		5%	Ovary
5%	Urinary	3%	Urinary
8%	Leukemia and lymphomas	7%	Leukemia and lymphomas
19%	All other	22%	All other

Figure 14-7. Estimated cancer mortality by site and sex, 1990. (After Silverberg E, Boring CC, Squires TS. Cancer statistics, 1990. CA 1991;40:9)

epithelium, florid, but not mild, hyperplasia is associated with a 1.5- to 2-fold increased risk of subsequent breast carcinoma (Fig. 14-8).

Metaplasia is a reversible transformation of one mature cell type to another in a given tissue. This is clearly demonstrated when the replacing mature cell type is present in tissue or in areas of tissue where it is not normally found. Proposed explanations of this poorly understood transformation include a redirection of stem cell differentiation or the dedifferentiation of fully mature differentiated cells. Epithelial metaplasia secondary to chronic inflammation has been extensively investigated. In cases of chronic gastroesophageal reflux, the normal distal esophageal squamous cell mucosa may undergo metaplasia to a gastric-type columnar epithelium. In the respiratory tract, the normal pseudostratified columnar epithelium may be replaced by squamous cells. Animal studies have demonstrated reversal of this metaplasia by administration of vitamin A (Fig. 14-9). The molecular and cellular signals responsible for metaplasia are unknown.

Dysplasia is a term usually applied to epithelial tissues, characterized by altered cell size, shape, and organization. Dysplasia is classified as mild, moderate, or severe, depending on the degree of cellular dedifferentiation. The cause of dysplasia is often unknown but may be secondary to chronic inflammation or exposure to environmental toxins or irritants. The gastrointestinal tract, respiratory tree, urinary bladder, cervix, vagina, breast, and skin all can exhibit foci of dysplasia. Nuclear polymorphism and hyperchromatism are present and often accompanied by total loss of cellular and epithelial polarity. Mitoses are more frequently seen in the afflicted areas than in the surrounding normal epithelium. Although disordered growth of superficial tissue is present, there is no penetration of abnormal cells through the epithelial basement membrane (see Fig. 14-8). Carcinoma in situ demonstrates all of the above changes, with an increased number of mitoses, but it is still confined by the basement membrane and may be considered the most disordered extreme of dysplasia. Although the association of dysplasia and synchronous or metachronous invasive carcinoma frequently has been described, not all dysplastic tissue progresses to carcinoma. Many tissues may demonstrate a *field effect*, with multiple, patchy areas of dysplasia. Because it is impossi-

ble to predict which organs with demonstrated dysplasia will develop invasive cancer, clinicians have advocated either close visual, radiologic, or endoscopic surveillance, or consideration of prophylactic resection of all tissue at risk.

Progression to malignant disease presents a common challenge to homeostatic mechanisms of the host, characterized by (1) unresponsiveness to normal growth-regulatory controls within host tissue, (2) adaptation of an invasive phenotype, and (3) the confounding of host immunity that enables evasion of immune-mediated tumor destruction. This chapter addresses the causes, mechanisms of transformation and progression, and potential therapeutic modalities that address peculiar biologic characteristics of neoplastic cells.

CAUSES

Immunodeficiency

Immunodeficiency syndromes comprise a spectrum of afflictions that result in absence or decrease in one or more of the components of the immune system. Deficiencies are either inherited or acquired. Patients deficient in immunoglobulins may be maintained by passive administration of commercially prepared immune serum globulins. In contrast, those with defects in cellular immunity (eg, absence of T lymphocytes) require more vigorous treatments.

The role of the immune system in the prevention of neoplastic disease has been the subject of extensive debate. Clinical observations and the results from experimental animal models are not completely congruent. For example, patients with immune deficiency and immunosuppressed transplant recipients are at greater risk for neoplastic disease. Frequently, these are tumors of the lymphoreticular system, and only selected nonlymphoid tissues exhibit increased incidence of neoplasia. Patients with acquired immunodeficiency syndrome and some transplantation patients are at an increased risk for Kaposi sarcoma.

In contrast to the clinical observations, experiments with carcinogen-induced murine models suggest that loss of T lymphocytes does not significantly affect carcinogenesis but does diminish host response to transplantable tumors. Analysis of the immune cellular participants in the surveillance against neoplastic progression reveals that in the normal host, several lymphoid cell compartments participate in the destruction of aberrant cells. Proposed cellular mechanisms include T, B, and natural killer (NK) lymphocytes as well as macrophages cytotoxic to emerging transformed cells. Unlike chemical carcinogenesis, compromising cellular immunity significantly increases animal susceptibility to viral oncogenesis. Although the precise role of host immunity in tumor surveillance, whether in humans or in animals, is yet to be elucidated, evidence suggests that the immune system is important in the prevention of cancer and that the components of host immunity may be marshalled in the treatment of residual disease after surgery.

Familial and Ethnic Influences

Among the many factors contributing to the initiation and progression of cancer, some result from inherited characteristics, often modified by cultural influences. These influences may either confer the neoplasm (less frequent) or increase the risk for specific cancers. In this section, a few examples are presented to illustrate the diversity of influences that may increase the incidence of tumors in selected populations.

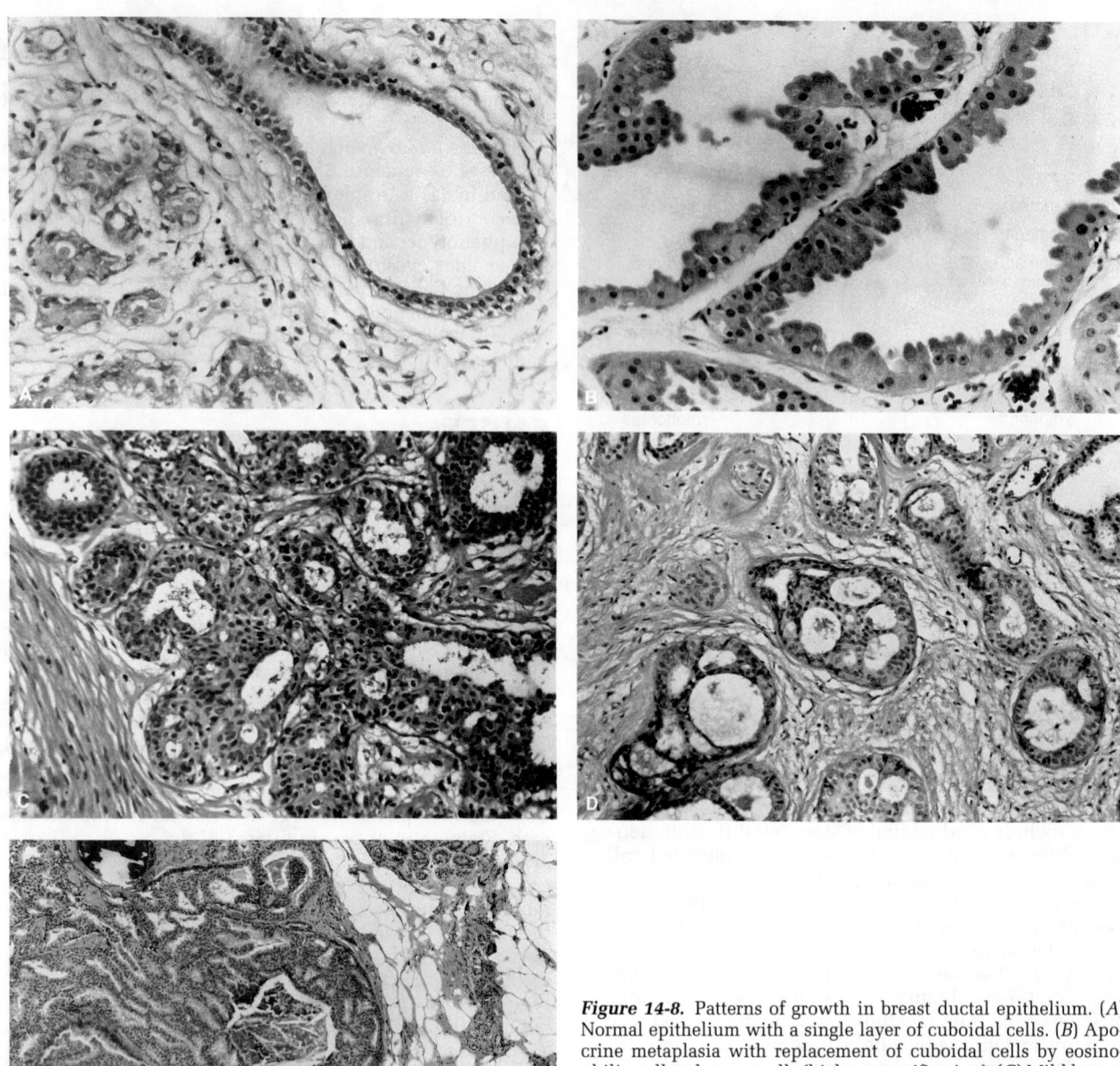

Figure 14-8. Patterns of growth in breast ductal epithelium. (*A*) Normal epithelium with a single layer of cuboidal cells. (*B*) Apocrine metaplasia with replacement of cuboidal cells by eosinophilic, tall, columnar cells (higher magnification). (*C*) Mild hyperplasia with three or four layers of cuboidal cells above the basement membrane with uniform nuclei. (*D*) Atypical hyperplasia (dysplasia) with more than one cell layer, variable size, chromatism of nuclei, and cribriform pattern. (*E*) Ductal carcinoma in situ with intraductal calcification and marked cellular replacement of the lumen. (Courtesy of Nour Sneige, MD, University of Texas M.D. Anderson Hospital and Tumor Institute, Houston)

Familial Breast Cancer

In the examination, diagnosis, and treatment of breast cancer, family medical history has become an important aspect in overall patient care. Investigation of family histories in breast cancer patients has revealed increased risks for not only breast cancer but also other neoplasms in first-degree relatives. Familial breast cancer is characterized by (1) early age of onset, (2) frequent bilateral disease, (3) genetic heterogeneity, and (4) vertical transmission, suggesting autosomal dominance. Ten to 15% of breast cancer cases display familial aggregation, but fewer meet all the criteria for familial breast cancer. Familial arrays can include men with breast cancer. Familial analysis reveals increased risk for other cancers, such as colon, ovarian, esophageal, stomach, and, to a lesser extent, sarcoma, lung

tumors, and adrenocortical carcinomas. Thus, it appears that a complex cancer syndrome may be manifest as a variety of neoplasms in a family.

Dysplastic Nevus

Familial melanomas are an uncommon occurrence. Between 4% and 10% of melanoma patients have a history of melanoma in first-degree relatives. The genetic basis of these observations is unknown. There is an autosomal dominant hereditary occurrence of melanoma, originally termed *B-K mole syndrome* and now called *dysplastic nevus syndrome*. Patients typically have between 10 and 100 pigmented lesions, usually larger than the junctional and compound nevi of childhood. Frequently, immunologic abnormalities are found in patients with familial mela-

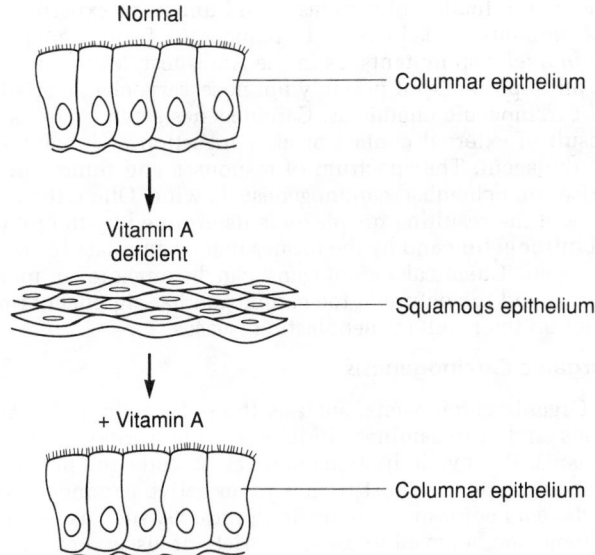

Normal

Columnar epithelium

Vitamin A
deficient

Squamous epithelium

+ Vitamin A

Columnar epithelium

Figure 14-9. Metaplasia of columnar epithelium to squamous epithelium in the presence of vitamin A deficiency and redifferentiation in the presence of vitamin A. (After Pitot HC. The language of oncology. In: Fundamentals of oncology, ed 3. New York, Marcel Dekker, 1986:24)

noma. Dysplastic nevi occur most frequently on the back and less commonly below the waist. The dysplasia may represent a stage of preneoplasia. Gross examination of a single lesion does not permit distinguishing dysplastic nevus from melanoma in situ. Nevertheless, it is believed that 40% of melanoma in situ began as dysplastic nevus.

Multiple Endocrine Neoplasias

Multiple endocrine neoplasia (MEN) occurs as one of three autosomal dominant familial cancer syndromes. Patients with MEN I, or Wermer syndrome, have multiple tumors of the anterior pituitary, parathyroids, and pancreatic islets. Cytogenetic analysis suggests that an allelic loss in chromosome bands 11q12 and 11q13 occurs in both the sporadic and familial form of MEN I. Other studies include losses on both chromosomes 11p and 11q. There may be linkage to the *int*-2 oncogene. MEN I patients have a basic fibroblast growth factor–like activity in their serum. The serum of normal subjects is devoid of such activity. Greater than half of patients with MEN I display adenomas in two or more different glands, and 20% have three or more glands involved. Hyperparathyroidism, pituitary adenomas, hypersecretion of gastrin or insulin, and adrenocortical hyperfunction are common characteristics. MEN I less frequently includes schwannomas, multiple cutaneous lipomas, thymomas, and bronchial or small intestinal carcinoids.

Patients with MEN II are subdivided into two subgroups, IIa and IIb. Patients in both subgroups have medullary thyroid carcinoma and pheochromocytomas. MEN IIa also includes parathyroid hyperplasia. MEN IIb includes mucosal neuromas, ganglioneuromatosis of the gastrointestinal tract, and a marfanoid habitus. MEN IIa is associated with losses in chromosomes 1 and 10, with the break for the deletion demonstrated at chromosome 1p32. Ascertaining genotype with a panel of restriction fragment-length polymorphism (RFLP) probes identified marker D10Z1, a pericentromeric region of chromosome 10, in medullary thyroid carcinoma in both MEN IIa and IIb. These results suggest possible loss of a tumor-suppressor gene and allelic

mutations in the same locus in the two different familial cancer syndromes. RFLP analysis may be useful in identifying patients at risk for MEN II.

Lynch Syndrome

Familial cancer trends are also manifest in colorectal cancers. The most widely investigated familial cancer of the colon is the hereditary nonpolyposis colorectal cancer (HNPCC). HNPCC syndrome is divided into two main categories: (1) hereditary site-specific colon cancer, or Lynch syndrome I, and (2) colorectal cancer in association with other forms of cancer, or Lynch syndrome II. The main features of Lynch syndrome I are an autosomal dominant model of heredity, no associated polyposis, right-sided colon cancers, multiple colon cancers, and long survival. In Lynch syndrome II, many of the characteristics are the same as in syndrome I, with the added burden of increased risk for endometrial, ovarian, stomach, and urinary tract tumors. Lynch syndrome II patients are at greater risk for recurrence. The HNPCC group constitutes nearly 5% of all colorectal cancers, and in some centers, this figure approaches 15% to 20%. The potential for control of this form of colorectal cancer lies in use of computer registries and clinical surveillance of the high-risk group.

Physical Carcinogenesis

Tumor induction by physical agents occurs by two mechanisms: (1) induction of cell proliferation over an extended period, thereby increasing the opportunity for events leading to transformation, and (2) physical agents that induce damage or changes in the fidelity of DNA replication. The former mechanism is demonstrated in experimental model systems, including implantation of essentially nondegradable objects such as urethan film. Clinically, oral prostheses, orthopedic prostheses, and self-induced chronic irritation have been observed to induce neoplasia in humans. The latter mechanism usually involves ionizing radiation or ultraviolet light. In either setting, the result is progressive neoplasms that in animals are usually immunogenic and display highly polymorphic tumor-associated antigens.

Foreign-Body Tumors

In humans, it is difficult to document the induction of a neoplasm due solely to the presence of a foreign body. Foreign bodies may act as cocarcinogens or promoters, or they may produce a chronic irritation that permits carcinogenesis by otherwise subtumorigenic doses of environmental agents. Alternatively, the foreign-body–induced irritation may only promote cellular proliferation but may thereby increase the possibility for errors in DNA replication that can lead to neoplastic transformation. The increased risk for cancer in patients with burns or with chemically induced irritations, such as irritation caused by ingestion of potassium hydroxide, provides an example of the close link between tumorigenesis and the induction of cell proliferation. Cellular accumulation and proliferation associated with chronic inflammatory conditions may contribute to carcinogenesis by increasing the probability for genetic changes that result in neoplastic transformation. An example may be the increased risk for cancer in patients with inflammatory bowel disease.

Response to foreign bodies often involves inflammation. The process results in the accumulation of infiltrating cells that elaborate factors that may affect other cells in situ. Such processes are fundamental to tumors resulting from introduction of foreign, ostensibly inert, material. An example may be the inflammatory tumor occurring in hip prostheses. In some instances, removal of the foreign body results in tumor regression, as in intracordal administration of Teflon prosthesis for paralytic dysphonia in human vocal cords.

Exposure to asbestos fibers or dust markedly increases the risk for neoplastic disease. Among the inorganic carcinogens, asbestos is unusual in its induction of otherwise rare mesotheliomas. In addition to the lung cancers, workers exposed to asbestos show increased incidence of bladder carcinoma, gastrointestinal tract neoplasms, and laryngeal and esophageal tumors. Clinical and experimental model investigations reveal that asbestos may act as a primary carcinogen or as a cocarcinogen. Thus, people who smoke tobacco and are exposed to asbestos fibers increase their risk beyond that associated with the individual susceptibilities.

In experiments with animals, brief exposure to croton oil followed by chronic (daily) abrasion with a wire brush induces tumors, many of which are fibrosarcomas. The chronic injury that occurs with limb prostheses can lead to development of superficial tumors that may become progressive in untreated patients. These observations strongly suggest that in the multistage process of tumorigenesis, the presence of foreign bodies may fulfill one or more of the critical steps necessary to induce a tumor.

Ionizing Radiation

When administered in experimental animals, α-, γ-, and x-irradiation, as well as ultraviolet light, induces tumors. Exposure of experimental animals to gamma or x-rays results in the induction of leukemia, lymphomas, thymomas, and to a lesser extent, brain and visceral tumors. Ultraviolet light is biologically significant in the 280- to 320-nm, or UVB, range. Ultraviolet light induces skin tumors (primarily sarcomas) and occasionally squamous cell carcinomas or melanomas in rodents. The mechanism of carcinogenesis usually involves chromosomal changes, induction of DNA adducts, mutations, altered DNA methylation, and activation of oncogenes. In the presence of oncogenic viruses, whether exogenous or endogenous, radiation may accelerate tumor induction. In addition to the direct effects on the tissue that lead to transformation, radiation is a potent immunosuppressive, thereby decreasing a potentially important tumor surveillance mechanism. Both gamma and x-rays directly and indirectly affect viability and function of lymphocytes. In contrast, ultraviolet light induces immunosuppression indirectly, possibly through release of biologically active substances from cells in the skin.

In humans, results of exposure and dose are time related. Both γ- and x-irradiation occur in carcinogenic doses as a consequence of occupational exposure and usually have significant impact on lymphogenesis. Resulting leukemia is progressive and lethal. Ultraviolet light from the UVB range may be responsible for induction or promotion of a number of human skin tumors. Among these are basal cell carcinoma, squamous cell carcinoma, and malignant melanoma. Basal and squamous cell carcinomas are found in greater prevalence on sun-exposed skin. A role for UVB in melanoma may be promotion rather than induction. Ultraviolet light may contribute an essential step to tumor development in various ways, including immunosuppression; damage to cells in the skin, such as keratinocytes and Langerhans cells; or induction of changes in cells that eventuate as tumor. Experimental evidence supports all three possibilities.

Chemical Carcinogenesis

Exposure to chemicals in the environment increases the risk for nearly all cancers. Designation of specific chemicals as carcinogens is based on two broad criteria: docu-

mented induction of neoplasms in humans or experimental animals and increased frequency of revertants of *Salmonella* sp mutants, as in the Ames test. Mutagenicity is an important, but possibly not necessary, characteristic of carcinogenic chemicals. Carcinogenesis can occur as a result of external contact or after ingestion or inhalation of the agent. The spectrum of responses and tumors that arise from chemical carcinogenesis is wide. Often, the nature of the resulting neoplasm is determined by the route of introduction and by the tissues that accumulate the carcinogen. Chemical carcinogens can be organic or inorganic, and the nature of the carcinogen has significant impact on the resultant neoplastic diseases.

Organic Carcinogenesis

Organic carcinogens, such as the polycyclic hydrocarbons and nitrosamines, induce a wide variety of neoplasms. Polycyclic hydrocarbons must undergo chemical transformation by host tissues to an active carcinogen to induce a neoplasm. Combustion products, such as benzopyrene, are believed to cause a variety of visceral cancers. In animals, these agents have been used to induce soft tissue and visceral tumors after relatively short exposures. In this experimental setting, the latent period (the time from exposure to the development of a tumor) for most organic carcinogens is inversely related to carcinogen dose. The time over which tumors arise and metastasize suggests that some tumors in humans may be the result of prolonged exposure to low doses of organic carcinogens.

The relation of rodent carcinogenesis to tumorigenesis in humans has been the subject of protracted controversy. The significance of a single bolus dose of carcinogen into an otherwise healthy host probably does not reflect the natural history of most human cancers. Nevertheless, the rodent models have enabled identification of some of the basic mechanisms by which organic carcinogens induce cancer.

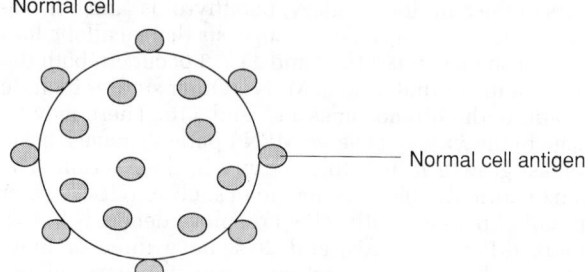

Figure 14-10. Although normal surface antigens may be reduced in malignant cells, they are not absent. Tumor-specific surface antigens may appear during transformation. (After McKhann CF. Tumor immunology. In: Immunology: a scope monograph. Kalamazoo. Upjohn, 1989:115)

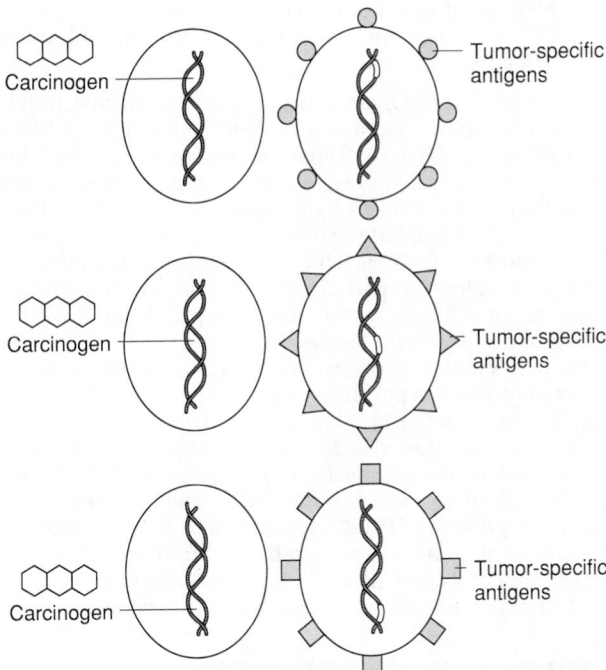

Figure 14-11. Chemical carcinogenesis results in production of tumor-specific antigens. Each tumor expresses antigenic specificity not shared by other neoplasms induced by the same chemical agent. (After McKhann CF. Tumor immunology. In: Immunology: a scope monograph. Kalamazoo, Upjohn, 1989:116)

Inorganic Carcinogens

Inorganic carcinogens are often heavy-metal compounds that result from fossil fuel combustion or industrial processes such as smelting. In humans, tumors are induced in the respiratory and urogenital system. In humans and rodents, compounds of nickel, cadmium, chromium, arsenic, and possibly lead induce a wide variety of neoplasms. Of the inorganic carcinogens, nickel is the most widely investigated. Insoluble forms of nickel, such as sulfides and subsulfides, are most carcinogenic. Exposure to the inorganic carcinogens is often occupational. Frequently, the exposure is chronic and in subtoxic doses. In humans, nickel smelting products induce nasopharyngeal carcinomas. In rodents, administration of insoluble nickel into the subcutis results in sarcomas. Intraocular injection induces sarcomas, carcinomas, and even melanomas. Metal carcinogens induce DNA adducts and DNA-protein cross-links

that decrease the fidelity of DNA replication. These DNA changes may increase the probability for transformation.

The biologic aspects of the host–tumor relation in tumors induced by inorganic carcinogens are unknown. Nevertheless, experimental tumors are immunogenic and, in many respects, indistinguishable from their histologically identical counterparts induced by organic carcinogenesis.

Immunology of Carcinogen-Induced Tumors

Tumors induced by carcinogens are moderately to strongly immunogenic. Experimental tumors induced by carcinogens display individually unique tumor antigens, which are designated as tumor-specific transplantation antigens (TSTA) because they are defined by induction of immunity to tumor transplant in inbred stocks of mice (Fig. 14-10). The extensive polymorphism is such that cross-reactivities occur at frequencies of less than 5%. Clonal analysis of chemically induced tumors reveals a low level of antigenic heterogeneity within a given tumor. (Figs. 14-11 and 14-12). Metastatic foci, however, may display significantly different TSTA than is found at the primary site. Immunity engendered by carcinogen-induced TSTA is mediated by T lymphocytes; serum antibody has a lesser role in tumor rejection. Despite the progression of the tumor at the primary site, the host may be systemically immune until the tumor achieves 5% of the body mass. Although most chemically induced tumors are solid, some are leukemia. The latter have polymorphic TSTA, and immunity may be mediated by antibody as well as T lymphocytes. Ultraviolet light–induced skin tumors have polymorphic TSTA that are so immunogenic that transplantation to syngeneic inbred stock requires immunosuppression.

The most compelling characteristics of tumors induced by carcinogenesis in experimental animals are the TSTA polymorphism and immunogenicity in the autochthonous host. These observations may also have relevance in humans. Investigations of the host–tumor relation in human melanoma have revealed that tumor-infiltrating lymphocytes (TILs) display autologous specificity in the lysis of tumor target cells, suggesting individually specific tumor antigens. Thus, adoptive therapy and active specific immunotherapy with vaccines must employ autologous agents. Vaccines may require preparations of each patient's own tumor cells and should accommodate the possibility of antigenic heterogeneity among tumor and metastatic sites.

Viruses

Induction of tumors by infectious agents was a long-disputed concept in the early part of this century. Today, it is unequivocal that both RNA and DNA viruses induce

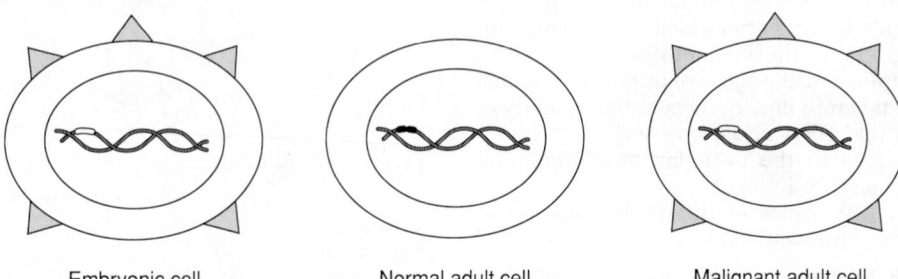

Figure 14-12. Eukaryotic cells contain functional genes for carcinoembryonic antigen (CEA) and normally express this molecule on their cell surfaces. In normal adult cells, the gene is repressed, and CEA is not present on the cell surface. In malignant cells, the gene is not repressed, and the gene product, CEA, is again present on the surface of the cell. (After McKhann CF. Tumor immunology. In: Immunology: a scope monograph. Kalamazoo, Upjohn, 1989:116)

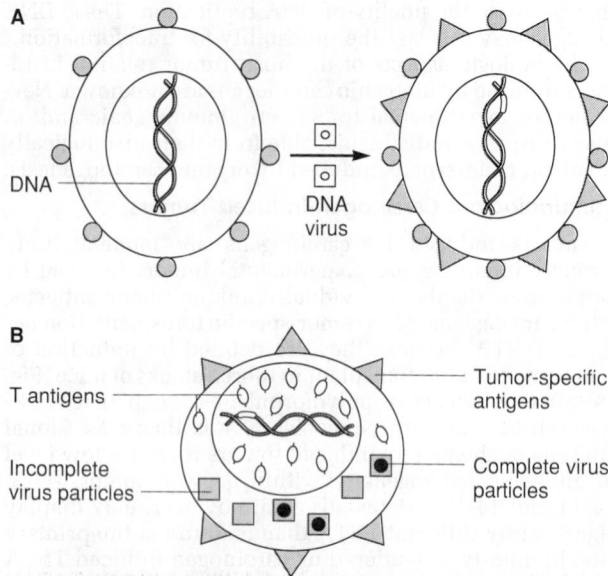

Figure 14-13. Viral transformation by an oncogenic virus can produce tumor-specific surface antigens (*A*) as well as intracellular antigens (T antigens) and new virus particles (*B*). (After McKhann CF. Tumor immunology. In: Immunology: a scope monograph. Kalamazoo, Upjohn, 1989:115)

tumors in animals from amphibians to primates. It has become accepted that this process also includes humans.[2] Oncogenic RNA viruses are subdivided into acute-acting types and chronic types. Acute-acting types induce sarcomas, leukemia, and lymphoid tumors in experimental animals. Chronic types induce leukemia and mammary tumors in animals and include human T-lymphotrophic viruses. The RNA viruses and the mechanisms of transformation of cells are discussed later. Oncogenesis by RNA virus results in the appearance of tumor-associated antigens on the surfaces of tumor cells (Fig. 14-13). A subset of the antigens may be shared among tumors induced by several different oncogenic viruses, whereas other tumor-associated antigens are unique to the individual oncogenic virus. All tumors induced by a single virus share the same virus-induced tumor antigens. In addition to the cell-surface antigens, antigens are expressed in the cytoplasm and in the nucleus.

Three groups of DNA viruses have oncogenic strains. The papovaviruses include the papilloma, polyoma, and simian viruses, which induce tumors in animals. Two others papovaviruses, JC and BK, were isolated from human tumors. The second group is made up of adenoviruses, and the third group comprises the herpesviruses. Adenoviruses were isolated from a variety of animal tumors; most of these are tumorigenic in newborn animals. An example of the herpesvirus group is the Epstein-Barr virus (EBV), which has been implicated as a cause of Burkitt lymphoma and nasopharyngeal carcinoma. An accumulating body of evidence suggests that DNA viruses, as well as RNA viruses, may participate in the initiation and promotion phases of tumorigenesis in humans.

Evidence for an EBV cause of Burkitt lymphoma includes the following observations:

1. Patients with EBV have higher titers of antibodies against the tumor-associated antigens and virus-determined antigens than unaffected people from the same family or age group.
2. Tumor cells have at least one copy of the viral DNA integrated into the host cell genome.

3. EBV transforms human cells in vitro.
4. EBV induces tumors after inoculation into subhuman primates.

The World Health Organization has indicated that previous and continued exposure to EBV results in high titers of antibody to the virus capsid antigen and a 30-fold increase in risk compared with control populations. Tumor induction does not occur by exposure to virus alone. EBV occurs world wide, but the tumor incidence is restricted to Africa and New Guinea. Thus, there are possibly climate-related cofactors or participating organisms endemic to these regions. These factors are no doubt layered over a background of genetic factors.

Herpes simplex virus type 2 (HSV-2) is the etiologic agent of genital herpes. Infected women with early sexual activity and a large number of sexual partners have significantly increased risk for cervical carcinoma. Women with invasive carcinoma have antibodies to HSV-2, and about 40% of cervical biopsies with severe dysplasia or carcinoma display HSV-2–specific DNA-binding protein. A similar relation has been established for human papovavirus (HPV). DNA of HPV-16 and HPV-18 have been demonstrated in cervical carcinoma biopsy specimens.

BIOLOGY OF ONCOGENESIS

Characteristics of the Transformed Cell

Inherent in the term *clonality* is the unicellular origin of a cell population (Fig. 14-14). Most hematopoietic and solid tumors arise from a single transformed cell. Whatever the causative agent leading to cellular transformation, not all cells exposed to that agent undergo transformation, and most transforming events are lethal. From the small surviving transformed cell population, some progress to terminal differentiation or apoptosis and are recognized as altered-self and eliminated by the host immune effector cells (Fig. 14-15).

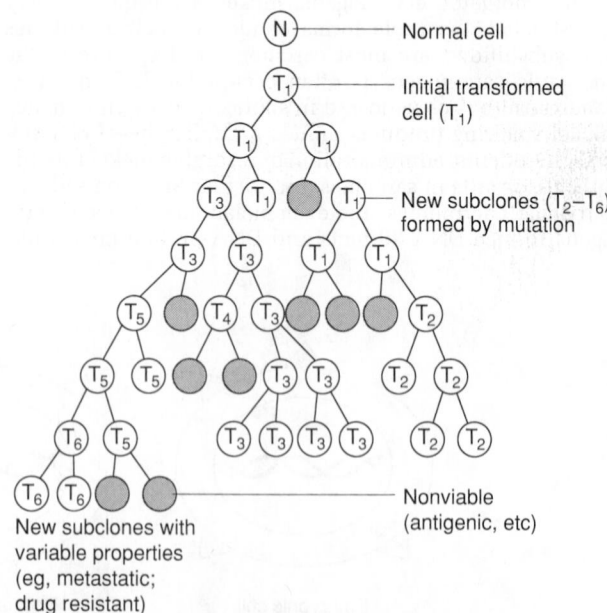

Figure 14-14. Clonal evolution of tumors. New subclones can emerge by mutation. Many mutations are fatal, and the subclones become extinct (*colored areas*); others provide growth advantages, and the subclones become dominant. (After Nowell PC. The clonal evolution of tumor cell populations. Science 1976;194:23)

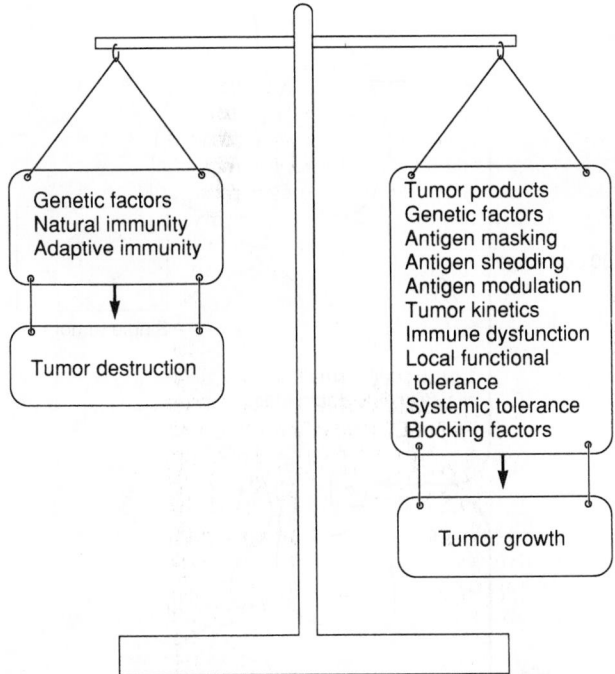

Figure 14-15. Tumor growth or destruction depends on a balance of factors within the host. (After Roitt IM, Brostoff J, Male DK. Immunology. St Louis, CV Mosby, 1985)

The two fundamental components of neoplastic tissue are heritable alterations in the genome and escape from normal regulation of growth. Laboratory models have used normal and neoplastic cells transformed by retroviruses or chemical and physical carcinogens. The spontaneous cause of cellular transformation to the malignant phenotype in humans is poorly understood.

Cellular transformation encompasses a variety of definitions. In vitro definitions include anchorage-independent growth (growth in soft agar) and loss of contact inhibition of growth in cell culture. Inherent in all definitions is a release or loss of normal growth regulation. Immortality in cell culture is characteristic of most transformed cells.

Nonneoplastic cells may also be transformed in vitro. One of the most frequent models of transformation uses simian virus 40 (SV40) transformed Swiss 3T3 mouse fibroblasts. These cells lose contact inhibition and continue to grow in multilayered mounds of cells. However, they rarely form tumors in vivo.

The definition of malignant or neoplastic transformation is much more strict and requires demonstration of tumorigenicity on inoculation of transformed cells into a living host. For human tumors growing in cell culture, this criterion requires the formation of transplantable tumors after inoculation into athymic, T-cell–deficient nude mice.

Many phenotypic, biochemical, and immunologic characteristics of cellular transformation have been described (Fig. 14-16). Transformed cells may exhibit changes in cellular morphology, such as cellular and nuclear pleomorphism, disordered arrangement of microfilament formation, and a variety of changes in cell-surface characteristics. Karyotypic changes are often evident in transformed cells, with an increase in aneuploid populations, frequent monosomy, trisomy, and other chromosomal aberrations. Cells transformed by chemicals or ultraviolet irradiation exhibit more antigenicity than spontaneously transformed cells, demonstrated by decreased tumorigenicity (ability to form tumors in nude mice), tumor regression, or tumor rejection after a second in vivo challenge.

Growth and Proliferation of Neoplastic Cells

Measurement of tumor growth has been hindered by the inability to follow changes in size of most human tumors over time. Most growth studies have used serial caliper

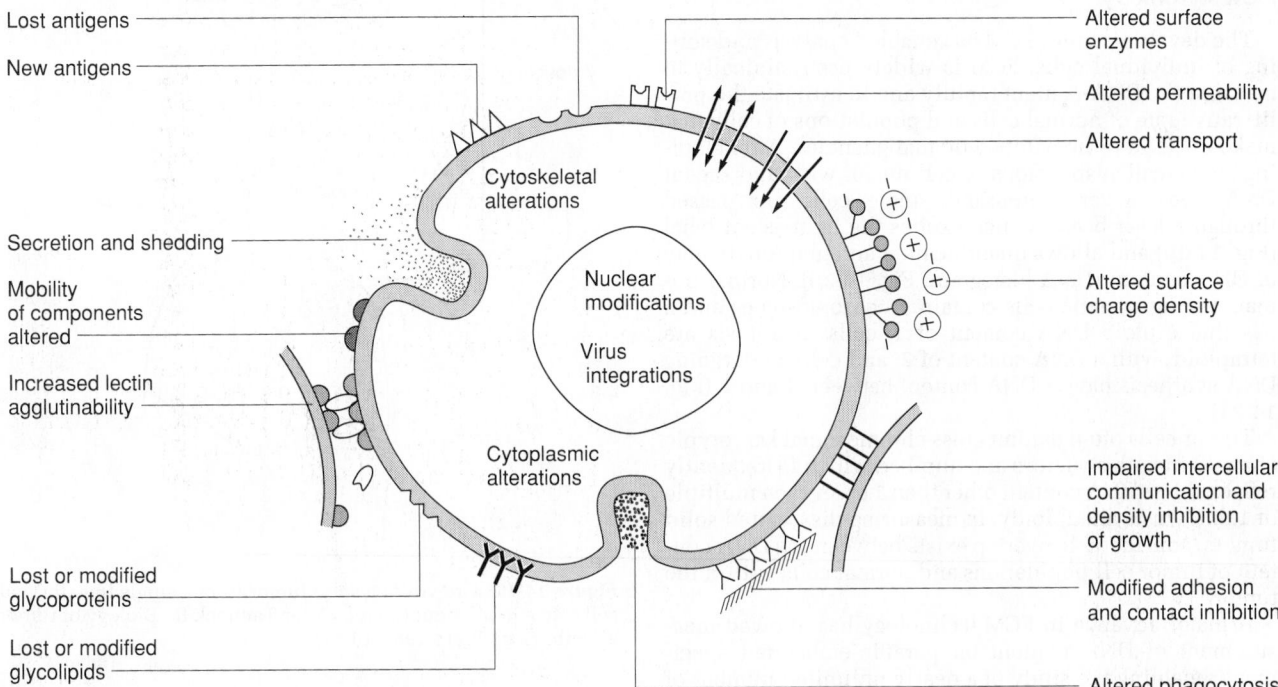

Figure 14-16. Alterations of cell structure and function that have been noted with neoplastic transformation. (After Nicolson GL. Trans-membrane control of the receptors on normal and tumor cells. II. Surface changes associated with transformation and malignancy. Biochim Biophys Acta 1976;458:1)

measurements of skin, subcutaneous, breast, and other body surface tumors, and serial chest radiography or computed tomography scanning of primary or metastatic pulmonary nodules, intraabdominal lesions, or other internal structures. From these measurements, one can calculate the time taken to increase the volume of the tumor cell mass two-fold, called the *volume doubling time* (T_D). In clinical practice, a frequently used measurement of change in size for an individual tumor mass is comparison of the product of the maximal perpendicular tumor diameters instead of the true three-dimensional tumor volume. Computed tomographic scanning and magnetic resonance imaging enable three-dimensional imaging and accurate computerized measurement of tumor volume.

Tumor Volume Doubling Time

A solid tumor originating from a single cell will have undergone about 30 volume doublings to reach 1 cm³ (1 g), the smallest clinically detectable size. Most tumors become lethal to the host at a mass of about 1 kg, which only requires an additional 10 doublings of cell mass (Fig. 14-17). Indeed, the duration of clinically apparent tumor represents only a fraction of that tumor's natural growth history. Although data from the preclinical growth phase of most human tumors is scarce, precluding reproducible mathematic models of tumor growth, it appears that most solid tumors do not exhibit exponential growth but instead demonstrate growth deceleration in later stages (Fig. 14-18). Suggested explanations include deprivation of an adequate blood supply to the tumor's core or depletion of host nutrients required to continue rapid growth above a certain size. Histologic sections of larger tumors often demonstrate central necrosis.

The measurement of tumor volume doubling time only provides a gross, and often late, estimate of tumor cell kinetics. A more accurate assessment of effects resulting from interventions requires a closer look at the individual components of growth kinetics.

Flow Cytometry

The development of FCM has enabled analysis and sorting of individual cells. FCM is widely used clinically to measure the DNA content rapidly and to estimate the proliferative rate of normal cells and populations of cells that make up solid or hematopoietic malignancies. After staining single-cell suspensions or cell nuclei with fluorescent DNA dyes, several thousand single cells are passed through a laser beam, which excites the fluorescent label (Fig. 14-19) and allows quantification and graphic display of DNA content (DNA histogram; Fig. 14-20). Normal human resting somatic cells contain 46 chromosomes and a baseline diploid DNA content of 1; cells in mitosis are tetraploid, with a DNA content of 2; and cells undergoing DNA synthesis have a DNA content between 1 and 2 (Fig. 14-21).

Tumor cells often exhibit gross chromosomal karyotypic changes in both structure and number, which is frequently reflected in a DNA content other than 1 or an even multiple of 1, known as aneuploidy. In measuring dissociated solid tumors, considerable overlap exists between the DNA content of tumor cell populations and normal cells within the tumor.

A major advance in FCM technology has allowed measurement of DNA content on paraffin-embedded specimens, enabling the study of a nearly unlimited number of archival pathologic specimens of all tumor types. Three limitations exist to evaluating paraffin specimens:

1. Prior fixation leads to alterations in binding of fluorescent dyes, which precludes use of an external dip-

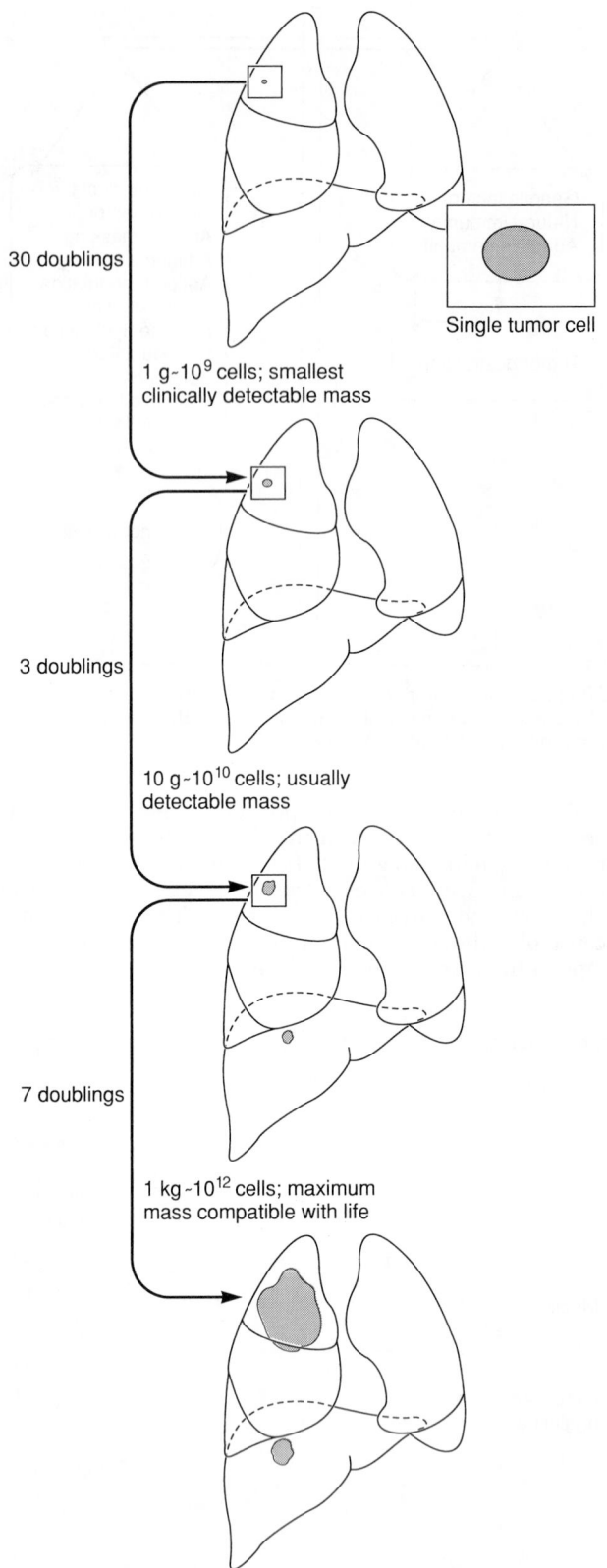

Figure 14-17. Growth of a solid tumor from a single transformed cell into a lethal tumor mass. (After Tannock IF. Biology of tumor growth. Hosp Pract 1983;18:81)

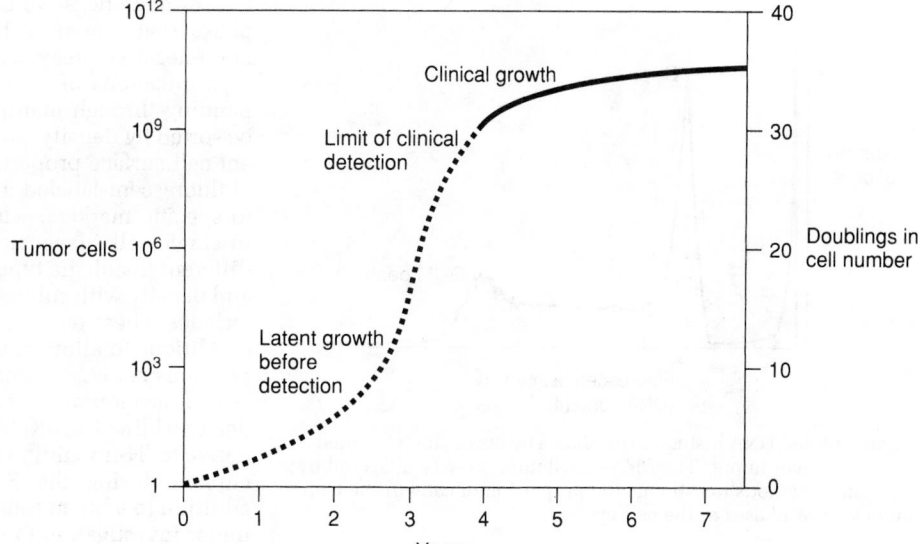

Figure 14-18. Theoretic growth curve for human tumors. Growth rates slow as tumors approach lethal mass. (After Tannock IF. Principles of cell proliferation: cell kinetics. In: DeVita VT, Hellman S, Rosenberg SA, eds. Cancer: principles and practice of oncology, ed 3. Philadelphia, JB Lippincott, 1989:4)

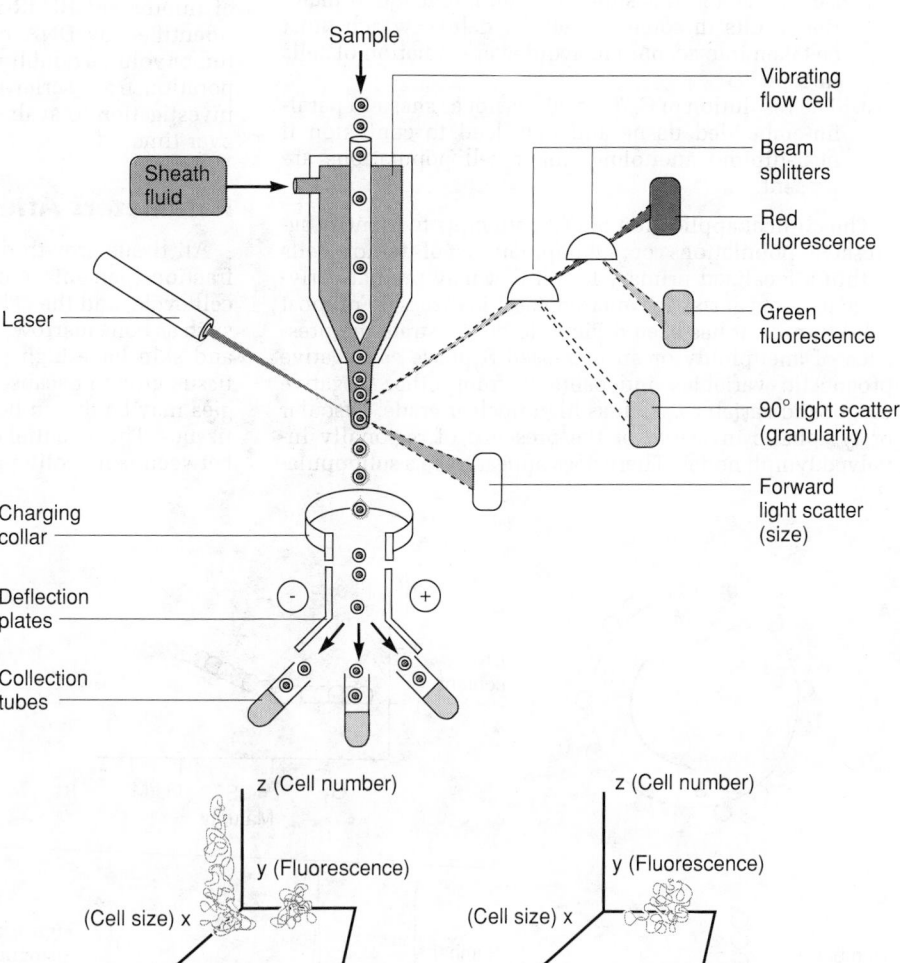

Figure 14-19. Schematic diagram of fluorescence-activated cell sorter. Cells within the sample are labeled with specific fluorescent reagents to detect surface antigens and then are introduced individually into a flow chamber. Each cell is illuminated by laser and measured for cell size (forward light scatter), for granularity (90-degree light scatter), and for two surface markers (red and green fluorescence). The cell stream breaks into charged droplets that are guided by deflection plates under computer control into appropriate collection tubes. Three-dimensional plots may be developed to describe the cell populations collected. (After Steward M, Male D. Immunologic techniques. In: Roitt IM, Brostoff J, Male DK, eds. Immunology, ed 2. New York, Gower, 1989:25)

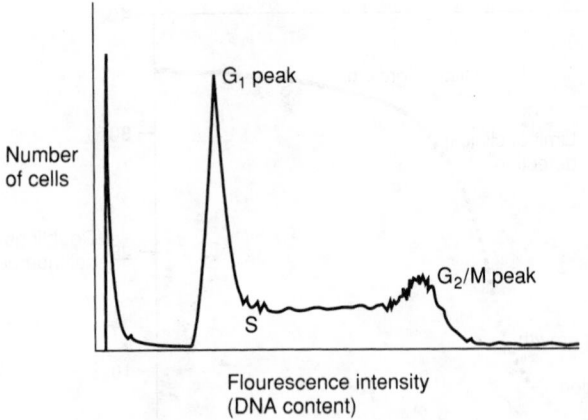

Figure 14-20. DNA histogram produced by flow cytometric analysis of a human tumor. The DNA distribution may be analyzed by computer methods to estimate the proportion of cells in the G, S, and G_2 to M phases of the cell cycle.

loid standard to identify the gap 0/gap 1 (G_0/G_1) diploid peak, and which relies on the presence of normal cells within the study sample.

2. Dewaxing and digestion of paraffin-embedded material results in some subcellular debris, which must be taken into account to avoid overestimation of cells in S phase.

3. The resolution of G_0/G_1 peaks is not as sharp in paraffin-embedded tissue and may lead to confusion if near-diploid aneuploid tumor cell populations are present.

The clinical application of FCM attempts to identify aggressive populations or subpopulations of tumor cells within a localized primary lesion that may predict early-stage patients at risk for micrometastatic disease. For most solid tumors, it has been difficult to demonstrate the presence of aneuploidy or an increased S phase as negative prognostic variables independent from other negative prognostic variables, such as high nuclear grade, vascular or lymphatic invasion, or the presence of regionally involved lymph nodes. There does appear to be a subpopula-

tion of node-negative breast cancer tumors with a high S phase that are more biologically aggressive than other node-negative breast cancers.

Applications of FCM in the laboratory are rapidly expanding through manipulations of cell sorting. Cells can be sorted by density, size, and electric charge. Also, different cell-surface properties have allowed preassay binding of fluorescent-labeled monoclonal antibodies or vital dyes to specific markers, which can be recognized and sorted in single-cell suspensions. This allows sorting of cells of different histologic type and sorting of cells of similar size and density with subtle and nonvisible cell-surface characteristics. These techniques can be carried out under sterile conditions to allow clonal expansion of selected cell suspensions collected after sorting.

The development of a monoclonal antibody to bromodeoxyuridine (BUdR) has provided a nonradioactive alternative to ³H-thymidine to study incorporation of DNA precursors during the S phase of proliferating cells. In addition to a broad range of in vitro applications, BUdR is under investigation to study in vivo human tumor growth rates before surgical biopsy. BUdR is administered intravenously, and tumor tissue from a surgical biopsy is removed several hours later and digested, and the resultant single-cell suspension is analyzed by FCM. Cells that have incorporated BUdR are recognized by fluorescent-labeled antibodies to BUdR. Two-parameter FCM allows correlation of fluorescent BUdR-incorporated cells through S phase (identified by DNA content) to calculate an estimate of tumor volume doubling time. Measurement of BUdR incorporation from serial surgical biopsy specimens is under investigation to evaluate tumor responsiveness to therapy over time.

Parameters Affecting Tissue Growth

All tissue growth depends on three factors: the growth fraction (percentage of cycling cells), the duration of the cell cycle, and the cell-loss fraction. Many normal tissues, such as bone marrow, intestinal crypt epithelium, gametes, and skin have high proliferative rates but very little net tissue growth because of rapid cell turnover. Many analogies may be drawn between growing tumors and renewal tissues. The essential difference in tumors is an imbalance between cell proliferation and loss.

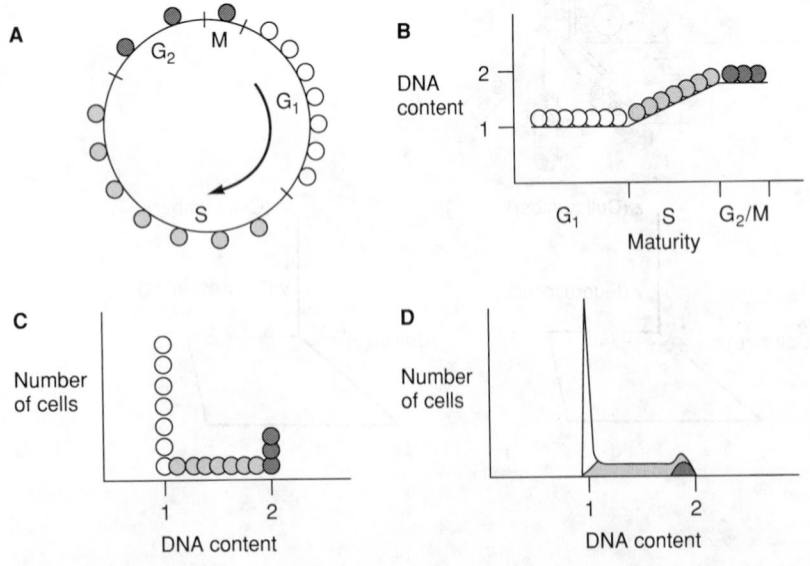

Figure 14-21. Illustration of generation of DNA histogram. (*A*) Distribution of cells around cell cycle for asynchronous population. (*B*) Relation between DNA content and position in cell cycle. (*C*) DNA distribution for cell population illustrated in B. (*D*) DNA histogram for hypothetical distribution illustrated in C. (After Tannock I. Cell kinetics and chemotherapy: a critical review. Cancer Treat Rep 1978;62:1117)

Tumor Growth Fraction

The growth fraction consists of the proportion of the total cell mass undergoing replication at a point in time. Primary tumors often consist of many cell types in addition to tumor cells. Fibroblasts; infiltrating host immune effector cells, such as lymphocytes, macrophages, and neutrophils; normal parenchymal cells from the involved organ or tissue; neurons; and normal vascular and lymphatic endothelial cells may all be present in various proportions within a tumor. Most cells that compose human neoplasms do not undergo cell division. The growth fraction of tumors can be measured using the ^{3}H-thymidine–labeling index or FCM, both of which can be used to determine the percentage of cells undergoing DNA synthesis. Table 14-3 demonstrates a range of 4% to 24% for several solid tumors. Even in clinically aggressive solid tumors, a growth fraction of about 10% is not uncommon. An important distinction must be made between potential and actual cell proliferation. The proliferative rate for normal and neoplastic tissues is dynamic and is influenced by regulation and entry of normally quiescent cells into the cell cycle to increase cell number through cell division. It is likely that the growth fraction fluctuates over the natural history of most solid tumors. A maximum growth fraction of about 37% occurs during the exponential, linear segment of the typical tumor growth curve seen in Figure 14-18. Indeed, an equal or higher growth fraction can be demonstrated for some normal tissues, for which the ^{3}H-thymidine–labeling indices for normal bone marrow and gastrointestinal crypt stem cells range from 30% to 70% and 12% to 18%, respectively.

Tumor Cell Cycle

The cell cycle may be simply defined as the sequence of events involved in the growth and division of one cell into two daughter cells with identical chromosomal number and composition. The fate of these daughter cells may take three directions: (1) reentry into a new cell cycle, resulting in two new identical progeny; (2) early cell death; or (3) entry into a permanent or reversible quiescent phase with no increase in cell number (Fig. 14-22). Cells participating in the cell cycle are known as *cycling* or *proliferating* cells. The cell cycle has been classically described by time intervals involved in DNA synthesis (S phase), mitosis (M phase), and the gaps of time between these events— G_1 phase before DNA synthesis and G_2 between DNA synthesis and mitosis. A G_0 phase has been described for cells

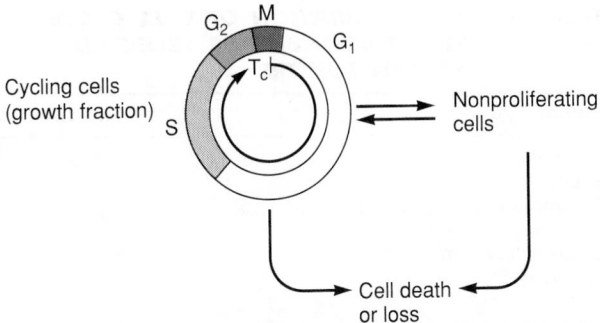

Figure 14-22. Model of tumor cell cycle including both proliferating cells (growth fraction) and nonproliferating cells. (After Ruddon RW. Cancer biology, ed 2. New York, Oxford University Press, 1987:142)

not actively proliferating but capable of undergoing cellular division after an appropriate signal.

The duration of the cell cycle is remarkably similar for most tumors, ranging from 2 to 4.5 days, regardless of the marked variation in clinical growth rates of the same tumors (Table 14-4). Differences in normal or neoplastic growth rates are minimally affected by the cell cycle time.

Tumor Cell Death or Cell Loss

The primary determinant of neoplastic tissue growth and progression is a discordance between the growth fraction and the cell loss fraction. The high proliferative rate of normal bone marrow and gastrointestinal stem cells is tightly balanced with the high cell loss of these tissues, manifested by a short life-span and high-volume mucosal cell slough, respectively. In tumors, the slight increase in growth fraction is not compensated by a proportional increase in cell death or cell loss. The loss of growth regulation has been linked to abnormalities in growth factor expression and alterations in specific cellular growth-regulatory genes known as *protooncogenes.*

ONCOGENES

Carcinogenesis is a complex, multistep process. Malignant tumors are presumed to arise after accumulation of specific changes in the normal regulation of growth and differentiation. Research has enabled recognition of some of the molecular, genetic, and chromosomal alterations that compose the basis of multistep tumorigenesis.[3,4] Oncogenesis occurs in three distinct steps: initiation, promotion, and progression. Each stage is the result of a series of changes in many of the underlying molecular mechanisms governing normal cellular differentiation and growth. These regulatory mechanisms may include growth factors and their receptors, signal transduction molecules, oncogenes, and antioncogenes. When a cell accumulates a critical number of perturbations in the expression or function of these molecules, it may then undergo morphologic malignant transformation. Elucidation of the changes attendant to malignant transformation is noted in the investigation of chemical and viral oncogenesis.

Many of the recent advances in molecular oncology stem from the discovery of tumor viruses and the ensuing discovery of retroviral oncogenes, the presence of which was hypothesized more than 25 years ago. The relation of oncogenes to tumorigenesis was not substantiated until molecular analysis of viral oncogenesis was achieved. This was the initial step in understanding the role of specific genes in neoplastic transformation.

Table 14-3. PROPORTION OF S-PHASE CELLS IN SELECTED TYPES OF HUMAN TUMORS

Tumor Type	Labeling Index (% Using ^{3}H-Thymidine)	S Phase (% by Flow Cytometry)
Breast		
Primary	4	8
Metastatic	9	10
Colorectal	11	18
Squamous cell	13	19
Sarcomas	5	11
Lymphomas		
Low grade		4
Intermediate grade	21	9
High grade		24

(Adapted from Wolberg WH, Ansfield FJ. The relationship of thymidine labeling index in human tumors in vitro to the effectiveness of 5-fluorouracil chemotherapy. Cancer Res 1971;31:448)

Table 14-4. MEAN DURATION OF CELL CYCLE TIME OBTAINED FOR SELECTED HUMAN TUMORS

Tumor Type	Cycle Time (d)
Melanoma	2.5
Breast	2.5
Squamous cell of head and neck	2.5
Lung	4.5
Colon and rectum	3.0
Lymphomas	2.0
Acute leukemia	2.5

A virus consists of a small package of genetic information, either in the form of DNA or RNA, wrapped in a structural protein coat. In the lytic infection cycle in cells, the viral genome controls replication of the genetic package, synthesis of viral proteins, and formation of new viral particles. In nonlytic conditions, viruses may also insert their genetic material into the genome of host cells and induce changes consistent with neoplastic transformation.

There are six basic families of DNA tumor viruses. Virus DNA may be replicated epigenetically, or incorporated into the host cell genome and subsequently replicated. Depending on several host cell factors, viral DNA induces transformation. Among RNA viruses, hepatitis B virus is strongly associated with the development of hepatocellular carcinoma, and more than 80% of cervical carcinomas evidence papillomavirus infection. Of the spectrum of RNA viruses, only the retrovirus family is associated with oncogenesis. The role of RNA retroviruses in human cancers is less evident than their role in rodent leukemia and adenocarcinomas and in avian leukemia and sarcomas.

The molecular basis for the oncogenic potential of the DNA viruses has been difficult to define, largely because the viral genes are involved in the expression and replication of viral DNA without integration into the host genome. DNA viruses also typically result in lysis of the host cell with release of the progeny virus. In vitro models of SV40 and polyomavirus indicate that DNA viruses may regulate host cell transcription and create a state of continued proliferation without completion of the normal lytic cycle.

The discovery of the RNA retroviruses, the first isolated by Rous in 1911 from chicken sarcoma, led to our present understanding of oncogenes and their normal precursors, the protooncogenes. When a retrovirus infects a cell, the viral RNA is reverse-transcribed into a double-stranded DNA by the viral enzyme reverse transcriptase. The viral DNA is then integrated into the host chromosomal DNA, forming a DNA provirus. During transcription of chromosomal DNA, viral DNA is also transcribed by host cell RNA polymerase, producing copies of the viral genome and messenger RNA (mRNA). The mRNA is then translated into proteins for viral progeny. New virus particles are then released by budding from the plasma membrane without cell lysis or death (Fig. 14-23).

In oncogenic retroviruses, viral gene expression results in neoplastic transformation of cells in vitro and tumor induction in vivo. All the transforming retroviruses contain at least one gene that is not involved in the viral replication process and that instead participates in transformation. Retroviral oncogenes are designated by three-letter names, often representing the tumors induced or the cell line from which the oncogene has been isolated. Rous sarcoma virus contains the *src* gene, which encodes a membrane-associated enzyme responsible for phosphorylation of cellular proteins. The products of oncogenes differ in their cellular locations, functions, and proposed mechanisms for transformation. In some systems, the genes may be expressed as a distinct translational product with transforming potential or as a fusion of a viral replicative sequence and the transforming sequence. In all retroviruses, oncogenes are an integrated part of the viral genome, not involved in replication, but essential for the malignant potential of the virus.

Retroviral oncogenes originate from normal cellular genes called *protooncogenes*.[1] Protooncogenes are incorporated into the viral genome during recombination events between the virus and host DNA. During this transduction process, the normal genes may be rearranged or mutated. The altered forms of the protooncogenes may differ in terms of their regulatory or protein-coding sequences. Indeed, these alterations are responsible for the transforming potential of the retroviruses. Oncogenes isolated from viruses are designated with the letter v (v-*src*), and oncogenes isolated from the host cellular DNA are designated with the letter c (c-*fos*).

Identification of cellular oncogenes by gene transfer experiments advanced our understanding of the molecular basis of cancer. DNA isolated from human tumors and transferred to recipient cells induced transformation. The cellular oncogenes were identified as altered forms of the normal protooncogenes, which had become activated by point mutations or DNA rearrangements. Additionally, some cellular oncogenes are homologous to the viral oncogenes found in retroviruses. For example, v-*mos* and c-*mos* sequences differ at only 25 positions out of 1157 nucleotides, and the corresponding proteins differ by only 11 amino acids.

Substantial evidence supports the hypothesis that human tumors can arise consequent to cellular oncogene activation. The first line of investigation that supports this concept is elucidation of the normal roles of the protooncogenes. Many of the protooncogenes are expressed during periods of proliferation, development, and differentiation. Thus, the cellular protooncogenes may be key regulatory components in cell growth. Abnormal protooncogene function or activation may, therefore, result in the deregulated proliferation and dedifferentiation characteristic of the neoplastic state.

Various activation mechanisms can change a normal gene into an oncogene. Point mutations (single nucleotide changes in DNA) are one such mechanism. For example, members of the *ras* gene family are some of the most frequently activated oncogenes in solid human tumors. The *ras* gene products are plasma membrane proteins capable of binding guanosine triphosphate (GTP). As discussed later, these proteins, called *G proteins,* are involved in intracellular signal transduction. Research from several laboratories reveals that in tumors with *ras* activation, the difference in the oncogene compared with the normal gene is a single nucleotide change. Point mutations resulting in single amino acid substitutions in the ras protein change a normal protein into one with transforming activity.

Another important mechanism of oncogene activation is chromosomal translocation, the shifting of a segment of one chromosome to another chromosome. One of the most well-known examples is the formation of the Philadelphia chromosome in chronic myelogenous leukemia. The protooncogene c-*abl* is translocated from chromosome 9 to the *bcr* locus on chromosome 22. Transcription of the new *bcr/abl* locus results in the formation of a fusion protein. This new protein has enhanced tyrosine kinase activity and transforming capabilities (Fig. 14-24). Burkitt lymphoma is characterized by the translocation of c-*myc* protooncogene from chromosome 8 to either chromosome 2, 14, or 22. The protooncogene thus becomes positioned

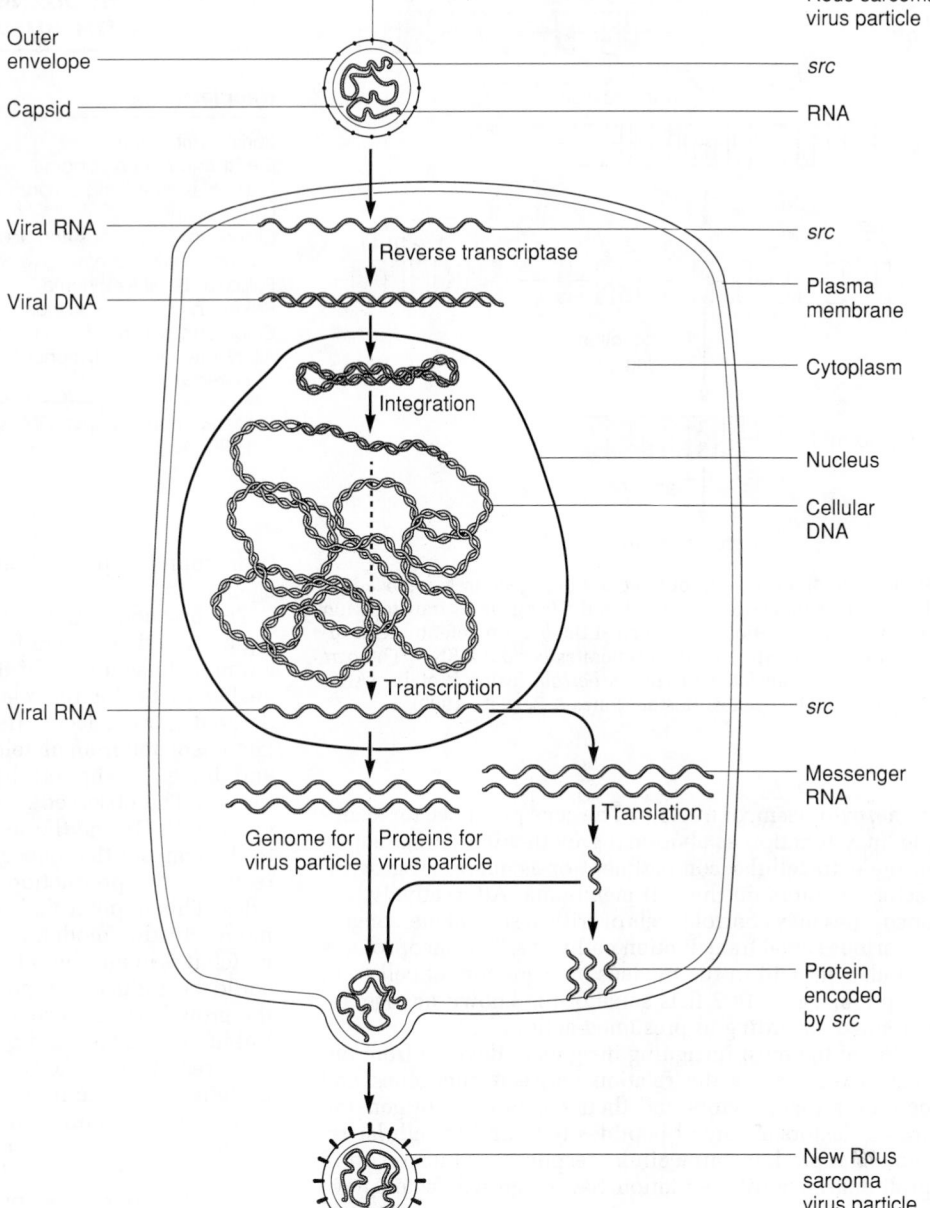

Outer
envelope

Capsid

Viral RNA

Viral DNA

Reverse transcriptase

Integration

Transcription

Viral RNA

Genome for | Proteins for
virus particle | virus particle

Translation

Rous sarcoma
virus particle

src

RNA

src

Plasma
membrane

Cytoplasm

Nucleus

Cellular
DNA

src

Messenger
RNA

Protein
encoded
by *src*

New Rous
sarcoma
virus particle

Figure 14-23. Neoplastic transformation by Rous sarcoma virus. When the Rous sarcoma retrovirus infects a cell, viral RNA is copied into double-stranded DNA by viral reverse transcriptase. After forming a circle, the viral DNA becomes integrated into the host cell DNA. Transcription of host DNA also results in transcription of viral DNA. Some viral RNA copies are included in new viral particles. Translation of viral RNA provides several proteins for inclusion into virus particles. Translation of viral RNA also produces the V-*src* gene product, which is not a component of the virus particle. The *src* gene product is a protein kinase, localized to the inner surface of the plasma cell membrane, which phosphorylates intracellular proteins. Protein phosphorylation results in cellular proliferation. (After Bishop JM. Oncogenes. Sci Am 1982;246:80)

near highly transcribed genes involved in immunoglobulin production. Probably because of its proximity, the translocation results in a deregulation of c-*myc* expression.

In other tumors, an oncogene may be found in an increased number of gene copies per cell, termed *amplification.* DNA amplification results in an increased level of gene expression (Fig. 14-25). Amplification of N-*myc* has been found to correlate with prognosis in patients with neuroblastoma. Patients demonstrating N-*myc* amplification, even in early-stage tumors, have biologically more aggressive tumors. Clinically, the observation of N-*myc* amplification translates into a higher incidence of tumor recurrence, progression, and resistance to chemotherapy. A partial list of frequent oncogenes and their mechanisms of activation is shown in Table 14-5.

In addition to the activation of oncogenes, studies of certain inherited tumors suggest that a loss of specific chromosomal regions may play a permissive role in the development of a neoplasia. Usually, the losses involve only one of the two parental chromosomes present in normal cells. The lost genes are presumed to encode growth-inhibitory signals. In somatic cell hybridization experiments, the fusion of a normal cell and a tumor cell yields a nontumorigenic hybrid, presumably as a result of the replacement of a lost tumor-suppressor gene in the transformed cell. Tumor-suppressor genes, or *antioncogenes,* are often described as acting recessively at the cellular level, referring to the ability of the cell to maintain a normal phenotype in the presence of one normal parental gene or wild-type allele. A second genetic event or mutation in the normal allele would thus result in transformation to the cancerous phenotype. Table 14-6 lists several tumor-suppressor genes or chromosomal losses found in human neoplasms.

Despite the ever-increasing number of oncogenes identified, many of these genes can be classified according to the actions of their encoded proteins. These groupings are based on the action of the oncogene protein in the mem-

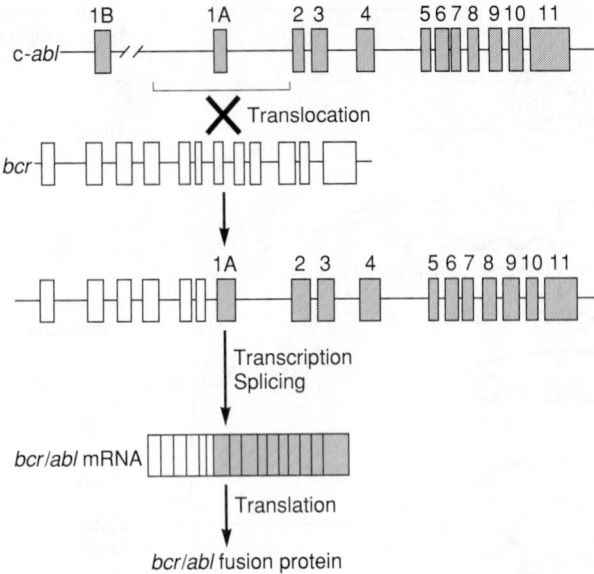

Figure 14-24. Activation of the c-*abl* oncogene by translocation. The c-*abl* protooncogene is fused to the *bcr* gene by translocation such that transcription is initiated at the *bcr* promoter but continues through *abl*. Splicing then generates *bcr/abl* mRNA. The *bcr/abl* mRNA is translated to yield a *bcr/abl* fusion protein. (After Cooper GM. Oncogenes. Boston, Jones & Bartlett, 1990)

brane, cytoplasm, or nucleus. The gene products, for example, may function as abnormal growth-stimulating factors in the extracellular compartment or as abnormal growth-factor receptors on the cell membrane. Alternatively, the oncogenes may control levels of critical second messengers in various signal transduction pathways. The oncoproteins can also act within the nucleus as regulators of cell transcription. Table 14-7 lists some of the known oncogenes, classified according to presumed action.

One of the most intriguing insights to develop from oncogene research is the relation between oncogenes and peptide growth factors and their receptors.[5,6] In general, growth factors are small peptides that bind to cellular receptors to produce intracellular responses, which result in proliferation or differentiation. Several growth factors have

Table 14-5. ONCOGENE ACTIVATION ASSOCIATED WITH HUMAN NEOPLASMS

Neoplasm	Oncogene	Activation Mechanism
Burkitt lymphoma	c-*myc*	Translocation
Breast and lung carcinoma	c-*myc*	Amplification
Neuroblastoma, lung carcinoma	N-*myc*	Amplification
Lung carcinoma	L-*myc*	Amplification
Chronic myelogenous and acute lymphocytic leukemia	*abl*	Translocation
Follicular B-cell lymphoma	*bcl*-2	Translocation
Breast and ovarian carcinoma	*erb* B-2	Amplification
Colon and pancreatic carcinoma	K-*ras*	Point mutation
Acute myeloid and lymphoid leukemia	N-*ras*	Point mutation

(Adapted from Cooper GM. Oncogenes. Boston, Jones & Bartlett, 1990)

been found experimentally to function as transforming agents.

The first correlation between an oncogene and a physiologically active growth factor was demonstrated when the amino acid sequence of the sis oncogene product was revealed to be highly related to the β chain of platelet-derived growth factor (PDGF). PDGF is a major growth factor isolated from platelets, used by fibroblasts in culture, and thought to support the growth of several mesenchymal tissues. The observed sequence homology between the β chain of PDGF and the sis oncogene product lends support to the concept that oncogene transformation could be the result of the production of extracellular mitogenic peptides. This hypothesis is called the *autocrine stimulation model*. In this model, a cell produces a growth factor to which it responds by cell proliferation. Cell transformation could be induced by continual autocrine stimulation of the growth factor receptor (Fig. 14-26). Further evidence linking oncogenes and growth factors is provided by the discovery that the oncogenes *int*-2, *hst*, and *fgf*-5 encode proteins related to fibroblastic growth factor.

Autocrine stimulation by growth factors is dependent on the presence of the growth factor receptors on the cell surface. Oncogenes may be responsible for altered growth factor receptor expression and activity. Increased numbers

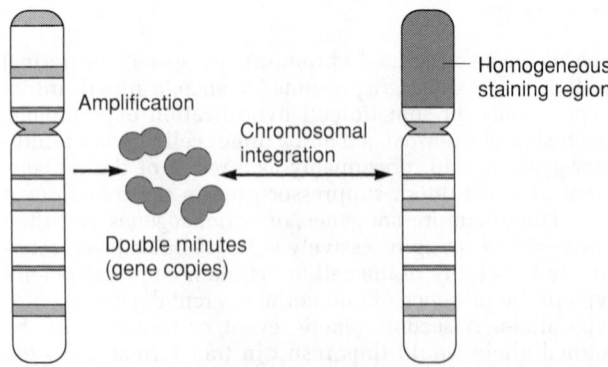

Figure 14-25. Oncogene activation through amplification. A gene locus can be amplified by repeated DNA replication. Recombination yields tandem arrays of amplified DNA, which form double minutes when excised from the chromosome. Integration of the double minutes into another chromosome forms a homogeneous staining region. (After Cooper GM. Oncogenes. Boston, Jones & Bartlett, 1990)

Table 14-6. TUMOR-SUPPRESSOR GENE LOSS REPORTED IN HUMAN NEOPLASMS

Tumor-Suppressor Gene or Chromosome	Neoplasm
Rb (Chromosome 13)	Retinoblastoma; osteosarcoma; breast, bladder, and small cell lung carcinoma
p53 (Chromosome 17)	Lung and colon carcinoma
Chromsome 1	Neuroblastoma
Chromosome 3	Lung and renal cell carcinoma
Chromosome 5	Colon carcinoma
Chromosome 11	Wilms tumor, hepatoblastoma, adrenal carcinoma, rhabdomyosarcoma, bladder and breast carcinoma
Chromosome 18	Colon carcinoma
Chromosome 22	Acoustic neuroma, meningioma

(Adapted from Cooper GM. Oncogenes. Boston, Jones & Bartlett, 1990)

Table 14-7. ONCOGENES AND ASSOCIATED NEOPLASMS

Category	Oncogene	Homologous Cellular Gene	Associated Neoplasm
Growth factors	*sis*	PDGF	
	int-2	FGF	Breast carcinoma
Transmembrane growth factor receptors	*erbB*	EGF receptor	
	neu		Breast carcinoma
	fms	M-CSF receptor	
	ros, kit		
Membrane-associated tyrosine kinases	*abl*		Chronic myelogenous leukemia, acute lymphocytic leukemia, acute myelogenous leukemia
Membrane-associated guanine nucleotide–binding proteins	K-, N-, and H-*ras*		Colorectal, lung, or prostate carcinoma
	src		
	fes, fps		
Cytoplasmic serine and threonine kinases	*raf/mil, mos*		
Cytoplasmic hormone receptors	*erb* A	Thyroid hormone receptor	
Nuclear factors	*c-myc*		Burkitt lymphoma
	N-*myc*		Neuroblastoma
	L-*myc*		Small cell lung carcinoma
	fos		Osteosarcoma
	jun		
	myb, ets, ski		
Antioncogenes	*Rb, p53, p21, pcc, mcc*		Retinoblastoma
Others	*bcl-2*		Non-Hodgkin's lymphomas
	bcl-1, int-1		Breast carcinoma

PDGF, platelet-derived growth factor; FGF, fibroblast growth factor; EGF, epidermal growth factor; M-CSF, mononuclear colony-stimulating factor.
(Adapted from Ducker BJ, Mamon HV, Roberts U. Oncogenes, growth factors and signal transduction. N Engl J Med 1989;321:1383)

of receptors or receptors with unusually high affinity could have proliferative effects similar to increased levels of the growth factor. Indeed, tumors with extremely high numbers of receptors for epidermal growth factor (EGF) have been described in head and neck squamous cell carcinomas, colon tumors, and breast cancers. In breast cancer, EGF receptor status has been correlated with early recurrence and disease-free survival.

Growth factor receptors have related structural and functional characteristics. These receptors consist of three distinct domains or regions, each with its own function. First, there is an amino-terminal, extracellular, ligand-binding domain. Second, there is a sequence of hydrophobic amino acids creating the transmembrane domain, which anchors the protein and may modify signal transduction. Third, the carboxy-terminal portion is on the cytoplasmic side of the membrane and is the tyrosine kinase domain. This tyrosine kinase domain works to phosphorylate tyrosine residues on cellular proteins, which are thought to function subsequently as important second messengers (Fig. 14-27).

A relation between oncogenes and growth factor receptors was noted in 1984 as sequence homology between the receptor for EGF and the v-*erb*-B oncogene. The major areas of homology include the transmembrane and tyrosine kinase domains. The ligand-binding domain is deleted in the erb-B oncogene product (Fig. 14-28). This truncated receptor is believed to be constitutively active and is able to generate a mitogenic signal in the absence of EGF binding.

Several other receptors encoded by oncogenes demonstrate deletions of the ligand-binding domains. These include the *kit, ros, met, ret,* and *trk* oncogenes. The loss of the extracellular domain results in a truncated receptor that may lack normal regulatory controls. Thus, the receptor may express unregulated tyrosine kinase activity with resultant signals for uncontrolled cellular proliferation (Fig. 14-29).

The binding of growth factors to receptors has also been shown to control the expression of certain oncogenes. Specifically, binding of PDGF results in increased expression of the oncogenes, c-*myc* and c-*fos*. These latter two oncogenes encode nuclear proteins that may play a role in control of cell cycle and mitotic regulation.

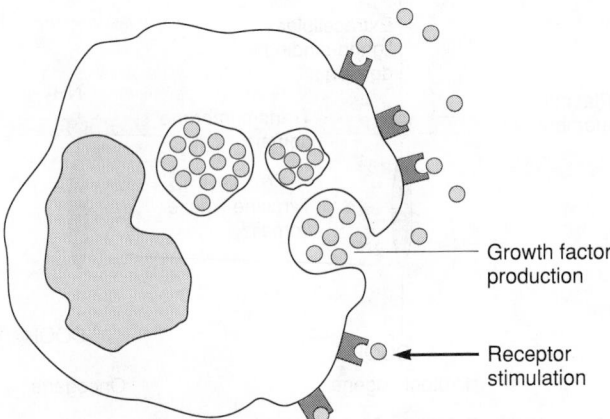

Growth factor production

Receptor stimulation

Figure 14-26. Autocrine stimulation of cellular proliferation involves the production by a cell of a growth factor to which it also responds. The autostimulation results in continuous cell proliferation. (After Cooper GM. Oncogenes. Boston, Jones & Bartlett, 1990)

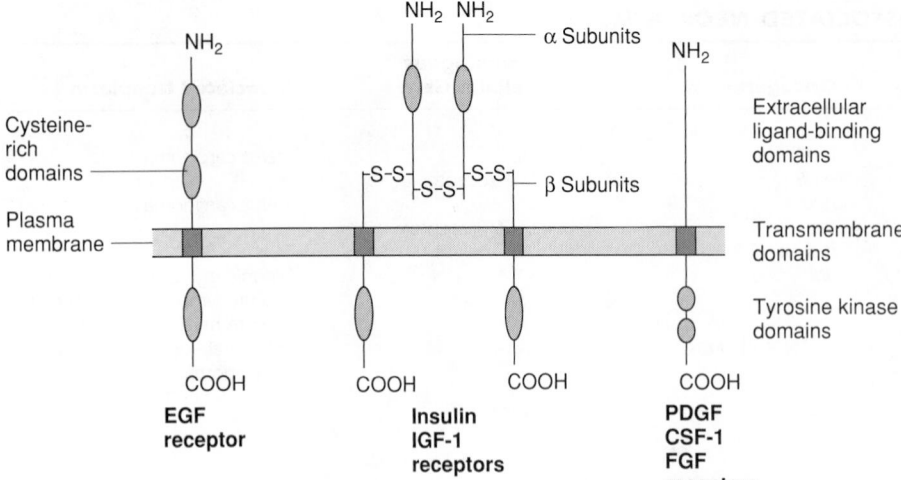

Figure 14-27. Schematic diagram of tyrosine kinase receptor organization. In each instance, the receptors contain amino-terminal extracellular ligand-binding domains, a transmembrane domain, and a carboxy-terminal intracellular tyrosine kinase domain. PDGF, platelet-derived growth factor; CSF-1, colony-stimulating factor 1; FGF, fibroblastic growth factor. (After Cooper GM. Oncogenes. Boston, Jones & Bartlett, 1990)

As evident in the previous discussion, there are several levels of interaction of growth factors and oncogenes. Oncogenes may encode proteins that function in an autocrine manner to stimulate cell proliferation. Oncogenes may also result in the expression of altered growth factor receptors with abnormal signal transduction activity. Growth factors may also exert effects through the activation of certain protooncogenes. This close relation between growth factors and oncogenes has led to new theoretic modalities for cancer treatment. Monoclonal antibodies to growth factor receptors have been developed and demonstrate activity against cell lines in vitro. Specific tyrosine kinase inhibitors are also in developmental stages.

The largest group of known oncogenes encode proteins associated with the inner surface of the cell membrane. These membrane-associated molecules may transmit signals from growth factor receptors on the cell surface to secondary cytoplasmic messengers, leading to cell proliferation.[7] The generation of intracellular signals in response to the action of extracellular factors at the cell surface is termed *signal transduction*. The *src* and *ras* families of oncogenes are representative of membrane-associated proteins involved in signal transduction. The *src* family has tyrosine kinase activity, and the *ras* proteins are characterized by binding of the guanine nucleotides, guanosine diphosphate (GDP) and GTP.

Phosphorylation of proteins on specific tyrosine residues is a key regulatory mechanism. As previously discussed, many of the growth factor receptors are in fact tyrosine kinases. In many cases, tyrosine phosphorylation has a profound stimulatory effect on enzyme activity of the phosphorylated protein. Tyrosine kinases include members of the *src* family, *abl* and *fps* oncogenes. The physiologic stimuli responsible for activation of the nonreceptor kinases are not clearly defined. Thus, their roles in signal transduction pathways are not as well described as the receptor kinases. Despite this, evidence shows that control of nonreceptor tyrosine kinase activity plays a key role in multiple cellular processes involving cellular metabolism, cytoskeletal integrity, and cellular proliferation.

Tyrosine kinases, such as the src protein, may be regulated by phosphorylation. The activity of the src gene product is thought to be distinctly elevated in colon adenocarcinomas relative to normal colon epithelial cells. In a normal cell, the phosphorylation of an enzyme is a transient, regulatory event. In the case of an oncoprotein, the enzyme may be constitutively activated, resulting in the unregulated transfer of phosphate to tyrosine residues on targeted proteins. These targets, or effector proteins, subsequently may be responsible for sending abnormal or uncontrolled mitogenic signals to the cell nucleus. Identifying these effector proteins is the basis of much molecular research. Characterization of these molecular messengers will help clarify signal transduction pathways. These secondary messengers may serve as targets for specific chemotherapeutic inhibitors of tyrosine kinase function.

As mentioned previously, proteins known to bind GTP are referred to as G proteins. Binding of GTP results in increased enzyme activity. Enzyme activity is also regulated by the length of time GTP remains bound before it is degraded to GDP. Stimulation of a cell-surface receptor results in an exchange of GDP for GTP, with the G protein converted to an activated configuration. While in the active state, secondary messengers are generated in specific signal transduction pathways, such as the phosphotidylinositol and protein kinase C systems (Fig. 14-30).

Hormonal activation of adenylate cyclase is an example of such a system. Binding of hormone to the β-adrenergic receptor results in activation of the G protein, Gs. The

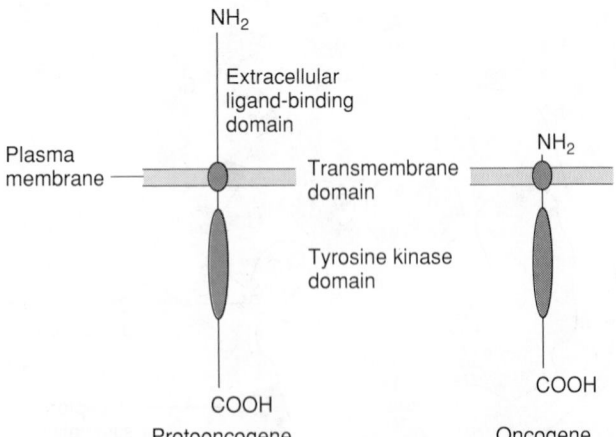

Figure 14-28. Relation of *erb* B protooncogene to the *erb* B oncogene. The *erb* B protooncogene includes an extracellular ligand-binding domain, a transmembrane domain, and an intracellular tyrosine kinase domain. The extracellular ligand-binding domain is truncated or absent in the *erb* B oncogene. (After Cooper GM. Oncogenes. Boston, Jones & Bartlett, 1990)

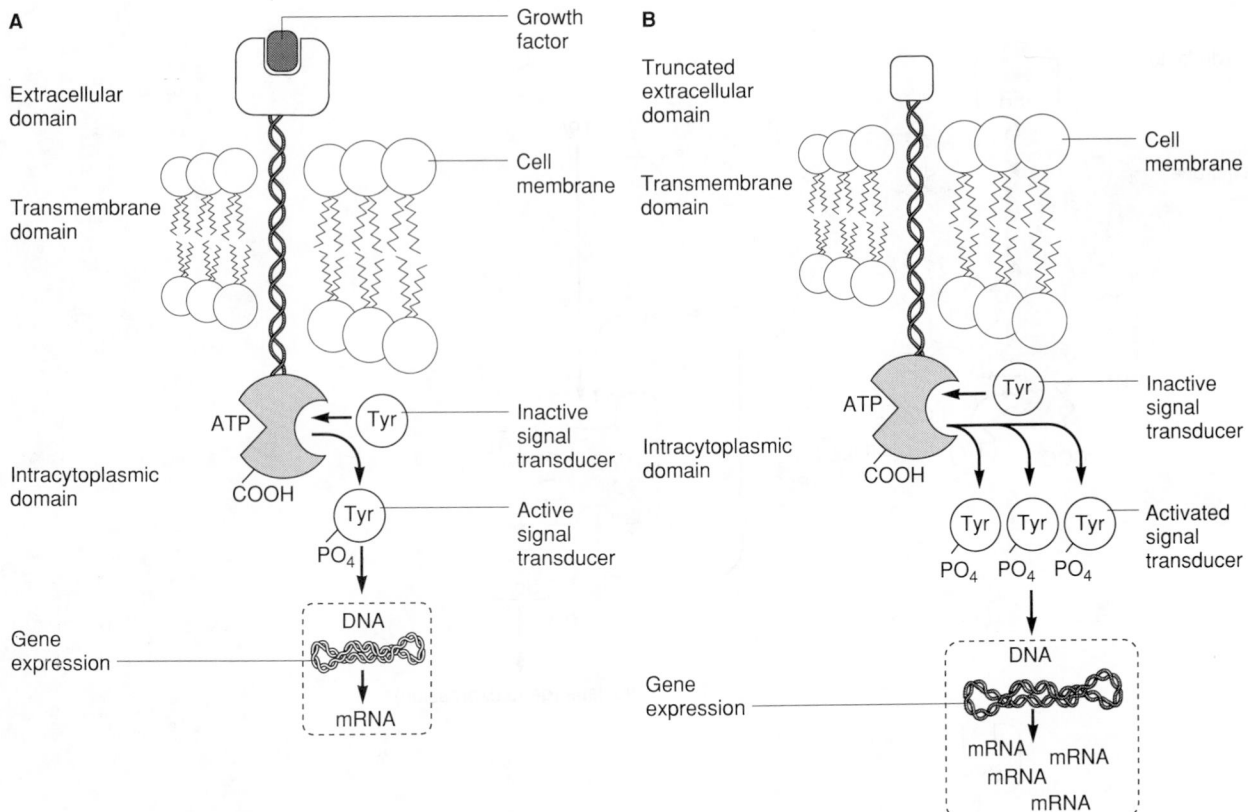

Figure 14-29. Schematic representation of growth factor receptors and intracellular events that follow ligand binding. (*A*) Normal growth factor receptors contain extracellular domains that bind the growth factor, a domain that spans the cell membrane, and an intracytoplasmic domain that acts as a tyrosine (Tyr) kinase for substrate proteins. Tyr phosphorylation, using ATP, activates intracellular proteins that in turn cause increased gene transcription. (*B*) Mutated growth factor receptors can lose a portion of the extracellular domain, resulting in continuous activation of the Tyr kinase intracellular domain. Continuous tyrosine phosphorylation results in a constant proliferative signal transmitted from the cell membrane to the nucleus. (After Arbeit JM. Molecules, cancer, and the surgeon. Ann Surg 1990;212:3)

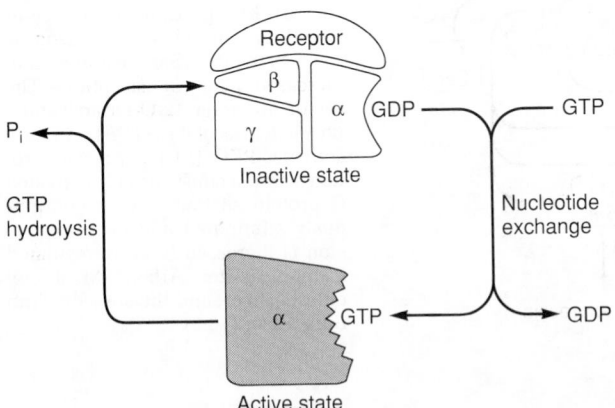

Figure 14-30. Regulation of membrane G proteins by guanine nucleotide binding. In the inactive state, the G protein α, β, and γ subunits are bound in a complex with GDP. Binding of a ligand to a cell-surface receptor induces the exchange of GTP for GDP. The β and γ subunits dissociate, and the activated γ unit interacts with its target molecule. Hydrolysis of GTP to GDP terminates a subunit activation. (After Cooper GM. Oncogenes. Boston, Jones & Bartlett, 1990)

activated Gs stimulates adenylate cyclase, which catalyzes the conversion of ATP to cAMP, a key second messenger.

The principal G proteins belong to the *ras* family of protooncogenes. Three members of the *ras* family have been identified and are designated as c-H-*ras*, c-K-*ras*, and c-N-*ras*. These genes encode related proteins localized to the inner surface of the cell membrane. As noted, activation of these proteins by cell-surface receptors results in the exchange of GDP for GTP and conversion to the activated state, with the generation of phospholipid-derived second messengers. A major component of this signal transduction process is the phosphotidylinositol system.

Activated G proteins may phosphorylate and activate phospholipase C, which splits phosphatidylinositol 4,5-biphosphate into inositol triphosphate and diacylglycerol. Inositol triphosphate stimulates release of calcium from intracellular stores, and diacylglycerol activates the protein kinase C in conjunction with released Ca^{2+}.

Activated protein kinase C results in a multitude of intracellular responses. Activated protein kinase C phosphorylates proteins on serine and threonine residues. There is also an increase in c-*fos* and c-*myc* expression, nuclear oncogenes thought to encode important mitogenic regulators. Protein kinase C phosphorylates and subsequently modulates the activity of growth factor receptors. The ability to activate, either directly or indirectly, the phosphotidylinositol system, protein kinase C, or both pathways is

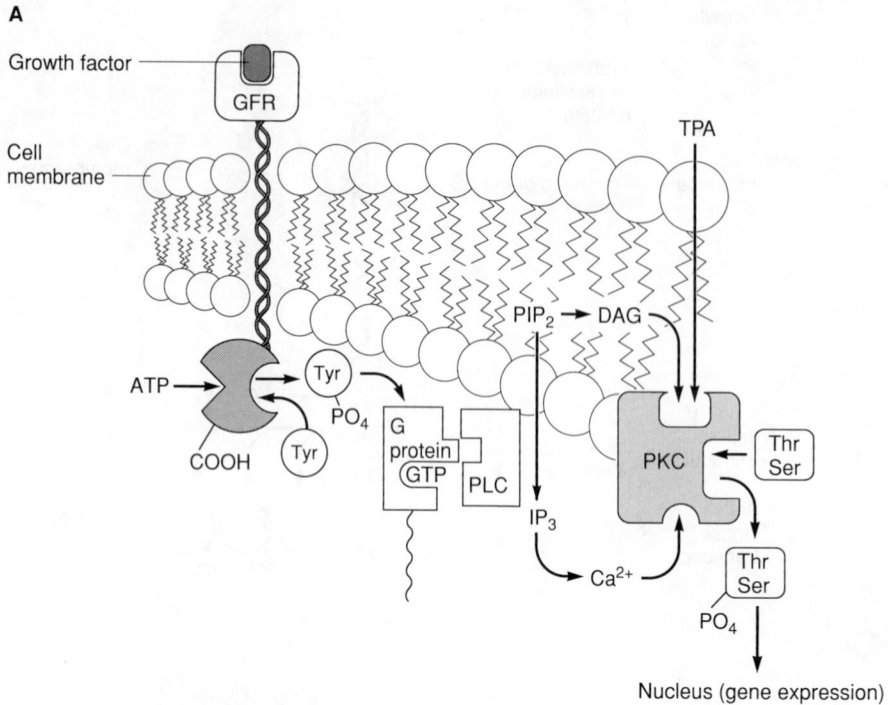

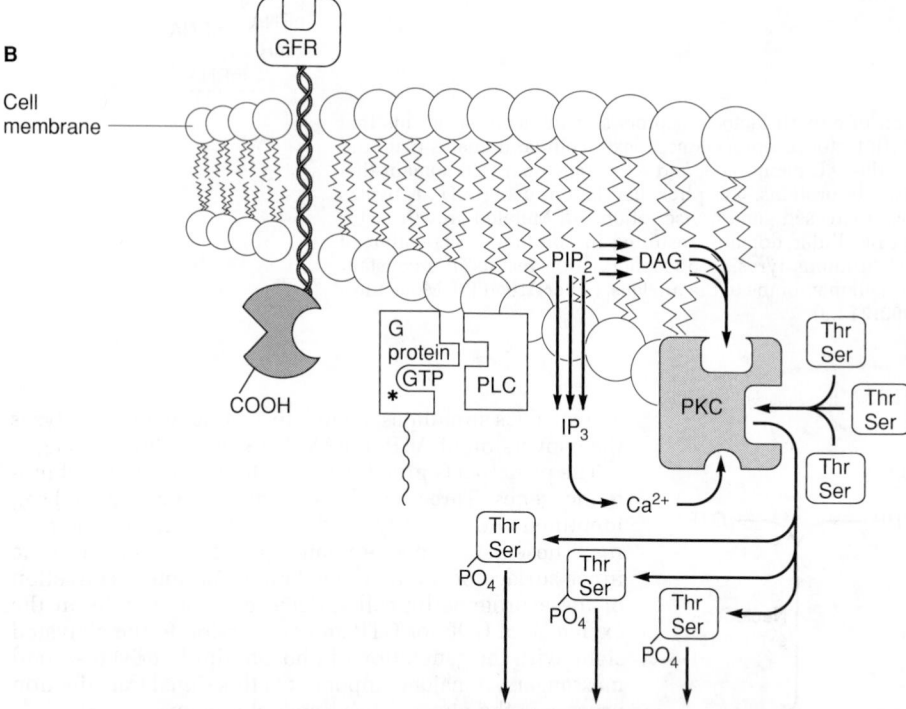

Figure 14-31. (*A*) Growth factor receptor (GFR) occupation can activate phospholipase C (PLC) by means of stimulatory G proteins. Hydrolysis of IP_2 by PLC results in subsequent activation of protein kinase C (PKC), phosphorylation of intracellular proteins on threonine (Thr) or serine (Ser) residues, and increased gene transcription. The tumor promoter 12-O-tetradecanoyl phorbol-13-acetate (TPA) directly activates PKC. (*B*) The *ras* oncoprotein acts as a constitutively activated G protein so that PKC is continuously stimulated and gene expression is increased in an unregulated fashion. (After Arbeit JM. Molecules, cancer, and the surgeon. Ann Surg 1990;212:3)

shared by a number of receptor kinases, nonreceptor tyrosine kinases, and G proteins (Fig. 14-31).

Thus, the abnormal expression or activation of the receptors or any of the molecules within the signal system may be responsible for transformation of the cell. An example of this concept is the characteristic point mutations of the *ras* gene, which result in a constitutively activated protein. Mutations at positions 12, 13, or 61 within the *ras* gene result in proteins capable of increasing the rate of GDP–GTP exchange or decreasing hydrolysis of GTP and conversion of the enzyme to its inactive state (Fig. 14-32). The

protein kinase C system thus receives continual proliferative signals, ultimately leading to cell transformation.

Proteins with serine and threonine kinase activity have also been identified. Members of the *raf* gene family are thought to play a role in the signal transduction of several growth factor systems. Unlike most of the tyrosine kinases, these oncogene products are found as soluble cytoplasmic proteins. The raf proteins may be intermediate cytoplasmic signal transducers, coupling signals originating at the cell membrane to the final consequences of gene expression within the nucleus. Other proteins with serine–threonine

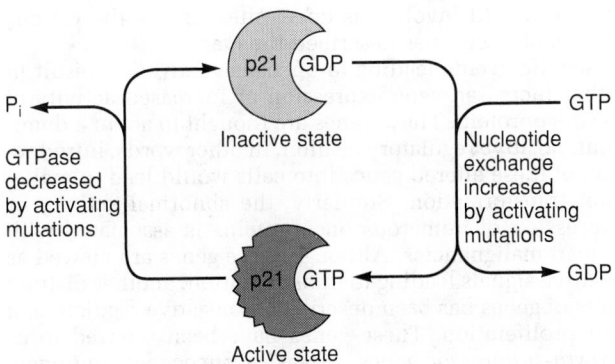

Figure 14-32. The *ras* protein (p21) is maintained in an abnormally activated state by mutations that increase exchange of GDP for GTP or decrease GTPase activity. (After Cooper GM. Oncogenes. Boston, Jones & Bartlett, 1990)

kinase activity include members of the protein kinase C family, c-*mos*, and c-*pim*-1. As seen repeatedly throughout this discussion, altered or abnormal expression of a normal protooncogene results in the production of an oncoprotein with transforming potential. This also applies to the protein–serine–threonine kinases. Deletion of a normal amino-terminal regulatory domain results in a constitutively activated protein with full transforming ability.

It becomes clear that many of the protooncogenes function normally as integrated members of precise signal transduction pathways. Malignant transformation must ultimately involve abnormal mitogenic signals transmitted to the cell nucleus and the subsequent loss of the normal gene expression. Therefore, it is logical to expect some oncogenes to encode proteins that are localized to the nucleus. These genes are termed *nuclear oncogenes* (Table 14-8): c-*fos*, c-*jun*, c-*myb*, c-*myc*, and n-*myc*. They function as transcriptional regulatory molecules. The c-erb-a protein is a thyroid hormone receptor whose function may be to serve as a negative regulator of thyroid-induced cell proliferation.

The c-fos and c-jun oncogene products are components of a transcriptional activator termed AP-1. Binding of the fos and jun proteins forms a heterodimer with enhanced DNA-binding affinity. This heterodimer binds to an AP-1 target site on the DNA, with the ultimate result being increased transcription of the AP-1 target genes (Fig. 14-33). Interestingly, the role of c-fos and c-jun products as transcriptional activators is regulated by protein kinase C activity. As previously discussed, protein kinase C is important in growth factor signal transduction pathways and is itself a potential oncogene. Thus, transcriptional factors such as c-*fos* and c-*jun*, which are influenced by protein kinase C activity, may represent the nuclear component of a signal pathway initially starting with a ligand-binding event at the cell surface.

The transforming potential of these nuclear oncogenes would presumably result as an alteration of their normal role in signal transduction systems leading to cell proliferation. The constitutive expression of these transcriptional activators could thus represent one potential mechanism of malignant transformation.

The c-*erb*-A gene functions as a thyroid hormone receptor. Its ability to function as an oncogene results from a somewhat different mechanism than that discussed for c-*fos* and c-*jun*. Normally, the gene product is thought to repress transcription in the absence of hormone. Binding of thyroid releases this negative regulation, resulting in transcription of the target genes. Evidence from several laboratories indicates that the c-*erb*-A oncoprotein has lost the ability to bind thyroid hormone. The oncoprotein is thus functioning as a constitutive, hormone-independent repressor of thyroid hormone-inducible genes. This loss of normal function leads to increased transforming potential (Fig. 14-34).

Nuclear oncogenes in the *myc* family, as noted previously, are activated in a wide variety of human malignancies. The exact mechanism of malignant transformation as a result of *myc* activation remains to be elucidated. It appears that changes in cell cycle regulation may be involved. Oncoproteins from c-*myc* may stimulate cells to progress from G_1 into S phase (DNA synthesis), resulting in persistent cellular proliferation by inducing the target gene expression.

The review of oncogenes has thus far emphasized their various biochemical and structural characteristics. It becomes clear that most of these protooncogenes function normally as specific components in elegant signal trans-

Table 14-8. **NUCLEAR ONCOGENE PRODUCTS**

Protooncogene	Protein Molecular Weight
Thyroid hormone receptor (*erb*)	52,000
myc Family	
c-*myc*	64,000
L-*myc*	66,000
N-*myc*	64,000
Transcription factor AP-1 components	
c-*jun*	47,000
jun-B	40,000
jun-D	40,000
c-*fos*	62,000
fra-1	38,000
fos-B	45,000
Other nuclear oncogenes	
myb	75,000
ets-1	51,000
ets-2	56,000
ski	60,000
rel	68,000

(Adapted from Cooper GM. Oncogenes. Boston, Jones & Bartlett, 1990)

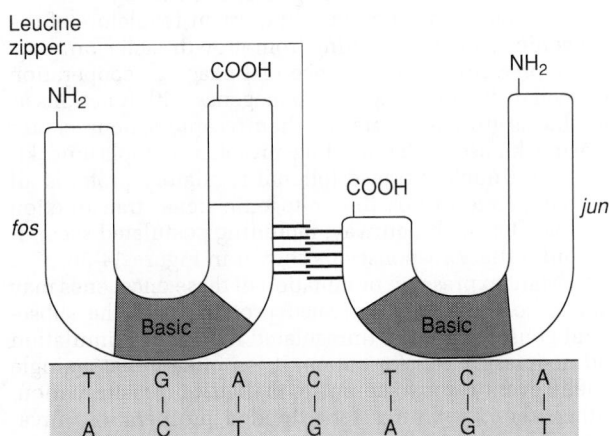

Figure 14-33. Interdigitation of leucine side chains of *jun* and *fos* form a leucine zipper. The *jun–fos* heterodimer binds to an AP-1 target site to provide transcriptional regulation. (After Cooper GM. Oncogenes. Boston, Jones & Bartlett, 1990)

Thyroid hormone receptor

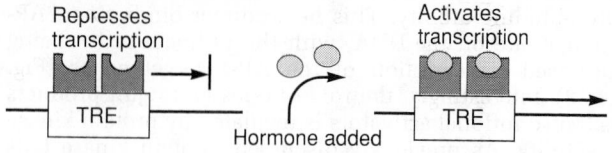

erb **A oncogene**

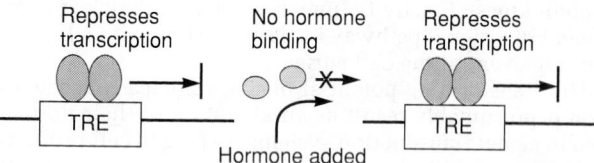

Figure 14-34. The thyroid hormone receptor (*erb* A protoonco-gene) binds to the thyroid hormone response element (TRE) to repress transcription. Thyroid hormone binding converts the receptor to a transcriptional activator, and target genes are expressed. The *erb* A oncogene has lost the ability to bind thyroid hormone and therefore acts as a constitutive repressor of thyroid hormone responsive genes. (After Cooper GM. Oncogenes. Boston, Jones & Bartlett, 1990)

duction pathways. In the normally regulated cell, binding of extracellular ligands by specific cell membrane receptors is ultimately transmitted as a mitogenic signal to the cell nucleus. The final response involves increased transcription of target genes, DNA synthesis, and cell proliferation. It has been demonstrated that many of the protooncogenes are linked and act in a cooperative fashion involving signal transduction. For example, binding of PDGF at its receptor on fibroblasts results in increased transcription of the c-*myc* gene (Fig. 14-35). Examples of binding of specific growth factors and activation of the receptor with subsequent changes in activity or expression of linked protooncogene products have been demonstrated in several systems.

As discussed, activation of PDGF and EGF receptor tyrosine kinases results in increased activation of the phosphotidylinositol and protein kinase C systems. Similarly, PDGF binding may result in tyrosine phosphorylation of the c-*raf* kinase, with subsequent increase in its enzyme activity. Growth factor stimulation may also regulate the transcription of nuclear oncogenes, such as c-*fos* and c-*jun*. These in turn function as important regulators of the mitogenic signals originating from growth factor binding. This represents clear evidence of linkage or cooperation between different oncogenes. Oncogenes with functions as variable as growth factors and their receptors, nonreceptor tyrosine kinases, GTP-binding proteins, cytoplasmic kinases, and nuclear transcriptional regulatory proteins all may cooperate in possible mitogenic signal transduction circuits. One such pathway, including postulated secondary and tertiary responses, is shown in Figure 14-36.

Aberrant expression or mutation of these oncogenes may lead to constitutively activated proteins with the subsequent consequences of unregulated mitogenic stimulation and neoplastic transformation. It is unlikely that a single genetic event leads to complete malignant transformation. Rather, the capabilities for extended proliferation, invasion of adjacent tissues, and metastasis are probably acquired as a sequence of genetic events. Multiple changes in the elaborate biochemical circuitry would require abnormal expression or activation of several cooperating oncogenes. The gradual acquisition of these molecular

changes could involve, as target sites, any of the various classes of oncogenes described thus far.

Genetic events leading to oncogene activation result in either increased gene expression or increased activity of the oncoprotein. These genes are thought to act in a dominant, positive regulatory fashion. In other words, introduction of these altered genes into cells would lead to malignant transformation. Similarly, the abnormal activity or expression of numerous oncoproteins is associated with human malignancies. Although these genes are viewed as positive signals leading to transformation, another distinct class of genes has been described as negative regulators of cell proliferation. These genes have been referred to as *growth-suppressor genes, recessive oncogenes, antioncogenes,* or *tumor-suppressor genes.* The loss of these genes would allow tumor development. The loss of tumor-suppressor genes is a recessive change in the sense that the loss of function leads to the loss of normal growth-inhibitory signals. Tumor-suppressor genes may function as governors of growth and proliferative signals, and actually suppress malignant transformation.

Evidence of tumor-suppressor genes is derived from several lines of investigations.[8] Karyotype analysis revealed that certain malignancies have characteristic losses of specific chromosomes, and the technique of chromosomal banding demonstrated the deletion of particular chromosomal bands in other diploid cancers. More detailed information about the existence of tumor-suppressor genes developed from cell hybridization experiments, the study of familial cancers, and the loss of heterozygosity in tumors. Experiments involving fusion between malignant and normal cells yielded hybrids that were nontumorigenic. Tumorigenicity was thought to be suppressed in the hybrids by the addition of genetic material that was absent in the original malignant cells (Fig. 14-37).

If genetic changes are fundamental to the cancer process, then certain malignancies should have congenital patterns of expression. Genetic analysis of families with hereditary and sporadic retinoblastomas has provided evidence for the role of tumor-suppressor genes in human tumors. In inherited retinoblastomas, an abnormal retinoblastoma (*Rb*) gene is transmitted to half the offspring. As long as a normal allele is present, the tumor does not develop, and the abnormal germ-line mutation behaves in a recessive fashion; however, a second mutation of the normal allele (somatic cell mutation) may occur in a retinal cell, leading to the development of the tumor. Thus, loss of both parental alleles of the suppressor gene results in malignant trans-

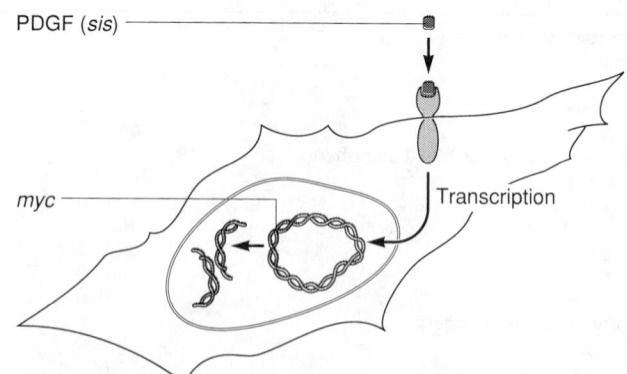

Figure 14-35. Protooncogenes can act cooperatively in proliferative signal transduction. Stimulation of quiescent fibroblasts with platelet-derived growth factor (PDGF; *sis* protooncogene product) stimulates c-*myc* transcription. (After Cooper GM. Oncogenes. Boston, Jones & Bartlett, 1990)

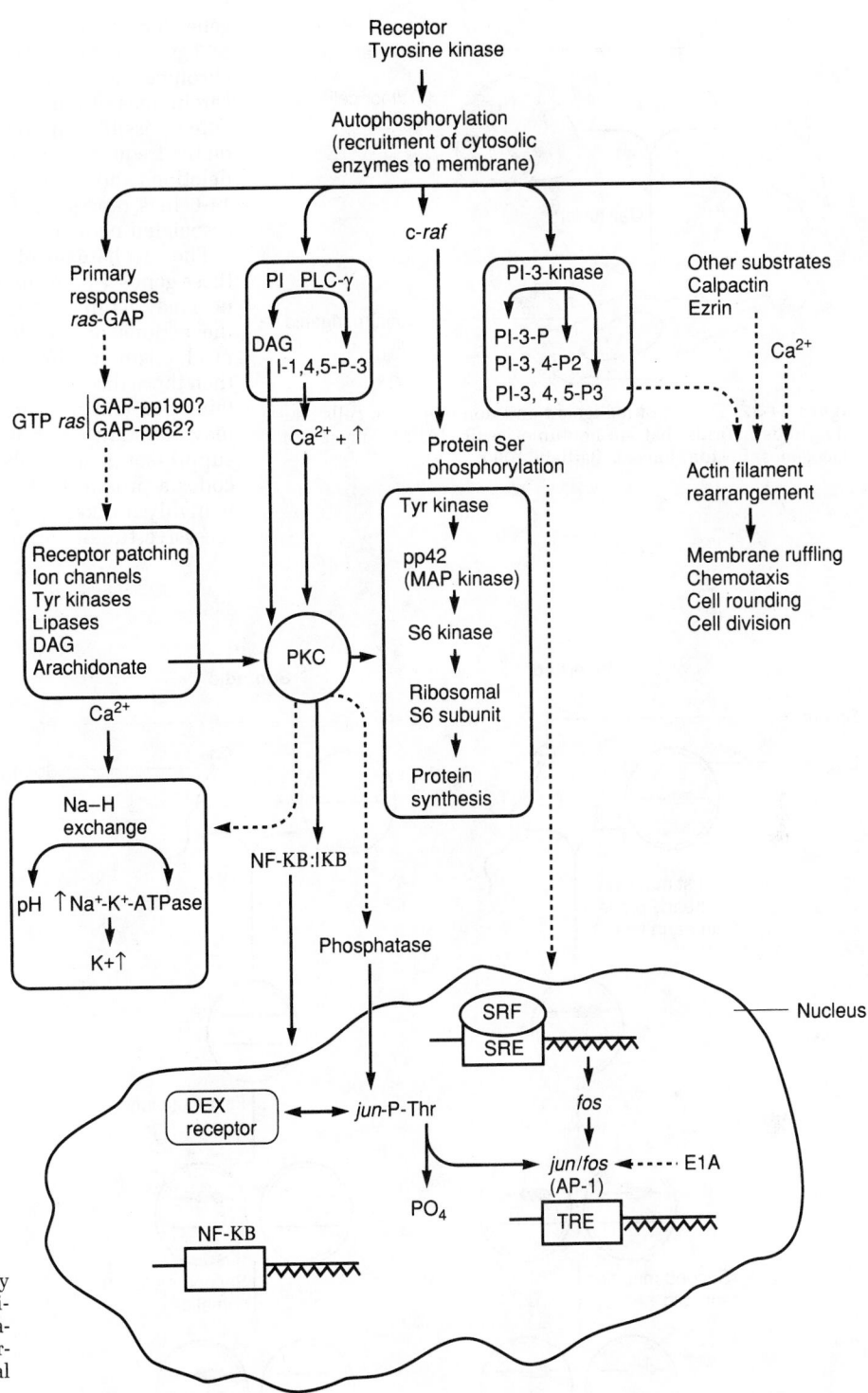

Figure 14-36. A cascade of primary and secondary responses can be initiated by receptor tyrosine kinase activation. (After Cantley LC, Auger KR, Carpenter C, et al. Oncogenes and signal transduction. Cell 1991;64:281)

formation of the retinal cell. In sporadic retinoblastomas, development of a tumor requires two somatic mutations (Fig. 14-38). In either case, the result is the loss of any normal allele capable of inhibiting tumor formation. The genetic loss in retinoblastomas involves deletion of chromosome 13q14.

Using the technique of RFLP, tumor-suppressor genes can be identified through the loss of heterozygosity of the allele in question or a specific marker associated with that allele. Heterozygosity refers to the presence of two different alleles for a given gene. RFLP allows the identification of these different alleles based on differences in the restriction sites of DNA-digesting enzymes. After treatment with the restriction endonucleases, the DNA can be hybridized with a polymorphic gene probe (Fig. 14-39). This reveals the differences in the alleles for the gene locus in question. In the *Rb* gene example, presence of heterozygosity at the *Rb* locus prevents tumor development because of the influence of the normal wild-type allele. Loss of this wild-type allele in a second genetic event results in the absence of a normal tumor-suppressor gene product and the subsequent development of tumor formation (Fig. 14-40).

The *Rb* gene is only one example of a tumor-suppressor

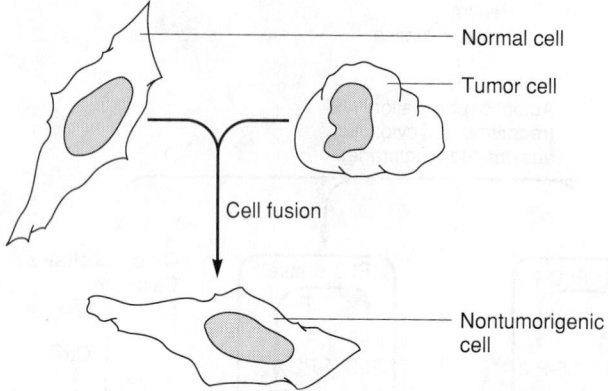

Figure 14-37. Fusion of malignant and nonneoplastic cells usually yields hybrids that are nontumorigenic. (After Cooper GM. Oncogenes. Boston, Jones & Bartlett, 1990)

gene thought to be involved in human malignancies. The *p53* gene, named for the protein it encodes and located on chromosome 17q12, is a suppressor gene implicated in carcinomas of the breast, lung, colon, and osteosarcomas. Other possible suppressor genes are thought to exist based on the frequency and consistency of specific chromosomal deletions and rearrangements in certain neoplasms. Table 14-6 lists representative tumor-suppressor genes and the associated neoplasms.

The mechanism of action of the proteins encoded by these genes is being examined. In general, these gene products may act in a coordinated, balanced fashion to regulate the actions of the dominantly transforming genes. The mechanisms to do so may be even more widely ranging than those discussed for the dominant oncogenes. The proteins p53 and p105-Rb are nuclear phosphoproteins that may function as transcriptional regulators. The tumor-suppressor gene involved in neurofibromatosis type 1 encodes a protein that may regulate several ras proteins. It is highly unlikely that any of the dominant oncogenes or recessive tumor-suppressor genes would function in any

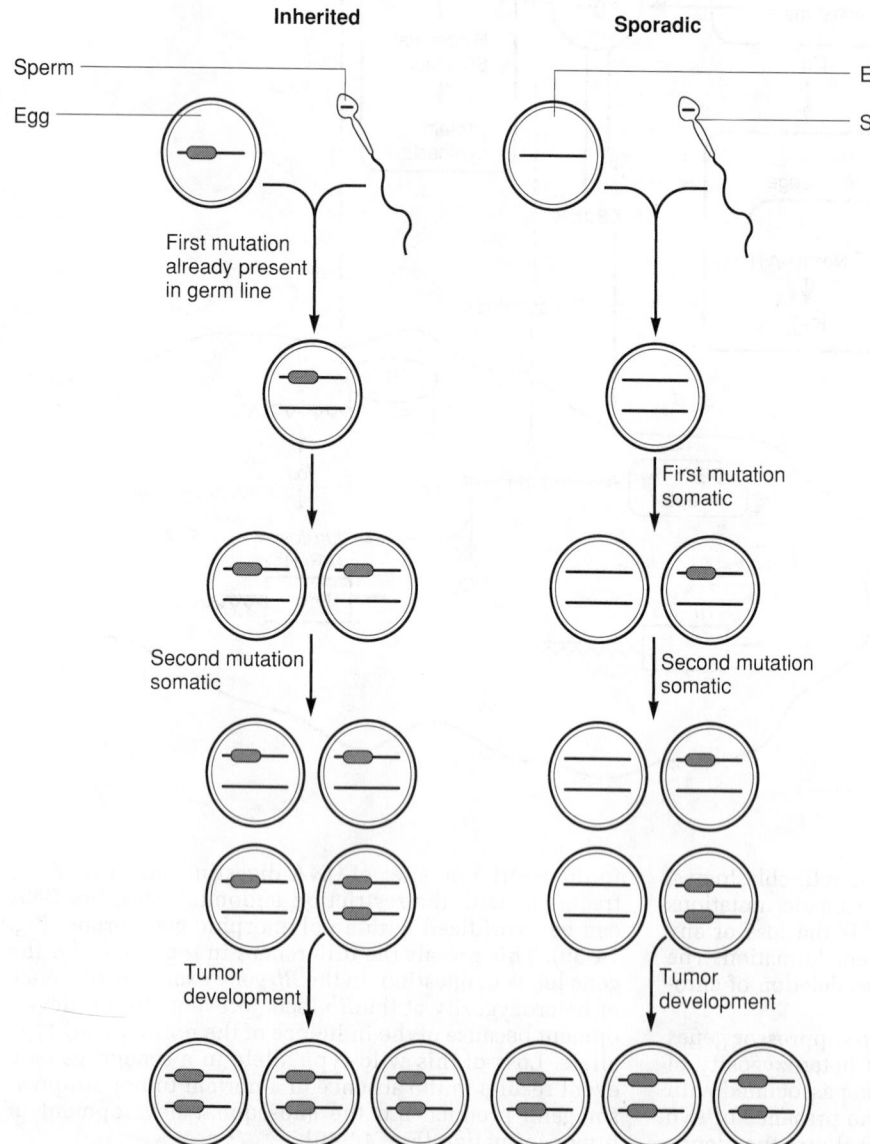

Figure 14-38. The model for development of retinoblastoma has served as a model for tumor-suppressor gene function. In inherited retinoblastoma, a mutation is transmitted through the gene line of the affected parent. The second mutation occurs somatically in a retinal cell. The second mutation leads to the development of a tumor. In sporadic retinoblastoma, two somatic mutations precede tumor development. (After Cooper GM. Oncogenes. Boston, Jones & Bartlett, 1990)

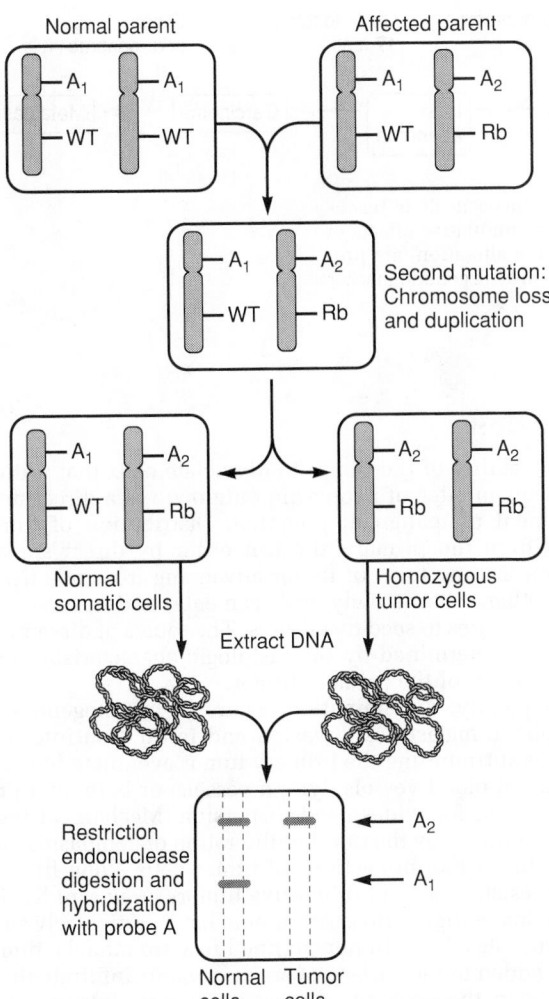

Figure 14-39. Restriction fragment-length polymorphism can be used to detect loss of normal allele in retinoblastoma tumor cells. A retinoblastoma (Rb) mutation is linked to marker A_2, and affected patients are heterozygous at this locus, with somatic cells containing both A_1 and A_2. After a somatic mutation causing loss of A_1, tumor cells become heterozygous for the A_2 marker. This homozygosity can be detected by restriction endonuclease digestion and hybridization with probe A. (After Cooper GM. Oncogenes. Boston, Jones & Bartlett, 1990)

mutually exclusive fashion. Rather, these genes are likely to function in a precise, coordinated biochemical circuit of elaborate checks and balances.

Carcinogenesis is thought to be a progressive accumulation of unique genetic alterations.[9] These changes result ultimately in the loss of normal regulation of growth and differentiation. Models proposing specific genetic changes related to the particular steps of initiation and progression have been developed. Each step in the process is associated with the acquisition of additional neoplastic characteristics. Thus, the capability of unregulated proliferation, invasiveness, and metastasis may be the result of specific molecular alterations. Most of the evidence linking specific genetic lesions to the steps in this progression is empiric. As the functions of the tumor-suppressor genes are defined and integrated with the proposed roles of the dominant oncogenes, a cohesive mechanistic and biochemical pattern of malignant transformation may emerge.

A genetic model for colorectal tumorigenesis has been proposed[10] (Fig. 14-41) that includes the following salient features:

1. Colorectal tumors appear to arise as a result of the mutational activation of dominant oncogenes coupled with the mutational inactivation of tumor-suppressor genes.
2. Mutations in at least four or five genes are required for full malignant transformation. It is the total accumulation of changes rather that the sequence of the accumulation that is important.
3. Mutant tumor-suppressor genes may predispose to further genetic changes even when present in the heterozygous state.

Metastatic ability is likely to be related to the acquisition of other, as yet undefined, alterations.

This discussion has outlined remarkable advances in understanding the molecular basis of human malignancies. These discoveries include the activation of dominant oncogenes and the loss of tumor-suppressor genes. It is becoming clear that these genes play fundamental roles not only in the pathogenesis of neoplastic cells but also in the development, differentiation, and growth of normal cells. The future holds promise that these revelations of molecular biology will become useful in the care of the cancer patient. Application of this knowledge may prove benefi-

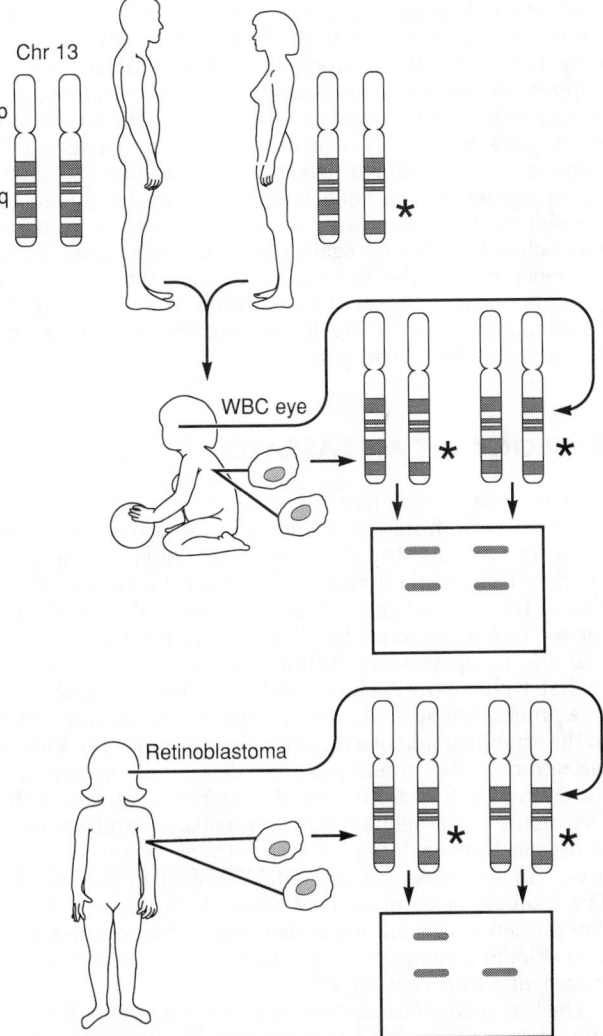

Figure 14-40. The tumor-suppressor gene paradigm as illustrated by the retinoblastoma gene. (After Arbeit JM. Molecules, cancer, and the surgeon. Ann Surg 1990;212:3)

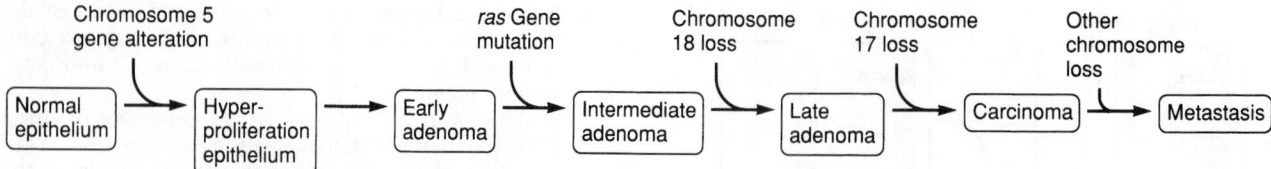

Figure 14-41. Model of colorectal tumorigenesis proposed by Vogelstein. Oncogenesis is postulated to be a multistep process involving a series of genetic alterations. The cumulative effects of oncogene activation and tumor-suppressor gene loss, but not the order of the alteration, are proposed to be crucial for neoplastic transformation. (After Fearen ER, Vogelstein B. A genetic marker for colorectal tumorigenesis. Cell 1990;61:759)

cial in terms of diagnosis, prognosis, and treatment. As noted, identification of allelic deletions in the *Rb* gene can be used in screening to detect high-risk people. Deletions of chromosome 5 have been identified in patients with the hereditary familial polyposis syndrome. The use of oncogenes as prognostic indicators is also continuing to evolve. For example, amplification of the *her-2/neu* gene in breast cancer is associated with both an increased frequency of lymph node metastasis and decreased disease-free survival. Similarly, amplification of N-*myc* in neuroblastomas is predictive of rapid disease progression and unresponsiveness to chemotherapy.

More challenging is the development of molecular antineoplastic therapy. The most direct therapeutic application would be the introduction of functional tumor-suppressor genes into neoplastic cells. Unfortunately, this would require the formidable task of introducing the desired gene into every cancer cell. A more reasonable approach may involve targeting the protein products of oncogenes. Exceptional specificity may be gained by developing unique tyrosine kinase inhibitors or by using monoclonal antibodies against overexpressed growth factor receptors. In the future, the surgeon who wishes to provide optimal care will be required to understand the molecular events affecting the presentation, prognosis, and treatment of the cancer patient.[11]

BIOLOGY OF METASTASIS

Metastasis is the active or passive dissemination of neoplastic disease from the site of origin to a distant site or organ in the host. In cancer, the primary site undergoes changes that enable tumor cells to enter the microcirculation (intravasation) and thereafter increases the possibility for seeding distal sites. Seeding follows the traversing of vascular compartments, followed by adherence to endothelial walls, extravasation, and invasion of the stroma. The process has several critical steps that ultimately result in the establishment of a metastatic site (Fig. 14-42). Vascularization of the tumor provides the initial opportunity for entry into the circulation. As tumor cells traverse the vasculature, microemboli may trap cells in capillary beds of organs, thus enabling adherence to the vessel wall, followed by extravasation and establishment in the stroma. The biologic basis of each of these stages remains to be determined, but as our understanding of this complex process emerges, we are presented with more possibilities for therapeutic intervention.

The treatment of cancer encompasses surgery, radiotherapy, chemotherapy, and immunotherapy. Singly, none of these modalities offers cure in most instances. Usually, treatment includes several approaches. In nearly all instances, the objective is eradication of metastatic seedings.

Invasion

The ability of the tumor to dissociate cells that initiate subsequent sites of neoplastic outgrowth is a direct measurement of malignant potential. Distribution of tumor cells from the primary site can occur by direct spread, with a leading front of tumor advancing from one tissue to another. Alternatively, cells can enter and traverse coelomic cavities to seed distal sites. The routes of dissemination are determined by the histologic characteristics and the location of the primary tumor.

Frequently, dissemination occurs as hematogenous or lymphatic metastases. Invasion and infiltration into host tissues surrounding the primary tumor eventuate in penetration of blood vessels, lymph vessels, or both, and provide access for widespread dispersion. Mechanical pressure produced by the rapid proliferation of neoplasms may force finger-like projections of tumor cells along lines of least resistance. Not all invasive tumors grow rapidly; indeed, many highly invasive tumors have particularly slow growth rates. Even in nonconfined in vitro models, tumor cells added to the surface of organ explants infiltrate these tissues in the absence of pressure factors. Intrinsic cell motility may play a role in tumor cell invasion. The rates of migration of tumor cells and homologous normal cells are assayed primarily by in vitro techniques. In these systems, an association exists between increased cell motility and tumorigenic potential.

Normal cells grown in monolayer culture are contact-inhibited with regard to directional locomotion. Malignant cells do not demonstrate contact inhibition. If a similar lack of constraint is displayed within three-dimensional structures, then invasive cells may demonstrate considerable mobility. Tumor cells possess the organelles necessary for active locomotion and can form cellular cytoplasmic processes, indicative of motility, during the invasive process. Inhibition of cell motility prevents invasion in some in vitro models. For example, treatment of tumor cells with cytoskeleton-disrupting agents before introduction into experimental animals alters metastatic patterns. Little correlation is seen, however, between the absence of contact inhibition in tumor cells growing as monolayer cultures and their invasive behavior when implanted in vivo. Cell motility is only one of a number of conditions that must be present before tumor cells can successfully invade distant tissues.

Evidence for the involvement of tissue-degradative enzymes in neoplastic invasion is convincing. The production and activation of specific tissue-destructive enzymes such as lysosomal hydrolases and collagenases has been documented in tumor invasion. Destruction of host tissue by hydrolytic enzymes, aided by pressure atrophy and the occlusion of blood and lymph vessels by an expanding tumor mass, facilitates infiltration of neoplastic tissue. Histologic examination of tissues obtained from sites of tumor

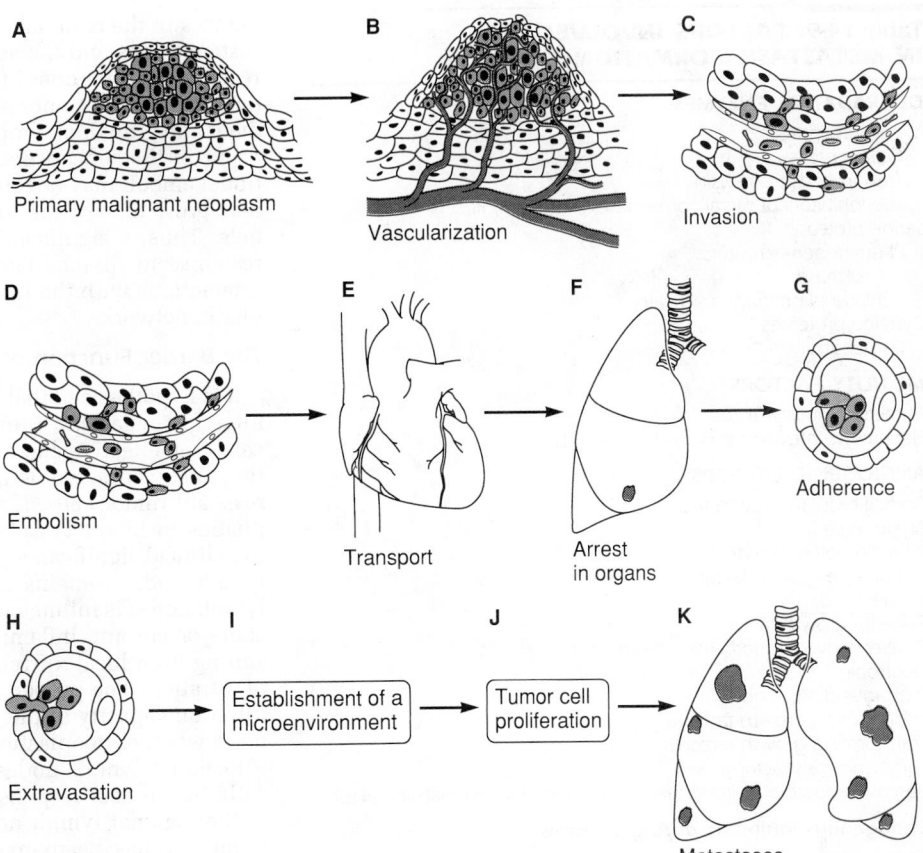

A
Primary malignant neoplasm

B
Vascularization

C
Invasion

D
Embolism

E
Transport

F
Arrest in organs

G
Adherence

H
Extravasation

I
Establishment of a microenvironment

J
Tumor cell proliferation

K
Metastases

Figure 14-42. Steps in the formation of metastatic cancer. (After Fidler IJ, Balch CM. The biology of cancer metastasis and implications for therapy. Curr Probl Surg 1987;24:136)

invasion displays considerable variation in the degree of tissue damage, and many human and animal malignant neoplasms express higher levels of lytic enzymes than benign tumors or corresponding normal tissues. Lysosomal catheptic activities are elevated within some tumor tissues, and increased production of cathepsin B in breast carcinomas has been observed compared with that in normal or benign tissue.

Enhanced production and secretion of the serine protease plasminogen activator has been associated with the neoplastic transformation of a variety of cell types. A major focus of investigation is the possible role of this enzyme in invasion and metastasis. Many normal cells produce high levels of plasminogen activator, and variants of murine melanoma cell lines with different invasive capacities show no consistent correlation between malignant behavior in vivo and plasminogen activator production or secretion. Clearly, the relative importance of different enzymes could vary from one tumor system to another.

Invasion of normal tissues, intercellular matrices, and vascular basement membranes by metastatic cells requires the active participation of hydrolytic enzymes. Connective tissue proteins are classified into four major groups: collagen, elastin, glycoproteins, and proteoglycans. The distribution of each protein varies among different tissues. The constituents of the extracellular matrix are stabilized and organized by interactions among the tissue proteins, and the stability is easily disordered by degradative enzymes released from tumor cells.

Both intravasation and extravasation are pivotal in hematogenous, systemic metastasis. In either instance, the tumor cells are confronted with a barrier significantly composed of type IV collagen. Type IV collagen is a major structural protein of basement membranes between paren-

chymal cells and the connective tissue on which cells rest. A strong correlation exists between the ability of murine tumor cells to produce spontaneous metastases and their ability to produce increased levels of collagenase IV. Tumor cells that invade blood vessels or leave capillaries of distant organs in which they have lodged must penetrate the basement membrane. Dissolution of the basement membrane, suggestive of enzymatic action, has been observed in areas adjacent to arrested tumor cells.

The collagenase prepared from metastatic murine tumor cells preferentially digests this basement membrane collagen. Cells recovered from the venous effluent of a murine fibrosarcoma, potentially the invasive population, solubilized basement membrane collagen to a significantly greater extent than cells from the parent population. It appears that metastatic tumor cells exhibit a preferential attachment to type IV collagen substrates. Because tumor cells can lodge selectively in areas of endothelial damage, the possession of high levels of collagenase type IV may be fundamental to invasion and metastasis (Table 14-9).

Lymphatic and Hematogenous Spread

Clinical observations give the impression that carcinomas spread by the lymphatic route and mesenchymal tumors spread by means of the bloodstream. This impression is erroneous. Lymphatic and vascular systems have numerous connections. Experimentally, it has been shown that disseminating tumor cells can pass from one system to another. The two systems are inseparable, and the division into lymphatic spread and hematogenous spread is an arbitrary one used only for the sake of academic discussion. The next sections treat the vascular and lymphatic dissemination of neoplastic cells separately, with no intent to associate tumor histiotype with the routes of migration.

Table 14-9. FACTORS INVOLVED IN METASTASIS FORMATION

DEGRADATIVE ENZYMES

Metalloproteinases
  Collagenases
  Transin and stromelysin
Tissue inhibitors of metalloproteinases (TIMP) I, II, III
Serine proteases
  Plasminogen activators
    Urokinase
    Tissue plasminogen activator
Cysteine proteases
  Cathepsins

MOTILITY FACTORS

Autocrine motility factor
Hepatocyte growth factor and scatter factor

ANGIOGENIC FACTORS

Acidic fibroblast growth factor
Angiogenin
Basic fibroblast growth factor
Hepatocyte growth factor
Interleukin-8
Placenta growth factor
Platelet-derived endothelial cell growth factor
Pleotropin
Prostaglandin E_1 and E_2
Transforming growth factor α
Transforming growth factor β
Tumor necrosis factor α
Vascular endothelial growth factor and vascular permeability factor

Endogenous Inhibitors of Angiogenesis

Angiostatin
Cartilage-derived inhibitor
Heparinase
Interferon
Platelet factor 4
Prolactin fragment
Protamine
Thrombospondin
Tissue inhibitor of metalloproteinase

ADHESION MOLECULES

Carcinoembryonic antigen
Proteoglycans
Intercellular adhesion molecule 1
Selectins
CD43
CD44
E-cadherin
P-cadherin
Integrins

Lymphatic Dissemination

The process of infiltration and expansion into host tissues results in the penetration of small lymphatic vessels by tumor cells. Tumor cell emboli in the vessels are responsible for initiation of lymphatic metastases. Tumor emboli may be trapped in the first lymph node encountered. Metastatic emboli may traverse lymph nodes or even bypass them to form distant nodal metastases (*skip metastasis*).

Lymph nodes are immunologically responsive in patients with neoplasms. Lymph nodes in the area of a primary neoplasm are often enlarged and clinically palpable, signifying hyperplasia of lymph node follicles accompanied by proliferation of reticulum cells and sinus endothelium or growth of tumor cells. Tumor presence stimulates the activation, proliferation, and release of immunocompetent cells in the lymphoreticular system. The reaction commences in the regional lymph nodes and later proceeds to distant nodes and the spleen. Proliferative changes in the regional lymph nodes often precede the spread and subsequent growth of tumor emboli within them. Initial entrapment and growth of lymphatic-borne tumor emboli usually occur in the subcapsular sinus of the lymph node. Additional emboli may be released from the sinus, or the tumor may grow toward the hilar region and the efferent channels. Thus, a significant proportion of the host immune response to disseminated tumor growth occurs through interactions with the immune cells in the peripheral lymphatic network.

The Barrier Function of Lymph Nodes

It is hypothesized that lymph nodes serve as a temporary filter for metastatic tumor cells. Although lymph nodes can be an effective, but temporary, barrier to tumor spread, they also can serve as a repository for immunoselected, resistant tumor cells. If tumor cells translocate from lymphatics to blood vessels and back with great ease, then the clinical significance of malignant cells trapped within lymph nodes remains a question. Filtration capacity of lymph nodes is influenced in several ways. Tumor growth, acute or chronic inflammatory reactions, and fibrosis resulting from local x-irradiation may reduce the efficiency of filtration. The properties of tumor cells, rather than the filtration capacity of the lymph node, may actually determine whether neoplastic cells are trapped and destroyed.

Regional lymph nodes may be involved immunologically in the host response to neoplasms. The importance of the regional lymph nodes to the initiation of systemic immunity has been investigated in a series of models. Adoptive transfer of regional lymph node cells by intraperitoneal administration from tumor-bearing animals to normal animals induces tumor allograft immunity. Furthermore, skin allografts lacking lymphatic connections are tolerated only until restoration of the lymphatic system occurs. Construction of skin pedicles in guinea pigs lacking afferent lymphatics leads to indefinite retention of skin allografts.

Twenty years ago, the classic concept of en bloc resection of primary tumors of the breast and their regional lymph nodes was challenged. The retention of the regional lymph nodes free of metastatic cells was hypothesized to be important in maintaining a high level of systemic tumor immunity to aid in preventing growth of disseminated micrometastases. Subsequent clinical trials comparing simple and radical mastectomy showed no improvement in survival rates of patients and an increased incidence of axillary lymph node metastasis in the patients who underwent simple mastectomy.

Studies in animals revealed that the regional lymph nodes may be important for the initiation of immunity against a transplantable syngeneic tumor in mice. The effect is dependent on the antigenicity of the tumor. Immunogenicity is assessed based on the ability of the tumor to induce complete protection against transplant challenge in syngeneic hosts. In weakly immunogenic tumors, regional lymph nodes were important in the initiation of systemic immunity, but strongly immunogenic tumors induced systemic immunity independent of the presence of the regional lymph nodes.

The contradictory findings on the role of the regional lymph nodes in controlling cancer metastasis are consistent with our knowledge of the heterogeneity of tumor cells, metastases, antigens, and host models. Different tumor models, and especially differences in experimental conditions, indeed influence the relative biologic behavior of tumor cells. In animal tumor models, melanoma cells implanted intradermally arrive at a draining lymph node before production of metastases in visceral organs. Mouse melanoma cells injected intramuscularly (quadriceps femoris) produce metastases in visceral organs without necessarily involving draining lymph nodes. In human cutaneous melanoma, there is extensive involvement of local and regional lymphatics. In contrast, human ocular melanoma and mucosal melanoma show early metastasis to visceral organs and no lymph node metastases.

Hematogenous Metastasis

Although most research in oncology pertains to the prevention and treatment of primary tumors, metastasis is what most often leads to the ultimate demise of the patient. Understanding the biology of metastasis is essential so that the surgeon can do the following:

- Identify patients at high risk for metastasis
- Identify common patterns of failure so that the timing and selection of appropriate diagnostic studies are performed
- Determine appropriate treatment modalities for established metastasis
- Select adjuvant therapies after surgical treatment
- Integrate other therapeutic modalities in the treatment of metastasis
- Select appropriate palliative treatment options
- Develop new treatment strategies, either in the adjuvant setting or for established metastasis

The Metastatic Cascade

Tumor metastasis is a highly selective, nonrandom process, consisting of a series of linked, sequential steps, that favors the survival of a subpopulation of metastatic cells preexisting within the primary tumor mass. The mere presence of tumor cells in the circulation does not predict that metastasis will occur because most tumor cells that enter the bloodstream are rapidly destroyed. By 24 hours after entry into the circulation, less than 1% of radiolabeled tumor cells are still viable; and less than 0.1% of tumor cells introduced into the circulation survive to produce metastases.[12,13] For a tumor cell to be able to form a clinically relevant metastasis, it must express a complex phenotype that requires that the balance of positive and negative regulators of the metastatic cascade be in favor of metastatic survival and growth.

The process of metastasis begins with tumor cell invasion of the surrounding normal stroma. This process requires the production of degradative enzymes facilitating dissolution of the basement membrane, with or without a concomitant decrease in expression of inhibitors of degradation. An increase in tumor cell proliferation without invasion of the basement membrane theoretically leads to carcinoma in situ. Once the invading cells penetrate the vascular or lymphatic channels, a single cell or clump of cells may detach and be transported within the circulatory system. The rapid death of most circulating tumor cells is probably due to the traumatic nature of blood turbulence. Tumor cells may aggregate with other tumor cells (homotypic aggregation) or blood components such as platelets and lymphocytes (heterotypic aggregation), providing a protective mechanism against turbulence or immune surveillance. Tumor emboli must arrest in the capillary bed of compatible organs, necessitating the expression of appropriate cell-surface adhesion molecules (Fig. 14-43). Exposure of the capillary basement membrane is a result of the normal and continuous physiologic process of endothelial cell shedding and may allow adhesion of tumor emboli. Platelet adherence to damaged areas followed by degranulation causes further retraction of endothelial cells and augments attachment of tumor emboli or platelet–tumor cell emboli.

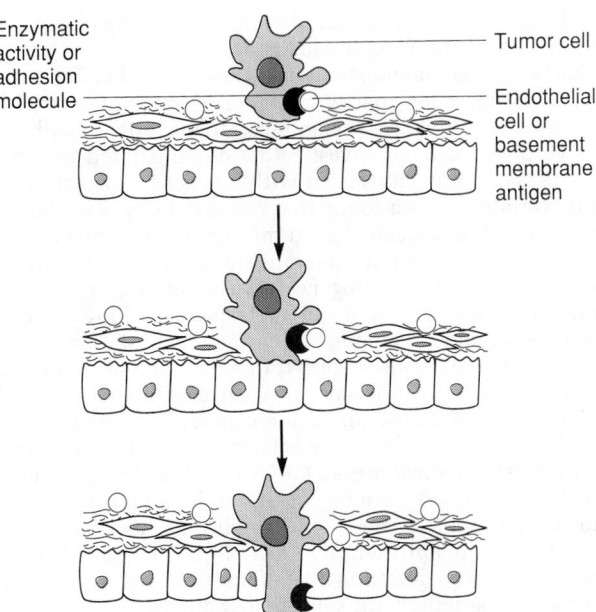

Figure 14-43. Adhesion and extravasation of tumor cells at the site of metastasis.

Extravasation into the organ parenchyma requires both degradative enzymes and motility factors. The next requirement in the process of producing clinically relevant metastasis is the ability to proliferate. Tumors may grow to a size of 1 to 2 mm based on the limits of oxygen diffusion, but continued growth requires the acquisition of a blood supply. Failure to complete one or more steps of the process eliminates the cells. To produce clinically relevant metastases, the successful metastatic cell must therefore exhibit a complex phenotype that is regulated by transient or permanent changes in different genes at the DNA or mRNA level.[14,15]

The Role of Angiogenesis in Metastasis

Angiogenesis is essential for both primary and metastatic tumor growth.[16] The greater the vascularization of a tumor, the greater is the chance of distant metastases.[17,18] This phenomenon is due to two processes: (1) increased vascular proliferation in tumors is associated with a larger tumor mass releasing a greater number of cells into the circulation, thus increasing the probability of metastasis; and (2) the increase in vasculature in highly angiogenic tumors increases the surface area that tumor cells may use to enter the circulation. The molecular determinants that regulate angiogenesis in the process of metastasis have only recently been investigated.

Tumor angiogenesis is not a passive process. Specific factors must be expressed, and the appropriate receptors must be present on the target endothelium to initiate basement membrane degradation, endothelial cell proliferation and migration, and capillary tubule formation. The dynamic process of angiogenesis is regulated by a balance of positive and negative regulators. Angiogenic factors may be released by tumor cells or the cells inhabiting the organ of metastasis, such as mast cells and macrophages.

Although tumor cells are constantly shed from a primary tumor and enter the circulation, only a small percentage actually form a metastasis. It follows that the greater the number of cells released into the circulation, the greater is the chance that a cell will possess the phenotype necessary to form a metastasis. As tumors increase in size, they shed more cells into the circulation; this finding correlates closely with microvessel density.[19]

Early studies demonstrated an association between the degree of tumor vascularity and metastases in patients with intermediate-thickness melanoma.[18] In 49 patients with invasive breast cancer, investigators demonstrated that tumor vessel counts correlated with metastasis formation; a multivariate analyses found that vessel density was a better predictor of metastasis than tumor grade or tumor size.[20] Other investigators have demonstrated a positive correlation between tumor angiogenesis (vessel counts or density) and tumor aggressiveness or metastases in lung cancer, prostate cancer, squamous cell carcinoma of the head and neck, central nervous system tumors, testicular germ cell tumors, bladder carcinoma, ovarian carcinoma, cervical carcinoma, melanoma, and colon cancer.[21–28] In the collective literature examining the relation between vascularity and metastasis, greater than 90% of studies demonstrate a positive correlation. An angiogenic index of a primary tumor may become a means by which patients will be selected for adjuvant therapy. Phase I and II clinical trials are underway examining the efficacy of antiangiogenic therapy in patients with solid malignancies.[29]

Host Factors and Metastasis

Metastasis depends on the interaction of favored tumor cells with a compatible milieu provided by a particular organ environment. In humans and in experimental rodent systems, numerous examples have shown malignant tumors to metastasize to specific organs. Two arguments were advanced to explain organ-specific metastasis. In 1889, Paget[30] proposed that the growth of metastases is influenced by the interaction of particular tumor cells (the "seed") with unique organ environments (the "soil"), and that metastases result only when the seed and soil are compatible. Forty years later, Ewing[31] challenged Paget's seed and soil theory and hypothesized that metastatic dissemination occurs by purely mechanical factors that are a result of the anatomic structure of the vascular system. These explanations have been evoked separately or together to explain the secondary site preference of certain types of neoplasms. In a review of clinical studies on secondary site preferences of malignant neoplasms, it was concluded that regional metastasis can be attributed to anatomic or mechanical considerations, such as efferent venous circulation or lymphatic drainage to regional lymph nodes, but that distant organ colonization by metastatic cells depends on unique patterns of site specificity.[32]

These observations have been confirmed both experimentally and clinically. The microenvironment of each organ can influence the implantation, invasion, survival, and growth of particular tumor cells, with the importance of each individual interaction varying among different tumor systems.

Heterogeneity of Metastasis

In neoplasia, heterogeneity is carried to its largest exponent.[33] The differences due to histology, anatomic location, and cellular ploidy all have an impact by multiplying the possibilities for heterogeneity. It has been demonstrated that great heterogeneity exists within a single neoplasm. Diversity is manifest in malignant potential, quantitative expression of cell-surface histocompatibility antigens, and antigenic specificities expressed by cells within a tumor or between primary and metastatic cells. The following discussion addresses the aspects of heterogeneity that impact the biology of metastasis.

To produce a clinically apparent metastasis, malignant tumor cells must pass through a sequence of potentially lethal interactions with host homeostatic mechanisms, not the least of which is avoidance of recognition and destruction by host defense. Failure to complete any step in the metastatic program results in elimination of the errant tumor cell. This complexity explains, in part, why the process is inefficient. For example, the presence of tumor cells in the circulation does not predict that clinical metastasis will occur because most tumor cells that enter the bloodstream are rapidly destroyed. By 24 hours after entry into the circulation, less than 1% of radiolabeled tumor cells are still viable, and less than 0.1% of tumor cells introduced into the circulation survive to produce metastases. The 0.1% of circulating cells responsible for the development of metastases either survived by random chance or were selected for survival and growth from preexistent subpopulations of cells.

At the time of diagnosis, many human and animal neoplasms are composed of subpopulations of cells with distinctly different biologic properties. Cells isolated from individual neoplasms differ in morphology, karyotype, growth rate, antigenicity and immunogenicity, cell-surface receptors for lectins, hormone receptors, response to therapies, and potential for invasion and metastasis. During the last decade, the concept that neoplasms are heterogeneous and contain multiple subpopulations of cells with different biologic properties has gained wide consensus. An appreciation of biologic diversity within tumors has suggested three important principles for metastatic development. First, the process of metastasis is not random. Second, neoplasms are not uniform entities but rather contain cells exhibiting heterogeneous metastatic capabilities. Third, the outcome of metastasis depends on the properties of both tumor cells and host factors; the balance of these contributions varies among tumors arising in different tissues and even among tumors of similar histologic origin in different patients.

The specificity with which metastatic tumor cells display predilection for selected target organs suggests a molecular recognition system whereby tumor cells are able to bind specifically to target tissues to establish the mechanism of residence. Cell-surface molecules, some of which may be integrins or ligands of integrins, may assign organ specificity to the metastatic phenotype. Further study of these molecules will elucidate the mechanisms of organ or tissue predilection in metastasis and also afford a biologic basis for novel strategies to prevent establishment of metastases.

Primary Tumors

Cells with a spectrum of metastatic potential may be isolated from parent tumor lines (animals) or primary tumors (humans). Most cells do not evidence metastatic behavior. Two broad strategies have been advanced to isolate metastatic cells that differ from the parent neoplasm. First, tumor cells are selected in vivo in a cyclic selection protocol. Tumor cells are implanted subcutaneously or intramuscularly or injected intravenously into mice, and dissemination is allowed to occur. The metastatic lesions are harvested from target organs or sites, and the cells recovered are then expanded in culture or immediately reselected in vivo using the same protocol. The cycle is repeated several times. The proportion of metastatic foci that occurs from inoculation of cycled cells is compared with that of the cells from the parent tumor to document the selection of cells with enhanced metastatic capacity for tissue sites. The increase in metastatic capacity of the recovered cells is a selection and does not result from the adaptation of tumor cells to preferential growth in a particular organ. This procedure was originally used to obtain a highly metastatic line from transplantable murine melanomas. The selection process has been adapted to isolation of metastatic tumor cell lines from many of the experimental tumors.

Assessment of metastatic potential in human tumors is now performed in vivo in congenitally athymic nu/nu (nude) mice. These animals have severely impaired cell-mediated immunity and are incapable of rejecting foreign tissue transplants, thereby affording an in vivo setting to assess malignant potential and metastatic proclivity. Within this system, several human tumor lines and primary tumors display subpopulations of cells with widely differing metastatic properties.

Origin of Cellular Diversity

Different metastatic propensities among tumor cells of an individual neoplasm are no longer controversial. Three aspects of the extensive cellular heterogeneity are the subject of ongoing investigation in tumor biology laboratories: timing of variant appearance, origin of diversity, and regulation of variant expression. Do metastatic variants arise in a primary tumor early or late in the development of the primary neoplasm? Once metastatic cells develop in a neoplasm, is there a growth advantage over nonmetastatic cells so that with the passage of time metastatic cells constitute most cells in a neoplasm? How is the proportion of metastatic cells to nonmetastatic cells regulated? As answers to these questions emerge, they may help surgeons in making decisions critical to the timing and sequence of multimodality treatments for primary tumors and metastases.

The first question seeks a fundamental aspect of carcinogenesis. Whether of unicellular or multicellular origin, most tumors are heterogeneous and contain subpopulations of cells with differing biologic behavior. Tumors may arise as the result of a rare event, somatic mutation, wherein the origin is presumed unicellular. Indeed, substantial evidence from studies using a marker immunoglobulin or glucose-6-phosphate dehydrogenase in women with X-chromosome–inactivation mosaicism suggests that chronic myelogenous leukemia, Burkitt lymphoma, and multiple myeloma arise from a single cell. In contrast, hereditary trichoepithelioma and colon carcinoma are presumed multicellular in origin. Some of the most widely investigated animal model tumors, such as chemically induced murine fibrosarcomas, are also multicellular in origin.

Cellular diversity is consistent with neoplasms that are multicellular in origin. Such tumors are probably populated by the progeny of several transformed cells. In chemically induced sarcomas, cells obtained from different areas of the tumor differed in their growth rate, susceptibility to cytotoxic drugs, and antigenicity. Tumors that are unicellular in origin are also not uniform. The evidence that diversity is continually generated is substantial.

Tumors undergo a series of changes as part of the natural history of the disease. For example, tumors initially diagnosed as benign may, over a period of many months or even years, assume a malignant phenotype. Acquired genetic variability within developing clones of tumors, coupled with host selection pressures, results in new clonal sublines of increased growth autonomy or malignancy.

This hypothesis predicts that progression toward malignancy is accompanied by increased genetic instability of the malignant cells. In four different experimental tumor models, highly metastatic cells were less phenotypically stable than their nonmetastatic counterparts isolated from the same single neoplasm. The rapid generation of diversity is presumed the product of increased genetic instability. Highly metastatic clones exhibit a higher rate of spontaneous mutation than the cells from poorly metastatic lines. These results are in accord with the hypothesis that tumor progression occurs as a result of acquired genetic alterations. Additional evidence that genetic mechanisms are responsible for tumor progression comes from experiments using mutagens, such as nitrosoguanidine or ultraviolet radiation. Treatment of tumor cell populations with mutagens induces variants with (1) increased tumorigenicity, (2) metastatic capacities, (3) decreased tumorigenic potential, and (4) increased immunogenicity. The more metastatic a tumor cell population, the greater is the likelihood that the constituent cells will undergo spontaneous mutations that result in rapid phenotypic diversification and increased opportunities for escape from therapeutic modalities. Diversification may be further exaggerated by the mutagenic action of many of the cytotoxic antineoplastic drugs used in therapy.

Tumors of unicellular origin may exhibit metastatic heterogeneity very early in development. This conclusion is based on the in vivo behavior of murine fibroblasts transformed by an oncogenic virus. Six colonies of murine embryo fibroblasts, each derived from a single cell, were infected in vivo with murine sarcoma virus and then propagated as pedigree cell lines. Intravenous injection of viable cells from each clone resulted in marked differences among the clones with regard to colonization of the lung. Because the parent cell population was derived from a single transformed cell, the differences resulted from rapid phenotypic diversification. Similarly, when the clones from two colonies (one of high and one of low experimental metastatic capacity) were subcloned and evaluated in the same manner, both clones exhibited a pattern of metastatic heterogeneity. As indicated earlier, the more metastatic tumors display greater heterogeneity. The clone with higher metastatic capacity exhibited a greater degree of variability than the clone with lower metastatic capacity. Despite the single-cell origin, diversification occurred during the 6 weeks after the subcloning, yielding cells with different metastatic properties. Generation of metastatic heterogeneity in neoplasms does not require a prolonged latent period (Fig. 14-44).

Cells within the tumor mass are not autonomous units but are regulated by the proximity of other neoplastic cells. Different subpopulations of mammary tumor cells affect the growth patterns and chemosensitivity of other groups of cells. Similar regulatory control may exist for the metastatic phenotype of different cells within a mixed tumor. To test for this regulatory control, two poorly metastatic clones and two highly metastatic clones were isolated from the B16-F10 melanoma line. These clones were cultured in vitro or in vivo for 5, 10, or 20 weeks, and then subclones derived at each of these intervals were reassessed for their metastatic ability. After only 10 in vitro passages, many subclones that differed significantly from the parent clone were isolated. Continued cultivation introduced more variability such that by 20 and 40 passages, most clones tested differed significantly from their parent clones. In marked contrast, the metastatic phenotype of the uncloned B16 melanoma lines B16-F1 and B16-F10 remained remarkably stable for 30 in vivo passages or 60 in vitro passages. Similar stability was attained when different clones were mixed together and cocultivated as polyclonal populations; however, the subsequent removal of all but one clone led to the rapid generation of biologic diversity in the remaining clone.

The instability of metastatic properties in clones is not limited to cell lines that have been serially passed in vitro or in vivo for considerable periods. The same phenomenon has been identified in clones isolated from newly induced

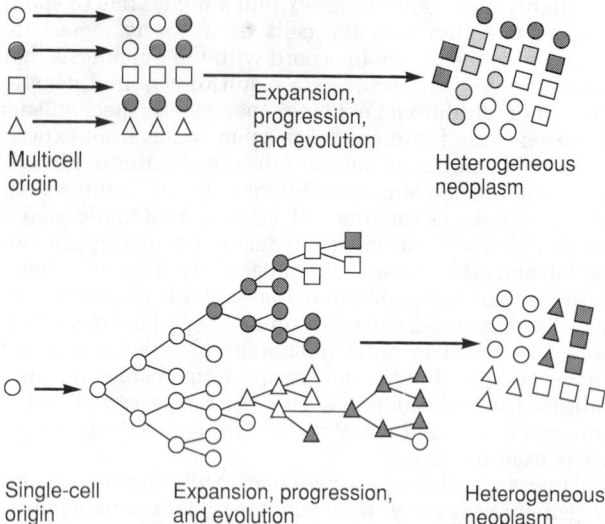

Figure 14-44. Pathways for generation of biologic diversity in neoplasms. Neoplasms developing from a multicell origin and from a single-cell origin both demonstrate biologic diversity when they attain clinically detectable size. (After Hellman S. Principles of radiation therapy. In: DeVita VT, Hellman S, Rosenberg SA, eds. Cancer: principles and practice of oncology, ed 3. Philadelphia, JB Lippincott, 1989:247)

tumors and subjected to a minimum period of cultivation before assay of their metastatic properties. Clones isolated from several ultraviolet radiation–induced fibrosarcomas and methylcholanthrene-induced tumors that were excised within 3 months of their initial detection each contained a small fraction of clones with unstable metastatic properties. The fraction of unstable clones in these populations increased during further passage in culture and serial transplantation in syngeneic mice. The proportion of unstable clones is significantly higher in cell populations harvested from tumors that had been allowed to reach an advanced stage of progression before excision. This indicates that unstable clones evolve in situ and that the proportion of such clones increases with tumor progression.

These data provide evidence that different subpopulations of tumor cells stabilize their relative proportions and thereby impose an equilibrium on the combined population. Removal of the stabilizing effect, by isolating clones or by applying a strong selection pressure such as chemotherapy, leads to rapid diversification in the resurgent populations. Although the nature of these stabilizing influences and their modes of action are not yet understood, their existence argues against randomness in tumor development. Rather, the society of tumor cells imposes regulatory constraints on its individual members to maintain cellular diversity and its concomitant benefits for tumor survival. Certainly, this phenomenon, irrespective of its underlying mechanisms, further complicates attempts to understand the process of tumor progression toward malignancy.

Origin of Heterogeneity in Metastases

Although the concept of site-specific metastasis has only recently been investigated in the laboratory, clinicians readily recognize that certain tumors metastasize preferentially to specific sites. For example, it is well known that renal cell carcinoma tends to metastasize to the lung, ocu-

lar melanoma and colon cancer metastasize to the liver, and breast cancer and prostate cancer selectively metastasize to bone. Although the site of metastasis may appear to be due to venous drainage patterns, it cannot be denied that environment is an important component of the metastatic process. Understanding the patterns of site-specific metastasis from primary tumors is necessary to develop appropriate clinical follow-up strategies.

Therapeutic regimens that cure tumors in mice are ineffective in the treatment of malignancies in humans. In mice, tumors are inoculated in the subcutaneous tissues despite the fact that these tumors rarely, if ever, are found in subcutaneous tissues in humans. Investigators have advocated the use of orthotopic implantation of tumor cells as a model for studying the natural history of tumor growth. Models have been developed in which colon cancer cells are injected into the wall of the colon, bladder cancer is injected into the bladder wall, and renal cell carcinoma is injected into the parenchyma of the kidney. After orthotopic implantation of tumor cells, metastatic patterns differ greatly depending on the site of implantation of a primary tumor. Colon cancer tumor cells injected into the subcutaneous tissues rarely metastasize, whereas colon cancer cells injected into the wall of the cecum or beneath the capsule of the spleen (portal vein injection) metastasize to the liver. Colon cancer injected into the kidney does not form metastasis. Tumor cell gene expression is regulated in part by the environment. The expression of the *mdr* gene is higher in tumor cells implanted in the colon than in those implanted in the subcutaneous tissues.

It is likely that many factors govern site-specific metastasis. The endothelium that lines the organ of metastasis must express the appropriate receptors for tumor cells to attach. The environment within the organ of metastasis must express growth factors that serve as ligands for specific growth factor receptors on the membrane of tumor cells. An interesting study that demonstrated this phenomenon used tumor cells injected into the subcutaneous tissues at the time of partial hepatectomy or nephrectomy. After partial hepatectomy, subcutaneous colon cancer inoculations increased in size, whereas there was no increase in growth of subcutaneous colon cancer cells in mice that underwent partial nephrectomy. After partial hepatectomy, regenerative factors within the liver were also found in the peripheral circulation. Such growth factors as hepatocyte growth factor or TGF-α may bind to receptors that are found on colon cancer cells.

Investigation of the biologic and biochemical properties of human tumors was formerly restricted largely to in vitro analyses. For obvious and ethical reasons, in vivo human investigations are not consistent with patient care standards. The development of congenitally athymic nude mice enabled investigation of human tumor progression in vivo. The nude mouse is homozygous for nu determining thymic aplasia and absence of hair. Heterozygotes (nu−/+) are euthymic. The nude mice have severely impaired cellular immune responses and are thus incapable of (1) resisting infection with a variety of bacteria, fungi, viruses, and protozoan organisms and (2) rejecting foreign tissue grafts. Human tumors readily propagate in various organs and tissues of the nude mouse, with growth dependent on the route of introduction. Assessment of malignant potential as reflected in the number and location of metastases is possible. The heterogenous nature of metastatic human neoplasms may be investigated under defined conditions in nude mice. Factors such as tumor heterogeneity, stage of differentiation, expression of protooncogenes, expression of cell-surface enzymes, and adhesion molecules may be correlated with the metastatic potential of tumor cell populations in the intact host.

The nude mouse model has been employed to investigate the metastatic proclivity of human tumors to specific sites. In addition, the nude mouse has served as a method for propagation of tumor tissue from neoplasms that adapt poorly to in vitro culture. The inability to reject foreign tissue allows not only transplantation of tumor xenografts but also adoptive transfer of human lymphocytes into tumor-bearing nude mice to determine the therapeutic potential of ex vivo propagated lymphocytes.

Other strains of immunocompromised mice are increasing the ability to investigate xenotransplanted tumors and lymphoid cells. Severe combined immunodeficient mice have impaired cell-mediated and humoral immune responses. These mice may prove to be superior to nude mice in the analysis of host–tumor interactions using lymphocytes and tumor from the same human donor.

PRINCIPLES OF SURGICAL ONCOLOGY

The practice of radical surgery in an effort to improve survival has been replaced with multimodality anticancer treatment regimens. A greater understanding of the biology of cancer has revealed that malignancies do not always spread in a stepwise, sequential fashion, that is, first to lymph nodes and then to distant sites. Most tumors metastasize to numerous and distant sites independent of whether the regional nodal basin is involved. Lymph node involvement is a marker of systemic disease and provides the clinician with the knowledge that the tumor possesses the phenotype capable of producing metastasis. As a general rule, the survival of patients with lymph node metastases is half that of patients with node-negative malignancies, despite the fact that nodal metastases have been resected. In many circumstances, extensive surgery offers no benefit to the patient with cancer, yet it may subject the patient to the morbidity and mortality associated with radical procedures. Although survival from solid malignancies has not improved a great deal in the recent past, the true advances in oncologic surgery relate to the fact that similar overall survival can be obtained with less surgery. In addition, multimodality treatment may improve quality of life in patients with cancer. As an example, chemoradiation for rectal cancer has a marginal impact on overall survival but has decreased local recurrence rates in the pelvis from between 25% and 50% to between 0% and 12%. Improvements in our ability to detect patients likely to harbor micrometastatic disease should improve the efficacy of adjuvant therapy. Furthermore, new treatment regimens based on correction of molecular alterations in malignancies should improve survival. The oncologic surgeon must be able not only to perform surgery safely but also to integrate properly other treatment modalities in the care of the cancer patient.

The Surgeon in the Treatment of Cancer

Screening for malignancies is an integral part of the clinician's goal in minimizing the morbidity and mortality of cancer. Successful screening programs employ a cost-effective method for early detection in high-risk groups. Early detection affords the advantages of more conservative therapy with potentially less morbidity and significantly increased surgical cure rates. Screening programs should encompass people with genetic predisposition for cancer. Among these are people with a family history of breast cancer, colon cancer, or medullary thyroid cancer, and those with predisposing characteristics such as dysplastic nevus syndrome and polyposis of the colon. It is necessary for the surgeon to be aware of germ-line markers that may detect patients with an increased risk of malignancy, such those with loss of the *apc* gene (familial polyposis coli) or those with von Hippel–Lindau disease.

The surgeon now has a number of options for surgical treatment of individual patients with local, locoregional, and metastatic disease. Selection requires that the surgeon knows (1) the natural history of the neoplasm, (2) patterns of metastasis specific to the cancer, (3) the goals of the operation for a particular stage (cure, local disease control, palliation, or staging), and (4) the risk of the surgery for the individual patient. The present and future directions of cancer care involve the appropriate integration of all available treatments—surgery, radiotherapy, chemotherapy, hormone therapy, biologic therapy, and possibly gene therapy. Integrated therapy offers numerous combinations because each modality offers an ever-increasing number of options. Further considerations include the sequence, dosage, interval, and duration of therapeutic administrations. The surgeon must be an effective partner in the multidisciplinary care of cancer patients to ensure administration of adjuvant therapy consistent with the needs of the individual cancer patient. Although the surgeon may not personally deliver these other cancer treatments, he or she should be thoroughly knowledgeable about their indications, risks, and benefits. The surgeon should know how to coordinate these adjuvant treatments in the surgical patient with the proper dose, timing, and sequence to ensure the maximum probability for cure, local disease control, and function, in addition to the best cosmetic result and lowest morbidity. For the most part, deployment of these treatments must be based on information from controlled clinical trials demonstrating the value of each combination of therapy or sequence of treatment. Cost-effectiveness of treatment and diagnostic studies will play a major role in patient care in the future.

Preoperative chemotherapy is an example of multidisciplinary cancer care in which there have been significant advances. There is sufficient evidence to justify preoperative chemotherapy for selected patients with a variety of histologic types of tumor, including osteogenic sarcoma, soft tissue sarcomas of the extremities, testicular carcinoma, esophageal cancer, gastric carcinoma, lung cancer, and locally advanced breast carcinoma. The advantages of preoperative chemotherapy are two-fold. First, in some patients, it may reduce the bulk of the tumor (including those tumors that are unresectable or borderline resectable), thereby enabling a more complete, safer operation with less risk of local or regional failure. Second, preoperative chemotherapy permits the physician to assess responsiveness to that form of chemotherapy. For patients who have a major response, continuing the same chemotherapy regimen postoperatively to maximize cure rates is justified, based on the assumption that the microscopic tumor that cannot be seen is also susceptible to the chemotherapy regimen.

Postoperative chemotherapy or hormonal therapy is being used effectively as an adjunct to standard treatment for cancer patients. One example of benefit for such treatment is the improved survival rates for patients with stage II breast cancer who undergo adjuvant chemotherapy (premenopausal women) or hormonal therapy (postmenopausal women). The preliminary results of several studies of these treatments for high-risk node-negative breast cancer patients have also shown improved disease-free survival rates. Other studies demonstrated improved survival rates in Duke stage C rectal carcinoma patients using a combination of chemotherapy and radiotherapy.

The surgeon must know not only how to integrate other treatment modalities with surgery in the care of the cancer patient but also when not to operate. For example, squamous cell carcinoma of the anus can be adequately treated by chemoradiation regimens alone in 85% of patients. Patients with greater than four liver metastasis from colorectal cancer rarely survive 5 years, and thus, outside of a protocol, resection is contraindicated.

Intraoperative treatment modalities should be reviewed before subjecting a patient to surgery. Knowledge of the benefits of intraoperative radiotherapy or brachytherapy is essential in treating patients with a high likelihood of local recurrence, such as those with sarcomas of the extremities. Furthermore, indications for intraoperative adjuvants, such as isolated limb perfusions, should be considered in patients with extremity melanoma with in-transit disease. Lymphatic mapping for melanoma and breast cancer is being studied to determine the appropriateness of selective lymphadenectomy for these cancers.

Surgeons have a definite but limited role in excising isolated distant metastatic lesions, especially those in the brain, lung, liver, and soft tissues. It must be emphasized that patient selection is critical, and such operations should be performed only when the potential benefits clearly outweigh the risks. The best results are obtained when surgical excision of metastatic lesions can be combined with effective chemotherapy. Several institutions have demonstrated a 20% to 30% 5-year survival rate in selected patients whose pulmonary metastases from sarcomas, melanomas, colon cancers, and testicular carcinomas have been resected. In a national survey of patients undergoing liver resection for colorectal metastases, the overall 5-year survival rate was 33%. Excision of metastatic tumors to the brain is also indicated in selected patients, especially when combined with irradiation. In the future, excision of surgically accessible metastatic lesions will increase, especially in those patients who have had a significant response to systemic therapy.

Reducing Surgical Mortality, Morbidity, and Cost

Although the primary goals of cancer surgery are increasing life-span and maximizing local disease control, it is also important to minimize surgical mortality, morbidity, and cost. Several technologic advances, such as laparoscopy, intraoperative ultrasonography, lasers, intraoperative radiotherapy, and implantable drug infusion devices, can substantially reduce morbidity and even mortality.

Laparoscopy has been applied to the treatment of patients with malignancies. Laparoscopic colectomies, abdominoperineal resections, nephrectomies, pancreatectomies, splenectomies, lung resections, and numerous other diagnostic procedures have been performed. The use of laparoscopy as a staging tool for patients with pancreatic and gastric malignancies and lymphoma often can save a patient from unnecessary surgery. In addition, laparoscopy is being used to place gastrostomy and jejunostomy feeding tubes at the time of staging so that patients may better tolerate neoadjuvant therapy. There are anecdotal reports of patients developing port-site recurrences, but this phenomenon occurs no more frequently than wound recurrences in patients who have undergone open procedures. The specific indications for the use of laparoscopy in cancer patients are still being defined, although certainly the use of laparoscopy for staging is appropriate.

Intraoperative ultrasonography has enabled more precise and safer operations in several areas. In liver tumors (both primary and metastatic), it allows the surgeon to detect previously unrecognized lesions (found in about 10% of patients), define the relation of the tumor to such vital structures as the hepatic and portal veins, and in some instances, perform segmental resections instead of lobar resections. Patient selection is improved, and morbidity and mortality rates may be reduced. The brain and pancreas are other areas in which intraoperative ultrasonography is useful in localizing and identifying adjacent vital structures. It is also being used in selected patients with clinically occult breast masses as a substitute for needle localization to reduce the amount of breast tissue excised during the biopsy.

Laser surgery can reduce surgical morbidity and the duration of hospital stay in selected instances. Therapeutic laser endoscopy represents a significant advance for patients with obstructing carcinomas involving the rectum, esophagus, or bronchus because these tumors can be vaporized to reestablish a patent lumen. This nonoperative approach improves the patient's ability to eat or breathe without emergency surgery. Later, elective surgery can sometimes be performed on these patients, who would otherwise have faced multiple operations and a higher complication rate from urgent surgery in a debilitated state. In one series of patients, more than 95% of obstructing rectal carcinomas were relieved of bleeding or obstruction with therapeutic laser endoscopy, which obviated the need for emergency colostomy. Lasers are also being used in selected patients with multiple metastatic pulmonary nodules (especially sarcomas) so that less lung tissue is removed; this is an especially important consideration in patients who might have marginal pulmonary reserves after more extensive surgery.

Bladder cancers are another disease for which lasers have had a beneficial impact. Bladder fulgeration with electrocautery generally requires several days of hospitalization and a bladder catheter. With the use of a Yag laser, however, the same procedure can be done on an outpatient basis without a bladder catheter and with less bleeding, a faster recovery, and lower cost.

The cost of medical care increases by 8% to 10% a year nationally. Minimizing this cost is an important physician responsibility when cost-containment measures do not compromise the quality of patient care. Methods by which the surgeon can reduce the cost of cancer care include (1) more outpatient procedures (eg, biopsies, venous access), (2) reduced hospitalization, and (3) fewer diagnostic surveys. Costs incurred in the care of the cancer patient are closely scrutinized by insurers and third-party providers, and the surgeon must be able to substantiate all costs incurred in the process of treating the cancer patient.

It is becoming increasingly clear that the type and frequency of metastatic evaluations for the symptomless cancer patient can be reduced because the yield of occult metastases is too low to justify the expense. A study from the National Surgical Adjuvant Breast Project involving almost 8000 bone scans yielded only 35 bone metastases in symptomless patients. Another study demonstrated that survival rates in breast cancer patients were not significantly improved with extensive metastatic surveys in symptomless patients. A national survey of metastatic evaluations for melanoma demonstrated a lack of benefit from metastatic evaluation by radionuclide scanning in symptomless surgical patients. The value of carcinoembryonic antigen as a marker of recurrence in patients with colon cancer has been well documented, but whether detection of an elevated carcinoembryonic antigen level impacts on survival has been questioned. Metastatic studies should be used judiciously in symptomless patients to reduce medical costs.

Cancer Rehabilitation

Rehabilitation of patients physically, emotionally, and socially is a vital part of cancer management, and the surgeon has an important role in these areas. The use of plastic and reconstructive surgery techniques has vastly improved the quality of life for many patients after ablative surgery. An excellent example is the availability of breast reconstructive surgery (using a TRAM flap, latissimus flap, or implantable prosthesis) for patients who need a total mastectomy; this field has made significant strides in achieving excellent cosmetic results. Limb salvage techniques that employ combinations of chemotherapy, radiotherapy, and surgery for patients with bone and soft tissue sarcomas have significantly reduced the need for major limb amputations. Prosthetic devices, including artificial joints, have greatly improved the functional rehabilitation of patients with extremity sarcomas who would otherwise face the prospect of an amputation. Another significant area of advancement has been in microvascular surgery and the use of free composite grafts. For example, free flaps from the iliac crest have been used for mandibular reconstruction in patients with extensive head and neck cancers.

Palliative Care

Despite our best efforts, the 5-year survival rate for cancer patients is still 50%. Thus, the oncologic surgeon must have a thorough understanding of methods to provide palliative care to the patient who has unresectable disease. This may involve performing surgical bypass to relieve bowel obstruction, stenting a strictured bile duct, or merely providing pain control and comfort. The surgeon must refrain from operating strictly for diagnostic purposes or simply to observe. Diagnostic imaging should be used before considering any invasive procedure to obtain a diagnosis. Surgery in the patient with unresectable disease is often followed by complications such as dehiscence or pneumonia. These patients have decreased immune function and wound healing capacity. When surgery is warranted in such patients, wound closure should be meticulous and pulmonary toilet aggressive.

Patients with end-stage malignancy may require pain control beyond the scope that a surgeon can deliver. Integration with the anesthesia and pain service is essential to manage adequately the pain of a patient with end-stage malignancy. Pain management can range from optimization of oral medications to nerve blocks and epidural infusions. Bone pain may be decreased with palliative radiation. Pain from expansion of Glisson capsule due to a liver tumor may be decreased with transarterial embolization. The oncologist must also work closely with Social Services in arranging the appropriate hospice care.

Clinical Research

All surgeons should participate in clinical trials, either through institutional studies or cancer cooperative groups, whenever possible. Clearly, the quality and quantity of clinical research today will be reflected in the standard treatment tomorrow. It is important that surgeons be even more knowledgeable in such areas as clinical biostatistics, use of computers for data management, writing of protocols for prospective studies, organization of an infrastructure for conducting clinical research (ie, research nurses and data managers), and scientific communications. These basic tools and principles should also be fully incorporated into surgical training programs.

During the 1980s, the knowledge necessary to achieve optimal management of the surgical patient with cancer greatly expanded. The role of the surgeon now integrates a range of treatment options that in many instances address both locoregional and systemic disease control. The goal in managing the surgical patient with cancer is a full implementation of multidisciplinary cancer care to provide the highest quality of care with maximum rehabilitation at the lowest possible cost, maximizing both duration and quality of life.

PRINCIPLES OF RADIATION BIOLOGY AND RADIOTHERAPY

The clinical practice of oncology involves three major therapeutic modalities: surgery, chemotherapy, and radiotherapy. The surgeon-in-training becomes progressively more skilled in performing complex oncologic resections and reconstructions. During this time, the surgeon has a modicum of exposure to chemotherapeutic principles and practice. Even more lacking is the development of any clear understanding of radiation biology and radiotherapy. The need to rectify this deficiency becomes clear when one considers that more half of all cancer patients receive some form of ionizing radiation.[34]

Ionizing Radiation

Ionizing radiation is energy that is absorbed by tissue. The absorption of this energy results in the excitation and ejection of an orbital electron, thus creating ionized atoms and molecules. Radiation can be categorized as particulate or electromagnetic. Particulate radiation consists of subatomic particles, such as electrons, protons, and neutrons. Roentgen rays (x-rays), derived from electrical machines and linear accelerators, and gamma rays, originating from the decay of radioisotopes, represent the electromagnetic form of ionizing radiation. The energy released by electromagnetic radiation has the characteristics of a wave or a packet of energy, the photon. The ability to quantify the intensity of the ionizing radiation allows for an understanding of tissue absorption and penetration. Essentially, as the energy of the radiation is increased, the depth of penetration through tissues is increased (Fig. 14-45). Additionally, the absorption mechanisms differ at varying intensities. At the high intensities described as supervoltage or megavoltage, the full energy of the radiation is not transferred to the tissue until some distance is reached. Therefore, high-energy radiation penetrates through skin and other superficial structures, but its full ionizing potential is not obtained until it reaches the deeper target tissues. This is considered a *skin-sparing effect*.

The clinical description of this absorbed energy is based on the amount of energy absorbed per unit mass. Previously, this was described as the rad, with 100 rads equaling 1 J/kg. Currently, dosages are described as grays, and 1 Gy equals 100 rad. The ranges of electromagnetic radiation used are depicted in Figure 14-45.

Radiation Techniques: Brachytherapy and Teletherapy

Two general types of radiation techniques are used clinically. *Brachytherapy* is the technique in which the source of the radiation is adjacent to or within the targeted tissue. In this method, isotopes such as gold-198 and iodine-125 are placed in special catheters, the positioning of which

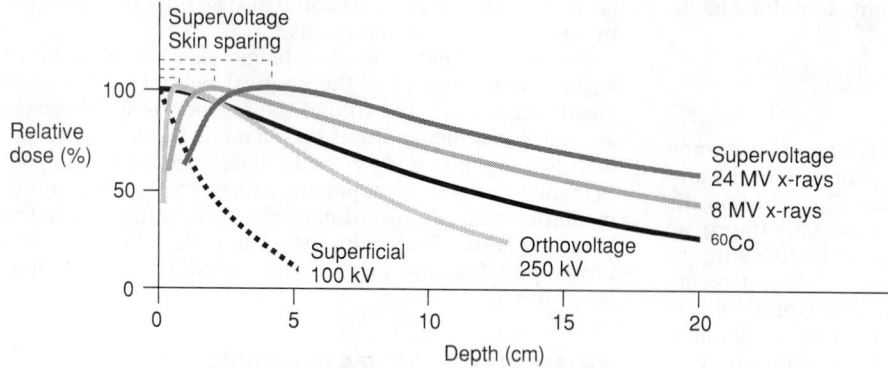

Figure 14-45. Radiation doses at various tissue depths for differing types of ionizing radiation. (After Hellman S. Principles of radiation therapy. In: DeVita VT, Hellman S, Rosenberg SA, eds. Cancer: principles and practice of oncology, ed 3. Philadelphia, JB Lippincott, 1989:247)

is based on precise geometric considerations. The placement of the radiation source is critical because, in principle, a high dose of energy is delivered to the immediate vicinity of the target and then decreases rapidly with distance. The advantage of this technique is the ability to deliver high, concentrated doses to the target while limiting damage to nearby normal tissue. Clinical applicability is somewhat limited, but there is considerable experience with brachytherapy in the treatment of some oral tumors, gynecologic malignancies, and soft tissue tumors of the extremities.

The other common technique in clinical practice is *teletherapy*. In this method, orthovoltage or supervoltage machines, such as cobalt machines, electrical machines, and linear accelerators, are used to deliver high-energy electromagnetic beams. The source of the radiation is removed from direct physical contact with the patient. The absorbed dose is determined by a number of factors, including geometric and tissue characteristics of the target and the energy of the radiation. The radiation beam can be modified using various methods, such as filters and collimators, to deliver a maximum dose to targeted tissues while minimizing the effects on the transited normal tissues. The importance of this principle is obvious when considering the potential hazards of inappropriately applied radiotherapy for the treatment of pelvic or pulmonary malignancies.

Radiation Biology

Having outlined the clinical methods used to deliver ionizing radiation, we next consider the interaction of radiation with living cells. In essence, the goal of radiotherapy is to render the malignant cell incapable of further proliferation. This is accomplished by causing irreparable damage to key biologic molecules within the cell. Some of the biologic damage produced by ionizing radiation is due to a direct effect on DNA. High-energy radiation can cause direct breaks in chromosomal DNA, rendering it incapable of replication. Most of the biologic effects, however, are due to an indirect action mediated by free radicals. These free radicals are generated by the interaction of the ionizing radiation with water. The free radicals have an extremely short half-life but, while present, can cause damage to DNA and other key intracellular molecules. This indirect component of radiation damage can be enhanced by the presence of molecular oxygen, which helps to explain why cells deficient in oxygen are relatively radioresistant.

Adverse Effects and Biology of Normal Tissue

The sensitivity of mammalian cells to ionizing radiation is described in survival curves (Fig. 14-46). These curves describe the fraction of cells surviving a given dose of

radiation. The general form of the dose–response curve has a relatively shallow initial slope, or shoulder region. The survival curve then becomes steeper at higher doses. The shoulder region represents a measure of the ability of cells to repair damaged DNA at sublethal doses. The steeper portion of the curve reflects the radiosensitivity of cells at the usual clinical doses delivered. In cell culture, no difference exists between the dose–response curves of normal cells and those of neoplastic cells of the same histologic origin; therefore, survival curves cannot fully explain the differences in clinical effects.

The radiosensitivity of cells also depends on their position within the cell cycle. Cells in the mitotic phase are most sensitive. In addition, normal tissues and tumors differ in their responses to fractionated irradiation. At the time of any given dose, only a fraction of cells are in a vulnerable position within the cell cycle. Subsequently, the sensitivity of the tumor compared with normal tissue depends on the ability of cells to redistribute and repopulate within the radiated volume. In tumors that are particularly radiosensitive, this balance between cell killing and repopulation favors the normal tissues over the tumor. The ability to recruit cells from adjacent undamaged areas should also favor normal tissues.

As noted, the presence or absence of molecular oxygen greatly influences the proportion of cells killed by a given

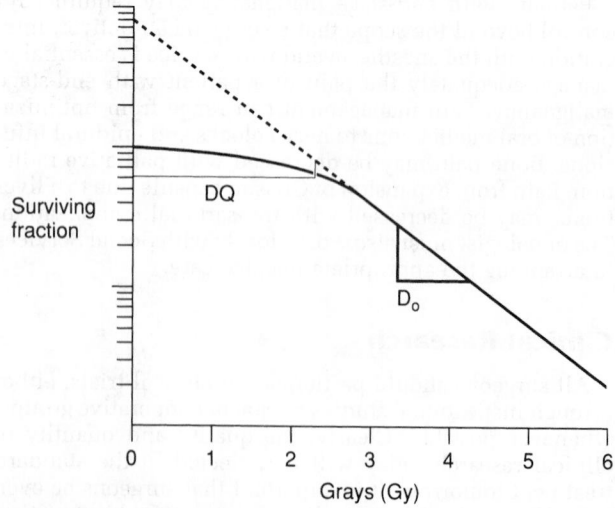

Figure 14-46. Radiation survival curve. DQ, threshold dose for radiation-induced cell death; D_o, exponential portion of the survival curve. (After Hellman S. Principles of radiation therapy. In: DeVita VT, Hellman S, Rosenberg SA, eds. Cancer: principles and practice of oncology, ed 3. Philadelphia, JB Lippincott, 1989:247)

dose of radiation. It is clearly the most important biologic response modifier for enhancing the formation and prolonging the survival of free radicals. Therefore, radiosensitivity of cells within a given tumor varies based on their location relative to oxygen-carrying capillaries (Fig. 14-47). Cells in hypoxic regions of a tumor may escape the effects of radiation. As conditions change with progressive cell killing, fewer cells theoretically exist in hypoxic regions, and oxygen may become more evenly distributed within the tumor volume. Obviously, this principle of reoxygenation is not always clinically efficient, as evidenced by the relative radioresistance of larger tumors compared with smaller or earlier lesions of the same histologic origin.

Pharmacologic Modification

The key role of molecular oxygen has served as a stimulus for developing pharmacologic response modifiers. This research has demonstrated that the response of cells and tissues can be altered by chemical agents. Nitroimidazoles are compounds with electron-affinity compounds that can substitute for oxygen and serve as hypoxic cell sensitizers. Halogenated pyrimidines, such as BUdR and IUdR, can be incorporated into DNA and increase sensitivity to the ionizing effects of radiation (Fig. 14-48). On the other hand, sulfhydryl compounds scavenge free radicals and act as radioprotective agents.[35]

Tumor Biology

Clearly, the goal of radiotherapy is to obtain tumor control while balancing the complications and adverse effects on normal tissue. The probability of obtaining adequate tumor control with a given total dose of radiation can be described as a sigmoid curve (Fig. 14-49). The risk of developing major complications is similarly related to total dose. There exists a range in which tumor control is improved with increasing

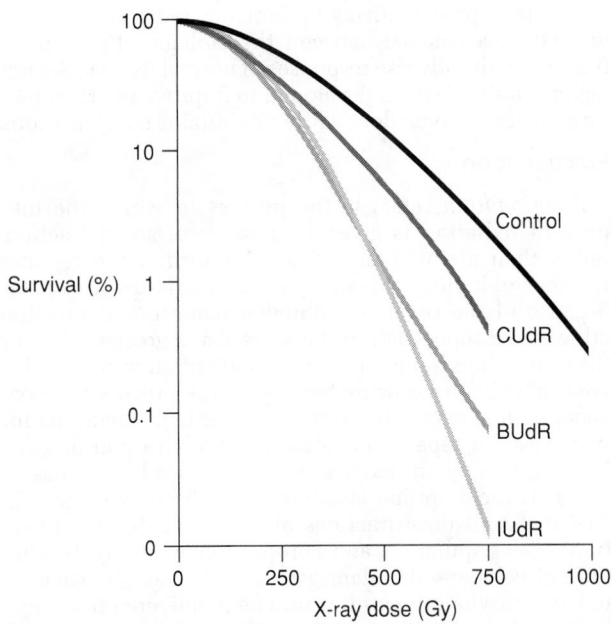

Figure 14-48. Incorporation of halogenated pyrimidines increases sensitivity of tumor cells to the lethal effects of radiation. (After Hellman S. Principles of radiation therapy. In: DeVita VT, Hellman S, Rosenberg SA, eds. Cancer: principles and practice of oncology, ed 3. Philadelphia, JB Lippincott, 1989:247)

total dose while the probability of major complications is low. At progressively higher doses, however, little is gained in terms of tumor control, while the risk of significant complications is markedly increased. These curves are determined by characteristics of the tumor and the transited normal tissues. The adverse effects on organ function of normal tissue depend on the reproductive requirements of the irradiated cells. Tissues such as skin, gastrointestinal mucosa, and bone marrow are particularly sensitive to the effects of ionizing radiation. In contrast, tissues such as liver and bone, which have lower rates of cell turnover and proliferation, do not demonstrate radiation damage unless called on to repair injury or increase mitotic rate. Germ-line cells, therefore, are also at increased risk for radiation damage. Increasing therapeutic doses for malignancy results in a higher incidence of mutagenesis or sterility.

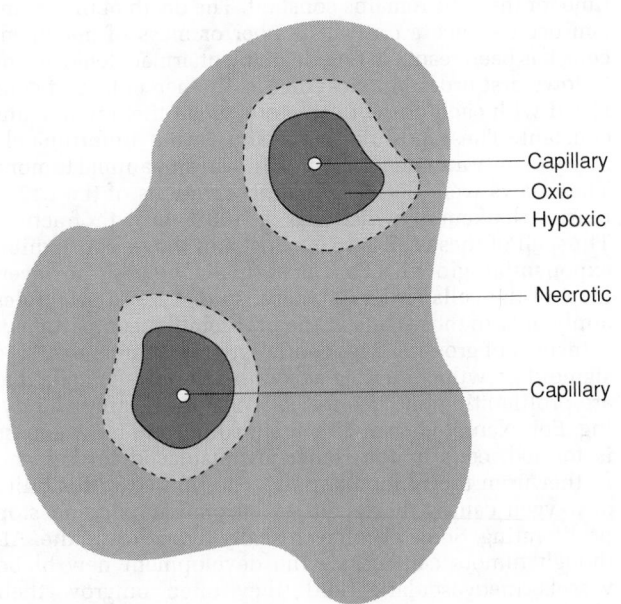

Figure 14-47. Tumors contain regions that are anoxic, hypoxic, and well-oxygenated and that vary with the distance from capillaries. The response to ionizing radiation varies with the degree of tissue oxygenation. (After Hellman S. Principles of radiation therapy. In: DeVita VT, Hellman S, Rosenberg SA, eds. Cancer: principles and practice of oncology, ed 3. Philadelphia, JB Lippincott, 1989:247)

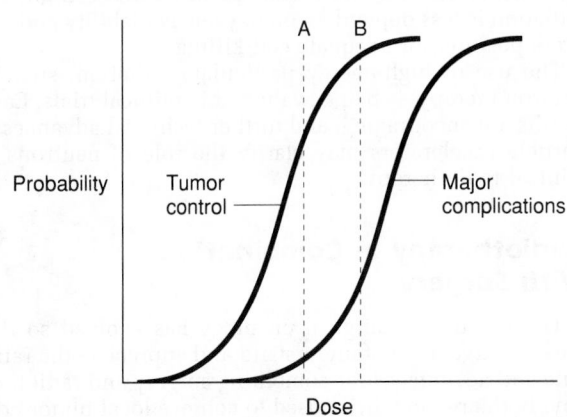

Figure 14-49. Probability curves for tumor control and complications associated with radiotherapy. The area between A and B represents the desired therapeutic dose range in which probability of tumor control is maximized with a low complication risk.

The therapeutic effects of ionizing radiation must be viewed as a balance between the biologic effect on the tumor and the adverse responses of normal tissues. Several techniques have been developed to improve the therapeutic gain at any given dose while minimizing complications.

Fractionation

Fractionation refers to the process in which the total dose of radiation is given in a series of small fractions rather than a single large dose. A multifraction regimen has several biologic advantages. Normal tissues are spared because of the repair of sublethal damage and the time allowed for repopulation. There is also a greater effect on the tumor than if the same amount of radiation were delivered in a single exposure because of the process of reoxygenation that occurs between dose fractions. Fractionation increases the separation between acutely responding and late-responding normal tissues. As discussed, these tissues differ in their normal steady-state proliferative rate (Fig. 14-50). Small dose fractions allow lethal damage to the tumor cell population, and a proportion of rapidly dividing normal cells are also damaged. The damage, however, is not as overwhelming as it would be if delivered in a single large dose, and the responding tissue is able to repair with rapid repopulation. In addition, slowly proliferating tissues are spared irreparable damage, and the late complications of radiotherapy are decreased.

Extensions of these principles have led to the development of new application schemes described as *hyperfractionation* and *accelerated fractionation*. Accelerated treatment plans compress the overall treatment time for tumors that are rapidly dividing by giving the same total number of fractions but giving them two or three times per day. Normal-sized fractions are usually between 1.8 and 2.5 Gy. Hyperfractionation schemes give multiple smaller fractions several times per day. The overall time period is similar, but theoretically the late effects are further reduced (see Fig. 14-50A).

High Linear Energy Transfer Radiation

Another attempt to increase the therapeutic effectiveness of radiation has been the development of high linear energy transfer (LET) radiation. Conventional radiation employs photons and electrons, which are relatively sparsely ionizing. Therefore, the relative biologic effectiveness is higher at any given dose (Fig. 14-51).

High LET radiation has other biologic advantages. For example, the accumulation and repair of sublethal damage and potentially lethal damage with LET is less important than with conventional radiation. In addition, high LET radiation is less dependent on oxygen availability and cell cycle position for adequate cell killing.

The use of high-energy particulate radiation, such as neutron therapy, is being evaluated in clinical trials. Early results are encouraging, and further technical advances in particle accelerators may clarify the role of neutrons in clinical radiotherapy.

Radiotherapy in Combination With Surgery

The practice of surgical oncology has evolved so that today's surgeon must understand and appreciate the rationale and advantages for combining surgery and radiotherapy. Both are modalities used to achieve local tumor control. Surgery offers the advantage of removing the principal tumor mass but is limited by the extent of peripheral margins obtainable. To achieve microscopically clear margins often necessitates more radical resection, with its attendant increases in morbidity and mortality. Radiotherapy, on the other hand, rarely fails at the periphery of tumors. As noted, however, radiotherapy is limited by the larger tumor mass that contains cells existing in various stages of the cell cycle and in a relatively hypoxic environment. To achieve macroscopic tumor control often requires higher doses and more widely applied radiotherapy. As expected, this results in a higher incidence of major complications. Thus, the rationale for combining the two modalities is that lower doses of radiation can be used to eradicate microscopic tumor extensions, while surgery, which is usually more conservative, removes the principal mass. This combination has yielded higher local success rates with less radical surgery and lower doses of radiation.[36]

Successful examples of this strategy already exist in clinical practice. Treatment of early-stage breast carcinoma by lumpectomy and postoperative radiotherapy gives equal rates of local control and overall survival to mastectomy. Similarly, soft tissue sarcomas can often be treated with combined modalities, thus reducing the need for amputation.

PRINCIPLES OF ANTINEOPLASTIC CHEMOTHERAPY

Most of the chemotherapeutic agents available were discovered more by trial and error, rather than by design, although certain exceptions exist. For example, 5-fluorouracil and cytosine arabinoside were synthesized to interfere directly with the function and synthesis of nucleic acids. Likewise, melphalan (phenylalanine mustard) was synthesized to treat melanoma because phenylalanine is a precursor of melanin, although this drug has limited activity against this tumor when administered in a standard fashion (Table 14-10).

Analysis of tumor biology has allowed the derivation of principles of growth kinetics. The first principles state that for any group of proliferating cancer cells, the doubling time for the cells remains constant. The death of the organism occurs once a critical number or mass of malignant cells has been reached. Cell death by pharmacologic means follows first-order kinetics; that is, the percentage of cells killed with each dose or cycle of a given therapy remains constant. These postulates are simple but unfortunately apply to only a small number of human and animal tumors. These laws were derived from observations of the L1210 murine leukemia, which has a 100% growth fraction. Thus, all of these cells are cycling, and the tumors exhibit exponential growth. For most malignancies, however, most of the cells are in G_0 phase, so that these principles apply only to those cells in the proliferating compartment.

Instead of growing exponentially, most tumors exhibit a sigmoid growth curve that accounts not only for cells that are proliferating but also for cells that are resting and dying. For example, even with small solid tumors, as a mass is formed, cells in the center are displaced further and further from their blood supply. The limited diffusibility of oxygen causes these cells to become anoxic and stop proliferating. Some become critically hypoxic and die. Although tumors can induce the development new blood vessels (neovascularization), they often outgrow their blood supply, leading to necrosis. In addition, even though the growth fraction of a small tumor is high, the total number of cells actually dividing is small. The growth rate is at a maximum because of the efficient delivery of oxygen and nutrients to all cells within the microscopic focus. Rapid expansion of the tumor is followed by a gradual reduction in the growth rate as the tumor enlarges and

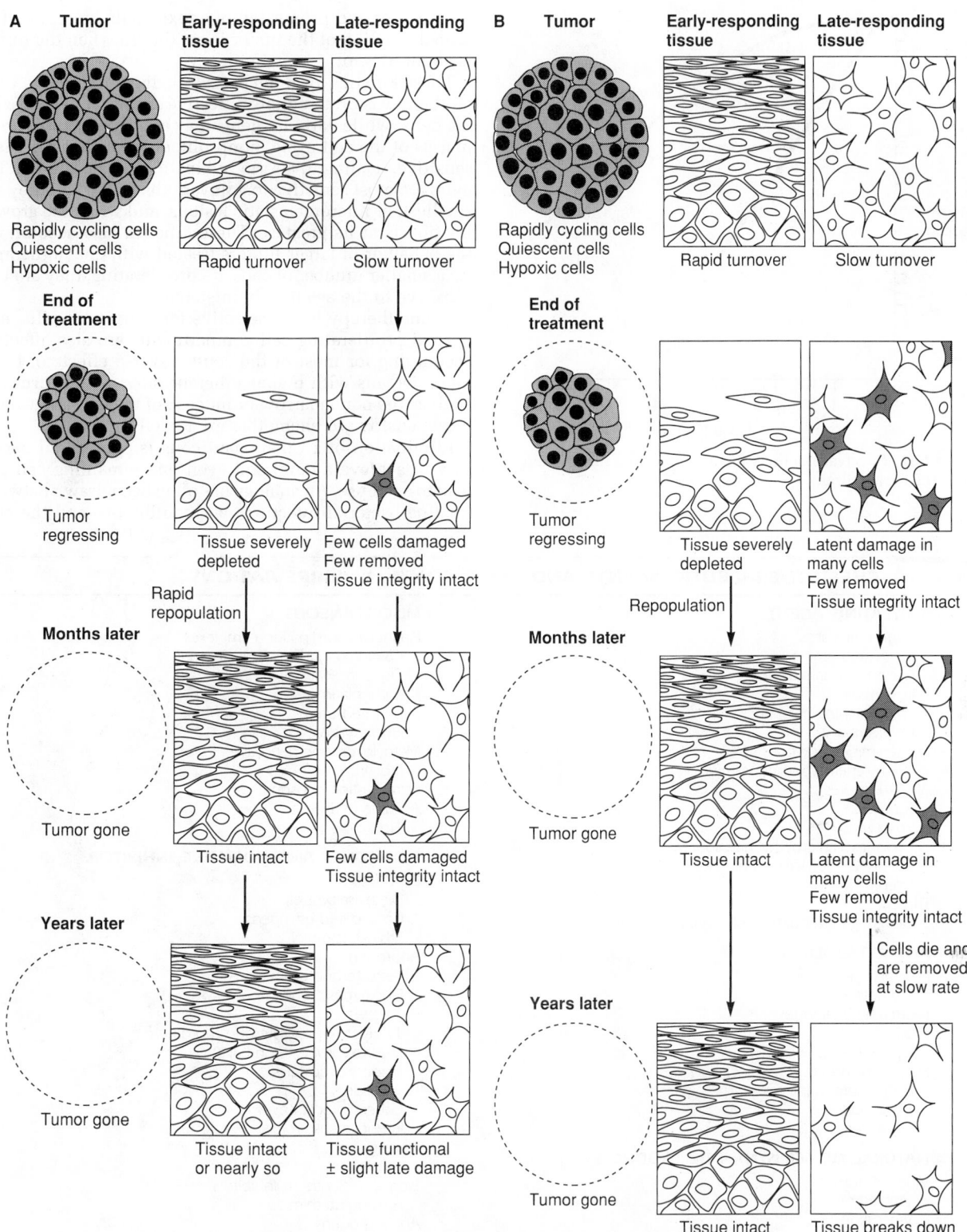

Figure 14-50. Patterns observed after delivery of radiation dose in many small fractions (*A*) and a few large fractions (*B*). Smaller dose fractions produce less damage to late-responding tissues than to early-responding tissues; larger fractions produce relatively more damage to late-responding tissues than to early-responding tissues. With smaller fractions, early-responding tissues can repair and repopulate by cell division. With larger-dose fractions, early-responding tissues repair and repopulate as with smaller fractions. However, late-responding tissues are damaged to a greater extent and exhibit this damage after a latent period when cells in these tissues begin to turn over. (After Hall EJ. Radiation biology. CA 1985;55:2051)

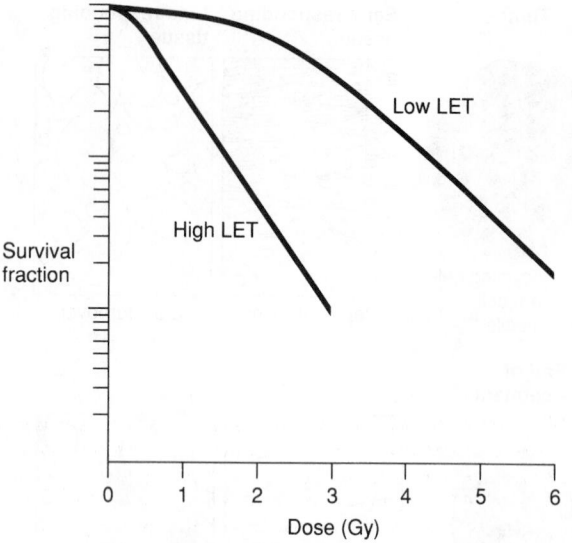

Figure 14-51. Survival fractions for high and low linear energy transfer (LET) radiation.

the number and proportion of anoxic cells increases. The growth fraction of the tumor is maximum when the tumor is about 37% of its maximum size.

These kinetics form the basis for adjuvant therapy. Chemotherapy is preferentially effective against actively dividing cells; while various agents may affect cells in different phases of the cell cycle, nonproliferating cells are far less sensitive, leading to a form of kinetic drug resistance. Tumors are most sensitive to adjuvant therapy when they are smallest, or micrometastatic lesions, and when the growth fraction is at its greatest. These kinetics also account for the behavior of larger tumors treated with chemotherapy. As a smaller number of cells are proliferating, they are less sensitive to the agents administered.

Chemotherapy is not selective for neoplastic cells, and normal proliferating cell compartments are also affected, accounting for most of the acute adverse effects of treatment. Organs with higher inherent rates of cell turnover, such as the bone marrow or mucosa of the gut, are usually most sensitive to chemotherapy toxicity.

Elimination of all malignant cells is considered necessary to achieve a cure, and even one remaining cell can lead to a relapse. An analogy has often been drawn between treating bacterial infections with antibiotics and the che-

Table 14-10. CHEMOTHERAPEUTIC AGENTS AND THEIR COMMON ABBREVIATIONS

ALKYLATING AGENTS

Nitrogen mustards
  Mechlorethamine
  Cyclophosphamide
  Ifosfamide
  Phenylalanine mustard
  Chlorambucil
Ethylenimine derivatives
  Triethylenethiophosphoramide
Alkyl sulfonates
  Busulfan
Nitrosoureas
  Cyclohexyl-chloroethyl nitrosourea
  1,3-Bis-[2-chloroethyl]-1-nitrosourea
  Streptozotocin
Triazenes
  Dimethyl triazenoimidazole carboxamide

ANTIMETABOLITES

Folic acid analogues
  Methotrexate
Pyrimidine analogues
  5-Fluorouracil
  Cytosine arabinoside
Purine analogues
  6-Mercaptopurine
  6-Thioguanine
  Deoxycoformycin

NATURAL OR SEMISYNTHETIC PRODUCTS

Vinca alkaloid
  Vinblastine
  Vincristine
Antibiotics
  Doxorubicin
  Mitoxantrone
  Daunorubicin
  Bleomycin
  Dactinomycin
  Mithramycin
  Mitomycin C
Enzymes
  L-Asparaginace
Epipodophyllotoxins
  Etoposide
  Teniposide

MISCELLANEOUS

Platinum coordination complexes
  Cis-diamminedichloroplatinum II
  Cisplatin (Platinol)
  Carboplatin
Substituted urea
  Hydroxyurea
Methylhydrazine derivative
  Procarbazine
Estramustine phosphate
Acridine derivative
  Amsacrine

HORMONES AND HORMONE INHIBITORS

Estrogens
  Diethylstilbestrol
  Conjugated estrogens
  Ethinyl estradiol
Androgens
  Testosterone propionate
  Fluoxymesterone
Progestins
  17-Hydroxyprogesterone caproate
  Medroxyprogesterone acetate
  Magestrol acetate
Leuprolide
  Goserelin acetate
Adrenocorticosteroids
Antiestrogens
  Tamoxifen
Hormone Synthesis Inhibitors
  Aminoglutethimide
Antiandrogens
  Flutamide

motherapeutic treatment of malignancies, and these comparisons often influenced the design of the earliest of clinical trials of chemotherapeutic agents. A major difference between the end points of either therapy lies in the role of the immune system. Successful antimicrobial treatment reduces the bacterial load or inhibits growth of the organisms until the body is able to recognize them as foreign and mount a sufficient immune response. By comparison, while immunity undoubtedly has a role in inhibiting malignant tumor growth, as witnessed by the aggressiveness of such lesions in immunosuppressed patients, the immune system is not always capable of recognizing residual disease below some threshold and destroying the malignant clones.

For example, suppose a drug regimen produces a 1-log kill of cells each time it is administered, or a 90% reduction in disease with each dose. A 1-cm lesion that is barely clinically detectable contains 10^9 cells, and in practice, there are usually many such lesions. For a hypothetical patient, we may suppose 10 such lesions for a body tumor burden of 10^{10} cells. Assuming no resistance and a 100% growth fraction within the tumor, six cycles of therapy will produce a 6-log kill, or 99.9999% elimination of the malignancy (Fig. 14-52). Each lesion will still have 10^3 cells, however, and despite the fact that the patient will have a complete clinical remission, he or she will not be cured. This situation does not always portend rapid demise. With the increase in sensitivity of detection techniques such as those based on the polymerase chain reaction, it is often possible to detect the presence of remaining malignant clones, even though the disease is otherwise clinically occult. The impact of a persistently positive polymerase chain reaction in a patient who otherwise appears to be in complete clinical remission remains unknown.

Malignant Cell Resistance

In the example cited earlier, a truly idealized situation was depicted, assuming three things: (1) that all of the cells were progressing through the cell cycle, (2) that all of the cells were equally sensitive to the regimen prescribed, and (3) that the patient found the regimen tolerable enough to undergo six cycles. Such a situation is usually unrealistic because although clinicians are able to make adjustments and ameliorate adverse effects, they are unable to affect the first two factors. In human tumors, all cells are not

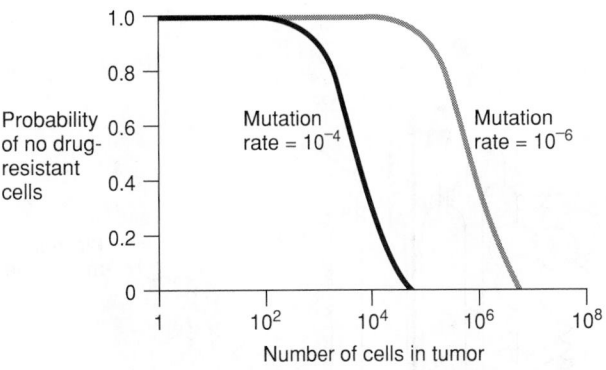

Figure 14-53. The probability of no drug-resistant cells existing within a neoplasm depends on the number of cells within the tumor and on the rate of mutation to the drug-resistant state, expressed as the mutations per cell division. (After Goldie JH, Coldman AJ. A mathematical model for relating the drug sensitivity of tumors to their spontaneous mutation rate. Cancer Treat Rep 1979;63:1727)

continuously cycling, and all cells are not equally sensitive to the therapy. In addition to kinetic resistance, malignant cells are often inherently resistant to the chemotherapeutic agents used, and this form of resistance usually results in the ultimate failure of the treatment regimen. In animal tumor models, spontaneous mutation rates of 10^{-7} to 10^{-4} have been observed and can account for the development of such resistance (Fig. 14-53). Although the spontaneous mutation rate within human tumors is unknown, it is probably within this range. Tumors are not composed of monotonous clones of one cell, but of subpopulations. Most tumors consist of at least 2, and in some cases as many as 15, subpopulations. As the number of tumor cells increases, the likelihood of resistant clones developing increases in turn.

According to mathematic models, malignant cells mutate to acquire drug resistance at a rate commensurate with the amount of genetic instability inherent to any particular neoplasm. Mutations begin before a neoplasm is clinically detectable. For example, if a 1-g tumor nodule containing 10^9 cells has a spontaneous mutation rate of about 10^{-5}, it would contain 10^4 cells resistant to any particular agent at the time of its detection. Treatment of such a tumor would lead to a complete clinical response, although the lesion would recur, an observation similar to that noted with lesions that are sensitive to chemotherapy but not curable, such as small cell carcinomas or metastatic adenocarcinomas of the breast. De novo resistance to two different drugs should be far less likely and would be observed in only one cell out of 10^{10} malignant cells, or one cell in a 10-g malignant mass. If this is true, the use of multidrug therapy should be much more effective than single-agent therapy. In many malignancies, this hypothesis is confirmed by therapeutic results. Exceptions include adenocarcinomas of the pancreas and colorectum and choriocarcinoma. The increase in response rates observed with multiagent chemotherapy, however, often do not translate into increases in patient survival. With rare exceptions, single agents do not produce durable remissions or cures.

The resistance that becomes clinically manifest during the administration of chemotherapy often affects drugs of different classes, with a variety of presumed intracellular targets. Such resistance, a function separate from the state of proliferation of the malignant cells, may exist to an agent a priori (intrinsic resistance) or may develop after an initial response to therapy (acquired resistance). One form of this

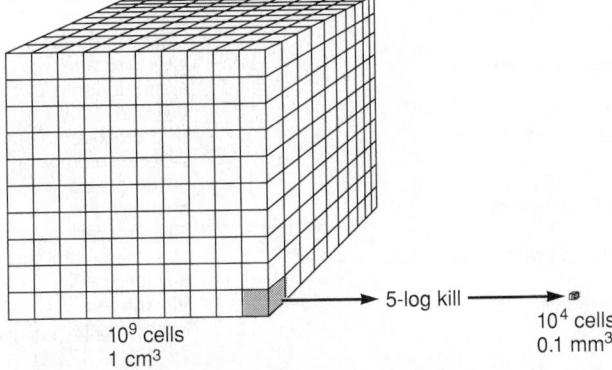

Figure 14-52. Effective chemotherapy resulting in a 5-log kill eliminates 99.999% of tumor cells but still leaves 10^4 viable cells and fails to cure the neoplasm. (After Fidler IJ, Balch CM. The biology of cancer metastasis and implications for therapy. Curr Probl Surg 1987;24:137)

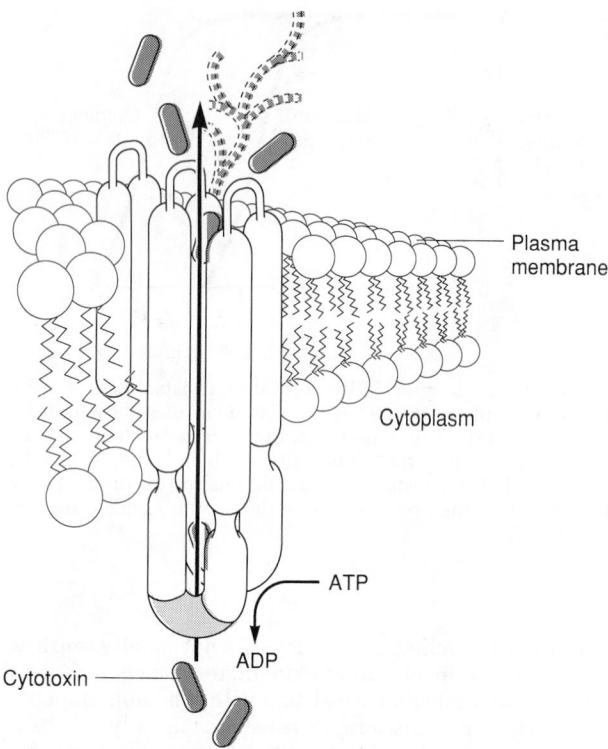

Figure 14-54. The P-glycoprotein product of the multidrug-resistant gene is a transport protein localized to the cytoplasmic membrane. This pump uses the energy provided by ATP to transport cytotoxins out of the cell. (After Burt RK, Fojo AT, Thorgeirsson SS. Multidrug resistance due to P-glycoprotein. Hosp Pract 1990:67)

resistance to diverse agents has been termed *pleiotropic* or *multidrug resistance*. Classic or typical resistance is exhibited by tumors, often after an initial response to chemotherapy with any of a variety of naturally occurring antitumor products. This form of resistance is mediated by the cell-surface protein, P-glycoprotein, a product of the *mdr*-1 gene. A magnesium-dependent ATPase, P-glycoprotein acts as a transmembrane efflux pump and appears to serve as a cellular detoxifier and possibly as a chloride pump. P-glycoprotein causes the extrusion of diverse agents such as anthracyclines, epipodophyllotoxins, *Vinca* alkaloids, and actinomycins, out of the cell before they are able to reach their intracellular targets (Fig. 14-54). The *mdr*-1 gene appears to have been conserved through evolution, even to the extent that it shares significant nucleotide homology with several bacterial wall efflux pumps, such as pstB, hisP, malK, oppD, and hlyB. The protein is normally found on the luminal surface of such organs as the colon and rectum, small intestine, proximal tubules of the kidney, and gravid uterus; the acinar and bile canalicular surfaces of pancreatic and hepatic parenchymal cells, respectively; and in cells of the adrenal cortex, where there is no polarity to the cell-surface location. P-glycoprotein has likewise been found in tumors derived from these organs.

P-glycoprotein can be induced in vitro by exposing cell lines to increasing concentrations of various agents, a phenomenon that also extends to tissues and cell lines not known normally to express significant amounts of P-glycoprotein, such as melanoma, ovarian carcinoma, small cell carcinoma of the lung, and adenocarcinoma of the breast. The activity of P-glycoprotein can be inhibited by different agents, such as calcium-channel blockers, cardiac antiarrhythmic drugs, and monoclonal antibodies. Unfortu-

nately, there has been little clinical success in attempting to inhibit P-glycoprotein during the administration of chemotherapy. This failure may be due to the inability to achieve inhibition in vivo but is more likely due to the presence of additional mediators of resistance. There are myriad additional mechanisms to account for the failure of an antineoplastic agent, including inactivation of a drug before reaching the target, conjugation of the agent by glutathione, enhanced target repair, mutations in targets, or alterations in the amount of an intracellular target (Table 14-11).

Because cells that are resistant to any particular agent are likely to be present within a malignancy at the time of diagnosis, combination chemotherapy is used in an attempt to provide antineoplastic therapy that encompasses all potential tumor clones while minimizing toxic adverse effects. If possible, drugs with known single-agent efficacy, different modes of action, and nonoverlapping side effects are used at maximal or near-maximal doses. Significant reduction in drug dosages is often associated with suboptimal responses.

Dose Intensity

For most drugs, there exists a dose–response curve, such that a reduction in dose leads to a predictable decrease in curability. Although complete responses may still be observed with a small reduction in delivered dose, true cures are unlikely because some cells remain viable. In some models, a 20% decrease in dose leads to a 50% de-

Table 14-11. MECHANISMS OF DRUG RESISTANCE

Mechanism	Agent
Multidrug resistance	*Vinca* alkaloids
	Antitumor antibiotics
	Etoposide
Transport defect	Methotrexate
	Melphalan
	Nitrogen mustard
	Cytosine arabinoside
Poor activation	Cytosine arabinoside
	5-Azacitidine
	5-Fluorouracil
	6-Thioguanine
	6-Mercaptopurine
	Methotrexate
	Doxorubicin
Drug inactivation	Cytosine arabinoside
	Alkylating agents
	6-Thioguanine
	6-Mercaptopurine
Improved DNA repair	Alkylating agents
	Antitumor antibiotics
	Cisplatin
Gene amplification	Methotrexate
	2-Deoxycoformycin
	5-Fluorouracil
Alternate pathways	Methotrexate
	5-Fluorouracil
Altered pools of competing substrate	Cytosine arabinoside
	5-Fluorouracil
Target alterations	Vincristine
	Methotrexate
	5-Fluorouracil
	Hydroxyurea
	Steroids

(Adapted from DeVita VT. Principles of chemotherapy. In: DeVita VT, Hellman S, Rosenberg SA, eds. Cancer: principles and practice of oncology, ed 3. Philadelphia, JB Lippincott, 1989:279)

crease in cure rate, although complete responses are still noted at the same frequency. When computing the dose to be administered, the physician must account for the patient's performance status, comorbid diseases that may be affected by the potential toxicities of the regimen, or prior organ dysfunction that may significantly enhance the toxicities of the regimen by virtue of alterations of drug metabolism (such as anthracycline use in the setting of hepatic insufficiency or cisplatin use in patients with renal insufficiency). Usually, if such drugs must be used with curative intent, dosage reductions are unavoidable.

It is important not only to deliver adequate doses with each treatment cycle but also to deliver them in a timely fashion. The interval between each treatment cycle is determined by the toxic effects experienced by normal tissues and the amount of time required for resolution of the effects. The scheduling of treatment courses is crucial. If a course follows too closely on the preceding one, additive toxicities are noted, much to the detriment of the patient, and often the ability to deliver further therapy is at least temporarily compromised. For most agents, the dose-limiting toxicity is myelosuppression, usually leukopenia or thrombocytopenia. Nadir blood counts are reached about 14 days after the initiation of each cycle and begin to improve 3 to 5 days later, often with complete resolution by day 28. The resiliency of the bone marrow reserve is dependent on prior chemotherapy and radiotherapy. Agents such as busulfan, mitomycin C, procarbazine, and the nitrosoureas display delayed myelosuppression, often occurring up to 4 weeks after the initiation of therapy and lasting several weeks. Therapy with these drugs may be delivered only every 6 to 8 weeks; furthermore, therapy with these agents may lead to chronic cumulative myelosuppression and, in some cases, marrow failure.

The implications for clinical practice are profound in that patient survival may be compromised if suboptimal therapy is delivered. A strong argument can be made for providing near-maximal intensity of regimen for potentially curative lesions such as Hodgkin disease, aggressive non-Hodgkin lymphomas, or testicular carcinomas. Most solid tumors are not presently curable, however, even with the extremely high dosages used with autologous bone marrow transplantation. Other modulations of therapy, such as administering the drugs as a protracted continuous infusion, as multiple daily doses, or as an infusion modulated by circadian patterning, have reduced toxicity or increased response rates but have yet to impact patient survival. Pushing a regimen to maximal intensity with a lesion such as a metastatic colorectal or non–small cell lung carcinoma, neither of which is yet considered a curable lesion, makes little sense. When chemotherapy is delivered with palliative rather than curative intent, toxicities assume paramount importance, because the sole purpose of therapy is preservation of the quality of life.

Administration of Chemotherapy

The treatment of most solid neoplasms and lymphomas requires a multimodality approach, incorporating locoregional and systemic approaches. An example is the treatment of a locally advanced rectal cancer, with the concomitant administration of chemotherapy and radiotherapy either before or after surgical resection. Usually, it is either the surgical resection of all gross disease, or irradiation of the same, which is considered to be the definitive therapy. With the exception of chemotherapy administered with radiotherapy in an effort to boost the efficacy of the radiotherapy, the timing of the chemotherapy depends on the clinical situation and the goal of treatment. For example, after removal of all visible disease from patients with cer-

tain lesions, such as breast or colorectal carcinoma or osteosarcoma, who are at high risk for systemic disease, chemotherapy is offered in an effort to eradicate the micrometastatic disease that is presumed to remain. Known as adjuvant therapy, the goal is neither palliation of symptoms nor reduction of obvious masses, but rather is the increase in overall survival and in disease-free survival and a reduction in relapse rates. The agents used are frequently the same as those offered for the palliative therapy of obvious metastatic disease. Certain exceptions exist, such as the use of levamisole for Duke stage C colon cancer, although it has no role in the treatment of metastatic colon cancer. Usually, adjuvant therapy is administered for a defined period of time, often several months to a year.

Chemotherapy can also be administered before definitive local therapy, referred to as *neoadjuvant* or *primary therapy*. In theory, neoadjuvant therapy reduces the primary lesion and allows for a less extensive resection; it may also treat micrometastatic disease before it is clinically apparent. With an evaluable primary lesion, it may be possible to determine the efficacy of a particular chemotherapy regimen, so that it may be continued after resection of the lesion as adjuvant therapy. The major disadvantage associated with neoadjuvant therapy is the potential for the chemotherapy to have no effect on the primary lesion, with a marginally resectable lesion becoming unresectable in the interim.

In most instances, chemotherapy is administered as the only treatment for advanced disease, with metastases in multiple sites that cannot be resected simultaneously for cure or safely encompassed in a radiotherapy port. This has been referred to as *induction* or *first-line chemotherapy*. If a patient's disease progresses through this regimen, any other treatments used are known as *salvage regimens*. In general, salvage regimens are less active than first-line regimens, and responses tend to be of shorter duration.

Most chemotherapy is administered intravenously, although some drugs, such as etoposide and cyclophosphamide, are absorbed well enough to be offered orally. Other agents, such as tamoxifen and hydroxyurea, are available only in an oral preparation. The systemic administration of chemotherapy in this fashion addresses metastatic disease throughout the body, although cytotoxic concentrations of drugs may not be achieved in all areas. Such regions are known as *sanctuary sites* and include the testis and central nervous system.

Often, malignant disease is limited to one organ or site, and techniques have been devised to deliver therapy solely or predominately to the affected areas. One example of this is intraarterial chemotherapy, which has been used with some success to treat neoplasms limited to the liver, head and neck, pelvis, or a limb. Limb-only therapy most frequently employs complete vascular isolation of the limb, sometimes in conjunction with hyperthermia. In a similar manner, chemotherapy can be given into the abdominal cavity to treat peritoneal disease, and intrathecal therapy can be used to treat leptomeningeal carcinomatosis. Higher tissue concentrations of chemotherapy may be achieved by the regional approach, and most studies cite higher response rates than when the same, or similar, drugs are administered systemically. Regional administration of an agent does not always reduce adverse systemic effects because many drugs do not remain confined to the zone of perfusion, and in some cases, such as fluoropyrimidine-induced biliary sclerosis associated with hepatic arterial therapy, novel toxicities emerge. Some techniques, such as hepatic arterial chemotherapy for metastatic colon cancer with liver-only disease or intraperitoneal therapy for ovarian cancer, have become standard practice. Due to a lack of carefully controlled randomized clinical trials, it has been difficult to demonstrate superiority of these approaches in terms of patient survival. Many patients are not cured by these treatments because of progression either at the target site or at regions outside of the zone of perfusion. Because the administration of regional therapy is technically demanding, until a survival benefit is demonstrated by a randomized trial, most types of regional therapy should be available on an investigational basis only.

Therapeutic Responses and Toxicity

Before incorporation as part of a regimen for a particular tumor, a drug's efficacy must be demonstrated, usually by eradicating physically evaluable disease. This is often accomplished through phase II and phase III trials. Phase I trials are designed to evaluate a drug or regimen for the determination of a maximally tolerated dose, toxicities, and potential treatment schedules. Phase II studies provide an estimate of the activity of a drug or regimen against a specific tumor, usually with small numbers of patients (often less than 40). Phase III studies are usually randomized trials to determine whether a drug with known activity in a particular setting is beneficial to patients with the malignancy being investigated. Phase III studies are usually much larger trials that often require extensive coordination between multiple clinical centers.

A *partial response* is regarded as a 50% to 99% reduction in all bidimensionally measurable disease, lasting at least 4 weeks or one treatment cycle. A *complete response* is defined as a total disappearance of all signs and symptoms associated with all malignant lesions, and complete resolution of all laboratory parameters associated with the disease, lasting at least 4 weeks or one treatment cycle. A *minor response* is a reduction of less than 50% of all bidimensionally measurable disease, or a reduction of 50% or greater that does not last at least 4 weeks or one treatment cycle. A minor response is not considered significant, although it may indicate potential biologic activity. Neither a minor nor a partial response is curative, although they may be associated with palliation of symptoms. The presence of a residual mass does not always indicate viable disease because it may be composed of necrotic or fibrotic tissues.

The administration of chemotherapy is virtually always associated with side effects. In some instances, especially when therapy is being offered with a significant chance for cure, patients should be supported to the utmost while attempting to deliver as much of the planned chemotherapy as possible. This includes the use of antiemetics, blood products and hematologic growth factors, antibiotics, intravenous fluids, and occasionally intravenous hyperalimentation. It is difficult to justify the morbidity of such intensive therapy to patients, or the financial and emotional cost, if no curative treatment exists for a lesion, such as a metastatic pancreatic or renal cell carcinoma.

Although any drug can cause a diverse array of toxicities, most classes of drugs are known for particular adverse effects. These are often graded by their severity from 0 (no toxicity) through 4 (life-threatening toxicity); grade 5 toxicity is equivalent to death. Most therapies allow for dosage reductions for toxicities greater than grade 2 or 3; one exception is the therapy of acute leukemia, for which a grade 4 hematologic toxicity is expected. Some of the most common toxicities are listed in Table 14-12. Some toxicities are only observed with prolonged drug administration, such as anthracycline-induced cardiotoxicity, bleomycin- and nitrosourea-related pulmonary fibrosis, or secondary leukemias associated with nitrosoureas, etoposide, or mechlorethamine (nitrogen mustard), or when drugs are given at very high doses (nitrosourea-related hepatic venoocclusive disease) or are given regionally (chemical peritonitis, arteritis, or biliary sclerosis).

Until more effective treatments are devised for most malignancies, the main goal of therapy is to preserve quality of life (Table 14-13). Many clinical trials are beginning to address this issue, and some newer agents, such as gemcitabine in the therapy of advanced adenocarcinoma of the pancreas, have demonstrated benefit in terms of improving the quality of life when compared with the standard treatment of 5-fluorouracil alone. It is likely that this aspect of clinical trials will be further integrated into active practice. As always, nothing substitutes for an open physician–patient relationship, with a well-informed patient acting as both partner and manager of his or her health care team.

PRINCIPLES OF IMMUNOTHERAPY

A role is emerging for adaptation of basic and clinical immunologic principles to the treatment of human cancers. The rapidly evolving advances in our understanding of the basic mechanisms of cell-mediated immunity in turn have provided new strategies involving biologic therapy based on a concept that the host immune system may be manipulated in vivo and ex vivo to cause rejection of neoplastic growth. The development of molecular biology and cell cloning techniques during the past decade has provided novel and valuable tools for investigation of the biology of host-tumor relations and for administration of biologic agents to cancer patients. Prototypic strategies reveal a prospect for the future of biotherapy that is very encouraging. Considering the possibilities for biologic and molecular genetic approaches to modulate host immunity, present clinical trials constitute only a small fraction of the available options. This section discusses recent advances that have evolved into exciting treatment strategies that employ biologic modulation of host-tumor immune responses. The efficacy of these strategies is a forthcoming issue that awaits implementation.

Host Immune Response

Previous immunologic investigation in cancer patients was founded on circulating antibody levels and cytotoxic lymphocytes in human blood; however, demonstration of antibodies against human cancers is infrequent. Most immunoglobulins in the blood are not involved in immune response directed against tumor-associated antigens. Additionally, most peripheral blood lymphocytes (T cells and K cells) have either a low or undetectable level of cytotoxicity against autologous and heterologous tumor targets. Only NK cells have consistently demonstrated cytotoxicity against human tumors, but the level of cytotoxicity usually does not correlate with prognosis. Thus, the immune effector mechanisms in the peripheral circulation may not be appropriate for assessment of the tumor–host interactions. Alternatively, the lymphocytes and immune effectors at the site of the neoplasm provide a new opportunity for exploration of the tumor–host relation.

Important new information has emerged from investigations of the nature and function of TILs that emigrate directly into human cancers. Functional analysis of TILs in melanoma and renal cell carcinoma has resulted in a two-compartment model of host immune response in which (1) the host immune defense in the vascular compartment is primarily composed of antibodies and NK cells that destroy tumor cells in transit within the circulatory system, and (2) the tissue level defenses use cytotoxic T lymphocytes and macrophages as the primary effector cells responsible for eliciting an immune rejection response.

Table 14-12. **COMMON CHEMOTHERAPEUTIC AGENTS**

Drug	Indication	Toxicities
ALKYLATING AGENTS: transfer alkyl groups to nucleic acids and other biologically important molecules		
Busulfan	Chronic myelogenous leukemia, myeloproliferative disorders	Myelosuppression, pulmonary fibrosis, gonadal dysfunction, marrow failure
Chlorambucil	Chronic lymphocytic leukemia, Waldenström macroglobulinemia	Myelosuppression, gonadal dysfunction, secondary leukemia
Cyclophosphamide	Hematologic malignancies, Hodgkin's disease, non-Hodgkin's lymphomas, carcinomas of the breast and ovary, sarcomas, small cell lung cancer, pediatric malignancies	Leukopenia, cystitis, nausea and vomiting, alopecia, cardiac necrosis, gonadal dysfunction, SIADH
Ifosfamide	Carcinomas of the breast, ovaries, lung, testicles; lymphomas; sarcomas	Myelosuppression, cystitis, nephrotoxicity, hepatotoxicity, lethargy and confusion
Dacarbazine	Hodgkin's disease, non-Hodgkin's lymphomas, melanoma, sarcomas	Nausea and vomiting, flu-like syndrome, myelosuppression, hepatotoxicity
Cisplatin	Carcinomas of the ovary, testis, cervix, head and neck, bladder, lung (small and non–small cell), esophagus; lymphomas	Nausea and vomiting, nephrotoxicity, neurotoxicity, hearing loss, electrolyte imbalance
Carboplatin	Carcinoma of the ovary, bone marrow transplantation	Myelosuppression, nausea and vomiting
Melphalan	Multiple myeloma, ovarian cancer	Myelosuppression, anorexia, nausea and vomiting
Mechlorethamine	Lymphomas, Hodgkin's disease	Myelosuppression, secondary leukemia, severe vesicant, nausea and vomiting, alopecia, rash, gonadal dysfunction, neurotoxicity
Nitrosoureas (Carmustine, BCNU; lomustine, CCNU)	Lymphomas, Hodgkin's disease, brain cancer, bone marrow transplantation	Myelosuppression, secondary leukemia, hepatotoxicity, pulmonary fibrosis, nausea and vomiting, nephrotoxicity, confusion
Streptozocin	Neuroendocrine tumors	Nephrotoxicity, nausea and vomiting, myelosuppression, hepatotoxicity, hypoglycemia
Procarbazine	Hodgkin's disease, lymphomas, brain cancer	Myelosuppression, monoamine oxidase inhibition, nausea and vomiting, lethargy, myalgias, arthralgias, neurotoxicity, dermatitis
Mitomycin C	Carcinomas of the breast, lung, gastrointestinal tract, cervix, bladder	Myelosuppression, severe vesicant, weakness, anorexia, hemolytic anemia, renal insufficiency, nausea and vomiting
ANTIMETABOLITES: interfere with nucleic acid synthesis and are cell cycle specific		
Cytosine arabinoside	Acute myelogenous leukemia, leptomeningeal carcinomatosis, lymphomas	Myelosuppression, ischemic bowel, stomatitis, nausea and vomiting, hepatotoxicity, cerebellar toxicity
5-Fluorouracil	Carcinomas of the breast, cervix, head and neck, gastrointestinal tract; nonmelanoma skin cancer	Mucositis, diarrhea, myelosuppression, dermatitis, hepatotoxicity (intraarterial therapy), nausea and vomiting
Floxuridine	Hepatic arterial therapy	Mucositis, biliary sclerosis, nausea and vomiting, abdominal pain
6-Mercaptopurine	Acute lymphoblastic leukemia	Myelosuppression, cholestasis, rash, anorexia, nausea and vomiting
Methotrexate	Carcinomas of the breast, head and neck, esophagus; choriocarcinoma; leptomeningeal carcinomatosis; osteogenic sarcoma	Myelosuppression, stomatitis, diarrhea, intestinal bleeding and perforation, arachnoiditis, hepatic dysfunction, cirrhosis, radiation recall, pneumonitis, renal dysfunction
Gemcitabine (Difluorodeoxycytidine)	Experimental	Myelosuppression, weakness
Pentostatin	Hairy cell leukemia, T-cell lymphomas	Nephrotoxicity, risk of severe infections without neutropenia, lethargy, hepatotoxicity, mild myelosuppression
Fludarabine	B-cell chronic lymphocytic leukemia	Myelosuppression, tumor lysis syndrome, weakness, neurotoxicity, edema, pneumonitis, nausea and vomiting, anorexia, gastrointestinal bleeding, stomatitis, diarrhea

(continued)

Analysis of TILs in these two human neoplasms has revealed (1) impairment of lymphocyte function at the tumor site, (2) a strategy for reinstating immune function ex vivo, (3) potential diversity in the nature and function of TILs from histologically different tumors, and (4) in TILs, a lack of correlation between phenotypic expression and function of T lymphocytes.

Extraordinary diversity may be present in effector cell type and function among different human cancers. Investi-gations of human TILs have identified several populations of cytotoxic T lymphocytes recovered from melanoma and renal cell carcinoma that differ in expression of class I major histocompatibility complex and in response to tumor-associated antigens. Prominent differences are evident on comparison of the lymphocyte populations of TILs that marginate into melanoma and renal cell carcinoma. Melanoma TILs have cytotoxic lymphocytes that proliferate in the presence of interleukin-2 (IL-2) and antigens.

Table 14-12. COMMON CHEMOTHERAPEUTIC AGENTS (Continued)

Drug	Indication	Toxicities
PLANT ALKALOIDS		
Epipodophylotoxins: topoisomerase II inhibition		
Etoposide (VP-16)	Acute myelogenous leukemia, testicular cancer, small cell lung cancer	Myelosuppression, nausea and vomiting, alopecia, ileus, hypotension
Teniposide (VM-26)	Pediatric leukemia	Same as etoposide
Taxanes: excessive microtubule polymerization		
Paclitaxel (Taxol)	Carcinomas of the breast, ovary, head and neck, esophagus; lymphomas	Myelosuppression, alopecia, cardiac arrhythmias, neurotoxicity, abdominal pain, muscular cramps and myalgias
Docetaxel (Taxotere)	Experimental	Same as paclitaxel, fluid third spacing (vascular leak syndrome)
Vinca Alkaloids: microtubule disruption		
Vincristine	Acute lymphocytic leukemia; Hodgkin's disease; lymphomas; sarcomas; carcinomas of the breast, bladder, lung; Wilms tumor	Mild myelosuppression, neuropathy, ileus, SIADH
Vinblastine	Carcinomas of the breast and testis, Hodgkin's disease, lymphomas, neuroblastoma, choriocarcinoma	Myelosuppression, mild neuropathy, ileus, abdominal pain, nausea and vomiting
Camptothecins: topoisomerase I inhibition		
Topotecan Irinotecan (CPT-11) 9-Aminocamptothecin	Experimental	Myelosuppression, diarrhea (CPT-11), nausea and vomiting, pulmonary toxicity, weakness
ANTIBIOTICS		
Anthracyclines: Topoisomerase II inhibition		
Doxorubicin Daunorubicin Idarubicin	Acute leukemias (daunorubicin, idarubicin); multiple myeloma; lymphomas; Hodgkin's disease; carcinomas of the breast, liver, stomach, bladder, lung (small cell); sarcomas; neuroblastoma; Wilms tumor	Myelosuppression, cardiomyopathy, alopecia, nausea and vomiting, mucositis, radiation recall, severe vesicant
Bleomycin: DNA strand scission	Lymphomas; Hodgkin's disease; carcinomas of the head and neck, testis	Pneumonitis, pulmonary fibrosis, fever and chills, anaphylaxis, dermatitis, mild myelosuppression
Actinomycin D: RNA synthesis inhibition	Choriocarcinoma, sarcomas, neuroblastoma, Wilms tumor	Myelosuppression, nausea and vomiting, mucositis, dermatitis, alopecia, diarrhea, severe vesicant, radiation recall
MISCELLANEOUS AGENTS		
Mitoxantrone—*topoisomerase II inhibitor*	Acute leukemias, lymphomas	Myelosuppression, nausea and vomiting (mild), minimal cardiotoxicity, alopecia (mild), blue sclera and nails
Mitotane—*blocks adrenocorticoid synthesis*	Adrenal carcinoma	Nausea and vomiting, depression, dermatitis, lethargy
Hydroxyurea—*blocks nucleotide reductase, inhibits DNA synthesis*	Chronic myelogenous leukemia	Myelosuppression, nausea and vomiting, increased blood urea nitrogen, headaches, dermatitis
Amsacrine—*Topoisomerase II inhibition*	Acute myelogenous leukemia	Myelosuppression, vesicant, phlebitis, alopecia, stomatitis, hepatotoxicity, neurotoxicity
L-Asparaginase—*depletes extracellular asparagine stores*	Acute lymphoblastic leukemia	Allergic reactions, nausea and vomiting, anorexia, hepatitis, pancreatitis, coagulopathy (usually subclinical), lethargy, depression, glucose intolerance
Tamoxifen—*estrogen receptor antagonist*	Breast carcinoma	Thrombophlebitis, vaginal bleeding, endometrial carcinoma, tumor flare, nausea, hot flashes
Estrogens—*androgen antagonists*	Prostate carcinoma, breast carcinoma	Thromboembolic events, gynecomastia, fluid retention, vaginal bleeding, increased cardiovascular deaths, hypercalcemic flare
Aminoglutethimide—*aromatase inhibitor*	Breast carcinoma	Dermatitis, somnolence, ataxia, nystagmus

SIADH, syndrome of inappropriate antidiuretic hormone secretion.

Table 14-13. **TWO PERFORMANCE STATUS SCALES**

KARNOFSKY PERFORMANCE STATUS SCALE

Definition	Percentage	Status
Able to carry on normal activity; no special care is needed	100	Normal; no complaints; no evidence of disease
	90	Able to carry on normal activity; minor signs of symptoms of disease
	80	Normal activity with effort; some signs of symptoms of disease
Unable to work; able to live at home; cares for most personal needs; a varying amount of assistance is needed	70	Cares for self; unable to carry on normal activity or do active work
	60	Requires occasional assistance but is able to care for most needs
	50	Requires considerable assistance and frequent medical care
Unable to care for self; requires equivalent of institutional or hospital care; disease may be progressing rapidly	40	Disabled; requires special care and assistance
	30	Severely disabled; hospitalization is indicated although death not imminent
	20	Very sick; hospitalization is necessary
	10	Moribund; fatal processes progressing rapidly
	0	Dead

EASTERN COOPERATIVE ONCOLOGY GROUP PERFORMANCE STATUS SCALE

Status	Definition
0	Normal activity
1	Symptoms, but ambulatory
2	In bed less than 50% of time
3	In bed more than 50% of time
4	100% bedridden

The ex vivo propagated melanoma TILs kills only autologous cells and not allogeneic tumor cells. On the other hand, TILs from human renal cell carcinomas have the capacity to kill both autologous and allogeneic human cancer cells after IL-2 activation. Initially, it was concluded that the unrestricted cytotoxicity of renal cell carcinoma by TILs was due to predominance of NK cells known to lyse a vast array of allogeneic targets. Phenotypic analysis of TILs separated by a fluorescence-activated cell sorter, however, revealed an anomalous T cell that was cytotoxic in vitro for both autologous and allogeneic targets. The novel modality of T-cell–mediated tumor lysis in the absence of major histocompatibility complex compatibility may suggest (at least in renal cell carcinoma) the possibility of producing antitumor T cells from allogeneic donors.

The function of human TILs need not correlate with the phenotypic (cluster designate, CD) marker expression as ascribed to T cells in murine tumor model systems. In mice, $CD3^+CD4^+$ lymphocytes are predominantly associated with helper T-cell function, whereas $CD3^+CD8^+$ T lymphocytes have cytotoxic or suppressor cell function. Experiments using cloned human TILs showed no correla-

tion between the CD4 or CD8 expression and the functional capacity of cloned $CD3^+$ T cells. Thus, $CD4^+$ cells, otherwise known as T_H lymphocytes, enigmatically possess cytotoxic capabilities, and $CD8^+$ cells produce different cytokines, such as IL-2 and IL-4, functions usually ascribed to $CD4^+$ helper cells.

Biologic Therapy

The major premises of biologic therapy are that (1) cancer progression results from failure of the host immune defenses to recognize and reject the tumor, and (2) biologic agents, either alone or in combination, augment the immune response and thereby elicit a rejection response that reverses the imbalance in tumor–host relations and blunts tumor progression. A variety of biologic therapy agents are available for clinical trials. The objective in the clinical trials is to stimulate effector cell function, including T lymphocytes, NK cells and cytotoxic macrophages, and B lymphocytes. The choice of agent depends on many variables. Most important are the lymphocyte populations sought for augmentation. Thus, therapy may invoke vaccines, cytokines, drugs, and adoptively transferred lymphocytes.

Tumor Cell Vaccines

Immunization of cancer patients against tumor-associated antigen has been attempted during the past decade. Some vaccines clearly elicit an antibody response against tumor-associated agents, but evocation of T-cell–mediated immunity has been difficult. Moreover, it is much more difficult to demonstrate an individual immune response in peripheral blood in patients who have received tumor immunizations, probably because of their compromised immune function.

One approach is to combine the tumor cells with a strong antigen such as a nonpathogenic virus in the form an oncolysate. In experimental models, the addition of virus antigens to tumor promotes an associative immune recognition that affords stronger host immunity to tumor-associated antigens. The use of the nononcogenic viruses available as attenuated vaccines enables rapid adaptation to therapy in humans. Phase I and II studies of polyvalent oncolysate-cultured melanoma cells demonstrated that more than 70% of patients were immunized, as evidenced by a new serum antibody against tumor-associated antigens. The toxicity was minimal, and survival rates were improved in the phase II study as compared with computer-matched historical controls. Other vaccine protocols are undergoing clinical trial for melanoma, colon carcinoma, renal cell carcinoma and ovarian carcinoma. These strategies include the use of autologous tumor cell vaccines, subcellular fractions, and isolated or synthetic tumor antigens. Each modality offers the prospect of vaccine preparations that activate tumor-specific immunity with specific emphasis on activation of cell-mediated immunity and antitumor antibody.

Recombinant Cytokines

Advances in molecular biology have provided therapeutic quantities of a variety of interleukins and interferons (IFNs) for administration of pharmacologic doses of pure material in a quantity sufficient to assess efficacy in cancer treatment. The availability of recombinant pure cytokines enables clinical trials that address specific biologic questions, provide interpretable analyses, and offer a potentially more effective form of treatment. For example, composite results of early trials with nonrecombinant IFN in patients with advanced melanoma only demonstrated a 4% major response rate. Several years later, trials using

Table 14-14. GENE DELIVERY SYSTEMS

Method	Ex Vivo	In Vivo	Expression
Direct injection of DNA	+	++	Transient
Electroporation	++	—	Stable after selection
Calcium phosphate precipitation	+	—	Stable after selection
Liposomes	+	++	Transient
Ligand DNA conjugates	—	++	Transient
Complex ligand DNA conjugates	—	++	Transient
Viral delivery			
Retrovirus	++	++/?	Stable
Adenovirus	+	++	Transient
Adeno-associated virus	++	?	Stable
Vaccinia virus	+	++	Transient
Herpesvirus	+	++	?

(After Lyerly HK, Dimaio MJ. Gene delivery systems in surgery. Arch Surg 1993;128:1197)

recombinant IFN-α for metastatic melanoma showed a major response rate of about 23% (range, 14% to 28%). IL-2, the T-cell growth factor, induces a major response, particularly in patients with metastatic melanoma and metastatic renal cell carcinoma, but not in patients with breast cancer, colon cancer, or lymphoma. Some responses are dramatic, including significant regression in major organs such as liver and lung. The intravenous administration of the cytokines is not without significant toxicity, however. It is clear that they trigger a cascade of effects that result in other lymphocyte activities in addition to the direct effects of IL-2 on other tissues. Some of the side effects are similar to those seen with septic shock.

Adoptive Cellular Therapy

The initial strategy of adoptive cellular therapy used ex vivo–prepared lymphokine-activated killer (LAK) cells in combination with high doses of IL-2. The LAK cells were prepared from peripheral blood lymphocytes. Although major response rates of 18% to 20% were seen, it was not clear whether the major contributor to the response was the IL-2 or LAK cells. Subsequent studies suggest that IL-2 and not LAK cells may be the major contributor to the responses. Some evidence suggests that LAK cells may be

more important for renal cell carcinoma than for melanoma. Subsequently, the methodology was developed for isolating TILs from human melanoma and renal cell carcinoma. After proliferation ex vivo in the presence of IL-2, the TILs were returned to the patients along with concurrent IL-2 therapy. In preliminary studies, response rates of up to 40% were obtained. Thus, unlike LAK cells, TILs may have an important role in the therapy of locoregional disease. LAK cells may remain useful in treatment of hematogenous dissemination and in some renal cell carcinomas.

Multiagent Biologic Therapy

Combination biologic therapy is undergoing clinical trials for treatment of most major cancers in humans. The multiagent concept is plausible because (1) multiple immune abnormalities are likely to occur in cancer patients; (2) there is heterogeneity in immune responses relative to the site of the metastases; and (3) combinations of agents with different mechanisms of action are more likely to augment individual aspects of immune response additively or synergistically in a diverse population of cancer patients. For example, combinations of IL-2 plus IFN-α elicit a higher rate and more durable response time for metastatic melanoma than either cytokine alone. Combinations of tumor antigen, lymphokines, and cyclophosphamides are intended to activate tumor-specific immunity, promote effector T-cell proliferation, and down-regulate suppressor T cells.

New Approaches to Delivering Biologic Therapy

As discussed previously, significant toxicity is associated with intravenous administration of cytokines to cancer patients. Cytokines must be administered frequently because of their short half-lives in blood. In addition, cytokines are not always distributed to all areas of the body and often do not traverse the blood–brain barrier. In a pilot study, investigators adapted an innovative approach by delivering IL-2 intrathecally to patients with metastatic disease in the meninges.

Another innovative approach is incorporation of IFN and adjuvants into liposomes, thereby directing the cytokine to a specific host cell population. In animal models, liposomes are ingested by macrophages. Degradation of the packaged therapy results in intracellular release of adju-

Table 14-15. CHARACTERISTICS OF VIRAL VECTORS FOR GENE THERAPY

Virus	Advantages	Disadvantages
Retrovirus	Extensive experience using this virus is available; efficient; integrates genome	Need for active cell replication; potential risk of insertional mutagenesis; potential for development of replication-competent (helper) virus (depending on the construct)
Adenovirus	Able to concentrate to high titers; can infect nonreplicating cells; no packaging cell lines	Presence of many adenoviral genes in vectors can stimulate immunity, affecting ability to give repeated doses
Adeno-associated virus	Less risk of insertional mutagenesis; nonpathogenic (ubiquitous in humans); can infect nonreplicating cells	Lack of information on long-term consequences of integration and gene expression from the adeno-associated virus provirus; requires coinfection with helper adenovirus or herpesvirus for replication
Herpesvirus	Can infect nonreplicating cells; large genome (150 kb), can potentially transfer large, intact genes	Little information on long-term fate or stability of gene expression; could potentially become latent in neural cells
Hepatitis B virus (hepadnavirus)	Hepatotropic; tendency to integrate in vivo	Little information or experience with its usage

(After Chang AGY, Wu GY. Gene therapy: applications to the treatment of gastrointestinal and liver diseases. Gastroenterology 1994;106:1076)

vants, such as muramyl tripeptides and IFN, which then activate macrophages to become cytotoxic against cancers. A randomized study in canine osteogenic sarcoma showed significantly greater response and survival rates when animals received the muramyl tripeptide liposomes as compared with those that received empty liposomes. This novel approach has been extended to human studies, beginning with a pilot study of patients with osteogenic sarcoma and melanoma.

Gene Therapy for Cancer

We now have a better understanding of the molecular alterations that occur in the progression to malignant disease. Current hypotheses dictate that multiple genetic aberrations are necessary for a cell to become malignant. Correction of any one of these aberrations may return the cell to the normal state or may induce apoptosis. Methods to correct the genetic aberrations within a tumor cell involve the delivery of normal genes to those cells. The field of gene therapy opens new avenues for the treatment of malignant disease but, at the same time, involves ethical issues and the development of new toxicities that are inherent to the delivery systems.

Gene therapy can be separated into in vitro and in vivo components. In vitro gene therapy involves the removal of cells from a patient. Numerous methods have been developed by which genes can be introduced into cells in vitro (Table 14-14). All of these methodologies involve introduction of cDNA into the target cell in the appropriate orientation with functional promoters. Examples of the usefulness of in vitro gene therapy include the transfer of cytokine genes to T lymphocytes and of the *mdr* gene to bone marrow progenitor cells.

The use of in vivo gene therapy is significantly more complex. Although calcium phosphate coprecipitation, particle bombardment, liposomal transfer, and receptor-mediated ligand transfer have all been attempted, the mainstay of investigations in gene therapy involves the use of viral vectors (Table 14-15). The viral vectors used are replication-deficient vectors; therefore, they are thought not to be dangerous outside of the host.

Clinical protocol studies are investigating several distinct areas in which gene therapy may be applicable, including the following:

1. Transfer of cytokine genes into tumor cells that are irradiated before administration. Typically, tumors are excised for biopsy, and the cells are grown in vitro. Gene transfer is then performed in vitro, and the cells that secrete the cytokine of interest are irradiated to prevent further proliferation. These cells are then inoculated back into the cancer patient with the hope of inducing an immune response initiated by the increased level of cytokine secretion.
2. Up-regulation of *hla* genes in a tumor mass to be recognized by the immune system.
3. Insertion of a suicide gene into tumor cells, such as the *hsv* thymidine kinase gene. This involves the transfer of the thymidine kinase gene from the herpesvirus into cancer cells. Retroviral vectors are used because these vectors only transfer genes into dividing cells (such as cancer cells). Once the gene is introduced into a cell, ganciclovir is delivered, initiating autologous killing of the tumor cell.
4. Replacement of certain tumor-suppressor genes, such as the *p53* tumor suppressor gene, may allow a tumor cell to progress to apoptosis. Likewise, inhibiting the activity of a mutated gene, such as k-*ras,* with anti-

sense infection may decrease the growth of tumor cells carrying this genetic mutation.
5. Insertion of the *mdr* gene into progenitor bone marrow cells allows higher-dose chemotherapy to be delivered to patients with malignancies. This would protect the bone marrow and hematopoietic system from cytotoxic agents normally destructive to such cells.

Clinical trials using gene therapy technology undergo a rigorous review by the National Institutes of Health and the Food and Drug Administration. Unfortunately, early results from preliminary trials have not been as promising as expected. As always, there are no simple answers to complex questions, and the role of gene therapy in the treatment of malignant disease remains to be defined and refined.

REFERENCES

1. Bishop JM. Molecular themes in oncogenesis. Cell 1991; 64:235.
2. Bishop JM. Cellular oncogenes and retroviruses. Annu Rev Biochem 1983;52:301.
3. Arbeit JM. Molecules, cancer, and the surgeon. Ann Surg 1990;212:3.
4. Brown JM, Harken AH, Sharefkin JB. Recombinant DNA and surgery. Ann Surg 1990;212:178.
5. Ducker BJ., Mamon HJ, Roberts M. Oncogenes, growth factors, and signal transduction. N Engl J Med 1989;321:1383.
6. Cross M, Dexter TM. Growth factors in development, transformation, and tumorigenesis. Cell 1991;64:271.
7. Cantley LC, Auger KR, Carpenter C, et al. Oncogenes and signal transduction. Cell 1991;64:281.
8. Marshall CJ. Tumor suppressor genes. Cell 1991;64:313.
9. Hunter T. Cooperation between oncogenes. Cell 1991;64:249.
10. Fearon ER, Vogelstein B. A genetic model for colorectala tumorigenesis. Cell 1990;61:759.
11. Weinberg RA. A molecular basis of cancer. Sci Am 1983; 249:126.
12. Liotta LA, Steeg PS, Stetler-Stevenson WG. Cancer metastasis and angiogenesis: an imbalance of positive and negative regulation. Cell 1991;64:327.
13. Fidler IJ, Balch CM. The biology of cancer metastasis and implications for therapy. Curr Probl Surg 1987;24:137.
14. Fidler IJ, Radinsky R. Genetic control of cancer metastasis. (Editorial) J Natl Cancer Inst 1990;82:166.
15. Radinsky R, Fidler IJ. Regulation of tumor cell growth at organ-specific metastases. In Vivo 1992;6:325.
16. Folkman J. What is the evidence that tumors are angiogenesis dependent? J Natl Cancer Inst 1989;82:4.
17. Weidner N. Tumor angiogenesis: review of current applications in tumor prognostication. Conference proceedings. New cancer strategies: angiogenesis antagonists. Washington, DC, Cambridge Healthtech Institute, 1995.
18. Srivastava A, Laidler P, Davies RP. The prognostic significance of tumor vascularity in intermediate thickness (0.76–4.0 mm thick) skin melanoma: a quantitative histologic study. Am J Pathol 1988;133:419.
19. Liotta LA, Kleinerman J. Saidel GM. Quantitative relationships of intravascular tumor cells, tumor vessels, and pulmonary metastases following tumor implantation. Cancer Res 1974;34:997.
20. Weidner N, Semple JP, Welch WR, Folkman J. Tumor angiogenesis and metastasis-correlation in invasive breast cancer. N Engl J Med 1991;324:1.
21. Gasparini G, Weidner N, Bevilacqua P. Intratumoral microvessel density and p53 protein: correlation with metastasis in head-and-neck squamous-cell carcinoma. Int J Cancer 1993;55:739.
22. Weidner N, Carroll PR, Flax J. Tumor angiogenesis correlates with metastasis in invasive prostate carcinoma. Am J Pathol 1993;143:401.
23. Macchiarini P, Fontanini G, Hardin M, Squartini F, Angeletti C. Relation of neovascularisation to metastasis of non-small-cell lung cancer. Lancet 1992;340:145.

24. Li VW, Folkerth RD, Watanabe H. Microvessel count and cerebrospinal fluid basic fibroblast growth factor in children with brain tumors. Lancet 1994;334:32.

25. Olivarez D, Ulbright T, DeRiese W, et al. Neovascularization in clinical stage A testicular germ cell tumor: prediction of metastatic disease. Cancer Res 1994;54:2800.

26. Weidner N, Tumor angiogenesis: review of current applications in tumor prognostication. Conference proceedings. New cancer strategies: angiogenesis antagonists. Washington, DC, Cambridge Healthtech Institute, 1995.

27. Graham CH, Rivers J, Kerbel RS, Stankiewicz KS, White WL. Extent of vascularization as a prognostic indicator in thin (<0.76) malignant melanomas. Am J Pathol 1994;145:510.

28. Takahashi Y, Kitadai Y, Bucana C, Cleary KR, Ellis LM. Expression of vascular endothelial growth factor and its receptor (KDR) correlates with vascularity, metastasis and proliferation of human colon cancer. Cancer Res 1995;55:3964.

29. Kerbel RS. Growth dominance of the metastatic cancer cell: cellular and molecular aspects. Adv Cancer Res 1990;55:87.

30. Paget S. The distribution of secondary growths in cancer of the breast. Lancet 1889;1:571.

31. Ewing J. Neoplastic diseases. Philadelphia, WB Saunders, 1928.

32. Sugarbaker EV. Patterns of metastasis in human malignancies. Cancer Biol Rev 1981;2:235.

33. Nicolson GL. Oncogenes, genetic instability, and evolution of the metastatic phenotype. Adv Viral Oncol 1987;6:143.

34. Hall EJ. Radiation biology. Cancer 1985;55:2051.

35. Fu KK. Biological basis for the interaction of chemotherapeutic agents and radiation therapy. Cancer 1985;55:2123.

36. Suit HD, Todoroki T. Rationale for combining surgery and radiation therapy. Cancer 1985;55:2246.

SURGERY: SCIENTIFIC PRINCIPLES AND PRACTICE, Second Edition, edited by Lazar J. Greenfield, Michael W. Mulholland, Keith T. Oldham, Gerald B. Zelenock, and Keith D. Lillemoe. Lippincott–Raven Publishers, Philadelphia, © 1997.

CHAPTER 15

HUMAN GENE THERAPY

STEVEN E. RAPER

Why do surgeons need to know about gene therapy? The simplest answer is that all major advances in clinical medicine become a part of the armamentarium of the surgeon. On another level, surgical procedures are needed to deliver genetically modified cells or vectors into hosts, whether in preclinical animal trials or in human patients. Throughout this chapter, the contribution of surgeons to the delivery of genes in the various organ systems is emphasized.

The new disciplines of molecular medicine and gene therapy are now clinical realities that will revolutionize the practice of medicine. Only a fraction of the human genome has been cloned, sequenced, and mapped to individual chromosomes. As genes become known, their roles in the pathogenesis of disease can be studied, and rational preventive, diagnostic, and therapeutic strategies can be developed. The regulatory process leading to approval of diagnostic and treatment protocols has been designed to ensure maximum safety to experimental subjects as well as those involved in the care of these medical pioneers. The first gene therapy protocols have been directed toward the hematopoietic system, the respiratory tract, and the liver. Other organs and organ systems are amenable to such treatments, including the heart, skeletal muscle, skin, kidney, and pancreas. Recombinant retroviruses were the first to be exploited for their ability to stably integrate foreign genetic matter, but a low rate of gene transfer has led to the search for other gene transfer vectors with a higher level of efficiency. Recombinant adenoviruses appear most promising. Adeno-associated viruses (AAV), liposomes, DNA–protein complexes, and other viruses are also being evaluated.

The ability to recombine DNA fragments resulted from the identification of restriction enzymes capable of precisely cutting DNA molecules at defined locations. Initially, DNA engineering was difficult, and nonviral approaches to gene transfer were attempted. Human β-globin and bacterial xanthine-guanine phosphoribosyl transferase were introduced into deficient cells by the technique of calcium phosphate precipitation and were shown to reverse biochemical defects. At the same time, the ability of tumor viruses, the papovaviruses, to transform cells to a malignant phenotype was found to be due to stable, heritable integration of viral genes into the host cell genome. This strategy was used in 1972 to transfer foreign bacterial and bacteriophage genes into mammalian cells using recombinant simian virus 40.

Due to a rapidly expanding ability in the scientific community to perform genetic manipulation, ethical and safety concerns about the new technology arose. In 1974, planning for oversight of recombinant DNA studies began. The Recombinant DNA Advisory Committee (RAC) was formed.[1] During the ensuing years, preclinical data was collected, and the first gene marking study, evaluating the presence of tumor infiltrating lymphocytes transduced with a retrovirus containing a neomycin resistance gene neo[r] was begun in 1989. The first therapeutic protocol, involving the treatment of children with severe combined immunodeficiency by transducing autologous lymphocytes with a retrovirus containing the gene for adenosine deaminase (ADA), was begun in 1990. In the United States, 37 protocols were approved by the RAC in 1992, 64 in 1993, and 89 in 1994.[2] Another 15 or so have been approved outside of the United States, and more than 300 patients have been enrolled and treated.

Gene therapy protocols are first reviewed by local institutional review boards, which determine whether the protocols meet federal standards for protection of human subjects, and institutional biosafety committees, which supervise safety procedures of the protocols. Proposals are then reviewed by the RAC, which determines the feasibility of safety of the protocol. Once approved by the RAC, a protocol is sent to the director of the National Institutes of Health. The Food and Drug Administration then ensures that the biologic agents used in the proposed trial are reasonably safe for human subjects[3] (Fig. 15-1).

THE HUMAN GENOME PROJECT

The US Human Genome Project was organized to assist in a large-scale international effort to sequence the human genome (genetic material). The first goal, which should be achieved by the end of 1997, is to develop a genetic map of the entire human genome, accurate to within 2 to 5 centimorgans. The centimorgan, named for the great geneticist T. H. Morgan, is a unit of genetic distance between two positions on a chromosome, defined as a 1% chance of recombination during a given meiotic event.[4] The second goal is to have a physical map with a resolution of 100 kb (1 kb equals 1000 nucleotide base pairs) by 1998. Third, a complete sequence of the entire human genome, using the physical map just described, is to be developed by the year 2005. Finally, all genes contained in the human genome will be identified, a process which will continue well into the 21st century.

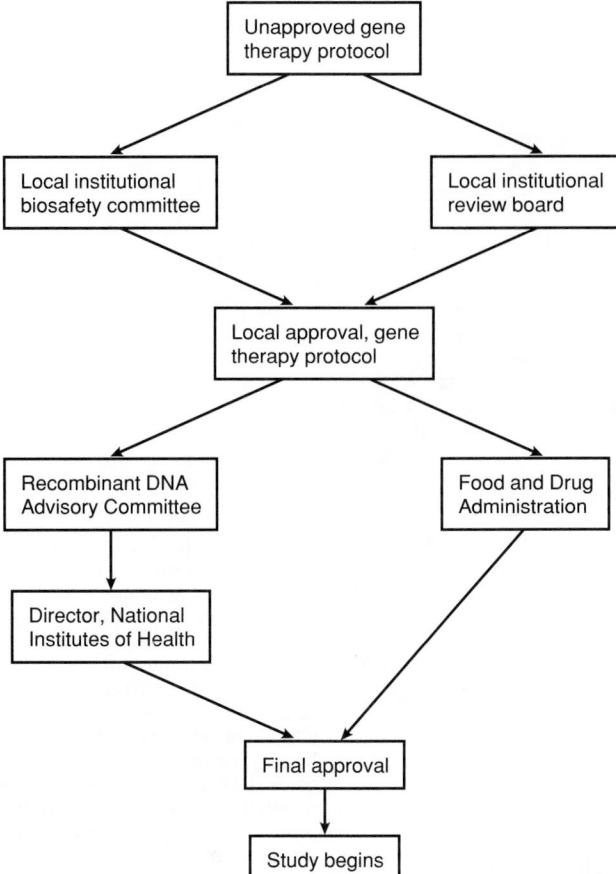

Figure 15-1. Pathway taken for approval of gene therapy protocols. On May 9, 1996, the RAC was dissolved. Gene therapy protocols no longer require sign-off by the Director of NIH. These responsibilities were assumed by the FDA.

A major unsolved question is how many genes the human genome contains. If one defines a gene as a distinct transcriptional unit that may be translated into one or a set of related proteins, estimates set the number at 60,000 to 70,000.[5] Defined in this way, more genes are likely to be discovered than with the traditional definition: a mappable locus that can be mutated to a detectable phenotype. The relation of total genes to detectable phenotypes is obscured by the fact that different mutations of a single gene may result in multiple phenotypes. Physical analysis and sequencing have identified more than twice as many genes as would be predicted from mutagenesis studies. One hypothesis is that many mutations in important genes result in embryonic mortality.

The US Human Genome Project also includes development of computer technology to assist in the storage of the massive amounts of data generated; analysis of the ethical, social, and legal implications of the genetic data base; and education of new investigators. The project has already had a major impact on biomedical research. Genes associated with Huntington disease, neurofibromatosis, amyotrophic lateral sclerosis, myotonic dystrophy, and fragile X syndrome have been identified. Genes associated with more common diseases, such as colon and breast cancer, hypertension, diabetes, and Alzheimer disease, have also been identified.

GENERAL APPROACHES TO GENE THERAPY

The development of gene therapy protocols requires an understanding of the gene defect, biology of the target cell population, pathobiology of the disease, and the required

technologies. Two general strategies are considered when planning treatment of diseases with somatic gene therapy. The approach used frequently in the earliest human trials is referred to as *ex vivo gene therapy*. Ex vivo gene therapy involves harvesting autologous cells, modifying the cells ex vivo, and subsequently transplanting genetically modified autologous cells back into the patient from whom they were derived.[6] A variety of somatic cells have been studied for ex vivo somatic gene transfer, including hematopoietic stem cells,[7] lymphocytes,[8,9] hepatocytes,[10] endothelial cells,[11] and fibroblasts.[12] Two advantages to this approach are that gene transfer can be accomplished efficiently in vitro, and the genetically modified cells can be characterized before transplantation. Ex vivo gene therapy generally requires two invasive procedures: target cell harvest and genetically altered cell reinfusion. Efficacy depends on the number of cells that can be harvested and the titer and efficiency of infection of the target cells by the chosen vector. Recombinant retroviruses have been the preferred vectors for most ex vivo gene therapy trials.

A second approach to gene therapy is direct delivery of the therapeutic genes to cells in vivo. This approach requires gene transfer vectors capable of targeting the correct cell type and transporting the gene to the nucleus where it is expressed. A wide array of gene transfer substrates is available, including respiratory airway epithelial cells,[13] myocytes,[14,15] synovium,[16] and brain.[17] Approaches for in vivo gene transfer include adenoviruses,[18,19] AAV,[20] herpes simplex virus,[17] hybrid viruses,[21] nonviral substrates such as liposomes,[22,23] and DNA–protein complexes.[24] For a summary of the available vectors and their suitability for various gene therapy strategies, refer to Table 15-1.

HEMATOPOIETIC SYSTEM
Recombinant Retroviruses

Recombinant retroviruses have been used for almost all trials of hematopoietic gene transfer, both to mark cells and to treat diseases. Retroviruses assumed an important early role in gene therapy trials for two reasons: the genome is relatively easy to manipulate, and the virally encoded genes integrate into host chromosomes. Retrovirus particles are composed of a ribonucleic acid (RNA) genome encapsidated into a complex virus particle structure containing both viral and cellular components (Fig. 15-2). The virus enters cells primarily on the basis of interactions between viral coat proteins and complementary proteins on the host cell membrane.[25] Once internalized, the viral RNA is converted to a double-stranded DNA sequence, the provirus. The proviral DNA is integrated into the host chromosome by means of an integrase protein using provi-

Table 15-1. VECTORS IN GENE THERAPY

Vector	Application to Gene Therapy		
	Ex Vivo	In Situ	Expression
Retrovirus	Yes	No	Stable
Adenovirus	No	Yes	Transient
Adeno-associated virus	Yes	Yes	Stable
Herpes simplex virus	No	Yes	Latent
Vaccinia virus	No	Yes	Transient
Liposomes	Yes	Yes	Transient
DNA–protein complexes	No	Yes	Transient
DNA injection	No	Yes	Transient
CaPO4 precipitation	Yes	No	Transient
DEAE dextran	Yes	No	Stable

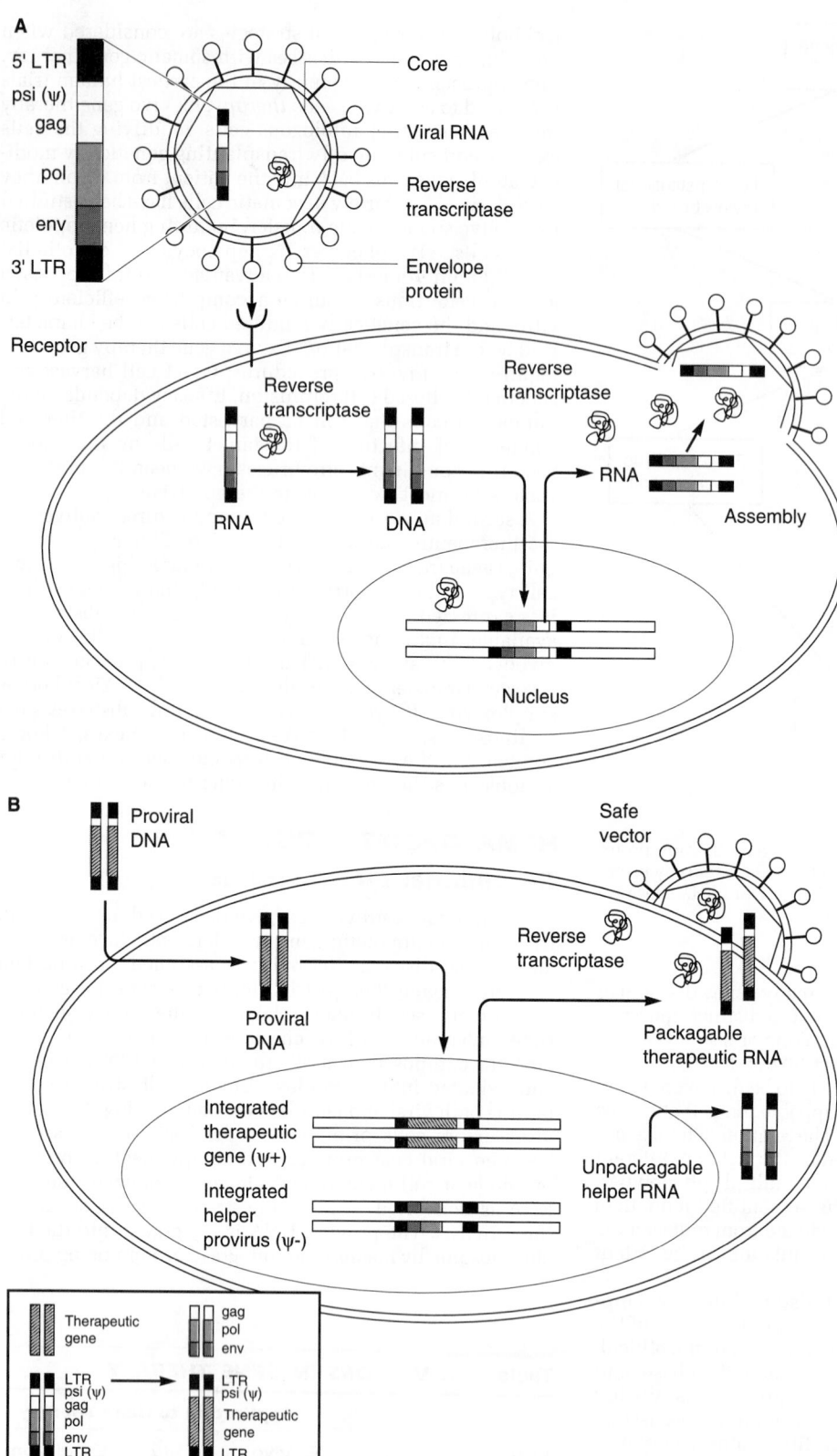

Figure 15-2. (*A*) Processes used in the construction of a retroviral vector. The schematic drawing represents the key features of a retroviral particle. Envelope (env) proteins are important in binding and uptake of the virus by the host cell. Viral reversed transcriptase allows conversion of viral RNA to a DNA provirus. Long terminal repeats (LTRs) are essential for viral integration into the host chromosome. The ψ sequence is necessary for packaging of RNA molecules into virions before budding from the host cell membrane. pol, reverse transcriptase; gag, core proteins.

(*B*) Steps in the life cycle of a retrovirus. The envelope glycoproteins bind to specific cell-surface proteins and allow fusion of the virus with the cell membrane, permitting entry of virion particles. Once in the cell, molecules of viral reverse transcriptase convert RNA to DNA. Proviral DNA integrates randomly into the genome of the proliferating host cell. Retroviral progeny are synthesized using host cell mechanisms. Packaging of infectious RNA requires ψ sequences.

(*C*) Steps in construction of therapeutic proviral DNA. Using standard DNA cloning techniques, one may substitute a therapeutic gene, along with desired promoters, enhancers, and selectable markers, for endogenous retroviral structural sequences, such as gag, pol, and env. By making the therapeutic DNA provirus ψ-positive, subsequent therapeutic RNA molecules can be selectively packaged. *(continues)*

ral DNA sequences known as *long terminal repeats*.[26] An important point is the need for host cell replication for successful proviral DNA integration.[27]

Retroviruses used in gene therapy protocols are required to be replication defective; that is, they should be able to infect host cells and produce the protein of interest, but

not produce more retroviruses. These replication-defective retroviruses are produced by a packaging cell line. A packaging cell line is engineered to produce proteins necessary to assemble retroviral particles. It lacks the packaging sequence ψ, however, and is therefore unable to produce RNA molecules that encode complete retroviral genomes

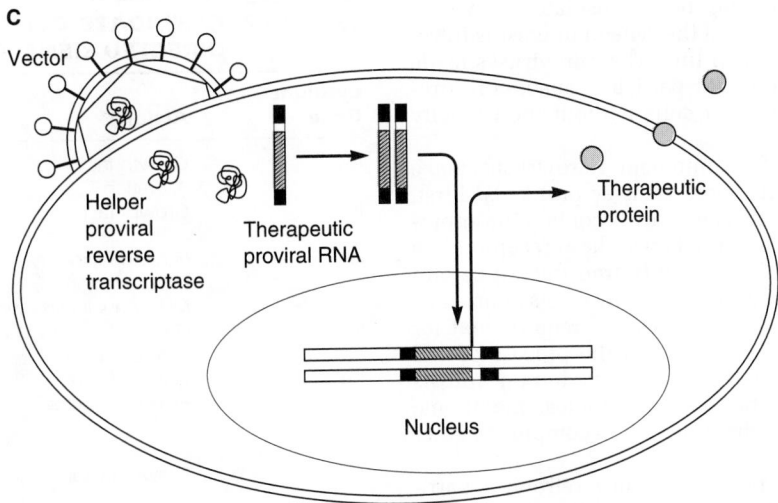

Figure 15-2. *(Continued)*

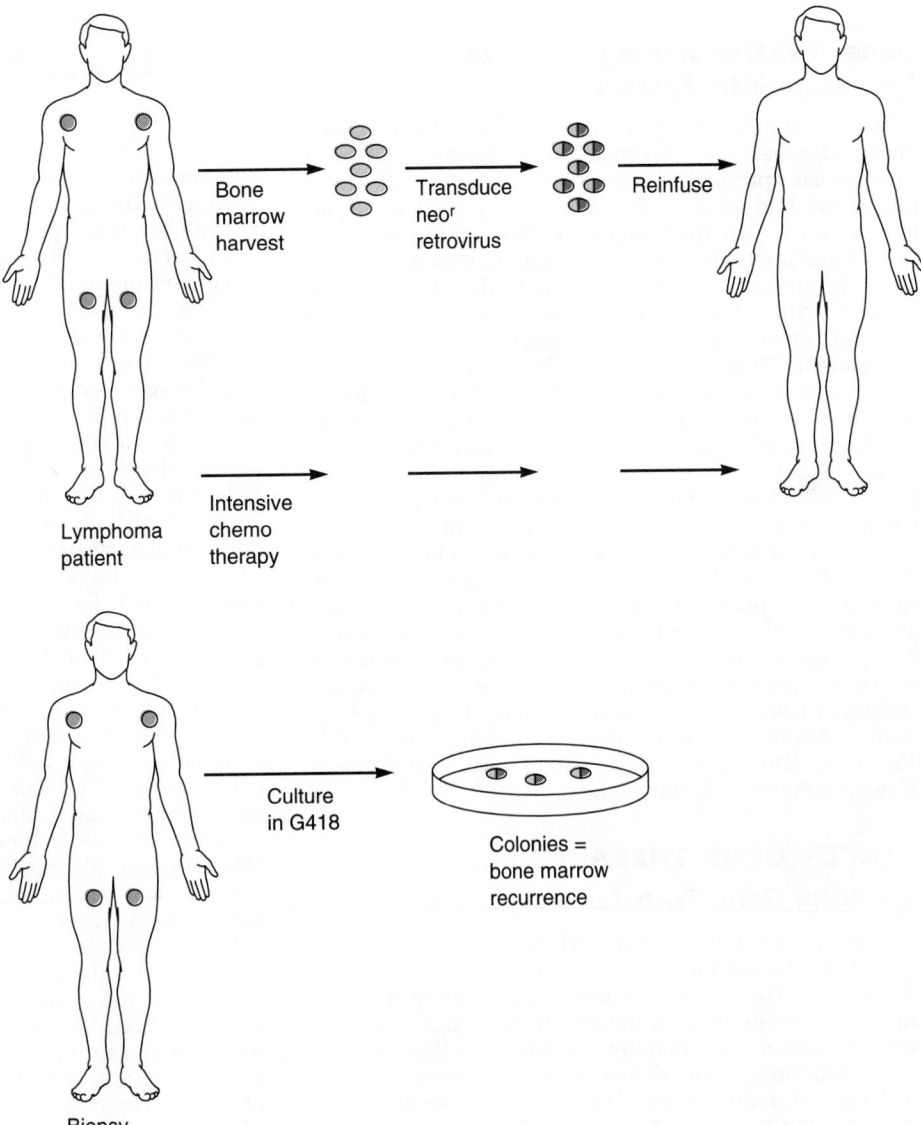

Figure 15-3. Use of a retroviral vector containing the neomycin resistance gene in marker studies for treatment of lymphoma patients. Presence of colonies later containing the neomycin resistance gene, surviving in the presence of the antibiotic G418, indicates bone marrow recurrence of the malignant cells.

nor RNA molecules that may be encapsulated. A vector containing the ψ sequence and the gene of interest is introduced into the packaging cell line. The retroviruses made are replication-defective vector particles capable of introducing their genes into target cells without the capacity for replication.

Several limitations of recombinant retroviruses make them unsuitable for some gene transfer protocols. First, retrovirus entry requires that target cells contain the appropriate viral receptor.[28] In many cases, these receptors are not known. Difficulties in efficiently transducing certain target cell populations may be due to low levels or absence of appropriate virus receptors. A second requirement for efficient retroviral gene integration is the process of cell proliferation.[29] The dependence of integration on mitosis is thought to be due to the need for nuclear membrane breakdown to enable the viral integration complex to enter the nucleus.

Production is another problem because retrovirus particles are relatively labile when compared with other viruses. In general, retroviruses cannot be purified without significant loss of infectivity. Media from packaging cell lines must be plated directly onto cultures of target cells. Titers of infectious retrovirus are in the range of 10^6 to 10^7 particles per milliliter, 5 to 6 logs lower than that of adenoviruses.

Gene Transfer Strategies in the Hematopoietic System

Marker studies attempt to show the location of transduced or genetically modified cells. The first approved gene transfer protocol involved a marker study of tumor infiltrating lymphocytes (TILs) and their trafficking patterns in vivo. TILs are lymphocytes that are found within tumors and are thought to facilitate an increased immune-mediated tumor destruction. In the trial, TILs from five patients with advanced melanoma were transduced in vitro with an antibiotic resistance gene and reinfused back into patients. Some cells isolated from subsequent tumor biopsies of these patients were TILs that had antibiotic resistance. Transduced cells were demonstrated in the tumor for up to 64 days and in the peripheral circulation for up to 189 days.[30–32] Similar marker studies were used in patients with lymphoma who underwent intensive chemotherapy and autologous bone marrow transplantation.

Marker studies are also useful for studies of relapse of a variety of lymphoid tumors. Autologous bone marrow and mobilized peripheral blood cells may both contain progenitor (stem) cells. Before bone marrow ablation by chemotherapy and radiation, bone marrow cells are transduced with neo^r expressing retroviruses. If tumor recurs after autologous transplantation, lesions undergo biopsy and examined for the presence of neomycin-resistant tumor cells (Fig. 15-3). This approach has confirmed that the source of relapse is the transplanted bone marrow.[33]

CANCER GENE THERAPY

Cytokine Gene Transfer

Given the diversity of proposed targets for cancer therapy, opportunities for cancer gene therapy trials abound (Table 15-2). The four general categories of cancer-directed therapy are cytokine gene transduction, oncogene and tumor suppressor gene therapy, suicide gene therapy, and cell surface antigen–mediated immune response.

The genetic modification of tumor cells to secrete certain cytokines has been shown to diminish tumor growth and enhance host immune response in animal models. Many

Table 15-2. CANDIDATE CYTOKINES FOR CANCER-DIRECTED GENE THERAPY

Cytokine Gene	Action	Target Cells
IL-2	Growth factor Activation	T and B lymphocytes
IL-3	Growth factor	Stem cells Progenitor cells
IL-4	Growth factor Differentiation MHC class II expression	B and T lymphocytes (IgG1 and IgE) Macrophages
IL-6	Growth factor Differentiation	B and T lymphocytes Antibody-forming cells
IL-7	Growth factor Activation factor	Pre–B lymphocytes T lympyhocytes Macrophages Thymocytes
IL-12	Growth factor	Cytotoxic and natural killer cells T lymphocytes
Interferon-γ	MHC class I expression Immunoregulation B-cell differentiation Antiviral	Lymphocytes Monocytes
Tumor necrosis factor α	Inflammation Catabolism Cytokine production Adhesion molecule production	Fibroblasts Endothelium

cytokine genes have been used with different tumor models in preclinical trials. A recurring theme in these studies is that host cell response varies depending on the cytokine used and the inherent immunogenicity of the native tumor.

Tumors modified to secrete cytokines are used to upregulate the host immune response against tumors. Because some cytokines have considerable toxicity when administered systemically, cytokine secretion of the tumor can theoretically attain maximal effects where it matters most, while minimizing side effects. Interleukin-2 (IL-2) is one such cytokine (Fig. 15-4). At least 10 trials have been approved by the RAC for IL-2 gene therapy of cancer.[2] Preclinical studies in animal models showed that tumor secretion of IL-2 resulted in tumor rejection in immunocompetent hosts using various tumor models (sarcoma, colon cancer, plasmacytoma, adenocarcinoma, lung cancer, glioblastoma). Tumor rejection has been ascribed to CD8-positive lymphocytes, natural killer cells, and polymorphonuclear leukocytes.[34–37]

IL-4 is also being tested in human trials. IL-4 has been shown in animal models to have a significant antitumor activity (plasmacytoma, renal cell cancer, melanoma, mammary cancer). Evidence supports a role for granulocytes (eosinophils) and CD8-positive lymphocytes in the immune response mediated by IL-4.[38–40]

Tumor necrosis factor α secretion by murine tumor lines (fibrosarcoma, plasmacytoma, lymphoma, mammary adenocarcinoma) caused rejection of the primary tumor inoculum. Immune response has been attributed to CD4+ and CD8+ cells as well as to macrophages.[41,42]

Interferon-γ (IFN-γ) secretion by tumor either retards or prevents tumor growth, depending on the tumor system being studied. Macrophages and CD8+ cells have been implicated in antitumor effects of IFN-γ in the tumor models. IFN-γ also up-regulates major histocompatibility complex class I expression by tumor cells. This may also contribute to increasing immunogenicity of the tumor.[43–45]

Tumor necrosis factor α, IFN-γ, granulocyte-macrophage

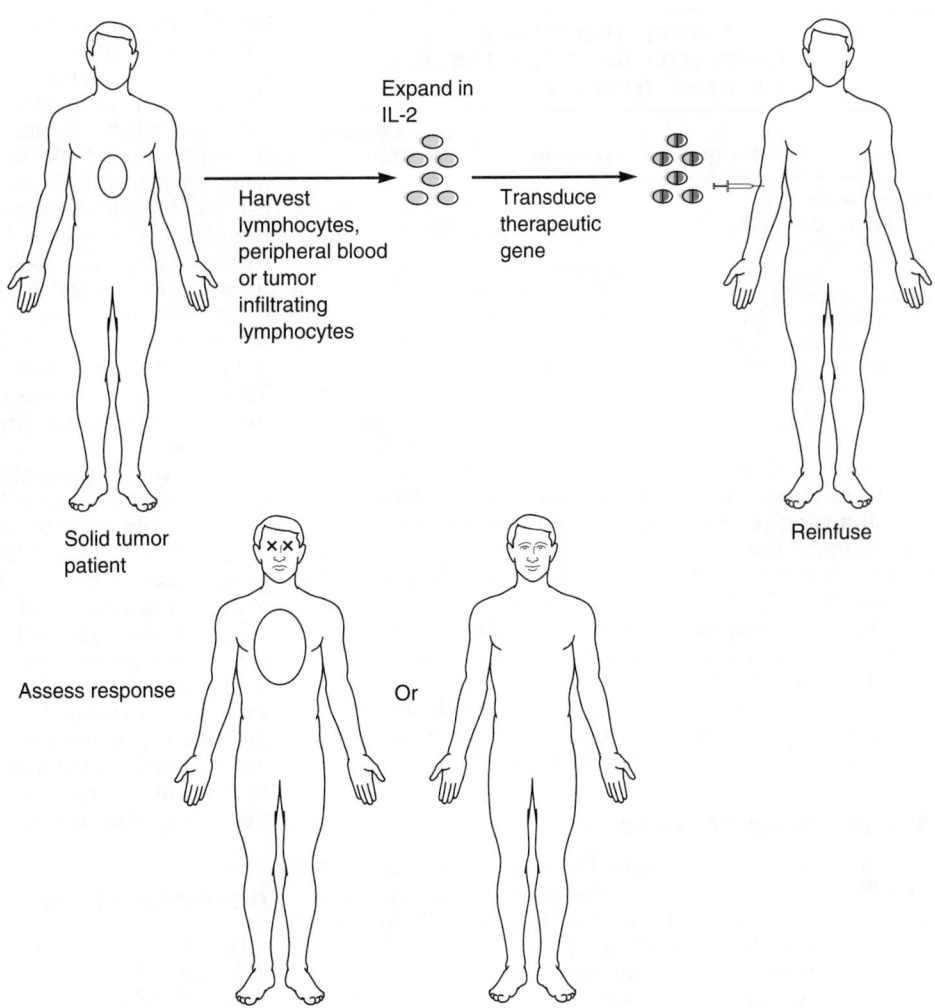

Expand in
IL-2

Harvest
lymphocytes,
peripheral blood
or tumor
infiltrating
lymphocytes

Transduce
therapeutic
gene

Reinfuse

Solid tumor
patient

Assess response   Or

Figure 15-4. An example of the use of adoptive immunotherapy. Interleukin-2 (IL-2) and major histocompatibility complex antigen has been shown in animal models to augment native immune responses to solid organ tumors.

colony-stimulating factor, and IL-12 are also being tested in clinical trials involving patients with metastatic disease. A common objective with these trials is to enhance the immune system of the host against autologous tumors.

Gene Mutation–Directed Therapy

Probably the most mechanistic strategy to combat cancer involves manipulation of mutant genes responsible for unrestrained growth of tumors. The genes that have been identified as associated with carcinogenesis fall broadly into two categories: protooncogenes and tumor-suppressor genes (Table 15-3). Protooncogenes encode for proteins that participate in normal cellular proliferation. Protooncogenes can be altered to become oncogenes whose products allow unrestrained proliferation in a permissive physiologic milieu. Tumor-suppressor genes encode proteins that inhibit cellular proliferation and promote cellular differentiation. In general, oncogene mutations are dominant in that only one mutant allele is required for the development of a malignant phenotype.[46] In contrast, tumor-suppressor mutations are generally recessive; one normal allele maintains normal growth control and differentiation. Important exceptions are known for both oncogenes and tumor-suppressor genes. In the gene encoding a nuclear DNA binding protein, p53, the presence of mutant p53 alleles acts as a dominant negative mutation by the formation of heterodimers. Not only must normal protein be

present, but abnormal protein production must be suppressed[47] (Fig. 15-5). The ras oncogene has been shown to be associated with the highest mutation rate of any oncogene studied thus far. Mutations of ras are found in 30% of small cell tumors of the lung and in 75% to 90% of pancreatic cancers.[48]

Many strategies for oncogene-directed cancer therapy involve the use of antisense oligodeoxynucleotides.[49,50] Instead of engineering a virus or other gene delivery vehicle, a piece of DNA is inserted that is complementary to messenger RNA molecules. The antisense molecules bind to the sense mRNAs so that mRNA translation cannot occur (Fig. 15-6). If the bound mRNA subsequently escapes its antisense partner, translation can proceed. Antisense molecules are essentially drugs that do not require virus-mediated gene transfer. The oligonucleotides can be made resistant to nuclease degradation.[51]

Ribozymes are molecules that bind to mRNA, much like antisense molecules. Ribozymes are catalytic, however, and can cause structural modifications in the mRNA, effectively blocking transcription. The ability of ribozymes to catalyze posttranscriptional RNA modifications may also be exploited in attempts to repair mutant RNA molecules and to revert them to correct message[52] (Fig. 15-7).

For tumor-suppressor gene therapy, the gene encoding p53 is the most actively studied molecule. Human trials have been approved by the RAC for non–small cell lung cancer. In preclinical animal models, non–small cell lung

Table 15-3. ONCOGENES AND TUMOR SUPPRESSOR GENES AS TARGETS FOR GENE THERAPY

Gene	Designation	Function	Chromosome Location
Adenomatous polyposis coli	APC	Cytoskeletal	5q
Rous-associated sarcoma	K-*ras*-2	G protein	12p
Nuclear protein	*p53*	Cell cycle control	17p
Retinoblastoma	Rb	Cell cycle control	13q
Deleted in colon carcinoma	DCC	Cell adhesion	18q

cancer cells were retrovirally transduced with wild-type p53, inducing programmed cell death or apoptosis. Further, intratracheal instillation of the retrovirus–p53 construct prevented the growth of these cells.[53] The p53 gene transduction also caused suppression of growth of osteosarcoma and neuroepithelioma cells.[54] Two other genes have been tested against tumors in animal studies. The DCC (deleted in colon carcinoma) gene, which encodes for a cell adhesion molecule, and nm23, which encodes a nucleotide diphosphate kinase, have both been shown to suppress tumor formation or metastasis.[55,56]

Suicide Drug Therapy

A different strategy, originally used in the treatment of brain tumors, is based on the selective introduction of the herpes simplex thymidine kinase (HSVtk) gene into tumor cells.[57] Addition of the drug ganciclovir leads to synthesis of toxic nucleotides, which are incorporated into newly synthesized DNA, resulting in cell death. The HSVtk and ganciclovir therapy also demonstrated a poorly understood phenomenon, the "by-stander" effect, whereby both transduced and nontransduced cells are killed with the addition of ganciclovir in vivo. Hypotheses on this phenomenon include leak-age of toxic nucleotides through intercellular communications with other cells, and destruction of the blood supply of the tumor when transduced endothelial cells are killed. This by-stander effect can be advantageous, especially when technical limitations dictate that only a fraction of the tumor cells can be transduced. Human trials are being developed for mesothelioma, lymphoma, ovarian cancer, and hepatic metastases.[58–62] The varicella-zoster virus thymidine kinase gene has also been used to treat hepatoma cells by using liver-specific (α-fetoprotein, albumin) transcriptional regulatory sequences.[63]

Cytosine deaminase is another enzyme that being used as a suicide gene. Cytosine deaminase converts nontoxic 5-fluorocytosine to the antineoplastic drug 5-fluorouracil. Transduction of tumors in vivo with this gene has caused tumor regression and protection against wild-type tumor challenge.[64]

The reverse approach to tumor killing has also been tried. Instead of selectively targeting tumor cells for suicide therapy, attempts to protect normal tissues with the multidrug resistance gene (MDR1) have been made. The MDR1 gene encodes a protein, P-glycoprotein, which is capable of exporting a variety of chemotherapeutic agents from the cell, protecting the cells from destruction. Clinical trials using retroviruses expressing the MDR1 gene to target and thus protect bone marrow cells during therapy for breast and ovarian cancer have been approved. A drawback of the MDR1 gene therapy strategy is that the P-glycoprotein is not capable of pumping alkylating agents out of the cell. MDR1 gene therapy is therefore not useful for tumors when treatment relies on alkylating drugs.[65]

Adenosine Deaminase Deficiency

Deficiency of ADA results in severe combined immunodeficiency. The first therapeutic human gene therapy trial, initiated at the National Cancer Institute, involved retroviruses that expressed ADA. In September 1990, a 4-year-old girl with severe combined immunodeficiency received infusions of autologous culture-expanded peripheral blood T lymphocytes. The T cells had been corrected in vitro by transduction with a retrovirus expressing the gene for

p53 function: Dominant negative

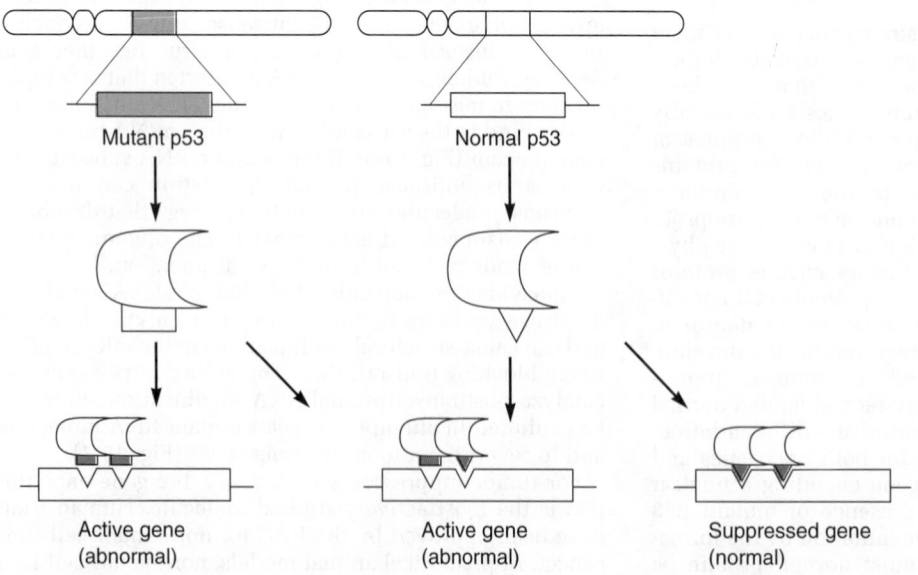

Active gene (abnormal)

Active gene (abnormal)

Suppressed gene (normal)

Figure 15-5. The gene p53 functioning as a dominant negative mutation. The mutant p53 may form a heterodimer with normal p53. The formation of a heterodimer in this manner fails to suppress gene transcription appropriately. Formation of a normal homodimer suppresses transcription.

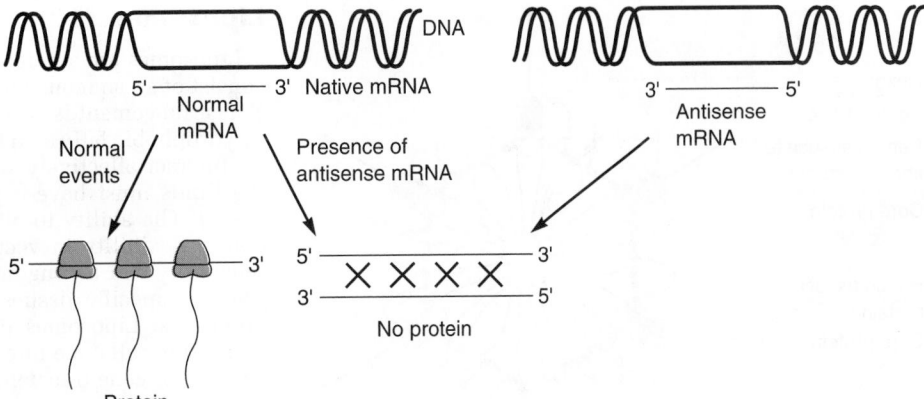

Figure 15-6. Diagrammatic representation of the use of antisense mRNA to block translation. The antisense mRNA is complementary to, and binds with, the targeted mRNA. Formation of a stable antisense mRNA–native mRNA complex prevents protein formation.

ADA.[66] Despite the need for repeated infusions (about three a year), the patient has been clinically normal, even to the extent of growing tonsils. A second patient was treated in 1991 and is also well.

RESPIRATORY TRACT

Adenoviruses

Recombinant adenoviruses represent an important technology for in vivo gene therapy of pulmonary diseases.[67,68] There are more than 40 human adenovirus serotypes, many of which are pathogenic in humans. Diseases caused by adenoviruses include hepatitis, conjunctivitis, upper respiratory tract infection, and diarrhea.[69] Many episodes of the childhood common cold are the result of adenoviral infections. Multiple exposures to adenoviruses throughout life result in the development of humoral immunity.

Human adenovirus contains 36 kb of double-stranded DNA that undergoes an intricately regulated program of gene expression during the viral life cycle.[69,70] The genomic organization of human adenovirus and the general strategy for recombinant virus production are presented in Figure 15-8 and 15-9, respectively. Adenoviruses are internalized by receptor-mediated endocytosis and transported to the nucleus where the immediate early genes, E1a and E1b, are expressed. The products of these genes subsequently regulate expression of a variety of host genes and activate the expression of early delayed genes, which include E2, E3, and E4. These early gene units express a

variety of proteins involved in the regulation and control of the viral life cycle. The concerted activities of the early genes contribute to initiation of the late phase of viral replication, whose hallmark is the onset of DNA replication and activation of expression from a major late promoter. A large mRNA produced from this major late promoter undergoes extensive posttranscriptional processing, leading to expression of five sets of late proteins (L1 through L5) that constitute the structural components of the virion.

The initial strategy for the development of recombinant adenoviruses for gene therapy was based on the hypothesis that deleting the E1a and E1b region genes would render the recombinant virus unable to replicate[71] (see Fig. 15-9). Production of the virus, which can be grown in large quantities and highly purified, is relatively easy. Administration of the virus in vivo has been associated with high-level gene expression in several animal models.[72]

A number of investigators have observed that expression of a gene delivered in a recombinant adenovirus is transient and usually associated with the development of inflammation at the site of transgene expression.[73–76] The prevailing hypothesis is that the infected cells express viral antigens and are targeted for destruction by the host immune system.[77] Cellular immune responses to the genetically modified cells result in destruction and replacement with non–transgene-containing cells. The problem of transient expression and tissue injury is an area of investigation. In the future, it is hoped that recombinant viruses will be engineered to subvert the immune system.[78,79]

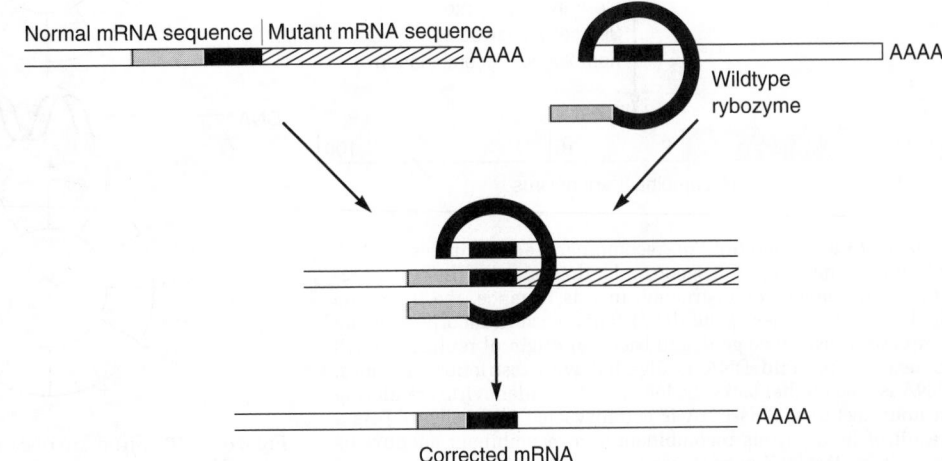

Figure 15-7. Use of ribozymes to correct mutant mRNA. The ribozyme binds to the mutant strand of mRNA, as does an antisense mRNA molecule, but the ribozyme is also capable of editing the mRNA strand and correcting the mutant sequences.

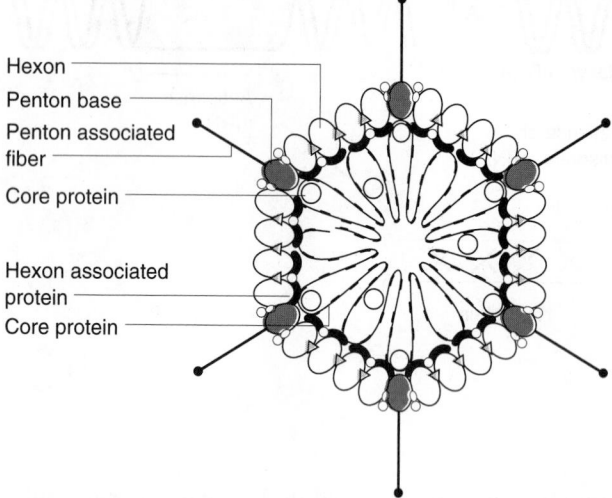

Figure 15-8. Schematic representation of adenovirus structure. Proteins designated by II, III, IV, VI, VIII, and IX are subunits of the viral capsid. The core contains proteins V and VII and a terminal protein covalently linked at each of the 5′ ends of the linear DNA.

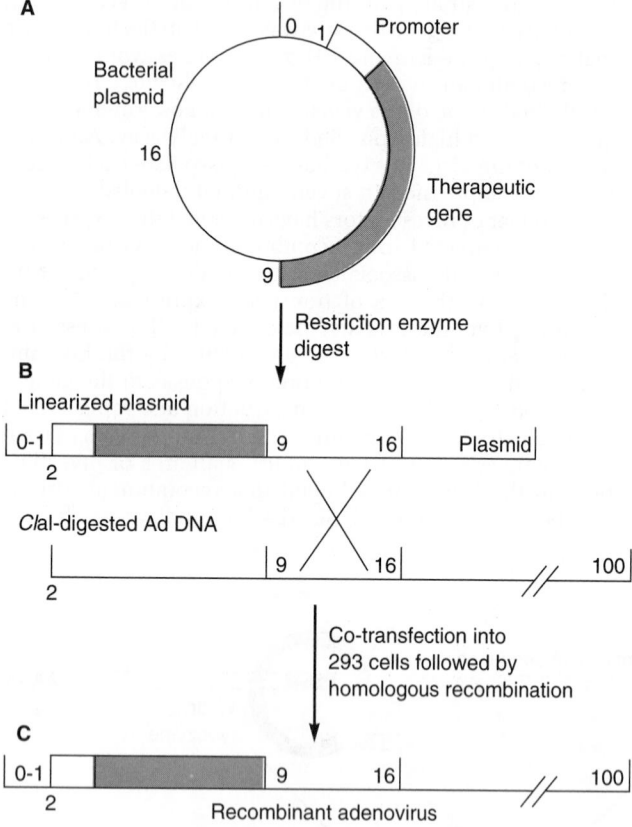

Figure 15-9. Generation of recombinant adenoviruses. (*A*) A plasmid-containing a transgene under the control of the cytomegalovirus promoter is constructed. In this instance, the transgene is the β-galactosidase gene (lacZ). This plasmid incorporates the ampicillin-resistance gene and bacterial origin of replication. (*B*) Linearized plasmid DNA is digested with restriction enzymes. DNA is created that lacks the left end of the adenovirus, rendering it noninfectious. This DNA is cotransvected into cells. (*C*) As a result of homologous recombination, a recombinant adenovirus containing the lacZ gene is produced.

Liposomes

Liposomes are a heterogeneous class of substances that consist of an aqueous interior delimited by a lipid bilayer. This arrangement is accomplished by phospholipids with a hydrophobic fatty acid tail and a hydrophilic head group. To interact effectively with the negative charge of DNA, the lipids must have a positive cationic charge[80,81] (Fig. 15-10). The ability to alter the formulation of liposomes allows flexibility in vector design. Temperature and pH sensitivity can be engineered, and liposomes can be targeted to specific tissues or made to mimic cell surface properties. Liposomes can be designed to be degraded within the cell once internalized. The use of liposomes as vectors for gene transfer is illustrated in Figure 15-11.

For optimal performance, liposome preparations should specifically target cells where the delivered gene will be maximally active and minimally toxic. One approach has been to evade cells of the reticuloendothelial system with liposomes coated with sialic acid residues, which are not ingested by tissue macrophages.[82] Alterations to minimize phagocytosis and avoid tissue macrophages include the use of lipids, such as GM1 monosialoganglioside and cholesterol.[83] Liposome design to increase specifically transcriptional activity of hepatocyte-directed liposomes has used a basic protein associated with transcriptionally active chromatin, high-mobility group protein 1 (HMG1). Incorporation of HMG1 into liposomes resulted in a threefold increase in activity over liposomes that did not use HMG1.[84]

Cystic Fibrosis

Cystic fibrosis is a lethal autosomal recessive disorder caused by mutations of the cystic fibrosis transmembrane conductance regulator (CFTR) gene. The CFTR gene encodes a 170-kd protein that functions as a cyclic adenosine monophosphate–regulated chloride channel on the apical surface of epithelial cells. Seven human gene therapy studies for cystic fibrosis are being performed throughout the world, involving more than 50 patients. Gene therapy for cystic fibrosis serves as the paradigm for in vivo human

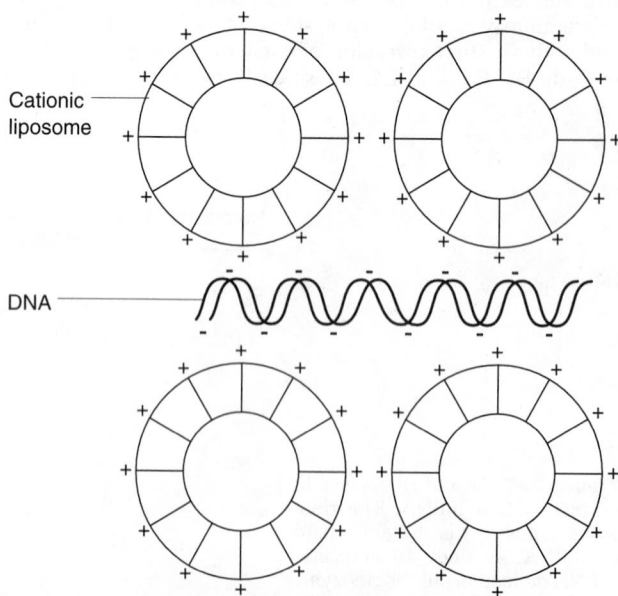

Figure 15-10. Structure of cationic liposome and contained plasmid DNA.

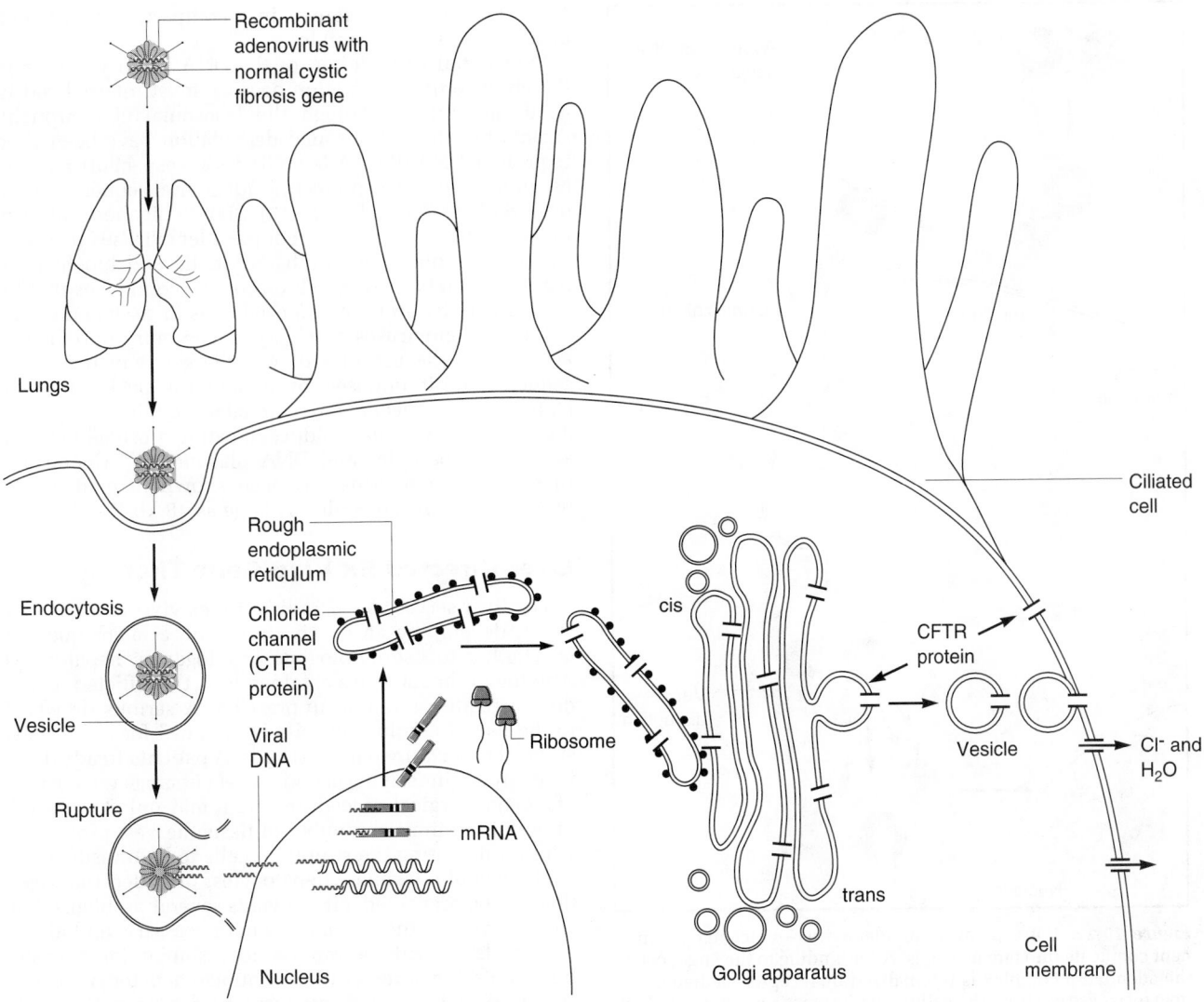

Figure 15-11. Schematic depiction of a planned experiment to use altered adenoviruses carrying the normal cystic fibrosis gene as a treatment for the disease. The adenoviruses are injected in the bronchiole lumen and penetrate the epithelial cell by endocytosis. Within the cell, viral DNA escapes and penetrates the nucleus, and mRNA formation begins on viral DNA. This mRNA leaves the nucleus and forms the cystic fibrosis transmembrane conductance regulator (CFTR) protein within the endoplasmic reticulum. The CFTR protein (chloride channel) is passed to the Golgi apparatus for further processing and then leaves the Golgi apparatus on a vesicle. The vesicle fuses with the cell membrane, and a functioning chloride channel, produced by the CFTR gene, is in place. The channel permits secretion of chloride and water to dilute excess mucus and to clear the airway.

gene therapy. As opposed to ex vivo gene therapy, which has exploited the use of recombinant retroviruses, in vivo gene therapy has so far used predominantly adenoviruses or cationic liposomes (Fig. 15-12).

In three recent studies, two using adenovirus type 2 and one using liposomes, CFTR cDNA was expressed in vivo in nasal mucosa or bronchial epithelium. The first trial documented correction of the CFTR-mediated chloride transport defect in nasal epithelium in three patients.[85] In a separate trial, a recombinant adenovirus, AdCFTR, was administered to the nasal and bronchial epithelium of four patients with cystic fibrosis. No recombination, complementation, or virus shedding was noted. A transient systemic and pulmonary syndrome was observed in one patient.[67] In the third study, designed to circumvent the inflammation associated with

adenovirus-mediated gene transfer, 15 patients were treated with either liposome carrier or liposome complexed to DNA encoding the CFTR protein. No inflammation was noted, and a partial, transient correction of the chloride secretion deficit was seen.[86]

LIVER

A number of inborn errors of metabolism due to single gene defects are known that primarily affect the liver or its secreted proteins.[87,88] Table 15-4 lists diseases that can be treated by liver-directed gene therapy trials. A number of nonmetabolic diseases are candidates for liver-directed gene therapy as well. Allograft rejection, cancer, and viral infection, common problems when compared with the primary metabolic diseases, are included in this group.

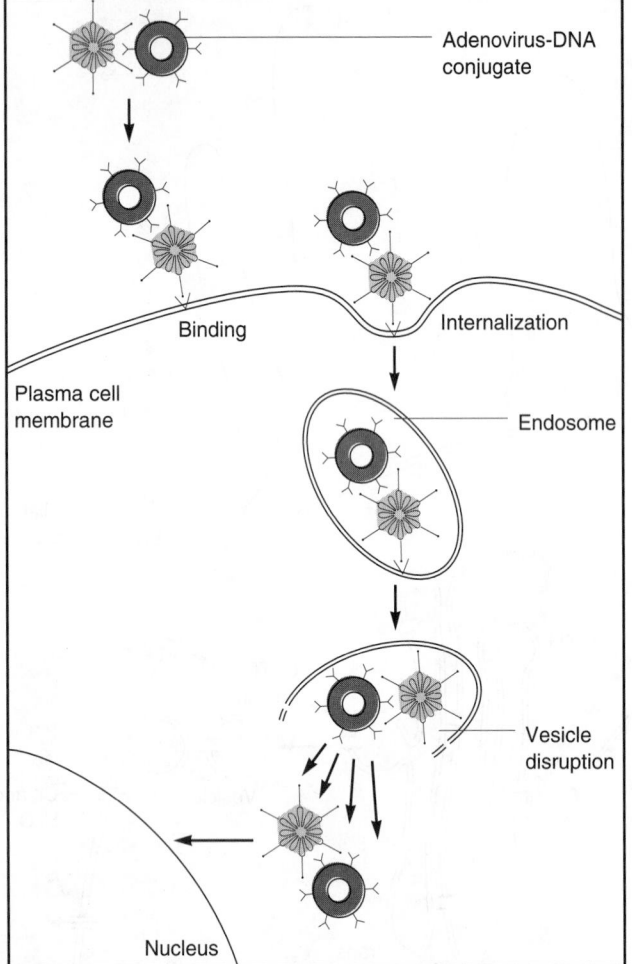

Figure 15-12. Entry pathway of adenovirus–molecular component conjugate into targeted cells. After binding to the target cells, the adenoviral complex is internalized by receptor-mediated endocytosis. Escape from the cellular endosome is accompanied by adenovirus-mediated disruption of the vesicle. This disruption allows the complex to enter the cytosol, where it has access to nuclear pores. The adenovirus may pass the nuclear pores to an intranuclear position.

DNA–Protein Complexes

Using the receptor-mediated endocytosis pathway, non-viral strategies are being developed to accomplish gene transfer in the liver. Advantages include specific targeting of a defined cell population, physiologic means of cell entry, and the possibility of repetitive treatment with the therapeutic gene. Although DNA–protein complex administration is associated with gene transfer efficiencies similar to viral vectors, several problems remain. The number of cell surface receptors that could be targeted is small. For liver, these are limited to asialoglycoprotein and transferrin receptors.[89–91] A polypeptide ligand for the hepatocyte-specific asialoglycoprotein receptor, asialoorosomucoid, was mixed with a plasmid-based expression DNA vector. The DNA–protein complex was internalized in a specific, saturable manner, and transient gene expression was noted.[89,92] In some cases, novel mechanisms appear to allow transgene persistence in vivo after DNA complex–mediated gene transfer.[93] The molecular state of the liver-associated transgene after DNA complex administration was predominantly episomal, suggesting that the

viral DNA may be retained in a compartment in which degradation is not possible.

Substantial degradation of the DNA usually occurs in the absence of proliferation because most internalized ligands are routed through the lysosomal compartment. Agents to inhibit lysosomal degradation have been used to prolong DNA life.[94] Adenoviruses are especially adept at escaping lysosomes, protecting adenoviral sequences from degradation[95,96] (see Fig. 15-12). Simple biochemical reactions can be carried out to couple adenoviruses to DNA–polylysine complexes. Both enzymatic and biochemical reactions can be performed to produce complexes that infect essentially 100% of exposed cells in tissue culture.[97]

Using adenoviruses passively to gain entry into the cell also allows the use of sequences larger than the 7.5-kb sequence limit imposed by adenovirus packaging constraints. Virus-specific monoclonal antibodies can be conjugated to polylysine residues, creating a bridge between adenovirus particles and DNA plasmids.[95,98] Chemically inactivated adenovirus has been shown to mediate the transfer of DNA molecules as large as 48 kb.[99]

Liver-Directed Ex Vivo Gene Therapy

The liver serves as a paradigm for ex vivo gene therapy. When developing an ex vivo protocol, a major question is whether to use autologous or allogeneic hepatocytes. Autologous hepatocytes obtained from the afflicted patient do not require immunosuppression. A serious drawback to the use of autologous cells is the need for an invasive surgical procedure to harvest cells. A patient already debilitated by an underlying genetic defect is subject to the risks of a major surgical procedure, and it may only be possible to perform a limited number of tissue harvest procedures without depleting the supply of cells to be transduced.

The use of allogeneic hepatocytes, provided that rejection can be prevented, circumvents several problems. Surgical harvest in the recipient is not necessary, and allogeneic cells provide a renewable resource for repeated treatments. Cryopreservation of human hepatocytes can be accomplished. Isolated, cryopreserved human liver cells were injected intraperitoneally into Gunn rats (hepatic bilirubin uridine diphosphoglucuronosyltransferase deficient) and Nagase analbuminemic rats. Rats of both strains were made immunodeficient by back-crossing with

Table 15-4. GENETIC DISEASES THAT ARE POTENTIAL LIVER-DIRECTED EX VIVO GENE THERAPY CANDIDATES

Disease	Gene Defect
Familial hypercholesterolemia	Low-density lipoprotein receptor
Cystic fibrosis	Cystic fibrosis transmembrane conductance regulator
Neonatal hyperammonemia	Ornithine transcarbamylase
Hemophilia A	Factor VIII
Hemophilia B	Factor IX
Mucopolysaccharidosis type I	α-L-Iduronidase
Mucopolysaccharidosis type VII	β-glucuronidase
Crigler-Najjar syndrome type I	Uridine diphosphoglucuronate–bilirubin glucuronosyltransferase
Hereditary tyrosinemia type I	Fumarylacetoacetate hydrolase
Citrullinemia	Argininosuccinate synthetase

athymic (inherited T-cell deficient) strains. No histologic evidence of rejection was seen in the athymic rats, but the immunocompetent rats did exhibit rejection. Importantly, there was evidence of partial correction of both genetic defects.[100–102]

Cultured hepatocytes provide several challenges as targets for virus-mediated gene transfer. Although it is possible to isolate relatively pure fractions of hepatocytes and to establish primary cultures, hepatocytes are difficult to maintain for extended periods and cannot be passaged. Furthermore, hepatocytes begin to lose differentiated function within several days of isolation. Efficient transduction must therefore be achieved by a single, relatively short exposure to virus soon after the cells are isolated.

Another consideration is the site of transplantation. For hepatocytes, the extracellular matrix of the liver is best able to support the hepatocyte, and only in the liver are hepatocytes able to develop polarity and to secrete bile. Because the liver is the recipient of all portal venous blood, and because thrombosis is a potentially disastrous complication, the volume and number of cells to be infused is an important issue.[103] A high-flow system, such as the portal vein, appears best for uniform dissemination of cells into the liver.

Gene transfer studies with amphotropic recombinant retroviruses have been performed in hepatocytes from a variety of species. Using highly enriched populations of hepatocytes cultured from rats, the β-galactosidase gene from *Escherichia coli* was efficiently and stably transduced using a retroviral vector. Presence of the gene, not found in mammalian cells, was demonstrated by histochemical staining and DNA analysis.[10] An efficiency of infection of about 25% was obtained with the virus. Analysis showed that 95% of the cells present in culture were hepatocytes by enzyme cytochemistry and peroxidase immunohistochemistry. Similar results have been obtained by other investigators in rats, newborn and adult mice, newborn and adult rabbits, and baboons.

Human hepatocytes can also be cultured, and procedures have been developed for the efficient transduction of primary cultures of human hepatocytes with retroviral vectors.[104] Gene transfer using a recombinant retrovirus containing the gene for the human low-density lipoprotein (LDL) receptor has been accomplished.[105]

Direct reinfusion of autologous human hepatocytes into a tributary of the portal venous system is the preferred approach to hepatocyte transplantation. The ability to leave an indwelling catheter at the time of hepatocyte harvest allows the readministration of autologous hepatocytes without the need for further surgery or anesthesia. The vessels can be studied radiologically immediately before hepatocyte reinfusion to ensure that the vessel is open and that hepatopetal flow is present. Transcatheter delivery was developed in animal models and has been adapted for use in humans.[106]

Portal vein thrombosis remains the most potentially morbid complication of the intraportal administration of autologous hepatocytes. Portal hypertension with the development of ascites or variceal hemorrhage may cause clinical deterioration in patients with already diminished physiologic reserve. In a patient who may require liver transplantation to correct liver failure from a metabolic disease, the development of infection may cause an urgently needed transplantation to be deferred, with a potential negative impact on patient well-being. Complete thrombosis with organized clot adherent to the endothelium of the portal vein may also preclude subsequent liver transplantation. There are no data on the incidence of portal vein thrombosis after the intraportal transplantation of autologous hepatocytes, but crude pancreatic tissue preparations have been associated with a 4% incidence of portal vein thrombosis.[107] Similar data have been published for the intraportal infusion of highly purified islet cell preparations.[108] The incidence of portal vein thrombosis after infusion of autologous hepatocytes is expected to be lower because the infusate contains a purified suspension of disaggregated cells rather than tissue fragments.

Other strategies for the infusion of genetically altered hepatocytes into the portal vein may be appropriate in selected cases. One approach, used in islet cell transplantation, is to cannulate the umbilical vein remnant in the falciform ligament. Although no clinical studies using hepatocytes have been performed, injection of highly purified pancreatic islets has been done without evidence of portal vein thrombosis.[108] Several drawbacks exist. The umbilical vein remnant may be atretic, and the infusion volume may be limited. Prior upper abdominal surgery may have resulted in the surgical division of the falciform ligament. If the patient has portal hypertension, hepatofugal flow might result in shunting of transplanted cells away from the liver.

Another approach to hepatocyte delivery is intrasplenic transplantation. Transduced hepatocytes have been intrasplenically transplanted in animal models. By in situ analysis, transgenic cells could be seen in the intrahepatic portal spaces, and at longer times as a part of the periportal hepatic lobule, with more than half of the cells that were originally transplanted into the spleen engrafted permanently into the liver.[109] The ability of intrasplenically transplanted hepatocytes to function in a liver-specific manner has been shown to occur by the maintenance of P450, albumin, and α-fetoprotein gene expression.[110] A report has been made on the feasibility of intrasplenic human hepatocyte transplantation.[110a]

Familial Hypercholesterolemia

The molecular basis of familial hypercholesterolemia (FH) is a mutation in the gene that encodes the LDL receptor. Patients who inherit one abnormal allele have moderate elevations in plasma LDL and suffer premature coronary heart disease. The prevalence of heterozygotes in most populations is 1 in 500, representing about 5% of patients younger than 45 years who suffer myocardial infarction. Patients with two abnormal LDL receptor alleles have severe FH and life-threatening coronary artery disease. Characterization of mutant alleles has revealed a variety of mutations, including deletions, insertions, missense mutations, and nonsense mutations.[111,112] Class 1 mutations are associated with no detectable protein and are often caused by gene deletions. Class 2 mutations lead to abnormalities in intracellular processing of the protein. Class 3 mutations specifically affect binding of the ligand LDL, and class 4 mutations encode receptor proteins that do not internalize within hepatocytes.

The hepatocyte is the preferred target cell for gene therapy of FH.[111,113] The liver modulates cholesterol homeostasis through a variety of metabolic functions that are uniquely expressed in its parenchymal cells. LDL is the primary carrier of cholesterol in the plasma. Hepatic LDL receptors contribute to more than 90% of the high-affinity uptake and degradation of LDL in vivo.[114,115] A complete deficiency of LDL receptor activity in FH leads to a metabolic state in which the catabolism of LDL and its precursor, intermediate density lipoprotein, is decreased, resulting in massive hypercholesterolemia.[116]

The liver is the only organ capable of excreting cholesterol from the body.[115] Cholesterol excretion is accomplished, in part, through the conversion of free cholesterol to bile acids.

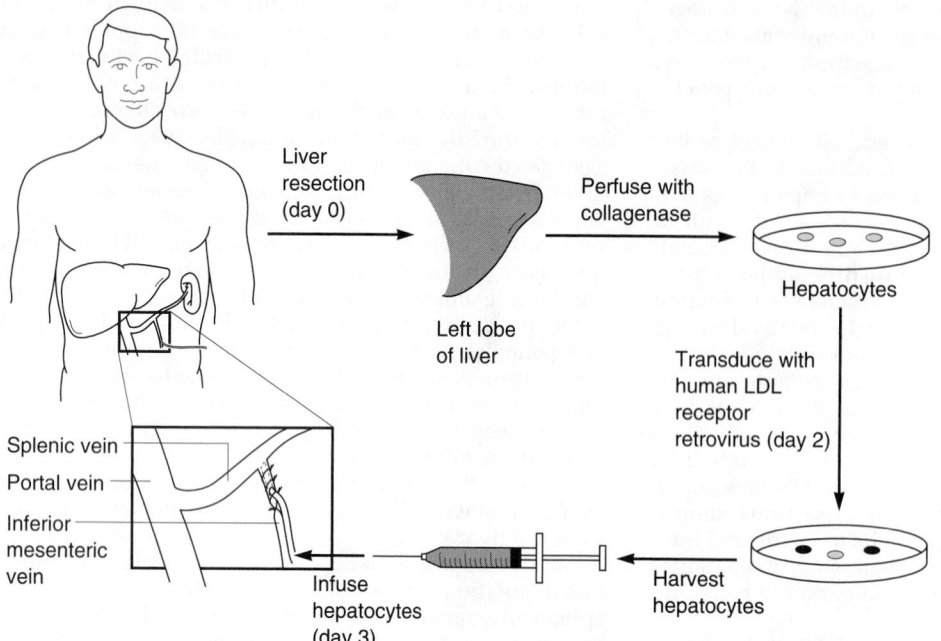

Figure 15-13. Strategy of ex vivo gene therapy for familial hypercholesterolemia. LDL, low-density lipoprotein.

Biliary cholesterol is formed by de novo synthesis and by receptor-mediated degradation of lipoproteins.[116] In humans, 1 g of cholesterol is excreted per day by this route.[115]

The Watanabe heritable hyperlipidemic (WHHL) rabbit has been used as an animal model in FH. The WHHL rabbit has an LDL receptor gene mutation that renders the receptor nonfunctional and leads to accelerated atherosclerosis and premature cardiovascular death.[117] In a prelude to human gene therapy, liver tissue was removed from WHHL rabbits and used to isolate hepatocytes and establish primary cultures. Hepatocytes transduced with a gene encoding the human LDL receptor expressed supranormal levels of functional protein.[102] Transplantation of genetically corrected cells into the animal from which they were derived was associated with a 30% to 40% decrease in serum cholesterol and detectable recombinant LDL receptor expression for up to 6 months.[118]

Based on rabbit and nonhuman primate studies, a clinical protocol was initiated to treat five homozygous FH patients by ex vivo gene therapy.[119] Eligible patients were subjected to a two-step procedure in which a portion of liver was removed and hepatocytes isolated and cultured (Fig. 15-13). Recombinant retroviruses were used to transduce a normal LDL receptor gene into the cultured hepatocytes, which were harvested on day 3 and infused into the portal circulation through an indwelling catheter. The patients were evaluated for engraftment of corrected hepatocytes through a series of metabolic and molecular biologic studies. Three months after gene therapy, a small amount of liver tissue was harvested by percutaneous biopsy and analyzed for the presence of recombinant-derived DNA and RNA. The first patient was an FH homozygote with symptomatic coronary artery disease.[120] Four additional patients, including children and adults, were treated and have done well. The therapy is viewed as an adjunct to more traditional therapies, such as plasmapheresis and cholesterol-lowering drugs.

Ornithine Transcarbamylase Deficiency

Ornithine transcarbamylase (OTC) deficiency is one of five documented diseases related to disruption of the urea cycle. The urea cycle is responsible for the conversion of nitrogenous compounds into urea as well as the de novo synthesis of arginine. OTC deficiency is inherited as an X-linked disorder and is characterized by neonatal encephalopathy, hypothermia, apnea, and markedly elevated plasma ammonia levels in men. The OTC enzyme product is found almost exclusively in mitochondria of the liver, making OTC deficiency a candidate for liver-directed gene therapy.

The human OTC gene has been mapped to the short arm of the X chromosome.[121] The gene is subject to X inactivation in women, and mosaicism of the liver in heterozygous women has been observed.[122] Even partial restoration of OTC activity corrects severe disease to a mild or asymptomatic form. The active enzyme functions in the mitochondria, where targeting is accomplished by an OTC precursor leader peptide sequence cleaved in the mitochondrial matrix.[123]

Therapy is nonspecific and involves protein intake restriction and activation of other pathways for the metabolism of waste nitrogen. Supplementation with sodium benzoate and sodium phenylacetate causes the synthesis of hippurate and phenylacetylglutamine, which can serve as alternate sources of excretable nitrogen.[124] Anecdotal reports have been made of liver transplantation for intractable coma caused by OTC deficiency. Protocols involving the use of both adenoviruses and retroviruses for reestablishing OTC activity in affected female heterozygotes and male hemizygotes are proposed.

Hepatic Bilirubin Uridine Diphosphoglucuronate Glucuronyl Transferase

Bilirubin, the pigment derived from the reticuloendothelial system degradation of heme proteins, is a lipophilic molecule in its unconjugated state and can cause neonatal kernicterus in high concentrations. Two molecules of circulating bilirubin are bound to one albumin, and bilirubin is avidly cleared in the liver by a mechanism that is carrier mediated and liver specific.[125] Inside the hepatocyte, bilirubin binds to ligandin, a form of glutathione-S-transferase, and is subsequently conjugated to a number of polar molecules, usually glucuronic acid. The conjugation reaction is catalyzed by hepatic bilirubin uridine diphosphoglucuronate (UDP) β-D-glucuronosyltransferase, a microsomal enzyme. The conjugated bilirubin pigments are subsequently excreted into the bile.

A congenital deficiency of hepatic bilirubin UDP β-D-glucuronosyltransferase has been identified as the cause of Crigler-Najjar syndrome type I.[126] The trait is inherited as an autosomal recessive characteristic, occurs in all races, and is often associated with consanguinity.[127]

Conventional therapy attempts to reduce bilirubin levels by nonenzymatic means, such as phototherapy or plasmapheresis. Phototherapy is helpful in the neonatal population, but becomes impractical for patients older than 3 years because body mass increases relative to surface area, and the skin becomes thicker and more heavily pigmented. Plasmapheresis works by removing circulating bilirubin bound to albumin from the plasma and is the most effective means of acutely decreasing bilirubin. Liver transplantation has also been performed for Crigler-Najjar syndrome type I.[128]

An important factor in considering Crigler-Najjar syndrome type I for gene therapy is the presence of an animal model for disease, the Gunn rat. Gunn rats exhibit nonhemolytic unconjugated hyperbilirubinemia. Heterozygote animals are clinically normal, but homozygotes have unconjugated bilirubin levels between 3 and 20 mg/dL, pale bile, and frequently kernicterus. The gene coding for the defective isoform of the enzyme has been cloned and provides the basis for consideration of gene therapy.[129,130]

α_1-Antitrypsin Deficiency

α_1-Antitrypsin (α_1-AT) is a plasma protease inhibitor with elastase as a major physiologic substrate. Synthesis, posttranslational modification, and secretion occur primarily in the hepatocyte. Disease-causing alleles are inherited in an autosomal recessive manner. Homozygotes have only 15% to 20% of the normal plasma levels of α_1-AT. The α_1-AT mutation leads to a single lysine for glutamic acid substitution at position 342, disrupting a salt bridge and altering the three-dimensional structure of the protein. Defects in normal α_1-AT expression and processing, due to a mutation, can lead to pathology in the lung and liver. Diminished levels of α_1-AT in the blood result in an imbalance between proteases and protease inhibitors, allowing destruction of lung parenchyma. Chronic obstructive pulmonary disease is the most common clinical manifestation of α_1-AT deficiency, with basal lung parenchyma most severely affected.

In nonsmokers, the onset of clinical symptoms occurs between the ages of 45 and 50 years. Elements in tobacco smoke enhance oxidation and inactivation of residual α_1-AT. Smokers have onset of symptoms in their mid-30s, an increased rate of progression of disease, and poorer survival rates. There is also a sex difference in survival. In one series, 98% of nonsmoking women and 65% of nonsmoking men with α_1-AT deficiency were alive at 55 years of age. In the same study, only 30% of smoking women and 18% of smoking males were alive at 55 years of age, with most succumbing to end-stage chronic obstructive pulmonary disease.[131]

The liver is the primary site of α_1-AT biosynthesis. In some cases, alteration in the protein sequence of α_1-AT prevents normal posttranslational processing and results in the intracellular accumulation of large quantities of abnormal protein, detectable as intracytoplasmic inclusions.[132] One pathologic consequence of abnormal protein accumulation is the development of liver injury. In one series of patients with homozygous α_1-AT deficiency, 5%

had cirrhosis, with the incidence increasing to 15% in male patients older than 51 years.[133,134]

The introduction of a normal copy of the α_1-AT gene into the hepatocyte is not likely to correct liver disease. The secretion of increased levels of normal α_1-AT into the plasma, however, should ameliorate obstructive lung disease, which is the predominant clinical manifestation of the mutant gene. Replacement therapy of α_1-AT may also decrease the progression of liver disease, if elevated plasma levels exert negative feedback on hepatic transcription and translation of aberrant alleles.[135] Orthotopic liver transplantation is the only form of therapy capable of correcting both the hepatic and pulmonary manifestations of α_1-AT deficiency. At least 39 patients have undergone liver transplantation for α_1-AT deficiency, with a 5-year actuarial survival approximating 70%.[136]

The administration of exogenous α_1-AT appears to restore antineutrophil elastase defenses to normal.[137,138] A number of experimental models using gene transfer to correct α_1-AT deficiency have been reported. A retroviral vector was used to insert human α_1-AT cDNA into the genome of mouse fibroblasts, resulting in α_1-AT secretion.[139] Recombinant human α_1-AT cDNA has been successfully transferred to human umbilical vein endothelial cells.[140] Primary rat hepatocyte cultures infected with a recombinant adenovirus containing a human α_1-AT cDNA synthesized and secreted human α_1-AT for 4 weeks with no evidence of toxicity. Intraportal infusion of recombinant adenovirus resulted in the production of α_1-AT, without histologic evidence of liver injury.[141] A canine model of liver-directed ex vivo gene therapy using retrovirally altered autologous hepatocytes has also been performed.[142]

Hemophilia B

Hemophilia B is an X-linked chromosomal blood-clotting disorder that results when the gene encoding factor IX is deficient or functionally defective. The enzyme is synthesized in the liver, and the existence of animal models for this genetic disease have permitted the development of somatic gene therapy protocols aimed at transfer of functional copies of the factor IX gene into the liver. A recombinant retroviral vector was used for the transfer of human factor IX cDNA in rabbit hepatocytes. The infected rabbit hepatocytes produced human factor IX that was indistinguishable from functional protein derived from human plasma.[143]

Factor IX hepatic gene transfer has also been accomplished in vivo by the direct infusion of recombinant retroviral vectors into the portal vasculature. Canine factor IX cDNA was transduced directly into the hepatocytes of affected dogs in vivo. The expression of the recombinant retrovirus was dependent on a partial (two thirds) hepatectomy to induce liver cell mitosis. The dogs transduced with canine factor IX recombinant retrovirus constitutively expressed canine factor IX for 5 months after the procedure at a high enough concentration to improve the whole-blood clotting time and partial thromboplastin time.[144] Other cell types have been studied for systemic factor IX replacement, including primary myoblasts, capillary endothelial cells, and primary skin fibroblasts.[145–147]

VASCULAR SYSTEM

Atherosclerosis is a complex, polygenic disease that, by virtue of its impact on public health, is a desirable target for gene therapy intervention. Gene therapy strategies for vascular disease are being developed that should be useful for coronary arteries, aorta, and peripheral vessels. Target cells for atherosclerosis-mediated gene therapy include the endothelial cell and smooth muscle cell. A variety of genes have been proposed and have been used with success in vitro and in vivo in animal models, although no human trials have yet been approved (Table 15-5).

Preclinical Models

Gene transfer into endothelial cells and smooth muscle cells has been shown in a variety of species, including rats, rabbits, dogs, sheep, and humans.[11,148–150] Retroviruses, adenoviruses, and liposomes have all been shown to be efficient gene-transfer vectors for these two vascular cell types.[149,151–153] Although direct plasmid DNA gene transfer has also been used in vitro, success has been only modest.[154] Given the tight junctions and small fenestrations of capillaries, successful gene transfer strategies for the vascular tree in situ have been slow to develop. The most promising approach has involved localized temporary occlusion of the circulation to allow transduced endothelial cells or the gene transfer vector enough time to deposit on the vessel surface.

The first successful in vivo study was performed in a minipig model. Endothelial cells were retrovirally transduced with marker genes in vitro and then allowed to come in contact with a balloon-injured femoral arterial segment. The vessel was then removed and studied for the presence of gene transfer.[155] Subsequent studies showed that it was not necessary to denude the capillary endothelium to allow genetically modified endothelial cells to express transgene constructs.[156] The long-term stability of the retrovirally transduced vascular cells was confirmed in an animal model in which transgene-expressing cells persisted for more than 12 months.[157]

Because damaging vessels to promote healing is not appropriate, methods for direct in vivo gene transfer have also been developed. Using a double-balloon catheter to administer recombinant retroviruses to an isolated segment of iliofemoral artery, persistent gene transfer could be detected for up to 21 weeks.[158] All cell types found in the arterial wall were transduced in this system. Liposomes have also been used to effect gene transfer into arteries. Low-level gene transfer is seen with liposomes in normal arteries; increased expression is seen with cell proliferation.[159]

Recombinant adenoviruses have also been used to target the vascular system. In the carotid artery or jugular vein, recombinant adenoviruses expressing α_1-AT show high-level but temporary gene expression.[152] The presence of endothelial disruption appears to increase gene transfer to the media.[160,161] In another study, adenovirus gene delivery could be detected in endothelial cells, intima, and adventitia, where the route of delivery appeared to be through the adventitia.[162]

In an attempt to study pathobiology of the arterial system, DNA liposomes and a recombinant retrovirus were constructed to express the human major histocompatibility antigen molecule HLA-B7. Transduction of the HLA-B7 molecule into vessels by either vector resulted in autoimmune vasculitis.[163] Transduction of the genes for acidic fibroblast growth factor, platelet-derived growth factor, or transforming growth factor β results in intimal smooth muscle hyperplasia and angiogenesis.[164]

Vascular smooth muscle cell proliferation in response to injury is an important etiologic factor in vascular proliferative disorders, such as occlusion after peripheral arterial bypass and restenosis after coronary grafting. Two new approaches suggest that gene therapy can be used to inhibit the process of intimal hyperplasia. Recombinant adenovirus-mediated HSVtk gene transfer into balloon-injured arteries followed by systemic ganciclovir treatment resulted in significant decreases in intimal hyperplasia in swine.[165] Using recombinant adenoviruses expressing the tumor-suppressor retinoblastoma gene (Rb), similar inhibition of neointima proliferation was seen in models of arterial injury.[166]

MUSCLE

In the development of gene therapy strategies for muscle, uniform delivery of genes is of prime importance. For inherited diseases such as muscular dystrophy, all muscle fibers should be treated to restore function, although certain muscles such as the diaphragm are critical to survival. Similarly, gene transfer into the myocardium in the case of cardiomyopathy would need to be global.

Muscular Dystrophy

Two forms of muscular dystrophy exist, the most severe form being the Duchenne variant, which occurs in about 1 in 3500 live male births. Duchenne muscular dystrophy is inherited as an X-linked recessive trait and causes progressive muscle weakness leading to confinement in a wheel chair and death from respiratory failure. Duchenne muscular dystrophy is due to complete absence of dystrophin from the muscle cell surface. Histologically, affected muscle is characterized by fiber necrosis, fibrosis, and fatty infiltration.[167] A milder form of the disease is caused by a defective gene that encodes only half the full-size protein. The dystrophin gene is one of the largest human genes isolated.[168] The actual function of dystrophin is not known, but its large size (427 kd) indicates that it is most likely a structural protein.[169]

Recombinant retroviruses have been engineered to express a 6.3-kb dystrophin minigene. Injection of the retroviral vector into tibialis anterior resulted in the expression of transgene.[170] Adenovirus-mediated dystrophin transfer has also been shown to enhance the number of

Table 15-5. STRATEGIES FOR PERIPHERAL VASCULAR GENE THERAPY

Gene Product	Abbreviation	Action	Cell Type
Fibroblast growth factor	FGF	Induction of intimal hyperplasia	Smooth muscle cells
Platelet-derived growth factor	PDGF	Induction of intimal hyperplasia	Smooth muscle cells
Factor IX	FIX	Anticoagulation	Endothelial cells
Tissue plasminogen activator	tPa	Clot lysis	Endothelial cells
Herpes simplex virus thymidine kinase	HSVtk	Inhibition of intimal hyperplasia	Smooth muscle cells
Retinoblastoma protein	Rb	Inhibition of intimal hyperplasia	Smooth muscle cells
Vascular endothelial growth factor	VEGF	Arterial collateral development	Endothelial cells
Renin	—	Vascular smooth muscle growth	Smooth muscle cells
Angiotensin-converting enzyme	ACE	Vascular smooth muscle growth	Smooth muscle cells

positive muscle fibers.[171] In this study, 6% to 50% of biceps femoris fibers were positive for dystrophin for up to 98 days.

The difficulties involved in working with the full-length dystrophin gene were overcome by using direct DNA injection into skeletal and cardiac muscle. Although not generally applicable due to low transfer efficiency (1%), the ability to inject large genes may be of some interest in the future.[172] The direct injection of DNA into cardiac muscle may be a potential strategy for ventricular aneurysms and other focal defects, although delivery strategies must still be developed.[15]

Muscle Cells as Delivery Vehicles for Secreted Proteins

Use of myoblasts, or muscle precursor cells, as factories for the production and secretion of serum proteins has generated a great deal of interest. Mature multinucleated skeletal muscle fibers are formed during growth and development by the fusion of mononucleated precursor cells (myoblasts). Myoblasts can be isolated from adult skeletal muscle, cultured, transduced, and then returned to the host, where they fuse with existing muscle fibers.[173] A myocyte cell line has been transduced with both human growth hormone and factor IX, with biochemical evidence of the secretion of both proteins in the serum.[174,175]

CENTRAL NERVOUS SYSTEM
Herpes Simplex Virus

The ability to manipulate the expression of genes in the mammalian brain leads to opportunities to treat neurologic disorders. DNA viruses have been used for most attempts at gene therapy of nonmalignant central nervous system disease. Herpes simplex virus type I has been used extensively because of its neurotropic host cell range.[176,177] Like adenoviruses, recombinant herpes simplex virus vectors retain functional viral genes that may be cytotoxic or that may reactivate preexisting latent virus in recipient cells.[178] To circumvent these problems, defective herpes simplex viruses have been engineered to eliminate viral genes while retaining certain recognition sequences.[179]

Adeno-Associated Viruses

Adeno-associated virus is a human parvovirus that can propagate as a lytic infection or integrate into the host genome as a provirus. In general, AAV requires the presence of a helper virus, usually adenovirus, to initiate productive infection. Five serotypes of AAV have been identified, but AAV-2 is the most extensively characterized. AAV-2 DNA is a single-strand linear molecule about 4.7 kb in length.[180,181] In the presence of adenovirus helper function, infectious AAV plasmids may be able to express transiently much larger foreign sequences.[182,183] Integration of AAV is targeted to a site on the distal portion of the long arm of chromosome 19, decreasing the risk of insertional mutagenesis from random integration.[184]

These unique aspects of AAV have led to its use as a transduction vector for nervous tissues. Successful gene transfer with transduction frequencies as high as 80% have been demonstrated in human erythroid cells and lymphocytes.[9,185,186]

Parkinson Disease

Parkinson disease is caused by loss of the nigrostriatal pathway and is responsive to therapies that facilitate dopaminergic transmission in the caudate and putamen of the basal ganglia. One therapeutic approach is to transduce cells with the enzyme tyrosine hydroxylase, which synthesizes L-dopa. In an animal model of Parkinson disease, fibroblasts were modified with a recombinant retrovirus expressing tyrosine hydroxylase. Phenotypic return to normal behavior was noted.[187] Recombinant AAVs expressing tyrosine hydroxylase have also been used, with significant behavioral recovery noted for up to 4 months.[188]

PANCREAS

The pancreas is a good candidate organ for gene therapy. In addition to being a target for cancer therapy and immune modulation for allograft transplantation, pancreatic manifestations of diabetes and cystic fibrosis are important metabolic diseases that may be treatable by genetic modification.

The two types of diabetes mellitus are insulin-dependent (type I) and non–insulin-dependent (type 2) diabetes. Failure of insulin secretion in response to elevated plasma glucose levels and resistance of peripheral tissues to the cellular effects of insulin characterize type I or type II diabetes, respectively. Type I diabetes, usually affecting the young, is now known to result from autoimmune attack against the islets of Langerhans. Type II diabetes, usually affecting adults, is composed of a variety of defects related to impaired insulin secretion and insulin insensitivity of target tissues, such as skeletal muscle.

Type I Diabetes

Gene therapy for diabetes presumes that suitable genes could be identified as targets. Substantial progress has been made in identifying the genetic contribution to type I diabetes.[189] Members of a family affected with diabetes are at increased risk for development of the disease. In humans, two chromosome regions show linkage to insulin-dependent diabetes mellitus: (1) the human major histocompatibility complex, HLA, on chromosome 6p21, also known as IDDM1; and (2) the insulin gene region on 11p15, or IDDM2.[190] Other diabetes susceptibility genes, named IDDM3, IDDM4, and IDDM5, have been identified by high-resolution genetic linkage maps.[191]

The finding of a major gene linkage with HLA on chromosome 6 fits well with the known mechanism of type I diabetes: autoimmune destruction of insulin-producing pancreatic β cells. Histologically, a chronic mononuclear infiltration consisting of T lymphocytes is seen, as islet function is gradually destroyed.[192] Data suggest an inductive role for enteroviruses in initiating attack on islet peptides.

Type II Diabetes

The predominant phenotype in type II diabetes consists of obesity, arterial hypertension, dyslipidemia, and atherosclerotic coronary artery disease.[193] The incidence is 3% in Western populations but may be 10% to 20% in subjects older than 60 years.[194] As in type I diabetes, type II diabetes is strongly inherited, but the mode of inheritance is not known. The concordance rate in monozygotic twins is 70% to 80%, while dizygotic twins have a rate of 10% to 20%. In offspring and siblings of type II diabetes patients, the lifetime risk of developing clinically overt disease is 40%.[195]

Genes proven to play a role in type II diabetes include the insulin gene,[196] the insulin receptor gene,[197] a mitochondrial leucine tRNA gene,[198] the glucokinase gene,[199] the GLUT2 glucose transporter gene,[200] and a gene tightly linked to ADA on chromosome 20.[201] In the maturity-onset diabetes of the young subtype, 40% of patients may have glucokinase gene mutations, suggesting that gene therapy ex vivo to transfer the correct gene into islets could be an option. In the insulin receptor defect and insulin resistance syndromes, correcting the defect by gene transfer would presumably involve most cells of the body, but especially skeletal muscle, fat, and liver.

Islet Transplantation

Islet transplantation has been shown to be a viable clinical approach to rendering diabetic patients euglycemic. Initial work in animals demonstrated that islets could be isolated and transplanted as isografts. Islet isografts were shown to reverse the diabetic state when transplanted into sites such as the liver.[202–204] In addition to rendering diabetic animals euglycemic, islet transplants could prevent or reverse early diabetic complications.[205]

The realization that human diabetes is not easily modeled in large animals led to human clinical trials. Human islet allografts have been shown to maintain normoglycemia without exogenous insulin therapy in diabetic patients receiving immunosuppression. The ultimate goals are early transplantation of islets to prevent diabetes-related complications and avoidance of immunosuppression.

The autoimmune attack on autologous β cells in type I diabetic patients, as well as rejection of allogeneic islets, may be ameliorated by immunomodulation of the islet, the recipient, or both. In transgenic models of type I diabetes, antibody depletion experiments prevented the development of diabetes.[206] These types of models suggest that, by using various immunoinhibitory cytokines to generate local unresponsiveness to antigens, type I diabetes could be prevented.

Gene Transfer in Islets of Langerhans

Plasmid DNA has been used in vitro in transient transfection protocols to elucidate the mechanisms of transcriptional regulation of the insulin gene.[207] Multiple sequence elements appear to be involved. Recombinant adenoviruses have been shown to accomplish gene transfer efficiently into freshly isolated rat islets of Langerhans.[208] Gene expression in cultured islets was noted for up to 21 days, and analysis of sections demonstrate that 60% to 70% of the islets cells were targeted.[209] Using a functional virus expressing hexokinase I, basal levels of insulin release and glucose usage were increased.[209]

The ability to engineer adenoviruses will allow investigation of regulatory enzymes in the pathway of glucose metabolism. Viruses expressing antisense oligodeoxynucleotides to these enzymes and tissue-specific or inducible promoter and enhancer constructs can also be developed to gain insight into the basic mechanisms of insulin release.

Cystic Fibrosis

Exocrine pancreatic insufficiency is present in most cystic fibrosis patients from birth.[210] Pathology is caused by obstruction of ducts by abnormally thick, inspissated secretions. This results in dilation of secretory ducts and flattening of the cuboidal epithelium. There is widespread loss of acini and intraluminal calcifications, as seen with other types of chronic pancreatitis. The islets of Langerhans are preserved until late, but eventually progressive scarring of the gland is associated with the development of diabetes.

Clinically, pancreatic enzyme deficiency results in protein and fat malabsorption. The stools are greasy, bulky,

and foul-smelling. Fat loss may be as high as 70% and is accompanied by deficiency of the fat-soluble vitamins A, D, E, and K. In the first 6 months of life, protein malabsorption can be so severe that it leads to hypoproteinemia and anasarca. With increasing age, low growth rates due to malnutrition, the vitamin deficiency states of xerophthalmia and night blindness (vitamin A), diminished bone density (vitamin D), and coagulopathy (vitamin K) are seen. Recombinant adenoviruses have been used to transduce genes encoding for pancreatic lipase as a way of treating pancreatic enzyme deficiency.[211]

REFERENCES

1. President's Commission for the Study of Ethical Problems in Medicine and Biomedical and Behavioral Research. Splicing life: the social and ethical issues of genetic engineering with human beings. Washington, DC, US Government Printing Office Stock No. 83-600500, 1982.
2. Anderson WF. End-of-the-year potpourri. Hum Gene Ther 1994;5:1431.
3. Kessler DA, Siegel JP, Noguchi PD, Zoon KC, Feiden KL, Woodcock J. Regulation of somatic-cell therapy and gene therapy by the Food and Drug Administration. N Engl J Med 1993;329:1169.
4. Collins F, Galas D. A new five year plan for the U.S. Human Genome Project. Science 1993;262:43.
5. Fields C, Adams MD, White O, Venter JC. How many genes in the human genome? Nature Genet 1994;7:345.
6. Cepko CL, Roberts BE, Mulligan RC. Construction and applications of a highly transmissible murine retrovirus shuttle vector. Cell 1984;37:1053.
7. Williams DA, Lemischka IR, Nathan DG, Mulligan RC. Introduction of new genetic material into pluripotent hematopoietic stem cells of the mouse. Nature 1984;310:476.
8. Culver K, Cornetta K, Morgan R, et al. Lymphocytes as cellular vehicles for gene therapy in mouse and man. Proc Natl Acad Sci USA 1991;88:3155.
9. Muro-Cacho CA, Samulski RJ, Kaplan D. Gene transfer in human lymphocytes using a vector based on adeno-associated virus. J Immunother 1992;11:231.
10. Wilson JM, Jefferson DM, Choudhury JR, Novikoff PM, Johnston DE, Mulligan RC. Retrovirus-mediated transduction of adult hepatocytes. Proc Nat Acad Sci USA 1988;85:3014.
11. Wilson JM, Birinyi LK, Salomon RN, Libby P, Callow AD, Mulligan RC. Implantation of vascular grafts lined with genetically modified endothelial cells. Science 1989;244:1344.
12. Axelrod JH, Read MS, Brinkhous KM, Verma IM. Phenotypic correction of factor IX deficiency in skin fibroblasts of hemophilic dogs. Proc Natl Acad Sci USA 1990;87:5173.
13. Rosenfeld MA, Yoshimura K, Trapnell BC, et al. In vivo transfer of the human cystic fibrosis transmembrane conductance regulator gene to the airway epithelium. Cell 1992;68:143.
14. Wolff JA, Malone RW, Williams P, et al. Direct gene transfer into mouse muscle in vivo. Science. 1990;247:1465.
15. Lin H, Parmacek HS, Morle G, Bolling S, Leiden JM. Expression of recombinant genes in myocardium in vivo after direct injection of DNA. Circulation 1990;82:2217.
16. Roessler BJ, Allen ED, Wilson JM, Hartman JW, Davidson BL. Adenoviral-mediated gene transfer to rabbit synovium in vivo. J Clin Invest 1993;92:1085.
17. Palella TD, Hidaka Y, Silverman LJ, Levine M, Glorioso J, Kelley WN. Expression of human HPRT mRNA in brains of mice infected with a recombinant herpes simplex virus-1 vector. Gene 1989;80:137.
18. Burns JC, Friedmann T, Driever W, Burrascano M, Yee JK. Vesicular stomatitis virus G glycoprotein pseudotyped retroviral vectors: concentration to very high titer and efficient gene transfer into mammalian and nonmammalian cells. Proc Nat Acad Sci USA 1993;90:8033.
19. Ghosh-Choudhury G, Graham FL. Stable transfer of a mouse dihydrofolate reductase gene into a deficient cell line using human adenovirus vector. Biochem Biophys Res Commun 1987;147:964.
20. Rosenfeld MA, Siegfried W, Yoshimura K, et al. Adenovirus-

mediated transfer of a recombinant a1-antitrypsin gene to the lung epithelium in vivo. Science 1991;252:431.

21. Samulski RJ, Chang LS, Shenk T. Helper-free stocks of recombinant adeno-associated viruses: normal integration does not require viral gene expression. J Virol 1989;63:3822.

22. Felgner PL, Gadek TR, Holm M, et al. Lipofection: a highly efficient, lipid-mediated DNA-transfection procedure. Proc Natl Acad Sci USA 1987;84:7413.

23. Nicolau C, Legrand A, Grosse E. Liposomes as carriers for in vivo gene transfer and expression. Methods Enzymol 1987; 149:157.

24. Wu GY, Wu CH. Receptor-mediated in vitro gene transformation by a soluble DNA carrier system. (Published erratum appears in J Biol Chem 1988;263:588) J Biol Chem 1987; 262:4429.

25. Varmus H, Swanstrom R. Replication of retroviruses. In: Weiss R, Teich N, Varmus H, Coffin J, eds. RNA tumor viruses. New York, Cold Spring Harbor Press, 1984:369.

26. Mulligan RC. Gene transfer and gene therapy: principles, prospects, and perspective. In: Lindsten J, Pettersson U, eds. Etiology of human disease at the DNA level. New York, Raven Press. 1991:143.

27. Miller DG, Adam MA, Miller AD. Gene transfer by retrovirus vectors occurs only in cells that are actively replicating at the time of infection. Mol Cell Biol 1990;10:4239.

28. Miller AD. Retrovirus packaging cells. Hum Gene Ther 1990;1:5.

29. Roe TY, Reynolds TC, Yu G, Brown PO. Integration of murine leukemia virus DNA depends on mitosis. EMBO J 1993; 12:2099.

30. Rosenberg SA, Spiess P, Lafreniere R. A new approach to the adoptive immunotherapy of cancer with tumor infiltrating lymphocytes Science 1986;223:1318.

31. Fisher B, Packard BS, Read EJ, et al. Tumor localization of adoptively transferred indium-111 labelled tumor infiltrating lymphocytes in patients with metastatic melanoma. J Clin Oncol 1989;7:250.

32. Rosenberg SA, Aebersold PM, Cornetta K, et al. Gene transfer into humans: immunotherapy of patients with advanced melanoma, using tumor infiltrating lymphocytes modified by retroviral gene transduction. N Engl J Med 1990;323:570.

33. Brenner MK, Rill DR, Moen RC, et al. Gene marking to trace origin of relapse after bone marrow transplantation. Lancet 1993;341:85.

34. Haddada H, Ragot T, Cordier L, Duffour MT, Perricaudet M. Adenoviral interleukin-2 gene transfer into P815 tumor cells abrogates tumorigenicity and induces antitumoral immunity in mice. Hum Gene Ther 1993;4:703.

35. Vieweg J, Rosenthal FM, Bannerji R, et al. Immunotherapy of prostate cancer in the Dunning rat model: use of cytokine-modified tumor vaccines. Cancer Res 1994;54:1760.

36. Gansbacher B, Zier K, Daniels B, Cronin K, Bannerji R, Gilboa E. Interleukin-2 gene transfer into tumor cells abrogates tumor immunogenicity and induces protective immunity. J Exp Med 1990;172:1217.

37. Karp SE, Farber A, Salo JC, et al. Cytokine secretion by genetically modified non-immunogenic murine fibrosarcoma: tumor inhibition by IL-2 but not tumor necrosis factor. J Immunol 1993;150:896.

38. Golumbek PT, Lazenby AJ, Levitsky HI, et al. Treatment of established renal cancer by tumor cells engineered to secrete interleukin-4. Science 1991;254:713.

39. Tepper RI, Pattengale PK, Leder P. Murine interleukin-4 displays potent antitumor activity *in vivo*. Cell 1989;57:503.

40. Tepper RI, Coffmen RL, Leder P. An eosinophil-dependent mechanism for the antitumor effect of IL-4. Science 1992; 257:548.

41. Teng MN, Park BH, Koeppen HKW, Tracey KJ, Fendly BM, Schreiber H. Long-term inhibition of tumor growth by tumor necrosis factor in the absence of cachexia or T-cell immunity. Proc Nat Acad Sci USA 1991;88:3535.

42. Blankenstein T, Qin Z, Uberla K, et al. Tumor suppression after tumor-cell targeted tumor necrosis factor gene transfer. J Exp Med. 1991;173:1047.

43. Rosenthal FM, Cronin K, Bannerji R, Golde DW, Gansbacher B. Augmentation of antitumor immunity by tumor cells transduced with a retroviral vector carrying the interleukin-2 and interferon-g cDNAs. Blood 1994;83:1289.

44. Restifo NP, Spiess PJ, Karp SE, Mule JJ, Rosenberg SA. Non-immunogenic sarcoma transduced with the cDNA for interferon-g elicits CD8+ T cells against the wild-type tumor: correlation with antigen presentation capability. J Exp Med 1992;175:1423.

45. Colombo MP, Ferrari G, Stoppacciaro A, et al. Granulocyte colony-stimulating factor gene transfer suppresses tumorigenicity of a mouse adenocarcinoma in vivo. J Exp Med 1991;173:889.

46. Bishop JM. Molecular themes in oncogenesis. Cell 1991; 64:235.

47. Kern SE, Pietenpol JA, Thiagalingam S, et al. Oncogenic forms of p53 inhibit p53-regulated gene expression. Science 1992;256:827.

48. Motojima K, Urano T, Nagata Y, Shiku H, Tsurifune T, Kanematsu T. Detection of point mutations in the kirsten ras oncogene provides evidence for the multicentricity of pancreatic carcinoma. Ann Surg 1993;217:138.

49. Ratajczak MZ, Kant JA, Luger SM, et al. In vivo treatment of human leukemia in a *scid* mouse model with c-myb antisense oligodeoxynucleotides. Proc Nat Acad Sci USA 1992;89:11823.

50. Funato T, Yoshida E, Jiao L, Tone T, Kashani-Sabett M, Scanlon KJ. The utility of an anti fos ribozyme in reversing cisplatin resistance in human ovarian carcinomas. Adv Enzyme Reg 1992;32:195.

51. Zon G, Stec WJ. Phosphorothioate oligonucleotides. In: Eckstein F, ed. Oligonucleotides and analogues: a practical approach. Oxford, UK, Oxford University Press, 1991:87.

52. Sullenger BA, Cech TR. Ribozyme-mediated repair of defective mRNA by targeted trans-splicing. Nature 1994;371:616.

53. Fujiwara T, Grimm EA, Mukhopadhyay T, Cai DW, Owen-Schaub LB, Roth JA. A retroviral wild-type p53 expression vector penetrates human lung cancer spheroids and inhibits growth by inducing apoptosis. Cancer Res. 1993;53:4129.

54. Chen YM, Chen P-L, Anvaiz N, Goodrich D, Lee WH. Expression of wild-type p53 in human A573 cells suppresses tumorigenicity but not growth rate. Oncogene 1991;6:1799.

55. Cai DW, Mukhopadhyay T, Liu Y, Fujiwara T, Roth JA. Stable expression of the wild-type p53 gene in human lung cancer cells after retrovirus-mediated gene transfer. Hum Gene Ther 1993;4:617.

56. Fujiwara T, Grimm EA, Mukhopadhyay T, Zhang WW, Owen-Schaub LB, Roth JA. Induction of chemosensitivity in human lung cancer cells in vivo by adenovirus mediated transfer of the wild type p53 gene. Cancer Res 194;54:2287.

57. Culver KW, Ram Z, Walbridge S, Ishii H, Oldfield EH, Blaese RM. In vivo gene transfer with retroviral vector-producer cells for treatment of experimental brain tumors. Science 1992;256:550.

58. Moolten FL, Wells JM. Curability of tumors bearing herpes thymidine kinase genes transferred by retroviral vecttors. JNCI 1990;82:297.

59. Ram Z, Walbridge S, Shawker T, Culver KW, Blaese RM, Oldfield EH. The effect of thymidine kinase transduction and ganciclovir therapy on tumor vasculature and growth of 9L gliomas in rats. J Neurosurg 1994;81:256.

60. Ram Z, Walbridge S, Oshiro EM, et al. Intrathecal gene therapy for malignant leptomeningeal neoplasia. Cancer Res 1994;54:2141.

61. Smythe WR, Kaiser LR, Hwang HC, et al. Successful adenovirus-mediated gene transfer in an in vivo model of human malignant mesothelioma. Ann Thor Surg 1994;57:1395.

62. Caruso M, Panis Y, Gagandeep S, Houssin D, Salzmann JL. Regression of established macroscopic metastases after in situ transduction of a suicide gene. Proc Nat Acad Sci USA 1993;90:7024.

63. Huber BE, Richards CA, Krenitsky TA. Retroviral-mediated gene therapy for the treatment of hepatocellular cancer: an innovative approach for cancer therapy. Proc Nat Acad Sci USA 1991;88:8039.

64. Mullen CA, Coale MM, Lowe R, Blaese RM. Tumors expressing the cytosine deaminase suicide gene can be eliminated in vivo with 5-fluorocytosine and induce protective immunity to wild-type tumor. Cancer Res 1994;54:1503.

65. Kerr WG, Mule JJ. Gene therapy: current status and future prospects. J Leukocyte Biol 1994;56:210.

66. Blaese RM. Development of gene therapy for immunodeficiency: adenosine deaminase deficiency. Pediatr Res 1993; 33(Suppl 1):S49.

67. Crystal RG, McElvaney NG, Rosenfeld MA, et al. Administration of an adenovirus containing the human CFTR cDNA to the respiratory tract of individuals with cystic fibrosis. Nature Genet 1994;8:42.

68. Yang YY, Raper SE, Cohn JA, Engelhardt JF, Wilson JM. An approach for treating the hepatobiliary disease of cystic fibrosis by somatic gene transfer. Proc Nat Acad Sci USA 1993;90:4601.

69. Horwitz MS. Adenoviridae and their replication. In: Fields BN, Knipe CN, eds. Fundamental virology. New York, Raven Press, 1991:1679.

70. Shenk T, Williams J. Genetic analysis of adenoviruses. Curr Top Microbiol Immunol 1984;111:1.

71. Graham FL, Smiley J, Russell WC, Nairn R. Characteristics of a human cell line transformed by DNA from human adenovirus 5. J Genet Virol 1977;36:59.

72. Kozarsky KF, Wilson JM. Gene therapy: adenovirus vectors. Curr Opin Genet Dev 1993;3:499.

73. Simon RH, Engelhardt JF, Yang Y, et al. Adenovirus-mediated transfer of the CFTR gene to lung of non-human primates: toxicity study. Hum Gene Ther 1993;4:771.

74. Engelhardt JF, Simon RH, Yang Y, et al. Adenovirus-mediated transfer of the CFTR gene to lung of non-human primates: biological efficacy study. Hum Gene Ther 1993;4:771.

75. Zabner J, Petersen DM, Puga AP, et al. Safety and efficacy of repetitive adenovirus-mediated transfer of CFTR cDNA to airway epithelia of primates and cotton rats. Nature Genet 1984;66:17.

76. Bout A, Perricaudet M, Baskin G, et al. Lung gene therapy: in vivo adenovirus-mediated gene transfer to rhesus monkey airway epithelium. Hum Gene Ther 1994;5:3.

77. Yang Y, Nunes FA, Berencsi K, Furth EE, Gönczöl E, Wilson JM. Cellular immunity to viral antigens limits E1-deleted adenoviruses for gene therapy. Proc Natl Acad Sci USA 1993;91:4407.

78. Engelhardt JH, Yang Y, Stratford-Perricaudet LD, et al. Direct gene transfer of human CFTR into human bronchial epithelia of xenografts with E1-deleted viruses. Nature Genet 1994; 4:27.

79. Yang Y, Nunes FA, Berencsi K, G94ncz94l E, Engelhardt JF, Wilson JM. Inactivation of E2a in recombinant adenoviruses limits cellular immunity and improves the prospect for gene therapy of cystic fibrosis. Nature Genet 1994;7:362.

80. Smith JG, Walzem RL, German JB. Liposomes as agents of DNA transfer. Biochim Biophys Acta 1993;1154:327.

81. New RRC. Liposomes: a practical approach. In: Rickwood D, Hames BD, eds. The practical approach series. Liverpool, IRL Press, 1990.

82. Lasic DD, Martin FJ, Gabizon A, Huang SK, Papahadjopoulos D. Sterically stabilized liposomes: a hypothesis on the molecular origin of the extended circulation times. Biochim Biophys Acta 1991;1070:187.

83. Hug P, Sleight RG. Liposomes for the transformation of eukaryotic cells. Biochim Biophys Acta 1991;1097:1.

84. Kato K, Nakanishi M, Kaneda Y, Uchida T, Okada K. Expression of hepatitis B virus surface antigen in adult rat liver. Co introduction of DNA and nuclear protein by a simplified liposome method. J Biol Chem 1991;266:3361.

85. Zabner J, Couture LA, Gregory RJ, Graham SM, Smith AE, Welsh MJ. Adenovirus-mediated gene transfer transiently corrects the chloride transport defect in nasal epithelia of patients with cystic fibrosis. Cell 1993;75:207.

86. Caplen NJ, Alton EWFW, Middleton PG, et al. Liposome-mediated CFTR gene transfer to the nasal epithelium of patients with cystic fibrosis. Nature Med 1995;1:39.

87. Horwitz AL. Inherited hepatic enzyme defects as candidates for liver-directed gene therapy. Curr Top Microbiol Immunol 1991;168:185.

88. Bilheimer DW, Goldstein JL, Grundy SM, Starzl TE, Brown MS. Liver transplantation to provide low density lipoprotein receptors and lower plasma cholesterol in a child with homozygous familial hypercholesterolemia. N Engl J Med 1984;311:1658.

89. Wu GY, Wu CH. Receptor-mediated in vitro gene transformation by a soluble DNA carrier system. J Biol Chem 1987;262:44299.

90. Fisher KJ, Wilson JM. Biochemical and functional analysis of an adenovirus-based ligand complex for gene transfer. Biochem J 1994;299:49.

91. Michael SI, Curiel DT. Strategies to achieve targeted gene delivery via the receptor-mediated endocytosis pathway. Gene Ther 1994;1:223.

92. Wu GY, Wilson JM, Shalaby F, Grossman M, Shafritz DA, Wu CH. Receptor-mediated gene delivery in vivo: partial correction of genetic analbuminemia in Nagase rats. J Biol Chem 1991;266:14338.

93. Wilson JM, Grossman M, Cabrera JA, Wu CH, Wu GY. A novel mechanism for achieving transgene persistence in vivo after somatic gene transfer into hepatocytes. J Biol Chem 1992;267:11483.

94. Perales JC, Ferkol T, Beegen H, Ratnoff OD, Hanson RW. Gene transfer in vivo—sustained expression and regulation of genes introduced into the liver by receptor-targeted uptake. Proc Nat Acad Sci USA 1994;91:4086.

95. Seth P, Fitzgerald D, Ginsberg H, Willingham M, Pastan I. Evidence that the penton base of adenovirus is involved in potentiation of toxicity of Pseudomonas exotoxin conjugated to epidermal growth factor. Mol Cell Biol 1984;4:1528.

96. Curiel DT, Agarwal S, Wagner E, Cotten M. Adenovirus enhancement of transferrin-polylysine-mediated gene delivery. Proc Natl Acad Sci USA 1991;88:8850.

97. Wagner E, Zatloukal K, Cotten M, et al. Coupling of adenovirus to transferrin-polylysine/DNA complexes greatly enhances receptor-mediated gene delivery and expression of transfected genes. Proc Nat Acad Sci USA 1992;89:6099.

98. Cotten M, Wagner E, Zatloukal K, Phillips S, Curiel DT, Birnstiel ML. High-efficiency receptor-mediated delivery of small and large (48 kilobase) gene constructs using the endosome-disruption activity of defective or chemically inactivated adenovirus particles. Proc Nat Acad Sci USA 1992;89:6094.

99. Moscioni AD, Roy-Choudhury J, Barbour R, et al. Human liver cell transplantation: prolonged function in athymic-Gunn and athymic-analbuminemic hybrid rats. Gastroenterology 1989;96:1546.

100. Patel A, Hardy MA, Roy-Choudhury N, et al. Long-term correction of genetic defect of liver function in rat by transplantation of liver cells after ultraviolet irradiation. Mol Biol Med 1989;6:187.

101. Wilson JM, Johnston DE, Jefferson DM, Mulligan RC. Correction of the genetic defect in hepatocytes from the Watanabe heritable hyperlipidemic rabbit. Proc Nat Acad Sci USA 1988;85:4421.

102. Farney AC, Sutherland DER. Islet autotransplantation. In: Ricordi C, ed. Pancreatic islet cell transplantation. Austin, RG Landes, 1992:291.

103. Grossman M, Raper SE, Wilson JM. Towards liver-directed gene therapy: retrovirus-mediated gene transfer into human hepatocytes. Somatic Cell Mol Genet 1991;17:601.

104. Raper SE, Wilson JM, Grossman M. Retroviral-mediated gene transfer in human hepatocytes. Surgery 1992;112:333.

105. Grossman M, Raper SE, Wilson JM. Transplantation of genetically-modified autologous hepatocytes into non-human primates: feasibility and short-term toxicity. Hum Gene Ther 1992;3:501.

106. Memsic L, Busuttil RW, Traverso LW. Bleeding esophageal varices and portal vein thrombosis after pancreatic mixed-cell autotransplantation. Surgery 1984;95:238.

107. Scharp DW, Lacy PE, Santiago JV, et al. Results of our first nine intraportal islet autografts in type 1 insulin-dependent diabetic patients. Transplantation 1991;51:76.

108. Gupta S, Aragona E, Vemuru RP, Bhargava KK, Burk RD, Choudhury J-R. Permanent engraftment and function of hepatocytes delivered to the liver: implications for gene therapy and liver repopulation. Hepatology 1991;14:144.

109. Maganto P, Traber PG, Rusnell C, Dobbins WO III, Keren D, Gumucio JJ. Longterm maintenance of the adult pattern of liver specific expression for P-450b, P-450e, albumin and

alpha-fetoprotein genes in intrasplenically transplanted hepatocytes. Hepatology 1990;11:585.

110. Goldstein JL, Hobbs H, Brown MS. Familial hypercholesterolemia: lipoprotein and lipid metabolism disorders. In: Scriver CR, Beaudet AL, Sly WS, Valle D, eds. Metabolic basis of inherited disease, vol 2, ed 7. 1995:1981.

110a. Mito M, Kusano M, Kawaura Y. Hepatocyte transplantation in man. Transplant Proc 1992;25:3052.

111. Russell DW, Esser V, Hobbs HH. Molecular basis of familial hypercholesterolemia. Arteriosclerosis 1989;9(Suppl 1):I8.

112. Brown MS, Goldstein JL. A receptor-mediated pathway for cholesterol homeostasis. Science 1986;232:34.

113. Lodstein JL, Dana SE, Brown MS. Esterification of low density lipoprotein cholesterol in human fibroblasts and its absence in homozygous familial hypercholesterolemia. Proc Natl Acad Sci USA 1974;71:4288.

114. Glickman RM, Sabesin SM. Lipoprotein metabolism. In: Arias IM, Boyer JL, Fausto N, Jakoby WB, Schachter D, Shafritz DA, eds. The liver: biology and pathobiology, ed 3. New York, Raven Press, 1994:391.

115. Goldstein JL, Kita T, Brown MS. Defective lipoprotein receptors and atherosclerosis: lessons from an animal counterpart of familial hypercholesterolemia. N Engl J Med 1983;309:288.

116. Robins SJ, Fasulo JM, Collins MA, Patton GM. Evidence for separate pathways of transport of newly synthesized and preformed cholesterol into bile. J Biol Chem 1985;260:6511.

117. Watanabe Y. Serial inbreeding of rabbits with hereditary hyperlipidemia (WHHL rabbit). Atherosclerosis 1980;36:261.

118. Roy-Choudhury J, Grossman M, Gupta SJ, Roy-Choudhury N, Baker JR, Wilson JM. Long-term improvement of hypercholesterolemia after *ex vivo* gene therapy in LDLR deficient rabbits. Science 1991;254:1802.

119. Wilson JM, Grossman M, Raper SE, et al. Clinical protocol: ex vivo gene therapy of familial hypercholesterolemia. Hum Gene Ther 1992;3:179.

120. Grossman M, Raper SE, Kozarsky K, et al. Successful ex vivo gene therapy directed to liver in a patient with familial hypercholesterolaemia. Nature Genet 1994;6:335.

121. Lindgren V, DeMartinville B, Horwich AL, Rosenberg LE, Francke U. Human ornithine transcarbamylase locus mapped to band Xp21.1, near the Duchenne muscular dystrophy locus. Science 1984;226:698.

122. Ricciuti FC, Gelehrter TD, Rosenberg LE. X-chromosome inactivation in human liver: confirmation of X-linkage of ornithine transcarbamylase. Am J Hum Genet 1976;28:332.

123. Mori M, Miura S, Tatibana M, Cohen PP. Characterization of a protease apparently involved in processing of pre-ornithine transcarbamylase in liver mitochondria. Mol Cell Biochem 1982;49:97.

124. Brusilow SW, Horwich AL. Urea cycle enzymes. In: Scriver CR, Beaudet AL, Sly WS, Valle D, eds. Metabolic basis of inherited disease, vol 1, ed 7. New York, McGraw Hill, 1995:1187.

125. Scharschmidt BF, Waggoner JG, Berk PD. Hepatic organic anion uptake in the rat. J Clin Invest 1975;56:1280.

126. Crigler JF, Najjar VA. Congenital familial non-hemolytic jaundice with kernicterus. Pediatrics 1952;10:169.

127. Roy-Choudhury J, Wolkoff AW, Arias IM. Hereditary jaundice and disorders of bilirubin metabolism. In: Scriver CR, Beaudet AL, Sly WS, Valle D, eds. Metabolic basis of inherited disease, vol 2 ed 7. New York, McGraw-Hill, 1995:2161.

128. Kaufman SS, Wood RP, Shaw BW, et al. Orthotopic transplantation for type I Crigler-Najjar syndrome. Hepatology 1986;6:1259.

129. Bosma PS, Seppen J, Goldhoorn B, et al. Bilirubin UDP glucuronyltransferase I is the only relevant bilirubin glucuronidating isoform in man. J Biol Chem 1994;269:17960.

130. Bosma PJ, Glodhoorn B, Sinaasappel M, Oostra B, Oude Elfrink RPJ, Jansen PLM. A Crigler-Najjar family type 2 study indicating B-UGT-1 as the physiologically important bilirubin UDP glucuronosyl transferase form. Hepatology 1992;16:79A.

131. Cox DW. Alpha-1-antitrypsin deficiency. In: Scriver CR, Beaudet AL, Sly WS, Valle D, eds. Metabolic basis of inherited disease, vol 3, ed 7. New York, McGraw Hill, 1995;4125.

132. Bathurst IC, Travis J, George PM, Carrell RW. Structural and functional characterization of the abnormal Z α-1-antitrypsin isolated from human liver. FEBS Lett 1984;177:179.

133. Cox DW, Smyth S. Risk for liver disease in adults with a-1-antitrypsin deficiency. Am J Med 1983;74:221

134. Eriksson S, Carlson J, Velez R. Risk of cirrhosis and primary liver cancer in α-1-antitrypsin deficiency N Engl J Med 1986;314:736.

135. Birrer P, McElvaney NG, Chang-Stroman LM, Crystal RG. Alpha 1-antitrypsin deficiency and liver disease. J Inherit Metab Dis 1991;14:512.

136. Esquivel CO, Vicente E, Van Thiel D, et al. Orthotopic liver transplantation for alpha-1-antitrypsin deficiency: an experience in 29 children and ten adults. Transplant Proc 1987; 19:3798.

137. Hubbard RC, Brantly ML, Sellers SE, Mitchell ME, Crystal RG. Anti-neutrophil-elastase defenses of the lower respiratory tract in alpha-1-antitrypsin deficiency directly augmented with an aerosol of alpha-1-antitrypsin. Ann Intern Med 1989;111:206.

138. McElvaney NG, Hubbard RC, Birrer P, et al. Aerosol alpha 1-antitrypsin treatment for cystic fibrosis. Lancet 1991; 337:392.

139. Garver RI, Chytil A, Courtney M, Crystal RG. Clonal gene therapy: transplanted mouse fibroblast clones express human a1-antitrypsin gene in vivo. Science 1987;237:762.

140. Lemarchand P, Jaffe HA, Danel C, et al. Adenovirus-mediated transfer of a recombinant human alpha-1-antitrypsin cDNA to human endothelial cells. Proc Natl Acad Sci USA 1992;89:6482.

141. Jaffe HA, Danel C, Longenecker G, et al. Adenovirus-mediated in vivo gene transfer and expression in normal rat liver. Nature Genet 1992;1:372.

142. Kay MA, Baley P, Rothenberg S, et al. Expression of human alpha 1-antitrypsin in dogs after autologous transplantation of retroviral transduced hepatocytes. Proc Natl Acad Sci USA 1992;89:89.

143. Armentano D, Thompson AR, Darlington G, Woo SL. Expression of human factor IX in rabbit hepatocytes by retrovirus-mediated gene transfer: potential for gene therapy of hemophilia B. Proc Nat Acad Sci USA 1990;87:6141.

144. Kay MA, Rothenberg S, Landen CN, et al. In vivo partial correction of hemophilia B: sustained partial correction in factor-IX deficient dogs. Science 1993;262:117.

145. Axelrod JH, Read MS, Brinkhous KM, Verma IM. Phenotypic correction of factor IX deficiency in skin fibroblasts of hemophilic dogs. Proc Nat Acad Sci USA 1990;87:5173.

146. Dai Y, Roman M, Naviaux RK, Verma IM. Gene therapy via primary myoblasts: long-term expression of factor-IX protein following transplantation in vivo. Proc Nat Acad Sci USA 1992;89:10892.

147. Yao SN, Wilson JM, Nabel EG, Kurachi S, Hachiya HL, Kurachi K. Expression of human factor IX in rat capillary endothelial cells. Proc Nat Acad Sci USA 1991;88:8101.

148. Zweibel JA, Freeman SM, Kantoff PW, et al. High-level recombinant gene expression in rabbit endothelial cells transduced by retroviral vectors. Science 1989;243:220.

149. Dichek DA, Nussbaum O, Degen SJF, Anderson WF. Enhancement of the fibrinolytic activity of sheep endothelial cells by retroviral mediated gene transfer. Blood 1991;77:533.

150. Lynch CM, Clowes MM, Osborne WRA, Clowes AM, Miller AD. Long-term expression of human adenosine deaminase in vascular smooth muscle of rats: a model for gene therapy. Proc Nat Acad Sci USA 1992;89:1138.

151. Podrazik RM, Whitehill TA, Ekhterae D, Williams WD, Messina LM, Stanley JC. High level expression of recombinant human tPA in cultivated canine endothelial cells under varying conditions of retroviral gene transfer. Ann Surg 1992;216:446.

152. Lemarchand P, Jaffe HA, Danel C, et al. Adenovirus-mediated transfer of a recombinant human α-1-antitrypsin cDNA to human endothelial cells. Proc Nat Acad Sci USA 1992: 89:6482.

153. Pickering JG. Jekanowski J, Weir L, Takeshita S, Losordo DW, Isner JM. Liposome-mediated gene transfer into human vascular smooth muscle. Circulation 1994;89:13.

154. Etchberger KJ, Taylor MW. Transfection with bacterial genes

as a marker for cells seeded on vascular flow surfaces. Ann Vasc Surg 1989;3:123.

155. Nabel EG, Plautz G, Boyce FM, Stanley JC, Nabel GJ. Recombinant gene expression in vivo within endothelial cells of the arterial wall. Science 1989;244:1342.

156. Messina LM, Podrazik RM, Whitehill TA, et al. Adhesion and incorporation of lacZ transduced endothelial cells into the intact capillary wall of the rat. Proc Nat Acad Sci USA 1992;89:12018.

157. Clowes MM, Lynch CM, Miller AD, Miller DG, Osborne WRA, Clowes AM. Long-term biological response of injured rat carotid artery seeded with smooth muscle cells expressing retrovirally introduced human genes. J Clin Invest 1993; 93:644.

158. Nabel EG, Plautz G, Nabel GJ. Site-specific gene expression in vivo by direct gene transfer into the arterial wall. Science 1990;249:1285.

159. Takeshita S, Gal D, Leclerc G, et al. Increased gene expression after liposome-mediated arterial gene transfer associated with intimal smooth muscle cell proliferation: in vitro and in vivo findings in a rabbit model of vascular injury. J Clin Invest 1994;93:652.

160. Lee SW, Trapnell BC, Rabe JJ, Virmani R, Dichek DA. In vivo adenoviral vector-mediated gene transfer into balloon-injured rat carotid arteries. Circ Res 1993;73:797.

161. Guzman RJ, Lemarchand P, Crystal RG, Epstein SE, Finkel T. Efficient and selective adenovirus-mediated gene transfer into vascular neointima. Circulation 1993;88:2838.

162. Rome JJ, Shayani V, Newman KD, et al. Adenoviral vector-mediated gene transfer into sheep arteries using a double balloon catheter. Hum Gene Ther 1994;5:1249.

163. Nabel EG, Plautz G, Nabel GJ. Transduction of a foreign histocompatibility gene into the arterial wall induces vasculitis. Proc Nat Acad Sci USA 1992;89:5157.

164. Nabel EG, Yang Z, Plautz G, et al. Recombinant fibroblast growth factor-1 promotes intimal hyperplasia and angiogenesis in arteries in vivo. Nature 1993;362:844.

165. Ohno T, Gordon D, San H, et al. Gene therapy for vascular smooth muscle cell proliferation after arterial injury. Science 1994;265:781.

166. Chang MW, Barr E, Seltzer J, et al. Cytostatic gene therapy for vascular proliferative disorders with a constitutively active form of the retinoblastoma gene product. Science 1995; 267:518.

167. Moser H. Duchenne muscular dystrophy: pathogenic aspects and genetic prevention. Hum Genet 1984;66:17.

168. Koenig M, Hoffman EP, Bertelson CJ, Monaco AP, Feener C, Kunkel LM. Complete cloning of the Duchenne muscular dystrophy (DMD) cDNA and preliminary genomic organization of the DMD gene in normal and affected individuals. Cell 1987;50:509.

169. Blau HM. Muscling in on gene therapy. Nature 1993; 364:673.

170. Dunckley MG, Wells DJ, Walsh FS, Dickson G. Direct retroviral mediated transfer of a dystrophin minigene into mdx mouse in vivo. Hum Mol Genet 1993;2:717.

171. Ragot T, Vincent N, Chafey P, et al. Efficient transfer of a human dystrophin minigene to skeletal muscle of mdx mice. Nature 1993;361:647.

172. Dickson G, Love DR, Davies KE, Wells KE, Piper TA, Walsh FS. Human dystrophin gene transfer: production and expression of a functional recombinant DNA-based gene. Hum Genet 1991;88:53.

173. Salminen A, Elson HF, Mickley LA, Fojo AT, Gottesman MM. Implantation of recombinant rat myocytes into adult skeletal muscle: a potential gene therapy. Hum Gene Ther 1991;2:15.

174. Barr E, Leiden JM. Systemic delivery of recombinant proteins by genetically modified myoblasts. Science 1991;254:1507.

175. Dai Y, Roman M, Naviaux RK, Verma IM. Gene therapy via primary myoblasts: long-term expression of factor IX protein following transplantation in vivo. Proc Nat Acad Sci USA 1992;89:10892.

176. Ho DY, Mocarski ES, Sapolsky RM. Altering central nervous system physiology with a defective herpes simplex vector expressing the glucose transporter gene. Proc Nat Acad Sci USA 1993;90:3655.

177. Glorioso JC, Goins WF, Meaney CA, Fink DJ, Deluca NA. Gene transfer to brain using herpes simplex virus vectors. Ann Neurol 1994;35:S28.

178. Johnson PA, Myanohara A, Levine F, et al. Cytotoxicity of a replication-defective mutant of herpes simplex virus 1. J Virol 1992;66:2952.

179. Kaplitt MG, Kwong AD, Kleopoulos SP, et al. Preproenkephalin promoter yields region-specific and long-term expression in adult brain after direct in vivo gene transfer via a defective herpes simplex viral vector. Proc Natl Acad Sci USA 1994;91:8979.

180. Srivastava A, Lusby EW, Berns KI. Nucleotide sequence and organization of the adeno-associated virus 2 genome. J Virol 1983;45:555.

181. Muzyczka N. Use of adeno-associated virus as a general transduction vector for mammalian cells. Curr Top Microbiol Immunol 1992;158:97.

182. Wondisford FE, Usala SJ, DeCherney GS, et al. Cloning of the human thyrotropin β-subunit gene and transient expression of biologically active human thyrotropin after gene transfection. Mol Endocrinol 1988;2:32.

183. Srivastava CH, Samulski RJ, Lu L, Larsen SH, Srivastava A. Construction of a recombinant human parvovirus B19: adeno-associated virus 2 (AAV) DNA inverted terminal repeats are functional in an AAV-B19 hybrid virus. Proc Nat Acad Sci USA 1988;86:8078.

184. Samulski RJ, Zhu X, Xiao X, et al. Targeted integration of adeno-associated virus (AAV) into human chromosome 19. EMBO J 1991;10:3941.

185. Samulski RJ, Chang LS, Shenk T. Helper-free stocks of recombinant adeno-associated viruses: normal integration does not require viral gene expression. J Virol 1989;63:3822.

186. Walsh CE, Liu JM, Xiao X, Young NS, Nienhuis AW, Samulski RJ. Regulated high level expression of a human gamma-globin gene introduced into erythroid cells by an adeno-associated virus vector. Proc Nat Acad Sci USA 1992; 89:7257.

187. Wolff JA, Fisher LJ, Xu L, et al. Grafting fibroblasts genetically modified to produce L-dopa in a rat model of Parkinson's disease. Proc Nat Acad Sci USA 1989;86:9011.

188. Kaplitt MG, Leone P, Samulski RJ, et al. Long-term gene expression and phenotypic correction using adeno-associated virus vectors in the mammalian brain. Nature Genet 1994;8:148.

189. Todd JA, Aitman TL, Cornall RJ, et al. Genetic analysis of autoimmune type 1 diabetes mellitus in mice. Nature 1991;351:542.

190. Morton NE, Green A, Dunsworth T, et al. Heterozygous expression of the insulin dependent diabetes mellitus (IDDM) determinants in the HLA system. Am J Hum Genet 1983; 35:201.

191. Davies JL, Kawaguchi Y, Bennett ST, et al. A genome-wide search for human type 1 diabetes susceptibility genes. Nature 1994;371:130.

192. Roep BO, Arden SD, DeVries RR, Hutton JC. T-cell clones from a type I diabetes patient respond to insulin secretory granule proteins. Nature 1990;345:632.

193. Reaven GM. Role of insulin resistance in human disease. Diabetes 1988;37:1595.

194. Harris MI, Hadden WC, Knowler WC, Bennett PH. Prevalence of diabetes and impaired glucose tolerance and plasma glucose levels in US populations aged 20-74 yr. Diabetes 1987;36:523.

195. Granner DK, O'Brien RM. Molecular physiology and genetics of NIDDM. Diabetes Care 1992;15:369.

196. Kishimoto M, Sakura H, Hayashi K, et al. Detection of mutations in the human insulin gene by single strand conformation polymorphisms. J Clin Endocrinol Metab 1992;74:1027.

197. Menzel S, Neumer C, Zorad S, et al. Restriction fragment length polymorphisms of the insulin receptor gene, type 2 diabetes, and insulin binding. Diabetes Metab 1991;17:391.

198. Kadowaki T, Kadowaki H, Mori Y, et al. A subtype of diabetes mellitus associated with a mutation of mitochondrial DNA. N Engl J Med 1994;330:962.

199. Froguel P, Zouali H, Vionnet N, et al. Familial hyperglyce-

mia due to mutations in glucokinase: definition of a subtype of diabetes mellitus. N Engl J Med 1993;328:697.

200. Unger RH. Diabetic hyperglycemia: link to impaired glucose transport in pancreatic β-cells. Science 1991;251:1200.

201. Bell GI, Xiang KS, Newman MV, et al. Gene for non–insulin dependent diabetes mellitus (maturity-onset diabetes of the young subtype) is linked to DNA polymorphism on human chromosome 20q. Proc Nat Acad Sci USA 1991;88:1484.

202. Lacy PE, Kostianovsky M. A method for the isolation of intact islets of Langerhans from the rat pancreas. Diabetes 1967;16:35.

203. Reckard CR, Barker CF. Transplantation of isolated pancreatic islets across strong and weak histocompatibility barriers. Transplant Proc 1973;5:761.

204. Kemp CB, Knight MJ, Scharp DW, Ballinger WF, Lacy PE. Effect of transplantation site on the results of pancreatic islet isografts in diabetic rats. Diabetologia 1973;9:486.

205. Mauer S, Sutherland DER, Steffes MW, et al. Pancreatic islet transplantation: effects on the glomerular lesions of experimental diabetes in the rat. Diabetes 1974;23:748.

206. Ohashi PS, Oehen S, Buerki K, et al. Ablation of tolerance and induction of diabetes by virus infection in viral antigen transgenic mice. Cell 1991;65:305.

207. German MS, Wang J. The insulin gene contains multiple transcriptional elements that respond to glucose. Mol Cell Biol 1994;14:4067.

208. Csete ME, Afra R, Mullen Y, Drazan KE, Benhamou PY, Shaked A. Adenoviral-mediated gene transfer to pancreatic islets does not alter function. Transplant Proc 1994;26:756.

209. Becker TC, BeltrandelRio H, Noel RJ, Johnson JH, Newgard CB. Overexpression of hexokinase I in isolated islets of Langerhans via recombinant adenovirus: enhancement of glucose metabolism and insulin secretion at basal but not stimulatory glucose levels. J Biol Chem 1994;269:21234.

210. DiSant'agnese PA, Hubbard VS. The pancreas. In: Taussig LM, ed. Cystic fibrosis. New York, Thieme-Stratton, 1984:230.

211. Maeda H, Danel C, Crystal RG. Adenovirus-mediated transfer of human lipase complementary DNA to the gallbladder. Gastroenterology 1994;106:1638.

CHAPTER 16

TRANSPLANTATION AND IMMUNOLOGY

JONATHAN S. BROMBERG, JEFFREY D. PUNCH,
ROBERT M. MERION, MITCHELL L. HENRY,
RONALD M. FERGUSON, DARRELL A. CAMPBELL, JR.,
JOHN M. HAM, JEREMIAH G. TURCOTTE, SARA J. SHUMWAY,
R. MORTEN BOLMAN III, LARRY R. KAISER,
AND LAWRENCE ROSENBERG

Transplant Immunology

JONATHAN S. BROMBERG

The major impediment to universal, long-term allograft function in transplant recipients is the host immune response. Various manifestations of host antidonor immune reactivity result in allograft dysfunction and loss. To prevent these adverse outcomes, systemic immunosuppression is required. Current immunosuppression, however, is not completely reliable in preventing or reversing rejection, and immunosuppression itself results in several undesirable complications. To control the events that occur during clinical organ allografting, it is important to understand the processes of antigen recognition, the effector mechanisms of immune reactivity, and the cellular and molecular interactions that control and regulate the fate of antigen.

INITIATION OF THE IMMUNE RESPONSE

Recognition of Antigen

For allografts to be recognized as foreign and subsequently rejected, or as self and therefore accepted, the potential antigenic determinants of the graft must come into contact with a variety of specific receptors of the immune system. Antigen–receptor interactions are the first steps in a series that ultimately determine the fate of an antigen or an organ. The molecular and cellular participants in these processes are the immunoglobulin receptors of B cells, the antigen or T-cell receptors (TCRs) of T cells, and major histocompatibility complex (MHC) antigens of antigen-presenting cells (APCs).

Direct Recognition of Antigen by Immunoglobulin

Conceptually, the easiest interaction to understand is the direct binding of antigen to immunoglobulin. In this case, antigen can be any cellular constituent (eg, protein, carbohydrate, lipid, nucleic acid) that is bound by high affinity to a specific immunoglobulin, or antibody. Antibody molecules generally comprise two heavy (H) chains and two light (L) chains. Each chain has an amino-terminal variable (V) region domain, which differs from antibody to antibody. Each chain also has a few to several carboxy-terminal constant (C) region domains, which different antibody molecules may share. There are several different classes of immunoglobulins. The typical IgG dimer, comprising two L chains and two H chains, is shown in Figure 16-1. Other classes of antibodies differ from IgG in their polymeric structure, number of H-chain constant region domains, and soluble or cell membrane location of the molecules. These features are listed in Table 16-1. Membrane-bound immunoglobulin generally serves as an antigen-specific receptor for stimulating naive or memory

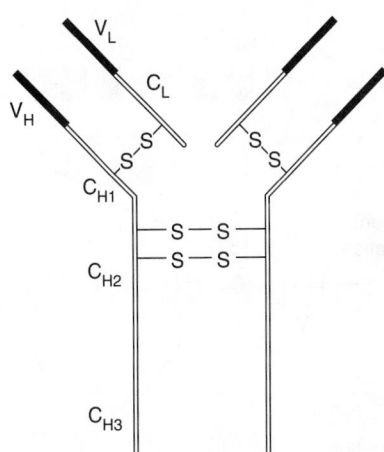

Figure 16-1. Structure of immunoglobulin (IgG). Variable (V) and constant (C) regions of heavy (H) and light (L) chains are joined by disulfide bonds.

Table 16-1. STRUCTURAL PROPERTIES OF IMMUNOGLOBULIN CLASSES AND SUBCLASSES

IMMUNOGLOBULIN	IgD	IgM	IgG	IgA	IgE
SUBCLASSES	—	—	G1, G2, G3, G4	A1, A2	—
MOLECULAR WEIGHT (kd)	184	970	146–170	160	188
POLYMERIC STRUCTURE	Dimer	Pentamer	Dimer	Monomer, dimer, or trimer	Dimer
ADDITIONAL CHAINS	—	J chain	—	J chain	—
FUNCTIONAL ASSOCIATIONS	Membrane-bound receptor	Primary antibody; membrane receptor	Secondary antibody	Muscosal antibody	Immediate hypersensitivity

B cells, whereas soluble antibodies generally perform effector functions of antigen recognition, opsonization, complement-mediated lysis, or activation of effector cells through Fc-receptor interactions. The generation of membrane versus soluble forms of immunoglobulin is usually the result of alternative splicing of mRNA.

Genetic analysis of immunoglobulin gene structure reveals several features that demonstrate how antibody diversity is generated and maintained. The H-chain gene complex is encoded on chromosome 14 in humans; κ L chains are encoded by chromosome 2 and λ L chains by chromosome 22. A single B cell can produce only a single type of L chain from only one of its chromosomes, a process termed *allelic exclusion*. The molecular determinants of allelic exclusion are just beginning to be elucidated. There appears to be a complex interaction between positive and negative regulatory transcription factors at the level of chromatin structure, and these factors are in turn regulated by membrane-initiated signaling events in response to specific antigens.[1]

H- and L-chain loci have a common structural motif of the V regions located upstream, or 5′, of the C region. Furthermore, there are many V regions. These have been sequenced and further subdivided into unique or related classes and subclasses. Presumably, these multiple V region families arose by an evolutionary process of gene duplication followed by mutation of individual family members. Further analysis has shown that between the V and C regions are multiple additional genetic elements that provide further structural variation. These elements are termed *joining* (J) and *diversity* (D) regions. J regions are present in both H- and L-chain genes, whereas D regions are present only in H-chain genes. During the process of B-cell maturation, these separate regions are physically brought together in a stochastic process that excises the intervening DNA sequences, including other V, D, and J genes (Fig. 16-2). Because there are many different V-, D-, and J-region genes for each H and L chain locus, which all may independently associate, the combinatorial possibilities are extremely large, showing why the immune system is able to generate antibodies for virtually all known antigenic determinants. The general process of gene rearrangement in B cells involves the complex interaction of membrane-initiated differentiating signals, cytoplasmic transcriptional factors, and nucleic acid excisional machinery at the level of chromatin structure.[1-4]

Further diversity is also generated by the nucleic acid

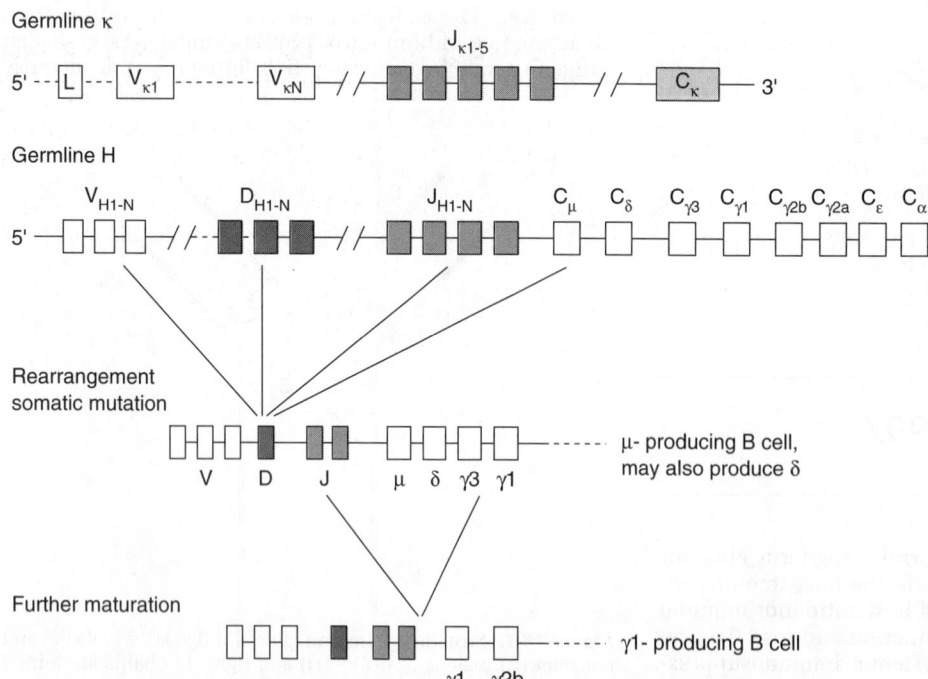

Figure 16-2. Structure of germline immunoglobulin heavy and light chain loci showing V, D, J, and C region genes. Maturation results in approximation of specific genes.

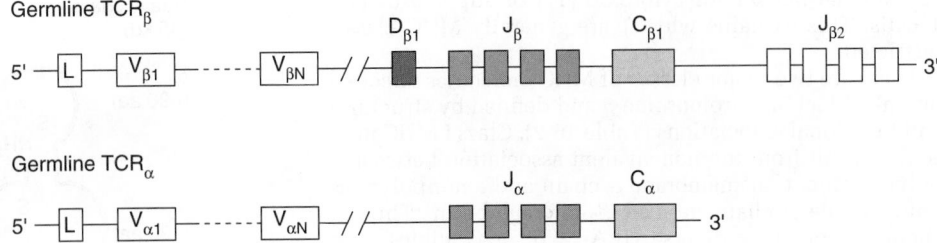

Figure 16-3. Structure of TCR β- and α-chain loci.

template-independent addition of nucleotides (N regions) at the V–D, V–J, and D–J junctions. N regions increase the diversity of immunoglobulin sequences and antibody specificity by another few orders of magnitude. Thus, what is known about the immunoglobulin gene structure explains the presence of diversity at the protein level. Importantly, the regions of greatest nucleotide diversity correspond to the three hypervariable regions of the antibody molecule, which are the amino acid contact residues responsible for direct antigen–antibody or receptor–ligand interactions.

It was previously concluded that a single B cell expresses only a single isotype, or H chain. However, molecular analysis shows that alternative mRNA splicing may allow a single B cell to express different H chains. It was also previously considered that membrane-bound forms of immunoglobulin functioned independently as antigen receptors. However, biochemical analysis demonstrates that at least three invariant chains, Ig-α, Ig-β, and Ig-γ, must associate with surface immunoglobulin for efficient expression and signal transduction.[5,6]

Recognition of Antigen by the T-Cell Receptor in the Context of the Major Histocompatibility Complex

T cells do not bind and recognize antigen directly. T cells recognize a complex composed of a peptide fragment of antigen bound to an MHC molecule. In other words, T cells recognize antigen in the context of MHC, a process termed *MHC restriction*. Structural and genetic analysis of the TCR reveals that it shares many principles with B-cell immunoglobulin receptors. The TCR is composed of separate α and β chains encoded by loci on chromosomes 14 and 7, respectively. Each locus is comprised of a series of V, D, J, and C segments (Fig. 16-3). The α-chain locus has only V and J genes, whereas the β locus has D regions. These loci undergo rearrangements during T-cell development, maturation, and differentiation, following the principles of gene rearrangement and allelic exclusion. This results in the generation of enormous receptor diversity and the potential to recognize the entire universe of antigens. Diversity is further increased by the insertion of N regions at V-D-J junctions.

T cells may also express alternative TCR γ and δ chains encoded on chromosomes 7 and 14, respectively. These chains are similar to α and β but show somewhat less diversity and are structurally more similar to immunoglobulins than $\alpha\beta$ TCR. Further, $\gamma\delta$ T cells recognize not only peptide but also nonpeptide antigens,[7] and they may play unique roles in recognizing certain intracellular pathogens (eg, mycobacteria, listeria).[8,9] TCR $\gamma\delta$ T cells are particularly concentrated among intraepithelial lymphocytes of the gastrointestinal tract, further reinforcing the notion that $\gamma\delta$ T cells perform functions related to surveillance of certain pathogens. Soluble forms of the TCR exist, resulting

from alternative mRNA splicing or from proteolytic cleavage of surface receptors. The function of soluble TCR is not understood; studies show these molecules behaving as suppressor factors or proinflammatory mediators.

As for surface immunoglobulin, the TCR is not expressed alone in the membrane. The TCR requires the coexpression of a complex of invariant chains termed *cluster determinant 3* (CD3). CD3 is a complex of five transmembrane proteins (γ, δ, ε, ζ, η), as shown in Figure 16-4, which are important for the assembly of the TCR and its transport and insertion into the cell membrane. The CD3 complex plays an essential role in signal transduction by the TCR, particularly the cytoplasmic domains of the ζ and η chains.[10] Additional molecules also function in tandem with the $\alpha\beta$ TCR. In particular the CD4 and CD8 molecules, transmembrane proteins that are likewise members of the immunoglobulin gene superfamily, physically associate with the $\alpha\beta$ TCR and bind to the same MHC molecules as the TCR. This association increases the affinity and avidity of TCR and T cells for antigen. CD4 binds to class II MHC (ie, HLA-DR, DP, and DQ) and is generally considered a cell surface marker for helper T cells (T$_H$). This explains why T$_H$ are MHC class II restricted. CD8 binds to class I MHC (ie, HLA-A, B, and C) and is generally considered a

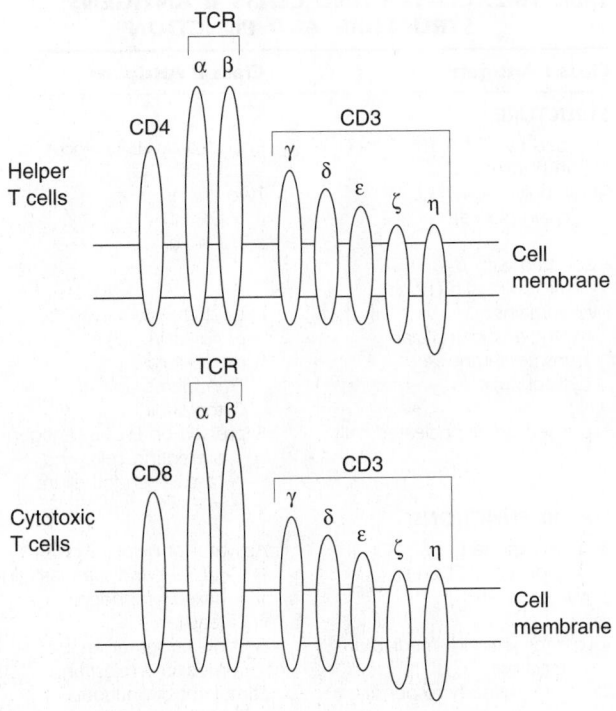

Figure 16-4. TCR complex in the cell membrane composed of TCR $\alpha\beta$, CD3, CD4, and CD8 chains.

cell surface marker for cytotoxic (T_c) or suppressor (T_s) T cells. This explains why T_c are generally MHC class I restricted.

There are two major classes of MHC molecules encoded by linked loci on chromosome 6 and defined by structural and functional associations (Table 16-2). Class I MHC molecules result from the noncovalent association between a polymorphic, transmembrane α chain and a nonpolymorphic soluble β chain, termed β_2-microglobulin. Thus, α chains encoded by diverse HLA-A, B, or C alleles each associate with β_2-microglobulin on the cell surface (Fig. 16-5). Class II molecules result from the noncovalent association of polymorphic transmembrane α and β chains encoded by HLA-DP, HLA-DQ, or HLA-DR (Fig 16-6). There are separate α and β chains encoded within each separate class II subregion. Despite some structural differences, these class I and II dimers all have four major extracellular domains with two of the domains contributing the major amino acid side chains to the walls of the peptide binding groove.

The TCR binds to a complex of MHC plus antigen. X-ray crystallography has determined the three-dimensional structure of these complexes and provided a firm structural and biochemical basis for understanding the cellular process of MHC restriction.[11,12] Figure 16-7 shows that the α_1 and α_2 domains of an MHC class I molecule form a groove on the surface of the MHC molecule. Peptide antigens are loaded into this groove when the functions of antigen processing and presentation are performed. The α_1 and β_1 domains of class II MHC perform a similar function. The TCR residues come in contact with residues of both antigen and MHC. Therefore, polymorphisms of the TCR generated by gene arrangement, and polymorphisms of MHC resulting from allelic variation within the population and the expression of several different class I or II molecules, provide the structural variation required to accommodate the potential universe of antigenic determinants. Some of the most important recent advances in immunol-

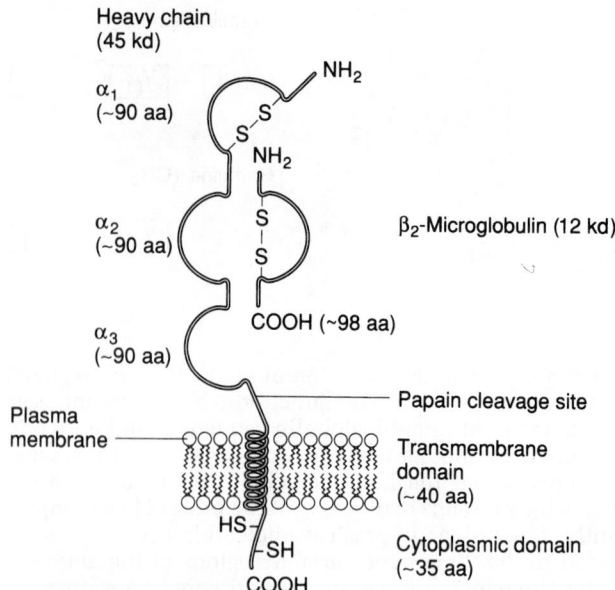

Figure 16-5. HLA class I molecule. The polymorphic heavy chain (45 kd) of the class I polypeptide is noncovalently bound to the invariant light chain, β_2-microglobulin (12 kd). The heavy chain consists of five domains—three extracellular domains (α_1, α_2, and α_3), a transmembrane domain, and a cytoplasmic domain. The α_1 and α_2 domains contain the most polymorphic residues responsible for antigen binding and form the side walls of the peptide binding groove; the transmembrane portion anchors the molecule to the plasma membrane; and the β_2-microglobulin stabilizes the conformation of the extracellular domains.

ogy have been the determination of the three-dimensional structure of the MHC, peptide binding groove, and TCR and the unequivocal demonstration of the loading of peptide antigen into the MHC molecules. Precise, structurally based approaches to altering the T cell's initial recognition of antigen are now possible and are being investigated ex-

---

Table 16-2. CLASS I AND CLASS II ANTIGENS: STRUCTURE AND FUNCTION

Class I Antigens	Class II Antigens
STRUCTURE	
Encoded by HLA-A, -B, -C loci in humans	Encoded by HLA-D locus (DR, DP, DQ)
Single polymorphic heavy chain (45 kd)	Two chains α (29 kd) β (34 kd)
Associated with β_2-microglobulin (12 kd)	—
Five domains α_1, α_2, α_3 extracellular Transmembrane Cystoplasmic	Four domains α_1, α_2 or β_1, β_2 extracellular Transmembrane Cytoplasmic
Expressed on all nucleated cells	Expressed on B cells, antigen-presenting cells, and vascular endothelium
MAJOR FUNCTIONS	
Activator and target for cytotoxic T (CD8+) lymphocytes	Activator of helper T cells (CD4+) and stimulator in mixed lymphocyte reaction
Target for antibody-mediated rejection	Possible target for antibody-mediated rejection
Stimulate antibody response	Stimulator of antibody response (unknown significance)

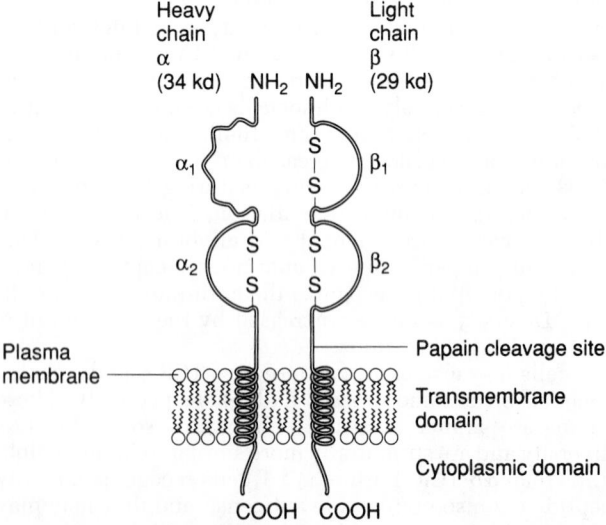

Figure 16-6. HLA class II molecule. The two chains, α (29 kd) and β (34 kd), are noncovalently associated and are made up of four domains—two extracellular domains, a transmembrane domain, and a cytoplasmic domain. Most of the allelic variance is contained in the β chain. The peptide binding site is believed to be in the groove between the α_1 and β_1 domains.

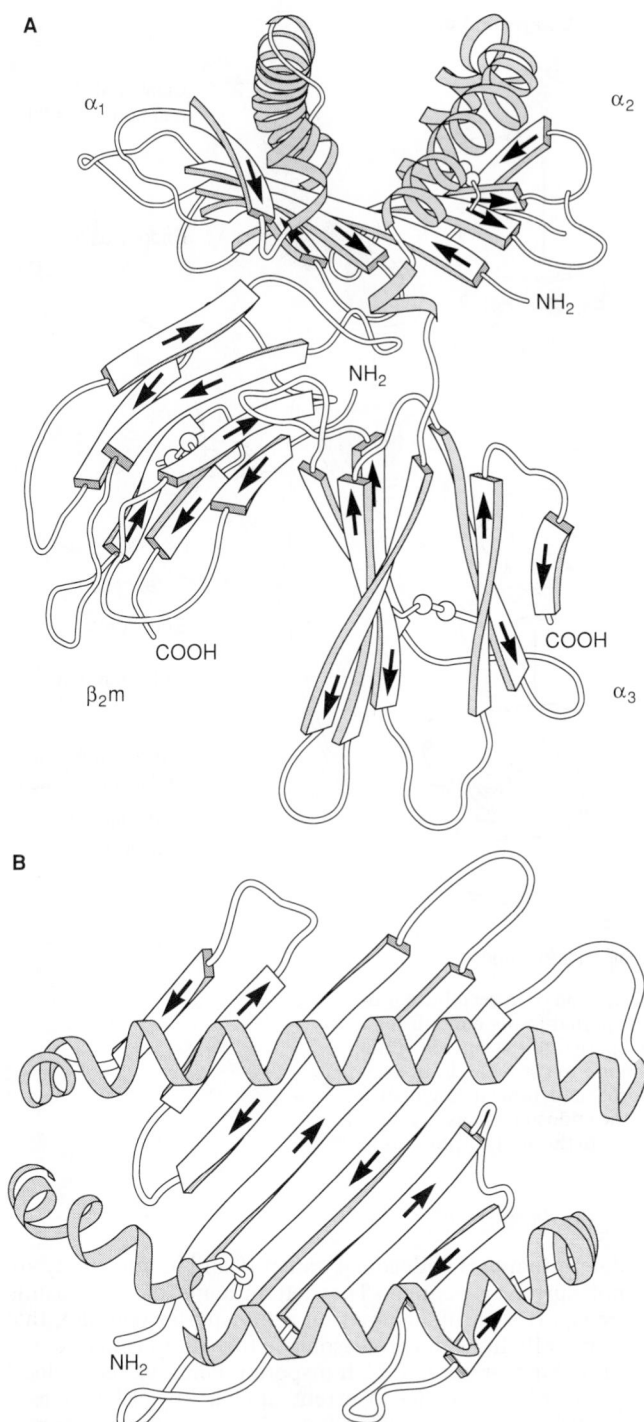

Figure 16-7. Human HLA-A2 class I molecule. (*A*) There are four domains with the polymorphic α_1 and α_2 on top presenting themselves to the T-cell-receptor and α_3 and β_2 below close to the cell membrane. (*B*) Looking at the top of the molecule, the peptide binding groove is shown as made up of the α_1 and α_2 domains forming the side walls and the β pleated sheet forming the floor.

perimentally to determine their application to clinical transplantation.

Antigen Processing

Identifying the MHC–antigen complex structure has also initiated much recent study toward defining the pathways by which antigen is loaded onto MHC molecules. The path-

ways of antigen processing encompass a wide variety of cellular functions, including the receptor-mediated endocytosis of antigen, transfer of cytoplasmic or endosomal antigen to proteolytic organelles, translocation of proteolyzed peptide into the endoplastic reticulum to nascent "naked" MHC molecules, correct folding of new MHC molecules around antigen, transport of antigen–MHC via the *cis-* and *trans-*Golgi apparatus to the cell surface, and recycling of cell surface MHC molecules to endosomal and Golgi compartments to exchange one antigenic peptide for another (Fig. 16-8). This brief list of some of the defined steps of antigen processing and presentation reveals that many of the normal cellular housekeeping processes are co-opted during the handling of antigen. These processes include vesicle transport and fusion, microtubule and microfilament function, correct folding and localization of nascent polypeptides coming off the ribosome by chaperonins, and control of intracellular proteolysis. Therefore, the study and eventual understanding of antigen processing and presentation requires knowledge of most normal cellular functions. Immunosuppression may eventually be directed not at T cells or B cells, as is currently the case, but may alter the functions of chaperones, Golgi apparatus, or proteolytic controls.

Figure 16-8 provides a general picture of the major processes, which include antigen uptake, proteolysis, translocation to the endoplasmic reticulum or Golgi, and presentation on the cell surface.[13-36] A number of important features should be mentioned. The source of antigen determines how and where it comes into contact with the processing machinery and onto which MHC molecules it is loaded. Thus, endogenously synthesized proteins, such as self-proteins or viral antigens in the cytoplasm, are degraded in the cytoplasm, transported to the endoplasmic reticulum, and loaded onto nascent class I MHC. Conversely, exogenously synthesized antigens are taken up in endosomes through receptor-mediated processes, degraded within an endosomal compartment (eg, lysosome, Golgi apparatus, or a unique structure), transported to the Golgi, and loaded onto nascent class II MHC. Although this general scheme for the processing and presentation of endogenous versus exogenous antigens will likely remain intact, there are numerous exceptions where endogenous antigens may be presented by class II MHC or exogenous antigens presented by class I MHC. This undoubtedly reflects the incomplete understanding of vesicle transport, proteolytic control, partitioning of molecules to various endosomal compartments, and the molecular control of MHC folding and peptide loading.

Proteolytic degradation of antigens may be accomplished either in endosomal compartments, probably through fusion with lysosomes, or in the cytoplasm. The latter process seems to be accomplished by a large multi-protein complex called the *proteasome*. In addition, some of the proteasome subunits are encoded within the MHC region. Thus, the MHC provides the information to degrade antigen and to determine the carrier onto which antigenic peptides are loaded. The control of proteolysis is currently poorly understood; it is not clear if all cellular constituents have equal access to proteolytic components or if antigens are somehow preferentially shunted into the system. Proteolytic enzymes have specificity for particular peptide bonds; therefore, not all proteins should be equally susceptible to the processing apparatus and some should make "better" antigens than others. This has been confirmed experimentally using amino acid substituted antigens. In addition, there is allelic variation among the MHC-encoded proteasome subunits so that antigen is processed into different peptides by different alleles. Allelic variation within MHC class I and II peptide binding grooves also determines what set

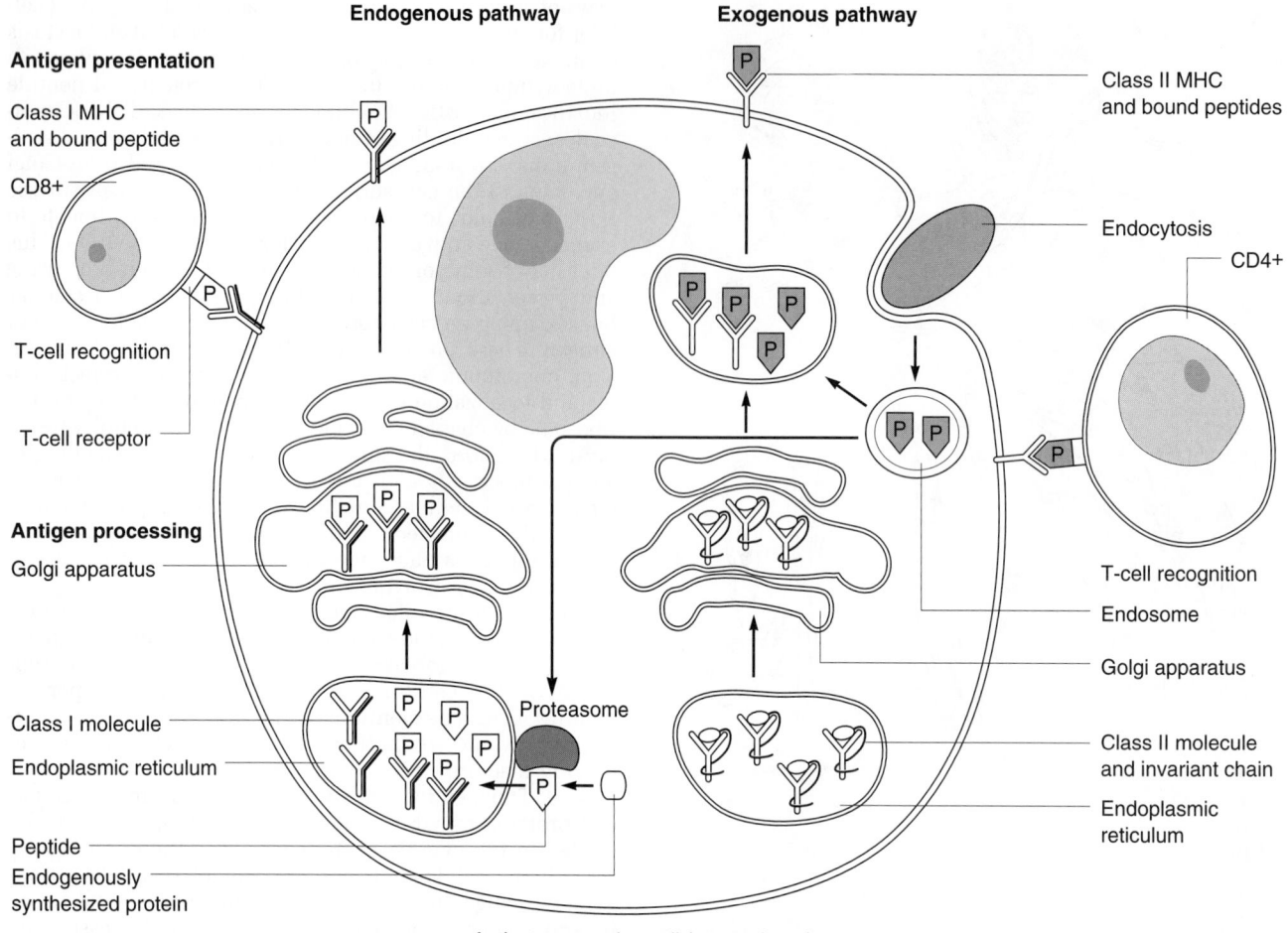

Figure 16-8. Antigen processing and presentation. Endogenously synthesized or intracellular proteins (eg, viral gene products) are degraded into peptides that are transported to the endoplasmic reticulum. These peptides bind to class I MHC molecules and are transported to the surface of the antigen-presenting cell. CD8+ T cells recognize the foreign peptide bound to class I MHC by way of the TCR complex. Exogenous antigen (eg, bacterial) is endocytosed and broken down into peptide fragments in endosomes. Class II molecules are transported to the endosome in association with the invariant chain, bind the peptide, and are delivered to the surface of the antigen-presenting cell, where they are recognized by CD4+ cells.

of peptides can be bound by MHC molecules. Thus, heterogeneity of antigens, proteolytic enzymes, and MHC molecules all determine the nature of the peptide ultimately presented to the TCR.

Further molecular analysis demonstrates that the MHC class I peptide binding groove is a fairly closed structure and can accommodate peptides of a relatively restricted size, ranging from 8 to 10 amino acids in length. Conversely, the class II groove is larger and more open ended. It can tolerate more length heterogeneity in the peptide that it binds so that a modal distribution of 12 to 24 amino acids is found loaded onto these molecules. These structural constraints suggest that certain types of antigens may be presented only by certain MHC molecules. Indeed, there is evidence that certain microbial antigens are preferentially presented by class I MHC.[37,38] This example also represents one exception where exogenously synthesized antigens are presented by class I. While the discussion to this point has focused on protein antigens, it is not currently known if or how nonprotein antigens are loaded into the antigen binding groove of MHC molecules.

Another important issue is how antigen is transported into the endoplasmic reticulum or Golgi apparatus. The determinants of endosomal transport and its specificity are not currently defined. The determinants of cytoplasmic transport seem dependent on a transporter complex that physically links the proteasome to the endoplasmic reticulum. Furthermore, this transporter complex is at least partly MHC encoded. Current models suggest that as a peptide antigen is degraded, it is immediately transported from the proteasome to the lumen of the endoplasmic reticulum where it is loaded onto class I MHC. The facts that the MHC encodes the transporter and that allelic variation is also present in these molecules provide another level of variation in the ability to ultimately recognize any antigen.

Another noteworthy issue is how peptide is loaded into the binding groove of MHC molecules. Experimental evidence suggests that class I and II dimers are incompletely assembled in the endoplasmic reticulum and are also bound by chaperone proteins. In the case of class II MHC, this chaperone is called the *invariant chain.* Failure to load peptide results in retention of MHC molecules within the endoplasmic reticulum and markedly decreases cell surface MHC expression. Loading of peptide causes the release of MHC by chaperones, completion of folding and assembly, and transport to the cell surface. A related issue is the fate and recycling of cell surface antigen–MHC complexes. There is evidence of endocytosis and reloading of both class I and II molecules with new peptide antigens. The molecular determinants of these processes are still poorly defined.

Antigen Presentation and Antigen-Presenting Cells

Based on the previous discussion, it is apparent that antigen processing and presentation depend on a large number of coordinated intracellular events. Many of these events, however, seem to depend on normal cellular processes of transport, proteolysis, and posttranslational modification of proteins. Antigen presentation also depends on the expression of MHC-encoded class I, class II, proteasome, and transporter molecules. All nucleated cells express MHC class I, and many cell types can also express the other loci. This suggests that many different cell types are capable of presenting antigens. In fact, this has been proved in a number of experimental and clinical analyses. Nonetheless, certain cell types are more efficient at processing and presenting antigen and are localized to certain tissues or organs that increase the likelihood that they will participate in antigen presentation. These so-called professional APCs are generally considered to be monocytes and macrophages. In addition, putatively closely related interstitial dendritic cells and Langerhans cells of the dermis are extremely efficient APCs. These cells constitutively express class I and II MHC and the other MHC-encoded components. All these products can be up-regulated in response to proinflammatory cytokines, such as interferon-γ (IFN-γ). These cells are also localized to regions, such as the lymph nodes, spleen, and skin, where they are most likely to encounter antigen. Other cell types, such as vascular endothelium, organ parenchymal cells, and tumor cells, can act as APCs under many conditions. The nature of the responding T cell, the cytokine milieu, and the expression of other cell surface adhesion receptors determine APC function.

Alloreactivity

The discussion to this point has centered on general considerations of antigenic recognition. In transplantation, the response to alloantigens is most germane. The immune response to alloantigens is extraordinarily strong and the immune system seems obsessed by allelic variations in MHC antigens. Thus, in a culture of human T lymphocytes stimulated with a purified protein antigen (eg, murine cytochrome C), far less than 1% of the T cells respond to the antigen. Conversely, if the same culture is stimulated with human allogenic cells expressing different MHC alleles, up to 10% of the T cells respond to the antigenic stimulation. In terms of clinical transplantation, this suggests that the immune system is specifically directed against foreign MHC and that any attempts to improve immunosuppression, prevent rejection, and prolong allograft survival depend on a detailed understanding of alloreactivity.

Current cellular and molecular models of alloreactivity rely on the understanding of TCR and MHC structural interactions. The TCR does not recognize MHC alone but as a complex of antigen plus MHC. During T-cell maturation, autoreactive T cells are eliminated or tolerized (see Development of Lymphocytes). Thus, T cells that recognize self-peptides loaded into self-MHC are no longer present or able to respond to antigen. The remaining T cells have TCR specificities that enable them to recognize foreign peptides loaded onto self-MHC molecules, a concept termed *recog-*

nition of altered self. These same T cells may also fortuitously recognize foreign peptides loaded onto allo-MHC or even self-peptides loaded onto allo-MHC. The reason for these other types of recognition is that TCR–antigen–MHC interactions ultimately rely on the three-dimensional interaction of amino acid side chains of the molecules.

Figure 16-9 shows these potential TCR–MHC interactions, including recognition of self-peptides on self-MHC, or an autoimmune response, and various types of alloantigenic responses. The recognition of foreign or self-peptides loaded onto allo-MHC is termed *direct recognition* because intact allo-MHC is being recognized. The response to foreign MHC peptides loaded onto self-MHC is termed *indirect* recognition since intact allo-MHC is not being recognized. These terms and concepts apply to both class I and class II MHC as well as CD4+ and CD8+ T cells. Most alloreactivity is due to allogenic cells of the donor organ acting as APCs and presenting endogenous peptides in the context of allogenic class I MHC to host CD8+ T cells. However, all permutations of self and foreign peptides and MHC, and class I and II MHC, have been demonstrated to occur experimentally or clinically. A single T cell may be capable of recognizing one peptide in the context of self-MHC and another peptide in the context of allo-MHC.

Antigenicity

The structural and cellular information in the previous section provides a foundation for considering what determines whether a molecule is perceived as an antigen and how strong an immune response it elicits. In the case of a protein antigen, it must be correctly transported, proteolyzed, loaded onto MHC molecules, and interact with the

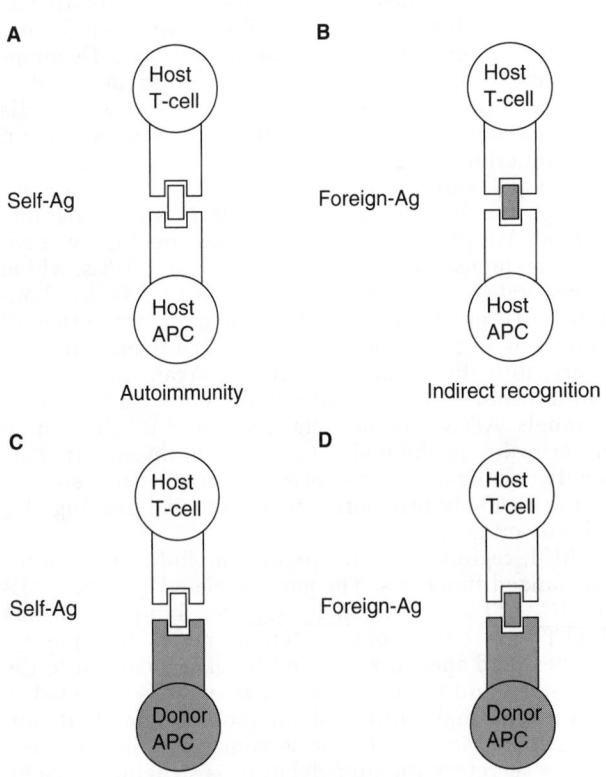

Figure 16-9. TCR recognition of self- and foreign peptide antigen in the context of self or foreign MHC molecules. *A* represents autoimmunity. *B, C,* and *D* are aspects of alloimmunity.

TCR. Failure to achieve any one of these steps may prevent an appropriate immune response. Immunosuppressive strategies based on this new information are currently being experimentally evaluated and are discussed later in this chapter. There are many other determinants of antigenicity, such as antigen quartenary structure,[39] location of cell types involved in presenting antigen,[40] the types of T cells present, and the types of cytokines present during the response. These issues are also discussed later in this chapter. The molecular pathways for antigen processing and presentation are defined for *peptide* antigens. Pathways for carbohydrates, lipids, nucleic acids, or derivatives of these are currently undefined and may have novel interactions with APC pathways or be incapable of eliciting T-cell immunity. The complexity of the response to antigen demonstrates that many potential loci for immunosuppression exist and that to achieve timely effective immunosuppression, many of these loci may have to be simultaneously disrupted.

Sites of Antigen Recognition

Anatomic Organization of the Immune Response

In vitro experimental studies of immune function often juxtapose stimulator and responder cells in an environment where all possible cellular interactions may take place more or less equally. In vivo, the situation is quite different because cells and antigen are sequestered or compartmentalized. Thus, interactions among cells are more restricted, resulting in a channeling of immune responses in certain directions. There are several intersecting levels of anatomic organization of the immune system. First, immature T cells, B cells, and APCs arise centrally in the bone marrow. The initial interaction of T and B cells with the bone marrow microenvironment may determine if these cells are tolerized to self-antigens expressed in the bone marrow. T cells undergo further maturation and selection in the thymus (see Development of Lymphocytes). Interactions with thymic medullary and cortical tissues determine that self-reactive cells are tolerized while altered-self reactive cells remain fully functional.

Second, mature cells circulate in the periphery through the lymphatic and vascular systems, passing through lymph nodes. Lymph nodes are highly organized juxtapositions of T cells, B cells, and APCs, which concentrate antigen in the vicinity of responding lymphocytes. For example, a wound infection or a skin graft introduce bacterial antigens or alloantigens, respectively, into the dermis. Antigen is taken up by APCs and transported to regional lymph nodes via lymphatic channels. APCs present antigen to T and B cells, which either reside in the node or recirculate through it. This highly organized and stereotyped sequence of events result in antibody production by B cells and priming of T cells to antigen.

Third, regional collections of lymphoid tissue serve specialized functions. The gut-associated lymphoid tissue (GALT) and bronchial-associated lymphoid tissue (BALT) are collections of lymph nodes (eg, Peyer's patches) and specialized T and B cells, localized to the gut lumen and tracheobronchial tree, areas expected to have a very high burden of antigen and microbial contamination. Most B cells can secrete IgA in these tissues. IgA, or secretory immunoglobulin, is structurally capable of retaining its functions of opsonization and antimicrobial activity within gut and bronchial secretions. There are also intraepithelial TCR $\gamma\delta$ T cells of the gut. As mentioned earlier, these cells may have specialized roles in responding to certain microorganisms by virtue of TCR specificity for evolutionarily conserved microbial antigens. The signals that localize IgA+ B cells or $\gamma\delta$+ T cells or that induce cells already present in these regions to express the relevant receptors are not currently understood.

Fourth, there is a division between the function of central and peripheral lymphoid tissue. Antigen presented peripherally (ie, subcutaneously or intradermally) localizes to regional lymph nodes and induces long-lived T- and B-cell immunity. Antigen presented centrally (ie, orally, intrabronchially, or intravenously) may induce transient or local immunity (eg, intestinal IgA secretion) but also tends to induce systemic unresponsiveness or tolerance to the antigen. This may be an adaptive response to prevent severe debilitating inflammatory responses to what we ingest or breathe. From the standpoint of transplantation, it may be possible to take advantage of this central versus peripheral difference in antigen presentation to help induce tolerance. What determines this difference is currently unknown. The possibility that the nature of the APC in central compartments (eg, liver, spleen, BALT, GALT) is different than in the peripheral lymph node has been considered. No such differences, however, have been unequivocally demonstrated. More recent inquiries suggest that the microenvironment differs between central and peripheral compartments (eg, cytokine levels) and that this interacts with APCs to channel immune responses in various directions.

Homing and Trafficking

It has long been known that lymphocytes traffic between the vascular and lymphatic compartments and localize to sites of inflammation and that specialized subsets can home to specific anatomic sites (eg, IgA+ B cells to the gut). Recently, many of the determinants of lymphocyte homing and trafficking have been defined by molecular and cellular techniques, and the physiologic roles of these components is now a much more tractable problem. The major issue to understand in homing and trafficking is leukocyte–vascular endothelial cell interactions. This is the initial interaction required in any immune or inflammatory response. It is not possible for a lymphocyte to home, localize, or circulate without first passing through the vascular endothelial layer. Studies using videomicroscopy and blocking specific molecules with antibodies or genetic techniques have shown that this initial interaction can be divided into several steps.[41] Many of these studies have examined neutrophils and monocytes in addition to lymphocytes. In the first step, leukocytes come in contact with the vascular endothelium and adhere to the surface. The cell attaches then rolls over the endothelial surface as a result of hemodynamic shear forces. In the second step, the leukocyte is activated to express other receptors and secretes cytokines. The endothelial cell may also become activated and alter receptor expression and cytokine production. In the third step, the leukocyte stops on the endothelial surface, and the adhesive interaction between the cells increases. The final step is transendothelial cell migration.

Each step is associated with several specific interactions between receptors on the leukocyte cell surface and ligands on the endothelial surface or with soluble cytokine ligands. Because so many cytokines and surface receptors or ligands have now been identified, with many more reported regularly in the literature,[42,43] the current challenge is to understand how all these signals are integrated in a coherent and specific fashion. Current modeling suggests that specific classes of molecules are associated with each

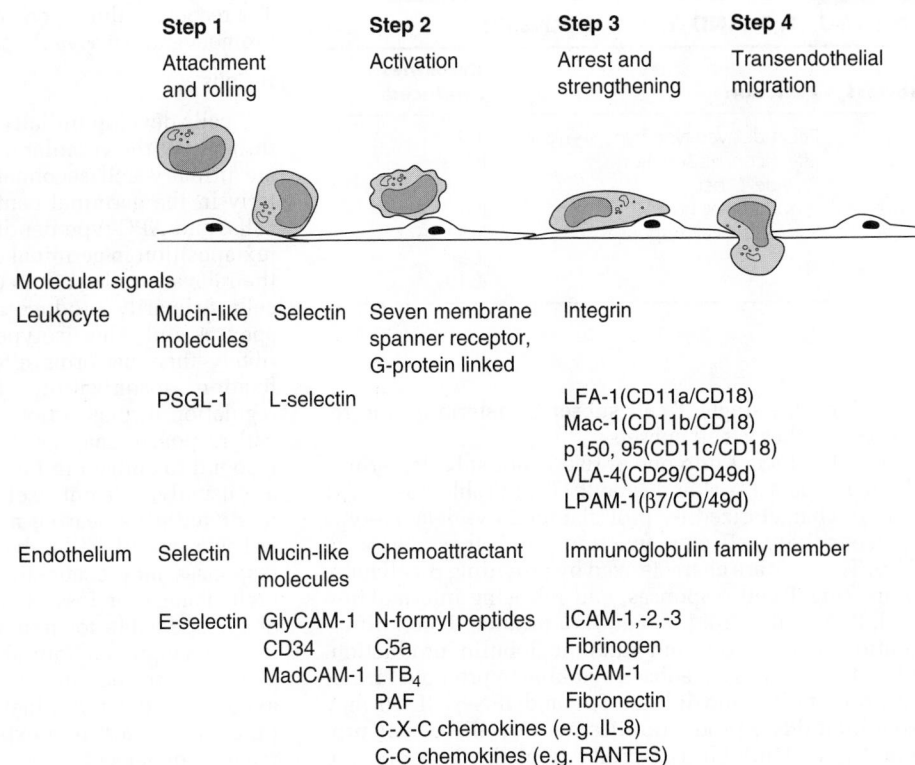

	Step 1 Attachment and rolling	Step 2 Activation	Step 3 Arrest and strengthening	Step 4 Transendothelial migration

Molecular signals

Leukocyte	Mucin-like molecules	Selectin	Seven membrane spanner receptor, G-protein linked	Integrin
	PSGL-1	L-selectin		LFA-1(CD11a/CD18) Mac-1(CD11b/CD18) p150, 95(CD11c/CD18) VLA-4(CD29/CD49d) LPAM-1(β7/CD/49d)

Endothelium	Selectin	Mucin-like molecules	Chemoattractant	Immunoglobulin family member
	E-selectin	GlyCAM-1 CD34 MadCAM-1	N-formyl peptides C5a LTB$_4$ PAF C-X-C chemokines (e.g. IL-8) C-C chemokines (e.g. RANTES)	ICAM-1,-2,-3 Fibrinogen VCAM-1 Fibronectin

Figure 16-10. Model of leukocyte–vascular endothelial cell interactions important for specific trafficking and homing. The three major classes of cellular adhesion receptors—selectins, integrins, immunoglobulin gene superfamily members—play distinct temporal and functional roles.

of the first three steps of the trafficking process and that these molecules are restricted by cell type.[41] The result is a three-digit "zip code," which may specifically direct neutrophils, monocytes, or lymphocytes to the correct anatomic location. This model is illustrated in Figure 16-10. Different subsets of lymphocytes or other leukocytes can express different receptor and cytokine arrays. Likewise, different subsets of endothelial cells also express different molecular arrays. These differences could account for fine tuning and further specificity of the system.

Cells and Molecules That Participate in Antigen Recognition

T Cells

The central paradigm for the initiation of an immune response is that antigen is taken up by an APC, processed, and then presented to a T cell (Fig. 16-11). The T cell is activated in response to appropriately processed and presented antigen. The activated T cell may become an effector T cell and may also provide help to B cells, other T cells, or even macrophages, which then proceed to act as immune effectors. In this paradigm, the T cell plays a central and indispensable role. For this reason, much of transplantation immunology is directed toward understanding and manipulating T-cell responses.

T cells are divided into two main subclasses: CD4+ and CD8+. CD4+8+ double-positive cells are usually immature T cells or thymocytes, whereas the fully differentiated T cell is usually single positive. Because of the molecular interactions described earlier,[44,45] CD4+ T cells are restricted to recognizing antigen in the context of class II MHC and usually perform roles related to B-cell help, T-cell help, and inflammatory responses, such as delayed and contact hypersensitivity. CD8+ T cells are restricted to class I MHC and often perform cytotoxicity. Under certain circumstances, particularly experimental conditions with

transgenic or knock-out derived cells, CD4+ cells can be class I restricted or perform cytotoxic functions. Conversely CD8+ cells can be class II restricted or perform helper or inflammatory functions. These findings suggest there is sufficient plasticity in TCR structure and in cellular programming so that a single T-cell subset can perform the functions of other subsets. This may also imply that blocking or ablating the function of a single T-cell subset may not provide reliable immunosuppression from the standpoint of clinical transplantation. However, the complexity of immunoregulatory systems might permit the ma-

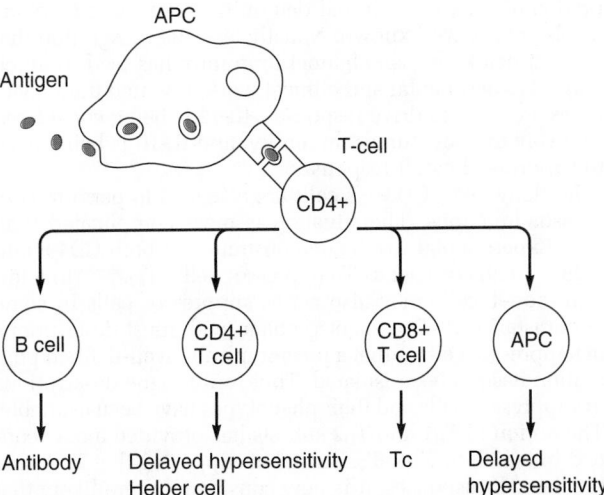

Figure 16-11. Central paradigm for cellular initiation of an immune response. CD4+ T cells respond to appropriately presented antigen on antigen-presenting cells (APCs) and in turn help other T cells, B cells, and APCs.

Table 16-3. T$_H$1 AND T$_H$2 SUBCLASSES

Subclass	Function	Cytokines Produced
T$_H$1	Effect delayed-type hypersensitivity	IL-2
	Effect contact sensitivity	IFN-γ
	Provide T$_c$ help	(Respond to IL-12)
T$_H$2	Provide B-cell help	IL-2
	Suppress T-cell responses	IL-4
		IL-5
		IL-10

nipulation of a single T-cell subset to determine the responses of other T-cell subsets.

CD4+ T cells fall into one of two major subsets, termed T helper type 1 (T$_H$1) and type 2 (T$_H$2) (Table 16-3). T$_H$1 cells are characterized by proinflammatory, delayed-type hypersensitivity effector functions and the release of IFN-γ. T$_H$2 cells are characterized by providing B-cell help, suppressing T-cell responses, and releasing interleukin-4 (IL-4), IL-5, and IL-10. IL-4 and IL-5 promote B cell differentiation, maturation, and immunoglobulin production, and IL-4 may act as a feedback cytokine to promote further T$_H$2 proliferation and inhibit T$_H$1 and IFN-γ. IL-10 may also inhibit IFN-γ production. Conversely, IFN-γ may promote T$_H$1 and inhibit T$_H$2 production. Furthermore, the potent macrophage-derived T-cell stimulatory cytokine, IL-12, also promotes T$_H$1 production. Current models suggest that T$_H$1 and T$_H$2 form a regulatory circuit in which one subset inhibits the activity of the other (Fig. 16-12). These models imply that the channeling of an immune response occurs early and is determined by the relative balance of T$_H$ subsets and their cytokines.

Several uncertainties about the T$_H$1/T$_H$2 model remain. Although these subsets have been repeatedly demonstrated in murine experimental systems, it is not clear if the human subsets are so well defined and compartmentalized. There may be more overlap in humans. Second, it is not clear if T$_H$1 and T$_H$2 interconvert or if their phenotype represents terminal differentiation. A related issue is whether T$_H$1 and T$_H$2 are derived from a common T$_H$0 precursor or if they represent more distant and distinct lineages. Third, the amount and ratio of IL-12, IL-4, IL-2, and IFN-γ at the initiation of an immune response determine whether T$_H$1 or T$_H$2 predominate, yet the initial determinants of these cytokine levels are not well known. Nonetheless, the recognition that distinct cytokines can channel immunity has lead to much current experimental and clinical work in which these cytokines are used to drive responses. IL-12 is being considered as a way to boost tumor immunity, and IL-10 is being used to suppress allograft responses.

In many texts, CD8+ T cells are also said to perform suppressor functions. The situation is more complicated than this. Experimental results demonstrate that both CD4+ and CD8+ T cells can act as T suppressor cells (T$_s$).[46-50] In addition, non-T cells may also act as suppressor cells in some circumstances.[51] The major problem with most descriptions of suppressor cells is that a phenotypically well-defined population has not been isolated. Thus, only vague descriptions of suppressor cells and their phenotypes have been available. The notion of T$_H$1 and T$_H$2 subsets has provided a new context in which to view T$_s$. Instead of supposing that T$_s$ down-regulate all responses, it is now considered more likely that T$_s$ channel immunity in one direction or another. Thus, T$_H$2 cells suppress T$_H$1 and T$_c$ function while supporting B cell responses. Current models suggest that T$_H$2 cells are the relevant T$_s$ of cell-mediated immunity, and attempts to boost

T$_H$2 responses during organ allografting are seen as a way to promote graft survival.[47]

B Cells

B cells develop initially in the bone marrow, recirculate throughout the vascular and lymphatic systems, and initiate primary and secondary antibody responses, particularly in the germinal centers of lymph nodes. B cells, T cells, and APC-type dendritic cells are brought into close juxtaposition in germinal centers, concentrating antigen to the relevant cells and receptors of the immune system. B cells primarily produce antibody—IgM for primary responses and other isotypes for secondary responses. Antibody then performs effector functions of complement fixation, opsonization, clearance, or feedback immune regulation through idiotype–anti-idiotype interactions. B cell responses may be *T independent*, in which B cells respond to antigen in the absence of helper T cells. These are usually, but not exclusively, IgM responses to polymeric antigens bearing multiple identical epitopes, such as bacterial cell wall polysaccharides. T cell–independent responses may occur after transplantation and result in graft damage or loss. T call–independent responses are also responsible for much of the natural antibody found in graft recipients. Natural antibody is preformed immunoglobulin directed toward alloantigens, despite no previous exposure of the individual to the alloantigen. The antibody putatively arises from exposure to cross-reactive environmental antigens.

T-dependent responses require the T cell–APC–B cell interaction. This interaction requires coordinated signaling among these cells of numerous cell surface and soluble ligands. The specificity of the interaction is assured by the specificity of the T- and B-cell receptors for antigen. Thereafter, a series of nonclonally distributed receptors and ligands interact to amplify and modulate these signals. Figure 16-13 shows some of the important cell surface receptor interactions that take place during T-cell stimulation of B cells. Because so many potential interactions may occur, it is unclear which signals are absolutely required or how any one receptor or group of receptors may alter the function of other receptors. Nonetheless, current models[52-56] suggest that the interactions of primary importance are as follows:

- TCR–antigen–class II MHC–CD4
- Antigen–sIgM (B-cell antigen receptor)
- CD28–CD80 (B7/BB1)
- CD40–CD40L

Failure to engage these receptors severely or completely inhibits appropriate responses. Secondary receptor–ligand interactions of importance include CD11a/18 (LFA-1)–CD54 (ICAM-1), CD2–CD58 (LFA-3), and CD19–

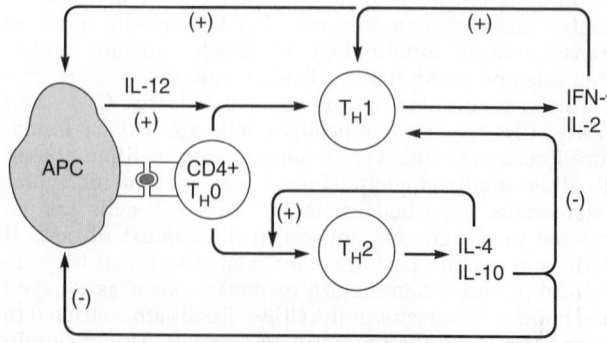

Figure 16-12. T$_H$1/T$_H$2 paradigm of CD4+ T-cell subsets.

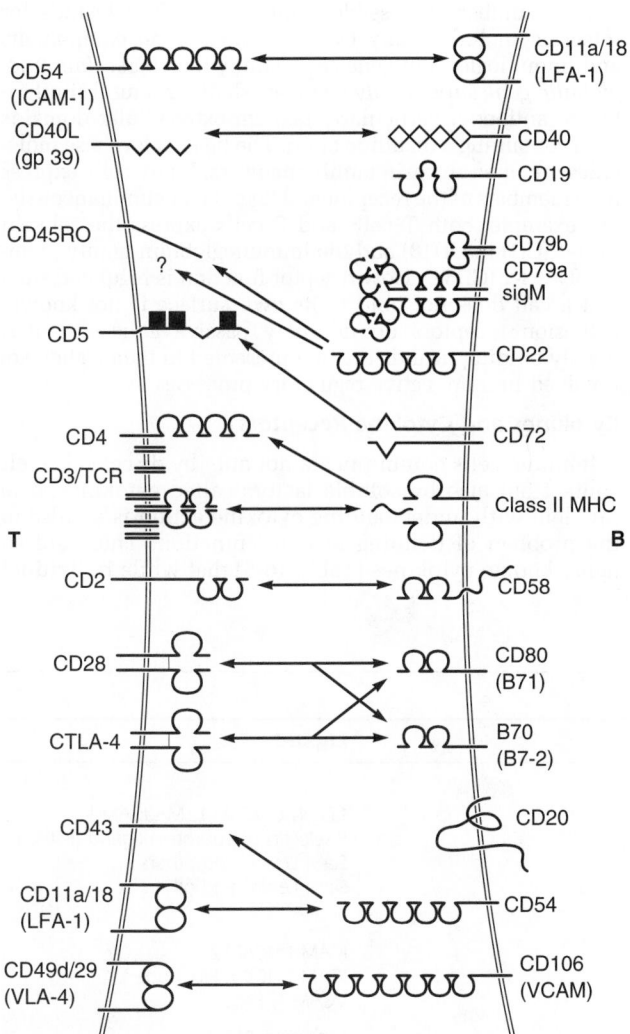

Figure 16-13. Adhesion receptors that may mediate interactions between CD4+ T cells and B cells.

16-13 shows, B cells express the relevant ligands and receptors for direct T-cell interactions. Thus the T–APC–B ternary complex may really be a T–B binary complex. This is probably the major interaction during secondary responses when T and B cells are already partially activated and express many of the relevant receptors. For primary responses, CD40L, CD80, CTLA4, and other receptors are not yet up-regulated, and direct T–B interactions are less efficient. In this case, professional APCs are likely required to initiate appropriate immunity.

Antigen-Presenting Cells

It has already been mentioned that virtually any cell type may perform the functions of an APC because many of the steps of processing and presentation take advantage of ubiquitous, constitutive cellular pathways. Most frequently, the term *APC* is applied to monocyte/macrophage or dendritic cells because both express class I and class II MHC, the cells are specialized to take up extracellular components and catabolize them, and these cells are histologically and anatomically located at sites most relevant for antigen entry and recognition. Based on these criteria, B cells are also efficient APCs and are generally most relevant for secondary responses when T cells are already primed or partially activated.

Another cell type of major importance for APC function, particularly in organ allografting, is the vascular endothelial cell.[57-64] As discussed earlier, this is the cell that the immune system first comes in contact with and that directs the homing, trafficking, and egress of lymphocytes into regions of inflammation. Vascular endothelial cells are dynamic in their ability to process and present antigen and to direct lymphocyte function. Quiescent endothelial cells are far less efficient and active with these processes than activated cells. Activation usually occurs as a result of antigen nonspecific signals during inflammation. Trauma, burns, ischemia, infection, allografting, or any other proinflammatory condition can activate endothelial cells. The signals most relevant for endothelial activation are the cytokines IL-1 and IL-4, tumor necrosis factor (TNF), and bacterial lipopolysaccharide. In turn, activated endothelial cells produce cytokines (IL-1, IL-6, IL-8, IFN-γ, and TGFβ) and display cell surface receptors important for presentation or trafficking (class II MHC, increased class I MHC, VCAM-1, ELAM-1, and P-selectin). From the standpoint of transplantation, nonimmunologic events, such as prolonged cold ischemic time or the type of preservation solution, can profoundly affect endothelial cell function and integrity and subsequent lymphocyte–endothelial cell interactions. Despite close tissue matching and good immunosuppression, these nonimmunologic events can activate endothelium, which in turn activates lymphocytes and other leukocytes and facilitates the development of antigen-dependent, immunologic organ rejection.

Adhesion Receptors

An essential feature of lymphocyte communication is the interaction of cell surface receptors with specific ligands.[65-71] As shown in Figures 16-10 and 16-13, a large number of potential interactions among T cells, B cells, APCs, and vascular endothelial cells can occur. Several features are important. First, although these molecules have often been called adhesion molecules, most are transmembrane proteins linked to cytoplasmic second messengers. Therefore, receptor engagement is likely to lead to a series of second signals that may alter the transcriptional activation of a wide array of genes and subsequently cellular function. Adhesion is only one function of these molecules.

While it is possible to describe in detail the individual function of any single receptor–ligand pair, the issue of un-

(unknown ligand). Failure to achieve these interactions, however, does not necessarily inhibit the B-cell response. Cytokines also required for T–B interactions include IL-4 and IL-5, which promote immunoglobulin class switching to IgE and IgG4 production, and IL-10 and IL-12, which promote switching to IgG1, IgG2, IgG3, and IgA.

The molecular signaling between T and B cells demonstrates that the B cell is not a passive member of the pair that merely receives T-cell–derived signals and then secretes immunoglobulin. As T cells become activated, they express CD40 ligand (CD40L), which binds to CD40 on B cells and activates B cells. B cells in turn then express more CD80 (B7/BB1) which binds to the T-cell CD28 receptor. CD28 ligation provides a potent costimulatory signal to T cells, which synergizes with TCR/CD3-derived activational signals. Therefore, there is important bidirectional T–B communication. B-cell–derived immunoglobulins may also regulate T and B immunity through idiotype–anti-idiotype interactions. In this case an antibody recognizes and binds to the polymorphic antigen binding region of B- or T-cell antigen receptors. The interaction can positively or negatively regulate immunity. Lastly, the B cell itself may act as an APC. The ability of surface immunoglobulin to bind low concentrations of antigen with high affinity makes B cells particularly efficient APCs. As Figure

derstanding the integration of many different signals has been a less tractable problem. Figure 16-10 shows current models that assign these receptors to a few related molecular groups and to a few functionally separate steps. Clearly, the immune system has an extraordinary amount of redundancy so that if a single pathway or receptor–ligand pair is compromised, it is likely other processes circumvent the block.

Adhesion receptors are classified into three major groups based on structural similarities. The *selectins* are transmembrane glycoproteins. The amino-terminal domain is lectin-like in structure. Lectins are molecules that bind carbohydrates. The amino-terminal domain is followed by a domain with homology to epidermal growth factor. This domain is followed by two to nine repeated domains with homology to complement binding proteins. The ligands for selectins are mucin-like molecules containing large amounts of carbohydrate presumably bound by the lectin domain. Distinct selectins are recognized on leukocytes, platelets, and endothelial cells and termed L-selectins, P-selectins, and E-selectins (Table 16-4). *Integrins* are heterodimeric transmembrane proteins. There are at least eight known integrin β chains that can associate with a wide variety of α chains, generating a large number of possible combinations. The ligands for integrins include many basement membrane components and immunoglobulin gene superfamily members. *Immunoglobulin gene superfamily* members share structural similarities to antibody, particularly tandem extracellular domains each containing a disulfide bond. The ligands for these molecules are often integrin family members. Many cells express both members of the receptor and ligand pair simultaneously. For example, both T cells and B cells express the selectin LFA-1 (CD11a/CD18) and the immunoglobulin family member ICAM-1 (CD54). How receptor function is regulated such that a cell does not bind to its own surface is not known. Adhesion receptors do not play passive adhesive roles, merely binding ligands that are presented to them. They are involved in more active regulatory processes.

Cytokines and Cytokine Receptors

Immune cells communicate not only by direct cell–cell contact but also by soluble factors called cytokines. The problem with understanding cytokine action is similar to the problem of defining receptor function. There are so many known cytokines (Table 16-5) that while individual

Table 16-4. ADHESION RECEPTORS

Molecule	Primary Expression	Ligand
SELECTINS		
L-selectin (CD62L)	PMN, lymphocytes	CD34, GlyCAM-1, MAdCAM-1
P-selectin (CD62P)	EC, platelets	P-selectin glycoprotein ligand (PSGL-1) Sialyl Lewis^x and others
E-selectin (CD62E)	EC	Sialyl Lewis^x and others
INTEGRINS		
LFA-1 (CD11a/CD18) (β_2, αL)	PMN, lymphocytes	ICAM-1, ICAM-2
Mac-1 (CD11b/CD18) (β_2/αM)	PMN	ICAM-1, iC3b, Fibrinogen, LPS
VLA-4 ($\alpha_4\beta_1$ integrin)	Eosinophils, lymphocytes	VCAM-1, FN

Integrin Subunits		Ligands and Counterreceptors	Integrin Name
β_1	α_1	Collagens, laminin	VLA-1
	α_2	Collagens, laminin	VLA-2
	α_3	Fibronectin, laminin, collagens	VLA-3
	α_4	Fibronectin, VCAM-1	VLA-4
	α_5	Fibronectin	VLA-5
	α_6	Laminin	VLA-6
	α_7	Laminin	VLA-7
	α_8	?	
	α_v	Vitronectin, fibronectin	
β_2	α_L	ICAM-1, ICAM-2, ICAM-3	LFA-1
	α_M	iC3b, fibrinogen, factor X, ICAM-1	Mac-1
	α_x	Fibrinogen	p150, 95
β_3	α_{IIb}	Fibrinogen, fibronectin, von Willebrand factor, vitronectin, thrombospondin	
	α_v	Vitronectin, fibrinogen, von Willebrand factor, thrombospondin, fibronectin, osteopontin, collagen	
β_4	α_6	?	
β_5	α_v	Vitronectin	
β_6	α_v	Fibronectin	
β_7 (=β_P?)	α_4	Fibronectin, VCAM-1, MAdCAM-1	LPAM-1
	α_{IEL}	?	
β_8	α_v	?	

IMMUNOGLOBULIN SUPERFAMILY		
ICAM-1 (CD 54)	Lymphocytes, EC	LFA-1, Mac-1
ICAM-2 (CD102)	Lymphocytes, EC	LFA-1
VCAM-1 (CD106)	EC	VLA-4
PECAM-1	EC, PMN, lymphocytes, platelets	?
MAdCAM-1	EC	LPAM-1
CD28	T	CD80 (B7/BB1)
CTLA4	T	CD80, B70/B7-2, B7-3
CD2	T, NK, some B	CD58 (LFA-3), possibly CD59

PMN, polymorphonuclear cell; EC, endothelial cells; T, T cells; NK, natural killer cells; B, B cells.

Table 16-5. CYTOKINE AND CYTOKINE RECEPTORS

	Origin	Responding Cells
CYTOKINE		
IL-1α or -β	Monocytes, EC	T, B, EC
IL-2	T, B	T, B, monocytes, EC
IL-3	T	T
IL-4	T	T, B, monocytes, mast cells, EC, eosinophils
IL-5	T	T, B, eosinophils
IL-6	T, B, monocytes, EC	T, B, EC
IL-7	T	T, B, monocytes
IL-8	T, EC, monocytes	T, EC, neutrophils
IL-9	T	T, mast cells
IL-10	T	T, B, monocytes
IL-11	Fibroblasts	B, megakaryocytes
IL-12	Monocytes	T, B, NK
IL-13	?	B, monocytes
IL-14	?	B
IFN-α or -β	EC	T, B, EC
IFN-γ	T, B	T, B, EC
TNF-α	T, B, EC	T, B, EC
TNF-β	T	T, B, EC
G-CSF	Fibroblasts, osteoblasts	Granulocytes
GM-CSF	T	Granulocytes, monocytes
M-CSF	Fibroblasts, monocytes	Monocytes
Classic Chemoattractants		
N-formyl peptide	Bacterial	Monocytes, granulocytes
C5a	Complement activation	Monocytes, granulocytes
LTB4	Arachidonate metabolism	Monocytes, neutrophils
PAF	Phosphotidylcholine metabolism	Monocytes, granulocytes
C-X-C Chemokines		
IL-8	T, EC, monocytes	T, EC, neutrophils
β-Thromboglobulin	Platelets	T, granulocytes
C-C Chemokines		
MCP-1	T, EC, monocytes	Monocytes
MIP-1α,β	T, monocytes	T, monocytes, granulocytes
RANTES	T, platelets	Monocytes

CYTOKINE RECEPTORS

Type I Cytokine Receptors (Hematopoietin Receptors)

IL-2, -4, -7, -9, -13, -15 receptors (share γ-chain)
IL-3, -5, GM-CSF receptors (share KH97 subunit)
LIF, OSM, CNTF, IL-6, IL-11 receptors
   (share gp130 subunit)
GH, PRL
EPO, G-CSF

Type II Cytokine Receptors

IFN-α, -β, -γ

TNF-Like Receptors

TNF-α, TNF-β receptors
gp39 (CD30-L)
CD27-L, CD30-L
NGF, 4-1BB
Fas

TGF-β Receptor Family

TGF-βI, TGF-βII receptors (share common TSR-I subunit)
Activin receptor-II, -IIβ

IL-8 Receptor Family (Seven-Membrane Spanner, G-Linked Proteins)

IL-8R
C5a-R
PAF-R
fMLP-R

EC, endothelial cells; T, T cells; B, B cells.

detailed actions are defined, many of these actions overlap and it is not yet possible to integrate these signals into a unified model.[72-95] Furthermore, many different cell types are capable of expressing each cytokine or cytokine receptor. This makes it difficult to define any specificity of cytokine function. Nonetheless, several generalizations have practical implications.

First, the chemoattractant cytokines are important for leukocyte homing and trafficking (see Fig. 16-10). Table 16-5 shows that these molecules are categorized according to structural criteria.

Second, the central paradigm of T cell–APC–B cell interactions (see Fig. 16-11) relies on the production of a few cytokines (Fig. 16-14). The initial CD4+ T cell–APC interaction results in IL-1 production by APCs, which stimulates CD4+ T cells. These cells then produce IL-2, IL-4, and IL-5. IL-2 and IL-4 help stimulate CD8+ T cells and B cells or even self-stimulate CD4+ T cells by a mechanism termed *autocrine stimulation*. IL-5 primarily helps B cells. Many other cytokines, however, are involved even in this central paradigm (see Fig. 16-12). Blockade of any single cytokine rarely impairs the stimulatory process because other cytokines tend to be redundant.

Third, the distinction between receptors and cytokines is often blurred. Alternative mRNA splicing, posttranslational modifications, or cell surface endopeptidases can convert cell bond receptors into soluble mediators or vice versa. For example, TNF-α can be found as a soluble or cell surface molecule. Cytokine receptors can be processed into soluble fragments that still bind the relevant cytokine. In this case, the soluble receptor may act as an inhibitor of cytokine function because it prevents the interaction of the cytokine with its specific cell surface receptor. Alternatively, these same soluble receptors may prolong the serum half-life of cytokines by preventing proteolytic degradation and may transport the active cytokine to regions of inflammation or antigen presentation. In this case, the soluble receptor potentiates rather than inhibits cytokine function. This situation occurs with a soluble TNF receptor. Soluble forms of the TCR and class I MHC molecules have also been described. While their physiologic roles are uncertain, both suppressor and activator functions have been ascribed to these molecules. Likewise, B cell immunoglobulin may be cell bound and act as the B-cell antigen specific receptor or circulate freely as soluble antibody performing a variety of immune regulatory or effector functions.

Fourth, cytokine receptors are often heteromeric complexes sharing common subunits with other cytokine re-

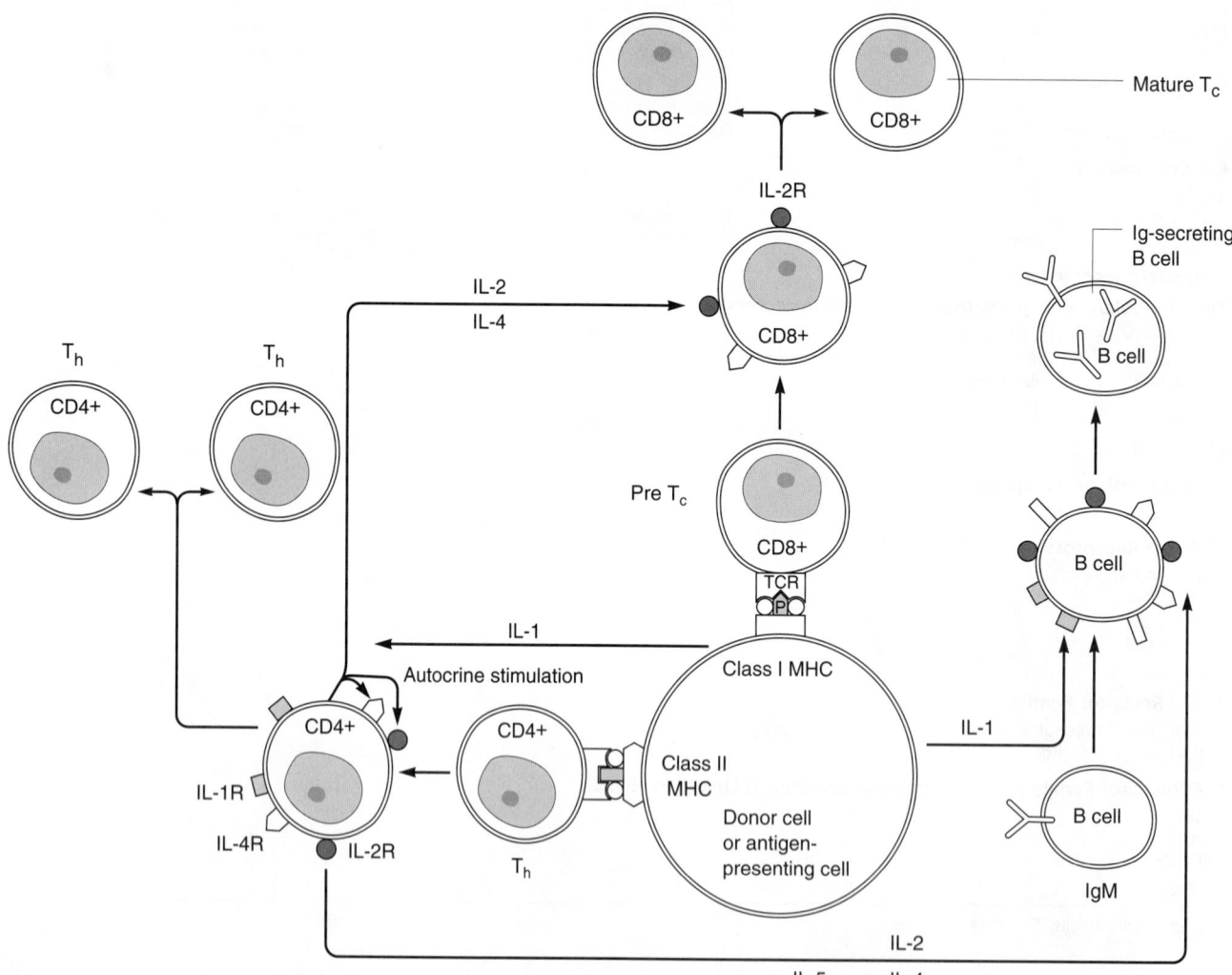

Figure 16-14. T- and B-cell activation. Two signals are required. First, alloantigen binds to antigen-specific receptors—the TCR (T cells) or surface IgM (B cells). The second, or costimulatory, signal is provided by IL-1 released by the antigen-presenting cell. CD4+ T_h release IL-2, IL-4, and IL-5, which provide help for CD8+ T_c and for B-cell activation.

ceptors and possessing unique, but related, subunits that confer specificity for an individual cytokine. Genetic or pharmacologic interference with receptor function may therefore impair the effects of only one or of several cytokines. For example, the IL-2, IL-4, IL-7, IL-9, IL-13, and IL-15 receptors all have related cytokine specific subunits and share a common γ subunit. The same is true for the IL-6, IL-11, leukemia inhibitory factor (LIF), oncostatin M (OSM), and ciliary neurotrophic factor (CNTF) receptors; and the IL-3, IL-5, and granulocyte-monocyte colony stimulating factor (GM-CSF) receptors.

EFFECTOR MECHANISMS OF THE IMMUNE RESPONSE

Cellular Effectors

Once primed and activated, T cells, B cells, and APCs perform the effector functions of graft rejection.[96–103] B cells secrete specific antibody that binds to the allograft cell surface and can kill cells by complement-mediated lysis. Antibody may also alter graft cell function by binding to and cross-linking important cell surface receptors, causing receptor blockade, receptor activation, or inappropriate cellular responses. Antibody may also direct other cells, which possess receptors for the constant region of the immunoglobulin molecule, termed *Fc receptors* (FCRs), to the allogenic cells. Many cell types express FcRs, including T cells, APCs, natural killer (NK) cells, and granulocytes. These FcR+ cells may damage or kill cells with antibody bound to the cell surface by a process called *antibody dependent cellular cytotoxicity* (ADCC).

Monocytes and macrophages, the prototypical APCs, become activated by CD4+ T cells during the initial encounter with antigen (see Fig. 16-11). These activated APCs can then cause local tissue destruction through direct cell lysis and phagocytosis or indirectly through release of cytotoxic cytokines (eg, TNF and lymphotoxin). CD4+ T cells can also generate local tissue destruction through inflammatory processes similar to delayed-type hypersensitivity. Cytotoxic lymphokines are released, and other inflammatory cells, such as APCs, are recruited to the local environment.

Cytotoxic CD8+ T lymphocytes kill target cells through direct cell contact. Killer T cells have cytoplasmic granules containing a series of cytotoxic proteins. Contact with a target cell causes the release of these granules onto or into the target. Granule contents include perforins, which assemble to form pores in the target cell membrane, making the cells leaky and susceptible to osmotic death. Granzymes are a series of serine proteases that can disrupt normal intracellular proteins. Cytotoxic T cells also kill cells by engaging a target cell surface receptor called *Fas,* a member of the TNF-receptor family (see Table 16-5). The interaction of the Fas ligand on the T-cell surface with Fas on the target cell surface leads to apoptotic target cell death. Fas and Fas ligand are distributed not only throughout the immune system but also on many other cell types. It is probably a general mechanism for determining cellular responses to development, immune activation, and oncogenesis. The regulation and control of the cellular response to engagement of Fas by its ligand involves a poorly understood series of cytoplasmic events comprising second messenger pathways and transcriptional regulators. Delineation of these events will probably lead to important methods for controlling cytotoxic responses.

In addition to the above mentioned cells, a number of other cell types probably also participate in the process of graft destruction and rejection, although their precise roles are not well understood. NK cells are large granular lymphocytes lacking immunoglobulin and most T-cell surface markers.[104,105] They do, however, express CD2 (characteristic of T cells) and a subclass of FcR known as CD16, which is characteristic of some B cells. NK cells also express the IL-2 receptor, secrete numerous cytokines (IL-1, IL-2, IL-3, IL-4, IL-6, GM-CSF, TNF, IFN-α, IFN-γ), and produce cytotoxic granzymes and phospholipases. NK cells function by lysing target cells. The mechanism by which NK cells recognize targets is still controversial. The receptor molecules and target molecules are still not known, although some evidence suggests that cells lacking class I MHC are susceptible to NK-mediated lysis. Likewise, the precise role of NK cells in allograft rejection is not understood, but these cells may be found infiltrating rejecting grafts, and it is presumed they are recruited to the inflammatory site.

Eosinophils are classically found throughout acutely rejecting allografts. Their role and function in graft rejection is also not understood, but they do perform potent cytotoxic effector function. IL-5, which is secreted by CD4+ T_H2 cells, is a potent trophic cytokine for eosinophils. The process of T-cell activation may therefore recruit eosinophils to rejecting grafts.

Other cell types, including neutrophils, basophils, and mast cells, can also be found in rejecting grafts or other inflammatory processes.[107,108] These cells are presumably recruited to regions of inflammation by cytokines and changes in vascular endothelium. These cells have direct cytotoxic effects, produce cytotoxic cytokines, and recruit additional cells to their locality.

Soluble Effectors

The soluble cytokines have been discussed thus far in terms of promoting homing and trafficking, inducing antigen-specific immunity, and amplifying immune responses. Cytokines also participate directly in the process of inflammation or graft destruction.[109–117] TNF-α and TNF-β have direct cytotoxic effects on parenchymal cells and may help mediate the final effector pathway. Many other cytokines (eg, IL-2, IL-4, IL-5, IL-6, IL-10, and IFN-γ) can be found within rejecting allografts. These cytokines are probably not directly cytotoxic but recruit additional cells and amplify those already present.

Many other soluble mediators are probably also involved in allograft destruction. Antibody-directed, complement-mediated lysis is an important mechanism in hyperacute and some forms of acute rejection.[118] Clotting factors are activated when vascular endothelium is compromised by antibody, cytokines, or cell-mediated injury. Obviously, vascular thrombosis is lethal to vascularized organ allografts. Injured vessels may also release the potent vasoconstricting peptide endothelin, further decreasing blood flow to injured grafts.[119] Kinins, prostaglandins, and prostacyclins may all participate in the effector stage of the inflammatory response, serving to potentiate cellular injury or recruit more proinflammatory cells.[120] Oxygen intermediates, such as nitric oxide and oxygen free radicals, are also likely important mediators of tissue destruction in transplantation.[121–124] So many potential mediators of cellular death make it difficult to control the process at the effector stage. Strategies that interfere with only a single cytotoxic pathway are unlikely to have major therapeutic effects. It will be necessary to subvert many effector pathways or to block initiation processes further upstream of effector mechanisms.

Clinical Syndromes

The wide variety of immune effector mechanisms results in a limited number of defined presentations in clinical transplantation (Figs. 16-15 to 16-18). *Hyperacute rejection*

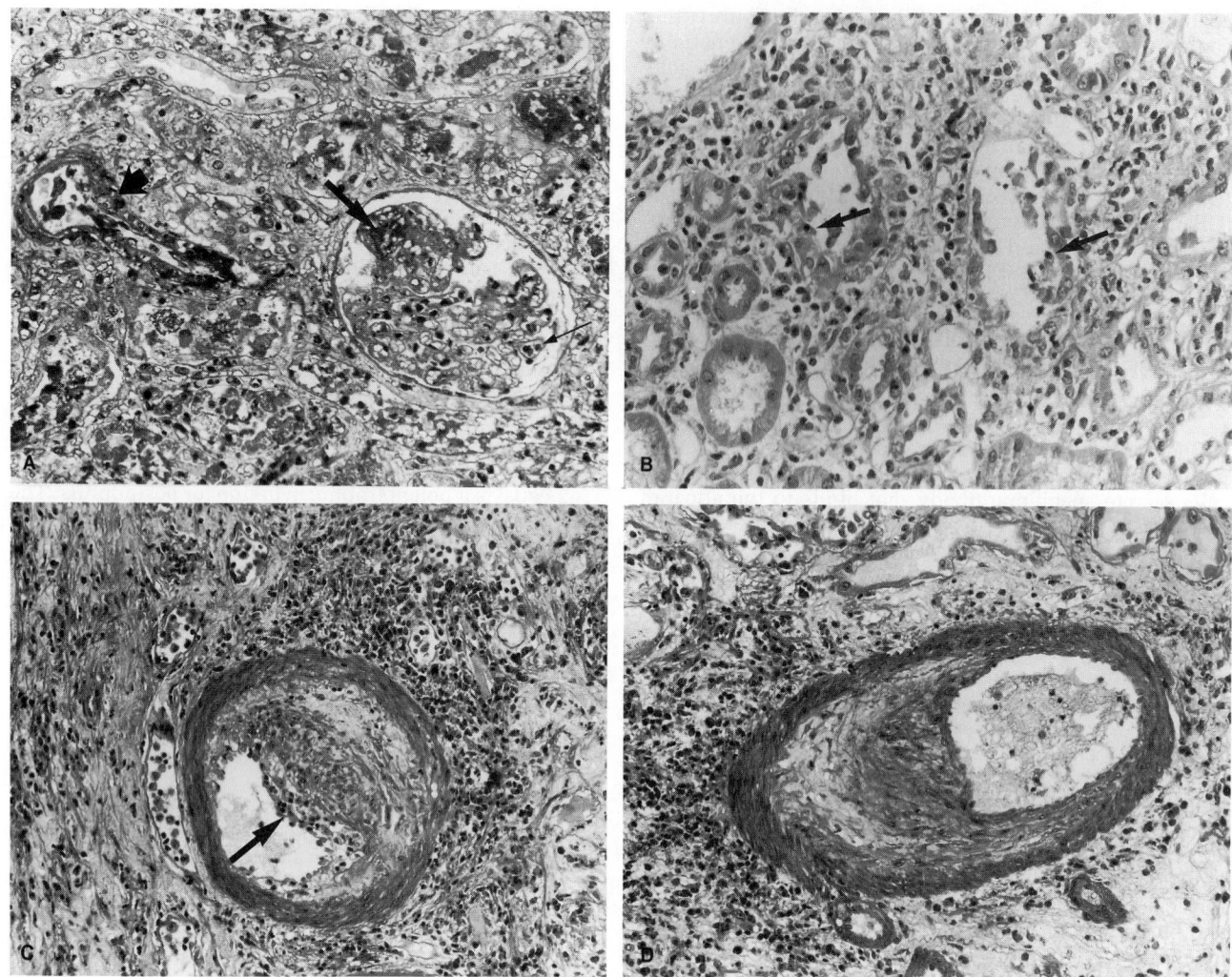

Figure 16-15. Kidney rejection. (*A*) Hyperacute rejection characterized by microthrombi in the glomerular capillaries (*large arrow*), infiltration with neutrophils (*small thin arrow*), and endothelial destruction (*thick arrow*). (*B*) Acute tubulointerstitial rejection showing an interstitial lymphocytic infiltrate, interstitial edema, and infiltration of lymphocytes into the epithelium of the tubules (tubulitis; *arrow*). (*C*) Acute vascular rejection with a subendothelial lymphocytic infiltrate (*arrow*), along with some evidence of chronic vascular rejection. (*D*) Chronic rejection with severe proliferative endarteritis. (Courtesy of Roger D. Smith, MD)

is the result of preformed antibody binding to the allograft at the time of revascularization in the operating room. Complement is activated, resulting in endothelial cell destruction, vascular leak, recruitment of platelets and neutrophils, thrombosis of vessels, and destruction of the graft within minutes to hours. Hyperacute rejection can occur if transplants are performed across an ABO incompatibility or if the recipient possesses high titer antidonor class I HLA antibodies.[125] Since current clinical protocols test for the presence of such incompatibilities or antibodies (see Important Aspects of Antigenicity and Immunity for Clinical Transplantation), hyperacute rejection should not occur. Kidney, heart, pancreas, and lung allografts are all susceptible to hyperacute rejection; however, liver grafts are relatively resistant to this process and are often transplanted across antibody differences (termed a *positive crossmatch*) and even across an ABO difference. The reason for this resistance is not understood but may relate to the large mass of hepatic parenchyma and its ability to absorb antibody and complement or to the way antibody and complement interact with hepatic endothelium and its dual blood supply. In addition, hyperacute rejection is

responsible for the major barrier to xenotransplantation (across species barrier).[126] Most mammals have high titer, preformed antibodies directed against cell surface antigens of other species. The current challenge in experimental xenotransplantation is to control antibody, complement function, and prevent hyperacute rejection.

Acute rejection usually occurs days to weeks after transplantation; it rarely occur months or years later. It is initiated by T-cell–dependent immunity and is characterized microscopically by a lymphocytic infiltrate accompanied by plasma cells, eosinophils, and a few mast cells or neutrophils. In the kidney, the infiltrate is in the tubular interstitium, causing a tubulitis. Particularly severe forms also cause a vasculitis or vascular rejection. Hepatic acute cellular rejection is typically a mixed cellular infiltrate in the portal triad with eosinophils, disruption of biliary endothelium, and portal venous endothelialitis. The heart demonstrates an interstitial lymphocytic myositis, while the lung shows varying degrees of peribronchiolar and perivascular lymphocytic infiltration. Most current clinical immunosuppressive agents are directed toward T cells and preventing or treating acute rejections.

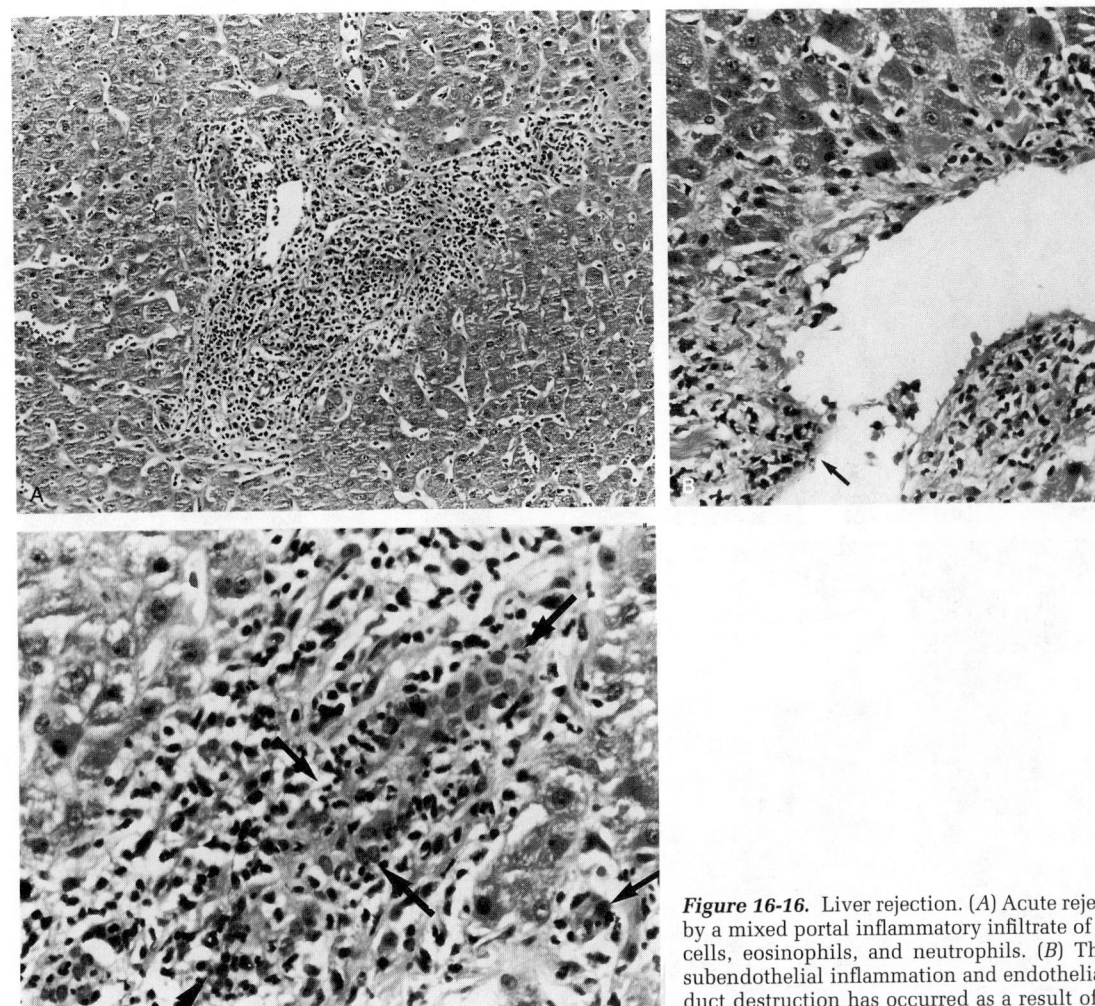

Figure 16-16. Liver rejection. (*A*) Acute rejection is characterized by a mixed portal inflammatory infiltrate of lymphocytes, plasma cells, eosinophils, and neutrophils. (*B*) The portal vein shows subendothelial inflammation and endothelialitis (*arrow*). (*C*) Bile duct destruction has occurred as a result of infiltrating mononuclear cells. (Courtesy of Makunda Ray, MD)

Chronic rejection usually occurs months to years after transplant. It is characterized by loss of normal histologic structure, fibrosis, and atherosclerosis. Renal chronic rejection demonstrates interstitial fibrosis, tubular and glomerular loss, and vascular obliteration. Hepatic chronic rejection is characterized by portal fibrosis and the disappearance of bile ducts (ductopenia or vanishing bile duct syndrome). Accelerated graft atherosclerosis is the cardinal manifestation with hearts, and bronchiolitis obliterans indicates chronic pulmonary rejection. Chronic rejection is a major cause of graft failure and patient loss with all organs.[127] The problem with understanding and eventually treating and preventing chronic rejection is that it undoubtedly represents the final common pathologic pathway of a variety of insults. Thus, repeated bouts of rejection, drug toxicity, recurrent infections (eg, pneumo-

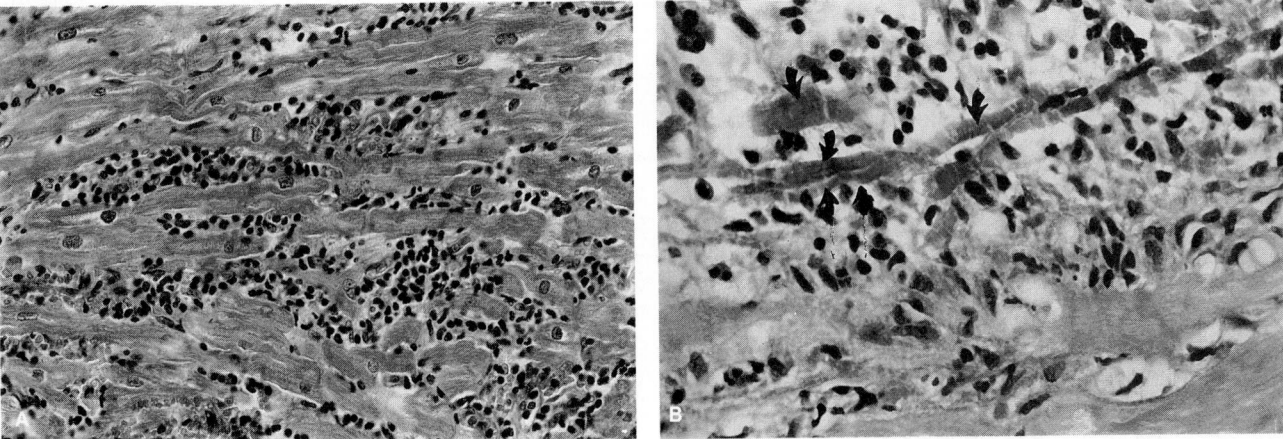

Figure 16-17. Heart rejection. Severe rejection manifests as a diffuse lymphocytic infiltrate with neutrophils and hemorrhage in the interstitium and myocyte necrosis (*arrows*). (Courtesy of Jeff Safitz, MD)

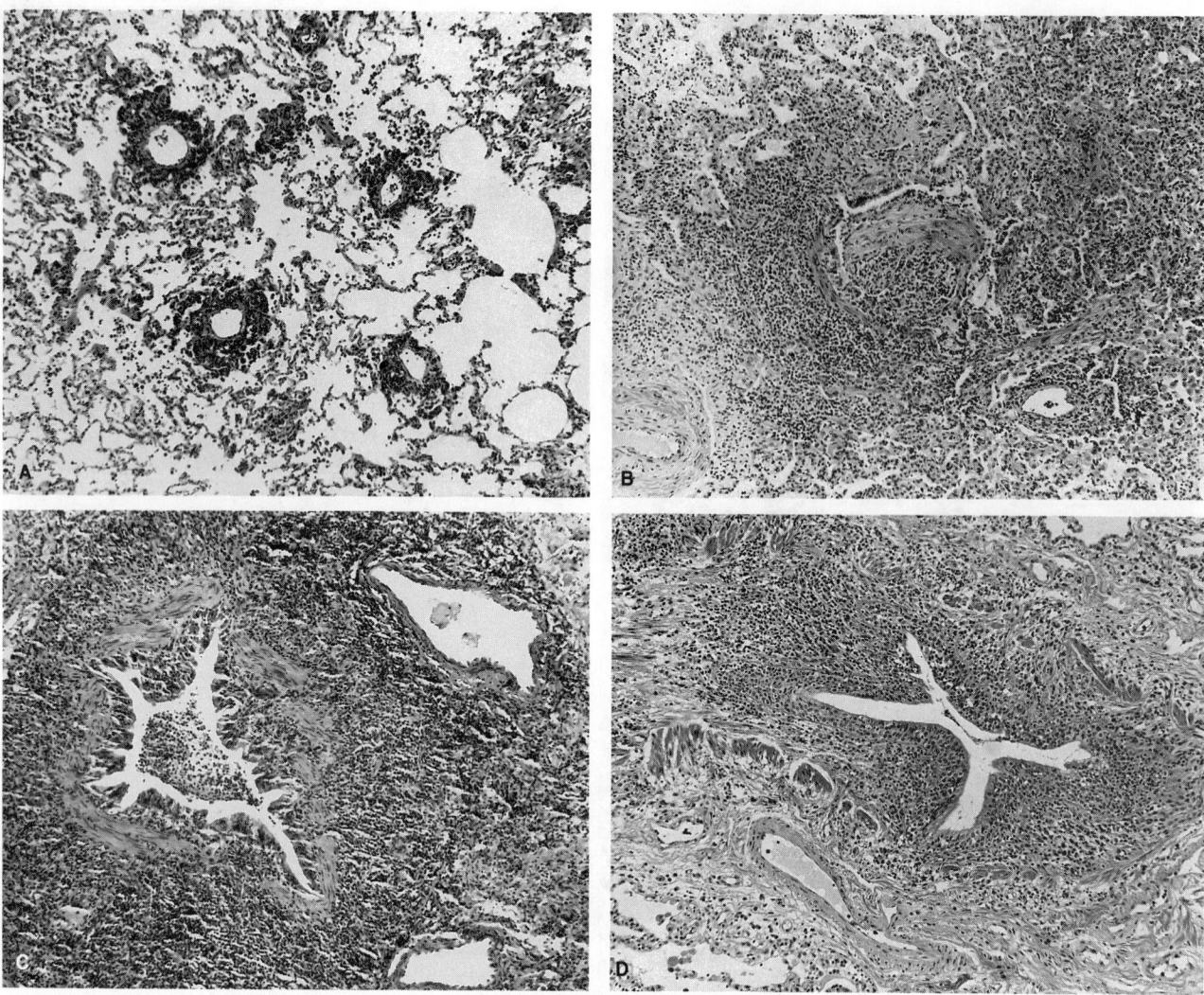

Figure 16-18. Lung rejection. (*A*) Mild acute rejection with a perivascular mononuclear infiltrate around small venules and arterioles. (*B*) With progression to moderate rejection, extension of the infiltrate into the alveolar septa occurs. (*C*) In severe rejection, there is a diffuse perivascular, interstitial, and peribronchiolar infiltrate with abundant fibrin, red blood cells, and neutrophils in the air spaces. (*D*) Bronchiolitis obliterans is the result of chronic rejection and is characterized by narrowing of the bronchioles from scarring. A mild mononuclear infiltrate is still present. (Courtesy of Samuel A. Yousem, MD, University of Pittsburgh, Pittsburgh)

nias in lung transplants or cholangitis in liver transplants), chronic obstruction (ureter, bile ducts, pancreatic duct), severe ischemic damage to donor organs at the time of transplant, use of older or suboptimal organ donors, or patient noncompliance with the immunosuppressive regimen can all contribute to a pathologic diagnosis of chronic rejection. Preventing chronic rejection requires attention to each of these problems. Nonetheless, a feature common to all types of chronic rejection is vascular atherosclerosis and obliteration with intragraft expression of certain cytokines and adhesion molecules, such as IL-1, IL-6, TNF-α, and ICAM-1.[128] Methods to prevent chronic rejection may come from a better understanding of vascular biology and how cytokines affect the process of atherosclerosis.[129]

REGULATION OF THE IMMUNE RESPONSE
Development of Lymphocytes

The preceding sections have outlined the major molecular and cellular interactions that occur on primary antigenic stimulation and show that different responses, cell types, and molecular entities may be involved. Superimposed on these pathways, however, are several layers of complex immune regulation that result from a variety of cellular interactions. It is important not only that the immune system responds to antigen but also that the response is of the appropriate magnitude, type, and duration and that responses to self (ie, autoimmunity) are avoided. The regulatory processes that control these parameters have important implications for transplantation tolerance and immunosuppression.

The primary determinants of T- and B-cell receptor specificity occur during early lymphocyte development in the bone marrow and thymus.[130–136] When developing, immature T or B cells come in contact with self-antigen in these compartments, antigen binds to those cells that possess receptors for self, and the cells are tolerized. The next problem to consider is what happens to cells that are not exposed to self-antigens in these central lymphoid compartments because the antigen is expressed only in the periphery. When lymphocytes mature, migrate to the periphery, and come in contact with these antigens, what prevents subsequent autoimmune responses? There are several levels of control of this process. First, newly emerging lymphocytes are susceptible to tolerizing signals in the periphery, so contact with self-antigen shortly after egress from the bone marrow or thymus can also lead to appropriate nonresponsiveness. Second, because B-cell responses are T-cell dependent, if the T cell is tolerant, the B cell does not respond to the autoantigen. Third, many autoantigens are not expressed on, and therefore not presented by, professional APCs. This results in a failure of appropriate presentation so that T cells cannot "see" the antigen; TCR may be engaged but tolerance, instead of immunity, ensues.

The problem of T-cell maturation is actually more complex than what was discussed earlier in this chapter. As noted, the T-cell receptor is selected to recognize altered self or a foreign peptide loaded into the antigen binding groove of class I or class II self-MHC. The cellular and molecular processes by which this occurs are the subject of intense current investigations and represent one of the major intellectual challenges in immunology. As T cells mature in the thymus, they sequentially acquire TCRβ, TCRα, plus CD4 and CD8 cell surface receptors. This is accompanied by migration from medullary to cortical regions of the thymus and by extensive proliferation and *loss* of most thymocytes. Numerous experimental studies have revealed that the maturing T cell expresses TCRs of multitudinous specificities and that these cells interact with class I and class II molecules on the thymic epithelium. A very strong interaction between a developing T cell and the thymic epithelium indicates autoimmunity and leads to negative selection of those T cells by a process called programmed cell death, or *apoptosis*. This is probably responsible for the massive thymocyte loss seen in the normal thymus. Alternatively, complete failure of the T cell to interact with the thymic epithelium probably also results in negative selection by failure to stimulate these developing T cells.

However, a low-affinity interaction between the T cell and the thymic epithelium results in T-cell stimulation, positive selection, and proliferative expansion of those T cells. Thus, these regulatory processes select T cells that have a low affinity for self-peptides and self-MHC (Fig. 16-19). Presumably then, these cells have a higher affinity for allogenic peptides and self-MHC and are able to respond appropriately to antigen. These same cells are also able fortuitously to recognize self-peptides in the context of allo-MHC and allogenic peptides in the context of allo-MHC. This focuses attention again on the fact that T cells are obsessed with the MHC and on why such a high percentage of T cells in an unselected population respond to a single allogenic MHC.

A major unresolved issue in thymic selection of T cells is TCR expression. The process of assortment and rearrangement of α and β V-D-J regions, accompanied by the addition of N regions, must interact with the maturation, proliferation, and selection processes at the level of the thymic epithelium. It is unclear whether TCR expression is an entirely random, stochastic process with subsequent positive or negative selection of T cells or whether there may be an instructional component such that as TCRβ and the TCRα chains are expressed, they interact with epithelial ligands and direct further assortment and rearrangement of receptor genes. There is evidence for both of these mechanisms; however, a definitive answer requires a more detailed understanding of the precise regulatory and transcriptional mechanisms that connect cell surface TCR receptors to TCR gene rearrangements and expression in the nucleus.

Receptor Driven Stimulation of T and B Responses

The ultimate control of all antigen and developmentally driven responses depends on a series of receptor–ligand interactions at the cell surface. For B cells, this comprises

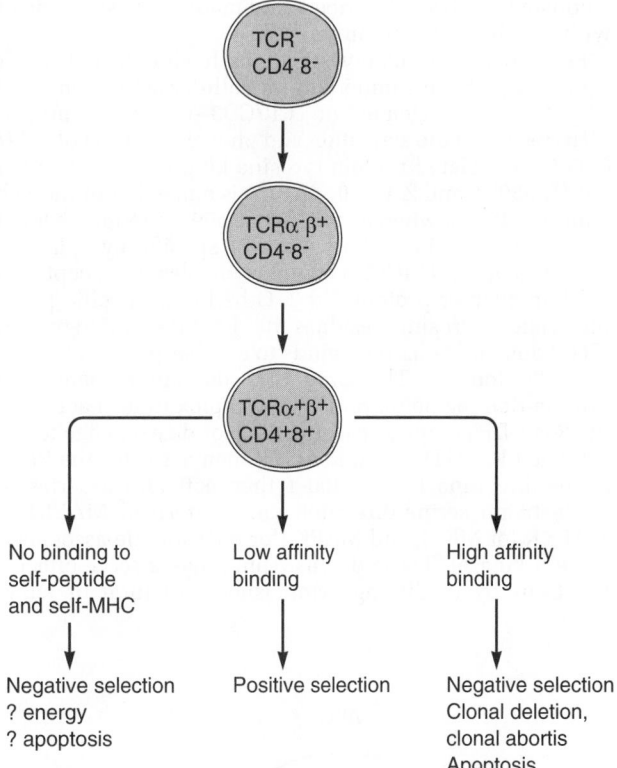

Figure 16-19. Thymic selection of developing T cells.

antigen and cell surface immunoglobulin. For T cells, this includes antigen, TCR, MHC, and CD4 and CD8 interactions. However, these signals are generally not enough to completely stimulate T- and B-cell proliferation, maturation, and effector function. B cells require additional ligands, such as the soluble cytokines IL-2, IL-4, and IL-5. Likewise, T cells also require cytokines, such as IL-1, IL-2, IL-4, IFN-γ, IL-10, and IL-12 (see Figs. 16-12 and 16-14). T cells also require the simultaneous or sequential engagement of multiple coreceptors (see Fig. 16-13) to become fully activated. CD4 and CD8 are the primary coreceptors, and their engagement is usually absolutely required for T-cell responses. Another major coreceptor is CD28 and the closely related receptor CTLA4.[137,138] The ligands for these receptors are CD80 (B7/BB1) and B70/B7-2. Both receptors can bind both ligands. Blockade of these particular receptor–ligand interactions can prevent T-cell stimulation and cause tolerance to antigen. These pathways are being investigated as a way to produce clinical transplantation tolerance. Additional coreceptors that are important for activation include CD2, CD29/CD49d (VLA-4) and CD11a/CD18 (LFA-1). Their ligands are CD58(LFA-3), VCAM-1, and CD54 (ICAM-1), respectively. Despite the description of a large number of important receptor–ligand interactions, there is no unified view of hierarchy among the receptors or of combinations of stimulated receptors that may eventuate in a given type of response.

Understanding receptor-driven stimulation and engagement of multiple coreceptors is ultimately the biochemical problem of elucidating the cytoplasmic second messenger pathways and transcriptional transactivators and repressors activated by each receptor or receptor combination. Numerous second messenger pathways, including G proteins, phospholipid and inositol phosphate metabolism, calcium currents, protein phosphorylation, and cAMP metabolism have been described, and many of these are dealt with in other chapters in this text.

For T cells, recent investigations have outlined major signaling pathways important for cellular activation[139-142] (Fig. 16-20). Engagement of TCR/CD3–CD4/8 by antigen-MHC results in the activation and phosphorylation of TCR/CD3 by associated protein tyrosine kinases (PTKs) called p56[lck], p59[fyn], and ZAP-70. ZAP-70 is a member of the Syk family of PTKs, whereas p56[lck] and p59[fyn] are members of the Src family. Phosphorylation of specific cytoplasmic tyrosines of the TCR/CD3 complex enables the receptor to bind an adapter protein, Grb2. Grb2 binds specific phosphorylated tyrosine residues by its Src-homology two (SH2) domain. Grb2 then binds to another protein, Sos, by its SH3 domain. The Grb2 SH3 domain recognizes a proline-rich region on Sos. This complex in turn activates the Ras-GDP complex, causing nucleotide exchange to the activated Ras-GTP form. Ras-GTP then activates the Raf-1 serine-threonine kinase. Raf-1 then activates a series of downstream serine-threonine kinases termed MAPKKK, MAPKK (or MEK), and MAPK (for microtubule-associated protein kinase). These downstream kinases serve effector functions by modifying cytoplasmic structural or enzymatic proteins or modifying cytoplasmic transcriptional factors that subsequently translocate to the nucleus. Several levels of control of this cascade are beginning to be elucidated, in particular cAMP negatively regulates Raf-1 kinase. Thus, two major signaling systems are linked by this recently described interaction. Once an understanding is achieved about what signaling pathways are activated by each T-cell coreceptor, then a hierarchy or classification scheme may be possible in which blockade or activation of particular receptors or combinations of receptors will reliably produce specific gene activation or inactivation and tolerance.

It is also worth noting that the PTKs activate phospholipase Cg1 (PLC-g1), which catalyzes the hydrolysis of phosphatidyl-inositol-biphosphate (PIP_2) to inositol-triphosphate (IP_3) and diacyl glycerol (DG). IP_3 increases intracellular calcium and activates the cytoplasmic protein tyrosine phosphatase, calcineurin. Calcineurin dephosphorylates tyrosines on the inactive cytoplasmic nuclear factor of activated T cells ($NF\text{-}AT_c$). The now activated, dephosphorylated $NF\text{-}AT_c$ is translocated to the nucleus where it complexes with nuclear subunits (NF-ATn) and acts as a transcriptional regulator. This pathway is not

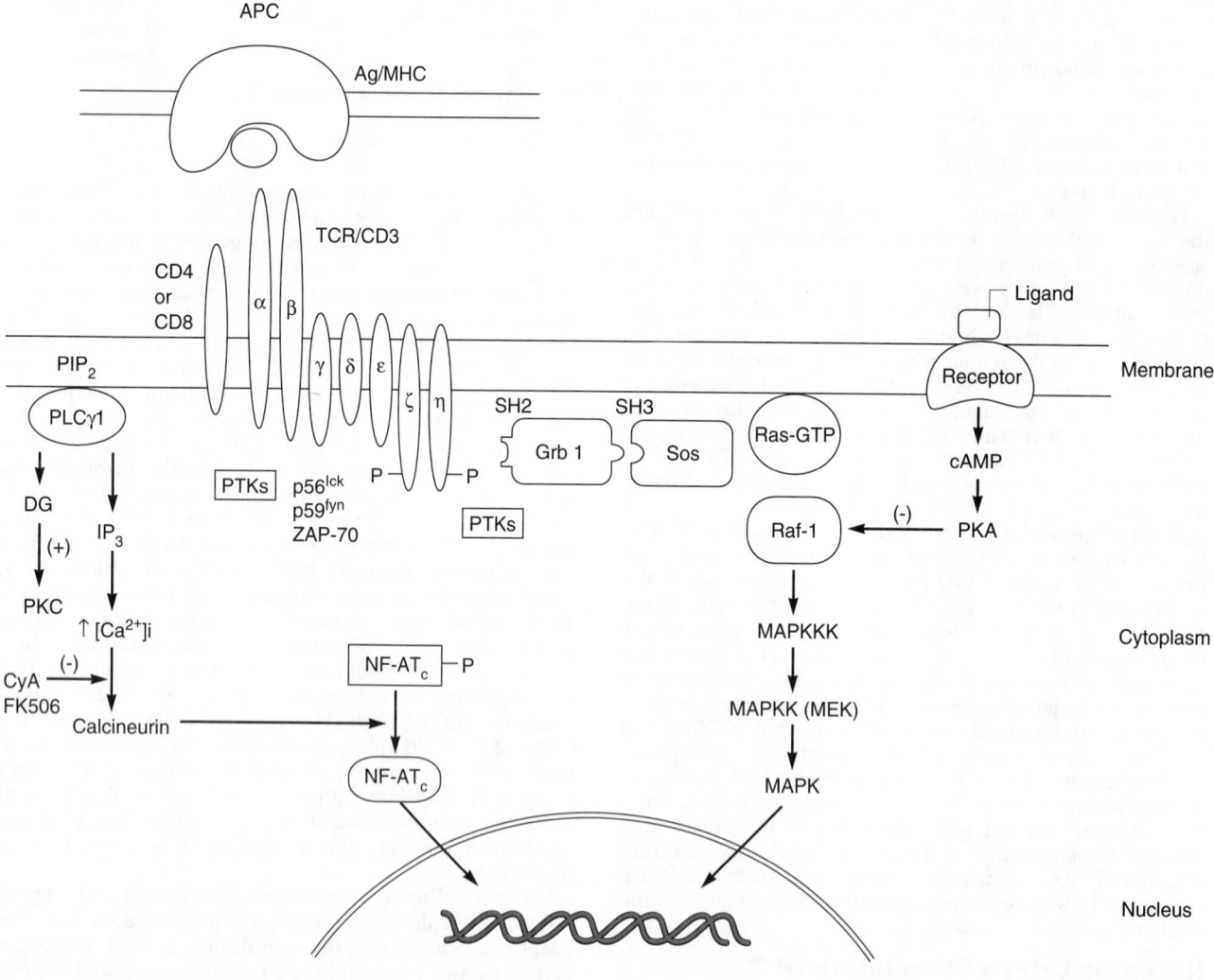

Figure 16-20. Signaling pathways of activated T cells.

only linked to the other important pathways but is also blocked by the immunosuppressive agents cyclosporine and FK 506.

Tolerance

The term tolerance is applied to a variety of different circumstances and therefore presents a semantic problem depending on context. Tolerance usually refers to whole animal or organism responses observed experimentally or clinically. It is a functional and not a mechanistic observation. The usual criteria for tolerance include long-term graft acceptance without the need for chronic immunosuppression. In addition, a second donor-specific allograft (ie, of the same MHC type as the original donor) should also be accepted without the need for additional immunosuppression. The most desirable endpoint from a clinical view would be true tolerance; however, this is virtually never achieved clinically and achieved only with difficulty experimentally. From a practical standpoint, long-term graft acceptance with minimal chronic immunosuppression, regardless of responses to subsequent second grafts, would be highly desirable and of enormous clinical benefit.

When the term *tolerance* is applied to cellular analyses of lymphocytes, it is again a functional and not a mechanistic description. T and B lymphocytes can be tolerant or nonresponsive to antigen in a variety of specific ways.[143-150] *Clonal abortion* refers to the developmental process whereby nascent T- and B-cell clones that recognize autoantigen with high affinity are eliminated. Evidence suggests that at this developmental stage, high-affinity engagement of the antigen-specific receptor and coreceptors leads to second messenger events resulting in apoptosis. In the case of T cells, the complete failure to engage the TCR/CD3 complex may likewise lead to apoptotic clonal elimination.

Clonal deletion can encompass the process of clonal abortion, but it also refers to the elimination of mature T- and B-cell clones. There are probably several specific cellular and molecular mechanisms responsible for this process. Prolonged or excessive stimulation of the antigen receptor can eventually cause lymphocyte death. Antiidiotype antibodies can eliminate idiotype-positive clones. Suppressor cells may kill or deliver cytotoxic signals to certain antigen reactive clones.

Clonal anergy is a state in which potentially reactive clones and their receptors are physically present but fail to respond to antigen. Anergy may also be the result of several distinct mechanisms including prolonged receptor stimulation, receptor down-modulation, idiotype–antiidiotype interactions, suppressor cells, and inappropriate APC function in which coreceptor or cytokine function is blocked.

Suppression generally refers to an active process in which a leukocyte or its soluble products inhibit the development or effector function of immune lymphocytes. CD8+ T cells, CD4+ T cells, B cells, macrophages, NK cells, and other cell types have all been shown to act as suppressor cells in certain experimental systems. Given the cellular interactions that can take place during lymphocyte recruitment (see Figs. 16-11 and 16-14), it could be anticipated that each interactive site could be a locus for suppression. Given the number of mechanistic possibilities for clonal deletion and clonal anergy, it is also likely that numerous cells could be involved in suppression. Current models of immune regulation suggest that the T_H1/T_H2 dichotomy (see Fig. 16-12) may explain much of suppression and be used in practical clinical settings. Thus, IL-10 can be used to suppress allograft responses, and IL-12 can be used to boost anticancer responses.

The term *split tolerance* is used to describe a state in which some responses to alloantigen are suppressed or deleted while other responses remain intact. This is likely a reflection of more detailed cellular analyses of tolerant states where anergy or suppression are dominant mechanisms. Likewise, T cells may proliferate or produce some cytokines, such as IL-2, in response to specific alloantigen but may be unable to generate cytotoxic effector cells because of anergy.

The major problem in clinical transplantation is that despite the detailed description of a large number of potential molecular and cellular mechanisms for inducing and maintaining tolerance, or some type of relative nonresponsiveness, it is not yet possible to reliably and reproducibly control any of these mechanisms in clinical settings. Our ability to induce tolerance will likely rely on a complete understanding of intracellular activational pathways (see Fig. 16-20).

Potential Loci for Inducing Nonresponsiveness

The molecular, cellular, and tissue-specific organization of immune development and responses suggests there are a number of discrete steps suitable for interventions designed to promote tolerance or immunosuppression. The thymus is the primary site for T-cell development and for positive and negative selection of specific T-cell clones, depending on the clonotypic expression of the TCR. If specific alloantigen could be placed in the thymus, this could redirect TCR selection and produce tolerance. This has been achieved in experimental models by injecting the recipient thymus with donor-derived cells.[151-153] The problem with applying this to humans is the relatively involuted characteristic of the adult thymus. This may be approachable with thymotrophic hormones. Nonetheless, the principle remains that thymic presentation of alloantigen "teaches" developing T cells to recognize that alloantigen as self.

The bone marrow is the primary site for B-cell development, and there is some evidence that precursor T cells can be tolerized to some antigens at this stage. In addition, bone marrow precursors populate the thymus. Protocols that attempt to replace part or all of the bone marrow stem cell and precursor population with donor-derived cells should induce tolerance to donor alloantigen.[154] In addition, partial replacement of the stem cell compartment results in chimerism, or a state in which both donor- and recipient-derived cells coexist in lymphoid organs. There is much current interest in protocols that combine parenchymal organ grafting with bone marrow or stem cell transplantation. While these approaches are still experimental, there is evidence that some patients with very long surviving allografts, who receive minimal or no immunosuppression, have stable low-level chimerism of lymphoid cells.[154]

The APC is an absolute requirement for proper T-cell activation. Techniques that alter APC function may induce T_H2 suppressor cells, anergy, or tolerance rather than T_H1 help cells, CD8+ cytotoxic T cells, or graft rejection. One approach to this is the isolation of specialized APC subpopulations that channel T-cell responses in one direction or another.[155] Another approach is the use of ultraviolet B irradiation, which can disrupt APC function and produce suppression or anergy. The problem with both of these methods is that it is not possible to replace, or expose to physical agents, all the APCs in an individual. A more rational approach will be the use of APC receptor–ligand disrupting agents.

The major intellectual and scientific directions in immunology have been the understanding of the molecular events of receptor–ligand interactions, second messenger pathways, and transcriptional regulation. New immunosuppressive drugs will likely be designed to interact with these pathways. For example, it is now known that cyclosporine and FK 506 act primarily by inhibiting the NF-AT transcriptional activator. Other agents under development are molecules that block the major CD28/CTLA4–B7-1/B7-2 costimulatory pathway of T cells, support the preferential production of the T_H2 immunosuppressive cytokine IL-10, or disrupt the TCR–antigen–MHC interaction.

Clinical Immunosuppression

Despite the tremendous knowledge of immune regulation, current immunosuppressive regimens used for clinical transplantation are based on empirically derived protocols, using agents such as azathioprine and corticosteroids developed in the 1960s or cyclosporine A developed in the 1970s (Table 16-6). Newer, more rationally designed drugs are currently being subjected to clinical trials and several may soon receive approval. Protocols for immunosuppression vary widely from one transplant center to another and even within a center from one organ to another. The major principle of immunosuppression is to *induce* the patient with high doses of drugs at the time of allografting to prevent rejection. The drugs are then reduced rapidly, within days to weeks, to less toxic *maintenance* levels. Patients are examined frequently, and multiple laboratory tests are obtained to detect rejection or organ dysfunction early for effective treatment. Induction regimens rely on three or four drugs (azathioprine, corticosteroids, cyclosporine, antibodies), whereas maintenance regimens rely on two or three of these drugs. Treatment of first or mild rejections is usually accomplished with high-dose "pulse" steroids, whereas steroid-unresponsive, very severe, or secondary rejections are often treated with antibodies, especially OKT3.

The antimetabolites include azathioprine and cyclophosphamide (Cytoxan). By interfering with nucleic acid metabolism, these agents inhibit proliferation and clonal expansion of activated lymphocytes, limiting alloantigen-specific immune responses. Many immunosuppressive regimens employ these drugs during induction immunosuppression at the time of allografting or for maintenance immunosuppression. They are most useful for preventing rejection but have little role for treating an acute, ongoing rejection. A more recent pharmaceutical, the morpholino-ethyl ester of mycophenolic acid, also called RS-61443, inhibits purine metabolism. It may be more potent and lymphocyte selective than azathioprine. Current experimental data suggest it has important roles in inducing and maintaining immunosuppression and treating ongoing, particularly resistant rejections.

Glucocorticoids are mainstays of virtually all immunosuppressive regimens and are used for inducing, maintaining, and treating rejections. Glucocorticoids are primarily transcriptional regulators, binding to cytoplasmic steroid receptors, which are then translocated to the nucleus where the complex binds specific gene promoters and other regulatory regions. The glucocorticoids all have similar immunosuppressive actions, and none is more effective than any other at equipotent doses. The relative potency on a milligram basis for the most commonly used drugs are hydrocortisone and cortisol, 1 mg; prednisone, 4 mg; and prednisolone and methylprednisolone, 5 mg. Steroid use is associated with several significant complications and side effects (see Table 16-6), and at equipotent doses all have equivalent toxicities. While the use of multi-ple-drug regimens has decreased the overall dosing of glucocorticoids, the goal of steroid-free regimens for inducing and maintaining immunosuppression and for treating rejection in all patients has not been achieved.

Cyclosporine is a hydrophobic, cyclic undecapeptide that binds to a cytoplasmic protein, cyclophilin. Cyclophilin is a peptide-prolyl isomerase, or rotamase, an enzyme with the ability to alter protein conformations by inducing *cis-trans* rotation around proline amino acid residues. Cyclosporine inhibits the rotamase activity of cyclophilin. The major immunosuppressive activity of cyclosporine appears to be related to the ability of the cyclosporine–cyclophilin complex to bind and inhibit the cytoplasmic protein tyrosine phosphatase calcineurin (see Fig. 16-20). This in turn inhibits activation of the $NF-AT_c$ transcriptional factor. In essence, cyclosporine is a transcriptional regulator. It is an integral part of all immunosuppressive regimens for induction and maintenance therapy but seems to have little role in reversing an ongoing acute rejection. The addition of cyclosporine to routine immunosuppressive regimens in 1983 has allowed for the exponential growth of transplantation over the last decade. The 1-year graft and patient survival rates for the various organs increased from the 30% to 60% range to the 70% to 90% range. Cyclosporine has several significant toxicities (see Table 16-6), but attempts to design congeners with less toxicity but equal immunosuppression have not been successful.

The search for additional immunosuppressive agents lead to the discovery of tacrolimus, or FK 506, approved by the FDA in 1994. This macrolide antibiotic binds to a series of related cytoplasmic receptors termed FK binding protein (FKBP). FKBP is a peptide-prolyl isomerase distinct from cyclophilin. FK 506 inhibits the rotamase activity of FKBP, and the FK 506–FKBP complex inhibits calcineurin. Thus cyclosporine and FK 506 have similar mechanisms of action. FK 506 is 10 to 100 times more potent than cyclosporine on a molar basis, but it too is associated with a number of significant and similar toxicities (see Table 16-6). FK 506 has roles in inducing and maintaining immunosuppression and may also be particularly useful for treating resistant rejections. A structurally similar compound, called rapamycin, is currently undergoing clinical trials. This macrolide binds to and inhibits FKBP; however, it does not complex to calcineurin. Its molecular mechanism is currently under investigation. The existence of compounds such as cyclosporine, tacrolimus, and rapamycin suggest that there must be normal cellular constituents that regulate calcineurin function. These regulatory factors are currently unknown; their purification and isolation will presumably lead to more rational drug design for immunosuppression.

Antimetabolites, glucocorticoids, and rotamase inhibitors are universally applied both to induction and to maintenance immunosuppression, and any of these agents may be administered chronically to patients. The fourth major group of reagents is antibodies. These may be given for only short periods of time because of their extreme potency and because of host antiimmunoglobulin responses that limit their efficacy. Antibodies are used for induction to prevent rejection and for treatment of acute, ongoing rejections. There are two major types of antibody preparations (Table 16-7). Polyclonal antibodies, such as antilymphocyte (ALG) or antithymoctye globulin (ATG), are prepared by immunizing animals with human lymphocytes or lymphoid lines, bleeding the animals to obtain serum, and purifying whole immunoglobulin from serum. These preparations are directed primarily against many different antigens present on T cells (eg, CD2, CD3, CD4, CD8) but also recognize B-cell, monocyte, platelet, and granulocyte anti-

Table 16-6. CURRENTLY APPROVED IMMUNOSUPPRESSIVE AGENTS

Agent (Brand Name)	Mechanism of Action	Dosage	Monitoring	Clinical Uses	Adverse Effects
Azathioprine (Imuran)	Inhibits purine synthesis via active metabolites 6-thioinosinic acid (via conversion to 6-MP) and 6-thioguanine nucleotides; inhibits DNA and RNA synthesis; has greater effect on T cells than B cells	1–3 mg/kg/d IV or PO	Maintain WBCs >3000/μL	Part of regimens to lower doses of cyclosporine or prednisone	Myelosuppression (leukopenia, occasionally thrombocytopenia and megaloblastic anemia), hepatitis, cholestatis, hepatic vein thrombosis, pancreatitis dermatitis, alopecia, increased susceptibility to infections
Cytoxan	Alkylates DNA	0.5–1.5 mg/kg/d	Maintain WBCs >3000/μL	Substitution for azathioprine if adverse effects occur	Leukopenia, thrombocytopenia, hemorrhagic cystitis, nausea, vomiting, increased susceptibility to infections
Glucocorticoids	Complex; affects T cells and macrophages; has little effect on antibody production by B cells. Steroid-receptor complex binds to DNA; alters transcription and translation of genes responsible for cytokine synthesis; blocks MLR and development of CTL; inhibits IL-1 and IL-6 synthesis	Prednisolone, 1–2 mg/kg/d induction; 0.1–0.2 mg/kg/d maintenance bid, qd, or qod dosing Prednisolone, 2 mg/kg/d for rejection; tapering schedule Solu-Medrol 5–15 mg/kg/d IV for rejection	No objective means to monitor; adjustment done by protocol; adverse effects	Foundation of most multidrug protocols; treatment of rejection	Cushingoid features (moon facies, acne, centripetal obesity, striae), hypertension, weight gain (increased appetite), hyperglycemia, osteoporosis, type II diabetes, poor wound healing, pancreatitis, peptic ulcer, colonic perforation, psychosis, increased susceptibility to infections
Cyclosporine (Sandimmune)	Binds to cyclophilin; blocks transcription of several early T-cell activation genes, including IL-2, IL-3, IL-4, and IFN-γ; inhibits IL-1 production by macrophages	8–10 mg/kg/d PO qd, bid, or tid or 2.5–3 mg/kg/d IV	Trough levels (usually 12 h); serum creatinine; mg/kg dose (protocol); biopsy (histologic evidence of cyclosporine toxicity)	Induction therapy with prednisolone or azathioprine in most multidrug regimens	Nephrotoxicity, hypertension, hyperkalemia, hyperuricemia and gout, gingival hypertrophy, hepatotoxicity, hirsutism, tremors, seizures, hyperglycemia, hemolytic uremic syndrome, increased susceptibility to infection
FK 506, Tacrolimus (Prograf)	Similar to cyclosporine (10–100 times more potent); binds to FKBP; blocks expression of IL-2 receptors on allostimulated T cells	0.15 mg/kg/d PO qd or bid or 0.075 mg/kg IV q 12 h	Trough levels; serum creatinine; dose mg/kg dose (protocol); adverse effects (neurologic)	Induction therapy with prednisone; treatment of rejection; maintenance without prednisolone	Nephrotoxicity, headache, weight loss, tremors, paresthesia, increased sensitivity to light, insomnia and mood changes, increased susceptibility to infections

MLR, mixed lymphocyte response; CTL, cytotoxic T lymphocytes.

Table 16-7. POLYCLONAL AND MONOCLONAL ANTIBODIES

Antibody	Source	Mechanism of Action	Dosage	Monitoring	Clinical Uses	Adverse Effects
ALG or ATG	Horse, goat, rabbit	Depletes T cells more than B cells as a result of complement-dependent lysis and opsonization	10–30 mg/kg/d IV qd over 6 h; must be given in central line	Peripheral T-cell levels; monitor for antihorse or antigoat antibody development; platelets; WBC count	Induction with azathioprine or prednisone as part of triple or quadruple therapy protocols; treatment of rejection with or without steroids	Fever, chills, leukopenia, thrombocytopenia, nausea, vomiting, diarrhea, arthralgia, headache, myalgia, rash, pruritus, urticaria, chest pain, phlebitis, rarely anaphylaxis or serum sickness
OKT3	Mouse	Reacts with CD3 recognition complex on T cells; blocks recognition of class I or II antigens; inhibits generation and function of effector T cells; opsonizes CD3+ cells; modulates CD3 antigen-recognition complex; renders T cells anergetic or kills them by apoptosis	2.5–10 mg/d IV over 30 min; can be given in peripheral vein	Peripheral CD3 levels; monitor for antimouse antibody development	Same as ALG, ATG	Usually with first dose: fever, chills, diarrhea, headache, nausea, vomiting dyspnea, wheezing, pulmonary edema, tachycardia, hypotension, aseptic meningitis, seizures, coma; markedly reduced with pretreatment with steroids, acetaminophen, indomethacin, and diphenhydramine hydrochloride

gens. Polyclonal antibodies are very useful for induction but tend to be less effective for treatment of acute rejection. They are associated with a number of side effects related either to their depleting effect on cell populations (leukopenia, thrombocytopenia) or allergic reactions related to host antiimmunoglobulin responses (urticaria, rash, pruritus).

The second type of antibody preparation is monoclonal antibody, derived from cloned hybridoma cells of a single specificity. The only monoclonal currently commercially available is OKT3, approved by the FDA in 1985. It is a mouse monoclonal directed against the nonpolymorphic ε chain of the CD3 complex of the TCR. It therefore recognizes all T cells (both $\alpha\beta$ TCR and $\Gamma\delta$ TCR) and interferes with their antigen recognition functions in the context of either class I or class II MHC. OKT3 is used for both induction and the treatment of rejection. It is the most efficacious agent currently available for the treatment of rejection. It is used either as first-line treatment for rejection or as treatment for rejections unresponsive to high-dose steroids or polyclonal antibodies.

It has previously been considered that polyclonal or monoclonal antibodies function by inhibiting T-cell function either through opsonization, complement-mediated lysis, or steric hindrance of the TCR. Although these mechanisms certainly do occur, it is now clear that other effects may be even more important for immunosuppression. When OKT3 is first administered to a patient, a significant clinical response often occurs within 30 minutes to 4 hours, consisting of fevers, chills, rigors, myalgias, arthralgias, and vascular leak. This has been called the *cytokine syndrome* and is due to OKT3 binding to and cross-linking T-cell CD3, which activates all T cells thereby causing massive release of IL-2. The IL-2 in turn causes other cells to release IL-1, IL-6, INF-γ, and TNF-α. These cytokines can be found at very high concentrations throughout the serum, and blocking cytokine production or action can ameliorate the cytokine syndrome. When T cells are stimulated, they lose cell surface CD3, CD4, and CD8 as a result of the antibody. This process is termed *antigenic modulation* and results in naked T cells that are refractory to antigenic stimulation because they lack receptors. Because OKT3 binds CD3 in the absence of other T-cell costimulatory signals (eg, CD28, CD2, CD29/49d, CD11a/18), this is the equivalent of inappropriate antigen presentation, which experimentally can result in anergy or apoptosis. There is now evidence that because of OKT3, these T cells may also be rendered anergic or even killed by apoptotic mechanisms. The effects of cytokine stimulation, antigenic modulation, anergy, and apoptosis may be separable, and experimental work to produce a form of OKT3 that lacks the clinically deleterious cytokine-inducing properties while preserving the other immunosuppressive characteristics is of significant current interest. Polyclonal antibodies also have anti-CD3 specificities and may therefore have a similar mechanism of action. In addition, because polyclonals have many other antireceptor specificities, they may produce a variety of other effects related to receptor cross-linking, antigenic modulation, anergy, and apoptosis.

Many other monoclonal antibodies are undergoing clinical evaluation, including anti-CD4, anti-CD8, and anti–IL-2. All seem to have some efficacy, but none have proved superior to OKT3. Consideration has also been given to toxin-conjugated monoclonal antibodies, but none has reached phase II or III clinical transplant trials.

Several dozen other compounds of diverse structure and mechanistic activity have been or are being evaluated in experimental and clinical allografting protocols. Several, discussed here briefly, will likely be approved during the next decade. The bacterial product 15-deoxyspergualin (DSG) is a potent immunosuppressive with mild side effects including neurotoxicity, anorexia, and bone marrow depression.[156] Its mechanism may be related to binding to cytoplasmic members of the heat shock protein 70 (Hsp 70) family.[157] Hsp members are often involved as chaperones in protein folding and transport; therefore, DSG may interfere with antigen presentation. Leflunomide, an isoxazol derivative, has potent immunosuppressive activities and synergizes with cyclosporine.[158,159] Its mechanism may be related to inhibiting intracellular messengers and second signals generated by IL-2 and costimulatory receptors such as CD28. This suggests that leflunomide may inhibit protein kinases. Molecules aimed at effector mechanisms of cellular destruction have also had some activity in experimental analyses. Thus, inhibitors of complement, platelet-activating factor, nitric oxide synthesis, superoxide synthesis, granzymes, perforins, and interleukins can all prolong graft survival. These latter agents will probably have only adjunctive roles since the most important processes to regulate are probably the initiation of immune responses, immunological priming, and immunologic memory.

Recent investigations have focused on the design of soluble molecules that mimic various parts of the TCR–antigen–MHC–CD4/CD8 complex. A molecule with high enough affinity for the recognition complex could inhibit T-cell activation and immunity. Analogues of CD4 can perform such function.[160] Likewise, analogues of peptide antigen seem to complete with antigen at the level of binding to the peptide groove of MHC. Furthermore, antigen analogues may induce a negative regulatory signal in T cells and actually anergize T cells as a result of altered receptor affinities and kinetics.[161–163] This form of immunosuppression also has the advantage of being strictly antigen specific. One envisions transplanting a patient and then injecting the individual with mimics of the immunodominant peptides corresponding to the mismatched MHC molecules of donor origin to promote selective anergy.

A variety of physical methods have been considered for immunosuppression. Total lymphoid irradiation is successful in experimental transplantation.[164] It ablates much of the immune system and also seems to generate suppressor cells. There is concern that total lymphoid irradiation markedly increases the risk of systemic infection and lymphoid malignancies. It has been known since the early 1970s that prior blood transfusions are associated with a decreased risk of renal allograft rejection and increased graft survival.[165] Furthermore, donor-specific transfusions have an antigen-specific protective effect. The cellular and molecular consequences of transfusion or donor-specific transfusion are not certain; however, the presentation of antigen to central lymphoid compartments (eg, intravenous injection of cells) can generate suppression, anergy, and tolerance (see Sites of Antigen Recognition). Problems with transfusion include the fact that 10% to 30% of transfused recipients develop high-titer anti-HLA antibodies. These highly sensitized recipients cannot be transplanted. In this respect, transfusions may merely be "selecting" potential high- versus low-reacting recipients. Transfusions and donor-specific transfusions were widely used until the 1980s. The advent of cyclosporine erased much of the benefit that transfusions conferred; they are now only rarely employed. Oral feeding of antigen or peptide can also produce suppression, anergy, and tolerance.[166,167] A trial of oral peptides in multiple sclerosis patients suggested they conferred some clinically beneficial immunosuppressive effect.[166] It remains to be seen if the same can be accomplished with clinical allografting.

Complications of Immunosuppression

The therapeutic index for immunosuppressives is very low. As a result, numerous toxicities and adverse effects occur, and they are an integral part of treating transplant patients (see Tables 16-6 and 16-7). The most obvious complication is infection. As immunosuppression becomes stronger and more effective, the recipient's ability to resist infection diminishes. Allograft recipients are susceptible both to typical bacterial infections (eg, urinary tract infection, pneumonia, wound infections) and to infections with unusual organisms (eg, fungus, virus, atypical bacteria). Immunosuppressives also blunt the inflammatory response to infection so that patients present with very subtle signs and symptoms or very late in the infectious process. The tenets of patient care are the judicious management of immunosuppression to prevent infectious complications, the use of prophylactic antibiotics (ie, acyclovir or ganciclovir for herpesviruses; sulfamethoxazole for pneumocystis; and nystatin, clotrimazole, or fluconazole for candidiasis), and a low index of suspicion to examine, culture, and treat patients for suspected infections.

Figure 16-21 diagrams the typical transplant-related infections and when they occur. Of particular concern is cytomegalovirus (CMV). CMV, a member of the herpes family, can infect any cell in the body and produce cytopathic effects. CMV infection in immunocompetent individuals is often clinically inapparent and results in the viral genome persisting in the patient's lymphocytes for life. As a result, organ transplantation almost invariably results in the transfer of viral genomes to the recipient. Evidence of past infection is indicated by elevated serum IgG anti-CMV titers; about 70% of the population is CMV seropositive. When seropositive (ie, previously infected) patients are transplanted and immunosuppressed, CMV virus from their own lymphocytes may be reexpressed and reactivate disease. Reactivation disease is generally mild and self-limited and presents about 6 weeks after transplant as fevers, myalgias, arthralgias, leukopenia, mild elevation of liver enzymes, and mild nonspecific abdominal complaints. A more serious situation occurs when a previously uninfected CMV-seronegative patient receives an organ from a CMV-seropositive donor. This situation occurs in 10% to 30% of transplant patients. The recipient has almost a 100% chance of developing CMV infection and greater than a 70% chance of developing clinically significant or even life-threatening disease, including CMV encephalitis, pneumonitis, hepatitis, and necrotizing gastroenteropathy with perforation and bleeding. Effective prophylactic regimens now include the following: acyclovir, 800 mg four times a day PO for 3 months; ganciclovir, 2.5 mg/kg twice a day IV for 2 weeks; and CMV hyperimmune globulin, 150 mg/kg for 5 doses over 6 to 8 weeks. Therapeutic regimens for established disease include ganciclovir and CMV IgG.

Another complication in allograft recipients is malignancy. There is an increased incidence for only a few histologic types of tumors. The immunosuppressive drugs do not appear to be directly mitogenic or transforming, but rather suppress immune mechanisms that keep transformed cells in check. Squamous cell carcinomas of the exposed areas of the skin are by far the most common. These are generally not aggressive or invasive tumors and can be cured with simple local excision. Avoiding UV exposure from the sun is the best preventive measure.

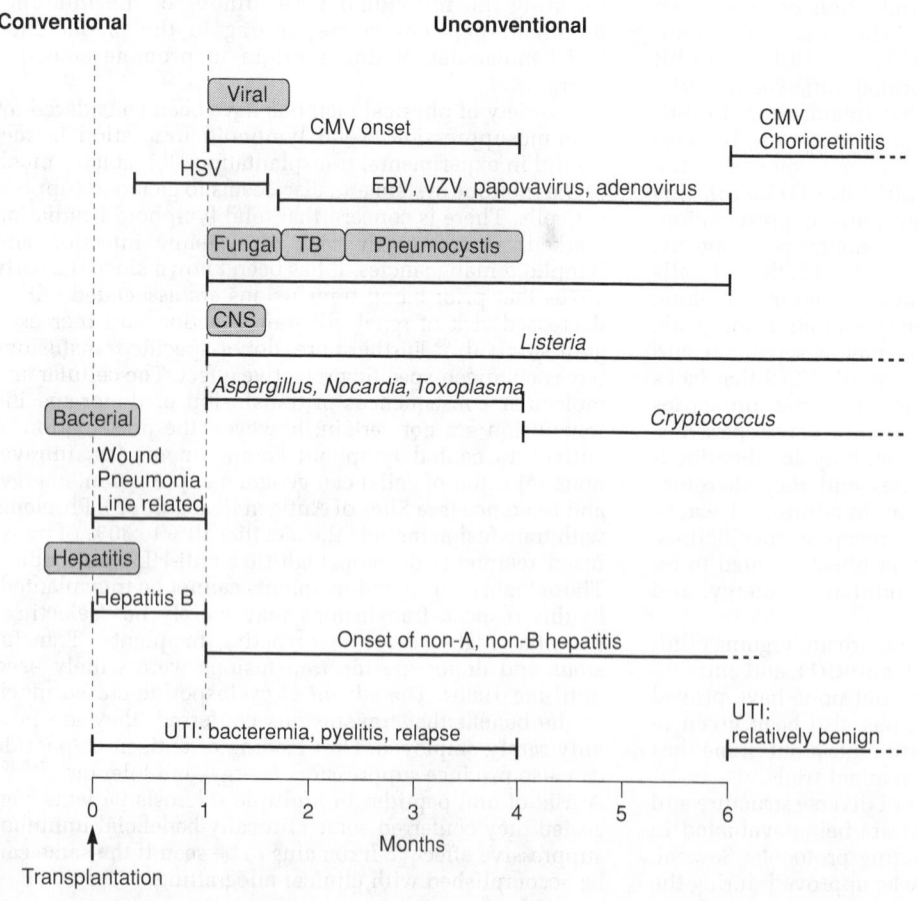

Figure 16-21. Timing of posttransplantation infections. (After Rubin RH, Wolfson JS, Cosimi AB, et al. Infection in the renal transplant patient. Am J Med 1981;70:405)

Lymphomas are the next most common tumor and are 10 to 100 times more common in transplant recipients than in the general population. These are usually non-Hodgkin's B-cell lymphomas and are often related to malignant transformation by Epstein-Barr virus (EBV). In immunocompetent individuals, EBV normally infects B cells and causes polyclonal proliferation of infected cells. The infection is eventually controlled by cytotoxic CD8+ T cells, which recognize and kill viral antigens on the surface of infected B cells. In immunosuppressed patients, T-cell–mediated immunity is impaired, allowing EBV directed polyclonal B-cell proliferation to continue. Some of the B-cell clones eventually acquire additional mutations, and a benign polyclonal expansion of B cells becomes a more aggressive oligoclonal proliferation. One of these clones can accumulate even more mutations and become an autonomous, monoclonal lymphoma. At this stage, the lymphoma may even lose viral antigens and become insusceptible to immune control. The incidence of lymphoma is directly related to the amount of immunosuppression received over time. Thus, avoiding overimmunosuppression prevents this malignancy. Management of established disease consists primarily of reducing or withdrawing immunosuppression, even to the point of allograft rejection and loss. While this latter maneuver is possible with renal and pancreatic transplants where the patient may return to dialysis or insulin, it is not possible with hepatic or cardiac grafts. High-dose intravenous acyclovir is sometimes effective for treatment and may have a role in prophylaxis. Conventional chemotherapy for lymphoma is generally ineffective for these tumors.

Other tumors with a higher incidence in transplant patients include Kaposi sarcoma and a slight increase in cervical carcinoma. The etiology of Kaposi sarcoma is not known but may be related to a virus or other microorganism. Cervical carcinomas are related to papilloma viruses. This association suggests that immunosuppression primarily interferes with normal antiviral responses in the case of some tumors. Common neoplasms, such as breast, lung, and colon cancer, are *not* more common in transplant patients than in the general population, suggesting that immune mechanisms are generally irrelevant for these tumors. The effect of immunosuppression on the recurrence of a preexisting or a previously treated cancer is controversial. Data suggest that immunosuppression either has no effect or may slightly increase the incidence of recurrent carcinoma. Current clinical recommendations suggest that following a curative resection, patients should wait at least 2 years before undergoing transplant.[168] It is also possible to transplant a tumor to a recipient from a donor with metastatic disease. Therefore, a history of malignancy excludes potential organ donors. The one exception to this rule is malignant CNS tumors that usually do not metastasize. Unfortunately, even these tumors have been transferred by organ transplantation despite no clinical evidence of metastatic disease.[169]

Tables 16-6 and 16-7 also show a large number of drug specific toxicities, many of which are clinically common. This again stresses the point that the therapeutic index for immunosuppression is very narrow and that frequent monitoring of laboratory tests is required for patients receiving these agents. Of particular concern is atherosclerotic vascular disease. During the past two decades, organ failure and infection have become less significant causes of morbidity and mortality while various manifestations of vascular disease have become more important. In fact, coronary artery disease is the primary cause of mortality in the renal transplant population. Many factors related to immunosuppression contribute to vascular disease. Glucocorticoids alter serum lipid components and ratios to unfavorable varieties. They also promote glucose intolerance and insulin resistance. Cyclosporine unfavorably alters serum lipids and contributes to insulin resistance. It also causes hypertension by mechanisms related to vascular endothelial cell–induced release of endothelin and interferes with renal function by altering glomerular hemodynamics and renal prostaglandin production. Prolonged cyclosporine administration may lead to permanent renal damage and eventually the need for dialysis. Rapamycin and FK 506 share the same toxicities as cyclosporine, causing hypercholesterolemia, insulin resistance, hypertension, and renal insufficiency. Renal insufficiency itself further contributes to hypertension and dyslipidemia. All these variables contribute to atherosclerosis of cerebral, coronary, renal, and peripheral vascular beds. The care of transplant patients now requires careful monitoring of individual drug doses and levels to reduce their toxicities. Close attention to serum lipid profiles, hypertension, weight, diet, and exercise are also major factors in the long-term treatment of these patients.

Another complication of organ allografting is graft-versus-host disease (GVHD). All vascularized allografts contain lymph nodes and mature lymphocytes. These donor-derived T and B cells can be stimulated by host alloantigen and transiently repopulate the host. The anti-host reactive cells can cause T-cell–mediated lesions, such as hepatitis, dermatitis, or gastrointestinal mucosal lesions as seen in bone marrow transplant recipients with GVHD. The B cells can produce antihost antibodies; if there is an ABO incompatibility this can even result in a hemolytic anemia. GVHD is usually self-limited as the donor cells are eliminated either by immunosuppression or host anti-donor responses.

Important Aspects of Antigenicity and Immunity for Clinical Transplantation

Current clinical protocols determine a limited number of variables and parameters for matching and allocating donor organs to potential recipients. ABO compatibility is obviously required for successful transplantation. Placing an A donor organ in an O recipient results in hyperacute rejection due to the presence of preformed anti-A antibodies. It is possible to transplant A2 donor organs into O recipients because most anti-A antibodies do not bind to the A2 ligand. It is also possible to place O organs into A or B recipients; however, because of the severe organ shortage and long waiting lists, this is not usually performed.

The central position of MHC in immune regulation suggests that HLA matching is very important for allografting. Significant data prove that HLA matching is important for kidney and pancreas transplantation. A well-matched organ has up to a 10% long-term survival advantage over a poorly matched graft. However, as the overall success rate for renal allografting approaches 90%, there is currently debate over the magnitude of this advantage and what defines poor versus good matching. Good data show that HLA matching is *not* important for liver transplantation and does not affect graft survival. The immunologic reasons for this are not known. The data for cardiac grafting are more controversial; there is probably a small advantage for HLA matching with this organ.

Most laboratories currently use serologic-based, or antibody-based, techniques to type potential donors and recipients for HLA. The main loci typed are HLA-A, HLA-B, and HLA-DR. For a normal completely heterozygous individual, this results in six antigens typed, and a complete donor-recipient match is referred to as a six-antigen match.

Newer nucleic acid- and polymerase chain reaction-based techniques are being used by an increasing number of HLA laboratories. This technology is more accurate than serologic-based techniques and types for additional loci, including HLA-DP and HLA-DQ and separate α and β chains. Typing for more loci may allow for better matching. Conversely, because HLA heterogeneity is so enormous and because there is such a severe shortage of donor organs, technical advances in typing may confer no benefit on clinical results.

An important test for graft compatibility is the crossmatch. This assay determines if there are preformed antibodies in the potential recipient's serum that react with antigens on the cell surface of the potential donor's lymphocytes (Fig. 16-22). A positive crossmatch means that such antibodies are present and that hyperacute rejection will ensue if the transplant is performed. Appropriate controls are always performed to exclude autoantibodies. Crossmatching is important for kidney, pancreas, lung, and heart allografting, whereas hepatic allografts resist hyperacute rejection. The reasons for this resistance are not known but may relate to the large mass of hepatic tissue that can absorb antibody and complement and still preserve sufficient functioning cellular mass.

Figure 16-22 shows that the standard crossmatch detects high-titer complement-fixing antibodies. If the recipient

has antidonor antibodies that inefficiently fix complement, a positive crossmatch could be missed. Some laboratories use enhancing techniques, such as a secondary antibodies or fluorescent flow cytometry, to increase the sensitivity of the crossmatch. The problem with these modifications is that increased sensitivity is accompanied by decreased specificity; therefore, some positive crossmatches could be clinically acceptable. Clinical experience has shown that positive crossmatches from IgG antibodies are the most significant, whereas positive testing from IgM antibodies is not clinically relevant. IgM antibodies can be eliminated from serum specimens by adding a reducing agent such as dithiothreitol.

Figure 16-22 also shows that the standard crossmatch tests donor-derived lymphocytes for the presence of antigen. Since the most relevant antibodies are anti-HLA and since HLA is expressed by essentially all cell types, the experimental design is appropriate. However, if the recipient has antibodies that are cell- or organ-specific, these antibodies may be missed by the standard crossmatch. Some recipients do occasionally possess cell- or organ-specific antibodies, and hyperacute or severe accelerated acute rejection can ensue in these situations. Experimental studies have also demonstrated a distinct vascular endothelial cell–specific antigen system, which can be a target for hyperacute rejection. This endothelial cell system is, however, still poorly defined and reagents are not available for widespread clinical use. The practical consequences of all these limitations is that hyperacute rejections rarely occur due to noncomplement fixation or antibodies with unusual specificities. Conversely, some positive crossmatches, which have precluded a transplant, may have been determined by too sensitive a technique.

Another important test that also reflects the presence of host antidonor antibodies is the panel reactive antibody (PRA). Most recipients on transplant waiting lists send serum samples to the transplant center on a regular basis. These sera are then periodically tested against a panel of typing cells of known HLA specificities using techniques identical to those for the crossmatch (see Fig. 16-22). The percentage of cells with which recipient serum reacts is determined and this number is the PRA. Most normal individuals have no anti-HLA antibodies and a low PRA (0% to 5%). Patients who have been transfused, pregnant, previously transplanted, or have an autoimmune disorder that induces a lot of antibodies may have a high PRA (50% to 99%). The presence of a very high PRA suggests a patient is likely to have a positive crossmatch. This information is useful for determining the logistics of organ allocation when cadaveric donor organs become available and have to be transplanted within a short time frame.

A matching technique used in living-related transplantation is the mixed lymphocyte culture or mixed lymphocyte reaction. Lymphocytes are isolated from peripheral blood specimens from both donor and recipient. The donor cells are γ-irradiated to prevent mitosis, and the two cell populations are placed in culture together. Recipient cells recognize donor antigen in culture, are activated, and proliferate rapidly. After a few days of culture, the amount of proliferation is measured by incorporating radiolabeled nucleic acids into the cells. The amount or degree of proliferation compared to appropriate positive and negative controls is assumed to represent the potential for a host antidonor response and the chance of allograft rejection. Unfortunately, the correlation between the mixed lymphocyte reaction and clinical outcome is poor and most centers no longer use this test. Further, because this assay requires several days to complete it is not useful for cadaveric grafting.

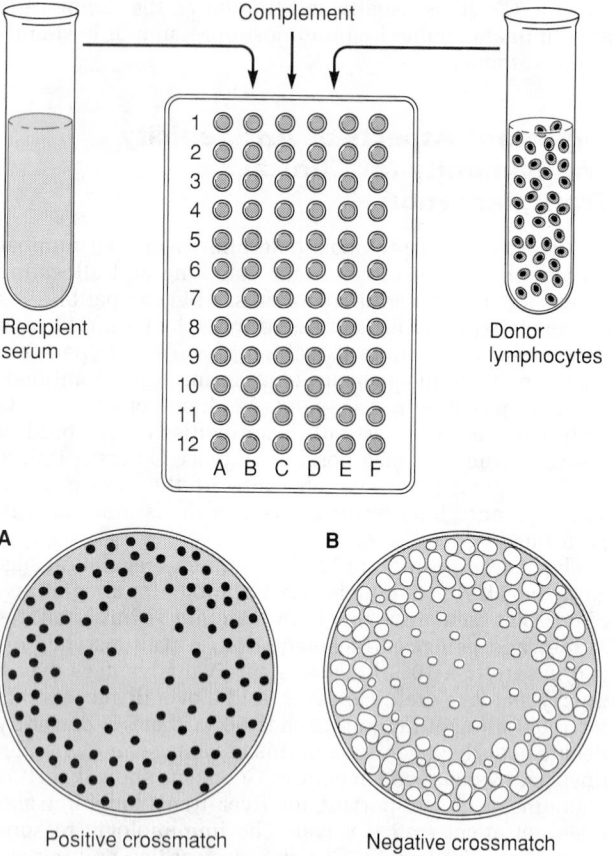

Figure 16-22. Lymphocytotoxicity crossmatch. Recipient serum is incubated with donor lymphocytes and complement in microtiter plates. If donor-specific lymphocytotoxic antibodies are present in the recipient serum, antibody binding results in complement fixation and lysis of the donor lymphocytes. This is detected by the addition of a dye that is taken up through the damaged cell membrane, and a positive crossmatch is noted (A). If no antibodies are present, cells remain viable and do not take up the dye (B). This is a negative crossmatch.

FUTURE DIRECTIONS

Xenotransplantation

The most critical problem in clinical transplantation is the shortage of donor organs. There has been continued liberalization of criteria for acceptable cadaveric donors and improvements in operative techniques and preservation solutions. Still, only about 20% to 30% of potentially suitable donors are ever used. At the same time, the increasing success of organ transplantation has increased indications for transplantation and demands for organs. As a result, the number of people waiting for organs in the United States is currently more than 30,000 and growing by 10% to 15% each year. Societal enforcement of mandatory seatbelt and helmet laws and reduced tolerance for drunk driving have substantially reduced the available donor pool. One approach to this shortage is xenotransplantation, the use of organs from different species. The successful application of this modality could provide an unlimited supply of organs and make all transplant operations elective procedures. There are a number of significant issues, however.

The choice of donor species is limited. Primate donors are scarce, expensive, and many species are even endangered. In addition, transmission of simian retroviruses to humans could be life-threatening. It is currently considered that the pig would be a good donor because of size, physiology, acceptance by public opinion, the substantial knowledge of porcine genetics, and the ability to make inbred and transgenic animals.

The major current barrier to xenotransplantation is hyperacute rejection.[170] Most mammals have high-titer antibodies directed against multiple cell surface antigens of other species. These antibodies may arise through environmental or food-borne exposures to antigens or represent cross reactions with other environmental antigens. Humans have multiple antiporcine antibodies[171] and pig-to-human transplantation results in hyperacute rejection.[172] Approaches to this problem are under investigation. One approach, consisting of methods to deplete serum antibody by plasmaphoresis and concurrently suppress B-cell function, works only transiently in animal models. A second approach, to understand the cellular and molecular process of antibody-antigen binding, complement fixation, and cellular death, is more promising. This work suggests that depleting or negatively regulating complement function may be practical and successful.[173] Means to regulate complement function include soluble inhibitors of complement or the construction of transgenic pig donors that have human complement regulatory proteins engineered into the cell membranes. A third approach is to enumerate the targets of antibody recognition. There is some indication that xenoreactive antibodies of most humans recognize only a limited number of molecules and that many individuals in a population share these same antibody specificities.[171] It may therefore be possible to generate transgenic pigs that have the relevant target molecules either "knocked out" or replaced with the human counterpart. Such "humanized" organs may be immunologically equivalent to allografts instead of xenografts.

Another problem with xenotransplantation is the transmission of unusual pathogenic organisms, or zoonoses. As mentioned, primates may be particularly unsuitable because of transmission of retroviruses. Presumably porcine retroviruses are less likely to produce stable infections in human hosts; however, even this may not be true in an immunosuppressed recipient. Bacterial, protozoal, fungal, helminth, and nonlysogenic viral pathogens are all potential problems, particularly in an immunocompromised individual. The subject of zoonoses in transplantation is currently in its infancy, and extensive studies must be performed to devise appropriate clinical protocols for prophylaxis, monitoring, and treatment of infections.

Gene Therapy

Technical advances in the delivery and expression of exogenous genetic elements have made gene transfer and gene therapy practical approaches to managing many diseases. In transplantation, gene therapy has at least two potential roles. First, liver transplantation is performed for a number of inborn errors of metabolism (eg, Wilson disease). If these diseases are diagnosed prior to irreversible liver damage, then the missing enzyme could be transfected into the patient's own liver and the disease cured without the need for transplantation. The newly introduced gene may be immunogenic and represent an autoantigen or alloantigen. In that case, the patient would still require immunosuppression but probably not of the magnitude normally administered to organ recipients. A variation in this approach is to remove tissue from the patient, grow single cell suspensions in culture, stably transfect the cells in culture, and return the cells to the patient. Fibroblasts, vascular endothelial cells, lymphocytes, and hepatocytes are all good candidates for this technique and have proved successful in experimental protocols. The second role for gene therapy is in the actual delivery of immunosuppression. Cytokines, receptors, antisense RNA, or transcriptional regulators could all be engineered into appropriate delivery vectors and introduced directly into the graft. Experimental protocols have successfully demonstrated the utility of these approaches in animals.

Gene transfer and gene therapy are such new modalities that it is not yet clear how they will eventually be used. A number of difficult technical problems remain to be solved. Current transfer vectors result in only transient, low-level expression of the transferred gene within a few cells in the target organ. Sustained, high-level gene expression throughout the graft has not yet been reliably achieved in any system. The transfer vectors and the transferred gene may be highly immunogenic. Additional immunosuppressive strategies are therefore required to circumvent those responses that would limit gene transfer efficacy. The transfer vectors also have potential pathogenic effects that may limit their utility. For example, adenoviral vectors can induce direct cytopathic effects by disrupting lysosomal membranes. Retroviral vectors can incorporate into genomic DNA and therefore have the potential for malignant transformation. Candidate genes for gene therapy have been evaluated in experimental systems, but it is not certain which will be most useful. For example, TGFβ is a soluble immunosuppressive cytokine; however, it can also induce exuberant fibrosis of the vasculature. IL-10, another immunosuppressive cytokine, can also activate T and B cells in some circumstances. Cytoplasmic or membrane-bound gene transfer products may be better candidates, but unless they can be expressed uniformly throughout the graft, their utility is doubtful. Some of the problems with gene transfer may make it particularly suited to transplantation. The transient expression of an immunosuppressive molecule within a graft at the time of transplantation may be the immunoregulatory signal that would permit the induction of tolerance without the need for long-term, systemic administration of conventional immunosuppression. Low-level expression of gene transfer products may also limit the immunosuppressive effect solely to the target organ, preventing systemic immunosuppression and its deleterious side effects.

Cellular Transplants

There are several situations in which cellular transplantation would better serve the potential recipient than whole organ transplantation. As mentioned earlier, liver transplantation for certain inborn errors of metabolism could be supplanted by providing a specific gene product. This could be accomplished by infusing liver cells from a normal donor into the portal vein of the recipient and allowing them to populate the recipient liver. Such protocols have been successful in experimental models but would require conventional immunosuppression. In addition, the ability to detect rejection would be difficult by either biochemical or histologic means. An alternative is to obtain recipient hepatocytes by partial liver resection, grow them in culture, stably transfect with the appropriate gene or genes, and reinfuse them into the recipient portal circulation. Immunosuppression may be required since the new gene product may be recognized as foreign. Similar approaches with fibroblasts, smooth muscle, skeletal muscle, lymphocytes, and vascular endothelial cells have been demonstrated in experimental models.

Pancreas transplantation is performed for type I diabetes, so only the endocrine tissue is required by the recipient. The exocrine tissue in conventional whole organ pancreas transplantation is often the source of a variety of complications related to the exocrine secretions. Therefore, pancreatic islet transplantation would be preferable. Some islet transplants have been performed in humans, and the overall success rate for this highly experimental process is still poor, although there are a few notable exceptions. There are two major barriers to islet cell transplantation. First, the physical and mechanical means to separate islets from the whole organ are expensive and inefficient. With current technology, it may be necessary to use several donors for each recipient. With the current donor shortage, this is not a long-term solution to the problem. Xenotransplantation, with the use of porcine islets, may circumvent this problem but introduces the immunologic difficulties of xenoantigens. The second major barrier is immunosuppression and rejection. The success of any organ or cell transplant relies on the ability to detect rejections at an early stage with a simple biochemical or histologic test. None are known for islet transplants and this is hampering current attempts to provide appropriate immunosuppression for these patients. These issues will likely yield to further experimental endeavors, islet transplantation will likely supplant whole organ pancreas transplantation eventually.

Organ Preservation

JEFFREY D. PUNCH AND ROBERT M. MERION

PATHOPHYSIOLOGY OF ORGAN PRESERVATION INJURY

The removal, storage, and transplantation of a solid organ from a cadaveric donor profoundly alters homeostatic control of that organ's milieu interior. These effects manifest according to how long the return to normal organ function is delayed or prevented once the transplantation procedure is completed. The injury sustained by an organ during procurement, preservation, and transplantation occurs primarily as a result of ischemia and hypothermia.

Ischemic injury is customarily classified as either warm or cold ischemia. Warm ischemia and its consequences are associated with normothermic events that occur before the organ is removed from the body. Cold ischemia refers to events occurring during the interval between initial organ cooling and revascularization in the recipient.

The principles of modern organ preservation are to provide for hypothermia, prevent cellular swelling, and avoid of biochemical injury.[178] These principles are based on known physiologic events that occur during organ storage and result in loss of cellular integrity, changes in ionic composition, and disruption of cellular energy systems. The following sections describe these phenomena. Finally, the effects of oxygen derived free radicals, cytokines, and nitric oxide at the time of reperfusion are discussed.

Structural Integrity

The cell membrane plays a crucial physical protective role for the cell and also provides an active interface with the extracellular environment. Receptors, ion regulation, and enzyme systems linked to the cell membrane complex contain extracellular, transmembrane, and intracellular components essential to their function. The interrelation of such systems with the membrane itself is highly dependent on a stable configuration of the lipid bilayer and on tight control of temperature, pH, and osmolarity. Organ ischemia and preservation disrupt all these relations. Lowering the temperature through the phase transition of lipids profoundly changes the conformation and stability of the membrane and drastically alters the function of membrane-bound enzymes. Physicochemical membrane changes induced by hypothermia result in increased permeability, which in turn adds to the burden of maintaining a stable intracellular environment and contributes to cell swelling. Organ preservation solutions are therefore hypertonic in order to minimize these alterations.

Ionic Composition

The foregoing membrane changes are compounded by crippling of the Na^+-K^+-ATPase pump, production of excess hydrogen ion, and the influx of calcium ions. Aside from maintaining membrane potential, the Na^+-K^+-ATPase pump is primarily responsible for regulating the intracellular concentrations of sodium and potassium. Hypothermia paralyzes this ion pump, allowing potassium to pass out of the cell and down its concentration gradient to the extracellular environment and allowing sodium, which is normally kept at a low concentration in the cell, to pour into it. Current preservation solutions have electrolyte compositions similar to the high potassium and low sodium concentrations in the cell. Osmotic gradients are therefore minimized, and the cellular ionic charge remains relatively constant.

Hydrogen ion production continues in ischemic organs and may result in cellular damage. Intracellular pH gradually falls without replenishment of buffering capabilities, and under conditions requiring a switch from aerobic to anaerobic glycolysis, the production of lactic acid also increases. The liver appears to be especially susceptible to this type of injury. A plausible mechanism has been described whereby glucokinase in the liver phosphorylates glucose (endogenous or provided in preservation solution) to glucose-6-phosphate.[179] The normal metabolic pathway for glucose-6-phosphate results in production of pyruvate and ultimately lactate by lactic dehydrogenase (Fig. 16-23). Unlike the kidney, the hepatic isozyme of lactic dehydrogenase, M4, functions particularly well under aci-

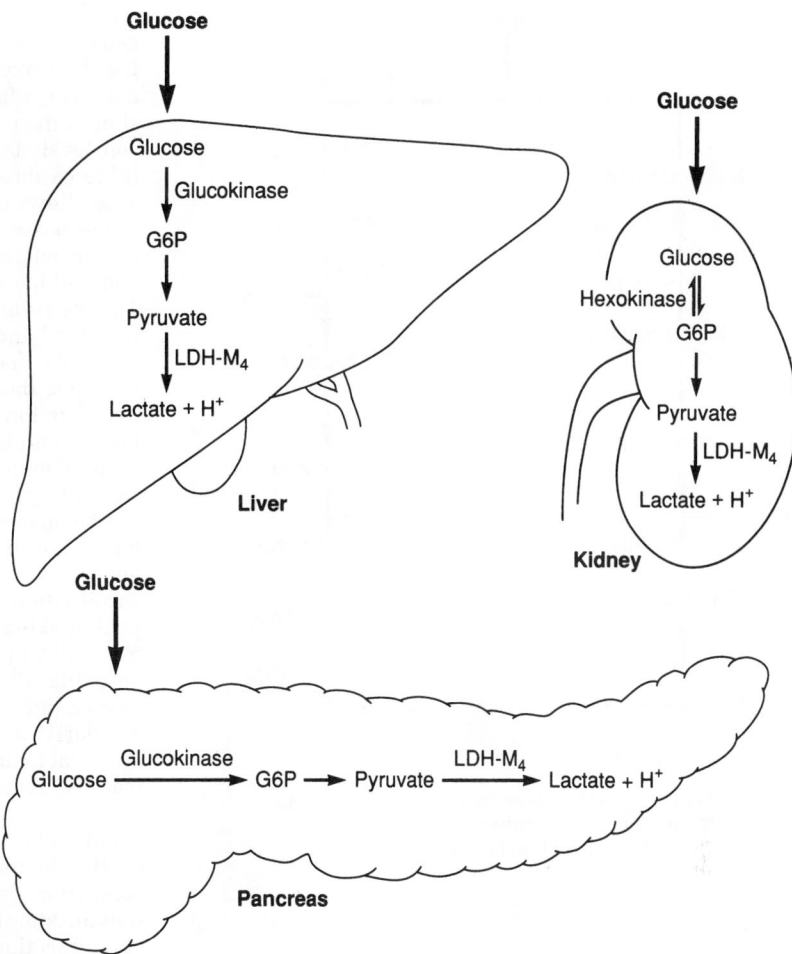

Figure 16-23. The effects of acidosis on glucose metabolism are organ specific. For example, the M_4 isozyme of lactic acid dehydrogenase (LDH) functions well in an acidotic environment in the presence of high concentrations of lactic acid. (After Belzer FO, Southard JH. Principles of solid-organ preservation by cold storage. Transplantation 1988;45:673)

dotic conditions in the presence of high concentrations of lactic acid.

Calcium-ion permeability increases with ischemia, and a rapid influx of calcium may overwhelm mitochondrial buffering capacity. There is increased activity of calmodulin, a cytoplasmic calcium-binding protein. A cascade of enzyme activation events, including the up-regulation of phospholipases and subsequent production of prostaglandin derivatives, results in mitochondrial and cell membrane injury. Vascular smooth muscle myofibrillar contraction may be initiated by increased cellular calcium concentrations, with the resulting vasospasm contributing to ischemic damage. Endothelin, a 21–amino acid peptide with potent vasoconstrictor properties, may also play a major role in ischemia because of vasospasm in this setting.[180]

Cellular Energy

The energy that aerobic cells require is provided by a combination of the enzymatic breakdown of glucose (glycolysis) and by the process of cellular respiration, encompassing the transfer of electrons from organic molecules to molecular oxygen (electron transport and oxidative phosphorylation; Fig. 16-24). Hypothermia decreases metabolic rate and slows the rate at which enzymes degrade cellular components, but metabolism is not completely suppressed. It has been calculated that cooling from 37° to 0°C results in a 12-fold reduction of cellular metabolism.[178] Although metabolism and utilization of cellular energy

stores are slowed, ATP and ADP, the major sources of cellular metabolic energy, are gradually depleted during hypothermia. This is presumably due to residual energy requirements that exceed the capacity of the cell to produce ATP.

During ischemia and organ preservation, the glycolytic pathway is sidetracked to lactate production as the Krebs tricarboxylic acid cycle and mitochondrial respiration are impaired. Although some of the enzymes of the Krebs cycle can be found in the extramitochondrial cytoplasm, the enzymatic reactions of the cycle occur in the inner compartment. Mitochondrial dysfunction, therefore, is responsible for most of the changes in cellular energy associated with ischemia and organ preservation.

Hypothermic preservation results in reduced activity of mitochondrial enzymes. Cellular respiration, which requires adenine nucleotide substrates, is reduced. For adenosine diphosphate to be transported into the mitochondrion as a substrate for conversion to the high-energy adenosine triphosphate, a membrane adenine nucleotide translocase is required. Hypothermia unfavorably alters the relation between the enzyme and the inner mitochondrial membrane where it resides, reducing substrate delivery.[181] Phospholipid hydrolysis by phospholipases increases levels of free fatty acids, acyl derivatives of which may also affect membrane structure and the function of the translocase. Cannibalization of adenosine diphosphate that is sequestered in the extramitochondrial cytoplasm by adenylate kinase for conversion to adenosine triphosphate results in accumulation of adenosine monophosphate as a

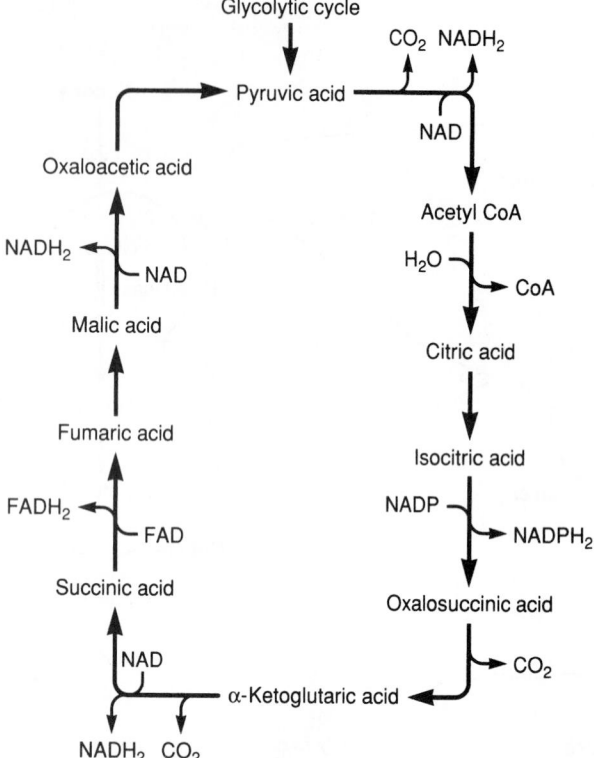

Figure 16-24. Cellular energy requirements are met largely through the processes of glycolysis, the Krebs tricarboxylic acid cycle, and oxidative phosphorylation.

by-product. This reduces purine synthesis and results in the loss of adenosine triphosphate precursors from the cell.

Reperfusion Injury

It is now apparent that much of the injury to transplanted organs actually occurs not during the ischemia per se but on organ reperfusion. This realization has led to many advances in organ preservation aimed at preventing such injury. Furthermore, some of the events that occur during reperfusion may result in enhanced immunogenicity of the graft. A better understanding of these events will hopefully lead to the development of preservation methods that decrease the propensity for allograft rejection.

Oxygen Free Radical-Mediated Effects

Fundamental work during the 1970s and 1980s established the mechanisms by which reactive species of oxygen are produced in biologic systems and documented the effects of these molecules on various cells and tissues.[182] The best studied model involves the production of super-oxide anion (O_2^-) as a by-product of the enzymatic catabolism of the purine metabolites, hypoxanthine and xanthine, to uric acid by xanthine oxidase (Fig. 16-25). During ischemic states, cytosolic enzyme is activated by increased intracellular calcium resulting in the conversion of xanthine dehydrogenase to xanthine oxidase. Both xanthine dehydrogenase and xanthine oxidase catabolize hypoxanthine and xanthine to uric acid. Xanthine oxidase uses molecular oxygen as an electron acceptor, forming O_2^- as a result. Superoxide anion rapidly reacts with itself to form hydrogen peroxide, a potent oxidant capable of injuring the cell by oxidizing lipid membranes and cellular pro-

teins. Hydrogen peroxide then produces a cascade of oxygen free radicals that are even more potent oxidants including hydroxyl radical (OH•) and singlet oxygen. The damaging effects of oxygen free radicals begin on reperfusion of the organ. During ischemic conditions, tissue oxygen levels fall below the threshold needed to allow xanthine oxidase to metabolize xanthine and hypoxanthine. This allows the intracellular concentration of these metabolites to rise. On reperfusion, oxygen is suddenly available and metabolism proceeds rapidly resulting in a dramatic and sudden production of reactive oxygen intermediates. The cellular defenses against peroxidation are overwhelmed and injury occurs.[183]

Agents that reduce oxygen free radical generation, or scavenge them once they are formed are able to decrease peroxidation caused by oxygen free radicals during reperfusion, and have been used to determine the contribution of these molecular species to preservation-related reperfusion injury. Allopurinol, an inhibitor of xanthine oxidase, has been shown to have protective effects when used before the ischemic insult in a variety of experimental systems. Unfortunately, allopurinol has other effects, such as vasodilation and preservation of the purine nucleotide pool, making it a less-than-ideal agent for defining oxygen free radical effects. Other, more specific studies using superoxide dismutase have clearly demonstrated a role for oxygen radicals in reperfusion injury in transplantation.[184] Similarly, desferrioxamine, an iron chelator, removes an essential metal cofactor for the generation of the extremely reactive hydroxyl radical resulting in decreased oxidative injury.

Indirect evidence of oxygen free radical effects is based on the documentation of lipid peroxidation. In this process, interaction of highly reactive oxygen species with polyunsaturated fatty acids in the cell membrane starts a chain reaction that may ultimately destroy cellular integrity and result in cell death. The products of this reaction can be measured by several different assays. The magnitude of lipid peroxidation appears to be inversely related to levels of glutathione, which functions as an endogenous free radical scavenger. Glutathione and other agents that protect against peroxidation are therefore useful in organ preservation solutions to attenuate reperfusion injury.

Production of oxygen free radicals also initiates production of prostaglandins, including leukotriene B_4, by direct activation of phospholipase A_2. This chemoattractant causes leukocyte adherence to vascular endothelium. These neutrophils may contribute to local injury by plugging the microcirculation and by degranulation resulting in proteolytic damage to the organ.

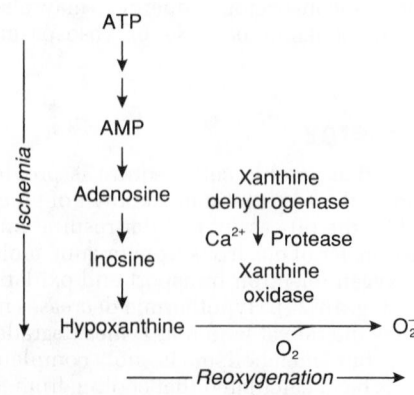

Figure 16-25. The classic pathway of superoxide anion generation by the metabolism of purines by xanthine oxidase.

Cytokine-Mediated Effects

Cytokines are a recently described group of intercellular messenger molecules that may be produced in a variety of normal and pathophysiologic states. Ischemia and reperfusion are known to be associated with a marked release of tumor necrosis factor-α, a cytokine with profound systemic effects.[185] Other cytokines, including interferon-γ, interleukin-1 and interleukin-8 (neutrophil chemotactic factor) may also be released during organ reperfusion and up-regulate adhesion molecule expression on vascular endothelium. These changes may lead to leukocyte adherence, platelet plugging, and ultimately failure of the graft following revascularization. Furthermore, adhesion molecule up-regulation makes the organs more immunogenic, leading to a greater probability of rejection at a later date.

Nitric Oxide-Mediated Effects

Nitric oxide is an extremely labile autocoid generated by nitric oxide synthase from L-arginine. It has potent vasodilatory effects on microvasculature and is responsible for a wide variety of physiologic effects. Evidence suggests that production of nitric oxide is induced by inflammatory cytokines, including tumor necrosis factor-α, interferon-γ, and interleukin-1. In the setting of ischemia-reperfusion, nitric oxide may therefore directly mediate injury to organs as a result of cytokine release. Increased synthesis also correlates with acute rejection.[186]

CONTEMPORARY CLINICAL PRACTICE

The science of transplantation has developed rapidly during the past 30 years. Improved understanding of the immune response to allografts and better appreciation of the complexity of organ ischemia and preservation-related injury have contributed to greatly improved graft and patient survival results. Most solid-organ transplants are now performed as the therapeutic option of choice, and in many cases transplantation offers the only definitive treatment for a given disease entity. As a result, an ever-widening list of indications for solid-organ transplantation has emerged, placing increasing pressure on an already limited supply of donor organs. For example, as of May 1994, 25,500 patients were awaiting cadaveric renal transplantation in the United States, compared with 17,500 patients 4 years earlier. During this same period, the number of patients waiting for cardiac, pulmonary, hepatic, and pancreatic transplants jumped from 3500 to more than 8500.[187] Each year, more patients are placed on waiting lists than are transplanted, causing the waiting time to continually increase.

Longer waiting time for organ recipients means that many patients die before receiving a life-saving organ. This shortage has prompted an extensive effort to increase the available supply of organs. Part of this effort is aimed at improving public knowledge of the critical need for donor organs through the national media. An equally important component is directed at increasing the number of medical professionals who seek organ donations from potential donors' next of kin; one of the major reasons potential organs are lost is that so many medical staff members fail to request these consents. Legislative efforts are also underway in many states that either would automatically make every resident an organ donor, unless they provide a written statement indicating they do not want to donate, or that would require citizens to decide if they want to be organ donors each time they renew their driver's license.[188] It is hoped that these measures will ease the shortage of organs. Finally, transplant surgeons are examining methods to ex-

tend the pool of existing organ donors to include elderly donors, donors with known disease processes that would have previously excluded them from consideration, and non-heartbeating donors.

Determination of Suitability for Cadaveric Organ Donation

General Considerations

The characteristics of a suitable cadaveric organ donor can be divided into those that are general in nature and those that are organ-specific. Broadly stated, the general attributes of an acceptable organ donor include a diagnosis of brain death, previously good general health, and relative hemodynamic stability maintained from the time of the event that precipitated brain death until organ procurement is complete. Informed consent from the donor's next of kin is required before organ procurement. Brain death is discussed in detail later in this chapter. A detailed understanding of this condition and its associated pathophysiology is essential for successfully procuring and transplanting solid organs from cadaveric donors. The circumstances that lead to a diagnosis of brain death usually occur in a setting not conducive to the taking of a detailed medical history. Nevertheless, an effort should be made to contact family members or friends of the potential donor. In this way, the presence of any contraindications to donation can be identified early, and the next of kin can be spared the difficulties of a decision about donation. Cardiorespiratory arrest per se should not preclude consideration for organ donation, particularly if the arrest was witnessed, cardiopulmonary resuscitation was instituted promptly, and restoration of effective cardiac hemodynamics was successful.

Age

As experience has been gained with donors considered less than ideal, it has become apparent that arbitrarily defined age limits for organ donors are unnecessary. Ample evidence supports the relaxation of upper age limits for most abdominal organs. For example, renal procurement from cadaveric donors up to age 65 years is now routinely considered, and successful renal transplantation has been reported from a cadaveric donor of 84 years.[189] Donor age has been similarly deemphasized in some hepatic transplantation programs, in which donors up to age 70 years have been used, and almost 10% are older than 50 years. The acceptable upper age limit of donors for cardiac transplantation has been cautiously but steadily increased, and occasional heart donors older than 45 years have been used after careful screening.

Transplantation of organs from very young donors is usually successful, particularly if the recipient is also a child. Examples include pediatric hepatic and cardiac transplantation. Although the former case is amenable to a reduced size allograft from an adult as an alternative, no such option exists for the child requiring cardiac replacement. Considerable controversy exists with regard to the advisability of transplanting kidneys from infants and children under age 5 years[190,191] (Fig. 16-26). Lower graft survival have been reported when kidneys from very young donors have been transplanted, especially when the recipients are adults.[191] Some centers, however, have recently reported extremely good short-term results using en bloc transplantation of both kidneys from pediatric donors to adults.[192]

Overall Premorbid Health

Because most cadaveric organ donors have acute cerebral trauma or intracerebral catastrophe as the cause of brain death, serious associated systemic diseases are rela-

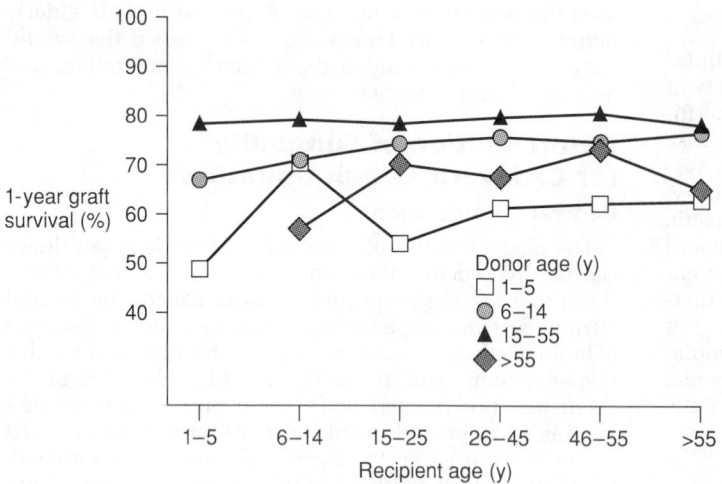

Figure 16-26. Relation between donor and recipient age and 1-year kidney graft survival. (After Zhou YC, Cecka JM. Effect of age on kidney transplants. In: Terasaki PI, ed. Clinical transplantation 1989. Los Angeles, UCLA Tissue Typing Laboratory, 1989:369)

tively uncommon in this population. Nevertheless, careful screening to ensure that the donor was previously in good health is mandatory. Common disorders, such as hypertension and diabetes mellitus, do not automatically disqualify a person from organ donation, but the duration, severity, and treatment of such conditions should be evaluated for their potential effects on individual organs.

Hemodynamic Stability

Cardiovascular instability and eventual cardiopulmonary collapse occur in all brain-dead patients. Thus, hemodynamic management is one of the most important aspects of donor management once brain death has been established and consent for organ donation has been obtained. As stated previously, many potential organ donors sustain significant hypotension or even cardiac arrest during the initial stages of their illness or as the presenting signs of intracerebral catastrophe. Knowledge of the course and management of these episodes is helpful in predicting damage to the various organs and in guiding the workup of the donor for suitability of the organs for transplantation. In terms of specific organs, the kidneys appear to tolerate transient hypotension best, whereas the liver and pancreas may be more severely damaged by such episodes. The cardiac response to hypotension or actual cardiac arrest depends on the cause of the hemodynamic instability and the magnitude of direct cardiac injury sustained as a result of cardiac compressions during cardiopulmonary resuscitation.

Contraindications

Sepsis. Active systemic infection is an absolute contraindication to organ donation. Documented positive blood cultures or known systemic infection that has not been completely eradicated rule out a potential organ donor because of the risk transmitting infection to an immunosuppressed recipient. The risk of infection rises with the duration of donor hospitalization before organ donation. A history of diseases such as tuberculosis or human immunodeficiency viral infection would render a person unsuitable for donation. A question frequently arises as to the advisability of transplanting organs from a donor with pneumonia or urinary tract infection.[193] In most cases, simple bacteriuria accompanying catheter drainage of the bladder without evidence of invasive cystitis should not deter the use of cadaveric kidneys, but attention should be paid to ureteral cultures taken at the time of organ procurement. Colonization of the respiratory tract is an invari-

able consequence of endotracheal intubation in modern intensive care units (ICUs) and, in the absence of necrotizing pneumonitis, does not contraindicate organ donation. In all cases, appropriate antibiotic therapy should be initiated before the procurement procedure.

Viral Infection. All potential organ donors, regardless of whether they are considered high-risk, should be tested for evidence of infection with human immunodeficiency virus. Under most circumstances, this test is carried out using an enzyme-linked immunosorbent assay. Although the incidence of false-positive results is somewhat of a problem, the high sensitivity of the test ensures that the risk of transmitting this virus is minimized. Testing is also routinely done for evidence of hepatitis B and C. History of viral hepatitis or serologic evidence of past infection have previously been considered absolute contraindications to organ donation. Many centers are now reconsidering this issue in selected situations. Although a percentage of organs from donors who have evidence of past infection with the hepatitis B virus are able to transmit the virus, these organs may be considered for recipients that have long-standing infection with this virus or have received the recombinant hepatitis B vaccine and have demonstrated serologic immunity. Similarly, organs from donors with evidence of past infection with the hepatitis C virus are possible sources of infectious virus. The risk of infection is small however, and these organs are now being considered for patients with known preexisting exposure to the hepatitis C virus.[194]

Other viral titers that are frequently determined during workup of a donor include members of the herpesvirus family, such as cytomegalovirus, Epstein-Barr virus, and herpes simplex virus. Evidence of previous infection with these viruses does not ordinarily preclude organ donation but may call for additional therapy in the recipient, such as hyperimmune globulin administration in the case of cytomegalovirus, since this agent can be transmitted with the donor organ.

Cancer. Whether treated or not, cancer has long been considered to contravene organ donation. This tenet of organ transplantation is based on the knowledge that tumor cells can circulate widely throughout the body even in patients with malignant lesions thought to be localized. Transplanting even a small number of malignant cells into a recipient who is heavily immunosuppressed carries the threat of dissemination of malignancy and a disastrous outcome. The only exception to this rule has been the donor with a primary malignancy of the central nervous system (CNS). It has long been thought that as long as the blood–brain barrier is intact, these tumors are rarely capable of systemic spread. Although the transmission of a CNS tumor of donor origin to a liver transplant recipient has been reported, the rate of transmission depends on the organ transplanted and the type of malignancy involved.[195] These cases must be considered on an individual basis.

History of Substance Abuse. Unfortunately, the use of alcohol and illicit drugs, such as marijuana, cocaine, amphetamines, barbiturates, and various narcotics, including heroin, is not uncommon. Although casual use of these substances, excluding intravenous use, does not necessarily rule out organ donation, one must be mindful of the tendency to underreport substance abuse and its potential impact on specific organ systems. Although most organ procurement organizations accept some donors with a history of substance abuse, all are wary of the possibility of associated conditions, end-organ damage, and the potential risk of infectious disease transmission.

Specific Organ Dysfunction

The condition of particular organs greatly dictates their individual suitability for transplantation. With appropriate emphasis on the overall maintenance of donor homeostasis, however, most, if not all, transplantable organs should be procured from most donors. A history of long-standing hypertension may result in fixed damage to the kidneys as a result of hypertensive scarring and secondarily to the effects of aortic and renal atherosclerosis. Similarly, insulin-dependent diabetes mellitus produces a well-known renal lesion. These changes may be reversible after transplantation into a nondiabetic recipient.[196] The kidneys are relatively resilient organs, and simple measures usually suffice to identify serious renal dysfunction. Measurements of hourly urinary output, coupled with determinations of the central venous pressure, are useful for monitoring the adequacy of volume repletion in potential donors. Significant volume depletion occurs during the course of many disorders that lead to brain death. This is the combined result of intentional volume contraction to treat cerebral edema and the effects of diabetes insipidus accompanying lethal brain injury. Serum creatinine should be measured as a global, if imperfect, measure of renal function. Significant elevation of the serum creatinine level during the donor's hospitalization may be a sign of renal injury, predisposing to delayed graft function after transplantation. If necessary, an abbreviated form of a creatinine clearance measurement can be made on a 4-hour urine sample.

Preexisting hepatic disease usually can be identified before organ procurement. A history of hepatitis or cirrhosis of any kind precludes donation. Although calculous biliary tract disease would appear to be a contraindication to hepatic procurement, prior cholecystectomy for uncomplicated cholelithiasis is not an absolute contraindication to liver donation. Standard liver function tests, such as serum alanine aminotransferase, aspartate aminotransferase, alkaline phosphatase, and bilirubin, may be helpful in identifying gross injury to the donor liver resulting from traumatic, metabolic, or hemodynamic causes. The absolute levels of these tests, however, are poor indicators of the likelihood of immediate, life-sustaining graft function in the recipient. Hepatic synthetic function as assessed by prothrombin time may also be deceiving because of the effects of severe brain injury on the coagulation cascade.[197]

The pancreas may be difficult to assess until the time of organ procurement. Hyperglycemia and hyperamylasemia are common in patients who sustain brain death, particu-

larly if the cause is traumatic. A careful history to establish the absence of preexisting diabetes mellitus and pancreatitis provides the most useful information. A history of alcohol abuse alone does not correlate well with the finding of chronic pancreatitis pathology at laparotomy. Computed tomographic examination of the abdomen may be indicated if the donor sustained any abdominal injury, but the decision to exclude a potential donor should not be made lightly because of the critical shortage of organs. It is more appropriate to examine the organ at the time of multiple organ harvesting to determine if it is suitable for transplantation rather than to make a decision based on historical or laboratory information alone.

Cardiac dysfunction resulting in arrhythmia or the need for inotropic support suggest that the heart is unsuitable for transplantation. Transient supraventricular tachycardia, ventricular arrhythmia associated with severe hemodynamic instability, or cardiac arrest require thorough investigation before acceptance as a cardiac donor. Significant valvular disease and wall motion abnormalities can be readily identified by a bedside echocardiograph, a study that is routinely obtained by many transplant centers. In many cases, the fluid management of the donor radically affects the apparent cardiac function, since overhydration or underhydration markedly reduces effective cardiac output. Urine output can be extremely misleading because of the loss of antidiuretic hormone secretion from the hypothalamus. Measurements of central venous pressure or pulmonary artery wedge pressure may allow for more accurate management of fluid replacement. Determining cardiac output using a flow-directed balloon-tipped pulmonary artery catheter is also helpful and complements echocardiograph findings. In questionable cases, cardiac catheterization may be required to exclude significant coronary artery disease.

Brain Death

Definition

The concept of brain death was first detailed in the 1968 Report of the Ad Hoc Committee of Harvard Medical School developed to examine the definition of brain death.[198] This document established the following clearly defined criteria that reliably predicted irreversibility: (1) unreceptivity and unresponsivity; (2) absence of spontaneous muscular movement; (3) absence of reflexes; and (4) silent electroencephalogram. Since the publication of the so-called Harvard Criteria, the prerequisites for diagnosing brain death have been refined. Most hospitals have assembled a Brain Death Committee that is responsible for making uniform determinations of brain death according to locally established specific criteria, while conforming generally to the Harvard Criteria. At the University of Michigan Medical Center, the following requirements must be met to make a firm diagnosis of brain death:

1. The presence of reversible causes of coma should be excluded.
2. To establish the loss of all functions of the entire brain, the following clinical criteria must be met:
   Deep coma
   Absence of brain-stem function
   Absence of spontaneous respiration
3. A confirmatory diagnostic test must be carried out.

Reversible causes of coma include sedation, hypothermia below 32.2°F (8°C), neuromuscular blockade, and shock. Coma should be deep and fixed, without perception or response to external stimuli, including deep pain. Decerebrate and decorticate responses should not be present. Occasionally, spinal reflexes may be present. Absence of brain-stem function can be documented by confirming the absence of pupillary light response, corneal reflex, oculocephalic reflex, oculovestibular reflex, and spontaneous respiration.

An apnea test can be performed to assess spontaneous respiration. Ventilating the patient with 100% oxygen for 10 minutes before the test reduces the risk of hypoxemia and subsequent cardiovascular collapse. After preoxygenation, passive flow of oxygen into the endotracheal tube is continued, and the patient is monitored for evidence of respiratory effort. During this interval, hypercarbia with a $PaCO_2$ greater than 60 mmHg should be documented by arterial blood gas testing.

The confirmatory test of choice is an electroencephalogram documenting electrocerebral silence. This may be done 6 hours after the initial clinical determination of brain death and, when accompanied by a second clinical determination, is diagnostic of brain death. Alternatively, four-vessel cerebral arteriography demonstrating cessation of blood flow to the brain may be used within an hour of the clinical brain death declaration. Nuclear scintigraphic determination of brain blood flow has been recognized as a satisfactory method to definitively confirm brain death. The advantage of this test is that it can be done as a portable examination at the patient's bedside in the ICU or emergency department, avoiding the risk of transporting a potentially unstable patient.

Etiology

Any condition that results in an overwhelming cerebral insult may be sufficient to cause brain death. In general, these conditions fall into the broad categories of subarachnoid hemorrhage, direct cerebral trauma, primary malignancy of the CNS, and other rare and miscellaneous entities. Subarachnoid hemorrhage may result from rupture of an intracranial aneurysm or other cerebrovascular accident leading to lethal intracerebral hemorrhage. This entity is responsible for most cases of brain death that lead to organ donation. Brain injury after vehicular trauma is also common. Automobile drivers and passengers, pedestrians, bicyclists, and boaters may be involved in accidents that result primarily in injuries to the brain and brain stem, leading to brain death with maintenance of other organ system function. Patients with firearms injuries, including those that are self-inflicted, represent about 10% of all organ donors. Primary CNS malignancies account for about 1% of all organ donors. As mentioned, the transplantation of extrarenal organs from patients with these types of cancer may be unwise in view of recent evidence that such tumors can be transmitted to hepatic transplant recipients.

Pathophysiology

Cardiovascular Instability.   During the events that lead to brain death, there is usually progressive intracranial hypertension. Important pathophysiologic responses are evident before the actual occurrence of brain death, including the development of marked systemic hypertension associated with vastly increased sympathetic activity and the massive release of catecholamines. Arrhythmia may become manifest at any time during the process of tentorial herniation. Bradyarrhythmia may be associated with the systemic hypertensive response to intracranial hypertension (Cushing reflex), but ventricular and supraventricular tachyarrhythmia may also be seen in the presence of high levels of catecholamines.

Once herniation is complete and brain death has occurred, a high proportion of donors manifest a hypotensive response related to the loss of sympathetic tone and the failure to maintain circulating catecholamine levels. It has been reported that 62% of brain-dead patients sustain cardiac arrest within 24 hours and 87% by 72 hours in the absence of specific donor maintenance measures.[199] Even with aggressive donor support, about 10% of donors manifest cardiopulmonary arrest during the interval between the determination of brain death and the procurement of organs.[200]

Central Hormonal Failure.   As the brain and brain stem cease to function, failure of the central hormonal axis occurs. Pituitary hormones cease to be produced, and diabetes insipidus ensues. Without antidiuretic hormone, urinary output may increase to astonishing rates, sometimes well in excess of 1 L/h. The urine becomes extremely dilute, resulting in increasing serum osmolarity and hypernatremia. The resultant hypovolemia may contribute to cardiovascular collapse if untreated.

The influence of other aspects of central hormonal function are less well understood. There is experimental evidence of reduced circulating levels of triiodothyronine, cortisol, and insulin after brain death in pigs and baboons.[201,202] These factors may contribute to the hemodynamic instability, cardiovascular collapse, and hyperglycemia so often seen in association with brain death and have led some to advocate using combinations of these compounds before organ procurement. Confirmatory studies in humans have not shown that these hormonal systems play major roles in the pathophysiology of hypotension following brain death.

Request for Permission From Next of Kin

Most states, as well as the federal government, have passed legislation requiring that relatives of deceased patients be asked whether they are willing to permit organ or tissue donation. Unfortunately, the contribution of such laws to an increase in the actual supply of donor organs is not clear. Far more important than a legislated request requirement is the careful training, uniform deployment, and empathic demeanor of the individuals who actually approach the family. In many hospitals, trained donor coordinators are on call to discuss the option of organ donation with bereaved families. These people can come from a variety of fields, including medicine, nursing, social work, or pastoral care. Increasingly, it appears that refusal by the family is one of the biggest stumbling blocks toward increasing the supply of organs actually donated. It is also clear that any discussion of possible organ donation should occur at a time subsequent to and separate from when the family is informed of the patient's death.

The use of the term brain death may be confusing to lay people and professionals alike, perhaps implying that brain death is different from other kinds of death. Obviously, the distinction is intended to differentiate this way of dying from cardiac death but not to indicate that the person is any less dead. Phrases such as "keeping the organs alive so they can be transplanted" are as misleading and confusing as they are incorrect.

According to the Uniform Anatomical Gift Act, a signed and witnessed organ donor card is a legally binding indication of the decedent's wishes, but throughout North America and most European countries, the family's consent is routinely obtained before organ procurement. Although it is desirable that the entire family agree about donating, the legal next of kin is required to agree to the donation and grant signed permission. The hierarchy for permission from next of kin is as follows:

1. Spouse
2. Adult son or daughter

3. Either parent
4. Adult brother or sister
5. Guardian
6. Any other person authorized to dispose of the body

Non-Heartbeating Organ Donors

The profound shortage of organs has led some transplant centers to initiate efforts aimed at using organs from patients who are declared dead in the emergency department and who do not have effective cardiac function. Once the patient is declared dead, the organ procurement team is notified and the organs are rapidly cooled by infusing ice-cold preservation fluids into percutaneously placed cannulae in the aorta and the peritoneal cavity. Generally, this occurs within minutes of arriving in the emergency department and before the family has been notified of the patient's demise. Before procuring the organs for transplantation, permission is obtained from the patient's next of kin. In some instances, the family refuses donation, in which case the cannulae are removed and the organs are left in place. The rationale behind this approach is based on the realization that many patients die in the emergency department before organ donation can be undertaken. This approach is controversial since many transplant surgeons believe it may produce negative publicity from families who are angry to discover that their family member was prepared for organ donation minutes after arrival at the hospital without their permission. Limited experience with this technique indicates that results obtained when organs are transplanted from non-heartbeating donors are inferior to those when conventional donors are used, but that many functional organs, especially kidneys, can be salvaged by this approach.

Donor Maintenance

Tissue Perfusion

Since most donors have been maintained with a minimum of fluids to prevent increased cerebral edema, one of the first priorities in donor maintenance should be to promptly restore intravascular volume. Depending on the duration of the donor's underlying illness, this may require from 3 to 10 L of volume resuscitation. In general, the dosage of pressor agents required to support blood pressure can be progressively decreased as the central venous pressure is raised to 10 to 12 cm H_2O. Crystalloid may be used, and lactated Ringer solution is often given because its slightly lower sodium concentration counteracts the sodium-concentrating effects of diabetes insipidus. If the latter condition has resulted in severe hypernatremia, the addition of free water may be necessary. Colloid and blood should be used to restore and maintain osmotic pressure and normovolemia. The hematocrit should be kept around 35 to replace traumatic losses and to maintain oxygen-carrying capacity. Enough volume should be administered to achieve a urine output of at least 100 mL/h and a systolic arterial pressure of 90 to 120 mmHg. Higher levels of arterial blood pressure are usually unnecessary because of the loss of sympathetic tone accompanying brain death.

If diabetes insipidus is severe, exogenous vasopressin must be given. Desmopressin acetate, a synthetic analogue of 8-arginine vasopressin that is available in a variety of forms, appears to have the least splanchnic vasoconstrictive effect relative to its antidiuretic action. This agent can be given by a variety of routes, including intranasally, subcutaneously, or intravenously. The usual dosage is 20 mg intranasally or 2 to 4 mg intravenously or subcutaneously.

Oxygenation and Ventilation

Arterial blood gases should be checked regularly and appropriate adjustments of the ventilator made to optimize gas exchange and acid–base balance. Oxygen supply should be adequate to maintain an arterial oxygen saturation of greater than 95% and, if available, a mixed venous oxygen saturation above 70%. Low levels of positive end-expiratory pressure may facilitate achieving a balanced oxygen supply and demand.

Inotropic Support

Most donors are hypovolemic at the time of brain death and are receiving inotropic support in lieu of volume to support their blood pressure. Dopamine hydrochloride is the most commonly used agent. The need for dosages of this drug in excess of 10 mg/kg/min usually indicates persistent hypovolemia, and the restoration of normovolemia is almost always accompanied by a reduction in dopamine requirements. High doses of dopamine maintained for long periods before organ procurement may be associated with increased rates of acute tubular necrosis and hepatic allograft failure. Cardiac procurement is often abandoned if high doses of inotropic support are required despite adequate volume status.

Other inotropic agents, such as isoproterenol, epinephrine, norepinephrine, and Neo-Synephrine, are occasionally used, but this should be discouraged because of their peripheral vasoconstrictive effects. Dobutamine is occasionally used in conjunction with low doses of dopamine.

Prevention of Hypothermia

Thermoregulatory homeostatic mechanisms are destroyed when brain death occurs, and severe hypothermia may lead to ventricular arrhythmia and cardiac arrest. Warming blankets should be placed over and under the donor to keep body temperature above 35F8C, and exposure for examination or intervention should be kept to a minimum. If maintaining normal body temperature is a problem, intravenous fluids may be prewarmed before administration, and a heated humidifier circuit can be added to the ventilator.

Multiple-Organ Procurement

United Network for Organ Sharing and the Coordination of Teams

When brain death has been declared, the person has been identified as a suitable organ donor, and permission has been given by the next of kin, the logistics of organ procurement must be arranged. Since passage of the National Organ Transplantation Act, a national organ procurement and transplantation network has been organized. The federal contract for this important function has been awarded to the United Network for Organ Sharing (UNOS). UNOS is responsible for the fair and equitable distribution of cadaveric donor organs throughout the United States. The 50 states are divided into 11 regions of about equal population (Fig. 16-27). Within each region, UNOS-certified local organ procurement organizations (OPOs) are responsible for maintaining the list of potential recipients for their respective catchment areas. All potential recipients in the United States are entered into the UNOS computer system, and a point allocation system is used to determine, within any given OPO, the appropriate recipient for a given donor organ. If a particular organ cannot be used by a recipient in the OPO, the next suitable recipient in the region is offered the organ. Finally, if no recipients in the OPO region can be found, the organ is offered to any recipient in the nation. In each case, recipient priority

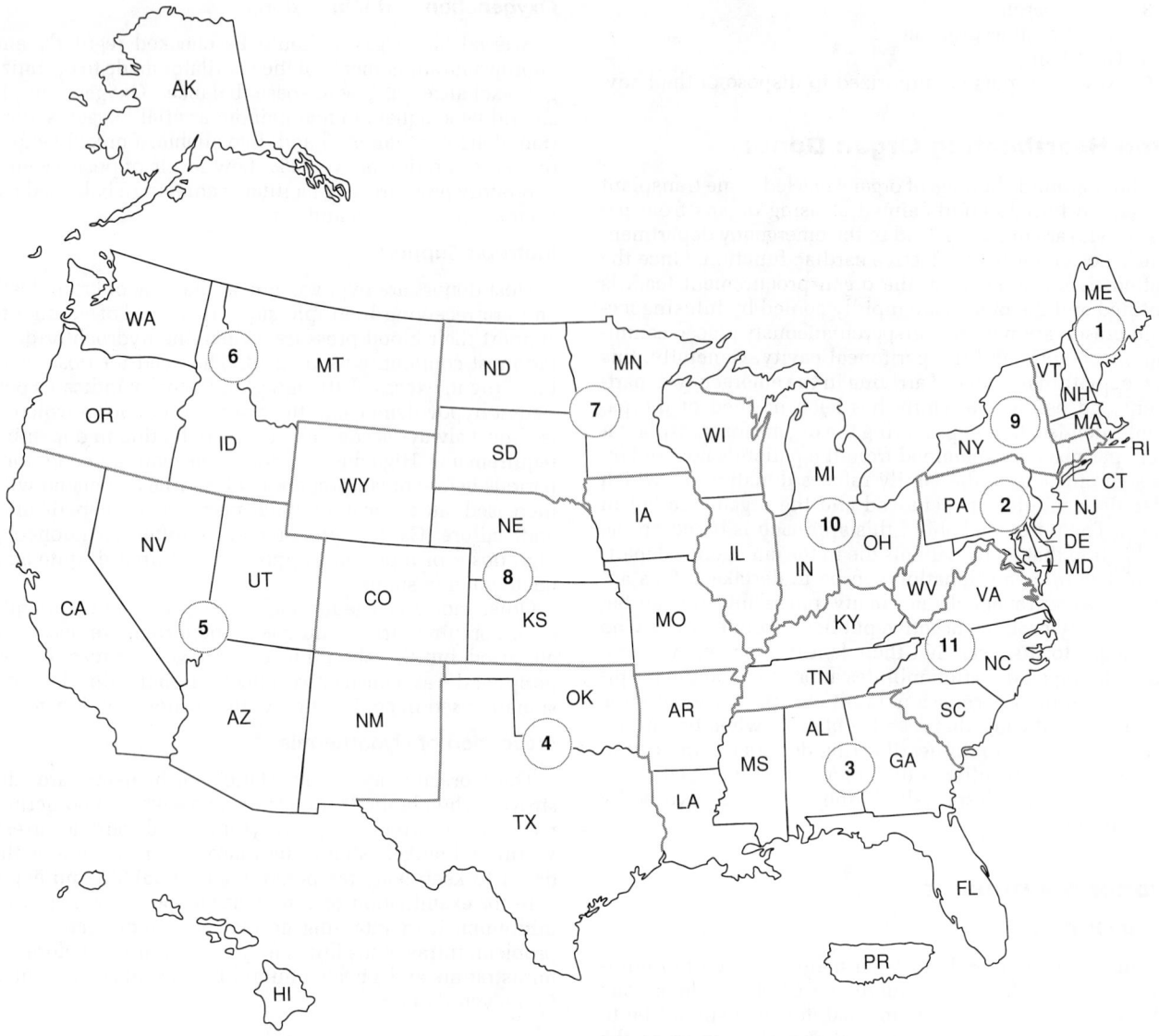

Figure 16-27. The United Network for Organ Sharing has divided the 50 United States into 11 regions of about equal populations for purposes of administration of organ procurement, distribution, and educational objectives.

is ranked by the existing point allocation system. The only exception to these general rules relates to renal transplant recipients who share six antigens with the donor. These kidneys are automatically shared nationwide even if suitable local recipients are available.

Recipients of the various organs may reside in geographically distant locations. Because the recipient transplantation teams must be given considerable detailed information about the donor to decide whether to use a particular organ for a particular recipient, a finite period of time is required to assemble the necessary donor retrieval teams. When all teams are on site at the donor hospital, the donor is transferred to the operating room for the actual procurement procedure.

Surgical Technique for Multiple Organ Procurement

Techniques of multiple organ procurement allow for the removal of the heart, lungs, kidneys, liver, and pancreas from a single donor for transplantation into six or more recipients. The following discussion details the methods used to remove all these organs from a donor.

The heartbeating donor is brought to the operating room from the ICU or emergency department with appropriate hemodynamic and electrocardiographic monitoring. Oxygen is delivered by hand bagging at 100% inspired concentration. Inotropic drug infusions are continued during transport and procurement. The anesthesiologist should maintain close communication with the procurement teams to avoid the development of cardiac arrhythmia, hypotension, and hypoxemia.

The steps in the procedure can be categorized as follows: (1) incision; (2) exploration and inspection; (3) individual organ mobilization; (4) in situ perfusion; (5) removal of organs; and (6) closure of the incision. Postprocurement processing, packaging, and transport to the recipient centers are the final steps.

The entire torso is prepared with an iodine-containing solution, and a field is draped from the neck to the pubis. A long, midline incision is made from the suprasternal notch to the pubis. The sternum is split with an electrical or air-powered saw if available, although manual methods using a Lebsche knife or Gigli saw also work well. Exposure of the abdominal organs may be facilitated by adding cruciate incisions (Fig. 16-28). A general exploration is carried out to ensure that no unexpected conditions are present that would preclude donation, such as tumor, infection, or specific organ damage. In general, a no-touch technique is used to minimize trauma to the organs during the procurement procedure.

For the so-called rapid technique of organ procurement, little in the way of mobilization of individual organs is necessary. Preparation for in situ perfusion consists of a complete Kocher maneuver, with mobilization of the right colon, duodenum, and small intestine in a cephalad direction to the patient's left (Fig. 16-29). The aorta is exposed from the bifurcation distally to the level of the left renal vein proximally. The inferior mesenteric artery is divided. Lumbar branches may be ligated and divided at this point. The inferior vena cava is similarly exposed. Next, the left triangular ligament of the liver is taken down, exposing the crural muscle at the aortic hiatus. The aorta is encircled with a tape at the diaphragm (Fig. 16-30A). These maneuvers can be accomplished in about 15 minutes and allow for immediate in situ perfusion through the distal aorta and crossclamping of the proximal aorta in the event that the donor becomes hemodynamically unstable or sustains

cardiac arrest. Warm ischemia is completely prevented by in situ perfusion.

Stable donors offer the luxury of further preparation before in situ flushing. The inferior mesenteric vein is isolated as it enters the retroperitoneum behind the pancreas. This vein provides convenient access for in situ portal flushing using a small catheter, such as a Javid shunt. The pars flaccida of the lesser omentum should be inspected for evidence of a replaced left hepatic artery arising from the left gastric artery, and minimal dissection of the hepatic artery is necessary (see Fig. 16-30B). The portal triad should be palpated for evidence of a replaced right hepatic artery arising from the superior mesenteric artery. This vessel, when present, can be felt as it courses toward the liver posterior to the common bile duct and along the right side of the portal vein as it emerges from its origin off the superior mesenteric artery posterior to the pancreas (Fig. 16-31).

If the pancreas is to be donated, a total gastrectomy greatly facilitates atraumatic mobilization of the gland. After administration of 250 mL of an iodine-containing solution, followed by a similar volume of amphotericin B solution (50 mg/L), the nasogastric tube is removed and

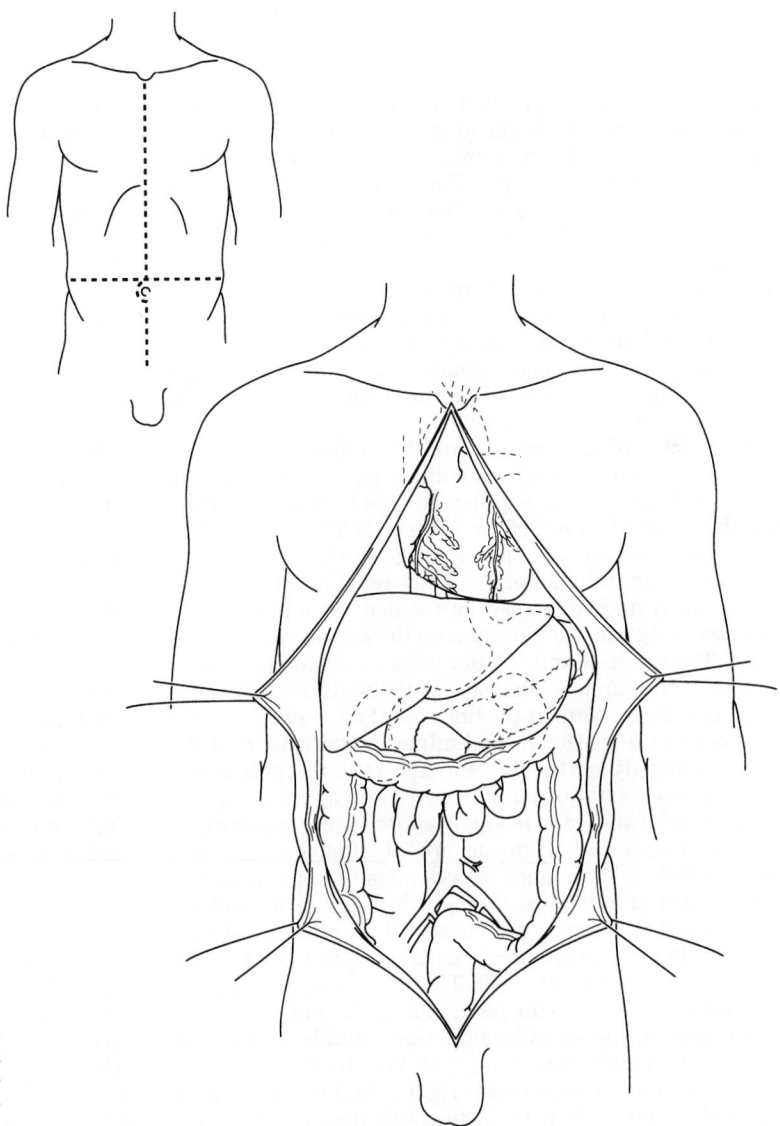

Figure 16-28. A complete midline incision from suprasternal notch to pubis is made for multiple organ procurement. The sternum is split. If necessary, cruciate abdominal incisions are added to facilitate exposure of the intraabdominal organs.

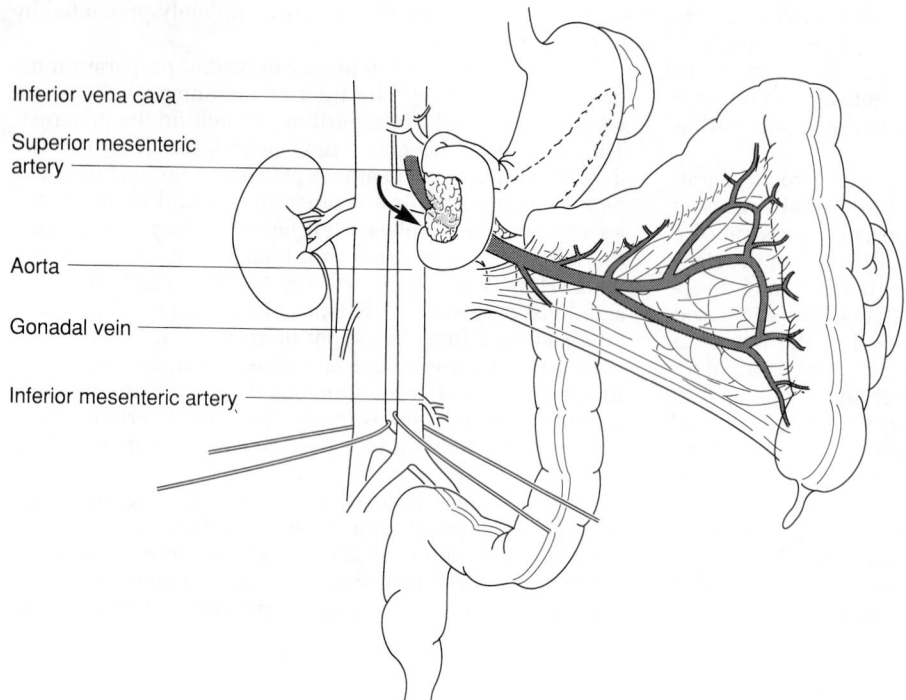

Inferior vena cava

Superior mesenteric artery

Aorta

Gonadal vein

Inferior mesenteric artery

Figure 16-29. The Kocher maneuver is used to completely mobilize the right colon and duodenum, exposing the retroperitoneum, including the aorta, from the level of the superior mesenteric artery to the bifurcation and the inferior vena cava from the iliac veins to the edge of the liver.

the gastroesophageal junction is divided with a stapling device. After the gastrocolic omental tissue is divided, the short gastric vessels are carefully divided between ligatures or hemostatic clips. The left and right gastric branches to the stomach are then divided. Finally, a stapling device is applied just beyond the pylorus, and the stomach is removed (Fig. 16-32). The spleen is delivered anteriorly, dividing its attachments to the body wall and diaphragm. Using the spleen as a handle, the retroperitoneal attachments of the pancreas are divided from lateral to medial, until the major superior mesenteric vessels are reached (Fig. 16-33). The distal duodenum is likewise divided near the Treitz ligament.

The course of the ureters should be identified. The Gerota fascia is widely incised to allow topical cooling with iced slush solution to supplement the in situ perfusion. Complete mobilization of the kidneys before in situ flushing is unnecessary and risks damage to the renal vessels or inadvertent division of accessory renal arteries.

The heart and lungs can be readied for removal by a team working simultaneously with the abdominal retrieval team. The superior and inferior vena cavae are mobilized, and the aortic arch is dissected sufficiently for the placement of a crossclamp at the time of infusion of aortic root cardioplegia (Fig. 16-34). Preliminary mobilization of the lungs is usually performed, and access to the pulmonary artery is necessary for pulmonary preservation.

When all teams are ready, a coordinated sequence of events ensures that all organs are simultaneously cooled and protected. The donor is systemically heparinized. A Javid shunt is advanced through the inferior mesenteric vein near the pancreas and advanced into the portal vein (Fig. 16-35*A*). A cardioplegia needle is positioned in the aortic arch (see Fig. 16-35*B*). The distal abdominal aorta is cannulated for in situ perfusion of the kidneys, liver, and pancreas, and an exsanguination cannula is placed in the distal inferior vena cava (see Fig. 16-35*C*). Alternatively, the inferior vena caval–right atrial junction may be divided in the chest with suction catheters placed in the

caval lumen and right thoracic cavity to decompress the venous circulation at the moment of aortic crossclamping.

The aortic arch and the abdominal aorta at the diaphragm are simultaneously crossclamped. Cardioplegia solution is infused under pressure into the aortic root, perfusing the coronary arteries and arresting the heart. Ventilation is ceased. Portal and distal aortic perfusion are initiated with ice-cold preservation solution. Topical iced slush is placed in the abdomen and chest to assist the cooling process. The heart and lungs are then removed. The clamp is removed from the distal vena caval cannula for exsanguination and preclusion of venous congestion.

The liver and pancreas are removed en bloc. The diaphragm surrounding the suprahepatic inferior vena cava and adjacent to the bare area of the liver is divided. The infrahepatic inferior vena cava is divided just cephalad to the left renal vein. The liver and pancreas unit is now attached only by the distal superior mesenteric vessels coursing to the small bowel and by the aortic origins of the superior mesenteric artery and celiac axis. The superior mesenteric branches emerging from the uncinate process are ligated and divided, and a cylinder of aorta is removed encompassing the superior mesenteric artery and celiac axis. The liver and pancreas are separated as a bench procedure, retaining the celiac axis with the liver (Fig. 16-36). The splenic artery is divided at its origin. This vessel and the superior mesenteric artery are reconstructed with a bifurcated donor iliac artery graft. The portal vein is divided about 1 cm from the pancreas. The common bile duct is divided at the superior edge of the pancreas.

The kidneys are also removed en bloc. The ureters are given wide berth to avoid devascularization and are divided near their entrance into the bladder. Dissection is carried out posterior to the aorta and vena cava in the plane of the prevertebral fascia. Once removed, the left renal vein is divided flush with the vena cava (Fig. 16-37). The aorta is opened in the midline to identify the orifices of the renal arteries from within the lumen. In this way, multiple renal arteries can be readily identified and kept on a single aortic

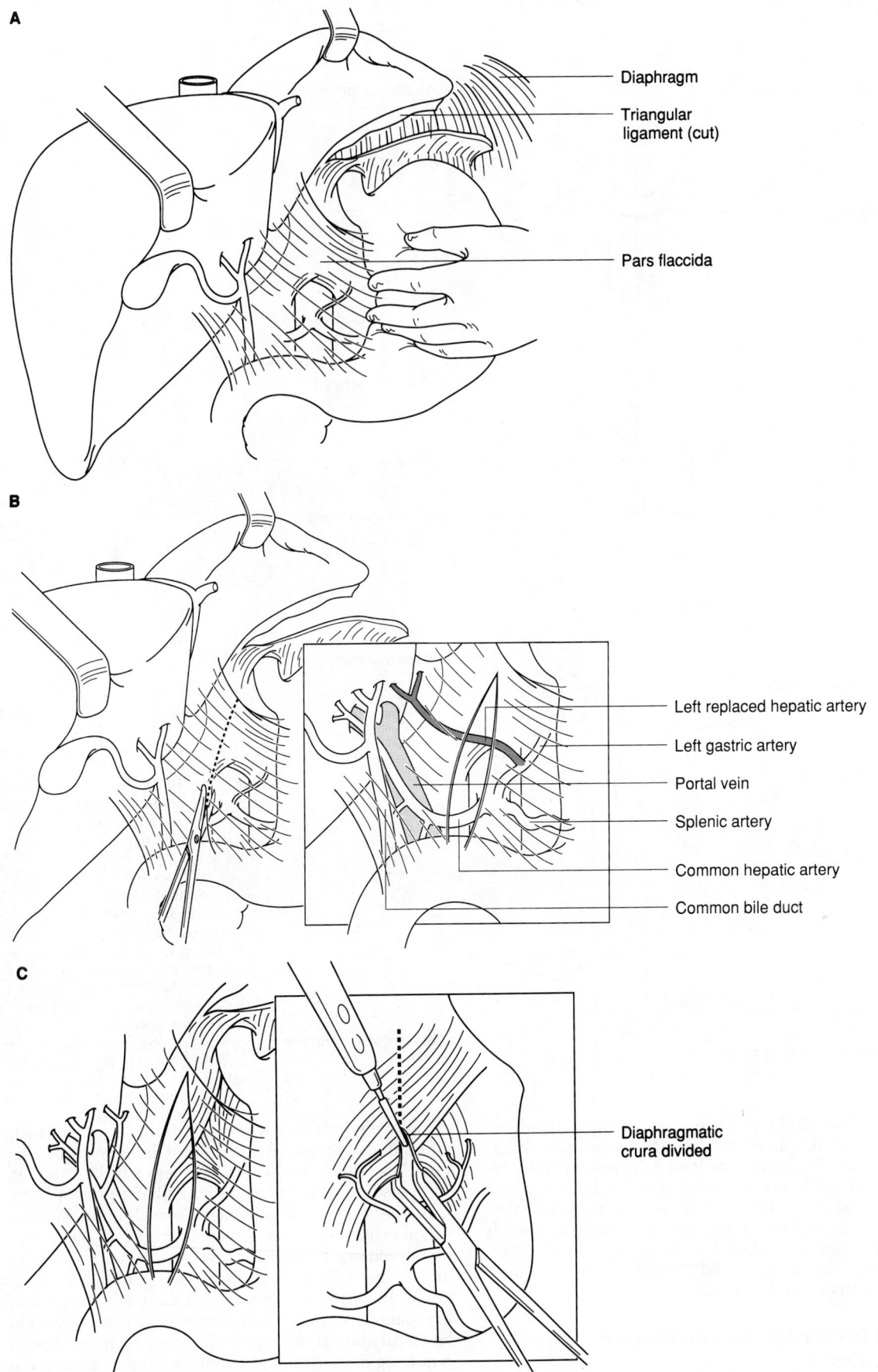

Figure 16-30. (A) The left triangular ligament is divided and the left lateral segment of the liver is retracted to expose the esophagus and aortic hiatus. (B) The pars flaccida of the lesser omentum is widely opened after checking for the presence of a replaced left hepatic artery arising from the left gastric artery. (C) After division of the diaphragmatic crura, the supraceliac aorta is encircled at the level of the diaphragm.

Labels in figure:

A:
- Diaphragm
- Triangular ligament (cut)
- Pars flaccida

B:
- Left replaced hepatic artery
- Left gastric artery
- Portal vein
- Splenic artery
- Common hepatic artery
- Common bile duct

C:
- Diaphragmatic crura divided

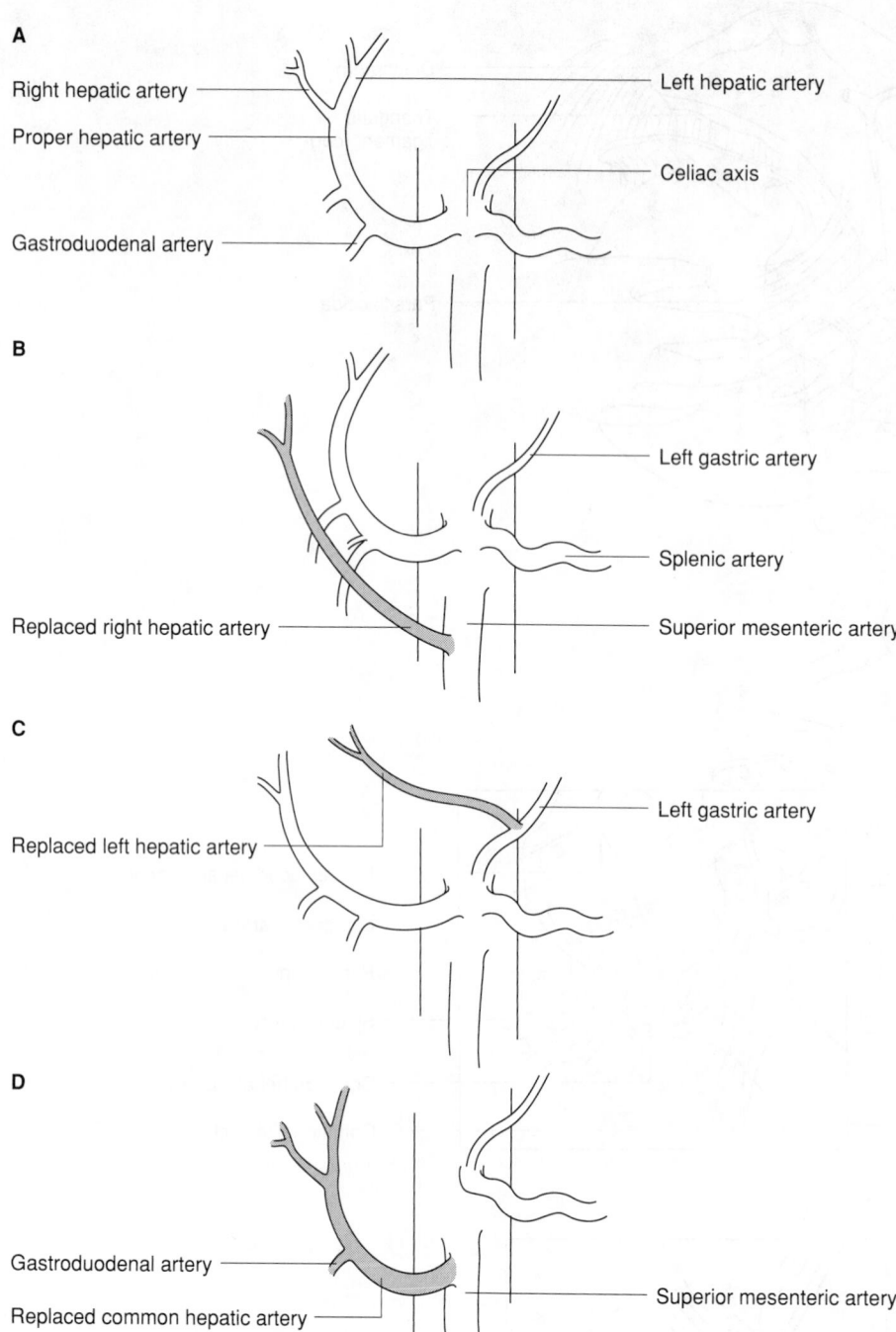

Figure 16-31. (*A*) Standard hepatic arterial anatomy, arising as a single vessel as a branch of the celiac axis. (*B*) Aberrant hepatic arterial anatomy, with a replaced right hepatic artery arising from the superior mesenteric artery and ascending posterior to the common bile duct and anterolateral to the portal vein. (*C*) A replaced left hepatic artery arising from the left gastric artery is usually visible and palpable crossing the pars flaccida of the lesser omentum from the lesser curvature of the stomach. (*D*) A completely replaced common hepatic artery arising from the superior mesenteric artery.

Carrel patch. Most kidneys are stored by simple hypothermia rather than the more cumbersome technique of machine perfusion.[203] Studies indicate that posttransplantation renal allograft function is similar regardless of the technique used (Fig. 14-38). Once the abdominal and thoracic organs have been removed, samplings of lymph nodes and spleen are taken for tissue typing and cross-match testing. The chest and abdomen are closed, and standard postmortem care is given.

Current Preservation Techniques and Results

Kidney, Liver, and Pancreas

Until relatively recently, the primary solution used for cold-storage preservation of the kidneys was Euro-Collins solution (Table 16-8). This formulation provides a hyper-osmolar environment with intracellular electrolyte composition that is intended to reduce cellular swelling. In combination with hypothermia, kidneys can be safely stored in this solution for 36 to 48 hours before transplantation.

In the 1980s, the advent of new immunosuppressive agents, such as cyclosporine, meant that for the first time, extrarenal organs could be transplanted with good success, and the need for more effective preservation became apparent. Cold ischemia limitations of about 8 hours for the liver and pancreas meant that donor and recipient teams had to be exquisitely coordinated. Complex recipient operations requiring a multitude of ancillary support services had to be organized in the middle of the night, and all personnel involved in the procedure, including the surgeons, started the operation in a fatigued condition.

At the University of Wisconsin (UW), a solution was developed that has totally transformed the practice of hepatic and

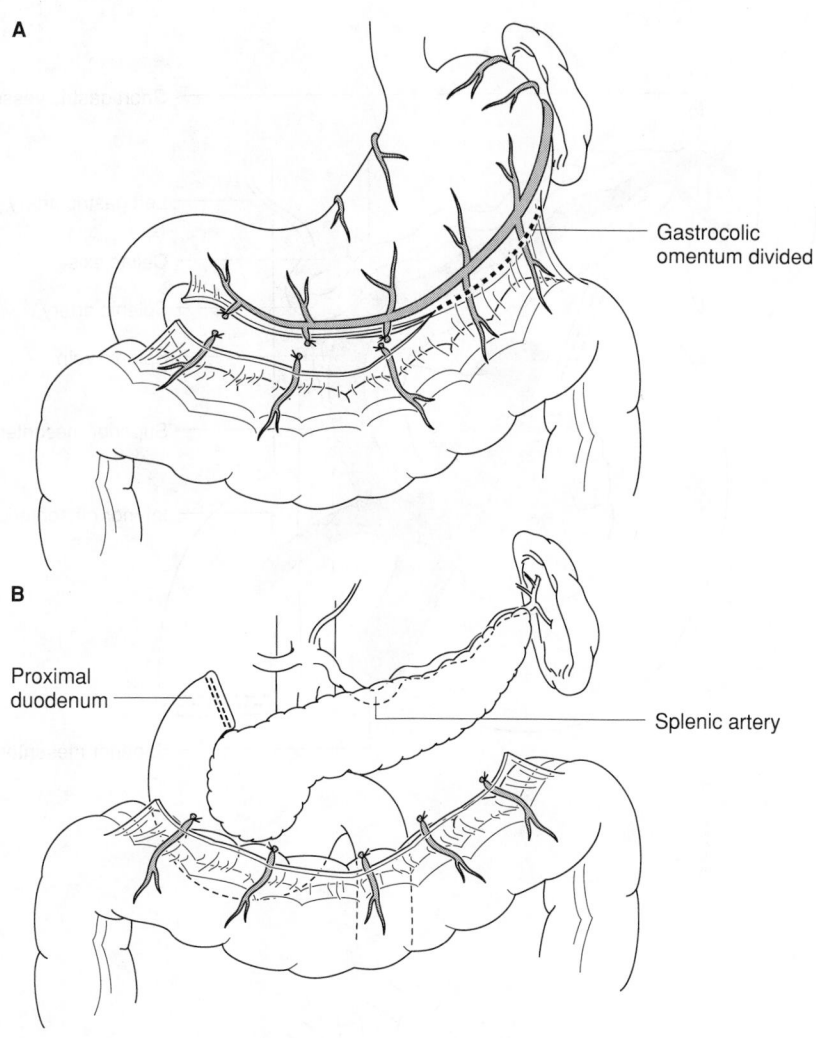

A

Gastrocolic
omentum divided

B

Proximal
duodenum

Splenic artery

Figure 16-32. (*A*) Division of the gastrocolic omentum exposes the pancreas. The short gastric vessels are ligated and divided, separating the spleen from the stomach. (*B*) After completion of devascularization, the stomach is stapled proximally and distally and removed to facilitate exposure and mobilization of the pancreas.

pancreatic transplantation at most centers in North America and Europe. The new solution, termed UW cold-storage solution, is based on the use of lactobionate, raffinose, hydroxyethyl starch, and a host of other ingredients designed to provide high-energy phosphate precursors, hydrogen-ion buffering capacity, and antioxidant properties. It is unclear how many of these components are truly necessary. Lactobionate, an impermeant anion to prevent cellular swelling, is used in place of the glucose contained in Euro-Collins solution. Raffinose, a naturally occurring trisaccharide of fructose, glucose, and galactose, which is abundant in sugar beets, provides additional osmotic activity. Hydroxyethyl starch is a colloid intended to prevent an increase in the extracellular space.[178] UW solution is used as the preservation method of choice by nearly all programs performing hepatic and pancreatic transplantations. Both organs can be reliably stored for 24 hours (Fig. 16-39), and isolated clinical cases with total cold ischemia times in excess of 30 hours have been reported.[204,205] Although these livers function in terms of hepatocellular metabolism, evidence is accumulating that cold ischemia longer than 12 hours may be associated with a higher incidence of biliary strictures.

It is not clear whether the UW cold-storage solution has any significant advantages over Euro-Collins solution for preserving kidneys. In a large, randomized, multicenter European trial, patient and graft survival rates were similar among recipients of the two solutions, but the incidence of delayed graft function requiring dialysis was reduced by about one third in the UW group. The results of other ongoing trials are needed before a definitive statement can be made about the relative merits of the two solutions in renal preservation.

Heart and Lungs

Cardiac preservation has changed relatively little in recent years. Hyperkalemic, crystalloid cardioplegia solution is used at 4F8C, and 4 hours is the generally accepted limit of cold ischemia. For this reason, donor and recipient operations must be precisely coordinated.

A comprehensive review of pulmonary preservation has recently been published.[206] Hypothermia is used along with intracellular-type solutions. Pulmonary inflation also appears to be important. The optimal vascular perfusate for the lungs remains unknown, however, and results with pulmonary transplantation are still limited by deficiencies in the quality and duration of preservation.

Small Intestine

The transplantation of small bowel segments with or without concomitant liver transplant is being performed with increasing regularity as the treatment of choice for short-gut syndrome. The bowel is generally preserved with UW solution, although experimental evidence does not indicate that this solution offers any advantage over simple hypothermia.[207] Most small bowel procurements, however, are from donors

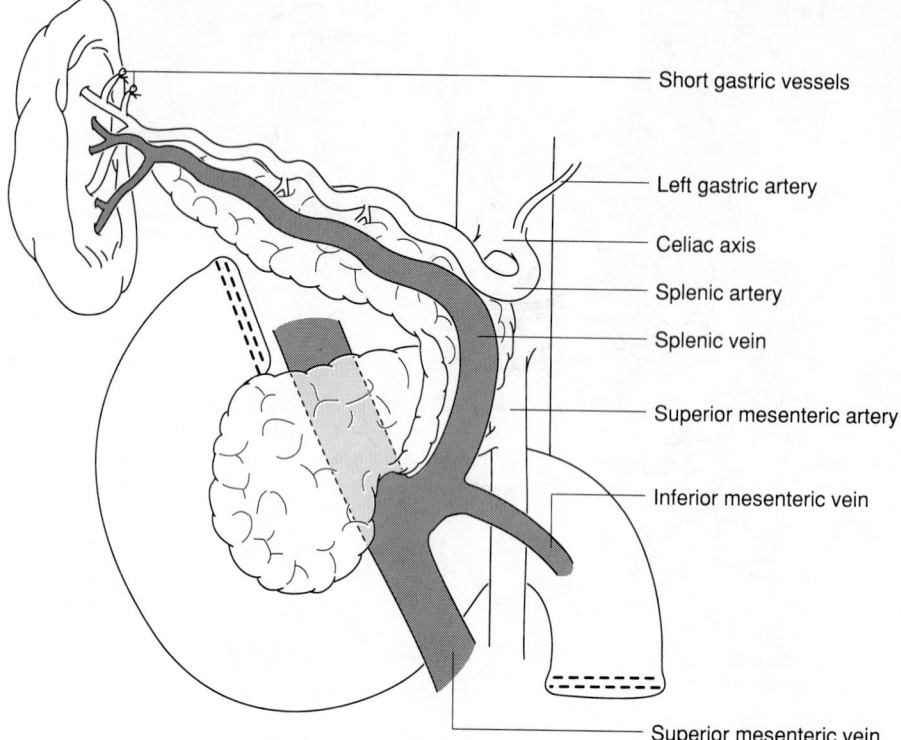

Short gastric vessels

Left gastric artery

Celiac axis

Splenic artery

Splenic vein

Superior mesenteric artery

Inferior mesenteric vein

Superior mesenteric vein

Figure 16-33. The pancreas is reflected anteriorly and to the right to the level of the superior mesenteric vein near the confluence with the splenic vein. The aortic origins of the celiac axis and superior mesenteric arteries are identified.

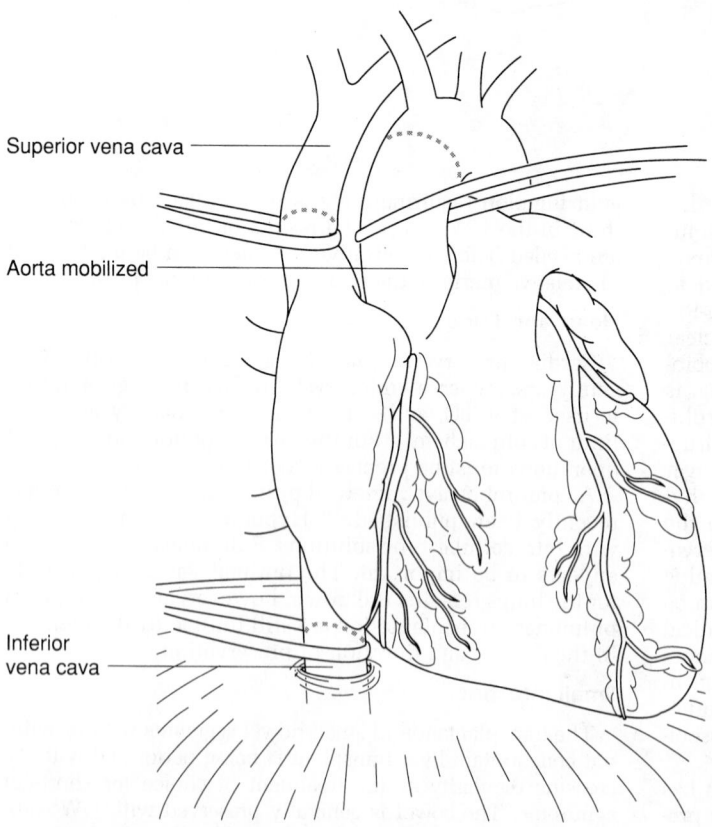

Superior vena cava

Aorta mobilized

Inferior vena cava

Figure 16-34. Preparation of the heart for cardioplegia. Minimal dissection is necessary. The venae cavae are encircled, and the aorta is separated from the pulmonary artery.

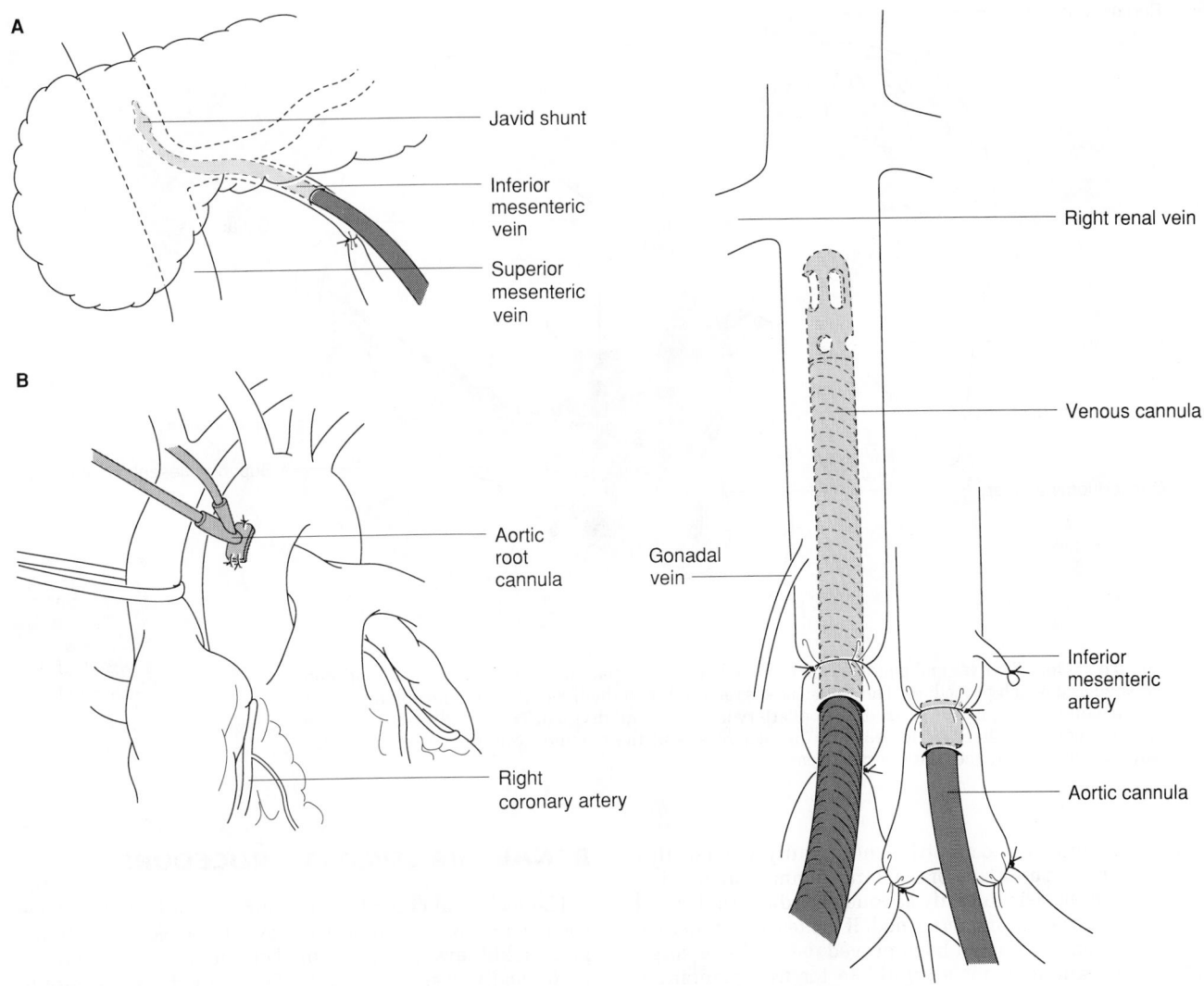

Figure 16-35. In situ perfusion set-up. (*A*) A cannula is placed into the portal vein through the inferior mesenteric vein for portal venous perfusion. (*B*) A needle is placed in the aortic root for perfusion of the coronary arteries with cardioplegia solution. (*C*) A cannula is placed in the distal aorta for retrograde perfusion with cold preservation solution. Another cannula is placed in the distal vena cava for venous decompression and exsanguination.

that have multiple useful organs, hence the use of standard intraaortic preservation techniques. The current limit of cold ischemia time for the small intestine is about 12 hours.[208]

Renal Transplantation

MITCHELL L. HENRY AND RONALD M. FERGUSON

INDICATIONS

The indication for renal transplantation is basically the presence of end-stage renal disease (ESRD). Improvements in pharmacologic immunosuppression, rejection therapy, management of infectious complications, and preoperative and postoperative care have made renal transplantation the primary therapeutic modality for ESRD. If logistic problems can be addressed, transplantation can be performed before the institution of dialysis. Excellent short- and long-

term results can be achieved regardless of the cause of the renal failure (Table 16-9). For example, although renal failure secondary to diabetes was once thought to contraindicate renal transplantation in the early years of clinical transplantation, it is now the single most common disease requiring renal transplantation in the United States, constituting up to 25% of cases.

The most pragmatic method for identifying patients with renal failure who might benefit from transplantation is identification of contraindications rather than indications. Absolute contraindications include systemic malignancy, active infections (including human immunodeficiency virus), and the inability to comprehend the procedure, its ramifications, or follow-up requirements.

An outline of the workup of a potential recipient is presented in Table 16-10. The evaluation identifies coexisting problems or disease entities that need be addressed to improve the procedure's outcome. In particular, screening tests are done to identify bacterial or viral infections, which, if untreated, might complicate the posttransplantation course. Curative treatment before transplantation, whether with antimicrobials or surgery, is important. If

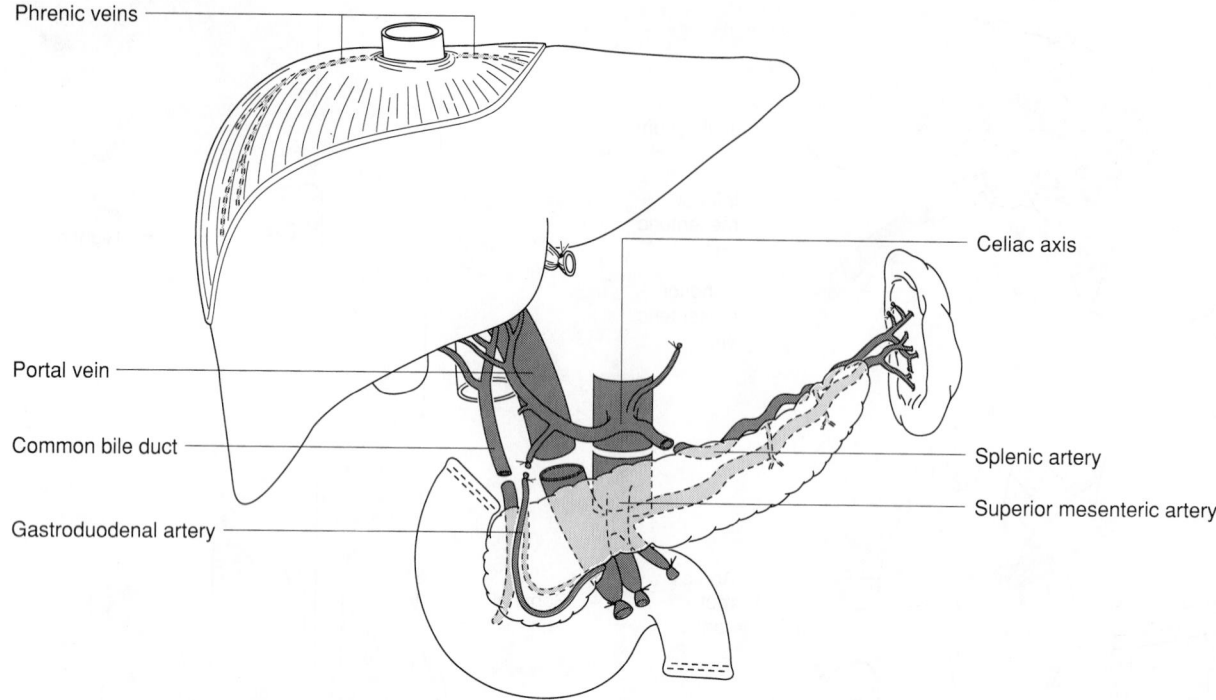

Figure 16-36. The liver and pancreas are removed en bloc. Separation of the two organs is accomplished as a bench procedure. The celiac axis is retained with the liver, dividing the splenic artery just beyond its origin. The gastroduodenal artery is ligated and divided. The portal vein is divided about 1 cm from the superior edge of the pancreas, and the common bile duct is divided just superior to its entrance into the pancreas.

a patient's infection cannot be successfully treated, that patient is not a candidate for renal transplantation. In addition, screening tests to verify adequate cardiovascular and pulmonary reserves are performed. If the tests demonstrate poor function that cannot be improved medically or surgically, the patient is not a candidate for transplantation. Age is not a determining factor per se, but older patients are more likely to have significant cardiovascular or pulmonary disease, making them poor candidates.

RENAL TRANSPLANT PROCEDURE

The technical considerations for renal allografting have become relatively standardized over time. Nearly all transplanted kidneys (except in small children) are placed retroperitoneally in the iliac fossa. This provides proximity to usable vasculature and the bladder, fixes the kidney anatomically, and does not violate the abdominal cavity. A lower abdominal incision is made, the abdominal muscu-

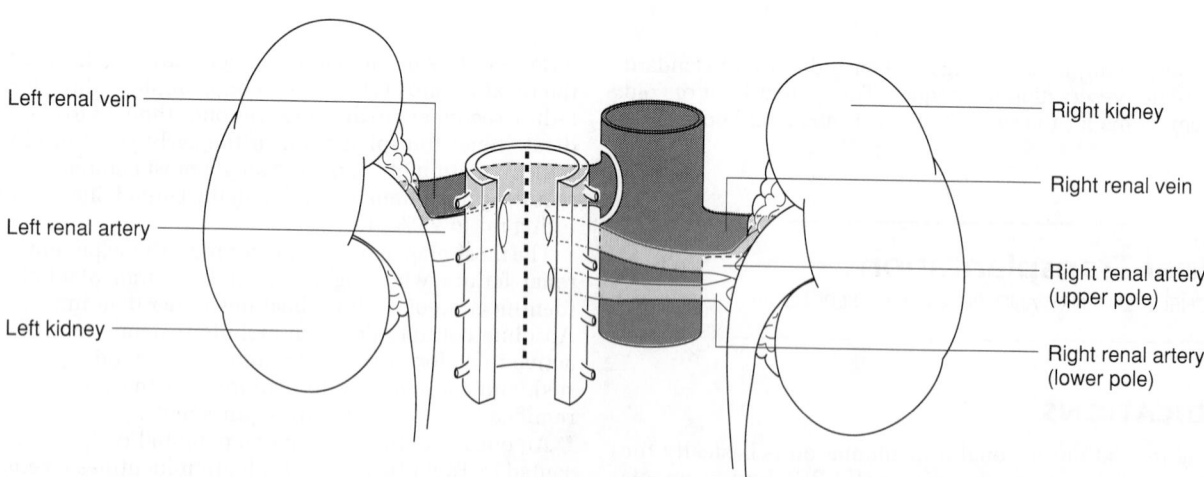

Figure 16-37. The kidneys are removed en bloc and separated on the back bench. Safe division is ensured by viewing the kidneys posteriorly. The aorta is divided between the paired lumbar arteries, and renal arterial orifices can be viewed directly from within the aortic lumen. This avoids any hilar dissection with the accompanying risk of injury to renal arteries. The left renal vein is divided at its entrance to the inferior vena cava, leaving the entire cava with the shorter right renal vein.

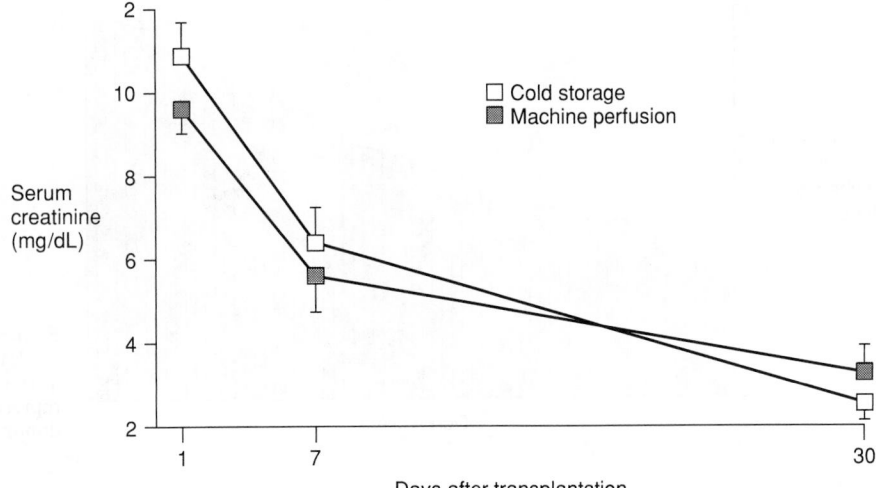

Figure 16-38. Machine perfusion and simple hypothermic storage preservation of cadaveric kidneys results in nearly identical return of renal function after transplantation. (After Merion RM, Oh HK, Port FK, Toledo-Pereyra LH, Turcotte JG. A prospective randomized trial of cold-storage versus machine-perfusion preservation in cadaveric renal transplantation. Transplantation 1990;50:230)

lature is divided, and the peritoneum is mobilized medially, exposing the iliac vessels. Overlying lymphatics are ligated and divided to avoid lymphatic leaks and subsequent lymphoceles. The external iliac artery and vein are mobilized to serve as donor vessels. The internal iliac artery, previously the preferred arterial supply, is now used only in special circumstances. Use of the internal iliac vessels requires more dissection. The artery is prone to develop occlusive atherosclerotic disease at its origin, and its use may impair important collateral circulation, especially in the elderly and in diabetics. The renal vein and arteries are anastomosed to the external iliac vein and artery, respectively, with fine polypropylene sutures.

The ureter is anastomosed to the bladder directly. The standard Ledbetter-Politano ureterocystostomy, in which the ureter is tunneled submucosally, has been gradually replaced by an extravesicular method. The ureterocystostomy is performed by first placing a small incision in the anterolateral aspect of the bladder. After spatulation of the ureter, construction of a direct mucosa-to-mucosa anastomosis is performed using fine monofilament absorbable sutures. The seromuscular layers of the bladder are then reapproximated over the ureter, creating a short tunnel to prevent reflux.

LIVING DONORS

Despite efforts to increase the supply of cadaveric donor organs, the number of donated organs has reached a plateau over the last several years. With increasing numbers of ESRD patients referred for transplantation, efforts to increase a patient's ability to receive a transplant have emphasized the use of living donors. Advantages of living donor transplantation include the following:

- Improved short- and long-term graft survival
- Routine immediate allograft function
- Planned operative timing, allowing for optimization of the medical condition of the recipient and, in many cases, avoidance of dialysis
- Fewer rejection and infectious episodes
- Shorter hospital stays

Inherent in the use of living donors is the concept of safety, in both the short and long term, for the donor. Although perioperative morbidity and mortality are extremely low, an exhaustive preoperative work-up is mandatory to rule out both intrinsic renal disease (or systemic

diseases that may cause renal insufficiency) and preexisting cardiovascular or pulmonary abnormalities that would compromise the potential donor. In the absence of positive findings, several studies have demonstrated the short- and long-term safety of live renal donations.[209,210]

Most living donors are close relatives of the recipient. Parent–child or sibling combinations are most common. The use of haploidentical or identical combinations has received the most attention and study.

Transplantation in this setting has allowed excellent results in both short- and long-term follow-up. One-year graft survival for recipients of living, related donor organs during the past 10 years has been above 80% and has exceeded that of recipients of cadaveric transplants (primary and repeated transplants) at all time points (Fig. 16-40). Nearly all transplantation centers that perform living, related donor transplantations report 1-year graft survival rates of over 90%. Although uniform success using living, related donors has not always been the case, by preconditioning the recipient with the use of donor-specific blood transfusions from their living donor, graft survival in single-

Table 16-8. COMPOSITION OF HYPOTHERMIC ORGAN PRESERVATION SOLUTIONS

Component	Amount per Liter
EURO-COLLINS SOLUTION	
KH_2PO_4	2.05 g
K_2HPO_4	7.4 g
KCl	1.12 g
$NaHCO_3$	0.84 g
Glucose	35 g
UW SOLUTION	
K^+-lactobionate	100 mmol
KH_2PO_4	25 mmol
$MgSO_4$	5 mmol
Raffinose	30 mmol
Adenosine	5 mmol
Glutathione	3 mmol
Insulin	100 IU
Penicillin	40 IU
Dexamethasone	8 mg
Allopurinol	1 mmol
Hydroxyethyl starch	50 g

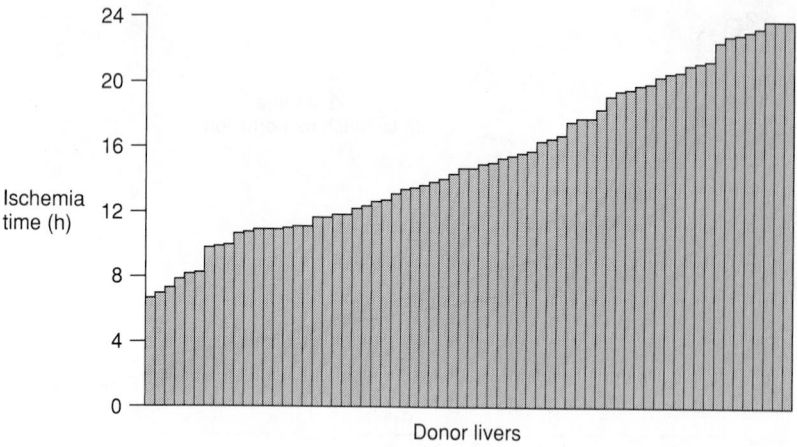

Figure 16-39. Distribution of ischemia times using UW solution for liver transplant preservation at the University of Michigan. Each vertical bar represents the preservation time for an individual donor liver.

haplotype matches compares favorably with identically matched donor–recipient pairs (90% to 95% 1-year graft survival rate).[211]

The major drawback with this maneuver is the development of recipient antidonor antibodies (sensitization), which occurs in nearly one third of recipients. The development of sensitizing antibodies eliminates the use of that donor. In response to this problem, concurrent administration of azathioprine has been used in association with donor-specific transfusions, decreasing the incidence of sensitization to about 10%.[212] With the introduction of cyclosporine in the early 1980s, the use of donor-specific transfusions with subsequent immunosuppression using azathioprine and prednisone was compared with results in nontransfused recipients treated with cyclosporine and prednisone.[213] Graft survival has been excellent in long-term follow-up (Fig. 16-41). The use of cyclosporine without transfusions avoids the issue of sensitization, however, and no potential donors are lost simply as a result of the transfusion. Most centers have now adopted this position, and routine donor-specific transfusions are seldom performed in adults.

The identically matched donor-recipient–sibling combination is a unique one. Graft survival rates are uniformly excellent, approaching 95% at 1 year, with an immunosuppressive protocol consisting only of azathioprine and prednisone. Most clinicians believe this is the maximal survival rate possible and that the use of cyclosporine, with its side effects, is not indicated. Cyclosporine monotherapy has also been successfully used in this group of patients to avoid corticosteroid use.[214]

In an effort to expand the donor pool, the use of living, nonrelated donors and ABO-incompatible donors is being investigated. Although still controversial in some areas, spousal donors and other highly motivated people have been used successfully as nonrelated donors. Ethical questions have limited the wide applicability of this group of donors. Excellent graft survival rates have been demonstrated in spousal combinations using donor-specific transfusion protocols (93% 4-year graft survival rates).[215] Experimental protocols examining the use of ABO-incompatible renal donors have been performed. One report suggests 1- and 2-year graft survival rates of 88% in 17 patients undergoing living, related, ABO-incompatible transplantation (with all patients having preoperative plasmapheresis and concurrent splenectomy).[216]

CADAVERIC RENAL TRANSPLANTATION

As the success of renal transplantations improved in the early era of the procedure, new sources of organs for transplantation were needed to meet the demand for transplants. The concept of cadaveric donors and the uses of cadaveric organs were easily appreciated, but actually defining and implementing the use of these donors required

---

Table 16-9. CAUSES OF RENAL FAILURE IN RENAL TRANSPLANTATION

Congenital	Aplasia, obstructive uropathy
Hereditary	Alport syndrome, polycystic disease, tuberous sclerosis
Metabolic	Amyloidosis, cystinosis, nephrocalcinosis, oxalosis
Neoplasms	Renal cell carcinoma, Wilms tumor
Progressive	Diabetic nephropathy, chronic pyelonephritis, Goodpasture syndrome, hypertension, membranous glomerulonephritis, lupus nephritis, nephrotic syndrome, obstructive uropathies, scleroderma
Trauma	Vascular occlusion, parenchymal destruction

Table 16-10. PRETRANSPLANTATION WORKUP OF POTENTIAL RENAL RECIPIENTS

INITIAL WORKUP

History and physical examination
Laboratory analyses: serum electrolytes, calcium, magnesium, phosphorus, complete blood count, platelets, AST, APT, alkaline phosphatase, prothrombin time, partial thromboplastin time, viral serologies (including herpes simplex, cytomegalovirus, HIV, and hepatitis A, B, and C), urinalysis and urine culture, ABO and HLA typing, serum for frozen storage

ROUTINE EXAMINATIONS

Dental
Pap smear
Ophthalmologic (diabetic patients)
Psychosocial

SECONDARY WORKUP (BASED ON PRELIMINARY FINDINGS)

Cardiac: Stress ECG, stress MUGA, echo, coronary angiography
Gastrointestinal: upper and lower endoscopy, gallbladder echo
Genitourinary: voiding cystourethrogram, cystoscopy, retrograde ureterography
Pulmonary: arterial blood gases, pulmonary functions

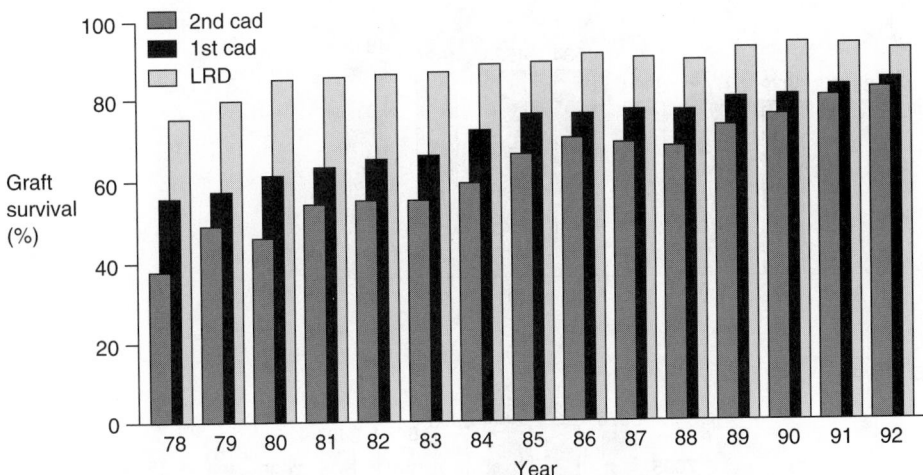

Figure 16-40. Graft survival from 1978 through 1992 by type—first cadaveric recipient, second cadaveric recipient, or living related donor (LRD) recipient.

much thought and refinement over time. Initially, donors in whom cardiopulmonary function had ceased were used, but results were not optimal because of poor kidney function. Recipient treatment nearly always required postoperative dialysis. Restricting organ donation to brain-dead, heartbeating patients improved early organ function and overall success. The recognition that brain death means the patient is dead and the development of objective criteria for diagnosing brain death have led to an increased availability of cadaveric organs. Specific medical criteria have been developed and, with strict adherence to these criteria, identification of suitable organ donors is possible. Needy recipients can now be candidates for renal transplantation, even though they do not have an appropriate living donor.

The development of potent and effective chemical immunosuppression has allowed further expansion of cadaveric renal transplantation. Through the 1960s and 1970s, the use of azathioprine and prednisone in combination, with or without the use of antilymphocyte preparations, allowed the field of renal transplantation to continue to grow, with improved results over time. A notable upswing in activity in the early to mid-1980s (Fig. 16-42*B*) coincided with the introduction of cyclosporine. This agent inhibits alloresponsiveness at sites within the immune cascade that previous medications did not. Use of cyclosporine has led to an explosion of activity in both renal and nonrenal solid-organ transplantation because of successes associated with its use.

With this increase in transplantation activity, the major problem has become the lack of an adequate donor pool for potential recipients. Unfortunately, the donor supply has not met these increasing requirements. From 1982 through 1993, the number of cadaveric kidneys transplanted in the United States remained remarkably constant, while the number of potential recipients grew linearly. Limits on transplantation activity are directly related to the inability to increase the number of cadaveric organs (see Fig. 16-42*A*). Studies have shown that the potential donor pool may be nearly three times larger than realized. Many attempts to improve the number of organs, including legislated request requirements, appear to have failed. Ongoing efforts continue, especially education of the public and medical personnel, and concepts such as "decoupling"[217] have led to improved consent rates although they have not increased the number of total donors significantly. This has led to the acceptance of marginal donors, such as older or hemodynamically compromised donors. The return to the non-heartbeating donor may also increase the total number of organs available for transplantation.

PRESERVATION

One of the major advances in the field of transplantation in the 1980s was the development of a new preservation solution, the University of Wisconsin (UW) solution. Its impact on kidney, pancreatic and hepatic preservation is well documented. Studies demonstrate that it is more efficacious than its predecessor, Collins solution.[218]

The kidney is the most successful of all the solid organs transplanted, at least in terms of our ability to keep organs viable for prolonged periods. Hypothermia allows for a remarkable, yet incomplete, diminution in the metabolic needs of the stored organ. Simple cold storage may maintain the viability of a kidney for up to 48 hours, and pulsatile preservation is effective for up to 72 hours. The goals of each method are to maintain both structural and metabolic integrity and to minimize reperfusion injury.

One of the remaining controversies in kidney preservation is the use of simple cold storage relative to cold pulsa-

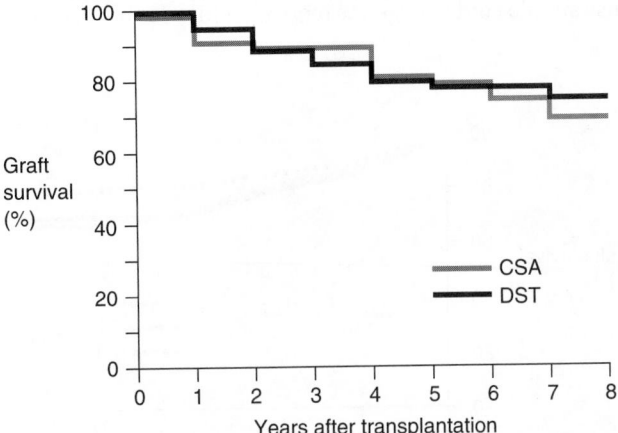

Figure 16-41. Graft survival over 8-year period comparing patients undergoing cyclosporine-based (CSA) therapy with those undergoing donor-specific transfusions (DST) without cyclosporine.

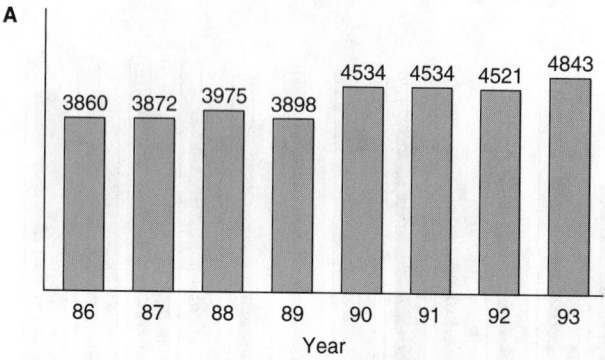

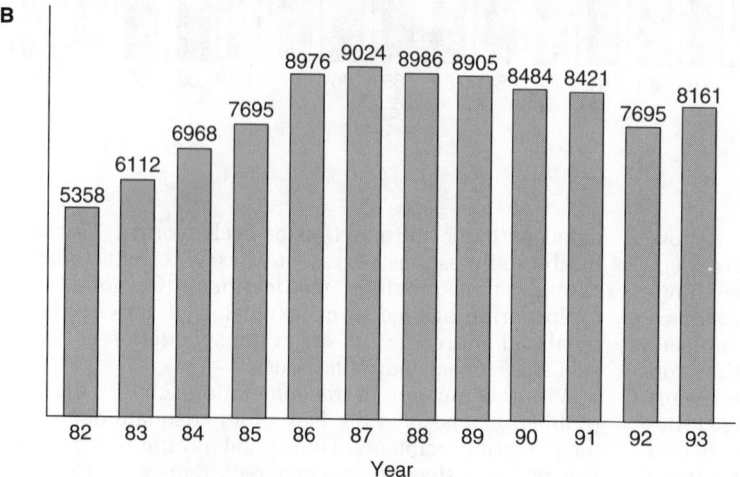

Figure 16-42. (A) Number of cadaveric donors from 1986 to 1993. (B) Number of cadaveric kidney transplants performed from 1982 to 1993.

tile preservation. Simple cold storage involves perfusing the surgically excised kidney with a preservation solution (Collins or UW solution) and then immersing the organ in a cold fluid-filled container maintained at about 4°C. The perfusate solution is a complicated electrolyte solution that mimics intracellular electrolyte concentrations and that is adjusted to be slightly hyperosmolar. Pulsatile perfusion uses a mechanical device that perfuses the cannulated renal artery with a cold perfusate under pulsatile pressure. Advocates of each method note certain advantages. Simple cold storage is an inexpensive, operator-independent, simplified method. Pulsatile preservation allows for prolonged preservation, the ability to perfuse and monitor the microcirculation during preservation (by

observing pressures, flows, and thus resistance), and perhaps the ability to alter these characteristics with pharmacologic agents. With newer preservation solutions, pulsatile preservation can improve the "metabolic integrity" of the kidney, demonstrated by improving the concentrations of high-energy phosphate compounds found in the cortex over the time of perfusion. The drawback to the continuous perfusion technique is the reliance on mechanical devices, the need to monitor the device, and greater expense. Several prospective studies comparing these two methods have demonstrated a lower incidence of early graft dysfunction in kidneys preserved with pulsatile perfusion.[219,220] Despite these studies, most centers continue to use simple cold storage. As more marginal donors and non-

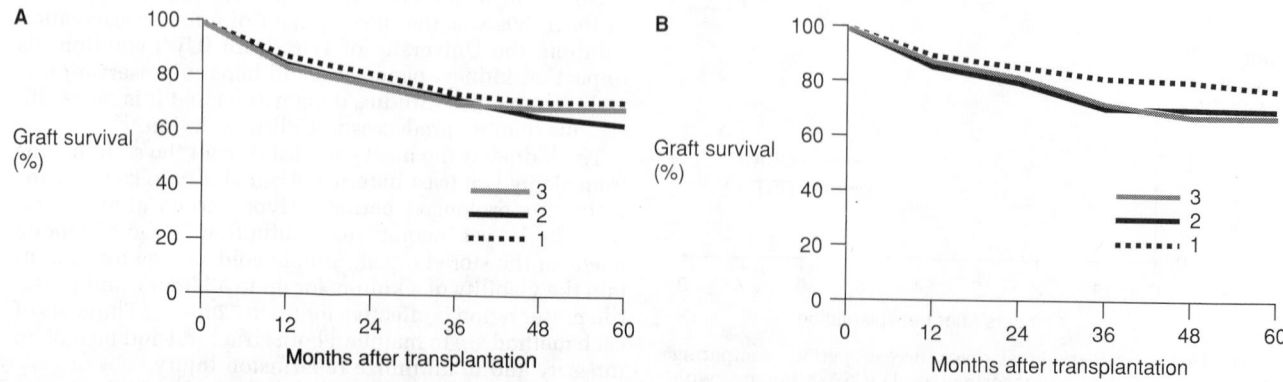

Figure 16-43. Graft survival rates over time of centers 1 through 3 (A) and centers 4 through 6 (B) of the Transplant Information Share Group.

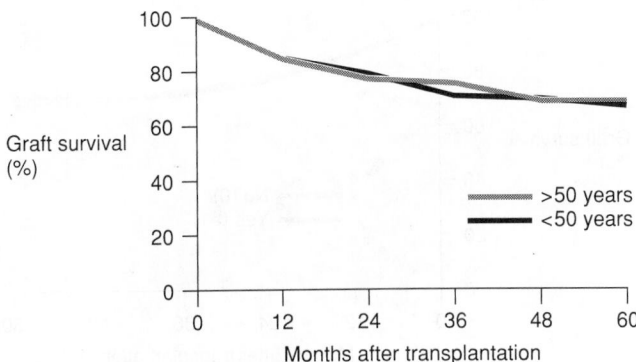

Figure 16-44. Outcome in first cadaveric renal transplant recipients stratified by age.

heartbeating donors are used, the use of machine preservation, to maintain the viability of these organs, may increase.

IMMUNOSUPPRESSION

The success of renal allografting using only azathioprine and prednisone was modest compared with current outcomes. Figure 16-40 outlines the outcomes of recipients of cadaveric transplants treated with azathioprine and prednisone by year through 1983. It also illustrates that beginning in 1984, graft survival improved notably with the introduction of cyclosporine. Outcomes were significantly improved not only in patients receiving their first allografts but also in recipients of repeated transplants in the CSA era (see Fig. 16-41). Several prospective studies have demonstrated statistically improved graft outcomes using this agent. Even in studies that have not demonstrated improvement, the use of cyclosporine has provided the following positive benefits over azathioprine-based immunosuppression:

- Decreased incidence of rejection episodes
- Decreased incidence of infection (particularly CMV)
- Lower cost associated with transplantation
- Shorter hospital stay and fewer readmissions

A number of side effects are associated with the use of cyclosporine. Nephrotoxicity, hypertension, and metabolic effects (including hyperuricemia, hyperkalemia, hypercholesterolemia, and hirsutism) have all been attributed to cyclosporine use. The potent nephrotoxic effects of cyclosporine are the most problematic. In early trials

with cyclosporine, a high incidence of early and prolonged graft dysfunction was recognized. Up to 40% of recipients required dialysis after transplantation. This was coupled with a high incidence of primary nonfunction (ie, grafts that never functioned after transplantation). Additionally, the early baseline graft function of kidneys treated with cyclosporine in the immediate postoperative period was consistently poorer, as reflected by serum creatinine, than baseline function of those treated with azathioprine. From these observations, it was concluded that kidneys already injured by procurement, preservation, and reperfusion were especially vulnerable to cyclosporine nephrotoxicity. As a result, a modification of the posttransplantation immunotherapy that withheld cyclosporine in the early postoperative period was developed. This was termed *sequential therapy*. An antilymphocyte preparation, along with azathioprine and prednisone, was administered initially after transplantation and was followed in sequence by cyclosporine, when acceptable graft function was established. The first report on the outcome of sequential therapy demonstrated excellent graft survival of 89% at 1 year, coupled with a low incidence of immediate renal dysfunction (9%) without any increase in infectious complications (particularly cytomegalovirus) or neoplasms.[221]

Several long-term follow-up studies using the sequential protocol have been reported, and a large multicenter study has confirmed this protocol's efficacy. The Transplant Information Share Group (TISG) is a six-center collaborative study group that examined the outcome of nearly 1000 first cadaveric renal transplantations immunosuppressed with the sequential protocol.[222] The study's purpose was to identify the influence on graft survival of HLA matching and transfusion, using a uniform immunosuppressive protocol designed to maximize immunosuppression and minimize immunologic factors affecting graft survival. The outcome demonstrated excellent patient and graft survival in first-time recipients of cadaveric organs (Fig. 16-43). In addition, the study demonstrated that many previously important risk factors could be abrogated by the judicious use of cyclosporine, especially the need for HLA matching and pretransplantation blood transfusion.

HIGH-RISK GROUPS

In the azathioprine and prednisone era, several immunologic and nonimmunologic risk factors were identified as having an adverse effect on graft outcome. These risk factors included increased age, diabetes, lack of pretransplantation blood transfusions, poor HLA donor–recipient matching, early dysfunction, and retransplantation. With the introduction of cyclosporine, the relevance of these

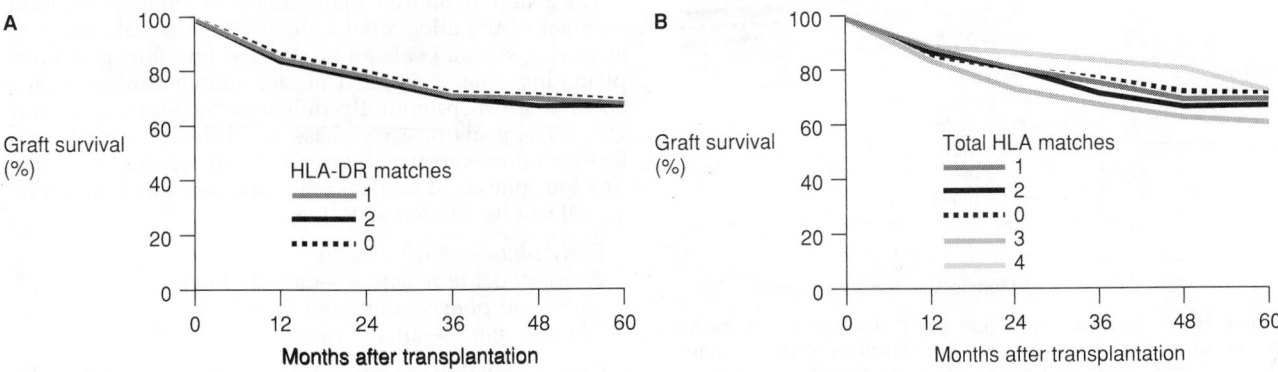

Figure 16-45. Graft survival according to HLA-DR matches (*A*) and total HLA matches (*B*).

risk factors to successful outcome was reevaluated. Historically, renal allograft recipients older than 50 years did poorly compared with their younger counterparts. Much of the graft loss was found to be associated with patient deaths, usually as the result of overwhelming infection. With the cautious use of cyclosporine and prednisone, however, excellent patient and graft survival rates have been reported.[223] With the use of cyclosporine, older patients appear to have fewer rejection episodes, even in the presence of less immunosuppressive medication, which perhaps reflects a less avid immune system. The TISG has demonstrated nearly identical outcomes when graft survival is examined according to age (Fig. 16-44). A careful dosing regimen associated with the more selective immunosuppressive actions of cyclosporine has allowed older patients to receive transplants successfully.

In the first two decades of clinical renal transplantation, diabetes was considered a contraindication to renal transplantation. Current reports demonstrate acceptable patient and graft survival and show that, compared with hemodialysis treatment of diabetic ESRD, patient survival with transplantation is markedly improved. With the introduction of cyclosporine, no difference in outcome was reported when diabetic recipients were compared with nondiabetic recipients.[224] Other large studies have also demonstrated good outcome in diabetic renal allograft recipients. More recently, combined kidney/pancreas transplantation has provided excellent patient and graft survival associated with normalized glucose metabolism and renal function.

A more controversial question deals with the issue of prospective donor–recipient HLA matching. Clear evidence supports a beneficial effect of HLA matching when using immunosuppression confined to azathioprine and prednisone.[225] This benefit is not so clear-cut, however, when cyclosporine is the primary immunosuppressant. Multicenter data demonstrated advantageous posttransplantation outcomes when very well-matched recipients were compared with less well-matched recipients. On the other hand, the TISG and several smaller single-center studies have not demonstrated any clear advantage to matching (Fig. 16-45). It is not easy to explain the disparity between these different studies; however, the best survival in older series (the best-matched group) is relatively equivalent to the overall survival in the TISG and single-center data (Fig. 16-46). This suggests that as graft survival continues to improve, the influence of previously important variables will be more difficult to demonstrate. It also is reasonable to postulate that the use of cyclosporine in protocols

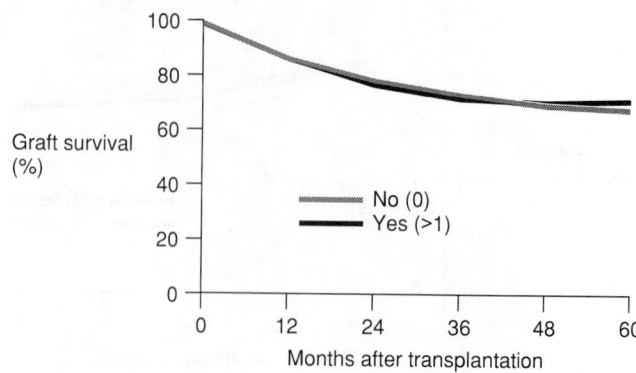

Figure 16-47. Graft survival of Transplant Information Share Group population by presence (Yes) or absence (No) of pretransplantation blood transfusion.

designed to maximize its efficacy (eg, sequential therapy) may override those previously important variables.

Less controversial is the issue of pretransplantation random blood transfusions. Data from the azathioprine and prednisone era show a clear-cut benefit and improved graft survival after multiple random blood transfusions. The TISG and other studies, however, could find no advantage to blood transfusions when cyclosporine is used (Fig. 16-47). Transfused patients have a risk of developing anti-HLA antibodies, making it much more difficult for them to undergo organ transplantation in a timely fashion.

An evolving concept is that the organ's quality the time of transplantation has an important impact on graft survival. A kidney suffering from early dysfunction, as defined by the lack of sustaining renal function in the final posttransplantation week necessitating dialysis, has significantly poorer 1-year graft survival than those with immediate function[222] (Fig. 16-48). This effect has been demonstrated in other large data bases.[226] Black recipients have also been demonstrated to have poorer graft survival than white recipients, even when treated with identical immunosuppressive regimens. This disparity in single-center studies has been wide, and in the UNOS database (multicenter data collection), outcome in black patients is up to 13% poorer at 3 years posttransplantation. Most recently, investigators have shown that graft survival in the black recipient with poorly controlled blood pressure is notably worse than in blacks with normal blood pressure or whites with or without abnormal blood pressure[227] (Fig. 16-49). This study suggests that poorly controlled blood pressure may adversely impact the black recipient.

OUTCOME

The goal of renal transplantation is to achieve long-term survival of the allografted kidney. The clinical course to achieving such a goal can be divided into four posttransplantation phases. In each phase, unique clinical events occur that can profoundly influence long-term graft survival. The goals of each phase are different in that each focuses on preventing and treating a unique set of events. The four phases of clinical renal posttransplantation (Fig. 16-50) can be defined as follows:

Early phase—days 0 to 30
Phase of acute rejection—days 31 to 180
Quiescent phase—days 180 to 365
Chronic phase—after 1 year

Graft survival of the transplanted kidney is traditionally expressed in a graphic demonstration of actuarial probabil-

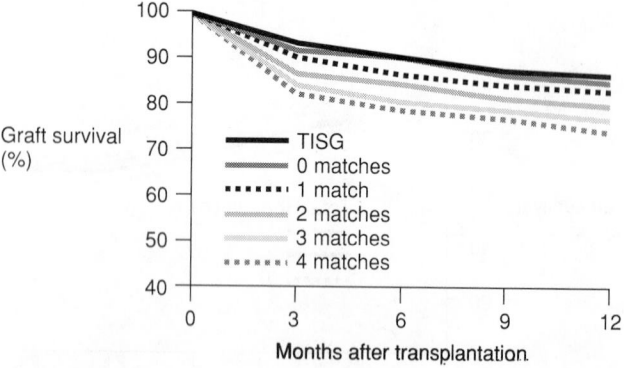

Figure 16-46. Comparison of graft survival in the Collaborative Transplant Study by match versus graft survival of entire Transplant Information Share Group (TISG) population regardless of match.

ity as first described by Kaplan and Meier. There are two ways to lose a graft—either by graft failure alone or by death of the patient regardless of the degree of graft function at the time of death. A review of 607 first cadaveric renal transplantations determined the incidence and timing of graft and patient loss. A total of 146 losses were recorded during a posttransplantation follow-up of between 1 and 8 years. Of these, 70 were graft losses alone and 76 were patient losses, 85% of whom died with normal or near-normal functioning kidneys. More than half the deaths were due to cardiovascular complications, not related to immunosuppression but closely related to comorbid cardiovascular variables present at the time of transplantation. Less than 25% of the deaths were related to immunosuppression.

When the timing, or phase, of graft loss and patient loss are examined in the posttransplantation clinical course, an interesting pattern emerges. Two thirds of all graft losses alone (without death) occur from 1 to 6 months after transplantation. Only 14% of all graft losses occur after 1 year (Table 16-11). In contrast, half of the patient losses (most dying with functioning grafts) occur more than 1 year after transplantation. In the first year after transplantation, graft loss due to rejection is the most common cause of loss. More than 1 year after transplantation, the most common cause of graft loss is patient death. Patient death results primarily from cardiovascular causes, with the graft functioning.

Phase 1

In the first several weeks after transplantation, there are four goals of patient care:

- To prevent patient mortality in the immediate postoperative period
- To achieve immediate function of the transplanted kidney
- To establish a baseline of stable renal function as close to normal as possible
- To prevent an early acute rejection episode

To accomplish these goals, many centers have adopted an immunosuppressive protocol that delays the institution of the nephrotoxic immunosuppressant, cyclosporine, until a baseline of renal function has been established. This usually occurs between 5 and 7 days after transplantation in kidneys transplanted with immediate function. During the first week, a course of prophylactic antilymphocyte globulin (ALG) in conjunction with tapering doses of oral prednisone and azathioprine is often used. Cyclosporine

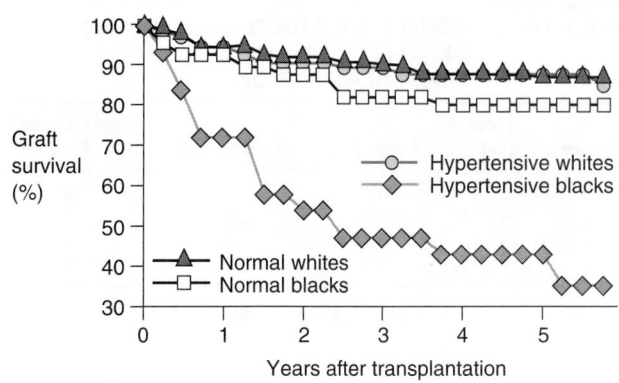

Figure 16-49. Graft survival of cadaveric recipients as function of race and presence or absence of hypertension.

is then begun when the serum creatinine is less than 2.5 mg/dL, usually by the fifth to the seventh day after transplantation. At this time, ALG is discontinued, and the patient is maintained on cyclosporine, prednisone, and azathioprine as a triple maintenance immunosuppression (Fig. 16-51). This protocol accomplishes the goals of achieving good immediate function and preventing early rejection.

The goal of achieving immediate function of the transplanted kidney is very important for several reasons. First, immediate function of the kidney allows a shorter initial hospital stay and greater ease in diagnosing and managing any intervening acute rejection as well as any nephrotoxic side effects of cyclosporine. Second, as previously noted, immediate function is associated with significantly improved short- and long-term graft survival. Therefore, optimal kidney procurement and preservation techniques to achieve immediate function are important determinants of both short- and long-term graft survival.

Phase 2

The period between 1 and 6 months after transplantation is the most active and crucial time in the clinical course of a renal transplant patient. During this time, 63% of all graft losses, 22% of deaths, and 74% of all acute rejection episodes occur (Fig. 16-52). An acute rejection episode in a renal allograft recipient is the single most important clinical event determining both short-term (1-year) and long-term (5-year) graft survival. The incidence of acute rejection using the immunosuppressive protocol described previously is shown in Table 16-12. Two thirds of recipients of first cadaveric renal grafts never have an acute rejection episode, 17% have only one rejection episode, and

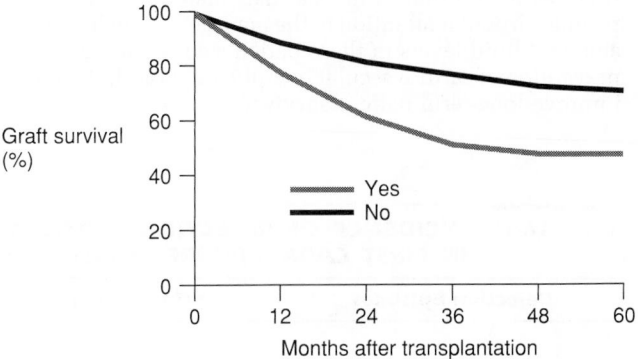

Figure 16-48. Outcome based on the need for (Yes) or lack of (No) hemodialysis after transplantation.

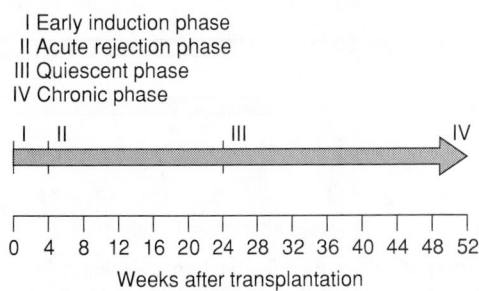

Figure 16-50. Timeline outlining posttransplantation phases.

Table 16-11. TIMING OF GRAFT LOSSES AND DEATHS AFTER RENAL TRANSPLANTATION

Phase	Time (wk)	Total (%)	Deaths (%)	Graft Losses (%)
1	0–4	13	12	14
2	4–24	42	22	63
3	24–48	12	16	9
4	48→	33	50	14

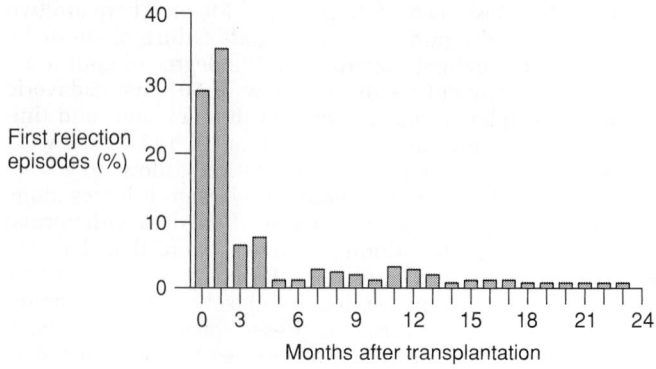

Figure 16-52. Timing of acute rejection episodes.

19% have two or more. Fortunately, acute rejection can be diagnosed and successfully treated in over 80% of cases. The impact of this clinical event, however, is substantial (Fig. 16-53). The 1-year graft survival for patients having no rejection episode is 90%; for those who have only one rejection episode, it is 67%; and for those having two or more rejection episodes, it is 60%. Although there is an impact on short-term survival, the influence of acute rejection is also evident in long-term graft survival. For the 64% of patients who never experience an acute rejection episode, 5-year graft survival is 87%. For those patients having only one rejection episode that is successfully treated, the graft survival (see Fig. 16-53) drops to 50%. For those with two or more acute rejection episodes, there is only 20% graft survival at 5 years. Thus, the occurrence an acute rejection episode during phase 2 is a highly significant determinant of long-term graft survival despite the ability to successfully treat the episode.

It appears that *chronic rejection,* the slowly progressive loss of renal function that happens over months, occurs predominately in patients who have had a previous, successfully treated acute rejection episode.[228,229] The incidence of graft loss due to chronic rejection in patients who had two or more acute rejection episodes is apparent (see Fig. 16-53).

The manner in which a single acute rejection episode is treated can significantly influence the subsequent degree of chronic graft loss experienced over the next several years (Fig. 16-54). The three treatment modalities commonly used in one study were oral high-dose prednisone alone, oral prednisone with ALG, and oral prednisone with OKT3.[230] ALG is made from equine serum that has been hyperimmunized to human lymphocytes. OKT3 is a murine monoclonal antibody that is a pure IgG with exquisite specificity for the human CD3 complex, an integral part of

the human T-cell receptor. The 1-year graft survival of those treated with prednisone alone is about 72%, with survival for prednisone and ALG at 69%. Patients treated with OKT3 and prednisone have an 88% 1-year graft survival rate. This difference is amplified at 3 years, with the OKT3 and prednisone group having an 82% 3-year graft survival rate compared with 55% and 50% graft survival rates for those treated with prednisone alone or prednisone in combination with ALG, respectively.

These data suggest that the events of phase 2, although occurring in the first few months after transplantation, have far-reaching implications. The occurrence of an acute rejection episode and the manner in which it is treated profoundly influence the long-term fate of an allografted kidney.

Phase 3

Phase 3 is the posttransplantation period that begins at 6 months and continues to the 1-year mark. This often is a quiescent time with few influential clinical events. During this period, only 9% of all graft losses and 9% of all acute rejection episodes occur.

Phase 4

The fourth phase after renal transplantation is the chronic phase, which begins at 1 year after transplantation and continues thereafter. The most characteristic feature of this period is the low frequency of acute rejection: only 7% of all acute rejection episodes occur after 1 year. In addition, only 14% of all graft losses (alone) occur after 1 year. The most prominent feature of this phase is patient loss. Half of all deaths after transplantation occur after 1 year, making death of the recipient the most common cause of graft loss in this period. Because most posttransplantation deaths are due to myocardial infarction and stroke, paying particular attention to the management of hypertension and lipid levels in these patients could influence the prevention of cardiovascular complications and, therefore, improve long-term patient survival.

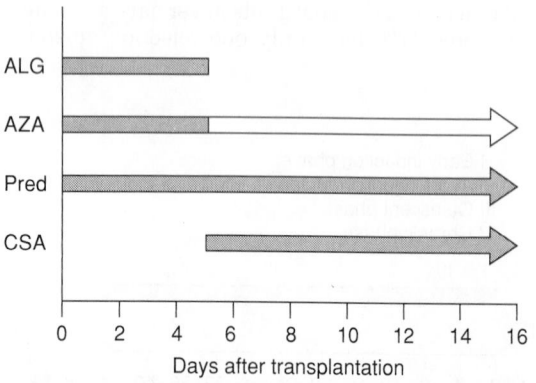

Figure 16-51. Outline of sequential immunotherapy by days after transplantation. ALG, antilymphoblast globulin; AZA, azathioprine; pred, prednisone; CSA, cyclosporine.

Table 16-12. INCIDENCE OF REJECTION EPISODES IN FIRST CADAVERIC RECIPIENTS

Rejection Episodes	Incidence (%)
0	64
1	17
>1	19

COMPLICATIONS

Posttransplantation complications can be categorized as early or late. Most early complications are caused by infections, which range from simple wound infections to overwhelming bacterial or fungal sepsis. The scourge of transplantation over the years has been cytomegalovirus infection. This virus has a host of presentations, from mild temperature elevations to deadly multisystem involvement. In the cyclosporine era, the incidence of infection with this virus appears to have decreased. Newer management strategies using prophylactic acyclovir also have been found to decrease the occurrence of this virus. The development of ganciclovir, with specific efficacy against cytomegalovirus, has also lowered the overall impact of established cytomegalovirus infections.

Other early problems include urologic complications, which occur in about 3% to 5% of cases. These are usually urine leaks associated with either distal ureteral necrosis or bladder leaks or ureteral obstruction secondary to a lymphocele. The former can often be handled conservatively with percutaneous ureteral drainage and stenting or Foley catheter drainage. Ureteral obstruction requires drainage of the isolated retroperitoneal lymph collection into the abdominal cavity by creating a peritoneal window. This decompresses the ureter and normalizes renal function.

The major late complication is renal artery stenosis. Renal artery stenosis may be heralded by uncontrolled hypertension and is diagnosed by renal transplantation angiography. Percutaneous balloon angioplasty or operative repair can be employed to correct the abnormality.

CONCLUSION

Renal transplantation in the latter half of the 1990s has a favorable outlook. Living, related donor–recipient combinations have been liberalized to increase the donor pool. Cadaveric transplantation continues with graft and patient survival improving as the subtleties of immunosuppression are more fully recognized. Preservation modalities continue to demonstrate increasing prolongation of graft viability and improvement in the incidence of early dysfunction. Previously important high-risk variables have been abrogated as the result of a better understanding of clinical care of the renal transplant recipient. Newer, novel immunosuppressants and the impact on graft and patient outcome are undergoing rigid clinical testing. The clinical course of the recipient continues to be defined and refined by large clinical experiences.

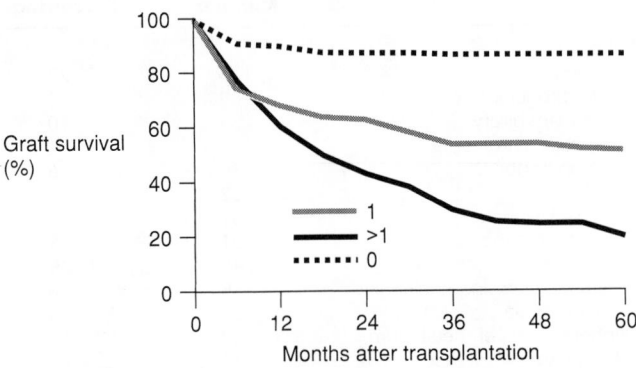

Figure 16-53. Impact of the number of rejection episodes on graft survival.

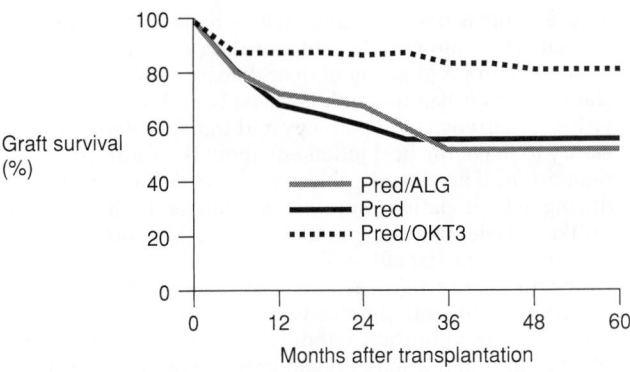

Figure 16-54. Outcome of first rejection episode by treatment modality. OKT3, murine monoclonal antibody; pred, prednisone; ALG, antilymphoblast globulin.

Hepatic Transplantation

DARRELL A. CAMPBELL, JR., JOHN M. HAM,
JEREMIAH G. TURCOTTE, AND ROBERT M. MERION

The evolution of hepatic transplantation has been remarkably rapid. Only within the past decade have technical and immunologic problems been surmounted to the extent that a high level of success with this procedure is now achieved. Among the many pioneers in this area, Thomas Starzl from the University of Pittsburgh and Roy Calne from Cambridge University stand out. Starzl developed the modern transplantation technique and its clinical application, and Calne was responsible for introducing cyclosporine into clinical practice with parallel development of operative technique. The information presented here derives directly or indirectly from information originally contributed by these two people.

INDICATIONS FOR HEPATIC TRANSPLANTATION

General Considerations

The most common indication for hepatic transplantation is end-stage liver disease (ESLD), which typically results in the demise of the patient within 1 year and for which no other therapy is effective or suitable. Attempting hepatic transplantation thus entails making two determinations. First, it must be determined that the patient actually has ESLD, and second, it must be determined when, in the course of the end-stage disease, transplantation should be done. In practice, the first determination is considerably easier than the second.

The term *end-stage* refers to the culmination of a variety of pathologic processes that leave the damaged liver with minimal function and no potential for recovery. This important assessment is made primarily on a histologic basis and supplemented by clinical information. For example, the patient presenting with liver failure and a history of alcoholism might have ESLD or might suffer instead from acute alcoholic hepatitis, a reversible disorder. The distinction could be made by biopsy and would be confirmed by improvement in the absence of alcohol. Many other clinical situations occur in which ESLD must be accurately distinguished from acute liver failure with a reversible component, particularly acute viral hepatitis or drug toxicity.

The rate of progression of liver disease from a functional state to invalidism to death is variable and may be several years. Experience in hepatology and transplantation is necessary to make the best judgment about the timing of transplantation. The overall objective is to define the period during which patient survival for longer than 1 year is unlikely. Delaying transplantation until this point assumes that maximum benefit will be obtained from the native liver and also recognizes that best results are obtained if transplantation is done electively, not in an emergency.

How is the important window of opportunity for transplantation determined? Considerable experience with the complications of liver failure have pointed to certain ominous predictors of reduced (6 months or less) survival. Such factors include rapidly deepening jaundice, diuretic-resistant ascites, spontaneous hepatic encephalopathy, recurrent sepsis (including spontaneous bacterial peritonitis), recurrent variceal hemorrhage, and prolongation of the prothrombin time to more than 8 seconds above control values in spite of adequate vitamin K replacement.[231] Emergence of any such condition makes the decision for transplantation relatively clear-cut. If one is to err in this decision-making process, it should be toward earlier transplantation, since inordinate conservatism usually results in the calamitous occurrence of all complications of liver failure at once, with predictable results. Another factor that supports earlier transplantation candidacy is the unpredictable nature of donor organ availability.

The important but intangible indication of patient fatigue often enters into the decision to perform the transplantation procedure. Severe fatigue is a common complaint of the patient with ESLD. Inability to perform activities of daily living and resultant depression are indications for surgery. No great benefit is obtained by postponing transplantation if the patient is left with a miserable, dependent life-style. Similarly, intractable pruritus associated with severe liver disease is occasionally the primary indication for transplantation because the resultant impairment of the patient's quality of life is so profound.

Although these considerations apply to the more chronic forms of liver failure, important emergency decisions about transplantation must be made when the patient presents with fulminant hepatic failure, defined as the progression from good health to liver failure with hepatic encephalopathy within 8 weeks. A certain percentage of these patients recover spontaneously but most do not. The decision to perform transplantation is based on clinical grounds. The most important consideration is the rate of neurologic deterioration. Surgery is indicated if the patient progresses to stage III (stuporous) or IV (unresponsive) coma with documentation of severe hepatic insufficiency, the most reliable indicator being a factor V level of less than 20%.

The number of absolute contraindications to hepatic transplantation has decreased during the past several years as experience with the procedure has increased. The absolute contraindications for transplantation are inability to withstand the operative procedure, usually for cardiovascular or pulmonary reasons, recent intracranial hemorrhage or irreversible neurologic impairment, active substance abuse, intractable hypotension requiring pressor support, evidence of infection with human immunodeficiency virus, ongoing bacterial infection, and extrahepatic malignancy.

A number of medical conditions are no longer considered absolute contraindications to hepatic transplantation. For instance, a thrombosed portal vein is no longer a contraindication to transplantation because techniques have been devised to bypass or disobliterate the obstructed seg-

ment. The associated comorbidity of juvenile-onset diabetes mellitus formerly precluded transplantation. In current practice, this is not necessarily the case, depending on the patient's physiologic status at the time of evaluation. Renal insufficiency, either end-stage or relative, clearly increases the morbidity of the hepatic transplantation but is not a contraindication. Renal transplantation can be done at the time of hepatic transplantation, and some degree of preoperative renal insufficiency often is reversible after successful hepatic transplantation. Advanced age (more than 70 years) is a relative contraindication to surgery, but in most centers, the physiologic state of the patient is a more important consideration than the chronologic age.

Specific Diseases for Which Transplantation Is Appropriate

In the absence of contraindications, virtually any disease resulting in liver failure is amenable to treatment. The causes of liver failure in 539 patients undergoing hepatic transplantations are shown in Table 16-13. A brief description of some of the more common diseases encountered in an hepatic transplantation center follows.

Primary Biliary Cirrhosis

Primary biliary cirrhosis, thought to be autoimmune in nature, has a relatively predictable clinical course, characterized by gradually increasing serum bilirubin levels and progressive fatigue. Early stages of the disease are usually asymptomatic, and disease progression may evolve over 20 years. Transplantation is commonly considered appropriate when the serum bilirubin reaches 10 mg/dL.

Primary Sclerosing Cholangitis

Primary sclerosing cholangitis is a common indication for transplantation since there is no other effective treatment. In addition to the usual considerations about the timing of transplantation, two other features are important. First, recurrent cholangitis should speed the decision to transplant since a chronically infected liver makes the transplantation process more difficult and dangerous. Second, primary sclerosing cholangitis is often indistinguishable from cholangiocarcinoma, and any doubt about the

---

Table 16-13. CAUSES OF LIVER FAILURE IN 539 PATIENTS UNDERGOING PRIMARY HEPATIC TRANSPLANTATIONS

	Number	Percentage
Cirrhosis		
Laennec	125	23
Cryptogenic	69	13
Primary biliary	55	10
Hepatitis, chronic		
Non-A, non-B	30	6
B	22	4
C	31	6
Autoimmune	31	6
Fulminant	49	9
Primary sclerosing cholangitis	35	6
Biliary atresia	31	6
Inborn errors of metabolism	32	6
Neoplasm	17	3
Budd-Chiari syndrome	10	2
Iatrogenic	2	—

diagnosis warrants earlier consideration of transplantation. In most cases, colectomy for associated inflammatory bowel disease is done after successful transplantation since the failing liver would make the patient a poor candidate for a large abdominal procedure. Because transplantation is successful treatment, preoperative management should be limited to percutaneous methods of biliary decompression and stricture dilatation. Operative biliary decompression is usually no more effective than percutaneous techniques, and it increases the risk of subsequent transplantation by producing adhesions in the right upper quadrant.

Non-A, Non-B Hepatitis

Hepatitis C is probably the most common cause of the disorder referred to as non-A, non-B hepatitis, but other as yet uncharacterized viruses undoubtedly play a role as well. Recurrence of viral hepatitis in the transplanted liver occurs, but it usually follows an indolent course. Results of transplantation for this disease are comparable to the other noninfectious conditions.

Biliary Atresia

Biliary atresia is by far the most common indication for hepatic transplantation in pediatric patients. Recommended treatment includes creation of a portoenterostomy (Kasai procedure), if this can be done before 3 months of age. After this point, success rates diminish markedly. Five-year survival rates after a Kasai procedure range from 37% to 50%.[232] Growth and nutritional failure, the development of portal hypertension with variceal hemorrhage, and recurrent cholangitis are indications for hepatic transplantation. In patients with an unsatisfactory course, multiple revisions of the portoenterostomy should be avoided to facilitate subsequent transplantation.

Inherited Metabolic Disorders

Among the more interesting indications for transplantation are the inherited metabolic disorders. Some enzymatic deficiencies in this group result in destruction of the liver so transplantation may resolve the liver failure as well as supply the missing enzyme. Disorders in this category are Wilson disease, α_1-antitrypsin deficiency, tyrosinemia, and type I glycogen storage disease. In other cases, the liver is not affected by the disease, and transplantation is undertaken solely as enzyme replacement therapy. Diseases that have been cured by hepatic transplantation in this category are hemophilia A or B, homozygous familial hypercholesterolemia, Niemann-Pick disease, and oxalosis.

Fulminant Hepatic Failure

The most common causes of fulminant hepatic failure are non-A, non-B hepatitis, hepatitis B, and various drug toxicities. In the latter group, acetaminophen toxicity is particularly prominent.

Budd-Chiari Syndrome

Budd-Chiari syndrome is characterized by obliteration of the hepatic veins and presents as the triad of right upper quadrant pain, hepatomegaly, and ascites. A side-to-side portocaval shunt, in which the portal vein serves as an outflow tract for the congested liver, is the preferred therapy for cases not yet complicated by the development of cirrhosis. Transplantation is reserved for cases that present as liver cell failure, cases in which preoperative studies document no significant pressure gradient between portal vein and the inferior vena cava, and cases in which there is associated portal vein or inferior vena caval thrombosis.

Alcoholic Liver Disease

In some centers, a great reluctance exists toward transplantation of patients who have a long history of alcoholism. On a clinical level, the concern has been that these patients may relapse into alcoholism after transplantation, with medical noncompliance and consequent graft failure. On a broader level, concern has been expressed that society should not pay for expensive treatments for diseases caused by self-destructive behavior. With more experience in this area, it has been recognized that the incidence of recidivism after transplantation is low, and results in this category are as good as for non–alcohol-related categories. With regard to social policy, firm guidelines have not yet been established, but two points seem relevant. First, society already supports the concept of medical care for other types of self-destructive behavior, such as for the complications of cigarette smoking. Second, transplantation costs for treating alcoholics do not seem as expensive when viewed in the context of obligatory costs for other treatments for the same disorder, such as portocaval shunting. The decision to perform liver transplantation for an alcoholic patient should be made only after careful examination by an experienced substance abuse specialist, including documentation of adequate patient insight and family support.

In a medical context, alcoholic patients considered for transplantation are those who have failed sclerotherapy and who are in Child classification B or C. Child class A patients suffering from alcoholism are usually treated with a distal splenorenal shunt if sclerotherapy has failed. An alcoholic patient with life-threatening variceal hemorrhage that did not respond to sclerotherapy or other nonoperative measures should undergo a mesocaval shunt if transplantation is contemplated. This type of decompressive procedure effectively controls variceal hemorrhage but does not distort right upper quadrant anatomy such that subsequent transplantation is made more difficult.

Primary Liver Tumors

Primary hepatic malignancy, most often hepatoma or cholangiocarcinoma, is sometimes an indication for transplantation, but the results are substantially worse than in most other disease states because of recurrent disease. Transplantation is justified in the occasional case in which the tumor is central but relatively small, the patient is otherwise healthy, and there is no evidence of extrahepatic disease after exhaustive evaluation. Typically, a back-up recipient is in the hospital available for transplantation if it is not possible to proceed with the planned transplantation.

Hepatitis B

All patients with hepatitis B who undergo transplantation become reinfected. The progression of the disease varies, ranging from the asymptomatic carrier state of chronic antigenemia to early cirrhosis and death. Transplantation for this indication carries a poorer prognosis than for most other indications but is still done in most centers because the patients are usually young and there is no acceptable alternative. A lower percentage of patients survive for long periods.

PREOPERATIVE ASSESSMENT AND MANAGEMENT

Urgent Transplantation

The patient with an acutely failing liver presents with varying degrees of hemodynamic instability and multiorgan failure. It is possible to achieve good transplantation results if the process has not progressed too far before admission and if aggressive treatment strategies are employed.

On first assessment, a careful neurologic examination must be done, and the coma grade should be determined. Patients in grade IV coma (unresponsive) benefit from constant monitoring of intracranial pressure (ICP). An ICP monitor may be placed in the subdural space in the operating room. An epidural location is chosen if bleeding is excessive. An attempt is made to keep cerebral perfusion pressure (mean arterial blood pressure minus intracranial pressure) above 60 mmHg. A low mean arterial blood pressure is treated with pressors, and elevation of ICP is treated with hyperventilation and mannitol. Severe elevations of ICP may result in brain death. Hemodynamic stability is maintained by monitoring intravascular volume. Expansion of the intravascular volume may be limited by considerations about ICP, in which case temporary inotropic support is required. Acute renal failure is managed with continuous arteriovenous hemofiltration with or without dialysis, and this may be continued intraoperatively. Because the acutely failing liver produces an acutely failing reticuloendothelial system, florid sepsis often ensues, and broad-spectrum antibiotics are required. Pulmonary insufficiency is a common accompaniment of liver failure and is managed with intubation, high concentration of inspired oxygen, and, if necessary, positive end-expiratory pressure.

Elective Transplantation

Under elective conditions, the potential candidate for hepatic transplantation is usually presented to a multidisciplinary committee for evaluation. Assuming an acceptable indication and no contraindications, attention is directed to the patient's psychological profile and family support resources. These factors are of immense importance because the transplantation process requires a lifelong commitment to a complex medical regimen that involves daily immunosuppression and follow-up care. A history of substance abuse requires careful evaluation by specialists. Demonstrated noncompliance with other types of medical therapy, lack of insight and willingness to confront the issue of substance abuse, and lack of a satisfactory support structure are factors that may make transplantation a poor choice for a patient.

After a decision for hepatic transplantation is made, it is common to wait for several months for a suitable donor organ to become available. During this interval, surveillance of the patient by the transplantation team is required so that rapid deterioration is recognized and treated. Encephalopathy is treated with lactulose and protein restriction, variceal hemorrhage with sclerotherapy, and refractory ascites with large-volume paracentesis. Spontaneous bacterial peritonitis requires hospital admission and antibiotic therapy.

HEPATIC TRANSPLANTATION PROCEDURE

Anesthetic Management

Because most patients report for hepatic transplantation procedures without an opportunity for extensive preoperative preparation, induction of anesthesia is conducted, assuming that the patient has a full stomach, with rapid sequence technique and cricoid pressure. After intubation, anesthesia is maintained with a combination of inhalation agent and intravenous infusions of paralytic and analgesic drugs. Patients at high risk for cardiovascular problems are often treated with high-dose narcotic technique. Multiple vascular access lines are then placed for monitoring and administration of blood and blood products. Two 8.5F cannulas are placed in the central venous system by internal jugular or subclavian puncture for transfusion through a rapid infusion device. A balloon-tipped flow-directed pulmonary artery catheter is also inserted. Two arterial lines are placed, one in the radial artery for continuous arterial blood pressure monitoring and a second in the right femoral artery for periodic blood sampling.

Intraoperative Management of Coagulopathy

Bleeding during hepatic transplantation ranges from trivial to torrential. For the most part, administration of blood and blood products during the procedure is dictated more by the central filling pressures, as indicated by the pulmonary artery diastolic pressure, than by estimated blood loss on the operative field. The latter is notoriously inaccurate, and updated estimates lag behind the patient's needs. Early in the operation, preexisting coagulopathy may dictate the use of fresh frozen plasma, cryoprecipitate, and platelet transfusions, but usually these components are reserved for use later in the procedure. Packed red blood cells (RBCs) are generally required during the preliminary dissection of the diseased recipient liver.

Evaluating the patient's coagulation status during the transplantation procedure requires frequent determinations of standard parameters, such as prothrombin time, partial thromboplastin time, factor levels, and platelet count. These are determined every hour or two. The use of intraoperative thromboelastography facilitates decision making by rapidly identifying which components of the coagulation cascade are deficient and by easily identifying the presence of a fibrinolytic state. This technique relies on measurements of the resistance to movement of a fine wire traveling through a defined arc in a sample of blood.[233] A strain gauge connected to a strip recorder provides a record of changes over time as blood coagulation occurs, and a variety of measurements are made on the tracing (Fig. 16-55). A range of normal and abnormal thromboelastography tracings is shown in Figure 16-56.

Starting with the anhepatic phase, when the recipient liver is devascularized, a period of fibrinolysis and coagulation failure occurs. This failure is due to the complete cessation of production of hepatic coagulation proteins and fibrinolysis inhibitors and to the inability of the liver to metabolize profibrinolytic compounds. Replacing coagulation factors with fresh frozen plasma and cryoprecipitate is important during this phase.

After revascularization of the donor liver, surgical bleeding may occur. Once this is controlled, a second period of coagulopathy, also characterized by fibrinolysis, may occur. This second fibrinolytic phase results from products of the ischemia and reperfusion injury sustained by the donor organ. This phase usually develops within 1 or 2 hours after revascularization and may be severe, although spontaneous resolution is the rule rather than the exception. When fibrinolysis is unusually severe or persistent, antifibrinolytic therapy with ϵ-aminocaproic acid is helpful. A loading dose of 5 g is given intravenously, and further doses of 1 g/h may be given if necessary until the period of fibrinolysis has

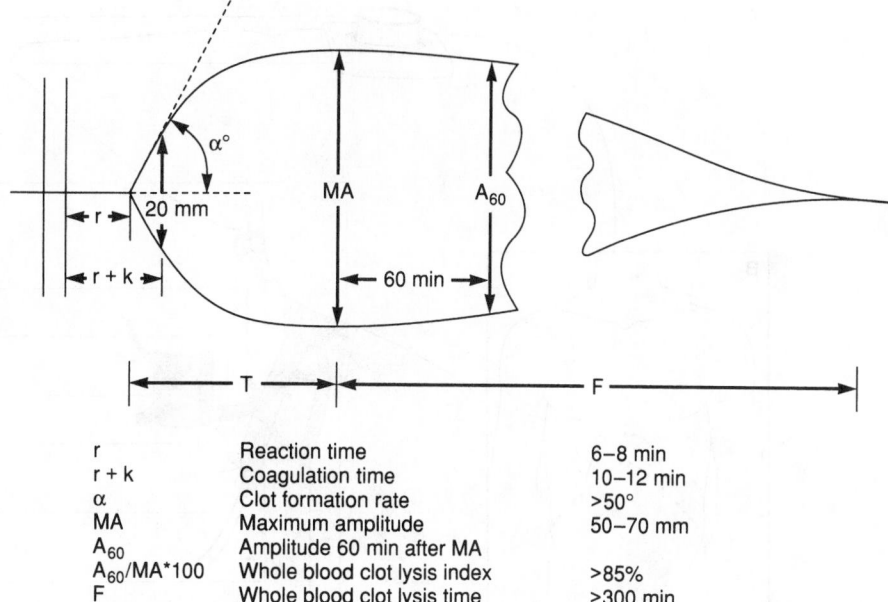

Figure 16-55. Schematic tracing of thromboelastogram. Reaction time (r) represents the initiation of coagulation through the intrinsic system, primarily reflecting the activity of factors XII, XI, and VIII. Coagulation time (r+k) adds the effects of platelets and fibrinogen. Maximum amplitude (MA) is a qualitative measure of clot quality and is mainly affected by platelets, fibrinogen, and factor XIII. Any marked reduction from MA to A_{60} is indicative of clot lysis.

r	Reaction time	6–8 min
r + k	Coagulation time	10–12 min
α	Clot formation rate	>50°
MA	Maximum amplitude	50–70 mm
A_{60}	Amplitude 60 min after MA	
A_{60}/MA*100	Whole blood clot lysis index	>85%
F	Whole blood clot lysis time	>300 min

passed. It is important to discontinue ε-aminocaproic acid therapy as soon as possible to avoid the potential complications of intravascular thrombus formation or complete thrombosis of major vessels.

Surgical Technique

Transplantation of the liver is one of the most technically demanding surgical procedures.[234] Conceptually, hepatic transplantation may be thought of as comprising three distinct sequential phases. The first phase involves the preliminary dissection and skeletonization of the recipient's diseased liver. The second phase, known as the anhepatic phase, refers to the period starting with devascularization of the recipient's liver and placement of the patient on venovenous bypass and ending with revascularization of the newly implanted organ. The third phase is the period after revascularization that includes biliary reconstruction and abdominal closure. The following sections describe the surgical technique of hepatic transplantation, emphasizing the potential pitfalls and detailing various strategies for circumventing the many technical challenges that may confront the transplantation surgeon during this formidable procedure.

Dissection of Recipient Liver

After the anesthetic preparation, the patient's chest, abdomen, left axilla, and left groin are prepared with a povidone-iodine solution and draped as a single large surgical field. The most commonly employed incision is a bilateral subcostal incision with an upper midline extension to the xiphoid process (Fig. 16-57). The incision is carried into the peritoneal cavity and is held open with a mechanical retractor, providing excellent exposure of the entire upper abdomen. Accumulated ascitic fluid is aspirated and sent for cell count and culture. The ligamentum teres hepatis is carefully divided between clamps, and sutures are transfixed because a large recanalized umbilical vein is often present in patients with severe portal hypertension.

After inspection of the liver for unforeseen abnormalities, such as an unsuspected hepatoma in a cirrhotic liver, attention is directed to dissecting and skeletonizing the

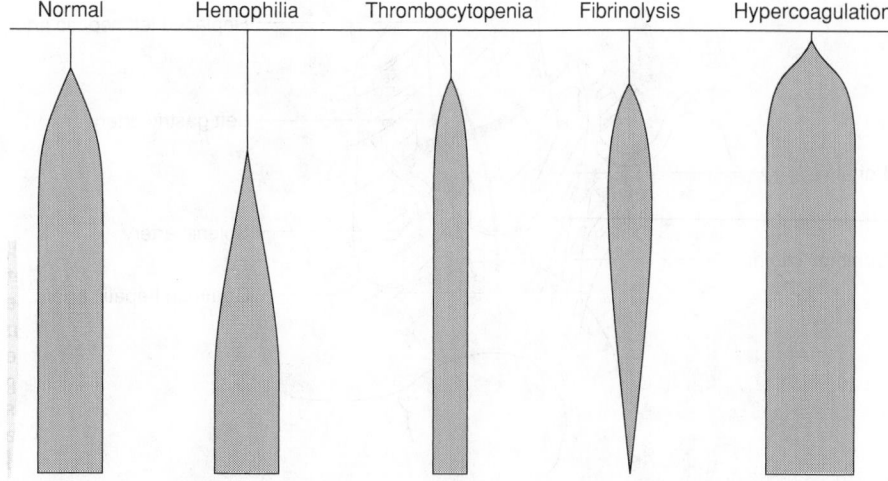

Figure 16-56. Thromboelastogram patterns. The characteristics of a normal thromboelastogram tracing is shown at left. Also shown are various disease states representing specific factor deficiency (hemophilia), insufficient numbers of platelets (thrombocytopenia), clot lysis (fibrinolysis), and a hypercoagulable state.

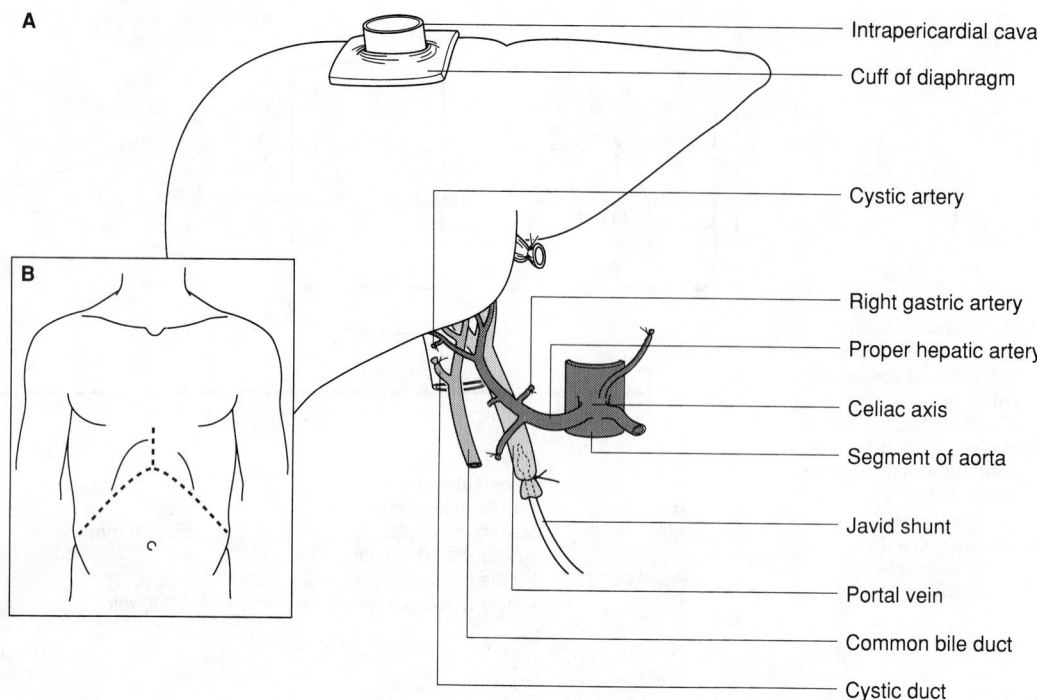

A

B

- Intrapericardial cava
- Cuff of diaphragm
- Cystic artery
- Right gastric artery
- Proper hepatic artery
- Celiac axis
- Segment of aorta
- Javid shunt
- Portal vein
- Common bile duct
- Cystic duct

Figure 16-57. (*A*) The donor liver after excision and before transplantation. (*B*) Bilateral subcostal incision with a subxiphoid extension.

structures of the portal triad. The hepatic artery can be palpated in the anteromedial aspect of the portal triad. Palpation posterior to the common bile duct and lateral to the portal vein reveals the presence of a replaced right hepatic artery. Inspection of the pars flaccida of the lesser omentum along the lesser curvature of the stomach demonstrates a replaced left hepatic artery arising from the left gastric artery (Fig. 16-58). The proper hepatic artery is freed from the gastroduodenal artery to its bifurcation into the left and right hepatic arterial branches.

The common bile duct is dissected from below the level of the cystic duct entrance to the bifurcation of the com-

mon hepatic duct in the hilum of the liver. The cystic duct and proximal common hepatic duct are divided. Frequently, collateral venous channels are present running along the course of the bile duct. Care must be exercised during dissection in this area, or significant hemorrhage may occur. In addition, the major blood supply to the distal recipient common bile duct comes from branches of the hepatic artery, so extensive skeletonization of the distal duct should be avoided.

Once the bile duct and the hepatic artery are freed from surrounding tissues, the portal vein can be easily approached from its anterior, medial, and lateral aspects. An-

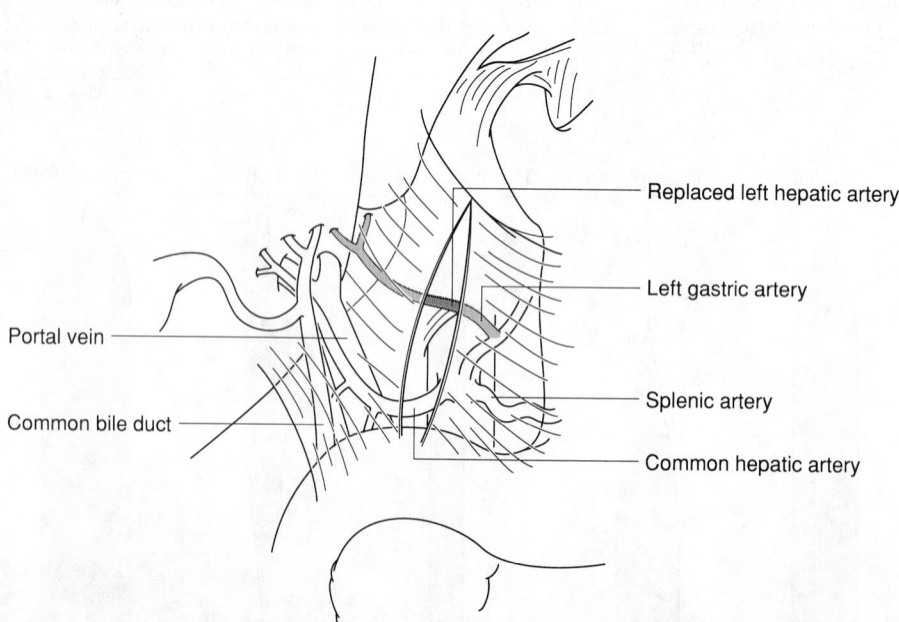

- Replaced left hepatic artery
- Left gastric artery
- Splenic artery
- Common hepatic artery

Portal vein

Common bile duct

Figure 16-58. A replaced left hepatic artery usually arises as a branch of the left gastric artery, traversing the pars flaccida of the lesser omentum from left to right toward the left lobe of the liver.

terior branches are rarely found in the portal vein, even in the presence of severe portal hypertension. Thus, dissection is commenced anteriorly between the bile duct and the hepatic artery. The portal vein should be freed over most of its length from the pancreas to the bifurcation in the hepatic hilum to facilitate placement of the venovenous bypass cannula, described later. Dissection to the confluence of the superior mesenteric and splenic veins may be necessary if the main portal vein is thrombosed and cannot be disobliterated.

Next, the infrahepatic inferior vena cava is mobilized in the retroperitoneum. Large collateral veins may be encountered, and care must be exercised to prevent injury to the renal veins as they enter the vena cava. An avascular plane is generally present behind the vena cava in the segment between the renal veins and the right adrenal vein where it enters the retrohepatic vena cava (Fig. 16-59). Patients with cirrhosis, and especially those with Budd-Chiari syndrome, may have a greatly enlarged caudate lobe, increasing the difficulty of surrounding the vena cava below the liver. Individual hepatic veins draining the caudate lobe may need to be divided to increase the length of infrahepatic vena cava.

The remaining ligamentous attachments of the liver are then divided. The falciform and left triangular ligaments are divided. The coronary ligaments and bare area of the liver are dissected, with care taken to avoid injury to the phrenic or hepatic veins, eventually freeing the suprahepatic inferior vena cava where it traverses the diaphragm. During mobilization of the bare area, the right lobe of the liver is displaced medially to expose, ligate, and divide the right adrenal vein as it enters the retrohepatic vena cava. In some cases, most commonly with Budd-Chiari syndrome, the bare area of the liver and the area around the suprahepatic vena cava may be so densely fibrotic and filled with collaterals that safe dissection is impossible. Transdiaphragmatic exposure of the intrapericardial por-

tion of the inferior vena cava is recommended under these circumstances[235] (Fig. 16-60).

Anhepatic Phase and Implantation of the Donor Liver

At this stage, the liver has been skeletonized sufficiently to permit its rapid removal, and preparations are made for venovenous bypass. Although venovenous bypass is not used routinely by some centers performing hepatic transplantation, this technique has many advantages, and most hepatic transplantation groups advocate its use.[236] Maintenance of venous return from the kidneys and lower extremities during the anhepatic phase results in a smoother hemodynamic course for most patients, allowing time for a more deliberate approach to hemostasis of the right upper quadrant after recipient hepatectomy and before implantation of the hepatic allograft. Renal functional abnormalities also appear to be less common in recipients transplanted under the protection of venovenous bypass.

Venovenous bypass is accomplished from the portal vein and inferior vena cava (Fig. 16-61). Cannulas are placed percutaneously in the femoral and internal jugular vein and advanced into the inferior and superior vena cava, respectively. Inferior vena caval blood is delivered to the superior vena cava by a centrifugal pump. The cannulas, tubing, and centrifugal pump head undergo a heparin-bonding process to reduce the chances of thrombus formation and subsequent embolism, and flow rates of 1 to 2 L/min are usual. Once venovenous bypass has been established, the recipient hepatectomy is completed. After division of the left and right hepatic arteries, the portal vein is divided, and the splanchnic side of the portal vein is added to the venovenous bypass circuit using a Y connection. This results in total bypass flow rates of 2 to 3 L/min. Flow rates greater than 3 L/min may be associated with an increased risk of RBC hemolysis. At this point, the anhepatic phase begins.

The recipient hepatectomy is continued by dividing the

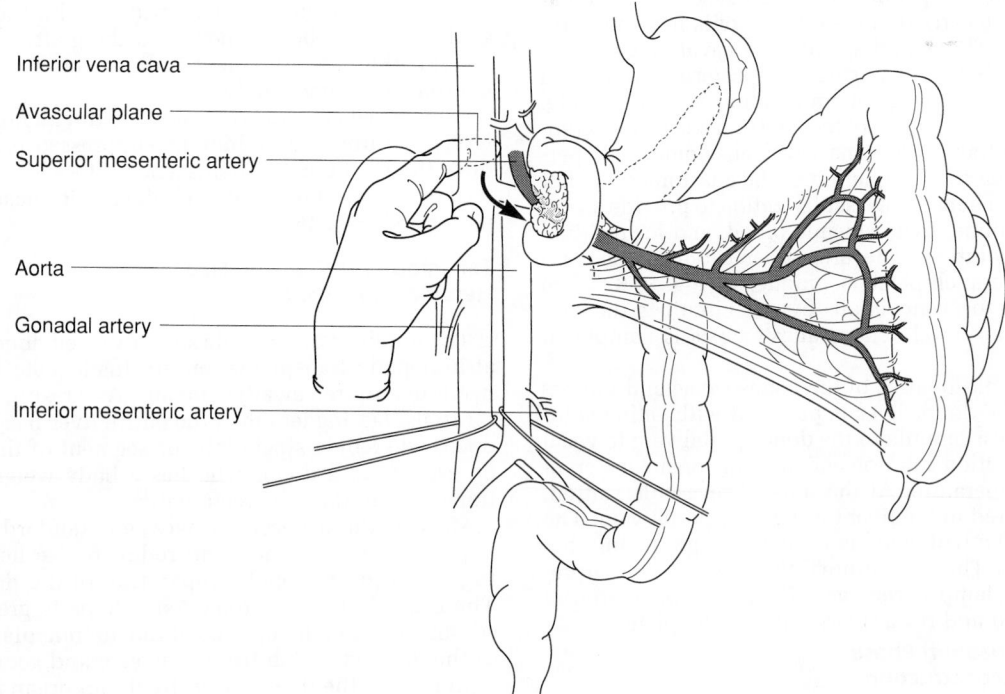

Figure 16-59. A finger is gently used to dissect bluntly in the avascular plane behind the inferior vena cava, superior to the right renal vein and inferior to the right adrenal vein.

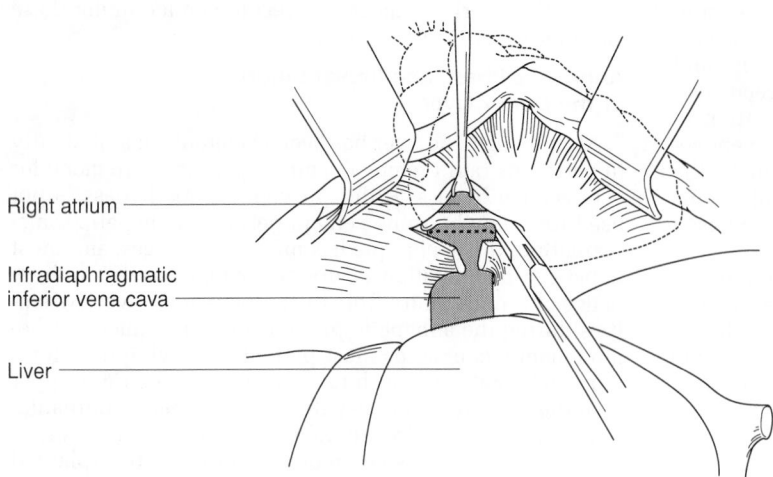

Right atrium

Infradiaphragmatic
inferior vena cava

Liver

Figure 16-60. If the suprahepatic vena cava cannot be safely dissected, the intrapericardial segment of the inferior vena cava can be easily exposed by incising the diaphragm. A clamp is placed at the junction between the right atrium and inferior vena cava.

infrahepatic inferior vena cava between vascular clamps. Hepatectomy is completed by placing a sturdy clamp on the suprahepatic inferior vena cava as it passes through the diaphragm and excising the diseased liver. The hepatic veins are divided within the substance of the liver to allow the creation of a large suprahepatic cuff comprised of the left, middle, and right hepatic veins (Fig. 16-62).

After removal of the recipient liver, the right upper quadrant is carefully inspected, and hemostasis is obtained. Complete hemostasis in the bare area is essential since this region is relatively inaccessible once the donor liver is implanted. Reperitonealization of the bare area can be accomplished using the posterior peritoneum, and it tamponades venous oozing that may occur after transplantation.

The donor liver is brought to the operative field. Bench preparation performed previously includes meticulous ligation of tributaries of the vena cava (right adrenal and phrenic veins), portal vein, and hepatic artery. A Carrel patch of donor aorta is used for the arterial anastomotic site (Fig. 16-63). The gallbladder is removed. The vascular anastomoses are carried out using monofilament polypropylene suture. The suprahepatic vena caval anastomosis is performed first by suturing the posterior wall from within the lumen using an imbricating technique (Fig. 16-64). The anterior aspect of the anastomosis is then completed. The infrahepatic vena caval anastomosis is performed next, but the completion of the anastomosis is left until the time of hepatic revascularization to provide a vent for air, for acidotic, hyperkalemic blood, and for residual preservation solution. The arterial anastomosis is completed using a branch-patch technique (see Fig. 16-63). The portal limb of the venovenous bypass circuit is then removed, and the portal venous anastomosis is completed end to end.

During the anastomoses of the venae cavae and the hepatic artery, the donor liver is perfused with saline solution at 4°C by a cannula in the donor portal vein to wash out the preservation solution and keep the organ at a cryoprotective temperature. At the time of revascularization, inflow is restored to the liver through the portal vein. The first 200 to 300 mL of blood is vented through the infrahepatic vena cava. The final suture is then tied, and the suprahepatic caval clamp is removed. Finally, hepatic arterial flow is restored and revascularization is complete.

Postrevascularization Phase and Biliary Reconstruction

After revascularization, the donor liver usually assumes a normal color and consistency within 10 to 15 minutes. Identifying and controlling surgical bleeding entails a me-

ticulous examination of each of the vascular anastomoses as well as a search for unligated branches of the major vessels. The femoral bypass cannula is removed at this stage and the internal jugular cannula is removed on the first postoperative day.

Biliary reconstruction can use any of several options. The most common biliary anastomosis is a choledochocholedochostomy. This anastomosis is carried out using interrupted absorbable monofilament suture with spatulation of the donor and recipient ducts. The anastomosis is stented with a T tube that exits through the recipient common bile duct or with a smaller straight tube introduced through the donor cystic duct and advanced across the anastomosis (Fig. 16-65). Patients with a diseased biliary tract, such as those with primary sclerosing cholangitis or those who have a recipient duct of inadequate size or quality, require reconstruction with a choledochoenteric anastomosis. Most commonly, a standard Roux-en-Y choledochojejunostomy is carried out. No attempt is made to stent the anastomosis and, if possible, a retrocolic loop is used. In selected patients, especially children, the donor gallbladder can be retained with the graft and used as a conduit (Fig. 16-66). Under ordinary circumstances, bile is produced immediately.

Abdominal closure is accomplished with nonabsorbable fascial suture in these immunosuppressed patients to reduce the likelihood of dehiscence. Closed-suction peritoneal drains are only used if a bilioenteric anastomosis was performed (Fig. 16-67).

Technique for Reduced-Size Hepatic Transplantation

The numbers of available suitably sized donors for pediatric hepatic transplantation are inadequate to meet the needs of children awaiting organs. As a result, a technique for transplanting less than the entire liver has been developed, whereby a single lobe or segment of the liver may be used from a donor who has a body weight up to 10 times greater than the recipient.[237]

Most of the differences between standard orthotopic hepatic transplantation and reduced-size hepatic grafting relate to the bench preparation of the donor organ. The crucial step in reduced-size hepatic grafting is assessing how much hepatic volume to transplant. Because of the marked variability in the size and geometric configuration of the liver, the entire donor organ is generally brought to the recipient's operating room. Careful comparison of donor and recipient dictates the segment or lobe that is chosen (Fig. 16-68). In general, donors

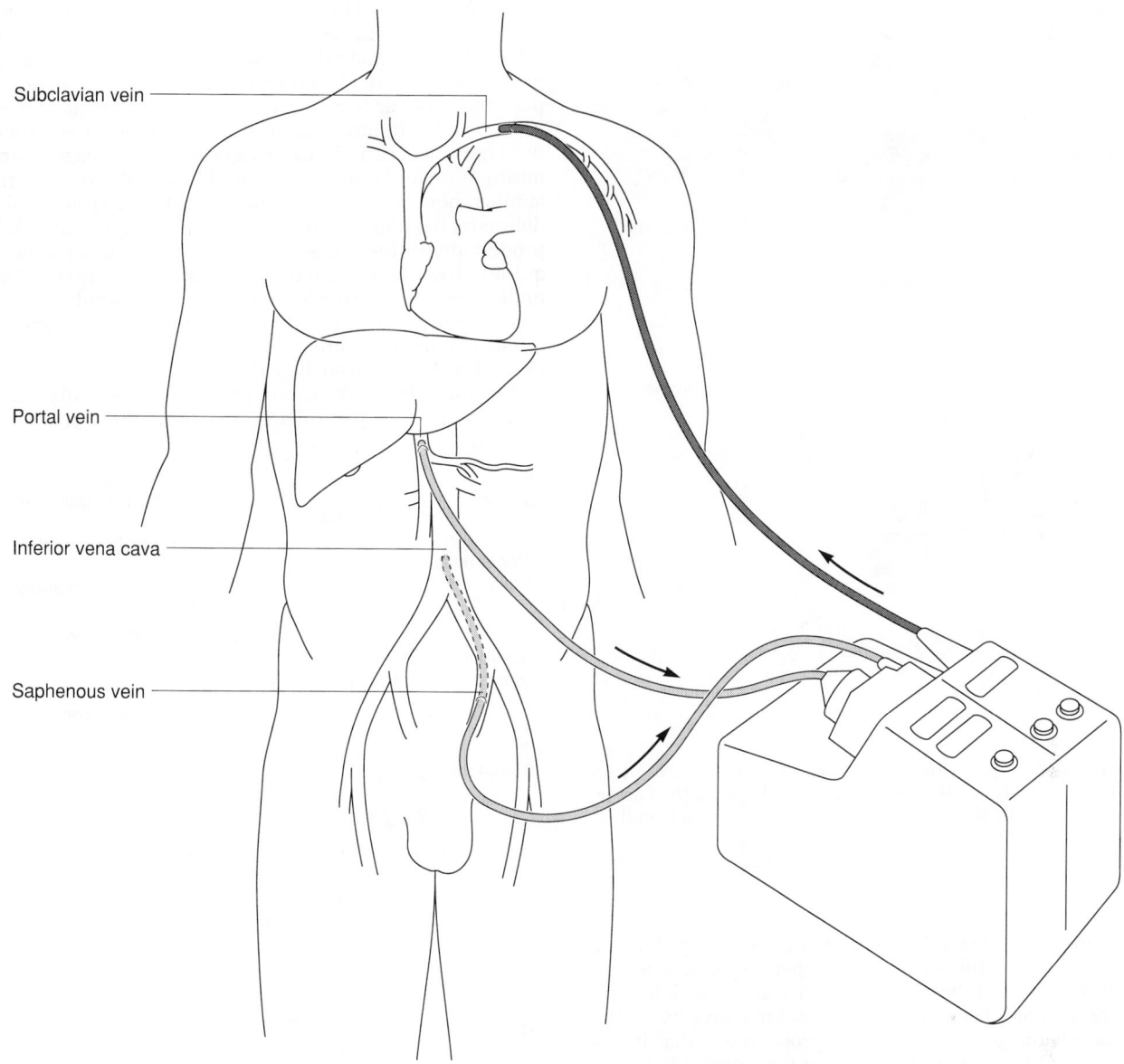

Subclavian vein

Portal vein

Inferior vena cava

Saphenous vein

Figure 16-61. Set-up for venovenous bypass during hepatic transplantation. Cannulas are placed into the portal vein to decompress the splanchnic bed and inferior vena cava (through the greater saphenous vein) to decompress the lower extremities and kidneys during the anhepatic phase of the transplant. A centrifugal pump is used to deliver bypassed blood to the central circulation by means of a cannula passed into the axillary vein.

weighing two to three times more than the recipient can provide a right-lobe graft. Donors who are more than three but less than six times the recipient's weight can be used for a left-lobe graft, and larger donors necessitate the use of the left lateral segment.

In all cases, the main portal vein, hepatic artery, and bile duct of the donor are retained, and the branches to the unused segments or lobes are ligated and divided. The hepatic parenchyma is divided sharply along anatomic planes, and vascular and biliary structures along the cut surface are meticulously suture ligated. Biologic glues are not necessary if this step is assiduously completed. The entire inferior vena cava is retained with most lobar grafts. Longitudinal tapering can be performed if there is a large size discrepancy between the diameters of the donor and recipient venae cavae. In the case of a left lateral segment

graft, the recipient retrohepatic vena cava is left in place, and the left hepatic vein of the segmental graft is anastomosed to a cuff fashioned from the recipient's hepatic veins (Fig. 16-69).

Orientation of the graft lobe or segment is important. Right-lobe grafts can be placed in the usual anatomic position. Left-lobe and left lateral segment grafts must be rotated about 45 degrees in the transverse plane to place hepatic parenchyma in the empty hepatic fossa.

Auxiliary Liver Transplantation

Under some circumstances, there is a good rationale for placing the donor allograft in an heterotopic rather than orthotopic position, leaving the diseased liver in place. This procedure is referred to as an *auxiliary liver transplant*. It is used occasionally for cases in which trans-

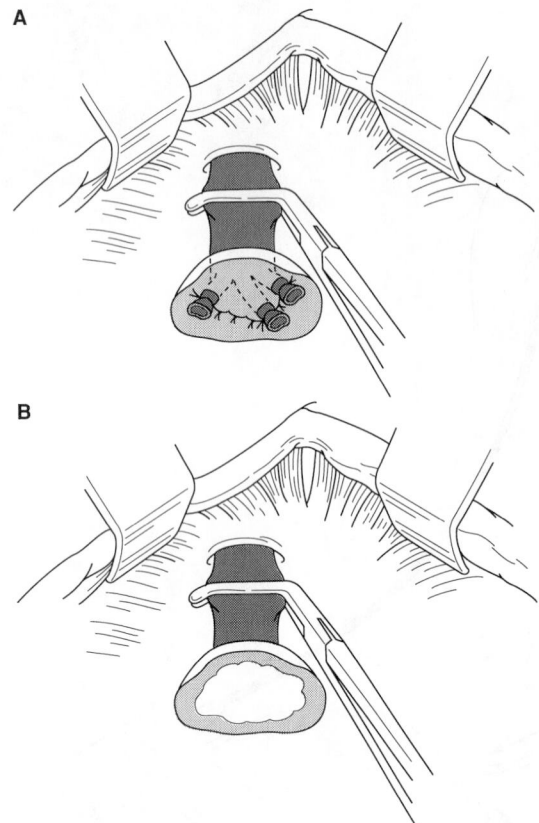

Figure 16-62. (*A*) The diseased recipient liver is removed by incising the liver below the level of the hepatic veins. (*B*) The hepatic veins are then opened to form a large suprahepatic cuff for anastomosis.

plantation is indicated for enzymatic deficiency, but the native liver functions well in all other respects. It is also used in cases of fulminant hepatic failure in which there is a reasonable chance for recovery of the native liver. The major advantage of the auxiliary procedure is that it is a procedure of lesser magnitude than the orthotopic procedure. Success rates of the auxiliary transplant have improved as technical refinements have occurred and are comparable to success rates for orthotopic transplantation. Figure 16-70 demonstrates the technique used in one institution.

POSTOPERATIVE COMPLICATIONS

The degree of preoperative debilitation and the complexity of the operative procedure make complications following hepatic transplantation a certainty. As always, prompt recognition and treatment are essential. In transplantation, however, the additional burden of early, heavy immunosuppression predisposes to problems not usually encountered in other areas of surgery. Complications associated with immunosuppression, which are predominantly infectious, were detailed earlier. In the following sections, some of the major surgical complications that occur after hepatic transplantation are described.

Primary Nonfunction

For reasons that are poorly understood, about 5% to 10% of transplanted livers function so poorly in the immediate postoperative period that death is likely in the absence of

retransplantation. This is referred to as primary nonfunction of the allograft. Clearly, most cases of nonfunction are related to inadequate tissue preservation in ice storage or to occult organ dysfunction in the donor, but a sizable percentage of cases may arise from immunologic mechanisms, probably humoral. In the worst cases, the patient does not regain consciousness, a coagulopathy ensues, and multiple organ failure develops. Typically, liver enzyme studies show hepatocellular injury, with SGOT and SGPT determinations in the 5000 to 10,000 range, and little bile production. In these cases, urgent retransplantation is required. Because of the tenuous condition of the recipient under these circumstances, however, the morbidity rate is high, usually about 50%. Even when the patient survives retransplantation, neurologic injury is common. When one examines the removed hepatic transplant, major arterial and venous blood vessels are patent; histologically, however, there is complete disruption of the normal lobular

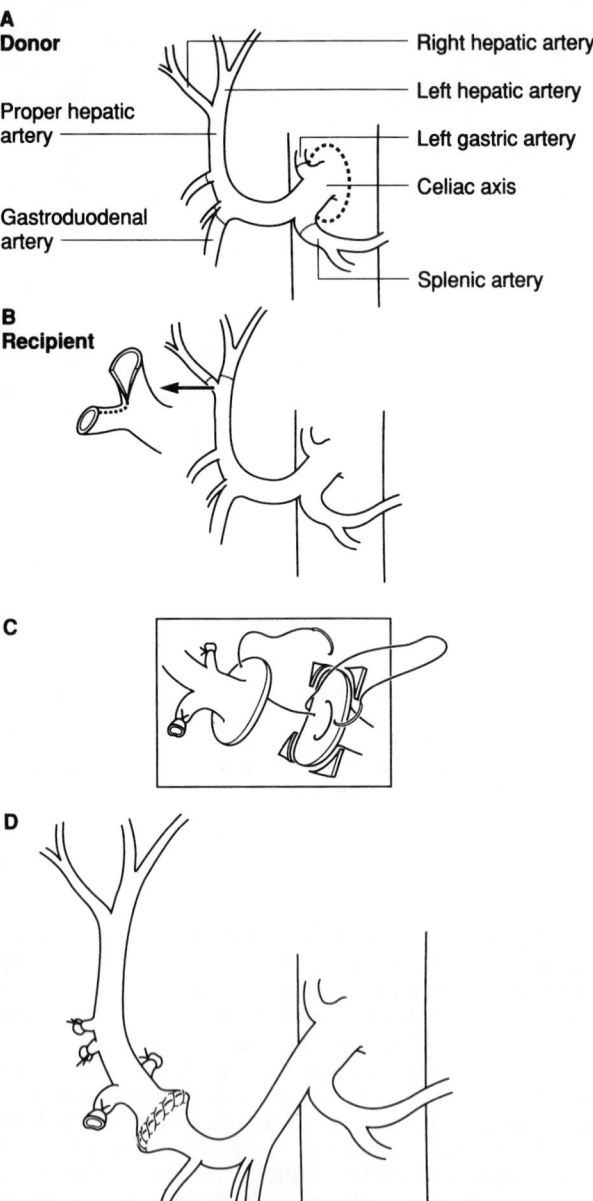

Figure 16-63. (*A*) The donor hepatic artery is procured with a Carrel patch of aorta. (*B*) The recipient hepatic artery bifurcation is used to fashion a branch patch for a larger anastomosis. (*C*) The anastomosis is carried out using continuous monofilament suture material. (*D*) The completed anastomosis.

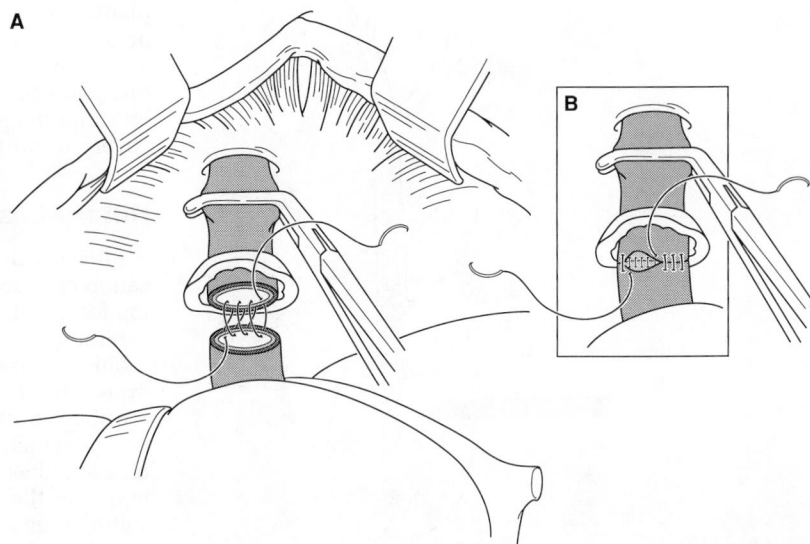

Figure 16-64. The suprahepatic vena caval anastomosis. (*A*) Posterior suture line. (*B*) Anterior suture line.

architecture, with obliteration of sinusoids by RBCs, fibrin, and neutrophils. The clinical definition of primary nonfunction of hepatic allografts is as follows:

Essential Characteristics
Occurrence within 96 hours after the operation
Patent portal vein and hepatic artery

Three of Four Characteristics Required
Bile output below 20 mL in 12 hours
Bilirubin level greater than 10 or rising 5 mg/d or more
PT/PTT ratio of 1.5 or greater
Factors V and VIII less than 25% of normal

Nonspecific Cholestasis

In 15% of cases, early postoperative function of the liver is sufficient to sustain life but imperfect in that progressive cholestasis develops.[238] This development is often referred to as nonspecific cholestasis syndrome or delayed function and is defined as the progressive rise in bilirubin past the third postoperative day in the absence of identifiable causes of cholestasis. This syndrome is the result of ischemic injury to the liver in the course of harvesting and preservation in ice. In this respect, it is analogous to the development of acute tubular necrosis after renal trans-

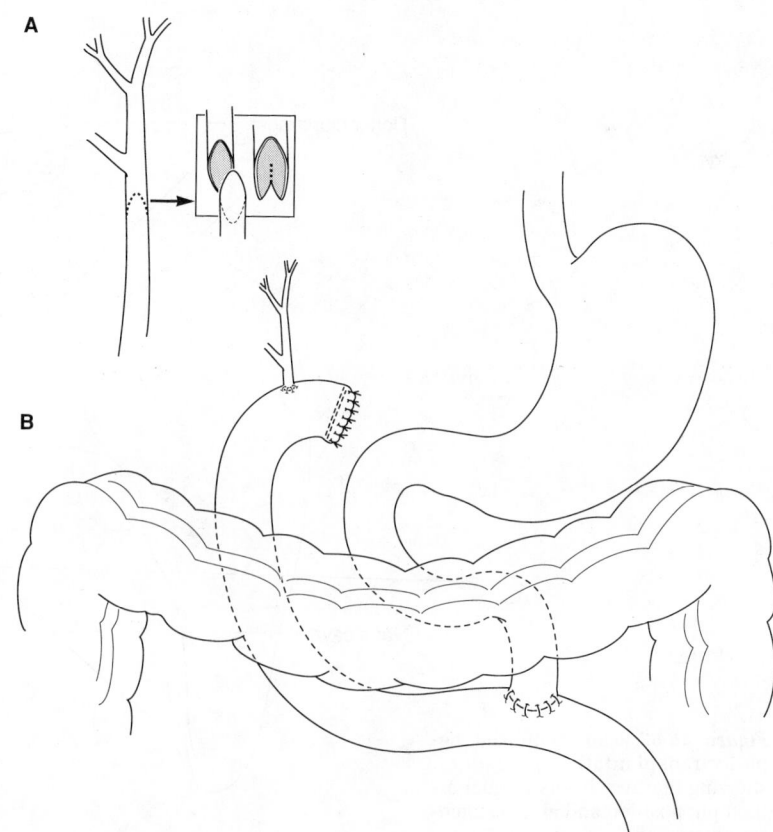

Figure 16-65. (*A*) In most cases, a spatulated choledochocholedochostomy is performed over a small drainage tube introduced through the donor cystic duct. (*B*) Patients with diseased or unsuitable common bile duct require biliary reconstruction with a Roux-en-Y choledochoenterostomy.

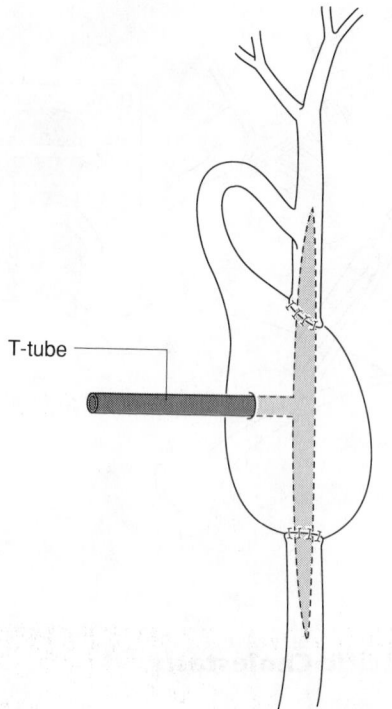

Figure 16-66. The Calne biliary conduit. In this procedure, described by Sir Roy Calne, the donor gallbladder is interposed between donor and recipient bile ducts to provide added length to the donor biliary tree.

plantation. Typically, synthetic function is preserved, but no bile is produced. Serum bilirubin levels often exceed 30 mg/dL for 2 to 3 weeks. The syndrome must be accurately distinguished from rejection; this is usually accomplished by serial biopsy. In the absence of rejection, complete recovery usually occurs.

Biliary Leak or Obstruction

Biliary leak or obstruction is a common surgical complication encountered after hepatic transplantation, accounting for about 20% of postoperative surgical problems.[239]

Biliary obstruction presents as an unexplained rise in bilirubin and alkaline phosphatase determinations and is confirmed by T-tube cholangiography or by a percutaneous transhepatic cholangiogram. Early strictures do not cause biliary dilatation and are not usually identified by abdominal ultrasound examinations. The most common site of obstruction is at the level of the choledochocholedochostomy, resulting from ischemia, kinking, or technical factors. Because the blood supply of the terminal portion of the donor bile duct derives solely from the hepatic artery, any stricture of the bile duct should prompt an investigation into the patency of the hepatic artery. Strictures of the biliary tree after hepatic transplantation are first treated by balloon dilation using percutaneous techniques. This is usually successful, but if not, operative revision is necessary.

Biliary leakage is a feared complication, with a high (50%) mortality rate.[240] Most frequently, leakage develops in the third or fourth postoperative week. The high mortality rate may be the result of concomitant hepatic arterial thrombosis, infection of the leaked bile, or the difficulty of bile duct repair in an area of inflamed tissue. Biliary leaks may also occur when the operatively placed T tube is removed 3 to 6 months

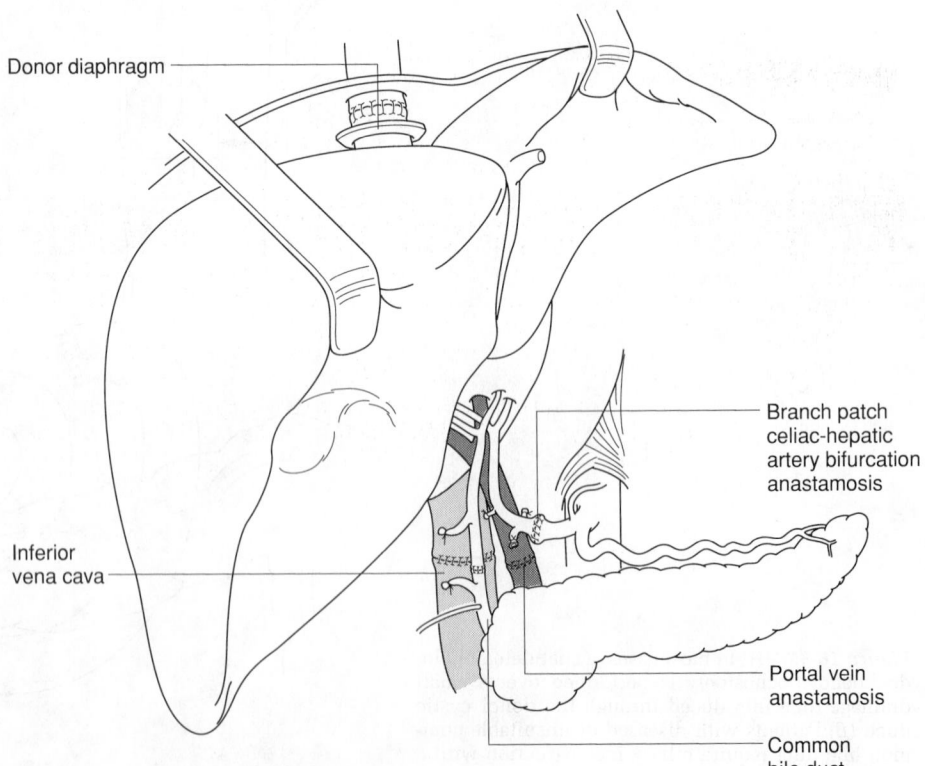

Figure 16-67. The completed hepatic transplantation procedure, showing the liver in the normal orthotopic position and all anastomoses completed.

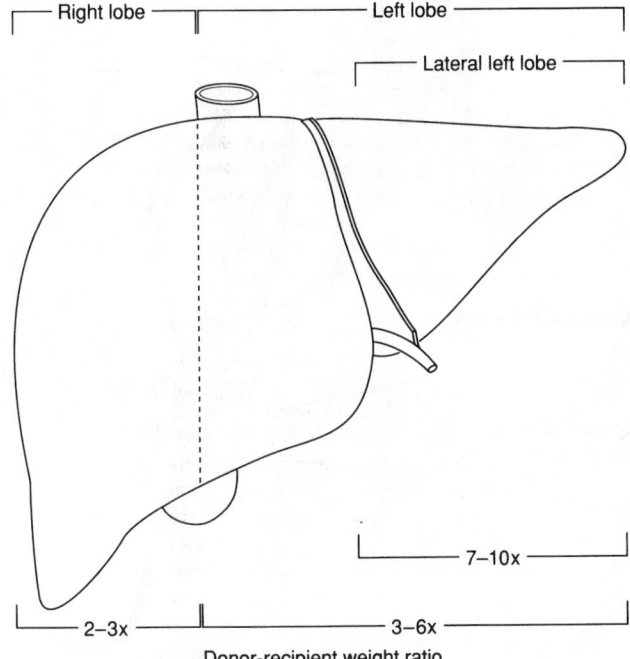

Figure 16-68. Reduced-size hepatic transplantation is accomplished by dividing the liver along established surgical anatomic planes. The choice of segment is based on the size discrepancy between the donor and recipient.

after surgery. In these cases, immunosuppression prevents host mechanisms from isolating the T-tube tract with scar tissue. Removal of the T tube leads to free spill of bile into the peritoneal cavity, an occurrence that is rare in the nontransplantation setting (Fig. 16-71). Late bile leakage from the T-tube site in a transplantation patient is less dangerous than leakage in the immediate postoperative period and is usually treated by hospitalization and intravenous antibiotics or by placement of a nasobiliary stent inserted retrograde into the common duct by endoscopy.

Hemorrhage

Laparotomy to control postoperative bleeding is required in 15% of cases.[240] In about half of reoperations, a specific bleeding point is identified. The survival rate is higher in these cases, in contrast to those in which diffuse bleeding is encountered, presumably because the latter circumstance is usually associated with poor allograft function and resultant coagulopathy. If significant bleeding occurs after hepatic transplantation, a common and sensible policy is to transfuse the patient until hypothermia and coagulopathy are corrected, with subsequent (1 to 3 days) evacuation of blood from the peritoneal cavity. Evacuation of clot is done to relieve intraabdominal pressure and to reduce the chance of intraabdominal infection.

Hepatic Artery Thrombosis

Hepatic artery thrombosis occurs in 5% of adult hepatic transplantation cases and in up to 25% of pediatric cases.[241] Technical factors, the flow rate of arterial blood past the anastomosis, and factors causing hypercoagulability all appear to contribute to the overall incidence of this complication.

As in any type of arterial surgery, meticulous technique is essential, and small imperfections may result in catastrophe.

The requirement for a complex interposition graft between donor and recipient vessel and the intraoperative revision of the arterial anastomosis are both associated with an increased incidence of thrombosis. In most cases of hepatic artery thrombosis, no obvious technical flaw is detected.

The rate of arterial blood flow in the reconstructed hepatic artery is an important determinant of long-term patency with reduced flow. Children are predisposed to hepatic artery thrombosis because they have smaller vessels and lower mean arterial blood pressure than adults. In pediatric cases, an arterial diameter of less than 3 mm is associated with a

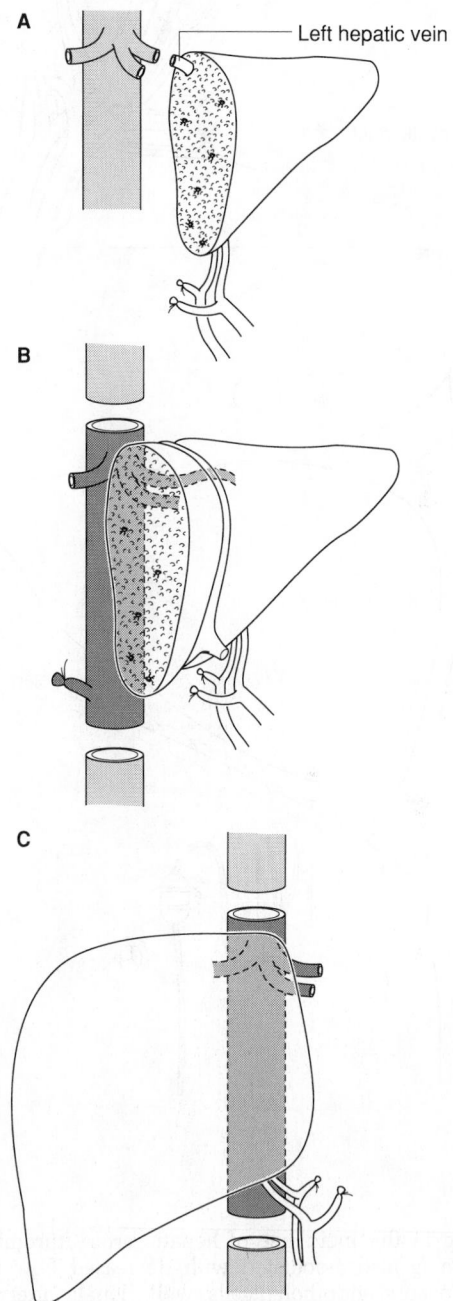

Figure 16-69. Prepared lobar grafts. (*A*) A left lateral segment graft is performed using the donor left hepatic vein. The recipient vena cava is left in situ. (*B*) A left lobe graft is transplanted with the entire donor vena cava. The graft must be rotated 45 to 90 degrees in the transverse plane to place hepatic parenchyma in the hepatic fossa and to prevent kinking. (*C*) A right lobe graft is placed in the usual anatomic position.

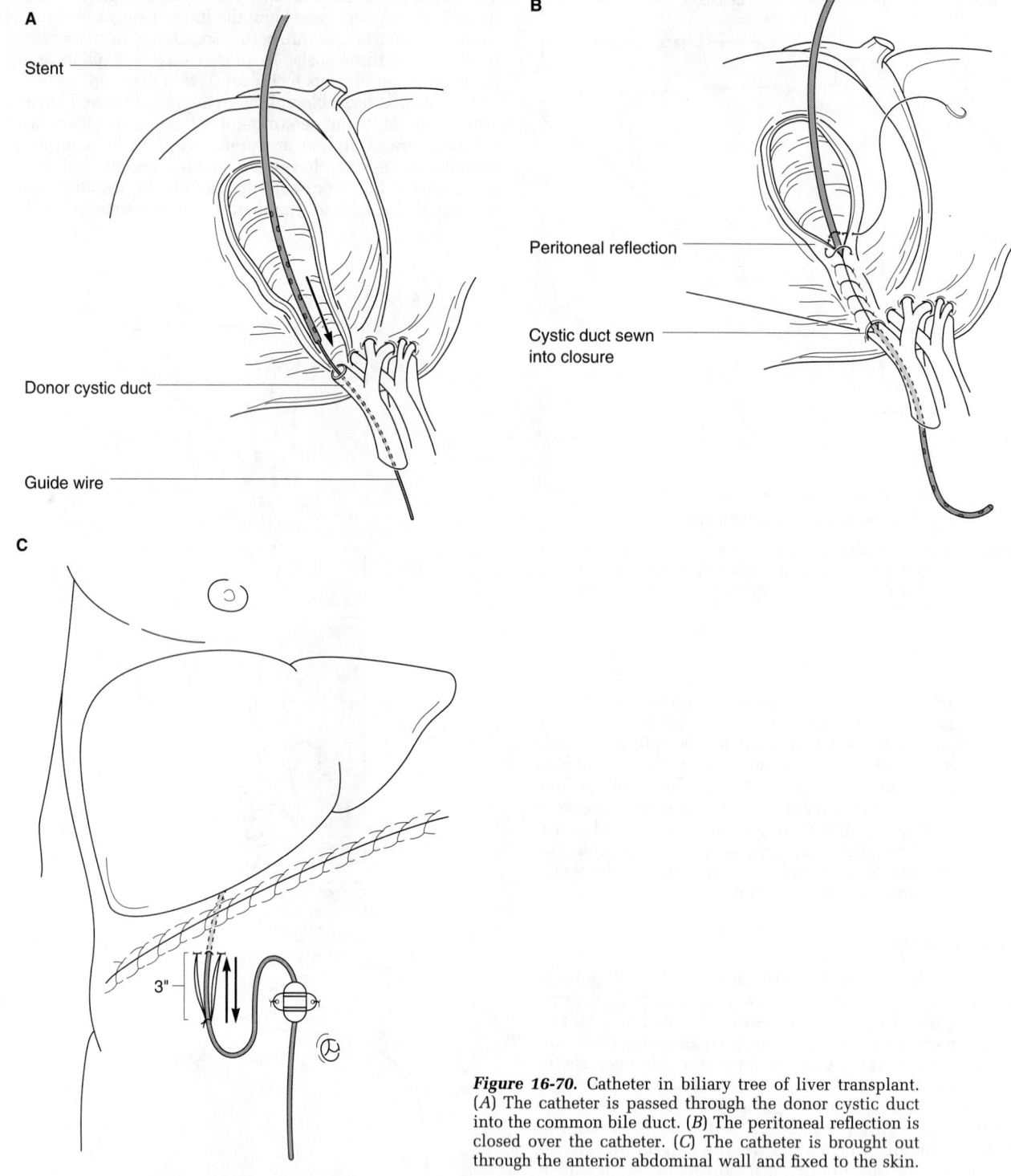

A

Stent

Donor cystic duct

Guide wire

B

Peritoneal reflection

Cystic duct sewn
into closure

C

3"

Figure 16-70. Catheter in biliary tree of liver transplant. (*A*) The catheter is passed through the donor cystic duct into the common bile duct. (*B*) The peritoneal reflection is closed over the catheter. (*C*) The catheter is brought out through the anterior abdominal wall and fixed to the skin.

doubling in the incidence of hepatic artery thrombosis.[242] Rejection is also associated with decreased flow because when it occurs, endothelial cells swell. Hepatic artery thrombosis occurs more commonly in association with rejection.

A postoperative hypercoagulable state associated with hepatic transplantation may predispose to hepatic artery thrombosis. Recent information indicates that relatively poor hepatic production of natural regulatory anticoagulants, such as proteins C and S and antithrombin III, immediately after transplantation promotes coagulation because production of

procoagulant factors, such as factor V and VII, occurs more rapidly after revascularization.[239] This observation has prompted some centers to administer fresh frozen plasma as a source of antithrombin III and proteins C and S in the postoperative period. Most centers recommend prophylactic aspirin to prevent hepatic artery thrombosis in children.

In adults, hepatic artery thrombosis usually presents as a marked rise in prothrombin time determination and transaminases. Occasionally, the first manifestation is biliary stricture or leakage. Immediate thrombectomy with re-

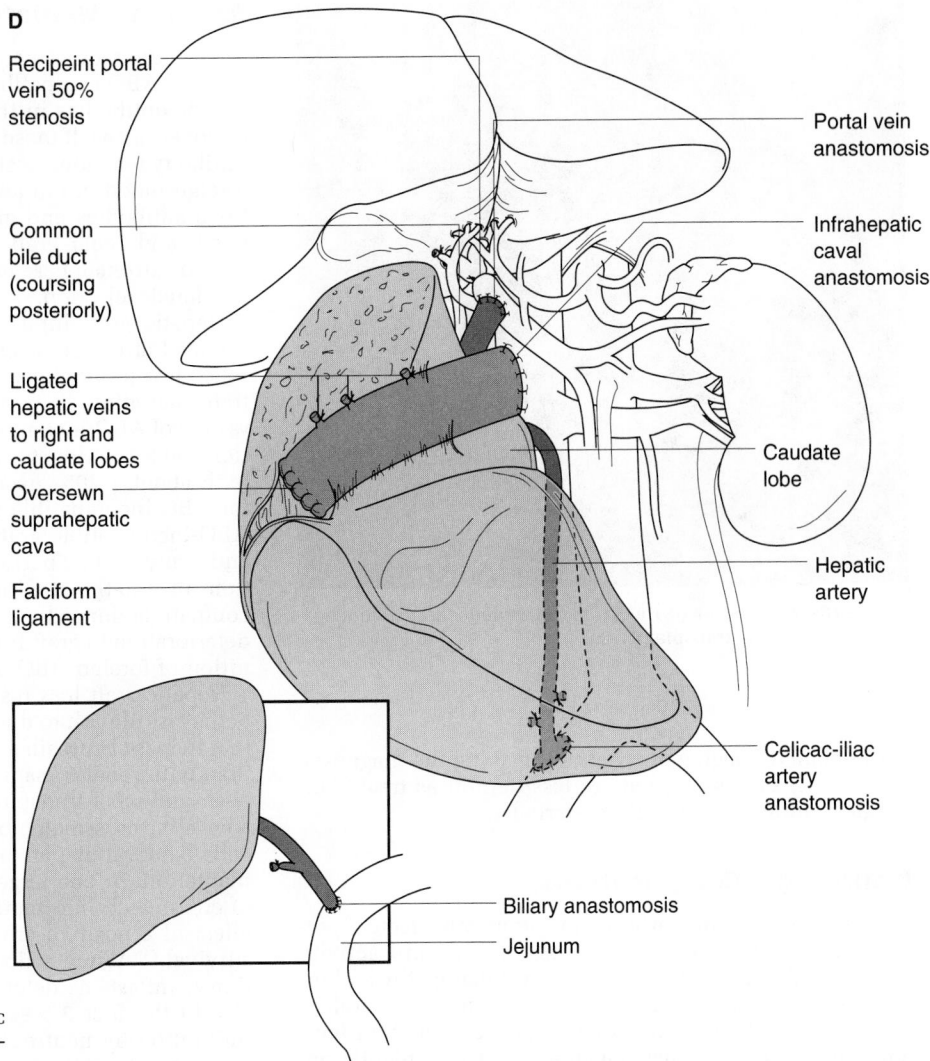

D

Recipeint portal vein 50% stenosis

Common bile duct (coursing posteriorly)

Ligated hepatic veins to right and caudate lobes

Oversewn suprahepatic cava

Falciform ligament

Portal vein anastomosis

Infrahepatic caval anastomosis

Caudate lobe

Hepatic artery

Celicac-iliac artery anastomosis

Biliary anastomosis

Jejunum

Figure 16-70. *(Continued)* Heterotopic auxillary liver transplant using a reduced-size allograft.

vision of the arterial anastomosis has been successfully accomplished on occasion, but more often repeat transplantation is needed. In children, the presentation of this complication is more varied and ranges from fulminant hepatic failure to isolated biliary leak to focal intraparenchymal abscess to no detectable abnormality. The important determinants dictating one outcome versus another are not known.

Portal Vein Thrombosis

Postoperative portal vein thrombosis is much less common than hepatic artery thrombosis, occurring in 2% to 3% of cases.[241] As for hepatic artery thrombosis, the most important predisposing factors relate to the size of the native portal vein and to the rate of blood flow through the native portal vein. The size of the portal vein is influenced by the patient's age and by the presence of previous thrombus, which results in a reduced luminal diameter. Blood flow through the portal vein may be low as a result of the preoperative development of retroperitoneal collaterals from the portal venous system to the renal vein and inferior vena cava. A previous surgically created splenorenal shunt must be disconnected at the time of transplantation since it usually is associated with reduced flow through the portal vein.

Portal vein thrombosis typically presents with marked elevation of enzyme and prothrombin time determinations and progressive liver failure. Occasionally, liver failure does not develop. In this case, the clinical course is one of recurrent variceal hemorrhage, which can be treated by a distal splenorenal shunt.

Vena Caval Thrombosis

Because of the large luminal diameter of the vena cava and its high flow rate, thrombosis of the vena cava rarely occurs after hepatic transplantation and is reported in less than 1% of cases.[241]

Intraabdominal Sepsis

Intraabdominal sepsis presents as diffuse peritonitis or localized abscess and occurs in about 5% of cases.[240] Peritonitis is the result of infection of ascitic fluid, the leakage of infected bile, or leakage of enteric contents into the peritoneum from gastrointestinal perforation. Abscesses develop most commonly in the peritransplant area, but they also develop between loops of small bowel. As would be expected in a frail patient population treated with immunosuppression, mortality from this complication is high (60%). Percutaneous techniques used in association

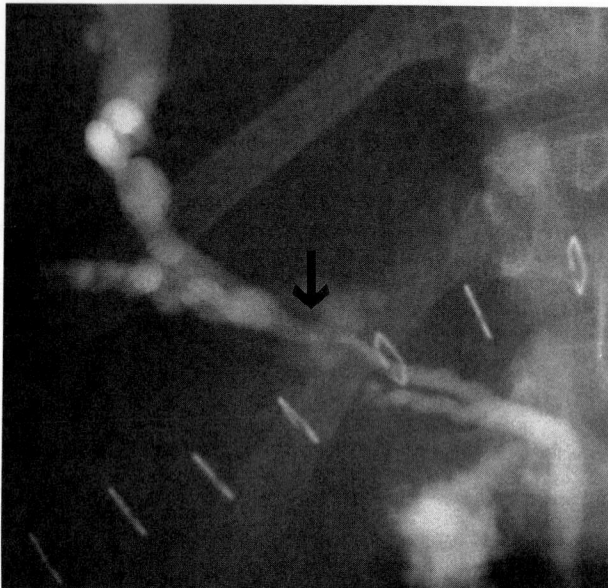

Figure 16-71. Bile leak (*arrow*) from the choledochocholedochostomy after hepatic transplantation.

with detailed imaging are useful in making the diagnosis, particularly of abscess, but are less helpful as treatment. Surgical drainage is usually preferred.

Neurologic Complications

A number of preoperative and postoperative factors predispose to impaired consciousness and seizure activity after transplantation. Preoperative encephalopathy and intraoperative hypotension or anoxia result in cerebral edema, which is worsened by massive resuscitation with administration of intravenous fluids after transplantation. Occasionally, air embolism occurs at the time of revascularization of the transplant, causing neurologic dysfunction. If the patient fails to awaken promptly after transplantation, and particularly if the transplant is functioning well, an urgent computed tomographic scan of the head should be obtained to rule out intracranial hemorrhage and to assess the degree of cerebral edema.

Seizures are common after transplantation and result from any of the factors listed previously as well as from drugs administered, particularly cyclosporine and trimethoprim-sulfamethoxazole. A history of seizures or preoperative encephalopathy greatly predisposes to postoperative seizure activity. Seizures are treated with diazepam and phenytoin and careful monitoring of cyclosporine levels. Rarely, a syndrome similar to progressive multifocal leukoencephalopathy develops, with progressive mental deterioration and death. This is thought to be due in part to the pronounced central nervous system toxicity of cyclosporine.[243]

REJECTION AND IMMUNOSUPPRESSION

Immunosuppressive treatment of the hepatic transplant recipient is similar to intraoperative technical management in that even a small error may be detrimental. Two issues are of prime importance—recognizing rejection in its many guises and choosing an immunosuppressive response appropriate to the type of rejection encountered.

Antibody-Mediated Rejection

Absolute requirements for successful renal transplantation are ABO compatibility and the absence of lymphocytotoxic antibodies in the recipient capable of recognizing donor antigens. If these requirements are not met, antigen–antibody reactions occur involving either isoantibodies to foreign blood group antigens of the graft or lymphocytotoxic antibodies and graft HLA antigens. Complement is fixed, and renal graft destruction ensues within hours. This occurrence is referred to as hyperacute, or antibody-mediated, rejection.

Hepatic graft injury from preexisting host antibodies directed at donor ABO determinants does occur but in a much less pronounced fashion than in the context of renal transplantation. Large series have documented that overall results of ABO-incompatible donor–recipient transplantations are inferior to ABO-compatible transplantations, with about a 20% decrease in 1-year graft survival rates for ABO-incompatible grafts. A substantial percentage of ABO-incompatible grafts function long term,[244] however, and many centers perform ABO-incompatible transplantation in life-threatening situations in which no ABO-compatible donor liver is available. It is assumed that the deterioration in graft function relates to isoantibody recognition of foreign ABO antigens on liver tissue.

Hepatic graft loss resulting from lymphocytotoxic antibodies is difficult to document, but most observers believe that it does occur, albeit in a much less predictable fashion than with renal transplantation.[245] It is a rare event, however, and most transplantation programs do not insist on a negative crossmatch between recipient serum and donor cells before transplantation, as is the case in renal transplantation. In one large series, a retrospective evaluation of crossmatch information failed to show any deleterious effect of a positive crossmatch on ultimate hepatic graft survival.[246] When it does occur, antibody-mediated rejection manifests as deterioration of allograft function, usually in the first 3 weeks postoperatively. Biopsy reveals infiltration by neutrophils, endothelial cell hypertrophy, and focal deposits of fibrin. Immunofluorescence studies may show antibody and complement in the vessel wall.

Why the liver is less susceptible to antibody-mediated destruction than the kidney is not clearly understood but probably relates to two factors. First, the liver has a vastly different microcirculation than does the kidney, with a preponderance of sinusoidal channels and a smaller capillary network. It is probable that antibody-mediated injury affects blood flow through the delicate capillary network of the kidney more than it does liver sinusoids. In addition, each hepatocyte is exposed to two sinusoidal channels, presumably permitting survival if only one sinusoid is occluded. Finally, differences in HLA antigen expression are known to exist in the two organs, with the kidney the more antigenic of the two.

Cell-Mediated Rejection

Acute, or cell-mediated, rejection occurs frequently but is effectively blunted by antirejection therapy. Acute rejection occurs most commonly in the first 2 postoperative months. In modern practice, cell-mediated rejection is a less common cause of graft loss than are primary nonfunction or hepatic artery thrombosis. Still, the effectiveness of antirejection treatment assumes a relatively early diagnosis, which is in turn the result of careful monitoring by the transplantation physician.

The diagnosis of cell-mediated rejection is made on clinical as well as histologic grounds. Clinical features include fever and a decrease in bile output or a change in consis-

Table 16-14. DIAGNOSIS OF HEPATIC ALLOGRAFT REJECTION

CLINICAL
Fever
Jaundice
Decrease in bile output
Change in consistency of bile

LABORATORY
Leukocytosis
Eosinophilia
Elevation of transaminases
Elevation of serum bilirubin
Elevation of prothrombin time

BIOPSY
Portal lymphocytosis
Endothelitis
Bile duct infiltration by cells, with duct injury

tency and color of bile from deep green to a watery light green. Laboratory evaluation of peripheral blood demonstrates leukocytosis and occasionally eosinophilia. Biochemical changes include elevated levels of serum transaminases, alkaline phosphatase, serum prothrombin time, and serum bilirubin. Any of these findings should prompt a biopsy (Table 16-14). Typical biopsy findings in cases of cell-mediated rejection are a triad of portal lymphocytosis, endotheliitis (subendothelial deposits of mononuclear cells), and bile duct infiltration and damage (Figs. 14-72 and 14-73). Various classification schemes have been devised to grade the severity of the rejection process based on the degree of cellular involvement or injury in these areas. Cell characterization studies have documented that the cells in the portal triads are primarily T cells, with fewer macrophages and neutrophils. Bile duct epithelial cells appear to be a prime target of immune attack, and they are known to express large amounts of class II HLA antigen.

In contrast to biopsy evaluation of renal allografts, in which small arteries are frequently seen, the peripheral biopsy of the hepatic transplant rarely includes a sizable artery. Thus, valuable information about vascular injury by lymphocytes is not available to the hepatic transplantation pathologist. Although small arteries are clearly targets in hepatic as well as renal transplantation, the only manifestation of this process may be centrilobular necrosis of cells, a typical ischemic change.

Occasionally, a biopsy done on a routine or protocol basis shows histologic evidence of rejection in the absence of clinical or biochemical evidence of rejection. Treatment of this finding is controversial and ranges from full antirejection therapy to no therapy. Spontaneous disappearance of such findings has been reported. Most transplantation specialists would at least perform frequent follow-up biopsies in such cases.

Chronic Rejection

Chronic rejection is characterized by relentless immune attack on small bile ducts. Clinically, the pattern is one of gradual biliary obstruction, with elevation of alkaline phosphatase and bilirubin, in the absence of abnormalities in large bile ducts. Histologically, small bile ducts are obliterated or completely absent, with a less pronounced cellular infiltrate than is seen with acute rejection. The loss of small bile ducts is partly the result of lymphocytes' direct immune-mediated attack on biliary epithelium. Relative to other cells in the liver, biliary epithelium tends to express more class I antigen. Class II antigen expression is induced as the result of an episode of acute rejection. Thus, biliary epithelial cells are vulnerable targets for host attack because of their antigenicity. Loss of bile ducts may also occur indirectly as the result of ischemia secondary to immune-mediated obliteration of small to medium arteries. Vanishing bile duct syndrome, defined as absence of bile ducts in 15 of 20 portal triads examined,[247] is produced by chronic rejection but could also conceivably be the result of ischemia or other mechanisms. This syndrome is commonly encountered after transplantation of the liver into a patient with antidonor lymphocytotoxic antibodies.[248] Vanishing bile duct syndrome also has been seen with increasing frequency in patients recovering from cytomegalovirus infection.[249] As in the case of renal trans-

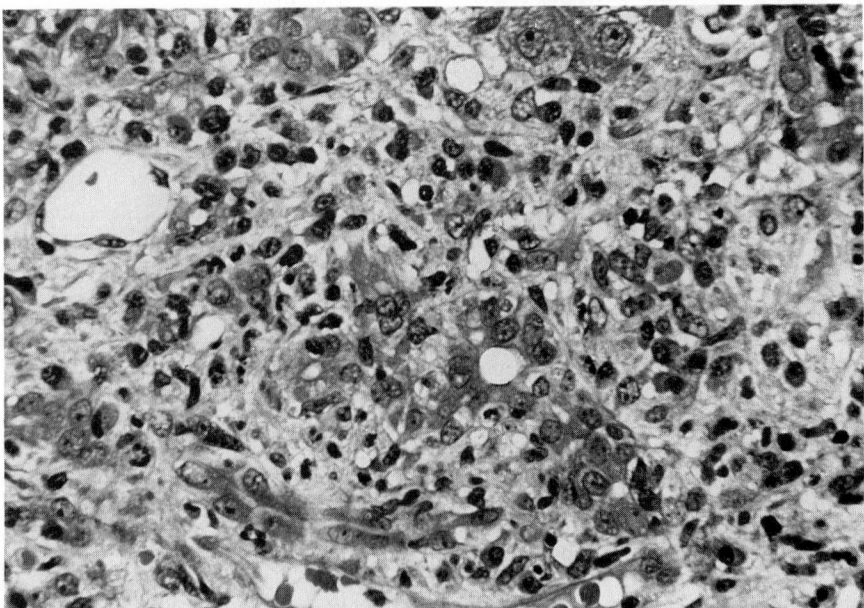

Figure 16-72. Histologic findings in hepatic transplant rejection—bile duct injury. The bile duct (*center*) is infiltrated by lymphocytes.

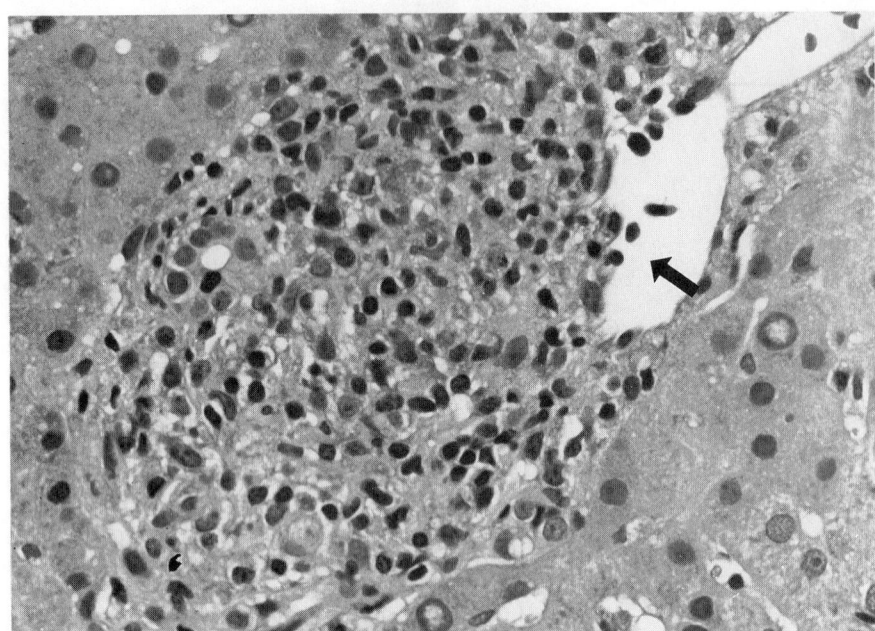

Figure 16-73. Histologic findings in hepatic transplant rejection—portal tract lymphocytosis and endotheliitis. The portal triad (*center*) shows a dense cellular infiltrate. The arrow indicates endotheliitis.

plantations, chronic rejection responds poorly to increases in immunosuppressive medication, and retransplantation is usually required.

Immunosuppression Induction and Maintenance

A common immunosuppressive protocol used in hepatic transplantation consists of an initial 1- to 2-week course of antithymocyte globulin, high doses of prednisone with a rapid taper, azathioprine, and cyclosporine. This therapy regimen has evolved to its present form for several reasons. First, an important principle contends that more drugs in smaller doses are safer and more effective than larger doses of fewer drugs. This increased efficacy probably relates to the different mechanisms of actions of the drugs involved, which have synergistic effects. Second, it was necessary to devise a protocol that would not produce nephrotoxicity in the first few posttransplantation days, a time when the kidneys are recovering from ischemia associated with a long and difficult operative procedure. Prophylactic administration of antithymocyte globulin, starting at the first posttransplantation day, provides effective immunosuppression without nephrotoxicity. Cyclosporine, a nephrotoxic drug, can then be added to the immunosuppressive regimen when renal function is clearly improving, usually after 5 to 7 days.

Cyclosporine is the mainstay of treatment, and maintenance of drug levels in a therapeutic range is an important element of patient management. Daily monitoring of serum levels is necessary in the initial postoperative period because many of the drugs used for other reasons affect cyclosporine levels and because bile is necessary for efficient cyclosporine absorption. Hepatic production of bile may be variable in the first few postoperative weeks as the result of rejection or ischemia.

Because immunosuppression predisposes to infection, prophylactic antiviral and antibacterial drugs are usually administered. A typical regimen includes trimethoprim-sulfamethoxazole and acyclovir for the first postoperative month. The former is particularly useful in the prevention of *Pneumocystis carinii* infection, and the latter decreases the incidence of herpesvirus infection. Many centers ad-

minister prophylactic high-titer antibody to cytomegalovirus as well.

Treatment of Acute Rejection

Despite the overall effectiveness of the regimen described, acute rejection does occur and must be treated promptly. On establishment of the diagnosis, high doses of methylprednisolone are administered (usually 500 mg to 1 g) intravenously on a daily basis for 3 days. This treatment is effective in reversing 50% to 75% of acute rejection episodes. Steroid-resistant rejection is treated with Orthoclone OKT3, a monoclonal antibody directed at the T3 determinant common to all mature T cells. OKT3 is administered daily for 10 to 14 days with close monitoring of the number of T cells in the peripheral blood. Treatment is highly effective, and it is unusual to lose an allograft secondary to acute rejection.

RESULTS

Generally accepted rates for 1- and 5-year survival after hepatic transplantation are 75% and 65%, respectively. One of the most important determinants of success is the status of the patient at the time of transplantation. The patient survival rate after transplantation was 42% for patients taken to surgery directly from an intensive care unit, but 84% for patients not taken from an intensive care setting.[250] The following four specific preoperative risk factors have been identified that correlate with survival: (1) the degree of preoperative neurologic impairment; (2) the degree of malnutrition, (3) the serum bilirubin level; and (4) the degree of prolongation of the serum prothrombin time.[251] Using a scoring system based on these parameters, patients in the low-risk category had a 96% chance of 6-month survival, and patients in the high-risk category had a 22% chance of 6-month survival.

In contrast to the patient's condition at the time of transplantation, the precise cause of liver failure in most cases is not an important determinant of success. Thus, 5-year survival is not significantly different for liver failure brought on by postnecrotic cirrhosis, primary biliary cirrhosis, alcoholic cirrhosis, primary sclerosing cholangitis, or biliary atresia. These indications comprise the great majority of transplantations done in this country.

Transplantation for three specific disease categories, however, results in significantly reduced 5-year survival rate. In the first of these, fulminant hepatic failure, reduced success is the result of the precarious clinical circumstances at presentation. This is largely unavoidable because of the rapid progression of disease. Little controversy exists about this indication for transplantation once irreversibility has been established. The 5-year survival rate for fulminant hepatic failure was recently reported to be 59.6%. Transplantation for hepatitis B and hepatic neoplasm, however, results in a predictable recurrence of disease, and substantial decrements in patient survival. Reported 5-year survival rates for these indications are 31.9% and 33.6%, respectively. These findings have generated controversy about the appropriateness of transplantation for these indications.

Hepatitis B recurs in the transplant in over 90% of cases and may result in a rapid clinical deterioration, with cirrhosis and death occurring within months. In other cases, the hepatitis B virus develops a more benign, commensal-type relationship with the host, resulting in chronic hepatitis B antigenemia (the carrier state) but little apparent liver disease. Most cases fall between these extremes, but the factors that account for one clinical course or the other are completely unknown. Despite the reduced overall success, the young age of the transplant patient, the invariable failure of nonoperative treatment, and the unpredictable nature of posttransplantation disease progression makes withholding transplantation extremely difficult. Repeat transplantation for recurrent hepatitis B is generally not performed.

Although the reported survival of patients undergoing liver transplantation for hepatic neoplasm is low overall, increasing experience in this area indicates that certain well-defined subgroups of patients may achieve acceptable survival rates particularly in association with adjuvant chemotherapy. For hepatoma, favorable prognostic features include relatively small tumor size, favorable histology, absence of vascular invasion, and the absence of lymph node metastases to the portal triad. Such patients have a 5-year survival rate in excess of 60%. Adjuvant chemotherapy with doxorubicin (Adriamycin) appears to confer additional benefit. Results following transplantation for cholangiocarcinoma are invariably poor, and this is an uncommon indication for transplantation. Transplantation has been successfully used in hepatoblastoma, hemangioendothelioma, and some metastatic neuroendocrine tumors. Transplantation is unsuccessful in patients with metastatic colorectal or breast neoplasm.

Age is an important factor influencing results. Results in patients transplanted at 1 year of age or less are inferior to those obtained in older patients, largely for technical reasons.[252] Survival is markedly reduced in patients who undergo transplantation after age 65 years.[253]

Cardiac Transplantation
SARA J. SHUMWAY AND R. MORTON BOLMAN III

HISTORY

Cardiac transplantation became a clinical reality on December 3, 1967. The way had been paved, however, by a number of experimental studies as well as by the clinical application of other solid-organ transplantations, such as kidney and liver.

The first experimental cardiac transplantation was performed by Carrel and Guthrie at the University of Chicago in 1905.[254] A small dog's heart was reimplanted heterotopically in the neck of a larger dog. The exact anastomoses are not known, but the transplant apparently functioned for a time. The technique for the anastomoses was established early. Demikhov performed more heterotopic cardiac transplants from 1940 to 1962.[255] The longest graft survival was 32 days with an intrathoracic heart that beat in a nonfunctioning capacity. Experimental orthotopic cardiac transplantation was performed successfully in 1958.[256]

In 1960, Lower and Shumway combined several new advances to achieve short-term survival in dogs receiving orthotopic cardiac transplants.[257] The recipient underwent surface cooling to 28°C while on cardiopulmonary bypass; the donor heart was placed in iced saline at 4°C for 5 minutes; and the total organ ischemia time averaged about 1 hour requiring four anastomoses (two atrial and two great vessel). The survival time before rejection caused graft failure was 6 to 21 days. Five years later Lower, Dong, and Shumway reported long-term survival of 250 days in a dog that had undergone cardiac transplantation.[258] Rejection episodes had been detected by a drop in voltage on electrocardiogram (ECG). Treatment with azathioprine and methylprednisolone restored the ECG to normal.

The first clinical cardiac transplantation was greeted with a great deal of enthusiasm. One year later, 102 cardiac transplantations had been done in 17 countries. By 1970, however, several centers had called for a moratorium because of poor survival. A few centers persisted, including Stanford University, Medical College of Virginia, and Groote Schuur Hospital in Capetown, South Africa.

From 1968 to 1978, the 1-year survival rate improved from 22% to 65% at Stanford.[259] Rabbit antithymocyte globulin was added to the immunosuppressant armamentarium.[260,261] The technique of endomyocardial biopsy was pioneered by Caves in 1974.[262] Billingham developed a histologic system for grading rejection based on the endomyocardial biopsy specimens.[263] By the end of the 1970s, cyclosporine added a new dimension to immunosuppression.

Cardiac retransplantation became an option in 1977 for failing grafts or graft atherosclerosis.[264] A second wave of enthusiasm for cardiac transplantation occurred in the 1980s, brought on largely by greater success with cyclosporine added to the immunosuppression protocol. In 1989, at least 2450 cardiac transplants were performed.[265]

INDICATIONS

The primary indication for cardiac transplantation is end-stage heart disease in a patient who is not expected to survive more than 6 months to 1 year. Additionally, no other medical or surgical treatment option is available to help the patient.

Most candidates for cardiac transplantation are New York Heart Association class 3 or 4 as a result of a cardiomyopathy. In one series of 311 patients, the age range was 6 days to 67 years at the time of transplantation. About 75% of patients have either an idiopathic or ischemic cardiomyopathy; these two groups are almost equal in size (slightly more have ischemic cardiomyopathy). The indications for the other 25% include congenital heart disease, valvular heart disease, viral cardiomyopathies, and failed initial cardiac transplant, as well as familial and restrictive cardiomyopathies.

PREOPERATIVE EVALUATION AND SELECTION CRITERIA

The ideal surgical candidate for cardiac transplantation is an emotionally stable patient with a supportive family who is highly motivated to take good care of his or her new heart. Toward that end, every potential recipient is evaluated for about a week. This can be done on an outpatient basis if the patient is reasonably stable.

Each patient undergoes a complete history and physical examination. Any history or evidence for malignancy or ongoing infection must be noted and pursued. Any other end-stage organ disease is at least a relative contraindication. Potential problems with compliance are a great concern, and the referring physician can be helpful. We insist that all potential recipients be nonsmokers who do not consume alcohol and are at an appropriate weight for their height and body build. If obesity is a problem, a reasonable weight loss program is initiated provided there is enough time.

The standard barrage of tests are obtained (Table 16-15). The inpatient cost of this series of tests and evaluations is about $8000, but the outpatient cost is only about $5000. The purpose of all this testing is to rule out any of the relative or absolute contraindications to cardiac transplantation. Relative contraindications include the following:

- Age greater than 65 years
- History of malignancy (not cured)
- Ongoing infection
- Systemic disease
- Irreversible hepatic, pulmonary, or renal damage
- Recent cerebrovascular or neurologic deficit
- Pulmonary embolus within 6 weeks

Table 16-15. PRETRANSPLANTATION TESTS AND EVALUATIONS

History and physical examination
Obstetric and gynecologic consultation for female patients, including Pap smear, herpes culture, and birth control counseling
Laboratory analyses
  Hematology: complete blood count, platelet count, coagulation battery, fibrinogen, factor V
  Chemistry: blood urea nitrogen, creatinine, electrolytes, calcium, PO_4, fasting, blood sugar, serum electrophoresis, cholesterol, triglycerides, amylase, SGOT, bilirubin, alkaline phosphatase, thyroid index, hepatitis profile, lipoprotein screen, creatinine clearance
  Microbiology: cytomegalovirus, Epstein-Barr virus, varicella-zoster, herpes simplex virus titers
  Immunology: ABO type and screen (this is double-checked), HLA-A, B, C, and DR typing and antileukocyte antibody screening, quantitative immunoglobulins, and human immunodeficiency virus (patient gives verbal consent)
Tests seen by nurse clinician, transplantation cardiologist, and transplantation cardiac surgeon)
  Chest radiograph, posteroanterior and lateral
  Bilateral mammogram for female patients
  Stool guaiac (three tests)
  12-lead electrocardiogram
  Cardiac catheterization, including pulmonary artery pressures and resistance
  MUGA scan; right and left ejection fractions or echo, or both
  Spine (thoracic, lumbar) and hip radiographs
  Pulmonary function tests, including lung volumes and DLCO
  Ventilation–perfusion lung scan
  Head CT scan without contrast
  Bone age for children
  Neuropsychologic evaluation
  Cardiopulmonary exercise test

- Active ulcer or bleeding diathesis
- Smoking, drinking, or recreational drug use
- Poorly controlled diabetes mellitus
- Pulmonary vascular resistance greater than 6 to 8 Wood units (480 to 640 dyne/s/cm^5)
- Psychologically unstable, unreliable, or history of poor compliance

The patient is seen by a clinical psychologist and a social worker in addition to the team composed of a nurse clinician, transplant cardiologist, and transplant cardiac surgeon. Once patients are involved in testing, they are invited to attend a cardiac transplantation support group session.

OPERATIVE TECHNIQUE

Cardiac transplantation depends on careful organization and timing of the operation. The donor procurement team checks the donor's blood type, serology tests, chest radiograph, and ECG. The recipient team does not anesthetize the patient until a report is received from the donor team indicating that the donor heart looks fully functional. Usually the recipient heart is not excised until the donor heart arrives in the operating room.

At the donor operation, the superior vena cava is mobilized circumferentially, and the inferior vena cava is mobilized to a lesser degree. The ascending aorta is separated from the main pulmonary artery. Once the other organs are ready for procurement, the donor is fully heparinized. The superior vena cava is divided between 0 silk ties, and a stapler may also be used after removal of any central lines. The inferior vena cava is divided just above the diaphragm. The heart is allowed to beat until empty (three to five beats). The aortic cross-clamp is applied at the level of the innominate artery, and 1 L of cold potassium cardioplegic solution is administered into the aortic root. We use Stanford cardioplegia. Pediatric hearts receive 15 to 20 mL/kg of cardioplegia. Cold topical saline is also applied. Once the cardioplegia has been delivered, the pulmonary veins are divided flush with the pericardium. The main pulmonary artery is divided at the level of its bifurcation. The aorta is divided at the level of the arch beyond the take-off of the innominate artery. The heart is then stored in cold saline solution in a sterile container at about 4°C.

Orthotopic Transplantation

When orthotopic cardiac transplantation is performed, the recipient heart is excised along the atrioventricular groove beginning in the right atrium (Fig. 16-74). The appendage is usually excised, and the incision extends posteriorly through the coronary sinus. The great vessels are divided just above the sinuses of Valsalva. The size of the left atrial cuff is determined by the pulmonary veins. If the left atrial appendage is preserved, the left pulmonary veins are usually in no way compromised. Once the heart has been excised, the left atrial appendage can be amputated separately. The donor heart is carefully examined for a patent foramen ovale and abnormal coronary artery branching. The pulmonary veins are connected to create a large posterior atrial cuff. The sinus node is visualized; a curvilinear incision is made from the inferior vena cava toward the right atrial appendage avoiding the sinus node area. The aorta and pulmonary artery are separated and cleaned of any debris.

The left atrial anastomosis is performed first with the heart wrapped in a cold saline sponge. Usually, 3-0 monofilament polypropylene suture is used in an adult and 4-0 polypropylene in a child (Fig. 16-75). The left atrium is filled with cold saline before completion of this suture

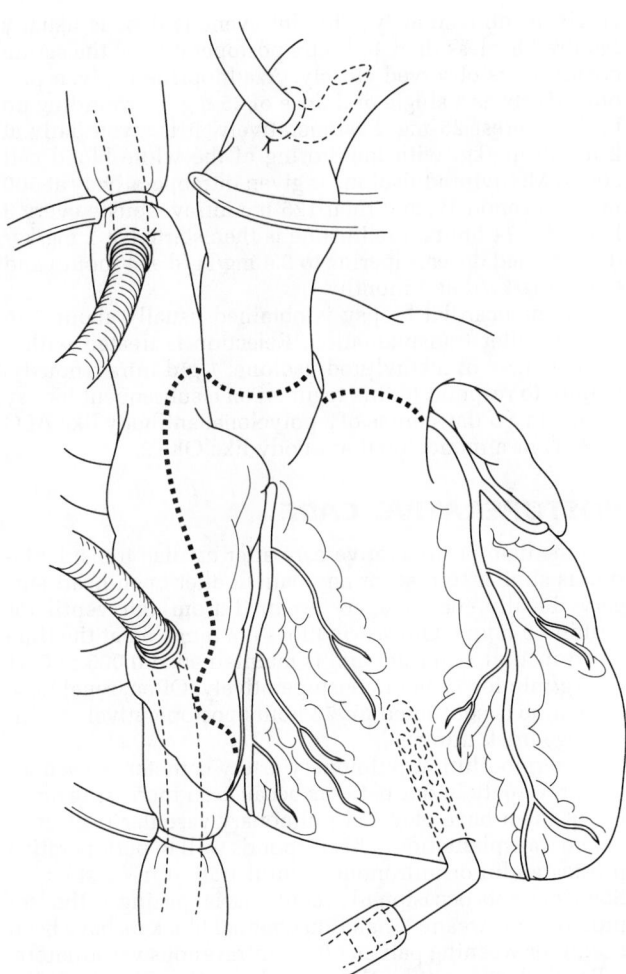

Figure 16-74. First phase of cardiac transplantation operation—excision of the recipient heart. The incision runs along the atrioventricular groove, beginning in the right atrium. The pulmonary artery and aorta are incised as marked by the dashed line.

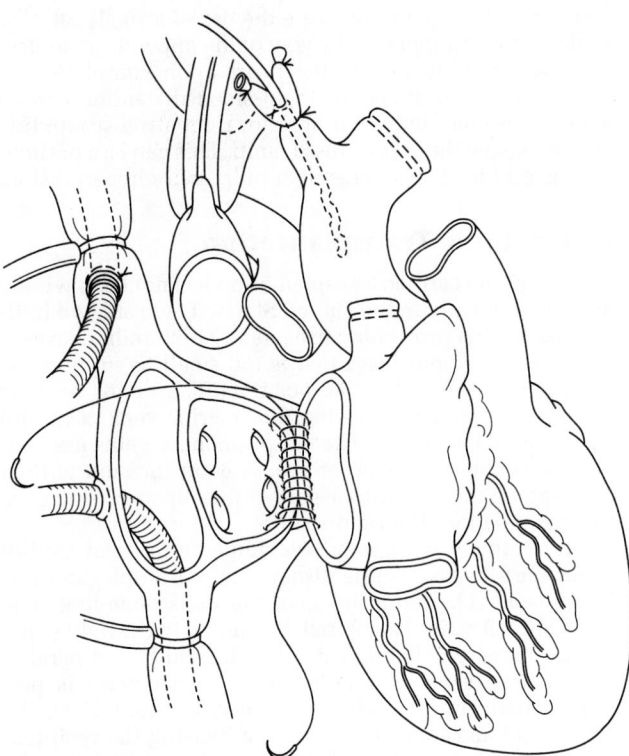

Figure 16-75. Anastomosis of the donor heart to the recipient left atrium.

line. The heart has topical cold saline running over it for the remainder of the implantation. The right atrial anastomosis is performed next, and care is taken to avoid any impingement of the sinus node or coronary sinus by this suture line. Before completion of this suture line, the oximetric thermodilution catheter is passed into the right ventricle and out the pulmonary artery.

The pulmonary artery anastomosis is then performed end-to-end with running 4-0 monofilament suture. The pulmonary arteries should be trimmed and approximated so that kinking is not a possibility. A significant kink in a newly constructed pulmonary artery can cause right-sided heart failure. Finally, donor and recipient aortas are sewn end-to-end with running 4-0 monofilament suture (Fig. 16-76). The anastomosis should allow enough mobility for visualization of the posterior surface of the aortic suture line. The aortic cross-clamp is released after deairing maneuvers, and these maneuvers are continued. Ventricular pacing wires are placed on the donor right ventricle, and atrial pacing wires are secured to the donor right atrium.

The preferred donor heart ischemia time should be less than 4 hours if possible.[265] To achieve this goal, it is sometimes necessary to perform the left atrial anastomosis, followed by the aortic anastomosis. The aortic cross-clamp is then released, and the right atrial and pulmonary arterial anastomoses are performed as the heart is being reper-

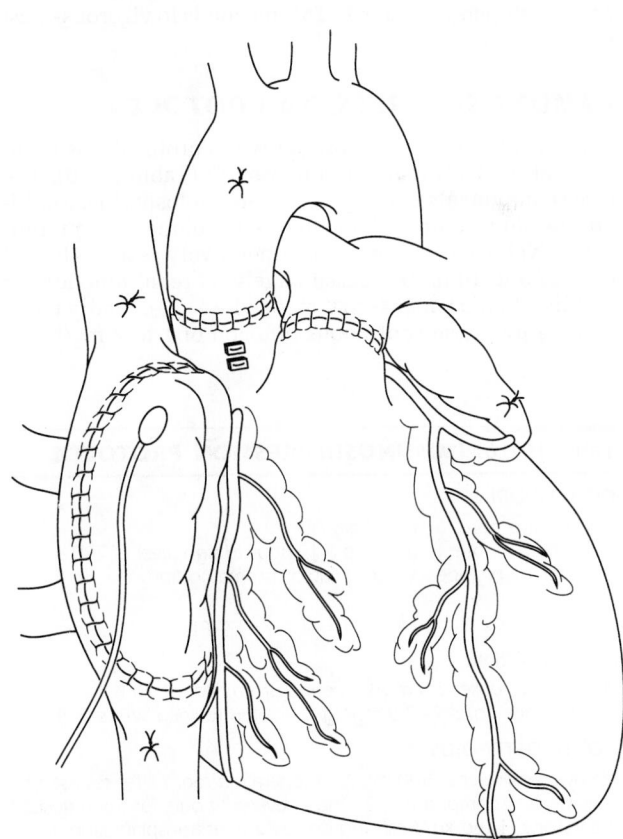

Figure 16-76. Completed cardiac graft operation with epicardial pacemaker in place.

fused. Some surgeons advocate the use of a small catheter in the left atrium, placed by way of the appendage, to drip cold saline solution into the heart upon completion of the left atrial anastomosis. Right-sided distention can be avoided by completing the anterior right atrial suture line after releasing the aortic cross-clamp. This can be a particularly good idea for patients with pulmonary hypertension.

Heterotopic Transplantation

Heterotopic cardiac transplantation has not been widely applied clinically in the United States. There are two indications for this procedure: irreversibly high pulmonary resistance or a donor heart that is too small to support the recipient in the orthotopic position. The donor heart is prepared by first oversewing the inferior vena cava and right pulmonary veins. The left pulmonary veins are connected to create a single orifice. A 6-cm incision is then made along the posterior aspect of the superior vena cava that extends into the right atrium.

The recipient aorta is cross-clamped after total cardiopulmonary bypass is established, and cardioplegic arrest is achieved. The left atrial anastomosis is done first. The recipient left atrium is incised, beginning in the right superior pulmonary vein and extending inferiorly and parallel to the atrial septum. The left atrial anastomosis is performed with running 3-0 polypropylene suture. Next, the right atrial anastomosis is done by incising the recipient superior vena cava for a distance of about 6 cm into the right atrium. The posterior wall of this suture line is done first, again with running 3-0 suture. The aortic anastomosis is then performed end to side with running 4-0 suture. The pulmonary artery anastomosis is the last to be completed, also end to side, but this often requires an interposition graft of 20-mm woven Dacron.

Right lower lobe atelectasis is a common problem in the early postoperative course. This responds to vigorous chest physiotherapy.

IMMUNOSUPPRESSION PROTOCOL

The triple-drug immunosuppression protocol was pioneered at the University of Minnesota[266] (Table 16-16). The three components of this protocol are cyclosporine, azathioprine, and combined methylprednisolone and prednisone. Cyclosporine is given preoperatively as a single oral dose of 6 to 10 mg/kg, based largely on renal function. In addition to the usual 4- to 6-mg/kg dose given orally twice daily, a low-dose continuous infusion of 1 to 2 mg/h can

Table 16-16. IMMUNOSUPPRESSION PROTOCOL

CYCLOSPORINE

Preoperative dose: 6–10 mg/kg PO
Maintenance dose: targeted to a 12-hour trough level of 200 ± 25 ng/mL by high-performance liquid chromatography during the first 6 months
After 6 months: trough level of 100 ± 25 ng/mL

AZATHIOPRINE

Preoperative dose: 2.5 mg/kg (round up to nearest 25 kg)
Maintenance dose: 2–2.5 mg/kg/d (titrated to keep WBCs ≥ 4000)

CORTICOSTEROIDS

Methylprednisolone, 500 mg IV, in operating room after release of aortic crossclamp, then 125 mg IV every 8 hours for three doses
Prednisone, 1 mg/kg/d starting on day 2 after transplantation, in divided doses, with tapering to 0.3 mg/kg/d by 3 months
0.15–0.10 mg/kg/d by the end of the first year

be given intravenously. This intravenous dose is usually required for less than 48 hours postoperatively; the serum creatinine is observed closely. Azathioprine is given preoperatively as a single oral dose of 25 mg/kg, rounding up to the nearest 25 mg. Postoperatively, it is given daily at 2 to 2.5 mg/kg, with monitoring of the white blood cell count. Methylprednisolone is given intraoperatively at 500 mg intravenously, and then 125 mg intravenously every 8 hours for 24 hours. Prednisone is then started at 1 mg/kg/d in divided doses, tapering to 0.4 mg/kg/d at 1 month and to 0.3 mg/kg/d at 3 months.

Endomyocardial biopsy is obtained usually about 7 to 10 days after transplantation. Rejection is treated with a 3-day course of methylprednisolone, 1 g/d intravenously. Failure to respond to this regimen on a subsequent biopsy results in a 5-day course of a polyclonal antibody like ALG or ATG or a monoclonal antibody like OKT3.

POSTOPERATIVE CARE

Immediate postoperative care after cardiac transplantation is similar to that for any patient after open heart surgery. Ideally, patients are weaned from the ventilator within 48 hours. Orogastric tubes are removed at the time of extubation. Isoproterenol is maintained at 0.005 to 0.01 mg/kg/min for 72 hours postoperatively. Often, renal dose dopamine is continued for 72 hours postoperatively to encourage brisk diuresis.

A thermodilution pulmonary artery catheter is used almost routinely in our patients because an increasing number of them have elevated pulmonary vascular resistance before transplantation. This responds well to perioperative prostaglandin or milronone administration in most cases. Some patients occasionally require atrial pacing as the isoproterenol is weaned. Calcium channel blockers have been useful for weaning patients from intravenous vasodilators.

Prophylactic antibiotics are discontinued when the chest tubes are removed, usually on the second postoperative day. Oral diet usually is started after chest tube removal on the second postoperative day. Endomyocardial biopsy is performed 7 to 10 days after transplantation, and pacing wires are often removed at that time.

Preoperative recipient and donor titers are obtained for cytomegalovirus, herpes simplex virus, varicella zoster virus, and Epstein-Barr virus. These titers are repeated before patient discharge. All patients receive trimethoprim-sulfamethoxazole at a dosage of two tablets daily for a creatinine less than 3 and only one tablet daily for a creatinine greater than 3. Pentamidine inhaler is given monthly to the few patients who are allergic to sulfa drugs. Acyclovir is given prophylactically to prevent viral infections. It is given as 10 mg/kg intravenously every 8 hours, and when patients can tolerate the oral medication, it is given as 800 mg every 6 hours. Acyclovir therapy is continued as long as the patient does not experience any alteration in liver or renal function.

REJECTION

The diagnosis of rejection is based on endomyocardial biopsies. Biopsies are routinely performed 7 to 10 days after transplantation and then every 2 weeks for 3 months, once a month for 6 months, and then once every 3 months. After 2 years, biopsies are performed annually. A recent review of experience in pediatric cardiac transplant patients has shown that surveillance biopsies during the first 6 months after transplantation may show clinically unsuspected rejection. After 6 months, rejection discovered on biopsy in the absence of symptoms is rare.

The standardized grading system was proposed by the

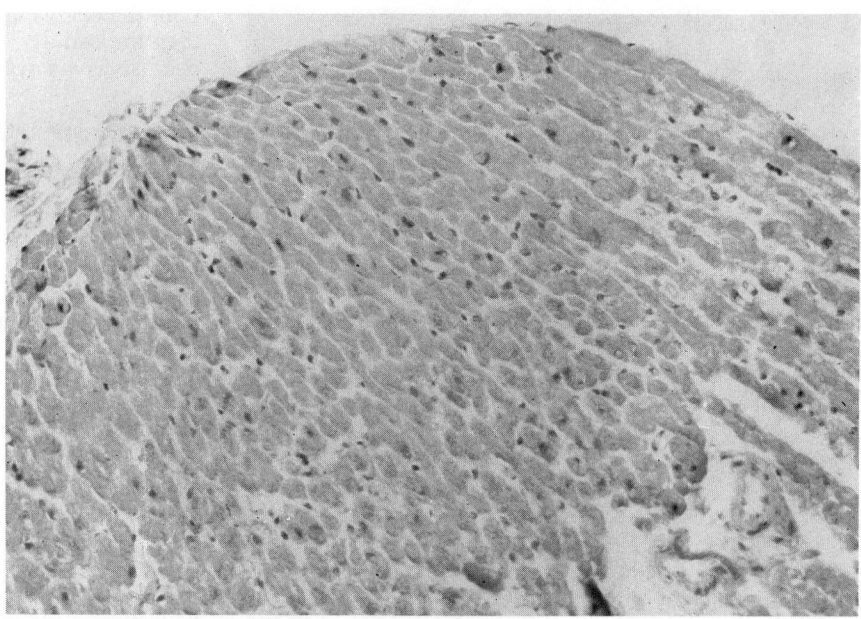

Figure 16-77. Endomyocardial biopsy specimen demonstrating normal myocardial tissue.

International Society for Heart and Lung Transplantation in 1990.[267] Normal endomyocardium on a biopsy specimen is demonstrated in (Fig. 16-77). Grade 0 is no evidence of rejection. It should be used when there is neither evidence of acute rejection nor a cellular infiltrate or any other histopathologic change. Grade 1A is mild acute rejection (Fig. 16-78). It represents a distinct perivascular infiltrate of large activated lymphocytes in one or two locations within a single biopsy fragment or several biopsy pieces. Myocyte damage is not seen. Plump endothelial cells should be differentiated from a perivascular infiltrate. Grade 1B is diffuse, mild acute rejection (Fig. 16-79). This is a sparse but more diffuse infiltrate of activated lymphocytes extending into the interstitium between the myocytes. Again, myocyte necrosis is not seen. This sparse infiltrate may be seen in one or several pieces of the biopsy tissue. Grade 2 is focal, moderate acute rejection (Fig. 16-80). This is the

situation where a single large circumscribed infiltrate of activated lymphocytes, with or without eosinophils, and with focal myocyte damage is seen. This grade exists to evaluate the need for therapy in patients with one focus of myocyte damage on a cardiac biopsy. Grade 3A is multifocal, moderate acute rejection (Fig. 16-81). This represents multifocal lymphocytic infiltrates with or without eosinophils with two or more foci causing myocyte necrosis or obvious myocyte replacement. Lymphocytes indent or overlap myocytes and so cause partial or total myocyte damage. Free myocyte nuclei, the remnants of myocyte damage, may be seen within these infiltrates. Grade 3B is diffuse or borderline severe acute rejection (Fig. 16-82). This is a more diffuse aggressive inflammatory infiltrate within several pieces of the biopsy tissue. Myocyte damage is obvious, as well as definite myocyte replacement by inflammatory cells. Eosinophils and occasional neutro-

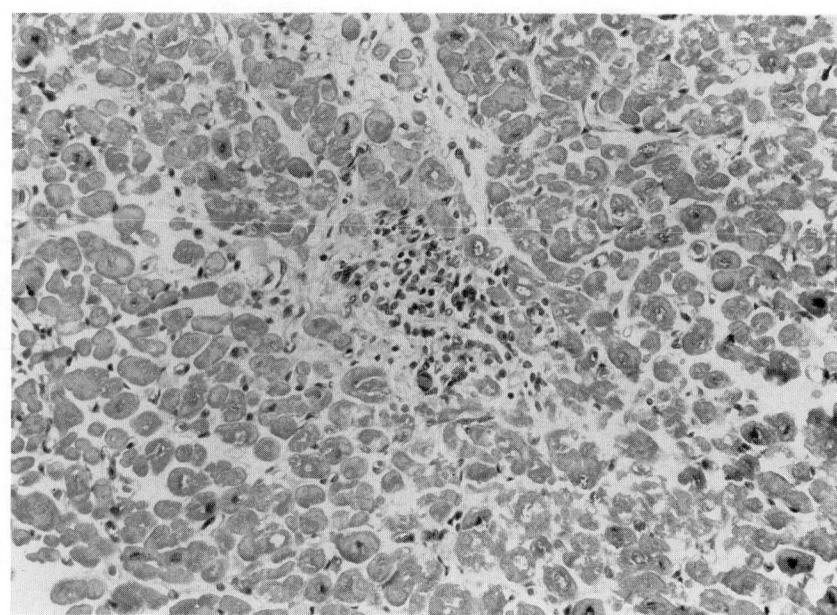

Figure 16-78. Histologic appearance of mild cardiac rejection.

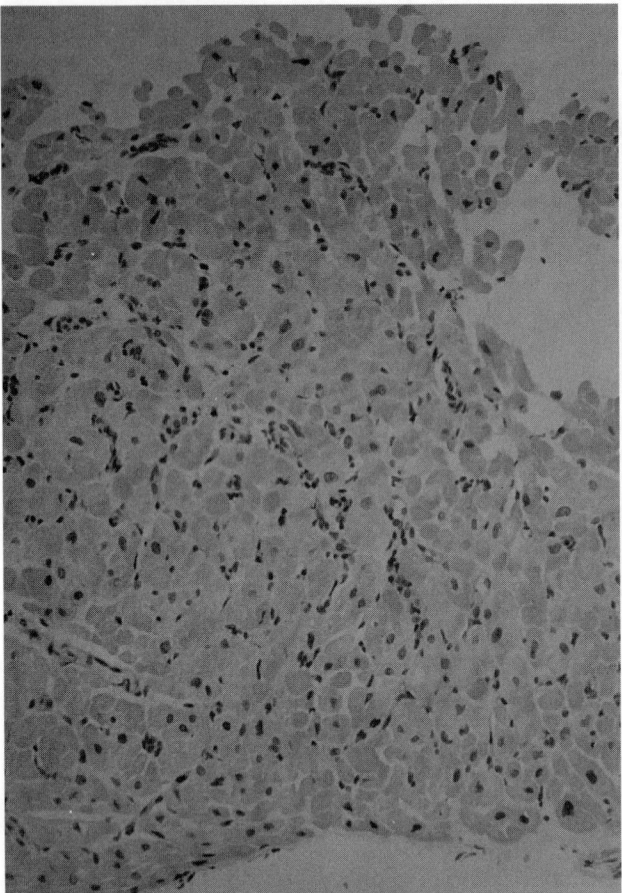

Figure 16-79. Grade 1B—diffuse, mild acute rejection.

phils may be present. Hemorrhage is not seen, and if present, is focal. Grade 4 is severe acute rejection. The inflammatory infiltrate is polymorphous including neutrophils and eosinophils. It should be in more than one piece of the biopsy. Often, superimposed vasculitis resulting in interstitial hemorrhage is seen. Edema may also be present. When the patient has been treated for ongoing acute rejec-

tion, the edema and hemorrhage may be more prominent than the cellular infiltrate. This is the situation in which necrosis is always present.

PEDIATRIC CARDIAC TRANSPLANTATION

Pediatric cardiac transplantation became a real clinical entity in 1984.[268] This brought national attention to the need for donors in the pediatric and even the neonatal age group. Cardiac transplantation is now an accepted therapy for infants and older children with severe congenital heart disease and cardiomyopathy. Most children undergoing heart transplants have end-stage cardiomyopathy. Congenital heart disease is a growing indication. The only absolute contraindication to pediatric heart transplantation is severely elevated pulmonary vascular resistance, usually greater than 8 Wood units. Other absolute contraindications are the same as for adults, namely irreversible renal or hepatic disease, active systemic infection, and uncured malignancy.

The donor operation in a pediatric case proceeds much as it does in the adult. In patients who have had Fontan procedures, additional length of superior vena cava is needed.[269] Patients with pulmonary atresia require additional pulmonary artery. Patients with hypoplastic left heart syndrome require procurement of the entire aortic arch and part of the descending thoracic aorta.[270] Recent reports suggest that Roe's solution may be superior to Stanford cardioplegia in pediatric cardiac transplantation.[271] The recipient operation proceeds much the same way as it does for the adult, however, more complex reconstruction may be necessary in patients who have had previous congenital heart surgery or who present with hypoplastic left heart syndrome. Some controversy exists about whether it is better to do the first stage of the Norwood operation and then the heart transplant, or to do the heart transplant first.

Overall, patient survival in pediatric heart transplantation has not changed much since 1984. The 2-year survival rate is better in patients older than 5 years. In our own series of 25 patients, aged 7 days to 18 years, 7 have died. Four deaths were early, three were related to donor organ failure, and one was due to multiorgan system failure. All

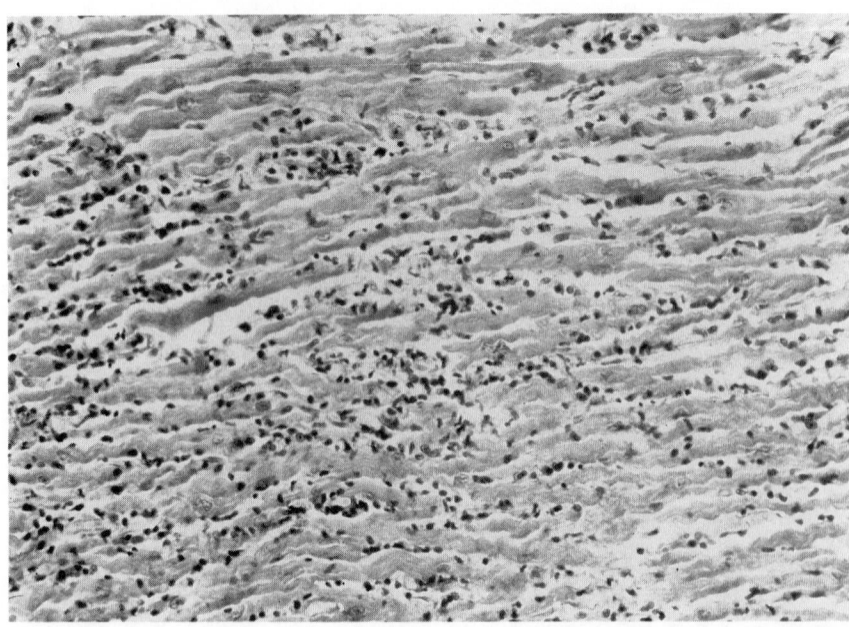

Figure 16-80. Grade 2—focal, moderate acute rejection.

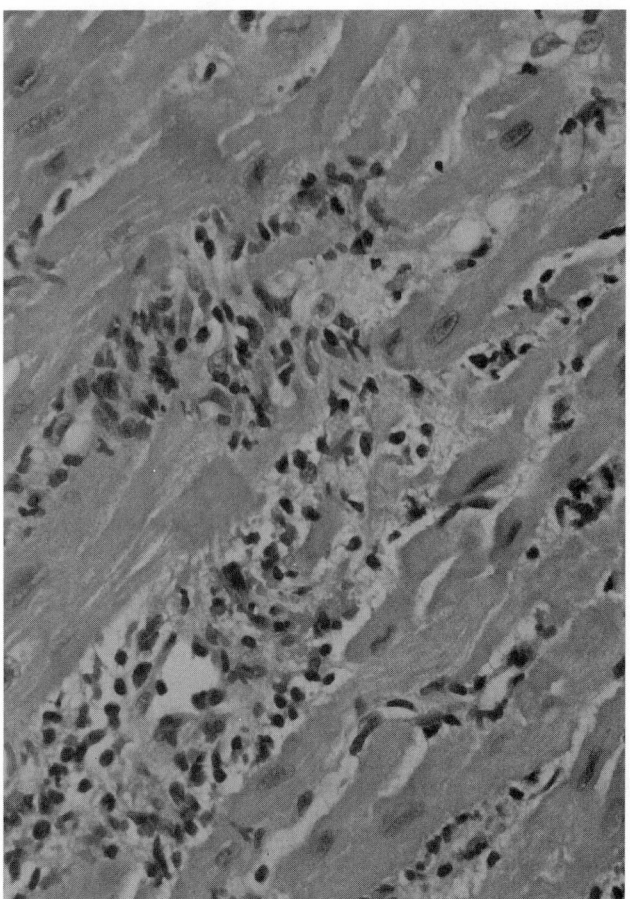

Figure 16-81. Grade 3A—multifocal, moderate acute rejection.

three of the late deaths were related to acute rejection and two of these were in teenagers who became noncompliant with their immunosuppression.

GRAFT ATHEROSCLEROSIS

Graft atherosclerosis is a serious complication of cardiac transplantation. It is thought to be the result of chronic vascular rejection, which occurs more than 6 months after transplantation. Isolated lesions have been successfully treated with percutaneous transluminal coronary angioplasty and even with coronary artery bypass grafting. Diffuse disease requires retransplantation. Certain risk factors for graft atherosclerosis may include older donor heart, cytomegalovirus infection, elevated serum triglyceride levels (over 280 mg/dL) at 1 year, and two or more acute rejection episodes.[272]

The pathophysiology of this form of arterial disease is selective involvement of the graft arterial tree without involvement of the recipient native vessels. This suggests its immunologic or injury-related basis. There are two schools of thought regarding its pathogenesis. One school believes that it represents an exaggeration of the immune mechanism involved in spontaneous atherogenesis. The other believes that the disease may be the result of endothelial injury related to cooling the heart to 4°C at procurement, and subsequent reperfusion injury. There are four categories of graft coronary atherosclerosis—fibrous intimal thickening, atheromatous plaque, intermediate lesions, and diffuse necrotizing vasculitis. In one series, it was found that by the fifth year after transplantation, graft atherosclerosis was a major cause of graft failure.[273]

Once the diagnosis is made, the therapeutic approach to graft atherosclerosis is neither satisfying nor effective. Multivessel angioplasty has been used. Discrete proximal lesions in patients have been successfully treated with angioplasty. This is thought to be only palliative, however. The definitive therapy remains retransplantation and, of course, graft atherosclerosis does recur. The overall 1-year survival rate for retransplantation, as reported by the Registry of the International Society of Heart and Lung Transplantation, is only 54.4%.[274]

RESULTS AND SURVIVAL

The Registry of the International Society for Heart Transplantation has collected data on 26,704 heart transplants from 251 centers.[275] The overall 1-year survival rate is 80%. The overall 5-year actuarial survival rate is about 65%. Since 1983, however, the actuarial survival rate at 1 year for these patients has been 86%. Survival in patients receiving heterotopic cardiac transplants is significantly lower than in patients receiving hearts in the orthotopic position.

In the pediatric age group, the actuarial survival rate at 2 years is 80% in our own series and 76% at 5 years.[276] Infection and rejection are just as significant problems to manage in this age group. Because congenital heart disease is often the reason for transplantation in these patients, right ventricular dysfunction resulting from preexisting pulmonary hypertension has occurred.

RESEARCH AND FUTURE CONCERNS

Research is directed toward several areas in cardiac transplantation, including graft atherosclerosis, less invasive rejection detection, new immunosuppressants, xenografts, and totally implantable artificial devices.

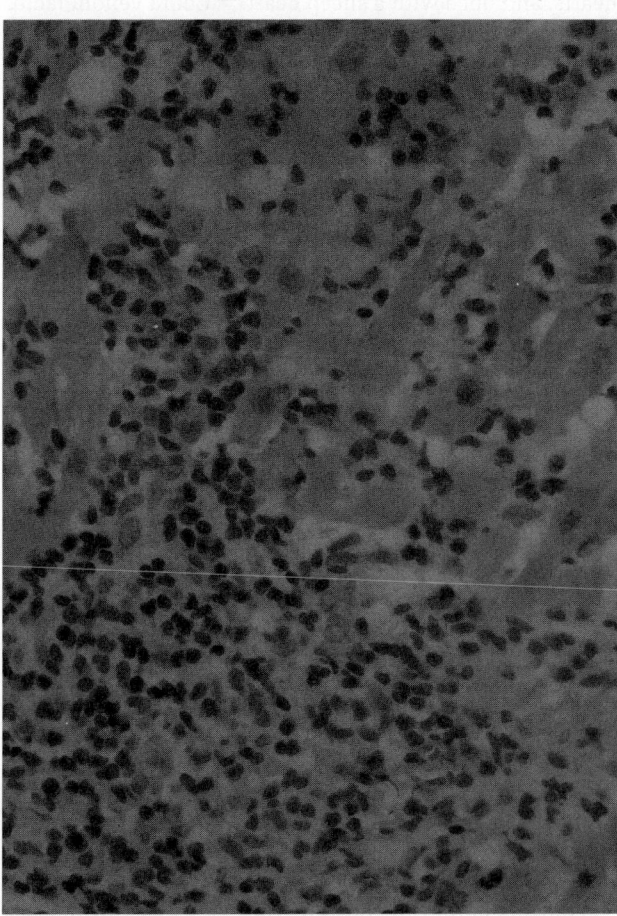

Figure 16-82. Grade 3B—diffuse or borderline severe acute rejection.

Despite careful diet control and the use of aspirin and dipyridamole, graft atherosclerosis continues to be a problem. At 3 years after transplantation, some degree of coronary artery disease was present in 29% of our recipients. Better control of rejection and fewer cytomegalovirus infections may help prevent this complication. Invasive approaches to combat this are percutaneous coronary transluminal angioplasty, coronary artery bypass graft, and retransplantation. Graft atherosclerosis does recur.

Frequent endomyocardial biopsies can lead to sampling error and the presence of scar or fibrosis instead of reasonable endomyocardial tissue for examination. Magnetic resonance (MR) imaging has been shown to be useful in the noninvasive diagnosis of cardiac transplant rejection in the acute phase.[277] Myocardial rejection has had a high correlation with increased myocardial thickness, wall motion abnormalities, and prolonged T_2 relaxation times. T_2 relaxation time measurements are known to increase with increasing tissue water content. MR imaging has been used most extensively with pediatric patients who are too small to provide frequent endomyocardial biopsy specimens. More work needs to be done to develop greater confidence in this technique. Work with a canine model appears to offer hope of detecting early rejection using strategically positioned electrodes placed at the time of cardiac transplantation.[278]

FK 506 has been demonstrated to be an effective immunosuppressant in cardiac transplantation.[279] Mycophenolate mofetil is currently in clinical trials in the United States.[280]

Xenografts have been used clinically as cardiac transplants without success at least five times from 1964 to 1985—twice with chimpanzee hearts, twice with baboon hearts, and once with a sheep heart.[281] Cobra venom factor has been used to inactivate complement, and experimental animal recipients have undergone plasmapheresis, but severe graft rejection is an established outcome in a short time in discordant models.[282] The best concordant model in primates boasts a graft survival time of 77 days.[283]

If xenografts were to be used now, they would be used as bridges to transplantation. Totally implantable left ventricular assist devices will soon be available to act in that capacity. The Novacor device is undergoing clinical trials to obtain FDA approval for that use. Good results have been obtained with the Novacor and with the Thermetics pump as bridges to transplantation.[284,285] The total artificial heart in the form of the Jarvik pneumatically driven artificial heart has been shelved.

Over 90% of all cardiac transplant recipients are totally rehabilitated and can resume normal active lives. Unfortunately, only 46% to 56% are able to return to full-time work, usually because of problems related to insurance and disability incomes. Over 95% of cardiac transplant recipients surveyed do not regret their decision and said they would have a cardiac transplantation again.[286] The first adult cardiac transplant recipient in the United Stated died of a "galaxy of complications" in January 1968.[287] Now, 28 years later, cardiac transplantation is an accepted, often routine therapeutic option for selected patients with end-stage heart disease.

Pulmonary Transplantation

LARRY R. KAISER

Transplantation of the lung represents one of the last horizons in solid-organ transplantation. After an initial effort at human pulmonary transplant in 1963, there was considerable excitement but little activity in this area until 1967, when a flurry of pulmonary transplantations followed the first successful human cardiac transplantation. The longest lung transplant survivor during this early period lived 10 months, most of that time spent in the hospital. The major problems preventing successful pulmonary transplantation have been the failure of the airway anastomosis to heal, infection, and rejection.[288]

Unlike other solid organs, the lung has no systemic arterial supply that can be reconnected. Bronchial artery anatomy varies greatly, and the size of bronchial arteries, even when they can be identified, precludes direct anastomosis. Therefore, the bronchial anastomosis is ischemic after the operation, and airway dehiscence may occur about 3 weeks after transplantation. The combination of anastomotic ischemia and other factors, including the susceptibility of the lung to infection because of its direct contact with the outside environment via the airway, prevented successful transplantation despite the efforts of many investigators.[289]

The first combined heart and lung transplantation was performed successfully in 1981, but the procedure sometimes required removal of an otherwise normal heart from the recipient. Combined cardiac and pulmonary transplantation introduced a series of new problems related to transplanting two organs, including those associated with heart transplantation and especially accelerated coronary artery atherosclerosis. With combined cardiac and pulmonary transplantation, however, healing of the tracheal anastomosis presents less of a problem, probably because the bronchial artery collaterals in the subcarinal space are preserved.

Recognizing the potential advantage of single-lung transplantation, investigators experimentally defined the factors contributing to failure in pulmonary transplantation.[290] They demonstrated the significant detrimental effect that corticosteroids exert on airway healing and showed that cyclosporine did not have this adverse effect. Delaying the administration of maintenance corticosteroids proved advantageous. The investigators also demonstrated that wrapping the bronchial anastomosis with a pedicle of gastrocolic omentum resulted in early capillary ingrowth and revascularization of the airway, promoting healing.

Another significant factor contributing to the improved success of single-lung transplantation was the recognition that careful recipient selection is crucial. Initially, it was felt that the ideal candidate for single-lung transplantation was an individual with end-stage restrictive disease (pulmonary fibrosis), a situation that would lead to preferential ventilation and perfusion of the graft because of the increased compliance and relatively decreased pulmonary vascular resistance of the transplanted lung. In addition, although almost all previous attempts at pulmonary transplantation involved desperately ill, ventilator-dependent patients, lung replacement in a moribund patient who has already suffered significant nutritional depletion and muscle wasting is likely to fail. It is important to select individuals who are ambulatory and to place potential recipients in an intense pretransplantation pulmonary rehabilitation program to further increase the likelihood of a successful outcome. Improvement in patient selection may indeed be the single most important factor responsible for the success of pulmonary transplantation, even though indications for pulmonary transplantation have broadened considerably.

INDICATIONS

Pulmonary transplantation is offered to patients with irreversible end-stage pulmonary disease (ESPD) whose life expectancy is 1 year or less. Patients with ESPD are classified according to the physiologic derangement, regardless of the initial cause. Patients usually have either predominantly obstructive or restrictive disease, although occasionally they may have a mixed defect. Those with end-stage obstructive physiology may demonstrate changes of emphysema, either nonbullous or bullous, or changes secondary to chronic infection (bronchitic). Patients with cystic fibrosis fall into the latter category, their lung disease resulting from the ravages of chronic, persistent infection (bronchiectasis; Fig. 16-83A). Patients with cystic fibrosis may also present with a mixed obstructive–restrictive picture. Those with idiopathic pulmonary fibrosis have restrictive physiology (see Fig. 14-82B). Patients with a congenital deficiency of the α_1-antitrypsin protease commonly present with bullous emphy-

sema, most noticeable at the lung bases (see Fig. 14-82C). A number of patients also have radiographic and physiologic changes that are similar to those seen in α_1-antitrypsin deficiency but their levels of α_1-antitrypsin are normal, suggesting the absence of other, as yet undescribed, proteases.

Patients with pulmonary vascular disease are a separate and distinct group. Those with end-stage disease have either primary pulmonary hypertension, a disease of unknown cause, or secondary pulmonary hypertension, resulting from increased pulmonary perfusion caused by a shunt at the cardiac or supracardiac level. When pulmonary vascular resistance increases sufficiently, the resul-

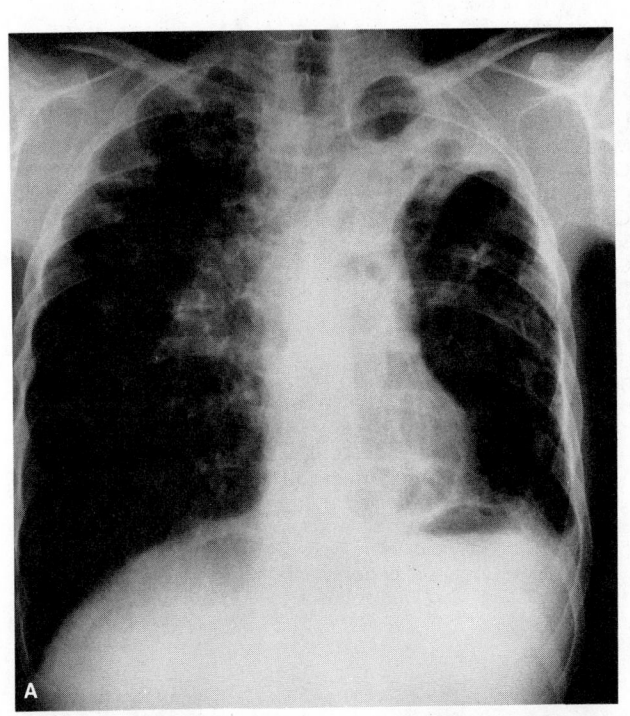

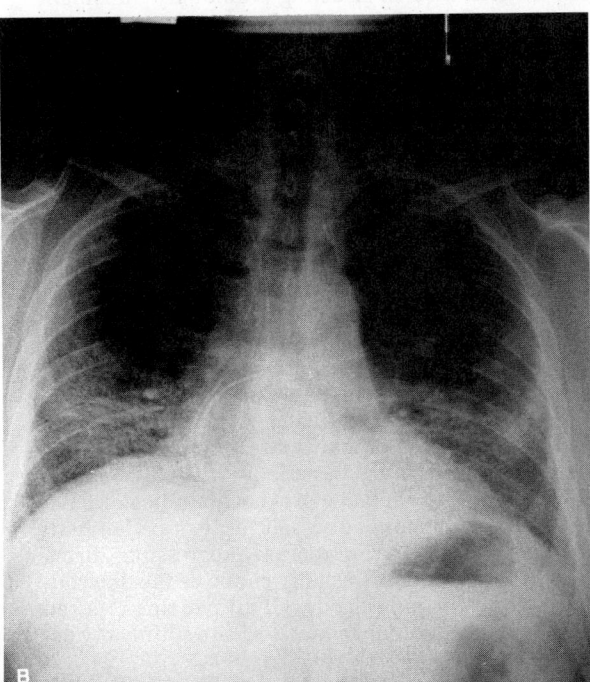

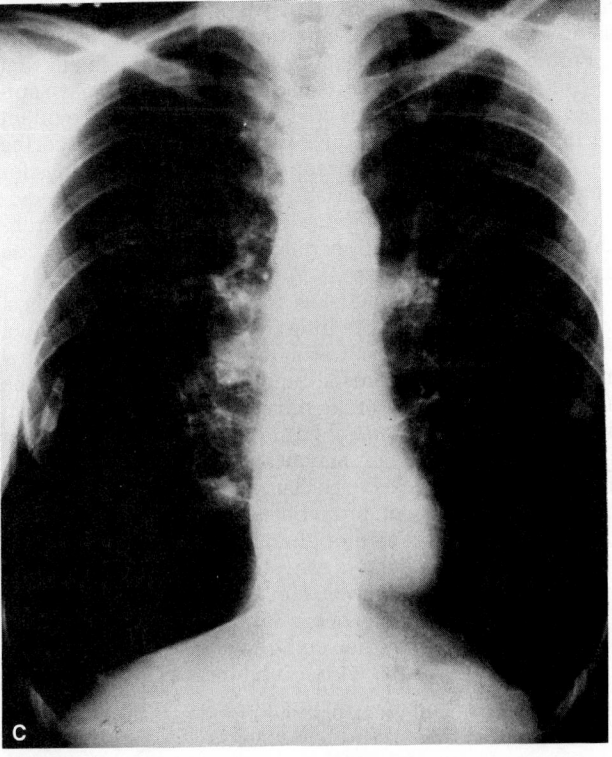

Figure 16-83. (A) Chest radiograph of a patient with cystic fibrosis showing typical changes caused by infection that results in a mixed obstructive-restrictive picture. Hyperexpansion of the lungs and evidence of bronchiectasis are apparent. (B) Chest radiograph of a patient with idiopathic pulmonary fibrosis. The lungs demonstrate a diffuse interstitial pattern with a distinct reduction in size. (C) Chest radiograph of a patient with end-stage emphysema caused by α_1-antitrypsin deficiency. There is a paucity of lung markings, and marked bullous changes can be seen at the bases. The lungs are markedlyhyperinflated with downward displacement of both hemidiaphragms.

tant increase in pulmonary artery pressure reverses shunt flow from right to left. This is known as *Eisenmenger syndrome*. When shunt reversal occurs, patients are typically considered inoperable because at this point, the mortality associated with primary cardiac operations is prohibitive. Theoretically, it is feasible to close the cardiac shunt if one inserts a new lung or lungs, thus unloading the right ventricle with the subsequent decrease in pulmonary vascular resistance to normal levels and the improvement of right ventricular function.

Because of problems with donor availability, lung transplantation is limited to those patients 60 years old or younger (with some flexibility) who have no other systemic disease and who have no significant coronary artery disease. The criteria used in selecting pulmonary transplant recipients are as follows:

- ESPD with life expectancy of less than 18 months
- No other systemic disease
- No significant coronary artery disease
- No significant psychiatric disorder
- No contraindication to immunosuppression
- Age 60 years or under (with some flexibility)
- Adequate psychosocial support system

Candidates for pulmonary transplantation ordinarily have significant functional impairment that interferes with activities of daily living. In those patients with restrictive or obstructive disease, abnormal gas exchange is the major problem, and essentially they all require supplemental oxygen 24 hours a day. In patients with pulmonary vascular disease, the manifestations of right ventricular failure predominate. These latter patients may or may not require oxygen.

Predicting life expectancy in patients with ESPD is difficult since there are no reliable prognostic indicators that provide reliable estimates of how long a given patient will live. Documented evidence of disease progression during the previous 6 to 12 months usually supports the determination of limited life expectancy. Of all patients referred for transplant consideration, about 30% are ultimately accepted (Table 16-17).

Potential candidates need to be extremely well motivated to cope with the stresses associated with both the pretransplantation and posttransplantation periods and with the lifelong care they require after transplantation. Transplantation trades one chronic disease for another—the posttransplantation state. Patients require daily medication to maintain their transplanted organ and are constantly at risk for infection.

DONOR CONSIDERATIONS

Unlike other solid organs for transplantation, potential donor lungs may be assessed by plain radiographs. In addition, bronchoscopy provides a way to directly examine the potential donor organs and to collect material for culture and Gram stain, the results of which may influence later treatment of the recipient. No other organ has the same risk of infection; a pulmonary infiltrate may preclude the use of a lung. A small infiltrate in one lung without evidence of purulent secretions may still allow this lung to be used in a double-lung transplant. Likewise, a pulmonary infiltrate does not necessarily preclude use of the contralateral lung for single-lung transplant. Unfortunately, the lungs of a particular donor may not be suitable when all other organs are acceptable. Because all brain-dead patients have endotracheal tubes and are on mechanical ventilation, there is a high likelihood that the airway is either colonized with bacteria or that there is ongoing invasive infection. With pulmonary infection, an infiltrate is often present on the chest radiograph. Even with a clear chest

Table 16-17. DE NOVO TUMORS IN ORGAN TRANSPLANT RECIPIENTS

Type of Cancer	Patients*
Cancers of skin and lips	978
Lymphomas	341†
Carcinomas of uterus	
Cervix	146
Body	17
Carcinomas of lung	116
Kaposi sarcoma	93
Carcinomas of colon and rectum	92
Carcinomas of breast	80
Carcinomas of vulva, perineum, penis, or scrotum	70
Carcinomas of kidney	
Host kidney	61
Allograft	6
Carcinomas of head and neck (excluding thyroid, parathyroid, and eye)	65
Leukemias	61
Metastatic carcinoma (primary site unknown)	58
Carcinomas of urinary bladder	47
Carcinomas of liver and bile ducts	39
Carcinomas of thyroid	37
Soft tissue sarcomas	32
Cancers of stomach	30
Testicular carcinomas	28
Ovarian cancers	25
Carcinomas of prostate gland	24
Cancers of the pancreas	21
Brain neoplasms	14
Miscellaneous tumors	37
TOTAL	2518

* There were 2353 patients, of whom 157 (6.7%) had more than one type of tumor affecting different organs. Of these patients, 8 each had three different types of cancer.
† One patient had two different types of lymphoma. (Penn I. Development of new tumors after transplantation. In: Cerelli GJ, ed. Organ transplantation and replacement. Philadelphia, JB Lippincott, 1988:439)

radiograph, however, purulent secretions contraindicate using the lungs for transplantation.

Problems with the lungs may begin when the insult that results in brain death occurs because the patient may aspirate gastric contents. Signs of aspiration may not be evident on the chest radiograph for 24 to 48 hours, underscoring the importance of bronchoscopy before accepting lungs for transplantation. Characteristic early bronchoscopic evidence of aspiration includes erythematous tracheobronchial mucosa, purulent secretions, and occasionally the presence of food particles.

Major pulmonary contusion resulting from blunt chest trauma also may eliminate lungs from donor consideration, but minor to moderate contusion unilaterally may still allow use of the lungs in a bilateral lung recipient. Evaluating the full extent of contusion at the time of donor retrieval is often difficult because the interval from injury to determination of brain death and donation may be short. Although the detrimental effect on gas exchange caused by a pulmonary contusion is usually transient, further bleeding into the lung parenchyma could occur if cardiopulmonary bypass is required to perform the transplantation, as would be the case in a recipient with pulmonary hypertension.

Pulmonary edema may occur as a result of massive head injury and may be further complicated by certain donor management protocols, which include the following:

- Maintenance of mean arterial blood pressure above 70 mmHg

- Preference of inotropic support over massive volumes of crystalloid solution to maintain blood pressure (dopamine, 2.5 to 10 µg/kg/min)
- Replacement of fluid at the rate of the previous hour's urine output plus 100 mL
- Maintenance of normothermia
- Maintenance of positive end-expiratory pressure at 5 cm
- Frequent endotracheal suctioning
- Gram staining of sputum
- Monitoring of arterial blood gases every 2 hours

Traditionally, renal transplantation teams have tried to ensure that adequate urine output is preserved; therefore, they preferentially infuse large volumes of crystalloid solutions. Cardiac transplantation teams prefer to avoid using high doses of inotropic agents to maintain blood pressure and also tend to administer large amounts of crystalloid solutions (Fig. 16-84). The importance of coordinating donor management to prevent "flooding" of the lungs, which are much more susceptible to the development of edema after significant cerebral insult, cannot be overstated if lungs are to be available for transplantation. Whether such edematous lungs may be "dried out" when in place in the recipient remains to be determined. The contribution of pulmonary lymphatics, of necessity severed during the donor retrieval at the time of bronchus division, to the clearing of edema in the pulmonary parenchyma is unknown.

A recent review of experience with lung donors shows that in 1 year, 174 potential donors were identified. Of these, 128 were rejected outright. After the retrieval team reached the donor hospital, 14 more were refused for a variety of reasons (Fig. 16-85). Most commonly, the lungs were refused after an initial acceptance because bronchoscopy was abnormal or because arterial blood gases significantly deteriorated between the time of acceptance and the time the retrieval team reached the donor hospital. Size of the donor lungs is less important when the recipient suffers from emphysema, in which each hemithorax is very large, compared with pulmonary fibrosis, in which the hemithorax is contracted. The most important size consideration is a reasonable match between donor and recipient height.

LUNG PRESERVATION

An important area of investigation involves optimal preservation of the ischemic lung. The donor lung must not only remain viable; it must also participate actively in gas exchange immediately after implantation. A protocol is employed that uses both a flush technique with cold crystalloid solution and topical cooling to 4°C by immer-

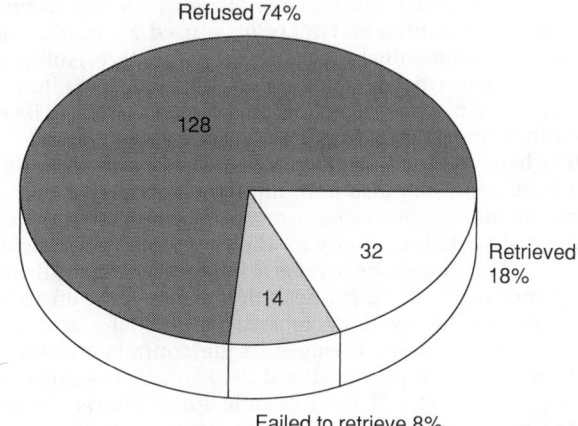

Figure 16-85. Summary of pulmonary donor referrals during a 12-month period. Of 174 referrals, 128 (74%) were refused outright, and 32 (18%) went on to transplantation. On 14 occasions, a team was sent to a donor institution only to find that the lungs were not suitable.

sion. At the time of donor lung retrieval, just before cross-clamping of the aorta, prostaglandin E₁ is injected directly into the pulmonary artery to vasodilate the pulmonary vascular bed. Vasodilation allows for more uniform distribution of the flush solution and for more uniform and rapid cooling. Prostaglandin E₁ may also serve a cytoprotective role by a mechanism yet to be determined. Crystalloid solution (Euro-Collins) at 4°C is rapidly flushed into the pulmonary artery. After removal of the donor heart, leaving a cuff of left atrium around the pulmonary veins, the lungs are removed by dividing the trachea above the carina and the pulmonary artery just proximal to the bifurcation.

The maximal safe interval for the lung to remain ischemic even when cooled has not been defined. Based on empiric observation, 6 hours has been selected as the limit. This time constraint places limits on the distance that one may travel to procure lungs. The limits of donor lung ischemia have been expanded because of efforts to develop bilateral, sequential lung replacement. The second lung to be implanted perforce is ischemic for a longer time because the lungs are not implanted simultaneously. The longest cold ischemic time has been in the range of 9 to 10 hours, and the lung functioned well within 24 hours after implantation. Although donor lung dysfunction occasionally occurs (5% to 10% incidence), manifest by abnormally high oxygen requirements, prolonged need for mechanical ventilation, and persistent infiltrates on chest radiograph, it is usually reversible. Also, the development of this problem has not correlated with prolonged donor lung ischemic time.

Whether one type of solution used for flushing the lungs is better than another remains to be determined. Experimentally, a low potassium dextran (LPD) solution may be better for early lung function than the standard Euro-Collins solution. Using both an isolated perfused rabbit lung model and a canine model, the LPD solution was superior to other solutions in terms of gas exchange during the early posttransplantation period. With the LPD solution used for preservation, bilateral, sequential pulmonary transplantations have been performed in baboons using lungs with ischemic times of 16 to 18 hours, and excellent gas exchange has been noted immediately after implantation and again at 72 hours postoperatively. Other methods of preservation have also been used experimentally. Core cooling of the donor with an extracorporeal circuit has

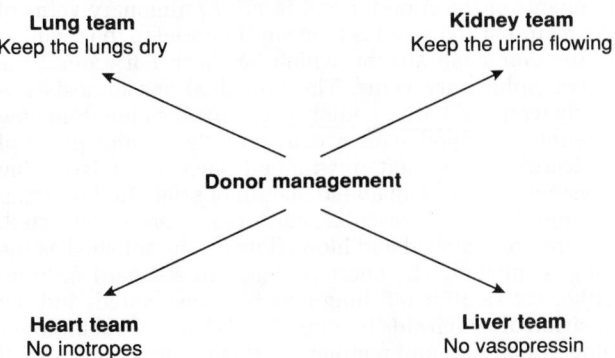

Figure 16-84. Each organ retrieval team has its own set of donor management protocols that often conflict.

been used extensively in Great Britain for cardiopulmonary transplantation. Others have used an immersion technique without flushing the pulmonary artery. Autoperfusion of the cardiopulmonary block represents an alternative method of heart and lung preservation and has been used in some centers.

It is believed that lung injury results not only from the ischemic insult but also from injury occurring at the time of reperfusion of the ischemic organ. Several experimental models of acute lung injury implicate oxygen free radicals as a factor in the genesis of reperfusion injury. A significant early increase in lung permeability is seen after an ischemic period followed by reperfusion, which improves within several hours. Changes in the contralateral, nonischemic lung are presumably due to substances released during reperfusion of the ischemic lung. Efforts are directed at identifying techniques to attenuate the reperfusion injury.

Most experimental studies in lung preservation to date have been largely empiric, evaluating the effects of various techniques on subsequent lung function. Further progress requires a more detailed understanding of events at the cellular level during ischemia and reperfusion so that a rational approach to reduce or eliminate these changes may evolve. Satisfactory preservation techniques must protect not only cell structure and metabolism, but also functional integrity of the lung as a whole to maintain normal gas exchange. In addition, methods of preservation that allow for a prolonged ischemic time must also preserve the viability and microcirculation of the airway to prevent subsequent complications of airway healing. It would serve no useful purpose to extend the ischemic time only to have the airway fail to heal because of thrombosis in small vessels. Given the ability to safely preserve livers and kidneys for 24 hours or longer, it seems likely that donor lung preservation times will be extended in the near future.

TRANSPLANTATION OPERATION

Whether one lung or both lungs are replaced depends on recipient factors, including the cause of the ESPD as well as donor lung availability. It is clear that patients with chronic infection, such as cystic fibrosis, require replacement of both lungs. Patients with restrictive physiology (pulmonary fibrosis) do well with single-lung replacement. The situation in patients with end-stage obstructive disease, specifically emphysema, offers considerably more variability. Early in the pulmonary transplantation experience, it became evident that problems resulted from leaving the native emphysematous lung in situ. Specifically, air trapping in the remaining native lung, with resultant mediastinal shift, significantly crowded the transplanted lung, resulting in poor expansion and minimal function. Ventilation (V̇) preferentially went to the overly compliant native lung, while most of the perfusion (Q̇) went to the newly transplanted lung, creating a significant V̇/Q̇ mismatch that further worsened an already precarious situation. Despite these concerns, it has been conclusively demonstrated over the past few years that single-lung transplantation not only is an acceptable operation for patients with emphysema, but may be the operation of choice for patients over age 50.[291] From a donor standpoint, single-lung transplantation, when acceptable, is a more efficient use of donor organs. The decision to use single-lung transplantation for emphysema evolved mainly from experience with the original en bloc double-lung operation, which involved a tracheal anastomosis and routine cardiopulmonary bypass and resulted in significant perioperative cardiac morbidity and mortality.

Replacement of both lungs, when indicated, was greatly simplified by the development and refinement of the bilateral, sequential lung transplant procedure. Using a bilateral thoracosternotomy incision ("clamshell" procedure) permits easier completion of the recipient pneumonectomies than is achieved using median sternotomy, and replacing the lung sequentially usually avoids the need for cardiopulmonary bypass. Even previous chest operations are not contraindications for this procedure. This operation has replaced the original en bloc double-lung procedure and the heart–lung transplantation as the operation of choice for patients with ESPD who need both lungs and for those with pulmonary vascular disease.

In patients with pulmonary hypertension, it is questionable whether to replace one or both lungs. Originally single-lung transplantation was chosen because replacing one lung allowed adequate unloading of the right ventricle with immediate improvement in right ventricular function and normalization of pulmonary artery pressures. It soon became apparent, however, that replacing both lungs in this patient population offers a better margin of safety in the perioperative period and probably results in better hemodynamics in the long term. Whether replacement of both lungs is absolutely required remains to be determined but currently is preferred in most transplant centers for patients with pulmonary hypertension, despite the donor limitations.

OPERATIVE TECHNIQUE

Single-Lung Transplantation

The performance of the donor operation does not vary since one always attempts to use both lungs, either for single-lung replacement on two recipients or for distribution to another transplant medical center. This practice provides the most efficient use of limited donor organs. In the recipient operation, a standard posterolateral thoracotomy is performed, with dissection of the hilar structures as usual for a pneumonectomy (Fig. 16-86). The dissection mobilizes the main pulmonary artery, both superior and inferior pulmonary veins, and the mainstem bronchus. When the donor lung arrives in the operating room, the recipient pneumonectomy is performed by dividing the hilar vessels as far distally as possible and the bronchus at the level of the upper lobe take-off.

The implantation operation begins with construction of an anastomosis between the donor and recipient bronchus done in a telescoping fashion with one end brought up inside the other by placing horizontal mattress sutures using nonabsorbable material. This is followed by anastomosis of the pulmonary artery. Instead of individual venous anastomoses, a new left atrial cuff is constructed from the remnants of the superior and inferior pulmonary veins of the recipient. This cuff is then anastomosed to the remnant of the donor left atrium, which has been left around the donor pulmonary veins. The bronchial anastomosis formerly wrapped with a pedicle of gastrocolic omentum now is either wrapped with a conveniently located piece of pericardial fat or left unwrapped since the telescoping anastomosis offers an added margin of safety for bronchial healing. Once the vascular anastomoses are constructed, clamps are removed and blood flow is reestablished as the lung is inflated. The chest is closed in standard fashion. Either the right or left lung may be transplanted, and the decision of which side to transplant is based on both donor lung availability and recipient perfusion lung scan data. If one lung receives most of the perfusion, the opposite lung is transplanted.

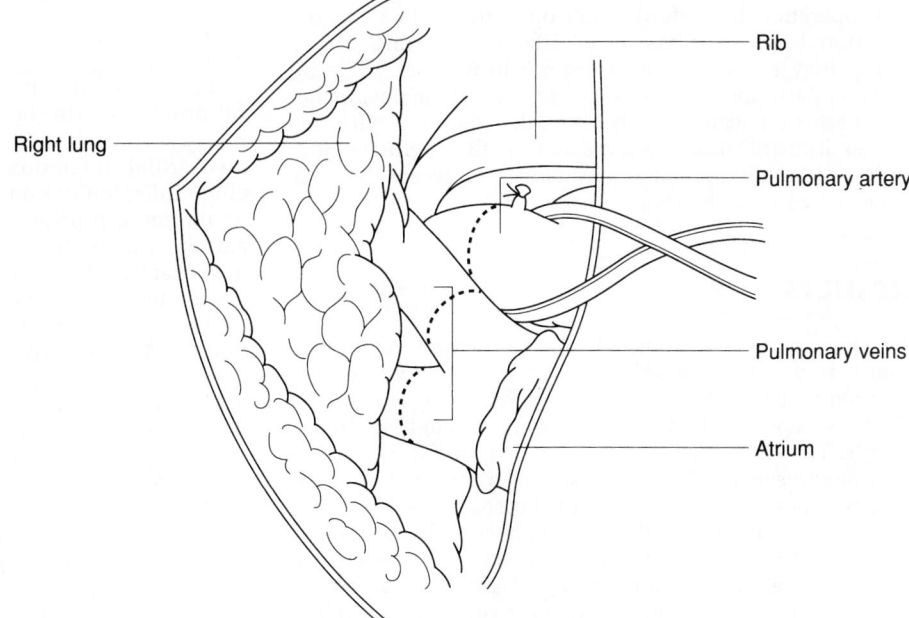

Figure 16-86. Mobilization of the hilum of the right lung demonstrating the encircled pulmonary artery with the first branch ligated and divided. The superior and inferior pulmonary veins have been exposed. Both the artery and veins are taken as close to the lung as possible. The bronchus is divided at the level of the take-off of the upper lobe.

Double-Lung Transplantation

The technique of double-lung transplantation has evolved considerably since the late 1980s. The favored approach is essentially bilateral, sequential lung replacement.[292] With the patient in the supine position, this operation is performed through a bilateral thoracosternotomy (clamshell) incision that includes anterolateral thoracotomies and a transverse sternotomy (Fig. 16-87). The thoracosternotomy incision provides excellent access to both hemithoraces, facilitating dissection and mobilization of hilar structures. This exposure is particularly important in recipients with diffuse dense adhesions between the visceral and parietal pleural surfaces as is often seen in patients with "infected" ESPD, such as cystic fibrosis.

Although both lungs are replaced, the operation can usually be performed without cardiopulmonary bypass. By first replacing the lung with the least function, the oxygenation and ventilation is maintained by the lung that receives the major fraction of perfusion. If the patient is unable to tolerate single-lung ventilation because of inadequate gas exchange or because of rising pulmonary artery pressures with right ventricular dysfunction, then cardiopulmonary bypass is instituted. The donor lungs are separated as for single-lung transplantation, leaving a cuff of left atrium around the pulmonary veins on each side. The recipient pneumonectomy is carried out with the patient maintained on one-lung ventilation. Each donor lung is implanted using essentially the same technique as described for single-lung transplantation. The bronchial anastomosis is completed first, followed by the pulmonary arterial and then the left atrial anastomoses. Flow and ventilation are restored to the newly implanted lung, and the patient is then supported by this lung while the opposite lung is removed and the second lung is implanted. Although all cardiac output is going through the newly implanted lung once the opposite pulmonary artery is ligated, clinically significant pulmonary edema has not been a problem. Both thoracotomies are then closed, and the sternum is approximated with wire sutures.

Other than procedures performed in patients with pulmonary hypertension, essentially all of these procedures

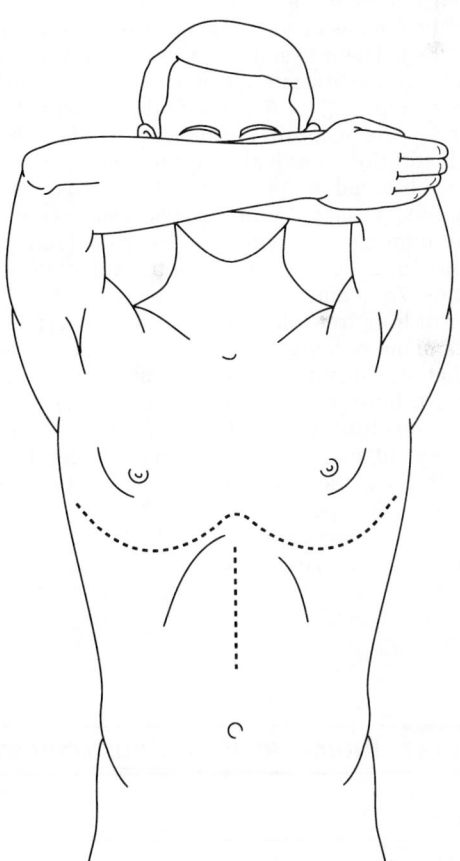

Figure 16-87. The position of the patient on the operating table before the start of the bilateral, sequential pulmonary transplantation operation. The chest incision, a bilateral thoracosternotomy, is seen, as is the separate midline incision used to expose the omentum. The sternum is divided transversely, and the fifth intercostal space on each side is entered.

are done without the need for cardiopulmonary bypass. The operation has afforded the opportunity to compare function between lungs with different ischemic times. Lungs may remain ischemic from 7 to 9 hours and still actively participate in gas exchange. Immediate postoperative perfusion scans usually show that the lung with the longer ischemic time receives less of the perfusion initially, although perfusion normalizes between the two lungs by 24 to 48 hours.

RESULTS

In just over 10 years since the first successful lung transplant, some 3000 transplants have been performed, according to a 1994 St Louis International Lung Transplant Registry report. Of these, 1960 were single-lung transplants. The single most common indication for transplant was emphysema either as a result of α_1-antitrypsin deficiency (411 cases) or idiopathy (911 cases). Most of the so-called idiopathic cases of emphysema are related to cigarette smoking. Pulmonary fibrosis, the indication first treated successfully by lung transplantation accounted for 523 transplants. Other indications are summarized in Table 16-18.

The overall 1-year actuarial survival rate following lung transplant is about 70% (single, 70%; bilateral, 74%). At 2 years, the survival rate drops to 63% (single, 61%; bilateral, 68%). At 1 and 2 years, patients with emphysema have the best survival rate, whereas those with pulmonary hypertension have the worst (77% versus 61%). Patients with cystic fibrosis do almost as well as those with emphysema (72%). There is some continued fall off in survival at 3 years with an overall rate of 57%, which drops to 51% at 4 years and 46% at 5 years. Only 44 patients were at risk for 5 years according to the registry data. In a given single institution, survival data may be somewhat better than that observed in the Registry Data. At Barnes Hospital in St Louis, 1- and 2-year survival rates were 87% for patients undergoing single-lung transplantation between 1988 and 1992. For bilateral lung transplantation, the figures were 76% and 73%, respectively.[293] Only a small number of lung transplant patients have survived as long as 7 years, but one needs to remember that it was only in 1988 that significant numbers of transplants began to be performed. Improved results have been seen since 1990, both as a result of technical refinements in the operation and transplant surgeons who are overcoming the learning curve. The postoperative care of these patients has also improved with experience.

The long-term outlook for patients undergoing lung transplantation remains unknown, but some insight can be gained by examining the factors responsible for long-term morbidity and mortality in this patient population.

COMPLICATIONS

Complications resulting from pulmonary transplantation occur frequently, may be severe, and occasionally result in death. Intraoperative complications include technical problems with the vascular or bronchial anastomoses, injury to the phrenic or recurrent laryngeal nerves, and myocardial infarction. Postoperative complications include infection of viral, bacterial, or fungal causes related to immunosuppression, problems with airway healing, and intraabdominal complications. Wound infection is noted rarely, although overriding of the sternal edges after double-lung transplantation is not uncommon. Table 16-19 summarizes the major complications encountered during 35 consecutive pulmonary transplantations.

Causes of recipient death can be categorized according to the time frame in which they occur. Early deaths (sooner than 90 days following transplant) most commonly result from bacterial infection. Primary donor organ failure accounts for the next largest group of deaths followed by heart failure. Rejection accounts for only 6% of deaths in the early posttransplantation period. Hemorrhage and airway dehiscence each are responsible for 6% of early postoperative deaths.

Infection accounts for about a third of late deaths (after 90 days) following transplantation. A similar percentage results from manifestations of chronic rejection and obliterative bronchiolitis. Respiratory failure and malignancy are the next most common causes of late mortality, each accounting for about 6% of deaths. Despite the major strides made in the operation itself and early postoperative care, the complications resulting from chronic immunosuppression continue to plague the transplant recipient.

Immunosuppression begins immediately after completion of the transplant operation. Patients are initially begun on intravenous cyclosporine at a dosage that maintains a cyclosporine blood level between 300 and 400 ng/mL. Immunosuppression also includes azathioprine and antilymphocyte globulin. Administration of the latter is usually begun the day after transplantation and is maintained for 7 to 10 days. Maintenance steroid administration begins on or about posttransplantation day 7.

With few exceptions, acute rejection episodes occur soon after transplantation, usually between posttransplantation days 5 and 7. Usually, two or three rejection episodes occur within the first month. Rejection may be heralded by mild temperature elevation, perihilar fluffy infiltrates, or a minimal decrease in blood oxygenation as measured by arterial oxygen tension. Because rejection occurs so frequently during this period, the distinction between infection and rejection may be difficult. Often, the distinguishing factor between these two entities is that rejection noticeably responds positively to the administration of corticosteroids. Treatment of early rejection episodes involves the use of bolus corticosteroid administra-

---

Table 16-18. INDICATIONS FOR PULMONARY TRANSPLANTATION*

Diagnosis	Total	Single-Lung (n = 1960)	Bilateral Lung (n = 1012)
Chronic obstructive pulmonary disease	877	725	152
α_1 = Antitrypsin deficiency	384	272	112
Cystic fibrosis	419	1	418
Primary pulmonary hypertension/Eisenmenger syndrome	327	220	107
Idiopathic pulmonary fibrosis	510	466	44
Other	455	276	179

* St Louis International Lung Transplant Registry, September 1994 report)

Table 16-19. MAJOR COMPLICATIONS DURING 35 CONSECUTIVE PULMONARY TRANSPLANTATIONS

	FEV$_1$ (%)		FVC	
	Pretransplantation	Posttransplantation	Pretransplantation	Posttransplantation
SINGLE-LUNG				
Emphysema	19	61	52	78
Pulmonary fibrosis	48	69	46	68
BILATERAL LUNG	20	101	57	92

FEV$_1$, forced expiratory volume in 1 second; FVC, forced vital capacity.
(Adapted from Davis RD, Pasque MK. Pulmonary transplantation. Ann Surg 1995;221:14)

tion given on three consecutive days. Within 12 to 18 hours after the first corticosteroid dose, symptoms relating to rejection usually resolve, including clearing of infiltrates on chest radiograph.

The diagnostic experience using transbronchial biopsy to diagnose and monitor rejection at some centers after cardiopulmonary transplantation is impressive, but the number of biopsies required to maximize specificity is large. One group recommends obtaining 18 separate transbronchial biopsy specimens to achieve a 95% specificity. The risks and potential complications of transbronchial lung biopsy do not justify their routine performance because suspected rejection episodes respond so well to corticosteroids. Transbronchial lung biopsy can be used when the issue of rejection versus infection is not resolved after steroid administration. Flexible bronchoscopy can be performed at the bedside, and 6 to 10 separate biopsies can be obtained under fluoroscopic guidance. When symptoms or signs of rejection persist despite adequate treatment, open lung biopsy may be considered.

Infection in the posttransplantation period continues to be a significant cause of morbidity as well as mortality. Bacterial pneumonias usually respond to appropriate antibiotic therapy, and patients are maintained on specific antibiotics as dictated by sputum culture and results of bronchial washings obtained at bronchoscopy. Antibiotic administration is particularly important if one predominant organism is grown from the donor lung cultures obtained at organ harvest. If a specific organism is grown from donor bronchial washings, the recipient is maintained on an appropriate antibiotic or combination of antibiotics for at least 1 week. The most common organism recovered from donor bronchial washings is *Staphylococcus aureus*. In a series of 32 transplantations, this organism was recovered from donors 11 times and subsequently from 4 transplant recipients. Other commonly recovered pathogens include *Enterobacter* species and *Candida albicans*. The presence of organisms cultured from donor bronchial washings, however, does not absolutely predict the development of invasive infection in recipients. Less than half of recipients from whom organisms were recovered went on to develop invasive infection.

The second most significant pathogen is cytomegalovirus (CMV). The diagnosis of CMV is usually made from culture of bronchoalveolar lavage fluid or tissue obtained from transbronchial lung biopsy. In the pulmonary transplantation population, CMV pneumonitis is the predominant form of CMV infection, although CMV enteritis and retinitis also occur. This experience corresponds to that seen in cardiac and cardiopulmonary transplant recipients. About half of lung recipients develop documented CMV infection. Ganciclovir has proved particularly effective and is the drug of choice for CMV infection in this

circumstance. The drug is well tolerated in most patients, with neutropenia accounting for most of the toxicity. The mortality rate from life-threatening CMV infections treated with ganciclovir has been reported at 10%,[294] far better than the 40% or greater mortality reported before this agent was available. Major difficulties with life-threatening CMV infection have occurred in CMV-negative recipients who receive a lung from a CMV-positive donor (primary infection) or in recipients already CMV-positive (secondary infection). Current practice is to attempt to place only a CMV-negative donor lung in a CMV-negative recipient, but this often proves to be unrealistic given the shortage of donor organs. Despite initial thoughts to the contrary, data from the St Louis International Lung Transplant Registry fails to demonstrate any survival advantage at 1 or 2 years posttransplantation by avoiding donor–recipient CMV mismatching. Cytolytic therapy especially with OKT3 is associated with an increased risk and severity of CMV infection. CMV prophylaxis with ganciclovir is used in some centers for CMV-positive recipients or in those recipients who receive a lung from a CMV-positive donor. The way the drug is given for prophylaxis varies since there is no established regimen that all treating physicians follow.

Other than infection, a major concern after pulmonary transplantation is airway anastomotic healing. During the early pulmonary transplantation experience, problems with airway healing resulted in a significant percentage of deaths. Patients often did well for the first 3 weeks after transplantation, and then the bronchial anastomosis split, often with erosion into the pulmonary artery. Bronchial anastomotic healing initially was facilitated by withholding maintenance corticosteroids until after the first posttransplantation week and using an omental pedicle wrapped around the anastomosis. Historically, most problems with airway healing occurred after the en bloc double-lung operation, which involves a tracheal anastomosis. Double-lung transplantation required extensive dissection in the subcarinal space, resulting in the disruption of a number of bronchial collateral vessels. Since this operation was modified to one involving bilateral, sequential lung replacement using two bronchial anastomoses, airway problems have been infrequent and now are rarely if ever implicated in recipient deaths. Partial bronchial dehiscences often heal without sequelae. The use of a telescoping bronchial anastomosis, in which the donor bronchus is intussuscepted into the recipient bronchus or viceversa, obviates the need for the omental pedicle wrap, allows for immediate use of corticosteroids, and has essentially eliminated anastomotic healing problems.

About 20% of pulmonary transplant recipients develop progressive deterioration in pulmonary function because of obliterative bronchiolitis. The incidence of this complication reportedly approaches 50% after heart–lung trans-

Table 16-20. HEMODYNAMIC DATA FOR SINGLE-LUNG TRANSPLANTATIONS IN PATIENTS WITH PULMONARY HYPERTENSION

Measurement	Pretransplantation	Posttransplantation
Pulmonary artery pressure		
Mean	58 mmHg	16 mmHg
Systolic	94 mmHg	28 mmHg
Right ventricular ejection fraction	25%	52%
Cardiac output	4 L/min	7 L/min
Pulmonary vascular resistance	1302 dyne/cm/s^5	161 dyne/cm/s^5

plantation. This complication is seen following pulmonary transplantation as well. The lesion is characterized histologically by progressive small airway destruction, filling of these small airways with an inflammatory exudate and finally fibrosis and is first manifested clinically by a subtle decrease in pulmonary function reflected in a decreased forced expiratory volume in 1 second (FEV$_1$). This complication is likely a form fruste of chronic rejection although its exact etiology remains unknown. A good animal model of obliterative bronchiolitis does not exist, making study of this entity difficult. If diagnosed early, enhancing immunosuppression may either halt the process or slow the progression. It has been hypothesized that the development of obliterative bronchiolitis in cardiopulmonary transplantation patients is related to an A2 antigen mismatch. Others postulate that CMV infection may be implicated. Once diagnosed, it is imperative to increase immunosuppression to prevent what is usually an insidiously progressive disorder. Unfortunately, in patients who have developed obliterative bronchiolitis and then undergo retransplantation, the lesion has redeveloped in the newly transplanted lungs.

POSTTRANSPLANTATION PHYSIOLOGY

Pulmonary transplantation has afforded an opportunity to observe changes in pulmonary physiology that are not seen under ordinary circumstances. It is important to examine these changes relative to the type of transplantation operation.

The development of bilateral, sequential lung replacement provides the opportunity to indirectly assess lung function by perfusion lung scan. Because the newly implanted lungs have different ischemic times, the immediate posttransplantation perfusion scan would be expected to demonstrate less perfusion to the side with the longer ischemic time. Indeed, this situation does occur, especially when ischemic times exceed 6 hours; however, the relative perfusion to each side usually equalizes within 24 to 48 hours.

Performing single-lung transplantations in patients with pulmonary hypertension has been particularly illustrative in demonstrating the potential for reversing right ventricular dysfunction. As soon as the lung is implanted, the morphology of the right ventricle changes significantly, as assessed by transesophageal echocardiography. The intraventricular septum, previously bulging into the left ventricle, immediately assumes a normal position. An increase in contractility of the right ventricle occurs with significant decrease in dilatation. The pulmonary artery pressure immediately decreases and is essentially normal by the time the patient leaves the operating room (Table 16-20). Late catheterization studies (2 years posttransplantation) in pa-

tients undergoing this operation show continued normal hemodynamics.

The situation after single-lung transplantation in patients with emphysema is also illustrative. One would expect a significant $\dot{V}/\dot{Q}$ mismatch to occur, with ventilation to the native lung occurring preferentially because the native lung is significantly more compliant. Conversely, perfusion should preferentially go to the newly transplanted lung because of lower pulmonary vascular resistance. Despite this occurrence, patients undergoing this operation do well from a functional standpoint (Fig. 16-88). Early data show that physiologic dead space (V_D/V_T) decreases with work, with a shift in ventilation toward the transplanted side. By 3 months after transplantation, the ventilation–perfusion mismatch narrows (Fig. 16-89). Despite the mismatch, no patient has demonstrated carbon dioxide retention.

From a clinical standpoint, improvement in pulmonary function is seen almost immediately after transplantation. The measurement most often used is FEV$_1$, and marked improvement is seen within 2 weeks. The FEV$_1$ essentially triples and then remains fairly stable (Fig. 16-90). This observation holds true for both single- and double-lung replacement in patients with obstructive disease. Improvement after bilateral lung replacement is slightly better.

Likewise, exercise studies show significant improvement after lung transplantation. Though patients who receive two lungs may do better on pulmonary function studies, this benefit is not translated into significantly better exercise capability. Maximum oxygen consumption, maximum work, peak ventilation, and anaerobic threshold are increased after lung transplantation but remain well below normal values. This may be due in large part to an accompanying abnormal cardiovascular response to exercise.

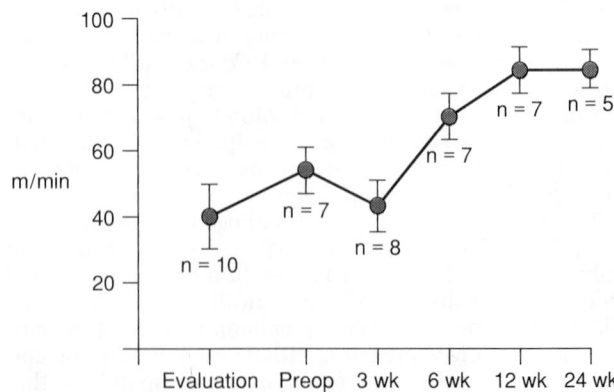

Figure 16-88. Mean 6-minute walk data for a group of patients undergoing single-lung transplantations for emphysema. Marked improvement is seen at the 6-week level, with continued improvement at 12 weeks.

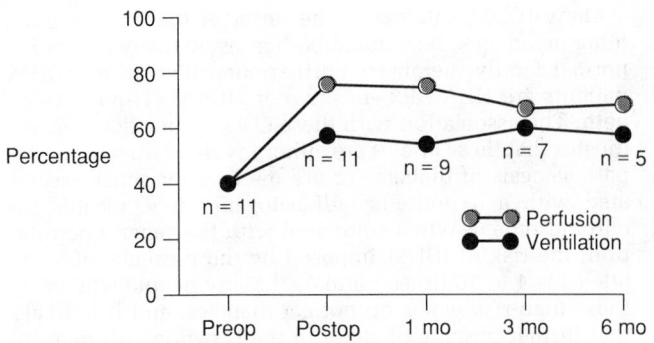

Figure 16-89. Mean values for ventilation and perfusion for patients undergoing single-lung transplantation for emphysema. Note the ventilation–perfusion mismatch that occurs, as expected, after transplantation.

When exercise testing is performed, no difference is noted between emphysema patients who receive one lung. This may be due to the fact that emphysema sufferers receiving a single lung do better than we would predict because of the effect of the transplant operation on the remaining native lung. Specifically, the shift in the mediastinum toward the transplanted side results in a relative "volume reduction" on the contralateral side with repositioning of the contralateral hemidiaphragm to a more normal location and to a normal concave configuration. This reconfiguration of the hemidiaphragm allows for significantly better diaphragm excursion and improved lung mechanics and gas exchange.

FUTURE CONSIDERATIONS

Pulmonary transplantation has slowly evolved from an experimental therapy. The number of these transplantations performed is still small compared with other solid-organ replacements, but this is rapidly changing. Donor availability is still a major issue and will likely continue as an obstacle. Questions about long-term follow-up and preservation of lung function also remain to be answered. Pulmonary transplantation has joined other solid-organ transplantations as a viable alternative in patients with end-stage disease. Cost considerations and managed care will likely have a significant impact on trans-

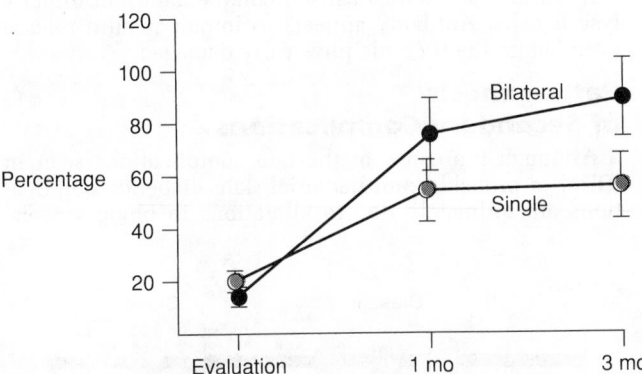

Figure 16-90. Comparison of percentage of predicted FEV_1 in 14 patients undergoing single and 10 patients undergoing bilateral sequential pulmonary transplantation for chronic obstructive pulmonary disease.

plantation as we enter the next century despite the accomplishments of the past 20 years.

Pancreatic and Islet Transplantation

LAWRENCE ROSENBERG

THE NATURE OF DIABETES

Diabetes mellitus has been classified as type I, or insulin-dependent diabetes mellitus (IDDM) and type II, or non–insulin-dependent diabetes mellitus (NIDDM). NIDDM patients have been subdivided further into the following categories: nonobese (possibly IDDM in evolution), obese, and maturity onset (in young patients). Among the population with diabetes mellitus, about 20% suffer from IDDM. Diabetes develops either when a diminished insulin output occurs or when a diminished sensitivity to insulin cannot be compensated for by an augmented capacity for insulin secretion. In patients with IDDM, a decrease in insulin secretion is the principal factor in the pathogenesis, whereas in patients with NIDDM, a decrease in insulin sensitivity is the primary factor.

IDDM is ketosis prone and affects primarily young people. It appears to develop after a prodrome of autoimmunity directed toward islet cells, which is characterized by islet cell antibodies, insulin autoantibodies, or antibodies against a human islet protein that has recently being identified as glutamic acid dehydrogenase (GAD65 or GAD67).[295,296] At the time of clinical diagnosis, a major portion of the B cells have been destroyed, and the islets of Langerhans have been infiltrated by inflammatory cells. It is believed that islet destruction is caused by a viral infection superimposed on a susceptible genetic background with subsequent autoimmune attack of the islets. Patients with IDDM may develop retinopathy leading to blindness; peripheral and autonomic neuropathy resulting in loss of sensation in the extremities, orthostatic hypotension, delayed gastric emptying, and tachycardia; and nephropathy culminating in renal failure. Pregnancy is associated with a significant infant mortality, and life expectancy is shortened.

Symptoms of IDDM often appear only 1 to 2 months before diagnosis is made. Polyuria, polydipsia, weight loss, and fatigue are the cardinal symptoms.

The level of glycosylated hemoglobin (HbA_{1c}) can be used to evaluate the patient's overall metabolic state, since HbA_{1c} reflects the average blood level of glucose during the preceding 1 to 2 months. A long-term increase in the blood level of glucose leads to the nonenzymatic glycosylation of polypeptides and proteins such as hemoglobin. Although less than 20% of patients have ketoacidosis when diabetes is first diagnosed, HbA_{1c} is over 10% in most cases. Determination of C-peptide levels in the blood is one of the best means of directly evaluating B-cell function because the secretion of C-peptide is dependent on blood glucose concentrations.

After initial insulin therapy, many patients become asymptomatic, and after several weeks, up to 25% of patients undergo a remission. This remission usually lasts less than a year.

Fifteen to 20 years after onset of IDDM, asymptomatic manifestations of microangiopathy are found in nearly all patients. Only about 40% of patients, however, have lesions that progress to cause the well-characterized secondary complications of diabetes.

Exogenous insulin therapy prevents diabetic ketoacidosis and keeps patients with IDDM alive, but even with multiple injections, insulin pump therapy, careful attention to diet, and judicious use of exercise, achieving normoglycemia is difficult. Transplanting an effective islet cell mass reestablishes a euglycemic state, enhances the quality of life, and yields the best possible chance for preventing, stabilizing, or reversing the secondary complications. Islet replacement can be provided by transplanting a vascularized graft of the pancreas or a nonvascularized graft of islet tissue.

Prevalence and Incidence

Diabetes has a tremendous impact not only on the health of the patient but also on the function of health care systems. According to the National Diabetes Data Group report of 1984,[297] about 6 million people in the United States have been diagnosed with diabetes, and an additional 4 to 5 million people have undiagnosed diabetes. Despite a falling incidence, from a peak of 300 per 100,000 population in 1973 to 230 per 100,000 in 1981, the prevalence continues to increase due to a 19% decline in deaths caused by diabetes since 1970. About 10,000 people in the United States develop IDDM each year. It has been predicted that the size of this population will double in 15 years.

Late Complications

Diabetes mellitus is directly responsible for about 38,000 deaths each year in the United States. Because vascular complications are so common in this patient population, this disease may contribute to 300,000 deaths annually, which makes it the third leading cause of death in the United States. Diabetes is the major cause of new cases of blindness in this country. Diabetics are 25 times more likely than nondiabetics to develop blindness, 17 times more likely to develop renal disease, 20 times more likely to develop gangrene, and twice as likely to develop heart disease or to suffer stroke.[298] About 10% of diabetics undergo a major amputation during their lifetime, and over 80% of the major amputations performed in the United States occur in diabetics. Fourteen percent of diabetics are bedridden for an average of 6 weeks per year.[297]

In addition to 5800 new cases of blindness, 4500 perinatal deaths, 40,000 lower-extremity amputations, and 3000 deaths due to diabetic coma, about 4000 new cases of end-stage renal disease are caused by diabetes annually, and it has been said that diabetes is the most important cause of end-stage renal disease in the Western world. Diabetes mellitus is the cause of renal failure in up to 40% of new patients admitted to US dialysis centers, and renal failure due to diabetic nephropathy is the indication for about 25% to 30% of renal transplantations. The cumulative incidence of diabetic nephropathy after 40 years of diabetes is 45%. The total annual economic impact of diabetes mellitus was estimated at more than $14 billion dollars in 1989, including medical expenses, lost time from work, and so forth.

Pathogenesis

The pathogenesis of the loss of pancreatic B cells remains obscure. Both humoral and cellular anti–B-cell activities have been documented, suggesting autoimmunity as a cause of the disease. Antibodies directed against GAD may act either by mediating complement-dependent cytotoxicity or by inhibiting B-cell function or replication.[299]

Many IDDM patients at the onset of the disease have other organ-specific autoantibodies, as do many otherwise normal family members. Furthermore, 95% of all IDDM patients are HLA-DR3–positive or HLA-DR4–positive or both. The association with these class II specifications indicates that these alleles are either involved directly in the pathogenesis of diabetes or are markers for genes associated with a hypothetical diabetogenic gene located on chromosome 6. When compared with the general population, the risk of IDDM imposed by the presence of these alleles is 4 to 10 times normal.[301] Many people who carry these high-risk genes do not get diabetes, and it is likely that further probing of genes in the D region will identify the actual gene imparting risk (Fig. 16-91). The D region of the major histocompatibility complex can be further divided into the DP, DQ, and DR regions, and the susceptibility gene may be more closely linked to the DQ region. Antibodies to GAD have been correlated with HLA-DQB1 alleles and genotypes, as determined by sequence-specific oligonucleotide hybridizations after polymerase chain reaction was applied to exon 2 of the DQ beta 1 gene. HLA-DQ2 was significantly increased in IDDM patients with antibodies to GAD.[299]

Viral infection of the B cell is believed to be an important inciting event in the pathogenesis of diabetes. This has been hypothesized to occur by either direct inflammatory disruption of the islets or induction of an immune response. In animal models, activated T lymphocytes infiltrate islets before or at the same time as the diabetes develops. Lymphocytes are also found in the islets of young people dying from new-onset diabetes. Conversion of the B cell from self to nonself is also a necessary step in the course of events leading to diabetes. An increase occurs in the ratio of helper to suppressor T cells in the circulation, which is likely caused by a decrease in the number of suppressor T lymphocytes. An unbalanced helper T lymphocyte population could predispose to enhanced antibody production on exposure to foreign antigen. The activation of helper T cells requires the presence of a class II molecule and a foreign or alloantigen on the surface of an antigen-presenting cell. Normal islet cells do not express HLA antigens on the cell membrane, but class II HLA molecules appear on the surface of B cells early in the onset of diabetes. This could occur in response to viral infection (through the production of interferon-γ) and in turn render the cell potentially recognizable as nonself. The susceptibility is linked to the fit between the newly appearing class II molecule, the membrane antigen (foreign or autologous), and a particular T-cell receptor on the helper cell.

The final step, the destruction of B cells, probably involves both humoral and cell-mediated mechanisms. Islet cell–surface antibodies can fix complement and directly lyse B cells. Antibody appears to impair insulin release even before the B cell is physically damaged.

Pathogenesis of Secondary Complications

Although the cause of the late complications seen in IDDM is probably multifactorial, late diabetic complications are ultimately due to alterations in blood vessels,

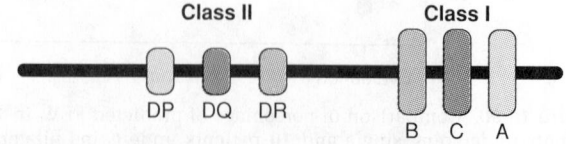

Figure 16-91. Major histocompatability complex on the long arm of the human chromosome 6.

nerves, and connective tissue. The importance of the polyol pathway, wherein glucose is reduced to sorbitol by aldol reductase, has recently been recognized. Sorbitol appears to be a tissue toxin and is implicated in the pathogenesis of retinopathy, neuropathy, cataracts, nephropathy, and aortic disease.[302] Sorbitol accumulation leads to a reduction in the cellular content of myoinositol, abnormal phosphoinositide metabolism, and a reduction in Na^+-K^+-ATPase activity. In the experimental setting, aldol reductase inhibition can prevent cataract formation and retinopathy.

The nonenzymatic glycosylation of proteins such as Hb A_{1c}, albumin, lens protein, fibrin, collagen, and lipoproteins is yet another mechanism that may lead to alterations of normal physiology. Glycosylated low-density lipoproteins are not recognized by the low-density lipoprotein receptor, and the plasma half-life is therefore elevated. Conversely, glycosylated high-density lipoproteins turn over more rapidly than native high-density lipoproteins, and consequently, cholesterol transport is decreased.

Macroangiopathy is manifested by atherosclerosis associated with intimal proliferation and medial calcification, which result in luminal narrowing. Nonenzymatic glycosylation of lipoproteins may play an important role, leading to widely distributed arteriosclerosis at an earlier stage.

Diabetic microangiopathy is characterized by excessive thickening of capillary basement membranes. The thickness increases with the duration of disease and with increasing age. Increased intercapillary pressure as well as metabolic abnormalities are probably influential factors in the pathogenesis of basement membrane thickening. Alterations in capillary permeability are also required for the progression of clinically significant lesions. The cause of increased capillary permeability is not known, but genetic, metabolic, and hemodynamic factors all play a role.

After about 20 years of diabetes, background retinopathy is present in 80% to 100% of patients. These alterations do not cause visual disturbances, but the changes progress and lead to impaired vision in 30% of cases. An increase in capillary permeability is the earliest sign of retinal change and is followed by an occlusion of retinal capillaries with subsequent formation of aneurysms and arteriovenous shunts. Hypoxia secondary to occlusion acts as a stimulus for new vessel formation. These newly formed vessels are extremely fragile, due in part to a lack of adjacent pericytes; therefore, bleeding may occur in the retina and into the vitreous body. Five years after the onset of proliferative retinopathy, half of untreated patients become blind in both eyes.

Diabetic nephropathy consists of a glomerulopathy (diffuse or nodular glomerulosclerosis and exudative lesions), arteriolar hyalinization, and tubular lesions, such as atrophy and basement membrane thickening. Clinical nephropathy is characterized by persistent proteinuria (greater than 0.5 g/24 h), decreased glomerular filtration rate, and increased blood pressure. The glomerular lesions result from the accumulation of basement membrane–like material in the mesangium. Glomerular sclerosis is found in most IDDM patients after 15 years of diabetes, but clinical nephropathy develops in only 40% of these patients. Seven years after the onset of persistent proteinuria, the mortality rate for untreated patients is 50%.

An elevated glomerular filtration rate and enlargement of the whole kidney and glomerulus are abnormalities that are noted consistently in IDDM before any clinical nephropathy is manifest. Glomerular filtration rate is usually above the normal range for years before any sign of renal failure. Leakage of small amounts (30 to 299 mg/d) of urinary albumin, so-called microalbuminuria, presages subsequent renal failure and, in fact, predicts the development of clinical nephropathy. Microalbuminuria identifies a group of diabetics who progress to renal failure within 10 years. The risk of developing end-stage diabetic nephropathy is increased 20-fold in diabetics with even small amounts of urinary albumin compared with those free of this finding. Proteinuria greater than 1 g/d in IDDM heralds impending azotemia within 1 to 5 years. Should a patient remain free of proteinuria for 30 years, the subsequent risk of clinical nephropathy is minimal.

The importance of capillary hypertension and hyperglycemia are only now being appreciated fully. Recurrent glomerulosclerosis and renal failure can destroy kidneys obtained from nondiabetic organ donors when placed into diabetic recipients. Kidneys transplanted into recipients who have become diabetic only after transplantation (steroid diabetes) may subsequently show characteristic nodular glomerulosclerosis. Early glomerulopathy is reversible in a euglycemic environment, as shown by the disappearance of glomerulosclerosis in cadaveric donor kidneys from a diabetic donor after transplantation into nondiabetic recipients.

Diabetic neuropathy is characterized by axonal degeneration and segmental demyelinization, perhaps due to alterations in axonal transport caused by accumulation of sorbitol in the tissues. The cumulative incidence of polyneuropathy is 100%. Symptoms manifest symmetrically in the distal part of the body, the legs, and different parts of the autonomic nervous system. Symptoms may include paresthesia, altered cutaneous sensitivity, pain, and paresis. Autonomic neuropathy may lead to disturbances of gastric emptying and severe, often nocturnal diarrhea. Autonomic neuropathy of the cardiovascular system can result in orthostatic hypotension and sudden death from arrhythmia. The urinary system may also be affected, resulting in bladder dysfunction.

PANCREATIC TRANSPLANTATION

The discovery of insulin laid the foundation for the modern management of diabetes mellitus.[303] Insulin has prevented the early mortality associated with the metabolic derangements of diabetes and dramatically extended the life span of diabetics. Before the discovery of insulin, the secondary complications of diabetes were rarely seen because most patients at risk did not survive sufficiently long for them to appear. After the discovery of insulin, the secondary complications of diabetes became the major cause of diabetic morbidity and mortality. Investigation and treatment of the primary defect in diabetes became sidetracked as efforts focused on treating the secondary complications of the disease. Such treatments, however, did not solve the basic problem of the deranged metabolism of diabetes, and a few researchers continued to pursue pancreatic transplantation in the experimental setting.

Pancreatic transplantation is performed to provide an endogenous source of insulin and other islet hormones. It functions in a physiologic manner to restore normal metabolism, with the ultimate goal being to prevent, stabilize, or reverse the degenerative complications of diabetes.

Exogenous insulin administered by standard techniques cannot reliably prevent wide variations of plasma levels of glucose.

The Diabetes Complications and Control Trial (DCCT) has reported that intensive conventional therapy using multiple injections of insulin and close monitoring of blood glucose, can control the level of blood glucose, allow glycosylated hemoglobin to approach but not reach normal levels, increase nerve conduction velocity, and decrease blood lipids.[304] Nevertheless, dangerous hypoglycemic episodes, a high patient dropout rate, and poor control of "brittle" diabetes suggest that this therapy is an incomplete solution to the problems posed by IDDM.

Evidence from both animal and human studies suggests that kidneys transplanted from normal donors to diabetic recipients develop lesions of diabetic nephropathy. Conversely, such lesions in kidneys taken from diabetic donors regress after transplantation into nondiabetic recipients. The microscopic lesions of diabetic nephropathy have also been observed to regress in the native kidneys of recipients of a successful pancreatic transplantation. The extent to which pancreatic transplantation can favorably influence established pathologic lesions is not fully known. Results of animal experiments suggest that these lesions probably need to be at an early stage of development.

The history of clinical pancreatic transplantation revolves around the investigation and introduction of new, and at times ingenious, surgical techniques.[305] Starting in the latter half of the 20th century, Brooks and Gifford[306] were the first to describe pancreatic transplantation in a large animal model. Their studies yielded two important pieces of information. First, in principle, pancreatic transplantation was technically feasible, and second, failure of the graft was usually due to thrombosis or complications from the exocrine part of the gland. The first clinical pancreatic transplantation was undertaken at the University of Minnesota in 1966. The first 12 pancreaticoduodenal grafts were anastomosed to a Roux-en-Y loop of recipient jejunum. Only one of these initial 12 grafts functioned for longer than 1 year. In 1978, Dubernard and colleagues[307] reported that exocrine secretions of the segmental allograft could be ablated before transplantation by injecting a synthetic polymer into the duct. This new technique of segmental pancreatic transplantation with occlusion of the pancreatic duct was proven safe, and it ushered in a resurgence of interest in vascularized pancreatic grafts. Through the late 1970s and early 1980s, there was a return to the original method of whole-organ pancreatic transplantation with a segment of donor duodenum anastomosed to a loop of recipient intestine, but this was still associated with a significant morbidity and mortality. In 1985, Sollinger and colleagues[308] reported a modification of this technique that involved anastomosing the donor pancreas to the urinary bladder of the recipient using a button of donor duodenum. In 1986, Nghiem and associates[309] reported a further modification in which a composite pancreaticoduodenal graft from the donor was anastomosed to the recipient urinary bladder using a segment of duodenum. Currently, these are the most popular techniques for pancreatic transplantation: (1) polymer injection (used mainly in Europe), (2) enteric drainage (used mainly in Europe), and (3) bladder drainage (used mainly in North America). A technique of pancreatic transplantation with no negative and only positive features has yet to be described.

Indications

Pancreatic transplantation can be applied to three categories of patients. In the first category are diabetic patients who already have undergone successful renal transplantations. In the patient with a functioning renal transplant, the need for long-term immunosuppression, the demonstration of prior allograft acceptance, and the continued risk for recurrent diabetic nephropathy are all compelling reasons to offer pancreatic transplantation. The second group of patients are those with ESRD requiring renal transplantation. These people may benefit either from simultaneous or sequential renal–pancreatic transplantation. The final group of patients are nonuremic diabetics with other complications of their disease. This group rep-

resents potentially the largest number of IDDM patients who could benefit from pancreatic transplantation. The specific selection criteria for pancreatic transplantation are as follows:

- IDDM, as documented by an absence of circulating C-peptide
- Age between 18 and 50 years
- Microalbuminuria with a creatinine clearance greater than 60 to 70 mL/min (pancreas alone)
- Microalbuminuria with a creatinine clearance less than 60 mL/min (consider for simultaneous renal–pancreatic transplantation)
- Proteinuria with a projected requirement for dialysis or established end-stage diabetic nephropathy (consider for simultaneous renal–pancreatic transplantation)
- Autonomic neuropathy (not an independent inclusion criterion)
- Retinopathy (not an independent inclusion criterion)
- Labile diabetes and failure of medical management (may be an independent criterion for pancreatic transplantation alone)
- Sufficient cardiac reserve
- Psychosocial fitness
- Thorough understanding or risks and benefits
- Absence of usual transplant recipient exclusion criteria

Simultaneous Renal–Pancreatic Transplantation

The advantages of simultaneous renal–pancreatic transplantation compared with the sequential procedure (renal followed by pancreatic) include the following: (1) the recipient's need to accept only one set of donor antigens; (2) the ability to monitor rejection of the pancreas by identifying the well-recognized signs of renal allograft rejection; (3) the immunosuppressive effect of uremia; (4) transplantation in patients who have not been maintained on chronic immunosuppression; and (5) a single, albeit longer, anesthetic exposure. Of these advantages, the most important is the use of renal function as an early indicator of pancreatic graft rejection. Moreover, the early diagnosis of renal rejection after simultaneous renal–pancreatic transplantation reduces the number of subsequent pancreas rejections. Hyperglycemia is a late sign of rejection in the pancreatic transplant recipient—usually too late to effectively reverse rejection because 90% to 95% of the islet cell mass will have already been eliminated. The disadvantages of simultaneous renal–pancreatic transplantation are extensive surgery in a uremic diabetic patient and potential adverse effect on the renal allograft as a result of a pancreatic complication.

By transplanting a renal graft with a pancreatic graft, several of the problems associated with each of the grafts are addressed. These include the recurrence of diabetic nephropathy in the transplanted kidney, diagnosis of pancreatic rejection, and stabilization or prevention of late diabetic complications of diabetes mellitus. For patients who are determined to be candidates for renal transplantation and immunosuppression, adding a pancreatic graft appears to be a logical approach to treating diabetes and the attendant renal failure at the same time. Patients undergoing the simultaneous transplantation procedure do not die of complications related exclusively to the pancreatic allograft, nor does the presence of the pancreas and its associated problems prejudice the survival of the renal allograft. In most centers, the immunosuppression regimen is the same for both organs as it is for the kidney alone.

Pancreatic Transplantation Alone

Candidates for a pancreatic transplantation alone can be divided into two groups—those already possessing a renal allograft and those with no or only early diabetic nephropathy. Ideally, pancreatic transplantations should be performed in patients who do not yet have, but are destined to develop, secondary complications of diabetes that are more serious than the potential side effects of immunosuppression. There is no way to predict which patients will develop these late complications before the earliest lesions appear. In recipients of a pancreas after a kidney, only the surgical risks need to be considered since immunosuppression is obligatory.

The selection process must be more rigorous for the nonuremic, nonrenal transplantation patient who does not yet have end-stage diabetic nephropathy. In such candidates, both the surgical and the immunosuppressive risks must be balanced against the possible benefits of pancreatic transplantation. The potential for benefit, however, is greater in this than in any other group of diabetic patients. If any lesions do exist, they should be at a stage at which progression to a level more serious than the potential side effects of antirejection treatment would occur if diabetes were not corrected. In other words, the risks of immunosuppression, as well as the surgical risks of transplantation, should be less than the risks of remaining diabetic.[310]

Pancreas Procurement

Donor Assessment

Most pancreatic transplantations have been performed with organs from cadaveric donors. The donors are previously healthy people who developed global cerebral infarction (ie, brain death) and are maintained on ventilatory support. General contraindications to organ donation include the presence of malignant disease (with the exception of intracerebral tumors that do not disseminate) and generalized infections. Positive serology for hepatitis B or human immunodeficiency virus are also contraindications to organ donation.

Absolute contraindications for cadaveric pancreatic organ donation include the presence of diabetes mellitus, chronic pancreatitis, and pancreatic damage secondary to trauma. Relative contraindications include a history of alcohol abuse and relapsing pancreatitis. With special regard to pancreatic transplantation, blood glucose and serum amylase levels should be examined in cadaveric donors. Hyperglycemia, if present, may be due to the intravenous infusion of large amounts of glucose-containing solutions. Cerebral infarction may alter blood glucose homeostasis and result in hyperglycemia, possibly by decreasing peripheral insulin levels. Hyperamylasemia may also exist in the donor, and in the absence of intraabdominal trauma, it has been suggested that this may be a consequence of cerebral infarction. The final decision concerning the suitability of the pancreas for transplantation is made during its actual removal.

Vascular Anatomic Considerations

The arterial supply to the pancreas is derived from the celiac axis through the gastroduodenal and splenic arteries and from the superior mesenteric artery (SMA). The final reconstruction of the vascular anatomy of the transplant varies depending on the type of pancreatic graft that is procured from the donor. The whole-organ graft is composed of the entire pancreas with or without a segment of adjacent duodenum. With the whole graft, the arterial supply is by way of the celiac axis and the SMA, and usually these two vessels are removed together on an aortic patch (Fig. 16-92), which is anastomosed end-to-side to a recipient artery. The venous outflow of the graft is by the portal vein. If the liver is to be harvested from the same donor, the common hepatic artery usually is required for the vascular pedicle of the liver. In this case, the gastroduodenal artery is ligated, and the pancreatic head and duodenum then derive their arterial supply from the inferior pancreaticoduodenal artery arising from the SMA. If the celiac axis is also taken with the liver, the severed splenic artery can be anastomosed end-to-side to the SMA (Fig. 16-93). Alternatively, an extension graft fashioned from the bifurcation of a donor common iliac artery can be used to join the SMA and the splenic artery. When a segmental pancreatic graft is being procured, the blood supply is derived from the splenic vessels.

No-Touch Technique of Dissection

One of the keys to successful pancreatic transplantation is avoiding injury to the donor pancreas during dissection to minimize postischemic pancreatitis in the recipient. This can best be accomplished by using a so-called no-touch technique when removing the pancreas from the donor. The spleen, which is harvested along with the pancreas, can be used as a handle to manipulate the graft during both the procurement and the transplantation. Minimizing posttransplantation pancreatitis reduces the risk of developing intragraft thrombosis and subsequent organ loss. Additional important maneuvers should include ligating the large lymphatic channels along the aorta to prevent subsequent ascites or lymphatic fistula in the recipient and dividing the portal vein on commencing the flush-out to avoid parenchymal damage resulting from a buildup of pressure in the portal vein.

Organ Preservation

Pancreatic graft procurement is performed using in situ perfusion techniques. The goal of preservation technique is to subject the organ to as little damage as possible during the period of hypothermic ischemia to achieve optimal graft function. The major problems associated with preserving the pancreas relate to its peculiar microarchitecture: (1) edema develops rapidly even after minor surgical manipulation; (2) the blood flow through the vasculature of the parenchyma is not high, and an elevation in the perfusion pressure during flushing can readily cause edema and disruption of vascular endothelium; and (3) the exocrine tissue appears to be more susceptible to preservation injury than the endocrine tissue.

Organ preservation techniques are designed to reduce the metabolic rate. Oxygen consumption, which is mandatory for energy supply, is significantly diminished under hypothermic conditions. Maintaining the ionic balance between the intracellular and extracellular spaces is of primary importance. To conserve this state, an electrochemical potential gradient exists across the cell membrane, mainly supported by energy-rich phosphates, the most important of which is ATP. Hypothermia reduces the level of ATP, which in turn leads to inactivity of the ionic pump and subsequently to cell swelling. Cell injury during hypothermia causes a no-reflow phenomenon in that on revascularization of the graft, blood flow through capillaries and small blood vessels of the graft is prevented.

The following components of a suitable pancreatic preservation solution are thought to be particularly important:

Hyperosmolar solutions reduce cell swelling but may also lead to cell shrinkage during preservation so that on reperfusion, there is a rapid rebound swelling to equilibrate intracellular and extracellular osmolality. This could lead to capillary compression and diminished blood flow.

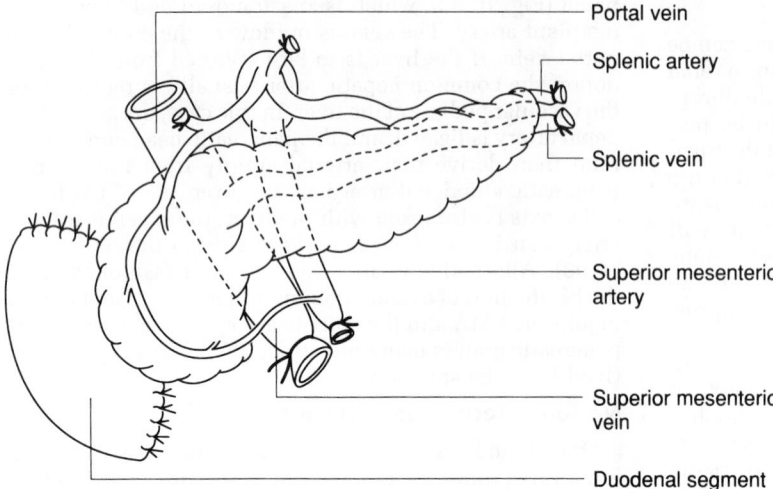

Portal vein

Splenic artery

Splenic vein

Superior mesenteric artery

Superior mesenteric vein

Duodenal segment

Figure 16-92. The whole-organ composite pancreaticoduodenal graft with the arterial supply derived from the celiac axis and superior mesenteric artery. The venous outflow is through the portal vein.

Impermeants prevent cell swelling.

Hyperkalemia may prevent cellular potassium loss.

Methylprednisolone is thought to stabilize cell membranes, thereby preventing release of lysosomal enzymes.

Osmotically active ions (eg, $MgSO_4$) within the extracellular space may act as metabolic inhibitors and membrane stabilizers and help preserve intracellular potassium.

The volumes of solution used and the pressures generated in the parenchyma of the gland are probably of crucial importance for proper functioning of the graft in the immediate posttransplantation period. Thrombosis appears to occur, in part as a result of an intraglandular process involving the pancreatic microvasculature. Therefore, a low-pressure, low-volume flush to avoid intravascular damage to the gland is important.

Operative Technique

Anatomic and Physiologic Bases

A main obstacle to successful pancreatic transplantation has been the anatomic architecture of the pancreas, which comprises about 2 million endocrine islets randomly distributed in an organ that consists mainly of exocrine tissue. Technical problems of transplanting endocrine pancreatic tissue chiefly concern the exocrine part of the gland but also relate to the predisposition of the graft to vascular thrombosis. Surgical considerations in pancreatic transplantation include the following:

- Whole-organ versus segmental grafts
- Inclusion of the donor duodenum
- Ductal filling or exocrine diversion
- Exocrine diversion to intestine or bladder
- Intraperitoneal or extraperitoneal placement of the graft
- Systemic or splanchnic insulin delivery

There are, in principle, three options for managing the exocrine secretions. The first option involves maintaining exocrine secretion by internal drainage of the exocrine pancreas, which can be achieved by anastomosing the ductal system to either the intestinal tract (stomach, small intestine) or the urinary tract (ureter, bladder). These techniques are the most commonly used today and have provided the best overall results. The second technique, free drainage of the pancreatic juice into the peritoneal cavity, is certainly the least technically demanding method of transplantation. It is, however, associated with many other complications. Ablation of exocrine secretion, the third option, can be accomplished by two techniques. The first, duct ligation, has been associated with exocrine atrophy

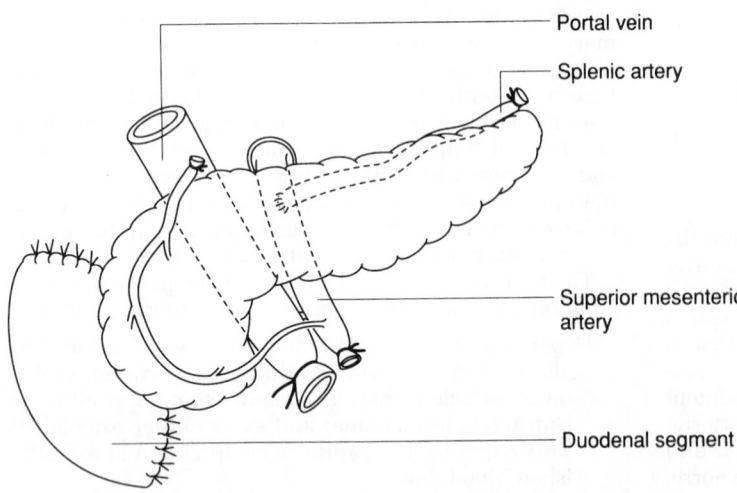

Portal vein

Splenic artery

Superior mesenteric artery

Duodenal segment

Figure 16-93. The arterial reconstruction of a whole-organ composite graft when the celiac axis and hepatic artery have been procured for a renal allograft.

and extensive fibrosis, resulting eventually in endocrine insufficiency. Ductal ligation has also had unpredictable effects on the exocrine tissue, associated with a high risk of acute pancreatitis and peripancreatic sepsis. The other method of ductal ligation involves injecting the pancreatic duct system with a synthetic polymer that solidifies within several minutes, completely blocking exocrine secretion as a result.

Whole-Organ, Composite Pancreaticoduodenal Graft

There are some inherent advantages to using the whole organ rather than a segment for grafting. A larger mass of islet tissue can be transplanted, and the blood flow across the anastomosis is greater, a factor that may reduce the risk of thrombosis. The whole pancreas can be procured alone or en bloc with the second portion of the duodenum, which in turn can be anastomosed to the recipient urinary bladder or jejunum.

The enterically drained pancreas (without duodenum) has in the past been associated with a significant incidence of anastomotic leakage, leading to pancreatic fistula, perigraft abscess, and systemic sepsis. Many of these allografts had to be removed. These problems can be obviated to a large extent if the donor duodenum (removed en bloc with the pancreas) is used to establish the anastomosis. Alternatively, the pancreaticojejunostomy can be drained externally by a catheter placed in the pancreatic duct. This provides a means of diverting exocrine secretions during healing of the anastomosis.

Several important features of the recipient operation of bladder drainage are worth emphasizing. First, when the duodenal segment is removed en bloc with the pancreas from the donor using a stapling instrument, it is necessary to invert the stapled ends with nonabsorbable suture before transplantation. Second, the right iliac fossa is the preferred location for the pancreatic allograft. The portal vein–iliac vein anastomosis is accomplished first and is placed low on the external iliac vein to avoid creating an acute angle at the portal vein–splenic vein junction. Third, the spleen is removed after the pancreas is revascularized. Finally, the bladder–duodenum anastomosis is performed in two layers (Fig. 16-94).

The bladder drainage technique greatly facilitates the early diagnosis of rejection by providing a means to measure the output of amylase from the graft, as reflected by the urinary amylase activity. This is expressed as units per hour or units per liter. In a stable graft, the day-to-day variability is in the range of 5000 to 10,000 IU/h. Potentially deleterious by-products of bladder drainage include the following: (1) persistent bleeding from the duodenal segment with subsequent ulceration; (2) persistent metabolic acidosis secondary to the continued excretion of pancreatic bicarbonate in the urine; and (3) urethritis and balanitis. These complications are uncommon and are probably related to the activation of pancreatic enzymes in the urine secondary to urinary tract infection.

Segmental Graft

One perceived advantage to using a segmental graft is that it makes the harvesting of a liver and a pancreas from the same cadaver donor less cumbersome because there is no conflict over the arterial supplies to the organs. This technique can be applied to living, related donors. Exocrine secretion can be maintained by anastomosing the pancreas to a Roux-en-Y limb of recipient jejunum, or secretion can be obliterated by polymer duct injection. If exocrine drainage is maintained, a catheter can be left in the pancreatic duct and brought out through the abdominal

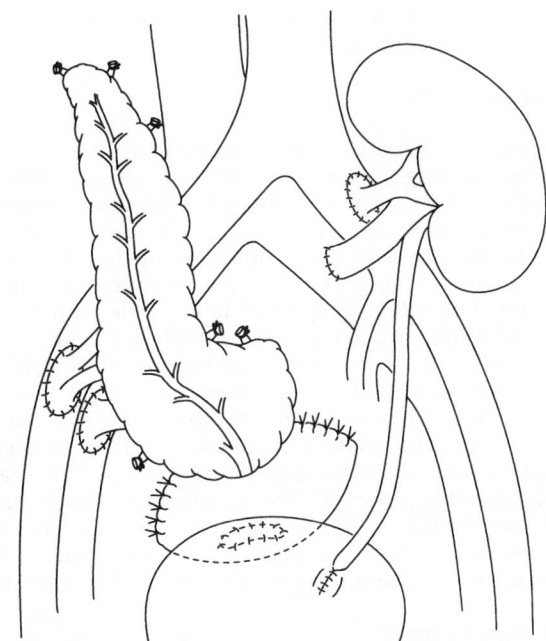

Figure 16-94. The whole-organ composite pancreaticoduodenal graft placed in the right iliac fossa and anastomosed to the urinary bladder, with a cotransplanted kidney placed in the left iliac fossa. (After Terasaki PI, ed. Clinical Transplantation 1989. Los Angeles, UCLA Tissue Typing Laboratory, 1989)

wall to temporarily divert secretions to permit healing of the anastomosis.

Duct injection of a polymer substance is the simplest means of controlling exocrine pancreatic secretion, but shortly after transplantation, many patients so treated develop exocrine leakage and wound complications. Most of these fistulas heal, however, and the infection risk has been low. The major concern with the ductal injection technique is whether the resultant fibrosis will eventually cause a cessation of endocrine graft function. A number of grafts have ceased function for no apparent cause, and there has been a significant rate of allograft thrombosis using this technique. Finally, enthusiasm for the use of this technique has been tempered by recent findings indicating that monitoring of exocrine secretion is crucial for the early diagnosis of allograft rejection.

Regardless of the type of graft transplanted, most agree that the grafts should be placed intraperitoneally. The extensive surface area of the peritoneum is probably of considerable help in absorbing the exudate that escapes from the surface of the pancreas. The incidence of anastomotic leaks and wound complications has been greatly reduced with the intraperitoneal placement of grafts.

Perioperative Management Issues

Immunosuppression

The immunosuppression regimen at most centers in North America involves an induction phase and quadruple immunosuppression with either ALG/ATG or monoclonal OKT3, prednisone, cyclosporine, and azathioprine. OKT3 or ALG/ATG is usually continued for 10 to 14 days, and steroids are tapered to about 30 mg/d. Cyclosporine is administered orally in the range of 5 to 6 mg/kg, depending on renal function, and the dosage of azathioprine is 1 to 2 mg/kg orally or intravenously. This regimen has produced excellent patient and allograft survival with a minimum of infection-related morbidity.

Anticoagulation

Vascular thrombosis of the pancreas is the most common cause of sudden graft loss in the early postoperative period. Therefore, some form of perioperative anticoagulation is recommended. Suggested protocols include aspirin alone, subcutaneous heparin plus aspirin, systemic heparinization, and dextran 40, begun intraoperatively and continued at a rate of 10 mL/h for 48 to 72 hours, plus aspirin, 325 mg/d, plus subcutaneous heparin, 5000 IU subcutaneously three times daily. The risk of thrombosis must be weighed against the risks of intraoperative and postoperative hemorrhage. With the recognition that thrombosis is related in large part to manipulation of the gland during the donor operation, techniques of organ procurement have been changed, and together with the introduction of better preservation solutions, the incidence of thrombosis has been reduced from 25% to less than 10%. At the least, aspirin is recommended for all pancreatic transplant recipients.

Endocrine Function

Successful pancreatic transplantation restores the plasma level of glucose to normal. Glucose levels fall by as much as 2.7 to 5.5 mmol/L/h (50 to 100 mg/dL/h) from the time of vascular unclamping. Peripheral glucose sensitivity may be decreased postoperatively by the hormonal response to surgical stress, the inappropriate release of glucagon, and high doses of steroids. The increased levels of glucagon do not seem to be the result of corticosteroid or anesthetic drugs administered during surgery, since hyperglucagonemia does not occur in uremic, nondiabetic recipients of renal allografts alone. C-peptide levels are often difficult to interpret because of the altered urinary C-peptide clearance of kidneys that may not be functioning optimally.

There is a significant diurnal variation in blood level of glucose, especially in the first week after transplantation. This change may be as great as 3 to 5 mmol/L (54 to 90 mg/dL), with the blood glucose rise beginning in the early afternoon. This rise in blood glucose needs to be distinguished from other causes of hyperglycemia that require urgent attention, such as venous thrombosis.

Exocrine Function

The function of the exocrine part of the gland is judged by the serum amylase as well as by the enzyme concentration and volume of the graft secretions. These can be monitored easily if exocrine drainage has been diverted to the urinary bladder or to the intestine when a drainage catheter has been left in the pancreatic duct and brought out externally. In the case of pancreaticocystostomy, urinary pH is an additional measurement that can be useful.

To reduce local complications attributed to continued exocrine secretion in the early posttransplantation period, some have recommended the use of octreotide (Sandostatin), a long-acting synthetic analogue of the potent inhibitory hormone, somatostatin. Although pancreatic fistulas have been treated successfully with octreotide, this drug can interfere with the absorption of orally administered cyclosporine, resulting in subtherapeutic serum levels of cyclosporine.[311] When administered in a prophylactic manner before the induction of pancreatitis, octreotide produces a much more severe form of inflammation and tissue injury.[312]

Postoperative Complications

Complications of pancreatic transplantation include the following:

Immunologic
Rejection
Recurrence of diabetes

Nonimmunologic
Thrombosis
Bleeding
Pancreatitis
Anastomotic failure
Sepsis
Pancreatic ascites, pseudocyst
Pancreatic fistula
Intestinal obstruction, perforation (intestinal drainage)
Metabolic acidosis (bladder drainage)
Urethritis, balanitis, cystitis (bladder drainage)

The complications that are responsible for graft failure and the frequency of their occurrence are summarized in Table 16-21.

Immunologic

The main problem with pancreatic transplantation is the lack of an easy, reliable technique for the early diagnosis of rejection, particularly in separate renal–pancreatic transplantations in which the only valid parameter has been an increase in plasma concentration of glucose. A rise in plasma glucose levels is a late indicator of rejection. By the time hyperglycemia is evident, 90% of the islet mass may be destroyed, and antirejection therapy cannot reverse the process. The clinical features of pancreatic rejection often are extremely difficult to differentiate from the development of local complications resulting in graft failure. In the patient undergoing simultaneous renal–pancreatic transplantation, the development of renal rejection, which is easily identified by a rising serum creatinine, has been taken as an index of active and concomitant pancreas rejection.

Urinary diversion has the advantage of allowing exocrine pancreatic function to be assessed directly by measurement of pancreatic enzymes in the urine. With a well-functioning whole-organ graft, urinary amylase levels between 2000 and 10,000 IU/L by the first posttransplantation day, 10,000 to 20,000 IU/L by day 3, and more than 30,000 IU/L by 2 weeks can be expected. A decrease of 30% to 50% in the output of urinary amylase appears to be a good indicator of pancreatic rejection. Urinary pH has proved to be an easy screening test for rejection, which patients can use at home. Urine pH after pancreatic transplantation with urinary diversion should be above 7 because of secretion of pancreatic bicarbonate into the urine. An early finding in rejection is a decrease in bicarbonate

---

Table 16-21. TECHNICAL FAILURES IN PANCREATIC TRANSPLANTATION

Complication	SPK (n = 2112)	PAK (n = 205)	PTA (n = 147)
Thrombosis	132 (6.3%)	26 (12.7%)	16 (10.9%)
Bleeding	16 (0.8%)	2 (1.0%)	1 (0.7%)
Infection	43 (2.0%)	8 (3.9%)	3 (2.0%)
Anastamotic leak	9 (0.4%)	2 (1.0%)	—
Pancreatitis	39 (1.8%)	6 (2.9%)	5 (3.4%)
TOTAL	239 (11.3%)	44 (21.5%)	25 (17.0%)

SPK, simultaneous pancreas and kidney transplantation; PAK, pancreas after kidney; PTA, pancreas transplantation alone.

output associated with a significant fall in urinary pH. A similar indication of early rejection may be a decrease in the requirement for oral bicarbonate replacement in a recipient who previously had taken bicarbonate for the treatment of a metabolic acidosis caused by the urinary loss of pancreatic graft bicarbonate.

An increase in the serum level of pancreatic anodal trypsinogen is a sensitive, specific, early marker of pancreas rejection,[313] and is beginning to be adopted at many centers. The use of anodal trypsinogen should allow for the proper timing of graft biopsies and the judicious use of immunosuppressive agents, which result in increased allograft survival for pancreas after kidney and pancreas-alone allografts.

Cytologic examination of pancreatic juice from enterically diverted grafts, in which a pancreatic duct drainage catheter has been placed, has demonstrated that an increase in the number of inflammatory cells is an early and sensitive marker for pancreatic allograft rejection. Application of this technique, however, is limited. Percutaneous fine-needle aspiration of the pancreas for cytologic examination or biopsy of the pancreas by open or percutaneous means for histology can also be helpful in establishing the diagnosis of rejection. These techniques have not been applied widely, however, because of the risk of fistula formation and the difficulty in their interpretation. Serum levels of tumor necrosis factor and both serum and urine levels of interleukin-2 receptor are being investigated as sensitive, albeit less specific, markers of pancreatic allograft rejection.

The more traditional, nonspecific indicators of allograft rejection include fever, leukocytosis, and an increased serum amylase level. The use of these indices, however, does not permit the early diagnosis of pancreas rejection at a stage when it would be easily reversible.

Pancreatic allograft rejection appears to be more difficult to treat successfully than renal graft rejection. This difficulty probably relates to our inability to make a diagnosis at an early stage. A rejection episode can be treated initially with steroid pulse therapy, 250 to 500 mg/d of methylprednisolone intravenously, for 1 to 3 days. Many recommend that a pancreatic rejection, because of its vigorous nature, be treated immediately with either monoclonal OKT3 or a polyclonal antilymphoblast globulin.

Recurrence of autoimmune isletitis has been described in identical-twin and other related-donor pancreatic grafts after transplantation to nonimmunosuppressed or minimally immunosuppressed recipients. Recurrence of disease can be prevented by administering adequate immunosuppression.

Nonimmunologic

Graft Thrombosis.   Thrombosis and subsequent ischemic necrosis of the graft are complications that have contributed to graft failure in a substantial number of patients. The high incidence of this problem has been explained by the fact that the pancreas is a so-called low-flow organ. Removal of the spleen in combination with postclamping edema, which to a varying degree always follows ex vivo organ preservation, may be sufficient to facilitate the occurrence of thrombosis.

As mentioned previously, it appears that the most important preventive factor is meticulous surgical technique. This includes an appreciation for the eventual vascular anatomic reconstruction and extremely careful handling of the pancreatic graft during organ procurement to minimize the chance for postoperative pancreatitis and postischemic swelling. Precise vascular technique to avoid irregularities of suture lines and kinking of vessels is of critical importance.

Graft thrombosis usually presents in the initial 12 to 24 hours after transplantation and is signaled by the sudden elevation in the serum glucose level or by the failure of the glucose level to fall toward normal. The diagnosis can be confirmed by a radionuclide perfusion scan to delineate flow to the pancreas. If the diagnosis is confirmed, the graft must be removed expeditiously to prevent septic or vascular complications.

Graft Pancreatitis.   This complication may occur early as well as late after pancreatic transplantation. Early postoperative pancreatitis is usually a consequence of injury to the pancreas during procurement and preservation. After transplantation, there is inevitably a rise in the serum amylase level, which usually peaks after 24 to 48 hours. Hyperamylasemia may or may not be associated with abdominal pain and clinical signs of peritonitis. Treatment of pancreatitis in this setting is the same as that for any other form of acute pancreatitis. Pancreatitis in the early posttransplantation period is usually self-limited. Should pancreatitis progress, however, thrombosis may ensue, necessitating removal of the graft. The inflamed pancreas may become the focus of a septic process, resulting in pancreatic abscess, anastomotic failure, peripancreatic abscess, peritonitis, and pancreatic fistula. Any one of these complica-

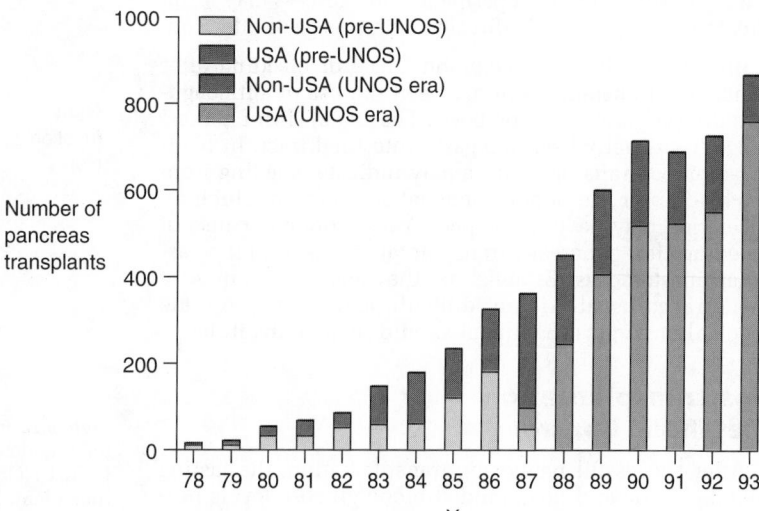

Figure 16-95. Number of transplants tabulated by the International Pancreas Transplant Registry between 1966 and 1993 includes figures from before and since formation of the United Network for Organ Sharing (UNOS) in 1987. The reporting for 1993 is incomplete. The total cases for the United States (USA) was 3662 (45 clusters) and for the non-USA was 1832 (1 cluster). The world total with cluster cases included was 5540.

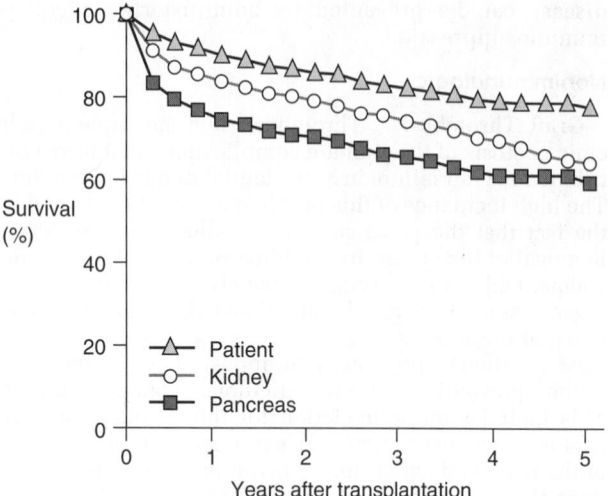

Figure 16-96. Patient, kidney, and pancreas graft survival rates in recipients of bladder-drained simultaneous pancreas and kidney transplants from cadaveric donors reported to IPTR/UNOS, 1987–1992.

tions could prompt early removal of the graft, and abdominal ultrasonography or computed tomographic scanning should be performed early to help confirm the diagnosis of pancreatitis and to identify complications.

Anastomotic Failure. This may occur if the exocrine secretion of the graft has been preserved and diverted to either the intestine or the urinary bladder. With the introduction of a pancreatic duct catheter to direct pancreatic secretions away from the anastomosis during the time of healing, the incidence of anastomotic failure for intestinally drained allografts has been reduced significantly. Bladder drainage of the pancreatic allograft has always been associated with an extremely low incidence of anastomotic leakage. Anastomotic leak is a potentially life-threatening complication. When it is diagnosed, early reoperation is the treatment of choice. If a leak cannot be repaired, the graft usually must be removed.

Sepsis. Most intraabdominal septic complications occur in the first few weeks after transplantation. Sepsis is almost always related to the development of graft pancreatitis or anastomotic failure. When a leak occurs in a graft that has been placed intraabdominally, a fistula may not always develop; rather, a peripancreatic abscess may form. Treatment is specifically directed at the cause of infection.

Bleeding. The most common cause of bleeding after pancreatic transplantation has been the use of anticoagulant drugs to prevent thrombosis. The actual site of hemorrhage has usually been the gastrointestinal tract. In bladder-drained grafts, hematuria may indicate bleeding from the bladder or the donor duodenal segment, in which an ulceration may have developed. A less common cause of bleeding after pancreatic transplantation has been the vascular anastomoses. Establishing the cause and source of hemorrhage usually is not difficult, and the appropriate medical or surgical treatment should then be instituted.

Posttransplantation Metabolic Control

After successful pancreatic transplantation, the fasting blood glucose and postprandial blood glucose levels normalize within hours. Hb A_{1c} levels eventually normalize

in most patients and are only slightly elevated in a few patients. The 24-hour metabolic glucose profile demonstrates no difference when compared with nondiabetic kidney recipients on similar immunosuppression regimens.

Hyperinsulinemia with elevated levels of C-peptide is found in most pancreatic transplant recipients due to the systemic venous drainage of the graft. Some evidence indicates that there is increased insulin production secondary to reduced insulin sensitivity associated with steroids. Insulin release during arginine and tolbutamide administration is usually normal or near-normal, and hepatic glucose regulation is also normal. The results of oral and intravenous glucose tolerance tests are mixed, in part because of the varying mass of islet tissue transplanted. Most centers report that these studies are normal in at least 80% of recipients with functioning grafts.

Late Complications

The major reason to perform pancreatic transplantation is to prevent the appearance, halt the progression, or induce regression of the secondary complications of diabetes. If pancreatic transplantation does not influence the course of secondary complications, it probably should not be applied, at least not in nonuremic, nonrenal transplant recipients, until fully effective, nontoxic immunosuppression is available. In patients with end-stage diabetic nephropathy who undergo renal transplantation, immunosuppression is obligatory, and pancreatic transplantation is justified to avoid the need for insulin and to improve the life-style that ensues, even if other secondary complications are advanced. Even in these patients, however, secondary complications may be favorably influenced.

A review of the effects of pancreatic transplantation on secondary complications is difficult and complex. There have been no randomized studies to date, and there have been only a few studies in which patients with failed grafts have been used as controls. The severity of complications in a given organ system has in many instances been advanced, and therefore, a beneficial effect would not be anticipated.[314]

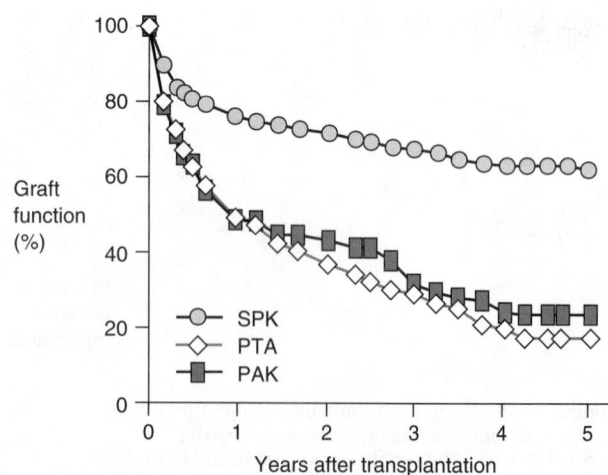

Figure 16-97. Graft functional survival rates by recipient category for bladder-drained cadaveric pancreas transplants reported to IPTR/UNOS, 1987–1993. SPK, simultaneous pancreas and kidney transplant; PAK, pancreas after kidney transplant; PTA, pancreas transplant alone.

Table 16-22. RESULTS OF RISK FACTOR ANALYSIS FOR US PANCREAS TRANSPLANTS

	Relative Risk			
	ALL (n = 2062)	SPK (n = 1757)	PAK (n = 178)	PTA (n = 127)
PAK vs SPK	2.62			
PTA vs SPK	2.43			
Recipient age				
≥45 y vs <45 y	1.18	1.08	1.60	1.50
Preservation time				
Categories 1–4*	0.87	0.84	1.94	1.02
ALG/ATG				
Yes versus no	0.91	0.91	1.12	0.15
OKT3				
Yes versus no	0.93	0.89	1.9	0.18
Mismatches				
0–6 (stepwise)	0.96	0.90	1.11	1.31
Retransplantation versus primary	1.43	1.09	1.51	1.70
Era				
1990–1993 versus 1987–1989	0.99	0.99	0.98	0.95

SPK, simultaneous pancreas and kidney transplantation; PAK, pancreas after kidney; PTA, pancreas transplantation alone; RR, relative risk.
* Category 1: <12 h; category 2: 12–23 h; category 3: 24–29 h; category 4: ≥30 h.

Nephropathy

If a renal graft from a nondiabetic donor is placed in a diabetic patient, morphologic signs of diabetic nephropathy develop as early as 2 years after transplantation. In contrast, in patients who have undergone simultaneous renal–pancreatic transplantation, renal graft biopsy specimens obtained 2 to 4 years after transplantation show no light-microscopic changes suggestive of diabetic nephropathy. These findings suggest that normoglycemia achieved by a pancreatic transplantation prevents diabetic nephropathy.

Whether already established renal diabetic lesions are reversible by pancreatic transplantation is crucial for the timing of the intervention. In renal transplant recipients who have biopsy evidence of mild diabetic nephropathy at the time of pancreatic transplantation, follow-up renal biopsies did not reveal progression of the renal disease. In patients who underwent pancreatic transplantation alone, with mild nephropathy in the native kidneys, renal function remained stable after several years of follow-up. These findings suggest that preexisting diabetic lesions may be halted by pancreatic transplantation. In patients with functioning pancreatic grafts, renal biopsies have shown a decreased glomerular mesangial volume compared with diabetic controls.

Successful pancreatic transplantation prevents recurrence of diabetic nephropathy in a transplanted kidney. Pancreas transplantation alone, in nonuremic, nonrenal transplant recipients, can induce regression of microscopic lesions of diabetic nephropathy. Evidence suggests that in most patients with early nephropathy, progression to renal failure is avoided by a successful pancreatic transplantation.

Neuropathy

For the most part, the subjective signs of peripheral neuropathy (paresthesia, muscle weakness, leg cramps) and autonomic dysfunction (gastroparesis, constipation, diarrhea, orthostatic hypotension) improve remarkably after pancreatic transplantation. Objectively, the somatic motor and sensory systems appear to be favorably influenced by a functioning pancreatic transplant, with stabilization of evoked muscle amplitude potentials and improvement in some other parameters of nerve function. Autonomic function remains stable. Although this evidence suggests that the progression of diabetic polyneuropathy can be halted and slightly improved by successful pancreatic transplantation, the degree of improvement is small, probably because of established structural damage to the peripheral nervous system.

Retinopathy

Almost all recipients of pancreatic transplants who have been studied had advanced retinopathy. In recipients of pancreatic transplants alone, the course of retinopathy, at least during the first year after transplantation, is similar for those with and without sustained graft function. Deterioration in retinopathy grade occurred in about 30% of the recipients by 3 years, whether the graft functioned continuously or failed early. Thereafter, retinopathy in patients

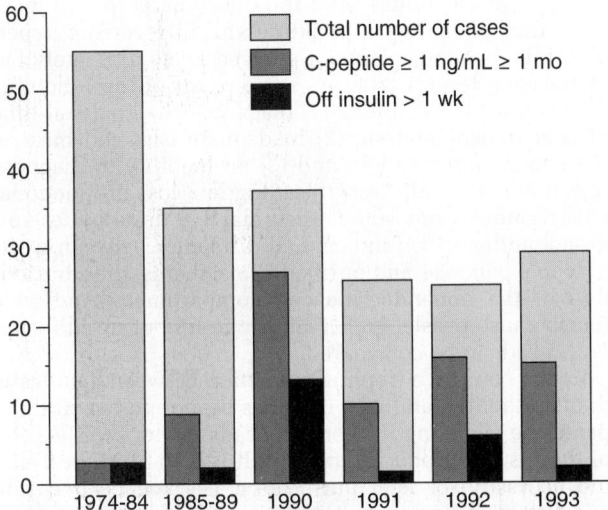

Figure 16-98. Insulin independence and basal C-peptide after adult islet allotransplantation through 1993. (After Int Islet Transplant Registry Newslett 1994;4)

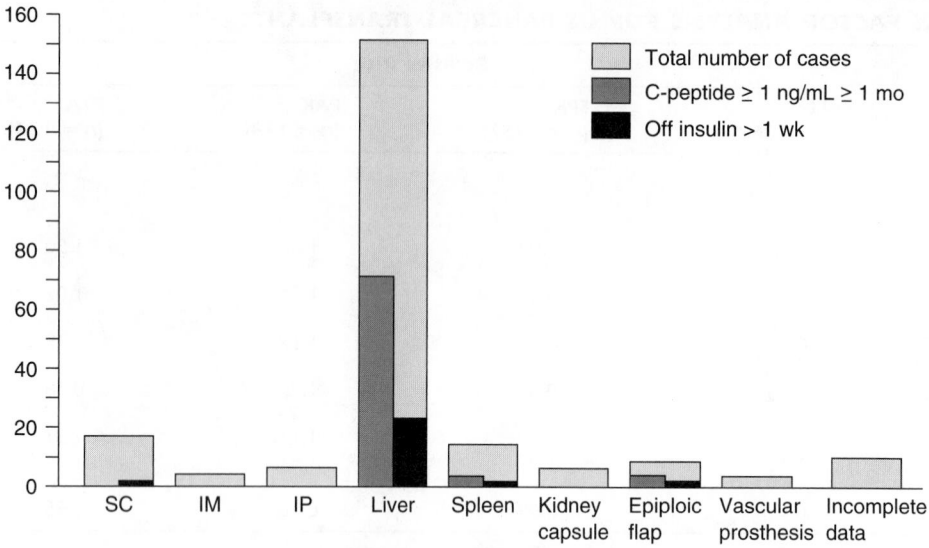

Figure 16-99. Insulin independence and basal C-peptide after adult islet (and one xenograft) through 1993, according to site of implantation. (After Int Islet Transplant Registry Newslett 1994;4)

with functioning grafts remained stable, unlike those with failed grafts, in whom deterioration continued.

Results

At the end of 1993, 5540 pancreatic transplantations had been reported to the International Pancreas Transplant Registry (Fig. 16-95). Since 1987, the Registry has also collected data on United States transplantations for the United Network for Organ Sharing (IPTR/UNOS). The overall patient and graft (pancreas and kidney) survival rates are shown in Figure 16-96.

The overwhelming number of pancreas transplantations are whole organs drained into the urinary bladder. At 1 year, the overall graft survival rate is 76%, regardless of whether a kidney transplant has also been done. When these data are analyzed further by recipient category (pancreatic transplantation alone, simultaneous renal–pancreatic transplantation, pancreatic after renal), it becomes clear that the best pancreatic allograft function rate is achieved when simultaneous renal–pancreatic transplantation is performed (Fig. 16-97).

A summary of the factors that may influence the successful outcome of pancreatic transplantation is shown in Table 16-22.

ISLET TRANSPLANTATION

Exocrine pancreatic replacement is not the purpose of pancreatic transplantation. The exocrine tissue, which constitutes 95% of the gland, to a large extent is responsible for the many complications associated with pancreatic transplantation. The objective of islet transplantation is the provision, early enough in the course of diabetes, of an effective islet cell mass that would function in a physiologic manner to either prevent, stabilize, or reverse the secondary complications of the disease. Much enthusiasm has been generated for islet transplantation, but it is clearly in the early investigative stage compared with whole-organ pancreatic transplantation.

The isolation and purification of sufficient numbers of human islets of Langerhans has improved with the introduction of techniques that involve intraductal perfusion of the pancreas with specific collagenase-containing solu-

tions. Major efforts are now underway in various centers to bring islet transplantation to clinical fruition (Fig. 16-98).

Because the mass of islet tissue transplanted and surviving is the critical determinant of ultimate allograft function, some important issues remain to be resolved. Earlier work suggested that islet transplantation into diabetic rodents prevented or stabilized the late complications of the disease, but more recent work suggests that only whole-organ pancreatic transplantation is capable of permanently reversing the diabetic state and preventing secondary complications. In rodent and large animal studies, islet recipients showed progressive loss of graft function in the long term.

The clinical experience with the transplantation of purified islets, regardless of the recipient site, also continues to be disappointing (Fig 16-99). An unexpectedly large islet mass is required to achieve demonstrable serum levels of C-peptide, let alone successful restoration of normal glucose homeostasis with insulin independence. As a consequence, more than one pancreas is required to produce a graft of sufficient cell mass. Furthermore, it is becoming clear that the inability to sustain graft survival may represent a major unforeseen problem.

These shortcomings pose the question as to why pancreas transplantation is so successful in reversing hyperglycemia, but transplants of purified islets ultimately fail in the long term. Certainly, some or all of the following factors must be pertinent: (1) inadequate cell mass at time of islet transplantation; (2) inadequate islet cell mass at the site of implantation; and (3) an inability to diagnose rejection sufficiently early, leading to a loss of functional islet tissue. As relevant as they may be, these issues still do not address the fundamental difference between grafts of whole pancreas and purified islets, that is, the contribution of the nonendocrine cell compartment. And so a fourth cause of islet graft failure, the loss of trophic support, needs to be considered.

In this context, a trophic interaction between pancreatic duct epithelium and islet cells has been reported, and the paracrine signaling that occurs leads to the proliferation of the insulin-producing cells.[315] It is also of interest that the necessity for islet purification has been called into question,[316,317] and that at least one group has successfully transplanted human recipients with unpurified islets from a single donor.[318]

The recognition and prevention of rejection also remain

limiting factors for islet transplantation. Single-drug immunosuppressive therapy with cyclosporine, a known islet cell toxin, has been predictably disappointing, as have early clinical trials using a triple-drug regimen. Methods for the immunologic isolation of the graft, therefore, are presently being pursued aggressively. If shown to be practical and effective, these might obviate the requirement for immunosuppressive agents.

REFERENCES

1. Eckhardt LA. Immunoglobulin gene expression only in the right cells at the right time. FASEB J 1992;6:2553.
2. Komori T, Okada A, Stewart V, et al. Lack of N regions in antigen receptor variable region genes of TdT-deficient lymphocytes. Science 1993;261:1171.
3. Gilfillan S, Dierich A, Lemeur M, et al. Mice lacking TdT: mature animals with an immature lymphocyte repertoire. Science 1993;261:1175.
4. Aldhouse P. Transgenic mice display a class (switching) act. Science 1993;262:1212.
5. Cambier JC, Campbell KS. Membrane immunoglobulin and its accomplices: new lessons from an old receptor. FASEB J 1992;6:3207.
6. Clark MR, Campbell KS, Kazalauskas A, et al. The B cell antigen receptor complex: association of Ig-a and Ig-b with distinct cytoplasmic effectors. Science 1992;258:123.
7. Constant P, Davodeau F, Peyrat M, et al. Stimulation of human gdT cells by nonpeptidic mycobacterial ligands. Science 1994;264:267.
8. Momvaerts P, Arnoldi J, Russ, F, et al. Different roles of and T cells in immunity against an intracellular bacterial pathogen. Nature 1993;365:53.
9. Schild H, Mavaddat N, Litzenberger C, et al. The nature of major histocompatibility complex recognition by gd T cells. Cell 1994;76:29-37.
10. Weiss A. T cell antigen receptor signal transduction: a tale of tails and cytoplasmic protein-tyrosine kinases. Cell 1993;73:209.
11. Williams AF, Beyers AD. At grips with interactions. Nature 1992;356:746.
12. Barinage M. Getting some "backbone": how MHC binds peptides. Science 1992;257:880.
13. Germain RN. MHC-dependent antigen processing and peptide presentation: providing ligands for T lymphocyte activation. Cell 1994;76:287.
14. Townsend A. A new presentation pathway? Nature 1992;356:386.
15. Schmid SL, Jackson MR. Making class II presentable. Nature 1994;368:103.
16. Howard JC, Seelig A. Peptides and the proteasome. Nature 1993;365:211.
17. Powis SJ, Deverson EV, Coadwell WJ, et al. Effect of polymorphism of an MHC-linked transporter on the peptides assembled in a class I molecule. Nature 1992;357:211.
18. Lanzavecchia A, Reid PA, Watts C. Irreversible association of peptides with class II MHC molecules in living cells. Nature 1992;357:249.
19. Peterson M, Miller J. Antigen presentation enhanced by the alternatively spliced invariant chain gene product p41. Nature 1992;357:596.
20. Malnati MS, Marti M, LaVaute T, et al. Processing pathways for presentation of cytosolic antigen to MHC class I–restricted T cells. Nature 1992;357:702.
21. Riberdy JM, Newcomb JR, Surman MJ, et al. HLA-DR molecules from an antigen-processing mutant cell line are associated with invariant chain peptides. Nature 1992;360:474.
22. Eisenlohr LC, Bacik I, Bennink JR, et al. Expression of a membrane protease enhances presentation of endogenous antigens to MHC class I–restricted T lymphocytes. Cell 1992;71:963.
23. Kaer LV, Ashton-Rickardt PG, Ploegh HL, et al. TAP-1 mutant mice are deficient in antigen presentation, surface class I molecules, and $CD4^-8^+$ T cells. Cell 1992;71:1205.
24. Pfeifer JD, Wick MJ, Roberts RL, et al. Phagocytic processing of bacterial antigens for class I MHC presentation to T cells. Nature 1993;361:359.
25. Michalek MT, Grant EP, Gramm C, et al. A role for the ubiquitin-dependent proteolytic pathway in MHC class I–restricted antigen presentation. Nature 1993;363:552.
26. Germain RN, Rinker AG. Peptide binding inhibits protein aggregation of invariant-chain free class II dimers and promotes surface expression of occupied molecules. Nature 1993;373:725.
27. Driscoll J, Brown MG, Finley D. MHC-linked LMP gene products specifically alter peptidase activities of the proteasome. Nature 1993;365:262.
28. Gaczynska M, Rock KL, Goldberg AL. γ-Interferon and expression of MHC genes regulate peptide hydrolysis by proteasomes. Nature 1993;365:264.
29. Heemels MT, Schumacher TN, Wonigeit K, et al. Peptide translocation by variants of the transporter associated with antigen processing. Science 1993;262:2059.
30. Jackson MR, Cohen-Doyle MF, Peterson PA, et al. Regulation of MHC class I transport by the molecular chaperone, calnexin (p88, IP90). Science 1994;263:384.
31. Chicz RM, Urban RG, Lane WS, et al. Predominant naturally processed peptides bound to HLA-DR1 are derived from MHC-related molecules and are heterogeneous in size. Nature 1992;358:764.
32. Momburg F, Roelse J, Howard JC, et al. Selectivity of MHC-encoded peptide transporters from human, mouse and rat. Nature 1994;367:648.
33. Bodmer H, Viville S, Benoist C, et al. Diversity of endogenous epitopes bound to MHC class II molecules limited by invariant chain. Science 1994;263:1284.
34. Ortmann B, Androlewicz MJ, Cresswell P. MHC class I/β_2-microglobulin complexes associate with TAP transporters before peptide binding. Nature 1994;368:864.
35. Suh WK, Cohen-Doyle MF, Fruh K, et al. Interaction of MHC class I molecules with the transporter associated with antigen processing. Science 1994;264:1322.
36. Hunt DF, Michel H, Dickinson TA. Peptides presented to the immune system by the murine class II major histocompatibility complex molecule I-A^d. Science 1992;256:1817.
37. Kurlander RJ, Shawar SM, Brown ML, et al. Specialized role for a murine class I-b MHC molecule in prokaryotic host defenses. Science 1992;257:678.
38. Rotzschke O, Falk K, Stevanovic S, et al. Qa-2 molecules are peptide receptors of higher stringency than ordinary class I molecules. Nature 1993;361:642.
39. Bachmann MF, Rohrer UH, Kundig TM, et al. The influence of antigen organization on B cell responsiveness. Science 1993;262:1448.
40. Guymer RH, Mandel TE. A comparison of corneal, pancreas, and skin grafts in mice. Transplantation 1994;57:1251.
41. Springer TA. Traffic signals for lymphocyte recirculation and leukocyte emigration: the multistep paradigm. Cell 1994;76:301.
42. Malinowski K, Waltzer WC, Jao S, et al. Homing of CD8CD57 T lymphocytes into acutely rejected renal allografts. Transplantation 1992;54:1013.
43. Turunen JP, Mattila P, Halttunen, et al. Evidence that lymphocyte traffic into rejecting cardiac allografts is CD11a- and CD49d-dependent. Transplantation 1992;54:1053.
44. Parham P. The box and the rod. Nature 1992;357:538.
45. Konig R, Huang L, Germain RN. MHC class II interaction with CD4 mediated by a region analogous to the MHC class I binding site for CD8. Nature 1992;356:796.
46. Reiner SL, Wang Z, Hatam F, et al. T_H1 and T_H2 cell antigen receptors in experimental leishmaniasis. Science 1993;259:1457.
47. Takeuchi T, Lowry RP, Konieczny B. Heart allografts in murine systems. Transplantation 1992;53:1281.
48. Gaur A, Haspel R, Mayer J, et al. Requirement for $CD8^+$ cells in T cell receptor peptide-induced clonal unresponsiveness. Science 1993;259:91.
49. LaRosa FG, Smilek D, Talmage DW, et al. Evidence that tolerance to cultured thyroid allografts is an active immunological process. Transplantation 1992;53:903.
50. Qin S, Cobbold SP, Pope H, et al. "Infectious" transplantation tolerance. Science 1993;259:974.

51. Halwani F, Guttmann RD, Ste. Croix H, et al. Identification of natural suppressor cells in long-term renal allograft recipients. Transplantation 1992;54:973.
52. Clark EA, Ledbetter JA. How B and T cells talk to each other. Nature 1994;367:425.
53. Marx J. Cell communication failure leads to immune disorder. Science 1993;259:896.
54. Hill A, Chapel H. The fruits of cooperation. Nature 1993; 361:494.
55. Tsubata T, Wu J, Honjo T. B-cell apoptosis induced by antigen receptor crosslinking is blocked by a T-cell signal through CD40. Nature 1993;364:645.
56. Carter RH, Fearon DT. CD19: lowering the threshold for antigen receptor simulation of B lymphocytes. Science 1992; 256:105.
57. Mantovani A, Bussolino F, Dejana E. Cytokine regulation of endothelial cell function. FASEB J 1992;6:2591.
58. Gerritsen ME, Bloor CM. Endothelial cell gene expression in response to injury. FASEB J 1993;7:523.
59. Willebrand E, Salmela K, Isoniemi H, et al. Induction of HLA class II antigen and interleukin-2 receptor expression in acute vascular rejection of human kidney allografts. Transplantation 1992;53:1077.
60. Fuggle SV, Sanderson JB, Gray DW, et al. Variation in expression of endothelial adhesion molecules in pretransplant and transplanted kidneys: correlation with intragraft events. Transplantation 1993;55:1170.
61. Wuthrich RP, Jenkins TA, Snyder TL. Regulation of cytokine-stimulated vascular cell adhesion molecule-1 expression in renal tubular epithelial cells. Transplantation 1993;55:172.
62. Pelletier RP, Morgan CJ, Sedmak DD, et al. Analysis of inflammatory endothelial changes, including VCAM-1 expression, in murine cardiac grafts. Transplantation 1993;55:315.
63. Hoffmann MW, Wonigeit K, Steinhoff G, et al. Production of cytokines (TNF-alpha, IL-1-beta) and endothelial cell activation in human liver allograft rejection. Transplantation 1993;55:329.
64. Morgan CJ, Pelletier RP, Hernandez CJ, et al. Alloantigen-dependent endothelial phenotype and lymphokine mRNA expression in rejecting murine cardiac allografts. Transplantation 1993;55:919.
65. Albelda SM, Smith CM, Ward PA. Adhesion molecules and inflammatory injury. FASEB J 1994;8:504.
66. Hynes RO. Integrins: versatility, modulation, and signaling in cell adhesion. Cell 1992;69:11.
67. Lasky LA. Selectins: interpreters of cell-specific carbohydrate information during inflammation. Science 1992; 258:964.
68. Shimizu Y, Shaw S. Mucins in the mainstream. Nature 1993;366:630.
69. Baumhueter S, Singer MS, Henzel W, et al. Binding of L-selectin to the vascular sialomucin CD34. Science 1993; 262:436.
70. Berg EL, McEvoy LM, Berlin C, et al. L-selectin–mediated lymphocyte rolling on MAdCAM-1. Nature 1993;366:695.
71. Taylor PM, Rose ML, Yacoub MH, et al. Induction of vascular adhesion molecules during rejection of human cardiac allografts. Transplantation 1992;54:451.
72. Paul WE, Seder RA. Lymphocyte responses and cytokines. Cell 1994;76:241.
73. Nowak R. Bubble boy paradox resolved. 1993;262:1818.
74. Kondo M, Takeshita T, Higuchi M, et al. Functional participation of the IL-2 receptor γ chain in IL-7 receptor complexes. Science 1994;263:1453.
75. Kishimoto T, Akira S, Taga T. Interleukin-6 and its receptor: a paradigm for cytokines. 1992;258:593.
76. Kishimoto T, Taga T, Akira S. Cytokine signal transduction. Cell 1994;76:253.
77. Taga T, Kishimoto T. Cytokine receptors and signal transduction. FASEB J 1993;7:3387.
78. Stahl N, Yancopoulos GD. The alphas, betas, and kinases of cytokine receptor complexes. Cell 1993;74:587.
79. Hunter T. Cytokine connections. Nature 1993;366:114.
80. Stahl N, Boulton TG, Farruggella T, et al. Association and activation of Jak-Tyk kinases by CNTF-LIF-OSM-IL-6 β receptor components. Science 1994;263:92.
81. Ramsay AJ, Husband AJ, Ramshaw IA, et al. The role of interleukin-6 in mucosal IgA antibody responses in vivo. Science 1994;264:561.
82. Scott, P. IL-12: initiation cytokine for cell-mediated immunity. Science 1993;260:496.
83. Afonso LC, Scharton TM, Vieira LQ, et al. The adjuvant effect of interleukin-12 in a vaccine against leishmania major. Science 1994;263:235.
84. Massague J. Receptors for the TGF-β family. Cell 1992;69:1067.
85. Wrana JL, Attisano L, Carcamo J, et al. TGFβ signals through a heteromeric protein kinase receptor complex. Cell 1992; 71:1003.
86. Barral-Netto M, Barral A, Brownell CE, et al. Transforming growth factor-β in leishmanial infection: a parasite escape mechanism. Science 1992;257:545.
87. Attisano L, Carcamo J, Ventura F, et al. Identification of human activin and TGFβ type I receptors that form heteromeric kinase complexes with type II receptors. Cell 1993;75:671.
88. Smith CA, Farrah T, Goodwin RG. The TNF receptor superfamily of cellular and viral proteins: activation, constimulation, and death. Cell 1994;76:959.
89. Cohen J. New protein steals the show as "costimulator" of T cells. Science 1993;262:844.
90. Beutler B, van Huffel C. Unraveling function in the TNF ligand and receptor families. Science 1994;264:667.
91. Suda T, Takahashi T, Golstein P, et al. Molecular cloning and expression of the Fas ligand, a novel member of the tumor necrosis factor family. Cell 1993;75:1169.
92. Barinaga M. Interfering with interferon. Science 1993;259: 1693.
93. Huang S, Hendriks W, Althage A, et al. Immune response in mice that lack the interferon-γ receptor. Science 1993;259:1742.
94. Darnell JE, Kerr IM, Stark GR. Jak-STAT pathways and transcriptional activation in response to IFNs and other extracellular signaling proteins. Science 1994;264:1415.
95. Wu CJ, Lovett M, Wong-Lee J, et al. Cytokine gene expression in rejecting cardiac allografts. Transplantation 1992;54:326.
96. Halloran PF, Broski AP, Batiuk TD, et al. The molecular immunology of acute rejection: an overview. Transplant Immunol 1993;1:3.
97. Bishop DK, Shelby J, Eichwald E. Mobilization of T lymphocytes following cardiac transplantation. Transplantation 1992;53:849.
98. Doherty PC. Cell-mediated cytotoxicity. Cell 1993;75:607.
99. Kagi D, Vignaux F, Ledermann B, et al. Fas and perforin pathways as major mechanisms of T cell–mediated cytotoxicity. Science 1994;265:528.
100. Mueller C, Shao Y, Altermatt HJ, et al. The effect of cyclosporine treatment on the expression of genes encoding granzyme A and perforin in the infiltrate of mouse heart transplants. Transplantation 1993;55:139.
101. Clement MV, Legros-Maida S, Isreal-Bib D, et al. Perforin and granzyme B expression is associated with severe acute rejection. Transplantation 1994;57:322.
102. Clark WR. The hole truth about perforin. Nature 1994;369: 16-17.
103. Kagi D, Ledermann B, Burki K, et al. Cytotoxicity mediated by T cells and natural killer cells is greatly impaired in perforin-deficient mice. Nature 1994;369:31.
104. Whiteside TL, Herberman RB. Role of human natural killer cells in health and disease. Clin Diagn Lab Immunol 1994;1:125.
105. Raulet DH. A sense of something missing. Nature 1992; 358:21.
106. Martinez OM, Ascher NL, Ferrell L, et al. Evidence for a nonclassical pathway of graft rejection involving interleukin 5 and eosinophils. Transplantation 1993;55:909.
107. Zhang Y, Ramos BF, Jakschik BA. Neutrophil recruitment by tumor necrosis factor from mast cells in immune complex peritonitis. Science 1992;258:1957.
108. Baggiolini M, Boulay F, Badwey JA, et al. Activation of neutrophil leukocytes: chemoattractant receptors and respiratory burst. FASEB J 1993;7:1004.
109. Morel D, Norman E, Lemoine C, et al. Tumor necrosis factor alpha in human kidney transplant rejection: analysis by in situ hybridization. Transplantation 1993;55:773.
110. Pizarro TT, Malinowska K, Kovacs E, et al. Induction of

TNFα and TNFβ gene expression in rat cardiac transplants during allograft rejection. Transplantation 1993;56:399.

111. Saito R, Prehn J, Zuo X, et al. The participation of tumor necrosis factor in the pathogenesis of lung allograft rejection in the rat. Transplantation 1993;55:967.

112. Martinez OM, Villanueva JC, Lake J, et al. IL-2 and IL-5 gene expression in response to alloantigen in liver allograft recipients and in vitro. Transplantation 1993;55:1159.

113. Merville P, Pouteil-Noble C, Wijdenes J, et al. Detection of single cells secreting IFN-gamma, IL-6, and IL-10 in irreversibly rejected human kidney allografts, and their modulation by IL-2 and IL-4. Transplantation 1993;55:639.

114. Kopf M, Baumann H, Freer G, et al. Impaired immune and acute-phase responses in interleukin-6–deficient mice. Nature 1994;368:339.

115. Blancho G, Moreau JF, Chabannes D, et al. HILDA/LIF, G-CSF, IL-1b, and TNFα production during acute rejection of human kidney allografts. Transplantation 1993;56:597.

116. Bentouimou N, Moreau JF, Peyrat MA, et al. The effects of cyclosporine on HILDA/LIF gene expression in human T cells. Transplantation 1993;55:163.

117. Blotnick S, Peoples GE, Freeman MR, et al. T lymphocytes synthesize and export heparin-binding epidermal growth factor-like growth factor and basic fibroblast growth factor, mitogens for vascular cells and fibroblasts: differential production and release by CD4$^+$ and CD8$^+$ T cells. Proc Natl Acad Sci USA 1994;91:2890.

118. Johnston PS, Wang MW, Lim SM, et al. Discordant xenograft rejection in an antibody-free model. Transplantation 1992;54:573.

119. Stansby G, Fuller B, Jeremy J, et al. Endothelin release:a facet of reperfusion injury in clinical liver transplantation? Transplantation 1993;56:239.

120. Spurney RF, Ibrahim S, Butterly D, et al. Leukotrienes in renal transplant rejection in rats. J Immunol 1994;152:867.

121. Langreher JM, Hoffman RA, Lancaster JR, et al. Nitric oxide: a new endogenous immunomodulator. Transplantation 1993;55:1205.

122. Xenos ES, Stevens RB, Sutherland DE, et al. The role of nitric oxide in IL-1b–mediated dysfunction of rodent islets of langerhans. Transplantation 1994;57:1208.

123. Connor HD, Gao W, Nukina S, et al. Evidence that free radicals are involved in graft failure following orthotopic liver transplantation in the rat: an electron paramagnetic resonance spin trapping study. Transplantation 1992;54:199.

124. Land W, Schneeberg H, Schleibner S, et al. The beneficial effect of human recombinant superoxide dismutase on acute and chronic rejection events in recipients of cadaveric renal transplants. Transplantation 1994;57:211.

125. Alexandre GP, Latinne D, Gianello P, et al. Preformed cytotoxic antibodies and ABO-incompatible grafts. Clin Transpl 1991;5:583.

126. Bach FH. Xenotransplantation: problems for consideration. Clin Transpl 1991;5:595.

127. Paul LC, Fellstrom B. Chronic vascular rejection of the heart and the kidney: have rational treatment options emerged? Transplantation 1992;53:1169.

128. Hancock WH, Whitely WD, Tullius SG, et al. Cytokines, adhesion molecules, and the pathogenesis of chronic rejection of rat renal allografts. Transplantation 1993;56:643.

129. Hajar DP, Pomerantz KB. Signal transduction in atherosclerosis: Integration of cytokines and the eicosanoid network. FASEB J 1992;6:2933.

130. Weissman IL. Developmental switches in the immune system. Cell 1994;76:207.

131. vonBoehmer H. Positive selection of lymphocytes. Cell 1994;76:219.

132. Nossal GJ. Negative selection of lymphocytes. Cell 1994; 76:229.

133. Allen PM. Peptides in positive and negative selection: a delicate balance. Cell 1994;76:593.

134. Marrack P, Parker DC. A little of what you fancy. Nature 1994;368:397.

135. Janeway CA. Thymic selection: two pathways to life and two to death. Immunity 1994;1:3.

136. vonBoehmer H, Kisielow P. Lymphocyte lineage commitment: instruction versus selection. Cell 1993;73:207.

137. Schwartz RH. Costimulation of T lymphocytes: the role of CD28, CTLA-4, and B7/BB1 in interleukin-2 production and immunotherapy. Cell 1992;71:1065.

138. Harding FA, McArthur JG, Gross JA, et al. CD28-mediated signalling co-stimulates murine T cells and prevents induction of anergy in T-cell clones. Nature 1992;356:607.

139. McCormick F. How receptors turn Ras on. Nature 1993; 363:15.

140. Marx J. Two major signal pathways linked. Science 1993;262:988.

141. Weiss A, Littman DR. Signal transduction by lymphocyte antigen receptors. Cell 1994;76:263.

142. Hall A. A biochemical function for Ras: at last. Science 1994;264:1413.

143. Jenkins MK, Miller RA. Memory and anergy: challenges to traditional models of T lymphocyte differentiation. FASEB J 1992;6:2428.

144. Sprent J. T and B memory cells. Cell 1994;76:315.

145. vonBoehmer H. Tolerance by exhaustion. Nature 1993; 362:696.

146. Ferber I, Schonrich G, Schenkel J, et al. Levels of peripheral T cell tolerance by different doses of tolerogen. Science 1994; 263:674.

147. Critchfield JM, Racke MK, Zuniga-Pflucker J, et al. T cell deletion in high antigen dose therapy of autoimmune encephalomyelitis. Science 1994;263:1139.

148. Ramsdell F, Fowlkes BJ. Maintenance of in vivo tolerance by persistence of antigen. Science 1992;257:1130.

149. Lombardi G, Sidhu S, Batchelor R, et al. Anergic T cells as suppressor cells in vitro. Science 1994;264:1587.

150. Araten DJ, Lawton T, Ferrara J, et al. In vitro alloreactivity against host antigens in an adult HLA-mismatched bone marrow transplant recipient despite in vivo host tolerance. Transplantation 1993;55:76.

151. Posselt AM, Barker CF, Friedman AL, et al. Prevention of autoimmune diabetes in the BB rat by intrathymic islet transplantation at birth. Science 1992;256:1321.

152. Campos L, Alfrey EJ, Posselt AM, et al. Prolonged survival of rat orthotopic liver allografts after intrathymic inoculation of donor-strain cells. Transplantation 1993;55:866.

153. Markmann JF, Odorico JS, Bassiri H, et al. Deletion of donor-reactive T lymphocytes in adult mice after intrathymic inoculation with lymphoid cells. Transplantation 1993;55:871.

154. Starzl TE, Demetris AJ, Trucco M, et al. Chimerism and donor-specific nonreactivity 27 to 2 years after kidney allotransplantation. Transplantation 1993;55:1272.

155. Fuchs EJ, Matzingert P. B cells turn off virgin but not memory T cells. Science 1992;258:1156.

156. Morris RE. ±15-Deoxyspergualin: a mystery wrapped within an enigma. Clin Transpl 1991; 5:530.

157. Nadler SG, Tepper MA, Schacter B, et al. Interaction of the immunosuppressant deoxyspergualin with a member of the Hsp70 family of heat shock proteins. Science 1992;258:484.

158. Chong AS, Finnegan A, Jiang X, et al. Leflunomide, a novel immunosuppressive agent. Transplantation 1993;55:1361.

159. Williams JW, Xiao F, Foster P, et al. Leflunomide in experimental transplantation. Transplantation 1994;57:1223.

160. Jameson BA, McDonnell JM, Marini JC, et al. A rationally designed CD4 analogue inhibits experimental allergic encephalomyelitis. Nature 1994;368:744.

161. Travers P. Immunological agnosia. Nature 1993;363:117.

162. Weber S, Traunecker A, Oliveri F, et al. Specific low-affinity recognition of major histocompatibility complex plus peptide by soluble T-cell receptor. Nature 1992;356:793.

163. Sloan-Lancaster J, Evavold BD, Allen PM. Induction of T-cell anergy by altered T-cell–receptor ligand on live antigen-presenting cells. Nature 1993;363:156.

164. Roslin MS, Tranbaugh RE, Panza A, et al. One-year monkey heart xenograft survival in cyclosporine-treated baboons. Transplantation 1992;54:949.

165. Hardy MA, Reed E, Suciu-Foca N. Antiidiotypic antibodies and pretreatment with blood transfusions in organ transplantation. Clin Transpl 1991; 5:501.

166. Weiner HL, Mackin GA, Matsui M, et al. Double-blind pilot trial of oral tolerization with myelin antigens in multiple sclerosis. Science 1993;259:1321.

167. Hancock WW, Sayegh MH, Kwok CA, et al. Oral, but not

intravenous, alloantigen prevents accelerated allograft rejection by selective intragraft TH2 cell activation. Transplantation 1993;55:1112.

168. Penn I. The effect of immunosuppression on pre-existing cancers. Transplantation 1993;55:742.

169. Colquhoun SD, Robert ME, Shaked A, et al. Transmission of CNS malignancy by organ transplantation. Transplantation 1994;57:970.

170. Leventhal JR, Matas AJ. Xenotransplantation in rodents: a review and reclassification. Transplantation Reviews 1994;8:80.

171. Gorski A, Grieb P, Makula J, et al. Human xenoreactive natural antibodies: avidity and targets on porcine endothelial cells. Transplantation 1993;56:1251.

172. Chari RS, Collins BH, Magee JC, et al. Treatment of hepatic failure with ex vivo pig-liver perfusion followed by liver transplantation. N Engl J Med 1994;331:234-237.

173. Dalmasso AP, Platt JL. Prevention of complement-mediated activation of xenogeneic endothelial cells in an in vitro model of xenograft hyperacute rejection by C1 inhibitor. Transplantation. 1993;56:1171.

174. Michaels MG, Simmons RL. Xenotransplant-associated zoonoses. Transplantation 1994;57:1.

175. Shaked A, Csete ME, Shiraishi M, et al. Retroviral-mediated gene transfer into rat experimental liver transplant. Transplantation 1994;57:32.

176. Fedoseyeva EV, Li Y, Huey B, et al. Inhibition of interferon-γ—mediated immune functions by oligonucleotides. Transplantation 1994;57:606.

177. Ramanathan M, Lantz M, MacGregor RD, et al. Inhibition of interferon-γ—induced major histocompatibility complex class I expression by certain oligodeoxynucleotides. Transplantation 1994;57:612.

178. Belzer FO. Evaluation of preservation of the intra-abdominal organs. Transplant Proc 1993;25:2527.

179. Belzer FO, Southard JH. Principles of solid-organ preservation by cold storage. Transplantation 1988;45:673.

180. Simonson MS, Dunn MJ. Endothelins: a family of regulator peptides. Hypertension 1991;17:856.

181. Southard JH, Senzig KA, Belzer FO. Effects of hypothermia on canine kidney mitochondria. Cryobiology 1980;17:148.

182. McCord JM. Oxygen-derived free radicals in postischemic tissue injury. N Engl J Med 1985;312:159.

183. Clavien PA, Harvey RP, Strasberg SM. Preservation and reperfusion injuries in liver allografts. Transplantation 1992;53:957.

184. Koyama I, Bulkley GB, Williams GM, et al. The role of oxygen free radicals in mediating the reperfusion injury of cold preserved ischemic kidneys. Transplantation 1985;40:590.

185. Colletti LM, Burtch GD, Remick DG, et al. The production of tumor necrosis factor alpha and the development of a pulmonary capillary injury following hepatic ischemia/reperfusion. Transplantation 1990;49:268.

186. Devlin J, Palmer RMJ, Gonde CE,et al. Nitric oxide generation. Transplantation 1994;58:592.

187. UNOS Update 1994;7:37.

188. Council on Ethical and Judicial Affairs, American Medical Association. Strategies for cadaveric organ procurement. JAMA 1994;272:809.

189. The 11th report of the human renal transplant registry. JAMA 1973;226:1197.

190. Zhou YC, Cecka JM. Effect of age on kidney transplants. In: Terasaki PI, ed. Clinical transplants 1989. Los Angeles, UCLA Tissue Typing Laboratory, 1989:369.

191. Wengerter K, Tellis VA, Soberman R, et al. Transplantation of pediatric donor kidneys to adult recipients: is there a critical donor age? Ann Surg 1986;204:172.

192. Bergmeijer JH, Cransberg K, Nijman JM, et al. Functional adaptation of en-bloc—transplanted pediatric kidneys into pediatric recipients. Transplantation 1994;58:623.

193. Belzer FO, Kountz SL. Criteria for selection of cadaver donors. Transplant Proc 1972;4:591.

194. Roth D, Fernandez JA, Babischkin S, et al. Detection of hepatitis C virus among cadaver organ donors: evidence for low transmission of disease. Ann Intern Med 1992;117:470.

195. Morse JH, Turcotte JG, Merion RM, et al. Development of a malignant tumor in a liver transplant graft procured from a donor with a cerebral neoplasm. Transplantation 1990;50:875.

196. Abouna GM, Al-Adnani MS, Kremer GD. Reversal of diabetic nephropathy in human cadaveric kidneys after transplantation into non-diabetic recipients. Lancet 1983;2:1274.

197. Kaufman HH, Hui KS, Mattson JC, et al. Clinicopathologic correlations of disseminated intravascular coagulation in patients with head injury. Neurosurgery 1984;15:34.

198. A definition of irreversible coma: report of the Ad Hoc Committee of Harvard Medical School to examine the definition of brain death. JAMA 1968;205:337.

199. Jorgensen EO. Spinal man after brain death. Acta Neurochir (Wien) 1973;28:259.

200. Emery RW, Cork RC, Levinson MM, et al. The cardiac donor: a six-year experience. Ann Thorac Surg 1986;41:356.

201. Novitzky D, Wicomb WN, Cooper DKC, et al. Electrocardiographic, hemodynamic and endocrine changes occurring during experimental brain death in the Chacma baboon. Heart Transplant 1984;4:63.

202. Novitzky D, Wicomb WN, Cooper DKC, et al. Improved cardiac function following hormonal therapy in brain dead pigs: relevance to organ donation. Cryobiology 1987;24:1.

203. Merion RM, Oh HK, Port FK, et al. A prospective randomized trial of cold-storage versus machine-perfusion preservation in cadaveric renal transplantation. Transplantation 1990;50:230.

204. Todo S, Nery J, Yanaga K, et al. Extended preservation of human liver grafts with UW solution. JAMA 1989;261:711.

205. D'Alessandro AM, Sollinger HW, Hoffmann RM, et al. Experience with Belzer UW cold storage solution in simultaneous pancreas-kidney transplantation. Transplant Proc 1990;22:532.

206. Haverich A, Scott WC, Jamieson SW. Twenty years of lung preservation: a review. Heart Transplant 1985;4:234.

207. Kokudo Y, Furuya T, Takeyochi I, et al. Comparison of University of Wisconsin, Euro-Collins, and lactated Ringer's solutions in rat small bowel preservation for orthotopic small bowel transplantation. Transplant Proc 1994;26:1492.

208. Furukawa H, Casavilla A, Abu-Elmagd K, et al. Basic considerations for the procurement of intestinal grafts. Transplant Proc 1994;26:1470.

209. Anderson CF, Velosa JA, Frohnert PP, et al. The risks of unilateral nephrectomy: status of kidney donors 10 to 20 years postoperatively. Mayo Clin Proc 1985;60:367.

210. Hakim RM, Goldazer RC, Brenner BM. Hypertension and proteinuria: long-term sequelae of uninephrectomy in humans. Kidney Int 1984; 25:930.

211. Salvatierra OJ, Vincenti F, Amend W, et al. Deliberate donor specific blood transfusions prior to living related renal transplantation. Ann Surg 1980;192:543.

212. Anderson CB, Sicard GA, Etheredge EE. Pretreatment of renal allograft recipients with azathioprine and donor-specific blood products. Surgery 1982;92:315.

213. Sommer BG, Ferguson RM. Mismatched living related donor renal transplantation: A prospective randomized study. Surgery 1985;98:267.

214. Kahan BD, Kerman RH, Wideman CA, et al. Impact of cyclosporine on renal transplant practice at the University of Texas Medical School at Houston. Am J Kidney Dis 1985;5:288.

215. Sollinger HW, Kalayoglu M, Belzer FO. Use of DST protocol in living unrelated donor-recipient combinations. Ann Surg 1986;204:315.

216. Alexandre GPJ, Squifflet JP, DeBruyere M, et al. Present experiences in a series of 26 ABO-incompatible living donor renal allografts. Transplant Proc 1987;19:4538.

217. Garrison RN, Bentley FR, Raque GH, et al. There is an answer to the shortage of organ donors. Surg Gynecol Obstet 1991;173:391.

218. Ploeg RJ. Kidney preservation with the UW and Euro-Collins solutions. Transplantation 1990;49:281.

219. Mozes MF, Finch WT, Reckard CR, et al for the Study Committee of the Illinois Transplant Society. Comparison of cold storage and machine perfusion in the preservation of cadaver kidneys: a prospective, randomized study. Transplant Proc 1985;17:1474.

220. Halloran P, Aprile M. A randomized prospective trial of cold

storage versus pulsatile perfusion for cadaver kidney preservation. Transplantation 1987;43:827.

221. Ferguson RM, Sommer BG. Cyclosporine (CsA) in renal transplantation: a single institution experience. Am J Kidney Dis 1985;5:296.

222. Ferguson RM for The Transplant Information Share Group. A multicenter experience with sequential ALG/cyclosporine therapy in renal transplantation. Clin Transpl 1988;2:285.

223. Sommer BG, Ferguson RM, Davin TD, et al. Renal transplantation in patients over 50 years of age. Transplant Proc 1981;13:33.

224. Sutherland DER, Fryd DS, Strand MH, et al. Results of the Minnesota randomized prospective trial of cyclosporine versus azathiprine-antilymphocyte globulin for immunosuppression in renal transplant recipients. Am J Kidney Dis 1985;5:318.

225. Ting A, Morris PJ. Powerful effect of HLA-DR match on survival of cadaveric renal allografts. Lancet 1980;2:282.

226. Cecka JM, Terasaki PI. The UNOS Scientific Renal Transplant Registry—1990. In: Terasaki P, ed. Clinical transplants 1990. Los Angeles, UCLA Tissue Typing Laboratory, 1991:2.

227. Cosio FG, Dillon JJ, Falkenhain ME, et al. Racial differences in renal allograft survival: the role of systemic hypertension. Kidney Int 1995;47:1136.

228. Tesi RJ, Henry ML, Elkhammas EA, Davies EA, Ferguson RM. The frequency of rejection episodes after combined kidney–pancreas transplant: the impact on graft survival. Transplantation 1994;58:424.

229. Almond PS, Matas A, Gillingham K, et al. Risk factors for chronic rejection in renal allograft recipients. Transplantation 1993; 55:752.

230. Tesi RJ, Elkhammas EA, Henry ML, et al. OKT3 for primary therapy of first rejection episode in kidney transplants. Transplantation 1993;55:1023.

231. Sherlock S. Chronic hepatitis and cirrhosis. Hepatology 1984;4:255.

232. Alagile D. Extrahepatic biliary atresia. Hepatology 1984; 4:75.

233. Hartert H. Blutgerinnungstudien mit der Thromboelastographie einem neuen Untersuchingsverfahren. Klin Wochenschr 1948;16:257.

234. Calne RY, ed. Liver transplantation. New York, Grune & Stratton, 1983.

235. Burtch GD, Merion RM. Transdiaphragmatic exposure for direct atrial-caval anastomosis in liver transplantation for Budd-Chiari syndrome. Transplantation 1989;47:161.

236. Griffith BP, Shaw BW, Hardesty RL, et al. Venovenous bypass without systemic anticoagulation for transplantation of the human liver. Surg Gynecol Obstet 1985;160:271.

237. Broelsch CE, Emond JC, Whitington PF, et al. Reduced size liver transplantation. Ann Surg 1990;212:368.

238. Williams JW, Vern S, Peters TG. Cholestatic jaundice after transplantation. Am J Surg 1986;151:65.

239. Stahl R, Duncan A, Hooks M, et al. A hypercoagulable state follows orthotopic liver transplantation. Hepatology 1990;12:553.

240. Lebeau G, Yanaga K, Marsh J, et al. Analysis of surgical complications after 397 hepatic transplantations. Surg Gynecol Obstet 1990;3:317.

241. Lerut J, Tzakis A, Boon K. Complications of venous reconstruction in human orthotopic liver transplantation. Ann Surg 1987;205:404.

242. Mazzaferro V, Esquivel C, Makowka L. Hepatic artery thrombosis after pediatric liver transplantation: a medical or surgical event? Transplantation 1989;47:971.

243. deGroen P, Aksamit A, Rakela J. Central nervous system toxicity after liver transplantation. N Engl J Med 1986;317:861.

244. Gordon R, Iwatsuki S, Esquivel C. Liver transplantation across ABO blood groups. Surgery 1986;100:342.

245. Haub D, Shover D, Norsen HJ, et al. Hyperacute rejection of a human orthotopic liver allograft in a presensitized recipient. Clin Transplant 1987;1:304.

246. Gordon R, Rung J, Markus B, et al. The antibody crossmatch in liver transplantation. Surgery 1986;100:705.

247. Ludwig J, Wiesner R, Balts KP. The acute vanishing bile duct syndrome (acute irreversible rejection) after orthotopic liver transplantation. Hepatology 1987;7:476.

248. Balts K, Moore B, Perkins J. Influence of positive lymphocyte crossmatch and HLA matching in vanishing bile duct syndrome in human liver allografts. Transplantation 1988; 45:376.

249. O'Grady J, Sutherland S, Harvey F. Cytomegalovirus infection and donor/recipient HLA antigens: interdependent cofactors in pathogenesis of vanishing bile duct syndrome after liver transplantation. Lancet 1988;2:302.

250. Starzl TE, Iwatsuki S, Van Thiel DH, et al. Evolution of liver transplantation. Hepatology 1982;2:614.

251. Shaw B, Wood P, Gordon R. Influence of selected patient variables and operative blood loss on six-month survival following liver transplantation. Semin Liver Dis 1985;5:385.

252. Starzl T, Demetrius A. Liver transplantation: a 31-year perspective. Curr Probl Surg 1990;27:4.

253. Annual Report on the US Scientific Registry for Organ Transplantation and the Organ Procurement and Transplantation Network, 1988 and 1989.

254. Carrel A, Guthrie CC. The transplantation of veins and organs. Am J Med 1985;10:1101.

255. Demikhov VP. Experimental transplantation of vital organs. New York, New York Consultants Bureau, 1962.

256. Goldberg M, Berman EF, Akman CC. Homologous transplantation of the canine heart. J Int Coll Surgeons 1958; 30:575.

257. Lower RR, Shumway NE. Studies in orthotopic homotransplantation of the canine heart. Surg Forum 1960;11:18.

258. Lower RR, Dong E Jr, Shumway NE. Long-term survival of cardiac homografts. Surgery 1965;58:110.

259. Baumgartner WA, Reitz BA, Oyer PE, et al. Cardiac homotransplantation. Curr Probl Surg 1979;16:1.

260. Griepp RB, Stinson EB, Dong E Jr, et al. The use of antithymocyte globulin in human heart transplantation. Circulation 1972;45/46(Suppl 1):147.

261. Bieber CP, Griepp RB, Oyer PE, et al. Use of rabbit antithymocyte globulin in cardiac transplantation. Transplantation 1976;22:478.

262. Caves PK, Billingham ME, Stinson EB, et al. Serial transvenous biopsy of the transplanted human heart: improved management of acute rejection episodes. Lancet 1974;2:821.

263. Billingham ME. Diagnosis of cardiac rejection by endomyocardial biopsy. J Heart Transplant 1982;1:25.

264. Copeland JG, Griepp RB, Bieber CP, et al. Successful retransplantation of the human heart. J Thorac Cardiovasc Surg 1977;73:242.

265. Heck CF, Shumway SJ, Kaye MP. The Registry of the International Society for Heart Transplantation: sixth official report, 1989. J Heart Transplant 1989;8:271.

266. Bolman RM, Elick B, Olivari MT, et al. Improved immunosuppression for heart transplantation. J Heart Transplant 1985;4:315.

267. Billingham ME, Cary NRB, Hammond ME, et al. A working formulation for the standardization of nomenclature in the diagnosis of heart and lung rejection: heart rejection study group. J Heart Transplant 1990;9:587.

268. Bailey LL, Nehlsen-Cannarella SL, Concepcion W, Jolley WE. Cardiac xenotransplantation in a neonate. JAMA 1985;254:3321.

269. Menkis AH, McKenzie FN, Novick RJ, et al. Special considerations for heart transplantation in congenital heart disease. J Heart Transplant 1990;9:602.

270. Bailey LL, Gundry SR, Razzouk, et al. Bless the babies: one hundred fifteen late survivors of heart transplantation during the first year of life. J Thorac Cardiovasc Surg 1993;105:805.

271. Kawauchi M, Gundry SR, de Begona JA, et al. Prolonged preservation of human pediatric hearts for transplantation: correlation of ischemic time and subsequent function. J Heart Lung Transplant 1993;12:55.

272. McDonald K, Rector TS, Braunlin EA, et al. Association of coronary artery disease in cardiac transplant recipients with cytomegalovirus infection. Am J Cardiol 1989;64:359.

273. Gao SZ, Schroeder JS, Alderman EL, et al. Prevalence of accelerated coronary artery disease in heart transplant survivors. Circulation 1989;80(Suppl 3):3.

274. Kaye MP. The registry of the International Society for Heart

and Lung Transplantation: tenth official report—1993. J Heart Lung Transplant 1993;12:541.

275. Hosenpud JD, Novick RJ, Breen TJ, et al. The registry of the International Society for Heart and Lung Transplantation: eleventh official report—1994. J Heart Lung Transplant 1994;13:561.

276. Slaughter MS, Braunlin EA, Bolman RM III, et al. Pediatric cardiac transplantation: results of 2- and 5-year follow-up. J Heart Lung Transplant 1994;13:624.

277. Lund G, Morin RL, Olivari MT, et al. Serial myocardial T_2 relaxation time measurements in normal subjects and heart transplant recipients. J Heart Transplant 1988;7:274.

278. Irwin ED, Bianco RW, Clack R, et al. Use of epicardial electrocardiograms for detecting cardiac allograft rejection. Ann Thorac Surg 1992;54:669.

279. Armitage JM, Fricker FJ, del Nido P, et al. A decade (1982 to 1992) of pediatric cardiac transplantation and the impact of FK 506 immunosuppression. J Thorac Cardiovasc Surg 1993;105:464.

280. Taylor DO, Ensley RD, Olsen SL, et al. Mycophenolate mofetil (RS-61443): preclinical, clinical, and three-year experience in heart transplantation. J Heart Lung Transplant 1994;13:571.

281. Pierson RN, Reemtsma K, Rose EA. Cardiac xenografting. In: Baumgartner WA, Reitz BA, Achuff SA, eds. Heart and heart–lung transplantation. Philadelphia, WB Saunders, 1990:303.

282. Adachi H, Rosengard BR, Hutchins GM, et al. Effects of cyclosporine, aspirin, and cobra venom factor on discordant cardiac xenograft survival in rats. Transplant Proc 1987;19:1145.

283. Kurlansky PA, Sadeghi AM, Michler RE, et al. Comparable survival of intra-species and cross-species primate cardiac transplants. Curr Surg 1986;43:413.

284. Portner PM, Oyer PE, Pennington DG, et al. Implantable electrical left ventricular assist system: bridge to transplantation and the future. Ann Thorac Surg 1989;47:142.

285. Frazier OH, Rose EA, McManus Q, et al. Multicenter clinical evaluation of the Heartmate 1000 IP left ventricular assist device. Ann Thorac Surg 1992;53:1080.

286. Lough ME, Lindsey AM, Shinn JA, et al. Life satisfaction following heart transplantation. J Heart Transplant 1985;4:446.

287. Shumway NE. Palo Alto Times, January 22, 1968.

288. Egan TM, Kaiser LR, Cooper JD. Lung transplantation. Curr Probl Surg 1989;10:681.

289. Wildevuur CR, Benfield JR. A review of 23 human lung transplants done by 20 surgeons. Ann Thorac Surg 1970;9:489.

290. Lima O, Golberg M, Peters WS, et al. Effects of methylprednisolone and azathioprine on bronchial healing following lung transplantation. J Thorac Cardiovasc Surg 1981;83:211.

291. Kaiser LR, Cooper JD, Trulock EP, et al. The evolution of single lung transplantation for emphysema. J Thorac Cardiovasc Surg 1991;102:333.

292. Pasque MK, Cooper JD, Kaiser LR, et al. Improved technique for bilateral lung transplantation: rationale and initial clinical experience. Ann Thorac Surg 1990;49:785.

293. Davis RD, Pasque MK. Pulmonary transplantation. Ann Surg 1995;221:14.

294. Keay S, Peterson E, Icenogle T, et al. Ganciclovir treatment of serious cytomegalovirus infection in heart and heart-lung transplant recipients. Rev Infect Dis 1988;10:5563.

295. Michelsen B, Grove A, Vissing H, et al. Modern concepts of diabetes and its pathogenesis. In: Dubernard JM, Sutherland DER, eds. International handbook of pancreas transplantation. Boston, Kluwer Academic Publishers, 1989:13.

296. Kaufman DL, Erlander MG, Clare-Salzler M, et al. Autoimmunity to two forms of glutamate decarboxylase in insulin-dependent diabetes mellitus. J Clin Invest 1992;89:283.

297. Davidson MB. Preface. In: Diabetes mellitus: diagnosis and treatment. New York, John Wiley & Sons, 1981:v.

298. National Diabetes Data Group. Diabetes in America: diabetes data compiled 1984. Washington, DC, US Department of Health and Human Services, 1984. US Dept of Health, Education, and Welfare publicaiton 85-1468.

299. Serjeantson SW, Court J, Mackay IR, et al. HLA-DQ genotypes are associated with autoimmunity to glutamic acid decarboxylase in insulin-dependent diabetes mellitus patients. Hum Immunol 1993;38:97.

301. Nerup J, Mandrup-Poulsen T, Molvig J. The HLA-IDDM association: implications for etiology and pathogenesis of IDDM. Diabetes Metab Rev 1987;3:779.

302. Greene DA, Lattimer S, Ulbrecht J, et al. Glucose-induced alterations in nerve metabolism: current perspective on the pathogenesis of diabetic neuropathy and future directions for research and therapy. Diabetes Care 1985;8:290.

303. Bliss M. A long prelude. In: The discovery of insulin. Chicago, University of Chicago Press, 1982:20.

304. Orchard TJ. From diagnosis and classification to complications and therapy: Diabetes Control and Complications Trial. Diabetes Care 1994;17:326.

305. Najarian JS. Landmarks in clinical pancreas transplantation. In: Groth CC, ed. Pancreatic transplantation. Philadelphia, WB Saunders, 1988:15.

306. Brooks JR, Gifford GH. Pancreatic homotransplantation. Transplant Bull 1959;6:100.

307. Dubernard JU, Traeger J, Neyra P, et al. A new method of preparation of segmental pancreatic grafts for transplantation: trials in dogs and in man. Surgery 1978;84:633.

308. Sollinger HW, Kalayoglu M, Hoffman RM, Belzer FO. Results of segmental and pancreatico-splenic transplantation with pancreatico-cystostomy. Transplant Proc 1985;17:360.

309. Nghiem DD, Beutel WD, Corry RJ. Duodenocystostomy for exocrine pancreatic drainage in experimental and clinical pancreaticoduodenal transplantation. Transplant Proc 1986; 18:1762.

310. The University of Michigan Pancreas Transplant Evaluation Committee. Pancreatic transplantation for IDDM: proposed candidate criteria before end-stage diabetic nephropathy. Diabetes Care 1988;11:669.

311. Rosenberg L, Dafoe DC, Schwartz R, et al. Administration of somatostatin analog (SMS 201-995) in the treatment of a fistula occurring after pancreas transplantation: interference with cyclosporine immunosuppression. Transplantation 1987;43:764.

312. Metrakos P, Rosenberg L, Duguid WP, et al. Prophylactic sandostatin potentiates acute pancreatitis. Surg Forum 1990;41:160.

313. Perkal M, Marks C, Lorber MI, et al. A three-year experience with serum anodal trypsinogen as a biochemical marker for rejection in pancr eatic allografts: false positives, tissue biopsy, comparison with other markers, and diagnostic strategies. Transplantation 1992;53:415.

314. Sutherland DER, Dunn DL, Goetz FC, et al. A 10-year experience with 290 pancreas transplants at a single institution. Ann Surg 1989;210:274.

315. Metrakos P, Yuan S, Agapitos D, Rosenberg L. Intercellular communication and maintenance of islet cell mass: implications for islet transplantation. Surgery 1993;114:423.

316. Rosenberg L. In vivo cell transformation: neogenesis of beta cells from pancreatic ductal cells. Cell Transplant 1995; 4:371.

317. Gores P, Sutherland DER. Pancreatic islet transplantation: is purification necessary. Am J Surg 1993;166:538.

318. Gores PF, Najarian JS, Stephanian E, et al. Insulin independence in type I diabetes after transplantation of unpurified islets from single donor with 15-deoxyspergualin. Lancet 1993;341:19.

TWO

SURGICAL PRACTICE

SURGERY: SCIENTIFIC PRINCIPLES AND PRACTICE, Second Edition, edited by
Lazar J. Greenfield, Michael W. Mulholland, Keith T. Oldham, Gerald B. Zelenock,
and Keith D. Lillemoe. Lippincott–Raven Publishers, Philadelphia, © 1997.

CHAPTER 17

HEAD AND NECK

JAMES P. NEIFELD

Although the head and neck make up a small part of the total body area in adults, many organ systems are present in this area, and both benign and malignant diseases occur in all these organ systems. This chapter focuses on extracranial diseases of the head and neck and their effects on normal physiology.

Thorough knowledge of the anatomy of the head and neck area is an essential prerequisite to treatment of diseases in this area. The oropharynx and hypopharynx provide a common pathway for both the digestive and respiratory systems. The nasal cavity and paranasal sinuses represent a continuum to the oropharynx; inspired air is warmed and filtered in these areas. Air enters the glottis and then proceeds down into the lungs. During swallowing, the respiratory system is separated from the digestive system by elevation of the larynx and closure of the glottis, preventing aspiration. Thus, anything that inhibits movement of the larynx also causes the glottis to be unable to close during deglutition. These inhibitors include benign and malignant disease processes, as well as iatrogenic factors, such as the performance of a tracheostomy.

DIAGNOSTIC APPROACH

The initial evaluation of patients with head and neck complaints starts with a proper history and physical examination. Important factors in the history include site and duration of symptoms and exacerbating or ameliorating factors. The patient's complaints can indicate the site of the abnormality. A patient complaining of difficulty eating may have a tumor of the oral cavity; hoarseness suggests a laryngeal abnormality; and dysphagia may suggest pharyngeal or cervical esophageal cancer. A patient can present with a neck mass and no complaints relating to the mucosal surfaces; the site of the mass may suggest the area to investigate for a possible primary tumor. Other important aspects of the history include cigarette smoking and alcohol ingestion; these factors are rarely absent in head and neck cancer.

Physical examination includes inspection, palpation, and indirect laryngoscopy. Careful intraoral examination requires the use of a headlight, removal of any dentures or other prostheses, and careful palpation of all surfaces that can be reached by the examining finger. Many lesions of the head and neck are submucosal, and even mucosal tumors can have a large amount of submucosal spread. Palpation of the neck is important for delineation of the size, consistency, and extent of any masses. Indirect laryngoscopy is essential to view the vocal cords, supraglottic larynx, and piriform sinus areas. The use of a flexible laryngoscope may be necessary in patients who are uncooperative or in whom adequate visualization cannot be obtained with use of a mirror and headlight.

Patients presenting with head and neck complaints must also have an adequate general physical examination. Cancers of the lung, breast, or digestive tract, and genital or urinary tract tumors can present as neck masses. Careful physical examination may detect blood in the stool, a breast mass, a rectal mass, or a testicular mass, which would greatly affect the subsequent diagnostic workup.

If the results of the physical examination are normal (with the exception of the head and neck area), a biopsy of the primary site must be performed to determine the histologic character of the lesion. In patients who have cancer, a panendoscopy should be performed because of the high incidence of associated second head and neck primary cancers, esophageal cancers, or lung cancers. If the patient has a neck mass and no primary site of tumor is evident, biopsy of the neck mass should be performed. At institutions with experienced cytologists, fine-needle aspiration biopsy is preferable to open biopsy to avoid potential contamination of the planes for a subsequent definitive operation. If adequate cytology is not available, incisional biopsy for large masses or excisional biopsy for small masses may be necessary after endoscopy has ruled out an upper aerodigestive tract tumor. If the patient has a neck mass and an obvious cancer in the oral cavity, pharynx, or larynx, the mass in the neck should be assumed to be a metastasis, and biopsy should not be performed.

BENIGN LESIONS

Tumors

The most common benign tumor of the head and neck is benign lymphadenopathy. The causes for this are almost innumerable. In children, lymphadenopathy is often the result of viral infections or tonsillitis. In adults, carious teeth are a common cause of enlarged lymph nodes in the upper neck. Mononucleosis, other viral diseases, sinusitis, tonsillitis, periodontal disease, and skin disease are other common causes of lymphadenopathy. The underlying cause is usually evident, but when it is not, biopsy can sometimes be performed. The treatment for benign lymphadenopathy is directed toward the underlying disease. When the primary disease is controlled, or any infection is eradicated, lymphadenopathy often regresses but frequently does not totally disappear.

Infections

Infections in the head and neck can be simple or complex. Sinusitis is a common infection that is usually self-limited with infrequent complications. Sinusitis can develop secondary to allergies, viruses, or bacteria. Fungal infections are less frequent and more often seen in diabetics or immunosuppressed patients. Most cases of sinusitis can be treated well with antibiotics (Fig. 17-1), but if they do not respond, other complications can result and surgery may be necessary. Complications of maxillary sinusitis are rare because most of these infections respond to antibiotics. Ethmoid sinusitis can develop secondary to maxillary sinusitis and may be complicated by orbital cellulitis. When this occurs, it is usually well treated by antibiotics. Frontal sinusitis may be more severe and may cause meningitis or epidural abscess. When frontal sinusitis does not respond to systemic antibiotics, the sinus must be opened and irrigated. Removal of the infected mucosa may be necessary to control infection. Chronic maxillary sinusitis that cannot be controlled by antibiotics may require a Caldwell-Luc operation, which involves an incision between the upper lip and upper gum to make an entrance into the maxillary sinus (Fig. 17-2). Curettage of the maxillary sinus and formation of a nasoantral window facilitate drainage and should control any remaining infection. Chronic ethmoid sinusitis may require ethmoidectomy to remove nasal polyps and other epithelial debris.

Peritonsillar abscesses are complications of acute tonsillitis. Infection is deep to the tonsillar capsule, and pus forms between the tonsillar capsule and the superior constrictor muscle. Massive edema of the entire soft palate can develop, as well as edema of the lateral pharyngeal wall. When this occurs, inflammation of the pterygoid

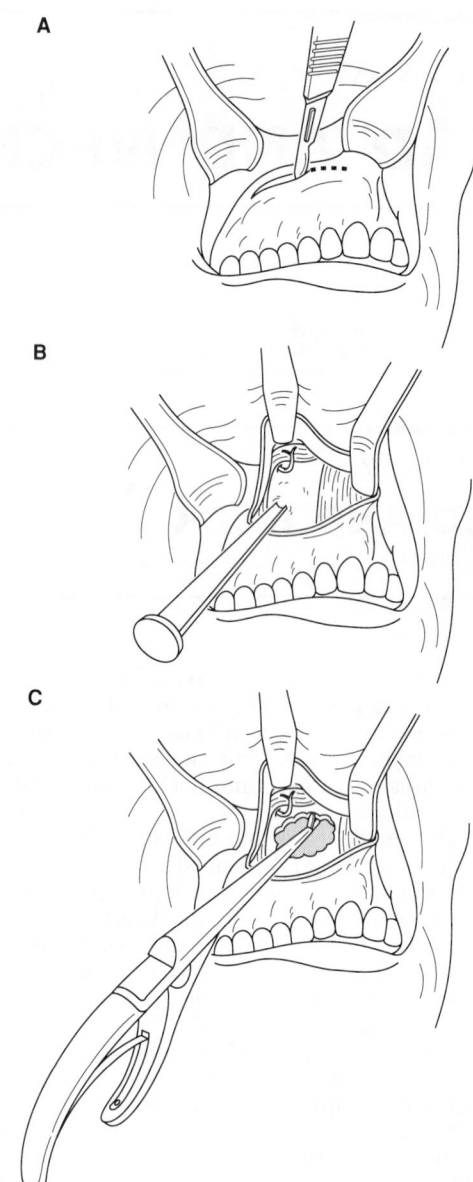

Figure 17-2. Caldwell-Luc procedure. (*A*) Incision between upper lip and gum. (*B*) Entrance made into maxillary sinus. (*C*) Curettage and débridement performed through hole made in anterior wall of the maxilla.

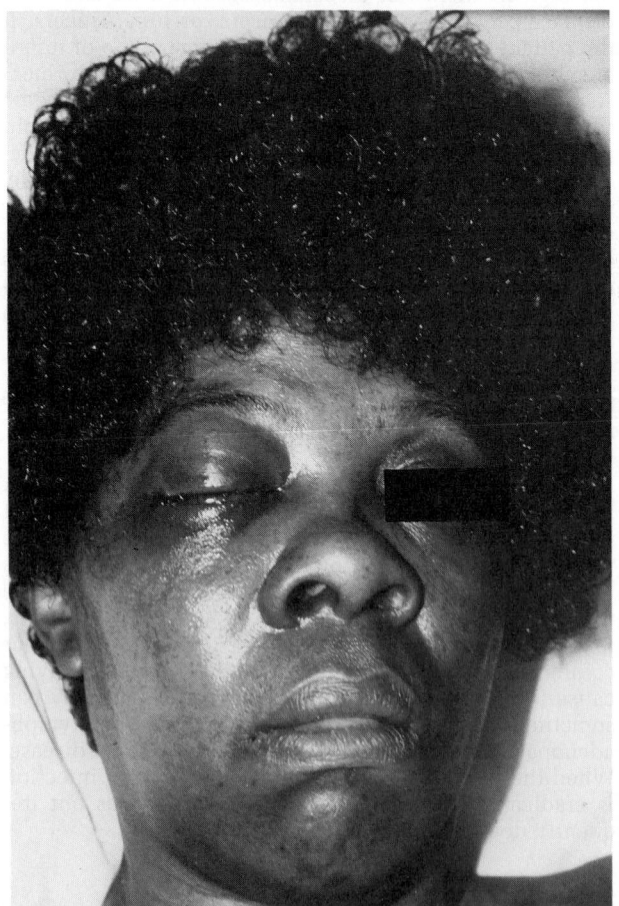

Figure 17-1. Maxillary sinusitis with periorbital cellulitis and proptosis secondary to dental caries. Intravenous antibiotics cured this infection.

muscles can result in trismus. In late cases there may be so much edema and the abscess may be so large that the airway is compromised. Tracheostomy may be necessary before it is safe to drain the abscess. In cases of cellulitis, high doses of penicillin usually result in a rapid response. If pus is present, however, incision and drainage may be necessary. This is done through a transoral approach, with an incision along the anterior tonsillar pillar. The abscess cavity subsequently drains when the patient swallows. Because these abscesses recur frequently, they are an indication for tonsillectomy.

Parapharyngeal infections and abscesses are unusual in adults. Parapharyngeal abscesses can be secondary to tonsillitis or pharyngitis, and they often present as marked swelling in the anterior cervical triangle between the carotid sheath and superior constrictor muscles. Penicillin is the antibiotic of choice, since most of these infections are streptococcal in origin. Because of the proximity of the carotid artery, these infections should be drained extra-orally through an incision anterior to the border of the sternocleidomastoid muscle. Retropharyngeal infections are unusual in adults and can be caused by tumor perforation or perforation by a foreign body. They are best drained by means of an incision through the posterior wall of the pharynx; concomitant administration of antibiotics is a necessity.

Salivary gland infections are unusual and most often are seen in patients with poor dental care. Acute inflammation may be seen when the salivary duct is obstructed, as with a stone. Infection in this circumstance is usually self-limited and controlled with antibiotics and removal of the stone. When patients do not respond to antibiotics, excision of the necrotic gland may be necessary. When patients require resection of the parotid gland, infection and marked inflammation can make preservation of the facial nerve difficult. The submandibular gland is intimately associated with the ramus mandibularis branch of the facial nerve as well as with the lingual nerve; operating on this gland when it is acutely infected can result in damage to either or both of these nerves. Thus, antibiotics should be used as the initial treatment of infections in the salivary glands.

Hemorrhage

Upper airway hemorrhage can be due to benign or malignant processes. Most upper airway hemorrhage is caused by bleeding from the nose. Epistaxis can be caused by tumor, infection, or trauma. The most common site is the plexus of vessels in the inferior portion of the nasal septum, which is superficial and easily traumatized. Bleeding from the anterior portion of the nose can usually be controlled by simple pressure. If this is not sufficient, a topical vasoconstrictor can be applied, or the bleeding point can be cauterized. Bleeding from the posterior portion of the nose is much more difficult to control. The posterior portion of the nasal cavity may require obstruction with a Foley catheter balloon or a posterior nasal pack. Patients who receive this type of therapy should also receive prophylactic antibiotics to prevent the development of sinusitis. Bleeding from this area may require control by ligation of the internal maxillary artery as it passes behind the maxillary sinus. Through a Caldwell-Luc approach, both the anterior and posterior walls of the maxillary sinus are removed, and the maxillary artery is dissected free from tissue in the pterygomaxillary fossa and clipped. This method has the advantage of obviating a posterior nasal pack and should also prevent recurrent bleeding.

Other sites of massive upper airway hemorrhage are unusual. Malignancies usually are the cause of these bleeds because of involvement of a branch of the carotid artery, erosion of tumor into the carotid artery, or bleeding from an ulcerated tumor bed. Treatment depends on whether the tumor can be resected and what structures are involved. Bleeding from the carotid artery requires ligation of the artery; bleeding from an ulcerated tumor can be temporarily controlled by packing.

Upper Airway Obstruction

Upper airway obstruction can be secondary to benign or malignant processes. Although epiglottitis is frequently thought to be a disease of infants and children, it can also be found in adults and can be life threatening. Epiglottitis is usually the result of a bacterial infection, the treatment of which consists of antibiotics and humidification of the air. If respiratory distress continues, intubation should be performed, always in the operating room with a tracheostomy tray available for use if necessary. Patients usually require intubation for a short time. Acute epiglottitis does not tend to be a recurring problem.

Upper airway obstruction can also be due to trauma. Trauma to the larynx can require emergency cricothyroidotomy in the field or tracheostomy immediately on arrival in the emergency department. Generally, oral intubation should not be attempted in these patients, because it can precipitate total airway obstruction.

Patients who present with tumors causing upper airway obstruction also should be evaluated in the operating room. Indirect laryngoscopy or fiberoptic laryngoscopy can precipitate obstruction of the airway and emergency tracheostomy. Thus, the patient should be brought to the operating room, local anesthesia should be used, and a laryngoscope should be gently introduced. If the airway is extremely narrow, a tracheostomy should be performed. Some patients can be temporized by laser treatment of the tumor to open the airway before definitive treatment of the cancer.

MALIGNANT LESIONS

Cancers arising in the head and neck are fairly common, with more than 40,000 new squamous cell carcinomas diagnosed in the United States each year. Mucosal cancers are unusual in patients under 40 years of age and are much more common in men than in women. A common predisposing factor in the development of these cancers is tobacco.[1] The combination of cigarette smoking and alcohol ingestion is synergistic and also appears to be dose dependent in terms of both cigarette smoking and alcohol ingestion. With the increasing use of chewing tobacco in the United States, there has been an increasing frequency of buccal mucosal cancers at the site where the chewing tobacco rests intraorally. These cancers also are becoming more common in younger patients. Young people who chew tobacco develop premalignant changes in the oral mucosa at an early age; this suggests that cancer will ultimately develop if these people continue to use chewing tobacco. Lip cancer has also been associated with pipe smoking; the typical pipe smoker keeps the pipe in one place on the lips, and cancer can develop in response to the heat of the pipe on the lower lip. Thus, head and neck cancers appear to arise as a response to tobacco in general, not just cigarette smoking.

Molecular Biology

Recent studies have investigated the molecular biology and genetics of head and neck cancer.[2] Amplification of the epidermal growth factor receptor gene has been demonstrated in both cell culture and fresh tissues; it is expressed in higher levels in tumor than in normal mucosa and in increasing levels in poorly differentiated tumors as compared with well-differentiated tumors. The tumor suppressor gene p53 has been extensively studied in head and neck cancer. Abnormal p53 function has been detected in 33% to 100% of specimens; it does not appear to correlate with tumor size. The correlation of p53 mutations with prognosis has yielded conflicting results. Even fewer data have been reported from investigations of the c-*erbB*-2 oncoprotein, the c-*myc* gene family of nuclear proteins, the *ras* oncogene, and other less-studied gene products. Future investigations may describe the correlations of these (or other) oncogenes or gene products with carcinogenesis and prognosis. Ultimately, the development of strategies to overcome gene mutations may help prevent the development of head and neck cancer.

Staging

Before treating patients with head and neck cancer, clinical staging is mandatory. After the complete history, physical examination, indirect laryngoscopy, and panendoscopy, the patient can be staged according to the TNM system (Tables 17-1 and 17-2). Panendoscopy is mandatory before staging, because second primary cancers develop in about 15% of patients. Of these, about one third are second head and neck cancers, one third are primary lung cancers, and one third are primary esophageal cancers. This should not be unexpected, since the same factors that cause head and neck cancer also cause lung and esophageal cancer. Lung and esophageal cancers occur concomitantly with head and neck cancer in 5% of patients; the other 10% develop these cancers later.

The TNM system for head and neck cancer is similar to that for other sites: *T* relates to the size of the primary tumor, *N* to the size and extent of lymph node metastases, and *M* to distant disease. The staging for head and neck cancer is somewhat different from that for other cancers in several aspects. First, it varies according to the primary site. For example, cancers of the oral cavity are staged according to size, whereas cancers of the larynx are staged according to involvement of one or both vocal cords, fixation of cords, and deep extension. Cancers of the paranasal sinuses are staged according to whether they are localized to the sinus and how deeply they invade. Cancers of the hypopharynx and nasopharynx are staged according to the number of subsites involved. Unlike the typical staging of other cancers, labeling cancers of the head and neck as stage IV may not necessarily denote distant disease, and the regional lymph nodes may not even contain metastatic tumor. A T4 cancer is a stage IV cancer. Thus, a cancer that is T4, N0, M0 is classified as a stage IV cancer even though it is purely a local tumor; this is because the prognosis is poor for patients with such advanced local tumors. A stage IV head and neck cancer can be an advanced tumor confined to the primary site, a tumor with large regional lymph nodes, or a tumor that has spread to distant metastatic sites. A summary of survival rates correlated with primary site and stage is shown in Table 17-3.

Preoperative evaluation of patients with head and neck cancer, in addition to history, physical examination, and panendoscopy, should include routine laboratory work and a chest radiograph. If the patient has any dysphagia, a barium swallow may also be indicated. Routine use of computed tomographic (CT) scans, magnetic resonance imaging (MRI), or other imaging techniques is not indicated. MRI and CT are indicated for tumors that encroach on the base of the skull or that are difficult to assess clinically. Laryngeal tumors that appear small and confined on clinical examination may have cartilage invasion demonstrated on CT scan performed as preradiotherapy planning; this can change the planned treatment. If a neck mass seems to involve the carotid artery, angiography to study intracerebral cross-circulation is indicated if carotid artery resection is contemplated. Thus, the workup should be individualized according to the site and size of the tumor.

Mucosal Cancers

Oral Cavity

The oral cavity can be divided into several primary sites: the oral tongue, which includes the anterior two thirds of the tongue; floor of the mouth; alveolar ridge; hard palate; and buccal mucosa. Cancers arising in these areas tend to produce symptoms that include difficulty eating, oral bleeding, and soreness. Because of the insidious onset of symptoms, patients with cancers of the oral cavity may lose a great deal of weight before they seek medical attention. They may find it is easy to change their diets from regular food to soft food and then to liquids, thus preventing pain that occurs with chewing. Caloric intake may greatly diminish before presentation to a physician. Cancers in these areas tend to spread first to lymph nodes in the submental and submandibular areas and then to the mid-jugular chain.

Cancers of the anterior two thirds of the tongue usually produce a chronic, nonhealing ulcer. During the course of the disease, more than two thirds of patients with tongue cancer develop cervical lymph node metastases. Small cancers of the tongue have an excellent prognosis. Over 80% of patients survive 5 years free of disease if the cancer is found when it is less than 2 cm (T1). Once cervical lymph nodes are involved, however, the prognosis is markedly worsened, with only 30% to 40% of patients alive and free of disease after 5 years.

The floor of the mouth is the area between the tongue and the inner surface of the mandible. Cancers commonly develop in the anterior floor of the mouth and can involve either or both Wharton ducts, resulting in marked submandibular gland enlargement and pain. Despite the large size of these glands, they may represent only benign swelling rather than metastatic spread of cancer of the floor of the mouth. Treatment depends on the size of the tumor. Small tumors are well treated with either surgery or radiotherapy, but larger tumors should be treated surgically along with the regional lymph nodes, usually by radical neck dissection. Survival rates are similar to those for tongue cancer.

The gingiva and hard palate are uncommon sites for the development of squamous cancers. Cancers in the minor salivary glands are more frequent than squamous cancers arising on the hard palate, but both tumors are treated in a similar fashion. Surgery is the preferred treatment because cancers that involve bone respond less favorably to radiotherapy than do cancers that have no bony involvement. Spread to the lymph nodes from these primary sites is unusual.

Buccal mucosal cancers are relatively uncommon in the United States. They are much more common in areas where chewing tobacco and betel nuts are common, such as India. These cancers tend to be slower-growing and better differentiated, and they have a lower rate of lymph node metastasis than other oral cancers. An uncommon variant of squamous cell carcinoma, verrucous cancer, is a well-differentiated malignancy characterized by benign-appearing histology and exophytic, frondlike growth. These cancers rarely spread to lymph nodes and commonly arise from the buccal mucosa. Verrucous tumors are less responsive to radiotherapy than more invasive, less differentiated squamous cell carcinomas. Cancers in this area often require full-thickness resection of the cheek. Flap closure may be necessary.

The treatment of oral cavity cancers includes wide resection, and if the tumor is large (T2 or greater) or is associated with clinically positive nodes, a radical neck dissection should be performed simultaneously.[3] Lymph node metastases are uncommon for small tumors but can occur in up to 60% of patients with clinically normal neck examinations when the primary tumor is staged T2 or greater. Survival rates for cancers of the hard palate are slightly lower than those for other cancers of the oral cavity because of the difficulty in obtaining adequate margins.

Pharynx

The pharynx can be divided into three areas: the nasopharynx, the area above the soft palate; the oropharynx, the area between the upper portion of the epiglottis and

Table 17-1. TNM CLASSIFICATION FOR STAGING OF CANCER OF THE HEAD AND NECK

PRIMARY TUMOR

Oral Cavity

TX	Primary tumor cannot be assessed
T0	No evidence of primary tumor
Tis	Carcinoma in situ
T1	Tumor 2 cm or less in greatest dimension
T2	Tumor more than 2 cm but not more than 4 cm in greatest dimension
T3	Tumor more than 4 cm in greatest dimension
T4	Tumor invades adjacent structures

Oropharynx

T1	Tumor 2 cm or less in greatest dimension
T2	Tumor more than 2 cm but not more than 4 cm in greatest dimension
T3	Tumor more than 4 cm in greatest dimension
T4	Tumor invades adjacent structures (eg, cortical bone, soft tissues of neck, deep [extrinsic] muscle of tongue)

Hypopharynx

T1	Tumor limited to one subsite of hypopharynx
T2	Tumor invades more than one subsite of hypopharynx or adjacent site, without fixation of hemilarynx
T3	Tumor invades more than one subsite of hypopharynx or adjacent site, with fixation of hemilarynx
T4	Tumor invades adjacent structures (eg, cartilage, soft tissues of neck)

Nasopharynx

T1	Tumor limited to one subsite of nasopharynx
T2	Tumor invades more than one subsite of nasopharynx
T3	Tumor invades nasal cavity or oropharynx
T4	Tumor invades skull or cranial nerve

Maxillary Sinus

T1	Tumor limited to antral mucosa, with no erosion or destruction of bone
T2	Tumor with erosion or destruction of infrastructure, including hard palate or middle nasal meatus
T3	Tumor invades any of following: skin of cheek, posterior wall of maxillary sinus, floor or medial wall of orbit, anterior ethmoid sinus
T4	Tumor invades orbital contents or any of the following: cribriform plate, posterior ethmoid or sphenoid sinuses, nasopharynx, soft palate, pterygomaxillary or temporal fossae, base of skull

Supraglottis

T1	Tumor limited to one subsite of supraglottis, with normal vocal cord mobility
T2	Tumor invades more than one subsite of supraglottis or glottis, with normal vocal cord mobility
T3	Tumor limited to laynrx, with vocal cord fixation, or invades postcricoid area, medial wall of piriform sinus, or preepiglottic tissues
T4	Tumor invades thyroid cartilage or extends to other tissues beyond larynx (eg, oropharynx, soft tissue of neck)

Glottis

T1	Tumor limited to vocal cord (may involve anterior or posterior commissures), with normal mobility
T1a	Tumor limited to one vocal cord
T1b	Tumor involves both vocal cords
T2	Tumor extends to supraglottis or subglottis or with impaired vocal cord mobility
T3	Tumor limited to larynx with vocal cord fixation
T4	Tumor invades thyroid cartilage or extends to other tissues beyond larynx (eg, oropharynx, soft tissues of neck)

Subglottis

T1	Tumor limited to subglottis
T2	Tumor extends to vocal cord, with normal or impaired mobility
T3	Tumor limited to larynx, with vocal cord fixation
T4	Tumor invades through cricoid or thyroid cartilage, or extends to other tissues beyond larynx (eg, oropharynx, soft tissues of neck)

REGIONAL LYMPH NODE INVOLVEMENT

NX	Regional lymph nodes cannot be assessed
N0	No regional lymph node metastasis
N1	Metastasis in single ipsilateral lymph node, 3 cm or less in greatest dimension
N2	Metastasis in single ipsilateral lymph node, more than 3 cm but not more than 6 cm in greatest dimension; or in multiple ipsilateral lymph nodes, none more than 6 cm in greatest dimension; or in bilateral or contralateral lymph nodes, none more than 6 cm in greatest dimension
N2a	Metastasis in single ipsilateral lymph node, more than 3 cm but not more than 6 cm in greatest dimension
N2b	Metastasis in multiple ipsilateral lymph nodes, none more than 6 cm in greatest dimension
N2c	Metastasis in bilateral or contralateral lymph nodes, none more than 6 cm in greatest dimension
N3	Metastasis in lymph node, more than 6 cm in greatest dimension

DISTANT METASTASIS

MX	Presence of distant metastasis cannot be assessed
M0	No distant metastasis
M1	Distant metastasis

Table 17-2. STAGING OF HEAD AND NECK CANCER

Stage	Stage Grouping
0	Tis, N0, M0
I	T1, N0, M0
II	T2, N0, M0
III	T3, N0, M0
	T1, N1, M0
	T2, N1, M0
	T3, N1, M0
IV	T4, N0–1, M0
	Any T, N2–3, M0
	Any T, any N, M1

the nasopharynx; and the hypopharynx, the area below the epiglottis extending to the cervical esophagus. Although these areas are defined anatomically, they represent a continuum, and cancers from one area frequently involve another site of the pharynx.

Cancers of the nasopharynx involve a wide spectrum of diseases, unlike most areas of the head and neck. The most common malignant tumors of the nasopharynx include squamous cell carcinoma, lymphoepithelioma, and lymphoma. The lymphoepithelioma is a poorly differentiated squamous cell carcinoma that spreads early to lymph nodes. Cancers of the nasopharynx can present with nasal or eustachian tube obstruction, epistaxis, bloody rhinorrhea, decreased hearing, or cranial nerve involvement. In addition, they can present as (often bilateral) lymph node metastases along the spinal accessory lymph node chain. These cancers are associated with elevated levels of anti–Epstein-Barr virus antibodies. These antibodies are present in 45% to 100% of affected patients, depending on the stage of the tumor. Treatment is by radiotherapy, and surgery is usually reserved for lymph node metastases that have not been controlled by radiation. Chemotherapy, especially in childhood and adolescent lymphoepitheliomas, often produces dramatic regression of the tumor before the administration of radiotherapy. The role of chemotherapy in adults is less clear, and it does not seem to have made a major impact on survival. The overall survival rate at 5 years is about 30% to 35%.

The oropharynx includes the tonsil, soft palate, base of the tongue, and posterior pharyngeal wall. Most cancers in this area originate in the tonsil or in one of the tonsillar pillars, and most are squamous cell carcinomas. These cancers can be exophytic or deeply invasive. Patients usually complain of a sore throat, ear pain, or a mass in the neck. Both radiotherapy and surgery are used with similar efficacy for these cancers, although very large cancers are probably better treated by aggressive surgery when adequate margins can be obtained.

The hypopharynx includes the piriform sinus area, an outpouching of the pharyngeal mucosa adjacent to the larynx; the postcricoid area; and the inferior wall of the posterior pharynx. The hypopharynx is richly supplied by lymphatics and hypopharyngeal cancers, and piriform sinus cancers spread to lymph nodes early in their course. It is rare to find a hypopharyngeal cancer early, and even very small primary cancers can cause massive lymph node metastasis. Surgery is the optimal treatment for these cancers, because radiotherapy alone rarely controls local disease. Many believe that postoperative radiotherapy is mandatory even after adequate resection of cancers of the hypopharynx. Cancers of the hypopharynx usually require a laryngectomy to obtain a margin around the tumor, be-

cause the anterior wall of the hypopharynx and the medial wall of the piriform sinus are composed of the larynx. Because of the propensity of these tumors to spread to the regional lymph nodes, ipsilateral radical neck dissection is mandatory even when nodes are not clinically palpable. The survival rate depends on the stage of cancer and usually ranges from 20% to 40%.

Larynx

The larynx is most commonly divided into the supraglottis (epiglottis, aryepiglottic fold, and false vocal cords), glottis (true vocal cords), and subglottis (the area below the true vocal cords). Symptoms depend on where in the larynx the cancer arises.

Supraglottic cancers can cause hoarseness when they reach a large size, or, because of involvement of the epiglottis, they can make swallowing difficult and allow aspiration. These cancers spread to regional lymph nodes at an earlier stage than do other cancers of the larynx, and radical neck dissection is usually performed in combination with laryngectomy. Unlike cancers of the intrinsic larynx, supraglottic cancers frequently spread to the submental or submandibular lymph nodes, which must be removed during lymph node dissection. Small cancers of the supraglottic larynx can be treated by partial laryngectomy, and radiotherapy is often given after surgery. Cancers of the glottis usually present early, with patients seeking medical attention for hoarseness. A patient who is hoarse with no other cause, has hoarseness that does not resolve, or has hoarseness that does not improve during the day should undergo indirect and, if this is normal, direct laryngoscopy. Small cancers (T1 or T2) can be treated with radiotherapy, with an 80% to 95% 5-year disease-free survival rate. Small recurrences after radiotherapy can be treated with cordectomy; cervical lymph node metastasis for early-stage laryngeal carcinoma is uncommon. Larger cancers, including T3 (cord fixation) or T4 (deep invasion) cancers, are best treated by surgery. There has been a resurgence in interest in radiotherapy for these more advanced cancers, but little progress in the way of long-term improvement.

Subglottic cancers are difficult to diagnose and can cause

Table 17-3. CORRELATION OF PRIMARY SITE AND STAGE OF HEAD AND NECK CANCER WITH SURVIVAL RATES

Primary Site	Survival Rate (%)*			
	Stage I	Stage II	Stage III	Stage IV
ORAL CAVITY				
Tongue	70	50	40	20
Floor of mouth	70	50	25	10
Buccal mucosa	75	65	30	20
Alveolar ridge	80	65	35	15
PHARYNX				
Nasopharynx	80	60	40	20
Oropharynx	80	60	30	20
Hypopharynx	60	50	30	10
LARYNX				
Supraglottic	75	60	50	25
Glottic	95	80	50	30
Subglottic†				

* These numbers represent approximate averages; wide ranges have been reported for all sites and stages.
† Too rare for meaningful survival data.

hoarseness or dyspnea. Metastasis is more common than with glottic cancers.[4] The optimal treatment is a laryngectomy with resection of lymph nodes in the tracheoesophageal grooves.

Paranasal Sinuses

Sinus cancers are unusual, difficult to diagnose, and difficult to treat.[5] They occur most commonly in the maxillary sinuses; the ethmoid sinuses are the second most frequent place of occurrence, and their occurrence in the frontal and sphenoid sinuses is extremely uncommon. These cancers can present as nasal stuffiness, as epistaxis, or, when more advanced, as a bulging cheek, nose, or forehead, or they can present with proptosis. Cranial nerve involvement may be evident in patients with maxillary sinus cancers, with a loss of sensation in the branch of the trigeminal nerve supplying the face. More advanced cancers can be associated with deficits in the extraocular muscles due to invasion through the floor of the orbit. Actual loss of vision is rare and suggests invasion through the skull base to involve an optic nerve, or gross destruction of the globe itself.

Cancers arising in the paranasal sinuses include squamous cell carcinomas and minor salivary gland cancers, especially adenoid cystic carcinomas (cylindromas).[6] Lymphomas can also arise in these areas. Treatment depends on the stage of the disease. Small cancers can be treated with radiotherapy alone or by surgery. Surgery for maxillary sinus cancers includes maxillectomy, but more advanced cancers are better treated with more aggressive therapy. Surgical therapy requires resection with a margin of normal tissue around the tumor; for cancers that encroach on the base of the skull, this can include a combined intracranial–extracranial (craniofacial) resection. In these instances, a craniotomy is performed to push the brain out of the way, thereby protecting it and making resection of the skull base a safe procedure. When resection cannot be performed, high-dose radiotherapy is associated with excellent response rates. Complications from this therapy include loss of vision as well as radiation osteomyelitis. Mucosal melanomas arising within the paranasal sinus have also been reported. These melanomas are extremely rare and are best treated operatively. Even with adequate margins, however, they often spread early, and the prognosis is dismal.

Salivary Gland Tumors

The salivary glands can be subdivided into three major glands and innumerable smaller, or minor, salivary glands. The major salivary glands are the parotid, submandibular (submaxillary), and sublingual glands; thousands of minor salivary glands are found throughout the oral cavity, the pharynx, and the paranasal sinuses. Tumors that arise in the salivary glands are both benign and malignant. The larger the salivary gland, the more likely a tumor arising within it will be benign.[7] Conversely, the smaller the salivary gland, the more likely a tumor arising within it will be malignant. Tumors of the parotid gland are about 80% benign and 20% malignant; tumors of the submandibular gland about 50% benign and 50% malignant; and over 50% of tumors of the minor salivary glands are malignant. A large number of both benign and malignant tumors can be found in the salivary glands, and treatment varies with the histology.

The most common benign tumor of the salivary glands is the benign mixed tumor (pleomorphic adenoma; Table 17-4). This tumor has both epithelial and mesenchymal components, has a wide variety of patterns, and can (rarely) dedifferentiate into a malignant tumor. Treatment

Table 17-4. BENIGN SALIVARY GLAND TUMORS

Type	Approximate Percentage
Pleomorphic adenoma (benign mixed tumor)	90
Papillary cystadenoma lymphomatosum (Warthin tumor)	10
Oncocytoma	<1
Monomorphic adenoma	<1

is by excision, with a margin of normal tissue in all directions around the tumor. For parotid tumors, the most common site is in the superficial lobe. Resection usually involves a superficial (or lateral) parotid lobectomy because removal without exposure and preservation of the facial nerve endangers the facial nerve. Recurrence rates should be close to zero when the lesion is removed properly with a margin of normal tissue around the tumor. After enucleation or tumor spillage, recurrence rates are high, and another resection may be necessary, which might include the facial nerve. For recurrent tumors or tumors with inadequate margins, postoperative radiotherapy has proved effective in preventing further recurrences.

Warthin tumors (papillary cystadenoma lymphomatosum) are unusual tumors that occur in the parotid glands. They usually occur in males, about 10% are bilateral, and they are composed of lymphoid tissue containing germinal centers. If the diagnosis is made preoperatively, enucleation suffices to treat these tumors, but patients require follow-up for observation of the contralateral gland. If the tumor is not diagnosed preoperatively, then parotid lobectomy is indicated.

Other benign tumors of the salivary glands are rare. Diffuse enlargement of the salivary glands can be seen in Sjögren syndrome, in viral diseases such as mumps, or with inflammation due to ductal obstruction from a sialolith. Cysts of the parotid glands are rare, and they may represent cysts of the first branchial cleft. These also should be removed surgically by parotid lobectomy.

Malignant tumors of the salivary glands are uncommon. The most frequent site is the parotid gland. The most common cancer arising in the salivary glands is the mucoepidermoid cancer (Table 17-5). This tumor contains both epidermoid cells and mucus-containing cells and can be of two types—low-grade or high-grade. Low-grade tumors are treated by wide excision; in the parotid gland this is usually superficial parotid lobectomy, and in the submandibular gland this is resection of that gland. High-grade tumors must be treated more aggressively because they frequently spread to lymph nodes. Radical neck dissection is often indicated even in the absence of clinically palpable nodes.

The adenoid cystic carcinoma (cylindroma) is a slow-growing tumor that spreads along nerve sheaths. It can be difficult to determine the extent of tumor, and it is not infrequent that an apparent wide excision has positive margins. High-dose radiotherapy is often effective in controlling local disease, but the tumor usually spreads late in its course, and pulmonary metastases 8 or more years after initial treatment are not uncommon. These patients have high 5-year survival rates, but most eventually develop metastatic disease.

Other cancers of the salivary glands include acinic cell carcinoma, a low-grade tumor that grows slowly and is best treated by local surgery. Adenocarcinomas and malignant mixed tumors are unusual tumors of the salivary glands and are treated by wide excision; some surgeons advocate

Table 17-5. MALIGNANT SALIVARY GLAND TUMORS

	Percentage of Cancers			5-Year Survival Rate (%)
	Parotid	Submandibular	Minor	
Mucoepidermoid				
Low-grade	30	20	16	90
High-grade				40
Adenoid cystic				
(cylindroma)	11	33	39	61
Acinic cell	12	<1	<1	80
Malignant mixed	15	20	3	40
Squamous cell	7	11	3	20
Adenocarcinoma	12	12	32	40
Others	12	2	15	

Table 17-6. MOST COMMON PRIMARY SITES IN PATIENTS PRESENTING WITH NECK MASSES

Nodal Level	Primary Site
I	Anterior tongue
	Floor of mouth
	Anterior alveolar ridge
II	Oropharynx
	Nasophaynx
III	Hypopharynx
	Larynx
	Lateral tongue
IV	Usually subclavicular
V	Scalp
	Nasopharynx
	Parotid gland

prophylactic radical neck dissection. Less than 1% of cancers of the salivary glands are epidermoid cancers, but these tend to be aggressive, and prophylactic radical neck surgery is generally recommended. Lymphomas and sarcomas can arise within salivary glands and are treated like similar tumors elsewhere in the body.

Other Tumors

Patients can present with metastatic tumor within a cervical lymph node but with no known primary site of tumor. These cancers are usually squamous cell epitheliomas and constitute about 5% of all head and neck cancers. The primary site may be suspected from the location in the neck of the nodal metastasis (Fig. 17-3 and Table 17-6). If the evaluation for the primary site is unrevealing (including panendoscopy and random biopsies of the nasopharynx, tonsil, and hypopharynx), radical neck dissection or radiotherapy can be used to treat the neck metastasis. The primary site subsequently becomes evident in only about 25% of such patients.

Many other tumors can arise in the head and neck. Soft tissue sarcomas are discussed in detail elsewhere, but the head and neck area presents several anatomic problems in resecting these tumors. The general principle for the resection of soft tissue sarcomas is to obtain a normal tissue plane in all directions around the tumor. Because of the proximity of vital structures, this is often difficult if not impossible in the head and neck area. Thus, many patients with soft tissue sarcomas can undergo a resection with

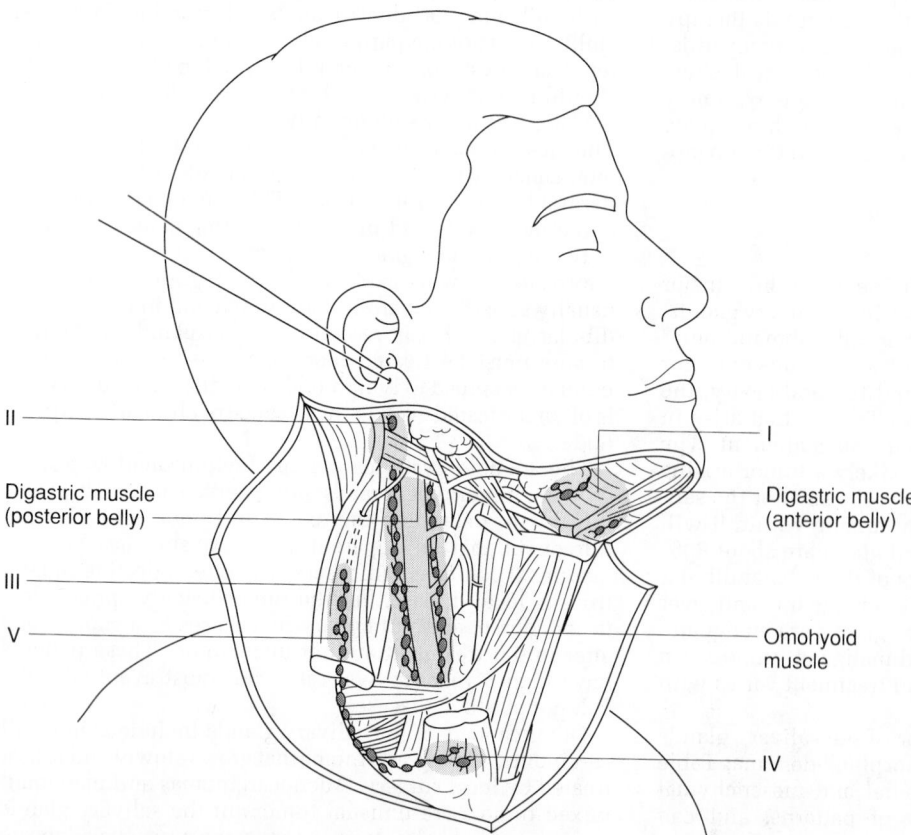

Figure 17-3. Lymphatic drainage of the head and neck. Level I includes the submental and submandibular lymph nodes. Level II includes the upper jugular chain (jugulodigastric) lymph nodes. Level III includes the middle jugular chain lymph nodes (those between the digastric muscle superiorly and the omohyoid muscle inferiorly). Level IV includes the lower jugular chain lymph nodes (below the omohyoid muscle). Level V includes the posterior triangle, or spinal accessory chain, lymph nodes.

minimal or positive margins and should be considered candidates for postoperative radiotherapy or the use of interstitial implants or brachytherapy.

Melanomas frequently arise in the head and neck, and they are treated in a manner similar to that for melanomas elsewhere in the body, except for melanomas arising within the mucosa. Mucosal melanomas are rare, have a poor prognosis, and often present at an advanced stage. They often originate in the paranasal sinuses, nasopharynx, or oral cavity, and they spread hematogenously earlier than cutaneous melanomas, probably because there is no basement membrane in oral mucosa as there is in skin. The mucosa is richly supplied with blood vessels and lymphatics, and adequate margins around a primary tumor may not be sufficient to prevent regional lymph node spread or systemic metastases. No adjuvant therapy has proved beneficial.

The most common site for Hodgkin disease is the neck. Patients with cervical masses, especially posterior cervical masses, and no obvious epithelial malignancy should be seriously considered for lymphoma. If the rest of the examination is unremarkable, a fine-needle aspiration biopsy, open biopsy, or both should be performed. Non-Hodgkin lymphoma arises in cervical lymph nodes less commonly than does Hodgkin disease, and the surgeon's role here is also one of diagnostician.

Tumors that arise from the chromaffin tissues (chemodectoma, paraganglioma) are rare and most commonly originate in the carotid body or along the vagus nerve. Intracranial tumors also arise from this tissue and are termed *glomus jugulare* tumors. Ninety percent are benign, but 10% are malignant and can spread hematogenously or to regional lymph nodes. These are vascular tumors, and an arteriogram of a carotid body tumor can be considered diagnostic. Most chemodectomas arise in the carotid body in elderly patients, and they grow slowly. Symptoms usually consist of a mass in the neck; if the patient has other concomitant medical problems and is asymptomatic, the chemodectoma may be observed and not treated. For symptomatic or rapidly growing tumors, resection should be considered. When tumors develop in the carotid body, a subadventitial plane can usually be obtained on the carotid artery and the tumor resected without sacrificing the artery. Occasionally, large tumors require carotid resection and arterial reconstruction.

Vagal paragangliomas require resection of the vagus nerve; resulting disability consists of recurrent laryngeal nerve paralysis. Tumor histology does not differentiate benign from malignant processes, and only the clinical behavior of the tumor can be used to determine if the tumor is malignant. The presence of regional lymph node metastases signifies a malignant tumor. No adjuvant therapy is known to be beneficial.

SURGICAL CONSIDERATIONS

A large number of procedures make up the armamentarium of surgeons operating on the head and neck. General indications were described previously, and further details follow.

Tracheostomy

Tracheostomy is a frequently performed operation that has a low morbidity if performed correctly. The most common indications are upper airway obstruction, prolonged dependence on a ventilator, and use as protection for major head and neck surgery. Tracheostomy is performed through either a vertical or horizontal incision made at the

level of the second tracheal ring (Fig. 17-4); the isthmus of the thyroid usually needs to be retracted caudally. A small flap of anterior tracheal cartilage should be sutured to the skin to allow access to the trachea if the tube is dislodged before maturation of the tract. Meticulous hemostasis is mandatory to prevent postoperative bleeding.

Complications of tracheostomy are infrequent but include bleeding and infection. Long-term complications can include erosion of the innominate artery, especially when a hard-cuffed tracheostomy tube is used.

Cervical Lymph Node Biopsy

Enlarged cervical lymph nodes may require biopsy at almost any site within the neck. Thorough knowledge of anatomy is necessary to avoid complications. Posterior (spinal accessory chain) lymph nodes are superficial and easily excised, but the surgeon must remember at all times that the spinal accessory nerve lies adjacent to these nodes. Damage to this nerve must be carefully avoided, because the disability can be severe. Lymph nodes in this area are best excised by carefully teasing the node away from surrounding tissue, avoiding damage to any tubular structure.

Supraclavicular, or scalene, lymph node biopsy must be performed with care to avoid injury to the structures in the carotid sheath (medial to the scalene triangle), thoracic duct (medial and deep), phrenic nerve (deep), brachial plexus (deep and lateral), and transverse cervical vessels (superior). The lymph nodes removed in this operation are between the omohyoid muscle, sternocleidomastoid muscle, subclavian vein, and internal jugular vein (Fig. 17-5).

Submandibular nodes are in proximity to the ramus mandibularis branch of the facial nerve. Care must be taken to visualize this small nerve, retract it (usually superiorly), and thereby prevent damage, which can result in a marked cosmetic deformity with an inability to lift the corner of the mouth.

Parotid Gland

Operations on the parotid gland must be performed without paralyzing the patient. The facial nerve runs between the two anatomic lobes of the parotid gland and must be preserved unless involved by tumor. If the patient is not paralyzed, proximity to the nerve can be easily demonstrated during the course of the dissection by stimulating the main trunk or its branches. The usual incision is preauricular, carried in front of the external auditory canal, then curved anteriorly below the angle of the mandible. The digastric muscle is exposed, and the main trunk of the facial nerve can be identified between the digastric muscle and the external auditory canal. The gland is retracted superiorly and anteriorly, and the nerve is traced distally (Fig. 17-6). All branches of the nerve should be identified and traced from proximal to distal until the superficial lobe of the gland is removed. For the rare tumor that arises within the deep lobe of the parotid gland, the superficial lobe should be removed before dissecting the posterior aspect of the branches of the facial nerve in order to retract and protect them, thus facilitating removal of the deep lobe of the gland. Most malignant tumors in the deep lobe of the parotid gland require facial nerve resection. Fortunately, most tumors (both benign and malignant) within the parotid gland arise in the superficial lobe.

When branches of the facial nerve or the main trunk itself are resected, nerve grafting is often used. Both the sural nerve and the greater auricular nerve are excellent conduits, and the facial nerve has the highest success rate for peripheral nerve grafting (about 90%). It can take 6 months or more for function to be restored after grafting.

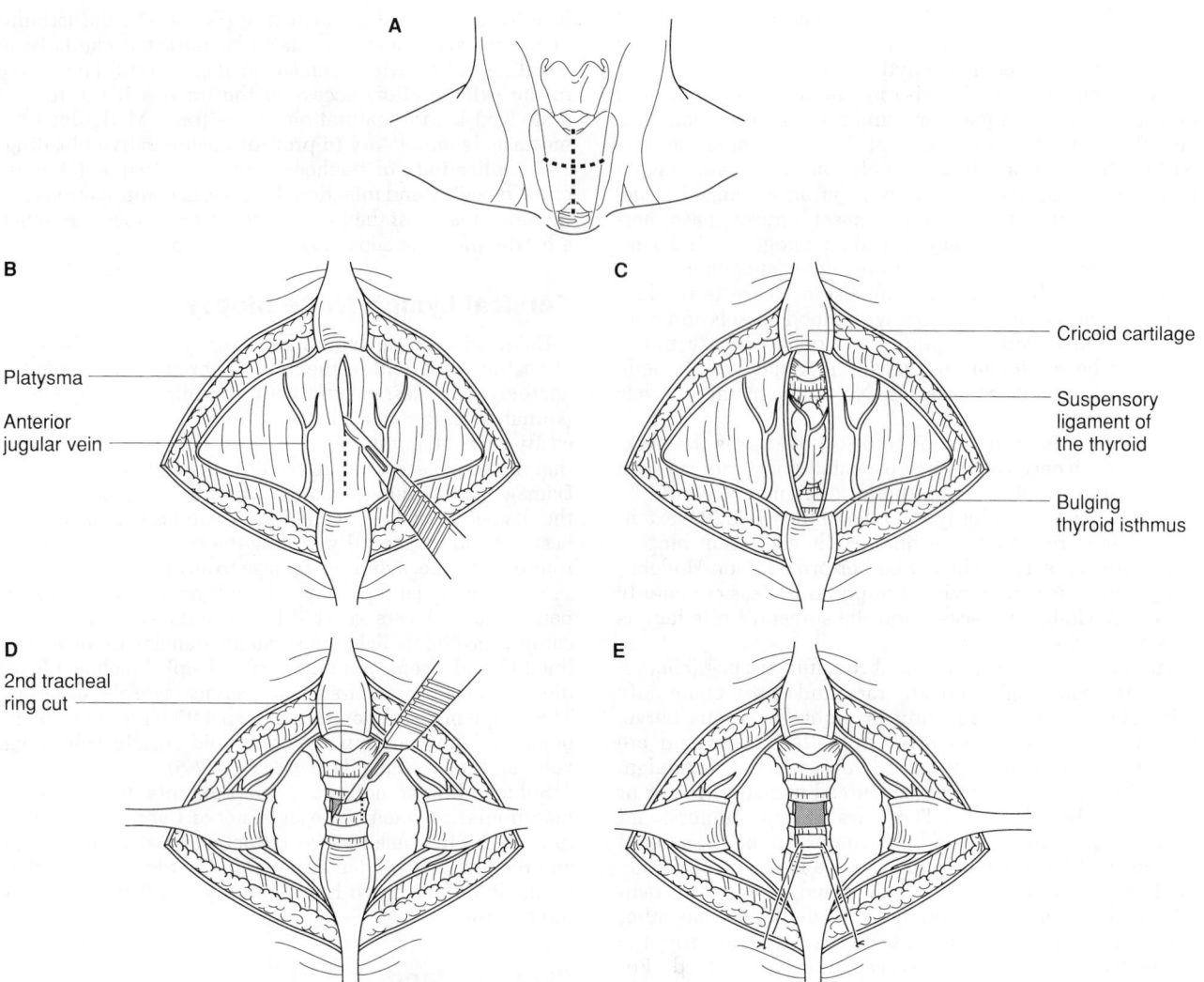

Figure 17-4. Tracheostomy. (*A*) Incision is usually made transversely for elective tracheostomy, but a vertical incision allows for less bleeding when the procedure must be performed emergently. (*B*) The strap muscles are separated in the midline. The thyroid isthmus may bulge into the wound (*C*), necessitating inferior retraction (*D*). (*E*) After the second tracheal ring is cleaned off, an inferiorly based flap is developed in the tracheal wall and sutured to the skin to allow easy access to the trachea while the tract is maturing.

In addition, the facial nerve may not work normally for a prolonged period of time even if all branches have been observed and preserved throughout their course. A rare complication of dissection of the facial nerve, gustatory sweating (Frey syndrome), is related to the fact that the auriculotemporal nerve runs with the facial nerve. Damage to this small branch, with subsequent reinnervation of the skin, results in sweating on that side of the face whenever a patient eats. This happens less frequently than once in 1000 parotidectomies. Other complications are even more unusual.

Submandibular Gland

Resection of the submandibular gland is usually performed through a submandibular incision that is carried through the subcutaneous tissue and platysma (Fig. 17-7). Care must be taken to identify the ramus mandibularis branch of the seventh nerve to avoid damage resulting in an inability to smile or raise the commissure of the lip on that side. The lingual nerve is deep to the submandibular gland and must be identified before division of deep blood supply to the gland. The chorda tympani nerve comes off the lingual nerve and is necessarily divided during resection of the submandibular gland. The hypoglossal nerve is deep to the submandibular gland, usually is not seen during excision of the submandibular gland, and should not be damaged during resection of the gland. Complications of removal of this gland include damage to the nerves mentioned, with resulting loss of motor function (due to damage to the ramus mandibularis branch of the seventh nerve) or loss of taste (due to damage to the lingual nerve).

Radical Neck Dissection

Removal of the lymph node–bearing tissue in the neck is important for the control of most epithelial cancers. Many different incisions have been used for radical neck dissection (Fig. 17-8). These depend on the experience of the surgeon, the site of the tumor, and whether a previous incision was made in the neck. If an open biopsy was performed, the biopsy site needs to be excised during the

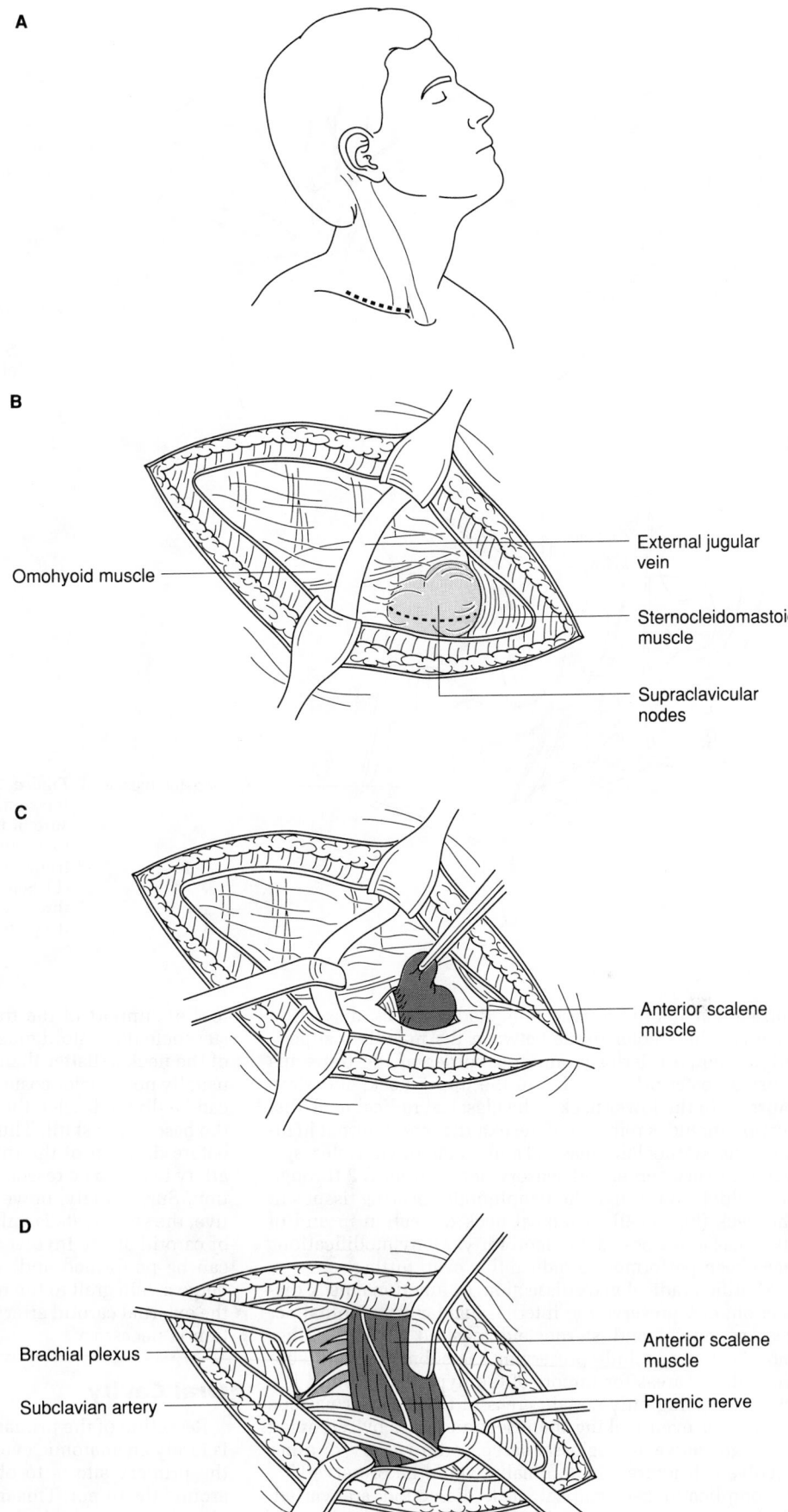

A

B

Omohyoid muscle

External jugular vein

Sternocleidomastoid muscle

Supraclavicular nodes

C

Anterior scalene muscle

Figure 17-5. Supraclavicular (scalene) node biopsy. (*A*) An incision is made over the lateral edge of the sternocleidomastoid muscle, with some extension further laterally. (*B*) After the platysma is incised, the areolar tissue containing the lymph nodes is exposed. (*C*) The areolar tissue between the omohyoid muscle (superiorly), external jugular vein (laterally), carotid sheath (medially), and clavicle (inferiorly) is dissected free. (*D*) Completed dissection, demonstrating the anterior scalene muscle, brachial plexus, and phrenic nerve at the base of the dissection.

D

Brachial plexus

Subclavian artery

Anterior scalene muscle

Phrenic nerve

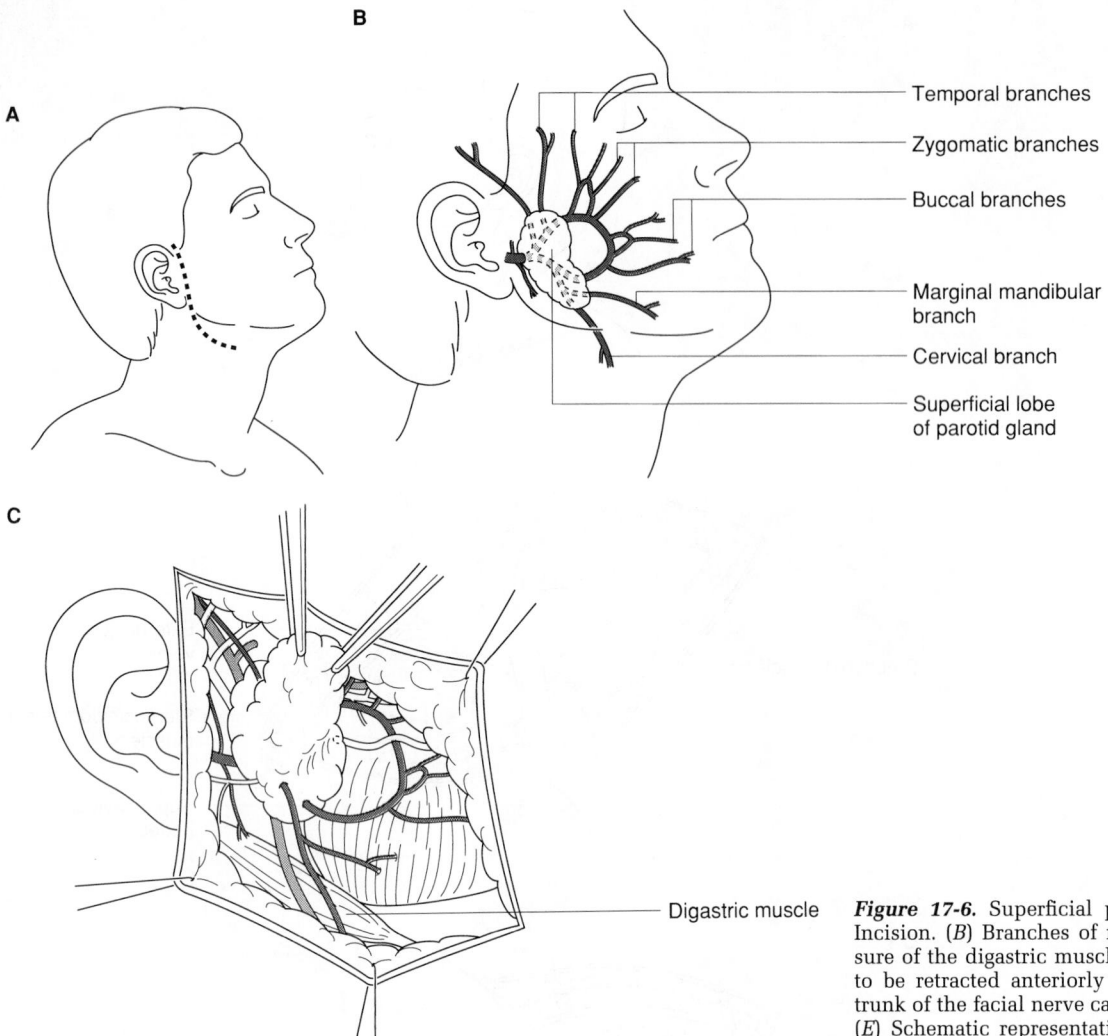

Figure 17-6. Superficial parotidectomy. (*A*) Incision. (*B*) Branches of facial nerve. Exposure of the digastric muscle allows the gland to be retracted anteriorly (*C*) and the main trunk of the facial nerve can then be seen (*D*). (*E*) Schematic representation of facial nerve through the parotid gland, separating it into deep and superficial lobes. (*continues*)

subsequent definitive resection. Radical neck dissection removes the areolar tissue between the mandible superiorly, clavicle inferiorly, anterior border of the trapezius muscle posteriorly, midline in the upper neck, and strap muscles in the lower neck.[8] The classical radical neck dissection includes removal of the external and internal jugular veins, sternocleidomastoid and omohyoid muscles, spinal accessory nerve, and sensory nerves from C-2 through C-5, which go through the lymph node–bearing tissues in the neck (Fig. 17-9). A radical neck dissection in and of itself has a low associated morbidity. Many modifications have been performed to reduce this even further.

Modified radical neck dissection, or functional neck dissection, can preserve the internal jugular vein, spinal accessory nerve, and sternocleidomastoid muscle. Other modifications include preserving the submental and submandibular areas for tumors of the hypopharynx and larynx, dissecting only certain areas of the neck for various tumors, or even making the resection larger by removing the vagus nerve, hypoglossal nerve, carotid artery, or other involved structures that normally would be preserved.

Complications of radical neck dissection are varied. Drainage catheters are left in place for several days, and if they are removed too soon, a seroma can develop, with resultant infection. If the spinal accessory nerve is resected, a winged scapula and shoulder drop caused by the loss of support of the trapezius muscle result. When the sternocleidomastoid muscle is removed, the involved side of the neck is flatter than the contralateral side, but this is usually not a major cosmetic defect. The hypoglossal nerve can be divided when the internal jugular vein is ligated at the base of the skull. Thus, this nerve should be identified before division of the internal jugular vein. If the carotid artery needs to be resected, a stroke is a possible complication. Surprisingly, however, when this procedure is elective, the stroke rate is only 5% to 10%. If there is suspicion of carotid artery involvement before surgery, flow studies can be performed and, if necessary, the patient can undergo a vein graft to the resected area of the carotid. If only the external carotid artery must be resected, no reconstruction is necessary.

Oral Cavity

Resection of the primary cancer arising in the oral cavity is rarely an anatomic event. The basic principle in treating the primary site is to obtain a wide margin (1 to 2 cm) around the tumor. This may necessitate resection of a margin of the mandible (marginal mandibulectomy) or removal of a segment of the mandible (segmental mandibulectomy) when the bone is invaded by tumor. When a segment of the mandible is resected, it should be recon-

D

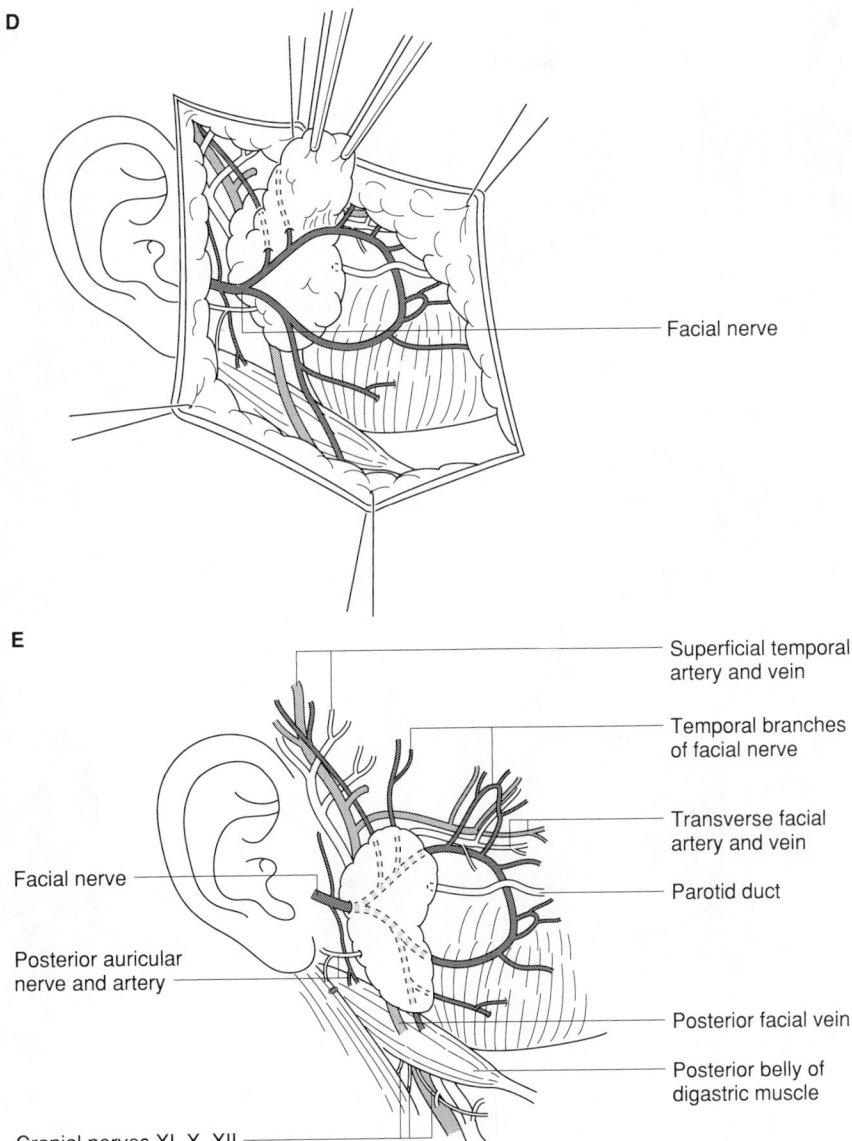

Facial nerve

E

Superficial temporal
artery and vein

Temporal branches
of facial nerve

Transverse facial
artery and vein

Parotid duct

Facial nerve

Posterior auricular
nerve and artery

Posterior facial vein

Posterior belly of
digastric muscle

Figure 17-6. (*Continued*)   Cranial nerves XI, X, XII

structed to provide the best possible functional and cosmetic result. When sufficient soft tissue is present to cover the defect, mandibular reconstruction can be with a metal plate. When both soft tissue and bone are required for reconstruction, use of a myocutaneous flap (usually trapezius, using the wing of the scapula) or a free osteo(myo)cutaneous flap with microvascular anastomoses gives the best results.

Larynx

Total laryngectomy is performed for advanced cancers of the larynx and for those that recur after irradiation; removal of one lobe of the thyroid gland (the lobe on the same side of the larynx as the tumor) is usually performed in continuity with laryngectomy. Laryngectomy can be done in continuity with the radical neck dissection. Several features of laryngectomy are extremely important. As little pharyngeal mucosa as necessary should be removed. This facilitates pharyngeal closure, decreases the incidence of stricture, and decreases the need for flap closure. Subsequent swallowing is facilitated by a widely patent pharynx. The parathyroid glands should not be resected

during a laryngectomy; by preserving one lobe of the thyroid gland with its blood supply, the chance of removing all functioning parathyroid tissue is small. The permanent tracheostomy must also be done with a great deal of care; use of a double Z-plasty produces a widely patent tracheostomy and decreases the risk of tracheostomal stenosis.

The most significant early complication after laryngectomy is breakdown of the pharyngeal closure. This results in a wound infection in the neck and often results in a pharyngocutaneous fistula. Most fistulas close with conservative care, but an occasional fistula requires subsequent operative closure. The treatment for pharyngeal breakdown with neck infection is to open the neck to facilitate drainage; frequent wound care is necessary because the area is constantly bathed by saliva. If this is not performed expeditiously, infection can involve the wall of the carotid artery, and a carotid rupture can ensue.

Other important immediate complications were alluded to earlier. Hypoparathyroidism is an infrequent but potentially devastating complication. Serum calcium should be checked frequently for the first 2 or 3 days after surgery. A long-term complication of laryngectomy is pharyngeal stricture. Most pharyngeal strictures

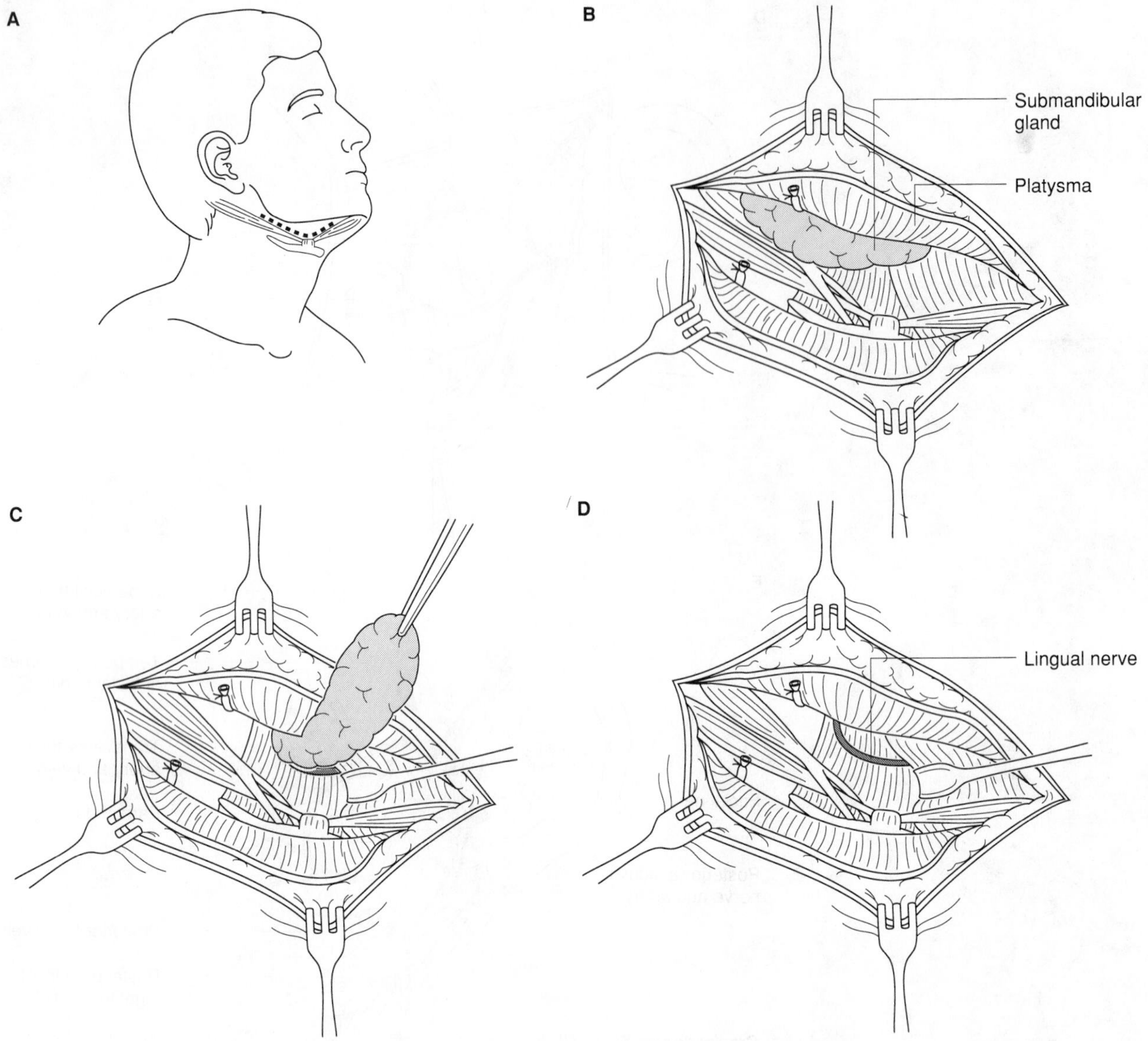

A

B

Submandibular
gland

Platysma

C

D

Lingual nerve

Figure 17-7. Resection of submandibular gland. (*A*) Skin incision, usually placed in a skin crease. (*B*) After division of platysma, the ramus mandibularis is identified and retracted superiorly. (*C*) Elevation of the gland allows identification of the lingual nerve. (*D*) After removal of the gland, the lingual nerve is in the base of the wound.

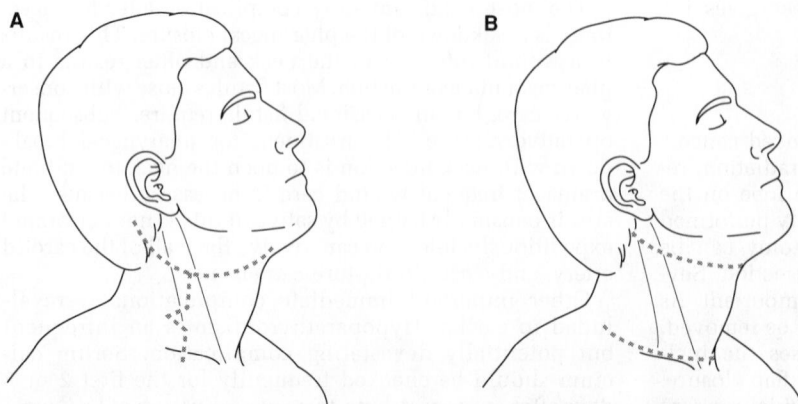

A

B

Figure 17-8. Frequently used incisions for radical neck dissection.

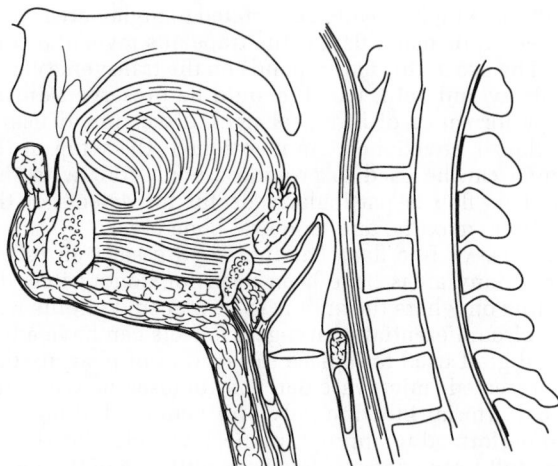

Figure 17-10. Cross section demonstrating proximity of hypopharynx to larynx. The posterior wall of the larynx is the hypopharyngeal mucosa.

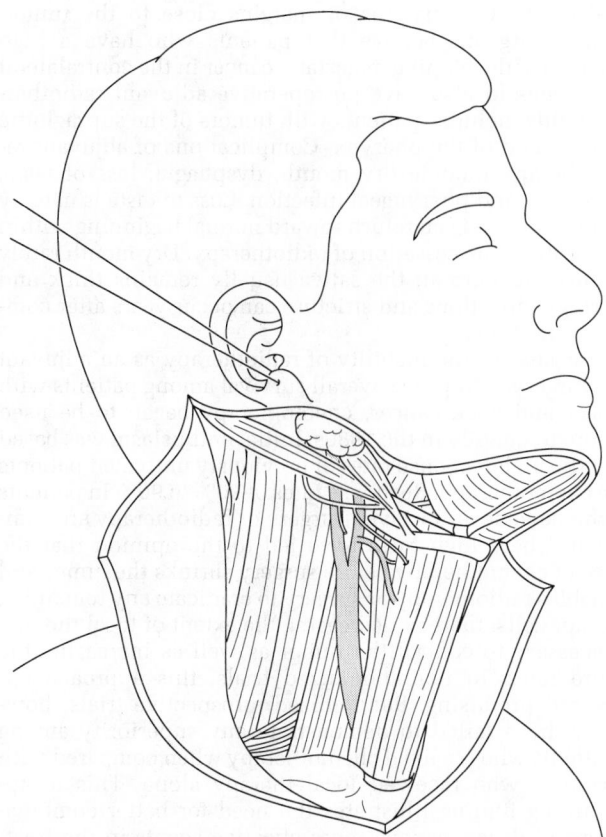

Figure 17-9. Schematic representation of operative field after radical neck dissection.

are soft and can be dilated with flexible dilators; occasional strictures may not respond to this therapy and may require revision of the closure. Tracheostomal stenosis is infrequent; when it occurs early after surgery, it should be treated by progressively enlarging the lumen with larger tracheostomy tubes. The largest tube possible should be left in place for many months. If restenosis follows this procedure, tracheostomal revision is necessary; performing a double Z-plasty is an excellent way to decrease the chance of recurrence of the stenosis. Patients with late-onset tracheostomal stenosis should undergo operative intervention because the conservative method of dilation is unlikely to be successful.

Pharynx

Operations on the pharynx vary depending on where in the pharynx the tumor arises. Tumors in the hypopharynx usually require laryngectomy (Fig. 17-10) to obtain an adequate margin. The resulting pharyngeal defect is often too large to close with local tissue, and rotation of outside tissue (such as a pectoralis major myocutaneous flap) or use of a free tissue transfer (such as a jejunal free flap with use of microvascular anastomosis) may be necessary to provide a widely patent pharynx for swallowing. Pharyngeal tumors often involve the parapharyngeal and retropharyngeal lymph nodes; thus, to remove potentially involved lymph nodes, pharyngectomy should include removal of all tissue to the prevertebral fascia.

Reconstruction

Major advances in reconstruction after resection of head and neck cancers began in the late 1970s.[9] The most important advance is the use of the pectoralis major

myocutaneous flap (Fig. 17-11). This flap consists of anterior chest wall skin, subcutaneous tissue, and pectoralis major muscle with its underlying blood supply. The thoracoacromial artery and vein, which are branches of the axillary artery and vein, run along the underside of the pectoralis major muscle. The artery gives off branches through the muscle to the skin, and by rotating the skin island with its underlying muscle and blood supply, a vascularized section of tissue can be used to reconstruct defects in the head and neck. This flap provides excellent tissue for closure of defects in the pharynx, floor of the mouth, and skin. When used to line the floor of the mouth or pharynx, the epithelium eventually develops a mucosa-like appearance as a result of its constant bathing in saliva. Thus, even when the patient has a great deal of hair growing on the skin that has been rotated, the hair eventually stops growing, and the skin appears similar to normal mucosa.

Another excellent flap for use in head and neck recon-

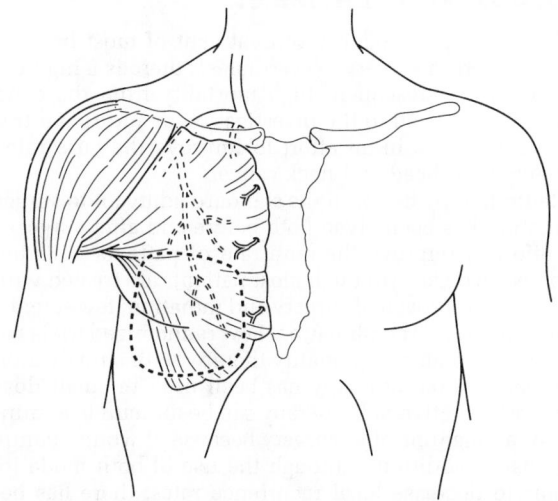

Figure 17-11. Pectoralis major myocutaneous flap. The skin "paddle" can be tailored to the defect it is designed to occupy. The myocutaneous flap rotates on the axis of the thoracoacromial vessels.

struction, which can often be rotated to higher areas than the pectoralis major flap, is the trapezius myocutaneous flap. The use of this flap depends on the transverse cervical artery and vein, which should be preserved during the performance of a radical neck dissection if use of this flap is envisioned. As mentioned, the wing of the scapula can be used to provide a bone graft with this flap. This flap is particularly useful for defects of the mandible, maxilla, and temporal bone area.

The use of free flaps has increased greatly in recent years. Many areas have been used for donor sites, depending on where the graft is to be placed. Patients who have circumferential pharyngeal defects can have a free jejunal graft used to replace the section of pharynx that was resected; microvascular anastomoses between the jejunal arterial blood supply and venous drainage are then performed to appropriate neck vessels. For skin or other soft tissue defects, free flaps with use of the radial forearm, the latissimus dorsi, the circumflex iliac, or even the transverse rectus abdominis muscle (with the epigastric vessels sutured to the cervical vessels) can be used. These flaps are particularly useful for skin defects, mucosal defects, or combined defects. The success rate of free flaps is about 90%, and most of the unsuccessful 10% retain at least a part of the flap. Complications are related to vascular anastomoses and venous congestion.

Rehabilitation

Patients undergoing large resections in the head and neck area must be evaluated and treated by use of a team approach. Speech therapists are extremely important in developing or improving speech after surgery as well as in helping the patient to relearn swallowing. Physical therapy is important for patients who undergo radical neck dissections, especially when the spinal accessory nerve is resected or damaged. Other members of the rehabilitation team include prosthodontists, who may be necessary for fitting a maxillary prosthesis or facial prosthesis, or for dental restoration. Long-term rehabilitation may also necessitate continued plastic surgical interventions and should always be tailored to the patient's needs and desires. Oral surgeons, neurosurgeons, and occupational therapists also are important members of the rehabilitation team for selected patients.

ADJUVANT TREATMENT

The principal modality of treatment of most head and neck cancers is surgery. Nevertheless, there is a high morbidity and a subsequent high mortality from the cancer itself. This has led to the investigation of additional treatment modalities in an effort to improve the cure rate of patients with head and neck cancer.

Radiotherapy has been the standard adjuvant to surgery. Radiation has been given both before and after surgery in an effort to improve the cure rate of patients with head and neck cancer. Although most patients are treated with a combined approach of surgery and radiation, few scientific data support this combination. Few randomized trials have compared combined modality therapy with surgery alone. Preoperative radiotherapy has been used in small doses, and postoperative radiotherapy can be difficult to administer for a long time after surgery because of wound complications. In addition, although the use of both modalities seems to decrease local recurrence rates, there has been no improvement in overall survival among patients treated with both surgery and radiation when compared with patients treated with surgery alone. Radiation treatment appears to be indicated for patients who have microscopically involved margins or margins close to the tumor. Many surgeons believe that patients who have a high chance of developing metastatic cancer in the contralateral neck should also have postoperative adjuvant radiotherapy; this includes patients with tumors of the supraglottic larynx and of the pharynx. Complications of adjuvant radiotherapy include dry mouth, dysphagia, loss of taste, stricture, and pharyngeal infection. Loss of taste is usually temporary and can return toward normal beginning within a month of the cessation of radiotherapy. Dry mouth rarely returns to normal; the saliva usually remains thick and stringy. Infections and stricture can occur years after completion of therapy.

Because of the inability of radiotherapy as an adjuvant to surgery to improve overall survival among patients with head and neck cancer, chemotherapy began to be used more frequently in the 1980s. Initial enthusiasm was based on the high response rates of previously untreated patients to chemotherapy. Response rates of 70% to 90% in patients who have never received surgery or radiotherapy are common. These high rates have led to the opinion that the use of chemotherapy before surgery shrinks the tumor and enables radiotherapy or surgery to eradicate any remaining tumor cells, thereby decreasing the extent of local therapy necessary to control the tumor as well as increasing the cure rates. In nonrandomized trials, this approach appeared promising. Randomized, prospective trials, however, have failed to demonstrate any superiority among patients who received chemotherapy when compared with patients who received local therapy alone. This disappointing finding illustrates the need for better combinations of drugs or new, more effective agents in the treatment of these cancers.

Another type of systemic therapy is immunotherapy. Head and neck cancers are easy to reach, easy to dissect, and easy to inject. With the use of animal models, evidence has accumulated that direct injection of an immunopotentiating agent into the tumor itself may enable a more profound host response to the tumor, thereby enabling the host to develop an immunity to his or her own tumor cells. Randomized, prospective trials using both *Corynebacterium parvum* and bacillus Calmette-Guerin have been unsuccessful in demonstrating any significant improvement in either disease-free or overall survival rates with this approach. Other types of immunotherapy have been attempted in nonrandomized trials and have not been successful in improving survival.

Intraarterial chemotherapy has been used to shrink large, unresectable tumors. This approach has the advantage of delivering high chemotherapy doses directly into the tumor, with the potential for dramatic shrinkage of the tumor. Unfortunately, randomized prospective trials have not been performed to further evaluate this costly, time-consuming approach.

Another approach, which has not been evaluated in randomized, prospective trials, is brachytherapy. Patients who undergo resection have afterloading catheters left in

Table 17-7. SINGLE-AGENT CHEMOTHERAPY*

Drug	Response Rate (%)
Methotrexate	42
Cisplatin	34
5-Fluorouracil	27
Bleomycin	26

* More than 100 reported patients for each single agent; drugs tested on fewer than 100 patients not listed.

Table 17-8. COMBINATION CHEMOTHERAPY FOR SQUAMOUS CELL CARCINOMA OF THE HEAD AND NECK

Treatment Regimen	Response Rate (%)		Complete Response Rate (%)	
	Previously Treated Patients	Untreated Patients	Previously Treated Patients	Untreated Patients
Cisplatin, bleomycin, methotrexate	45	77	12	21
Cisplatin, bleomycin	32	76	5	23
Cisplatin, methotrexate		60		0
Cisplatin, 5-fluorouracil		93		54

areas of the tumor bed that are thought to be at high risk for developing local recurrence. When sufficient wound healing has occurred, usually after 7 to 10 days, radioactive pellets are placed into these catheters and left for a period calculated to deliver a high dose of radiotherapy to the local area. This approach appears promising because it can control local disease, but it has the drawback that only a limited area can be irradiated.

Thus, although a large number of different approaches are being tried, combined modality therapy has yet to provide a significant advantage over surgery alone—or, in the case of small tumors, radiotherapy alone—in the management of head and neck cancers. Newer approaches include new combinations of chemotherapy, intraarterial chemotherapy, brachytherapy, and hyperfractionated or accelerated radiotherapy. In the absence of a controlled clinical trial, however, it is difficult to advocate any of these approaches.

METASTATIC DISEASE

Treatment of metastatic disease is generally unsatisfactory for patients with head and neck cancer. When patients experience a recurrence in the neck, surgery is the best way to control the tumor locally. If the recurrence is not resectable, radiotherapy can be beneficial for those patients not previously irradiated. Hyperfractionation, administering the radiation in two or more doses per day, and radiation associated with hyperthermia are under investigation in patients with recurrent head and neck cancer as attempts to improve the therapeutic efficacy of radiation.

Frequently, metastasis to the lung occurs. When solitary, it can be difficult to determine if the mass is metastatic disease or represents a primary lung cancer. More than half of solitary pulmonary nodules that develop in patients with histories of head and neck cancer actually represent primary pulmonary cancers. Thus, the workup for a solitary nodule in the lung should be identical to that for a patient with a primary lung cancer, and the patient should be treated accordingly.

When patients have metastatic disease outside the confines of surgery or irradiation, chemotherapy is the only systemic modality with a significant chance of objective tumor response. Among patients with head and neck cancer, the response rates to single agents are low (Table 17-7) and response durations are short, averaging about 4 months. Combination chemotherapy has higher response rates (40% to 50%; Table 17-8), but response durations are also short. In randomized, prospective trials, survival is no longer than that achieved with single-agent chemotherapy. Patients undergoing chemotherapy are frequently elderly, have other medical problems, and are unable to tolerate the most active drugs. For example, patients with impaired renal function should not receive cisplatin, and bleomycin should not be given to patients who have chronic obstructive pulmonary disease. Therefore, chemotherapy must be tailored not just to the tumor but to the patient's underlying medical status. Although response rates are higher with combination chemotherapy, the incidence of side effects is also much higher than with single-agent chemotherapy. Because there is no improvement in response duration and overall survival is not affected, combination chemotherapy for recurrent and metastatic head and neck cancer should be reserved for clinical trials.

REFERENCES

1. Blot WJ, McLaughlin JK, Winn DM, et al. Smoking and drinking in relation to oral and pharyngeal cancer. Cancer Res 1988; 48:3282.
2. Brachman DG. Molecular biology of head and neck cancer. Semin Oncol 1994;21:320.
3. Jacobs CD, Goffinet DR, Fee WE. Head and neck squamous cancers. Curr Probl Cancer 1990;14:1.
4. Candela FC, Shah J, Jaques DP, Shah JP. Patterns of cervical node metastases from squamous carcinoma of the larynx. Arch Otolaryngol Head Neck Surg 1990;116:432.
5. Ketcham AS, VanBuren JM. Tumors of the paranasal sinuses: a therapeutic challenge. Am J Surg 1985;150:406.
6. Spiro JD, Soo KC, Spiro RH. Squamous carcinoma of the nasal cavity and paranasal sinuses. Am J Surg 1989;158:328.
7. Attie JN, Sciubba JJ. Tumors of major and minor salivary glands: clinical and pathologic features. Curr Probl Surg 1981; 18:68.
8. DeSanto LW, Beahrs OH. Modified and complete neck dissection in the treatment of squamous cell carcinoma of the head and neck. Surg Gynecol Obstet 1988;167:259.
9. Coleman JJ. Reconstruction of the pharynx after resection for cancer: a comparison of methods. Ann Surg 1989;209:554.

SURGERY: SCIENTIFIC PRINCIPLES AND PRACTICE, Second Edition, edited by
Lazar J. Greenfield, Michael W. Mulholland, Keith T. Oldham, Gerald B. Zelenock,
and Keith D. Lillemoe. Lippincott–Raven Publishers, Philadelphia, © 1997.

CHAPTER 18

ESOPHAGEAL ANATOMY AND PHYSIOLOGY, AND GASTROESOPHAGEAL REFLUX

PETER F. CROOKES AND TOM R. DEMEESTER

ANATOMY

A detailed knowledge of the esophagus and its relations to other structures is essential for the surgeon to identify the sites and significance of lesions by indirect studies such as endoscopy, barium roentgenography, and computed tomography. This knowledge is also critical to the surgeon's ability to perform esophageal surgical procedures safely.[1] In this section, the embryology of the esophagus is first described, then the topographic relations of the esophagus are reviewed, and finally the conduct of investigations that yield anatomic information is detailed.

Embryology

The embryology of the esophagus is important to an understanding of the pathogenesis of congenital malformations of the esophagus and trachea. The embryonic esophagus forms when paired longitudinal grooves appear on each side of the laryngotracheal diverticulum. These grooves subsequently grow medially and fuse to form the tracheoesophageal septum. This septum divides the foregut into the ventral laryngotracheal tube and the dorsal esophagus. Incomplete fusion of the two lateral grooves was thought to be the major factor in the pathogenesis of congenital tracheoesophageal fistula, but the anomaly is now attributed to abnormal growth and differentiation of the lung buds. Initially, the esophagus is short, but elongation occurs rapidly, and the final relative length is attained by the 7th gestational week. This is followed by endodermal proliferation, resulting in near obliteration of the esophageal lumen and subsequent recanalization as large vacuoles develop and coalesce. The striated muscle of the upper esophagus is derived from the caudal branchial arches and is innervated by the vagus nerve and its recurrent laryngeal branches. The smooth muscle of the lower esophagus arises from splanchnic mesenchyme and is supplied by a visceral nerve plexus derived from neural crest cells. The adult position of the vagus nerves on the esophagus is the result of unequal growth of the greater curve of the stomach relative to the lesser curve, resulting in rotation of the left vagus anteriorly and the right vagus posteriorly.

Cervical Esophagus

The cervical esophagus begins below the cricopharyngeus muscle, which is a continuation of the inferior constrictor of the pharynx. The potential space between these muscles posteriorly is the site where a Zenker diverticulum develops. The adult cervical esophagus is about 5 cm long. It begins at the level of the C-6 vertebra and extends to the lower border of T-1, curving slightly to the left in its descent. Anteriorly, it abuts the trachea and the posterior larynx and can be dissected away from both organs if necessary. Posteriorly, the retroesophageal space is continuous above with the retropharyngeal space and below with the superior mediastinum. Laterally, the omohyoid muscle crosses it obliquely and is usually divided to gain access to the esophagus. The carotid sheaths lie laterally, and the lobes of the thyroid and the strap muscles lie anteriorly. The recurrent laryngeal nerves lie in the posterolateral grooves between the esophagus and the trachea. The right recurrent nerve runs a more oblique course and is more prone to anatomic variance. Consequently, although the surgical approach to this portion of the esophagus may be from either side of the neck through an incision along the anterior border of sternocleidomastoid muscle, the left side is chosen if possible.

Thoracic Esophagus

The thoracic esophagus in its upper part is closely related to the posterior wall of the trachea. This close relation is responsible for the early spread of cancer of the upper esophagus into the trachea, and it limits the ability of the surgeon to perform an en bloc resection of such a tumor. Above the level of the tracheal bifurcation, the esophagus passes to the right of the descending aorta. It then moves to the left, passes behind the tracheal bifurcation and the left main bronchus, and descends to the diaphragm. In its lower third, the esophagus courses anteriorly and to the left to traverse the diaphragmatic hiatus. The lower esophagus is covered only by mediastinal pleura on the left; this portion is the most common site of perforation in Boerhaave syndrome. The azygos vein is closely related to the esophagus as it arches from its paraspinal position over the right main bronchus to enter the superior vena cava. The thoracic duct ascends posterior and to the right of the distal esophagus, but at the level of T-5, it passes dorsal to the aorta and ascends on the left side of the esophagus and posterior to the left subclavian vein.

Throughout its length, the attachments of the esophagus to its adjacent structures other than the posterior trachea are weak. This accounts for the ease with which the esophagus can be bluntly mobilized out of the mediastinum during transhiatal esophagectomy. In general, the lower esophagus is most easily approached through the left chest, but access to the supraaortic esophagus is restricted. Thus,

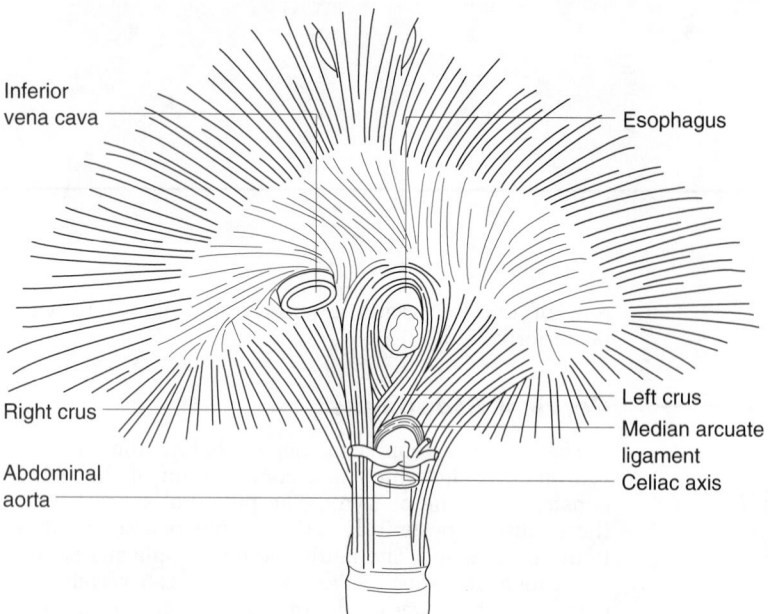

Inferior
vena cava

Esophagus

Right crus

Left crus

Median arcuate
ligament

Celiac axis

Abdominal
aorta

Figure 18-1. Diaphragm and esophageal hiatus seen from below.

a left thoracotomy is most useful for performing a Heller myotomy, transthoracic fundoplication, or resection of an epiphrenic diverticulum. Access to the entire thoracic esophagus can be obtained only from the right chest, but access to the intraabdominal organs is restricted by the liver and normally requires a separate upper abdominal incision.

Abdominal Esophagus

The abdominal esophagus begins as the esophagus enters the abdomen through the diaphragmatic hiatus (Fig. 18-1). It is surrounded by a fibroelastic membrane, the phrenoesophageal membrane, which arises from the subdiaphragmatic fascia (Fig. 18-2). The lower limit of the phrenoesophageal membrane anteriorly is marked by a prominent fat pad, which corresponds to the gastroesophageal junction. The lower esophageal sphincter (LES) is a zone of high pressure, 3 to 5 cm long in adults, at the lower end of the esophagus. Although it does not correspond to any macroscopic anatomic structure, its function appears to be related to the microscopic architecture of the muscle fibers. The esophageal hiatus is formed by the right and left crura, which form a sling of muscular fibers arising by

tendinous bands from the anterolateral surface of the first four lumbar vertebrae. The relative contribution of the right and left crura to the sling is variable. Surgeons name the crura from their relation to the esophagus, whereas anatomists name them from their relation to the aorta. Thus, both right and left "surgical" crura originate from the right "anatomic" crus. Caudally, the crura are united by a tendinous arch, the median arcuate ligament, just anterior to the aorta at the level of the celiac axis.

Blood Supply and Venous Drainage

The blood supply and venous drainage are largely segmental. The inferior thyroid artery provides the main blood supply to the cervical portion of the esophagus. This becomes important in a patient with a previous thyroidectomy, although ligation is usually performed distal to the esophageal branch. The thoracic portion of the esophagus receives its blood supply from two sources. Usually, branches from two to three bronchial arteries provide the proximal arterial supply, and branches directly from the aorta supply the more distal thoracic esophagus. The upper of these aortic branches arises between the sixth and seventh thoracic vertebrae; the lower one arises between the

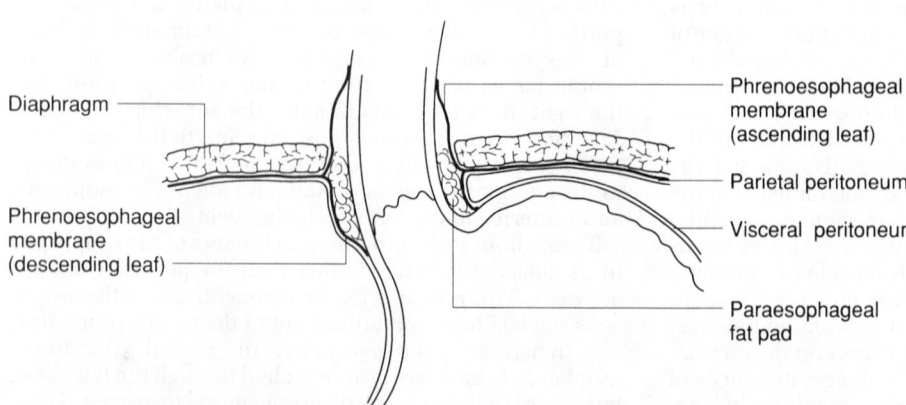

Diaphragm

Phrenoesophageal
membrane
(descending leaf)

Phrenoesophageal
membrane
(ascending leaf)

Parietal peritoneum

Visceral peritoneum

Paraesophageal
fat pad

Figure 18-2. Attachments of the phrenoesophageal membrane.

eighth and ninth thoracic vertebrae. Intrathoracic mobilization of the esophagus during the performance of antireflux procedures often requires ligation of these branches. The abdominal esophagus receives its blood supply from branches of the left gastric artery and inferior phrenic arteries (Fig. 18-3). A particularly constant artery at the base of the left surgical crus connects the inferior phrenic artery to branches of the left gastric artery and is sometimes called the *Belsey artery*. It is often seen during the crural dissection in performing laparoscopic fundoplication. Once the vessels have entered the muscular wall of the esophagus, branching occurs at right angles to provide a longitudinal vascular plexus. This anatomic arrangement allows for mobilization of the esophagus from the stomach to the aortic arch without ischemic injury.

A venous plexus in the submucosa collects capillary blood and delivers it into a periesophageal venous plexus. From this plexus, esophageal veins arise that empty into the inferior thyroid vein proximally; into the bronchial, azygos, or hemiazygos veins in the thorax; and into the left gastric vein in the abdominal region (Fig. 18-4). The left gastric vein, or coronary vein, provides the principal collateral in portal hypertension when esophageal varices develop. The submucosal veins become much more superficial in the most distal esophagus, 1 to 2 cm above the gastroesophageal junction, and are consequently the most common site of bleeding in portal hypertension. The continuity between the submucosal venous networks of the esophagus and stomach provides an additional collateral pathway for portal blood to enter the superior vena cava through the azygos vein in patients with portal hypertension.

Lymphatics

The lymphatics of the esophagus forms a rich submucosal network draining into regional lymph nodes in the periesophageal connective tissue[2] (Fig. 18-5). There is thus little barrier to longitudinal spread of cancer in the esophagus; it is estimated that for every 1 cm of axial spread, there is 6 cm of longitudinal spread. Lymphatic drainage from the upper two thirds of the esophagus is usually ceph-

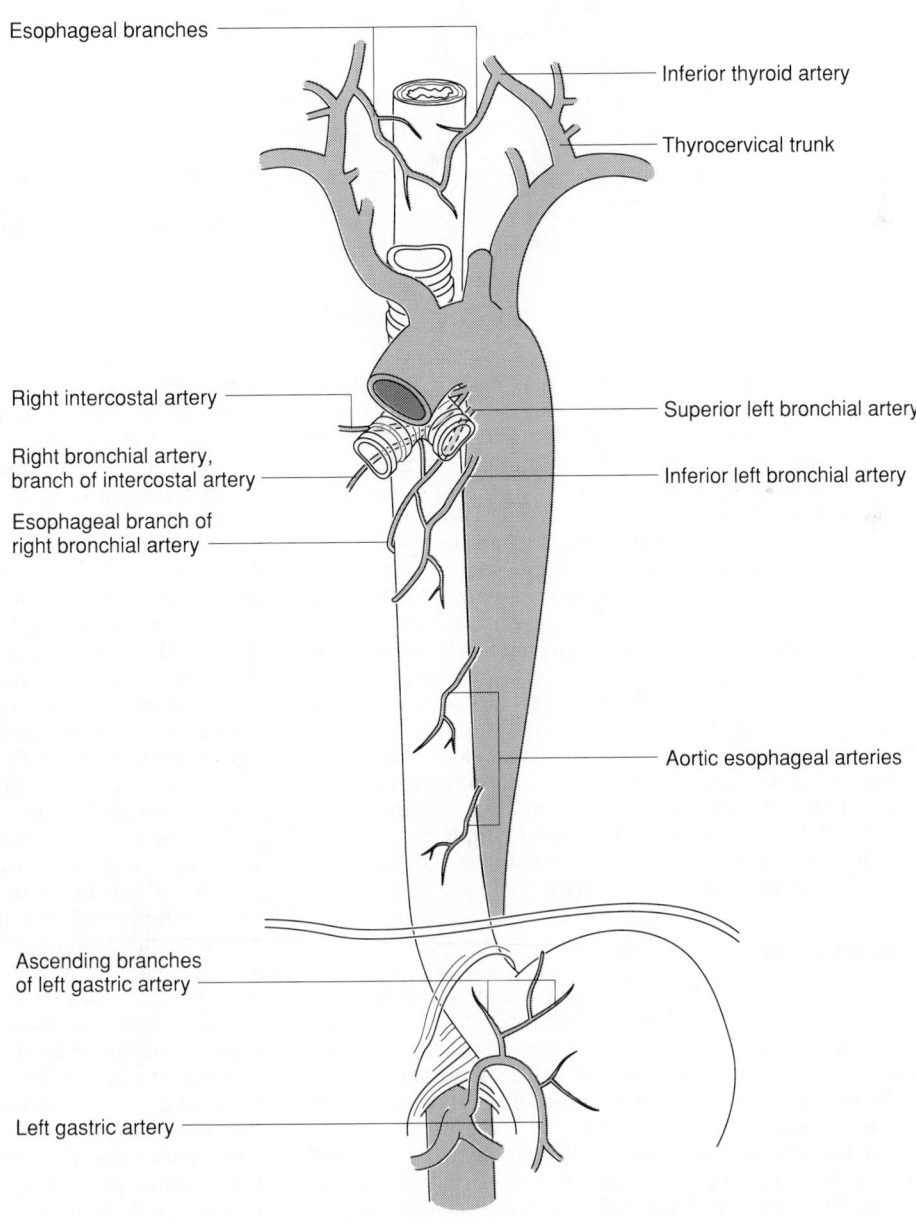

Figure 18-3. Arterial blood supply of the esophagus.

Esophageal branches

Inferior thyroid artery

Thyrocervical trunk

Right intercostal artery

Superior left bronchial artery

Right bronchial artery, branch of intercostal artery

Inferior left bronchial artery

Esophageal branch of right bronchial artery

Aortic esophageal arteries

Ascending branches of left gastric artery

Left gastric artery

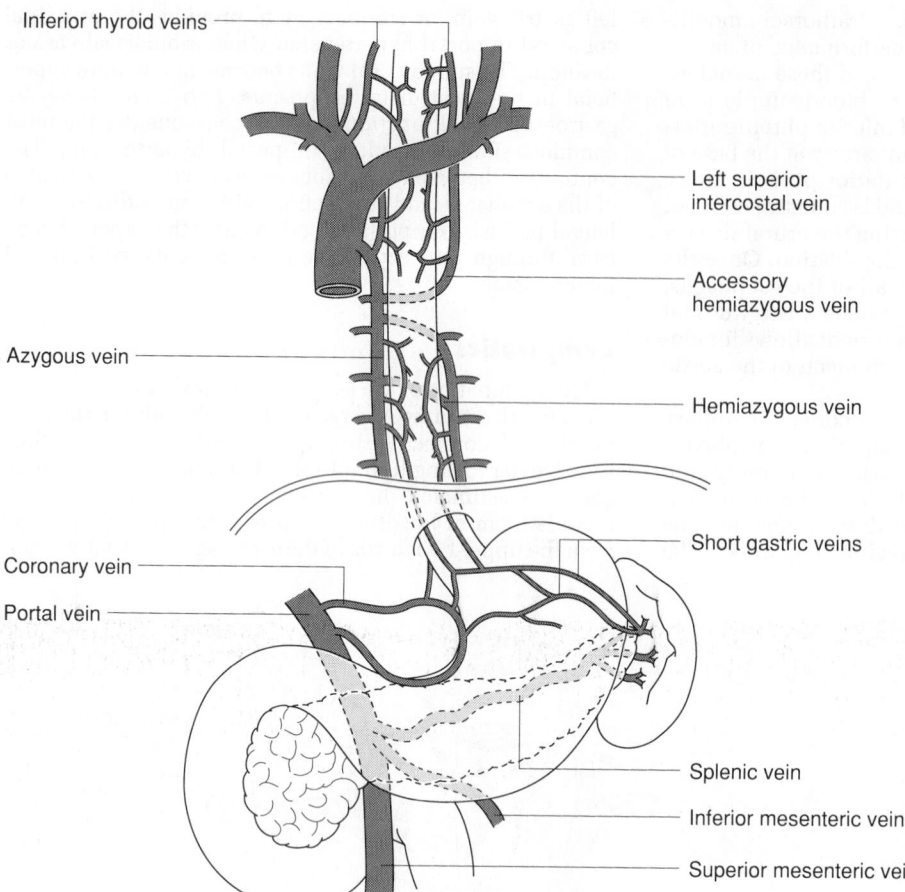

Figure 18-4. Venous drainage of the esophagus.

alad, but drainage from the lower one third is in both directions. In the cervical region, esophageal lymphatic drainage is toward the internal jugular and upper tracheal nodes. Posterior mediastinal nodes drain the thoracic portion of the esophagus dorsally. Drainage from the anterior portion of the thoracic esophagus is most often to tracheal nodes superiorly and subcarinal and paraesophageal nodes inferiorly. In the abdomen, the esophageal lymph drains to cardiac and celiac nodes, which may eventually drain into the cisterna chyli or the thoracic duct. Although lymphatic metastases in the esophagus generally involve the regional nodes in proximity, nodal involvement can occur several centimeters away from the primary lesion because of the rich intramural lymphatic anastomotic channels.[1] When a carcinoma is limited to the mucosa (above the muscularis mucosae), the incidence of lymphatic metastases is low, but once into the submucosa, the incidence rises to 60%. The results of three-field lymph node dissection for esophageal carcinoma have emphasized the widespread lymphatic connections within the esophagus.

Innervation

The innervation of the cricopharyngeal sphincter and cervical portion of the esophagus is from both the right and left recurrent laryngeal nerves. These nerves, arising from the vagus, travel dorsally around the subclavian artery on the right and the arch of the aorta on the left. Branching to both the esophagus and trachea occurs as these nerves ascend in the tracheoesophageal groove. The nerve may be injured during dissection of the upper esophagus in the neck, or during the mediastinal dissection in transhiatal esophagec-

tomy. Although much attention is given to the vocal cord dysfunction that accompanies recurrent laryngeal nerve damage, it is also clear that cricopharyngeal sphincter dysfunction and motility problems of the cervical esophagus can occur with injury to these nerves. Serious aspiration after recurrent nerve injury is caused not only by cricopharyngeal dysfunction but also by the additional morbidity incurred because of inability to close the glottis during swallowing and loss of the protection afforded by effective coughing.

Branches from the left recurrent laryngeal nerve and from both vagus nerves provide innervation of the upper thoracic esophagus. The esophageal plexus on the anterior and posterior wall of the esophagus provides innervation for the lower esophagus. The esophageal plexus also receives fibers from the thoracic sympathetic chain. The single trunks located distally contain fibers from both right and left original vagus nerves.

Efferent preganglionic sympathetic fibers supplying the esophagus arise from the fourth to sixth spinal cord segments and terminate in the cervical and thoracic sympathetic ganglions. Fibers from the superior cervical ganglion arrive at the pharyngeal plexus by way of vagal nerves. The postganglionic fibers reach the esophagus by branches from the cervical and thoracic sympathetic chain. The distal esophageal segments also receive direct sympathetic fibers from the celiac ganglion.

Afferent visceral sensory pain fibers from the esophagus terminate without synapsing in the first four segments of the thoracic spinal cord, following both sympathetic and vagal pathways. Pain fibers from the heart also travel in these same pathways, explaining the similarity of the symptoms in many esophageal and cardiac diseases.

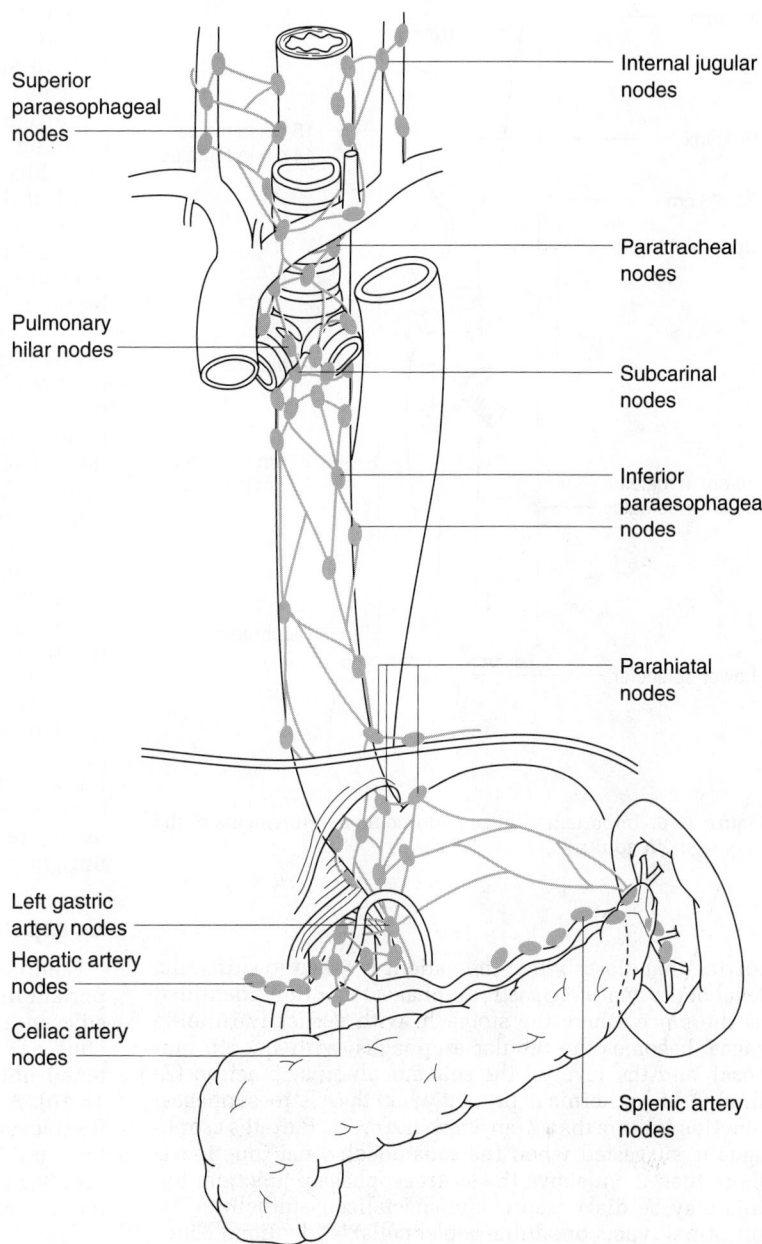

Figure 18-5. Lymphatic drainage of the esophagus.

INVESTIGATION OF STRUCTURAL ABNORMALITIES

Endoscopy

Endoscopy is generally the first investigation in patients with foregut symptoms. The exception is when the patient's chief complaint is dysphagia, when preliminary anatomic information should first be obtained by barium swallow. Endoscopy allows visualization of a wide range of disease processes and permits both diagnostic and therapeutic measures. The chief risks are oversedation, aspiration, and instrumental perforation.

Most patients are adequately prepared with topical anesthesia and intravenous sedation. Monitoring of heart rate and pulse oximetry must be carried out, and resuscitation equipment must be available. The endoscope is introduced through a mouth guard into the pharynx. Entry into the esophagus is aided by having the patient swallow. The locations of esophageal landmarks are measured endo-

scopically from the incisor teeth (Fig. 18-6). The cricopharyngeus is normally at 15 cm in adults. The tracheal bifurcation and indentation of the aortic arch is between 24 and 26 cm from the incisor teeth. This landmark is helpful in localizing intraluminal lesions. The position of the gastroesophageal junction is best identified during the initial endoscope introduction, before it is advanced into the stomach, to avoid reducing a sliding hiatal hernia. Once in the stomach, the scope is directed toward the pylorus and advanced into the second part of the duodenum. The duodenum and stomach are then systematically inspected as the scope is withdrawn. Turning the lens of the scope a thorough 180 degrees (retroflexion) allows inspection of the fundus and cardia. Attention is paid to the frenulum of the gastroesophageal junction and to the closeness with which the cardia grips the scope. The instrument is then straightened and withdrawn through the cardia and esophagus. Three landmarks are measured in the region of the cardia: the level of the crura (observed as a slitlike nar-

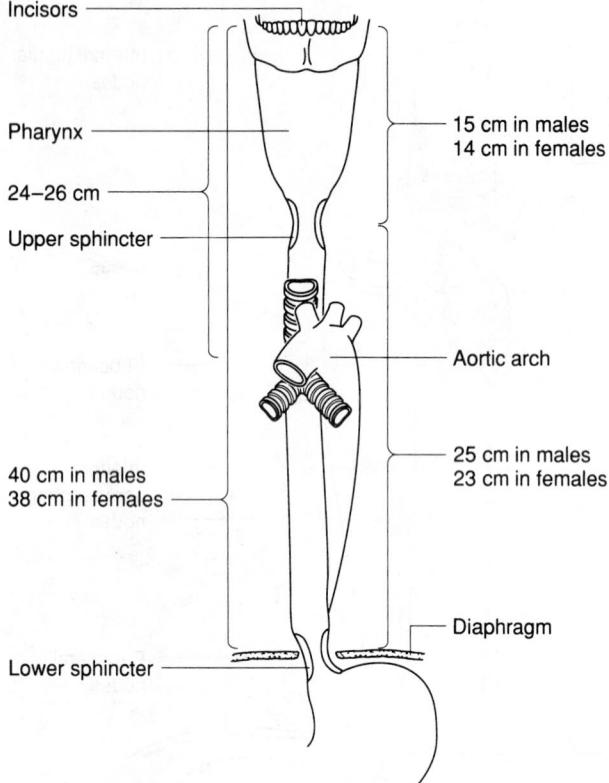

Figure 18-6. Important clinical endoscopic measurements of the esophagus in adults.

rowing that closes when the patient is asked to sniff), the level of the anatomic gastroesophageal junction (identified as the place where the stomach, with vertically running rugae, becomes the tubular esophagus, with smooth mucosa), and the level of the squamocolumnar junction (Z-line). A hiatal hernia is present when the gastroesophageal junction is more than 2 cm above the crura. Barrett's esophagus is suggested when the squamocolumnar junction is more than 2 cm above the gastroesophageal junction, but this may be diagnosed if any specialized epithelium (ie, intestinal type, containing goblet cells) is identified above the gastroesophageal junction histologically, regardless of the measured length of the columnar segment.[3] Esophagitis is recognized by the presence of redness, linear erosions, or ulceration of the mucosa and is generally classified on a graded scale of severity, such as the Savary-Miller classification (Table 18-1). The most recent modification of this classification recognizes that Barrett's mucosa can coexist with any degree of esophagitis.[4]

Barium Studies

A barium esophagogram complements endoscopy in providing both structural and functional information, especially when the entire examination is recorded on videotape. The esophagus begins as a continuation of the pharynx, the transition occurring at the lower border of the sixth cervical vertebra (Fig. 18-7). Topographically, this corresponds to the cricoid cartilage anteriorly and the transverse processes of the sixth cervical vertebra, which can be palpated laterally. The esophagus ends at the cardia of the stomach at the level of the 11th thoracic vertebra. The esophagus is relatively fixed at its upper and lower ends, and during swallowing, these points of fixation move

1 to 2 cm cranially. Three areas of esophageal narrowing are noted on both barium esophagogram and endoscopy (Fig. 18-8). The first narrowing is at the site of the cricopharyngeus muscle, which often causes difficulty in introducing a rigid esophagoscope, and is consequently the most common site of endoscopic perforation. The left main bronchus and aortic arch cause narrowing of the middle third of the esophagus. The most distal narrowing of the esophagus is at the diaphragmatic hiatus and is caused by the LES mechanism. These normal points of narrowing tend to retard swallowed foreign objects. Also, corrosive liquid ingestion results in prominent mucosal injury at these sites since the liquid is slowed in passage.

The pharyngoesophageal region is evaluated in the upright position. Movement of the hyoid and larynx, epiglottis, soft palate, and tongue are easily identified, and their relation to cricopharyngeal opening determined. Aspiration, if observed, can be timed and residual barium remaining after a swallow identified. Esophageal body peristalsis is studied with the patient in the horizontal–prone–oblique position. A swallowed bolus normally generates a stripping wave (primary peristalsis), which clears the bolus completely. Residual material may stimulate a secondary peristaltic wave in the absence of a swallow. Motility disorders characterized by disorganized activity with simultaneous contractions give rise to tertiary waves, often with a segmented appearance to the barium column, sometimes described as a "rosary beading" or "corkscrew" appearance. A hiatal hernia, best seen with the patient in the horizontal position, may be found to be reducible in the upright position. Barium studies are of little value in detecting reflux unless spontaneous reflux is observed in the upright position.

Computed Tomography

Computed tomographic scanning of the esophagus is important in delineating the relation of esophageal lesions to adjacent structures, especially the trachea, left main bronchus, and aorta. The esophagus normally appears as a flattened hollow structure with a thin wall (Figs. 18-9 and 18-10). A more circular cross-sectional appearance with a fluid level is evidence of distal obstruction. The computed tomographic scan gives important information in staging esophageal tumors because it can demonstrate involvement of adjacent structures (eg, the trachea), involvement of lymph nodes, and distant metastases.

PHYSIOLOGY

Although the gastrointestinal tract is a continuous hollow tube with similar structural features, its different functions related to ingestion, digestion, absorption of chemical energy, and elimination of residue are performed

---

Table 18-1. **SAVARY-MILLER CLASSIFICATION OF REFLUX ESOPHAGITIS**

Grade	Description
1	Single or multiple erosions on a single fold: erosions may be erythematous or exudative
2	Multiple erosions affecting multiple folds: erosions may be confluent
3	Multiple circumferential erosions
4	Ulcer, stenosis, or esophageal shortening
5	Barrett's epithelium; columnar metaplasia in the form of noncircular (islands or tongues) or circular extensions

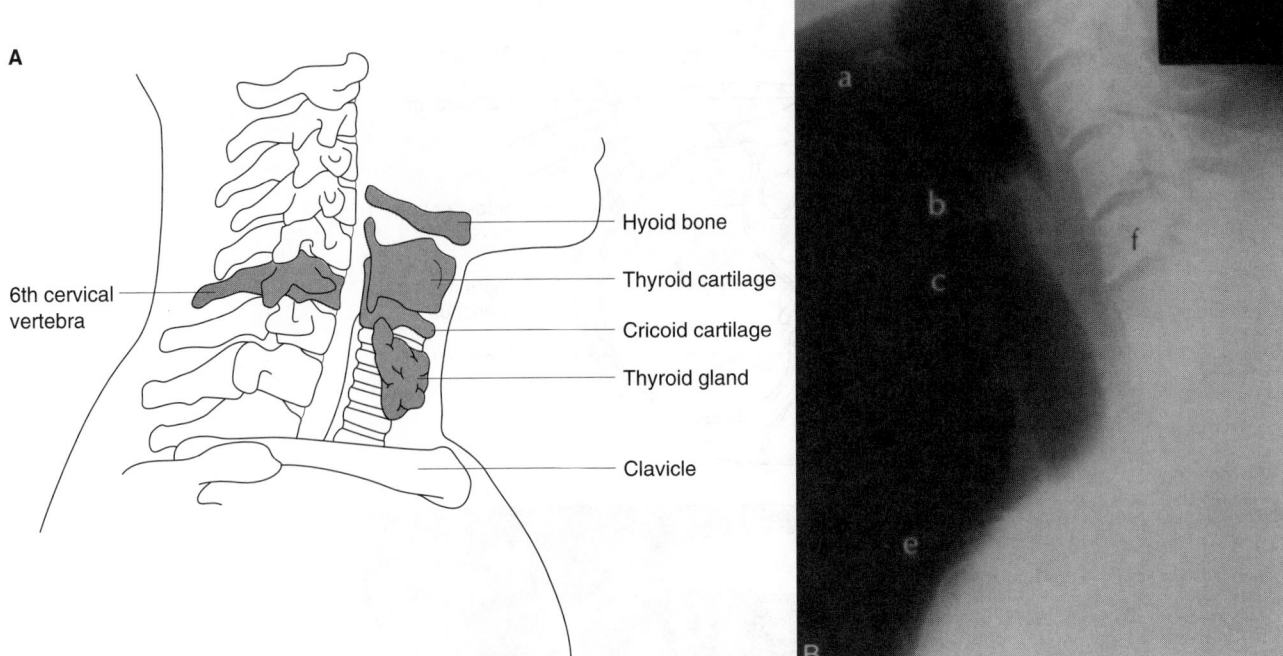

Figure 18-7. (*A*) Topographic relations of the cervical esophagus. (*B*) The corresponding lateral radiographic appearance: a, hyoid bone; b, thyroid cartilage; c, cricoid cartilage; e, sternomanubrial joint; f, C-6.

separately in different compartments (Fig. 18-11). Common to each compartment is the presence of a sphincter to separate it from adjacent compartments, a pumping mechanism to propel contents into the next most distal compartment, and the ability to maintain a distinct chemical and metabolic environment appropriate to its function. The motor activity of each functional compartment generally has three components: a pump, a valve, and a receptacle (reservoir). Proximally, the pharynx functions as a pump, the upper esophageal sphincter (UES) and soft palate and epiglottis as the valve, and the upper esophagus as the receptacle. The distal esophagus is characterized by higher amplitude contractility and pumps food through the valve (the LES) into the proximal stomach, which acts as a reservoir. The distal antrum behaves as a pump, propelling chyme through a valve (the pylorus) into the duodenum. Similarly, the small intestine pumps its contents through the ileocecal valve into a capacitance organ, the cecum. Throughout the smooth muscle portion of the gastrointestinal tract, the valves are not one-way flap valves,

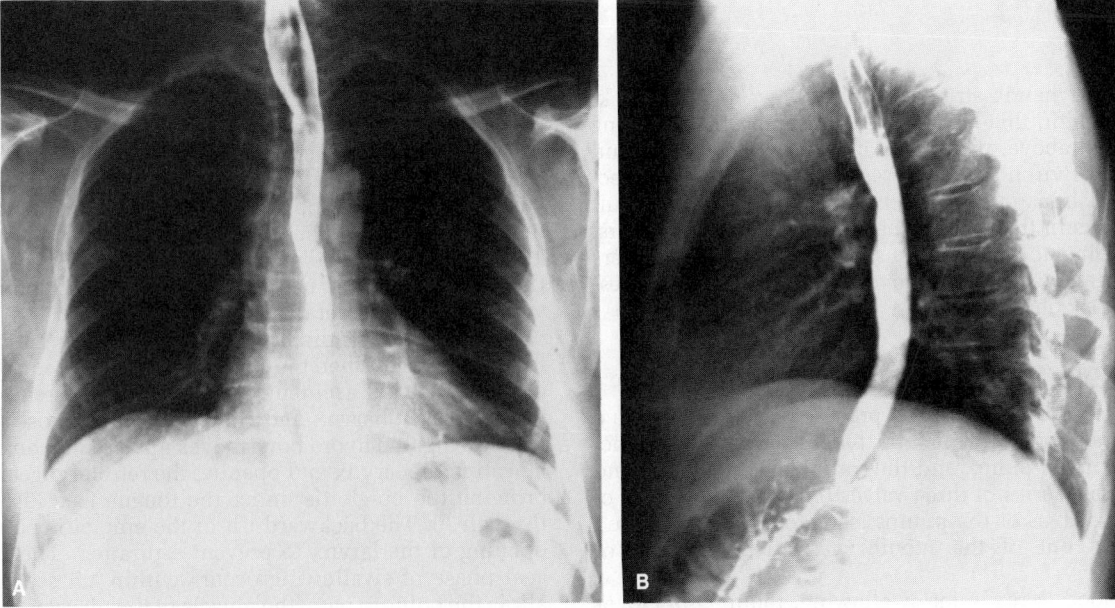

Figure 18-8. Barium esophagogram. (*A*) Anteroposterior view. (*B*) Lateral view.

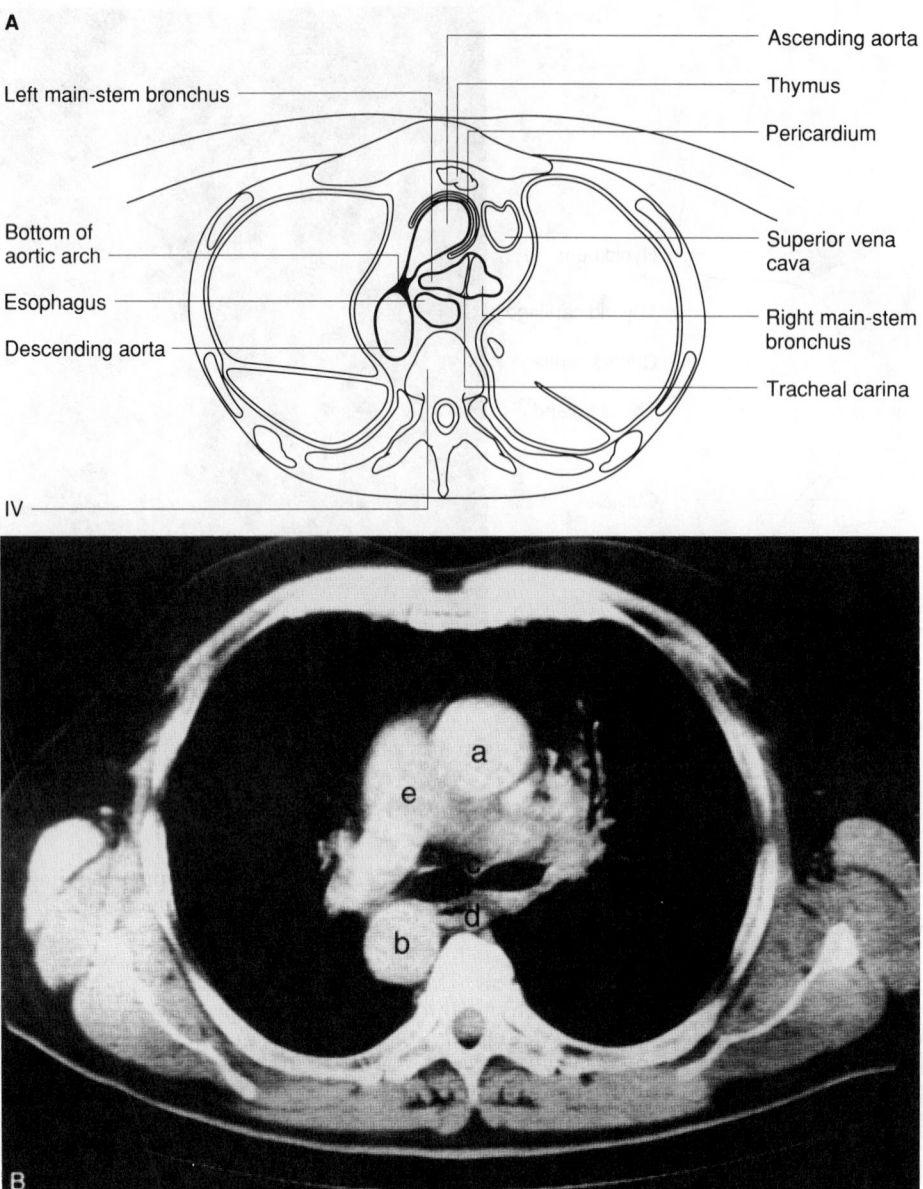

A

Left main-stem bronchus

Bottom of aortic arch

Esophagus

Descending aorta

IV

Ascending aorta

Thymus

Pericardium

Superior vena cava

Right main-stem bronchus

Tracheal carina

B

Figure 18-9. (A) Cross section of the thorax at the level of the tracheal bifurcation viewed from above. IV, T-4. (B) CT appearance viewed from above. a, ascending aorta; b, descending aorta; c, carina; d, esophagus; e, pulmonary artery.

but rather dynamic structures that allow episodic backflow. In health, this backflow is limited by the pumping action from above, thus maintaining the unique pH and enzymatic environment. In disease, however, both ineffective aboral transport and pathologic backflow can result from defects in the pumps, the valves, and the reservoirs. When applied to the esophagus, this general schema offers a simple framework for understanding the diverse manifestations of esophageal disease.

Pharyngoesophageal Segment

It is useful to visualize the process of swallowing as a mechanical model in which the tongue and pharynx function as a piston pump, and the soft palate, epiglottis, and UES act as a series of three valves (Fig. 18-12). Failure of either the valves or the pumps leads to difficulty in food propulsion out of the mouth, nasal regurgitation, or aspiration.

When food is ready for swallowing, the tongue moves the bolus into the posterior oropharynx and forces it into the hypopharynx (see Fig. 18-12A through D). Immobility of the tongue from scarring secondary to radiation or chemical burns or from paresis due to neuromuscular disease can produce great difficulty in the pharyngeal phase of swallowing. As the tongue's contact with the hard palate moves posteriorly, the soft palate is elevated (see Fig. 18-12C through H), thereby closing the passage between the oropharynx and nasopharynx. This partitioning prevents pressure generated in the oropharynx from being dissipated through the nose. This pressure is normally at least 60 mmHg. When the soft palate is paralyzed, as after a cerebral vascular accident, food is commonly regurgitated into the nasopharynx and comes out of the nose. During swallowing, the hyoid bone moves upward and anteriorly, elevating the larynx and opening the retrolaryngeal space, bringing the epiglottis under the tongue (see Fig. 18-12I through P). The backward tilt of the epiglottis covers the opening of the larynx to prevent aspiration. The pharyngeal phase of swallowing occurs within 1.5 seconds. To allow the bolus to pass, the muscle of the pharyngoesophageal segment must be compliant. Reduction in compliance

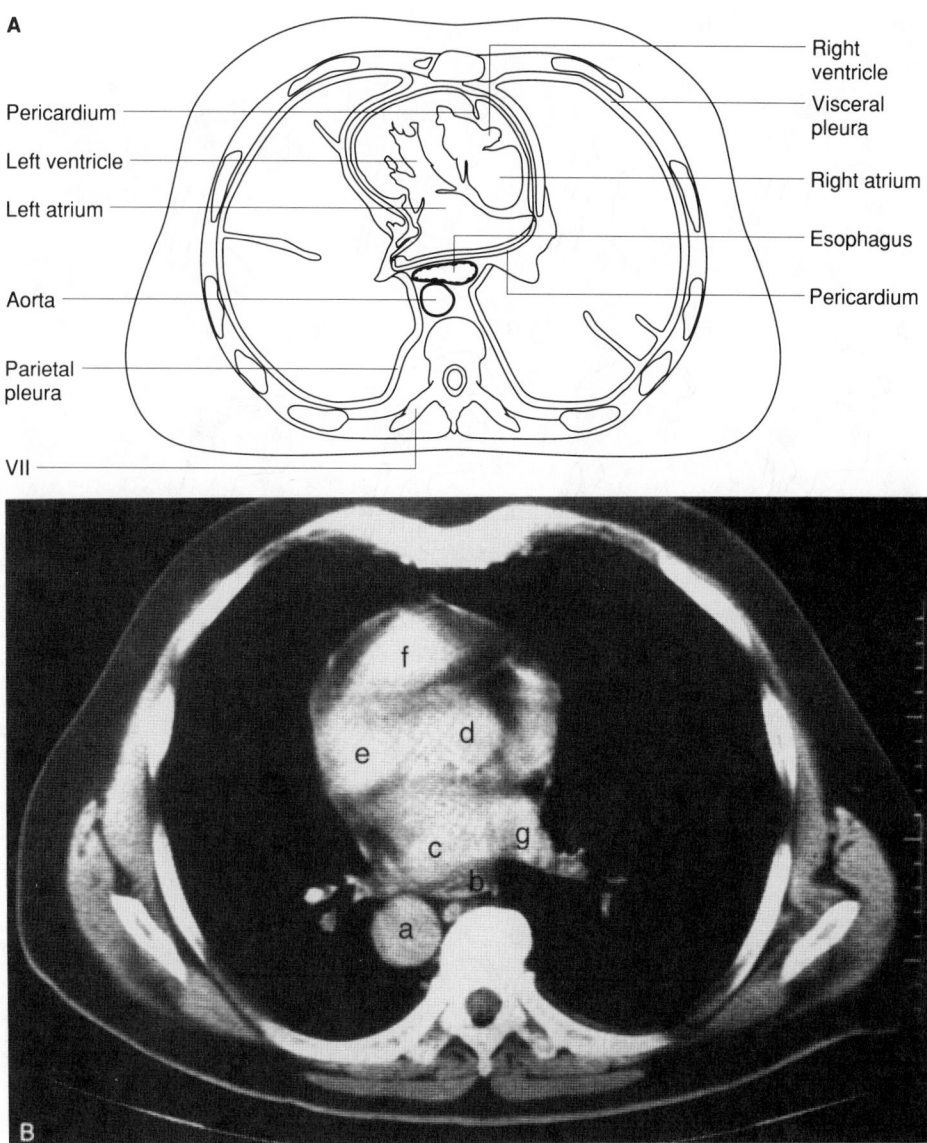

Figure 18-10. (*A*) Cross section of the thorax at mid-atrial level viewed from above. VII, T-7. (*B*) CT appearance viewed from above. a, aorta; b, esophagus; c, left atrium; d, right atrium; e, left ventricle; f, right ventricle; g, pulmonary vein.

leads to increased resistance to emptying of the pharynx. In stroke patients, loss of compliance results from denervation of the skeletal muscle and subsequent fibrosis.

Esophageal Body

The pressure gradient across the UES is accentuated by the subatmospheric environment of the cervical esophagus. Intraesophageal pressure becomes increasingly negative until the mid-esophagus is reached. Thereafter, bolus transport by peristalsis must overcome a pressure gradient

and propel the bolus into the positive-pressure environment of the stomach (Fig. 18-13). The peristaltic wave generates an occlusive pressure varying from 30 to 120 mmHg, and its amplitude increases from the mid-esophagus to the cardia (Fig. 18-14). It travels down the esophagus at 2 to 4 cm/s and reaches the distal esophagus about 7 seconds after swallowing starts. A velocity of 20 cm/s or greater is defined as a simultaneous wave, although waves at speeds of 7 to 10 cm/s are of no propulsive value.

To be effective, peristaltic contractions must be both of sufficient amplitude to generate an occlusive contraction

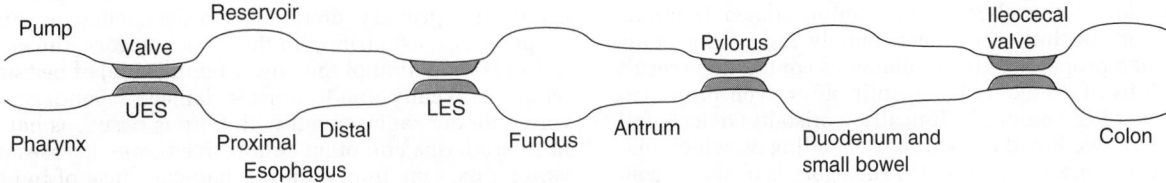

Figure 18-11. Schematic representation of different functional units of the gastrointestinal tract. LES, lower esophageal sphincter; UES, upper esophageal sphincter.

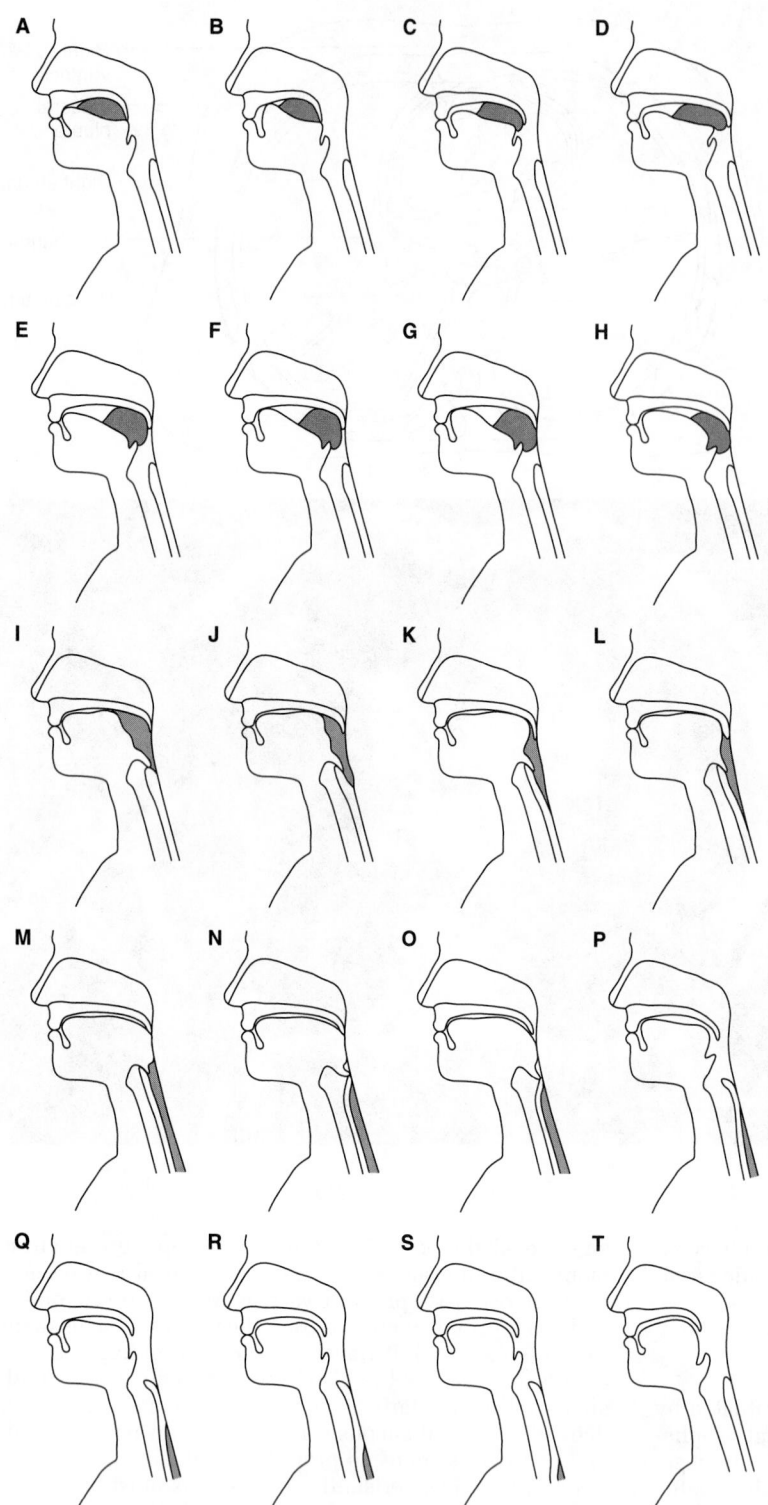

Figure 18-12. Sequence of events during the pharyngeal phase of swallowing, showing the action of the tongue coordinated with the movement of soft palate, larynx and epiglottis during a swallow. (Davenport HR. Physiology of the digestive tract, ed 5. Chicago, Yearbook, 1982:37)

and sufficiently organized for the wave of contraction to propel a food bolus aborally. Low-amplitude contractions that do not occlude the lumen merely indent the bolus rather than propel it, and simultaneous contractions result in portions of the bolus being split off or even propelled back toward the mouth.[5] Clinically, peristaltic defects fall into one of two broad categories, depending on which major feature is most impaired. One category is characterized by defect in organization of peristaltic waves and is primarily a neural phenomenon. This is recognized by the presence of simultaneous waves on motility studies and is typical of the primary motility disorders, such as diffuse esophageal spasm (DES). In the other category, the notable defect is reduction of the power (amplitude) of peristalsis, which is usually due to muscle damage secondary to severe reflux or replacement with fibrous tissue, as happens in scleroderma and other connective tissue diseases or severe reflux. One important mechanical cause of impaired motility occurs when the esophagus is not anchored at its distal end. Loss of this inferior anchor occurs with a large

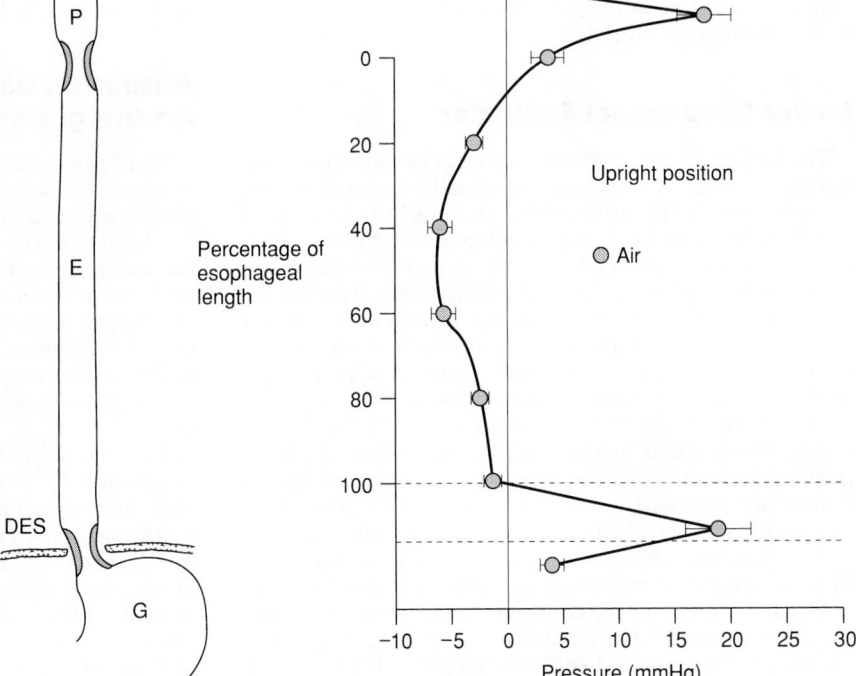

Figure 18-13. Resting pressure profile the foregut showing the atmospheric pressure in the pharynx (P), the subatmospheric mid-esophageal pressure (E), and the superatmospheric intragastric pressure (G), with the interposed high-pressure zones of the upper and lower esophageal sphincters. DES, lower esophageal sphincter. (After Waters PF, DeMeester TR. Foregut motor disorders and their surgical management. Med Clin North Am 1981;65:1237)

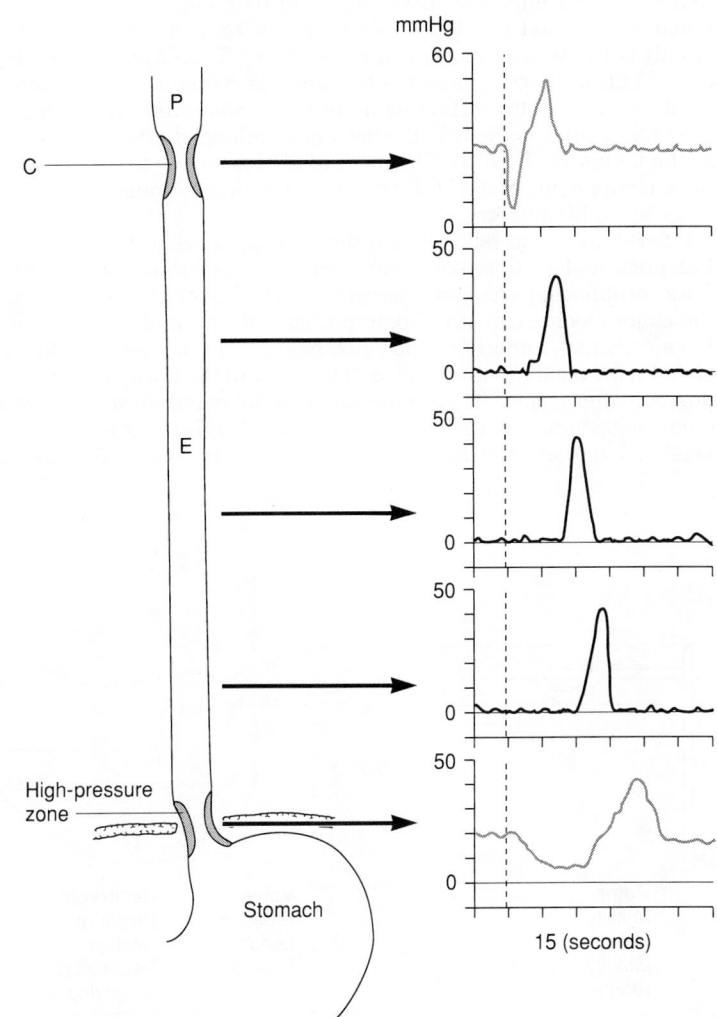

Figure 18-14. Intraluminal esophageal pressure changes in response to swallowing. (After Waters PF, DeMeester TR. Foregut motor disorders and their surgical management. Med Clin North Am 1981;65:1238)

sliding hiatal hernia; it sometimes produces a "concertina" appearance of the esophagus on roentgenography and can lead to inefficient propulsion.

Lower Esophageal Sphincter

The LES provides a pressure barrier between the esophagus and stomach. The sphincter normally remains actively closed to prevent reflux of gastric contents into the esophagus. Relaxation of the LES is mediated by inhibitory neurons. It occurs either to allow entry of food or to allow exit of air during belching. The LES relaxes shortly after the initiation of a swallow. Incomplete relaxation is characteristic of achalasia and after excessively tight or improperly constructed fundoplication, and contributes to the patient's dysphagia in both these situations.

The ability of the LES to remain closed in the face of a pressure gradient tending to promote reflux of gastric contents from the positive-pressure environment of the abdomen into the negative-pressure environment of the chest depends on several features. The most significant is the *resting pressure*. Of equal importance is the ability of the LES to respond to variations in intraabdominal pressure associated with daily activities. These elevations normally are transmitted to the sphincter, causing it to collapse and remain closed, provided sufficient length of the sphincter remains exposed to abdominal pressure and the compressive effect of the crura. This *abdominal length* is often reduced in hiatal herniation because of attenuation of the phrenoesophageal membrane.[6] The *overall length* of the LES is also an important determinant of its competence, much as the total resistance of a series of resistors in a circuit is the sum of individual resistances.[7] This feature of the LES protects against the tendency to reflux after a meal because gastric filling tends to cause shortening of the LES, similar to the way the neck of a balloon shortens as the balloon is inflated. The method of measuring these three components of the LES is discussed under Stationary Esophageal Manometry.

Gastric juice also refluxes into the esophagus when the LES pressure falls to zero for short periods. These *transient lower esophageal sphincter relaxations* are thought to be the major mechanism of reflux in normal subjects and are the mechanism underlying the belch reflex. They are associated with vagal function and tend to occur in the upright position after meals.[8] Their importance in the pathophysiology of gastroesophageal reflux disease (GERD) is controversial, but they are likely to be important in patients whose manometric sphincter characteristics are normal, and this tends to be the case in early disease.

Antireflux Barrier: An Integrated Concept

Protection against reflux of gastric juice depends on the integrated effect of the LES, the esophageal body, and the gastric reservoir (Fig. 18-15). The competence of the LES is related to the resting pressure, the abdominal length, and the overall length, as discussed earlier. A mechanically defective sphincter is not always associated with increased esophageal acid exposure because it may be compensated by the clearance function of the esophageal body. Abnormalities of the esophageal body and the stomach contribute to the development and progression of GERD, discussed next.

The role of the *esophageal body* in limiting acid reflux is related to its ability to clear the esophagus of acid. Clearance has two components: volume clearance, which requires peristalsis; and chemical clearance, which requires saliva. After a reflux episode, the bulk of the acid is cleared by an oncoming peristaltic wave. Small residual amounts of acid on the mucosal surface are neutralized by saliva. Defective contractility and defective saliva production both tend to increase esophageal acid exposure. Clearance is aided by gravity and is thus more impaired in the recumbent position. Clearance is also impaired in hiatal herniation, when loss of fixation of the gastroesophageal junction leads to refluxing of gastric acid from the supradiaphragmatic pouch of stomach into the esophageal body.

Abnormalities of the *gastric reservoir* that predispose to gastroesophageal reflux include gastric dilation, increased intragastric pressure, persistent gastric reservoir, and increased gastric acid secretion. The effect of *gastric dilation* is to shorten the overall length of the LES, resulting in a decrease in the sphincter resistance to reflux. It most commonly results from aerophagia, which may be due to an unconscious increase in swallowing in an effort to improve esophageal clearance. Each swallow results in the propulsion of 1 to 2 mL of air into the stomach. This accounts for the symptom of bloating often seen in these patients. *Increased intragastric pressure* occurs because of loss of active relaxation as the stomach fills; it occurs after vagotomy or in diabetic gastroparesis. A *persistent gastric reservoir* results from delay in gastric emptying. It is caused by myogenic abnormalities, such as gastric atony in advanced diabetes, diffuse neuromuscular disorders,

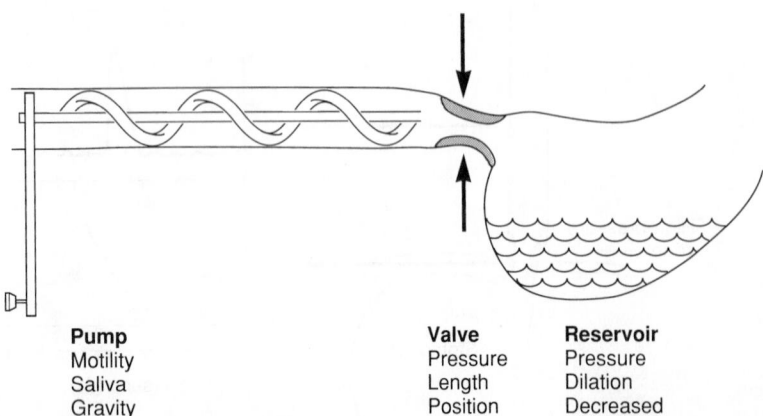

Pump	Valve	Reservoir
Motility	Pressure	Pressure
Saliva	Length	Dilation
Gravity	Position	Decreased
Anatomy		emptying
		Secretion

Figure 18-15. Mechanical model of the antireflux mechanism showing the esophageal body acting as a pump, the lower esophageal sphincter as a valve, and the stomach as a reservoir. (After DeMeester TR, Attwood SE. Gastroesophageal reflux disease, hiatus hernia, achalasia of the esophagus in spontaneous rupture. In: Schwartz SI, Ellis H. eds. Maingot's abdominal operations, vol 1, ed 9. Norwalk, CT, Appleton-Century-Crofts, 1989:514)

anticholinergic medications, and postviral infections. Nonmyogenic causes are vagotomy, antropyloric dysfunction, and duodenal dysmotility. *Gastric hypersecretion* can increase esophageal exposure to gastric acid juice by accentuation of physiologic reflux of acid. This may be due either to increased concentration of acid or increased resting volume of gastric secretions.

In a patient with a normal esophageal body and LES, the underlying cause for excessive gastroesophageal reflux is likely to be an abnormality of gastric function.

INVESTIGATION OF FUNCTIONAL ABNORMALITIES

Fundamental to understanding disorders of esophageal function are assessment of the contractility of the esophageal body and sphincters and measurement of esophageal acid exposure. These key investigations form the basis for rational therapy in most benign esophageal diseases.

Stationary Esophageal Manometry

Stationary esophageal manometry is an investigative tool in which a catheter containing pressure sensors is inserted into the esophagus to measure pressures in the esophageal body and sphincters at rest and in response to swallowing. It is indicated in the following clinical situations:

Nonobstructive dysphagia: Patients with dysphagia in whom a structural (mechanical) cause has not been identified by endoscopy or esophagogram are likely to have a motility disorder, which can be detected only by manometry.

Noncardiac chest pain: Retrosternal chest pain in the absence of coronary artery disease is a frequent cause of morbidity and anxiety. Every year, it is estimated that 180,000 patients with central chest pain are found to have negative coronary angiography. Of these, 20% to 40% have a motility abnormality.

Gastroesophageal reflux disease: The indications for manometry in patients with suspected GERD are chiefly to assess the status of the LES and to identify a motility disorder of the esophageal body. A defective sphincter is predictive of a poor long-term response to medical therapy but of a good response to surgery. The presence of a motility defect profoundly alters the operative strategy in patients with GERD and should always be excluded by manometry before operative therapy.

Manometry is also known to be the most accurate way of locating the LES before placement of a pH electrode for 24-hour pH monitoring in patients suspected of having GERD. Finally, postoperative manometry objectively assesses if the goal of the operation has been attained and encourages the surgeon to modify the technique in light of the results.

The test is performed by passing the lubricated manometric catheter through the anesthetized nostril into the pharynx. The neck is then flexed, and the patient takes a swallow of water as the catheter is advanced through the relaxed cricopharyngeal sphincter into the esophagus. It is further advanced until all recording ports are in the stomach. A manometric study consists of four components, described in the following sections.

Assessment of the LES. As the catheter is slowly withdrawn in 1-cm increments, the high-pressure zone of the LES is reached by the uppermost transducer. The lower (distal) border of the LES is the point where the resting pressure rises above gastric baseline, and the upper border

the point where it reaches esophageal baseline. Between these two points is the respiratory inversion point (RIP), where the positive deflections with inspiration change to negative deflections, the functional division between the abdomen and chest. Three components of the LES are measured:

1. The *resting pressure* is the pressure above gastric baseline measured in mid-respiration at the RIP. The pressures in the high-pressure zone are a combination of the intrinsic pressure of the LES, the applied pressure of the intraabdominal environment, and compression by the crura of the diaphragm. Generally, the applied intraabdominal pressure is equal to the intragastric pressure and thus is usually disregarded.
2. The *overall length* of the sphincter is the distance from the distal border to the proximal border.
3. The *abdominal length* is the distance from the distal border of the LES to the RIP and represents the portion of the LES subject to fluctuations in intraabdominal pressure. In hiatal herniation, the diaphragmatic and intrinsic components are sometimes separated rather than superimposed, resulting in a long high-pressure zone described as a double hump. The effect of applied intraabdominal pressure is negated if the abdominal length is too short.

These features are illustrated in the tracing in Figure 18-16. The values for each of these components from each transducer are expressed as an average. The lower limits of normal (fifth percentile) are a resting pressure of less than 6 mmHg, an overall length of less than 2 cm, or an abdominal length of less than 1 cm. If any one component is below normal, the sphincter is mechanically defective. A defect in one or even two components of the LES may be compensated by good esophageal body function, but when all three components are defective, excessive esophageal acid exposure is almost inevitable.[9]

All the pressures measured along the length of the sphincter and around its circumference during the pull-through may be treated as vectors having both magnitude and direction, and hence integrated into a three-dimensional image, the volume (vector volume) of which is a measure of LES resistance (Fig. 18-17). A vector volume below the fifth percentile of normal is a more sensitive measure of mechanical deficiency of the LES than the parameters described earlier. The prevalence of a defective LES increases with increasing severity of GERD; it is lowest in patients without evidence of endoscopic injury and highest in patients with stricture or Barrett's esophagus.[10]

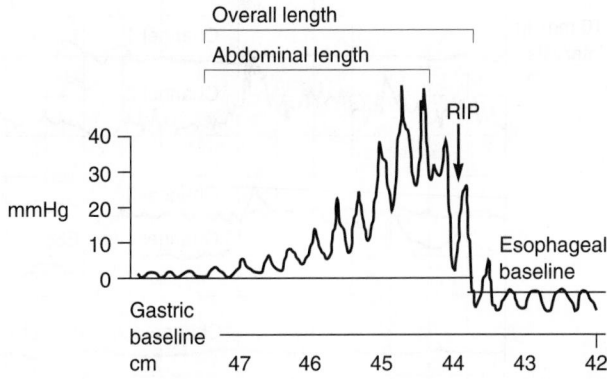

Figure 18-16. Manometric tracing as a transducer is pulled across the lower esophageal sphincter, showing the pressure, overall length, and abdominal length. RIP, respiratory inversion point.

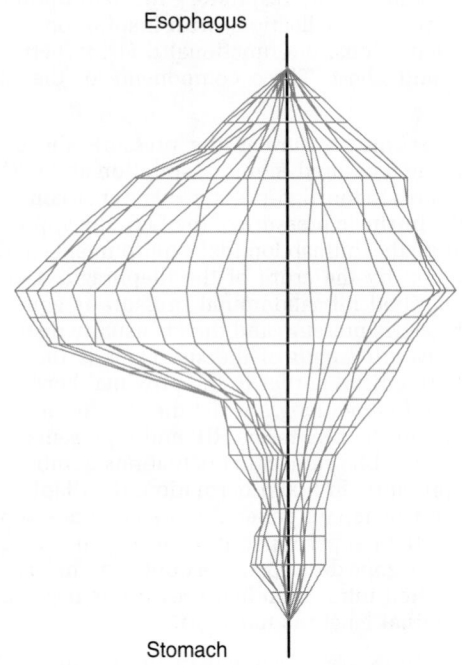

Figure 18-17. Three-dimensional representation of the lower esophageal sphincter.

Measurement of LES Relaxation.   The catheter is positioned with a transducer in the LES, and a series of swallows are obtained by giving 5-mL boluses of water. The LES pressure normally drops to gastric baseline immediately after the swallow, before the oncoming peristaltic wave reaches the lower esophagus (Fig. 18-18).

Esophageal Body Manometry.   After the LES study, the catheter is positioned so that the transducers span the length of the esophageal body, and the peristaltic response to 10 swallows of 5 mL of water is measured. The features of individual contractions are the amplitude, duration, slope, and morphology (ie, whether single, double, or triple peaked). Transmission of waves from one level to the next is assessed by the speed of wave propagation and by noting any interruption of wave progression. Most commercially available manometric systems automatically measure these features and relate the results to those of normal subjects (Fig. 18-19).

Assessment of the UES.   The position, length, and resting pressure of the UES and its relaxation with swallowing are assessed with a technique similar to that for the LES. The key features to be assessed are the adequacy of pharyngeal contraction and the timing and extent of UES relaxation. An indirect measure of UES stiffness or loss of compliance is the intrabolus pressure, which appears as a small, separate prepharyngeal wave, or a shoulder on the upstroke of the pharyngeal contraction wave.[11]

Measurement of Esophageal Acid Exposure: 24-Hour pH Monitoring

The development of 24-hour pH monitoring was a major advance in unraveling the pathophysiology of GERD. All previous tests had relied on the production of reflux by some kind of provocative maneuver, which often had little relevance to the patient's daily activities. The 24-hour pH monitoring has made it possible to quantify the degree of reflux in normal subjects and to categorize different patterns of reflux in patients with GERD.

Indications

Although 24-hour pH monitoring logically precedes manometry in the work-up of suspected GERD, it is usually performed after the LES has been located by manometry. It is the principal method in the diagnosis of GERD and has effectively replaced all other methods of measuring esophageal acid exposure. It is indicated in any patient with symptoms suggestive of GERD, unless the symptoms

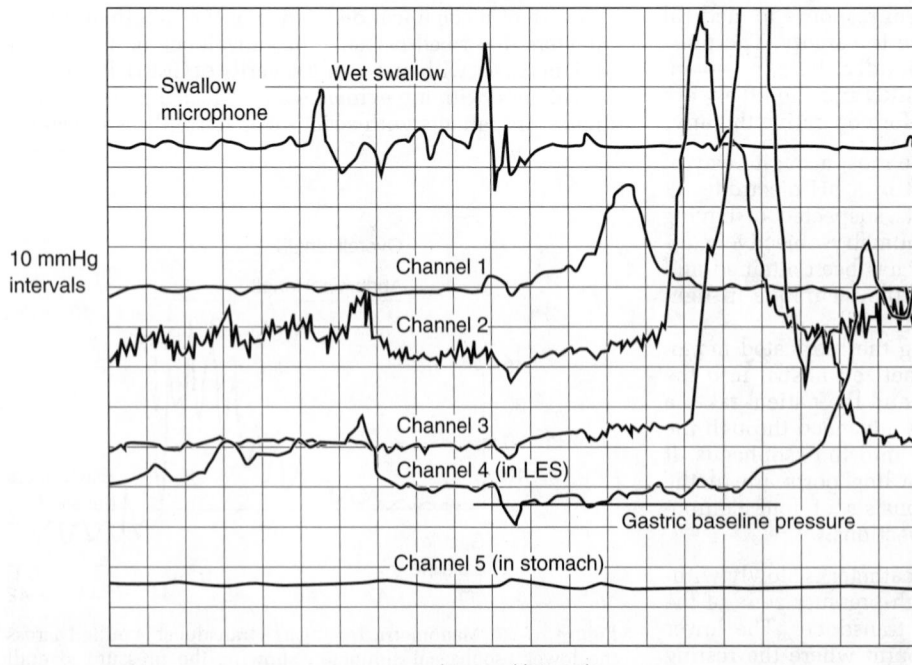

Figure 18-18. Relaxation of the lower esophageal sphincter (LES) in response to a swallow.

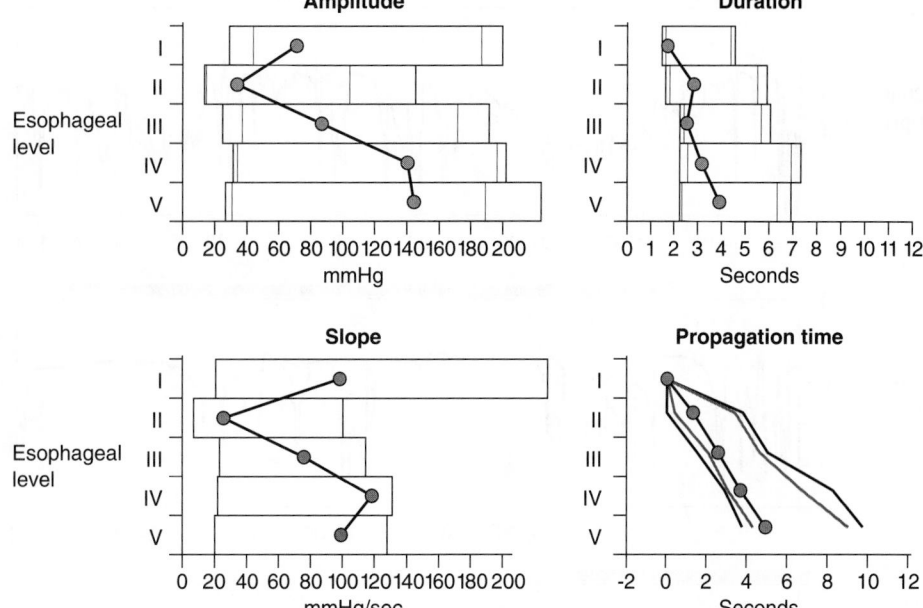

Figure 18-19. Typical results from esophageal body obtained during stationary manometry in a normal subject. Analysis is based on mean values from 10 swallows of 5 mL water. The five boxes represent values from each of the five transducers spanning the length of the esophageal body from above downward. The line represents the patient's values. The outer lines of the boxes show the 5th and 95th percentiles of normal, and the inner dotted lines represent the 10th and 90th percentiles.

are trivial or permanently abolished by a 12-week course of acid-suppression therapy. The need for continued acid suppression should stimulate objective study. This is especially important in patients who are being considered for antireflux repair. Atypical presentations of GERD are also common. They include noncardiac chest pain (after a negative cardiac evaluation) and several respiratory conditions, especially adult-onset asthma, aspiration, nocturnal wheezing, and chronic laryngitis. In children, persistent neonatal vomiting, apparent life-threatening events, and failure to thrive may all be due to reflux. Twenty-four hour pH monitoring in such patients allows the opportunity to confirm or refute the diagnosis of GERD and to relate the patient's symptoms during the monitored period to episodes of reflux.[12]

Twenty-four–hour esophageal pH monitoring is simply a measure of esophageal acid exposure, and an abnormal test should not be equated with the presence of GERD. Rather, it should stimulate a search for the cause of the excessive acid exposure.

Technique

Medications such as H_2 blockers and prokinetics should be discontinued for 48 hours before the procedure. Omeprazole can produce prolonged acid suppression and should be stopped for 2 weeks before pH monitoring. Glass pH electrodes are more accurate than antimony electrodes, especially for pH 6.0 to 7.0. All pH probes should be calibrated before and after the test in buffer solutions at pH 1.0 and 7.0, and the drift in pH must be within of 0.2 units of the standard for accurate interpretation of the results. In adults, the pH probe is placed 5 cm above the manometrically determined upper border of the LES. The catheter is taped to the nostril and looped behind the ear to maintain a stable position with minimal patient discomfort. The pH values are recorded by a digital storage device strapped to the patient's side. The patient returns home and is instructed to carry out normal daily activities but to avoid strenuous exertion. During the day, the patient should remain in the upright position and follow the prescribed diet,

which includes a wide range of foods with a pH of 5.0 to 7.0. Smoking and alcohol consumption are prohibited during the test. The patient notes in a diary the times of meals, retiring for sleep, and rising the following morning as well as the presence and duration of any symptoms.

Interpretation

Reflux episodes are defined as periods when the esophageal pH is less than 4.0. Normal (physiologic) reflux occurs in the form of short, rapidly cleared postprandial episodes. Abnormal esophageal acid exposure can be defined as that exceeding the 95th percentile of healthy subjects. A typical tracing of a patient with excessive reflux is shown in Figure 18-20.

A few episodes of long duration are more injurious than many brief episodes, even though the total acid exposure time may be similar. Thus, a composite scoring system has been derived that integrates several different features of the pH record into a single measurement of esophageal acid exposure. The score is calculated from the six parameters shown in Table 18-2 and is produced by most commercially available computer software packages. When measured in the this way, esophageal acid exposure in normal subjects is independent of nationality or dietary habits, and when the composite score is used, it is also independent of gender. In addition to quantifying the actual time the esophageal mucosa is exposed to gastric acid, it gives a measure of the ability of the esophagus to clear refluxed acid and correlates esophageal acid exposure with the patient's symptoms.

In addition to the measurement of acid exposure, pH monitoring can also be used to detect excessive alkaline exposure (pH higher than 7.0) in the esophagus. This is important clinically because it may be an indirect indication that the refluxing gastric juice is mixed with duodenal contents. A more direct measure of duodenogastric reflux (DGR) is available using the bile probe (see later). Evidence is emerging that components of bile and duodenal juice are important in the pathogenesis of Barrett's esophagus and its complications.[13]

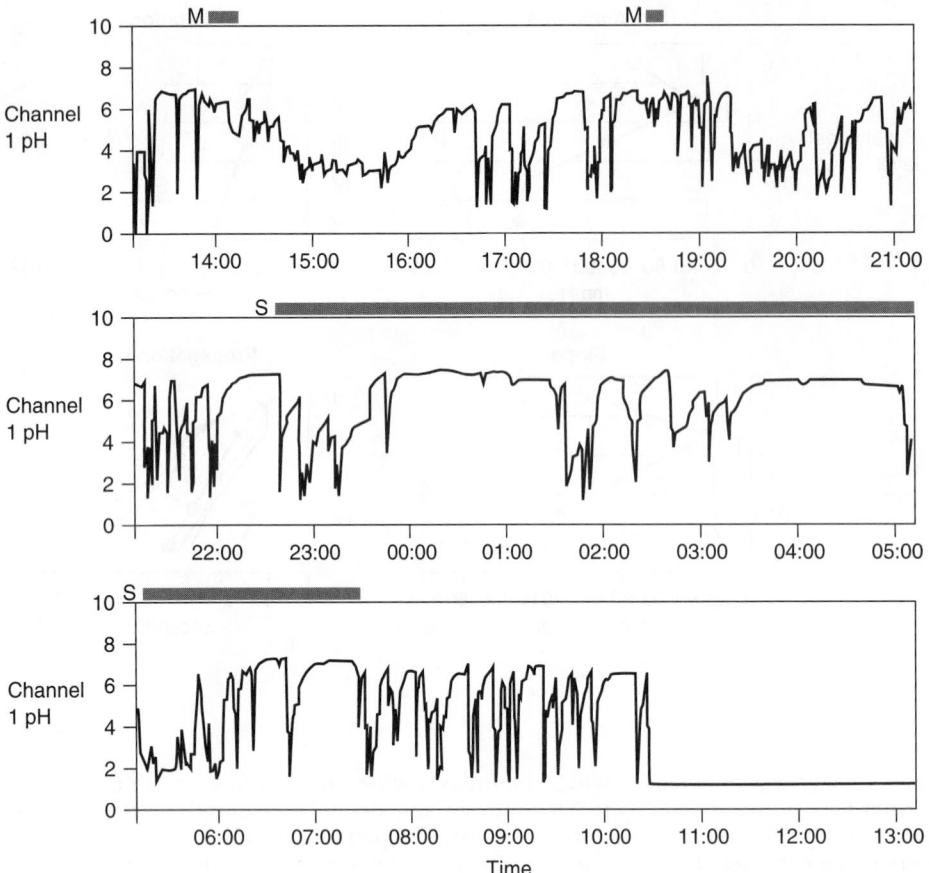

Figure 18-20. Typical 24-hour esophageal pH record from a patient with both upright and supine reflux. Each of the three panels represents an 8-hour period. Note frequent and prolonged drops in esophageal pH to less than 4.0. M, meal period; S, supine period.

Additional Tests for the Investigation of Esophageal Disease

Dual Esophageal pH Monitoring

Investigation of patients who have respiratory symptoms such as nocturnal cough, wheeze, asthma, or recurrent pneumonia may include pH monitoring of both proximal and distal esophagus. Two pH electrodes are positioned in the esophagus, one 5 cm above the upper border of the LES and the other 1 cm below the lower border of the UES. A key feature of this test is the correlation between reflux episodes and subsequent respiratory symptoms experienced by the patient. If a clear relation can be established, and there is no motility defect in the esophagus, then abolition of reflux by surgery should be followed by good symptomatic relief.

Provocative Testing

In the standard acid reflux test, the stomach is loaded with HCl, and reflux in response to various straining maneuvers is detected by an esophageal pH probe. This test still has a place in patients with hypochlorhydria and a history suggestive of GERD.

The Bernstein test, in which hydrochloric acid is dripped into the esophagus through a nasogastric tube, is sometimes used to determine whether a patient's symptoms are reproduced by acid exposure. It is basically a measure of esophageal mucosal sensitivity. It has been largely superseded by the use of 24-hour pH monitoring.

The edrophonium test is occasionally performed in patients with central chest pain with a suspected esophageal cause. Although edrophonium often causes marked increases in peristaltic amplitude, the end-point of the test

Table 18-2. VALUES OF 24-HOUR ESOPHAGEAL pH MONITORING IN 50 HEALTHY ADULT VOLUNTEERS FOR pH LESS THAN 4.0

Measures	pH Values					
	Mean	SD	Median	Minimum	Maximum	95th Percentile
Total time pH <4 (%)	1.5	1.4	1.2	0.0	6.0	4.5
Upright time pH <4 (%)	2.2	2.3	1.6	0.0	9.3	8.4
Supine time pH <4 (%)	0.6	1.0	0.1	0.0	4.0	3.5
Episodes	19.0	12.8	16.0	2.0	56.0	46.9
Episodes ≥5 min	0.8	1.2	0.0	0.0	5.0	3.5
Longest episode (min)	6.7	7.9	4.0	0.0	46.0	19.8
Composite score	6.0	4.4	5.0	0.4	18.0	14.7

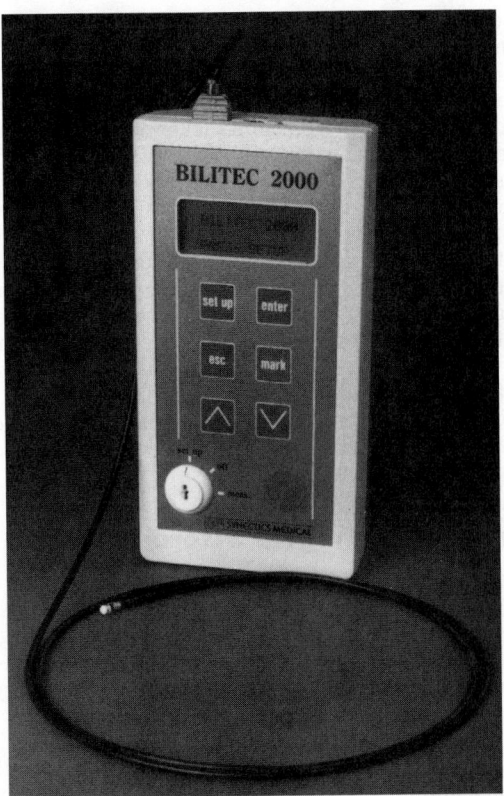

Figure 18-21. The esophageal bile probe system.

is reproduction of the patient's typical symptoms rather than the generation of a specific motility abnormality.

Ambulatory (24-Hour) Esophageal Manometry

The ambulatory esophageal manometry technique assesses esophageal body peristalsis during a 24-hour period. It is performed with a solid-state catheter that has miniature transducers located at three levels in the esophageal body and a proximal sensor situated in the pharynx to flag swallows. The great advantage of ambulatory motility is the ability to record esophageal function during the patient's normal daily activities, especially during meals. It provides a much more comprehensive picture of esophageal function than is possible by stationary manometry. In normal subjects, the esophagus becomes progressively more organized from the supine to the upright to the meal period, a feature that is reflected in the higher prevalence of effective peristaltic waves during meals. Loss of this improved organization of esophageal activity during mealtimes is a subtle sign of motility disorder, and when fewer than half of waves during the meal period are effective and peristaltic, there is a significant correlation with the presence of dysphagia.[14]

Esophageal Bile Probe

The esophageal bile probe is a portable spectrophotometric device capable of continuously detecting the presence of bilirubin during a 24-hour period in the ambulatory setting. A fiberoptic cable is connected to a light source and a digital storage device and is worn on the patient's side (Bilitec 2000; Fig. 18-21). The light source emits light at the wavelength of maximum absorbance of bilirubin (453 nm). The light is transmitted across a 2 mm space to a white Teflon reflector, which reflects the light back to

the probe (Fig. 18-22). The absorbance of light at this wavelength indicates the presence of bilirubin, and the amount of light reflected back to the probe is proportionally reduced. A sentinel beam is also incorporated into the fiberoptic assembly to detect when loss of signal is due to a food particle blocking the reflectance of emitted light. The catheter bearing the bile probe is passed into the esophagus and positioned 5 cm above the upper border of the LES. One potential pitfall is that the yellow colorings in foodstuffs (eg, butter) may give falsely high values, and this type of food should not be consumed during monitoring.[15]

Tests of Gastric Function

The function of the esophageal body and LES are affected by abnormalities in the stomach, as described earlier. The ability to study the stomach has lagged behind that of the esophagus because of the greater complexity of its functions.

Gastric Emptying

Gastric emptying is affected by the composition and consistency of the ingested meal. Protein empties faster than fats, and liquids empty faster than solids. Delayed gastric emptying may be an important etiologic factor in patients with GERD and a normal LES. Mild delay is likely to be corrected by Nissen fundoplication.

Gastric emptying is quantitatively assessed using radionucleide techniques. After ingestion of a labeled meal, anterior and posterior images of the area of interest are obtained by a gamma camera collimator for a period of 60 seconds every 15 minutes. Studies are best performed with patients in the upright position, but the patient must remain still during the entire study. Abnormalities in gastric emptying may be identified when the value is outside the normal range, and are conventionally described as rapid or delayed. More information may be obtained by plotting the patient's emptying curve against the normal values to see if and when the patient falls outside the normal range.

A new technique to evaluate gastric emptying in an ambulatory setting is available. A portable geiger counter is connected to a preamplifier and a digital storage device, which can collect counts for 24 hours. The probe is passed transnasally and positioned in the proximal stomach 5 cm distal to the lower border of the LES. The patient then ingests up to three labeled meals during the ensuing 24 hours. This gives three measurements of gastric emptying and can be used to study the effect of posture, movement, and food composition. In addition, the gastric emptying probe can be combined with gastric pH monitoring or antroduodenal manometry.

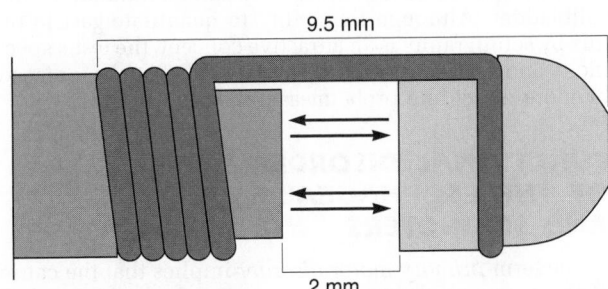

Figure 18-22. Schematic view of the bilirubin sensor. Light is emitted from the probe and passes across a 2-mm space to a Teflon reflector, which reflects the nonabsorbed light back to the probe.

Ambulatory (24-Hour) Gastric pH Monitoring

Gastric pH monitoring can be useful in identifying DGR. Relative gastric alkalinization gives an indirect measure of DGR. The study is conducted similarly to that of esophageal pH monitoring, except that the pH probe is positioned in the fundus 5 cm below the lower border of the LES. More direct evaluation of DGR can be obtained by use of the gastric bile probe (see below).

Gastric Acid Analysis

Gastric acid analysis is the traditional method for diagnosing gastric acid hypersecretion. The analysis is performed after an overnight fast in patients who have been off all antisecretory medications for 48 hours and omeprazole for 2 weeks. The stomach is intubated with a nasogastric tube, and basal acid output is determined by collecting gastric secretions for four 15-minute periods. The maximal acid output is determined by collecting 15-minute aliquots of gastric secretions over a 1-hour period after stimulation of the gastric secretory state with intravenous pentagastrin in doses of 6 μg/kg. The peak acid output is determined by selecting the two consecutive highest stimulated periods. The values obtained are usually expressed as milliequivalents per hour (mEq/h). Hypersecretion is present when basal acid output is more than 5 mEq/h, maximal acid output is more than 20 mEq/h, or peak acid output is more than 35 mEq/h.

Gastric Bile Probe

The gastric bile probe can be used to detect bile in the stomach. The probe is positioned 5 cm below the lower border of the LES. It is a more direct measure of DGR than gastric pH monitoring. Early studies have indicated that gastric exposure to bilirubin (above the absorption threshold of more than 0.2) occurs up to 15% of the time in normal subjects. The technique is promising, and its role in the investigation of patients with suspected DGR is the subject of several ongoing studies.

Antroduodenal Motility Assessment

Antroduodenal motility assessment is the technique used to study the motor function of the antrum and duodenum in response to a meal. Short-term studies (2 to 4 hours) can be performed with water-perfused catheters, but ambulatory studies with solid-state catheters are now possible. Computerized analysis is still being developed, and the method is likely to be valuable for investigation of gastroparesis and postoperative emptying disorders of the stomach.

Cholescintigraphy

Scintigraphic imaging of bile reflux into the stomach can be performed after intravenous injection of 5 mCi of technetium-99m iminodiacetic acid derivatives such as disofenin, followed by cholecystokinin stimulation of the gallbladder. Although the ability to quantitate gastric reflux by scintigraphy is an attractive concept, the test's specificity and sensitivity are low, and it is likely to be replaced by more direct bile probe measurement in future.

FUNCTIONAL DISORDERS OF THE ESOPHAGEAL BODY AND SPHINCTERS

The term *primary motor disorder* implies that the cause of the muscular defect is not known, whereas *secondary motor disorders* are the result of some systemic disease affecting the esophagus. In practice, the most common secondary motor disorder is the hypoperistalsis associated with complicated GERD, but the term usually refers to a systemic connective tissue or neuromuscular disease, such as scleroderma or polymyositis.

There are four identifiable categories of primary motor disorders: achalasia, DES, nutcracker esophagus, and hypertensive LES. A fifth category is termed *nonspecific motor disorder* and includes those patients whose motor function is clearly abnormal but who do not fall into one of the four major categories. These five categories are derived from the manometric features on stationary motility. The advent of ambulatory motility assessment, however, has shown that these categories may not be as distinct as the classification implies. For example, intermediate forms exist. It is nevertheless convenient to use these categories until a broadly based consensus is achieved.

For convenience, all disorders of the pharyngoesophageal phase of swallowing are discussed in this section, although they arise from a variety of causes.

Pharyngoesophageal Disorders

Disorders of the pharyngoesophageal phase of swallowing result from a discoordination of the neuromuscular events involved in chewing, initiation of swallowing, and propulsion of the material from the oropharynx to the cervical esophagus. The most common causes of pharyngoesophageal dysphagia are neuromuscular diseases. The most important are cerebrovascular disease, myasthenia gravis, Parkinson disease, motor neuron disease, multiple sclerosis, and muscular diseases such as myotonic dystrophy and polymyositis. Other important causes are structural lesions, including tumors, Zenker diverticula, and scarring of the tongue or pharynx from caustic injury, previous surgery, or radiotherapy. Rarely, pharyngoesophageal dysphagia is caused by extrinsic compression from goiter or cervical spine osteophytes.

Pathophysiology

All the diseases mentioned earlier produce their effects by disrupting one or more of the components of the pharyngeal mechanism illustrated in Figure 18-23.

Weakness or immobility of the tongue produces difficulty in thrusting the bolus into the oropharynx, thus compromising oropharyngeal transfer. Paralysis of the soft palate prevents the oropharynx from being partitioned off from the nasopharynx, preventing pressurization of the pharynx. This accounts for the frequent occurrence of nasal regurgitation and the nasal quality to the voice in these patients. If the larynx cannot be elevated, there is loss of airway protection, and patients are prone to aspiration. The UES may relax either incompletely, prematurely, or both. If pharyngeal pressure overcomes any residual pressure in the UES, swallowing may be normal, but incomplete UES relaxation in the face of inadequate pharyngeal pressure causes poor pharyngeal clearance of the bolus. Further, when the swallow is complete and the larynx and epiglottis have returned to their resting position, residual material in the hypopharynx is aspirated. Studies in which videoroentgenography and manometry were combined demonstrated that in certain patients with pharyngeal swallowing disorders, notably Zenker diverticulum or cricopharyngeal bar, the UES relaxes manometrically, but there is roentgenographic evidence of diminished opening and increased pressure in the bolus. This intrabolus pressure (Fig. 18-24), recognized as a small wave just before the pharyngeal wave, is thought to reflect the compliance of the pharyngoesophageal segment and is elevated in the presence of muscle pathology, indicating reduced compliance.

Careful questioning elicits a history of difficulty in trans-

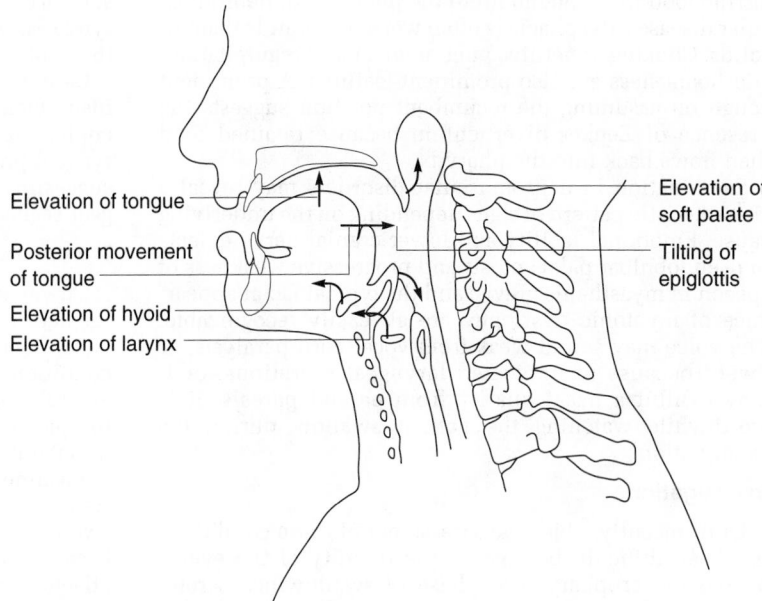

Figure 18-23. Sequence of events during the oropharyngeal phase of swallowing.

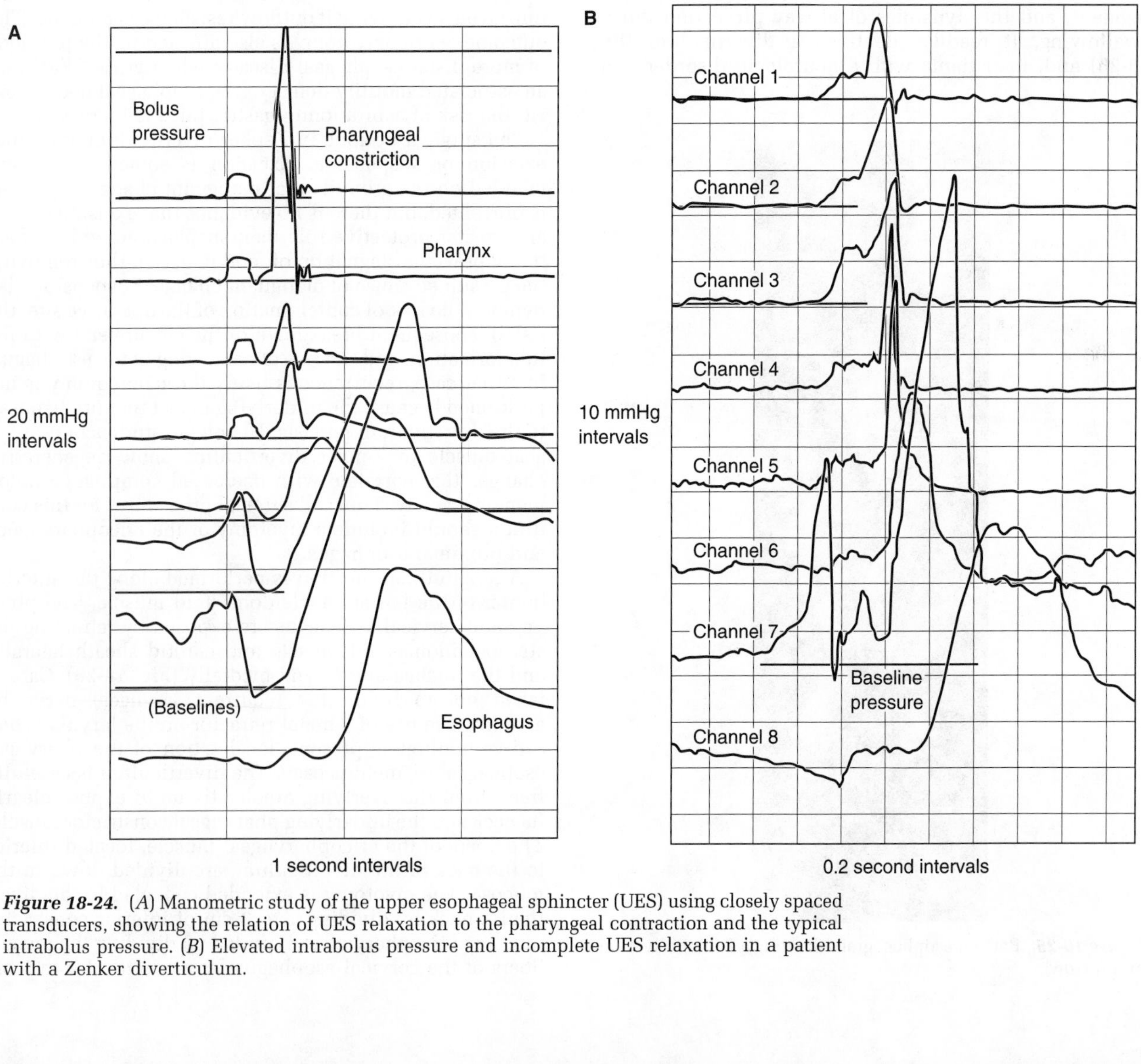

Elevation of tongue

Posterior movement of tongue

Elevation of hyoid

Elevation of larynx

Elevation of soft palate

Tilting of epiglottis

A

Bolus pressure

Pharyngeal constriction

Pharynx

20 mmHg intervals

(Baselines)

Esophagus

1 second intervals

B

Channel 1

Channel 2

Channel 3

Channel 4

Channel 5

Channel 6

Channel 7

Channel 8

10 mmHg intervals

Baseline pressure

0.2 second intervals

Figure 18-24. (*A*) Manometric study of the upper esophageal sphincter (UES) using closely spaced transducers, showing the relation of UES relaxation to the pharyngeal contraction and the typical intrabolus pressure. (*B*) Elevated intrabolus pressure and incomplete UES relaxation in a patient with a Zenker diverticulum.

ferring food from the mouth to the pharynx. In neuromuscular diseases, dysphagia is often worse for liquids than for solids. Choking, repetitive pneumonia, nasal regurgitation, and hoarseness are also prominent features. A prominent cough on assuming the recumbent position suggests the presence of Zenker diverticulum because retained food then flows back into the pharynx.

Examination in neuromuscular disorders may reveal a characteristic pattern of signs depending on the underlying cause. Emotional lability and lower cranial nerve defects in pseudobulbar palsy, ptosis and progressive weakness of speech in myasthenia gravis, and the typical facial appearance of myotonic dystrophy are all easily recognizable. The voice may sound weak from vocal cord paralysis, or "wet" because of uncleared laryngeal secretions, or it may exhibit a nasal quality from palatal paresis. It is worthwhile watching the patient swallow during the examination.

Investigation

Until recently, objective assessment of these conditions has been difficult, because of the rapidity of the events during the oropharyngeal phase of swallowing. Careful analysis of videoroentgenographic studies, esophagoscopy, manometry with specially designed catheters, and 24-hour esophageal pH monitoring can identify the cause of a pharyngoesophageal dysfunction in most of the conditions described. Videoroentgenography is the most objective test to evaluate oropharyngeal bolus transport, pharyngeal contraction, relaxation of the pharyngoesophageal segment, and the dynamics of airway protection during swallowing. It readily identifies a diverticulum (Fig. 18-25) and, in patients with a neurologic disorder, may

show a cricopharyngeal bar, indicating a failure of the pharyngoesophageal segment to relax completely, or stasis of the contrast medium in the valleculae.

Carefully performed motility studies may demonstrate insufficient relaxation or premature contraction of the cricopharyngeus, high sphincter pressure, inadequate pharyngeal pressurization, or an elevated intrabolus pressure suggesting decreased compliance of the pharyngoesophageal segment.

Treatment

Therapeutic options in all these diseases are limited by the nature of the pathology. In practice, medical treatment is confined to (1) drug treatment for a specific neurologic condition (eg, myasthenia gravis or Parkinson disease), and (2) therapy from a speech pathologist designed to train the patient to maximize residual function. Patients with unilateral brain-stem or cranial nerve lesions can be taught to swallow better by turning the head to the affected side. Aspiration can also be reduced by training the patient to swallow against a closed glottis, and if this is impossible because of vocal cord paresis, a Teflon injection into the affected vocal cord may allow improvement.

The surgeon's role is to reduce outflow resistance by performing cricomyotomy. Initially, this was recommended only for patients with demonstrable failure of UES relaxation. More recently, a number of reports indicate that a wide variety of neuromuscular diseases may be improved by cricomyotomy.[16] This is because a weak or uncoordinated pharyngeal contraction may be sufficient to permit improved swallowing if outflow resistance is reduced. The outcome of cricomyotomy is also affected by the presence of more distal esophageal disease; when gross GERD and an associated motility defect of the esophageal body coexist, the risk of aspiration of gastric juice is increased.

The surgical options in Zenker diverticulum are either excision or suspension. Excision is sometimes recommended on the grounds that malignant change in the sac is prevented, but there is no evidence that excision carries any greater protective role than suspension, which effectively prevents stagnation of food material, thus removing the presumed cause of malignant change. Suspension also removes the risk of contamination of the operative site, the risk of subsequent breakdown of the closure site with fistula formation, and the risk of narrowing of the esophagus. In either case, recurrence is likely if cricomyotomy is not performed because the underlying defect that predisposed to the diverticulum persists. Histologic studies of esophageal muscle in Zenker diverticulum show degenerative changes that correlate with decreased compliance noted manometrically. Thus, all surgical procedures for this condition should include a myotomy or the cricopharyngeus and proximal esophagus.

A longitudinal incision is performed along the anterior border of the left sternocleidomastoid muscle. The pharynx and cervical esophagus are exposed by retracting the sternocleidomastoid muscle and carotid sheath laterally and the trachea and larynx medially (Fig. 18-26). Care is taken not to injure the recurrent laryngeal nerve by avoiding the use of a metal retractor on the larynx. When a diverticulum is present, localization of the pharyngoesophageal segment is easy. The diverticulum is carefully freed from the overlying areolar tissue to expose clearly its neck and the underlying pharyngeal constrictor muscle. The fibers of the cricopharyngeal muscle, located inferior to the neck of the diverticulum, are divided down to the mucosa. The myotomy is extended cephalad to the diverticular neck by dividing 1 to 2 cm of inferior constrictor muscle of the pharynx and caudad by dividing the muscle fibers of the cervical esophagus for a length of 4 to 5 cm

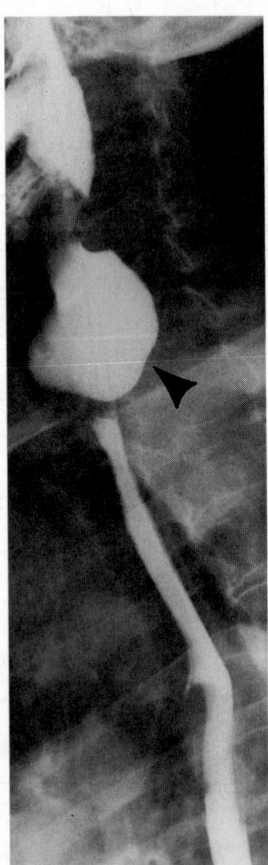

Figure 18-25. Barium esophagogram showing a Zenker diverticulum (*arrow*).

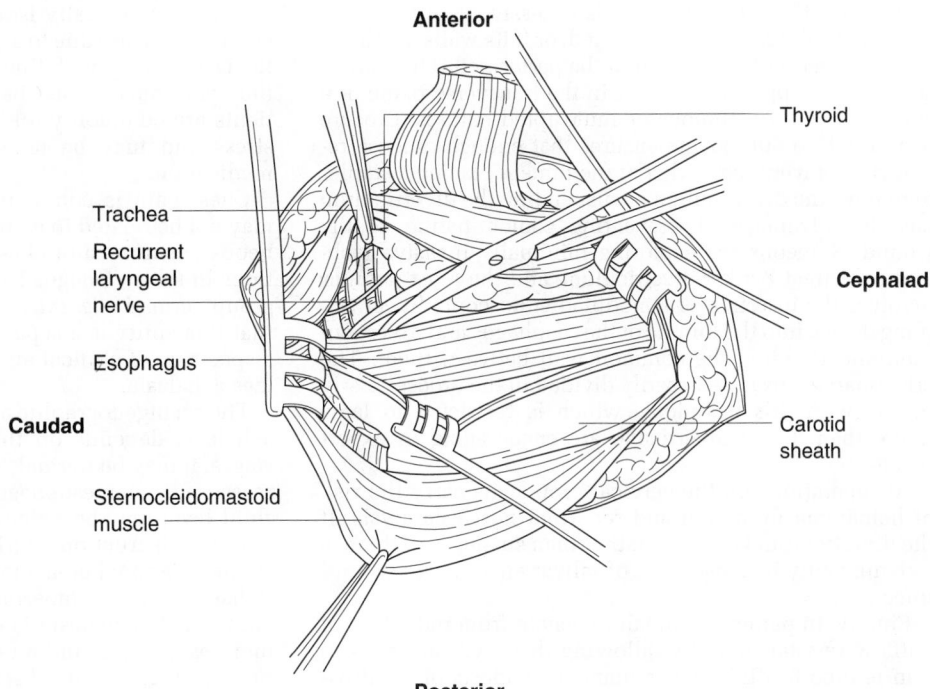

Figure 18-26. Initial exposure of the cricopharyngeal segment and cervical esophagus through a left neck incision.

(Fig. 18-27). It can be difficult to identify the cricopharyngeus muscle in the absence of a diverticulum. When local anesthesia is used, the patient can be asked to swallow, which usually shows an area of persistent narrowing at the pharyngoesophageal junction. The myotomy is started in the easily identifiable cervical esophageal wall and extended cephalad 1 cm into the posterior pharyngeal muscle above the pharyngoesophageal junction. Critical in the performance of this operation is the maintenance of meticulous hemostasis. The venous pumping action of the lung can cause the development of a large hematoma in the mediastinum postoperatively, which at best delays the improvement in the patient's dysphagia, and may result in laryngeal edema and the need for tracheostomy. The cervical wound is then closed without drainage, and oral alimentation is started the next day. The patient is usually discharged on the first or second postoperative day.

If the diverticulum is large enough to persist after myotomy, it can be suspended by suturing its apex to the prevertebral fascia using a nonabsorbable suture, that is, diver-

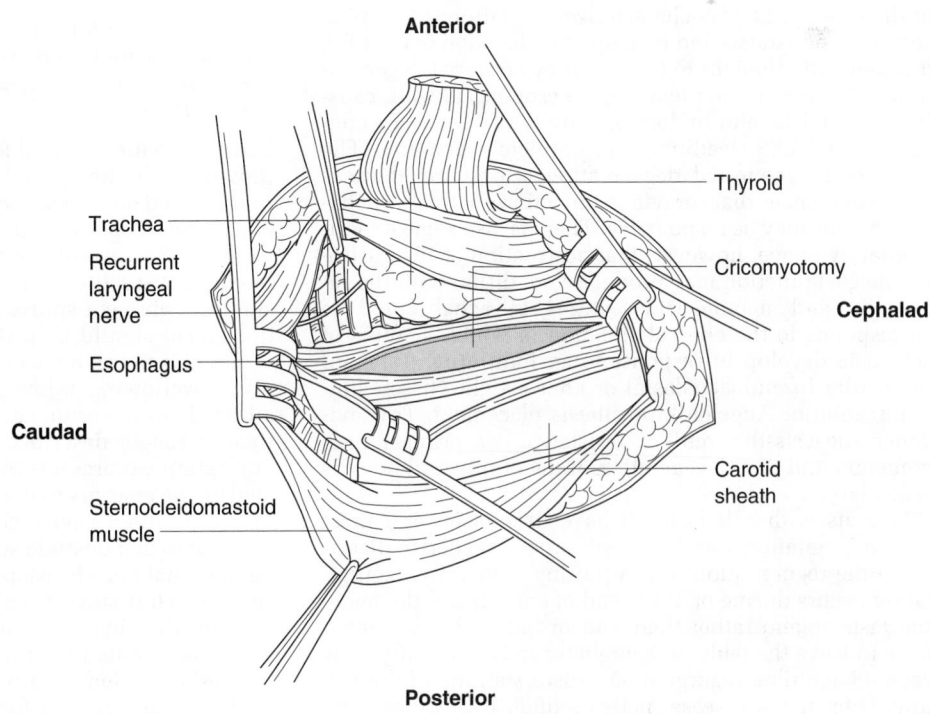

Figure 18-27. Completed cricomyotomy.

ticulopexy. If the diverticulum is excessively large so that it would be redundant if suspended, or if its walls are thickened, a diverticulectomy should be performed. This can be achieved by applying a stapler in the transverse plane or a single layer of continuous or interrupted sutures. Closure over a 35F to 40F bougie ensures that enough mucosa remains to prevent narrowing of the lumen. Placing a stapler to remove the diverticulum or suspending the diverticulum has the advantage of preventing contamination of the wound. Surgeons are exploring minimally invasive techniques to treat Zenker diverticulum, and the most popular involves the insertion of a modified endoscopic linear stapling device into the lumina of the esophagus and diverticulum, and dividing the common wall between them. The cricopharyngeus is necessarily divided in the process. Early results with this technique, which is restricted to large (more than 3 cm) diverticula, are encouraging in expert hands.

All operations on the cervical esophagus carry the risk of hematoma formation and recurrent nerve paralysis. If the diverticulum is opened rather than suspended, there is a significantly increased risk of salivary fistula and wound infection.

Finally, in patients who fail to benefit from reduction of outflow resistance and swallowing therapy, the only option is tube feeding. A percutaneous endoscopic gastrostomy is inserted, and liquid feedings are given either through a continuous pump or by bolus injection. If aspiration of tube feedings from gastroesophageal reflux is a problem, a tube can be inserted through the percutaneous endoscopic gastrostomy and fed into the distal duodenum under endoscopic control, but sometimes the upward angulation of the gastrostomy causes the duodenal tube to flip back into the stomach. A formal jejunostomy is the most trouble-free solution but requires a general anesthetic.

Primary Motor Disorders of the Esophageal Body

Achalasia

Achalasia is the best known primary motility disorder of the esophagus. It is characterized by failure of esophageal body peristalsis and incomplete relaxation of the LES. It is generally thought to be caused by neuronal degeneration in the myenteric plexus of the esophageal wall, causing aperistalsis, and by loss of activity of inhibitory neurons in the LES, leading to incomplete relaxation. The cause of the neuronal degeneration is obscure; there is some evidence that previous infection with varicella-zoster virus may be responsible. There is also some experimental evidence, however, that obstruction at the gastroesophageal junction may produce a condition with the radiologic and manometric features of achalasia. This corresponds to the clinical situation in which features of achalasia develop in response to an infiltrating tumor of the cardia (pseudoachalasia) or after a tight Nissen fundoplication or Angelchik prosthesis placement. This evidence suggests that outflow resistance is a primary phenomenon and that degeneration of the esophageal body is secondary.

Patients with achalasia all have dysphagia, and most have regurgitation. Careful questioning is needed to distinguish the regurgitation from vomiting. Generally, regurgitation occurs during or at the end of a meal, and the material tastes bland rather than sour or bitter. Patients often have to leave the table to regurgitate, and are usually slow eaters. Nighttime regurgitation causes staining of the pillow. Late in the disease, patients often lose weight and may become socially isolated. Respiratory symptoms are common and are due to aspiration. One further characteristic is the length of time, frequently several years, that the symptoms persist before the diagnosis is made. Patients are commonly told that their symptoms are due to stress and may be taking antidepressant or anxiolytic medication.

Chest pain is common in patients with achalasia and may not be related to eating. In some patients, the simultaneous occurrence of chest pain and manometric contractions in the esophagus has led to the description of a subgroup termed *vigorous achalasia*. Evidence casts doubt that this entity is a separate disease; it is more likely that a spectrum of clinical and manometric findings characterizes achalasia.

The roentgenographic appearance of the esophagus with achalasia depends on the stage of the disease. In early stages, it may be normal, and these patients may be falsely reassured. Later, esophageal dilation develops, and an air–fluid level may be noted. Both of these findings indicate outflow obstruction. Barium is rarely seen to enter the stomach, and when a good view of the cardia is obtained, it has a narrow, tapering, bird's beak appearance (Fig. 18-28). Late achalasia is characterized by a tortuous, sigmoid esophagus, and an epiphrenic diverticulum may be present (Fig. 18-29). Absence of the gastric air bubble may be noted and is due to the inability to propel swallowed air into the stomach.

Endoscopy frequently reveals residual liquid or food in the esophagus. Unlike a stricture, the narrowing at the lower end permits the passage of the endoscope, usually with a characteristic popping sensation. In untreated cases, mild esophagitis may be observed, sometimes attributable to fermentation or stagnation of esophageal contents. When the patient has had previous treatment for achalasia, such inflammation is likely to be caused by gastroesophageal reflux. In every patient with presumed achalasia, it is important to view the cardia from below with the endoscope retroflexed because a small infiltrating gastroesophageal tumor may otherwise be missed.

Manometry is required to establish the diagnosis of achalasia. The following are classic features (Fig. 18-30) of achalasia seen at stationary manometry:

- Elevated LES pressure
- Incomplete LES relaxation
- Absence of esophageal body peristalsis
- Positive intraesophageal body pressure

Not every patient has all four features. Sometimes, the LES pressure is in the normal range, but it is never subnormal in untreated achalasia. Care is needed in interpreting LES relaxation. If the transducer is positioned in the lower part of the LES, upward movement of the LES during swallowing causes the transducer to be momentarily in the stomach, giving a spurious impression of relaxation. The transducer should be positioned in the proximal portion of the LES to ensure accuracy.

On swallowing, a low-pressure wave is usually seen at all levels in the esophagus simultaneously. This is sometimes wrongly described as a simultaneous contraction, but it simply represents transmission of the pressure generated by the pharynx to the esophageal body, which behaves as a fluid-filled cavity closed at its lower end. It is not unusual to demonstrate some peristaltic activity in the upper (skeletal muscle) esophagus. The intraesophageal pressure, which is subatmospheric in normal subjects, is typically positive in achalasia, reflecting resistance to outflow.

Data are limited with regard to 24-hour pH and motility studies in patients with achalasia. Generally, excessive acid exposure is rare before dilation or operation. A charac-

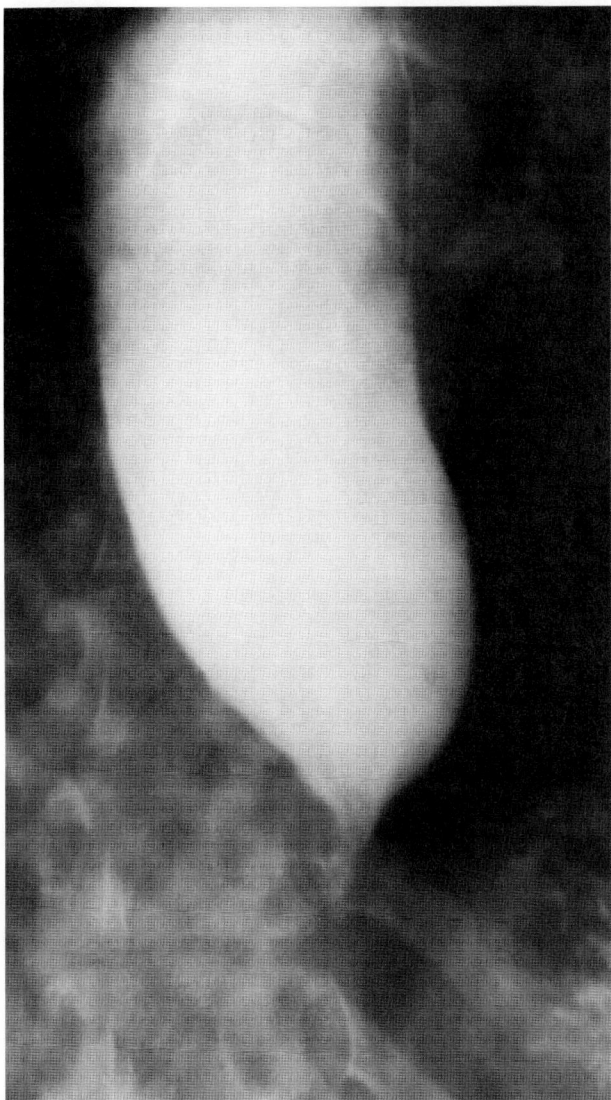

Figure 18-28. Barium esophagogram demonstrating a dilated esophagus and the characteristic bird's beak deformity in a patient with achalasia. (Waters PF, DeMeester TR. Foregut motor disorders and their surgical management. Med Clin North Am 1981;65:1244)

ranges from 2% to 10%. Some patients can be treated conservatively after perforation, but most need emergency thoracotomy for closure. The risk of gastroesophageal reflux after dilation is not known because large studies of 24-hour pH monitoring after dilation are lacking, but the risk of clinically significant symptoms appears to be low.

All surgical procedures employ a variant of Heller myotomy, in which the circular muscle of the lower esophagus is divided. In the United States, most myotomies are carried out through the chest, but the abdominal route is favored in Europe. Regardless of the route chosen, the four important principles are (1) adequate myotomy, (2) minimal hiatal disturbance, (3) antireflux protection without the creation of obstruction, and (4) prevention of closure of the myotomy with healing. The advent of minimally invasive surgery has led to the development of thoracoscopic and laparoscopic myotomies, and these are widely performed with comparable results to open surgery. There is broad agreement that if the myotomy is performed through the abdomen, an antireflux procedure should be added, and that a full Nissen wrap, however floppy, leads to long-term failure.[17] Either a posterior (Toupet) or anterior (Dor) hemifundoplication should be used. When approached through the chest, there is controversy about the need for an antireflux procedure; it has been suggested that less hiatal disturbance and a more limited myotomy are possible by this route. Our preference is to add a partial fundoplication of the Dor type when performing open transthoracic myotomy, but not when performing it thoracoscopically, because the enhanced view enables a more precise determination of the distal limit of the myotomy to be made.

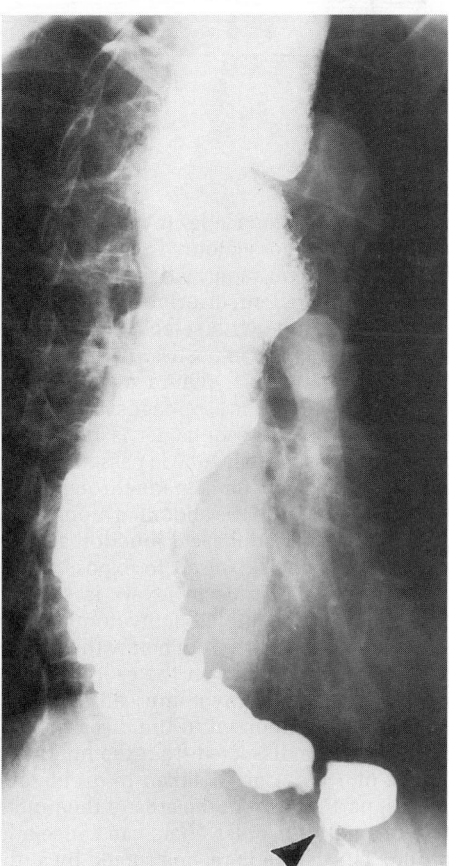

Figure 18-29. Barium esophagogram in a patient with advanced achalasia showing a dilated sigmoid esophagus and an epiphrenic diverticulum (*arrow*).

teristic pattern is the gradual fall in pH over a period of hours, and this may represent fermentation of residual food material because it clears after swallowing water. When true reflux episodes occur, they are prolonged because of the absence of peristalsis.

Treatment.   Although some patients show a short-lived symptomatic and manometric response to calcium-channel blocking agents, the mainstay of treatment for achalasia is either balloon dilation or surgery. The description of botulinum toxin injection has created much interest, but the reduction in LES pressure obtained by the investigators is small and the follow-up short. Its role is therefore unproven.

Balloon dilation has the advantages that it can be done on an outpatient basis and has minimal recovery time. It is less likely to be effective than surgical treatment and frequently needs to be repeated. The risk of perforation of the lower esophagus is higher with this procedure than with any other form of esophageal instrumentation and

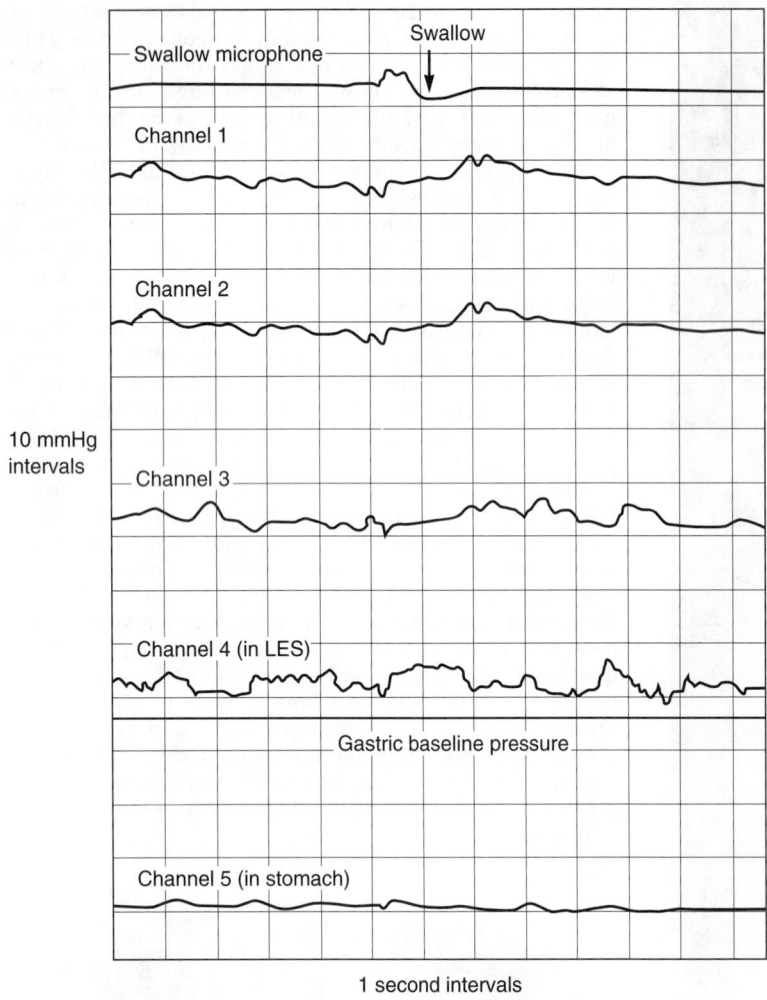

Figure 18-30. Manometric tracing in a patient with achalasia showing nonrelaxation of the lower esophageal sphincter and absent peristalsis.

Technique.   A modified Heller myotomy is usually performed through a left thoracotomy in the seventh intercostal space. The inferior pulmonary ligament is divided, and the left lung is retracted superiorly. The use of a double-lumen endotracheal tube with selective ventilation of the right lung greatly aids the exposure. An incision is made in the posterior mediastinal pleura over the esophagus, and the left lateral wall of the esophagus is exposed. Unless absolutely necessary, the esophagus is not circumferentially dissected. A nasogastric tube is passed to decompress the stomach. A 2-cm incision is made through the phreno-esophageal membrane into the abdomen along the left crus. This exposes the gastroesophageal junction and its associated fat pad. The latter is excised to expose the junction. A myotomy through all muscle layers is started on the esophageal body. The completed myotomy extends distally over the stomach to 1 to 2 cm below the gastroesophageal junction and proximally on the esophagus for 4 to 5 cm (Fig. 18-31). A longer myotomy can be performed if there is a vigorous component to the disease.

The muscle layer is dissected from the mucosa laterally for a distance of 1 cm. Care is taken to divide all minute muscle bands, particularly in the area of the junction. The persistence of small muscular fibers can cause a failure of the operation. The cardia is reconstructed by suturing the gastric fundic flap to the margins of the myotomy for a distance of 4 cm (Fig. 18-32) to prevent healing of the myotomy site and to provide reflux protection in the area

of the divided sphincter. If an extensive dissection of the cardia has been done, or if return of the cardia to the abdomen causes angulation, a more formal Belsey repair is performed. The gastric fundic flap is allowed to retract into the abdomen and is maintained there by passing the tails of the tied apical sutures of the flap through the diaphragm (Fig. 18-33).

Before closure, the myotomy site is checked for perforation by insufflating air into the nasogastric tube, with the myotomy site submerged in normal saline. If the mucosa is perforated at surgery, it should be carefully repaired using fine nonabsorbable sutures. The mucosa usually is covered by the tongue of gastric fundus brought up to perform the antireflux procedure. The same principles are followed exactly when performing the myotomy thoracoscopically, but the operator is aided by an assistant performing simultaneous endoscopy to visualize the gastroesophageal junction from within. This allows precise delineation of the extent of myotomy.

Performance of the procedure thoracoscopically is done through ports placed as shown in Figure 18-34. The rigidity of the thoracic cavity obviates the need for gas insufflation. The principles of operation are the same except that the hiatal dissection is less extensive. An L-shaped electrocautery hook is used to perform the myotomy, and the lower limit of the incision is defined with the help of intraoperative flexible esophagoscopy to visualize the gastroesophageal junction. At the end of the procedure, the tho-

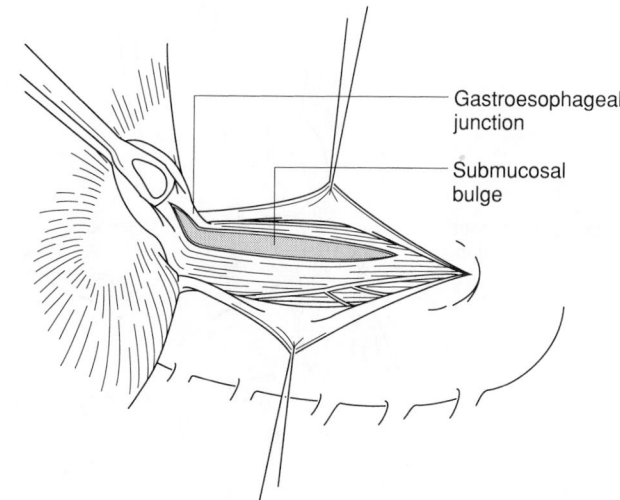

Figure 18-31. Myotomy of the lower esophageal sphincter, extending from below the aortic arch proximally and 1 to 2 cm beyond the gastroesophageal junction on to the stomach.

racic cavity is filled with water, and air is insufflated through the endoscope to confirm mucosal integrity. No nasogastric tube is used after thoracoscopic myotomy.

Attention in the early postoperative period is directed to the chest. The nasogastric tube is removed when the risk of gastric distention has passed, as judged by scanty aspirate and passage of flatus and active bowel sounds. This is usually by the 3rd or 4th day after open surgery. An esophagogram on the 5th to 7th postoperative day should demonstrate unimpaired passage of contrast into the stomach without extravasation. Wound infections should be rare because the gastrointestinal tract is not opened. Mucosal perforations are usually easily seen and repaired at the time of surgery, but an unrecognized perforation is a serious complication and should be suspected in a patient with continuing fever or chest signs.

Late complications include the persistence of dysphagia, due either to an inadequate myotomy or a complete fundic wrap, or the recurrence of dysphagia, due either to a reflux-induced stricture or closure of the myotomy. When due to reflux, the patient usually has associated severe heartburn. The treatment of these patients is problematic. In general,

the shorter the interval between primary surgery and recurrence of symptoms, the more likely the cause is a technical failure. In such patients, repeat myotomy or conversion of the fundoplication to a partial type has a good chance of success. When symptoms recur after several years, repeat myotomy is less likely to be successful, and esophageal replacement may be required (see later).

Many workers describe an increased incidence of squamous carcinoma of the esophagus in achalasia. It is not clear what the risk is, or whether effective treatment of achalasia prevents it. All patients with achalasia should be followed endoscopically at least every 2 years. Experienced surgeons believe that the development of a "tree-bark" appearance to the mucosa is consistent with a greater risk of developing carcinoma.

Outcome. A single pneumatic dilation achieves adequate relief of dysphagia and pharyngeal regurgitation in about 60% of patients with achalasia. Repetitive dilations increase this figure to about 70%. Close follow-up is required, and if dilation fails, myotomy is indicated. For a dilated or tortuous esophagus, balloon dilation is potentially dangerous, and surgery is the better option. Whether to treat newly diagnosed esophageal achalasia by forceful dilation or by operative cardiomyotomy remains controversial from the standpoint of patient comfort, but the long-term outcome data support surgery. Only one controlled randomized study[18] comparing the two modes of therapy has been performed. The results showed a clear advantage for surgery. The study was criticized because the method of dilation was thought to be inadequate, but the surgical outcome remained favorable when the dilation technique was changed. Several large series retrospectively describe the results obtained with the two modes of treatment, and their conclusions similarly support the superiority of surgical treatment over balloon dilation. Despite objections regarding variations in surgical and dilation techniques and the number of physicians performing the procedures, these collective data appear to support operative myotomy as the initial treatment of choice. Although it has been reported that a myotomy after previous balloon dilation is more difficult, this has not been our experience unless the cardia has been ruptured. In this situation, operative intervention either immediately or after healing can be difficult.

Diffuse Esophageal Spasm

Diffuse esophageal spasm is an esophageal motor disorder characterized clinically by substernal chest pain or dysphagia. DES differs from classic achalasia in that it

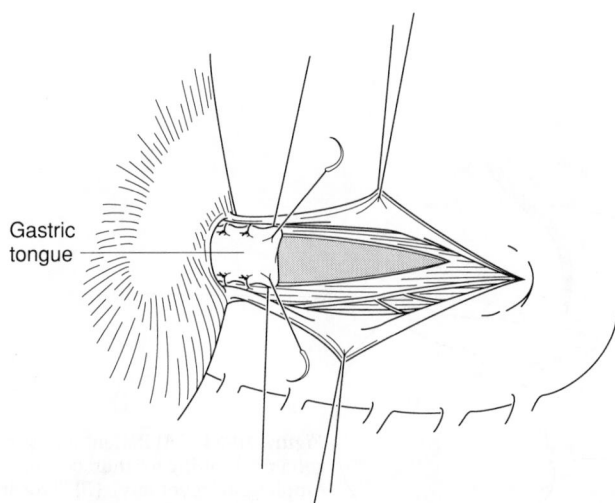

Gastric tongue

Figure 18-32. Reconstruction of the cardia after a myotomy, illustrating the gastric flap covering the distal 4 cm of the myotomy.

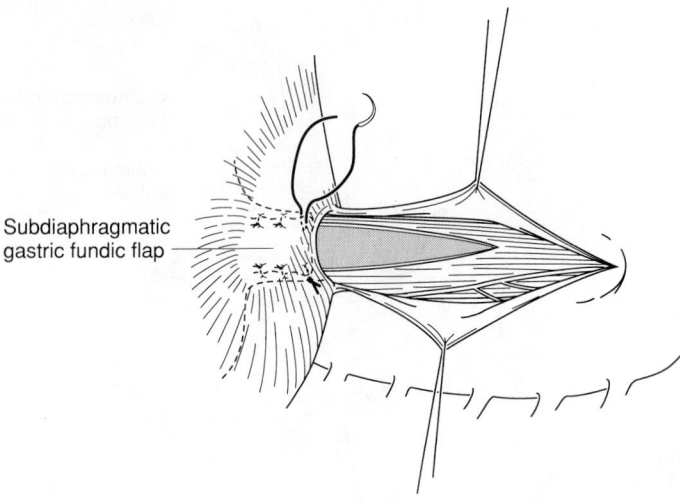

Subdiaphragmatic gastric fundic flap

Figure 18-33. Completed reconstruction of the cardia after myotomy of the body and lower esophageal sphincter, illustrating the subdiaphragmatic position of the gastric fundic flap. The tails of the tied apical sutures of the flap have been passed through the diaphragm and tied 2 cm apart at the margins of the myotomy.

A

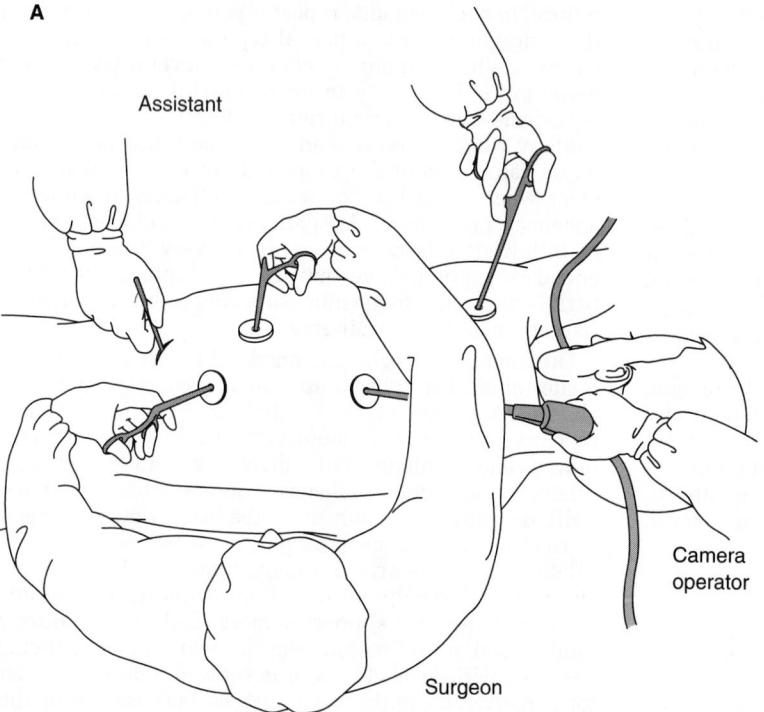

Assistant

Camera operator

Surgeon

B

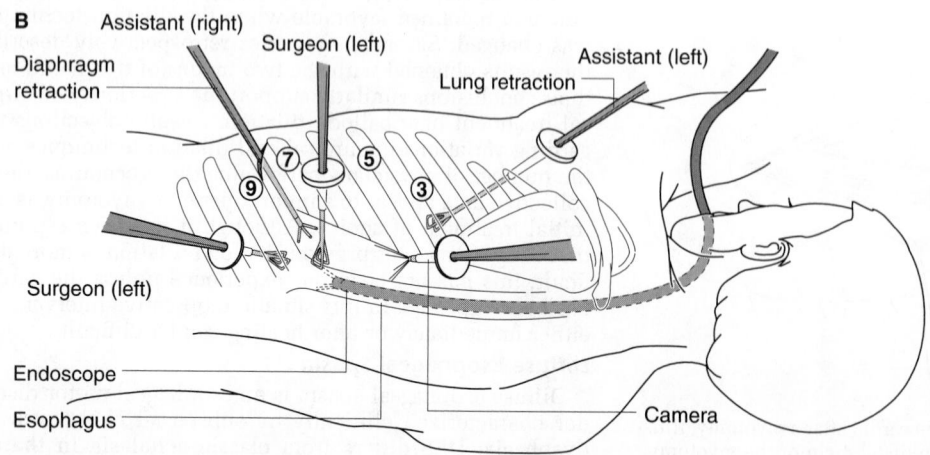

Assistant (right)

Surgeon (left)

Assistant (left)

Diaphragm retraction

Lung retraction

⑨ ⑦ ⑤ ③

Surgeon (left)

Endoscope

Esophagus

Camera

Figure 18-34. (A) Patient and surgeon positioning for thoracoscopic esophageal myotomy. (B) Trocar placement. Four 10-mm ports and a single 2- to 3-inch incision are used.

represents a primary disease of the esophageal body, produces less dysphagia, causes more chest pain, and has less effect on the patient's general condition. True symptomatic DES is more rare than achalasia. Roentgenographic abnormalities, such as segmental spasm with compartmentalization of the esophagus or formation of a diverticulum, are the anatomic correlates of the disordered motility function. The abnormal motility disorder usually occurs before the development of the roentgenographic abnormalities. The development of a diverticulum may temporarily alleviate the symptom of initial dysphagia, replacing it with postprandial symptoms of pain and regurgitation of undigested food, suggesting achalasia. In most patients with diverticula, simultaneous contractions of the esophageal body can be identified manometrically. If not, a traction-related cause of the diverticulum should be sought.

Manometric abnormalities in DES can be present over the total length of the smooth muscle portion of the esophageal body. In segmental esophageal spasm, the manometric abnormalities are confined to a short segment of the esophagus. The classic manometric finding in these patients is the frequent occurrence of simultaneous and repetitive esophageal contractions, which may be of abnormally high amplitude or long duration. Key to the diagnosis of DES is that the esophagus retains a degree of peristaltic ability, in contrast to that of achalasia. A criterion of 20% or more simultaneous contractions in 10 wet swallows has been used to define DES. This figure, however, is arbitrary and controversial. More useful criteria may be developed based on ambulatory motility studies.

The LES in patients with DES usually shows normal resting pressure and relaxation on deglutition. A hypertensive sphincter with poor relaxation may also be present and may represent early achalasia. In patients with advanced disease, the radiographic appearance of tertiary contractions appears helical and has been termed *corkscrew esophagus* or *pseudodiverticulosis* (Fig. 18-35).

DES is a benign disease that rarely causes nutritional problems and does not lead to life-threatening complications. For this reason, symptom control is the only significant goal of treatment. Medical treatment for DES is designed to abolish strong simultaneous contractions and generally employs calcium-channel blockers or long-acting nitrates. The surgical option is to perform myotomy of the esophageal body. Surgery for DES is not as successful as for achalasia and is considered only when medical treatment is ineffective. In general, the higher the incidence and extent of simultaneous contractions, the more successful is the myotomy. This is because the myotomy effectively abolishes the beneficial peristaltic contractions as well as the simultaneous contractions. Generally, if more than 70% of the esophageal contractions are simultaneous on ambulatory motility assessment, the benefits of myotomy outweigh the loss of residual peristaltic waves.[19] Esophageal body myotomy should always be accompanied by myotomy of the LES (with partial fundoplication if performed by open surgery) because even a normal LES can impose an outflow resistance too great for the myotomized body to overcome.

Nutcracker Esophagus

This term *nutcracker esophagus* is used to describe a manometric abnormality in which the amplitude of esophageal body peristalsis is greater than 2 standard deviations above normal. It was first recognized when increasing numbers of patients with noncardiac chest pain were investigated by esophageal manometry, and is the most common primary motility disorder of the esophagus. Ambulatory motility studies, however, have shown that many of these patients are either normal or have features of diffuse

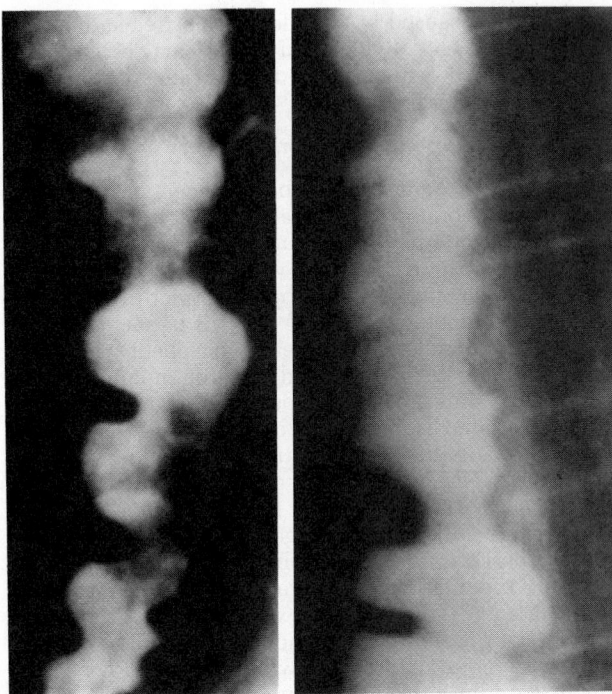

Figure 18-35. Barium esophagograms of two patients with diffuse esophageal spasm, showing corkscrew esophagi with multiple contractions. (Waters PF, DeMeester TR. Foregut motor disorders and their surgical management. Med Clin North Am 1981;65:1249)

spasm or a nonspecific esophageal motor disorder; therefore, this disease may not be a pathologic entity.

The dominant symptom of this condition is central crushing chest pain. It may have no relation to food ingestion but differs from angina in that it more frequently comes on at rest. Dysphagia or classic heartburn may be present, but this tends to be overshadowed by the chest pain.

Patients with nutcracker esophagus are usually referred from cardiologists with normal coronary angiograms and a request for esophageal motility testing. Barium radiography and endoscopy are not usually helpful. The pathognomonic feature on manometry is the presence of prolonged high-amplitude waves, with a peak of more than 180 mmHg. The numeric threshold depends on the methodology of each laboratory. The waves are normally peristaltic. Many patients with noncardiac chest pain are found to have increased esophageal acid exposure, and this subgroup is important to identify because they respond well to fundoplication.

Myotomy for isolated nutcracker esophagus with symptoms of chest pain has a low success rate, and the mainstay of treatment for these patients is muscle relaxants, such as nitrates and calcium-channel blockers. If features of DES are discovered on ambulatory manometry, myotomy is more likely to be successful.

Hypertensive Lower Esophageal Sphincter

Hypertensive LES is characterized by an elevated basal pressure of the LES (more than 95th percentile of normal). Patients typically present with chest pain and dysphagia. In about half of patients with this manometric abnormality, the LES relaxation and esophageal body peristalsis are normal, but the remainder have associated motility disorders of the esophageal body, particularly hypertensive peristalsis and simultaneous contractions. Symptoms in these patients may be caused by a prolonged postrelaxation contraction of the LES. Myotomy of the LES may be indicated for dysphagia in patients who do not respond to medical therapy or dilations.

Nonspecific Esophageal Motor Disorders

Many patients complaining of dysphagia or chest pain of noncardiac origin demonstrate a variety of esophageal contraction patterns on esophageal manometry that are clearly out of the normal range but that do not meet the criteria of a classic primary esophageal motility disorder. Esophageal manometry in these patients frequently shows an increased number of multipeaked or repetitive contractions, contractions of prolonged duration, nontransmitted contractions, interruption of a peristaltic sequence at various levels of the esophagus, or contractions of low amplitude. These motility abnormalities have been termed *nonspecific esophageal motility disorders*. The significance of these abnormal contractions in the cause of chest pain or dysphagia is still unclear. Surgery plays no role in treatment of these disorders unless there is an associated diverticulum, in which case the diverticulum is suspended or resected, and distal myotomy extending across the LES is performed. The finding of a nonspecific motor disorder may be important in a patient with proven GERD because it may warn the surgeon of future trouble after a complete 360-degree Nissen fundoplication.

Making a clear distinction between the classic primary esophageal motility disorders and the nonspecific esophageal motility disorders is often not possible. Patients diagnosed as having a nutcracker esophagus often have only nonspecific esophageal motility abnormalities when studied repeatedly, and progression from a nonspecific esophageal motility disorder to classic DES during the course of the disease has been demonstrated. The finding of a nonspecific esophageal motility disorder, therefore, may represent only a manometric marker of an intermittent, more severe esophageal motor abnormality. Combined ambulatory 24-hour esophageal pH and motility monitoring has shown that increased esophageal exposure to gastric juice is common in patients diagnosed as having a nonspecific esophageal motility disorder. Furthermore, respiratory symptoms associated with GERD are increased in the presence of a nonspecific esophageal motility disorder. In some situations, the motor abnormalities may be induced by the irritation of refluxed gastric juice; in other situations, it may be a primary event unrelated to the presence of reflux. The distinction is important because correction of the reflux by total fundoplication cures the patient if the reflux is primary, but if the motility disorder is primary, it may result in failure to improve the respiratory symptoms and in deterioration of the esophageal body.

Secondary Motor Disorders of the Esophagus

Many connective tissue and neuromuscular diseases affect the esophageal body, but the most significant is scleroderma because most patients with this condition develop dysphagia. The loss of esophageal function is caused by replacement of the muscle of the lower esophagus and LES by fibrous tissue. The manometric hallmark of the condition is absence of LES pressure and severely impaired contraction amplitude in the smooth muscle portion of the esophagus. The grossly defective LES allows superimposed reflux-induced injury to occur, accelerating the loss of body function. Many patients experience esophageal strictures. Antireflux surgery in this situation must involve a partial fundoplication, but some patients eventually require esophageal replacement. Sometimes, the situation is compounded by a severe delay in gastric emptying, and patients are greatly improved by performing total gastrectomy and reconstruction with a Hunt-Lawrence jejunal pouch in a Roux-en-Y fashion.

Surgical treatment of motor disorders by myotomy cannot normally reverse the disease process; rather, it creates a defect to overcome an existing defect. In advanced disease when residual esophageal function has been destroyed, myotomy is ineffective. Further, the superimposition of an esophageal stricture on top of a primary motor disorder makes any procedure aimed at preserving the esophagus unlikely to succeed. If more than one myotomy has been attempted in the past, it is highly unlikely that any procedure short of esophagectomy will provide symptomatic relief. The indications and choice of esophageal substitute are considered in the section on esophageal replacement in benign disease.

GASTROESOPHAGEAL REFLUX DISEASE

Gastroesophageal reflux is a normal phenomenon. Most normal people experience short episodes of reflux, usually after meals. Gastroesophageal reflux *disease* occurs when esophageal acid exposure exceeds that of a normal population. This can be measured only by 24-hour pH monitoring. Other definitions used in the past were either nonspecific (eg, symptoms of heartburn or regurgitation) or indirect (eg, the presence of a hiatal hernia), or they detected the disease only when complications such as esophagitis were present. The ready availability of 24-hour esophageal pH monitoring allows the physician to quantitate the abnormality, to assess objectively the response to treatment, and to formulate a logical approach to therapy.

Symptoms attributed to GERD are common, as judged from sales of prescribed and over-the-counter antacids. It is estimated that 7% of Americans suffer from daily heartburn, and up to 30% use antacids at least once a month. Most people whose symptoms are controlled by such means do not consult a physician, and of those who do, few are referred to surgeons. The spectrum of patients seen by a surgeon is thus variable and depends on local referral patterns.

Pathophysiology

Pathologic gastroesophageal reflux may result from a defect in the LES, the esophageal body, or the stomach, as discussed earlier. The most important clinical cause of GERD is a mechanically defective LES. This accounts for about 50% to 60% of patients with increased esophageal acid exposure. It is important to identify these patients because they generally have a good outcome after antireflux surgery but a poor response to medical treatment. The other two causes of increased esophageal acid exposure are inefficient esophageal clearance of refluxed gastric juice and abnormalities of the gastric reservoir that augment physiologic reflux.

Clinical Features

Symptoms can be classified as either typical (ie, heartburn and regurgitation) or atypical (ie, noncardiac chest pain, pulmonary problems such as asthma, recurrent pneumonia or progressive fibrosis, laryngeal symptoms such as hoarseness and aspiration, and loss of dental enamel).

Heartburn is the most common symptom associated with GERD, usually occurring 30 to 60 minutes after meals.

Heartburn exacerbated by lying flat or bending over suggests a profound weakness of the LES. It may be associated with belching and regurgitation of acid into the throat. If the regurgitated material comes from the esophagus, it tastes bland and suggests a motor disorder, and if it regurgitates from the stomach and tastes bitter, it suggests DGR.

If the regurgitation is associated with aspiration, a variety of respiratory symptoms may result. Sometimes, the picture resembles asthma, and GERD should always be considered in managing this condition. A history of isolated episodes of pneumonia or frequent bouts of wheezing and coughing at night is also suggestive of GERD. Hoarseness may be present from laryngeal irritation.

Dysphagia resulting from GERD is usually insidious and results from a motility disorder secondary to esophagitis, loss of esophageal compliance, or stricture formation. Patients usually localize dysphagia to the level of the lower sternum, but we have found that cervical dysphagia is common in GERD. Patients' localization of the site of obstruction is not always reliable; generally, an obstructing lesion does not cause symptoms to be perceived distal to the lesion. It is common to find that heartburn ceases to be a prominent symptom when a stricture has developed. By contrast, the sudden development or rapid progression of dysphagia suggests a tumor. In the absence of a history of heartburn, a squamous cancer of the esophagus is likely, but if heartburn was prominent, the most common cause is adenocarcinoma arising in Barrett's esophagus.

Angina-like chest pain, sometimes called *noncardiac chest pain,* is frequently caused by GERD. These patients often describe other classic symptoms of GERD, which tend to be mild and overshadowed by the chest pain. Of patients with angiographically negative chest pain, 20% to 50% have an esophageal cause, and of these, 50% have increased esophageal acid exposure. On the other hand, patients with angiographic lesions may have two causes for their chest pain, and some patients whose angina is poorly responsive to medical treatment may fall into this category.

Epigastric pain and nausea may be associated with other symptoms of GERD and usually result from pathologic DGR or delayed gastric emptying. It is important to recognize these symptoms before offering a patient antireflux surgery because they may persist after operation, and the patient should be warned of their presence and the possibility of future medical or surgical therapy.

Bloating is mainly a gastric symptom suggesting gastric dilation secondary to aerophagia or delayed gastric emptying. It may be accompanied by adaptive relaxation of the abdominal muscles causing visible distention. Although sometimes thought to result from fundoplication, bloating is also a common complaint in medically treated disease.

Investigation

As outlined earlier, the initial investigations in most patients with foregut symptoms include a barium esophagogram and upper gastrointestinal endoscopy. In patients with GERD, these only uncover a pathologic lesion if a complication of the disease, such as esophagitis, stricture, or Barrett's esophagus, or a potentially related condition, such as hiatus hernia, is present. The next step in investigation is physiologic testing of the esophagus and stomach using esophageal manometry and pH monitoring. Additional tests depend on the abnormalities revealed by these basic assessments. Combined pH monitoring and chest roentgenography is helpful if there are respiratory symptoms; and gastric emptying tests, gastric acid analysis for hypersecretion, and esophageal and gastric bile probe monitoring may be required to elucidate gastric symptoms.

Ambulatory esophageal motility may help define an esophageal motility disorder if stationary manometry is equivocal.

As a result of this process of investigation, a comprehensive understanding of esophageal function will be reached, enabling the physician to identify the etiologic factor responsible and predict the outcome of alternative treatments.

Complications

Complications of GERD are defined by the presence of tissue injury and include esophagitis, stricture, and Barrett's esophagus. One of the most detailed studies of the natural history of GERD comes from Lausanne, Switzerland. In this study, intensive endoscopic follow-up of a defined population for 30 years has shown that in about 45% of patients, the esophagitis develops as an isolated episode that does not return (Fig. 18-36). In the 55% of patients with recurrent disease, however, progression to more severe disease occurs in 42% (about 23% of the total). Why some patients experience complications and others do not is not known, but several factors appear to be associated:

1. The status of the LES has emerged as a significant factor in several long-term studies, and LES dysfunction predicts a poor response to medical treatment. Table 18-3 shows the relation of a defective sphincter to complications in 150 consecutive adult patients with proven gastroesophageal reflux. Note that Barrett's esophagus is almost always associated with a mechanically defective sphincter. Figure 18-37 shows the relation of LES resistance as measured by the vector volume technique to the degree of acid exposure for patients with and without injury. A clear inverse relation between acid exposure and LES resistance is demonstrated even in patients without tissue injury. This is further evidence that LES failure is an early event in the pathogenesis of GERD and that patients with tissue injury have more profound impairment of LES function.

2. Any defect of esophageal clearance that prolongs the contact time between the refluxate and the mucosa is likely to lead to increased esophageal injury. This may be due to failure of esophageal propulsion, as in primary motor disorders. More commonly, the defect in clearance is secondary to reflux-induced damage, creating a vicious cycle of increasing esophageal injury. Patients with strictures and Barrett's esophagus may thus have a profound defect in esophageal contractility. When the injury extends beyond the mucosa, the consequent interference with esophageal function may not revert to normal when the mucosa has healed. It is worth emphasizing that although the mucosa may heal by intensive acid-suppression therapy, the abnormalities in the LES and esophageal body generally do not. This is because the mucosa is repeatedly being renewed, whereas muscle cells once damaged are unlikely to recover.

3. The presence of a hiatal hernia is also associated with more complications of GERD. The cause-and-effect relation between hiatal herniation and GERD is controversial. Early workers used the terms *hiatal hernia* and *reflux esophagitis* as near synonyms, whereas later studies showed that the feature that distinguished pathologic from physiologic reflux was not the presence of a hiatal hernia but rather the LES pressure. As the diagnosis of hiatal herniation has become more standardized, it has become clear that

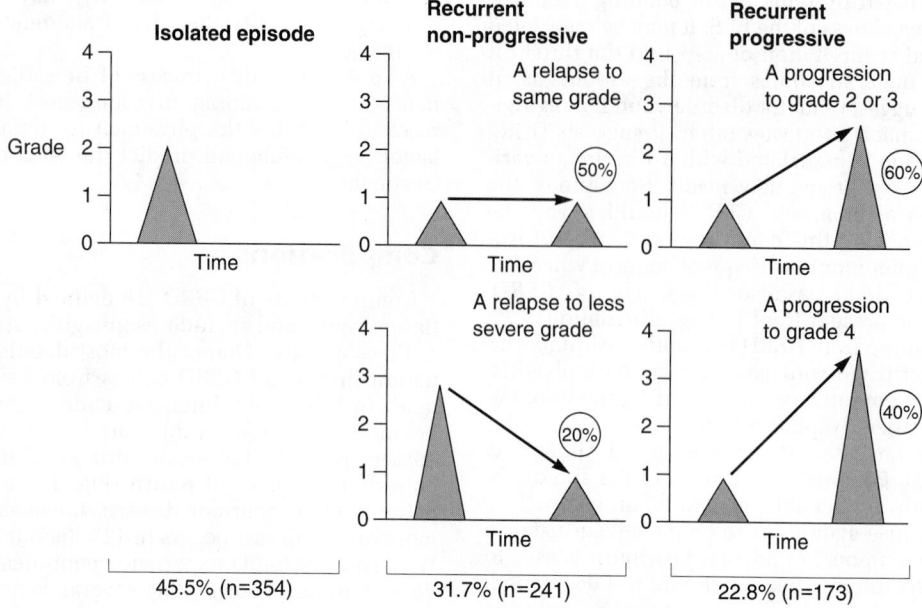

Figure 18-36. The natural history of erosive esophagitis in patients with gastroesophageal reflux disease. This study was carried out in Lausanne, Switzerland, with a relatively stable population of patients who underwent serial endoscopy by the same team over a period of several years. (Monnier P, Ollyo J-B, Fontolliet C, Savary M. Epidemiology and natural history of reflux esophagitis. Semin Lap Surg 1995;2:2).

the presence of a hiatal hernia interferes with the emptying of the distal esophagus and causes a defect in acid clearance.[20] Thus, patients with GERD associated with a hiatal hernia have more complications of the disease than those without. Conversely, the prevalence of hiatal herniation in patients with GERD increases as the complications become more severe. Most patients with Barrett's esophagus or stricture have a hiatal hernia.

4. The composition of the refluxed material also has an effect on the development of complications. The injurious effect of refluxed gastric juice depends on a number of factors. Pepsin-induced mucosal damage is likely only at a pH of 1.0 to 2.5, but in the presence of bile salts and a higher pH, trypsin may be more important. Not only is trypsin activated at a pH higher than 5.0, but the solubility of potentially injurious bile salts is greatest at neutral pH. In the clinical situation, complications of GERD are more common when there is an alkaline component to the refluxate (Fig. 18-38). In Barrett's esophagus, the development of complications such as stricture and ulceration is strongly associated with increased alkaline exposure. The presence of acid or alkaline reflux and the pres-

ence of a mechanically defective sphincter are independent determinants of mucosal damage, and when combined, the effects are additive. A patient with both features has a 95% incidence of complications.[21]

Esophagitis

Esophagitis is usually diagnosed by the presence of macroscopic mucosal erosions at endoscopy. Mere erythema of the mucosa is subjective, especially on a video screen, and is consequently of little significance. Erosions first appear on the apex of distal mucosal folds and progress to affect multiple folds, eventually becoming confluent. Histologically, erosions are characterized by loss of surface epithelium and neutrophil infiltration. Histologic abnormalities of esophagitis when the epithelium is visually normal are of uncertain relevance. Increased height of the basal cell layer of the squamous epithelium and increased depth of the papillae are now thought to be too nonspecific to be diagnostically useful. Rather, neutrophil infiltration is the hallmark of histologic esophagitis. Other markers include eosinophil infiltration or the presence of degenerate balloon cells in the epithelium. As many as half of patients with symptoms and proven GERD have no evi-

Table 18-3. COMPLICATIONS OF GASTROESOPHAGEAL REFLUX DISEASE IN 150 CONSECUTIVE ADULT PATIENTS

Complication	Patients	Normal LES (%)	Defective LES (%)
None	59	58	42
Esophagitis	47	23*	77
Stricture	19	11	89
Barrett's esophagus	25	0	100

LES, lower esophageal sphincter.
* Grade of esophagitis more severe with defective LES.

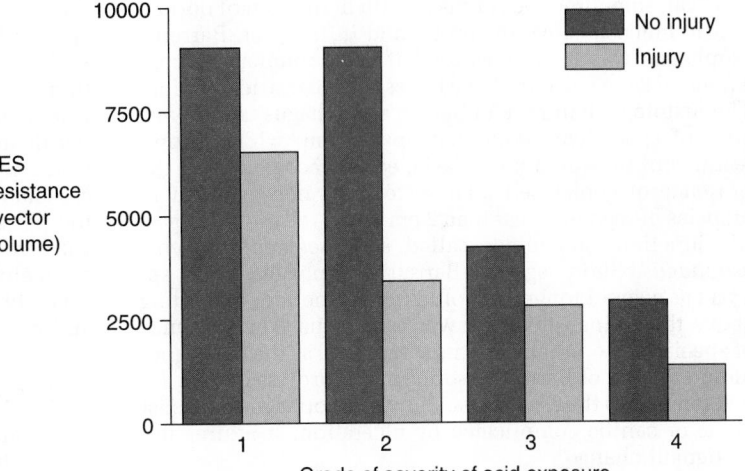

Figure 18-37. Summary of the relation between a defective sphincter and esophageal acid exposure. The resistance of the lower esophageal sphincter (LES), measured by the vector volume technique, is shown on the Y axis, and increasing severity of acid exposure is depicted on the X axis. For the pH severity score, grade 1: the percentage of total time that the pH is less than 4 is 0%–4%; grade 2 is 4%–8%; grade 3 is 8%–12%; and grade 4 is more than 12%. Even in patients without injury (*dark bars*), the inverse relation is present, suggesting that failure occurs early in the history of gastroesophageal reflux disease.

dence of esophagitis on endoscopy. Acid reflux is not the only cause of esophagitis; caustic ingestion is obvious from the history, and viral or fungal infection have specific histologic features, but pill-induced injury is an important nonreflux cause that has no specific histologic appearance. This emphasizes the importance of documenting esophageal acid exposure before making the diagnosis of GERD.

Esophageal Ulceration

Historically, esophageal ulcers were the first clinical manifestation of GERD to be described. They resemble peptic ulcers in the stomach or duodenum in that they have a tendency to penetrate deeply and lead to bleeding or perforation. They are found most commonly in association with Barrett's esophagus, often near the squamocolumnar junction and, when healed, may lead to the high midesophageal stricture characteristic of that condition.

Esophageal Stricture

More severe esophagitis causes circumferential changes that can cause fibrosis in the deeper layers, leading to stricture and esophageal shortening. Strictures have an in-

flammatory component as well as fibrous replacement of muscle. Improvement in the former is partly responsible for diminished dysphagia after corrective antireflux surgery or intensive medical treatment. Most reflux strictures occur in the distal esophagus unless Barrett's esophagus is present, in which case the stricture is often more proximal. The development of a reflux stricture causes slowly progressive dysphagia for solids, usually after a long history of heartburn and regurgitation. Rapidly progressive dysphagia or severe weight loss are uncommon and suggest malignancy.

Barrett's Esophagus

The condition in which the esophagus is lined with columnar epithelium was first described by Norman Barrett in 1950, although he incorrectly believed it to be congenital in origin. It is now realized that it represents advanced GERD. In most practices, Barrett's esophagus is found in 7% to 10% of patients with GERD. It is characterized endoscopically by the presence of velvety orange-red mucosa that lines the esophagus, and histologically by the presence of columnar epithelium. The visual appearance at endos-

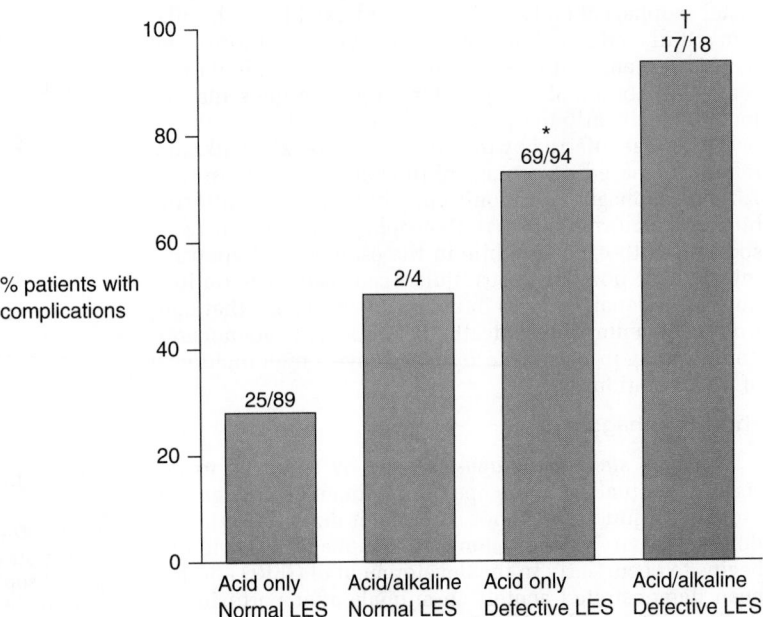

Figure 18-38. The prevalence of complications in patients with gastroesophageal reflux disease and acid or acid–alkaline reflux with and without a mechanically defective sphincter. *$P < .01$ versus patients with normal lower esophageal sphincter (LES). †$P < .05$ versus patients with only acid reflux and a defective LES.

copy can sometimes be confused with herniation of normal gastric mucosa above the crura, and in the past, Barrett's esophagus was only diagnosed if the columnar mucosa extended 2 cm or more above the esophagogastric junction. The histologic hallmark of Barrett's esophagus is the presence of specialized columnar epithelium, which shows features of intestinal metaplasia, easily recognized by the presence of goblet cells. These features may be seen in biopsies of segments less than 2 cm above the esophagogastric junction, sometimes called *short-segment Barrett's esophagus*. Short-segment Barrett's esophagus often appears as a small tongue of columnar epithelium extending above the Z-line into the lower esophagus. The presence of specialized epithelium is now regarded as the pathognomonic feature of Barrett's esophagus regardless of how far it extends into the esophagus. Barrett's esophagus can exist alone or can be complicated by ulceration, stricture, and malignant change.

Once Barrett's epithelium is present, medical therapy or antireflux surgery rarely causes it to regress. Unless it is actually ablated (eg, with laser therapy), it persists. The most significant feature of Barrett's esophagus is its malignant potential. The metaplastic epithelium usually undergoes dysplastic change before becoming frankly neoplastic, but the changes may be focal and thus missed on biopsy. Most pathologists distinguish only two grades of dysplasia: low grade and high grade. High-grade dysplasia is synonymous with carcinoma in situ, and up to half of esophagi removed for such a condition demonstrate foci of invasive carcinoma. The exact magnitude of the risk of malignancy is debated and ranges from 1 per 50 to 1 per 150 patient-years. Even the most conservative estimates indicate a risk 40 times that seen in the general population. Adenocarcinoma of the esophagus is rapidly increasing in most Western countries, and Barrett's esophagus is the only known risk factor. In the United States, adenocarcinoma accounted for about 3% of esophageal cancers between about 1930 and 1970; since the mid-1970s, its incidence has risen by 10% per year. It now accounts for almost 50% of all esophageal cancers. The ratio of white to black patients is 7:1, and the male/female ratio is 5:1. At least some genetic factors are thought to account for this predilection for white male patients. On the other hand, the increase in incidence suggests an environmental cause.

Physiologic dysfunction in Barrett's esophagus is characteristic of advanced reflux disease; a defective LES, poor distal esophageal body peristalsis, and fixed hiatal herniation are all common. Mucosal insensitivity to acid-induced pain is present and may explain why many patients present late. Abnormal composition of gastric juice may be found, specifically the presence of duodenal juice. In the past, this was inferred by the presence of so-called alkaline reflux (increased percentage of time at a pH of more than 7.0) on esophageal pH monitoring, but reports monitoring bilirubin confirm that Barrett's esophagus is frequently associated with excessive bile in the esophagus. Repetitive injury from noxious gastric juice can lead to mutations during the repair process in the p53 gene, a gene that controls programmed cell death. Patients with adenocarcinoma arising in Barrett's esophagus have a high incidence of p53 mutations.

Short Esophagus

The term *short esophagus* is used by surgeons to describe the situation in the operating room when the gastroesophageal junction cannot be brought down into the abdominal cavity without tension. Esophageal shortening begins to occur early in the development of GERD and has been demonstrated acutely in animals after perfusion of the esophagus with acid. Manometric studies demonstrate that shortening of the esophageal body increases as complications become more severe (Fig. 18-39). It is associated with shortening of the longitudinal muscle, hiatal herniation, and periesophageal inflammation. Radiologically, it is associated with fixation of the hiatal hernia; that is, the hernia does not reduce in the upright position after a swallow. Any hernia greater than 5 cm in length is likely to be associated with esophageal shortening. Manometrically, the peristaltic amplitude in the distal esophagus is often subnormal. If this condition is detected only at the time of an abdominal fundoplication, the surgeon's options are severely limited. It is much better to detect it ahead of time and plan the operative strategy accordingly.

Surgical Treatment

The aim of surgery is to restore the patient to a life free of symptoms, without the need to take regular medications, and without undue social, dietary, or other lifestyle restrictions. The status of a patient whose reflux symptoms must be controlled by taking regular acid suppression therapy, taking prokinetic agents, avoiding late meals and rich or spicy food, eschewing tea, coffee, alcohol, tobacco, chocolate, and peppermint, wearing only loose clothes, and sleeping with the head of the bed elevated cannot be considered ideal. The social and domestic disruption imposed by these restrictions is considerable and leads to noncompliance. Only two randomized trials have compared the relative merits of medical versus surgical treatment. Both showed a clear advantage for surgical treatment, but some are reluctant to accept this conclusion, arguing that the medical treatment in both did not include omeprazole.[22] An ongoing trial comparing laparoscopic Nissen fundoplication with proton pump inhibitors may provide a conclu-

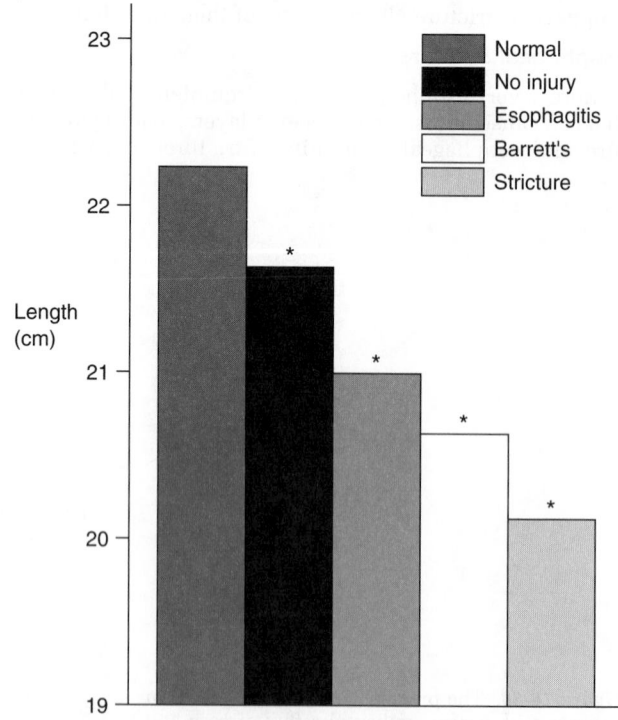

Figure 18-39. Manometric length of the esophagus in patients with gastroesophageal reflux disease compared with normal subjects. Esophageal length progressively shortens as the complications of the disease become more severe. *$P < .001$ versus normal subjects.

sion more relevant to current practice. There is no doubt that proton pump inhibitors represent a great advance in the medical treatment of GERD, but until recently, long-term use was discouraged by the US Food and Drug Administration. Serum gastrin levels are usually raised in patients on long-term omeprazole, and there are theoretic and experimental reasons to believe that the trophic effect of long-term gastrin elevations may predispose to neoplasia. In rats, gastric carcinoid tumors have been reported. Long-term omeprazole use in patients with severe esophagitis generally heals the esophagitis if a high dose is given but is associated with atrophic gastritis. No reports of cancer in humans attributable to omeprazole have been made. A limiting factor in the medical treatment of GERD is that treatment addresses only acid suppression, ignoring the other potentially injurious components of the refluxate, which continue to cause damage despite symptomatic relief.

The traditional reasons for an internist to refer a patient with GERD for surgery are an unsatisfactory response to medical treatment and the development of uncontrollable complications. These end-points are subjective and likely to be influenced by gatekeeper policies in a managed care environment. An approach that aims to make the diagnosis and elucidate the pathophysiology at an early stage is preferred. This allows more accurate prognostic information to be given to the patient and the appropriate selection of rational and cost-effective therapy.

Operative Indications

The first requirement in the consideration of antireflux surgery is objective demonstration of the presence of GERD by 24-hour pH monitoring. Second, the patient must have either symptoms or complications of the disease. Third, the disease should be caused by a defect remediable by surgical therapy, such as a mechanically defective LES. Studies have indicated that a Nissen fundoplication has beneficial effects in addition to restoring the characteristics of the LES. It may accelerate gastric emptying and reduce the frequency of transient LES relaxations. Consequently, even in patients without defective sphincters, there are situations in which a Nissen fundoplication can correct the underlying abnormality. The algorithm in Figure 18-40 summarizes the approach to selecting patients with suspected GERD for surgery.

Although it is usually straightforward to categorize patients in accordance with this scheme, the following alternative scenarios should also be noted:

1. If 24-hour esophageal pH monitoring is normal in a patient with unequivocal endoscopic esophagitis, the possibilities of alkaline, drug-induced, or retention esophagitis should be considered. If the patient also has a defective LES and a hiatal hernia, the circumstances of the pH test should be reviewed. Sometimes, patients have not stopped acid-suppression medication in time, or have eaten so little during the test that it does not reflect normal daily life. Pure alkaline reflux occasionally occurs in the absence of acid reflux and may be detected by ambulatory bile probe monitoring.

2. If the sphincter is manometrically normal in a patient with increased esophageal exposure to gastric juice, the patient should be evaluated for an esophageal or gastric cause of increased acid exposure. In this situation, the most common abnormality is gastric hypersecretion.

3. Some patients with increased acid exposure and a mechanically defective sphincter but no complications of the disease respond well to medical therapy but require long-term medication for continued relief. These patients should be given the option of surgery as a cost-effective alternative. At current (1995) prices, omeprazole 20 mg daily costs about $220 per month, and many patients need double or even triple this dose to achieve a clinical response.

4. Symptoms of reflux, such as respiratory manifestations, often respond well to antireflux surgery. Patients often record that omeprazole reduces heartburn but not regurgitation and coughing attacks. When respiratory symptoms are combined with typical symptoms such as heartburn and regurgitation, the results

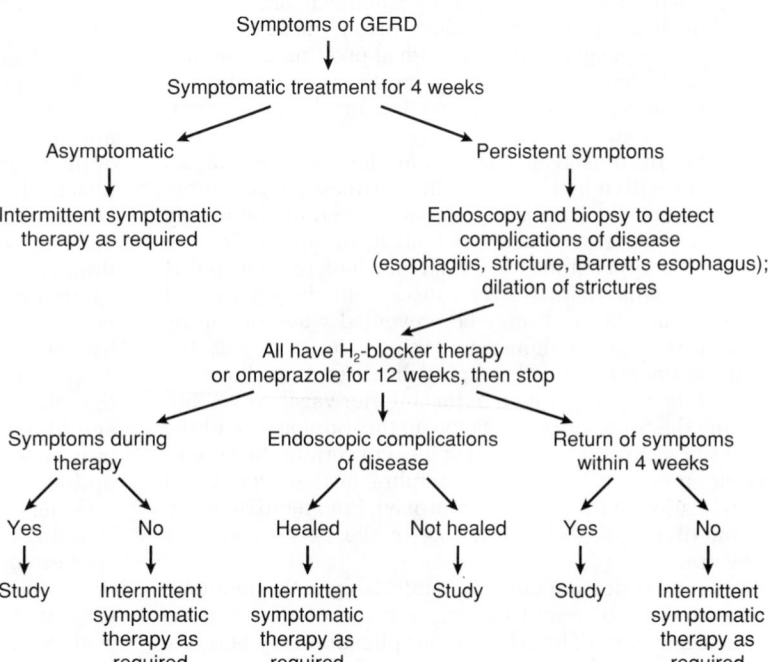

Figure 18-40. Algorithm for selecting patients with symptoms suggestive of gastroesophageal reflux disease (GERD) for further study.

of antireflux surgery are generally good. When the respiratory symptoms are the only manifestation of GERD (ie, in the absence of heartburn), the results of surgery are less beneficial. This is because many of these patients have an associated motor disorder that encourages the retrograde transport of saliva even in the absence of gastroesophageal reflux, or because the long-standing lung disease actually is primary and the reflux secondary.

5. Complaints of epigastric pain, nausea, vomiting, and loss of appetite may be due to excessive DGR, which occurs in about 11% of patients with GERD. This problem is usually confined to patients who had previous upper gastrointestinal surgery. The coexistence of these gastric symptoms in a patient who also has typical symptoms of GERD should prompt a thorough evaluation of the stomach using the bile probe, 24-hour pH monitoring, or radionuclide scanning. In these patients, correction of only the incompetent cardia can result in continued nausea and epigastric pain on eating. In rare cases, surgery is necessary to control severe DGR by performing a bile diversion procedure. When the symptoms emerge after antireflux repair, the administration of sucralfate (Carafate) may be helpful.

Several important principles underlie antireflux surgery that, if ignored, risk failure of the operation and result in unwanted postoperative symptoms. When faced with a number of potential operative solutions, adherence to underlying principles guides the surgeon to make a rational decision. Almost all antireflux operations involve plicating the lower esophagus with fundus. One notable exception is the Hill operation, but it requires intraoperative manometry and is not widely used. The Hill operation may be most valuable in patients who previously underwent gastric surgery. Other operations, such as those that use a ligamentum teres sling or that involve the creation of a lesser-curve gastroplasty tube, are rarely used.

Only the fundus, and not the upper body of the stomach, should be used to construct the fundoplication. The fundus should be fully mobilized by dividing the short gastric arteries. The surgeon should take advantage of the ability of the fundus to relax in concert with the LES after a swallow. If the fundus is not adequately mobilized, or is twisted round the lower esophagus under tension, the risk of postoperative dysphagia is high. The ideal position of the fundus is such that the anterior lip and the posterior lip envelop the lower esophagus, meeting in about the right lateral position.

The fundus must be placed around the lower esophagus. In patient with a hiatal hernia, the gastroesophageal junction may not be obvious. An inexperienced operator may mobilize the lesser curve and create a fundoplication around the upper stomach, which may look tubular in this situation. This serious error causes both dysphagia and recurrent heartburn. It may be prevented when operating through the open abdomen by taking care to identify the gastroesophageal fat pad, keeping the dissection above the level of the hepatic branch of the anterior vagal nerve, and placing the fundoplication between the esophagus and the posterior vagus nerve. This is of less concern in the laparoscopic approach because the diaphragm is elevated and visualization of the cardia is improved. Preoperative recognition of esophageal shortening is the best preventive measure.

The fundoplication must lie comfortably in the abdomen without tension, requiring only closure of the crura to maintain it there. The whole fundoplication may herniate into the chest if the crura are not closed, if there is tension on the fundoplication because of undetected esophageal shortening, or both. This creates an iatrogenic paraesophageal hernia. Although the fundoplication functions as an antireflux barrier even in the intrathoracic situation, the patient experiences postprandial chest pain as the fundoplication is distended with air, and the risks of ulceration and hemorrhage from the herniated pouch of stomach are substantial.

In creating an antireflux barrier, the surgeon is to some extent trading off the risk of dysphagia against the risk of recurrent reflux. The Nissen fundoplication as originally described protected against reflux effectively, but at the expense of a substantial incidence of dysphagia and gas-bloat syndrome. The modern version of the adult Nissen operation, using a short, 1- to 2-cm fundoplication constructed over a 60F bougie and using fully mobilized fundus to envelop the lower esophagus, has to a great extent overcome these early problems. Partial fundoplications, such as the Belsey operation, produce a less resistance to outflow and are therefore appropriate for patients with poor esophageal body motility. The long-term recurrence rate is higher, however, after the Belsey operation. There has been a resurgence of interest in partial fundoplications done through the abdomen because of the perceived risk of dysphagia and gas-bloat syndrome after the 360-degree Nissen fundoplication. These operations are named after their originators (eg, Toupet, Dor, Watson, and Lind operations). Several randomized studies comparing partial and total fundoplications have found that partial fundoplications produce a lower incidence of early dysphagia and bloating, but the differences disappear with follow-up. Because the principles underlying the construction of these various partial fundoplications are similar to those for the Belsey operation, long-term failure may be a problem. Rather than adopt a blanket policy of performing partial fundoplications in all cases, it makes more sense to uncover the dominant physiologic abnormality and tailor the operation accordingly.

Tailored Antireflux Operation

Patients with normal esophageal length and normal esophageal body motility are best served by a transabdominal Nissen fundoplication. This is normally done using laparoscopy. Usually, this situation is found in early disease, before severe complications have developed. If the patient is obese or requires concomitant surgery of the lung or esophageal body, the transthoracic route is preferable.

The presence of a motility disorder alters the operative strategy. If the peristaltic amplitude is low (less than 20 mmHg) in the distal third of the esophagus, a Nissen fundoplication creates excessive resistance and leads to dysphagia. In this situation, the Belsey fundoplication is a better choice. Moreover, it allows the surgeon to mobilize the esophagus to a much greater extent than is possible through the abdomen. Usually, some degree of esophageal shortening is present when distal esophageal peristalsis is poor. In addition to extensive mobilization, a Collis gastroplasty can be created to produce an extra 5 cm of neoesophagus around which a Belsey wrap can be added. In the relatively rare situation in which low distal peristaltic amplitude is associated with normal esophageal length, a transabdominal partial fundoplication is a reasonable option.

Generally, if the motor disorder is secondary to long-standing reflux, a good result can be expected. The results are less good if the motor disorder is primary. This distinction is sometimes difficult, but usually reflux-induced motor damage is associated with a defective LES and esophageal body shortening. The combination of GERD and a named primary motor disorder, such as achalasia or DES,

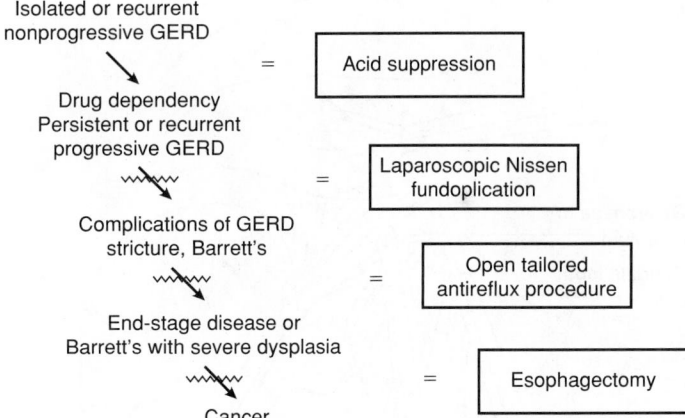

Figure 18-41. Conceptual scheme of the appropriate treatment at each stage of the spectrum of gastroesophageal reflux disease (GERD).

is rare unless myotomy or balloon dilation has been performed. In these circumstances, the primary motor disorder should be treated by myotomy of the body, LES, or both.

End-stage reflux disease (eg, with undilatable stricture, after previous unsuccessful antireflux operations, or when Barrett's esophagus leads to high-grade dysplasia) is best served by esophageal replacement. The most durable substitute is the colon, and the functional results are especially good if the vagus nerves are intact. Figure 18-41 summarizes the operative treatment of GERD depending on the stage of the disease.

Nissen Fundoplication

The essential elements for the performance of a transabdominal fundoplication are common to both the laparoscopic and open procedures and include the following:

- Crural dissection; identification and preservation of both vagi and the anterior hepatic branch
- Circumferential dissection of the esophagus
- Crural closure
- Fundic mobilization by division of short gastric vessels
- Creation of a short, loose fundoplication by enveloping the anterior and posterior wall of the fundus around the lower esophagus

Laparoscopic fundoplication has become commonplace and may soon replace traditional open Nissen fundoplication as the procedure of choice.[23] The patient should be placed supine in a modified lithotomy position, with the head of the table elevated 30 to 45 degrees. The knees should be only slightly flexed. When the legs are sharply flexed at the knees, they interfere with the mobility of the instruments during the course of the procedure. Five 10-mm ports are used, as indicated in Figure 18-42. The camera is placed above the umbilicus, one third of the distance to the xiphoid process. The right-sided liver retractor is best placed immediately subcostal to the right of the xiphoid. This allows an acute angle toward the left lateral segment of the liver and the ability to push the instrument toward the operating table, lifting the liver. A second retraction port is placed laterally toward the left flank at the level of the umbilicus. The operating ports are placed in the right and left mid-clavicular lines, 2 inches below the costal margin. Placing the operating trocars on either side of the midline allows triangulation between the camera and the two instruments, avoiding the difficulty associated with the instruments being in direct line with the camera. The falciform ligament hangs low in many patients and

provides a barrier around which the left-handed instrument must be manipulated. We use a 12-mm universal port in the left mid-clavicular position to allow unhampered use of instruments of different diameters.

One of the most important elements of laparoscopic surgery is adequate retraction and safe exposure of the necessary structures. Laparoscopic fundoplication begins with exposure of the esophageal hiatus. A fan retractor is placed into the perixiphoid port to hold the left lateral segment of the liver toward the anterior abdominal wall. A Babcock clamp is placed into the left anterior axillary port, and

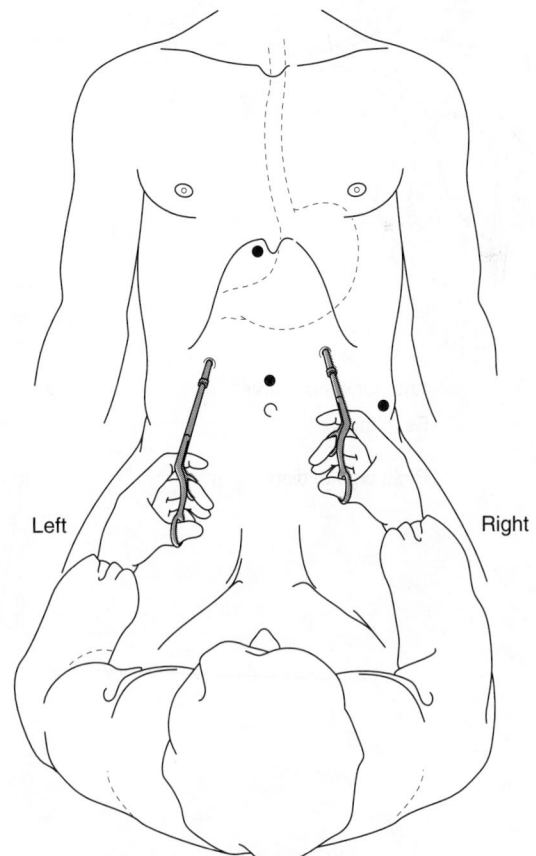

Figure 18-42. Positioning of the patient and trocars for laparoscopic antireflux surgery. The patient is placed with the head elevated 45 degrees in the modified lithotomy position.

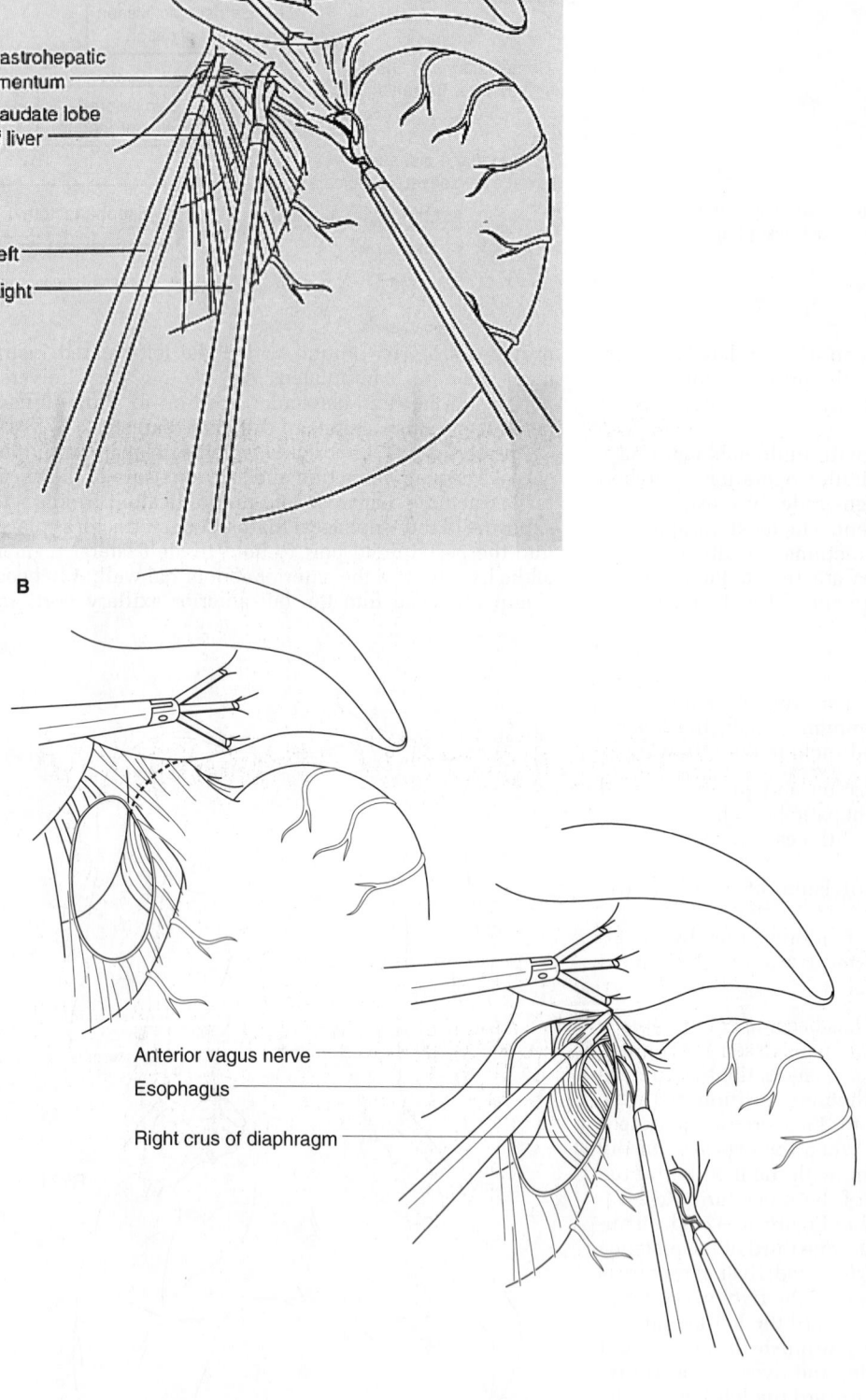

A

Gastrohepatic omentum

Caudate lobe of liver

Left

Right

B

Anterior vagus nerve

Esophagus

Right crus of diaphragm

Figure 18-43. Initial retraction for exposure of the esophageal hiatus. A fan retractor is placed below the left lateral segment of the liver to retract it anteriorly. (*A*) The gastrohepatic omentum is incised above the hepatic vagal branches, and the right crus is exposed. (*B*) The dissection is carried anteriorly toward the superior margin of the left crus.

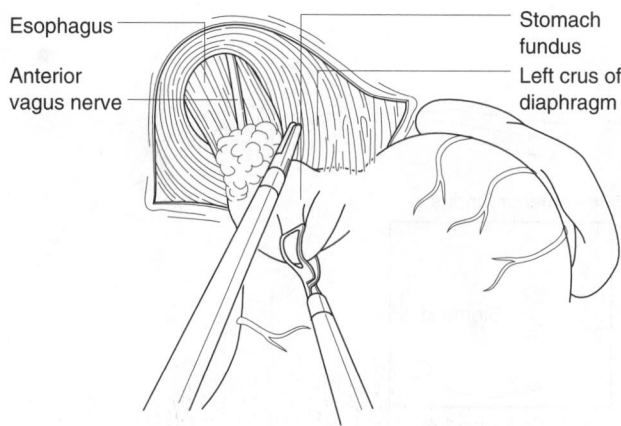

Esophagus

Anterior
vagus nerve

Stomach
fundus

Left crus of
diaphragm

Figure 18-44. Dissection of the left crus and the angle of His. A complete dissection of the left side is the key to safe encirclement of the esophagus.

the stomach is retracted caudad, exposing the esophageal hiatus. Commonly, a hiatal hernia needs to be reduced.

The key to the hiatal dissection is identification of the crura. In all except the most obese patients, there is a thin window in the gastrohepatic omentum overlying the caudate lobe of the liver. Dissection is begun by incision of this window above the hepatic branch of the anterior vagal nerve (Fig. 18-43). A large left hepatic artery arising from the left gastric artery is present in up to 25% of patients. It should be identified and avoided. Once the gastrohepatic omentum is opened, the lateral aspect of the right crus becomes evident. The peritoneum overlying the anterior aspect of the right crus is incised. The medial portion of the right crus leads into the mediastinum and is entered by blunt dissection with both instruments. At this juncture, the esophagus usually becomes evident. The right crus is retracted laterally, and the posterior or right vagus is identified and kept with the esophagus. The anterior or left vagus is left undisturbed.

Lifting the esophagus with a blunt-tipped grasper placed within the esophageal hiatus, the dissection is carried inferiorly and laterally, exposing the medial and lateral aspects of the right crus. A large hiatal hernia often makes this portion of the procedure easier because it accentuates the diaphragmatic crura. On the other hand, dissection of a large mediastinal hernial sac can be difficult.

After dissection of the right crus, attention is turned toward the angle of His, and a complete dissection of the

lateral and inferior aspect of the left crus and the fundus of the stomach is performed (Fig. 18-44). This dissection is the key maneuver, allowing circumferential mobilization of the esophagus. Failure to do so results in difficulty encircling the esophagus, particularly if approached from the right. Repositioning of the Babcock retractor toward the fundic side of the stomach facilitates retraction for this portion of the procedure.

The esophagus is mobilized by careful dissection of the anterior and posterior soft tissues within the hiatus. This can be difficult if the operating ports are placed too medially. In the presence of severe esophagitis and transmural inflammation, esophageal dissection may be particularly difficult. After this dissection, a grasper is passed by the surgeon's left-handed port behind the esophagus and over the left crus. A Penrose drain is placed around the esophagus to facilitate further dissection and crural closure (Fig. 18-45).

The crura are dissected inferiorly to expose the V-shaped decussation. The esophagus is held anterior and to the left and the crura approximated with three or four interrupted 1-0 silk sutures, starting just above the aortic decussation and working anteriorly.

Complete fundic mobilization is necessary for construction of a tension-free fundoplication. The liver retractor is replaced with a second Babcock forceps to retract the upper stomach. The gastrosplenic omentum is suspended anteroposteriorly in a clothesline fashion using both Babcock forceps, and the lesser sac is entered about one third the distance down the greater curvature of the stomach. The short gastric vessels are sequentially dissected, doubly clipped, and divided (Fig. 18-46). With caution and meticulous dissection, the fundus can be completely mobilized in most patients.

The posterior wall of the mobilized fundus is gently brought behind the esophagus to the right side. The anterior wall of the fundus is brought anterior to the esophagus above the supporting Penrose drain (Fig. 18-47). Both posterior and anterior fundic lips are manipulated to allow the fundus to envelop the esophagus without twisting (Fig. 18-48). The laparoscopic visualization has a tendency to exaggerate the size of the posterior opening that has been dissected. If the right lip of the fundoplication has a bluish discoloration, the stomach should be returned to its original position and the posterior dissection enlarged. Once adequately placed, a 60F bougie is passed. The fundoplication is sutured with a single U-stitch of 2-0 Prolene buttressed with felt pledgets. The most common error is an attempt to grasp the anterior portion of the stomach to construct the fundoplication rather than the posterior fun-

A   **B**

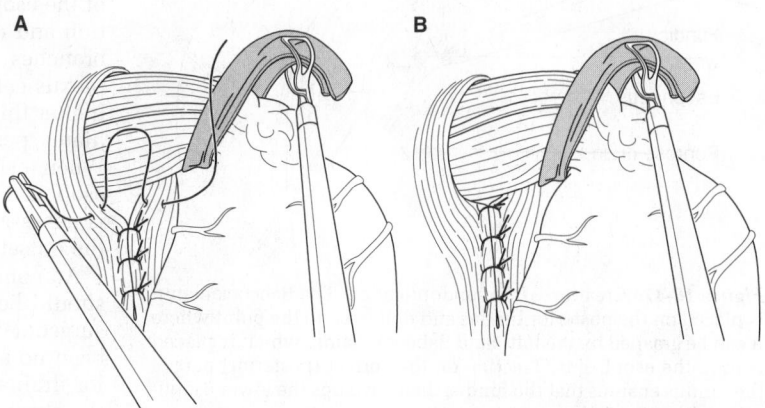

Figure 18-45. A Penrose drain is placed around the esophagus to facilitate exposure for crural closure. (*A*) Three or four sutures are placed to close the crura. (*B*) The completed closure.

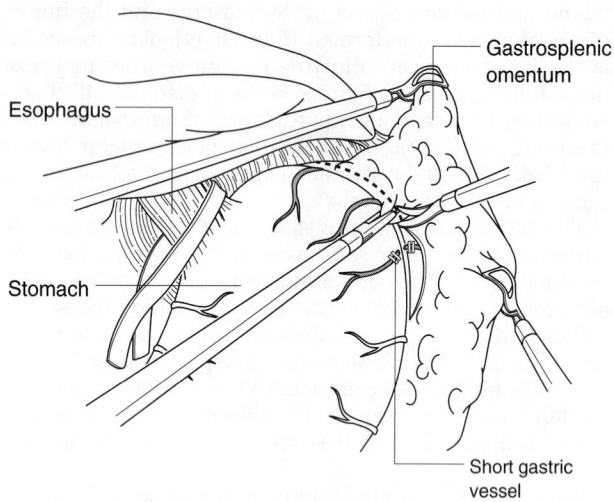

Figure 18-46. Retraction of the gastrosplenic omentum facilitates division of the short gastric arteries.

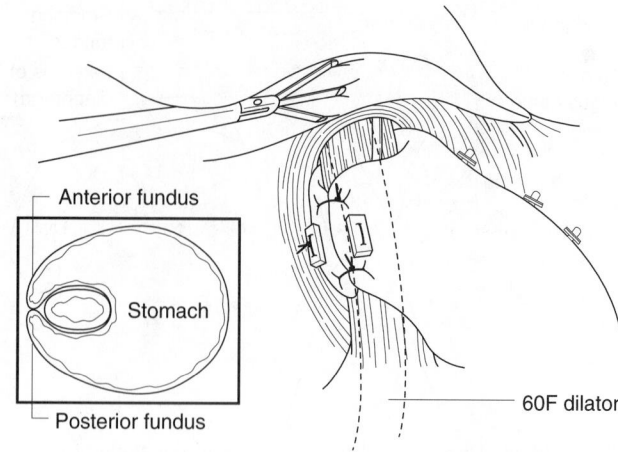

Figure 18-48. Fixation of the fundoplication. The fundoplication is sutured in place with a single U-stitch of 2-0 Prolene reinforced by Teflon pledgets on the outside.

dus. The esophagus should comfortably lie in the untwisted fundus before suturing. Two anchoring sutures of 3-0 silk are placed above and below the U-stitch to complete the fundoplication. When finished, the suture line of the fundoplication should be facing in a right lateral direction. The bougie is replaced with a nasogastric tube, which should pass easily into the stomach. If it does not, intraoperative endoscopy should be performed.

Open Nissen Fundoplication

The open Nissen fundoplication performed less often now, but it is still easier when other complex procedures, such as highly selective vagotomy or a bile diversion procedure, are combined with the Nissen fundoplication. Operating on a patient who underwent several previous upper abdominal operations may be more difficult using the laparoscopic approach. The principles of the open operation are identical to those enumerated earlier. Exposure is aided

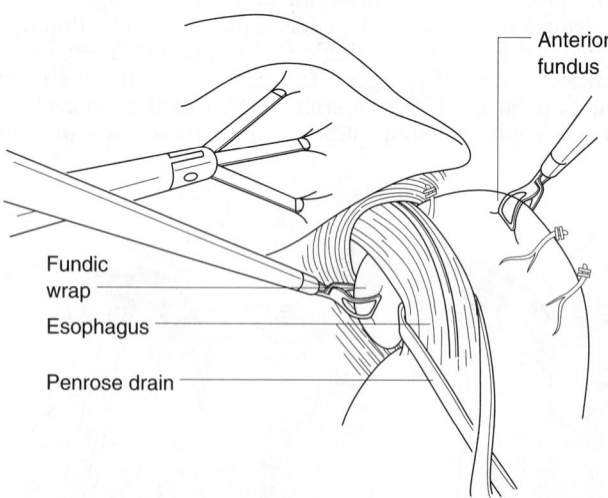

Figure 18-47. Creation of the fundoplication. The Babcock clamp is placed on the posterior fundus and delivered to the point where it can be grasped by the left-hand Babcock clamp, which is placed behind the esophagus. Traction on the correct (posterior) part of the fundus ensures that the fundus then envelops the lower esophagus without twisting.

by putting the patient in the reverse Trendelenburg position and using a sternal retractor to elevate the liver and costal margin. For accurate positioning of the fundoplication, its posterior lip is passed between the posterior vagus nerve and the esophageal wall.

For the transthoracic approach, a left posterolateral thoracotomy is placed through the sixth intercostal space. Reoperations are easier through the seventh intercostal space. This allows better exposure of the abdomen through a peripheral diaphragmatic incision, in which the diaphragm is incised circumferentially 2 to 3 cm from the chest wall for a distance of about 10 to 15 cm. An adequate rim of diaphragm must be preserved along the chest wall for reapproximation of the muscle after the fundoplication is complete. If further abdominal exposure is necessary, the thoracic incision can be extended diagonally across the rectus muscle to the abdominal midline, dividing the costal margin and the bridge of diaphragmatic muscle. Exposure is greatly facilitated by the use of a double-lumen endotracheal tube, allowing selective deflation of the left lung.

The principles of creating and securing the fundoplication are the same regardless of whether the approach is abdominal or thoracic, including fundic mobilization by division of the short gastric vessels and closure of the hiatus. Before creating the fundoplication, it is important to ensure that the gastroesophageal junction can be placed below the hiatus without tension. Several steps may be necessary to achieve this: the first is thorough mobilization of the esophagus up to the aortic arch. This involves ligation and division of the two bronchial arteries. Next, the branches of the left vagus nerve to the left pulmonary plexus can be divided in an effort to reduce the tension. If after this maneuver the tendency to ride up through the hiatus persists, a Collis gastroplasty is done (see later). When a short fundoplication of 1 to 2 cm is used and the esophagus has been adequately mobilized, this step rarely is necessary in patients in whom it was not planned from the outset.

At completion of the procedure, a nasogastric tube should be able to be passed, without guidance from the surgeon, directly into the stomach to ensure that there has been no angulation of the distal esophagus. A chest tube for drainage of the pleural cavity is properly placed and the chest incision closed.

Belsey Mark IV Repair

The techniques of the Belsey Mark IV and the transthoracic Nissen operations are similar, differing only in the construction of the gastric fundoplication. The steps are illustrated in Figure 18-49. To perform the Belsey Mark IV reconstruction, the esophagus and cardia are mobilized, and the fundus of the stomach is freed by dividing the short gastric vessels as it is brought up through the hiatus into the chest. The fundus is held in place by two rows of three horizontal mattress sutures placed equal distances between the seromuscular layers of the stomach and the muscular layers of the esophagus. Each suture should obtain a firm grip of the esophageal wall. The first row of sutures is placed 1.5 cm above the external gastroesophageal junction and is tied only tightly enough to obtain tissue apposition without disrupting the muscle fibers of the esophagus. A second row of sutures is placed 1.5 to 2 cm above the first row, using the position of the previously placed sutures in the first row as a guide. Once again, the sutures in the second row are tied carefully to achieve tissue apposition without strangulation. The tails of these sutures are not cut, but are separately rethreaded on a large,

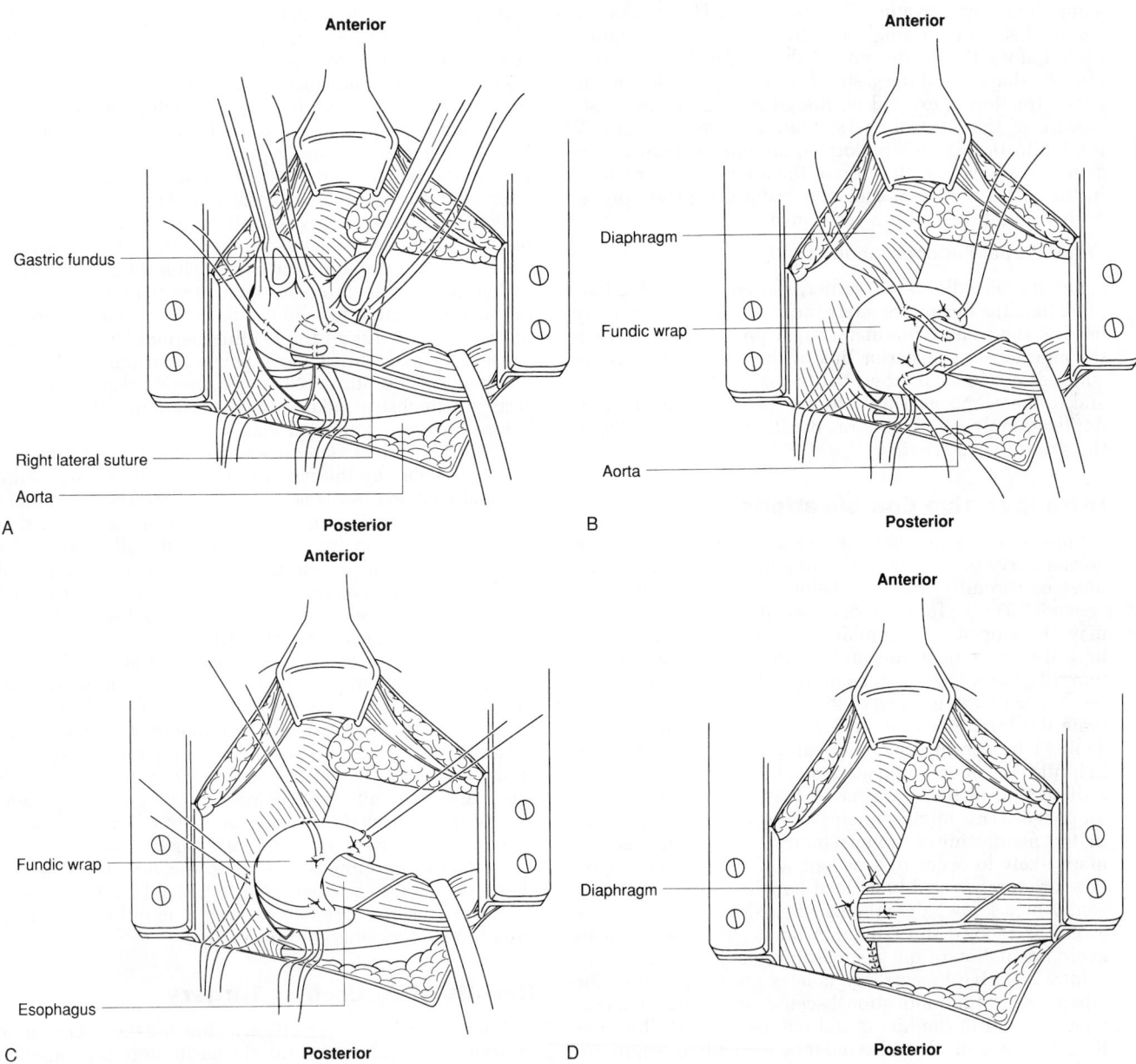

Figure 18-49. Construction of a Belsey partial fundoplication. (*A*) Placement of the first row of sutures 1.5 cm above the gastroesophageal junction. Particular attention must be given to the placement of the right lateral suture. (*B*) Placement of the second row of sutures 1.5 to 2 cm above the previously tied sutures of the first row. (*C*) Placement of the tails of the previously tied second row of sutures through the diaphragm, 0.5 cm apart and 1 to 1.5 cm from the edge of the hiatus. The sutures are placed at the 4-, 8-, and 12-o'clock positions on an imaginary clock face oriented with the 6-o'clock position posterior to the hiatus and anterior to the aorta. (*D*) Completed procedure, showing the right and left crura approximated by tying the previously placed sutures. The position of the tied holding sutures is shown. (After DeMeester TR. Transthoracic antireflux procedures. In: Nyhus LM, Baker RJ, eds. Mastery of surgery. Boston, Little, Brown, 1984:386)

thin Ferguson needle and passed 0.5 cm apart from each other through the diaphragm from the abdominal to the thoracic surface, 1 cm from the edge of the hiatus. These sutures must be carefully positioned so that the fundoplication is anterior and not lateral to the esophagus. Their placement is facilitated by the use of a spoon retractor to protect abdominal structures. The needle is guided along the inner surface of the spoon before passing it through the diaphragm. The fundoplication is gently replaced in the abdomen and the diaphragmatic sutures carefully tied.

Collis Gastroplasty

The gastroplasty is best performed through the chest. A 4- to 5-cm gastric tube is created over a 48F bougie placed along the lesser curvature of the stomach. This can be accomplished with a single application of a GIA stapler placed along the fundic side of the bougie. To achieve a uniform diameter of the gastric tube throughout its length, gentle traction is exerted on the greater curvature before closure of the jaws of the stapler. The Belsey Mark IV fundoplication is then performed around the gastric tube as described earlier. Because of the absence of peristalsis in the gastric neoesophagus, we prefer the Belsey procedure to minimize outflow resistance.

Other Partial Fundoplications

For reasons discussed earlier, partial fundoplications other than the Belsey are rarely indicated. The most widely used is the transabdominal Toupet procedure, in which the anterior and posterior lips of the fundoplication are sutured, not to each other, but to the right and left crura and to the esophageal wall, to produce a 270-degree fundoplication. It can be performed without having to divide the short gastric arteries.

Intraoperative Complications

Splenic injury can occur from excessive traction on the greater curve of the stomach, and adhesions to the spleen must be carefully dissected before the fundoplication is created. Bleeding from minor or peripheral splenic injuries may be stopped by a combination of electrocautery and topical hemostatic agents and should not require splenectomy. The esophagus can be injured during the hiatal dissection or by the passage of the large bougie used to calibrate the fundoplication. The first type of injury can be avoided by careful dissection under direct vision. It is helpful if the operator conceives of the dissection as being a dissection of the crura rather than a dissection of the esophagus. This mind set helps establish the correct plane in the mediastinum. Bougie injury of the esophagus is more likely to occur in a patient with severe esophagitis or a stricture. A well-lubricated bougie should be passed gently by a knowledgeable anesthesiologist after the surgeon has relaxed the retraction on the Penrose drain to avoid angulation of the gastroesophageal junction.

Intraoperative hemorrhage creates great difficulties for laparoscopic fundoplication because accumulated blood tends to pool in the hiatus and reduces overall illumination. The surgeon should avoid it by meticulous technique and avoid the use of irrigation when possible. Hemorrhage that endangers safe dissection by obscuring the surgeon's view is an indication for conversion to an open procedure.

Pneumothorax occasionally occurs if the mediastinal pleura is breached and the insufflated gas enters the pleural cavity. It is first manifested by an increase in peak inspiratory pressures. Ventilation may be improved by reducing the CO_2 insufflation pressure, but if this cannot be done without impairing exposure, the procedure should be converted to an open fundoplication.

If the patient is selected correctly, the surgeon should not encounter the unfortunate situation of performing an abdominal fundoplication but being unable to reduce the gastroesophageal junction into the abdomen. The options in this difficult predicament include conversion to a transthoracic approach or the transabdominal creation of a Collis gastroplasty tube by making a window with the EEA stapler and firing the GIA stapler between the window and the angle of His. Neither of these is ideal, and it is much better to anticipate the problem and plan the procedure accordingly.

Postoperative Management

After laparoscopic surgery, recovery is generally speedy. The nasogastric tube can be removed the morning after surgery and liquids commenced. If no dysphagia is experienced, soft foods are introduced later that day, and the patient can go home on the second postoperative day. As experience in laparoscopic fundoplication is gained, earlier discharge is becoming possible, and some surgeons have performed it as a day case. No practice is yet standard. After open surgery, return of gastric and intestinal function is slower, and respiratory complications are more frequent because of the decreased ventilation caused by the pain of the long upper abdominal incision. Thus, after either open abdominal or transthoracic repair, the patient is kept on nasogastric suction for about 5 days to prevent distention of the stomach during the healing period. Distention can cause a breakdown of the repair. A barium swallow is obtained on the 6th or 7th postoperative day to demonstrate the unobstructed passage of barium into the stomach before starting a solid oral diet.

In the first 2 weeks after operation, slight dysphagia may be experienced by the patient, but this disappears as the traumatic edema resolves. During this period, the patient should avoid swallowing large boluses of solid food that might stress the repair. Dysphagia occasionally persists for a longer period if an intramural hematoma at the site of the fundoplication has developed. This usually is absorbed within 4 to 6 weeks, and the dysphagia then subsides. Persistent dysphagia after this time in a patient with a previous stricture usually responds to a single dilation. Other important but preventable causes of prolonged postoperative dysphagia are the presence of a motility defect and technical errors. One of the immediate benefits of an antireflux procedure is that immediately after recovering from anesthesia, the patient experiences relief from heartburn and regurgitation. Before discharge, the patient should be counseled that until the habit of air swallowing is broken, increased flatus and mild gastric distention may occur due to trapping of the air in the stomach. The patients also should be instructed to take all medications in liquid or crushed form for at least 6 months to avoid a drug-induced esophageal injury.

Results of Antireflux Surgery

When patients are correctly selected and the operation is performed in conformity with the basic surgical principles outlined earlier, long-term relief of symptoms is achieved by more than 90% of patients.[24] Most patients experience some increase in flatulence and abdominal distention, but in most, it quickly resolves. The open Nissen fundoplication has been most extensively studied both clinically and physiologically. Results show actuarial freedom from symptoms in 91% of patients at 10 years, and the operation achieves this result by restoring the mechanical characteristics of the LES, that is, the overall length, intraabdominal length, and resting pressure. The effect of successful surgery can be visualized by three-dimensional representation of the LES (Fig. 18-50).

The outcome of complicated reflux disease is more variable and depends on residual esophageal function. Paradoxically, the outcome after a Collis-Belsey operation tends to be better than after a Belsey operation alone. This is probably because patients suitable for the Belsey procedure have normal esophageal length but poor contractility. Therefore, the motility disorder is primary rather than secondary to reflux and does not improve after surgery. Most patients with strictures who have a good symptomatic response to dilation respond well to fundoplication. In Barrett's esophagus, the ability of effective antireflux surgery to protect against the development of cancer is still not proved. Most clinical experience, however, indicates that Barrett's esophageal cancers are exceedingly rare after fundoplication, most commonly occurring in patients treated medically for an extended period. The American College of Gastroenterology keeps a registry of Barrett's esophagus patients who are followed after both medical and surgical treatment, and the incidence of dysplasia and cancer is significantly higher in the medically treated group. Thus, the weight of evidence strongly suggests that timely fundoplication is protective against cancer. Better still would be a policy of prevention.

Failed Antireflux Repairs

Patients with one or more previous unsuccessful antireflux operations constitute a particularly challenging group. In these patients, it is especially important to obtain the fullest possible information about esophageal function. The reasons for a poor result may be either because of technical errors in performing the operation or because of inappropriate indications for operation. Several typical patterns are discernible:

1. The so-called slipped Nissen fundoplication may develop when the upper stomach passes cephalad through the fundoplication and causes both dysphagia and heartburn. It is more likely that the condition

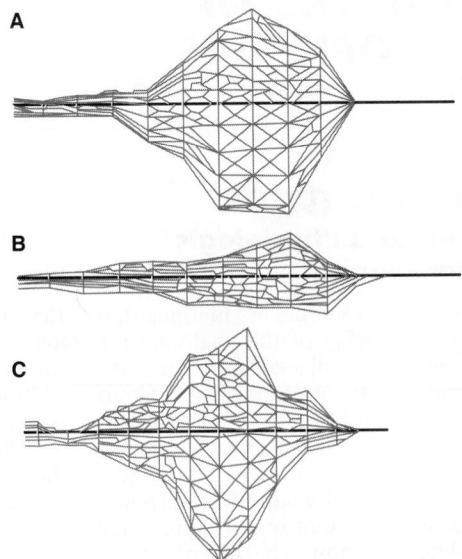

Figure 18-50. Three-dimensional representation of the lower esophageal sphincter in a normal volunteer (*A*), in a patient with Barrett's esophagus (*B*), and in the same patient 1 year after Nissen fundoplication (*C*).

was created at the time of surgery because of inadequate mobilization of the fundus or because unrecognized esophageal shortening and limited visualization of the gastroesophageal junction resulted in a fundic wrap around the upper stomach rather than the lower esophagus. This problem usually necessitates that a Collis-type gastroplasty be combined with a Belsey repair to ensure that the fundoplication sits below the diaphragm without tension.

2. If the fundoplication is too tight, the patient develops dysphagia immediately after operation. Manometry shows a high-pressure, nonrelaxing sphincter and may also show high-pressure simultaneous waves in the esophageal body, making it difficult to distinguish it from vigorous achalasia. These cases highlight the importance of obtaining manometry on all patients before proceeding to antireflux surgery. In a patient with normal preoperative motility, the cause is usually a technical fault and can be prevented by constructing the fundoplication over a 60F bougie, as described earlier. Surgical correction involves the creation of a looser fundoplication. If prospective manometry was not performed, the surgeon must assess this clinically from a history of preoperative dysphagia suggesting an underlying motility disorder. The treatment of such a disorder must include a myotomy and partial fundoplication, as described in the section on primary motor disorders of the esophageal body.

3. Disruption of the fundoplication manifested clinically and physiologically by recurrent reflux has at least three predisposing causes:
   a. Inadequate suture technique: taking inadequate bites of tissue, or the use of flimsy or quickly absorbable material.
   b. Choice of operation: all partial fundoplications, such as the Toupet procedure, are more prone to disruption than a Nissen fundoplication. This is because the integrity of the repair depends on sutures to the esophageal wall and because all of these repairs require much more abdominal length of esophagus than a Nissen repair, therefore placing the repair under tension.
   c. Unrecognized esophageal shortening leads to tension on the wrap, which may then become undone.

Individual case reports of other complications after antireflux repairs include anatomic aberrations, such as the development of paraesophageal hernia, and fistulous complications from gastrointestinal tract perforation and sepsis. Examples of the latter are gastropleural and gastrobronchial fistulas.

Inappropriate patient selection also can lead to patient dissatisfaction after the operation. This most often occurs when the cause of the reflux is primarily a defect in the esophageal body or the gastric reservoir, or when the operation has been performed for symptoms in the absence of objective documentation of the disease. Careful study of all patients before considering antireflux surgery minimizes the incidence of such problems.

The principles underlying treatment of these patients rely on the physiologic assessment of residual esophageal function. Generally, if a clear reason for the failure can be identified, and the patient has undergone only one or two previous attempts at repair, then a good result can be expected. Multiple previous operations or the presence of complex motility patterns should suggest the need for esophageal replacement, generally with colon.

Esophagectomy and esophageal replacement are occasionally indicated in the treatment of advanced GERD. To perform this operation safely and with good functional results requires the advantages of a specialist center where expertise in assessment, operative skill, and intensive care are readily available. In the absence of these facilities, the temptation to persist with ineffective medical treatment or to try yet another antireflux operation is strong. The indications for esophagectomy are Barrett's esophagus with high-grade dysplasia and what is generally described as *burned-out esophagus*. Additional indications are failure of a third antireflux operation, severe coexistent motility disorder, or the presence of an undilatable stricture. Either colon or stomach can be used to replace the esophagus. Colonic replacement is more difficult, requiring three anastomoses rather than one, but it has superior functional long-term results, particularly if it opens into a vagally innervated stomach. This is more likely to be the case in severe primary motility disorders because after multiple operations at the gastroesophageal junction, the vagus nerves are unlikely to be intact. In this eventuality, the proximal stomach, if left in situ, would be a nonfunctioning, atonic bag, thereby contributing to upper abdominal discomfort. Therefore, the proximal stomach is removed and the colon graft anastomosed to the antrum.[25]

REFERENCES

1. Rothberg M, DeMeester TR. Surgical anatomy of the esophagus. In: Shields TW, ed. General thoracic surgery, ed 3. Philadelphia, Lea & Febiger, 1989.
2. DeMeester TR, Barlow AP. Surgery and current management for cancer of the esophagus and cardia, parts I and II. Curr Probl Surg 1988;25:477.
3. Schnell TH, Sontag SJ, Chejifec G. Adenocarcinoma arising in tongues or short segments of Barrett's esophagus. Dig Dis Sci 1992;37:137.
4. Monnier P, Ollyo J-B, Fontolliet C, Savary M. Epidemiology and natural history of reflux esophagitis. Semin Lap Surg 1995;2:2.
5. Kahrilas PJ, Dodds WJ, Hogan WJ. Effect of peristaltic dysfunction on esophageal volume clearance. Gastroenterology 1988;94:73.
6. DeMeester TR, Wernly JA, Bryant GH, Little AG, Skinner DB. Clinical and in vitro analysis of determinants of gastroesophageal competence. Am J Surg 1979;137:39.
7. Bonavina L, Evander A, DeMeester TR, et al. Length of the distal esophageal sphincter and competency of the Cardia. Am J Surg 1986;151:25.
8. Dent J, Dodds WJ, Friedman RH, et al. Mechanism of gastroesophageal reflux in recumbent asymptomatic human subjects. J Clin Invest 1980;65:256.
9. Zaninotto G, DeMeester TR, Schwizer W, et al. The lower esophageal sphincter in health and disease. Am J Surg 1988;155:104.
10. Stein HJ, DeMeester TR, Naspetti R, Jamieson J, Perry RE. Three-dimensional imaging of the lower esophageal sphincter in gastroesophageal reflux disease. Ann Surg 1991;214:374.
11. Cook IJ, Dodds WJ, Dantas RO, et al. Opening mechanisms of the human upper esophageal sphincter. Am J Physiol 1989;257G748.
12. DeMeester TR, Wang CI, Wernly, JA et al. Technique, indications and clinical use of 24-hour esophageal pH monitoring. J Thorac Cardiovasc Surg 1980;79:656.
13. Attwood SEA, DeMeester TR, Bremner CG, et al. Alkaline gastroesophageal reflux: implications in the development of complications in Barrett's columnar-lined lower esophagus. Surgery 1989;106:764.
14. Stein HJ, DeMeester TR, Eypasch EP, Klingman RP. Ambulatory 24-hour esophageal manometry in the evaluation of esophageal motor disorders and non-cardiac chest pain. Surgery 1991;110:753.
15. Bechi P, Pucciani F, Baldini F, et al. Long-term ambulatory enterogastric reflux monitoring: validation of a new fiberoptic technique. Dig Dis Sci 1993;38:1297.
16. Duranceau A. Pharyngeal and cricopharyngeal disorders. In: Pearson FG, ed. Esophageal surgery. New York, Churchill Livingstone, 1995:389.
17. Andreollo NA, Earlam RJ. Heller's myotomy for achalasia: is an added antireflux procedure necessary? Br J Surg 1987;74:765.
18. Csendes A, Braghetto I, Henriquez A, Cortes C. Late results of a prospective randomised study comparing forceful dilatation and oesophagomyotomy in patients with achalasia. Gut 1989;30:299.
19. Eypasch E, DeMeester TR, Klingman R, Stein HJ. Physiological assessment and surgical management of diffuse esophageal spasm. J Thorac Cardiovasc Surg 1992;104:859.
20. Sloan S, Rademaker AW, Kahrilas PJ. Determinants of gastroesophageal junction incompetence: hiatal hernia, lower esophageal sphincter or both? Ann Intern Med 1992;117:977.
21. Stein HJ, Barlow AP, DeMeester TR, Hinder RA. Complications of gastroesophageal reflux disease: role of the lower esophageal sphincter, esophageal acid and acid/alkaline exposure, and duodenogastric reflux. Ann Surg 1992;216:35.
22. Spechler SJ, and the VA Gastroesophageal Reflux Study Group. A prospective trial of medical and surgical therapies for gastroesophageal reflux disease. N Engl J Med 1992;326:786.
23. Peters JH, Heimbucher J, Kauer WKH, Incarbone R, Bremner CG, DeMeester TR. Clinical and physiologic comparison of laparoscopic and open Nissen fundoplication. J Am Coll Surg 1995;180:385.
24. DeMeester TR, Bonavina L, Albertucci M. Nissen fundoplication for gastro-esophageal reflux disease: evaluation of primary repair in 100 consecutive patients. Ann Surg 1986;204:9.
25. DeMeester TR, Johansson K-E, Franze I, et al. Indications, surgical technique, and long-term function results of colon interposition or bypass. Ann Surg 1988;208:460.

SURGERY: SCIENTIFIC PRINCIPLES AND PRACTICE, Second Edition, edited by Lazar J. Greenfield, Michael W. Mulholland, Keith T. Oldham, Gerald B. Zelenock, and Keith D. Lillemoe. Lippincott–Raven Publishers, Philadelphia, © 1997.

CHAPTER 19

TUMORS, INJURIES, AND MISCELLANEOUS CONDITIONS OF THE ESOPHAGUS

MARK B. ORRINGER

ESOPHAGEAL TUMORS
Anatomic and Physiologic Considerations

Most esophageal tumors are malignant; less than 1% are benign. A knowledge of the anatomic relations between the esophagus and adjacent structures is important both in understanding the presentation of esophageal tumors at various levels and in planning therapy. For example, tumors involving the cervicothoracic esophagus (the segment from the cricopharyngeal sphincter to the thoracic inlet at the level of the suprasternal notch) often involve the larynx and therefore require a laryngopharyngectomy for complete resection. The magnitude of this operative undertaking, combined with a pharyngeal anastomosis to reestablish alimentary continuity, is far greater than that typically faced by the surgeon performing the usual palliative esophageal resection for carcinoma of the intrathoracic esophagus. The upper thoracic esophagus is contiguous with the posterior membranous trachea anteriorly and the aortic arch and great vessels. Thus, patients with cancer involving the upper thoracic esophagus should routinely undergo preoperative bronchoscopy to rule out invasion of the posterior membranous trachea, which would preclude resection. When resecting an upper thoracic esophageal tumor through a thoracotomy, the approach is a *right* fourth or fifth interspace incision because the aortic arch interferes with mobilization of the upper thoracic esophagus through the left chest. Mid-thoracic esophageal tumors can involve the carina or proximal main-stem bronchus, particularly where the esophagus passes behind the left main-stem bronchus, the common site for presentation of a malignant tracheoesophageal fistula. Once again, because of its anatomic proximity to the tracheobronchial tree, a mid-thoracic esophageal tumor may require a *right* thoracotomy, which provides optimal exposure to the carina and proximal bronchi. Distal esophageal tumors are approached transthoracically through a *left*-sided approach because the most distal esophagus and esophagogastric junction cannot be adequately visualized through the right chest.

Another important anatomic consideration when performing esophageal resection is the unique submucosa of the esophagus, the unusual fat content of which allows a great deal of mobility of the overlying mucosa. Unless great care is taken to ensure that every anastomotic stitch transfixes the submucosa, an anastomotic leak may occur as a result of the mucosa retracting proximally and accurate apposition of the mucosa not being achieved.[1] The esophagus is a mucosa-lined muscular tube that lacks a serosa. It is surrounded by adventitia, or mediastinal connective tissue, which is a loose fibroareolar layer. Transmural invasion by esophageal carcinomas is exceedingly common, the tumor not being limited by overlying pleura, in contrast to intestinal cancers, which often extend to, but not through, the adjacent peritoneum.

Although it has a segmental blood supply, the esophagus is well vascularized by numerous arteries and has an extensive collateral circulation. The cervical esophagus receives blood supply from the superior and inferior thyroid arteries, both communicating through collaterals. Four to six aortic esophageal arteries supply the intrathoracic esophagus and anastomose through collaterals with the inferior thyroid, intercostal and bronchial, inferior phrenic, and left gastric arteries. Anatomic studies of the esophageal blood supply indicate that the esophageal arteries terminate in fine capillary networks before actually penetrating the esophageal muscle layer.[2] In the process of transhiatal blunt esophageal mobilization, therefore, if the dissection is kept close to the esophageal wall, the risk of serious hemorrhage from a sizable vessel is minimal.

An understanding of esophageal innervation is important in explaining the effect on swallowing of tumors and operations involving the cervicothoracic esophagus.[3] The esophagus is innervated through the visceral autonomic nervous system. Efferent sympathetic innervation, concerned with vasoconstriction, peristalsis, contraction of the sphincters, and muscular wall relaxation, is through the cervical and thoracic sympathetic chain. Afferent parasympathetic innervation controls increases in glandular and peristaltic activity and is through the vagus nerves, which also carry some sensory fibers. The superior laryngeal nerves arise from the vagus nerves in the neck and divide into external and internal laryngeal branches. Both the cricothyroid muscle, which is the tensor of the vocal cords, and a portion of the inferior pharyngeal constrictor are supplied by the external laryngeal nerve, while the internal laryngeal nerve provides sensory innervation of

the larynx above the vocal cords and the base of the tongue. The parasympathetic innervation of the cervical esophagus, as well as innervation to the upper esophageal sphincter, is provided by the recurrent laryngeal branches of the vagus nerves. Therefore, injury to the recurrent laryngeal nerve during construction of a cervical esophagogastric anastomosis (or any cervical or thoracic operation) may produce not only hoarseness but also upper esophageal sphincter dysfunction with incapacitating and life-threatening aspiration on swallowing. This is a disastrous complication in a patient undergoing an operation to reestablish the ability to swallow comfortably. Similarly, delayed gastric emptying due to impaired motility or pylorospasm after division of the vagus nerves during performance of an esophagectomy for cancer may result in catastrophic regurgitation and aspiration.

Finally, gastroesophageal reflux plays an important role not only in the development of adenocarcinoma of the lower esophagus but also in the immediate and long-term functional results of an esophagogastric anastomosis. The relation among severe gastroesophageal reflux, the development of Barrett's mucosa, and subsequent adenocarcinoma has been well described. After esophageal resection for both benign and malignant esophageal disease, gastroesophageal reflux continues to play an important role. In constructing a low intrathoracic esophagogastric anastomosis, the surgeon relegates the patient to almost certain gastroesophageal reflux due to the iatrogenic hiatal hernia that is created. The higher the esophagogastric anastomosis within the thorax, the lower is the incidence of subsequent gastroesophageal reflux. With a cervical esophagogastric anastomosis, in which virtually the entire stomach is in the thorax and none is below the diaphragmatic hiatus, clinically significant gastroesophageal reflux is rare. Gastroesophageal reflux is also one of the important factors responsible for the morbidity of an intrathoracic esophagogastric anastomotic leak. The resultant mediastinitis and empyema are due not only to the extravasation of saliva and oral bacteria but also to the chemical effects of refluxed bile and gastric acid draining through the anastomosis.

Benign Esophageal Tumors and Cysts

Benign tumors of the esophagus are rare, constituting only 0.5% to 0.8% of esophageal neoplasms.[4] They are classified into two major groups: epithelial (mucosal) and intramural (extramucosal)[5] (Table 19-1). Even more rare are heterotopic collections of tissue within the esophageal wall.

Leiomyomas

Leiomyomas represent the most common benign intramural esophageal tumor and characteristically occur in patients between 20 and 50 years of age. The tumors are multiple in 3% to 10% of patients, have no established gender preponderance, and can occur at any level within the esophagus but rarely occur in the cervical segment. More than 80% of esophageal leiomyomas occur in the middle and lower thirds of the esophagus. Because calcification can occur within a leiomyoma, this must be considered in the differential diagnosis of a calcified mediastinal mass. Histologically, leiomyomas are composed of interlacing bundles of smooth muscle cells. Tumors less than 5 cm in diameter rarely cause symptoms. When larger than this, dysphagia, retrosternal pressure, and pain are the common complaints. Most reported leiomyomas have been incidental autopsy findings and were asymptomatic. When a leiomyoma virtually encircles the esophageal lumen, obstruction and regurgitation can occur. Bleeding more often occurs with the malignant form of the tumor, leiomyosar-

Table 19-1. CLASSIFICATION OF BENIGN ESOPHAGEAL TUMORS

EPITHELIAL TUMORS

Papillomas
Polyps
Adenomas
Cysts

NONEPITHELIAL TUMORS

Myomas
  Leiomyomas
  Fibromyomas
  Lipomyomas
  Fibromas
Vascular tumors
  Hemangiomas
  Lymphangiomas
Mesenchymal and other tumors
  Reticuloendothelial tumors
  Lipomas
  Myxofibromas
  Giant cell tumors
  Neurofibromas
  Osteochondromas

HETEROTOPIC TUMORS

Gastric mucosal tumors
Melanoblastic tumors
Sebaceous gland tumors
Granular cell myoblastomas
Pancreatic gland tumors
Thyroid nodules

(Nemir P Jr, Wallace HW, Fallahnejad M. Diagnosis and surgical management of benign disease of the esophagus. Curr Probl Surg 1976;13:1)

coma. Malignant degeneration of leiomyomas is exceedingly rare, with fewer than 10 reported cases. Occasionally, large, confluent leiomyomas involve the lower esophagus and cardia. Most leiomyomas, however, are solitary and vary from 2 to 5 cm in diameter. Another interesting variation of this tumor is diffuse leiomyomatosis of the esophagus, in which there is extensive infiltration of the entire esophagus as well as multiple leiomyomas of the stomach, uterus, major airways, and ureters. This condition has occurred in children as young as 7 years of age, tends to occur in families, and may also be associated with hypertrophy of the vulva and clitoris, cataracts, and deafness.

Esophageal leiomyomas produce a characteristic smooth, concave submucosal defect with sharp borders and abrupt sharp angles where the tumor meets the normal esophageal wall on barium swallow examination. The tumor often appears to lie half within and half outside the esophagus (Fig. 19-1). As with every esophageal tumor, esophagoscopy is indicated to exclude the presence of carcinoma. If the radiologic impression of a leiomyoma is confirmed endoscopically, a biopsy of the mass should *not* be performed so that subsequent extramural resection is not complicated by scarring at the biopsy site. At esophagoscopy, these tumors are characteristically mobile, have an intact overlying mucosa, and can be displaced by the advancing esophagoscope. Endoscopic ultrasonography has provided a new means for evaluating the esophageal leiomyoma, which is seen as a distinct intramural mass of characteristic low echodensity.[6]

An asymptomatic leiomyoma or one discovered incidentally on a barium swallow examination can be safely observed and followed with periodic barium esophagograms and endoscopic ultrasonography. Although excision of the esophageal mass provides the only definitive tissue diagnosis, the characteristic radiographic appearance, slow growth rate, and low risk of malignant degeneration, as well as the ability to follow leiomyomas with endoscopic ultrasonography, justify conservative management. Tumors that are symptomatic or larger than 5 cm in diameter should be excised. Tumors of the middle third of the esophagus are approached through a right thoracotomy, while those in the distal third are approached through a left thoracotomy. Once the esophagus is encircled and the tumor located, the overlying longitudinal muscle is split in the direction of its fibers. The tumor is then gently dissected away from the contiguous underlying submucosa and adjacent muscle. When enucleation of the tumor is complete, the longitudinal esophageal muscle is reapproximated, although a large extramucosal defect may be left without complication. Giant leiomyomas of the cardia and adjacent stomach may require esophageal resection for their removal (Fig. 19-2). Alternatively, multiple enucleations may be performed. When resection is complete, leiomyomas virtually never recur.

Polyps

Benign polyps of the esophagus are rare and typically arise in the cervical esophagus. Traction on these polyps caused by repeated peristaltic contractions results in pro-

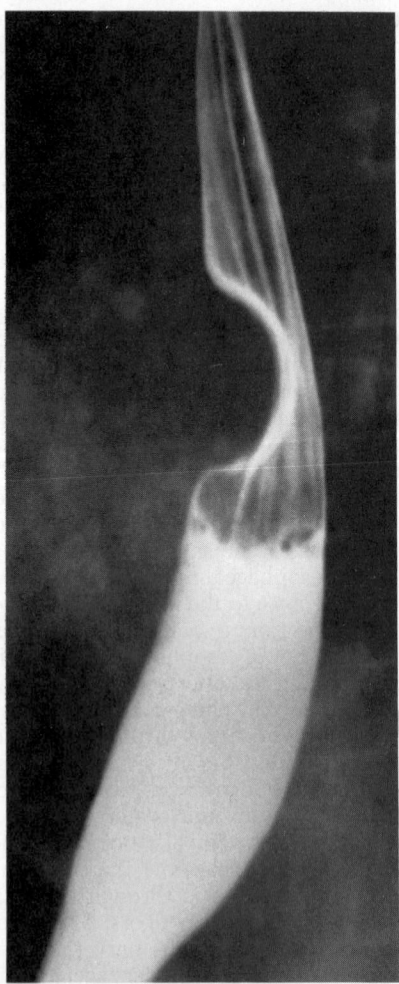

Figure 19-1. Esophagogram showing a leiomyoma with the typical acute angle at its junction with the esophageal wall. (Orringer MB. Tumors of the esophagus. In: Sabiston DC Jr, ed. Textbook of surgery, ed 13. Philadelphia, WB Saunders, 1986:736)

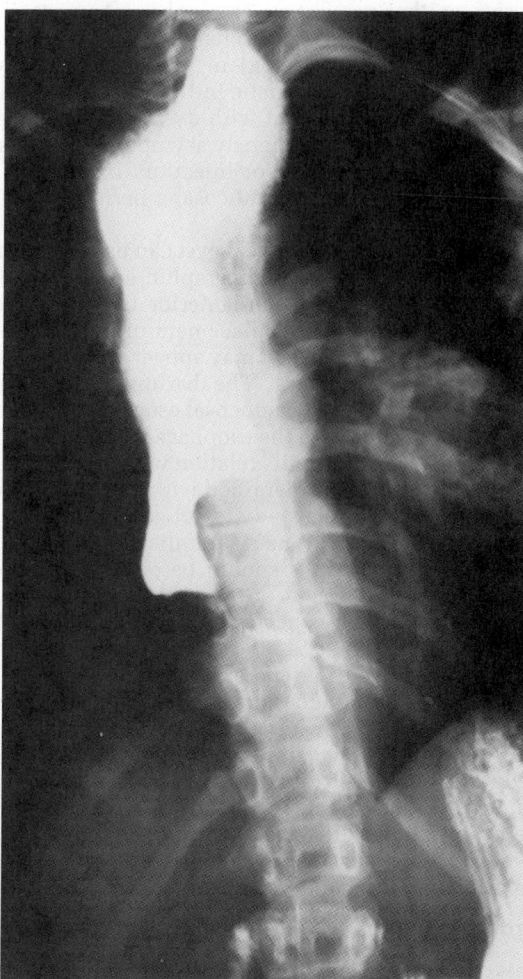

Figure 19-2. Esophagogram showing a giant leiomyoma that involved the distal half of the esophagus and esophagogastric junction and that necessitated an esophagectomy for its removal. (Orringer MB. Tumors of the esophagus. In: Sabiston DC Jr, ed. Textbook of surgery, ed 13. Philadelphia, WB Saunders, 1986:737)

gressive lengthening of their pedicles. This may be responsible for their dramatic presentations, at times intermittently extruding into and even out of the mouth or producing asphyxia as the upper airway becomes obstructed. Most benign polyps occur in older men, and these frequently are attached to the cricoid cartilage. The tumors typically produce dysphagia, but hematemesis or melena may occur if the overlying mucosa becomes ulcerated. These polyps tend to be solitary with a long, cylindric configuration that may produce marked esophageal dilation. Histologically, they are composed of fibrovascular tissue with varying amounts of associated fat. Barium swallow findings may be nondiagnostic or inaccurately interpreted in these patients. The polyp may be overlooked as an air bubble or may be misdiagnosed as a carcinoma, or even as a foreign body or achalasia if it has caused marked esophageal dilation (Fig. 19-3). Similarly, esophagoscopy may fail to define the polyp, particularly if the pedicle is not demonstrated and the mucosa overlying the polyp is normal. The endoscopist simply passes the lesion, which is soft and easily displaced with the esophagus. Although esophageal polyps have been removed endoscopically by electrocoagulation of the pedicle, the recommended approach is resection through a lateral cervical esophagotomy, delivering the polyp from the esophagus, resecting

its mucosal base of origin, and repairing the defect under direct vision (Fig. 19-4).

Hemangiomas

Esophageal hemangiomas are rare, constituting 2% to 3% of benign tumors. Although they are generally asymptomatic, they can be responsible for periodic gastrointestinal bleeding or even massive and fatal hematemesis. Asymptomatic lesions discovered incidentally during performance of an esophagoscopy should be followed with periodic endoscopy. Those that have bled require treatment, and although resection has been the standard approach, laser endoscopy provides an effective alternative for control of the small bleeding sites visualized through the esophagoscope.

Miscellaneous Benign Tumors

Benign esophageal tumors other than leiomyomas and polyps are extremely rare. *Granular cell myoblastomas* actually arise from Schwann cells, not muscle as their name implies. They produce dysphagia, retrosternal pain, nausea, and vomiting. They are difficult to diagnose endoscopically because of their submucosal location and have a

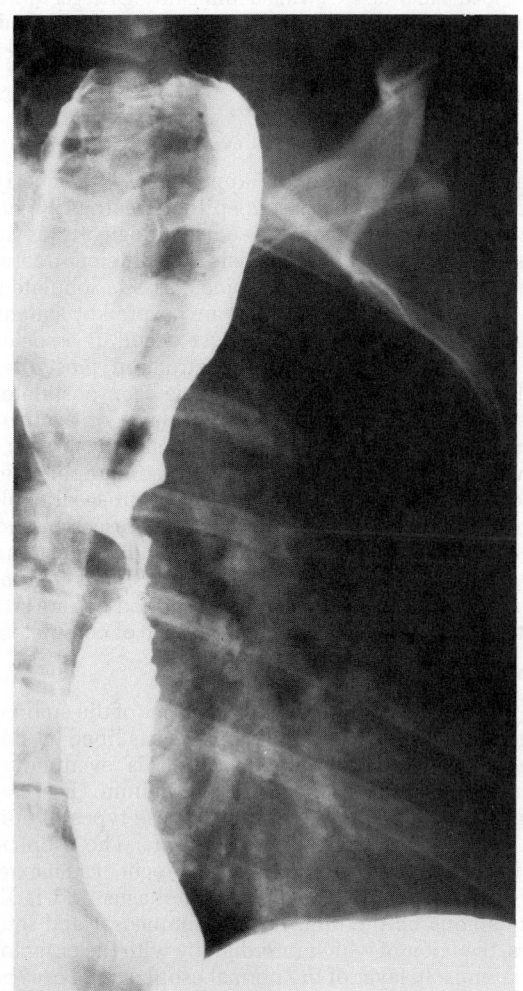

Figure 19-3. Barium esophagogram of a patient with a giant benign fibroepithelial polyp, showing a large intraluminal mass distending the cervical and upper thoracic esophagus. (Orringer MB. Miscellaneous conditions of the esophagus. In: Orringer MB. Zuidema GD, eds. Shackelford's surgery of the alimentary tract. Philadelphia, WB Saunders, 1991:460)

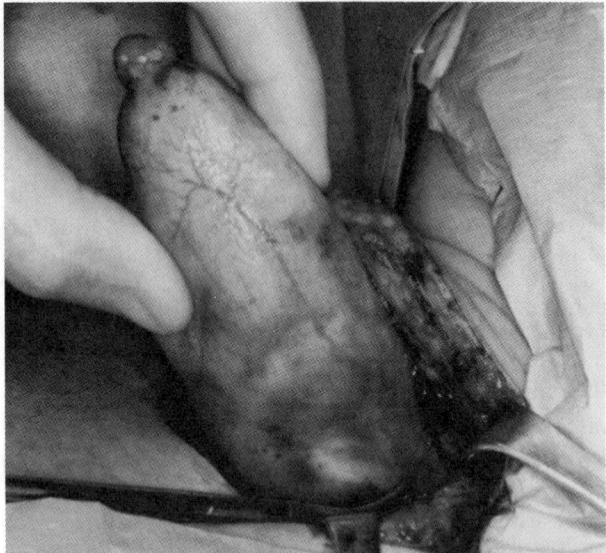

Figure 19-4. Operative photograph of the patient shown in Figure 19-3. The giant polyp has been delivered out of the cervical esophagus through a left-sided neck incision. The patient's head is toward the right, and the retractors are against the sternocleidomastoid muscle. The hemostat indicates the base of the polyp, which was divided and oversewn without difficulty. (Orringer MB. Miscellaneous conditions of the esophagus. In: Orringer MB, Zuidema GD, eds. Shackelford's surgery of the alimentary tract. Philadelphia, WB Saunders, 1991:470)

characteristic grayish yellow appearance. The overlying mucosa typically shows pseudoepitheliomatous hyperplasia, which may be misdiagnosed histologically as squamous cell carcinoma. Local excision is sufficient treatment of symptomatic tumors. *Papillomas,* sessile lobulated tumors that have a fibrous core and are covered by squamous mucosa, have been reported. Most occur in association with some degree of esophageal obstruction, most often in the distal esophagus. Papillomas have been postulated to represent localized epithelial hyperplasia or even to be premalignant lesions, but their true significance is unknown. On the basis of their size and radiographic configuration, papillomas at times warrant esophageal exploration to exclude malignancy, but a major resection should be avoided because local excision is adequate therapy. *Esophageal adenomas, carcinoid tumors,* and *inflammatory pseudotumors* also have been reported but are so rare that they are mentioned only for the sake of completeness.

Cysts

Esophageal cysts arise as outpouchings of the embryonic foregut. Embryologically, the esophagus is lined by simple columnar ciliated epithelium, which is eventually replaced by stratified squamous epithelium. Esophageal cysts can therefore contain both of these types of epithelium as well as fat and smooth muscle. The esophageal duplication cyst is a variation of the foregut cyst; it extends along the length of the thoracic esophagus and is lined by squamous epithelium. It has submucosal and muscle layers, the latter of which interdigitate with the outer longitudinal muscle layer of the normal esophagus. Three quarters of esophageal duplication cysts present in childhood, and more than 60% are located along the right side of the esophagus. As is the case with other foregut cysts, esophageal duplication cysts are frequently associated with vertebral anomalies (Klippel-Feil deformity or spina bifida) and spinal cord abnormalities. More than 60% of esophageal

cysts cause either respiratory or esophageal symptoms in the first year of life. Those located in the upper third of the esophagus tend to present in infancy, while lower-third cysts may be asymptomatic initially and present later in childhood. Adults present with dysphagia, choking, or retrosternal pain when previously asymptomatic cysts enlarge as a result of bleeding or infection. In the rare cyst that contains ectopic gastric mucosa, a perforation of the cyst may occur.

The diagnosis of an esophageal cyst can usually be made on the basis of its typical radiographic appearance (Fig. 19-5). On the standard posteroanterior chest roentgenogram, the cyst may cause displacement of the trachea; on lateral chest roentgenogram, it may appear as a retrocardiac posterior mediastinal mass. The barium esophagogram demonstrates a smooth extramucosal esophageal mass that rarely communicates with the esophageal lumen. The cystic nature of the lesion and its relation with adjacent mediastinal structures may be identified with computed tomography (CT), although this study is not generally necessary to make the diagnosis. When a duplication cyst is suspected, spinal radiographs should be obtained preoperatively to identify an origin of the cyst in the notochord. Because esophageal cysts have a predilection for bleeding, ulceration, perforation, and infection, excision is generally recommended. This can generally be achieved with low morbidity by an extramucosal resection. In the rare event that the wall of the cyst cannot be separated from the common esophageal wall, it can be left behind, but the mucosa of the cyst should be stripped away to prevent recurrence. Alternative surgical treatments, such as marsupialization of the cyst, internal drainage, or cauterization of the mucosa, do not represent optimal management. Recurrence of the cyst after complete excision is rare.

Heterotopic Tumors

Islets of columnar mucosa may be found lining the pharynx and esophagus. These islets are much more common near the upper end than the lower end of the esophagus. Endoscopically, they are described as an *inlet patch* of columnar mucosa. Given the embryologic replacement of the initial columnar ciliated epithelium by stratified squamous epithelium, the occurrence of preserved inlet patches of columnar epithelium is readily explained. This tissue is not to be confused with Barrett's mucosa and has little, if any, premalignant disposition. There have also been isolated reports of sebaceous gland tumors as well as ectopic pancreatic and thyroid tissue within the esophagus. These are primarily autopsy reports that have little clinical significance.

Malignant Esophageal Tumors

Squamous Cell Carcinoma

World-wide, 95% of all esophageal cancers are squamous cell carcinomas. In the United States and Europe, however, the incidence of adenocarcinoma arising in Barrett's mucosa is increasing at an alarming rate and in many areas surpasses that of squamous cell tumors. There is wide variation in the incidence of squamous cell carcinoma of the esophagus throughout the world. Among the white populations of the United States, Canada, Israel, Nigeria, and throughout Europe, the incidence is relatively low (3 or 4 per 100,000 population). In contrast, in high-risk areas of northeastern Iran, Transkei in South Africa, Linxian county in Hunan province in northern China, and certain areas of southern Russia that border on the Caspian Sea, the incidence is more than 35 per 100,000 population and is as high as 53 to 800 per 100,000 population in

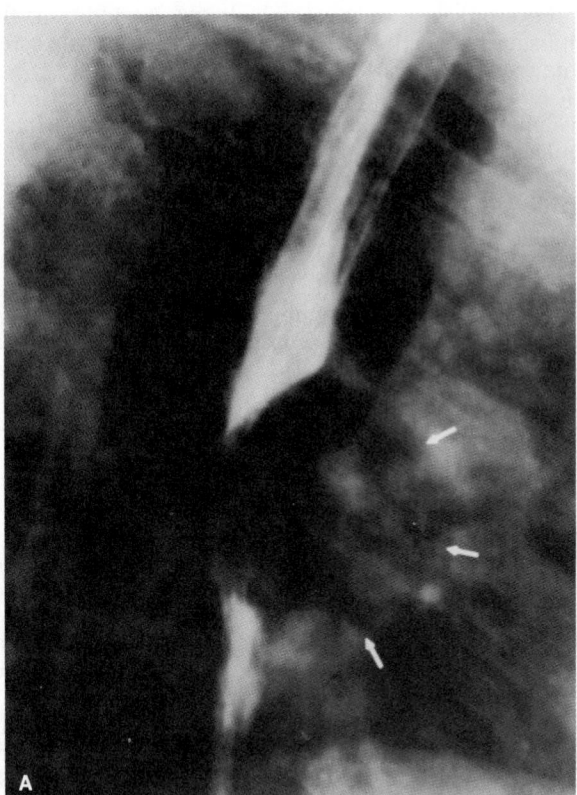
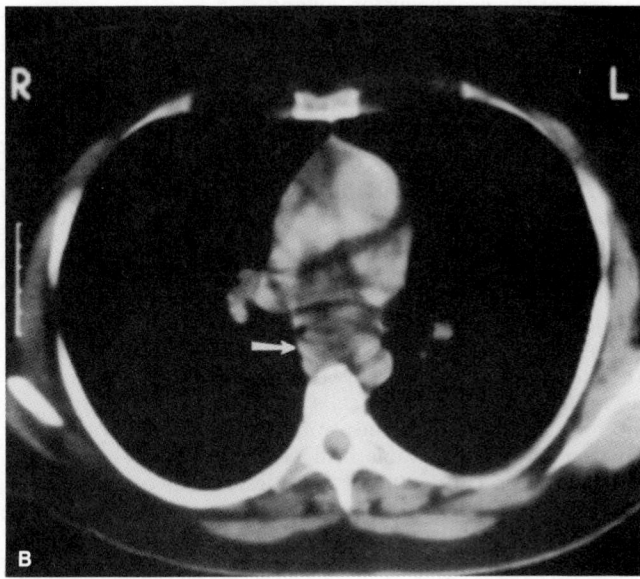

Figure 19-5. Esophageal duplication cyst presenting as a high posterior mediastinal mass. (*A*) Barium esophagogram showing the intramural, extramucosal esophageal mass. (*B*) CT scan showing the cystic nature of the lesion (*arrow*).

people older than 50 years of age.[7,8] This disease occurs most commonly in the seventh decade of life and generally is 1.5 to 3 times more common in men than in women. The predilection for men, however, is reversed in those regions with a high incidence of Plummer-Vinson syndrome, which more commonly affects women.

The cause of esophageal carcinoma is unknown. It is thought to occur most often as a result of prolonged exposure of the esophageal mucosa to noxious stimuli in patients who have a genetic predisposition to the disease. Epidemiologic studies in endemic areas of China, for example, suggest that the presence of large amounts of carcinogenic nitrosamines in the soil, the contamination of foods by mutagenic fungi, most often *Geotrichum candidum*, and yeast are responsible for the high incidence of this tumor. In northeast Iran, esophageal carcinoma is primarily a condition of the poorest social stratum, and the use of opium, which contains pyrolysates, and the ingestion of very hot tea are believed to result in repeated esophageal mucosal injury and eventual malignant degeneration. Chewing tobacco with or without betel nut, betel leaf, slaked lime, or a resin from the acacia has been linked to the development of esophageal carcinoma in India, Pakistan, and Sri Lanka. In Singapore, ingestion of burning-hot beverages and the use of Chinese tobacco and wine are believed to be etiologic factors. The increased incidence of esophageal carcinoma among the south African Bantus and Zulus has been linked to the high nitrosamine content of their soil as well as to the contamination of their food by molds, especially the *Fusarium* species, which produces carcinogens. The most consistent risk factors among populations from Normandy, Brittany, Europe, and the United States are alcohol consumption and cigarette smoking. Carcinomas of the hypopharynx and the cervical esophagus occur almost as of-

ten in women as they do in men, probably as the result of the greater incidence of Plummer-Vinson syndrome in woman. In Sri Lanka, esophageal carcinoma is primarily a disease of women and is the most commonly encountered gastrointestinal tract malignancy. Alcohol, tobacco, zinc, nitrosamines, malnutrition, vitamin deficiencies, anemia, poor oral hygiene, dental caries, previous gastric surgery, and chronic ingestion of hot foods or beverages have all been linked to the development of esophageal cancer. In addition, certain premalignant esophageal conditions are well recognized and are discussed later.

Pathologically, esophageal carcinoma occurs over a spectrum that ranges from the early lesion (also termed *early carcinoma, superficial spreading carcinoma, intramucosal carcinoma,* or *carcinoma in situ*), which is limited to the mucosa, to the more advanced form, in which the tumor penetrates the muscle layers of the esophagus or beyond. Carcinoma in situ typically is found in patients between 40 and 50 years of age and gradually progresses to invasive squamous cell carcinoma over 2 to 4 years. Microscopically, early esophageal carcinoma is defined in terms of the depth of tumor involvement, either intraepithelial (carcinoma in situ), intramucosal (limited to the lamina propria), or submucosal. The histologic features of esophageal dysplasia resemble those seen in the uterine cervix, and as dysplasia becomes severe, histologic differentiation from carcinoma in situ becomes difficult. Once dysplastic cells are seen traversing the basement membrane and extending into the underlying connective tissue, the diagnosis of early invasion is made. Carcinoma in situ of the esophagus tends to be multifocal. Early esophageal carcinoma has been well documented in China, where the high incidence of esophageal carcinoma has justified mass screening techniques, and the disease is frequently detected before it has advanced enough to cause symptoms. Thus, several macroscopic growth patterns have been defined: a coarsely granular, reddish, slightly raised, plaque-like type; an erosive type; the occult form, which is not apparent on gross inspection of the esophagus; and the papillary type, in which a slightly polypoid lesion of less than 3 cm is seen. Advanced squamous cell carcinoma of the esophagus is defined as a tumor that involves the muscle layers of the esophagus or beyond.

In the TNM classification for staging esophageal cancer, the esophagus is divided into four main sections: (1) the *cervical* (from the lower border of the cricoid cartilage to the thoracic inlet, or 15 to 18 cm from the upper incisor teeth); the *upper thoracic* (from the thoracic inlet to the level of the carina at about 24 cm at endoscopy); the *middle third* (from the carina to half the distance to the esophagogastric junction, or about 32 cm); and the *lower* (to the esophagogastric junction at 40 cm).[9] Using this arbitrary division of the esophagus, 8% of squamous cell carcinomas occur in the cervical esophagus, 55% in the upper and mid-thoracic segments, and 37% in the lower thoracic segment. Microscopically, most squamous cell carcinomas of the esophagus are moderately differentiated and contain islands of atypical squamous cells that infiltrate the underlying adjacent normal tissues and contain keratin pearl formation and intercellular bridges between the tumor cells. Macroscopically, 60% of these lesions are fungating intraluminal growths, 25% are ulcerative lesions associated with extensive infiltration of the adjacent esophageal wall, and 15% are infiltrating. Esophageal carcinoma tends to be multifocal, and a patient who survives treatment of one carcinoma has at least twice the risk of developing a second primary esophageal neoplasm than the normal population.

Esophageal carcinoma is notorious for its aggressive biologic behavior. It tends to infiltrate locally, involving adjacent lymph nodes and spreading along the extensive submucosal esophageal lymphatic channels. Lack of an esophageal serosa favors tumor extension into adjacent structures such as the pericardium, aorta, tracheobronchial tree, diaphragm, stomach, and left recurrent laryngeal nerve. Mediastinal, supraclavicular, or celiac lymph node metastases are present in at least 75% of patients with esophageal cancer at the time of initial diagnosis. Cervical esophageal cancers tend to drain to the deep cervical, paraesophageal, posterior mediastinal, and tracheobronchial lymph nodes, while the lower esophageal tumors spread to paraesophageal, celiac, and splenic hilar lymph nodes. Distant spread to the liver and lungs is seen in 90% of cases at autopsy. The overall prognosis of invasive squamous cell carcinoma is dismal, with 5% to 12% of patients surviving 5 years. Unfortunately, extraesophageal tumor extension is present in 70% of cases at the time of diagnosis, and when lymph node metastases are present, 5-year survival is only 3%, compared with 42% when there is no lymph node spread.

Adenocarcinoma

Adenocarcinomas account for 2.5% to 8% of primary esophageal cancers, but in the United States and Europe, the frequency of this tumor is increasing at a rate surpassing that of any other cancer.[10,11] This increase is largely the result of the growing prevalence of adenocarcinoma arising in Barrett's mucosa. Adenocarcinomas most often involve the distal third of the esophagus, have a peak incidence in the sixth decade of life, and are three times more common in men than in woman. Esophageal adenocarcinoma has three potential origins: (1) the malignant degeneration of metaplastic columnar epithelium (Barrett's mucosa), (2) heterotopic islands of columnar epithelium, or (3) the esophageal submucosal glands. In addition, the esophagus may be involved secondarily by a gastric carcinoma growing upward.

Severe gastroesophageal reflux is a major factor in the development of a columnar epithelium–lined (Barrett's) esophagus.[12] Refluxed gastric acid, proteases, and bile erode the normal squamous epithelium, and the residual pluripotential basal cells may differentiate along multiple cell lines, producing a variety of columnar epithelial cell types. The diagnosis of Barrett's esophagus is established at endoscopy by histologic documentation of columnar mucosa extending into the tubular esophagus at least 2 cm above the anatomic esophagogastric junction. This metaplasia may extend up to the thoracic inlet, and it has been estimated that patients with Barrett's esophagus are 40 times more likely to develop adenocarcinoma than the general population. The true incidence of Barrett's esophagus in the general population is unknown, but it is estimated that adenocarcinoma arises in up to 8% to 15% of patients with a columnar epithelium–lined esophagus.

Barrett's mucosa occurs in three characteristic histologic patterns:

Gastric fundus-type epithelium, which has a foveolar surface pattern (no villi), but contains glands with parietal cells, chief cells, and mucous cells

Junctional-type epithelium, in which there are no villi present and in which cardiac-type mucous glands without parietal or chief cells are seen. The mucosa has a foveolar pattern that is flat and typically is seen in normal colon, gastric cardia, and villous atrophy of the small bowel.

Specialized columnar epithelium, which is typically characterized by villiform folds lined by a single layer of glycoprotein-secreting columnar cells and mucus-secreting goblet cells. Cryptlike glands between the villi are also lined by columnar and goblet cells and contain few if any parietal or chief cells. This epithelium has also been termed *incomplete intestinal metaplasia* because only the goblet cell component of intestinal epithelium is present (Fig. 19-6).

The latter specialized or intestinal type of metaplasia has the highest association with carcinoma. The gastric fundus-type epithelium is found closest to the stomach, the junctional mucosa proximal to the fundus type, and the specialized epithelium adjacent to the squamous epithelium, which is proximal to it. Dysplasia occurs to varying degrees in Barrett's mucosa, and dysplasia clearly is a premalignant esophageal lesion. The histologic features of dysplasia are an increased nuclear/cytoplasmic ratio, loss of the basilar orientation of the epithelial cells along the basement membrane, irregular chromatin clumping, hyperchromatic nuclei, and prominence of the nucleoli (Fig. 19-7). Severe dysplasia is almost always associated with carcinoma in situ and mandates aggressive therapy.

As is true of squamous cell carcinoma, esophageal adenocarcinoma has an aggressive biologic behavior that is characterized by frequent transmural invasion and lymphatic spread. Because many of these tumors arise in the lower third of the esophagus, paraesophageal, celiac axis, and splenic hilum lymph node metastases are common. The lung and liver are the visceral organs most frequently involved by metastases. Esophageal adenocarcinoma is associated with a 5-year survival rate of 0% to 7%. Without lymph node involvement, survival of 5 years is possible, compared with an average survival of only 9 months in patients with lymph node involvement.

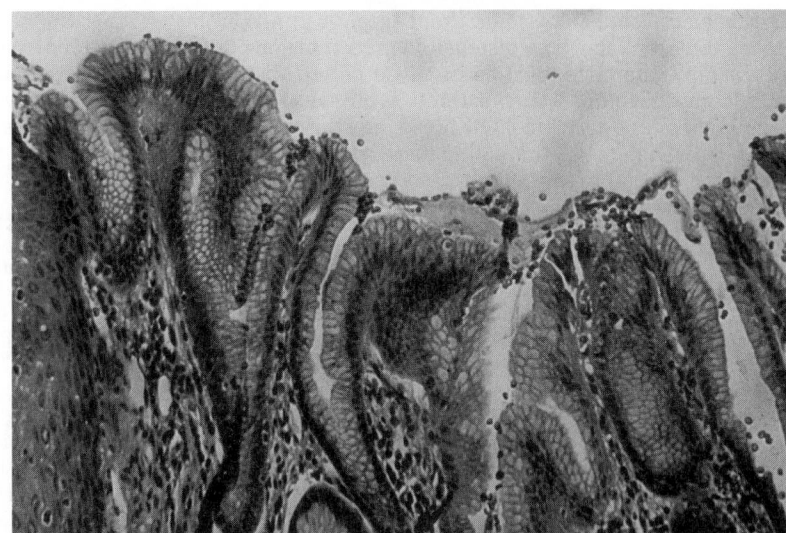

Figure 19-6. Photomicrograph of esophageal biopsy showing Barrett's mucosa with intestinal metaplasia and no dysplasia. Note the villiform folds lined by uniform goblet cells, all with their nuclei basally oriented.

Other Malignancies

Anaplastic small cell (oat cell) carcinoma arises in the esophagus from the same argyrophilic cells that give rise to this tumor in the lung. As is the case with their pulmonary counterparts, these tumors contain neurosecretory granules on electron microscopy. They are extremely aggressive tumors, they are commonly associated with distant spread at the time of diagnosis, and survival beyond 1 year is rare.[13]

Adenoid cystic esophageal carcinoma is another rare lesion, and fewer than 50 cases have been reported. These tumors typically occur in the middle third of the esophagus, are discovered late in their course, metastasize widely, and are associated with a median survival of only 9 months.[14]

About 100 cases of malignant melanoma of the esophagus have been reported, and these rare lesions constitute less than 0.1% of esophageal malignancies. Malignant melanoma may involve the esophagus either as a primary tumor or as a secondary metastasis. In the former situation, it is thought to arise from melanocytes that occur in the esophagus. These tumors typically present as large (7 cm or more) polypoid masses, which may or may not be pigmented. The average survival is only 13.4 months, and less than 5% survive 5 years. Metastasis to liver, lymph nodes, lung, and brain is common.[15]

Carcinosarcoma describes a lesion of the esophagus that has histologic features of both squamous cell carcinoma and malignant spindle cell sarcoma. These typically polypoid tumors generally occur in the distal two thirds of the esophagus, grow to large size (10 to 15 cm), and have a poor prognosis, with 2% to 6% of patients surviving 5 years.[16,17]

Pathophysiology of Esophageal Neoplasms

Local Effects

Symptoms from esophageal carcinoma may be insidious in onset, beginning as nonspecific retrosternal discomfort, indigestion, or transient dysphagia. Early esophageal carcinoma that is limited to the mucosa or submucosa may be completely asymptomatic or may produce localized spasm

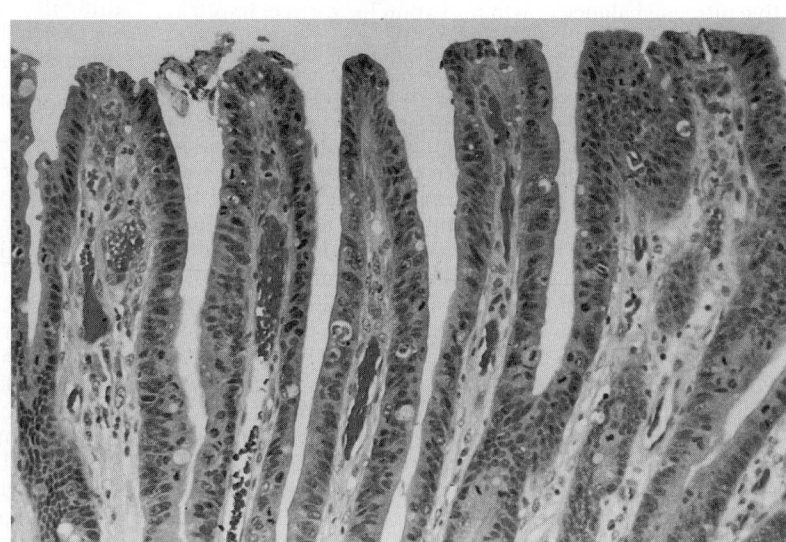

Figure 19-7. Photomicrograph of esophageal biopsy showing Barrett's mucosa with intestinal metaplasia and high-grade dysplasia. In contrast to the Barrett's mucosa shown in Figure 19-6, the basilar orientation of these epithelial cells along the basement membrane has been lost, the nuclei are of varying sizes and are hyperchromatic, and the nucleoli are prominent.

that is manifested as periodic esophageal obstruction. Because the esophagus is a distensible tube, a major portion of the circumference must be involved before obstructive symptoms develop. Many patients who sense difficulty swallowing a bolus of meat or bread subconsciously alter their eating habits by eliminating these coarse foods, chewing their food more thoroughly, and using more liquids to wash down food. By the time of presentation to a physician with a complaint of dysphagia, symptoms have often been present for 6 to 8 months.

Dysphagia is the most common presenting symptom of esophageal carcinoma. It develops in 90% of patients and is the primary manifestation of the disease in more than 80%. Dysphagia may present in several ways. It may be a subtle retrosternal discomfort as a bolus of food is swallowed, a transient feeling of retrosternal discomfort with swallowing that may not recur for several weeks or months, painful swallowing (odynophagia), or complete esophageal obstruction. *Weight loss* is the next most common symptom and is present in about 40% of patients with esophageal carcinoma. *Pain* is the initial symptom in 10% of patients. It may be precordial, retrosternal, epigastric, or intrascapular. Transient retrosternal pain radiating to the back or neck as the solid bolus of food passes through the tumor and causes local distention or muscle contraction has a much different implication than constant, boring retrosternal or epigastric pain, which more often represents local invasion by the tumor. *Regurgitation* of undigested food that has not passed through the esophagus should not be confused with the vomiting of gastric contents. *Respiratory symptoms* may be due either to aspiration or to direct invasion of the tracheobronchial tree by the tumor. These symptoms include cough, dyspnea, pleuritic pain, or hemoptysis. *Hematemesis* is a rare, early symptom of esophageal carcinoma, but bleeding from an esophageal malignancy is seldom of sufficient quantity to cause melena. *Hoarseness* from recurrent laryngeal nerve involvement is an ominous sign of unresectability. The course of the left main-stem bronchus anterior to the esophagus at the level of the carina is significant in the patient with a mid-esophageal tumor because the common wall between the esophagus and left main-stem bronchus may become involved with tumor and lead to the development of a malignant tracheoesophageal fistula.

Systemic Effects

Although the systemic effects of esophageal carcinoma are less well recognized than the local effects, they may have important clinical significance. Weight loss and negative nitrogen balance due to starvation have direct implications on the morbidity and mortality of esophageal resection in these patients. Virtually every patient with advanced esophageal obstruction is dehydrated and total body volume depleted from impaired oral intake. The patient with esophageal obstruction is prone to the development of severe hypokalemia with secondary muscle weakness. One to 2 L of saliva is produced each day, and the concentration of potassium within saliva (20 mEq/mL) is higher than that in any other gastrointestinal secretions. Patients who are unable to swallow their saliva, therefore, may present with marked hypokalemia. Fever and systemic toxicity may be due to aspiration from the obstructed esophagus.

The production of parathormone by some squamous cell esophageal carcinomas has been documented and may result in hypercalcemia, even in the absence of bone metastases. Preoperative hypercalcemia in the patient with esophageal carcinoma and no demonstrable bone metastases has been suggested to be a poor prognostic sign. The occurrence of hypertrophic osteoarthropathy with carcinoma of

the esophagus has been reported. Dermatomyositis has a frequent association with underlying malignancy and has occurred in patients with occult esophageal carcinoma. Apparently a vagal nerve–mediated response, the occurrence of "swallow syncope" has been reported in a few patients with esophageal obstruction due to carcinoma.

Diagnostic Investigations

History and Physical Examination

Because more than 90% of patients with esophageal carcinoma experience dysphagia as their primary presenting symptom,[18] a complaint of dysphagia in any adult cannot be taken lightly. In most cases, particularly in patients 50 years of age or older, a complaint of dysphagia warrants *both* a barium swallow examination and an endoscopic evaluation to rule out the presence of carcinoma. The combination of esophageal biopsy and brushings for cytologic evaluation establishes a diagnosis of carcinoma in 95% of patients with malignant strictures. Patients with long-standing reflux symptoms that have been well controlled with medical therapy who then develop an increase in retrosternal discomfort should not be presumed to have esophagitis. Rather, they should undergo appropriate radiographic and endoscopic evaluation. Aside from evidence of weight loss, most patients with esophageal carcinoma have few objective findings on physical examination to aid in the diagnosis. Nonetheless, careful examination for cervical or supraclavicular lymph node metastases, abdominal masses, and liver nodularity is warranted. The finding of a hard, supraclavicular lymph node in the patient with an intrathoracic esophageal carcinoma warrants fine-needle aspiration biopsy. If metastatic disease is documented, the presence of a stage IV tumor has been established. Resectional therapy of the esophageal tumor in this situation is seldom justified because the patient's expected survival is so poor. Laboratory studies should include a complete blood count, blood urea nitrogen, and serum creatinine to assess the state of hydration, as well as liver function tests, including total protein and albumin levels to assess nutrition. Serum electrolytes, particularly potassium and calcium levels, should also be obtained.

In obtaining a history from the patient who complains of dysphagia, the physician should ask the patient to localize with one finger on the anterior chest or neck the point at which food lodges when swallowing. The patient with a mechanical esophageal obstruction such as a carcinoma is able to localize the consistent point of obstruction without difficulty. This is in contrast to the patient with neuromotor obstruction, who may only sense slow esophageal emptying diffusely in the retrosternal area.

Radiographic Studies

A *barium swallow* examination is the first study that should be obtained in a patient who complains of dysphagia. Tumors of the cervical esophagus are most difficult to identify by barium swallow examination, and carcinoma of the cardia may be confused with achalasia, a benign stricture, or esophageal spasm. Nevertheless, the barium swallow examination localizes obvious esophageal pathology in preparation for subsequent esophagoscopy and allows the endoscopist to predict the level at which the tumor is located and the area that requires the most careful examination. The typical esophageal carcinoma presents radiographically as an irregular, rigid narrowing of the esophageal wall (Fig. 19-8). The normal mucosal pattern is frequently destroyed. Polypoid fungating tumors present as irregular filling defects with ulcerated borders within the esophagus. An old dictum relates that an esophagus

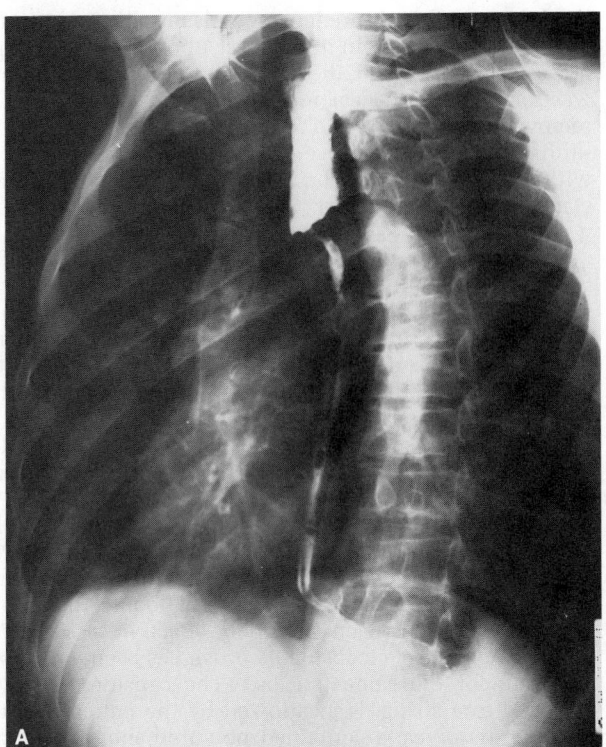 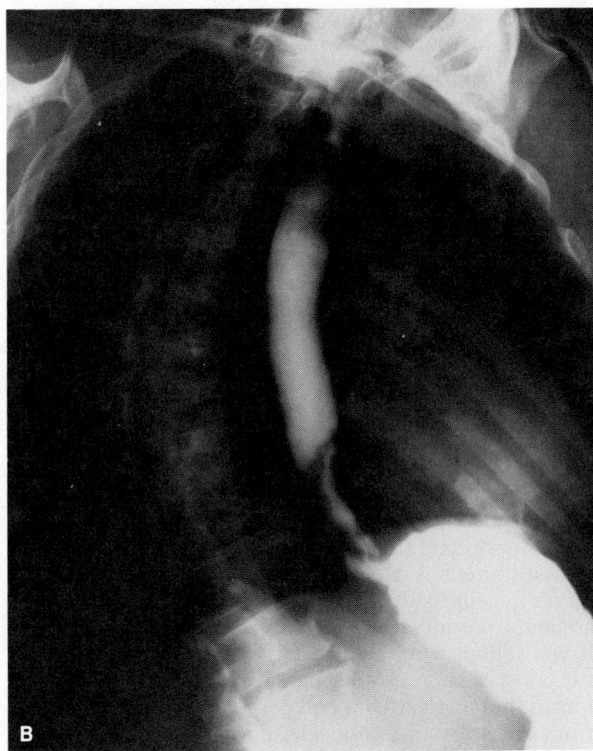

Figure 19-8. (*A*) Barium esophagogram showing an upper esophageal squamous cell carcinoma at the level of the aortic arch. Note the mucosal irregularity and shelf of tumor, which is characteristic of carcinoma. (*B*) Esophagogram showing a distal esophageal adenocarcinoma presenting as a characteristic apple-core constriction above the esophagogastric junction. (Orringer MB. Tumors of the esophagus. In: Sabiston DC Jr, ed. Textbook of surgery, ed 13. Philadelphia, WB Saunders, 1986:736)

that is dilated proximal to a stenosis is most indicative of a benign chronic obstruction, whereas an esophagus proximal to a carcinoma has "not had enough time" to dilate. This observation has proved to be incorrect on numerous occasions. Similarly, although a smooth, tapered radiographic esophageal stricture supposedly reflects benign disease, *any* stenosis merits esophageal biopsy and brushings for cytologic evaluation to rule out carcinoma. The barium swallow examination may also show a soft tissue mass adjacent to the esophageal tumor indicative of extraesophageal local invasion. In only half of patients with esophageal carcinoma is the plain *chest radiograph* abnormal, the most common findings being an air–fluid level in the obstructed esophagus, a dilated esophagus, abnormal mediastinal soft tissue representing adenopathy, pleural effusions, or pulmonary metastases.

The *chest and upper abdominal CT scan* is the standard radiographic technique for staging esophageal carcinoma. Normal esophageal wall thickness should not exceed 5 mm on CT scanning, which is also helpful in demonstrating regional adenopathy or pulmonary, liver, adrenal, or distant nodal metastasis. When distant metastases (eg, to liver or lung) are suspected on CT scan, tissue diagnosis with fine-needle aspiration biopsy is warranted. A positive histologic diagnosis of stage IV carcinoma translates to an average survival of only 6 to 12 months, and therefore an operation of the magnitude of esophagectomy is contraindicated. Several investigators have reported the value of CT in evaluating resectability of esophageal carcinoma. Gastric invasion, however, is difficult to detect with CT because gastric folds usually collapse, and the coexistence of a hiatal hernia renders evaluation of both tumor length and gastric extension by CT difficult. It has also been

shown that CT is not useful in assessing aortic invasion by the tumor because contiguity of the esophageal mass with the aorta does not prove invasion, and resection is often possible even in patients with greater than 90 degrees of contact between the esophagus and aorta.[19]

Bronchoscopy. Bronchoscopy should be performed in patients with carcinoma of the upper and middle thirds of the esophagus to exclude invasion of the posterior membranous trachea or main-stem bronchi, which precludes a safe esophagectomy.

Other Studies. Magnetic resonance imaging to evaluate mediastinal invasion has not gained widespread popularity. Bone scan is not warranted unless the patient has specific complaints suggesting that bone metastases exist. Similarly, routine brain scans are not indicated because brain metastases from carcinoma of the esophagus are uncommon (less than 4% in patients being evaluated for esophagectomy).[20]

Esophagoscopy

Esophagoscopy is one of the most important diagnostic tools in the assessment of the patient with esophageal symptoms from any cause. The flexible fiberoptic esophagoscope permits endoscopic assessment with greater ease than was possible with the rigid instruments. Unfortunately, as esophagoscopy has become a more commonly performed procedure, a rather cavalier attitude has emerged. Esophagoscopy, particularly for evaluation of an obstructing lesion, is a potentially dangerous undertaking, and a perforation in the patient with cancer is of tremendous gravity. Certain basic principles regarding esophagoscopy should always be borne in mind.

Basic Principles and Anatomic Relations. The safe performance of esophagoscopy requires familiarity with normal esophageal anatomy, particularly the three areas of naturally occurring anatomic narrowing: (1) the cervical constriction at the level of the cricopharyngeal sphincter; (2) the bronchoaortic constriction at the level of the fourth thoracic vertebra behind the tracheal bifurcation, where the left main-stem bronchus and aortic arch cross the esophagus; and (3) the diaphragmatic constriction, where the esophagus traverses the diaphragm. As a general rule, elective esophagoscopy should not be performed without a prior barium esophagogram displayed in view of the endoscopist during the procedure. Knowledge of the existing esophageal abnormality from the barium esophagogram assists the endoscopist in planning the procedure. It is useful to relate an esophageal abnormality on a barium swallow examination to certain anatomic landmarks and then to extrapolate from this assessment the approximate level within the esophagus at which the abnormality should be seen. The upper esophageal sphincter is typically seen on the barium esophagogram at the level of the seventh cervical or first thoracic vertebral bodies, or about 15 cm from the upper incisor teeth at esophagoscopy in the adult. The sternomanubrial junction (angle of Louis) on the anterior chest wall aligns with the tracheal bifurcation, which is seen in most barium esophagograms at the level of about the fourth thoracic vertebra and corresponds to a point 25 cm from the upper incisors. The normal esophagogastric junction is typically seen endoscopically 40 cm from the upper incisors at the level of the eleventh or twelfth thoracic vertebra. With these landmarks in mind, a mid-esophageal tumor located at the level of the tracheal bifurcation on a barium esophagogram, for example, should be anticipated to be seen endoscopically at a point about 25 cm from the upper incisor teeth.

The patient suspected of having esophageal carcinoma is most often evaluated with the flexible fiberoptic esophagoscope using local anesthesia and sedation. The endoscopic assessment of an obstructing esophageal lesion may be uncomfortable for the patient, and one should not persist with attempts to obtain a biopsy to or dilate the stenosis in a patient who is anxious, combative, or uncooperative; at times, general anesthesia may be required. Fungating exophytic carcinomas are readily diagnosed endoscopically with biopsies. Constricting esophageal tumors, however, may narrow the esophageal lumen so that only normal proximal esophageal mucosa is evident at the site of the stricture. In such cases, gentle dilation of the stricture followed by biopsies from within the stenosis as well as brushings for cytologic evaluation generally establish the malignant nature of the obstruction.

Vital Staining and Ultrasound. Vital staining of the esophageal mucosa is a technique that is useful in detecting dysplastic esophageal lesions that are not obvious on direct endoscopic assessment.[21,22] Carcinoma in situ (intraepithelial carcinoma) or microinvasive carcinoma may appear endoscopically as flat, nondescript lesions (leukoplakia or erythroplakia) and therefore can be difficult to diagnose. Lugol (3% iodide) solution or 2% toluidine blue may be applied through the esophagoscope to the esophageal mucosa. Lugol solution stains normal glycogenic esophageal mucosa brown, while abnormal mucosa (early carcinoma, esophagitis, Barrett's mucosa) remains unstained. A swab of Lugol solution applied through the rigid esophagoscope stains the normal areas of esophageal mucosa and shows the endoscopist the nonstaining, abnormal areas that should be obtained at biopsy. Alternatively, toluidine blue is a metachromatic stain with affinity for cell nuclei. Therefore, tissues with a high cellu-

lar density and high nucleus/cytoplasm ratio take up the stain quickly and retain it for about 1 hour. This technique is performed through the rigid esophagoscope, initially washing the esophageal mucosa with 1% acetic acid to remove excess mucus and food particles, applying 1% toluidine blue for 1 minute, and then washing the stain away with 1% acetic acid. The areas of mucosa that remain stained are sampled for biopsy and are likely to be neoplastic.

Endoscopic ultrasound is being used with increasing frequency as an adjunct to the standard radiologic and endoscopic assessment of esophageal disease.[6] It offers the potential for more sensitive staging of esophageal carcinoma by detecting the depth of invasion and the presence of abnormal mediastinal adenopathy. Ultrasound permits the endoscopic delineation of the mucosa, submucosa, and muscular layers of the esophagus as well as adjacent tissues. Lymph nodes as small as 5 mm can be recognized with this instrument.

Cytologic screening of large populations at high risk for developing esophageal carcinoma is possible using a number of readily available outpatient techniques. In China, abrasive cytology using a swallowed balloon catheter (balloon cytology) has been extremely effective in screening for carcinoma. An encapsulated brush has been developed in Japan for the same purpose. The capsule, which is attached to a string, is swallowed by the patient. As the capsule dissolves, a contained polyurethane sponge ball expands, and as it is withdrawn through the esophagus, abrasive cytology is made possible. Combining abrasive cytology with vital staining of the esophageal mucosa may prove to yield the best sensitivity and specificity for screening populations.

Premalignant Esophageal Lesions

As indicated previously, chronic irritation of esophageal mucosa by a variety of noxious stimuli (alcohol, tobacco, hot foods and liquids) eventually may lead to the development of esophageal carcinoma. A variety of esophageal lesions have a recognized premalignant nature. The patient who survives the initial injury long enough to develop a caustic esophageal stricture has a 1000-fold increased risk of developing carcinoma compared with the normal population. This is but one reason that the esophagus that is strictured after caustic ingestion should be resected rather than bypassed, particularly in young patients.

The premalignant nature of Barrett's esophagitis was discussed earlier. When a fundoplication is performed to relieve reflux symptoms in the patient who has Barrett's mucosa, the columnar epithelium within the esophagus rarely regresses. For this reason, periodic surveillance endoscopy should be performed. In the patient with Barrett's mucosa with no or mild dysplasia, endoscopy at 1- to 2-year intervals is probably adequate. In the patient with moderate dysplasia, surveillance endoscopy and biopsy at 6-month intervals is appropriate. As indicated earlier, severe dysplasia in the patient with Barrett's mucosa is virtually synonymous with carcinoma in situ and is an indication in most instances for esophageal resection.

Because reflux esophagitis constitutes a chronic chemical injury of the esophageal mucosa, it is regarded as a potentially premalignant abnormality of the esophagus that requires aggressive medical therapy or surgical control.

About 10% to 12% of patients with achalasia of the esophagus who are observed for 15 years or longer develop esophageal carcinoma. The cause is thought to be related to the irritating effects of the fermenting intraesophageal contents on the adjacent esophageal mucosa. These tumors are typically squamous cell carcinomas located in the middle third of the esophagus and frequently at the site of the air–fluid level seen in the obstructed organ on barium swallow examination. The diagnosis of carcinoma in these patients is typically made when tumors are far advanced because the patient with chronic dysphagia from underlying achalasia does not detect a change in swallowing as the tumor enlarges within the dilated esophagus. The prognosis for esophageal cancer in the patient with achalasia is poor. Patients who have carried a diagnosis of achalasia for 15 years or more should undergo surveillance endoscopy, perhaps with the addition of vital staining, because of their risk for developing carcinoma.

Plummer-Vinson syndrome (Paterson-Kelly syndrome or sideropenic dysphagia) is a premalignant esophageal condition. The term *sideropenic dysphagia* refers to the development of cervical dysphagia in patients who have iron-deficiency anemia. These patients are typically elderly women who are edentulous and have atrophic oral mucosa with glossitis and koilonychia (brittle, spoon-shaped fingernails). Associated cervical esophageal webs are common (Fig. 19-9). The incidence of this syndrome is high in Scandinavia and Great Britain. Treatment consists of esophageal dilation to disrupt the web and correction of the nutritional deficiency. About 10% of patients develop squamous cell carcinoma of the hypopharynx, oral cavity, or esophagus.

An increased incidence of esophageal carcinoma is found in patients who have familial keratosis palmaris et plantaris (tylosis), which is inherited as an autosomal dominant trait.

This condition is characterized by hyperkeratosis of the interphalangeal epithelium and soles of the feet, fissures and scaling of the thickened skin of the palms and soles, and disordered sweating. Esophageal cancer occurs in these families at an earlier age than in the normal population.

Patients who have experienced radiation esophagitis during the course of treatment for lymphoma, lung, breast, or other mediastinal malignancies are at increased risk for developing esophageal carcinoma years later.

Finally, several isolated reports have been made of esophageal carcinomas that have been found incidentally within esophageal diverticula, presumably as a result of the irritating effects on the mucosa of stagnant, putrefying food within the pouch. Esophageal diverticula are therefore also regarded as premalignant esophageal lesions, although this occurrence is extremely rare.

Treatment of Esophageal Cancer

Therapy of esophageal carcinoma is influenced by the knowledge that in most of these patients, local tumor invasion or distant metastatic disease precludes cure. Neither chemotherapy, radiotherapy, nor surgery alone has achieved significant and consistent long-term survival in patients with esophageal carcinoma. Although certain chemotherapeutic agents, such as cisplatin, 5-fluorouracil, bleomycin, and methotrexate, either alone or in combination, have been associated with partial responses of some of these tumors, long-term remission has not been the rule.[23]

Radiation

Although squamous cell carcinoma is generally regarded as a radiosensitive and therefore potentially curable tumor, radiotherapy has not achieved cure in most of these patients.[24] Radiotherapy is used in the treatment of esophageal carcinoma to provide either palliation or cure or as an adjunct to esophagectomy. Palliative radiotherapy in the range of 4000 to 5000 cGy over 3 to 4 weeks relieves dysphagia sufficiently in nearly half of patients with advanced metastatic carcinoma and severe dysphagia to allow them to swallow liquids and diet supplements. "Curative" supervoltage radiotherapy is delivered in doses of 5000 to 7000 cGy over 5 to 7 weeks, using rotational and oblique ports to avoid spinal cord injury. Unfortunately, the average 5-year survival after such treatment is between 6% and 10% in most series because radiation fails to control either the primary tumor or distant metastatic disease.

Similarly, although surgical treatment most effectively relieves the esophageal obstruction, resectional therapy is local therapy, and unfortunately, esophageal carcinoma in most patients is a systemic disease when it is diagnosed. Thus, reported 5-year survival rates after esophageal resection for carcinoma usually average between 10% and 15%, with more than 80% of patients dying within 1 year of diagnosis. Several Japanese reports indicate 5-year survival rates of 25% to 38%, with combined preoperative radiotherapy followed by resection. Such results have not been duplicated in Western cultures, where until recently, the aim of therapy has been palliation.

Intubation

A variety of endoesophageal tubes (Celestin, Fell, Mackler, Mousseau-Barbin, Souttar, Wilson-Cook) have been used to provide palliation in patients with esophageal carcinoma.[25] Basically, these tubes are divided into two types—the *pulsion* tubes, which are pushed through the tumor with the aid of an esophagoscope; and the *traction* or pull-through tubes, which are pulled into place by downward traction through a gastrotomy. As is the case with many conceptually simple procedures, implementa-

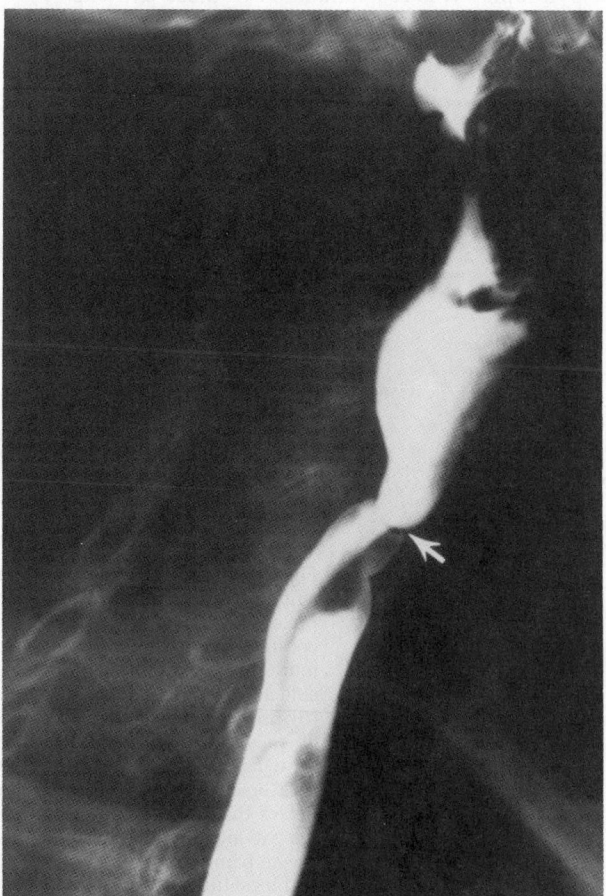

Figure 19-9. Typical cervical esophageal web (*arrow*) extending from the anterior esophageal wall. (Orringer MB. Diverticula and miscellaneous conditions of the esophagus. In: Sabiston DC Jr, ed. Textbook of surgery, ed 13. Philadelphia, WB Saunders, 1986:726)

tion in the clinical setting is problematic. Transoral esophageal intubation is associated with an overall mortality rate of 14% and a complication rate of at least 25%, the latter due to perforation of the esophagus, migration of the tubes, or obstruction of the tubes by food or tumor overgrowth. Although patients may be better able to handle their saliva after intubation of their esophageal tumors, oral intake must be restricted to a semiliquid diet, and palliation is far from optimum (Fig. 19-10). Palliative intubation for esophageal carcinoma is associated with an average survival of less than 6 months. This technique is reserved almost exclusively for patients with malignant tracheoesophageal fistulas, in whom the tube is used to occlude the esophageal side of the fistula while allowing oral alimentation.

A variety of expandable intraesophageal metallic stents have been used to achieve palliation in patients with unresectable esophageal carcinoma.[26,27] These stents are easier to insert than the older plastic tubes, have a larger lumen, and theoretically, carry less risk of perforation. They are inserted under fluoroscopy using a flexible esophagoscope. Additional experience with this technique is rapidly being acquired, and a multiinstitutional trial evaluating expandable metallic stents is underway in the United States.

Laser

Endoscopic laser fulgurating of esophageal carcinoma, particularly with the Nd:YAG laser, has been used to achieve temporary relief of the esophageal obstruction in patients with unresectable tumors.[27] Generally, multiple sessions are required to resect sufficient tumor to achieve an adequate lumen, and functional success with restoration of comfortable swallowing is achieved in 75% to 80% of patients.[28]

Bypass

A variety of surgical procedures, such as substernal gastric or colon bypass, have been developed as palliative internal bypasses of unresectable esophageal carcinomas. Because survival in patients with unresectable esophageal carcinoma averages less than 6 months, it is difficult to justify such bypass operations, which are associated with a mortality rate between 15% and 25%.[29,30] This is simply too large an operation for a patient with so advanced a malignancy. Similarly, reversed gastric (Heimlich) tubes are associated with a 25% to 40% mortality rate.

Resection

Transthoracic Resection. For most patients with localized esophageal carcinoma, resection provides the most effective and reliable palliation of dysphagia. The traditional surgical approach to distal esophageal carcinoma is a left thoracoabdominal incision (Fig. 19-11). After resecting the distal esophagus, proximal stomach, and adjacent lymph nodes, an intrathoracic esophagogastric anastomosis is performed. Tumors involving the mid-esophagus are resected through either a thoracoabdominal or separate thoracic and abdominal incisions, and a high intrathoracic esophagogastric anastomosis is performed (Fig. 19-12). Because a truncal vagotomy is an inevitable accompaniment of esophageal resection for carcinoma, and delayed gastric emptying occurs in 15% to 30% of patients after a truncal vagotomy, a drainage procedure, either a pyloromyotomy or pyloroplasty, is recommended in these patients.

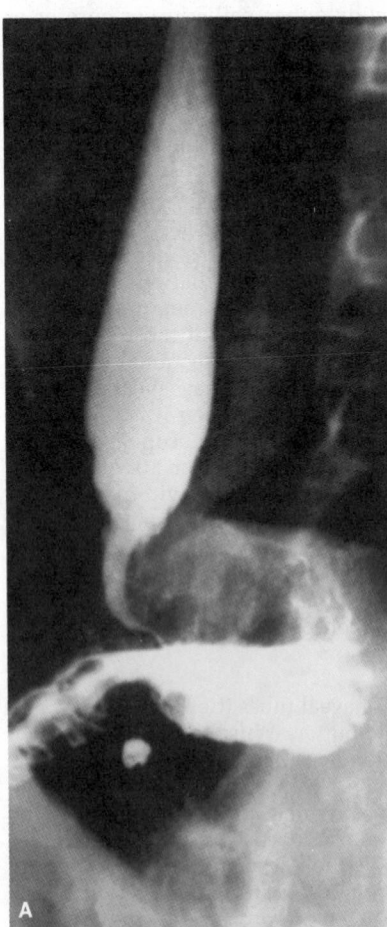
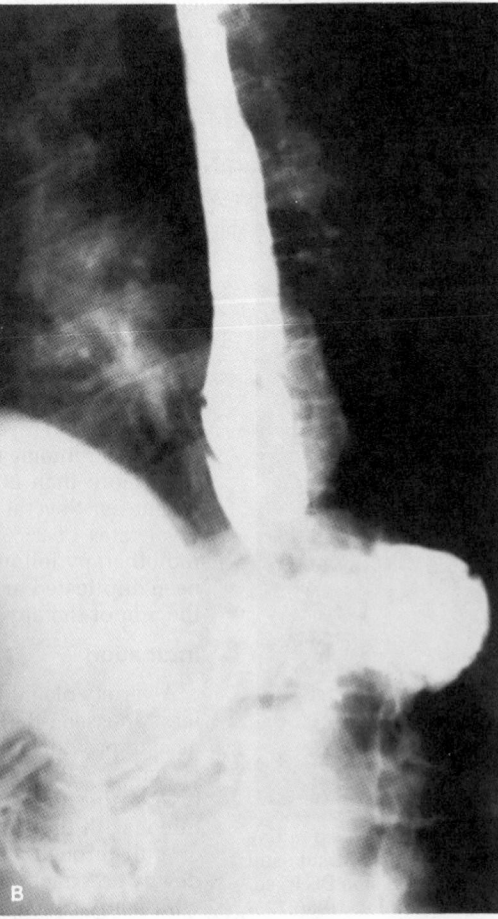

Figure 19-10. (*A*) Distal esophageal stricture that was erroneously interpreted as being due to spasm because of its smooth, tapered contour. This proved to be an unresectable adenocarcinoma of the cardia. (*B*) Esophagogram after placement of a Celestin intraesophageal tube showing free passage of barium into the stomach. Despite the relative relief of the esophageal obstruction, the patient continued to experience severe pain from esophageal spasm and local tumor invasion. Adequate palliation was not achieved. (Orringer MB. Tumors of the esophagus. In: Sabiston DC Jr, ed. Textbook of surgery, ed 13. Philadelphia, WB Saunders, 1986:736)

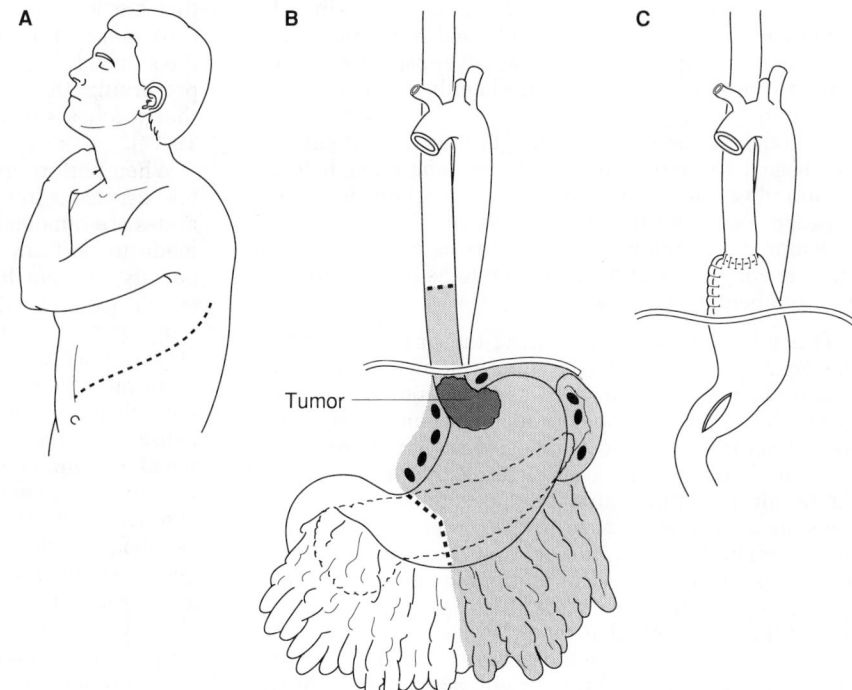

Figure 19-11. Standard thoracoabdominal esophagogastrectomy for carcinomas of the distal esophagus and cardia. (*A*) Thoracoabdominal incision. (*B*) Tissue to be resected (*colored area*). (*C*) Completed reconstruction after intrathoracic esophagogastric anastomosis and either pyloromyotomy or pyloroplasty to prevent postvagotomy pylorospasm. (After Ellis FH Jr. Treatment of carcinoma of the esophagus and cardia. Mayo Clin Proc 1960; 35:653)

Unfortunately, the standard right or left transthoracic esophagectomy and intrathoracic esophagogastric anastomosis have significant disadvantages. Weakened patients with esophageal obstruction may have difficulty tolerating combined thoracic and abdominal operations, and resulting postoperative incisional pain and inability to breathe deeply may lead to atelectasis and respiratory insufficiency that require mechanical ventilatory assistance and often result in pneumonia.

The second disadvantage of the standard operations is the potential for disruption of the intrathoracic esophageal anastomosis with resulting mediastinitis and sepsis, a fatal complication in half of patients in whom it occurs. These two factors, the physiologic impact of a combined thoracoabdominal operation and the disastrous results of an intrathoracic esophageal anastomotic disruption, are responsible for reported operative mortality rates for this operation that during the past decade have ranged from 15% to 40% and average 30%.[31] In several more modern series[32-34] of transthoracic esophageal resection and reconstruction for carcinoma reported by highly experienced surgical teams, operative mortality rates in the range of 3% have been achieved.

A further disadvantage of the standard intrathoracic esophagogastric anastomosis is inadequate long-term relief of dysphagia owing either to tumor recurrence at the anastomotic suture line or to the development of reflux esophagitis above the anastomosis. Because of the notorious spread of esophageal carcinoma in submucosal lymphatics well beyond the gross extent of the tumor, a 10-cm proximal

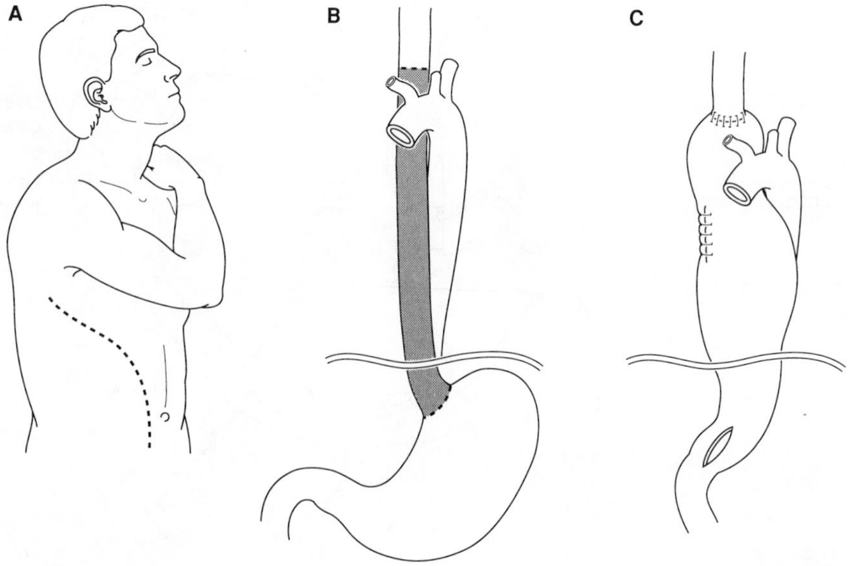

Figure 19-12. Standard thoracoabdominal esophagogastrectomy for tumors of the upper and middle thirds of the thoracic esophagus. (*A*) Either the continuous thoracoabdominal incision or separate thoracic and abdominal incisions are used. (*B*) Portion of esophagus to be resected (*colored area*). (*C*) Completed reconstruction with high intrathoracic esophagogastric anastomosis and gastric drainage procedure. (After Ellis FH Jr. Treatment of the esophagus and cardia. Mayo Clin Proc 1960;35:653)

margin of resection is advocated whenever possible. Patients who undergo a major esophageal resection and reconstruction only to have recurrent dysphagia from tumor at the anastomosis several months later have received poor palliation.

Although it has long been taught that the patient with esophageal carcinoma does not live long enough to develop reflux esophagitis after a low intrathoracic esophagogastric anastomosis, this is clearly not the case, and the development of reflux in these patients can produce not only severe pyrosis and reflux symptoms but also dysphagia from benign stenosis.

Transhiatal Resection.   During the past two decades, the technique of transhiatal esophagectomy without thoracotomy has been popularized as an operation that minimizes the factors responsible for most poor results from traditional transthoracic esophageal resection and reconstruction.[35] In this operation, irrespective of the level of the tumor, the entire intrathoracic esophagus is resected, the stomach is repositioned in the posterior mediastinum in the original esophageal bed, and the gastric fundus is anastomosed to the cervical esophagus above the level of the clavicles. The operation is performed through an upper-midline abdominal incision and a cervical incision, eliminating the need for a thoracotomy. The properly mobilized stomach, based on the right gastric and right gastroepiploic vascular arcades, readily reaches above the level of the clavicles for a cervical anastomosis. A generous Kocher maneuver to mobilize the pyloroduodenal junction, pyloromyotomy, and feeding jejunostomy are performed routinely (Fig. 19-13). The thoracic esophagus is mobilized through the diaphragmatic hiatus and a neck incision (Fig. 19-14). For distal-third esophageal tumors

that are localized to the cardia, instead of resecting the proximal half of the stomach, the high lesser curvature of the stomach is divided 4 to 6 cm beyond the gross tumor, preserving the point along the high greater curvature that reaches superiorly to the neck (Figs. 19-15 through 19-17).

When performing a transhiatal esophagectomy, accessible cervical, intrathoracic, and intraabdominal lymph nodes are removed for staging purposes, but no attempt is made to perform an en bloc resection of the esophagus and its adjacent lymph node–bearing tissue. Transhiatal esophagectomy without thoracotomy and a cervical esophagogastric anastomosis have the following advantages: (1) a thoracotomy in a debilitated patient is avoided; (2) an intrathoracic esophageal anastomosis is avoided, and if a cervical anastomotic leak occurs, the resulting salivary fistula is easily managed by opening the neck wound and packing it and is not a fatal complication; (3) intraabdominal or intrathoracic gastrointestinal suture lines are avoided; and (4) subsequent clinically significant gastroesophageal reflux is rare. This operation has been criticized because of its limited exposure of the intrathoracic esophagus through the diaphragmatic hiatus and, therefore, the risk of intraoperative bleeding from the divided aortic esophageal branches. In addition, one cannot carry out a complete mediastinal lymph node dissection through the diaphragmatic hiatus for purposes of staging or potential cure.

Among 423 consecutive patients with carcinoma of the thoracic esophagus and cardia, transhiatal esophagectomy without thoracotomy was possible in 417 (97%). Of the 417 resected tumors, 23 (5%) were located in the upper third, 115 (28%) in the middle third, and 279 (67%) in the

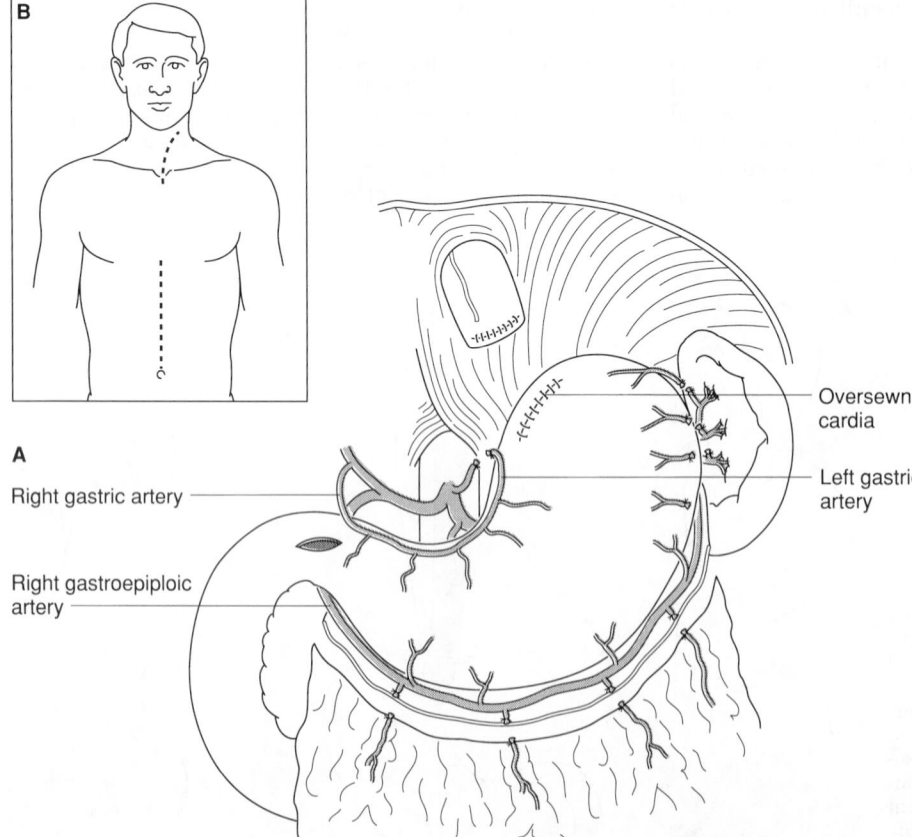

Right gastric artery

Right gastroepiploic artery

Oversewn cardia

Left gastric artery

A

B

Figure 19-13. (*A*) Standard mobilization of the stomach for esophageal replacement either in the posterior mediastinal or substernal position. The left gastric artery and left gastroepiploic vessels have been divided. The mobilized stomach is based on the remaining right gastric and right gastroepiploic arteries that are preserved. A pyloromyotomy and generous Kocher maneuver are performed. (*B*) Left cervical incision and upper midline abdominal incision used for transhiatal esophagectomy and esophageal replacement with stomach in the posterior mediastinum. (After Orringer MB, Sloan H. Substernal gastric bypass of the excluded thoracic esophagus for palliation of esophageal carcinoma. J Thorac Cardiovasc 1975;70:836)

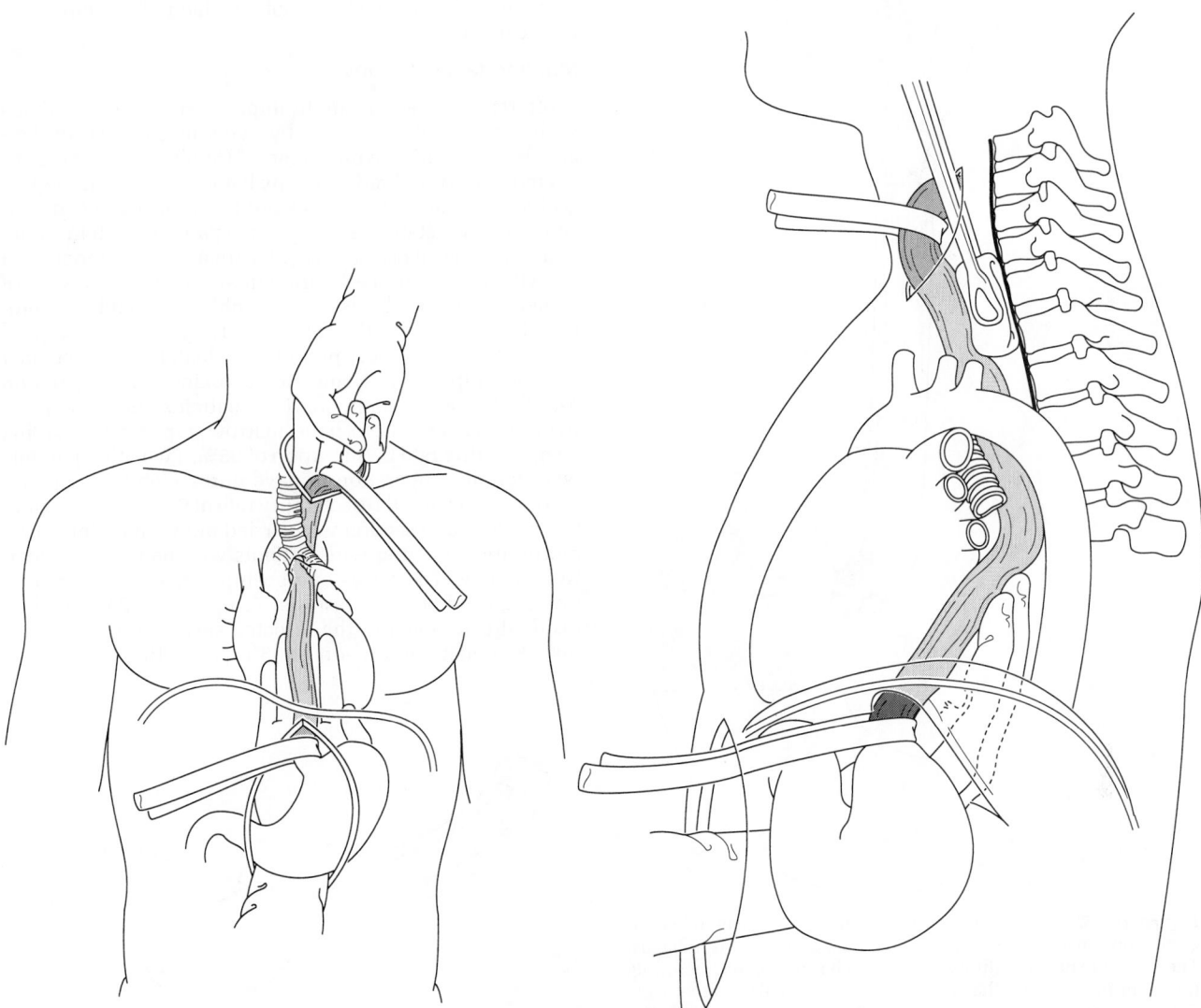

Figure 19-14. (A) Transhiatal mobilization of the thoracic esophagus from the posterior mediastinum using blunt dissection and traction on rubber drains placed around the esophagogastric junction and the cervical esophagus. The volar aspects of the fingers are kept against the esophagus to reduce the risk of injury to adjacent structures. (B) Lateral view showing transhiatal mobilization of the esophagus away from the prevertebral fascia using a half sponge on a stick inserted through the cervical incision and advanced until it makes contact with the hand inserted from below through the diaphragmatic hiatus. Arterial pressure is monitored as the heart is displaced forward by the hand in the posterior mediastinum. (After Orringer MB. Surgical options for esophageal resection and reconstruction with stomach. In: Baue AE, Geha AS, Hammond GL, eds. Glenn's thoracic and cardiovascular surgery, ed 5. Norwalk, CT, Appleton & Lange, 1990)

lower third of the esophagus. One-hundred and forty-eight of the tumors (35%) were squamous cell carcinomas, and 256 (62%) were adenocarcinomas. A cervical esophagogastric anastomosis was possible in 408 (98%) of these patients, a colon interposition being required in 9 patients who had undergone prior gastric resections for peptic ulcer disease. This experience clearly has demonstrated that the normal stomach, when properly mobilized, readily reaches to the neck for construction of a cervical esophagogastric anastomosis.

The postsurgical TNM staging system for esophageal carcinoma is shown in Table 19-2. Of the 417 carcinomas resected using the transhiatal approach, 200 (48%) were either transmurally invasive or metastatic beyond regional lymph nodes (stage III or IV tumors). Only 42 (10%) patients had tumors confined to the mucosa (stage I). There

was one intraoperative death from mediastinal hemorrhage, and intraoperative blood loss averaged less than 1000 mL. The hospital mortality rate was 5%. The overall 2-year survival rate was 41%, and the 5-year survival rate, 27%. These survival data, although comparable to those reported in most series of transthoracic resections, were obtained with less postoperative morbidity and mortality. On the basis of this experience, a transhiatal esophagectomy without thoracotomy is advocated whenever possible for resectable esophageal carcinomas. This approach should not be used for tumors that are judged on palpation through the diaphragmatic hiatus to have invaded the aorta or the tracheobronchial tree.

Radical Resection. At the other end of the spectrum from transhiatal resection for esophageal carcinoma is the

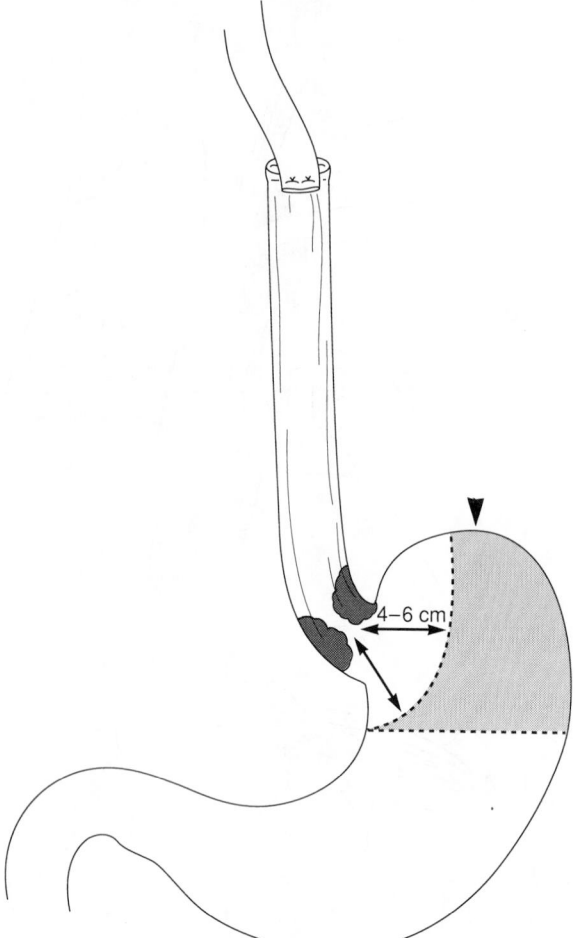

Figure 19-15. Transhiatal esophagectomy and proximal partial gastrectomy used for lesions of the cardia and distal esophagus. The entire greater curvature of the stomach is preserved, including the point (*arrowhead*) that will reach most cephalad to the neck, A 4- to 6-cm gastric margin is obtained while preserving the entire greater curvature. The colored area indicates that portion of the stomach that is usually resected in a standard hemigastrectomy used for a distal esophageal carcinoma. Such a resection, however, eliminates the possibility of a cervical esophagogastric anastomosis. (After Orringer MB, Sloan H. Esophagectomy without thoracotomy. J Thorac Cardiovasc Surg 1978;76:643)

radical transthoracic esophagectomy with en bloc dissection of contiguous lymph node–bearing tissues. This is a much more formidable operation, the results of which, when compared with those of transhiatal esophagectomy without thoracotomy and *no* formal lymph node dissection, are not significantly different (Table 19-3). These data indicate that survival after resection of esophageal carcinoma is more a function of the extent and stage of the tumor than of the size of the specimen or number of lymph nodes removed. Skinner and associates[36] have reported on a group of 31 patients, half with adenocarcinoma and half with squamous cell carcinoma, undergoing radical esophagectomy under more stringent selection criteria. The overall 1- and 2-year survival rates were 65% and 32%, respectively. As a general rule, the stomach is the preferred visceral esophageal substitute, being far more resilient than intestine and readily reaching to the neck for replacement of the entire esophagus. Colonic interposition is a major operative undertaking in patients with esophageal carcinoma and should be used only in selected cases

in which the stomach is not available for esophageal replacement.

Multimodality Therapy

Efforts have been made to improve survival in patients with esophageal carcinoma by using multimodality therapy in combination with surgery.[18] Combined preoperative chemotherapy and radiotherapy before transhiatal esophagectomy for carcinoma, for example, has provided encouraging survival statistics. Forty-three patients with intrathoracic esophageal carcinoma (21 with adenocarcinoma and 22 with squamous cell carcinoma) received 3 weeks of chemotherapy with cisplatin, vinblastine, and 5-fluorouracil, concurrent with 3750 to 4500 cGy of radiotherapy.[37] After a 3-week recovery period, transhiatal esophagectomy was accomplished. Hematologic toxicity and radiation esophagitis were common. Two patients died preoperatively of sepsis due to bone marrow suppression, giving an operability rate in this group of 95%. Two other patients were found at operation to have unresectable tumors, resulting in an overall resectability rate of 91%. The transhiatal esophageal resection was carried out with no increased morbidity compared with patients who had no preoperative therapy. There was one postoperative death from an unrecognized brain metastasis. Ten patients (24%) had no residual carcinoma in the resected specimen (T0, N0 status). At a mean follow-up of 36 months, the median sur-

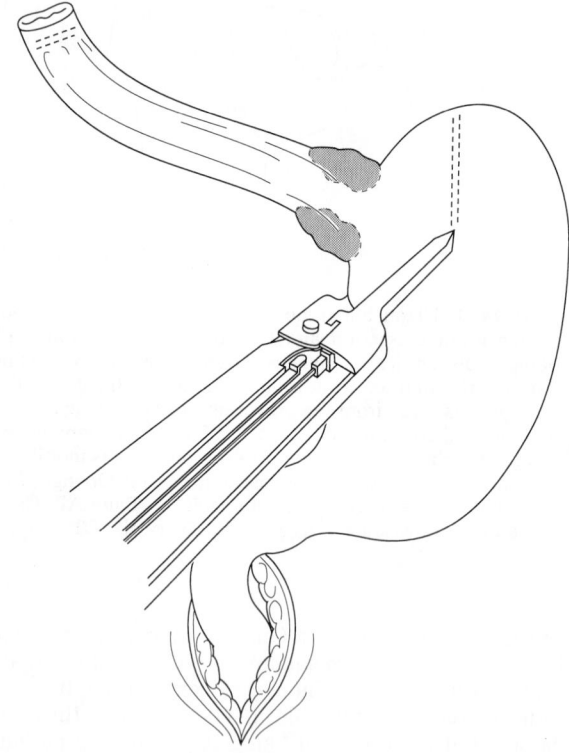

Figure 19-16. Gastric division after transhiatal mobilization of the intrathoracic esophagus for a carcinoma of the cardia. The mobilized stomach and attached distal esophagus have been delivered from the abdominal incision and are retracted superiorly as the surgical stapler is applied, beginning along the lesser curvature and proceeding toward the high greater curvature (*dashed line*). This is the standard method used to prepare the stomach for esophageal replacement after transhiatal esophagectomy. The remaining gastric "tube" readily reaches to the neck for a cervical anastomosis. (After Orringer MB, Sloan H. Esophageal replacement after blunt esophagectomy. In: Nyhus LM, Baker RJ, eds. Mastery of surgery. Boston, Little, Brown, 1984:426)

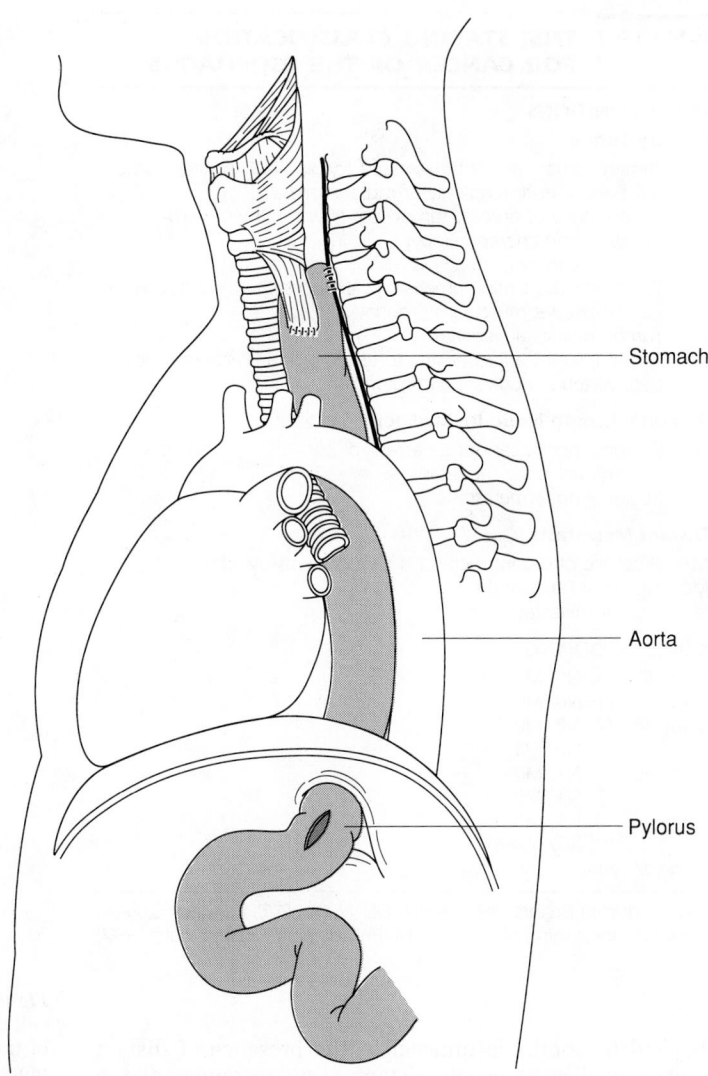

Stomach

Aorta

Pylorus

Figure 19-17. Final position of the mobilized stomach in the posterior mediastinum after transhiatal esophagectomy and cervical esophagogastric anastomosis. The gastric fundus has been suspended from the cervical prevertebral fascia, and an end-to-side cervical esophagogastrostomy has been performed. The pylorus is now located several centimeters below the level of the diaphragmatic hiatus. (After Orringer MB, Sloan H. Esophagectomy without thoracotomy. J Thorac Cardiovasc Surg 1978;76:643)

vival time for all 43 patients was 29 months (Kaplan-Meier estimate), a clear improvement over the 12-month median survival time with transhiatal esophagectomy alone. All 10 patients with T0, N0 status (complete responders) were alive and tumor free at a median follow-up of 36 months. At a median follow-up of 78.7 months, the 5-year survival rate of all 43 patients was 34%, and that of the complete responders, a gratifying 60%. The overall 1- and 2-year survival rates in this group of 72% and 60%, respectively, compare favorably with the 65% and 32% figures referred to earlier reported by Skinner and associates after radical esophagectomy. These preliminary results have generated hope that it may be possible to alter the natural history of esophageal carcinoma and achieve long-term survival, not just palliation, in some of these patients. They have justified a phase III prospective randomized trial that was just completed at the University of Michigan and is being analyzed.

CERVICOTHORACIC ESOPHAGEAL CARCINOMAS

Carcinomas that involve the cervicothoracic esophagus and the adjacent larynx either primarily or secondarily require esophageal reconstruction after laryngopharyngectomy.[38,39] Concomitant radical neck dissection may also

be required because of regional lymph node involvement. Resection of these tumors may require division of the high retrosternal trachea, which is facilitated by removal of the anterior breast plate and construction of a mediastinal tracheostomy (Figs. 19-18 through 19-22). Replacement of the pharynx and cervical esophagus may also be achieved with skin tubes, rotated myocutaneous flaps, and isolated, free jejunal grafts anastomosed to a cervical arterial blood supply and venous drainage with microvascular technique. These operations, however, are often multistaged, prolonged, and fraught with technical problems. Therefore, a laryngopharyngectomy for cervicothoracic esophageal tumors and a concomitant transhiatal esophagectomy without thoracotomy can provide the maximum distal esophageal margin while restoring alimentary continuity using stomach anastomosed to the pharynx. Such a one-stage resection and reconstruction for these carcinomas has obvious advantages in that it avoids staged procedures, multiple intestinal anastomoses, and prolonged hospitalization.

Once the diagnosis of esophageal carcinoma has been established, a staging CT scan of the chest and abdomen should be obtained to rule out distant metastatic disease (eg, pulmonary, hepatic, or retroperitoneal lymph node metastases), which would preclude even a palliative resection. Fine-needle aspiration is required to document distant metastases suspected on the CT scan. Because survival

Table 19-2. TNM STAGING CLASSIFICATION FOR CANCER OF THE ESOPHAGUS

TNM DEFINITIONS

Primary Tumor

TX   Primary tumor cannot be assessed (cytologically positive tumor not evident endoscopically or radiographically)

T0   No evidence of primary tumor (eg, after treatment with radiation and chemotherapy)

Tis   Carcinoma in situ

T1   Tumor invades lamina propria or submucosa, but not beyond it

T2   Tumor invades muscularis propria

T3   Tumor invades adventitia

T4   Tumor invades adjacent structures (eg, aorta, tracheobronchial tree, vertebral bodies, pericardium)

Regional Lymph Node Involvement

NX   Regional nodes cannot be assessed

N0   No regional node metastasis

N1   Regional node metastasis

Distant Metastasis

MX   Presence of distant metastasis cannot be assessed

M0   No distant metastasis

M1   Distant metastasis

STAGE GROUPING

Stage 0   Tis, N0, M0
Stage I   T1, N0, M0
Stage IIA T2, N0, M0
           T3, N0, M0
Stage IIB T1, N1, M0
           T2, N1, M0
Stage III T3, N1, M0
           T4, any N, M0
Stage IV   Any T, any N, M1

(Adapted from Beahrs OH, Henson DE, Hutter RVP, Kennedy BJ, eds. Manual for staging of cancer, ed 4. Philadelphia, JB Lippincott, 1992)

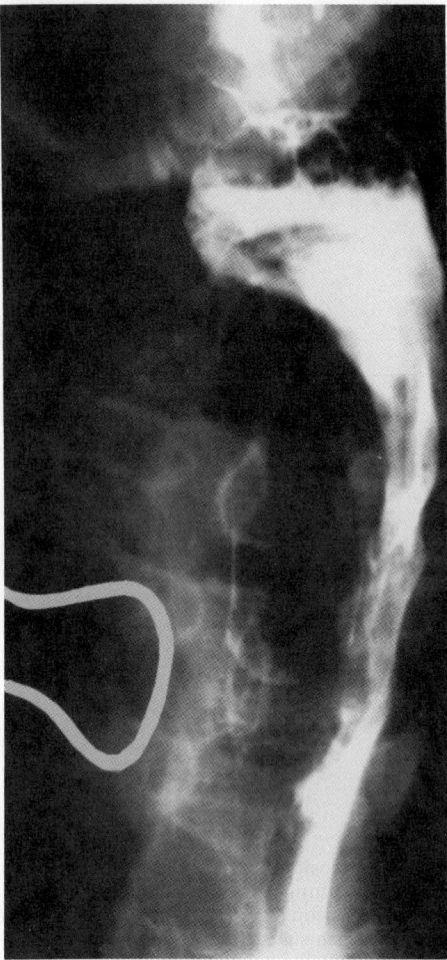

Figure 19-18. Barium esophagogram showing a large squamous cell carcinoma involving the cervicothoracic esophagus. The head of the clavicle has been highlighted to emphasize how such tumors can straddle the thoracic inlet and involve the trachea behind the sternum. (Orringer MB. Transhiatal esophagectomy without thoracotomy. In: Orringer MB, ed. Shackelford's surgery of the alimentary tract, vol 1. The esophagus. Philadelphia, WB Saunders, 1991:428)

beyond 6 months is unusual in the presence of distant metastatic disease, esophagectomy is not recommended in the patient with proved pulmonary or hepatic metastases (stage IV disease). Patients with upper- or middle-third esophageal tumors require bronchoscopy to exclude tracheobronchial invasion that contraindicates resection. Brain and bone scans are done only in patients with specific complaints suggesting metastases in these sites.

Vigorous preoperative pulmonary physiotherapy is essential to minimizing postoperative pulmonary complica-

Table 19-3. EFFECT ON SURVIVAL OF EXTENT OF ESOPHAGEAL RESECTION FOR CARCINOMA

Esophageal Tumor Site	3-Year Actuarial Survival Rate*	
	Radical Esophagectomy With En Bloc Lymph Node Dissection†	Transhiatal Esophagectomy Without Formal Lymph Node Dissection‡
Middle third	14% (29)	17% (40)
Lower third	33% (37)	31% (47)

* Number of patients in each group is given in parentheses.

† From Skinner DB. En bloc resection for neoplasms of the esophagus and cardia. J Thorac Cardiovasc Surg 1983;85:59.

‡ From Orringer MB. Transhiatal esophagectomy without thoracotomy for carcinoma of the esophagus. Ann Surg 1984;200:282.

tions. Abstinence from cigarette smoking for at least 2 weeks before operation is mandatory, and use of an incentive spirometer for 2 weeks before surgery conditions the patient for postoperative breathing exercises. Patients who are dehydrated or catabolic from their inability to eat have a nasogastric feeding tube placed for enteral nutrition and are permitted to nourish themselves at home with diet supplements through the feeding tube, providing 2000 to 3000 kcal/d. Intravenous hyperalimentation is rarely used. Carious teeth should be removed or repaired preoperatively to minimize the infectious complications that can result from anastomotic disruption and swallowed oral bacteria. If the stomach is not normal because of a history of gastric surgery or caustic injury, a barium enema should be obtained to assess the suitability of the colon as an esophageal replacement, and the colon is prepared in the event that a colonic interposition is needed.

CAUSTIC INJURY

Caustic ingestion occurs in two broad categories of patients—children younger than 5 years of age who accidentally swallow these agents and adults who are attempting

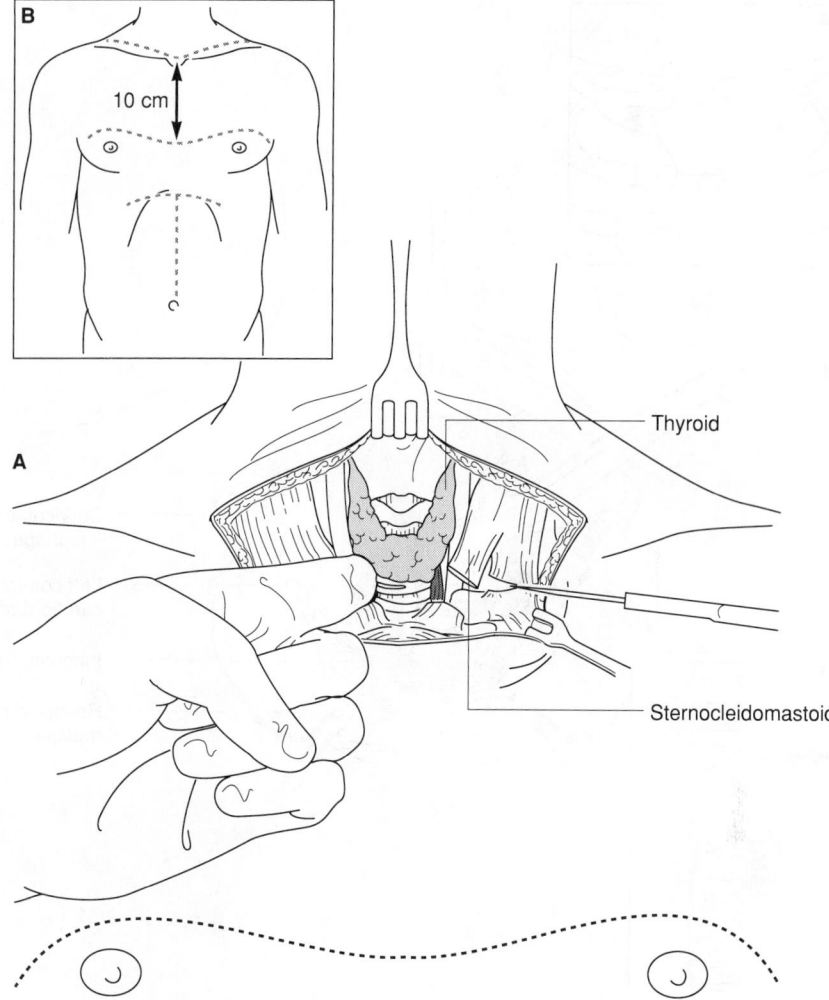

Figure 19-19. (*A*) Extended collar incision used to determine if the cervicothoracic esophageal tumor of the type shown in Figure 19-18 is not invading the adjacent prevertebral fascia or carotid vessels. If the tumor is resectable, the anterior cervical skin and platysma flap are elevated, and the origin of the sternocleidomastoid muscles is divided from the clavicles with electrocautery. (*B*) Bipedicled upper thoracic apron flap that may be used for subsequent anterior mediastinal tracheostomy. In most cases, vigorous downward retraction of the anterior upper thoracic skin permits resection of the anterior breast plate without the need for the additional transverse incision shown. (After Orringer MB, Sloan H. Anterior mediastinal tracheostomy. J Thorac Cardiovasc Surg 1979; 78:850)

suicide. More than 5000 caustic ingestions occur annually in the United States. The most common agents responsible for caustic esophageal injuries are alkalis, acids, bleach, and detergents containing sodium tripolyphosphate. Ingestion of detergents and bleach virtually always causes only mild esophageal irritation, which heals without significant adverse sequelae. Acids and alkalis, on the other hand, may have devastating effects that range from acute multiorgan necrosis and perforation to chronic esophageal and gastric strictures. Alkalis are more destructive, producing liquefaction necrosis, which almost ensures deep penetration, whereas acids usually cause coagulation necrosis that in part limits the depth of the injury.

In 1967, the introduction in the United States of concentrated liquid alkali preparations (eg, Drano, Liquid Plumber) dramatically altered the nature and extent of caustic esophageal injuries. Before that time, alkali (lye) was typically available only in solid form, in which lye crystals tend to adhere to the mucosa of the oropharynx and upper esophagus, producing burns in patches or linear streaks. Thus, solid alkali rarely reached the stomach in sufficient quantity to damage it. In contrast, the high viscosity of the liquid alkali preparations prolongs contact between these substances and the mucous membranes and also facilitates their rapid transit into the stomach. Resulting severe damage to the esophagus and stomach, as well as to adjacent organs, such as the trachea, colon, small bowel, pancreas, and aorta, is common. Ingested acids typ-

ically pass through the esophagus, quickly producing major gastric injury with relative sparing of the esophagus, although significant esophageal damage can occur.

In response to either ingested acid or alkali, reflex pyloric spasm occurs, with resultant pooling of these agents in the gastric antrum. Resulting antral stenosis produces a typical hourglass-like deformity (Fig. 19-23). Laboratory studies using the canine model have shown that both cricopharyngeal and pyloric spasm occur when concentrated lye enters the esophagus and stomach.[40] The esophagus contracts vigorously, propelling the caustic into the stomach. Pyloric and gastric contraction follows and propels the caustic agent back up into the esophagus. This seesaw movement of the caustic agent between the esophagus and stomach occurs for several minutes until both gastric and esophageal atony occur as the result of extensive damage to both organs.

Clinical Features

The clinical manifestations of caustic ingestion are directly related to the amount and character of the agent ingested.[41] There may be virtually no symptoms from mild pharyngeal, esophageal, or gastric burns.[42] Solid alkali typically causes burns of the mouth, pharynx, and upper esophagus. The resulting severe pain usually causes immediate expectoration so that relatively little of the caustic agent is swallowed. These burns usually induce excessive

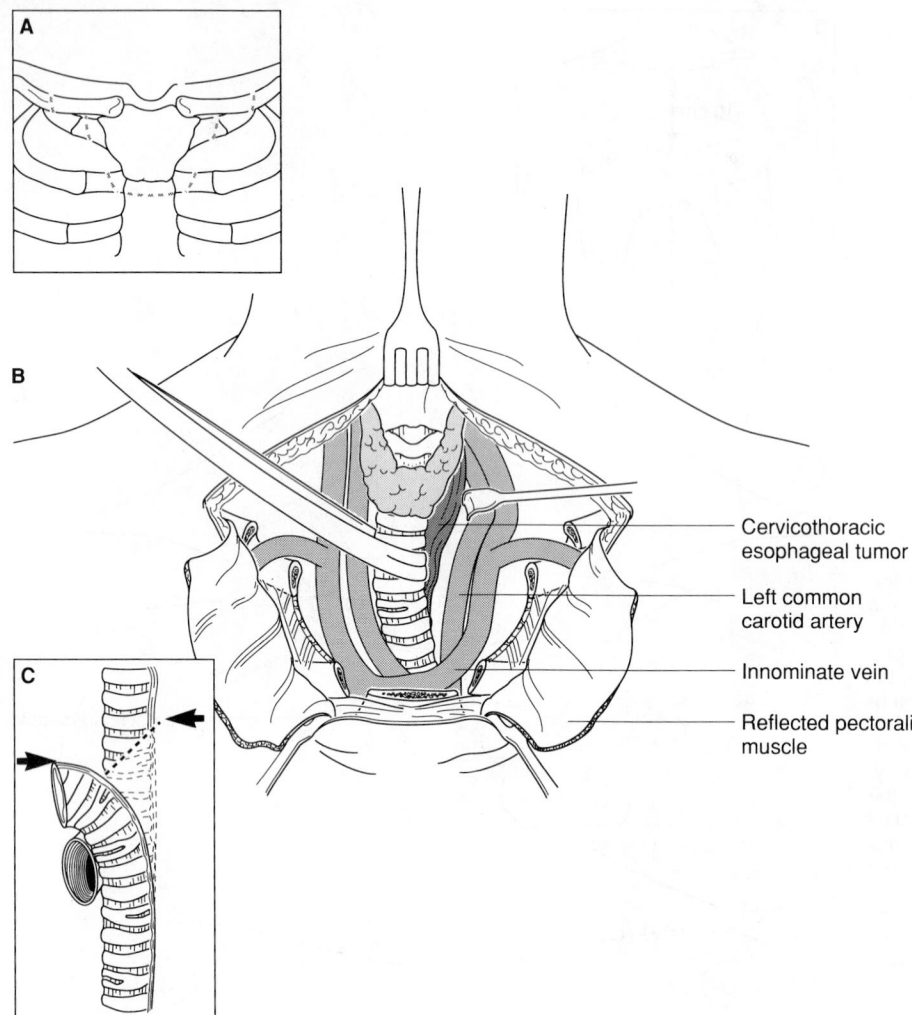

Cervicothoracic
esophageal tumor

Left common
carotid artery

Innominate vein

Reflected pectoralis
muscle

Figure 19-20. (*A*) Removal of the anterior thoracic breast plate, consisting of medial clavicles and short segments of upper manubrium and adjacent first and second ribs, provides exposure of the superior mediastinum and its contents. (*B*) The cervicothoracic esophagus with its contained tumor separated from the great vessels of the neck. (*C*) Oblique division of the trachea, preserving as much of the posterior membranous portion (*arrows*) as possible in preparation for construction of the anterior mediastinal tracheostomy. The trachea is brought forward over the innominate artery and sutured to the skin. (After Orringer MB, Sloan H. Anterior mediastinal tracheostomy. J Thorac Cardiovasc Surg 1979;78: 850)

salivation. On examination, the mucosa of the mouth and oropharynx shows patchy areas of white to gray-black pseudomembranes. Patients may also present with hoarseness, stridor, aphonia, and dyspnea from laryngotracheal edema or destruction. At the other end of the spectrum is liquid alkali ingestion. This form of alkali is usually swallowed quickly, producing less injury to the mouth and pharynx but more damage to the esophagus, stomach, or both, than its solid counterpart. Patients may present with dysphagia, odynophagia, and aspiration. Severe retrosternal, back, or abdominal pain and signs of peritoneal irritation suggest that mediastinitis or peritonitis resulting from esophageal or gastric perforation has occurred. With acid ingestion, gastric injury is more common; therefore, signs and symptoms are frequently localized to the abdomen.

When esophageal or gastric perforation results from caustic ingestion, patients demonstrate progressively severe sepsis and hypovolemic shock until appropriate resuscitative measures are instituted. In the absence of gastric or esophageal perforation, the acute clinical manifestations typically resolve within several days, with clinical improvement lasting for several weeks. After this, symptoms due either to esophageal or gastric stricture formation begin. Although only 10% to 25% of adult patients who ingest solid alkali develop strictures, most patients who ingest liquid alkali have severe esophageal and usually gastric injury that often results in stricture formation. Children with limited exposure from accidental ingestions

are less likely to have severe injuries. Acid ingestion most often results in stricture or contracture of the antrum or pylorus.

Immediate Diagnosis and Treatment

Acute caustic ingestion is an indication for hospitalization. Initial management centers on stabilizing the patient and assessing the severity of the injury. Vomiting should not be induced. Because caustic injuries produce almost instantaneous tissue damage, attempts to dilute the agent by having the patient drink water are futile. In fact, this may only aggravate the problem by producing increased gastric distention and vomiting. Oral intake should be withheld and hypovolemia corrected with intravenous fluids. Careful observation for evidence of airway obstruction is mandatory. Endotracheal intubation or tracheostomy may be required if there is significant laryngeal edema or actual laryngeal destruction. Broad-spectrum antibiotics are indicated once the diagnosis of substantial esophageal injury has been established to diminish the risk of pulmonary infection from aspiration as well as bacterial invasion through the damaged esophageal wall. Although corticosteroids have been advocated in the acute phase of caustic ingestion to minimize subsequent stricture formation, their efficacy has not been established.[43,44] Because corticosteroids may mask signs of sepsis and visceral perforation and impair healing, their use in caustic esophageal

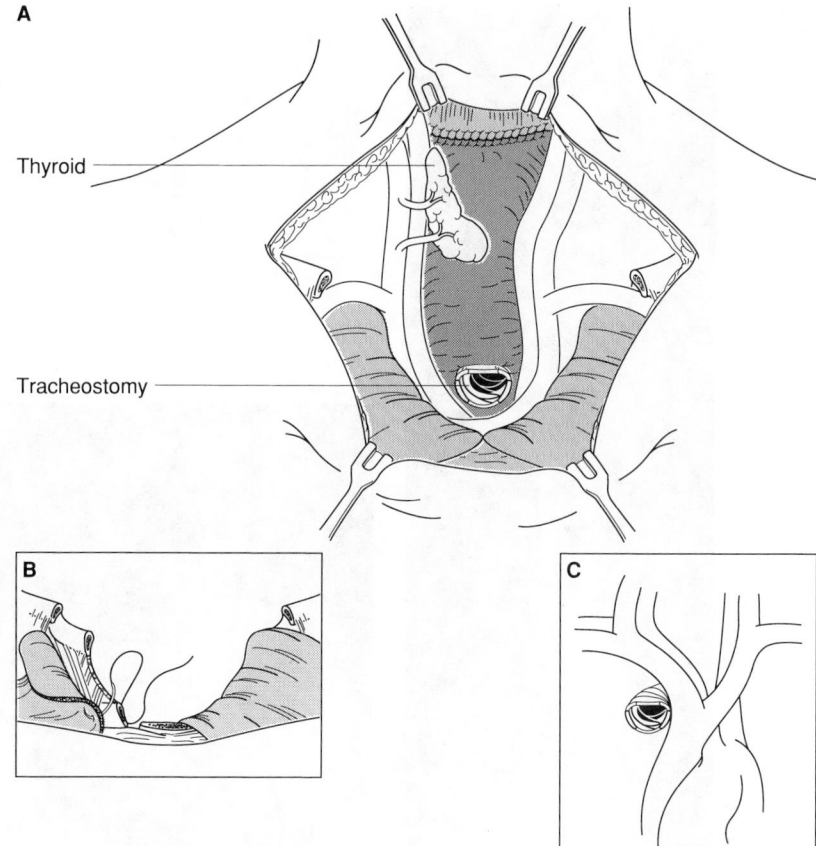

Figure 19-21. (*A*) After resecting the larynx, pharynx, and attached esophagus, the stomach is mobilized through the posterior mediastinum in the original esophageal bed and anastomosed to the pharynx as shown. Thyroid and parathyroid tissue are preserved whenever possible. The divided trachea is positioned over the innominate artery for construction of the mediastinal tracheostomy. (*B*) Covering the divided edge of the divided bony chest wall with remaining pectoralis muscle. (*C*) Transposition of the remaining trachea inferiorly and to the right of the innominate artery and vein to minimize tension and the risk of a possible innominate artery erosion when the trachea is sewn to the skin. (After Orringer MB, Sloan H. Anterior mediastinal tracheostomy. J Thorac Cardiovasc Surg 1979;78:850)

injury is potentially deleterious and is therefore not recommended.

A relatively urgent contrast examination of the esophagus may provide important information in the patient with a caustic injury.[45] Radiographically, acute mucosal esophageal injuries are seen as blurred irregular margins with linear streaking of contrast in deeper ulcers. Submucosal edema may be manifest by scalloped or straightened esophagogastric junction margins. Dilation of the esophagus and stomach, gastric ulcerations, air in the gastric wall, and frank extravasation of contrast material from the esophagus or stomach are common. A contrast esophagogram is the best way to make the diagnosis of esophageal perforation and should be performed if the diagnosis is suspected either at the time of admission or in subsequent follow-up. Identification of the site of perforation is vitally important in the planning of subsequent intervention. The initial esophagogram in these patients can be performed with a water-soluble agent (eg, Gastrografin), but dilute barium provides much better mucosal detail and should be used if the diagnosis of perforation is suspected.

Management

Esophagogastroscopy should be performed soon after admission to establish whether significant esophageal injury has occurred and to permit grading of the severity of the injury (Table 19-4). Endoscopic evaluation alone, however, cannot determine with certainty the actual depth of the injury. The risk of perforation may be minimized by using a small-caliber, flexible pediatric endoscope and adequate sedation to prevent retching and movement by the patient. Although in the past it was taught that the endoscope should not be advanced beyond the first burned area, more recently, complete examination of the esophagus and stomach has been recommended, especially if severe burns are not detected proximally. This can be accomplished safely.

After the initial resuscitative and diagnostic measures are performed, patients with caustic injuries must be observed carefully. Those with no more than first-degree burns require no other specific therapy for 24 to 48 hours. The incidence of subsequent esophageal stricture is low in patients with such injuries. Those who have second- or third-degree burns require careful and more prolonged observation for evidence of esophageal or gastric necrosis during the acute phase of the injury. Full-thickness necrosis of the esophagus, stomach, or other organs requires emergent resection. It is extremely difficult to determine on the basis of clinical, endoscopic, and radiographic information whether full-thickness necrosis has occurred. Patients with free intraperitoneal air, mediastinal air, extravasation of contrast material from the stomach or esophagus, peritonitis, or abdominal or mediastinal sepsis require immediate surgical exploration. Similarly, exploration is indicated in patients with severe persistent back or retrosternal pain suggesting mediastinitis and in those with metabolic acidosis suggesting visceral necrosis. The finding of a gastric pH greater than 7 has been suggested as an indicator of severe gastric damage and the need for exploration. Unfortunately, this is not a reliable finding, particularly in the presence of gastric blood. Clinical evidence of peritonitis remains a much more sound indication for abdominal exploration in these patients.

Patients with caustic liquid ingestion necessitating operative intervention are generally best explored through the abdomen. This approach permits assessment of the injury to the intraabdominal organs as well as resection of areas

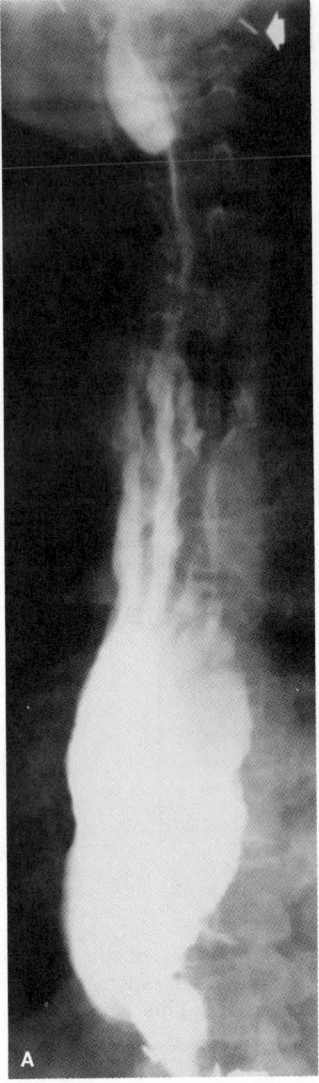

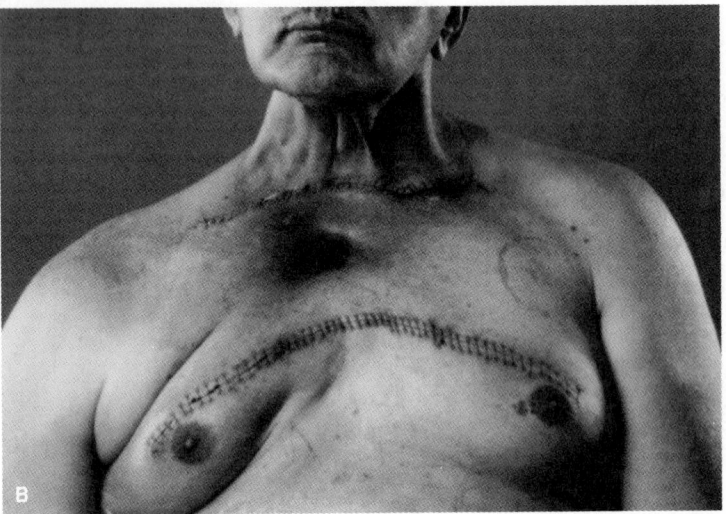

Figure 19-22. (*A*) Postoperative barium esophagogram in patient shown in Figure 19-18 after laryngopharyngectomy, transhiatal esophagectomy, pharyngogastric anastomosis, and anterior mediastinal tracheostomy. Large arrow marks the pharyngogastric anastomosis. Small arrow is at level of the pyloromyotomy. (*B*) Appearance of anterior mediastinal tracheostomy. This tracheostomy is located several centimeters inferior to the traditional permanent cervical tracheostomy in the suprasternal notch.

of full-thickness gastric necrosis. Although only the lower portion of the esophagus is well visualized through the diaphragmatic hiatus, if an esophageal resection is required, transhiatal esophagectomy without thoracotomy is readily performed by the addition of a cervical incision.[46,47] Before beginning the abdominal exploration, therefore, the operative field should be prepared and draped to include the area from the mandible to the pubis and anteriorly to both mid-axillary lines. In patients who have sustained an acute caustic esophageal injury necessitating a resection, the surrounding periesophageal edema resulting from the caustic burn often facilitates transhiatal dissection.

When esophageal or gastric resection for acute caustic injury is required, restoration of alimentary continuity should be deferred until the patient has recovered from the acute insult and the development of chronic stricture formation in retained organs can be evaluated. As a rule, when the injury resulting from acid or alkali ingestion is severe enough to warrant gastric resection, esophageal resection is usually required as well. Even if the esophagus has been spared, it is usually unwise to simply close off the distal esophagus and leave it as a blind pouch within the mediastinum. It is safer to perform a transhiatal dissection of the esophagus at the time of the gastrectomy. The mobilized thoracic esophagus is then delivered out of the cervical incision, and only the necrotic portion is resected,

sparing as much potentially viable esophagus as possible. The remaining esophageal stump is then tunneled subcutaneously for construction of an esophagostomy on the lower neck or, preferably, on the anterior chest wall (described later).

In contrast to the approach just described, Estrera and associates[48] have advocated a much more aggressive protocol in which all patients with second- or third-degree caustic injuries identified at endoscopy undergo immediate exploratory laparotomy. Those who are found to have full-thickness injuries are treated by resection, typically esophagogastrectomy, and those without full-thickness injuries have placement of a silicone stent, which is left in the esophagus for 3 weeks to prevent stricture formation. Greater experience with this approach is needed before it can be advocated routinely.

Esophageal stricture formation after second- and third-degree burns is the rule, and dilation therapy has been the traditional therapy for chronic caustic esophageal strictures. Dilation therapy should not be instituted until at least 6 to 8 weeks after the injury, when reepithelialization is complete, to minimize the risk of esophageal perforation (Fig. 19-24). If a caustic esophageal stricture is perforated during dilation, esophagectomy and visceral esophageal substitution is the best approach because repair of a perforation proximal to a stricture is rarely successful. Strictures

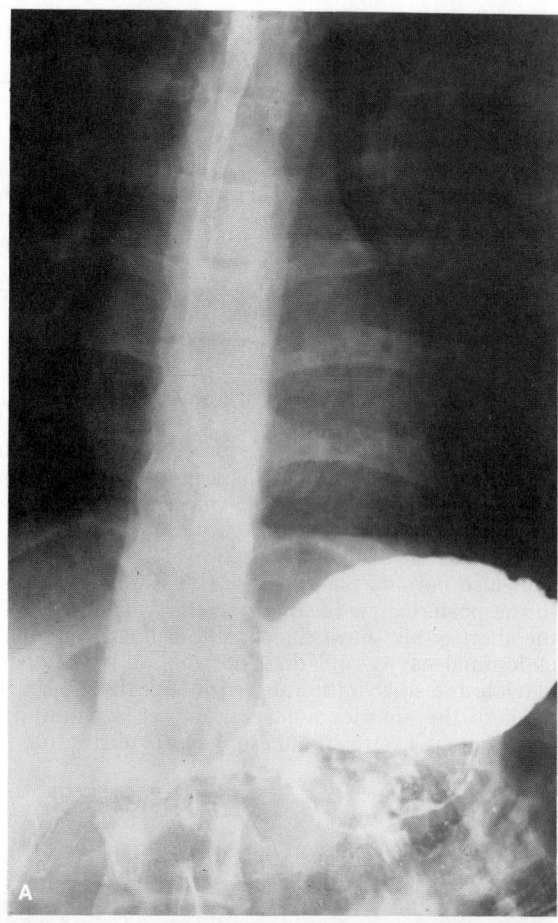

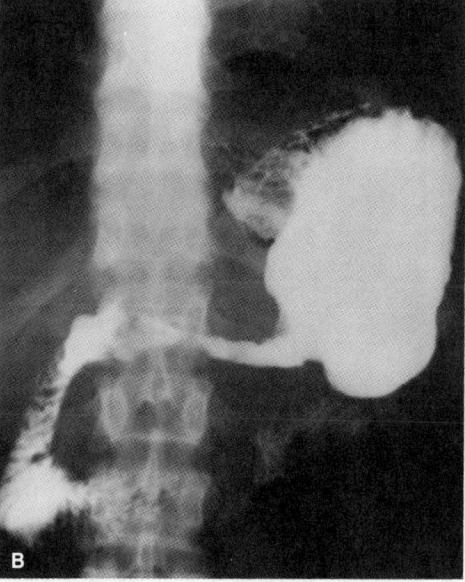
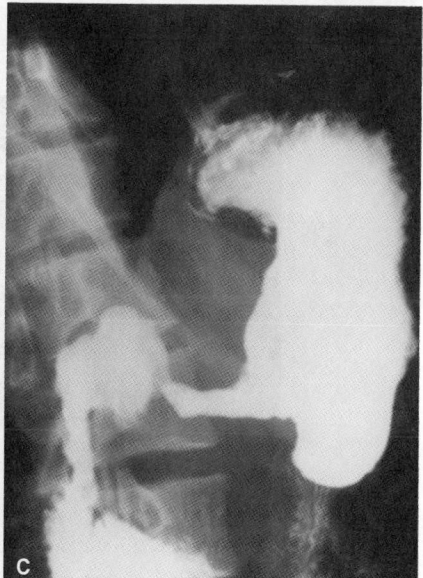

Figure 19-23. (*A*) Caustic stricture of the esophagus and stomach. (*B* and *C*) Detail of stomach showing the typical hourglass deformity due to severe antral stenosis with sparing of the body of the stomach and duodenum.

that cannot be adequately dilated (to a 46F dilator or larger for adults) and those that remain refractory to dilation after 6 to 12 months require esophageal substitution, usually with colon. The stomach is the preferred esophageal substitute, but its use in these patients may be precluded by gastric scarring and contracture secondary to the original injury.

Severe esophageal strictures resulting from caustic ingestion have been managed in the past by retrosternal colonic interposition, leaving the native, destroyed esopha-

gus in situ in the posterior mediastinum. Recent data, however, favor resection of the damaged esophagus in virtually every case, for several reasons. First, the retained obstructed esophagus can develop into a posterior mediastinal retention cyst or abscess. Second, caustic injuries may result in destruction of the lower esophageal sphincter as fibrosis of the esophagogastric junction occurs, and resulting reflux esophagitis in the retained esophagus can occur if the esophagus is still in continuity with the stomach. Finally, the risk of esophageal carcinoma developing

Table 19-4. ENDOSCOPIC GRADING OF CAUSTIC ESOPHAGEAL INJURY

Severity of Injury	Endoscopic Findings
First-degree	Mucosal hyperemia and edema
Second-degree	Mucosal ulceration with vesicles and exudates; pseudomembrane formation
Third-degree	Deep ulceration with charring and eschar formation; severe edema obliterating the lumen

after a caustic injury is about 1000 times the usual risk, with an incidence of 0.8% to 4%, typically after a latent period of 20 to 40 years. Therefore, a young patient whose caustic esophageal stricture is simply bypassed must be followed indefinitely for the development of carcinoma in the native esophagus, contrast studies of which are virtually impossible to obtain. Resection of the strictured esophagus also permits placement of the esophageal substitute in the posterior mediastinum in the original bed. This is the shortest and most direct route between the neck and abdominal cavity and does not require resection of the clavicle and adjacent sternum to enlarge the superior opening into the anterior mediastinum, as is required when carrying out a retrosternal esophageal substitution.

ESOPHAGEAL PERFORATION

Esophageal perforation has a variety of causes[49] (Table 19-5). Regardless of the specific cause, however, the pathophysiology and consequences of the resulting mediastinitis share common features that demand prompt recognition and treatment of the esophageal disruption.[1] Unless the perforation is contained by preexisting periesophageal fibrosis, saliva and gastric contents dissect into the fascial plains of the neck and mediastinum, and mediastinitis ensues. Except in edentulous patients, the presence of oral bacteria in these fluids initiates an infection. Esophageal and gastric contents are sucked into the mediastinum by respiratory movements and negative intrathoracic pressure. As salivary enzymes, gastric acid, bile, and food enter the mediastinum, the fulminant inflammatory response progresses. This mediastinal "burn" produces massive fluid accumulation, which can displace the trachea, heart, or lungs. Just as may be the case with blunt chest trauma and pulmonary contusion, the tracheobronchial tree may respond to the surrounding inflammation with a reflux bronchorrhea that results in copious pulmonary secretions and noisy, wet respirations centrally, with relatively clear breath sounds peripherally. As circulating extracellular fluid volume is lost into the mediastinum, neck, or adjacent pericardial, pleural, or peritoneal spaces, hypovolemia and respiratory distress become manifest. The entire process is aggravated if there is preexisting esophageal disease causing obstruction distal to the perforation.

Clinical Features

Patients with esophageal perforation characteristically present with cervical or thoracic pain or difficulty swallowing, respiratory distress, and fever. Perforations of the cervical or upper thoracic esophagus generally cause cervical or high retrosternal pain, while those of the middle or distal esophagus produce anterior thoracic, posterior thoracic, interscapular, or epigastric pain. Upper thoracic esophageal perforations may produce signs of right pleural

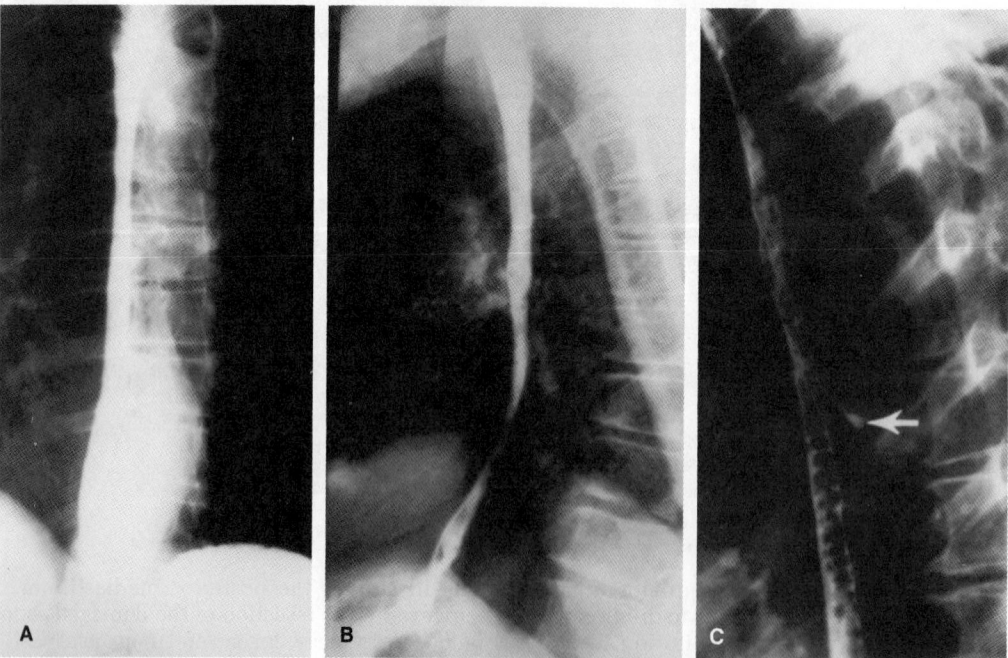

Figure 19-24. Posteroanterior (*A*) and lateral (*B*) views from Gastrografin swallow in a patient who complained of chest pain after dilation of his caustic esophageal stricture, which was incorrectly and prematurely dilated within 10 days of ingesting Drano, before reepithelialization of the esophagus was complete. No perforation was seen with this study. (*C*) Barium esophagogram demonstrates a perforation (*arrow*) in the middle third of the thoracic esophagus. (Orringer MB. Complications of esophageal surgery and trauma. In: Greenfield LJ, ed. Complications in surgery and trauma, ed 2. Philadelphia, JB Lippincott, 1990:302)

Table 19-5. CAUSES OF ESOPHAGEAL PERFORATION

INSTRUMENTAL
Endoscopy
Dilation
Intubation
Sclerotherapy
Laser therapy

NONINSTRUMENTAL
Barogenic trauma
  Postemetic (Boerhaave syndrome)
  Blunt chest or abdominal trauma
  Other (eg, labor, convulsions, defecation)
Penetrating neck, chest, or abdominal trauma
Operative trauma
  Esophageal reconstruction (anastomotic disruption)
  Vagotomy, pulmonary resection, hiatal hernia repair, esophagomyotomy
Corrosive injuries (acid or alkali ingestion)
Erosion by adjacent infection
Swallowed foreign body

effusion, while distal esophageal perforation is associated with left pleural effusion.

Diagnosis

Pain or fever after esophageal instrumentation or operation is indicative of an esophageal perforation until proved otherwise and is an indication for an immediate contrast esophagogram. Because the morbidity and mortality rates associated with esophageal perforation are directly related to the time interval between diagnosis of the injury and its repair or drainage, an aggressive attitude toward diagnosing a perforation must be adopted. When the diagnosis is considered, a water-soluble contrast agent should be administered. If this study is negative, dilute barium should be administered. Barium is relatively inert, and the fear of barium extravasating into the mediastinum through the site of injury and producing a severe reactive mediastinitis is unfounded. The risk of barium leaking into the mediastinum is far less than that of failing to recognize the perforation in a timely fashion. Also, because barium provides far better mucosal detail than water-soluble agents, only if barium has been used for the esophagogram should this study in search of a perforation be termed negative (see Fig. 19-24).

If there is concern about the possibility of a perforation after esophagoscopy, a chest roentgenogram may help to confirm the diagnosis by demonstrating air in the soft tissues of the neck or mediastinum or a hydrothorax or pneumothorax. A normal chest roentgenogram, however, does not rule out an esophageal perforation. If a perforation is suspected or considered, a contrast study of the esophagus is mandatory both to establish the diagnosis and to demonstrate the exact site of the injury. In the exceedingly rare instance in which the esophagogram is equivocal or clinical suspicion overrides a negative study, a contrast-enhanced CT scan may lead to the diagnosis.[50]

Management

The initial treatment of an acute esophageal perforation focuses on decreasing bacterial and chemical contamination of the mediastinum and restoring intravascular volume losses. Oral intake is withheld, and the patient is instructed not to swallow saliva. A disposable oral dental suction at the bedside is often helpful for evacuating oral secretions. Broad-spectrum intravenous antibiotics with activity against oral flora are administered using a combination of a cephalosporin (cefazolin or cefamandole), 1 g/4 h, and an aminoglycoside (gentamicin or tobramycin), 1 to 1.5 mg/kg/8 h. Nasogastric tube decompression of the stomach is instituted to minimize possible gastroesophageal reflux and further soiling of the mediastinum. In the patient with a well-contained proximal perforation, however, a nasogastric tube may only interfere with the ability to breathe deeply, without providing any additional protection. Therapy of esophageal perforation is influenced by the location of the tear, its size and cause, the length of delay in diagnosis, the extent of mediastinal and pleural contamination, and the presence of intrinsic esophageal disease. Treatment must therefore be individualized.

Nonoperative Therapy

Although most esophageal perforations require operative intervention, selected patients may be managed nonoperatively with cessation of oral intake, administration of antibiotics, and intravenous hydration until the disruption heals or the small contained cavity begins to decrease in size.[51,52] Criteria for nonoperative therapy of an esophageal perforation include the following: (1) a local, contained disruption without evidence of pleural contamination (hydrothorax or pneumothorax), (2) a walled-off extravasation in which contrast material drains back into the esophagus, (3) minimal or no symptoms, and (4) minimal or no evidence of systemic infection (fever or leukocytosis). The usual clinical settings in which such perforations are encountered are cervical esophageal tears caused by esophagoscopy; intramural dissections that have occurred during dilation of a stricture or pneumatic dilation for achalasia; and an asymptomatic esophageal anastomotic disruption discovered on a routine postoperative contrast study. When treating such perforations conservatively, oral hygiene should be optimized to minimize further contamination by oral bacteria by having patients brush their teeth four to six times a day. A nasogastric tube is seldom helpful. Nutrition may be maintained by a nasogastric feeding tube, gastrostomy, or jejunostomy or by intravenous hyperalimentation until oral intake can be resumed, usually 1 to 3 weeks after the injury.

When selecting patients for nonoperative therapy of esophageal perforations, one must be certain that any cavity resulting from the tear is well contained and well drained internally into the esophagus. In patients who present within 24 hours of their esophageal injury, it may not be possible to determine whether the leak is well contained, and delay in surgical intervention may only allow mediastinal sepsis to progress. Therefore, nonoperative therapy of esophageal perforations is best suited for patients presenting more than 24 hours after the injury with no systemic evidence of sepsis and clearly demonstrable, contained, internally drained leaks on barium esophagogram. Infants with iatrogenic perforation can often be successfully managed without operation. Perforations complicating pneumatic dilation for achalasia occur in 4% to 6% of patients, and most are small and well-managed medically with antibiotics and intravenous hyperalimentation.[53-55] For the remainder of patients with perforations, operative therapy is generally indicated.

Operative Therapy

Cervical and Upper Thoracic Esophageal Perforations. Cervical esophageal perforations lead to progressive contamination of the mediastinum as infection descends dependently along the fascial planes from the neck. Unless adequate drainage is accomplished, death from mediastinitis follows. Most cervical and upper thoracic perforations (to the level of the carina or the fourth thoracic vertebral body) may be adequately drained through a cervical approach, placing drains in the retroesophageal space (Fig. 19-25). An incision is made parallel to the anterior border of the sternocleidomastoid muscle, which is retracted laterally along with the carotid sheath and its contents. The trachea, thyroid gland, and strap muscles are retracted medially. It may be necessary to divide the omohyoid muscle, middle thyroid vein, and occasionally the inferior thyroid artery to reach the prevertebral fascia. Once this is identified, blunt finger dissection into the prevertebral space gives access to the abscess cavity, and appropriate drains are placed and brought out through the skin incision.

In most situations, because of the overlying trachea and larynx, it is not possible to identify the cervical esophageal tear for direct suture closure. This is seldom a problem, however, because spontaneous healing of a well-drained cervical esophageal perforation generally occurs within several days. Insufflation of air into the esophagus through a nasogastric tube or small flexible esophagoscope may be useful in identifying the tear and permitting direct closure if it is accessible. Nutrition during the first few days can be maintained with a small nasogastric feeding tube. Oral liquids can be resumed within 5 to 7 days of the injury if the fistula output is minimal. When a cervical esophageal perforation extends into either pleural cavity or the lower mediastinum, the cervical approach is inadequate, and transthoracic drainage is required.

Thoracoesophageal Perforations.   The earlier an esophageal perforation is recognized and treated, the better is the chance for successful primary repair. Historically, it has been taught that delay of repair beyond 6 to 8 hours of the injury is frequently associated with so much local inflammation that the torn esophageal wall is simply not amenable to suture repair. As a general rule, early esophageal perforations are those diagnosed well within 24 hours of the injury. Most agree that such perforations that are not associated with intrinsic esophageal disease are best treated with primary repair of the tear combined with wide mediastinal drainage. Mediastinal drainage is achieved by opening the mediastinal pleura from the level of the tear to the thoracic inlet superiorly and the diaphragm inferiorly, irrigating the mediastinum, and placing a large-bore chest tube that allows transpleural drainage. Perforations of the lower third of the esophagus are approached through a left thoracotomy in the sixth or seventh interspace, while more proximal thoracic esophageal tears are approached through a right thoracotomy. Perforations of the intraabdominal esophagus unassociated with pleural contamination are approached through the abdomen.

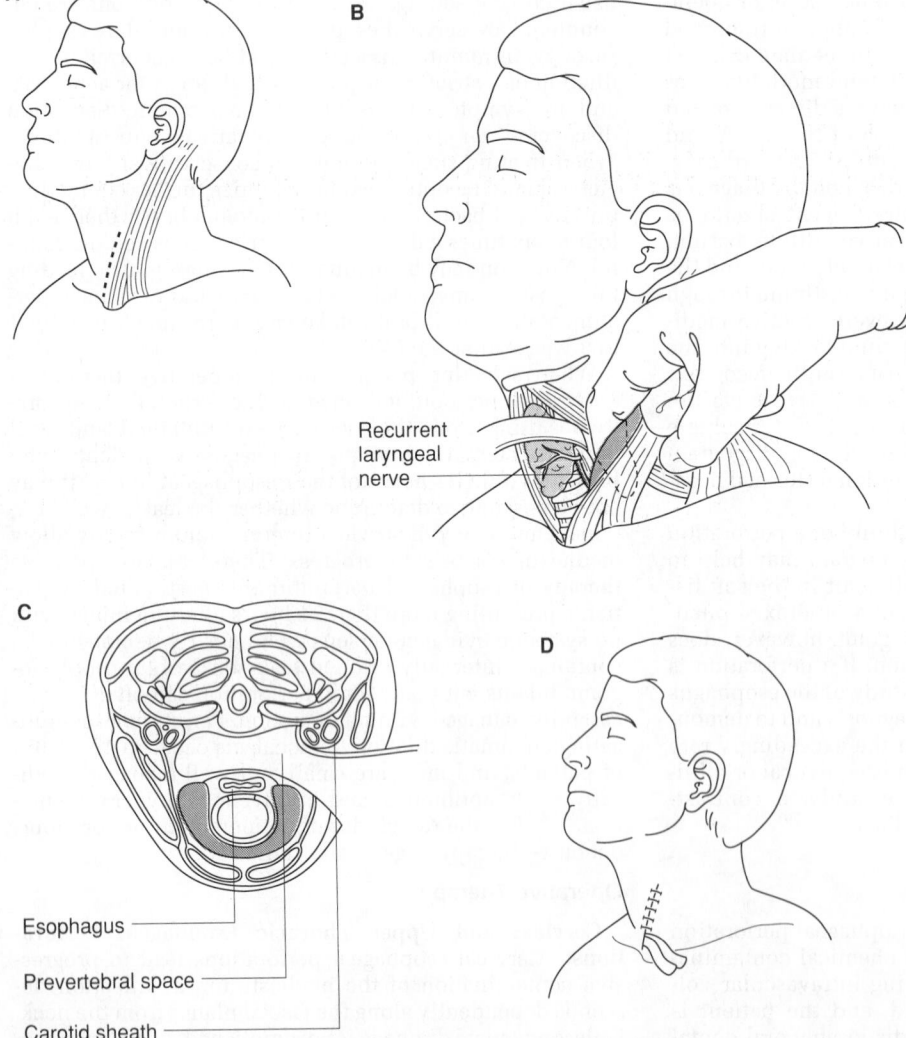

Recurrent
laryngeal
nerve

Esophagus

Prevertebral space

Carotid sheath

Figure 19-25. Approach for drainage of a cervical esophageal perforation. (*A*) Skin incision parallel to the anterior border of the left sternocleidomastoid muscle, extending from the level of the cricoid cartilage to the sternal notch. (*B*) With the sternocleidomastoid muscle and carotid sheath retracted laterally, and the trachea and thyroid gland medially, blunt disection along the prevertebral fascia in the superior mediastinum is carried out. Injury to the recurrent laryngeal nerve in the tracheoesophageal groove must be avoided. (*C*) Schematic drawing of the prevertebral space drained by this cervical approach. (*D*) Two 1-inch rubber drains placed into the superior mediastinum are brought out through the neck wound and allow establishment of an esophagocutaneous fistula, which usually heals spontaneously. (After Orringer MB. The mediastinum. In: Nora PH, ed. Operative surgery, ed 3. Philadelphia, WB Saunders, 1990:370)

A change in philosophy has occurred regarding the application of primary repair to perforations occurring in an otherwise normal esophagus *regardless of the duration of the injury*. It has now been documented that with meticulous technique, the results are good.[56-58] The entire length of the mucosal injury must be exposed by extending the muscle defect 1 to 2 cm beyond the extent of the mucosal tear (Fig. 19-26). With a 40F or larger dilator within the esophagus to prevent undue narrowing, an endo-GIA stapler is applied, and the defect is closed. The staple suture line is reinforced by approximating adjacent muscle (Fig. 19-27). The perforation repair can then be reinforced with a pedicled flap of normal tissue (eg, parietal pleura, anterior mediastinal fat, gastric fundus, intercostal muscle), but this is not essential if the repair has been well performed. After repair of perforations of the lower esophagus (eg, after post-emetic rupture), a fundoplication around the repair is ideal for reinforcement of the suture line (Fig. 19-28). This fundoplication, however, should not be left in the chest to avoid subsequent complications of a paraesophageal hernia. More proximal esophageal repairs can be buttressed with intercostal muscle or parietal pleura. The intercostal muscle reinforcement should be carried out as an onlay patch rather than encircling the esophagus to avoid subsequent esophageal obstruction that may occur as periosteum is regenerated. Omentum may be mobilized into the chest to reinforce an esophageal suture line at virtually any level. The parietal pleura must be inflamed and thickened if it is to provide adequate support of the suture line.

After repair and drainage of the esophageal tear, a nasogastric tube is used to treat postoperative ileus, and thereafter, nasogastric tube feedings can be instituted until oral intake is resumed. It is wishful thinking to assume that the patient who is swallowing no food has a "protected" suture line because saliva containing digestive enzymes and oral bacteria is traversing the esophagus from the moment the patient awakens from general anesthesia. Therefore, once the postoperative ileus has subsided, oral liquids may

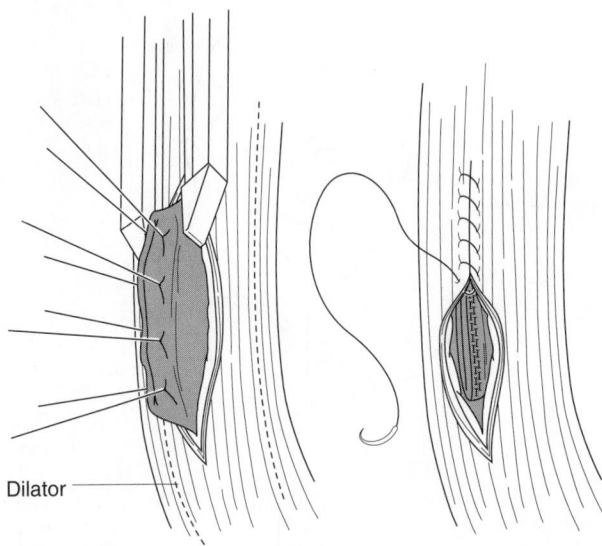

Figure 19-27. Primary repair of esophageal perforation (continued). (*Left*) Stay sutures placed into inflamed pouting mucosa elevate normal submucosa into jaws of an endo-GIA stapler. The stapler is applied below inflamed edematous mucosal edges (*dashed line*). (*Right*) After amputation of the pouting mucosal edge, the staple suture line is supported by approximating the adjacent muscle with a running suture. (After Whyte RI, Iannettoni MD, Orringer MB. Intrathoracic esophageal perforation: the merit of primary repair. J Thorac Cardiovasc Surg 1995;109:140)

be resumed. There appears to be no evidence that swallowing a liquid diet results in a higher incidence of subsequent suture line disruption. A barium esophagogram is obtained 10 days after the repair to document the integrity of the esophagus, and the chest tube is not removed until after this examination. If disruption of the esophageal repair occurs, the resulting esophagopleural cutaneous fistula should heal spontaneously if external drainage through the chest tube is adequate and there is no associated distal esophageal obstruction. Such fistulas do not necessarily contraindicate oral alimentation if they are small and well drained.

Esophageal Perforation Associated With Intrinsic Disease. Perforations associated with distal obstruction from intrinsic esophageal disease constitute a much more challenging problem because breakdown of an attempted repair is common in the presence of distal obstruction. It is therefore important that the associated obstruction be relieved at the time of repair and drainage. For example, the patient with achalasia who sustains a distal perforation during balloon dilation should be treated with suture repair, esophagomyotomy to relieve the distal obstruction, and a partial fundoplication to buttress the tear if possible. A patient who sustains a small perforation during dilation of a "soft" dilatable reflux stricture may be treated successfully with repair of the tear, dilation of the stricture to relieve the obstruction, and an antireflux operation.

Patients with intrinsic esophageal disease that cannot be treated effectively by more conservative means (eg, esophageal carcinoma; nondilatable, "hard" benign stricture; caustic injury; or extensive esophageal devitalization associated with high-velocity gun-shot wounds) are best treated by esophageal resection. Improvements in techniques of esophageal replacement have resulted in a general philosophy that it is unwise to attempt to salvage a diseased esophagus simply because esophagectomy is re-

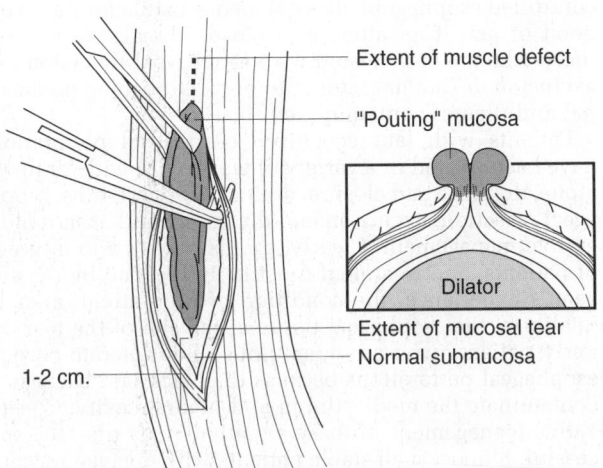

Figure 19-26. Primary repair of esophageal perforation. The edematous mucosa pouting through the muscular defect (*inset*) is grasped with Allis clamps and elevated. A 1-cm vertical esophagomyotomy is made at either end of the muscular defect to expose the entire limits of the tear. This is facilitated by using a right-angle clamp to direct muscularis away from underlying submucosa around the entire circumference of the tear. The result of this mobilization is exposure of a circumferential rim of normal submucosa that can then be closed. (After Whyte RI, Iannettoni MD, Orringer MB. Intrathoracic esophageal perforation: the merit of primary repair. J Thorac Cardiovasc Surg 1995;109:140)

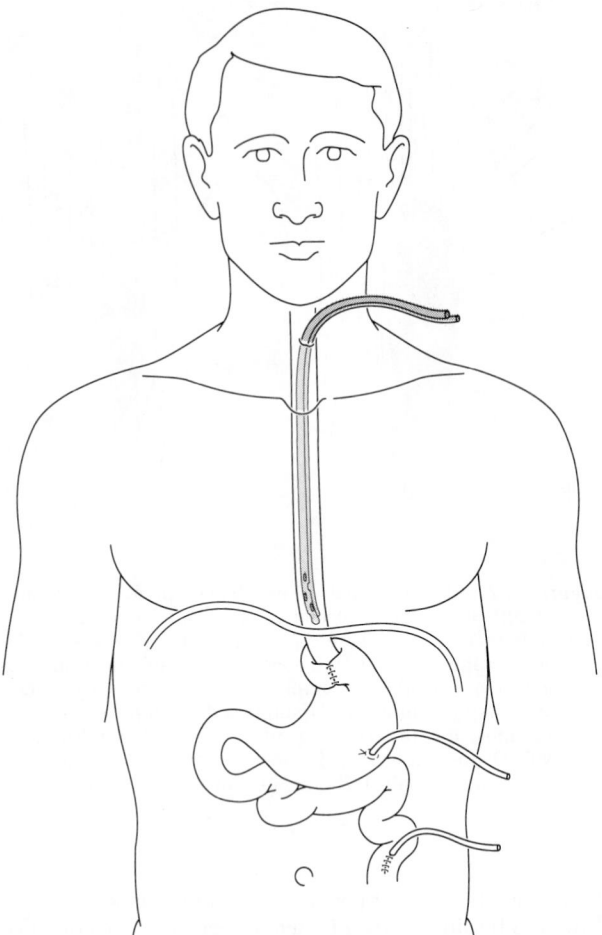

Figure 19-28. Repair of distal esophageal perforation and reinforcement with a fundoplication. To avoid potential complications of a paraesophageal hernia, the fundoplication should not be left in the chest. A decompressing gastrostomy and feeding jejunostomy, in addition to drainage of the esophagus with a nasogastric sump drain, are used. (After Orringer MB. Complications of esophageal surgery and trauma. In: Greenfield LJ, ed. Complications in surgery and trauma, ed 2. Philadelphia, JB Lippincott, 1990:302)

garded as too major an undertaking. If an esophagectomy is necessary in a patient with a perforated and diseased esophagus, a total thoracic esophagectomy has the advantages of eliminating the source of mediastinal and pleural contamination as well as permitting a cervical esophageal anastomosis, which has far less morbidity than an intrathoracic one.[59]

If the esophageal perforation is diagnosed promptly and mediastinal contamination is not excessive, immediate restoration of alimentary continuity can be achieved at the time of esophagectomy. This is the best approach when the stomach is healthy and available for esophageal substitution and a cervical esophagogastric anastomosis. Although immediate esophageal substitution with unprepared colon has been used successfully, it is not the preferred alternative. Patients with esophageal perforations caused by caustic ingestion and those who are unstable or severely ill should undergo esophagectomy and cervical esophagostomy followed by later reconstruction. The preferred approach for immediate reconstruction after esophagectomy is to position the mobilized stomach in the posterior mediastinum in the native esophageal bed (see Fig. 19-17). A feeding jejunostomy tube is used routinely

for postoperative nutritional support until oral intake is adequate.

In situations in which immediate esophageal reconstruction is not possible, the stomach is divided from the esophagus, the cardia is oversewn, and the esophageal hiatus is closed to avoid herniation of abdominal viscera into the chest. The intrathoracic esophagus is then mobilized through the diaphragmatic hiatus and a cervical incision, delivering the entire thoracic esophagus through the neck wound and placing it on the anterior chest wall. Only devitalized or extensively damaged esophagus should then be resected; the remaining esophageal stump is tunneled subcutaneously on the anterior chest wall, and a low cervical or high anterior thoracic esophagostomy is constructed (Fig. 19-29). The mediastinum can be copiously irrigated through the cervical incision and the diaphragmatic hiatus at the time of esophagectomy (Fig. 19-30). An anterior thoracic esophagostomy is much easier to care for than an esophagostome in the usual location in the supraclavicular fossa, and the extra length of remaining esophagus may facilitate later retrosternal esophageal reconstruction with stomach or colon. A feeding jejunostomy is used for enteral alimentation until reconstruction is performed several weeks later. A gastrostomy tube should also be inserted in the event that gastric atony or pylorospasm follow the vagotomy that accompanies esophagectomy. If the stomach empties well after several days, gastrostomy feedings may be used in preference to jejunostomy tube feedings, which are less amenable to bolus administration and are therefore not as convenient for the patient.

Late Esophageal Perforation. The longer the time interval between the occurrence of the perforation and operative treatment, the more inflamed are the tissues adjacent to the tear and, at least theoretically, the greater is the risk of failure of primary suture repair. Although this is may be the case, as discussed earlier, it is not the rule, and it is well worth inspecting every esophageal tear to ascertain if primary repair might be feasible. The most difficult decision involves distinguishing between patients with delayed esophageal perforations who are best treated with a controlled esophagopleural cutaneous fistula (or the likelihood of one if an attempt at closure breaks down) and those who are best treated with esophageal diversion and exclusion or esophagectomy to prevent ongoing mediastinal and pleural contamination.

Patients with late-recognized esophageal perforations have been treated in a variety of ways, with wide drainage alone, drainage and closure, drainage over a T-tube, esophageal resection, exclusion and diversion, and even nonoperative management. Clearly, this is not a uniform group of patients, and treatment must be influenced by the surgeon's experience, the condition of the patient, and the quality of the esophageal tissue at the site of the tear. Elderly patients who are edentulous often tolerate chronic esophageal perforations because they lack oral bacteria to contaminate the mediastinum and pleural cavity. Conservative management in these situations may often be successful. In most such stable patients with delayed recognition of esophageal perforations, a feeding jejunostomy and a decompressing gastrostomy to prevent gastroesophageal reflux are useful. Distal esophageal obstruction must be relieved, if necessary, by continuing dilations until the fistula closes. Well-drained esophagopleural cutaneous fistulas almost always heal spontaneously if there is no distal obstruction.

As discussed earlier, late recognized esophageal perforations may be successfully closed with meticulous technique.[56] With chronic esophageal defects that are too large to permit direct closure without tension, pedicled pleural

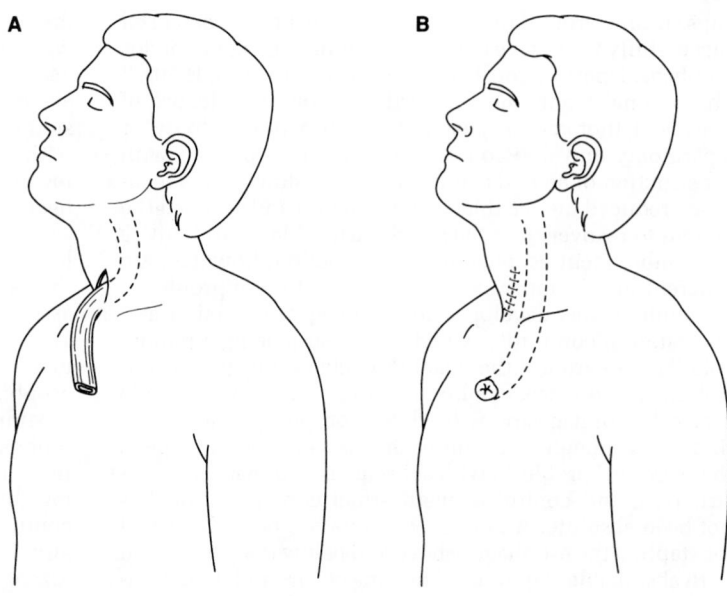

Figure 19-29. Construction of an anterior thoracic esophagostomy instead of the traditional end cervical esophagostomy in the supraclavicular fossa. (*A*) The thoracic esophagus has been delivered out of the neck wound and is placed on the anterior chest wall. Devitalized esophagus is resected, leaving as much remaining normal esophagus as possible and locating its distal extent for construction of the stoma. (*B*) The remaining esophagus has been tunneled subcutaneously and the end sutured to the skin. Stomal appliances are readily applied to the flat surface of the anterior chest; and when performing a colon interposition at a later time, an additional 7 to 12 cm of esophageal length is available for the reconstruction. (After Orringer MB. Complications of esophageal surgery and trauma. In: Greenfield LJ, ed. Complications in surgery and trauma, ed 2. Philadelphia, JB Lippincott, 1990:302)

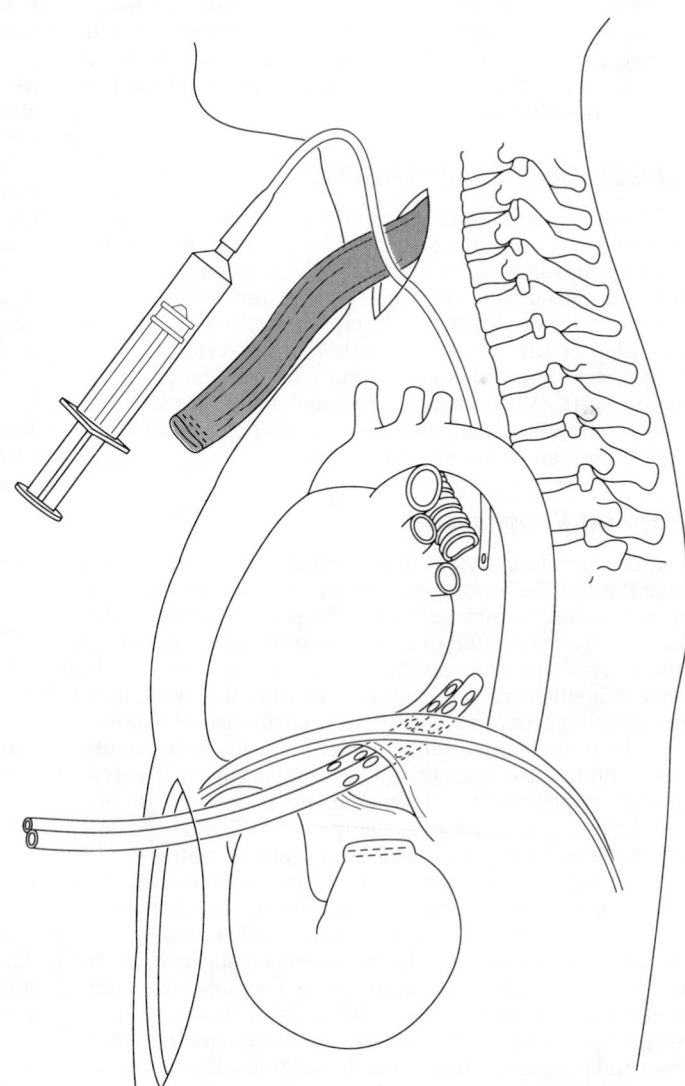

Figure 19-30. Irrigation of the posterior mediastinum after transhiatal esophagectomy for irreparable esophageal disruption. After several liters of irrigation and placement of bilateral chest tubes to drain the intentionally opened mediastinal pleura, an anterior thoracic esophagostomy (as shown in Fig. 19-29) is constructed.

flaps sutured around the edges of the defect have been used successfully to achieve closure.[60] Esophageal exclusion for esophageal perforation has been used since the 1950s.[61] The original technique involved division and closure of the distal thoracic esophagus through a thoracotomy or laparotomy and division of the cervical esophagus with construction of an end cervical esophagostomy. This technique reduced mediastinal contamination and allowed the patient to recover from the septic insult. Major difficulties with subsequent esophageal reconstruction, however, are inherent in this approach. To circumvent these problems, a technique was developed for esophageal diversion and exclusion in continuity, which involved placing a removable ligature around the distal thoracic esophagus to control gastroesophageal reflux and then performing a side cervical esophagostomy to divert oropharyngeal secretions.[62] Although this approach has conceptual appeal, there are still problems with subsequent esophageal reconstruction, and control of mediastinal contamination has not been absolute. A newer technique has been described for stapling the esophagus above and below the perforation with absorbable staples until healing occurs and then dilating the esophagus to disrupt the staple line and restore continuity of the lumen at a later date. Further experience with this technique is needed before its efficacy is established.

As a general rule, most patients with esophageal perforation require surgical intervention. Nonoperative therapy is contraindicated in most patients with esophageal tears, and an aggressive approach, using an esophagectomy if necessary, is often less radical treatment and more reliable in the long run than conservative techniques intended to preserve the esophagus.

INFECTIOUS ESOPHAGITIS

Chronic debilitation, immunosuppression, and prolonged use of antibiotics predispose to the development of infectious esophagitis, *Candida albicans* being the most common cause. The epidemic of acquired immunodeficiency syndrome (AIDS), however, has resulted in a variety of esophageal infections due to other fungi (*Torulopsis* and *Histoplasma* spp), viruses (cytomegalovirus, herpes simplex virus [HSV], human immunodeficiency virus [HIV], and Epstein-Barr virus), mycobacteria, and protozoa (*Cryptosporidium* and *Pneumocystitis* spp).[63]

Monilial Esophagitis

C albicans is a fungus that normally is a commensal inhabitant of the mouth, oropharynx, and gastrointestinal tract. This fungus may become pathogenic in patients who are severely debilitated or immunosuppressed. The use of potent broad-spectrum antibiotics, immunosuppression in organ transplant recipients, and the wide use of chemotherapeutic agents have resulted in an increased number of patients with monilial esophagitis. In its initial acute phase, monilial esophagitis with oropharyngeal involvement causes painful swallowing. As the disease progresses into the thoracic esophagus, abnormal esophageal peristalsis (decreased frequency and amplitude of primary and secondary peristaltic waves) and spasm may be seen. Radiographically, a characteristic cobblestone-like pattern of luminal nodulation is seen as a result of inflammation and edema of the submucosa. In the advanced stages of acute monilial esophagitis, the radiographic findings on barium swallow are those of mucosal ulceration, with an irregular, shaggy-appearing, narrowed esophageal lumen due to mucosal and submucosal edema and pseudomembrane formation. The initial endoscopic findings are those of an erythematous, nonulcerated mucosa with an overlying whitish, cheesy exudate or pseudomembrane. The mucosa becomes granular and friable as the inflammatory reaction extends into the wall of the esophagus. Transmural invasion of the esophageal wall occurs and can be controlled with antifungal therapy if the patient survives the underlying disease, but chronic stricture formation may result after healing of the acute esophagitis. A characteristic radiographic pattern of intramural esophageal pseudodiverticulosis occurs as the result of dilation and outpouching of the esophageal submucosal glands that are inflamed from associated infection, stasis, or distal obstruction (Fig. 19-31). These esophageal submucosal glands are more numerous in the upper half of the esophagus, where monilial esophageal strictures are also encountered.[64]

Minimally compromised patients with mild monilial esophagitis should receive oral nystatin suspension, 1 million to 3 million units every 6 hours, or clotrimazole, 100 mg three to five times a day. This treatment should be continued for 1 to 3 weeks, although the infection generally subsides within 7 to 10 days. Oral amphotericin B lozenges, ketoconazole, or fluconazole may be used as an alternative. More immunosuppressed patients (eg, those with AIDS) or those with more severe cases warrant high-dose fluconazole, 100 to 200 mg orally once a day, and ketoconazole, 400 to 800 mg orally once a day. Intravenous fluconazole or amphotericin B are used in granulocytopenic patients.[65] Because esophageal stricture formation may result from a bout of acute monilial esophagitis, patients who recover from the acute episode should be followed with periodic barium swallows during the first year to ensure the earliest possible detection of a developing stricture and prompt institution of dilation therapy if needed.

Viral esophagitis is the second most common cause of infectious esophagitis, HSV being the most common infection in immunosuppressed transplant recipients and cytomegalovirus in HIV-positive patients.[63] Viral esophagitis produces mucosal ulceration, and patients present with dysphagia and odynophagia. The esophageal ulcers associated with viral infections appear on barium esophagogram as large lesions in cytomegalovirus disease and smaller (less than 1.5 cm) ulcers in HSV. The diagnosis is established endoscopically by biopsy, brushings, and washings for cytology, histology, and viral culture. HSV is diagnosed by isolation of the virus and identification in tissue culture, although the demonstration of multinucleated giant cells on Wright- or Giemsa-stained scrapings from the vesicles are presumptive evidence. The infection generally responds well to treatment with acyclovir.

Other Infections

Sporadic cases of infectious esophagitis due to syphilis and tuberculosis have been reported. Crohn's disease of the esophagus has also been reported as a rare cause of esophagitis. Tuberculosis of the esophagus is rare, and reported cases have invariably occurred in patients with advanced pulmonary tuberculosis who swallow copious sputum that is heavily laden with tubercle bacilli. Esophageal involvement can occur in several ways: from implantation of swallowed bacilli, direct extension from adjacent lung or subcarinal lymph nodes, lymphatic spread from infection elsewhere, or hematogenous spread from a distant site. The mid-thoracic esophagus at the level of the carina is most frequently involved, probably as a result of spread from tuberculous paratracheal and subcarinal lymph nodes. Tuberculous esophagitis occurs in one of three forms: ulcerating, hypertrophic (stricture formation), or miliary. Esophageal symptoms may be totally absent or

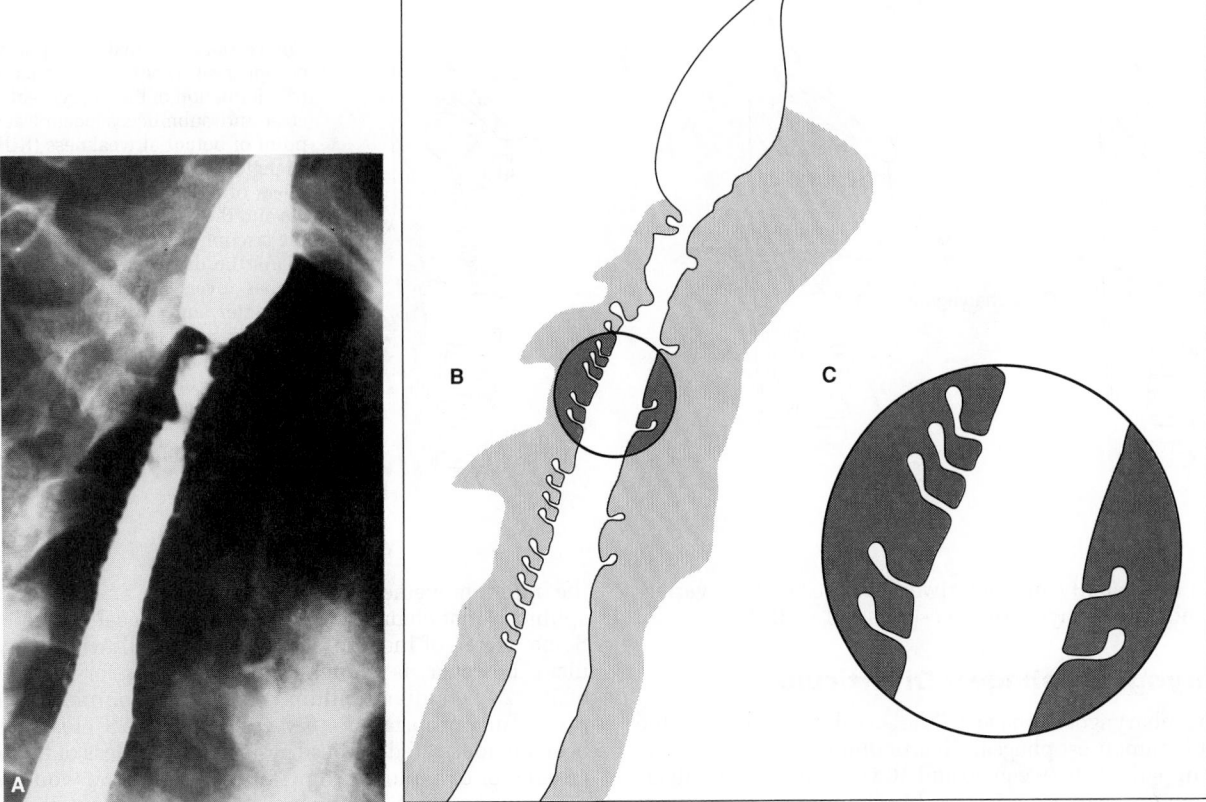

Figure 19-31. Esophagogram (*A*) and drawing (*B* and *C*) of an irregular upper thoracic esophageal stricture due to monilial esophagitis. The characteristic pattern of intramural pseudodiverticulosis is due to dilated submucosal esophageal glands. (*B* and *C* after Orringer MB, Sloan H. Monilial esophagitis: an increasingly frequent cause of esophageal stenosis? Ann Thorac Surg 1978;36:364)

may range from intense pain on swallowing in the ulcerative form of the disease to dysphagia in the hypertrophic form. The barium esophagogram frequently fails to demonstrate the ulcerative or miliary forms of the disease, but the hypertrophic form appears as a mid-esophageal stenosis. Fiberoptic esophagoscopy with biopsy of the stenosis establishes a diagnosis of esophageal tuberculosis by demonstrating the characteristic mucosal patterns and by retrieving the organisms that are identified with appropriate stains. The treatment of esophageal tuberculosis, like that of tuberculosis elsewhere in the body, is appropriate antituberculosis chemotherapy. Involvement of the esophagus in tuberculosis frequently occurs at an advanced stage of systemic disease that responds poorly to antituberculosis drugs. It may be necessary to dilate the stenosing hypertrophic form of esophageal tuberculosis. Rarely, obstruction of the mid-esophagus by a mass of enlarged subcarinal or paraesophageal lymph nodes may occur, requiring resection of these nodes to reestablish comfortable swallowing.

Syphilis of the esophagus is extremely rare and occurs in three forms—a primary chancre in the esophageal mucosa, a secondary stage that appears as an esophageal erosion or diffuse esophagitis and may be associated with cutaneous manifestations, and a tertiary stage in which a gumma appears as a submucosal mass that enlarges into the lumen of the esophagus, ulcerates, and results in stricture formation or perforation. Syphilis of the esophagus has a predilection for normally narrow areas of the esophagus and may result in either an esophagorespiratory tract fistula or aortic erosion. The treatment of syphilis of the esophagus, like that of the systemic disease, is high-dose

penicillin. Both the systemic disease and esophageal lesions typically respond dramatically to this treatment.

DIVERTICULA

An esophageal diverticulum is an epithelial-lined mucosal pouch that protrudes from the esophageal lumen. Most esophageal diverticula are acquired, and they occur predominantly in adults. Esophageal diverticula may be classified according to their location, the extent of wall thickness that accompanies them, or their presumed mechanism of formation.[66] Pharyngoesophageal (Zenker) diverticula occur at the junction of the pharynx and esophagus; parabronchial (mid-esophageal) diverticula occur in proximity to the tracheal bifurcation; and epiphrenic (supradiaphragmatic) diverticula occur in the distal 10 cm of the esophagus. Diverticula containing all layers of the normal esophageal wall (mucosa, submucosa, and muscle) are termed *true* diverticula, while those consisting of only mucosa and submucosa are *false* diverticula. Most esophageal diverticula arise because elevated intraluminal pressure forces the mucosa and submucosa to herniate through the esophageal musculature; these are false diverticula. On the other hand, traction diverticula result from external inflammatory reaction in adjacent mediastinal lymph nodes that adhere to the esophagus and pull the wall toward them as healing and contraction occurs, and these are true diverticula. Pharyngoesophageal and epiphrenic diverticula are pulsion diverticula that are generally associated with abnormal esophageal motility. Parabronchial diver-

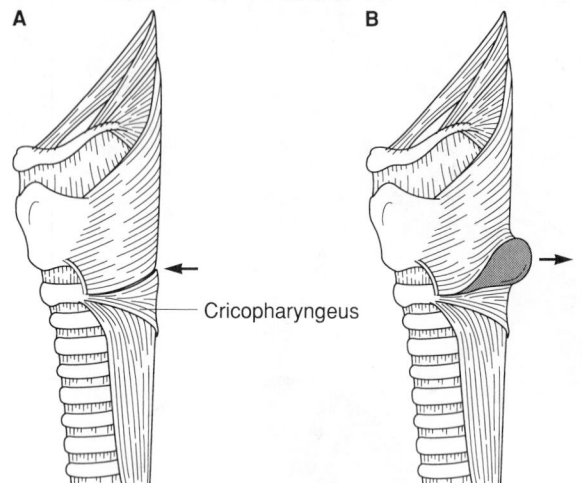
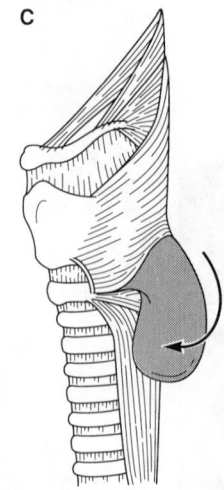

Cricopharyngeus

Figure 19-32. Formation of pharyngoesophageal (Zenker) diverticulum. (*A*) Herniation of the pharyngeal mucosa and submucosa occurs at the point of potential weakness (Killian triangle; *arrow*) between the oblique fibers of the thyropharyngeus muscle and the more horizontal fibers of the cricopharyngeus muscle. (*B* and *C*) As the diverticulum enlarges, it drapes over the cricopharyngeus sphincter and descends into the superior mediastinum in the prevertebral space. (After Orringer MB. Diverticula and miscellaneous conditions of the esophagus. In: Sabiston DC Jr, ed. Textbook of surgery, ed 13. Philadelphia, WB Saunders, 1986:726)

ticula are usually but not always of the traction variety and include all layers of the esophageal wall.

Pharyngoesophageal Diverticulum

The pharyngoesophageal (Zenker) diverticulum is the most common esophageal diverticulum and typically occurs in patients between 30 and 50 years of age. The diverticulum consistently arises within the inferior pharyngeal constrictor muscle, between the oblique fibers of the thyropharyngeus muscle and the more horizontal fibers of the cricopharyngeus muscle, the upper esophageal sphincter (Fig. 19-32). The point of transition in the direction of these muscles (Killian triangle) represents an area of potential weakness in the posterior pharynx and is the site of formation of the diverticulum. Manometric measurement of upper esophageal sphincter function is difficult with existing standard recording equipment, which may not document

the rapid movements of swallowing in an asymmetric sphincter that changes position with laryngeal excursions. Some degree of incoordination in the swallowing mechanism, however, is thought to be the basis for formation of the Zenker diverticulum. Pharyngeal contraction that occurs inappropriately *after* cricopharyngeal closure has been demonstrated in these patients. Regardless of the precise motor dysfunction, a pulsion diverticulum would not occur in these patients unless there were some reason for unusually elevated esophageal pressures. As the swallowed bolus exerts pressure within the pharynx, mucosa and submucosa herniate through the anatomically weak area above the cricopharyngeus muscle. The diverticulum gradually enlarges with time, extending over the cricopharyngeus muscle, and dissects downward in the prevertebral space posterior to the esophagus and occasionally into the superior mediastinum.

Patients with pharyngoesophageal diverticula character-

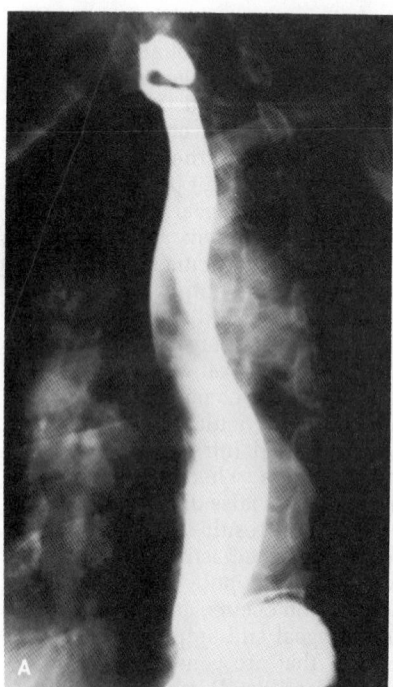
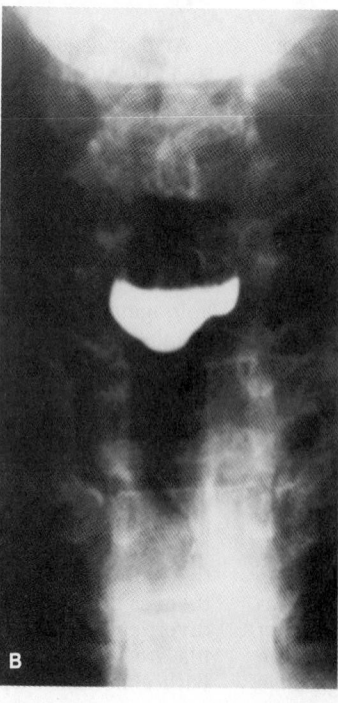

Figure 19-33. Small Zenker diverticulum. (*A*) The 2.5-cm pouch and the esophageal narrowing distal to it representing the tight cricopharyngeus sphincter. (*B*) Detail of pouch showing retained barium. (Orringer MB. Extended cervical esophagomyotomy for cricopharyngeal dysfunction. J Thorac Cardiovasc Surg 1980;90:669)

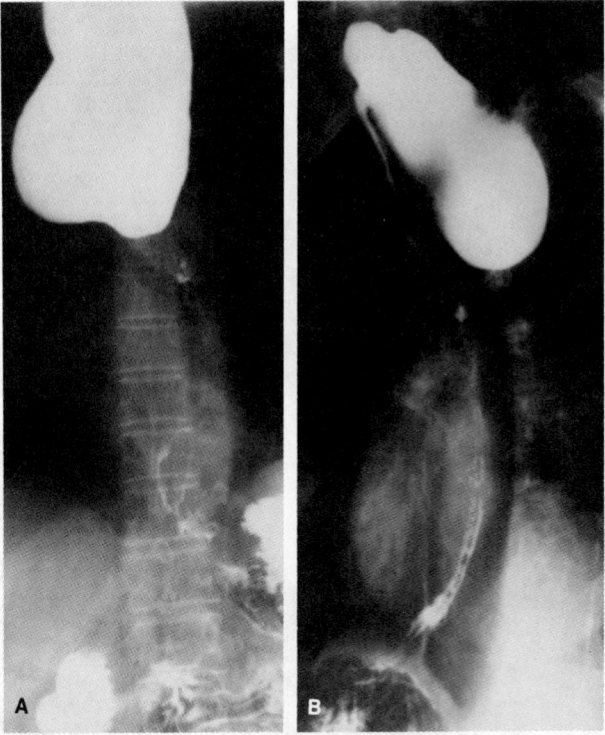

Figure 19-34. Posteroanterior (*A*) and oblique (*B*) views from barium esophagogram in an elderly woman presenting with cervical dysphagia and a 40-lb weight loss that were initially thought to be secondary to an esophageal malignancy. This 15-cm pharyngoesophageal diverticulum was treated successfully with diverticulectomy and cervical esophagomyotomy. (Orringer MB. Diverticula and miscellaneous conditions of the esophagus. In: Sabiston DC Jr, ed. Textbook of surgery, ed 13. Philadelphia, WB Saunders, 1986:726)

istically present with complaints of cervical dysphagia, effortless regurgitation of undigested food or pills, a gurgling sensation in the neck on swallowing, periodic choking, and aspiration (Fig. 19-33). Marked weight loss and dysphagia in an elderly patient may be misdiagnosed as an esophageal malignancy (Fig. 19-34). The diagnosis of a Zenker diverticulum is established with a barium esophagogram. In evaluating the patient with a Zenker diverticulum, it must be realized that it is the degree of upper esophageal sphincter muscle dysfunction, not the absolute size of the pouch, that determines the severity of symptoms experienced by these patients. That is, a patient with a 5-mm Zenker diverticulum may have as many or more symptoms than a patient with a 3-cm pouch. In most patients with symptoms, surgical treatment is indicated regardless of the size of the pouch to prevent additional complications (aspiration and nutritional impairment). As is the case with every pulsion diverticulum, the proper surgical treatment of a Zenker diverticulum must be directed at relieving the underlying neuromotor abnormality responsible for the increased pharyngeal pressure.

The first surgical approaches to Zenker diverticula involved simply excising the pouch and suturing the pharyngeal defect. The underlying upper esophageal sphincter dysfunction was not appreciated, and there was a high incidence of suture line disruption with resulting cervical and mediastinal infection. Currently, a cricopharyngeal myotomy, which relieves the relative obstruction distal to the pouch, is regarded as the most important aspect of surgical treatment in these patients (Fig. 19-35). This operation is performed through a left cervical incision that parallels the anterior border of the sternocleidomastoid muscle. The sternocleidomastoid muscle and carotid sheath and its contents are retracted laterally, and the thyroid and trachea medially. The inferior thyroid artery is an important anatomic landmark in this operation. Once it is

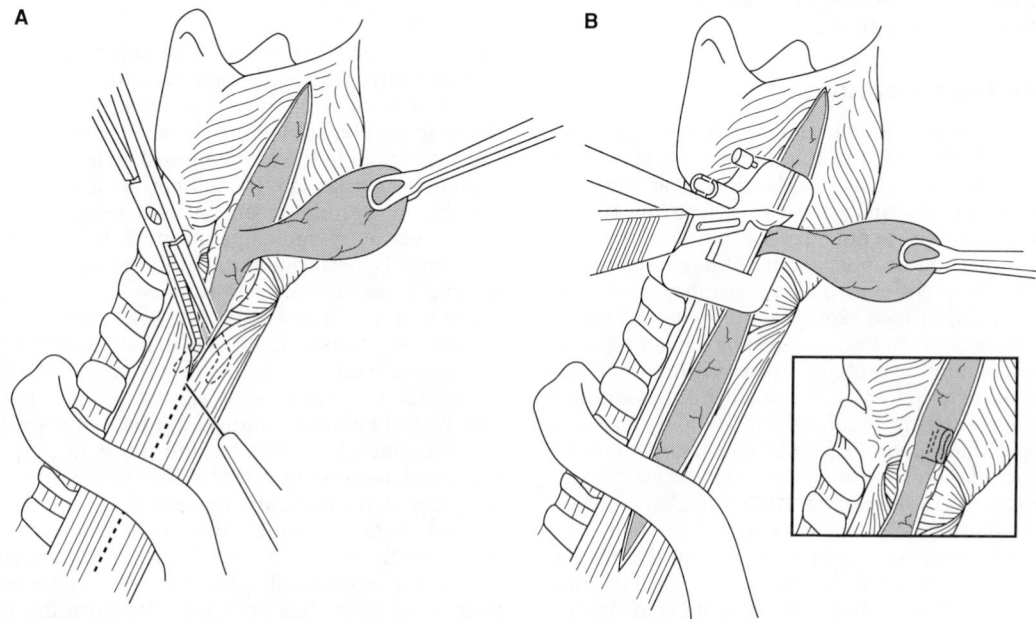

Figure 19-35. Cervical esophagomyotomy and concomitant pharyngoesophageal diverticulum resection. (*A*) An esophagomyotomy is performed for several centimeters in either vertical direction from the base of the mobilized diverticulum. (*B*) After completion of the esophagomyotomy, the base of the pouch is crossed with a TA-30 stapler and amputated. (After Orringer MB. Extended cervical esophagomyotomy for cricopharyngeal dysfunction. J Thorac Cardiovasc Surg 1980; 80:669)

divided, the diverticulum is consistently found beneath it. The diverticulum is identified and dissected to its base, and an extramucosal esophagomyotomy is performed in either vertical direction for several centimeters from the base of the pouch to ensure that all cricopharyngeal muscle fibers are divided. Pouches of up to 3 cm simply are incorporated with the mucosa and submucosa, which bulge through the divided muscle at the site of the esophagomyotomy, and no resection of the pouch is needed. Larger pouches are excised using the surgical stapler. The results of treatment are excellent, and recurrence is rare if the relative obstruction distal to the pouch has been relieved by complete division of the upper esophageal sphincter. An alternative approach is diverticulopexy, which involves mobilizing the pouch, inverting it, and suspending it from adjacent tissues so that the mouth is dependent. This operation is successful only if combined with a cervical esophagomyotomy. Endoscopic division of the common wall between the diverticulum (internal pharyngoesophagomyotomy, or the Dohlman procedure) has been used with success by a small number of surgeons for treatment of Zenker diverticulum.[67]

Mid-Esophageal Traction Diverticulum

Mediastinal granulomatous disease (eg, tuberculosis or histoplasmosis) is the common cause of mid-esophageal traction diverticulum. This type of diverticulum is much smaller than the pulsion diverticulum and has a characteristic blunt tapered tip that points toward the adjacent subcarina and parabronchial lymph nodes to which it adheres (Fig. 19-36). It is typically diagnosed as an incidental finding on a barium esophagogram and almost always is asymptomatic. No specific treatment is indicated. At times, however, inflammatory necrosis of the granulomatous reaction may produce a fistula between the esophagus and the tracheobronchial tree, requiring division of the fistula and interposition of normal tissues. Mid-esophageal traction diverticula must be differentiated from pulsion diverticula, which may also occur in this location and are associated with neuromotor esophageal dysfunction, as is the case with epiphrenic diverticula.

Epiphrenic Diverticulum

An epiphrenic or supradiaphragmatic diverticulum occurs within the distal 10 cm of the thoracic esophagus. It is a pulsion diverticulum that arises because of abnormally elevated intraluminal esophageal pressure (see Fig. 19-36). Although many patients do not have symptoms at the time of diagnosis on barium esophagogram, others have symptoms from the frequently associated esophageal conditions: hiatal hernia, diffuse esophageal spasm, achalasia, reflux esophagitis, and carcinoma. Dysphagia and regurgitation are the common symptoms of an epiphrenic diverticulum, and retrosternal pain may occur from associated diffuse esophageal spasm. Esophageal manometry and acid reflux testing in these patients should be performed to define the associated motor abnormality and to assess competence of the lower esophageal sphincter mechanism (see Chap. 18). Pouches smaller than 3 cm and causing little or no symptoms require no treatment. Severe dysphagia, chest pain, or an anatomically dependent or enlarging pouch are indications for repair. Unless there is an associated distal esophageal stricture or tumor, it must be inferred that the patient with an epiphrenic diverticulum has abnormally elevated intraesophageal pressure that has produced the pouch and is the result of neuromotor dysfunction. This can be documented manometrically.

The surgical approach to epiphrenic diverticula is

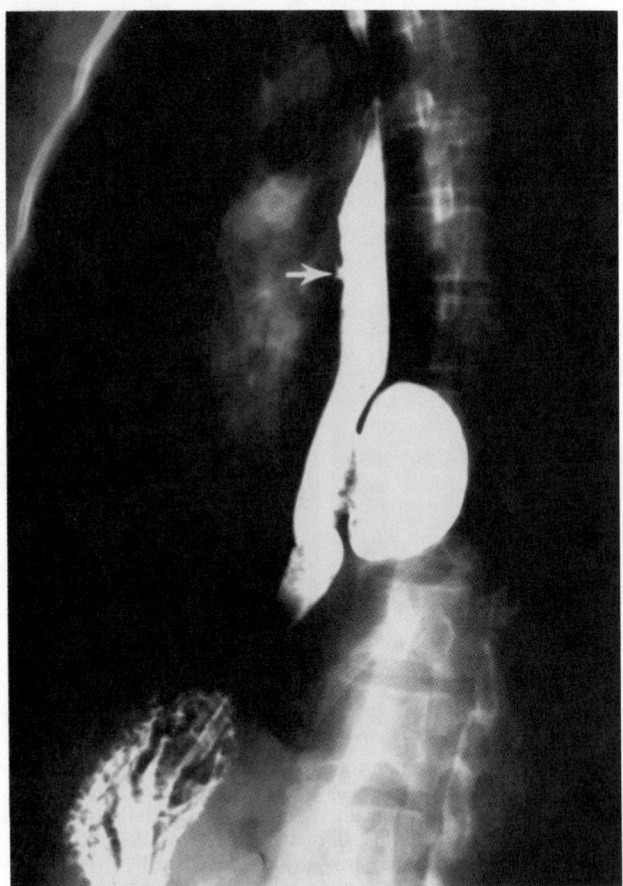

Figure 19-36. Barium esophagogram showing an epiphrenic diverticulum as well as a small traction diverticulum (*arrow*) of the middle esophagus. (Orringer MB. Diverticula and miscellaneous conditions of the esophagus. In: Sabiston DC Jr, ed. Textbook of surgery, ed 13. Philadelphia, WB Saunders, 1986:726)

through a left sixth or seventh interspace posterolateral thoracotomy. This is the case even for diverticula that present to the right of the esophagus. A long extramucosal thoracic esophagomyotomy is performed from the level of the aortic arch to the esophagogastric junction (Fig. 19-37). If there is an associated hiatal hernia or incompetent lower esophageal sphincter, an antireflux operation should be carried out at the same operation. If an adequate esophagomyotomy is performed, and the abnormally elevated intraesophageal pressure is thus relieved, suture line disruption and recurrence of the diverticulum are rare. Controversy exists about the distal extent of the muscle incision as well as about the requirement for a concomitant antireflux operation. One school argues that the lower esophageal sphincter should not be disturbed if preoperative esophageal manometry and reflux testing show that it is normal. Others argue that to relieve completely the distal esophageal obstruction, the esophagomyotomy must be carried distally through the lower esophageal sphincter and onto the stomach for 1.5 cm. The resulting incompetent lower esophageal sphincter necessitates routine addition of an antireflux operation. Because the myotomized esophagus does not have normal propulsive force, when adding an antireflux procedure, a partial, 240-degree Belsey fundoplication, rather than a 360-degree Nissen fundoplication, is preferred so that functional obstruction is avoided. A Mayo Clinic report cites a 9% operative mortality rate associated with diverticulectomy and esophagomy-

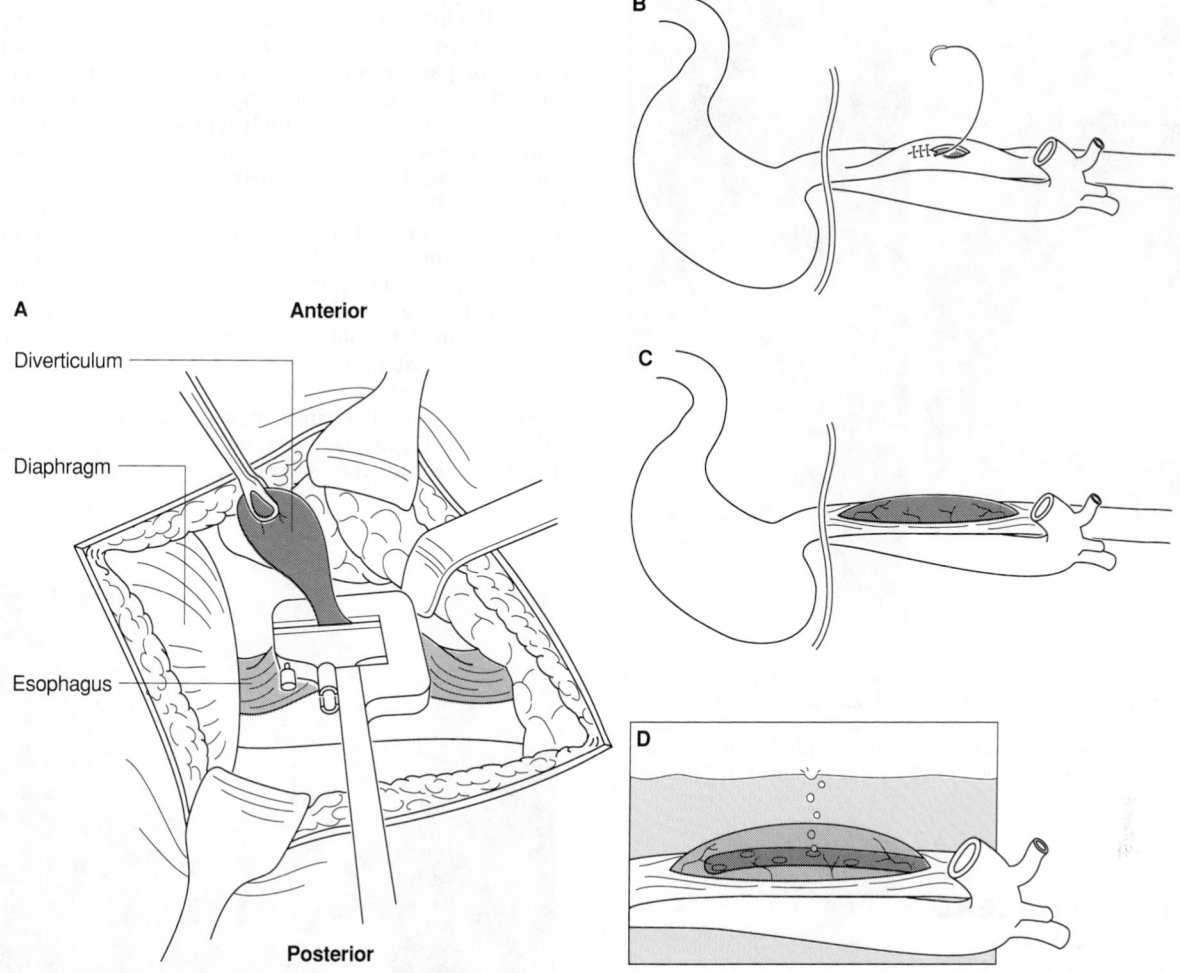

Figure 19-37. Technique of resection of epiphrenic diverticulum and concomitant esophagomyotomy. (*A*) The diverticulum is mobilized to its base and amputated with a TA-30 surgical stapler. (*B*) The staple suture line oversewn. (*C*) A long esophagomyotomy is performed from the esophagogastric junction to the aortic arch 180 degrees on the opposite wall of the esophagus. (*D*) Air is insufflated through an intraesophageal nasogastric tube, with the esophagus submerged under saline to be certain that integrity of the mucosa has been maintained. (After Orringer MB. Complications of esophageal surgery and trauma. In: Greenfield LJ, ed. Complications in surgery and trauma, ed 2. Philadelphia, JB Lippincott, 1990:302)

otomy, emphasizing that minimally symptomatic diverticula should not be operated on.[68]

DISTAL ESOPHAGEAL WEB (SCHATZKI RING)

A Schatzki ring is an annular constriction of the distal esophagus that occurs at the esophagogastric junction in a patient with a sliding hiatal hernia. The ring characteristically projects into the lumen at a right angle to the long axis of the esophagus (Fig. 19-38). The incidence of Schatzki ring is unknown because most patients with this abnormality do not have symptoms. Although periodic dysphagia may be experienced when the ring measures 20 mm or less on barium swallow examination, the diameter at which dysphagia almost always is experienced is 13 mm or less. The cause of a Schatzki ring is not established. The ring occurs precisely at the squamocolumnar epithelial junction. Microscopically, it is covered by squamous epithelium over its upper surface and columnar epithelium on the gastric side. This is not a true fibrotic stricture be-

cause there may be minimal submucosal fibrosis and no involvement of the esophageal muscle. Schatzki ring can be seen only radiographically on a barium esophagogram because the squamocolumnar junction is above the diaphragm, that is, because there is a hiatal hernia. The presence of a Schatzki ring indicates that a hiatal hernia is present, but it is *not* indicative of either associated gastroesophageal reflux or esophagitis. It may be difficult to differentiate a Schatzki ring from a localized stricture due to gastroesophageal reflux.

In patients with dysphagia from Schatzki ring but no associated reflux symptoms, an excellent response often is obtained with periodic esophageal dilations. In patients who have both dysphagia and reflux symptoms, periodic dilations and an antireflux medical regimen are required. A few patients have persistent dysphagia or severe reflux symptoms despite medical therapy, and in this group, intraoperative dilation to disrupt the ring, in combination with an antireflux operation, gives good results. Resection of the distal esophageal ring alone, without repair of the associated hiatal hernia, is not adequate treatment.

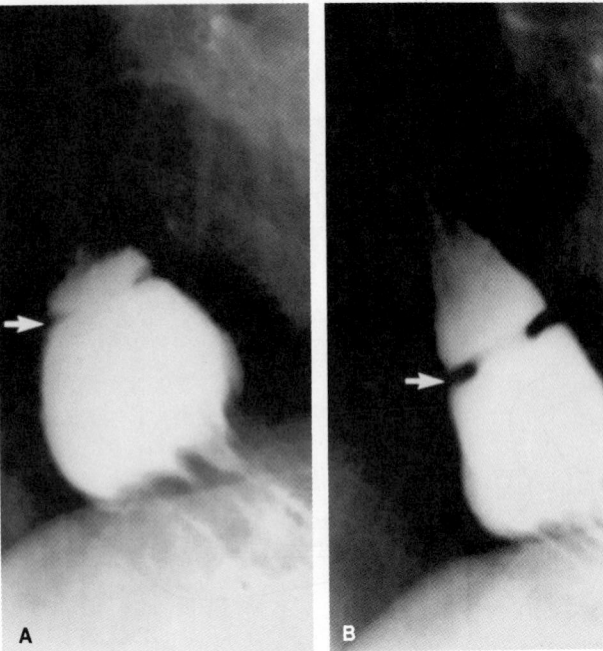

Figure 19-38. Esophagogram showing a typical distal esophageal web (Schatzki ring; *arrows*) that projects into the lumen at right angles to the axis of the esophagus and occurs at the esophagogastric junction above a sliding hiatal hernia. (Orringer MB. Diverticula and miscellaneous conditions of the esophagus. In: Sabiston DC Jr, ed. Textbook of surgery, ed 13. Philadelphia, WB Saunders, 1986:726)

RARE ESOPHAGEAL ABNORMALITIES

Esophageal Involvement in Dermatologic Disorders

A variety of dermatologic conditions also involve squamous epithelium of the esophagus.[69] The development of vesicles and the subsequent formation of thin esophageal webs have been reported in pemphigus vulgaris, bullous pemphigoid, and benign mucous membrane pemphigoid. These vesicles rupture, leaving denuded areas of superficial ulceration that may become secondarily infected and heal with fibrosis. In patients with pemphigus, the mucosal surfaces most commonly involved are those of the oral cavity and vagina; occasionally, the larynx, nose, and anus, and least frequently, the esophagus, are involved. The characteristic bullae on the cutaneous and mucosal surfaces are diagnostic, and confirmation is made on examination of biopsy specimens. When these patients complain of dysphagia or painful swallowing, dilation therapy should be instituted early in the course of the disease to prevent the subsequent development of severe strictures. Epidermolysis bullosa dystrophica is a rare genetic skin disease that, unlike other bullous dermatoses, is inherited and generally begins early in life. The condition may be associated with severe blistering of the mucous membrane and can result in perforation or stricture formation.[70] As with the other dermatoses, dilation therapy is effective in maintaining comfortable swallowing in these patients.

Other Conditions

Certain rare conditions occasionally may have to be considered in the differential diagnosis of patients with dysphagia. Marked cardiomegaly, hepatomegaly displacing the esophagus against the diaphragmatic hiatus, and tortuosity of the thoracic aorta resulting in esophageal compression all have been reported to cause dysphagia. Aberrant thyroid or parathyroid tissue may produce cervical dysphagia (Fig. 19-39). The development of cervical vertebral body osteophytic spurs, which typically involve the fifth, sixth, and seventh cervical vertebral interspaces, may displace the esophagus anteriorly and produce dysphagia (Fig. 19-40). It is important, particularly in elderly patients, to assess the cervical spine when evaluating the esophagogram before endoscopy because the presence of exostoses makes esophagoscopy more dangerous and warrants use of a pediatric flexible fiberoptic esophagoscope to exclude carcinoma in these patients with dysphagia. At times, removal of the osteophyte through an anterior cervical approach may produce excellent results.

Congenital vascular rings may compress the esophagus and produce dysphagia. The most common type of vascular ring is an aberrant right subclavian artery, which arises as

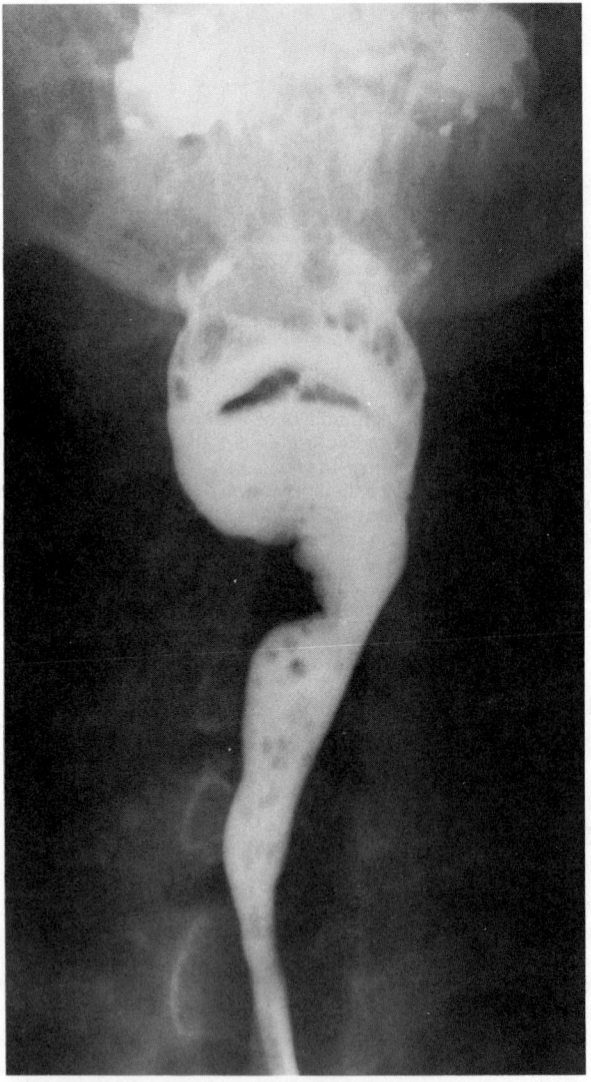

Figure 19-39. Cervical esophagogram showing an intrinsic right lateral mass that proved to be an aberrantly located right lobe of the thyroid gland posterolateral to the esophagus. A right thyroid lobectomy relieved the patient's dysphagia. (Orringer MB. Diverticula and miscellaneous conditions of the esophagus. In: Sabiston DC Jr, ed. Textbook of surgery, ed 13. Philadelphia, WB Saunders, 1986:726)

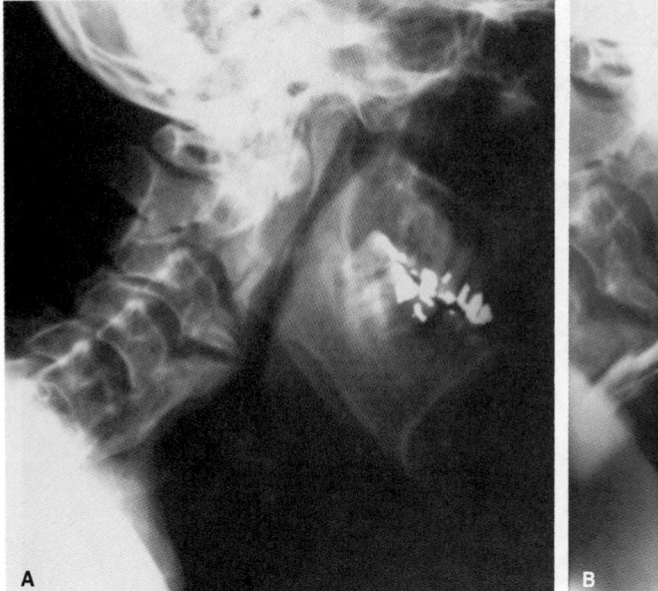

Figure 19-40. Cervical osteophytes displacing the esophagus anteriorly. (*A*) Soft tissue radiograph of the neck. (*B*) Displacement of the barium-filled esophagus by the osteophytes. (Orringer MB. Diverticula and miscellaneous conditions of the esophagus. In: Sabiston DC Jr, ed. Textbook of surgery, ed 13. Philadelphia, WB Saunders, 1986:726)

the fourth branch of the aortic arch. This condition is usually asymptomatic, but it can produce esophageal obstruction in infancy or childhood or be responsible for dysphagia lusoria in adults. The classic finding on barium swallow examination is indentation of the posterior esophageal wall high in the thorax, caused by the aberrant right subclavian artery. Angiography is usually used to confirm the diagnosis. Other causes of dysphagia, especially gastroesophageal reflux with secondarily induced motor dysfunction, must be excluded. In infants, the vascular ring is approached through a left thoracotomy, and the vessel is divided and oversewn at its origin from the aortic arch. The retroesophageal portion of the vessel is oversewn and allowed to retract. In adults, this lesion has more recently been approached through a median sternotomy instead of a left thoracotomy. The origin of the aberrant right subclavian artery is identified, and the vessel is ligated and divided. The retroesophageal segment of the vessel is used for vascular reconstruction either by creating an anastomosis to the right common carotid artery or by interposing a 10-mm vascular prosthesis between the end of the divided subclavian artery and the arch of the aorta.

The esophagus may be involved secondarily by metastases to mediastinal lymph nodes from other sites.[71] Virtually any malignant tumor may metastasize to mediastinal lymph nodes, but carcinomas of the breast, lung, esophagus, and stomach predominate. Mediastinal lymphatics communicate extensively with the esophagus, and therefore, any of these tumors may invade the esophageal wall from without and cause extrinsic obstruction. This is difficult to diagnose histologically with an esophageal biopsy because the tumors are submucosal. Bronchogenic carcinoma metastatic to subcarinal lymph nodes may produce dysphagia from marked displacement of the esophagus (Fig. 19-41). Similarly, metastases to mediastinal lymph nodes from breast carcinoma may displace the esophagus and cause dysphagia. Therefore, any woman with a history of breast cancer, no matter how remote, who complains of dysphagia should be evaluated for possible mediastinal lymph node metastases.

ACQUIRED TRACHEOESOPHAGEAL FISTULAS
Nonmalignant Fistulas

Only 10% of acquired fistulas between the esophagus and tracheobronchial tree are due to benign disease.[72] These nonmalignant fistulas result from erosion by contig-

uous infected subcarinal or mediastinal lymph nodes (eg, tuberculosis, histoplasmosis, syphilis, or actinomycosis); trauma (eg, caustic injury, penetrating or blunt chest trauma, intubation, erosion of aspirated foreign body, dilation of esophageal stricture); late sequelae of chronic midesophageal traction diverticulum; or erosion by an endotracheal or tracheostomy tube cuff in a patient requiring prolonged ventilatory support. Patients present with characteristic paroxysmal coughing while eating as swallowed food or liquid enters the tracheobronchial tree. In patients who are mechanically ventilated, tracheal secretions may be reported to be excessive, there may be difficulty with ventilation because of loss of inspired air into the gastrointestinal tract or out of the mouth, or gastric distention may occur. Regurgitation of gastric contents into the esophagus through the fistula and into the lungs may cause fulminant aspiration pneumonia.

The diagnosis should generally be established with a contrast esophagogram. Because water-soluble contrast agents are hygroscopic and may have irritating pulmonary effects, dilute barium should be used for this study. Barium is inert and causes no harm to the lungs in small amounts. Bronchography may be useful in delineating the site of the fistula and defining diseased pulmonary parenchyma that may need to be resected at the time of repair of the fistula. A CT scan is used to define mediastinal adenopathy and to exclude the presence of a mediastinal tumor mass. Endoscopy should be performed to exclude the presence of malignancy and to assess the size and location of the fistula. Small fistulas may be difficult to localize endoscopically, and simultaneous esophagoscopy and bronchoscopy performed while insufflating air through the flexible esophagoscope may be helpful in identifying the fistula along the posterior membranous trachea, which is inspected for bubbles of air. Biopsy specimens and brushings are taken from the tracheal and esophageal sides of the fistula for cytologic evaluation.

Benign acquired fistulas due to mediastinal granulomatous disease are approached through a right posterolateral thoracotomy in the fourth or fifth intercostal space. The fistula is identified and divided, and the opening in the esophagus is débrided and closed. The tracheal or bronchial defect is similarly closed. Occasionally, communications with a segment of lung may necessitate a limited

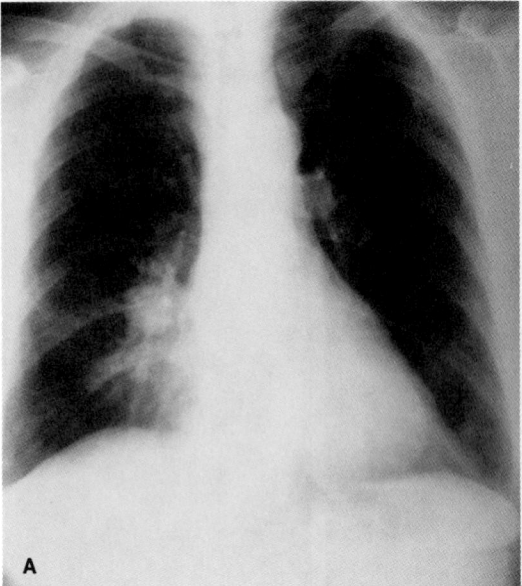
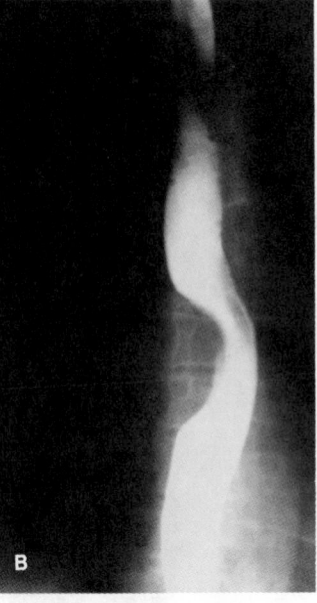

Figure 19-41. (*A*) Chest roentgenogram of a 60-year-old smoker who presented with dysphagia and a right infrahilar lung mass (*arrow*). Bronchogenic carcinoma was diagnosed. The patient had metastases to subcarinal lymph nodes that were displacing the mid-esophagus, as seen on the barium esophagogram (*B*). (Orringer MB. Miscellaneous conditions of the esophagus. In: Orringer MB, ed. Shackelford's surgery of the alimentary tract, vol 1. The esophagus. Philadelphia, WB Saunders, 1991:460)

pulmonary resection. To prevent recurrence of the fistula, viable adjacent tissue, such as mediastinal fat, pleura, pericardium, or a rotated intercostal muscle pedicle, should be interposed between the tracheobronchial and esophageal suture lines. Long-term results are excellent, and the recurrence of properly repaired fistulas is rare.[73]

Mechanically ventilated patients who develop a tracheoesophageal fistula are faced with a disastrous complication. Repair of the fistula is best deferred until the patient has been weaned from the ventilator. The fistula is managed initially by removing any nasogastric tube that is present and replacing the endotracheal or tracheostomy tube with another that has a large-volume, low-pressure cuff that is inflated below the fistula if possible. The stomach is decompressed with a gastrostomy, and a feeding jejunostomy tube is inserted for alimentation. Diversion of swallowed saliva by means of a cervical esophagostomy should be avoided if possible because this greatly complicates subsequent esophageal reconstruction.

Small fistulas, such as those resulting from an endotracheal intubation injury, are approached through a cervical collar or oblique incision anterior to the sternocleidomastoid muscle. The fistula is localized by carefully dissecting in the tracheoesophageal groove. The tracheal and esophageal openings are closed with interrupted 4-0 absorbable sutures, and the adjacent sternohyoid muscle is detached from the hyoid bone, rotated between the two suture lines, and sutured in place to prevent fistula recurrence.

Endotracheal or tracheostomy tube cuff injuries usually produce circumferential tracheal damage that necessitates a tracheal resection. This is performed through a cervical collar incision. The damaged short segment of trachea is resected, and the distal end is intubated to permit ventilation, while the esophageal fistula is sutured closed and covered with mobilized sternocleidomastoid muscle. After resecting the damaged segment of trachea, a primary tracheal anastomosis is performed. It is preferable to leave no tracheal tube in place postoperatively. The results of such repair are excellent in the patient who is no longer dependent on mechanical ventilation. Several reports have described successful endoscopic closure of tracheoesophageal fistulas, but the technique is not yet widely used.[74,75]

Malignant Tracheoesophageal Fistulas

Ninety percent of acquired fistulas between the esophagus and tracheobronchial tree in adults are the result of malignant disease (Fig. 19-42). Tracheoesophageal fistulas complicate the course of disease in about 5% of patients who have esophageal carcinoma, 0.2% of patients with lung cancer, and 15% of patients with tracheal cancer.

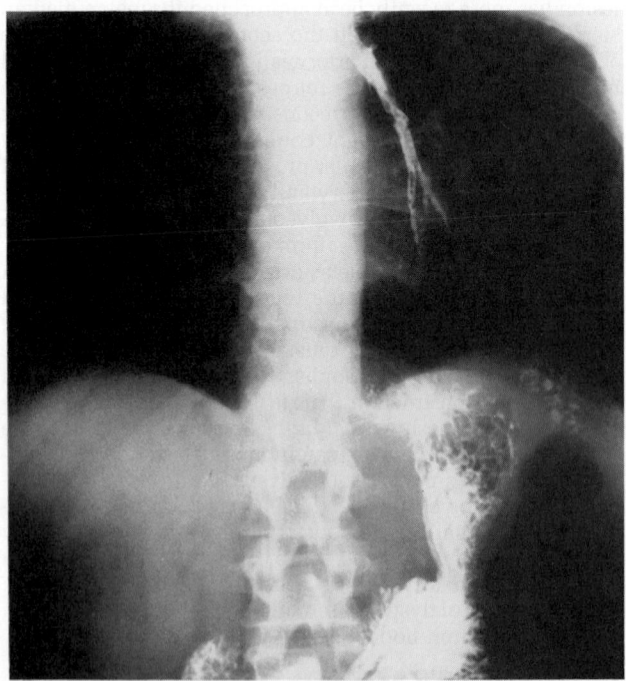

Figure 19-42. Barium esophagogram in a patient with a malignant tracheoesophageal fistula, showing the typical simultaneous opacification of the left main-stem bronchus and the gastrointestinal tract. (Orringer MB, Sloan H. Substernal gastric bypass of the excluded thoracic esophagus for palliation of esophageal carcinoma. J Thorac Cardiovasc Surg 1975;70:836)

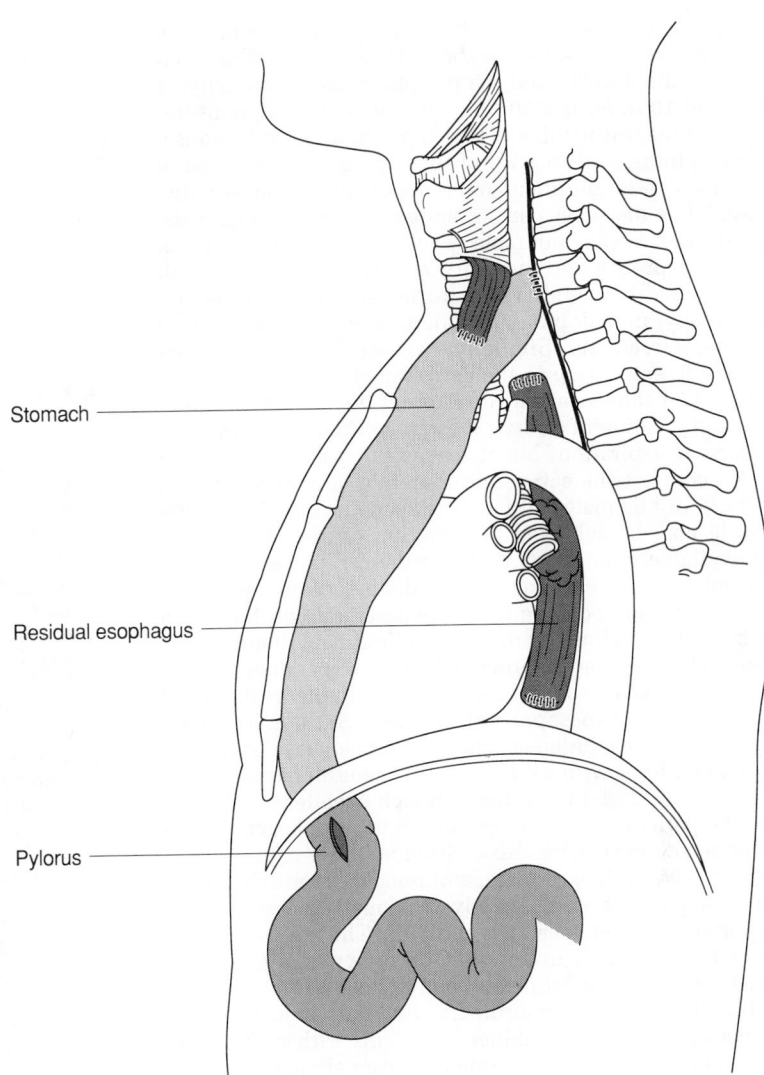

Stomach

Residual esophagus

Pylorus

Figure 19-43. Lateral view after substernal gastric bypass of the excluded thoracic esophagus for a malignant tracheoesophageal fistula. After dividing and closing the cervical esophagus and esophagogastric junction, thereby excluding the diseased esophagus in the posterior mediastinum, the stomach is mobilized retrosternally in the anterior mediastinum, and an end-to-side cervical esophagogastric anastomosis is constructed. Secretions produced by the esophagus are vented into the tracheobronchial tree and periodically expectorated. (After Orringer MB, Sloan H. Substernal gastric bypass of the excluded thoracic esophagus for palliation of esophageal carcinoma. J Thorac Cardiovasc Surg 1975;70:836)

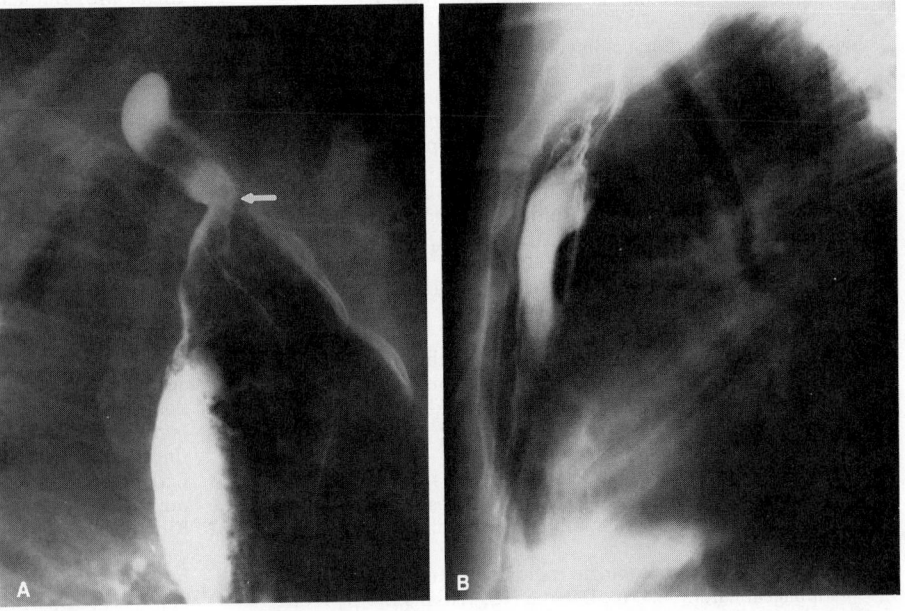

Figure 19-44. Postoperative barium esophagogram after substernal gastric bypass of the malignant tracheoesophageal fistula shown in Figure 19-42. (*A*) The cervical esophagus angulates anteriorly at the thoracic inlet to meet the retrosternal stomach (arrow indicates the esophagogastric anastomosis). (*B*) Lateral view shows the retrosternal stomach in the anterior mediastinum. (Orringer MB, Sloan H. Substernal gastric bypass of the excluded thoracic esophagus for palliation of esophageal carcinoma. J Thorac Cardiovasc Surg 1975;70:836)

Malignant fistulas between the esophagus and respiratory tree involve the trachea in about 55% of cases, the bronchus in about 40%, and the peripheral lung parenchyma in about 10%. Nearly 80% of patients with malignant tracheoesophageal fistulas die within 3 months of the onset of symptoms, and in 85% of these patients, the cause of death is aspiration pneumonia, not distant metastatic disease.[76] For the most part, a malignant tracheoesophageal fistula represents incurable disease for which resection carries a prohibitive mortality and is seldom indicated. Because palliative relief of recurrent aspiration is the aim of therapy, insertion of a feeding tube does not constitute adequate treatment. Similarly, because these patients are unable to eat, owing to the paroxysmal coughing that occurs when they swallow, division of the cervical esophagus and creation of a cervical esophagostomy may prevent recurrent aspiration, but it leaves the patient unable to enjoy comfortable eating and therefore fails to satisfy the criteria of adequate palliation. Effective occlusion of the fistula may be achieved by insertion of one of a variety of available endoesophageal prostheses. These tubes are placed into the esophagus with the aid of an esophagoscope and may occlude the esophageal side of the fistula sufficiently to allow swallowing of liquids without aspiration into the tracheobronchial tree. Expandable metal stents also have been used successfully in the treatment of malignant tracheoesophageal fistulas.[77] Substernal gastric bypass of the excluded esophagus has been used for palliation in patients with a malignant tracheoesophageal fistula (Figs. 19-43 and 19-44). Even though excellent palliation for the patient with a malignant tracheoesophageal fistula may be achieved with this technique, these patients usually survive only 6 months, and operative mortality rates in these patients who have advanced malignancy has been reported to be between 20% and 60%. The results of using long segments of jejunum or colon to bypass a malignant tracheoesophageal fistula are equally dismal. It is therefore difficult, except in extraordinary situations, to justify these major operative undertakings in patients with such a short life expectancy.[29] Often, supportive care alone is the most humane treatment for these patients.

REFERENCES

1. Orringer MB. Complications of esophageal surgery and trauma. In: Greenfield LJ, ed. Complications in surgery and trauma, ed 2. Philadelphia, JB Lippincott, 1990:302.
2. Liebermann-Meffert DMI, Leuscher U, Neff V, et al. Esophagectomy without thoracotomy: is there a risk of intramediastinal bleeding? Ann Surg 1987;206:184.
3. Liebermann-Meffert D, Duranceau A. Anatomy and embryology. In: Orringer MB, Zuidema GD, eds. Shackelford's surgery of the alimentary tract, ed 4, vol 1. The esophagus. Philadelphia, WB Saunders, 1996:3.
4. Postlethwait RW, Lowe JE. Benign tumors and cysts of the esophagus. In: Orringer MB, Zuidema GD, eds. Shackelford's surgery of the alimentary tract, ed 4, vol 1. The esophagus. Philadelphia, WB Saunders, 1996:369.
5. Nemir P Jr, Wallace HW, Fallahnejad M. Diagnosis and surgical management of benign disease of the esophagus. Curr Probl Surg 1976;13:1.
6. Tio TL. Endoscopic ultrasonography in the evaluation of smooth muscle tumors of the upper gastrointestinal tract: a comparison with computed tomography, endoscopy, and barium meal. In: Tio TK, ed. Endosonography in gastroenterology. Bolivia, Springer-Verlag, 1988:104.
7. Devitt PG, Iyer PV, Rowland R. Pathogenesis and clinical features of cancer of the esophagus. In: Jamieson GG, ed. Surgery of the esophagus. Edinburgh, Churchill Livingstone, 1988:551.
8. Duranceau A. Epidemiologic trends and etiologic factors of esophageal carcinoma. In: Delarue NC, Wilkins EW Jr, Wong J, eds. International trends in general thoracic surgery, vol 4. Esophageal cancer. St Louis, CV Mosby, 1988:3.
9. Beahrs OH, Henson DE, Hutter RVP, Kennedy BJ, eds. Manual for staging of cancer, ed 4. Philadelphia, JB Lippincott, 1992:57.
10. Blot WJ, Devesa SS, Kneller RW, Fraumeni JF Jr. Rising incidence of adenocarcinoma of the esophagus and gastric cardia. JAMA 1991;265:1287.
11. Hesketh PJ, Clapp RW, Doos WG, Spechler SJ. The increasing frequency of adenocarcinoma of the esophagus. Cancer 1989;64:526.
12. Spechler SJ, Goyal RK, eds. Barrett's esophagus: pathophysiology, diagnosis, and management. New York, Elsevier, 1985.
13. Ibrahim NBN, Briggs JC, Corbishley CM. Extrapulmonary oat cell carcinoma. Cancer 1984;54:1645.
14. Epstein JI, Sears DL, Tucker RS, Eagan JW. Carcinoma of the esophagus with adenoid cystic differentiation. Cancer 1984;53:1131.
15. Chalkiadakis G, Wihlm, JM, Morand G, Weill-Bousson M, Witz JP. Primary malignant melanoma of the esophagus. Ann Thorac Surg 1985;39:472.
16. Xu L, Sun C, Wu L, Chang Z, Liu T. Clinical and pathological characteristics of carcinoma of the esophagus: report of four cases. Ann Thorac Surg 1984;37:197.
17. Burt M. Unusual malignancies. In: Pearson FG, Deslauriers J, Ginsberg RJ, Hiebert CA, McKneally MF, Urschel HC Jr, eds. Esophageal surgery. New York, Churchill Livingstone, 1995:629.
18. Ferguson MK, Skinner DB. Carcinoma of the esophagus and cardia. In: Orringer MB, Zuidema GD, eds. Shackelford's surgery of the alimentary tract, ed 4, vol 1. The esophagus. Philadelphia, WB Saunders, 1996::305.
19. Quint LE, Glazer GM, Orringer MB, Gross BH. Esophageal carcinoma: CT findings. Radiology 1985;155:171.
20. Gabrielsen TO, Eldevik OP, Orringer MB, Marshall BL. Esophageal carcinoma metastatic to the brain: clinical value and cost-effectiveness of routine enhanced CT before esophagectomy. Am J Neuroradiol 1995;16:1915.
21. Endo M. Special techniques in the endoscopic diagnosis of esophageal carcinoma. In: Delarue NC, Wilkins EW Jr, Wong J, eds. International trends in general thoracic surgery, vol 4. Esophageal cancer. St Louis, CV Mosby, 1988:45.
22. Shiozaki H, Tahara H, Kobayashi K, et al. Endoscopic screening of early esophageal cancer with Lugol dye method in patients with head and neck cancers. Cancer 1990;66:2068.
23. Roth JA, Lichter AJ, Putnam JB, Forastiere AA. Cancer of the esophagus. In: Devita VT, Hehman S, Rosenberg SA, eds. Cancer principles and practice of oncology, ed 4:FN2Grace: colon missing in this title? Philadelphia, JB Lippincott, 1993:776.
24. Turrisi AT. Esophageal cancer: the role of radiation. In: Orringer MB, Zuidema GD, eds. Shackelford's surgery of the alimentary tract, ed 4, vol 1. The esophagus. Philadelphia, WB Saunders, 1996:333.
25. Game PA, Devitt PG. Intubation for carcinoma of the esophagus. In: Jamieson GG, ed. Surgery of the esophagus. Edinburgh, Churchill Livingstone, 1988:805.
26. Reed CE. Comparison of different treatments for unresectable esophageal cancer. World J Surg 1995;19:828.
27. Barnett JL. Esophageal carcinoma: palliation with intubation and laser. In: Orringer MB, Zuidema GD, eds. Shackelford's surgery of the alimentary tract, ed 4, vol 1. The esophagus. Philadelphia, WB Saunders, 1996:358.
28. Narayan S, Sivak MV. Palliation of esophageal carcinoma: laser and photodynamic therapy. Chest Surg Clin North Am 1994;4:347.
29. Orringer MB. Substernal gastric bypass of the excluded esophagus: results of an ill-advised operation. Surg 1984;96:467.
30. Postlethwait RW. Oesophageal bypass using the colon. In: Jamieson GG, ed. Surgery of the oesophagus. Edinburgh, Churchill Livingstone, 1988:727.
31. Earlam R, Cunha-Melo JR. Oesophageal squamous cell carcinoma. I. A initial review of surgery. Br J Surg 1980;67:381.
32. King RM, Pairolero PC, Trastek VF, et al. Ivor Lewis esophagogastrectomy for carcinoma of the esophagus: early and late functional results. Ann Thorac Surg 1987;44:119.
33. Lazac'h P, Topart P, Etienne J, Charles LF. Ivor Lewis opera-

tion for epidermoid carcinoma of the esophagus. Ann Thorac Surg 1991;52:1154.

34. Mathisen DJ, Grillo HC, Wilkins EW Jr, et al. Transthoracic esophagectomy: a safe approach to carcinoma of the esophagus. Ann Thorac Surg 1988;45:137.

35. Orringer MB, Marshall B, Stirling MC. Transhiatal esophagectomy for benign and malignant disease. J Thorac Cardiovasc Surg 1993;105:265.

36. Skinner DB, Ferguson MK, Soriano A, Little AG, Starszak VM. Selection of operation for esophageal cancer based on staging. Ann Surg 1986;204:391.

37. Forastiere AA, Orringer MB, Perez-Tamayo C, et al. Preoperative chemoradiation followed by transhiatal esophagectomy for carcinoma of the esophagus: final report. J Clin Oncol 1993;11:1118.

38. Grillo HC, Mathisen DJ. Cervical exenteration. Ann Thorac Surg 1990;49:401.

39. Orringer MB. Anterior mediastinal tracheostomy with and without cervical exenteration. Ann Thorac Surg 1992;54:628.

40. Kirsh MM, Ritter F. Caustic ingestion and subsequent damage to the oropharyngeal and digestive passages. Ann Thorac Surg 1976;21:74.

41. Goldman LP, Weigert JM. Corrosive substance ingestion: a review. Am J Gastroenterol 1984;79:85.

42. Gorman RL, Khin-Maung-Gyi MT, Klein-Schwartz W, et al. Initial symptoms as predictors of esophageal injury in alkaline corrosive ingestions. Am J Emerg Med 1992;10:189.

43. Anderson KD, Rouse TM, Randolph JG. A controlled trial of corticosteroids in children with corrosive injury of the esophagus. N Engl J Med 1990;323:637.

44. Howell JM, Dalsey WC, Hartsell FW, Butzin CA. Steroids for the treatment of corrosive esophageal injury: a statistical analysis of past studies. Am J Emerg Med 1992;10:421.

45. Kuhn JR, Tunell WP. The role of initial cineesophagography in caustic esophageal injury. Am J Surg 1983;146:804.

46. Gossot D, Sarfati E, Celerier M. Early blunt esophagectomy in severe caustic burns of the upper digestive tract. J Thorac Cardiovasc Surg 1987;84:188.

47. Orringer MB. Transhiatal esophagectomy for benign disease. J Thorac Cardiovasc Surg 1985;90:649.

48. Estrera A, Taylor W, Mills LJ, et al. Corrosive burns of the esophagus and stomach: a recommendation for an aggressive surgical approach. Ann Thorac Surg 1986;41:276.

49. Jones WG II, Ginsberg RJ. Esophageal perforation: a continuing challenge. Ann Thorac Surg 1992;53:534.

50. White CS, Templeton PA, Attar S. Esophageal perforation: CT findings. AJR 1993;160:767.

51. Michel L, Malt RA, Grillo HC. Operative and non-operative management of esophageal perforation. Ann Surg 1981;194:57.

52. Cameron JL, Kieffer RH, Hendrix TR, et al. Selective nonoperative management of contained intrathoracic esophageal disruptions. Ann Thorac Surg 1979;27:404.

53. Barnett JL, Eisenman R, Nostrant TT, Elta GH. Witzel pneumatic dilation for achalasia: safety and long-term efficacy. Gastrointest Endosc 1990;36:482.

54. Parkman HP, Reynolds JC, Ouyang A, et al. Pneumatic dilatation or esophagomyotomy treatment for idiopathic achalasia: clinical outcomes and cost analysis. Dig Dis Sci 1993;38:75.

55. Lo AY, Surick B, Ghazi A. Nonoperative management of esophageal perforation secondary to balloon dilatation. Surg Endosc 1993;7:529.

56. White RI, Iannettoni MD, Orringer MB. Intrathoracic esophageal perforation: the merit of primary repair. J Thorac Cardiovasc Surg 1995;109:140.

57. Wright CD, Mathisen DJ, Wain JC, et al. Reinforced primary repair of thoracic esophageal perforation. Ann Thorac Surg 1995;60:245.

58. Ohri SK, Liakakos TA, Pathi V, et al. Primary repair of iatrogenic thoracic esophageal perforation and Boerhaave's syndrome. Ann Thorac Surg 1993;55:603.

59. Orringer MB, Stirling MB. Esophagectomy for esophageal disruption. Ann Thorac Surg 1990;49:35.

60. Grillo HC, Wilkins EW. Esophageal repair following late diagnosis of intrathoracic perforation. Ann Thorac Surg 1975;20:387.

61. Johnson J, Schwegman CW, Kirby KK. Esophageal exclusion for persistent fistula following spontaneous rupture of the esophagus. J Thorac Surg 1956;32:827.

62. Urschel HC, Razzuk MA, Wood RE, et al. Improved management of esophageal perforation: exclusion and diversion in continuity. Ann Surg 1974;179:587.

63. Wilcox MC. Esophageal disease in the acquired immunodeficiency syndrome: etiology, diagnosis, and management. Am J Med 1992;92:412.

64. Orringer MB, Sloan H. Monilial esophagitis: an increasingly frequent cause of esophageal stenosis? Ann Thorac Surg 1978;26:364.

65. McDonald GB. Esophageal disease caused by infection, systemic illness, medications, and trauma. In: Sleisenger MS, ed. Gastrointestinal disease, ed 5. Philadelphia, WB Saunders, 1993:427.

66. Pairolero PC, Trastek VF. Surgical management of esophageal diverticula. In: Orringer MB, Zuidema GD, eds. Shackelford's surgery of the alimentary tract, ed 4, vol 1. The esophagus. Philadelphia, WB Saunders, 1996:285.

67. van Overbeck JJM, Hoeksema PE. Endoscopic treatment of the hypopharyngeal diverticulum: 211 cases. Laryngoscope 1982;92:88.

68. Benacci JC, Deschamps G, Trastek VF, et al. Epiphrenic diverticulum: results of surgical treatment. Ann Thorac Surg 1993;55:1119.

69. Sherertz EF, Jorizzo JL. Cutaneous disease of the esophagus In: Castell DO, ed. The esophagus. Boston, Little, Brown, 1992:793.

70. Horan TA, Urschel JD, MacEachern NA, et al. Esophageal perforation in recessive dystrophic epidermolysis bullosa. Ann Thorac Surg 1994;57:1027.

71. Herrara JL. Benign and metastatic tumors of the esophagus. Gastroenterol Clin North Am 1991;20:775.

72. Gudovsky LM, Koroleva NS, Biryukov YB, et al. Tracheoesophageal fistulas. Ann Thorac Surg 1993;55:868.

73. Mathisen DJ, Grillo HC, Wain JC, Hilgenberg AD. Management of acquired nonmalignant tracheoesophageal fistula. Ann Thorac Surg 1991;52:759.

74. Antonelli M, Cicconetti F, Vivino G, Gasparetto A. Closure of a tracheoesophageal fistula by bronchoscopic application of fibrin glue and decontamination of the oral cavity. Chest 1991;100:578.

75. Vandenplas Y, Helven R, Derop H, et al. Endoscopic obliteration of recurrent tracheoesophageal fistula. Dig Dis Sci 1993;38:374.

76. Burt M, Diehl W, Martini N, et al. Malignant esophagorespiratory fistula: management options and survival. Ann Thorac Surg 1991;52:1222.

77. Do YS, Sond HY, Lee BH, et al. Esophagorespiratory fistula associated with esophageal cancer: treatment with a Gianturco stent tube. Radiology 1993;187:673.

SURGERY: SCIENTIFIC PRINCIPLES AND PRACTICE, Second Edition, edited by Lazar J. Greenfield, Michael W. Mulholland, Keith T. Oldham, Gerald B. Zelenock, and Keith D. Lillemoe. Lippincott–Raven Publishers, Philadelphia, © 1997.

CHAPTER 20

ENDOSURGICAL PRINCIPLES

STEVE EUBANKS

Endosurgery has revolutionized the contemporary surgical management of a number of disease processes. For certain procedures, clear benefit is apparent, but for many, the risk/benefit analysis is incomplete. Few surgical procedures have escaped the scrutiny of laparoscopic and thoracoscopic surgeons. Many diseases and their surgical management are undergoing careful comparison of pain, morbidity, cosmetic outcome, cost-effectiveness, length of hospital stay, and degree of interference with the patient's normal activities.

Although the modern era of endosurgery began in 1987 with the introduction of laparoscopic cholecystectomy, laparoscopy has been performed for more than 90 years. Diagnostic endoscopy can be traced to the work of Bozzini in 1806.[1,2] He developed the first endoscope, the *Lichtleiter,* which used candlelight transmitted through a tin tube. For decades, gynecologists used laparoscopy for sterilization procedures and diagnostic examinations. Intermittent reports of successful general surgical applications of laparoscopic techniques appeared during the past 80 years. However, endosurgery was not widely accepted until modern video technology, high-flow insufflation, and Hopkins rod-lens telescopes scopes combined to allow an operative team to work together and a surgeon to work with both hands. Application to many common surgical problems followed. Implementation occurred at a rate unprecedented in the history of surgery.

Endosurgery refers to operations performed with visualization provided through a telescope placed into a body space. Although endosurgery is used in virtually all surgical subspecialties, this review emphasizes endosurgical principles as they apply to abdominal endosurgery (laparoscopy) and thoracoscopy.

LAPAROSCOPY

Access

The abdominal wall is a barrier between the surgeon and a large variety of disease processes. It is a major source of pain and morbidity in open operations, since it must be violated to repair or remove diseased tissue within the peritoneal cavity. The laparoscopic surgeon attempts to effect a cure while minimizing collateral damage to the healthy abdominal wall.

The initial access to the peritoneal cavity during laparoscopic surgery is accomplished within seconds. Unfortunately, this act has been the source of many complications and several deaths. Placement of the primary trocar or Veress needle is the source of most major complications in laparoscopic surgery.[3]

The Veress needle is the device used most frequently for initial access to the abdominal cavity. The needle is placed into the peritoneal cavity through a small (less than 2 mm) skin incision by either gradual advancement of the needle or a short dartlike motion. Most insertions are safe and uneventful, but the potential for harm is great. The needle can be placed inadvertently within the bowel lumen or major blood vessels. Bowel injury, hemorrhage, exsanguination, and fatal air emboli have been reported.

A small number of surgeons begin the laparoscopic procedure by blindly placing a 5- or 10-mm trocar into the peritoneal cavity without previous establishment of a pneumoperitoneum.[4] Most endosurgeons consider this blind-insertion technique an ill-advised approach with unnecessary risk.

An open technique for abdominal access was described by H.M. Hasson in 1971.[5] This approach is the most commonly used alternative to the Veress needle. The differences between the Hasson and Veress techniques are analogous to the differences between the open and closed techniques for diagnostic peritoneal lavage. The open technique for trocar insertion uses a 10- to 12-mm skin incision within the umbilicus or in the periumbilical area. Dissection of the subcutaneous tissue is accomplished with sharp dissection or electrocautery. The fascia is identified, grasped between clamps, and incised. The underlying peritoneum is elevated and incised under direct vision. The initial abdominal access port is then placed into the peritoneal cavity.

Complications can occur with any of the techniques described. Those associated with the open technique are almost always limited to superficial bleeding or minor injury to the intestine. The Veress technique and the blind trocar insertion have a small but documented risk of serious intestinal injury, vascular trauma, and death. Experience and training must guide the surgeon in the choice of access route for an individual patient.

After the establishment of pneumoperitoneum and placement of the initial trocar, the laparoscopic telescope is placed into the abdominal cavity; all subsequent trocars enter the abdomen under direct visualization. The J-maneuver is frequently used for the placement of secondary ports (Fig. 20-1).

Proper positioning of the trocars through the abdominal wall is crucial for the successful completion of the laparoscopic operation. Triangulation of the trocars allows convergence of the telescope and instrument tips on the target organ while minimizing extracorporeal interference between instruments (Fig. 20-2).

In adults, the trocars should be placed a minimum of 8 cm apart so that a wide range of extracorporeal manipulation is possible. Ideal placement of trocars and equipment allows the surgeon to squarely face the operative site and television monitor. Trocar positions should allow the surgeon's hands and arms to work from a comfortable, ergonomically correct position.

Three to five trocars are used to accomplish most laparoscopic operations. The exact number of trocars placed is guided by standard, proven techniques, as well as by individual anatomic and pathologic variations. The safety of any given procedure must not be compromised in an attempt to avoid an additional 5- or 10-mm wound. Conversely, an excessive number of trocars may lead to injury due to instrumentation interference or lack of coordinated movements by team members.

Physiology

Reduced tissue trauma and carbon dioxide (CO_2) pneumoperitoneum are the two factors that account for the principal physiologic effects of laparoscopy. Reduced abdominal wall retraction, decreased manipulation of abdominal viscera, and lack of exposure of the viscera to room air during laparoscopy may be important secondary factors that contribute to improved postoperative gastrointestinal function when compared with an open surgical procedure. Most physiologic effects of CO_2 pneumoperitoneum are detrimental; however, these are generally limited to the intraoperative period and are easily managed if anticipated. An optical cavity (or working space) is required for laparoscopy. This is most commonly created by insufflation of CO_2 under pressure into the peritoneal cavity.

Alternatives to CO_2 include gases such as helium and argon. Inert gases potentially reduce many of the adverse hemodynamic and metabolic effects of CO_2 absorption.[6,7] Nitrous oxide appears promising as an alternative to CO_2 in early studies. Alternative gases do not, however, eliminate adverse effects related to elevations in abdominal pressure. CO_2 is preferred because of its low cost, ready availability, rapid absorption and physiologic elimination, and noncombustible nature.

Gasless laparoscopy is an effective alternative to pneumoperitoneum in some circumstances, although experience is more limited. Gasless laparoscopy provides exposure using an internal retracting device placed through a

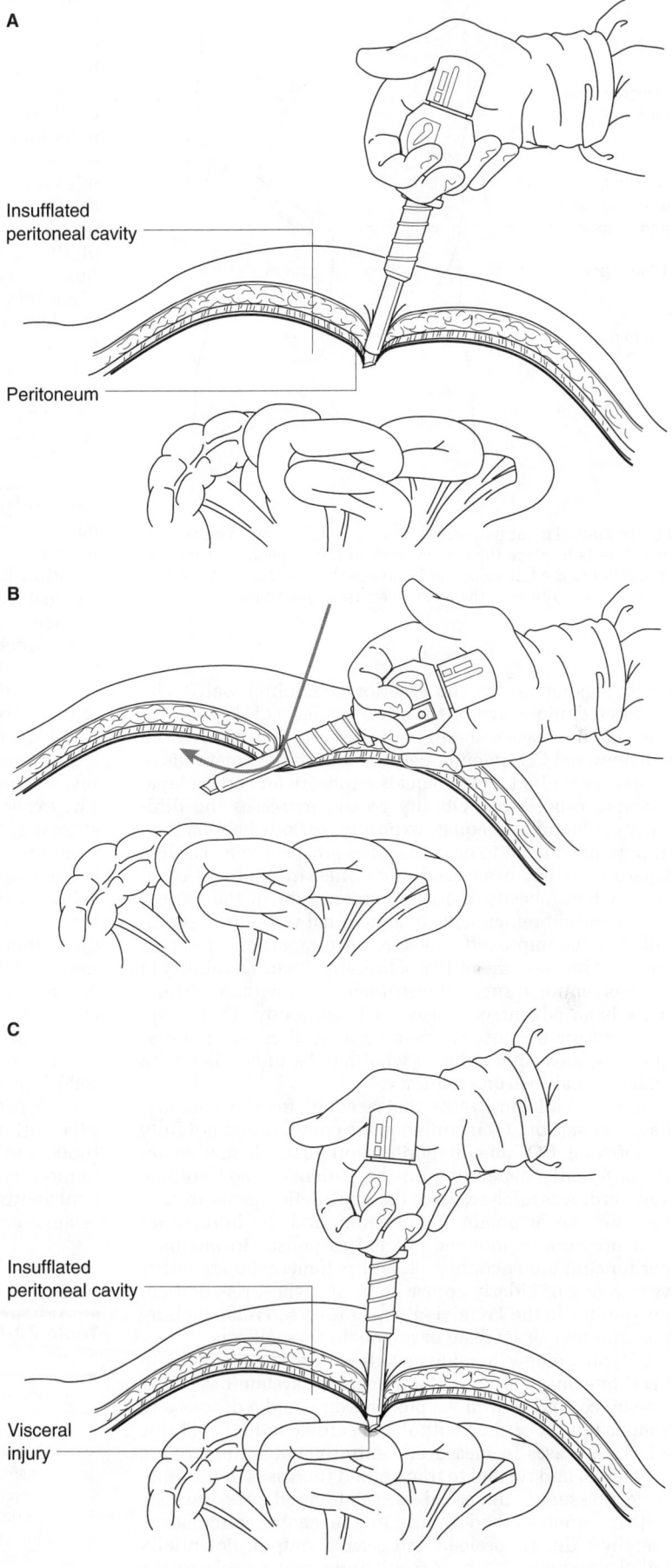

Figure 20-1. (*A*) A laparoscopic trocar is placed into the peritoneal cavity under direct vision after insufflation. (*B*) It can be placed safely using a J-maneuver as shown to direct the sharp tip tangentially away from the underlying viscera after penetration of the abdominal wall. This is done under visual control. (*C*) Laparoscopic port placement can lead to visceral injury if done without appropriate caution.

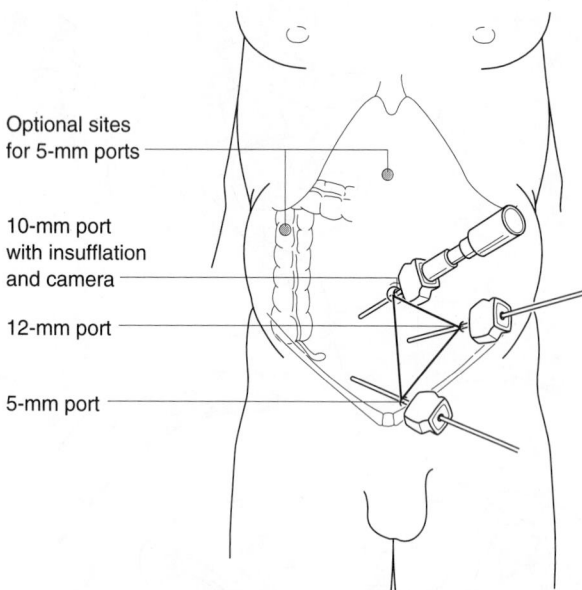

Optional sites
for 5-mm ports

10-mm port
with insufflation
and camera

12-mm port

5-mm port

Figure 20-2. Trocar placement for a right colectomy. The general principle is to place the camera port so the surgeon's visual axis is parallel to the telescope, and to place the working ports so that the operative site is at the apex of an isosceles triangle.

small incision to lift the anterior abdominal wall.[8] The gasless technique avoids the adverse effects of CO_2 absorption and increased abdominal pressure that result from conventional CO_2 pneumoperitoneum. Gasless methods of access are limited by inadequate exposure for certain laparoscopic procedures. Obesity greatly increases the difficulty of obtaining adequate exposure, so body habitus is an important concern to be considered prospectively. Gasless laparoscopy has been used more often in Asia and other areas where obesity is less common than in the United States. Recent refinements in abdominal wall–lifting technology have improved exposure of intraperitoneal organs and may increase the utility of this approach. The ability to use conventional surgical instrumentation without airtight ports is an advantage of gasless laparoscopy. This is appealing from the cost perspective, as well as for the infrequent laparoscopic surgeon who may be unfamiliar with endosurgical instrumentation.

The physiologic events that account for the hemodynamic effects of CO_2 insufflation are complex and not fully understood. CO_2 pneumoperitoneum affects hemodynamics differently depending on the patient's blood volume and cardiovascular reserve, the anesthetic agents in use, the duration of pneumoperitoneum, and the intraperitoneal pressure maintained. Varied responses to pneumoperitoneum are encountered, and patients who are either very young or elderly appear to be at highest risk. Patient positioning in the Trendelenburg or reverse Trendelenburg position may exacerbate or attenuate these effects.

CO_2 pneumoperitoneum usually results in an increase in heart rate, mean arterial blood pressure, systemic vascular resistance, and central venous pressure, and a decrease in venous return, cardiac output and cardiac index[9–12] (Table 20-1). Increases in measured central venous pressure are artifactual and related to transmitted increases in intrathoracic pressure.[13] Increased intraabdominal pressure may impair venous blood return to the central circulation, thereby reducing preload and cardiac output. Potentially lethal dysrhythmias may result from hypercarbia or the vagal response to parietal peritoneal stretching.[14–16] In-

creased cardiac work results from elevated vascular resistance, and this can raise myocardial oxygen demand, predisposing patients with coronary artery occlusion disease to myocardial infarction.[17,18]

Cardiac complications are the most common cause of death after cholecystectomy.[19] A recent comparison of the outcomes for matched patients undergoing 1107 laparoscopic cholecystectomies with 1283 open cholecystectomies revealed significantly fewer cardiac complications in the laparoscopic group (0.06% versus 1.4%).[20] Despite the use of historical control patients in this study, the benefit of the laparoscopic approach on postoperative cardiac function is significant. The postoperative cardiac benefits of a minimally invasive operation must be weighed against the detrimental intraoperative effects of CO_2 pneumoperitoneum on cardiac output.

Intraoperative physiologic effects of CO_2 pneumoperitoneum on pulmonary function are undesirable yet well tolerated by most patients without serious preexisting pulmonary disease. CO_2 insufflation to 10 to 15 cm H_2O predictably diminishes oxygenation and impairs ventilation because lung volumes are reduced as a result of cephalad displacement of the diaphragm.[21,22] Reduced pulmonary compliance and increased airway resistance result from the pneumoperitoneum as well.[23] Systemic CO_2 absorption leads to hypercarbia, and acidosis is a potential adverse effect of CO_2 insufflation. Hypercarbia is easily reversed or prevented in most patients with normal pulmonary function by increasing minute ventilation. An increase of 20% to 25% is commonly required, and end tidal CO_2 monitoring is often helpful in this regard. Patients with preexisting pulmonary disease pose more difficult problems and require prospective anesthesia planning.

The postoperative pulmonary benefits of a minimally invasive operation over an open operation are significant. The expected reduction in forced expiratory volume in 1 second (FEV_1) and forced vital capacity (FVC) after an open operation are attenuated when the operation is performed laparoscopically.[24] Observed reduction in FVC and FEV_1 on the first postoperative day are 20% lower after laparoscopic cholecystectomy compared with open cholecystectomy.[25] Immediate postoperative spirometry is less impaired following laparoscopic cholecystectomy when compared with open cholecystectomy.[26,27] An excellent comparison of the pulmonary effects of open and closed cholecystectomy demonstrated a significant improvement in oxygen saturation, maximal voluntary ventilation, and total lung capacity for the laparoscopic technique.[28]

Postoperative ileus is a major factor in the length of hospitalization after open operations. Postoperative ileus is thought to result from sympathetically mediated inhibition of motility, primarily affecting the colon.[29,30] Other factors contributing to ileus include bowel manipulation, stress-related hormones other than catecholamines (eg, vaso-

Table 20-1. PHYSIOLOGIC EFFECTS OF PNEUMOPERITONEUM

Parameter	Effect
Mean arterial pressure	Increased
Systemic vascular resistance	Increased
Pulmonary vascular resistance	Increased
Heart rate	Increased
Central venous pressure	Increased
Venous return	Decreased
Cardiac output	Decreased
Cardiac index	Decreased

pressin), and postoperative narcotic usage. Several clinical studies have demonstrated earlier return of bowel function after laparoscopic surgery compared with open surgery.[31-33] Rapid return of colonic electrical activity and preservation of small bowel motility after laparoscopic cholecystectomy have been shown using a canine model.[34] The degree to which these effects are attributable to a reduction in narcotic usage is not known.

The endogenous response to injury involves adaptive mechanisms by which the body attempts to maintain homeostasis. These biologic responses may be excessive and maladaptive when local factors enter the systemic circulation. The systemic inflammatory response precipitated by multisystem trauma, severe infection, or major elective operation can lead to increased microvascular permeability, a hypermetabolic state, capillary thrombosis, and, subsequently, multiple-system organ failure. The ability of the patient to tolerate these events depends primarily on the magnitude of the precipitating stimulus and the previous health status of the individual. Recent and ongoing attempts to modulate the response to injury have failed to provide reliable therapy in this clinical setting. Theoretically, laparoscopic surgery may avoid a maladaptive stress response by minimizing the initial injury stimulus resulting from an operative procedure.

Elevations in serum catecholamine, cortisol, and glucose levels in postoperative patients who have had laparoscopic cholecystectomy are significantly diminished and return to normal more quickly than in patients who have undergone open cholecystectomy.[35] The systemic cytokine response to laparoscopy is significantly attenuated when compared with open laparotomy. Serum interleukin-6 (IL-6) and C-reactive protein levels, erythrocyte sedimentation rate, and circulating white blood cell count are all more normal after laparoscopic cholecystectomy than after open cholecystectomy.[36-40] Thus, an attenuated neuroendocrine and cytokine response to elective surgery is expected when a less invasive approach is taken, although the physiologic importance of these findings has yet to be defined.

Preservation of immunocompetence is a desired result of a minimally invasive operation. After laparotomy, the delayed hypersensitivity response is normally significantly diminished. It was recently shown that the response of animals undergoing peritoneal insufflation with CO_2 is significantly retained after identical skin antigen testing.[41] These findings are consistent with the observation that T-cell function in pigs undergoing laparoscopic colon resection is more normal than for animals undergoing the same operation by laparotomy.[42] A comparison of tumor growth in mice undergoing laparotomy with those undergoing peritoneal insufflation demonstrated a permissive effect of laparotomy on tumor growth rates.[43,44] In humans, IL-6 serum levels and circulating white blood cell counts on postoperative days 1 and 6 after laparoscopic cholecystectomy are normal, whereas significant increases occur for patients who undergo open cholecystectomy.[45] Additionally, monocyte HLA-DR expression, an important correlate of antigen presenting ability, is significantly reduced in the open cholecystectomy group but preserved in the laparoscopic group. Significant decreases in monocyte and neutrophil superoxide anion generation, the neutrophil chemotactic response, tumor necrosis factor serum levels, and the peripheral white blood cell count are reported in laparoscopic patients compared with patients undergoing open cholecystectomy.[46] It is premature, however, to extrapolate from these findings that fewer infections and decreased tumor recurrence rates can be expected from the preserved immune function observed with laparoscopy. These issues are the focus of substantial and ongoing investigation.

Advantages and Disadvantages

Many of the advantages of laparoscopy are attributable to the physiologic findings described earlier. Other advantages include reduced pain, a shorter hospital stay, fewer wound complications, and cosmetic improvement. Cost savings are realized with many operations when laparoscopic techniques are used instead of laparotomy. Conversely, laparoscopy may increase the cost of treatment if no diagnostic or therapeutic maneuvers are averted by the laparoscopic procedure. For example, hospital and operating room costs are higher for laparoscopic hernia repair than for open hernia repair.[47] The laparoscopic approach must be justified by outcome and long-term quality-of-life studies when increased costs are incurred.

The disadvantages of laparoscopy are partially due to changes in the operating environment. The need for an optical cavity is resolved by creating a CO_2 pneumoperitoneum; however, this has negative physiologic sequelae. The technical challenges of operating with two-dimensional visualization on a television monitor require familiarization. Working against the fulcrum of the abdominal wall and using long, unfamiliar instruments can lead to frustration and fatigue. Different technical skills are required for proficiency at laparoscopy than open surgery. Fortunately, the same standards of surgical judgment apply to both procedures, despite the technical differences.

Laparoscopy permits the surgeon to assess only surface anatomy. This disadvantage can be partially overcome with intraoperative ultrasonography to evaluate the internal anatomy of certain target organs. Tactile feedback is rudimentary with laparoscopic instruments compared with conventional open palpation. Inability to manually manipulate viscera makes procedures such as splenectomy and nephrectomy more difficult technically using the laparoscopic approach.

Laparoscopy, like any emerging area of medicine, is vulnerable to criticism that long-term follow-up is lacking. Indeed, it is premature to make definitive statements about cancer recurrence rates for laparoscopic oncology procedures. Likewise, most laparoscopic hernia series have less than 5-years of follow-up for recurrence and late complications. The durability of laparoscopic antireflux operations has not been established. Well-designed long-term clinical outcome studies are mandatory to place these procedures in the correct overall context.

Current Status

Laparoscopy is fundamental to the contemporary practice of general surgery. Laparoscopic techniques are used variably, depending on the training, experience, technical skills, and type of surgical practice of the surgeon. In addition, opinions about the best treatment options for individual patients and specific disease entities vary. Laparoscopic cholecystectomy is now widely accepted as the gold standard for the treatment of calculous gallbladder disease.[48] The safety of laparoscopic cholecystectomy is well documented.[49] The efficacy and importance of diagnostic laparoscopy is established for the diagnosis of acute processes as well as the staging of malignancies.[50] The laparoscopic technique is preferred by many surgeons for the operative treatment of gastroesophageal reflux disease. Laparoscopic appendectomy is routinely performed in adult patients, although benefit is most apparent for women of child-bearing age with an uncertain diagnosis, when an exploratory laparotomy can be avoided.

Many other procedures can be safely and successfully performed by expert laparoscopists. Some of these procedures are technically difficult and time-consuming; some oncologic procedures have not been proved to be equivalent to open resections; some lack sufficient documentation of benefit to justify additional costs. Examples of these technically feasible procedures include colectomy, inguinal hernia repair, treatment of ulcer disease, splenectomy, adrenelectomy, and bypass procedures for pancreatic malignancy. The place of these procedures by laparoscopic means is still controversial.

Procedures that are not currently accepted as appropriate by laparoscopic approach include pancreaticoduodenectomy, the resection of masses that necessitate a large incision for specimen removal, and major hepatic resections. Laparoscopically assisted vascular procedures are currently performed in an investigational setting.

Surgical subspecialty enthusiasm for endosurgery is rapidly expanding. Laparoscopic and thoracoscopic spinal surgery is emerging as a potentially significant improvement in the management of back disease. Laparoscopy for the evaluation of trauma patients was promoted by Berci and colleagues[51] in the early 1980s with modest success; but renewed enthusiasm is apparent now with contemporary techniques.[52] Endosurgical procedures for plastic and reconstructive surgeons have been developed. The performance of balloon-assisted tissue dissection has proved feasible.[53] Pediatric surgeons, like adult general surgeons, have made good use of laparoscopic techniques for a wide variety of problems.

Complications

Of course, complications occur with laparoscopic procedures. Some complications, such as bile duct injuries, have received extensive publicity and provided the basis for early criticism of laparoscopy. Multiple large series from the gynecology literature have reported extremely low complication rates before the era that began with laparoscopic cholecystectomy in the late 1980s[54-61] (Table 20-2). Current complication rates for advanced laparoscopic operations are significantly higher than for large series. Factors that led to the low complication rates in these studies include limitation to relatively simple operations of short duration (primarily sterilization procedures), minimal tissue dissection, and a young, otherwise healthy patient population.

Many complications associated with advanced laparoscopic operations are inherent to the operative procedure, regardless of approach. Anastamotic leak after bowel resection is an intrinsic risk of intestinal surgery that is not demonstrably altered by the route of access if appropriately

done. Other risks are related to comorbid disease processes, such as diabetes mellitus, immunosuppression, and coronary artery disease. Certain risks, however, are uniquely attributable to the laparoscopic technique, including trocar injury to viscera or vascular structures, air embolus, trocar site hernia, injury from laparoscopic instrumentation, and complications caused by CO_2 pneumoperitoneum.

The Future

The future of laparoscopic surgery is one of new applications, technical refinement, improved educational methods, and the development of a credible research foundation. The last is necessary for the survival and growth of this field of medicine. Outcomes research involving cost/benefit analysis will play an increasingly important role in determining therapeutic options. Procedures that add significantly to the cost of patient care without providing objective improvement over current therapy will perish.

The interaction between industry and medicine has been precedent setting in the evolution of laparoscopy. Academic and commercial relationships have facilitated the development and production of enabling technologies and instrumentation. The importance of these relationships will be magnified as research is increasingly funded by corporate sponsors.

Laparoscopic education is an essential component of surgical resident education. The integration of laparoscopy into medical school and residency curricula has diminished the importance of the weekend course. Brief courses for the education of practicing surgeons will continue but without the burden of providing the educational foundation in laparoscopy for the next generation of surgeons.

Emerging technologies such as CD-ROM interactive programs, Internet access, and virtual reality simulation will play an adjunct role in the future training of laparoscopic surgeons. Telemedicine is used currently to provide educational programs and remote consultation. Telesurgery, operating at a location remote from the patient through fiberoptic connections and robotic effectors, is an area of interest to military surgeons. Telesurgical projects currently receive significant research support in the United States and abroad.

The most critical aspect for laparoscopy in the future is the expansion of research efforts. Opportunities abound for basic physiologic and metabolic study, outcomes research, prospective clinical trials, retrospective reviews, and the development of instrumentation and techniques. The

---

Table 20-2. REVIEW OF SEVERAL LARGE LAPAROSCOPIC SURVEYS

Investigators	Procedures	Major Complications (%)	Total Complications (%)	Death Rate (per 100,000 cases)
Loffler and Pent[54]	32,719	—	2.40	—
Riedel et al.[55]	292,462	0.19	0.19	5.1
Henning[56]	36,207	0.18		
	94,382	—		64.0
RCOG enquiry[57]	50,247	—	3.50	8.0
Phillips et al (1975 national survey)[58]	298,029	0.46 (D)	0.41	5.2 (D)
		0.37 (S)		2.5 (S)
Peterson et al (1988 AAGL survey)[59]	36,928	1.5	0.15	5.4
Phillips et al (1975 AAGL survey)[60]	117,705	0.31 (D)	0.29	4.2 (total)
Phillips et al (1982 AAGL survey)[61]	125,560	0.14 (S)	0.14	

D, diagnostic; S, sterilization.
Bailey RW. General considerations. In: Bailey RW, Flower JL, eds. Complications of laparoscopic surgery. St Louis, Quality Medical Publishing, 1995:4)

foundation on which laparoscopy will rest has yet to be completed.

THORACOSCOPY

Benefits of thoracoscopy were demonstrated in the early 20th century; like laparoscopy, however, these techniques were applied only infrequently until recently. Hans Christian Jacobaeus (1879–1937) devoted much of his career to the development of thoracoscopy and provided a foundation of thoracoscopic theory and technique on which subsequent generations of surgeons would build.[62–65] In 1910, Jacobaeus theorized that thoracoscopy could be applied to the diagnosis and treatment of pulmonary tuberculosis.[66]

Thoracoscopy is now used more widely than at any other point in history. The benefits of minimally invasive procedures demonstrated by orthopedists, general surgeons, and gynecologists have prompted thoracic surgeons to apply less invasive techniques for patients with pulmonary and pleural diseases. Improvements in instrumentation, optics, and anesthetic techniques have driven the resurgence of interest.

Anesthesia Considerations

Thoracoscopic procedures are successfully performed using local anesthesia, regional anesthesia with and without intravenous sedation, and general anesthesia. Most thoracoscopic operations employ general anesthesia with a dual-lumen endotracheal tube or some other strategy to provide independent lung ventilation. General anesthesia with a double-lumen endotracheal intubation provides continuous airway control, allows single-lung ventilation, decreases the risk of contralateral lung contamination, and obviates the need for patient cooperation.

A thorough preoperative evaluation of the patient with pulmonary disease is routinely performed before elective thoracoscopy. Baseline arterial blood gases and pulmonary function studies provide important prognostic information about a patient's ability to tolerate single-lung ventilation. Optimization of preoperative pulmonary function is accomplished by cessation of smoking, eradication of infection, chest physiotherapy, and treatment with bronchodilators or steroids when indicated. Improvement of pulmonary status reduces the incidence of postoperative pulmonary complications and enhances tolerance of general anesthesia.

Proper patient positioning is important for adequate surgical exposure and for the prevention of position-related injuries. The lateral decubitus position is routinely used for thoracoscopy. Positioning is essentially identical to that used for an open thoracotomy. Padding or "beanbag" positioning is used to secure the patient to the operating table. Pressure points are padded to prevent pressure necrosis, and the extremities are positioned and secured in a manner that avoids excessive stretch or pressure that might lead to neurologic injury. A roll of padding under the dependent axilla decreases the pressure on the neurovascular supply of the dependent arm. Sequential compression stockings placed on the lower extremities decrease the risk of deep venous thrombosis. Additionally, the intermittent inflation shifts the pressure points and may aid in the prevention of pressure-induced ischemic necrosis. Complications such as ischemic necrosis, neurovascular stretch or compression injury, and deep venous thrombosis occur infrequently but may lead to devastating problems.

The physiologic changes that occur during thoracoscopic procedures are not analogous to those of laparoscopy. Whereas many of the physiologic changes during laparoscopy occur as a result of insufflation of CO_2 into the peritoneal cavity, it is unusual to use pressurized gases during thoracoscopy. Most physiologic changes during thoracoscopy are the result of a pneumothorax, single-lung ventilation, patient positioning, and the response to anesthesia. The degree of tissue trauma caused by thoracoscopy is generally substantially diminished when compared with that of open thoracotomy.

The decreased physiologic insult associated with thoracoscopy may lead to more outpatient thoracic procedures or minimal hospital stays. The advantages offered by thoracoscopy also allow the surgical management of severely ill patients who would have previously been considered to be prohibitive or poor surgical risks.

Technical Considerations

Access to the thoracic cavity is gained by a technique similar to the placement of a chest tube. A 1- to 2-cm skin incision is placed on the lateral thorax. Electrocautery is used to divide the subcutaneous tissues and a clamp is used to spread muscle fibers and is bluntly advanced through the parietal pleura. A fingertip is placed into the pleural space and a 360-degree sweep is done to ensure that the lung is not at risk for injury. A thoracic cannula is placed over a blunt obturator and left in place throughout the procedure for instrument and telescopic access to the pleural cavity. The intercostal space selected for access is located directly beneath the skin incision. Using an intercostal space one or two ribs cephalad to the skin incision limits movement of the instruments to an unacceptable degree.

The principle of *triangulation* applies to thoracoscopy as it does to laparoscopy (Fig. 20-3). The operative target site serves as the apex of the triangle, whereas the telescope and other cannulas provide points that converge on the target. A diamond configuration of cannula placement on the lateral chest wall is frequently useful for thoracoscopic operations. Alternatively, a curvilinear array of access sites can be used.

The surgeon stands facing the operative site with a television monitor directly in the line of sight. Cannula sites are selected at locations that allow the surgeon and assistant to work parallel to the visual axis of the endoscope. Manipulation of instruments against the direction of the visual axis provides a mirror-image view and is to be avoided.

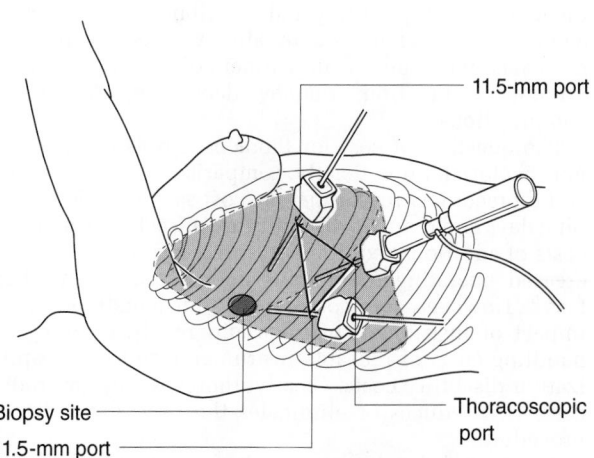

11.5-mm port

Biopsy site

11.5-mm port

Thoracoscopic port

Figure 20-3. Example of endosurgical port placement. Positioning varies for individual need, but the principle of triangulation used for laparoscopic surgery is equally applicable in the thorax.

The optical cavity within which the thoracoscopic surgeon operates is provided by collapse of the ipsilateral lung. The cavity is maintained by the fixed structure of the thoracic cage. Rarely, pressurized gas (usually CO_2) is instilled to facilitate collapse of the lung. Generally, inexpensive, nonsealing cannulas are used for thoracoscopy, since there is rarely a need to maintain a pressurized closed space. Some surgeons use no other cannulas than the one through which the scope is placed. Additional instruments may be placed directly through thoracic wall incisions. Limiting the number of cannulas can decrease cost slightly and allow the use of conventional instruments but can also lead to increased tissue trauma and bleeding at access sites.

Specialized thoracoscopy instruments with single-use and reusable designs enhance the ability of the surgeon to perform complex operations through small incisions. The endoscopic linear stapler is of great importance since it allows rapid, safe, and hemostatic division of lung parenchyma. Advances in optics and imaging provide magnified, high-resolution images that make possible the identification of very small structures and that allow safe dissection of tissue planes.

Thoracoscopy cannula sites, usually between one and five, are closed in layers at the conclusion of the procedure. A chest tube is routinely placed within the pleural cavity through one cannula site before inflation of the ipsilateral lung. A chest tube can be omitted if the procedure performed incurs minimal or no risk of a postoperative air leak.

Advantages and Disadvantages

The potential advantages of thoracoscopy over an open procedure are many:

- Less pain
- Shorter hospital stay
- Faster return to normal activities
- Decreased tissue trauma
- Reduced costs (fewer hospital days, reduced disability, avoidance of other diagnostic and therapeutic procedures)
- Improved cosmesis

The reduction of tissue trauma and pain with thoracoscopy when compared with thoracotomy is remarkable in most patients. The morbidity of a thoracotomy, regardless of the operation performed, is significant although not easily quantified. Postoperative pain and the attendant reduction in respiratory effort are significant factors that determine the length of hospital stay and contribute to postoperative complications. Thoracoscopy allows an earlier return to normal activity and less impairment of early postoperative pulmonary function, thereby decreasing the risk of complications.

The question of cost for thoracoscopy is complex and multifactorial. Superficially, comparisons of thoracoscopy and thoracotomy reveal that the cost savings of fewer hospital days and reduced disability are offset by the increased costs of additional equipment, single-use instruments, increased operating room time, and increased anesthesia fees.[67] However, few comparisons adequately assess the impact of instrument upgrade and repair, cleaning and handling costs of reusable instruments and posthospitalization disability costs. Clearly, thoracoscopy can reduce costs if it reduces or eliminates the need for additional procedures.

A potential disadvantage of thoracoscopy is the loss of direct tactile feedback. The surgeon must rely on endoscopic visualization and crude palpation with instruments. Therefore, detection of unsuspected deep parenchymal lesions is difficult with this approach. Many technical maneuvers are more difficult using an endosurgical approach. Suturing, anastamosis formation, and ligation of blood vessels are examples of routine operative skills that can be more tedious and time-consuming by means of thoracoscopy. The loss of three-dimensional visualization accentuates the difficulty of performing precise surgical maneuvers. The lack of long-term follow-up studies of thoracoscopy is also disturbing.

Current Status

Thoracoscopic techniques are widely used for diagnostic and therapeutic purposes. Indications for diagnostic thoracoscopy include the assessment of pleural effusions, diffuse interstitial lung disease, isolated pulmonary infiltrates, solitary pulmonary nodules, mediastinal lymphadenopathy, mediastinal cysts, neurogenic tumors, mediastinal masses, and other lesions.[68] Therapeutic thoracoscopy is used for many diseases of the lung, pleura, mediastinum, and pericardium. Limited cardiac applications, including single-vessel coronary artery bypass grafting, have been done as well. Several successful series of video-assisted thoracoscopic surgery (VATS) for pulmonary resection have been reported.[69–74] (Table 20-3). These combined reports include more than 1200 patients and demonstrate a rate of conversion to open thoracotomy of 4.4%.

Conversion from a thoracoscopic procedure to a thoracotomy is sometimes necessary to provide hemostasis, improve visability, safely perform the procedure, or manually palpate pathology that is difficult to visualize. The safety of the patient and the adequacy of the operation should never be compromised to avoid conversion to a conventional open operation. Complications occur during thoracoscopic operations but should not be more frequent than with open operations. Complications of thoracoscopic pulmonary resection are summarized in Table 20-4.[75]

The Future

The future of thoracoscopic surgery is difficult to predict. It has been greeted with less enthusiasm than has modern laparoscopy, although certain individuals and institutions have developed considerable experience and expertise. A new generation of thoracic surgeons exposed to minimally invasive procedures throughout training are more likely to pursue thoracoscopy aggressively. The economics of health care is certain to significantly affect the future role of thoracoscopy. Research is greatly needed to define the appropriate applications of these techniques on

Table 20-3. RESULTS OF THORACOSCOPIC PULMONARY RESECTION

Investigators		Patient	Conversion to Open Procedure
Mack et al.[69]	1993	300	2 (0.001%)
Landreneau et al.[70]	1992	85	0 (0%)
Allen et al.[71]	1993	118	35 (30%)
Kaiser and Bavaria[72]	1993	266	11 (4.1%)
Santambrogio et al.[73]	1995	22	1 (5%)
DeCamp et al.[74]	1995	425	5 (1.42%)
TOTAL		1216	53 (4.4%)

(Modified from Mault JR, Harpole DH, Douglas JM. Thoracoscopic pulmonary resection. In: Pappas TN, Schwartz LB, Eubanks S, eds. Atlas of laparoscopic surgery. Philadelphia, Current Medicine, 1996:26.10)

Table 20-4. POTENTIAL COMPLICATIONS OF THORACOSCOPIC PULMONARY RESECTION

Pneumothorax	Inadequate margin of resection
Persistent air leak	Lung injury
Hemorrhage	Intercostal neurovascular bundle injury
Air embolism	Equipment malfunction
Diaphragmatic perforation	Infection

(Modified from Mault JR, Harpole DH, Douglas JM. Thoracoscopic pulmonary resection. In: Pappas TN, Schwartz LB, Eubanks S, eds. Atlas of laparoscopic surgery. Philadelphia, Current Medicine, 1996;26:10)

the basis of objective evidence. Outcome studies are necessary to assess whether the theoretic benefits of thoracoscopy are clinically and statistically significant. Cost/benefit analysis is needed to determine whether the increased intraoperative costs are offset by shortened hospitalizations, fewer complications, and a more rapid return to work. A need exists for further development of instruments to facilitate difficult techniques, such as suturing and dissecting small structures. Palpation cannot be adequately replaced by technology in the forseeable future, but the addition of imaging modalities, such as intraoperative ultrasonography for parenchymal and mediastinal masses, may partially compensate. The convergence of these technologies with excellent training is likely to result in improvements in patient care and quality of life.

REFERENCES

1. Davis CJ, Filipi CJ. A history of endoscopic surgery. In: Arregui ME, Fitzgibbons RJ, Katkhouda M, McKernan JB, Reich H. eds. Principles of laparoscopic surgery: basic and advanced techniques. New York, Springer-Verlag, 1995:3.
2. Kelling G. Ueber oesophagoskopie, gastrokopie und kolioskopie. Munch Med Wochenschr 1902;1:21.
3. Oshinsky GS, Smith AD. Laparoscopic needles and trocars: an overview of designs and complications. J Laparoendosc Surg 1992;2:117.
4. Jarrett II JC. Laparoscopy: direct trocar insertion without pneumoperitoneum. Obstet Gynecol 1990;75:725.
5. Hasson HM. Open laparoscopy: modified instrument and method for laparoscopy. Am J Obstet Gynecol 1971;110:886.
6. Leighton TA, Liu S, Bongard FS. Comparative cardiopulmonary effects of carbon dioxide versus helium pneumoperitoneum. Surgery 1993;113:527.
7. Eisenhauer DM, Saunders CJ, Ho HS, Wolfe BM. Hemodynamic effects of argon pneumoperitoneum. Surg Endosc 1993;8:315.
8. Smith RS, Fry WR, Tsoi EKM, et al. Gasless laparoscopy and conventional instruments: the next phase of minimally invasive surgery. Arch Surg 1993;128:1102.
9. Ho HS, Gunther RA, Wolfe BM. Intraperitoneal carbon dioxide insufflation and cardiopulmonary functions: laparoscopic cholecystectomy in pigs. Arch Surg 1992;127:928.
10. Mclaughlin JG, Scheeres DE, Dean RJ, Bonnell BW. The adverse hemodynamic effects of laparoscopic cholecystectomy. Surg Endosc 1995;9:121.
11. Ortega AE, Peters JH. Physiologic alterations of endosurgery. In: Peter JH, DeMeester RT, eds. Minimally invasive surgery. St Louis, Quality Medical Publishers, 1994:23.
12. Safran DB, Orlando R. Physiologic effects of pneumoperitoneum. Am J Surg 1994;167:281.
13. Marathe US, Lilly RE, Silvestry SC, Davis JW, Schauer PR, Glower DD. Left ventricular contractility is not altered during carbon dioxide pneumoperitoneum. Surg Endosc 1996.
14. Shantha TR, Harden J. Laparoscopic cholecystectomy: anesthesia-related complications and guidelines. Surg Laparosc Endosc 1991;1:173.
15. See WA, Monk TG, Weldon BC. Complications of laparoscopy: strategies for prevention. In: Soper NJ, Odem RR, Clayman RV, McDougall EM, eds. Essentials of laparoscopy. St Louis, Quality Medical Publishing, 1994:215.
16. Carmichael DE. Laparoscopy-cardiac considerations. Fertil Steril 1971;22:69.
17. Safran D. Sgambati S, Orlando R. Laparoscopy in high-risk patients. Surg Gynecol Obstet 1993;176:548.
18. Westerband A, Van De Water J, Amzallag M, et al. Cardiovascular changes during laparoscopic cholecystectomy. Surg Gynecol Obstet 1992;175:535.
19. Deziel DJ. Complications of cholecystectomy: incidence, clinical manifestations, and diagnosis. Surg Clin North Am 1994;74:809.
20. Williams LF, Chapman WC, Bonau RA, McGee EC, Boyd RW, Jacobs JK. Comparison of laparoscopic cholecystectomy with open cholecystectomy in a single center. Am J Surg 1993;165:459.
21. Chui PT, Gin T, Oh TE. Anaesthesia for laparoscopic general surgery. Anaesth Intens Care 1993;21:163.
22. Wittgen CM, Andrus CH, Fitzgerald SD, Dahms TE, Kaminski DL. Analysis of the hemodynamic and ventilatory effects of laparoscopic cholecystectomy. Arch Surg 1991;126:997.
23. Farouck O, Saba A, Fath J, et al. Increases in intra-abdominal pressure affect pulmonary complicance. Arch Surg 1995;130:544.
24. Goodale RL, Beebe D, McNevin MP, Boyle M, et al. Hemodynamic, respiratory, and metabolic effects of laparoscopic cholecystectomy. Am J Surg 1993;166:544.
25. Frazee RC, Roberts RW, Okeson GC, Symonds RE, Snyder SK, Hendricks JL, Smith RW. Open vs. laparoscopic cholecystectomy: a comparison of postoperative pulmonary function. Ann Surg 1991;213:651.
26. Peters JH, Ortega A, Lehnerd SL, Campbell AJ, Schwartz DC, Ellison EC, Innes JT. The physiology of laparoscopic surgery: pulmonary function after laparoscopic cholecystectomy. Surg Laprosc Endosc 1993;3:370.
27. Putensen-Himmer G, Putensen C, Lammer H, Lingnau W, Aigner F, Benzer H. Comparison of postoperative respiratory function after laparoscopy or open laparotomy for cholecystectomy. Anesthesiology 1992;77:675.
28. Schauer PR, Luna J, Ghiatas A, Glen ME, Warren JM, Sirinek KR. Pulmonary function after laparoscopic cholecystectomy. Surgery 1993;114:389.
29. Bollinger SH, Quigley EMM. Disordered gastrointestinal motility. In: Quigley EMM, Sorrell MF, eds. The gastrointestinal surgical patient: preoperative and postoperative care. Baltimore, Williams & Wilkins, 1994:157.
30. Livingston EH, Passaro EP. Postoperative ileus. Dig Dis Sci 1990;35:121.
31. Litwin DEM, Girotti MJ, Poulin EC, Mamazza J, Nagy AG. Laparoscopic cholecystectomy: trans-Canada experience with 2201 cases. Can J Surg 1992;35:291.
32. Hoffman GC, Baker JW, Fitchett CW, Vansant JH. Laparoscopic-assisted colectomy: initial experience. Ann Surg 1994;219:732.
33. Senagore AJ, Luchtefeld MA, Mackeigan JM, Mazier WP. Open colectomy versus laparoscopic colectomy: are there differences? Am Surg 1993;56:549.
34. Schmieg RE, Schirmer BD, Combs MJ, Edwards M, Fariss A. Recovery of gastrointestinal motility after laparoscopic cholecystectomy. Surg Forum 1993;44:135.
35. Schauer PR, Sirinek KR. The laparoscopic approach reduces the endocrine response to elective cholecystectomy. Am Surg 1995;61:106.
36. Joris J, Cigarini I, Legrand M, et al. Metabolic and respiratory changes after cholecystectomy performed via laparotomy or laparoscopy. Br J Anaesth 1992;69:341.
37. Mealy K, Gallagher H, Traynor O, Hyland J. Physiological and metabolic responses to open and laparoscopic cholecystectomy. Br J Surg 1992;79:1061.
38. Dominioni L, Cuffari S, Giudce G, Carcano G, Nicora L, Dionigi R. The acute phase response after laparoscopic cholecystectomy and after open cholecystectomy. HPB Surgery 1993;6:65.
39. Roumen RMH, van Meurs PA, Kuypers HHC, Kraak WAG, Sauerwein RW. Serum interleukin-6 and C reactive protein

responses in patients after laparoscopic or conventional cholecystectomy. Eur Surg Res 1992;158:541.

40. Cho JM, LaPorta AJ, Clark JR, Schofield MJ, Hammond SL, Mallory PL. Response of serum cytokines in patients undergoing laparoscopic cholecystectomy. Surg Endosc 1994;8:1380.

41. Trokel MJ, Bessler M, Treat MR, Whelan RL, Nowygrod R. Preservation of immune response after laparoscopy. Surg Endosc 1994;8:1385.

42. Bessler M, Whelan RL, Halverson A, Treat MR, Nowygrod R. Is immune function better preserved after laparoscopic versus open colon resection? Surg Endosc 1994;8:881.

43. Allendorf JDF, Bessler M, Kayton ML, Whelan RL, Nowygrod R. Tumor growth after laparotomy or laparoscopy: a preliminary study. Surg Endosc 1995;9:49.

44. Allendorf JDF, Bessler M, Kayton ML, Oesterling SD, et al. Increased tumor establishment and growth after laparotomy vs laparoscopy in a murine model. Arch Surg 1995;130:649.

45. Kloosterman T, von Blomberg MBE, Borgstein P, Cuesta MA, Scheper RJ, Meijer S. Unimpaired immune function after laparoscopic cholecystectomy. Surgery 1994;115:424.

46. Redmond HP, Watson RWG, Houghton T, Condron C, Watson RGK, Bouchier-Hayes D. Immune function in patients undergoing open vs. laparoscopic cholecystectomy. Arch Surg 1994;129:1240.

47. Payne JH, Grininger LM, Izawam T, et al. Laparoscopic or open inguinal herniorrhaphy? A randomized prospective trial. Arch Surg 1994;129:973.

48. Soper NJ, Stockmann PT, Dunnegan DL, Ashley SW: Laparoscopic cholecystectomy: the new "gold standard"? Arch Surg 1992;127:917.

49. Meyers WC, Branum GD, Farouk M. A prospective analysis of 1518 laparoscopic cholecystectomies. N Engl J Med 1991;324:1072.

50. Eubanks S: The role of laparoscopy in diagnosis and treatment of primary or metastatic liver cancer. Semin Surg Oncol 1994;10:404.

51. Berci G, Dunkelman D, Michael S, et al. Emerging minilaparoscopy in abdominal trauma. Am J Surg 1983;146:261.

52. Smith RS, Tsoi EKM, Fry WR, et al. Laparoscopy is cost effective in the evaluation of abdominal trauma. Surg Endosc 1993;7:137.

53. Levin LS, Rehnke R, Eubanks S. Endoscopy of the upper extremity. Hand Clin 1995;11:59.

54. Loffler FD, Pent D. Indications, contraindications, and complications of laparoscopy. Obstet Gynecol Surv 1975;30:407.

55. Riedel HH, Lehmann-Willenbrock E, Conrad P, Semm K. German pelviscopic statistics for the years 1978–1982. Endoscopy 1986;18:219.

56. Henning H. The Dallas report on laparoscopic complications. Gastrointest Endosc 1985;31:104.

57. Chamberlain G, Carron-Brown J. Gynaecological Laparoscopy: the report of the working party of the confidential enquiry into gynaecological laparoscopy. London, Royal College of Obstetrics and Gynaecology, 1978.

58. Phillips J, Hulka J, Keith D, Hulka B, Keith L. Laparoscopic procedures: a national survey for 1975. J Reprod Med 1977;18:219.

59. Peterson HB, Hulka J, Phillips JM. American Association of Gynecologic Laparoscopists 1988 membership survey on operative laparoscopy. J Reprod Med 1990;35:587.

60. Phillips JM, Hulka B, Hulka J, Keith D, Keith L. Laparoscopic procedures: the American Association of Gynecologic Laparoscopists membership survey for 1975. J Reprod Med 1977;18:227.

61. Phillips JM, Hulka JF, Peterson HB. American Association of Gynecologic Laparoscopists 1982 membership survey. J Reprod Med 1984;29:592.

62. Jacobaeus HC. Possibility of the use of the cystoscope for investigation of serous cavities. Munch Med Wochenschr 1910;57:2090.

63. Jacobaeus HC. Endopleural operations by means of a thoracoscope. Beitr Klin Tuberk 1915;35:1.

64. Jacobaeus HC. The practical importance of thoracoscopy in surgery of the chest. Surg Gynecol Obstet 1922;34:209.

65. Jacobaeus HC. The cauterization of adhesions in pneumothorax treatment of tuberculosis. Surg Gynecol Obstet 1921;32:493.

66. Smythe WR, Kaiser LR. History of thoracoscopic surgery. In: Kaiser LR, Daniel TM, eds. Thorascopic surgery. Boston, Little, Brown, 1993:5.

67. Miller JI. Economics of thoracoscopic surgery. In: Kaiser LR, Daniel TM, eds. Thorascopic surgery. Boston, Little, Brown, 1993:255.

68. Johnson SH, Douglas JM. Diagnostic thoracoscopy. In: Pappas TN, Schwartz LB, Eubanks S, eds. Atlas of laparoscopic surgery. Philadelphia, Current Medicine, 1996:24.3.

69. Mack MJ, Shennib H, Landreneau RJ, Hazelrigg SR. Techniques for localization of pulmonary nodules for thoracoscopic resection. J Thorac Cardiovasc Surg 1993;106:550.

70. Landreneau RJ, Hazelrigg SR, Ferson PF, et al. Thoracoscopic resection of 85 pulmonary lesions. Ann Thorac Surg 1992;54:415.

71. Allen MS, Deschamps C, Lee RE, et al. Video-assisted thoracoscopic stapled wedge excision for indeterminant pulmonary nodules. J Thorac Cardiovasc Surg 1993;106:1048.

72. Kaiser LR, Bavaria JE. Complications of thoracoscopy. Ann Thorac Surg 1993;56:796.

73. Santambrogio L, Nosotti M, Bellaviti N, Mezetti M. Videothoracoscopy versus thoracotomy for the diagnosis of the indeterminant solitary pulmonary nodule. Ann Thorac Surg 1995;59:868.

74. DeCamp MM, Jaklitsch MT, Mentzer SJ, Harpole DH, Sugarbaker DJ. The safety and versatility of video-thoracoscopy: a prospective analysis of 895 cases. J Am Coll Surg 1995;181:113.

75. Mault JR, Harpole DH, Douglas JM. Thoracoscopic pulmonary resection. In: Pappas TN, Schwartz LB, Eubanks S, eds. Atlas of laparoscopic surgery. Philadelphia, Current Medicine, 1996;26:10.

STOMACH AND DUODENUM

SURGERY: SCIENTIFIC PRINCIPLES AND PRACTICE, Second Edition, edited by
Lazar J. Greenfield, Michael W. Mulholland, Keith T. Oldham, Gerald B. Zelenock,
and Keith D. Lillemoe. Lippincott–Raven Publishers, Philadelphia, © 1997.

CHAPTER 21

GASTRIC ANATOMY AND PHYSIOLOGY

MICHAEL W. MULHOLLAND

GROSS ANATOMY

The stomach and duodenum, along with the esophagus, liver, bile ducts, and pancreas, are derived from the embryonic foregut. During the 5th week of gestation, the future stomach is marked as a dilation in the caudal portion of the foregut. Cranial to this dilation, the trachea forms as a bud from the future esophagus. At this time, the primitive stomach is invested with both ventral and dorsal mesenteries. The embryonic ventral mesentery is represented in postnatal life by the falciform ligament and by the gastrohepatic and hepatoduodenal mesenteries that form the lesser omentum. The celiac artery, the major blood supply to the foregut, passes within the dorsal mesentery. The primitive dorsal mesentery ultimately forms three structures—the gastrocolic ligament, the gastrosplenic ligament, and the gastrophrenic ligament.

During the 6th and 7th weeks of gestation, the typical morphology of the stomach is established. Accelerated growth of the left gastric wall, relative to the right, establishes the greater and lesser curvatures. This unequal growth also rotates the stomach and causes the left vagal nerve trunk to assume its anterior position, whereas the right vagal trunk is located posteriorly. The growth of structures cephalad to the stomach cause the organ to descend. During the 6th week, the primitive stomach lies between the 10th and 12th thoracic segments. By the 8th week, the stomach is located between the 11th thoracic and the 4th lumbar segments. In adult life, the stomach is most commonly located between the 10th thoracic and the 3rd lumbar vertebral segments.

The stomach can be divided into anatomic regions based on external landmarks (Fig. 21-1). Although this division is commonly referred to in surgical texts and is useful in discussing gastric resective procedures, it does not necessarily reflect the secretory or motor functions of the mucosal and muscular layers of the stomach. The gastric cardia is the region of the stomach just distal to the gastroesophageal junction. The fundus is the portion of the stomach above and to the left of the gastroesophageal junction. The corpus constitutes the region between the fundus and the antrum. The margin between corpus and antrum is not distinct externally, but can be defined arbitrarily by a line from the incisura angularis on the lesser curvature to a point one fourth of the distance from the pylorus to the esophagus along the greater curvature. The gastric antrum is bounded distally by the pylorus, which can be appreciated by palpation as a thickened ring of smooth muscle.

The stomach is mobile in most individuals and is fixed at only two points—proximally by the gastroesophageal junction and distally by the retroperitoneal duodenum. Therefore, the position of the stomach varies and depends on the habitus of the person, the degree of gastric distention, and the position of the other abdominal organs. Anteriorly, the stomach is in contact with the left hemidiaphragm, the left lobe and the anterior segment of the right lobe of the liver, and the anterior parietal surface of the abdominal wall. The posterior surface of the stomach is related to the left diaphragm, the left kidney and left adrenal gland, the neck, tail, and body of the pancreas, the aorta and celiac trunk, and the periaortic nerve plexuses. The greater curvature of the stomach is in proximity to the transverse colon and the transverse colonic mesentery. The concavity of the spleen contacts the left lateral portion of the stomach.

The stomach is an extremely well-vascularized organ, supplied by a number of major arteries and protected by a large number of extramural and intramural collaterals. Gastric viability can be preserved after ligation of all but one primary artery, an advantage that can be exploited during gastric reconstructive procedures. The rich network of anastomosing vessels also means that gastric hemorrhage cannot be controlled by the extramural ligation of gastric arteries. Most gastric blood flow is ordinarily derived from the celiac trunk (Fig. 21-2). The lesser curvature is supplied by the left gastric artery, which is the first major branch of the celiac trunk, and by the right gastric artery, which is derived from the hepatic artery. Branches of the left gastric artery also supply the lowermost portion of the esophagus. The greater curvature is supplied by the short gastric and left gastroepiploic arteries, which are branches of the splenic artery, and by the right gastroepiploic artery, a branch of the gastroduodenal artery. In instances of celiac trunk occlusion, gastric blood flow is usually maintained from the superior mesenteric artery collaterally by way of the pancreaticoduodenal arcade. In general, venous effluent from the stomach parallels the arterial supply. The venous equivalent of the left gastric artery is the coronary vein.

As a first approximation, the lymphatic drainage of the stomach parallels gastric venous return (Fig. 21-3). Lymph from the proximal portion of the stomach along the lesser curvature first drains into superior gastric lymph nodes surrounding the left gastric artery. The distal portion of the lesser curvature drains through suprapyloric nodes. The proximal portion of the greater curvature is supplied by lymphatic vessels that traverse pancreaticosplenic nodes, whereas the antral portion of the greater curvature drains into the subpyloric and omental nodal groups. Secondary drainage from each of these systems eventually traverses nodes at the base of the celiac axis. These discrete anatomic groupings are misleading. The lymphatic drain-

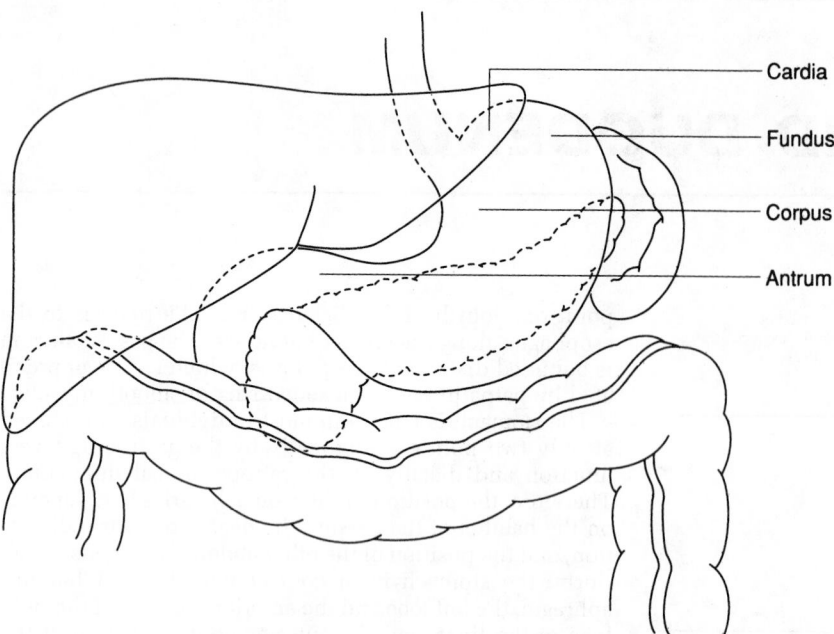

Figure 21-1. Topographic relations of the stomach.

age of the human stomach, like its blood supply, exhibits extensive intramural ramifications and a number of extramural communications. As a consequence, disease processes that involve the gastric lymphatics often spread intramurally beyond the region of origin and to nodal groups at a distance from the primary lymphatic zone.

The left and right vagal nerves descend parallel to the esophagus within the thorax before forming a periesophageal plexus between the tracheal bifurcation and the diaphragm. From this plexus, two vagal trunks coalesce before passing through the esophageal hiatus of the diaphragm

(Fig. 21-4). The left vagal trunk is usually closely applied to the anterior surface of the esophagus, whereas the posterior vagal trunk is often midway between the esophagus and the aorta. The anterior vagus supplies a hepatic division, which passes to the right in the lesser omentum before innervating the liver and biliary tract. The remainder of the anterior vagal fibers parallel the lesser curvature of the stomach, branching to the anterior gastric wall. The posterior vagus nerve branches into the celiac division, which passes to the celiac plexus, and a posterior gastric division, which innervates the posterior gastric wall.

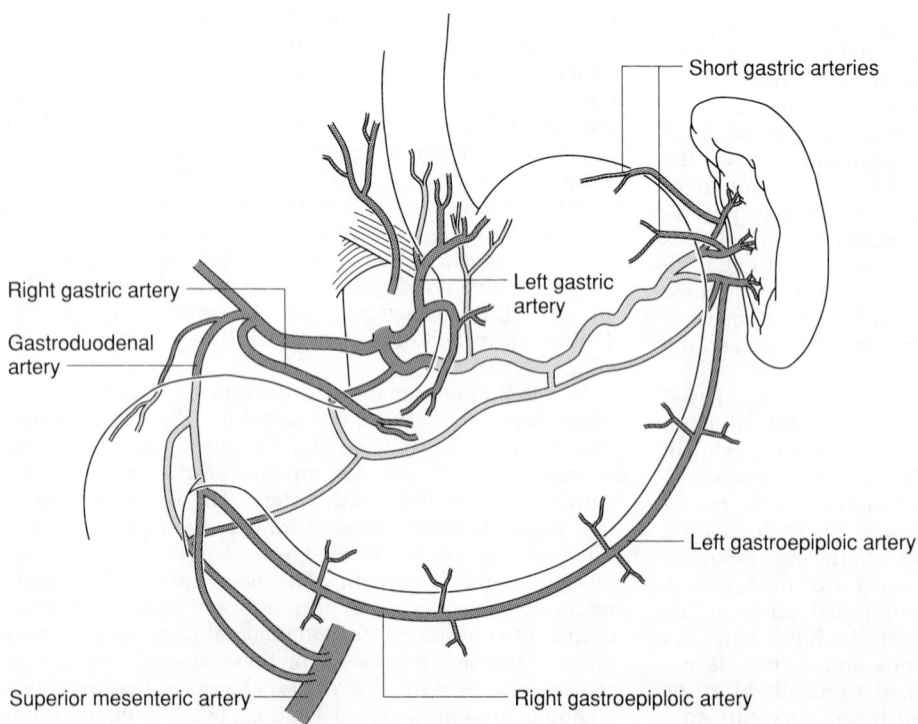

Figure 21-2. Arterial blood supply of the stomach.

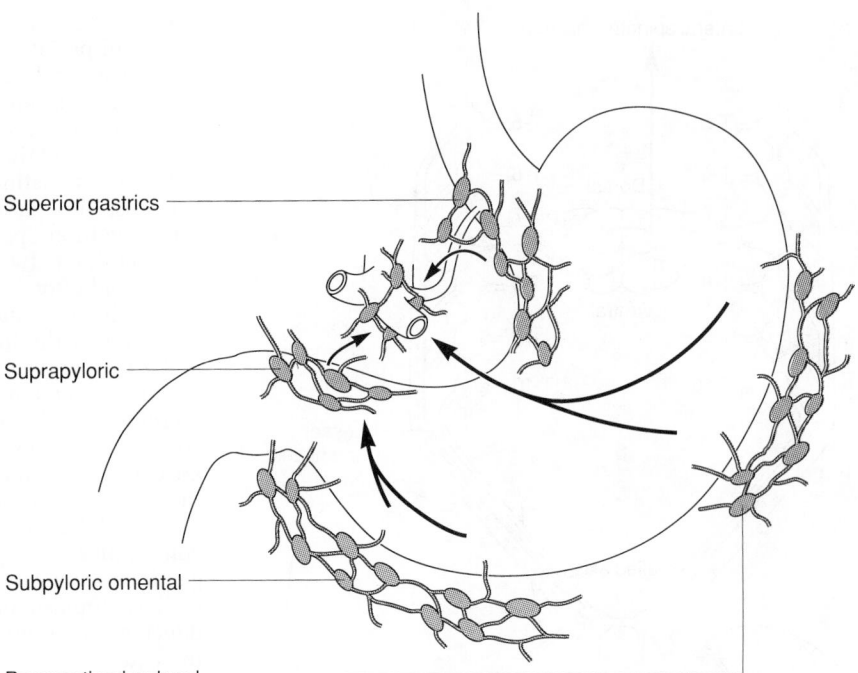

Superior gastrics

Suprapyloric

Subpyloric omental

Pancreaticoduodenal

Figure 21-3. Lymphatic drainage of the stomach.

About 90% of the fibers in the vagal trunks are afferent, transmitting information from the gastrointestinal tract to the central nervous system. Parasympathetic afferent fibers are not responsible for the sensation of gastric pain. Surprisingly, only 10% of vagal nerve fibers are motor or secretory efferents. Parasympathetic efferent fibers contained in the vagus originate in the dorsal nucleus of the medulla. Vagal efferent fibers pass without synapse to contact postsynaptic neurons in the gastric wall in the myenteric and submucous plexuses. Secondary neurons directly innervate gastric smooth muscle or epithelial cells. Acetylcholine is the neurotransmitter of primary vagal efferent neurons.

The gastric sympathetic innervation is derived from spinal segments T-5 through T-10. Sympathetic fibers leave the corresponding spinal nerve roots by way of gray rami communicantes and enter a series of bilateral prevertebral ganglia (Fig. 21-5). From these ganglia, presynaptic fibers pass through the greater splanchnic nerves to the celiac plexus where they synapse with secondary sympathetic neurons. Postsynaptic sympathetic nerve fibers enter the stomach in association with blood vessels. Afferent sympathetic fibers pass without synapse from the stomach to dorsal spinal roots. Pain of gastroduodenal origin is sensed through afferent fibers of sympathetic origin.

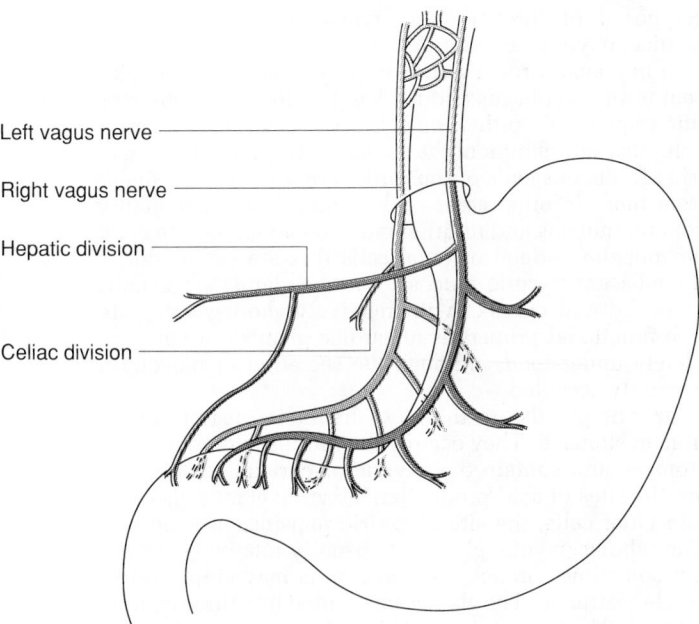

Left vagus nerve

Right vagus nerve

Hepatic division

Celiac division

Figure 21-4. Vagal innervation of the stomach.

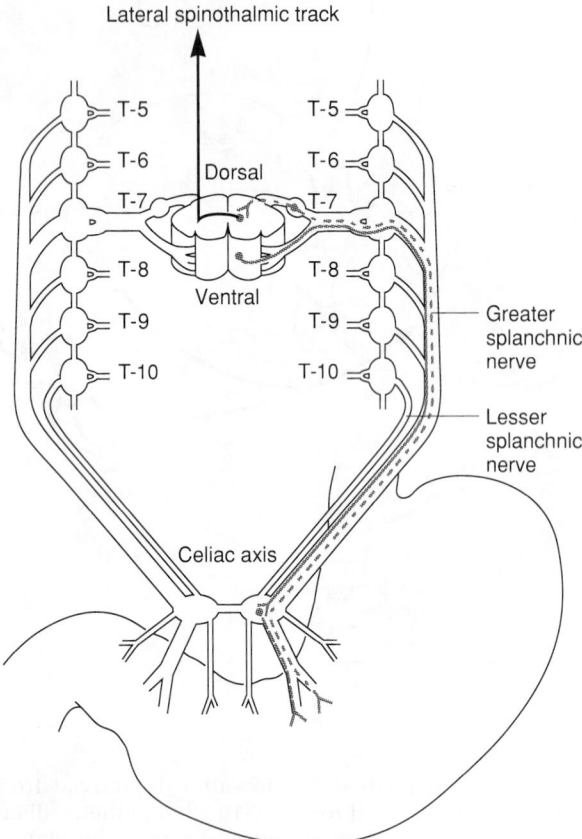

Figure 21-5. Derivation of gastric sympathetic innervation.

MICROSCOPIC ANATOMY

The glandular portions of the stomach are lined by a simple columnar epithelium composed of surface mucous cells. The luminal surface, visualized by scanning electron microscopy, appears cobblestoned, interrupted at intervals by gastric pits. Opening into the gastric pits are one or more gastric glands that impart functional significance to the gastric mucosa. The mucosa of the human stomach is composed of three distinct types of gastric glands—cardiac, oxyntic, and antral.

In humans, cardiac glands occupy a narrow zone adjacent to the esophagus and mark a transition from the stratified squamous epithelium of the esophagus to the simple columnar epithelium of the stomach. The surface and gastric pit mucous cells of the cardia are not distinguishable from those in other areas of the stomach. Cardiac glands contain mucous and undifferentiated and endocrine cells, but not the parietal or chief cells that are prominent in the adjacent oxyntic mucosa. Cardiac glands are usually branched and connect with relatively short gastric pits. The functional properties of cardiac glands are not completely understood, although the secretion of mucous is generally accepted.

Oxyntic glands are the most distinctive feature of the human stomach. They occupy the fundus and body of the stomach and contain the oxyntic or parietal cells, which are the sites of acid production. Oxyntic glands also contain chief cells, the site of gastric pepsinogen synthesis. The tubular oxyntic glands are usually relatively straight but sometimes branch; several glands may empty into a single gastric pit. The glands are divided into three regions: (1) the isthmus, containing surface mucous cells and a few

scattered parietal cells; (2) the neck, with a heavy concentration of parietal cells and a few neck mucous cells; and (3) the base of the gland, containing chief cells, undifferentiated cells, a few parietal cells, and some mucous neck cells. Endocrine cells are scattered throughout all three regions of oxyntic glands.

The most distinctive cell of the gastric mucosa is the acid-secreting parietal cell. Parietal cells have an unusual ultrastructural specialization in the form of intracellular canaliculi, a network of clefts extending to the basal cytoplasm and often encircling the nucleus, which is continuous with the gland lumen (Fig. 21-6). The surface area provided by the intracellular secretory canaliculi is large and is further magnified by microvilli lining the canaliculi. In parietal cells that are not stimulated to secrete acid, the secretory canaliculi are collapsed and inconspicuous. On stimulation, a several-fold increase in canalicular surface area occurs, the intracellular clefts become prominent, and the communication with the luminal surface is readily identified. These changes create an intracellular space in communication with the gastric lumen into which hydrogen ions are secreted at high concentration.

The cytoplasm of the parietal cell also contains an abundance of large mitochondria. Mitochondria are estimated to occupy 30% to 40% of the cytoplasmic volume of un-

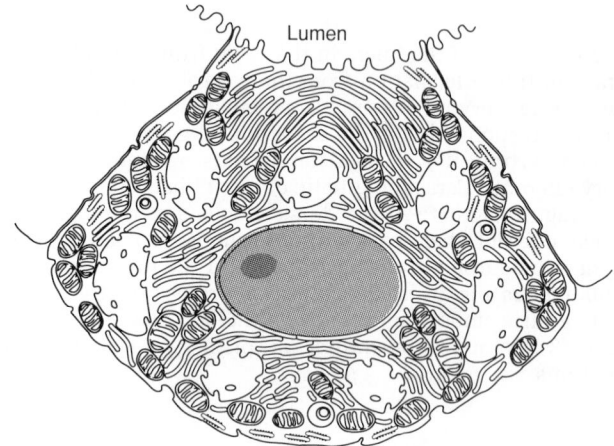

Nonsecreting parietal cell

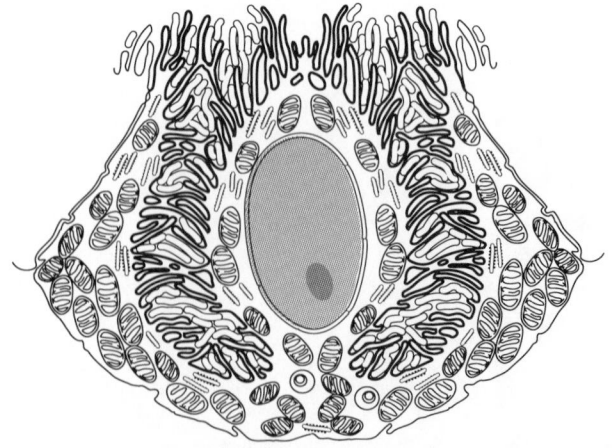

Acid-secreting parietal cell

Figure 21-6. Resting and stimulated parietal cell, emphasizing morphologic transformation with increase in secretory canalicular membrane surface area that occurs with acid secretion.

stimulated parietal cells, reflecting the extremely high oxidative activity of these cells. The oxygen consumption rate of isolated parietal cells is about five times higher than that of gastric mucous cells. The cytoplasm also contains a limited amount of rough endoplasmic reticulum, presumed to be the production site of intrinsic factor, which is also secreted by parietal cells.

In addition to parietal cells, the oxyntic glands also contain the gastric chief cells, which synthesize and secrete pepsinogen. Chief cells are most abundant in the basal region of the oxyntic glands. The cells have a morphology typical of protein-secreting exocrine cells and are similar in ultrastructural appearance to pancreatic acinar cells. Rough endoplasmic reticulum is abundant in the cytoplasm and extends between secretory granules. Zymogen granules containing pepsinogen are most concentrated within the apical cytoplasm. Pepsinogen is released by exocytosis from secretory granules at the apical surface of chief cells.

Antral glands occupy the mucosa of the distal stomach and pyloric channel. Antral glands are relatively straight and often empty through deep gastric pits. Although most cells within the antral glands are mucus secreting, gastrin cells are the distinctive feature of this mucosa. Gastrin cells are pyramid shaped, with a narrow area of luminal contact apically and a broad surface overlying the lamina propria basally (Fig. 21-7). Gastrin cells are identified immunocytochemically by the presence of the peptide. Granules ranging from 150 to 400 nm in diameter are the sites of gastrin storage and are most numerous in the basal cytoplasm. Gastrin is released by exocytotic fusion of the secretory granule with the plasma membrane. In contrast to secretion from chief cells, emptying of gastrin-containing granules occurs at the basal membrane rather than at the apical region of the cell. Gastrin thus released diffuses to and enters submucosal capillaries in close apposition to the lamina propria.

GASTRIC PEPTIDES

The stomach contains a number of biologically active peptides in nerves and mucosal endocrine cells including gastrin, somatostatin, gastrin-releasing peptide, vasoactive intestinal polypeptide (VIP), substance P, glucagon, and calcitonin gene–related peptide (CGRP). The two peptides with the greatest importance to human disease and to clinical surgery are gastrin and somatostatin.

Gastrin

The synthesis, secretion, and action of gastrin have been extensively studied, and many aspects of the biology of gastrin appear to be shared by other gastrointestinal peptide hormones.[1] The gene that encodes for gastrin has been isolated using a human DNA library. The human gene encompasses about 4100 base pairs and directs the synthesis of a peptide of 101 amino acids (Fig. 21-8). The resulting peptide, preprogastrin, contains the sequence of gastrin within its amino acid sequence. Preprogastrin consists of a signal peptide of 21 amino acids, an intervening peptide of 37 amino acids, the 34-residue region of the gastrin molecule, and a carboxy-terminal extension of 9 amino acids. Gastrin is derived from its preprohormone by the sequential enzymatic cleavage of the signal peptide, the intervening peptide, and the carboxy-terminal extension.

The signal peptide region of preprogastrin consists of a series of hydrophobic amino acids that direct the nascent peptide into the endoplasmic reticulum as it is translated from messenger RNA. After directing the preprogastrin molecule into the rough endoplasmic reticulum, the signal peptide is removed. The remaining peptide is termed *progastrin*. Progastrin is further processed as it traverses the endoplasmic reticulum to mature secretory vesicles. Enzymatic cleavage at a pair of basic amino acid residues proximal to the gastrin 34 (G_{34}) sequence removes the interven-

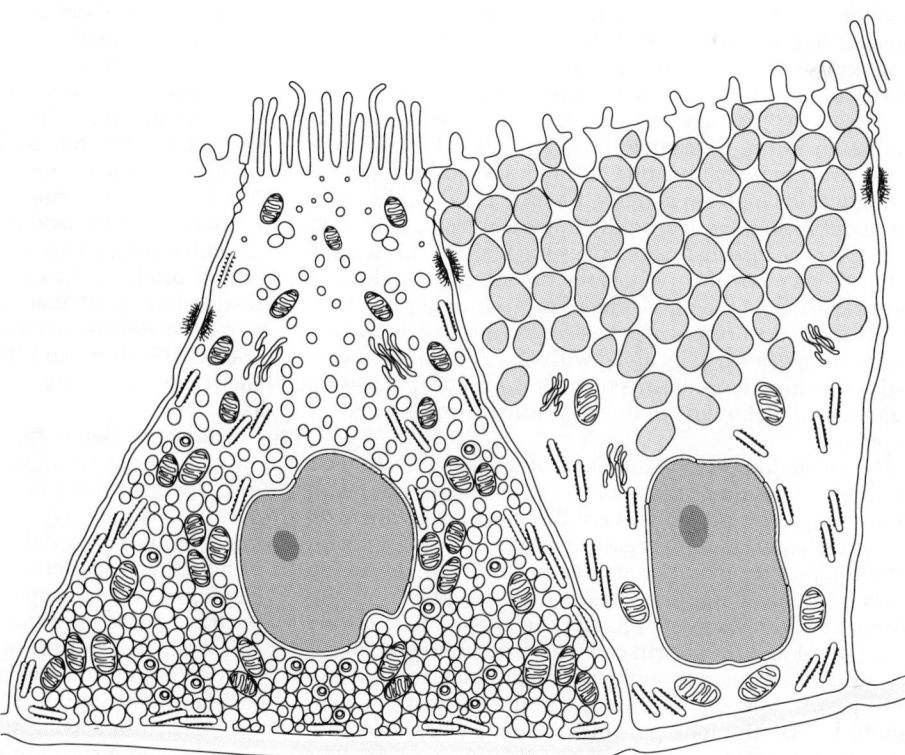

Figure 21-7. Contrasting morphology of antral gastrin cell (*left*) with basally oriented secretory granules and gastric mucous cell (*right*) with apical mucous granules.

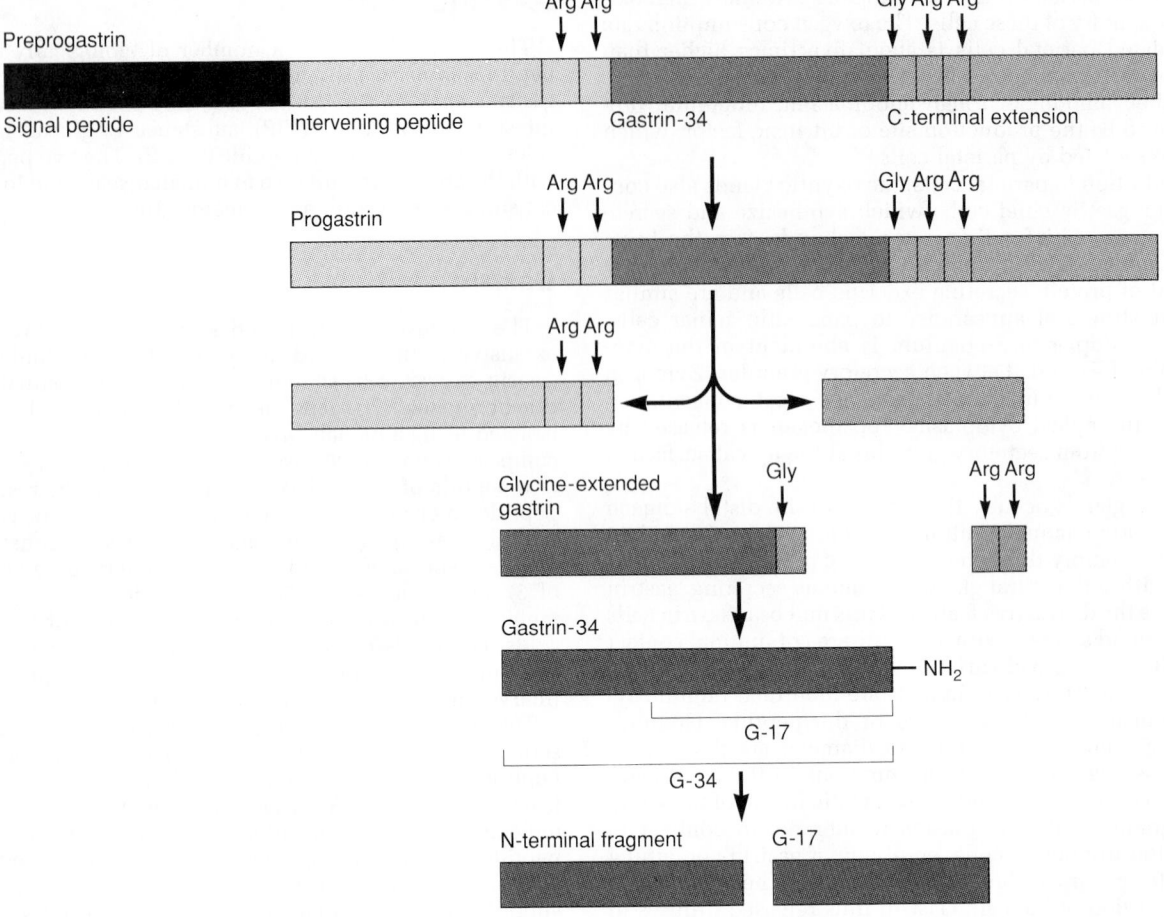

Figure 21-8. Sequential processing of preprogastrin molecule.

ing peptide. A similar cleavage removes a 6–amino acid fragment at the carboxy-terminal end. The peptide that remains has a Gly-Arg-Arg sequence at the carboxy end. Carboxypeptidase cleaves the Arg residues, and the peptide that results is termed *glycine-extended gastrin*. G_{34} is formed by cleavage of the Gly-Arg-Arg sequence and amidation of the C-terminal phenylalanine. Gastrin, like most gastrointestinal peptide hormones, requires terminal amidation for biologic activity. Gastrin 17 (G_{17}), the most abundant form of gastrin in the human antrum, is formed by further processing that removes the first 17 amino acids at the N-terminus of G_{34}. G_{34} is the predominate molecular form of gastrin in the duodenum. The various peptide fragments formed during the processing of progastrin are released from gastrin cells along with G_{17}. A number of biologic activities have been postulated for the processing fragments, although their physiologic relevance is unproved.

The most important stimulant of gastrin release is a meal. Small peptide fragments and amino acids that result from intragastric proteolysis are the most important food components that stimulate gastrin release. The most potent gastrin-releasing activities are demonstrated by the amino acids tryptophan and phenylalanine. Ingested fat and glucose do not cause gastrin release. Dietary amino acids are transported into the gastrin cell where decarboxylation enzymes convert them to amines. Intracellular amines promote gastrin release. Conditions that increase intracellular amine levels stimulate gastrin secretion, whereas conditions that prevent entry of amino acids into gastrin cells

inhibit release of the hormone. Gastric distention by a meal activates cholinergic neurons and stimulates gastrin release. As the meal empties and distention diminishes, VIP-containing neurons are activated, which stimulate somatostatin secretion, and thus attenuate gastrin secretion.

Postprandial luminal pH also strongly affects gastrin secretion. Gastrin release is inhibited when acidification of an ingested meal causes the intraluminal pH to fall below 3.0. Conversely, maintaining intragastric pH above 3.0 potentiates gastrin secretion following ingestion of protein or amino acids. Pernicious anemia and atrophic gastritis, which produce chronic achlorhydria, are associated with fasting hypergastrinemia and an exaggerated gastrin meal response. Release of mucosal somatostatin occurs with gastric acidification, and this peptide has been implicated in the inhibited gastrin release that occurs when luminal pH falls.

The vagus nerve appears to both stimulate and inhibit gastrin release. In humans, vagally mediated stimulation of gastrin release can be demonstrated by sham feeding, insulin-induced hypoglycemia, and administration of the vagal stimulant, γ-aminobutyric acid. In contrast to these stimulatory vagal effects, hypergastrinemia, observed following vagotomy, suggests that inhibitory vagal effects on gastrin release may also exist. Cholinergic neurons stimulate gastrin secretion directly by actions on gastrin cells. By decreasing somatostatin secretion, cholinergic neurons also indirectly stimulate gastrin release. Neurons that contain gastrin-releasing peptide stimulate gastrin secretion directly and also inhibit somatostatin release. In contrast,

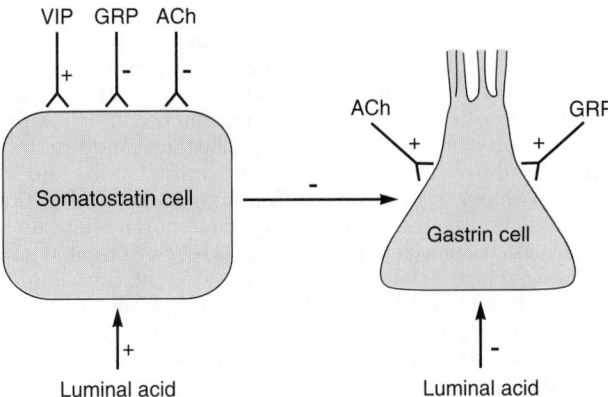

Figure 21-9. Interactions between somatostatin- and gastrin-producing cells of the gastric antrum.

neurons containing VIP stimulate secretion of somatostatin and thereby down-regulate gastrin release (Fig. 21-9). Adrenergic stimulation also increases gastrin release.

In addition to stimulating acid secretion from gastric parietal cells (detailed later in this chapter), gastrin has important physiologic actions in the control of gastrointestinal mucosal growth. The acid-secreting oxyntic mucosa is particularly sensitive to the trophic actions of gastrin, but the mucous membranes of the duodenum, colon, and pancreatic parenchyma are also affected. In animals, removing endogenous gastrin through antrectomy results in mucosal atrophy. Mucosal hypoplasia can be prevented by administering exogenous gastrin. Responsiveness to the trophic effects of gastrin is not present at birth because of the lack of mucosal gastrin receptors. Development of mucosal receptors occurs at the time of weaning and corresponds to the development of responsiveness to the trophic effects of the hormone. Stimulation of mucosal growth by gastrin is enhanced by the presence of solid food in the diet. The 17– and 34–amino acid forms of gastrin are equipotent in stimulating mucosal growth. In humans, the relative importance of gastrin and other influences, such as the composition and form of the diet and the actions of other trophic hormones, have not been completely established. Prolonged stimulation by high levels of gastrin, as seen in the Zollinger-Ellison syndrome, is associated with hypertrophy of the gastric mucosa. Smaller increases in circulating gastrin, such as those that follow vagotomy, do not cause mucosal hypertrophy.

Somatostatin

Somatostatin, like gastrin, is very significant in gastric physiology and has been investigated considerably. In addition, somatostatin and its biologically active analogues have important therapeutic applications in the treatment of digestive diseases and in gastrointestinal surgery. Somatostatin was first isolated from hypothalamic tissues and was named for its ability to inhibit the release of growth hormone. The peptide has subsequently been localized in neurons in central and peripheral nervous systems, and in endocrine cells in the pancreas, stomach, and intestine. The wide tissue distribution of somatostatin has suggested important regulatory functions, a concept validated by many investigations.

The human somatostatin gene is located on chromosome 3 and encodes for a precursor of 116 amino acids (Fig. 21-10). The somatostatin molecule is contained in the carboxy-terminal sequence of this preprohormone.[2] The first 24 amino acids of the amino terminus of preprosomatostatin constitute a signal peptide; cleavage of this signal peptide leaves prosomatostatin. Enzymatic cleavage of an additional 64–amino acid segment from prosomatostatin forms somatostatin 28.[3] Further processing of somatostatin 28 to somatostatin 14 is tissue-specifically regulated. In the stomach, most somatostatin exists as the shorter peptide.

Gastric somatostatin release responds to luminal, hormonal, and neural signals. Luminal acidification is associated with increased somatostatin release, whereas somatostatin release decreases when luminal pH is increased. A number of peptides have been demonstrated experimentally to release somatostatin from the stomach, including gastrin, cholecystokinin, and secretin. β-Adrenergic agonists have also been shown to release somatostatin. In contrast, electrical stimulation of vagal nerves inhibits somatostatin release, as does the cholinergic agonist, methacholine. By means of a paracrine feedback loop, gastrin also appears to stimulate somatostatin secretion.

The most important gastric function of somatostatin appears to be regulation of acid secretion and gastrin release. Circulating somatostatin appears to be important in modulating gastric acid secretion; locally released somatostatin

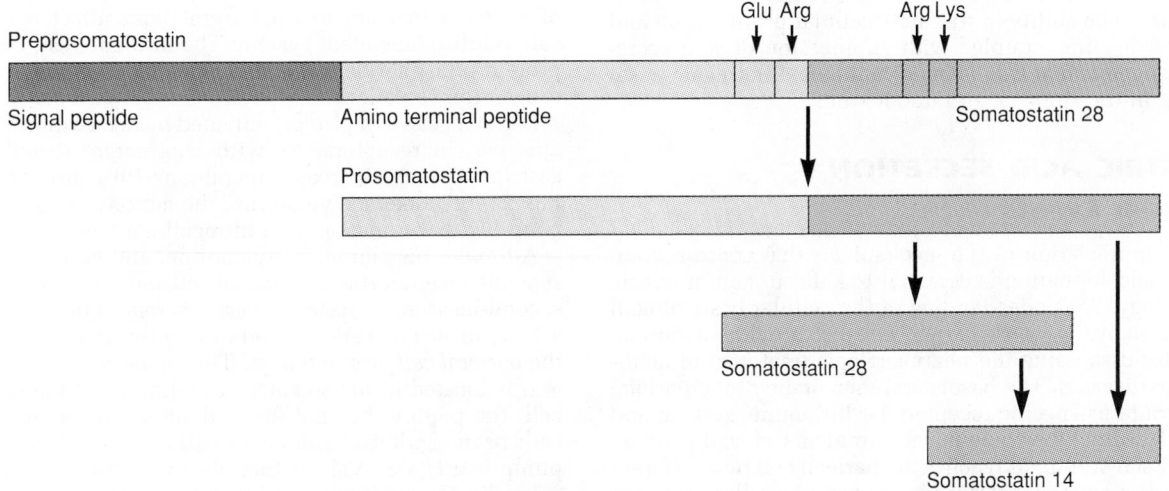

Figure 21-10. Derivation of somatostatin 14 from preprosomatostatin precursor.

functions to regulate gastrin release. In each instance, somatostatin serves an inhibitory function, decreasing acid secretion and diminishing the release of gastrin. In animals, antral or duodenal acidification has been associated with an increase in circulating somatostatin. Increases in circulating somatostatin are followed, in turn, by decreased gastric acid secretion. Infusion of exogenous somatostatin in doses that produce somatostatin levels similar to those observed postprandially has also been shown to inhibit acid secretion. In humans, concentrations of somatostatin capable of inhibiting acid secretion can do so without altering serum gastrin levels, indicating a direct action on the acid-secreting fundic mucosa.

Somatostatin is crucial in modulating gastrin release. Somatostatin is believed to influence gastrin secretion through a locally active intramucosal mechanism. Local actions of somatostatin are supported by ultrastructural studies of antral somatostatin cells, which demonstrate long cytoplasmic processes that make intimate cell-to-cell contact with antral gastrin cells. The presence of somatostatin at these sites of cellular contact imply that somatostatin cells influence the function of gastrin cells through local release of the peptide. Somatostatin can also reach neighboring gastrin cells through diffusion or local blood flow. A number of experiments have suggested that release of somatostatin and gastrin are functionally, although reciprocally, linked. For example, in anesthetized animals, increases in gastric pH or ingestion of a meal are associated with increases in gastrin and decreases in somatostatin in antral venous blood. Cholinergic agents stimulate gastrin release while inhibiting somatostatin release. Prostaglandin E_2, in contrast, inhibits gastrin release and stimulates somatostatin secretion. These and similar observations suggest that increases in somatostatin release are often associated with decreased gastrin secretion. The cellular mechanisms by which somatostatin inhibits gastrin release from antral gastrin cells have not been fully characterized.

EPIDERMAL GROWTH FACTOR

Epidermal growth factor (EGF) is a 53–amino acid peptide, synthesized by salivary and Brunner glands and secreted into the lumen of the digestive tract. EGF shares sequence homolgy with transforming growth factor-α and occupies the same cell surface receptor. EGF is a mitigen and stimulates proliferation of gastric and duodenal epithelial cells. EGF increases cellular proliferation through a transmembrane receptor with tyrosine kinase activity. EGF has also been reported to induce angiogenesis. Importantly, the peptide also inhibits gastric acid secretion in humans. The ability to stimulate cellular proliferation and wound healing, coupled with suppression of acid secretion, suggests that EGF is important in facilitating mucosal repair in the stomach and duodenum.

GASTRIC ACID SECRETION
Cellular Events

An appreciation of the mechanisms that control stomach's acid formation is essential to a discussion of gastric pathology. An understanding of the cellular basis of acid secretion by the gastric parietal cell also provides a foundation for discussing the pharmacologic treatment of acid–peptic diseases. The basolateral membrane of the parietal cell contains specific receptors for histamine, gastrin, and acetylcholine, the three major stimulants of acid production. Each stimulant reaches the parietal cell by a different route. Histamine is released from mast-like cells within the lamina propria and diffuses to the mucosa; acetylcholine is released in close approximation to the parietal cells from cholinergic nerve terminals; and gastrin is delivered by the systemic circulation to the fundic mucosa from its source in the antrum and proximal duodenum (Fig. 21-11).

Histamine receptors in the gastric mucosa are classified pharmacologically as H_2 receptors because they may be stimulated by agonists such as 4-methylhistamine and selectively blocked by agents such as cimetidine. Occupation of the histamine receptor activates a membrane-bound enzyme called adenylate cyclase (Fig. 21-12). Activated adenylate cyclase catalyzes the conversion of intracellular ATP to cyclic AMP (cAMP), and enhancement of cAMP production by histamine is closely linked to stimulation of parietal cell acid production. cAMP mediates histamine-stimulated acid production by activating protein kinases, which in turn catalyze protein phosphorylation.[4] The target protein molecule for this phosphorylation and the mechanism by which this activated product stimulates acid production have yet to be defined. Evidence suggests that occupation of the H_2 receptor also activates inositol triphosphate-dependent pathways and induces increases in intracellular calcium concentrations, an example of "cross talk" among signal transduction system.[5]

Acetylcholine and related cholinergic agonists activate parietal cells after binding to muscarinic receptors. The stimulatory effects of acetylcholine and its congeners can be abolished by atropine. Studies suggest that cholinergic stimulation of parietal cell function is coupled to enhanced mobilization of intracellular calcium. The resultant transient increases in intracellular calcium activate mechanisms that stimulate acid secretion (see Fig. 21-12). Evidence also indicates that occupation of acetylcholine receptors increases turnover of specific membrane phospholipids termed *phosphatidylinositides*.[6] Based on findings in a number of cell types, acetylcholine-receptor binding is postulated to be followed by activation of membrane-associated phospholipase C. Phospholipase C acts on phosphatidylinositol-4,5 bisphosphate (PIP_2) within the plasma membrane to liberate water-soluble inositol triphosphate (IP_3) and diacylglycerol (DAG). A major action of IP_3 is to increase intracellular calcium, mainly from intracellular stores in the endoplasmic reticulum. The resulting increased cytosolic calcium interacts with calmodulin or other calcium-binding proteins. Intracellular calcium in this form is postulated to modulate parietal cell function through protein phosphorylation or enzyme activation. DAG, the second product released by hydrolysis of PIP_2, activates a class of protein kinases that are phospholipid dependent and Ca^{2+}-activated protein kinase C. Protein kinase C in turn acts to phosphorylate a set of proteins that are distinct from those affected by the calmodulin-dependent system. The ultimate result of this protein phosphorylation is parietal cell activation and hydrogen ion secretion.

Parietal cells can also be activated by occupation of specific gastrin receptors. As with cholinergic stimulation, gastrin exposure increases membrane PIP_2 turnover (see Fig. 21-12). Like acetylcholine, the actions of gastrin depend highly on increases in intracellular calcium.[7]

Although histamine, acetylcholine, and gastrin occupy separate receptors on the parietal cell and activate differing second-messenger systems, each secretagogue ultimately acts by means of a specialized ion transport system called the *parietal cell proton pump*.[8] This membrane-bound protein is located in the secretory canaliculus of the parietal cell; the peptide has not been identified in other gastric cells or in significant amounts in other organs. The proton pump is a H^+-K^+-ATPase that electroneutrally exchanges cytosolic H^+ for luminal K^+. Hydrogen ions are concentrated 2.5-million–fold within the secretory canaliculus,

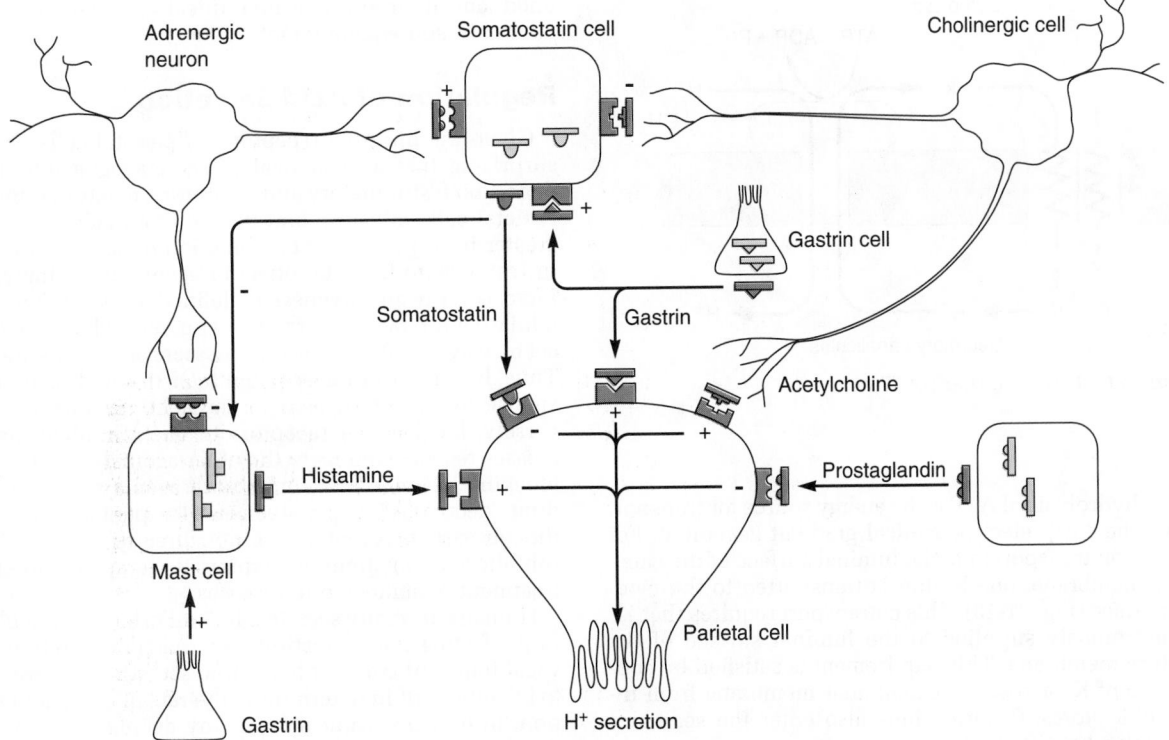

Figure 21-11. Interactions of cell types that affect parietal cell acid secretion.

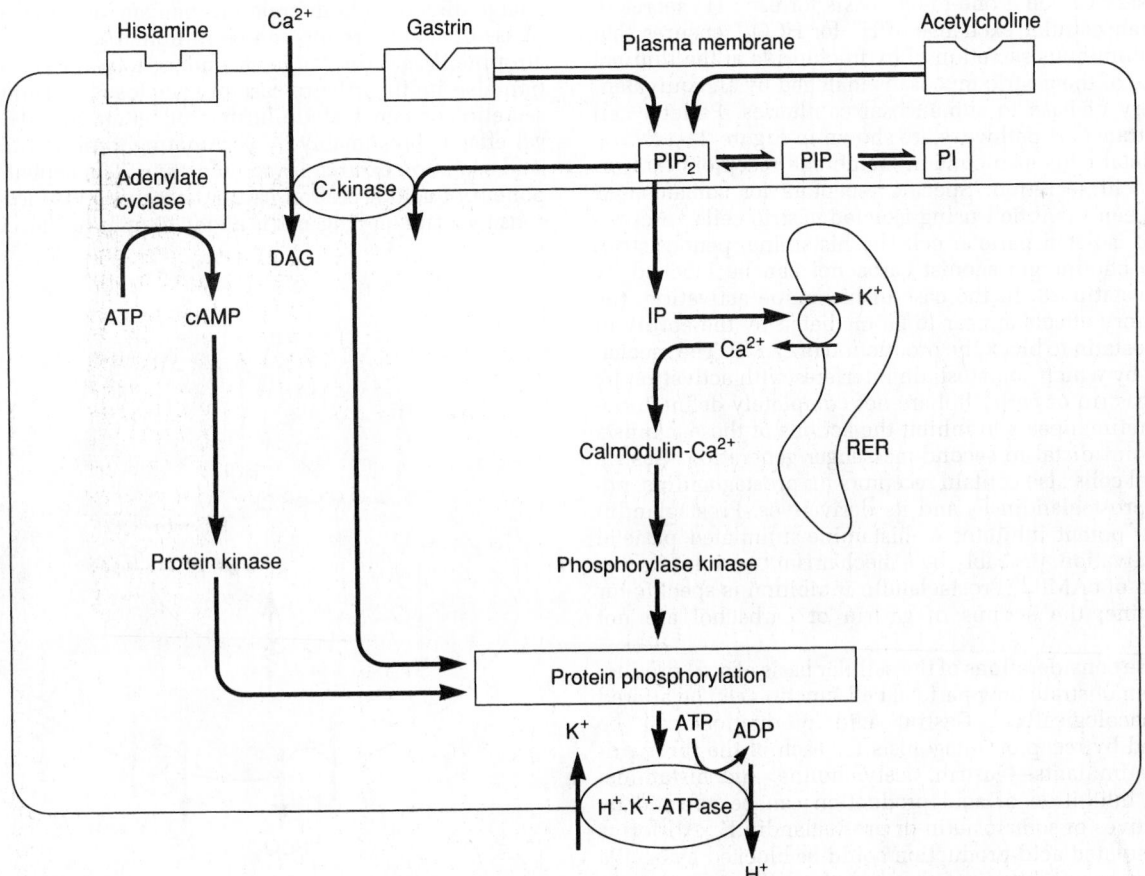

Figure 21-12. Cellular mechanisms controlling parietal cell acid secretion.

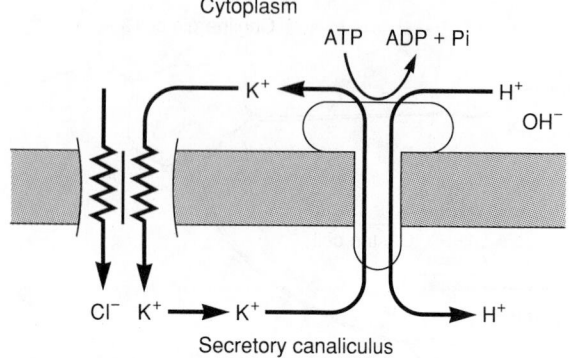

Figure 21-13. Gastric H^+-K^+-ATPase.

and the hydrolysis of ATP is the energy source for transport against the steep electrochemical gradient generated. For each H^+ ion transported to the luminal surface of the canalicular membrane, one K^+ ion is transported to the cytosolic surface (Fig. 21-13). This cotransport requires that K^+ be continuously supplied to the luminal surface of the secretory membrane. This requirement is satisfied by conductance of K^+ across the canalicular membrane from intracellular stores. Chloride ions also enter the secretory canaliculus by diffusion.

Activation of the H^+-K^+-ATPase significantly increases intracellular OH^- generation, with potential cellular toxicity. Carbonic anhydrase, which is associated with the canalicular membrane, converts OH^- to HCO_3^-. The HCO_3^- produced is disposed of by exchange for Cl^- at the basolateral membrane. Intracellular Cl^- thus acquired supplies the necessary Cl^- on a one-to-one basis for each H^+ secreted. The transcellular exchange of H^+ for HCO_3^- ensures that the voluminous secretion of hydrochloride at the luminal surface of the gastric mucosa is matched by an equivalent delivery of base to submucosal capillaries. Parietal cell ionic transport pathways are shown in Figure 21-14.

Parietal cells also contain membrane receptors that inhibit acid secretion. Specific receptors for somatostatin have been identified using isolated gastric cells.[9] Activation of isolated parietal cells by histamine, pentagastrin, or the cholinergic agonist carbachol can be blocked by somatostatin 28. In the case of histamine activation, the inhibitory effects appear to be mediated by the ability of somatostatin to block the production of cAMP. The mechanisms by which somatostatin interferes with activation by pentagastrin or carbachol are not completely defined. Somatostatin appears to inhibit the actions of these agonists at a point distal to second-messenger generation. Gastric parietal cells also contain receptors for prostaglandins, notably prostaglandin E_2 and its derivatives. Prostaglandin E_2 is a potent inhibitor of histamine-stimulated parietal cell activation, probably by a mechanism that inhibits formation of cAMP.[10] Prostaglandin inhibition is specific for histamine; the actions of gastrin or carbachol are not affected.

These considerations of the cellular basis of acid production demonstrate how parietal cell function can be altered pharmacologically.[11] Gastric acid production can be blocked by receptor antagonists for each of the three primary stimulants—gastrin, acetylcholine, and histamine. Direct inhibition of acid production can be affected by derivatives of somatostatin or prostaglandin E_2. All forms of stimulated acid production could be blocked by agents that act as inhibitors of the parietal cell proton pump. Agents that act at each of these points have been developed, and their appropriate clinical applications are discussed in subsequent chapters.

Regulation of Acid Secretion

Given the multiple receptors on parietal cells, it is not surprising that a great deal of secretagogue interdependence, both stimulatory and inhibitory, exists in humans.[12] Parietal cell activation and the resultant acid secretion is greater in response to a combination of agonists than it is in response to the total effect of agents used singly. This increase in responsiveness is defined as *potentiation*. Potentiating interactions are most apparent when agents that act by way of different second-messenger systems are used. Thus, histamine strongly potentiates the acid secretory response to pentagastrin or to carbachol in humans. Conversely, blockade of receptors to one stimulant also decreases responsiveness to the other agonists. For example, blocking histamine receptors with agents such as cimetidine decreases responsiveness to pentagastrin, even though gastrin receptors are not directly affected. These inhibitory interactions are exploited therapeutically in the treatment of acid–peptic diseases.

Humans normally secrete 2 to 5 mEq/h of hydrochloride in the fasting state, constituting basal acid secretion. Both vagal tone and ambient histamine secretion are presumed to be important in determining the rate of basal acid secretion. In humans, truncal vagotomy decreases basal secretion by about 85%. Similarly, H_2-receptor antagonists also inhibit basal acid secretion by about 80%. Gastrin does not have an important role in determining basal acid secretion in normal persons.

Stimulated acid secretion begins with the thought, sight, or smell of food (Fig. 21-15). This cephalic phase of gastric acid secretion is mediated by the vagus nerve. Vagal discharge directs a cholinergic mechanism, and the cephalic phase of acid secretion can be inhibited by administering atropine. Vagal discharge secondary to cephalic stimulation also inhibits the release of somatostatin. Diminished secretion of somatostatin further augments stimulatory vagal effects, presumably by eliminating tonic inhibition of acid secretion exerted by somatostatin. The cephalic component of acid secretion can be measured in normal persons by sham feeding and is about 10 mEq/h. The cephalic

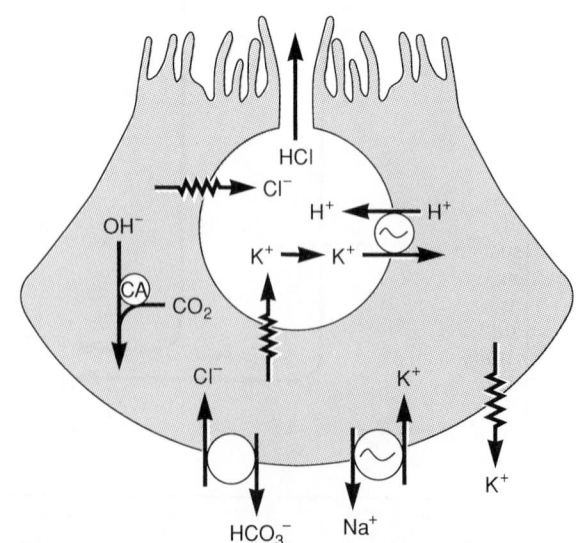

Figure 21-14. Ionic fluxes associated with acid secretion by the parietal cell.

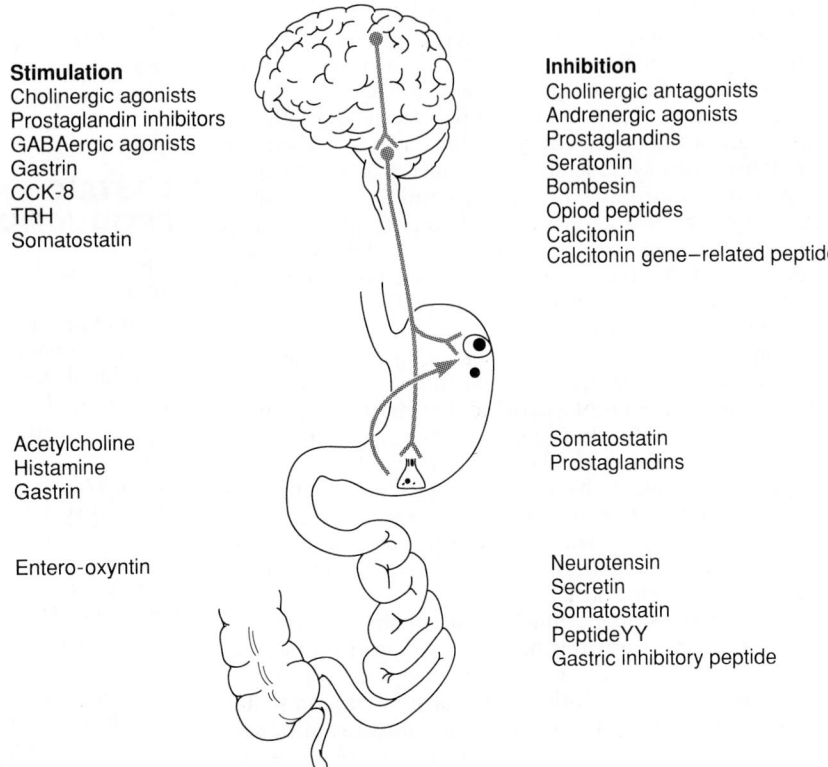

Stimulation
Cholinergic agonists
Prostaglandin inhibitors
GABAergic agonists
Gastrin
CCK-8
TRH
Somatostatin

Inhibition
Cholinergic antagonists
Andrenergic agonists
Prostaglandins
Seratonin
Bombesin
Opiod peptides
Calcitonin
Calcitonin gene–related peptide

Acetylcholine
Histamine
Gastrin

Somatostatin
Prostaglandins

Entero-oxyntin

Neurotensin
Secretin
Somatostatin
PeptideYY
Gastric inhibitory peptide

Figure 21-15. Regulation of acid secretion in vivo.

phase approximates 40% of the maximal acid secretory response to gastrin infusion.

The gastric phase of acid secretion begins when food enters the stomach. The presence of partially hydrolyzed food constituents, gastric distention, and the buffering capacity of food all stimulate acid secretion. Gastrin is the most important mediator of the gastric phase of acid secretion. In normal humans, acid secretory rates following a mixed meal average 15 to 25 mEq/h, about 75% of the maximal response achieved with infusion of exogenous gastrin or histamine. The meal response is less than the maximal response to exogenous stimulants because food also causes the release of somatostatin and initiates other inhibitory responses.

The inhibitory regulation of gastric acid secretion is accomplished by central nervous system, gastric, and intestinal mechanisms. Stimulated acid secretion can be inhibited experimentally by administering various neuropeptides into the lateral cerebral ventricles. These include gastrin-releasing peptide (bombesin), corticotropin-releasing factor, and CGRP. Although the relevance of these observations to human physiology remains to be determined, it is likely that central nervous system inhibition of acid secretion exists in humans. In this regard, the vagus nerve has both a stimulatory and an inhibitory role in acid secretion and gastrin release. Vagotomy causes fasting and postprandial hypergastrinemia, indicating that an inhibitory regulation of gastrin release normally exists. Hypergastrinemia is sustained long term after vagotomy by hyperplasia of antral gastrin cells. The vagal fibers to the oxyntic region of the stomach appear to mediate this inhibitory effect.

In humans, the most important and clearly established gastric inhibitory influence is the suppression of gastrin release when the antral mucosa is exposed to acid. When luminal pH falls to 2.0, gastrin release stops. Antral acidification also suppresses the gastrin response to an ingested

meal. Somatostatin acting locally within the gastric mucosa as a paracrine agent may mediate this important inhibitory response. Release of gastric somatostatin is reciprocally linked to that of gastrin; acidification of the antrum causes increases in somatostatin release and decreases in gastrin secretion. Antral distention also inhibits stimulated acid secretion, but it is not known whether this inhibition is neurally or hormonally mediated.

The entry of digestive products into the intestine begins intestinal phase inhibition of gastric acid secretion. Acidification of the duodenal bulb inhibits acid secretion, and although exogenous secretin also can inhibit acid secretion, this effect appears to be independent of the release of secretin from the duodenal mucosa. Hyperosmolar solutions and those containing fat also potently inhibit acid secretion. Several peptides, including secretin, somatostatin, peptide YY, gastric inhibitory peptide, and neurotensin, have been proposed as mediators of the intestinal phase effects. Each inhibits acid secretion experimentally. Their physiologic relevance remains to be determined.

PEPSIN

Pepsins are a heterogeneous group of proteolytic enzymes that are secreted by the gastric chief cells. Pepsin is derived under acidic conditions from pepsinogen by the autocatalytic loss of a variable N-terminal sequence of the parent compound. This conversion occurs slowly at pH values of 5.0 to 6.0 and occurs rapidly when luminal pH approximates 2.0. Pepsin catalyzes the hydrolysis of a wide variety of peptide bonds that contain acidic residues, with a pH optimum for hydrolysis between 1.5 and 2.5. Once activated, pepsin is sensitive to ambient pH values; it is irreversibly denatured at pH 7.0 or greater. In mammals, there are at least seven distinct pepsinogens, distinguished by electrophoretic mobility and representing varying isozymes of the enzyme. The pepsinogen isozymes can be distinguished in plasma and urine, and substantial effort has been expended to identify patterns of pepsinogen secretion in human disease. To date, such measurements have not been of significant clinical value.

The most important stimulus for pepsinogen secretion is cholinergic stimulation. Acetylcholine and its derivatives stimulate pepsinogen secretion by a mechanism that can be antagonized by atropine, indicating a muscarinic receptor. The receptor appears to have a high affinity for the selective muscarinic antagonist, pirenzepine, and therefore appears to be an M_1 type. Endogenous cholinergic stimulation through the vagal nerve results in the formation of a gastric secretion that is rich in pepsin. Although both exogenous histamine and gastrin can stimulate pepsin secretion, their actions appear to be indirectly due to the concomitant secretion of gastric acid rather than to direct stimulation of chief cells. Chief cells have also been shown to possess cholecystokinin receptors, and cholecystokinin-like peptides appear to have a direct stimulatory action on chief cells. The oxyntic mucosa contains somatostatin cells in proximity to chief cells. Pepsinogen secretion in response to a variety of stimuli has been demonstrated to be inhibited by somatostatin.

The major physiologic function of pepsin is to initiate protein digestion. Pepsin is highly active against collagen and may be important in the digestion of animal protein. Intragastric protein hydrolysis by pepsin is incomplete, and relatively large peptides enter the intestine, although amino acids and small peptide fragments are released. These products of partial hydrolysis are important signals for gastrin and cholecystokinin release, which in turn regulate digestive processes. In this way, pepsin also contributes to the overall coordination of the digestive process.

INTRINSIC FACTOR

The gastric mucosa is also the site of production of intrinsic factor, which is necessary for the absorption of cobalamin from the ileal mucosa. Total gastrectomy is regularly followed by cobalamin malabsorbtion, as is resection of the proximal stomach or atrophic gastritis that involves the oxyntic mucosa. Autoradiographic and immunocytochemical techniques have confirmed the parietal cell as the site of intrinsic factor synthesis and storage in humans. Intrinsic factor secretion, like acid secretion, is stimulated by histamine, acetylcholine, and gastrin. Unlike acid production, intrinsic factor secretion peaks rapidly after stimulation and then returns to baseline. The amount of intrinsic factor secreted usually greatly exceeds the amount needed to bind and absorb available dietary cobalamin. The role of intrinsic factor in cobalamin physiology is discussed in greater detail in Chapter 26.

GASTRIC BICARBONATE PRODUCTION

It is generally agreed that the gastric mucosa secretes HCO_3^- in addition to acid. The cells responsible for HCO_3^- production are presumed to be the surface mucous cells facing the gastric lumen, and HCO_3^- transport has been postulated to protect against damage from luminal acid.[13] In theory, H^+ ions diffusing from luminal bulk fluids toward the gastric mucosa could be neutralized by secreted HCO_3^- in close proximity to the surface (Fig. 21-16). In this way, nearly neutral pH could be maintained at the mucosal surface, even if the total amount of hydrochloride secreted greatly exceeded gastric HCO_3^- production. The occurrence of pH gradients at the surface of the gastric mucosa have been demonstrated in humans using microelectrodes. Drugs or chemicals that inhibit bicarbonate secretion result in acidification of the mucosal surface.

The degree of luminal acidity, reflected by pH, required to stimulate bicarbonate secretion is greater in the stomach than in the duodenum. Direct exposure of the gastric mucosa to pH levels of 2.0 or more increases bicarbonate secretion. In the duodenum, exposure of the mucosa to pH 5.0 doubles bicarbonate secretion, while exposure to pH 2.0 increases alkaline secretion 10-fold.

Local neural reflexes are important in mediating gastroduodenal bicarbonate secretion. Destruction of afferent (sensory) gastric neurons by the toxin capsaicin decreases the alkaline response to acid as does blocking intramural neural transmission with the ganglionic blocker called hexamethonium. In humans, vagally-stimulated duodenal bicarbonate secretion is not affected by atropine. The active vagal transmitter has not been identified with certainty, but appears to be VIP.

Therapeutically important inhibitors of gastric acid secretion, such as omeprazole or the H_2-receptor antagonists, do not affect gastroduodenal bicarbonate secretion. Sucralfate and other aluminum-containing compounds have been reported to increase bicarbonate secretion in humans.

Cholinergic agonists, vagal nerve stimulation, and sham feeding have all been shown to increase gastric HCO_3^- production. The effects of cholinergic stimulation can be

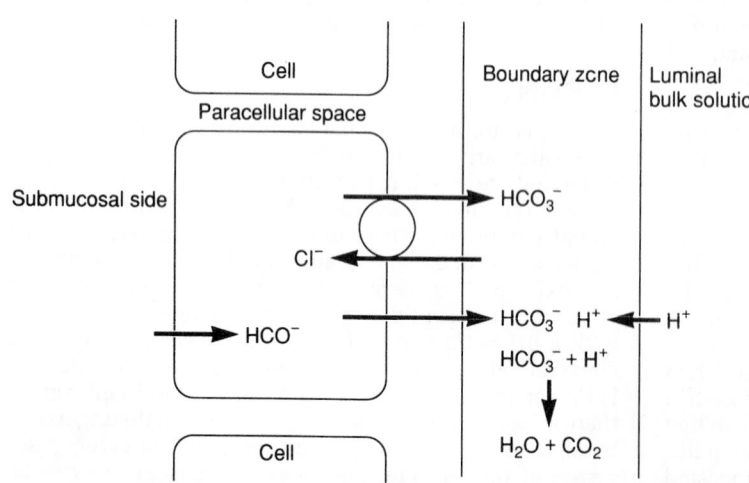

Figure 21-16. Schematic representation of mucosal bicarbonate secretion, showing neutralization of luminal hydrogen ions immediately above the mucosal surface.

blocked by atropine. In the human stomach, exposure to luminal perfusates at pH 2.0 has been associated with increased release of prostaglandin E_2. Prostaglandin E_2 and its synthetic derivatives are also potent stimulants of gastric bicarbonate secretion. Because mucosal bicarbonate production can be decreased in experimental models by indomethacin, endogenous prostaglandins are thought to be important in the mucosal alkaline response.

GASTRIC BLOOD FLOW

Because the gastric mucosa is metabolically highly active, control of mucosal blood flow is of great physiologic importance. In addition, studies have implicated perfusion abnormalities in the development of mucosal lesions during periods of stress. Mucosal blood flow is regulated by neural, hormonal, and locally active influences.[14]

Postganglionic sympathetic nerve fibers reach the stomach in association with its blood supply and richly innervate small mucosal arteries. Mucosal capillaries do not receive adrenergic innervation. Electrical stimulation of sympathetic nerves supplying the stomach is followed by decreased total gastric blood flow, decreased flow within celiac and gastroepiploic vessels, and diminished blood flow to the mucosa. With prolonged sympathetic stimulation, blood flow gradually increases to a new steady-state level. This phenomenon represents a partial escape from the vasoconstrictive adrenergic influence. Studies in animals demonstrate that vasoconstriction of the gastric vascular bed is mediated by α-adrenergic receptors, and that vasodilation, including adrenergic escape, is mediated by β-adrenergic receptors.

Stimulation of the vagus nerve is followed by a prompt increase in blood flow, suggesting a dilatory effect of parasympathetic nerves. The finding that vagotomy is accompanied by modest decreases in total gastric blood flow and mucosal blood flow is consistent with this concept. The effects of vagal stimulation on mucosal blood flow are complicated by accompanying increases in acid secretion. Almost all stimuli that increase acid production also increase blood flow secondarily. Because it is a potent stimulant of acid secretion, gastrin also increases mucosal blood flow.

The gastric mucosa and submucosa are richly supplied by nerve fibers that innervate submucosal blood vessels. The fibers contain a number of peptides including VIP, neurokinin A, substance P, and CGRP. CGRP is the most potent gastric vasodilator. Recent evidence suggests that CGRP-induced vasodilation involves endogenous nitric oxide. Nitric oxide, formed from L-arginine by the action of nitric oxide synthetase, diffuses to adjacent vascular smooth-muscle cells. Within smooth-muscle cells, nitric oxide activates guanylate cyclase. Increased cellular levels of cGMP mediate the vasodilatory properties of nitric oxide.

Nitric oxide modulates basal gastric vascular tone and controls gastric vasodilation and hyperemia. Nitric oxide mediates the hyperemic response that accompanies increases in acid secretion although the molecule has no direct stimulatory role in acid production.

Prostaglandins are important mucosally produced compounds that have clear effects on the gastric vasculature. Prostaglandins of the E class have been shown in animals and in humans to increase gastric blood flow at doses that decrease acid secretion. Indomethacin, in doses sufficient to inhibit prostaglandin formation, decreases the diameter of submucosal blood vessels and reduces basal blood flow. Complete inhibition of cyclooxygenase activity causes an approximate 50% reduction in resting blood flow. These studies suggest that endogenous, locally produced prostaglandins are crucial to maintaining basal gastric blood flow

in humans and probably act in concert with endogenous nitrous oxide.

GASTRIC MOTILITY
Gastric Smooth Muscle

Consideration of gastric motility requires that the stomach be viewed in functional terms as two different regions—the proximal one third and the distal two thirds. These areas are distinct in terms of smooth muscle anatomy, electrical activity, and contractile function. The regions do not correspond to the traditional anatomic divisions of fundus, corpus, and antrum.

In the proximal stomach, three layers of gastric smooth muscle can be distinguished—an outer longitudinal layer, a middle circular layer, and an inner oblique layer. In the distal two thirds of the stomach, the longitudinal layer is most clearly defined and the inner oblique layer is usually not distinct. The gastric smooth muscle ends at the pylorus. A septum of connective tissue marks the change from pylorus to duodenum, separating longitudinal and circular smooth muscle bundles and providing a point of electrical and mechanical transition (Fig. 21-17).

The smooth muscle of the proximal stomach is electrically stable, whereas the smooth muscle of the distal stomach demonstrates spontaneous, repeated electrical discharges. These electrical differences can also be demonstrated using intracellular recordings from isolated gastric smooth muscle cells, indicating that gastric smooth muscle cells are somehow programmed in terms of electrical activity. Extracellular electrical recording from the serosal surface of the stomach also demonstrates the intrinsic electrical activity of the distal stomach in the form of pacesetter potentials. Pacesetter potentials reflect partial depolarization of the gastric smooth muscle cell and are recorded during relatively long periods (2 or 3 seconds). Pacesetters originate along the greater curvature at a point in the proximal third of the stomach. Pacesetter potentials, discharging at a rate of three times per minute in humans, drive cells located distally. Spread of the pacesetter potentials is faster along the greater curvature, so that a ring of electrical activity reaches the pylorus simultaneously along both curvatures. The pacesetter potentials do not result in smooth muscle contraction, unless an additional depolarization is superimposed in the form of an action potential. When action potentials occur, a ring of smooth muscle contraction moves peristaltically along the distal stomach toward the pylorus. Gastric smooth muscle is affected by several neurohumoral agents that modulate contractility, both positively and negatively:

STIMULANTS

Acetylcholine
G_{17}
Cholecystokinin 8
Substance P
Dynorphin
Leucine enkephalin
Methionine enkephalin

INHIBITORS

VIP
Secretin
Glucagon

The smooth muscle activity of the proximal stomach is fundamentally different from that of the distal stomach. There are no pacesetter or action potentials in the proximal stomach. As a result, peristalsis does not occur. Proximal

Longitudinal muscle
of the stomach

Circular muscle
of the pylorus

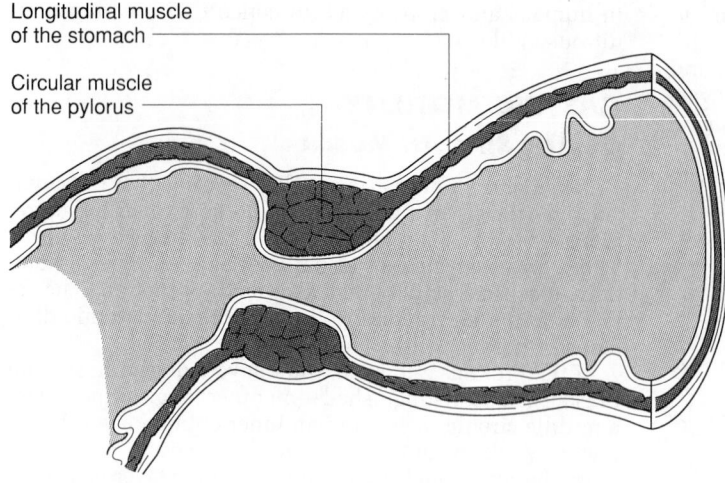

Figure 21-17. Cross-sectional anatomy of pyloric sphincter.

gastric contraction is tonic and prolonged, with increases in luminal pressure often sustained for several minutes.

Coordination of Contraction

Important vagally mediated reflexes influence intragastric pressure, presumably by affecting contractile activity of smooth muscle in the proximal stomach. The most important reflex is termed *receptive relaxation* and occurs with ingestion of a meal. Increasing gastric volumes are accommodated with little increase in intragastric pressure by relaxation of the proximal stomach. This receptive relaxation allows the proxial stomach to act as a storage site for ingested food in the immediate postprandial period. Afferent impulses, presumed to originate from stretch receptors in the gastric wall, are carried along vagal fibers; efferent vagal discharges are inhibitory. Receptive gastric accommodation is lost following either truncal or proximal gastric vagotomy. After the meal has been ingested, proximal contractile activity increases; alterations in proximal gastric tone cause the compressive movement of gastric content from the fundus to the antrum.

Food that enters the antrum from the proximal stomach is propelled peristaltically toward the pylorus. A number of observations indicate that the pylorus closes 2 or 3 seconds before the arrival of the antral contraction ring. This coordinate closing of the pylorus allows a small bolus of liquid and suspended food particles to pass while retropulsing the main mass of gastric contents back into the proximal antrum. The churning action that results mixes ingested food particles, gastric acid, and pepsin, and contributes to the grinding function of the stomach. Solid food particles do not ordinarily pass the pylorus unless they are no larger than 1 mm.

A consistent finding in humans ingesting a mixed solid-liquid meal is that liquids empty more quickly than solids. Characteristically, solid food empties only after a lag period, whereas liquid emptying begins almost immediately. A traditional interpretation of these human observations has been that the proximal stomach is the dominant force in determining how quickly a liquid meal empties by the gastroduodenal pressure gradient generated by proximal gastric contractions. The actions of the proximal stomach in liquid emptying are also regulated by the sieving actions of the antropyloric segment and are modified by the nutrient composition of the ingested meal. The distal gastric segment has been postulated to control solid emptying through its grinding and peristaltic actions. This traditional concept of the two-component stomach is useful in considering observations in humans that have undergone gastric operative procedures. Subjects who have undergone proximal gastric vagotomy exhibit accelerated emptying of liquids but have normal solid emptying. Because of loss of receptive relaxation, the denervation of the proximal stomach is presumed to increase intragastric pressure and accelerate liquid emptying while leaving the distal gastric segment unaffected. Conversely, vagal denervation of the antrum interrupts gastric emptying of solids to a greater degree than liquids. Although this model of gastric emptying oversimplifies the many mechanisms (gastric, pyloric, and intestinal) that work in concert to control gastric emptying, it provides a useful framework for considering the effects of gastric surgical procedures.

REFERENCES

1. Mulholland MW, Debas HT. Physiology and pathophysiology of gastrin: a review. Surgery 1988;103:135.
2. Dixon JE, Andrews PC, Collier K, et al. Cloning and biosynthetic studies of rat somatostatin. Scand J Gastroenterol 1983;82(Suppl):25.
3. Andrews PC, Dixon JE. Biosynthesis and processing of the somatostatin family of peptide hormones. Scand J Gastroenterol 1986; 21(Suppl):22.
4. Malinowski D, Sachs G, Cuppoletti J. Gastric H^+ secretion: histamine (cAMP-mediated) activation of protein phosphorylation. Biochim Biophys Acta 1988;972:95.
5. DelValle J, Wang L, Gantz I, Yamada T. Characterization of H_2 histamine receptor: linkage to both adenylate cyclase and $[Ca^{2+}]$i signaling systems. Am J Physiol 1002;263:G967.
6. Puurunen J, Schwabe U. Effect of gastric secretagogues on the formation of inositol phosphates in isolated gastric cells of the rat. Br J Pharmacol 1987;90:479.
7. Chew CS, Nakamura K, Ljungstrom M. Calcium signaling mechanisms in the gastric parietal cell. Yale J Biol Med 1992; 65:561.
8. Prinz C, Kajimura M, Scott D, et al. Acid secretion and the H, K ATPase of stomach. Yale J Biol Med 1992;65:577.
9. Park J, Chiba T, Yamada T. Mechanisms for direct inhibition of canine gastric parietal cells by somatostatin. J Biol Chem 1987; 262:14190.
10. Chen M, Amirian DA, Toomey M, et al. Prostanoid inhibition of canine parietal cells: mediation by the inhibitory guanosine triphosphate-binding protein of adenylate cyclase. Gastroenterology 1988;94:1121.
12. Debas HT, Mulholland MW. Drug therapy in peptic ulcer disease. Curr Probl Surg 1989;26:1.

13. Allen A, Flemstrom G, Garner A, Kivilaakso E. Gastroduodenal mucosal protection. Physiol Rev 1993;73:823.
14. Tepperman BL, Whittle BJR. Endogenous nitric oxide and sensory neuropeptides interact in the modulation of rat gastric microcirculation. Br J Pharmacol 1992;105:171.

SURGERY: SCIENTIFIC PRINCIPLES AND PRACTICE, Second Edition, edited by Lazar J. Greenfield, Michael W. Mulholland, Keith T. Oldham, Gerald B. Zelenock, and Keith D. Lillemoe. Lippincott–Raven Publishers, Philadelphia, © 1997.

CHAPTER 22

DUODENAL ULCER

MICHAEL W. MULHOLLAND

EPIDEMIOLOGY

Peptic ulceration remains a major public health problem in Western countries.[1] Some 300,000 new cases of peptic ulcer are diagnosed in the United States each year, and 4 million people receive some form of ulcer treatment. Overall, ulcer mortality and hospitalization rates have fallen during the past 20 years, but physicians are treating older patients with frequent comorbidity and ulcer disease of greater chronicity. Mortality attributed to peptic ulceration remains substantial: ulcer disease is listed as a contributing cause of death in more than 10,000 cases annually.

Treatment of peptic ulcer has changed dramatically within the past decade. A number of powerful antisecretory drugs have been introduced into clinical practice. Medical, endoscopic, and surgical therapies are frequently integrated in the care of individual patients. New insights into disease pathogenesis, especially the realization that gastric infection has a role in many cases of peptic ulceration, have been especially exciting.

No clear racial predilection for the development of duodenal ulceration exists, but genetic factors can be important. Hyperpepsinogenemia I, with autosomal dominant inheritance, is common in duodenal ulcer, although the relation of this trait to the development of ulceration remains obscure. A number of rare familial syndromes associated with peptic ulceration have been described.

PATHOPHYSIOLOGY

The pathogenesis of peptic ulceration is complex, multifactorial, and incompletely understood. The development of peptic ulceration is often depicted as a balance between acid–peptic secretion and mucosal defense, with the equilibrium shifted toward disease. Although large increases in acid secretion alone can occasionally cause ulceration, and although acid–peptic secretion is crucial in the development of ulcers, usually a defect in mucosal defense also exists to tip the balance away from health. Because of the multiple factors necessary to maintain mucosal health, the identification of a single pathogenetic defect resulting in ulceration has not been possible (Table 22-1).

Environmental Factors

Substantial evidence implicates cigarette smoking as a major risk factor in the development of duodenal ulcers.[2] Cigarette smoking patterns parallel ulcer hospitalization and mortality rates. The sharp decline in smoking rates recorded in middle-aged American men during the past 20 years has been accompanied by a decline in ulcer incidence in this group. Unhappily, increased cigarette smoking in young and middle-aged women has been mirrored by increased peptic ulceration in the female population. Cigarette smoking impairs ulcer healing and increases the recurrence of ulcers. Continued smoking attenuates the effectiveness of active ulcer therapy. Cigarette smoking increases both the probability that surgery will be required and the risks of operative therapy. A variety of mechanisms have been proposed to account for the deleterious effects of smoking, including decreased prostaglandin production, increased bile reflux, stimulation of acid production, and alterations in mucosal blood flow. The actions of cigarette smoke on gastroduodenal mucosa are not yet clear and may be multifactorial. Cessation of smoking is a key element of antiulcer therapy.

The belief is widespread that diet and environmental stress are important in the development of ulcers. Systematic study of these factors has been difficult, and supportive evidence is slim. No rigorous evidence exists to suggest that alterations in diet accelerate healing of ulcers. Caffeine has not been demonstrated to be detrimental. The role of alcohol is unsettled. In experimental models, direct application of alcohol to gastroduodenal mucosa induces injury, but in humans, alcohol consumption has been variously reported to impair and to increase ulcer healing. Although cirrhosis has been associated with an increased incidence of peptic ulceration, alcohol consumption in moderation has not definitely been shown to be harmful.

Nonsteroidal antiinflammatory drugs (NSAIDs) have emerged in the past several years as a significant risk factor for the development of acute ulceration.[3] Although acute mucosal injury caused by NSAIDs is more common in the stomach than in the duodenum, NSAID-induced ulcer complications occur with equal frequency in these two sites. NSAIDS produce a variety of lesions, ranging from hemorrhage, to superficial mucosal erosions, to deeper ulcerations. In the duodenum, it appears likely that invasive, NSAID-associated ulcers result from underlying peptic ulcer diathesis compounded by the direct injurious effects of the drugs.

The ulcerogenic actions of NSAIDs have been attributed to their systemic suppression of prostaglandin production. Numerous experimental models have demonstrated the ability of NSAIDs to injure the gastroduodenal mucosa. Ulcers resembling those caused by NSAIDs can be produced experimentally by antibodies to prostaglandins. Conversely, NSAID-associated gastric ulcers can be prevented by the coadministration of prostaglandin ana-

Table 22-1. POSTULATED PATHOGENETIC FACTORS IN PATIENTS WITH DUODENAL ULCER

ACID SECRETION
Increased acid secretory capacity
Increased basal secretion
Increased pentagastrin-stimulated output
Increased meal response
Abnormal gastric emptying

ENVIRONMENT
Cigarette smoking
Nonsteroidal antiinflammatory drug
Helicobacter infection

MUCOSAL DEFENSE
Decreased duodenal bicarbonate production
Decreased gastric mucosal prostaglandin production

logues. Ulcers associated with NSAIDs usually heal rapidly when the drug is withdrawn, corresponding to the reversal of antiprostaglandin effects. All available NSAIDs appear to possess the hazard of gastroduodenal ulceration. Clinically important ulceration (of both the stomach and duodenum) is estimated by the Food and Drug Administration to occur at a rate of 2% to 4% per patient-year. The risks inherent with NSAID use appear to be further increased by a history of peptic ulcer disease, by cigarette smoking, and by alcohol use. The incidence of NSAID-caused ulcer complications is highest in older patients, as is the attendant mortality.

Helicobacter pylori

Helicobacter pylori infection of the gastroduodenal mucosa has been implicated in the development of duodenal ulcers.[4,5] The relation between *H pylori* infection and ulceration must be considered very strong but inferential; a causal relation between *H pylori* infection and peptic ulceration has not been tested directly. Because *H pylori* infection is difficult to eradicate with certainty, and because of the potentially serious consequences of infection, the intentional exposure of humans to the organism to establish such a relation is not justified.

Several lines of circumstantial evidence establish *H pylori* as a factor in the pathogenesis of duodenal ulceration:

1. *H pylori* is the primary cause of chronic active gastritis, characterized by nonerosive inflammation of the gastric mucosa. Antral gastritis is nearly always present histologically in patients with duodenal ulcer, and *H pylori* can be isolated from gastric mucosa in almost all cases.
2. Gastric metaplasia is extremely common in duodenal epithelium surrounding areas of ulceration. *H pylori* binds only to gastric-type epithelium, regardless of location; metaplastic gastric epithelium can become colonized by *H pylori* from gastric sources.
3. Eradication of *H pylori* with antimicrobials that have no effect on acid secretion leads to ulcer healing rates equivalent to those seen with H_2-receptor antagonists.
4. Therapy with bismuth compounds, which eradicate *H pylori,* is associated with reduced rates of ulcer relapse relative to conventional therapy.
5. Relapse of duodenal ulcer after antimicrobial therapy is preceded by reinfection of the gastric mucosa by *H pylori.*

However, half of patients evaluated for dyspepsia, but without ulceration, have histologic evidence of mucosal bacterial infection. Furthermore, 20% of healthy volunteers harbor the bacteria; the incidence of the bacteria in the healthy, asymptomatic population increases with age. The occurrence of peptic ulcers in only a small proportion of individuals who carry the organism suggests that other factors must also act to induce ulceration.

The cellular mechanisms by which *H pylori* infection might cause ulceration have not been elucidated. Disruption of mucosal defense mechanisms by local inflammatory responses to the organism and mucosal injury by bacterial toxins have been postulated but not proved.

Acid Secretory Status

The formation of duodenal ulcers is dependent on gastric secretion of acid and pepsin. The dictum "no acid—no ulcer" properly focuses on the importance of luminal acid in the development of the disease, although a more complete statement might be "no acid and no *H pylori*—no ulcer." As a group, patients with duodenal ulcers have an increased capacity for gastric acid secretion relative to normal individuals (see Table 22-1). The maximal acid output of normal men is approximately 20 mEq/h in response to intravenous histamine stimulation, whereas duodenal ulcer patients secrete an average of about 40 mEq/h. Considerable overlap exists between these two groups, and the values for most individuals with duodenal ulcer fall within the normal range. The increase in acid secretion in some duodenal ulcer patients has been postulated to be due to an increase in the mass of parietal cells within the acid-secreting gastric mucosa or to an increased sensitivity to circulating gastrin. Both explanations remain controversial. *H pylori*–infested patients demonstrate increased postprandial gastrin release. Exaggerated gastrin secretion has been postulated to be caused by mediators of inflammation, such as interleukin-2.

Groups of duodenal ulcer patients demonstrate a prolonged and larger acid secretory response to a mixed meal than do groups of normal subjects. As with histamine-stimulated acid output, overlap between duodenal ulcer patients and normals exists. Disturbances in gastric motility can exacerbate meal-stimulated acid secretory abnormalities. Patients with duodenal ulcer have accelerated emptying of gastric contents, particularly liquids, after a meal, and duodenal acidification fails to slow emptying appropriately. In such individuals, the duodenal mucosa can be exposed to low pH for prolonged periods of time relative to normals.

Groups of patients with duodenal ulcer also demonstrate increased basal secretion of acid. Increased basal secretion can be demonstrated by nocturnal collection of gastric secretions. Although the mechanism responsible for increased basal secretion is not known, increased vagal discharge has been postulated. In support of this contention, basal acid secretion in duodenal ulcer patients correlates with circulating concentrations of vagally released pancreatic polypeptide. In addition, sham feeding, which is vagally mediated, does not increase acid output above basal secretion in these patients.

No strong evidence exists for endocrine abnormalities in the pathogenesis of peptic ulceration (excluding ulceration occurring as a result of the Zollinger-Ellison syndrome). Basal gastrin levels are normal in patients with duodenal ulcer. Tissue gastrin content is not increased. Although acidification of the antral lumen is less effective in inhibiting gastrin release in duodenal ulcer patients than in normal subjects, defects in stimulated gastrin release do not seem to be crucial in the development of ulcer disease. Circulating levels of somatostatin are normal in ulcer patients, although this observation may be of limited value, given the postulated local actions of mucosal somatostatin. Furthermore, exogenously administered somatostatin is normally effective in inhibiting gastrin release and in suppressing acid secretion.

Mucosal Defense Against Peptic Injury

Increasingly, attention has focused on the ability of the duodenal mucosa to resist the injurious effects of luminal acid and pepsin. Because many patients with duodenal ulcer secrete normal amounts of acid and pepsin, it is attractive to postulate that abnormalities of mucosal defense might result in ulceration. Several agents that are useful in the treatment of peptic ulceration are also cytoprotective, which is defined as the ability to protect the mucosa from injury at doses lower than the threshold dose needed to inhibit acid secretion. The ability of cytoprotective agents to heal ulcers has suggested that abnormalities in mucosal defense are responsible for some instances of ulceration. Most investigative efforts have focused on the role of mucosally secreted bicarbonate and on mucosal prostaglandin production.

Gastric surface epithelial cells secrete mucus and bicarbonate, creating a pH gradient within the mucus layer that is nearly neutral at the mucous cell surface, even when the lumen is highly acidic. Failure of normal bicarbonate secretion locally would, in theory, result in exposure of surface epithelial cells to the peptic activity of gastric secretions at low pH. Patients with duodenal ulcers have been demonstrated to have significantly lower basal bicarbonate secretion in the proximal duodenum than normal subjects.[6,7] Additionally, in response to a physiologically relevant amount of hydrochloric acid instilled into the duodenal bulb, stimulated bicarbonate output was about 40% of the normal response. If confirmed, these results suggest one mechanism by which ulceration could occur, even in individuals secreting normal amounts of acid.

Diminished mucosal prostaglandin production has also been proposed to exist in subsets of patients with duodenal ulcer. Prostaglandins and prostaglandin analogues have been shown to exert cytoprotective effects, to accelerate healing of established duodenal ulcers, and to decrease acid secretion. In the duodenum, locally produced prostaglandins stimulate mucosal bicarbonate secretion. In patients with active duodenal ulceration, gastric mucosal production of prostaglandin E_2 and other prostanoids has been shown to be diminished. An increase in prostanoid synthesis within the gastric mucosa characterized ulcer healing. A recent report suggests that duodenal bicarbonate responses to prostaglandin E_2 are impaired in duodenal ulcer patients.

DIAGNOSIS

The cardinal feature of duodenal ulceration is epigastric pain. The pain is usually confined to the upper abdomen and is described as burning, stabbing, or gnawing. Unless perforation or penetration into the head of the pancreas has occurred, referral of pain is not common. Many patients report pain on arising in the morning. Ingestion of food or antacids usually provides prompt relief. In uncomplicated cases, abnormal physical findings are minimal. The differential diagnosis is broad and includes a variety of diseases originating in the upper gastrointestinal tract. The most common disorders to be distinguished include nonulcerative dyspepsia, gastric neoplasia, cholelithiasis and related diseases of the biliary system, and both inflammatory and neoplastic disorders of the pancreas. In dyspeptic patients, the principal diagnoses that must be differentiated definitively are peptic ulceration and gastric cancer.

The evaluation of patients with suspected peptic ulceration usually involves either barium contrast examination of the stomach and duodenum or endoscopy. In most circumstances, endoscopy is the preferred method and has become the standard against which other diagnostic modalities are measured. Endoscopy is recommended because it eliminates the need for radiation, is safe, is preferred by elderly patients, and permits biopsy of the esophagus, stomach, and duodenum. In a controlled trial[8] comparing endoscopy and barium radiography, endoscopy was both more sensitive (92% versus 54%) and more specific (100% versus 91%) than radiographic examination. Endoscopy must be recommended with discretion because of associated morbidity (about 1 per 5000 cases) and higher costs.

Duodenal ulcer is characterized by lesions that are erosive to the bowel wall. When viewed endoscopically, the ulcers have a typical appearance. The edges are usually sharply demarcated, and the underlying submucosa is exposed. The ulcer base is often clean and smooth, although acute ulcers and those with recent hemorrhage can demonstrate eschar or adherent exudate. Surrounding mucosal inflammation is common. The most frequent site for peptic ulceration is the first portion of the duodenum, with the second portion less commonly involved. Ulceration of the third or fourth portions of the duodenum is unusual, and its occurrence should arouse suspicion of an underlying gastrinoma. Ulceration within the pyloric channel or in the prepyloric area is similar in endoscopic appearance to duodenal ulceration, and ulcers in these areas demonstrate other clinical features similar to duodenal ulcers.

Barium meal radiographs demonstrate retention of contrast in the ulcer. When viewed in profile, the ulcer can be seen to project beyond the level of the duodenal mucosa. Distortion of the duodenal bulb by spasm or cicatrization is a secondary sign of current or previous ulceration.

The hallmarks of the histologic appearance of duodenal ulcers are chronicity and invasiveness. Chronic injury is suggested by surrounding fibrosis; collagen is deposited within the submucosa during each round of ulcer relapse and healing. The adjacent mucosa often demonstrates evidence of chronic injury with infiltration of acute and chronic inflammatory cells. Gastric metaplasia, in which the duodenum exhibits histologic features of gastric mucosa, is common in the surrounding nonulcerated mucosa. The ulcer can extend for a variable distance through the wall of the duodenum, including the full thickness of the bowel in cases of perforation.

DRUG TREATMENT OF ULCER DISEASE

A consideration of the cellular mechanisms regulating the production of acid by the gastric parietal cell suggests several potential sites of action for drugs that act to inhibit acid secretion (Fig. 22-1). Receptor antagonists for histamine, gastrin, or acetylcholine, or antagonists of the parietal cell proton pump, might be expected to have therapeutic potential. In addition, agents that supplement or restore mucosal defenses might also have therapeutic importance in peptic diseases (Fig. 22-2). A number of compounds are available that have these characteristics.[9] Their use has dramatically altered the primary treatment of uncomplicated ulcer disease and has greatly changed the role of operative therapy in the treatment of patients with peptic ulceration. An appreciation of the uses and limits of drug therapy is necessary for all surgeons who treat patients with duodenal ulcer (Table 22-2).

Histamine-Receptor Antagonists

Histamine, released into the interstitial fluid by cells within the fundic mucosa, diffuses to the mucosal parietal cell. Histamine stimulates acid production by occupying a membrane-bound receptor and activating parietal cell adenylate cyclase. Histamine is released in response to a number of physiologic stimuli; blockade of histamine receptors inhibits most forms of stimulated acid secretion in humans. Parietal cell histamine receptors are classified as H_2 receptors because they are activated by agonists such as 4-methylhistamine and are selectively blocked by agents such as cimetidine. Some H_2-receptor antagonists also possess nongastric actions by binding to androgen receptors, by interacting with the hepatic microsomal oxidase system, and by crossing the blood–brain barrier. All clinically

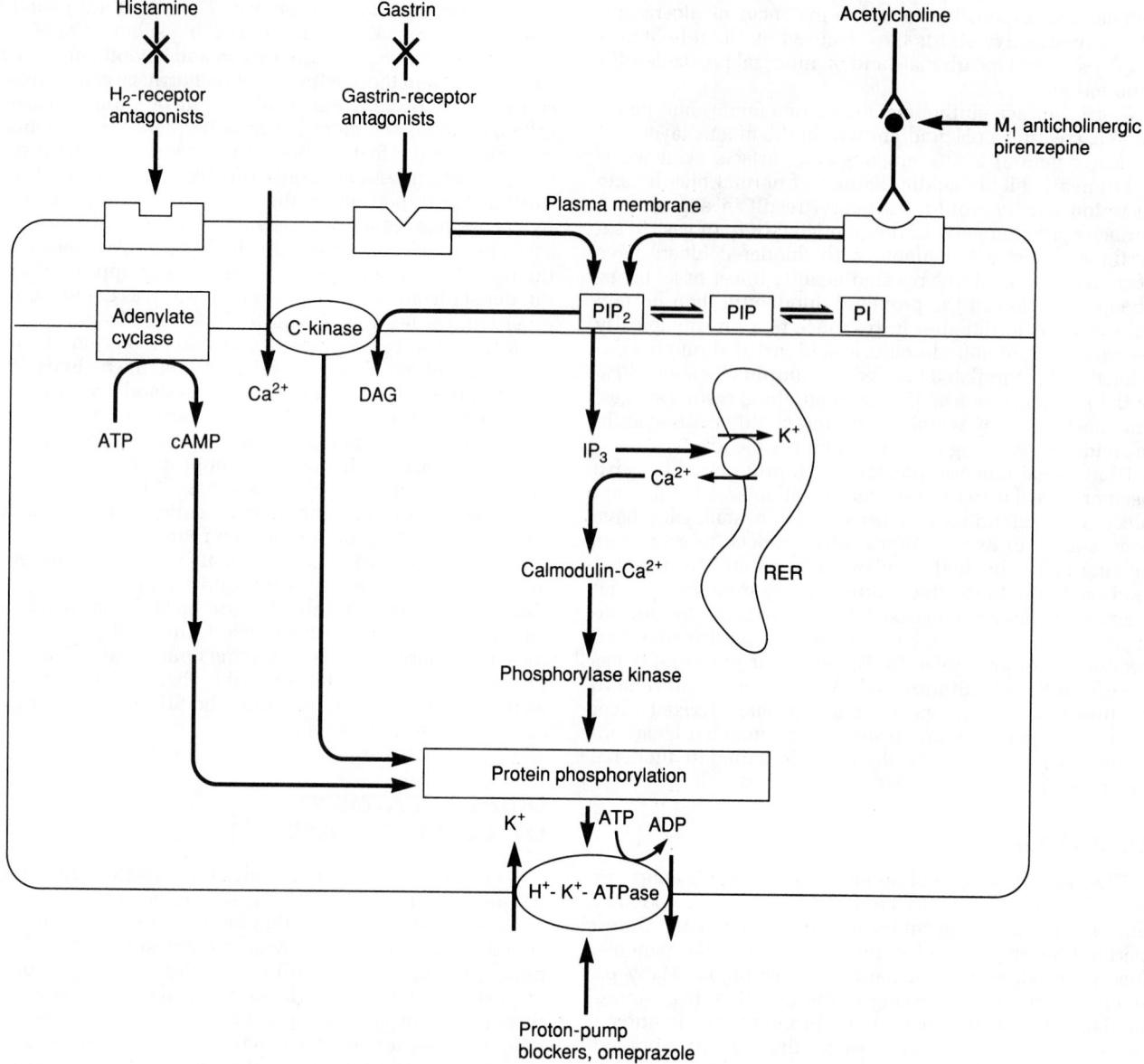

Figure 22-1. Antisecretory drugs that act on the gastric parietal cell and that are potentially useful in the treatment of duodenal ulcer. RER, rough endoplasmic reticulum; DAG, diacrylglycerol.

useful gastric histamine-receptor antagonists are of the H_2 type.

Cimetidine, ranitidine, famotidine, and newer H_2-receptor antagonists bind competitively to parietal cell H_2 receptors to produce a reversible inhibition of acid secretion. Cimetidine shares the imidazole ring of histamine; in ranitidine, the imidazole ring has been replaced with an alkyl furan ring (Fig. 22-3). In second-generation H_2-receptor antagonists, increasing structural differences compared with the parent compound have been introduced. As a result of these rearrangements, a series of compounds with increasing potency has been produced. There are two pharmacologic results: increased duration of action up to and beyond 24 hours, and improved specificity because of decreased interactions with receptors in nongastric tissues.

The pharmacokinetic profiles of cimetidine and ranitidine are similar. Peak plasma concentrations of cimetidine and ranitidine are achieved 1 to 3 hours after oral ingestion; elimination half-lives approximate 2 to 3 hours. Both cimetidine and ranitidine, along with their metabolic

products, are secreted in the urine, and renal failure significantly prolongs plasma clearance. On a molar basis, ranitidine is six to eight times more potent than cimetidine. In practice, this difference is not important; equipotent doses of these agents produce equivalent degrees of acid suppression.

An enormous, worldwide experience has been accumulated with the use of H_2-receptor antagonists. The agents are effective and safe when used in the treatment of peptic ulcer. The various compounds have similar efficacy in terms of ulcer healing when used in doses that produce similar reductions in acid output. When endoscopic criteria are used to determine healing, about 70% of patients are ulcer-free within 4 weeks of therapy. By 8 weeks, 85% to 90% of patients are pain-free and without endoscopic evidence of ulceration. Most studies of maintenance therapy have used single nocturnal doses of cimetidine or ranitidine; ulcer relapse during maintenance therapy occurs in about 15% of patients under these circumstances. It has become increasingly clear that H_2-receptor blockers do not

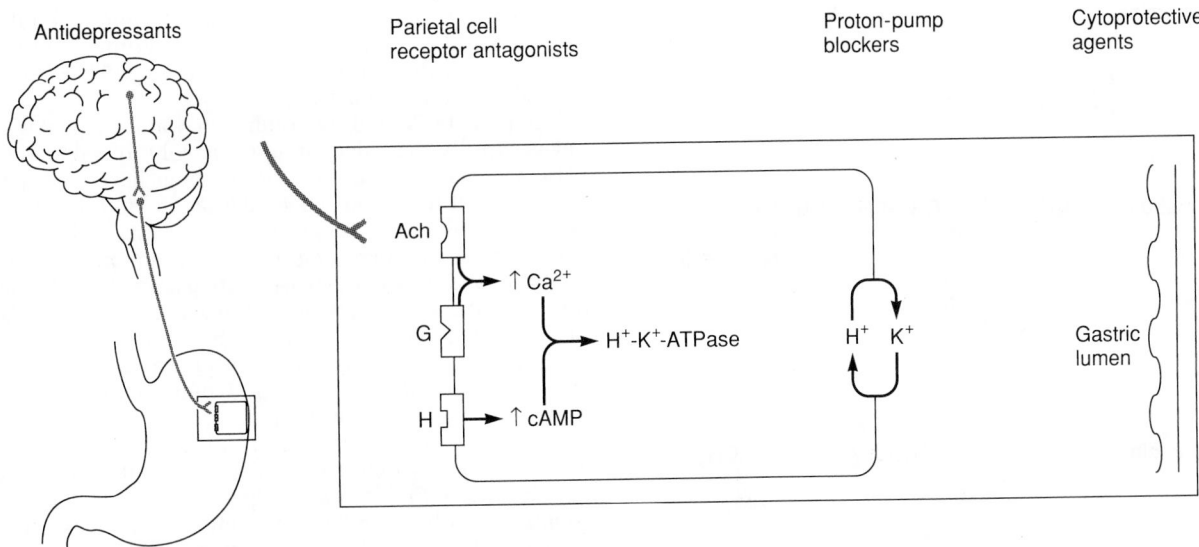

Figure 22-2. Overview of the sites of action of drugs with antiulcer activities.

affect the underlying ulcer diathesis; if H_2-receptor antagonists are stopped, recurrent ulceration occurs in greater than half of patients within 1 year.[10]

Although a variety of side effects have been reported, adverse reactions are infrequent (4% to 5%) and can usually be reversed by discontinuing the drug or reducing the dosage. Because cimetidine and ranitidine interact with the hepatic microsomal enzyme system, the agents can increase blood levels and pharmacologic effects of drugs that depend on hepatic metabolism. The most common medications that can be affected by coadministered H_2-receptor antagonists are warfarin, phenytoin, diazepam, propranolol, and theophylline. A number of neuropsychiatric effects have been reported with cimetidine, including agitation, confusion, and lethargy. These effects are most common in elderly patients or those with renal impairment, in whom alterations of drug metabolism might be expected. Symptoms rapidly clear with dose reduction or drug withdrawal. Gynecomastia has been reported in male patients taking high-dose cimetidine for prolonged periods.

Famotidine is representative of the second generation of H_2-receptor antagonists.[11] Famotidine has the advantages of greater potency and longer duration of action than either cimetidine or ranitidine. Pentagastrin-stimulated gastric acid secretin can be expected to be inhibited by 50% as long as 12 hours after an oral dose of 20 mg of famotidine.

Famotidine does not appear to interact with the hepatic microsomal enzyme system, nor does it appear to alter metabolism of hepatically eliminated drugs. Differences in pharmacokinetics do not translate into improved efficacy in the healing of ulceration. Doses of famotidine that cause equivalent acid suppression, compared with cimetidine or ranitidine, produce similar ulcer healing rates. It is anticipated that other, newer H_2-receptor antagonists will offer differences in pharmacokinetics, but not improved efficacy in ulcer healing.

Anticholinergic Drugs

Anticholinergic drugs block acid secretion by occupying muscarinic receptors for acetylcholine. Although most antimuscarinic agents potently inhibit acid secretion in humans, nonselective anticholinergic drugs such as atropine have frequent and unpleasant side effects, such as dry mouth, blurred vision, and urinary retention. For atropine, these limiting side effects occur at doses lower than necessary to significantly inhibit acid secretion. Selective anticholinergic agents have been developed that specifically interact with muscarinic receptors on postganglionic nerves of the stomach (M_1 receptors) and have less effect on classic (M_2) receptors present on parietal cells and on muscle cells of the pupil, bladder, and heart. Pirenzepine, a selective M_1 anticholinergic drug, thus inhibits vagally

Table 22-2. PHARMACOLOGIC PARAMETERS OF COMMONLY USED ANTIULCER DRUGS

Agent	Ulcer Therapy (Daily Dose)	Bioavailability (%)	Major Route of Excretion	Most Frequent Side Effects	Important Drug Interactions
Cimetidine	800–1200 mg	70	Renal	Neuropsychiatric effects, endocrine disorders	Hepatically metabolized drugs
Ranitidine	300–400 mg	70	Renal	Neuropsychiatric effects	Warfarin
Famotidine	40 mg	70	Renal	Nonspecific	
Prenzepine	100–150 mg	25	Feces	Dry mouth	
Omeprazole	20–30 mg	40–50	Renal	Nonspecific	
Sucralfate	4 g	Unabsorbed	Unabsorbed	Constipation	
Microprostol	800 μg	—	Tissue metabolism	Diarrhea	

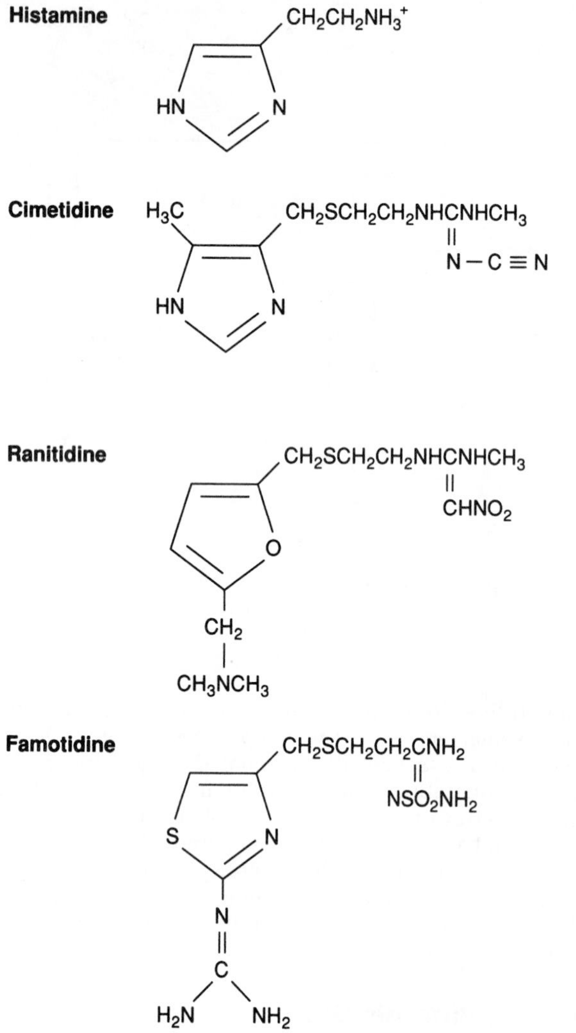

Figure 22-3. Chemical structures of selected H_2-receptor antagonists and their relation to histamine.

stimulated acid secretion while having minimal undesirable visual, urinary, or cardiac effects.[12]

Proton-Pump Blockers

Acid secretion by the gastric parietal cells is due to the active transport of hydrogen ions from the parietal cell cytoplasm into the secretory canaliculus in exchange for potassium. Because this so-called proton pump is tissue specific, being present only in gastric mucosa, its blockade would be expected to minimally affect nongastric functions. Omeprazole is representative of a family of compounds that selectively block the parietal cell proton pump.[13]

Omeprazole is a weak base, with a pKa of approximately 4. The drug is nonionized and lipid soluble at neutral pH, but it becomes ionized and activated at a pH of less than 3. In its activated state, omeprazole binds to the membrane-bound H^+-K^+-ATPase of the parietal cell. Because the compound is a weak base, omeprazole accumulates selectively within the acidic environment of the parietal cell secretory canaliculus; 4 hours after administration, the drug is detectable in appreciable quantities only in the gastric mucosa. If enough drug is administered to occupy all parietal cell binding sites, anacidity can be produced. Omeprazole,

in doses from 20 to 30 mg, causes nearly complete inhibition of stimulated gastric acid secretion within 6 hours. At 24 hours after drug administration, 60% to 70% reduction in acid secretion persists.

Omeprazole is slightly soluble in water of neutral pH but is rapidly degraded in aqueous solutions of reduced pH. As a result, various oral formulations have been developed to limit intragastric degradation and to improve systemic bioavailability. Repeated daily dosing with omeprazole results in increasing inhibitory action on gastric secretion and thus in decreased intragastric degradation of the drug. Acid suppression stabilizes after about 3 days. Because of tissue accumulation, the secretory actions of omeprazole do not correlate with plasma levels. Urinary excretion accounts for 75% to 80% of metabolic clearance; about 20% is detectable in the feces.

Omeprazole accelerates the healing of ulcers and provides superior symptomatic relief in patients with duodenal ulceration. Endoscopically proven ulcers demonstrate complete healing in 80% of patients after 2 weeks and in 95% of patients after 4 weeks when omeprazole is administered once daily. Several studies have demonstrated a significant inhibition of peak acid output, marked relief of epigastric pain, and decreased use of supplemental antacids during omeprazole therapy. Direct comparisons with H_2-receptor antagonists have generally favored omeprazole in terms of pain relief and the rate of ulcer healing. The use of omeprazole for long-term maintenance therapy has not been accepted because of concerns about the effects of chronically sustained hypergastrinemia. Peptic ulceration recurs in a high proportion of patients after cessation of omeprazole therapy, similar to recurrence rates observed with H_2-receptor antagonist therapy.

Toxicologic studies in animals have shown that omeprazole in high doses can produce histologic abnormalities in the gastric mucosa. Hyperplasia of enterochromaffin-like cells has been seen in chronically achlorhydric animals; the histologic changes correlate with circulating gastrin levels. Enterochromaffin-like cell hyperplasia is believed to be induced by the trophic effect of elevated gastrin. In humans, only patients with Zollinger-Ellison syndrome have received continuous high-dose omeprazole therapy, and hyperplasia of enterochromaffin-like cells has not been observed. Concerns about the development of enterochromaffin-like cell hyperplasia with long-term omeprazole use appear to have been overstated.

An additional objection to the long-term use of omeprazole has been bacterial overgrowth in the achlorhydric stomach. Although there have been no reports of illness due to bacterial overgrowth in individuals receiving this drug, increased bacterial counts have been observed in patients receiving higher dosages. When long-term omeprazole therapy is necessary, dosages should be adjusted to achieve an acid production of about 10 mEq/h in the hour before the next dose. Continuous anacidity is potentially deleterious and is not necessary to achieve ulcer healing. Omeprazole interferes with the oxidative metabolism of some drugs cleared by the hepatic microsomal enzyme system, although to a lesser extent than cimetidine.

Sucralfate

Sucralfate is the aluminum salt of sulfated sucrose. In the acidic environment of the stomach, sucralfate polymerizes, becoming viscous and adhering to the gastroduodenal mucosa. Coating of the ulcer base by the polymer has been claimed to provide a protective barrier, binding bile salts and inhibiting the actions of pepsin. Sucralfate also stimulates the production of mucus. Sucralfate stimulates increased mucosal prostaglandin E_2 production and increases bicarbonate secretion. Sucralfate binds epidermal growth factor and may protect the mitogen from acid degradation. Sucralfate stimulates epithelial proliferation at the ulcer margin. The drug has almost no buffering capacity. Virtually no systemic absorption occurs, and because of this property, sucralfate is the recommended agent for the treatment of peptic ulcer in pregnancy.

Sucralfate is effective in promoting the healing of acute duodenal ulceration. When sucralfate is administered at a dose of 1 g four times daily, over 80% of ulcers heal by 6 weeks, a rate that is roughly equivalent to that achieved with the use of H_2-receptor antagonists.[14] Pain relief with sucralfate is achieved less quickly than with antisecretory drugs. Side effects are infrequent and mild, and constipation is the most frequent complaint. The lack of systemic absorption and the low incidence of side effects make sucralfate attractive for long-term maintenance therapy.

Prostaglandin Analogues

Prostaglandins are 20-carbon oxygenated fatty acids synthesized from dietary fatty acids through the actions of cyclooxygenase. All prostaglandins have a cyclopentane ring and, depending on the structure of the ring, are classified as prostaglandin A, B, C, D, E, or F (Fig. 22-4). Analogues of the E_1 and E_2 type have been synthesized for clinical use. Prostaglandins have cytoprotective properties and, at higher doses, also have antisecretory actions. Antisecretory doses are required to heal ulcers. Native prostaglandins have short circulating half-lives and are metabolized locally by enzymes in a variety of tissues. Synthetic derivatives are useful because they resist degradation.

Misoprostol, the most widely used prostaglandin analogue, causes endoscopic healing of duodenal ulcers in over 60% of patients at 4 weeks when administered at 200 mg four times daily. Direct comparisons of misoprostol and H_2-receptor antagonists have generally shown comparable efficacy in the healing of acute duodenal ulcers.[15]

The major side effect of prostaglandin derivatives has been diarrhea. In 30% to 40% of treated patients, a change in stool character is seen, with frank diarrhea in 5%. In most cases, diarrhea stops even though drug administration is continued. Uterine bleeding has been reported in some women receiving the drug. The drug also has potential abortifacient properties.

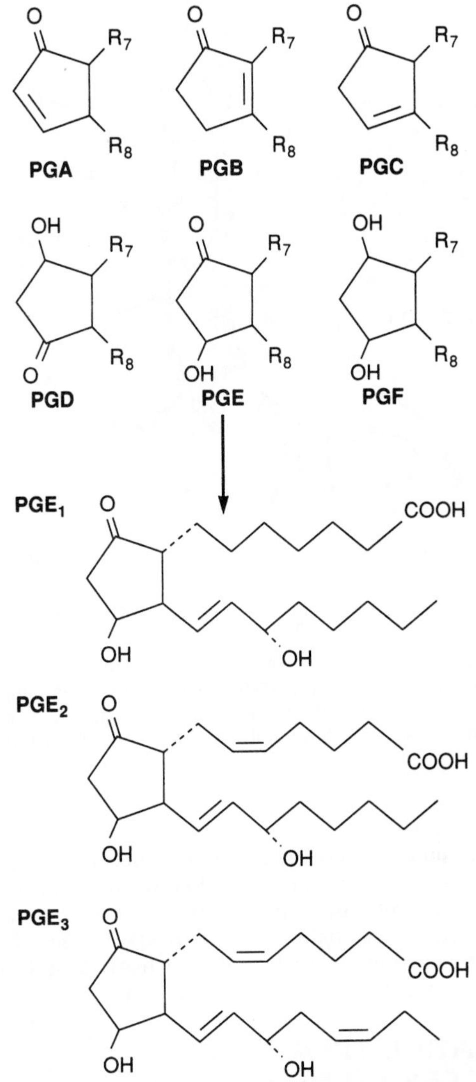

Antacids

The availability of compounds that effectively suppress acid production, combined with their greater convenience, has greatly reduced the use of antacids as the primary treatment for acute ulceration. Nonetheless, when properly used, antacids can effectively heal ulcers. Intensive treatment of acute ulcers with antacids (30 mL of liquid antacid taken seven times daily, providing about 1000 mEq of buffering capacity) has been shown to heal ulcers in 78% of patients at 4 weeks.[16] Although this rate compares favorably with the healing rates observed with other forms of therapy, the large and frequent dosages are unacceptable to many patients. In addition, a significant proportion of patients have diarrhea on such a regimen. Surprisingly, low-dose antacid regimens that deliver less than 200 mmol/d also promote ulcer healing. More palatable alternatives with equivalent effectiveness include low-dose antacid therapy and the use of antacids as supplements to other acid-suppressive agents.

Antimicrobial Therapy

The realization that *H pylori* infection has an important role in ulcer pathogenesis has led to the development of antimicrobial therapy for ulceration. One-agent, two-agent,

Figure 22-4. Prostaglandins are designated A through F based on the structure of the cyclopentane ring of the molecule. The lengths of the upper and lower carbon side chains are designated R_7 and R_8, respectively. Prostaglandins of the E class have been used clinically.

and triple therapy have all been used. Most successful regimens are based on a bismuth compound (colloidal bismuth subsalicylate or colloidal bismuth subcitrate) plus metronidazole, alone or in combination with amoxicillin or tetracycline. An effective combination is outlined below:

- Bismuth subsalicylate (Pepto-Bismol), two tablets with meals and at bedtime for 6 weeks
- Metronidazole, 250 mg three times a day for 2 weeks
- Amoxicillin, 500 mg three times a day, or tetracycline hydrochloride, 500 mg three times a day, for 2 weeks

Bismuth compounds act locally and achieve gastric concentrations above the minimum inhibitory concentration (MIC) for 90% of *H pylori* isolates. Metronidazole is secreted into the stomach at high concentration. The in vivo activity of mitronidazole is not diminished by gastric acidity. Triple therapy with bismuth, metronidazole, and tetracycline or amoxicillin eradicates *H pylori* in 90% of cases, compared with 0% eradication with ranitidine. Inclusion of an H_2-receptor antagonist or omeprazole has been re-

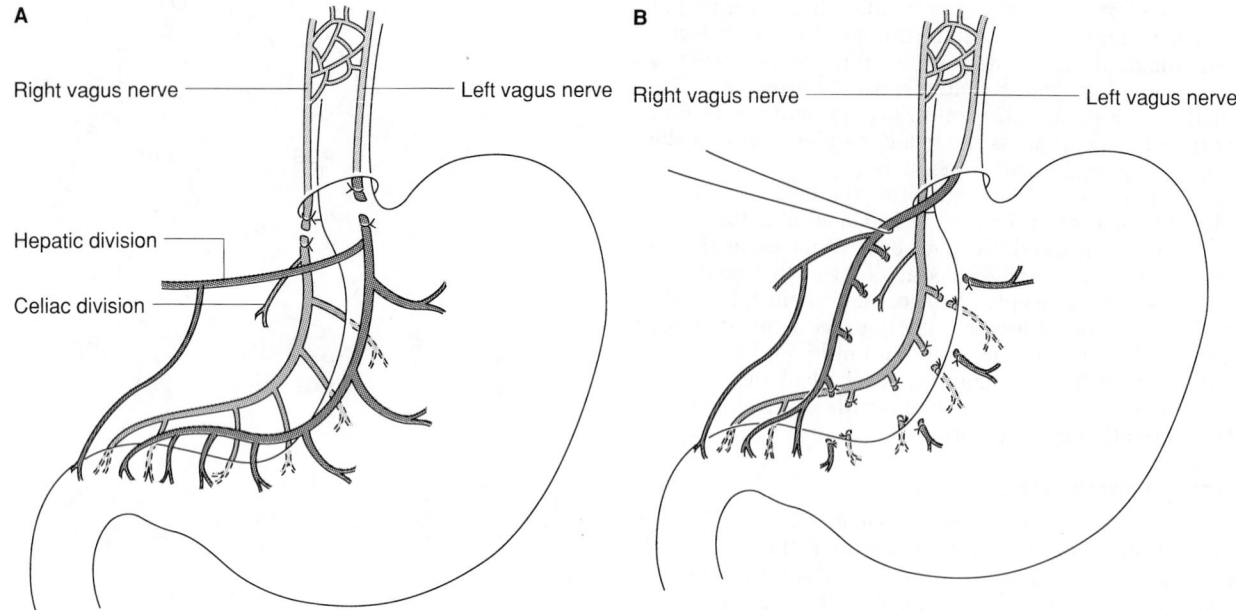

A

Right vagus nerve — Left vagus nerve

Hepatic division

Celiac division

B

Right vagus nerve — Left vagus nerve

Figure 22-5. Truncal vagotomy and proximal gastric vagotomy. (*A*) With truncal vagotomy, both nerve trunks are divided at the level of the diaphragmatic hiatus. (*B*) Proximal gastric vagotomy involves division of the vagal fibers that supply the gastric fundus. Branches to the antropyloric region of the stomach are not transected, and the hepatic and celiac divisions of the vagus nerves remain intact.

ported to increase the efficacy of antimicrobial therapy in some series.[17,18] Antimicrobial therapy has been recommended for peptic ulcer disease resistant to conventional therapy, including patients with ulcer relapse while on maintenance therapy and failure to heal in spite of H_2-receptor antagonist or omeprazole therapy.

OPERATIVE TREATMENT OF ULCER DISEASE

Surgical Goals

Operative intervention is reserved for the treatment of complicated ulcer disease. Four complications are most common and constitute the classic indications for peptic ulcer surgery—intractability, hemorrhage, perforation, and obstruction. The first goal in the surgical treatment of the complications of ulcer disease should be alteration of the ulcer diathesis so that ulcer healing is achieved and recurrence is minimized. The second goal is treatment of coexisting anatomic complications, such as pyloric stenosis or perforation. The third major goal should be patient safety and freedom from undesirable chronic side effects. To achieve these goals, the gastric surgeon can direct therapy via endoscopic, radiologic, or operative means, the appropriate choice depending on the clinical circumstances.

Operative Procedures

A number of operative procedures have been used to treat peptic ulcer, but three procedures—truncal vagotomy and drainage, truncal vagotomy and antrectomy, and proximal gastric vagotomy—are most widely used. In the operative treatment of peptic ulcer disease, vagotomy has a central role. Division of both vagal trunks at the esophageal hiatus—truncal vagotomy—denervates the acid-producing fundic mucosa as well as the remainder of the vagally supplied viscera (Fig. 22-5). Because denervation impedes

A

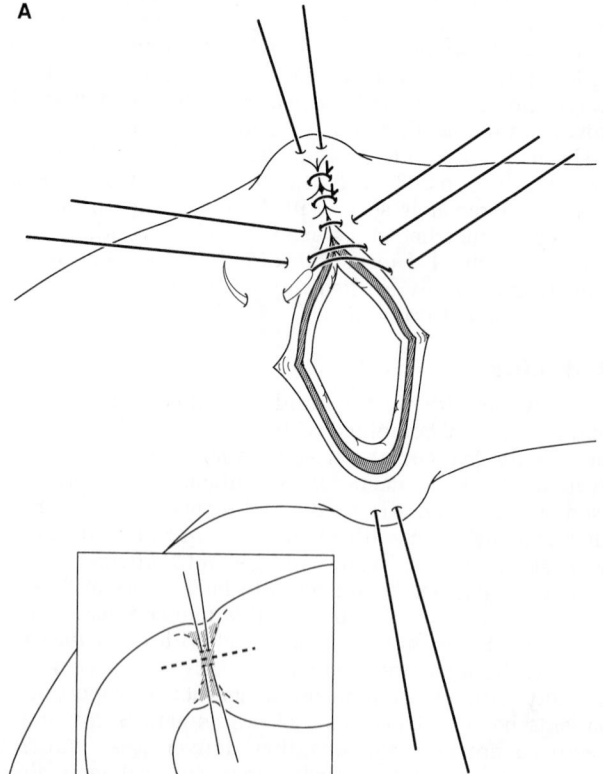

Figure 22-6. Pyloroplasty formation. A Heineke-Mikulicz pyloroplasty (*A*) involves a longitudinal incision of the pyloric sphincter followed by a transverse closure. The Finney pyloroplasty (*B*) is performed as a gastroduodenostomy with division of the pylorus. The Jaboulay pyloroplasty (*C*) differs from the Finney procedure in that the pylorus is not transected. (*continues*)

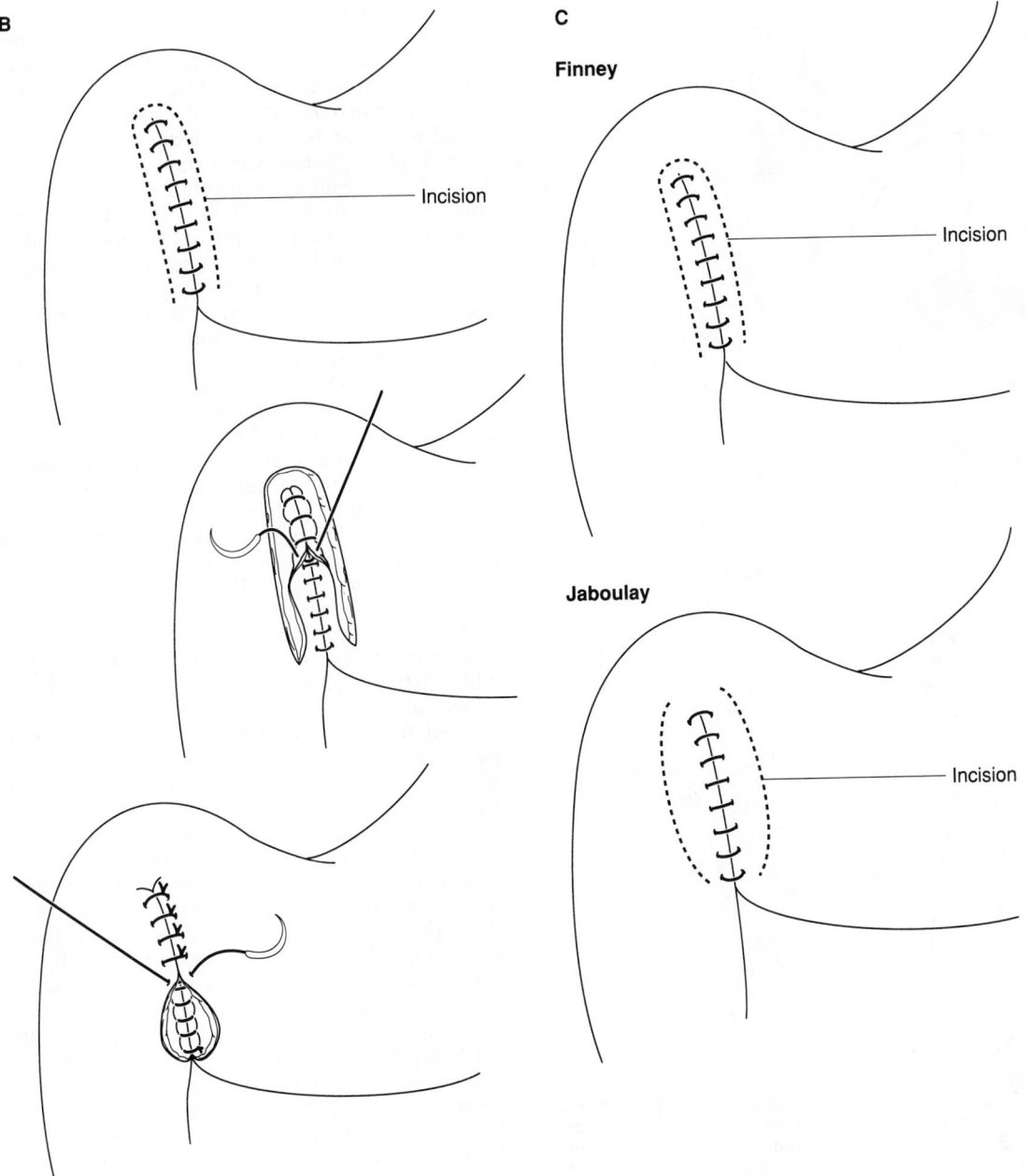

B

C

Finney

Jaboulay

Incision

Figure 22-6. (Continued)

normal pyloric coordination and can result in impairment of gastric emptying, truncal vagotomy must be combined with a procedure to eliminate pyloric sphincteric function. Usually, gastric drainage is ensured by performance of a pyloroplasty. Several methods of pyloroplasty have been described; often they are referred to eponymously (Fig. 22-6). The Heineke-Mikulicz pyloroplasty is performed by making a longitudinal incision of the pyloric sphincter extending into the antrum and the duodenum for about 2 cm on either side. The incision is closed transversely, thereby increasing the lumen of the pyloric channel. A Finney pyloroplasty is formed as a gastroduodenostomy with transection of the pyloric sphincter. The inner curve of the duodenum is approximated to the dependent aspect of the antrum and pyloric channel. A U-shaped incision is then made, crossing the pylorus. The pyloroplasty is completed by suturing the anterior duodenal wall to the antrum. For some cases in which severe pyloric scarring makes division of the pyloric channel difficult or hazardous, a side-to-side gastroduodenostomy can be used; this so-called Jaboulay procedure differs from the Finney pyloroplasty only in that the incision is not completed across the pyloric sphincter.

Truncal vagotomy can also be combined with resection of the gastric antrum to effect a further reduction in acid secretion, presumably by removing antral sources of gastrin. The limits of antral resection are usually defined by external landmarks, rather than the histologic transition from fundic to antral mucosae. The stomach is divided proximally along a line from a point above the incisura angularis to a point along the greater curvature midway from the pylorus to the gastroesophageal junction. Restoration of gastrointestinal continuity via a gastroduodenostomy is termed a Billroth I reconstruction. A Billroth II procedure uses a gastrojejunostomy (Fig. 22-7).

Proximal gastric vagotomy differs from truncal vagotomy

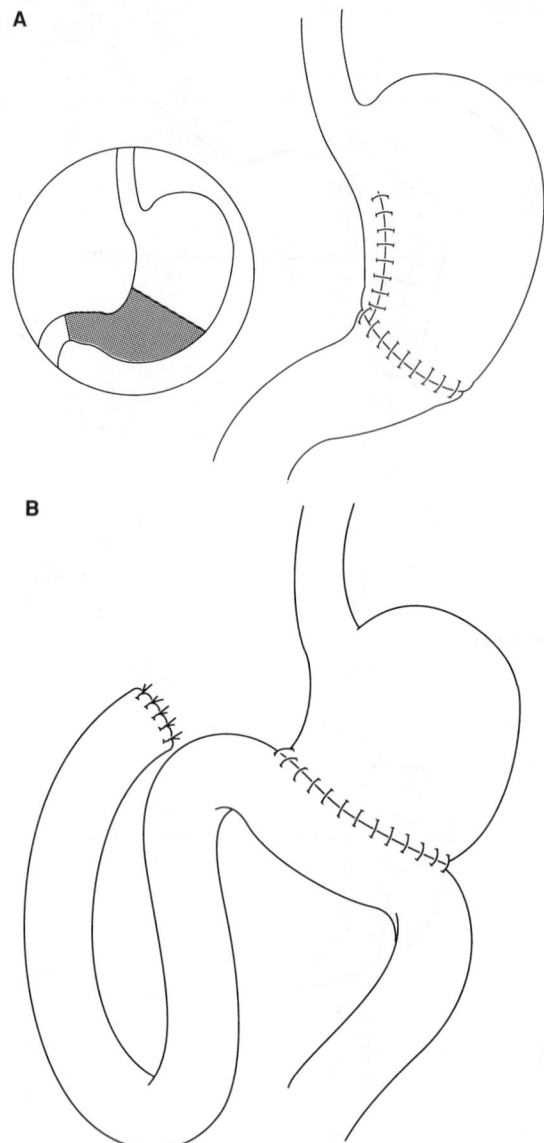

A

B

Figure 22-7. Antrectomy involves resection of the distal stomach (*blue area in inset*). Restoration of gastrointestinal continuity may be accomplished as a Billroth I gastroduodenostomy (*A*) or Billroth II gastrojejunostomy (*B*) reconstruction.

in that only the nerve fibers to the acid-secreting fundic mucosa are divided (see Fig. 22-5). Vagal nerve fibers to the antrum and pylorus are left intact, and the hepatic and celiac divisions are not transected. The denervation begins about 5 cm from the pylorus and extends proximally along the lesser curvature. In proximal gastric vagotomy, the distal esophagus is also skeletonized for a distance of 5 to 7 cm to divide any vagal fibers traveling to the fundus intramurally within the esophagus. The operation has also been called parietal cell vagotomy to emphasize its most important functional consequence.

Physiologic Consequences of Operation

Division of efferent vagal fibers directly affects acid secretion by reducing cholinergic stimulation of parietal cells. In addition, vagotomy also diminishes parietal cell responsiveness to gastrin and histamine. Basal acid secre-

tion is reduced by about 80% in the immediate postoperative period. Basal acid secretion increases slightly within months of operation but remains unchanged thereafter. The maximal acid output (MAO) in response to exogenously administered stimulants such as pentagastrin is reduced by about 70% in the early period after operation. After 1 year, pentagastrin-stimulated MAO rebounds to 50% of prevagotomy values but remains at this level on subsequent testing. Acid secretion due to endogenous stimulation by a liquid meal is reduced by 60% to 70% relative to normal subjects. The acid-reducing properties of proximal gastric vagotomy and truncal vagotomy are roughly equivalent in most series (Table 22-3).

The inclusion of antrectomy with truncal vagotomy causes further reductions in acid secretion. Pentagastrin-stimulated MAO is reduced by 85% relative to values recorded preoperatively. Little rebound in acid secretion occurs with the passage of time.

Truncal vagotomy and proximal gastric vagotomy both cause postoperative hypergastrinemia. Fasting gastrin values are elevated to about twice preoperative levels, and the postprandial response is exaggerated. Immediately after vagotomy, hypergastrinemia appears to be due to decreased luminal acid, with loss of feedback inhibition of gastrin release. Loss of vagal inhibitory pathways can also be important. Chronic hypergastrinemia, sustained long-term in most cases, is caused by gastrin cell hyperplasia in addition to loss of inhibitory feedback. When antrectomy is added to vagotomy, circulating gastrin levels are decreased. Basal gastrin values are reduced by about half and postprandial gastrin levels by two thirds. The major form of circulating hormone after antrectomy is gastrin 34, released from the duodenum.

Operations that involve vagotomy alter gastric emptying. Proximal gastric denervation abolishes vagally mediated receptive relaxation. Thus, for any given volume ingested, the intragastric pressure rise is greater and the gastroduodenal pressure gradient higher than in normals. As a result, emptying of liquids, which depends critically on the gastroduodenal pressure gradient, is accelerated after proximal gastric vagotomy. Because nerve fibers to the antrum and pylorus are preserved, the function of the distal stomach to mix and triturate solid food is preserved, and emptying of solids is nearly normal in patients who have undergone proximal gastric vagotomy. Truncal vagotomy affects the motor activities of both proximal and distal stomach. Solid and liquid emptying rates are usually increased when truncal vagotomy is accompanied by pyloroplasty.

Table 22-3. PHYSIOLOGIC ALTERATIONS CAUSED BY TRUNCAL VAGOTOMY

GASTRIC EFFECTS

Decreased basal acid output
   Reduced cholinergic input to parietal cells
Decreased stimulated maximal acid output
   Diminished sensitivity to histamine gastrin
   Decreased meal-induced acid secretion
Increased fasting and postprandial gastrin
Gastrin cell hyperplasia
Accelerated liquid emptying
Altered emptying of solids

NONGASTRIC EFFECTS

Decreased pancreatic exocrine secretion
   Decreased pancreatic enzymes and bicarbonate
Decreased postprandial bile flow
Increased gallbladder volumes
Diminished release of vagally mediated peptide hormones

Truncal vagotomy affects a number of other gastrointestinal functions because of the removal of efferent vagal innervation. Pancreatic exocrine secretion in response to a meal is diminished, with decreased bicarbonate and enzyme outputs. Postcibal biliary secretion is decreased, and gallbladder distention is observed. Fecal fat excretion doubles after truncal vagotomy, although clinical steatorrhea is unusual. Stimulated release of a number of gastrointestinal hormones—including pancreatic polypeptide, cholecystokinin, and secretin—is decreased. In most instances, these extragastric alterations in digestive function are subclinical in nature. Proximal gastric vagotomy, in which the vagal innervation to nongastric viscera is preserved, produces fewer physiologic alterations than does truncal vagotomy.

INTRACTABILITY

From the patient's perspective, the most important therapeutic issue is usually pain relief. In common usage, the term *intractability* has referred to ulcers that cause chronic pain because of failure to heal or because of relapse. With newer agents, such as omeprazole, pain relief can be achieved in most patients (up to 90%) within 2 weeks of beginning therapy, and pain is now infrequently a motive for operative intervention. Pain relief should not be equated with complete healing of ulcers, nor does absence of symptoms eliminate the risk of additional complications. A more useful definition of intractability would be mucosal healing refractory to medicinal treatment. Ulcers are considered refractory if they meet any of the following criteria:

1. Initial healing is delayed, so that ulceration persists at 3 months despite active drug therapy.
2. Ulcers recur within 1 year of initial healing despite maintenance therapy.
3. The ulcer disease is characterized by cycles of prolonged activity with brief or absent remissions.[19]

Intractability, in these terms, is an indication for operation.

When intractability is the reason for operation, the surgical recommendation should focus on safety, freedom from long-term disability, and avoidance of recurrent ulcer. In this circumstance, proximal gastric vagotomy is often considered the operation of choice. Proximal gastric vagotomy has the lowest operative mortality rate, the lowest incidence of postoperative symptoms, and an acceptable risk of recurrent ulcer. Collected series of proximal gastric vagotomies have reported an operative mortality rate of less than 0.05%,[20] lower than the reported mortality rate for any other gastric procedure for peptic ulcer. Truncal vagotomy and pyloroplasty performed for intractability has a reported mortality rate of 0.5% to 0.8%, whereas the mortality rate after truncal vagotomy and antrectomy approximates 1.5%.

A number of prospective, randomized trials have compared the various surgical options in terms of postoperative symptoms, including dumping, diarrhea, weight loss, and disturbance of life-style (Table 22-4). In most comparisons, proximal gastric vagotomy has proved superior to other operations in these measures. Dumping, a postprandial symptom complex of abdominal discomfort, weakness, and vasomotor symptoms of sweating and dizziness, occurs in 10% to 15% of truncal vagotomy and antrectomy patients in the early postoperative period and is chronically disabling in 1% to 2%. After truncal vagotomy and pyloroplasty, dumping is present initially in 10%, and remains severe in about 1%. Permanent symptoms of dumping are rare after proximal gastric vagotomy. The incidence of diarrhea, which is presumably caused by denervation of

Table 22-4. CLINICAL RESULTS OF DUODENAL ULCER SURGERY

	PGV (%)	TV + P (%)	TV + A (%)
Mortality rate	0	0.5–1	1–2
Acid reduction			
Basal	80	70	85
Stimulated	50	50	85
Ulcer recurrence	10	12	1–2
Gastric emptying			
Liquids	Accelerated	Accelerated	Accelerated
Solids	No change	Accelerated	Slowed
Dumping			
Mild	<5	10	10–15
Disabling	0	1	1–2
Diarrhea			
Mild	<5	25	20
Disabling	0	2	1–2

PGV, proximal gastric vagotomy; TV + P, truncal vagotomy and pyloroplasty; TV + A, truncal vagotomy and antrectomy.
(Adapted from Mulholland MW, Debas HT. Chronic duodenal and gastric ulcer. Surg Clin North Am 1987;67:489)

the pylorus and small bowel and by elimination of pyloric function, parallels the incidence of dumping after truncal vagotomy and antrectomy or pyloroplasty. Persistent or disabling diarrhea is present in less than 1% of patients after proximal gastric vagotomy. After truncal vagotomy, weight loss averages 2 kg in the first postoperative year, whereas with proximal gastric vagotomy, a weight gain is recorded. Reoperation after proximal gastric vagotomy is rarely needed for symptoms resulting from the operation.

The lower incidence of postoperative symptoms is obtained at the cost of a higher postoperative ulcer recurrence rate. The reported recurrence rates for proximal gastric vagotomy are variable, probably reflecting differences in experience and individual surgical skill. Although recurrence rates as low as 5% have been reported, a more generally accepted figure would be 10%. This rate is similar to that after truncal vagotomy and drainage (about 12%) but considerably greater than that reported after truncal vagotomy and antrectomy (1% to 3%). The reported ulcer recurrence rates after proximal gastric vagotomy can be adversely affected by the inclusion of prepyloric and pyloric channel ulcers. For reasons that are not clear, proximal gastric vagotomy is significantly less effective when used to treat ulcers in this position than when used for duodenal ulceration.

HEMORRHAGE

Hemorrhage is the leading cause of death associated with peptic ulcer, and the incidence of this complication has not changed since the introduction of H_2-receptor antagonists.[21] The lifetime risk of hemorrhage for duodenal ulcer patients who have not had surgery and who do not receive continuing maintenance drug therapy approximates 35%. Most hemorrhages occur during the initial episode of ulceration or during a relapse, and patients who have hemorrhaged previously have a higher risk of bleeding again. Patients with recurrent hemorrhage and elderly patients are at greatest risk of mortality, and these two groups should be resuscitated vigorously, investigated promptly, and treated aggressively.[22]

Upper gastrointestinal endoscopy is the appropriate initial diagnostic test when hemorrhage from duodenal ulceration is suspected. Endoscopy can correctly determine the site and cause of bleeding in over 90% of patients. An ulcer should be accepted as the bleeding source only if it has one of the stigmata of active or recent hemorrhage. Active hemorrhage is defined by an arterial jet, active oozing, or oozing beneath an adherent clot. The signs of recent hemorrhage include an adherent clot without oozing, an adherent slough within the ulcer base, or a visible vessel within the ulcer. The ability of these endoscopic findings to accurately predict recurrent hemorrhage has been extensively reported but remains controversial. About 30% of patients who have stigmata of recent hemorrhage experience rebleeding, and most of the patients who experience recurrent hemorrhage require emergency operation. These stigmata are not sufficiently accurate to be used alone as indications for operation. Rather, they serve as a warning that aggressive therapy is needed and close follow-up mandatory. The occurrence of hypovolemic shock and a posteroinferior location of the ulcer are additional clinical features that have been associated with increased risks of recurrent bleeding.

The ability to visualize bleeding duodenal ulcers endoscopically has led to attempts to treat hemorrhage endoscopically. There are many different methods of endoscopic therapy, but the most established consist of thermal coagulation. Thermal coagulation can be achieved by laser photocoagulation, bipolar electrocoagulation, or direct application of heat through a heater probe.[23] Unequivocal proof of efficacy, in the form of lowered rebleeding rates and avoidance of operation, has also been difficult to obtain. The analysis of reports of endoscopic treatment of hemorrhage is complicated by the 70% rate of spontaneous, though sometimes temporary, cessation of bleeding without intervention. An NIH Consensus Development Conference has recommended endoscopic hemostatic therapy in selected patients. Hemodynamic instability, need for continuing transfusion, red stool or hematemesis, age over 60, and serious medical comorbidity are clinical features that mandate endoscopic therapy. Rebleeding during hospitalization and the endoscopic findings of visible vessel, oozing, or bleeding associated with an adherent clot are other indications for endoscopic hemostasis. Ulcers with clean bases probably require no treatment. Failure of endoscopic hemostasis is usually due to inaccessibility because of scarring, to rapid active bleeding, or to an adherent clot. Patients treated endoscopically should be observed closely for further hemorrhage.

Operative intervention is appropriate for the following:

- Massive hemorrhage leading to shock or cardiovascular instability
- Prolonged blood loss requiring continuing transfusion
- Recurrent bleeding during medical therapy or after endoscopic therapy
- Recurrent hemorrhage requiring hospitalization

Operative therapy should consist of duodenotomy with direct ligation of the bleeding vessel within the ulcer base followed by a procedure to effect permanent reduction in acid production. Truncal vagotomy and pyloroplasty or truncal vagotomy and antrectomy have most commonly been used for this purpose. The need for emergency operation significantly increases surgical risks; mortality rates are increased about 10-fold.

PERFORATION

The lifetime risk for perforation in individuals with duodenal ulceration not receiving therapy approximates 10%. In contrast, ulcer perforation is unusual during maintenance therapy if initial ulcer healing has been achieved.

Perforation of a duodenal ulcer is usually accompanied by sudden and severe epigastric pain. The pain, caused by the spillage of highly caustic gastric secretions into the peritoneum, rapidly reaches peak intensity and remains constant. Radiation to the right scapular region is common because of right subphrenic collection of gastric contents. Occasionally, pain is sensed in the lower abdomen if gastric contents travel caudally through the paracolic gutter. Peritoneal irritation is usually intense, and most patients avoid movement to minimize discomfort.

Physical examination reveals low-grade fever, diminished bowel sounds, and rigidity of the abdominal musculature. Usually, upright abdominal radiographs reveal pneumoperitoneum, but up to 20% of perforated ulcers do not show free intraperitoneal air. Upper gastrointestinal contrast studies performed with water-soluble contrast agents can occasionally be helpful if pneumoperitoneum is not demonstrated but perforation is still suspected.

Although occasional reports have described the nonoperative treatment of this complication, perforation remains a strong indication for operation in most circumstances. Laparotomy affords the opportunity to relieve intraperitoneal contamination caused by the perforation and to provide permanent reduction in acid production.

Signs of antecedent duodenal ulceration, in terms of both history of prior symptoms and anatomic evidence of duodenal scarring, should be sought. Simple omental closure of duodenal perforation resulting from chronic ulceration does not provide satisfactory long-term results; up to 80% of patients so treated have recurrent ulceration, and 10% experience reperforation if untreated. About two thirds of all patients with perforation have chronic symptoms and therefore are at risk of recurrent disease. In these patients, the performance of a definitive antiulcer operation should be considered in addition to closing the perforation (Fig. 22-8). Recent reports suggest that patients without antecedent symptoms are also at risk for recurrent ulceration. By 5 to 6 years, symptomatic ulcer recurrence in patients with acute ulcer perforation is similar to that for patients with chronic disease. Definitive ulcer operation should therefore also be considered for patients with perforated acute ulcers.

A definitive ulcer operation should be performed in patients with perforation if the following circumstances apply[24]: there has been no preoperative shock; no life-threatening medical illness coexists; and the perforation has been present for less than 48 hours. If these criteria are not met, simple omental patching of the perforation and peritoneal débridement are usually safer; definitive therapy, if necessary, can be performed at a later date, when the patient has recovered. In addition, the antiulcer operation should ideally add no additional risk of long-term sequelae and should provide excellent protection against future ulceration.

For most patients receiving prompt surgical attention, definitive antiulcer therapy can be performed with a risk equivalent to that of simple closure. The risk of recurrent ulcer and the incidence of unpleasant postoperative symptoms are similar to those seen when operation is performed electively for intractability. The choice of antiulcer operation, therefore, depends on functional considerations similar to those for intractability. Proximal gastric vagotomy with patch closure of the perforation is an attractive alternative in this circumstance and has been shown to be both safe and effective in preventing ulcer relapse. Incorporation of the perforation as part of a pyloroplasty or resection of the site of perforation during antrectomy can also be combined with truncal vagotomy with favorable results.

OBSTRUCTION

Gastric outlet obstruction can occur acutely or chronically in patients with duodenal ulcer disease. Acute obstruction is caused by edema and inflammation associated

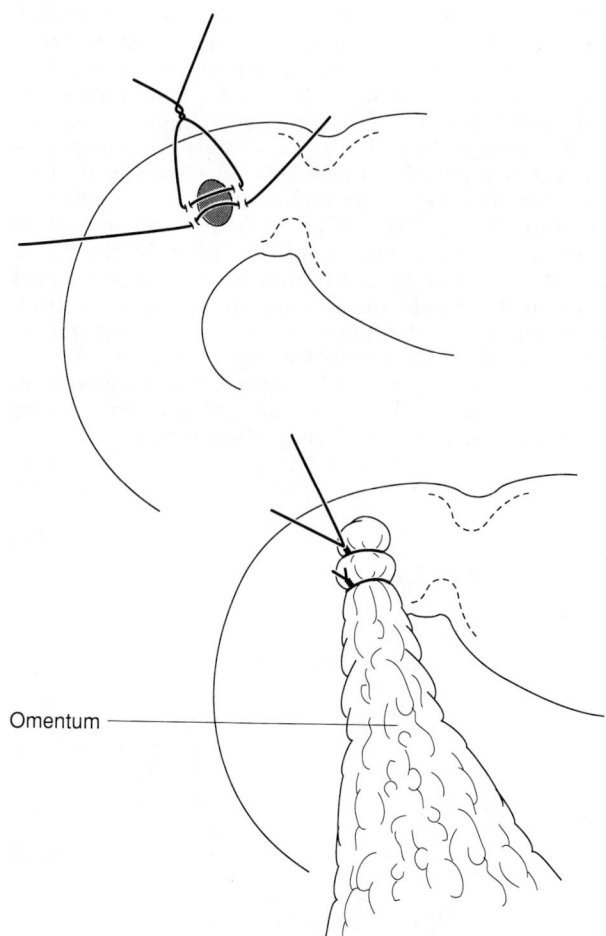

Figure 22-8. Omental patching of perforated duodenal ulcer.

with ulcers in the pyloric channel and the first portion of the duodenum. Pyloric obstruction is suggested by recurrent vomiting, dehydration, and hypochloremic alkalosis due to loss of gastric secretions. Acute gastric outlet obstruction is treated with nasogastric suction, rehydration, and intravenous administration of antisecretory agents. In

most instances, acute obstruction resolves with such supportive measures within 72 hours.

Repeated episodes of ulceration and healing can lead to pyloric scarring and a fixed stenosis with chronic gastric outlet obstruction. In cases of untreated duodenal ulceration, the lifetime risk of chronic pyloric stenosis approximates 10%.

Upper endoscopy is indicated to confirm the nature of the obstruction and to exclude neoplasm. Endoscopic hydrostatic balloon dilatation of pyloric stenoses can also be attempted at this time (Fig. 22-9). About 85% of pyloric stenoses are technically amenable to dilatation; 80% of treated patients report immediate symptomatic improvement.[25] Only 40% of patients with gastric stenoses have sustained improvement by 3 months after balloon dilatation. Recurrent stenoses are presumably due to residual scarring within the pyloric channel. Thus, although pyloric dilatation is occasionally palliative, in most cases operative correction is required.

Operative management of gastric outlet obstruction should include treatment of the underlying ulcer disease and relief of the anatomic abnormality. Truncal vagotomy with antrectomy and truncal vagotomy with drainage have both been used with success in this circumstance, with ulcer recurrence rates similar to those for intractability and with satisfactory restoration of gastric emptying. There is considerable interest in the use of proximal gastric vagotomy and duodenoplasty or dilatation for the treatment of pyloric stenosis, and the experience to date must be considered promising. Ulcer recurrence rates are not reported to be increased when proximal gastric vagotomy is used in this circumstance, which is surprising in view of the higher recurrence rates associated with pyloric channel ulcers.

POSTGASTRECTOMY SYNDROMES

A number of syndromes have been described that are associated with distressing symptoms after gastric operations performed for peptic ulcer or gastric neoplasm. The occurrence of severe postoperative symptoms is fortunately low, perhaps 1% to 3% of cases, but the disturbances can be disabling. The two most common postgastrectomy syndromes, categorized according to predomi-

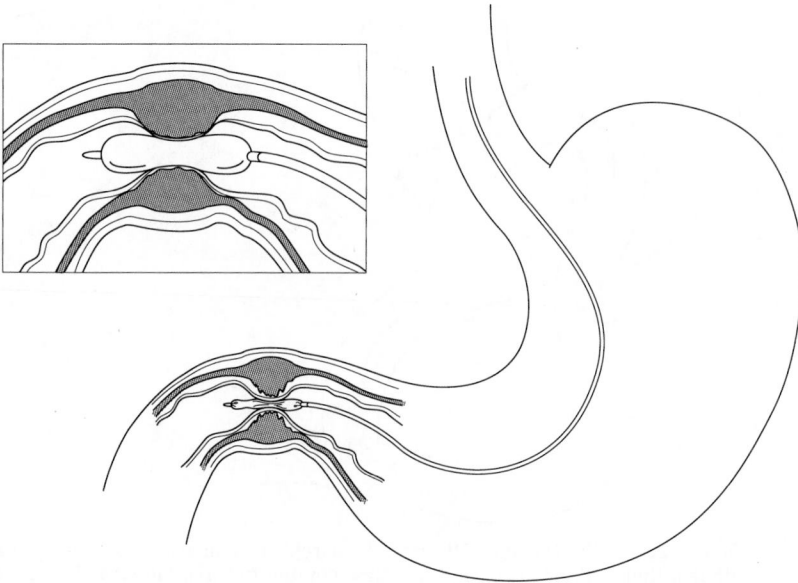

Figure 22-9. Schematic representation of balloon dilation of pyloric stenosis.

nant manifestation, are dumping and alkaline reflux gastritis.

Dumping

The term *dumping* denotes a clinical syndrome with both gastrointestinal and vasomotor symptoms. The precise cause of dumping is not known but is believed to relate to the unmetered entry of ingested food into the proximal small bowel after vagotomy and either resection or division of the pyloric sphincter. Early dumping symptoms occur immediately after a meal and include nausea, epigastric discomfort, borborygmi, palpitations, and, in extreme cases, dizziness or syncope. Late dumping symptoms follow a meal by 1 to 3 hours and can include reactive hypoglycemia in addition to the above symptoms.

Although a relatively large number of patients experience mild dumping symptoms in the early postoperative period, minor dietary alterations and the passage of time bring improvement in all but about 1%. The somatostatin analogue octreotide has been reported to improve dumping symptoms when 50 to 100 μg is administered subcutaneously before a meal.[26] The beneficial effects of somatostatin on the vasomotor symptoms of dumping are postulated to be due to pressor effects of the compound on splanchnic vessels. In addition, somatostatin analogues inhibit the release of vasoactive peptides from the gut, decrease peak plasma insulin levels, and slow intestinal transit, all effects that might be expected to ameliorate dumping symptoms. Octreotide administration before meal ingestion has been shown to prevent changes in pulse, systolic blood pressure, and packed red cell volume during early dumping and blood glucose levels during late dumping.

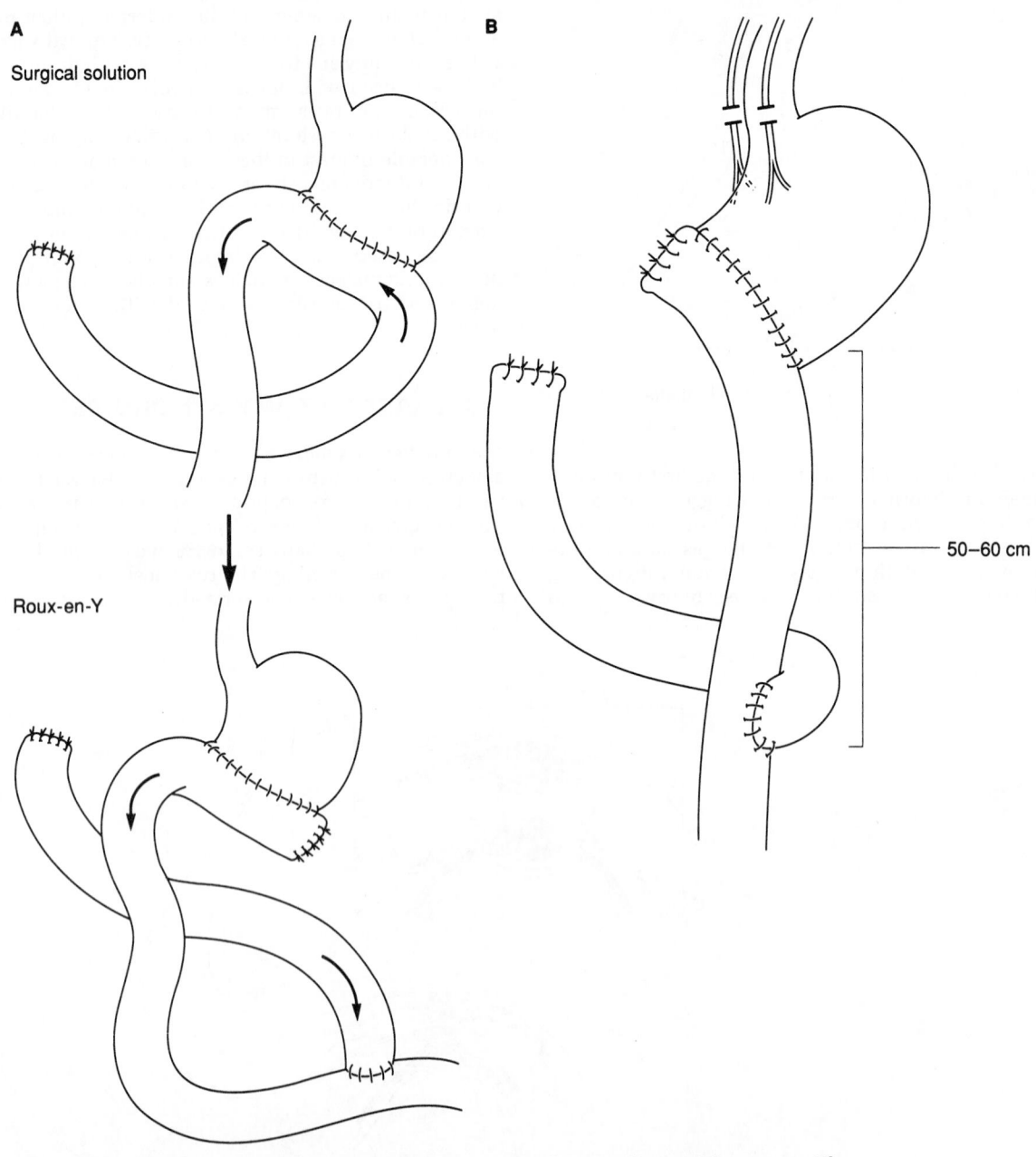

A Surgical solution

Roux-en-Y

B 50–60 cm

Figure 22-10. Conversion of Billroth II gastrojejunostomy to Roux-en-Y gastrojejunostomy. The afferent limb is divided (*A*), and intestinal continuity is reestablished by anastomosis 50 to 60 cm downstream from the original gastrojejunostomy (*B*).

Alkaline Reflux Gastritis

The term *alkaline reflux gastritis* should be reserved for patients who demonstrate the clinical triad of postprandial epigastric pain often associated with nausea and vomiting, evidence of reflux of bile into the stomach, and histologic evidence of gastritis. One or more of these findings occur transiently in 10% to 20% of patients after truncal vagotomy and drainage or resection, but they persist in only 1% to 2%.

The differential diagnosis for a patient with postoperative epigastric pain includes recurrent ulceration, biliary and pancreatic disease, afferent loop obstruction, and esophagitis in addition to alkaline reflux gastritis. Gastric acid analysis shows basal hypochlorhydria with little increase with pentagastrin stimulation. Serum gastrin measurements should be determined to exclude Zollinger-Ellison syndrome and retained gastric antrum. Endoscopic examination is essential to exclude recurrent ulcer. Endoscopy shows reflux of bile into the stomach. Quantitative assessment of enterogastric reflux can be obtained by intravenously injected radionuclides such as ^{99m}Tc HIDA. The radionuclide is excreted in the bile, and external scintigraphy over the abdomen can be used to measure reflux of bile into the stomach.

Endoscopically, the gastric mucosa appears red, friable, and edematous. Gastric inflammation is patchy and nonulcerative. Histologic examination shows mucosal and submucosal edema and infiltration of acute and chronic inflammatory cells into the lamina propria. Glandular atrophy and intestinal metaplasia are frequent accompaniments.

No perfect solution to alkaline reflux gastritis exists. Antacids, H_2-receptor antagonists, bile acid chelators, and dietary manipulations have not been demonstrated to be definitely beneficial. The only proven treatment for alkaline reflux gastritis is operative diversion of intestinal contents from contact with the gastric mucosa. The most common surgical procedure used for this purpose is a Roux-en-Y gastrojejunostomy with an intestinal limb of 50 to 60 cm constructed to prevent reflux of intestinal contents (Fig. 22-10). This procedure is effective in eliminating bilious vomiting (nearly 100%), but recurrent or persistent pain is reported in up to 30% of patients, and up to 20% of patients are troubled with delayed gastric emptying postoperatively.[27,28]

REFERENCES

1. Glise H. Epidemiology in peptic ulcer disease: current status and future aspects. Scand J Gastroenterol 1990;25(Suppl 175):13.
2. Sontag S, Graham DY, Belsito A, et al. Cimetidine, cigarette smoking, and recurrence of duodenal ulcer. N Engl J Med 1984;311:689.
3. Soll A. Pathogenesis of peptic ulcer and implications for therapy. N Engl J Med 1990;322:909.
4. Dooley CP, Cohen H. The clinical significance of *Campylobacter pyloris*. Ann Intern Med 1988;108:70.
5. Ateshkadi A, Iam NP, Johnson CA. *Helicobacter pylori* and peptic ulcer disease. Clin Pharmacol 1993;12:34.
6. Isenberg JI, Selling JA, Hogan DL, Koss MA. Impaired proximal duodenal mucosal bicarbonate secretion in patients with duodenal ulcer. N Engl J Med 1987;316:374.
7. Bukhave K, Rask-Madsen J, Hogan DL, Koss MA, Isenberg JI. Proximal duodenal prostaglandin E_2 release and mucosal bicarbonate secretion are altered in patients with duodenal ulcer. Gastroenterology 1990;99:951.
8. Dooley CP, Larson AW, Stace NH, et al. Double-contrast barium meal and upper gastrointestinal endoscopy: a comparative study. Ann Intern Med 1984;101:538.
9. Debas HT, Mulholland MW. New horizons in the pharmacologic management of peptic ulceration. Am J Surg 1986;151:422.
10. Sontag S. Current status of maintenance therapy in peptic ulcer disease. Am J Gastroenterol 1988;83:607.
11. Debas HT, Mulholland MW. Drug therapy in peptic ulcer disease. Curr Probl Surg 1989;26:9.
12. Carmine AA, Brogden RN. Pirenzepine: a review of its pharmacologic and pharmacokinetic properties and therapeutic efficacy in peptic ulcer disease and allied diseases. Drugs 1985;30:85.
13. Massoomi F, Savage J, Destache CJ. Omeprazole: a comprehensive review. Pharmacotherapy 1993;13:46.
14. Lykkegaard Nielsen MC, Vagn Nielsen O, Moesgaard F. Ulcer healing after treatment with sucralfate emulsion or ranitidine: randomized controlled study in peptic ulcer disease. J Clin Gastroenterol 1988;10:377.
15. Nicholson PA. A multicenter international controlled comparison of two dosage regimes of misoprostol and cimetidine in the treatment of duodenal ulcer in out-patients. Dig Dis Sci 1985;30:171S.
16. Berstad A, Weberg R. Antacids in the treatment of gastroduodenal ulcer. Scand J Gastroenterol 1986;21:385.
17. Labenz J, Gyenes E, Ruhl GH, Borsch G. Omeprazole plus amoxicillin: efficacy of various treatment regimens to eradicate *Helicobacter pylori*. Am J Gastroenterol 1993;88:491.
18. Labenz J, Gyenes E, Ruhl GH, Borsch G. Amoxicillin plus omeprazole versus triple therapy for eradication of *Helicobacter pylori* in duodenal ulcer disease: a prospective, randomized, controlled study. Gut 1993;34:1167.
19. Netchvolodoff CV. Refractory peptic lesions. Postgrad Med 1993;93:143.
20. Schirmer BD. Current status of proximal gastric vagotomy. Ann Surg 1989;209:131.
21. Christensen A, Bousfield R, Christiansen J. Incidence of perforated and bleeding peptic ulcers before and after the introduction of H_2-receptor antagonists. Ann Surg 1988;207:4.
22. Branicki FJ, Boey J, Fok PJ, et al. Bleeding duodenal ulcer: a prospective evaluation of risk factors for rebleeding and death. Ann Surg 1990;211:411.
23. Goh P, Tekant Y. Endoscopic hemostasis of bleeding peptic ulcers. Dig Dis 1993;11:216.
24. Boey J, Wong J, Ong GB. A prospective study of operative risk factors in perforated duodenal ulcers. Ann Surg 1982;195:265.
25. Hogan RB, Hamilton JK, Polter DE. Preliminary experience with hydrostatic balloon dilation of gastric outlet obstruction. Gastrointest Endosc 1986;32:71.
26. Lamers CBHW, Bijlstra AM, Harris AG. Octreotide, a long-acting somatostatin analog, in the management of postoperative dumping syndrome. Dig Dis Sci 1993;38:359.
27. Ritchie WP. Alkaline reflux gastritis: late results of a controlled trial of diagnosis and treatment. Ann Surg 1986;203:537.
28. Mulholland MW, Debas HT. Chronic duodenal and gastric ulcer. Surg Clin North Am 1987;67:489.

SURGERY: SCIENTIFIC PRINCIPLES AND PRACTICE, Second Edition, edited by Lazar J. Greenfield, Michael W. Mulholland, Keith T. Oldham, Gerald B. Zelenock, and Keith D. Lillemoe. Lippincott–Raven Publishers, Philadelphia, © 1997.

CHAPTER 23

STRESS ULCER AND GASTRIC ULCER

GORDON L. KAUFFMAN, JR., AND ROBERT L. CONTER

GASTRIC MUCOSAL DEFENSE

Gastric mucosal injury and ulceration originate with damage to the surface epithelium. Although patients with duodenal ulcer tend to have higher rates of acid secretion than nonulcer patients, this does not seem to be the case for patients with stress ulceration or gastric ulcer. Although a large body of evidence suggests that aggressive factors within the gastric lumen can predispose to ulceration, it has become clear that endogenous mucosal defense factors play an important role in maintaining gastric mucosal integrity and that mucosal injury can occur when these defenses are defective or altered. For better understanding of the pathophysiology of gastric mucosal injury, a contemporary view of mucosal defensive factors is presented in Figure 23-1. Much of the information related to these mechanisms has been derived from animal investigation; in many instances, however, verification of similar functions in humans has been described.

The concept of the gastric mucosal barrier has been proposed to describe the observation that the gastric mucosal epithelium could maintain a significant proton gradient without the occurrence of damage. No true, morphologically defined entity has been identified as this barrier; rather, it is believed to be a property of both gastric mucus and an intact monolayer of surface epithelial cells. Barrier function can be made defective by the intraluminal application of aspirin, bile acids, ethanol, and lysolecithin. Protons then diffuse down the concentration gradient from the lumen into the mucosa. Net flux of protons into the mucosa is associated with a concomitant movement of sodium, water, glucose, and protein from the mucosa into the lumen. Coinciding with these changes in permeability is a fall in the transmucosal electric potential difference and a release of histamine into the mucosa, enhancing blood flow. The end result is both macroscopic and microscopic evidence of mucosal damage with gross hemorrhage.

EPITHELIAL RESTITUTION

The gastric epithelium turns over more rapidly than any other epithelial surface in the body, being entirely replaced every 2 to 3 days.[1] Mucous neck cells, found at the junction of the gastric pit and gland, become surface epithelial cells by migration toward the luminal surface. This rapid epithelial replacement probably serves as the first line of defense against toxic substances and mechanical trauma.

During stress, widespread disruption of surface epithelial cells can occur in a matter of minutes. If the damage is superficial, it can be repaired rapidly (in 15 to 60 minutes) through the process of reepithelialization or restitution.[2] Epithelial damage results in a release of mucus from desquamated as well as viable cells and the formation over the site of injury of a "mucosal cap" whose other components are cellular debris and fibrin. This cap provides the epithelial cells with a microenvironment of relatively high pH attributable, in part, to a leakage of plasma from the damaged mucosal capillaries. The mucus cap is thought to retard acid back-diffusion into the mucosal defect.

Epithelial cells that remain viable flatten out and spread across denuded areas; however, no new cells are formed during this process. An intact muscularis mucosae is essential for restitution to occur. Cellular regeneration of epithelial cells and fibroblasts, along with angiogenesis, then initiates the healing process.

Another characteristic of the gastric mucosal surface epithelium that appears to render it less susceptible to injury is hydrophobicity.[3] Experimentally, administration of surface-active phospholipids that act as surfactants protects the gastric mucosa against acid-induced injury. Compounds that denature surfactant, such as ethanol and aspirin, are associated with gastric mucosal injury. Exogenous administration of prostaglandins, which are associated with protection, enhances the production of these surfactant components. Gastric gel mucus is most likely the major contributor to this property. Human gastric epithelium is more hydrophobic than duodenal or rectal epithelium.[4] No observation of this property of the gastric epithelium has been reported in patients predisposed to develop stress ulcer or in those with gastric ulcer.

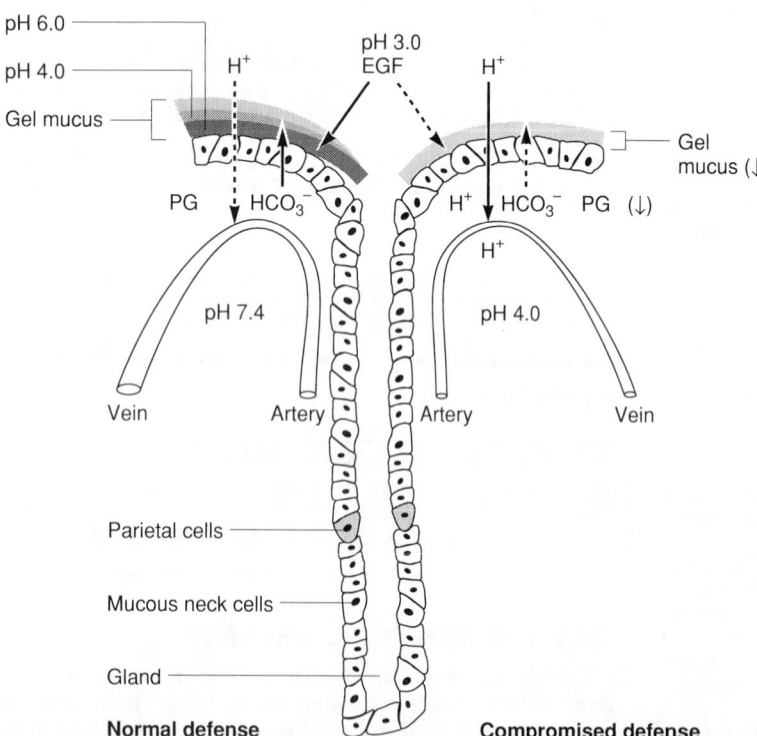

Figure 23-1. Schematic diagram of normal and compromised defense conditions. Abnormally low mucosal blood flow allows protons (H^+) to remain in the mucosa, resulting in an acidic pH. Gel mucus concentration and thickness may be reduced, as may HCO_3^- secretion. Endogenous prostaglandins (PG) in the mucosa and epidermal growth factor (EGF) may exert a lesser effect on mucosal function. As a result of barrier compromise, a greater mass of H^+ diffuses down the concentration gradient into the mucosa.

Mucus and Bicarbonate Secretion

Gastric mucus is produced by the surface epithelial cell. In addition to serving as a lubricant, mucus also enhances mucosal defense by forming an unstirred layer overlying the epithelial surface. This layer of gel mucus is dynamic, constantly released from the surface epithelial cell and degraded by proteolytic compounds such as pepsin. In humans, the thickness of this gel layer has been reported to be about 500 μm. The vacuoles containing mucus in the cytosol of the surface epithelial cell are released by cholinergic stimulation and intraluminal application of acetylcholine and prostaglandins. Synthesis and release are inhibited by aspirin-like compounds that inhibit cyclooxygenase. Gel mucus retards proton mobility by a factor of only three or four, a degree that is inadequate to maintain a near neutral pH at the apical membrane of the surface epithelial cell during luminal acidification. It is possible that larger molecules such as bile salts, lysolecithin, and pepsin, each of which can cause mucosal injury, can be significantly retarded by gel mucus. Gastric erosions develop after the removal of mucus from the mucosa. Evidence suggests that the depletion of gastric mucus hexosamine precedes the development of gastric ulcers in fasting experimental animals.

In addition to producing mucus, the gastric surface epithelial cells secrete a bicarbonate-rich fluid. Reported concentrations of bicarbonate range from 8 to 18 mmol/L, and the amount of bicarbonate secreted is about 5% to 10% of the amount of acid that the same surface of mucosa can produce. The magnitude of gastric bicarbonate secretion in humans ranges from approximately 0.5 to 2.6 mmol/h. As with mucus, bicarbonate secretion is stimulated by cholinergic agents and prostaglandins, and inhibited by cyclooxygenase inhibitors.

The release of bicarbonate into the gel mucus provides a significant mucosal defense by maintaining a near neutral acid–base milieu at the apical membrane of the surface epithelial cells. When luminal fluid pH is between 3.0 and 6.0, a pH gradient can be measured with a microelectrode.[5] When the luminal pH is around 3.0, the apical membrane of the surface epithelial cell can be exposed to a pH of about 5.0.

Mucosal Blood Flow

Maintenance of gastric mucosal blood flow enhances mucosal defense. In addition to providing the surface epithelial cells with nutrients and oxygen, blood flow serves as a sink for the removal of protons that have diffused across the epithelial membrane. The gastric mucosa becomes much more susceptible to injury when the submucosal pH falls below 4.0. By removing protons from the interstitial fluid, a near neutral pH is maintained as a defense against injury. Adequate mucosal blood flow also aids in preventing the formation of oxygen-derived free radicals.[6] These toxic reactive species of oxygen are lipid peroxidases and are generated when ischemia is followed by tissue reperfusion.

There is general agreement that mucosal ischemia plays a role in the development of stress gastritis. In the clinical setting, most patients who develop stress gastritis have experienced an episode of shock from sepsis, hemorrhage, or cardiac dysfunction. Gastric mucosal blood flow falls during hemorrhagic shock. It has been proposed that the relation between ischemia and stress gastritis can be explained by the depletion of high-energy phosphate compounds such as adenosine triphosphate from the gastric epithelium. Mucosal energy deficit, usually greater in the fundic mucosa than in the antrum, can result in cell death.

Patients in the intensive care unit setting with cardiovascular instability probably have fluctuations in gastric mucosal blood flow, although this has not been unequivocally demonstrated. A period of relative ischemia followed by reperfusion is likely to be associated with the generation of reactive oxygen species. As a consequence, cellular plasma membranes and subcellular organelles are injured and the integrity of the gastric epithelium destroyed. The importance of maintaining adequate mucosal blood flow in these precarious patients cannot be overemphasized.

Gastric mucosal ischemia is also believed to be a factor in the pathogenesis of chronic gastric ulcers. Patients with benign gastric ulcer have lower basal mucosal blood flow along the lesser curve than along the greater curve, the former being the location most often associated with gastric ulcer. As might be expected, blood flow in the base of an ulcer is lower than in normal-appearing mucosa. At the healing edge, flow is higher. It has also been suggested that prominent muscle bundles at the incisura compromise local mucosal blood flow during contraction, thereby rendering the mucosa susceptible to ulceration. Gastric contractions can reduce mucosal blood flow in the corpus by as much as 50% in some animals.

The factors that mediate gastric mucosal blood flow are poorly understood. Epidermal growth factor has been shown to have a protective effect on ethanol-induced mucosal injury by the enhancement of gastric blood flow. Dopaminergic agonists decrease gastric mucosal injury, whereas their antagonists aggravate stress- or ethanol-induced gastric injury, presumably by their respective maintenance or reduction of gastric blood flow. The effects of these and other potential systemic or locally produced mediators on gastric blood flow remain to be clearly defined.

Endogenous Prostanoids

The primary prostanoids produced in the gastric mucosa from the metabolism of arachidonic acid are prostaglandin E_2 (PGE_2) and prostacyclin (PGI_2).[8] Given exogenously, both inhibit acid secretion, stimulate the secretion of mucus and bicarbonate, and are vasodilators, enhancing mucosal blood flow. Given these observations and the knowledge that inhibitors of cyclooxygenase produce mucosal injury, much effort has gone into the study of potential aberrations in endogenous prostaglandin activity in patients with gastric ulcer disease. There is no clear pattern of aberrations in prostaglandin activity with respect to stress gastritis or chronic gastric ulcer.

The effects of inhibiting endogenous prostaglandin synthesis on mucosal integrity are well established. Inhibition of cyclooxygenase results in gastric mucosa devoid of PGE_2 and PGI_2. Cyclooxygenase inhibition is not sufficient to produce a mucosal injury unless a harmful intraluminal agent, such as aspirin, ethanol, bile salts, or lysolecithin, is present.[9] The degree of ulceration produced by any standard experimental ulcerogen is potentiated when endogenous cyclooxygenase activity is reduced by at least 80%.

Stress ulcers induced in experimental animals can be prevented by the administration of exogenous prostaglandins at doses that do not inhibit gastric acid secretion. Although the endogenous prostaglandin activity is reduced by 30% during experimental stress in rats, no studies have examined endogenous prostaglandins in patients predisposed to develop stress ulceration. Exogenous prostaglandins (E_2) as therapeutic agents can accelerate ulcer healing rates.

Trophic Peptides

Large doses of gastrin given over a long period of time produce macroscopically and microscopically evident trophic effects on the gastric mucosa. Incorporation of tritiated thymidine is also enhanced by exogenous or endogenous chronic hypergastrinemia. Any direct clinical correlate of these observations is not applicable to most patients with peptic ulcer disease other than patients with gastrinomas, who exhibit a hypertrophied gastric mucosa.

Epidermal growth factor (EGF) is a peptide produced by the salivary glands and Brunner glands within the duodenum. Given exogenously, EGF is antisecretory and stimulates ornithine decarboxylase activity and polyamine biosynthesis. Surgical removal of the salivary glands results in a loss of salivary EGF from the luminal fluid, which bathes the stomach and duodenum.[10] Sialoadenectomized animals have higher rates of gastric acid secretion and a gastric mucosa that is susceptible to injury produced by standard ulcerogens compared with control rats. Although no studies demonstrate a deficiency of EGF concentration in the luminal fluid in humans with gastric ulcer or stress gastritis, a case can be made for the role of EGF as a chronic trophic peptide that, acting luminally, enhances mucosal defense.

STRESS GASTRITIS

In the past decade, significant advances have been made in identifying the basic events that can culminate in life-threatening gastric bleeding from stress gastritis. Despite this progress, ambiguity and confusion exist with respect to the classification and pathophysiology of this disease process. Stress-gastritis lesions have been referred to as stress ulcers, stress erosive gastritis, and hemorrhagic gastritis.

Acute stress gastritis, by definition, occurs after major physical trauma, shock, sepsis, hemorrhage, respiratory failure, or severe burns. It is characterized by multiple superficial (nonulcerating) erosions that begin in the proximal or acid-secretory portion of the stomach and progress distally. Acute gastritis can also occur as a result of central nervous system disease (Cushing ulcer) or as a result of a thermal burn of greater than 35% of the body surface area (Curling ulcer). Drug-related gastritis can have different morphologic characteristics and a different cause than those lesions that develop after trauma or multiple organ system failure.

Definition of Lesions

Endoscopic studies demonstrate that the lesions of stress gastritis change with time. They have been detected within a few hours of the onset of injury, and acute mucosal erosions can be considered as early lesions if they occur within the first 24 hours and if they appear as multiple, shallow, discrete (1 to 2 mm) areas of erythema along with focal hemorrhage or an adherent clot. Frank bleeding occurs only after the gastric mucosa has eroded into the submucosa, which contains the blood supply. In some cases, a central area of pallor is surrounded by erythema rather than intramucosal bleeding, suggesting ischemia and reperfusion. Histologically, early stress lesions are wedge-shaped mucosal hemorrhages with coagulation necrosis of the superficial mucosal cells. In less aggressive forms, the surface epithelium is intact and scattered leukocytes are seen within the lamina propria. In the aggressive form, a more pronounced inflammatory cellular infiltrate and coagulation necrosis are observed. Fibrosis and scarring are not found in these acute lesions. The injury almost always begins in the proximal stomach and is only rarely (5%) seen in the antrum.

Acute stress-related gastritis can be classified as late if there is tissue reaction, organization around a clot, or an inflammatory exudate. This histologic picture can be seen 24 to 72 hours after injury. In contrast to the intensely erythematous appearance of early lesions, these late lesions have an appearance identical to that of regenerating mucosa around a healing gastric ulcer. Hemorrhage, inflammatory cell infiltration, and coagulation necrosis extend into the deeper (muscularis mucosa) layers of the gastric wall. The demonstration of early or late lesions is a function of the timing of endoscopy and the presence of ongoing acute mucosal injury of greater than 72 hours' duration. Both types of lesions can be seen endoscopically.

Predisposing Factors

Although the precise mechanisms responsible for the development of stress gastritis remain to be defined, current evidence[11] would support a multifactorial etiology: the presence of luminal acid, gastric mucosal permeability to protons, reduced gastric mucosal blood flow, reduced gastric mucus and bicarbonate synthesis and secretion, systemic acidosis, abnormal epithelial cell renewal, and altered production of endogenous prostaglandins. The end result is decreased gastric mucosal defense that, under physiologic conditions, protects against acid and pepsin aggression (Table 23-1).

Luminal Acid Secretion

There is little evidence suggesting that increased gastric acid secretion is the sole cause of stress gastritis. The presence of luminal acid appears to be necessary for this form of gastritis to occur. Complete neutralization of luminal acid or inhibition of gastric acid secretion precludes the development of experimental stress gastritis. It is likely that a critical concentration of luminal protons is required to initiate injury. Gastric mucosal ulceration develops when the pH in the lamina propria falls under conditions of increased proton back-diffusion. Although the absolute concentration of acid required to induce stress gastritis can vary, the pathogenesis of stress ulceration can be the result

---

Table 23-1. PREDISPOSING FACTORS FOR STRESS GASTRITIS

GASTRIC CONDITIONS

Luminal acid secretion
Mucosal permeability
Mucosal blood flow
Mucus and bicarbonate production
Epithelial cell renewal
Endogenous prostaglandins
Systemic acid–base status

CLINICAL CONDITIONS

Multiple trauma
Hypotension
Sepsis
Adult respiratory distress syndrome
Major burn
Oliguric renal failure
Hepatic dysfunction
Prolonged surgical procedures
Massive transfusion requirements
Extended intensive care stay

of a relatively small amount of luminal acid combined with alterations in gastric mucosal defense mechanisms.

Predisposing Clinical Conditions

Most gastrointestinal surgeons believe that the frequency of life-threatening hemorrhage from stress gastritis is diminishing, although this has not been documented epidemiologically. This decrease can be related to the improved quality of care provided to the critically ill patient. As a result, there are few well-designed, prospective, randomized, endoscopically controlled studies, using life-threatening hemorrhage as the end point, addressing the issues of prophylaxis, medical therapy, and surgical therapy. Instead, recommendations are based on studies with a limited number of patients in whom a fall in hematocrit or bloody nasogastric tube aspirate were considered to be end points. Several risk factors or predisposing clinical conditions have been identified. Specific risk factors include adult respiratory distress syndrome, multiple trauma, major burn of over 35% of the body surface area, oliguric renal failure, large transfusion requirements, hepatic dysfunction, hypotension, prolonged surgical procedures, and sepsis from any source. A direct correlation has been shown between acute upper gastrointestinal hemorrhage and the severity of critical illness.

Clinical studies that have not relied on endoscopy probably underestimate the true incidence of stress gastritis, because one endoscopically controlled study has shown that gastric erosions are present in all patients with life-threatening injuries. Sepsis appears to be the major predisposing condition. In another study, endoscopic examinations were performed on 30 critically ill patients; of 14 patients with sepsis, 4 had minor lesions and 10 had severe bleeding gastric erosions. Repeated endoscopy 4 days later revealed that the minor lesions had progressed to a more severe form of injury. In the 16 patients without sepsis, only 7 had minor ulcerations that did not progress, and no patient had severe gastritis.

Patients who have sustained a major thermal burn of 35% or more of their body surface area are at a predictably high risk for the development of gastric erosions and hemorrhage. Endoscopy has demonstrated that gastric erosions are present in 93% of these patients, whereas the occurrence of severe acute upper gastrointestinal hemorrhage in severely burned patients ranges between 25% and 50%. Histologically, this form of gastritis has the same appearance as that found in septic patients.

Conversely, Cushing ulcer, which can occur with intracranial tumors or after intracranial surgery or head trauma, can develop as a result of hypergastrinemia and gastric acid and pepsin hypersecretion. This ulcer tends to be single and deep and is found anywhere in the upper gastrointestinal tract. Perforation is a more common complication in Cushing ulcer than other forms of stress-related injury.

Presentation and Diagnosis

At least 60% of patients at risk develop stress erosions within 1 to 2 days of the precipitating event. Painless upper gastrointestinal bleeding may be the only clinical sign. The onset of hemorrhage is often delayed, usually occurring 3 to 10 days after the onset of the primary disease. The initial presentation may be the detection of only a few flecks of blood in the nasogastric tube or an unexplained drop in the hematocrit. Characteristically, the bleeding is slow and intermittent, but it can be rapid, heralded by hypotension and hematemesis. Guaiac-positive stools are usually found early; melena and hematochezia occur infrequently.

Esophagogastroduodenoscopy is the diagnostic modality of choice to confirm the diagnosis and to differentiate stress erosion from other sources of upper gastrointestinal hemorrhage. Correct identification of the bleeding source is made in over 90% of instances. If endoscopy is not diagnostic, visceral angiography through selective catheterization of the left gastric or splenic vessels can provide information regarding the primary vessel supplying the bleeding site. In contrast, barium examinations are usually of little value because of the superficial nature of stress erosions, and in fact they can be detrimental by interfering with the interpretation of subsequent arteriography. Analysis of gastric luminal contents does not aid in the diagnosis of gastric erosions because the rates of acid secretion vary greatly.

Medical Treatment

Immediate and definitive resuscitation is essential in all patients with established hemorrhage from erosive stress gastritis. Hypovolemic shock should be corrected with whole blood replacement, and any specific clotting abnormalities should be corrected with fresh frozen plasma, platelets, or both. Vigorous efforts should be made to identify a source of sepsis, and appropriate antibiotic therapy in conjunction with definitive surgical drainage of the septic focus should be completed. Percutaneous drainage of the abscess can be considered. Control of the gastric lesion depends on adequate drainage of the abscess.

The initial effort to control gastric hemorrhage consists of gastric saline lavage through a large-bore nasogastric tube. Lavage serves to fragment existing clots and to remove any pooled blood, reducing fibrinolysis at bleeding sites. Nasogastric decompression prevents gastric distention and the stimulus to gastrin release while removing bile and pancreatic juice that may have refluxed across the pylorus. Over 80% of patients who present with upper gastrointestinal hemorrhage stop bleeding with this approach.

Once acute bleeding has ceased, intragastric fluid should be maintained at a pH greater than 5.0 with antacids, H_2-receptor antagonists, the H^+-K^+-ATPase inhibitor, omeprazole, or combination therapy. Definitive treatment of ongoing acute active stress bleeding by antacids is largely unsuccessful. The administration of H_2-receptor blocking agents once active gastrointestinal bleeding has commenced is also usually ineffective as a definitive form of therapy. No evidence exists to suggest that the newer H_2-receptor antagonists are any more effective than cimetidine in arresting bleeding.

Endoscopic Therapy

The endoscope has become a valuable therapeutic and diagnostic instrument with electrocautery and laser photocoagulation capabilities. The effectiveness of endoscopic therapy is established with respect to electrocoagulation control of active bleeding from chronic gastric ulcers. Laser photocoagulation is equally effective but carries a 1% to 2% incidence of full-thickness perforation. Only a small number of patients with stress gastritis have been treated with these modalities, and the reports of effectiveness are anecdotal.

Angiographic Therapy

Selective angiographic catheterization of the splanchnic arterial circulation offers an additional means for the control of bleeding. Acute gastric bleeding can be effectively controlled by selective infusion of vasopressin into the splanchnic circulation through the left gastric artery. Vasopressin is administered by continuous infusion through the catheter at a rate of 0.2 to 0.4 IU/min for a maximum of 48 to 72 hours. Vasopressin should not be used in patients with ischemic cardiac disease or liver disease. Although effective in controlling blood loss, the use of selective intraarterial infusion of vasopressin is not associated with an improved survival rate. An additional angiographic technique that can be used to control acute bleeding is transcatheter embolization with Gelfoam, metal coils, or autologous blood clot. The extensive plexus of submucosal arterial vessels within the stomach can preclude definitive control of acute hemorrhage with this approach.

Surgical Therapy

About 10% to 23% of patients with acute stress ulcers continue to bleed or have recurrent bleeding despite aggressive medical, endoscopic, or angiographic therapy. A definitive operative approach should effectively control bleeding and carry the lowest possible mortality and the lowest rate of recurrent hemorrhage. The procedure that best fulfills these requirements is a matter of controversy. Vagotomy and drainage, vagotomy and antrectomy, vagotomy and subtotal gastrectomy, total gastric resection, and gastric devascularization have all been used in this context.[11,12] There are no prospective randomized clinical tests that confirm the superiority of one procedure over another. Some investigators have recommended total gastrectomy based on a mortality of 17%; others have reported mortality rates approaching 100% with subtotal or total gastric resection. In general, mortality rates for acute stress-induced hemorrhage range from 30% to 60% regardless of the surgical procedure used. Gastric devascularization in which the entire blood flow supply to the stomach is provided by means of the short gastric vessels has a recurrent bleeding rate of only 9% but a mortality rate comparable to that for other procedures.

For these reasons, it is prudent in this high-risk population to consider vagotomy and pyloroplasty with oversewing of isolated actively bleeding erosions. In patients with diffuse mucosal bleeding, either vagotomy and partial gastrectomy or gastric devascularization is most appropriate. In the unfortunate few patients with massive, life-threatening hemorrhage, total gastrectomy may be the only viable alternative.

Prophylaxis

Because of the high mortality rate in patients with active hemorrhage from acute stress-related mucosal lesions, high-risk patients should be treated prophylactically (Table 23-2).

Antacid Prophylaxis. The hourly administration of antacid (30 to 60 mL) by nasogastric tube, maintaining the gastric luminal fluid at a pH above 3.5, has proved to be effective prophylaxis.[13] If intragastric pH can be maintained above 5.0, over 99.9% of acid is neutralized and pepsin is inactivated. In a study of 100 seriously ill patients who were randomly assigned to receive placebo or antacid

Table 23-2. MEDICAL PROPHYLAXIS FOR STRESS GASTRITIS

Agent	Efficacy (%)
Antacid	>96
H₂ antagonists	>97
Sucralfate	96–100
Prostaglandins	<50

prophylaxis, bleeding was detected in 24.5% of patients given no prophylaxis, compared with 3.9% of patients given antacids through the nasogastric tube. In a review of data derived from 16 prospective trials (2133 patients) comparing antacid prophylaxis, cimetidine prophylaxis, and placebo, when occult blood detection was used as the minimal criterion for gastrointestinal bleeding, 3.7% of patients given antacids had evidence of blood loss versus 17.4% given cimetidine and 27.3% given placebo. When overt bleeding manifested by melena, hematemesis, or transfusion requirement was used as the minimum criterion, there was no significant difference in risk of bleeding when antacids and cimetidine were compared, with 3.3% and 2.7% of patients, respectively, developing significant bleeding; the placebo bleeding rate was 15%. Others have suggested that there is no strong justification to choose antacids over cimetidine to prevent stress-related hemorrhage. With endoscopic evidence of mucosal damage used as the end point, it has been suggested that cimetidine is as effective as antacids in preventing stress ulcerations. Although compelling evidence exists that H₂ blockers can prevent acute mucosal bleeding, their superiority to antacids continues to be debated. In contrast, most studies have demonstrated that it is easier to titrate gastric pH (higher than 5.0) with antacids than with the standard intermittent dose regimens of H₂-receptor antagonists.

Histamine-Receptor Antagonists. The preceding discussion suggests that H₂-receptor antagonists are as effective as antacids with respect to prophylaxis. Data suggest that continuous infusions of any of the H₂-receptor antagonists provide more consistent maintenance of an intraluminal gastric pH greater than 3.5 than do the standard intermittent-infusion regimens. Advantages of continuous infusion of these agents include a potential reduction in toxicity, decreased pharmacy costs and nursing duties, and possible enhancement of therapeutic benefit. Whether continuous infusion of H₂-receptor antagonists results in better clinical outcome or improved drug safety has yet to be determined.

Sucralfate Prophylaxis. Another additional antiulcer agent that has been evaluated for prophylaxis against stress ulceration is sucralfate. Sucralfate is not absorbed from the gastrointestinal tract and preferentially binds to areas in which the epithelium has become denuded. Controlled trials suggest that sucralfate, 1 g every 6 hours, can be as effective as antacids or cimetidine prophylactically.[14] In 100 critically ill patients, bleeding occurred in 6% of patients receiving antacids or cimetidine, whereas none of the 34 patients receiving sucralfate bled. Other investigators have concluded that sucralfate is as effective as antacid for the prevention of bleeding in critically ill patients. This form of protection, which is not antisecretory, prevents bacterial overgrowth by allowing the intragastric pH to remain low. Critically ill, intubated patients receiving sucralfate prophylactically have a lower incidence of pneumonia-related deaths than do patients receiving prophylactic antisecretory agents.

Prostaglandin Prophylaxis. Given exogenously, natural or synthetic prostaglandins of the E, F, and I series inhibit gastric acid secretion. Few studies have investigated the prophylactic use of prostaglandins in critically ill patients. One group compared the efficacy of 15(R)-15 dimethyl PGE₂ given at antisecretory doses with the efficacy of antacids and found that stress-related bleeding occurred in 50% of patients given the synthetic prostaglandin derivative compared with only 13.6% of patients receiving antacids. Another randomized prospective study compared a fixed dose of a PGE₁ synthetic analogue (misoprostol) with antacids and found them to be equally effective at preventing gastric mucosal injury as assessed endoscopically.

GASTRIC ULCER
Definition of Lesion

Clinically, it is often impossible to differentiate between gastric carcinoma and benign gastric ulcer because their symptoms are quite similar. Macroscopically, the classic gastric ulcer is a circular area devoid of mucosa, with a fibrous base, and lined by granulation tissue (Fig. 23-2). When seen on upper gastrointestinal barium studies, a sign of benign gastric ulcer is a radiolucent line, usually about 1 mm in width, partially or completely traversing the orifice of an ulcer. The line occurs because of the thin, underlying marginal mucosa of the ulcer crater. A second and more frequent sign of a benign gastric ulcer is the appearance of mucosal folds that radiate to the edge of the ulcer crater. Another finding on barium study that suggests benign gastric ulcer is spasm of gastric circular muscles on the gastric wall opposite the ulcer.

The most reliable radiographic sign of a malignant process is the demonstration of a tumor in the vicinity of the ulcer or a mass with central ulceration. Abnormal mucosal folds near the base of the crater or folds that are interrupted near the ulcer also suggest malignancy. A nodular or irregularly shaped ulcer base is consistent with malignant disease. Some patients with gastric carcinoma do not have radiographically obvious ulcers but present with nondistensible stomachs indicative of a diffusely spreading carcinoma (linitis plastica).

Endoscopic Identification

Most clinicians rely on upper gastrointestinal endoscopy as the modality of choice for diagnosing gastric ulcer. The differentiation of benign from malignant ulcers can be performed by examination of the ulcer base, the margin of the crater, the relation of the margin to the surrounding mucosal folds, and the size of the ulcer. The ulcer base is usually smooth and flat and covered by a gray to white fibrinous exudate. The ulcer crater can be linear but is usually round or oval in appearance. The margin of a typical benign ulcer is slightly raised, erythematous, and smooth. If the ulcer is benign, the mucosal folds are symmetric and taper smoothly to the edge of the ulcer. The

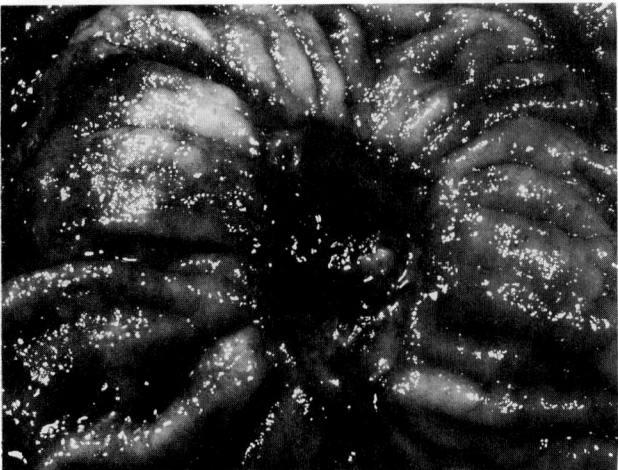

Figure 23-2. Gastric ulcer in resected specimen.

size of a gastric ulcer can also be a factor in differentiation of a benign from a malignant lesion: ulcers smaller than 1 cm are associated with only a 5% risk of malignancy.

Histologic Appearance

A gastric ulcer is a macroscopic defect that extends through the muscularis mucosa. Healing is dependent on the migration of adjacent mucosal cells to cover the defect. The histologic appearance varies with the chronicity and degree of healing. In an active ulcer, the four following zones are detectable histologically:

- The base of the ulcer, which is covered with a thin layer of fibrinous material
- A region of intense cellular (neutrophil) infiltrate immediately beneath this fibrinous material
- A region of active granulation tissue characterized by a mononuclear leukocytic infiltrate
- A region of fibrous or collagenous scar in the deepest tissue

Location

Gastric ulcers can occur anywhere in the stomach, although they usually present on the lesser curvature near the incisura angularis (Fig. 23-3). About 60% are located at or slightly above the angularis. Fifteen percent to 23% of gastric ulcers are distal to the incisura, and 10% are above this region, high on the lesser curvature. Only 5% of gastric ulcers are found on the greater curvature.

In addition, 97% of all gastric ulcers occur within 2 cm of the junctional zone between fundic and antral mucosa. Gastric ulcers appear at different distances from the pyloric sphincter because the antrum extends for variable (2 to 16 cm) distances from the pylorus. With increasing age, this junctional zone moves proximally along the lesser curvature, as does the incidence of gastric ulcer. Although a large gastric ulcer is more likely to be malignant than a small one, most are benign. In contrast to older teachings and opinions, most ulcers on the greater curvature of the stomach prove to be benign; the incidence of malignancy in an ulcer on the greater curve is 12% to 15%.

Gastric ulcers are divided into three categories, based on their location and gastric acid secretory status. A type I gastric ulcer is an ulcer in the body of the stomach, usually along the lesser curvature; it is associated with large volumes of secretion with a low to normal acid output (Fig. 23-4). Type I ulcers are not associated with duodenal, pyloric, or prepyloric mucosal abnormalities. In most reported series, 50% to 60% of patients have type I ulcers that arise within 1.5 cm of the histologic transition zone between the fundic and antral mucosa. There is a slight predominance of blood group A in patients with this type of gastric ulcer.

Type II gastric ulcer is located in the body of the stomach in combination with a duodenal ulcer (Fig. 23-5). These patients are usually acid hypersecretors. Duodenal ulcer usually precedes the development of gastric ulcer. About 23% to 25% of gastric ulcers are type II. A high percentage of these patients are of blood group O.

A type III gastric ulcer is characterized as a prepyloric ulcer and accounts for about 23% of lesions (Fig. 23-6). Patients with this lesion are typically acid hypersecretors and tend to be of blood group O.

Type IV gastric ulcer can be characterized as occurring high on the lesser curvature near the gastroesophageal junction (Fig. 23-7). In the United States, the incidence of type IV gastric ulcer is less than 10%.

A type V gastric ulcer can occur anywhere in the stom-

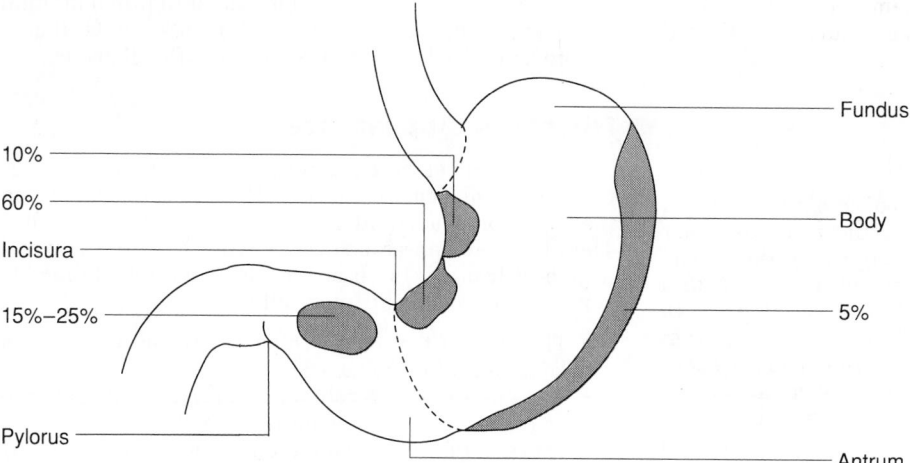

Figure 23-3. Location of gastric ulcers.

ach and occurs as a result of chronic ingestion of aspirin or nonsteroidal antiinflammatory agents.

Incidence

The incidence of gastric ulcer differs in various parts of the world. In Japan, gastric ulcers occur 5 to 10 times more often than duodenal ulcers. Gastric ulcer is twice as common as duodenal ulcer among the Chinese. In the Peruvian Andes, 96% of peptic ulcers are gastric, whereas at sea level in Peru, the usual ratio of duodenal to gastric ulcer prevails. In the United States, gastric ulcer is more common in men and elderly patients than in women and younger patients. In elderly patients, 30% to 50% of peptic ulcers are gastric as opposed to duodenal. Gastric ulcers rarely develop before age 40 years; the peak incidence occurs between ages 55 and 65; they are two to five times more common in the lower than in the higher socioeconomic classes; and they are slightly more common in the nonwhite than in the white population. Almost 90,000 new gastric ulcers are diagnosed each year. About 3000 patients die each year as a direct result of gastric ulcer

disease. Predisposing factors associated with gastric ulcers are shown in Table 23-3.

Acid and Pepsin Secretion

The role of abnormalities in acid and pepsin secretion in the pathogenesis of gastric ulcer is less clear than in duodenal ulcer. Although the presence of acid is essential to the production of gastric ulcer, the total secretory output is less important. Patients with ulcers in the body of the stomach (type I) tend to have acid secretory rates that are lower than normal, whereas patients with combined gastric and duodenal ulcers (type II) or prepyloric ulcers (type III) tend to have acid secretory rates that are higher than normal. Some critical concentration of gastric acid is required to participate in the cascade of events resulting in ulcer formation. Under conditions of increased hydrogen ion back-diffusion, mucosal ulcerations have been observed when the pH at the lamina propria falls from 6.7 to 6.5. Pepsin secretion usually parallels that of acid; the luminal concentration of pepsin, which has been shown to digest mucus effectively, can be elevated in patients

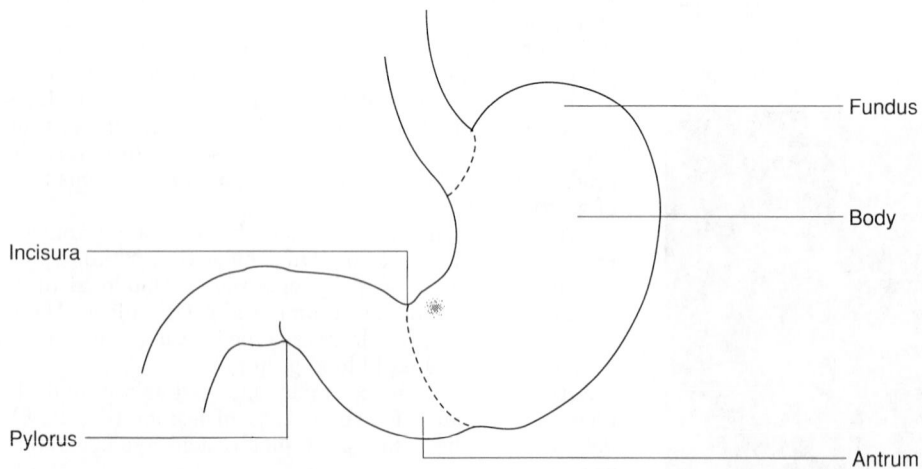

Type I Gastric Ulcer
Gastric body usually lesser curvature
Normal or low acid secretion
Hemorrhage infrequent, penetration common
Blood group A

Figure 23-4. Location of type I gastric ulcer with associated conditions.

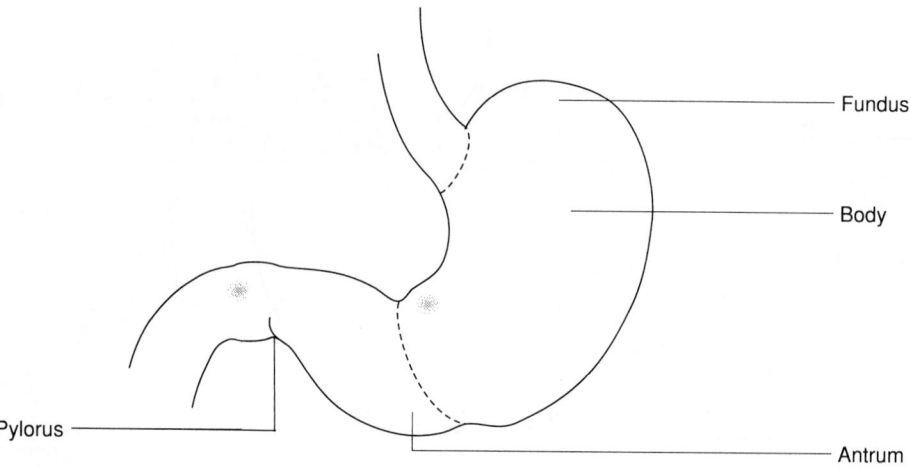

Type II Gastric Ulcer
Gastric body and duodenal ulcer
Hypersecretion of acid
Hemorrhage, obstruction, and perforation frequent
Blood group O

Figure 23-5. Location of type II gastric ulcer with associated conditions.

with gastric ulcer. The gastric epithelium produces two distinct pepsinogens, PGI and PGII. PGI is primarily synthesized by the chief cells in the fundic mucosa, whereas PGII is found in the pylorus, antrum, and fundic glands. Both pepsinogens are elevated (PGII greater than PGI) in the serum of some patients with peptic ulcer disease, yet the ratio of PGI to PGII that has been proposed as a potential risk factor for gastric ulceration is lower in patients with gastric ulcer than in those with duodenal ulcer. A clear cause-and-effect relationship has not been established for pepsinogen in ulcer disease.

Gastric Motility

Alterations in gastric motility can contribute to the formation of gastric ulcers. Gastric stasis with antral food retention could lead to increased gastrin release and a sub-

sequent increased rate of acid secretion. Delayed gastric emptying can also prevent clearing of refluxed duodenal contents. Other motility defects that have been proposed include an incompetent pyloric sphincter mechanism, the presence of prominent muscle bands near the incisura, alterations in the migrating motor complex, prolonged high-amplitude gastric contractions, and chronic mesenteric ischemia with resultant gastroparesis. Aberrant gastric motility has been found in only a small subset of patients with gastric ulcer.

Environmental Factors

Numerous environmental factors have been implicated in the pathogenesis of gastric ulceration. Nonsteroidal anti-inflammatory drugs (NSAIDs), aspirin, alcohol, tobacco,

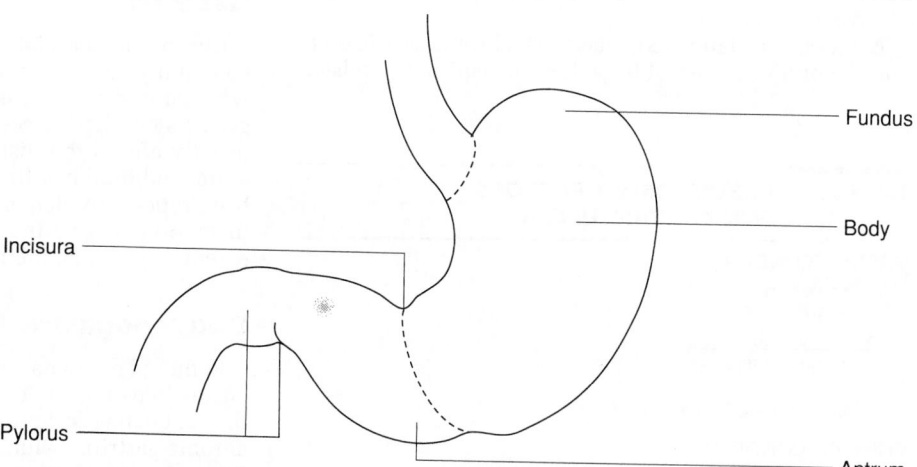

Type III Gastric Ulcer
Prepyloric
Hypersecretor of acid
Hemorrhage and perforation frequent
Blood group O

Figure 23-6. Location of type III gastric ulcer with associated conditions.

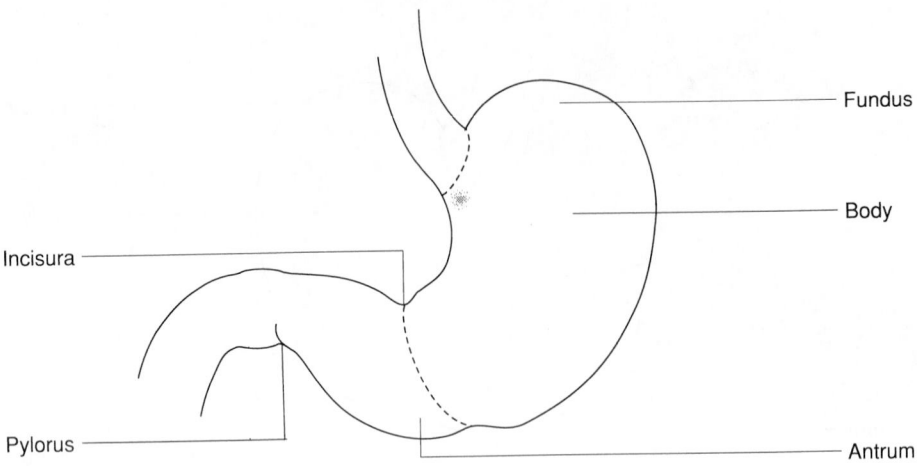

Type IV Gastric Ulcer
High on lesser curvature
Low acid secretion
Hemorrhage common, penetration frequent
Blood group O

Figure 23-7. Location of type IV gastric ulcer with associated conditions.

steroids, and stress have all been implicated as possible etiologic factors.

The incidence of symptomatic gastric ulcer in patients taking NSAIDs has been reported to be 5.5%. Recent reports have documented a clear association between NSAIDs and the endoscopic occurrence of gastric ulcer.[15] The prevalence of ulcers in the stomach or duodenum has been reported to range from 10% to 30% in patients receiving NSAIDs chronically. The mechanism by which these lesions occur is thought to be due, in part, to the inhibitory effect on gastric mucosal cyclooxygenase and hence prostaglandin synthesis. This is most likely a systemic effect rather than a local response of the gastric mucosa to exposure to NSAIDs. A direct luminal toxic effect of NSAIDs on the surface epithelium also contributes to damage. The gastric epithelial surface of most mammalian species is hydrophobic, a property primarily of the secreted gel mucus. Aspirin causes this hydrophobic surface layer to become more hydrophilic, resulting in altered ion transport and reduced transmucosal potential difference, which predispose to ulceration.

A strong association exists between chronic gastric ulcer and the prolonged use of large doses of aspirin (acetylsalicylic acid; ASA). Intragastric and parenteral ASA are known to produce significant gastric mucosal damage experimentally. In an endoscopically controlled study involving 82 patients with rheumatoid disease taking at least 8 ASA tablets each day, 17% had gastric ulcers and 40% had severe erosions. The cause-and-effect relationship between cyclooxygenase inhibition and gastric mucosal damage is supported by several other reports documenting prevention of gastric mucosal damage by the administration of oral prostaglandins.

Cigarette smoking also contributes to the development of gastric ulceration. Smoking is thought to decrease prostaglandin synthesis, enhance acid secretion, promote pyloric incompetence, increase duodenogastric reflux, and impede gastric mucosal blood flow. Alcohol is known to be a gastric mucosal irritant and, in large quantities, can cause acute gastritis. Whether alcohol is a risk factor for gastric ulceration remains uncertain.

Gastritis

Chronic superficial gastritis and atrophic gastritis are commonly associated with gastric ulcer. It is not known whether gastric ulcer is the initial event with subsequent gastritis or whether gastritis precedes ulceration. Gastritis usually affects the distal gastric mucosa but can be both antral and fundic or limited to the area of ulceration. It has been repeatedly demonstrated that the location of gastric ulceration reflects the extent of gastritis; the greater the extent of gastritis, the more proximal the ulcer.

Duodenogastric Reflux

Reflux of duodenal contents into the stomach frequently occurs in patients with gastric ulcer. Some have postulated that duodenogastric reflux is the primary event leading to chronic gastritis, which in turn predisposes to ulceration. Bile salts, lysolecithin, and pancreatic secretions are injurious to gastric mucosa. Damage is the direct result of a change in gastric mucosal barrier function and alterations in the mucus gel layer, making the mucosa more permeable to proton back-diffusion. Although these hypotheses are intriguing and are supported by some experimental evi-

---

Table 23-3. PREDISPOSING FACTORS FOR GASTRIC ULCER

GASTRIC CONDITIONS
Acid and pepsin
Gastric stasis
Coexisting duodenal ulcer
Duodenogastric reflux
Gastritis
Infection with *Helicobacter pylori*

CLINICAL CONDITIONS
Chronic alcohol use
Nonsteroidal antiinflammatory drugs
Smoking
Long-term corticosteroid therapy
Infection
Intraarterial chemotherapy

dence, several observations suggest that reflux of duodenal contents may not lead to ulcer formation. Medical regimens associated with ulcer healing do not alter bile reflux. Patients with type I gastric ulcers have neither decreased gastric emptying nor increased duodenogastric reflux. After antrectomy, reflux of bile and pancreatic juice is common, often leading to gastritis; however, gastric ulceration is rare.

Infection

Helicobacter pylori is a spiral organism that has been shown to colonize the antral mucosa of most patients with peptic ulcer disease. The organism survives in the mucus overlying the gastric antral mucosal epithelium perhaps because of the production of urease, which gives it a near neutral acid–base environment, even in the presence of intraluminal protons. Investigators recently isolated the organism and demonstrated that its presence highly correlated with the appearance of antral gastritis as well as gastric and duodenal ulcer. Nearly all *H pylori*–positive patients have antral gastritis that resolves with antibiotic therapy appropriate to eradicate the organism.

At least 50% of the adult population is colonized with *H pylori*. The diagnosis of *H pylori* colonization is made by any of a variety of techniques. Endoscopically obtained biopsy specimens can be subjected to histologic evaluation for the presence of the organism by use of either Giemsa or Warthin-Starry stains. The presence of urease-producing organisms can also be detected. The diagnostic sensitivity and specificity of these two modalities are greater than 90% and are higher than culture of the organism, which is no greater than 80% to 90%. Another technique used to diagnose colonization by *H pylori* is the urea breath test, which is available in only a few institutions because it requires mass spectrophotometric analysis of ^{14}C. The advantage of this diagnostic test is that it is noninvasive and allows repeated measurements on the same subject. Of the serologic diagnostic tests available, which include hemagglutination, complement fixation, and enzyme-linked immunosorbent assay, the last is the most frequently used.

A strong association exists between the presence of gastritis and colonization with *H pylori*, a combination that occurs in 70% to 90% of patients. *H pylori* colonization has been reported to occur in 80% to 100% of patients with duodenal ulcer and 80% of patients with gastric ulcer. Colonization in the duodenum occurs only in mucosa that has undergone intestinal metaplasia. Complete understanding of the mechanisms involved in ulcerogenesis associated with the presence of this organism remains elusive.

Although a direct cause-and-effect relationship between peptic ulcer disease and *H pylori* colonization has not been established, circumstantial evidence is rather convincing. In two prospective studies of patients with duodenal ulcer, eradication of *H pylori* infection with antibiotics in 74% to 88% of patients was associated with a decreased rate of duodenal ulcer recurrence compared with antisecretory therapy alone. Recurrence rates within 12 months of treatment ranged from 76% to 86% in patients treated with antisecretory therapy, compared with recurrence rates of 6% to 25% for those treated with eradication of *H pylori* with bismuth and antibiotic therapy in conjunction with antisecretory therapy. In a 7-year follow-up study of patients with duodenal ulcer treated with *H pylori* eradication, active duodenal ulcer was found in 23% of those remaining positive for *H pylori*, in contrast to only 3% of those remaining negative for *H pylori*. Similarly, in a study of 66 patients with duodenal ulcer who were positive for *H pylori* initially, the recurrence rate (6 to 33 months) was

2.4% in those rendered negative for *H pylori* compared with 62.5% in those in whom *H pylori* was not eradicated. No bleeding relapses occurred in patients who were negative for *H pylori*, but they occurred in 37.5% of patients remaining positive for *H pylori*. Moreover, patients with recurrent duodenal ulceration demonstrate persistent or recurrent *H pylori* colonization nearly 100% of the time. Similar evidence suggests that antimicrobial therapy reduces recurrence rates of gastric ulceration in patients whose gastric antrum is colonized by *H pylori*.[16]

There is no information regarding the role of *H pylori* in the predisposition to develop complications of peptic ulcer disease, such as bleeding and perforation, or in marginal ulceration following gastrectomy. It seems prudent, however, to continually assess patients with these conditions for the presence of the organism and, if present, to include an antimicrobial regimen with antisecretory therapy in the postoperative period.

Intraarterial Chemotherapy

Gastric and duodenal ulcers have been found to occur in some patients receiving hepatic artery infusion chemotherapy, usually 5-fluorouracil as a single agent or in combination with cisplatin, Adriamycin, and mitomycin C. A direct toxic effect of these chemotherapeutic agents on the nutrient side of the gastric mucosa has been suggested, because symptoms improve when chemotherapy is suspended.

Natural History

Symptomatically, gastric ulcers are characterized by recurrent cycles of quiescence and relapse. Of patients treated with a placebo, about 60% are pain free at 6 weeks, and 67% of gastric ulcers are healed after 3 months. When patients are maintained on a placebo for a year, recurrence can be demonstrated in 55% to 89%. In the Veterans Administration cooperative study, 377 patients whose gastric ulcers healed completely were observed for 2 years. Forty-two percent of these patients developed recurrent ulcers, and 50% of the recurrences occurred in the first 6 months. Recurrent gastric ulcers usually recur in the same area as the initial ulcer.

In addition to causing pain, gastric ulcers can bleed, obstruct, or perforate. Rarely, benign gastric ulcers have been associated with spontaneous gastrocolic fistulas. Complications requiring surgical intervention occur in 8% to 23% of these patients. Hemorrhage occurs at some time during the course of the gastric ulcer in 35% to 40% of patients. As a rule, patients with significant hemorrhage from gastric ulcer are older, are less likely to stop bleeding, and have higher morbidity and mortality rates than patients bleeding from duodenal ulcer. Hemorrhage occurs most frequently in patients with type II and III ulcers. Patients with a type IV ulcer can also present with massive, life-threatening hemorrhage.

Perforation is the most common complication of gastric ulcer. Most occur along the anterior or anterosuperior aspect of the lesser curvature. Generally, the older the patient, the higher the perforation; the larger the ulcer tends to be, the greater the associated morbidity and mortality.

Gastric outlet obstruction is most common in patients with a type II or III gastric ulcer. A differentiation must be made between benign obstruction and antral carcinoma. Type I ulcers can interfere with gastric motility but usually do not cause obstruction.

Presentation

The usual symptoms produced by a chronic gastric ulcer include abdominal pain described as gnawing, dull, or burning and localized to the midline or the left upper quadrant. Pain can be aggravated or precipitated by the ingestion of food. The pattern of the pain is usually less rhythmic or periodic than that described for duodenal ulcer. Other reported symptoms of gastric ulcer include nausea, vomiting, anorexia, and weight loss, which can occur in the absence of pyloric obstruction. Patients may not eat and lose weight because of a fear of postprandial symptoms. The physical examination may show epigastric tenderness. Laboratory studies are usually normal.

Acute gastric ulceration can present with either hemorrhage or perforation. It is unusual for an acute ulcer to present with obstruction. Asymptomatic or silent ulcers can be discovered in elderly patients with no prior history of ulcer disease and appear to be more severe and life threatening in patients taking NSAIDs.

The natural history of benign gastric ulcer is one of healing and recurrence. Rates of relapse, most of which are asymptomatic, are as high as 70% within 1 year of healing. The recurrent ulcer usually occurs near the site of the original ulcer. The most important prediction of recurrence is slow healing of the index ulcer. Benign recurrent ulcers heal on medical therapy as readily as the initial ulcer.

Diagnosis

The history and physical examination may be of limited value in distinguishing gastric from duodenal ulceration. The two principal means of diagnosing gastric ulcer are upper gastrointestinal radiographs and fiberoptic endoscopy. Contrast radiography is less expensive, and with a dedicated radiologist, 90% of gastric ulcers can be diagnosed accurately. About 5% of ulcers appearing radiographically benign are malignant.

Gastroscopy is the most reliable method of diagnosing a gastric ulcer, with an accuracy of over 97%. If multiple biopsies and brushings for cytology are performed, the probability of detecting a carcinoma is also in excess of 97%. Clinical features prompting early endoscopic evaluation include major weight loss, symptoms of gastric outlet obstruction, a palpable abdominal mass, and stool Hemoccult positivity or blood loss anemia. Endoscopic features that suggest malignancy include an exophytic mass, abnormal or disrupted mucosal folds, a necrotic ulcer crater, bleeding from the edge of the ulcer crater, a stepwise depression of the ulcer edge, heaped-up margins, and small extensions of the ulcer that blur a portion of the ulcer wall. If initial biopsies do not demonstrate malignant cells but the endoscopic appearance strongly suggests that a carcinoma is underlying the ulcer, repeat endoscopy with deeper biopsies should be performed.

Acid Secretory Studies

In the past, gastric secretory studies were commonly used in the evaluation of patients with gastric ulcer. Most patients with gastric ulcer have acid secretory rates within the normal range. In patients with histamine- or pentagastrin-fast achlorhydria or hypochlorhydria, the diagnosis of carcinoma should be considered, because 23% to 25% of patients with gastric cancer are achlorhydric.

Medical Therapy

Antacids

Antacids reduce gastric acidity and the enzymatic activity of pepsin by neutralizing protons. Gastric ulcers require a longer time to heal than duodenal ulcers, and the larger the gastric ulcer, the longer treatment is required for healing. Two problems associated with prolonged antacid use can decrease patient compliance—frequent dosing and unpleasant side effects such as diarrhea, constipation, and alkalosis.

Histamine-Receptor Antagonists

Histamine-receptor antagonists are the most commonly prescribed antisecretory drugs used to treat patients with benign gastric ulcer (Table 23-4). These compounds block the H_2-receptor on parietal cells and thereby reduce all forms of stimulated gastric acid secretion. Five H_2-receptor antagonists are available—cimetidine, ranitidine, famotidine, nizatidine, and roxatidine. In general, gastric ulcer healing rates can be expected to exceed 80% after 8 weeks of therapy with these agents. There does not seem to be any significant difference in efficacy among the five H_2-receptor antagonists with respect to healing, yet each is significantly more effective than placebo. Recent clinical studies suggest that a single nocturnal dose of an H_2-receptor antagonist is as effective as multiple-dose regimens for acute healing. The choice of agent for the treatment of gastric ulcer should be based on compliance, cost, and side-effect profile.

Omeprazole

Omeprazole appears to be superior to ranitidine in the treatment of benign gastric ulcer because healing is more rapid, as is symptomatic relief.[17] Omeprazole also promotes healing of gastric ulcer in patients who continue to use NSAIDs. Ulcer recurrence after initial therapy is not greater than that observed with H_2-receptor antagonist–induced healing. Similar findings have been observed in the treatment of prepyloric (type III) ulcers and acute gastric ulcers in randomized prospective studies.

Anticholinergics

Pirenzepine and telenzepine are relatively selective muscarinic (M_1) inhibitors that block acid secretion to a greater extent than they inhibit cardiac, smooth muscle, and salivary gland function. The efficacy of pirenzepine approximates that of the H_2-receptor antagonists in gastric ulcer healing. Although healing rates for gastric ulcer are somewhat lower than they are for duodenal ulcer, several clinical trials suggest that pirenzepine can be as effective as cimetidine in treating patients with gastric ulcers.

Sucralfate

Sucralfate is the aluminum salt of sucrose octasulfate. At a pH below 3.5, sucralfate polymerizes to form a gel that binds to proteins in ulcerated or eroded mucosa as well as to normal mucosa. This gel forms complexes with

Table 23-4. MEDICAL TREATMENT OF GASTRIC ULCER

Agent	Mechanism of Action
Antacids	Neutralize gastric acidity and decrease activity of pepsin
H_2 antagonists	Block parietal cell H_2 receptor
Omeprazole	Inhibits H^+-K^+-ATPase pump
Anticholinergics	Block specific M_1 (muscarinic) receptor blocker in stomach wall
Sucralfate	Complexes with pepsin and bile salts and binds to proteins in mucosa
Prostaglandins	Inhibit acid secretion, increase endogenous mucosal defense

pepsin and bile salts adhering to the denuded ulcer base. Sucralfate has been suggested to enhance mucosal defense by stimulating prostaglandin synthesis, stimulating secretion of bicarbonate and mucus, and delivering epidermal growth factor, which binds to it, to the ulcer base. Sucralfate heals gastric ulcers as effectively as cimetidine.

Prostaglandins

Prostaglandins A, E, and I are produced by the gastric and duodenal mucosa. In addition to their antisecretory effects, they exert an important protective effect on the mucosa. Prostaglandin analogues include rioprostil, enprostil, arbaprostil, enisoprost, and trimoprostil. Although experimental evidence suggests that these compounds enhance mucosal defense at nonantisecretory doses, clinically they are used at antisecretory doses. Healing appears to be due to antisecretory as well as other effects. Prostaglandins are as effective as H_2-receptor antagonist for healing gastric ulcers.[18]

Dietary Considerations

Patients with peptic ulcers were frequently placed on a bland diet, a concept that was not based on any rigorous scientific data. Dietary restrictions do not appear to enhance the healing rate of gastric ulcers. Patients can be advised to avoid alcoholic beverages, chocolate, and fatty meals, which tend to decrease lower esophageal sphincter pressure and promote reflux of gastric acid into the esophagus. Furthermore, patients should be advised to stop smoking, not only because of its effect on decreasing esophageal sphincter tone but also because it is associated with failure of medical therapy for gastric ulcer.

Treatment of *Helicobacter pylori* Infection

Patients with gastric ulcer should be assessed for the presence of *H pylori* by one of the available tests. If colonization is present, an antibiotic regimen should be used in addition to antisecretory therapy. The regimen of triple antimicrobial agents, bismuth, subsalicylate, tetracycline, and metronidazole has been the most extensively studied. Amoxicillin can be substituted for tetracycline or metronidazole with only a slight reduction in efficacy. Another regimen has suggested the combination of ranitidine, metronidazole, and amoxicillin as being equally effective. Eradication rates in excess of 90% can also be anticipated with these regimens with a 23% ulcer recurrence rate after discontinuation of this medical therapy.

Treatment of NSAID-Induced Mucosal Injury

The treatment of ulcers in patients taking NSAIDs is complicated by the fact that many of these ulcers are clinically silent and may not respond to standard therapeutic regimens. Several reports have suggested that H_2-receptor antagonists fail to prevent the occurrence of NSAID ulcers. In addition, although sucralfate reduces superficial damage from NSAIDs, there is no convincing evidence that it prevents NSAID-induced ulceration.

In a controlled, randomized study, NSAID-induced gastric ulcers healed more rapidly in patients treated with omeprazole than in those treated with ranitidine, even with continued NSAID therapy. In a different controlled, randomized study, a synthetic prostaglandin analogue reduced the frequency of gastric ulceration from 4% per

month to 0.2% per month despite continued NSAID therapy.

The ideal medical therapy for NSAID-induced gastric mucosal injury has not been clearly established, although the synthetic prostaglandins appear to have a role in the prevention and treatment of this form of mucosal injury. If possible, the use of NSAIDs should be discontinued, because these lesions heal rapidly once the agent is withdrawn. If it is clinically inappropriate to stop NSAID therapy, cotherapy with either omeprazole or a synthetic prostaglandin should be prescribed.

Surgical Therapy

Indications

The indications for elective surgical treatment of gastric ulcer include failure of a newly diagnosed ulcer to heal completely within 12 weeks of medical therapy, failure of a recurrent ulcer to respond to medical therapy or recurrence after two initial courses of successful treatment, and the inability to exclude malignant disease. Although numerous surgical procedures have been described for each classification of gastric ulcer, the choice should, at the very least, allow for total excision of the ulcer for histologic evaluation and for reduction in gastric secretion. Patients considered for elective surgery should probably discontinue H_2-receptor antagonist therapy for about 72 hours before operation to restore gastric acidity and to minimize bacterial overgrowth.

Surgical Treatment of Type I Gastric Ulcer

A distinction should be made among the different types of gastric ulcer in selecting the most appropriate operative procedure, because treatment varies according to location, coexistent duodenal ulcer disease, and acid secretory status. The elective operation of choice for a type I benign gastric ulcer is a distal gastrectomy with gastroduodenal (Billroth I) anastomosis[19] (Fig. 23-8). Gastrojejunostomy (Billroth II) is an acceptable alternative, although this form of reconstruction is less physiologic. The ulcer should be included in the antrectomy specimen. The operative mortality rate associated with this procedure is 2% to 3%, the recurrence rate is 3%, and a good to excellent clinical result can be anticipated in over 90% of patients. The addition of truncal vagotomy does not appear to diminish the

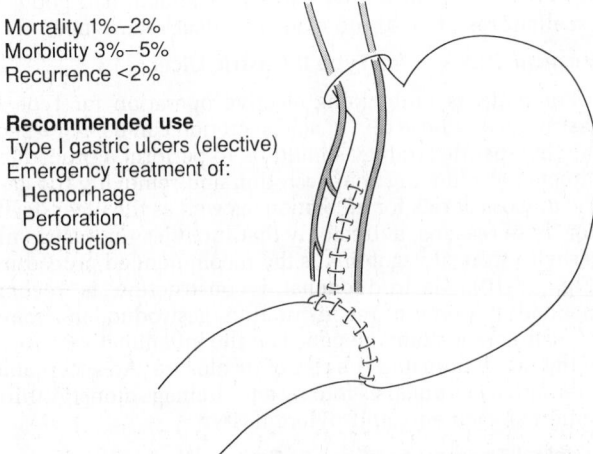

Mortality 1%–2%
Morbidity 3%–5%
Recurrence <2%

Recommended use
Type I gastric ulcers (elective)
Emergency treatment of:
  Hemorrhage
  Perforation
  Obstruction

Figure 23-8. Distal gastrectomy (without vagotomy), with associated morbidity, mortality, and recurrence rates, as well as indications.

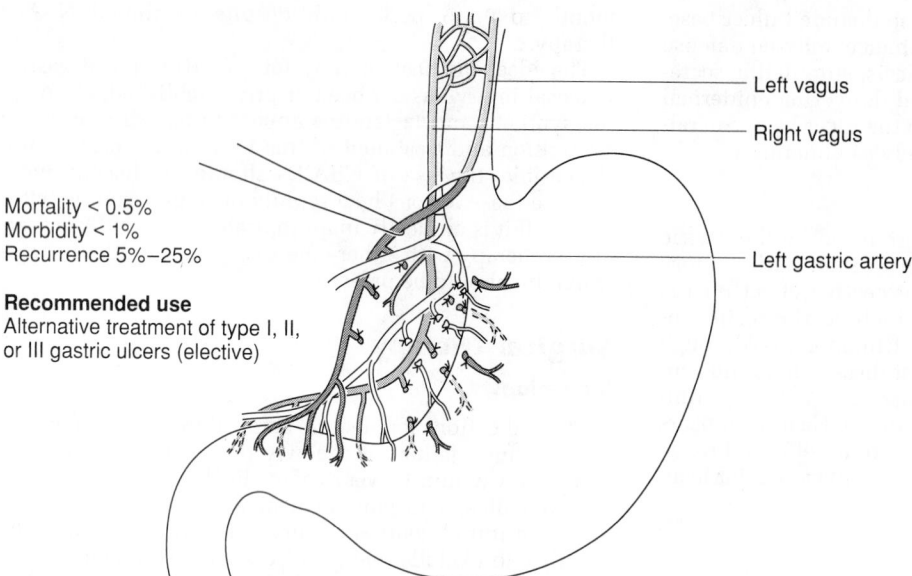

Left vagus

Right vagus

Left gastric artery

Mortality < 0.5%
Morbidity < 1%
Recurrence 5%–25%

Recommended use
Alternative treatment of type I, II,
or III gastric ulcers (elective)

Figure 23-9. Proximal gastric vagotomy, with associated morbidity, mortality, and recurrence rates, as well as indications.

recurrence rate but can increase the occurrence of postvagotomy diarrhea.

An alternative surgical procedure for type I gastric ulcer is a proximal gastric vagotomy (highly selective or parietal cell vagotomy) and excision of the ulcer (Fig. 23-9). In prospective studies of patients observed for short periods, and in a subsequent 10-year follow-up after this form of operative therapy, no difference between proximal gastric vagotomy and gastrectomy with gastroduodenal reconstruction has been observed.[20] The incidence of recurrent gastric ulceration ranges from 5% to 25%, averaging about 15% after proximal gastric vagotomy and ulcer excision. One drawback of this approach, depending on the size of the ulcer and the degree of surrounding inflammation, is that excision of the ulcer may not be technically feasible. The role of proximal gastric vagotomy and ulcer resection in the surgical treatment of gastric ulcer has yet to be fully evaluated.

Other procedures have been evaluated for the treatment of type I gastric ulcers. One group recommends removal of only the distal 4 or 5 cm of the stomach with the pylorus and incorporation of a tongue of gastric tissue along the lesser curvature to include the ulcer. In a 6- to 13-year follow-up, 87% of the 64 patients available had good to excellent results with no objective ulcer recurrence.

Surgical Therapy for Type II Gastric Ulcer

For patients undergoing elective operation for type II gastric ulcer whose rate of acid secretion can be increased, the therapeutic strategy should be to perform a procedure directed at reducing acid secretion and removing the gastric mucosa at risk for ulceration, as well as the ulcer itself. For these reasons, antrectomy that includes the gastric ulcer with truncal vagotomy is the recommended procedure (Fig. 23-10). Gastroduodenal reconstruction is recommended; the type of reconstruction, gastroduodenostomy or gastrojejunostomy, depends on the inflammatory nature of the duodenum and the risk of its closure. An acceptable alternative is truncal vagotomy and drainage alone. A third option is vagotomy and pyloroplasty.

Surgical Therapy for Type III Gastric Ulcer

Patients with type III (pyloric and prepyloric) gastric ulcers also tend to have higher rates of gastric acid secretion, often because of larger parietal cell masses, than pa-

tients with type I gastric ulcers. These patients should be approached surgically, as are patients with type II gastric ulcers or duodenal ulcers. The procedure of choice is vagotomy and antrectomy to include the ulcer. Recurrence rates of less than 2% are reported (see Fig. 23-10). A number of reports evaluating the role of proximal gastric vagotomy for type III ulcers indicate a recurrence rate for pyloric and prepyloric ulcers ranging from 12% to 44%.

Surgical Treatment of Type IV Gastric Ulcer

Patients with type IV or high-lying gastric ulcers near the gastroesophageal junction present a difficult management problem. The choice of surgical treatment depends on the ulcer's size, the distance from the gastroesophageal junction, and the degree of surrounding inflammation. Whenever possible, excision of the juxtaesophageal ulcer should be performed. The most aggressive technique described for the treatment of a type IV ulcer is a generous distal gastrectomy including a small portion of the esophageal wall and ulcer with a Roux-en-Y esophagogastrojejunostomy to restore continuity.[21]

A less aggressive procedure for type IV ulcers located 2 to 5 cm from the gastroesophageal junction is a distal gastric resection with a vertical extension of the resection to include the lesser curvatures with the ulcer. After resection, bowel continuity is restored with an end-to-end gastroduodenostomy.

Another described approach is a transgastric approach to the juxtaesophageal gastric ulcer. The procedure requires an 8-cm gastrotomy over the anterior gastric wall parallel to and just below the esophagus. The left gastric vessels are ligated close to the stomach, and a generous wedge resection of the anterior and posterior walls of the lesser curvature is completed to include the ulcer. The defect is closed transversely and a pyloroplasty is performed.

Surgical Therapy for Type V Gastric Ulcer

In a patient who is believed to have a type V gastric ulcer and who does not heal rapidly with cessation of the offending agent and institution of antisecretory therapy, an underlying malignancy must be considered. In general, except for cases of perforation or unrelenting hemorrhage, operation for chemically induced ulceration is not required.

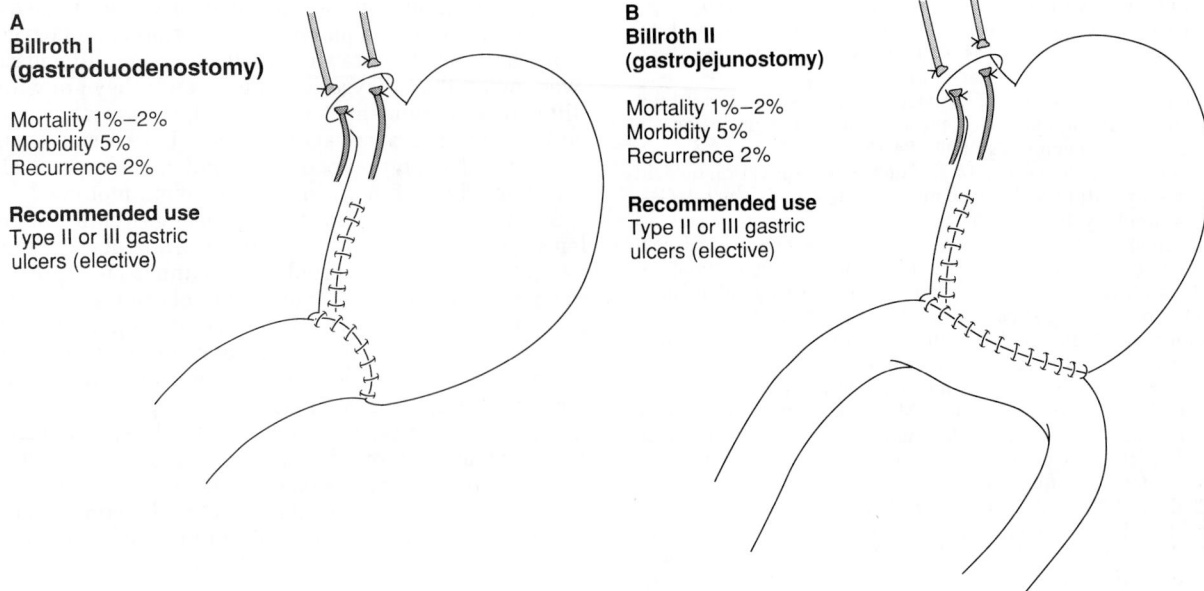

Figure 23-10. Vagotomy and antrectomy, with associated morbidity, mortality, and recurrence rates, as well as indications.

Surgical Therapy for Complications of Gastric Ulcer

Hemorrhage, perforation, and obstruction are the three most common complications of gastric ulcer. The indications for emergency operative therapy for benign gastric ulcer include hemorrhage and perforation. Gastric outlet obstruction is more common with type III ulcers but can occur in patients with type II ulcers. Obstruction is an unusual presentation in type I gastric ulcers, and its presence should suggest an underlying malignancy. All patients with gastric outlet obstruction should undergo preoperative gastric decompression for several days, correction of fluid and electrolyte imbalance, and endoscopy with biopsies before surgical intervention.

Definitive treatment for each of these complications is accomplished by a procedure designed to correct the emergent aspect of presentation and prevent recurrent ulceration. An antrectomy, which includes the ulcer with gastroduodenostomy, could be considered the procedure of choice for surgical treatment of each complication. The quoted operative mortality rates in this setting range from 10% to 40%.

In the presence of life-threatening hemorrhage, vagotomy plus pyloroplasty with suture ligation of the ulcer is an acceptable alternative. If possible, multiple biopsy specimens should be taken to exclude the presence of malignant disease. This procedure has been associated with rates of rebleeding approaching 30% to 40%.

In the extremely high-risk patient, acceptable alternative procedures include vagotomy and excision of the ulcer or biopsy and simple closure of a perforated ulcer with an omental patch. Care must be taken to avoid gastric outlet obstruction at the site of closure. Although recurrence rates (over 23%) and reoperative rates (about 25%) for both of these lesser procedures are high, they may serve as the only viable alternative in a severely ill patient.

Although most patients who present with obstruction from a gastric ulcer are amenable to antrectomy and gastroduodenostomy, scarring can be so severe as to preclude a safe anastomosis. If the resection can be performed but a gastroduodenostomy is deemed risky, a gastrojejunostomy should be undertaken.

Giant Gastric Ulcer

A giant gastric ulcer is defined as an ulcer whose diameter is 3 cm or greater. The lesser curvature is the most common site, with only 3% to 4% occurring along the greater curvature. Gastric ulcers often penetrate into contiguous structures such as spleen, pancreas, liver, and transverse colon and can be falsely diagnosed as nonresectable malignancies despite normal biopsy results. Most reports cite an incidence of malignancy ranging from 6% to 30%, increasing with the size of the ulcer. Because of the high likelihood of complications from giant gastric ulcer, early operation is thought to be the treatment of choice. The operation of choice is resection, including the ulcer, with vagotomy for type II or type III ulcers. If the ulcer has penetrated adjacent structures and cannot be dissected free, the stomach wall can be incised circumferentially, leaving the ulcer intact and behind, and the gastric resection completed. In poor-risk patients with significant underlying disease, a local excision combined with vagotomy and pyloroplasty can be considered.

REFERENCES

1. Johnson LR. Regulation of gastrointestinal growth. In: Johnson LR, Alpers DH, Christensen J, Jacobson ED, Walsh JH, eds. Physiology of the gastrointestinal tract, ed 2. New York, Raven Press, 1987:301.
2. Ito S, Lacey ER. Morphology of rat gastric mucosal damage, defense, and restitution in the presence of luminal ethanol. Gastroenterology 1985;88:250.
3. Lichtenberger LM. Ulcer disease: new aspects of pathogenesis and pharmacology. Boca Raton, CRC Press, 1989:447.
4. Spychal RT, Marrero JM, Savery-Muttu SH, et al. Measurement of surface hydrophobicity of human gastrointestinal mucosa. Gastroenterology 1989;97:104.
5. Takeuchi K, Magee D, Kritslow J, et al. Role of pH gradient of mucus in protection of gastric mucosa. Gastroenterology 1983;84:331.
6. Parks DA. Oxygen radicals: mediators of gastrointestinal physiology. Gut 1989;30:293.
7. Davenport HW, Warner HA, Code CF. Functional significance of gastric mucosal barrier to sodium. Gastroenterology 1964;47:142.

8. Whittle BJR, Vane JR. Prostanoids as regulators of gastrointestinal function. In: Johnson LR, Alpers DH, Christensen J, Jacobsen ED, Walsh JH, eds. Physiology of the gastrointestinal tract, ed 2. New York, Raven Press, 1987:143.

9. Ligumsky M, Golanska E, Hansen D, et al. Aspirin can inhibit gastric mucosal cyclo-oxygenase without causing lesions in the rat. Gastroenterology 1983;84:756.

10. Skinner KA, Tepperman BL. Influence of desalivation on acid secretory output and gastric mucosal integrity in the rat. Gastroenterology 1981;81:335.

11. Marrone GO, Silen W. Pathogenesis, diagnosis and treatment of acute mucosal lesions. Clin Gastroenterol 1984;13:635.

12. Hubert JP Jr, Kiernan PD, Welch JS, et al. The surgical management of bleeding stress ulcers. Ann Surg 1980;191:672.

13. Zinner MJ, Zuidema GD, Smith PL, et al. The prevention of upper gastrointestinal tract bleeding in patients in an intensive care unit. Surg Gynecol Obstet 1981;153:214.

14. Tryba N, Zeuvonou F, Torok M, et al. Prevention of acute stress bleeding with sucralfate, antacids or cimetidine: a controlled study with pirenzepine as a basic medication. Am J Med 1985;79(Suppl):21.

15. Craham DY, Smith JL. Gastroduodenal complications of chronic NSAID therapy. Am J Gastroenterol 1988;83:1081.

16. Forbes GM, Glaser ME, Cullins DJE. Duodenal ulcer treated with Helicobacter pylori eradication: seven year follow-up. Lancet 1994;343:258.

17. Walan A, Baclar JP, Classen M, et al. Effect of omeprazole and ranitidine on ulcer healing and relapse rates in patients with benign gastric ulcer. N Engl J Med 1989;320:69.

18. Herting RL, Nissen CH. Overview of misoprostol clinical experience. Dig Dis Sci 1986;31(Suppl):47S.

19. Thomas WEG, Thompson MH, Williamson RCN. The long-term outcome of Billroth I partial gastrectomy for benign gastric ulcers. Ann Surg 1982;189:189.

20. Emas S, Grupcev G, Eriksson B. Ten-year follow-up of a prospective, randomized trial of selective proximal vagotomy with ulcer excision and partial gastrectomy with gastroduodenostomy for treating corporal gastric ulcer. Am J Surg 1994;167:596.

21. Csendes A, Calvo M, Bragetto I. A surgical technique for high cardial or juxta-cardial benign chronic gastric ulcer. Am J Surg 1978;135:857.

SURGERY: SCIENTIFIC PRINCIPLES AND PRACTICE, Second Edition, edited by Lazar J. Greenfield, Michael W. Mulholland, Keith T. Oldham, Gerald B. Zelenock, and Keith D. Lillemoe. Lippincott–Raven Publishers, Philadelphia, © 1997.

CHAPTER 24

MORBID OBESITY

HARVEY J. SUGERMAN

Morbid obesity has been arbitrarily defined as 100 lb above ideal body weight, as defined actuarially by the Metropolitan Life Insurance Company. Morbid obesity is the degree of overweight that is clearly associated with increased disability and mortality (Fig. 24-1). Severe obesity (more than 244 lb for men or more than 225 lb for women) has been estimated to be present in 4.9% (2.8 million) of men and 7.2% (4.5 million) of women in the United States. The causes of morbid obesity are unknown but probably include genetic factors, abnormalities of neural or humoral transmitters to the hypothalamic hunger or satiety centers, dysfunction of the hypothalamic centers themselves, and psychologically induced oral dependency drives. Morbidly obese adults have been found to have a lower basal energy expenditure.[1] A genetic predisposition to obesity has been reported in several studies. In adopted children, the severity of obesity was more concordant with the natural than the adoptive parents.[2] Furthermore, monozygotic twins have much more similar weights, including marked overweight, than dizygotic twins, even if they grow up in different environments.[3] Other studies have shown that children born to overweight mothers have a significantly lower basal energy expenditure and more rapid weight gain than children born to normal-weight mothers.[4]

Severe obesity is associated with a large number of problems that give rise to the term morbid obesity (Table 24-1). Several of these problems are underlying causes for the earlier mortality associated with obesity; they include coronary artery disease, hypertension, impaired cardiac ventricular function, adult-onset diabetes mellitus, obesity hypoventilation and sleep apnea syndromes, hypercoagulability leading to an increased risk of pulmonary embolism, necrotizing panniculitis, diverticulitis, and necrotizing pancreatitis. Morbidly obese patients can also die as a result of difficulties in recognizing the signs and symptoms of peritonitis. Premature death is much more common: there is a 12-fold excess mortality in morbidly obese men in the 25- to 34-year age group.[5]

CENTRAL VERSUS PERIPHERAL OBESITY

A number of obesity-related problems may not be associated with death but can lead to significant physical or psychologic disability. These include degenerative osteoarthritis, pseudotumor cerebri, cholecystitis, skin infections, chronic venous stasis ulcers, stress overflow urinary incontinence, gastroesophageal reflux, sex hormone imbalance with dysmenorrhea, hirsutism, infertility, and an increased risk of uterine and breast cancer. Many morbidly obese patients suffer from severe psychologic and social disability.

Central obesity (android, or "apple," distribution of fat) is associated with a significantly greater morbidity than peripheral obesity (gynoid, or "pear," distribution of fat), and this increased morbidity is secondary to the increased metabolism of visceral fat. This increased visceral metabolism leads to increased blood glucose levels, hyperglycemia, increased insulin secretion, insulin-induced sodium reabsorption leading to hypertension, and increased fatty acid and cholesterol turnover with an increased risk of atherosclerosis and gallstones. This combination of problems is called syndrome X.[6] another major complication of central obesity is increased intraabdominal pressure, which can lead to venous stasis disease, gastroesophageal reflux, stress or urge urinary incontinence, obesity hypoventilation syndrome, nephrotic syndrome, incisional and inguinal hernia, and elevated pleural pressures that can markedly increase pulmonary artery and pulmonary capillary wedge pressures. The latter may be responsible for pseudotumor cerebri seen in morbid obesity. The increased central obesity has been assessed as an increased waist-to-hip ratio. However, severely obese patients often have both central and peripheral obesity, which cancel each other out; thus, waist-to-hip ratios can underestimate the severity of central obesity. Recent studies have shown that sagittal abdominal diameter is a more accurate reflection of central obesity.[7]

CARDIAC DYSFUNCTION

Morbid obesity is sometimes associated with cardiomegaly and impaired left ventricular function.[8] Severe obesity can be associated with a high cardiac output and a low systemic vascular resistance, leading to eccentric left ven-

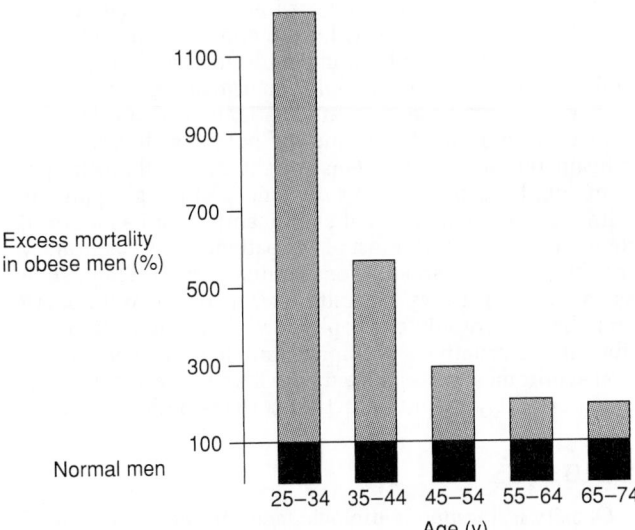

Figure 24-1. Percentage of excess probability of dying among morbidly obese men as computed for decades relative to mortality of US men as a whole. (After Drenick EJ, Bale GS, Seltter F, et al. Excessive mortality and causes of death in morbidly obese men. JAMA 1980;243:443)

tricular hypertrophy. Obesity is also frequently associated with hypertension, which leads to concentric left ventricular hypertrophy. This combination of obesity and hypertension, with left ventricular hypertrophy, can lead to left ventricular failure. Correction of morbid obesity improves cardiac function in these patients.[8] Morbid obesity is also associated with an accelerated rate of coronary atherosclerosis.[9] These patients often have hypercholesterolemia and an elevated ratio of high-density lipoprotein to low-density lipoprotein. Obese women with a body mass index (BMI; measured as weight [kg]/height [m]²) greater than 29 (BMI in morbid obesity greater than 35) have a significantly increased incidence of angina or myocardial infarction.[9]

Table 24-1. MORBIDITY OF SEVERE OBESITY

Cardiovascular dysfunction
  Hypertension
  Coronary artery disease
  Heart failure
Non–insulin-dependent diabetes mellitus (adult onset or type II)
Respiratory insufficiency of obesity (pickwickian syndrome)
  Obesity hypoventilation syndrome
  Obstructive sleep apnea syndrome
Increased intraabdominal pressure
  Stress overflow urinary incontinence
  Gastroesophageal reflux
  Venous disease
    Thrombophlebitis
    Stasis ulcers
    Pulmonary embolism
Nephrotic syndrome
Pseudotumor cerebri
Degenerative osteoarthritis
Cholelithiasis
Infectious complications
  Difficulty recognizing peritonitis
  Necrotizing subcutaneous infections
  Wound infections or dehiscence
Sexual hormone dysfunction
  Amenorrhea
  Infertility
  Hirsutism
  Endometrial cancer
  Breast cancer
Colon cancer
Psychosocial impairment

Respiratory insufficiency associated with morbid obesity can result in hypoxemic pulmonary artery vasoconstriction, which can lead to right-sided heart failure in severe cases. Correction of respiratory insufficiency after surgically induced weight loss improves the pulmonary artery hypertension within 3 months to 1 year.[8] Severe obstructive sleep apnea syndrome can be associated with prolonged sinus arrest, premature ventricular contractions, and sudden death.

PULMONARY DYSFUNCTION

Respiratory insufficiency of obesity is associated with either obesity hypoventilation syndrome, obstructive sleep apnea syndrome, or a combination of the two, commonly called the pickwickian syndrome. The obesity hypoventilation syndrome arises from the increased weight of the chest wall and increased intraabdominal pressure leading to a high-riding diaphragm. As a result, the lungs are squeezed, producing a restrictive pulmonary defect. These patients have markedly decreased expiratory reserve volume as well as smaller reductions in all other lung volumes. They have hypoxemia and hypercarbia while awake and a blunted ventilatory response to carbon dioxide. Chronic hypoxemia leads to pulmonary artery vasoconstriction and both right and left heart failure, as well as an increased risk of fatal arrhythmias and pulmonary embolism.

The obstructive sleep apnea syndrome is associated with severe obesity and is due to both depression of the normal genioglossus reflex, possibly secondary to a large, heavy tongue, and deposition of fat within the hypopharynx with narrowing of the airway. These patients snore while asleep and suffer from severe daytime somnolence with tendencies to fall asleep while driving or at work. The daytime somnolence is probably secondary to impaired nighttime stage III, IV, and REM sleep. The diagnosis of obstructive sleep apnea is suggested by a history of severe daytime somnolence, frequent nocturnal awakening, loud snoring, and morning headaches; it is confirmed with sleep polysomnography. This technique documents cessation of airflow during sleep associated with persistent respiratory efforts. This syndrome can be associated with sudden death and should always be considered in trauma victims who have fallen asleep while driving. Twelve percent of patients in one series who underwent gastric surgery for morbid obesity had respiratory insufficiency. Of the affected individuals, 25% had sleep apnea syndrome, 25% had obesity hypoventilation syndrome, and 50% had both.[10] Obesity is not the only factor causing respiratory embarrassment, because many patients who underwent surgery for morbid obesity and did not have clinically significant pulmonary problems weighed more than the patients with respiratory insufficiency, although patients with this problem weighed significantly more as a group than those without it. Most of the patients with respiratory insufficiency had an additional pulmonary problem, such as sarcoidosis, heavy cigarette use, recurrent pulmonary embolism, myotonic dystrophy, or idiopathic pulmonary fibrosis. Obstructive sleep apnea and obesity hypoventilation syndromes are associated with high mortality and serious morbidity; weight reduction corrects both.

DIABETES

Obesity is a frequent etiologic factor in the development of type II (adult-onset, non–insulin-dependent) diabetes mellitus (NIDDM). Morbidly obese patients can be resistant to insulin because of the marked down-regulation of insulin receptors. Most of these patients no longer require insulin after gastric surgery–induced weight loss.[11] The tendency toward hyperglycemia manifested by obese patients is another risk factor for coronary artery disease as well as for severe, even fatal, subcutaneous infections.

VENOUS STASIS DISEASE

Morbidly obese patients have an increased risk for deep venous thrombosis, venous stasis ulcers, and pulmonary embolism, secondary to the increased intraabdominal pressure associated with central obesity. Low levels of antithrombin III can increase their risk of blood clots. The increased weight within the abdomen raises inferior vena cava pressure and the resistance to venous return, increasing the tendency for thrombosis. A similar mechanism can be responsible for the increased risk of pulmonary embolism in patients with right heart failure secondary to hypoxemic pulmonary artery vasoconstriction. Stasis ulcers are common in morbidly obese patients. These can be incapacitating and extremely difficult to treat; weight reduction can be the critical factor, because pressure stockings and wound care are often ineffective.

DEGENERATIVE JOINT DISEASE

The increased weight in the morbidly obese leads to early degenerative arthritic changes of the weight-bearing joints, including the knees, hips, and spine. These patients are poor candidates for total joint replacement because of the inability of the artificial joint–bone interface to withstand the abnormal pressures. Many orthopedic surgeons refuse to insert total hip or knee prostheses in patients weighing more than 250 lb because of an unacceptable incidence of prosthetic loosening. Weight reduction following gastric surgery for obesity can permit subsequent successful joint replacement. In some instances, the decrease in pain after weight loss obviates the need for joint surgery.

OTHER OBESITY-RELATED CONDITIONS

Morbidly obese patients frequently suffer from gastroesophageal reflux. Women often have problems with stress overflow urinary incontinence. Both of these problems are probably related to an increased intraabdominal pressure. Pseudotumor cerebri, also known as idiopathic intracranial hypertension, can be associated with morbid obesity. Weight loss following gastric surgery for obesity is accompanied by a significant reduction in cerebrospinal fluid pressure and the associated headaches. Women often suffer from sexual dysfunction as a result of excessive levels of both the virilizing hormone androstenedione and the feminizing hormone estradiol. These can produce infertility, hirsutism, ovarian cysts (Stein-Leventhal syndrome), hypermenorrhea, and endometrial carcinoma. These hormonal abnormalities also resolve after weight loss.

DIETARY MANAGEMENT OF MORBID OBESITY

There are a number of dietary programs for weight reduction, including hospital-supervised programs, psychiatric behavioral modification programs, commercial organizations, commercial diets, protein-sparing fast programs, and diet pills. Unfortunately, no dietary approach has achieved uniform, long-term success for the morbidly obese. Although many individuals can lose weight successfully through dietary manipulation, the incidence of recidivism in the morbidly obese approaches 95%.[12] A National Institutes of Health (NIH) Technology Assessment Conference in 1992 concluded that dietary management of severe obesity, with or without behavioral modification, failed to provide acceptable evidence of long-term efficacy.[13]

SURGICAL MANAGEMENT OF MORBID OBESITY
Surgical Eligibility

According to a 1991 NIH Consensus Panel, patients are considered eligible if they have a BMI of 40 or over without comorbidity or a BMI of 35 or over with comorbidity (eg, diabetes, respiratory insufficiency, pseudotumor cerebri).

Jejunoileal Bypass

The first popular surgical procedure for morbid obesity was the jejunoileal bypass. This operation produced an obligatory malabsorption state through bypass of a major portion of the absorptive surface of the small intestine. The procedure connected a short length of proximal jejunum (8 to 14 inches) to the distal ileum (4 to 12 inches) as an end-to-end or end-to-side anastomosis. The end-to-end procedures, which were associated with a better weight loss, required decompression of the bypassed small intestine into the colon (Fig. 24-2). The jejunoileal bypass was associated with a number of early and late complications.[14] The most serious postoperative complication was cirrhosis due to either protein-calorie malnutrition or absorption of degradation products from bacterial overgrowth in the bypassed intestine. A rheumatoid-like arthritis also occurred as a result of absorption of bacterial products from the bypassed intestine; antigen–antibody complexes to bacterial antigens can be found in the joint fluid of affected individuals. Rapid weight loss, as well as malabsorption of bile salts, increased the risk of cholelithiasis because of the decrease in cholesterol solubility. Hypocalcemia was frequent because of chelation of calcium with bile salts, leading to severe osteoporosis. Multiple kidney stones were seen as a result of increased oxalate absorption from the colon, where it is normally bound to calcium. Intractable, malodorous diarrhea with associated potassium and magnesium depletion, metabolic acidosis, and severe malnutrition were common, as was vitamin B_{12} deficiency.

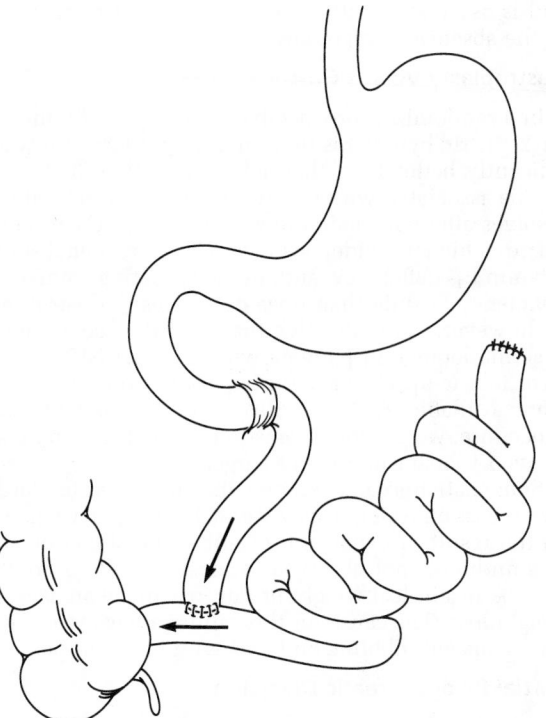

Figure 24-2. Schematic representation of jejunoileal bypass.

Bacterial overgrowth in the bypassed intestine also led to vitamin K deficiency, interstitial nephritis with renal failure, pneumatosis intestinalis and bypass enteritis associated with occult blood in the stools, and iron-deficiency anemia. Many of these problems, which are associated with bacterial overgrowth in the bypassed intestine, can be treated, at least temporarily, with metronidazole.

Some surgeons believe that all jejunoileal bypass procedures should be reversed because cirrhosis can develop insidiously in the absence of abnormal liver function tests. If the medical problems are severe (ie, progressive liver or renal dysfunction), the jejunoileal bypass can be reversed. Because these patients invariably regain their lost weight, conversion to a gastric procedure for obesity can be considered unless the patient is too ill (ie, severe cirrhosis with portal hypertension). Mechanical complications of the jejunoileal bypass include small bowel obstruction and intussusception of the bypassed intestine. Randomized, prospective studies have shown that the gastric bypass operation is associated with a comparable weight loss and a significantly lower complication rate than jejunoileal bypass.[15] Because of the significant complication rate, standard jejunoileal bypass should no longer be performed.

Gastric Procedures for Morbid Obesity

In 1969, investigators reported the results of weight loss following division of the stomach into a small upper pouch connected to a loop gastroenterostomy.[16] The concept for this procedure was based on the observation of weight loss that sometimes followed subtotal gastrectomy for duodenal ulcer disease. There was initial concern that peptic ulcers would develop in the bypassed stomach or duodenum, and although these have occurred, the incidence is low. The technique for gastric bypass was simplified with the use of stapling instruments. The concept of gastroplasty was then proposed as a safer, easier method for restricting food intake. In gastroplasty, the stomach is only stapled and not divided, leaving a small opening to permit the normal passage of food into the distal stomach and duodenum.

Gastroplasty

Gastroplasties have been performed with either horizontal or vertical placement of the staples. Horizontal gastroplasty usually requires ligation and division of the short gastric vessels between the stomach and spleen, and it carries the risk of devascularization of the gastric pouch or splenic injury. Horizontal gastroplasties included a single application of a 90-mm stapling device without suture reinforcement of the stoma between upper and lower gastric pouches, or a double application of staples with either a central or lateral Prolene-reinforced stoma. In one study, the failure rates (loss of less than 40% excess weight) for these three horizontal gastroplasty procedures were 71%, 46%, and 42%, respectively.[17] The vertical banded gastroplasty (VBGP) is a procedure in which a stapled opening is made in the stomach with the stapling device 5 cm from the cardioesophageal junction (Fig. 24-3). Two applications of a 90-mm stapling device are made between this opening and the angle of His, and a 1.5×5-cm strip of polypropylene mesh is wrapped around the stoma on the lesser curvature and sutured to itself but not to the stomach. Erosion of the mesh into the stomach has been an unusual complication of this procedure. Pouch enlargement is much less likely to occur with a vertical staple line in the thicker, more muscular part of the stomach (as compared with the horizontal gastroplasties), and the stomal diameter is fixed with the mesh band. The Silastic ring gastroplasty is a similar procedure (Fig. 24-4) that uses a vertical staple line and a Silastic tubing–reinforced stoma. Weight loss with vertical Silastic ring gastroplasty appears to be similar to that with VBGP. Use of the four-row parallel bariatric stapler has been associated with a 35% rate of staple line disruption, leading to failure of the operative procedure. Some surgeons now recommend transecting the stomach.

Gastric Bypass

Gastric bypass can also be performed with placement of the staples in a vertical or horizontal direction; the vertical direction is preferred because there is less risk of gastric pouch devascularization or splenic injury. Because of the high incidence of staple line disruption, some surgeons

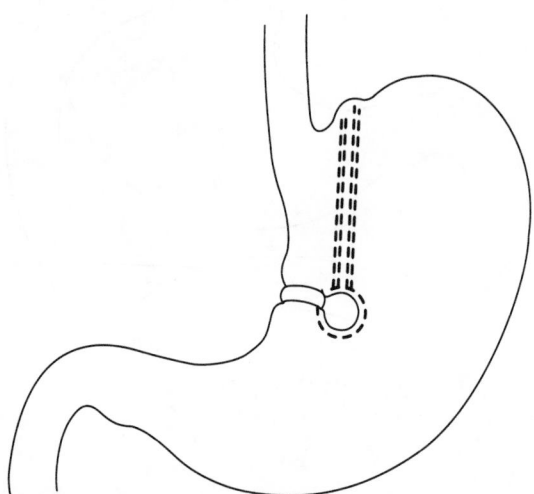

Figure 24-3. Vertical banded gastroplasty.

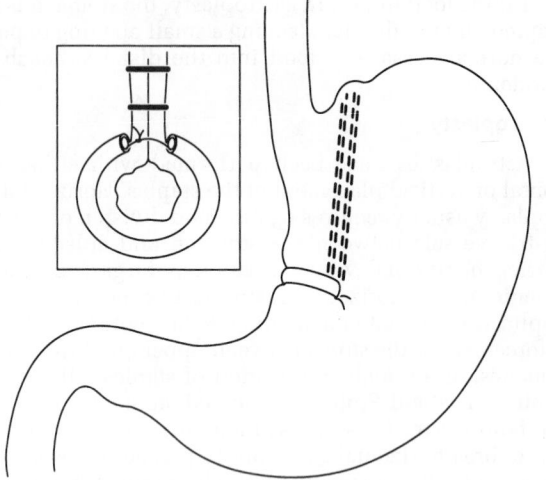

Figure 24-4. Vertical Silastic ring gastroplasty.

also recommend transecting the stomach for gastric bypass patients. However, with three superimposed applications of a 90-mm stapler, the incidence of staple line disruption has been less than 2%. The gastrojejunostomy used to drain the gastric pouch can be a loop, a loop with a jejuno-jejunostomy constructed below the gastrojejunostomy, or a Roux-en-Y limb. The latter two techniques prevent bile reflux into the gastric pouch. The length of the Roux-en-Y jejunal limb is usually 45 cm. However, superobese patients (BMI 50 kg/m² or greater) achieve a significantly better weight loss with a 150-cm Roux limb (long-limb gastric bypass).[18] The gastric pouch should be small (15 to 30 mL) and the stoma restricted to 1 cm (Fig. 24-5). The small gastric pouch has a limited volume of acid secretion

and is associated with a low incidence of marginal ulcer in the absence of vagotomy.

Gastroplasty Versus Gastric Bypass

In a randomized prospective trial (Fig. 24-6), the Roux-en-Y gastric bypass resulted in a weight loss that was significantly better than that achieved with VBGP.[19] VBGP can be associated with severe gastroesophageal reflux that resolves after conversion to gastric bypass. Gastric bypass carries a higher incidence of stomal ulcer, stomal stenosis, vitamin B_{12} deficiency, and, in menstruating women, iron-deficiency anemia than does gastroplasty. Gastric bypass is, however, more effective than VBGP in correcting glucose intolerance in patients without overt NIDDM. Long-term follow-up after gastric bypass has only recently become available. Although 10% to 15% of patients fail the procedure, weight loss seems to remain stable in most patients 5 years or more after surgery.[20]

Some patients can overcome the effect of a standard gastric bypass on weight loss. Although regained weight could be the result of expansion of either the stoma or pouch, this finding is not observed in most patients. About 10% to 15% regain lost weight or fail to achieve an acceptable weight loss. The cause for this failure appears to be excessive, constant nibbling on foods with high caloric density.

Partial Biliopancreatic Diversion

The partial biliopancreatic diversion was developed as both a gastric restrictive procedure and a malabsorptive procedure that does not have a blind intestinal limb for bacterial overgrowth.[21] In this operation, a subtotal gastrectomy is performed and the distal 2.5 m of small intestine is anastomosed with a large (2- to 3-cm) stoma to the proximal gastric remnant. The proximal, bypassed small intestine is reanastomosed to the distal ileum 0.5 m from the ileocecal valve. In this manner, the quantity of food ingested is partially restricted and then passes down the intestine mostly undigested and unabsorbed until it reaches the bile and pancreatic juices, 0.5 m from the ileocecal valve, where digestion and absorption take place. Treated patients usually pass four to six stools per day, which are foul smelling and float, reflecting malabsorption of fat. If the distal stomach is not resected, the operation is called a distal gastric bypass.

As with the proximal or standard gastric bypass, patients with the distal gastric bypass or partial biliopancreatic diversion are at risk for iron-deficiency anemia and vitamin

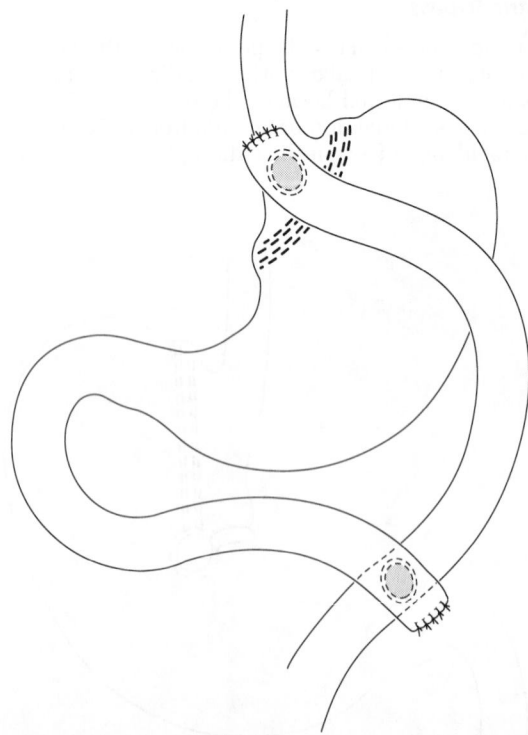

Figure 24-5. Proximal Roux-en-Y gastric bypass.

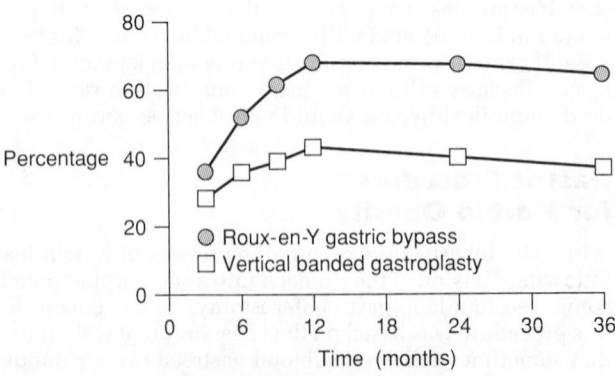

Figure 24-6. Percentage loss of excess weight over 3 years after Roux-en-Y gastric bypass compared with vertical banded gastroplasty. (After Sugerman HJ, Starkey J, Birkenhauer, R. A randomized prospective trial of gastric bypass versus vertical banded gastroplasty for morbid obesity and their effects on sweets versus non-sweets eaters. Ann Surg 1987;205:613)

B_{12} deficiency. In addition, they are also at risk for protein deficiency, osteoporosis secondary to calcium and vitamin D malabsorption, night-blindness and skin eruptions secondary to vitamin A deficiency, and problems with the other fat-soluble vitamins, E and K.[22]

Complications of Gastric Surgery for Morbid Obesity

The most feared complication of gastric surgery for morbid obesity is a postoperative gastric leak with the development of peritonitis. After gastroplasty, this can occur at the staple line, from the proximal gastric pouch or from the distal stomach. Many leaks were secondary to ischemic necrosis that occurs with horizontal stapling procedures, either gastroplasty or gastric bypass, after ligation of the short gastric vessels. Perforation of the distal stomach because of marked dilatation can occur after a gastric bypass operation as a result of afferent limb obstruction of a loop gastrojejunostomy or obstruction at the jejunojejunostomy of a Roux-en-Y procedure. This complication is usually heralded by frequent hiccups and can be diagnosed by noting a large gastric bubble on a plain abdominal roentgenogram. Impending gastric perforation requires urgent percutaneous or operative decompression. In patients converted from jejunoileal to gastric bypass or in patients with extensive adhesions from previous abdominal surgery, a gastrostomy tube should be inserted prophylactically for decompression. The gastrostomy tube also can be used for feeding until the patient's oral intake permits weight stabilization. A gastrostomy can also be used to feed patients who develop a leak from the proximal gastric pouch.

The most dangerous aspect of a gastric leak is the difficulty in recognizing the symptoms of peritonitis. By the third day after surgery, patients should have little pain. If postoperative gastric bypass or gastroplasty patients experience worsening pain and they complain of pain in the back or the left shoulder (consistent with inflammation of the left hemidiaphragm), urinary frequency, or rectal tenesmus (implying pelvic irritation), one must suspect a leak. Tachycardia, tachypnea, fever, and leukocytosis are usually also present. A leak can often be confirmed with an emergency upper gastrointestinal roentgenographic series using water-soluble contrast. If a leak is observed, or even if the study is negative but the suspicion is high, the patient's abdomen must be urgently reexplored. An attempt to repair the leak should be made, and a large sump drain should be placed nearby, because the repair frequently breaks down. This leads to a controlled fistula, which usually heals with total parenteral nutrition therapy or a distal, feeding jejunostomy.

A marginal ulcer develops in about 10% of gastric bypass patients. This usually responds to acid suppression therapy (H_2-receptor blocker or omeprazole). Stomal stenosis can develop in patients following Roux-en-Y gastric bypass or VBGP. Outpatient endoscopic balloon stomal dilation should be attempted. This is usually successful in gastric bypass patients but is effective in only half of stenoses in VBGP patients.

Rapid weight loss following either VBGP or gastric bypass is associated with a high incidence (32% to 35%) of gallstone formation with a 10% to 20% need for subsequent cholecystectomy for acute biliary colic or cholecystitis within 3 to 5 years of obesity surgery. Some surgeons recommend routine prophylactic cholecystectomy at the time of bariatric surgery; others perform cholecystectomy only with sonographic evidence of gallstones or biliary sludge. Prophylactic ursodeoxycholic acid, 300 mg orally twice daily, has been shown to reduce the risk of gallstone

formation from 32% to 2% when given for 6 months after gastric bypass surgery, and it has a very low risk of subsequent gallstone formation for the 6 months following discontinuation of the medication.[23]

A rare syndrome of polyneuropathy has occurred following gastric surgery for morbid obesity. This usually occurs in association with intractable vomiting and severe protein-calorie malnutrition. Acute thiamine deficiency has been thought to be responsible for this condition. Vitamin B_{12} deficiency has been observed following gastric bypass, and this mandates long-term follow-up of these patients with annual measurement of the vitamin B_{12} level. Deficiency of this vitamin is probably due to decreased acid digestion of vitamin B_{12} from food with subsequent failure of coupling to intrinsic factor. Iron-deficiency anemia can occur in menstruating women following gastric bypass. This can be refractory to supplemental ferrous sulfate, because iron absorption requires acid and takes place primarily in the duodenum and upper jejunum. Occasionally, iron-dextran injections may be necessary. All menstruating women should take two iron sulfate tablets (325 mg/d) by mouth after gastric bypass as long as they continue to menstruate.

Other complications, seen with any type of surgery in obese patients, include wound infection, wound dehiscence, incisional hernia, venous thrombosis, and pulmonary embolism. The incidence of lower leg venous thrombosis and pulmonary embolism can be significantly reduced with the use of intermittent venous compression boots. Early ambulation is also quite important. Pulmonary embolism is a not infrequent fatal complication in patients with heart failure associated with hypoxemic pulmonary hypertension and mean pulmonary artery pressure greater than 40 mmHg. It has been recommended that a vena cava filter be placed in these patients prophylactically at the time of obesity surgery. The operative mortality rate following gastric surgery for obesity is now about 0.5% in most series.

Failed Gastric Surgery for Obesity

Attempts to revise a failed gastroplasty are often unsuccessful because of recurrence of stomal dilation and problems with gastric emptying. Reoperation in these patients

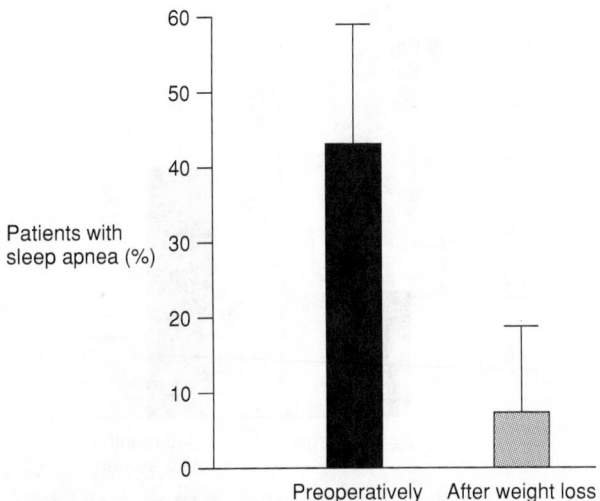

Figure 24-7. Reduction in percentage of sleep apnea (mean ± SD) in 22 patients with obstructive sleep apnea syndrome following weight loss induced by gastric surgery. (After Sugerman HJ, Fairman RP, Baron PL, Kwentus JA. Gastric surgery for respiratory insufficiency of obesity. Chest 1986;90:82)

is extremely difficult because of extensive adhesions to the liver and spleen. Results appear to be significantly better when these patients are converted to a Roux-en-Y gastric bypass. Because of the technical difficulties, these patients must understand that the risks of serious complications are far higher after a secondary than after a primary gastric bypass. It is probably inappropriate and dangerous to convert a failed gastric bypass to vertical gastroplasty. Furthermore, revision of a dilated gastrojejunal stoma has not been effective. Most patients who fail a gastric bypass do so as a consequence of excessive fat ingestion. If the patient has significant obesity comorbidity that has failed to resolve or has returned with weight regain, conversion to a malabsorptive distal gastric bypass (modified partial biliopancreatic diversion) can be performed; however, this can be associated with steatorrhea, fat-soluble vitamin deficiencies, and osteoporosis.

OVERVIEW OF GASTRIC SURGERY FOR MORBID OBESITY

Selectively applied gastric procedures for morbid obesity can yield a satisfactory weight reduction, with an average loss of one half to two thirds of excess weight within 1 to 1.5 years. Weight becomes stable at this level in most patients as the reduced caloric intake meets caloric expenditure. The patients must be followed carefully to ensure adequate protein, vitamin, and other micronutrient levels.

Weight loss completely corrects insulin-dependent diabetes in almost all cases, hypertension in 80%, and headaches associated with cerebrospinal fluid pressure elevation in pseudotumor cerebri. The obstructive sleep apnea syndrome resolves with weight loss (Fig. 24-7). Hypoxemia and hypercarbia seen in the obesity hypoventilation syndrome return toward normal with weight loss (Fig. 24-8). Elevated pulmonary artery and pulmonary capillary wedge pressures also improve significantly following weight loss with correction of abnormal arterial blood gases. The loss of weight usually corrects female sexual hormone abnormalities, permits healing of chronic venous stasis ulcers associated with venous insufficiency, prevents reflux esophagitis, relieves stress overflow urinary incontinence,

and improves low back pain, as well as joint-related pain. Weight loss can permit successful total artificial joint replacement. Patient self-image is often markedly improved after gastric surgery for obesity.

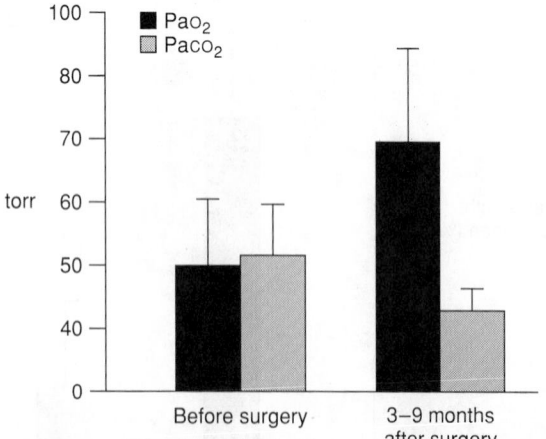

Figure 24-8. Significantly improved PaO₂ and PaCO₂ in 18 patients 3 to 9 months after gastric surgery–induced loss of 42%±19% excess weight. (After Sugerman HJ, Baron PL, Fairman RP, et al. Hemodynamic dysfunction in obesity hypoventilation syndrome and the effects of treatment with surgically induced weight loss. Ann Surg 1988;207:604)

REFERENCES

1. Ravussin E, Lillioja S, Knowler WC, et al. Reduced rate of energy expenditure as a risk factor for body-weight gain. N Engl J Med 1988;318:467.
2. Stunkard AJ, Sorensen TA, Hanis C, et al. An adoption study of human obesity. N Engl J Med 1986;314:193.
3. Stunkard AJ, Harris JR, Pedersen NL, McClearn GE. The body-mass index of twins who have been reared apart. N Engl J Med 1990;322:1483.
4. Roberts SB, Savage J, Coward WA, et al. Energy expenditure and intake in infants born to lean and overweight mothers. N Engl J Med 1988;318:461.
5. Drenick EJ, Bale GS, Seltter F, et al. Excessive mortality and causes of death in morbidly obese men. JAMA 1980;243:443.
6. Bjorntorp P. Abdominal obesity and the metabolic syndrome. Ann Med 1992;24:465.
7. Sjostrom L. A computer-tomography based multicompartment body composition technique and anthropometric predictions of lean body mass, total and subcutaneous adipose tissue. Int J Obes 1991;15(Suppl 2):19.
8. Sugerman HJ, Baron PL, Fairman RP, et al. Hemodynamic dysfunction in obesity hypoventilation syndrome and the effects of treatment with surgically induced weight loss. Ann Surg 1988;207:604.
9. Manson JE, Colditz GA, Stampfer MJ, et al. A prospective study of obesity and risk of coronary heart disease in women. N Engl J Med 1990;322:882.
10. Sugerman HJ, Fairman RP, Baron PL, Kwentus JA. Gastric surgery for respiratory insufficiency of obesity. Chest 1986;90:82.
11. Pories WJ, Caro JF, Flickinger EG, et al. The control of diabetes mellitus (NIDDM) in the morbidly obese with the Greenville gastric bypass. Ann Surg 1987;206:316.
12. Johnson D, Drenick EJ. Therapeutic fasting in morbid obesity. Arch Intern Med 1977;137:1381.
13. NIH Technology Assessment Conference Panel. NIH Conference: Methods for voluntary weight loss and control. Ann Intern Med 1992;116:942.
14. Hocking MP, Duerson MC, O'Leary JP, Woodward EF. Jejunoileal bypass for morbid obesity: late follow-up in 100 cases. N Engl J Med 1983;308:995.
15. Griffen WO, Young VL, Stevenson CC. A prospective comparison of gastric and jejunoileal bypass for morbid obesity. Ann Surg 1977;186:500.
16. Mason EE, Ito C. Gastric bypass. Ann Surg 1969;170:329.
17. Sugerman JH, Wolper JL. Failed gastroplasty for morbid obesity: revised gastroplasty versus Roux-en-Y gastric bypass. Am J Surg 1984;148:331.
18. Brolin RE, Kenler HA, Gorman JH, Cody RP. Long-limb gastric bypass in the superobese. A prospective randomized study. Ann Surg 1992;215:387.
19. Sugerman HJ, Starkey J, Birkenhauer R. A randomized prospective trial of gastric bypass versus vertical banded gastroplasty for morbid obesity and their effects on sweets versus non-sweets eaters. Ann Surg 1987;205:613.
20. Yale CE. Gastric surgery for morbid obesity: complications and long-term weight control. Arch Surg 1989;124:941.
21. Scopinaro N, Gianetta E, Civalleri D, Bonalum I, Bachi V. Two years of clinical experience with bilio-pancreatic bypass for obesity. Am J Clin Nutr 1980;33:506.
22. Clare MW. An analysis of 37 reversals on 504 biliopancreatic surgeries over 12 years. Obesity Surg 1993;3:169.
23. Sugerman HJ, Brewer WH, Shiffman ML, et al. Prophylactic ursodiol acid prevents gallstone formation following gastric bypass induced rapid weight loss: a multicenter, placebo controlled, randomized, double-blind prospective trial. Am J Surg (in press).

SURGERY: SCIENTIFIC PRINCIPLES AND PRACTICE, Second Edition, edited by
Lazar J. Greenfield, Michael W. Mulholland, Keith T. Oldham, Gerald B. Zelenock,
and Keith D. Lillemoe. Lippincott–Raven Publishers, Philadelphia, © 1997.

CHAPTER 25

GASTRIC NEOPLASMS

MICHAEL W. MULHOLLAND

Gastric cancer is a common, frequently lethal affliction and remains a serious and unsolved problem in general surgery. The disease often is not recognized until it is at an advanced stage. Gastric cancer usually cannot be controlled by operation alone, and surgical cure rates have not improved during the past 50 years. Technical innovations and basic scientific investigations continue to be applied to this disease, however, and cautious optimism for the future is appropriate.

ADENOCARCINOMA

Epidemiology

Between 1930 and 1980, the incidence of gastric cancer declined dramatically in the United States (Fig. 25-1). For men, the 1980 incidence of gastric cancer (10 cases per 100,000 of population) was about one fourth the incidence recorded in 1930. The incidence of the disease remained relatively constant from 1980 to 1994; some 23,000 new cases were reported in 1990.[1] Gastric cancer remains among the top 10 causes of cancer-related deaths for both men and women in the United States. The reasons for this early decline in the incidence of gastric cancer are unknown, and the factors contributing to its persistence in the latter decades have not been identified.

The worldwide incidence and death rates for gastric cancer vary markedly. The highest age-adjusted death rate for gastric cancer occurs in Japan, where the disease accounts for about 50% of cancer-related deaths in men and 40% of cancer deaths in women.[2] High incidence rates are also reported in Chile, Costa Rica, Hungary, Portugal, Singapore, and Romania, a geographically and ethnically diverse group (Fig. 25-2). It has been widely assumed that exposure to environmental carcinogens, probably in the diet, accounts for the increased disease frequency observed in these populations. This supposition is supported by studies of immigrant populations. Migration from an area at high risk to one at low risk is associated with a decreased probability of developing gastric cancer. In animal models, ingested nitrites and metabolic derivatives such as nitrosamines can promote gastric carcinogenesis. Although nitrites in the diet have been postulated to have a role in gastric carcinogenesis in humans, specific dietary constituents that promote tumor formation in humans have not been identified. Important new studies, outlined later, indicate that exposure to *Helicobacter pylori* can also have a role in the development of gastric carcinoma.

Premalignant Lesions

Gastric Polyps

The risk of developing gastric cancer is greater in stomachs that harbor polyps. This risk is related most closely to polyp histology, size, and number. Variations in these three factors account for the wide range in reported risk associated with gastric polyps. In terms of malignant potential, gastric polyps can be divided into two broad categories—hyperplastic polyps and adenomatous polyps.

Hyperplastic polyps are common, occurring in 0.5% to 1% of the general population and accounting for 70% to 80% of all gastric polyps.[3] The hyperplastic polyp contains an overgrowth of histologically normal-appearing gastric epithelium. Atypia is rare. Hyperplastic gastric polyps are considered to have no neoplastic potential.

Most individuals with hyperplastic polyps are asymptomatic. Dyspepsia and complaints of vague epigastric discomfort are the most common complaints, although coexistent gastroduodenal disease is also frequently identified. Complications are unusual, and gastrointestinal hemorrhage occurs in less than 20%. When hyperplastic polyps are discovered, endoscopic removal for histologic examination is indicated and is sufficient treatment.

Adenomatous polyps, in contrast, have a distinct risk for the development of malignancy.[3] Mucosal atypia is frequent, and mitotic figures are more common than in hyperplastic polyps. Dysplasia and carcinoma in situ have developed in adenomatous polyps observed over time. The risk for the development of carcinoma has been estimated at 10% to 20% and is greatest for polyps more than 2 cm in diameter. Multiple adenomatous polyps increase the risk of cancer. The presence of an adenomatous polyp is also a marker indicating an increased risk for the development of cancer in the remainder of the gastric mucosa.

Symptoms are similar to those for hyperplastic polyps. Endoscopic removal is indicated for pedunculated lesions

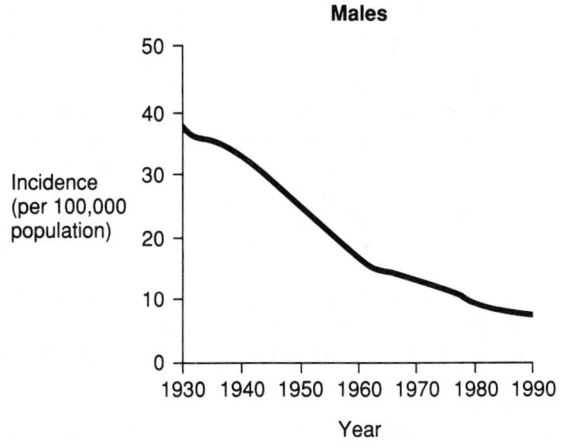

Males

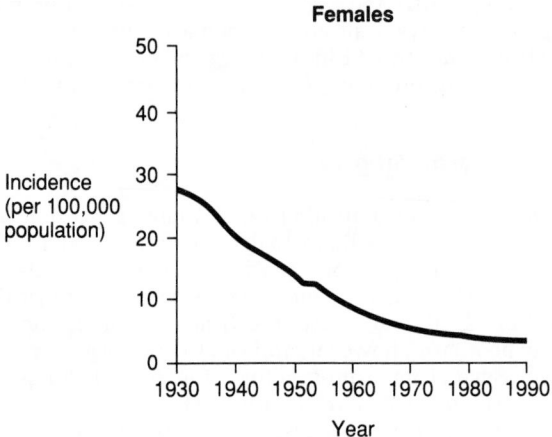

Females

Figure 25-1. Incidence of gastric cancer deaths in the United States.

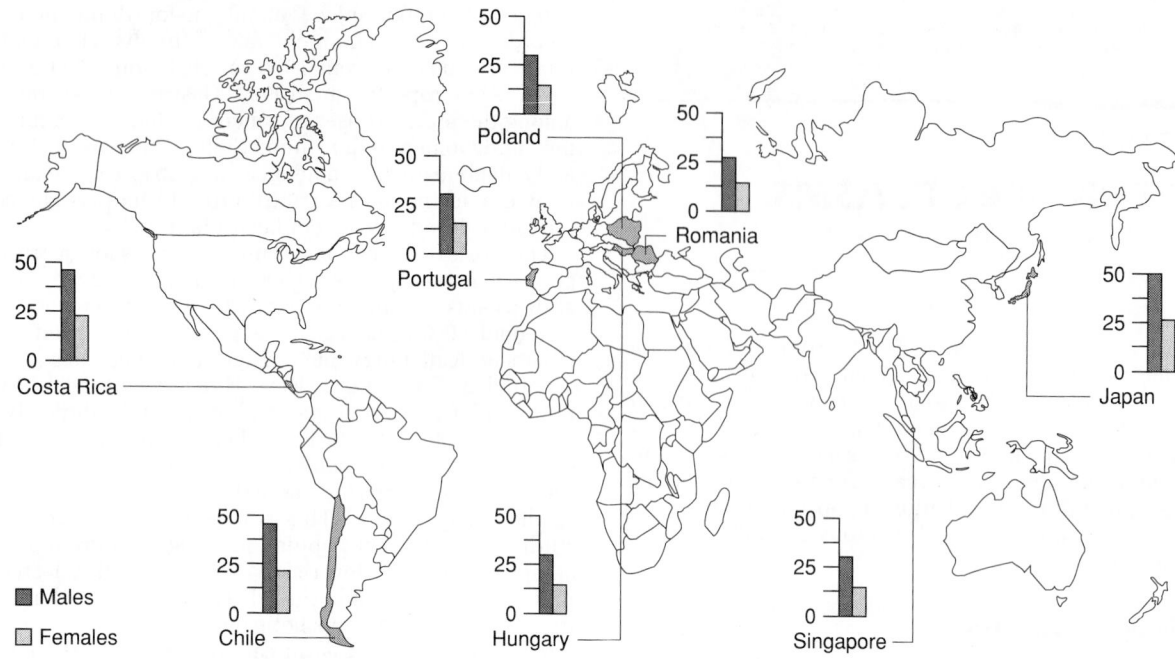

Figure 25-2. Worldwide incidence of gastric cancer.

and is sufficient if the polyp is completely removed and shows no evidence of invasive cancer on histologic examination. Operative excision is recommended for sessile lesions larger than 2 cm, for polyps with biopsy-proven invasive carcinoma, and for polyps complicated by pain or bleeding. After removal, endoscopic surveillance of the gastric mucosa is indicated.

Gastritis

The incidence of both gastric cancer and atrophic gastritis increases with age. Chronic gastritis is frequently associated with intestinal metaplasia and mucosal dysplasia, and these histologic features are often observed in mucosa adjacent to gastric cancer. Gastritis is frequently progressive and severe in the gastric mucosa of cancer patients.

A possible role for *H pylori* in gastric carcinogenesis has received considerable investigative attention.[4-6] The association of gastric cancer and chronic gastritis caused by *H pylori* is suggestive but is considerably weaker than evidence linking the organism to benign ulceration. If *H pylori* infestation is a precursor for gastric carcinoma, an increased prevalence of the organism would be expected in areas of high cancer incidence. In developed nations, the frequency of *H pylori* in patients with gastric adenocarcinoma ranges from 20% to 80%, similar to the incidence in age-matched controls. In contrast, a higher than expected prevalence has been reported in regions of China with a high incidence of gastric cancer as well as in other regions of the world with high cancer rates. Anti–*H pylori* anitbodies, presumed to be serologic evidence for prior infection, have also been reported in small groups of patients with gastric cancer. The strongest association appears to exist for patients with the intestinal subtype of gastric cancer, which is believed to develop in association with chronic gastritis.

Investigators have postulated that the reduction in gastric cancer in developed countries during this century may be due to a reduction in *H pylori* infestation secondary to improved nutrition and hygiene. Proof of an etiologic role for *H pylori* in gastric carcinogenesis will await the development of effective immunization followed by long-term population studies.

Gastric malignancy seems to be increased in patients with chronic gastritis associated with pernicious anemia, although the risk appears to have been overstated in the past. This disease, characterized by fundic mucosal atrophy, loss of parietal and chief cells, hypochlorhydria, and hypergastrinemia, is present in 3% of people older than 60 years. For individuals in whom pernicious anemia has been active for more than 5 years, the risk of gastric cancer is twice that of age-matched controls. Evidence also indicates an increased risk of gastric carcinoid development in patients with pernicious anemia. This increased risk warrants aggressive investigation of new symptoms in patients with long-standing pernicious anemia, but it is not high enough to justify repeated endoscopic surveillance. There is no evidence that antral gastritis, frequently observed in patients with peptic ulceration, has any malignant potential.

Intestinal metaplasia, the presence of intestinal glands within the gastric mucosa, is also commonly associated with both gastritis and gastric cancer. The evolution from metaplasia to dysplasia to carcinoma to invasive cancer has been demonstrated in other organs, but no direct evidence can be provided for this progression in gastric cancer.

Previous Gastric Surgery

A number of uncontrolled reports have suggested that gastric cancer is more likely to develop in individuals who have undergone previous partial gastrectomy. This so-called gastric remnant cancer has become, by repetitive reporting, a clinical entity; the true risk for developing gastric neoplasm, however, appears to have been overestimated. Several large prospective studies with long-term follow-up indicate that the relative risk is not increased for up to 15 years after gastric resection, with modest increases (three times the control value) observed only after 25 years.[7]

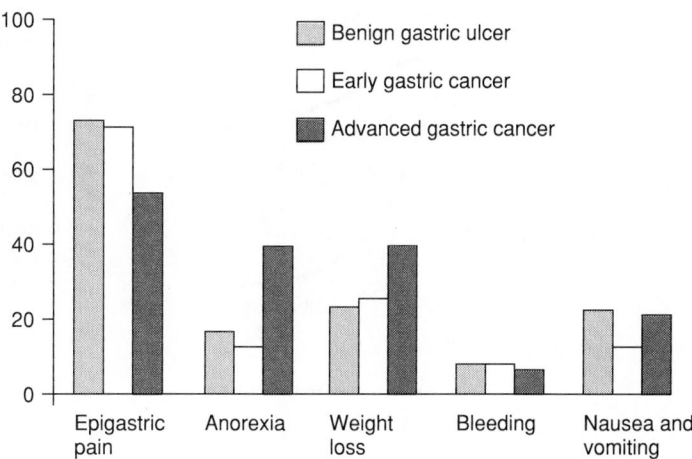

Figure 25-3. Clinical symptom frequency in benign gastric ulcer, early gastric cancer, and advanced gastric cancer. (After Meyer WC, Damiano RJ, Postlethwait RW, Rotolo FS. Adenocarcinoma of the stomach: changing patterns over the past four decades. Ann Surg 1987;205:18)

Clinical Features

The symptoms produced by gastric cancer are not specific and can unfortunately closely mimic those associated with a number of nonneoplastic gastroduodenal diseases, especially benign gastric ulcer (Fig. 25-3). In early gastric cancers, epigastric pain is present in over 70% of patients.[8] The pain is often constant, nonradiating, and unrelieved by food ingestion. In a surprising number of patients, pain can be relieved, at least temporarily, by antacids or gastric antisecretory drugs. Anorexia, nausea, and weight loss are present in less than 50% of patients with early gastric cancers but become increasingly common with disease progression. Dysphagia is present in 20% of patients with proximal gastric lesions. Melena occurs in 20% and acute upper gastrointestinal hemorrhage in 10%. Perforation is rare (1%).

In most patients with early gastric cancers, physical examination is normal. Stool is guaiac-positive in one third. Abnormal physical findings usually reflect advanced disease (Table 25-1). Cachexia, abdominal mass, hepatomegaly, and supraclavicular adenopathy usually indicate metastasis. There are no simple laboratory tests specific for gastric neoplasms.

Diagnosis and Screening

Fiberoptic endoscopy is the most definitive diagnostic method when gastric neoplasm is suspected. In the initial stages, gastric cancers can appear polypoid, as flat plaquelike lesions, or as shallow ulcers. Advanced lesions are typically ulcerated. The ulcer border can have an irregular, beaded appearance because of infiltrating cancer cells, and the base is frequently necrotic and shaggy. The ulcer can appear to arise from an underlying mass. Although each of these features suggests a malignant ulcer, differentiation of benign from malignant gastric ulcers can be definitively made only with gastric biopsy. Accuracy of diagnosis can exceed 95% if multiple biopsy specimens are obtained. False-negative results occur in approximately 10% of patients, usually as the result of sampling error; false-positive results are rare. Diagnostic accuracy can be further enhanced by the addition of direct brush cytology.

The ability to diagnose gastric adenocarcinoma endoscopically has prompted screening programs for populations at high risk. Mass screening has been performed in Japan since the 1960s with the use of fiberoptic endoscopy. By 1985, more than 5 million evaluations had been performed, with more than 6200 detections of gastric cancer. The overall yield for the Japanese screening program has been 0.12%.[2] The proportion of early cancers, defined as tumors whose growth is confined to the mucosa and submucosa regardless of the presence or absence of metastatic disease in the perigastric lymph nodes, steadily increased during the study period. From 1985 to 1986, 62% of gastric malignancies detected by this program were early cancers.[2] Early detection translates directly into improved survival (Fig. 25-4). The Japanese findings that early detection can improve survival have been confirmed by European investigations, in which patients with early gastric cancers had survival rates equivalent to those of patients with benign gastric ulcer[9] (Fig. 25-5). Mass screening for gastric adenocarcinoma has not been advocated in the United States or Canada. With incidence rates approximately one fifth of those observed in Japan, detection rates are too low to justify such a program economically.

Barium contrast radiographs have, in the past, been the standard method for diagnosing gastric neoplasm. Single-contrast examinations have a diagnostic accuracy of 80%. This diagnostic yield increases to about 90% when double-contrast (air and barium) techniques are used. Typical findings include ulceration, the presence of a gastric mass, loss of mucosal detail, and distortion of the gastric silhouette (Fig. 25-6).

Computed tomography (CT) has been used both as a primary diagnostic method and to assess extragastric spread. When performed with intraluminal contrast, CT can reliably demonstrate infiltration of the gastric wall by tumor, gastric ulceration, and hepatic metastasis (Figs. 25-7 and 25-8). The technique is less reliable with regard to invasion of adjacent organs or the presence of lymphatic metastases. In one series, involvement of adjacent organs was overestimated in 19% (false-positive). Conversely, me-

Table 25-1. COMMON SYMPTOMS AND PHYSICAL FINDINGS IN GASTRIC CANCER

Symptoms	Physical Findings
Weight loss	Guaiac-positive stool
Pain	Cachexia
Nausea and vomiting	Abdominal mass
Anorexia	Abdominal tenderness
Dysphagia	Hepatomegaly
Melena	—

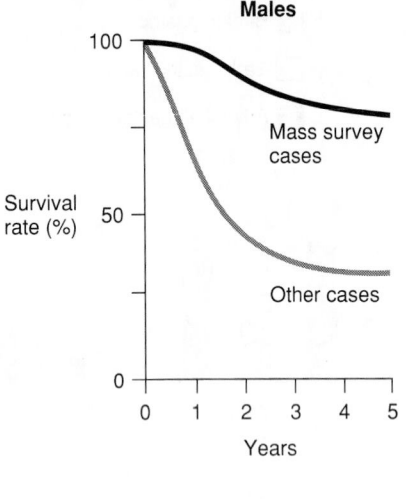

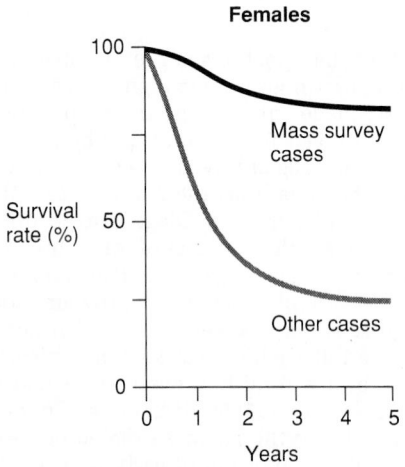

Figure 25-4. Early cancer survival rate in Japan.

tastases to regional or distant lymph nodes was underestimated in 37% (false-negative).[10] Because of these limitations, CT does not fulfill the requirements for a reliable staging method and usually does not eliminate the necessity for laparotomy.

Endoscopically directed ultrasound is another method

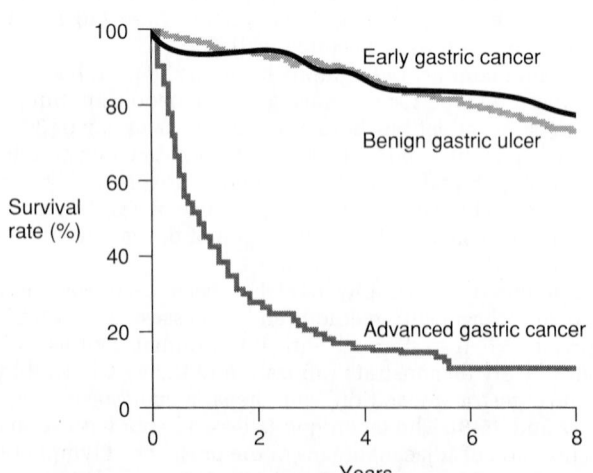

Figure 25-5. Early cancer survival rate in Europe.

of preoperative evaluation. Endoscopic ultrasound uses transducers with frequencies between 7.5 and 12 MHz. With such high frequencies, the gastric wall is visualized as a five-layered structure with alternating echogenic and low-echo layers. Acoustic coupling of the transducer to the mucosa is achieved by instillation of water into the stomach.

Endoscopic ultrasound is quite sensitive in evaluating gastric submucosal lesions and in differentiating them from gastric compression by adjacent organs or disease processes. Benign leiomyomas frequently do not cause erosion or ulceration of the overlying mucosa and appear as round, hypoechoic masses with smooth margins. The lesion is usually contiguous with muscularis propria. Malignant transformation is suggested by size (larger than 3 cm), irregular margins, destruction of normal wall layers, and hypoechoic foci caused by necrosis.

Gastric adenocarcinomas present several features that can be detected by endoscopic ultrasound. Ultrasound has been shown to accurately measure gastric wall thickness; increased wall thickness due to tumor infiltration has been confirmed histologically. The depth of gastric cancer invasion can be accurately determined in 80% of cases. Early gastric cancer, confined to the mucosa and submucosa, can be differentiated from advanced cancer in greater than 90% of examinations. In addition, gastric adenocarcinoma can be distinguished from gastric lymphoma based on ultrasonographic characteristics. Typically, scirrhous carcinoma demonstrates preservation of the normal five-layer structure with hypoechoic thickening of the third and fourth layers. With lymphoma, there is diffuse thickening of the gastric wall and blurring of the layered pattern.[11,12]

Endoscopic ultrasound is poor in nodal staging of gastric cancer, with an accuracy of 50% to 80%. Nodal size, although often used in ultrasound and CT to differentiate benign from malignant lymph nodes, is of little value. Eval-

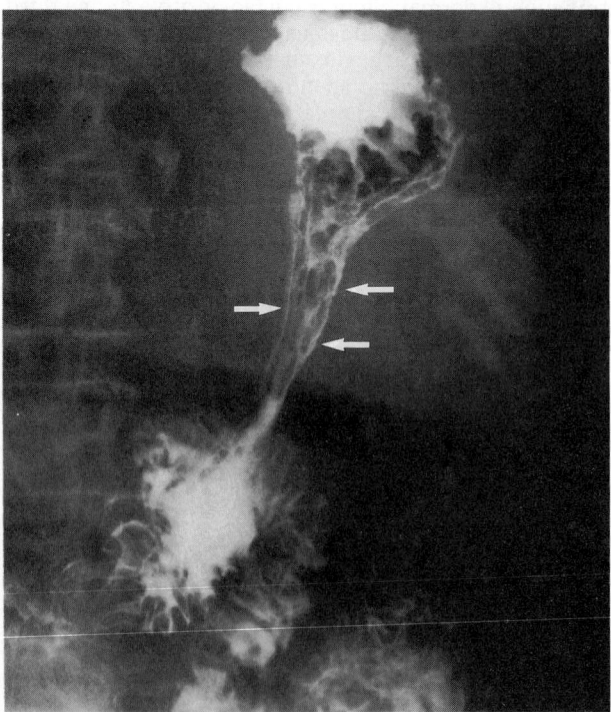

Figure 25-6. Barium contrast radiograph demonstrating extensive involvement of the gastric body by infiltrating adenocarcinoma (linitis plastica). The gastric silhouette is narrowed (*arrows*), and the stomach is nondistensible.

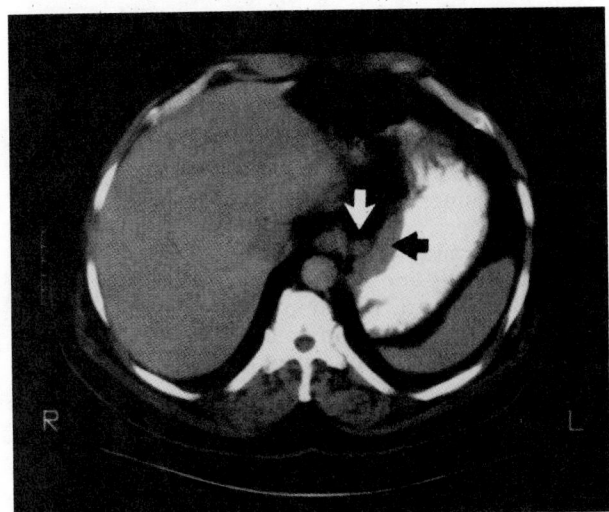

Figure 25-7. CT scan demonstrating mass along lesser curvature of the stomach (*black arrow*) and associated lymph node enlargement (*white arrow*).

mosome 17p at the site of the p53 tumor suppressor gene has also been reported.

Many gastric adenocarcinomas demonstrate increased expression of the K-*ras* protooncogene and the growth factor TGF-α. Increased expression correlates with advanced stage, grade, depth of invasion, lymphatic metastasis, and worsened prognosis. Mutations of the p53 tumor suppressor gene are found in a high proportion of human gastric cancers. Overexpression of the receptor for epidermal growth factor has been observed consistently.[13]

In the United States, gastric adenocarcinomas occur with equal frequency in the proximal and distal regions of the stomach. During the past 15 years, about 40% of cases have involved the proximal stomach, which is defined as the esophagogastric junction, fundus, or body, and an equal proportion have arisen in the antrum. In 15% of cases, the stomach is diffusely involved at the time of diagnosis. Proximal involvement is more common in elderly patients. The proportion of tumors involving the proximal stomach has dramatically increased over the past decades; in the 1960s, only 16% involved this region. Prognosis is distinctly less favorable for tumors arising from the proximal

uation for hepatic and distant metastasis requires computed tomography.

Pathology

Gastric adenocarcinoma occurs in two distinct histologic subtypes—intestinal and diffuse. These subtypes are characterized by differing pathologic and clinical features and by differing patterns of metastatic spread.[12]

In the intestinal form of gastric cancer, the malignant cells tend to form glands. The intestinal form of malignancy is more frequently associated with gastric mucosal atrophy, chronic gastritis, intestinal metaplasia, and dysplasia. Gastric cancer with intestinal histology is more common in populations at high risk (eg, Japan and China), and it occurs with increased frequency in men and older patients. Clinical studies suggest that this subtype more frequently demonstrates blood-borne metastases.

The diffuse form of gastric adenocarcinoma does not demonstrate gland formation and tends to infiltrate tissues as a sheet of loosely adherent cells. Lymphatic invasion is common. Intraperitoneal metastases are frequent. The diffuse form of gastric adenocarcinoma tends to occur in younger patients, in women, and in populations with a relatively low incidence of gastric cancer (eg, the United States). The prognosis is less favorable for patients with diffuse-subtype histology.

Efforts have been made to grade tumors on histologic criteria. Progressively anaplastic carcinomas are assigned higher grades. Not surprisingly, histologic grade correlates closely with 5-year survival; only 11% of grade IV patients survive 5 years, whereas 66% of grade I patients are alive 5 years after operation.

Gastric adenocarcinomas demonstrate a number of chromosomal and genetic abnormalities. Cytometric analysis reveals that gastric tumors with a large fraction of aneuploid cells (with a greater than normal amount of nuclear DNA) tend to be more highly infiltrative and have a poorer prognosis. Chromosomal abnormalities are relatively frequent in gastric adenocarcinomas. Deletion of chromosome 5q, corresponding to sites of the familial adenomatous polyposis coli (APC) gene and the in colon carcinoma (DCC) gene, has been reported in association with well-differentiated gastric cancers. A 60% allele loss on chro-

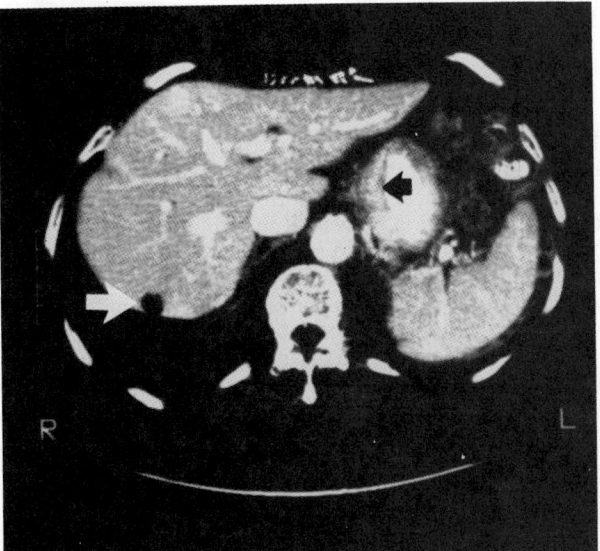

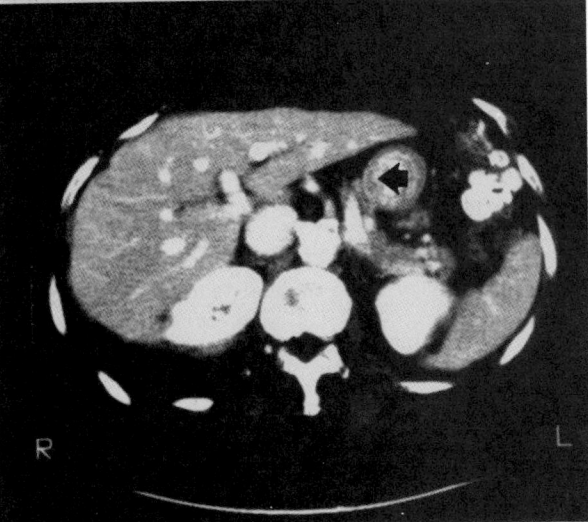

Figure 25-8. CT scans of the upper abdomen showing extensive thickening of the gastric wall (*black arrows*) caused by infiltrating adenocarcinoma and associated hepatic metastasis (*white arrow*).

Table 25-2. TNM CLASSIFICATION FOR STAGING OF GASTRIC CANCER

TNM DEFINITIONS

Primary Tumor

T1   Tumor confined to the mucosa
T2   Tumor involves the mucosa and submucosa, and extends to but does not penetrate serosa
T3   Tumor penetrates serosa with or without invasion of adjacent structures
T4   Diffuse involvement on gastric wall without obvious boundaries (linitis plastica)

Regional Lymph Node Involvement

N0   No nodal metastasis
N1   Metastasis to perigastric lymph nodes in immediate vicinity of tumor
N2   Metastasis to lymph nodes distant from primary tumor or along both curvatures of the stomach

Distant Metastasis

M0   No distant metastasis
M1   Metastasis beyond regional lymph nodes

STAGE GROUPING

Stage I   T1, N0, M0
Stage II   T2–3, N0, M0
Stage III   T1–3, N1–3, M0
Stage IV   Tumor unresectable or metastatic

---

stomach or for those with diffuse involvement of the organ relative to antral tumors.

The gastric cancer staging format used by the American Joint Commission is presented in Table 25-2. The staging system is oriented toward surgical and pathologic examinations but also accurately reflects prognosis (Fig. 25-9). A consideration of staging data illustrates the high frequency with which lymph node metastases are present at the time of diagnosis in the United States, and the severe impact this lymphatic involvement has on survival. Even early gastric cancers have a 15% prevalence of nodal metastasis.

Curative Treatment

Surgical resection is the only hope for cure in gastric cancer, and an advanced stage of disease at the time of diagnosis precludes curative resection for most patients. The surgical objectives in gastric cancer must, therefore, be to maximize chances for cure in patients with localized tumor and to provide effective and safe palliation to patients with advanced malignancy. Evolution of the surgical approach to gastric adenocarcinoma has focused on the following five issues:

- The extent of gastric resection needed for potentially curable lesions
- The role of perigastric lymphadenectomy
- The adequacy of proximal and distal resection margins
- The role of splenectomy
- The implications of involvement of adjacent organs

During the 1940s and 1950s, increasingly radical operations were advocated for the treatment of gastric cancer, including total gastrectomy, extended subtotal gastrectomy with en bloc resection of celiac and splenic lymph nodes, splenectomy, and distal pancreatectomy. With time, it became apparent that radical operations increased operative morbidity but did not improve survival. A prospective trial of various operations for the treatment of gastric cancer

has not been performed, but reports from a number of institutions allow a consensus. For early lesions (N0–1, M0) of the antrum or middle stomach, distal subtotal gastrectomy including 80% of the stomach provides satisfactory 5-year survival without increases in operative morbidity. Proximal gastric lesions or larger middle stomach lesions may require total gastrectomy or esophagogastrectomy to encompass the tumor (Figs. 25-10 and 25-11). Regardless of the extent of gastric resection, patients with more advanced tumors fare poorly because of the increased likelihood of lymphatic and hematogenous spread.

The extent of gastric resection is determined, in part, by the need to obtain a resection margin free of microscopic disease. Microscopic involvement of the resection margin by tumor cells is associated with poor prognosis. In one series, all patients with positive surgical margins developed recurrent disease, and histologically positive margins were strongly correlated with the development of anastomotic recurrence.[14] In contrast to colon cancer, gastric cancer frequently demonstrates extensive intramural spread. The propensity for intramural metastasis is related, in part, to the extensive anastomosing capillary and lymphatic network within the wall of the stomach. Retrospective studies suggest that a line of resection 6 cm from the tumor mass is necessary to ensure a low rate of anastomotic recurrence. Efforts to achieve larger margins have not translated into improved survival.

The value of extended lymphadenectomy in the treatment of gastric adenocarcinoma is controversial. The largest favorable experience has been reported by Japanese surgeons and the Japanese Research Society for Gastric Cancer.[15,16] Because the benefits of extended lymphadenectomy accrue only to patients with local or regional disease, intraoperative staging must be undertaken to exclude patients with spread to liver, peritoneum, or serosa of the stomach. In the Japanese system, resections are characterized as follows:

R1—resection of stomach, omentum, and perigastric lymph nodes
R2—resection of stomach and omentum, and en bloc removal of the superior leaf of the transverse mesocolon, the pancreatic capsule, and lymph nodes along the branches of the celiac artery and in the infraduodenal and supraduodenal areas
R3—resection of the above structures plus lymph nodes along the aorta and esophagus, along with the spleen and the tail of the pancreas

Only retrospective studies of extended perigastric lymph-

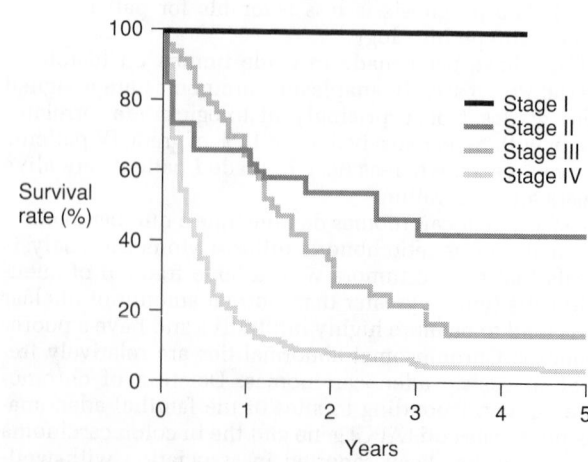

Figure 25-9. Survival rate of gastric cancer by stage.

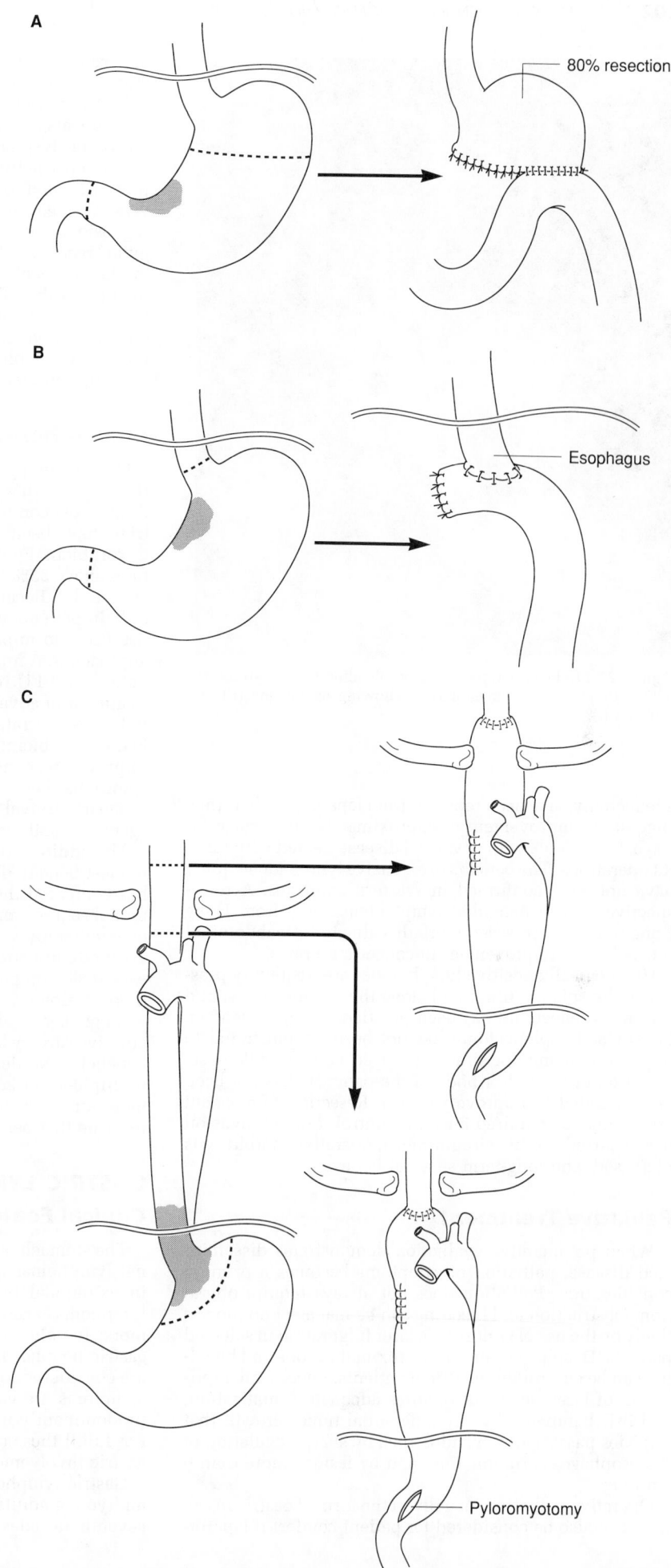

Figure 25-10. Surgical options for resection of gastric neoplasms. (*A*) Subtotal gastrectomy with gastrojejunal reconstruction. (*B*) Total gastrectomy with esophagojejunostomy. (*C*) Esophagogastrectomy with anastomosis in cervical or thoracic position.

A

80% resection

B

Esophagus

C

Pyloromyotomy

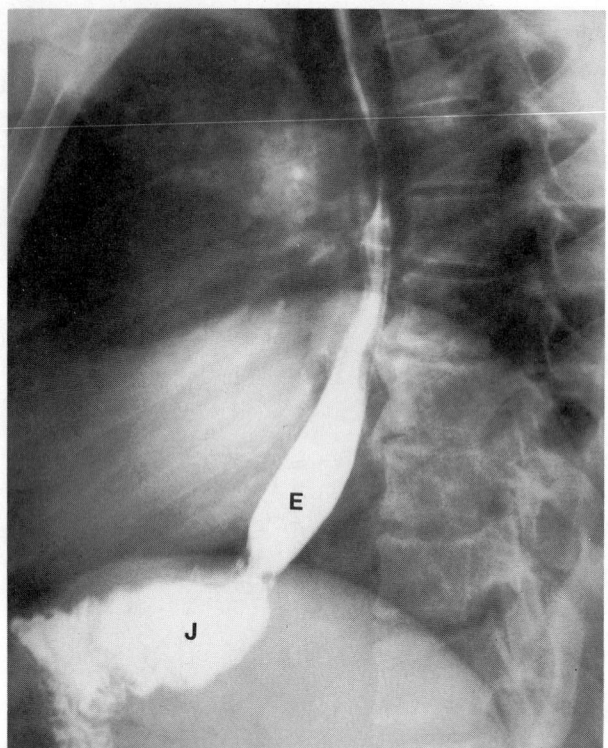

Figure 25-11. Postoperative radiograph after total gastrectomy with esophagojejunal anastomosis, showing esophagus (E) and jejunum (J).

adenectomy have been reported from Japan. Together, they suggest an improvement of approximately 10%, stage for stage, for patients with advanced disease treated with R2 or R3 operations. The benefits of extensive lymphadenectomy have not been confirmed in Western countries. A retrospective trial of extended lymphadenectomy from Hong Kong reported increased morbidity due to intraabdominal sepsis but no improvement in cancer cure rates.[17]

Histologically positive lymph nodes are frequently present in the splenic hilum and along the splenic artery, and routine splenectomy has been practiced in some centers. Prophylactic splenectomy has not been demonstrated to improve outcome for similarly staged patients. Likewise, resection of the tail or body of the pancreas has not been demonstrated to improve survival. Resection of adjacent organs may be required for local control if direct invasion has occurred. In this circumstance, operative morbidity is increased, and long-term survival is rare.

Palliative Treatment

When preoperative evaluation demonstrates disseminated disease, palliation of symptoms becomes a primary consideration. Palliation does not always require operation. Obstruction and bleeding can be managed nonoperatively by the use of endoscopic laser fulguration in selected patients. Dysphagia caused by proximal lesions and bleeding can be controlled in 80% of patients. Successful application of laser treatment requires adequate visualization, and it is hampered by circumferential tumor growth that impedes passage of the endoscope, by sharp angulation of the esophagogastric junction, and by lesions more than 6 cm long.

Operative palliation, usually in the form of gastric resection, can also be considered for patient comfort if laparot-

omy can be performed with acceptable morbidity and mortality. No prospective studies are available to suggest that palliative resection prolongs survival. Nonetheless, resection appears to provide superior relief of symptoms, particularly for dysphagia, compared with surgical bypass. Bypass of obstructing distal gastric lesions without resection provides relief to less than half of patients, and mean survival averages less than 6 months. For proximal obstructing lesions, total gastrectomy with Roux-en-Y esophagojejunal reconstruction may be necessary. An operative mortality rate of less than 5% has been reported, and introduction of the EEA stapler has reduced anastomotic leak rates to less than 5% in several series.[18] Mean survival after palliative gastric resection approximates 9 months. For nonresectable gastric adenocarcinomas, when dysphagia is present, radiation therapy may have a palliative role.

Chemotherapy

Chemotherapy has limited use in the treatment of patients with disseminated gastric adenocarcinoma. The drugs most commonly used in single-agent chemotherapy trials have been 5-fluorouracil (5-FU), mitomycin C, and doxorubicin. Few single-agent trials have partial response rates above 25% to 30%, and complete responses have not occurred.[19] Because long-term survival can be expected only in patients who experience complete response, there has been no impact on patient survival from single-drug approaches. A number of trials have used FAM (the combination of 5-FU, doxorubicin, and mitomycin C) for the treatment of advanced gastric cancer, with an overall partial response rate of about 33%. The combination of 5-FU, doxorubicin, and cisplatin has been associated with improved response rates in some series, and complete response has been seen in 12% of treated patients. Increases in mean survival have not yet been proved with multiple-agent chemotherapy.

The addition of radiation therapy to chemotherapy has modest benefit. The Gastrointestinal Tumor Study Group has compared therapy with 5-FU and radiation followed by subsequent maintenance with 5-FU/methyl CCNU to chemotherapy with methyl CCNU alone. The 5-year survival rate in patients treated with chemoradiation therapy was 16%, compared with 7% for the group with chemotherapy alone.[20]

Single-agent adjuvant chemotherapy after potentially curative surgery for gastric adenocarcinoma has not proved beneficial. No definitive data are available to suggest that multiple-agent adjuvant combinations based on 5-FU are more effective than single agents, although several trials indicate that benefit may exist.

GASTRIC LYMPHOMA
Clinical Features

The stomach is the site of more than half of gastrointestinal lymphomas and is the most common organ involved in extranodal lymphomas (see Chap. 29). Non-Hodgkin lymphomas account for about 5% of malignant gastric tumors; lymphoma represents an increasing proportion of gastric neoplasms diagnosed in the past decade. Patients are considered to have primary gastric lymphoma if initial symptoms are gastric and the stomach is exclusively or predominantly involved with the tumor. Patients who do not fulfill these criteria are considered to have secondary gastric involvement from systemic lymphoma.

Gastric lymphoma is distinctly uncommon in children and young adults. The peak incidence is in the sixth and seventh decades. Symptoms are indistinguishable from those of gastric adenocarcinoma. Epigastric pain, weight loss, anorexia, nausea, and vomiting are common.[21] Although gross bleeding is uncommon, occult hemorrhage and anemia are observed in more than half of patients.

Diagnosis

Radiologic findings are similar to those for adenocarcinoma. Endoscopic examination has become the diagnostic method of choice. Endoscopic biopsy, combined with endoscopic brush cytology and ultrasonography, provides positive diagnosis in 90% of cases. Submucosal growth without ulceration of the overlying mucosa can occasionally render endoscopic biopsy nondiagnostic. When gastric lymphoma is first diagnosed by endoscopic means, evidence of systemic disease should be sought. CT of the chest and abdomen (to detect lymphadenopathy), bone marrow biopsy, and biopsy of enlarged peripheral lymph nodes are all appropriate. A commonly used staging system is as follows:

Stage I—tumor confined to stomach
Stage II—tumor with spread to perigastric lymph nodes
Stage III—nodal involvement beyond perigastric lymph nodes (eg, paraaortic nodes)
Stage IV—tumor spread to other organs in the abdomen (spleen, liver)

Treatment

A multimodality treatment program is used in most centers for primary gastric lymphomas, with gastrectomy as the first step in the therapeutic strategy.[22] This approach has evolved empirically, and prospective data to support it are lacking. Several advantages of this approach have been cited:

1. More accurate histologic evaluation is possible.
2. In cases with localized tumor, the procedure can be curative.
3. Gastrectomy eliminates the risk of life-threatening hemorrhage or perforation, which attends the treatment of tumors involving the full thickness of the gastric wall.

The role of resection in the treatment of gastric lymphoma is controversial, and increasing numbers of patients are treated with chemoradiation therapy alone.

The risk of hemorrhage or perforation was frequently alluded to in the past and has probably been overstated. The risk of perforation in primary gastric lymphomas that are treated with cytolytic agents in unresected patients approximates 5%.[23] The use of endoscopic ultrasonography to detect full-thickness involvement of the gastric wall is being investigated to identify patients at risk for perforation.

If gastrectomy is performed before chemotherapy or radiotherapy, extended radical resections are not indicated. Unlike adenocarcinoma, microscopically positive resection margins do not predict local recurrence in cases of lymphoma when radiotherapy is administered postoperatively. The postoperative mortality rate is under 5% and has been 0% in several recent series. In a limited number of patients with stage I disease, surgery is considered curative and no further therapy is required. Many authors have reported retrospectively that postoperative radiation to the gastrectomy bed improves local and regional control.[24,25] With radiation doses ranging from 3500 to 4400 cGy, local recurrence was observed in less than 15% of treated patients.

In more than 30% of patients with stage II disease who undergo apparently adequate surgery and radiotherapy, the cancer will recur outside the treatment field. Patients with stage II primary gastric lymphoma should, therefore, be considered to have systemic disease and to require systemic therapy in addition to surgery or radiotherapy. The use of chemotherapy, either primarily or as postoperative adjuvant therapy, is rational and is supported by several retrospective reports. Survival for gastric lymphoma is closely linked to stage at diagnosis (Fig. 25-12).

GASTRIC CARCINOIDS

Gastric carcinoid tumors have been considered to be rare tumors, accounting for 3% to 5% of all gastrointestinal carcinoids, and only 0.3% of gastric neoplasms[26] (see Chap. 29). The number of gastric carcinoids may have been underestimated in the past because of confusion with gastric carcinoma. It has been recognized that in addition to an increased risk of adenocarcinoma, patients with pernicious anemia have an increased risk for development of gastric carcinoids. This association has suggested to several investigators that gastric carcinoids can develop as a result of chronic trophic stimulation by hypergastrinemia associated with pernicious anemia.[27] Carcinoid tumors associated with pernicious anemia have been located in the gastric body or fundus. Histologically, the tumors appear as nests of monotonous hyperchromatic cells originating in the submucosa or within the basal area of gastric glands. Invasion, uncommon in small tumors, occurs with increasing frequency in tumors larger than 2 cm.

Most patients with small gastric carcinoids are asymptomatic. When viewed endoscopically at an early stage, carcinoids are reddish pink to yellow submucosal nodules

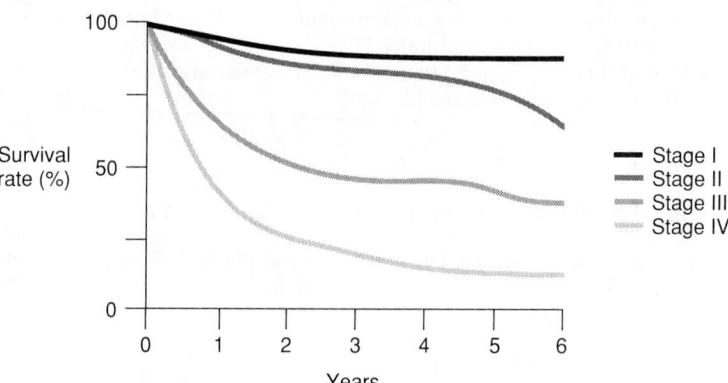

Figure 25-12. Survival of gastric lymphoma by stage.

in the proximal stomach. Tumors are frequently multiple. Larger tumors can cause ulceration of the overlying mucosa; symptoms are similar to those of gastric ulcer or gastric adenocarcinoma. Endoscopic biopsy is usually diagnostic if deep enough to sample submucosal tumor cells. Because of the potential for invasion, attempts at curative resection are indicated in almost all cases.

GASTRIC SARCOMAS

Sarcomas can arise from any of the mesenchymal components of the gastric wall, constituting about 3% of gastric malignancies. Leiomyosarcomas are predominant, whereas angiosarcomas and fibrosarcomas are rare. Leiomyosarcomas occur with equal frequency in both sexes in the sixth and seventh decades of life. The tumor frequently has prominent extraluminal growth and attains a large size before causing symptoms. Endoluminal growth or ulceration of the overlying mucosa due to ischemic necrosis can be associated with epigastric pain, weight loss, and gastrointestinal hemorrhage. Clinical symptoms are identical to those produced by adenocarcinoma. With large tumors, an epigastric mass can be detected by physical examination.

Leiomyosarcomas must be differentiated from their benign counterparts, leiomyomas. Benign smooth muscle tumors are often asymptomatic until they reach a large size. Symptoms related to mass effects with compression of adjacent structures are most frequent. Gastrointestinal hemorrhage can occur as a result of necrosis of overlying gastric mucosa. Endoscopic examination is usually normal if the major component of growth is extraluminal; umbilication of the mucosa can indicate an underlying mass. The presence and nature of symptoms should direct the need for surgical excision.

Grossly, the tumors are firm, gray-white masses; a pseudocapsule separating tumor from normal smooth muscle can occasionally be present. When the tumors reach a large size, central necrosis is common. Leiomyosarcomas are often graded histologically, with the frequency of mitotic figures the prime indicator of aggressive behavior. Lesions with more than 5 to 10 mitoses per 10 high-power fields demonstrate increased metastasis. With benign leiomyomas, mitoses are absent or rare.

Intraperitoneal sarcomatosis is frequent, as is local recurrence after resection. Metastasis occurs by way of the hematogenous route; thus, hepatic involvement is common. Lymphatic metastasis is observed in less than 10% of patients.

Leiomyosarcomas are not radiosensitive, and chemotherapy has not been shown to improve survival. Surgical resection has been the treatment of choice. En bloc resection of the tumor and involved structures should be attempted. Negative surgical margins must be ensured histologically, but extensive lymphadenectomy is not indicated because of the low frequency of lymphatic metastasis. The overall survival rate approximates 50%. Low-grade lesions have a significantly better prognosis (81% 5-year survival rate) than high-grade lesions (32%).[28]

REFERENCES

1. Silverberg E, Boring CC, Squires TS. Cancer Statistics, 1990. CA 1990;40:9.
2. Hisamichi S. Screening for gastric cancer. World J Surg 1989;13:31.
3. Harju E. Gastric polyposis and malignancy. Br J Surg 1986;73:532.
4. Correa P. Human gastric carcinogenesis: a multistep and multifactorial process: first American Cancer Society award lecture on cancer epidemiology and prevention. Cancer Res 1992;52:6735.
5. Wyatt JI. Gastritis and its relation to gastric carcinogenesis. Semin Diagn Pathol 1991;8:137.
6. Veldhuyzen van Zanten, Sherman PM. *Helicobacter pylori* infection as a cause of gastritis, duodenal ulcer, gastric cancer and nonulcer dyspepsia: a systematic overview. Can Med Assoc J 1994;150:177.
7. Toftgaard C. Gastric cancer after peptic ulcer surgery: a historic prospective cohort investigation. Ann Surg 1989; 210:159.
8. Meyers WC, Damiano RJ, Postlethwait RW, Rotolo FS. Adenocarcinoma of the stomach: changing patterns over the past 4 decades. Ann Surg 1987;205:1.
9. Heberer G, Teichmann RK, Kramling HJ, Gunther B. Results of gastric resection for carcinoma of the stomach: the European experience. World J Surg 1988;12:374.
10. Andaker L, Morales O, Hojer H, et al. Evaluation of preoperative computed tomography in gastric malignancy. Surgery 1991;109:132.
11. Nicholson DA, Shorvon PJ. Review article: endoscopic ultrasound of the stomach. Br J Surg 1993;66:487.
12. Boddie AW, McBride CM, Balch CM. Gastric cancer. Am J Surg 1989;157:595.
13. Wright PA, Williams GT. Molecular Biology and Gastric Carcinoma. Gut 1993;34:145.
14. Shiu MH, Moore E, Sanders M, ET AL. Influence of the extent of resection on survival after curative treatment of gastric cancer: a retrospective multivariate analysis. Arch Surg 1987;122:1347.
15. Maruyama K, Okabayashi K, Kinoshita T. Progress in gastric cancer in Japan and its limit of radicality. World J Surg 1987;11:418.
16. Noguchi Y, Imada T, Matsumoto A, et al. Radical surgery for gastric cancer: a review of the Japanese experience. Cancer 1989;64:2053.
17. Robertson CS, Chung SCS, Woods SDS, et al. A prospective randomized trial comparing R₁ subtotal gastrectomy with R₃ gastrectomy for antral cancer. Ann Surg 1994;250:176.
18. Wong J, Cheung H, Fan YW, et al. Esophagogastric anastomosis performed with a stapler: The occurrence of leakage and stricture. Surgery 1987;101:408.
19. Findlay M, Cunningham D. Chemotherapy of carcinoma of the stomach. Cancer Treat Rev 1993;19:29.
20. Gastrointestinal Tumor Study Group. A combination chemotherapy and combined modality therapy for locally advanced gastric carcinoma. Cancer 1982;49:1771.
21. Rao A, Kagan AR, Potyk D, et al. Management of gastrointestinal lymphoma. Am J Oncol 1984;7:213.
22. Shiu MH, Nisce LZ, Pinna A, et al. Recent results of multimodal therapy of gastric lymphoma. Cancer 1986;58: 1389.
23. Mittal B, Wasserman TH, Griffith RC. Non-Hodgkin's lymphoma of the stomach. Am J Gastroenterol 1983;78:780.
24. Gobbi PG, Dionigi P, Barbieri F, et al. The role of surgery in the multimodal treatment of primary gastric non-Hodgkin's lymphoma: a report of 76 cases and review of the literature. Cancer 1990;65:2528.
25. Bozzetti F, Audisio RA, Giardini R, Gennari L. Role of surgery in patients with primary non-Hodgkin's lymphoma of the stomach: an old problem revisited. Br J Surg 1993;80:1101.
26. Creutzfeldt W. The achlorhydria–carcinoid sequence: role of gastrin. Digestion 1988;39:61.
27. Borch K, Renvall H, Liedberg G. Endocrine cell proliferation and carcinoid development: a review of new aspects of hypergastrinaemic atrophic gastritis. Digestion 1986;35(Suppl 1): 106.
28. Shiu M, Farr G, Papachristou D. Myosarcomas of the stomach: natural history, prognostic factors and management. Cancer 1982;48:177.

SURGERY: SCIENTIFIC PRINCIPLES AND PRACTICE, Second Edition, edited by
Lazar J. Greenfield, Michael W. Mulholland, Keith T. Oldham, Gerald B. Zelenock,
and Keith D. Lillemoe. Lippincott–Raven Publishers, Philadelphia, © 1997.

CHAPTER 26

ANATOMY AND PHYSIOLOGY OF THE SMALL INTESTINE

WALTER A. KOLTUN AND THEODORE N. PAPPAS

The small intestine is the portion of the gastrointestinal (GI) tract that extends from the duodenal cap to the ileocecal valve. Historically, the small intestine was presumed to have only digestive and absorptive functions because of the presence of digestive enzymes, its long length, and its massive surface area. As knowledge of the anatomy and physiology of the small intestine has increased, it has become apparent that the small intestine is also the body's largest endocrine organ and the largest component of its immune system. The number of hormones and paracrine and neurocrine substances known to be produced in the small intestine has multiplied rapidly during the past decade. The small intestine is the largest body surface area that is exposed to the outside environment, and the immune system plays an important role in protecting the body from that environment.

GROSS ANATOMY

Duodenum

The duodenum is the first portion of the small intestine. Beginning at the duodenal cap just beyond the pylorus, it extends about 20 to 30 cm to the ligament of Treitz, the anatomic point where the jejunum begins. The duodenum is divided into four points—the bulb, followed by the second (descending), third (transverse), and fourth (ascending) portions.[1]

The duodenal cap, or bulb, is a triangular organ that projects slightly cephalad from the pylorus. It overlies the common bile duct and is the anchor point for the hepatoduodenal ligament. The cap is 5 cm long and is the site of over 90% of duodenal ulcers. The posterior wall of the first portion of the duodenum is directly adjacent to the head of the pancreas, and posterior penetrating ulcers in this area erode into the pancreas and the underlying gastroduodenal artery.

An endoscopic view of the duodenal cap reveals a small lumen. On immediate entry into the duodenal cap, the anterior wall is seen because the duodenum takes a slight posterior turn. Just past the pyloroduodenal junction are the fornices of the duodenal cap, which can be best seen by retroflexion. The surface of the duodenal cap is smooth until the distal bulb, where concentric Kerckring folds begin and continue to the descending duodenum.

The blood supply to the duodenal cap comes directly from the hepatic artery as a supraduodenal arterial branch. Additional vascularity to the duodenal cap comes from the gastroduodenal artery as it branches from the hepatic artery. The gastroduodenal artery sends branches posteriorly into the pancreas and anteriorly into the duodenal cap. The branches of the arterial supply of the second and third portion of the duodenum have been termed the *anterosuperior* and *posterosuperior pancreaticoduodenal arteries*, coming from the gastroduodenal artery, and the *anteroinferior* and *posteroinferior pancreaticoduodenal arteries*, coming from the superior mesenteric arteries. They anastomose and form a common supply to both duodenum and pancreas. The first jejunal branch of the superior mesenteric artery (SMA) supplies the jejunum just past the ligament of Treitz and sends small branches back to the fourth portion of the duodenum (Fig. 26-1).

The second (descending) portion of the duodenum courses posteriorly and caudally from the duodenal cap to the level of the first lumbar vertebra. During its course, it is attached to the head of the pancreas. The second portion of the duodenum becomes a retroperitoneal structure as it courses posteriorly. In this retroperitoneal position, the duodenum directly overlies Gerota fascia and, more medially, the inferior vena cava. At the junction between the duodenal cap and second portion of the duodenum, one can find the foramen of Winslow posterior to the hepatoduodenal ligament. The hepatic flexure of the colon is draped directly on the anterior surface of the second portion of the duodenum.

The descending duodenum is about 10-cm long. The obvious endoscopic feature of the second portion of the duodenum is the Kerckring folds, concentric mucosal folds about 1 to 2 mm thick and 2 to 4 mm high. They are separated by 2 to 4 mm of flat, smooth duodenal mucosa. The diameter of the second portion of the duodenum varies from 3 to 5 cm. The major papilla in the duodenum enters the midpoint of the second portion of the duodenum. The papilla (ampulla of Vater) appears anatomically as a hooded fold, marking the confluence of the common bile duct and the main pancreatic duct (duct of Wirsung) and is surrounded by the muscular sphincter of Oddi. In 50% to 60% of patients, an accessory pancreatic duct (the duct of Santorini) can be seen entering the duodenum proximal to the ampulla of Vater. Endoscopically, this lesser, or minor, papilla appears as a 1- to 3-mm sessile polypoid structure.

The duodenum's third (transverse) and fourth (ascending) portions complete the duodenum sweep. The third portion is almost entirely retroperitoneal. It is intricately attached to the uncinate process of the pancreas and extends from the second portion of the duodenum to the third lumbar vertebra directly over the aorta. The third portion of the duodenum is wedged between the SMA and the aorta. The transition between the third and fourth portion of the duodenum is found in the acute angle made by

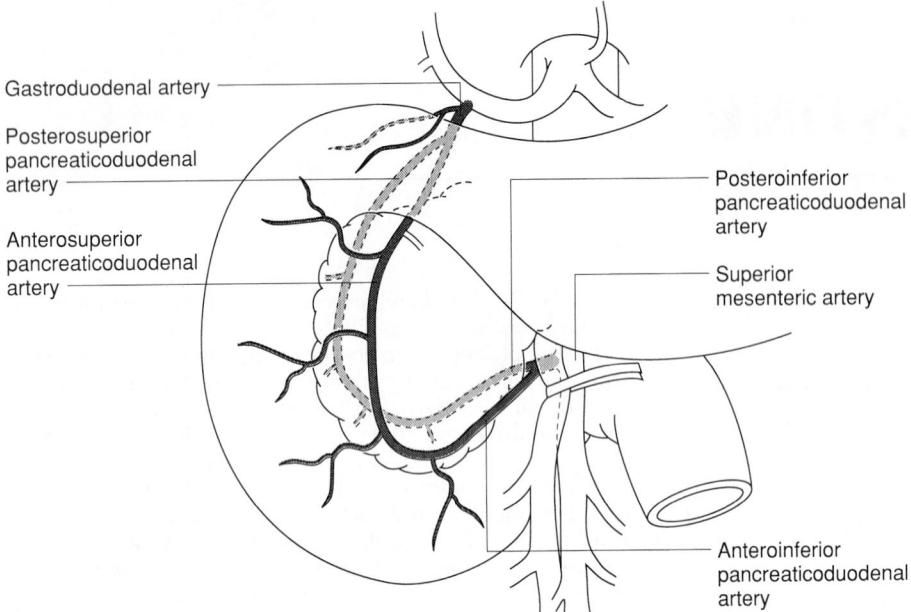

Figure 26-1. Arterial supply to the duodenum.

these two arteries. The fourth portion of the duodenum passes superiorly and obliquely to reach the ligament of Treitz. The ligament of Treitz is composed of a slip of striated muscle extending downward from the right crus of the diaphragm and a fibromuscular band passing from the duodenum toward the celiac axis. At the ligament, the jejunum passes directly forward and inferiorly and is no longer attached to the retroperitoneum.

The endoscopic appearance of the third and fourth portions of the duodenum is characterized by a continuing series of valvulae conniventes (Kerckring folds). It is unusual to traverse the third and fourth portions of the duodenum during a routine upper endoscopic examination unless a pediatric colonoscope is used.

Jejunum and Ileum

The jejunum is the portion of the small intestine that courses from the ligament of Treitz to an arbitrary point approximately two fifths of the distance to the ileocecal valve. The length of the jejunum has been estimated at 100 cm, although this distance can vary dramatically depending on the status of the small intestine. The jejunum is the widest portion of the small intestine, and the diameter progressively decreases as the ileocecal valve is approached.[2]

The ileum makes up the distal three fifths of the combined jejunoileal length. The ileum is about 100 to 150 cm long, although, as with the jejunum, the length varies. The lumen decreases in size as it progresses to its most terminal portion.

In contrast to the long jejunum and ileum, small intestinal mesentery has a short base of about 15 cm. The mesentery extends from the ligament of Treitz region left of the midline near the second lumbar vertebra, across the midline tangentially toward the right lower quadrant. The mesentery tethers the small intestine, preventing kinking of its blood supply. The mesentery also contains a large supply of lymphatics and fat.

The blood supply of the jejunum and the ileum originates from the SMA. The first jejunal branch of the mesenteric artery is found at the point where the SMA crosses the duodenum. After this, several jejunal and ileal branches emanate from the SMA during its course. The SMA circles along the length of the distal small intestine as a marginal artery before anastomosing with the ileal branch of the ileocolic artery. The arterial supply of the jejunum and ileum have distinct morphologies. The vasa recta supplying the jejunum are long end-arteries originating from short jejunal arcades. These vessels are often visible, because the mesenteric fat does not usually encroach on the mesenteric border of the intestine. In contrast, the vasa recta in the terminal ileum are small; the arterial arcades from the SMA approach the mesenteric border of the ileum. The ileal vasa recta are often obscured by fat, which covers the mesentery to the edge of the bowel (Fig. 26-2).

The mucosal surface of the jejunum is characterized by smooth surfaces interrupted by valvulae conniventes. These folds are taller and more numerous in the jejunum but become shorter and less frequent in the distal ileum. No other unique mucosal features in the jejunum and ileum are apparent to the naked eye.

HISTOLOGY

The wall of the small intestine is made up of three major layers—the mucosa, submucosa, and muscle. The mucosa, or inner lining, is responsible for absorption and secretion. Mucosal thickness varies from 500 to 900 μm, and multiple villi increase the surface area. The mucosal surface of the small intestine has both exocrine and endocrine functions. The submucosa, the layer just beneath the mucosa, has a rich network of blood vessels, lymphatics, and nerves.

There are two muscular layers of the small intestine, an inner circular layer and an outer longitudinal layer. These layers are responsible for intestinal motility. Within the muscular layers are the myenteric plexus of Auerbach and a plexus of ganglia for nonmyelinated nerve fibers. The serosa, or outer coat, of the small intestine is incomplete where the duodenum is a retroperitoneal structure, but it completely surrounds the jejunum and ileum.

Intestinal absorptive cells constitute most of the columnar cells of the villi.[3] Absorptive cells are 20 to 26 μm high, with basally placed nuclei. The intestinal absorptive

A

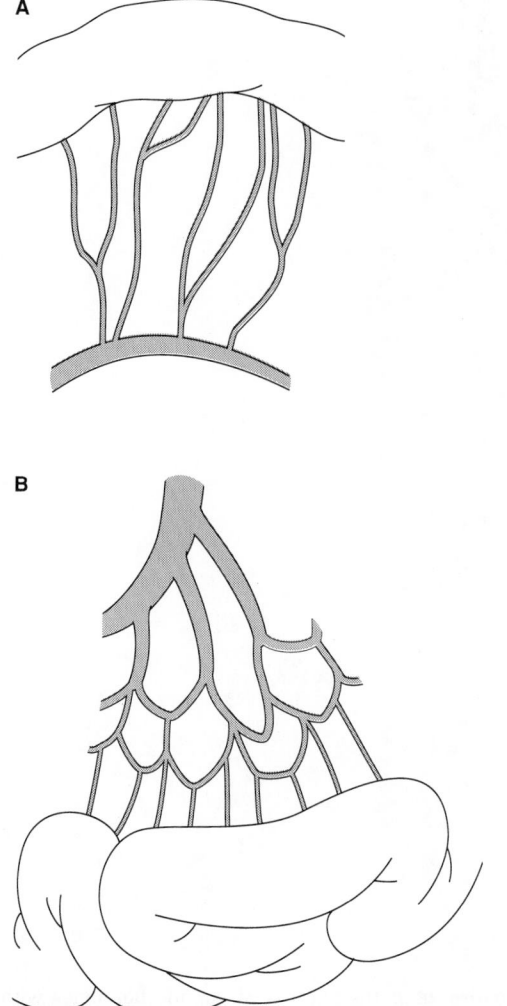

B

Figure 26-2. Contrasting vasa recta of jejunum (*A*) and ileum (*B*).

cells at the apex of the villi contain multiple microvilli, which increase the absorptive surface area of the small intestine. The surface of the microvilli is covered by a mucopolysaccharide coat termed the *glycocalyx*. Microvilli are approximately 1 μm long and 0.08 μm wide. On the surface of the microvilli are disaccharidases and peptidases, which are involved in the terminal digestion of nutrients. The microvilli also appear to have unique mechanisms for binding substances for absorption. The absorptive cells also contain lysosomes, which hold hydrolytic enzymes for digesting internal or external products. Abundant mitochondria are found in absorptive cells, as are a Golgi complex, a granular endoplasmic reticulum, and a basally placed nucleus.[4]

Goblet cells are exocrine secretory cells found in the absorptive epithelium. Goblet cells have a narrow base, a basally positioned nucleus, and a wide head filled with mucigen droplets. Mucigen is secreted by the goblet cell to lubricate the surface of the epithelium.

Paneth cells are found at the base of the villi in a region called the *crypts of Lieberkühn*. These pyramid-shaped cells contain secretory granules, which contain lysosomal enzymes.

Theliolymphocytes are distributed among absorptive cells in the mucosa. These lymphocytes are T cell in origin and have both suppressor and cytolytic activity.

Amine precursor uptake and decarboxylation (APUD) cells are dispersed throughout the mucosa of the small intestine. These endocrine cells produce hormones, neuropeptides, and paracrine agents. The most well known of these cells are the enterochromaffin cells, which occupy the basal portion of the crypts and are thought to secrete 5-hydroxytryptamine. Specific areas of the small intestine have higher concentrations of specific neuroendocrine cells than other areas (Fig. 26-3).

Submucosa

Brunner glands are found in the submucosa of the duodenum and upper jejunum. These glands are connected to the crypt of Lieberkühn by a small duct, which empties into the lumen of the small intestine. These glands produce a clear, viscous alkaline solution that is thought to protect the duodenal mucosa. Glucagon and secretin have been found to stimulate secretion from Brunner glands.

Peyer patches are also located in the submucosa and are found predominantly in the ileum. Peyer patches are 8 to 10 mm in diameter and consist of dense lymphatic tissue. A large number of lymphocytes usually surround these areas. The aggregates are more abundant during youth and tend to disappear with old age.

HORMONES, NEUROTRANSMITTERS, AND PARACRINE SUBSTANCES

Cholecystokinin (CCK) is a peptide and acts both as a neurotransmitter and as a true hormone. Molecular forms include peptides with 8, 33, 39, and 58 amino acids. CCK is found in high concentrations in both the brain and the gut. In the GI tract, CCK immunoreactive cells are primarily located in the mucosa of the duodenum and jejunum, and CCK is released from the mucosa in response to luminal fats and proteins. Following CCK release from the duodenum and jejunum, the gallbladder contracts and the sphincter of Oddi relaxes, emptying bile into the duodenum. CCK acts in a synergistic fashion with secretin to stimulate pancreatic exocrine secretion. Postprandial levels of CCK probably act in a physiologic way to delay gastric emptying.

Secretin is a 27–amino acid peptide in the same structural family as glucagon, vasoactive intestinal peptide (VIP), and gastric inhibitory peptide. Secretin is found in the S cells of the duodenum and jejunum. It is a true hormone, released in response to acid in the duodenum when luminal pH falls below 4.5. Intraduodenal secretion of pancreatic bicarbonate neutralizes duodenal pH, diminishing the release of secretin. The amount of secretin released after a meal is sufficient to stimulate pancreatic secretion. Other biologic functions of exogenously infused secretin appear to have little or no physiologic role.

Somatostatin is a paracrine peptide and occurs in two different forms: 14–amino acid and 28–amino acid peptides. Somatostatin has been localized in multiple areas of the central nervous system, peripheral nervous system, and gut. Somatostatin may act as a neurotransmitter and may also act as a paracrine agent in the pancreatic islets and in the mucosa of the stomach. Somatostatin-containing D cells have also been found in small quantities throughout the gut mucosa. It has been hypothesized that somatostatin has a regulatory role along with motilin in controlling motility by means of the migrating motor complex. It is believed that motilin activates the migrating motor complex and that this effect is counteracted by somatostatin. In addition, somatostatin is released during a meal and regulates the release of gastric acid and gastrin by a paracrine inhibitory mechanism. Somatostatin may also

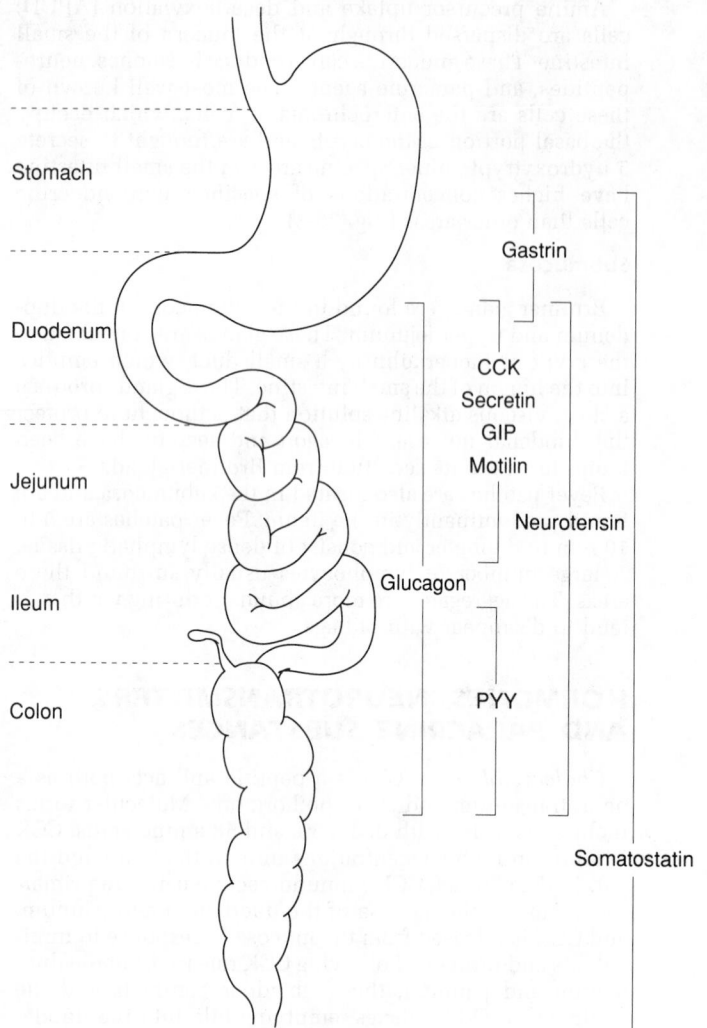

Stomach

Gastrin

Duodenum

CCK
Secretin
GIP
Motilin

Jejunum

Neurotensin

Glucagon

Ileum

PYY

Colon

Somatostatin

Figure 26-3. Distribution of peptide hormones within the gastrointestinal tract.

have a similar effect in autoregulating pancreatic exocrine secretion.

Gastric inhibitory polypeptide (GIP) is a 42–amino acid peptide that is structurally related to the glucagon family. GIP is thought to function as a true hormone and is localized in highest concentration in the mucosa of the duodenum and jejunum. GIP is also found in small quantities in the antrum and terminal ileum. Physiologically, GIP may regulate insulin release by augmenting the insulin response to an oral meal (incretion effect). It does not affect the insulin response to intravenous nutrients.

Motilin is a 22–amino acid peptide localized in enterochromaffin cells of the mucosa of the upper small intestine that may have a physiologic role in regulating the migrating motor complex. It is released during the fasting state, and increased levels correspond with the onset of the migrating motor complex. The initiation of motilin release during the migrating motor complex appears to be cholinergic dependent.

Neurotensin is a 13–amino acid neurotransmitter found in the central nervous system and gut. Specific endocrine cells, or N cells, that contain neurotensin are found in the ileal mucosa. Smaller quantities are found in the jejunum, stomach, duodenum, and colonic mucosa. Neurotensin is released by a mixed meal and fats, and carbohydrates and protein release much smaller increments. It has been proposed that neurotensin has a physiologic role in fat-initiated changes in gastric acid secretion, gastric emptying, pancreatic secretion, and intestinal motility.

Pancreatic glucagon and *enteroglucagon* belong to the family of peptides that includes secretin, VIP, and GIP. The smaller peptide, glucagon, has 29 amino acids, whereas the larger enteroglucagon molecule contains 37 amino acids. Both pancreatic and enteric glucagon are formed from a common prohormone, glicentin, which has 69–amino acid residues. Glucagon functions in opposition to insulin to promote glycogenolysis, lipolysis, gluconeogenesis, and ketogenesis. Glucagon may also be important in the stress response to trauma. Enteroglucagon is found in the ileum and colon and may regulate intestinal mucosa cell turnover.

Peptide YY (PYY) is a proposed hormone in the same family as neuropeptide Y and pancreatic polypeptide. It has 36–amino acid residues and is found predominantly in the mucosa of the terminal ileum and right colon. It is released in response to a mixed meal and to fats. Postprandial concentrations of PYY inhibit acid secretion, perhaps by blocking acetylcholine release at the vagal cholinergic nerve ending. It is not clear whether the action of PYY on pancreatic secretion or gastric emptying is truly physiologic.

IMMUNOLOGY

Both immunologic and nonimmunologic processes protect a person from the entry of noxious materials while allowing the gut to absorb needed nutrients. Nonimmunologic mechanisms of defense include the following:

- Gastric acidity and enteric proteolytic enzymes (including lysozymes), which degrade harmful toxins and organisms
- Production of mucin, which coats and protects the epithelium as well as inhibits the growth of bacteria
- Peristalsis, which can remove and clean the gut of macromolecules, microbes, and parasites
- Rapid epithelium turnover, which tends to dilute and exclude antigens attempting entry at the surface
- Competitive inhibition between endogenous and pathologic bacteria[5]

A significant component of enteric defense involves immunologic mechanisms. Gut-associated lymphoid tissue represents a major division of the immune system and is made up of aggregated (Peyer patches, lymphoid follicles, mesenteric lymph nodes) and nonaggregated (luminal, intraepithelial, and lamina propria leukocytes) cellular components.[6]

Nonaggregated Lymphoid Tissue

Lymphocytes, macrophages, and neutrophils in the bowel lumen are probably the first cells to encounter an antigenic challenge. Increased numbers of luminal lymphocytes are associated with Peyer patches during GI infection, and there is evidence of transepithelial migration of polymorphonuclear leukocytes into the intestine after antigenic and chemotactic stimuli. The luminal presence of such cells probably represents an effector function aimed at neutralizing the instigating antigen.

Intraepithelial lymphocytes are found between the epithelial cells lining the GI tract, abutting the basement membrane (Fig. 26-4). It is estimated that 15% to 25% of viable epithelial cells are immune-derived cells, such as lymphocytes, and various proportions of macrophages, mast cells, neutrophils, and eosinophils. Their number can be dramatically influenced by luminal passage of food and bacterial antigens, and increases in them probably represent increases in a differentiated population of cytolytic T cells. Intraepithelial lymphocytes appear to enter the epithelium through the blood stream at the level of the crypt, but they do not migrate in concert with epithelial cells. They probably avoid being sloughed and reenter the lamina propria after exposure to luminal antigens.

The lamina propria contains a wide array of nonaggregated lymphoid tissue, including B cells, T cells, macrophages, eosinophils, and mast cells. Some 80% to 99% of the B cells are active producers of immunoglobulin A (IgA). In comparison, only 2% to 5% of B cells found in other lymphoid tissues in the body secrete IgA. In contrast to intraepithelial lymphocytes, most T lymphocytes in the lamina propria have a helper–inducer function, with a smaller subset expressing cytolytic function. Mast cells and eosinophils constitute less than 1% of the lamina propria cell population. Mast cells and eosinophils can be activated by numerous stimuli, including IgG and IgE immune complexes, and they play a prominent role in GI allergy and hypersensitivity reactions.

Aggregated Lymphoid Tissue

The aggregated cellular portion of gut-associated lymphoid tissue consists of lymphoid follicles found throughout the small intestine, Peyer patches (which represent large collections of follicles usually found on the antimesenteric border of the ileum), and mesenteric lymph

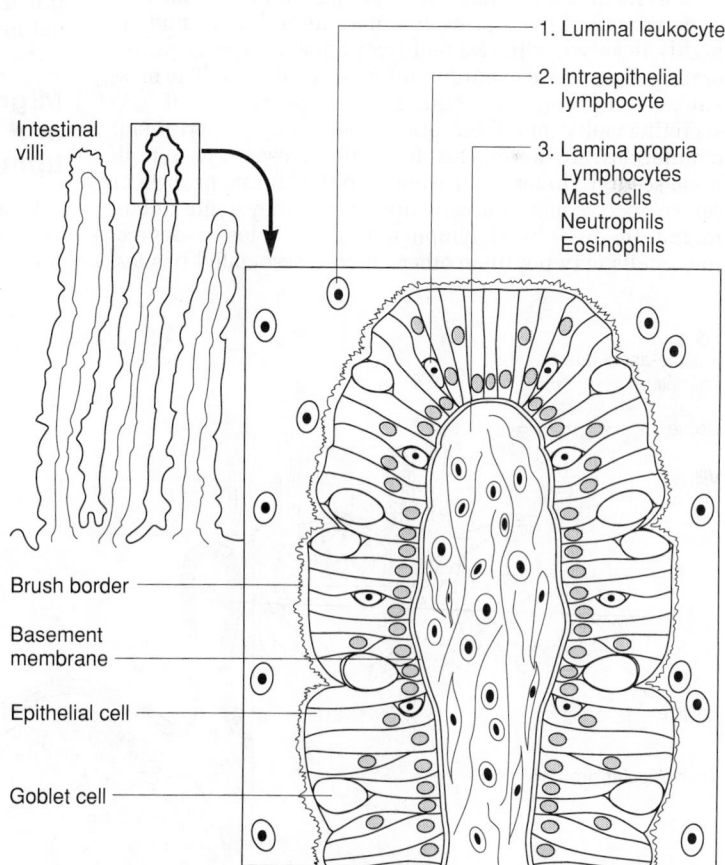

Figure 26-4. Small intestinal villus with associated immunologic cells.

nodes. The microscopic anatomy of the Peyer patch and its functional components have been extensively studied (Fig. 26-5). The Peyer patch represents a highly specialized structure centrally involved in the recognition and processing of antigen and the eventual expression of mucosal immunity. Follicles are separated by T-cell–dependent interfollicular areas and have specialized epithelium overlying their apical dome region. The follicles contain germinal centers and have high concentrations of B cells and some plasma cells. Although these B cells are readily identified as precursors to the IgA-secreting B cells of the lamina propria, they do not actively secrete IgA while residing in the germinal center. The interfollicular zone is populated predominantly by T cells, and it appears to play a part in regulating maturation and amplification of the B cells into competent antigen-specific, IgA-secreting cells.

The dome region of the follicle contains a high concentration of lymphocytes, macrophages, and plasma cells and is separated from the intestinal lumen by a follicle-associated epithelium that contains specialized M (membrane) cells. The M cell actively transports macromolecules and luminal particles transcellularly by a pinocytotic mechanism, presenting these antigens to the underlying cells. In this way, the M-cell and dome regions are believed to be a sampling and processing site for luminal antigen, allowing controlled entry of antigen into the Peyer patch. The maturation of B cells into antigen-specific IgA-secreting precursors takes place in the germinal center and is controlled by helper and suppressor T cells from the adjacent interfollicular areas. Activated T and B cells are drained by lymphatic means, pass through lymph nodes, and eventually enter the vascular circulation through the thoracic duct. They are then delivered to the lamina propria where they become capable of antigen-specific IgA production.

The mesenteric lymph node appears to be less specialized in its character than the Peyer patch. Populated by a wide variety of leukocytes, the mesenteric lymph node is highly reactive, with resident lymphocytes rapidly proliferating in response to enteric antigenic challenge. The mesenteric lymph node contains a higher proportion of IgA-secreting cells and their precursors than its peripheral counterpart. Lymphocytes from the mesenteric lymph node seem to preferentially home to the lamina propria or return to the mesenteric lymph node; they tend not to migrate to peripheral lymph nodes. To a lesser degree, these cells may populate other mucosa-associated tissues,

such as those in the lung or the salivary and mammary glands, where they participate in secretory immune function.

Secretory Immune System

The major immunoglobulin of the intestinal immune system is IgA. IgG-containing cells represent less than 5% of all immunoglobulin-containing cells of the gut. In the serum, IgA occurs largely in its monomeric form. In the GI tract (and other mucosal tissues), IgA exists as a dimer, complexed covalently with two additional molecules— the J chain that links the two IgA moieties and the secretory component that aids in transepithelial delivery. The entire complex is termed *secretory IgA*. The J chain is made by the same plasma cell that secretes the IgA, whereas the secretory component is a transmembrane glycoprotein produced by the intestinal epithelial cell.

The functional characteristics of IgA are unlike those of other antibodies. Unlike IgG or IgM, secretory IgA does not induce Fc-mediated inflammatory reactions. Antigen–IgA complexes do not activate the classic or alternate complement systems, nor does IgA promote the phagocytosis of bacteria by opsonization. Most of IgA's protective effect derives from its ability to bind the threatening antigen efficiently, while resisting enzymatic degradation by gut enzymes. The binding of antigen to IgA stimulates protective mucus secretion and can prevent the uptake of viruses and bacteria by promoting contact and entrapment within the epithelial mucus layer. Bacteria also can be immobilized by IgA attachment to pili or fimbriae, leading to impaired cellular division and enhanced degradation by luminal enzymes. Secretory IgA can bind to macromolecules and toxins, altering their biologic activity and impeding transmucosal entry. The facilitation of these rather unobtrusive defense mechanisms by IgA minimizes the need for an inflammatory response and so protects the fragile intestinal mucosa.

Migratory Pathways and Gastrointestinal Immunoresponsiveness

When an antigen is presented to the immune system, local immunity, systemic immunity, or tolerance can take place. The dose, time course, and route by which antigen

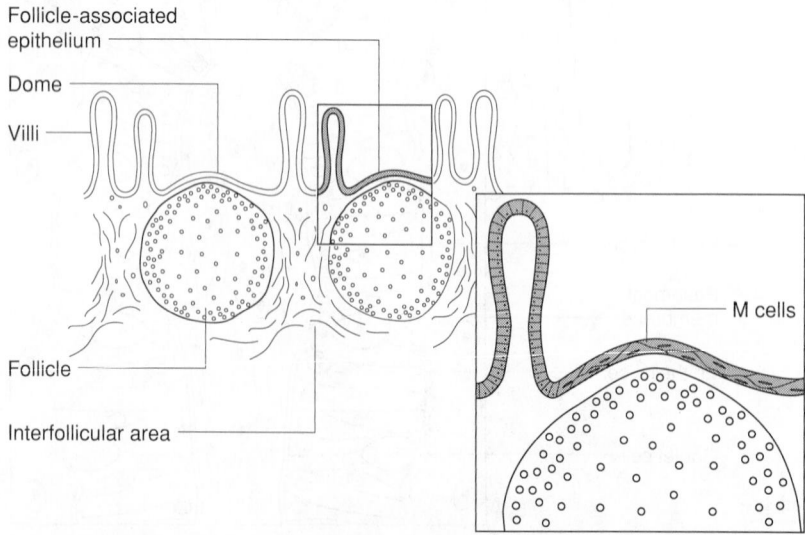

Figure 26-5. Epithelial anatomy in the area of Peyer patches.

is presented determine the type and degree of immune response. For example, parenteral immunization usually produces a systemic IgG response. An IgA effect frequently requires peroral gut inoculation. Systemic tolerance frequently means suppressor cell generation but may also involve local immunity (ie, inhibition of further antigen absorption by enteric IgA binding, minimizing systemic exposure to antigen). This distinction between systemic immunity, usually represented by an IgG response, and enteric immunity, associated with IgA production, partly explains variations in immunoresponsiveness. This model is further expanded by the observation that other mucosa-associated tissues share IgA, gut-initiated immunity. Thus, antigen-specific IgA is found in the GI tracts of offspring after postpartum maternal enteral immunization, having been transferred by consumption of IgA-containing breast milk.

The mechanism of mucosa-associated immunoresponsiveness is also related to the migratory pathways of stimulated GI lymphocytes. The migratory path of the enteric lymphocytes commences with exposure to antigen within the gut lumen. Small amounts of such antigen are sampled by the M cell and presented to the underlying antigen-processing cells, which then stimulate the IgA-bearing lymphocytes in the Peyer patch. In the Peyer patch, stimulated cells leave by way of the lymphatics, populate mesenteric lymph node, and eventually drain through the thoracic duct into the systemic circulation. They then migrate, or home, to the lamina propria or other mucosa-associated tissues, such as the mammary or salivary glands, cervix, and lungs. At these sites, final maturation takes place, and antigen-specific IgA production occurs.

This immunizing process can be affected by many factors. Migration of IgA-bearing cells to the mammary gland, for example, preferentially occurs during lactation or the late stages of pregnancy and can be reproduced experimentally by hormonal manipulation. Furthermore, specific IgA-secreting cells populate only those bowel segments that have continued exposure to antigen, as shown by isolated-loop immunization experiments. The recognition factors by which this homing mechanism exists may involve lymphocyte antigen recognition, specific receptors on the postcapillary venule, and the targeting of secretory component. Nutritional compromise, such as protein or vitamin-A deficiency, can also alter normal migrating patterns, presumably by affecting synthesis of membrane receptors. The interaction of IgA-bearing cells with the systemic immune system is poorly understood and probably involves a second set of recognition factors.

MOTILITY

The intrinsic motility of the small intestine aids the GI tract in its basic functions of digestion and absorption. Motile contractions promote contact of ingested material with enzymes, chyme, and gut mucosa and deliver food to various portions of the gut where specialized absorptive functions can take place. Motility also participates in enteric defense by evacuating offending ingested material, such as toxins and bacteria. Decreased bowel motility can lead to stasis and bacterial overgrowth, which can compromise absorption and nutrition.

Most information relating to motility correlates mechanical contraction with myoelectric activity, using electrodes placed along the intestinal wall. Smooth muscle depolarization acts through a calcium-dependent pathway to cause smooth muscle contractions. The longitudinal smooth muscle cells of the intestine facilitate aboral transmission of electrical depolarization through intercellular tight junctions. In addition to intrinsic electromechanical characteristics, motility is also affected by extrinsic electrical and hormonal factors.[7]

Intrinsic Electrical Activity

The smooth muscle cell of the gut has a resting membrane potential of 40 to 50 millivolts (mV) and varies in a cyclic fashion by about 5 to 15 mV. This variation results in phasic depolarization referred to as slow waves, basic electrical rhythm, pacemaker potential, or electrical control activity (Fig. 26-6). By itself, the slow wave does not cause a muscular contraction. It occurs at a uniform frequency for a given segment of intestine and decreases in frequency as one proceeds aborally. In the human duodenum, the slow wave frequency is 11 to 12 cycles/min; slow wave frequency decreases to 8 to 9 cycles/min in the ileum.[8] Because there is electrical coupling between the smooth muscle cells, the distal portions of the gut are entrained by the higher frequencies of the proximal gut. When the intestine is transected, the distal segment is released electrically and expresses its slower intrinsic frequency. From mid-jejunum distally, electrical coupling is incomplete; therefore, the slower frequencies are variably evident in the normal state. Because muscular contractions depend in part on slow wave frequency, proximal high frequencies cause more contractions, which tend to propel intestinal contents aborally.

A second electrical characteristic of the smooth muscle cell is the spike or action potential. The spike potential represents a rapid change in membrane potential. When it occurs repetitively during a slow wave depolarization, it elicits a mechanical contraction of the smooth muscle (see Fig. 26-6). Unlike slow waves, spike potentials only conduct over a short distance, leading to a discrete ringlike contraction of the intestine. Although slow waves are constantly present, spike potentials are not, and the bowel contracts only when the two are superimposed. Thus, the initiation, frequency, and migration of contractions largely depends on the slow wave, but contractions do not occur without spike potentials.[9]

Between the circular and longitudinal smooth muscle layers lies the myenteric nerve plexus. This plexus is the most prominent aggregate of the enteric neurons. The multitude of nerves within the intestinal wall have efferent, afferent, and intrinsic reflex functions. The intrinsic nervous control of motility is sophisticated. One neuron may have multiple dendritic processes that act relatively independently of each other. There are inhibitory and excit-

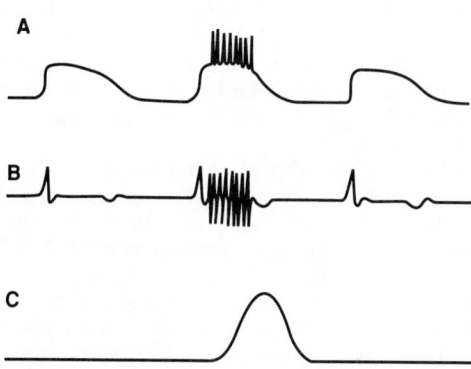

Figure 26-6. (*A*) Recording of transmembrane potential showing slow waves and superimposed spike potentials. (*B*) Extracellular recording of electrical activity represented in *A*. (*C*) Muscular contraction in response to electrical activity in *A*. (After Christensen J. The control of gastrointestinal movements: some old and new views. N Engl J Med 1971;285:85)

atory modulations and several different types of mechano-sensitive units that respond with various patterns of depolarization on stimulation. One such pattern results in the peristaltic reflex, contractions above and relaxation below a site of small bowel distention. Acetylcholine is the probable neurotransmitter of excitatory neurons. Inhibitory neurons are nonadrenergic and noncholinergic, and adenosine triphosphate (ATP), VIP, somatostatin, serotonin, and substance P have all been suggested as neurotransmitters.

Interdigestive Motility Pattern

During the fasting state, the well-defined pattern of small bowel electrical activity is referred to as the *interdigestive myoelectric complex*, the "intestinal housekeeper," or the *migrating motor complex* (MMC). This cyclic pattern of spike bursts and muscular contractions that migrate from duodenum to terminal ileum is divided into four phases:

Phase I—quiescence, with no spikes or contractions
Phase II—accelerating, irregular spiking activity
Phase III—activity front, a series of high-amplitude, rapid spikes corresponding to strong, rhythmic gut contractions
Phase IV—subsiding activity

In humans, the cycle lasts about 90 to 120 minutes. Each phase passes in sequence along the intestine, and when the terminal ileum is reached, the process resumes in the proximal gut. This interdigestive cycle is interrupted and replaced by rapid spiking activity (similar to phase II) when the gut receives a food bolus. The duration of this interruption depends on the volume and nature of the food stuffs, with fats causing the longest duration of rapid spiking.

The function of the interdigestive pattern is unclear. It has been considered a housekeeper because it periodically sweeps residual luminal contents, bacteria, desquamated cells, and other debris out of the small intestine, preventing bacterial overgrowth. Gut function varies during its different phases. Absorption is greatest during phase I and poorest in phase III, and transit is most rapid in phase III. The disruption of the MMC by feeding only occurs in those animals that bolus feed, such as humans and dogs. In animals that more or less eat constantly, such as sheep, the complex recycles continuously, uninterrupted by eating.

The myoelectric activity of the small intestine represents a delicate interplay of extrinsic and intrinsic neural, hormonal, and intraluminal factors. The initiation of the MMC front (phase III) does not depend on extrinsic innervation, since it is not abolished by vagotomy or interruption of the splanchnic nerves. It is likely that the orderly migration of the MMC is the responsibility of the extrinsic nervous system, and the initiation of the complex itself is either intrinsic or hormonal.

Blood levels of the GI peptide hormone motilin correlate closely with MMC activity, and exogenous motilin can induce the MMC front. Other hormones that have serum levels paralleling MMC activity are pancreatic polypeptide and somatostatin. Alternatively, the neural plexus present within the intestinal wall may well play a part in initiating the MMC by means of a spontaneous oscillator mechanism. Other substances that can initiate the MMC front include histamine, metoclopramide, and morphine.

The disruption of the MMC by feeding is at least partially hormonally mediated. In physiologic doses, neurotensin can interrupt the MMC by mimicking the feeding response. Gastrin, CCK, and insulin are also effective. Extrinsic innervation plays a role, since denervation can compromise,

but not totally abolish, the response. MMC activity can be disrupted by the sight or smell of food but not by parenteral nutrition. Orally consumed fats are much more effective at interrupting the MMC than equicaloric amounts of carbohydrate or protein.

Small bowel motility appears to result from intrinsic electromechanical characteristics of smooth muscle and from myenteric nerve plexuses, which are modulated to a large degree by extrinsic nerves and hormonal mechanisms. The interrelations of these factors and the coordinated movement of enteric contents continue to demand investigation.

DIGESTION AND ABSORPTION

The most obvious function of the GI tract is digestion and absorption of food for the continued growth and survival of the organism. The small intestine plays the largest role in absorption, with some preparation of ingested food performed in the stomach (excluding mastication and salivary enzyme effects). Gastric acid secretion and muscular contractions promote hydrolysis and mixing of chyme, which is then delivered for further digestion and absorption to the small intestine. Absorption begins in the duodenum, although this segment of intestine also plays a prominent endocrine role. Chyme stimulates the release of secretin and CCK from duodenal mucosa, both of which aid in digestion by promoting pancreatic secretion and gallbladder emptying.

The jejunum is the site of maximum absorption of all ingested material except for vitamin B_{12} (cobalamin). Although its mucosa contains numerous specific transport processes, the presence of large intercellular pores produces a permeable membrane and allows rapid passive transfer of solutes and water. The ileum is less permeable and makes greater use of active-transport mechanisms such as specific receptors for vitamin B_{12} and bile salts. The colon actively absorbs sodium, secretes potassium in response to aldosterone, and dehydrates the enteric material in preparation for elimination.[10]

Absorption of Water

The absorption of water is a dynamic process reflecting the net result of flux both into and out of the lumen of the gut. When a radioactively labeled bolus of water enters the intestine, there is 50% net absorption within 30 minutes, although 50% of the radioactive tracer is found in the blood within 2 to 3 minutes, reflecting a rapid bidirectional movement of water.

About 1 to 1.5 L of water is ingested each day, with another 5 to 10 L secreted by the GI tract in the form of salivary (1 to 2 L), gastric (2 to 3 L), biliary (0.5 L), pancreatic (1 to 2 L), and intestinal (1 L) secretions. About 80% of this fluid is reabsorbed by the small intestine. Because of this large bidirectional movement of water, a small alteration in intestinal permeability or transport rate can rapidly result in net secretion and diarrheal disease states.

Net water movement into or out of the lumen of the gut is determined largely by the tonicity of the enteric material. When a meal is ingested, a large volume of fluid is added by the salivary glands and stomach, and a hypotonic solution of chyme is deposited in the upper small intestine. In addition, the neutralization of stomach acid by bicarbonate from the pancreas decreases osmotic pressure by generating sodium chloride and water. Because of the large intercellular pores in the jejunum, water rapidly leaves the intestinal lumen, bringing enteric contents closer to isotonicity. In the more distal intestine, the intercellular channels are smaller (3 to 3.5 Å), creating a less porous membrane. Water absorption tends to depend more on following the active transport of solutes into the paracellular spaces. Of the original 6 to 11 L of water entering the duodenum in 24 hours, less than 1 L is delivered to the colon.

Absorption of Electrolytes

There are four basic mechanisms of sodium absorption: (1) simple electrogenic absorption, (2) non−electrolyte-stimulated absorption, (3) neutral absorption, and (4) solvent drag.[11] The first three depend on the presence of the Na$^+$-K$^+$-ATPase pump in the basolateral cell membrane. This process extrudes three Na$^+$ ions from the cell for every two K$^+$ ions that enter, using energy generated by hydrolysis of ATP. The pump maintains a low intracellular concentration of sodium, which assists several mechanisms of absorption present at the apical membrane.

Simple electrogenic absorption of sodium is an electrochemically favored process in which sodium leaves the electrically neutral, high-sodium concentration of the intestinal lumen and enters the negatively charged, low-sodium concentration of the cell interior (Fig. 26-7). This portion of the process does not require energy but rapidly halts if the Na$^+$-K$^+$-ATPase pump is inhibited with ouabain, reflecting its dependence on the energy-requiring maintenance of the electrochemical gradient at the basolateral membrane.

Non−electrolyte-stimulated sodium absorption involves the coupled absorption of sodium with an organic solute, such as glucose, and is mediated by a specific carrier molecule in the apical membrane. Sodium is transported down its electrochemical gradient, which provides energy for the uphill transport of the organic solute against a concentration gradient. A number of substances are absorbed in this fashion, including D-hexoses, L−amino acids, dipeptides, water-soluble vitamins, bile salts (in the ileum), and sodium.

Neutral sodium chloride absorption is a process that couples sodium and chloride transport in a fashion similar to nonelectrolyte absorption described earlier for glucose (Fig. 26-8). The uphill transport of chloride would be driven by the downhill passage of sodium. Alternatively, two neutral, ion countertransport mechanisms appear to exist—one exchanging hydrogen for sodium and another using chloride and bicarbonate. This exchange ultimately results in the absorption of sodium chloride and the luminal generation of water and carbon dioxide. The energetics of this exchange are not clear, but they depend in part on low intracellular concentrations of cyclic AMP and calcium.

Finally, a significant portion of sodium absorption, especially in the proximal intestine, depends on the phenomenon of solvent drag. When osmotic forces generate the rapid movement of water from the intestinal lumen through intercellular tight junctions into the interstitium, there is friction between the water and the dissolved electrolytes. This frictional force drags sodium ions along with the movement of water. In the jejunum, where intercellular junctions are large and osmotic forces greatest, solvent drag represents a significant portion of overall sodium absorption. Although the intestine has a high bidirectional sodium flux, it nonetheless is highly sodium preserving. Of the 250 to 300 mEq/d of sodium consumed by the average adult, over 95% is absorbed, with less than 5 mEq/d excreted in the stool.

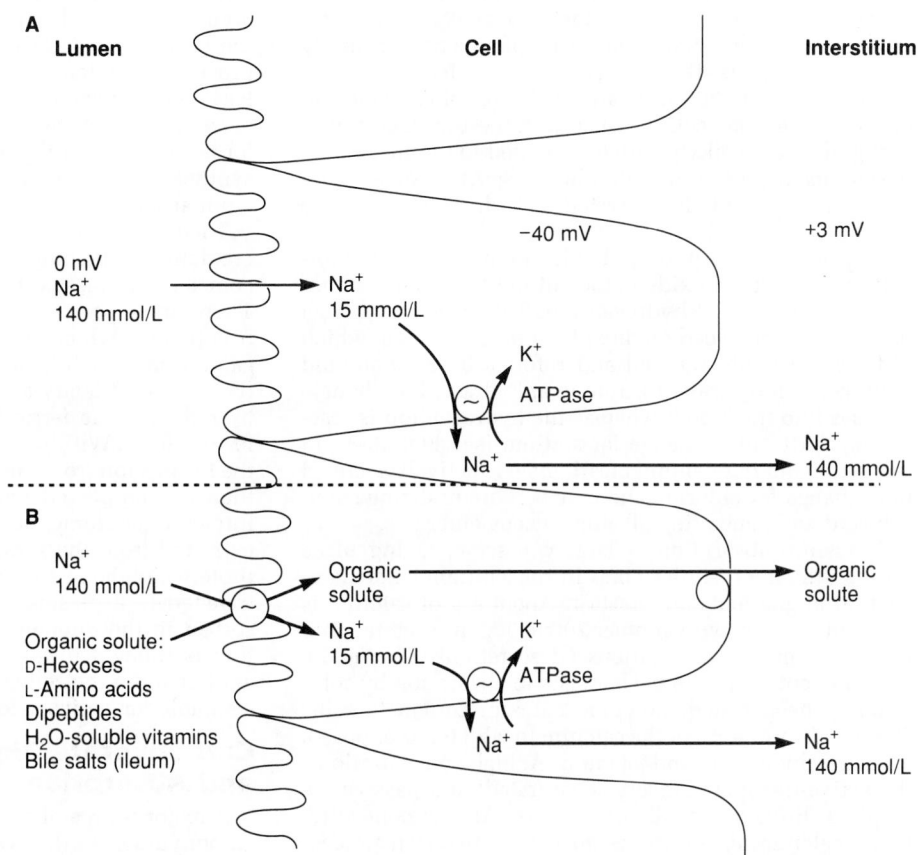

Figure 26-7. Two mechanisms of sodium absorption: electrogenic absorption (*A*) and non−electrolyte-stimulated absorption (*B*). (After Granger DN, Barrowman JA, Kuietys PR. Clinical gastrointestinal physiology. Philadelphia, WB Saunders, 1985:154)

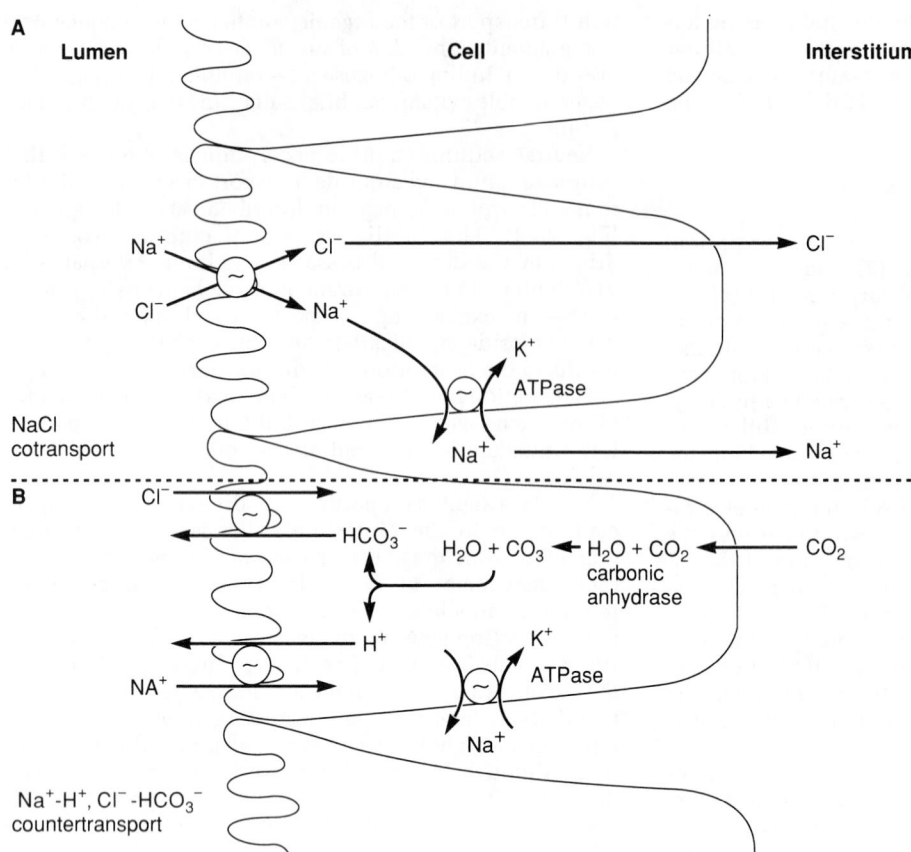

Figure 26-8. Two models of neutral sodium chloride absorption—the cotransport system (*A*), and the sodium–hydrogen, chloride–bicarbonate countertransport system that plays a part in chloride and bicarbonate absorption (*B*). (After Granger DN, Barrowman JA, Kuietys PR. Clinical gastrointestinal physiology. Philadelphia, WB Saunders, 1985:156)

Chloride ion absorption is managed both passively and actively. The active sodium chloride cotransport or countertransport process described earlier plays a role primarily in the ileum and is effective against a large electrochemical gradient (see Fig. 26-8). Passive diffusion of chloride can occur through paracellular spaces, since the interstitium is slightly electrically positive compared to the gut lumen. A significant portion of chloride transport involves reabsorption of chloride ion secreted as hydrochloric acid by the stomach.

Bicarbonate absorption in the jejunum involves the formation of carbon dioxide in the gut lumen from bicarbonate ion and secreted hydrogen ion. This generates a high partial pressure of carbon dioxide in the gut lumen, which diffuses back into the cell and reforms bicarbonate and hydrogen ion by way of carbonic anhydrase. Bicarbonate diffuses into the blood, whereas the hydrogen ion is resecreted, partly in exchange for sodium (see Fig. 26-8). In the ileum and duodenum, bicarbonate is actively secreted in exchange for chloride and assists in neutralizing stomach acid and generating alkaline succus entericus.

Potassium absorption is largely passive, taking place through the intercellular pores in the jejunum where concentration gradients are greatest. About 1 g of calcium is ingested per day, with another 200 to 300 mg secreted into the gut lumen by the various GI secretions. The acidic environment of the stomach assists in absorption by solubilizing the ingested, nonionic calcium carbonate salts. The gut absorbs 40% of the calcium to which it is exposed, all in the duodenum and jejunum. At high concentrations, the active-transport process is saturated, and passive absorptive diffusion of calcium occurs. At low concentrations, calcium absorption is an active, two-step process involving the capture of calcium by calcium-binding pro-

tein, facilitated by active transport across the apical membrane into the cell and active transport out of the cell at the basolateral surface using a Ca^{2+}-ATPase pump. This process is regulated by parathyroid hormone, which is released in low-calcium states and promotes the conversion of vitamin D to the active 1,25-dihydroxycholecalciferol form. The 1,25-dihydroxycholecalciferol increases the synthesis of calcium-binding protein and so increases calcium absorption.

The absorption of iron is a complex mechanism, and its regulation is incompletely understood. Most dietary iron comes from ingested meat as myoglobin and hemoglobin. There are separate transport mechanisms for complexed iron (heme), which is most rapidly absorbed, and for inorganic iron, which is preferentially absorbed in the ferrous (Fe^{2+}) form. Dietary ascorbic acid aids in iron absorption by reducing the ferric (Fe^{3+}) ion to the more absorbable ferrous form. Within the cell, enzyme mechanisms liberate the ferrous ion from the heme moiety. The ferrous iron can then be complexed with apoferritin to form ferritin, an intracellular storage form of iron. Alternatively, it can be extruded from the serosal surface of the cell by a carrier protein and then delivered to other tissues complexed with transferrin, a plasma transport protein. Most iron is absorbed in the duodenum and proximal jejunum. Regulation is thought to take place by modulating the level of apoferritin in the cell and so regulating the amount of iron available for delivery to the transferrin protein.

Carbohydrate Digestion and Absorption

A major source of caloric nutrition comes in the form of carbohydrate. In the Western diet, this is primarily made up of starch (about 60%), sucrose (30%), and lactose

(10%). The typical adult consumes an average of 400 g/d of carbohydrate, which yields about 1600 kcal (4 kcal/g) of energy.

The form of starch termed *amylopectin* is a polysaccharide made up of glucose linked in linear (1,4) fashion with branch points (1,6) at approximately every 25 glucose moieties (Fig. 26-9). Long linear starch molecules without branching are called *amylose*. Digestion of both amylose and amylopectin begins with salivary amylase and continues with pancreatic amylase, yielding maltose (glucose dimers, 1,4 linkage), maltotriose (glucose trimers, 1,4 linkage), and a combination of a-dextrins (such as isomaltose) averaging 6 glucose moieties incorporating the 1,6 branch points. This digestive process is usually complete by the time the carbohydrate load reaches the distal duodenum. These small oligosaccharides, along with sucrose (glucose–fructose dimer) and lactose (glucose–galactose), are then presented to the brush border of the jejunum to complete the digestion and absorption processes.

In the brush border of the small intestine, numerous specific enzymes catalyze the hydrolysis of these short-chain sugars into their component hexoses (glucose, galactose, and fructose). These monosaccharides are then absorbed into the cell. Glucose and galactose compete for the same carrier mechanism and require sodium for transport across the cell membrane (see Fig. 26-7). The sugar then exits the cell at the basolateral surface by facilitated diffusion with the cotransported sodium extruded by the Na^+-K^+-ATPase pump. Fructose is absorbed by a facilitated diffusion mechanism and is sodium independent.

Dietary fiber represents nondigestible carbohydrate, such as cellulose, and is poorly represented in the Western diet. Fiber is commonly found in all-bran cereals, beans, partially cooked vegetables, and raw pulpy fruits. High-fiber diets retain water within the intestinal lumen and significantly shorten intestinal transit time. Dietary fiber can adsorb organic materials, such as bile salts and lipids, and inorganic minerals, such as zinc, calcium, magnesium, and iron. How these properties affect carcinogenesis is controversial.

Protein Digestion and Absorption

Protein is an essential part of the daily diet. The average adult requires about 0.6 g/kg/d, although growing children and pregnant women require significantly more, on the order of 4 g/kg/d. A caloric energy source, amino acids represent the basic building blocks of necessary body proteins. In addition to dietary consumption, an almost equal amount of the protein load within the gut comes from enteric sources, such as secreted enzymes, desquamated cells, and plasma protein leakage. Ninety percent of this protein load is absorbed.

The hydrolysis of protein into its constituent amino acids starts in the stomach with the secretion and activation of pepsinogen into pepsin. In the duodenum, peptidases from the pancreas break down the large protein molecules into smaller peptide chains. Endopeptidases (eg, trypsin, elastase, chymotrypsin) hydrolyze peptide bonds between specific amino acids, whereas the exopeptidases (eg, carboxypeptidase A and B) hydrolyze amino acids from the C-terminal ends of the protein segments. About 30% of protein is digested to free amino acids, and the remainder to short oligopeptides of two to six amino acids.

Further hydrolysis of these short amino acid peptides occurs either at the brush border or within the cellular cytoplasm. In the apical cell, membrane transport mechanisms exist to transfer dipeptides or tripeptides into the cytosol, where specific peptidases further hydrolyze the peptides to their component amino acids. Larger peptides are first enzymatically cleaved in the brush border and absorbed as either dipeptides, tripeptides, or free amino acids.

There are at least four amino acid transport mechanisms, each based on the electrochemical characteristics of the amino acid to be transported—neutral, dibasic, acidic (or

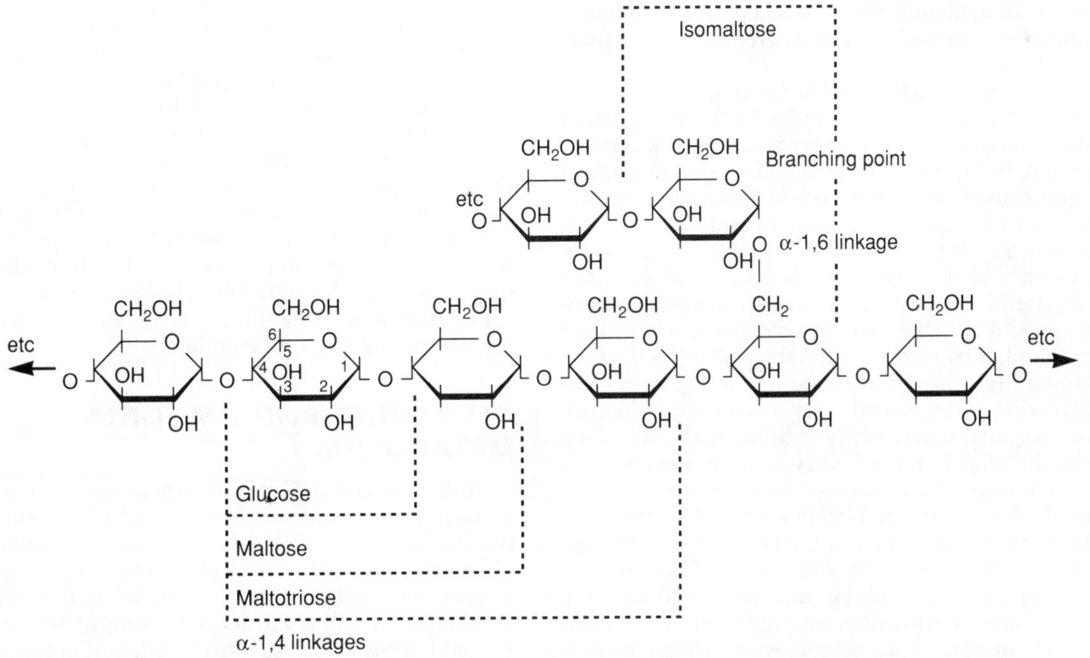

Figure 26-9. The structure of starch. Pancreatic and salivary amylase catalyze hydrolysis of the 1,4 linkages, yielding short-chain oligosaccharides that are then further hydrolyzed into monosaccharides in the brush border. (After Davenport HW. A digest of digestion, ed 2. Chicago, Year Book, 1978)

dicarboxylic), and imino. Energy for transport is derived from the cotransport of sodium and ultimately from the Na⁺-K⁺-ATPase pump. The absorption of dipeptides and tripeptides is more rapid than single amino acid absorption and accounts for the largest part of protein absorption. These transport processes similarly use sodium- and energy-dependent carrier mechanisms (see Fig. 26-7). After further digestion within the cell, free amino acids diffuse into the portal circulation.

Fat Digestion and Absorption

The average Western diet contains between 60 and 100 g of fat, 90% in the form of triglycerides, and the remainder in the form of cholesterol, phospholipids, and fat-soluble vitamins. Fat digestion and absorption begin with triglyceride digestion in the intestinal lumen. Lipase, a pancreatic enzyme, cleaves the fatty moieties at the 1 and 3 positions on the glycerol backbone, yielding two fatty acids and a monoglyceride (a fatty acid esterified to glycerol). The secretion of lipase (and its necessary cofactor, colipase) from the pancreas is stimulated by CCK, which is secreted by the duodenal mucosa in response to the presence of fatty acids in the duodenum.

After lipolysis, the free fatty acids and monoglycerides are solubilized in the aqueous contents of the intestine by forming bile micelles. Micelles are 50 to 400 Å in diameter and are aggregations of bile salts and fatty acids. The hydrophobic portions of the molecules face inward, and the hydrophilic portions face the outside aqueous phase. Other lipids, such as cholesterol, lecithins, and the fat-soluble vitamins (A, D, E, and K), can reside in the central hydrophobic core. Although micelles are many times larger than any one lipid molecule, their water-compatible nature allows them to traverse the unstirred water layer next to the brush border and to intimately approximate themselves and their component molecules to the mucosal cell for efficient absorption.

Absorption of micelle contents occurs by a process of dissolution in the lipid bilayer of the mucosal cell. This process does not require energy and is rapid. The emptied bile micelle is immediately ready to accept new lipid components from the aqueous phase and to repeat the transport process.

Once within the cell, fatty acids are transferred to the endoplasmic reticulum using a cytosolic carrier protein referred to as *fatty acid–binding protein*. In the endoplasmic reticulum, resynthesis of triglycerides takes place, and with the addition of phospholipid and a glycoprotein coat added in the Golgi apparatus, a chylomicron is formed. Chylomicrons are large particles, 750 to 6000 Å in diameter, that consist of 90% triglyceride and 10% phospholipid, cholesterol, and protein. They are packaged in secretory vesicles and exit the cell by exocytosis, where they enter the lymphatics through the terminal villus lacteal. Smaller lipoprotein particles containing a higher cholesterol/triglyceride ratio, called *very low-density lipoproteins*, are also manufactured by the mucosal cell. They seem to be the major route of entry into the bloodstream for dietary cholesterol.

Long-chain fatty acids are largely absorbed by this process and eventually gain entry to the bloodstream through the thoracic duct. Short-chain fatty acids (fewer than 8 carbon atoms) are water soluble and enter and exit the enterocyte by simple diffusion without need for bile micelles or chylomicrons. They are removed through the portal circulation without entering the lymphatics. Medium-chain triglycerides (6 to 14 carbon atoms) are absorbed and removed from the intestine by both simple diffusion and the absorptive process used by long-chain fatty acids. They need not be reesterified and can enter the portal circulation directly as free fatty acids.

Absorption of Bile Salts

Some 80% to 90% of secreted bile salts found in the micelle is reabsorbed and returned to the liver through the portal circulation. In the liver, bile salts are resecreted and stored in the gallbladder in preparation for the next meal. This circular flow of bile is termed *enterohepatic circulation*, and the small portion of bile lost in the feces (about 500 mg) is balanced by hepatic synthesis. The reabsorption of bile is both passive and active. Passive absorption occurs along the entire length of the small intestine and depends on the lipid solubility of the bile salt. Glycine bile conjugates are more soluble than taurine conjugates. As much as 50% of bile is passively reabsorbed.

Active absorption of bile occurs only in the terminal ileum, probably through a sodium-linked cotransport system (see Fig. 26-7). A small amount of bile escapes into the colon, where it is deconjugated by bacteria, promoting lipid solubility and further passive absorption. High colon concentrations of bile salts promote diarrhea by inhibiting sodium and water absorption. This commonly occurs in patients with ileal resections and can be treated with the bile-binding resin, cholestyramine. Compromised fat absorption for any reason can similarly decrease bile absorption by stabilizing the bile micelles. Long-chain fatty acid malabsorption can be treated by substituting medium- or short-chain fatty acids for long-chain species.

Vitamin Absorption

Fat-soluble vitamins (A, D, E, and K) are principally absorbed by micelles along with fats and exit the mucosal cell through chylomicrons to enter the lymph. Water-soluble vitamins are absorbed in the ileum and jejunum by various means. Vitamins C (ascorbic acid), B₁ (thiamine), B₁₂ (cobalamin), and niacin use active-transport mechanisms linked to sodium cotransport. Folic acid and vitamin B₂ (riboflavin) are absorbed by facilitated diffusion. Pyridoxine (B₆) is absorbed by simple diffusion.

Vitamin B₁₂ absorption requires a glycoprotein called *intrinsic factor*, which is produced by the parietal cells of the stomach. One intrinsic factor molecule binds two molecules of cobalamin, and this complex attaches to a specific receptor in the terminal ileum. Free cobalamin does not bind to the receptor, and any compromise of the production of intrinsic factor, as occurs in patients after proximal gastrectomy, decreases B₁₂ absorption. After absorption, the free vitamin is extruded from the cell and transported in the blood by B₁₂-binding proteins called *transcobalamins*. Vitamin B₁₂ is essential in DNA synthesis; deficiency leads to anemia.

GLUTAMINE AND AMMONIA METABOLISM

Glutamine is the most abundant amino acid in the blood as well as the major respiratory fuel of the enterocyte. It plays a key role in total body nitrogen and ammonia metabolism. Ammonia is part of all amino acids, proteins, and nucleic acids yet is relatively toxic when free in the blood. Glutamine provides for detoxification of ammonia in peripheral tissues, such as muscle, when it is generated from glutamate and ammonia by the enzyme glutamine synthetase. Glutamine leaves the muscle and is taken up by the kidneys and intestine, where it is deaminated. The liberated ammonia is then cleared by either hepatic ureagenesis or by renal excretion. The small intestine, with its portal circulation, is therefore well suited to use glutamine as its primary fuel. In the enterocyte, the regenerated glutamate enters the tricarboxylic acid cycle after further deamination to α-ketoglutarate but is also involved in the production of alanine and citrulline (Fig. 26-10). Twenty to 30% of circulating plasma glutamine is taken up by the small intestine and accounts for about 50% of the ammonia generated by the intestine. The remaining ammonia is largely the product of colonic bacteria metabolism. Decreasing ammonia levels in patients with hepatic insufficiency, therefore, involves modulating both small intestinal protein metabolism and colonic bacterial flora.

Glutamine can be taken up by the enterocyte from either the arterial circulation or the intestinal lumen. Orally administered glutamine decreases the arterial extraction of the amino acid, suggesting a common intracellular pool. During times of simple surgical stress, intestinal glutamine utilization is increased, resulting in depressed blood levels despite increased muscle synthesis. This effect can be mimicked by glucocorticoid administration. In contrast, severe sepsis is associated with decreased glutamine extraction by the intestine, resulting in normal or elevated blood glutamine levels. The consequences of inadequate glutamine supply or utilization can lead to a compromise in the intestine's bacterial barrier function and relate to the hypothesis that multiple organ system failure results from intestinal bacterial translocation and sepsis.

Numerous studies relate glutamine supplementation to improved intestinal morphology and function. Glutamine added to intravenous hyperalimentation solutions improves such parameters as intestinal villus height and DNA and protein content in animal models. Similarly, oral glutamine improves animal survival and intestinal morphology after various intestinal injuries, such as those seen after whole abdominal irradiation or intestinal transplantation. Surgical patients receiving glutamine-supplemented hyperalimentation solutions show improved nitrogen balance and protein metabolism, suggesting a decreased need for glutamine synthesis at the expense of skeletal muscle. Most standard hyperalimentation solutions do not contain glutamine because of its short shelf-life and its potential for ammonia toxicity. This can be circumvented by using glutamine dipeptides or adding glutamine at the time of administration of hyperalimentation solutions. Overall, however, human data confirming the beneficial effects of glutamine supplementation on both intestine and patient are relatively lacking. Early resumption of enteral feeding still provides the safest and most effective way to maintain a healthy intestinal mucosa.

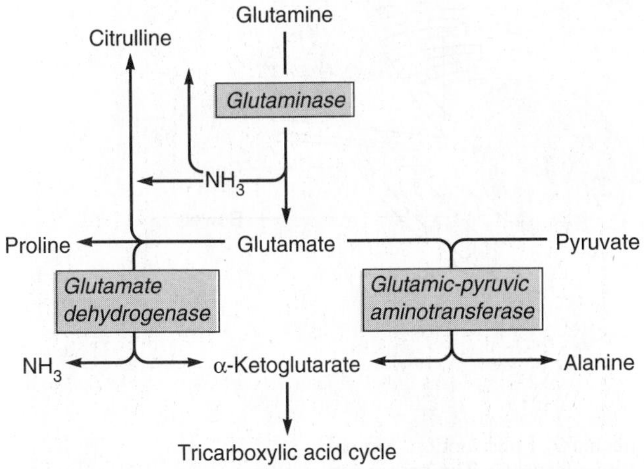

REFERENCES

1. Anderson JE. Grant's atlas of anatomy, ed 8, vol 2. Baltimore, Williams & Wilkins, 1983:46.
2. Haubrich WS. Gross anatomy of the small intestine. In: Berk JE, ed. Bockus gastroenterology, ed 4, vol 3. Philadelphia, WB Saunders, 1985:1479.
3. Shiner M. Microscopic anatomy of the small intestine. In: Berk JE, ed. Bockus gastroenterology, ed 4, vol 3. Philadelphia, WB Saunders, 1985:1485.
4. Faucett DW. A textbook of histology, ed 11. Philadelphia, WB Saunders, 1986:641.
5. Hanaver SB, Kraft SC. Intestinal immunology. In: Berk JE, ed. Bockus gastroenterology, ed 4, vol 3. Philadelphia, WB Saunders, 1985:1607.
6. Kagnoff MF. Immunology of the digestive system. In: Johnson LR, ed. Physiology of the gastrointestinal tract, ed 2. New York, Raven Press, 1987:1699.
7. Vantrappen GR, Janssens JP. Small bowel motility. In: Berk JE, ed. Bockus gastroenterology, ed 4, vol 3. Philadelphia, WB Saunders, 1985:1493.
8. Cohen S, Snape WJ. Movement of the small and large intestine. In: Sleisenger MH, Fordtran JS, eds. Gastrointestinal disease: pathophysiology, diagnosis, management, ed 4, vol 2. Philadelphia, WB Saunders, 1989:1088.
9. Weisbrodt NW. Motility of the small intestine. In: Johnson LR, ed. Physiology of the gastrointestinal tract, ed 2. New York, Raven Press, 1987:631.
10. Davenport HW. Physiology of the digestive tract, ed 5. Chicago, Yearbook, 1982.
11. Granger DN, Barrowman JA, Kuietys PR. Clinical gastrointestinal physiology. Philadelphia, WB Saunders, 1985.
12. Souba WW. The gut as a nitrogen-processing organ in the metabolic response to critical illness. Nutr Supp Serv 1988;8:15.

SURGERY: SCIENTIFIC PRINCIPLES AND PRACTICE, Second Edition, edited by Lazar J. Greenfield, Michael W. Mulholland, Keith T. Oldham, Gerald B. Zelenock, and Keith D. Lillemoe. Lippincott–Raven Publishers, Philadelphia, © 1997.

CHAPTER 27

ILEUS AND BOWEL OBSTRUCTION

DAVID I. SOYBEL

The modern approach to intestinal obstruction and ileus has paralleled the development of techniques for safe abdominal surgery. From 1880 to 1925, it was recognized that proximal intestinal decompression could provide relief from the symptoms of mechanical obstruction or ileus.[1-3] In 1933, investigators reported the efficacy of gastrointestinal intubation in relieving symptoms of intestinal distention caused by intestinal obstruction or by the ileus that resulted from laparotomy.[4,5] Subsequently, experimental evidence indicated that the source of gaseous distention in cases of obstruction or ileus was swallowed air.[6] The value of intravenous fluid resuscitation in experimental models of intestinal obstruction was recognized as early as 1912[7] and became a principle of care of patients with intestinal obstruction in the late 1920s. By 1920, plain abdominal radiographs were used in the diagnosis of intestinal obstruction.[3] Thus, the principles of early diagnosis,

Figure 26-10. Metabolism of glutamine within the enterocyte.

rapid intravenous fluid resuscitation, gastrointestinal decompression, and early operation to avoid intestinal gangrene and peritonitis were established well before the advent of antibiotic therapy, invasive hemodynamic monitoring, and parenteral nutrition.[8] These early developments were most important in reducing morbidity and mortality of mechanical intestinal obstruction and ileus.[9]

MECHANICAL OBSTRUCTION OF THE INTESTINE

Terminology and Classification

The term *mechanical obstruction* means that luminal contents cannot pass through the gut tube because the lumen is blocked. This contrasts with *neurogenic* or *functional* obstruction in which luminal contents fail to pass because of disturbances in gut motility that prevent coordinated peristalsis from one region of the gut to the next. This latter form of obstruction is commonly referred to as *ileus* in the small intestine and *pseudoobstruction* in the large intestine. In *simple* obstruction, the intestinal lumen is partially or completely occluded without compromise of intestinal blood flow. Simple obstructions can be *complete*, meaning that the lumen is totally occluded (Fig. 27-1), or *incomplete*, meaning that the lumen is narrowed but permits distal passage of some fluid and air. In *strangulation* obstruction, blood flow to the obstructed segment is compromised, and tissue necrosis and gangrene are imminent. Strangulation usually implies that the obstruction is complete, but some forms of partial obstruction can also be complicated by strangulation.

Obstruction is classified according to etiology and location of the obstructing lesion. As detailed in Table 27-1, distinctions are drawn between intraluminal foreign bodies or gallstones, intramural lesions such as tumors or intussusceptions, and extrinsic or extramural

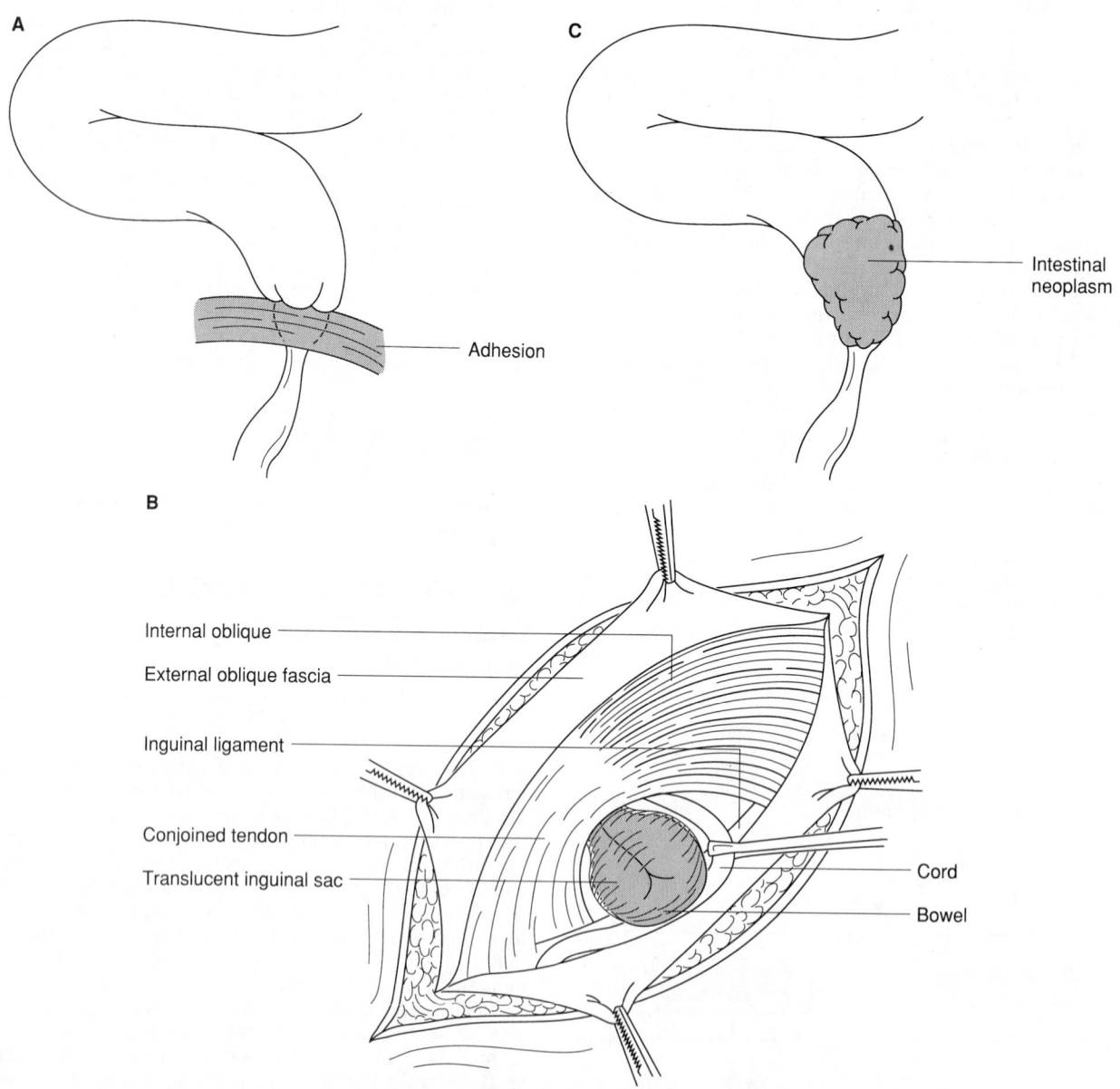

Figure 27-1. Schematic illustration of different forms of simple mechanical obstruction. Simple obstruction is most often due to adhesion (*A*), groin hernia (*B*), or neoplasm (*C*). The hernia can act as a tourniquet, causing a closed-loop obstruction and strangulation.

Table 27-1. CLASSIFICATION OF ADULT MECHANICAL INTESTINAL OBSTRUCTIONS

INTRALUMINAL

Foreign bodies
Barium inspissation (colon)
Bezoar
Inspissated feces
Gallston
Meconium (cystic fibrosis)
Parasites
Other (eg, swallowed objects,
    enteroliths)
Intussusception
Polypoid, exophytic lesions

INTRAMURAL

Congenital
    Atresia, stricture, or stenosis
    Web
    Intestinal duplication
    Meckel's diverticulum
Inflammatory process
    Crohn's disease
    Diverticulitis
    Chronic intestinal ischemia or
        postischemic stricture
    Radiation enteritis
    Medication induced (nonsteroidal
        antiinflammatories, postassium
        chloride tablets)
Neoplasms
    Primary bowel (malignant or benign)
    Secondary (metastases, especially
        melanoma)
Traumatic
    Intramural hematoma of duodenum

EXTRINSIC

Adhesions
Congenital
    Ladd or Meckel's
        bands
    Postoperative
    Postinflammatory
Hernias
    External
    Internal
Volvulus
External mass effect
    Abscess
    Annular pancreas
    Carcinomatosis
    Endometriosis
    Pregnancy
    Pancreatic pseudocyst

lesions such as adhesions. Proximal, or high, obstructions involve the pylorus, duodenum, and proximal jejunum. Intermediate levels of obstruction involve the intestine from the mid-jejunum to the mid-ileum. Distal levels of obstruction arise in the distal ileum, ileocecal valve, and proximal colon, whereas the most distant, or low, obstructions arise in regions beyond the transverse colon. As shown in Table 27-2, clinical symptoms and signs of obstruction (pain, vomiting, abdominal distention, gas pattern on abdominal radiographs) vary with the level of obstruction.

It is also important to distinguish *open-loop* from *closed-loop* obstructions. An open-loop obstruction occurs when intestinal flow is blocked but proximal decompression is possible through vomiting. A closed-loop obstruction occurs when inflow to the loop of bowel and outflow from the loop are both blocked. This permits gas and secretions to accumulate in the loop without a means of decompression, proximally or distally. Examples of closed-loop obstructions include torsion of a loop of small intestine around an adhesive band (Fig. 27-2), incarceration of bowel in a hernia, volvulus of the cecum or colon, and development of an obstructing carcinoma of the colon with a competent ileocecal valve. Closed-loop obstruction of the small intestine causes sudden, severe abdominal pain and vomiting, whereas obstructions of the large intestine cause pain and sudden abdominal distention. Pain often precedes associated findings of localized abdominal tenderness or involuntary guarding. When physical findings develop, viability of the bowel is often compromised.

Pathophysiology of Intestinal Obstruction

Local Effects of Bowel Obstruction

When a loop of bowel becomes obstructed, intestinal gas and fluid accumulate. The rate at which symptoms and complications develop depends on luminal volume, bacterial proliferation, and alterations in motility and perfusion.

Intestinal Gas. About 80% of the gas seen on plain abdominal radiographs is attributable to swallowed air.[6] About 70% of the gas in the obstructed gut is inert nitrogen.[10] Oxygen accounts for 10% to 12%, carbon dioxide 6% to 9%, hydrogen 1%, methane 1%, and hydrogen disulfide 1% to 10%. In the setting of acute pain and anxiety, patients with intestinal obstruction may swallow excessive amounts of air. Passage of such swallowed air distally is prevented by nasogastric suction.

Intestinal Flora. An important contribution to normal digestive function comes from the resident bacterial population. In patients with normal gastric acid secretion, the chyme entering the duodenum is nearly sterile. The small numbers of bacteria that are found in stomach and proximal intestine are aerobic, gram-positive species similar to those found in the oropharynx. Distally, in the ileum and colon, gram-negative aerobes are present, and anaerobic organisms predominate. Total bacterial counts in normal

Table 27-2. SYMPTOMS AND SIGNS OF BOWEL OBSTRUCTION

Symptom or Sign	Proximal Small Bowel (Open Loop)	Distal Small Bowel (Open Loop)	Small Bowel (Closed Loop)	Colon and Rectum
Pain	Intermittent, intense, colicky; often relieved by vomiting	Intermittent to constant	Progressive, intermittent to constant; rapidly worsens	Continuous
Vomiting	Large volumes, bilious and frequent	Low volume and frequency; progressively feculent with time	May be prominent (reflex)	Intermittent, not prominent; feculent when present
Tenderness	Epigastric or periumbilical; quite mild unless strangulation is present	Diffuse and progressive	Diffuse, progressive	Diffuse
Distention	Absent	Moderate to marked	Often absent	Marked
Obstipation	May not be present	Present	May not be present	Present

(Adapted from Schuffler MD, Sinanan MN. Intestinal obstruction and pseudo-obstruction. In: Sleisenger MH, Fordtran JS, eds. Gastrointestinal disease, ed 5. Philadelphia, WB Saunders, 1993:898)

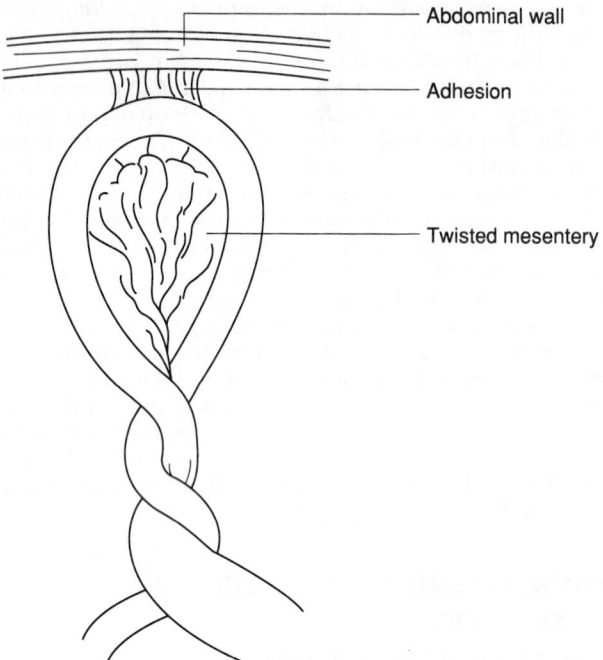

Abdominal wall

Adhesion

Twisted mesentery

Figure 27-2. Schematic illustration of a closed-loop obstruction. The small intestine twists around its mesentery, compromising inflow and outflow of luminal contents from the loop. Also, the vascular supply to the loop may be compromised because of the twisting of the mesentery. The risk of strangulation is high.

feces reach 10^{11} organisms per gram of fecal matter. Control of the bacterial populations depends on intact motor activity of the intestines and the interactions of all species present. This ecology can be disturbed by antibiotic therapy or surgical reconstructions that result in stasis within intestinal segments. Intestinal bacteria serve several functions, including the following:

- Metabolism of fecal sterols, releasing the short-chain fatty acids that are an important food source for colonocytes
- Metabolism of fecal bile acids, fat-soluble vitamins, and vitamin B_{12}
- Breakdown of complex carbohydrates and organic matter, leading to the formation of carbon dioxide, hydrogen, and methane gases[8]

Evidence suggests that the normal flora contributes to baseline levels of intestinal secretion and normal intestinal motility. The small intestines in germ-free animals are frequently dilated, fluid filled, and without peristalsis.[11,12]

In recent years, the role of bacterial toxins in mediating the mucosal response to obstruction has received increasing attention. In germ-free dogs, luminal accumulation of fluid is not observed, and absorption continues.[11] In addition, it is well recognized that bacterial endotoxins can stimulate secretion, possibly by means of release or potentiation of neuroendocrine substances and prostaglandins.[12] Because a substantial number of systemic microvascular and hemodynamic responses to endotoxemia appear to be attributable to heightened synthesis of nitric oxide,[13,14] it seems likely that mucosal responses to local inflammation and endotoxin release also are altered by conditions modifying the synthesis or activity of nitric oxide. The role of nitric oxide in mucosal fluid and electrolyte movements is under active investigation.[15,16]

Intestinal Fluid. Fluid accumulates intraluminally with open- or closed-loop small intestinal obstruction because of the following:

- Intraluminal distention and pressure
- Release of prosecretory and antiabsorptive hormones and paracrine substances
- Changes in mesenteric circulation
- Elaboration and luminal release of bacterial toxins[8,17]

Experimental studies and clinical investigation[18,19] demonstrated that elevation of luminal pressures above 20 cm H_2O inhibits absorption and stimulates secretion of salt and water into the lumen proximal to an obstruction. In closed-loop obstruction, luminal pressures can exceed 50 cm H_2O and may account for a substantial proportion of luminal fluid accumulation.[20] In simple open-loop obstruction, distention of the lumen by gas rarely leads to luminal pressures higher than 8 to 12 cm H_2O.[21] Thus, in open-loop obstruction, the contributions of high luminal pressures to hypersecretion may not be important.

The release of endocrine and paracrine substances is suggested to occur in mechanical bowel obstruction.[22,23] Vasoactive intestinal polypeptide may be released from the submucosal and myenteric plexuses within the gut wall, promoting epithelial secretion and inhibiting absorption.[22] Excess release of prostaglandins can also occur.[23]

Intestinal Blood Flow. Microvascular responses to intestinal obstruction also can play an important role in determining hydrostatic gradients for fluid transfer across the mucosa into the lumen. In response to heightened luminal pressure, total blood flow to the bowel wall may initially increase.[24] Enzymatic breakdown of stagnant intestinal contents leads to increased osmolarity of luminal contents. Along with secretory stimulation and absorptive inhibition of the mucosa, the simultaneous changes in hydrostatic and osmotic pressures on the blood and lumen sides of the mucosa favor flow of extracellular fluid into the lumen. Subsequently, blood flow is compromised as luminal pressures increase, bacteria invade, and inflammation leads to edema within the bowel wall.

Intestinal Motility. Obstruction of the intestinal lumen does not simply block distal passage of luminal contents. The accumulation of fluid and gas in the obstructed lumen also elicits changes in the myoelectrical function of the gut, proximal and distal to the obstructed segment. In response to this distention, the obstructed segment itself may dilate, a process known as receptive relaxation.[25] Such changes ensure that, despite accumulation of air and fluid, intraluminal pressures do not rise easily to the point of compromising blood flow to the intestinal mucosa. At sites proximal and distal to the obstruction, changes in myoelectrical activity are time dependent. Initially, there may be intense periods of activity and peristalsis. Subsequently, myoelectrical activity is diminished, and the interdigestive migrating myoelectrical complex pattern, is replaced by ineffectual and seemingly disorganized clusters of contractions.[26-28] Similar alterations have been observed in experimental models of large bowel obstruction.[29,30] Subsequent patterns of myoelectrical quiescence may correspond to an increasing accumulation of fluid and air proximally and the attempt to prevent luminal pressures from rising.

Complications of Bowel Obstruction

Closed-Loop Obstruction. The complications of closed-loop obstructions evolve rapidly. The reasons for this rapid evolution are best understood by considering the simplest and most common form of closed-loop obstruction, appendicitis. When a fecalith obstructs the blind-ended appendix, secretion of mucus and enhanced peristalsis represent the initial attempt to clear the blockage. Intense, crampy abdominal pain focused at the umbilicus results. Nausea and vomiting are not uncommon as a reflexive response to hyperperistalsis and stretching of the mesentery. During the next 8 to 18 hours, continued secretion of mucus leads to high intraluminal pressures, stasis, bacterial overgrowth, and mucosal disruption. When luminal pressure exceeds mural venous pressure and then capillary perfusion pressures, inflammatory cells are recruited from surrounding peritoneal structures. This sequence of events leads to intense inflammation, release of exudate in the area of the appendix, and the first localization of pain from the umbilicus to the area of peritoneum lying nearest the inflamed appendix. Peritoneal findings (localized tenderness, involuntary guarding, rebound or referred tenderness) and fever appear. Subsequently, 20 to 24 hours into the illness, the blood supply of the appendix is compromised. Gangrene and perforation follow, and if not contained by surrounding structures, free perforation leads to peritonitis. Toxins from necrotic tissue and bacterial overgrowth are released into the systemic circulation, and shock ensues. Torsion of a loop of small intestine around an adhesive band or inside a hernia leads to a similar sequence of events. Torsion of the large bowel is usually accompanied by massive distention of the loop by air and feces.

Open-Loop Obstruction. Complications of open-loop obstruction do not evolve as rapidly as those in closed-loop obstruction. Not uncommonly, an open-loop obstruction located in the proximal jejunum can be decompressed by the patient's ability to vomit. The obstruction is characterized by loss of gastric, pancreatic, and biliary secretions, with resulting electrolyte disturbances, including dehydration, metabolic alkalosis, hypochloremia, hypokalemia, and usually hyponatremia. In contrast, obstruction of the distal ileum may lead only to a slowly progressive distention of the small intestine, with accommodation by intestinal myoelectrical function and minor alterations in fluid and electrolyte balances. Open-loop obstruction located in the midgut is often characterized by events similar to those seen in closed-loop obstruction or combinations of events seen in high and low obstruction (see Table 27-2). Thus, patients with distal jejunal obstruction may present with a combination of complications resulting from loss of intestinal contents from vomiting, as well as distention and compromise of intestinal wall perfusion.

Clinical Presentation and Differential Diagnosis

The four key symptoms that are associated with acute mechanical bowel obstruction include abdominal pain, vomiting, distention, and obstipation. Colon obstruction is usually accompanied by varying levels of pain, with massive abdominal distention, and obstipation. Other abdominal conditions, such as appendicitis, diverticulitis, perforated peptic ulcer, cholecystitis, or choledocholithiasis, can usually be distinguished from small bowel obstruction by clinical examination and basic laboratory data. Bowel obstruction can complicate any of these abdominal conditions. The presence of another abdominal process does not exclude the complication of small bowel obstruction.

Numerous attempts have been made to use groupings of clinical criteria to establish the diagnosis of complete and irreversible intestinal obstruction, and to distinguish complete obstruction from partial intestinal obstruction. In recent studies, computer-assisted analysis has been used to identify such criteria.[31] Key factors in the history and clinical examination include the following:

- Previous abdominal surgery
- Quality of pain (colicky and intermittent versus steady)
- Abdominal distention
- Hyperactivity of bowel sounds

Not surprisingly, the use of such computer-assisted algorithms confirms that the most important clues to the diagnosis of simple obstruction of the small intestine result from a complete and careful history and physical examination. The role of plain abdominal radiographs and other imaging studies is to confirm the clinical diagnosis of *simple* obstruction. In simple obstruction, laboratory studies do not play a direct role in diagnosis but are helpful in understanding the extent of complications such as dehydration, strangulation, and sepsis.

Strangulation obstruction of the small or large intestine is accompanied by symptoms and signs that suggest peritonitis. Large fluid shifts and systemic toxicity are imminent or have already occurred. These signs include abdominal tenderness or involuntary guarding localized to the area of the strangulated loop of bowel, decreased urine output, fever, and tachycardia. There have been attempts to use common clinical and laboratory test criteria to identify the likelihood that the obstruction is associated with strangulation. Investigators have suggested that the risk of strangulation is low in patients with incomplete or complete small bowel obstruction as long as fever, tachycardia, localized abdominal tenderness, and leukocytosis are not present.[32] These researchers observed, however, in a setting consistent with bowel obstruction, that any one of these four cardinal signs indicates a small risk of strangulation. Any two of these signs together increase the risk of strangulation so high as to warrant immediate surgery. These and other authorities have stressed that when complete obstruction is present, no satisfactory criteria are available to reliably exclude the possibility of strangulation.[32–34] Metabolic acidosis and increases in serum amylase, inorganic phosphate, hexosaminidase, intestinal fatty acid–binding protein (I-FABP), and serum D-lactate levels have all been associated with intestinal ischemia.[35,36] Such laboratory abnormalities can be helpful in diagnosing established strangulation in a small group of patients in whom the diagnosis of necrotic bowel is not clear. A noninvasive and rapid test that can provide information to suggest that tissue necrosis is imminent but not yet established has not been developed, however.[37]

Radiographs and Imaging

Plain Films

The role of plain abdominal radiographs and imaging studies is to confirm the diagnosis of bowel obstruction, locate the site of obstruction, and provide insight into the lesion responsible for the obstruction. On plain radiographs of the abdomen, the findings that suggest the diagnosis of small bowel obstruction reflect the accumulation of air and fluid proximal to, and clearance of fluid and air distal to, the point of obstruction. Such findings include dilated loops of small bowel on the flat plate and multiple air-fluid levels located at different areas on the upright film or lateral decubitus film (Fig. 27-3). Dilated loops of small intestine are defined as those larger than 3 cm in diameter. Free air represents perforation of a viscus and mandates immediate operation. In general, colon loops do not contain air. If there is air in the colon, the obstruction may be complete but early, or it may be incomplete.

In the colon, tightly closed loop obstructions, such as

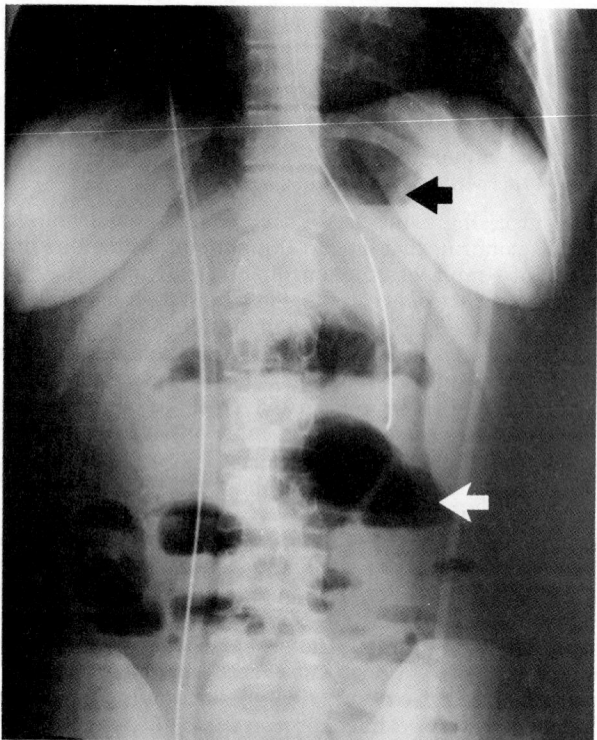

Figure 27-3. Plain upright abdominal film of a patient with small intestinal obstruction. There are air-fluid levels in the stomach (*black arrow*), multiple dilated loops of small intestine (*white arrow*), and no air in the colon or rectum.

Under some circumstances, contrast studies are unnecessary and may be contraindicated. For example, in the classic setting of abdominal pain, nausea, vomiting, and a plain film indicating multiple air-fluid levels in the small intestine and colonic collapse, the diagnosis of acute obstruction can be made clinically. Failure to improve in a short time mandates operation, and contrast studies are unnecessary. When strangulation or perforation is strongly suspected, contrast studies are contraindicated.

The choice of contrast materials includes water-insoluble suspensions of barium and water-soluble agents such as Gastrografin or Hypaque. Barium studies provide the clearest images in both small bowel studies, in which the contrast is given from above, and colorectal studies, in which the contrast is given by enema. If barium leaks into the peritoneum, it elicits intense peritonitis. If there is any possibility of bowel perforation or gangrene, barium should not be used. Water-soluble agents are hyperosmotic and can elicit fluid translocation into the gut. When the obstruction of the small intestine is incomplete, these agents can facilitate resolution.[38]

Computed Tomography and Other Imaging Modalities

The potential benefits of computed tomographic (CT) scanning in the diagnosis of bowel obstruction include the following:

1. With dilute barium used for luminal contrast, the obstructing segment can be localized and characterized as complete or incomplete.[39,40]
2. The nature of the obstructing lesion, especially if it is malignant, can be established.

volvulus of the cecum, transverse colon, and sigmoid colon, are accompanied by distention of the obstructed segment (Fig. 27-4). The proximal colon is considered dilated when it reaches 8 to 10 cm, and the sigmoid colon is dilated at 4 to 5 cm. In contrast, obstruction by carcinoma or diverticulitis presents with massive distention of the entire colon from the point of obstruction to the ileocecal valve. From this standpoint, any large bowel obstruction represents a closed loop as long as the ileocecal valve is competent. Although it is usually possible to differentiate obstruction of the small bowel from that of the large bowel, localizing the site of obstruction within these organs is not possible by the appearance of plain films alone.

One point needs to be stressed about the appearance of plain films in patients with closed-loop obstructions of the small intestine. Such a loop of bowel may contain fluid and very little gas. Thus, it may not be visible or only barely visible as a minimally dilated sentinel loop that remains unchanged in position on films that are performed in different projections. Also, because such patients generally present early after the onset of symptoms, the loops proximal to the closed loop will not have had time to fill with air, and the remainder of the abdomen may appear gasless.

Contrast Studies

Contrast studies (small bowel follow-through, enteroclysis, contrast enema) can provide specific localization of the point of obstruction and may identify the nature of the underlying lesion. When obstruction of the small intestine is not progressing or resolving, a small bowel follow-through is indicated to confirm the presence and location of the obstruction. Also, even under acute circumstances, diagnosis and management of colonic obstruction are generally enhanced by the use of a contrast enema.

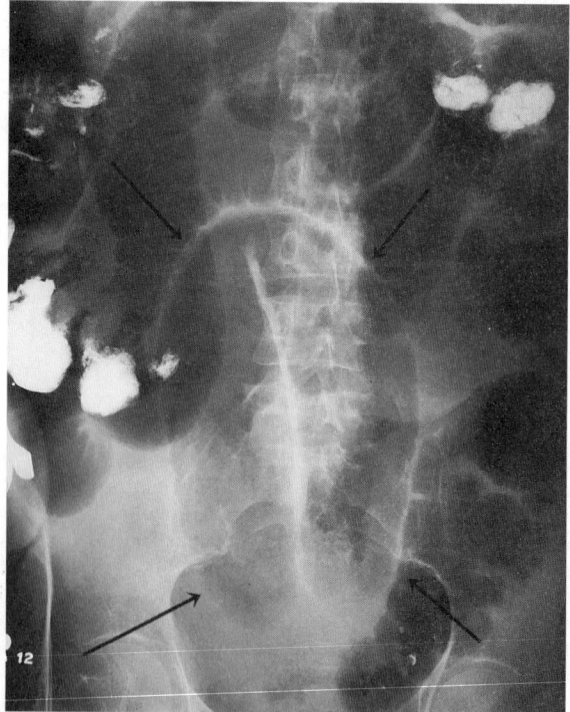

Figure 27-4. Plain supine abdominal film of a patient with sigmoid volvulus. The centrally located sigmoid loop is outlined by trapped air (*arrows*). The proximal small intestine is dilated as well, suggesting that the volvulus has been present for sufficient time to cause accumulation of air and fluid proximally. (Courtesy of John Braver, MD, Department of Radiology, Brigham and Women's Hospital, Harvard Medical School, Boston)

3. Additional abdominal pathology (eg, metastases, ascites, parenchymal liver abnormalities) can be identified.

Evidence also suggests that CT can improve preoperative detection of strangulation in certain circumstances.[41,42] Findings at the site of obstruction include beaklike narrowing, mesenteric edema or vascular engorgement, moderate to severe wall thickening, and intramural air (pneumatosis). A recent study also suggested that real-time abdominal sonography can aid in the diagnosis of strangulation obstruction. The presence of significant amounts of peritoneal fluid and of an akinetic and dilated loop of bowel is strongly associated with strangulation.[43] In 15 patients who had strangulation but who were thought to have simple obstruction only, these findings helped to make the preoperative diagnosis of infarction. The role of CT and real-time ultrasound in the early detection of strangulation seems promising. Again, when the clinical picture suggests strangulation, unnecessary imaging studies should not delay resuscitation or expeditious transfer to the operating room. Such studies are not necessarily helpful when clinical criteria and basic abdominal radiographs indicate the presence of a simple and complete obstruction. By itself, this diagnosis mandates urgent exploration, and the information sought should be weighed against the risk of delaying surgery.

General Considerations in Management of the Patient With Bowel Obstruction

The presentation of small bowel obstruction depends on the level of obstruction, the open- or closed-loop nature, and the interval since the onset of symptoms. Pain, vomiting, obstipation, and distention are present in variable degrees. Patients with obstruction of the large bowel present with abdominal pain, distention, and obstipation. Vomiting and acute fluid and electrolyte imbalances are sometimes prominent. Elderly patients are prone to dehydration. The overall picture, however, is usually one of a patient with abdominal symptoms that are evolving and getting worse. In the settings described here, the following questions must be addressed as expeditiously as possible:

1. Is the pain out of proportion to the physical findings?
2. How rapidly are the symptoms and signs evolving (minutes, hours, or more slowly)?
3. Does the patient suffer from dehydration and serum electrolyte and pH imbalances?
4. Is the obstruction complete or incomplete?
5. Is there a possibility of strangulation?

Clinical data and basic laboratory studies provide reliable information to answer the first three questions. Answering questions 4 and 5 often depends on close clinical observation and reexamination in the first hours or days after presentation. Abdominal radiographs and imaging studies are frequently used to provide additional information to help answer the last questions; they also provide information to identify the obstructing lesion.

The principles of diagnosis and management of bowel obstruction begin with clinical information. Laboratory studies and plain abdominal films are used to confirm the diagnosis of obstruction and to determine the extent of physiologic impairment. The patient's history and clinical course in the first few hours of observation are used to determine the likelihood of strangulation. Indications for surgery include rapid evolution of symptoms and signs and diagnosis that the obstruction is complete. Contrast or imaging studies are used only when symptoms are not

evolving rapidly and when identification of the underlying lesion might alter the operative strategy.

The initial management of all patients with suspected bowel obstruction includes restricting oral intake and starting infusion of intravenous isotonic Ringer or normal saline solution. Restoration of fluid and electrolyte balance is a priority, often requiring frequent evaluation of serum electrolytes and pH. In rapidly evolving cases or in patients with significant dehydration, an indwelling urinary catheter should be placed to monitor urine output. Invasive hemodynamic monitoring (eg, with a Swan-Ganz catheter) may be necessary to monitor the response to fluid resuscitation in patients with underlying cardiac, pulmonary, or renal insufficiency. Nasogastric decompression is indicated in all but the most mild cases. The nasogastric tube serves to prevent distal passage of swallowed air and minimizes the discomfort of refluxing intestinal content. The use of longer tubes has been advocated in certain settings, especially for patients with chronic but intermittent obstruction arising from Crohn's disease, peritoneal carcinomatosis, radiation enteritis, or many previous laparotomies for obstruction. The underlying rationale is that advancement of the tip of the long tube to the obstructed loop would permit more effective decompression, perhaps resulting in relaxation of the loop and relief of the obstruction. Although this concept is appealing, no well-designed trials have been performed to support the use of the long tube in such settings.[44]

Studies in humans have demonstrated that, even in simple obstruction, bacteria can translocate across the intestinal mucosa, passing into lymph channels.[45] Furthermore, experimental studies have demonstrated that germ-free animals can survive strangulation obstruction longer than normal animals and that luminal fluid taken from obstructed segments in germ-free animals is much less toxic than fluid taken from normal animals.[46,47] It is well established that perioperatively administered antibiotics reduce wound infection and abdominal sepsis rates in patients undergoing operation to relieve intestinal obstruction, simple or strangulated. Once the decision has been made to proceed with surgery, broad-spectrum antibiotics covering gram-negative aerobes and anaerobes should be administered. The use of antibiotics in patients who have not yet been committed to operation has not been evaluated systematically. Giving antibiotics to patients who are being observed can obscure the underlying process and, in the end, delay optimal therapy.

The decision to perform abdominal exploration to relieve intestinal obstruction should be made expeditiously, but not in the absence of critical information or before adequate resuscitation. When the diagnosis of bowel obstruction is likely or certain, indications for surgery include the following:

- Rapidly progressing abdominal pain or distention, with or without peritoneal findings
- Development of peritoneal findings, fever, diminished urine output, leukocytosis, hyperamylasemia, metabolic acidosis
- Failure of obstructive picture to resolve in 24 to 48 hours, even in the absence of evolving symptoms or peritoneal findings

Once a diagnosis of complete obstruction is made, whether simple or strangulated, operation should proceed without undue delay. It is reasonable to commit the patient to a period of observation if the diagnosis is uncertain, if there is a possibility of a nonsurgical diagnosis, or if the obstruction is not complete. A practical point is that obstruction occurring in a patient without a previous history of laparotomy is not likely to be caused by peritoneal adhesions.

This is known as de novo obstruction and, whatever the underlying cause, usually does not resolve without surgery.

Specific Types of Bowel Obstruction

Adhesions

Peritoneal adhesions account for more than half of small bowel obstruction cases. Lower abdominal procedures such as appendectomy, hysterectomy, and abdominoperineal resection are common precursor operations to adhesive obstruction. Adhesions form after any abdominal procedure, however, including cholecystectomy, gastrectomy, and abdominal vascular procedures. In long-term follow-up, about 5% of patients undergoing laparotomy develop adhesive obstruction; of these, 10% to 30% suffer additional episodes.[48] Simple adhesive obstruction is distinguished from most other forms of obstruction by its capacity to resolve without surgical intervention. According to recent surveys, up to 80% of episodes of small bowel obstruction caused by adhesions resolve nonoperatively.[32,33,38,42,44,49] This observation makes it difficult to distinguish a complete mechanical obstruction that resolves nonoperatively from a partial obstruction that never was complete. From a practical standpoint, the distinction does not matter. A history of a laparotomy simply provides a reasonable basis for expectant management of patients in whom it is not yet possible to diagnose a complete obstruction. Ultimately, patients who present with signs and symptoms of bowel obstruction are treated according to the clinical course.

The pathobiology of adhesion formation has been the subject of considerable investigation. Histologic examination of chronic adhesions reveals foreign-body reaction, usually to talc, starch, lint, intestinal content, or suture.

Talc and starch are found less often than previously because of improvements in the techniques of surgical glove manufacture and sterilization. Mesothelial cells are the presumed origin of tissue plasminogen activator (TPA). TPA binds fibrin and plasminogen, thereby preventing adhesion formation. Inflammatory cells, including mast cells, appear to be significant in the process that produces adhesions, but the cell biology of their contributions is not yet defined.[50] A number of experimental approaches have been tried to reduce adhesion formation, including peritoneal exposure to TPA, phosphatidylcholine, vitamin E, polyethylene glycol, high-molecular-weight dextrans, and polypentapeptide of elastin. The benefit of such strategies in reducing the incidence of small bowel obstruction has not been proved. The most reasonable approach to reducing adhesion formation includes meticulous attention to hemostasis, gentle surgical technique, and removal of foreign material from the peritoneal cavity. It is also possible that the use of monofilament sutures for fascial closure and avoidance of closure of the peritoneum as a separate layer lower the formation of adhesions between viscera and the abdominal wall.[51]

Early Postoperative Adhesions

Obstruction immediately after abdominal surgery is uncommon but occurs in up to 1% of patients during the 4 weeks after laparotomy. Adhesions are responsible for about 90% of such cases and hernias for about 7%. Intussusception, abscess, or technical errors are be responsible for the remainder of cases.[52,53] Most cases occur after surgery of the colon, especially abdominoperineal resections, or operations in the lower abdomen. It is rare for upper abdominal surgery to cause such obstructions. Patients with acutely evolving symptoms and signs represent cases

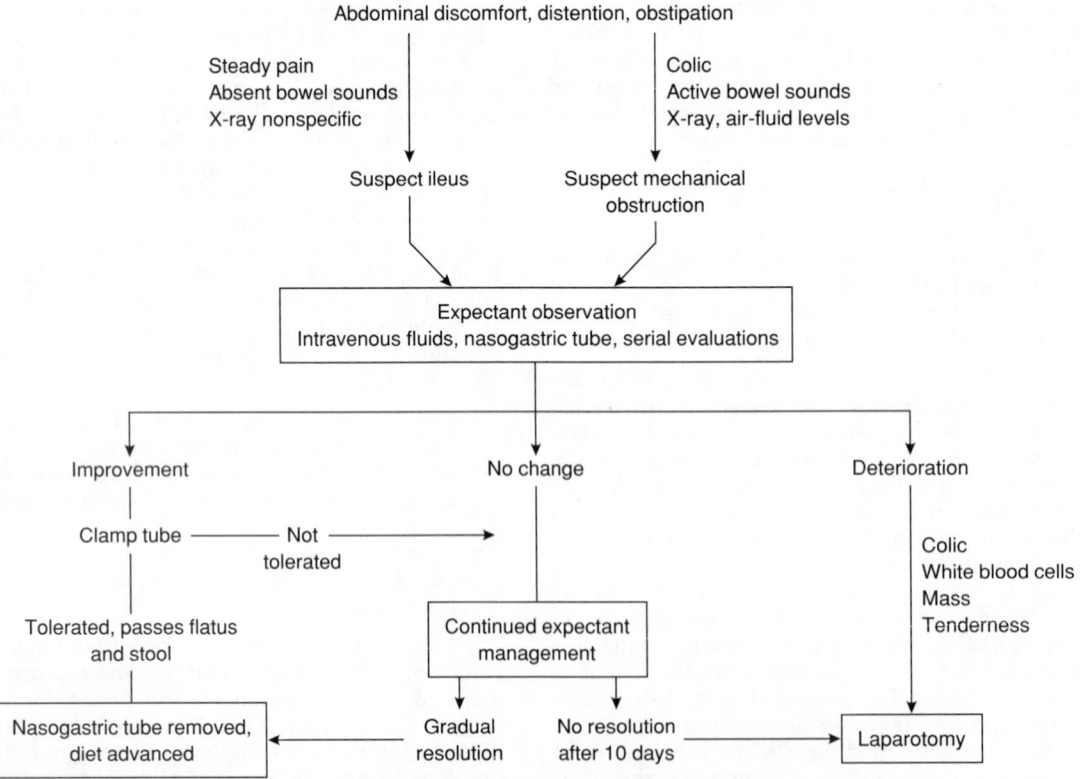

Figure 27-5. An approach to postoperative intestinal obstruction. (Adapted from Welch JP. Bowel obstruction: differential diagnosis and clinical management. Philadelphia, WB. Saunders, 1989)

of complete obstruction and should be treated as such. In this setting, the mortality rate may be as high as 15% because of delays in recognition and operative intervention. The loss of bowel sounds after a short period of normal or hyperactive activity is worrisome for ischemia of the obstructed segment. Most cases can be treated as partial intestinal obstruction; with use of nasogastric suction and intravenous fluids, symptoms usually resolve within a few days (Fig. 27-5). When the clinical course does not demand earlier intervention, a nonoperative approach can be tried for 10 to 14 days; this corrects the obstruction in over 75% of cases.[54,55]

Hernia

Hernias of all types are second only to adhesions as the most frequent causes of obstruction. External hernias, such as inguinal or femoral hernias, may present with the symptoms of obstruction. Femoral hernias are particularly prone to incarceration and bowel necrosis because of the small size of the hernia inlet.[56] Internal hernias, including obturator hernias, paraduodenal hernias, and hernias through the foramen of Winslow or mesenteries, are usually diagnosed at laparotomy for obstruction. When herniation is the cause of the obstruction, the patient is quickly resuscitated and taken to the operating room. The hernia is re-

duced and the viability of the bowel assessed. If viable, the bowel is left alone; if not, it is resected. The hernial defect is then repaired. One important consideration is the Richter hernia. In this variant, only a portion of the wall of the bowel is incarcerated. These hernias occur most frequently in association with femoral or inguinal hernias. Complete obstruction can occur if more than half to two thirds of the bowel circumference is incarcerated.

Gallstone Ileus

As a result of intense inflammation surrounding a gallstone, a fistula may develop between the biliary tree and the small or large intestine. Most fistulas develop between the gallbladder fundus and duodenum. If the stone is more than 2.5 cm in diameter, it can lodge in the narrowest portion of the terminal ileum, which is just proximal to the ileocecal valve. This complication is rare, accounting for fewer than 6 in 1000 cases of cholelithiasis and no more than 3% of cases of intestinal obstruction. Typically, the patient is elderly and presents with intermittent symptoms over several days, as the stone tumbles distally toward the ileum. The classic findings on plain radiographs include intestinal obstruction, a stone lying outside the right upper quadrant, and air in the biliary tree (Fig. 27-6).

Treatment includes removal of the stone and resection

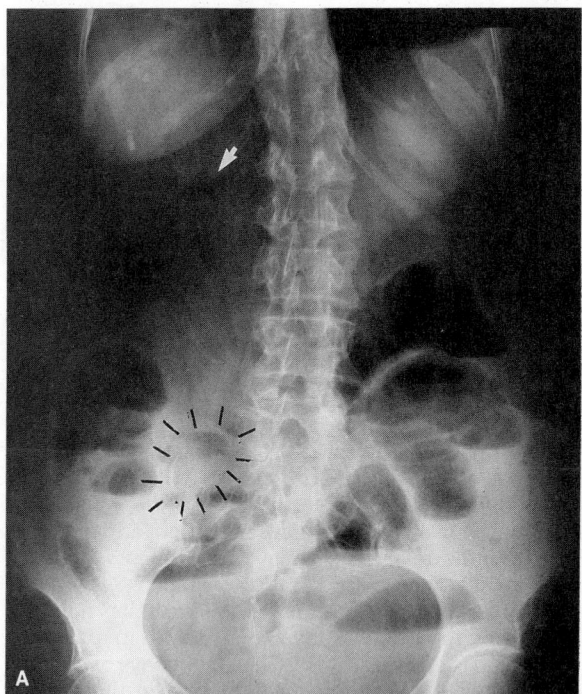

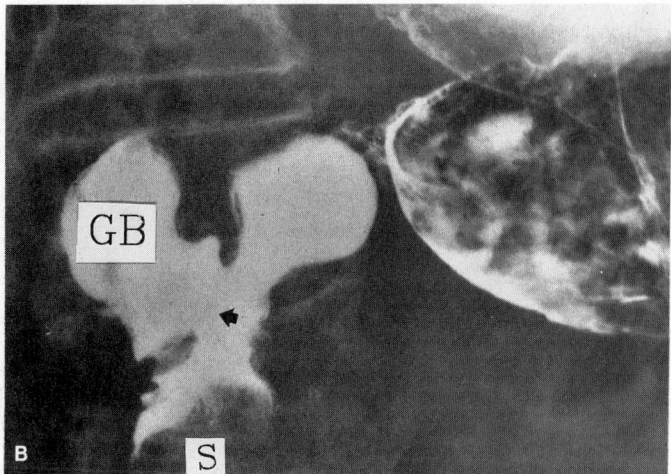

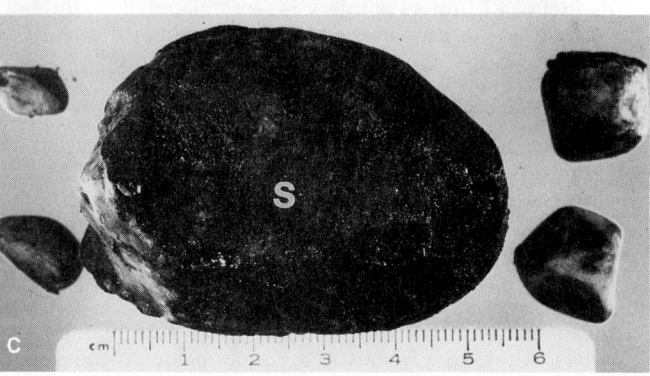

Figure 27-6. (*A*) Plain radiograph of a patient with gallstone ileus, showing air in the biliary tree (*arrows*) and a gallstone (*highlights*) outside the right upper quadrant. (*B*) Upper gastrointestinal radiograph showing a cholecystoduodenal fistula (*arrow*) with a large stone (S) obstructing the duodenum. (*C*) Stones recovered from the duodenum and mall stones found distally in the small intestine (*B* from Fromm D. Small intestine. In: Gastrointestinal surgery. New York, Churchill Livingstone, 1985)

of the obstructed bowel segment if there is evidence of tissue necrosis. The difficult decisions in management relate to the biliary tract. Arguments in favor of resecting the biliary fistula and removing the gallbladder include the possibility of recurrence of gallstone ileus and the risk of cholangitis because of reflux of intestinal content into the biliary tree. When operation on the biliary fistula is performed, the mortality rate doubles relative to that of simple removal of the gallstone. The long-term incidence of biliary tract infections has not been high enough to warrant an aggressive approach at the initial operation. Some investigators have advocated cholecystectomy at a second operation, especially if the patient is young and fit. Except in highly selected patients, cholecystectomy should not be performed at the initial operation for gallstone ileus. The entire intestine should be carefully searched to exclude the possibility of additional large stones. The risk of a recurrent gallstone ileus is about 5% to 10%.[57] Recurrences typically occur within 30 days of the initial episode and are usually caused by stones in the small intestine that were missed at the original operation.

Intussusception

About 5% of intussusception cases occur in adults. An intussusception occurs when one segment of bowel telescopes into an adjacent segment, resulting in obstruction and ischemic injury to the intussuscepting segment (Fig. 27-7). The obstruction may become complete, particularly if tissue inflammation and necrosis occur. Ninety percent of adult cases are associated with pathologic processes. Tumors, benign or malignant, act as the lead point of intussusception in over 65% of adult cases. A significant proportion of cases have been reported to occur after abdomi-

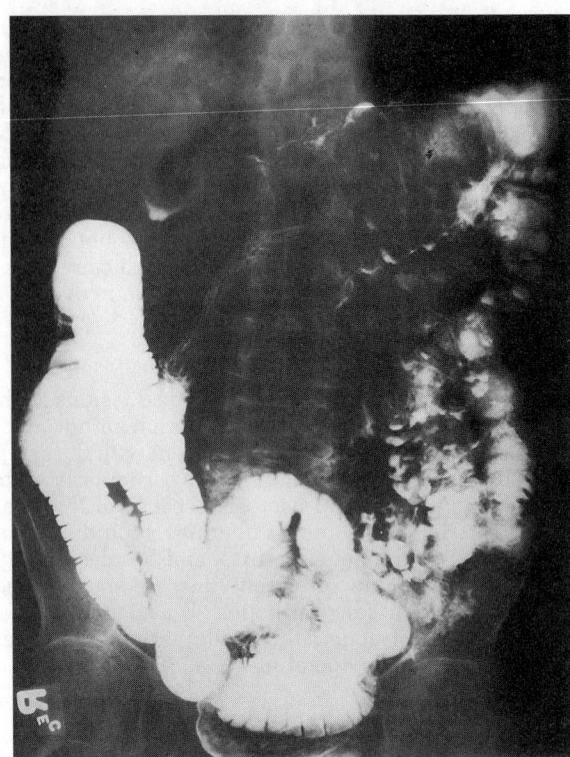

Figure 27-8. Barium enema showing intussusception of ileum (*arrows*) into ascending colon shortly after a cecectomy for tumor with ileal to ascending colon anastomosis. (Courtesy of John Braver, MD, Department of Radiology, Brigham and Women's Hospital, Harvard Medical School, Boston)

nal surgery for other lesions. In the postoperative period, 20% relate to the suture line, 30% to adhesions, and 50% to intestinal tubes.[58] Intussusception related to long tubes can occur when the tube is withdrawn but most frequently occurs with the tube in place. Perioperative intussusception frequently subsides without intervention.[58]

Four types of intussusception are recognized: enteric, ileocolic, ileocecal, and colonic. In the ileocolic form, the ileum telescopes into the colon past a fixed ileocecal valve. In the ileocecal form, the valve itself is the lead point of the intussusception.

Radiographic features of intussusception are not specific. Plain films reveal evidence of partial or complete obstruction. Occasionally, a sausage-shaped soft tissue density, outlined by two strips of air, is seen. It has recently been suggested that sonography may be useful in diagnosis in both pediatric and adult cases. The mainstays of diagnosis are contrast studies (Fig. 27-8). Because of the high incidence of tumors, surgery is recommended. Reduction by hydrostatic pressure, which is the standard of care in pediatric cases, should not be attempted.

Crohn's Disease

Intestinal obstruction is the most frequent indication for surgery in patients with Crohn's disease.[59,60] In this disease, obstruction occurs under two different sets of circumstances. When the disease flares acutely, the lumen may be narrowed by a reversible inflammatory process. The result is an open-loop obstruction that may respond to intravenous hydration and nasogastric decompression and to therapy with corticosteroids or other antiinflammatory drugs. Alternatively, obstruction can occur in the setting of a chronic stricture. Chronic strictures do not respond to

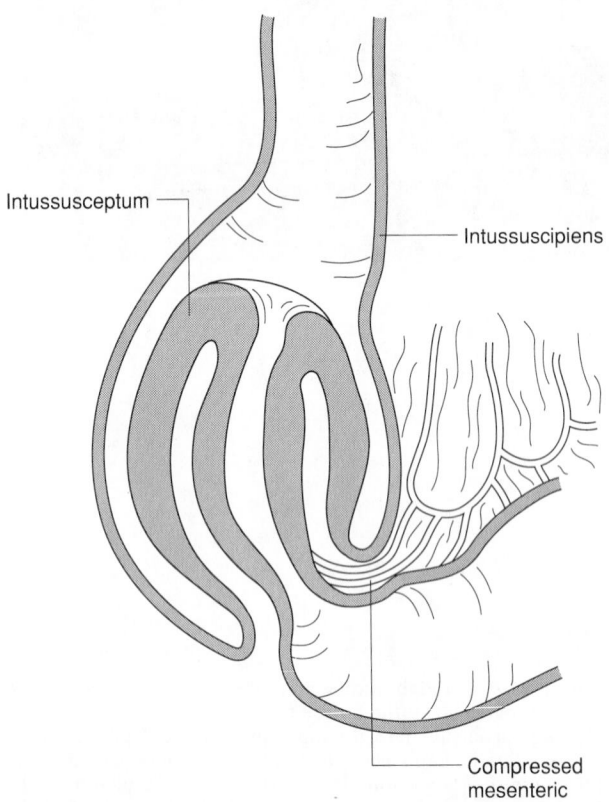

Figure 27-7. Anatomy of intussusception. The intussusceptum is the segment of bowel that invaginates into the intussuscipiens.

conservative measures; when they are diagnosed, operative therapy should not be delayed. Affected bowel may not dilate proximal to the obstruction but can develop a small perforation. Such a microperforation may not be large enough to be associated with free air on plain films. The patient may present with significant abdominal pain and tenderness. A CT scan is sensitive in differentiating conditions that require immediate surgery (closed-loop obstruction, microperforation) from simple obstruction that would otherwise be managed nonoperatively. In the absence of clinical progression of symptoms and signs, extended conservative management is warranted before the patient is committed to surgery.

Malignant Obstruction

Obstruction can complicate malignancies of the small and large bowel in a number of settings. Most commonly, a primary lesion such as an adenocarcinoma or a lymphoma enlarges until the lumen of the intestine is blocked. The lesion then presents with symptoms and signs associated with the level of obstruction. Another setting involves a patient who previously has undergone surgery for malignancy and now returns with evidence of bowel obstruction. The likelihood that the obstruction is caused by recurrent disease relates to several factors:

- The origin of the primary malignancy
- The stage of the primary malignancy
- The designation of the original surgery as curative or palliative

Gastric and pancreatic carcinomas often present with or are subsequently complicated by peritoneal carcinomatosis and ensuing obstruction. With respect to colon and rectal carcinomas, as many as half of cases of obstruction after resection of the primary tumor are caused by adhesions and not recurrent malignancy.[61] In addition, even if obstruction is caused by unresectable disease, significant palliation can be obtained through bypass or enterostomy in 75% of patients (Fig. 27-9).

Volvulus

The term *volvulus* indicates that a loop of bowel is twisted more than 180 degrees about the axis of its mesentery. Volvulus has been reported for the cecum, transverse colon, splenic flexure, and sigmoid colon. A special variant of volvulus, complicating a condition known as Chilaiditi syndrome, can occur when redundant loops of the transverse colon slip between the liver and diaphragm and then twist.[62] The most common site for volvulus is the sigmoid colon, accounting for 65% of cases.[63] By definition, a vol-

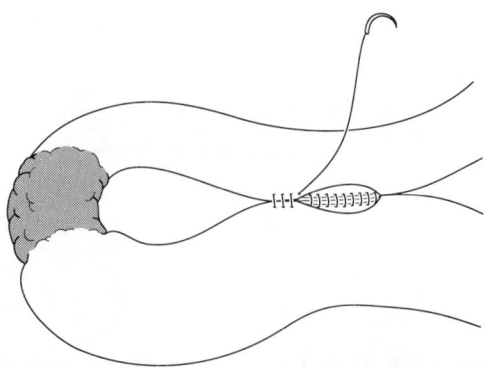

Figure 27-9. Significant palliation can be achieved in a patient with obstructing, but unresectable, malignancy. Enteroenterostomy is performed to bypass the obstructing segment.

vulus is a form of closed-loop obstruction of the colon. Volvulus of any segment of the colon is associated with abdominal distention and, usually, severe abdominal pain. As shown in Figure 27-4, the most common radiographic features include the bent inner tube appearance of the sigmoid. The preferred method of management involves endoscopic decompression. A flexible sigmoidoscope is advanced gently into the rectum until a rush of air and feces indicates that the loop has been detorsed. A rectal tube is then advanced into the loop as a stent to prevent twisting again. Gangrene of the colon does not usually develop if the patient is treated promptly. This conservative approach resolves the volvulus in 85% to 90% of cases, and elective resection of the redundant segment can then be planned. After endoscopic decompression, recurrence of the volvulus is higher than 60% if sigmoid resection is not performed.[64] Semielective operation to remove the sigmoid should be performed if the patient is fit for surgery.[64,65] Most of these patients are elderly and infirm; 15% have histories of psychiatric disorder. If the patient presents with peritoneal findings, sepsis, and shock, rapid resuscitation followed by urgent resection and colostomy is warranted. Other forms of volvulus generally cannot be detorsed without operation. Fixation of the twisted segment is generally a less satisfactory solution than resection of the involved segment.

Radiation Enteritis

Radiation injury elicits an underlying vasculitis and fibrosis that lead to chronic, recurring, low-grade partial obstruction of the small intestine or cicatrization and bleeding in the colon and rectum. Operation is indicated for incapacitating symptoms but is associated with increased risk. Attempts to suture scarred loops can result in chronic inflammation and the formation of interloop abscesses and fistulas. The incidence of suture line leak is high.

Role of Laparoscopy in the Management of Small Bowel Obstruction

Since the advent of laparoscopically assisted techniques for general abdominal surgery, a number of investigators have reported the feasibility of laparoscopic approaches to obstruction of the small or large bowel. Laparoscopy has been used for lysis of adhesions, enterolithotomy for gallstone ileus, and fixation of volvulus segments. Laparoscopic approaches to all forms of abdominal surgery have been advocated as a way of reducing the formation of adhesions and thus reducing the long-term risk for adhesive small bowel obstruction. This benefit has not yet been documented. In a number of anecdotal case reports, bowel obstruction has been observed as a complication of laparoscopic procedures. Specific lesions causing obstruction include Richter hernias resulting from entrapment of bowel in trocar entry sites or in unrecognized internal or abdominal wall hernias. The incidence of these complications in large series has not been published but should diminish with improvements in trocar design and operator experience.

ILEUS AND PSEUDOOBSTRUCTION
Ileus
Etiologic Factors

Ileus reflects underlying alterations in motility of the gastrointestinal tract, leading to functional obstruction. From a practical standpoint, ileus represents the interval between abdominal exploration and the reappearance of flatus and bowel movements. Our understanding of the

Table 27-3. POTENTIAL CONTRIBUTIONS TO PROLONGED ILEUS

NEUROGENIC

Spinal cord lesions or injury
Retroperitoneal process, hematoma, tumor
Ureteral colic

METABOLIC

Hypokalemia
Uremia
Ca^{2+}, Mg^{2+} imbalance
Hypothyroidism
Diabetic coma or ketoacidosis

PHARMACOLOGIC

Anticholinergics
Opiates
Autonomic blockers
Antihistamines
Psychotropics
Phenothiazines
Haloperidol
Tricyclic antidepressants
Clonidine
Vincristine

INFECTIOUS

Systemic sepsis
Pneumonia
Peritonitis
Herpes zoster
Tetanus
Bacterial overgrowth of bowel

physiology of ileus has been hindered by the insensitivity of techniques for studying gastrointestinal motility. Clinically, bowel sounds and passage of flatus have been used to follow postoperative progress. Electromyographic or intraluminal pressure recordings have proved to be reproducible and more objective but have not necessarily correlated with the ability of the different segments of the bowel to coordinate propulsion of gas and liquid from the stomach to the rectum. More recently, the distribution of radiolabeled $^{51}CrO_4$, as it is propelled aborally, has been used as a marker of intestinal transit. When radioactive markers are given orally after laparotomy, they remain in the stomach for 12 to 24 hours. Although such markers move into the small intestine rapidly, and electromyographic activity seems normal by 4 to 6 hours after laparotomy, the markers can remain in the small intestine for 3 to 5 days before moving to the transverse colon and beyond for defecation.[66] Peritonitis or spillage of noxious material (acid, bile, stool) leads to increases in delay of marker passage.

A number of factors have been implicated in the development and persistence of ileus (Table 27-3). These include sympathetic neuronal hyperactivity and increases in endogenous opioid release and other peptides, such as calcitonin gene-related peptide or motilin.[66-69] Use of anticholinergic medications and narcotics delays recovery from ileus.[70,71] In clinical studies, the use of patient-controlled analgesia delivered intravenously delays recovery from ileus compared with the intramuscular route.[71] Also implicated have been solute and electrolyte disturbances such as hypokalemia and hypercalcemia or hypocalcemia and hypomagnesemia, uremia, diabetic ketoacidosis, and metabolic conditions such as hypothyroidism. In the current era of laparoscopically assisted general abdominal surgery, it appears that less invasive access and manipulation of the bowel may decrease the interval between operation and the passage of flatus and stool.[72] There is also evidence that the interval to toleration of oral diets is shorter than previously thought for patients undergoing laparotomy or laparoscopy.[73]

Diagnosis

Because ileus is a predictable consequence of laparotomy, it is important to distinguish normal *postoperative* ileus from what some authors have termed *paralytic* ileus. The distinction is based on time since operation and clinical circumstances. For example, for a patient who has undergone elective cholecystectomy, the normal period for the ileus should not be more than 48 hours. For the patient who has undergone a low anterior resection of the colon, 3 to 5 days before passage of flatus would not be unexpected. Thus, the absence of bowel sounds, flatus, or bowel movements beyond the expected period indicates delayed resolution.

When the patient's postoperative ileus has extended beyond the expected period, plain films of the abdomen reveal gas in segments of both the small and large bowel (Fig. 27-10). The patient may experience discomfort and distention as swallowed air fills loops that do not have effective peristalsis. The differential diagnosis includes mechanical obstruction from early postoperative adhesions (see earlier). To differentiate early postoperative obstruction from ileus, contrast studies or a CT scan is help-

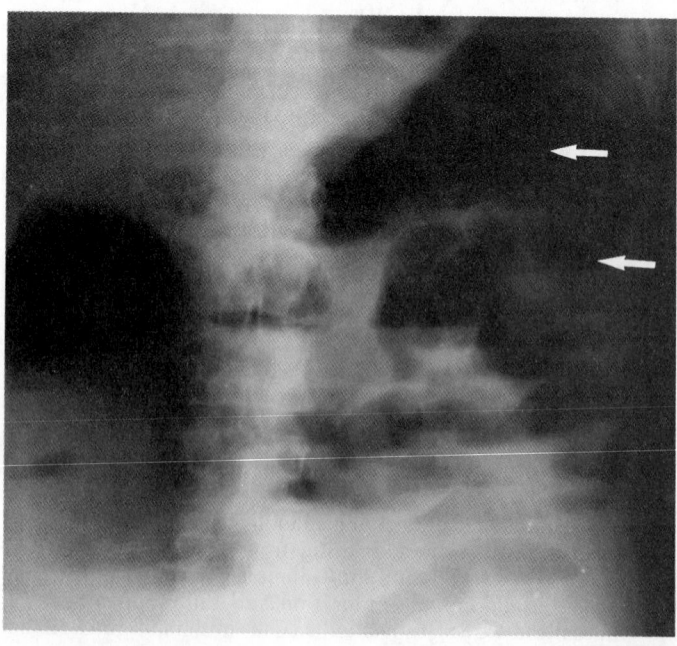

Figure 27-10. Plain upright abdominal radiograph of a patient with ileus. Air-fluid levels are present in the stomach and small intestine (*arrows*). Gas is seen in the colon. These findings are characteristic of, but not specific for, ileus.

ful. The latter may be useful if other abdominal pathology, such as an abscess, could be contributing to the clinical picture. The flow of contrast to the large bowel excludes the diagnosis of complete small bowel obstruction but does not necessarily exclude a partial obstruction.

Management

A number of interventions have been advocated for reducing the period of ileus. In recent years, prokinetic agents such as metoclopramide, cisapride, and erythromycin have been evaluated in this clinical setting. For certain forms of upper gastrointestinal ileus (eg, after a Whipple procedure), such medications may be effective in promoting gastric emptying.[74] There has been little success in using these agents to shorten recovery times after lower abdominal procedures.[75,76] Recent experimental studies have used pharmacologic interventions specifically directed at abnormal release of neurotransmitters or hormones that might prolong ileus. Agents as diverse as opioid antagonists, a somatostatin analogue, sympatholytic agents, local anesthetics, and nonsteroidal antiinflammatory drugs such as ketorolac promote faster recovery to normal myoelectric activity and shorten intestinal transit times.[67-69,72,77,78] Few of these interventions have been evaluated clinically. Measures to prevent prolongation of ileus include meticulous technique in the operating room, minimal use of narcotics for analgesia, correction of electrolyte or metabolic imbalances, and early recognition of septic complications that may contribute to prolongation beyond the expected period for ileus.

Colonic Pseudoobstruction

Etiologic Factors

Acute pseudoobstruction of the colon, also known as Ogilvie syndrome, is an often painless paralytic ileus of the large bowel characterized by rapidly progressive abdominal distention. Plain radiographs of the abdomen may reveal air in the small bowel and distention of discrete segments of the colon (cecum or transverse colon) or of the entire abdominal colon. Although the distention of the colon is not caused by mechanical obstruction, the wall of the bowel, particularly that of the cecum, can become sufficiently distended so that its blood supply is compromised. Gangrene, perforation, peritonitis, and shock can follow. Major risk factors for the development of Ogilvie syndrome include severe blunt trauma, orthopedic trauma or procedures, acute cardiac events or coronary bypass surgery, acute neurologic events or neurosurgical procedures, and acute metabolic derangements.[79] Only 5% of cases occur in the absence of other conditions. Several lines of evidence suggest that Ogilvie syndrome is related, at least partly, to sympathetic nervous overactivity or interference with sacral parasympathetic efferents.

Diagnosis

The diagnosis is usually apparent from plain films. In doubtful cases, and when bowel necrosis is not a significant worry, a gentle Hypaque contrast enema can establish the nonmechanical nature of the dilation. Colonoscopy can be both therapeutic and diagnostic. Features suggesting the complication of bowel ischemia include localized tenderness, leukocytosis, metabolic acidosis, evidence of sepsis, and a rapidly deteriorating clinical course.

Management

Initial management includes resuscitation and correction of underlying metabolic or electrolyte imbalances. A nasogastric tube is helpful if the patient is vomiting and

can prevent swallowed air from passing distally. When bowel ischemia is suspected, surgery is indicated. If bowel necrosis is found, the affected segment is resected and an ileostomy or colostomy established. If the bowel is viable, a cecostomy is placed to vent the colon and prevent distention.

If distention is painless and the patient shows no signs of toxicity or bowel ischemia, expectant management is successful in about 50% of cases.[80,81] If the distention worsens so that the cecal diameter increases beyond 10 to 12 cm, or if it persists for more than 48 hours, colonoscopy is recommended. Endoscopic decompression is successful in 60% to 90% of cases,[80,81] but colonic distention can recur in up to 40%. Rectal tubes are ineffective in managing distention of the proximal colon. Such tubes can be useful in promoting passage of air and feces after colonoscopy but should not be used as temporizing measures to avoid colonoscopic decompression. In anecdotal reports, prokinetic agents such as cisapride and erythromycin have been used to treat Ogilvie syndrome with success. Successful resolution of pseudoobstruction has been reported with sympatholytic agents or spinal sympathetic block. The efficacies of these modalities have not been systematically evaluated.

REFERENCES

1. Treves F. Intestinal obstruction: its varieties, with their pathology, diagnosis, and treatment. Philadelphia, HC Lea's Son, 1884
2. Ballantyne GH. The meaning of ileus: its changing definition over three millenia. Am J Surg 1984;148:252.
3. Welch JP. History. In: Bowel obstruction: differential diagnosis and clinical management. Philadelphia, WB Saunders, 1990:3.
4. Wangensteen OH, Paine JR. Treatment of acute intestinal obstruction by suction with a duodenal tube. JAMA 1933;101:1532.
5. Paine JR, Carlson HA, Wangensteen OH. Postoperative control of distension, nausea and vomiting: clinical study with reference to employment of narcotics, cathartics, and nasal catheter suction-siphonage. JAMA 1933;100:1910.
6. Wangensteen OH, Rea CE. The distension factor in simple intestinal obstruction: an experimental study with exclusion of swallowed air by cervical esophagostomy. Surgery 1939;5:327.
7. Hartwell HJ, Hoguet JP. Experimental intestinal obstruction in dogs with special reference to the cause of death and the treatment by large amounts of normal saline solution. JAMA 1912;59:82.
8. Milamed DR, Hedley-White J. Contributions of the surgical sciences to a reduction of the mortality rate in the United States for the period 1968–1988. Ann Surg 1994;219:94.
9. Wangensteen OH. Intestinal obstructions, ed 3. Springfield, IL, Charles C Thomas, 1955.
10. Ellis H. Pathology. In: Intestinal obstruction. New York, Appleton-Century-Crofts, 1982:11.
11. Heneghan J, Robinson J, Menge H, Winistorfer B. Intestinal obstruction in germ-free dogs. Eur J Clin Invest 1981;11:285.
12. Roscher R, Oettinger W, Berger HG, et al. Bacterial microflora, endogenous endotoxin, and prostaglandins in small bowel obstruction. Am J Surg 1988;155:348.
13. Stark ME, Szurszewski JH. Role of nitric oxide in gastrointestinal and hepatic function and disease. Gastroenterology 1992;103:1928.
14. Caplan MS, Hedlund E, Hill N, MacKendrick W. The role of endogenous nitric oxide and platelet-activating factor in hypoxia-induced intestinal injury in rats. Gastroenterology 1994;106:346.
15. Kubes P. Nitric oxide modulates epithelial permeability in the feline small intestine. Am J Physiol 1992;262:G1138.
16. Barry MK, Aloisi JD, Pickering SP, Yeo CJ. Nitric oxide modulates water and electrolyte transport in the ileum. Ann Surg 1994;219:382.

17. Shields R. The absorption and secretion of fluid and electrolytes by obstructed bowel. Br J Surg 1965;52:774.

18. Sung DT, Williams LF. Intestinal secretion after intravenous fluid infusion and small bowel obstruction. Am J Surg 1971;121:91.

19. Wright HK, O'Brien JJ, Tilson MD. Water absorption in experimental closed segment obstruction of the ileum in man. Am J Surg 1971;121:96.

20. Ruf W, Suehiro G, Suehiro A, Pressler V, MacNamara JJ. Intestinal blood flow at various intraluminal pressures in the piglet with closed abdomen. Ann Surg 1980;191:157.

21. Ohman U. Studies on small intestinal obstruction. I. Intraluminal pressure in experimental low obstruction in the cat. Acta Chir Scand 1975;141:413.

22. Basson M, Fielding LP, Bilchik A, et al. Does vasoactive intestinal polypeptide mediate the pathophysiology of bowel obstruction? Am J Surg 1989;157:109.

23. Ohman U. The effects of luminal distension and obstruction on the intestinal circulation. In: Shepherd AP, Granger DN, eds. Physiology of the intestinal circulation. New York, Raven Press, 1984:321.

24. Enochsson L, Nylander G, Ohman U: Effects of intraluminal pressure on regional blood flow in obstructed and unobstructed small intestines in the rat. Am J Surg 1982;144:558.

25. Fondacaro JD. Intestinal blood flow and motility. In: Shepherd AP, Granger DN, eds. Physiology of the intestinal circulation. New York, Raven Press, 1984:107.

26. Camilleri M. Jejunal manometry in distal subacute mechanical obstruction: significance of prolonged simultaneous contractions. Gut 1989;30:468.

27. Frank JW, Sarr MG, Camilleri M. Use of gastroduodenal motility to differentiate mechanical and functional intestinal obstruction: an analysis of clinical outcome. Am J Gastroenterology 1994;89:339.

28. Summers RW, Yanda R, Prihoda M, Flantt A. Acute intestinal obstruction: an electromyographic study in dogs. Gastroenterology 1983;85:1301.

29. Fraser I. Motility changes associated with large bowel obstruction and its surgical relief. Ann R Coll Surg Engl 1984;66:321.

30. Coxon JE, Dickson C, Taylor I. Changes in colonic motility during the development of large bowel obstruction. Br J Surg 1985;72:690.

31. Eskelinen M, Ikonen J, Liponen P. Contributions of history-taking, physical examination, and computer assistance to diagnose small bowel obstruction: a prospective study of 1333 patients with acute abdominal pain. Scand J Gastroenterol 1994;29:715.

32. Stewardson RH, Bombeck CT, Nyhus LM. Critical operative management of small bowel obstruction. Ann Surg 1978;187:189.

33. Sarr MG, Bulkley GB, Zuidema GD. Preoperative recognition of intestinal strangulation obstruction: prospective evaluation of diagnostic capability. Am J Surg 1983;145:176.

34. Pain JA, Collier DS, Hanka R. Small bowel obstruction: computer-assisted prediction of strangulation at presentation. Br J Surg 1987;74:981.

35. Murray MJ, Barbose JJ, Cobb CJ. Serum D-lactate levels as a predictor of acute intestinal ischemia in a rat model. J Surg Res 1993;54:507.

36. Gollin G, Marks WH. Early detection of small intestinal ischemia by elevated circulating intestinal fatty acid binding protein (I-FABP). Surg Forum 1991;42:118.

37. Kazmierczak SC, Lott JA, Caldwell JH. Acute intestinal infarction or obstruction: search for better laboratory tests in an animal model. Clin Chem 1988;34:281.

38. Assalia A, Schein M, Kopelman D, Hirschberg A, Hashmonai M. Therapeutic effect of oral Gastrografin in adhesive, partial small bowel obstruction: a prospective randomized trial. Surgery 1994;115:433.

39. Frager D, Medwid SW, Baer JW, Mollinelli B, Friedman M. CT of small bowel obstruction: value in establishing the diagnosis and determining the degree and cause. Am J Roentgenol 1994;162:37.

40. Balthazar EJ. Geore W. Holmes lecture: CT of small bowel obstruction. Am J Roentgenol 1994;162:255.

41. Smerud MJ, Johnson CD, Stephens DH. Diagnosis of bowel infarction: a comparison of plain films and CT scans in 23 cases. Am J Roentgenol 1990;154:99.

42. Ha HK, Park CH, Kim SK, et al. CT analysis of intestinal obstruction due to adhesions: early detection of strangulation. J Comput Assist Tomogr 1993;17:386.

43. Ogata M, Imai S, Hosotani R, Aoyama H, Hayashi M, Ishikawa T. Abdominal ultrasonography for the diagnosis of strangulation in small bowel obstruction. Br J Surg 1994;81:421.

44. Brolin RE, Krasna MJ, Mast BA. Use of tubes and radiographs in the management of small bowel obstruction. Ann Surg 1987;206:126.

45. Deitch EA. Simple intestinal obstruction causes bacterial translocation in man. Arch Surg 1989;124:699.

46. Cohn I Jr, Floyd CE, Dresden CF, et al. Strangulation obstruction in germ-free animals. Ann Surg 1962;156:692.

47. Amundsen E, Gustafsson BE. Results of experimental intestinal strangulation obstruction in germfree rats. J Exp Med 1963;117:823.

48. Landercasper J, Cogbill TH, Merry WH, Stolee RT, Strutt PJ. Long-term outcome after hospitalization for small bowel obstruction. Arch Surg 1993;128:765.

49. Krebs HB, Goplerud DR. Mechanical intestinal obstruction in patients with gynecological disease. Am J Obstet Gynecol 1987;157:577.

50. Liebman SM, Langer JC, Marshall JS, Collins SM. Role of mast cells in peritoneal adhesion formation. Am J Surg 1993;165:127.

51. O'Leary DP, Coakley JB. The influence of suturing and sepsis on the development of post-operative peritoneal adhesions. Ann R Coll Surg Engl 1992;74:134.

52. Coletti L, Bossart PA. Intestinal obstruction in the early postoperative period. Arch Surg 1989;55:385.

53. Stewart RM, Page CP, Brender J, et al. The incidence and risk of early post-operative small bowel obstruction: a cohort study. Am J Surg 1987;154:643.

54. Pickleman J, Lee RM. The management of patients with suspected early post-operative small bowel obstruction. Ann Surg 1989;210:216.

55. Serror D, Feigin E, Szold A, et al. How conservatively can post-operative small bowel obstruction be treated? Am J Surg 1993;165:121.

56. Chamary VL. Femoral hernia: intestinal obstruction is an unrecognized source of morbidity and mortality. Br J Surg 1993;80:230.

57. Reisner RM, Cohen JR. Gallstone ileus: a review of 1001 reported cases. Am Surg 1994;60:441.

58. Sarr MG, Nagorney DM, McIlrath DC. Post-operative intussusception in the adult. Arch Surg 1981;116:144.

59. Mekhijan HS, Switz DM, Watts HD, et al. National Cooperative Crohn's Disease Study: factors determining recurrence of Crohn's disease after surgery. Gastroenterology 1979;77:907.

60. Farmer RG, Whelan G, Fazio VW. Long-term follow-up of patients with Crohn's disease. Gastroenterology 1985;88:1818.

61. Soybel D, Bliss D, Wells S. Colorectal carcinoma. Curr Probl Cancer 1987;11:259.

62. Orangio GR, Fazio VW, Winkelman E, McGonagle BA. The Chilaiditi syndrome and associated volvulus of the transverse colon: an indication for surgical therapy. Dis Colon Rectum 1986;29:653.

63. Gibney EJ. Volvulus of the sigmoid colon. Surg Gynecol Obstet 1991;173:243.

64. Wertkin MG, Aufses AH. Management of volvulus of the colon. Dis Colon Rectum 1978;21:40.

65. Peoples JB, McCafferty JC, Scher KS. Operative therapy for sigmoid volvulus: identification of risk factors affecting outcome. Dis Colon Rectum 1990;33:643.

66. Nadrowski L. Paralytic ileus: recent advances in pathophysiology and management. Curr Surg 1983;40:260.

67. Zittel TT, Reddy SN, Plourde V, Raybould HE. Role of spinal afferents and CGRP in the postoperative gastric ileus in anesthetized rats. Ann Surg 1994;219:79.

68. Cullen JJ, Eagon JC, Kelly KA. Gastrointestinal peptide hormones during postoperative ileus. Dig Dis Sci 1994;39:1179.

69. Riviere PJ, Pascaud X, Chevalier E, et al. Fedotozine reverses ileus induced by surgery or peritonitis: action at peripheral kappa opioid receptors. Gastroenterology 1993;104:724.

70. Frantzides CT, Cowles V, Salaymeh B. Morphine effects on

riod. Am J Surg 1992;163:144.

71. Stamley BK, Noble MJ, Gilliland C, et al. Comparison of patient controlled analgesia vs. intramuscular narcotics in resolution of postoperative ileus after retropubic prostatectomy. J Urol 1993;150:1434.

72. Garcia-Caballero M, Vara-Thorbeck C. The evolution of postoperative ileus after laparoscopic cholecystectomy. A comparative study with conventional cholecystectomy. Surg Endosc 1993;7:416.

73. Binderow SR, Cohen SM, Wexner SD, Nogueras JJ. Must early post-operative intake be limited to laparoscopy? Dis Colon Rectum 1994;37:584.

74. Yeo CJ, Barry MK, Sauter PK, et al. Erythromycin accelerates gastric emptying after pancreaticoduodenectomy: a prospective, randomized, placebo-controlled trial. Ann Surg 1993; 218:229.

75. Bonacini M, Quiason S, Reynolds M, et al. Effect of intravenous erythromycin on postoperative ileus. Am J Gastroenterol 1993;88:208.

76. Cheape JD, Wexner SD, James K, Jagelman DG. Does metoclopramide reduce the length of ileus after colorectal surgery? Dis Colon Rectum 1991;34:437.

77. Cullen JJ, Eagon JC, Dozois EJ, Kelly KA. Treatment of acute post-operative ileus with octreotide. Am J Surg 1993;165:113.

78. Kelley MC, Hocking MP, Marchand SD, Sninsky CA. Ketorolac prevents postoperative small intestinal ileus in rats. Am J Surg 1993;165:107.

79. Vanek VW, Al-Salti M. Acute pseudoobstruction of the colon (Ogilvie's syndrome): an analysis of 400 cases. Dis Colon Rectum 1986;29:203.

80. Love R, Starling JR, Sollinger HW, et al. Colonoscopic decompression of acute colonic pseudo-obstruction (Ogilvie's syndrome). Gastrointest Endosc 1988;34:426.

81. Strodel WE, Nostrant TT, Eckhauser FE, Dent TL. Therapeutic and diagnostic colonoscopy in nonobstructive colonic dilation. Ann Surg 1983;197:416.

CHAPTER 28

CROHN'S DISEASE

WOLFGANG H. SCHRAUT AND DAVID S. MEDICH

Since the landmark publication by Crohn and associates in 1932,[1] regional enteritis, or *Crohn's disease,* has evolved from a seemingly rare intestinal affliction to one of the major digestive tract disorders encountered in clinical practice. Crohn's disease, which affects predominantly a young, economically productive patient population, is a chronic, intermittently exacerbating condition. It is unpredictable in its course, lacks a specific therapy, and requires frequent and repeated surgical intervention. The disease has a major impact on the patients' quality of life and socioeconomic well-being and, as a consequence, becomes important in terms of health care education, policies, and economics.

DEFINITION

Crohn's disease is a chronic, transmural inflammatory condition. The process can involve the entire alimentary tract, usually discontinuously, from the mouth to the anus. The terminal ileum and proximal colon are the sites most commonly affected. Involvement of extraintestinal tissues (eg, joints, skin, eyes) is common and indicates that Crohn's disease is a systemic disorder rather than a localized intestinal disease. The course of Crohn's disease is variable and characterized by waxing and waning of histopathologic and physiologic changes and related clinical manifestations.

The causes and pathogenesis of Crohn's disease have remained elusive. Many etiologic factors have been proposed, but no single cause has been delineated conclusively. Crohn's disease may be the common manifestation of several distinct causes or of a combination of several factors.

EPIDEMIOLOGY

Since the historic description of Crohn's disease in 1932, there has been a marked increase in its reported incidence. In part, this increase reflects changes in the availability of medical care and increased awareness of the disease with an increased rate of diagnosis. Demographic surveys conducted in Scandinavia, Great Britain, Central Europe, Israel, South Africa, and the United States documented increasing incidence during the 1950s and 1960s, with stabilization during the past decades in some geographic areas and further expansion in other areas. On the basis of these surveys, certain demographic features can be associated with Crohn's disease. The worldwide prevalence is estimated to be 10 to 70 cases per 100,000 population, with an incidence of 0.5 to 6.3 cases per 100,000 population per year. The disease is almost exclusively encountered in industrialized nations of Western Europe and the United States (recognizing the lack of studies from Africa, Asia, and South America), which suggests that environmental factors are important in the pathogenesis. Although Crohn's disease is prevalent in certain populations and ethnic groups, no groups are immune to the disease.[2] Jewish people are afflicted three to eight times more often than non-Jews, and Jewish people from different countries are not equally affected. A study of the Jewish population in Tel Aviv revealed that Ashkenazi Jews born outside of Israel had a four-fold increase in incidence compared with Ashkenazi Jews born in Israel (16.69 per 100,000 versus 4.19 per 100,000 population).

Aggregation in families can occur (10% to 30% according to different reports). First- and second-generation relatives of patients with Crohn's disease in Denmark have a 10- and 3-fold increased prevalence, respectively, compared with all inhabitants of that area.[3] Parent–child and sibling–sibling aggregation is more frequent than in less close relatives, suggesting that genetic factors play a role. Although familial aggregation is noted, there is no evidence for simple mendelian transmission. HLA typing, blood group determination, and association with genetic syndromes have not uncovered genetic links.

Crohn's disease arises most commonly between 15 and 30 years of age, with a second peak at 55 to 60 years of age. Men and women are equally affected. The disease is more commonly seen in urban residents than rural dwellers and is associated with higher levels of education. Perinatal and postnatal infections, especially diarrheal illness, are found to have occurred more frequently in patients with inflammatory bowel disease than in patients without. These infections might alter the immune response in genetically susceptible people, and further immunologically stressful events later in life might trigger the clinical onset of disease.

Cigarette smoking increases the risk for Crohn's disease and also hastens clinical, endoscopic and surgical recurrence after resection.[4]

ETIOLOGIC THEORIES

The cause or causes of Crohn's disease remain unknown, despite nearly 60 years of investigation. Detection of noncaseating granulomas in the inflamed tissues has suggested infectious causes; epidemiologic findings have prompted investigations into genetic, dietary, and environmental factors; clinical response to antiinflammatory and immunosuppressive agents has encouraged research to delineate immunologic causes. Two major hypotheses have evolved. The infectious theory contends that a still unidentified microbe or agent causes the disease and that the immune system responds appropriately to the invasion. The immunologic theory (the favored theory) suggests that the immune system reacts inappropriately to antigenic challenge. In both theories, the immune system plays a major role in pathogenesis.

Infectious Causes

Given the characteristic histologic findings of granuloma formation, which resemble intestinal tuberculosis, early investigations focused on bacterial causes of Crohn's disease, most notably infection with *Mycobacterium* sp. Several reports on the isolation of mycobacteria from mesenteric lymph nodes and intestine involved in Crohn's disease have supported, but not proved, a mycobacterial cause. Positive cultures have also been recovered from patients suffering from ulcerative colitis as well as from patients without inflammatory bowel disease. Only 23% of patients with Crohn's disease have elevated mycobacterial antibody levels, and similar levels have been detected in healthy controls with purified protein derivative–positive skin tests.[5]

Studies to detect a bacterial cause of Crohn's disease have shown that one third of patients have abnormal (qualitative and quantitative) microflora in the small bowel, most likely the result of inflammation and fecal stagnation.[6] Unusual bacterial species, cell wall defective variants, and L-forms have been implicated but not confirmed as causative agents. Multiple studies, however, demonstrate that the luminal bacterial flora or their products play an important role in perpetuating the inflammatory intestinal process.

Research into viral causes has been inconclusive. Viral pathogens have been isolated from tissue extracts of patients with Crohn's disease, but linkage to the induction or persistence of Crohn's disease has not been convincing.

Immunogenetic Causes

The frequent occurrence of Crohn's disease within families suggests that the development of the disease might be genetically determined. Because the immune system appears to play a major role in the pathogenesis, many investigations have sought a linkage between Crohn's disease and gene products that regulate immunity. Such an association has not been demonstrated.

Aberrations in the mechanisms of the intestinal mucosal immune system play a major role in the development and persistence of Crohn's disease. Intensive study of the overall immune competence of patients with Crohn's disease, of isolated aspects of the enteric immune system, and of the histopathology and immunopathology of tissues has documented many immunologic alterations. Some alterations may reflect a true causative defect, whereas others may be the result of the chronic debilitating disease and its treatment or a consequence of chronic inflammatory intestinal processes. A unifying concept tying all of these findings together has not evolved, although several working models designate Crohn's disease as a disorder of the intestinal immune system.

If Crohn's disease is considered an autoimmune process, the enterocyte would be the most likely target of the immune-mediated attack (Fig. 28-1). A number of reports describe antibody and lymphocyte reactivity to enterocytes. Circulating antibodies directed against colonic epithelial cells have been detected in the serum of patients with Crohn's disease. These antibodies were found to cross-react with *Escherichia coli* 014 polysaccharide, suggesting that sensitization against *E coli* antigens would precipitate an autoimmune process directed against enterocytes.[7] The presence of antibody could not be correlated with disease activity because antibodies were found in pa-

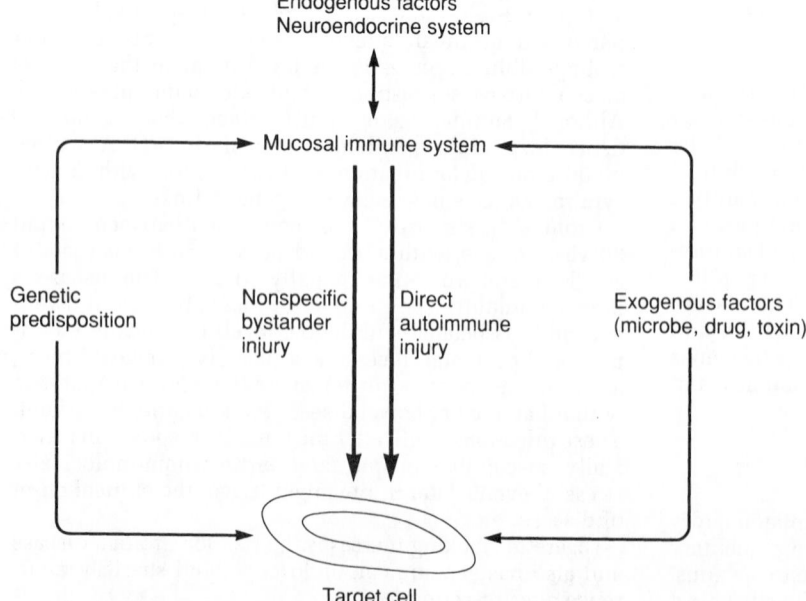

Figure 28-1. Overview of the elements that may contribute to the pathogenesis of inflammatory bowel disease. (After Shanahan F, Targan S. Immunology of inflammatory bowel disease. In: Shaffer E, Thomson ABR, eds. Modern concepts in gastroenterology, vol 2. New York, Plenum, 1989:293)

tients with other diseases and in healthy volunteers.[8] The antibodies were not found to be cytotoxic for colonic enterocytes in vitro and in vivo.[9] Lymphocyte-mediated cytotoxicity (requiring a serum immune complex or antibody) has been detected in patients with Crohn's disease, but it was directed against colonic cells and not small bowel epithelial cells, even in patients with disease limited to the small intestine.[10]

No primary defect in systemic or mucosal immunity has been identified in Crohn's disease, but numerous alterations have been reported, which indicate a disturbed immunoregulation. It is possible that an abnormal response of T cells to antigens, either an insufficient suppressor cell response or an excessive helper cell response, is important in the pathogenesis of Crohn's disease. The influence of suppressor cells has received much attention. It has been proposed that a decreased or blunted suppressor cell response to antigens results in an uninhibited immune response with elaboration of cell-, humoral-, and lymphokine-mediated tissue damage (Fig. 28-2). In this formulation, the intestinal epithelium is not the primary target but is injured as a bystander. Reports on peripheral blood and

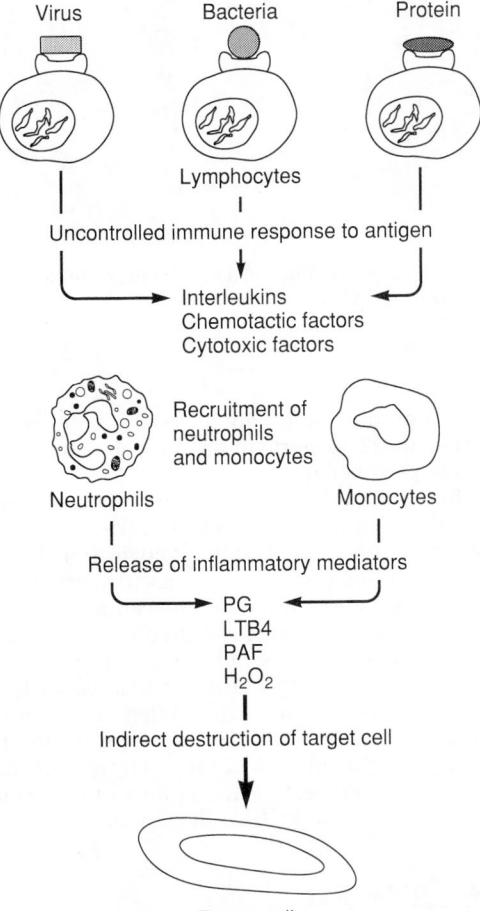

on mucosal suppressor cell activity have been contradictory, possibly because of differences in patient populations studied, variable cell tests used, and the presence of heterogeneous suppressor cell subpopulations.

In the lamina propria of intestine with active Crohn's disease, there is a two- to three-fold increase in total lymphocytes, with the greatest increase in immunoglobulin G (IgG)-producing B cells. The presence of IgG might facilitate an antigen-specific effector response with inflammatory tissue destruction. This destruction would be aided by the increase in mast cells and neutrophils. Alterations in immunoregulation involving the afferent limb have also been reported. The expression of major histocompatibility complex antigens by intestinal epithelial cells is increased in the presence of inflammation, and antigen presentation may be enhanced and may induce local mucosal immune responses to antigens that otherwise might not be processed.

Despite advances in epidemiology, bacteriology, virology, and immunology, the causes of Crohn's disease remain unknown. Although many alterations in cellular and humoral immune functions associated with Crohn's disease have been observed, no primary defect, either systemic or mucosal, humoral or cellular, has been identified. Ongoing and future research may identify the specific defects and antigens that, in concert, cause Crohn's disease. New rodent models of spontaneous colitis bring new insight into the pathogenesis question and should help to delineate further the intricacies of the mucosal immune system.[11]

PATHOLOGY

Crohn's disease can affect any part of the gastrointestinal tract. The most common site is the ileocecal region. The disease may be rapidly progressive or may run an indolent course with intermittent episodes of exacerbation. The acute, active phase is marked by aphthous mucosal ulcers, lymphoid aggregates, granulomas, and transmural chronic inflammation with fissures and fistulas. The quiescent or healing phase is characterized by fibrosis with stricture formation and chronic ulcers. The granulomatous inflammatory process may involve other tissues and organs. Histologic features include the following:

- Presence of granulomas away from ulcerations
- Presence of granulomas in lymph nodes or other organs
- Presence of lymphoid aggregates in submucosa and subserosa
- Fissures and ulcers extending into the muscularis propria
- Transmural inflammation

Macroscopic Appearance

Resected or in situ bowel segments involved by Crohn's disease are rigid and thickened as a result of fibrosis and inflammatory edema narrowing the bowel lumen. The mesenteric fat reaches over the antimesenteric bowel wall (Fig. 28-3). The serosa may be granular and dulled by exudate. The mesentery is foreshortened, thickened, and edematous and contains enlarged inflamed mesenteric lymph nodes. The inflammatory process may extend into adjacent tissues and structures, causing fistulas, abscesses, and sinus tracts. Inflammation and fibrosis often distort normal anatomic boundaries, causing ureteral deviation and obstruction or bowel obstruction with matting together of involved and uninvolved bowel loops. Fistulous communications are possible between the diseased bowel

Figure 28-2. Mucosal immune effector mechanisms that have been proposed as possible mediators of a direct specific attack against the putative target cell in inflammatory bowel disease. These may be generated in response to either an alteration in the target cell or an external agent, or they may arise from a breakdown in mucosal immune tolerance to normal host epithelial cells. PG, prostaglandin; PAF, platelet-activating factor. (After Shanahan F, Targan S. Immunology of inflammatory bowel disease. In: Shaffer E, Thomson ABR, eds. Modern concepts in gastroenterology, vol 2. New York, Plenum, 1989:293)

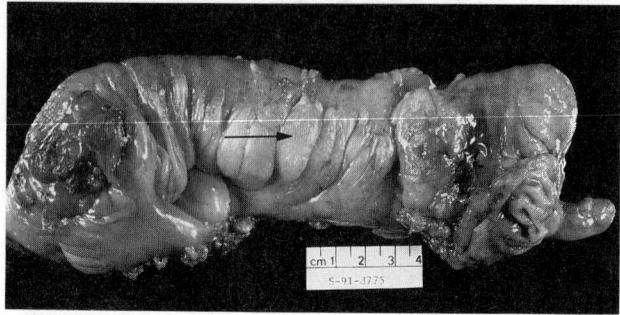

Figure 28-3. External appearance of Crohn disease involving the small intestine. The mesentery is thickened, and the mesenteric fat (*arrow*) extends over the lateral wall of the bowel (fat creeping).

and any intraabdominal and extraabdominal structure or organ.

Opening of an intestinal segment resected for Crohn's disease discloses thickening of the bowel wall, narrowing of the lumen, longitudinal ulcerations, cobblestoning, aphthoid ulcers, and dilation of proximal uninvolved bowel (Fig. 28-4).

Microscopic Features

The pathologic changes begin with a focal accumulation of inflammatory cells adjacent to a crypt. Localization at the crypt leads to aphthoid ulcers, fissure-like ulcers, and crypt abscesses (Fig. 28-5). Granulomas are localized, well-formed aggregates of epithelioid histocytes surrounded by lymphocytes and giant cells. Caseation is absent. Granulomas are not found in all patients with Crohn's disease, and the reported incidence varies greatly. On average, two thirds of patients with Crohn's disease demonstrate this finding. Fistulas and sinus tracts develop from confluent crypt abscesses and transmural inflammation. Transmural inflammation is characterized by lymphoid aggregates in a widened submucosa and similar accumulations external to the muscularis propria. Transmural inflammation is accompanied by serositis causing adherence to other loops of bowel or adjacent organs. Epithelial cell injury with necrosis is not the initial event but evolves as the inflammatory process matures. Often, the overlying mucosa is only edematous, whereas the submucosal compartment discloses edema and infiltration by lymphoid and inflammatory cells. The mature inflammatory lesion contains lymphocytes (more T cells than B cells), macrophages, and neutrophils. T cells consist of both suppressor and helper

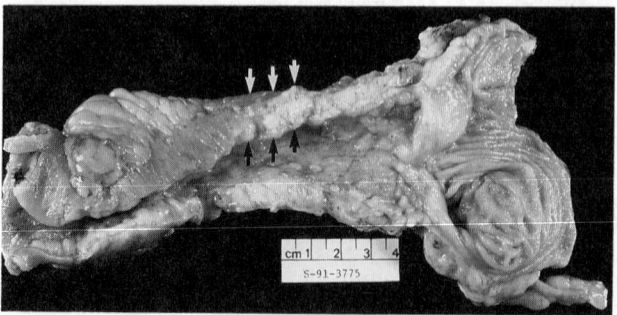

Figure 28-4. Narrow longitudinal stricture involving the ileum. Ulceration, bowel wall thickening (*arrows*), and proximal dilation of uninvolved bowel are visible.

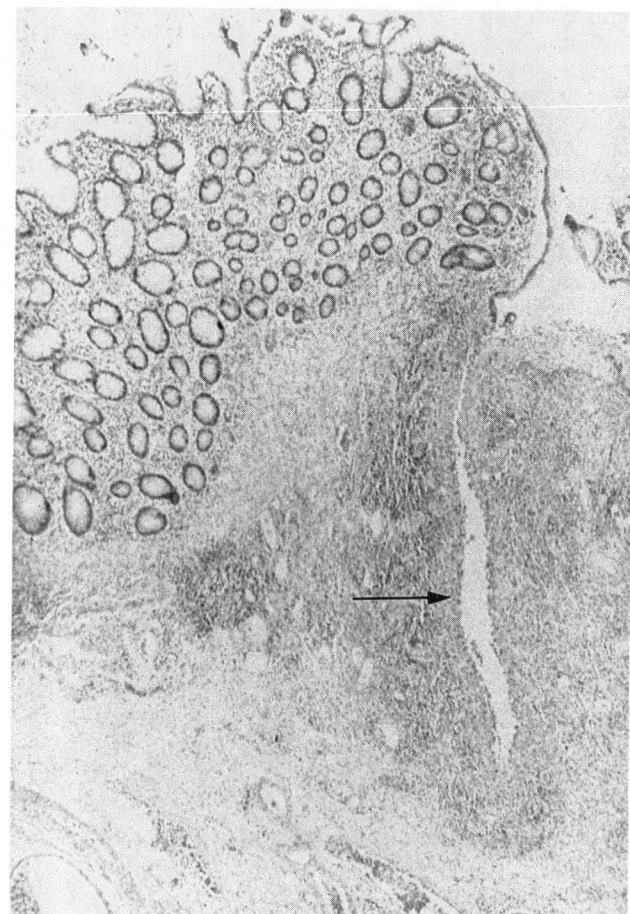

Figure 28-5. Fissure-like deep ulcer (*arrow*) surrounded by architecturally preserved villi and crypts.

cells. B cells producing IgG are more common than in the normal intestine. The most common B cell is normally the IgA-positive plasma cell.

The differentiation between Crohn's disease involving only the colon and ulcerative colitis is the most common diagnostic dilemma in the histopathologic and clinical diagnosis of inflammatory bowel disease. Ulcerative colitis is a mucosal disease that begins at the rectum and is contiguous, whereas Crohn's colitis can involve all layers of the bowel wall and is often discontinuous. Macroscopic and microscopic histopathologic features that aid differentiation are summarized in Table 28-1. When the diagnosis of either entity cannot be agreed on, the term *indeterminate colitis* is applied. About 10% of cases fall into the indeterminate category. In these instances, the clinical course of the disease determines the final diagnosis.

Clinical Features

Abdominal pain is a frequent complaint of the patient with Crohn's disease. Pain of an intermittent colicky nature is induced by distention and peristaltic contractions of the bowel as a consequence of a partial or complete bowel obstruction. A more constant pain is caused by parietal peritoneal irritation. A multifaceted approach is taken to treat the underlying problem: dietary measures relieve or avert obstruction; antiinflammatory agents decrease inflammation and edema of the diseased bowel; and antispasmodics allay cramping. A decrease of the inflam-

Table 28-1. HISTOPATHOLOGIC DIFFERENTIATION OF CROHN'S COLITIS AND ULCERATIVE COLITIS

Crohn's Colitis	Ulcerative Colitis
MACROSCOPIC	
Transmural involvement	Disease confined to mucosa except in toxic dilation
Segmental disease, fistulas	Rectum always involved
Thickened wall with "creeping fat"	Normal thickness of bowel wall
Occasional pseudopolyps	Pseudopolyps
Small bowel may be involved	Small bowel not involved (except as backwash ileitis)
Perianal disease common	Perianal disease less common
MICROSCOPIC	
Transmural inflammation and fibrosis	Inflammation of mucosa and submucosa
Crypt abscesses less common	Crypt abscesses common
Cobblestoning	Pseudopolyps
Narrow, deeply penetrating ulcers	Shallow, wide ulcers
Fissures, fistulas	
Granuloma common	Granuloma rare
Mucus secretion increased	Mucus secretion decreased

matory process is associated with lessened peritoneal irritation and pain.

Diarrhea is the result of multiple mechanisms. Mucosal inflammation decreases absorption and increases secretion. Decreased bile acid absorption (due to ileal disease or ileal resection) can lead to a diminished bile salt pool, which interferes with fat absorption. Free fatty acids decrease electrolyte and water absorption in the colon, and increased delivery of bile salts to the colon promotes osmotic diarrhea. The lack of the ileocecal valve can result in bacterial overgrowth of the small bowel, thus interfering with nutrient digestion and absorption. Complex carbohydrates reaching the colon are subject to fermentation, another potential cause of diarrhea. Several of these mechanisms may play a role in the development of diarrhea. Therapeutic approaches vary but nearly always involve dietary measures and antidiarrheals.

Anorexia, nausea, and vomiting may be precipitated by partial intestinal obstruction. The patient recognizes that these symptoms are intensified by oral intake and therefore eats less. The ensuing undernutrition reduces general health, further compromising food intake and well-being. Often, drug therapy impairs appetite and contributes to anorexia.

Nutritional deficits are not always clinically obvious, but they are usually present in the patient with Crohn's disease. Malnutrition may be global, as in caloric deficit, or may consist of isolated, specific deficits (eg, vitamins, trace elements, bile acids, electrolytes). Usually, nutritional impairment is caused by reduced or inadequate dietary intake due to anorexia, combined with disease-imposed dietary restrictions. In fact, most patients with Crohn's disease have a seemingly sufficient caloric intake, suggesting that other mechanisms play a role.[12] Inflammatory involvement of the bowel, bacterial overgrowth in partially obstructed segments, loss of absorptive surface from resections, and diarrhea may cause nutritional deficits. Caloric expenditure may be increased by chronic inflammation and superimposed infection. The catabolic effects of steroid therapy and the gastrointestinal side effects of sulfasalazine, long-term antibiotic therapy, and immunosuppressive regimens must be considered.

Clinical consequences of impaired absorption and resulting malnutrition are diverse and include the following:

- Diarrhea with dehydration and electrolyte loss
- Steatorrhea
- Gallstones
- Protein-losing enteropathy
- Growth retardation
- Anemia (microcytic, megaloblastic)
- Hypoproteinemia with edema
- Demineralization of bone
- Hypovitaminoses (B_{12}, folic acid)
- Renal oxalate stones

These consequences are particularly serious in children with Crohn's disease. Growth retardation and delayed maturation are found in 10% to 40% of children and adolescents with this disease but can be reversed or ameliorated by aggressive nutritional therapy.[13]

Patients with terminal ileal disease are prone to development of renal urate or oxalate stones. Urine volume decreases because of intestinal loss of water, and a mild ileostomy-associated metabolic acidosis leads to a lower urine pH. These changes decrease urate solubility and promote stone formation. A lack of unchelated intraluminal calcium, secondary to fatty acid saponification, enables free oxalate to reach the colon, where it is absorbed. Changes in urinary flow secondary to water loss due to diarrhea are cofactors in oxalate precipitation. Dietary measures and increased fluid intake are usually sufficient therapy. As a result of altered bile salt metabolism with the development of lithogenic bile, patients with ileal disease and ileal resections are also at risk for cholelithiasis.

The anatomic location of the disease within the gastrointestinal tract determines to a great extent the clinical features of Crohn's disease, the type of complications that occur, the indicated operative procedures, and the prognosis. Three major categories of disease are recognized—ileocolic (41% to 55%), small intestinal (30% to 40%), and colonic (14% to 26%). Certain features are linked more commonly to specific locations (Table 28-2). The following classification according to histopathologic and pathophysiologic criteria, rather than anatomic subgrouping, has been proposed:

- Stenosing, fibrosing, and stricturing Crohn's disease requiring and amenable to surgical therapy

Table 28-2. CLINICAL FEATURES OF CROHN'S DISEASE

Disease Manifestations	Site of Disease (%)		
	Small Intestine Only	Small Intestine and Colon	Colon Only
Diarrhea	87	92	88
Abdominal pain	78	79	74
Hematochezia	10	22	46
Intestinal obstruction	34	44	17
Fissures and fistulas			
Anal, perirectal	22	50	51
Internal, cutaneous	18	34	13
Systemic manifestations			
Arthritis, arthralgia	18	19	27
Iritis, uveitis	3	4	7
Liver disease	3	5	5
Skin lesions	3		8

(Donaldson RM Jr. Small and large intestine in Crohn's disease. In: Sleisinger MH, Fordtran JS, eds. Gastrointestinal disease, ed 4. Philadelphia, WB Saunders, 1989:1336)

Table 28-3. EXTRAINTESTINAL MANIFESTATIONS OF CROHN'S DISEASE

SKIN
Pyoderma gangrenosum
Erythema nodosum multiforme
Vasculitis
Aphthous stomatitis

EYES
Conjunctivitis
Iritis
Iridocyclitis, episcleritis
Uveitis
Vasculitis

JOINTS
Arthritis
Ankylosing spondylitis
Hypertrophic osteoarthropathy

LIVER
Sclerosing cholangitis
Pericholangitis (rare)
Granulomatous hepatitis (rare)

- Fistula- and abscess-forming disease approached by medical management, interventional radiology, and surgery
- Aggressive inflammatory form of disease, primarily addressed by antiinflammatory agents and immunosuppressive therapy

In most patients with Crohn's disease, the clinical picture centers around the triad of abdominal pain, diarrhea, and weight loss. These signs and symptoms have an insidious, gradual onset and are persistent and progressive, with a waxing and waning course that varies in intensity from patient to patient. The onset of Crohn's disease is nearly always obscure and poorly defined, and the diagnosis is often delayed. Vague abdominal symptoms may precede recognition and diagnosis by years. More specific complaints, such as intermittent abdominal pain, diarrhea, and episodic weight loss, usually predate a firm diagnosis by about 2 to 3 years.[14] In only 30% of patients is the diagnosis made within 1 year of the onset of symptoms. The range of ages at the time of diagnosis is wide, but 60% of cases develop before 40 years of age and 26% before 20 years of age.[14] The diagnosis is usually made during an acute exacerbation, but at times extraintestinal manifestations may be the initial clinical presentation.

More than 90% of patients with Crohn's disease have intermittent but progressive abdominal pain and diarrhea. Abdominal pain is due to partial obstruction and is worsened by oral intake. Pain is often accompanied by a tender mass in the right lower abdominal quadrant and by febrile episodes. Signs and symptoms may mimic acute appendicitis; not infrequently, they precipitate abdominal exploration to establish the diagnosis. A common manifestation of Crohn's disease is perianal disease, including anal fistulas with extension to adjacent organs and regions, fissures, and perirectal abscesses. Other common manifestations include the following:

Skin lesions

Erosion
Ulceration
Abscess
Skin tags
External hemorrhoids

Anal canal lesions

Ulcer
Stenosis
Abscess
Hemorrhoids
Fissure
Fistulas to skin
Fistulas to vagina

The prevalence of perianal disease is about 25% in patients with ileitis, 50% in patients with ileocolitis, and 40% in patients with isolated colonic involvement. Perianal disease is one of the initial signs of presentation in one third of patients.

Crohn's disease is frequently associated with extraintestinal manifestations. Infrequently, extraintestinal manifestations are the initial feature of Crohn's disease. The skin, eyes, and joints are the most common sites of extraintestinal disease, and the prevalence is higher with colonic than with small bowel disease (Table 28-3). Progressive and recurrent episodes are characteristic of Crohn's disease, and only about 20% of patients remain symptomless 10 to 20 years after the initial episode.[15] In most patients, the disease eventually advances to a stage requiring surgical intervention for alleviation of symptoms or to treat complications such as obstruction, fistula, or abscess.

Crohn's disease is a waxing and waning condition and cannot be cured by any available medical or surgical therapy. Recurrence of Crohn's disease is inevitable, given enough time, and is a major therapeutic dilemma. The definition of recurrence is variable and has included radiologic, endoscopic, pathologic, and clinical criteria as well as the need for reoperation. Using endoscopic evaluation with biopsy as the determinant of recurrent disease after resection, a recurrence rate of 79% after 1 year has been reported.[16] Not all patients have clinical symptoms or signs of a magnitude requiring reoperation.

The course of disease in children is the same as in adults, with the exception that it is frequently accompanied by growth retardation. Although Crohn's disease is progressive, the death rate is low. About 10% of affected patients die as a direct or indirect result of Crohn's disease.

COMPLICATIONS

The unpredictable chronic inflammatory process of Crohn's disease is associated with diverse complications. Small bowel obstruction is the most common complication of small bowel and ileocolonic disease. Obstruction is usually partial and intermittent in the early stages of the disease, but as inflammation and fibrosis progress, obstruction often becomes complete. Fistula formation between diseased bowel to nearly any conceivable organ or site is one of the pathognomonic features of Crohn's disease (Table 28-4). The development of fistulas is usually associated

Table 28-4. TYPES OF FISTULAS IN CROHN'S DISEASE

Type	Occurrence (%)
Enteroenteric	>20
Enterocutaneous	>20
Enterovesical, enteroureteral, enterourethral, ileosigmoid	2–6
Duodenoenteric	1–2
Enterorectal	1–2
Enterovaginal	3–5

with an inflammatory mass, fever, obstructive symptoms, and pain. Intraabdominal abscesses are classified as interloop, intramesenteric, retroperitoneal, ileopsoas, and enteroperitoneal (bounded by parietal peritoneum and abdominal viscera). These abscesses often accompany the development of a fistula and are clinically reflected by fever, onset of new or worsening abdominal pain, and an abdominal mass.

Toxic megacolon or toxic dilation is a serious complication and occurs in about 6% of patients with Crohn's disease. A similar condition has also been described for the ileum. Toxic dilation is postulated to be caused by severe submucosal inflammation, with destruction or impairment of the myenteric plexus and the muscularis propria, inducing muscular atony and bowel distention. The use of anticholinergics, antidiarrheals, and analgesics may precipitate toxic dilation. Diagnostic radiologic and endoscopic interventions are also potential risk factors for its development. The patients are acutely ill, febrile, and tachycardiac, and they have increasing abdominal pain, diarrhea, and progressive abdominal distention. An abdominal radiograph confirms the diagnosis (Fig. 28-6). Close clinical observation, repeated radiographs to detect worsening or resolution, and blood counts are recommended to time surgical intervention.

Perianal or anorectal disease can be viewed as a primary feature of Crohn's disease or as a complication. Anorectal disease has a major impact on patient well-being. Because of the lack of effective therapy, it is a particularly difficult and frustrating problem for both patient and attending physician. Fissures and edematous skin tags are most commonly seen. Fissures tend to be eccentrically situated and

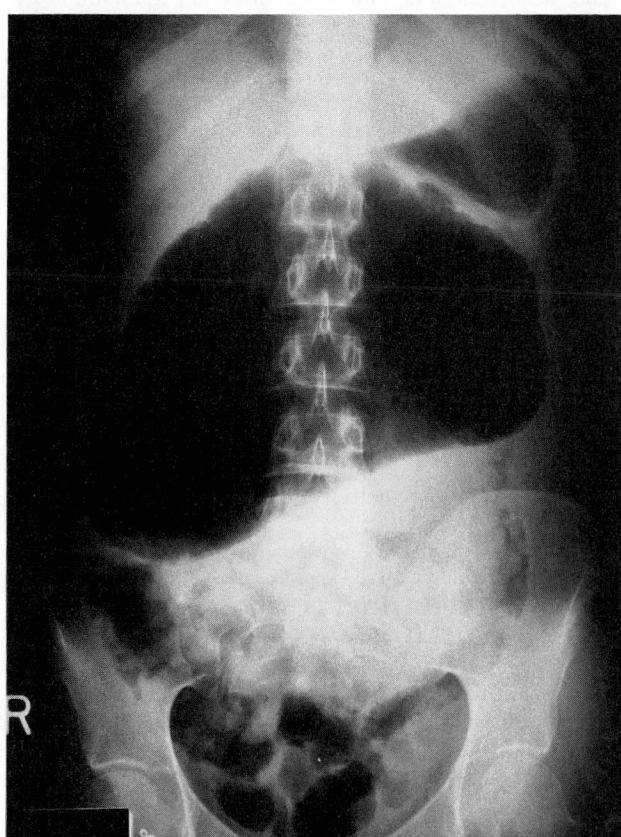

Figure 28-6. Radiograph showing toxic megacolon. Prominent dilation of the transverse colon is present. The descending colon is narrow and appears foreshortened.

surprisingly indolent given their degree of ulceration. Exacerbated by diarrhea, these lesions often progress to ulcerations, abscesses, and multiple fistulas; this may proceed to anal stricture and incontinence requiring proctectomy or diversion. Often, perianal disease is characterized by remission and recurrence, with intact anal function.

Free perforation with peritonitis, although rare, is an unequivocal indication for laparotomy. Massive intestinal bleeding, also uncommon, is caused by deep ulcerations eroding into a large submucosal vessel. Colonic disease is associated with a 20% to 30% incidence of chronic rectal bleeding. Insidious chronic blood loss leads to microcytic anemia without melena or hematochezia. In addition to these major gastrointestinal complications, a multitude of nutritional deficits and extraintestinal complications can occur. Furthermore, a number of conditions common to severely ill patients can evolve, such as thromboembolic phenomena and amyloidosis. Finally, the side effects and complications of drug therapy must be recognized.

The risk for small or large bowel carcinoma is increased in the patient with Crohn's disease. The diagnosis is often delayed because the signs and symptoms of an intestinal malignancy are similar to those of active Crohn's disease (eg, obstruction, mass, bleeding). The prognosis is usually poor by the time the carcinoma is diagnosed.

DIAGNOSIS

History and Physical Examination

A detailed history often reveals intermittent episodes of abdominal pain, diarrhea, and weight loss. Frequently, examination of the patient discloses undernutrition, pallor, and signs of malabsorption. The abdominal examination may disclose altered bowel sounds, distention, inflammatory mass or abscess, tenderness, and fistulas. Examination of the perineum and anorectum may demonstrate tender, ulcerated anal tags, eccentrically located fissures, fistulas, abscesses, rectal ulcers, and strictures. Fistulas are often extensive, with tracking into groin, genital organs, and gluteal regions.

No specific laboratory test for Crohn's disease is available. Anemia, leukocytosis, and hypoproteinemia are common. Serum orosomucoid levels, acute-phase protein levels, erythrocyte sedimentation rates, and other laboratory tests have not evolved as measures of disease activity and severity.

Endoscopic Examination

Endoscopic examination of the colon and rectum is often performed as a step in the diagnostic work-up. Colonoscopy determines the extent of the disease, confirms radiographic abnormalities, and permits biopsies of abnormal areas. Most patients have erythema and edema as a result of chronic diarrhea. In the presence of colorectal involvement by Crohn's disease, specific endoscopic features are encountered that usually allow a differentiation from ulcerative colitis—aphthous ulcers, linear ulcers, ulcers in otherwise normal-appearing mucosa, cobblestoning, and asymmetric and discontinuous involvement (Table 28-5).

Radiologic Examination

When Crohn's disease is suspected, contrast radiographs of the gastrointestinal tract are essential for differential diagnosis and delineation of the extent and severity of disease (Table 28-6). Radiologic examination is indicated for the patient with progressive disease who is ready for surgical therapy or who requires a major change in medical

Table 28-5. COLONOSCOPIC MUCOSAL FEATURES AND THEIR DIAGNOSTIC SPECIFICITY IN INFLAMMATORY BOWEL DISEASE*

Lesion	Ulcerative Colitis	Crohn's Disease
INFLAMMATION		
Distribution		
Colon		
Contiguous	+++	+
Symmetric	+++	+
Rectum	+++	+
Friability	+++ .	+
Topography		
Granularity	+++	+
Cobblestoned	+	+++
ULCERATION		
Location		
Overt colitis	+++	+
Ileum	0	++++
Discrete lesion	+	+++
Features		
Size > 1 cm	+	+++
Deep	+	++
Linear	+	+++
Aphthoid	0	++++
BRIDGING	+	++

* Specificity index range of 0 (not seen) to ++++ (diagnostic).
(Hogan WJ, Hensley GT, Geenen JE. Endoscopic evaluation of inflammatory bowel disease. Med Clin North Am 1980;64:1084)

management, and for the patient with recurrent symptoms after surgical resection. Barium contrast studies disclose a number of specific findings in patients with Crohn's disease (Fig. 28-7). The CT scan delineates masses and abscesses, and endoscopic retrograde cholangiopancreatography is used to diagnose hepatobiliary involvement (sclerosing cholangitis). A correlation between the extent of disease seen radiologically and the clinical symptoms does not exist.[17] Recurrent disease after surgical resection is often apparent radiologically (eg, stenosis, mucosal irregularity in the ileum proximal to the ileocolonic anastomosis) before the development of clinical signs and symptoms.

DIFFERENTIAL DIAGNOSIS

The signs and symptoms of Crohn's disease are nonspecific. A multitude of infections and other inflammatory conditions may warrant differential diagnostic consideration (Table 28-7). Most important is a differentiation between Crohn's disease and chronic ulcerative colitis, especially when the inflammation is limited to the colorectum. Differentiation between the two conditions does not rest on a single sign, symptom, or test result; rather, a multitude of findings are assembled that support one entity over the other. The histopathologic evaluation of biopsy material may be the diagnostic determinant in cases in which the disease is limited to the rectum. The initial diagnosis of ulcerative colitis is confirmed in 80% of instances, is changed to Crohn's colitis in 10% to 15%, and remains indeterminate in 5% to 10% when a definite diagnosis cannot be made by clinical, radiologic, and pathologic criteria. Patients with indeterminate colitis or proctitis may be assigned a determinate diagnosis by evolving signs, symptoms, and criteria characteristic of one or the other condition. Often, a long-term clinical course marked by

features of one disease more than the other permits diagnosis.

MEDICAL MANAGEMENT

Therapy for Crohn's disease includes supportive medical care with treatment of acute exacerbations and surgical therapy for complications of long-standing intestinal inflammation. The natural history of Crohn's disease, characterized by acute exacerbations and prolonged remissions, must be kept in mind in assessing the efficacy of drug therapy. Disease-specific treatment does not exist; thus, emphasis is placed on the alleviation of symptoms, nutritional support, and suppression of the inflammatory process.

Treatment of Symptoms

Abdominal Pain

Pain control by medication is frequently required as an adjuvant to therapies directed against the underlying inflammatory processes. Opiates and other analgesics must be used with great caution because these agents decrease bowel motility and increase the risk of ileus and obstruction. Antispasmodics may be used to decrease postprandial hypermotility, but extensive inhibition of peristalsis leading to an ileus or toxic dilation must be recognized and avoided.

Diarrhea

Most patients require treatment for diarrhea, a central clinical feature of Crohn's disease. Opiates and opiate derivatives have long been used, and most patients experience at least partial diminution of their symptoms. Codeine, diphenoxylate, and loperamide are the commonly used agents. They are most effective in patients whose diarrhea is caused by chronically active disease or intestinal resection. Their use during severe, acute flares has an undefined risk for developing toxic megacolon, dilation, and obstruction. Side effects are related to central nervous system depression. Loperamide is the best-tolerated drug because of its incomplete penetration of the blood–brain barrier. Cholestyramine is effective in patients with bile-salt–induced diarrhea secondary to ileal disease or resection. Dietary restriction of fats is effective for steatorrhea. In refractory cases of diarrhea, the administration of octreotide, a synthetic analogue of somatostatin, may be considered.

Nutritional Therapy

An association between diet and etiologic factors has not been documented, nor does direct evidence suggest that diet alters disease activity. Many patients report fewer

Table 28-6. RADIOLOGIC FINDINGS IN INFLAMMATORY BOWEL DISEASE

Crohn's Disease	Ulcerative Colitis
Segmental involvement	Contiguous involvement
Skip lesions	Rectum always involved
Cobblestoning	Pseudopolyps
Pseudodiverticula	Loss of haustral markings
Strictures	Strictures (cancer)
Toxic dilation rare	Toxic megacolon
Longitudinal ulcers	
Transverse fissures	
Intramural fistulas	

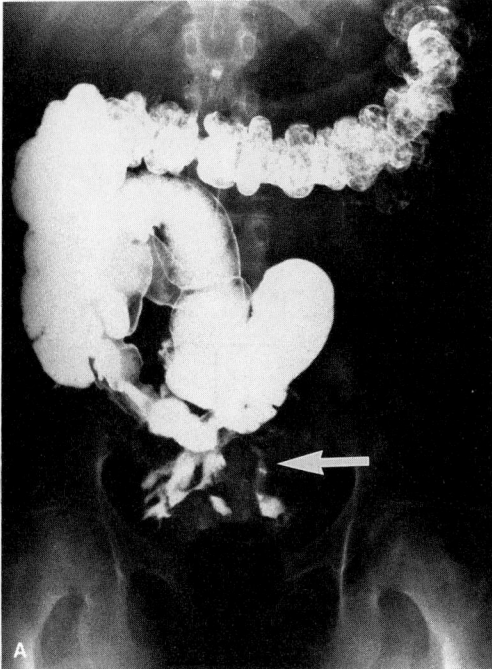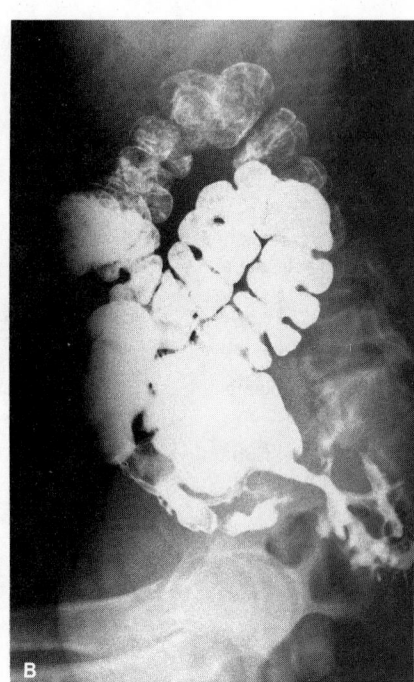

Figure 28-7. Radiographic studies (anteroposterior view in *A*, lateral view in *B*) showing fistulas extending into the presacral space (*arrow*). After percutaneous drainage with CT guidance, resection and primary anastomosis were performed without complications.

symptoms after an exclusion diet based on personal food experience, but this practice can lead to near-total food avoidance and severe malnutrition in the most severe cases.

Nutritional support of malnourished patients with Crohn's disease has been shown to increase nutritional parameters such as body weight, visceral protein status, and nitrogen balance. Bowel rest with total parenteral nutrition (TPN) or enterally fed elemental diets has been widely used to treat acute disease, both as supportive and primary therapy.[18] TPN is indicated to treat malnutrition, as preoperative therapy to replete the patient nutritionally, for short-gut syndrome, for fluid and electrolyte repletion of the patient with a jejunostomy, for chronic small bowel obstruction, and for growth retardation. Elemental formulas use simple compounds, which are absorbed in the proximal gut, effectively placing the distal small bowel and large intestine at rest. TPN has not been found more effective than enteral diets. Healing rates of fistulas using bowel rest and TPN as primary therapy are reported to be as high as 50% to 75%.

The use of long-term TPN to support patients with short-gut syndrome and high-output proximal fistulas has been shown to improve the quality of life but not to alter disease-related complications. The use of TPN to prepare a patient for planned surgical resection is controversial. The perioperative complication rate has not differed significantly between TPN-treated groups and untreated groups. Less small bowel (20 cm less on average) was resected in the TPN-treated group than in the untreated group. This reduction in bowel resected may reflect the beneficial effect of waiting until active disease becomes quiescent, or this finding may simply reflect an uncontrolled, unrandomized study. The length of hospital stay and, consequently, expense was significantly greater in the TPN-treated patients, suggesting that only those patients with the most severe disease or most profound nutritional deficits should be considered for preoperative TPN.[19]

Drug Therapy

Corticosteroids

Systemic corticosteroids have been used to treat Crohn's disease since the 1940s. The exact mechanism of action is not clear, but nonspecific immunosuppression is the likely effect (Fig. 28-8). The long-term risks of corticosteroid use are well known, making it prudent to administer systemic corticosteroids for the shortest time and at the lowest effective dose possible. Several well-designed trials have assessed the efficacy of corticosteroid use. The results indicate that prednisone (or an equivalent) at 0.5 to 0.75 mg/kg/d is significantly better than placebo in the treatment of acute exacerbations, with 60% of patients achieving and maintaining remission for the duration of the 17-week treatment, versus 30% for the placebo group.[20] Patients with quiescent disease and patients who achieved

Table 28-7. DIFFERENTIAL DIAGNOSIS OF CROHN'S DISEASE

INFECTIOUS CONDITIONS	OTHER CONDITIONS
Yersinia infection	Ulcerative colitis
Salmonellosis, shigellosis	Radiation enteritis
Campylobacter enteritis	Ischemic colitis
Tuberculosis	Irritable bowel disease
Pseudomembranous colitis	Diverticulitis
(*Clostridium difficile*)	Appendicitis
Staphylococcal enteritis	Behçet syndrome
Viral enteritis (lymphogranuloma	Sprue
venereum)	Sarcoidosis
Fungal Infections	**NEOPLASIA**
Histoplasmosis	Lymphoma
Candidiasis	Adenocarcinoma
	Polyposis syndromes
Protozoal Infections	
Amebiasis	
Lambliasis	
Giardiasis	
Schistosomiasis	

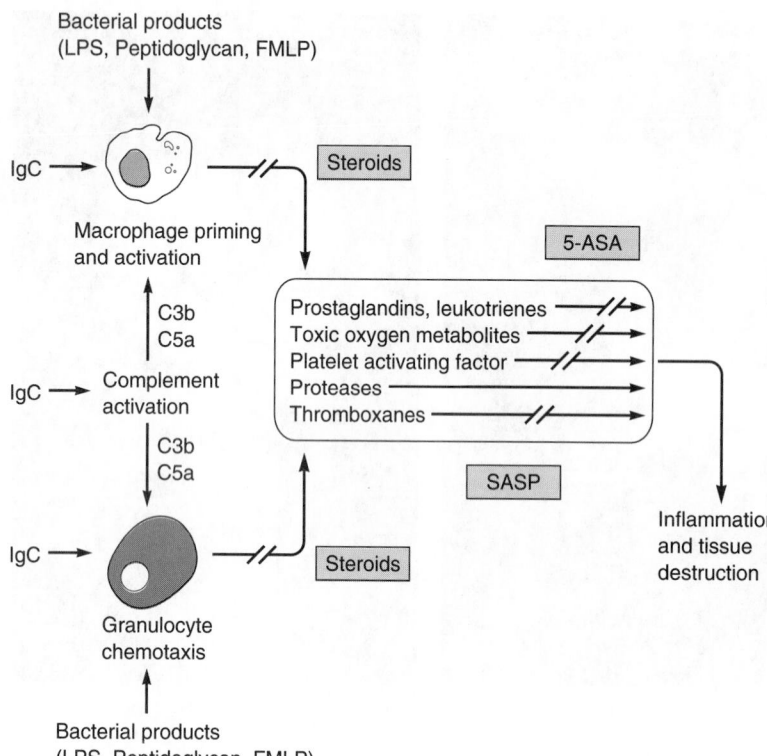

Figure 28-8. Mechanisms of tissue injury in inflammatory bowel disease. The events that initiate inflammatory bowel disease are largely undefined but involve activation of cells and initiation of the inflammatory cascade. Antibiotics may reduce the antigen load; steroids and immunosuppressive drugs block immunologic processes at various sites; 5-ASA compounds have inhibitory effects at multiple sites of the immune system. LPS, lipopolysarcharide; FMLP, formyl-methionyl-leucyl-phenylalanine; SASP, sulfasalazine. (After Hanauer SB. Highlights of controversies in IDB workshop. IBD Chronicle 1993;1:7)

remission through medical or surgical therapy, did not benefit from long-term continued corticosteroid treatment. The European Cooperative Crohn's Disease Study[21] compared prednisolone alone to the combination of prednisolone and sulfasalazine. This study found no benefit for combination therapy except in patients who had not received previous therapy or in patients with disease confined to the colon. Prednisone therapy caused significant side effects in more than half of the patients treated for acute exacerbations. Of patients treated prophylactically with low-dose corticosteroids, about one fourth required a dose readjustment or discontinuation of therapy.

Topical corticosteroids have been used with success in the treatment of distal colitis. Prednisolone metasulfobenzoate, beclomethasone, and budesonide are newer topical corticosteroids given as enemas or oral capsules. They have strong local antiinflammatory effects but are rapidly metabolized after absorption. These agents appear to be as effective as traditional corticosteroids without elevating serum cortisone levels or strongly suppressing the hypothalamic–pituitary–adrenal axis.[22]

Sulfasalazine

Sulfasalazine, like corticosteroids, was first used in the 1940s to treat Crohn's disease. Sulfasalazine consists of a sulfonamide moiety, sulfapyridine, which is linked to the aspirin analogue 5-aminosalicylate (5-ASA). Intestinal bacteria cleave the compound in the distal ileum and colon, allowing the sulfonamide portion to be absorbed. The 5-ASA moiety remains available to the intestinal mucosa in the lumen and is excreted intact. The mechanism of action is postulated to be due to inhibitory effects at several levels in the conversion pathway for arachidonic acid and its metabolites, prostaglandins (cyclooxygenase pathway) and leukotrienes (lipoxygenase pathway).[22] Sulfasalazine is more effective than placebo in achieving remission of acute disease. It is most effective in patients with predominantly

colonic disease and less effective than corticosteroids in treating patients with small bowel disease. Patients without symptoms do not appear to benefit from prophylactic treatment. Sulfasalazine is well tolerated, with only 4% of patients requiring discontinuation of the drug secondary to gastrointestinal side effects. Another benefit is that the drug is inexpensive.

The use of 5-ASA enemas to treat colonic disease was established by several trials, but 5-ASA is available to the mucosa only up to the splenic flexure, making this a well-tolerated, safe therapy that is ineffective for most patients with Crohn's disease. Preparations of 5-ASA that prevent absorption in the proximal gut have been developed. Encouraging data suggest that slow-release forms are effective in therapy of Crohn's disease of the small bowel and colon. Furthermore, commencement of oral 5-ASA compounds after curative resection reportedly reduces or postpones early recurrence, making these new agents the first possibly to have a prophylactic effect.[23,24]

Antibiotics

Broad-spectrum antibiotics are clearly indicated for septic complications of Crohn's disease. Their use as therapy for symptoms attributed to bacterial overgrowth is controversial. Broad-spectrum and antimycobacterial antibiotics have been tried as primary therapy without success. Metronidazole, originally used to treat anaerobic and parasitic infections, has been found to be effective in the treatment of selected patients with Crohn's disease. The Cooperative Crohn's Disease Study[25] in Sweden used the Crohn's disease activity index and plasma orosomucoid (an acute-phase reactant) levels to compare the efficacy of metronidazole to that of sulfasalazine in the treatment of symptomatic disease. Both drugs were equally effective, but more patients who failed with sulfasalazine improved when switched to metronidazole than conversely. Metronidazole is most often used in the treatment of perianal disease.

The side effects are dose related and include gastrointestinal upset, urticaria, reversible neutropenia, and peripheral neuropathy. Mutagenicity and chromosome aberration, observed in some animal studies, have not been demonstrated in humans at the recommended dosage. The mechanism of action is not clear but is considered to be related either to antianaerobic effects or to a direct immunosuppressive effect.

Azathioprine and 6-Mercaptopurine. The rationale for using immunosuppressive drugs in Crohn's disease is sound because the tissue injury is immune mediated. Azathioprine and its active metabolite, 6-mercaptopurine, are the most widely used and studied immunosuppressive agents administered to patients with Crohn's disease. Azathioprine is a purine analogue that inhibits nucleic acid metabolism. The drug alters the proliferation of chronic inflammatory cells and their mediators and requires an average of 3 months of treatment to be effective. Trials using long-term (at least 1 year) 6-mercaptopurine therapy, in addition to the drugs already taken by the study patients, demonstrate that 67% of patients improved, compared with 8% receiving placebo. A steroid-sparing effect was demonstrated because 75% of the patients receiving corticosteroids tolerated dose reduction or discontinuation of corticosteroids. During 3 to 4 years of chronic therapy, these agents were effective in decreasing disease activity, steroid requirements, and complications leading to surgery.[26] Thus, these agents, in contrast to corticosteroids and sulfasalazine, are effective in maintaining remission. The side effects are dose dependent; bone marrow suppression developed in 2% of the patients in one large series. Acute pancreatitis develops in 2% to 4% of patients but resolves when the drug is discontinued. There are extensive reports on the safety of these drugs.[27]

Methotrexate. Methotrexate is a folic acid inhibitor whose immunosuppressive and antiinflammatory effects have been shown to be of benefit in the treatment of autoimmune diseases such as rheumatoid arthritis, psoriasis, and Reiter syndrome. Data from large prospective control trials are not available, but in smaller series, some two thirds of patients with unresponsive, chronic inflammatory bowel disease responded to a 12-week course of methotrexate. Studies that assess the substantial risks and benefits of long-term methotrexate therapy are needed.

Cyclosporine. Cyclosporine is an immunosuppressant that has revolutionized organ transplantation. It is effective in preventing acute rejection by altering T-lymphocyte–mediated immune responses. After several retrospective series suggested that cyclosporine was effective in Crohn's disease, a randomized prospective trial was performed to compare cyclosporine to placebo. A 3-month course of cyclosporine versus placebo was used to treat 71 patients with chronically active Crohn's disease who were unresponsive to or intolerant of corticosteroid therapy. After 3 months of treatment at 5 to 7.5 mg/kg/d, 59% of the cyclosporine-treated group (versus 32% on placebo) improved; of responders, 38% maintained their remission for at least several months after cyclosporine was discontinued (statistically no difference from a control group). Unlike azathioprine, the beneficial effects of cyclosporine were noted within 2 weeks. During this short period, the side effects of cyclosporine were not serious. The Canadian Crohn's Relapse Prevention Trial[26] came to the conclusion that low-dose oral cyclosporine treatment conferred no therapeutic benefit for patients with both low and high disease activity and no reduction in the need for other forms of therapy.

Surgical Treatment

In view of the high rate of recurrence of Crohn's disease after surgical resection, surgical therapy is not curative but palliative. Operative therapy is reserved for complications of the disease, and bowel resection for patients with uncomplicated disease is justified only in unusual circumstances. Surgery is also indicated when medical therapy has failed and the patient is chronically debilitated on account of the disease. Failure of medical management includes intractability, suggesting that the patient's well-being, life-style, and employment are significantly impaired by unrelenting symptoms and debilitating side effects of medical therapy.

Preoperative Preparation

Preoperative preparation should include bowel cleansing with enemas, a clear liquid diet, and electrolyte catharsis given orally. If the patient has a stenotic lesion in the intestinal tract and a complete or partial small bowel obstruction, oral bowel preparation must be undertaken cautiously and may not be possible. Prophylactic parenteral antibiotics are administered perioperatively, but antibiotic coverage is continued postoperatively beyond the usual two doses only when there is obvious sepsis.

Technical Aspects of the Operative Procedure

Abdominal exploration must be complete and nearly always requires division of all adhesions. The site of disease or recurrence is assessed, and the length of the uninvolved proximal small intestine is estimated. A meticulous search for any skip lesion is undertaken. The colon is inspected for the presence or absence of Crohn's colitis.

The proposed sites of bowel transection are identified; these should be adjacent to the clinically obvious limits of involvement. The lines of resection should be chosen conservatively, only a few centimeters proximal and distal to the site of visible changes of Crohn's disease—narrowing of the intestinal lumen, thickening of the bowel wall, serositis, tortuosity of the serosal vessels, creeping fat over the intestinal surface, and thickening of the mesenteric margins of the bowel. The site for bowel transection is cleared of mesenteric tissues for about 1 cm, allowing a technically easy intestinal anastomosis. Microscopic evidence of Crohn's disease at the resection margins does not compromise safe anastomosis. Frozen-section examination of resection margins is not necessary. After anastomosis, the mesenteric rent is closed, the peritoneal cavity is irrigated, the retroperitoneum is again inspected for possible sites of bleeding, and the incision is closed in layers.

In a substantial number of patients, especially those undergoing reoperation, extensive mesenteric foreshortening with dense adherence of the diseased bowel to the retroperitoneum may be encountered in the region of the upper ureter, pancreas, and the third and fourth portions of the duodenum. In this situation, the risk of pancreatic, duodenal, and ureteral injury is substantial. There is also the risk of serious intraoperative hemorrhage if the foreshortened mesentery, which always contains enlarged and engorged mesenteric arteries and veins, is injured or torn.

Management of Fistulas and Abscesses

If a retroperitoneal fistulous tract is encountered in the course of mobilizing the diseased bowel segment, the diseased intestine is removed, and the fistulous tract is transected. When a fistulous tract is encountered or an abscess is opened, the contents are evacuated carefully by suction, and all necrotic tissue is excised. In the course of this retroperitoneal procedure, injury to the right ureter, the third and fourth portions of duodenum, and the inferior vena cava and superior mesenteric vein must be avoided.

In patients with duodenal fistulas, the duodenum is mobilized completely to allow safe excision of the margins of the duodenal fistula, followed by closure. If the fistulous communication between the diseased intestine and duodenum involves the mesenteric side of the duodenum, adjacent pancreatitis is always present to some degree. A fistulous communication between the intestine and the pancreatic ductal system is possible. Such a situation can be treated by ileocolonic resection of the primarily involved small and large bowel, supplemented by either a Roux-en-Y pancreaticojejunostomy or distal pancreatectomy.

After a diagnosis of a fistula, as soon as the extent of the fistulous tract and its communication to the various intraabdominal organs are determined, a surgical correction of the problem should be planned. A surgical procedure should be undertaken when the fistulous tracts are as clean as possible, at a time when active inflammatory processes are under control, and when the patient is in good nutritional condition and has an adequate bowel preparation. Enteroenteric fistulas, ileosigmoid fistulas, and minor enterocutaneous fistulas of low output do not always require operative repair if the fistulous tract is well established and does not cause bleeding, cause intermittent febrile episodes, or interfere with the patient's well-being. Once a fistula causes clinical symptoms or is associated with metabolic consequences, surgical correction is mandated.

In dealing with enterocutaneous fistulas, the patient is readied by bowel preparation, which, in the presence of complex, extensive fistulization, is best achieved by placing the patient on TPN. During this time, the fistulous tracts clear of fecal material, and the skin opening heals as much as possible. The bowel giving rise to the fistula is separated from surrounding loops of uninvolved intestine and resected. The fistulous tract is transected as it penetrates the abdominal wall. In most of these instances, spillage of purulent and fecal material is minimal, allowing a safe intestinal anastomosis. The tract through the abdominal wall is vigorously débrided, and the fistulous opening at the skin level is excised.

Fistulous communication to the sigmoid colon, the bladder, or any other intraabdominal organ not primarily involved by Crohn's disease is handled in a similar manner. The opening in the nondiseased organ is cleared and closed in layers. An ileosigmoid fistula is treated by resection of the diseased small bowel and wedge resection of the sigmoid, or by simple closure of the colonic defect.

A fistula coexisting with an inflammatory mass or abscess and leading to partial or complete bowel obstruction is a frequent reason for primary surgical procedures (up to 60%) and is equally often an indication for reoperation. The development of an enteric fistula, whether it communicates with another intraabdominal structure or with the skin, is associated almost invariably with an inflammatory mass. The mass consists of an inflamed mesentery containing markedly enlarged lymph nodes, loops of diseased and nondiseased intestine, and the parietal peritoneum. Frequently, there is purulent material within the interstices of the inflammatory mass, and, at times, there is a frank abscess. Percutaneous drainage of abscesses under sonographic or CT guidance is not always suitable for patients with Crohn's disease because multiple loops of diseased and nondiseased bowel have to be transgressed. Resection and drainage is safer in the management of these situations. Temporary closure of an enterocutaneous or enteroenteric fistula can sometimes be achieved by TPN and

bowel rest. A lasting closure is only possible by resection of the diseased intestine from which the fistula arises.

Stricture

Patients with recurrent Crohn's disease may experience multiple strictures of the small intestine, causing symptoms of partial obstruction and weight loss. Resection of multiple strictures can result in the short-gut syndrome and is, therefore, avoided. For short strictures, stricturoplasty is an excellent alternative to resection.

Stricturoplasty is achieved by placing a longitudinal incision across the short stenotic segment into the prestenotic and poststenotic bowel. For stricturoplasty, the longitudinal enterotomy is then converted into a transverse closure, analogous to the techniques of a Heinecke-Mikulicz pyloroplasty. The long-term results using this approach indicate that recurrence rates are not substantially increased with stricturoplasty, even though inflamed intestinal tissue is left in situ. In most cases, resection and stricturoplasty are complementary techniques and are not used in lieu of each other. Inflammatory changes at the margin of resection are acceptable and are compatible with a safe anastomosis. Consequently, histologic evaluation of the margins of resection by frozen section is not necessary.

Colonic Crohn's Disease

Some 68% of patients with Crohn's disease have inflammatory changes limited to the colon or have major colonic involvement.[28] Although disease in the colon is often segmental, colonic recurrences are frequent after limited segmental resections. A recurrence rate of 40% has been noted after right hemicolectomy for disease initially involving the right colon, and a rate of 30% after left hemicolectomy. The recurrence rate after total abdominal colectomy with ileorectal anastomosis is about 45%. In patients with diffuse disease of the colon and rectum, proctocolectomy with ileostomy is the treatment of choice. If the disease is less extensive and the rectum is spared, a limited resection with anastomosis is an acceptable approach.

Because recurrence after limited colonic resection for Crohn's colitis is frequent, reoperations on these patients are common. Therefore, the placement of the abdominal incision must be carefully planned, taking into account the likelihood of future intestinal stomas.

Dilemma of Recurrence

The incurability of Crohn's disease is a most frustrating aspect of managing this disease. Most patients whose disease is resected eventually have a recurrence. If recurrence is defined as alterations detected endoscopically, then 70% of cases recur within 1 year of surgery and 85% within 3 years.[16] A clinical recurrence (return of symptoms confirmed as Crohn's disease radiologically, endoscopically, or surgically) affects 20% of patients 2 years and 40% to 50% 4 years after surgery.[29] Reoperation becomes necessary in about 30% of patients by 5 years.

These statistics give impetus to maintain remission and prevent recurrence. Although it is common practice to stem recurrence with sulfasalazine, 5-ASA preparations, antibiotics, and possibly azathioprine, none of these (possibly excepting azathioprine) have definitely been proved effective. Aside from therapy-related risks, cost concerns must be considered.

Perianal Disease

Perianal disease is a frequent and recurrent manifestation of Crohn's disease and has a high morbidity but a low mortality rate. Perianal lesions can be viewed as primary lesions specific to Crohn's disease (eg, anal fissure, ulcerated hemorrhoidal tissues, cavitating intrarectal ulcer) and as secondary, nonspecific lesions (eg, subcutaneous fistulas, ulcerated external and internal hemorrhoids, anal stricture, and deep perianal abscesses and fistula).[30] Primary lesions are often accompanied by active disease in the proximal gastrointestinal tract.

A conservative surgical approach to these lesions is usually prudent. Many patients who have indolent anal fistulas can live comfortably with the disease for years. The development of an abscess, however, requires conventional drainage. If there is active proximal Crohn's disease and a concomitant flare of perianal disease, both entities must be treated. In the absence of Crohn's proctitis and during quiescence of proximal intestinal disease, an uncomplicated fistulous tract may be treated by standard surgical procedures; an anorectovaginal fistula can be treated under these circumstances by a rectal advancement flap, with a 50% to 70% success rate. Often, standard operations are impossible because of the transsphincteric nature of multiple interconnected fistulous tracts. A combination of partial excision, fistulotomy, and placement of drains may provide drainage and maturation of the fistulous tracts without leading to complete destruction of the sphincter mechanism. Patients with perianal disease in direct continuity with active rectal disease occasionally are considered for proctectomy. Fecal diversion by a proximal colostomy does not improve eventual healing but may provide relief of symptoms.

Extensive perineal sepsis complicating ischiorectal abscesses, rectocutaneous fistulas, or rectovaginal fistulas may involve the entire perineum and groin as a manifestation of Crohn's proctocolitis. In these patients, the perineum and the rectal sphincter are usually destroyed, and the rectum is extensively diseased. Proctocolectomy, performed in two stages, may be necessary. At the first operation, the entire abdominal colon is resected together with the upper two thirds of the rectum. An end-ileostomy is constructed, and the rectum is closed. At the termination of the first operation, the abscesses are drained, and the fistulous tracts are opened. Once suppuration has subsided, the rectum is resected using a perineal approach, residual fistulous tracts are excised, and vaginal defects are repaired. Extensive destruction of the posterior vaginal wall occasionally requires the use of a myocutaneous flap for repair. In 10% to 40% of patients, a persistent, nonhealing perineal wound develops.

Some persistent wounds are minor cutaneous sinuses, whereas others are large, infected cavities that destroy the perineum and adjacent tissue. Surgical treatment requires excision of the fibrous wall of the cavity and may also include the coccyx and portions of the sacrum. The wound is left open and heals secondarily in most instances.

Special Circumstances

The Elderly

Although the peak occurrence of Crohn's disease is before 35 years of age, there appears to be a second peak at 55 years of age.[14] Complications such as perforation, abscess formation, and hemorrhage appear more common. Colonic involvement is more common and requires a differential diagnosis from diverticulitis and from ischemic colitis, which may often be difficult.

Children

The clinical manifestations of Crohn's disease in children are similar to those in adults. The most discerning and disconcerting aspect is growth failure and related retardation of sexual development. Next to standard medical and surgical therapy, nutritional management plays a major role in the care of these patients.

Pregnant Women

Crohn's disease, if inactive at the time of conception, does not significantly affect the course of pregnancy or result in premature birth.[31] Active Crohn's disease, however, may be seriously detrimental. Pregnancy in patients with active Crohn's disease is twice as likely to end in spontaneous abortion as it is in patients with quiescent disease. Among patients with Crohn's disease, 63% of pregnancies associated with fetal complications occur in women with active disease. Disease activity rather than drug treatment is likely to be responsible for fetal complications. In women with active Crohn's disease at conception, or in those who require bowel resection during pregnancy, the risks of premature delivery are increased. Conversely, the notion that pregnancy may adversely effect the course of Crohn's disease has not been substantiated. Crohn and colleagues[32] reported a 16% rate of relapse of ileitis during pregnancy in patients in whom the disease was quiescent at conception. Among patients who had active disease, exacerbation occurred in 13%.

Surgical treatment of Crohn's disease during pregnancy is avoided, if possible. Indications for operation include failure of medical management, the presence of peritonitis, gastrointestinal hemorrhage, complete and persistent bowel obstruction, abdominal abscess and perforation, carcinoma, and enterocutaneous fistulas. Direct surgical intervention becomes necessary if its postponement jeopardizes mother and fetus. Often, a delaying strategy consisting of aggressive medical management with TPN is possible, and definitive surgical therapy can be performed during the postpartum period. The coincidence of pregnancy and acute Crohn's disease can be regarded as a complicating factor of either situation but is not a catastrophic event that precludes successful outcome of the pregnancy.

REFERENCES

1. Crohn BB, Ginsberg L, Oppenheimer GD. Regional ileitis: a pathological and clinical entity. JAMA 1932;99:1323.
2. Goldman CD, Kodner IJ, Fry RD, MacDermott RP. Clinical and operative experience with non-caucasian patients with Crohn's disease. Dis Colon Rectum 1986;29:317.
3. McConnell RB. Genetic aspects of idiopathic inflammatory bowel disease. In: Kirsner JB, Shorter RG, eds. Inflammatory bowel disease. Philadelphia, Lea & Febiger, 1988:87.
4. Cottone M, Rosselli M, Orlando A, et al. Smoking habits and recurrence in Crohn's disease. Gastroenterology 1994;106:643
5. Thayer WR, Coutu JA, Chiodini RJ, Van Kruiningen HJ, Merkal RS. Possible roll of mycobacteria in inflammatory bowel disease. II. Mycobacteria antibodies in Crohn's disease. Dig Dis Sci 1984;29:1080.
6. Vince A, Dyer NH, O'Grady FW, Dawson AM. Bacteriological studies in Crohn's disease. J Med Microbiol 1972;5:219.
7. Thayer WR Jr, Brown M, Sangree MH, et al. *Escherichia coli* 0:14 and colon hemagglutinating antibodies in inflammatory bowel disease. Gastroenterology 1969;57:311.
8. Strober W, James S. The immunologic basis of inflammatory bowel disease. J Clin Immunol 1986;6:415.
9. Rabin, BS, Rogers SJ. Nonpathogenicity of anti-intestinal antibody in the rabbit. Am J Pathol 1976;83:269.
10. Shorter RG, McGill DB, Bahn RC. Cytotoxicity of mononuclear cells for autologous colonic epithelial cells in colonic disease. Gastroenterology 1984;86:13.
11. Sartor RB. Insights into the pathogenesis of inflammatory bowel diseases provided by new rodent models of spontaneous colitis. Inflam Bowel Dis 1995;1:1:64.
12. Jones LA, Mathies AD, Rhodes J. Natural energy intake in undernourished patients with Crohn's disease. Br Med J 1984;288:193.
13. Motil KJ, Grand, RJ, David-Kraft E. The epidemiology of

growth failure in children and adolescents with inflammatory bowel disease. Gastroenterology 1983;84:1254.

14. Bayless TM, Yardley JH, Huang SS, et al. Crohn's disease. South Med J 1978;71:825.
15. Bergman L, Krause U. Crohn's disease: a long-term study of the clinical course of 186 patients. Scand J Gastroenterol 1977;12:937.
16. Rutgeerts P, Geboes K, Van Trappen G, et al. Predictability of the postoperative course of Crohn's disease. Gastroenterology 1990;99:956.
17. Goldberg HI, Caruthers SB Jr, Nelson JA, et al. Radiographic findings of the National Cooperative Crohn's Disease Study. Gastroenterology 1979;77:925.
18. Muller JM, Keller HW, Erasmi H, Pichlmaier H. Total parenteral nutrition initiation as the sole therapy in Crohn's disease: a prospective study. Br J Surg 1983;70:40.
19. Gouma D, von Meyerfeldt M, Rouflart M, Soeters P. Preoperative total parenteral nutrition (TPN) in severe Crohn's disease. Surgery 1988;103:648.
20. Summers R, Switz D, Sessions J, et al. National Cooperative Crohn's Disease Study: pursuits of drug treatment. Gastroenterology 1979;77:847.
21. Malchow H, Ewe K, Brandes T, et al. European Cooperative Crohn's Disease Study (ECCDS): results of treatment. Gastroenterology 1984;86:249.
22. Hanauer SB. Evolving medical therapies for inflammatory bowel disease. Progr Inflam Bowel Dis 1994;15:2.
23. Brignola C, Cottone M, Pera A, et al. Mesalamine in the pre-

24. vention of endoscopic recurrence after intestinal resection for Crohn's disease. Gastroenterology 1995;108:345.
24. McLeod RS, Wolff BG, Steinhart H, et al. Delayed recurrence following surgery for Crohn's disease. Gastroenterology 1994;106:A733.
25. Ursing B, Alm T, Barany F, et al. A comparative study of metronidazole and sulfasalazine for active Crohn's disease: the Cooperative Crohn's Disease Study in Sweden. Gastroenterology 1982;83:550.
26. Feagan BG, McDonald JWD, Rochon J, et al. Low-dose cyclosporine for the treatment of Crohn's disease. N Engl J Med 1994;330:1846.
27. Kornbluth A, George J, Sachar D. Immunosuppressive drugs in Crohn's disease. Gastroenterologist 1994;2:239.
28. Goligher JC. The outcome of excisional operations for primary and recurrent Crohn's disease of the large bowel. Surg Gynecol Obstet 1979;148:1.
29. Greenstein AJ, Sachar DB, Pasternack BS, et al. Reoperations and recurrences of Crohn's colitis and ileocolitis: crude and cumulative rates. N Engl J Med 1975;293:685.
30. Hughes LE, Jones IRG. Peri-anal lesions in Crohn's disease. In: Allan RN, Keighly MRB, Alexander-Williams J, Hawkins C, eds. Inflammatory bowel disease. Edinburgh, Churchill Livingstone, 1983:322.
31. Schraut WH. Inflammatory bowel disease in pregnancy. In: Cibils L, ed. Surgical diseases of pregnancy. New York, Springer-Verlag, 1989:252.
32. Crohn BB, Yarnis H, Korelitz BI. Regional enteritis complicating pregnancy. Gastroenterology 1956;31:615.

SURGERY: SCIENTIFIC PRINCIPLES AND PRACTICE, Second Edition, edited by Lazar J. Greenfield, Michael W. Mulholland, Keith T. Oldham, Gerald B. Zelenock, and Keith D. Lillemoe. Lippincott–Raven Publishers, Philadelphia, © 1997.

CHAPTER 29

SMALL INTESTINAL NEOPLASMS

MICHAEL G. SARR AND MICHEL M. MURR

Primary neoplasms of the small intestine are rare. This infrequent occurrence is especially intriguing when contrasted with the frequency of gastric and colonic neoplasms. Although the small intestine constitutes 75% of the total length of the gastrointestinal tract and over 90% of the mucosal surface area, less than 2% of all malignant neoplasms arise here. Benign neoplasms arising in the small intestine are more frequent, but they often remain asymptomatic and appear only at autopsy. The infrequency of small bowel neoplasms, the lack of pathognomonic symptoms, and the diversity of clinical presentations complicate the diagnosis and treatment.[1]

EPIDEMIOLOGY

Little is known about worldwide differences in incidence and prevalence of small intestinal neoplasms because of their infrequent occurrence. Some data suggest an increased incidence of small bowel cancer in developed Western countries and a positive correlation with prevalence rates of colonic carcinoma. Worldwide, primary small intestinal lymphomas differ in type, frequency, and incidence between the developed and underdeveloped nations, with a greater incidence of Mediterranean lymphoma (or α-chain disease) in the lower socioeconomic classes in North Africa and the Near East. In Japan, there

appears to be a geographic–ethnic variance; adenocarcinoma is more common and carcinoid tumors are rare in comparison to Western countries.[2] In the United States, there appears to be a slight male predominance in small bowel malignancy, with an overall incidence of 0.7 to 1.9 per 100,000 population. There is no clear-cut predilection for adenocarcinomas within racial groups or with urban versus rural distribution. In the United States, carcinoid tumors appear to be 70% more frequent in blacks, whereas lymphomas are twice as common in whites.

ETIOPATHOGENESIS

The mucosa of the small intestine is a rapidly regenerating tissue. As dying cells exfoliate, they are replaced by maturing enterocytes, which migrate in an axial direction from crypts where they have arisen from less-differentiated replicating stem cells. This self-renewal process normally cycles in 5 to 7 days and maintains the functional and structural integrity of the small intestine. It is striking that within this system of rapid turnover, which in theory creates a potential for erroneous cell replication, DNA duplication, and related mutational defects, mucosal neoplasms, unlike in the large bowel, are unusual. The interaction of factors involved in growth and differentiation, such as mitogens, polyamines, intraluminal nutrients, gastrointestinal hormones, and other growth and trophic factors (oncogenes, viruses, chemical carcinogens), is less frequently deranged than it is in the large intestine, despite the greater surface area of the small intestine.[3]

Although there have been many speculations about the interaction of carcinogens and the small bowel lumen, little is known about the causes of neoplastic induction in this tissue. In fact, most discussion has centered on explaining the infrequency of these neoplasms when compared with the stomach and large intestine. Several factors pertinent to the small intestinal milieu appear to be important. First, transit through the small intestine is comparatively rapid (about 1 to 2 hours), and exposure of any one area of the mucosa to ingested carcinogens is limited. Also, the alkaline pH and the decreased bacterial concentration in the lumen, when compared with the colonic lumen, minimize the formation of carcinogens from bile and ingested precarcinogens. Moreover, the high activity of the enzyme benzopyrene hydroxylase in the small intestinal mucosa detoxifies many carcinogens. These factors, in combination with rapid turnover of mucosal cells and the mechanically less irritating liquid content of small bowel chyme, are believed to limit neoplastic transformation within the mucosa.

Another factor of potential importance involves the humoral and cellular immune surveillance provided by the small intestine. Secretion of IgA into the lumen (secretory IgA) plays an important role in upper gut immune function. Similarly, the immunocompetent lymphoid tissue found within the wall of the more distal small bowel appears to provide an especially strong immunosurveillance mechanism against the development of malignancy. Defects in this immune surveillance system may explain the increased incidence of small bowel malignancies (especially lymphoma) in certain groups of immunocompromised patients, such as those with Crohn's disease, inherited immunodeficiency syndromes (eg, Wiskott-Aldrich syndrome, common variable immunodeficiency syndrome), and acquired immunodeficiency syndrome (AIDS). Posttransplantation lymphoproliferative diseases (PTLD), which have increased markedly since the introduction of cyclosporin A, appear to be closely linked to infection with the Epstein-Barr virus. PTLD are primarily monoclonal B-cell lymphomas and are associated with higher doses of immunosuppressive medications (particularly cyclosporin A). Similarly, patients with AIDS tend to develop B-cell lymphomas. The common underlying mechanisms point to a defect in immune surveillance that results in unchecked cellular replication and growth. The prevalence of α-chain lymphoma in geographic areas where parasitic intestinal infections are common is associated with defects in gut immune surveillance. Within this context, the concomitant occurrence of another independent neoplasm outside the gut in patients with primary small bowel malignancies is common, further supporting a theory of depressed overall immune surveillance.

Neoplasms of the small intestine have been induced in experimental animals by the administration of carcinogenic substances. Although some data suggest that these experimental tumors have a common *ras* gene mutation, the evidence is as yet unverified. Karyotype abnormalities, alterations in structural proteins and intestinal apomucins, and specific gene mutations or deletions in oncogenes or tumor suppressor genes are promising areas that require further investigation.[4] For instance, intestinal lymphomas, similar to non-Hodgkin lymphomas of other organs, show an increased expression of the protooncogene bCl_2 on chromosome 18; the significance of this finding is unknown but may prove to be of clinical significance in differentiating types of lymphoproliferative disease of the small intestine.

Clinical Presentation

Small intestinal neoplasms are somewhat unique in their insidious onset and nonspecific symptoms, virtually none of which is pathognomonic (Table 29-1). Although most benign tumors remain asymptomatic, malignant neoplasms eventually produce symptoms that vary according to the site and size of the tumor, the location and spread within the bowel wall, and the tendency to undergo necrosis and ulceration. Patients with cancers usually present with an element of weight loss and anorexia. Pain is the most common complaint, manifesting as either a dull ache

Table 29-1. CLINICAL PRESENTATION OF SMALL INTESTINAL NEOPLASMS

Findings	Occurrence (%)
BENIGN NEOPLASMS	
No symptoms	>50
Abdominal pain*	25
Intestinal obstruction	20
Hemorrhage	10
MALIGNANT NEOPLASMS	
Weight loss	90–100
Abdominal pain*	80
Intestinal obstruction	30
Abdominal mass	15
Perforation	10
Jaundice (periampullary neoplasms)	1–2

* Usually related to intermittent or incomplete mechanical obstruction

or, more commonly, a cramp related to underlying partial intestinal obstruction. Most malignant neoplasms cause pain by obstructing the lumen from circumferential growth; in contrast, intussusception can occur with benign or metastatic tumors. Kinking of the bowel wall and mesenteric fixation can lead to obstruction with the more locally based small carcinoids. Rarely, perforation occurs with lymphomas or leiomyosarcomas and presents as an acute abdomen. Bleeding is common with the epithelial lesions and hemangiomas, but it is usually occult; massive hemorrhage can occur with the more vascular leiomyosarcomas. Obstructive jaundice may herald the presence of a periampullary duodenal neoplasm. Malabsorption often coexists with extensive intestinal lymphomas, which present with steatorrhea. Extraintestinal symptoms of the carcinoid syndrome, in contrast to local intestinal symptoms, may be the first indication of the presence of a small bowel carcinoid tumor.

Physical findings are also vague. Adenocarcinomas can present with a complete small bowel obstruction (5% to 40% of patients), whereas lymphomas and leiomyosarcomas can manifest bulky abdominal masses. Usually, the physical examination is nonrevealing.

DIAGNOSIS

Many factors contribute to the delay in diagnosis of small bowel neoplasms. The insidious onset and vague character of the symptoms are often overlooked by patients and physicians alike, causing delays of up to 8 months from the onset of symptoms until diagnosis. Further delay can result from misinterpretation of subtle signs on radiographic imaging studies, especially if the treating physician and radiologist have a low index of suspicion for a small bowel neoplasm.

An objective preoperative diagnosis always requires the use of some imaging technique. Plain abdominal radiographs may show signs of intestinal obstruction but otherwise are usually nonspecific. Most commonly, the diagnosis is made by the presence of a filling defect, mass lesion, or intussusception on upper gastrointestinal barium examination with a small bowel follow-through. Some radiologists believe that a more sensitive technique is that of enteroclysis or small bowel enema, in which barium contrast is introduced directly into the proximal jejunum by an orojejunal tube. These gastrointestinal contrast studies allow visualization of the small bowel lumen. Computed tomography (CT), ultrasonography, and magnetic resonance imaging techniques can aid in the preoperative staging of patients by showing extraluminal extent as well as the presence of nodal or liver metastases. Endoscopy has proved beneficial in visualizing duodenal neoplasms and thereby helping to differentiate the possible causes of distal extrahepatic biliary obstruction secondary to a periampullary mass. This technique has replaced hypotonic duodenography. The ever-increasing advances in endoscopic technology, such as extended upper endoscopy or the introduction of Sunde-type enteroscopy, allow examination of most of the small bowel lumen; extended colonoscopy permits endoscopic examination of the distal 10 to 30 cm of the small intestine. Angiography is of occasional clinical value in diagnosing and localizing neoplasms of vascular origin such as hemangiomas or occasionally carcinoid tumors with a severe perivascular sclerosing reaction, but it has no role either as a screening test or in the staging of small bowel malignancies. Despite the variety and extent of imaging techniques, operative exploration usually serves as the definitive procedure necessary in most patients to establish the diagnosis and allow appropriate treatment.

BENIGN NEOPLASMS

Benign tumors arise from both epithelial and mesenchymal origins.[5] The most common lesions are adenomas, leiomyomas, and lipomas, but hamartomas, fibromas, angiomas, lymphangiomas, neurofibromas, and hemangiomas also occur (Table 29-2). The prevalence of these neoplasms varies between clinical and autopsy series.

Adenomas

Three types of adenomas occur—simple tubular adenomas, villous adenomas, and Brunner gland adenomas. Tubular adenomas occur most commonly in the duodenum and usually remain asymptomatic, but they occasionally bleed or cause obstruction. Because they are often pedunculated polyps with a low malignant potential, they are amenable to simple endoscopic polypectomy. If they are not, or if they are found in the jejunoileum, they can be treated with enterotomy or segmental intestinal resection.

Villous adenomas, in contrast to tubular adenomas, carry a distinct malignant potential similar to that of colonic villous adenomas. These neoplasms tend to occur most commonly in the duodenum and especially in the periampullary region. For unknown reasons, the inherited syndromes of colonic polyposis (familial polyposis, Gardner syndrome) have a special predilection for periampullary villous tumors in as many as 3% to 5% of patients.

Villous neoplasms can present with occult bleeding, gastric outlet obstruction, or biliary obstruction, depending on their anatomic location. Diagnosis is confirmed with endoscopic biopsy; however, because as many as 30% harbor adenocarcinoma, endoscopic biopsy does not ensure the absence of malignancy. Hence, removal is indicated, especially for lesions larger than 3 cm.[6] Endoscopic polypectomy is sufficient when no invasive carcinoma can be found in the polypectomy specimen; larger sessile lesions may require local operative resection. Invasive carcinoma necessitates a major resection to ensure a curative procedure, often involving pancreaticoduodenectomy for periampullary lesions.

Brunner gland adenomas represent hyperplasia of the exocrine glands of the proximal duodenal mucosa presenting as polypoid lesions of the first portion of the duodenum. Symptoms are unusual, and most of these tumors are found only incidentally. Occasionally they bleed. If the tumors are large, they can cause obstructive symptoms in rare cases. Because malignant transformation is unusual, treatment involves simple local resection either endoscopically or, rarely, by submucosal excision via duodenotomy.

Leiomyomas

The benign smooth muscle neoplasms, leiomyomas, are the most common symptomatic benign neoplasms. Leiomyomas occur most frequently in the jejunum as single, firm, gray-white lesions that microscopically show well-differentiated smooth muscle cells without mitoses. Radiographically, an ovoid, intraluminal filling defect with an intact overlying mucosa is highly suggestive of leiomyoma. Most leiomyomas enlarge extraluminally and can reach considerable, even palpable, size before recognition. They eventually outgrow their highly vascular blood supply, leading to central necrosis, ulceration, and intraluminal bleeding. Less commonly, their growth pattern is intraluminal, leading to mechanical intestinal obstruction. Smaller eccentric leiomyomas can cause intussusception. Treatment requires segmental resection. Differentiation of the larger lesion from its malignant counterpart, the leiomyosarcoma, can be difficult even after pathologic review. The presence of more than 2 mitotic figures per 50 high-power fields suggests a higher risk of local recurrence in symptomatic patients.

Lipomas

Lipomas occur predominantly in men and are found most commonly in the ileum and the duodenum arising from submucosal adipose tissue or mesenteric-based fat. Their extraluminal location leads to the appearance of an intramural or extramural mass with smooth borders, similar to a leiomyoma. CT can be pathognomonic by defining the density and thus confirming the diagnosis. Because lipomas have no malignant potential, excision is required only if the patient has symptoms. As with colonic lipomas, small intestinal lipomas found incidentally can safely be left untreated.

Peutz-Jeghers Syndrome

Peutz-Jeghers syndrome is an inherited syndrome of mucocutaneous melanotic pigmentation and multiple gastrointestinal polyps. It is transmitted as an autosomal dominant trait with a high degree of penetration. A single pleiotropic gene appears to account for both the gastrointestinal polyps and the melanin spots, which occur circumorally, on buccal mucosa and on the palms and soles of the feet. The polyps are really hamartomas and occur

Table 29-2. RELATIVE INCIDENCE OF BENIGN NEOPLASMS OF THE SMALL INTESTINE

Type	Occurrence (%)
Leiomyomas	18
Lipomas	15
Adenomas	15
Polyps (polyposis, Peutz-Jeghers)	15
Hemangiomas	13
Fibromas	10
Neurogenic tumors	7
Lymphangiomas	3
Myxomas	2
Other tumors	2

primarily in the jejunum and ileum, although half of patients have concomitant colorectal polyps and 25% have gastric polyps. For hamartomas, the progression of dysplasia to in situ carcinoma to invasive cancer is not a major concern. There have been a few reports, however, of presumed malignant transformation. More reports reveal an increased incidence of gastrointestinal and extraintestinal malignancies. Therefore, aggressive diagnostic and surveillance approaches should be followed for these patients.

These lesions most often present as intermittent intussusception. Occult hemorrhage occurs less frequently. Because of the widespread nature of their small intestinal involvement, extensive resection is not justified, and treatment should be limited to the segment producing complications. At the time of operative intervention, one should strongly consider the use of intraoperative enteroscopy to allow intraluminal polypectomies of other regions of the bowel as well.

Hemangiomas

Hemangiomas, true vascular neoplasms, constitute about 5% of small bowel tumors. They are often multiple and can involve the entire gastrointestinal tract, as in familial angiomatosis (Osler-Weber-Rendu disease). Hemangiomas vary in size from pinpoint lesions to more unusual large cavernous forms. Clinically, their significance lies in their propensity to cause occult or recurrent acute gastrointestinal blood loss. Diagnosis can be difficult and is revealed by angiography or endoscopy. Many are found at the time of exploration for gastrointestinal bleeding of unknown cause. If the tumors are small, treatment involves destruction by electrocauterization or laser therapy. Larger lesions may require segmental resection. Occasionally, multiple lesions can be isolated to the proximal small bowel and are thus amenable to an extensive proximal small bowel resection to prevent the need for frequent blood transfusions.

Endometriosis

Endometriosis is regarded as the presence of benign endometrial tissue in areas other than the uterus. The typical gross appearance of endometriosis of the small bowel involves puckered, bluish red, serosally based nodules found most commonly in the ileum. The adjacent bowel is often scarred, thickened, and adherent in reaction to the cyclic hormonal responses of the endometrioma. Rarely, this fibroinflammatory response accounts for obstructive symptoms secondary to a mechanical intestinal obstruction. Usually, endometriosis of the small intestine is found incidentally at celiotomy or laparoscopy and requires a simple biopsy to exclude metastatic malignancy. Treatment is conservative and noninterventional unless objective mechanical obstruction can be documented.[7] Hormonal suppression therapy can alter the functional behavior of the endometriosis and thereby prevent further gastrointestinal complications.

Conditions Mimicking Neoplasms

Congenital pancreatic rests appear as soft, yellowish nodules on the serosal surface of the small bowel. They require no treatment other than possibly biopsy to exclude malignancy. Splenosis follows previous splenic trauma in which splenic tissue has been dispersed by peritoneal seeding. These cherry-red nodules may be widespread throughout the peritoneal surfaces. Rarely, splenosis can cause a mechanical intestinal obstruction by fixation of adjacent segments of bowel. Enteric duplications of the gut can appear as mass lesions on preoperative imaging tests or as extrinsic or intramural cystic masses at exploration and require resection for diagnosis.

MALIGNANT NEOPLASMS

Unlike most other regions of the gut, several different types of malignant neoplasms of the small intestine occur with similar frequencies, including adenocarcinoma, leiomyosarcoma, lymphoma, and carcinoid tumors. The small bowel can also be the site of metastatic tumors, which can cause local complications mimicking primary tumors of the gut. The following sections address specific aspects of these separate neoplasms.

Adenocarcinoma

Adenocarcinomas are the most common small intestinal malignancy and constitute about 30% to 50% of all small bowel cancers. They tend to occur in patients in the sixth and seventh decade with a slight male predominance. Their incidence parallels that of colonic carcinomas worldwide, with a higher incidence in the more affluent Western nations. In the United States, the incidence is about 4 cases per 1,000,000 persons per year.

Origin

Adenocarcinomas arise from the epithelial cells of the small intestinal mucosa. Despite the vast length and surface area of the small intestine when compared with the large intestine, the incidence of small intestinal adenocarcinomas is surprisingly low. The reasons for the lack of malignant potential of the small bowel mucosa are unknown. Although there is a well-known malignant transformation to adenocarcinoma in previously benign periampullary villous adenomas, as occurs in the colonic polyposis syndrome, the polyp-to-cancer sequence is not well established for simple tubular adenomas of the small intestine. In contrast, in the Peutz-Jeghers syndrome, hereditary factors may play a role in malignant transformation. In Crohn's disease, the chronic inflammatory changes can predispose to the development of adenocarcinomas at a younger age, primarily in the ileum. Some studies have estimated that in patients with Crohn's disease, the risk of small bowel cancer may be 100 times that of the general population.

Anatomically, adenocarcinomas show a distinct polarity with decreasing frequency from duodenum to ileum. Given the difference in lengths between duodenum, jejunum, and ileum, the duodenal epithelium shows a substantially greater propensity toward malignant transformation (Fig. 29-1). Even within the duodenum, two thirds of the adenocarcinomas occur in the periampullary region, suggesting that the periampullary mucosa or luminal content (ingested potential carcinogens) interacts with pancreatobiliary secretions to induce local neoplastic changes.

Presentation and Diagnosis

Although the mode of presentation tends to vary with the anatomic location of the tumor in the small bowel, most adenocarcinomas present with weight loss and abdominal pain related to progressive intestinal obstruction. Obstructive jaundice is not an unusual presentation of periampullary adenocarcinomas. In contrast to the much more common cancer of the pancreas, which causes a relentless progression of jaundice, intermittent episodes of jaundice with cholangitis can occur with periampullary duodenal neoplasms secondary to intermittent ampullary obstruction related to tumor growth and subsequent necrosis. In the presence of hematochezia, this scenario raises

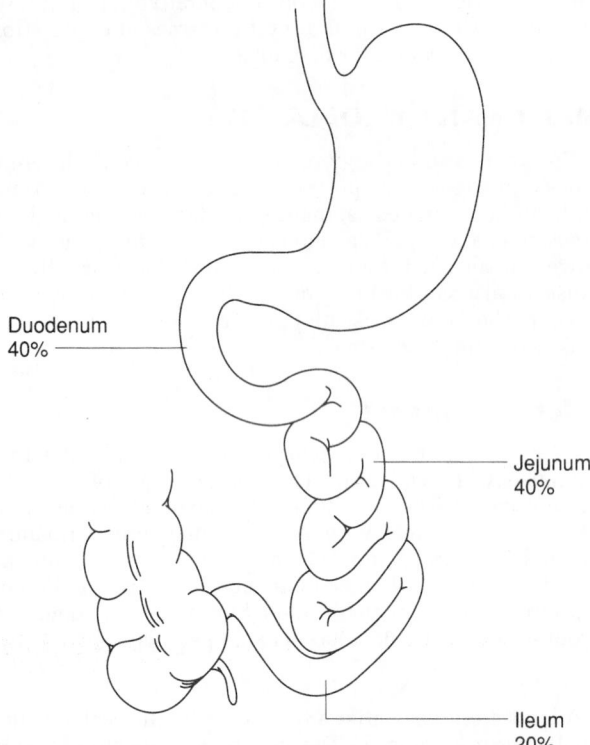

Figure 29-1. The duodenal mucosa has a substantially greater propensity for development of adenocarcinoma, especially considering its shorter length compared with the jejunum and ileum.

the possibility of a periampullary neoplasm. This distinction is important because periampullary duodenal malignancies are more frequently resectable for cure and have a favorable 5-year survival rate (approaching 40%), in contrast to a 5-year survival rate of no more than 10% with pancreatic cancer. Duodenal adenocarcinomas eccentric to the ampulla can reach considerable size before the duodenal lumen is compromised to the extent of causing mechanical obstruction.

In contrast, adenocarcinomas of the jejunoileum almost always present with a slowly progressive intestinal obstruction that is difficult to diagnose. The infiltrative nature of these neoplasms leads to typical apple-core defects with mucosal ulceration on gastrointestinal barium examinations (Fig. 29-2). When adenocarcinomas are located in the middle to distal small intestine, multiple loops of small bowel can overlap the lesion, making diagnosis difficult at an early stage. Blood loss is usually occult, although acute hemorrhage can occur. In contrast to lymphomas or leiomyosarcomas, a palpable mass or perforation is unusual. Unlike duodenal tumors, jejunoileal adenocarcinomas are not easily amenable to endoscopic diagnosis. The diagnosis of distal lesions is often made intraoperatively at the time of exploration for small intestinal obstruction of unknown cause. When extrahepatic biliary obstruction is seen on CT or ultrasonography, duodenal or ampullary adenocarcinomas are suspected by the presence of dilation of the intrapancreatic portion of the common bile duct. This dilation usually is absent in the more frequent pancreatic cancers, and the absence of a pancreatic mass suggests an ampullary level of obstruction. This distinction is important because one would be more aggressive surgically with duodenal or ampullary adenocarcinomas, which carry a much better prognosis with resection.

Treatment

Optimal operative treatment requires a wide, segmental resection including the draining nodal system. Most duodenal adenocarcinomas require a pancreaticoduodenectomy (Whipple resection) to incorporate the pertinent draining nodal basin. Small lesions in the first portion of the duodenum and distal cancers in the fourth portion of the duodenum can occasionally be removed by segmental resection depending on size, curative intent, and local findings. Isolated reports of successful transduodenal local resections of small invasive periampullary cancers have appeared, but this experience is anecdotal. Palliation of unresectable duodenal cancers causing intestinal obstruction can be obtained by gastrojejunostomy, provided that bleeding is not a prominent component of the tumor. If bleeding occurs, attempts at endoscopic palliation using laser photocoagulation can be of some short-lived benefit. Extrahepatic biliary obstruction can be palliated by operative biliary bypass or by endoscopic or percutaneous transhepatic biliary stent placement. Jejunoileal carcinomas are removed by segmental resections, with the proximal extent of the mesenteric lymphadenectomy limited by the superior mesenteric artery. Distal ileal lesions are best managed by a right hemicolectomy to include the relevant draining lymph nodes. Mid–small bowel adenocarcinomas can even be amenable to a laparoscopically assisted resection. Laparoscopic examination of the small bowel reveals the involved segment, and if the involved segment is mobile, an incision can be made overlying the mass just big enough to allow this segment to be exteriorized, and an extraabdominal resection can be performed (Fig. 29-3). This approach avoids a formal celiotomy.

Chemotherapy and Radiotherapy

The role of adjuvant or palliative chemotherapy is unclear. Response to 5-fluorouracil alone is poor (less than 20%), and experience with other agents of potential benefit is limited. There are no strong indications for chemotherapy. Because these mucin-producing adenocarcinomas are typically radioresistant, radiotherapy offers no significant benefit in treatment.

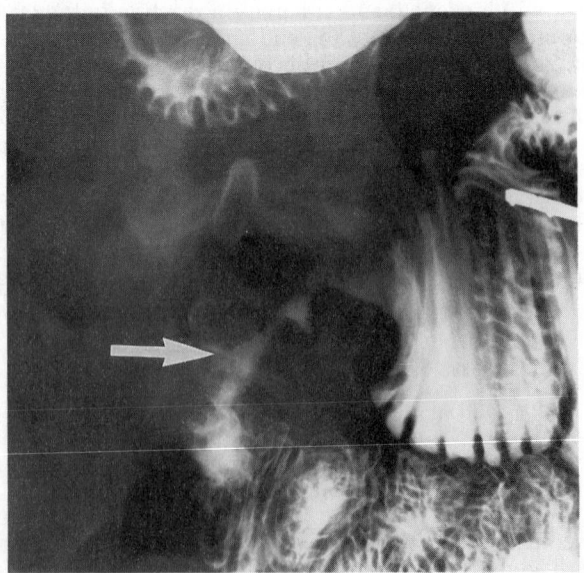

Figure 29-2. Characteristic apple-core lesion of primary small bowel adenocarcinoma.

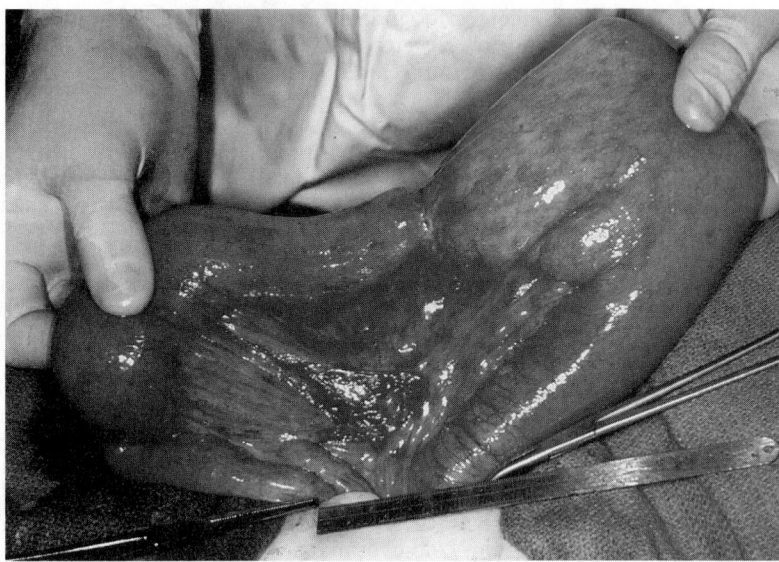

Figure 29-3. Laparoscopic-assisted extraabdominal resection of a small bowel neoplasm through a small incision.

Prognosis and Survival

The prognosis for small bowel adenocarcinomas is usually guarded because of their late, advanced presentation. Less than 50% of patients present with tumors confined to the bowel wall, and up to 25% have distant, nonnodal metastases. Overall 5-year survival rates range from 5% to 30%. Disease stage at the time of operation is the most crucial factor. In the absence of nodal involvement, the survival rate ranges from 50% to 70%; when lymph nodes are involved, the survival rate after curative resection is about 15%.

Leiomyosarcoma

Leiomyosarcomas account for 10% to 20% of all malignant neoplasms of the small intestine. Although they occur at all ages, the peak incidence is in the sixth decade with a slight male predominance.[8] There appears to be no association with geographic location, ethnic or racial background, occupational or industrial exposure, or hereditary factors.

Origin

Gut sarcomas can arise from any mesodermal component of the intestinal wall (eg, muscular, neural, connective tissue, vascular, or fat components). Leiomyosarcomas are by far the most common tumors; they arise from either the tunica muscularis or muscularis mucosa. Distinction between the malignant leiomyosarcomas and the benign leiomyomas can be difficult and is usually based on the number of mitoses per high-power microscopic field (more than two) and on concomitant cellularity, nuclear atypia, size of tumor, and presence of necrosis. This distinction is important because it determines prognosis. About 20% of these sarcomas are epithelioid leiomyosarcomas, characterized by bizarre pleiomorphic cells, which may have a somewhat better prognosis. The anatomic distribution of the leiomyosarcoma is roughly proportional to the length of the anatomic segment, with jejunoileal lesions the most common. Leiomyosarcomas arising in Meckel's diverticulum are disproportionately frequent for unknown reasons.

Presentation and Diagnosis

Unlike adenocarcinomas, leiomyosarcomas tend to grow extraluminally and obstruct the small intestine only late in their course. They often reach large sizes before causing objective symptoms warranting investigation. The mean duration of symptoms before diagnosis is about 1 year. Most commonly, patients present with abdominal pain and weight loss. Because of the highly vascular nature and large size of leiomyosarcomas, ischemia within the tumor causes areas of tumor necrosis, leading to hemorrhage (intraabdominal, gastrointestinal, or into the tumor) in about 66% of patients; intestinal perforation can present as an acute abdomen in up to 10% of patients. Intestinal obstruction can occur from external compression, less commonly from circumferential growth, and rarely from intussusception. A palpable abdominal mass can be evident in up to half of patients.

The diagnosis of leiomyosarcoma is often suspected by the presence of a mass effect causing obstruction on gastrointestinal barium examination. A barium-filled cavity indicative of an area of central necrosis suggests the diagnosis. Computed tomography may reveal a large, bulky, extraluminally based mass with central necrosis and occasionally with calcification (Fig. 29-4). Angiography can highlight a vascular mass that may suggest the diagnosis preoperatively. Celiotomy is usually required for both diagnosis and treatment.

Treatment

Optimal operative treatment requires a wide, en bloc segmental resection with the associated mesentery. Extended lymphadenectomy is not indicated because of the

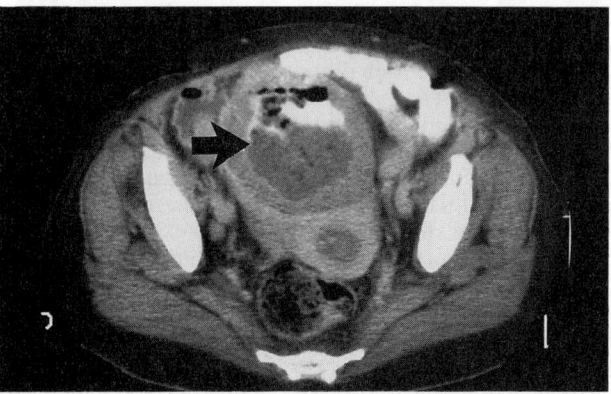

Figure 29-4. CT scan of leiomyosarcoma showing large size with central necrosis.

tendency of leiomyosarcomas to spread hematogenously as opposed to lymphatically. Nevertheless, up to 15% of specimens contain positive lymph nodes. Hepatic, intraperitoneal, and pulmonary metastases are present in 20% to 40% of patients at the time of celiotomy. For duodenal lesions, most resections involve a pancreaticoduodenectomy because of the bulky tumor size. Palliative bypass may be indicated in selected patients. Whether later resection of isolated hepatic or pulmonary metastases confers prolonged survival, as with other soft tissue sarcomas, is unknown, but an aggressive approach in appropriately selected patients probably should be considered.

Chemotherapy and Radiotherapy

Adjuvant chemotherapy or radiotherapy is of no benefit. There have been few trials of chemotherapy for recurrent or nonresectable disease, and objective response rates occurred in 10% to 40% of patients using combinations of doxorubicin (Adriamycin), cyclophosphamide (Cytoxan), and other agents. Palliation, however, is of short duration, and side effects are common. Leiomyosarcomas are radioresistant, and radiotherapy offers little therapeutic benefit.

Prognosis and Survival

The overall 5-year survival rate is about 40% to 50%. Surgical results correlate with both resectability (stage of disease) and histologic grade. The grade of the tumor is determined by the number of mitotic figures per high-power field (more than 10, high grade; less than 10, low grade); grade represents the single most important predictor of survival. The survival rate after curative resection of low-grade tumors is about 60% to 80%; after resection of high-grade neoplasms, it is less than 20%. Palliative resections (distant disease) of jejunoileal leiomyosarcomas are worthwhile, because up to 25% of patients live 5 years despite nonresected disease. Recurrent disease occurs both locally and through hematogenous routes such as the liver, lung, and brain.

Lymphoma

Lymphomas constitute about 10% to 15% of malignant small bowel neoplasms.[9,10] Small intestinal lymphomas occur as primary local neoplasms without concurrent peripheral lymphadenopathy or splenomegaly, or as secondary neoplasms presenting as part of a systemic disseminated lymphoma. Although primary gastrointestinal lymphomas are the most common form of extranodal lymphomas, they account for only 5% of all lymphomas. In developed Western countries, primary gastric involvement is most common, followed in incidence by the small intestine, the ileocecal area, and the colon. In the Mediterranean Basin and in socioeconomically underdeveloped countries, a form of lymphoma termed *immunoproliferative small intestinal disease* (IPSID) predominates. This latter condition is also called α-chain or heavy-chain disease because of the abnormal fragment of IgA heavy chain in the serum that is produced by diffuse infiltration of plasmacytoid lymphoma cells within the intestinal wall. Small intestinal lymphomas can occur in children younger than 10 years of age, usually as advanced, disseminated Burkitt lymphoma of the ileocecal region.[11] Small intestinal lymphomas most commonly occur during the fifth and sixth decades with a slight male predominance, and they can be multifocal in 15% of cases. Other conditions, such as celiac disease, Crohn's disease, and several forms of immunodeficiency syndromes, including the pharmacologically immunosuppressed patient, represent increased risk of developing extranodal gastrointestinal lymphomas. Some patients with AIDS have an aggressive form of lymphoma with predominant involvement of the gastrointestinal tract.[12]

Origin

Lymphomas arise from the lymphoid tissue within the wall of the small intestine. As might be expected, they predominate in the ileum, where the greatest concentration of gut lymphoid tissue occurs. These tumors previously were classified histomorphologically as lymphosarcomas or diffuse histiocytic lymphomas, but with current techniques of immunohistochemical staining of antigens specific for certain lymphoid cell populations, these terms are now obsolete. Experience with phenotypic surface-marker expression has shown that virtually all primary small bowel lymphomas are non-Hodgkin, B-cell lymphomas. They exhibit immunohistochemical characteristics similar to those of lymphomas in other parts of the body. T-cell varieties can occur sporadically or as a complication of celiac disease. Most small bowel lymphomas are intermediate or high-grade tumors with large-cell or immunoblastic features that have a diffuse rather than nodular growth pattern. Clinicopathologic staging is poorly standardized, controversial, and in a transition between phenotypic and histomorphologic criteria. Because the classic Ann Arbor staging system used with the more common peripheral nodal lymphomas has certain deficiencies with extranodal lymphomas, several other modified staging classifications have been proposed, but none is ideal or accepted by all groups (Table 29-3).

Presentation and Diagnosis

Patients with primary lymphomas of the small bowel usually present with nonspecific symptoms of fatigue, malaise, weight loss, and abdominal pain. In contrast to disseminated nodal lymphomas, fever, night sweats, pruritus, and cutaneous rashes are uncommon and suggest either a complication of the lymphoma or a secondary intestinal involvement from diffuse lymphoma. About 25% of patients present with an acute abdomen with perforation, obstruction, intussusception, or hemorrhage. Malabsorption can occur from diffuse mucosal involvement but is much less common with Western-type lymphomas than with the Mediterranean lymphoma. Although an abdominal mass may be evident, the physical examination is usually nonspecific, and diffuse lymphadenopathy is notably absent.

The diagnosis is usually suggested by findings on gastrointestinal contrast studies, including either submucosal nodules, mucosal ulcerations, or diffuse, coarse mucosal folds (Fig. 29-5). Other findings include fixation of involved intestinal loops or occasionally a characteristic aneurysmal dilation of the involved segment secondary to ulceration and necrosis of the tumor mass (Fig. 29-6). CT can help in diagnosis and staging by showing the presence of bulky mesenteric nodes in association with either dif-

Table 29-3. MODIFIED ANN ARBOR CLASSIFICATION OF PRIMARY NON-HODGKIN GASTROINTESTINAL LYMPHOMA

Stage	Description
IE	Tumor confined to small intestine
IIE	Spread to regional lymph nodes
IIIE	Spread to nonresectable nodal involvement beyond regional nodes
IVE	Spread to other organs within or beyond abdomen

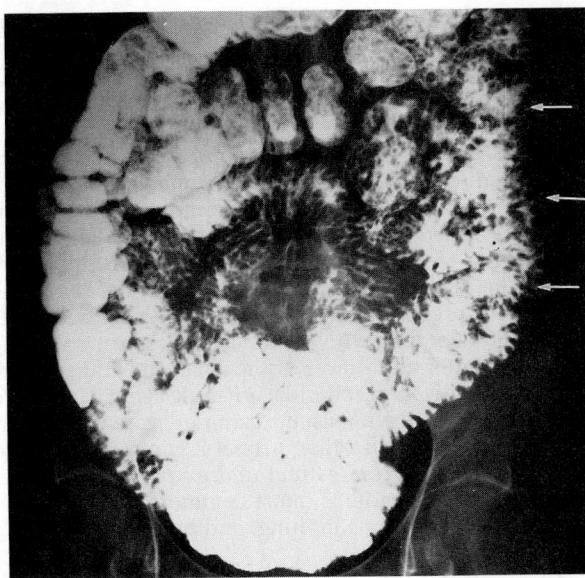

Figure 29-5. Gastrointestinal contrast study showing diffusely thickened folds of the small intestine secondary to small intestinal lymphoma.

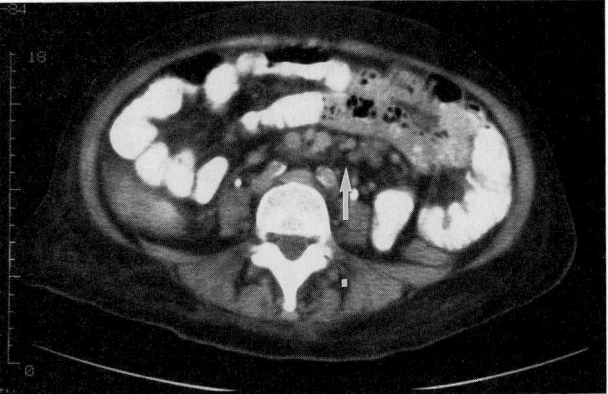

Figure 29-7. CT scan showing markedly enlarged mesenteric lymph nodes in a patient with small intestinal lymphoma.

fuse bowel wall thickening or a large tumor mass[13] (Fig. 29-7). Peroral or endoscopic biopsies are usually not worth pursing because of the anatomic location of most lymphomas in the distal small bowel.

Certain clinical settings are important. Intestinal lymphomas are known to be associated with several malabsorptive conditions. Clinical deterioration in a patient with previously controlled celiac disease should immediately suggest the diagnosis of lymphoma and may require celiotomy for confirmation. There also appears to be an increased incidence of lymphoma in Crohn's disease and dermatitis herpetiformis. Disorders of immunologic function have an increased incidence of extranodal intestinal lymphoma. These disorders include autoimmune diseases such as rheumatoid arthritis, Wegener granulomatosis, systemic lupus erythematosus, and congenital immunodeficiencies such as X-linked agammaglobulinemia and the Wiskott-Aldrich syndrome. Immunosuppressed patients after organ transplantation and patients treated with prolonged, high-dose chemotherapy are also at increased risk (up to 40- to 400-fold increase). AIDS has been associated with the development of aggressive, non-Hodgkin monoclonal B-cell lymphoma presenting with primary gastrointestinal involvement. This usually is a diffuse systemic disease, but extranodal lymphoma of the small bowel and anorectum has also been reported in AIDS patients. There are also a few reports of polyclonal and T-cell lymphomas in patients with AIDS.

Treatment

Most patients with intestinal lymphoma require operation, the goals of which include diagnosis, staging, relief of obstruction and perforation, and resection or debulking. Because intraoperative staging affects postoperative management, liver biopsy and sampling of paraaortic and mesenteric nodes outside the field of resection are important aspects of the operative management. When the lymphoma is localized, operative treatment should include aggressive resection with wide, en bloc lymphadenectomy. An exception is a primary duodenal lymphoma in which resection necessitates a Whipple procedure. This operative procedure as primary treatment for lymphoma remains controversial because it is a high-risk operation; however, this risk must be balanced against the known risk (estimated at 20%) of duodenal perforation or bleeding with combined curative radiotherapy and chemotherapy. Frequently, intestinal lymphomas are widespread or multicentric and are thus impossible to resect. Debulking, when feasible, should be considered, provided the overall health of the patient will not be jeopardized by removal of an excessive length of intestine.

Chemotherapy and Radiotherapy

The role of adjuvant therapy after curative resection for localized stage IE and IIE lymphomas is controversial and as yet undetermined (see Table 29-3). Nevertheless, most centers offer some form of chemoradiation regimen for these patients under the assumption that lymphomas are a systemic disease requiring adjuvant systemic therapy. When operative management has been directed at palliation or debulking, or with advanced disease (stage IIIE or IVE), a regimen of localized radiotherapy with combination cytotoxic chemotherapy is usually given. Although data are scant, the efficacy of such regimens appears to be limited, but they may provide worthwhile temporary responses.

Prognosis and Survival

The frequently widespread nature of primary small intestinal lymphomas makes their prognosis worse than that of gastric lymphomas. Prognosis depends primarily on

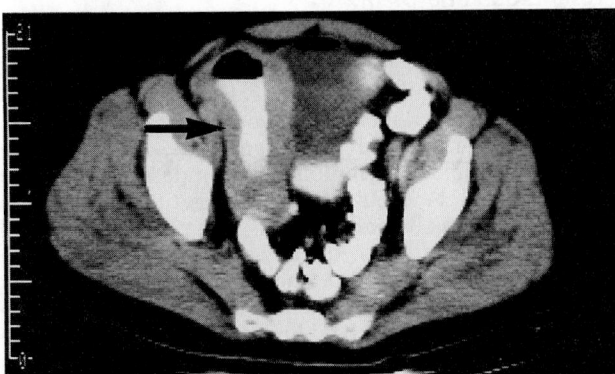

Figure 29-6. Aneurysmal dilation seen on gastrointestinal contrast study of a patient with a primary small intestinal lymphoma.

stage of disease at the time of diagnosis, but large size, multicentricity, local adjacent organ involvement, and associated complications such as perforation or malnutrition adversely affect prognosis. The overall 5-year survival rates range from 20% to 40%. With fully resected disease (stages I and II), the survival rate approaches 80%, but with stages III and IV, death usually ensues within 1 year of surgery.

Mediterranean Lymphoma

Mediterranean lymphoma is a variant of primary intestinal lymphoma and is most commonly found in lower socioeconomic populations in underdeveloped countries. This form of intestinal lymphoma has often been called α-chain or heavy-chain disease because of the predominance of an alpha heavy-chain protein in the serum, although recent reports from North Africa describe a nonsecreting variant. A more appropriate term for these variants of intestinal lymphomas is IPSID. IPSID occurs most commonly throughout the Mediterranean Basin and the Middle East, although sporadic cases appear in Western countries as well. IPSID affects primarily young adults, has a male predominance, and presents as weight loss, intestinal cramps, diarrhea, and steatorrhea. Clubbing of the fingers is often present. IPSID affects virtually the entire small intestine with predominant involvement of the jejunum and duodenum. Early on, the mucosa is infiltrated with benign-appearing plasma cells, but as the disease progresses, the cells assume a malignant, immunoblastic appearance with spread to nodal drainage areas.

The clinical course is generally one of escalating exacerbations and remissions; death results from progressive malnutrition or transformation to a disseminated, aggressive lymphoma. Rare cases of resolution with antibiotic treatment early in the course of the disease have been reported, although most patients experience a relentless downhill course. A combination of chemotherapy and radiotherapy results in an occasional response, but the ability to treat with a full dose regimen is limited by the associated malnutrition and malabsorption.

Posttransplant Lymphoproliferative Disease

Immunocompromised transplant patients are at a much greater risk of developing extranodal lymphomas characterized by their aggressive growth patterns and monoclonal nature. Early immunosuppressive regimens using very high doses of cyclosporin were associated not only with a very high incidence of these lymphomas (approximately 10%) but also with a markedly decreased time interval for their development after engrafting. Current regimens using lower doses have decreased the incidence of posttransplant lymphoproliferative disease, but it still occurs. It presents more commonly with intestinal bleeding and perforation. The mortality rate is high, and the surgeon should use all modalities of treatment, including a wide operative resection, chemotherapy or radiotherapy, or both, and, most important, reduction of the dosage of immunosuppression. The prognosis appears to be better in the less frequent polyclonal posttransplant lymphoproliferative disease. Chemotherapy combined with reduction of immunosuppression has little benefit in the monoclonal forms.

Carcinoid Tumors

Carcinoid tumors represent one of the most complex malignancies of the gut.[14] Our understanding of these often indolent neoplasms of variable malignant potential has evolved over the last several decades, especially with the recognition of their pleuripotential ability to secrete a number of heterogeneous endocrine and vasoactive substances, most commonly serotonin and the tachykinins (see Carcinoid Syndrome, later).

In most Western countries, carcinoids occur with a frequency similar to that of adenocarcinoma of the small intestine and thus represent one of the more common, clinically recognized small intestinal neoplasms. Incidence rates suggest about 600 new cases per year in the United States. The peak prevalence is in the sixth decade with a slight male predominance, but the age range (20 to 80 years) is broader than with the other small intestinal malignancies.[15] Carcinoid tumors of the small intestine, in contrast to appendiceal carcinoids, are multicentric in 30% of patients. For unknown reasons, carcinoids are well known to be associated with other primary, noncarcinoid neoplasms of both gastrointestinal and extraintestinal origin in 15% to 30% of patients, most commonly with carcinomas of the colon, stomach, lung, and breast.

Origin

Carcinoid tumors arise from Kulchitsky cells, a type of enterochromaffin cell in the crypts of Lieberkühn. These cells, referred to as argentaffin cells because of their affinity for silver stains, belong to the amine precursor uptake decarboxylase (APUD) system. The APUD concept was proposed originally to explain the existence of a related group of cells dispersed widely throughout the body that shared the ability to synthesize biogenic amines from an amine precursor. The APUD cells are a group of pleuripotential neuroendocrine cells presumably derived from the neural crest. These cells can synthesize a wide variety of vasoactive amines and regulatory peptides that can be demonstrated intracellularly by immunohistochemical techniques or by the presence of secretory granules on electron microscopy.

Histologically, carcinoids are very similar to islet cell carcinomas. They form a monotonous population of innocuous-appearing cells with uniform nuclei and cytoplasm and few mitoses. These findings led Oberndorfer to the term *karzioide,* or cancer-like, a misnomer because carcinoid tumors are true malignant neoplasms, although of variable malignant potential. Carcinoids are found in the foregut (usually stomach and duodenum), midgut (small bowel and appendix), and hindgut (rectum). Apart from the appendix, which harbors 85% of all carcinoids, the small intestine is the next most common site of origin (Fig. 29-8). Forty percent of small intestinal carcinoids are found within 2 feet of the ileocecal junction with multiple primary tumors occurring throughout the jejunoileum in 30% of patients.

Presentation and Diagnosis

Many small intestinal carcinoids and most appendiceal carcinoids are small and asymptomatic and are found only incidentally or at autopsy. Clinical symptoms can arise from the primary tumor, from the sequelae of metastatic disease, or from the carcinoid syndrome. As with other small bowel tumors, symptoms are nondescript. Because of the often indolent course of this tumor, the median duration of symptoms before diagnosis is 2 years. As the submucosal tumor infiltrates the bowel wall and beyond, the mesentery may become shortened, thickened, and fixed by an intense desmoplastic reaction characteristic of carcinoid tumors. This leads to kinking and angulation of intestinal loops. Thus, even though the diameter of the primary tumor is usually less than 2 cm and rarely mechanically compromises the lumen, this mesentery-based fixation can lead to symptoms of distal partial intestinal obstruction.

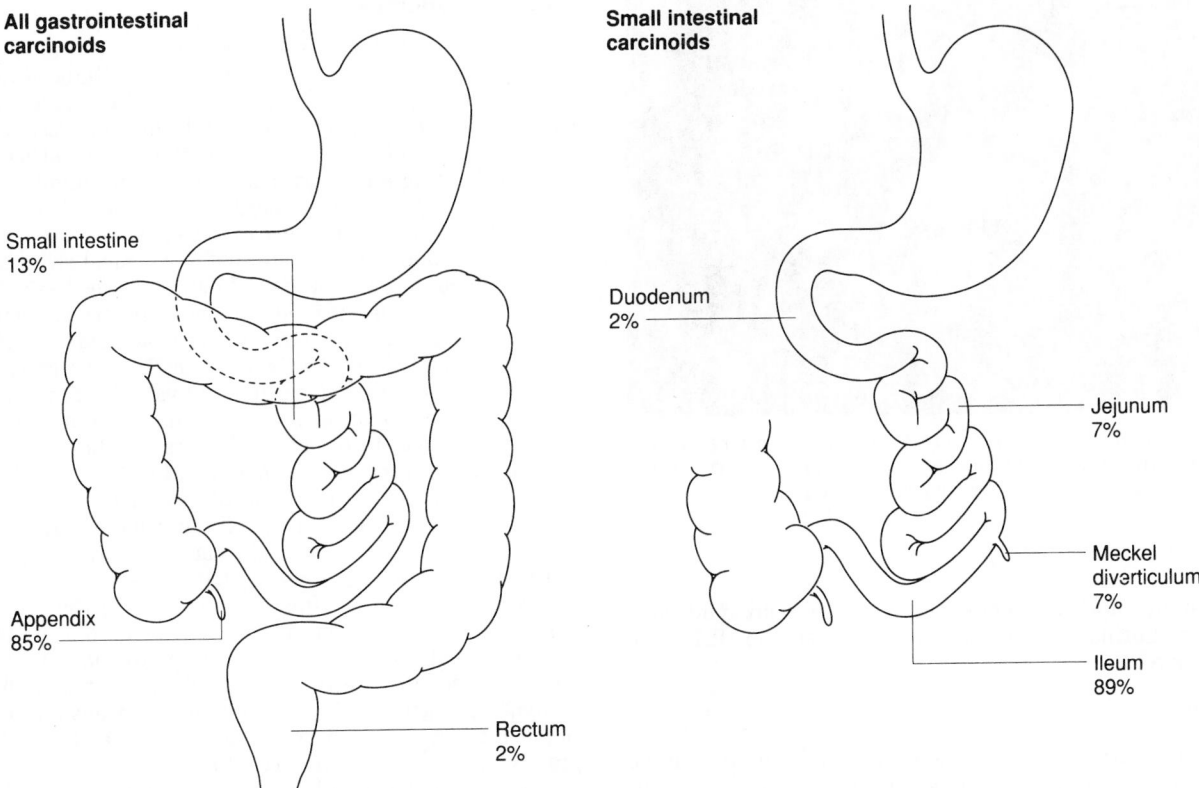

Figure 29-8. Relative incidence of gastrointestinal carcinoid tumors.

Although mucosal ulceration and bleeding can occur, as can intussusception, these symptoms are unusual. Intestinal ischemia or even infarction can occur secondary to a poorly understood type of mesenteric angiopathy, characterized by vascular thickening and sclerosis, that accompanies the desmoplastic mesenteric reaction. In addition to the carcinoid syndrome, another common clinical presentation involves constitutional symptoms of anorexia, weight loss, and fatigue related to the metastatic disease (nodal or hepatic), which is present in up to 90% of patients at the time of diagnosis. In many of these patients, the primary tumor remains asymptomatic.

Diagnosis requires a high index of suspicion. Differentiation from inflammatory processes such as Crohn's disease with gastrointestinal contrast studies can be difficult. Carcinoids more commonly show tethering and pleating of ileal folds with abrupt demarcation between stenotic tumor-involved ileum and normal adjacent bowel (Fig. 29-9). Associated submucosal nodules are occasionally present. Not uncommonly, the primary tumor may not be evident. CT may suggest carcinoid disease, not by recognition of the primary tumor but rather by demonstration of nodal metastases within the mesentery associated with a stellate pattern of soft tissue stranding (Fig. 29-10), or by the presence of multiple hepatic nodules, often involving a significant portion of the liver (Fig. 29-11). These hepatic metastases, also evident by ultrasonography, magnetic resonance imaging, and arteriography, may or may not function to produce vasoactive substances. Endoscopy is beneficial with the more unusual duodenal or rectal carcinoids but is of little diagnostic potential with small intestinal

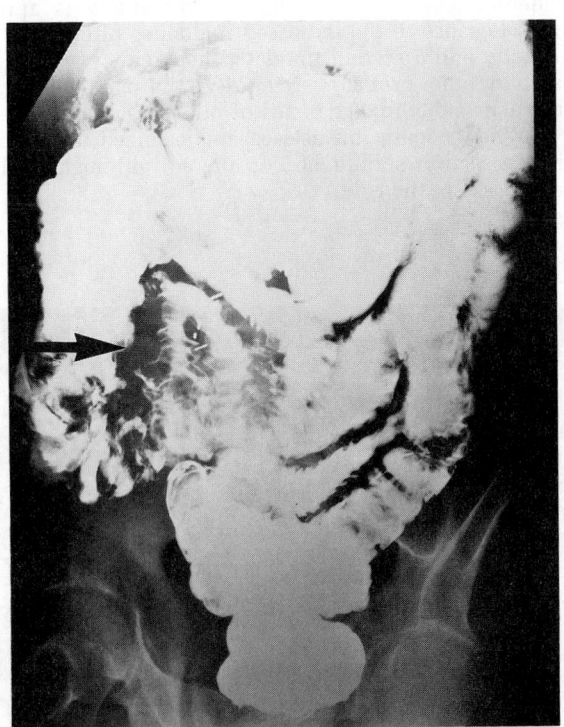

Figure 29-9. Small intestinal contrast study showing fixed areas of ileum involved by a carcinoid tumor.

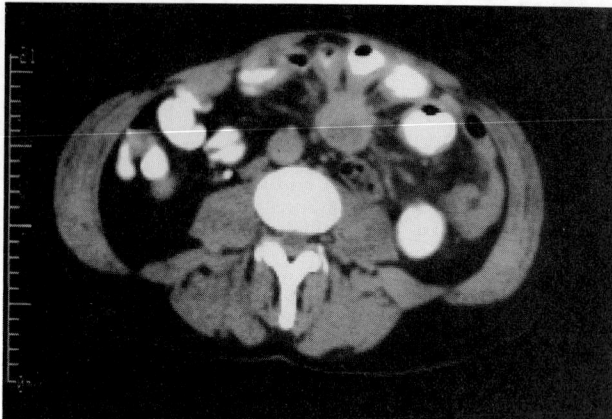

Figure 29-10. CT scan of a patient with an advanced carcinoid tumor. Stranding within mesentery is visible secondary to desmoplastic reaction to the primary tumor mass.

carcinoid tumors. In contrast to the carcinoid syndrome, levels of urinary 5-hydroxyindoleacetic acid (5-HIAA) are not increased.

Treatment

In the absence of the carcinoid syndrome, operative management of the primary small intestinal carcinoid tumor involves principles similar to those of other small bowel carcinomas. Wide en bloc excision should include as much of the nodal drainage pathways as possible because of their frequent involvement with metastatic tumor. In contrast to appendiceal carcinoids smaller than 2 cm, which are managed by simple appendectomy, appropriate treatment for most distal ileal carcinoids involves a right hemicolectomy. For more proximal tumors, a wedge-type segmental resection including the mesentery is appropriate. Because of the increased incidence of both multicentricity and a second unrelated malignancy, a diligent search for other primary carcinoids of the small bowel and for synchronous malignancies of other organs is imperative. When hepatic metastases are localized, a nonanatomic resection should be considered, although diffuse metastases are the rule.

Carcinoid Syndrome

Carcinoid syndrome is a spectrum of symptoms that manifests as late-stage disease with a large bulk of metastatic tumor deposits in the liver. When all the major clinical manifestations of carcinoid syndrome are present, the diagnosis is simple. The hallmark of the syndrome is intermittent flushing and diarrhea. The flushing involves the face, neck, and upper trunk and lasts for seconds or a few minutes. These symptoms can be provoked by certain foods, by alcohol, or by emotional or physical stress such as that encountered with the induction of anesthesia. Less common manifestations include bronchospasm, venous telangiectasia of the face and neck, and pellagra (characterized by dementia, dermatitis, and diarrhea). Heart failure that is secondary to endocardial and valvular fibrosis and is limited to the right heart is unusual at presentation but can develop later in the clinical course of the syndrome, presumably as a reaction to increased levels of circulating vasoactive amines in the blood of the inferior vena cava. The most dramatic and fortunately unusual manifestation of the carcinoid syndrome is the carcinoid crisis, a potentially life-threatening reaction that includes an intense, persistent, generalized flushing, severe diarrhea, and a spectrum of central nervous system symptoms ranging from mild light-headedness and vertigo to somnolence or coma. Associated cardiovascular abnormalities include tachycardia, arrhythmias, and either hypertension or hypotension. The carcinoid crisis requires an active and aggressive pharmacologic intervention.

The precise pharmacology and physiology of the mediators responsible for the symptoms of the carcinoid syndrome remain incompletely understood. Initially, serotonin was presumed to be the cause of the flushing and diarrhea; however, there is no predictable or consistent increase in blood serotonin concentrations during a flushing episode. Similarly, the other vasoactive substances commonly recognized to be produced by carcinoid tumors, including tachykinins (eg, substance P, neuromedin A), bradykinin, dopamine, histamine, and prostaglandins E and F, cannot be reliably implicated. Probably, the vasomotor sequelae are related to synergistic effects of several of these agents, most likely serotonin and bradykinin.

Confirmation of the clinical diagnosis of carcinoid syndrome is most readily obtained by evidence of serotonin overproduction.[14] An increased level of urinary 5-HIAA, a major metabolite of serotonin, is the most consistent find-

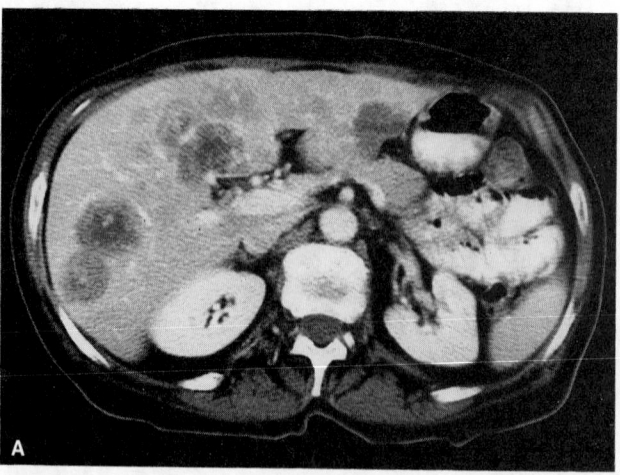

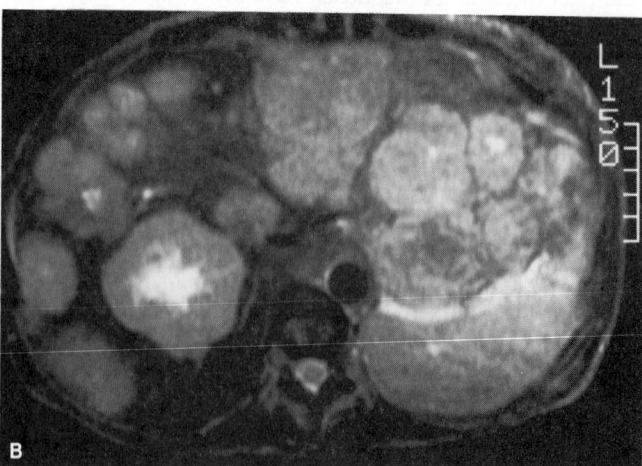

Figure 29-11. Massive involvement of liver with metastatic carcinoid tumor. (A) CT scan. (B) MRI scan.

ing, although alternate pathways for serotonin metabolism exist and may explain the rare patient with normal 5-HIAA levels. Normal 24-hour urinary 5-HIAA levels are less than 9 mg. Care must be taken in interpreting the results of this test because certain foods (eg, bananas, tomatoes, and pineapples) can increase urinary excretion of 5-HIAA. Several drugs (eg, phenothiazines) can also interfere with the assay. In the absence of the carcinoid syndrome, urinary 5-HIAA is usually normal in patients with carcinoid tumors lacking significant metastatic disease in the liver.

Treatment of the carcinoid syndrome is directed at relief or palliation of the symptoms. Although attempts at hepatic artery embolization and hepatic dearterializations are often effective, their durations of response are generally less than 4 months (sequential chemotherapy may improve tumor response after hepatic artery occlusion and prolong symptomatic relief). Hepatic transplantation has been performed in selected patients, but experience is limited. Operative debulking or attempts at curative resection of amenable liver metastases may offer a mean duration of relief of symptoms of up to 18 months.[16] The most efficacious treatment is pharmacologic. Trials of the serotonin antagonists cyproheptadine and methysergide and the histamine antagonists cimetidine and phenoxybenzamine (which prevents kallikrein release) may prove beneficial. The most active and effective agent in treatment of the carcinoid syndrome is the synthetic analogue of somatostatin, octreotide. Unlike the naturally occurring peptide, somatostatin, this long-acting analogue can be given subcutaneously and has biologic activity that lasts 8 to 12 hours. Octreotide decreases the concentration of circulating serotonin and urinary 5-HIAA in most patients, and it relieves or dramatically decreases flushing and diarrhea.[17] Tachyphylaxis occurs in some patients (median response, 4 months). Up to one third of patients achieve a long-lasting benefit for 2.5 years or more. Somatostatin or octreotide can also be life saving in patients with the carcinoid crisis and should be used when patients with the carcinoid syndrome are exposed to stressful situations such as operation or intense chemotherapy.

Chemotherapy and Radiotherapy

Chemotherapy of metastatic carcinoid tumor is of modest benefit. The most effective agents include doxorubicin, 5-fluorouracil, and streptozocin as single- or multiple-drug regimens. Responses occur in 20% to 30% of patients, but median durations of response are short-lived. Data suggest that chemotherapy may be more effective when combined with hepatic artery ligation or when the chemotherapeutic agent is incorporated into degradable starch microspheres, which are then embolized into the hepatic artery (most metastatic lesions have a primary arterial inflow). Preliminary results with immunotherapy of metastatic carcinoid tumors using recombinant α-interferons were encouraging, but larger studies have yielded disappointing results. Radiotherapy is of essentially no benefit. Although many metastatic carcinoid lesions take up the catecholamine analogue metaiodobenzyl guanidine, tagging it with iodine 131 as a therapeutic radionuclide has proved unrewarding.

Prognosis and Survival

Carcinoid tumors are slow growing. The overall 5-year survival rate is about 60%, but 5-year survival does not equal cure. Many patients live for extended periods of time with known nodal and liver metastases. Prognosis depends on the stage of the disease. With localized, nonmetastatic intestinal disease, the survival rate is no different from that of the general population. Nonmetastatic disease is unusual (below 10%). With resectable nodal disease, median survival is 15 years but decreases to 5 years with

nonresectable abdominal tumor, and to 3 years with liver metastases at the time of presentation. Patients with the carcinoid syndrome have a median survival of 38 months.

Metastatic Tumors

The small intestine can be the site of metastatic spread by means of direct extension or through peritoneal seeding from other intraperitoneal organs. Less commonly, hematogenous spread can occur from another primary neoplasm, such as melanoma or carcinoma arising in the breast, lung, stomach, or kidney. A long disease-free interval after treatment of the primary tumor can hinder diagnosis. Signs and symptoms of metastatic tumors are similar to those of primary small bowel malignancies, with pain and obstruction the most common symptoms. Treatment is palliative; if possible, limited resection is best to relieve symptoms, but bypass can be used if the disease is nonresectable. Prognosis is poor because this clinical situation represents distant metastatic disease. Metastatic melanoma in the small intestine deserves further discussion. Most of these metastatic foci remain asymptomatic and are best diagnosed by way of a contrast study. Concomitant distant metastasis decreases the mean survival to 12 months. Melanomas are particularly prone to mucosal erosion with intraluminal hemorrhage. If the patient has symptoms or if the intestinal metastases represent the only site of known metastasis, aggressive resectional therapy may be warranted in selected patients to improve the quality of life and possibly also the disease-free survival.

Incidental Small Intestinal Mass

Most incidentally discovered asymptomatic small bowel masses, whether single or multiple, are usually benign. Nevertheless, a diligent search should be conducted to exclude malignancy or intraperitoneal spread from elsewhere. When found at the time of gastrointestinal contrast study, further evaluation is often necessary. If in the duodenum, peroral endoscopy is the procedure of choice because if offers the possibility of biopsy. When the mass is in the jejunoileum, some form of operative evaluation may be required to exclude malignancy unless one can be assured that the mass is a lipoma. Operative evaluation is probably best undertaken not with a formal celiotomy but rather with a diagnostic (and potentially therapeutic) laparoscopy. The entire jejunoileum can be examined directly, and, when the mass is found, biopsy can be performed or the involved segment can be eviscerated through a small incision, allowing wedge resection or even segmental intestinal resection; this approach allows the diagnosis to be made without the morbidity of an exploratory celiotomy.

When a small intestinal mass is discovered incidentally at the time of abdominal operation for another condition, a frozen section biopsy should be performed whenever the diagnosis is in question. Certain conditions are characteristic, such as an ectopic pancreatic rest or splenosis, and may not require further investigation. In contrast, others, such as endometriosis, can mimic malignancy; biopsy may reveal their nature and avoid the need for a formal intestinal resection.

REFERENCES

1. Ashley SW, Wells SA Jr. Tumors of the small intestine. Semin Oncol 1988;15:116.
2. Kusumoto H, Takahashi I, Yoshida M, et al. Primary malignant tumors of the small intestine: analysis of 40 Japanese patients. J Surg Oncol 1992;50:139.

3. Townsend CM Jr, Beauchamp RD, Singh P, Thompson JC. Growth factors and intestinal neoplasms. Am J Surg 1988; 155:526.

4. Schmeisser HH, Janssen JWG, Lyons J, et al. Aristolochic acid activates *ras* genes in rat tumors at deoxyadenosine residues. Cancer Res 1990;50:564.

5. Morgan BK, Compton C, Talbert M, Gallagher WJ, Wood WC. Benign smooth muscle tumors of the gastrointestinal tract: a 24-year experience. Ann Surg 1990;211:63.

6. Bjorck KJ, Davis CG, Nagorney DM, Mucha P Jr. Duodenal villus tumors. Arch Surg 1990;125:961.

7. Prystowsky JB, Stryker SJ, Ujiki GT, Poticha SM. Gastrointestinal endometriosis: incidence and indications for resection. Arch Surg 1988;123:855.

8. Licht JD, Weissman LB, Antman K. Gastrointestinal sarcomas. Semin Oncol 1988;15:181.

9. Haber DA, Mayer RJ. Primary gastrointestinal lymphoma. Semin Oncol 1988;15:154.

10. Amer MH, El-Akkad S. Gastrointestinal lymphoma in adults: clinical features and management of 300 cases. Gastroenterology 1994;106:846.

11. Fleming ID, Turk PS, Murphy SB, Crist WM, Santana VM, Rao BN. Surgical implications of primary gastrointestinal lymphoma in children. Arch Surg 1990;125:252.

12. Friedman SL, Wright TL, Altman DF. Gastrointestinal Kaposi's sarcoma in patients with acquired immunodeficiency syndrome: endoscopic and autopsy findings. Gastroenterology 1985;89:102.

13. Dudiak KM, Johnson CD, Stephens DH. Primary tumors of the small intestine: CT evaluation. Am J Roentgenol 1989;152:995.

14. Moertel CG. An odyssey in the land of small tumors. J Clin Oncol 1987;5:1503.

15. Godwin JD II. Carcinoid tumors: an analysis of 2837 cases. Cancer 1975;36:560.

16. Que FG, Nagorney DM, Batts KB, Linz LJ, Kvols LK. Hepatic resection for metastatic neuroendocrine carcinoma. Am J Surg 1995;169:36.

17. Kvols LK, Moertel CG, O'Connell MJ, Schutt NJ, Rubin J, Hahn RG. Treatment of the malignant carcinoid syndrome: evaluation of a long-acting somatostatin analogue. N Engl J Med 1986;315:663.

SECTION E

PANCREAS

SURGERY: SCIENTIFIC PRINCIPLES AND PRACTICE, Second Edition, edited by
Lazar J. Greenfield, Michael W. Mulholland, Keith T. Oldham, Gerald B. Zelenock,
and Keith D. Lillemoe. Lippincott–Raven Publishers, Philadelphia, © 1997.

CHAPTER 30

PANCREATIC ANATOMY AND PHYSIOLOGY

DANA K. ANDERSEN AND F. CHARLES BRUNICARDI

ANATOMY

The pancreas is a retroperitoneal organ that lies behind the posterior peritoneal membrane at the level of the second lumbar vertebra (Fig. 30-1). The organ weighs 75 to 100 g and is 15 to 20 cm long. The pancreas is divided into three portions: (1) the head, which fits snugly into the duodenal C loop; (2) the neck, which lies over the superior mesenteric vessels; and (3) the body and tail, which are closely adherent to the posterior wall of the stomach and the spleen. Resection of the pancreas at the level of the neck results in a 50% reduction in pancreatic mass.

Embryology

The pancreas is of endodermal origin and arises from ventral and dorsal pancreatic buds. The ventral bud arises from the hepatic diverticulum, and the dorsal bud arises from the developing duodenum. During the fifth week of life, the dorsal bud appears first and grows rapidly. The ventral bud rotates clockwise behind the duodenum and fuses with the dorsal bud (Fig. 30-2). The ventral bud becomes the uncinate process and inferior head of the pancreas, whereas the dorsal bud becomes the neck, body and tail, and superior head of the pancreas. The ventral bud duct fuses with the dorsal bud to become the *main pancreatic duct,* or duct of Wirsung, which drains most of the pancreas. The proximal duct of the dorsal bud, known as the *lesser pancreatic duct,* or duct of Santorini, usually persists and drains into the duodenum through the lesser papilla (Fig. 30-3). Abnormalities in the rotation or fusion of the developing pancreas can result in specific congenital disorders.

Surgical Anatomy

Relations to Other Structures

The pancreas is almost entirely retroperitoneal and lies close to a number of organs (Fig. 30-4). The head of the pancreas fits closely into the curve of the duodenum and lies

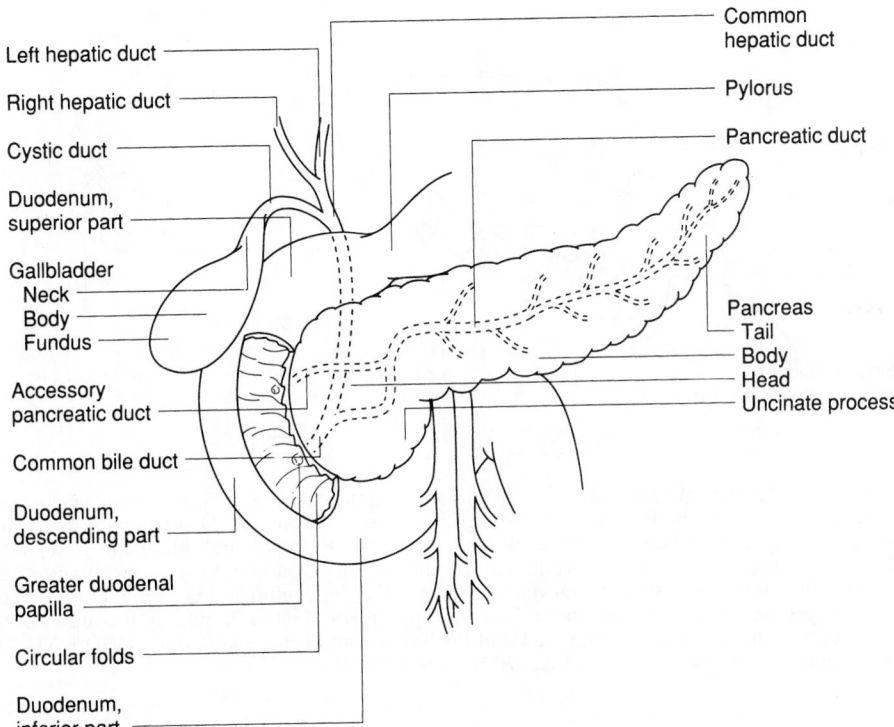

Figure 30-1. Relation of the pancreas to the duodenum and extrahepatic biliary system. (After Woodburne RT. Essentials of human anatomy. New York, Oxford University Press, 1973)

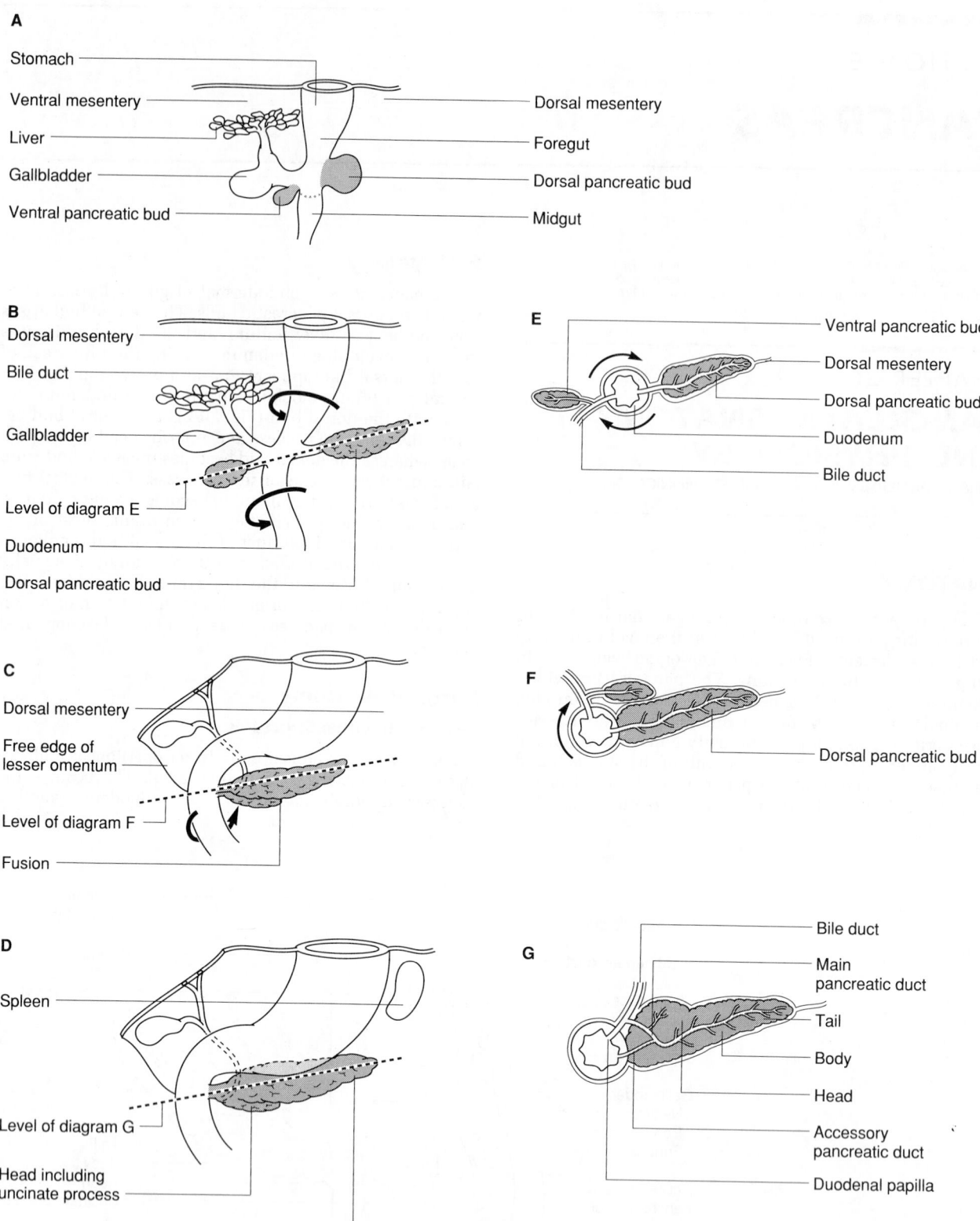

Figure 30-2. (*A* through *D*) Schematic drawings showing the successive stages in the development of the pancreas from the fifth through the eighth weeks. (*E* through *G*) Diagrammatic transverse sections through the duodenum and the developing pancreas. Growth and rotation (*arrows*) of the duodenum bring the ventral pancreatic bud toward the dorsal bud, and they subsequently fuse. The bile duct initially attaches to the ventral aspect of the duodenum and is carried around to the dorsal aspect as the duodenum rotates. The main pancreatic duct is formed by the union of the distal part of the dorsal pancreatic duct and the entire ventral pancreatic duct. (Moore KL. The developing human, ed 3. Philadelphia, WB Saunders, 1982)

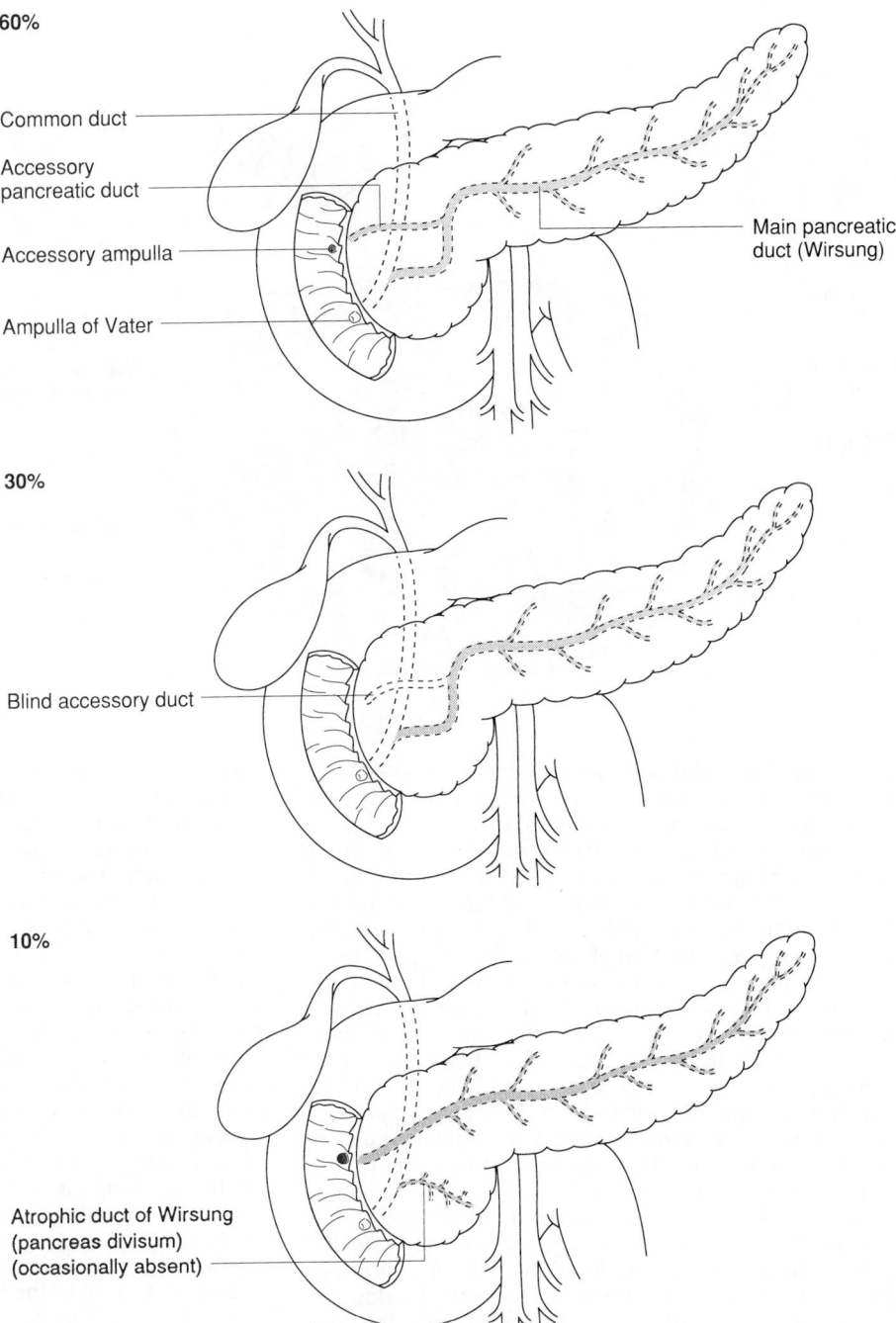

60%

Common duct

Accessory
pancreatic duct

Accessory ampulla

Ampulla of Vater

Main pancreatic
duct (Wirsung)

30%

Blind accessory duct

10%

Atrophic duct of Wirsung
(pancreas divisum)
(occasionally absent)

Figure 30-3. Anatomic configuration of the intrapancreatic ductal system. The lack of communication between the two ducts that occurs in 10% of cases is referred to as *pancreas divisum*. (After Silen W. Surgical anatomy of the pancreas. Surg Clin North Am 1964;44:1253)

to the right of the superior mesenteric vessels. The head is crossed anteriorly by the root of the transverse mesocolon and lies anterior and adjacent to the vena cava, the renal veins, and the right renal artery. The uncinate process, which is part of the head, wraps around and extends posteriorly to the superior mesenteric vessels. The common bile duct descends in the posterior surface of the pancreatic head to join the main pancreatic duct at the ampulla of Vater.

The neck is defined as that portion of the pancreas overlying the superior mesenteric vessels and is identifiable from the head of the pancreas by a notch that contains the superior mesenteric vessels. This part of the pancreas is sometimes referred to as the *incisura pancreatis*.

The body begins to the left of the neck. Its anterior surface is covered with peritoneum that forms the posterior floor of the lesser sac. The transverse mesocolon attaches

to its inferior margin. The body lies behind the posterior wall of the stomach and overlies the aorta at the origin of the superior mesenteric artery.

The small portion of the pancreas anterior to the left kidney is referred to as the *tail*. The tail of the pancreas lies close to the spleen, the left colic flexure, and the lienorenal ligament, making it susceptible to injury during splenectomy. An understanding of these complex relations can help to avoid injury while operating on the pancreas or on any of its adjacent organs and structures.

Pancreatic Ducts

The main pancreatic duct, or duct of Wirsung, runs the entire length of the pancreas and joins the common bile duct to empty into the duodenum at the ampulla of Vater. The duct usually lies in the center of the pancreas but

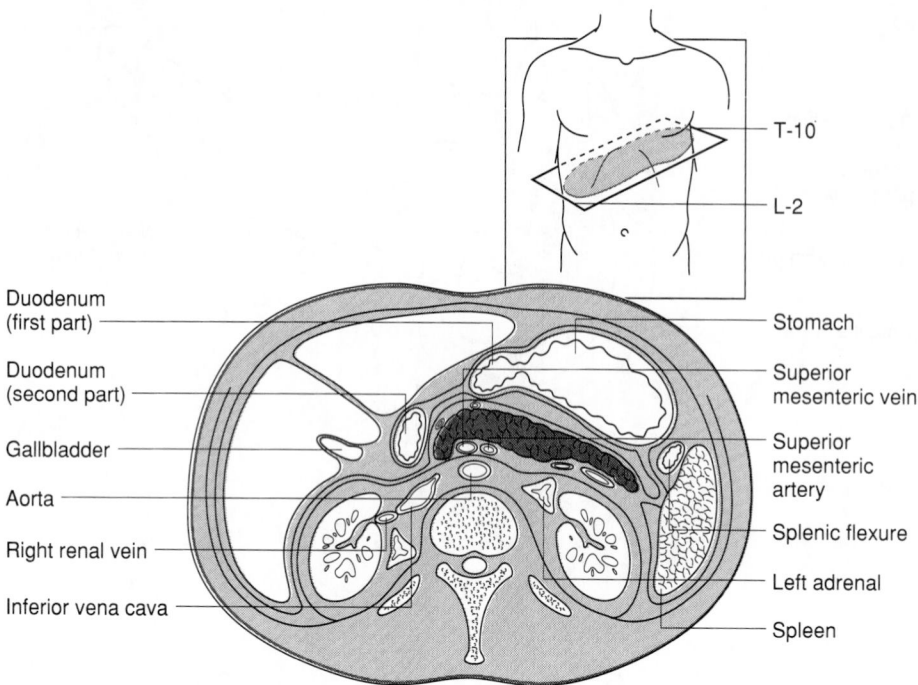

Figure 30-4. Cross-sectional relation of the pancreas to other abdominal structures in an oblique plane through the long axis of the pancreas extending from the level of L-2 on the right to T-10 on the left. (After Mackie CR, Moossa AR. Surgical anatomy of the pancreas. In: Moossa AR, ed. Tumors of the pancreas. Baltimore, Williams & Wilkins, 1980)

can be found near the posterior or anterior surfaces of the pancreas. The pancreatic duct is 2 to 3.5 mm in diameter and contains 20 secondary branches, which drain the tail, body, and uncinate process. Pancreatic ductal pressure is 15 to 30 mmHg, whereas that of the common bile duct is only 7 to 17 mmHg. The drainage of the lesser duct, or duct of Santorini, is variable. The lesser duct commonly drains the superior portion of the head of the pancreas. It empties separately into the second portion of the duodenum through the lesser papilla located 2 cm proximal to the ampulla of Vater. Usually, the lesser duct patently communicates with the main duct. When the ducts do not communicate, a connection is frequently present but nonpatent; less frequently, the lesser duct does not communicate at all with the major duct. Another variation is a lesser duct that empties into the main duct with no communication to the duodenum. All of the variations in the ductal system are secondary to differences in embryologic development and can be of clinical significance. Pancreas divisum results from an incomplete fusion of the ventral pancreatic duct with the dorsal duct during fetal development and is present in 5% of patients. In this anomaly, the lesser duct drains the entire pancreas; inadequacy of this pattern of drainage can result in chronic pain.

The main pancreatic duct joins with the common bile duct and empties at the ampulla of Vater. The surrounding sphincter of Oddi controls pancreatic and biliary secretions into the duodenal lumen. This sphincter is a complex set of muscular fibers surrounding the common bile duct and pancreatic duct and is regulated by neural and hormonal factors. The sphincter prevents reflux of duodenal contents into the ducts and can prevent reflux of bile into the pancreatic duct because of the differential in pancreatic and biliary ductular pressures. A short *common channel*, containing flow from both secretory systems, is seen in a significant number of patients (Fig. 30-5).

Arterial Supply

The pancreas receives its blood supply from a variety of major arterial sources. The celiac and superior mesenteric arteries supply blood to the pancreas through their major

branches (Fig. 30-6). In the head of the pancreas, there are arcades in the anterior and posterior surfaces, which generally collateralize. These arcades arise from branches of the gastroduodenal and superior mesenteric arteries. Just distal to the first portion of the duodenum, the gastroduodenal artery becomes the superior pancreaticoduodenal artery, which divides into anterior and posterior branches. The inferior pancreaticoduodenal artery is the first branch of the superior mesenteric artery and divides into anterior and posterior branches. The anterosuperior pancreaticoduodenal artery lies in the anterior head of the pancreas and collateralizes with the anteroinferior pancreaticoduodenal artery. The posterosuperior pancreaticoduodenal artery crosses the common bile duct and forms the posterior arcade with the posteroinferior pancreaticoduodenal artery. These arcades give off a rich vascular supply to the head and the second and third portions of the duodenum. The duodenum and head of the pancreas share a vascular supply; the two structures must be resected together. Twenty percent of patients have anomalies in the vascular supply to the head of the pancreas; the common hepatic, right hepatic, or gastroduodenal artery can arise from the superior mesenteric artery.

The body and tail of the pancreas are supplied by the splenic artery. The splenic artery arises from the celiac trunk and courses along the superior surface of the pancreas to the spleen. About 10 branches of the splenic artery supply the body and tail of the pancreas. Three of the larger branches are the following: (1) the dorsal pancreatic artery, which lies close to the celiac trunk; (2) the great pancreatic artery, or the pancreatica magna, which supplies the mid-portion of the body; (3) and the caudal pancreatic artery, which supplies the tail. These three arteries form channels that course through the length of the pancreas and collateralize with the inferior pancreaticoduodenal artery, which arises from the superior mesenteric artery.

Venous Drainage

The venous drainage of the pancreas and duodenum follows the arterial supply (Fig. 30-7). The veins are usually superficial to the arteries, and there is a similar frequency

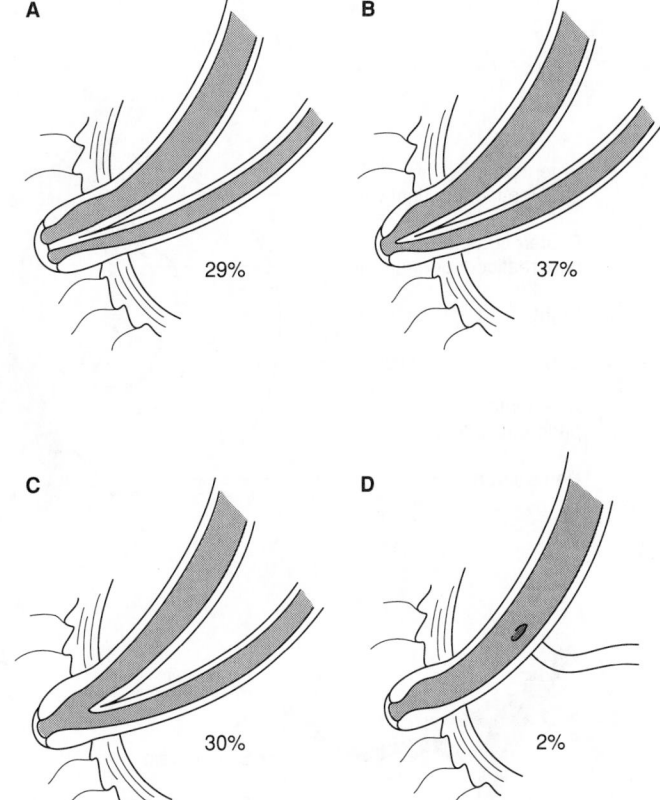

Figure 30-5. Variations in the relation between the intrapancreatic portion of the common bile duct and the main pancreatic duct at the ampulla of Vater. A common channel (*C*) is found in almost one third of subjects. (After Rienhoff WF Jr, Pickrell KL. Pancreatitis: anatomic study of pancreatic and extrahepatic biliary systems. Arch Surg 1945;51:205)

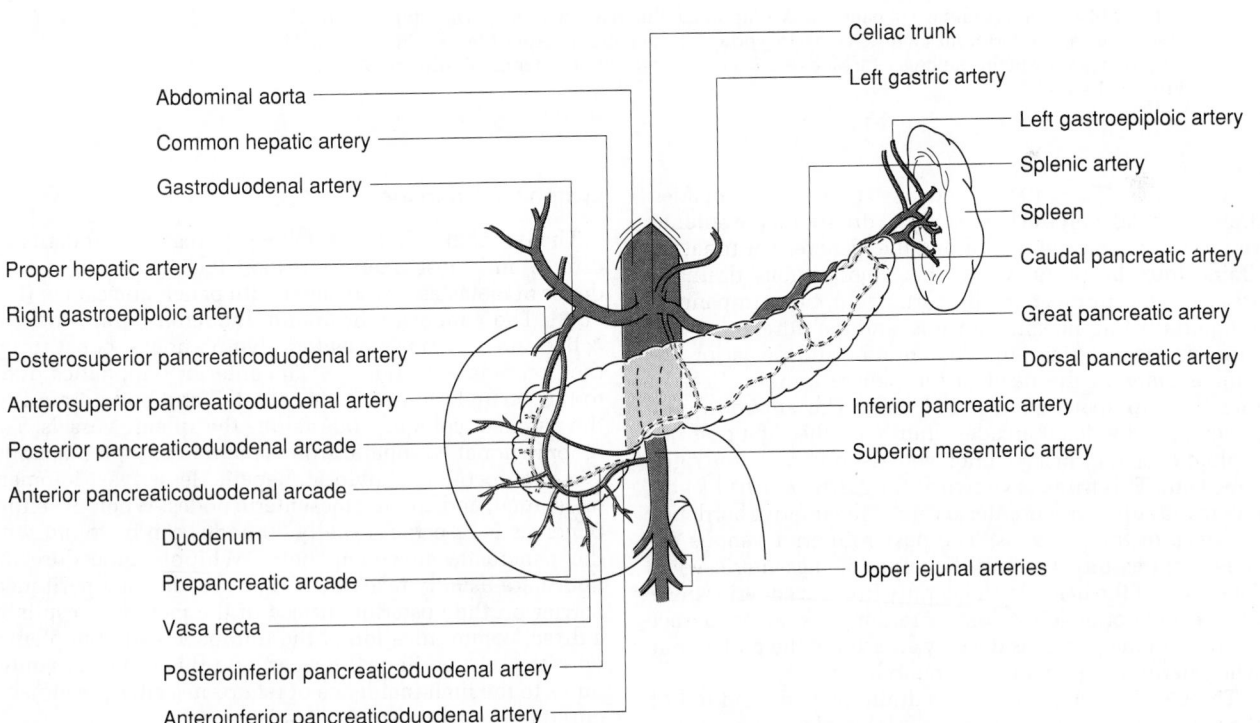

Figure 30-6. Arterial supply to the pancreas. (After Woodburne RT. Essentials of human anatomy. New York, Oxford University Press, 1973)

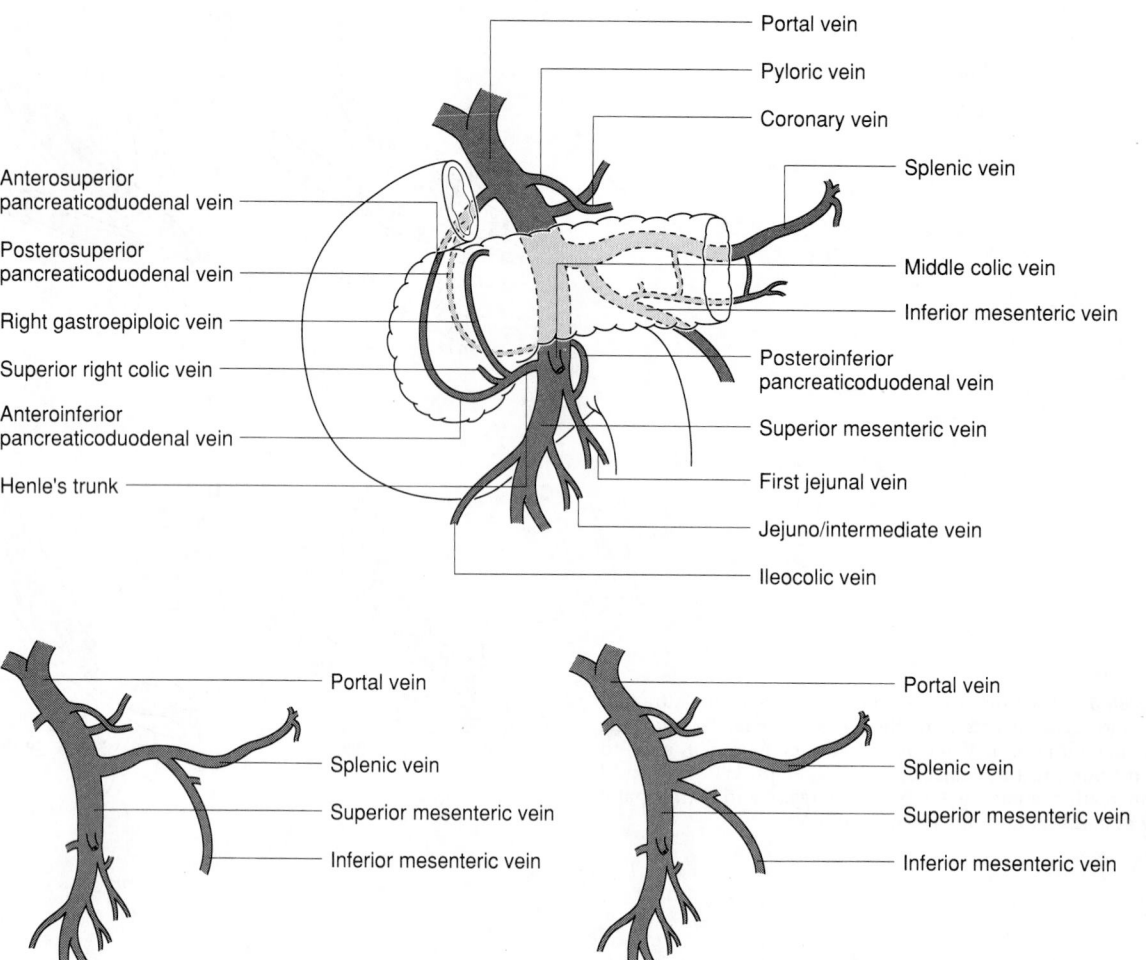

Anterosuperior
pancreaticoduodenal vein

Posterosuperior
pancreaticoduodenal vein

Right gastroepiploic vein

Superior right colic vein

Anteroinferior
pancreaticoduodenal vein

Henle's trunk

Portal vein

Pyloric vein

Coronary vein

Splenic vein

Middle colic vein

Inferior mesenteric vein

Posteroinferior
pancreaticoduodenal vein

Superior mesenteric vein

First jejunal vein

Jejuno/intermediate vein

Ileocolic vein

Portal vein

Splenic vein

Superior mesenteric vein

Inferior mesenteric vein

Portal vein

Splenic vein

Superior mesenteric vein

Inferior mesenteric vein

Figure 30-7. Venous drainage of pancreas. Variations in the relation of the portal, splenic, superior mesenteric, and inferior mesenteric veins are shown at the bottom. (After Mackie CR, Moossa AR. Surgical anatomy of the pancreas. In: Moossa AR, ed. Tumors of the pancreas. Baltimore, Williams & Wilkins, 1980)

of anomalies. The anterior and posterior venous arcades drain the head, and the body and tail drain into the splenic vein. All venous effluent from the pancreas ultimately drains into the portal vein. The major venous drainage areas are the suprapancreatic portal vein, the retropancreatic portal vein, the splenic veins, and the infrapancreatic superior mesenteric vein. The anterior and posterior venous arcades in the head of the pancreas drain directly into the suprapancreatic portal vein. The anteroinferior pancreaticoduodenal arcades drain with the right gastroepiploic vein to form a common venous trunk with the right colic vein. This trunk is known as the *gastrocolic trunk* and enters the superior mesenteric vein at the inferior border of the neck of the pancreas. The posteroinferior venous arcade empties directly into the superior mesenteric vein. The veins of the head drain laterally into the superior mesenteric and portal veins. For this reason, it is safe to dissect the neck of the pancreas directly anterior to the portal vein when performing a pancreaticoduodenectomy.

Three major venous branches drain the body and tail of the pancreas. These branches are (1) the inferior pancreatic vein, (2) the caudal pancreatic vein, and (3) the great pancreatic vein. All of these branches drain into the splenic vein. The inferior mesenteric vein courses behind the pancreas and either joins with the splenic vein or joins directly with the superior mesenteric vein.

Lymphatic Drainage

The lymphatic drainage of the pancreas is abundant and diffuse and most likely is responsible for the high incidence of metastases associated with pancreatic cancer (Fig. 30-8). The pancreatic head and duodenum drain into the celiac and superior mesenteric lymph nodes, constituting the predominant drainage. The anterior lymphatics drain to the peripyloric nodes, and the tail and body drain into the pancreaticolienal nodes along the splenic vessels. The other regional lymphatic groups include the splenic, transverse mesocolic, subpyloric, hepatic, lesser gastric omental, jejunal, and colonic mesenteric nodes. When the entire pancreas is resected, usually 70 nodes can be found with the pancreatic specimen. For a Whipple procedure, 35 nodes are usually recovered.[1] The absence of a peritoneal barrier on the posterior surface of the pancreas results in a direct communication of the intrapancreatic lymphatics with the retroperitoneal tissues, and this probably contributes to the high incidence of recurrence after presumably curative resections of pancreatic cancer.

Innervation

The exocrine and endocrine secretion of the pancreas is regulated by a rich neural supply that includes sympathetic fibers from the splanchnic nerves, parasympathetic

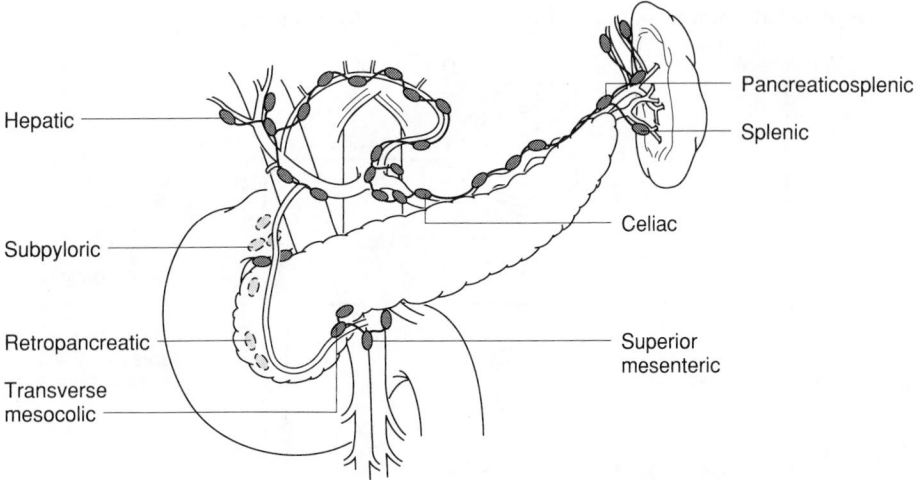

Figure 30-8. Lymph node groups receiving drainage from the pancreas. (After Mackie CR, Moossa AR. Surgical anatomy of the pancreas. In: Moossa AR, ed. Tumors of the pancreas. Baltimore, Williams & Wilkins, 1980)

fibers from the vagus, and peptidergic neurons, which secrete amines and peptides.[2] The sympathetic and parasympathetic fibers give rise to intrapancreatic periacinar plexuses, which send neural fibers to the bases of acinar cell groups (Fig. 30-9). The pancreatic islets are innervated by similar plexuses that communicate with both the islet vasculature and the islet cells. In general, parasympathetic fibers stimulate both exocrine and endocrine secretion, whereas sympathetic fibers have a predominantly inhibitory effect.[3] The peptidergic neurons that innervate the pancreas secrete hormones such as somatostatin, vasoactive intestinal peptide (VIP), calcitonin gene–related peptide (CGRP), and galanin. Although the peptidergic neurons influence exocrine and endocrine function, their precise physiologic role is unknown. The pancreas also has a rich afferent sensory fiber network, which probably contributes to intrinsic pancreatic pain associated with pancreatic cancer and chronic pancreatitis (Fig. 30-10). Although results have been equivocal, ganglionectomy or celiac ganglion blockage can be performed in an effort to interrupt these somatic fibers. The best results have been reported after combined bilateral thoracic sympathectomy and celiac ganglionectomy.[4]

STRUCTURE AND HISTOLOGY
Exocrine Structure

The two major components of the exocrine pancreas are the acinar cells and the ductular network. Together they constitute 80% to 90% of the pancreatic mass. The acinar cells secrete the enzymes responsible for digestion. The cells are pyramidal and have an apex that faces the lumen of the duct. Within the apex of the cell are numerous zymogen granules, which contain the digestive enzymes. Twenty to 40 acinar cells coalesce into a unit called the *acinus* (Fig. 30-11). A second cell type in the acinus is the centroacinar cell, which is responsible for fluid and electrolyte secretion by the pancreas. These cells contain carbonic anhydrase and other enzymes necessary for bicarbonate and electrolyte transport.[5]

The ductular system is composed of a network of conduits that carry the exocrine secretions into the duodenum. The acinus drains into small intercollated ducts. Several small intercollated ducts join to form an interlobular duct. The interlobular ducts contribute to fluid and electrolyte secretion along with the centroacinar cells. The interlobular ducts form secondary ducts that empty into the main

duct. The ductular network is progressively destroyed with recurrent episodes of pancreatitis, contributing in part to exocrine insufficiency and pain.

Endocrine Structure

Within the pancreas are small nests of cells that are responsible for the secretion of hormones that control glucose homeostasis. These nests are called *islets of Langerhans* and constitute 2% of the pancreatic mass. The islets contain an average of 3000 cells and range in diameter from 40 to 900 μm. The islets are composed of four major cell types—alpha (A), beta (B), delta (D), and pancreatic polypeptide (PP) or F cells, which secrete glucagon, insulin, somatostatin, and PP, respectively. The B cells are centrally located within the islet and constitute 70% of the islet mass, whereas the PP, A, and D cells are located at the periphery of the islet (Fig. 30-12). D cells have also been shown to be located within the core of human islets.[6] They constitute roughly 15%, 10%, and 5% of the islet cell mass, respectively. Islet cells can secrete more than one hormone. For example, in addition to insulin, the B cell secretes amylin, which can also regulate glucose metabolism.[7] The cellular composition of the islets varies throughout the pancreas. Islets in the uncinate process are rich in PP cells and poor in A cells, whereas the islets in the body and tail are rich in A cells and poor in PP cells (see Fig. 30-12). The B cells and D cells are evenly distributed throughout the pancreas.[8] The physiologic significance of this distribution remains largely unknown. As a consequence, certain operations can selectively remove a certain islet population. For example, pancreaticoduodenectomy removes 95% of the functioning PP cell mass, which can contribute to subsequent glucose intolerance.[9]

Islets contain small numbers of additional cells that secrete hormones such as VIP, serotonin, and pancreastatin. The islets also secrete numerous neuropeptides such as CGRP, neuropeptide Y, gastrin-releasing peptide, and somatostatin, which probably have local regulatory effects on endocrine and exocrine secretion. Islet cells are physiochemically distinct and are related to other neuroendocrine cells derived from the neural crest of the embryo. These groups of cells share the capacity of *a*mine *p*recursor *u*ptake and *d*ecarboxylation and can give rise to tumors called *APUDomas*.

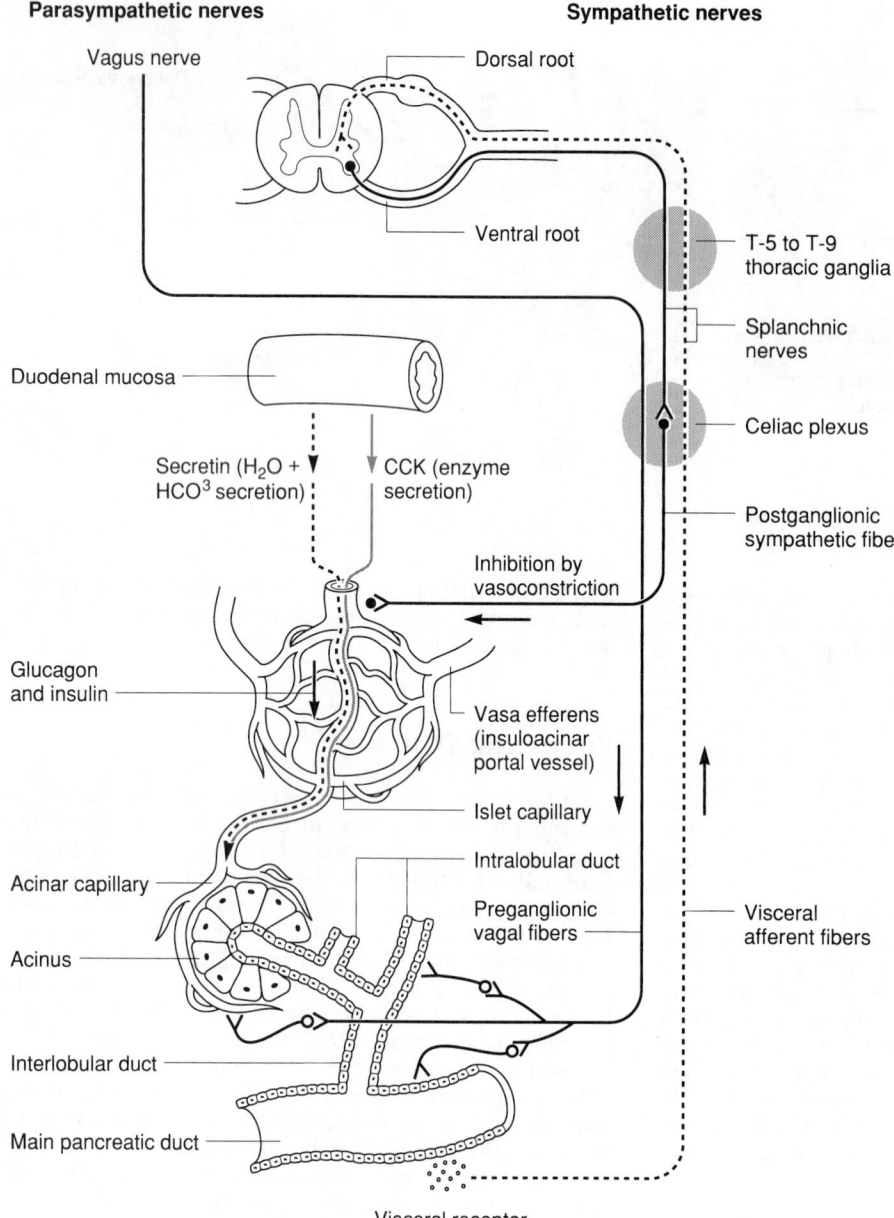

Figure 30-9. Schematic diagram of the neurohormonal control of the exocrine cells. Visceral receptors line the ductule system and carry the sensation of pain to the spinal cord. Sympathetic fibers first synapse in the celiac plexus after traveling through the thoracic ganglia and the splanchnic nerves. Postganglionic fibers then synapse on intrapancreatic arterioles. Parasympathetic preganglionic fibers travel through the celiac plexus after leaving the vagus nerves and course with vessels and ducts to synapse on postganglionic fibers near acinar cells, islet cells, and the smooth muscle of major ducts. Stimulation of these parasympathetic fibers results in an immediate release of pancreatic enzymes. Secretin and CCK first enter the pancreas through the capillary network of the islet cells, then enter the separate capillary network of the acinar tissue through the insuloacinar portal vessels. Glucagon, somatostatin, pancreatic polypeptide, and insulin from the islet cells reach the acinar tissue immediately after release. In this way, the islet cells can influence the acinar tissue responses to CCK and secretin. (After Tompkins RK, Traverso LW. The exocrine cells. In: Keynes WM, Keith RG, eds. The pancreas. New York, Appleton-Century-Crofts, 1981)

Intravascular Pattern

The blood flow to the pancreas has a distinctive pattern. The islets represent 2% of the pancreatic tissue but receive 20% to 30% of the pancreatic arteriolar flow. The distribution of blood flow can change after a meal, when blood flow to different parts of the pancreas is redirected.[10]

Research is examining the possibility of different microvascular patterns within the islets depending on location (periductular or intralobular). In one pattern, the arteriole of the islet penetrates into the islet and first perfuses the center, where the B cells are located.[11] The blood then flows toward the periphery, or mantel, of the islet, where the non-B cells are located, thus allowing high concentrations of insulin to modulate the secretion of the non-B cells through a paracrine action (Fig. 30-13). In another pattern, the arteriole perfuses the mantle, then the core.[12,13] The collecting vessels draining the islets then perfuse the acinar tissue. The perfusion of the acinar tissue with ve-

nous blood from the islet is known as the *insuloacinar portal system* and results in endocrine regulation of the exocrine pancreas. This regulation is principally due to insulin, but the other islet hormones, such as PP and somatostatin, are known to influence exocrine secretion.[14] Much of the acinar tissue is perfused directly by pancreatic arterial blood that bypasses the endocrine tissue.

PHYSIOLOGY
Exocrine Function

Early discoveries related to the exocrine pancreas were entirely separate from those involving the endocrine pancreas, as if the exocrine and endocrine pancreas were two separate organs.[15] Only recently has the intimate relation between exocrine and endocrine function been recognized. The pancreas secretes 500 to 800 mL/d of an alkaline fluid (or juice) that contains digestive enzymes. The alkaline pH

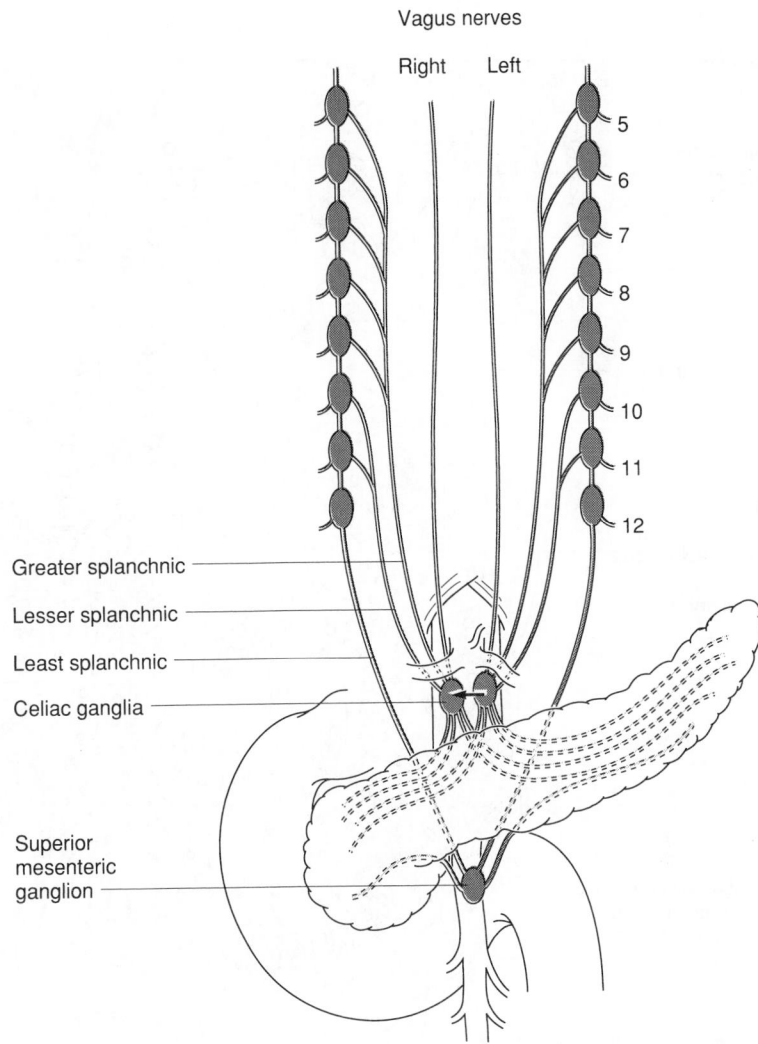

Figure 30-10. Diagram of the automomic nerve supply to the pancreas. (After Skandalakis JE, Gray SW, Rowe JS Jr, Skandalakis LJ. Anatomical complications of pancreatic surgery. Contemp Surg 1979; 15:17)

results from secreted bicarbonate, which serves to neutralize gastric acid and regulate the pH of the intestine, where the enzymes digest carbohydrates, proteins, and fats. Pancreatic fluid is colorless, odorless, and isosmotic. The pancreatic juice contains 0.2% protein, mostly enzymes such as amylase, lipase, and trypsinogen.

Bicarbonate Secretion

The centroacinar cells and ductular epithelium secrete fluid containing 20 mmol/L bicarbonate in the basal state and up to 150 mmol/L bicarbonate under maximal stimulation. The fluid has a pH that varies from 7.6 to 9.0, and it acts as a vehicle to carry inactive proteolytic enzymes to the duodenal lumen. Sodium and potassium concentrations are constant and equal those of plasma. Chloride secretion varies inversely with bicarbonate secretion, and the sum of these two cations remains constant and equal to that of plasma[16] (Fig. 30-14).

Bicarbonate is formed from carbonic acid by the enzyme carbonic anhydrase. Secretin, the major stimulant for bicarbonate secretion, is released from the duodenal mucosa in response to a duodenal luminal pH of less than 3.0. Cholecystokinin (CCK) only weakly stimulates bicarbonate secretion, whereas it potentiates secretin-stimulated bicarbonate secretion. Gastrin and acetylcholine are also weak stimulants of bicarbonate secretion.[17] Although choliner-

gic innervation appears to play a permissive role, bicarbonate secretion is inhibited by atropine and can be reduced 50% by a truncal vagotomy.[18]

Enzyme Secretion

The acinar cells secrete isozymes that fall into three major enzyme groups—amylases, lipases, and proteases. These enzymes include amylase, lipase, trypsinogen, chymotrypsinogen, procarboxypeptidases A and B, ribonuclease, deoxyribonuclease, proelastase, and trypsin inhibitor. The enzyme groups are not secreted in a fixed ratio, and specific nutrient stimulants can result in a relative increase of one enzyme over another. Dietary alterations can also result in changes in the relative amounts of amylases, lipases, and proteases secreted. When enzyme secretion is absent or impaired, malabsorption or incomplete digestion occurs, resulting in fecal losses of fat and protein.

Enzyme secretion is regulated primarily through hormonal and neural factors. The enteric hormone CCK is the predominant regulator and stimulates acinar cells through specific membrane-bound receptors. The intracellular effectors or second messengers are calcium and diacylglycerol. Acetylcholine strongly stimulates acinar cells when released from postganglionic fibers of the pancreatic plexus and acts in synergy with CCK to potentiate enzyme secretion (Fig. 30-15). Secretin and VIP weakly stimulate

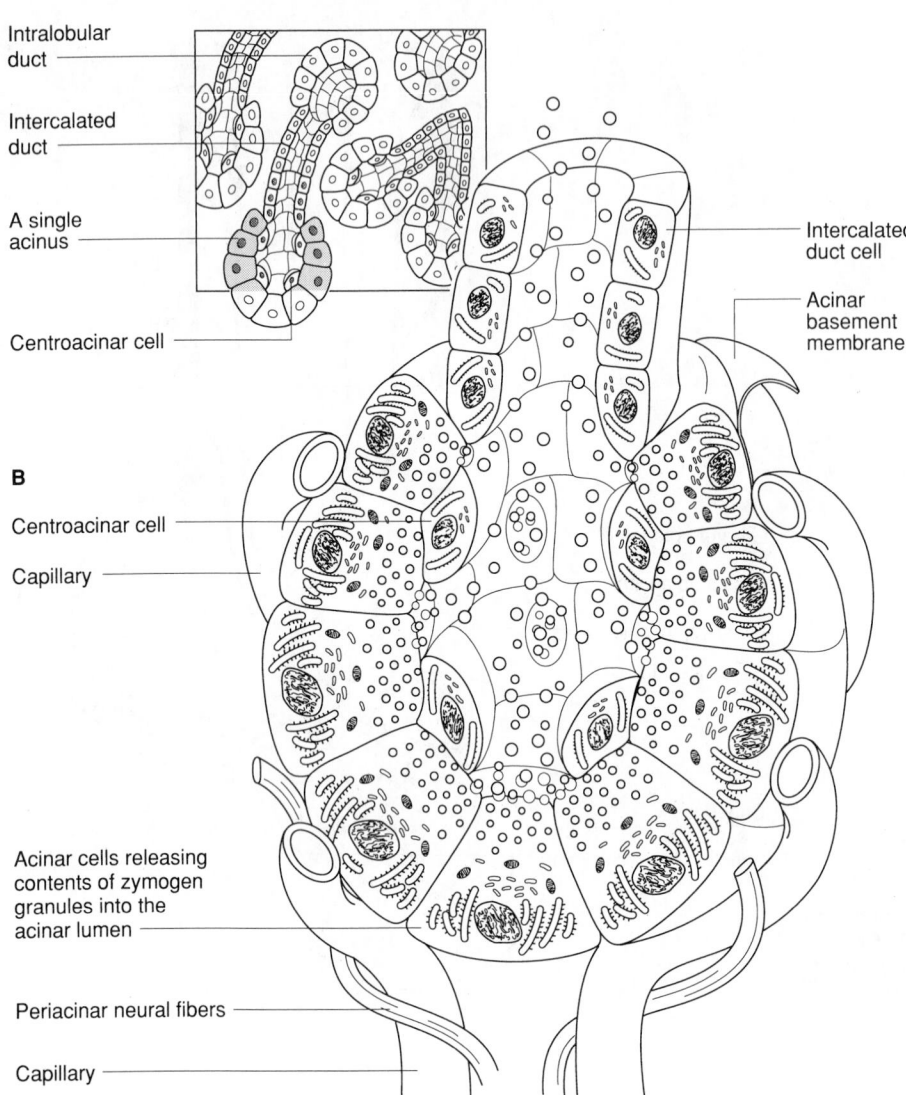

A

Intralobular duct

Intercalated duct

A single acinus

Centroacinar cell

Intercalated duct cell

Acinar basement membrane

B

Centroacinar cell

Capillary

Acinar cells releasing contents of zymogen granules into the acinar lumen

Periacinar neural fibers

Capillary

Figure 30-11. Histologic anatomy of the acinus. (*A*) Low-magnification view of a portion of the pancreas. (*B*) High-magnification view of a single acinus. (After Krstic RV. Die Gewebes des Menschen und der Saugetiere. Berlin, Springer-Verlag, 1978)

acinar cell secretion, but they also potentiate the effect of CCK on the acinar cells. Acinar cell secretion also is influenced by islet hormones by the insuloacinar portal system. The enzymes are synthesized in the endoplasmic reticulum of the acinar cells and are packaged in the zymogen granules. They are released from the apical portion of the acinar cells into the lumen of the acinus and are then transported into the duodenal lumen, where the enzymes are activated.

Enzyme Groups

Amylase is secreted within the human body from both pancreatic and salivary tissue. Pancreatic amylase represents isoamylase type P. A pancreatic source of excess levels of amylase, as in pancreatitis, can be determined by obtaining isoamylase studies. Amylase hydrolyzes starch and glycogen to glucose, maltose, maltotriose, and dextrins. Amylase is the only digestive enzyme secreted by the pancreas in an active form, although it functions optimally at a pH of 7.0.

Lipases emulsify and hydrolyze fat in the presence of bile salts. They hydrolyze insoluble esters of glycerol, alcohol esters, and water-soluble esters. Lipases func-

tion optimally at a pH of 7.0 to 9.0, and steatorrhea can result from over-acidification of the duodenum and jejunum, as occurs in gastric hypersecretory states. There are two phospholipases, A and B. Phospholipase A cleaves the fatty acid off lecithin or cephalin to form lysolecithin or lysocephalin. Phospholipase B cleaves the fatty acid off lysolecithin to form glycerol phosphatylcholine.

The proteolytic enzymes are essential for protein digestion. These enzymes are secreted as proenzymes and require activation for proteolytic activity. The proenzymes of trypsin and chymotrypsin are trypsinogen and chymotrypsinogen. They are activated primarily by a duodenal enzyme, enterokinase, which converts trypsinogen to trypsin. Trypsin, in turn, activates chymotrypsin, elastase, carboxypeptidase, and phospholipase. Trypsinogen can also be activated by a fall in pH below 7.0. Within the pancreas, enzyme activation is prevented by an antiproteolytic enzyme secreted by the acinar cells. This enzyme inactivates trypsin by direct binding, which protects the pancreatic tissue from autodigestion.

Trypsinogen is a 229–amino acid polypeptide that hydrolyzes proteins and also acts as a thrombokinase, ac-

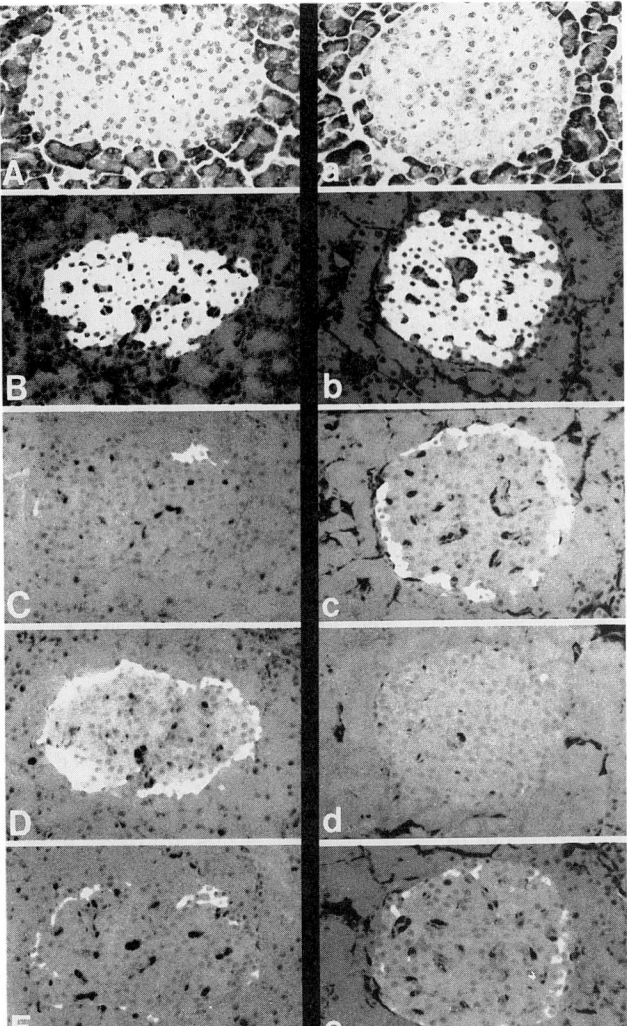

Figure 30-12. Histologic anatomy of the islet. Serial sections of a representative islet found in the ventral (*A* through *e*) and dorsal (*A* through *e*) portions of the pancreas. (*A* and *a*) Cells stained with hematoxylin-eosin. (*B* and *b*) B cells immunohistochemically stained with antiinsulin antisera. (*C* and *c*) A cells stained with antiglucagon antisera. (*D* and *d*) PP cells stained with antipancreatic polypeptide antisera. (*E* and *e*) D cells stained with antisomatostatin antisera. (Orci L. Macro- and micro-domains in the endocrine pancreas. Diabetes 1982;31:538)

celerating coagulation of the blood. Trypsinogen can convert spontaneously to trypsin, but the change is accelerated by enterokinase, by acid, or by active trypsin itself. Chymotrypsinogen is a 246–amino acid polypeptide. Chymotrypsinogen is converted to the active form, chymotrypsin, by trypsin or, indirectly, by enterokinase. The enzyme hydrolyzes proteins in a mechanism similar to that of trypsin but cleaves the proteins at a different site. The optimal activity of chymotrypsin and trypsin occurs at a pH of 8.0 to 9.0. Other proteolytic enzymes, such as carboxypeptidases A and B, are enzymes that further digest proteins that have been digested by trypsin and chymotrypsin. The nucleolytic enzymes, ribonuclease and deoxyribonuclease, hydrolyze nucleic acids into mononucleotides. Thus, through the secretion of the three classes of enzymes, the pancreas regulates complete digestion of fats, carbohydrates, and proteins.

Endocrine Function

Insulin Synthesis, Secretion, and Action

Insulin is a 56–amino acid polypeptide with a molecular weight of 6 kd. It consists of two polypeptide chains, an A and a B chain, joined by two disulfide bridges. Although species variation occurs in the amino acid sequence, the positions of the disulfide bridges are constant and important for biologic activity. Insulin is synthesized in the B cells of the islets of Langerhans. The B cells are destroyed in type I, or insulin-dependent, diabetes, leaving an absolute insulin deficiency. A considerable capacity exists for secretory reserves of insulin; 80% of the islet cell mass must be surgically removed before diabetes becomes clinically apparent.[19]

When the B cell is stimulated, a newly synthesized single chain peptide, proinsulin, is transported from the endoplasmic reticulum to the Golgi complex. At this site, proinsulin is packaged into granules and cleaved into insulin and a residual connecting peptide, or C peptide (Fig. 30-16). The granules then move toward the outer membrane by way of microtubules and are released into the intervascular space through emiocytosis. Defects in the synthesis and cleavage of insulin can lead to rare forms of diabetes mellitus, such as Wakayama syndrome and the proinsulin syndromes.[20]

Insulin is secreted in two phases. The first phase is a burst of stored insulin that lasts 4 to 6 minutes. This is followed by a second phase in which there is sustained secretion attributed to ongoing synthesis of insulin. The secretion of insulin is regulated by nutrient, neural, and hormonal factors. Glucose is the predominant nutrient regulator. The B cell is exquisitely sensitive to small changes in glucose concentration, with the maximal stimulation of insulin secretion occurring at a glucose concentration of 400 to 500 mg/dL.

Glucose is transported actively across cell membranes throughout the body by 55-kd membrane-bound facilitator peptides called *glucose transporters* (Fig. 30-17). Several classes of glucose transporters have been identified. The type of glucose transporter located on the B cell (GLUT-2) has a low affinity (or high K_m) for glucose, which results in modest transport of glucose at lower physiologic concentrations, but greater transport and therefore more subsequent insulin secretion at higher glucose concentrations.[21] Studies suggest that a loss of B-cell GLUT-2 glucose transporters can precede, and therefore contribute to, the development of diabetes.[22]

Orally administered glucose stimulates a greater insulin response than an equivalent amount of intravenous glucose through the release of enteric hormones that potentiate insulin secretion. This effect is known as the *enteroinsular axis*. Gastric inhibitory polypeptide (GIP) appears to be an important regulator of this incretion effect,[23] although other gut peptides, such as glucagon-like peptide-1, can contribute to this effect as well. Additional nutrients that regulate insulin secretion are amino acids, such as arginine, lysine, and leucine, and free fatty acids. Hormones that stimulate insulin secretion include glucagon, GIP, and CCK, whereas somatostatin, amylin, and pancreastatin are inhibitory. Insulin is also stimulated by sulfonylurea compounds, which act independently of the glucose concentration and form the basis of treatment of type II, or non–insulin-dependent, diabetes.

The B cell is neurally regulated by cholinergic fibers that stimulate insulin secretion. β-Sympathetic fibers are also stimulatory, whereas α-sympathetic fibers strongly inhibit insulin secretion. Loss of pancreatic innervation, which occurs after pancreatic transplantation, results in changes in the pattern or quantity of insulin secretion. Research is

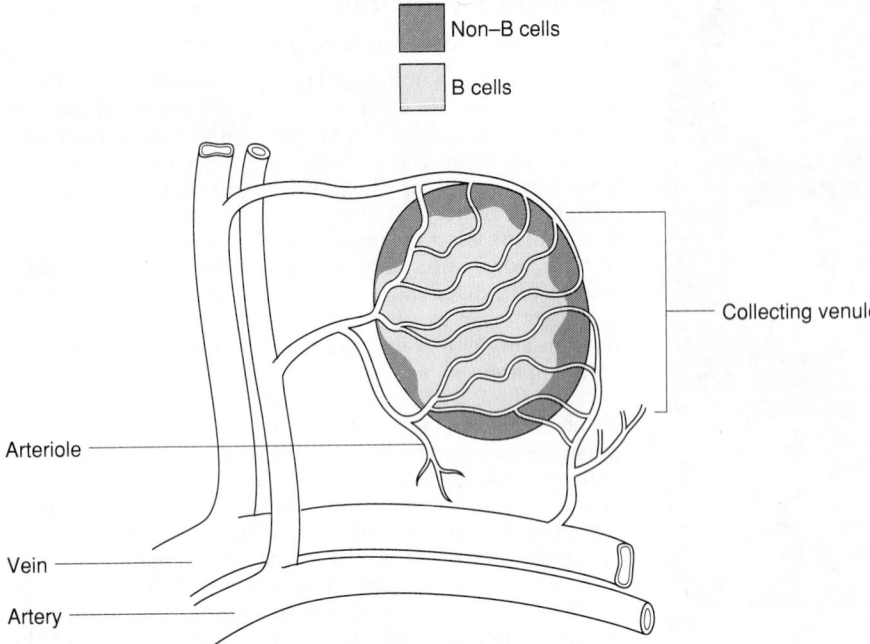

Figure 30-13. Diagram of a typical islet. Afferent arterioles enter the islet through discontinuities of the mantle of non–B cells and break into capillaries, most of which traverse the B-cell mass and pass through the mantle as efferent vessels. Occasionally a capillary passes at the interface of the B cells and non–B cells and never enters the B-cell core. In the larger islets, the efferent capillaries coalesce at the edge of the islet and pass along the mantle as collecting venules before draining in a vein. (After Bonner-Weir S, Orci L. New perspectives on the microvasculature of the islets of Langerhans in the rat. Diabetes 1982;31:883)

examining the role of neuropeptides such as CGRP and galanin in the regulation of insulin secretion.

Insulin is released in an oscillatory or pulsatile pattern and is controlled by an internal pacemaker, present even in isolated islets.[24] Once secreted, insulin has a half-life of 7 to 10 minutes and is metabolized primarily by the liver. Forty to 70% of insulin secreted into the portal vein is cleared by the hepatocytes during the first pass. The brain and red blood cells take up no insulin. The liver, kidney, and skeletal muscle slowly metabolize insulin and remove it from the circulation. Little insulin is excreted in the urine.

Insulin promotes glucose transport in all cells, except B cells, hepatocytes, and the central nervous system. Insulin-stimulated glucose transport in muscle and adipose tissue can also result from insulin regulation of membrane-bound glucose transporters. Insulin inhibits glycogenolysis, but stimulates protein synthesis. Insulin also inhibits fatty acid breakdown, and therefore inhibits ketone formation.

As with all endocrine systems, insulin binds to specific receptors. These receptors have been isolated and characterized. The insulin receptor is a glycoprotein with a molecular weight of 300 kd. The stimulation of the receptor depends on insulin concentration. Insulin resistance can be the result of either a decreased number of receptors or a decreased affinity for insulin, whereas excessive receptors can result in hypoglycemia. Defects in insulin receptors can lead to the insulin resistance seen in type II diabetes mellitus and in rare forms of diabetes, such as the type A syndrome, leprechaunism, and lipotrophic diabetes.[25]

Glucagon Synthesis, Secretion, and Action

Glucagon is a single-chain, 29–amino acid polypeptide with a molecular weight of 3.5 kd. Glucagon is secreted by the A cells of the islet and promotes hepatic glycogenolysis. Other forms of glucagon are released from the gut, including gastric glucagon, enteroglucagon, and glucagon-like peptides. Their physiologic role remains unclear.

Pancreatic glucagon secretion is controlled by neural, hormonal, and nutrient factors. Glucose is the primary regulator and has a potent suppressive effect on glucagon secretion. Glucagon and insulin respond in reciprocal fashion to changes in glucose concentrations; therefore, glucagon is considered a counterregulatory hormone to insulin. In a balance of actions, the two hormones work together to maintain basal glucose levels. Exaggerated or ex-

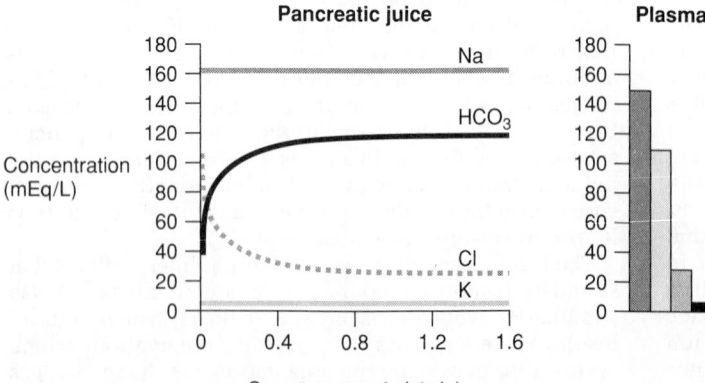

Figure 30-14. Relation of pancreatic secretion and concentration of electrolytes. (Bro-Rasmussen F, Kilman SA, Thaysen JH. Acta Physiol Scand 1956;37:97)

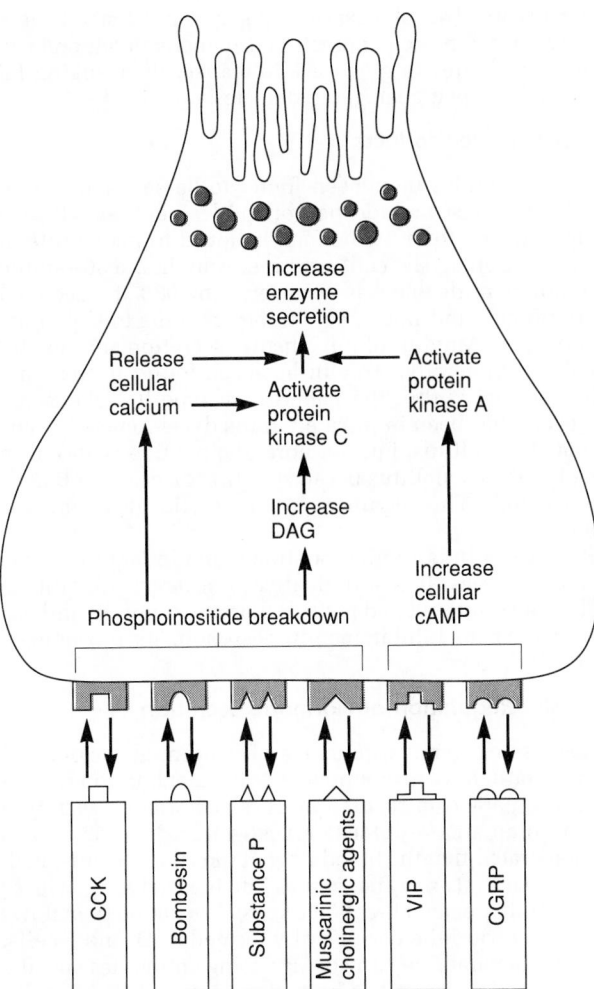

Figure 30-15. Schematic diagram of an acinar cell, demonstrating receptors for exocrine secretagogues and their intracellular bases of action. Six distinct classes of receptors are known, with principal ligands shown. CCK, cholecystokinin; VIP, vasoactive intestinal polypeptide; CRGP, calcitonin gene–related peptide; DAG, diacylglycerol.

cess glucagon secretion can contribute to hyperglycemia, whereas a failure of glucagon secretion or absence of glucagon-rich portions of the pancreas can contribute to profound hypoglycemia. Glucagon is stimulated by the amino acids arginine and alanine. Hormones such as GIP have been shown to have a stimulatory effect on glucagon secretion in vitro but not in vivo. Insulin and somatostatin have a potent suppressive effect on glucagon secretion and can regulate glucagon secretion through paracrine effects within the islet.

The neural regulation of glucagon is similar to that of insulin.[26] Cholinergic fibers have a strong stimulatory effect. α-Sympathetic fibers inhibit glucagon secretion, and β-sympathetic fibers are weakly stimulatory. The role of neuropeptides on glucagon secretion is unknown. Glucagon elevates blood glucose levels through the stimulation of glycogenolysis and gluconeogenesis. Along with epinephrine, cortisol, and growth hormone, glucagon is considered a stress hormone because it provides metabolic fuel during stress. The peptide is metabolized by the kidney and, to a lesser extent, by the liver.

Some authors consider dysfunctional A-cell secretion to play a major role in the elevation of blood sugar in diabetes. In the bidysfunction theory of diabetes, insulin secretion is absent or impaired and glucagon secretion is deranged, leading to hyperglycemia, ketoacidosis, and accelerated lipolysis.[27] Suppression of glucagon secretion with somatostatin has resulted in improved glucose homeostasis in insulin-dependent, type I diabetes.[28]

Somatostatin Synthesis, Secretion, and Action

In 1973, Brazeau and coworkers[28a] reported on the isolation of a hypothalamic peptide that inhibited the release of growth hormone (somatotropin) and named it *somatostatin*. Somatostatin is a 14–amino acid polypeptide that inhibits the release of almost all peptide hormones, as well as inhibiting gastric, pancreatic, and biliary secretion. Found in the D cell of the islet, the hormone's role within the pancreas remains unclear. Although exogenous infusion of somatostatin has been demonstrated to inhibit insulin, glucagon, and PP release, endogenous somatostatin has not been proved to influence the secretion of the other adjacent islet cells directly. Therefore, the D cell is probably responsible for paracrine regulation of islet cell hormone secretion.[29] Some researchers have suggested that the D cells regulate exocrine secretion as part of the insuloacinar portal system. Somatostatin has also been found

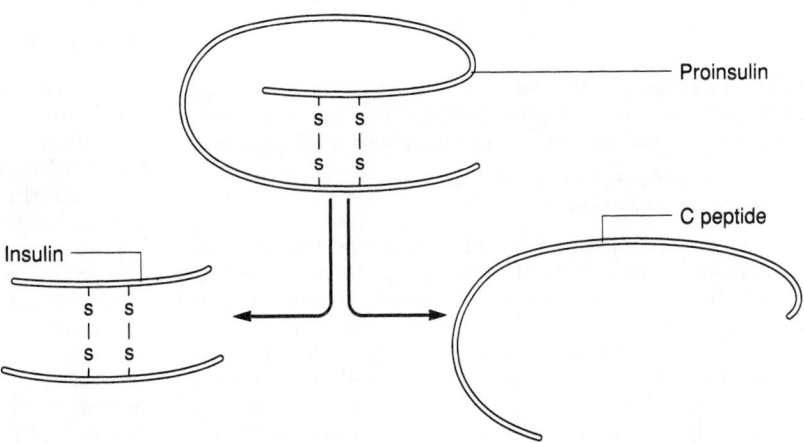

Figure 30-16. Synthesis of insulin. Proinsulin is synthesized by the endoplasmic reticulum and packaged within secretory granules of the B cell, where it is cleaved into insulin and C peptide. Equimolar amounts of insulin and C peptide are secreted into the bloodstream.

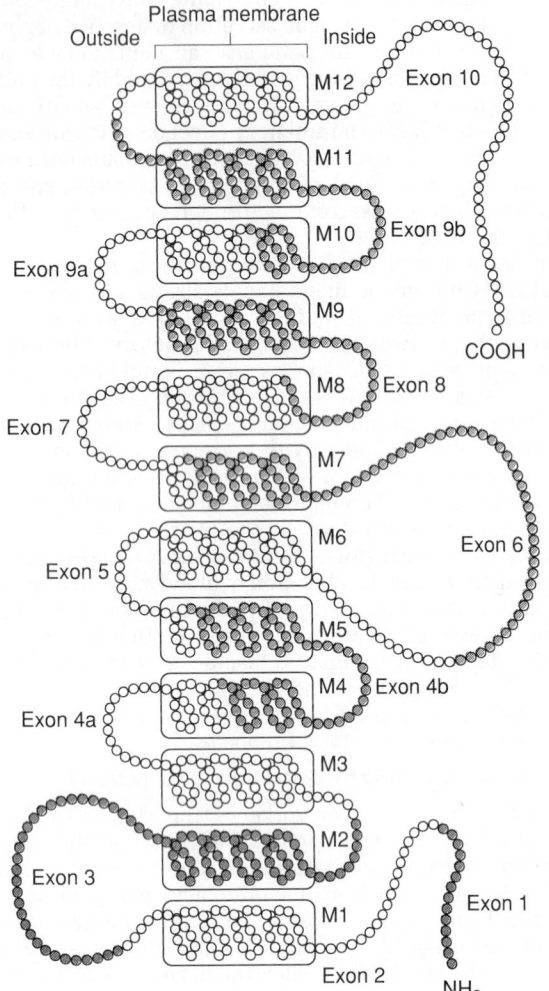

Figure 30-17. Model of basic structure of a membrane-bound glucose transporter peptide, encoded by a gene divided into 10 exon regions. Membrane-spanning β-helical peptide chains are numbered M1 to M12. Mutations of the promoter region of the gene or the synthesis of an abnormal form of the protein could result in altered transport of glucose. For the B-cell GLUT-2 transporter, this could cause reduced sensitivity to glucose. For the muscle and fat cell GLUT-4 transporter, this could result in decreased peripheral uptake of glucose. (After Bell GI, Kayano T, Buse JB, et al. Molecular biology of mammalian glucose transporters. Diabetes Care 1990;86:1615)

in the neurons of the islet and can act as an inhibitory neuropeptide. The peptide's potent inhibitory effect has been used to treat both endocrine and exocrine disorders.[30]

Pancreatic Polypeptide Synthesis, Secretion, and Action

Pancreatic polypeptide is a 36–amino acid peptide that is secreted by the F cells of the islet. The F cell is located predominantly in the uncinate process of the pancreas and represents 5% to 15% of the islet cell mass. The physiologic role of PP remains unclear. The peptide has been shown to inhibit exocrine secretion as well as choleresis and gallbladder emptying. Release of PP is regulated predominantly by cholinergic innervation. The rise in PP levels after a meal is ablated by vagotomy, and this can be used as a marker of completion of vagotomy. Circulating PP levels are increased in diabetes and in normal aging because of increased secretion. Other studies suggest that

PP is involved in glucose homeostasis and that PP deficiency after chronic pancreatitis or pancreaticoduodenectomy contributes to glucose intolerance, thus linking PP deficiency to pancreatogenic diabetes.[31]

Other Peptide Products

Other peptides have been found to be secreted within the islet. These include neuropeptides such as VIP, galanin, and serotonin, which are believed to play a role in the regulation of islet cell secretion. Amylin is a 36–amino acid polypeptide that was discovered in 1988. It is secreted by the B cell, but not in equimolar amounts to C peptide and insulin. Amylin inhibits insulin secretion and insulin uptake peripherally. Amylin has been found in the amyloid deposits within the pancreas of type II diabetic patients and has been implicated in the development of type II diabetes mellitus. Furthermore, the peptide is absent in type I diabetes mellitus because in this disease the B cells are ablated. The significance of amylin deficiency is unknown.

Pancreastatin is another peptide found in large amounts in the pancreas. It is a derivative of a larger, ubiquitous endocrine tissue-related peptide, chromogranin A, and has been shown to inhibit insulin secretion. Its physiologic role is unknown.

Intraislet Regulation of Hormone Secretion

Because exogenous infusions of insulin, glucagon, and somatostatin have profound effects on islet hormone secretion, the paracrine regulation of islet hormone secretion has been an area of intense investigation. In 1982, it was demonstrated that the blood flow of the islet is centripetal; that is, a central artery penetrates into the islet and perfuses the centrally located B-cell mass first. The blood then flows outward toward the peripherally located A, D, and F cells, allowing a paracrine cascade. By using antibodies specific for each hormone, it has been demonstrated that insulin secretion within the islet regulates the secretion of glucagon and somatostatin. This observation suggests that the suppression of glucagon during hyperglycemia is not regulated by glucose, but by an increase in insulin secretion (Fig. 30-18). Intraislet somatostatin is known to regulate insulin secretion.[29] The overall physiologic significance of the paracrine cascade is unknown, but it can result in the hyperglucagonemia and hypersomatostatinemia seen in insulin-dependent, type I diabetes.

Tests of Pancreatic Function

Exocrine Function

The secretin test is the classic test for pancreatic exocrine function.[32] After an overnight fast, the duodenum is intubated with a double-lumen tube. After 20-minute basal collections, an intravenous bolus of highly purified secretin, 2 U/kg, is administered, and four 20-minute collections of duodenal fluid are aspirated and analyzed for total volume, bicarbonate output, and enzyme secretion. The lower limits of normal for this study are 1.8 mL/kg/h of pancreatic fluid, 6.2 mEq/h of bicarbonate output, and 82 mEq/h of maximal bicarbonate content. Amylase secretion normally ranges from 6 to 18 IU/kg. The test is considered positive when abnormal values indicate there is exocrine pancreatic insufficiency (Table 30-1). In chronic pancreatitis, there is decreased bicarbonate secretion because of stasis in the ducts. In pancreatic malignancy, there is decreased volume because of replacement of the normal pancreas with cancer. After cholecystectomy, the pancreatic

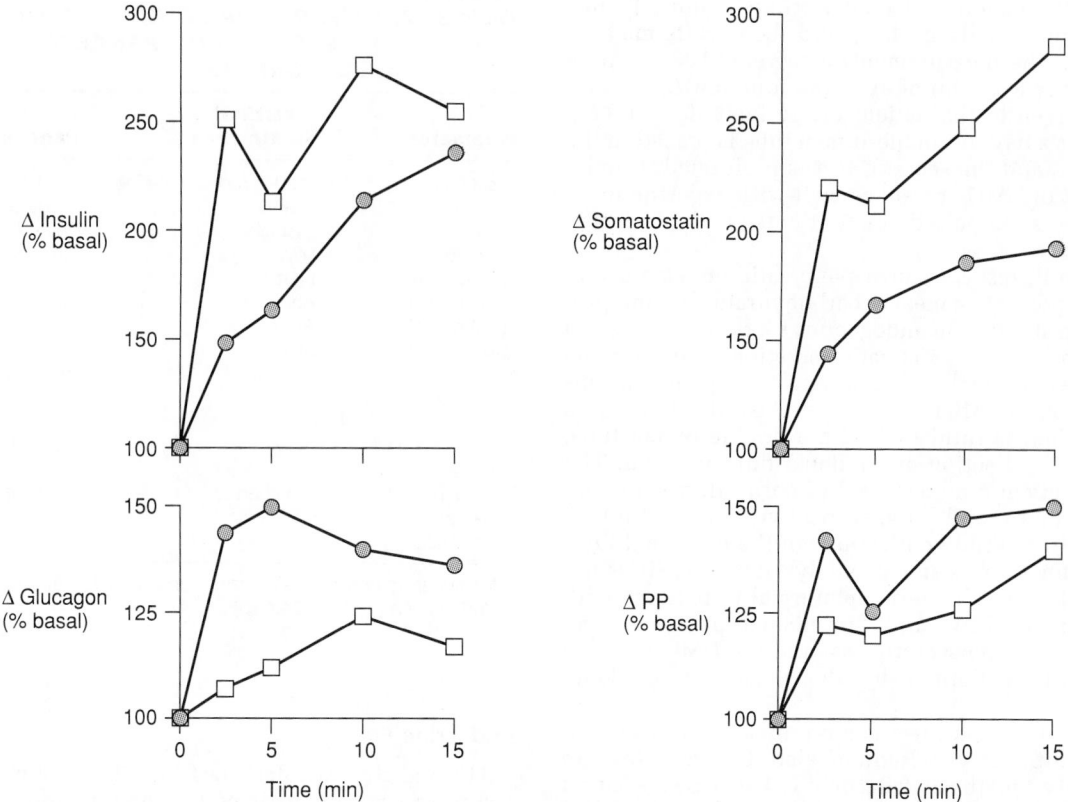

Figure 30-18. Paracrine modulation of islet secretion by insulin. The islet cell response to combined glucose (16 mmol) and GIP (1 nmol) perfusion in the isolated human pancreas is shown with (*circles*) and without (*squares*) the addition of 20 μU/mL insulin to the arterial circuit. Venous insulin concentrations ranged from 1500 to 3000 μU/mL. Insulin and somatostatin secretion are inhibited, whereas glucagon and PP secretion are enhanced. These data suggest that insulin exerts negative feedback on insulin secretion from the islet, and that insulin released from the B-cell core of the islet enhances somatostatin release from the D cells in the perimeter of the islet. (After Brunicardi FC, Druck P, Sun YS, et al. Regulation of pancreatic polypeptide secretion in the isolated perfused human pancreas. Am J Surg 1988;155:63)

juice can be diluted by bile, and results must be cautiously interpreted.

The fecal fat test is used to distinguish between pancreatic dysfunction and malabsorption secondary to enteric disease. Steatorrhea secondary to pancreatic disease is the result of lipase deficiency and is usually not present until lipase secretion is reduced by 90%. With a marked reduction of lipase secretion, there is an elevated 24-hour fecal fat content of greater than 20 g. Conversely, steatorrhea in the presence of low levels of fecal fat indicates intestinal dysfunction. A reduction in fecal fat indicates efficacy of pancreatic enzyme replacement in patients with exocrine insufficiency.

The dimethadione (DMO) test is based on the observa-

Table 30-1. CHARACTERISTIC RESULTS OF SECRETIN TESTING: FLOW, BICARBONATE, AND ENZYME CHANGES OBSERVED IN PATIENTS WITH VARIOUS PANCREATIC AND OTHER DISORDERS

Disorder	Pattern	Flow Rate	Maximum Bicarbonate Concentration	Enzyme Secretion
End-stage pancreatitis, advanced pancreatic cancer	Total insufficiency	Decreased	Decreased	Decreased
Chronic pancreatitis	Qualitative insufficiency	Normal	Decreased	Normal
Pancreatic cancer	Quantitative insufficiency	Decreased	Normal	Normal
Malnutrition*	Isolated enzyme deficiency	Normal	Normal	Decreased
Hemochromatosis, Zollinger-Ellison syndrome, various cirrhoses	Hypersecretion	Increased	Normal	Normal

* Sprue, ulcerative colitis, and regional enteritis
(Dreiling DA, Wolfson P. New insights into pancreatic disease revealed by the secretin test. In: Berk JE, ed. Developments in digestive diseases, vol 2. Philadelphia, Lea & Febiger, 1979:155)

tion that the pancreas degrades trimethadione (Tridione), an anticonvulsant drug, and secretes its metabolite, DMO. The measurement of secreted DMO can be used as an assessment of exocrine function. Trimethadione is given to the patient orally for 3 days, 0.45 g three times a day. A double-lumen tube is placed in the duodenum, and the secretin test is performed. Duodenal output of DMO correlates well with exocrine function and is impaired in patients with exocrine insufficiency.[33]

The Lundh test measures pancreatic enzyme secretion in response to a meal of carbohydrate, fat, and protein. The test relies on endogenous secretion of secretin and CCK as well as pancreatic secretion; therefore, the test can be abnormal in diseases involving the gastrointestinal mucosa. After an overnight fast, the duodenum of the patient is intubated with a double-lumen tube, and a basal collection of duodenal fluid is taken. The patient is given a mixed meal of corn oil, casein, and glucose, 18, 15, and 40 g, respectively, in 300 mL of water. Thirty-minute collections of the duodenal fluid are made for 2 hours and are analyzed for trypsin, amylase, and lipase. This test is abnormal in patients with chronic pancreatitis and diminished pancreatic reserve. As with the secretin test and the DMO test, the Lundh test is limited by the need for duodenal intubation.

The triolein breath test is a noninvasive test of exocrine insufficiency.[34] Radiolabeled triglycerides are given orally, and the metabolite, $^{14}CO_2$, can be measured in the breath. Corn oil, 25 g, containing 5 μCi of ^{14}C-triolein is given orally, and breath samples are obtained 4 hours later. The radioactivity of the breath samples is then measured. Patients with disorders of fat digestion or absorption exhale less than 3% per hour of the ^{14}C-triolein dose. The test is repeated after oral pancreatic enzyme replacement. Patients with exocrine insufficiency achieve a normal rate of $^{14}CO_2$ excretion, whereas patients with enteric disorders show no improvement.

The paraaminobenzoic acid (PABA) test is a second noninvasive test for determination of pancreatic insufficiency.[35] N-benzoyl-L-tyrosyl-paraaminobenzoic acid (BT-PABA) is cleaved by chymotrypsin to form PABA. PABA is excreted in the urine after being absorbed from the small intestine. One gram of BT-PABA in 300 mL of water is given orally, and urine collections are obtained for 6 hours. Patients with chronic pancreatitis excrete less than 60% of the ingested BT-PABA. This test is useful for moderate and severe pancreatic insufficiency.

The test-meal PP response allows confirmation of suspected pancreatic disease based on plasma levels of the islet hormone PP. Although no circulating peptide or compound changes specifically with pancreatic exocrine insufficiency, basal and meal-stimulated levels of plasma PP are reduced in severe chronic pancreatitis, or after extensive pancreatic resection. After an overnight fast, a test meal consisting of 20% protein, 40% fat, and 40% carbohydrate is ingested. Basal levels of immunoreactive PP (normal, 100 to 250 pg/mL) are frequently less than 50 pg/mL in severe chronic pancreatitis.[36] PP levels normally rise to 700 to 1000 pg/mL for 2 to 3 hours after the meal, but are reduced to 250 pg/mL or less in severe disease. Because PP release depends on intact pancreatic innervation, a depressed PP response can appear in cases of diabetic autonomic neuropathy or can follow truncal vagotomy or antrectomy (Table 30-2).

Table 30-2. DIFFERENTIAL DIAGNOSIS OF INTESTINAL AND PANCREATIC STEATORRHEA

Parameter	Intestinal Steatorrhea	Pancreatitis
Fecal fat	<20 g monoglycerides and diglycerides; soapy consistency	>20 g triglycerides; oily seepage
D-Xylose	Low	Normal
Secretin test	Normal	Abnormal
Small bowel series	Abnormal	Normal
Small bowel biopsy	Abnormal	Normal
Lundh meal	Normal	Abnormal
PABA test	Normal	Abnormal
PP response to test meal	Normal	Low
Vitamin B_{12} and folate	Low	Normal
Treatment with pancreatic enzymes	No change	Improvement

(Modified from Brandt LJ. Gastrointestinal disorders of the elderly. New York, Raven Press, 1984:470)

Endocrine Function

The oral glucose tolerance test is the most widely used test to assess pancreatic endocrine function. The test is an indirect assessment of the insulin response to an oral glucose load. After an overnight fast, the subject has two basal blood samples drawn for glucose determination. An oral glucose load, 40 g/m^2, is given over 10 minutes. Blood samples are drawn every 30 minutes for 2 hours (Table 30-3). This test is used to help confirm the diagnosis of diabetes.[37] Caution must be used in the interpretation of results because the oral glucose tolerance test measures the glucose profile and not the actual insulin response. The insulin response to oral glucose is affected by enteric factors, especially those hormones involved in the enteroinsular axis (eg, GIP, glucagon-like peptide 1, CCK). The test can also be affected by antecedent diet, drug use, exercise, and the age of the patient. Although a diagnosis of diabetes can be based on the oral glucose tolerance test, insulin secretion per se is but one factor that affects the test's performance.

The intravenous glucose tolerance test reflects the pancreatic endocrine response to a bolus of intravenous glucose.[38] The test measures the disappearance of plasma glucose after the glucose bolus, which indirectly reflects both insulin secretion and action. This test eliminates the gastrointestinal influences of glucose metabolism seen in the oral glucose tolerance test. After an overnight fast, two basal samples of blood are drawn. The patient is then given an intravenous bolus of glucose, 0.5 g/kg, over 2 to 5 minutes. Blood samples are drawn every 10 minutes for 1 hour. The decline in glucose concentration (percentage of disappearance per minute) is called the K value. A K value greater than or equal to 1.5 is normal. The intravenous glucose tolerance test response decreases with age, and results should be evaluated with age-adjusted criteria.

The intravenous arginine test is useful for the diagnosis of hormone-secreting tumors. The amino acid arginine stimulates the secretion of islet hormones. After an overnight fast, a 30-minute infusion of arginine, 0.5 g/kg, is given. Blood samples are taken every 10 minutes, and radioimmunoassays are performed for the specific

Table 30-3. INTERPRETATION OF ORAL GLUCOSE TOLERANCE TEST RESULTS

Interpretation	Fasting Glucose Value (mg/dL)		Intermediate Glucose Value (mg/dL)		2-Hour Glucose Value (mg/dL)
Normal	<115	*and*	All values < 200	*and*	<140
Impaired glucose tolerance	<140	*and*	Any value ≥ 200	*and*	140–199
Diabetic	≥140		(Glucose tolerance test		
	or		not necessary)		
	<140	*and*	Any value ≥200	*and*	≥200
Nondiagnostic	Any combination of glucose values that does not fit into another category				

(Modified from National Diabetes Data Group. Classification and diagnosis of diabetes mellitus and other categories of glucose intolerance. Diabetes 1979;28:1039)

hormones in question. This test is particularly useful for glucagon-secreting tumors, for which elevations of plasma glucagon over 400 pg/mL usually indicate a glucagonoma.

The tolbutamide response test is also useful in detecting hormone-secreting tumors. Tolbutamide is a sulfonylurea that stimulates insulin secretion. After an overnight fast, basal blood samples are drawn. One gram of sodium tolbutamide is given intravenously, and the blood glucose is monitored for 1 hour. Blood samples are also drawn for radioimmunoassay of insulin or other suspected hormones, such as somatostatin. In normal patients, the blood glucose falls to 50% of basal values after 30 minutes. Sustained hypoglycemia with hypersecretion of insulin is consistent with an insulinoma. In the case of a somatostatinoma, somatostatin levels are elevated to levels more than twice as high as the prevailing normal values for the particular somatostatin radioimmunoassay used.

REFERENCES

1. Cubilla AC, Fortner JC, Fitzgerald PJ. Lymph node involvement in carcinoma of the head of the pancreas area. Cancer 1978;41:880.
2. Ahren B, Taborsky GJ Jr, Porte D Jr. Neuropeptidergic versus cholinergic and adrenergic regulation of islet hormone secretion. Diabetologia 1986;29:827.
3. Havel PJ, Taborsky GJ Jr. The contribution of the autonomic nervous system to changes in glucagon and insulin secretion during hypoglycemic stress. Endocr Rev 1989;10:332.
4. Sadar ES, Cooperman AM. Bilateral thoracic sympathectomy-splanchnicectomy in the treatment of intractable pain due to pancreatic carcinoma. Cleve Clin Q 1974;41:185.
5. Gorelick FS, Jamieson JD. Structure-function relationship of the pancreas. In: Johnson LR, ed. Physiology of the gastrointestinal tract. New York, Raven Press, 1981:773.
6. Kleinman R, Gingerich R, Wong H, et al. The use of the Fab fragment for immunoneutralization of somatostatin in the isolated perfused pancreas. Am J Surg 1994;167:114.
7. Cooper GJ, Day AJ, Willis AC, et al. Amylin and the amylin gene: structure, function and relationship to islet amyloid and to diabetes mellitus. Biochem Biophys Acta 1989;1014:247.
8. Stefan Y, Orci L, Malaisse-Legae F, Perrelet A, Patel Y, Unger RH. Quantitation of endocrine cell content in the pancreas of non-diabetic and diabetic humans. Diabetes 1982;31:694.
9. Seymour NE, Brunicardi FC, Chaiken RL, et al. Reversal of abnormal glucose production after pancreatic resection by pancreatic polypeptide administration in man. Surgery 1988;104:119.
10. Jansson L, Hellerstrom C. Glucose-induced changes in pancreatic islet blood flow mediated by central nervous system. Am J Physiol 1986;25:E644.
11. Bonner-Weir S, Orci L. New perspectives on the microvasculature of the islets of Langerhans in the rat. Diabetes 1982;31:883.
12. Murakami T, Fujita T, Ohtsuka A, et al. The insulino-acinar portal and insulino-venous drainage systems in the pancreas of the mouse, dog, monkey and certain other animals: a scanning electron microscopic study of corrosion casts. Arch Histol Cytol 1993;56:127.
13. Liu Y, Guth PH, Kaneko K, et al. Dynamic in vivo observation of rat islet microcirculation. Pancreas 1993;8:15.
14. Lee W, Kazunori M, Funakoshi A. Effects of somatostatin and pancreatic polypeptide on exocrine and endocrine pancreas in the rats. Gastroenterol Jpn 1988;23:49.
15. Busnardo AC, Didio L, Tidrick R, Thomford N. History of the pancreas. Am J Surg 1983;146:539.
16. Davenport HW. Pancreatic secretion. In: Davenport HN, ed. Physiology of the digestive tract, ed 5. Chicago, Year Book Medical Publishers, 1982:143.
17. Valenzuela JE, Weiner K, Saad C. Cholinergic stimulation of human pancreatic secretion. Dig Dis Sci 1986;31:615.
18. Konturek SJ, Becker HD, Thompson JC. Effect of vagotomy on hormones stimulating pancreatic secretion. Arch Surg 1974;108:704.
19. Leahy JL, Bonner-Weir S, Weir GC. Abnormal glucose regulation of insulin secretion in models of reduced B-cell mass. Diabetes 1984;33:667.
20. Nanjo K, Sanke T, Mujano M, et al. Diabetes due to secretion of a structurally abnormal insulin (insulin Wakayama): clinical and functional characteristics of Leu-A3 insulin. J Clin Invest 1986;77:514.
21. Bell GI, Kayano T, Buse JB, et al. Molecular biology of mammalian glucose transporters. Diabetes Care 1990;13:198.
22. Orci L, Unger RH, Ravazzola M, et al. Reduced beta-cell glucose transporter in new onset diabetic BB rats. J Clin Invest 1990;86:1615.
23. Ebert R, Creutzfeldt W. Gastrointestinal peptides and insulin secretion. Diabetes Metab Rev 1987;3:1.
24. Opara EC, Atwater I, Go VLM. Characterization and control of pulsatile secretion of insulin and glucagon. Pancreas 1988;3:484.
25. Eisenbarth GS. Type I diabetes mellitus: a chronic autoimmune disease. N Engl J Med 1986;314:1360.
26. Brunicardi FC, Sun YS, Druck P, Elahi D, Andersen DK. Splanchnic neural regulation of insulin and glucagon secretion in the isolated perfused human pancreas. Am J Surg 1987;153:34.
27. Unger RH, Dobbs RE. Insulin, glucagon, and somatostatin in the regulation of metabolism. Ann Rev Physiol 1978;40:307.
28. Gerich JE. Somatostatin and diabetes. Am J Med 1981;70:619.
28a. Brazeau P, Vale N, Burgus R, et al. Hypothalamic polypeptide that inhibits the secretion of immunoreactive pituitary growth hormone. Science 1973;179:77.
29. Kleinman R, Watt P, Ohning G, et al. The regulatory role of intraislet somatostatin on insulin secretion in the isolated perfused human pancreas. Pancreas 1993;9:172.
30. Mulvihill SJ, Pappas TN, Passaro E, Debas HT. The use of somatostatin and its analogs in the treatment of surgical disorders. Surgery 1986;100:467.
31. Kennedy FP. Pathophysiology of pancreatic polypeptide secretion in human diabetes mellitus. Diabetes Nutr Metab 1990;2:155.

32. Dreiling DA, Wolfson P. New insights into pancreatic disease revealed by the secretin test. In: Berk JE, ed. Developments in digestive diseases, vol 2. Philadelphia, Lea & Febiger, 1979;155.

33. Noda A, Hayakawa T, Kondo T, Katada N, Kameya A. Clinical evaluation of pancreatic excretion test with dimethadione and oral BT-PABA test in chronic pancreatitis. Dig Dis Sci 1983;30:230.

34. Goff JS. Two-stage triolein breath test differentiates pancreatic insufficiency from other causes of malabsorption. Gastroenterology 1982;83:44.

35. Arvanitakis C, Greenberger NJ. Diagnosis of pancreatic disease by a synthetic peptide: a new test of exocrine pancreatic function. Lancet 1976;1:663.

36. Nealon WH, Beauchamp RD, Townsend CM, et al. Diagnostic role of gastrointestinal hormones in patients with chronic pancreatitis. Ann Surg 1986;204:430.

37. National Diabetes Data Group. Classification and diagnosis of diabetes mellitus and other categories of glucose intolerance. Diabetes 1979;30:1039.

38. Andres R, Tobin JD. Endocrine systems. In: Finch CE, Hayflick L. Handbook of the biology of aging. New York, Van Nostrand Reinhold, 1977:357.

SURGERY: SCIENTIFIC PRINCIPLES AND PRACTICE, Second Edition, edited by Lazar J. Greenfield, Michael W. Mulholland, Keith T. Oldham, Gerald B. Zelenock, and Keith D. Lillemoe. Lippincott–Raven Publishers, Philadelphia, © 1997.

CHAPTER 31
ACUTE PANCREATITIS
KAREN S. GUICE

Acute pancreatitis is a complex disorder of the exocrine pancreas characterized by acute acinar cell injury and both regional and systemic inflammatory responses. It is a common disease with a broad spectrum of clinical and pathologic findings that contribute to considerable morbidity and mortality. Because pathogenic mechanisms are unclear, specific treatment is not available. Empiric supportive care remains standard, and clinical outcomes have improved only to the extent that critical care has evolved in recent years. Most patients with acute pancreatitis have simple edematous pancreatitis, a self-limited and reversible process. In a small number of patients, fulminant or progressive disease develops, with pancreatic necrosis that can lead to multiorgan system failure or death. The problems related to acute pancreatitis pose a formidable challenge to both the clinical surgeon and the basic scientist.

PATHOLOGY

Normal pancreatic anatomy and physiology are presented in detail in Chapter 30. Relevant to this discussion are the features of acinar cell morphology and normal function, as shown schematically in Figure 31-1; the important ultrastructural features and the normal cytosolic processing of the digestive proenzymes are illustrated. The process is culminated by orderly apical discharge of zymogen granules into the acinar ductal lumen. Acute pancreatitis is characterized by alterations in acinar cell structure and function as well as by the development of acute regional and systemic inflammatory responses. The fundamental pathologic event is injury to the acinar cell.

Acute pancreatitis is characterized by interstitial edema formation. Grossly, the gland becomes enlarged and edem-atous, with small areas of focal necrosis involving either the pancreas or areas of adjacent retroperitoneal fat. Microscopically, edema is both interlobular and intralobular, and the acinar units appear dispersed within the relatively sparse fibrous matrix. Figure 31-2 illustrates the characteristic microscopic morphology of acute edematous pancreatitis.

Acute inflammation occurs rapidly. Experimentally, the process begins within minutes. The initial cellular response involves the infiltration of polymorphonuclear leukocytes into the perivascular regions of the pancreas. Within hours, mononuclear cells, including macrophages and lymphocytes, accumulate. Experimental evidence suggests that phagocyte-derived oxygen radicals and possibly other phagocytic products are involved in a primary injury to pancreatic capillary endothelial cells. The resulting increase in microvascular permeability facilitates access to the acinar cell microenvironment for circulating formed elements (additional neutrophils, monocytes, platelets) and humoral factors, such as complement products and cytokines. The relative importance of this inflammatory injury to the pancreatic microvasculature is unclear, but it provides one explanation for the process of local edema formation as well as for the systemic microvascular sequelae of acute pancreatitis.

Although clinical pancreatitis usually is a reversible disease characterized by acinar cell injury and edema formation, frank pancreatic necrosis develops in 5% to 10% of patients, which can lead to irreversible regional injury or multiorgan system failure. Predictably, this latter group of patients is the primary source of morbidity and mortality associated with acute pancreatitis. Histologic characteristics of advanced disease include extensive acinar cell necrosis, interstitial microabscess formation, extensive peripancreatic fat necrosis, microvascular thrombosis, and local hemorrhage. Pathologically, all these features appear to represent progression of processes already established with acute edematous pancreatitis.

PATHOPHYSIOLOGY

The cellular events that lead to acute pancreatitis may be initiated by a variety of different stimuli, and the process has been considered a final common pathway. Current data offer considerably more insight into the relevant pathogenic events than the simple historic concept that pancreatic autolysis occurs.

Acinar cell proteases (such as trypsin, chymotrypsin, carboxypeptidase, and elastase) and phospholipases are normally synthesized in an inactive zymogen form. Peptide synthesis is accomplished as depicted in Figure 31-1, and the proenzymes are packaged into cytoplasmic zymogen granules. After apical exocytosis into the acinar ductal lumen, these precursors are transported with water and bicarbonate through the pancreatic duct into the duodenum, where they are converted enzymatically into active forms by enterokinase, a brush-border enzyme. A variety of endogenous protease inhibitors (α_1-antitrypsin, β_2-macroglobulin, and pancreatic secretory trypsin inhibitor) are normally found in pancreatic tissue and pancreatic secretions, and in plasma in quantities sufficient to protect against premature or inappropriate activation of these digestive enzymes.[1]

Although the specific mechanisms that initiate human disease are not known, the normal orderly secretory sequence appears to be disrupted in acute pancreatitis.[2] Inappropriate protease activation overcomes endogenous antiprotease defenses. In experimental acute pancreatitis, zymogen granules become localized with lysosomes and fuse to form autophagic cytoplasmic vacuoles (zymogen

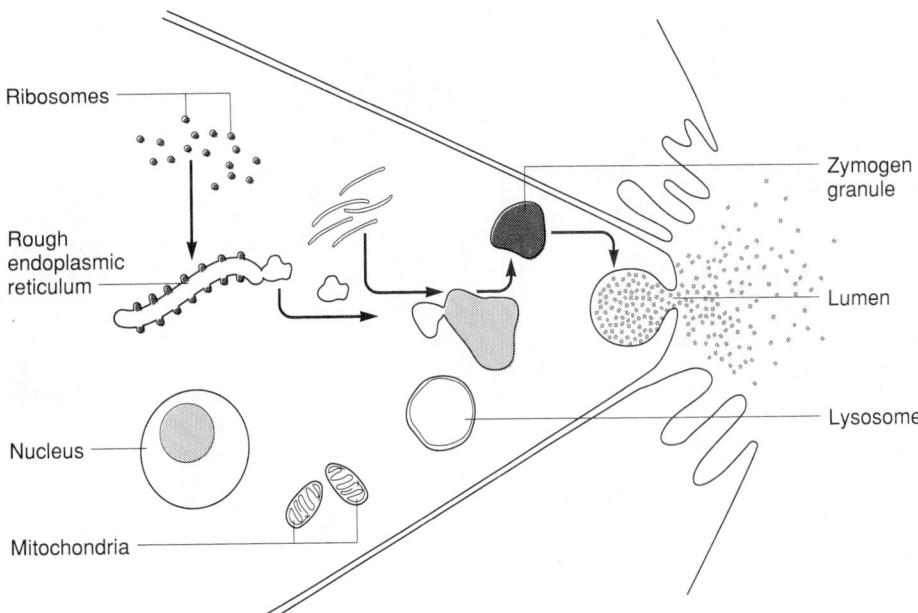

Figure 31-1. Normal acinar cell ultrastructure. Cytoplasmic processing of the proenzymes is depicted, with apical discharge into the acinar ductule by means of zymogen granule exocytosis.

lakes). These vacuoles move preferentially to the basolateral acinar cell cytoplasm, rather than to the luminal apex. Disordered discharge of the acinar cell contents through the basolateral cell membrane occurs. The mechanisms by which this cytoplasmic colocalization of zymogen granules and lysosomes occurs are not known, although evidence suggests that cytoskeletal alterations are associated with the loss of normal acinar cell polarity and loss of the ability to achieve apical exocytosis.[3]

Trypsinogen is normally a major constituent of the zymogen granules, whereas cathepsin B is usually abundant within the lysosomal fraction. Cathepsin B–induced trypsinogen cleavage is known to generate activated trypsin, which, in turn, is capable of further cytoplasmic proenzyme conversion.[1] The cytoplasmic liberation of activated proteases causes cell membrane injury, followed by the

disordered discharge of acinar cell contents through the basolateral cell membranes. This series of events is illustrated in Figure 31-3. Although many of the data for this concept are provided from experimental secretagogue-induced pancreatitis, other causes of acinar cell injury produce similar findings. For example, intracellular trypsinogen cleavage has been demonstrated after either hypoxia- or acidosis-induced acinar cell injury. Collectively, these findings suggest that the outcome of acinar cell injury involves intracellular activation of endogenous proteases, leading to further injury and the local extracellular discharge of acinar cell contents.

Once initiated, this process of protease release perpetuates acinar cell injury and initiates a regional acute inflammatory response, generating additional injury. Indeed, an important unanswered question is how endogenous

Figure 31-2. (*A* and *B*) Electron photomicrographs illustrating the histologic features of acute edematous pancreatitis. This rat specimen is from a model of cerulein-induced pancreatitis that is known to closely approximate human disease. There is extensive edema formation, acinar cell cytoplasm vacuolization, and polymorphonuclear cell (PMN) infiltration. Findings associated with experimentally induced acute edematous pancreatitis include the influx of PMNs, interstitial edema (int) and ductular dilation (d). Also visible is a zymogen granule (z) in *A*. Specimens from time-matched control animals (*C* and *D*) show normal pancreatic histology.

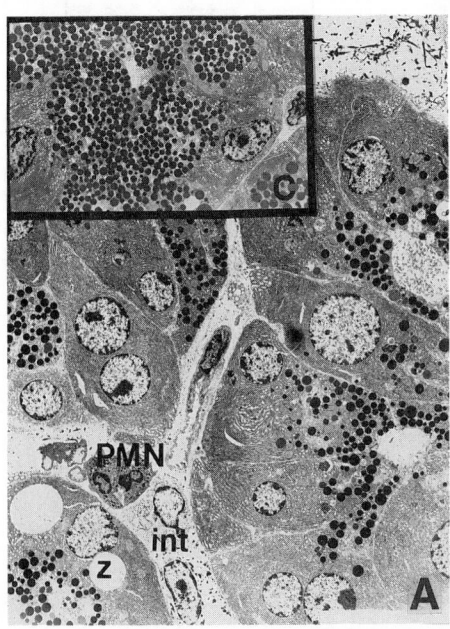
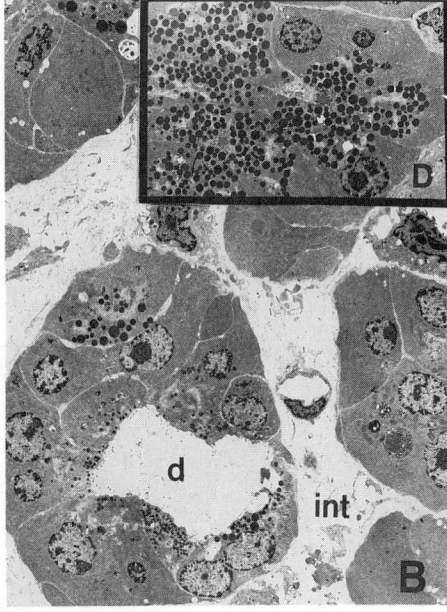

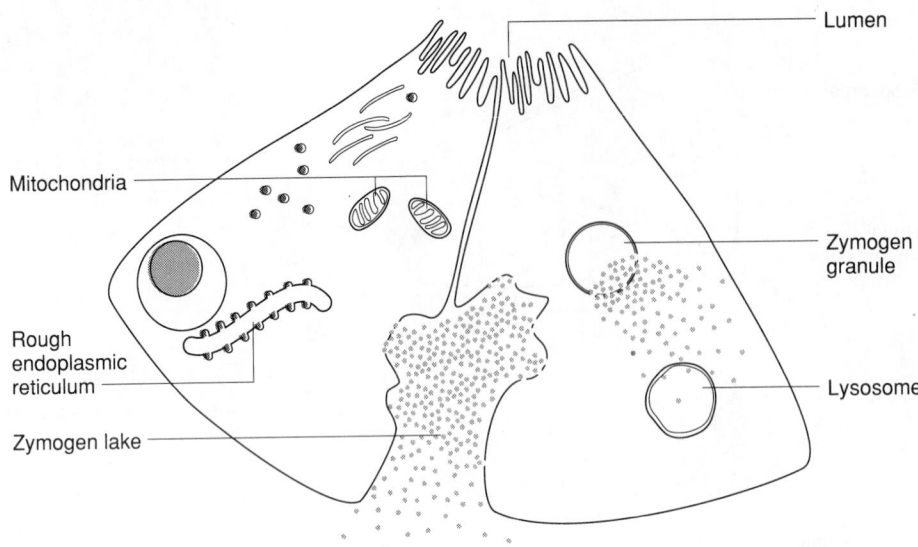

Figure 31-3. Schematic diagram illustrating the loss of acinar cell polarity and the process of cytoplasmic fusion of lysosomes and zymogen granules. Disordered basolateral discharge of activated proteases from the acinar cell follows.

control mechanisms prevent complete destruction of the acinar cell population once the process is triggered.

The endogenous inflammatory system participates early in the development of acute pancreatitis. Both humoral factors and cellular elements appear to be involved. Complement activation, histamine release, and bradykinin generation are demonstrable. Studies have suggested a role for cytokines in the acute inflammatory process of pancreatitis. Serum levels of tumor necrosis factor α, interleukin-6 (IL-6), and IL-1 are elevated in animals with experimental pancreatitis and in patients with systemic complications of acute pancreatitis.[4,5] Administration of an IL-1 receptor antagonist, even after the onset of acute pancreatitis, limited the degree of pancreatic inflammation.[4] The administration of anti–tumor necrosis factor antibody has both beneficial and deleterious effects on the development of local inflammation and may reflect the different experi-

mental models used.[6,7] Neutrophil-mediated pancreatic capillary endothelial injury appears to occur early, when the process is still reversible. NADPH oxidase–dependent oxygen radicals are directly implicated, whereas other phagocyte products, such as elastase, collagenase, cathepsin G and D, phospholipases A2 and C, DNAase, RNAase, glycosidases and other lysosomal hydrolases, platelet-activating factor, and myeloperoxidase, are all potential participants in both the acinar and endothelial cell injury processes. Chronic inflammatory cells, particularly macrophages, are recruited to the pancreas within hours and share many of the proinflammatory products noted earlier. The microvascular injury appears to amplify the inflammatory process (Fig. 31-4).

In addition to this localized pancreatic inflammation, evidence of a systemic response exists. Considerable data implicate the inflammatory process in the pathogenesis of

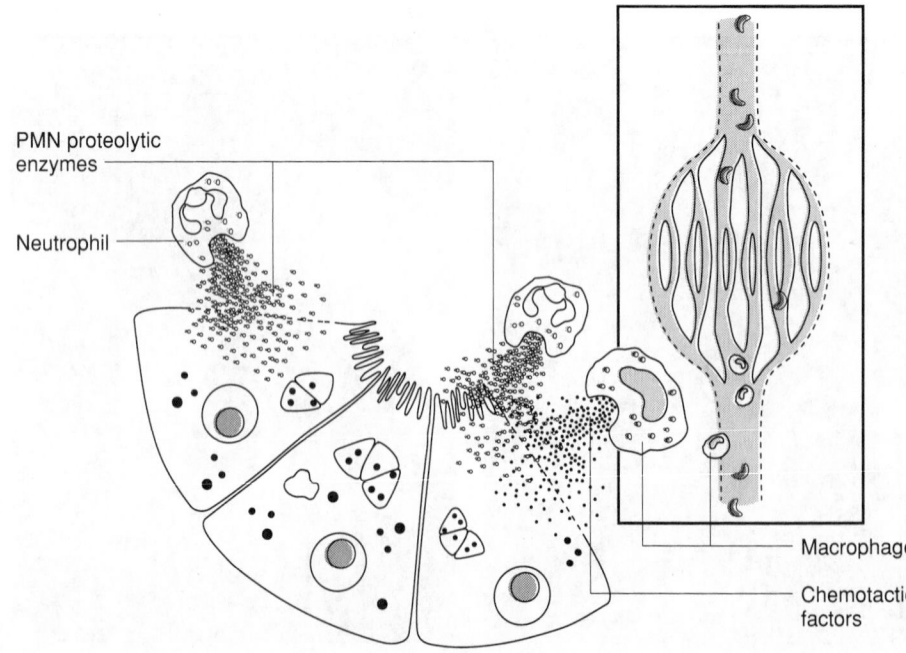

Figure 31-4. Schematic diagram illustrating the inflammatory response in acute pancreatitis. Inflammatory effector cells and plasma and tissue mediators are depicted. Increased microvascular permeability results from capillary endothelial cell injury.

pancreatitis-induced multiorgan system failure. The systemic distribution of activated neutrophils, mononuclear cells and macrophages, complement activation products, and other factors is clearly linked to remote organ dysfunction. A common event appears to be microvascular endothelial cell injury in diverse target organs. Pancreatitis-induced, polymorphonuclear leukocyte–dependent microvascular lung injury is one such example (Figs. 31-5 and 31-6). This pathologic process is a likely explanation for the frequent pulmonary symptoms and the occasional adult respiratory distress syndrome in patients with acute pancreatitis. Other target organs at risk for acute pancreatitis-induced injury are the liver, kidneys, and heart, although the mechanisms involved are less clear. Complications of acute pancreatitis include the following:

Early

Shock
Multiorgan failure
Encephalopathy
Coagulopathy
Sepsis
Hypocalcemia

Late

Pseudocyst
Diabetes
Abscess

Common clinical associations with acute pancreatitis include ethanol ingestion and pancreatic ductal obstruction. With regard to ethanol, a number of important observations

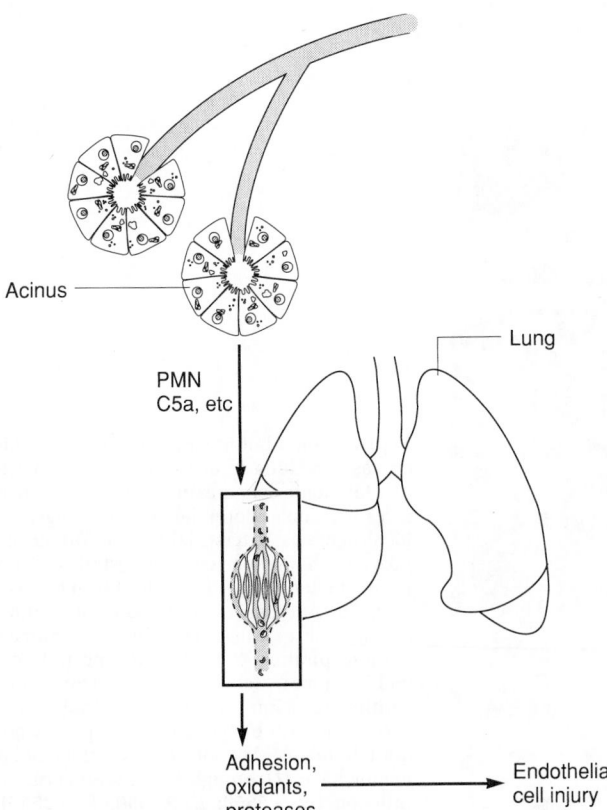

Figure 31-5. One consequence of the systemic inflammatory response associated with acute pancreatitis is neutrophil-dependent, oxygen radical–mediated alveolar capillary endothelial cell injury. PMN, polymorphonuclear leukocyte.

that are relevant to the pathogenic events are outlined in Figure 31-7. Acetaldehyde, the hepatic product of ethanol metabolism, is known to induce acinar cell cytoskeletal changes (microtubule disruption) as well as to increase acinar cell membrane permeability. Ethanol-induced elevations in plasma triglycerides provide a potential source of cytotoxic free fatty acids. In addition, endogenous trypsin-inhibiting capacity in both the pancreas and in pancreatic duct fluid is diminished after ethanol exposure. It appears that regional pancreatic blood flow is diminished after ethanol exposure, potentially adding ischemia to other acinar cell insults. The cytoskeletal disruption induced by acetaldehyde is consistent with the concept that the loss of acinar cell polarity and associated protein-processing abnormalities lead directly to ethanol-induced acute pancreatitis. Potentially important indirect ethanol effects include reduction in the level of protection afforded by the endogenous antiprotease system and hypoxic stress induced by diminished pancreatic microvascular blood flow.

Obstruction of the ampulla of Vater associated with pancreatic duct hypertension or increased permeability may also lead to extravasation of acinar cell contents into the pancreatic interstitium (Fig. 31-8). In this circumstance, the initial source of proenzyme cleavage is unknown because luminal small bowel contents have no access to this compartment. Neutrophil and macrophage products do provide a potential source of proteases for proenzyme cleavage and therefore represent a possible triggering mechanism. Experimentally, acute pancreatitis is reliably induced by bile duct or duodenal occlusion or by retrograde injection of substances such as bile, duodenal aspirate, drugs (including ethanol), and other substances into the pancreatic duct under pressure. Given the common clinical association of acute pancreatitis and gallstones or other occlusive lesions of the pancreatic duct, it is likely that these are relevant experimental observations.

The role of the microcirculation in the development of acute pancreatitis is poorly understood. In addition to increased permeability, microvascular thrombosis or obstruction by leukoaggregates may lead to local or regional tissue hypoxia. In nonacinar cell populations, it is well known that hypoxia-induced adenosine triphosphate depletion is associated with cytoskeletal (microtubule and microfilament) disruption. A similar finding in acinar cells would be consistent with the pathogenic scheme summarized earlier. Diminished microvascular blood flow occasionally initiates the process of acute pancreatitis. Clinically, hypoxic acinar cell injury is thought to be associated with events such as cardiopulmonary bypass, thromboembolic disease, and myocardial infarction.

CLINICAL FEATURES
Incidence and Demographics

The precise incidence of acute pancreatitis is difficult to determine because patients with mild pancreatitis may not seek medical care and because diagnostic criteria and reporting vary widely among institutions. For example, the incidence and mortality rates for acute pancreatitis from four separate areas within Great Britain are shown in Table 31-1.[4-7] Even with the benefits of a stable, relatively homogenous population and a nationalized reporting system, the incidence ranges from 53.8 to 238 cases per million population each year. In nonselected autopsy series, the evidence for past acute pancreatitis ranges from 0.14% to 1.3% (average, 0.31%). Variations among populations are highly dependent on social factors such as ethanol use and on environmental and hereditary determinants such as the incidence of gallstones.

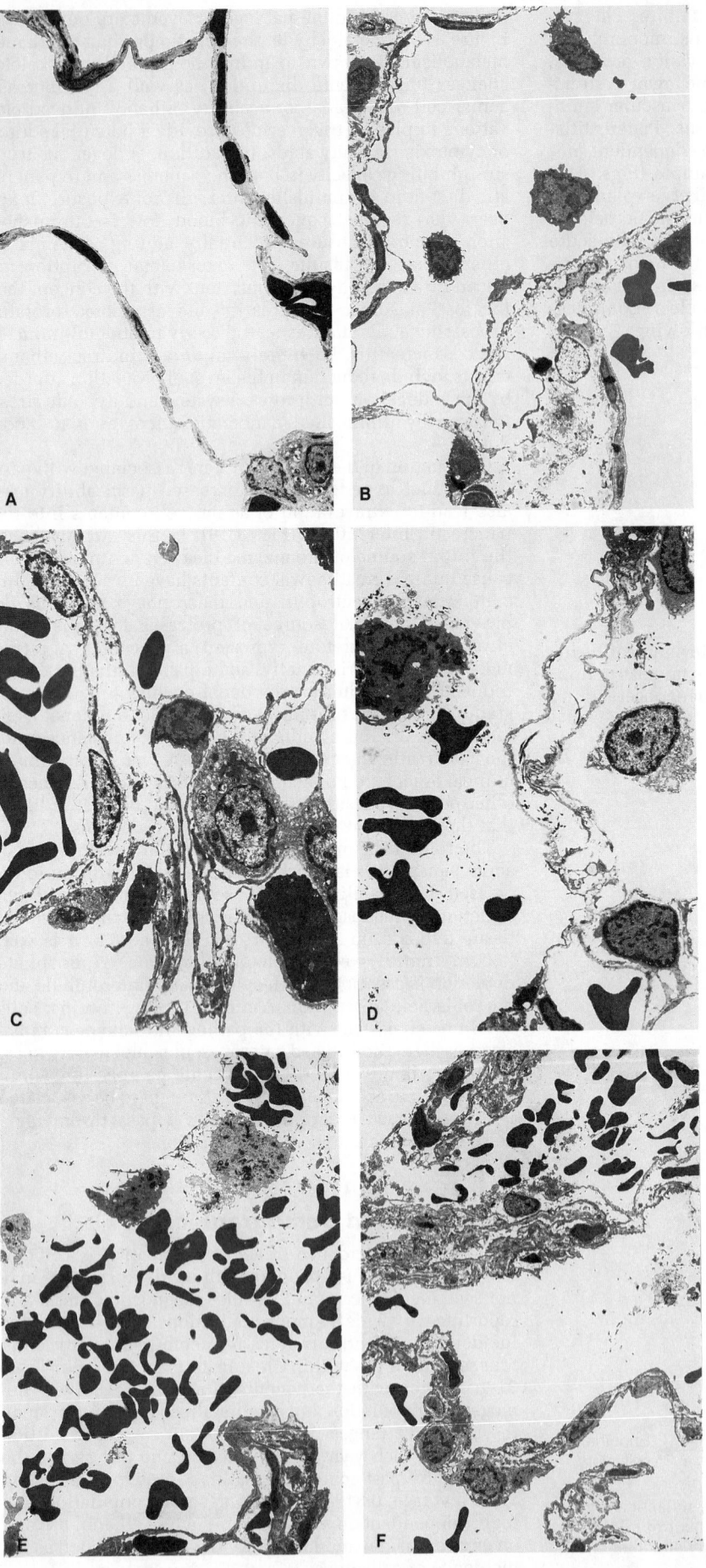

Figure 31-6. Photomicrographs of acute microvascular lung injury in rats with experimental acute pancreatitis. Histologic features include endothelial cell blebbing with focal necrosis, interstitial edema formation, polymorphonuclear cell sequestration, and intraalveolar hemorrhage with fibrin deposition. The microscopic features of this injury are similar to those seen in early human adult respiratory distress syndrome. (*A*) Normal rat lung ($\times$3400). (*B* and *C*) Three-hour cerulein infusion ($\times$3400). Interstitial edema is evident with blebbing of the capillary endothelial cells. Also present is intraalveolar hemorrhage. (*D* through *F*) Six-hour cerulein infusion (*D*, $\times$5650; *E*, $\times$2650; *F*, $\times$2550). Note the increase in intraalveolar hemorrhage and the presence of inflammatory cells within alveoli. Deposits of fibrin and interstitial edema are still evident.

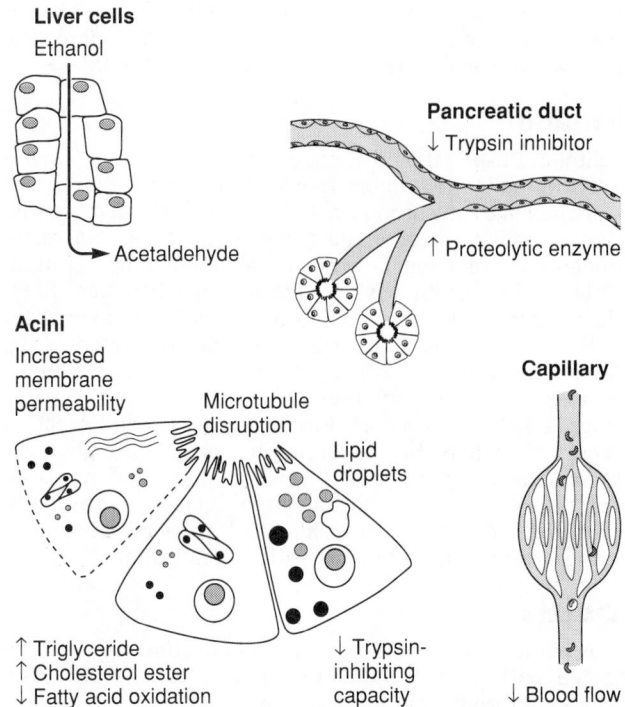

Figure 31-7. Ethanol- and acetaldehyde-induced changes in the pancreas include acinar cell microtubule disruption, increased cell membrane permeability, diminished trypsin-inhibiting capacity, and reduced regional blood flow. Each of these events may contribute to the pathogenesis of ethanol-related acute pancreatitis.

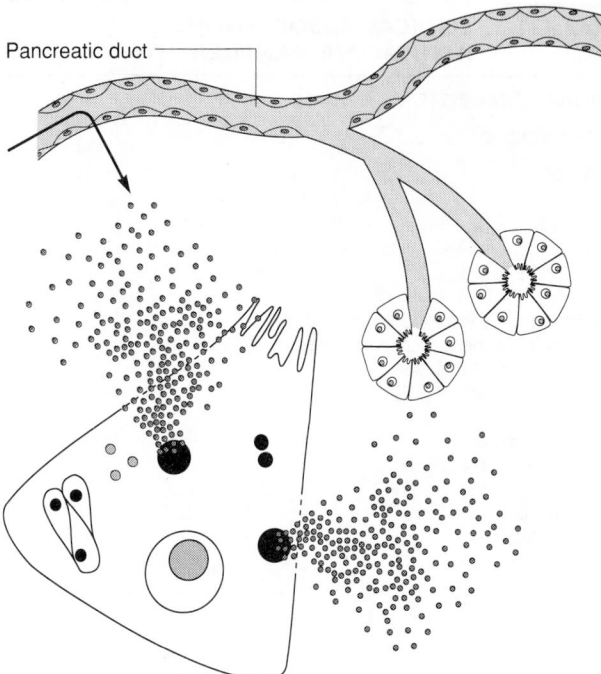

Figure 31-8. Pancreatic duct hypertension or reflux through the ampulla of Vater may lead to increased permeability of the pancreatic duct with leakage of activated proteases into the pancreatic interstitium. The result is self-perpetuating acinar cell injury.

Acute pancreatitis can occur at any age but is most common in adults between 30 and 70 years of age. In general, patients with gallstone-induced pancreatitis are older (age 40 to 60 years), whereas those with alcohol-associated pancreatitis are younger (age 30 to 40 years). There is considerable overlap. The sex distribution of acute pancreatitis depends on the clinical cause of the disease. In one report, women represented 68% of patients with gallstone-associated pancreatitis. Conversely, when alcohol is the primary association, most patients are men.

The mortality rates associated with acute pancreatitis range from 6% to 20.5%, depending on the particular study bias.[8–10] Acute hemorrhagic or necrotizing pancreatitis is associated with mortality rates of 50% or more. Necrotizing pancreatitis occurs in 5% to 10% of patients in most series of acute pancreatitis. More recent studies have reported lower mortality rates, reflecting advances in critical care, nutritional support, and antibiotic therapy.

Etiology and Clinical Associations

Clinical associations with acute pancreatitis can be divided into three broad categories—biliary stones, ethanol, and others (Table 31-2). Biliary tract stone disease and ethanol-induced pancreatitis account for most cases of acute pancreatitis reported worldwide. The particular distribution of causes reflects the source of the patient population evaluated. In a summary of 18 different reports of acute pancreatitis in the United States with a combined total of 7147 patients, 53% of patients were believed to have ethanol-induced disease, whereas 28% had proven biliary stones[11] (Table 31-3). In contrast, of 1539 cases reported on from Great Britain, 52% were gallstone related, 7% were ethanol related, and 34% had no identifiable

cause.[12] Table 31-3 includes data from collected series around the world.[13,14] The high incidence of idiopathic and other causes in India and Hong Kong may be related to endemic infestation with *Opisthorchis sinensis* in these geographic areas.

Biliary Tract Stone Disease

Because the intramural portion of the distal common bile duct is shared with the pancreatic duct (Fig. 31-9), pancreatic ductal hypertension may result when a gallstone obstructs the ampulla of Vater during passage into the duodenum, the classic common channel concept. If transient obstruction results in edema formation and ampullary dysfunction, reflux of bile or duodenal contents into the pancreatic duct may then initiate acute pancreatitis. If gallstone passage is arrested within the ampulla, pancreatic ductal hypertension may additionally contribute. Choledocholithiasis is not always demonstrable in cases of suspected biliary pancreatitis. In one review of

Table 31-1. INCIDENCE AND MORTALITY RATES FOR ACUTE PANCREATITIS FROM FOUR REGIONS WITHIN GREAT BRITAIN

Region (Year; Author)	Yearly Incidence (per Million)	Mortality Rate (%)
Leeds (1976; McMahon)	110	<10
West Lothian (1975–1977; Graham)	238	<10
Nottingham (1969–1976; Bourke)	56.9	16.3
Bristol (1950–1969; Trapnell)	53.8	20.5

Table 31-2. CLINICAL ASSOCIATIONS WITH ACUTE PANCREATITIS

BILIARY TRACT STONE DISEASE

ETHANOL

OTHER
Trauma
   Postprocedural
      Postoperative
      Post-ERCP
   Direct
   Mechanical (nongallstone) obstruction
      Tumors of the pancreas, duodenum, or bile duct
      Duodenal obstruction
      Pancreas divisum
Infection
Hyperlipidemia
Hyperparathyroidism
Drugs
   Steroids
      Estrogen
      Glucocorticoids
   Diuretics
      Furosemide
      Thiazides
      Ethacrynic acid
      Diazoxide
   Calcium
   Coumadin
   Cimetidine
   Quinidine
   Phenformin
   Azothioprine
   Mercuric chloride
   Paracetamol
   Sulfonamides
   Tetracyclines
   L-Asparaginase
   Methyldopa
   Clonidine
Pregnancy
Idiopathic

1450 patients with gallstone-associated pancreatitis, gallstone impaction at the ampulla of Vater was identified in only 2%. Simple cholelithiasis was found in 72%, choledocholithiasis in 20%, and cholecystitis without apparent gallstones in 8%.[15] Presumably, passage of a gallstone before diagnostic evaluation is routine. When stools are carefully screened in patients with suspected biliary pancreatitis, gallstones can be demonstrated in 85% to 94% of the patients within 10 days of the onset of disease.[16] Conversely, within a similar time frame, only 11% to 15% of patients with cholelithiasis but without acute pancreatitis pass gallstones through the gastrointestinal tract.[17]

Ethanol

Ethanol use is the most common cause of acute pancreatitis in the United States. In addition to the pathophysiologic mechanisms proposed earlier, it is likely that genetic, dietary, and environmental factors contribute. Pancreatic ductal hypertension is probable after ethanol ingestion. This may occur by several different mechanisms. First, the production and precipitation of protein (stone protein) within the pancreatic duct has been demonstrated[18] (Fig. 31-10). This process is coupled with an ethanol-induced increase in ampullary tension and therefore resistance (Fig. 31-11). Lastly, ethanol-induced gastric acid secretion increases pancreatic secretion indirectly through acid-mediated secretin release.[18] The combination of increased ampullary resistance and increased ductal flow results in pancreatic ductal hypertension and appears to enhance protease entry into the pancreatic interstitium.

Others

A wide variety of other clinical conditions may be associated with acute pancreatitis, as shown in Table 31-2. These are briefly summarized next.

Postprocedural Pancreatitis

Many surgical procedures in the upper abdomen are associated with postoperative pancreatitis. The incidence of acute pancreatitis after gastric resection is between 0.6% and 1.23%. After biliary tract surgery, particularly after common bile duct exploration, acute pancreatitis occurs with an incidence of 0.5% to 3%. Direct manipulation or retraction of the pancreas or pancreatic duct appears to be the most common cause. Acute pancreatitis develops in about 1% of patients after endoscopic retrograde cholangiopancreatography (ERCP).[19] This is a predictable event, and the risk can be minimized by limiting the pressure used for contrast injection of the pancreatic duct. Acute pancreatitis also occurs in patients after coronary artery bypass surgery and a variety of other procedures remote from the pancreas. Although pancreatitis in this circumstance is thought to result from ischemia, hypotension is not always noted. The systemic consequences of activation of the inflammatory system may contribute to changes in microvascular blood flow.

Abdominal Trauma

Acute pancreatitis occurs in about 1% to 2% of patients with abdominal trauma, whether blunt or penetrating. Contusion of the pancreatic parenchyma and pancreatic

Table 31-3. CLINICAL ASSOCIATIONS WITH ACUTE PANCREATITIS FROM COLLECTED REVIEWS AROUND THE WORLD

Country	Patients	Cause (%)			
		Biliary Stones	Ethanol	Idiopathic	Other
United States	7147	28	53	8	11
Great Britain	1539	52	7	34	7
Germany	279	51	22	24	3
France	294	34	33	—	—
Sweden	207	48	21	15	16
Denmark	163	33	42	21	4
India	42	17	23	31	29
Hong Kong	483	41	10	39	10

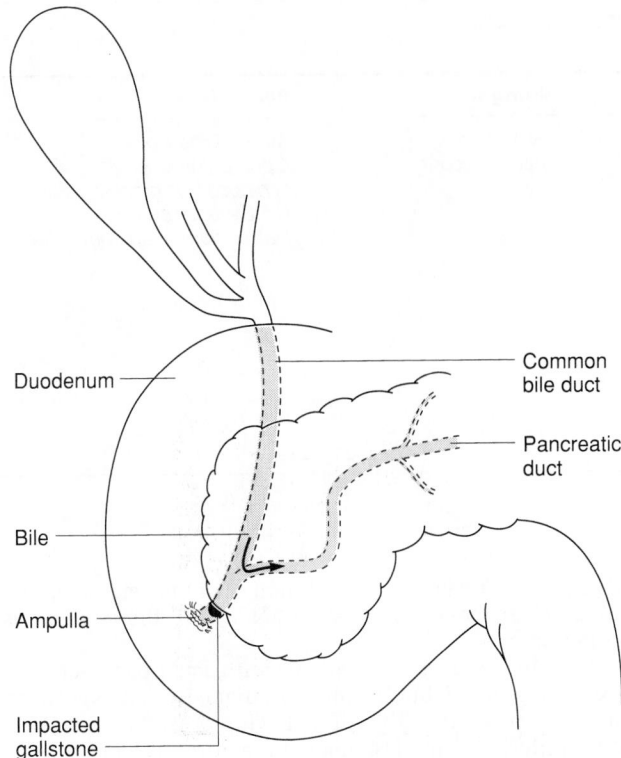

Figure 31-9. The common channel concept is illustrated as a gallstone at the ampulla of Vater leads to reflux of bile into the pancreatic duct.

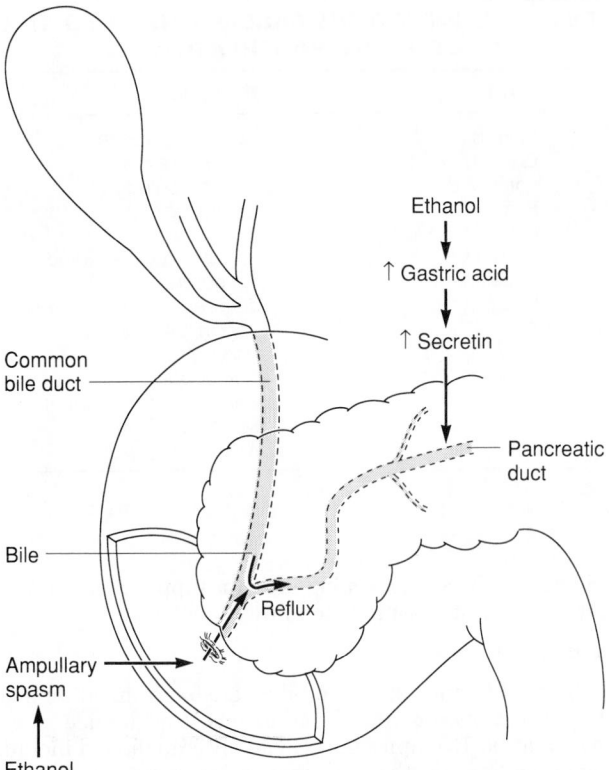

Figure 31-11. Ethanol-induced increases in ampullary resistance may exacerbate the reflux of bile into the pancreatic duct. Coupled with acid-stimulated, secretin-mediated increases in pancreatic secretion, this may contribute to pancreatic duct hypertension and the development of acute pancreatitis.

ductal injury both lead to extravasation of activated enzymes to initiate the process.

Hyperlipoproteinemia

Rare causes of acute pancreatitis are the hyperlipoproteinemias, types I and V.[20] The initial acinar cell injury is thought to result from the liberation of free fatty acids from

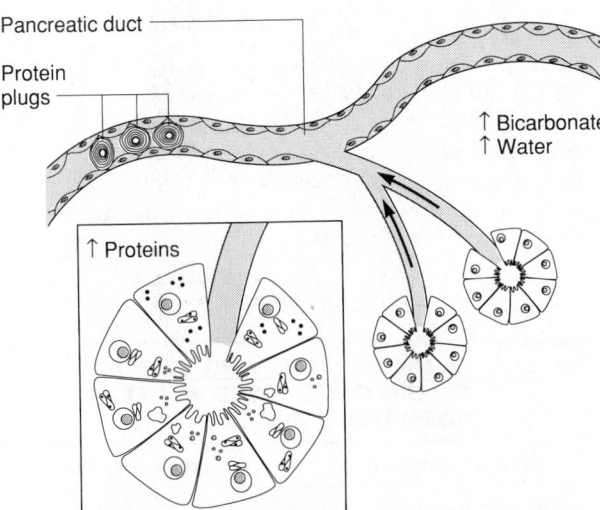

Figure 31-10. Ethanol induces the formation of protein (stone protein) plugs within the pancreatic ductules. These potentially obstructive deposits occur in conjunction with increased ampullary resistance (see Fig. 31-11) and increased pancreatic secretion of both water and bicarbonate.

circulating triglycerides by the local action of lipases within the pancreatic microcirculation. Physical disruption of the microvascular endothelium by cholesterol crystals may also occur.

Hyperparathyroidism

Acute pancreatitis is reported in 1% to 19% of patients with hyperparathyroidism. It is unclear whether increased circulating plasma levels of calcium or parathyroid hormone are primarily responsible. Hypercalcemia may be associated with the precipitation of calcium phosphate within the pancreatic duct as well as with pancreatic hypersecretion. The effects are similar to those illustrated in Figures 31-10 and 31-11. In addition, elevated parathyroid hormone levels may have a direct cytotoxic effect on acinar cells.

Drugs

Drug-induced acute pancreatitis is relatively common and has been reported in association with many pharmacologic agents. A partial summary is provided in Table 31-2. The mechanisms involved are largely unknown and are likely different among the offending drugs. The spectrum of potential pancreatic toxins includes simple physiologic secretagogues, such as cerulein (a cholecystokinin analogue), as well as exotic substances, such as scorpion (Tityus trinitatis) venom.

Infections

The development of acute pancreatitis has been reported after a variety of bacterial, fungal, parasitic, and viral infections (Table 31-4). Postulated mechanisms include direct

Table 31-4. INFECTIOUS CAUSES LINKED TO THE DEVELOPMENT OF ACUTE PANCREATITIS

Viral	Bacterial	Fungal	Parasitic
Mumps	*Staphylococcus* sp	Aspergillosis	*Ascaris lumbricoides*
Coxsackie B	*Escherichia coli*	Actinomycosis	*Opisthorchis sinensis*
Enterovirus	*Enterococcus* sp		*Echinococcus granulosus*
Epstein-Barr virus	*Enterobacter* sp		*Giardiasis lamblia*
Cytomegalovirus	*Proteus* sp		*Plasmodium falciparum*
Hepatitis B	*Pseudomonas aeruginosa*		
Hepatitis A	Spirochetes		
Hepatitis C	*Corynebacterium diphtheriae*		
	Legionnella spiro		
	Yersinia sp		
	Campylobacter sp		
	Salmonella typhimurium		
	Mycobacteria sp		
	Mycoplasma sp		

cytotoxic effects, coexisting immunosuppression, and alterations in pancreatic blood flow.

Vascular Disease

Impaired pancreatic blood flow arising from either anatomic lesions or functional events can induce acute pancreatitis. Examples not previously enumerated include embolization of the pancreaticoduodenal artery after translumbar aortography, celiac artery stenosis, ruptured abdominal aortic aneurysm, and myocardial infarction.

Immunologic Factors

Acute pancreatitis has been associated with systemic lupus erythematosus, rheumatoid arthritis, polyarteritis nodosa, and Be87het syndrome. Systemic vasculitis, the associated glucocorticoid use, and the presence of circulating antibodies to acinar cells are potentially related findings.

Obstruction of the Duodenum or the Pancreatic Duct

Intrapancreatic or duodenal tumors, parasitic obstruction of the pancreatic duct, other obstructions of the duodenum, and pancreas divisum are also associated with the development of pancreatic duct hypertension and acute pancreatitis.

Pregnancy

Acute pancreatitis has been linked to pregnancy with an incidence of 0.01% to 0.1%.[21] Because most reports include patients with gallstones, ethanol use, or other risk factors, it is unclear whether pregnancy is an independent risk factor.

Presentation

The cardinal clinical symptom for acute pancreatitis is epigastric pain that is visceral in character and radiates into the back. The degree of discomfort is variable. The pain may be similar to that of acute peritonitis and may mimic a perforated viscus. At the other extreme, pain may be minimal. Other common signs and symptoms are nonspecific (Table 31-5).

Clinical signs of complex disease or necrotizing pancreatitis include jaundice and hypotension. In addition, retroperitoneal hemorrhage associated with pancreatic necrosis may become apparent as blood dissects into the subcutaneous tissues, producing blue discoloration of the flanks (Grey Turner sign), the umbilicus (Cullen sign), or the inguinal ligament (Fox sign). None of these signs is common.[22]

The clinical course of patients with acute pancreatitis is exceedingly variable, seemingly enigmatic. The spectrum includes patients with minimal symptoms, few signs, and only mild hyperamylasemia who require little or no treatment and have few, if any, complications. The opposite end of the spectrum, without apparent differentiating risk factors, is fulminant pancreatic necrosis with hemorrhage and progressive, inexorable multisystem organ failure and death.

All prospective estimations of outcome are potentially flawed. Several grading systems have been developed, however, to estimate risks and outcomes based on the presenting clinical features, and the Ranson criteria are widely adopted. A patient with three or more of these findings has a mortality rate of about 30%.[23]

RANSON GRAVE PROGNOSTIC SIGNS ASSOCIATED WITH ACUTE PANCREATITIS

On Admission

Age above 55 years
White blood cell count above $16,000/\mu L$
Glucose level above 200 mg/dL
Lactase dehydrogenase level above 350 IU/L
Serum glutamic-oxaloacetic transaminase value above 250 IU/L

After 48 Hours

Hematocrit decrease of 10%
Blood urea nitrogen level increase of 5 mg/dL
Ca^{2+} level below 8 mg/dL

Table 31-5. COMMON SIGNS AND SYMPTOMS OF UNCOMPLICATED ACUTE EDEMATOUS PANCREATITIS

Sign or Symptom	Frequency (%)
Abdominal pain	85–100
Nausea and vomiting	54–92
Anorexia	83
Fever	12–80
Abdominal mass	6–20
Ileus	50–80

PaO$_2$ level below 60 mmHg
Base deficit value above 4 mEq/L
Fluid sequestration greater than 6 L

Pancreatitis-associated morbidity and mortality are directly correlated with the number of these criteria present. The mortality rate is 28% if three criteria are met, 40% for five or six, and 100% for seven or eight.[23] The APACHE II (Acute Physiology Score and Chronic Health Evaluation) scoring system for critically ill patients has also been applied.[24] Although not specific for acute pancreatitis, the APACHE score has some utility by predicting mortality rates in critically ill patients.

Diagnosis

The diagnosis of acute pancreatitis ultimately depends on a clinical judgment, generally based on the finding of appropriate epigastric abdominal pain and tenderness with the laboratory finding of hyperamylasemia. No single laboratory or physical finding is pathognomonic.

Imaging

Although a diffuse ileus and a solitary left upper abdominal sentinel loop are classic and are often seen on plain abdominal roentgenograms, neither is specific for acute pancreatitis. The psoas muscle margins may be obscured by retroperitoneal edema; pancreatic ascites may be apparent; pancreatic calcifications imply preexisting chronic disease. About one third of patients with acute pancreatitis have abnormal chest radiographs at the time of diagnosis. An upright chest radiograph may demonstrate segmental atelectasis, an elevated hemidiaphragm, pleural effusions, or the presence of early pulmonary parenchymal infiltrates. Barium studies of the gastrointestinal tract are seldom helpful for evaluating simple acute pancreatitis. If obtained, an upper gastrointestinal contrast study often demonstrates narrowing or spasm of the duodenum, with widening of the C loop secondary to pancreatic inflammation and edema formation.

Ultrasound provides a readily available, rapid, and non-invasive means of imaging the pancreas that is often helpful. In the case of simple acute pancreatitis, an enlarged, echolucent gland is typically seen. In addition, ultrasound examination yields information regarding cholelithiasis, choledocholithiasis, and the status of the intrahepatic and extrahepatic biliary ducts. The technique is also valuable for assessing and sequentially evaluating peripancreatic fluid collections or pancreatic pseudocysts. Computed tomography (CT) has similar capabilities to ultrasound, although sensitivity for detecting cholelithiasis is lower. Intraluminal contrast in the duodenum and small bowel is necessary to optimize CT imaging. Dynamic CT scanning with simultaneous intravenous contrast enhancement can give valuable information in evaluating regional pancreatic perfusion and may provide an estimate of the extent of pancreatic necrosis.

Either CT- or ultrasound-guided diagnostic needle aspiration allows access to peripancreatic or pancreatic fluid collections for diagnostic sampling or therapeutic drainage. Cultures may be obtained by this route, and, if appropriate, contrast injections can assess the relation of a pseudocyst or abscess cavity to the pancreatic duct. This latter information is important for any preoperative planning. Placement of therapeutic drainage catheters is routinely combined with CT- and ultrasound-directed imaging procedures.

The role of ERCP in the diagnostic evaluation of the patient with acute pancreatitis is severely limited because of the high risk of exacerbating existing inflammation.

ERCP is generally reserved for the evaluation of a patient with a suspected obstructive lesion and is timed to follow resolution of the acute phase of the illness. In addition, it is appropriate to obtain ERCP in a patient with idiopathic acute pancreatitis after a first recurrence of the disease. This strategy is designed to identify promptly anatomically correctable causes of acute pancreatitis. ERCP is also useful to delineate the pancreatic duct after injury, pseudocyst drainage, or the development of pancreatic ascites. Lastly, ERCP combined with urgent therapeutic sphincterotomy and gallstone extraction has been used for patients with impacted ampullary gallstones.

Biochemical Markers

Amylase. Amylase is released from the acinar cell into the pancreatic microcirculation in conjunction with the pathophysiologic events described earlier. The laboratory finding of hyperamylasemia in a patient with clinical signs and symptoms of acute pancreatitis is the usual means of confirming the diagnosis. Efforts to correlate the degree of hyperamylasemia with disease severity or prognosis have been consistently unsuccessful, and Ranson criteria are notable for the absence of serum amylase levels. An important reason for this relates to the relatively rapid clearance of amylase from plasma, the half-life being about 130 minutes. Pancreatitis resulting from a discrete event such as transient pancreatic duct obstruction with gallstone passage is characterized by a single serum amylase peak with a rapid rise and prompt clearance, both measured in terms of hours. Given the inherent delays in seeking clinical care and in obtaining diagnostic studies, this peak may have passed, and the serum amylase may be relatively normal within 24 hours of the event. A normal or minimally elevated serum amylase level may also be found in a patient with necrotizing pancreatitis or with chronic pancreatitis; in these instances, complete or nearly complete destruction of the acinar cell population may have occurred, reducing the plasma amylase level. Additionally, a number of nonpancreatic sources of amylase exist, so that hyperamylasemia may result from other pathology. Salivary glands, fallopian tubes, and the small bowel are important alternative amylase sources. Clinical conditions associated with hyperamylasemia include the following[25]:

- Salivary gland injury
- Burns
- Cerebral trauma
- Multiple trauma
- Diabetic ketoacidosis
- Macroamylasemia
- Renal transplantation
- Renal dysfunction
- Pneumonia
- Pregnancy
- Fallopian tube pathology
- Drugs
- Afferent loop syndrome
- Acute appendicitis
- Dissecting aortic aneurysm
- Small bowel injury
  Perforated ulcer
  Small bowel obstruction
  Mesenteric infarction

In the case of salivary gland disease, plasma amylase isoenzyme determinations differentiate the source. An accurate and more rapid amylase assay using a monoclonal antibody specific to salivary isoamylase has been described. Gastrointestinal tract pathology other than pancreatitis may lead to increased amylase absorption through the intestine or peritoneum and relatively mild elevations of pancreatic amylase in the circulation.

Because plasma amylase levels reflect renal clearance, renal dysfunction may also contribute to hyperamylasemia.[26] Indeed, determination of the ratio of amylase (A) clearance to creatinine (Cr) clearance is a potentially useful diagnostic test for acute pancreatitis. This fractional excretion calculation is shown:

$$Fe_A = \frac{(U_A) \times (S_{Cr})}{(U_{Cr}) \times (S_A)} \times 10$$

The normal fractional urinary excretion of amylase is between 1% and 4%. Clearance in excess of 4% to 4.5% is considered abnormal but is not specific for acute pancreatitis. Renal dysfunction, particularly with impaired tubular reabsorption, diabetic ketoacidosis, formation of amylase macroconjugates, and thermal injuries are clinical conditions that limit the specificity of this test. In the correct clinical setting, increased amylase clearance may provide a method of confirmation of hyperamylasemia that is useful after simple plasma elevations have been cleared.

Lipase. Lipase is derived primarily from pancreatic acinar cells, and its elevation is also taken as evidence of acinar cell injury in acute pancreatitis. Lipase is also nonspecific and has not proved more useful than serum amylase determinations in clinical use.

Other Serum Enzymes. Other acinar cell products, such as immunoreactive trypsin, chymotrypsin, elastase, ribonuclease, and phospholipase A2, may be detectable in plasma after the onset of acute pancreatitis. Measurement techniques are not in wide clinical use, but institutional enthusiasm for one particular assay or another has led to an abundant literature. None has overcome the limitations attending amylase determinations outlined earlier. Although it is appealing to consider that the pattern of enzyme release is related to the degree of acinar cell injury, experience with these markers is limited. Ribonuclease and phospholipase A2 plasma elevations may correlate with more complex disease.[27]

Methemalbumin. Methemalbumin results from the proteolytic conversion of hemoglobin into oxidized hematin that is conjugated with plasma albumin. Acinar cell protease release into the circulation increases red blood cell exposure to proteases and accelerates this process, so that methemalbumin plasma levels may be elevated with acute pancreatitis. A correlation between levels of methemalbumin and severity of pancreatic disease is proposed but unproved.[28]

Other Serum Abnormalities. Other characteristic but nonspecific biochemical features commonly associated with acute pancreatitis are summarized in Table 31-6. These may have both therapeutic and diagnostic relevance.

Management

Neither medical nor surgical treatment strategies provide specific therapy for the acinar cell injury characteristic of acute pancreatitis. Modern approaches provide general supportive care in the form of appropriate resuscitation, nutrition, and ventilation in the expectation that the cellular pathophysiologic processes will be self-limited. The closest approximations to specific therapy consist of elimination of pharmacologic stimuli, such as ethanol, or surgical relief of pancreatic ductal obstruction by procedures such as sphincterotomy. Empiric but successful treatments for specific complications such as pseudocyst or pancreatic abscess formation have been de-

Table 31-6. BIOCHEMICAL FEATURES OF ACUTE PANCREATITIS

INCREASED

Hematocrit, hemoglobin (hemoconcentration)
White blood cell count
Blood urea nitrogen
Creatinine
Bilirubin
Lipid, triglyceride levels
Glucose
Alkaline phosphatase
SGOT, SGPT

DECREASED

Hematocrit, hemoglobin (hemorrhage)
Calcium
Magnesium
PaO_2

OTHER

Respiratory alkalosis (early)
Metabolic alkalosis (early)
Consumptive coagulopathy
Metabolic acidosis (late)
Respiratory acidosis (late)

veloped. Rational treatment protocols using exogenous antiproteases, antioxidants, and other antiinflammatory agents may become available in the near future.

Medical Treatment

Conventional medical therapy for acute pancreatitis consists fundamentally of intravenous fluid resuscitation, nasogastric decompression, and monitoring of hematocrit, electrolytes, and blood gases. All are empiric and are not known to shorten or favorably alter the course of the disease.

Regional retroperitoneal inflammation and the systemic microvascular injury contribute to the loss of intravascular plasma volume. Hypovolemia may be mild or profound to the point of shock. A semiquantitative relation exists between the magnitude of extravascular fluid sequestration and the severity of the pancreatitis. This is recognized by inclusion of an estimated plasma volume deficit exceeding 6 L in the Ranson scoring system (see earlier list) as a grave prognostic sign. More than half of patients with acute pancreatitis have clinical evidence of inadequate end-organ perfusion. Resuscitation requires the intravenous administration of large volumes of isotonic crystalloid solution and the aggressive use of invasive hemodynamic monitoring devices.

Some degree of pulmonary dysfunction occurs in about two thirds of patients with acute pancreatitis. More than 70% of patients have evidence of transient hypoxemia, defined as a single PaO_2 of less than 70 mmHg.[29] Progression to acute respiratory failure requiring endotracheal intubation and mechanical ventilation carries a mortality rate of up to 75% but is a relatively uncommon event (about 5% of all cases).[30] Monitoring of pulmonary gas exchange with periodic arterial blood gases is standard in all patients with acute pancreatitis. Continuous transcutaneous monitoring of capillary hemoglobin saturation or measurement of mixed venous saturation is appropriate if evidence of acute respiratory distress develops. About one third of patients with acute pancreatitis have abnormalities on chest radiograph. Pleural effusion, pneumonia, and fully developed acute respiratory distress syndrome are all possible. The treatment of each is considered elsewhere.

Renal dysfunction is demonstrable in 40% to 80% of patients with acute pancreatitis. Therefore, renal function must be sequentially evaluated biochemically, and the urine output must be carefully monitored during the acute resuscitative phase of the illness. Early recognition of oliguria or azotemia allows correction. Hypovolemia is almost invariably the cause of the renal dysfunction and is therefore simply treated if recognized. The reported incidence of acute renal failure secondary to acute pancreatitis ranges from 2% to 20%. If required, dialysis, hemofiltration, and similar supportive measures are all associated with substantially increased mortality rates (up to 80%).[31]

Patients with acute pancreatitis share many hemodynamic and metabolic characteristics with septic patients. Glucose production is exaggerated, insulin resistance and pancreatic endocrine insufficiency may develop, and protein catabolism is marked. Nitrogen losses of as much as 40 g/d have been measured in patients with acute pancreatitis.[32] Nutritional support is a necessary feature of their care. It is appropriate to initiate nutritional support immediately after the acute resuscitation phase because of the unpredictable return of intestinal function and the extraordinary metabolic requirements.

Considerable debate has surrounded the selection of a nutritional route. A parenteral route is often required for hyperalimentation during the early postresuscitation period, because of the additional control of the intravascular compartment afforded and also because of persistent ileus. For patients with acute pancreatitis, it appears theoretically advantageous to minimize pancreatic secretion to avoid exacerbation of acute acinar cell injury. The administration of intravenous fat emulsions is known to increase pancreatic protein secretion in normal volunteers and is therefore potentially disadvantageous; there is no evidence that this is a clinically relevant concern.[33] Parenteral hyperalimentation is a mainstay in the treatment of these patients.

An enteral feeding route has the inherent advantages of maintaining more normal physiology, providing intestinal mucosal trophic support, and being less expensive. Although all enteral routes cause some peptide-mediated pancreatic secretion, this can be minimized with bypass of the stomach and duodenum using a jejunal feeding tube. Intraluminal fat in the jejunum provides a substantially diminished secretory stimulus to the pancreas when compared with more proximal feeding sites. The choice of route is less important than the need to provide adequate calories and to establish positive nitrogen balance.

Antibiotic therapy is reserved for specific infectious complications such as pneumonia or pancreatic abscess. Antibiotic use for simple acute edematous pancreatitis is contraindicated. Prospective randomized studies in patients with simple acute pancreatitis using ampicillin, lincomycin, and cephalothin have shown neither improvement in the clinical course nor a reduced likelihood of septic complications.

Specific metabolic complications such as hypokalemia, hypocalcemia, hemorrhage, and consumptive coagulopathy are treated with appropriate replacement products, such as potassium chloride, intravenous calcium gluconate or chloride, red blood cells, and fresh-frozen plasma. Hyperglycemia and glycosuria are the manifestations of altered carbohydrate metabolism in these patients. Hyperglycemia occurs in about 10% of patients and is generally a transient phenomenon. Permanent residual diabetes mellitus is much less frequent, occurring in fewer than 2% of patients. Treatment for the acute illness consists of the carefully titrated administration of exogenous glucose and insulin to maintain a euglycemic state.

Clinical evidence of encephalopathy is discernible in 4% to 20% of patients with acute pancreatitis. Symptoms may include disorientation, confusion, delirium, delusions, or hallucinations. Transient acute psychosis is also reported. Because ethanol ingestion and withdrawal also produce these symptoms, it is often difficult to distinguish the underlying cause. Cerebral edema, hemorrhage, and focal necrosis, presumably secondary to microvascular blood flow alterations, have all been associated with acute pancreatitis. Treatment is nonspecific and supportive.

Disorders of the coagulation system, particularly microvascular thrombosis and disseminated intravascular coagulopathy, are common in acute pancreatitis. Experimentally, decreased plasma levels of fibrinogen, factor VII, and platelets occur within hours after the onset of acute pancreatitis, consistent with the clinical observation that disseminated intravascular coagulopathy is normally an early event unless it occurs as a complication of late sepsis. At later times (6 or 7 days), clinical studies have shown hyperfibrinogenemia and increased platelet counts, suggesting enhanced thrombotic potential. Heparin, low-molecular-weight dextran, and fibrinolytic therapy have been shown to prevent microvascular thrombosis in experimental acute pancreatitis in dogs. In this favorable and controlled setting, these agents prevent the development of acute hemorrhagic pancreatitis. Other experimental interventions designed to increase regional blood flow, and therefore to minimize the extent of small vessel thrombosis, include surgical denervation of postganglionic sympathetic fibers to the pancreas or the use of pharmacologic ganglionic blockade. The latter approach has not undergone appropriate preclinical evaluation, and none of these anticoagulant strategies has proven clinical efficacy.

Hypocalcemia is relatively common (3% to 30%) in acute pancreatitis. The magnitude of the hypocalcemia correlates with the degree of illness. It appears that large quantities of calcium are bound in the tissues during the process of peripancreatic fat saponification. Other factors, such as changes in plasma levels of parathyroid hormone, glucagon, and calcitonin, may also contribute. Unattended, the hypocalcemia may progress to tetany. Periodic monitoring of serum calcium is standard practice during the acute illness. Treatment consists of intravenous replacement to maintain the serum calcium level within a normal range.

A variety of pharmacologic agents that directly or indirectly reduce acinar cell enzyme release or ductal secretion have undergone clinical evaluation for the treatment of acute pancreatitis, generally with unimpressive results. Among the first were anticholinergic drugs. Despite extensive experience over many years, no objective data have emerged to support their use. Clinical trials of glucagon and calcitonin based on the same principle have produced a similar lack of supportive data. A somatostatin analogue has been subjected to clinical trials for patients with acute pancreatitis. Somatostatin inhibits pancreatic enzyme and bicarbonate secretion by preventing the normal release of cholecystokinin, secretin, and other gut peptides. Despite the theoretic appeal, it has not been possible to demonstrate that somatostatin alters the natural history or prognosis of simple acute pancreatitis, although it diminishes pancreatic secretion.

Surgical Therapy

Surgical therapy for acute pancreatitis is reserved for specific complications and for those situations in which a correctable anatomic cause can be identified.

Endoscopic sphincterotomy is usually the initial therapeutic procedure for relief of biliary ductal obstruction when acute pancreatitis occurs in association with choledocholithiasis. The procedure reliably decompresses the ampulla of Vater, with overall clinical success for gallstone disimpaction or passage in 90% of patients.[34] This approach has greatly reduced the need for operative procedures designed to either divert or open and explore the common bile duct.

In the more usual circumstance, a patient who has simple cholelithiasis and an episode of acute pancreatitis is treated nonoperatively with resolution. The rate of recurrent biliary pancreatitis is as high as 34% to 56% within 6 weeks; therefore, an aggressive operative approach is appropriate. Cholecystectomy is often performed after the resolution of acute pancreatitis but before hospital discharge. Common bile duct instrumentation in this setting has a substantially increased risk of recurrent acute pancreatitis.

Anatomically correctable lesions that can cause acute pancreatitis include pancreas divisum, choledochal cysts (particularly a type III cyst or choledochocele), and pancreatic duct obstruction related to tumor, stricture, or injury. In the obstructive category, many patients have chronic pancreatitis or recurrent acute pancreatitis. Surgical therapy is directed at achieving adequate pancreatic duct drainage, usually by diversion into the jejunum for benign obstructions, or tumor resection if appropriate. Symptomatic pancreas divisum is best treated with operative transduodenal sphincteroplasty, whereas a type III choledochal cyst should be marsupialized into the duodenum.

Acute pancreatitis may be clinically indistinguishable at presentation from an acute abdomen related to other pathology. Perforated duodenal ulcer, acute appendicitis, and ruptured abdominal aortic aneurysms are sources of erroneous diagnoses. Virtually every experienced surgeon has performed an exploratory laparotomy for clinical evidence of peritonitis only to find simple acute edematous pancreatitis. In this situation, recognition of the correct diagnosis is crucial. It is important to avoid biopsy, resection, or other nontherapeutic procedures that carry significant risks. In the event that devitalized tissue or saponified retroperitoneal fat are present, careful débridement and external drainage may be appropriate.

Peritoneal lavage as a specific therapy for acute pancreatitis was proposed after experimental studies demonstrated improved survival in animals with fulminant pancreatitis. The concept was appealing in that activated proteases and other vasoactive substances identifiable in peritoneal aspirates from patients with pancreatitis would be removed, rather than systemically absorbed. Unfortunately, clinical trials using this approach have produced disappointing results, and the eventual overall mortality rate appears unchanged. Enthusiasm for this approach has diminished, although some continue to advocate its use.

Surgery is usually required for patients with necrotizing pancreatitis. When pancreatitis does not resolve spontaneously, diagnostic efforts are directed at distinguishing infected and noninfected areas of pancreatic necrosis. Needle aspiration of peripancreatic fluid collections at the time of CT or ultrasound scanning help to differentiate these possibilities. The presence of an infected sequestrum mandates operative exploration to débride devitalized tissue and to provide external drainage. Specific antibiotic coverage is essential and should be dictated by intraoperative cultures or aspirates from the necrotic tissue. Débridement is often required on multiple occasions, usually at 24- to 48-hour intervals, until the necrotic tissue is replaced by a granulating wound. Many strategies related to multiple operations with open and closed peritoneal drainage systems have been devised. The results of these methods are all comparable so long as colonized or infected devitalized tissue is not left in a closed abdominal cavity. For patients with apparently uninfected areas of pancreatic necrosis, operation may be deferred unless clinical evidence of deterioration develops. This is often a difficult judgment and is necessarily individualized for each patient.

Pancreatic Pseudocysts

A pancreatic pseudocyst is a fluid-filled cystic structure without a true epithelial lining that is associated with the pancreas or pancreatic duct (Fig. 31-12). True (epithelium-lined) cysts of the pancreas are rare, whereas pseudocysts are relatively common. Pancreatic pseudocysts account for fewer than 0.1% of all hospital admissions in the United States, but they occur in 2% to 10% of patients with pancreatic disease. The most common cause of pancreatic pseudocyst in the United States is ethanol-related chronic pancreatitis. Biliary and posttraumatic pancreatitis follow in frequency with regard to cause. The pseudocyst wall is composed of displaced adjacent viscera (often stomach, small bowel, or colon) and a fibrous capsule that has evidence of both acute and chronic inflammation. The thickness of this fibrous capsule is variable, depending on how long the pseudocyst has been present. The presence of a fibrous capsule becomes an important consideration in the timing and selection of drainage procedures. The fluid within the cyst cavity is usually serous in character and contains pancreatic secretions, including amylase and proteases, as well as albumin and inflammatory cells. The amylase content may be high; it is not unusual to see a level of several thousand international units in pseudocyst aspirates. If recent hemorrhage has occurred, bile pigment may also be present, and bacteria are cultured in about 35% of pseudocysts.[35]

The clinical presentation of a pancreatic pseudocyst is usually that of persistent visceral pain or ileus after an episode of acute pancreatitis. Fever, leukocytosis, and a palpable epigastric mass are common, nausea and vomiting less so. Jaundice suggests common bile duct obstruction from either intrinsic stones or extrinsic distortion. Most pseudocysts are unilocular and located in the head of the pancreas (Table 31-7). Pseudocysts can dissect essentially anywhere within the retroperitoneal space or mediastinum. Therefore, a variety of unusual presentations may occur, including intrathoracic or intraabdominal mass lesions. A left-sided pleural effusion is classic on chest radiograph. Splenic vein or portal vein thrombosis may occur with pseudocyst formation, resulting in so-called left-sided portal hypertension and bleeding esophageal varices.

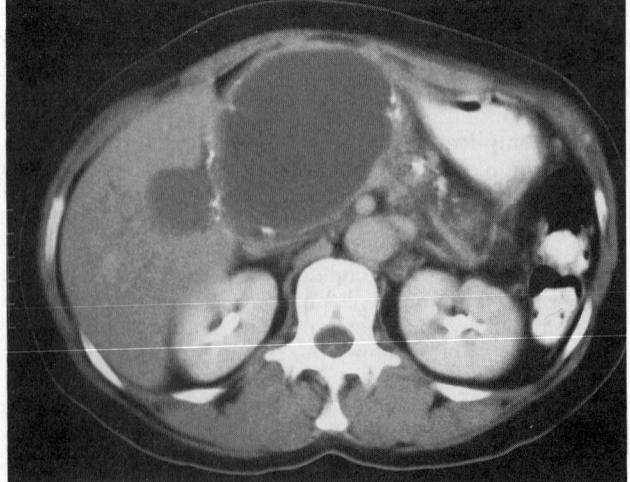

Figure 31-12. CT scan showing pancreatic pseudocyst.

Table 31-7. LOCATION OF PANCREATIC PSEUDOCYTS

Location	Incidence (%)
Head	45
Body	28
Tail	27

Initial management of pancreatic pseudocysts is based on whether the cyst is symptomatic. If the patient does not have symptoms and the cyst is small (less than 5 cm), it can be safely observed; many of these resolve over a period of weeks.[36] Concurrent chronic alcoholic pancreatitis, pseudocyst size greater than 5 cm, the presence of a multilocular or debris-filled pseudocyst cavity, and chronicity (longer than 6 weeks) are all factors that are associated with a lower probability of spontaneous resolution. If the cyst is large (more than 5 cm) or the patient does not have symptoms, ERCP is indicated to determine the pancreatic ductal anatomy. A pancreatic duct that communicates with the pseudocyst generally requires operative management. In some institutions, endoscopic placement of pancreatic stents to bridge the ductal disruption into the pseudocyst has been tried with moderate success.[37] If no ductal communication can be demonstrated by ERCP, a trial of percutaneous drainage may be attempted. For patients with infected pseudocysts, percutaneous drainage and intravenous antibiotics should be the initial management. Definitive management, based on ductal anatomy, is performed after resolution of the infection. Pseudocysts that present with bleeding or that develop bleeding as a complication during conservative treatment should undergo emergent angiography with embolization. If tumor is suspected, either percutaneous or intraoperative biopsy is indicated, with operative management based on the biopsy results and the location of the tumor. Timing for operative management is important. In general, a waiting period of 4 to 6 weeks from the onset of symptoms is appropriate to allow the pseudocyst wall to develop a thick fibrous capsule. If it is impossible to judge the date of pseudocyst formation, 4 to 6 weeks from the time of initial diagnosis is generally chosen, or the wall thickness may be estimated from an imaging study such as ultrasound or CT. A summary of the results of pseudocyst drainage is provided in Table 31-8.

Generally, a pancreatic pseudocyst can be observed for a period of weeks or months in an effort to allow for spontaneous resolution. Half or more of pseudocysts resolve spontaneously without complication.[36] Resolution may occur as a result of the reabsorption of cyst fluid, resolution of obstruction of the pancreatic duct, or rupture into an adjacent hollow viscus. Concurrent chronic alcoholic pancreatitis, pseudocyst size greater than 5 cm, the presence of a multilocular or debris-filled pseudocyst cavity, and chronicity (longer than 6 weeks) are all associated with a lower probability of spontaneous resolution. Indications for drainage include increasing size, infection, gastrointestinal tract obstruction, hemorrhage, spontaneous rupture, and failure to resolve.

Percutaneous ultrasound- or CT-directed aspiration or drainage catheter placement is an initial treatment option for these lesions. Experience is evolving, but it appears that the risk is low and that the recurrence rate is similar to that of open external drainage procedures. Simple aspiration is performed if the initial aspirate is sterile; if the aspirate is infected, a catheter or open drainage procedure is appropriate. Determination of pancreatic ductal anatomy is important whenever possible. Therefore, contrast injection into the pseudocyst at the time of aspiration should be considered to assess the possibility of pancreatic ductal communication and obstruction, or multiple cysts. The pseudocyst recurrence rate after simple aspiration is about 20% to 25%. Repeat aspiration has been successfully employed in the absence of infection or other symptoms.

The decision to proceed with an open surgical drainage procedure is usually reached because a complication develops. This may well be recurrence after repeated aspirations. Generally, a waiting period of at least 6 weeks is needed for the pseudocyst to resolve or for the wall to develop a thick fibrous capsule. If it is impossible to judge the date of pseudocyst formation, 6 weeks from the time of initial diagnosis is generally chosen; the wall thickness may be estimated from imaging studies such as ultrasound or CT.

The operative treatment for pseudocysts depends on the underlying cause of the cyst as well as the size, location, and maturity of the pseudocyst wall. Whenever possible, the status of the pancreatic duct should be assessed preoperatively, preferably by ERCP. Knowledge of the anatomy of the pancreatic duct allows design of an appropriate drainage plan. Operative drainage can be either external or internal. External drainage is chosen in the presence of infection or an immature capsule. The disadvantages of external drainage include the risk of pancreatic fistula formation and a pseudocyst recurrence. External drainage has been associated with a higher mortality rate, probably because it is used in patients at higher risk, especially those with sepsis, pancreatic abscesses, or ruptured pseudocysts.

The type of internal drainage procedure selected depends on the location of the pseudocyst and whether there is associated pancreatic ductal pathology. Cystogastrostomy is the simplest and safest alternative if the pseudocyst is appropriately adjacent to the posterior wall of the stomach. Cystojejunostomy using a Roux-en-Y or loop jejunostomy may also be appropriate, depending on the location and specific anatomy of the pseudocyst. Cystojejunostomy often requires a retrocolic approach through the transverse mesocolon to achieve truly dependent drainage. Pancreatic resection is associated with the lowest recurrence rate (3%), but is limited to pseudocysts occurring in the tail of the pancreas.

Pancreatic Abscess

The common causes of pancreatic abscess are an infected pancreatic pseudocyst and necrotizing pancreatitis. The diagnosis is suggested by persistent fever, leukocytosis,

Table 31-8. RESULTS OF PSEUDOCYST DRAINAGE PROCEDURES

Type	Complication Rate (%)	Recurrence Rate (%)	Mortality Rate (%)
Percutaneous aspiration	0	63	0
Percutaneous catheter	16	8	3
Surgical external drainage	35	20–25	7–27
Surgical internal drainage	25–35	5–9	3–9

and a palpable abdominal mass. Bacteremia and systemic toxicity are late clinical features. On imaging, debris within a cyst is more suggestive of an abscess; percutaneous aspiration with positive cultures is the definitive preoperative test. The diagnosis is facilitated by CT scanning or ultrasound-guided needle aspiration of suspicious peripancreatic fluid collections. The treatment of choice is wide surgical débridement with removal of all infected and devitalized tissues. Generous drainage is mandatory. Whether to leave the abdomen open and the choice of drainage systems remain controversial. Advocates of closed drainage (ie, placement of large, dependent drains and abdominal closure) report mortality rates of about 30%.[38] Use of open drainage or marsupialization with frequent dressing changes has a reported mortality rate of 10% to 15%. The important principles are to employ aggressive (often sequential) débridement, appropriate antibiotics, and effective external drainage. One of the major sources of morbidity and mortality in this situation is the late development of mycotic visceral pseudoaneurysms, particularly involving the splenic circulation. These may be complex management problems, requiring angiographic embolization or other innovative treatment strategies because standard operative surgical attack may be precluded. The overall mortality rate for pancreatic abscess is correlated with the Ranson criteria: 14% mortality if three risk factors are present, 100% mortality if five are present.[39]

REFERENCES

1. Rinderknecht H. Activation of pancreatic zymogens: normal activation, premature intrapancreatic activation, protective mechanisms against inappropriate activation. Dig Dis Sci 1986;31:314.
2. Steer ML, Meldolesi J. The cell biology of experimental pancreatitis. N Engl J Med 1987;316:144.
3. Saluja A, Hashimoto S, Saluja M, Powers RE, Meldolesi J, Steer ML. Subcellular redistribution of lysosomal enzymes during caerulein-induced pancreatitis. Am J Physiol 1987; 253:508.
4. Norman J, Franz M, Fabri PJ, Gower WR. Decreased severity of experimental acute pancreatitis by pre or post treatment with interleukin-1 receptor antagonist. Gastroenterology 1994;106:A311.
5. McKay C, Gallagher G, Baxter JN, Imrie CW. Systemic complications in acute pancreatitis are associated with increased monocyte cytokine release. Gut 1994;35:A575.
6. Grewal HP, El Din AM, Gaber L, Kotb M, Gaber AO. Amelioration of the physiologic and biochemical changes of acute pancreatitis using an anti−TNF-α polyclonal antibody. Am J Surg 1994;167:214.
7. Pollack AV. Acute pancreatitis: analysis of 100 patients. Br Med J 1959;1:6.
8. Imrie CW. Observations on acute pancreatitis. Br J Surg 1974;61:539.
9. Bourke JB, Giggs JA, Eldon DS. Variations on the incidence and the spatial distribution of patients with primary acute pancreatitis in the Nottingham area, 1969−1976. Gut 1979;20:366.
10. Trapnell JE, Duncan EHL. Patterns of incidence in acute pancreatitis. BMJ 1975;179:83.
11. Gliedman ML, Bolooki H, Rosen RC. Acute pancreatitis. Curr Probl Surg 1970;1:52.
12. Olsen H. Pancreatitis: a prospective clinical evaluation of 100 cases and review of the literature. Dig Dis 1974;19:1077.
13. Aldrete JS, Jimenez H, Halpern NB. Evaluation and treatment of acute and chronic pancreatitis: a review of 380 cases. Ann Surg 1980;191:664.
14. Howard JM. Pancreatitis in the United States of America. In: Howard JM, Jordan GL Jr, Reber HA, eds. Surgical diseases of the pancreas. Philadelphia, Lea & Febiger, 1987:231.
15. MacLaren IF. Pancreatitis in the British Isles. In: Howard JM, Jordan GL Jr, Reber HA, eds. Surgical diseases of the pancreas. Philadelphia, Lea & Febiger, 1987:234.
16. Cuilleret J, Guillemin G. Pancreatitis on the continent of Europe. In: Howard JM, Jordan GL Jr, Reber HA, eds. Surgical diseases of the pancreas. Philadelphia, Lea & Febiger, 1987:241.
17. Koo J, Ong GB. Pancreatitis in India and the Orient. In: Howard JM, Jordan GL Jr, Reber HA, eds. Surgical diseases of the pancreas. Philadelphia, Lea & Febiger, 1987:250.
18. Goebell H, Hotz J. Die Atiologie der akuten Pankreatitin. In: Forell MM, ed. Handbuch der Inneden Medizin, Band 3, Teil 6: Pankreas, 5: Auflage. Berlin, Springer-Verlag, 1976.
19. Acosta JM, Ledesma CL. Gallstone migration as a cause of acute pancreatitis. N Engl J Med 1974;310:484.
20. Kelly TR. Gallstone pancreatitis: local predisposing factors. Ann Surg 1984;200:479.
21. Cotton PB. Progress report: ERCP. Gut 1977;18:316.
22. Ditschuneit H. Hyperlipoproteinemia in the pathogenesis of acute pancreatitis. In: Beger HG, Buchler M, eds. Acute pancreatitis. Berlin, Springer-Verlag, 1987:32.
23. Hasselgren PO. Acute pancreatitis in pregnancy. Acta Chir Scand 1980;146:297.
24. Dickson AP, Imrie CW. The incidence and prognosis of body wall ecchymosis in acute pancreatitis. Surg Gynecol Obstet 1984;159:343.
25. Ranson JHC. Etiological and prognostic factors in human acute pancreatitis: a review. Am J Gastroenterol 1982;77:633.
26. Larvin M, McMahon MJ. Apache-II score for assessment and monitoring of acute pancreatitis. Lancet 1989;2:738.
27. Eckfeldt JH, Levitt MD. Diagnostic enzymes for pancreatic disease. Diagn Enzymol 1989;9:731.
28. Meshkinpour H, Vaziri ND. Interrelationship of renal and pancreatic disorders. Dig Dis Sci 1989;7:221.
29. Nevalainen TJ. Phospholipase A2 in acute pancreatitis. Scand J Gastroenterol 1988;23:897.
30. Geokas MC, Rinderknecht H, Walberg CB, Weissman R. Methemalbumin in the diagnosis of acute hemorrhagic pancreatitis. Ann Intern Med 1974;81:483.
31. Ranson JHC, Turner JW, Roses DF, Rifkind KM, Spencer FC. Respiratory complication in acute pancreatitis. Ann Surg 1974;179:557.
32. Jacobs ML, Daggett WM, Civetta JM, et al. Acute pancreatitis: analysis of factors influencing survival. Ann Surg 1977; 185:43.
33. Ettien JT, Webster PD III, eds. The management of acute pancreatitis. Chicago, Year Book, 1980:169.
34. Havala T, Shronts E, Cerra F. Nutritional support in acute pancreatitis. Gastroenterol Clin North Am 1989;18:525.
35. Kirby DF, Craig RM. The value of intensive nutritional support in pancreatitis. J Parenter Enter Nutr 1985;9:353.
36. Sanfrany L, Cotton PB. A preliminary report: urgent duodenoscopic sphincterotomy for acute gallstone pancreatitis. Surgery 1981;89:424.
37. Shatney CH, Lillehei RC. Surgical treatment of pancreatic pseudocysts: analysis of 119 cases. Ann Surg 1979;189:386.
38. Poston GJ, Williamson RCN. Surgical management of acute pancreatitis. Br J Surg 1990;77:5.
39. Huibregtse K, Smits ME. Endoscopic management of diseases of the pancreas. Am J Gastroenterol 1994;8:S66.

SURGERY: SCIENTIFIC PRINCIPLES AND PRACTICE, Second Edition, edited by
Lazar J. Greenfield, Michael W. Mulholland, Keith T. Oldham, Gerald B. Zelenock,
and Keith D. Lillemoe. Lippincott–Raven Publishers, Philadelphia, © 1997.

CHAPTER 32
CHRONIC PANCREATITIS
MICHAEL W. MULHOLLAND

CLASSIFICATION

Chronic pancreatitis is a disease characterized by progressive and permanent destruction of the pancreatic exocrine parenchyma associated with fibrosis of the gland. In contrast, acute pancreatitis is typified by lesions that may regress completely when the underlying cause is eliminated, such as edema, hemorrhage, and fat necrosis. Although both acute and chronic pancreatitis may be categorized into relapsing and nonrelapsing forms depending on their clinical presentation, progressive morphologic and functional derangement is demonstrated only by chronic pancreatitis. In chronic pancreatitis, fibrotic destruction of the exocrine gland is often also accompanied by endocrine dysfunction.

A number of international symposia have attempted to subcategorize forms of acute and chronic pancreatitis.[1] A major drawback of such classifications is the inability to distinguish reliably acute and chronic forms of the disease based on early clinical presentation. Because several years of observation may be necessary to distinguish recurrent attacks of acute pancreatitis and recurrent symptomatic chronic pancreatitis, the classification of pancreatitis is usually reduced to include only acute and chronic disease. Within chronic pancreatitis, calcifying chronic pancreatitis and obstructive chronic pancreatitis may be distinguished, with important functional and therapeutic implications (Fig. 32-1).

INCIDENCE

The incidence and prevalence of chronic pancreatitis, usually calculated from retrospective surveys, is not known with precision. In the United States and Western Europe, the incidence of new cases approximates 5 to 10 per 100,000 population per year, with a prevalence of about 25 cases per 100,000 inhabitants. Because alcohol consumption is the most important risk factor for the development of chronic pancreatitis, countries with low alcohol consumption rates generally have lower incidence rates of chronic pancreatitis. Correlation of alcohol intake with incidence of chronic pancreatitis within various populations has often been discrepant, however, suggesting that environmental or hereditary factors may also influence susceptibility to the disease.

CAUSES
Alcohol Consumption

Alcohol consumption is the major cause of chronic pancreatitis, with about 70% of cases attributable to this factor. Most patients with symptomatic chronic pancreatitis have consumed large volumes of alcohol for long periods of time. In one study, the average daily intake of alcohol in patients with alcoholic chronic pancreatitis was 150 to 175 g,[2] and the risk for development of chronic pancreatitis increased with increasing alcohol intake. The mean duration of alcoholism before recognition of chronic pancreatitis was 18 years for men and 11 years for women. The incidence of chronic pancreatitis in autopsy series of chronic alcoholics is as much as 50 times the rate of nondrinking controls. There does not appear to be a threshold for alcohol toxicity below which risk for chronic pancreatitis is absent. Abstainers are at a lower risk than people with low alcohol intake (1 to 20 g/d). Because only 10% of alcoholics develop chronic pancreatitis, however, factors other than long-term alcohol exposure may influence susceptibility. Diet may be important in this regard. In both experimental and clinical studies, the risk of alcohol-induced chronic pancreatitis is increased by high-protein, high-fat diets.

Heredity

The hereditary form of chronic pancreatitis is transmitted as an autosomal dominant trait of incomplete penetrance. Affected patients usually become symptomatic in childhood at an average age of 10 to 12 years. The clinical and histologic features of hereditary pancreatitis differ little from nonhereditary forms of the disease. The diagnosis may be made if several members of a family develop chronic pancreatitis in the absence of alcohol consumption or other known causes.

Hyperparathyroidism

Calcifying chronic pancreatitis may occur in the presence of long-standing untreated hyperparathyroidism. Because hyperparathyroidism is usually detected and treated at an early stage in Western countries, the incidence of associated chronic pancreatitis is decreasing, currently accounting for not more than 1% to 2% of cases. The pathogenesis of chronic pancreatitis in hyperparathyroidism is presumed to be due to injury caused by the unrelieved stimulation of acinar tissues attending elevated serum calcium levels. Acute elevation of serum calcium is a potent secretagogue for human pancreatic enzymes. In addition, intraductal precipitation of calcium in pancreatic secretions has been postulated in hyperparathyroidism.

Tropical Pancreatitis

Tropical chronic pancreatitis is a nutritional disease of importance in tropical Africa and Southeast Asia. The disease develops among juveniles and young adults in the setting of chronic malnutrition. Protein-calorie malnutrition and deficiencies of copper, zinc, and selenium have been associated with the disease. The precise cause remains elusive.

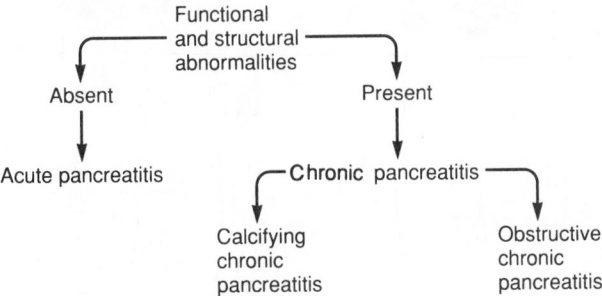

Figure 32-1. Classification of pancreatitis.

Duct Obstruction

Obstruction of the main pancreatic duct can cause a distinctive form of chronic pancreatic disease known as *obstructive pancreatitis.* Occlusion may be caused by tumors, congenital anomalies, scars from prior injury or inflammatory disease, or fibrosis of the ampulla of Vater. Although the gross alterations of the pancreas observed in obstructive pancreatitis are similar to those of other forms of chronic pancreatitis, microscopic changes are different. Obstruction causes diffuse atrophy of the exocrine tissue, whereas patchy atrophy is more common in early forms of nonobstructive chronic pancreatitis. Alternating areas of ductal stenosis and dilation are not seen; instead, the ductal system behind the obstruction is uniformly dilated. The ductal epithelium is preserved, and protein plugs and calcifications are unusual. Most notably, relief of obstruction can be followed by reversal of parenchymal fibrosis and atrophy. A restitution of pancreatic structure and function is not observed in other forms of chronic pancreatitis. Obstructive chronic pancreatitis is unusual, accounting for not more than 5% of cases.

Idiopathic Causes

The most common form of nonalcoholic calcifying pancreatitis in North America is idiopathic, a designation given to those cases with an unrecognized cause. Idiopathic pancreatitis accounts for about 15% of cases. Idiopathic pancreatitis has two peaks in incidence, suggesting that differing underlying causes may exist. The first peak occurs in young adulthood; the second type, termed *senile pancreatitis,* has a peak occurrence at 60 years of age.

PATHOGENESIS

The mechanisms by which alcohol consumption causes chronic pancreatitis are unknown. Most theories are inferences based on observations in acute or chronic animal models. Investigations have focused on direct toxic effects of alcohol on pancreatic exocrine cells, the effects of chronic alcohol intake on pancreatic protein secretion, and the role of calcium ions secreted into pancreatic juice.

Most investigators believe that the initial lesion in chronic pancreatitis is acinar cell injury.[3] The cellular mechanisms by which alcohol exerts toxic actions in acinar cells are discussed in detail in Chapter 31. A characteristic feature of early alcoholic chronic pancreatitis is a patchy distribution of normal acinar tissues in the midst of abnormal lobules. Microscopic examination shows irregular dilation of ductules, loss of ductal epithelium and acinar tissue, localized obstruction, and formation of small intraparenchymal cysts. Typically, precipitates of proteinaceous material are observed in intercalated and canalicular ducts. As the disease progresses, these protein plugs cause increasing ductal obstruction. Infiltration of the interstitium by inflammatory cells is followed by the deposition of fibrous tissue within and between lobules. In advanced stages, exocrine tissue is replaced by fibrosis. Endocrine islets survive in isolated nests in the midst of broad areas of scar tissue.

Increasing evidence indicates that abnormalities in pancreatic protein and calcium secretion may influence the development of chronic pancreatitis. In humans, chronic alcohol consumption is associated with a marked increase in total protein concentration in pancreatic secretions.[4] In addition, a markedly increased protein output in response to cholecystokinin may be observed in alcohol-fed dogs. The increased concentration of secretory enzymes is probably due to increased biosynthesis within acinar cells. In humans with chronic pancreatitis, abnormal proteins are detected in pancreatic secretions. Lactoferrin, not normally found in pancreatic secretions, may constitute up to 0.3% of total protein. This anionic molecule strongly associates with acidic molecules to form intraductal protein precipitates, postulated to be the basis for formation of pancreatic concretions.

A novel protein has been identified in the pancreatic secretions of normal controls and patients with chronic pancreatitis.[5] The association of this protein with pancreatic calculi led to its original designation as *pancreatic stone protein.* Pancreatic stone protein is now referred to as *lithostathine.* This phosphoglycoprotein has a molecular weight of 14,000. It has been localized immunohistochemically to zymogen granules in acinar cells, suggesting an exocrine secretory pathway paralleling digestive enzymes. Lithostathine is hydrolyzed by trypsin and cathepsin to lithostathine H1 and H2. Lithostathine H1 acts to inhibit pancreatic stone formation.[6] Lithostathine has the unique property of suppressing nucleation of calcium carbonate. Pancreatic secretions normally contain calcium at supersaturated concentrations, and the function of lithostathine is presumed to be inhibition of calcium carbonate crystal formation. Low levels of this protein could thus have a major influence on the development of calcific chronic pancreatitis.

Some patients with chronic pancreatitis have an elevated pancreatic ductal pressure. Sphincter of Oddi manometry is usually normal in such patients, suggesting that sphincteric dysfunction is not the cause of ductal hypertension.[7]

CLINICAL PRESENTATION
Pain

Pain is the predominant symptom in most patients with chronic pancreatitis. Pain associated with chronic pancreatitis is usually localized to the epigastrium, with radiation to the back in the region of the upper lumbar vertebrae (Fig. 32-2). The pain is usually dull rather than sharp and constant rather than intermittent or colicky. Radiation to

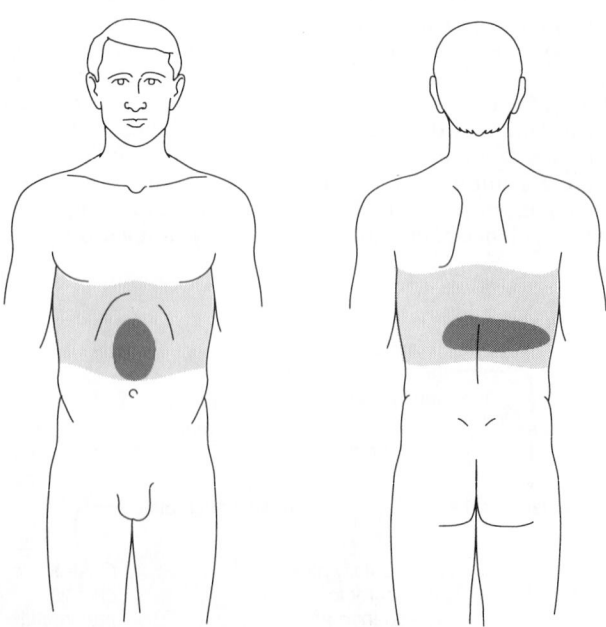

Figure 32-2. Topographic locations of pancreatic pain.

areas other than the back is distinctly unusual. The discomfort may occasionally be alleviated by bending forward and is worsened by the supine position. Ingestion of food or alcohol exacerbates the pain in many patients, usually immediately after eating. Most patients experience pain daily; occasionally, painful attacks are interposed by several pain-free days.

The mechanisms responsible for pain in chronic pancreatitis are incompletely understood. Possibilities include inflammation of the gland, damage to intrapancreatic nerves, increased pancreatic interstitial and intraductal pressure, and associated conditions such as pseudocysts, bile duct stenosis, or duodenal obstruction.

Intrapancreatic neural inflammation may be observed histologically in chronic pancreatitis. Intrapancreatic nerves usually remain viable while the parenchyma is replaced by fibrosis, but the nerves are retained in an abnormal condition. The nerves are larger and more numerous, and the organization of intraneural organelles is disturbed. The perineural sheath is disrupted so that it no longer forms a barrier to noxious substances. Foci of inflammatory cells are associated with nerves and ganglia; it has been postulated that degranulation of inflammatory cells in contact with nerves generates pain. Nerve bundles are edematous. The amount of neurotransmitters, such as substance P, in afferent neurons is increased, and it has been postulated that altered afferent nerves generate sustained painful signals.

Clinical studies suggest that continued pancreatic secretion in the presence of ductal obstruction by stricture or intraductal stone can result in elevated intrapancreatic pressure and thus pain. Several studies have shown that cessation of pancreatic pain occurs eventually in most patients with chronic pancreatitis.[8] Pain relief correlates closely with development of pancreatic insufficiency in these patients. These observations indicate that loss of exocrine function relieves pancreatic pain by reducing secretory ductal pressures. Direct measurement of ductal pressures, made in limited numbers of patients with chronic pancreatitis and dilated pancreatic ducts, supports this concept. In patients without pancreatic disease, intraductal pressures average 7 to 10 mmHg. In one study of eight patients with chronic pancreatitis, intraoperatively measured pancreatic tissue pressures averaged 17 mmHg.[9] In other studies of patients with dilated pancreatic ducts, direct-puncture pressure measurements made at surgery ranged from 18 to 48 mmHg.[10] Surgical decompression of dilated pancreatic ducts normalizes intrapancreatic pressure and is associated with immediate (but not necessarily permanent) pain relief in most patients.

Peripancreatic inflammation involving contiguous organs can cause painful symptoms localized to the affected region. The most commonly affected organs are the common bile duct and the duodenum. No strong evidence suggests that pancreatic ductal stones are a cause of pain in chronic pancreatitis, nor that their removal is therapeutic in this regard.

Malabsorption and Weight Loss

Malabsorption occurs when loss of functioning exocrine tissue is advanced, usually greater than 90%. Because pancreatic lipase secretion usually decreases before proteolytic enzymes, steatorrhea is often clinically apparent before azotorrhea. Steatorrhea occurs when lipase secretion falls below 5% to 10% of normal. Bulky, oily bowel movements and abdominal bloating are common complaints. Weight loss is nearly always observed. Deficiencies of fat-soluble vitamins are occasionally of clinical importance in patients with pancreatic insufficiency. Syndromes associ-

ated with deficiencies include coagulopathy (vitamin K), osteomalacia (vitamin D), neuropathy (vitamin E), night blindness (vitamin A), and dermatitis (essential fatty acids). In most patients with chronic pancreatitis, deficiencies of fat-soluble vitamins are subclinical, although body stores are decreased in a large proportion of patients.

Coincident with reduction of enzyme production, pancreatic bicarbonate secretion is diminished. As a result, postprandial duodenal pH may be decreased for prolonged periods. If duodenal pH is less than 4, acid denaturation of pancreatic enzymes may exacerbate malabsorption. Postprandial abdominal pain is common in patients with chronic pancreatitis, and the fear of this pain can lead to a further reduction in food intake.

Endocrine Insufficiency

Although the pathogenesis of chronic pancreatitis centers around the progressive destruction of exocrine tissues, the endocrine portion of the gland is inevitably affected as well. It has been common clinical teaching that exocrine insufficiency always precedes endocrine deficits in chronic pancreatitis. In fact, subclinical endocrine defects are common in the early stages of the disease. Altered insulin secretion has been consistently observed in these patients. Abnormal glucose tolerance can be demonstrated in 50% to 70% of patients with chronic pancreatitis; overt diabetes is present in 32% to 40%. Deficits are progressive; if individual patients are repetitively tested, progressive deterioration is observed.

Chronic pancreatitis produces a blunted insulin and C-peptide response to oral or intravenous glucose and reduced responsiveness to intravenous arginine, alanine, tolbutamide, or glucagon. Basal glucagon levels are usually normal, but glucagon responses to arginine, alanine, and insulin-induced hypoglycemia are often suppressed. Abnormal release of pancreatic polypeptide, gastric inhibitory peptide, and motilin have been reported.[11] A comparison of the endocrine and metabolic consequences of pancreatic diabetes and nonpancreatic forms of diabetes is presented in Table 32-1.

The long-term complications of pancreatic diabetes have not been well-studied, in part because long-term survival of patients with chronic pancreatitis has been poor. Although microvascular disease may be less common in pancreatic diabetes than in insulin-dependent diabetes mellitus, progressive changes occur over time. If patients with diabetes secondary to chronic pancreatitis survive long enough, the usual range of microvascular disorders proba-

Table 32-1. HORMONAL AND METABOLIC ASPECTS OF PANCREATIC DIABETES, IDDM, AND NIDDM

	Pancreatic Diabetes	IDDM	NIDDM
Insulin secretion	↓↓	↓↓↓	↓
Insulin sensitivity	N	↓	↓↓
Glucagon secretion	↓↓	↑/↓	↑/↓
Plasma amino acids	↑↑	↑ or N	↑ or N
Ketosis prone	↑↑	↑↑↑	↑
Glucose counterregulation	↓	N or ↓	N or ↓
Lipids	N	↑	↑↑

↑, Increased; ↓, decreased; N, normal; IDDM, insulin-dependent diabetes mellitus; NIDDM, non–insulin-dependent diabetes mellitus. (Adapted from Sjoberg RJ, Kidd GS. Pancreatic diabetes mellitus. Diabetes Care 1989;12:715)

bly will be observed. For example, retinopathy appears to occur at a rate equal to that of insulin-dependent diabetes mellitus.[12]

DIAGNOSIS

Routine Laboratory Tests

Routine tests of blood or serum are not helpful in making a diagnosis of chronic pancreatitis. Anemia is common but nonspecific. Leukocytosis is not observed unless acute disease is superimposed on chronic pancreatitis. Deficiencies of fat-soluble vitamins occur but are unpredictable after steatorrhea develops. Elevation of alkaline phosphatase may be observed if chronic fibrosis or compression by pseudocyst causes intrapancreatic biliary ductal obstruction.

Although serum amylase levels are almost always elevated in acute pancreatitis, amylase levels may be normal, elevated, or subnormal in chronic pancreatitis. Low values have been attributed to advanced loss of exocrine tissue, although total serum amylase is usually maintained near normal as a result of salivary amylase secretion. Persistently elevated amylase values in patients with chronic pancreatitis should suggest a superimposed attack of acute pancreatitis or the development of a complication, such as pseudocyst. Determination of urinary amylase secretion does not increase sensitivity, nor does assay for other pancreatic enzymes, such as lipase, elastase, isoamylase, or trypsin.

Tests of Pancreatic Exocrine Function

Tests of exocrine function may be divided into those that directly measure pancreatic secretion of enzymes or bicarbonate and those that indirectly measure the effects of secreted enzymes by assaying compounds that require pancreatic digestion before absorption.

Direct measurement of exocrine function requires collection of pancreatic secretions. This may be accomplished by direct cannulation of the pancreatic duct using endoscopic retrograde cholangiopancreatography (ERCP) or by using double-balloon tubes that isolate portions of the duodenum. Collection of pancreatic secretion is thus relatively invasive and uncomfortable. Appropriate corrections must be made for the effects of incomplete collection or dilution by gastric or intestinal secretions. Because basal pancreatic output in humans is variable, examination of secretion stimulated by intravenous cholecystokinin or secretin is necessary. Demonstration of subnormal pancreatic enzyme or bicarbonate secretion is diagnostic of chronic pancreatitis if pancreatic cancer has been excluded. Depressed secretion usually denotes advanced disease, however, because normal secretory values have been observed in patients with ERCP evidence of early chronic pancreatitis. In addition, direct measurement of pancreatic exocrine function is unreliable in patients with diabetes mellitus and cirrhosis. Because of the inability to detect early disease reliably and because of the attendant patient discomfort, direct measurements of exocrine function are not commonly performed.

Indirect tests of pancreatic function measure the absorption of some nutrient that first requires pancreatic digestion. Because clinically detectable malabsorption does not occur until 90% of exocrine function is lost, it is apparent that indirect tests of pancreatic function do not detect early stages of chronic pancreatitis. For all such tests, sensitivity is 90% to 100% for advanced disease but less than 50% for early chronic pancreatitis. False-positive tests may occur in other states that cause malabsorption (Crohn's disease, sprue, postgastrectomy states) or in association with diabetes mellitus, cirrhosis, or renal disease. In the bentiromide test, N-benzoyl-L-tyrosyl-p-aminobenzoic acid is digested by trypsin to release paraaminobenzoic acid. Free paraaminobenzoic acid, absorbed by the small intestine, is secreted by the kidney and assayed in urine. Fat malabsorption can be tested by feeding [^{14}C]olein and measuring exhaled $^{14}CO_2$.

Pancreatic Imaging Studies

Radiologic studies to define pancreatic structure have largely supplanted pancreatic functional tests in confirming the clinical diagnosis of chronic pancreatitis. The simplest confirmatory test for chronic pancreatitis is a plain abdominal film demonstrating calcification of the pancreas. This finding, present in 32% of patients, is pathognomonic of chronic pancreatitis.

Ultrasound is useful in initial evaluation of patients with suspected chronic pancreatitis. Supportive findings include atrophy of the gland, reduced echogenicity, dilation of the pancreatic duct to greater than 4 mm, and associated cystic lesions. Ultrasound examination of the pancreas may sometimes be compromised by overlying intestinal gas. Ultrasound has a reported sensitivity rate of about 60% for chronic pancreatitis and a specificity rate of 80% to 90%.

Computed tomographic (CT) examination of the pancreas is more sensitive than ultrasound in chronic pancreatitis, although CT examination involves ionizing radiation and is more expensive. CT findings consistent with this diagnosis include glandular atrophy, irregularity of the pancreatic outline, calcification, and ductal dilation (Figs. 32-3 and 32-4). Small cystic lesions are well demonstrated by CT. Sensitivity for CT approaches 75% to 90%, with a specificity of 85%.

ERCP has become widely recognized as the most sensitive and reliable method for diagnosing chronic pancreatitis. The sensitivity of ERCP approaches 90%, with equal specificity.[13] In earliest chronic pancreatitis, ductal changes are limited to secondary and tertiary ducts that show irregular dilation (Fig. 32-5). In moderate disease, the main pancreatic duct may be dilated with alternating areas of stenosis (Fig. 32-6). In advanced chronic pancreatitis, marked ductal changes may form a chain-of-lakes appearance (Fig. 32-7). ERCP is also useful in demonstrating associated anatomic abnormalities, such as common bile duct stenosis or pancreatic pseudocyst. Most studies comparing the sensitivity of ERCP and pancreatic secretory tests have found good correlation in advanced disease.[14] In earlier stages of chronic pancreatitis, correlation of morphologic changes and pancreatic function is often poor.

TREATMENT OF COMPLICATIONS

Pain

Abstinence

Management of pain in patients with chronic pancreatitis should begin with abstinence. With elimination of alcohol, 50% to 75% of patients have some decrease in pain, although most do not become pain free. Because alcohol is a secretagogue for pancreatic enzymes, pain relief is more likely in patients who retain some exocrine function.

Enzyme Replacement

Exogenous enzyme administration as a treatment for pain has been proposed, based on the concept of negative-feedback inhibition of pancreatic secretion.[15] In humans, the intraduodenal administration of trypsin or chymotryp-

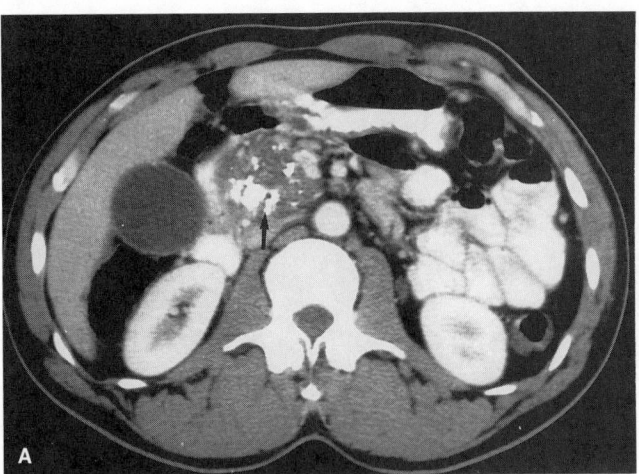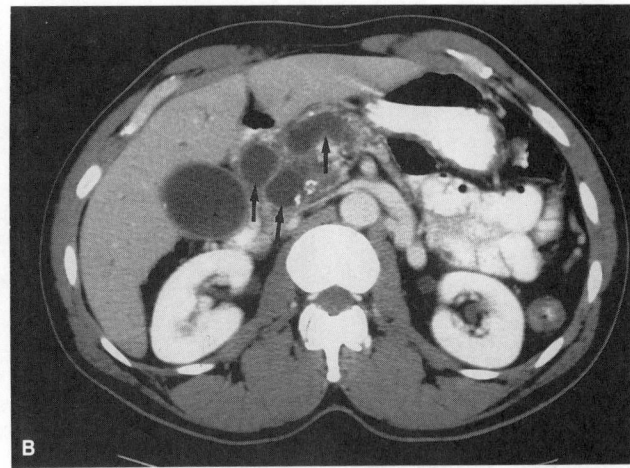

Figure 32-3. Abdominal CT scan demonstrating pancreatic calcifications (*arrow in A*) and associated cystic lesions (*arrows in B*).

sin inhibits pancreatic secretion, and diversion of pancreatic secretion from the duodenum stimulates secretion of digestive enzymes. It has been postulated that patients with chronic pancreatitis may have continuous stimulation by hormonal or neural pathways because of diminished secretion of digestive enzymes (Fig. 32-8). The increased stimulatory signals are presumed to cause or exacerbate pain. If this contention is correct, effective delivery of pancreatic enzymes to the duodenum will reduce chronic stimulation, decrease ductal pressure, and relieve pain. Although initial controlled trials suggested that improvement in pain can occur as a result of enzyme replacement, especially in patients with idiopathic pancreatitis, disappointing results have also been reported.[16,17] Enzyme replacement trials are difficult to interpret due to a high placebo effect rate (30%) in patients with chronic pancreatitis. Further studies are needed to evaluate this novel therapy. Cholecystokinin receptor antagonist and the somatostatin analogue octreotide have also been proposed for treatment of pain in chronic pancreatitis, but their efficacy is still unproved.

Endoscopic Therapy

The use of endoprostheses or stents placed into the pancreatic duct endoscopically has been proposed as a treatment for chronic pancreatitis complicated by ductal steno-

sis. About 30% to 75% of patients treated in this way had symptomatic improvement when observed for 14 to 36 months.[18-22] The use of pancreatic duct stents, however, is associated with a risk of pancreatic ductal injury and fibrosis. Because of this concern, many investigators recommend short-term use of stents to identify patients most likely to benefit from surgical drainage. The role of endoscopic removal of pancreatic ductal stones is unsettled. Fragmented by extracorporeal shock wave lithotripsy, stones can be extracted after sphincterotomy of the pancreatic duct. When stones are cleared, half of patients report long-term improvement in pancreatic pain.

Analgesics

Analgesics remain the mainstay for nonoperative treatment of pain in chronic pancreatitis. Nonnarcotic analgesics should be used initially. If pain is progressive, increases in dose or frequency of these agents should be attempted before narcotics are prescribed. Eventually, most patients with chronic pancreatitis require narcotic pain relief; addiction is common and makes evaluation of treatments aimed at pain relief difficult.

Percutaneous, radiologically guided injection of the celiac ganglia with neural ablative agents has been used in patients with chronic pancreatitis, based on the success

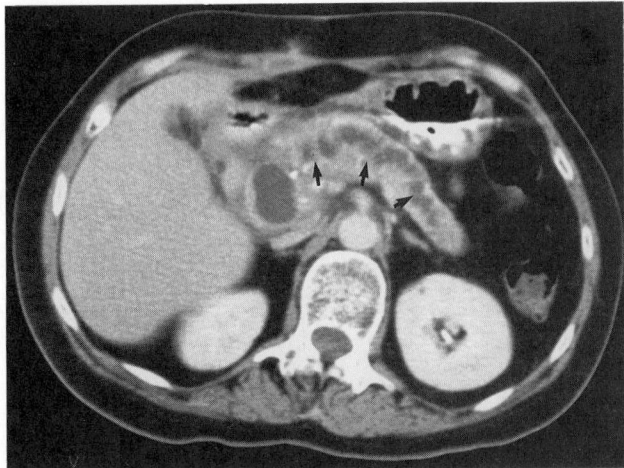

Figure 32-4. Abdominal CT scan in a patient with chronic pancreatitis, illustrating dilation of main pancreatic duct (*arrows*).

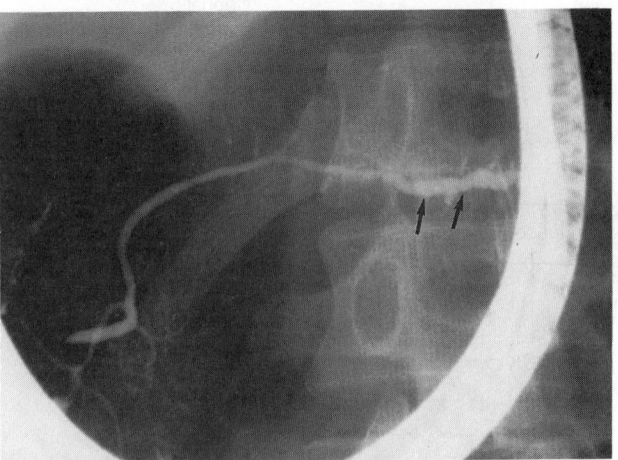

Figure 32-5. ERCP illustrating early changes of chronic pancreatitis with ductal ectasia confined to the pancreatic tail (*arrows*).

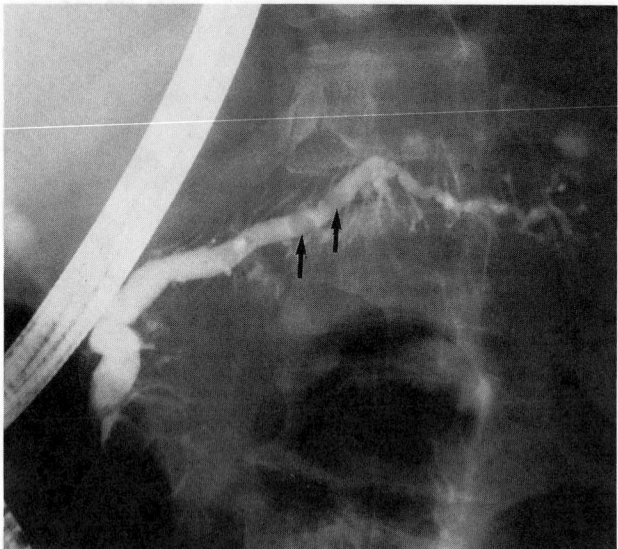

Figure 32-6. ERCP illustrating moderate dilation of the main pancreatic duct and ectasia of secondary ducts associated with moderately advanced chronic pancreatitis. Arrows indicate intraductal pancreatic stones.

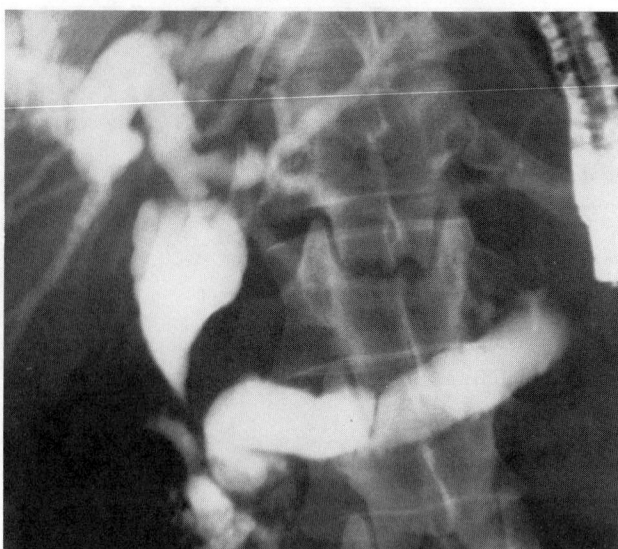

Figure 32-7. ERCP demonstrating florid pancreatic ductal dilation associated with end-stage chronic pancreatitis.

of this approach in patients with pancreatic cancer. The procedure is not usually effective long-term in chronic pancreatitis, with pain relief lasting 6 months in fewer than half of treated patients. Repeated injection is not usually successful.

Surgical Treatment

Intractable pain is the most frequent indication for operation in patients with chronic pancreatitis. Operation may be considered when pain is severe enough to interfere substantially with quality of life, to interrupt employment or normal family life, to affect general health by interfering with nutrition, or to cause narcotic addiction. All patients being considered for operative treatment should undergo CT examination of the pancreas to exclude pancreatic carcinoma and ERCP to evaluate pancreatic ductal anatomy.

Operative treatment for chronic pain associated with chronic pancreatitis can be broadly divided into ductal drainage procedures and resection procedures.

Pancreaticojejunostomy. When patients with chronic pancreatitis have pancreatic ducts dilated to more than 8 mm, ductal decompression using pancreaticojejunostomy (Puestow procedure) may be employed for relief of pain. The findings that ductal hypertension exists in patients with painful chronic pancreatitis and that surgical decompression reduces intrapancreatic pressure to normal provide the rationale for this operation. During operation, the entire anterior surface of the pancreas is exposed by separating the omentum from the transverse colon and entering the lesser sac (Fig. 32-9). The dilated pancreatic duct is palpated or is outlined using intraoperative ultrasound. The entire pancreatic duct is opened from the pancreatic tail to a point 1 cm from the duodenum; care is taken near

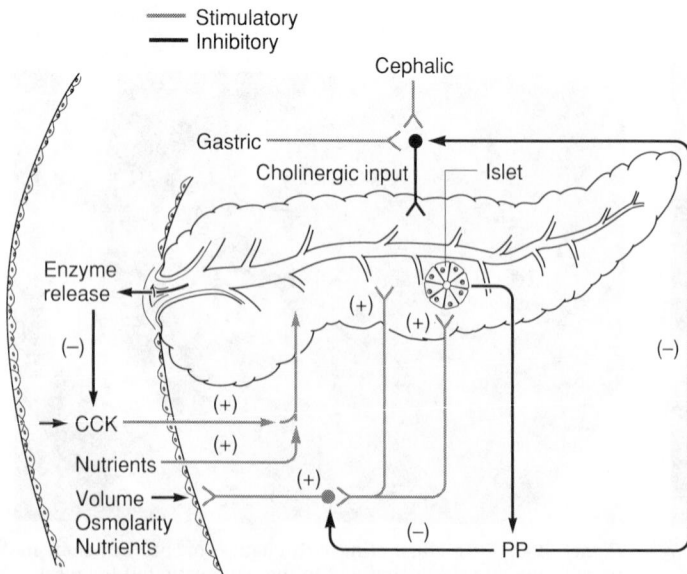

Figure 32-8. Schematic diagram of stimulatory and inhibitory influences on pancreatic exocrine secretion. CCK, cholecystokinin; PP, pancreatic polypeptide.

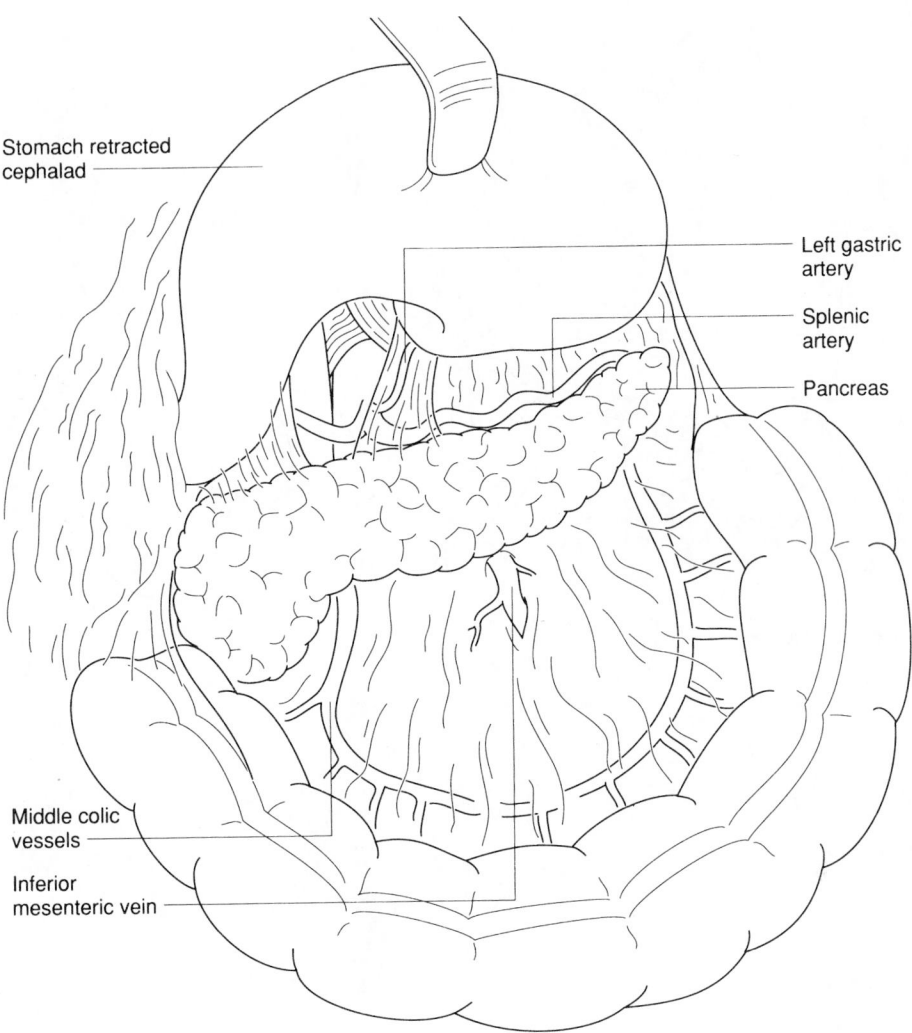

Stomach retracted
cephalad

Left gastric
artery

Splenic
artery

Pancreas

Middle colic
vessels

Inferior
mesenteric vein

Figure 32-9. Exposure of the anterior surface of the pancreas through the lesser sac.

the duodenal border not to injure the pancreaticoduodenal vessels (Fig. 32-10). A side-to-side anastomosis is then performed between the opened pancreatic duct and a loop of jejunum (Fig. 32-11). Removal of the spleen is not necessary.

The operative mortality of lateral pancreaticojejunostomy is low, with several series reporting in-hospital death rates of 0% to 4%.[23] Pancreaticojejunostomy does not remove pancreatic tissue and does not cause diabetes or worsen exocrine deficits. Conversely, operation does not result in improvement in malabsorption, although secretions can now empty freely through the pancreaticojejunostomy into the small intestine.[24] Usually, fibrotic replacement of pancreatic tissues continues postoperatively, although some evidence suggests that operation may slow this destructive process.[25]

About 80% of patients report complete or substantial improvement in pain soon after pancreaticojejunostomy.[23] Although pain recurs in some patients postoperatively, most patients remain pain free (Fig. 32-12). Recurrent or persistent pain after pancreaticojejunostomy requires reevaluation to exclude other disease processes, such as pancreatic carcinoma, peptic ulcer, calculous biliary disease, or bile duct stricture. If secondary disease processes are excluded, continued patency of the pancreaticojejunal anastomosis should be confirmed by ERCP examination.

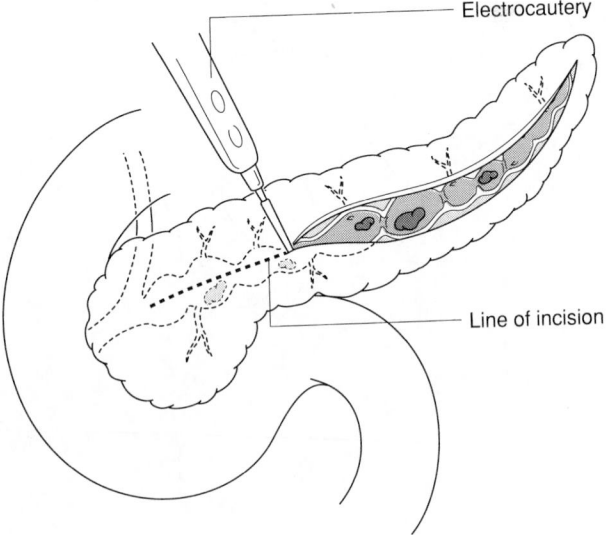

Electrocautery

Line of incision

Figure 32-10. Longitudinal incision of the main pancreatic duct preparatory to performing lateral pancreaticojejunostomy.

A

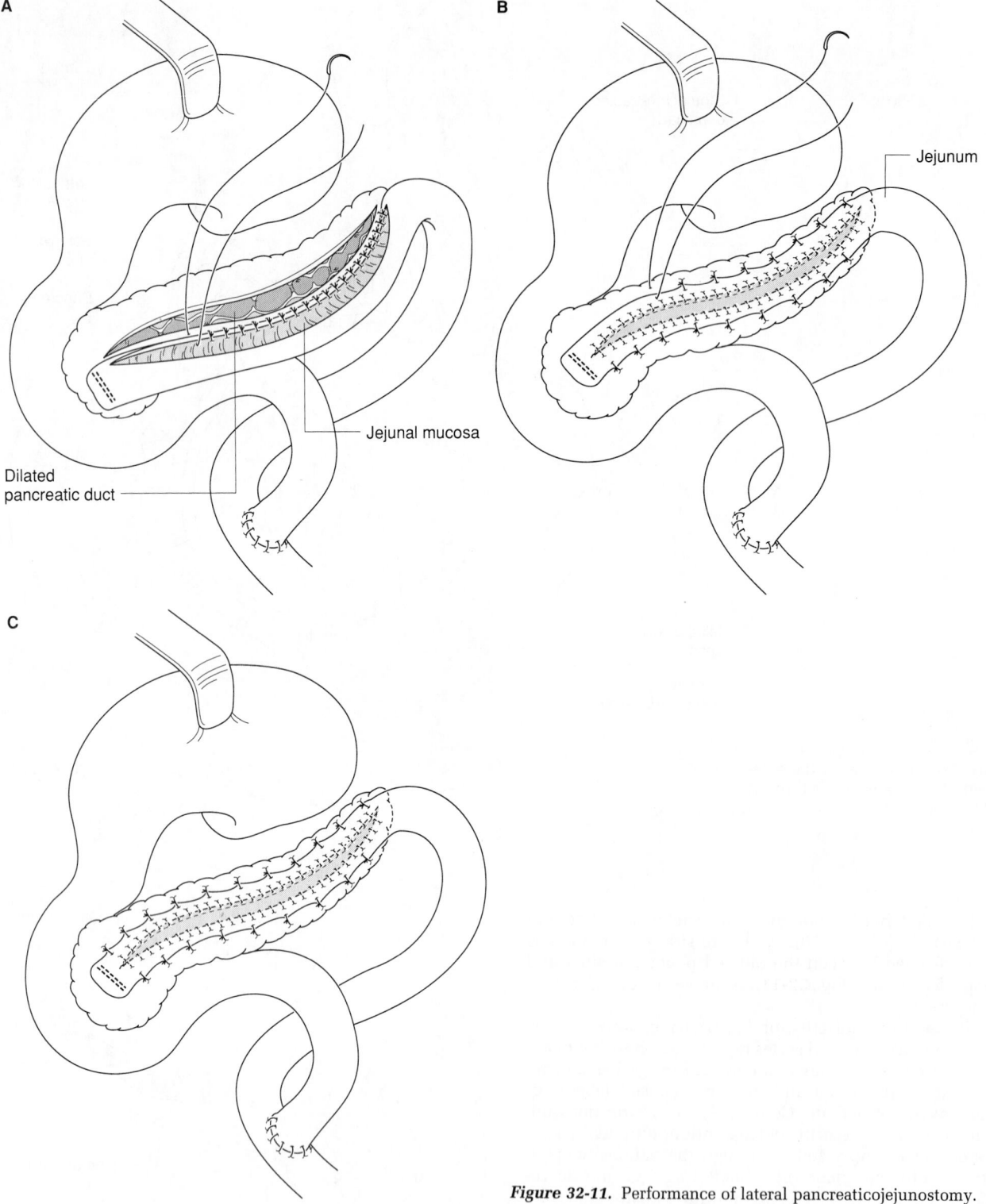

Dilated
pancreatic duct

Jejunal mucosa

B

Jejunum

C

Figure 32-11. Performance of lateral pancreaticojejunostomy.

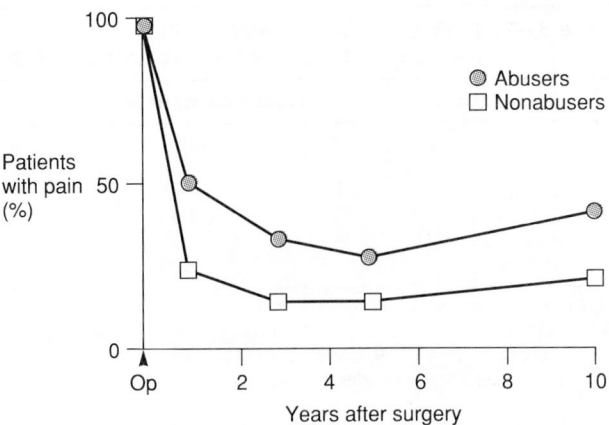

Figure 32-12. Long-term pain relief after pancreaticojejunostomy. (After Ihse I, Borch K, Larsson J. Chronic pancreatitis: results of operations for relief of pain. World J Surg 1990;14:53)

Pancreatic Resection. Pancreatic drainage is not feasible when pancreatic ducts are small or normal in diameter. Pancreatic resection may be considered when patients have small ducts, when the disease process involves primarily one portion of the gland and the remainder of the gland is nearly normal, or after a failed pancreaticojejunostomy. The rationale for pancreatic resection is that pain and risk of complications are reduced by removing the diseased portion of the gland.

Distal pancreatectomy may be performed when pathologic changes are confined to the tail or body of the pancreas. The proportion of pancreatic tissue that is resected is determined by the point of transection. For example, about half of pancreatic mass is removed when the gland is divided at the level of the superior mesenteric vessels; a 95% pancreatectomy leaves only a thin rim of pancreatic tissue within the duodenal C loop (Fig. 32-13). Pancreatic resection always reduces the amount of residual functioning endocrine and exocrine tissues. Postoperative diabetes occurs with a frequency proportionate to the degree of pancreatic resection and contributes substantially to late mortality after extended resections. Immediate pain relief is observed in about 80% of patients after distal pancreatectomy. Long-term palliation has been disappointing after distal pancreatectomy, and persistent pain relief is reported in fewer than two thirds of patients 5 to 10 years after surgery.[23]

Resection of the pancreatic head by pancreaticoduodenectomy (Whipple operation; see Chap. 33) may be appropriate in selected patients with disease confined predominantly to the head of the gland (Fig. 32-14). Indications for pancreaticoduodenectomy include (1) a chronic inflammatory mass involving primarily the head of the gland and the uncinate process, (2) a chronic inflammatory mass in the head of the pancreas associated with duodenal stenosis, (3) multiple pseudocysts confined to the head of the pancreas, and (4) failure of pancreaticojejunostomy secondary to inadequate drainage of the uncinate process.[23]

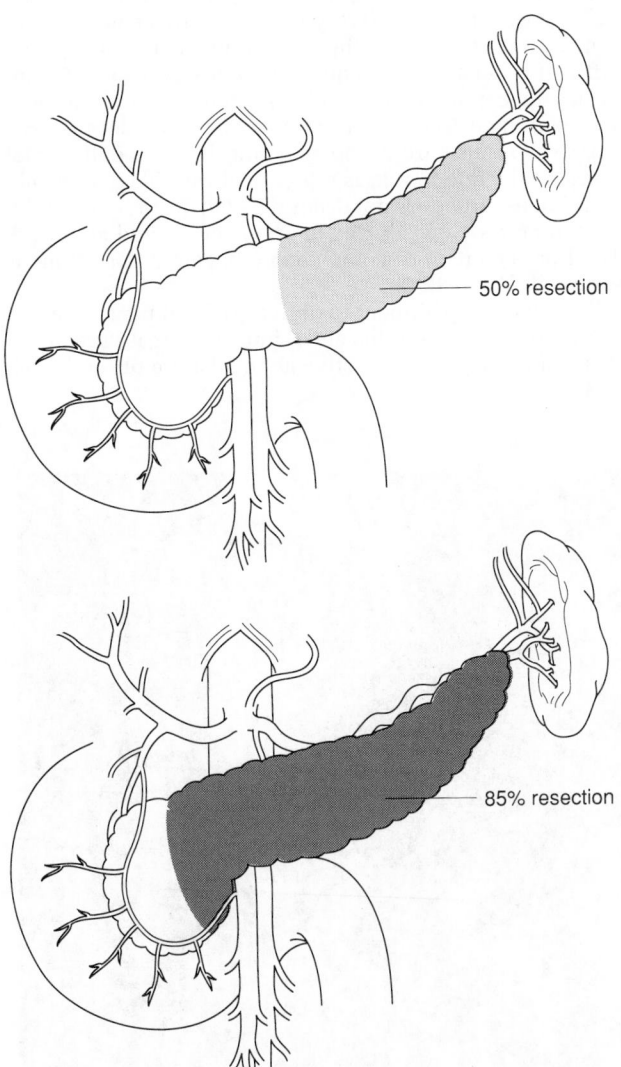

Figure 32-13. Points of parenchymal transection for 50% and 85% distal pancreatectomies.

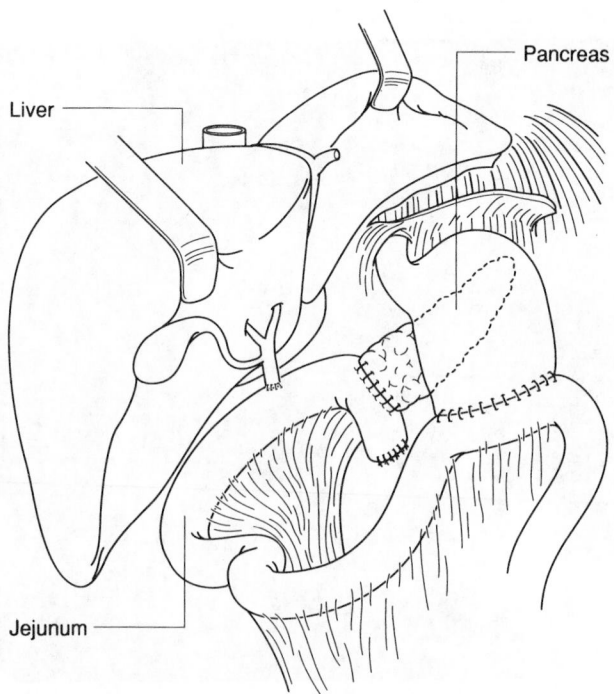

Figure 32-14. Reconstruction after standard pancreaticoduodenectomy.

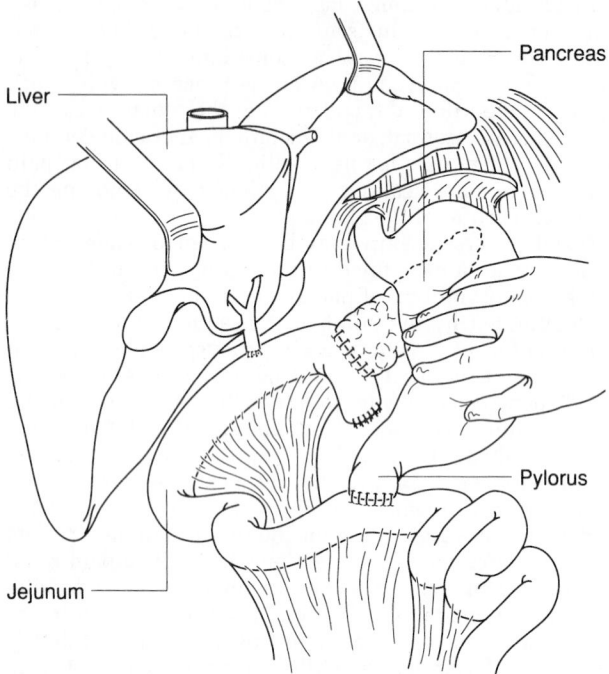

Figure 32-15. Reconstruction after pylorus-preserving pancreaticoduodenectomy.

Table 32-2. COMMERCIALLY AVAILABLE PANCREATIC ENZYME PREPARATIONS

Preparation*	Lipase Content (IU/pill)
Pancreatin	8000
Ilozyme	3600
Ku-Zyme HP	2300
Cotazym-S	2000
Pancrease	4500
Viokase	3800

* Each in capsule formulation.
(Adapted from Owyang C, Levitt M. Chronic pancreatitis. In: Yamada T, Alpers DH, Powell DW, Owyang C, Silverstein FE, eds. Textbook of gastroenterology. Philadelphia, JB Lippincott, 1991:1888)

A modification of the standard pancreaticoduodenectomy involving preservation of the gastric antrum and pylorus is also appropriate in these circumstances (Fig. 32-15).

Pancreaticoduodenectomy for chronic inflammatory disease has a mortality rate of less than 5% when performed in centers with substantial experience in pancreatic surgery. Pain relief occurs in 70% to 90% of patients in the first several years after operation and persists in about 80%

of long-term survivors. Diabetes occurs postoperatively in 10% to 25% of patients with chronic pancreatitis who undergo pancreaticoduodenectomy.

Malabsorption

Treatment of malabsorption secondary to pancreatic insufficiency requires delivery of exogenous pancreatic enzymes in active form to the duodenum. This goal is often difficult because of inadequate amounts of pancreatic enzymes in commercially available oral preparations and acid-peptic destruction of ingested enzymes. Because steatorrhea is most troublesome clinically, the delivery of lipase to the duodenum is the critical variable. Fat malabsorption usually does not occur if 25,000 IU of lipase activity can be provided during a 4-hour postprandial period. The lipase content of commercial enzyme preparations is shown in Table 32-2.

The major impediment to delivery of oral pancreatic enzymes to the postprandial small intestine is gastric acidity. Pancreatic enzymes are active at an alkaline pH and inac-

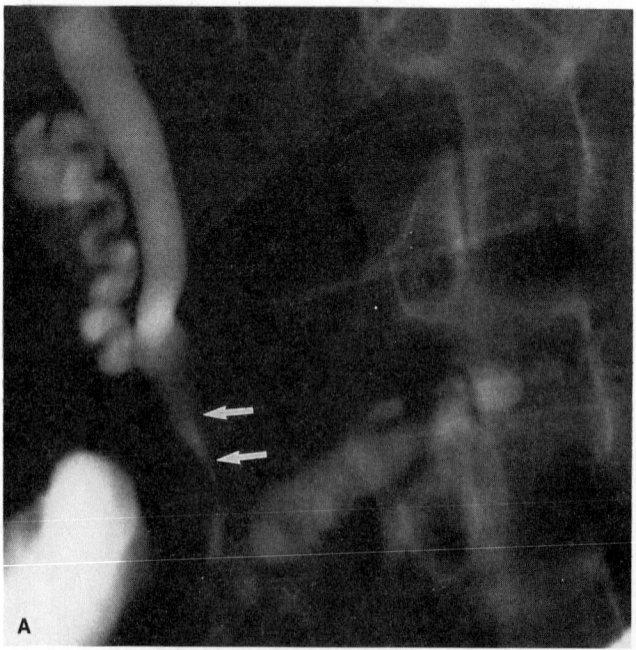
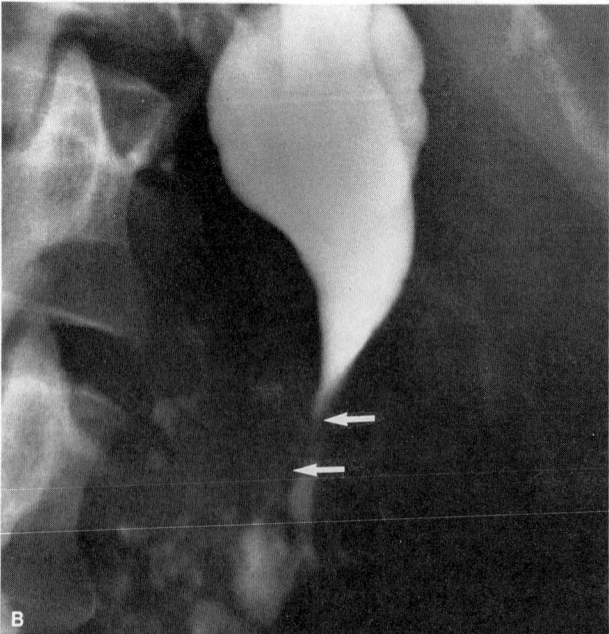

Figure 32-16. Endoscopic cholangiograms of early (*A*) and advanced (*B*) biliary stricture accompanying chronic pancreatitis. Smooth, tapering strictures (*arrows*) can be seen confined to the intrapancreatic portion of the bile duct.

tive at a pH of less than 5. Pancreatic lipase is irreversibly denatured at a pH of less than 4. Several approaches have been used to circumvent gastric effects. Large amounts of pancreatic enzymes have been given with meals in the hope that enough enzyme would survive gastric passage to digest the fat contained in a typical diet. Suppression of gastric acid production using histamine-2 (H_2) receptor antagonists or antacids are attempts to protect enzyme activity. Enteric-coated formulations of pancreatic enzymes have been prepared that resist acid but dissolve (and release their contents) on contact with the alkaline pH found in the small intestine. Finally, acid-stable forms of lipase with a wider pH range of activity, derived from *Aspergillus niger* and *Rhizopus arrhizus,* have been developed for human testing.[26]

A rational approach to treatment of pancreatic insuffi-

ciency begins with the administration of sufficient enzyme tablets to abolish azotorrhea and to reduce steatorrhea to tolerable levels. This often means ingesting several tablets with each meal. If symptoms persist, the number of tablets should be increased, or the fat content of meals may be decreased. H_2 receptor antagonists may be added for patients resistant to these measures. If steatorrhea persists, a search for other contributing causes (bacterial overgrowth, ileal disease) should be performed.

Biliary Complications

Biliary complications involving the common bile duct can occur in chronic pancreatitis because of the intimate association of that structure with the head of the pancreas. In two thirds of the population, the common bile duct

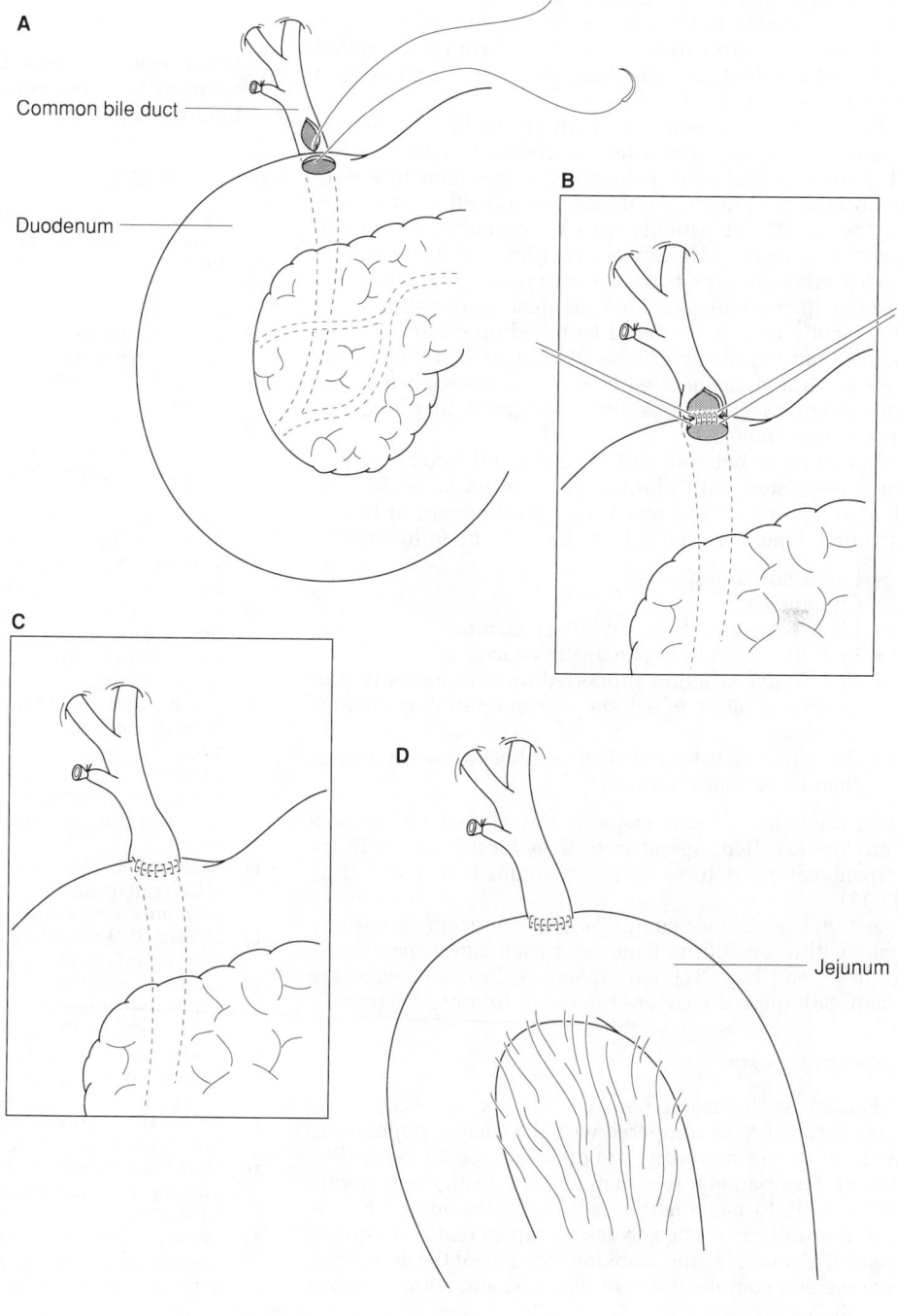

Figure 32-17. Operative construction of choledochoduodenostomy (*A* through *C*) and choledochojejunostomy (*D*).

traverses the pancreatic parenchyma; in about 25%, the common bile duct lies in a groove along the posterior surface of the pancreas; and in only 10%, the duct is extrapancreatic, always posterior to the gland. Thus, fibrosis associated with chronic pancreatitis can encase and compress the common bile duct.

Common bile duct stenosis is a relatively common complication of chronic pancreatitis, occurring in about 10% of cases observed long-term.[27] Alkaline phosphatase elevation is the most sensitive screening method for detection of biliary stenosis, and a larger proportion of patients demonstrate increases in alkaline phosphatase than develop jaundice or symptoms of biliary obstruction. Cholangiographic investigation of patients with common bile duct disease can be accomplished either by transhepatic or retrograde endoscopic routes. Because chronic pancreatitis patients with common bile duct disease frequently require treatment of concurrent pancreatic disease, examination of both systems is best accomplished by ERCP. Bile duct fibrosis typically results in long, gradually tapering strictures conforming to the intrapancreatic duct (Fig. 32-16). Malignant strictures usually result in abrupt termination of the biliary duct. The proximal suprapancreatic portion is variably dilated.

The most serious sequelae of unrelieved biliary obstruction are cholangitis and biliary cirrhosis. Collected series of chronic pancreatitis patients with common bile duct stenosis suggest that each of these complications develops in 7% to 10% of patients with radiographic abnormalities.[28] The degree of biliary obstruction as shown by cholangiography does not correlate with severity of pancreatic disease, liver histology, or biochemical abnormalities, and therapeutic decisions should be based on clinical factors rather than radiologic criteria. Persistent elevation of serum alkaline phosphatase (three to five times normal), although imperfect, is probably the best predictor of progressive biliary stenosis.[28]

Operation in patients with stricture of the common bile duct associated with chronic pancreatitis is justified to treat symptoms or to prevent the development of biliary cirrhosis. Operative indications include the following:

- Persistent jaundice
- Cholangitis
- Liver biopsy evidence of biliary cirrhosis
- Inability to exclude pancreatic cancer
- Progressive stricture supported by radiologically progressive dilation of extrahepatic and intrahepatic biliary ducts
- Persistent elevation of alkaline phosphatase at greater than three times normal

Both choledochoduodenostomy and choledochojejunostomy are excellent operative choices for patients with intrapancreatic strictures of the common bile duct[29] (Fig. 32-17).

A number of other complications can occur in chronic pancreatitis, including pancreatic pseudocyst, pancreatic ascites (see Chap. 31), and splenic vein thrombosis (see Chap. 38); these are covered in detail in other chapters.

PROGNOSIS

Patients with chronic pancreatitis have decreased long-term survival rates compared with the general population, with an excess mortality rate of 36% over 20 years (Fig. 32-18). Surprisingly, less than 20% of deaths are directly attributable to pancreatitis or its complications.[30] Excessive mortality is related to the extrapancreatic complications of alcoholism and smoking. Cancers of the aerodigestive system, complications of diabetes, and complications

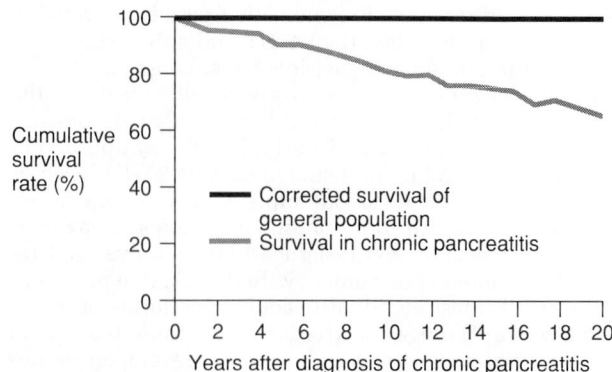

Figure 32-18. Long-term survival in patients with chronic pancreatitis. (After Petrozza JA, Sudhir KD, Latham PS, et al. Prevalence and natural history of distal common bile duct stenosis in alcoholic pancreatitis. Dig Dis Sci 1984;29:890)

of cirrhosis are the most frequent causes of death. Pancreatic cancer has been reported to occur in 4% of patients with chronic pancreatitis observed for 20 years.

REFERENCES

1. Gyr K, Singer M, Sarles H. Proceedings of the Second International Symposium on Pancreatitis. Amsterdam, Elsevier, 1984.
2. Sarles H, Cros RC, Bidart JM, et al. A multicenter inquiry into the etiology of pancreatic diseases. Digestion 1979;19:110.
3. Singh M, Simsek H. Ethanol and the pancreas. Gastroenterology 1990;98:1051.
4. Singh SM, Reber HA. The pathology of chronic pancreatitis. World J Surg 1990;14:2.
5. DeCaro A, Lohse J, Sarles H. Characterization of a protein isolated from pancreatic calculi of men suffering from chronic calcifying pancreatitis. Biochem Biophys Res Commun 1979;87:1176.
6. Sidhu SS, Tandon RK. The pathogenesis of chronic pancreatitis. Postgrad Med J 1995;71:67.
7. Steer ML, Waxman I, Freedman S. Chronic pancreatitis. New Engl J Med 1995;332:1482.
8. Ammann RW, Akovbiantz A, Largiader F, Schueler G. Course and outcome of chronic pancreatitis: longitudinal study of a mixed medical-surgical series of 245 patients. Gastroenterology 1984;86:820.
9. Ebbohoj N, Borly L, Madsen P, Svendsen LB. Pancreatic tissue pressure and pain in chronic pancreatitis. Pancreas 1986;1:556.
10. Okazaki K, Yamamoto Y, Kagiyama S, et al. Pressure of papillary sphincter zone and pancreatic main duct in patients with alcoholic and idiopathic pancreatitis. Int J Pancreatol 1988;3:457.
11. Nealon WH, Townsend CM, Thompson JC. The time course of beta cell dysfunction in chronic ethanol-induced pancreatitis: a prospective analysis. Surgery 1988;104:1074.
12. Sjoberg RJ, Kidd GS. Pancreatic diabetes mellitus. Diabetes Care 1989;12:715.
13. Caletti G, Brocchi E, Agostini D, et al. Sensitivity of endoscopic retrograde pancreatography in chronic pancreatitis. Br J Surg 1982;69:507.
14. Malfertheiner P, Buchler M. Correlation of imaging and function in chronic pancreatitis. Radiol Clin North Am 1989;27:51.
15. Folsch UR. Feedback regulation of pancreatic exocrine secretion in animals and man. Eur J Clin Invest 1990;20:S40.
16. Slaff J, Jacobson D, Tillman RC, et al. Protease-specific suppression of pancreatic exocrine secretion. Gastroenterology 1984;87:44.
17. Isaksson G, Ihse I. Pain reduction by oral pancreatic enzyme preparation in chronic pancreatitis. Dig Dis Sci 1983;28:97.
18. Partington PF, Rochelle REL. Modified Peustow procedure for

retrograde drainage of the pancreatic duct. Arch Surg 1960; 152:1037.

19. Grimm H, Meyer WH, Nam VC, Soehendra N. New modalities for treating chronic pancreatitis. Endoscopy 1989;21:70.

20. Geenen JE, Rolny P. Endoscopic therapy of acute and chronic pancreatitis. Endoscopy 1991;37:377.

21. Cremer M, Deviere J, Delhaye M, et al. Stenting in severe chronic pancreatitis: results of medium-term follow-up in seventy-six patients. Endoscopy 1991;23:171.

22. Huibregtse K, Schneider B, Vrij AA, Tytgat GN. Endoscopic pancreatic drainage in chronic pancreatitis. Gastrointest Endosc 1988;34:9.

23. Ihse I, Borch K, Larsson J. Chronic pancreatitis: results of operations for relief of pain. World J Surg 1990;14:53.

24. Bradley EL, Nasrallah SM. Fat absorption after longitudinal pancreaticojejunostomy. Surgery 1984;95:640.

25. Nealon WH, Thompson JC. Progressive loss of pancreatic function in chronic pancreatitis is delayed by main pancreatic duct decompression: a longitudinal prospective analysis of the modified Peustow procedure. Ann Surg 1993;217:458.

26. Roberts IM. Enzyme therapy for malabsorption in exocrine pancreatic insufficiency. Pancreas 1989;4:496.

27. Petrozza JA, Sudhir KD, Latham PS, et al. Prevalence and natural history of distal common bile duct stenosis in alcoholic pancreatitis. Dig Dis Sci 1984;29:890.

28. Frey CF, Suzuki M, Isaji S. Treatment of chronic pancreatitis complicated by obstruction of the common bile duct or duodenum. World J Surg 1990;14:59.

29. Eckhauser FE, Knol JA, Stroedel WE, et al. Common bile duct strictures associated with chronic pancreatitis. Am Surg 1983;49:350.

30. Levy P, Milan C, Pignon JP, et al. Mortality factors associated with chronic pancreatitis: unidimensional and multidimensional analysis of a medical-surgical series of 240 patients. Gastroenterology 1989;96:1165.

SURGERY: SCIENTIFIC PRINCIPLES AND PRACTICE, Second Edition, edited by Lazar J. Greenfield, Michael W. Mulholland, Keith T. Oldham, Gerald B. Zelenock, and Keith D. Lillemoe. Lippincott–Raven Publishers, Philadelphia, © 1997.

CHAPTER 33

NEOPLASMS OF THE EXOCRINE PANCREAS

RICHARD H. BELL, JR.

The management of neoplasms of the exocrine pancreas presents a major challenge to the surgeon. The most common of these tumors, ductal adenocarcinoma of the pancreas, has become the fifth most common cause of cancer death in the United States and continues for the most part to be recalcitrant to treatment. Other less common neoplasms of the pancreas can present formidable difficulties in diagnosis and treatment. The generally vague early symptoms of pancreatic disease, the inaccessibility of the organ to examination, the aggressiveness of most pancreatic tumors, and the technical difficulties associated with pancreatic surgery make pancreatic exocrine neoplasms among the most daunting diseases treated by surgeons. Nevertheless, progress has been made in our ability to manage pancreatic neoplasms.

DUCTAL ADENOCARCINOMA OF THE PANCREAS

Epidemiology and Etiology

The cause of pancreatic cancer is unknown. The most striking epidemiologic fact about pancreatic cancer is its steady increase in incidence during the 20th century, in contrast to declining or level rates for other gastrointestinal malignancies. Although the increase in pancreatic cancer has leveled off in the past decade or two, the current annual mortality rate in the United States of about 10 cases per 100,000 population is almost three times the rate in 1930 (Fig. 33-1). This rise in incidence parallels changes in the prevalence of cigarette smoking in the United States, and epidemiologic studies suggest that much of the increase in pancreatic cancer in recent decades is attributable to increased tobacco use.

Adenocarcinoma of the pancreas most commonly develops in the seventh decade of life and is rare before the age of 40 years. It occurs almost twice as often in American blacks as whites and is more common in men than in women by a ratio of 3:2.

Possible Etiologic Environmental Factors

The most consistently observed risk factor for pancreatic cancer is cigarette smoking. Most studies estimate that smoking doubles or triples a person's risk of developing pancreatic cancer. The mechanism is unknown, but carcinogens in cigarette smoke have been shown to produce pancreatic tumors in laboratory animals. Alcohol consumption has been implicated in some case-control studies of pancreatic cancer, but the overall evidence is inconsistent, and alcohol is not likely to be a major factor in the development of the disease. Although considerable public interest was focused on coffee consumption as a risk factor for pancreatic cancer, several case-control and cohort studies fail to support an association, and the overall evidence linking coffee consumption to pancreatic cancer is not compelling.

Although the details vary from study to study, several epidemiologic investigations point to the possible importance of diet in the development of pancreatic cancer. High dietary fat consumption is in general associated with an increased risk of pancreatic cancer, and this finding is consistent with the repeated demonstration that excess dietary fats, particularly unsaturated fats, promote carcinogenesis in animal models of pancreatic cancer. These findings do not mean that fatty foods contain carcinogens; it is more likely that fats promote the effects of carcinogens derived from other sources. Diets high in fruits and vegetables are associated with a lower incidence of pancreatic cancer.

Possible Etiologic Host Factors

Most cases of pancreatic cancer have no obvious predisposing host factors. This fact has clinical significance in the sense that, with the few exceptional situations men-

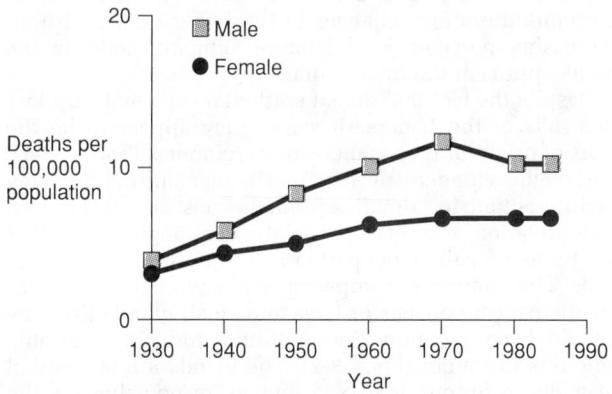

Figure 33-1. Age-adjusted death rates for pancreatic carcinoma. (After Silverberg E, Lubera J. Cancer statistics, 1987. CA Cancer J Clin 1987;37:2)

tioned later, there are no identifiable high-risk groups in whom screening of asymptomatic individuals is likely to be practical.

Abnormal glucose tolerance is present in about 80% of patients with pancreatic cancer, if carefully sought. Diabetes and pancreatic cancer occur together far more frequently than would be expected by chance. Studies suggest that people with long-standing diabetes are not at increased risk of developing pancreatic cancer. In most cases, diabetes manifests at about the same time as the pancreatic neoplasm; the onset of diabetes can be a early sign of pancreatic cancer. A diabetogenic substance may elaborated by pancreatic carcinomas; islet amyloid polypeptide has been proposed as a candidate peptide mediating glucose intolerance in patients with pancreatic tumors.

Chronic pancreatitis is a significant risk factor for the development of pancreatic cancer. It appears that all forms of chronic pancreatitis are associated with an increased risk of pancreatic cancer, suggesting that it is the pancreatitis and not the injuring agent (eg, alcohol) that is responsible for the augmented cancer risk. Studies indicate that patients who have previously undergone gastric resection are three to seven times more likely to develop pancreatic cancer as a control population. A few studies also suggest that women who have undergone cholecystectomy are at increased risk, although this observation has not been consistent.

Several reports have been made of familial clustering of pancreatic cancer. Epidemiologic studies suggest that about 7% of pancreatic cancer patients have a positive family history of the disease. Pancreatic cancer is also more common in a few rare autosomal dominant syndromes such as hereditary pancreatitis, multiple endocrine adenomatosis type I, and Gardner syndrome. For most cases, however, no hereditary basis for pancreatic cancer has been identified.

Pathology

The exocrine pancreas contains two major types of epithelium: acinar and ductal. The acinar cells of the pancreas are primarily concerned with the elaboration of digestive enzymes, whereas the ductal epithelium is responsible for the secretion of fluid and electrolytes and the conveyance of pancreatic juice to the duodenum. The ductal type of epithelium begins with the so-called centroacinar cells, which provide an interface to the acinar cells that cluster around them in a grapelike fashion. The smallest pancreatic ducts are lined by low cuboidal epithelium. As these ducts coalesce to form progressively larger conduits, the height of the lining cells increases; the epithelium becomes columnar in the main pancreatic duct. The character of the epithelium also changes in the larger ducts, with an increasing percentage of mucin-producing cells as the ducts approach the duodenum.

Despite the fact that ductal epithelial cells make up less than 5% of the pancreatic mass, they appear to be the cells of origin of most pancreatic carcinomas (Table 33-1). Although evidence suggests that acinar epithelium may dedifferentiate to a ductlike form, the most straightforward interpretation of human pancreatic carcinogenesis is that the tumors for the most part arise from preexisting ductal cells. The microscopic appearance of a typical ductal pancreatic cancer consists of large and small glands lined by cuboidal or columnar epithelium producing variable amounts of mucin (Fig. 33-2). The glands are embedded in a dense fibrous matrix, which is responsible for the scirrhous consistency of the tumors. The degree of differentiation of ductal carcinoma varies; poorly differentiated tumors demonstrate less gland formation and mucus pro-

Table 33-1. HISTOLOGIC CLASSIFICATION OF 645 CASES OF PRIMARY, NONENDOCRINE CANCER OF THE PANCREAS

Classification	Number
DUCT (DUCTULAR) CELL ORIGIN	572 (89%)
Duct cell adenocarcinoma	494
Giant cell carcinoma	27
Giant cell carcinoma (osteoid)	1
Adenosquamous carcinoma	20
Microadenocarcinoma	16
Mucinous (colloid) carcinoma	9
Cystadenocarcinoma (mucinous)	5
ACINAR CELL ORIGIN	8 (1%)
Acinar cell carcinoma	7
Cystadenocarcinoma (acinar cell)	1
UNCERTAIN HISTOGENESIS	61 (9%)
Pancreaticoblastoma	1
Papillary and cystic neoplasm	1
Mixed type—duct and islet cells	1
Unclassified	58
CONNECTIVE TISSUE ORIGIN	4 (1%)
TOTAL	645 (100%)

(Adapted from Cubilla AL, Fitzgerald PJ. Cancer [non-endocrine] of the pancreas: a suggested classification. In: Fitzgerald PJ. Morrison AB, eds. The pancreas. Baltimore, Williams & Wilkins, 1980:83)

duction and more epithelial anaplasia. Most patients with pancreatic cancer have an associated chronic obstructive pancreatitis, with duct dilation, atrophy and fibrosis of the acinar parenchyma, and varying degrees of chronic lymphocytic infiltration. About 10% of patients show histologic evidence of superimposed acute pancreatitis with a polymorphonuclear cell infiltrate; pseudocyst formation can occur in this group but is rare.

Precursor and Precancerous Lesions

Ductal carcinoma of the pancreas probably arises as a progressive process beginning with ductal hyperplasia, followed by the development of atypical hyperplasia, carcinoma in situ, and finally invasive carcinoma, as is the case for many neoplasms. Unfortunately, the study of preneoplastic lesions in the pancreas is confounded by the fact that the lesions are in general both asymptomatic and inaccessible. Papillary epithelial hyperplasia of the pancreatic ducts and atypical ductal hyperplasia have been found in the pancreata of patients with pancreatic cancer far more often than in controls. Cases of florid intraductal papillomatosis undergoing surgical resection have been analyzed and contain areas of atypical change. A few surgical specimens containing hyperplasia, carcinoma in situ, and invasive carcinoma have been reported. The interpretation of preneoplastic changes in the pancreas is made more difficult by the fact that coexistent obstructive pancreatitis can lead to hyperplastic changes near carcinomas and that intraductal spread of carcinoma can mimic multifocal atypia. Nevertheless, some form of progression of ductal changes is likely in the pathogenesis of pancreatic cancer. Its elucidation is of more than academic interest (witness the impact of colonoscopy and polypectomy in colon cancer) but awaits the technology for identifying it.

Site of Ductal Adenocarcinoma

Sixty to 70% of pancreatic ductal adenocarcinomas occur in the head of the gland. About 15% reside in the body of the gland, another 10% are in the tail, and the remaining

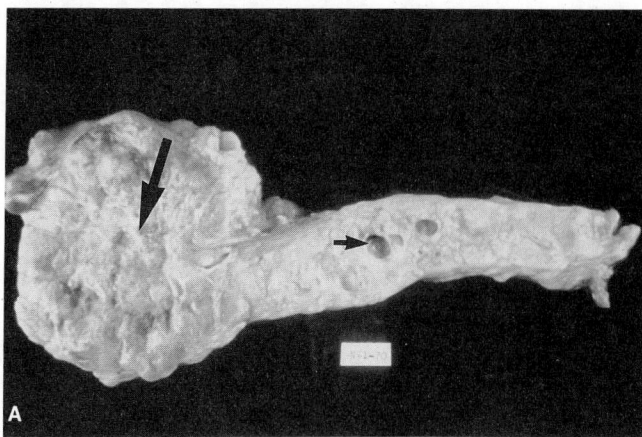
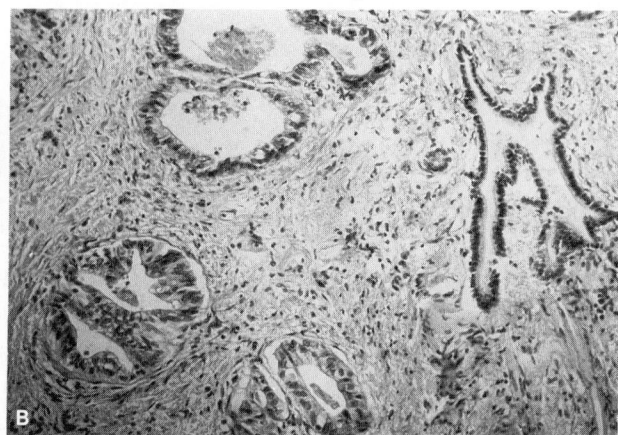

Figure 33-2. Gross and microscopic appearance of ductal adenocarcinoma of the head of the pancreas. In the gross specimen (*A*), the scirrhous reaction in the head of the pancreas (*arrow*) and the dilation of the main pancreatic duct in the body of the gland (*small arrow*) are notable. Microscopic section (*B*) demonstrates glands from a well-differentiated adenocarcinoma (*lower left*) embedded in a fibrous matrix. Some normal residual ductal structures remain (*right*).

5% to 15% are diffuse. The predilection of pancreatic cancer to develop in the head of the gland is unexplained. The practical consequence of this pattern is that tumors in the head are diagnosed earlier because they cause obstructive jaundice, whereas tumors in the body and tail tend to be more advanced at the time of symptomatic presentation. Tumors in the body and tail are typically larger at the time of diagnosis (average, 7 to 8 cm) than in the head (average, 4 to 5 cm).

Sites and Frequency of Local Extension

Extension beyond the confines of the pancreas is the rule rather than the exception in ductal carcinoma of the pancreas. The bile duct is invaded early in the course of the disease, and about 80% of patients with tumors in the head of the pancreas present with jaundice. Invasion of the first or second portion of the duodenum also occurs early in the course of the disease and is present in about 25% of cases. In most pancreatic cancers, there is early invasion of the retroperitoneum, either directly or along the course of autonomic nerves of the celiac plexus. Some degree of perineural invasion is present in 90% of cases. In about half of cases, the walls of the portal or superior mesenteric veins also are invaded, and complete transmural invasion can ultimately lead to thrombosis. Carcinoma of the body and tail can invade the splenic vein, with resultant thrombosis and development of gastric varices. Other sites of local invasion, which tends to occur later, include the superior mesenteric and splenic arteries, transverse mesocolon, stomach, kidneys, and left adrenal gland.

A few florid cases of extension of pancreatic cancer along the pancreatic duct into the tail of the gland have been described, occurring early in the course of the disease. There is considerable disagreement about how often intrapancreatic spread occurs. Several studies have addressed this question by searching for spread of carcinoma of the head of the pancreas to the body and tail in total pancreatectomy specimens. Using similar methods, these studies report widely divergent rates of extension beyond the standard pancreaticoduodenectomy margin, ranging from 10% to 70%. The explanation for these discrepancies is not clear. Most investigators agree that simultaneous multifocal origin of carcinoma in the human pancreas is rare.

Sites and Frequency of Metastatic Disease

The most common sites of metastatic spread from carcinoma of the pancreas are regional and juxtaregional lymph nodes and liver (Table 33-2). Lymphatic spread usually precedes hematogenous spread, and among patients undergoing resective surgery who appear to have no gross evidence of distant metastasis, the prevalence of lymph node metastasis on examination of the resected specimen is about 60%.

Knowledge of the route of lymph node metastasis of pancreatic carcinoma is important to the surgeon. Although the demonstration of lymph node involvement is not a contraindication to resection, the involved nodes must be included in the planned resection. The most common sites of lymph node involvement in pancreatic cancer

Table 33-2. SITES OF METASTASIS IN PANCREATIC CANCER

| | Site of Primary Carcinoma | | |
Site of Metastasis	Head (n = 106)	Body and Tail (n = 34)	Head, Body, and Tail (n = 24)
Regional lymph nodes	85	34	24
Juxtaregional lymph nodes	52	25	18
Liver	80	28	21
Stomach	15	7	13
Peritoneum	23	17	11
Lungs	28	8	7
Pleura	29	13	6
Pericardium	3	2	1
Colon	3	4	4
Spleen	6	11	4
Adrenal glands	15	9	5
Bones	13	5	3
Kidneys	9	7	6
Skin	1	1	2
No metastases	15	1	0

(Adapted from Kloppel G. Pancreatic, non-endocrine tumors. In: Kloppel G, Heitz PU, eds. Pancreatic pathology. New York, Churchill Livingstone, 1984:96)

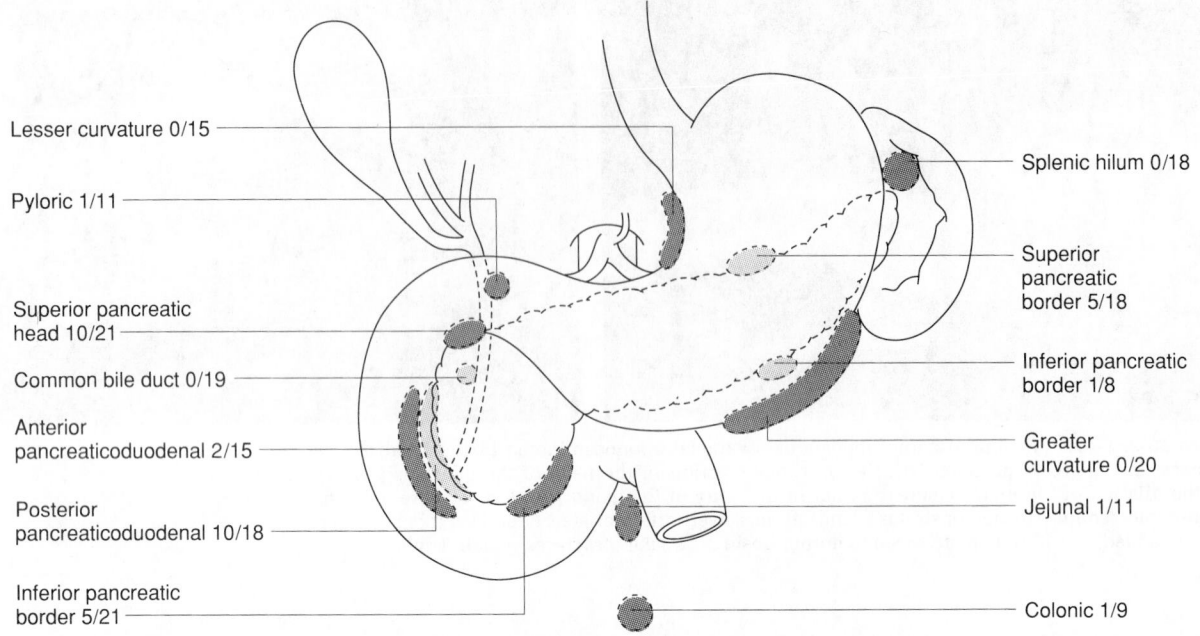

Figure 33-3. Lymph node involvement in duct cell carcinoma of the head of the pancreas in patients undergoing "curative" resection, most of whom were treated by total or regional pancreatectomy. The denominator indicates the number of patients in whom lymph nodes of that group were found, and the numerator indicates the number of patients in whom lymph nodes contained microscopically verified cancer. (After Cubilla AL, Fitzgerald PJ. Surgical pathology aspects of cancer of the ampulla-head-of-pancreas region. In: Fitzgerald PJ, Morrison AB, eds. The pancreas. Baltimore, Williams & Wilkins, 1980;72)

are the posterior pancreaticoduodenal nodes and the nodes along the superior margin of the pancreatic head (Fig. 33-3). Nodes along the superior mesenteric vein as it emerges from behind the neck of the gland should be included in the resection because they are frequently involved. Of considerable practical importance is the involvement of nodes along the body of the pancreas, even when the tumor arises in the head. These nodes are not removed in the course of a standard pancreaticoduodenectomy. At a minimum, therefore, this area should be carefully examined before resection. Some surgeons advocate a more extensive resection of the pancreas to include this area.

Staging of Pancreatic Cancer

Accurate pathologic staging of pancreatic cancer is important for a number of reasons. First and foremost, it has prognostic importance for the patient. Second, careful pathologic staging allows retrospective examination of the accuracy of diagnostic modalities such as computed tomography (CT). Finally, the results of therapeutic trials cannot be accurately judged or compared without detailed knowledge of the pathologic stage of the treated tumors. Table 33-3 shows a straightforward staging system oriented toward surgical resectability. Using this system, it was demonstrated in a total of 924 patients that the survival rate in stage I disease (33% at 1 year) was significantly higher than in stages II and III (combined 13% at 1 year). Survival rates were similar for cases of advanced direct extension (stage II, 15% at 1 year) and cases of lymph node metastases (stage III, 11% at 1 year). The survival rate for stage IV patients with distant metastases was significantly worse than in all other groups (5% at 1 year).

With improvements in diagnostic imaging, it has been possible to assess the natural history of small carcinomas

Table 33-3. TNM CLASSIFICATION FOR STAGING OF CANCER OF THE PANCREAS

TNM DEFINITIONS

Primary Tumor

T1 No direct extension of the primary tumor beyond the pancreas
T2 Limited direct extension (to duodenum, bile ducts, or stomach), still possibly permitting tumor resection
T3 Further direct extension, incompatible with surgical resection
TX Direct extension not assessed or not recorded

Regional Lymph Node Involvement

N0 Regional nodes not involved
N1 Regional nodes involved
NX Regional node involvement not assessed or not recorded

Distant Metastasis

M0 No distant metastasis
M1 Distant metastatic involvement
MX Distant metastatic involvement not assessed or not recorded

STAGE GROUPING

Stage I   T1, T2, N0, M0—No or limited direct extension to adjacent viscera, with no regional node extension and absence of distant metastases. Limited direct extension defined as involvement of organs adjacent to the pancreas that could be removed en bloc with the pancreas if a curative resection were attempted.

Stage II T3, N0, M0—Further direct extension of tumor into adjacent viscera, with no lymph node involvement and no distant metastases, which precluded surgical resection.

Stage III T1–3, N1, M0—Regional node metastases without clinical evidence of distant metastases.

Stage IV T1–3, N0–1, M1—Distant metastatic disease in liver or other sites.

(Adapted from Pollard HJ, et al. Staging of cancer of the pancreas. Cancer of the Pancreas Task Force. Cancer 1981;47:1631)

of the pancreas (2 cm or less). It is discouraging to find that these small tumors have already metastasized to lymph nodes in 30% to 40% of cases and that extrapancreatic invasion has occurred in about 30%. Less than half of patients with tumors 2 cm or smaller have stage I disease. The overall 5-year survival rate of patients with tumors of this size is about 30%.

Diagnosis

Many of the difficulties in the treatment of pancreatic cancer can be traced to our inability to diagnose the disease in its early stages. The vague early symptoms of pancreatic cancer are often minimized by both patient and physician, typically leading to a delay of months in making the diagnosis. It is ordinarily not until the patient develops jaundice or extreme weight loss that the diagnosis is made, and by this time the pancreatic tumor is typically large and has grown beyond the confines of the pancreas.

Clinical Symptoms and Signs

The most common presenting symptoms and signs of pancreatic cancer are listed in Tables 33-4 and 33-5. The most frequent symptom of pancreatic cancer is weight loss, which is usually substantial, averaging 10 kg. The weight loss can initially occur as an isolated symptom in the face of a seemingly normal appetite. Later, it is usually associated with anorexia. Unexplained documented weight loss should prompt a search for occult malignancy; in older adults, it is appropriate to perform a CT scan of the abdomen for this indication alone. Other digestive symptoms are common in pancreatic cancer and include nausea, vomiting, and change in bowel habits.

Table 33-4. SYMPTOMS OF PANCREATIC CANCER

Symptom	Patients (%)
HEAD	
Weight loss	92
Jaundice	82
Pain	72
Anorexia	64
Dark urine	63
Light stools	62
Nausea	45
Vomiting	37
Weakness	35
Pruritus	24
Diarrhea	18
Melena	12
Constipation	11
Fever	11
Hematemesis	8
BODY AND TAIL	
Weight loss	100
Pain	87
Weakness	43
Nausea	43
Vomiting	37
Anorexia	33
Constipation	27
Hematemesis	17
Melena	17
Jaundice	7
Fever	7
Diarrhea	3

(Adapted from Howard JM, Jordan GL Jr. Cancer of the pancreas. Curr Probl Cancer 1977;2:5)

Table 33-5. SIGNS OF PANCREATIC CANCER

Sign	Patients (%)
HEAD	
Jaundice	87
Palpable liver	83
Palpable gallbladder	29
Tenderness	26
Ascites	14
Abdominal mass	13
BODY AND TAIL	
Palpable liver	33
Tenderness	27
Abdominal mass	23
Ascites	20
Jaundice	13

(Adapted from Howard JM, Jordan GL Jr. Cancer of the pancreas. Curr Probl Cancer 1977;2:5)

Most patients with pancreatic cancer come to physicians because of jaundice. In people older than 60 years of age, the combination of jaundice and weight loss usually means carcinoma of the pancreas or periampullary region. The diagnosis is often evident, requiring only appropriate imaging studies for confirmation. The jaundice is progressive. It is associated with dark urine and light stools. Pruritus is present in about one fourth of jaundiced patients.

Although it is often taught that carcinoma of the pancreas presents with painless jaundice (to help distinguish it from choledocholithiasis), this aphorism is not accurate. Most patients do experience pain as part of the symptom complex of pancreatic cancer. It is usually perceived in the epigastrium but can occur in any part of the abdomen and can radiate to the back. Early on, it is often mild and vague, and it is in this phase that much of the delay in diagnosis occurs because patients are treated symptomatically without a vigorous diagnostic effort. In older adults, abdominal pain that persists and for which no reasonable explanation can be found merits a CT evaluation. Ultimately, 50% to 70% of patients with pancreatic cancer experience pain that they describe as moderate or severe; the prevalence is particularly high with tumors of the body and tail, probably because of invasion of the celiac plexus.

The most common presenting signs of pancreatic cancer are jaundice and hepatomegaly. When bilirubin levels are only minimally elevated, icterus may be confined to the sclerae, but most patients have cutaneous changes by the time of presentation. Hepatomegaly usually reflects congestion associated with biliary obstruction and does not imply the presence of metastatic disease unless the liver is nodular or hard. The obstructed gallbladder is palpable in about 25% of patients with pancreatic cancer. In most patients, the tumor itself is not palpable.

Ascites is present in about 15% of patients with pancreatic cancer. With large tumors, there can be gross or occult blood in the stool from invasion of the duodenum, stomach, or colon.

Laboratory Investigations

In carcinoma of the head of the pancreas, liver function tests typically reveal elevations in bilirubin (particularly the conjugated fraction) and alkaline phosphatase characteristic of extrahepatic biliary obstruction. The transaminases can also be elevated, but usually not to the extent of the alkaline phosphatase. If jaundice has been long-standing, the prothrombin time can be abnormally prolonged. Mild elevations of the serum amylase in the range of 300 U/L occur, but marked elevations of serum amylase are rare. Routine laboratory determinations add little to the diagnosis of pancreatic cancer other than reinforcing the suspicion of extrahepatic biliary obstruction.

Considerable effort has been expended to find serum markers of pancreatic cancer. Mucins are large glycosylated glycoproteins whose function appears to be protection and lubrication of epithelial cells. Mucin molecules are produced by most moderately well-differentiated pancreatic carcinomas. In the past few years, mucin-associated antigens have been isolated and purified, and monoclonal antibodies have been raised against these antigens. CA19-9 is an example of a mucin-associated carbohydrate antigen that can be detected in the serum of patients with pancreatic cancer. The CA19-9 antigen has been identified as sialosyl-fucosyl-lactotetrose, which corresponds to the sialylated Lewis[a] (Le[a]) blood group substance found on erythrocytes. About 5% of the Western population lacks the Lewis gene and therefore cannot make CA19-9. The CA19-9 antigen resides in cell membrane glycolipid and in mucin glycoprotein. CA19-9 can be detected in pancreatic juice, in serum, and in pancreatic tissue by immunohistologic techniques.

Serum levels of CA19-9 are elevated (above 37 U/mL) in about 75% of patients with pancreatic cancer. Unfortunately, CA19-9 is also elevated in about 10% of patients with benign diseases of the pancreas, liver, and bile ducts. The specificity of the CA19-9 test can be significantly improved by using a cutoff of 100 U/mL, but sensitivity is reduced to about 60%. CA19-9 is not sufficiently sensitive or specific to warrant its use by itself in population screening. The availability of CA19-9 also appears not to have led to earlier diagnosis of pancreatic cancer because most patients are symptomatic at presentation and CA19-9 is often not elevated in very small cancers. On the other hand, the use of CA19-9 with imaging studies improves overall diagnostic accuracy and can simplify the evaluation of patients with suspected pancreatic cancer.

Of potential diagnostic significance is the fact that about 90% of human pancreatic cancers contain the mutated c-K-*ras* oncogene. The c-K-*ras* gene is ordinarily present in human cells and encodes a membrane-bound protein that possesses high affinity for guanosine triphosphate and guanosine diphosphate and appears to be important for signal transduction across the cell membrane. The *ras* protein is active when bound to guanosine triphosphate but is inactive when bound to guanosine diphosphate. Certain mutations in the gene result in its transformation to an active oncogene. In the case of c-K-*ras,* a single point mutation at codon 12 is sufficient. As a result of the mutation, the level of activated *ras* protein rises, and high levels of active protein can contribute to unrestrained cellular growth by facilitating the transmission of growth factor signals across the cell membrane. The appeal of the detection of oncogenes or oncogene products as a diagnostic strategy is that they are likely to be specific for the premalignant or malignant state, in contradistinction to the tumor-associated antigens discussed earlier, which are also expressed to varying degrees in normal tissue and purely benign conditions. It has already been possible to detect the mutated c-K-*ras* gene in fine-needle cytologic aspirates, serum, stool, and pancreatic juice from patients with pancreatic carcinoma.

Radiologic Investigations

Imaging of the pancreas has dramatically improved with the development of ultrasonography, CT scanning, and endoscopic retrograde cholangiopancreatography (ERCP). With appropriate use of these studies, it should be possible to arrive at a radiologic diagnosis of pancreatic cancer in over 90% of patients presenting with the disease.

Standard transcutaneous ultrasonography is an appropriate first test in the evaluation of the patient with jaundice because the presence of a dilated common bile duct or intrahepatic bile ducts is essentially diagnostic of extrahepatic biliary obstruction. This finding directs the physician to a search for the cause of the obstruction. If the bile ducts are not dilated, mechanical obstruction is unlikely, and the diagnostic thrust should move toward hepatocellular disease. Ultrasonography is also the best test to determine whether gallstones are present; this is extremely important because choledocholithiasis is one of the conditions most likely to cause jaundice in the elderly population. If an ultrasound examination shows gallstones and no evidence of a pancreatic mass, the appropriate next step is ordinarily an ERCP (see later) to document common duct stones. On the other hand, if no gallbladder stones are present by ultrasonography, choledocholithiasis is unlikely, and a pancreatic or periampullary tumor or chronic pancreatitis becomes a more likely cause of the obstruction. Ordinarily, a CT scan is the most appropriate next test.

Ultrasonography reveals a pancreatic mass in 60% to 70% of patients with pancreatic cancer, but the sensitivity of ultrasound is slightly lower than that of CT, and the absence of a mass on ultrasound scan cannot be accepted as firm evidence against pancreatic cancer. Even if ultrasonography demonstrates a pancreatic mass, CT is usually appropriate to provide further evidence about the stage and extent of the tumor (see later). Additional potentially important findings that can be detected with ultrasonography are ascites and liver metastases. For patients suspected of having pancreatic cancer who present without jaundice (eg, with weight loss only), ultrasonography is not appropriate, and CT should be the first choice.

In most cases of pancreatic cancer, CT is the single most useful test. CT scanning not only usually detects the presence of the tumor mass but also provides important information about the extent of the tumor (Table 33-6 and Fig. 33-4). CT scans may miss tumors smaller than 2 cm. In such cases, the CT findings may be limited to pancreatic or bile duct dilation. Such findings are highly suspicious for pancreatic malignancy and should be further evaluated, ordinarily with ERCP. Dynamic CT scanning, in which high-speed scans are obtained during rapid intravenous administration of iodinated contrast material, and new techniques such as three-dimensional reconstruction from spiral scans provide excellent information about vascular invasion.

CT scans provide the best available radiologic information to determine whether or not a pancreatic neoplasm is resectable, but they cannot be considered absolutely de-

Table 33-6. CT FINDINGS IN PANCREATIC CANCER

Finding	Patients (%)
Pancreatic mass	96
Dilated pancreatic duct	68
Obstructive pseudocyst	11
Bile ducts dilated	58
Local tumor extension	68
Contiguous organ invasion	42
Vascular involvement	84
Liver metastases	36
Lymph node metastases	28
Ascites	8

(Adapted from Freeny PC, Marks WM, Ryan JA, Traverso LW. Pancreatic ductal adenocarcinoma: diagnosis and staging with dynamic CT. Radiology 1988:166:125)

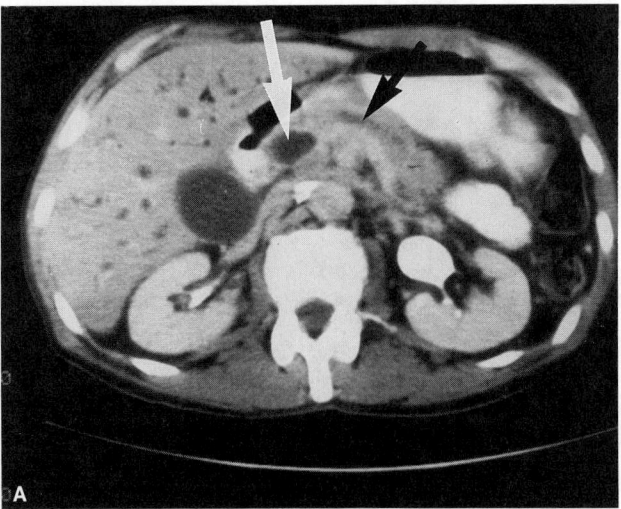
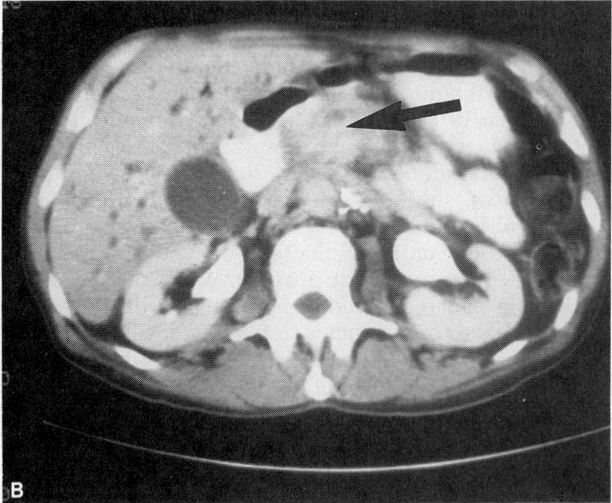

Figure 33-4. CT scan of the abdomen of a patient with ductal adenocarcinoma of the pancreas. (*A*) The obstructed and dilated common bile duct (*light arrow*) and pancreatic duct (*dark arrow*) can be seen. In an adjacent cross section (*B*), a large mass is present in the head of the pancreas (*arrow*).

finitive in this regard. Only about half of pancreatic tumors that appear to be confined to the pancreas on CT scan are found to be resectable in the operating room. CT scanning is more accurate in the diagnosis of unresectability. CT findings that indicate that the tumor is unlikely to be surgically curable include vascular invasion, enlarged lymph nodes outside the boundaries of resection, ascites, distant metastases (eg, liver), and distant organ invasion (eg, colon). When a CT scan shows distant metastases or extensive local invasion, the positive predictive value of the technique is high; some 90% of such patients have unresectable disease at laparotomy. *Resectability* is a relative term, the definition of which depends on how extensive a surgical resection is contemplated. For example, portal venous compression is typically considered a sign of unresectability, yet many surgical groups would consider performing a segmental resection of the portal vein if the tu-

mor otherwise appeared removable. Likewise, some groups advocate an extensive upper abdominal lymph node dissection, which encompasses nodes well away from the primary lesion.

Fine-needle aspiration biopsy of the pancreas under CT or ultrasound guidance is an important advance in the diagnosis of pancreatic cancer. A 22-gauge needle is passed directly into the pancreatic mass, and a cytologic examination is performed on aspirated cells (Fig. 33-5). The experience with this technique is extensive, and most centers report 70% to 80% sensitivity and 100% specificity. The technique is particularly useful in distinguishing chronic pancreatitis from pancreatic cancer and in providing a tissue diagnosis in patients with advanced disease who are not considered candidates for palliative or curative surgery.

ERCP is an excellent diagnostic test for pancreatic can-

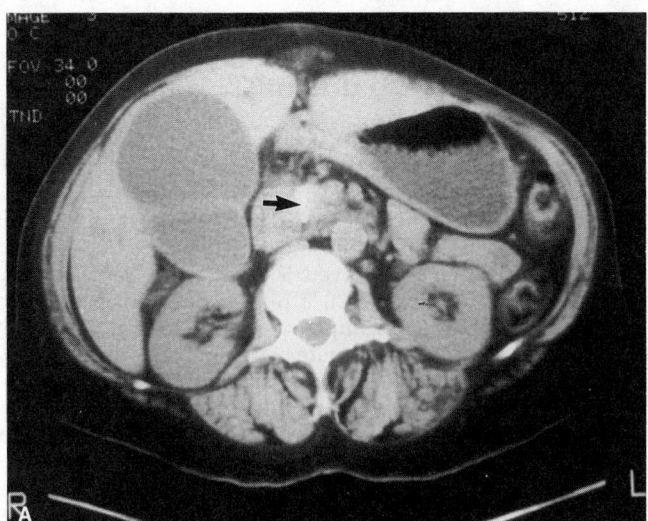
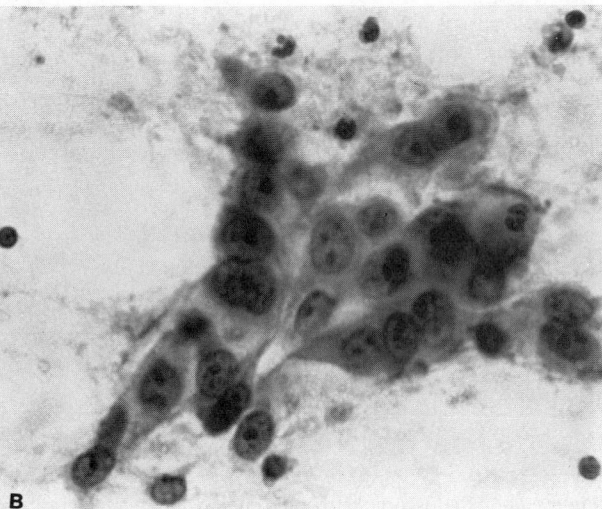

Figure 33-5. Percutaneous fine-needle aspiration biopsy of the pancreas. (*A*) A 22-gauge needle is passed into a mass in the head of the pancreas (*arrow*). (*B*) This stained aspirate is compatible with ductal adenocarcinoma of the pancreas.

cer, with sensitivities in the range of 90% (Fig. 33-6). ERCP does not provide any evidence about spread of disease beyond the pancreas. ERCP is indicated to resolve special problems in the diagnosis of pancreatic cancer. These include primarily cases with CT evidence of bile duct or pancreatic duct obstruction without a mass, cases in which the differentiation between chronic pancreatitis and pancreatic cancer is difficult, and cases of cholelithiasis and bile duct obstruction without a pancreatic mass on ultrasound. Findings on ERCP that suggest pancreatic cancer include irregular pancreatic duct narrowing, displacement of the main pancreatic duct, destruction or displacement of side branches of the duct, and pooling of contrast material in necrotic areas of tumor. In most cases, the bile duct portion of the study shows an irregular stenosis with proximal dilation. In cases in which the differential diagnosis lies between chronic pancreatitis and pancreatic cancer, the distinction can usually be made because chronic pancreatitis is characterized by multiple or long stenoses of the pancreatic duct. In contrast, pancreatic cancer typically causes an abrupt focal interruption of the duct.

Upper gastrointestinal endoscopy is a useful tool in the diagnosis of pancreatic cancer. Endoscopy can be valuable in finding tumors of the ampulla of Vater or duodenum, which have a considerably better prognosis than pancreatic cancers. It may be possible to obtain a tissue diagnosis of pancreatic cancer if there is invasion of the duodenum. Finally, it is possible to estimate the degree of duodenal obstruction in pancreatic cancer, which can have implications in choosing therapy.

An imaging technique that shows promise in the diagnosis and staging of pancreatic cancer is endoscopic ultrasonography. Rotating ultrasound probes at the tip of an upper gastrointestinal endoscope produce a 360-degree image. Pancreatic carcinomas appear as hypoechoic areas in the pancreatic substance (Fig. 33-7). Endoscopic ultrasonography appears to be more sensitive than transcutaneous ultrasound or CT in detecting tumors smaller than 2.5 cm.

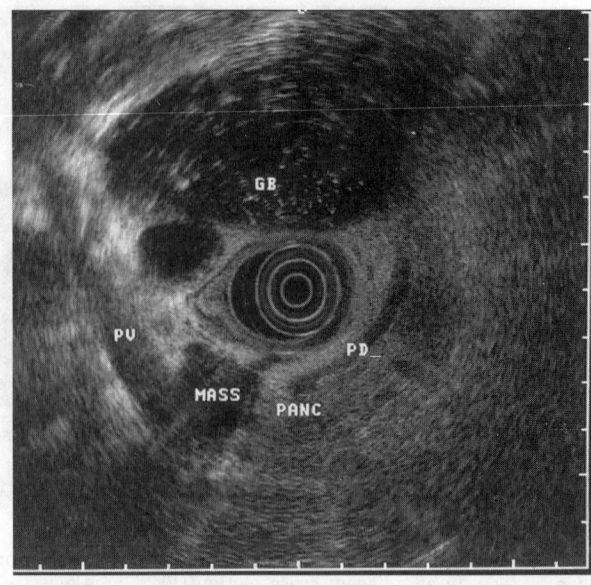

Figure 33-7. Endoscopic ultrasound of a 2.2-cm mass in the head of the pancreas (PANC). The transducer tip is located in the duodenal bulb. The dilated common bile duct and gallbladder (GB) can be seen at the top of the image. The pancreatic duct (PD) is also dilated. The mass involves the portal vein (PV), indicating an unresectable tumor, which was confirmed at laparotomy. (Courtesy of C. J. Lightdale, MD, Columbia-Presbyterian Medical Center, New York)

It is also sensitive tool for evaluating vascular invasion. It will probably assume a larger role in the diagnosis and staging of pancreatic cancer as experience increases.

The generally grim prognosis of pancreatic cancer has led to pessimism on the part of physicians evaluating elderly patients with jaundice. Because some jaundiced patients have nonmalignant diseases such as choledocholithiasis or fibrotic strictures of the bile duct due to chronic pancreatitis, and because some have tumors that carry a better prognosis than ductal carcinoma of the pancreas (such as carcinoma of the bile duct), it is inappropriate to provide only palliation of jaundice (eg, by endoscopic stent placement) without a tissue diagnosis. The tools are available to achieve a firm diagnosis in nearly all jaundiced patients and should be used.

Curative Treatment of Pancreatic Carcinoma

Surgery

Surgical resection is the only potentially curative therapy for pancreatic cancer. Unfortunately, few patients are actually cured of the disease. In one large review of about 37,000 cases of pancreatic cancer of all stages,[1] fewer than 1% of the patients survived 5 years after the diagnosis. Typically, only 10% to 20% of patients with pancreatic cancer can undergo attempted resection for cure, and that figure may be an overestimate because it is derived largely from patients referred to university surgical departments. Although the statistics are daunting, there have been some mildly encouraging improvements in surgical therapy for pancreatic cancer, and there are ongoing efforts to determine whether results can be improved by combining therapeutic modalities such as chemotherapy and radiotherapy with surgery.

Pancreaticoduodenectomy.   Most resectable carcinomas of the pancreas are located in the head of the gland,

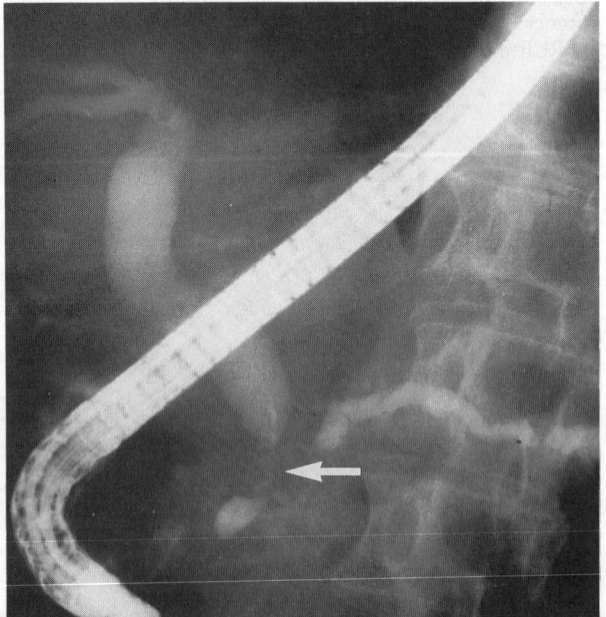

Figure 33-6. Endoscopic retrograde cholangiopancreatography in a patient with ductal adenocarcinoma of the pancreas, demonstrating circumferential stenosis of both the distal common bile duct and the pancreatic duct in the head of the pancreas. The location of the tumor is indicated by the arrow.

probably because the onset of jaundice results in earlier diagnosis than in tumors involving the body and tail of the gland. Whipple and colleagues[2] first described the operation of removal of the head of the pancreas and duodenum in 1935. The operation they described was a two-stage operation, actually performed for ampullary tumors, that differed in several technical respects from the pancreaticoduodenectomy of today. Nevertheless, Whipple described the essence of the operation, which continues to bear his name.

Pancreaticoduodenectomy is best performed through an upper abdominal incision (Fig. 33-8). On entering the abdomen, a thorough inspection of the entire peritoneal cavity should be made for evidence of metastatic disease, par-

ticularly concentrating on the liver, omentum, peritoneal surfaces, and subdiaphragmatic periaortic lymph nodes. If this exploration is negative, the head of the pancreas is mobilized by first reflecting the hepatic flexure of the colon downward and then mobilizing the head of the pancreas from the retroperitoneum. The tumor mass ordinarily is not difficult to feel because of its hardness in comparison with the rest of the pancreas and surrounding tissues. The pancreas away from the tumor can be somewhat firmer than usual because of the presence of obstructive pancreatitis, but it usually does not have the scirrhous consistency of the tumor itself. If the tumor mass can be palpated, the physician should attempt to obtain a tissue diagnosis. Fine-needle aspiration cytology can be performed with low

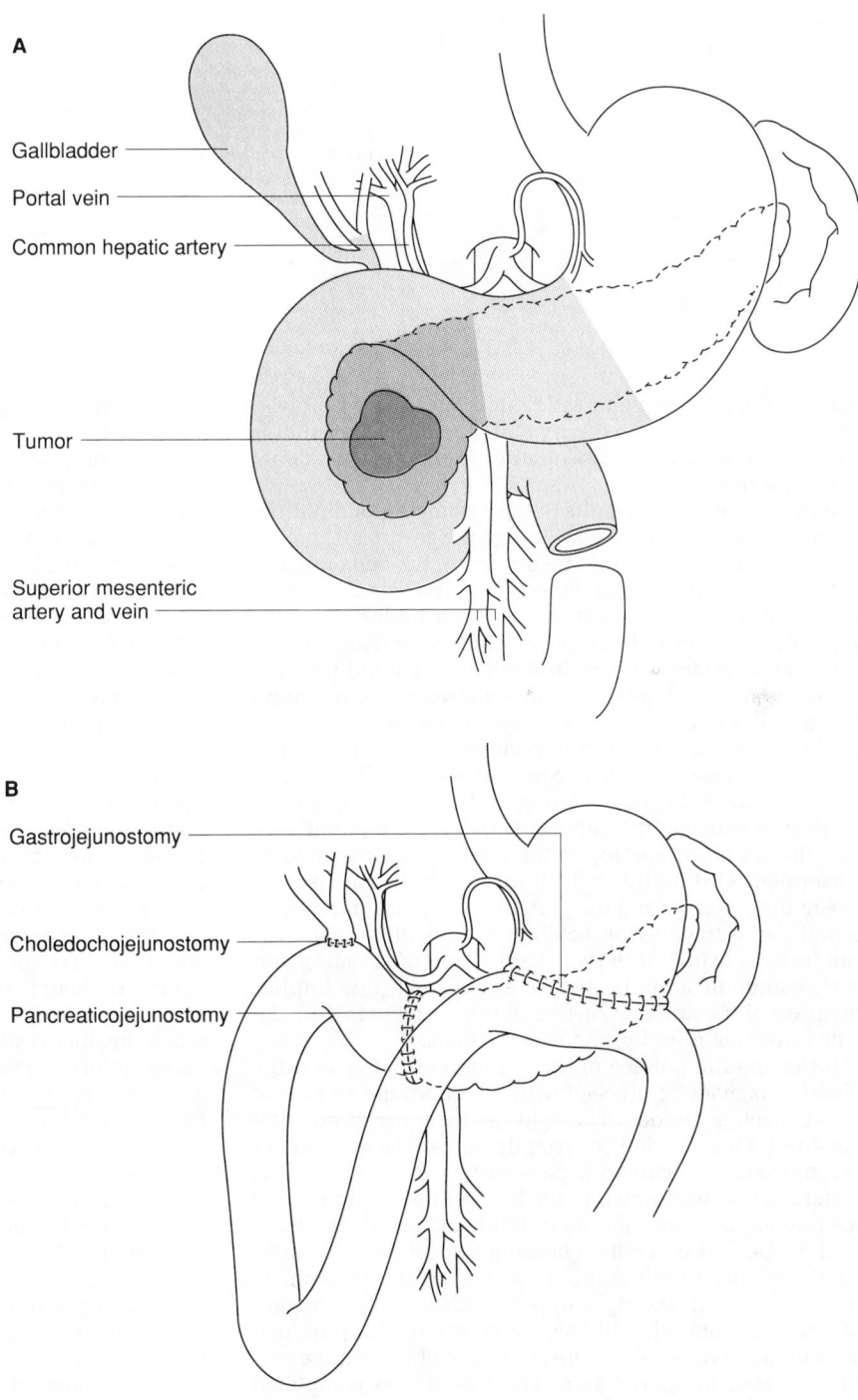

Figure 33-8. Pancreaticoduodenectomy. (*A*) The tissues to be resected in a standard pancreaticoduodenectomy are indicated. (*B*) Reconstruction after standard pancreaticoduodenectomy. (*C*) Reconstruction after pylorus-sparing variant of pancreaticoduodenectomy.

C

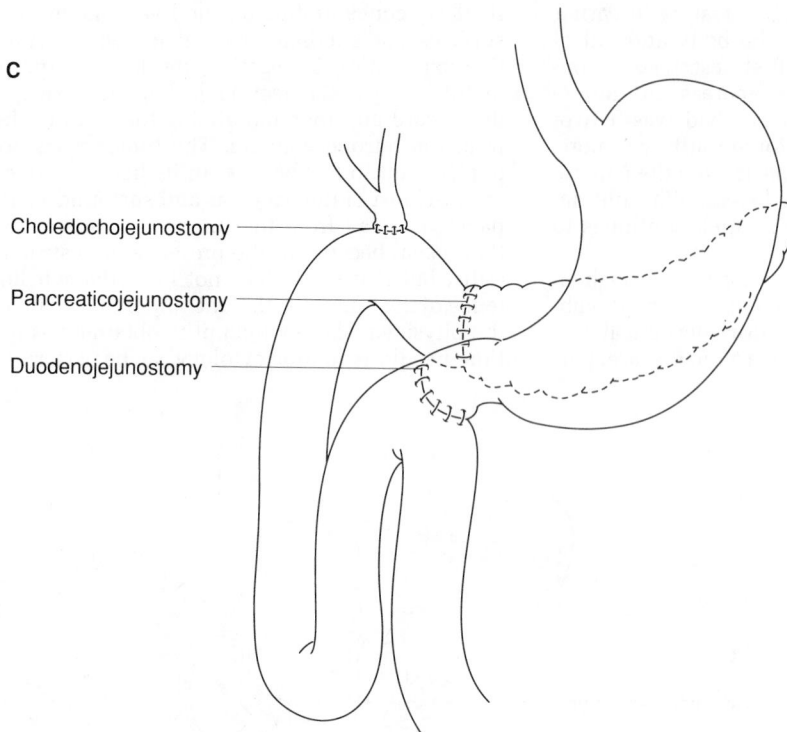

Choledochojejunostomy

Pancreaticojejunostomy

Duodenojejunostomy

Figure 31-7. (continued)

Figure 33-8. (continued)

risk of injury to the pancreatic duct; multiple passes can be easily made. The sensitivity of fine-needle aspiration is 70% or better and surpasses that of traditional incisional biopsy techniques.

While awaiting the results of the cytologic examination, the lesser sac is opened wide through the gastrocolic omentum. This maneuver allows inspection of the body and tail of the gland to determine the extent of the tumor involvement and allows examination of lymph nodes along the superior and inferior body of the pancreas and around the celiac axis. Enlarged nodes in these areas should undergo biopsy and be submitted for frozen-section examination because tumor in these areas is beyond the bounds of standard pancreaticoduodenectomy and constitutes a contraindication to resection (see Extended Radical Pancreatectomy). If there is no evidence of lymphadenopathy, a dissection between the anterior surface of the portal vein and the posterior surface of the neck of the pancreas is performed. Ordinarily, only thin areolar tissue lies between the pancreas and the portal vein, and a communication, inferior to superior, behind the neck of the pancreas can be established. If there is hard tissue intervening and such communication cannot be established, this implies invasion of the anterior surface of the portal vein and signals unresectability by standard methods.

If the anterior surface of the portal vein is free and the decision is made to proceed with resection, the antrum of the stomach is divided. The right gastric and gastroduodenal arteries are divided between ligatures. The gallbladder is removed, the common hepatic duct is divided, and the distal duct is freed down to the level of the upper edge of the duodenum. The jejunum is divided about 15 cm distal to the ligament of Treitz, choosing a location with sufficient mobility to allow the distal end of the jejunum to reach easily into the right upper quadrant. The ligament of Treitz is incised, and the mesentery of the proximal jejunum is divided. After this, the neck of the pancreas is divided over the portal vein. The resection is completed

by carefully ligating and dividing the branches of the portal vein emanating from the head of the pancreas. Finally, the uncinate process is dissected from beneath the portal vein. The inferior pancreaticoduodenal branch of the superior mesenteric artery supplies the uncinate process and is ligated in the course of this dissection.

After removal of the resected specimen, reconstruction requires three anastomoses. The pancreatic remnant ordinarily is anastomosed to the free end of the jejunum, the bile duct to the side of the jejunum, and the stomach to the side of jejunum downstream from the other anastomoses (see Fig. 33-8). The pancreaticojejunostomy is the most difficult anastomosis and the one most prone to disruption in the postoperative period. Several techniques have been described for the performance of this anastomosis, but the absence of a standard technique reflects the fact that no method is ideal. Some surgeons advocate direct mucosa-to-mucosa approximation of the pancreatic duct to the jejunum, with an outer layer joining the seromuscular layers of the bowel to the pancreatic capsule. Others prefer to anastomose the pancreas to the opened jejunum in such a way that the pancreatic remnant is invaginated into the jejunum. There is no evidence that one technique is superior to the other. The latter technique is easier to perform when the duct is small or the pancreas friable. The choledochojejunostomy is straightforward; either a single-layer anastomosis of nonabsorbable monofilament suture or a traditional two-layer anastomosis can be used. The gastrojejunostomy is performed in a standard fashion.

A modification of the standard pancreaticoduodenectomy to allow preservation of the antrum and pylorus of the stomach has become the procedure of choice in many institutions.[3] In this operation, no gastric resection is performed. The proximal duodenum is transected just distal to the pylorus and is anastomosed end-to-side to the jejunum (see Fig. 33-8). After recovery from surgery, emptying of liquids and perhaps solids from the stomach is improved compared with standard pancreaticoduodenectomy. Although patients with pylorus-preserving resections appear to regain weight better than historical controls with standard operations, the two procedures have not been rigorously compared. No major nutritional or symptomatic advantage can be unequivocally attributed to pylorus preservation. In fact, most patients even after standard pancreaticoduodenectomy do not suffer postgastrectomy symptoms. The prevalence of marginal ulceration after pylorus-preserving pancreaticoduodenectomy is reported to be less than 5%. On the negative side for pylorus preservation, return of gastric emptying in the immediate postoperative period appears to take longer than after standard operations; about half of patients experience at least 7 days of postoperative delay in gastric emptying, although nearly all cases ultimately resolve with conservative therapy.

Postoperative Course After Pancreaticoduodenectomy. Pancreaticoduodenectomy is a formidable operation, and the morbidity and mortality of this procedure have historically been high. Until recently, average operative mortality rates were reported to approximate 20%. In the past few years, several centers have reported large series with operative mortality rates lower than 5%. The reasons for this improvement are not clear but probably relate to improved general management of ill patients and to the concentration of these procedures in institutions with extensive experience.

The most dreaded complication of pancreaticoduodenectomy is disruption of the pancreaticojejunostomy, which occurs in about 10% of patients. Anastomotic breakdown can lead to the development of an upper abdominal abscess or can present as an external pancreatic fistula. In its most virulent form, disruption leads to necrotizing retroperitoneal infection, which can erode major arteries and veins of the upper abdomen, including the exposed portal vein or its branches or the stump of the gastroduodenal artery. Impending catastrophe is often preceded by a small herald bleed from the drain site. Such an event is an indication to return to the operating room to drain widely the pancreaticojejunostomy and to repair the involved blood vessel. Open packing of the wound may be necessary to control diffuse necrosis and infection. On rare occasions, completion pancreatectomy is required to control sepsis. Intraperitoneal hemorrhage is the most common cause of death from pancreaticoduodenectomy.

Upper gastrointestinal hemorrhage occurs in about 15% of patients in the immediate postoperative period after pancreaticoduodenectomy. The gastroenterostomy is the most common site of early postoperative bleeding. Bleeding also can occur in the gastric and jejunal mucosa. Sometimes bleeding from disruption of the pancreaticojejunostomy presents as gastrointestinal hemorrhage. It may be possible to treat punctate mucosal lesions with endoscopic cautery, but reoperation may be necessary to control bleeding. Alkalinization of the stomach throughout the perioperative period can help reduce the incidence of immediate postoperative bleeding.

Marginal ulceration occurs as a late complication in about 10% of patients undergoing pancreaticoduodenectomy. The ulcers usually occur within the first few months after surgery. The addition of truncal vagotomy to pancreaticoduodenectomy has been advocated, but in most reported series, vagotomy fails to reduce the incidence of stomal ulcer. Biliary fistulas occur in 5% to 10% of patients after pancreaticoduodenectomy. These are usually limited and respond to conservative management.

A common complication early after pancreaticoduodenectomy is delayed gastric emptying, particularly if the operation is of the pylorus-sparing variety. Gastric atony can require the institution of parenteral alimentation. Ordinarily, the gastric outlet obstruction is functional and

not anatomic, but occasionally abscess, inflammation, or scarring around the pancreas can cause a true mechanical obstruction of the overlying gastrojejunostomy. If, on barium swallow, contrast material enters the small bowel, conservative management is warranted. If no contrast enters the bowel, mechanical obstruction should be suspected; reoperation is usually necessary in the presence of complete outflow obstruction.

Results of Pancreaticoduodenectomy. In terms of cure, the results of standard pancreaticoduodenectomy are discouraging. On the one hand, most known cures of pancreatic cancer have been achieved with pancreaticoduodenectomy. On the other hand, survival figures indicate that relatively few patients undergoing pancreaticoduodenectomy are alive and free of disease 5 years after surgery. Some large centers have reported actuarial survival figures in the range of 20% after apparently curative pancreaticoduodenectomy.[4,5] Other centers with extensive experience continue, however, to report 5-year survival rates in the traditional range of 5% to 10%.[6] It is possible that we are beginning to see improvements in long-term cure rates, but actual 5-year survival in recent years (Table 33-7) indicates that relatively few patients treated by standard pancreaticoduodenectomy for carcinoma of the head of the pancreas are cured.

Autopsy studies reveal that pancreaticoduodenectomy often fails to control disease locally, resulting in retroperitoneal recurrence and regional lymphatic disease. In addition, most patients develop hematogenous metastases, most commonly in the liver but often in the lungs. Peritoneal implants, malignant ascites, and malignant pleural effusions are all common when disease recurs after surgery. The high incidence of local failure probably is due to a number of factors. These include inadequate tumor margins due to the proximity of vital structures (portal vein, superior mesenteric artery), failure to identify and resect regional lymphatic disease, unresected direct retroperitoneal extension, and unrecognized extension of disease into the remaining pancreas. Systemic failure is

Table 33-7. LONG-TERM SURVIVAL AFTER STANDARD PANCREATICODUODENECTOMY FOR PANCREATIC CANCER

Investigators	Patients Undergoing Pancreaticoduodenectomy	5-Year Survivors
Condie et al, 1989	13	1
Matsuno et al, 1988	28	2
Connolly et al, 1987	39	2
Grace et al, 1986	37	1
Parker & Postlethwait, 1985	10	0
Rosenberg et al, 1985	24	3
Jones et al, 1985	28	1
O'Brien & Mincey, 1985	26	3
Tsuchiya et al, 1985	163	4
Kuemmerle & Rueckert, 1984	39	9
Lerut et al, 1984	25	0
Warren et al, 1983	64	3
Cohen et al, 1982	36	0
Piorkowski et al, 1982	19	1
Herter et al, 1982	31	2
Bjorck et al, 1981	62	5
Edis et al, 1980	124	5
TOTAL	768	42 (5.4%)

presumably the result of unrecognized and untreated micrometastases at the time of surgery and spread of recurrent locoregional disease. Median survival after standard pancreaticoduodenectomy is about 1 year and reflects the inability to render patients disease free with standard surgery alone. Additional strategies must be developed to deal with these shortcomings. In general, two approaches have been taken: (1) increasing the extent of surgery to prevent local recurrence, and (2) using adjuvant chemoradiotherapy to improve local control and perhaps lessen systemic recurrence. These approaches are discussed later; the discussion is necessarily incomplete because many of these efforts are in the process of evaluation.

Total Pancreatectomy. In response to dissatisfaction with the results of standard pancreaticoduodenectomy for pancreatic cancer, several groups performed total pancreatectomy. The potential advantages of total removal of the pancreas are eradication of microscopic carcinoma extending beyond the standard pancreaticoduodenectomy margin and avoidance of the dangerous pancreaticojejunal anastomosis. Additionally, potentially involved lymph node groups along the body of the pancreas can be removed. The primary disadvantages of the operation are the resultant insulin-dependent diabetic state and complete pancreatic exocrine insufficiency, necessitating the oral administration of pancreatic enzymes.

The results of total pancreatectomy for pancreatic cancer have not proved to be superior to those for standard pancreaticoduodenectomy. In one report of 48 cases, mean survival was 12 months, similar to patients undergoing pancreaticoduodenectomy.[7] The 5-year survival rate was 14%. In another large study, the 5-year survival rate in 89 patients undergoing total pancreatectomy for ductal carcinoma of the pancreas was 7%, not a significant difference when compared with 4% in patients undergoing pancreaticoduodenectomy at the same institution.[8] Median survival was actually a few months shorter in total pancreatectomy patients, and the operative mortality rate was higher

than for pancreaticoduodenectomy (10% versus 4%). In most series, the mortality and morbidity rates from the two procedures have been equivalent or have been higher for total pancreatectomy. Diabetes resulting from total pancreatectomy is generally easy to manage, but in some cases the diabetic condition is brittle, and serious complications and deaths have occurred as a result. There also appears to be a higher incidence of marginal ulceration after total pancreatectomy than after pancreaticoduodenectomy. Few surgeons continue to advocate total pancreatectomy for adenocarcinoma of the pancreas.

Extended Radical Pancreatectomy. Because of the high incidence of direct retroperitoneal invasion and regional lymph node metastasis at the time of surgery, it has been argued that the scope of resection for pancreatic cancer should be enlarged to include a radical regional lymphadenectomy and resection of areas of retroperitoneal invasion. The operations generally include the following features:

- Extension of the pancreatic resection from the neck to the middle body of the pancreas
- Segmental resection and reanastomosis of the portal vein if necessary to achieve tumor-free margins
- Extensive lymphadenectomy to include the peripancreatic and celiac nodes
- Resection of retroperitoneal tissue, particularly in the right perinephric area and the region of the celiac plexus (Fig. 33-9)

Results with extended radical pancreatectomy have been inconsistent. In one series in which patients were treated with regional pancreatectomy for ductal carcinoma of the pancreas,[9] median survival (12 months) did not appear to be improved compared with the historical experience with pancreaticoduodenectomy. High operative morbidity and mortality rates have been reported by others. In sharp contrast are two publications from Japan that report 5-year survival rates of 33% and 29% after extended pancreatec-

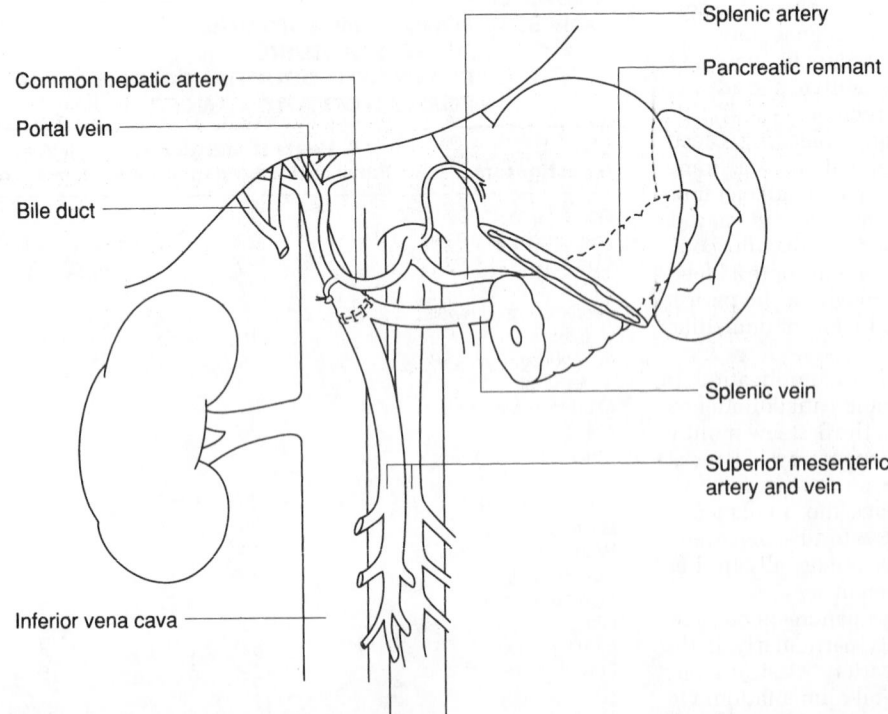

Common hepatic artery

Portal vein

Bile duct

Inferior vena cava

Splenic artery

Pancreatic remnant

Splenic vein

Superior mesenteric artery and vein

Figure 33-9. Extended radical pancreatectomy for pancreatic cancer, demonstrating extended pancreatic resection, retroperitoneal soft tissue dissection, lymphadenectomy, and segmental resection and reanastomosis of the portal vein.

tomy for ductal carcinoma of the pancreas.[10,11] The operative mortality rate was low (6%). In both series, survival rates represented a substantial improvement over historical survival rates with standard pancreaticoduodenectomy, which were 0% and 9%, respectively. Neither experience was a controlled trial. Additional reports suggest improved survival with the combination of radical pancreatectomy and intraoperative radiotherapy (IORT). Formal evaluation of extended pancreatectomy in controlled clinical trials is underway.

Surgery With Intraoperative Radiotherapy

The failure of pancreaticoduodenectomy consistently to control local disease in pancreatic cancer has led to the search for effective strategies to improve local control. IORT allows a full therapeutic dose of radiation to be rapidly delivered directly to the operative bed at the time of surgical resection. The potential advantage of such a technique is that therapy can be delivered immediately to areas where tumor margins may be inadequate, to local lymphatics, and to areas where tumor cells may have been spilled during the course of resection. At the same time, radiation doses to surrounding normal areas are minimized.

The technique of IORT is straightforward. Doses of about 2000 cGy are delivered through lucite cones that are chosen to best approximate the size and contour of the operative bed. The cones also displace neighboring organs, such as the colon and stomach, away from the radiation field. IORT is most conveniently delivered in a shielded dedicated operating room suite. In such circumstances, the patient is monitored and anesthesia administered from a side observation room during the 15 minutes that radiation is administered. If no such suite is available, the patient must be transported after resection (with portable anesthesia equipment) to the radiotherapy area and then transported back to the operating room for construction of the surgical anastomoses and wound closure.

The use of IORT as an adjuvant to surgical resection has been relatively limited, and insufficient information exists to judge its value. At the National Cancer Institute, patients with stages II to IV resectable pancreatic cancer were randomly assigned to receive either 2000-cGy IORT or conventional external-beam therapy.[12] The operative mortality was unusually high in the IORT group (5 of 13 patients). Analysis of the entire group revealed no advantage to the IORT treatment over external-beam radiotherapy. It is hoped that further experience in other controlled trials will demonstrate whether IORT will be of greater benefit as an adjuvant to surgical resection than conventional radiotherapy.

Surgery With Postoperative or Preoperative Adjuvant Chemoradiotherapy

The use of adjuvant radiation and chemotherapy after apparently curative resection of pancreatic carcinoma has been carefully evaluated in controlled trials performed by the Gastrointestinal Tumor Study Group.[13] This group initially reported that the use of 5-fluorouracil (5-FU) and external-beam radiotherapy after resection resulted in a therapeutic benefit (Fig. 33-10). Median survival rates were 21 months in the treatment group and 11 months in the control group; 40% of patients who received adjuvant therapy survived 2 years, in contrast with 9% of patients who received no further therapy. This advantage was confirmed in a subsequent study. The toxicity of the 5-FU irradiation regimen is limited; patients in these trials experienced leukopenia (20% prevalence), mucositis, and diarrhea, but there were no life-threatening complications. Because of demonstrated efficacy and low toxicity, this therapy

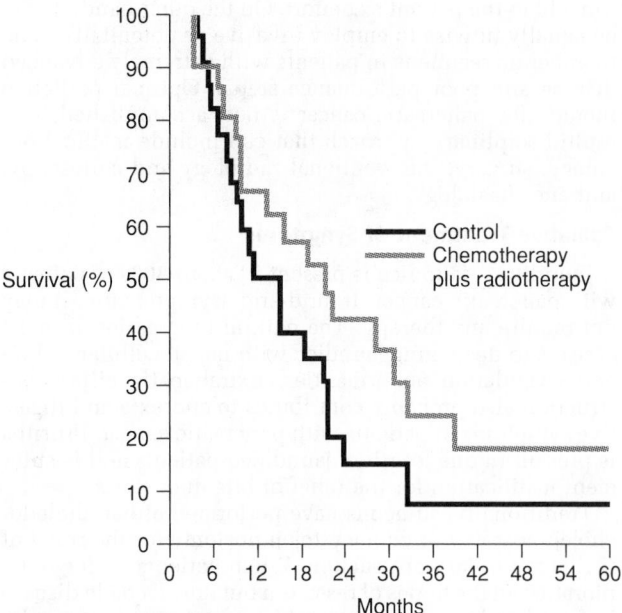

Figure 33-10. Comparison of survival in patients after resection of carcinoma of the pancreas who received either postoperative 5-fluorouracil and radiotherapy (21 patients) or no further treatment (22 patients). Survival was greater in the treated group than in the control group throughout the follow-up period ($P=.03$). (After Gastrointestinal Tumor Study Group, Ellenberg SS. Pancreatic cancer: adjuvant combined radiation and chemotherapy following curative resection. Arch Surg 1985;120:899)

should be advised for patients undergoing successful resection of a ductal carcinoma of the pancreas.

The rationale for preoperative chemoradiotherapy in pancreatic cancer arose from the observation in trials of postoperative therapy that many patients had radiotherapy delayed while recovering from surgery. The ability to palliate jaundice endoscopically has allowed patients with apparently resectable tumors to undergo preoperative treatment with 5-FU and radiotherapy, which nearly all patients are able to complete.[14] Patients are restaged after completion of radiotherapy. If no distant metastases are evident on restaging, laparotomy is performed; most of this selected group of patients have resectable tumors. Experience suggests that preoperative chemoradiotherapy is effective in preventing local recurrence and increases median survival to about two years, results similar to those with postoperative adjuvant therapy. Most patients ultimately fail systemically, and further improvements in adjuvant therapy need to be directed at the prevention of distant metastases.

Palliative Treatment of Pancreatic Carcinoma

Sadly, 85% to 90% of patients with pancreatic cancer have disease that is so extensive it precludes surgical resection. In addition, most patients who undergo apparently curative surgery eventually develop recurrent disease. Therefore, the palliative treatment of pancreatic cancer assumes the utmost clinical importance. General therapeutic guidelines are given later, but the appropriate palliative treatment of pancreatic cancer requires that the individual patient's outlook and clinical status be considered in the treatment decisions. Because of the generally poor prognosis of the disease, it is inappropriate to avoid therapy that can add to the patient's comfort. On the other hand, it may be equally unwise to employ invasive or potentially toxic therapeutic regimens in patients with extremely advanced disease and poor performance status. Optimal palliative therapy for pancreatic cancer is best accomplished by a multidisciplinary approach that can include medical oncology, surgery, interventional radiology and endoscopy, and anesthesiology.

Palliative Treatment of Symptoms

Jaundice. Jaundice is present in about 80% of patients with pancreatic cancer. If mild and asymptomatic, it may not require any therapy. The natural progression in most cases is to deepening jaundice with hepatocellular failure and coagulation abnormalities. Extrahepatic biliary obstruction also probably contributes to anorexia and digestive symptoms in patients with pancreatic cancer. Pruritus is present in one fourth of jaundiced patients and is sufficient justification for the relief of bile duct stasis.

Traditionally, surgeons have performed either choledochojejunostomy or cholecystojejunostomy for the relief of malignant biliary obstruction. When patients undergo exploration in the hopes of resection but unresectable disease is found, biliary bypass should be performed routinely. The jejunum is typically chosen as a conduit in preference to the duodenum because duodenal obstruction can occur as the tumor becomes more advanced. There has been much discussion about the use of the bile duct or the gallbladder for biliary decompression. Operative mortality and mean survival (about 6 months) do not differ between patients with cholecystojejunostomy and choledochojejunostomy.[15] Recurrent jaundice is more common after cholecystojejunostomy. Because recurrent jaundice constitutes a failure of palliation, the use of the common duct for biliary bypass is preferable in most patients. There are circumstances, however, in which it may be more appropriate to use the gallbladder. Such instances include patients with poor performance status, cases in which the tumor is bulky and invades the porta hepatis, or cases in which periductal varices have developed as a result of portal vein thrombosis. The suitability of the gallbladder as a biliary conduit must be proved intraoperatively. If, on aspiration, the gallbladder contains colorless fluid, the cystic duct can be assumed to be obstructed, and the gallbladder should be removed and not used for bypass. If there is green bile in the gallbladder, patency of the cystic duct should be proved by cholangiography before a bypass is performed. The cystic duct entrance into the bile duct should be at least 2 cm from any tumor. When such care is taken, cholecystojejunostomy provides adequate biliary decompression in 90% or more of patients so treated.

During the past several years, alternative nonsurgical techniques for the relief of biliary obstruction have been developed (Fig. 33-11). Either radiologic transhepatic drainage or retrograde endoscopic drainage can be successfully performed in most cases. The endoscopic route of placement appears to be superior to the transhepatic method when the two are compared directly and has become the preferred technique in most instances. If external transhepatic biliary drainage is performed radiologically, it is best, after a few days, to convert the external drain to an endoprosthesis so that the patient is not burdened with an external catheter.

Although endoscopic decompression of the bile duct can be accomplished initially in most patients, the durability of endoscopic stents is not as great as that of a surgically created bypass. The development of biliary sepsis and recurrent jaundice is more common in patients with stents in place than in surgically treated patients, and these episodes of sepsis frequently require hospitalization and stent

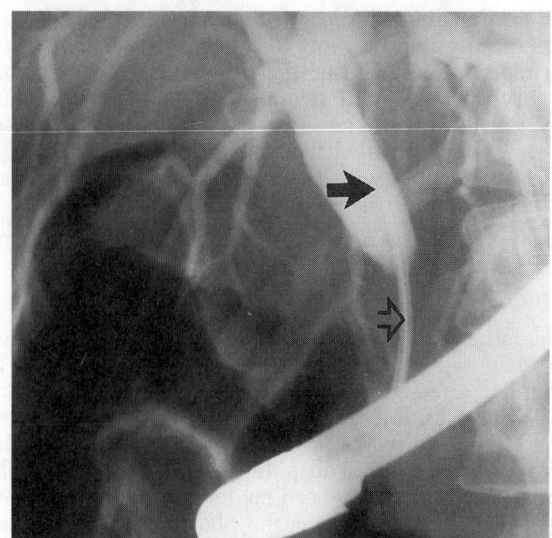

Figure 33-11. Endoscopic stent placement for common bile obstruction due to pancreatic cancer. A guide wire has been passed through the papilla of Vater and through the area of obstruction into the dilated common bile duct (*solid arrow*). A 10F plastic stent (*open arrow*) is piggybacked over the guidewire. The wire and endoscope are removed to complete the procedure.

changes that detract from the overall quality of palliation. On the other hand, the operation of choledochojejunostomy carries significant morbidity and mortality (about 20% of unselected patients die within 30 days of the procedure), and the nonsurgical methods of biliary decompression are generally associated with about 50% less initial mortality. Therefore, nonoperative methods are the best choice for patients with severe symptoms (eg, pruritus) but with advanced disease and poor performance status. Surgical bypass should be reserved for patients with an anticipated life expectancy of at least 3 months.

Vomiting and Duodenal Obstruction. Duodenal invasion of varying degree is present at the time of diagnosis in about one fourth of patients with pancreatic cancer. About 30% of all pancreatic cancer patients present with nausea and vomiting. Although it is not always possible to detect duodenal narrowing in these patients, many have motor abnormalities of the duodenum secondary to tumor involvement. In addition to patients who present with duodenal obstruction, 20% of patients treated with biliary bypass alone develop duodenal obstruction before death. There has been considerable debate about performing prophylactic gastroenterostomy in patients who do not demonstrate duodenal obstruction at the time of surgery. On the one hand, the performance of gastroenterostomy at the time of biliary bypass does not appear to add significantly to overall operative mortality, and the inclusion of gastroenterostomy avoids the necessity of a second operation in some patients. On the other hand, about 20% of patients experience prolonged delays in gastric emptying after gastroenterostomy, and this can be so protracted that it defeats the purpose of the operation. This is particularly the case in patients who are operated on with preexisting duodenal obstruction. The role of prophylactic gastroenterostomy thus remains controversial, but its routine use appears to be diminishing. It is certainly not indicated in asymptomatic patients whose jaundice is effectively palliated endoscopically. The incidence of marginal ulceration is low after gastroenterostomy; vagotomy is not recommended unless there is a history of ulcer diathesis.

Pain. Most patients with pancreatic cancer suffer from abdominal pain. It can be mild and manageable with oral medication, but 50% to 70% of patients ultimately develop moderate to severe pain that likely is due to invasion of retroperitoneal nerve trunks. Percutaneous chemical celiac plexus blockade in patients with advanced pancreatic cancer can provide substantial relief of pain. By infiltrating the retroperitoneal tissues around the body of the L-1 vertebra with 50 mL of 50% alcohol, it is possible to achieve good pain relief in 85% of patients; in about 75% of the successful cases, the relief lasts throughout the remainder of the patients' lives.[16] Ordinarily, a test block with local anesthetic is done 24 hours before the ablative block to determine whether a good response is likely. The most common complication is transient orthostatic hypotension lasting a few days, more common if patients have a history of hypertension or are hypovolemic. Although adverse neurologic sequelae have been reported, they are rare when careful technique is employed. Alcohol ablation of the celiac plexus at the time of surgery for biliary and gastric bypass can also be performed and has been shown to control pain effectively. The celiac plexus is located along the sides of the aorta just cephalad and posterior to the origin of the celiac artery and is directly injected by the surgeon.

Palliative Antineoplastic Therapy

5-Fluorouracil and External-Beam Radiotherapy. In a large controlled clinical trial,[17] the Gastrointestinal Tumor Study Group demonstrated that the combination of 5-FU and external-beam radiotherapy resulted in prolonged survival of patients with unresectable pancreatic cancer. Patients were randomly assigned to one of three treatment groups after exploration and surgical bypass: external-beam radiotherapy alone (6000 cGy), 5-FU plus 4000-cGy external-beam radiotherapy, or 5-FU plus 6000-cGy external-beam radiotherapy. The radiotherapy was administered in split courses of 2000 cGy each over 2 weeks, with 2-week rest periods between courses. The 5-FU was administered in a dose of 500 mg/m^2 on each of the first 3 days of each radiation cycle and then weekly after the completion of radiotherapy. The study demonstrated that patients who received combination therapy survived longer than patients who received radiotherapy alone, with median survival rates of 42 weeks for 5-FU with 4000 cGy, 40 weeks for 5-FU with 6000 cGy, and 23 weeks for 6000 cGy alone. External-beam radiotherapy and 5-FU should, therefore, be considered in all patients with unresectable disease. Although the toxicity of the regimen is mild, about 5% of patients develop severe thrombocytopenia or leukopenia. Nausea and vomiting are common. Because of toxic side effects, it may be inappropriate to recommend therapy for patients with widespread and extensive metastatic disease who have poor performance status.

Intraoperative Radiotherapy. It was hoped that IORT would be superior to external-beam radiotherapy for palliation of local disease in patients found to have unresectable pancreatic cancer. The potential advantage of IORT is the ability to deliver therapeutic doses of radiation to a narrow treatment port directly visualized at surgery and thus to avoid the morbidity of external-beam radiotherapy, which must be directed over a broader field. Early reports suggested that survival might be prolonged in comparison to historical controls, but a controlled trial failed to demonstrate any advantage of IORT over external-beam radiotherapy either in terms of survival or local disease control.[18] Other reports failed to demonstrate any survival advantage of IORT compared with concurrent nonrandomized patients receiving external-beam radiotherapy. Most groups evaluating IORT believe it has been effective in the amelio-

ration of pain, but the evidence suggests that IORT has little advantage over external-beam therapy in terms of tumor control.

OTHER EXOCRINE PANCREATIC NEOPLASMS

Solid and Cystic Tumor

Solid and cystic tumor of the pancreas is also referred to as *papillary–cystic neoplasm of the pancreas* or *papillary and solid neoplasm*. About 100 cases of this tumor have been reported, with a favorable outlook in comparison to many other pancreatic tumors.

Solid and cystic tumor is primarily a disease of adolescent and young women, with peak incidence between the ages of 10 and 35 years. Grossly, the tumors are rounded, soft, and light brown in color. The center of the tumor contains old blood and cystic spaces filled with necrotic debris. The rim of the tumor is fibrous and can contain calcifications. Histologically, the tumor consists of sheets of uniform cells with features of both endocrine and exocrine lineage, often arranged in pseudorosettes around fibrous stalks. The tumors are separated from surrounding normal pancreas by a fibrous capsule, but the capsule can be invaded by tumor. The histogenetic origin of the tumor is uncertain; it can arise from a primordial pancreatic stem cell. Reports indicate that some of the tumors have estrogen and progesterone receptors.

Solid and cystic tumors are usually large at the time of presentation, averaging 10 cm in diameter. Patients ordinarily present with an upper abdominal mass or abdominal pain. CT scanning is the most effective method for diagnosis, although findings are not specific. Scanning demonstrates a mass consisting of varying degrees of solid and liquefied material. Some tumors contain peripheral calcification. Despite the nonspecific appearance, a pancreatic mass of this sort in a young woman is most likely a solid and cystic tumor.

Treatment of solid and cystic tumor of the pancreas is surgical resection of the involved area of the pancreas. The tumors are most common in the tail of the gland, where they can be managed by distal pancreatectomy. The outlook after resection is good, and about 90% of patients appear to be cured by removal of the tumor.

Cystadenoma and Cystadenocarcinoma

Two uncommon cystic neoplasms of the pancreas have been described—serous cystadenoma (or microcystic adenoma) and mucinous cystic neoplasm (mucinous cystadenoma and mucinous cystadenocarcinoma). The distinction between the serous and mucinous types of cystic neoplasm is clinically significant because the serous variety is almost always a benign neoplasm, whereas the mucinous variety has clear malignant potential.

Serous Cystadenoma

Serous cystadenomas (Fig. 33-12) are usually large, well-circumscribed (average, 10 cm) tumors that occur most frequently in the body and tail of the pancreas. The tumors sometimes develop in the head of the pancreas and can present with obstructive jaundice owing to compression of the bile duct. They are slightly more common in women, and most occur in patients older than 50 years of age.

On cut section, the serous cystadenoma is multilocu-lated and consists of many small cysts ranging in diameter from 1 mm to 2 cm, arranged in a honeycomb pattern. The fluid in the cysts is clear and serous, and no mucin is

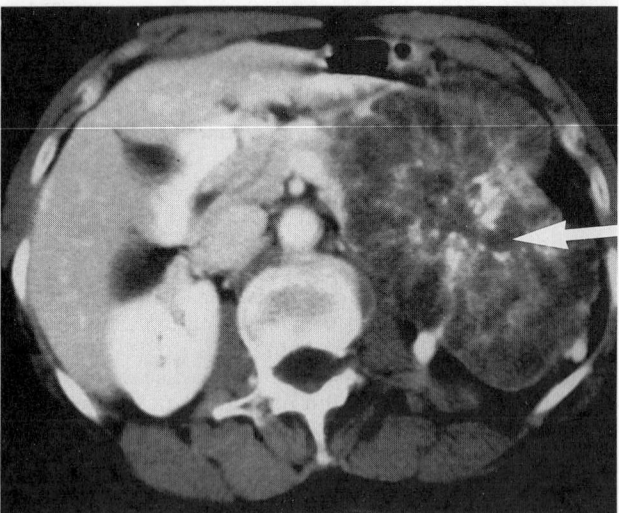

Figure 33-12. CT scan of large serous cystadenoma of the pancreas (*arrow*), demonstrating central stellate scar and tumor calcifications.

present. There is typically a stellate central core of fibrous tissue. Histologically, the tumor consists of multiple cystic spaces lined by bland cuboidal epithelium. The cells characteristically contain glycogen.

Serous cystadenoma usually presents as an abdominal mass or abdominal pain. The tumor also can be discovered as an incidental finding. CT scanning and ultrasonography are the most useful diagnostic tests and usually demonstrate a pancreatic mass. About 30% contain central calcifications. The cysts are often too small to appreciate radiologically. Serous cystadenoma is a benign neoplasm. Resection is usually indicated to differentiate the tumor from other, more dangerous pancreatic pathology, to eliminate discomfort, or occasionally to relieve biliary or intestinal obstruction. If removed with a small margin of surrounding normal pancreas, the tumor should not recur.

Mucinous Cystadenoma and Cystadenocarcinoma

In contrast to serous cystic neoplasms, the mucinous variety is potentially lethal. Nearly all cystic mucinous tumors of the pancreas contain at least focal areas of atypia

or frank carcinomatous transformation. Mucinous cystic neoplasms account for about 2% of pancreatic exocrine tumors.

The tumor occurs six times as often in females as in males. About 80% of the tumors are located in the body and tail of the pancreas. They present as large (average, 10 cm), soft, and somewhat irregular tumors. The cut appearance of the mucinous tumors is distinct from that of the serous cystic neoplasms in that the mucinous variety usually is unilocular or contains a few large cysts filled with thick mucus. There may be additional small cysts in the fibrous capsule of the tumor. Inspection of the lining of the large cyst cavities can reveal papillary epithelial ingrowths. Microscopically, the cysts are lined by columnar epithelium, which contains mucin. Although most of the cells may appear benign histologically, most tumors larger than 3 cm contain areas of premalignant or malignant change, and all mucinous cystic tumors should be considered to have malignant potential.

Most patients with mucinous cystic tumors present with abdominal pain or an abdominal mass. There may be associated weight loss, steatorrhea, or diabetes. The diagnosis is best made by CT and ultrasonography, which demonstrate a mass containing fluid-filled structures and internal septations (Fig. 33-13). Occasionally, it is possible to see the papillary tumor excrescences on the cyst walls. The fluid in mucinous tumors contains elevated levels of carcinoembryonic antigen, which may distinguish them from the serous variety. The proper treatment is surgical removal of the tumor; aggressive pancreatic resection, including pancreaticoduodenectomy, is appropriate. It is crucial to avoid mistaking a mucinous cystic tumor for a pancreatic pseudocyst. Internal drainage of a malignant mucinous cystic tumor results in catastrophic tumor dissemination and should never be performed. With appropriate treatment, all patients with histologically benign tumors should be cured; for tumors demonstrating malignant change, the 5-year survival rate after surgery is about 60%.

Pancreatic Lymphoma

Although lymphoma is not a pancreatic exocrine tumor in the true sense, it can arise in the pancreas and can present as a pancreatic mass lesion. About one third of all non-Hodgkin lymphomas include at least microscopic involvement of the pancreas, but the term *pancreatic*

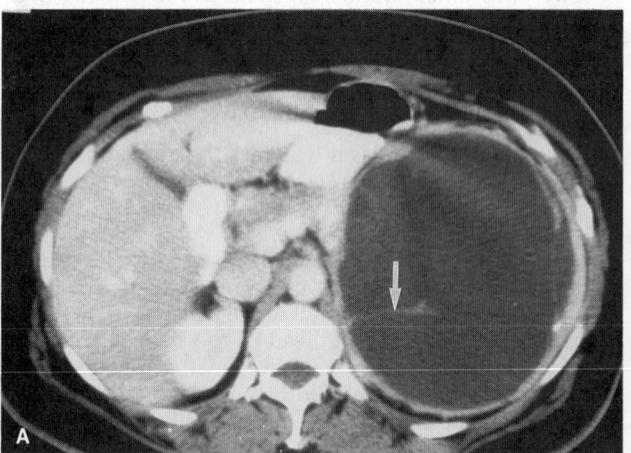
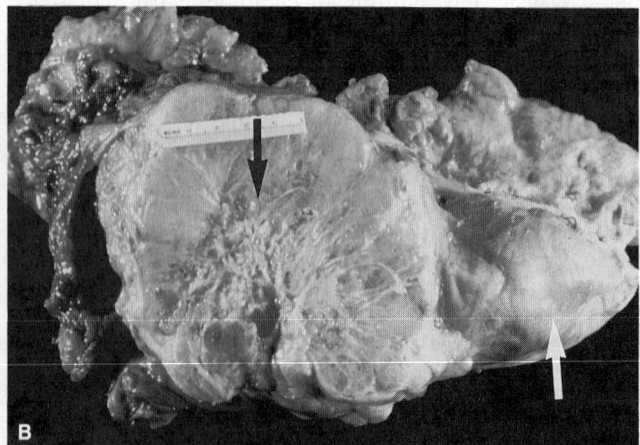

Figure 33-13. (*A*) CT scan appearance of mucinous cystadenocarcinoma of the pancreas. A large cyst with a single septation is visible (*arrow*). (*B*) A mucinous cystadenocarcinoma of the pancreas, which contains a large single cyst (*white arrow*) and an extensive solid component (*black arrow*).

lymphoma is reserved for those cases in which the lymphoma appears to have arisen in the pancreas and in which the bulk of the tumor burden is in the pancreas and peripancreatic tissues. Defined in this way, pancreatic lymphoma accounts for 1% to 2% of pancreatic neoplasms and about 1% of non-Hodgkin lymphomas.

Pancreatic lymphoma usually has a rapid onset, and the tumors attain large size quickly. At the time of presentation, pancreatic lymphomas are typically 6 to 10 cm. The clinical presentation is similar to that of ductal pancreatic cancer. Weight loss and jaundice are the most common symptoms. Pancreatic lymphoma may be difficult to distinguish from pancreatic carcinoma radiographically, except that the finding of a large tumor without vascular invasion and with extensive lymphadenopathy should raise the level of suspicion for lymphoma (Fig. 33-14).

When the diagnosis is suspected, percutaneous needle biopsy of the mass should be performed. If the diagnosis of lymphoma can be made unequivocally by percutaneous biopsy, and if there is sufficient tissue for cellular typing, laparotomy can be avoided because only rarely is it possible to resect the tumor, and jaundice usually resolves with chemotherapy. Most patients can be staged adequately with a CT scan and bone marrow biopsy. Surgical exploration is indicated if the diagnosis cannot be firmly established by needle biopsy, if additional tissue is believed necessary for adequate typing, or in the rare circumstance in which a small tumor might be completely resectable and the patient appears to have no disease outside the pancreas. Exploration for the purpose of biliary decompression alone is not ordinarily indicated. If the jaundiced patient is explored for another reason, cholecystojejunostomy is appropriate because the improvement in hepatic function allows the more rapid institution of multidrug chemotherapy. About half of patients undergo an initial complete remission with chemotherapy alone; long-term follow-up suggests, however, that most patients ultimately succumb to recurrent disease.

Other Pancreatic Exocrine Neoplasms

Because of the wide variety of cell types present in the normal pancreas, a broad spectrum of tumors can arise there. Among the many rare neoplasms of the exocrine pancreas is acinar cell carcinoma, which typically presents as a large tumor in the elderly. Some patients have an accompanying syndrome of metastatic fat necrosis with skin or bone and joint lesions, fever, and leukocytosis.

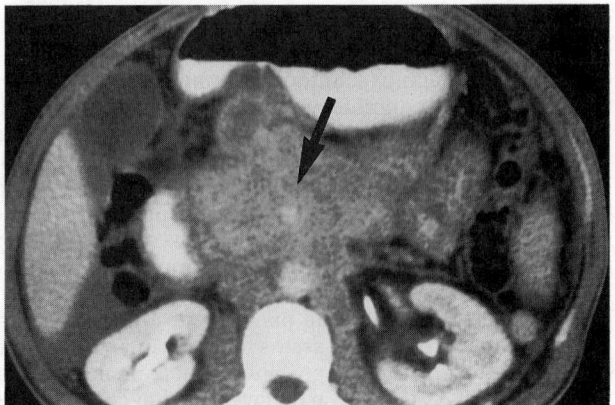

Figure 33-14. Pancreatic lymphoma. CT scan demonstrates a large mass virtually replacing the pancreas (*arrow*) and extensive peripancreatic lymphadenopathy.

Acinar tumors account for only about 1% of pancreatic exocrine neoplasms despite the fact that acinar cells are by far the most populous cell type of the normal pancreas. The rarity of acinar cell tumors is also surprising in view of the relative frequency of acinar tumors in some animal models of pancreatic cancer. Acinar cell tumors in humans can masquerade as islet tumors or undifferentiated tumors, but most form acinar structures and can be shown to contain zymogen granules by electron microscopy or to contain pancreatic enzymes by immunohistochemistry. The tumors are typically advanced at the time of presentation, with both lymphatic and hematogenous metastases present.

In addition to the usual moderately differentiated ductal tumors, other varieties of pancreatic carcinoma appear to arise from ductal epithelium. These include mucinous carcinoma, pleomorphic giant cell carcinoma, and adenosquamous carcinoma. Together they make up about 7% of pancreatic exocrine malignancies. They have no unique features from a diagnostic point of view, and their treatment and prognosis are similar to those of ductal carcinoma in general.

Although pancreatic exocrine neoplasms are rare in children, there are isolated reports of a tumor referred to as *pancreatoblastoma,* which contains both epithelial and mesenchymal elements. The epithelial component appears to arise from acinar cells. The tumors typically contain areas of degeneration and hemorrhage. Affected children usually present with an abdominal mass. CT scanning demonstrates a pancreatic mass that is not homogeneous. The tumors tend to be encapsulated, and the prognosis in the few cases reported appears to be favorable if the tumor can be resected. If nodal or hepatic metastases are present at presentation, the outlook is poor.

SUMMARY

The management of tumors of the exocrine pancreas remains a formidable problem. The last few years have seen improvement, particularly in the ability to detect pancreatic neoplasms radiologically but also in the safety of extirpative pancreatic surgery. Another important advance has been the firm demonstration that chemoradiotherapy is of value in the treatment of pancreatic cancer. The generally grim prognosis of pancreatic carcinoma relates primarily to the advanced stage of the tumors at the time of symptomatic presentation. The major challenges involve developing methods for earlier detection of pancreatic tumors, determining the optimal extent of surgery for pancreatic cancer, and developing adjunctive strategies to increase resectability and prevent tumor recurrence after surgery. Progress in meeting these goals has been slow, but some ground has been gained. In face of the increasing incidence of these tumors, it is important to continue to explore new possibilities in the hopes of further progress.

REFERENCES

1. Gudjonnson B. Cancer of the pancreas: 50 years of surgery. Cancer 1987;60:2284.
2. Whipple AO, Parsons WB, Mullins CR. Treatment of carcinoma of the ampulla of Vater. Ann Surg 1935;102:763.
3. Traverso LW, Longmire WP Jr. Preservation of the pylorus in pancreaticoduodenectomy. Surg Gynecol Obstet 1978;146:959.
4. Cameron JL, Crist DW, Sitzmann JV, et al. Factors influencing survival after pancreaticoduodenectomy for pancreatic cancer. Am J Surg 1991;161:120.
5. Trede M, Schwall G, Saeger HD. Survival after pancreatoduodenectomy. Ann Surg 1990;211:447.
6. Nitecki SS, Sarr MG, Colby TV, van Heerden JA. Long-term

survival after resection for ductal adenocarcinoma of the pancreas. Ann Surg 1995; 221:59.

7. Brooks JR, Brooks DC, Levine D. Total pancreatectomy for ductal carcinoma of the pancreas: an update. Ann Surg 1989;209:405.

8. Van Heerden JA, McIlrath DC, Ilstrup DM, Weiland LH. Total pancreatectomy for ductal adenocarcinoma of the pancreas: an update. World J Surg 1988;12:658.

9. Fortner JG. Regional pancreatectomy for cancer of the pancreas, ampulla, and other related sites: tumor staging and results. Ann Surg 1984;199:418.

10. Manabe T, Ohshio G, Baba N, et al. Radical pancreatectomy for ductal cell carcinoma of the head of the pancreas. Cancer 1989;64:1132.

11. Ishikawa O, Ohhigashi H, Sasaki Y, et al. Practical usefulness of lymphatic and connective tissue clearance for the carcinoma of the pancreas head. Ann Surg 1988;208:215.

12. Johnstone PA, Sindelar WF. Patterns of disease recurrence following definitive therapy of adenocarcinoma of the pancreas using surgery and adjuvant radiotherapy: correlations of a clinical trial. Int J Radiat Oncol Biol Phys 1993;27:831.

13. Kalser MH, Ellenberg SS. Pancreatic cancer: adjuvant combined radiation and chemotherapy following curative resection. Arch Surg 1985;120:899.

14. Rich TA, Evans DB. Preoperative combined modality therapy for pancreatic cancer. World J Surg 1995;19:264.

15. Sarr MG, Cameron JL. Surgical palliation of unresectable carcinoma of the pancreas. World J Surg 1984;8:906.

16. Brown DL, Bulley CK, Quiel EL. Neurolytic celiac plexus block for pancreatic cancer pain. Anesth Analg 1987;66:869.

17. Gastrointestinal Tumor Study Group. Therapy of locally unresectable pancreatic carcinoma: a randomized comparison of high-dose (6000 rad) radiation alone, moderate-dose radiation (4000 rad plus 5-fluorouracil), and high dose radiation plus 5-fluorouracil. Cancer 1981;48:1705.

18. Sindelar WF. Intraoperative radiotherapy in carcinoma of the stomach and pancreas. Recent Results Cancer Res 1988; 110:226.

SURGERY: SCIENTIFIC PRINCIPLES AND PRACTICE, Second Edition, edited by Lazar J. Greenfield, Michael W. Mulholland, Keith T. Oldham, Gerald B. Zelenock, and Keith D. Lillemoe. Lippincott–Raven Publishers, Philadelphia, © 1997.

CHAPTER 34

NEOPLASMS OF THE ENDOCRINE PANCREAS

CHARLES J. YEO

Neoplasms of the endocrine pancreas are rare, with an annual clinically recognized incidence in the United States of about 5 cases per million persons and per year. In unselected autopsy material, however, the prevalence of these tumors approximates 1 per 100 person-years and are typically noted as incidental findings. Cells of the pancreatic islets are presumed to originate from neural crest cells. Cells of this origin are called *amine precursor uptake and decarboxylation (APUD) cells*, indicating they have a high amine content of amine, are capable of amine precursor uptake, and contain an amino acid decarboxylase. A generalized derangement of the APUD system can cause abnormalities of multiple endocrine cells as is observed in multiple endocrine neoplasia (MEN) syndromes. Evidence suggests that some APUD cells may not originate from neural crest cells but rather have an endodermal origin.[1]

Neoplasms of the endocrine pancreas can be divided into functional and nonfunctional varieties. Most pancreatic endocrine neoplasms discovered clinically are functional, indicating that they elaborate one or more hormonal products into the blood, leading to a recognizable clinical syndrome. Functional tumors are named according to their predominate clinical syndrome and hormonal product (Table 34-1). Patients with endocrine tumors of the pancreas with no recognizable clinical syndrome and normal serum hormone levels (excluding pancreatic polypeptide) are considered to have nonfunctional pancreatic endocrine tumors.

All neoplasms of the endocrine pancreas have a similar light microscopic appearance. Routine histologic examination does not predict the biologic behavior or the endocrine manifestations of these neoplasms. Immunofluorescence techniques and the peroxidase-antiperoxidase procedure allow the demonstration of specific hormones within neoplastic cells. Malignancy is typically determined by the presence of local invasion that has spread to regional lymph nodes or by the existence of hepatic or distant metastases.

Recent observations in the fields of classic and molecular genetics have added to our knowledge of pancreatic endocrine neoplasms. For example, malignant pancreatic endocrine tumors have been found to have clonal chromosomal abnormalities in up to half of cases,[2] whereas *ras* oncogene mutations are absent in most of these tumors.[3] Gastrinoma has been shown to be associated with amplification of the *HER-2/neu* protooncogene,[4] and insulinoma has been shown to highly express mRNA for the a subunit of G_s protein.[5] Further, sporadic pancreatic endocrine tumors and tumors arising as a manifestation of MEN I have both been shown to have mutations leading to genetic loss on chromosome 11, thereby inactivating a putative tumor suppressor gene on that chromosome.[6]

Three general principles apply to the treatment of patients with suspected functional neoplasms of the endocrine pancreas. First is the recognition of the abnormal physiology or characteristic syndrome. Characteristic clinical syndromes are well described for insulinoma, gastrinoma, VIPoma, and glucagonoma. The somatostatinoma syndrome is nonspecific, much more difficult to recognize, and exceedingly rare. Second is the detection of hormone elevations in serum by radioimmunoassay. Radioimmunoassays are widely available for measuring insulin, gastrin, vasoactive intestinal peptide (VIP), and glucagon. Assays for somatostatin, pancreatic polypeptide, prostaglandins, and other hormonal markers are not widely available but can be obtained from certain laboratories and investigators. The third step in patient evaluation involves localizing and staging the tumor in preparation for possible operative intervention.

LOCALIZATION AND STAGING

The initial imaging technique recommended for localizing a pancreatic endocrine neoplasm is a dynamic abdominal computed tomographic (CT) scan with intravenous and oral contrast.[7-10] The accuracy of CT in detecting the primary islet cell tumor varies from about 35% to 85% and depends largely on the scanning technique and the size and location of the primary tumor (Fig. 34-1). The accuracy of the CT scan in tumor localization is improved by using both oral and intravenous contrast as well as focused dynamic scanning through the pancreas at 5-mm intervals. The CT scan is also used to assess for peripancreatic lymph node enlargement and the presence of hepatic metastases.

Should the CT scan fail to detect the primary tumor, the next step in radiograpic assessment is visceral angiography, focusing on the selective visualization of the arterial supply to the pancreas and peripancreatic regions.[11] The

Table 34-1. CLASSIFICATION OF FUNCTIONAL PANCREATIC ENDOCRINE TUMORS

Tumor (Syndrome)	Clinical Features	Extrapancreatic Location	Malignancy Rate
Insulinoma	Hypoglycemia	Rare	10%
Gastrinoma (Zollinger-Ellison)	Peptic ulcer Diarrhea	Frequent	50%
VIPoma (Verner-Morrison; watery diarrhea, hypokalemia, achlorhydria or hypochloride; pancreatic cholera)	Watery diarrhea Hypokalemia Achlorhydria	10%	Most
Glucagonoma	Hyperglycemia Dermatitis	Rare	Most
Somatostatinoma	Hyperglycemia Steatorrhea Gallstones	Rare	Most

accuracy of angiography in detecting the primary islet cell tumor varies from 45% to 85%, depending on radiographic technique and expertise, the selectivity of the contrast injection, and the size and neovascularity of the primary tumor (Fig. 34-2).

A newer technique that has shown clear promise for improving the preoperative localization of pancreatic endocrine neoplasms is endoscopic ultrasonography.[12-14] Rosch and colleagues[13] were able to correctly localize 32 of 39 tumors (82%) using endoscopic ultrasound after a CT scan had failed to locate the tumor (Fig. 34-3). In their experience, endoscopic ultrasonography was more sensitive than the combination of CT and visceral angiography. With further experience, endoscopic ultrasound may offer distinct advantages in evaluating patients with pancreatic endocrine neoplasms.

Another technique that holds promise for the imaging of pancreatic endocrine tumors is somatostatin receptor imaging. Early experience using whole body radionuclide scanning with iodine-labeled tyrosine³-octreotide has been reported with favorable results.[15] Additional studies have been reported using indium-labeled pentetreotide, an octreotide analogue.[16,17] These techniques rely on the presence of somatostatin receptors on many islet cell tumors[18] and have the potential to identify primary tumors as well as hepatic and extrahepatic metastases. A modification of the whole body technique has also been evaluated, using

a hand-held gamma-detecting probe intraoperatively along with intravenous injection of ¹²⁵I-tyrosine³-octreotide or lanreotide.[19,20] In addition to somatostatin-receptor imaging, the use of VIP-receptor imaging has been recently reported for patients with pancreatic endocrine neoplasms.[21]

In a minority of patients with pancreatic endocrine neoplasms, the primary tumor is not be localized with initial imaging studies such as CT, visceral angiography, or endoscopic ultrasound. This is most common in patients with insulinoma or gastrinoma. In these cases, performing selective transhepatic portal venous hormone sampling may help to assist in localizing the occult neoplasm.[22-26] This invasive technique is designed to demonstrate an increase in hormone concentration at the site where the tumor drains its hormonal product into the portal venous system (Fig. 34-4). The results of portal venous hormone sampling are used to define the region of the pancreas (or duodenum in the case of gastrinoma) that harbors the occult tumor. The overall accuracy of this test ranges from 70% to higher than 95% and depends on factors such as the number of portal venous samples obtained, the persistent autonomous production of the hormone by the tumor, and the careful handling and assaying of all specimens.

In addition to selective transhepatic portal venous hormone sampling, a newer technique has been described for localizing occult gastrinomas. This is called the *selective*

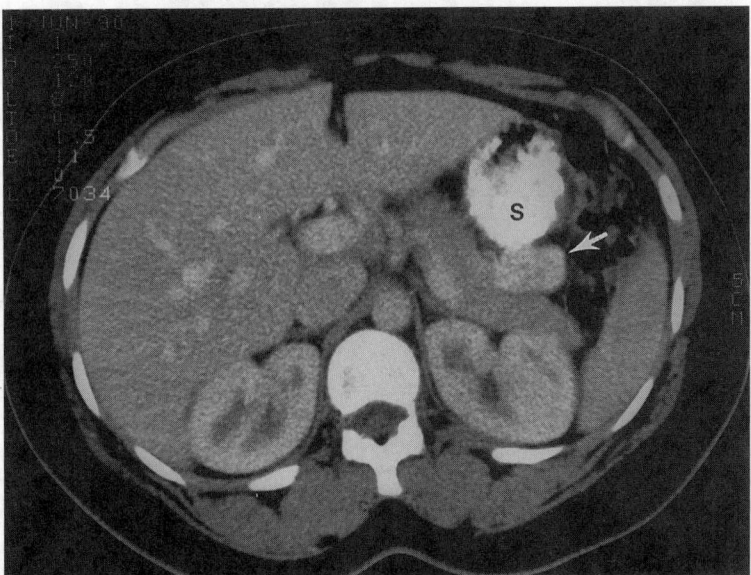

Figure 34-1. CT scan with oral and intravenous contrast in a patient with biochemical evidence of insulinoma. The neoplasm (*arrow*) is seen as a contrast-enhancing structure, 3 cm in diameter in the tail of the pancreas, posterior to the stomach (S). (Yeo CJ. Islet cell tumors of the pancreas. In: Niederhuber JE, ed. Current therapy in oncology. St Louis, Mosby– Year Book, 1993:272)

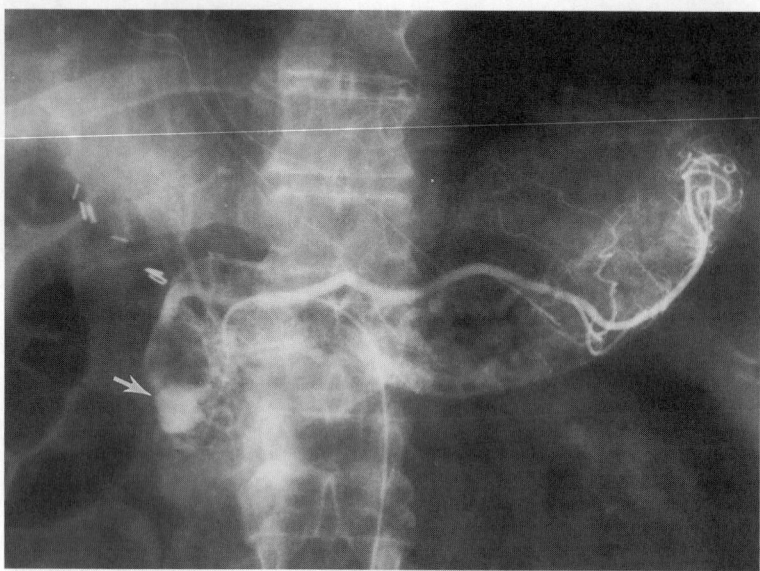

Figure 34-2. Selective celiac angiogram in a patient with gastrinoma. During the late phase of the angiogram a 2-cm neoplasm is demonstrated as a vascular blush (*arrow*). (Yeo CJ. Islet cell tumors of the pancreas. In: Niederhuber JE, ed. Current therapy in oncology. St Louis, Mosby–Year Book, 1993:272)

arterial secretin stimulation test. It involves selective visceral arterial secretin injection with concurrent hepatic venous sampling for gastrin.[27,28] This technique takes advantage of the unique biology of gastrinoma, in that gastrinoma cells are known to respond both in vitro and in vivo to secretin with the release of gastrin.[29,30] Secretin is serially injected through an arterial catheter into at least three sites—the splenic, gastroduodenal, and inferior pancreaticoduodenal arteries. Samples are drawn from an hepatic vein catheter before and immediately after these three or more arterial secretin injections. The arterial supply to the occult gastrinoma can be determined based on which selective secretin injection is followed by a large increment in hepatic vein gastrin concentration (Fig. 34-5). Using this

technique, the gastrinoma can be regionally localized either either within the duodenum and the head of the pancreas or, more uncommonly, in the body or tail of the pancreas. A recent prospective study compared selective transhepatic portal venous gastrin sampling with the selective arterial secretin stimulation test in 36 patients with gastrinoma.[31] In this study, the selective arterial secretin stimulation test was more sensitive than portal venous sampling in localizing gastrinomas, particularly small gastrinomas arising in the duodenum.

SURGICAL EXPLORATION

At the time of surgical exploration for pancreatic endocrine neoplasm, a complete evaluation of the pancreas and peripancreatic regions is performed. The body and tail of the pancreas are exposed by dividing the gastrocolic ligament. This portion of the pancreas can be partially elevated

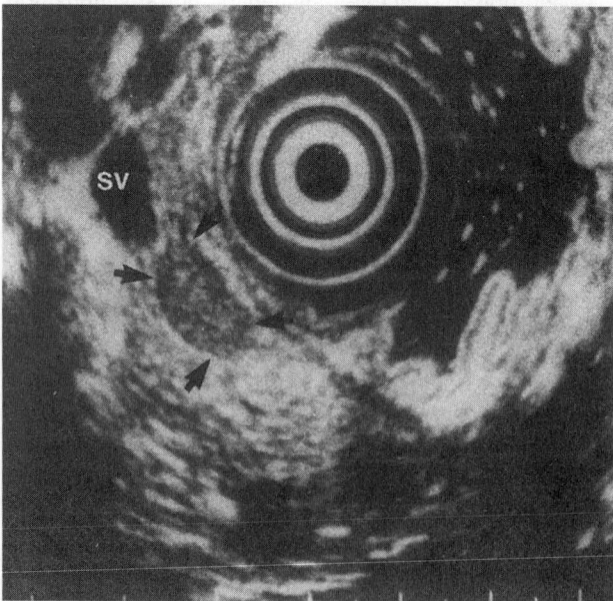

Figure 34-3. Endoscopic ultrasound image in a patient with an insulinoma (*arrows*) in the body of the pancreas. SV, splenic vein. (Rosch T, Lightdale CJ, Botet JF, et al. Localization of pancreatic endocrine tumors by endoscopic ultrasonography. N Engl J Med 1992;326:1721)

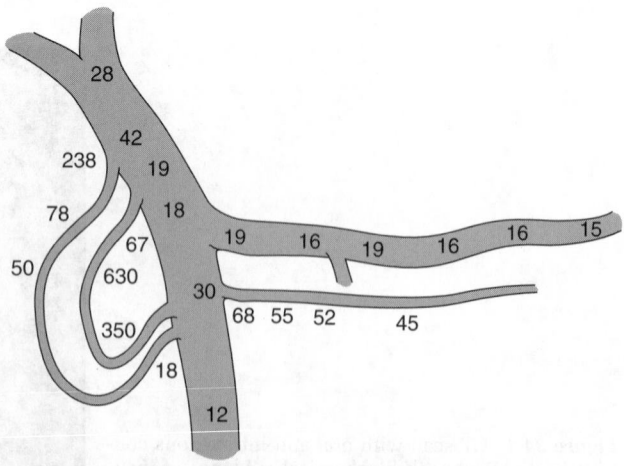

Figure 34-4. Schematic depiction of data from transhepatic portal venous insulin sampling in a patient with an insulinoma. Insulin levels are given in μU/mL. These data localize the neoplasm to the head of the pancreas. (After Norton JA, Sigel B, Baker AR, et al. Localization of an occult insulinoma by intraoperative ultrasonography. Surgery 1985;97:381)

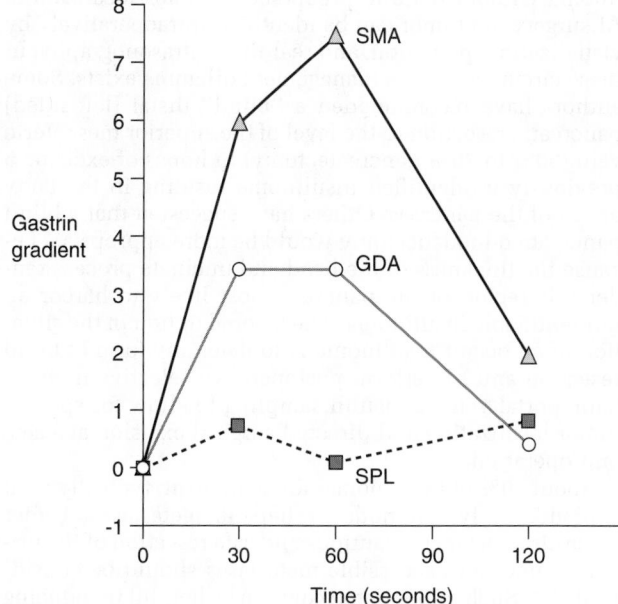

Figure 34-5. Graphic depiction of the results of a selective arterial secretin stimulation test in a patient with gastrinoma. The Y axis plots the rise in hepatic vein gastrin concentration (gastrin gradient) compared with basal values plotted on the X axis: 1 = 100% rise; 2 = 200% rise; and so forth. A rise in the hepatic vein gastrin concentration is observed following superior mesenteric artery (SMA) and gastroduodenal artery (GDA) secretin injections, localizing the neoplasm to the head of the pancreas or duodenum. SPL, splenic artery. (After Thom AK, Norton JA, Doppman JL, et al. Prospective study of the use of intraarterial secretin injection and portal venous sampling to localize duodenal gastrinomas. Surgery 1992;112:1002)

out of the retroperitoneum by dividing the inferior retroperitoneal attachments to the gland. After elevating the second portion of the duodenum out of the retroperitoneum using the Kocher maneuver, the pancreatic head and uncinate process are palpated bimanually. The liver is carefully assessed for evidence of metastatic disease. Potential extrapancreatic sites of tumor are evaluated in all cases, with particular attention paid to the duodenum, splenic hilum, small intestine and its mesentery, peripancreatic lymph nodes and the reproductive tract in women. One technique that provides additional information in the intraoperative setting is real-time ultrasonography, which can assist in tumor identification.[32,33] The goals of surgical therapy for pancreatic endocrine neoplasms include controlling symptoms from hormone excess, safely resecting maximal tumor mass, and preserving maximal pancreatic parenchyma. Management strategies, including preoperative, intraoperative, and postoperative considerations, vary for the different types of endocrine neoplasms of the pancreas.

INSULINOMA

Insulinoma is the most common neoplasm of the endocrine pancreas. The insulinoma syndrome is associated with the following, known as the Whipple triad: (1) symptoms of hypoglycemia during fasting; (2) documentation of hypoglycemia with serum glucose less than 50 mg/dL; and (3) relief of hypoglycemic symptoms following administration of exogenous glucose.[34] Autonomous insulin secretion from insulinomas leads to spontaneous hypoglycemia, with symptoms that can be characterized into two

groups (Table 34-2). Neuroglycopenic symptoms include confusion, seizure, obtundation, personality change, and coma. Hypoglycemia-induced catecholamine-surge symptoms include palpitations, trembling, diaphoresis, and tachycardia. In most cases, patients consume carbohydrate-rich meals and snacks to relieve or prevent these symptoms.

The Whipple triad is not specific for insulinoma. The differential diagnosis of adult hypoglycemia is extensive and includes the following:

- Reactive hypoglycemia
- Functional hypoglycemia associated with gastrectomy or gastroenterostomy
- Nonpancreatic tumors
    Pleural mesothelioma
    Sarcoma
    Adrenal carcinoma
    Hepatocellular carcinoma
    Carcinoid
- Hypopituitarism
- Chronic adrenal insufficiency
- Extensive hepatic insufficiency
- Surreptitious administration of insulin or ingestion of oral hypoglycemic agents

In some cases, nonendocrine tumors cause hypoglycemia,[35] with recent evidence implicating insulin-like growth factor II as one humoral causative factor.[36] Reactive hypoglycemia is the most common type of hypoglycemia, inducing symptoms of hypoglycemia 3 to 5 hours after meals, not typically after long periods of fasting.

A common mistake made in evaluating a patient with suspected insulinoma is to begin with an oral glucose tolerance test. Instead, insulinoma is most reliably diagnosed using a monitored fast. During a monitored fast, blood is sampled every 4 to 6 hours for glucose and insulin determinations and also at the time of symptom occurrence. Hypoglycemic symptoms typically occur when glucose levels are below 50 mg/dL, with concurrent serum insulin levels often exceeding 25 μU/mL. Additional support for the diagnosis of insulinoma comes from the calculation of the insulin/glucose ratio at different points during the monitored fast. Normal persons have insulin/glucose ratios less than 0.3, whereas patients with insulinoma typically demonstrate insulin/glucose ratios greater than 0.4 after a prolonged fast. Other measurable β-cell products synthesized in excess in patients with insulinoma include C peptide and proinsulin. Elevated levels of both are typically found in the peripheral blood of patients with insulinoma.

The possibility of surreptitious insulin or oral hypoglycemic agent administration should be considered in all patients with suspected insulinoma. C-peptide and proinsulin levels are not elevated in patients who self-adminis-

Table 34-2. **INSULINOMA**

Parameter	Description
Symptoms	
Neuroglycopenia causes	Confusion, personality change, coma
Catecholamine surge causes	Trembling, diaphoresis, tachycardia
Diagnostic tests	Monitored fast
	Insulin/glucose ratio
	C-peptide and proinsulin blood levels
Anatomic localization	Evenly distributed throughout pancreas

ter insulin. Additionally, patients self-administering either bovine or porcine insulin may demonstrate antiinsulin antibodies in circulating blood. Further, the presence of oral hypoglycemic agents such as sulfonylureas can be assessed using standard toxicologic screening.

After confirming the diagnosis of insulinoma by biochemical analyses, the appropriate localization and staging studies described earlier are performed. For insulinoma, the standard imaging studies include abdominal CT, endoscopic ultrasound, and visceral angiography. The treatment of insulinoma is surgical in nearly all cases. Insulinomas are found evenly distributed in the pancreas, with one third found in the head and uncinate process, one third in the body, and one third in the tail of the gland.[37] Of patients diagnosed with insulinoma, 90% are found to have benign solitary adenomas amenable to surgical cure. Less than 10% of patients with insulinoma have some form of the MEN I syndrome. In patients with MEN I, the possibility of multiple insulinomas must be suspected, and the recurrence rate is higher than in sporadic cases.[38] In about 10% of all cases, insulinoma is metastatic to peripancreatic lymph nodes or to the liver, justifying a diagnosis of malignant insulinoma.

During surgical exploration, the pancreas is assessed not only by operative palpation but also by intraoperative real-time ultrasonography to more thoroughly evaluate the entire pancreas and to search for the site of the primary tumor.[32,33] Small benign insulinomas not close to the main pancreatic duct can be removed by enucleation,[39] independent of their location in the gland (Fig. 34-6). In the body and tail of the pancreas, insulinomas more than 2 cm in diameter and those close to the pancreatic duct are most commonly excised by distal pancreatectomy. Large insulinomas deep in the head or uncinate process of the pancreas may not be amenable to local excision and may require pancreaticoduodenectomy.[40]

In rare instances, patients undergo exploration for insulinoma without definite preoperative tumor localization. At surgery, no tumor can be identified intraoperatively by visualization, palpation, and real-time ultrasonography. In these circumstances, a management dilemma exists. Some authors have recommended a "blind" distal (left-sided) pancreatic resection to the level of the superior mesenteric vein (60% to 70% pancreatectomy) in hopes of excising a previously unidentified insulinoma residing in the body or tail of the pancreas. Others have suggested that a blind pancreaticoduodenectomy would be more appropriate because the thickness of the head and uncinate process render this region of the pancreas most likely to harbor an unidentifiable insulinoma. The favored option in the situation of an occult insulinoma is to defer any form of blind resection and to perform postoperative selective transhepatic portal venous insulin sampling to allow for specific tumor localization and directed surgical excision at a second operation.[41]

About 10% of insulinomas are malignant, typically with evidence of lymph node or hepatic metastases. Under these circumstances, cautious and safe resection of the primary tumor and accessible metastases should be considered.[42–44] Such tumor debulking can be helpful in reducing hypoglycemic symptoms that can threaten long-term survival. The average patient survives several years after diagnosis and treatment of malignant islet cell tumors, indicating that the natural history of these malignant tumors typically follows an indolent course.[10,45] In patients with unresectable insulinoma, dietary manipulations to include judicious spacing of carbohydrate-rich meals and nighttime snacks can be helpful to minimize dangerous hypoglycemic episodes. Medications such as diazoxide and octreotide can be used to inhibit insulin release, raise serum glucose, and further minimize hypoglycemia. Chemotherapeutic agents with some efficacy against malignant insulinoma include streptozocin, dacarbazine, doxorubicin

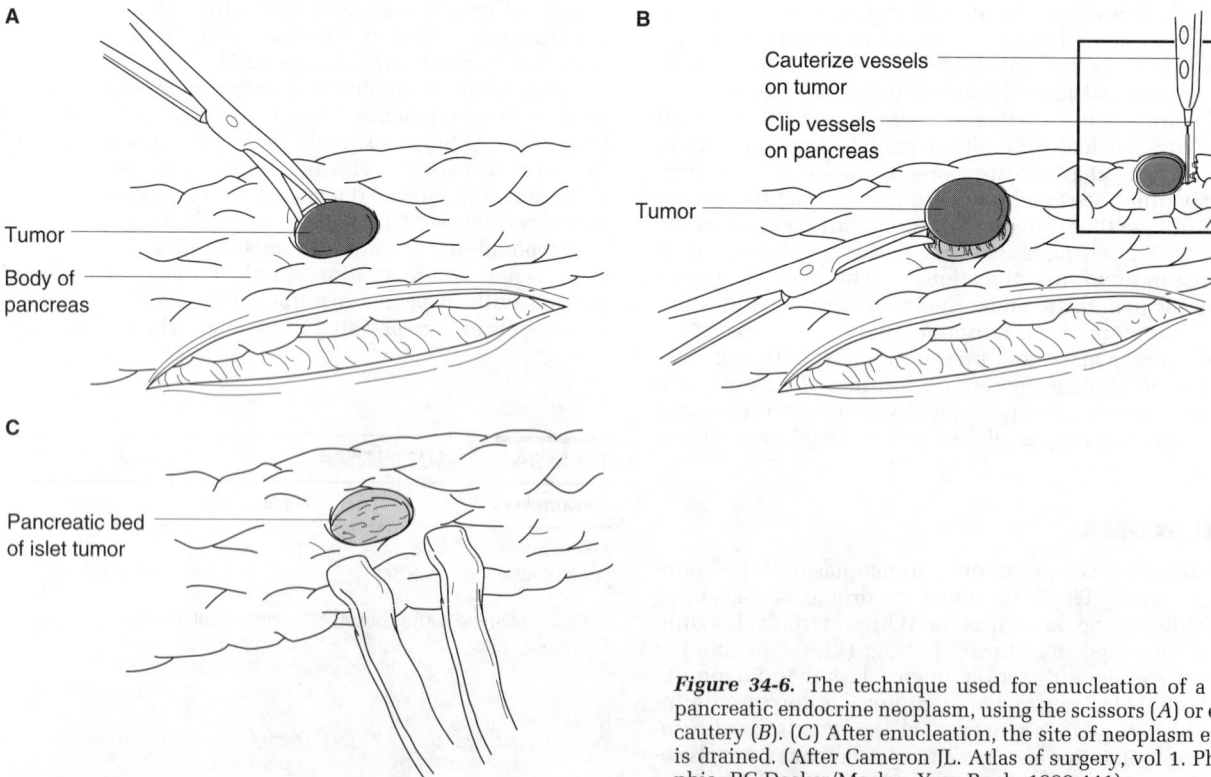

Figure 34-6. The technique used for enucleation of a benign pancreatic endocrine neoplasm, using the scissors (*A*) or electrocautery (*B*). (*C*) After enucleation, the site of neoplasm excision is drained. (After Cameron JL. Atlas of surgery, vol 1. Philadelphia, BC Decker/Mosby–Year Book, 1990:441)

Table 34-3. GASTRINOMA

Parameter	Description
Symptoms	Peptic ulcer disease
	Diarrhea
	Esophagitis
Diagnostic tests	Serum gastrin measurement
	Gastric acid analysis
	Secretin stimulation test
Anatomic localization	Duodenum and head of pancreas (gastrinoma triangle)

and 5-fluorouracil.[46-48] The highest response rates to chemotherapy have been observed using combination therapy.

GASTRINOMA (ZOLLINGER-ELLISON SYNDROME)

In 1955, Zollinger and Ellison described two patients with severe peptic ulcer disease and pancreatic endocrine tumors, postulating that an ulcerogenic agent originated from the pancreatic tumor.[49,50] It is currently estimated that 1 in 1000 patients with primary duodenal ulcer disease and 2 in 100 patients with recurrent ulcer after ulcer surgery harbor gastrinomas.[51] Seventy-five percent of gastrinomas occur sporadically, and 25% are associated with the MEN I syndrome. In the past, most gastrinomas were found to be malignant, based on the findings of metastatic disease at the time of workup or exploration. More recently, with increased awareness and earlier screening for hypergastrinemia, the diagnosis of gastrinoma is made earlier, leading to the discovery of a higher percentage of benign, curable neoplasms.[52,53] The clinical symptoms of patients with gastrinoma are a direct result of the circulating hypergastrinemia (Table 34-3). Abdominal pain and peptic ulceration of the upper gastrointestinal tract are seen in up to 90% of patients. Fifty percent of patients have some degree of diarrhea, and about 10% have diarrhea as the solitary symptom. Esophageal symptoms or endoscopic abnormalities from gastroesophageal reflux are seen in over 50% of patients, with esophagitis typically occurring in association with peptic ulcer disease or diarrhea.[54]

The diagnosis of gastrinoma should be suspected in several clinical settings, and the liberal use of serum gastrin measurement for screening is encouraged. The indications for measuring gastrin include the following:

- Peptic ulcer disease
  Initial diagnosis
  Recurrent ulcer
  Failure of medical therapy
  Postoperative ulcer
  Postbulbar ulcer
  Family history of ulcer disease
  Ulcer with diarrhea
- Prolonged undiagnosed diarrhea
- MEN I kindred
- Nongastrinoma pancreatic endocrine tumor (because of the high association of secondary hormone elevations)[55,56]
- Prominent gastric rugal folds on upper gastrointestinal series (reflecting the trophic effect of gastrin on the gastric fundus)

In most patients with gastrinomas, the fasting serum gastrin level is elevated to at least 200 pg/mL. Gastrin values over 1000 pg/mL are virtually diagnostic of gastrinoma, particularly when they are accompanied by hyperchlorhy-

dria or well-established ulcer disease. Fasting hypergastrinemia alone, however, is not sufficient for the diagnosis of gastrinoma. This is because hypergastrinemia can exist in other pathophysiologic states, since gastrin is the normal secretory product of antral G cells (Table 34-4). Gastric acid analysis is an important test in evaluating patients with suspected gastrinoma, because it can differentiate between ulcerogenic (high gastric acid) causes of hypergastrinemia and nonulcerogenic (low gastric acid) causes of hypergastrinemia. To obtain an accurate gastric acid analysis, patients must abstain from antisecretory medications, such as H_2 antagonists or omeprazole. The diagnosis of gastrinoma is supported by a basal acid output higher than 15 mEq/h in nonoperated patients, a basal acid output that exceeds 5 mEq/h in patients with previous vagotomy or antiulcer operations, or a ratio of basal to maximal acid output that exceeds 0.6.

Once it is documented that hypergastrinemia is associated with excessive acid secretion, provocative testing using secretin should be performed to differentiate between gastrinoma, antral G-cell hyperplasia or hyperfunction, and the other causes of ulcerogenic hypergastrinemia. The secretin stimulation test is done in the fasting state by obtaining peripheral serum samples for gastrin in the basal period, administering secretin, 2 U/kg, as an intravenous bolus, and obtaining serum samples for gastrin at 5-minute intervals for 30 minutes. An increase in the gastrin level of more than 200 pg/mL above the basal level supports the diagnosis of gastrinoma (Fig. 34-7). This conventional secretin stimulation test done on peripheral blood differs markedly from the doubly invasive selective arterial secretin stimulation test that is designed to localize the site of the primary tumor in patients with gastrinomas that have already been proved by biochemical testing.

After the biochemical confirmation of the diagnosis of gastrinoma, two steps are important in patient treatment. First, gastric acid hypersecretion is pharmacologically controlled. Omeprazole, 20 to 200 mg/d, is now considered the drug of choice for antisecretory therapy in patients with gastrinoma.[57,58] The dose is adjusted to achieve a nonacidic gastric pH during the hour immediately before the next dose of the drug. Second, after the initiation of omeprazole therapy, all patients with gastrinomas should undergo imaging studies to localize the primary tumor and to assess for metastatic disease. The modalities appropriate for localization and staging of gastrinoma patients have already been discussed and include dynamic abdominal CT scanning with intravenous and oral contrast, selective visceral angiography, endoscopic ultrasonography, somatostatin receptor imaging, percutaneous transhepatic portal venous sampling for gastrin, and the selective arterial secretin stimulation test.

Table 34-4. DISEASE STATES ASSOCIATED WITH HYPERGASTRINEMIA

NONULCEROGENIC CAUSES (NORMAL TO LOW ACID SECRETION)
Atrophic gastritis
Pernicious anemia
Previous vagotomy
Renal failure
Short-gut syndrome

ULCEROGENIC CAUSES (EXCESS ACID SECRETION)
Antral G-cell hyperplasia or hyperfunction
Gastric outlet obstruction
Retained excluded antrum
Zollinger-Ellison syndrome

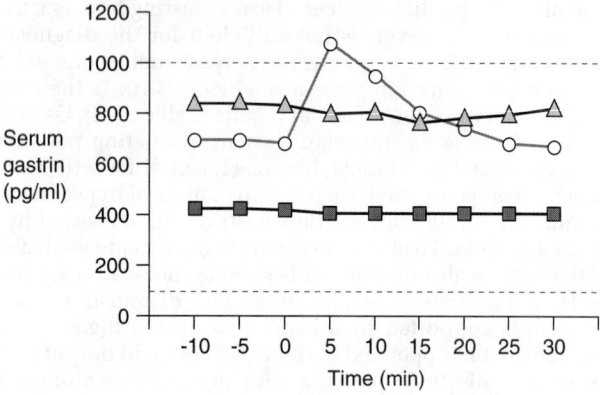

Figure 34-7. Results of intravenous secretin stimulation tests in patients with atrophic gastritis (*triangles*), gastric outlet obstruction (*squares*), and gastrinoma (*circles*). A positive test, consistent with the presence of gastrinoma, is indicated by an increase over basal serum gastrin levels of at least 200 pg/mL. (After Wolfe MM, Jensen RT. Zollinger-Ellison syndrome: current concepts in diagnosis and management. N Engl J Med 1987;317:1200)

Patients whose localization and staging studies indicate unresectable hepatic metastases should undergo percutaneous or laparoscopically directed liver biopsy for absolute histologic verification. If unresectable gastrinoma is confirmed, open surgical exploration is not performed, and the patient is maintained on long-term omeprazole therapy. Virtually all patients can be rendered achlorhydric with an appropriate dose of omeprazole. Noncompliant patients who refuse to take appropriate doses of omeprazole and who experience complications related to their ulcer diathesis may require total gastrectomy. Total gastrectomy removes the end organ (parietal cell mass) and was once the procedure of choice for gastrinoma. Today, its use in patients with gastrinomas has markedly declined.

In most patients, unresectable disease is not identified by staging studies, and patients should be offered surgical exploration with curative intent. At the time of exploration, the entire abdomen is carefully assessed for areas of extrapancreatic and extraduodenal gastrinoma.[59] Most gastrinomas are found to the right of the superior mesenteric vessels, in the head of the pancreas or the duodenum. This area is called the *gastrinoma triangle*[37,60] (Fig. 34-8). Intraoperative ultrasonography should be available to assist in tumor localization. In addition, intraoperative upper endoscopy may help by allowing transillumination of the duodenal wall and identification of small duodenal gastrinomas.[61,62] At exploration, any suspicious peripancreatic lymph nodes are excised and submitted for frozen section. Primary tumors located in the substance of the pancreas that are small (less than 2 cm) and well-encapsulated can be carefully enucleated. Pancreatic tumors without defined capsules or that are situated deep in the pancreatic parenchyma may require partial pancreatic resection by either distal pancreatectomy or pancreaticoduodenectomy.[40,63] In the absence of an identifiable pancreatic or duodenal tumor, a longitudinal duodenotomy can be performed at the level of the second portion of the duodenum to allow for eversion of the duodenum in a search for duodenal microgastrinomas.[61,64] Primary gastrinomas identified in the duodenal wall are resected locally with primary closure of the duodenal defect.[65,66] In a small percentage of patients, gastrinoma is found only in peripancreatic lymph nodes, with these lymph nodes harboring the primary tumor. Resection of these apparent lymph node primary gastrinomas has been associated with long-

term eugastrinemia and biochemical cure in up to half of cases.[67]

Occasionally, preoperative localization studies, such as portal venous gastrin sampling or the selective arterial secretin stimulation test, localize the tumor in the gastrinoma triangle; however, no tumor may be demonstrable at laparotomy. In the face of such a negative exploration, several surgical options are available. First, parietal cell vagotomy has been proposed as a way to reduce antisecretory drug dose requirements in patients on high-dose antisecretory drug therapy but without prior life-threatening complications.[68] The usefulness of parietal cell vagotomy in decreasing dose requirements has not been well established in patients treated with omeprazole, however, and such an operative procedure leaves behind potentially resectable gastrinoma. For these reasons, parietal cell vagotomy has lost favor as an option. The second surgical option for patients with negative results on exploration is total gastrectomy. Although total gastrectomy was the most reliable way to control ulcer diathesis in the past,[69] the introduction and availability of omeprazole has drastically reduced the need for total gastrectomy. There may still be a limited role for total gastrectomy in patients whose tumors cannot be localized if they cannot or will not take adequate doses of omeprazole. Unfortunately, like parietal cell vagotomy, total gastrectomy leaves the primary tumor behind with the potential for subsequent tumor growth, metastases, and patient death from tumor burden. A third, albeit controversial, surgical option in patients with clear-cut biochemical documentation of hypergastrinemia, hyperchlorhydria, and tumor localization in the gastrinoma triangle involves blind pancreaticoduodenectomy. In a small number of patients, these blind resections have yielded pathologically verified primary gastrinomas in the duodenal wall or the head of the pancreas which were not apparent at laparotomy. Blind resections should be performed as classic pancreaticoduodenectomies, including a distal gastric resection, because duodenal gastrinomas may arise close to the pylorus and be inadvertently left behind with pylorus-sparing pancreaticoduodenectomy. In a limited number of cases reported, patients have been rendered eugastrinemic

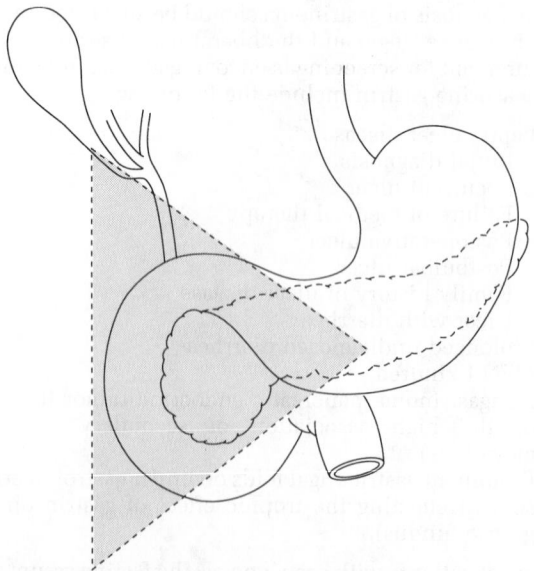

Figure 34-8. Most gastrinomas are found within the gastrinoma triangle. (After Stabile BE, Morrow DJ, Passaro E. The gastrinoma triangle: operative implications. Am J Surg 1984;147:26)

Table 34-5. VIPoma

Parameter	Description
Symptoms	Watery diarrhea
	Weakness
	Lethargy
	Nausea
Diagnostic tests	Hypokalemia
	Achlorhydria
	Serum vasoactive intestinal peptide levels
Anatomic localization	Most in body or tail of pancreas

by blind resection, and most continue to be eugastrinemic at postoperative follow-up.

The overall results in patients with gastrinoma have improved markedly since the initial description of the syndrome. In the 1950s and 1960s, most patients' gastrinomas were diagnosed late in the course of the disease, when the tumor burden was already significant. At that time, effective medical therapy for hyperchlorhydria was not available and sophisticated radiographic localization and staging techniques did not exist. Patients often suffered multiple ulcer complications, required total gastrectomy to control the ulcer diathesis, and typically succumbed to continued tumor growth following total gastrectomy. Recent reviews of gastrinoma patients treated surgically provide room for optimism.[51-53,70-72] Up to 35% of patients who undergo exploration for gastrinoma with curative intent have been rendered eugastrinemic at follow-up. When only those patients explored and thought to be successfully resected are considered, the cure rates approach 60% to 70%. These recent results represent a major improvement in the treatment of gastrinoma patients during the past few decades, and support the practice of initial pharmacologic control of gastric hypersecretion using omeprazole, followed by tumor localization and staging, in hopes of curative resection.

Most patients with incurable metastatic gastrinoma succumb to eventual tumor growth and dissemination. Multiple modalities have been used to treat patients with such metastatic gastrinoma. The overall objective response rate to chemotherapy appears to be less than 50%. A prospective study of monthly cycles of streptozocin, 5-fluorouracil, and doxorubicin in 10 patients with metastatic gastrinoma showed a partial response rate of 40%, with 60% having no response.[73] Chemotherapy did not improve the length of survival. Hormonal therapy with octreotide has been reported to improve symptoms, reduce hypergastrinemia, and diminish hyperchlorhydria in patients with metastatic gastrinoma.[74,75] Anecdotal reports suggest that octreotide may occasionally reduce tumor volume, although this response is clearly uncommon. The role of octreotide remains somewhat limited, however, because the drug must be parenterally administered and because omeprazole can control hyperchlorhydria and peptic symptoms in nearly all patients. Aggressive resection and palliative debulking of metastatic gastrinoma have been performed in a small number of patients, with apparent improvement in the clinical course.[42-44] Hepatic transplantation, hepatic artery embolization, and interferon therapy have all been used in a small number of patients with gastrinoma metastatic to the liver.[76-78] None of these therapies appears to be associated with reproducible improvements in survival.

Patients with gastrinoma associated with MEN I present difficult treatment issues. Omeprazole should be used to control gastric acid hypersecretion. Surgical treatment of hypercalcemia caused by parathyroid hyperplasia should preceed any surgical treatment of hypergastrinemia. MEN I gastrinoma typically involves multiple pancreatic or duodenal neoplasms,[79] and careful preoperative and intraoperative localization techniques are needed to guide resection. In limited numbers of patients, hypergastrinemia associated with MEN I gastrinoma has been corrected by surgical resection at short term follow-up. The overall cure rates with MEN I gastrinoma appear to be lower than those with sporadic gastrinoma.

VIPoma (VERNER-MORRISON SYNDROME)

Verner and Morrison are credited with the definition of this secretory-type diarrhea syndrome following their report of two cases in 1958.[83] Synonyms for this syndrome include the WDHA syndrome (watery diarrhea, hypokalemia, and either achlorhydria or hypochlorhydria) and the pancreatic cholera syndrome. Patients characteristically present with intermittent severe diarrhea, typically of a watery nature, averaging 5 L/d (Table 34-5). Malabsorption and steatorrhea are not common. Hypokalemia results from the fecal loss of large amounts of potassium (up to 400 mEq/d), and low serum potassium levels are associated with muscular weakness, lethargy, and nausea. Half of the patients have some degree of hyperglycemia and hypercalcemia, and cutaneous flushing can be observed in a minority. The diagnosis of VIPoma is typically made after excluding other more common causes of diarrhea (Table 34-6). The active agent in the VIPoma syndrome is usually VIP,[80] with a minority of patients having elevations of other candidate mediators such as peptide histidine-isoleucine or prostaglandins.[81] Because VIP secretion can be episodic in patients with VIPomas, several fasting VIP levels should be measured because a single low VIP level does not rule out the syndrome.

After biochemical documentation of elevated VIP levels, tumor localization and staging begins with dynamic abdominal CT scan with intravenous and oral contrast. In addition, because 10% of patients with VIPomas may have extrapancreatic tumors located in the retroperitoneum or thorax, a thoracic CT scan is indicated if the abdominal scan fails to identify a tumor. In most reported cases, the abdominal CT scan identified the tumor, and further im-

Table 34-6. VERNER-MORRISON SYNDROME: DIFFERENTIAL DIAGNOSIS

Entity	Workup
Villous adenoma	Lower GI endoscopy
Laxative abuse	Stool examination for phenolphthalein
Celiac disease	Fecal fat measurement
	D-Xylose tolerance test
	Small bowel biopsy
Parasitic and infectious diseases	Stool culture
	Ovum and parasite analysis
	Clostridium difficile toxin assay
Inflammatory bowel disease	Lower GI endoscopy
	Upper GI and small bowel series
Carcinoid syndrome	Urinary 5'-HIAA
	Upper GI and small bowel series
	Abdominal CT scan
	Serum serotonin measurement
Gastrinoma	Serum gastrin measurement
	Gastric acid analysis
	Secretin stimulation test

aging studies, such as visceral angiography or portal venous hormone sampling, were unnecessary.

In preparing patients with VIPomas for surgical exploration, fluid and electrolyte balances must be corrected by vigorous intravenous fluid administration and appropriate electrolyte replacement. Therapy with parenterally administered octreotide can be an important adjunct in the preoperative setting because octreotide leads to a reduction in circulating VIP levels with a resultant decrease in the volume of diarrhea. Before octreotide was available, corticosteroids and indomethacin were used preoperatively to control diarrhea and associated fluid and electrolyte losses.

Surgical excision of the VIPoma is appropriate in all patients with the Verner-Morrison syndrome. Most VIPomas have been located in the distal pancreas, where they are amenable to resection by distal pancreatectomy. If no tumor is found in the pancreas, a careful exploration of the retroperitoneum including both adrenals should be performed. Metastatic disease to the lymph nodes and the liver have been reported in half of all cases. In the presence of metastatic disease, safe palliative debulking of the metastatic tumor is indicated.[82]

In patients with recurrent or unresectable VIPoma, octreotide therapy is used to reduce circulating VIP levels and control diarrhea. Chemotherapy specific for VIPoma patients has not been studied prospectively, although small numbers of patients have appeared to partially respond to streptozocin, combination chemotherapy or interferon.

GLUCAGONOMA

The most common findings in the glucagonoma syndrome are severe dermatitis, mild diabetes, stomatitis, anemia, and weight loss[80] (Table 34-7). The dermatitis manifests as a characteristic skin rash termed necrolytic migratory erythema. This rash exhibits cyclic migrations with erythematous patches that spread serpiginously and central healing points of resolution. It has been theorized that the hypoaminoacidemia seen in patients with glucagonoma is responsible for the dermatitis. Because glucagon is a catabolic hormone, glucagonoma patients typically demonstrate malnutrition and hypoproteinemia.

The diagnosis of glucagonoma may be suggested by the clinical presentation and biopsy of the skin lesions but is secured by the documentation of elevated levels of fasting serum glucagon. Normal fasting levels of glucagon peak at 150 pg/mL. The diagnosis of glucagonoma can be confirmed by demonstration of hypoaminoacidemia, however, such testing is expensive and is not necessary in most cases.

Patients with biochemical documentation of hyperglucagonemia in the appropriate clinical setting should undergo radiographic localization and staging with dy-

Table 34-7. GLUCAGONOMA

Parameter	Description
Symptoms	Dermatitis manifested as necrolytic migratory erythema
	Stomatitis
	Weight loss
Diagnostic tests	Hyperglycemia
	Hypoproteinemia
	Serum glucagon measurement
	Serum amino acid profile
Anatomic localization	Most in body or tail of pancreas

Table 34-8. SOMATOSTATINOMA

Parameter	Description
Symptoms	Steatorrhea
	Right upper quadrant pain
Diagnostic tests	Hyperglycemia
	Hypochlorhydria
	Gallstones
	Serum somatostatin level
Anatomic localization	Most in head or uncinate process of pancreas

namic contrast-enhanced abdominal CT scan. Because these tumors are usually large and solitary, the CT scan localizes the tumor in most patients. Before exploration, attention should be given to managing the malnutrition. Total parenteral nutrition has been used to improve the catabolic state created by hyperglucagonemia, reverse the malnutrition, and improve the dermatitis. Octreotide has been used to reduce the circulating glucagon levels and to allow improved response to total parenteral nutrition.

Most glucagonomas have been located in the body and tail of the pancreas. These tumors are typically large and bulky, and surgical resection has required distal pancreatectomy. Metastases have been found in most patients, and safe debulking of these metastatic lesions should be considered.

Glucagonoma patients with incurable or recurrent disease appear to have low response rates to standard chemotherapeutic agents such as streptozocin and dacarbazine.[84] Octreotide can be successful in reducing elevated glucagon levels and in controlling the hyperglycemia and dermatitis associated with incurable glucagonoma.[85,86]

SOMATOSTATINOMA

The somatostatinoma syndrome is the least common of the five generally accepted functional pancreatic endocrine neoplasia syndromes, with an estimated annual incidence of less than 1 in 40 million people. The clinical features of the somatostatinoma syndrome are nonspecific and include steatorrhea, diabetes, hypochlorhydria, and cholelithiasis (Table 34-8). A fasting plasma somatostatin level can be used to confirm the diagnosis of a somatostatinoma. While the normal plasma level is below 100 pg/mL, patients with somatostatinoma have been found to have high levels of circulating somatostatin, often measurable in nanograms per milliliter.[87,88] Most somatostatinomas have been located in the head of the pancreas and the periampullary region. The most useful test for localization and staging is the abdominal CT scan, which has been used to identify and stage these typically large tumors. Preoperative treatment of patients with somatostatinoma involves treatment of hyperglycemia and malnutrition. Surgery resection for cure has been uncommon because of the presence of metastatic disease in most cases. Safe resection of the primary tumor and careful debulking of hepatic metastases appear to be indicated. At the time of exploration, cholecystectomy is indicated even in the absence of documented gallstones because of the concern about the development of cholelithiasis with persistently elevated somatostatin levels.

RARE CANDIDATE FUNCTIONAL PANCREATIC ENDOCRINE NEOPLASMS

There are several extremely rare clinical syndromes that have been proposed as candidate functional endocrine syndromes associated with pancreatic neoplasms (Table

34-9). These include calcitoninoma,[89,90] parathyrinoma,[91] GRFoma, ACTHoma and neurotensinoma.[92] Calcitonin-secreting pancreatic endocrine neoplasms are associated with watery diarrhea, whereas parathyrinomas are accompanied by elevations in PTH-related protein with clinical features of hypercalcemia. GRFoma is marked by elevations of serum growth hormone–releasing factor (GRF), with clinical features of acromegaly. ACTHoma has features of Cushing syndrome, with elevated serum adenocorticotropic hormone (ACTH). Neurotensinoma appears to be characterized by tachycardia, hypotension, and malabsorption, with elevation of serum neurotensin. As further cases are reported and clinical experience broadens, these rare and unusual functional pancreatic exocrine neoplasms and others may someday be recognized along with the classic five syndromes of insulinoma, gastrinoma, VIPoma, glucagonoma, and somatostatinoma.

NONFUNCTIONAL ISLET CELL TUMORS

In about a third of patients with neoplasms of the endocrine pancreas, there is no defined clinical syndrome and no lack of elevated serum insulin, gastrin, VIP, glucagon and somatostatin levels. These patients are considered to have nonfunctional endocrine neoplasms. The one hormone that may be elevated in the serum in these nonfunctional tumors is pancreatic polypeptide. It appears to be a marker for some pancreatic endocrine tumors without being the mediator of any specific pancreatic polypeptide–related clinical syndrome.[93] These nonfunctional endocrine neoplasms present with clinical manifestations such as abdominal pain, weight loss and jaundice resulting from space-occupying lesions in the pancreas.[94,95] These clinical manifestations are similar to those found in patients with ductal adenocarcinoma of the pancreas. Nonfunctional tumors are most commonly located in the head, neck, or uncinate process of the pancreas.[96] The malignancy rate for these tumors ranges from 50% to 90%. However, in contrast to the poor prognosis associated with ductal adenocarcinoma of the pancreas, these nonfunctional tumors tend to grow in a more indolent fashion and to be associated with a longer survival.

Localization and staging studies are performed in a similar fashion to those performed for patients with the more common diagnosis of ductal adenocarcinoma of the exocrine pancreas. The abdominal CT scan is used to evaluate the primary tumor and to assess for hepatic metastases. Preoperative cholangiography may be indicated in the setting of jaundice with the potential for imaging by endoscopic or percutaneous transhepatic routes. At surgery most of these nonfunctional neoplasms are larger than 2 cm and are not safely excised by local techniques. Tumors in the head, neck, or uncinate process of the pancreas typically require pancreaticoduodenectomy for safe resection, whereas tumors arising in the body or tail of the pancreas are treated by distal pancreatectomy. Patients with unresectable tumors in the head of the pancreas are candidates for surgical palliation of obstructive jaundice and gastric outlet obstruction by biliary-enteric and gastroenteric bypass, respectively. The overall 5-year survival rate in all patients with resected nonfunctional pancreatic neoplasms approaches 50%.[97]

In patients with unresectable disease, partial responses to combination chemotherapy have been reported. In a multicenter trial reported on by Moertel and associates,[46] 105 patients with advanced islet cell carcinoma, half of whom had nonfunctional tumors, were randomly assigned to one of three treatment regimens. The lowest response rate (30%) was seen in the group receiving chlorozotocin alone; an intermediate response rate of 45% was seen in patients receiving the combination of streptozocin plus 5-fluorouracil; and the highest response rate of 69% was seen in patients receiving streptozocin plus doxorubicin. The streptozocin-plus-doxorubicin therapy was associated with a significant survival advantage when compared to the other two treatments. The most common toxic reactions to the chemotherapy were nausea and vomiting, leukopenia, and mild renal insufficiency.

REFERENCES

1. Andrew A. Further evidence that enterochromaffin cells are not derived from the neural crest. J Embryol Exp Morphol 1974;31:589.
2. Long PP, Hruban RH, Lo R, et al. Chromosome analysis of nine endocrine neoplasms of the pancreas. Cancer Genet Cytogenet 1994;77:55.
3. Yashiro T, Fulton N, Hara H, et al. Comparisons of mutations of ras oncogene in human pancreatic exocrine and endocrine tumors. Surgery 1993;114:758.
4. Evers BM, Rady PL, Sandoval K, et al. Gastrinomas demonstrate amplification of the HER-2/neu protooncogene. Ann Surg 1994;219:596.
5. Zeiger MA and Norton JA. G$_s$ alpha: identification of a gene highly expressed by insulinoma and other endocrine tumors. Surgery 1993;114:458.
6. Eubanks PJ, Sawicki MP, Samara GJ, et al. Putative tumor-suppressor gene on chromosome 11 is important in sporadic endocrine tumor formation. Am J Surg 1994;167:180.
7. Fedorak IJ, Ko TC, Gordon D, Flisak M, Prinz RA. Localization of islet cell tumors of the pancreas: a review of current techniques. Surgery 1993;113:242.
8. Frucht H, Doppman JL, Norton JA, et al. Gastrinomas: comparison of MR imaging with CT, angiography, and US. Radiology 1989;171:713.
9. Wank SA, Doppman JL, Miller DL, et al. Prospective study of the ability of computed axial tomography to localize gastrinomas in patients with Zollinger-Ellison syndrome. Gastroenterology 1987;92:905.
10. Yeo CJ, Wang BH, Anthone GJ, Cameron JL. Surgical experience with pancreatic islet-cell tumors. Arch Surg 1993;128:1143.
11. Maton PN, Miller DL, Doppman JL, et al. Role of selective angiography in the management of patients with Zollinger-Ellison syndrome. Gastroenterology 1987;92:913.
12. Glover JR, Shorvon PJ, Lees WR. Endoscopic ultrasound for localisation of islet cell tumours. Gut 1992;33:108.
13. Rosch T, Lightdale CJ, Botet JF, et al. Localization of pancreatic endocrine tumors by endoscopic ultrasonography. N Engl J Med 1992;326:1721.
14. Thompson NW, Czako PF, Fritts LL, et al. Role of endoscopic ultrasonography in the localization of insulinomas and gastrinomas. Surgery 1994;116:1131.
15. Lamberts SWJ, Bakker WH, Reubi JC, Krenning EP. Somato-

Table 34-9. RARE FUNCTIONAL PANCREATIC ENDOCRINE NEOPLASMS

Tumor	Hormone/Candidate	Features
Calcitoninoma	Calcitonin	Secretory diarrhea
Parathyrinoma	PTH-related protein	Hypercalcemia Bone pain Normal serum PTH
GRFoma	Growth hormone releasing factor	Acromegaly
ACTHoma	Adrenocorticotropic hormone	Cushing syndrome
Neurotensinoma	Neurotensin	Tachycardia Hypotension Malabsorption

PTH, parathyroid hormone.

statin-receptor imaging in the localization of endocrine tumors. N Engl J Med 1990;323:1246.

16. Scherubl H, Bader M, Fett U, et al. Somatostatin-receptor imaging of neuroendocrine gastroenteropancreatic tumors. Gastroenterology 1993;105:1705.

17. Weinel RJ, Neuhaus C, Stapp J, et al. Preoperative localization of gastrointestinal endocrine tumors using somatostatin-receptor scintigraphy. Ann Surg 1993;218:640.

18. Reubi JC, Hacki WH, Lamberts SWJ. Hormone-producing gastrointestinal tumors contain a high density of somatostatin receptors. J Clin Endocrinol Metab 1987;65:1127.

19. Schirmer WJ, O'Dorisio TM, Schirmer TP, Mojzisik CM, Hinkle GH, Martin EW. Intraoperative localization of neuroendocrine tumors with ^{125}I-tyr^3-octreotide and a hand-held gamma-detecting probe. Surgery 1993;114:745.

20. Woltering EA, Barrie R, O'Dorisio TM, et al. Detection of occult gastrinomas with iodine^{125}-labeled lanreotide and intraoperative gamma detection. Surgery 1994;116:1139.

21. Virgolini I, Raderer M, Kurtaran A, et al. Vasoactive intestinal peptide-receptor imaging for the localization of intestinal adenocarcinomas and endocrine tumors. N Engl J Med 1994; 331:1116.

22. Norton JA, Shawker TH, Doppman JL, et al. Localization and surgical treatment of occult insulinomas. Ann Surg 1990; 212:615.

23. Vinik AI, Moattari AR, Cho K, Thompson N. Transhepatic portal vein catheterization for localization of sporadic and MEN gastrinomas: A ten year experience. Surgery 1990; 107:246.

24. Pedrazzoli S, Pasquale C, Miotto D, Feltrin GP, Petrin P. Transhepatic portal sampling for preoperative localization of insulinomas. Surg Gynecol Obstet 1987;165:101.

25. Vinik AI, Delbridge L, Moattari R, Cho K, Thompson N. Transhepatic portal vein catheterization for localization of insulinomas: a ten-year experience. Surgery 1991;109:1.

26. Fraker DL, Norton JA. Localization and resection of insulinomas and gastrinomas. JAMA 1988;259:3601.

27. Imamura M, Minematsu S, Suzuki T, et al. Usefulness of selective arterial secretin injection test for localization of gastrinoma in the Zollinger-Ellison syndrome. Ann Surg 1987;205:230.

28. Rosato FE, Bonn J, Shapiro M, Barbot DJ, Furnary AM, Gardiner GA. Selective arterial stimulation of secretin in localization of gastrinomas. Surg Gynecol Obstet 1990;171:196.

29. Gower WR Jr, Buzogany JA, Ellison EC, Knierim TH, Fabri PJ. Control of gastrin release in cultured gastrinoma-derived G cells. Surgery 1988;104:424.

30. Chiba T, Yamatani T, Yamaguchi A, et al. Mechanism for increase of gastrin release by secretin in Zollinger-Ellison syndrome. Gastroenterology 1989;96:1439.

31. Thom AK, Norton JA, Doppman JL, Miller DL, Chang R, Jensen RT. Prospective study of the use of intraarterial secretin injection and portal venous sampling to localize duodenal gastrinomas. Surgery 1992;112:1002.

32. Grant CS, van Heerden J, Charboneau JW, James EM, Reading CC. Insulinoma: the value of intraoperative ultrasonography. Arch Surg 1988;123:843.

33. Norton JA, Sigel B, Baker AR, et al. Localization of an occult insulinoma by intraoperative ultrasonography. Surgery 1985;97:381.

34. Whipple AO, Frantz VK. Adenoma of islet cells with hyperinsulinism: a review. Ann Surg 1935;101:1299.

35. Kahn CR. The riddle of tumour hypoglyceamia revisited. J Clin Endocrinol Metab 1980;9:335.

36. Daughaday WH, Emanuele MA, Brooks MH, et al. Synthesis and secretion of insulin-like growth factor II by a leiomyosarcoma with associated hypoglycemia. N Engl J Med 1988;319:1434.

37. Howard TJ, Stabile BE, Zinner MJ, Chang S, Bhagavan BS, Passaro E Jr. Anatomic distribution of pancreatic endocrine tumors. Am J Surg 1990;159:258.

38. Service FJ, McMahon MM, O'Brien PC, Ballard DJ. Functioning insulinoma: incidence, recurrence, and long-term survival of patients: a 60-year study. Mayo Clin Proc 1991;66:711.

39. Menegaux F, Schmitt G, Mercadier M, Chigott JP. Pancreatic insulinomas. Am J Surg 1993;165:243.

40. Udelsman R, Yeo CJ, Hruban RH, et al. Pancreaticoduodenectomy for selected pancreatic endocrine tumors. Surg Gynecol Obstet 1993;177:269.

41. Thompson GB, Service FJ, van Heerden JA, et al. Reoperative insulinomas, 1927 to 1992: an institutional experience. Surgery 1993;114:1196.

42. Carty SE, Jensen RT, Norton JA. Prospective study of aggressive resection of metastatic pancreatic endocrine tumors. Surgery 1992;112:1024.

43. Modlin IM, Lewis JJ, Ahlman H, et al. Management of unresectable malignant endocrine tumors of the pancreas. Surg Gynecol Obstet 1993;176:507.

44. McEntee GP, Nagorney DM, Kvols LK, et al. Cytoreductive hepatic surgery for neuroendocrine tumors. Surgery 1990;108:1091.

45. Thompson GB, van Heerden JA, Grant CS, Carney JA, Ilstrup DM. Islet cell carcinomas of the pancreas: a twenty-year experience. Surgery 1988;104:1011.

46. Moertel CG, Lefkopoulo M, Lipsitz S, et al. Streptozocin-doxorubicin, streptozocin-fluorouracil, or chlorozotocin in the treatment of advanced islet-cell carcinoma. N Engl J Med 1992;326:519.

47. Moertel CG, Hanley JA, Johnson LA. Streptozocin alone compared with streptozocin plus fluorouracil in the treatment of advanced islet-cell carcinoma. N Engl J Med 1980;303:1189.

48. Altimari AF, Badrinath K, Reisel HJ, Prinz RA. DTIC therapy in patients with malignant intra-abdominal neuroendocrine tumors. Surgery 1987;102:1009.

49. Zollinger RM, Ellison EH. Primary peptic ulcerations of the jejunum associated with islet cell tumors of the pancreas. Ann Surg 1955;142:709.

50. Zollinger RM, Ellison EC, Fabri PJ, et al. Primary peptic ulcerations of the jejunum associated with islet cell tumors: twenty-five-year appraisal. Ann Surg 1980;192:422.

51. Wolfe MM, Jensen RT. Zollinger-Ellison syndrome. Current concepts in diagnosis and management. N Engl J Med 1987;317:1200.

52. Yeo CJ. ZES: current approaches. Contemp Gastroenterol 1990;3:17.

53. Andersen DK. Current diagnosis and management of Zollinger-Ellison syndrome. Ann Surg 1989;210:685.

54. Miller LS, Vinayek R, Frucht H, et al. Reflux esophagitis in patients with Zollinger-Ellison syndrome. Gastroenterology 1990;98:341.

55. Chiang HCV, O'Dorisio TM, Huang SC, et al. Multiple hormone elevations in Zollinger-Ellison syndrome. Gastroenterology 1990;99:1565.

56. Wynick D, Williams SJ, Bloom SR. Symptomatic secondary hormone syndromes in patients with established malignant pancreatic endocrine tumors. N Engl J Med 1988;319:605.

57. Maton PN, Vinayek R, Frucht H, et al. Long-term efficacy and safety of omeprazole in patients with Zollinger-Ellison syndrome: a prospective study. Gastroenterology 1989;97: 827.

58. Metz DC, Pisegna JR, Fishbeyn VA, et al. Currently used doses of omeprazole in Zollinger-Ellison syndrome are too high. Gastroenterology 1992;103:1498.

59. Sawicki MP, Howard TJ, Dalton M, Stabile BE, Passaro E Jr. The dichotomous distribution of gastrinomas. Arch Surg 1990;125:1584.

60. Stabile BE, Morrow DJ, Passaro E Jr. The gastrinoma triangle: operative implications. Am J Surg 1984;147:25.

61. Sugg SL, Norton JA, Fraker DL, et al. A prospective study of intraoperative methods to diagnose and resect duodenal gastrinomas. Ann Surg 1993;218:138.

62. Frucht H, Norton JA, London JF, et al. Detection of duodenal gastrinomas by operative endoscopic transillumination: a prospective study. Gastroenterology 1990;99:1622.

63. Delcore R, Friesen SR. Role of pancreatoduodenectomy in the management of primary duodenal wall gastrinomas in patients with Zollinger-Ellison syndrome. Surgery 1992; 112:1016.

64. Thompson NW, Vinik AI, Eckhauser FE. Microgastrinomas of the duodenum: a cause of failed operations for the Zollinger-Ellison syndrome. Ann Surg 1989;209:396.

65. Farley DR, van Heerden JA, Grant CS, Thompson GB. Extra-pancreatic gastrinomas: surgical experience. Arch Surg 1994; 129:506.

66. Chiarugi M, Pucciarelli M, Goletti O, et al. Outcome of surgical treatment for extrapancreatic gastrinomas. Surg Gynecol Obstet 1993;177:153.

67. Arnold WS, Fraker DL, Alexander HR, et al. Apparent lymph node primary gastrinoma. Surgery 1994;116:1123.

68. Richardson CT, Peters MN, Feldman M, et al. Treatment of Zollinger-Ellison syndrome with exploratory laparotomy, proximal gastric vagotomy, and H_2-receptor antagonists: a prospective study. Gastroenterology 1985;89:357.

69. Thompson JC, Lewis BG, Weiner I, Townsend CM Jr. The role of surgery in the Zollinger-Ellison syndrome. Ann Surg 1983;197:594.

70. Norton JA, Doppman JL, Jensen RT. Curative resection in Zollinger-Ellison syndrome: results of a 10-year prospective study. Ann Surg 1992;215:8.

71. Fraker DL, Norton JA, Alexander HR, et al. Surgery in Zollinger-Ellison syndrome alters the natural history of gastrinoma. Ann Surg 1994;220:320.

72. Delcore R, Friesen SR. The place for curative surgical procedures in the treatment of sporadic and familial Zollinger-Ellison syndrome. Curr Opin Gen Surg 1994;2:69.

73. von Schrenck T, Howard JM, Doppman JL, et al. Prospective study of chemotherapy in patients with metastatic gastrinoma. Gastroenterology 1988;94:1326.

74. Mozell E, Woltering EA, O'Dorisio TM, et al. Effect of somatostatin analog on peptide release and tumor growth in the Zollinger-Ellison syndrome. Surg Gynecol Obstet 1990;170:476.

75. Mozell E, Cramer AJ, O'Dorisio TM, Woltering EA. Long-term efficacy of octreotide in the treatment of Zollinger-Ellison syndrome. Arch Surg 1992;127:1019.

76. Makowka L, Tzakis AG, Mazzaferro V, et al. Transplantation of the liver for metastatic endocrine tumors of the intestine and pancreas. Surg Gynecol Obstet 1989;168:107.

77. Ajani JA, Carrasco CH, Charnsangavej C, et al. Islet cell tumors metastatic to the liver: effective palliation by sequential hepatic artery embolization. Ann Intern Med 1988;108:340.

78. Pisegna JR, Slimak GG, Doppman JL, et al. An evaluation of human recombinant a interferon in patients with metastatic gastrinoma. Gastroenterology 1993;105:1179.

79. Pipeleers-Marichal M, Somers G, Willems G, et al. Gastrinomas in the duodenums of patients with multiple endocrine neoplasia type 1 and the Zollinger-Ellison syndrome. N Engl J Med 1990;322:723.

80. Rood RP, DeLellis RA, Dayal Y, Donowitz M. Pancreatic cholera syndrome due to a vasoactive intestinal polypeptide-producing tumor: further insights into the pathophysiology. Gastroenterology 1988;94:813.

81. Jaffe BM, Kopern DF, DeSchryver-Kecskemeti K, et al. Indomethacin-responsive pancreatic cholera. N Engl J Med 1977;297:817.

82. Nagorney DM, Bloom SR, Polak JM, Blumgart LH. Resolution of recurrent Verner-Morrison syndrome by resection of metastatic VIPoma. Surgery 1983;93:348.

83. Higgins GA, Recant L, Fischman AB. The glucagonoma syndrome: surgically curable diabetes. Am J Surg 1979;137:142.

84. Prinz RA, Badrinath K, Banerji M, et al. Operative and chemotherapeutic management of malignant glucagon-producing tumors. Surgery 1981;90:713.

85. Boden G, Ryan IG, Eisenschmid BL, et al. Treatment of inoperable glucagonoma with the long-acting somatostatin analogue SMS 201-955. N Engl J Med 1986;314:1686.

86. Altimari AF, Bhoopalam N, O'Dorisio T, et al. Use of a somatostatin analog (SMS 201-955) in the glucagonoma syndrome. Surgery 1986;100:989.

87. Ganda OP, Weir GC, Soeldner JS, et al. Somatostatinoma: a somatostatin-containing tumor of the endocrine pancreas. N Engl J Med 1977;296:963.

88. Kregs GJ, Orci L, Conlon JM, et al. Somatostatinoma syndrome. Biochemical, morphologic and clinical features. N Engl J Med 1979;301:285.

89. McLeod MK, Vinik AI. Calcitonin immunoreactivity and hypercalcitonemia in two patients with sporadic, nonfamilial, gastroenteropancreatic neuroendocrine tumors. Surgery 1992;111:484.

90. Howard JM, Gohara AF, Cardwell RJ. Malignant islet cell tumor of the pancreas associated with high plasma calcitonin and somatostatin levels. Surgery 1989;105:227.

91. Mao C, Carter P, Schaefer P, et al. Malignant islet cell tumor associated with hypercalcemia. Surgery 1995;117:37.

92. Meko JB, Norton JA. Endocrine tumors of the pancreas. Curr Opin Gen Surg 1994;2:186.

93. Langstein HN, Norton JA, Chiang HCV, et al. The utility of circulating levels of human pancreatic polypeptide as a marker for islet cell tumors. Surgery 1990;108:1109.

94. Kent RB III, van Heerden JA, Weiland LH. Nonfunctioning islet cell tumors. Ann Surg 1981;193:185.

95. Eckhauser FE, Cheung PS, Vinik AI, et al. Nonfunctioning malignant neuroendocrine tumors of the pancreas. Surgery 1986;100:978.

96. White TJ, Edney JA, Thompson JS, et al. Is there a prognostic difference between functional and nonfunctional islet cell tumors? Am J Surg 1994;168:627.

97. Evans DB, Skibber JM, Lee JE, et al. Nonfunctioning islet cell carcinoma of the pancreas. Surgery 1993;114:1175.

LIVER AND PORTAL VENOUS SYSTEM

SURGERY: SCIENTIFIC PRINCIPLES AND PRACTICE, Second Edition, edited by
Lazar J. Greenfield, Michael W. Mulholland, Keith T. Oldham, Gerald B. Zelenock,
and Keith D. Lillemoe. Lippincott–Raven Publishers, Philadelphia, © 1997.

CHAPTER 35

HEPATOBILIARY ANATOMY

DAVID R. BYRD

The general and hepatobiliary surgeon confronts the challenges of hepatic anatomy in one of four situations: (1) elective partial hepatic resection to remove a primary or secondary neoplasm; (2) elective or emergent decompression of portal venous hypertension or management of hepatic arterial aneurysms; (3) urgent total liver resection and reimplantation of a donor liver in a liver transplant recipient; and (4) emergent control of hemorrhage with or without liver resection in the patient with hepatic trauma.

Several unique anatomic features of the liver pose formidable obstacles to safe and successful surgery. The liver is a large, transversely oriented, fragile organ that is prone to fracture and bleeding with manipulation. A dual efferent blood supply is intertwined with delicate afferent biliary ducts in a crowded hepatic hilum. The three large hepatic veins that drain the liver empty directly into the inferior vena cava (IVC) posterior to the liver and are completely obscured from view without extensive retrohepatic dissection.

Every surgeon contemplating an operation that exposes or resects all or part of the liver should have a thorough understanding of the general hepatic anatomy and an absolute understanding of an individual patient's hepatic anatomy. This requires knowledge of segmental hepatic anatomy, relations of structures within the liver parenchyma, and correlation of preoperative imaging studies with an operative plan for each patient.

TOPOGRAPHIC ANATOMY AND RELATIONS TO PERIHEPATIC STRUCTURES

The normal adult liver is a large wedge-shaped organ occupying the right upper quadrant of the abdomen, extending vertically on the right side from the undersurface of the right hemidiaphragm to the anterior costal margin and horizontally to the left midclavicular line at the superior pole of the spleen. The anterior surface of the liver is invested by visceral peritoneum that extends to the anterior abdominal wall in the midline from the ligamentum teres or round ligament (the obliterated umbilical vessels) and by an obliquely oriented fusion of peritoneum known as the falciform ligament. Posteriorly, the investing peritoneum becomes contiguous with the peritoneum of the diaphragm at the coronary and triangular attachments, resulting in a rhomboidal retroperitoneal "bare area" not covered by peritoneum (Fig. 35-1). Glisson capsule is a thin fibrous covering that closely envelopes the entire liver deep to the peritoneum and sends thin fibrous septae into the hepatic parenchyma.

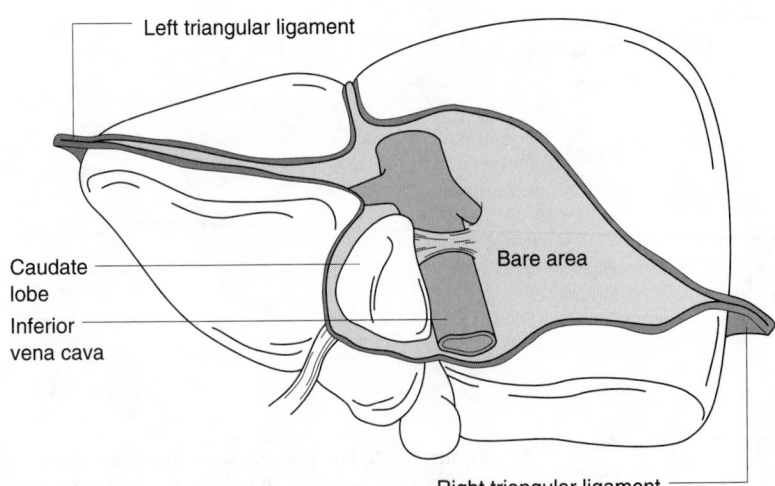

Figure 35-1. Posterior view of liver, showing the level of peritoneal reflections.

931

Ordinarily, the liver can be surgically separated from adjacent organs and structures by dividing areolar tissue planes (Fig 35-2). Neoplasms or inflammatory conditions in the liver or surrounding structures may obliterate these tissue planes and may be difficult to appreciate on preoperative imaging studies. Superiorly and anteriorly, the diaphragm or abdominal wall may be invaded by cancer or abscess. Posteriorly, neoplasms of the right adrenal gland or superior pole of the right kidney may densely adhere to the right hepatic lobe. Inferiorly, the gallbladder, hepatic flexure of the colon, duodenum, or periportal lymph nodes may be inseparable from the liver edge. On the left side, gastric or gastroesophageal junction cancers may invade the left hepatic lobe. Preoperative recognition of potential adjacent involvement is essential to help guide the choice of incision, to determine the preoperative function of both kidneys if nephrectomy becomes necessary, and to initiate a mechanical bowel preparation to allow a safe colon or gastric resection if required.

MORPHOLOGIC AND FUNCTIONAL ANATOMY

The description and definition of the anatomic divisions of the liver have been revised numerous times in the past 40 years. The revisions have been based on detailed autopsy studies and more recently on correlations with hepatic imaging by computed tomographic (CT) scanning and ultrasound. The original morphologic division of the liver into a right and left lobe based on separation by the falciform ligament has now been replaced by detailed descriptions of functional divisions based on hepatic venous drainage and portal pedicles (branches of the hepatic artery, portal vein, and bile duct) to individual segments. Extensively detailed descriptions and diagrams of hepatic anatomy form the modern understanding of the functional anatomy of the liver and should be carefully reviewed by all hepatic surgeons.[1–8]

Differences in the hepatic anatomic nomenclature in the English and French literature are confusing. Until recently, anatomic descriptions in the English literature began with the major divisions of the liver into a right and left hepatic lobe, separated by a vertical line drawn from the gallbladder fossa to the IVC (Fig. 35-3). The middle hepatic vein can be found within the hepatic parenchyma along this line, and there is little portal pedicle crossover using this division. The left lobe is further divided by the falciform ligament (continuous with the umbilical fissure) into a medial segment (quadrate lobe) and lateral segment. The main left hepatic vein courses to the left of the umbilical fissure. The right lobe is further divided into anterior and posterior segments by an intersegmental line, which has no reliable topographic landmarks and no intraparenchymal septae to allow easy identification. The caudate lobe is generally considered separately since it usually receives portal pedicle branches from both the right and left sides and has an isolated hepatic venous drainage through multiple short veins that enter directly into the IVC.

In the now widely accepted French nomenclature, the liver can be divided into eight discrete segments based on portal pedicle branches and hepatic venous drainage. The most surgically relevant rendition of Couinaud's "blow out" segmental diagram is shown in Figure 35-4. It demonstrates that segments VI and VII most accurately reside posteriorly in vivo but are often drawn to appear lateral in Couinaud's ex vivo description. In these descriptions, the left, middle, and right hepatic veins course in three vertical connective planes called *scissurae*, which divide the liver into four sectors, each receiving a major portal pedicle. The four sectors can be further subdivided into two additional segments each based on a transverse line drawn through the main right and left portal veins within these sectors known as the *transverse scissura*.

Enumeration of the segments begins left to right, beginning with segment I, the caudate lobe. The left lateral sector (lobe) consists of a superior segment II and an inferior segment III and is synonymous with the left lateral segment in older terminology. The left vertical scissura separates the left lateral sector from segment IV, which may be subdivided into a superior segment IVa and an inferior segment IVb, and is synonymous with the quadrate lobe or medial segment of the left lobe. The main scissura separates the right and left hepatic lobes. The right vertical scissura divides the right lobe into an anteromedial sector and a posterolateral sector. The anteromedial sector is further subdi-

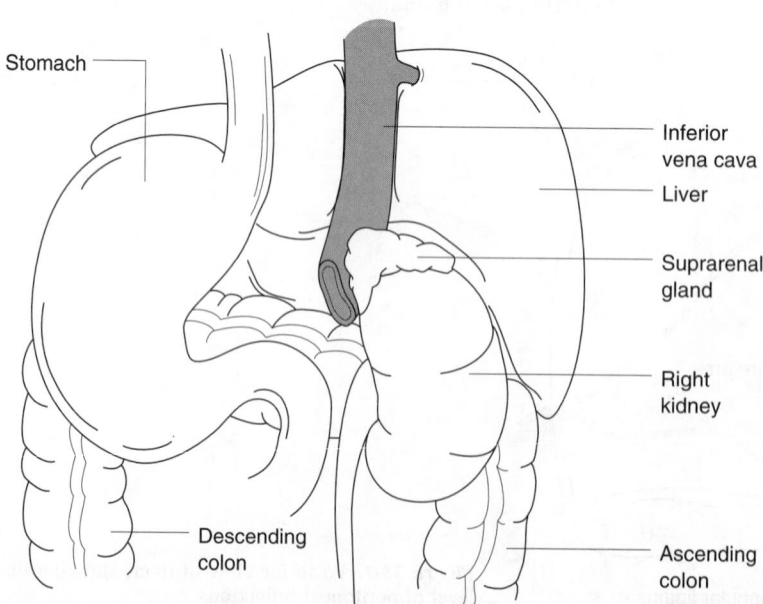

Stomach

Inferior vena cava

Liver

Suprarenal gland

Right kidney

Descending colon

Ascending colon

Figure 35-2. Posterior view of the liver, showing organs that produce impressions on the inferior surface of the liver.

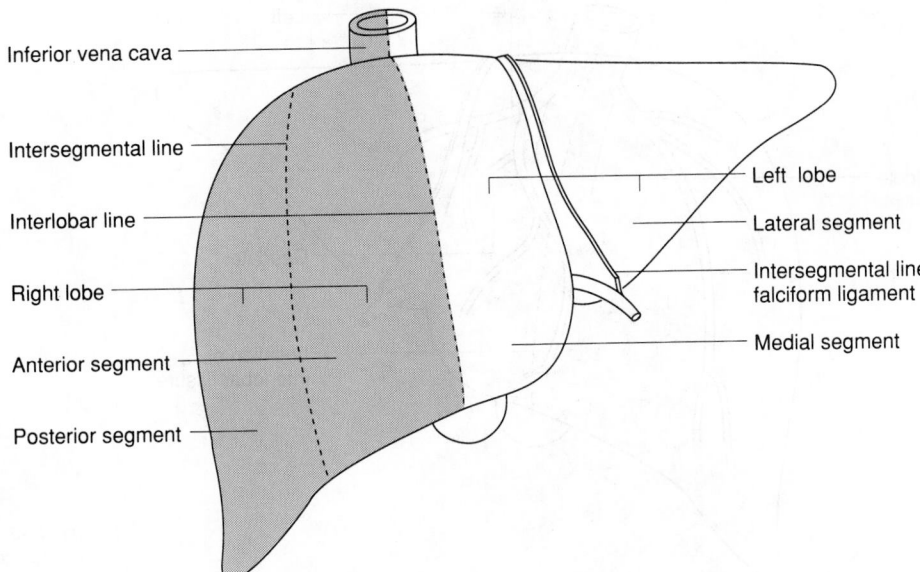

Figure 35-3. Anatomic division of liver into right and left lobes by a line extending from the gallbladder fossa posteriorly to the inferior vena cava.

vided into an inferior segment V and a superior segment VIII. The posterolateral sector is further subdivided into an inferior segment VI and a superior segment VII.

The major advantage of using this detailed segmental anatomy based on discrete portal pedicle branches is to accurately locate individual lesions in the hepatic substance by preoperative imaging and intraoperative ultrasound and to allow the possibility of less than lobar segmental anatomic resections that minimize blood loss and functional loss of hepatic reserve.

Hepatic Veins

Three major hepatic veins carry blood from the central veins of the hepatic substance to the IVC. Branches of these veins generally drain obliquely from inferior to superior and posterior within the hepatic parenchyma. In two thirds of patients, there is a single large right hepatic vein that joins the right anterior wall of the IVC and a middle and left hepatic vein that converge 1 to 2 cm from the IVC and

enter the left anterior wall of the IVC as a single vessel, adjacent to the right hepatic vein–IVC confluence (Fig. 35-5). In one third of patients, each major hepatic vein joins at the same horizontal level of the IVC as a separate trunk. In some patients, there is a short but definable extraparenchymal segment of one or more of the hepatic veins at the confluence with the IVC. More frequently, the entire length of the hepatic veins is intraparenchymal, which may preclude early, safe hepatic venous isolation during hepatic resection. These veins have a fragile, thin vessel wall, and inadvertent injury may result in rapid hemorrhage and considerable difficulty in isolating and controlling the injury.

The venous drainage of the liver begins in the central vein of the hepatic lobule. The left hepatic vein drains segments II, III, and IV. The middle hepatic vein drains a portion of segment IV and anterior segments V and VIII. The right vein drains the posterior segments VI and VII and a portion of the anterior segments.

Venous drainage of the caudate lobe occurs through mul-

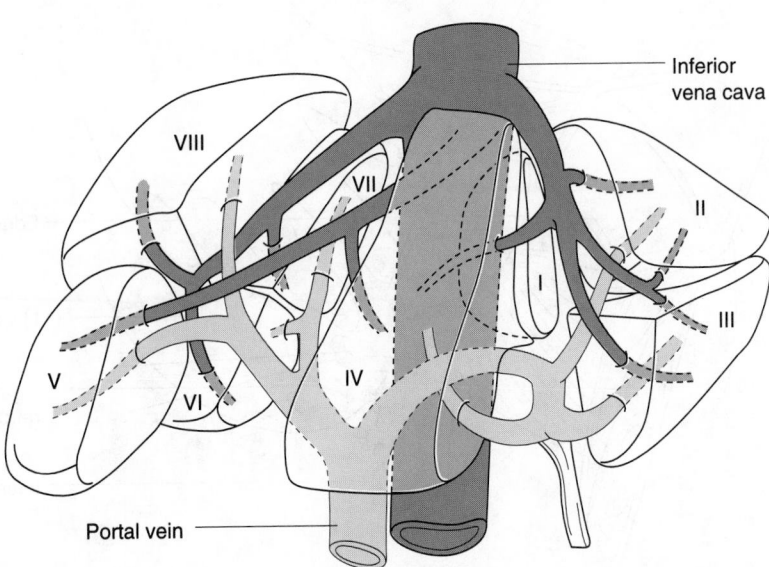

Figure 35-4. Functional division of the liver and the liver segments according to Couinaud's nomenclature.

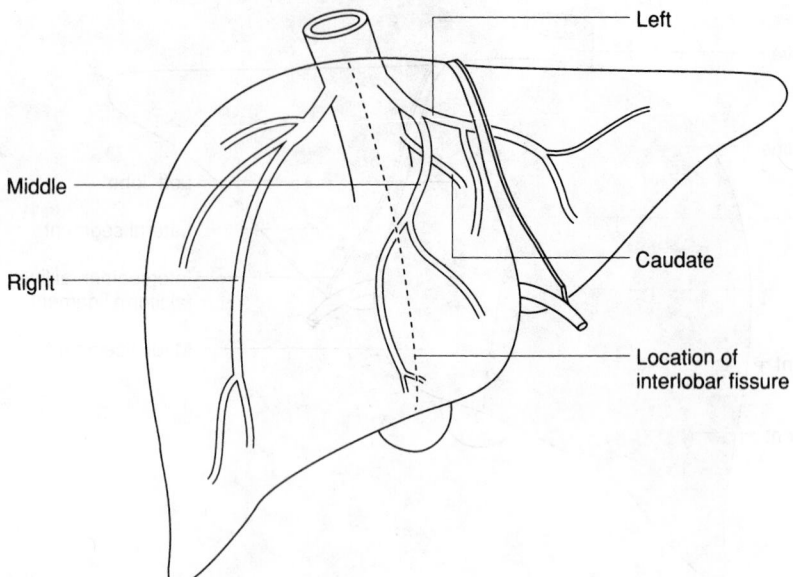

Figure 35-5. Three major hepatic veins drain the liver. The caudate segment of the liver usually drains directly into the inferior vena cava.

tiple short posterior veins that empty directly into the IVC. There are also several posterior accessory veins (up to 10) that drain the medial aspect of the right lobe and empty directly into the right anterior surface of the IVC (Fig. 35-6). Knowledge and identification of these accessory veins are essential during right hepatic lobectomy, caudate lobe resection, and right adrenalectomy.

Portal Veins

The origin of the main portal vein is formed by the confluence of the superior mesenteric and splenic veins posterior to the neck of the pancreas where it receives pyloric and coronary veins. It then courses cephalad and slightly obliquely to form the posteriormost structure within the hepatoduodenal ligament (portal triad), which is invested by leaves of the lesser omentum. In the hepatic hilum,

posterior to the hepatic duct and hepatic arterial bifurcations, there is an extrahepatic portal bifurcation into a short oblique right portal vein and a longer and more transverse left portal vein (Fig. 35-7). These branches become intraparenchymal and become invested along with the bile duct and hepatic arterial branches by extensions of Glisson capsule. There are usually one or two early, small posterior branches arising from both the right and left portal veins, providing a dual blood supply to the caudate lobe. The left portal vein then courses anteriorly in the pars umbilicus to give off a medial branch or branches to segment IV (quadrate lobe) and lateral branches to the left lateral sector, further subdividing into a superior branch to segment II and an inferior branch to segment III. The right portal vein further branches within 1 to 2 cm of the main portal bifurcation into an anterior division, which gives an inferior branch to segment V and a superior branch to segment

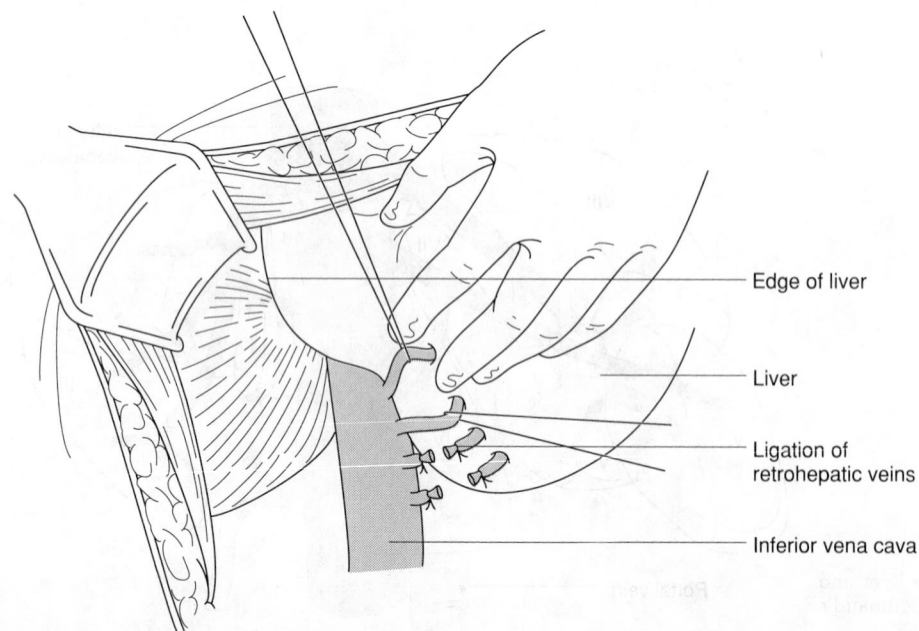

Figure 35-6. Retraction of right hepatic lobe medially exposes small venous tributaries that drain the right lobe directly into the retrohepatic vena cava. Several branches are undergoing ligation.

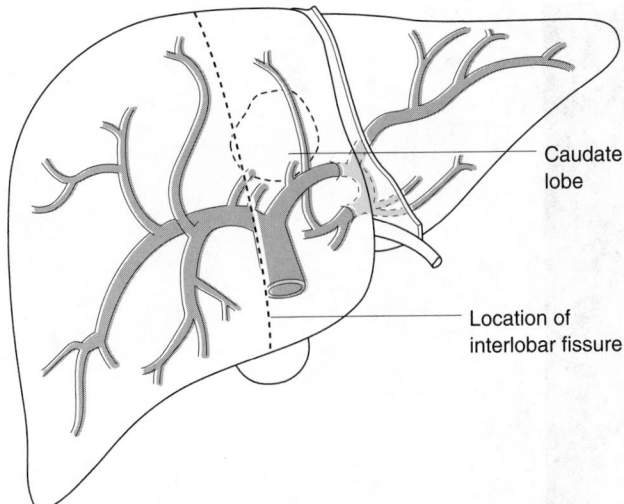

Figure 35-7. Intrahepatic divisions of the portal vein.

VIII, and a posterior division, which gives an inferior branch to segment VI and a superior branch to segment VII.

Hepatic Arteries

There is considerable variability in the origin and course of the right and left hepatic arteries. The most common finding is a transverse common hepatic artery from the celiac trunk that gives off the gastroduodenal, right gastric, and supraduodenal arteries and then courses obliquely in the left anterior aspect of the hepatoduodenal ligament as the proper hepatic artery. After giving off the cystic artery to the gallbladder, there is then a fairly low trifurcation into single right, middle, and left hepatic arteries. The middle hepatic artery may also arise from either the right or left hepatic arteries after a bifurcation of the proper hepatic artery. This arterial pattern is only found 55% of the time. The descriptions and frequency of hepatic arterial variants have been well characterized by Michels[5] (Table 35-1). Knowledge of the most common variations is extremely important since inadvertent division may occur during gastric, pancreatic, and hepatobiliary procedures. There may be a replaced or accessory left hepatic artery that arises from the left gastric artery and courses transversely in the lesser omentum (Fig. 35-8). With nearly equal frequency, there may be a replaced or accessory right hepatic artery from the superior mesenteric artery near its origin that courses posterior or through the head of the pancreas and obliquely along the right posterior border of the hepatoduodenal ligament. Within the hepatic parenchyma, the hepatic arterial branches course closely with bile duct branches and fairly closely with portal venous branches, invested by Glisson capsule, to supply portal pedicle branches to each hepatic segment (Fig. 35-9). Although original anatomic descriptions denied the existence of collateral vessels to the opposite hepatic lobe, imaged perfusion studies after ligation of main or replaced hepatic arteries have clearly demonstrated the presence of collateral flow to the deprived lobe, which can be demonstrated hours to days after ligation.

Details of biliary ductal anatomy are described in Chapter 40.

IMAGING OF THE LIVER
Ultrasonography

Ultrasound of the liver has been used for the past 20 years to identify lesions in the hepatic parenchyma, to describe the consistency and homogeneity of the liver (the fatty or cirrhotic liver), and to identify dilatation of the biliary tree and any abnormalities or stones in the gallbladder. In the past 10 years, detailed anatomic descriptions of the hepatic veins, portal pedicles, and IVC have been possible through the use of intraoperative ultrasound and advances in the resolution of ultrasound probes. Cooperation between radiologist and hepatic surgeon with the use of intraoperative ultrasound has enabled identification of lesions during surgery that were not visible by conventional transcorporeal ultrasound or CT scanning. Probes with horizontal or vertical orientation and different depths of resolution can be placed directly on the surface of the liver to allow complete definition of hepatic anatomy. Beginning superiorily at the IVC, the confluence and course of each of the hepatic veins can be easily determined (Fig. 35-10). More inferiorly, the main right and left portal pedicles can be seen coursing transversely in the transverse scissura. The left portal pedicle can be seen to course anteriorily as the pars umbilicus in the ligamentum teres. Portal structures are easily differentiated from hepatic veins by the hyperechoic extensions of Glisson capsule that surround these structures. If a circular structure is encountered and a mass or metastasis is suspected, scanning away from mass may reveal a tubular vascular shape that had been imaged in cross-section. Flattening a circular mass by external compression with the ultrasound probe differentiates a vascular structure from a solid mass.

Computed Tomography

The entire abdomen and pelvis cannot be imaged by ultrasound since there is distortion of some intraabdominal regions by gastric, small bowel, and colonic air. Thus, CT scanning has been increasingly used to screen for hepatic and other intraabdominal or retroperitoneal lesions. Conventional CT scanning includes 0.5- to 1-cm transectional images of the liver after oral administration of barium and bolus injection of intravenous contrast. Although resolution has improved, hepatic lesions smaller than 1 cm or lesions that are isodense with hepatic parenchyma may be missed.

Table 35-1. DESCRIPTION AND FREQUENCY OF HEPATIC ARTERIAL VARIATIONS

Description	Occurrence
Right, left, middle	55%
Right, middle, replaced left (off left gastric)	10%
Left, middle, replaced right (off superior mesenteric)	11%
Middle, replaced right and left	1%
Right, left, middle, accessory left	8%
Right, left, middle, accessory right	7%
Right, left, middle, accessory right and left	1%
Combined replaced right, accessory left or replaced left, accessory right	2%
No celiac trunk, common hepatic origin off superior mesenteric	2%
No celiac trunk, common hepatic origin off left gastric	0.5%

(After Michels NA. Newer anatomy of the liver and its variant blood supply and collateral circulation. Am J Surg 1966;112:337)

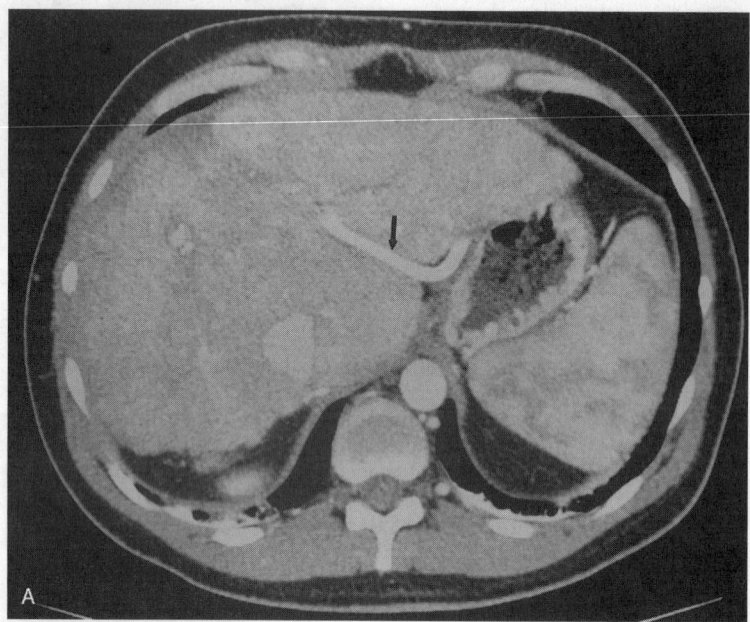

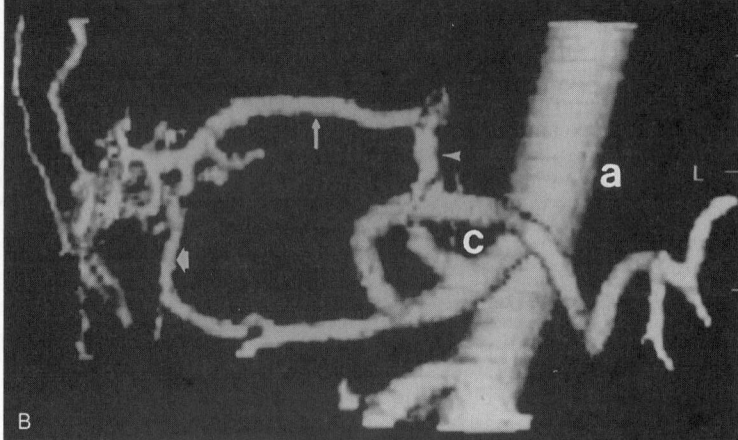

Figure 35-8. Replaced left hepatic artery arising from the left gastric artery. (*A*) Conventional transaxial images from a spiral CT scan during the arterial contrast phase, showing the replaced left hepatic artery (*dark arrow*) coursing in the lesser omentum. (*B*) Spiral CT imaging allows detailed visceral arterial reconstruction such as this oblique projection of the aorta (*a*) and celiac axis (*c*) which shows the replaced left hepatic artery (*thin arrow*) arising from the left gastric artery (*arrow head*) and the right hepatic artery coursing in the portal triad (*thick arrow*) (Courtesy of T. Winter, MD, Department of Radiology, University of Washington, Seattle)

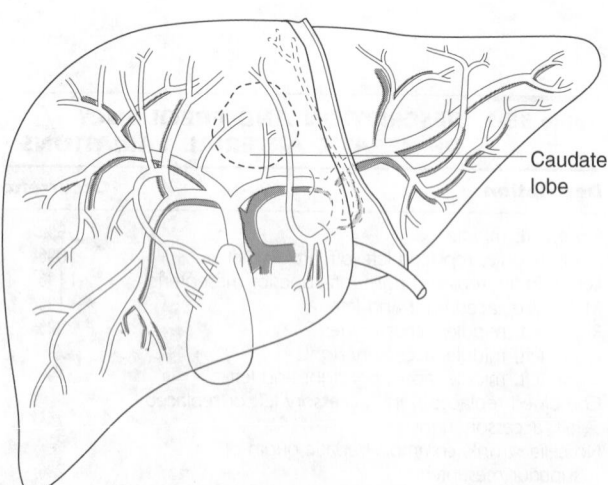

Figure 35-9. Intrahepatic divisions of bile ducts and hepatic arteries. Arterial and ductal supplies to liver parenchyma run in parallel.

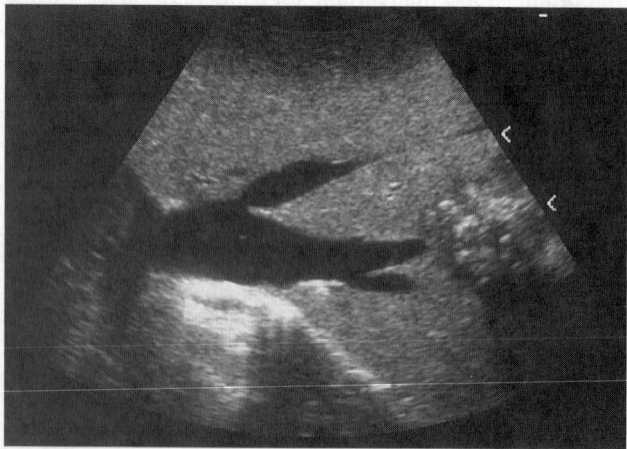

Figure 35-10. Intraoperative ultrasound of the liver depicting the middle and right hepatic vein confluence with the inferior vena cava. Hyperechoic parenchymal lesion can be seen straddling segments VII and VIII. (Courtesy of T. Winter, MD, Department of Radiology, University of Washington, Seattle)

Resolution of hepatic lesions has been greatly enhanced by the combination of visceral angiography and CT scanning, known as CT arterioportography. Most primary or secondary hepatic lesions are supplied mainly by branches of the hepatic artery. Immediate CT scanning after injection of contrast directly into the common hepatic artery (CT arteriography) may identify small hepatic lesions that usually show increased density relative to the surrounding hepatic parenchyma. CT portography includes direct injection of contrast into the splenic or superior mesenteric arteries, with CT imaging during the portal venous phase of this injection. Hepatic lesions supplied by the hepatic artery thus appear as discrete hypodense lesions surrounded by normal hepatic parenchyma enhanced by portal venous contrast. Anatomic relations between hepatic lesions and portal structures also become possible to aid in preoperative planning and determination of the feasibility of surgical resection. In many centers, CT portographic imaging of the liver is the gold standard before attempted resection of hepatomas or colorectal metastases to the liver. In other centers, conventional CT scanning followed by intraoperative ultrasound during exploration is preferred.

Double-helical (spiral) CT scanning is becoming more available and shows considerable promise to complement or replace CT arterioportography for preoperative imaging. This scanning technique allows total hepatic imaging in both the arterial and arteriovenous phases after a single rapid bolus injection of intravenous contrast during a single breath hold by the patient (Fig. 35-11). This technique also allows visualization of the portal structures and hepatic veins on a single scan and gives high resolution for small hepatic lesions. In addition, three-dimensional reconstructions in different planes can be created to further delineate hepatic parenchyma and demonstrate a CT-constructed hepatic arteriogram (see Fig. 35-8). This technique may completely replace the need for invasive angiography to fully characterize the blood supply to the liver before hepatic resection or after hepatic transplantation.

Magnetic Resonance Imaging

Magnetic resonance (MR) imaging of the liver has yielded results similar to CT scanning but has not demonstrated improvement sufficient to justify its higher cost. In addition, it does not provide optimal images of the intestine and retroperitoneum. Refinements in MR technique to increase resolution or decrease cost may increase its utility in the future.

Positron Emission Tomography Scanning

Recent advances in total body imaging using positron emission tomography scanning have enabled better resolution of hepatic primary and secondary tumors because of the increased metabolism in neoplasms of compounds such as glucose. By injecting radiolabeled glucose intravenously before scanning, areas of increased uptake may be imaged not only in the liver, but of equal importance, in areas outside of the liver, such as the primary tumor basin, regional nodes, or other distant sites, such as the lung. The current and future roles of this technique in the surgical management of hepatomas and metastatic lesions to the liver are under active investigation.

PREOPERATIVE EVALUATION OF HEPATIC RESERVE

Although the preoperative assessment and prediction of hepatic reserve after resection is critical in determining the safety, there has been only modest progress in

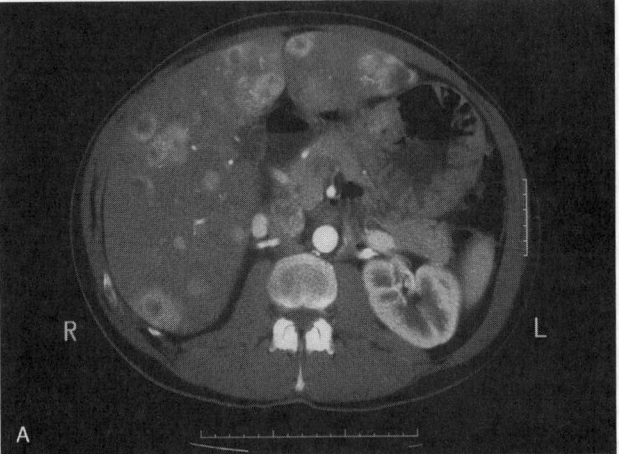

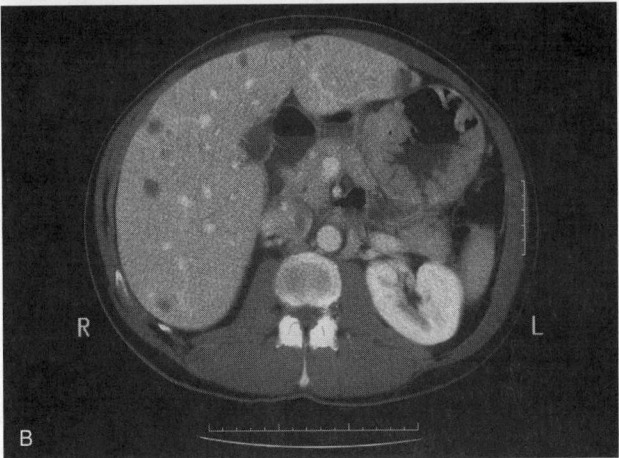

Figure 35-11. Double helical (spiral) CT scan in a 50-year-old man with hypervascular lesions from metastatic gastrinoma. (*A*) conventional venous contrast phase demonstrating a few poorly defined parenchymal lesions. (*B*) Hepatic arterial phase demonstrating clearer demarcation of lesions from surrounding normal parenchyma as well as several additional lesions. (Courtesy of T. Winter)

this measurement over the past 20 years. Liver function tests that measure the synthetic ability (albumin and prothrombin time), bile excretory function (total bilirubin and alkaline phosphatase), and prognostic scores (Child-Pugh score) have only been helpful to determine hepatic dysfunction before any intervention. More sophisticated dynamic tests include the following:

- Measurement of hepatic perfusion by the clearance of galactose or organic anionic dyes, such as indocyanin green and sulfobromophthalein
- Tests of microsomal function, such as the aminopyrine breath test, caffeine clearance, or lidocaine clearance
- Specific measurements of mitochondrial oxidative metabolism of the liver using ketone body ratio or redox tolerance index

None of these techniques has thus far proved to be universally accepted or reliable. The previous surgical dicta regarding the safety of resection are still reasonably accurate. In other words, resection of up to 75% to 80% of hepatic volume may be safely performed in the liver that has no evidence of hepatitis or cirrhosis. In the cirrhotic liver, wedge resections or segmental resections may be considered under some circumstances. Full lobar resection in the cirrhotic liver should be discouraged except in special circumstances and by experienced hepatic surgeons.

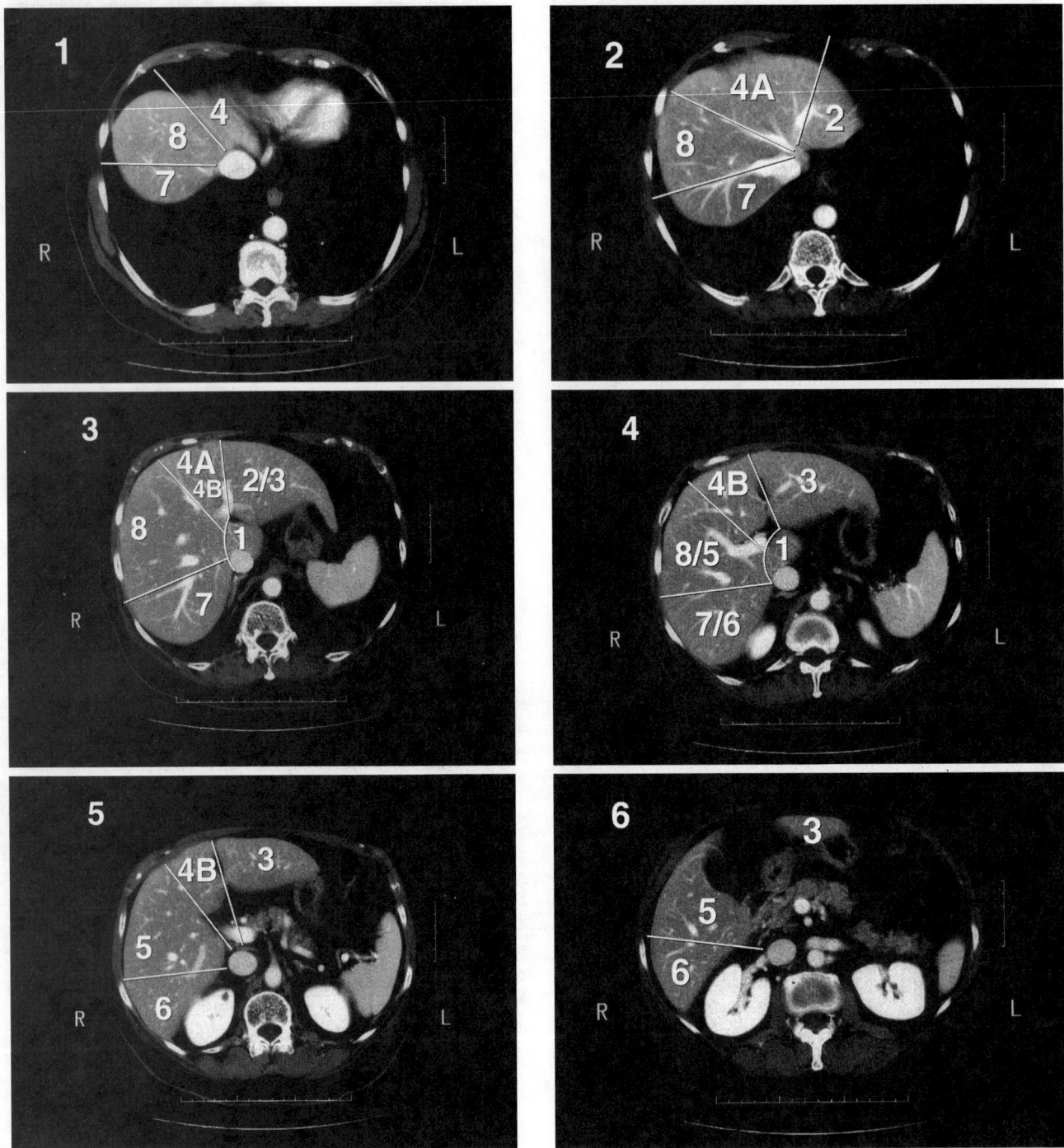

Figure 35-12. Transaxial CT image correlation of hepatic segmental anatomy by Couinaud's nomenclature. Note the posterior location of segments VI and VII, and compare with Figure 35-4.

Correlation of Computed Tomography With Segmental Anatomy

Preoperative CT scanning remains the primary imaging technique to determine the location of hepatic lesions and to estimate the extent of resection required to remove all disease. Very few descriptive reports are available that correlate the location of an hepatic lesion with photos of CT images. Figure 35-12 is provided to help guide the hepatic surgeon to the expected segment or segments of liver involved by a lesion and to provide an imaging technique that is complementary to intraoperative ultrasound in defining hepatic anatomy. Each sector of the liver can be easily defined by noting the location and course of the major hepatic veins that separate each sector. Individual segments within each sector may be identified by a superior or inferior location relative to the main portal structures within the transverse scissura. Some lesions may straddle two or more segments where a bisegmentectomy may be feasible.

Oncologic Considerations in Hepatic Resection

The goals in the operative management of primary or secondary neoplasms of the liver should be clearly delineated before any attempt at resection. Several questions should be answered: What is the diagnosis? What is the biology of the tumor in this patient? Is the goal of resection curative or palliative? Has other distant disease been excluded with a reasonable number of preoperative tests? What is the comorbid status of the patient? What other treatments are effective, and what is the optimal sequence of these treatments?

INTRAOPERATIVE ASSESSMENT

The principles of safe hepatic resection are simple: wide operative exposure with a generous incision and use of self-retaining retractors; a clear operative plan with capable surgical and anesthesia assistants; potential rapid control of vascular inflow and outflow; and the availability of autologous and banked blood products if necessary. The incisions most commonly used for major hepatic resections include an extended right subcostal incision with potential vertical or intercostal extensions if necessary (Fig. 35-13). A generous vertical incision is occasionally used for left-side resections and a right thoracoabdominal incision may be used for right-side resections. There are several current versions of self-retaining costal margin retractors that provide wide access to the entire subdiaphragmatic surface and may be combined with other self-retaining ringed retractors to keep the stomach, colon, and small bowel from the operative field.

For major resections or for complete intraoperative ultrasound, complete mobilization of the liver may be required. After detaching the hepatic flexure of the colon and ligation and dividing the falciform ligament, both the left and right triangular ligaments may be sharply taken down to fully mobilize the liver. During division of the left triangular ligament, care must be taken to avoid injury to the spleen, the left phrenic vein, the left hepatic vein, and the IVC. During division of the right triangular ligament, care must be taken to avoid injury to the right hemidiaphragm, the right adrenal gland and adrenal vein, the right phrenic vein, several moderate-sized accessory right hepatic veins draining into the right lateral wall of the vena cava, the main right hepatic vein, and the IVC. After mobilization,

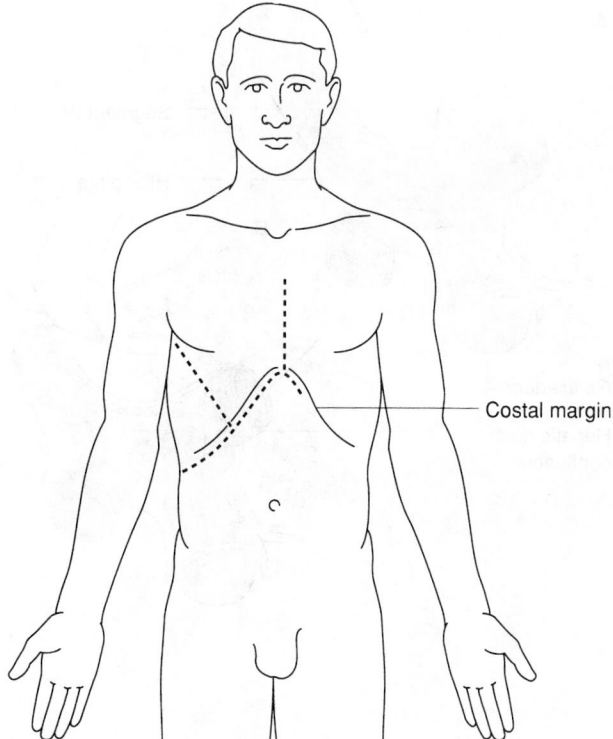

Figure 35-13. Incisions commonly used for hepatic resection.

digital and bimanual palpation is performed and intraoperative ultrasound may be performed.

Recognition of two of the three vertical scissurae is fairly reliable. The left lateral scissura courses just to the left of the umbilical fissure, and the main scissura courses along a line drawn from the gallbladder fossa anteriorly to the IVC posteriorly. The right vertical scissura is not reliably identified by external landmarks but has been described to begin at the anterior border of the liver, halfway from the distance between the right angle of the liver and the right side of the gallbladder bed, and as a vertical line coursing three fingerbreadths anterior and parallel to the right lateral edge of the liver.

Dissection of the porta hepatis is performed by many hepatic surgeons to identify the main bifurcations of the hepatic artery, bile duct, and portal vein. This allows individual ligation of unilateral branches of each of these structures during hepatic lobectomy but before parenchymal dissection. Ligation delineates the surface line of devascularization and eliminates the portal contribution of blood loss during parenchymal dissection. This technique requires tedious dissection and may take a considerable amount of time. An alternative approach has been recently described in which the main portal structures are left undisturbed and branches to a given lobe are ligated during parenchymal transection. Hemorrhage can be minimized by intermittent portal inflow occlusion by clamping or compressing the portal triad (Pringle manuever). Greater exposure of the superior aspect of the hepatic hilum and exposure of a high or intraparenchymal bifurcation of a portal structure may be aided by careful exposure of the hilar plate (Fig. 35-14) and division of Glisson capsule transversely at the inferiormost border of segment IV (the quadrate lobe). Details of this technique have been described elsewhere in the literature.[9]

There has been considerable debate over early versus late isolation and ligation of a given hepatic vein during

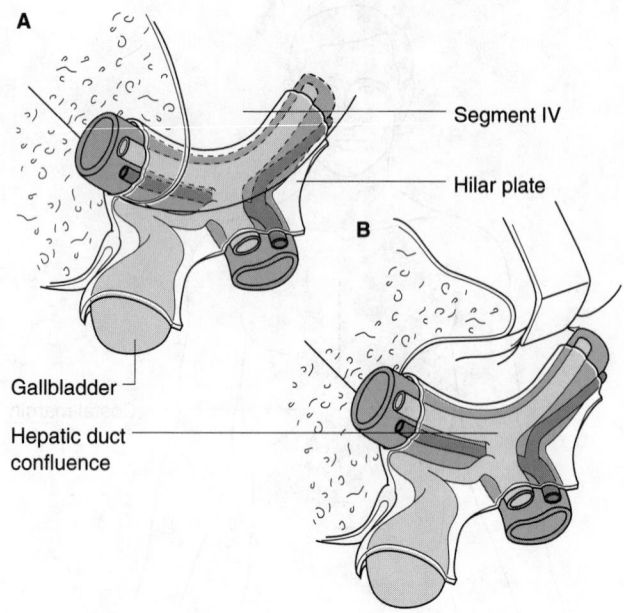

Figure 35-14. Lowering of the hilar plate. (*A*) The inferior border of segment IV (quadrate lobe) overlies the hepatic duct confluence. (*B*) Division of the connective issue investment allows elevation of segment IV, which results in a "lower" hilar plate and surgical exposure to the hepatic duct confluence. (After Blumgart LH, ed. Surgery of the liver and biliary tract New York, Churchill Livingstone, 1994)

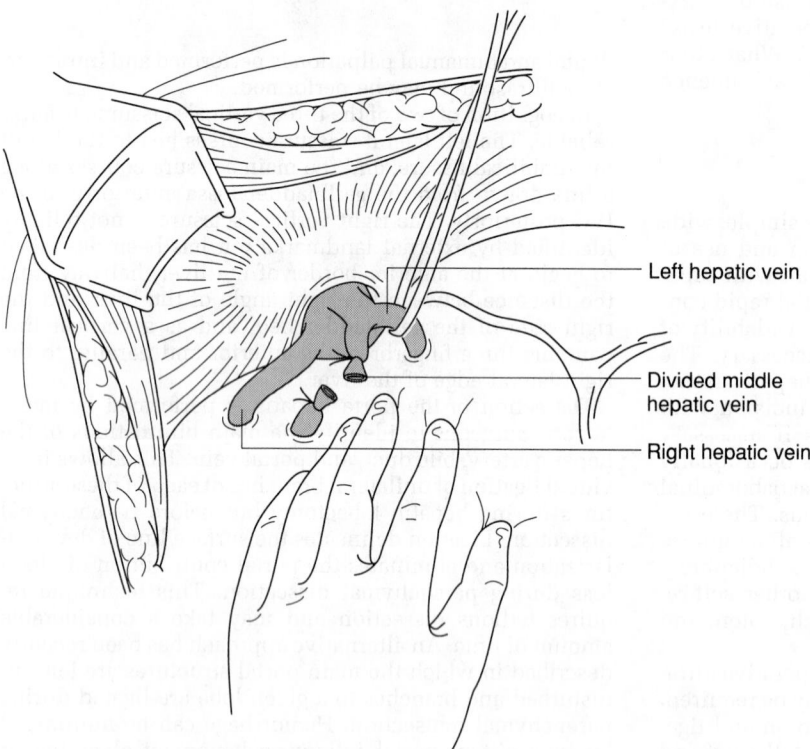

Figure 35-15. Caudal retraction of the left hepatic lobe with division of middle and left hepatic veins during left hepatic lobectomy.

lobectomy since the extraparenchymal component of hepatic vein may be quite short or absent. Because hemorrhage in this location may be difficult to expose and control, a safe strategy is always to avoid early isolation of a given hepatic vein or to attempt isolation only if a considerable length of vein is found on mobilization of the respective triangular ligament (Fig. 35-15).

MAJOR LOBECTOMY

Major lobectomy or hemihepatectomy includes segments V, VI, VII, and VIII (right hepatic lobectomy) or resection of segments II, III, and IV (left hepatic lobectomy). Extended resections of each major lobe have been described that include segments V, VI, VII, VIII, and IV (right trisegmentectomy in older nomenclature) or segments II, III, IV, and anterior segments V and VIII (left trisegmentectomy). The caudate lobe may or may not be included in the major resections, but care must be taken to preserve portal pedicle branches to this lobe if it is to be saved. A cholecystectomy is included in all of the above hepatic resections.

The steps involved in each of these major resections are similar and adhere to the tenets of optimal operative exposure and control of vascular inflow and outflow. In select circumstances, control of the vena cava may be desired. The infrahepatic vena cava may be safely encircled superior to the junction of the renal veins. The suprahepatic vena cava may be encircled with caution just inferior to the diaphragm or within the pericardium. Preparation for the Pringle maneuver is accomplished by encircling the main portal vein and proper hepatic artery using individual umbilical tape tourniquets or a noncrushing vascular clamp. Division of the hepatic parenchyma begins with scoring the Glisson capsule with cautery or knife and proceeds with dividing the hepatic substance using blunt dissection by finger fracture, the blunt end of an instrument or suction tip, or using an ultrasonic dessicator. Individual vessels and bile ducts are cauterized, sutured, or clipped in rapid succession from anterior to posterior. Constant reevaluation of the direction of transection prevents inadvertent division of vital vascular structures in adjacent segments. If temporary portal inflow occlusion is used, intermittent 10- to 20-minute intervals of clamping with 3 to 5 minutes to reestablish blood flow is recommended. The

hepatic veins are encountered in the hepatic substance near the vena cava and are carefully clamped and suture ligated to complete the resection. The raw hepatic surface is carefully inspected for bleeding and bile leaks that can be controlled by individual suture ligation, argon beam coagulator, or fibrin glue. The greater omentum can be used to buttress the transected liver edge. Perihepatic closed suction drains are often placed to monitor for unrecognized postoperative bile leaks.[10]

SEGMENTAL RESECTIONS

Recent hepatic resection stategies have focused on maximizing functional reserve without compromising safety. Segmental, bisegmental, and subsegmental or nonanatomic partial resections have been performed with increasing frequency and are now well described. An excellent monograph is available that shows detailed anatomy of segmental and bisegmental resections.[8] For example, Figure 35-16 demonstrates the vascular and biliary anatomy encountered during resection of segment VIII.

The caudate lobe (segment I) has several unique features that are important to consider before and during resection. This segment can essentially be thought of as a separate, smaller liver. Although segment I receives its afferent blood supply from both the right and left portal pedicles that arise early after the main portal bifurcation, the only parenchymal attachment to the remainder of the liver is via the thin caudate process, which extends from the posterior aspect of the right lobe (Fig. 35-17). The anterior surface of segment I is completely separated from the left lobe by the extension of the lesser omentum known as the *ligamentum venosum* (Fig. 35-18). There is a completely different route of hepatic venous drainage through multiple short veins passing directly posteriorly into the left and anterior surface of the vena cava. It is often unnecessary to remove this segment during hemihepatectomy unless its blood supply is compromised or there are oncologic reasons to remove it. Recently, isolated resection of segment I has been described for solitary lesions in this segment.[11]

Complete anatomic familiarity is essential for safe hepatic resection. The current standard for the performance of major hepatic resections should include a perioperative mortality rate of 5% or less, an infrequent need for blood

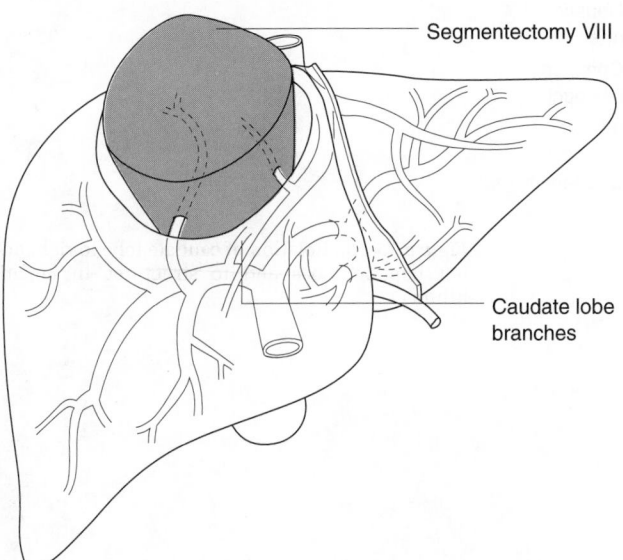

Figure 35-16. Isolated resection of segment VIII. The lack of dependable anterior topographic landmarks and the complex posterior relationships to the portal pedicles of segment I (caudate process and caudate lobe) render isolated resection of this segment extremely difficult.[8]

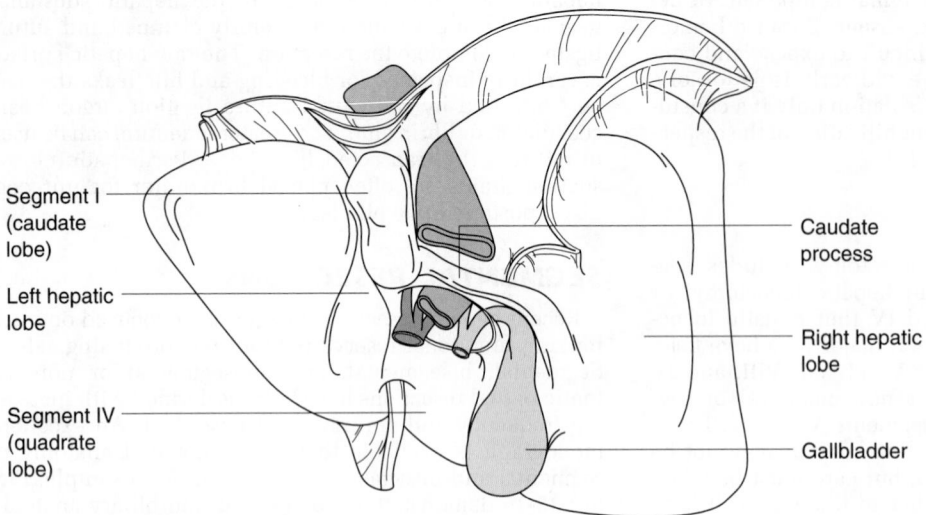

Segment I
(caudate
lobe)

Left hepatic
lobe

Segment IV
(quadrate
lobe)

Caudate
process

Right hepatic
lobe

Gallbladder

Figure 35-17. Inferior aspect of the liver, demonstrating relation of the caudate lobe to other hepatic structures.

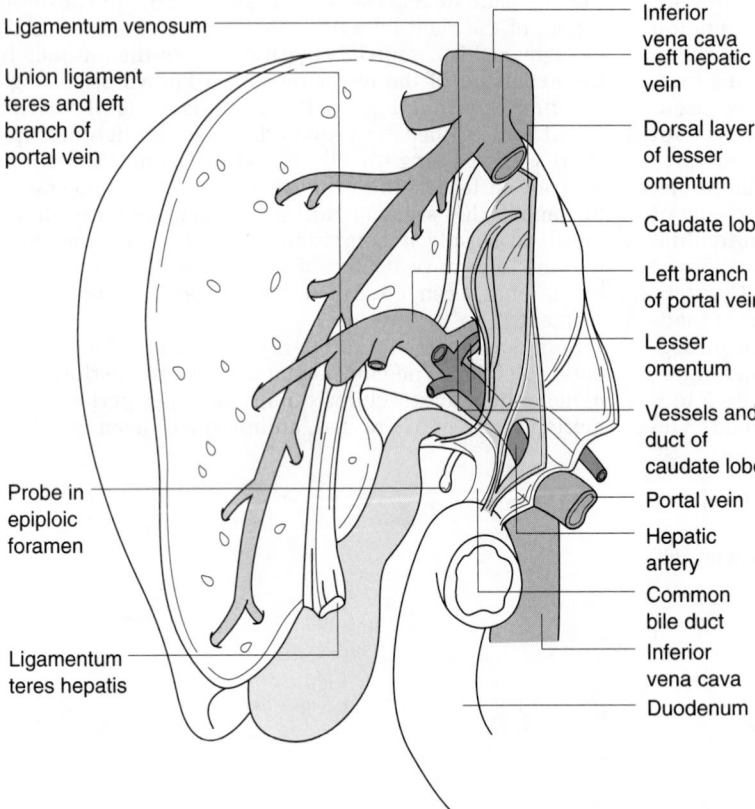

Ligamentum venosum

Union ligament
teres and left
branch of
portal vein

Probe in
epiploic
foramen

Ligamentum
teres hepatis

Inferior
vena cava
Left hepatic
vein

Dorsal layer
of lesser
omentum

Caudate lobe

Left branch
of portal vein

Lesser
omentum

Vessels and
duct of
caudate lobe

Portal vein

Hepatic
artery

Common
bile duct

Inferior
vena cava

Duodenum

Figure 35-18. Relation of caudate lobe to right and left hepatic lobes and to structures in hepatic hilum.

transfusions during or after straightforward hemihepatec-tomy, and the use of autologous blood replacement when needed and when prior donation is feasible. An interdisciplinary strategy is essential to define the goals of resection, the minimal volume of liver to be removed to accomplish those goals, and the most cost-effective use of preoperative and intraoperative imaging studies.

REFERENCES

1. Cantlie J. On a new arrangement of the right and left lobes of the liver. J Anat 1897;32:4.
2. McIndoe AH, Counseller VS. The bilaterality of the liver. Arch Surg 1927;15:589.
3. Goldsmith NA, Woodburne RT. The surgical anatomy pertaining to liver resections. Surg Gynecol Obstet 1975;105:310.
4. Healey JE Jr. Clinical anatomic aspects of radical hepatic surgery. J Int Coll Surg 1954;22:542.
5. Michels NA. Newer anatomy of the liver and its variant blood supply and collateral circulation. Am J Surg 1966;112:337.
6. Tung TT: Les résections majeures et mineures du foie. Paris, Masson, 1979.
7. Couinaud C. Le foie. Etudes anatomiques et chirurgicales. Paris, Masson, 1957.
8. Bismuth H, Houssin D, Castaing D. Major and minor segmentectomies "réglées" in liver surgery. World J Surg 1982;6:10.
9. Hepp J, Couinaud C. L'abord et l'utilisation du canal hépatique gauche dans les réparations de la voie biliaire principale. Presse Médicale 1956;64:947.
10. Adson MA, Beart RW. Elective hepatic resections. Surg Clin North Am 1977;57:339.
11. Yanaga K, Matsumata T, Hayashi H, et al. Isolated hepatic caudate lobectomy. Surgery 1994;115:757.

SURGERY: SCIENTIFIC PRINCIPLES AND PRACTICE, Second Edition, edited by Lazar J. Greenfield, Michael W. Mulholland, Keith T. Oldham, Gerald B. Zelenock, and Keith D. Lillemoe. Lippincott–Raven Publishers, Philadelphia, © 1997.

CHAPTER 36

HEPATIC PHYSIOLOGY

STEVEN E. RAPER

HISTOLOGIC ORGANIZATION OF THE LIVER

The free surface of the liver is lined by a single layer of mesothelial cells. Beneath this cell layer is the Glisson capsule, which is composed of collagen bundles, fibroblasts, and small blood vessels. At the hepatic hilus, the Glisson capsule joins with dense connective tissue inside the liver. Intrahepatic connective tissue provides support for the hepatic parenchyma; surrounds vessels, bile ducts, and nerves; and subdivides the parenchyma into its characteristic lobular structure. The dense connective tissue disappears within the lobules and is replaced by a more loosely organized reticular network, which provides a framework for orderly regeneration after hepatic injury.

The lobular structure of the mammalian liver has been recognized since the 17th century. In humans, the classic lobule, a polygonal or hexagonal arrangement of the sinusoids and their associated cell plates, is poorly defined. The smallest functional unit of the liver is the acinus.[1] The liver acinus is defined as a small oval or diamond-shaped mass of hepatic parenchyma. The apices of the acinus are the terminal hepatic venules, and its axis is formed by terminal branches of the portal vein, hepatic arteriole, and bile ductule (Fig. 36-1). The hepatocytes nearest the portal structures are the first to receive nutrients, the first to regenerate, and the last to die. Conversely, cells nearest the terminal hepatic venules receive blood of poorest quality and are less resistant to a variety of toxic injuries.

The hepatocyte is about 30 μm in diameter and constitutes 80% of the cell population of the adult human liver. The ability of individual hepatocytes to take up solute depends on the location of the hepatocyte within the lobule, the mechanism of solute uptake, and the affinity of the solute for albumin. This differential processing of solute within the lobule is called *hepatocyte heterogeneity*. Solutes that enter the cell by simple diffusion, such as ammonia, are taken up primarily in zone 1. Proteins taken up by receptor-mediated endocytosis, such as epidermal growth factor, also tend to be taken up in zones 1 and 2. Albumin-bound solutes, such as bilirubin, tend to be taken up by cells of all three zones because the large size of the albumin molecule allows it to distribute more evenly throughout the acinus.

PARENCHYMAL CELL ULTRASTRUCTURE
Plasma Membrane

The function of the hepatocyte is intimately related to structure. An understanding of the hepatocyte organelles that allow the liver to carry out its many metabolic missions is important (Fig. 36-2). The hepatocyte plasma membrane consists of a phospholipid bilayer in which hydrophobic fatty acid tails are oriented to the interior membrane and hydrophilic phospholipid head groups are oriented to the exterior (sinusoidal or cytoplasmic) membrane (Fig. 36-3). Within this phospholipid bilayer are proteins, often complexed with sugar molecules (glycoproteins), which serve either structural functions (eg, tight junctions) or metabolic functions (eg, receptor, carrier, or enzymatic). The hepatocyte plasma membrane is divided into three domains: (1) the sinusoidal domain, which is studded with microvilli to increase the absorptive area in contact with sinusoidal blood; (2) the basolateral domain, which is in contact with other liver cells; and (3) the bile canalicular domain, which under normal conditions is completely separated from the bloodstream by tight junctional complexes.[2]

Cell membranes, by virtue of their high lipid content, allow lipid-soluble molecules to enter the cell by simple diffusion. Polar molecules enter cells by membrane transport proteins (Fig. 36-4). Some transport proteins carry solute in a single direction and are called *uniports*. Cotransport carriers involve the transfer of a second solute. Two molecules transported in the same direction use a symport, whereas two molecules transported in opposite directions use an antiport. Passive transport can occur by simple or facilitated diffusion. Channel proteins allow molecules to diffuse simply into cells without binding, whereas carrier proteins first bind the solute and, by conformational change, allow it to be transported into the cell. The glucose carrier in hepatocytes is an example of carrier-facilitated diffusion. Active transport requires an energy source, usually adenosine triphosphate (ATP), to transport molecules against a thermodynamically unfavorable electrochemical or concentration gradient.

The various membrane regions are characterized by specific functions. The sinusoidal membrane is characterized by active bidirectional transport of proteins, water, and organic and inorganic solutes. Transport of large protein-bound substances into liver cells is facilitated by fenestra-

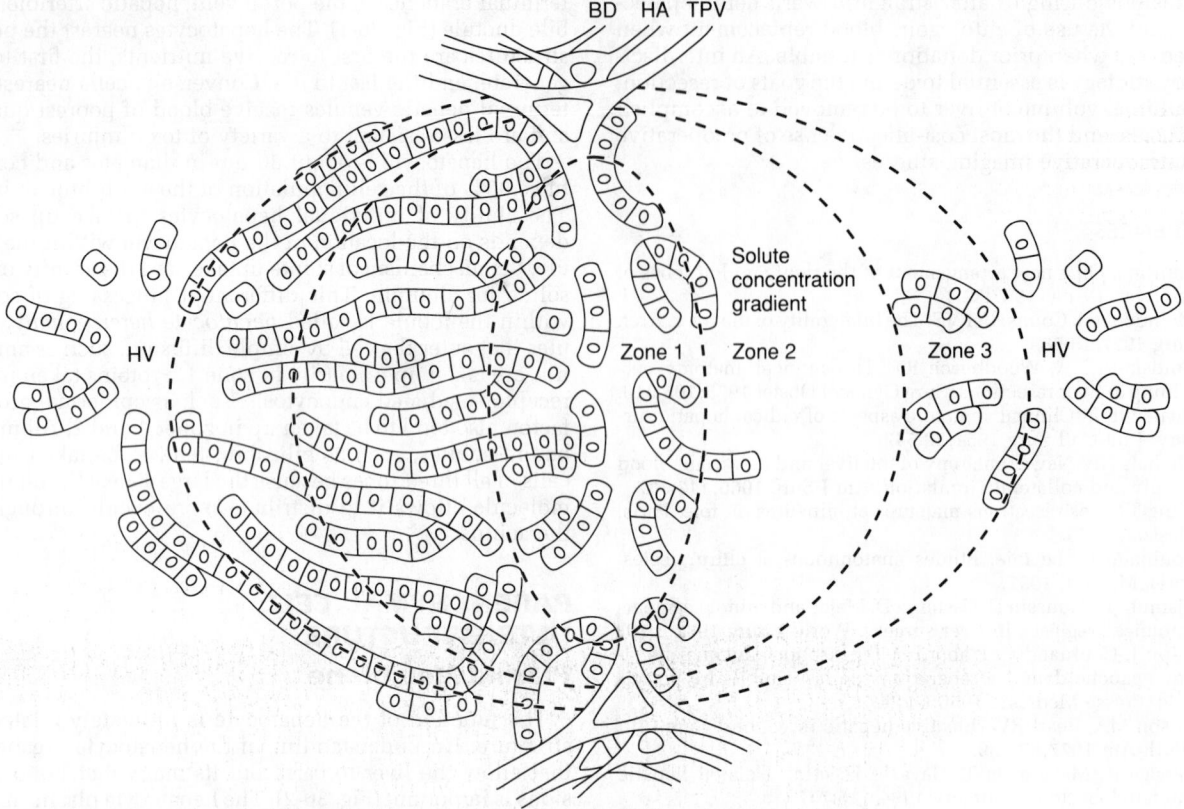

Figure 36-1. The hepatic acinus. Unidirectional perfusion of the hepatocytes within the acinus causes a gradient of solute concentration as blood moves from the terminal portal venule (TPV) to the hepatic venule (HV). Hepatocytes nearest the portal tract are labeled zone 1, mid-acinar cells are labeled zone 2, and centrilobular cells are zone 3. The TPV to HV oxygen gradient is 50 μmol/L. This implies that zone 1 cells have a higher oxygen tension than zone 3 cells. The concept of acinar zones fits well, therefore, with observations of histologic injury for a variety of toxins. BD, bile ductule; HA, hepatic arteriole. (After Rappoport AM. The acinus: microvascular unit of the liver. In: Lautt WW, ed. Hepatic circulation in health and disease. New York, Raven Press, 1981:175)

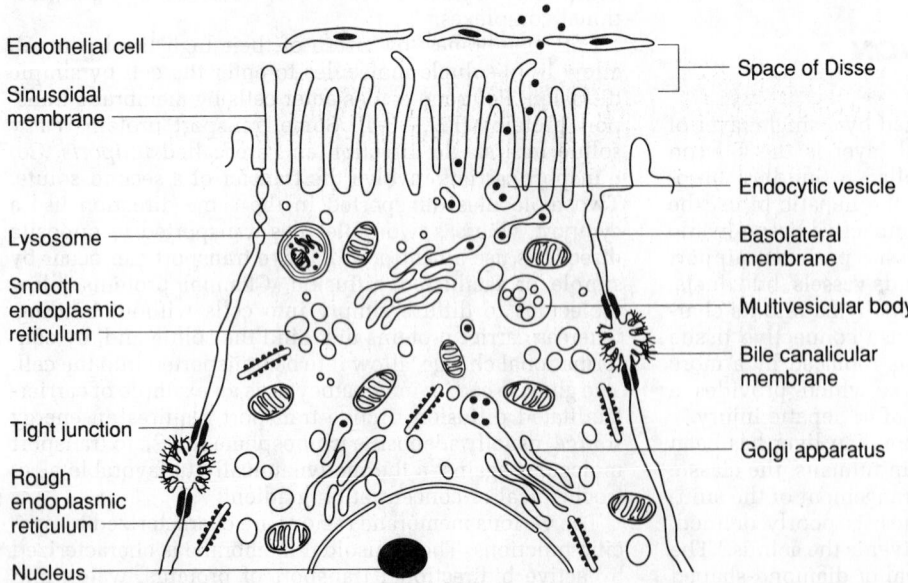

Figure 36-2. Major ultrastructural features of the hepatocyte.

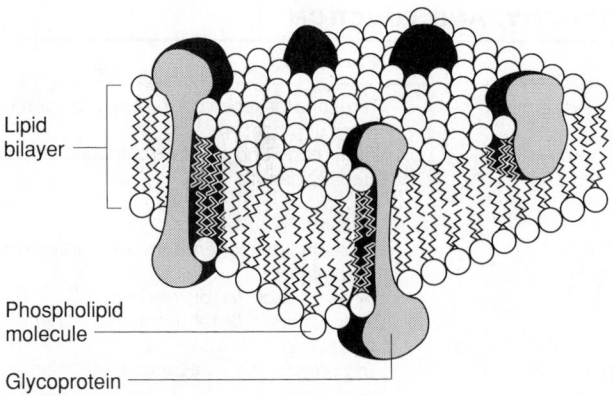

Figure 36-3. Schematic three-dimensional view of a small section of a hepatocyte membrane, illustrating the lipid bilayer and integral glycoproteins.

Lipid bilayer

Phospholipid molecule

Glycoprotein

tions of about 1000 nm in the endothelial cell membrane. The basolateral membrane extends from the sinusoid to the edge of the bile canaliculus. This portion of the membrane is almost flat and contains structural proteins that allow attachment and communication between cells. Tight junctional complexes separate the basolateral surface from the canalicular surface. Bile canalicular membrane surface area is also increased by the formation of microvilli. In humans, the total canalicular surface area can reach 10 m². The bile canalicular membrane is intimately associated with microfilaments, which appear responsible for canalicular shape and bile formation. Each plasma membrane do-

main contains characteristic membrane proteins. Alkaline phosphatase and 5′-nucleotidase are found predominantly in the canalicular membrane, whereas membrane receptors for various proteins are localized to the sinusoidal membrane.

The plasma membrane is also directly responsible for endocytosis, the process by which hepatocytes take up extracellular fluids and macromolecules. The three types of endocytosis are pinocytosis, phagocytosis, and receptor-mediated endocytosis. Pinocytosis is a process by which water and solute are nonspecifically taken up into vesicles of 0.1 to 0.2 μm. Phagocytosis involves the uptake of large particles, such as malaria sporozooites. Receptor-mediated endocytosis is a special form of pinocytosis and occurs when extracellular macromolecules bind to specific cell-surface receptors before internalization.

Cell-Surface Receptors

The sinusoidal membrane is studded with receptors, which are large glycoprotein molecules that span the plasma membrane lipid bilayer. A ligand-binding site of this receptor molecule projects into the space of Disse. When appropriate ligand-receptor binding occurs, the entire ligand can be internalized for intracellular degradation or biliary transport, or the ligand can transmit a signal to the interior of the hepatocyte by a number of intracellular second-messenger systems.[3] Table 36-1 lists known hepatocyte receptors, ligand specificity, and functions.

Although ligands undergo receptor binding and internalization at the plasma membrane, they can follow a number of different intracellular pathways (Fig. 36-5). In the intracellular compartments responsible for processing of

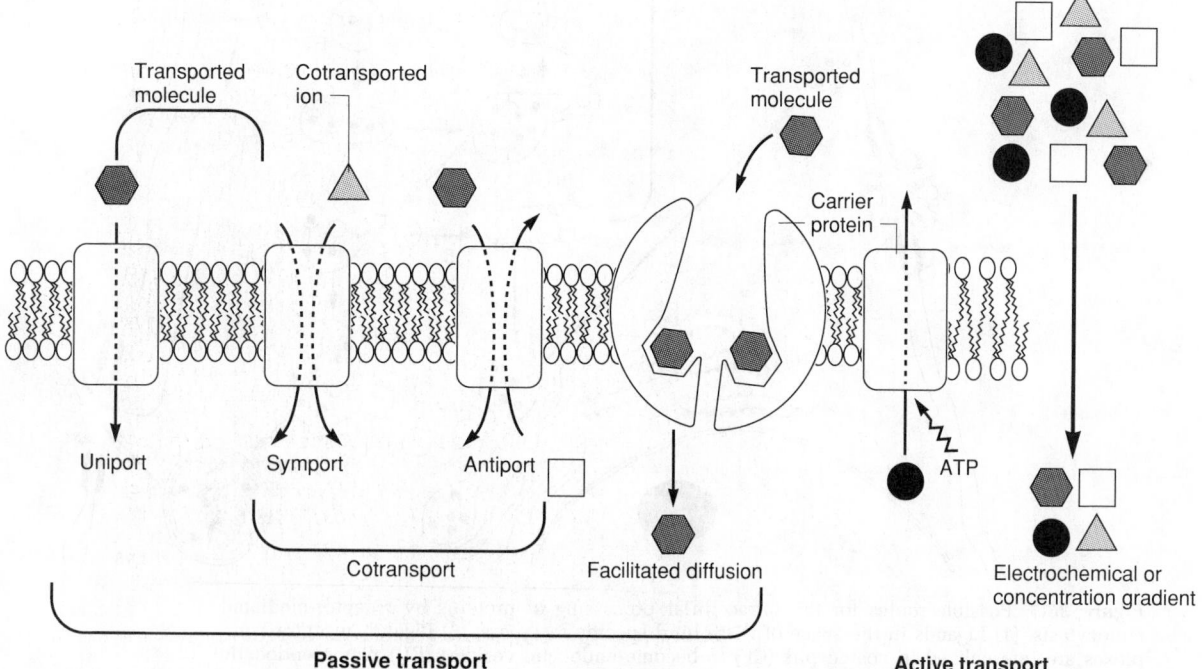

Transported molecule

Cotransported ion

Transported molecule

Carrier protein

Uniport   Symport   Antiport

Cotransport

Facilitated diffusion

ATP

Electrochemical or concentration gradient

Passive transport   **Active transport**

Figure 36-4. Schematic representation of the major types of membrane transport proteins, which are crucial for the transport of polar solutes. Passive transport involves passage of molecules in the direction of a concentration gradient. Uniports, symports, and antiports are examples of channel proteins, which allow molecules to pass by simple diffusion. Carrier proteins allow facilitated diffusion by specifically binding to individual molecules. Other carrier proteins actively transport molecules against a concentration or electrochemical gradient, a thermodynamically unfavorable event that requires ATP or some other form of exogenous energy.

Table 36-1. KNOWN HEPATIC RECEPTORS, LIGAND SPECIFICITY, AND FUNCTION

Receptor	Ligand	Function
Asialoglycoprotein	Desialylated proteins with exposed terminal galactose residues	Targeting of senescent proteins to lysomes for degradation
Chylomicron remnant	Lipoproteins containing apolipoprotein B-48	Triglyceride and cholesterol metabolism
Epidermal growth factor	Epidermal growth factor; transforming growth factor α	Hepatic growth
Growth hormone	Growth hormone	Hepatotrophic factor
Immunoglobulin A (IgA)	Polymeric IgA	Secretory component formation; intestinal immunity
Insulin	Insulin	Hepatotrophic factor; glycogenesis
Insulin-like growth factor 1 (IGF-1)	IGF-1	Hepatotrophic factor; lysosomal enzyme processing
	Lysosomal enzymes	
Low-density lipoprotein	Lipoproteins containing apolipoprotein B-100 or E	Triglyceride and cholesterol metabolism
Transferrin	Transferrin–iron complexes	Iron uptake and storage

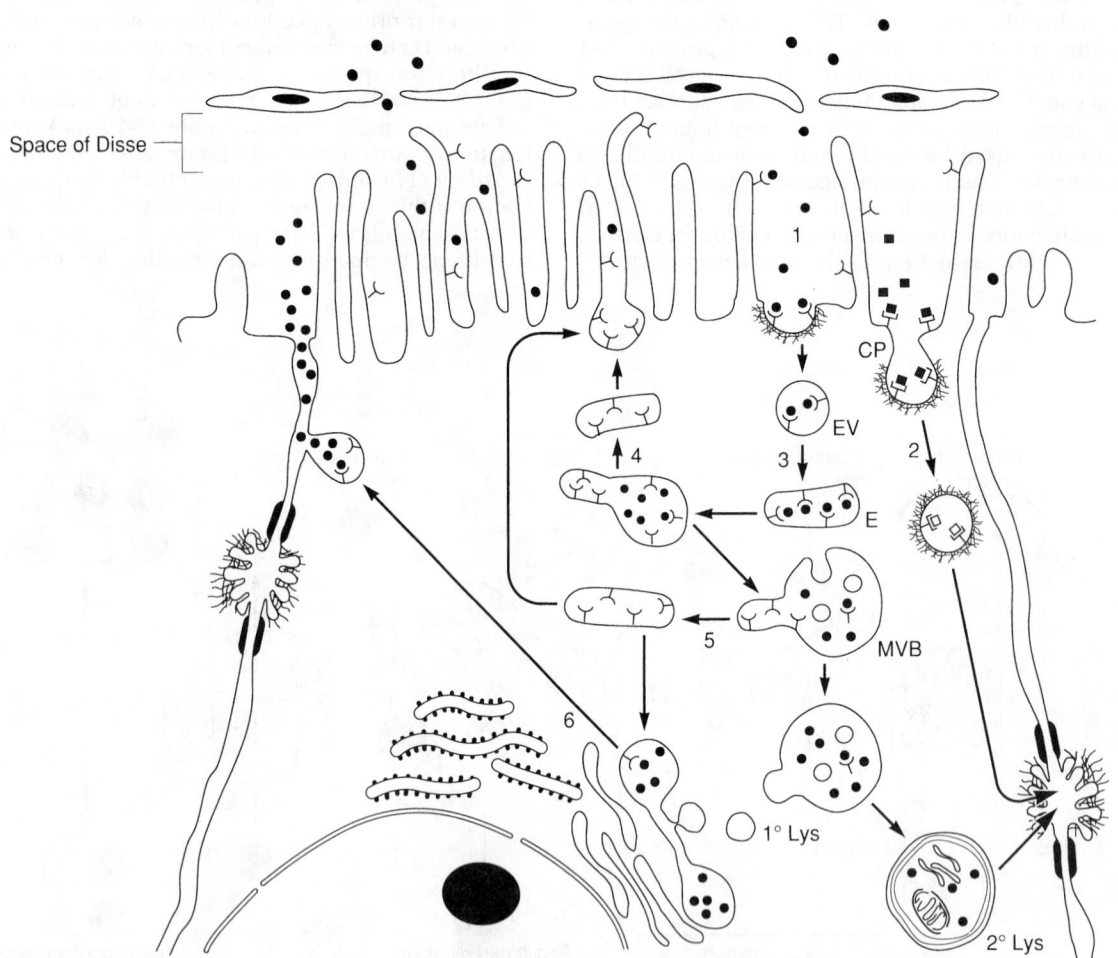

Figure 36-5. Possible routes for the intracellular processing of proteins by receptor-mediated endocytosis. (1) Ligands in the space of Disse bind specific receptors. (2) Ligand–receptor complexes are internalized in coated pits (CP) to become endocytic vesicles (EV). Some endocytic vesicles are transported directly to the bile canaliculus to secrete intact protein (ie, polymeric immunoglobulin A). (3) Other coated vesicles lose their clathrin coat and fuse to become endosomes (E). (4) Endosomes become acidified to become the compartment of uncoupling of receptor and ligand. Receptors are recycled to the plasma membrane, while the ligands remain in multivesicular bodies (MVBs). (5) MVBs fuse with primary lysosomes (1° Lys) to become secondary lysosomes (2° Lys), in which ligands are degraded and excreted into bile (ie, the asialoglycoproteins). (6) New receptors are synthesized in the rough endoplasmic reticulum and processed through the Golgi complex before insertion into the plasma membrane.

receptor-bound proteins, molecular sorting takes place, in effect targeting proteins to various intracellular destinations. Some of the ligand-receptor vesicles are coated with clathrin, a small protein that can encode sorting information.[4] Receptor phosphorylation may be another mechanism by which the liver can sort receptors to their final destinations.[5]

Some cell-surface receptors initiate a cascade of intracellular events by acting to generate intracellular second messengers, a process known as *signal transduction*. Such second messengers include cyclic adenosine monophosphate, inositol triphosphate, and diacylglycerol.[6] Each of these structurally simple chemicals can amplify cell membrane events and bring about major changes in cellular physiology (Fig. 36-6).

New methods of delivering biologic substances to intracellular targets are based on the use of receptor-mediated endocytosis. For example, by chemically coupling a biochemical antagonist to normally internalized proteins, normal liver cells can be protected from the toxic effect of a chemotherapeutic agent, while the malignant cells are killed.[7] Similarly, a DNA carrier system has been devised that can target selected DNA fragments to hepatocytes by way of the membrane asialoglycoprotein (ASGP) receptor. The DNA can be injected intravenously and selectively internalized by the liver, where gene expression may then occur.[8] These studies suggest that gene therapy in the future may be as simple as an intravenous injection. Such a strategy could conceivably replace liver transplantation for certain inborn errors of metabolism.

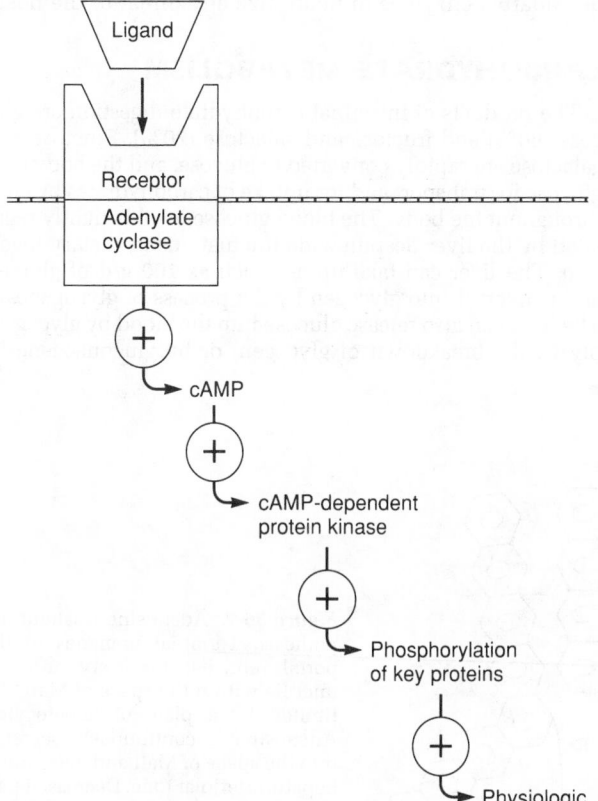

Figure 36-6. Role of cyclic adenosine monophosphate (cAMP)–dependent protein kinase in signal transduction. A single ligand–receptor interaction at the membrane is amplified many times by the stimulation of adenyl cyclase.

Mitochondria

Liver mitochondria are self-replicating organelles that contain an independent complement of DNA. The outer membrane is freely permeable to all molecules of 10 kd. The inner membrane contains the enzymes of the electron transport chain and ATP synthetase. The mitochondrial matrix contains hundreds of enzymes responsible for the interconversion of a wide variety of small molecules. Mitochondria are more numerous in the zone 1 cells, where oxygen tension is higher. The primary role of mitochondria is to generate large amounts of ATP through the citric acid cycle and oxidative phosphorylation. Electron transport enzymes of the inner membrane create a large electrochemical gradient, which drives ATP synthase to form new ATP.

Endosomes, Multivesicular Bodies, and Lysosomes

After the clathrin coat falls away from endocytosed vesicles, the vesicles coalesce to form endosomes.[4] The endosomal membrane contains an ATP-driven hydrogen ion pump that acidifies the endosome and thus causes dissociation of ligand and receptor. Endosomal components may return to the cell surface, in effect recycling receptors, or may enter multivesicular bodies, which are aggregates of endosomal remnants. Primary lysosomes are vesicles full of newly synthesized degradative enzymes capable of fusing with multivesicular bodies. Under acidic conditions, the lysosomal enzymes become active and result in secondary lysosomes, full of degraded intracellular components. Lysosomes are numerous in the liver and are found in the cytoplasm adjacent to the bile canaliculus and Golgi complex. Secondary lysosomes fuse with the bile canalicular membrane and discharge their contents into the bile (see Fig. 36-5).

Endoplasmic Reticulum and Golgi Complex

The liver is unique in that both smooth- and rough-surfaced endoplasmic reticula are well developed. The smooth endoplasmic reticulum (ER) is composed of a complex meshwork of branching tubules that communicate with the rough ER and the Golgi complex. Rough ER usually forms aggregates of parallel, flattened cisternae scattered throughout the cytoplasm. The granules that give the rough appearance to rough ER are ribosomes. The Golgi complex consists of three to five closely packed, parallel, smooth cisternae associated with some vesicular structures. The smooth ER, rough ER, and Golgi complex are collectively referred to as the *liver microsomal fraction*.

The liver microsomes are known to participate in the following mechanisms: (1) synthesis of albumin, fibrinogen, and other proteins destined for export to the plasma; (2) synthesis of cholesterol and bile salts; (3) glucuronidation of bilirubin, drugs, and steroids; (5) esterification of free fatty acids to triglycerides; and (6) glycogenolysis.

The Nucleus

The nucleus is the largest of the cellular organelles. It is separated from the cytoplasm by a nuclear envelope consisting of an inner and outer membrane. All of the chromosomal DNA is packaged into chromatin fibers in association with DNA-binding proteins called *histones*. Ribosomes are synthesized in the nucleolus to aid in protein synthesis. The cytoplasm and nucleus communicate through nuclear pores.

HEPATIC BLOOD FLOW
Control of Liver Blood Flow

The liver constitutes about 2.5% of the total body weight but receives 25% of the cardiac output. Total hepatic blood flow is 100 to 130 mL/min/kg. About two thirds of total hepatic flow is derived from the portal vein and one third from the hepatic artery. To a large extent, portal venous flow into the liver is regulated by extrahepatic factors such as the rate of flow from the intestines and spleen. Thus, hepatic flow might be expected to vary with the metabolic state of the organism. Blood flow in the liver, however, is remarkably unaffected by nutritional status. The constancy of total hepatic blood flow is due primarily to changes in hepatic arterial flow. Both intrinsic and extrinsic mechanisms of flow regulation are operative in the hepatic artery.[9]

Intrinsic flow regulation occurs through arterial autoregulation based on the local concentration of adenosine surrounding the hepatic arteriole and portal venule. Adenosine is a potent vasodilator of the hepatic arteriole. The vessels are surrounded by a limiting plate and a microenvironment called the *space of Mall* (Fig. 36-7). An increase in portal venous flow causes increased washout of adenosine and hepatic arteriolar constriction. If portal venous flow is reduced, local concentrations of adenosine increase and cause dilation of the hepatic arteriole, leading to a compensatory increase in hepatic arterial flow, and thus maintaining a constant level of total hepatic blood flow.[10]

Less is known about extrinsic flow regulation. Both humoral and neural mechanisms have been demonstrated. Although the hepatic artery can dilate in response to pharmacologic doses of many vasoactive compounds, the physiologic relevance is unknown. The hepatic artery does not constrict in the postprandial state despite marked increases in portal flow; some agents apparently can overcome the intrinsic regulatory control exerted by the adenosine washout response. Possible humoral mediators of extrinsic regulation include gastrin, glucagon, secretin, and bile salts. The hepatic artery is also densely innervated by sympathetic nerves, which are known to cause vasoconstriction mediated by α-adrenergic receptors.

Resistance to portal blood flow is thought to occur primarily across a distinct hepatic venous sphincter-like zone. Several investigators have documented histologically the presence of such sphincters in humans. This anatomic evidence is supported by detailed physiologic studies in several animal species. In normal liver, no resistance is attributable to either the portal venule or the sinusoid. The hepatic venous sphincters constrict in response to histamine, norepinephrine, angiotensin, and nerve stimulation (in cats and dogs).

The liver serves as a physiologic blood reservoir. About 25% to 30% of the liver volume is accounted for by blood; and in cases of acute blood loss, up to 30%, or as much as 300 mL, of the hepatic blood volume can be released into the systemic circulation without adverse effects on liver function. Conversely, in cases of right heart failure or other causes of systemic volume overload, as much as 1 L of extra blood can be stored in the liver before passive congestion and liver injury occur.

Blood Cleansing Function

Hepatic sinusoids are lined by an endothelium punctuated with pores that allow proteins as large as albumin to diffuse out of the vascular tree and into proximity with hepatocytes. Sinusoidal pressure is only 6 to 8 mmHg so that proteins can also diffuse back into the vasculature. Much of the extravasated protein enters the lymphatics, and hepatic lymph contains as much protein as plasma. This extreme permeability of the liver allows rapid exchange of a diverse number of nutrients, hormones, and environmental agents between the blood and the hepatocyte. The liver also acts as a filter for particulate debris, which enters the portal circulation through intestinal capillaries. Particles such as bacteria are ingested by Kupffer cells through the process of phagocytosis. Kupffer cells line the hepatic sinusoidal endothelium, where formed blood elements and particulate matter may be in direct contact with these phagocytic cells. Once particulate matter is internalized, Kupffer cells contain a wide variety of degradative enzymes to neutralize any threat to the host.

CARBOHYDRATE METABOLISM

The products of intestinal carbohydrate digestion are glucose (80%) and fructose and galactose (20%). Fructose and galactose are rapidly converted to glucose, and the body uses glucose for transport and for uptake of carbohydrates by cells throughout the body. The blood glucose level is tightly regulated by the liver despite wide fluctuations in dietary ingestion. The liver can take up as much as 100 g/d of glucose and convert it into glycogen by the process of glycogenesis. The liver can also release glucose into the blood by glycogenolysis, the breakdown of glycogen, or by gluconeogenesis,

A   B

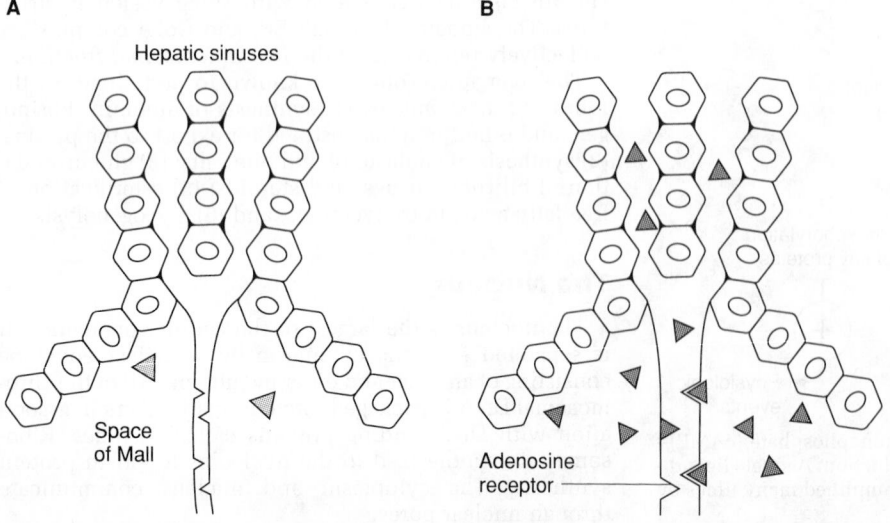

Figure 36-7. Adenosine washout hypothesis. Terminal branches of the portal vein, hepatic artery, and bile duct lie within the space of Mall, delimited by a plate of hepatocytes. Adenosine is continuously secreted into the space of Mall and determines hepatic arteriolar tone. Decreased portal vein flow causes increased levels of adenosine and hepatic arteriolar dilation. Increased flow decreases adenosine and causes vasoconstriction, the so-called hepatic arterial buffer response.

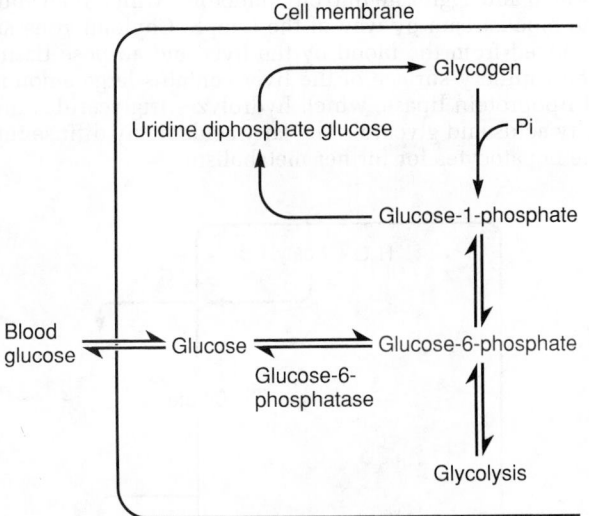

Figure 36-8. The chemical reactions of glycogenesis and glycolysis. Glucose-6-phosphatase allows hepatic glucose to be transported out of the hepatocyte for use in other tissues. Glucose-6-phosphate has a central role in carbohydrate metabolism.

the formation of new glucose from substrates such as alanine, lactate, glycerol, or certain dietary amino acids. Hormones play a key role in the hepatic regulation of glucose metabolism. Insulin, for example, stimulates glycogenesis, and glucagon stimulates glycogenolysis and gluconeogenesis. The liver metabolizes glucose primarily to provide substrates for biosynthetic reactions. Most other tissues use glucose to generate ATP for energy.[11]

Glycogen Storage and Metabolism

Glycogen is a complex polymer of glucose with an average molecular weight of 5 million. Liver cells can store up to 8% of their weight as glycogen. The first step in glycogen storage is the transport of glucose through the hepatocyte plasma membrane. About 90% of portal venous glucose is removed from the blood by liver cells through carrier-facilitated diffusion. Large numbers of carrier molecules on the sinusoidal domain of the hepatocyte are capable of binding glucose and transferring it to the cytoplasm. The rate of glucose transport is enhanced (up to 10-fold) by insulin.

Glycogenesis and Glycogenolysis

Once in the hepatocyte, glucose and ATP are converted by the enzyme glucokinase to glucose-6-phosphate (G6P), the first intermediate in the synthesis of glycogen (Fig. 36-8). Because complete oxidation of one molecule of G6P generates 37 molecules of ATP, and storage only uses one molecule of ATP, the overall efficiency of glucose storage in glycogen is a remarkable 97%.

Glycogenolysis does not occur by simple reversal of glycogenesis. Each succeeding glucose on a glycogen chain is released by glycogen phosphorylase (Fig. 36-9). Eventually, G6P is re-formed. G6P cannot exit from cells and must first be converted back to glucose. This reaction is catalyzed by glucose-6-phosphatase, found only in hepatocytes, kidney, and intestinal epithelial cells. Neither brain nor muscle cells, which use glucose as a primary fuel source, contain the phosphatase enzyme. This lack of glucose-6-phosphatase ensures a ready supply of glucose for the energy needs of brain and muscle. Liver does not use glucose primarily for fuel, but as a precursor for other molecules.

Glycolysis

Glycolysis is the pathway by which glucose is converted to two molecules of pyruvate (Fig. 36-10). This conversion has three effects: (1) a net gain of two ATP molecules, (2) generation of two molecules of nicotinamide adenine nucleotide, and (3) conversion of pyruvate to acetyl coenzyme A (CoA) and degradation of it in the citric acid cycle (see later). Glycolysis occurs in the cytoplasm, in contrast to the citric acid cycle, which occurs in the mitochondria (Fig. 36-11). During times of glucose excess, as in the fed state, the liver can use glycolysis as a means of generating energy in the form of ATP, but the oxidation of ketoacids is preferred.

Phosphogluconate Pathway

When glucose enters the liver, glycogen is formed until the hepatic glycogen capacity is reached (about 100 g). If excess glucose is still available, the liver converts it to fat by the phosphogluconate pathway (Fig. 36-12). Up to 30% of hepatic glucose metabolism occur by this pathway. Hydrogen atoms released in the phosphogluconate pathway combine with $NADP^+$ to form NADPH.[12]

Gluconeogenesis

When glucose becomes scarce, as in the fasting state, glycogenolysis occurs. Once glycogen stores have been depleted, the liver is capable of synthesizing new glucose by the process of gluconeogenesis. About 60% of the naturally occurring amino acids, glycerol, or lactate can be used as substrates for glucose production. Alanine is the amino acid easiest to convert into glucose. Simple deamination

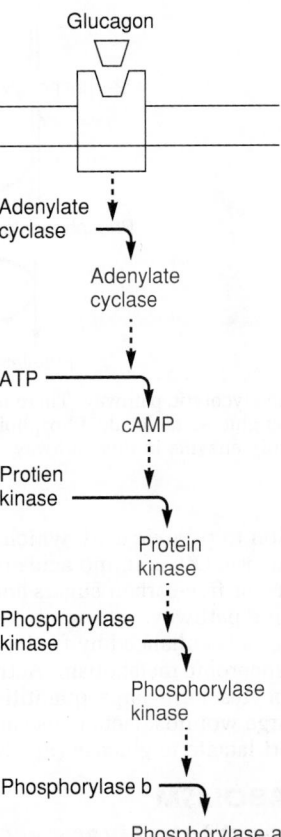

Figure 36-9. Glucagon-stimulated enzyme cascade responsible for control of glycogen metabolism. Inactive forms are shown in black, active forms in blue.

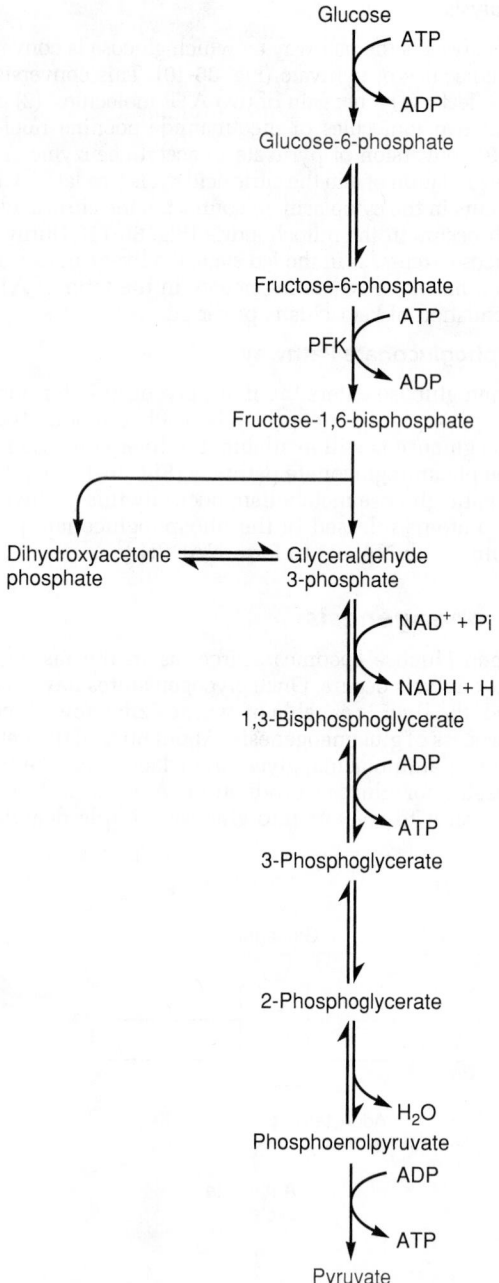

Figure 36-10. The glycolytic pathway. There is a net gain of two ATP molecules per glucose molecule. Phosphofructokinase (PFK) is the key regulatory enzyme in this pathway.

allows conversion to pyruvic acid, which is subsequently converted to glucose. Other amino acids can be converted into three-, four-, or five-carbon sugars and then enter the phosphogluconate pathway.

Gluconeogenesis is enhanced by fasting, critical illness, and periods of anaerobic metabolism. Active skeletal muscle and erythrocytes form large quantities of lactate. In patients with large wounds, lactate also accumulates. The liver can convert lactate to glucose (Fig. 36-13).

LIPID METABOLISM
Lipid Transport Into Liver

Dietary triglycerides are split into monoglycerides and fatty acids by the action of intestinal lipases. After absorption into the small intestinal cells, triglycerides are re-

formed and aggregate into chylomicrons, which then enter the bloodstream by way of the lymph. Chylomicrons are removed from the blood by the liver and adipose tissue. The capillary surface of the liver contains large amounts of lipoprotein lipase, which hydrolyzes triglycerides into fatty acids and glycerol. The fatty acids freely diffuse into the hepatocytes for further metabolism.

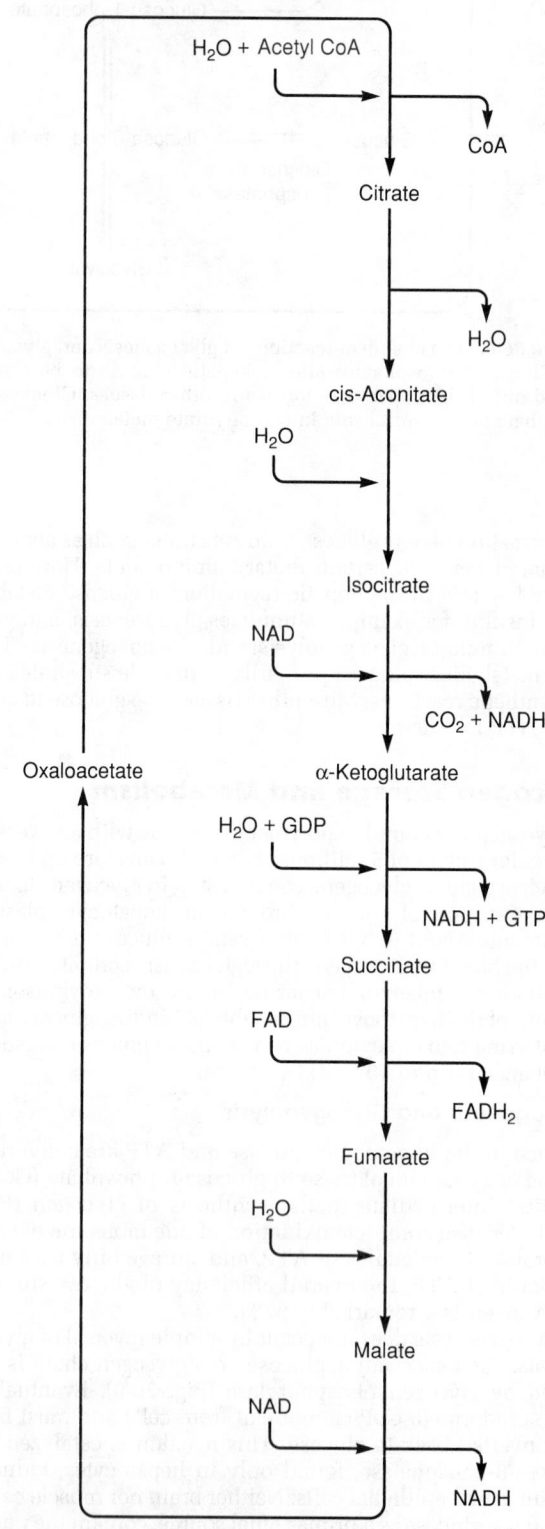

Figure 36-11. The citric acid cycle. NADH and FADH$_2$, formed in the citric acid cycle, are subsequently oxidized in mitochondria by means of the electron transport chain to generate ATP. Acetyl CoA plays a key role.

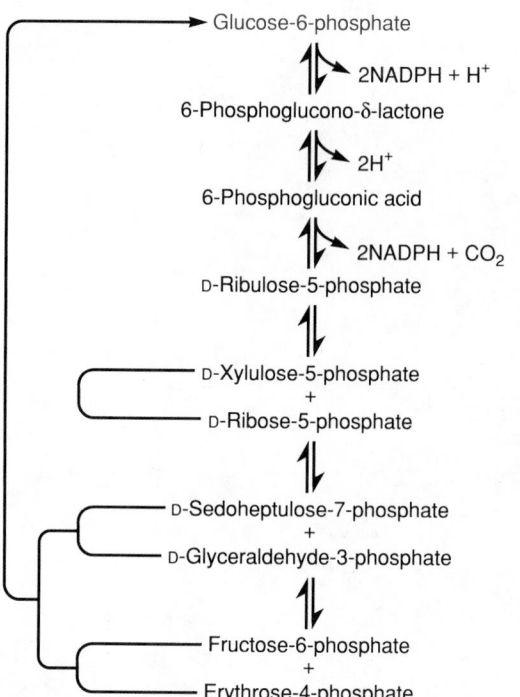

Glucose-6-phosphate

$\Updownarrow$ 2NADPH + H$^+$

6-Phosphoglucono-δ-lactone

$\Updownarrow$ 2H$^+$

6-Phosphogluconic acid

$\Updownarrow$ 2NADPH + CO$_2$

D-Ribulose-5-phosphate

$\Updownarrow$

D-Xylulose-5-phosphate
+
D-Ribose-5-phosphate

$\Updownarrow$

D-Sedoheptulose-7-phosphate
+
D-Glyceraldehyde-3-phosphate

$\Updownarrow$

Fructose-6-phosphate
+
Erythrose-4-phosphate

Figure 36-12. The phosphogluconate pathway. One of the major purposes of this pathway is to generate NADPH, which can serve as an electron donor and allows the liver to perform reductive biosyntheses.

The liver has a number of important functions in the metabolism of lipids, including the synthesis of apolipoproteins, the degradation of fatty acids into energy substrates, the synthesis of triglycerides from carbohydrates and proteins, and the synthesis of cholesterol and phospholipids from fatty acids.

Fatty Acid Metabolism

Most human fatty acids found in plasma are long-chain acids (C-16 to C-20). Because long-chain fatty acids are not readily absorbed by the intestinal mucosa, they must first be incorporated into chylomicrons. In contrast, short-chain and medium-chain fatty acids are absorbed directly into the portal circulation and are avidly taken up by hepatocytes. Free fatty acids in the circulation are noncovalently bound to albumin and are transferred to the hepatocyte cytosol by way of fatty acid–binding proteins. Under basal conditions, most free fatty acids are catabolized for energy by cardiac and skeletal muscle. Under conditions of adipocyte lipolysis, the liver can take up and metabolize fatty acids. The liver is unique in that it contains dehydrogenases that are capable of unsaturating essential dietary fatty acids. Structural elements of all tissues contain significant amounts of unsaturated fats, and the liver is responsible for the production of these unsaturated fatty acids. The best example is the production of the prostaglandin precursor, arachidonic acid. Dietary linoleic acid is elongated and dehydrogenated to arachidonic acid by the liver.

Fatty acid CoA esters are also synthesized in the cytosol after hepatic uptake. These fatty acid CoA esters can be converted into triglyceride, transported into mitochondria for the production of acetyl CoA and ATP, or stored in the liver as triglycerides. Figure 36-14 illustrates the essential pathways of hepatic lipid metabolism. The rate-limiting step in the synthesis of triglyceride is the conversion of acetyl CoA to malonyl CoA. Malonyl CoA in turn inhibits the mitochondrial uptake of fatty acid CoA ester.

Fatty acid CoA esters bind carnitine, a carrier molecule, and in the absence of cytosolic malonyl CoA, enter the hepatic mitochondria, where they undergo β-oxidation to acetyl CoA and ATP (see Fig. 36-14). Acetyl CoA can then take one of the following routes: (1) enter the tricarboxylic acid cycle and be degraded to CO_2; (2) be converted to citrate for fatty acid synthesis; or (3) be converted into 3-hydroxy-3-methylglutaryl CoA (HMG-CoA), a precursor of cholesterol and ketone bodies. The mitochondrial hydrolysis of fatty acids is a source of large quantities of ATP. The conversion of stearic acid to CO_2 and H_2O, for instance, generates 136 ATP molecules and demonstrates the highly efficient storage of energy in fat.

In times of unrestrained lipolysis, such as starvation, uncontrolled diabetes, or other conditions of triglyceride mobilization from adipocyte stores, the ability of liver to perform β-oxidation may be inadequate. Under such circumstances, significant hepatic storage of triglyceride or fatty infiltration of the liver can occur. Triglyceride storage by itself does not appear to be a cause of hepatic fibrosis or necrosis, but fatty infiltration may be a marker for derangement of normal processes by alcohol or drug toxicity, diabetes, chronic total parenteral nutrition, or morbid obesity. A specific type of microvesicular fatty accumulation is seen in a variety of diseases such as Reye syndrome and the acute fatty liver of pregnancy.

Cholesterol Metabolism

Cholesterol is an important regulator of membrane fluidity and is a substrate for bile acid and steroid hormone synthesis. Cholesterol may be available by dietary intake or by de novo synthesis. In mammals, about 90% of new cholesterol is synthesized in the liver from its precursor, acetyl CoA. Dietary cholesterol intake can suppress endogenous synthesis by inhibiting the rate-limiting enzyme in the cholesterol biosynthetic pathway, HMG-CoA reductase.[13] A competitive antagonist, lovastatin (Mevinolin), can also block HMG-CoA reductase and effectively lower plasma cholesterol by blocking cholesterol synthesis and stimulating low-density lipoprotein (LDL) receptor synthesis and allowing increased hepatic uptake and metabolism of cholesterol-rich LDL lipoproteins. The structure of the LDL receptor is known and serves as a model for other cell membrane receptors (Fig. 36-15).

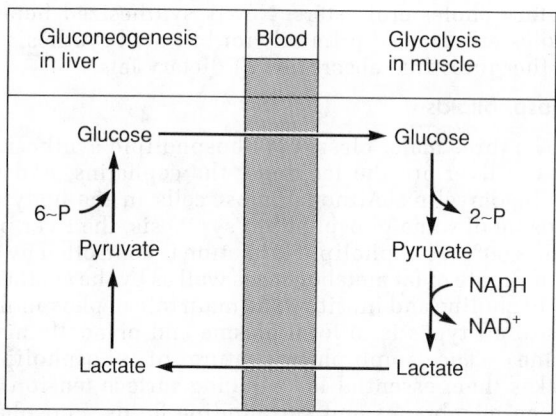

Figure 36-13. The Cori cycle, an elegant mechanism for the hepatic conversion of muscle lactate into new glucose. Pyruvate has a key role in this process.

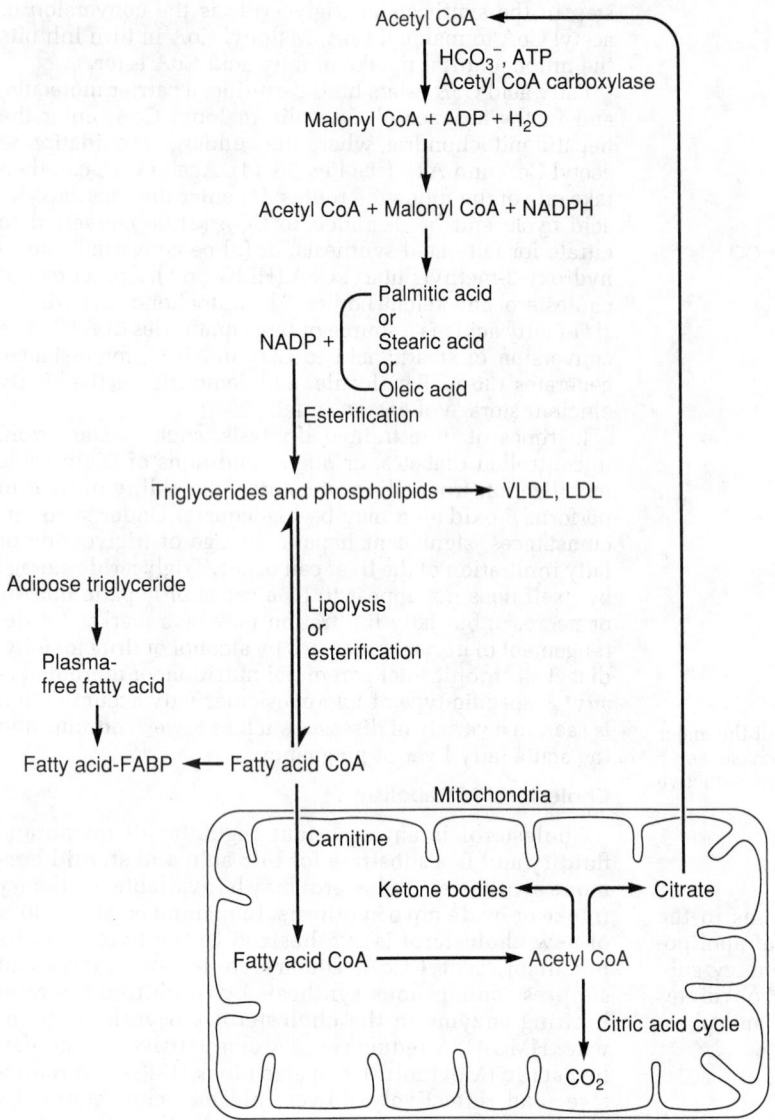

Figure 36-14. Diagram of hepatic fatty acid metabolism. Both dietary and newly synthesized fatty acids are esterified and subsequently degraded in the mitochondria for energy.

Cholesterol is lipophilic and hydrophobic, and most plasma cholesterol is found in lipoproteins esterified with oleic or palmitic acid. The liver can process cholesterol esters from all classes of lipoproteins. Hepatocytes can also take up chylomicron remnants containing dietary cholesterol esters. Newly synthesized hepatic cholesterol is used primarily for bile acid synthesis for further intestinal absorption of dietary fats.

Phospholipids

The three major classes of phospholipid synthesized by the liver are the lecithins, the cephalins, and the sphingomyelins. Although most cells in the body are capable of some phospholipid synthesis, the liver produces 90%. Phospholipid formation is controlled by the overall rate of fat metabolism as well as by the availability of choline and inositol. The main role of phospholipids of all types is to form plasma and organelle membranes. The amphiphilic nature of phospholipids makes them essential for reducing surface tension between membranes and surrounding fluids. Phosphatidylcholine, one of the lecithins, is the major biliary phospholipid and is important in promoting the secretion of free cholesterol into bile. Thromboplastin, one

of the cephalins, is needed to initiate the clotting cascade. The sphingomyelins are necessary for the formation of the myelin nerve sheath.

Protein Metabolism

Amino Acid Transport and Storage

Essentially all of the end products of dietary protein digestion are amino acids, which are absorbed by the enterocytes into the portal circulation in ionized states. Amino acids are taken up by hepatocytes by one of several active transport mechanisms (see Fig. 36-4). Amino acids are not stored in the liver but are rapidly used in the production of plasma proteins, purines, heme proteins, and hormones. Under certain conditions, the amine group is removed from amino acids, and the carbon chain is used for carbohydrate, lipid, or nonessential amino acid synthesis.

The ammonia formed as a result of deamination of amino acids is detoxified by one of two routes.[14] The most important pathway involves the conversion of ammonia to urea by enzymes of the Krebs-Henseleit cycle, found only in the liver (Fig. 36-16). A second route of ammonia metab-

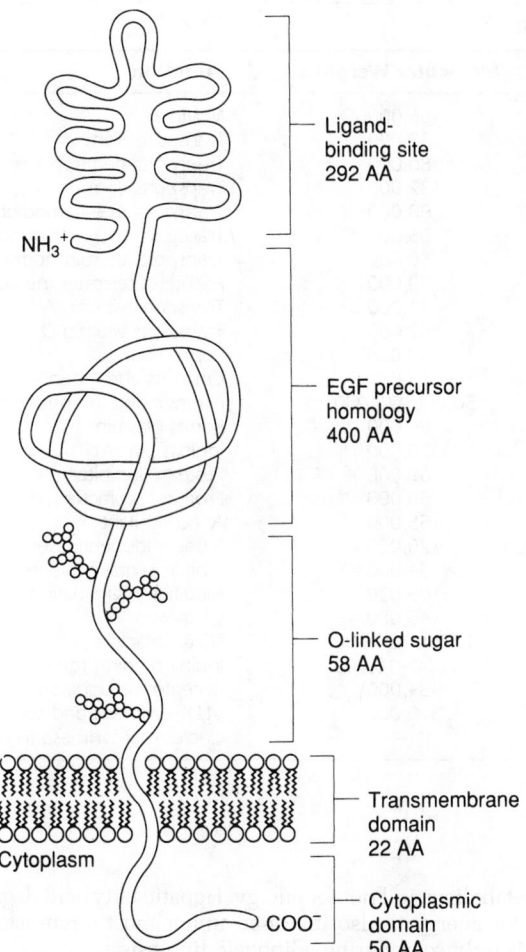

Figure 36-15. The low-density lipoprotein (LDL) receptor. An example of a transmembrane receptor that participates in receptor-mediated endocytosis. The LDL receptor specifically binds lipoproteins that contain apolipoprotein B-100 or E. Once internalized, the lipoproteins are degraded. Some receptors, such as the insulin receptor, have a larger cytoplasmic domain that is catalytically active. On binding insulin, the receptor is able to phosphorylate itself and other as yet unidentified proteins, leading to altered biologic activity. AA, amino acids.

olism involves deamination of L-glutamine by the kidney, with excretion of ammonia into the urine, important for urinary acidification.

Formation of Plasma Proteins

Essentially all albumin, fibrinogen, and apolipoproteins are derived from the liver, which can add up to 50 g of protein to the plasma a day. Of total hepatic protein synthesis, 75% is destined for export in plasma. Most newly synthesized proteins are not stored in the liver, and the rate of protein synthesis is primarily determined by the intracellular levels of amino acids. A partial list of major plasma proteins synthesized by the liver is found in Table 36-2.

The synthesis and export of albumin has been intensively studied. Human albumin is a single-chain polypeptide of 584 amino acids. The 17 disulfide bridges give albumin its tertiary structure and expose both electrostatic and hydrophobic binding sites, allowing albumin to bind with a variety of smaller molecules. Albumin does not contain terminal galactose residues and therefore is not rapidly cleared by ASGP receptors. As a result, the half-life of

albumin in plasma is 19 days.[15] Decreased hepatic protein synthesis is only partially responsible for the low plasma levels of albumin seen with cirrhosis or malnutrition. The long half-life of albumin makes it an insensitive indicator of hepatic synthetic function.

Many proteins undergo posttranslational modification of their tertiary structure after being synthesized in the liver rough ER. Glycosylation, or addition of carbohydrate moieties, occurs in the smooth ER. Sialation, or the addition of sialic acid, occurs in the Golgi. Glycosylation is important in allowing some proteins to bind with specific receptors for subsequent hepatic uptake and processing. Removal of sialic acid residues, or desialation, from the terminal galactose molecules of glycoproteins allows them to bind the ASGP receptor in the liver and undergo degradation. Desialation, therefore, is important in the clearance of senescent proteins from the plasma.

Protein Uptake and Degradation

Proteins such as ASGP are generally taken up by receptor-mediated processes. ASGPs are proteins that have undergone removal of sialic acid residues by tissue neuraminidases. Terminal galactose residues are exposed and are recognized by the ASGP receptor, allowing hepatic receptor-mediated endocytosis (see Fig. 36-5). Protein degradation occurs primarily in lysosomes. The lysosomal enzymes are nonselective in their activities; there are more than 20 known hydrolytic enzymes in lysosomes.

HEPATIC METABOLISM

Metabolic processes in the liver are essential for the production of fuel substrates for other organs. The liver, by virtue of its terminal position in the portal system, is the

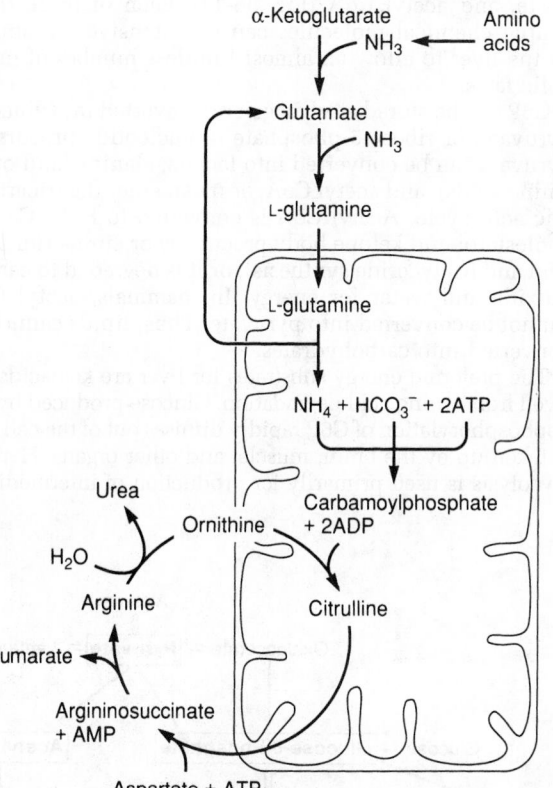

Figure 36-16. The urea cycle. Ammonia entering the urea cycle is derived from protein and amino acid degradation in tissues (endogenous) and colonic lumen (exogenous).

Table 36-2. MAJOR PROTEINS SYNTHESIZED BY THE LIVER

Broad Category	Protein	Molecular Weight	Function
Transport proteins	Albumin	66,000	Multiple
	Transferrin	57,000	Transports iron
	Hemopexin	80,000	Transports heme to liver
	Ceruloplasmin	132,000	Transports copper
	Haptoglobin	90,000	Transports free hemoglobin
	Thyroxine-binding globulin	55,000	Transports thyroid hormone
	Thyroxine-binding prealbumin	50,000	Transports thyroid hormone
	Testosterone–estradiol–binding globulin	90,000	Facilitates testosterone action
	Retinol-binding protein	21,000	Transports vitamin A
	Vitamin D–binding protein	52,000	Transports vitamin D
Coagulation proteins	Fibrinogen (factor I)	340,000	Forms fibrin
	Prothrombin (factor II)	73,000	Converts fibrinogen to fibrin
	Factors V, VII, IX, X, XI, XII	50,000–75,000	Extrinsic and intrinsic pathway
	Plasminogen	90,000	Forms plasmin
	α_2-antiplasmin	70,000	Inhibits plasmin
	Antithrombin III	60,000	Protease inhibitor
	Protein S	50,000	Protein C cofactor
	Protein C	55,000	Anticoagulant
Acute-phase reactants	α_2-macroglobulin	720,000	Binds endopeptidases
	α_1-antitrypsin	54,000	Inhibits serine proteases
	C-reactive protein	105,000	Modifies inflammation
	Orosomucoid	40,000	Unknown
Lipoprotein metabolism	Apolipoprotein AI, AII	17,000–30,000	LCAT cofactors
	Apolipoprotein CI, CII, CIII	6000–10,000	Inhibit binding to liver
	Apolipoprotein E	34,000	Receptor recognition
	Apo B100	510,000	VLDL synthesis and secretion
	LCAT	—	Cholesterol synthesis in blood

LCAT, lecithin–cholesterol acetyl transferase; VLDL, very-low-density lipoprotein.

organ that must regulate intestinally absorbed nutrients for tissue consumption or storage. The liver accomplishes its task by synthesizing three key metabolites—G6P, pyruvate, and acetyl CoA (Fig. 36-17). Each of these three simple chemical molecules can be extensively modified by the liver to allow an almost limitless number of metabolic fates.

G6P can be stored as glycogen or converted into glucose, pyruvate, or ribose-5-phosphate (a nucleotide precursor). Pyruvate can be converted into lactate, alanine (and other amino acids), and acetyl CoA, or it can enter the tricarboxylic acid cycle. Acetyl CoA is converted to HMG-CoA (a cholesterol and ketone body precursor) or citrate (for fatty acid and triglyceride synthesis), or it is degraded to carbon dioxide and water for energy. In mammals, acetyl CoA cannot be converted into pyruvate. Thus, lipids cannot be converted into carbohydrates.

The preferred energy substrates for liver are ketoacids derived from amino acid degradation. Glucose produced by the dephosphorylation of G6P rapidly diffuses out of the cell and is taken up by the brain, muscle, and other organs. Hepatic glycolysis is used primarily for production of intermediates

of metabolism and not for energy. Hepatic fatty acid degradation for energy is also inhibited under most circumstances and is only seen during adipocyte lipolysis.

BILE FORMATION

Composition and Secretion

The adult human liver secretes about 1.5 L of bile daily. Eighty percent of this volume is secreted by the hepatocytes (canalicular bile), and 20% is secreted by the bile duct epithelial cells (ductular bile). Solutes constitute about 3% of bile. The major solutes are conjugated bile acids, phosphatidyl choline, cholesterol, protein, and bilirubin. The organic solutes have transport systems, and the most important solutes are the bile acids. Bile acids are the main determinant of bile production, and canalicular bile flow is traditionally divided into bile acid–dependent and bile acid–independent components.

Bile acid–dependent flow is that portion of bile flow resulting from the active secretion of bile acids. Bile acid concentration in hepatic bile is usually between 1 and 5

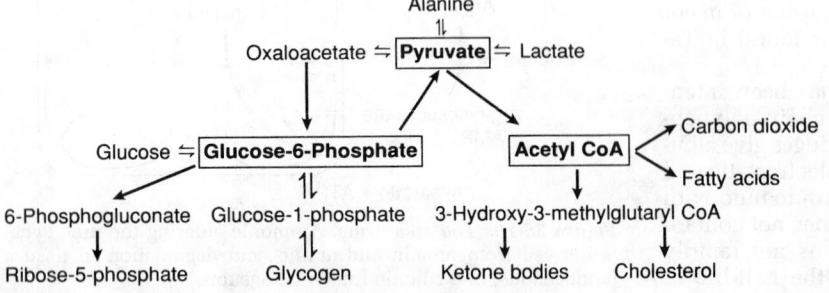

Figure 36-17. A summation of the key regulatory molecules the liver uses to perform its diverse metabolic duties. Essentially, any compound found in the body can be synthesized in the liver from glucose-6-phosphate, acetyl CoA, or pyruvate. The inability of mammalian liver to convert acetyl CoA to pyruvate means that fats cannot be converted to carbohydrates.

mmol. The concentration in plasma is 1 to 5 μmol, a 1000-fold difference. Bile flow is linearly related to bile acid output; hence, bile acids are one of the most important determinants of hepatic bile flow and account for about half of canalicular bile production.[16]

Conjugated bile acids enter the hepatocyte at the sinusoidal surface by a saturable membrane transport protein (see Fig. 36-4). The driving force for bile acid uptake is the electrochemical sodium gradient between sinusoidal blood and the cytoplasm. As sodium enters, conjugated bile acids passively move along with the sodium. Intracellular transport is less well understood than uptake of bile acids.

The ability of bile acids to stimulate bile acid–dependent flow depends on bile acid structure. Most bile acids form micelles when present in solution above a critical micellar concentration. When micelles form, the concentration of free, osmotically active bile acids decreases. Bile acids, such as dehydrocholate, that do not form micelles stimulate more bile flow than micelle-forming bile acids, such as taurocholate. Because bile formation is an active secretory process, bile secretory pressure can be higher than hepatic perfusion pressure. Bile, therefore, is fundamentally different than glomerular urine, which is essentially a pressure-driven ultrafiltrate of plasma.

The hepatic uptake of conjugated and unconjugated bilirubin, sulfobromophthalein, indocyanine green, and certain radiologic contrast media also appears to be carrier mediated. The process is saturable but does not appear to be sodium dependent, and these organic ions can compete with each other but not with bile acids for uptake. Unconjugated bilirubin is bound in plasma to albumin. Bilirubin is then released from albumin and subsequently internalized. After internalization, bilirubin binds to intracellular carrier proteins. Once in the hepatocyte, bilirubin is conjugated with glucuronic acid to bilirubin diglucuronide before biliary secretion. Less than 1% of biliary bilirubin is secreted in the unconjugated form.

Bile Acid Metabolism

In discussing bile acid metabolism, it is useful to distinguish primary from secondary bile acids. Primary bile acids are synthesized from cholesterol in the liver and, in humans, consist of cholic acid and chenodeoxycholic acid. Secondary bile acids are formed in the intestinal lumen by bacterial dehydroxylation and consist of deoxycholic

acid and lithocholic acid, from cholic acid and chenodeoxycholic acid, respectively. Essentially all the primary and secondary bile acids are conjugated with the amino acids glycine or taurine. Amino acid conjugation lowers the pKa of bile acids so that they remain ionized in the intestinal lumen and are not passively reabsorbed through nonionic diffusion. Conjugated bile acids also form micelles, which more effectively facilitate lipid digestion and absorption from the small intestine.[17]

The human liver synthesizes 300 to 400 mg/d of bile acids from cholesterol, or about 10% of the total bile salt pool. The rate of bile acid synthesis is tightly linked to bile acid loss through the colon. Bile acid synthesis is the major mechanism for cholesterol degradation in the body, and the rate-limiting enzymatic step is catalyzed by cholesterol 7-α-hydroxylase. By the dietary ingestion of resins that bind bile acids, such as cholestyramine, it is possible to increase the fecal excretion of bile acids and thus the degradation of cholesterol. Intestinal bile acids are efficiently (about 95%) taken up by the enterohepatic circulation (Fig. 36-18). Luminal bile acids are transported by carrier proteins in the distal ileum and appear in the portal venous effluent. The hepatocyte extracts more than 95% of portal venous bile acids for resecretion into the bile.

Biliary Lecithin and Cholesterol Secretion

The main biliary phospholipid is lecithin, or phosphatidyl choline. Lecithin is amphipathic, which means it contains both hydrophilic and hydrophobic domains. Lecithin serves two main purposes in bile—to solubilize free biliary cholesterol and to emulsify dietary fats in the intestines. Free cholesterol is not soluble in water or simple micelles of bile acids but is readily solubilized in mixed micelles of both bile acids and lecithin. Although most biliary cholesterol appears to be derived from plasma lipoproteins, biliary lecithin is predominantly synthesized in the liver. Biliary secretion of both lecithin and cholesterol is tightly linked to the rate of bile acid secretion, so that as bile acid output increases, so does biliary lipid secretion. Lecithin is also found in chylomicrons and other lipoproteins responsible for the intravascular transport of dietary lipids.

Biliary Proteins

Proteins constitute about 5% of the total biliary solute. Immunoglobulin A is an example of a protein that is secreted into bile intact. After binding to plasma membrane

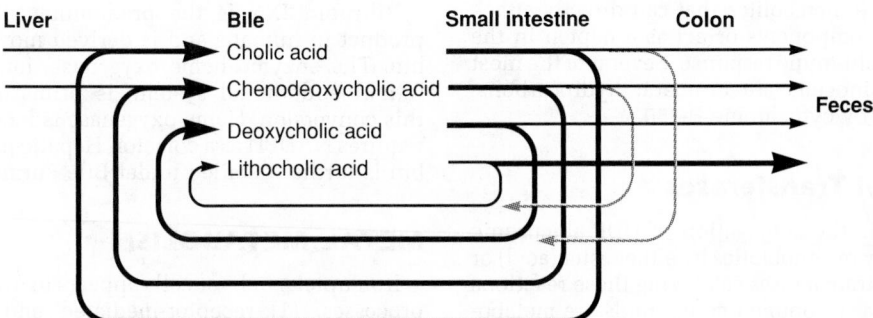

Figure 36-18. The enterohepatic circulation of bile acids. The primary bile acids—cholic acid and chenodeoxycholic acid—are synthesized in the liver from cholesterol. Deoxycholic acid and lithocholic acid are formed in the colon (*blue lines*) by bacterial degradation of the primary bile acids. All four bile acids are conjugated with glycine or taurine in the liver. Most of the lithocholic acid is also sulfated, which decreases reabsorption and increases fecal excretion. Bile acids are absorbed passively in the small and large intestinal epithelia and actively in the distal ileum.

receptors, undegraded proteins are transported through the hepatocyte in endocytic vesicles. The functions of intact proteins in bile can relate to intestinal immunity, as in secretory immunoglobulin A, or to the prevention of gallstone nucleation, as in apolipoproteins. A variety of proteins are also degraded in lysosomes before biliary excretion. This mechanism serves as a means of eliminating senescent plasma proteins, as in haptoglobin. Some regulatory peptides can use both pathways, for example, insulin and epidermal growth factor.[18]

HEPATIC BIOTRANSFORMATION

Biotransformation is defined as the intracellular metabolism of endogenous organic compounds (eg, heme proteins and steroid hormones) and exogenous compounds (eg, drugs and environmental compounds). The liver contains enzyme systems that can expose functional groups, such as hydroxyl ions (phase I reactions), or alter size and solubility of a wide variety of organic and inorganic compounds by conjugation with small polar molecules (phase II reactions). The general strategy of the liver is to convert hydrophobic, potentially toxic compounds into hydrophilic conjugates that can then be excreted into bile or urine.

The four general enzyme families responsible for hepatic biotransformation are the cytochromes P-450, the uridine diphosphate-glucuronyl (UDP-glucuronyl) transferases, the glutathione (GSH) S-transferases, and the sulfotransferases. Biotransforming enzymes are not distributed uniformly within the cells of the hepatic lobule. This heterogeneity may account for the ability of some drugs to cause damage preferentially in zone 3 hepatocytes (see Fig. 36-1).

Cytochromes P-450

The cytochromes P-450 are named for their ability to absorb light maximally at 450 nm in the presence of carbon monoxide. These enzymes are bound to the ER and collectively catalyze reactions by using NADPH and oxygen. The P-450 isozymes present in mammalian liver catalyze reactions such as oxidation, hydroxylation, sulfoxide formation, oxidative deamination, dealkylation, and dehalogenation. Such reactions allow further phase II conjugation with polar groups such as glucuronate, GSH, and sulfate.

The cytochromes P-450 can also create potentially toxic metabolites. Drugs such as acetaminophen, isoniazid, halothane, and the phenothiazines can be converted into reactive forms, causing cellular injury and death. The cytochromes also are responsible for the formation of organic free radicals, reactive metabolites that can directly attack and injure cellular components or act as a hapten in the generation of an autoimmune response. Several of the most potent known carcinogens are aromatic hydrocarbons, which are modified by cytochrome P-450.

UDP-Glucuronyl Transferases

Glucuronidation is the conjugation of UDP-glucuronic acid to a wide variety of xenobiotics by either ester (acyl) or ether linkages. The transferases catalyzing these reactions reside in the ER. Many common compounds are metabolized in this way, including bilirubin, testosterone, aspirin, indomethacin, acetaminophen, chloramphenicol, and oxazepam. Clinically significant loss of activity can occur with acute ethanol exposure or acetaminophen overdose, when formation of UDP-glucuronic acid from UDP-glucose is outstripped by use. Some acyl linkages lead to the generation of electrophilic centers that can react with other proteins. The covalent linkage of conjugated bilirubin to albumin is believed to occur by this mechanism.

Glutathione S-Transferases

The GSH transferases are more selective in the biotransformations they perform. GSH conjugation occurs only with compounds that have electrophilic and potentially reactive centers. The role of GSH conjugation catalyzed by the GSH S-transferases is best seen with acetaminophen. In this drug, cytochrome P-450 creates an electrophilic center that reacts with protein thiol groups or GSH. The presence of GSH S-transferase allows the preferential detoxification of acetaminophen rather than the potentially injurious binding to thiol groups. A class of GSH S-transferases, known is *ligandins*, appears to facilitate the uptake and intracellular transport of bilirubin, heme, and bile acids from plasma to liver. In addition to the detoxification of potential toxins, GSH is a substrate for GSH peroxidase, an enzyme important in the metabolism of hydrogen peroxide.

Sulfotransferases

The sulfotransferases catalyze the transfer of sulfate groups from 3′-phosphoadenosine-5′-phosphosulfate (PAPS) to compounds such as thyroxine, bile acids, isoproterenol, α-methyldopa, and acetaminophen. They are located primarily in the cytosol. Although many P-450 derivatives can be further conjugated by either the sulfotransferases or glucuronyl transferases, a limited ability of the liver to synthesize PAPS makes glucuronidation the predominant mechanism.

HEME AND PORPHYRIN METABOLISM

Heme is formed from glycine and succinate and is the functional iron-containing center of hemoglobin, myoglobin, cytochromes, catalases, and peroxidases. From glycine and succinate precursors, δ-aminolevulinic acid (δ-ALA) is synthesized by the rate-limiting enzyme ALA synthase. The porphyrinogens are intermediates in the pathway from δ-ALA to heme, and porphyrins are oxidized forms of porphyrinogen (Fig. 36-19). Inherited enzyme defects in the heme synthetic pathway cause the overproduction of various porphyrinogens, which can in turn cause clinical manifestations known as the *porphyrias*.[19] Acquired porphyria can occur as a result of heavy metal intoxication, estrogens, alcohol, or environmental exposure to chlorinated hydrocarbons.

Bilirubin IXα is the predominant heme degradation product in humans and is derived mostly from hemoglobin. The enzyme heme oxygenase, found in cells of the reticuloendothelial system, is primarily responsible for this conversion. Heme oxygenase is located in the ER and requires NADPH as a cofactor. Hepatic processing of bilirubin is further detailed under Bile Formation.

METAL METABOLISM

Iron uptake in liver cells appears to occur by two distinct processes: (1) receptor-mediated endocytosis of iron–transferrin complexes and (2) facilitated diffusion across the plasma membrane. More iron is taken up and stored by the liver than any other organ with the exception of the bone marrow. Transferrin is synthesized in the liver and has specific plasma membrane receptors on a number of different tissues. After endocytosis, the transferrin and iron dissociate and the transferrin and transferrin receptor

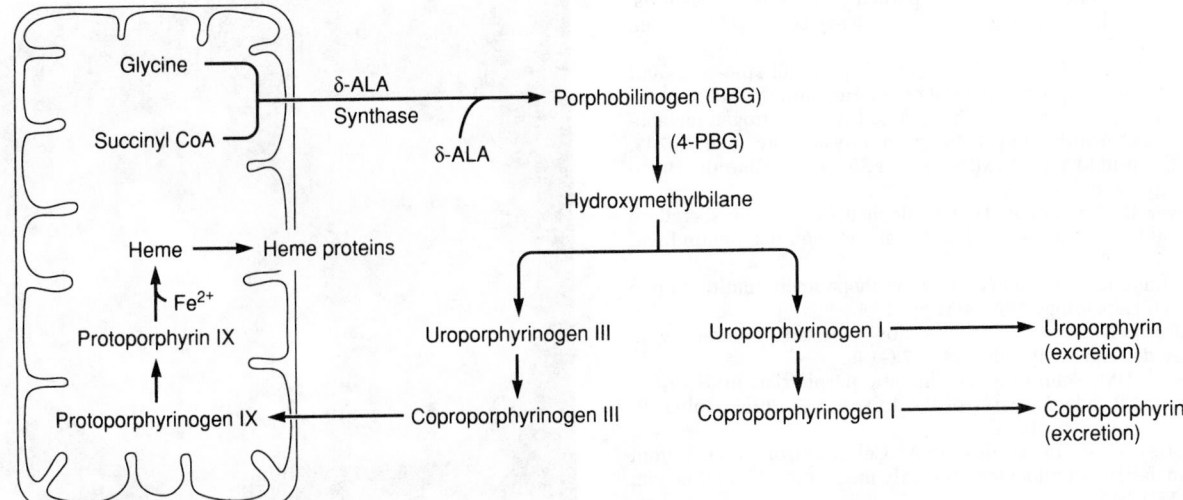

Figure 36-19. The heme biosynthetic pathway. Inherited defects of each of the heme biosynthetic enzymes except δ-ALA synthase have been described and lead to the clinical disorders known as the *porphyrias*.

return to the cell surface for recycling. A pathway appears to involve dissociation of iron and transferrin at the plasma membrane and subsequent internalization by carrier-mediated diffusion. Once internalized, iron is stored and complexed to apoferritin. Each apoferritin molecule is capable of storing several thousand iron molecules. The iron–apoferritin complex is called *ferritin* and under physiologic conditions is responsible for iron storage. Iron storage in a protein-bound form is essential because free iron can catalyze free radical formation, leading to cell injury.[20]

Copper is transported to the liver bound to albumin or histidine and enters the hepatocytes by a process of facilitated diffusion. Once inside the cell, copper can bind to several intracellular proteins for storage or as a necessary enzyme cofactor. Copper-binding proteins include metallothionein, monoamine oxidase, cytochrome C oxidase, and superoxide dismutase. *Ceruloplasmin* is a liver-derived protein that binds hepatic copper for transport to other tissues. The low levels of ceruloplasmin seen in patients with Wilson disease suggest a pathogenetic defect.

Zinc is taken up by and competes for the same binding sites as copper. In hepatocytes, zinc binds predominantly to metallothionein and is excreted into bile, where it undergoes enterohepatic circulation. Other metals, usually found in trace amounts, are lead, cadmium, selenium, mercury, and nickel. These metals are usually bound to metallothionein or GSH, and intoxication is associated with free radical formation and liver injury.

VITAMIN METABOLISM

The liver plays an important role in the metabolism of the fat-soluble vitamins A, D, and K. Hepatic bile salt secretion is necessary for solubilization and absorption of dietary fat-soluble vitamins from the intestine. The liver also stores significant amounts of the fat-soluble vitamins and synthesizes transport proteins for the various vitamins. Vitamin A is exclusively stored in the liver, and excessive ingestion of vitamin A can be associated with significant liver injury. Retinol-binding protein, synthesized by the liver, is responsible for the plasma transport of vitamin A.

Vitamin D must undergo metabolism in the liver to produce 25-hydroxyvitamin D, a necessary step in the conversion from dietary to biologically active vitamin D. Vitamin D undergoes biliary secretion, intestinal absorption, and hepatic uptake or enterohepatic circulation, similar to that seen in bile acid metabolism. Vitamin D–binding globulin is synthesized in the liver and is responsible for the transport of all forms of vitamin D. Vitamin K_1 is ingested with food, and vitamin K_2 is formed as a product of bacterial action in the gut lumen. Vitamin K is required for the the γ-carboxylation of glutamic acid residues, a necessary step in the hepatic synthesis of biologically active coagulation factors II, VII, XI, and X. Of the water-soluble vitamins, only vitamin B_{12} is stored to any appreciable extent in the liver.

REFERENCES

1. Rappaport AM. The acinus: microvascular unit of the liver. In: Lautt WW, ed. Hepatic circulation in health and disease. New York, Raven Press, 1981:175.
2. Jones AL, Spring-Mills E. The liver and gallbladder. In: Weiss L, ed. Histology: cell and tissue biology. New York, Elsevier, 1983:707.
3. Burwen SJ, Jones AL. Hepatocellular processing of endocytosed proteins. J Electron Microsc Tech 1990;14:140.
4. Geuze HJ, Van der Donk HA, Simmons CF, et al. Receptor mediated endocytosis in liver parenchymal cells. Int Rev Exp Pathol 1986;29:113.
5. Casanova JE, Breitfeld PP, Ross SA, Mostov KE. Phosphorylation of the polymeric immunoglobulin receptor required for its efficient transcytosis. Science 1990;248:742.
6. Bourne HR. Summary: signals past, present, and future. In: Cold Spring Harbor symposia on quantitative biology. LIII. Molecular biology of signal transduction. Cold Spring Harbor, NY, Cold Spring Harbor Laboratory, 1988:1019.
7. Wu GY, Wu CH, Stockert RJ. A model for the specific rescue of normal hepatocytes during methotrexate treatment of hepatic malignancy. Proc Natl Acad Sci USA 1983;80:3078.
8. Wu CH, Wu GY. Targeting genes: delivery and persistent expression of a foreign gene driven by mammalian regulatory elements in vivo. J Biol Chem 1989;264:16985
9. Lautt WW, Greenway CV. Conceptual review of the hepatic vascular bed. Hepatology 1987;7:952.
10. Lautt WW, Legare DJ, Ezzat WR. Quantitation of the hepatic arterial buffer response to graded changes in portal blood flow. Gastroenterology 1990;98:1024.
11. Hetenyi G, Perez G, Vranic M. Turnover and precursor-product relationships of non-lipid metabolites. Physiol Rev 1983;63:606.

12. Styrer L. Pentose phosphate pathway and gluconeogenesis. In: Styrer L, ed. Biochemistry, ed 3. New York, WH Freeman, 1988:427.

13. Havel RJ, Hamilton RL. Hepatocytic lipoprotein receptors and intracellular lipoprotein catabolism. Hepatology 1988;8:1689.

14. Meijer AJ, Lamers WH, Chamuleau RAFM. Nitrogen metabolism and ornithine cycle function. Physiol Rev 1990;70:701.

15. Rothschild MA, Oratz M, Schrieber SS. Serum albumin. Hepatology 1988;8:385.

16. Boyer JL, Gautam A, Graf J. Mechanisms of bile secretion: insights from the isolated rat hepatocyte couplet. Semin Liver Dis 1988;8:308.

17. Hoffman AF. Chemistry and enterohepatic circulation of bile acids. Hepatology 1984;4(Suppl 5):4.

18. LaRusso NF. Proteins in bile: how they get there and what they do. Am J Physiol 1984;247:G199.

19. Bissell DM, Schmid R. The hepatic porphyrias. In: Schiff L, Schiff ER, eds. Diseases of the liver, ed 5. Philadelphia, JB Lippincott, 1982:1061.

20. Morley CGD, Bezkorovainy A. Cellular iron uptake from transferrin: is endocytosis the only mechanism? Int J Biochem 1985;17:553.

SURGERY: SCIENTIFIC PRINCIPLES AND PRACTICE, Second Edition, edited by Lazar J. Greenfield, Michael W. Mulholland, Keith T. Oldham, Gerald B. Zelenock, and Keith D. Lillemoe. Lippincott–Raven Publishers, Philadelphia, © 1997.

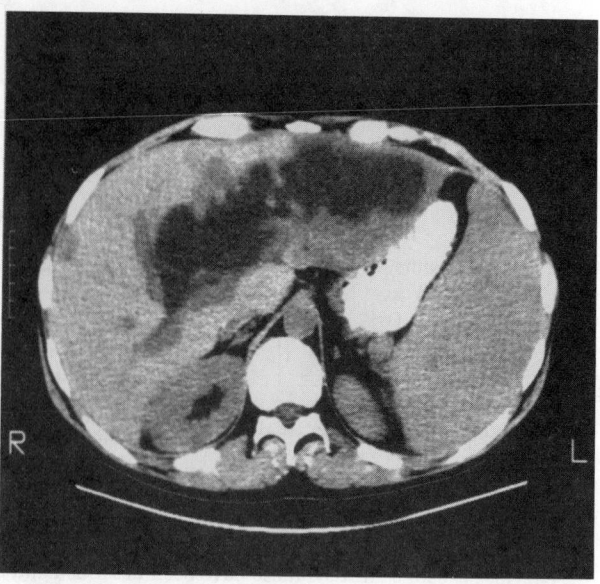

Figure 37-1. CT scan of a pyogenic hepatic abscess in a liver transplant recipient who developed an occlusion of the hepatic artery.

CHAPTER 37

HEPATIC INFECTION AND ACUTE HEPATIC FAILURE

MICHAEL R. LUCEY

PYOGENIC HEPATIC ABSCESS

Pyogenic hepatic abscesses are rare and account for less than 0.2% of adult admissions to hospitals in the United States, where most of these abscesses occur secondary to other infections.[1] Underlying causes of pyogenic hepatic abscess include benign or malignant biliary obstruction accompanied by cholangitis, extrahepatic abdominal sepsis, and trauma or surgery to the right upper quadrant. In special circumstances, pyogenic hepatic abscess is associated with hepatic arterial occlusion in liver transplant recipients (Fig. 37-1) or with the treatment of hepatoma by intraarterial chemotherapy or direct injection of ethanol. The method by which bacteria reach the hepatic parenchyma reflects these underlying causes. For example, in pyogenic hepatic abscess complicating biliary obstruction and cholangitis, bacteria spread directly through the biliary radicles to the hepatic parenchyma. Pyogenic hepatic abscess after intraabdominal sepsis (eg, diverticulitis) is most likely to be caused by a hematogenous spread through the portal bloodstream. Similarly, hematogenous spread by hepatic arterial inflow may occur in infectious endocarditis. Abscesses arising from hematogenous transmission are usually unifocal, whereas those resulting from biliary obstruction are more often multifocal. Metastatic cancer in the liver, diabetes mellitus, and alcoholism predispose patients to developing pyogenic hepatic abscess.

The organisms that predominate in pyogenic hepatic abscesses are gram-negative aerobic rods, streptococci, and anaerobes including *Bacillus fragilis*. When careful anaerobic cultures are performed, anaerobes or microaerophilic organisms are present in half of all pyogenic hepatic abscesses.

Pyogenic hepatic abscesses occur with equal frequency in men and women, and the median age at presentation is in the fifth decade. Pyogenic hepatic abscesses lead to death in about 15% of affected patients, usually as a result of uncontrolled sepsis. A typical presentation consists of fevers, chills, abdominal pain, and weight loss. Although 60% of patients have symptoms of 2 weeks' duration or less at diagnosis, delayed recognition is common because of the nonspecific symptoms. Some 40% of patients have abdominal tenderness. Overt jaundice is present in 20% of all cases. Almost all patients have a polymorphonuclear leukocytosis and nonspecific abnormalities of their biochemistry tests, including elevated alkaline phosphatase, elevated transaminases, and hypoalbuminemia.

The differential diagnosis is broad and includes ascending cholangitis, amebic hepatic abscess, and sepsis elsewhere in the body associated with hepatic dysfunction. It can sometimes be difficult to distinguish between pneumonia with accompanying abnormal liver tests and hepatic abscess with accompanying pulmonary changes. About 40% of patients with pyogenic hepatic abscess have right lower lobe abnormalities on chest radiograph, including atelectasis, pulmonary infiltrate, or elevated right hemidiaphragm.

The key to a correct diagnosis in suspected pyogenic hepatic abscess is the early use of appropriate hepatobiliary imaging tests. These tests include real-time ultrasonography, computed tomographic (CT) scans, radioisotope scans, and contrast-enhanced magnetic resonance imaging. Although a radioisotope scan is an accurate method of outlining abscesses larger than 2 cm in diameter, it is no longer the preferred test. Both ultrasonography and CT scanning more accurately define intrahepatic lesions, permit assessment of accompanying intraabdominal pathology, and allow needle aspiration of the abscess when appropriate. Real-time ultrasonography is the imaging test of choice for suspected pyogenic hepatic abscess. Because biliary obstruction and cholangitis are often part of the differential diagnosis, the hepatic parenchyma, biliary tree, and gallbladder should be inspected. Occasionally, the sonographic appearances of a pyogenic abscess are poorly defined early in the patient's clinical course and a second sonogram taken a few days later shows more characteristic features of an hepatic abscess. Sonography does not distinguish pyogenic from amebic abscess. CT scanning, especially with intravenous contrast, is as sensitive a diagnostic method as sonography and may be better in identifying an abscess in the area of the hepatic dome. Both real-time ultrasonography and contrast-aided CT scanning may fail to distinguish multiple microabscesses from hepatic parenchyma with diffuse fatty infiltration or from hepatic metastases. Contrast-aided magnetic resonance imaging promises to be an accurate method for recognizing hepatic abscesses.

Once a unifocal or multifocal hepatic abscess has been demonstrated on sonography or CT scanning, diagnostic percutaneous aspiration is advisable unless there are clear indications that the abscess may be amebic. Diagnostic aspiration allows the causative organism to be identified, even after antibiotics have been started. The antibiotic regimen can be modified based on subsequent culture results.

Although antibiotic therapy alone may be advisable for some patients in whom attempted drainage is judged to be excessively hazardous or in whom multiple abscesses appear small, antibiotics along with drainage is the preferred treatment for most pyogenic hepatic abscesses.[2] In many cases, percutaneous drainage under ultrasound or CT guidance is sufficient to evacuate pus. Surgical exploration is advised for unstable patients exhibiting signs of continued sepsis despite attempted nonsurgical treatment and for stable patients who have fevers that persist for longer than 2 weeks after percutaneous catheter drainage and the institution of appropriate antibiotics. Occasionally, surgical drainage is required if viscous pus cannot be aspirated percutaneously, if pus coexists with solid debris, or if the abscess is multilocular.

Before formal identification of the causative organism, antibiotic coverage should be started to treat aerobic gram-negative bacilli, microaerophilic streptococci, and anaerobic bacilli including *Bacteroides* sp. A commonly used combination is ampicillin, an aminoglycoside, with either metronidazole or clindamycin. Third-generation cephalosporins (eg, cephtriaxone) can be substituted for the aminoglycoside in patients at risk for renal toxicity. Once the causative organisms are identified, the antibiotic regimen should be modified to match their sensitivities. Intravenous antibiotics should be administered for 14 days and then replaced with oral preparations to complete a 6-week course. Defervescence occurs within the first week of intravenous antibiotics in most pyogenic hepatic abscesses, although up to 20% of cases are febrile into the second week of therapy. When possible, therapy directed at correcting the underlying pathology should be done simultaneously with antibiotics and drainage (eg, cholelithiasis and biliary ductal obstruction).

AMEBIC HEPATIC ABSCESS

Entamoeba histolytica is the only ameba that invades human tissue. The parasite is endemic throughout the world and is particularly troublesome in societies with poor sanitation. *E histolytica* exists in two forms—a cyst, which is the infective form, and a trophozoite. The infection is spread by the fecal–oral route. *E histolytica* causes two distinct clinical syndromes, amebic colitis and amebic hepatic abscess. About 10% of adults in the United States are entambic carriers who shed cysts in their feces without evidence of either colitis or abscess formation. This discussion is limited to amebic hepatic abscess.

Amebic hepatic abscess remains a diagnostic challenge. Effective therapy is available, and recovery is expected if therapy is started promptly. Amebic hepatic abscess can

have a presentation that is indistinguishable from pyogenic abscess with acute onset of fever, abdominal pain (often in the right upper quadrant), and disturbed liver chemistry tests. When this presentation occurs, liver sonogram and serologic tests for amebic infection can be used to make the diagnosis.[3] Some features that should prompt consideration of amebic hepatic abscess are a history of travel to or origin from a high-risk area or a history of alcoholism. Homosexual men are particularly at risk because they have a high frequency of bowel carriage of *E histolytica* and because they are at a higher-than-average risk for acquired immunodeficiency syndrome. About half of all patients presenting with amebic abscesses have abnormalities in the right lower lung field (eg, atelectasis, infiltrate, effusion, or elevated hemidiaphragm). The duration of illness at presentation of amebic hepatic abscess varies, and an acute form with symptoms that last for less than 2 weeks can be distinguished from a chronic form. Some chronic patients, nonetheless, have an acute decompensation that is then indistinguishable from typical acute cases. Although up to one third of patients with amebic hepatic abscess describe diarrhea, amebic colitis is rare.

Clinical examination does not separate amebic from pyogenic abscess.[3] Although subtle differences in the patterns of hematologic and liver tests between pyogenic and amebic abscess have been described, these are of little discriminatory value. Moderate elevations in the levels of serum amino transferases and alkaline phosphatase are common in both conditions. Significant increases in levels of serum bilirubin are uncommon in amebic hepatic abscess. A significant reduction in serum albumin levels (less than 3 g/dL) is rare in amebic hepatic abscess but is observed in half of patients with pyogenic hepatic abscess.

Liver ultrasonography is the initial imaging procedure of choice (Fig. 37-2A). No specific features reliably distinguish amebic abscess from pyogenic abscess. CT scanning is also an accurate method of detecting amebic hepatic abscess, although distinctive features have not been described (see Fig. 37-2B). Serologic tests for the presence of antibody to *E histolytica* (eg, indirect hemagglutination, enzyme-linked immunosorbent assay [ELISA], counterimmune immunofluorescence, and indirect immunofluorescence) are specific and sensitive in amebic hepatic abscess and are positive in 95% of cases. Antibody titers in invasive bowel disease without hepatic involvement can vary. A negative serologic test encountered in circumstances that are strongly suggestive of an amebic hepatic abscess may be due to a lack of a particular reactive epitope, and the diagnosis can then be made by using an alternative serologic test. The combination of an appropriate clinical setting, sonographic appearances of an hepatic abscess, and positive *E histolytica* serology confirm the diagnosis of amebic hepatic abscess and are sufficient to warrant proceeding immediately to medical therapy.

The drug of choice for amebic hepatic abscesses is metronidazole, 750 mg three times daily. Chloroquine phosphate can be added to metronidazole for acutely ill patients. Glucose-6-phosphate dehydrogenase activity should be checked before initiating chloroquine therapy. Alternative therapeutic regimens include dehydroemetrine, iodoquinol, and emetine. Most uncomplicated amebic hepatic abscesses do not require aspiration. Superinfection of an amebic abscess rarely occurs with this protocol and is usually a complication of invasive aspiration procedures or abscess rupture. Therapeutic aspiration should be performed to exclude pyogenic abscess in the occasional patient who is unresponsive to both metronidazole and chloroquine and in patients with large left lobe amebic abscesses that may rupture into the pericardium, a complication that is frequently fatal.

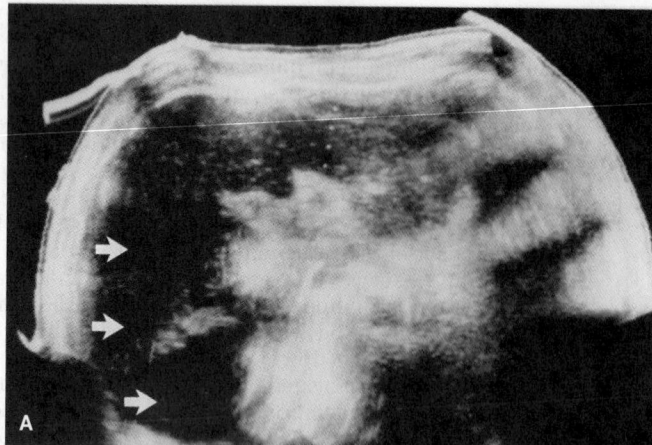
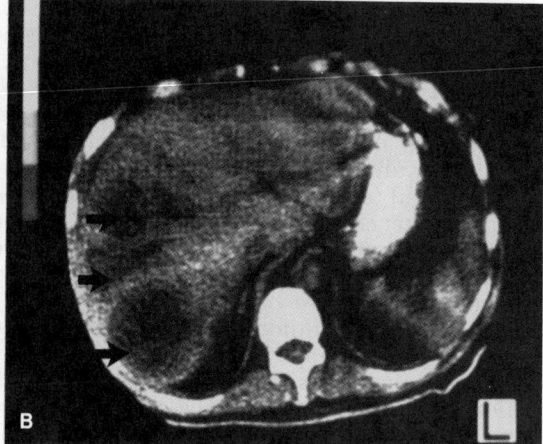

Figure 37-2. Sonogram (*A*) and CT scan (*B*) in a patient with multiple amebic abscesses (*arrows*).

HYDATID DISEASE OF THE LIVER

Echinococcosis in humans is caused by infection by the tapeworms *Echinococcus granulosis* and *Echinococcus multilocularis*. The more common pathogen in humans is *E granulosis*. Echinococcosis is a rare infection in North America. The dog is the definitive host, although the disease is endemic in sheep- and cattle-farming regions. Humans are intermediate hosts and acquire echinococcal eggs by ingesting contaminated food. The egg is digested in the duodenum and yields an embryo, which travels through the portal bloodstream and lodges in the liver. Occasionally, the echinococcal embryo may lodge in the lungs, spleen, central nervous system, or bone. An echinococcal embryo that has survived host defenses and is lodged in a capillary develops into an hydatid cyst. This slow-growing structure, which comprises the *Echinococcus* and host tissue, has three layers: (1) an outer pericyst, which is 2 to 4 mm thick and composed of fibroblasts that produce a capsule of fibrous and connective tissue; (2) a middle hyaline layer up to 2 mm thick and devoid of nuclei; and (3) an inner germinal layer from which the echinococcal scoleces develop. The life cycle of the organism is complete when the definitive host ingests infected viscera, thereby releasing the scoleces in its intestine, where they develop into adult worms.

Because hydatid cysts grow slowly, there is usually a protracted asymptomatic stage. Indeed, in endemic areas, many cases are discovered in persons without earlier symptoms. Symptoms, when they occur, are due to increases in cyst size leading to abdominal pain (the most common presenting symptom), biliary obstruction and jaundice, and, rarely, portal hypertension. Hydatid cysts may be associated with biliary tract pathology, either as a result of communication between the pericyst and biliary ducts or because of rupture of the cyst into the biliary tract. Communication with the biliary tract may lead to secondary bacterial infection of the cyst, cholangitis, or biliary obstruction. Occasionally, cysts spontaneously rupture into the peritoneal cavity and cause abdominal pain and anaphylaxis. Multiple intraabdominal cysts occasionally develop, presumably as the result of a previous unrecognized intraperitoneal leakage. Hepatic hydatid cysts may perforate the diaphragm and cause empyema, pulmonary cysts, biliobronchial fistulas, or pericardial collection. Alternatively, lung hydatid cysts can occur when the embryo migrates to the lung. The only typical clinical finding of hepatic hydatid cyst is a palpable hepatic mass.

Routine laboratory tests in patients with hydatid cysts may be normal or nonspecifically abnormal (eg, showing features of obstructive jaundice). Eosinophilia may be absent. Serologic tests (eg, indirect hemagglutination, complement fixation, dot immunobinding, and ELISA) are specific and sensitive, testing positive in 80% or more of hepatic hydatid cyst cases. Although routine chest or abdominal radiographs can show a mass, sometimes with a calcific rim, sonography and CT scans are favored for imaging hydatid cysts. The presence of calcification and daughter cysts within the parent cyst suggests echinococcosis.

In endemic areas, hydatid cyst disease should be considered before intervention is attempted, since percutaneous needling of hydatid cysts is unwise unless precautions against anaphylaxis are taken (see later discussion).[4] The cyst fluid is often under pressure, and needling can precipitate rupture with the potential for anaphylaxis or intraperitoneal seeding. Serologic testing should precede needling of any likely hydatid cyst.

The classic treatment of hydatid cysts is operative. The surgical aim is to remove any cysts without disseminating the organism.[5] At operation, the cyst is drained of fluid through a cannula, after carefully protecting the operative field from fluid leakage. If the aspirate is clear, a parasiticidal fluid (eg, ethyl alcohol or 20% sterile saline) is injected into the cyst to kill any adherent scoleces. If the cyst fluid is bilious, ethyl alcohol or hypertonic saline is not injected to avoid infusing irritant solution into the biliary tree. The cyst contents and pericystic wall is then removed with careful dissection.

Commonly, a surgical procedure is preceded by medical therapy to eradicate viable scoleces and reduce the risk of dissemination during the operation. Albendazole, 10 mg/kg/d for 3 months, has replaced mebendazole as the therapy of choice because of its superior absorption and distribution characteristics.[6] Percutaneous drainage of single or multiple hydatid cysts after treatment with albendazole is an alternative to surgical correction.[4] This should be attempted in carefully controlled circumstances only, with precautions against anaphylaxis such as serial monitoring of vital signs, placement of a running intravenous line, and ready availability of 1:10,000 adrenaline and resuscitation equipment. Hydrocortisone, 200 mg intravenously, is given as premedication.

SCHISTOSOMAL HEPATIC DISEASE

Schistosomiasis resulting from invasion by *Schistosoma mansoni* and *Schistosoma japonicum* is an important cause of portal hypertension worldwide. Two distinct syndromes can be recognized. Acute schistosomiasis occurs soon after cercariae enter the human host by penetrating the skin. Early manifestations include an irritating maculopapular rash that lasts for several days. After an incubation period of 1 to 2 months, a systemic syndrome of lassitude, anorexia, and gastrointestinal upset with intermittent fevers, chills, sweating, headache, diarrhea, muscle aches, and bronchospasm develops. In rare cases, there may be an acute abdomen and jaundice. On clinical examination, hepatomegaly, moderate splenomegaly, and generalized lymphadenopathy are recognized. Sigmoidoscopy shows a red edematous mucosa with fine granulation, petechiae, and ulcers. Diagnosis is established by revealing ova in the stool or ova trapped within the submucosa of the rectum. Acute syndromes are seen most frequently in nonimmune visitors to endemic areas. Occasionally, acute infection can produce widespread granulomatous necrosis and even death.

In contrast, chronic schistosomiasis is usually asymptomatic until variceal hemorrhage occurs. Ascites is less common. Hepatosplenomegaly is progressive, and the spleen can become large with resultant hypersplenism. The typical manifestations of chronic liver insufficiency (eg, jaundice, spider angiomas, palmar erythema, gynecomastia) are unusual with chronic schistosomiasis. Laboratory features include eosinophilia, hypoalbuminemia, hypergammaglobulinemia, and elevated serum alkaline phosphatase. Serum transaminases are usually normal. Inspecting the feces for ova is the diagnostic test of choice.

Praziquantel is the preferred agent for treating schistosomiasis in adults and children. Bleeding esophageal varices can be managed with variceal sclerotherapy. Portosystemic shunt surgery for managing recurrent variceal hemorrhage due to schistosomiasis is controversial.

VIRAL HEPATITIS

The five viruses that cause acute viral hepatitis are hepatitis A virus (HAV), hepatitis B virus (HBV), hepatitis C virus (HCV), which was formerly called non-A non-B (NANB) hepatitis, hepatitis D virus (HDV), formerly called delta hepatitis, and hepatitis E virus (HEV), formerly called epidemic waterborne NANB hepatitis. Table 37-1 summarizes the characteristics of these viruses, their modes of transmission, and the consequences of infection. Other viruses that can cause acute hepatitis (eg, Epstein-Barr virus [EBV], cytomegalovirus [CMV], herpes simplex virus [HSV], and varicella) are described in the section later in this chapter on hepatitis in immunocompromised hosts.

Hepatitis A Virus

Although epidemic community acquired jaundice was recognized centuries ago, HAV was not identified until 1973. Since then, HAV has been propagated in cell culture, and the complete genome has been cloned. HAV is a member of the picornavirus family, which also includes poliovirus, coxsackievirus, echovirus, and rhinovirus. HAV is a nonenveloped particle about 27 nm in diameter. It contains a single-stranded RNA genome, 7.5 kilobase (kb) in size, that encodes for a number of proteins. It is a robust virus and is stable at 60°C for 1 hour. There is only one known serotype for HAV.[7]

Humans appear to be the only host for HAV infection, although other primates have been infected experimentally. The principal mode of transmission of HAV infection is fecal–oral, although parenteral transmission is also possible. HAV replication occurs within the hepatocyte. Whether extrahepatic HAV replication occurs is unknown. HAV is thought to enter the hepatocyte after attaching to a viral receptor on the plasma membrane. It is unclear how the HAV particles leave the hepatocyte, although cell culture studies suggest that hepatocyte lysis is not required for HAV to egress from the hepatocyte. HAV particles may infect adjacent hepatocytes. Alternatively, vesicles containing HAV may be shed from the hepatocyte into the bile canaliculi, with passage of free virus into the feces. The mechanisms whereby HAV causes liver injury are incompletely understood. An initial phase of viral replication, in which the virus is not cytopathic, may be followed by a phase of immune-mediated liver injury associated with the emergence of anti-HAV immunoglobulin M (IgM) and a decline in HAV production.

HAV infections can produce either anicteric or icteric clinical syndromes (Fig. 37-3). In general, children have a greater frequency of anicteric infection than adults. Similarly, when children develop the icteric form of HAV infection, they often have a milder illness than adults. The incubation period is usually about 28 days. The initial prodrome consists of malaise, arthralgia, myalgia, anorexia, and loss of taste for food. In HAV infection, the prodrome may also include coryza, headache, photophobia, fever, and pharyngitis. Before the onset of jaundice, the patient may notice dark urine and pale stools. Many

Table 37-1. CHARACTERISTIC OF VIRUSES

Virus	Genus	Genome	Genome Length (kb)	Mode of Transmission	Incubation* (d) Mean	Incubation* (d) Range	Consequences of Infection Acute Hepatitis	Consequences of Infection Fulminant Hepatic Failure	Consequences of Infection Chronic Hepatitis	Consequences of Infection Hepatoma	Posttransplantation Infection Recipient to Allograft	Posttransplantation Infection New Acquisition
Hepatitis A	Picornavirus	RNA	7.5	Fecal–oral Parenteral	28	15–50	Yes	Yes	No	No	No	No
Hepatitis B	Hepadnavirus	DNA	3.2	Parenteral Venereal ? Fecal–oral	84	28–160	Yes	Yes	Yes	Yes	Yes	Yes
Hepatitis C	Flavivirus	RNA	10.2	Parenteral ? Venereal ? Fecal–oral	56	14–160	Yes	Probable	Yes	Yes	Yes	Yes
Hepatitis D	Viroid	RNA	1.67	Parenteral	—	—	Yes	Yes	Yes	No	Yes	Uncertain
Hepatitis E	Probably calicivirus	RNA	7.6	Fecal–oral	40	22–60	Yes	Yes†	No	No	Uncertain	No

* Time from exposure to clinical hepatitis.
† Especially in pregnant women in third trimester.

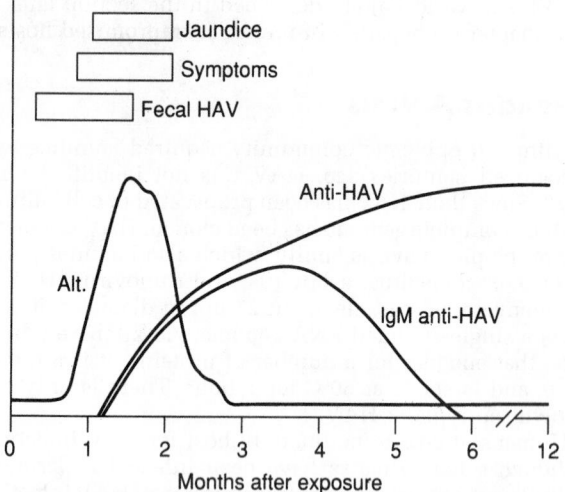

Figure 37-3. Clinical course of hepatitis A infection.

patients develop epigastric or right upper quadrant pain accompanied by diarrhea. This anicteric prodrome may persist from 2 days to 3 weeks. When it subsides without progression to overt jaundice, as it may in young patients, the illness is often attributed to influenza. With the onset of jaundice, the described constitutional features subside. On examination, the liver may be enlarged and slightly tender. Spider angiomas may develop acutely but disappear with the resolution of the hepatitis. Clinical jaundice persists for 1 to 6 weeks. Lassitude is commonly described in adults after hepatitis and may last for months.

Fecal shedding of HAV usually continues for about 7 to 10 days after the onset of jaundice (see Fig. 37-3). Measurement of serum transaminases usually reveals levels greater than 1000 IU/mL. The differential diagnosis includes any acute viral hepatitis and the many forms of acute toxic or ischemic hepatic injury. Serum anti-HAV IgM is usually detectable when jaundice appears and strongly indicates the diagnosis. Elevated titers of anti-HAV IgM may persist for months. The IgG fraction of anti-HAV rises as jaundice subsides, and this elevation persists for years. Liver biopsy is rarely required to make the diagnosis, but if performed, it demonstrates periportal and lobular infiltration by lymphocytes and macrophages associated with parenchymal injury. Hepatocellular injury is characterized by balloon degeneration of hepatocytes, acidophil bodies, and hepatocyte dropout. These changes lead to loss of the normal hepatic lobular architecture.

Serious consequences of HAV infections are uncommon. Patients with HAV infection rarely develop fulminant hepatic failure (see later discussion). Although occasional patients who have recovered from a typical HAV infection relapse 7 to 10 weeks after the initial rapid recovery, no chronic carrier state for HAV has been identified and HAV does not cause chronic active hepatitis or cirrhosis. HAV infection is not associated with the development of hepatoma. All that is required for treating most HAV patients is simple nursing care, adequate nutrition, and attention to hygiene after defecation.

A formalin-inactivated HAV vaccine, in which immunogenicity has been enhanced by conjugation with alum, has been licensed in many countries. Studies of this and another similar vaccine have shown that it is highly immunogenic, inducing an immune response in 95.7% and 99.8% of individuals after one and two doses, respectively.[8] The recommended dosage protocol is for two doses to be given 2 to 4 weeks apart. A booster injection given 6 to 12 months later provides longer protection, perhaps for many years. Field trials among at-risk children have shown that the vaccine is highly effective in preventing clinical HAV infection. The vaccine is safe; only minor side effects have been reported. The availability of HAV vaccination makes previous advice about HAV prophylaxis using immunoglobulin redundant. Vaccination should be recommended for travelers to endemic areas and for persons, such as sewage workers, whose occupation places them at high risk of exposure to HAV. The role of HAV vaccination in susceptible persons at a lower degree of risk, such as daycare personnel, intravenous drug abusers, and male homosexuals, has not been established.

Passive prophylaxis with intramuscular injection of immune globulin is recommended for susceptible (anti-HAV IgG–negative, anti-HAV IgM–negative) individuals, such as employees of daycare centers and custodial homes, where people with whom they have contact have been diagnosed with acute HAV. The Centers for Disease Control does not recommend administering immune globulin to susceptible persons more than 2 weeks after exposure.

Hepatitis B Virus

Hepatitis B virus is a member of the hepadnavirus family, which includes the closely related woodchuck hepatitis virus, ground squirrel hepatitis virus, and duck hepatitis virus. All hepadnaviruses contain a partially double-stranded DNA genome of 3200 base pairs and are packaged in a virion, which contains an outer surface coat and an inner core nucleocapsid.[9] HBV is similar to retroviruses in that viral replication is accomplished by a process in which viral DNA polymerase acts as a reverse transcriptase. As a result of overlapping reading frames, the genome encodes for multiple proteins including core protein (HBcAg), a serum marker of viral replication HBeAg, a surface coat protein (HBsAg), DNA polymerase, and a transactivating protein called *protein X* (Fig. 37-4). The initiation of transcription at one of two upstream initiation sites can generate longer forms of HBsAg—pre-S2, in which the HBsAg has an extra 88–amino acid segment, and pre-S1, which has an extra 128–amino acid segment. Both HBcAg and HBeAg are encoded by a common gene in which there are two initiation codons for protein synthesis. The product of protein synthesis initiated at the first, or pre-C, codon is HBeAg, which undergoes posttranslational processing in the endoplasmic reticulum and is then actively secreted out of the hepatocyte. In contrast, protein synthesis initiated at the second start codon, called the C codon, yields HBcAg which accumulates in the cytoplasm of the infected hepatocyte and is used for incorporation in complete virions. HBeAg is a marker for viral replication and therefore infectivity because its mRNA is coregulated with that of HBcAg, an essential constituent of virion formation.

Mutant HBVs arise from spontaneous alterations in the genome.[10] Perhaps the most frequently occurring mutation affects the precore region of the genome, sometimes called the *precore mutant virus*. In patients infected with precore mutant viruses, transcription of the precore region is prevented as a result of a base pair alteration in that region of the genome, and consequently, elaboration of HBeAg does not occur. Instead, anti-HBe antibody is usually present. Nonetheless, despite the precore mutation, as a result of the initiation of transcription at the C start codon, active viral replication occurs without formation of HBeAg. In these circumstances, active viral replication is recognizable, despite the absence of HBeAg, by the recognition of serum HBV DNA using standard hybridization methods. When precore (or HBeAg nonsecreting) viral mutants were

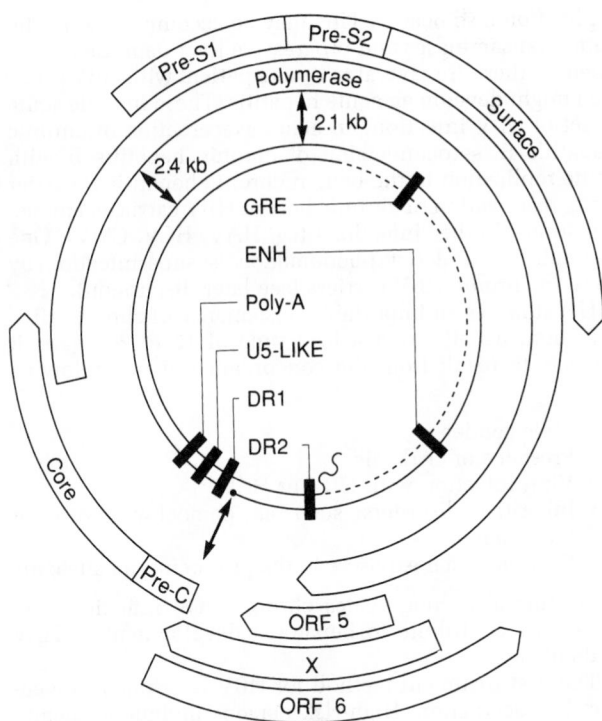

Figure 37-4. Hepatitis B viral genome.

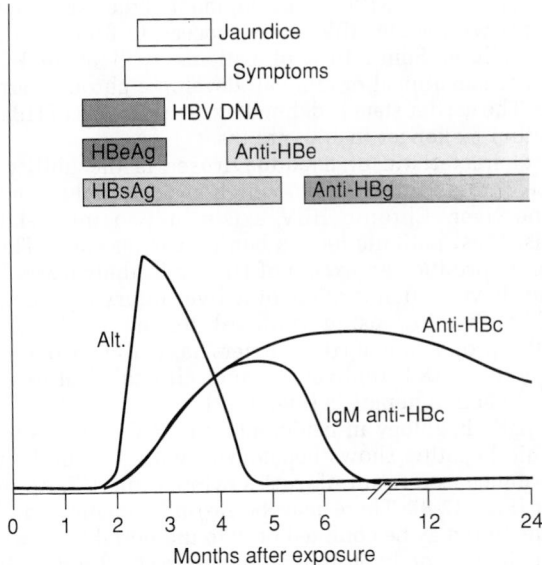

Figure 37-5. Clinical course of acute hepatitis B infection.

first identified, they were thought to be associated with aggressive hepatitis and fulminant hepatic failure. More recently, it has become clear that precore mutants are more widespread, frequently coexist with wild-type HBV forms, particularly during seroconversion from HBeAg-positive to anti-HBe–positive status.[10,11] Other mutant forms of HBV that involve mutation in the genome that encodes HBsAg have been described as occurring during "immune pressure" from passive or active immunization.[10]

HBV is spread by parenteral routes and by intimate personal contact. Vertical transmission from mother to infant is an important problem in the developing world. HBV is hepatotropic, and the hepatocyte is the principal site of viral replication. The mechanism whereby HBV enters the hepatocyte is unknown. Extrahepatic cellular infection can occur and may account for persistence of infection in some circumstances, such as after hepatic transplantation.[12] In general, HBV does not appear to be cytopathic to the hepatocyte. Rather, HBV hepatitis begins as an antigen-specific antiviral cellular immune response that initiates a sequence of nonspecific cellular and molecular immune effector mechanisms that combine to cause liver damage. Intense research is being focused on the currently unclear nature of the immune mechanisms that dictate the course of acute infection, the factors that influence the development of viral clearance or persistence, the progression to either benign chronic carriage of the virus or progressive injury including cirrhosis and/or hepatoma, and finally the genesis of escape mutants.[9] In some circumstances, such as hepatitis B in liver allografts, the virus appears to have a direct cytopathic effect.[13]

The onset of acute hepatitis B is often insidious (Fig. 37-5). Many cases are asymptomatic and are recognized by serologic survey of asymptomatic individuals during an outbreak. Commonly, a diagnosis of previous acute HBV is made in a patient with newly diagnosed chronic hepatitis B. The incubation of HBV is about 8 weeks. The first serum indicator of infection by HBV is serum HBsAg,

which may precede the onset of jaundice. When anicteric hepatitis develops, it is indistinguishable from acute HAV infection described previously. Acute HBV infection is accompanied by the certain serum and liver markers of viral replication: serum HBV DNA; serum HBV DNA polymerase; serum HBeAg; liver HBV DNA; and liver HBcAg. With the onset of clinical hepatitis, serum anti-HBc IgM becomes detectable. In most persons, when HBV infection is self-limited and does not progress to chronic hepatitis, anti-HBc IgM does not persist for more then 6 months after HBV is acquired. Thus, serum anti-HBc IgM is used to distinguish acute from chronic hepatitis B. Unfortunately, anti-HBcAb IgM occasionally persists for years after acute infection or may recur as an amnestic phenomenon in reactivating chronic active hepatitis B. It is, therefore, an imperfect marker for acute infection.

The outcome of acute hepatitis B infection of adults in the Western world (low carrier endemicity) is shown in Figure 37-6. Most patients have subclinical infections with complete recovery. About 25% experience clinical jaun-

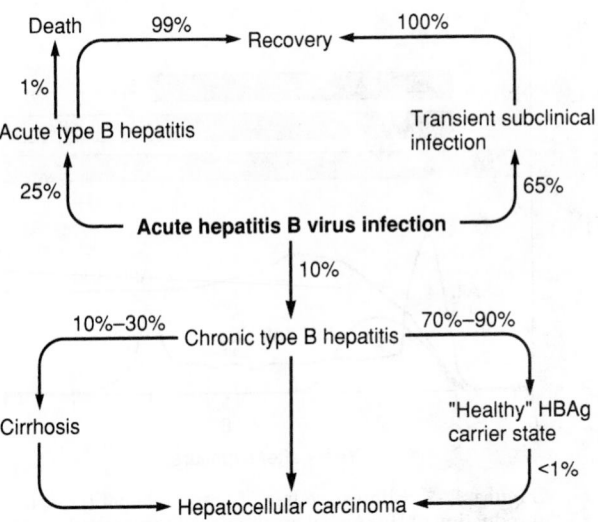

Figure 37-6. Common outcomes of acute hepatitis B.

dice that resolves without development of the carrier state. Patients with acute HBV rarely proceed to fulminant hepatic failure. Some 10% of patients with acute HBV, whether subclinical or clinical, develop a chronic carrier state. The carrier state is defined by the presence of HBsAg in serum for longer than 6 months.

A characteristic of hepadnaviruses is the ability to cause chronic infections in which viral particles persist in the liver. Chronic HBV exists in two interrelated forms. Most patients have a benign carrier state. These patients produce an excess of HBsAg in their livers but do not have evidence of ongoing liver injury or of active viral replication using standard testing methods. A smaller proportion of HBV carriers has evidence of ongoing active viral replication and clinical features of chronic active hepatitis (Fig. 37-7).

Hepatic histology in benign chronic HBV carriers with chronic hepatitis shows hepatocytes with a ground-glass appearance as a result of excess cytoplasmic HBsAg proteins (Fig. 37-8). There may be no inflammation, or inflammation may be confined only to the portal triad without evidence of liver injury. In contrast, chronic HBV carriers with progressive liver injury (previously called chronic active hepatitis) usually have serum markers of active viral replication (eg, HBeAg or HBV DNA), ongoing liver injury (eg, elevation of serum transaminase levels), and a histologic pattern of active inflammation. Molecular hybridization studies of liver tissue demonstrate HBV DNA sequences integrated into the native genome in benign chronic carriers. In contrast, in patients with chronic HBV associated with active replication and ongoing hepatitis, HBV sequences exist as free episomal HBV DNA in addition to genomic integration.

Chronic replicative hepatitis B can progress to cirrhosis. Patients with chronic hepatitis B can sometimes spontaneously become benign chronic carriers. This seroconversion is often accompanied by an acute exacerbation of hepatitis with a typical viral syndrome and elevated levels of transaminases. A similar phenomenon is observed when seroconversion is induced by interferon therapy. Spontaneous reactivation of chronic HBV infection resulting in seroconversion from the benign chronic carriage state to chronic liver injury with serum markers of active viral replication also occurs. This may be accompanied by elevated transaminases and progressive liver damage. Consequently, there are several reasons a patient with HBV infection might develop an acute hepatitis. These include acute onset of HBV infection, an acute exacerbation of chronic hepatitis B, seroconversion of chronic hepatitis B with acute replication to the benign chronic hepatitis B carrier state, reactivation of chronic benign HBV carriage, and acquisition of other infections (eg, HAV, HCV, CMV). One example of the latter phenomenon is superinfection by HDV in chronic HBV carriers (see later discussion).

Hepatoma is an important consequence of chronic HBV infection, usually after a lead time of 10 to 20 years. It appears to result from the concordance of the following factors:

- Male gender
- Presence of cirrhosis
- Viral infection with HBV or HCV
- Inherited disorders such as hemochromatosis or tyrosinemia
- Environmental exposure to the procarcinogen aflatoxin

Hepatoma also complicates chronic HCV infection, and HCV may contribute to hepatoma development in HBV endemic areas.

The best treatment method for HBV is primary prevention by vaccination. High-risk persons include all health care workers, those who have had sexual contacts with an acutely infected person or chronic carrier, those who share a household with persons who are at risk of parenteral exposure to HBV (eg, thalassemic persons, hemophiliacs, intravenous drug abusers), and visitors to areas of high endemicity. All people who have had susceptible household or sexual contact with a person with a positive serum test for HBsAg should be unequivocally advised to receive a full course of HBV vaccine, whether or not the index case expresses serum markers of viral replication. Sexual contacts of an index case should also receive passive prophylaxis with HB immunoglobulin (HBIG) and should use condoms during sexual intercourse until the contact has demonstrated adequate immune response to HBV vaccination. Similarly, susceptible contacts who have had a recent potential parenteral exposure (eg, accidental needlestick,

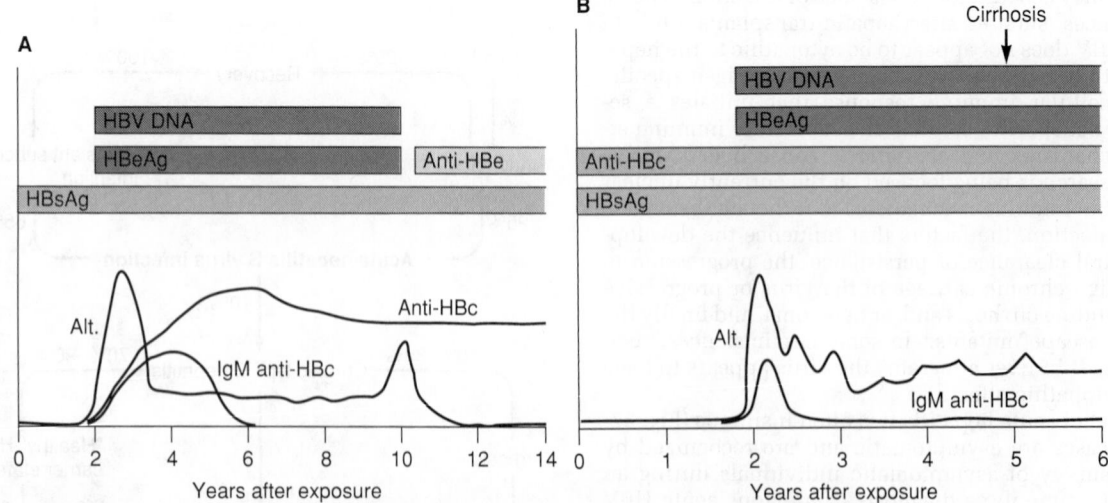

Figure 37-7. Clinical course of chronic hepatitis B. (*A*) A benign chronic carrier has continued production of HBsAg but an absence of serum markers of viral replication. (*B*) A pattern of continuing liver injury and serum markers of active viral replication.

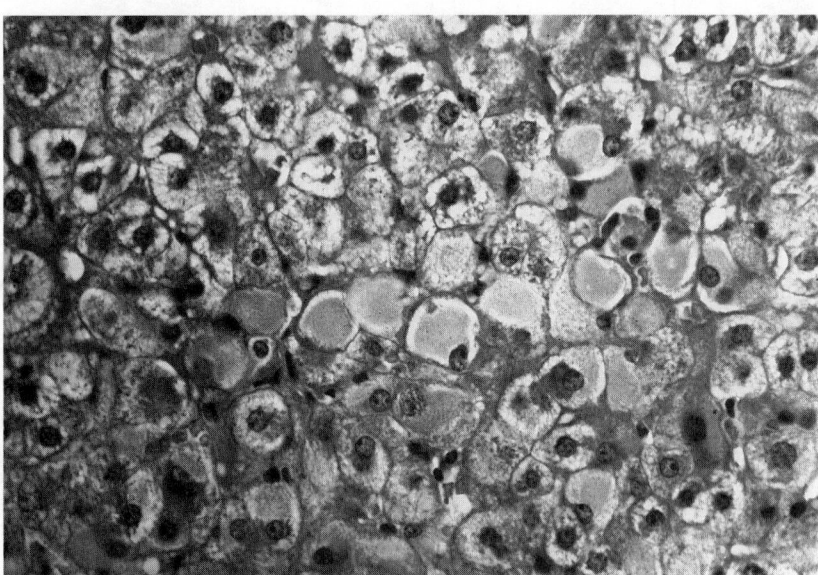

Figure 37-8. Photomicrograph of ground-glass hepatocytes (*arrows;* hematoxylin-eosin).

shared needles) should receive HBIG. The risk of transmitting HBV to intimate contacts from persons with serologic evidence of previous HBV infection but no markers of chronic carriage (ie, anti-HBsAb–positive, anti-HBcAb–positive, or HBsAg-negative status) are low. However, such previously exposed cases are potentially persistent carriers of minute amounts of HBV. Thus, vaccination for intimate contacts of these patients is also advised. Indeed, HBV vaccines are so safe and efficacious that some authorities have recommended universal HBV vaccination in North America. Vertical transmission from a chronically infected mother during parturition can almost always be prevented by early recognition of the mother's carrier status and administration of HBIG and vaccine to the newborn infant.

No established treatment strategies ameliorate acute HBV or prevent its progression to chronic infections. Patients with HBV-induced fulminant hepatic failure may require liver transplantation. Chronic HBV carriers with no markers of active viral replication should not receive interferon therapy. Clinical trials have demonstrated that interferon α, 5 million IU/d subcutaneously for 3 to 4 months, induces seroconversion from HBeAg-positive, HDV DNA–positive to anti-HBeAb–positive, HBV DNA–negative in about one third of stable patients with chronic active hepatitis B. In 10% of these patients, HBsAg is cleared from serum. An initial response is more common in patients with a moderate viral load, an active inflammatory response (ie, alanine aminotransferase [ALT] level higher than 200 IU/L), and an absence of human immunodeficiency virus (HIV). Asian patients with chronic HBV are infrequent responders to interferon α.

Hepatitis C

Hepatitis C virus is responsible for over 90% of posttransfusion NANB hepatitis and for most sporadic NANB hepatitis throughout the world. HCV is a lipid-enveloped, single-stranded positive-sense RNA virus with a genome of 9.4 kb.[14] It is closely related to pestiviruses and flaviviruses. A single, large open-reading frame encodes a large viral precursor polyprotein from which individual viral proteins are cleaved. These proteins are both structural and nonstructural. Based on nucleic acid sequencing, 6 major genotypes have been identified, with further subdivision into at least 15 subtypes.[15] There is worldwide geographic variation with regard to the predominant genotypic HCV forms in different areas. Furthermore, HCV genotypes may differ in their biologic characteristics, including severity of liver injury and responsiveness to interferon.

The most common identifiable sources of HCV acquisition in the United States are a prior transfusion of blood or blood-derived products and a history of illicit intravenous drug use. Sexual transmission of HCV is less commonly observed than with HBV. Indeed, its rarity makes it difficult to offer unequivocal advice to the spouse or sexual partner of an HCV-infected person. There is no evidence that using condoms reduces the already minuscule risk of sexual transmission of HCV.

Many uncertainties about HCV remain, including the mechanism of HCV entry into the hepatocyte, the life cycle of HCV in liver and other tissues, and the mechanism of HCV-related liver injury. About 70% of persons who contract posttransfusion HCV (and probably sporadic HCV as well) develop chronic hepatitis, and many progress to cirrhosis. The usual incubation period of posttransfusion HCV infection is from 5 to 10 weeks. The initial elevated ALT level ranges from 500 to 1000 IU/L and may be associated with little or no clinical disturbance.[16] Viral replication coincides with this initial episode of hepatitis, often with very high viral RNA titers (Fig. 37-9). Commonly, anti-HCV antibody does not appear till 18 weeks after the initial posttransfusion hepatic illness. In some persons, acute HCV hepatitis does not progress to chronic infection, and anti-HC antibody may or may not appear in the serum.[16] It is not clear whether there is a benign chronic carrier state for HCV. Chronic HCV infection is usually characterized by an indolent clinical syndrome in which the transaminases fluctuate from normal levels to 200 to 400 IU/L (Fig. 37-10), and at this time, viral replication is usually detectable by PCR amplification of HCV in serum. The quantitative levels of HCV RNA vary, however, and even qualitative HCV RNA can become undetectable for periods, only to later become positive again.[17] Consequently, a negative serum HCV RNA result in a previously positive person does not indicate invariably that the patient is no longer infected by the virus. Patients can harbor HCV for many years without apparent clinical ill effects, except for a history of fluctuating mild elevations in liver enzymes. A liver biopsy will show a spectrum of appear-

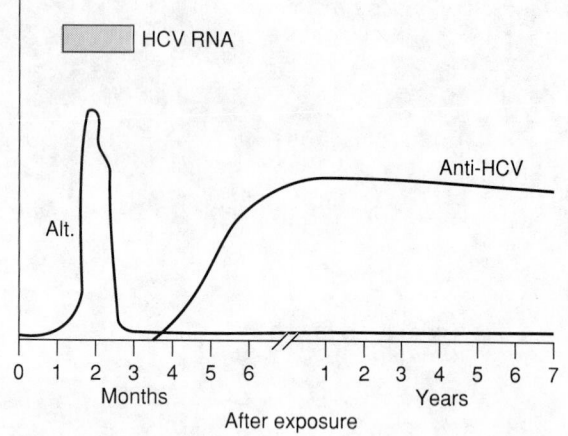

Figure 37-9. Clinical course in acute posttransfusion non-A, non-B hepatitis (hepatitis C).

ances ranging from normality, to a slight or more aggressive hepatitis, to cirrhosis. Typical histologic features of chronic HCV include a lymphocytic infiltrate in the portal triads, bile duct injury, acidophil bodies, and macrovesicular fat deposition. The natural history of chronic HCV has been difficult to define because of the extremely long interval between the time of acquisition and the manifestation of cirrhosis, often more than 20 years.[18] Hepatitis C does not appear to alter life expectancy, at least in the first 15 years of infection.[19] Once cirrhosis and end-stage liver disease develop, however, the clinical syndrome is indistinguishable from other forms of chronic liver failure.

Many factors can predispose a patient to the development of serious liver damage or hepatoma. HCV genotype is one candidate. Also, contemporaneous hepatic insults are important, especially chronic alcohol abuse or hemochromatosis. In some series, more than 40% of alcoholics with cirrhosis are infected with HCV.[20] Hepatitis C has been associated with many extrahepatic clinical phenomena, including the following:

- Membranoproliferative glomerulonephritis
- Mixed cryoglobulinemia
- Thyroiditis
- Sjögren syndrome
- Porphyria cutanea tarda
- Mooren ulcer
- Lichen planus

Interferon α is the only therapy for chronic HCV infection approved by the Food and Drug Administration. Some evidence suggests that early administration of interferons in acute HCV may reduce the risk of progression to chronic HCV. Interferon α, in the standard dosage schedule of 3 million IU given three times per week, reduces transaminases in about half of treated patients.[21,22] Restoring liver enzymes to the normal range may be accompanied by a loss of detectable HCV RNA in serum, using reverse transcription PCR to amplify the signal. This is associated with clinical improvement in extrahepatic manifestations, such as cryoglobulinemia or membranoproliferative glomerulonephritis. Unfortunately the biochemical response is usually transient, and the liver enzymes commonly relapse either during therapy or after interferon has been stopped. Similarly, a biochemical relapse is almost invariably associated with detectable serum HCV RNA.[17] No consensus exists on how best to proceed once an HCV-infected patient has relapsed or failed to respond to interferon. Some

experts advocate increasing the interferon dose or restarting or prolonging the duration of therapy. Good data to support these regimens are scanty, and these strategies raise important questions about the end points and objectives of interferon therapy in chronic HCV. As yet, there is no evidence that interferon alters the natural history of chronic HCV, or changes the incidence of cirrhosis or hepatoma. All HCV-infected persons should be advised to abstain from alcohol. Liver transplantation is the treatment of choice for patients with incapacitating liver failure due to chronic HCV, even though HCV usually infects the allograft.

Hepatitis D

Hepatitis D (or delta hepatitis) is caused by an incomplete virus-like particle similar to viroids and related satellite RNAs of plants. Like viroids, the genome of HDV is a covalently closed RNA circle consisting of 1.67 kb.[19] This is smaller than the genome of any conventional virus. HDV is found worldwide, and humans appear to be the only natural host.

Because of an association with HBV infection, HDV affects the same populations at risk for HBV. HDV requires simultaneous infection with HBV to complete its life cycle. HD antigen (HDAg) has been recovered from liver tissue infected by both viruses. Unlike HBV however, HDV infects only the hepatocyte, and no other sites of replication have been identified. When detectable in serum, HDAg exists within HBsAg particles. The mechanism by which HDV gains access to HBV-infected hepatocytes is unknown. Similarly, the mechanisms of HDV-induced liver injury are unknown. Curiously, HDV appears to suppress HBV replication.

HDV infection acquired simultaneously with HBV is termed *coinfection* (Fig. 37-11). HDV may also infect a host in whom HBV infection already exists. This is called *superinfection* (Fig. 37-12). In general, coinfection is a mild transient clinical phenomenon sometimes recognizable only by later detection of anti-HBcAb IgM and anti-HDV IgM. There may be a biphasic pattern of elevated transaminases, the first peak corresponding to acute HBV replication and the second peak corresponding to acute HDV replication. One circumstance in which the host would receive a large inoculum of HBV and HDV is acute coinfection among intravenous drug addicts. In two community-based studies of acute coinfection due to intravenous drug use, clinical hepatitis was common and some patients de-

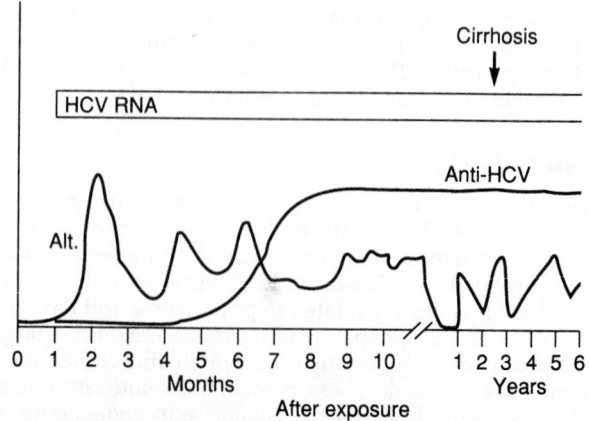

Figure 37-10. Clinical course in chronic posttransfusion non-A, non-B hepatitis (hepatitis C).

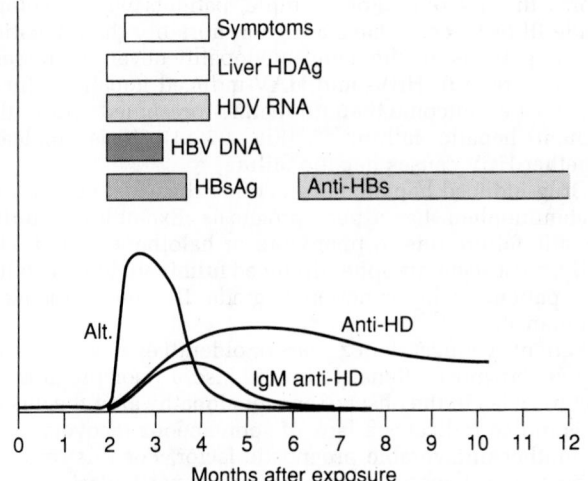

Figure 37-11. Synchronous infection with hepatitis B virus and hepatitis D virus.

veloped fulminant hepatic failure. Almost all patients with acute coinfection of HBV and HDV do not progress to chronic carriage of HDV, and some lose carriage of HBsAg as well. Similarly, reinfection often does not ensue following liver transplantation for fulminant hepatic failure due to HBV and HDV. This is probably because of the suppressant effect of HDV on HBV.

Superinfection by HDV is an important cause of acute hepatitis in persons already affected by chronic HBV infection. Superinfection may result from exposure to a small inoculum of HDV. Acquisition of acute HDV may result in seroconversion of HBsAg to anti-HBsAb and consequently loss of HDV infection also. Alternatively, chronic HDV and HBV infection may coexist (Fig. 37-13). Chronic hepatitis with progression to cirrhosis is one of the consequences of chronic HDV infection. Chronic hepatitis due to HDV is associated with persistent HDV replication, which may be accompanied by HDV-induced suppression of HBV replication. An association of HDV with primary hepatocellular carcinoma has not been found.

Tests for HDV infection are limited in most centers to measurement of anti-HDAb IgM and IgG. In research settings, HDAg and HDV RNA can be measured in the serum and liver. In typical cases, after an incubation period of 4 to 20 weeks, there is a short period of viral replication and shedding of HDAg into serum. Anti-HDAb IgM has been reported to give variable results in acute infection. Anti-HDAb IgG appears late in acute infection.

Interferon α has been used to treat chronic HDV infection.[23] It appears that eradication of HBV and HDV is rare even with high-dose therapy. A recrudescence of both viruses after stopping interferon is common, except in the rare instance that HBsAg is cleared during or soon after therapy. HDV and HBV coinfection can recur after liver transplantation, although this is less common than when patients infected with HBV alone undergo transplantation.[13]

Hepatitis E

Hepatitis E is a form of epidemic viral hepatitis previously called waterborne NANB hepatitis.[24] It is an ecologically determined disease associated with fecal contamination of drinking water. Large epidemics have been reported in the Indian subcontinent, Africa, and Central

America. Studies suggest that hepatitis E is caused by a unique virus with a single-stranded RNA genome of 7.6 kb and should probably be classified with caliciviruses. It does not appear to be related to HAV or other picornaviruses.

The usual incubation period is 40 days. Transient cholestatic jaundice develops, from which a complete recovery without chronic sequela occurs. An important exception is HEV infection during pregnancy. HEV has a predilection for pregnant women both in the frequency and severity of infection. Fulminant hepatic failure due to HEV is common in pregnant women during the third trimester. Providing clean water and hygienic disposal of excreta are important goals in controlling HEV infection.

ACUTE HEPATIC FAILURE

Fulminant hepatic failure is defined as the development of acute hepatic encephalopathy within 8 weeks of the onset of symptomatic hepatocellular disease in a previously healthy person.[25,26] Submassive hepatic necrosis denotes the development of acute hepatic encephalopathy within 9 to 24 weeks of the onset of symptomatic hepatocellular disease in a previously healthy person.[25,26]

Fulminant hepatic failure and its clinical variant, submassive hepatic necrosis, are clinical syndromes caused by the acute necrosis of a large proportion of hepatocytes. It is estimated that 2000 cases occur in the United States annually and that 80% of these patients die.[26] The key to the clinical definition is acute hepatic encephalopathy. Outcome is determined by the course of encephalopathy, which is measured on a four-grade scale as shown in Table 37-2. Cerebral edema, leading to increased intracranial pressure (ICP), is a common feature of severe fulminant hepatic failure and may cause permanent cerebral injury and death. Fulminant hepatic failure and submassive hepatic necrosis are always accompanied by severe coagulopathy.

The causes of fulminant hepatic failure are shown in Table 37-3. Fulminant hepatic failure may be subclassified histopathologically. In type I, transaminases are markedly increased and liver specimens show massive areas of confluent necrosis of hepatocytes.[26] Type II fulminant hepatic failure is associated with moderately elevated transami-

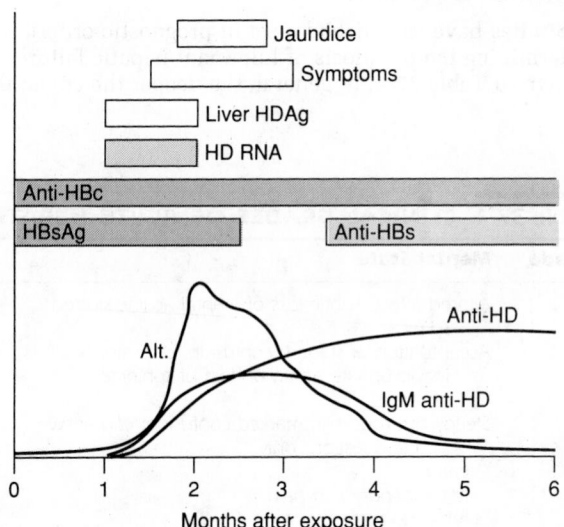

Figure 37-12. Superinfection of chronic hepatitis B carrier with hepatitis D.

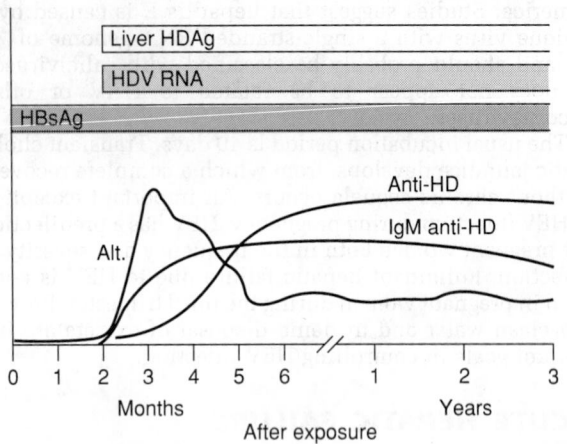

Figure 37-13. Clinical course of chronic hepatitis D infection.

nases, and pathology shows microvesicular fatty infiltration of hepatocytes without displacement of nuclei. It should be noted that chronic liver disease may present with an acute onset and mimic fulminant hepatic failure. Wilson disease is an exceptional example of this phenomenon and is usually included among the causes of fulminant hepatic failure. A history of heavy alcohol use also suggests chronic injury, even though alcoholics are at particular risk of acetaminophen-induced hepatic failure. A characteristic clinical scenario is the development of hepatic failure when an alcohol abuser stops drinking and 24 to 48 hours later develops abdominal pain due to gastritis, pancreatitis, or headache from a hangover. This person then takes a standard dose of acetaminophen to soothe symptoms, and unwittingly produces acute hepatic injury. When presented with an apparent case of acute hepatic injury, the physician must always answer two questions. Is this really an acute illness or rather the first presentation of a previously unrecognized chronic disorder? Are there single or multiple factors contributing to acute hepatic injury?

Predicting Outcome in Fulminant Hepatic Failure and Subacute Hepatic Necrosis

Studies have established a set of prognostic criteria for determining the prognosis of fulminant hepatic failure, as shown in Table 37-4. In general, the deeper the coma, the worse the outcome. For example, patients who develop grade III or IV coma have a higher mortality than hepatic failure patients in whom encephalopathy never progresses beyond grade II. HBV- and HAV-induced hepatic failure has a better outcome than idiopathic (presumed viral) fulminant hepatic failure[27,28] (Fig. 37-14). It is unclear whether HCV causes hepatic failure.

Drug-induced hepatic failure, other than that caused by acetaminophen, has a poor prognosis. Examples include hepatic failure due to phenytoin or halothane. Paradoxically, most acetaminophen-induced fulminant hepatic failure patients who experience grade III comas recover spontaneously.[27,28]

Patients younger than 2 years or older than 40 years have a poor prognosis. Renal failure is also a poor prognostic factor. Delay in the onset of encephalopathy after the onset of jaundice indicates a lack of spontaneous recovery and is another unfavorable prognostic factor. For this reason, submassive hepatic necrosis has a particularly poor outcome.

As mentioned, coagulopathy is always present. Some have recommended serum factor V levels as an indicator of when to proceed to transplant. A factor V level of less than 20% is a poor prognostic indicator.[29] Acidosis is a poor prognostic factor, particularly in acetaminophen-induced fulminant hepatic failure.

Management

All patients with fulminant hepatic failure should be transferred to an intensive care unit at a liver transplant center. Early transfer of patients with any degree of encephalopathy is crucial. Patients with acute hepatic injury that has not yet manifested encephalopathy can be treated in their local hospitals, but their physicians should alert a transplant center so that expeditious transfer can be arranged. Management should be directed toward the following:

Diagnosis: Anti-HBc antibody IgM, HBsAg, and anti-HAV IgM should be checked to identify patients with acute HBV and HAV. Antibodies to CMV, EBV, HSV, and varicella should also be checked. Serum ceruloplasmin levels should be determined, and eyes should be examined by slit lamp for corneal rings. A family history of early onset liver or neurological failure, or a history of gradual intellectual deterioration may be a clue to Wilson disease. An unusually low serum alkaline phosphatase level (lower than 80 IU) may also indicate underlying Wilson disease. The physician should look for toxic insults (eg, Amanita, drugs), and consider acute onset of chronic disease.

Table 37-2. CLINICAL GRADES OF ACUTE HEPATIC ENCEPHALOPATHY

Grade	Mental State	Tremor	Electroencephalogram Result
I	Altered affect, subtle loss of mental acuity, slurred speech	Slight or none	Normal
II	Accentuation of stage I, confusion, drowsiness, inappropriate behavior, loss of sphincter control	Easily elicited	Abnormal, generalized slowing
III	Sleepy but rousable, marked confusion, can answer simple questions only	Present when patient can cooperate	Always abnormal
IV	Coma IVa—responds to pain IVb—no response to pain	Cannot cooperate	Always abnormal

(Adapted from Jones EA, Schafer DF. Fulminant hepatic failure. In: Zakin D, Boyer TD, eds. Hepatology: a textbook of liver disease. Philadelphia, WB Saunders, 1990:320)

Table 37-3. CAUSES OF FULMINANT HEPATIC FAILURE

VIRAL INFECTION

Hepatitis A
Hepatitis B
Hepatitis D
Other viruses (less common)
    Cytomegalovirus
    Epstein-Barr
    Varicella
    Herpes

POISONS, CHEMICALS, AND DRUGS

Amanita phalloides
Acetaminophen
Tetracycline
Phosphorus
Halogenated volatile anesthetics (especially halothane)
Isomazid
Methyldopa
Valproate
Monoamine oxidase inhibitors

ISCHAEMIA AND HYPOXIA

Hepatic vascular occlusion
Acute circulatory stroke
Heat stroke
Gram-negative sepsis

MISCELLANEOUS

Acute fatty liver of pregnancy
Reyes syndrome
Wilson disease
Hodgkin and other lymphomas
Hereditary fructose intolerance
Galactosemia, tyrosinemia
Idiopathic (also called non-A non-B)

Specific therapy: Hepatic failure patients who have ingested acetaminophen should receive a full course of N-acetylcysteine.[30,31] There is unconfirmed evidence that N-acetylcysteine may be beneficial even in non–acetaminophen-related hepatic failure. Although there are considerable data to support a role for circulating benzodiazepines in the development of acute (and chronic) hepatic encephalopathy, there is no place for flumazenil in treating fulminant hepatic failure unless it is within a defined research protocol.

Avoidance of renal failure: Aminoglycosides, radiographic dye, and other potentially nephrotoxic agents should be used cautiously. Some practitioners advocate early introduction of dialysis for better management of fluid balance.

Metabolic fluxes: Hepatic failure may be complicated by hypoglycemia and coma, which could be misinterpreted as caused by to cerebral edema. Correcting hypoglycemia in hepatic failure may require large amounts of dextrose. Hypokalemia and acidosis may also complicate hepatic failure.

Hematologic stability: Coagulopathy should be corrected by fresh frozen plasma prior to invasive procedures (placement of central lines, placement of ICP monitor), or whenever there is evidence of hemorrhage (intracranial hemorrhage, gastrointestinal bleeding). In most circumstances, it is not necessary to give fresh frozen plasma simply to correct a prolonged prothrombin time of up to 30 seconds.

Hypotension is common in fulminant hepatic failure, despite high cardiac output, because of associated low systemic vascular resistance. Hypotension may exacerbate low cerebral perfusion pressure (CPP) consequent to raised ICP. Assisted ventilation should be undertaken in patients with grade IV coma or in patients with *any* evidence of hypoxia or respiratory distress because pulmonary edema and adult respiratory distress syndrome are features of deteriorating hepatic failure. Ventilation also maintains hypocapnea as an adjunct to controlling elevated ICP.

Patients with fulminant hepatic failure or subacute hepatic necrosis are at high risk for sepsis. Daily cultures of blood, urine, and other body fluids are advisable. This is particularly important because sepsis may prevent liver transplantation. The syndrome of high output hypotension mimics septicemia. Unexplained fever despite broad spectrum antibiotic coverage warrants consideration of an antifungal prophylaxis.

Cerebral edema is the single most dangerous complication of fulminant hepatic failure. Hepatic failure patients may have rapid and extreme changes in CPP precipitated by positional changes and movement. Acute elevation in ICP may present with seizures, changes in pupillary responses, and cerebral posturing. The immediate response to clinical signs of increased ICP should also exclude hypoglycemia. Hypoglycemia is a particular risk for patients with acetaminophen-related fulminant hepatic failure or patients with the microvesicular fat deposition disorders (eg, Reyes syndrome, acute fatty liver of pregnancy, valproate poisoning).

Only mannitol has been shown to offer a therapeutic benefit to the elevated ICP syndrome of hepatic failure. Dexamethazone is of no value. The ability of barbiturate coma and ventilator-driven hypocapnea to reverse ICP elevations associated with hepatic failure is unknown, but often tried on an empiric basis. Because ICP is subject to rapid changes, the use of ICP monitoring has increased in the treatment of severely ill patients with fulminant hepatic failure.[32,33] Monitoring ICP serves two purposes: (1) to guide attempts to reduce ICP and restore CPP; and (2) to recognize persistently elevated ICP and reduced CPP,

Table 37-4. PROGNOSTIC CRITERIA FOR PREDICTING REQUIRED LIVER TRANSPLANTATION IN PATIENTS WITH FULMINANT HEPATIC FAILURE

Cause of Liver Failure	Criteria
Acetaminophen toxicity	pH <7.3 (irrespective of grade of encephalopathy)
	or
	Prothrombin time >100 s and serum creatinine >3.4 mg/dL (300 μmol/L) in patients with grade III or IV encephalopathy
All other causes	Prothrombin time >100 s (irrespective of grade encephalopathy)
	or
	Any three of the following variables (irrespective of grade of encephalopathy):
	Age <10 years or >40 years
	Liver failure due to halothane or other drug idiosyncrasy or idiopathic hepatitis
	Duration of jaundice prior to encephalopathy >7 d
	Prothrombin time >50 s
	Serum bilirubin >17.5 mg/dL (300 μmol/L)

(Adapted from O'Grady JG, Alexander GJM, Hayllar KM, Williams R. Early indicators of prognosis in fulminant hepatic failure. Gastroenterology 1989;97:439)

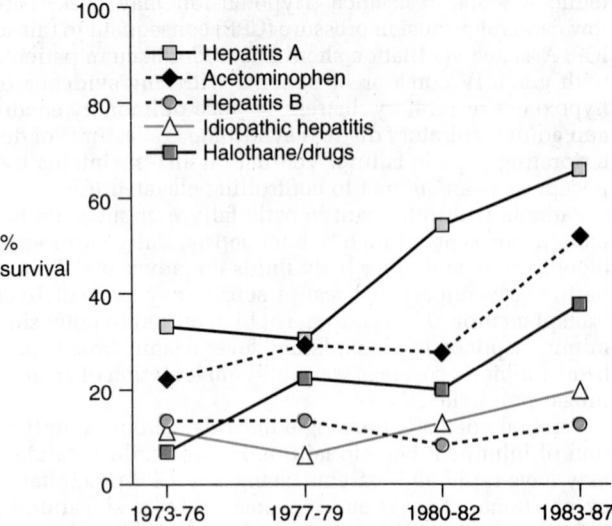

Figure 37-14. Survival of patients with fulminant hepatic failure leading to grade III or IV encephalopathy. Survival has improved over time for some causes, such as hepatitis A or B and acetaminophen-induced failure, but not for patients with halothane-induced or idiopathic hepatitis. (After O'Grady JG, Gimson AES, O'Brien CJ, Pucknell A, Hughes RD, Williams R. Controlled trials of charcoal hemoperfusion and prognostic factors in fulminant hepatic failure. Gastroenterology 1989;97:439)

which cause irreversible brain injury before the patient undergoes transplantation. The absolute thresholds that predict irreversible brain injury have been challenged recently.

ICP monitoring is *not* advised before the patient is transferred to a liver transplant center. Rather, early transfer before grade IV coma is recommended. Placement of an epidural catheter is indicated on the following conditions:

1. All eligibility criteria for transplant are met.
2. Patient is in grade IV coma with some brain stem function on neurologic examination.
3. Patient is receiving mechanical ventilation.
4. No evidence of intracranial bleeding is seen on head CT scan within 24 hours.
5. Mean arterial blood pressure exceeds 70 mmHg
6. Prothrombin time is 25 seconds or less, and the platelet count is 100,000 or lower after aggressive replenishment.
7. Family member is available for consent.

The final decision is made on a case-by-case basis in consultation with the neurosurgeon.

The goal of ICP monitoring is to maintain CPP of at least 60 mmHg. Treatment should begin when CPP falls below 60 mmHg. Treatment strategies to maintain an adequate CPP include the following:

- Manipulation of the height of the head to maximize CPP
- Pressor support to maintain mean arterial blood pressure 60 mmHg higher than the ICP, but a systolic arterial pressure no higher than 180 mmHg or a mean pressure of 120 mmHg
- Osmotic diuresis with 20% mannitol to maintain serum osmolality ideally at 300 to 310 mOsm but no more than 320 mOsm
- Hyperventilation to maintain $PaCO_2$ at 25 to 30
- Administration of an intravenous 50-mL bolus of 3% saline if serum sodium is less than 146 mEg/L and renal and cardiac parameters permit

- Avoidance of steroids
- Intracranial hemorrhages not evacuated

ICP monitoring should be discontinued in the following circumstances: a liver transplantation has been successfully completed and the coagulopathy and neurologic examinations are improving; the patient ceases to be eligible for liver transplantation; or clinically detectable brain stem function is absent, and either CPP falls below 30 mmHg for more than 6 hours or the ICP is greater than 60 mmHg for more than 6 hours.

Liver transplantation is a life-saving procedure for patients with hepatic failure or submassive hepatic necrosis that does not respond to medical management.[34] Notwithstanding the aforementioned prognostic factors, the most important indicators that the patient needs liver transplantation are the level of encephalopathy and the trend of change in encephalopathy. Unfortunately, because acute hepatic encephalopathy can vary between grades II and III in a matter of minutes, making a decision based on these factors remains difficult. For this reason, some clinicians have used coagulation factor levels, particularly a factor V level that is less than 20% of normal values, as indicators of when to transplant.[29] The decision to place a patient with fulminant hepatic failure on the transplant list is also confounded by the difficulty in procuring a suitable donor organ quickly. Even when listed as a highest emergency status, it is not unusual for a patient in North America to wait for 72 hours or longer for a suitable donor. During this time, further deterioration, especially worsening cerebral edema, may make transplantation impossible. For this reason, human heterotopic transplants, extracorporeal perfusion through human or pig livers or artificial hepatocyte perfusion devices, and xenografts have been attempted to sustain the patient until spontaneous recovery develops or a suitable organ is found.

The outcome of liver transplantation in patients with fulminant hepatic failure is somewhat worse than for that performed for other causes. One-year survival rates of 50% to 60% are common.

HEPATIC INFECTIONS ASSOCIATED WITH HUMAN IMMUNODEFICIENCY VIRUS OR AUTOIMMUNE DEFICIENCY SYNDROME

Asymptomatic patients who are positive for HIV antibody may present with abnormal liver chemistry tests. Liver disturbance in these patients may have many causes spanning the gamut of noninfectious liver diseases. Many asymptomatic patients who are positive for HIV antibody also have markers of exposure to HBV and HDV. HCV antibodies are common in hemophiliacs, a population that has been at higher-than-average risk for HIV infection. In contrast, the prevalence of HCV-positive serology in male homosexuals who are HIV-positive has been reported to be low. The investigation and management of abnormal liver tests for persons who are HIV Ab−positive without AIDS is no different than for persons who are HIV Ab−negative.

Many patients with clinically overt AIDS carry markers for exposure to viral hepatitis. In one large series of predominantly male homosexuals with AIDS, 89% had serologic evidence of previous exposure to HBV, whereas 10% were HBsAg-positive.[35,36] Only one of the HBsAg-positive patients developed chronic active hepatitis and none had cirrhosis, again suggesting that HBV may assume a benign course in patients with HIV infection.

AIDS may be accompanied by a host of opportunistic

infections that can localize to the liver. these include *Mycobacterium avium-intracellulare, Mycobacterium tuberculosis,* CMV, EBV, HSV, and fungal infections (eg, *Cryptococcus neoformans, Histoplasma capsulatum, Coccidioides immites, Candida albicans*). When these infections involve the liver, they share a common clinical presentation of fever, hepatomegaly, and abnormal liver chemistries. Usually, there is a disproportionate elevation in serum alkaline phosphatase, and jaundice is unusual. Liver histology may show nonspecific changes including granuloma formation. Specific features may also be found. Thus, *M avium-intracellulare* can often be identified by stains for acid-fast bacilli. Even when these are negative, *M avium-intracellulare* is usually cultured from infected liver tissue. CMV may produce large intranuclear and multiple smaller cytoplasmic inclusions within Kupffer cells, biliary duct epithelium, and occasionally hepatocytes, accompanied by periportal mononuclear inflammatory infiltrate and focal hepatocyte necrosis.

The presence of opportunistic viral bacterial or fungal infections in AIDS is usually a manifestation of disseminated infection in patients with advanced disease. Although hepatic pathogens have frequently been identified, they have rarely been implicated as the cause of death. Rather, they appear as a marker of end-stage AIDS. Similarly, effective therapy requires changing the underlying process of immunodeficiency. There is no effective therapy for hepatic *M avium-intracellulare. M tuberculosis* should be treated with antituberculosis chemotherapy. As stated, CMV hepatitis in AIDS is usually a component of systemic CMV infection and may respond to ganciclovir. Therapy for hepatic fungal infection may be attempted with amphotericin B and fluconazole.

HEPATIC INFECTIONS IN IMMUNOSUPPRESSED HOSTS

Persons receiving major immunosuppressive drugs are at risk for hepatic infections. This is particularly true for recipients of major organ transplants. The organisms that affect the liver in pharmacologically immunosuppressed persons are similar to those observed in patients immunosuppressed by HIV. HBV and HDV infection are well described in major organ transplant recipients.

When a patient with chronic HBV receives an orthotopic liver graft, infection of the grafted liver by HBV is almost invariable and often causes marked liver injury. Recent evidence suggests that frequent repeated administration of exogenous anti-HBsAg, so-called HBIG, significantly reduces the frequency and severity of recurrent HBV in the allograft.[37] HDV also recurs in the grafted liver but may have a less severe course. HCV commonly recurs in the grafted liver, although the natural history of HCV in liver allografts remains to be determined. A common viral infection of the grafted liver is caused by CMV. CMV infection of the liver graft is rarely disseminated and is often self-limited without treatment. Ganciclovir is effective when there is clinically significant hepatitis.

Similarly, renal graft recipients may develop HBV infections of their livers.[37] This usually represents HBV infection acquired before transplantation. In many instances, serum HBsAg is positive at the time of surgery. There is controversy about whether the presence of HBV should influence the decision to proceed to renal transplantation in a patient with end-stage renal failure. The consensus appears to be that HBV infection is not a contraindication to renal transplantation. Data on hepatic HCV infection in renal transplant patients are evolving. CMV hepatitis occurs in renal graft recipients and may be part of a disseminated CMV infection.[38] Just as in HIV infection, immunosuppressed patients may have systemic infections that affect the liver in addition to other tissues. These include *M tuberculosis,* CMV, varicella, and *C albicans.* Curiously, *M avium-intracellulare* has not been observed frequently in patients with major organ grafts. Hepatic abscess is also unusual in these patients. One exception, albeit a rare one, is pyogenic abscess in hepatic transplant recipients, which is often related to occlusion of the hepatic artery.

REFERENCES

1. Brandborg LL, Goldman IS. Bacterial and miscellaneous infections of the liver. In: Zakim D, Boyer TWB, eds. Hepatology: a textbook of liver disease, ed 2. Philadelphia, WB Saunders, 1990:1086.
2. Bertel CK, van Heerden JA, Sheedy PF. Treatment of pyogenic hepatic abscesses. Arch Surg 1986;121:554.
3. Barnes PF, DeCock KM, Reynolds TN, Ralls PW. A comparison of amebic and pyogenic abscess of the liver. Medicine 1987;66:472.
4. Khuroo M S, Dar MY, Yattoo GN, et al. Percutaneous drainage versus albendazole in hepatic hydatidatosis: a prospective randomized study. Gastroenterology 1993;104:1452.
5. Davidson RA. Issues in clinical parasitology: the management of hydatid cyst. Am J Gastroenterol 1984;79:397.
6. Gil-Grande LA, Rodriguez-Caabeiro F, Prieto JG, et al. Randomized controlled trial of efficacy of albendazole in intraabdominal hydatid disease. Lancet 1993;342:1269.
7. Cohen JI. Hepatitis A virus: insights from molecular biology. Hepatology 1989;9:889.
8. Innes BL, Snitbhan R, Kunasol P, et al. Protection against hepatitis A by an inactivated vaccine. JAMA 1994;271:1328.
9. Lau JYN, Wright TL. Molecular virology and pathogenesis of hepatitis B. Lancet 1993:342:1335.
10. Carman W, Thomas H, Domingo E. Viral genetic variation: hepatitis B virus as a clinical example. Lancet 1993:34;349.
11. Okamoto H, Yotsumoto Y, Akahane T, et al. Hepatitis B viruses with precore region defects prevail in persistently infected hosts along with seroconversion to the antibody against e antigen. J Virol 1990;64:1298.
12. Yoffe B, Burns DK, Bhatt HS, Combes B. Extrahepatic hepatitis B virus DNA sequences in patients with acute hepatitis B infection. Hepatology 1990;12:187.
13. Lucey MR, Graham DM, Martin P, et al. Recurrence of hepatitis B and delta hepatitis after orthotopic liver transplantation. Gut 1992;33;1390.
14. Choo QL, Kuo G, Weiner AJ, et al. Isolation of a cDNA clone derived from a blood-borne non-A, non-B viral hepatitis genome. Science 1989;244:359.
15. Simmonds P, Alberti A, Alter H, et al. A proposed system for the nomenclature of hepatitis C viral genotypes. Hepatology 1994;19:1321.
16. Farci P, Alter HF, Wong D, et al. A long-term study of hepatitis C virus replication in non-A, non-B hepatitis. N Engl J Med 1991;325:98.
17. Lau JYN, Mizokami M, Ohno T, et al. Discrepancy between biochemical and virological responses to interferon α in chronic hepatitis C. Lancet 1993;342:1208.
18. Takahashi M, Yamada G, Miyamoto R, Doi T, Endo H, Tsuji T. Natural course of chronic hepatitis C. Am J Gastroenterol 1993;88:240.
19. Sheef LB, Buskell-Bales Z, Wright EC, et al. Long-term mortality after transfusion-associated non-A, non-B hepatitis. N Engl J Med 1992;327:1906.
20. Pares A, Barrera JM, Bruguera M, et al. Hepatitis C antibodies in chronic alcoholic patients: association with severity of liver injury. Hepatology 1990;12:1295.
21. Davis GL, Balart LA, Schiff ER, et al. Treatment of chronic hepatitis C with recombinant interferon alfa. N Engl J Med 1989;30:1501.
22. Di Bisceglie AM, Martin P, Kassianides C, et al. Recombinant interferon alfa therapy for chronic hepatitis C. N Engl J Med 1989;321:1506.
23. Farci P, Mandas A, Coiana A, et al. Treatment of chronic hepatitis D with interferon alfa-2a. N Eng J Med 1994;330:88.

24. Krawczynski K. Hepatitis E. Hepatology 1993;17:932.
25. Lee WM. Acute liver failure. N Engl J Med 1993;329:1862.
26. Jones EA, Schafer DF. Fulminant hepatic failure. In: Zakin D, Boyer TD, eds. Hepatology: a textbook of liver disease. Philadelphia, WB Saunders, 1990:320.
27. O'Grady JG, Gimson AES, O'Brien CJ, Pucknell A, Hughes RD, Williams R. Controlled trials of charcoal hemoperfusion and prognostic factors in fulminant hepatic failure. Gastroenterology 1988;94:1186.
28. O'Grady JG, Alexander GJM, Hayllar KM, Williams R. Early indicators of prognosis in fulminant hepatic failure. Gastroenterology 1989;97:439.
29. Bismuth H, Samuel D, Gugenheim J, et al. Emergency liver transplantation for fulminant hepatitis. Ann Intern Med 1987;107:337.
30. Smilkstein MJ, Knapp GL, Kulig KW, Rumack BH. Efficacy of oral N-acetylcysteine in the treatment of acetaminophen overdose. N Engl J Med 1988;319:1557.
31. Harrison PM, Keays R, Bray GP, Alexander GJM, Williams R. Improved outcome of paracetamol-induced fulminant hepatic failure by late administration of acetylcysteine. Lancet 1990;335:1572.
32. Lidofsky SD, Bass NM, Prager MC, et al. Intracranial pressure monitoring and liver transplantation for fulminant hepatic failure. Hepatology 1992;16:1.
33. Blei AT, Olafsson S, Webster S, Levy R. Complications of intracranial pressure monitoring in fulminant hepatic failure. Lancet 1993;341:157.
34. Emond JC, Aran PP, Whitington PF, Broelsch CE, Baker AL. Liver transplantation in the management of fulminant hepatic failure. Gastroenterology 1989;96:1553.
35. Perrillo RP, Regenstein FG, Roodman ST. Chronic hepatitis B in asymptomatic homosexual men with antibody to the human immunodeficiency virus. Ann Intern Med 1986; 105:382.
36. Schneiderman DJ, Arenson DM, Cello JP, Margaretten W, Weber TE. Hepatic disease in patients with the acquired immune deficiency syndrome (AIDS). Hepatology 1987;7:925.
37. Samuel D, Muller R, Alexander G, et al. Liver transplantation in European patients with the hepatitis B surface antigen. N Engl J Med 1993;329:1842.
38. Degos F, Lugassy C, Degott C, et al. Hepatitis B virus and hepatitis B-related viral infection in renal transplant recipients. Gastroenterology 1988;94:151.

SURGERY: SCIENTIFIC PRINCIPLES AND PRACTICE, Second Edition, edited by Lazar J. Greenfield, Michael W. Mulholland, Keith T. Oldham, Gerald B. Zelenock, and Keith D. Lillemoe. Lippincott–Raven Publishers, Philadelphia, © 1997.

CHAPTER 38

CIRRHOSIS AND PORTAL HYPERTENSION

FREDERIC E. ECKHAUSER, STEVEN E. RAPER, AND JEREMIAH G. TURCOTTE

CIRRHOSIS

More than a century and a half has elapsed since Laennec first described the pathologic and clinical features of cirrhosis in 1826. He proposed the term *cirrhosis* to describe the orange or tawny appearance of the liver characteristic of this condition. Since that time, experts have argued about both the definition and pathogenesis of this disorder. Cirrhosis is defined as a chronic disease of the liver in which diffuse destruction and regeneration of hepatic parenchymal cells has occurred, and in which a diffuse increase in connective tissue has resulted in disorga-

nization of the lobular and vascular architecture.[1] The principal pathologic features of cirrhosis include hepatic parenchymal necrosis, regeneration, and scarring. From a clinical standpoint, distortion of the vascular architecture causes the most serious complications—portal hypertension with resulting ascites and variceal hemorrhage.

A wide variety of classifications of cirrhosis have been proposed. The lack of a uniform classification system is largely due to the inconsistent relations between the clinical, laboratory, and pathologic aspects of the disease. Simple systems distinguish between regular and irregular anatomic patterns of cirrhosis; however, the correlation between the anatomic classification of cirrhosis and its causes is poor. Furthermore, histologic lesions that are considered by pathologists as typical of the major types of cirrhosis frequently coexist within the same liver. No single classification system is ideal or entirely comprehensive, but the most useful classification categorizes cirrhosis by morphologic, histologic, and etiologic criteria (Table 38-1).

Morphologic Classification

Morphologic classifications of cirrhosis include micronodular, macronodular, and mixed forms. In many cases the gross appearance of the liver may be a more reliable indicator of the anatomic type of cirrhosis than a histologic sample. The pattern of nodularity and scars reflects the nature of the insult and the pattern of necrosis as well as the size of the necrotic zones. For example, uniform lobular insults generally lead to regular cirrhosis, and nonuniform confluent necrosis leads to irregular cirrhosis.

Micronodular cirrhosis is characterized by uniform nodules and scars. The nodules are usually less than 3 mm in diameter. They are formed from fragments of single liver lobules and lack normal lobular organization. This pattern is typical of Laennec or nutritional cirrhosis in alcoholics and of pigmentary cirrhosis in patients with hemochromatosis.

Macronodular cirrhosis is characterized by nodules and scars of varying sizes, and most of the nodules exceed 3 mm in diameter. Macronodular cirrhosis is categorized

Table 38-1. CLASSIFICATION OF CIRRHOSIS

MORPHOLOGIC	ETIOLOGIC
Macronodular	Alcohol
Micronodular	Viral hepatitis
Mixed	Biliary obstruction
	Primary
HISTOLOGIC	Secondary
Portal	Venoocclusive
Postnecrotic	Hemochromatosis
Posthepatitic	Wilson disease
Primary obstructive	Autoimmune
Primary	Syphilis
Secondary	Drugs and toxins
Venoocclusive	α_1-Antitrypsin deficiency
	Cystic fibrosis
	Glycogen storage disease
	Other metabolic diseases
	Sarcoidosis
	Copper
	Small bowel bypass
	Idiopathic

(Modified from Conn HO, Atterbury CE. Cirrhosis. In: Schiff L, Schiff ER, eds. Diseases of the liver, ed 6. Philadelphia, JB Lippincott, 1987:726)

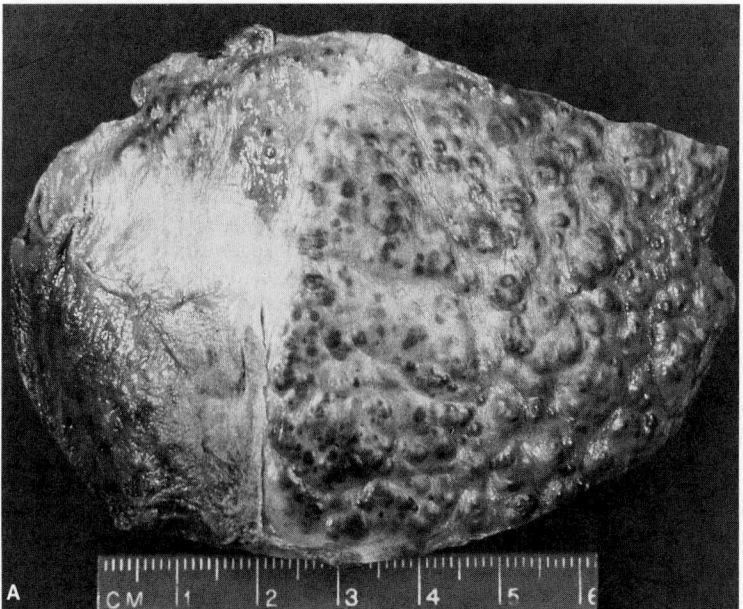
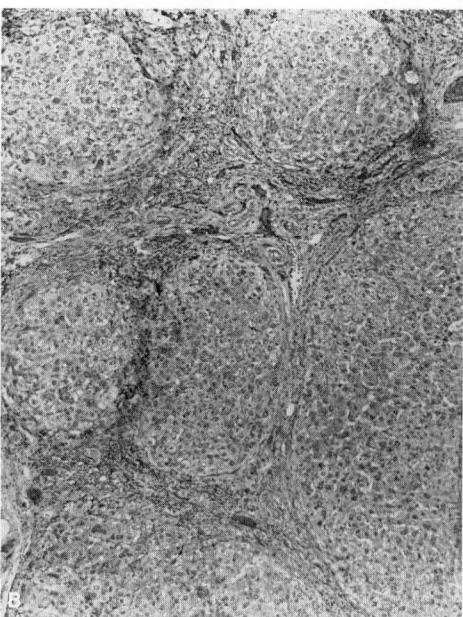

Figure 38-1. (*A*) Small, shrunken liver and a fairly regular pattern of nodularity. This appearance is fairly typical of end-stage cirrhosis, regardless of the cause. (*B*) Photomicrograph of cirrhotic liver showing irregular nodules of regenerating hepatocytes surrounded by scar (trichrome stain, × 60).

into two subtypes, postnecrotic and posthepatitic, which can be distinguished by the pattern of scar formation. Both anatomic forms are coarsely nodular in appearance. In posthepatitic cirrhosis, macronodules are separated by thin scars. This form is sometimes referred to as *septal* or *trabecular cirrhosis* and is typical of Wilson disease. In postnecrotic cirrhosis, the macronodules are separated by broad as well as thin scars. This pattern is frequently seen in patients with viral hepatitis. The macronodular pattern of cirrhosis may reflect end-stage disease (Fig. 38-1). In mixed cirrhosis, micronodular and macronodular patterns are equally represented in liver specimens.

Histologic Classification

Portal cirrhosis is typically observed in alcoholics and in patients with hemochromatosis. These livers vary in size depending on the severity and duration of the insult.

The surface is granular with fine nodules that are 1 to 5 mm in diameter and separated by thin septae or scars. Portal cirrhosis can usually be distinguished histologically by the presence of several specific hepatocellular alterations such as Mallory bodies and megamitochondria.

Mallory bodies occur in many forms of liver disease, including Wilson disease, primary biliary cirrhosis, and hepatocellular tumors. Centrilobular location usually connotes an alcoholic cause.[2] Mallory bodies are eosinophilic, intracytoplasmic inclusions that are classified most reliably by their electron microscopic appearance (Fig. 38-2). Mallory bodies are composed of hollow intermediate-sized tonofilaments that contain prekeratin and are most likely derived from the hepatocyte cytoskeleton. Depletion of intracellular filament protein weakens the cytoskeleton and results in loss of microvilli. The cell also changes to a spherical configuration (balloon degeneration), with disor-

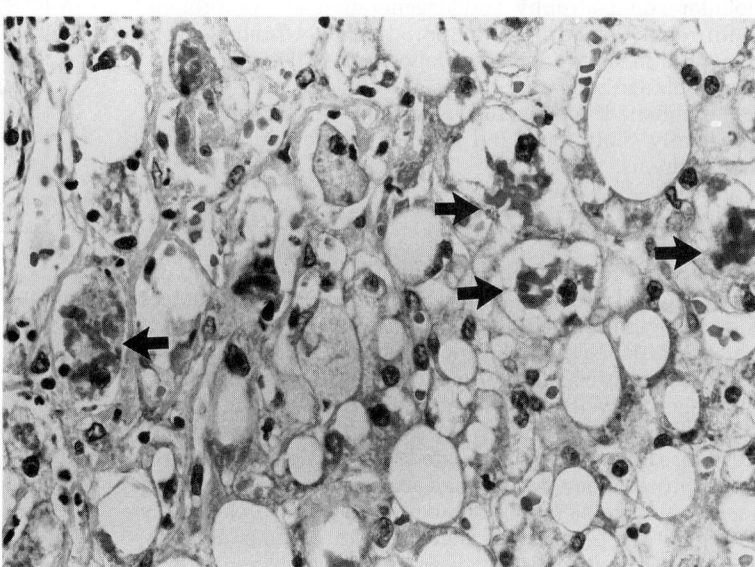

Figure 38-2. Alcoholic hepatitis. Mallory bodies (*arrows*) are evident within the swollen, clear cytoplasm of several hepatocytes. This hyaline material is chemotactic for leukocytes, and many are seen within the field (hematoxylin–eosin, × 470).

ganization of intracellular organelles and possible cell lysis due to disruption of the plasma membrane. Lesions that are immunologically and ultrastructurally similar to Mallory bodies can be produced experimentally in mice following administration of griseofulvin and dieldrin, both carcinogens capable of inducing hepatomas. This observation is intriguing because of the possible autoimmune and neoplastic implications.

Megamitochondria indicate alcoholic liver disease. The enlarged, spherical mitochondria, which are negative for periodic acid–Schiff stain, are found primarily in the centrilobular zone. Megamitochondria vary in size from 2 to 10 mm and are clearly distinguishable from Mallory bodies and lysosomes. They are more common than Mallory bodies, but the prognosis is not as poor.

Postnecrotic cirrhosis is characterized by large regenerating nodules separated by coarse, irregular scars. The scars, or *septae*, are composed of type I collagen, which is birefringent when viewed with polarized light. Regenerative nodules usually can be distinguished histologically from passive nodules formed by ingrowth of septae into normal lobules by the presence of double-cell rather than single-cell plates.[3] Piecemeal parenchymal necrosis is common in chronic active hepatitis and to some extent in acute viral hepatitis. This descriptor should be reserved to include hepatocellular necrosis with evidence of lymphocytic infiltration. Fatty infiltration and alcoholic hyaline (Mallory bodies) are rarely present.

Biliary cirrhosis is characterized by a coarsely granular or macronodular liver. This condition results from long-standing cholestasis secondary to obstruction of intrahepatic or extrahepatic bile ducts. Typical histologic findings of primary biliary cirrhosis include degeneration and necrosis of interlobular and septal bile ducts, portal granulomas, and portal aggregation of mononuclear cells.[4] Bile duct alterations are also common in secondary biliary cirrhosis. The most distinctive feature of large duct obstruction is the presence of bile lakes caused by rupture of a bile duct with extravasation of bile into the portal tracts.

Venoocclusive cirrhosis results from chronic, passive congestion of the liver. This congestion may be due to a central cardiac cause such as tricuspid insufficiency, to constrictive pericarditis, or to hepatic venous outflow occlusion associated with Chiari disease or the Budd-Chiari syndrome. Typically, the liver is enlarged with a nutmeg-like appearance. The central veins and draining sinusoids are uniformly congested. In severe cases, frank hemorrhage with focal hepatic necrosis is observed. Significant centrilobular zonal atrophy and degeneration are prominent, with relative sparing of the portal zones. Unrelieved obstruction leads to increased deposition of collagen in the centrilobular zone and sclerosis of central veins. In cases of established venoocclusive cirrhosis, maximal fibrosis is usually centrizonal and nodular regeneration is rarely conspicuous.

Pathogenesis

Cirrhosis begins with an insult that results in hepatic parenchymal necrosis. A large number of etiologic factors have been implicated, including alcohol consumption, viral hepatitis, toxins, chronic biliary obstruction, genetically transmitted metabolic disorders such as hemochromatosis and Wilson disease, and possibly malnutrition. Regardless of the underlying cause, the normal hepatic response to necrosis is attempted regeneration. This restorative process may be impaired in several ways, including destruction of the reticulin framework about which orderly regeneration progresses, alterations in cellular and humoral immunity, disturbances in vascular ingrowth to

areas of potential regeneration, associated malnutrition, and possibly humoral growth inhibitors (Fig. 38-3).

Fibrogenesis occurs in the nonregenerating areas of necrosis producing scars. The collagen types present in normal livers (I, III, IV, V, and VI) increase proportionately in cirrhotic livers, suggesting coordinated regulation of collagen gene expression. Recent evidence suggests that noncollagen extracellular matrix proteins, such as fibronectin, laminin, and the proteoglycans, may play an important modulating role in hepatic fibrogenesis by binding directly to collagen, blocking collagen degradation, or acting as chemoattractants for inflammatory cells.[5] Inflammation is also an important modulator of fibrogenesis and appears to stimulate collagen production either directly or by the action of inflammatory mediators, such as monokines and lymphokines, that stimulate cell proliferation.

As attempted restoration continues, fibrotic zones connect to produce septae, which surround the residual parenchyma. Proliferation of residual parenchyma is limited by the enveloping scars and leads to nodular areas that are differentiated morphologically by size. The process of destruction, scarring, and nodularity results in distortion of the vascular architecture and leads to venous obstruction, portal hypertension, and formation of intrahepatic arterioportal and portal-hepatic venous shunts that adversely affect sinusoidal perfusion and hepatocyte function.

Etiologic Factors

The precise causes of cirrhosis are unknown, but it is clear that multiple factors are involved. Liver cells are sensitive to a variety of physical, microbiologic, and chemical

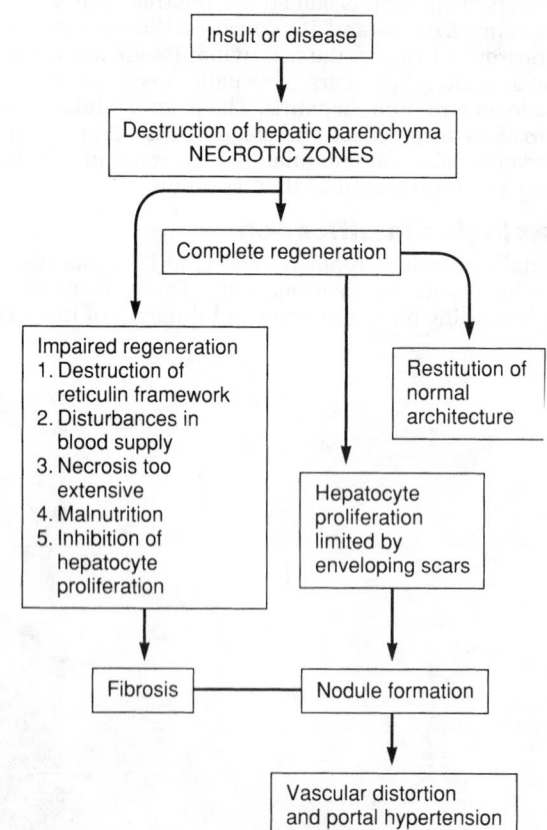

Figure 38-3. The evolution of cirrhosis. Fibrosis occurs in nonregenerative necrotic areas, producing scars. The pattern of nodularity and scars reflects the type of response to injury (eg, uniform versus nonuniform necrosis) and the extent of injury.

agents, all of which may produce cellular injury. The eventual development of cirrhosis is determined by the nature and severity of the cellular injury and the liver's ability to regenerate.

Microbiologic Injury

Most infectious hepatitides are viral in origin. Hepatitis A is caused by an RNA virus that replicates in the cytoplasm. There is no documentation that this form of viral hepatitis progresses to cirrhosis, possibly because the cytopathic effect of this virus on the hepatocyte is not mediated through an immunologic mechanism. Hepatitis B is a DNA virus that replicates in the cell nucleus. Progression to chronic active hepatitis, characterized histologically by periportal inflammation or confluent necrosis, is unusual. Among patients with chronic active hepatitis, however, the risk of developing cirrhosis may be as high as 70%. Non-A, non-B (NANB) hepatitis also exhibits a propensity to become chronic. The prevalence of cirrhosis among patients with this form of viral hepatitis ranges from 5% to 10%. Immunologic factors have been suggested to explain the cellular injury pattern seen in patients with chronic active (NANB and type B) hepatitis. Hepatocyte membrane proteins may serve as antigens to elicit an immunologic response in which antibody-dependent cytotoxicity is the main effector mechanism.[6]

Chemical Injury

The mechanisms of chemical hepatotoxicity include direct and indirect actions. Agents such as cyanide and arsenite directly affect enzymatic pathways and mitochondrial energy production, altering cellular homeostasis. Indirectly acting agents cause injury either by producing a toxic intermediate during biotransformation of the parent compound or by causing deletion of a crucial intracellular component. For example, carbon tetrachloride is metabolized in the liver by the cytochrome P-450 pathway to form a toxic, electrophilic metabolite that causes cell necrosis by combining covalently with cell proteins. Acetaminophen is detoxified chiefly by conjugation with glucuronic acid or sulfate. A minor portion is metabolized by the P-450 pathway to form a toxic intermediate. Under ordinary circumstances, these toxic metabolites react with glutathione and are excreted in the urine as mercapturic acid derivatives. Saturation of the glucuronic pathway with large doses of acetaminophen results in progressive depletion of intracellular glutathione stores, accumulation of toxic intermediates, and eventual cell necrosis.

The actions of agents such as carbon tetrachloride and acetaminophen are predictable and generally related to dose. Other classes of drugs (eg, anticonvulsants such as phenytoin) cause unpredictable or idiosyncratic reactions thought to be immunologically mediated. These patients frequently present with serum sickness-like features such as malaise, fever, maculopapular rash, and lymphadenopathy. Laboratory evidence of marked leukocytosis with atypical lymphocytes and an absolute eosinophilia suggests drug hypersensitivity.

Epidemiologic studies in humans show a close association between alcohol consumption and the incidence of death from cirrhosis. Several studies have related the development of liver injury to the degree and chronicity of alcohol consumption. Only a small percentage of chronic alcohol abusers actually develop cirrhosis. Among these patients, multiple factors are responsible for the development of cirrhosis, including environmental, genetic, nutritional, and other factors that modify the individual's susceptibility to liver damage. Malnutrition and the type of alcoholic beverage consumed appear to be less important than the degree and duration of alcohol consumption.

Alcohol can affect liver cell function in a number of ways (Table 38-2). Like many hepatotoxins, the toxic effects of alcohol are caused indirectly by reactive intermediates. Alcohol metabolism is complex and involves at least three pathways, including an alcohol dehydrogenase pathway in the cytosol, a cytochrome P-450 microsomal pathway in the endoplasmic reticulum, and a catalase pathway in peroxisomes. Acetaldehyde is the principal reactive compound generated by alcohol metabolism. The hepatotoxicity of acetaldehyde is related to its binding affinity for sulfhydryl and amino groups as well as for phosphatidylethanolamine, a major constituent of cellular membranes. Binding with intracellular proteins and phospholipids alters membrane integrity and enzymatic function, frequently to the detriment of the cell. Alcohol has also been shown experimentally to alter mitochondrial structure and function, hepatic protein synthesis, and metabolism of cofactors necessary for intracellular enzyme activity.

Biliary Ductal Obstruction

Any disease that causes chronic obstruction of the extrahepatic biliary tract can potentially lead to the development of secondary biliary cirrhosis. Less than 10% of patients with biliary obstruction develop cirrhosis, and the time course varies, ranging from 3 to 12 months or longer.[7] The precise pathogenesis of biliary cirrhosis is not known. The early microscopic features of the disease include periportal necrosis, formation of bile lakes, and portal scarring. Disease progression results in a pattern that may be histologically indistinguishable from other forms of cirrhosis.

Primary biliary cirrhosis is a chronic liver disease characterized by progressive inflammation and obliteration of intrahepatic bile ducts. The disease classically presents in middle-aged females with fatigue, pruritus, jaundice, hepatomegaly, and abnormal liver function studies. Serologic markers such as antimitochondrial antibodies are present in most cases. Histologically, there may be evidence of bridging fibrosis, canalicular cholestasis, and a virtual absence of interlobular bile ducts. The disease is relentlessly progressive, but survival ranges from 5 to 20 years. Decreased survival correlates with advanced age, symptoms, hepatosplenomegaly, degree of bilirubin elevation, and the extent of hepatic fibrosis. Conventional therapy is directed toward relieving pruritus, malabsorption, and bone disease. Experimental studies using D-penicillamine are inconclusive, and the high incidence of adverse drug effects and the lack of any demonstrable survival ben-

---

Table 38-2. EFFECTS OF ALCOHOL ON LIVER CELL FUNCTION

Disorganizes the lipid portion of cell membranes, leading to adaptive changes in their composition
Alters capacity of cells to cope with environmental toxins
    Biotransformation to create toxic intermediates
    Interference with normal detoxifying mechanisms
    Increased synthesis of endogenous toxins
Oxidation of alcohol produces acetaldehyde, a toxic and reactive intermediate
Inhibits protein export from liver
Modifies hepatic protein synthesis in fasted animals
Alters structure and function (energy production) of mitochondria
Alters metabolism of cofactors essential for enzyme activity (pyridoxine, folate, choline, vitamin E)
Alters oxidation reduction potential of liver cell

(Modified from Zakim D, Boyer TD. Hepatology: a textbook of liver disease. Philadelphia, WB Saunders, 1982:759)

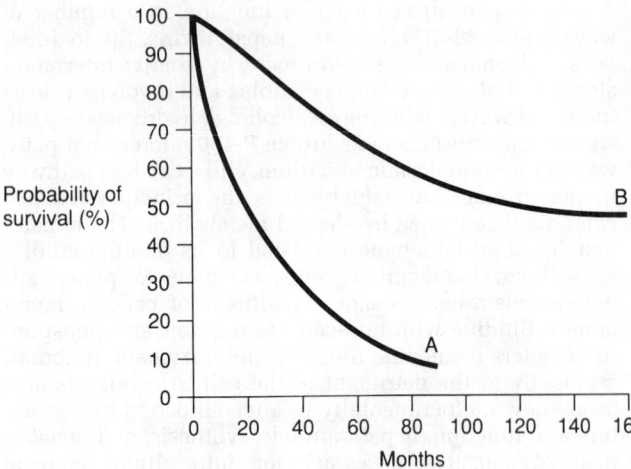

Figure 38-4. Curve A represents the probability of survival after the appearance of the first major complication of the disease in 121 test patients who developed decompensated cirrhosis. Curve B represents the probability of survival after diagnosis in all cases studied. (After Gines P, Quintero E, Arroyo V, et al. Compensated cirrhosis: natural history and prognostic factors. Hepatology 1987;7:122)

efit in treated patients creates limited enthusiasm for this therapeutic approach.[8]

Venous Outflow Obstruction

Cardiac cirrhosis is seen most frequently in the clinical setting of long-standing cardiac decompensation secondary to tricuspid insufficiency or constrictive pericarditis. Both the condition and its correct ante mortem diagnosis are uncommon. Early morphologic changes include centri-

lobular congestion, hemorrhage, and necrosis combined with phlebosclerosis of central veins and scars connecting centrizonal areas. These changes are fairly specific for cardiac cirrhosis, although the specificity may be lost as the condition progresses.

Hepatic venous outflow obstruction (Budd-Chiari syndrome) may cause a lesion that is microscopically similar to cardiac cirrhosis. Despite the histologic similarities, this condition can generally be differentiated from cardiac cirrhosis on the basis of normal cardiovascular function and hemodynamic evidence of normal intracardiac pressures.

Natural History

Recent studies have analyzed the natural history of cirrhosis as a function of the degree of hepatic decompensation at the time of diagnosis. A high proportion of patients with compensated cirrhosis remain well for many years after diagnosis. In these studies, the probability of remaining compensated 10 years after diagnosis was 42%, and the survival probability of compensated patients was 47%.[9] The prognosis worsened considerably once patients developed clinical evidence of hepatic decompensation (eg, ascites, jaundice, encephalopathy or gastrointestinal [GI] hemorrhage). Among these patients, the probability of 5-year survival was only 16% (Fig. 38-4). Useful predictors of survival include serum bilirubin, γ-globulin, prothrombin time, alkaline phosphatase, hepatic stigmata of cirrhosis, sex, and age.

The effect of alcohol consumption or abstinence on the natural history of cirrhosis remains unclear. In one study, the overall 5-year survival was 63% for abstainers versus 40.5% for those who continued to drink.[10] The effect of alcohol on survival may have been less important than the degree of hepatic compensation at the time of inclusion in

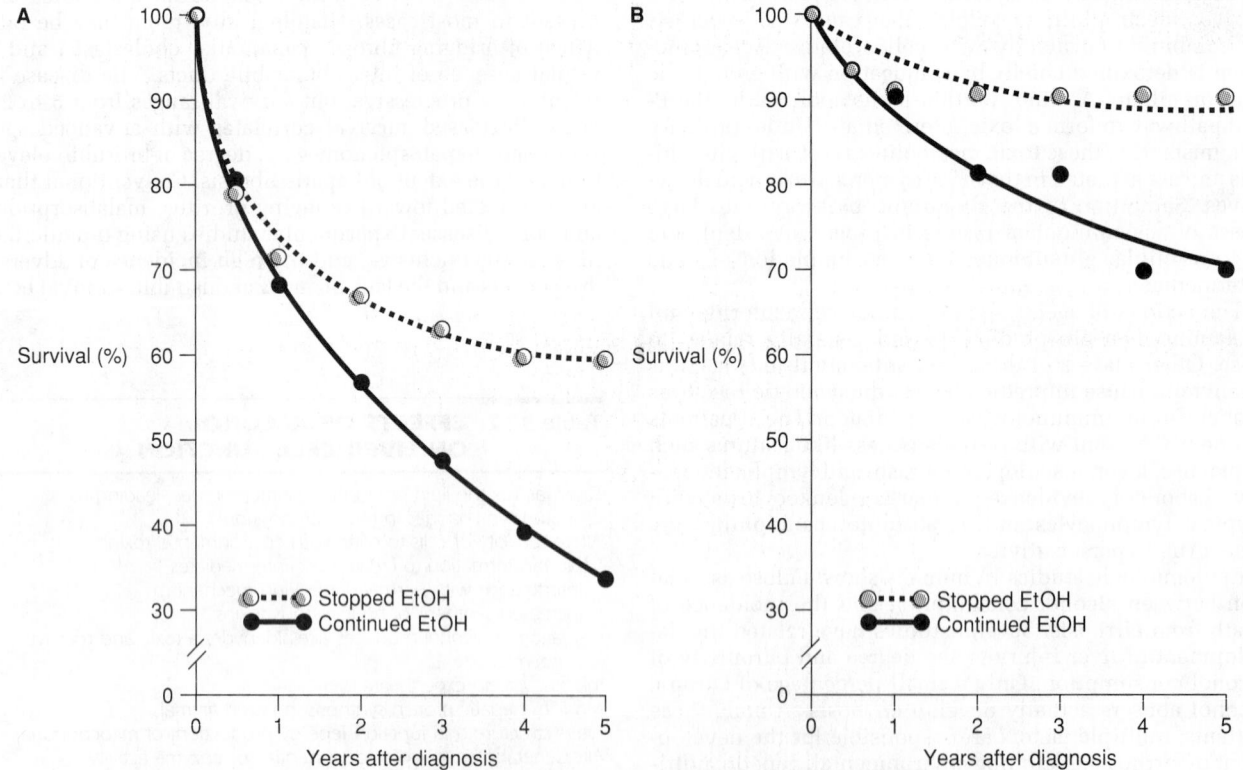

Figure 38-5. (*A*) Survival rates of patients with alcoholic cirrhosis and jaundice, ascites, or hematemesis. (*B*) Survival rates of patients with alcoholic cirrhosis who lacked jaundice, ascites, or histories of gastrointestinal bleeding. EtOH, ethyl alcohol. (After Powell WJ, Klatskin G. Duration of survival in patients with Laennec's cirrhosis. Am J Med 1968;44:406)

the study (Fig. 38-5). Continued alcohol consumption may have less of an effect on survival than the intensity of alcohol consumption.

Decompensated cirrhosis has an ominous prognosis. Ascites is the most common manifestation of hepatic decompensation, but variceal bleeding is without question the most clinically conspicuous complication. Until recently, attempts to analyze survival data after variceal hemorrhage have been thwarted by a lack of information concerning the natural history of this complication. We know from previous studies of compensated patients with cirrhosis that the probability of developing a major complication such as GI bleeding, ascites, or encephalopathy approaches 50% and that bleeding occurs as a primary manifestation in about 25% of patients. The early mortality rate for variceal hemorrhage approximates 40%. The risk of death depends more on the severity of the underlying liver disease than on the type of therapy (medical versus surgical). Physiologic predictors such as the Child hepatic risk classification system are useful indicators of early survival but appear to have less long-term predictive value than the patient's ability to survive the early posthemorrhage period. Because the risk of dying or of rebleeding appears to be highest immediately after an acute hemorrhage and to decrease thereafter, newer therapeutic interventions aimed at reducing overall mortality risks must focus on the early posthemorrhage period.

Clinical Features

The clinical features of cirrhosis can vary considerably depending on whether the disease is latent (compensated) or active (decompensated). Latent cirrhosis may be discovered during a routine physical examination for fairly nondescript complaints such as fatigue, anorexia, and weight loss. Physical findings such as palmar erythema, spider angiomas, Dupuytren contractures, and hepatosplenomegaly may be helpful diagnostic signs. Ascites and dilated abdominal wall veins indicate portal hypertension. Biochemical studies may be normal or abnormal in these patients. Subtle changes in serum transaminases, hypoalbuminemia, and hyperglobulinemia may be the earliest biochemical clues to the diagnosis of latent cirrhosis. In the clinical setting, the diagnosis can only be made with certainty by liver biopsy. Patients with compensated cirrhosis usually remain asymptomatic for many years, but eventually, most develop complications related either to hepatic failure or portal hypertension (eg, variceal bleeding, ascites, or encephalopathy). The course may vary considerably depending on the causes of the underlying liver disease.

Patients with decompensated cirrhosis usually manifest failing general health, with muscle wasting, jaundice, and ascites with or without peripheral edema. Several factors may precipitate acute decompensation, including exposure to potential hepatotoxins, such as alcohol, certain drugs and anesthetic agents, GI bleeding, electrolyte imbalances such as hypokalemia, and intercurrent infections. Unexplained fever or sepsis may result from spontaneous bacterial peritonitis or may develop secondary to altered hepatic reticuloendothelial function and intrahepatic portal systemic shunting. Mental aberrations, a flapping tremor, and fetor hepaticus may be present in patients with severe decompensation. Jaundice is common, and its intensity correlates roughly with the severity of hepatic dysfunction. The physical findings observed most frequently in patients with cirrhosis are listed in Table 38-3.

Abnormal laboratory findings include elevated levels of serum bilirubin, alkaline phosphatase, and γ-globulin. Hypergammaglobulinemia is probably related to increased

Table 38-3. PHYSICAL FINDINGS IN CIRRHOSIS

Physical Findings	Cases (%)
Palpable liver	96
Jaundice	68
Ascites	66
Spider angiomas	49
Dilated abdominal wall veins	47
Palpable spleen	46
Testicular atrophy	45
Palmar erythema	37
Noninfectious fever	22
Hepatic coma	18
Gynecomastia	15
Dupuytren contractures	5

(Powell W, Klatskin G. Duration of survival in patients with Laennec's cirrhosis. Am J Med 1968;44:406)

serum levels of antibody directed against intestinal antigens such as *Escherichia coli* that are not cleared by the damaged liver. Anemia is a frequent finding and may indicate recent GI blood loss. Hypersplenism with increased sequestration and destruction of blood elements may result in leukopenia or thrombocytopenia. The prothrombin time is frequently prolonged and, in severe cases, may be unresponsive to parenteral vitamin K administration.

ACUTE (FULMINANT) HEPATIC FAILURE

The diagnosis of acute (fulminant) hepatic failure is based on the development of encephalopathy within 8 weeks of the onset of symptoms. The overall prognosis is poor, but the hepatic lesions are potentially reversible, and recovery can lead to restoration of normal liver function. Conventional therapy should therefore include providing temporary hepatic support and treating expected complications. Recent advances in hepatic transplantation also have significant therapeutic implications for patients with acute hepatic failure.

Etiologic Factors and Pathogenesis

The most frequent cause of acute hepatic failure worldwide is NANB viral hepatitis. A variety of other viral agents, including herpes simplex and cytomegalovirus, can cause massive hepatic necrosis in patients with an altered immunologic status. Less frequent causes include hepatotoxins such as anesthetic agents, antiinflammatory and antidepressant drugs, carbon tetrachloride poisoning, acetaminophen overdose, and alcoholic hepatitis. On rare occasions, fulminant hepatic failure occurs as a complication of eclampsia, acute Wilson disease, or acute circulatory failure due to sepsis or a primary cardiac event.

From a clinicopathologic standpoint, fulminant hepatic failure can be classified into two major types (Table 38-4). The type I lesion is characterized histologically by patchy areas of massive, confluent hepatic necrosis. This type is associated with viral and drug etiologies. The early clinical course is characterized by high serum aminotransferase levels. The type II lesion is typically associated with fatty liver of pregnancy, Reye syndrome, and alcoholic hepatitis. Histologically, microvesicular fatty infiltration of hepatocytes is much more prominent than hepatocellular necrosis. The lack of necrosis accounts for the low serum aminotransferase levels observed with this type of hepatic failure.

Table 38-4. CLINICOPATHOLOGIC CLASSIFICATION OF ACUTE HEPATIC FAILURE

	Type I	Type II
Serum aminotransferase	Markedly elevated	Elevated
Hepatic histology	Patchy areas of confluent necrosis	Microvesicular fatty infiltration
Causes	Hepatitis viruses	Pregnancy
	Halothane	Tetracycline
	Acetaminophen	
	Isoniazid	

(Zakim D, Boyer TD. Hepatology: a textbook of liver disease. Philadelphia, WB Saunders, 1982:417)

No reliable criteria predict outcome and response to treatment. Higher grades of encephalopathy (depth of coma) on admission are associated with a worse prognosis. For example, of patients admitted with stage IV encephalopathy (deep coma with variable responsiveness to painful stimuli), about 30% die within 2 days, and 70% to 80% ultimately die regardless of treatment. In patients with lower grades of encephalopathy, however, survival rates of 50% or higher are common. Other variables have been correlated with survival, including age, cause of acute hepatic failure, and major complications such as respiratory or renal failure. Survival is higher among young patients, partly because they rarely have systemic disorders that accompany aging, and partly because their livers are better able to regenerate after a severe injury.

Routine laboratory tests and other diagnostic studies such as electroencephalography have limited predictive value. Liver function studies such as serum aminotransferases, bilirubin, and albumin are unreliable.

Clinical Features

The diagnosis of fulminant hepatic failure is based on clinical findings of hepatic encephalopathy in the absence of stigmata of chronic liver disease. Early features of encephalopathy may include personality changes, restless delirium, and uncooperative or violent behavior. Asterixis and fetor hepaticus may be subtle at this stage and frequently are overlooked. Routine biochemical studies commonly reflect hepatic dysfunction, but elevated bilirubin levels and jaundice do not correlate with neuropsychiatric changes. The later stages of encephalopathy are characterized by convulsions, altered consciousness, dysconjugate eye movements, and decerebrate posturing with plantar flexor responses. These late changes indicate depressed brain-stem function, which may progress to circulatory failure and frank respiratory arrest. Some 80% of patients with acute hepatic failure die of well-recognized complications such as cerebral edema, hemorrhage in the GI tract, and sepsis.

Management

General Supportive Measures

Management should include general supportive measures and specific treatments for hepatic encephalopathy, cerebral edema, electrolyte and metabolic disturbances (eg, hypoglycemia and hyponatremia), infection, and bleeding. Complications should be aggressively treated. Patients should be transferred to an intensive care unit where specialized personnel and monitoring equipment are readily available.

The level of hepatic encephalopathy should be monitored frequently using a coma profile that appraises forebrain and brain-stem functions. Most profiles assess verbal response, eye opening, pupil reactivity, oculocephalic and oculovestibular reflexes, motor responses, and respiratory activity. The profile used should be simple and should provide semiquantitative data about the patient's neurologic status. Sedatives should be used judiciously to avoid worsening the coma.

The ante mortem diagnosis of cerebral edema can be difficult to establish in these patients. The clinical diagnosis should be suspected in any patient who exhibits a deteriorating level of consciousness, sluggish pupillary reflexes, or decerebrate posturing. Although direct monitoring of intracranial pressure is not endorsed uniformly, it may be the only objective measure of cerebral edema in patients with acute hepatic failure. The importance of such monitoring in head trauma patients has been confirmed by findings that intracranial pressure levels higher than 60 mmHg, even for short periods, are associated with a poor prognosis.[11] Intracranial pressure monitoring also permits measurement of the baseline intracranial pressure-volume relation and of the response to therapeutic interventions such as hyperventilation and administration of hypertonic solutions and glucocorticoids.[12]

Hypoglycemia is an unusual complication of liver disease except in patients with acute hepatic failure or hepatic neoplasms. The liver's enormous reserve capacity accounts for the rarity of hypoglycemia except as a preterminal event. If unexpected, hypoglycemia can develop rapidly and cause sudden death in a small percentage of these patients. This complication can be prevented by frequent monitoring of blood glucose levels and continuous administration of a 10% dextrose solution.

The combination of central respiratory depression and an impaired gag reflex results in a high incidence of pulmonary complications in patients with acute hepatic failure. Chest radiograph abnormalities, including atelectasis, lobar consolidation, and pulmonary edema, are observed in up to half of patients. Because of the high incidence of aspiration pneumonia in patients with severe encephalopathy (stage IV coma), many authors advocate elective endotracheal intubation and, when appropriate, mechanical ventilation. Frequent sputum cultures and chest radiographs should be obtained along with serial blood cultures. Aggressive but directed antibiotic treatment is warranted if the patient develops bacteriologic, radiographic, or clinical evidence of progressive pulmonary infection.

Bleeding is a frequent cause of death in patients with acute hepatic failure. Hypoprothrombinemia due to depressed liver synthesis of clotting factors II, VII, IX, and X and qualitative or quantitative platelet disorders contribute to abnormal hemostasis in these patients. Intravascular coagulopathies may be difficult to diagnose and frequently are multifactorial. A variety of mechanisms have been implicated, including systemic endotoxemia, impaired clearance of activated clotting factors, and elaboration by the diseased liver of thromboplastin-like substances that activate the extrinsic coagulation pathway.

Local factors may contribute significantly to the bleeding diathesis observed in these patients. In this context, preventive measures may play an important role. For example, patients with acute hepatic failure are known to be at high risk for upper GI tract bleeding, and prophylaxis with H_2-receptor antagonists is indicated. Vitamin K should be administered intravenously to encourage carboxylation of factor II, VII, IX, and X precursors to moieties with coagulant activity.

Artificial Hepatic Support

The rationale for artificial liver support systems in patients with fulminant hepatic failure is that the liver injury may be potentially reversible; therefore, improved survival may be expected if patients can be supported long enough for hepatic regeneration to occur. Unfortunately, there is no controlled evidence that any artificial support system improves survival in patients with acute hepatic failure once they have progressed to deep coma. The dilemma is compounded by a lack of criteria to reliably predict the outcome of acute hepatic failure, although the expected survival rate for this condition is 15% to 20%.

A variety of artificial liver support systems have been devised in the past 15 to 20 years, but none is optimal because of technological limitations related to problems of bioincompatibility (Table 38-5). This failure is due to an incomplete understanding of the biochemical disturbances occurring in acute hepatic failure that need to be corrected. Ideally, the procedure adopted should remove toxins from the blood and provide factors normally synthesized by a healthy liver. Procedures such as charcoal hemoperfusion or hemodialysis over polyacrylonitrile membranes are effective for removing small and middle-molecular-weight substances from the blood, but they are designed strictly for that purpose. Cross-circulation and perfusion procedures using humans or primates efficiently remove toxins and provide deficient factors synthesized by the liver, but they can be criticized as unethical. Only one method of artificial liver support, exchange blood transfusion, has been subjected to a rigorous controlled trial, with no apparent survival benefit compared with conventional measures.[13]

Orthotopic Liver Transplantation

The lack of definitive medical treatment for acute hepatic failure makes liver transplantation seem attractive, especially for patients with little or no chance of recovering normal liver function. The adoption of this form of therapy must be viewed with caution. Improved intensive care, continuous monitoring of intracranial pressure, vigorous treatment of cerebral edema with mannitol and respirator-controlled hypoventilation, and careful attention to potential complications have improved survival rates to almost 50% in some centers (Fig. 38-6). Preliminary evidence also suggests that prostaglandin E may improve the outcome of patients with acute hepatic failure by preserving the integrity of the hepatic microcirculation and the reticulin network needed for hepatic regeneration.[14]

Perhaps the most significant drawback to widespread acceptance of liver transplantation for acute hepatic failure is the lack of criteria to reliably predict which patients

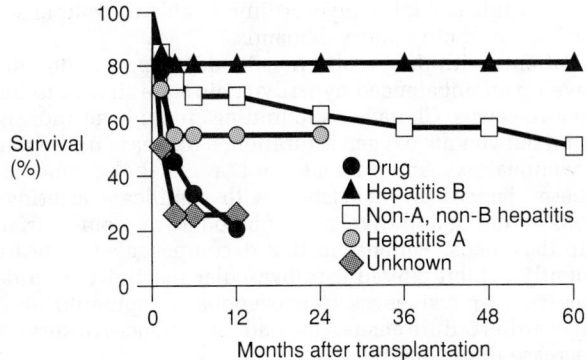

Figure 38-6. Patient survival (life table method) after liver transplantation in adults and children for fulminant hepatic failure. Included are 9 cases of drug-related liver failure, 13 cases of acute hepatitis A, and 4 cases of unknown cause. (After Turcotte JG. Portal hypertension as I see it. In: Child CC III, ed. Portal hypertension. Philadelphia, WB Saunders, 1974:84)

are likely to benefit from operation. Patients with mild to moderate degrees of coma (grades I and II) are likely to recover spontaneously without the need for liver transplantation. Rapid deterioration of neurologic status to grade III or IV coma and coagulation factor V levels less than 20% of normal are associated in some centers with a mortality rate of over 95%. Another variable in the survival equation appears to be the cause of acute hepatic failure. Spontaneous recovery after acetaminophen overdose or hepatitis A infection is far more likely to occur than after hepatitis B, NANB hepatitis, or other drug-induced reactions.

CHRONIC LIVER DISEASE

Systemic Manifestations

Hepatic failure has a profound effect on virtually every organ system in the body. It can occur as a rapidly progressive lesion in the absence of preexisting liver disease or as a terminal event in patients with chronic active hepatitis or end-stage cirrhosis. The clinical presentation and treatment of hepatic failure are similar, regardless of the cause. Excluding the syndrome of acute, fulminant hepatic failure discussed previously, there is no definite relation between hepatic pathology and the clinical manifestations of hepatic failure. The syndrome of chronic hepatic failure should therefore be viewed as a series of functional rather than anatomic consequences of disordered liver function.

Cardiorespiratory Manifestations

The survival of cirrhotic patients after any major stress, such as operation or a major GI hemorrhage, is determined by the extent of their underlying liver disease and by the adequacy of the cardiovascular response to the increased circulatory demands. Careful studies have identified patterns of cardiovascular compensation in cirrhotic patients. The basal state is characterized by increased cardiac output and no peripheral vascular or pulmonary dysfunction. The balanced hyperdynamic response state is associated with enhanced myocardial function (increased cardiac output and heart rate), no change in oxygen consumption or mixed venous Po_2, and no evidence of acidosis. This state can be recognized clinically by the presence of bounding peripheral pulses, warm extremities, and occasional club-

---

Table 38-5. TESTED METHODS OF TEMPORARY LIVER SUPPORT

Exchange blood transfusion*
Plasmaphoresis
Total-body washout
Cross-circulation with humans or baboons
Hemoperfusion through human cadaveric liver or isolated animal liver
Hemodialysis using conventional or polyacrylonitrile membranes
Hemoperfusion of charcoal or albumin-coated resins

* Only this modality was tested with a randomized controlled trial. The mortality rate was unchanged compared with conventional treatment.

bing. In this state, the myocardium is able to compensate for increased circulatory demands.

Patients with progressive hepatic decompensation often develop an unbalanced hyperdynamic state similar to that seen in sepsis. Characteristic findings include an increase in mixed venous oxygen saturation, a decrease in the arteriovenous oxygen gradient, and a metabolic acidosis. These changes are consistent with significant arteriovenous shunting and diversion of blood away from nutrient capillary beds. Patients in this decompensated state frequently exhibit altered cardiovascular reactivity with decreased responsiveness to exogenous norepinephrine. If myocardial failure ensues, the patient's chances of survival decrease dramatically.

Pulmonary Manifestations

The pulmonary manifestations of cirrhosis can include dyspnea, cyanosis, clubbing, and arterial oxygen desaturation. Dyspnea is uncommon in the absence of ascites. Arterial oxygen desaturation is seen in about half of all decompensated cirrhotic patients. Many pathophysiologic processes have been proposed to explain this observation, including right-to-left shunts through pulmonary arteriovenous anastomoses, altered ventilation-perfusion ratio, alveolar hypoventilation, impaired pulmonary diffusing capacity, and altered oxyhemoglobin dissociation. Pulmonary arteriovenous anastomoses have been demonstrated in the lungs of cirrhotic patients and along the pleural surfaces. These microcirculatory shunts may be accompanied by larger collaterals, including periesophageal veins that bridge the portal and pulmonary venous circulations by anastomosing with mediastinal, bronchial, and azygous veins. Significant right-to-left shunting does not commonly occur in the absence of elevated portal pressures and esophageal varices.

Abdominal distention due to ascites may produce areas of pulmonary collapse and alter the ventilation-perfusion relation in some cirrhotic patients. Nonuniform ventilation may also result from pleural effusions, which occur in a small percentage of cirrhotic patients. The presence of altered ventilation-perfusion ratio in cirrhotic patients without ascites suggests that additional factors may be important. Premature airway closure with air trapping in the lower lung fields and inappropriate pulmonary microvascular vasodilation have both been implicated in this process.

Alveolar hypoventilation is an unlikely cause of oxygen desaturation, because most decompensated cirrhotic patients exhibit an increased respiratory drive that has been attributed to elevated blood ammonia levels. Reduced pulmonary diffusing capacity has been measured in up to 20% of cirrhotic patients. Rightward shifts in the oxyhemoglobin dissociation curve may decrease oxygen affinity and contribute to hypoxemia.

The role of each of these factors are unclear, partly because they are difficult to measure in a clinical setting. Poor oxygen exchange and impaired myocardial function alone portend a poor prognosis in decompensated cirrhotic patients, and the combination of the two is invariably lethal unless corrected in a short period. Table 38-6 summarizes the cardiorespiratory abnormalities observed in cirrhotic patients and lists the pathophysiologic processes thought to be responsible for each abnormality.

Renal Manifestations

The association between liver disease and renal function abnormalities has been recognized for many years. Many of the observed alterations in renal function and electrolyte

Table 38-6. CARDIORESPIRATORY ABNORMALITIES IN CIRRHOSIS

Abnormality	Pathophysiology
↓ Arterial P_{O_2}	Portopulmonary and intrapulmonary shunts
↓ Arteriovenous O_2 difference	Arteriolar and capillary shunts
↓ Peripheral resistance	Systemic-splanchnic arteriovenous shunts
↑ Cardiac output	Low peripheral resistance
↑ Plasma volume	Increased whole body sodium and water secondary to hyperaldosteronism Low peripheral resistance

metabolism are a direct consequence of primary liver disease and have important clinical implications.

Sodium Handling

The clinical course of patients with decompensated cirrhosis is frequently characterized by progressive impairment of renal sodium handling, leading to the development of ascites and peripheral edema. These patients avidly retain sodium and can excrete urine that is virtually free of sodium. In general, ascites accumulation and weight gain continue as long as sodium ingestion exceeds the kidney's ability to excrete sodium. The pathogenesis of this disorder remains controversial. The more traditional theory suggests that the primary abnormality is diminished effective plasma volume, leading to reduced tubular reabsorption of sodium, expanded extracellular fluid volume, and ascites formation. A more recent hypothesis suggests that the primary event is inappropriate retention of sodium by the kidney with secondary expansion of plasma volume, leading to an accumulation of ascites and peripheral edema.[15] Although there is evidence to support each of these principal hypotheses, other factors have been implicated, including enhanced tubular reabsorption of sodium and increased sympathetic activity leading to decreased renal blood flow. The role of hyperaldosteronism has also been debated. Elevated plasma aldosterone levels are frequently observed in cirrhotic patients and have been attributed to increased adrenal secretion and decreased hepatic degradation. Other possible mechanisms include alterations in renal prostaglandins and abnormal synthesis or degradation of a humoral natriuretic factor or factors.

Water Handling

Impaired water excretion is also encountered in cirrhotic patients and has important therapeutic implications. The hyponatremia observed in these patients is dilutional in origin and invariably responds to water restriction, regardless of its severity. Even moderate hyponatremia (serum sodium levels below 125 mEq/L) should be treated in these patients to prevent neurologic damage. The two mechanisms proposed to explain impaired water homeostasis in cirrhotic patients include enhanced antidiuretic hormone activity and decreased delivery of glomerular filtrate to the diluting segments of the nephron. The relative importance of each is not clear.

Hepatorenal Syndrome

Progressive oliguric renal failure is frequently seen in patients with advanced liver disease. To make this diagnosis with certainty, one must exclude all other known causes of renal failure. The syndrome is marked by variability in both its presentation and clinical course. Virtually all patients have clinical evidence of ascites and other stigmata of advanced hepatic disease. The syndrome can also occur in patients with mildly impaired hepatic function. Most patients who develop hepatorenal syndrome ultimately die. These patients exhibit renal function abnormalities that differ considerably from acute renal failure but may be indistinguishable from prerenal azotemia (Table 38-7).

The precise pathogenesis of hepatorenal syndrome is not known. Experimental and pathologic evidence suggests that the syndrome is primarily functional in nature. Reduced renal perfusion with intrarenal blood flow redistribution resulting in cortical ischemia has been cited as the chief cause, but other mechanisms have been proposed, including inappropriate activation of the renin-angiotensin system, altered prostaglandin activity, and systemic endotoxemia due to spontaneous portosystemic shunting.

Proper treatment of acute oliguria occurring in a cirrhotic patient is predicated on establishing an accurate diagnosis. The most consistent finding in patients with hepatorenal syndrome is a strikingly low urine sodium concentration (usually less than 10 mEq/L and frequently less than 5 mEq/L) and well-maintained urine concentrating ability (urine osmolality at least 100 mOsm/L greater than plasma osmolality). In comparison, the urine sodium concentration in patients with acute renal failure usually exceeds 30 mEq/L, and the urine osmolality is equal to that of plasma. Hepatorenal syndrome can readily be distinguished from acute renal failure, but differentiation from prerenal azotemia can be more difficult. Prerenal azotemia occurs commonly in cirrhotic patients who require diuretic therapy for treatment of ascites and peripheral edema. Overzealous diuretic therapy in this setting may result in contraction of the intravascular volume with renal hypoperfusion and azotemia.

Therapy consists of eliminating diuretics and other drugs that may adversely affect renal function, ensuring a satisfactory intravascular volume, and vigorously treating suspected septicemia. Volume expanders may have transient benefit but do not affect outcome. Specific therapeutic measures such as ascites ultrafiltration and reinfusion and hemodialysis have not proved effective in managing hepatorenal syndrome. Implantable peritoneovenous shunts have been advocated in some centers, but careful studies of patients with documented hepatorenal syndrome are rare.[16] Despite what sometimes appear to be heroic efforts, the outlook for patients with hepatorenal syndrome remains grim. Hyponatremia and hypotension in these patients presage death and are unresponsive to virtually all forms of therapy.

Disorders of Glucose Homeostasis

The liver plays a pivotal role in carbohydrate homeostasis. Under normal fasting conditions, hepatic glucose production is necessary to supply glucose as an energy source for obligate glucose-metabolizing tissues, such as red blood cells and the central nervous system (CNS). The liver produces 150 to 200 g/d of glucose, of which 75% is derived from breakdown of hepatic glycogen stores and 25% is derived from gluconeogenesis. Glycogenolysis is regulated by several factors, including changes in portal venous glucose concentration and insulin and glucagon secretion by the pancreas. Because fasting hepatic glycogen stores are depleted within 24 hours, prolonged fasting or stress require that an increasing proportion of hepatic glucose production must come from gluconeogenesis.

Glucose intolerance is seen in patients with chronic forms of cirrhosis, hemochromatosis, and acute hepatitis. Several studies have demonstrated abnormal glucose tolerance in about half of patients with chronic liver disease.[17] Fasting blood glucose is normal in most of these patients, and the 2-hour postprandial blood glucose level rarely exceeds 200 mg/dL. Despite abnormal glucose tolerance, these patients do not appear to be at risk for the microvascular diseases (nephropathy and retinopathy) seen in diabetes.

The precise pathophysiologic alterations responsible for glucose intolerance in patients with chronic liver disease are not known. Hormonal imbalances may play an important role. Elevated peripheral blood insulin levels are commonly observed in cirrhotic patients. Enhanced pancreatic secretion or decreased hepatic degradation of insulin are possible explanations. Hyperglucagonemia has also been implicated as a cause of glucose intolerance in cirrhotic patients. Because there is no evidence of altered glucagon degradation in cirrhotic patients, hypersecretion of glucagon by the pancreas appears to be the cause of elevated glucagon.[18] Peripheral hyperglucagonemia occurs only in patients with evidence of portosystemic shunting, and levels of glucagon are highest in patients with large, surgically created shunts. The precise mechanism by which elevated glucagon levels contribute to glucose intolerance is unknown, but one hypothesis suggests that hyperglucagonemia may affect glucose homeostasis by enhancing gluconeogenesis.

Growth hormone has also been implicated in the glucose intolerance of chronic liver disease. In addition to decreased hepatic degradation, growth hormone secretion appears to be enhanced by several factors, including thyrotropin releasing hormone and oral ingestion of glucose. Other hormones, such as cortisol, estrogens, androgens, and prolactin, influence glucose metabolism but appear to play a limited role in the glucose intolerance of chronic liver disease.

Hepatic Encephalopathy

Hepatic encephalopathy is a poorly explained neuropsychiatric syndrome characterized by diverse neurologic abnormalities, histopathologic evidence of nonspecific structural changes in neurons, and a variable prognosis.

Table 38-7. DIFFERENTIAL DIAGNOSIS OF ACUTE AZOTEMIA IN PATIENTS WITH LIVER DISEASE

	Prerenal Azotemia	Hepatorenal Syndrome	Acute Renal Failure
Urinary sodium	<10 mEq/L	<10 mEq/L	>30 mEq/L
Urine/plasma creatinine ratio	>30:1	>30:1	<20:1
Urine osmolality	100 mOsm or more than plasma osmolality	100 mOsm or more than plasma osmolality	Equal to plasma osmolality
Urine sediment	Normal	Normal	Casts; cellular debris

(Zakim D, Boyer TD. Hepatology: a textbook of liver disease. Philadelphia, WB Saunders, 1982:460)

Pathogenesis

Several hypotheses to explain the pathogenesis of hepatic encephalopathy have been proposed:

- Presence of putative toxins such as ammonia, mercaptans, phenols, and fatty acids
- Amino acid imbalance and false neurotransmission
- γ-Aminobutyric acid (GABA) neuroinhibitory system
- Synergism of putative neurotoxins
- Metabolic and other abnormalities including alkalosis, hypoxia, electrolyte imbalance, hypotension, infection

Considerable controversy surrounds each hypothesis. The most plausible explanation suggests that the pathogenesis of hepatic encephalopathy is related to impaired hepatic extraction and metabolism of neuroactive metabolites that result in neural inhibition.[19]

Ammonia has been widely implicated in the pathogenesis of hepatic encephalopathy despite conflicting evidence. Ammonia is derived from the breakdown of proteins and purines in the GI tract. Under normal circumstances, ammonia is converted to urea and glutamine in the liver. In the presence of acute hepatic parenchymal damage or extensive portal systemic shunting, ammonia bypasses the liver, leading to increased levels in peripheral blood. Blood ammonia levels correlate poorly with the stage of encephalopathy. Furthermore, electrophysiologic evidence suggests that high concentrations of ammonia decrease rather than increase neural inhibition.[9] Increased seizure activity would be an expected consequence of decreased neural inhibition; however, seizure activity is uncommon with encephalopathy related to acute or chronic forms of liver disease. A variation of the ammonia hypothesis suggests that multiple neurotoxins, including ammonia, mercaptans, short-chain fatty acids, and possibly phenol, act synergistically to produce hepatic encephalopathy. The only evidence to support this hypothesis has been measurement of these putative neuroactive metabolites in the plasma, cerebrospinal fluid, blood, and brain of affected individuals. Until additional data are available, this explanation must remain suspect.

One of the more popular hypotheses has implicated false neurotransmitters in the pathogenesis of hepatic encephalopathy. This theory suggests that neural inhibition is the result of depletion of normal CNS neurotransmitters, such as norepinephrine and dopamine, and replacement with false neurotransmitters, such as octopamine, serotonin, and phenylethanolamine. The factors that predispose a patient to this abnormal state include plasma amino acid imbalance (increased ratio of aromatic to branched-chain amino acids) with net influx of aromatic amino acids into the brain and net efflux of glutamine from the brain. Tryptophan accumulation in the CNS leads to increased synthesis of false neurotransmitters and depression of CNS function.

Much of the evidence supporting the false neurotransmitter hypothesis is circumstantial. Plasma amino acid imbalances in cirrhotic patients with encephalopathy are well documented, but there is a poor correlation between the ratio of branched-chain to aromatic amino acids and the level of encephalopathy. Elevated serum levels and 24-hour urinary excretion of octopamine (a putative false neurotransmitter) have been demonstrated in cirrhotic patients with encephalopathy and reported as evidence to support this hypothesis.[9] Clinical efforts to treat hepatic encephalopathy by administering solutions of branched-chain amino acids or dopaminergic drugs, such as L-dopa and bromocriptine, have failed to show any consistent benefit.[20] Furthermore, autopsy studies of cirrhotic patients with encephalopathy have demonstrated normal brain levels of norepinephrine and dopamine and decreased levels of octopamine.[19] These findings are opposite those predicted by the false-neurotransmitter theory.

GABA is a neutral amino acid found in high concentrations throughout portions of the brain and is considered the principal inhibitory neurotransmitter in the vertebrate

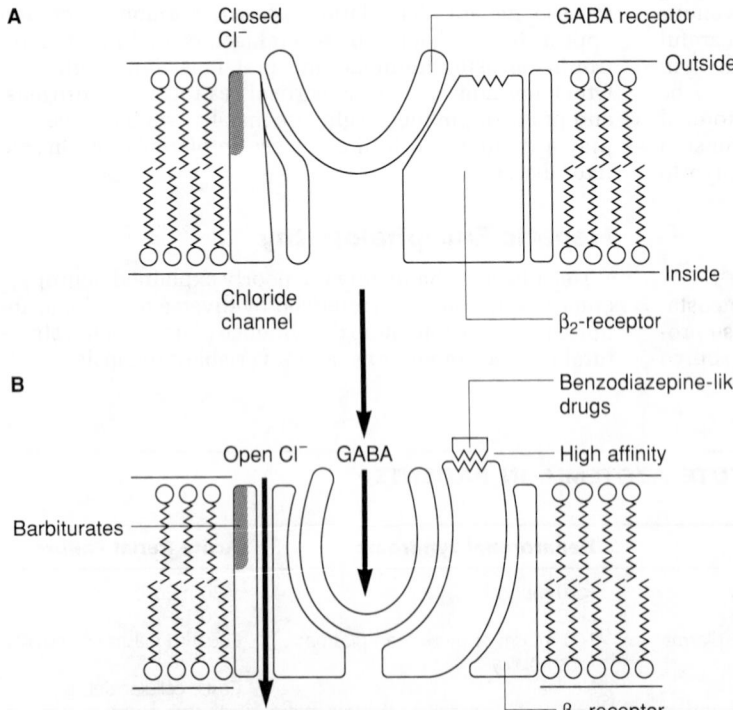

Figure 38-7. Diagrammatic representation of GABA–benzodiazepine chloride ionophore receptor complex in the surface membrane of a postsynaptic neuron. (*A*) The receptor complex in an unactivated state. (*B*) The receptor complex in an activated state with the chloride channel open. Activation of the receptor complex causes opening of the chloride channel and hyperpolarization of the cell membrane. (After Jones EA, Gammal SH. Hepatic encephalopathy. In: Arias IM, Jakoby WB, Popper H, Schachter D, Shafritz DA. The liver: biology and pathobiology, ed 2. New York, Raven Press, 1988:988)

brain. Evidence suggests that activation of the GABA system may be important in the pathogenesis of hepatic encephalopathy. GABA is synthesized in the brain from glutamate and is stored in cytoplasmic vesicles. After stimulation, GABA is released in the synaptic cleft and binds to specific postsynaptic receptors, generating an inhibitory potential. The GABA receptor binds several classes of ligands, including GABA and drugs such as benzodiazepines and barbiturates. The GABA neuroinhibitory system mediates the sedative-hypnotic effects of these classes of drugs (Fig. 38-7). For reasons that are unclear, hepatic failure appears to increase the brain density of GABA receptors.[7] This observation may explain the increased sensitivity to benzodiazepines and other inhibitory neurotransmitters observed among patients with chronic liver disease.

Clinical Features

Patients with hepatic encephalopathy present with variable obtundation and mental confusion. Stigmata of chronic liver disease are frequently apparent. In the absence of a history of liver disease or clinical findings compatible with acute hepatic parenchymal injury or cirrhosis, differentiation from other neuropsychiatric disorders can be difficult. Simple psychometric testing may detect subtle intellectual deficits and can be performed in the office. Comparing samples of the patient's writing over time or asking the patient to perform simple mathematical tasks such as serial sevens may provide early clues of progressive intellectual deterioration. Progression of encephalopathy is characterized by the development of asterixis (a coarse, flapping hand tremor elicited best by asking the patient to hyperextend the wrist) and fetor hepaticus (a distinct breath odor probably related to pulmonary excretion of mercaptans).

Laboratory studies are nonspecific and reflect only the presence of advanced liver disease. Measurements of blood ammonia correlate poorly with the severity of encephalopathy. Electroencephalographic abnormalities associated with hepatic encephalopathy are nonspecific and may be observed in patients with other metabolic disorders and altered mental status.

Management

Treatment of hepatic encephalopathy includes general supportive measures, diet manipulation, and specific therapies to decrease ammonia absorption from the gut and reverse plasma amino acid imbalances (Table 38-8).

Acute deterioration in a patient with compensated cirrhosis warrants thorough investigation of possible precipitating factors. Well-recognized precipitating factors include GI bleeding, constipation, hypokalemic metabolic alkalosis, hypotension, dehydration, and infection. The patient should be questioned about ingestion of sedative-hypnotic drugs (eg, barbiturates and benzodiazepines) that may exacerbate encephalopathy. The lungs and urinary tract should be carefully evaluated for the possibility of an infectious etiology. In patients with ascites, diagnostic paracentesis should be performed to rule out spontaneous bacterial peritonitis. The possibility of an unsuspected hepatocellular carcinoma should be considered, especially in patients with long-standing cirrhosis.

Dietary protein should be temporarily withheld and gentle purgatives should be given to eliminate nitrogenous materials from the GI tract. Intravenous glucose solutions should be administered to prevent dehydration and to minimize endogenous protein breakdown. As the encephalopathy clears, oral feeding of protein can be resumed in small increments of 10 to 20 g/d as tolerated. In patients with

Table 38-8. TREATMENT OF HEPATIC ENCEPHALOPATHY

Identify precipitating factors
  Disordered carbohydrate metabolism
  Narcotics
  Infection
  Hypotension
  Hypoxia
  Excess exogenous protein
  Gastrointestinal bleeding
  Electrolyte abnormalities
  Alkalosis
Supportive therapy
  Eliminate dietary nitrogen
  Purge gastrointestinal tract to remove blood and other
    nitrogenous compounds
  Nonabsorbable antibiotics (neomycin or metronidazole)
  Lactulose or lactilol
Dopamine receptor agonists
  L-Dopa and bromocriptine*
Branched-chain amino acids†
Temporary liver support
Orthotopic liver transplantation

* Arousal effect in selected patients may be due to enhanced renal
  function.
† High cost and equivocal benefits of intravenous amino acid mixtures
  make it difficult to justify routine use.

chronic encephalopathy, long-term protein restriction is often necessary to control symptoms.

Measures to decrease ammonia absorption from the gut include oral administration of nonabsorbable antibiotics and lactulose. Neomycin reduces ammonia formation by decreasing the bacterial flora responsible for the hydrolysis of intraluminal proteins. Initially, 4 to 6 g should be administered in divided doses. Ototoxicity and nephrotoxicity are uncommon because only 1% to 3% of the drug is systemically absorbed after oral administration. Neomycin is effective in the long term and is considered by many to be the drug of choice for acute and chronic encephalopathy. Alternative antibiotics such as tetracycline and metronidazole are suboptimal because of limited effectiveness or potential CNS toxicity.

Lactulose is a synthetic disaccharide that is not hydrolyzed in the upper GI tract and reaches the colon virtually intact. In the colon, it is broken down by bacteria into galactose and fructose, which are then metabolized to a mixture of organic acids. Acidification of the fecal stream suppresses ammonia-forming organisms such as Bacteroides and favors conversion of ammonia to the less diffusible ammonium ion. Lactulose also produces an osmotic catharsis that aids fecal excretion of nitrogenous compounds. The dosage varies from 15 to 30 mL three times a day and should be titrated to produce two or three semisolid stools a day. Side effects such as diarrhea, flatulence, and electrolyte abnormalities are uncommon but can be managed by decreasing the daily dose.

Dopamine agonists such as L-dopa and bromocriptine have been used with variable success. The mechanism of action is thought to involve displacement of false neurotransmitters in the CNS, with restoration of normal levels of excitation and inhibition. Several groups have reported temporary arousal after administering L-dopa to patients with acute encephalopathy resistant to neomycin and lactulose, but one controlled trial concluded that the drug was ineffective.[19]

Plasma amino acid imbalances have been implicated in the pathogenesis of hepatic encephalopathy. The rationale for administering solutions rich in branched-chain amino acids has been to normalize the ratio of branched-chain to aromatic amino acids and thereby prevent accumulation of false inhibitory neurotransmitter substances in the CNS. Early work suggested that intravenously administered mixtures of branched-chain amino acids would correct plasma amino acid abnormalities and ameliorate hepatic encephalopathy.[20] Controlled clinical trials failed to confirm this conclusion. Considering that these intravenous amino acid mixtures are costly, it is difficult to justify their use, especially since their effectiveness is not proved.

Other therapies such as temporary liver support have a limited role in the management of chronic hepatic encephalopathy and should be viewed as a possible bridge to hepatic transplantation. The efficacy and results of orthotopic hepatic transplantation for acute hepatic encephalopathy are discussed in the section on acute hepatic failure.

PORTAL HYPERTENSION

The standard anatomy of the liver and its vasculature have been well described. Certain variations in this anatomy are pertinent to the pathophysiology associated with portal hypertension and cirrhosis and the feasibility of constructing portosystemic shunts. With mesenteric angiography, many vascular variations can be identified preoperatively. Renal vein and vena caval variations are also common, and it is helpful to visualize these structures when planning a portosystemic shunt.

Standard hepatic arterial anatomy is present in only about half of patients. The origin of the right hepatic artery is either totally or partially replaced to the superior mesenteric artery in 18% of patients. This artery courses behind the head of the pancreas and behind the common bile duct. Unless care is taken, the artery is easily injured when dissecting the hepatoduodenal ligament to fashion a portacaval shunt. The portal vein crosses the artery anteriorly near its origin from the superior mesenteric artery. When the portal vein is stretched posteriorly to construct a portacaval shunt, the vein may be kinked as it crosses the artery and portal hypertension may persist.[21] The origin of the left hepatic artery is totally or partially replaced to the left gastric artery with a frequency of 25%. Ligating the left gastric artery when performing a distal splenorenal shunt or a gastric devascularization procedure carries the risk of compromising the arterial supply to the left lobe of the liver.

The three major splanchnic veins are the portal vein and its two major tributaries, the superior mesenteric and splenic veins. One of the veins must be patent and of adequate size to construct one of the standard portosystemic shunts. With portal hypertension, one of the veins is often thrombosed. Additionally, many variations in the anatomy of the splenic–superior mesenteric vein confluence exist and may preclude fashioning some types of portosystemic shunts. A fairly common variation is the absence of a superior mesenteric vein trunk; instead, three or more smaller mesenteric veins may merge with the splenic vein to form the origin of the portal vein. With this variation, construction of an adequate mesocaval shunt may not be possible.

An abundance of potential hepatic arterial and portal venous collaterals has been identified.[22,23] Venous collaterals often course through the hepatoduodenal ligament, and large submucosal varices are sometimes present in the gallbladder with portal hypertension and especially with portal vein thrombosis. Portoazygous and portopulmonary venous collateral shunts course through the diaphragm, the splenophrenic ligament, and the bare area behind the spleen. The presence of this rich collateral network frequently adds to the blood loss and morbidity associated with cholecystectomy or splenectomy in patients with portal hypertension.

The ligament of the vena cava courses posterior to the vena cava, just caudad to the caval ostium in the diaphragm. The ligament attaches to the posterior aspect of segment I (caudate lobe) and segment VIII (posterosuperior) of the right hepatic lobe. When these segments enlarge with cirrhosis or Budd-Chiari syndrome, the vena cava may be entrapped and narrowed, and the venous pressure in the cava is high. This may preclude construction of a standard portosystemic shunt anastomosed to the infrahepatic cava for outflow.

Physiology

Portosystemic Collaterals and the Hyperdynamic State

If portal pressure is elevated, spontaneous portosystemic collaterals develop in an attempt to decompress the portal system. Such collaterals increase venous return to the heart and increase cardiac output. In humans, the most important collaterals develop as tributaries of the coronary, short gastric, and paraesophageal veins, the intercostal, esophageal, and azygous veins, the superior, middle, and inferior hemorrhoidal veins, and the paraumbilical plexus. Retroperitoneal veins and veins draining abdominal viscera in contact with the abdominal wall through so-called bare areas, and connections to the left renal vein from the splenic, adrenal, and gonadal veins may also serve as sites for the development of venous collaterals (Fig. 38-8). In addition, an area of distal esophagus extends 5 cm from the gastroesophageal junction in which the veins course primarily in the lamina propria rather than in the submucosa. Postmortem studies have demonstrated an increase in vessel size in the distal esophagus in patients with portal hypertension. Such studies support the concept that portosystemic collaterals and varices are formed by dilatation of preexisting channels and provide a structural basis for the predominantly distal location of esophageal varices.

Most clinical and laboratory reports support the concept of a hyperdynamic circulation in patients with portal hypertension. Rats with portal vein stenosis develop portal hypertension with a collateral pattern similar to that seen in humans. With portal vein stenosis, blood flow increases in all segments of the GI tract, muscle, and kidney, primarily as a result of precapillary vasodilation. Peripheral vasodilation leads to increased venous return, decreased systemic vascular resistance, and increased cardiac output.[24] Cardiac output increases for about 4 days and then plateaus, suggesting that a critical level of portosystemic shunting is required to maintain the hyperdynamic state.

Portosystemic shunting as well as humoral factors may be responsible for portal hypertension-induced splanchnic hyperemia and increases in portal blood flow. The existence of arteriovenous connections in the normal GI tract have been identified both in the gastric submucosa of humans with cirrhosis and portal hypertension, as well as in animal models of portal hypertension. The identification of arteriovenous connections in the gastric submucosa may also be related to the development of portal hypertensive gastropathy. Arteriovenous connections have also been identified in the small intestine. Another explanation for the increased splanchnic flow seen in portal hypertension is the release of vasodilatory metabolites from the tissues. Acute portal hypertension has been shown to increase oxygen consumption in the small intestine of a number of animal preparations.

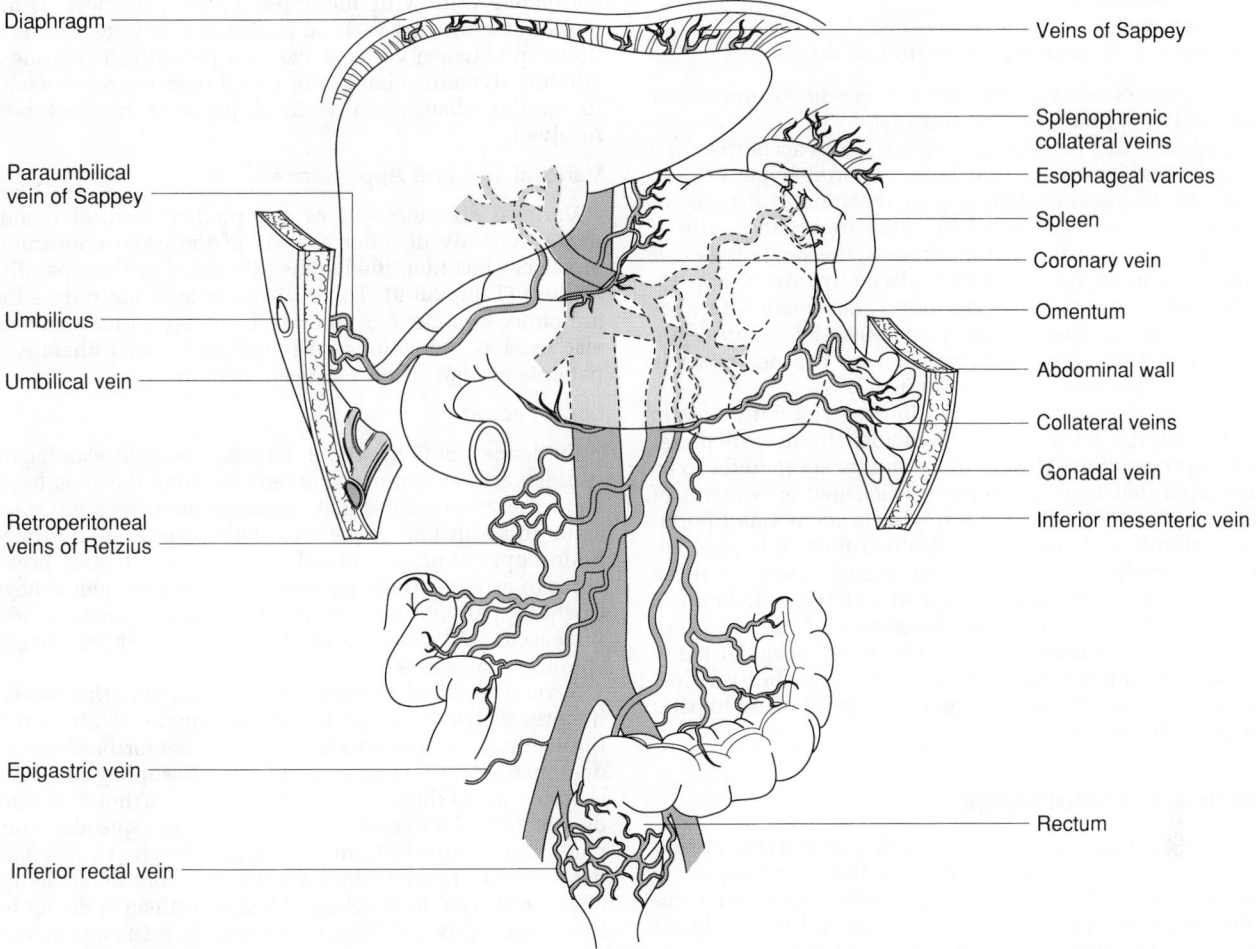

Figure 38-8. Potential venous collaterals that develop with portal hypertension. The veins of Sappey drain portal blood through the bare areas of the diaphragm and through paraumbilical vein collaterals to the umbilicus. The veins of Retzius form in the retroperitoneum and shunt portal blood from the bowel and other organs to the vena cava.

Changes in Blood Volume and Hepatic Resistance

Increased intravascular volume may play a significant role in precipitating variceal hemorrhage. Increased plasma volume has been noted in patients with cirrhotic and noncirrhotic portal hypertension and in cirrhotic patients with acute variceal hemorrhage compared with those without hemorrhage. The role of acute volume expansion as a precipitating factor is also suggested by clinical reports noting variceal hemorrhage after the administration of contrast media for angiography, during pregnancy, and after the surgical placement of a peritoneal venous shunt to reduce ascites. In a vessel at the limits of compliance, such as an esophageal varix, a small increase in volume causes a disproportionately large increase in wall tension and results in rupture. Injudicious volume overexpansion may therefore precipitate variceal bleeding.

Intrinsic flow is thought to be regulated by the hepatic arterial buffer response. Both the portal venous and hepatic arterial vascular beds also may be regulated by a modulating myogenic mechanism. The myogenic theory postulates that stretch receptors are present in the vessel wall and can sense changes in transmural wall tension. According to the law of Laplace, tension across a vessel wall is the product of pressure and radius. The myogenic response, then, causes vasoconstriction (a decrease in the radius of the vessel) as vessel pressure increases to maintain a constant tension.[24]

Extrinsic neurohumoral mechanisms also exist to control resistance of the hepatic vasculature. The splanchnic viscera are densely innervated by sympathetic vasoconstrictor fibers found predominantly in the arterioles. Parasympathetic innervation also exists, but the role of these vagally derived fibers is debated. The following endogenous compounds are capable of modulating hepatic resistance:

Agents That Increase Splanchnic Flow

Bile acids
Bradykinin
Cholecystokinin
Epinephrine
Gastrin
Glucagon
Histamine
Neurotensin
Prostaglandins PGI_2, PGE_1, PGA_1, and PGA_2
Vasoactive intestinal peptide (in high doses)

Agents That Decrease Splanchnic Flow

Epinephrine (in high doses)
Norepinephrine
Prostaglandins PGF_{2a} and PGD_2

Thromboxane B$_2$
Somatostatin
Vasoactive intestinal peptide (in low doses)

These compounds can directly act on smooth muscle or indirectly modulate neural pathways.

Anatomic and pathophysiologic changes accompanying hepatic cirrhosis also contribute to portal hypertension. The ratio of presinusoidal to postsinusoidal resistance in the normal liver is almost 50:1, compared with a ratio of 5:1 for skeletal muscle. With cirrhosis, the single liver cell plates of normal sinusoids are replaced by rows of hepatocytes that are two or more cells thick. The hepatic arterioles and the presinusoidal and postsinusoidal venules are trapped within bridging fibrous septa. The net effect is increased pressure across the sinusoid.

Another characteristic alteration observed with hepatic cirrhosis is the development of vascular shunts from portal to hepatic venules. Most of these shunts are thought to be sinusoids that have dilated and thickened as a result of hepatocyte loss. These atypical vessels act as small portacaval shunts that permit portal blood flow to bypass hepatic parenchymal cells. The fenestrated character of the endothelial cell membrane is also lost with cirrhosis, a phenomenon known as *capillarization* of the sinusoid. Normally, these fenestrations allow free passage of many proteins required for homeostasis, and this ability is lost in cirrhosis. Shunts between hepatic arterioles and hepatic venules also occur but are rare.

Variceal Hemorrhage

About two thirds of patients with portal hypertension develop varices; of these, only two thirds subsequently experience a variceal hemorrhage. Such observations emphasize the need to identify patients most likely to bleed from esophageal varices and to provide a rationale supporting prophylactic and therapeutic intervention. The factors that are most important in the pathogenesis of variceal hemorrhage are portal pressure, intravariceal pressure, variceal size and structure, and other local factors.

Portal and Variceal Pressure

There appears to be a minimum threshold of portal pressure required for the development of esophageal varices. In patients with intrahepatic portal hypertension, usually due to alcoholic cirrhosis, variceal hemorrhage rarely occurs when the portal pressure gradient (portal minus free hepatic venous pressure) is less than 12 mmHg. Patients with portal pressure gradients above this level do not invariably develop varices.

A number of clinical observations emphasize the importance of the relationship between elevations of portal pressure and hemorrhage. A higher mean portal pressure has been noted in patients who manifest variceal hemorrhage. When measured 48 hours after an episode of hemorrhage, patients with higher portal pressures had a significantly higher mortality. In some patients with varices who have undergone visceral angiography, higher portal and azygous pressures, as a result of volume expansion caused by administration of angiographic dye, have been associated with rebleeding. Cirrhotic patients with newly developed hepatocellular carcinoma often present with variceal hemorrhage, presumably as a result of tumor-induced arteriovenous shunting and increased portal flow.

The measurement of portal pressure has been traditionally used to estimate the risk of variceal hemorrhage and the response to therapy. Such a relationship assumes that portal pressure is directly proportional to variceal pressure. Endoscopic measurements of variceal pressure have correlated well with measured portal pressures. Direct measurement using variceal puncture also suggests a relationship between variceal size and pressure. The issue of whether dynamic changes in portal pressure are reflected in similar changes in variceal pressure has not been resolved.

Variceal Size and Appearance

Variceal size alone does not predict variceal hemorrhage. A study of other aspects of the gross appearance of varices has identified signs associated with impending rupture (Table 38-9). These visual criteria not only allow judicious treatment of acutely bleeding varices, but are also used as indications for prophylactic sclerotherapy in patients at high risk for variceal hemorrhage.[25]

Local Factors

Evidence conflicts about whether erosive esophagitis causes variceal rupture. The erosion hypothesis is based on postmortem studies that document acute erosive esophagitis in about half of patients with variceal hemorrhage. Endoscopic studies routinely document a higher prevalence of esophagitis in patients with variceal hemorrhage. Cirrhotic patients with ascites have been shown to have increased acid reflux and decreased lower esophageal sphincter pressures.

Several lines of evidence do not support the erosion hypothesis. Histology of biopsy specimens obtained during evaluation of patients with variceal hemorrhage has not documented an increased incidence of esophagitis. When esophageal pH monitoring is performed, cirrhotic patients do not have increased numbers of reflux episodes compared with controls. Control of acid reflux by H$_2$ blockade has not been shown to decrease the incidence of rebleeding after esophageal hemorrhage. Most investigators do not believe that reflux esophagitis is a significant factor in variceal rupture.

ASCITES

Pathophysiology

The main factors that control fluid exchange between the intravascular and tissue spaces are the capillary hydrostatic pressure and the colloid osmotic pressure. In patients with cirrhosis, colloid osmotic pressure is frequently low because of defective albumin synthesis. The scarring and regeneration that typifies cirrhosis ultimately causes distortion of intrahepatic vascular architecture, with elevation of hepatic sinusoidal and intestinal capillary pressures. These factors contribute to transudation of fluid into the peritoneal cavity. Ascitic fluid is a mixture of hepatic

---

Table 38-9. ENDOSCOPIC SIGNS THAT CORRELATE WITH RISK OF VARICEAL RUPTURE

Category	Subcategory
Basic color	White varices
	Blue varices
Signs	Red color sign
	Red wale marking
	Cherry red spot
	Hematocystic spot
	Diffuse redness
Form	Linear
	Tortuous
	Large

(Japanese Research Society for Portal Hypertension)

and splanchnic lymph and varies in protein concentration, depending on the site of origin. Splanchnic lymph is low in protein. The protein concentration in hepatic lymph is high because of increased permeability of the sinusoidal bed compared with other capillary systems. Increased hepatic lymph production in cirrhotic patients also contributes to ascites formation.

The pathogenesis of ascites formation in cirrhosis has not been fully elucidated. The underfill theory postulates that ascites accumulation and splanchnic venous pooling lead to contraction of the effective circulating plasma volume. The resulting alterations in renal perfusion then lead to sodium retention by stimulation of the renin–angiotensin–aldosterone system and other less well-defined mechanisms. Investigators using a water immersion model that reproducibly increases central blood volume have demonstrated normalization of renal sodium handling with marked natriuresis and kaliuresis in a group of decompensated cirrhotic patients.[26] These studies support the importance of diminished effective plasma volume in ascites formation.

The mechanism by which diminished effective plasma volume leads to avid sodium retention has been investigated extensively. Reduced mean renal blood flow and intrarenal redistribution of blood flow from cortical to juxtamedullary nephrons has been demonstrated in cirrhotic patients using tracer techniques such as xenon washout. These pathologic abnormalities have been attributed to a variety of factors, including alteration in endogenous prostaglandin production, disequilibrium of the kallikrein-kinin system, and hyperaldosteronism.[26] Evidence suggests that hyperaldosteronism plays a permissive rather than primary role in the abnormal renal sodium handling associated with cirrhosis. Atrial natriuretic factor and other humoral factors have also been implicated. No single mechanism satisfactorily explains the pathologic sodium retention observed in cirrhotic patients with ascites. Rather, the cause appears to involve complex interrelations between the following neural, humoral, and vascular factors; the predominant factor may vary as the severity of liver disease progresses[27]:

Hormonal

Hyperaldosteronism
Alterations in renal prostaglandins
Alterations in kallikrein-kinin system
Increased estrogens
Prolactin
Humoral natriuretic factor

Neural and Hemodynamic

Alterations in intrarenal blood flow distribution
Increased sympathetic nervous system activity

The overflow theory suggests that inappropriate sodium and water retention with expansion of the plasma volume is the primary event in ascites formation.[28] The initiating cause of sodium retention is unknown, but suggested mechanisms include increased renal tubular sensitivity to endogenous aldosterone or elaboration of a nonaldosterone sodium-retaining factor. Expansion of the extracellular fluid compartment leads to suppression of the renin–angiotensin–aldosterone system with the establishment of a new sodium equilibrium at a higher than normal level. With advancing cirrhosis and the development of hypoalbuminemia and portal hypertension, the expanded extracellular and plasma compartments overflow into the peritoneal cavity.

A unitary hypothesis has been presented to explain the pathogenesis of ascites in cirrhosis.[29] In stage I (preascitic underfill phase), increased hepatic sinusoidal resistance leads to splanchnic pooling and reduced effective intravascular volume (EIV). This activates regulatory mechanisms that cause sodium and water retention with restoration of normal EIV. In stage II (overflow phase), the rate of lymph production increases. Ascites is not detectable clinically as long as the absorptive capability of hepatic and splanchnic transport mechanisms is not exceeded. By this time, a well-defined circulatory disorder has been established, with a large splanchnic venous pool, multiple portosystemic venous collaterals, and arteriovenous fistulas in the lungs, liver, skin, and other organs. Circulatory efficiency is compromised by reduced peripheral resistance and diversion of splanchnic arterial flow through newly formed arteriovenous anastomoses. If cardiac reserve is not sufficient to meet these increased circulatory demands, renal perfusion may be decreased with further sodium and water retention. In stage III (advanced overflow phase with tense ascites), high intraabdominal pressure interferes with lymph reabsorption and reduces venous return and cardiac function.

Clinical and Laboratory Features

Ascites may develop abruptly or slowly over the course of several months. The onset of ascites usually indicates the presence of advanced liver disease. Rapid-onset ascites are usually related to some precipitating event, such as upper GI hemorrhage, excessive diuretic therapy with dehydration, electrolyte imbalance, exposure to hepatotoxins, or growth of a cirrhosis-associated hepatic tumor. The short-term prognosis in such situations is reasonably good if the underlying cause can be corrected.

Cirrhotic patients with ascites exhibit many common physical findings. Temporal and peripheral muscle wasting are prominent features along with conspicuous abdominal distention. Increased intraabdominal pressure predisposes the patient to hernias in the umbilical and inguinal regions. Associated portal hypertension may cause recanalization of the umbilical vein with distention of periumbilical collaterals to form a caput medusa. Sometimes, a thrill can be palpated and a bruit heard over the epigastrium from high-velocity flow in the portal systemic collaterals (Fig. 38-9).

A pleural effusion is present in up to 10% of cirrhotic patients with ascites; in most, the effusion occurs in the right pleural cavity. The effusion results from movement of ascites fluid from the peritoneal cavity into the pleural space through small peritoneopleural communications in the diaphragm. Effective ascites management usually controls the pleural effusion. Peripheral edema involving the lower extremities is usually symmetrical and can be ascribed to increased fluid retention, often with coexisting hypoalbuminemia and declining renal function.

Diagnostic paracentesis should always be performed to confirm the cause of ascites. Bowel perforation and hemorrhage, especially from dilated abdominal wall collaterals, are potential complications but can be avoided by careful attention to detail. The abdominal wall should be surveyed with a pocket Doppler to identify sites of high flow, indicating the presence of nearby dilated collaterals or the epigastric vessels. Whenever possible, the paracentesis should be performed in the midline, midway between the umbilicus and the pubic tubercle. A 22-gauge needle should be used. The patient should always be asked to void before paracentesis to avoid inadvertent injury to the urinary bladder.

Cirrhotic ascites is usually straw colored, clear, or greenish. Blood-staining indicates the possibility of an underlying malignancy. Protein concentration rarely exceeds 2 g/dL, except in cases of malignancy, infection, or pancreatic duct disruption with release of pancreatic enzymes into

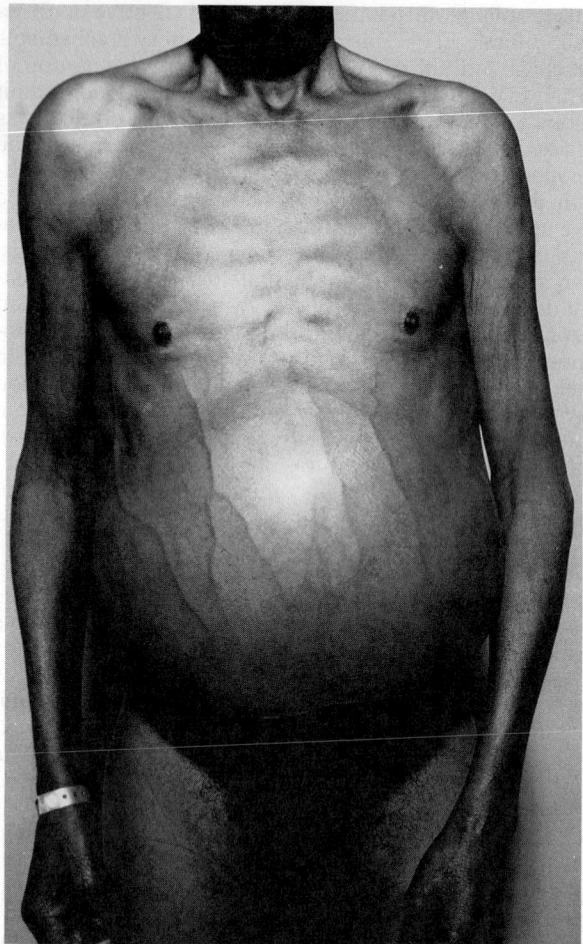

Figure 38-9. Man with hepatic cirrhosis and tense ascites, showing prominent abdominal wall collateral veins. The pattern of collateral flow in relation to the umbilicus may provide useful information about the site of venous obstruction. For example, with portal vein obstruction, collateral flow is centrifugal, or away from the umbilicus. Conversely, with obstruction of the inferior vena cava, flow is centripetal, or toward the umbilicus.

the peritoneal cavity. To help distinguish among the various causes, an aliquot of ascites should be sent routinely for measurement of ascitic fluid protein, red blood cell count, white blood cell count and differential, amylase, pH, glucose, and culture and sensitivity (Table 38-10).

Complications

Spontaneous bacterial peritonitis (SBP) occurs as a complication of cirrhotic ascites in up to 10% of patients. SBP is defined as infected ascitic fluid with no other demonstrable site of infection.[30] This is a serious complication, with reported in-hospital mortality rates of 60% to 90%. The pathogenesis of SBP is not entirely clear, but the source of contamination appears to be hematogenous in origin. Recently, translocation of bacteria through the intestinal wall has been implicated in the pathogenesis. In most patients with SBP, the infection is monomicrobial, and about two thirds of organisms are enteric, primarily *E coli* (Table 38-11).

The clinical features and laboratory findings of SBP may vary widely. Fever and abdominal pain are common, but objective evidence of peritonitis may be absent or subtle. At times, a patient may be asymptomatic. Many authorities

Table 38-10. DIFFERENTIAL DIAGNOSIS OF ASCITES

PORTAL HYPERTENSION

Cirrhosis and other intrahepatic diseases
Hepatic congestion
  Congestive heart failure
  Constrictive pericarditis
  Inferior vena cava obstruction
  Budd-Chiari syndrome
Portal vein occlusion

HYPOALBUMINEMIA

Nephrotic syndrome
Protein-losing enteropathy
Malnutrition

MISCELLANEOUS DISORDERS

Myxedema
Ovarian disease (Meig syndrome, struma ovarii)
Peritoneal carcinomatosis
Pancreatic ascites
End-stage renal disease
Chylous ascites
Bile ascites
Urine ascites

(Sleisenger MH, Fordtran JS. Gastrointestinal disease: pathophysiology, diagnosis and management, ed 4. Philadelphia, WB Saunders, 1989:433)

believe that a Gram stain is inaccurate for diagnosing SBP and recommend initial broad-spectrum antibiotic treatment until the results of culture and sensitivity testing are available.

Peripheral leukocytosis is common in patients with SBP, and blood cultures are positive in nearly half of cases.[30] In up to 30% of patients, peritoneal fluid cultures are negative. Therefore, the diagnosis of SBP is often based on examination of the ascitic fluid. The fluid is usually clear but may be cloudy or turbid. A presumptive diagnosis of SBP can be made when the white cell count in the ascitic fluid exceeds $500/\mu L$ and more than 50% of the leukocytes are polymorphonuclear. Some authors would diagnose SBP when the white cell count exceeds $250/\mu L$. A variety of metabolic markers induced by bacterial infection have been suggested to aid the diagnosis of SBP, but the polymorphonuclear leukocyte count appears to be the most useful test.[31]

SBP must be differentiated from other causes of bacterial peritonitis (Table 38-12). With appropriate antibiotics, a

Table 38-11. BACTERIOLOGY OF SPONTANEOUS BACTERIAL PERITONITIS

Organisms	Percentage of Total
Escherichia coli	40
Pneumococci	15
Streptococci	14
Klebsiella	7
Pseudomonas	3
Proteus	3
Staphylococci	3
Anaerobes	5
Other	20
Multiple isolates	10

(Adapted from Targan S, Chow A, Gluze L. Role of anaerobic bacteria in spontaneous peritonitis of cirrhosis. Am J Med 1977;62:397)

Table 38-12. DIFFERENTIAL DIAGNOSIS OF SPONTANEOUS BACTERIAL PERITONITIS AS DISTINGUISHED FROM NONSPONTANEOUS BACTERIAL PERITONITIS

Feature	Spontaneous	Nonspontaneous
History of GI disease	Usually negative	Often positive
Abdominal examination	Positive rebound	Pain, rigidity
Pneumoperitoneum	Absent	Often present
Appearance of fluid	Frequently clear	Cloudy to purulent
Ascites fluid pH	7.0–7.4	6.5–7.3
Ascites fluid glucose	Same as blood	Lower than blood
Species of bacteria	Single	Multiple
Anaerobes	Rare	Common
Blood in ascites fluid	Rare	Common

(Adapted from Schiff L, Schiff ER. Diseases of the liver, ed 6. Philadelphia, JB Lippincott, 1987:83)

successful outcome can be expected in 60% of patients. Despite this favorable initial response, the overall prognosis is grave. Only one third of surviving patients live 1 year; of these, half have recurrent SBP with a mortality risk approaching 50%.[31] Successful treatment must be prompt and aggressive. Broad-spectrum cephalosporins are recommended to avoid the potential nephrotoxicity associated with aminoglycosides. SBP is an indicator of advanced liver disease, and patients who otherwise qualify should be considered for hepatic transplantation. Prophylactic antibiotics are frequently recommended after the first episode, especially in patients awaiting hepatic transplantation.

Umbilical and other abdominal wall hernias occur in nearly 20% of cirrhotic patients with ascites. They result from increased intraabdominal pressure and wasting of abdominal wall fascia and muscles. Common complications include incarceration, leakage, and rupture. These hernias should be repaired electively. The operative mortality rate for emergency herniorrhaphy approaches 15% to 30%.[32] Discoloration, ulceration, leakage, or a rapid increase in the size of the hernia herald impending rupture and are indications for prompt repair.

Treatment

A rational approach to treating ascites often requires a balance between what is optimal and what is practical. Modern medical therapy is often effective. Refractory ascites—that is, ascites unresponsive to medical therapy—is usually a manifestation of end-stage liver disease. The most expedient solution would be orthotopic hepatic transplantation. Although attractive, this solution is not feasible for many patients, and there are insufficient numbers of livers available to treat the large numbers of US patients with end-stage liver disease.

Sodium and Fluid Restriction

The mainstay of therapy is sodium restriction. To be effective, daily sodium intake should be restricted to 40 mEq or less. Recumbency decreases sympathetic nervous system activity and increases portal blood flow and renal perfusion relative to an upright position. Therapy with bed rest and sodium restriction results in spontaneous diuresis in 5% to 15% of patients. Several factors can be used to predict early responders, including 24-hour urine sodium excretion of more than 10 mEq, normal creatinine clearance, reversible disease, such as acute fatty liver in an

alcoholic, and identification of treatable predisposing conditions, such as excess sodium intake, infection, or GI bleeding.[33] The remaining 85% to 95% of patients require additional therapy with diuretics, carefully monitored fluid restriction, intermittent large-volume paracentesis, peritoneovenous shunting, or in a few instances, portosystemic decompression or orthotopic hepatic transplantation.

Diuretics

Diuretic therapy is intended to restrict the ability of the nephron to conserve sodium. The two most commonly used classes of drugs act at different sites in the nephron. Spironolactone is an aldosterone antagonist that is weakly natriuretic, conserves potassium, and acts primarily on the distal tubule. Spironolactone has been recommended as the first diuretic to use. The usual starting dose is 50 mg every 8 hours; up to 100 mg every 6 hours may be indicated if tolerated. Gynecomastia in men, metabolic acidosis, and hyperkalemia are complications of spironolactone therapy. Complications are usually dose related.

Between 25% and 50% of patients treated initially with spironolactone require a second diuretic for a satisfactory response. In most cases, a thiazide or more potent loop diuretic, such as furosemide, bumetanide, or muzolimine, is used. These agents are potent natriuretics that act on the proximal nephron. By using spironolactone to block distal sodium reabsorption, the effectiveness of these natriuretics is enhanced. Loop diuretics can cause significant complications, including azotemia, hypokalemia that is unrelated to the diuretic response, hyponatremia, and encephalopathy. The maximum amount of fluid that can translocate from the peritoneal cavity into the vascular space has been estimated to be 900 mL/d. In patients with peripheral edema, fluid is more readily mobilized from the interstitial space into the vascular space. Intravascular volume contraction can be avoided if the rate of diuresis is limited to a weight loss of 0.5 to 0.75 kg/d in patients without peripheral edema and to 1 to 2 kg/d in patients with edema.

Therapeutic Paracentesis

Therapeutic, as opposed to diagnostic, paracentesis is usually limited to patients with tense or symptomatic ascites. Several studies have shown that repeated paracentesis in stable cirrhotic patients may be as safe and effective as medical therapy and shortens the length of hospitalization.[34] One advantage of therapeutic paracentesis is that fluid is removed directly from the peritoneal cavity rather than first depleting the intravascular space to shift fluid from the abdomen or peripheral interstitial space. In general, intravenous albumin should be administered to maintain circulating blood volume and avoid renal impairment. The recommended dosage of albumin replacement is 10 g for each liter of ascites removed. Single large-volume paracentesis has also been reported to be effective and safe. Up to 10 L of ascitic fluid can be removed in 1 hour if salt-poor albumin is administered simultaneously. Paracentesis is usually contraindicated in the presence of hepatorenal syndrome, a severe coagulopathy, or progressive acute encephalopathy.

Surgery

In a small percentage of patients, surgical implantation of a peritoneovenous shunt may be advisable. A variety of shunts have been developed since their introduction in 1974.[35] All of these shunts result in unidirectional flow of ascites from the peritoneal cavity into the venous

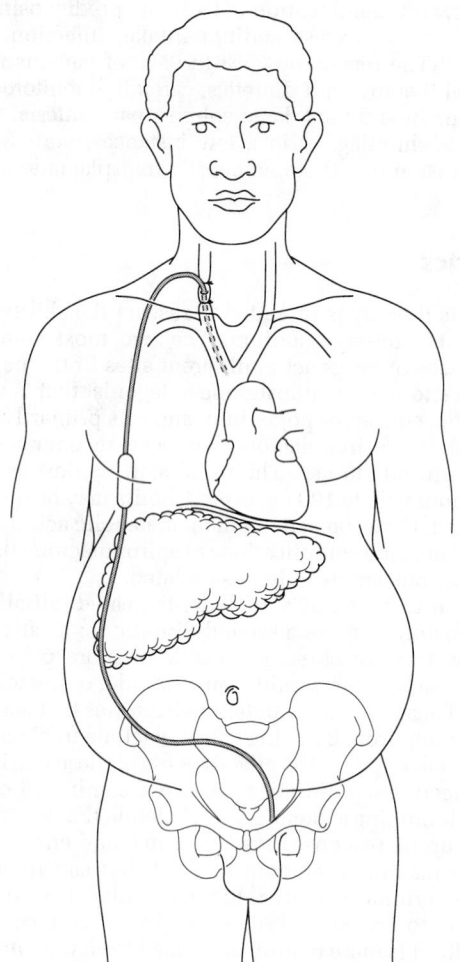

Figure 38-10. LeVeen peritoneovenous shunt used for routing ascites fluid into the systemic circulation. The shunt consists of fenestrated tubing for insertion into the peritoneal cavity, a one-way valve, and a length of venous tubing for insertion into the superior vena cava.

circulation (Fig. 38-10). The principal indication for using a peritoneovenous shunt is disabling ascites that is refractory to conventional medical treatment and therapeutic paracentesis. Contraindications include liver failure, severe coagulopathy, bacterial peritonitis, cardiac failure, and a recent history of hemorrhage from esophageal or gastric varices. Early technical problems related to shunt malposition or occlusion are unusual. Despite the simplistic nature of this device, postoperative mortality and morbidity rates of 20% and 60%, respectively, have been reported.[36] The precipitation of disseminated intravascular coagulopathy, variceal hemorrhage, or hepatic failure may require eliminating measures designed to augment shunt flow, the use of ε-aminocaproic acid, and shunt ligation.

Reaccumulation of ascites after peritoneovenous shunt placement suggests shunt occlusion. To correct the problem, it is important to accurately determine the site of obstruction. This can be done in a stepwise fashion using Doppler ultrasound, technetium colloid scintigraphy, and direct contrast injection of the venous tubing.[37] Up to 25% of patients develop shunt malfunction as a result of partial or complete occlusion 5 years or longer after shunt insertion. Only half of these patients require shunt revision to control their ascites. Bacterial

peritonitis may occur with the shunt in place and many times occludes the shunt. Treatment consists of systemic antibiotics and shunt removal, but despite these measures the mortality rate has been reported to be nearly 60% with this complication. The survival after peritoneovenous shunting has been compared with conventional medical therapy in four randomized trials.[38] The combined results indicate that peritoneovenous shunting does not prolong survival compared with conventional therapy. The shorter length of hospitalization required for treatment and the palliation achieved may justify the use of this operation in selected patients.

Peritoneovenous shunting has also been compared with high-volume paracentesis combined with albumin infusion to define the relative merits of these two treatments. In one recent study, patients were randomly assigned to undergo either paracentesis with albumin infusion or peritoneovenous shunting. Outcome variables included mortality and morbidity rates, the duration of the results of initial hospitalization, and the need for rehospitalization.[39] Comparable numbers of patients in the two groups required readmission to the hospital during follow-up. Complications requiring readmission (encephalopathy, bacterial infection, and GI bleeding) were also similar in the two groups. However, the overall number of hospital readmissions was higher in the paracentesis group than in the peritoneovenous shunt group. Twenty shunt obstructions requiring readmission to the hospital developed in 15 patients (31%) with peritoneovenous shunts. The probabilities of developing shunt obstruction after 1 and 2 years were 40% and 52%, respectively. The probability of survival at 2 years was similar for the paracentesis group and the peritoneovenous shunt group.

The clinical results of peritoneovenous shunting have not been entirely satisfactory despite improved renal function and decreased ascites.[40] Modifying the shunt by adding a titanium tip to the venous tubing of the valve reduced the risk of venous thrombosis at 1 and 2 years to acceptable levels (5% and 12%, respectively). Short-term prophylactic antibiotic therapy and evacuation of ascites at the time of shunt placement are currently advocated to decrease the risk of infectious complications and postshunt coagulopathy. Predictors of poor outcome include a history of previous variceal bleeding and spontaneous bacterial peritonitis. Both of these factors significantly decrease the probability of short- and long-term survival after peritoneovenous shunting.[40]

Transjugular intrahepatic portosystemic shunts (TIPS) effectively control variceal bleeding by reducing portal pressures below critical threshold values. TIPS are hemodynamically similar to a side-to-side portacaval shunt and should also provide effective control of ascites in patients refractory to conventional medical therapy. In one recent study, 22 patients with refractory ascites underwent TIPS.[41] Of the 15 patients who survived more than 30 days after TIPS, ascites was improved in 14 patients (93%). The pre-TIPS level of hepatic dysfunction, judged by the Child-Pugh score, correlated accurately with post-TIPS survival. Patients with poor hepatic reserve (Child-Pugh score higher than 10) all died after TIPS if orthotopic liver transplantation was not performed. By comparison, most patients with good or moderate hepatic reserve (Child-Pugh score below 10) survived for at least 6 months. In a similar study, investigators showed that TIPS are effective for refractory ascites in class B but not in class C patients. These results suggest that control of ascites and survival in poor-risk cirrhotic patients may require orthotopic liver transplantation to correct the underlying disorder.[42]

BUDD-CHIARI SYNDROME AND VENOOCCLUSIVE DISEASE

Definition and Pathogenesis

Budd-Chiari syndrome is an uncommon condition caused by obstruction of venous outflow from the liver. The pathologic lesions responsible for this condition include endophlebitis obliterans of the hepatic veins and occlusion of the hepatic veins or suprahepatic inferior vena cava from thrombosis or obstructing webs.

The causes of Budd-Chiari syndrome vary widely (Table 38-13). The most common causes of thrombotic occlusion of the hepatic veins are hematologic disorders, including polycythemia vera and paroxysmal nocturnal hemoglobinuria.[43] Among Asian Americans, membranous obstruction of the suprahepatic inferior vena cava accounts for most cases. In 20% to 30% of cases, no cause can be readily identified.[44]

Venoocclusive disease of the liver accounts for a small percentage of Budd-Chiari syndrome cases. The chief pathologic findings of venoocclusive disease are central vein dilation, centrilobular necrosis, and concentric luminal narrowing of terminal hepatic venules. Venoocclusive disease has been described after ingestion of pyrrolizidine alkaloids and after chemotherapy for various malignancies.

Clinical Course

Typically, patients with Budd-Chiari syndrome present with right upper quadrant pain, hepatomegaly, and ascites. A small percentage of patients present with fulminating hepatic failure. Most patients develop a slowly progressive disease with ascites and peripheral muscle wasting. In most cases, routine determinations of liver function, including serum aminotransferases, and alkaline phosphatase are only moderately abnormal; the serum bilirubin concentration rarely exceeds 5 mg/dL.[44]

Technetium colloid hepatic scintiscans usually show diffuse, nonhomogeneous uptake in the periphery of the liver, with pronounced concentration centrally over the

---

Table 38-13. ETIOLOGIC FACTORS IN BUDD-CHIARI SYNDROME

Idiopathic
Hematologic disorders
  Polycythemia vera
  Paroxysmal nocturnal hemoglobinuria
  Myeloproliferative disorders
  Antithrombin III deficiency
  Circulating lupus anticoagulants
Oral contraceptives
Pregnancy and postpartum
Tumors
  Hepatocellular carcinoma
  Renal cell carcinoma
  Adrenal carcinoma
  Leiomyosarcoma of the inferior vena cava
Vena caval webs
Infections
  Amebic abscess
  Aspergillosis
  Hydatid cyst
Phlebitis
Trauma
Venoocclusive disease

(Adapted from Maddrey WS. Hepatic vein thrombosis [Budd-Chiari syndrome]. Hepatology 1984;4:44S)

---

caudate lobe.[45] This tracer uptake pattern is thought to result from sparing of the caudate lobe, which has hepatic veins that drain separately into the inferior vena cava. Vena caval and hepatic vein catheterization remains the gold standard for diagnosing Budd-Chiari syndrome.[44]

Liver biopsy should be obtained whenever possible. Typical features include centrilobular congestion, sinusoidal dilation, and cell dropout in the absence of a marked inflammatory response.[44] Fibrosis occurs as part of the reparative process associated with parenchymal necrosis and usually indicates a more advanced stage of the disease.

Most untreated patients with Budd-Chiari syndrome eventually die of hepatic failure or complications of cirrhosis. In one recent series of 19 untreated patients, 17 (89%) died within 3.5 years of the onset of symptoms.[45] Intensive medical treatment with diuretics and anticoagulants may relieve symptoms but does not appear to confer any additional survival benefit. Thrombolytic therapy with streptokinase or urokinase is usually ineffective.

Treatment

Surgery plays the major role in treatment of Budd-Chiari syndrome. Medical therapy, including fluid restriction, diuretics, injection of thrombolytic agents, and balloon angioplasty, has not demonstrated a long-term benefit in most cases. Peritoneovenous shunts relieve ascites but fail to decompress the liver or halt the progression of liver injury. Effective surgical approaches consist of construction of portosystemic shunts, resection of membranous webs, and orthotopic hepatic transplantation.

A portal decompressive procedure should be the first surgical option considered for treating Budd-Chiari syndrome. Conventional portosystemic shunts, all of which use the infrahepatic vena cava as an outflow tract, are only feasible when the vena cava is not obstructed by the hypertrophied caudate lobe or a vena caval web.[46] Postshunting encephalopathy does not appear to be a problem. Traditionally, side-to-side portacaval shunts have been constructed when the vena cava is not obstructed. Success rates in these circumstances approximate 75%. When the inferior vena cava is obstructed, short-term satisfactory decompression has been achieved with mesoatrial, portoatrial, and splenoatrial shunts.[47] There has been a high incidence of late thrombosis with these shunts, and modified direct atrial shunts are under investigation. Transatrial resection of constricting webs in the vena cava, dilatation of webs, and direct reconstruction of the retrohepatic cava are other options that have been reported in a few cases.[48-51]

Orthotopic hepatic transplantation is indicated when the operations described earlier are not feasible or have failed or when there is evidence of severe progressive hepatic fibrosis on biopsy and laboratory evidence of deteriorating liver function. Transplantation may be complicated by the coexistence of a hypercoagulable state that may cause recurrent hepatic vein thrombosis. This complication has largely been avoided by using long-term anticoagulation therapy.[52] Some clinicians advocate the use of chemotherapy when a myeloproliferative disorder causes hepatic vein thrombosis. Figure 38-11 presents a logical treatment algorithm for managing Budd-Chiari syndrome.

DIFFERENTIAL DIAGNOSIS OF PORTAL HYPERTENSION

Portal hypertension is a clinical manifestation of many different disease states. The causes of portal hypertension can be divided into disorders that increase resistance and disorders that increase flow (Table 38-14). Causes of in-

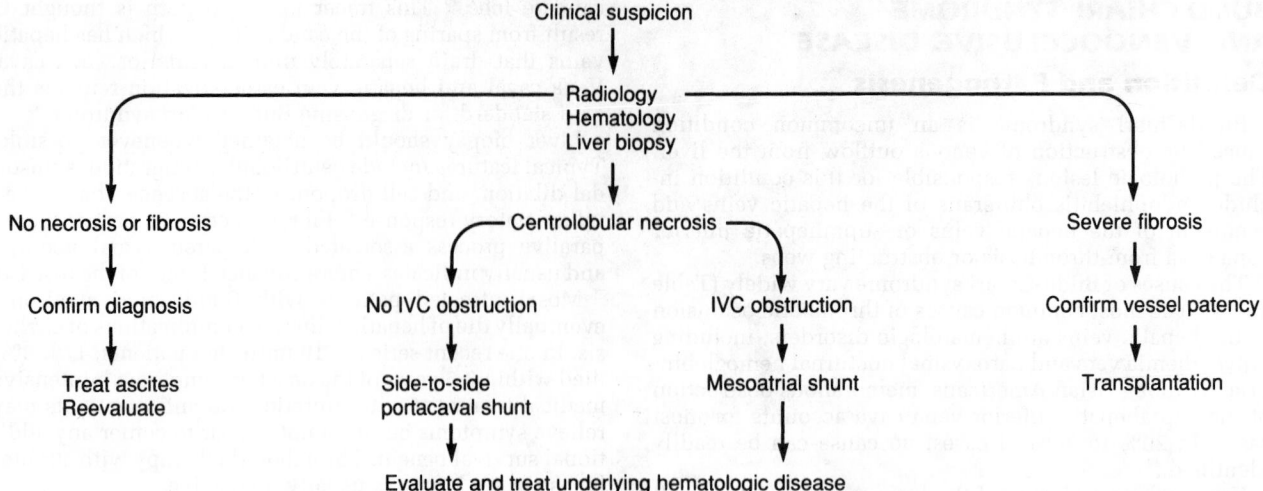

Figure 38-11. Algorithm for treating patients with Budd-Chiari syndrome. IVC, inferior vena cava. (After Henderson JM, Warren WD, Millikan WJ, et al. Surgical options: hematologic evaluation and pathologic changes in Budd-Chiari syndrome. Am J Surg 1990;1959:41)

Table 38-14. COMMON CAUSES OF PORTAL HYPERTENSION

DISORDERS THAT PRIMARILY INCREASE RESISTANCE TO FLOW

Prehepatic

Congenital atresia
Extrinsic compression
Portal, superior mesenteric, or splenic vein thrombosis

Hepatic

CIRRHOSIS

α_1-Antitrypsin deficiency
Cryptogenic cirrhosis
Cystic fibrosis
Hemochromatosis
Nutritional (alcoholic)
Posthepatic
Wilson disease

CONGENITAL HEPATITIC FIBROSIS

Focal regenerative hyperplasia
Hepatic venoocclusive disease
Idiopathic
Metastatic carcinoma
Sarcoidosis
Schistosomiasis
Toxin and drug injuries

ACUTE DISEASE

Acute fatty liver
Alcoholic hepatitis
Fulminant hepatic failure

Posthepatic

Budd-Chiari syndrome
Chronic heart failure
Constrictive pericarditis
Vena caval webs

DISORDERS THAT PRIMARILY INCREASE FLOW

Arterioportal Fistula

Hepatocellular carcinoma
Mesenteric arteriosclerotic or aneurysmal vascular disease
Osler-Weber-Rendu syndrome

Splenomegaly

creased resistance to flow are more common and can be categorized as prehepatic, hepatic, or posthepatic. Prehepatic (commonly referred to as extrahepatic) causes of portal hypertension are due to obstruction of one or more of the major splanchnic veins. The most common prehepatic cause of portal hypertension and the most common overall cause of portal hypertension in young children is thrombosis of the extrahepatic portal vein. Thrombosis is thought to be induced by omphalitis, intraabdominal infection, or other endophlebitides of unknown cause. In adults, extrinsic compression secondary to metastatic cancer is the most common cause of extrahepatic portal vein obstruction, but pancreatitis, polycythemia vera, lymphadenopathy, and an idiopathic variety have all been described as causes. Patients with extrahepatic obstruction generally have normal liver function, and their prognosis as a group is better than patients with portal hypertension secondary to intrahepatic disease. Splenic vein thrombosis may cause left-sided portal hypertension, leading to esophageal varices. Cancer, pancreatitis, and trauma are common causes of splenic vein thrombosis.

Hepatic diseases causing portal hypertension may be acute or chronic. Acute portal hypertension secondary to acute fatty liver or acute alcoholic hepatitis may subside with treatment of the underlying disease. Cirrhosis of the liver, the most common chronic intrahepatic disease leading to portal hypertension, can result from many distinct causes. Alcohol is the most common etiology of cirrhosis in the United States. Workplace chemicals that may cause liver injury include carbon tetrachloride, vinyl chloride, copper sulfate, and arsenicals. Common inborn errors of metabolism that lead to cirrhosis of the liver are Wilson disease, hemochromatosis, and α_1-antitrypsin deficiency. Nonalcoholic causes of portal hypertension are many, and include posthepatitic cirrhosis, sclerosing cholangitis, other diseases that chronically obstruct the biliary tree, and sarcoidosis. Schistosomiasis is thought to be the most common cause of portal hypertension in the world.

Idiopathic portal hypertension, previously included in the nonspecific category of diagnoses referred to as Banti syndrome, is now defined as portal hypertension and splenomegaly in the absence of portal vein occlusion or demonstrable liver disease. Nodular regenerative hyperplasia of the liver and metastatic cancer both cause portal hypertension, presumably by mechanical compression of the intrahepatic portal venous branches. Hepatic venoocclusive disease is caused by obliteration of small hepatic venules. This process is seen in about 20% of patients who undergo bone marrow transplantation with ingestion of pyrrolizidine alkaloids, as a consequence of hepatic irradiation, and with urethane exposure.

The posthepatic causes of portal hypertension comprise a group of diseases that obstruct outflow of blood from the liver. Budd-Chiari syndrome is the occlusion of extrahepatic hepatic veins. A Budd-Chiari–type syndrome can also be caused by membranous webs in the vena cava. Such webs are more common in Asian Americans and are usually found at the point where the embryologic ductus venosus inserts into the fetal vena cava. Restrictive pericarditis, tricuspid valve stenosis, and other cardiac lesions associated with chronic elevation of right heart pressure may cause hepatic congestion and portal hypertension. The histologic picture is similar to that seen in Budd-Chiari syndrome.

Portal hypertension may also be caused by supraphysiologic flow into the liver. Congenital arteriovenous fistulas occur in Osler-Weber-Rendu syndrome or are acquired as a result of liver biopsy, hepatic trauma, or rupture of a hepatic or mesenteric artery aneurysm. Patients with arterioportal fistulas rarely develop congestive heart failure because of resistance across the hepatic vascular bed. Nonportal hypertensive splenomegaly may also cause increased portal flow and is seen in diseases such as myelofibrosis, polycythemia rubra vera, Gaucher disease, and lymphoreticular malignancies. The onset of variceal hemorrhage or increase of ascites in a known cirrhotic patient should provoke a search for hepatocellular carcinoma. Arterioportal shunts in the hepatoma are thought to exacerbate preexisting portal hypertension.

TREATMENT OF GASTROESOPHAGEAL VARICEAL HEMORRHAGE
Choice of Therapy

The proper choice of therapy for elective treatment of individual patients depends on several important considerations. The natural history of the disease causing the portal hypertension, residual hepatic function, the presence of associated disease, continuing drug or alcohol abuse, the availability of patent major splanchnic veins, and the location of the varices causing the bleeding are factors that influence prognosis and choice of therapy.

Several systems have been devised to estimate hepatic reserve, postoperative mortality, and long-term prognosis. Unfortunately, no single liver function test is available that consistently correlates with residual hepatic function or estimates prognosis. Five laboratory and clinical factors have been used to categorize patients into three risk categories before they undergo portosystemic shunts[53] (Table 38-15). This system, which has been adopted by many groups, is known as the Child or Child-Turcotte risk classification method.[54] The method is simple and has proved to reliably estimate prognosis, especially early postoperative mortality. Other systems or modifications of the Child-Turcotte system have also been used, but no great advantage has been documented. The presence of Mallory bodies in the liver is an independent prognostic indicator. If many Mallory bodies are seen on liver biopsy in patients with cirrhosis, the prognosis is poor regardless of the Child-Turcotte risk category.[55]

The most common location of bleeding varices is in the esophagus. Sclerotherapy is usually the first line of definitive treatment for esophageal varices. Ten to 15%

Table 38-15. CHILD-TURCOTTE HEPATIC RISK CLASSIFICATION*

Parameter	Category		
	A	B	C
Bilirubin (mg/dL)	<2	2–3	>3
Albumin (g/dL)	>3.5	3–3.5	<3
Ascites	None	Treatable	Refractory
Encephalopathy	None	Minimal	Severe
Nutrition (muscle mass)	Normal	Fair	Poor

* This system correlates with operative mortality and long-term prognosis after construction of portosystemic shunts and has been used to estimate hepatic reserve and prognosis in many other clinical settings. Five variables are included because no single test reliably estimates operative mortality or long-term prognosis. Some judgment is needed in applying this system, because patients' laboratory studies or clinical status frequently overlap into more than one risk category.
(Wantz GE, Payne MA. Experience with portacaval shunt for portal hypertension. N Engl J Med 1961;265:721.)

of patients also have gastric varices that often cannot be treated effectively with sclerotherapy. The site of bleeding varices is rarely the duodenum, ileum, bladder, or colostomy or ileostomy stomas. In recent years, portal hypertensive gastropathy, as distinct from other causes of gastritis, has also been recognized as an important cause of bleeding secondary to portal hypertension. Decompressing the portal hypertension with a portosystemic shunt is the most feasible therapy for bleeding varices distal to the esophagus and for portal hypertensive gastropathy, provided the patient has good or moderate hepatic reserve. So-called left-sided portal hypertension is caused by thrombosis of the splenic vein. Splenectomy is the treatment of choice for this relatively uncommon cause of variceal bleeding.

Most patients with bleeding varices who have good or moderate hepatic function (Child-Turcotte A or B) are candidates for a trial of serial sclerotherapy. If sclerotherapy fails or is not feasible, a portosystemic shunt should be considered. Patients with poor liver function (Child-Turcotte C and some B) or with rapidly progressive liver disease are candidates for hepatic transplantation, provided they meet the other criteria necessary for successful transplantation. Devascularization and transection procedures have a limited and somewhat controversial role in the management of bleeding varices. The individual types of medical and surgical treatment available are discussed in more detail in the next sections.

Medical Management of Bleeding Varices
Vasopressin

Vasopressin (antidiuretic hormone) is a peptide derived from the posterior pituitary. The synthetic analogue, 8-arginine vasopressin, is frequently used to treat acute variceal hemorrhage and acts by decreasing portal venous pressure or flow through splanchnic vasoconstriction. Vasopressin constricts the arterioles and venules of the splanchnic bed, but also is capable of constricting esophageal smooth muscle. Vasopressin is usually administered as a continuous infusion into a peripheral vein at 0.2 to 0.6 IU/min. Vasopressin alone has been reported to temporarily control acute variceal hemorrhage in 50% to 75% of patients.[56] Complications include cardiac and peripheral extremity cutaneous ischemia. Simultaneous administration of nitroglycerin reduces the incidence of these complications. Portal or mesenteric venous thrombosis has also been reported, presumably from reduced flow.

Somatostatin

Somatostatin is a tetradecapeptide with many inhibitory actions in the GI tract. In pharmacologic doses, it acts as a vasoconstrictor to reduce splanchnic blood flow. Two trials have demonstrated that intravenous somatostatin has similar efficacy in controlling acute hemorrhage when compared with vasopressin, but does not cause the cardiovascular side effects.[56] The ability to use octreotide, a longer-acting analogue of somatostatin, may further improve the results of somatostatin therapy in acute variceal hemorrhage.

Propranolol

Propranolol, a synthetic β-adrenergic receptor blocking agent, lowers portal pressure and reduces liver blood flow and cardiac output. Not all patients respond to propranolol with clinically detectable decreases in portal pressure. Propranolol has been shown to prevent recurrent variceal bleeding in a large, placebo-controlled trial of compensated cirrhotic patients observed for 2 years.[57] Other investigators have not been able to reproduce these results. The data do not justify the routine use of propranolol.

Balloon Tamponade

Balloon tamponade is generally used for temporary control of acute variceal hemorrhage that is unresponsive to vasopressin or sclerotherapy. Compressing the gastroesophageal junction and esophageal wall with the balloons controls bleeding by tamponading and compressing the submucosal veins. The most frequently used devices have two balloons—one for the stomach to compress the gastroesophageal junction and one for the esophagus. The Sengstaken-Blakemore tube has three lumens—two to inflate the balloons and one to evacuate the gastric contents (Fig. 38-12). The Minnesota tube has a fourth lumen to evacuate oropharyngeal secretions above the inflated balloons.

Initial control of acute variceal hemorrhage occurs in about 80% of patients, but bleeding recurs promptly on deflation of the balloons in more than 50%. Serious complications occur in about 10% of patients and may include esophageal rupture, esophageal pressure necrosis, tracheal obstruction from balloon migration, and aspiration pneumonia. To avoid complications, patients requiring balloon tamponade should be in an intensive care unit for monitoring and have an endotracheal tube inserted to prevent aspiration pneumonia. A nasogastric tube can also be positioned above the esophageal balloon to help aspirate oropharyngeal secretions.

Endoscopic Sclerotherapy

Type of Scope

Endoscopic sclerotherapy was initially performed with the rigid esophagoscope. Most endoscopists now prefer to use a flexible endoscope.[58] Flexible endoscopy can be performed without general anesthesia, and the equipment is easily transported to the bedside. Modern therapeutic endoscopes have two ports—one for the sclerotherapy needle and one for aspiration of blood and secretions.

A number of modifications of the flexible endoscope have been described. An oversheath allows rapid passage from the oropharynx to the distal esophageal junction. Some oversheaths have a slotted end to allow the varix to prolapse into the lumen of the scope. Some endoscopes also are equipped with balloons to occlude the stomach and esophagus. These balloons are designed to decrease active hemorrhage but may interfere with visualization of the varices and precise variceal injection.

Techniques of Injection

The basic goal of sclerotherapy is to obliterate the variceal lumen or induce sclerosis of the submucosa, where varices usually arise. *Freehand variceal injection* is most frequently practiced and is the term given to the injection of sclerosant without the aid of an oversheath.

Several techniques of sclerosant injection have been described (Fig. 38-13). In the United States and Great Britain, intravariceal sclerotherapy is practiced widely. This direct attack on the varix is associated with the best rates of control of acute bleeding. Paravariceal injection is commonly practiced in Europe and Japan, and involves submucosal injections of sclerosant between varices. The goal is to eradicate the submucosal space and compress the varices extrinsically. This approach may take several days to be effective and is not suited for controlling acute hemorrhage. One recent prospective study combining both techniques has been associated with promising results and a low incidence of local complications.[59]

Choice of Sclerosant

The ideal sclerosant has not been developed. The fatty acid–based sclerosants, such as sodium morrhuate and ethanolamine oleate, have a higher incidence of minor complications, such as fever, chest pain, and pleural effusion. Morrhuate is probably the most commonly used

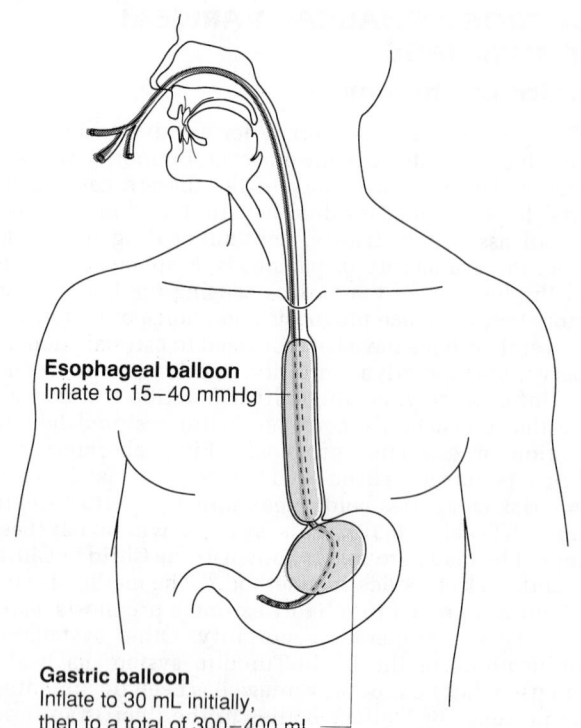

Esophageal balloon
Inflate to 15–40 mmHg

Gastric balloon
Inflate to 30 mL initially,
then to a total of 300–400 mL

Figure 38-12. The Sengstaken-Blakemore tube is used to tamponade acutely bleeding gastroesophageal varices. The tube has three lumens—one to aspirate the stomach, another to inflate the gastric balloon, and a third to inflate the esophageal balloon. Patients treated with balloon taponade should be in an intensive care unit, and almost all should have endotracheal tubes in place to avoid aspiration.

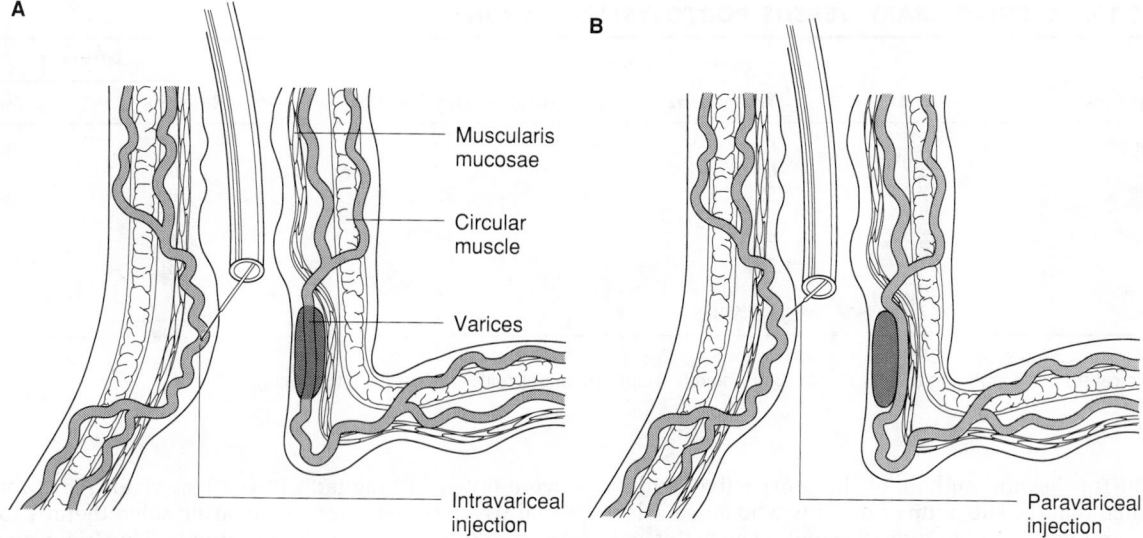

Figure 38-13. Techniques of intravariceal (*A*) and paravariceal (*B*) injection of esophageal varices.

sclerosant in the United States, whereas ethanolamine oleate is widely used in Europe. In a canine model of portal hypertension, 95% ethanol was shown to be associated with the highest incidence of injury to normal esophageal tissue.[59] The trend is toward the development of combination agents, such as a combination of sodium tetradecyl sulfate, ethanol, and cefazolin.[59]

Complications

Transient substernal chest pain is the most common esophageal complication of sclerotherapy and is thought to be caused by either esophageal spasm or mediastinitis. The treatment is expectant management. Dysphagia is relatively common and is usually associated with a distal esophageal stricture. No increase in gastroesophageal reflux has been detected. Stricture occurs in as many as 25% of sclerotherapy patients and is almost always treatable with esophageal dilatation.

The incidence of ulceration depends on the reporting criteria. When small areas of superficial mucosal slough are included, the incidence may be as high as 75%. Symptomatic ulcers, as defined by bleeding or delayed perforation, are much less common. Esophageal perforation is the most feared complication of sclerotherapy and comprises a spectrum of injury ranging from a localized injection site leak to a delayed postnecrotic perforation with pleural and mediastinal sepsis. Although the incidence of postnecrotic perforation is only 1%, the mortality rate is higher than 50%. The incidence of injection site leaks is about 8%, and these lesions can usually be treated with parenteral antibiotics and parenteral nutrition. Traumatic perforation has been rare since the advent of the flexible endoscope. Sclerotherapy-associated portal and mesenteric venous thrombosis does occur and must be considered when deciding whether to perform sclerotherapy in a patient who may subsequently require a portacaval shunt or hepatic transplantation.[60]

Cardiac complications, either caused by or associated with sclerotherapy, are rare but include cardiac arrest, coronary spasm, and tamponade. Pulmonary complications include asymptomatic pleural effusions, aspiration pneumonia, and acute respiratory diseases (ARDS). Aspiration pneumonia is common and is minimized by appropriate airway protection and minimal sedation. Sodium morrhu-

ate may cause an idiosyncratic pulmonary injury leading to ARDS in some patients. This dreaded complication presents as fulminant respiratory failure and may be confused with massive gastric aspiration.

Bacteremia may occur during sclerotherapy. Reported rates of bacteremia are as high as 16%.[60] Spontaneous bacterial peritonitis may occur after sclerotherapy, and patients with ascites should probably receive antibiotic prophylaxis. Perinephric abscess, brain abscess, and bacterial endocarditis have also been reported. Prophylactic parenteral antibiotics should be used for patients with prosthetic valves, previous endocarditis, rheumatic valvular disease, idiopathic hypertrophic subaortic stenosis, patent ductus arteriosus, ventricular septal defect, and tetralogy of Fallot.

Sclerotherapy Versus Medical Management With Vasopressin and Balloon Tamponade

At least three clinical trials have demonstrated that emergent sclerotherapy is able to halt active variceal bleeding that fails to respond to more conservative measures.[61] Early mortality rates are generally decreased in sclerotherapy-treated patients. Sclerotherapy has proved more effective than balloon tamponade and vasopressin therapy in two trials and equally effective in a third. In one study, sclerotherapy provided an nearly 100% improved protection rate against recurrent variceal bleeding compared with balloon tamponade and was associated with fewer complications. The data suggest that sclerotherapy is more effective than conservative medical therapy, with no increase in the frequency or severity of complications.

Sclerotherapy Versus Surgery

Four prospective randomized trials have compared the relative efficacy of portosystemic shunting with sclerotherapy for controlling variceal hemorrhage. In a group of actively bleeding Child-Turcotte C patients, nonselective portal decompression or sclerotherapy was performed.[62] The other three trials compared shunting with sclerotherapy in an elective setting and included class A, B, and C patients.[63-65] The incidence of early rebleeding after treatment was clearly higher in the sclerotherapy group. Early survival was not influenced, but patients who received portacaval shunts generally died of hepatic failure, whereas sclerotherapy patients died primarily of bleeding

Table 38-16. SCLEROTHERAPY VERSUS PORTOSYSTEMIC SHUNT*

Investigators	Patients	Treatment	Rebleeding Rate (%)	Survival Rate (%)	Months
Warren et al[62]	36	ES	53	84	24
	35	DSRS	3	59	24
Cello et al[61]	32	ES	50	28	18
	32	PCS	19	13	18
Teres et al[64]	55	ES	38	71	24
	57	DSRS	14	68	24
Rikkers et al[63]	30	ES	57	61	25
	27	DSRS/PCS	19	65	25

ES, endoscopic sclerotherapy; DSRS, distal splenorenal shunt; PCS, portacaval shunt.
* From clinical studies comparing the results of portal systemic shunt operations with endoscopic sclerotherapy.

(Table 38-16). Several authors of the prospective studies commented that the subgroup of patients who failed sclerotherapy and proceeded to surgery actually had better survival rates than patients who were originally randomized to surgery. The ability of patients to survive a portosystemic shunt after sclerotherapy may be due to an improvement in hepatic risk status or to self-selection, because these patients have survived for a time and tolerated additional hemorrhage. A retrospective study of patients undergoing distal splenorenal shunting confirmed that hepatic risk status could be improved before surgery. Long-term survival was related to the hepatic risk status at the time of the index bleed, whereas operative mortality correlated with hepatic risk status at the time of surgery.[66]

The somewhat diminished survival of patients who underwent distal splenorenal shunting was attributed to the gradual development of hepatofugal flow through the portosystemic collaterals as measured by a decrease in galactose elimination capacity.[63] Prograde portal flow was maintained in the sclerotherapy patients.

Trials have been conducted comparing sclerotherapy with esophageal transection.[66] The risk of rebleeding was higher in the sclerotherapy patients, but no differences were noted in long-term (2-year) survival. A randomized trial was also performed comparing sclerotherapy to transection in high-risk cirrhotic patients. This trial also found that early mortality was higher in patients with transection but that long-term mortality was the same.[67] It appears that in terms of early mortality and potential resources saved, sclerotherapy is preferable to esophageal transection.

Long-Term Survival

The long-term survival of patients treated with sclerotherapy continues to be debated. Of five major randomized trials designed to study the outcome of sclerotherapy, only one showed a significant increase in survival. The Copenhagen multicenter trial suggested that sclerotherapy can reduce long-term mortality by more than 60%. This survival benefit was seen only in Child-Turcotte class A and B patients and was presumably due to the ability of sclerotherapy to decrease rebleeding.[68] Improved long-term survival has also been noted when sclerotherapy was compared with distal splenorenal shunt, presumably because sclerotherapy maintained prograde portal flow.[63] Metaanalysis has been performed on the data from seven randomized clinical trials evaluating the effect of repeated sclerotherapy on long-term survival. Metaanalysis demonstrated that sclerotherapy reduced the number of deaths by 25%.[69] In summary, the available data support the use of sclerotherapy as an effective way to prolong survival in patients who have experienced variceal hemorrhage.

Prophylaxis Against Variceal Hemorrhage

Mortality rates as high as 40% have been associated with the first episode of variceal hemorrhage and have prompted the study of measures to prevent the first hemorrhage.[70,71] In the 1960s, several prospective studies were published in which patients were assigned to to undergo either a portacaval shunt or to be treated expectantly. All patients with varices that had not yet bled were included, although we now know that one third to one half of these patients probably would have never bled. No benefit was seen with prophylactic shunts, and they are no longer performed.

Two multicenter, randomized trials have investigated propranolol administration to prevent the first episode of variceal hemorrhage in cirrhotic patients; both were associated with encouraging results. After a 2-year observation period, cumulative patient survival was better in the propranolol group than in the placebo group.[72] An American trial also showed decreased bleeding in patients treated with propranolol, but no improvement in survival was

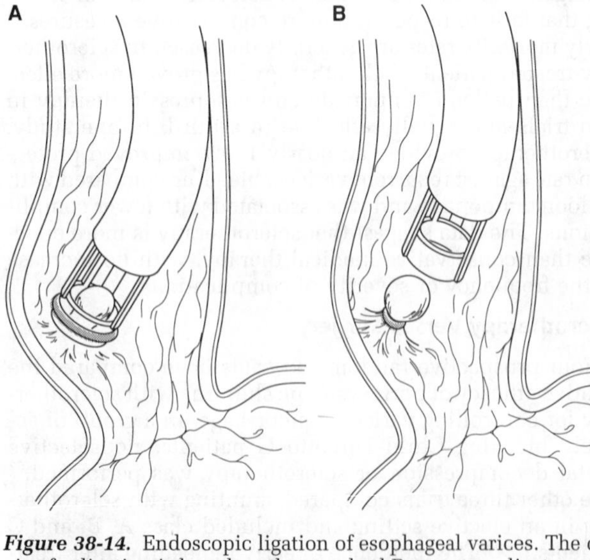

Figure 38-14. Endoscopic ligation of esophageal varices. The device for ligation is based on the standard Barron-type ligater used in the treatment of anal hemorrhoids. The esophageal varix is drawn up into the ligating device with suction (*A*), and the base of the varix is ligated with an O-ring (*B*). Up to six varices can be treated at a single session.

seen.[73] Such positive early results must be tempered with caution because recent studies suggest that propranolol has a minimal effect even in patients who have already bled.

A number of prospective, controlled trials of prophylactic sclerotherapy have been done and suggest that sclerotherapy in appropriately selected patients can prevent the risk of hemorrhage. A group of 109 patients with cirrhosis and endoscopically proven varices were randomly assigned to treatment with or without sclerotherapy. The frequency of bleeding was diminished from 57% to 9%.[74] A series of 95 patients, predominantly Child-Turcotte class C with large varices, were randomly assigned to receive sclerotherapy or no treatment.[75] With an average follow-up of 13 months, bleeding occurred in 53% of controls but in only 22% of sclerotherapy-treated patients. Some of the

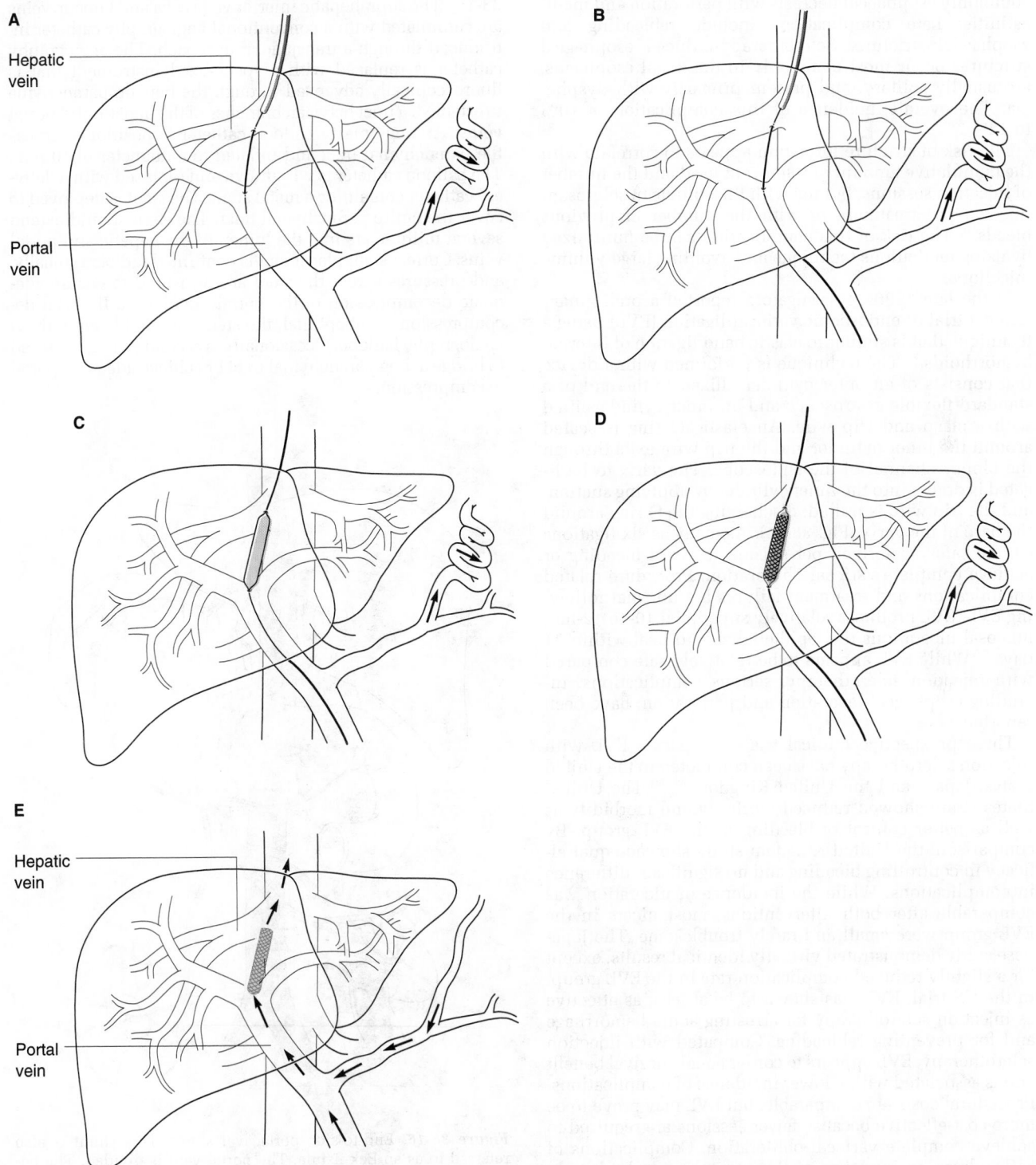

Figure 38-15. Schematic representation of steps used to create a transjugular intrahepatic portosystemic shunt. (After Zemel G, Katzen BT, Becker GJ, Benanati JF, Sallee S. Percutaneous transjugular portosystemic shunt. JAMA 1991;266:390)

beneficial effect of sclerotherapy appears to be lost as mean follow-up time extends beyond 36 months.

Endoscopic Variceal Ligation

Sclerotherapy is an effective treatment for variceal bleeding and, when used in conjunction with other medical measures, improves long-term survival compared with medical therapy alone. Early complications of sclerotherapy occur in about 30% of patients, including retrosternal pain, fever, hemorrhage from the injection site, and less commonly esophageal necrosis with perforation and mediastinitis. Late complications include rebleeding and esophageal stricture. Sclerotherapy-induced esophageal strictures occur most commonly in the distal esophagus, are usually solitary, and present primarily with dysphagia. The overall incidence of this complication is 10% to 12%.[69]

The risk of stricture formation appears to correlate with the cumulative amount of sclerosant used and the number of injection sessions, but not with the volume of sclerosant injected per treatment or with the number of previous bleeds.[76] The risk of this complication can be minimized by using meticulous technique and avoiding large-volume injections.

In the late 1980s, investigators reported a preliminary clinical trial of endoscopic variceal ligation (EVL) using a technique that is similar to elastic band ligation of internal hemorrhoids.[77] The technique is performed with a device that consists of an outer cylinder affixed to the end of a standard flexible gastroscope and an inner cylinder fitted with a clasp and trip wire. An elastic O ring is seated around the inner cylinder and the trip wire exits through the biopsy channel of the endoscope. The varix to be ligated is drawn into the inner cylinder by applying suction, and the trip wire is pulled, discharging the O ring around the base of the varix (Fig. 38-14). As many as six ligations can be safely performed per session to arrest bleeding or achieve complete variceal obliteration. Procedure-related complications and treatment failures are unusual following EVL. EVL produces relatively superficial 10- to 12-mm mucosal ulcerations that epithelialize and heal within 21 days.[77] While EVL appears to be relatively safe compared with injection sclerotherapy, serious complications, including esophageal laceration and perforation, have been reported.

Three prospective clinical trials comparing EVL with injection sclerotherapy have been conducted in the United States, Japan, and the United Kingdom.[78-80] The United States study showed reduced mortality and morbidity as well as better control of bleeding in the EVL group. By comparison, the United Kingdom study showed equal efficacy in controlling bleeding and no significant difference in complications. While the incidence of ulceration was comparable after both interventions, most ulcers in the EVL group were small and rarely troublesome. The Japanese study demonstrated virtually identical results, except for a slightly reduced complication rate in the EVL group. In the US trial, EVL was shown to be at least as effective as injection sclerotherapy for arresting acute hemorrhage and for preventing rebleeding. Compared with injection sclerotherapy, EVL appears to confer equal survival benefit and is associated with a lower incidence of complications. Procedural costs are comparable, but EVL may prove to be more cost-effective because fewer sessions are required to achieve complete variceal obliteration. Complications of EVL related to insertion of the overtube can be largely overcome by introducing it over a tapered dilator rather than an endoscope.

TIPS is a new investigational therapy that has shown considerable promise for managing variceal hemorrhage. The concept of creating an intrahepatic portosystemic shunt by establishing an artificial fistula between branches of the the portal vein and the systemic circulation was proposed 20 years ago and has since undergone many modifications and improvements.[81] Early efforts were complicated by a high incidence of stenosis despite repeated attempts at balloon dilation.

The development of an implantable, expandable metal stent enhanced the applicability of TIPS in humans.[82] More recently, the TIPS technique has been standardized[83] (Fig. 38-15). The suprahepatic inferior vena cava and hepatic veins are cannulated with a conventional angiography catheter introduced through a transjugular approach. The angiography catheter is replaced with a specialized instrument that is fluoroscopically advanced through the hepatic parenchyma to establish a tract between branches of the hepatic and portal veins. An angioplasty balloon catheter is positioned across the parenchymal tract and inflated to a diameter of 10 mm. The balloon catheter is withdrawn and replaced with a delivery catheter containing a metal stent. The stent is deployed to cover the entire parenchymal tract. The stent should extend several millimeters into the lumen of the hepatic and portal veins. Correct stent placement is confirmed radiographically, and pressures across the stent are measured to ensure adequate decompression of the portal circulation. If portal decompression is suboptimal, the stent can be dilated with an angiography balloon. Occasionally, a second stent is required to bridge a long parenchymal tract or achieve adequate portal decompression.

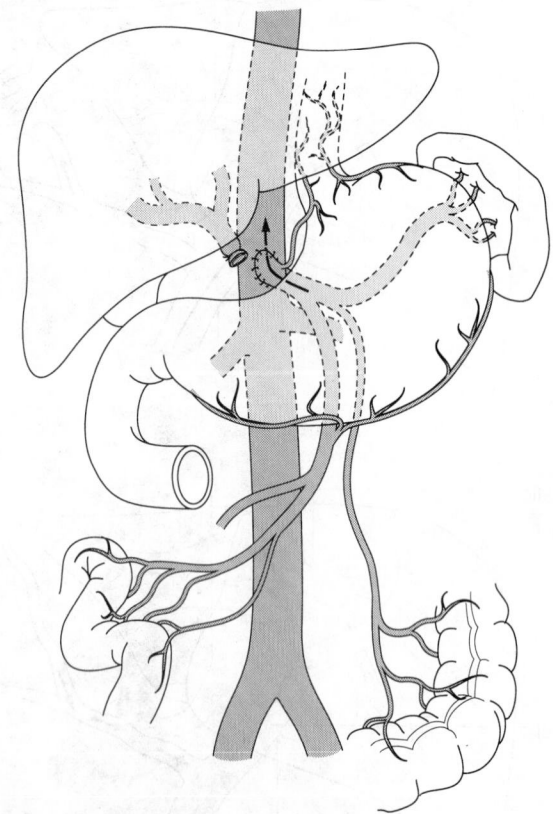

Figure 38-16. End-to-side portacaval shunt. This shunt is also referred to as an Eck fistula. The portal vein is divided. The hepatic limb of the portal vein is ligated. The splanchnic end of the portal vein is anastomosed end to side to the vena cava. All portal blood is necessarily diverted into the cava, and the hepatic limb of the portal vein cannot serve as an outflow track.

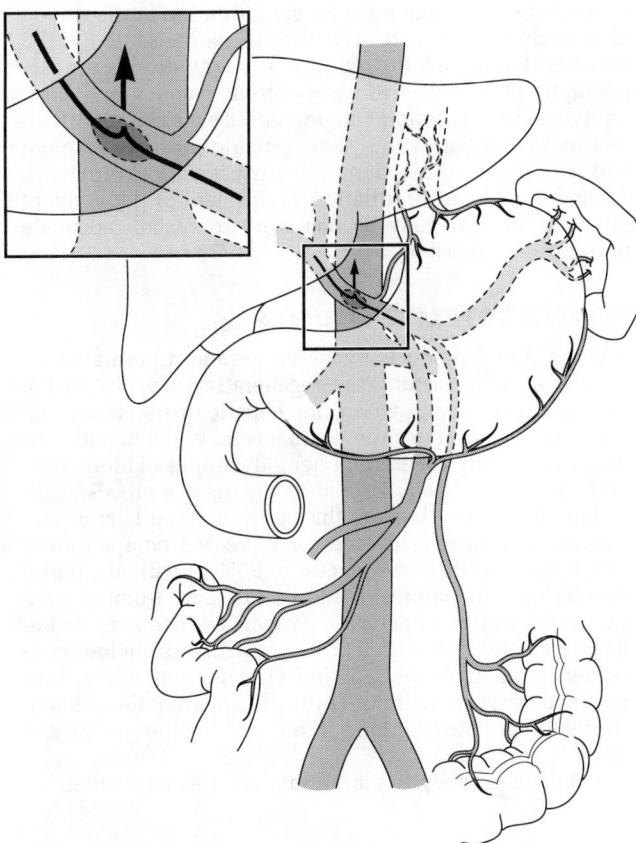

Figure 38-17. Side-to-side portacaval shunt. An anastomosis is made between the side of the portal vein and the side of the inferior vena cava. With a standard diameter shunt, almost all splanchnic blood is diverted around the liver into the low-pressure vena cava. The hepatic limb of the portal vein serves as an outflow track from the liver toward the low-pressure vena cava.

A number of studies have demonstrated the efficacy and safety of TIPS in patients with portal hypertension and variceal bleeding. Stents can be implanted successfully in about 90% of patients with a procedure-related mortality rate of less than 10%.[84] Significant reduction of portal pressure (more than 50%) is usually achieved and provides immediate and sustained control of variceal bleeding. Because TIPS is hemodynamically similar to a side-to-side portosystemic shunt, it has proved to be of practical benefit to selected patients with ascites or hydrothorax that are unresponsive to conventional treatment.[85] Although most patients become more responsive to diuretic therapy, a significant number die or develop disabling encephalopathy, thus detracting from the overall efficacy of the procedure. TIPS has also been used successfully to treat patients with Budd-Chiari Syndrome.[86] The role of TIPS in this setting is less clear because portacaval or mesoatrial shunts and orthotopic liver transplantation have been used with success. TIPS may be useful in selected patients with high-grade obstruction of the retrohepatic inferior vena cava or mesenteric venous anatomy that precludes standard portacaval or mesoatrial shunts.

Firm clinical data indicate that TIPS effectively controls acute variceal hemorrhage in patients with portal hypertension, regardless of the etiology of the underlying liver disease or the degree of hepatic decompensation. Protracted bleeding with hemodynamic instability, progressive coagulopathy, and visceral hypoperfusion invariably lead to liver failure and death. TIPS may be life-saving, especially if conventional treatment fails to adequately control variceal bleeding. Liver transplantation in this setting is associated with prohibitve morbidity and mortality rates.[87] In this setting, TIPS can be performed with greater ease and safety than a portosystemic shunt.

TIPS has also been used for preoperative portal decompression to facilitate orthotopic liver transplantation. Liver transplantation in the presence of a portosystemic shunt is associated with longer operating time, increased operative blood loss, longer hospital stay and possibly decreased survival.[88] Pretransplant TIPS should reduce portal pressure, thereby reducing operative time and blood loss. In practice, TIPS has been shown to have only a limited impact in this group of patients.[88] TIPS also must be used cautiously in transplant candidates with poor liver function to avoid the potential risk of accelerated hepatic dysfunction due to decreased portal perfusion. In one recent study of TIPS patients evaluated for orthotopic liver transplantation, only 50% required transplantation within 2 months of portal decompression. Of the remaining patients, one third remained as potential transplant candidates and two thirds were well and did not require transplantation.[88]

The major complications of TIPS include encephalopathy and stenosis or occlusion of the stent. Encephalopathy occurs in 10% to 20% of patients after TIPS and is managed with dietary protein restriction and lactulose.[89] This complication appears to correlate with increasing age of the patient and increased shunt diameter and shunt flow.

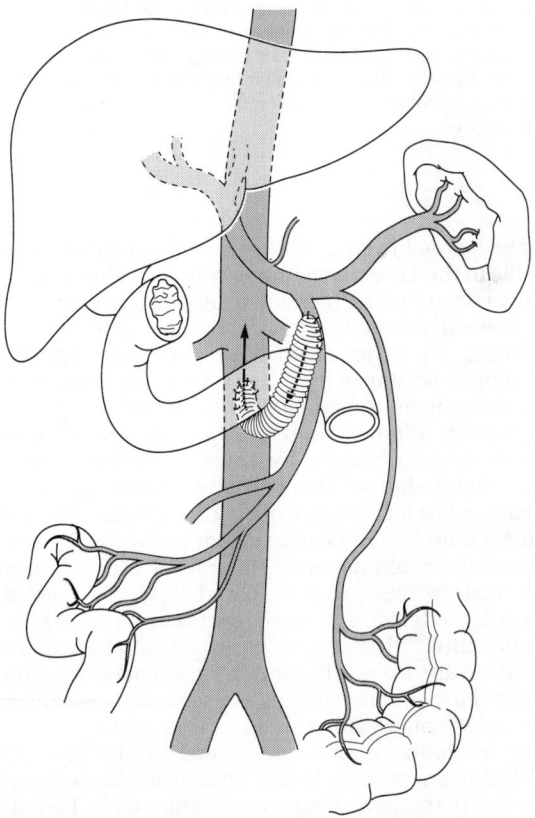

Figure 38-18. Interposition mesocaval shunt. A plastic prosthesis or an autogenous internal jugular vein is used for the shunt. One end is anastomosed to the inferior vena cava, and the other end is anastomosed to the trunk of the superior mesenteric vein. The shunt curves around the lower edge of the third portion of the duodenum and is sometimes called a C shunt.

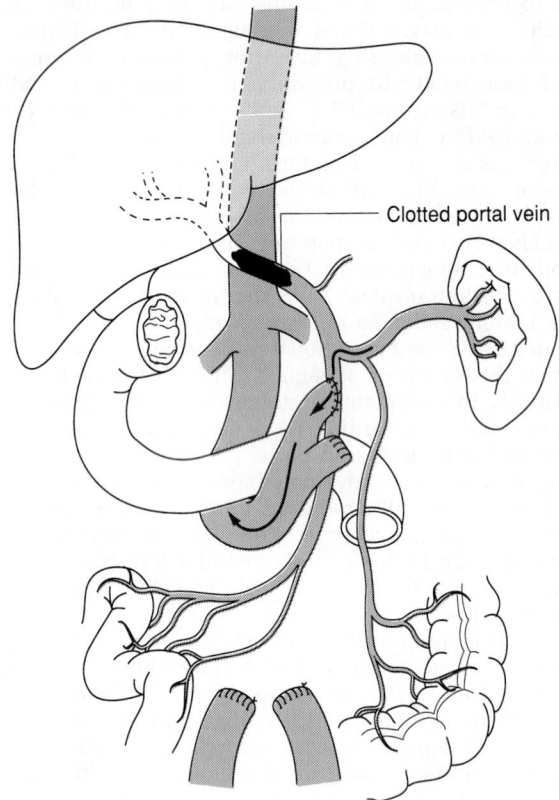

Figure 38-19. Marion-Clatworthy cavomesal shunt. This shunt was designed for use in small children with thrombosed portal veins. The distal end of the vena cava or the limbs of the iliac veins are divided. The proximal end of the iliac vein or cava are then anastomosed to the side of the trunk of the superior mesenteric vein. Small children can tolerate division of the cava without developing chronic lower extremity edema or chronic venous insufficiency.

Lessons learned from portosystemic shunt surgery are applicable to the TIPS procedure as well. Initially, total surgical diversion of portal blood flow into the systemic circulation seemed desirable to minimize the risk of variceal rebleeding. However, about 40% of patients undergoing total shunts developed disabling symptoms of encephalopathy. Subsequent experience with "selective" portal decompression afforded by the distal splenorenal shunt or "partial" portal diversion by a small-caliber interposition H-graft shunt showed that partially preserving portal hypertension has a protective effect on liver function. Shunt diameter must be sufficient to reduce portal pressure below a critical threshold necessary to prevent variceal bleeding while maintaining prograde portal flow and mesenteric venous hypertension, thereby decreasing the risk of encephalopathy.[90] Radiologically placed intrahepatic stents generally vary from 7 to 10 mm in diameter and appear to have the same physiologic consequences as surgically constructed small-caliber interposition grafts.

The development of pseudointimal hyperplasia following TIPS is unpredictable and often leads to stenosis and occlusion of the stent. Progressive reduction in TIPS diameter increases the portosystemic pressure gradient and the risk of variceal rebleeding. Color duplex ultrasonography has been shown to be a reliable noninvasive method for assessing TIPS patency and blood flow. In one study of TIPS patients evaluated prospectively with color duplex ultrasonography, progressively decreasing flows or flow

reversal indicated the need for stent dilation or placement of a second stent in nearly 20% of patients.[91] All TIPS patients should be followed carefully with duplex ultrasonography at intervals to assess shunt patency and flow. Equivocal results prompt angiographic evaluation with direct measurement of the portosystemic pressure gradient and with contrast injection to identify technical problems. As mentioned earlier, dilation of the stent or deployment of a second stent may be necessary to sustain adequate portal decompression.

PORTOSYSTEMIC SHUNTS

When portal blood is bypassed around a normal liver, hepatic atrophy occurs, the regenerative capacity of the liver is impaired, and with time, hepatic insufficiency, encephalopathy, and usually death ensue. When hepatic cirrhosis is present, the normal hemodynamics of blood flow to the liver are already altered by the disease process. Portal blood bypasses the liver through venous collaterals and varices, and varying degrees of increased compensatory hepatic arterial flow may occur. In 20% of patients, portal flow becomes hepatofugal, and portal vein thrombosis occurs in 5% to 10% of patients. Patients with hepatic cirrhosis tolerate diverting surgical shunts with less obvious consequences than do normal individuals, and many have survived for years without clinically apparent detrimental effects after construction of an end-to-side portacaval shunt.[92]

Although portosystemic shunts are the most effective

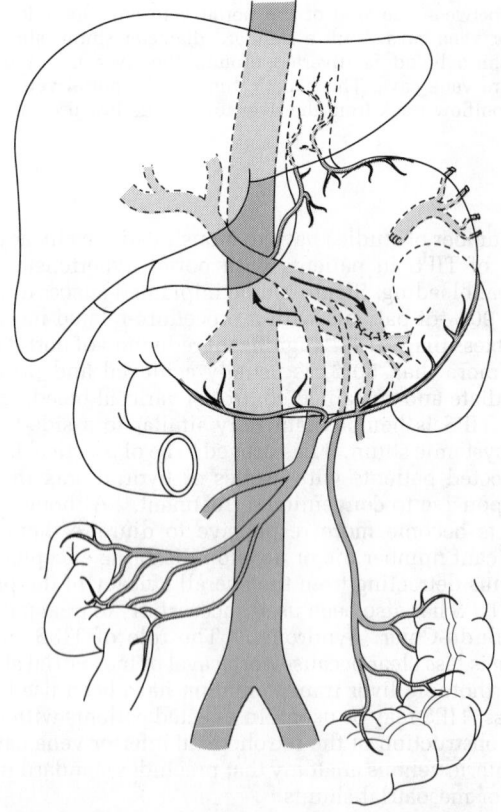

Figure 38-20. Central splenorenal shunt after the spleen is excised. A splenectomy is performed and the splenic vein is mobilized. The central (proximal) end of the splenic vein is anastomosed to the side of the renal vein. The portal system is decompressed through the splenic vein into the left renal vein and vena cava.

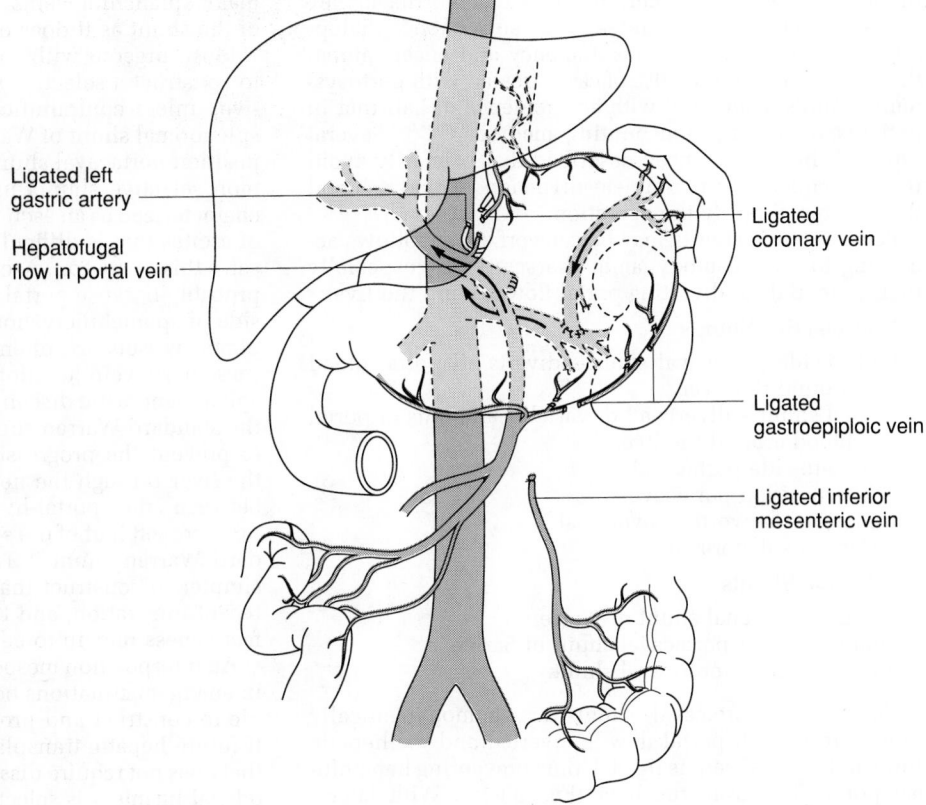

Figure 38-21. Distal splenorenal Warren shunt. The splenic vein is divided near its junction with the superior mesenteric vein. The distal end of the splenic vein is anastomosed to the renal vein. Varices are selectively decompressed through the stomach and short gastric veins into the splenic vein and then into the vena cava through the renal vein. Portal hypertension is maintained in the portal and superior mesenteric vein to provide enough pressure to drive portal blood through the diseased liver.

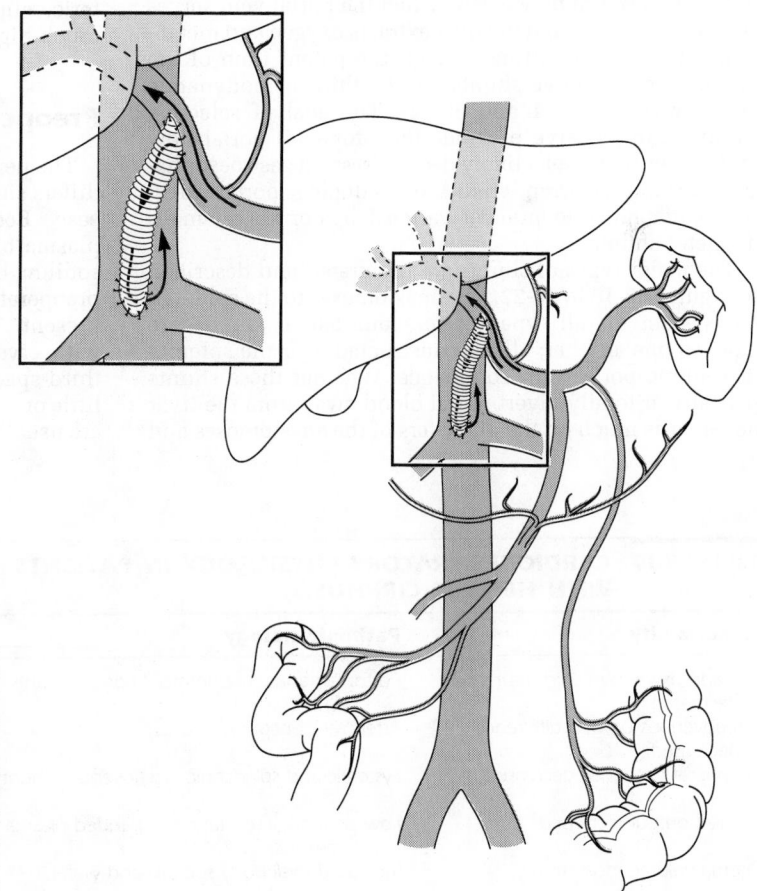

Figure 38-22. Small-diameter interposition portacaval Sarfeh shunt. A vascular prosthesis measuring 8 to 10 mm in diameter is interposed between the side of the vena cava and the side of the portal vein. The goal is to partially reduce portal pressure and thereby prevent variceal hemorrhage but still maintain sufficient pressure to permit prograde flow of portal blood to the liver. This procedure is simpler to perform than that for the Warren shunt and theoretically avoids the problem of an increasing proportion of portal blood being diverted away from the liver over time, as occurs with the Warren shunt.

therapy for preventing recurrent variceal hemorrhage, they are associated with an increased incidence of encephalopathy. Progressive hepatic insufficiency and encephalopathy are seen in 30% to 50% of cases treated with portosystemic shunts, compared with an incidence of half that in patients treated by nonshunting methods.[61,63,64] Several types of shunts have been described that primarily avoid the consequences of complete diversion of portal blood flow or that simplify the operation.

Portosystemic shunts may be categorized as follows according to their hemodynamic characteristics, especially their potential for diverting portal flow around the liver:

Nonselective Shunts

End-to-side portacaval shunt—diverts all portal blood around the liver
Lateral shunt—diverts all or variable amounts of portal blood around the liver
   Side-to-side portacaval
   Interposition portacaval
   Marion-Clatworthy cavomesal
   Central splenorenal

Selective Shunts

Distal splenorenal shunt of Warren
Small-diameter portacaval shunt of Sarfeh
Small-diameter mesocaval shunt

End-to-side portacaval shunts are hemodynamically unique in that all portal flow is diverted and the hepatic limb of the portal vein is ligated, thus preventing hepatofugal portal flow from the liver (Fig. 38-16). With lateral shunts, a direct or indirect side-to-side lateral connection is constructed between the splanchnic and systemic systems, and the hepatic limb of the portal vein remains patent (Figs. 38-17 to 38-20). A greater compensatory increase in hepatic arterial flow occurs when the portal vein serves as an outflow tract and the liver extracts oxygen and metabolites from blood exiting through the patent limb of the portal vein. Selective shunts are the third hemodynamic category (Figs. 38-21 and 38-22). The goal of selective shunts is to preserve prograde (hepatopedal) portal flow to the liver while selectively decompressing gastroesophageal varices (Warren shunt) or reducing portal pressure sufficiently to prevent variceal hemorrhage (small-diameter shunts).

The major types of shunts are illustrated and described in Figures 38-16 to 38-22. The anastomoses to the splanchnic system for all types of the four lateral shunts are close to one another; all are constructed near the splenic-mesenteric-portal vein confluence. Whether these shunts partially or totally divert portal blood away from the liver depends as much on the diameters of the anastomoses and

major splanchnic veins and the details of the construction of the shunt as it does on the type of lateral shunt.

Most surgeons with a special interest in this field attempt to construct a selective shunt when the operation is elective, unless contraindications are present.[63,93] The distal splenorenal shunt of Warren and the small-diameter interposition portacaval shunt of Sarfeh are the two most common selective shunts used. The Warren shunt has been characterized as an ascitogenic operation, and the presence of ascites that is difficult to control medically contraindicates this operation. Ascites may increase postoperatively, probably because portal hypertension persists in the right side of splanchnic venous system and because large lymphatic vessels are often divided near the splenic vein–mesenteric vein junction during the dissection. Complete splenopancreatic disconnection is a recent modification of the standard Warren shunt. This modification is designed to prevent the progressive shunting of blood away from the liver through the new collaterals that form over time between the portal-hypertensive right and the low-pressure left half of the splanchnic venous bed after a standard Warren shunt.[94] The Sarfeh shunt, although much simpler to construct than a Warren shunt, is a relatively recent innovation, and the long-term patency rate and effectiveness remain to be determined.[95]

An interposition mesocaval shunt is frequently preferred in emergent situations because the shunt is relatively simple to construct and promptly halts variceal hemorrhage. If future hepatic transplantation is contemplated, a shunt that does not require dissection in the area of the hepatoduodenal ligament is selected. A distal splenorenal shunt in elective circumstances or an interposition mesocaval shunt to halt acute variceal hemorrhage is recommended.[96] Other types of shunts, usually using smaller splanchnic veins such as the left gastric (coronary) or inferior mesenteric vein, have been described, but the thrombosis rate is much higher than with a standard shunt.

Preoperative and Postoperative Care

The perioperative care of patients with hepatic cirrhosis differs significantly from that of patients without liver disease. Because these patients already have expanded plasma and interstitial spaces and increased total body sodium, both sodium and water replacement are restricted preoperatively and postoperatively, especially if ascites is present. Third-space losses are replaced conservatively with crystalloid in the early postoperative phase. After third-space fluid sequestration has been replaced, usually little or no additional sodium is administered. The patients are usually receiving sufficient sodium because most drugs

---

Table 38-17. CARDIORESPIRATORY PHYSIOLOGY IN PATIENTS WITH HEPATIC CIRRHOSIS

Abnormality	Pathophysiology	Physical Signs
Po₂ and oxyhemoglobin saturation decreased	Portopulmonary and intrapulmonary shunts	Cyanosis, clubbing of fingers
Arteriovenous oxygen difference decreased	Arteriolar or capillary shunts	Palmer erythema, spider telangiectasia
Peripheral resistance decreased	Systemic and splanchnic arteriovenous shunts	Tendency to hypotension, hypertension unusual, widened pulse pressure
Cardiac output increased	Low peripheral resistance, expanded plasma volume	Systolic ejection murmur, short occlusion time, rapid pulse
Plasma volume increased	Increased total body sodium and water, secondary aldosteronism	Edema, ascites, high-output cardiac failure if severe

are in the form of a sodium salt and all blood products contain substantial quantities of sodium. Patients with cirrhosis tend to be deficient in total body potassium. Proper management requires careful monitoring and generous replacement of this electrolyte.

Most patients with liver disease have significant alterations in their cardiorespiratory physiology (Table 38-17). Arterial oxygen pressure tends to be low, cardiac output may be high, peripheral resistance can be as low as one third of normal, and plasma volume is often expanded. The baseline values for blood gas and Swan-Ganz pressure and cardiac output determinations may vary substantially from normal ranges. These baseline deviations from normal should be corrected when severe and need to be taken into account when interpreting blood gas and pulmonary artery studies both before and after operation.

Most patients with significant liver disease have abnormalities in their coagulation systems. If secondary hypersplenism is also present, the platelet count as well as the red and white blood cell counts may be low. Generous replacement with fresh frozen plasma, platelets, and cryoprecipitate (factor VIII) is almost always needed intraoperatively and should be continued postoperatively until the coagulation status has stabilized and all bleeding has halted. Coagulation factors should be replaced prophylactically rather than risking major hemorrhage. If therapy is withheld until the coagulation studies are severely abnormal or until bleeding occurs, the abnormalities are difficult to correct and often more blood and blood components are consumed than if prophylactic treatment had been instituted.

Many patients with cirrhosis are protein depleted and malnourished. Special attention to nutrition is indicated. As much as twice the normal caloric intake may be needed to achieve caloric balance. Most patients tolerate intravenous hyperalimentation, provided that excessive amounts of protein or amino acids are not infused. Early enteral feeding is also desirable to help avoid infection secondary to bacteria translocated from the gut. Vitamin deficiencies, especially of vitamins A, D, K, and B, may be present and extra supplementation is recommended. Magnesium, zinc, calcium, or phosphorous may be low. These should be monitored and replaced if needed. Some surgeons administer extra glucose and insulin, so-called hepatotrophic factors, in an attempt to prevent the onset of hepatic failure.

Results of Decompressive Operations

Postoperative mortality and long-term prognosis in patients with bleeding varices are directly related to the natural history of the underlying liver disease and the hepatic

Table 38-18. RESULTS OF PORTAL DECOMPRESSION WITH FOUR DIFFERENT TYPES OF SHUNTS

Investigators	Type of Shunt	Patients	Operative and Long-Term Mortality Rate
Henderson et al[94]	Distal splenorectal shunt with pancreatic disconnection	78	30%
Pacquet et al[97]	Mesocaval	100	35% (5 y)
Turcotte et al[98]	Portacaval	146	49% (3 y)
Malt et al[99]	Central splenorenal	52	52% (3 y)

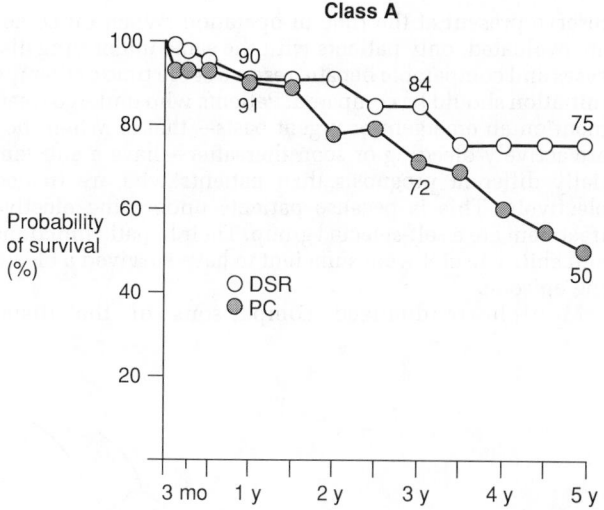

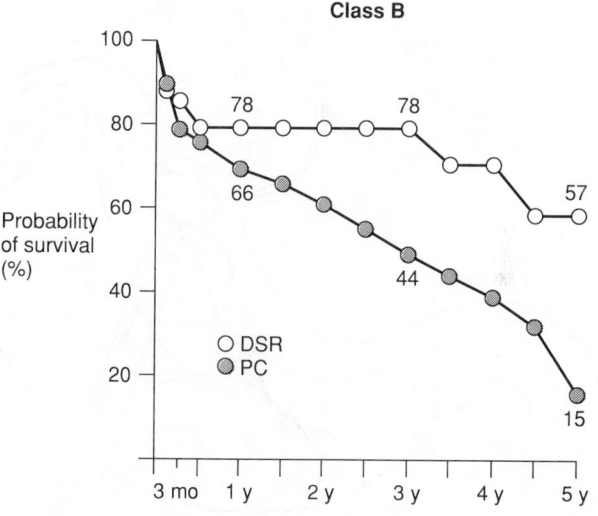

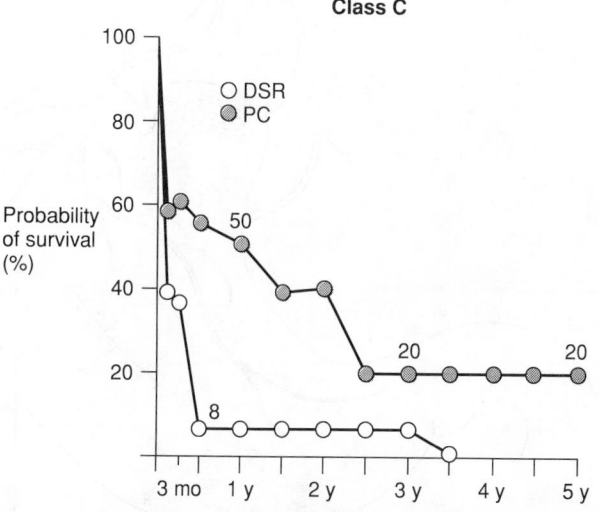

Figure 38-23. Comparison of distal splenorenal (DSR) shunts with elective portacaval (PC) shunts. Almost all of the patients had hepatic cirrhosis, and most had alcoholic cirrhosis. Operative mortality is included in these actuarial survival probabilities. Classes A, B, and C refer to the Child-Turcotte hepatic risk classification.

reserve present at the time of operation. When outcomes are evaluated, only patients with the same underlying diseases and comparable hepatic reserve at the time of therapy initiation should be compared. Patients who undergo treatment on an emergent or urgent basis—that is, when they are actively bleeding or soon thereafter—have a substantially different prognosis than patients who are treated electively. This is because patients undergoing elective treatment are a self-selected group. Their hepatic functions and ability to clot were sufficient to have survived a bleeding episode.

Multiple randomized comparisons of the distal

splenorenal shunt with other types of portosystemic shunts have been reported. Operative mortality and long-term prognosis are similar, but patients undergoing distal splenorenal shunts develop less encephalopathy. Less encephalopathy is also seen after the selective Sarfeh shunt and after nonshunting procedures, such as sclerotherapy or devascularization. When comparing shunts with nonshunting procedures, only minor differences in long-term survival are reported, but the mode of death usually changes. With nonshunting procedures, a greater proportion of patients die of recurrent hemorrhage. After construction of a shunt, a greater

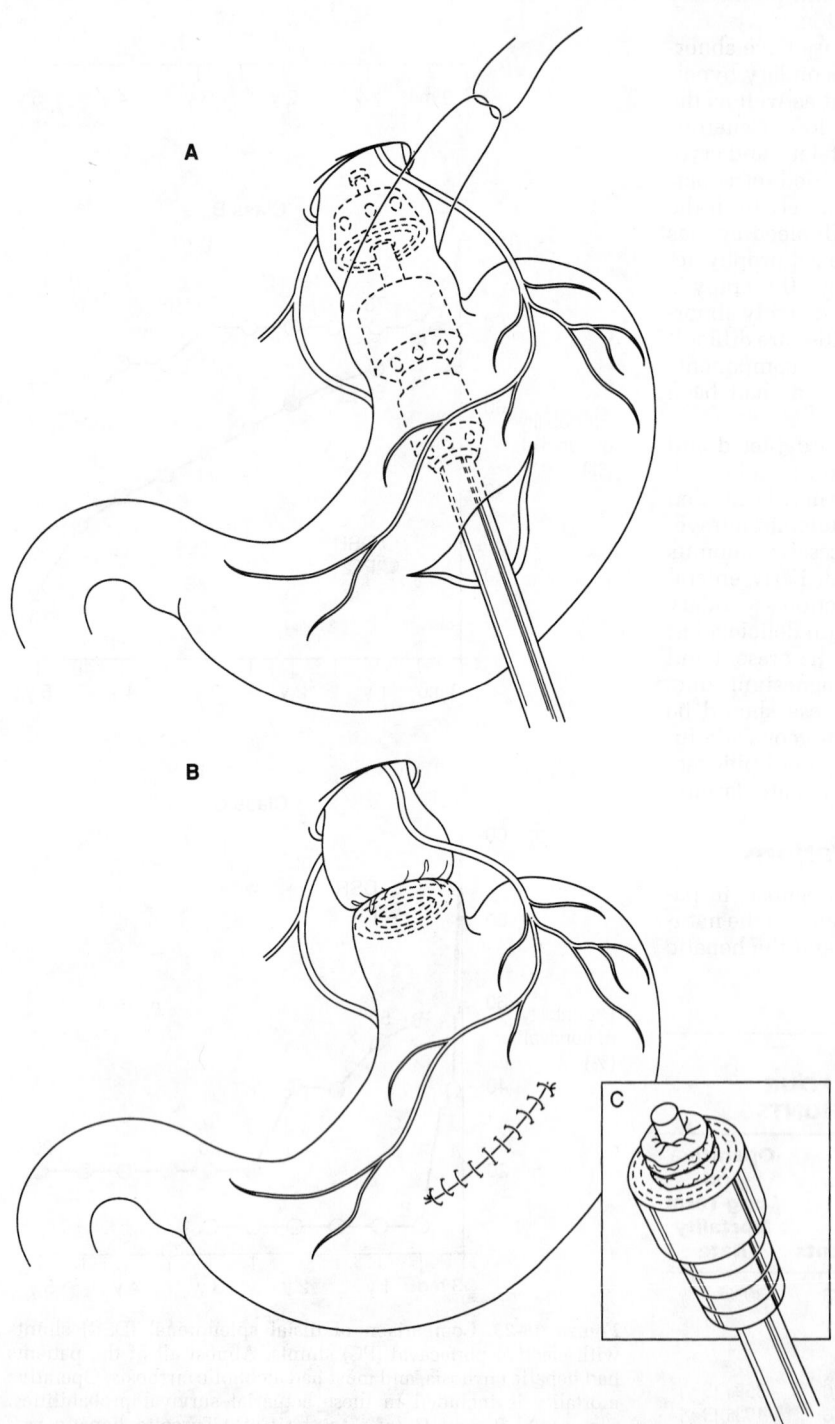

Figure 38-24. Transection and reanastomosis of the distal esophagus with the stapling device to control variceal hemorrhage. (*A*) A stapling device is inserted through a small gastrotomy incision. (*B*) When the device is fired, the esophagus is simultaneously transected and reanastomosed with staples. (*C*) If the device fires correctly, a complete ring of esophageal tissue is excised.

proportion die of hepatic failure. Table 38-18 summarizes the results of some major series on the different types of shunts. Figure 38-23 compares the results of portacaval shunts with distal splenorenal shunts. The class-A patient's 3-year actuarial survival rate, including operative mortality, is 83.6% for distal splenorenal shunts; for class B, it is 77.8%. This is a substantial improvement over previous experience with portacaval shunts. The results with a distal splenorenal shunt in class-A and -B patients are probably better than could be achieved with hepatic transplantation.

DEVASCULARIZATION AND TRANSECTION PROCEDURES

A wide variety of nonshunting procedures to treat gastroesophageal hemorrhage have been described. These range from simple transection or stapling of the esophagus or proximal stomach to extensive esophagogastric devascularization and splenectomy. At times, esophagogastric resection with jejunal or colonic interposition has been used. Transection of the esophagus or stomach interrupts the submucosal as well as the intermuscular venous collateral vessels. Splenectomy eliminates the splenic component of portal blood flow that may temporarily lower portal pressure.

Esophageal or Gastric Transection Alone

Most esophageal or gastric transection procedures are now performed with stapling devices. An end-to-end stapling instrument can be introduced into the esophagus through a small gastrotomy incision. The distal esophagus is both transected and reanastomosed with staples when the device is triggered (Fig. 38-24). Straight stapling devices can be used to divide and staple the stomach. Urgent

or emergent esophageal transection is associated with a mortality rate of 28% to 60%.[97] Perioperative complications include leaks due to faulty technique, ischemia, and stenosis of the anastomosis. Late complications of esophageal transection are stricture formation and recurrence of variceal bleeding. Recurrent variceal bleeding occurs in 15% to 50% of patients. Some patients with recurrent varices can be treated successfully with sclerotherapy.

In the 1970s, Sugiura and Futagawa[98] described an extensive devascularization and transection procedure performed through separate abdominal and thoracic incisions (Fig. 38-25). The excellent results achieved by these authors have not been duplicated by Western surgeons. The results of Sugiura and Futagawa are difficult to apply to experience in the United States, because only 25% of their patients had hepatic cirrhosis. The procedure is only used selectively in the United States. Key elements of the operation are devascularization of the distal 6 to 8 cm of esophagus, devascularization of the greater curve of the stomach to the level of the incisura, highly selective or parietal cell vagotomy, transection and reanastomosis of the esophagus, and splenectomy.

The precise role of devascularization and transection procedures is unclear. Some surgeons believe that devascularization and transection procedures should be considered in selected, good-risk patients in whom sclerotherapy is not feasible or has failed, and especially in patients in whom the three major splanchnic veins (portal, splenic, and superior mesenteric) are thrombosed, thus precluding the construction of a standard shunt.

PORTAL HYPERTENSION IN CHILDREN

The cause of portal hypertension in children differs significantly from adults. Portal vein thrombosis accounts for about half of the cases. Posthepatitic cirrhosis or chronic

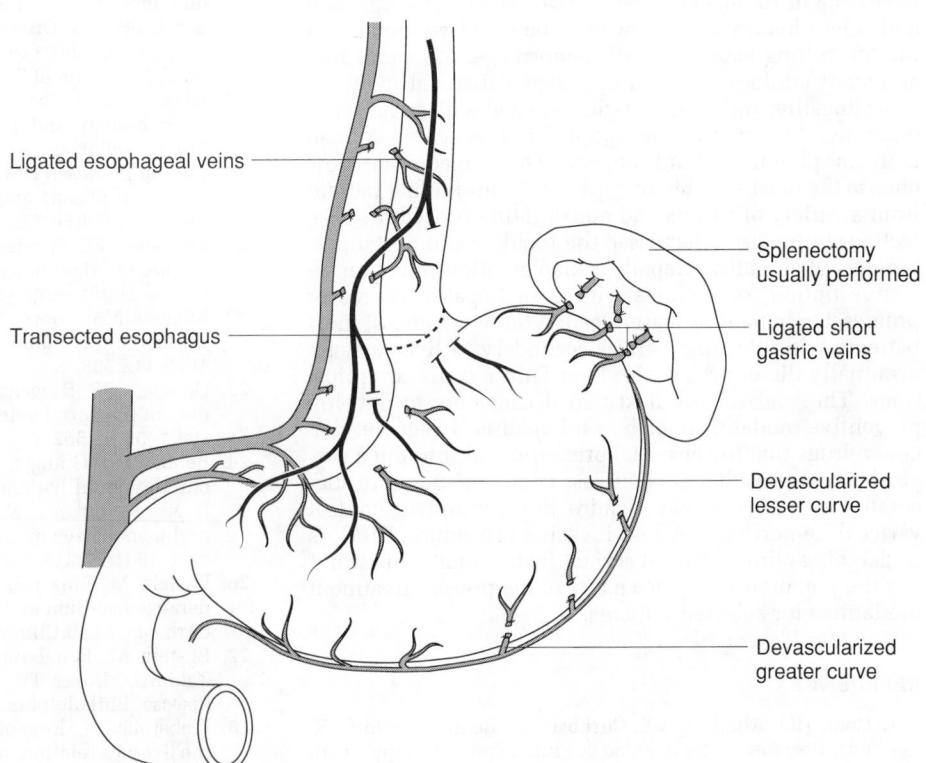

Ligated esophageal veins

Transected esophagus

Splenectomy usually performed

Ligated short gastric veins

Devascularized lesser curve

Devascularized greater curve

Figure 38-25. Sugiura esophageal transection and devascularization operation.

active hepatitis is the second most common cause. Various congenital defects, such as congenital hepatic fibrosis, may also cause portal hypertension. Inborn errors of metabolism that lead to cirrhosis or abnormal deposition of lipid in the liver are occasionally seen. Some of these latter patients are best treated with hepatic transplantation if the inherited disease is known to be progressive or fatal, and especially if the transplant also corrects the genetic enzymatic or metabolic defect. Common causes in adults also occur in children. Frequently, a liver biopsy is necessary to differentiate the underlying hepatic disease and select the appropriate treatment.

In children, sclerotherapy has almost completely replaced other forms of treatment for bleeding varices. Long-term success rates in over 90% of patients have been reported.[99] Shunts are indicated for the few sclerotherapy failures or when the family may be noncompliant with the follow-up necessary for successful serial sclerotherapy. Excellent survival without significant encephalopathy can be achieved in children with noncirrhotic forms of portal hypertension. The Marion-Clatworthy cavomesal shunt was specifically designed for the small child with a thrombosed portal vein. The relatively large diameter of this shunt avoids the high thrombosis rate accompanying central splenorenal shunts. Improvements in technique and instrumentation have made the central splenorenal shunt more successful in children in recent years, but the requirement for splenectomy is a major disadvantage of this shunt. In Europe, and increasingly in the United States, a popular shunt for small children with thrombosed portal veins is the jugular vein interposition mesocaval shunt.[100] This procedure avoids dividing the cava or implanting a plastic prosthesis. The shunt is quite feasible in small children because the internal jugular vein is relatively larger in this age group. Some surgeons prefer a distal splenorenal shunt if the splenic vein is at least 5 mm in diameter or a mesocaval jugular vein shunt when the splenic vein is less than 5 mm in diameter.

Major advances in the management of portal hypertension have been introduced in the past two decades. Vasopressin and sclerotherapy have proved to be effective modalities for controlling acute variceal hemorrhage. Most children and many adults with bleeding varices can avoid an operation altogether and be successfully treated with serial sclerotherapy. Mesenteric angiography has provided a road map for planning shunt surgery. The surgeon can now choose the most suitable therapy for the individual patient from a variety of shunts and nonshunting procedures. Selective shunts have decreased the incidence of postshunting encephalopathy. Hepatic transplantation offers an effective option for patients with poor hepatic reserve or progressive hepatic disease. Despite these advances, most patients with bleeding varices secondary to liver disease eventually die of progressive liver failure or its complications. The goals of the next two decades are to develop preventive modalities, such as a hepatitis B vaccine, discover drugs that lower portal pressure, and introduce surgical procedures that are both less complex and more successful for patients who require intervention to control variceal hemorrhage. A less invasive procedure, TIPS, is undergoing clinical trial at several institutions. This shunt has the potential to replace many of the present treatment modalities for selected patients.

REFERENCES

1. Conn HO, Atterbury CE. Cirrhosis. In: Schiff L, Schiff ER, eds. Diseases of the liver, ed 6. Philadelphia, JB Lippincott, 1987:725.
2. Gerber MA, Popper H. Relation between central canals and portal tracts in alcoholic hepatitis. Hum Pathol 1972;3:199.
3. Popper H. Pathologic aspects of cirrhosis: a review. Am J Pathol 1977;87:228.
4. Beswick DR, Boyer JL. Primary biliary cirrhosis. Hepatology 1984;4:295.
5. Chojkier M, Brenner DA. Therapeutic strategies for hepatic fibrosis. Hepatology 1988;8:176.
6. Sherlock S. Chronic hepatitis. In: Sherlock S, ed. Diseases of the liver and biliary system. London, Blackwell, 1989:348.
7. Ferenci P, Riederer P, Jellinger K, et al. Changes in gamma-aminobutyric acid receptors in patients with hepatic encephalopathy. Gastroenterology 1983;84:1381.
8. Dickson ER, Fleming CR, Ludwig J. Primary biliary cirrhosis. Perspect Liver Dis 1979;6:487.
9. Gines P, Quintero E, Arroyo V, et al. Compensated cirrhosis: natural history and prognostic factors. Hepatology 1987;7:122.
10. Powell WJ, Klatskin G. Duration of survival in patients with Laennec's cirrhosis. Am J Med 1968;44:406.
11. Harrid MA, Daries M, Mellon PJ, et al. Clinical monitoring of intracranial pressure in fulminant hepatic failure. Gut 1980;21:866.
12. Miller JD. Clinical aspects of intracranial pressure-volume relationships. In: McLaurin RL, ed. Head injuries. New York, Grune & Stratton, 1976:239.
13. O'Grady JG, Alexander GJM, Hayllar KM, et al. Early indicators of prognosis in fulminant hepatic failure. Gastroenterology 1989;97:439.
14. Sinclair SB, Greig PD, Blendis LM, et al. Biochemical and clinical response of fulminant viral hepatitis to administration of prostaglandin E. J Clin Invest 1989;84:1063.
15. Lieberman FL, Denison EK, Reynolds TB. The relationship of plasma volume, portal hypertension, ascites and renal sodium retention in cirrhosis: the overflow theory of ascites formation. Ann NY Acad Sci 1970;170:202.
16. Epstein M. Peritoneovenous shunt in the management of ascites and the hepatorenal syndrome. Gastroenterology 1982;82:790.
17. Feingold KR, Siperstein MD. Abnormalities of glucose metabolism in liver disease. In: Zakim D, Boyer TWD, eds. Hepatology: a textbook of liver disease. Philadelphia, WB Saunders, 1982:499.
18. Van Thiel DH, Stone BG, Schade RR. The liver and its effect on endocrine function in health and diseases. In: Schiff L, Schiff ER, eds. Diseases of the liver, ed 6. Philadelphia, JB Lippincott, 1987:148.
19. Jones EA, Gammal SH. Hepatic encephalopathy. In: Aria IM, Jakoby WB, Popper H, Schachter D, Shafritz DA, eds. The liver: biology and pathobiology, ed 2. New York, Raven Press, 1988:994.
20. Fischer JE, Rosen HM, Ebeid AM, et al. The effect of normalization of plasma amino acids on hepatic encephalopathy. Surgery 1976;80:77.
21. Eckhauser FE, Strodel WE, Thompson NW, Turcotte JG. The "replaced" right hepatic artery: a technical dilemma in portacaval shunt surgery. Surg Gynecol Obstet 1980;151:533.
22. Michels NA. Newer anatomy of the liver and its variant blood supply and collateral circulation. Am J Surg 1966;112:338.
23. Douglass BE, Baggenstoss AH, Hollinshead WH. The anatomy of the portal vein and its tributaries. Surg Gynecol Obstet 1950;91:562.
24. Benoit JN, Granger DN. Splanchnic hemodynamics in chronic portal hypertension. Semin Liver Dis 1986;6:287.
25. Beppu K, Inokuchi K, Koyanagi N, et al. Prediction of variceal hemorrhage by esophageal endoscopy. Gastrointest Endosc 1981;27:213.
26. Epstein M, Pins DS, Schneider H, et al. Determinants of deranged sodium and water homeostasis in decompensated cirrhosis. J Lab Clin Med 1976;87:822.
27. Epstein M. Renal function abnormalities in cirrhosis. In: Zakim D, Boyer TD, eds. Hepatology: a textbook of liver disease. Philadelphia, WB Saunders, 1982:449.
28. Lieberman FL, Reynolds TB. Plasma volume in cirrhosis of the liver: its relation to portal hypertension, ascites and renal failure. J Clin Invest 1967;46:1297.

29. Stanley MM. Pathogenesis of ascites in cirrhosis: a unitary hypothesis. ASAIO Trans 1989;35:161.

30. Hoefs JC, Canawati HN, Sapico FL, et al. Spontaneous bacterial peritonitis. Hepatology 1982;2:399.

31. Garcia-Tsao G. The diagnosis of bacterial peritonitis: comparison of pH, lactate concentration, and leukocyte count. Hepatology 1985;5:91.

32. Lemmer JH, Strodel WE, Knol JA. Management of spontaneous umbilical hernia rupture in the cirrhotic patient. Ann Surg 1983;198:30.

33. Sherlock S. Ascites. In: Sherlock S, ed. Diseases of the liver and biliary system, ed 8. Oxford, UK, Blackwell, 1989;129.

34. Gines P, Arroyo V, Quintero E, et al. Comparison of paracentesis and diuretics in the treatment of cirrhotics with tense ascites. Gastroenterology 1987;92:234.

35. LeVeen HH, Christoudias G, Ip M, et al. Peritoneo-venous shunting for ascites. Ann Surg 1974;180:580.

36. Greig PD, Langer B, Blendis LM, et al. Complications after peritoneovenous shunting for ascites. Am J Surg 1980;139:125.

37. LeVeen HH, Vujic I, D'Ovidio NG, et al. Peritoneovenous shunt occlusion: etiology, diagnosis and therapy. Ann Surg 1984;200:212.

38. Stanley MM. Randomized trials of treatment of ascites in alcoholic cirrhosis. ASAIO Trans 1989;35:174.

39. Gines P, Arroyo V, Vargas V, et al. Paracentesis with intravenous infusion of albumin as compared with peritoneovenous shunting in cirrhosis with refractory ascites. N Engl J Med 1991; 325:829.

40. Hillaire S, Labianca M, Borgonovo G, et al. Peritoneovenous shunting of intractable ascites in patients with cirrhosis: improving results and predictive factors of failure. Surgery 1993;113:373.

41. Benner KG, Sahagun G, Saxon R, Barton RE, et al. Selection of patients undergoing transjugular intrahepatic portosystemic shunting for refractory ascites. Hepatology 1994;20:69A.

42. Lebrec D, Giuily N, Hadeneque A, et al. Transjugular intrahepatic portosystemic shunt vs paracentesis for refractory ascites: results of a randomized trial. Hepatology 1994;20:417A.

43. Maddrey WC. Hepatic vein thrombosis (Budd-Chiari syndrome). Hepatology 1984;4:44S.

44. Mitchell MC, Boitnott JK, Kaufman S, et al. Budd-Chiari syndrome: etiology, diagnosis and management. Medicine 1982;61:199.

45. Tavill AS, Wood EJ, Kreel L, et al. The Budd-Chiari syndrome: correlation between hepatic scintigraphy and the clinical, radiological and pathological findings in 19 cases of hepatic venous outflow obstruction. Gastroenterology 1975;68:509.

46. Orloff MJ, Johansen KH. Treatment of Budd-Chiari syndrome by side-to-side portacaval shunt: experimental and clinical results. Ann Surg 1978;188:494.

47. Franco D, Vons G, Lecompte Y, et al. Portoatrial shunt in Budd-Chiari syndrome. Surgery 1986;99:388.

48. Chang CH, Lee MC, Shieh MJ, et al. Transatrial membranotomy for Budd-Chiari syndrome. Ann Thoracic Surg 1989;48:409.

49. Senning A. Transcaval posterocranial resection of the liver as treatment of the Budd-Chiari syndrome. World J Surg 1983;7:632.

50. Turcotte JG, O'Neal RM, Zuidema GD, et al. The effect of splenic transposition on portal circulation. J Surg Res 1961;1:299.

51. Akita H, Sakoda K. Portopulmonary shunt by splenopneumopexy as a surgical treatment of Budd-Chiari syndrome. Surgery 1980;87:85.

52. Campbell DA, Rolles K, Jamieson N, et al. Hepatic transplantation with perioperative and long-term anticoagulation as treatment for Budd-Chiari syndrome. Surg Gynecol Obstet 1988;166:511.

53. Wantz GE, Payne MA. Experience with portacaval shunt for portal hypertension. N Engl J Med 1961;265:721

54. Child CG, Turcotte JG. Surgery and portal hypertension. In: Child CG III, ed. Major problems in clinical surgery: the liver and portal hypertension, vol 1. Philadelphia, WB Saunders, 1964:1.

55. Eckhauser FE, Polley T, Bloch D, Appelman H, O'Leary Turcotte JG. Hepatic pathology as a determinant of prognosis after portal decompression. Am J Surg 1980;138:105.

56. Kraveta D, Bosch J, Teres J, Bruix J, Rimola A, Rodes J. Comparison of intravenous somatostatin and vasopressin infusions in treatment of acute variceal hemorrhage. Hepatology 1984;4:442.

57. Villeneuve J-P, Pomier-Layrargues G, Infante-Rivard C, et al. Propranolol for prevention of recurrent variceal hemorrhage: a controlled trial. Hepatology 1986;6:1239.

58. Bornman PC, Kahn D, Terblanche J, Worthley C, Spence RAJ, Krige JJEJ. Rigid versus fiberoptic endoscopic injection sclerotherapy. Ann Surg 1988;208:175.

59. Jensen DM. Sclerosants for injection sclerosis of esophageal varices. Gastrointest Endosc 1983;29:315.

60. Hunter GC, Steinkirchner T, Burbige EJ, Guernsey JM, Putnam CW. Venous complications of sclerotherapy for esophageal varices. Am J Surg 1988;156:497.

61. Infante-Rivard C, Esnaola S, Villeneuve JP. Role of endoscopic variceal sclerotherapy in the long-term management of variceal bleeding: a meta-analysis. Gastroenterology 1989;96:1087.

62. Cello JP, Grendell JH, Crass RA, Weber TE, Trunkey DD. Endoscopic sclerotherapy versus portacaval shunt in patients with severe cirrhosis and acute variceal hemorrhage: long term follow-up. N Engl J Med 1987;316:11.

63. Warren WD, Henderson JM, Millikan WJ, et al. Distal splenorenal shunt versus endoscopic sclerotherapy for long term management of variceal bleeding: preliminary report of a prospective randomized trial. Ann Surg 1986;203:454.

64. Rikkers LF, Burnett DA, Volentine GD, Buchi KN, Cormier RA. Shunt surgery versus endoscopic sclerotherapy for long-term treatment of variceal bleeding: early results of a randomized trial. Ann Surg 1987;206:261.

65. Teres J, Bordas JM, Bravo D, et al. Sclerotherapy vs distal splenorenal shunt in the elective treatment of variceal hemorrhage: a randomized, controlled trial. Hepatology 1987;7:430.

66. Pomerantz RA, Eckhauser FE, Knol JA, Guice K, Raper SE, Turcotte JG. Operative timing and patient survival following distal splenorenal shunt. Am Surg 1989;55:333.

67. Teres J, Baroni R, Bordas JM, Visa J, Pera C, Rodes J. Randomized trial of portacaval shunt, stapling transection, and endoscopic sclerotherapy in uncontrolled variceal bleeding. J Hepatol 1987;4:159.

68. Sorensen TIA. Sclerotherapy after first variceal hemorrhage in cirrhosis: a randomized multicenter trial. N Engl J Med 1984;311:1594.

69. Infante-Richard C, Esnaola S, Villeneuve JP. Role of endoscopic variceal sclerotherapy in the long-term management of variceal bleeding: a meta-analysis. Gastroenterology 1989;96:1087.

70. Paquet KJ, Koussouris P. Is there an indication for prophylactic endoscopic paravariceal injection sclerotherapy in patients with liver cirrhosis and portal hypertension. Endoscopy 1986;18(Suppl 2):32.

71. DeFranchis R. Prediction of the first variceal hemorrhage in patients with cirrhosis of the liver and esophageal varices: a prospective multicenter study. N Engl J Med 1988;319:983.

72. Pascal J-P, Cales P. Propranolol in the prevention of first upper gastrointestinal-tract hemorrhage in patients with cirrhosis of the liver and esophageal varices. N Engl J Med 1987;317:856.

73. Conn HO, Grace ND, Bosch J, Groszmann RJ, et al. Propranolol in the prevention of the first hemorrhage from esophagogastric varices: a multicenter randomized clinical trial. The Boston—New Haven—Barcelona Portal Hypertension Study Group. Hepatology 1991;13:902.

74. Witzel L, Wolbergs E, Merki H. Prophylactic endoscopic sclerotherapy of oesophageal varices: a prospective controlled study. Lancet 1985;1:773.

75. Santangelo WC, Dueno MI, Estes BL, Krejs GJ. Prophylactic sclerotherapy of large esophageal varices. N Engl J Med 1988;318:814.

76. Guynn TP, Eckhauser FE, Knol JA, et al. Sclerotherapy-induced esophageal strictures; risk factors and prognosis. Am Surg 1991;53:567.

77. Stiegmann GV, Goff JS. Endoscopic esophageal varix ligation: priliminary clinical experience. Gastrointest Endosc 1988;34:113.

78. Stiegmann GV, Goff JS, Michaletz-Onody PA, et al. Endoscopic sclerotherapy compared to endoscopic ligation for bleeding esophageal varices. N Engl J Med 1992;326:1527.

79. Hashizume M, Ohta M, Ueno K, et al. Endoscopic ligation of esophageal varices compared with injection sclerotherapy: a prospective, randomized trial. Gastrointest Endosc 1993;39:123.

80. Gimson AE, Ramage JK, Panos MZ, et al. Randomized trial of variceal band ligation versus injection sclerotherapy for bleeding esophageal varices. Lancet 1993;342:391.

81. Rosch J, Hanafee WN, Snow H. Transjugular hepatic venography and radiological portosystemic shunt: an experimental study. Radiology 1969;92:1112.

82. Palmaz J, Sibbitt RR, Reuter SR, et al. Expandable intrahepatic portacaval stents: early experience in the dog. Am J Roentgenol 1985;145:821.

83. Ring EJ, Lake JR, Roberts JP. Using transjugular intrahepatic portosystemic shunts to control variceal bleeding before liver transplantation. Ann Intern Med 1992;16:304-09.

84. Conn HO. Transjugular intrahepatic portal-systemic shunt: the state of the art. Hepatology 1993;17:148-58.

85. Pomier-Layrargues G, Legault L, Roy L, et al. TIPS for treatment of refractory ascites: a pilot study. Hepatology 1993; 18:187A.

86. Lopez RR, Benner KC, Hall L, et al. Expandable venous stents for treatment of Budd-Chiari Syndrome. Gastroenterology 1991;100:1435.

87. Wood RP, Shaw BW, Rikkers LF. Liver transplantation for variceal hemorrhage. Surg Clin North Am 1990;70:449.

88. Somberg KA. Transjugular intrahepatic portosystemic shunts have a limited impact on the liver transplant operation. Gastroenterology 1994;106:990A.

89. Somberg KA, Lake JR, Doherty MM, et al. The clinical course following TIPS in liver transplant candidates. Hepatology 1993;18:186.

90. Sarfeh IJ, Rypins EB, Mason GR. A systematic appraisal of portocaval H-graft diameters: clinical and hemodynamic perspective. Ann Surg 1986;204:356.

91. Haag K, Noeldge G, Sellinger M. Transjugular portosystemic shunt: monitoring of function by color duplex ultrasonography. Gastroenterology 1992;102:817A.

92. Collini FJ, Brener B. Portal hypertension (collective review). Surg Gynecol Obstet 1990;170:177.

93. Langer B, Taylor BR, MacKenzie DR, Gilas T, Stone RM, Blendis L. Further report of a prospective randomized trial comparing distal splenorenal shunt with end-to-side portacaval shunt: an analysis of encephalopathy, survival and quality of life. Gastroenterology 1985;88:424.

94. Henderson JM, Warren WD, Millikan WJ, Galloway JR, Kawasaki S, Kutner MH. Distal splenorenal shunt with spleno-pancreatic disconnection: a 4-year assessment. Ann Surg 1989;210:332.

95. Sarfeh IJ, Rypins EB, Mason GR. A systematic appraisal of portocaval H-graft diameters: clinical and hemodynamic perspectives. Ann Surg 1986;204:356.

96. Brems JJ, Hiatt JR, Klein AS, et al. Effect of a prior portosystemic shunt on subsequent liver transplantation. Ann Surg 1989;209:51.

97. Spence RAJ, Johnson GW. Results in 100 consecutive patients with stapled esophageal transection for varices. Surg Gynecol Obstet 1985;160:323.

98. Sugiura M, Futagawa S. Esophageal transection with paraesophagogastric devascularization in the treatment of esophageal varices. World J Surg 1984;8:673.

99. Hill ID, Bowie MD. Endoscopic sclerotherapy for control of bleeding varices in children. Am J Gastroenterol 1991; 86:472.

100. Gauthier F, De Dreuzy O, Valayer J, Montupet PH. H-type shunt with an autologous venous graft for treatment of portal hypertension in children. Pediatr Surg 1989;24:1041.

SURGERY: SCIENTIFIC PRINCIPLES AND PRACTICE, Second Edition, edited by Lazar J. Greenfield, Michael W. Mulholland, Keith T. Oldham, Gerald B. Zelenock, and Keith D. Lillemoe. Lippincott–Raven Publishers, Philadelphia, © 1997.

CHAPTER 39

HEPATIC NEOPLASMS

JOHN B. HANKS AND W. SCOTT ARNOLD

DIAGNOSTIC EVALUATION

The goals of the evaluation of a liver mass are to establish the diagnosis, to determine whether surgical treatment is warranted, and, if so, to judge resectability with an appropriate procedure. The diagnosis of a liver mass can often be achieved with knowledge of possible pathologies, a complete history and examination, and a logical cost-effective and efficient application of modern radiologic and laboratory tests (Fig. 39-1). Lesions that can present as hepatic masses are outlined in Table 39-1.

The patient's age, medical history, and exposure history are particularly important. For example, a patient with a history of a colon resection for adenocarcinoma is clearly at risk for metastatic disease. Fever, weight loss, and malaise associated with right upper quadrant pain can be an indication of primary tumors or abscesses. Particularly relevant is a history of hepatitis, alcoholism, or hereditary or metabolic causes of cirrhosis, all of which are associated with an increased risk of malignancy and may affect later choices of major hepatic resection. Family history may reveal a hereditary polycystic disorder or an uncommon entity such as neurofibromatosis with its increased risk of hepatic sarcoma. A history of exposure to hepatotoxins such as Thorotrast, arsenic, aflatoxin, or vinyl chloride should be explored. A history of hormone ingestion or possible hormonal excess is also important, given the relation between sex steroids and both hepatic adenoma and hepatocellular carcinoma (HCC). A history of human immunodeficiency virus infection or immunosuppression increases the likelihood of infectious masses as well as primary hepatic lymphoma. Physical examination should include an evaluation of the sequelae of hepatic dysfunction, such as spider telangiectasia, easy bruisability, and palmar erythema. A thorough physical examination, with careful evaluation of the skin, eyes, heart, colon, and rectum, may identify sources of primary tumor that have metastasized.

There are four roles for the radiologic evaluation of liver masses: screening of high-risk populations, such as patients with chronic hepatitis or patients before and after resection of colon cancer; detection of a suspected liver mass based on laboratory or physical examination; further diagnostic evaluation of a known mass; and, finally, preoperative or intraoperative evaluation of anatomy and resectability. Tests commonly used in the evaluation of hepatic masses include the following:

- Dynamic computed tomography (CT) scan
- Magnetic resonance (MR) imaging
- Transabdominal, endoscopic, and intraoperative ultrasound
- Radionuclide studies (Tc^{82n} sulfur colloid scan, tagged red blood cell scan)
- CT angiography

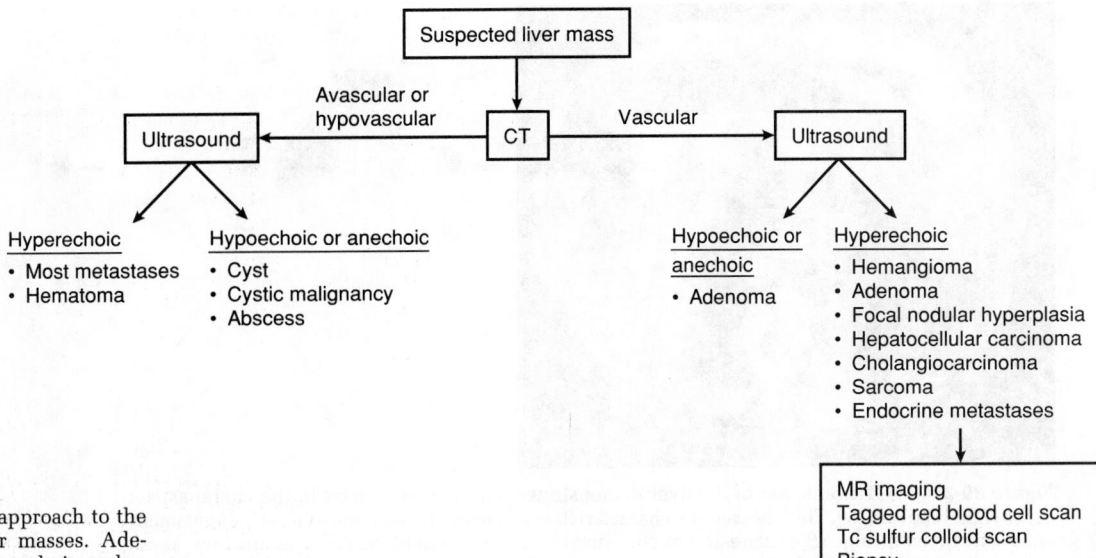

Figure 39-1. One approach to the evaluation of liver masses. Adenoma may be hyperechoic or hypoechoic on ultrasound.

- Angiography
- Guided fine-needle aspiration or core needle biopsy
- Endoscopic retrograde cholangiopancreatography and percutaneous transhepatic chemangiography

In the Western world, the tests most often used for screening, detection, and diagnosis are dynamic bolus-

Table 39-1. CLASSIFICATION OF HEPATIC MASS LESIONS

BENIGN
Adenoma
Focal Nodular Hyperplasia
Benign Macronodular Regeneration
Cystic Diseases
Acquired (false or pseudocysts, with no true epithelial lining)
    Abscesses
        Pyogenic
        Parasitic
    Benign cystadenoma
    Posttraumatic cysts
Congenital
    Solitary (unilocular or multilocular)
    Polycystic disease
    Caroli disease (multiple cystic dilatations of intrahepatic bile ducts)
    Solitary dilation of an intrahepatic duct

Vascular Tumors
Cavernous hemangioma
Other: capillary hemangioma, intermediate-grade lesions such as hemangioendothelioma and epithelioid hemangioendothelioma

Bile Duct Adenoma
Other: Fibroma, Lipoma, Teratoma, Hemartoma, Angiomyolipoma
MALIGNANT
Metastatic Disease
Primary Malignancy
Hepatocellular carcinoma
Angiosarcoma
Cholangiocarcinoma (intrahepatic)
Hepatoblastoma
Undifferentiated carcinoma
Other: fibrosarcoma, liposarcoma, carcinosarcoma, lymphoma
Cystic degeneration of above malignancies

enhanced CT, MR imaging, and ultrasound. CT and MR imaging have comparable sensitivities of about 90% and are often complementary in the evaluation of a mass. Ultrasound is only slightly less sensitive and is operator dependent, but it is a cost-effective procedure that adds useful information to the evaluation of a mass.[1,2] The most sensitive tests for the detection of liver masses are CT angioportography (CTAP) and intraoperative ultrasound, the latter with a sensitivity of about 96%.[3] Like angiography, they are generally reserved for preoperative or intraoperative evaluation of resectability. Dynamic CT scanning remains the dominant imaging modality for routine screening and diagnosis because it is sensitive, is widely available, provides helpful anatomic information, and allows the evaluation of other intraabdominal structures and the detection of extrahepatic disease. Dynamic bolus-enhanced CT scanning involves rapid intravenous injection of contrast material followed immediately by rapid scans of contiguous levels. The rate and pattern of enhancement allow a reasonable distinction to be made between hypovascular and hypervascular lesions. CT scanning often yields qualitative information sufficient to make a diagnosis. For example, cavernous hemangiomas often have a characteristic enhancement pattern that obviates the need for angiography (Fig. 39-2).

Hepatic MR imaging is evolving rapidly and has become a useful tool in the detection and diagnosis of liver lesions. It has a sensitivity equal to that of CT.[1,2] Although anatomic resolution is lower, expense is greater, and availability is less than that of CT, MR with T1- and T2-weighted images with gadolinium enhancement can aid in the differential diagnosis of a mass. For example, MR imaging is now considered a test of choice for distinguishing hemangiomas from other mass lesions (see later).

Transabdominal ultrasound remains extremely useful in the evaluation of liver masses and is often the initial imaging procedure performed. Intraoperative ultrasound (Fig. 39-3) ranks with CTAP in terms of sensitivity and is often considered the gold standard (short of resection with pathologic evaluation) in the evaluation of liver lesions. Additionally, intraoperative ultrasound can be used to guide surgical resections by clarifying the proximity of the portal and hepatic venous branches.[4]

Radionuclide imaging is less sensitive and specific than CT, MR imaging, and ultrasound and has a high percentage

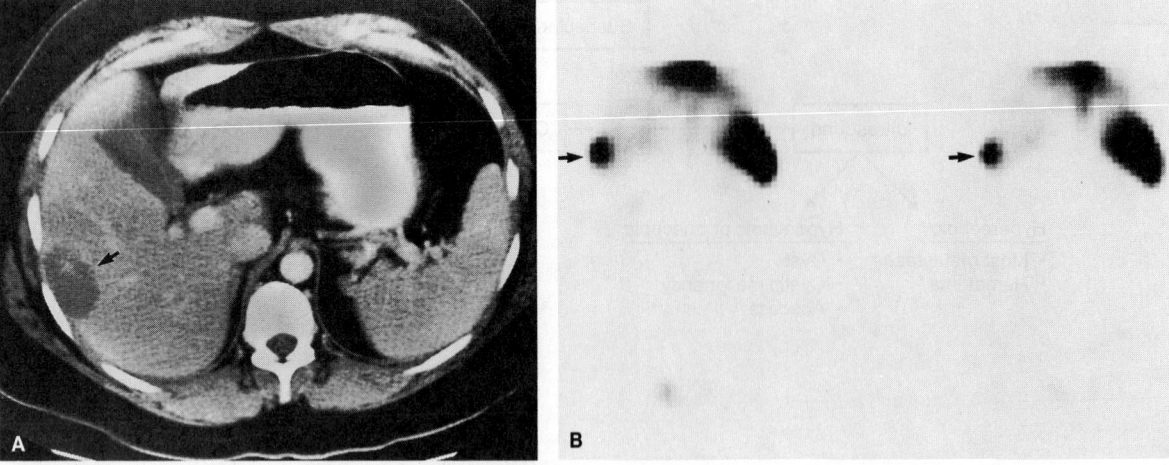

Figure 39-2. (*A*) CT evaluation of the liver demonstrated a 3- to 3.5-cm mass in the lateral aspect of the right lobe (*arrow*). This showed the characteristics of a hemangioma (peripheral enhancement with centripetal filling). (*B*) Diagnosis was confirmed by a tagged red blood cell scan (*arrow*). These two confirmatory tests obviate the need for arteriographic evaluation of these lesions.

of false-positive and false-negative results. The lower limit of detectability is about 2 cm. Nuclear medicine scans have a limited role in modern screening and detection, but they can help differentiate discrete masses. There are various radionuclides, each of which has a different role in imaging. Technetium-99m–labeled sulfur colloid is taken up by the reticuloendothelial cells (Kupffer cells) of the liver and spleen and provides structural rather than functional information. Technetium pertechnetate is useful in evaluating vascular lesions. Gallium 67 is taken up more readily by malignant and inflammatory cells than by hepatocytes. For example, a primary liver tumor should be a relatively cold spot on sulfur colloid scan, a positive image with pertechnetate because of its vascularity, and a hot spot on gallium scan. Focal nodular hyperplasia (FNH) has Kupffer cells and does not produce a defect on sulfur colloid scan, as do adenomas. A newly developed and promising field is radioimmunologic imaging, in which radiolabeled monoclonal antibodies to specific tumor antigens are injected and imaged. Initial results with monoclonal antibody to a colorectal carcinoma antigen as well as with anti–α-fetoprotein antibodies in HCC have been promising.[5,6]

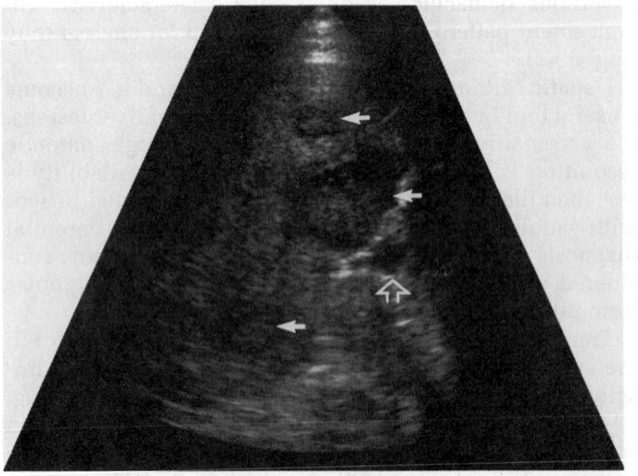

Preoperative evaluation of a liver mass addresses specific surgical issues such as vascular and biliary anatomy and the detection of additional small lesions or significant vascular involvement that would render a patient unresectable. Tests used preoperatively include arteriography and CT arteriography (CTA) or CTAP. Arteriography, often performed in concert with CTAP, remains valuable as a preoperative study to define vascular anatomy. Arteriography is also helpful in detecting and defining small hypervascular lesions, such as HCCs (Fig. 39-4), and endocrine metastases. Arteriography is less helpful in detecting hypovascular lesions such as colorectal metastases. CTAP involves the direct injection of contrast into the hepatic artery (CTA) or superior mesenteric artery with delayed films to demonstrate the portal vein (CTAP).

Biopsy of a liver mass may be performed percutaneously (with or without CT or ultrasound guidance), laparoscopically, or at laparotomy. The biopsy may be for cytology only (fine-needle aspiration [FNA]) or for histology (larger-bore core biopsy). Guided FNA has an overall sensitivity of 77% to 94% and may allow a distinction between primary and secondary malignancy[7] (Fig. 39-5). The risks associated with needle biopsy include bleeding, infection, needle track seeding of tumor, and sampling errors. For example, cells from an adenoma may resemble normal liver cells, or a portion of a hemangioma may resemble a scar. Hypervascular masses, coagulopathy, and ascites are contraindications to percutaneous core biopsy. FNA biopsy is generally safe under these circumstances.

In the evaluation of any liver mass, percutaneous biopsy should be performed only if it can reasonably be expected to obviate the need for exploratory laparotomy. Most patients with symptomatic masses should be considered for laparotomy, thereby making preoperative histology superfluous. Biopsy of a suspected primary or metastatic malignancy with clinical indications of unresectability may spare the patient an unnecessary laparotomy. Laparoscopy with biopsy has been used to evaluate liver masses and to avoid laparotomy.

BENIGN LIVER DISEASE

Although benign tumors of the liver have traditionally been considered a rare entity, they have recently assumed importance because of the association between adenomas

Figure 39-3. Intraoperative ultrasound is becoming increasingly important in the evaluation of the extent of hepatic metastases. The high-quality resolution of this modality demonstrates multiple metastases (*closed arrows*) throughout all segments and in continuity with the major vascular and biliary structures. Open arrow indicates portal vein.

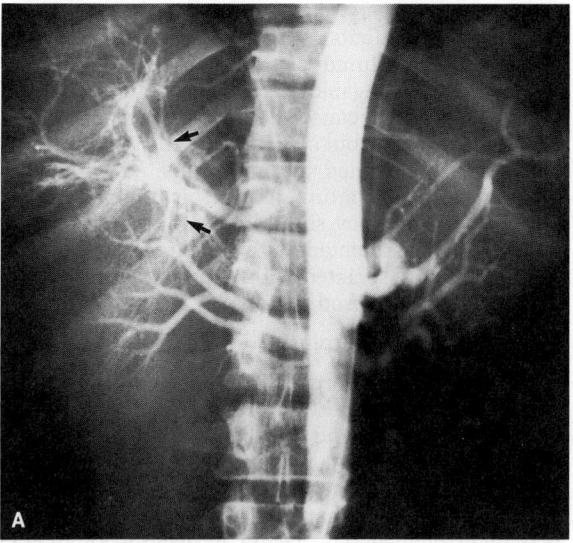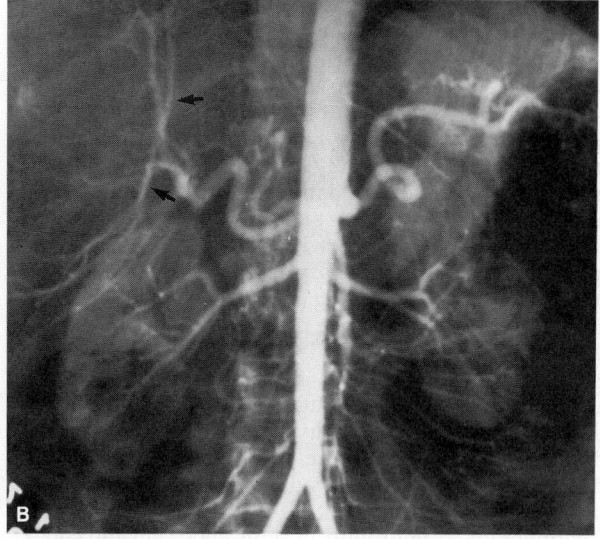

Figure 39-4. (*A*) Arteriogram of a hypervascular right lobe lesion arising from the right hepatic artery (*arrow*). A diagnosis of a hepatoma is suggested because of the evidence of neovascularity in this area. (*B*) Arteriogram from a patient who presented with a mass in the right lobe of the liver after resection of a colorectal primary lesion. The bowing of the arterial supply from the right hepatic artery (*arrow*) is consistent with a hypovascular lesion, which was later confirmed to be a 10-cm metastasis from the original colorectal primary lesion.

and oral contraceptives and because of increased incidental detection.

Benign Solid Tumors

Hepatocellular Adenoma

Hepatocellular adenoma is clearly linked with the use of oral contraceptive medications. The increased incidence of adenomas can be traced from the early 1960s, when the use of birth control medication became common. Although adenomas can occur in men and children, over 90% occur in women (usually between the ages of 20 and 40 years), most of whom have a history of oral contraceptive use.[8] Adenomas have been associated with both types of syn-

thetic estrogen and all forms of progesterone used in oral contraceptives. Estrogens may be etiologically more important because adenomas can occur in patients receiving conjugated estrogens and in those with estrogen-producing tumors. The likelihood of developing a hepatic adenoma appears to be related to the duration and dosage of estrogens and is greater at ages over 30 years. Although adenomas can occur in patients in the absence of hormone excess, suspicion of a hepatic adenoma should prompt a check for increased exogenous hormone ingestion or endogenous steroid production. Adenoma has also been associated with glycogen storage disease type 1 and anabolic steroid use. In 25% of men with hepatic adenomas, there is a history of androgen use. Most (75%) of these lesions occur in the right lobe of the liver.

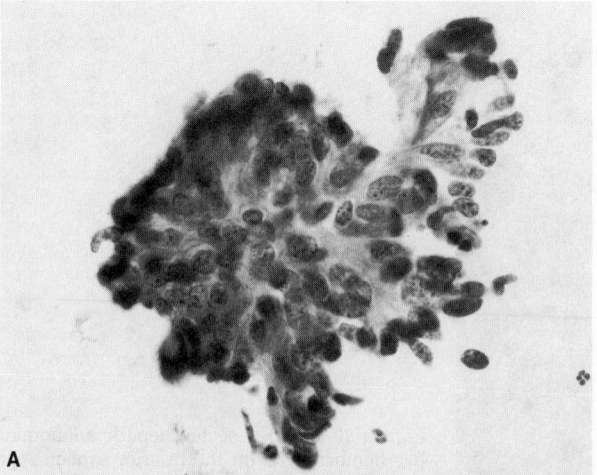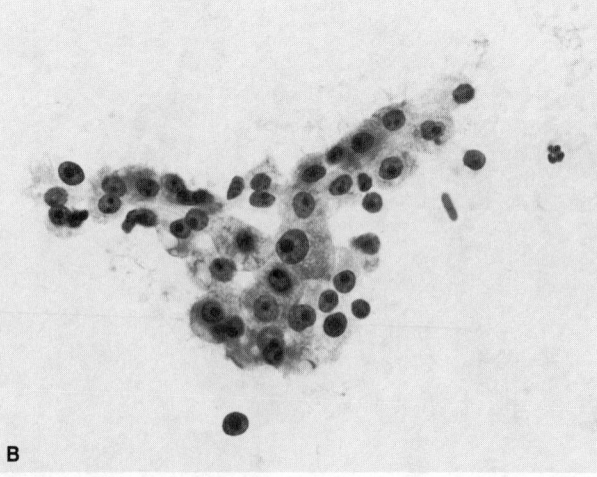

Figure 39-5. (*A*) The cells of a needle aspiration of a metastasis from a colonic adenocarcinoma. The cells are columnar and are arranged in a thick cluster (Papanicolaou stain, ×500). (*B*) Fine-needle aspiration of a primary hepatocellular carcinoma. The cells in this lesion have enlarged nuclei with macronucleoli and dense, granular cytoplasm (Papanicolaou stain, ×500).

Pathologically, the adenoma consists of benign normal-appearing hepatocytes that are usually well circumscribed and distinguishable from normal parenchyma by a distinct lack of bile duct architecture. Adenomas are generally believed not to be premalignant.

Although adenomas may be asymptomatic, most patients have symptoms (usually abdominal pain, which occurs in as many as 50% of patients). Ten percent to 33% of patients present with acute signs and symptoms secondary to bleeding or rupture with intraperitoneal hemorrhage[9,10] (Fig. 39-6). Laboratory tests are usually normal unless there has been bleeding. Hepatomegaly or an upper abdominal mass is a common physical finding.

No radiologic test is specific for adenomas. CT is the most useful preliminary test and often reveals areas of hemorrhage and necrosis. Angiography may add to CT findings by demonstrating a hypervascular tumor with a peripheral blood supply. ^{99m}Tc sulfur colloid scans show a cold spot that distinguishes adenoma from FNH but not from other solid masses.

Treatment for patients with an acute abdomen and shock is emergent surgery. For asymptomatic or less acutely symptomatic patients, surgery is also the treatment of choice, given the tumor's tendency to bleed and the small chance of coexisting malignancy. Birth control pills should be discontinued because they not only increase the incidence of adenomas but also increase the complication rate. If resection is deemed too hazardous, conservative management with discontinuation of birth control pills is in order, and pregnancy should be avoided. Although pregnancy is not associated with an increased incidence of adenoma, it is associated with tumor growth, tumor symptoms, and an increased incidence of tumor rupture.

Focal Nodular Hyperplasia

Focal nodular hyperplasia should not be confused with adenoma. Although FNH predominantly affects young women, it is also found in men and children. Unlike adenomas, there is no clear relation between oral contraceptives and the development of FNH. FNH is usually asymptomatic and does not have a propensity to bleed or undergo malignant change. The lesion is usually found inciden-

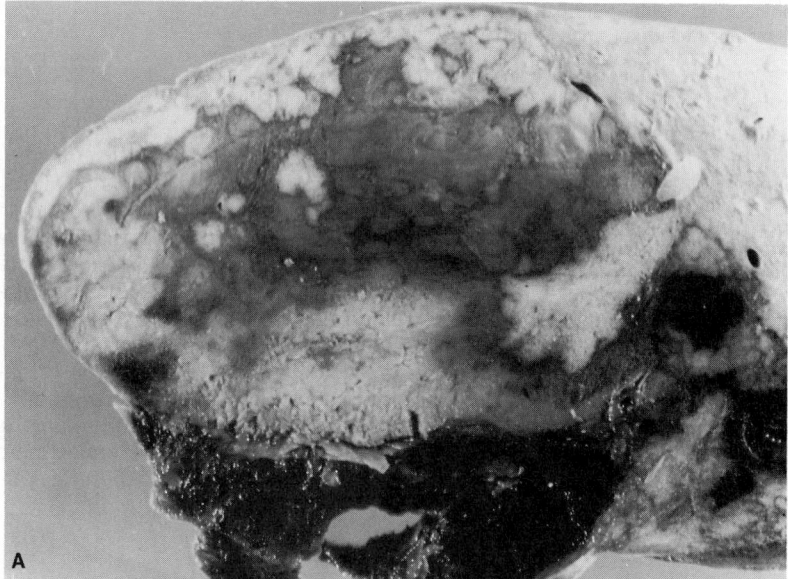

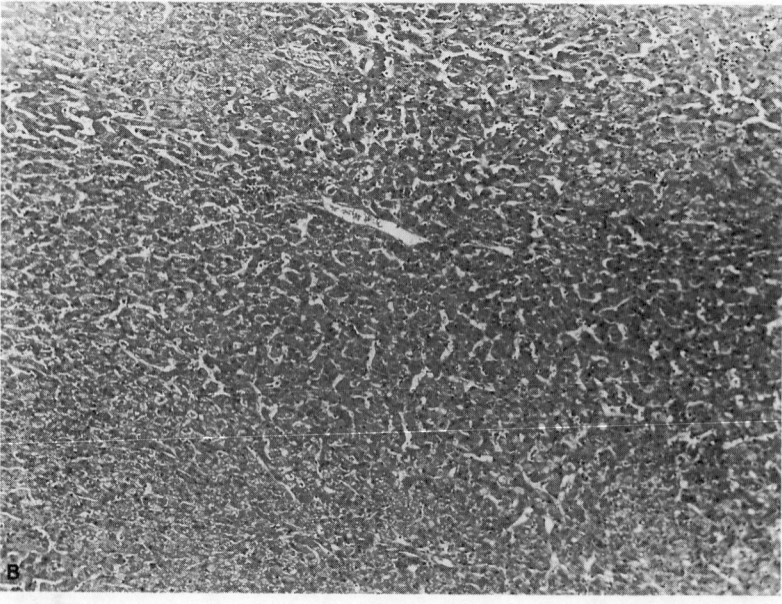

Figure 39-6. (*A*) Resected hepatic adenoma that has hemorrhaged on the inferior aspect. A large amount of clot is protruding through the ruptured capsule of the liver. (*B*) Microscopy of the adenoma reveals the rather uniform appearance of the hepatocytes and no evidence of biliary architecture.

tally. Patients with symptoms generally complain of abdominal discomfort. A few patients have hepatomegaly, a mass, or tenderness on examination. Instances of bleeding are rare.

Grossly, the lesion's most characteristic difference from adenomas is its lobulation. Larger lesions also tend to develop a central stellate scar. Histologically, FNH contains normal-appearing hepatocytes, bile ducts, and Kupffer cells, unlike adenomas.

Laboratory tests are normal in patients with FNH. CT, MR imaging, and ultrasound are sensitive for FNH but are often not diagnostically specific. The presence of a central scar is helpful but uncommon. Angiography is sensitive, and the appearance is that of a hypervascular mass similar to adenomas. Radionuclide imaging can be useful, because FNH is the only lesion that contains Kupffer cells and therefore appears isodense rather than as a defect. The combination of CT, ultrasound, and radionuclide scan often reveals FNH but is not always unequivocally diagnostic.

Treatment of asymptomatic patients is conservative when the diagnosis is clear. If there is any doubt regarding the diagnosis, an excisional biopsy is indicated for small, easily removed lesions. An incisional or percutaneous core biopsy may be performed for large or inaccessible lesions. Therapy for symptomatic patients should be individualized, because the risk of removing a large mass may be greater than the risk of observation.

Bile Duct Hamartomas and Adenomas

The terms *bile duct hamartoma* and *bile duct adenoma* are often used synonymously, but they actually describe two separate and uncommon entities. Hamartomas are more common. Both are small, incidental findings that derive their importance from their confusion with metastatic or primary malignancy.

BENIGN VASCULAR LESIONS

Hemangiomas

Cavernous hemangiomas of the liver are the most common benign hepatic tumor and are detected in 2% to 7% of autopsies. They are the second most common hepatic tumor, exceeded only by metastases.[10] Although capillary hemangiomas exist in the liver, they are rare, small, and of minimal clinical significance. Cavernous hemangiomas consist histologically of cystically dilated, endothelium-lined vascular spaces. They occur in all age groups and are seen most commonly in females. Hemangiomas are not premalignant and have no definable etiologic factors in their development. Many believe they are benign congenital hamartomas.

Less than half of affected patients have symptoms. Those with symptoms usually have large masses. Symptoms commonly include vague right upper quadrant discomfort, pain, fullness, early satiety, and sometimes nausea, vomiting, and fever. Physical examination may be notable for hepatomegaly, mass, or bruit. Complications are rare but include obstructive jaundice, gastric outlet obstruction, and a consumptive coagulopathy (Kasabach-Merritt syndrome) initiated by thrombosis within the large hemangiomas. Spontaneous rupture or hemorrhage is infrequent.[10]

There are usually no laboratory abnormalities in patients with hemangiomas. The most useful radiologic tests for diagnosing hemangiomas are MR imaging, CT, and tagged red blood cell scanning. These tests have largely replaced angiography (Fig. 39-7). CT often demonstrates a diagnostically characteristic enhancement pattern. Gadolinium-enhanced MR imaging has been shown to be sensitive and specific in the diagnosis of hemangioma and has better resolution than the tagged blood cell scan.[11] FNA biopsy of suspected hemangiomas can be performed; however, this procedure can and should be avoided if the diagnosis is secure with less-invasive procedures. A particularly common clinical dilemma is distinguishing an incidentally discovered hemangioma from malignancy. If the lesion has an appearance on CT compatible with hemangioma, the next confirmatory test should be tagged blood cell scanning or MR imaging.

Given the benign natural history of hemangioma and its low risk of rupture, observation is indicated for asymptomatic patients, especially for lesions smaller than 4 cm. Surgical excision is the only consistently effective treatment for symptomatic masses and should be performed if the lesion is localized and accessible with an acceptable operative risk. Treatment for the unusual unresectable, symptomatic hemangiomas may include radiation therapy, corticosteroids, and embolization, although these are only modestly effective.

BENIGN CYSTIC DISEASES

There are many varieties of hepatic cysts. Most cystic liver lesions are benign and uncommon. They are being diagnosed with increasing frequency with the advent of more sophisticated radiologic techniques.

Congenital Hepatic Cysts and Related Diseases

Congenital hepatic cysts are uniformly benign, may be single or multiple, and are uncommon, with a prevalence of 0.14% to 0.3% in autopsy series. Solitary cysts are more common than polycystic disease. The pathogenesis of congenital hepatic cysts is unclear, but they most likely result from failure of intralobular bile ducts to fuse with interlobular bile ducts because of dysgenesis, stenosis, or obstruction. An alternative theory is that they are caused by congenital lymphatic obstruction.

Solitary Congenital Hepatic Cysts

The symptomatic solitary cyst may cause vague right upper quadrant discomfort or pain, a sensation of epigastric fullness or heaviness, early satiety, and sometimes nausea and vomiting from pressure of the cyst on adjacent viscera. Most cases are asymptomatic. Hepatomegaly or a palpable mass is not uncommon, and respiratory symptoms may occur if the cyst is large. Complications are rare but include hemorrhage into the cyst, secondary bacterial infection, torsion (if pedunculated), and obstructive jaundice from compression of extrahepatic ducts. In the absence of complications, laboratory abnormalities are uncommon. Cysts are somewhat more common in females (about 3:1), usually occur in the right lobe, and are more often multilocular than unilocular. There is no apparent genetic transmissibility or association with renal cysts. They are lined by cuboidal epithelium resembling bile duct epithelium and are filled with fluid that can be clear, mucoid, bloody, or bilious (Fig. 39-8). Carcinoma can occur in a liver cyst but is extremely uncommon.

If the patient has no symptoms, the cyst was discovered incidentally, and there is no evidence of infection or malignancy, one may observe the patient. Neither percutaneous aspiration nor surgery is indicated. Cysts nearly always recur after simple aspiration. If there are internal echoes, however, the cyst should be aspirated under ultrasound or CT guidance for culture and cytology. If the cyst is discovered incidentally at laparotomy or laparoscopy, it should be aspirated (for

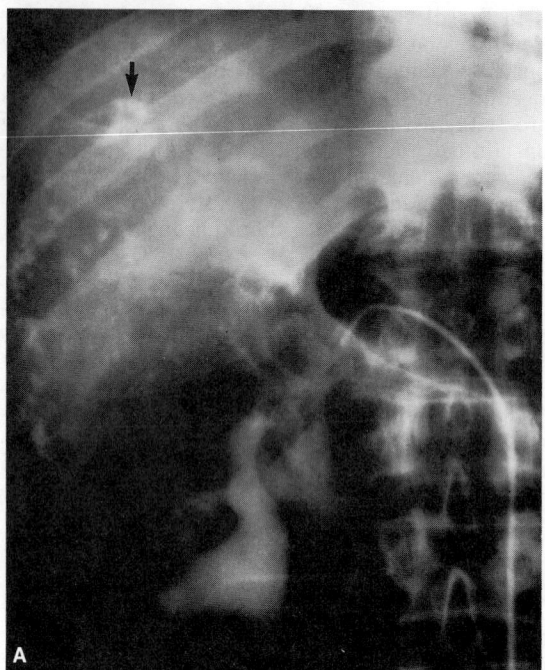

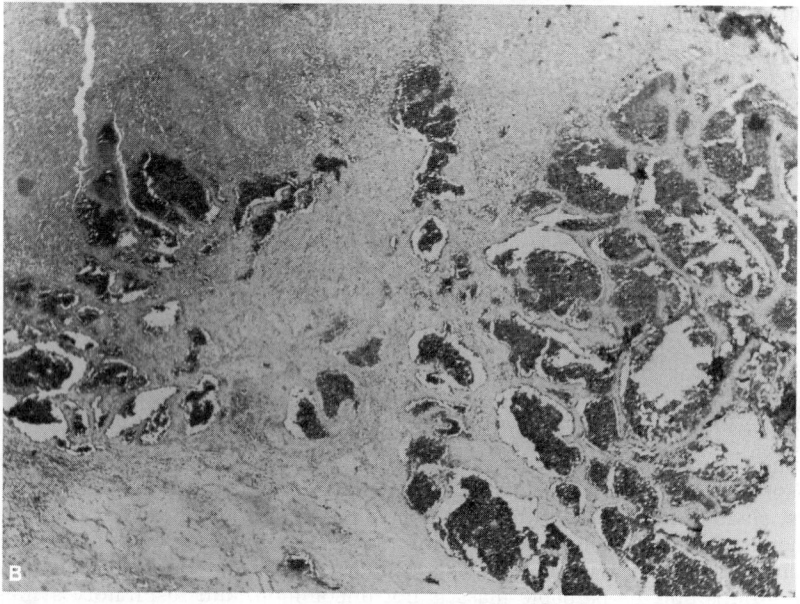

Figure 39-7. (*A*) Arteriographic evaluation of a mass seen on ultrasound. A diagnosis of hemangioma can be made from this arteriogram because of the extent of neovascularity and early venous filling (*arrow*). (*B*) The endothelium-lined sinus cavities have thickened septae that are diagnostic of the cavernous hemangioma. (Hanks JB, Jones RS. The liver. In: Fromm P, ed. Gastrointestinal surgery. New York, Churchill Livingstone, 1985)

Gram stain, culture, and cytology). If not infected, it should be left alone unless easily resectable. Treatment of symptomatic cysts is surgical. Indications for surgery include symptoms, rupture, hemorrhage, and infection.

A symptomatic, uninfected simple cyst is best treated by excision, if possible. Larger cysts may be unroofed with free peritoneal drainage unless there is a history of hemorrhage or evidence of biliary communication. If the cyst communicates with the biliary system (grossly or by cholangiogram), the leak may be oversewn or the cyst drained by Roux-en-Y cystojejunostomy. Infected cysts should be drained externally and resected later or marsupialized. Aspiration with injection of sclerosants has met with some clinical success but should not be performed in the setting of infection, hemorrhage, or biliary communication.

Polycystic Disease

Polycystic liver disease is associated with polycystic kidney disease. Infantile polycystic disease is an autosomal recessive disorder of the renal and hepatic compo-

nents with a spectrum of severities. Hepatic involvement is usually present, but children with severe perinatal and neonatal forms often die of renal failure. If they survive, the hepatic disease predominates as congenital hepatic fibrosis. Adult polycystic disease is the most common cystic disease. It has autosomal dominant transmission with an incidence of 1:1000. About half of patients with adult polycystic liver disease have renal involvement, and hepatic involvement occurs in 15% to 75% of patients with renal disease.[12] Ten percent to 30% of patients with adult polycystic disease also have intracranial arterial aneurysms.

Hepatic polycystic disease is most often bilobar, it may be microscopic or large, and the cysts generally contain clear fluid. Hepatic cysts in infantile forms may be discovered incidentally in a workup for renal symptoms or may present as congenital hepatic fibrosis. Adult polycystic liver disease is frequently asymptomatic and may be discovered during evaluation of renal symptoms. If symptomatic, cysts cause disturbances similar to those of solitary cysts. Treatment is reserved for patients with symptoms

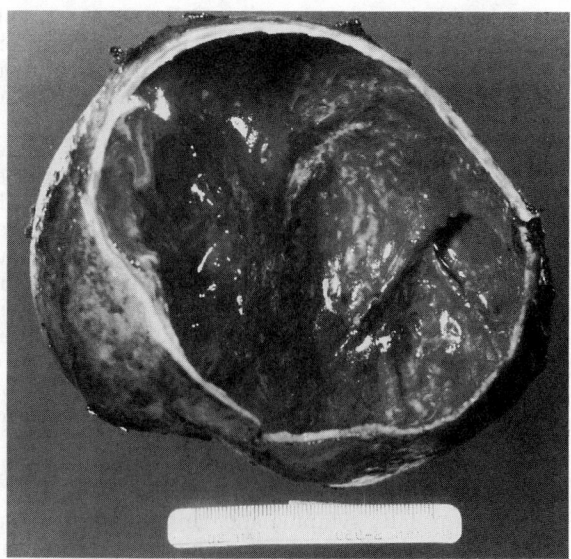

Figure 39-8. A large unilocular congenital hepatic cyst. (Hanks JB, Jones RS. The liver. In: Fromm P, ed. Gastrointestinal surgery. New York, Churchill Livingstone, 1985)

or complications and consists of unroofing or excising accessible cysts or fenestration to drain deeper cysts into more superficial cysts. Extensive and unresectable disease has recently been treated with liver transplantation.

Acquired Hepatic Cysts

Traumatic hepatic cysts are false cysts (they have no true epithelial lining) that result from a resolved subcapsular or intraparenchymal hematoma. These cysts lack a capsule, a history of trauma, and have a fibrotic wall that contains hemosiderin, but otherwise they are similar to solitary congenital cysts and should be treated in a conservative fashion.

Neoplastic cysts of the liver can be primary biliary cystadenomas or cystadenocarcinomas but more commonly are metastases from primary tumors, such as pancreatic or ovarian carcinomas. Alternatively, they may represent cystic degeneration of a solid primary or metastasis. Such malignancies taking a cystic form are uncommon but need to be considered in the workup of cystic hepatic disease.

PRIMARY HEPATIC MALIGNANCY

In North America and western Europe, most liver malignancies are metastases; primary liver cancers are less common. Worldwide, primary liver cancer is more common, especially in equatorial areas (Southeast Asia, Japan, and Africa). Primary cancers of the liver are predominantly of four histologic types:

- HCC, which constitutes nearly three fourths of all cases
- Cholangiocarcinoma, a malignancy of the intrahepatic bile duct epithelium (see Chap. 42) that makes up 5% to 30% of all cases
- Angiosarcoma
- Hepatoblastoma

There are many less common pathologies, such as mixed HCC–cholangiocarcinoma, fibrosarcomas, rhabdomyosarcomas, leiomyosarcomas, teratocarcinomas, adenosquamous carcinomas, hepatic neurofibromatosis, and, with the increasing incidence of acquired immunodeficiency

syndrome and immunosuppressive drugs, primary hepatic lymphoma and Kaposi sarcoma. HCC, the most prevalent of these classifications, has been discussed using various terms, including *primary liver cancer* and *hepatoma*. Because it has a defined epidemiology as well as a partially understood etiology and pathogenesis, there is cautious optimism concerning future treatment and prevention.

Hepatocellular Carcinoma

Epidemiology, Etiology, and Pathogenesis

Hepatocellular carcinoma has three well-known epidemiologic associations—hepatitis B virus (HBV) infection, cirrhosis, and various hepatotoxins, most notably aflatoxin B1. The geographic distribution of cases correlates with the prevalence of associated risk factors. Even correcting for HBV carriage rates, HCC occurs two to three times more commonly in men and is more common among cirrhotic men than among cirrhotic or noncirrhotic women. Race is a less clearly defined risk factor. The tumor is especially prevalent among Asians and African blacks, but this may represent the higher prevalence of HBV in those countries. Other risk factors for HCC include type 1 glycogen storage disease, α_1-antitrypsin deficiency, hemochromatosis, tyrosinemia, and use of androgens (and, to a much lesser extent, oral contraceptives). Wilson disease is apparently not a risk factor.

HCC is strongly associated with HBV infection. There is no link between HCC and hepatitis A virus, but there does appear to be a link between HCC and hepatitis C virus.[13] In the United States and Europe, where HBV carriage is less than 1%, HCC represents only 2% to 3% of all cancers, with a prevalence at autopsy of 0.25%.[14] In high-incidence areas such as Africa and Southeast Asia, where the HBV carriage rate is 10%, HCC constitutes nearly 40% of all cancers, with a 2% to 8% prevalence. In one study from Asia, 87% of patients with HCC were HB$_s$Ag-positive.[15] The risk of developing HCC is related to the chronicity of HBV infection. When HBV is acquired vertically (mother to child), as often occurs in endemic areas, there is a 200-fold increase in HCC prevalence compared with noncarriers and a 50% lifetime risk. When HBV is acquired as an adult, which is usual in the West, it infrequently progresses to HCC.

HBV appears to be important in hepatocellular oncogenesis. Insertion of the viral genome into the host DNA is probably an initiating event. Both HBV DNA and HBV RNA have been found in HCC tissue. The virus seems to integrate at random into the host genome, and the viral DNA is both transcribed and translated. Although both asymptomatic carriers and patients with chronic hepatitis have viral integration, HCC is more likely to develop in patients with high levels of replication, such as those with chronic active hepatitis. Integration of a gene-promoter sequence may activate a cellular oncogene (a growth factor, second messenger, or receptor), or the integration may destroy an antioncogene. Studies have shown a high level of HBV surface antigen gene-promoter integration and a low level of the core gene integration. No specific oncogene product has yet been firmly implicated.

Cirrhosis is a frequent result of HBV infection and an independent risk factor for HCC. Cirrhosis associated with HCC is predominantly the macronodular (postnecrotic, posthepatic) type, and it has about a 10% risk of progressing to HCC. Nevertheless, the micronodular form is more common in early alcoholic cirrhosis and progresses to HCC in about 2% to 3% of cases.[16] Thus, HCC may develop in patients with HBV and cirrhosis, with HBV alone, or with cirrhosis (from any cause) alone, or it may develop secondary to toxin exposure. Worldwide, cirrhosis is present in 60% to 90% of cases of HCC. In the United States, only 5% to 15% of patients with cirrhosis develop HCC. Cirrhosis and hepatotoxins cause chronic regeneration and nuclear activity and therefore may act as direct promoters or may increase cellular susceptibility to other toxins. In any event, cirrhosis associated with malignancy significantly lowers the survival rate after resection.

Finally, aflatoxin B1, a mycotoxin from the fungus *Aspergillus flavus*, is a potent carcinogen and may play a role in the development of HCC in areas where foodstuffs are frequently contaminated with the fungus.

Pathology

Hepatocellular carcinoma exists grossly as a unifocal, multifocal, or infiltrative mass (Fig. 39-9). Involved hepatocytes may be well differentiated or poorly differentiated. Well-differentiated forms may be difficult to distinguish from normal liver or from an adenoma. Poorly differentiated forms may appear as giant cells, small cells, or spindle cells (mimicking a sarcoma). There is also a clear cell morphology of HCC. The clear cell type and HCC with a lymphocytic infiltrate have better prognoses. There is no clearly premalignant lesion, although the cells on the well-differentiated end of the spectrum of cellular atypia may

closely resemble hepatic adenomas. Cellular components of HCC may have sex steroid receptors, and these receptors may have implications for hormonal therapy. The tumors frequently stain positive for AFP, α_1-antitrypsin, and sometimes carcinoembryonic antigen (CEA).

The fibrolamellar variant of HCC has a distinctly better prognosis, with a 5-year survival rate after resection of 50% to 60% versus 25%[17] (Fig. 39-10). It occurs primarily in younger patients (90% are younger than 25 years old) and has a slight female predominance. Fibrolamellar tumors are usually associated with normal AFP levels and are infrequently associated with HBV or cirrhosis (less than 10% and 5%, respectively). The tumor is composed of polygonal cells growing in nests or cords separated by fibrous stroma. Because of its better prognosis, consideration of surgical resection should be more aggressive for fibrolamellar HCC.

Clinical Presentation

Patients are usually symptomatic. Unfortunately, symptoms are often masked by background hepatitis or cirrhosis, and the only sign may be sudden clinical deterioration. Rarely, it may present as metastatic disease with a pulmonary lesion or bone pain. The classic finding is painful hepatomegaly, with or without nodular enlargement. Right up-

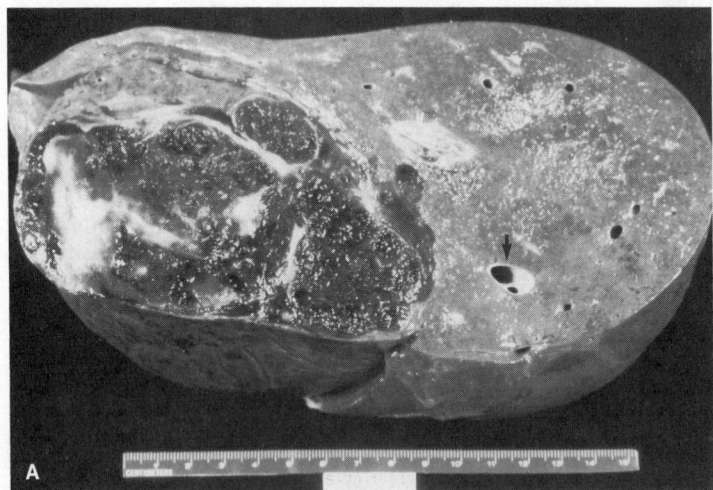

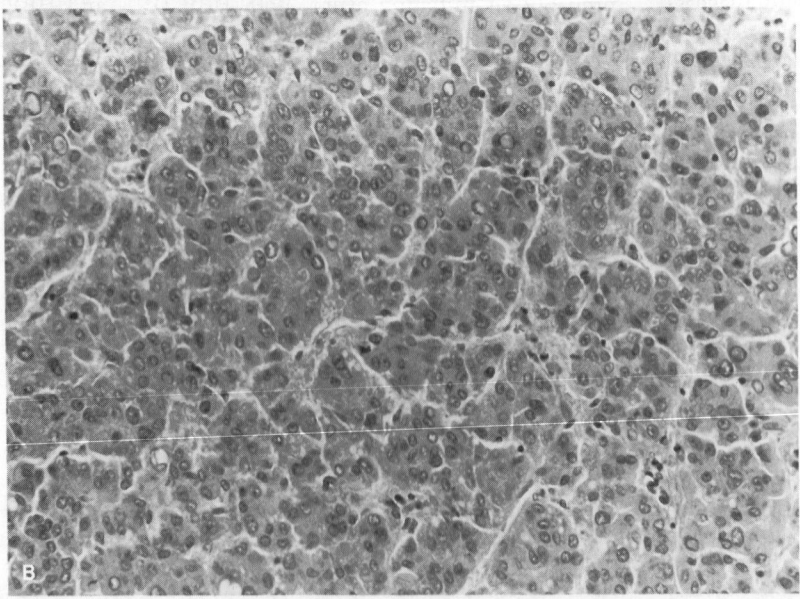

Figure 39-9. (*A*) A 9-cm hepatocellular carcinoma in the right lobe of the liver. Note the pseudoencapsulation of the lesion and its proximity to a 1-cm right hepatic vein (*arrow*). (*B*) The microscopic anatomy with hepatocytes of varying sizes and altered nuclear morphology.

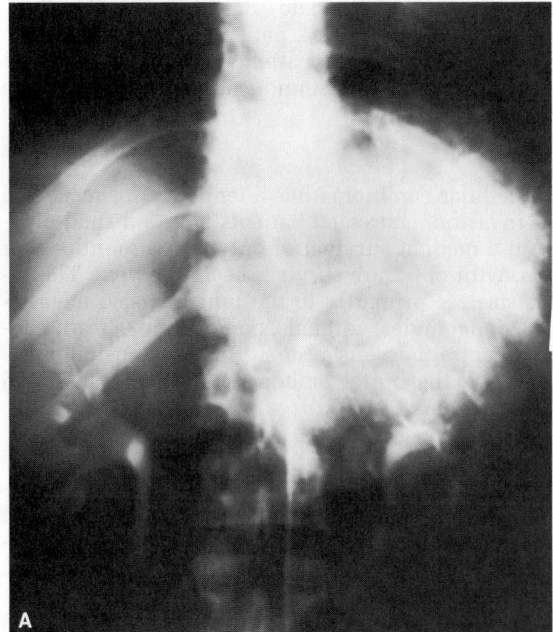

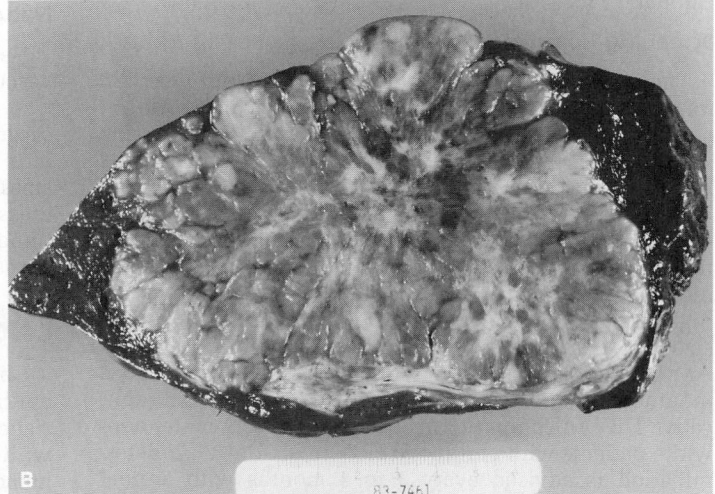

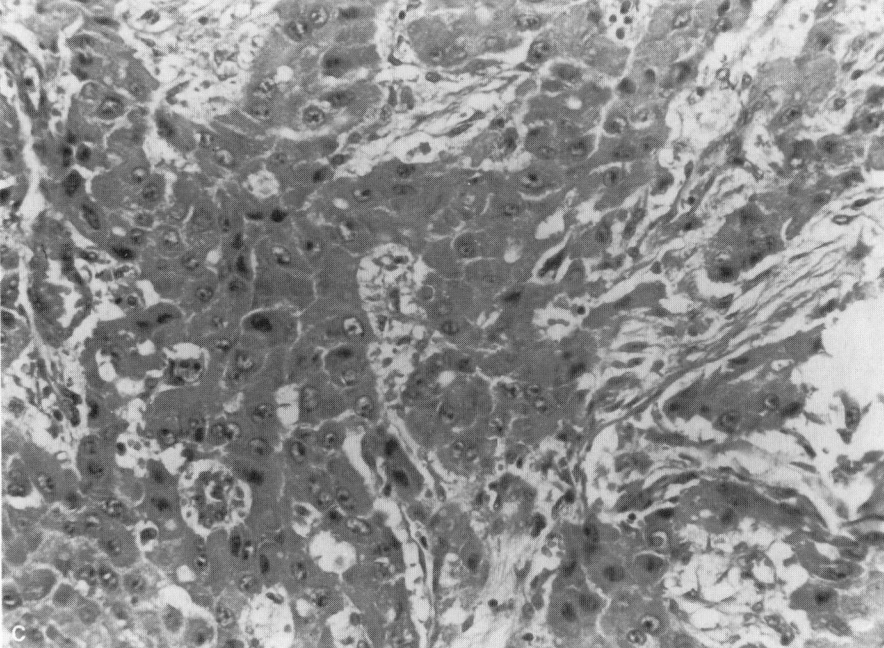

Figure 39-10. Arteriography of left hepatic mass demonstrates an interesting variant in which the left hepatic artery arises from the left gastric artery. (*A*) A tumor blush is demonstrated in a large 10-cm lesion. (*B*) The gross lesion, in contrast to Figure 39-9, shows a more fibrous component grossly. (*C*) Histologic examination shows widely variant hepatocellular morphology with distinct fibrous ingrowth. This lesion is a fibrolamellar hepatoma.

per quadrant pain is present in more than one half of cases, and a palpable mass is present in more than 30%. Weight loss, anorexia, and malaise occur in 25% to 30% of cases. Fever is not uncommon. Patients may also develop splenomegaly and varices as well as ascites. Severe, sudden abdominal pain may indicate hemorrhage into the mass. Intraperitoneal bleeding occurs in 10% of patients. Jaundice occurs in 10% to 40% of cases but is rarely due to biliary obstruction. Anemia often occurs with HCC. Paraneoplastic syndromes are also possible and include erythrocytosis, dysfibrinogenemia, hypoglycemia, hypercalcemia, hypertension (from angiotensin production), and diarrhea (from vasoactive intestinal peptide or gastrin production).

Diagnosis

Abdominal CT is the radiologic test used most often to evaluate suspected HCC. This imaging modality yields good anatomic resolution and can detect extrahepatic dis-

ease. Percutaneous FNA or core biopsy can be used to obtain tissue diagnosis. Other, more sensitive tests for the detection of HCC, sometimes used preoperatively, include CTAP, CT with iodized oil injection, and angiography. Laparotomy remains the best method for determining extrahepatic disease spread. The role of laparoscopy as a preoperative staging modality is evolving. Intraoperative ultrasound is another method for guiding resection. Patients should additionally have a chest radiograph and cytologic evaluation of any ascites present to rule out metastatic disease. Levels of AFP, an embryonal and fetal α_1-globulin derived from embryonic foregut cells, are elevated in 70% to 95% of patients with HCC.[18] Standard liver enzymes may be abnormal but are nonspecific, often reflecting underlying liver disease. Levels of serum AFP generally correlate with tumor size. AFP values can be falsely elevated in cases of pregnancy, yolk sac tumors, and hepatitis. Nevertheless, a persistently elevated AFP should alert the clinician to the possibility of tumor. A new laboratory test, des-γcarboxyprothrombin, is reportedly 75% to 90% sensitive.[19] There are also early studies of the detection of tumor-specific antigens with monoclonal antibodies. Urinary pseudouridine is under investigation as a biochemical marker for HCC.

Screening Recommendations

The TNM (tumor, node, metastasis) classification system for HCC is presented in Table 39-2. If HCC is to be found at a small, asymptomatic, and potentially surgically curable stage, an effective screening program for high-risk patients is necessary. An accepted and successful screening regimen used in Asia consists of interval testing for AFP in combination with ultrasound examination. Because the tumor median doubling time is 4 months (range, 1 to 14 months), screening should be done every 4 months for high-risk patients if the tumors are to be detected at a small size (1 to 3 cm). One proposed screening regimen includes AFP every 3 to 4 months with ultrasound every 4 to 6 months for high-risk patients (defined as those with replicative HBV infection or cirrhosis, particularly male, non-white patients with childhood HBV infection). AFP determination is advised every 3 to 4 months with annual ultrasound for patients at moderate risk (those who have nonreplicative HBV infection or adult HBV infection and those who are white and female). Screening is not considered cost-effective for low-risk patients (no HBV infection or cirrhosis). Postoperative patients should be followed with regular AFP and ultrasound examination, as is done for high-risk patients.

Natural History

Hepatocellular carcinoma has a tendency for local and vascular invasion. Untreated patients have a dismal prognosis with a median survival of only 3 to 4 months after diagnosis, with only rare survival beyond 1 year. The tumor metastasizes primarily to the lung but also metastasizes to regional nodes, adrenals, bone, kidney, heart, pancreas, and central nervous system. Direct extension of the tumor through the portal or hepatic venous system can occasionally occur.

CHOLANGIOCARCINOMA

Cholangiocarcinoma is a malignancy of the bile duct epithelium and may have either an intrahepatic or an extrahepatic location. Cholangiocarcinomas are associated with infestation of *Clonorchis* species, ulcerative colitis, hemochromatosis, chronic cholangitis, and cystic diseases with areas of bile stasis (choledochoceles). Intrahepatic cholangiocarcinoma is much less common than extrahepatic cholangiocarcinoma. Intrahepatic cholangiocarcinoma is usually discovered on workup of a liver mass. A primary hepatic malignancy known as *cholangiohepatocellular carcinoma* has features of both cholangiocarcinoma and HCC.

Principles of diagnosis and treatment of intrahepatic cholangiocarcinoma follow those described for HCC. Cholangiocarcinoma is fully discussed in Chapter 42, and hepatoblastoma is discussed in Chapter 105.

PRIMARY HEPATIC SARCOMAS

Primary hepatic sarcomas are rare. The most common and best studied hepatic sarcoma is angiosarcoma, which has been associated with the following carcinogens—vinyl chloride monomer, a volatile chemical used in the plastics industry; Thorotrast, a radiologic contrast medium used between 1928 and 1950; and arsenic. Exposure to androgens such as methyltestosterone is also a risk factor. There is a long latent period between exposure and development of malignancy. The tumor is highly malignant with significant metastatic potential, locally invasive, and rapidly fatal. Another sarcoma of the liver is epithelioid hemangioendothelioma, an intermediate-grade neoplasm that is the malignant counterpart of pediatric hemangioendothelioma. Treatment of epithelioid hemangioendothelioma is not well defined, but the lesion should be regarded as malignant and treated as such. Although the sarcomas are usually primary, they are sometimes metastatic. An examination of the retroperitoneum should be performed to exclude metastatic spread to the liver.

Table 39-2. TNM CLASSIFICATION FOR STAGING OF LIVER TUMORS

TNM DEFINITIONS

Primary Tumor

TX Primary tumor cannot be assessed
T0 No evidence of primary tumor
T1 Solitary tumor 2 cm or less in greatest dimension without vascular invasion
T2 Solitary tumor 2 cm or less in greatest dimension with vascular invasion, or
    Multiple tumors limited to one lobe, none more than 2 cm in greatest dimension, without vascular invasion, or
    A solitary tumor more than 2 cm in greatest dimension without vascular invasion
T3 Solitary tumor more than 2 cm in greatest dimension with vascular invasion, or
    Multiple tumors limited to one lobe, none more than 2 cm in greatest dimension, with vascular invasion, or
    Multiple tumors limited to one lobe, any more than 2 cm in greatest dimension, with or without vascular invasion
T4 Multiple tumors in more than one lobe, or tumor involves a major branch of portal or hepatic veins

Lymph Node Involvement

NX Regional lymph nodes cannot be assessed
N0 No regional lymph node metastasis
N1 Regional lymph node metastasis

Distant Metastasis

MX Presence of distant metastasis cannot be assessed
M0 No distant metastasis
M1 Distant metastasis

STAGE GROUPING

Stage I	T1,	N0,	M0
Stage II	T2,	N0,	M0
Stage III	T1,	N1,	M0
	T2,	N1,	M0
	T3,	N0,	M0
	T3,	N0,	M0
Stage IVA	T4, any N, M0		
Stage IVB	Any T, any N, M1		

(Union Internationale Contra le Cancer)

Therapeutic Options for Primary Hepatic Malignancies

Curative Therapy

Surgical resection offers the only chance for cure of primary hepatic malignancy, and survival is better if tumors are small and asymptomatic. Unfortunately, few primary adult hepatic malignancies are resectable, usually because of cirrhosis, extensive involvement of structures at the porta hepatis, and metastasis. Cirrhosis limits the liver's ability to regenerate after resection and therefore increases the risk of postoperative hepatic failure. Limited hepatic resection has been successful for selected patients with small tumors who also have cirrhosis and decreased liver function.

Small tumors can be removed with wedge resection or segmentectomy, but larger tumors generally require formal lobectomy. Surgery is often aided by intraoperative ultrasound. The 5-year survival rate after resection for cure averages 25% for HCC, with an operative mortality rate of 4% to 9%. Lower mortality and better survival can be expected for patients with small, asymptomatic tumors and no cirrhosis. Survival is worse and operative mortality is higher in patients with cirrhosis, larger tumors, invasive tumors, or more poorly differentiated tumors, and with poor performance status. Five-year survival for the fibrolamellar variant is significantly better.

Most patients who undergo resection have recurrence. Usually, recurrence is local and occurs at the margin of resection or within the parenchyma of the residual lobe. For patients undergoing a limited resection for a small tumor, the extent of tumor margin has not been associated with increased recurrence. For tumors larger than 4 cm, a tumor-free margin of more than 1 cm is required to limit recurrence.[20] Treatment for recurrences is often limited by the reduced liver mass. Repeat surgery is the first choice but often is not possible. Palliative hepatic artery embolization may be recommended for unresectable HCC but is subject to the constraints of decreased hepatic reserve. When resection is not possible, chemotherapy, immunotherapy, and transplantation become alternative treatments.

Transplantation for Primary Hepatic Malignancy

The role of orthotopic liver transplantation (OLT) for HCC continues to evolve. Partial hepatic resection is the treatment of choice for patients with resectable lesions with minimal to moderate liver dysfunction. However, for patients with severe hepatic dysfunction, larger or centrally located tumors, or bilobar tumors, OLT may be the preferred approach. Extrahepatic disease with lymph node involvement is a contraindication to resection or transplantation. Patients with high-risk tumors (greater than 5 cm, not encapsulated, or associated with vascular invasion) should be considered for neoadjuvant or adjuvant multimodality therapy.[21]

Palliative Therapy

Chemotherapy. No single-agent or multiagent chemotherapy is particularly effective in treating HCC. Doxorubicin is the recommended agent, with combination therapy showing no advantage. Regional chemotherapy involves surgical or percutaneous placement of a hepatic arterial catheter and a continuous infusion pump. The response to doxorubicin that is given by hepatic artery catheter (nearly 50%) is better than the response to doxorubicin that is given systemically.[22] The long-term advantage of hepatic arterial versus peripheral delivery has not been conclusively proved. The drugs 5-fluorouracil, fluorodeoxyuridine, cisplatin, and mitomycin are under investigation for use in regional chemotherapy. Despite tumor responses, systemic and regional chemotherapy do not significantly increase survival.

Ischemic Therapy. The rationale for treating vascular liver tumors, both primary and secondary, with arterial obstruction is the derivation of nutrient blood flow of liver tumors from the hepatic artery. Hepatic artery ligation, alone or in combination with regional chemotherapy, has been shown to be ineffective for primary liver cancer. Hepatic artery ligation has a high complication rate and often

cannot be used in patients with compromised liver function caused by cirrhosis. Hepatic artery embolization for primary hepatic malignancy has shown some palliative benefit, especially in combination with regionally delivered doxorubicin or cisplatin. Both hepatic artery ligation and embolization can be used for acute control of tumor rupture.

Radiation Therapy. Radiation therapy for the treatment of primary hepatic malignancy has been limited by a dose-related hepatitis that occurs after 2500 to 3000 cGy. Nevertheless, it remains useful for acute palliation, and when it is used in combination with systemic chemotherapy it may be equivalent or superior to intraarterial chemotherapy.

METASTATIC LIVER DISEASE
Biology of Hepatic Metastases

The liver is a common site for metastatic deposits, particularly from abdominal primaries, because of its dual blood supply (75% from the portal vein, 25% from the hepatic artery) and histologic filtering structure. Tumor emboli are commonly seen in the portal venules at autopsy, and it is estimated that hepatic metastases occur in at least 50% of patients in whom the primary tumor drains into the portal vein. Other factors are also important. There is a definite biologic predilection of cancers for various organs, probably based on cell–cell interactions and other homing mechanisms. Successful evasion of the host immune response is also required. Once settled in the liver, the tumor secretes various proteolytic enzymes and angiogenesis factors. The establishment of an independent blood supply allows metastases to develop.

Colorectal, breast, lung, melanoma, and pancreatic islet cell tumors, as well as other visceral adenocarcinomas and carcinoid tumors, frequently metastasize to the liver. Nasopharyngeal carcinoma and lymphomatous and leukemic metastases may also occur. There has been little enthusiasm for resection of liver metastases from nonportal tumors (eg, breast, lung, melanoma) because of the probability of systemic metastasis. Only colorectal, pancreatic, and carcinoid tumors have a reasonable chance of being liver-only metastases. Of these, only colorectal cancer has been extensively studied because it occurs frequently enough and with sufficiently limited hepatic involvement.

Natural History of Metastatic Colorectal Cancer

Liver metastases are first noted at laparotomy during primary cancer resection in 8% to 30% of patients.[23] If present, symptoms and signs may include malaise, fever, weight loss, right upper quadrant pain or fullness, a palpable mass, and occasionally ascites or splenomegaly. Jaundice is infrequent and may be due to metastatic obstruction of the biliary tract, or it may occur late in the course of disease as a result of loss of parenchyma and cholestasis. Metastases are usually asymptomatic and are discovered by biochemical and radiologic evaluation (Fig. 39-11).

Of the 150,000 cases of colorectal primaries resected each year, about 60,000 (40%) recur at some site. Of patients in whom disease recurs, 20% apparently have only hepatic metastases. It is this subgroup that is potentially surgically curable.

Studies consistently report an operative mortality rate of less than 5% and 5-year survival rates averaging 25% for hepatic resection for colorectal metastases (Table 39-3). Those who survive beyond 5 years seem to do well,

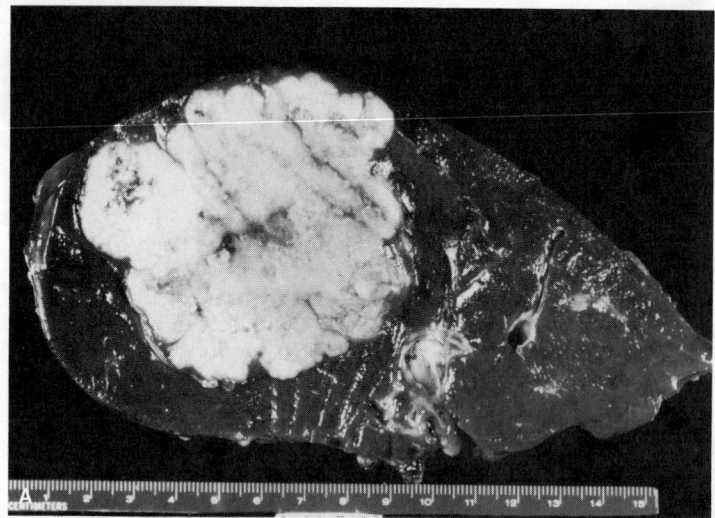

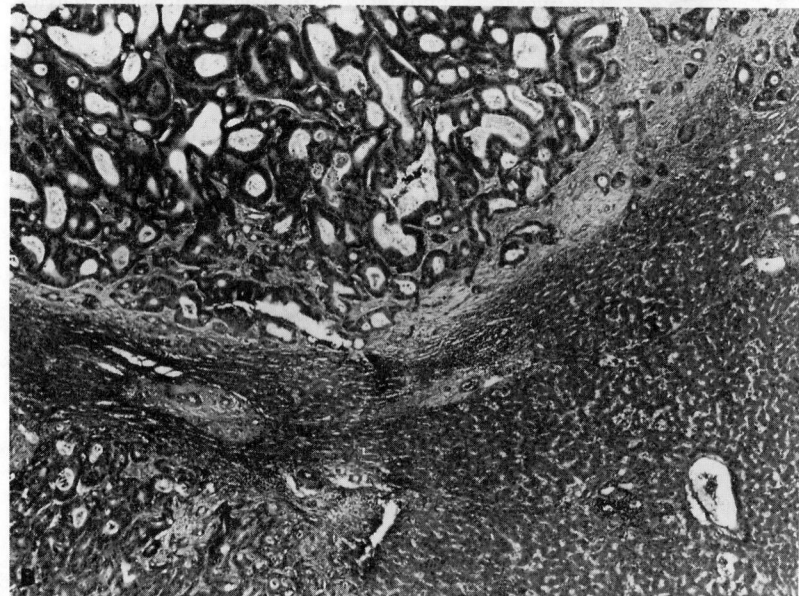

Figure 39-11. (*A*) A 7-cm single colorectal metastasis demonstrated within a surgical specimen. (*B*) Under microscopy, a moderately differentiated adenocarcinoma of the colon is shown adjacent to an area of pseudoencapsulation and normal hepatic parenchyma. (Hanks JB, Jones RS. Curr Probl Cancer 1986;10:245)

with only an additional 5% dying of recurrence during the next 5 years. These results suggest a survival advantage when compared with the natural outcome of untreated hepatic metastases. The median survival of patients with untreated metastases is 3 to 10 months, with only 20% surviving past 1 year.

Evaluation

No laboratory test is sufficiently specific or sensitive to be used exclusively for the detection of hepatic metastases. No test is greater than 65% accurate, and although many studies favor a specific test, there is no consensus. The most useful tests include CEA determination (for colorectal metastases), alkaline phosphatase, serum glutamic oxaloacetic transaminase, γ-glutamyltransferase, lactate dehydrogenase, and 5′-nucleotidase (Table 39-4). Although the more conventional laboratory tests such as CEA are helpful, they are often not elevated until disease is extensive. Therefore, they should not be used alone for the evaluation of metastatic disease. Preoperative evaluation is often done with CT, ultrasound, and angiography to define vascular anatomy (Fig. 39-12). Additionally, a patient with suspected colorectal metastases after previous resection should undergo colon evaluation, because metachronous colon cancer develops in 3% of patients, and suture line recurrence should be excluded.

Treatment

Surgery

The preoperative evaluation of a patient with liver metastases must have as its goals determination of resectability and identification of favorable prognostic factors. The following are relevant prognostic factors.

Extrahepatic Disease. In patients with extrahepatic disease, the 5-year disease-free survival rate is only 4%. Extrahepatic disease is a consistently negative prognostic factor and should be considered a contraindication to further surgery.

Margin of Resection. Overall survival is significantly improved (44% 5-year survival rate) with margins greater than 1 cm. Survival is decreased in patients with positive margins or margins of up to 1 cm. Thus, the inability to obtain adequate margins of resection can be considered a contraindication to resection.

Table 39-3. SURVIVAL WITH RESECTED COLORECTAL HEPATIC METASTASES

Investigators	Patients	Operative Mortality Rate (%)	Survival Rate (%) 1 Year	Survival Rate (%) 5 Years
Adson et al, 1981	141	2		25
August et al, 1985	33	0		
Bengmark et al, 1982	39	6	80	10
Cady et al, 1984	23	0		
Coppa et al, 1985	25	4		25
Ekberg et al, 1986	72	6		16
Fortner et al, 1987	65	7	89	
Flanagan and Foster, 1987	45			23
Hughes et al, 1989	>800			32
Iwatsuki et al, 1986	60			45
Kortz et al, 1984	16	6	75	29
Morrow et al, 1982	29			27
Rajpal et al, 1982	34	12	80	

Number of Metastases. The number of metastases is a less consistent but statistically significant factor. Patients with four or more metastases have a poorer prognosis. The existence of this many metastases can be considered a contraindication to resection, when taken in the context of other prognostic factors.

Size of Metastases. The absolute size of metastases is not a significant factor except that greater total liver volume of metastasis requires a larger hepatic resection. Large size may preclude adequate margins and may indicate a longer development time with an increased likelihood of micrometastases.

Intrahepatic Distribution. The survival curves for patients with multiple unilobar versus multiple bilobar metastases are identical. Thus, bilobar metastases amenable to a parenchyma-sparing resection with adequate margins are not a contraindication to surgery.

Other. Anatomic resections appear to have an advantage over wedge resections because of their better ability to obtain margins. The Dukes stage of the primary lesion clearly does have implications for prognosis. Patients with

Dukes C lesions do not fare as well as those with Dukes A and B lesions. Patients with Dukes C tumors have an increased incidence of extrahepatic recurrence despite complete resection of the primary and hepatic metastases. The influence of grade or differentiation of the primary has not been well studied, but there are indications that measures such as tumor DNA content predict prognosis.[24] Neither patient age nor sex is prognostic.

The proportion of patients with hepatic metastases who could be considered resectable is about 5% to 10%. If patients are properly selected and undergo surgery with a mortality rate less than 5%, about 25% can be expected to be 5-year survivors. This figure can approach 40% in patients with a good prognostic profile. Resection is a reasonable procedure given its low risk, the lack of curative medical therapeutic options, and the dismal prognosis without surgery.

Surgical Options

Patients may undergo nonanatomic wedge resection for peripherally located lesions, newer anatomically based segmentectomies that allow good margins and sparing of uninvolved parenchyma, or classic lobectomies or triseg-

Table 39-4. LABORATORY EVALUATION IN PATIENTS WITH SUSPECTED HEPATIC METASTASES

Test	Results	Description
CEA		
CEA alone	86% sensitivity	CEA is used in the detection of colorectal cancer and its metastatic spread.
CEA & LDH together	87% sensitivity	Although not specific for colorectal cancer, serial CEA levels are sensitive for
	47% specificity	disease recurrence in patients with colorectal cancer.
AP		
AP	77% sensitivity	AP is an enzyme with distribution in the liver, bile duct, bone, placenta, kidney,
AP with positive CEA	88% sensitivity	and WBCs. Like GGT and 5'-nucleotidase, it is elevated in cases of biliary
	12% false-positive	obstruction or infiltrating diseases more than with hepatocellular injury.
GGT	97% sensitivity	GGT is found in the liver, kidney, pancreas, heart, brain, and spleen. It has been most consistently sensitive, alone and in combination with AP, in hepatic metastatic disease.
5'-NUCLEOTIDASE	65% sensitivity	Despite a wide tissue distribution, increased serum levels occur only with hepatobiliary disease. Its values correlate closely with AP and GGT. Compared with AP, GGT, and SGOT, it had the lowest false-positive rate and best positive predictive value.

AP, alkaline phosphatase; CEA, carcinoembryonic antigen; GGT, γ-glutamyltransferase; LDH, lactate dehydrogenase; WBCs, white blood cells.

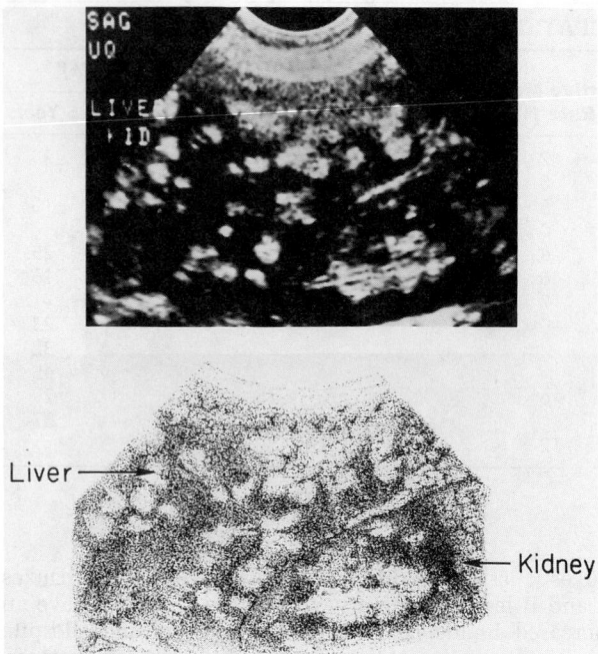

Figure 39-12. Abdominal ultrasound reveals multiple metastatic deposits within the liver. (Hanks JB, Jones RS. Curr Probl Cancer 1986;10:245)

mentectomy. The best technique is that which allows the best margins with sparing of the liver mass. Moderate success with repeat hepatic resection for recurrent colorectal metastases has been reported.[25]

About 80% of patients have recurrence after resection of colorectal liver metastases, with 65% having liver involvement. When patients with inadequate resection margins are discounted, the liver-only recurrence rate is reduced. Thus, most patients with recurrence after adequate resection have disease spread beyond the liver at the time of hepatic resection, and recurrence is likely because of missed occult metastases.

Palliative options for patients with unresectable metastases are limited to systemic or regional chemotherapy, hepatic artery ligation, cryosurgery, percutaneous ethanol injection, chemoembolization, immunotherapy, and radiation therapy.

REFERENCES

1. Ferrucci JT. Liver tumor imaging. Cancer 1991;67:1189.
2. Wernecke K, Rummeny E, Bongartz G, et al. Detection of hepatic masses in patients with carcinoma. Am J Radiol 1991;157:731-739.
3. Soyer P, Levesque M, Elias D, et al. Detection of liver metastases from colorectal cancer: comparison of intraoperative ultrasound and CT during arterial portography. Radiology 1992;183:541.
4. Bismuth H, Castaing O, Garden OJ. The use of operative ultrasound in surgery of primary liver tumors. World J Surg 1987;11:610.
5. Cohn KH, Welt S, Banner WP, et al. Localization of radioiodinated monoclonal antibody in colorectal cancer: initial dosimetry results. Arch Surg 1987;122:1420.
6. Goldenberg DM, Goldenberg H, Higginbotham-Ford E, et al. Imaging of primary and metastatic liver cancer with ^{131}I monoclonal and polyclonal antibodies against alpha-fetoprotein. J Clin Oncol 1987;5:1827.
7. Sautereau O, Vire O, Cazes PY, et al. Value of sonographically guided fine needle aspiration biopsy in evaluating the liver with sonographic abnormalities. Gastroenterology 1987;93:715.
8. Rooks JB, Ory HW, Ishak KG, et al. Epidemiology of hepatocellular adenoma. JAMA 1979;242:644.
9. Kerlin P, Davis GL, McGill DB, et al. Hepatic adenoma and focal nodular hyperplasia: clinical, pathologic, and radiologic features. Gastroenterology 1983;84:994.
10. Nichols FC, vanHeerden JA, Weiland LH. Benign liver tumors. Surg Clin North Am 1989;69:297.
11. Nelson RC, Chezmar JL. Diagnostic approach to hepatic hemangiomas. Radiology 1990;176:11.
12. Doty JE, Tompkins RK. Management of cystic diseases of the liver. Surg Clin North Am 1989;69:285.
13. Johnson PJ. Hepatic viruses, cirrhosis, and liver cancer. J Surg Oncol 1993;3(Suppl):28.
14. Lefkowitch JH. The epidemiology and morphology of primary malignant liver tumors. Surg Clin North Am 1981;61:169.
15. Lee CS, Sung JL, Hwang LY, et al. Surgical treatment of 109 patients with symptomatic and asymptomatic hepatocellular carcinoma. Surgery 1986;99:481.
16. Oberfield RA, Steele GD, Gollan JL, Sherman D. Liver cancer. CA Cancer J Clin 1989;39:212.
17. Berman MM, Libbey NP, Foster JH. Hepatocellular carcinoma: polygonal cell type with fibrous stroma—an atypical variant with a favorable prognosis. Cancer 1980;46:1448.
18. Okuda K. The liver cancer study group of Japan: primary liver cancers in Japan. Cancer 1980;45:2663.
19. Solier J-P, Gozin D, Lefrere JJ, et al. A new method to assay des-gamma-carboxyprothrombin: results obtained in 75 cases of hepatocellular carcinoma. Gastroenterology 1986;91:1258.
20. Yoshida Y, Kanematsu T, Matsumata T, et al. Surgical margins and recurrence after resection of hepatocellular carcinoma in patients with cirrhosis: further evaluation of limited hepatic resection. Ann Surg 1989;209:297.
21. Farmer DG, Rosove MH, Shaked A, et al. Current treatment modalities for hepatocellular carcinoma. Ann Surg 1994;219:236.
22. Balch CM, Urist MM. Intraarterial chemotherapy for colorectal liver metastases and hepatomas using a totally implantable drug infusion pump. Recent Results Cancer Res 1986;100:234.
23. Saenz NC, Cady B, McDermott WV, Steele GO. Experience with colorectal cancer metastatic to the liver. Surg Clin North Am 1989;69:361.
24. Kokal WA, Duda RB, Azumi N, et al. Tumor DNA content in primary and metastatic colorectal carcinoma. Arch Surg 1986;121:1434.
25. Ekberg H, Tranberg KG, Anderson R, et al. Patterns of recurrence in liver resection for colorectal secondaries. World J Surg 1987;11:541.

SURGERY: SCIENTIFIC PRINCIPLES AND PRACTICE, Second Edition, edited by Lazar J. Greenfield, Michael W. Mulholland, Keith T. Oldham, Gerald B. Zelenock, and Keith D. Lillemoe. Lippincott–Raven Publishers, Philadelphia, © 1997.

CHAPTER 40

BILIARY ANATOMY AND PHYSIOLOGY

NATHANIEL J. SOPER

EMBRYOLOGY

The primordial anlagen of the liver, extrahepatic bile ducts, gallbladder, and ventral part of the pancreas are evident in the human embryo at about the fifth week of intrauterine life or when the embryo is about 3 mm long (Fig. 40-1A). This anlage is a thickened area of entoderm on the ventral surface in the caudal portion of the foregut where it joins the midgut.[1,2] Superior and inferior caudal buds form as the hepatic diverticulum grows out into the ventral mesogastrium. The cranial sacculation of the diverticulum migrates ventrally and superiorly into the septum transversum, which separates the thoracic and the abdominal cavities. The solid mass of endodermal cells spreading with this cephalic bud forms the right and left lobes of the liver. The superior growth of the cranial portion of the hepatic diverticulum, which extends from the duodenum to the liver, results in the formation of the hepatic, common hepatic, and common bile ducts. The caudal portion of the hepatic diverticulum develops into the gallbladder and cystic duct. The lobes of the liver and a solid cylinder of entoderm cells, which eventually form the extrahepatic biliary tract and the gallbladder, are evident when the embryo is 5 mm long (see Fig. 40-1B). Vacuolization takes place in this cylindrical mass, forming the lumen of the common bile duct, the hepatic and cystic ducts, and the gallbladder, starting at 7 weeks' gestation. The common bile duct is attached to the ventral aspect of the duodenum and is in close contact with the ventral pancreatic bud. With rotation of the duodenum and ventral pancreatic bud, the proximal portion of the extrahepatic tract also rotates, and the common bile duct enters into the left posterior surface of the duodenum. This rotation occurs when the fetus reaches the 7-mm stage (see Fig. 40-1C), and by the 12-mm stage (see Fig. 40-1D), the bile ducts and gallbladder are in normal position. At the terminal end of the common duct, the musculature of the sphincter of Oddi arises de novo from mesenchyme, appearing about 5 weeks after development of the duodenal muscles.

ANATOMY

Gallbladder

The gallbladder is a pear-shaped organ bound to a fossa on the right inferior surface of the liver by connective tissue and vessels, and it lies between the right, left, and quadrate hepatic lobes[1-3] or hepatic segments IV and V (Fig. 40-2). The gallbladder occasionally has a complete peritoneal covering and true mesentery predisposing to torsion. Rarely, the organ is located so deeply within the liver parenchyma that it can be reached from the outside only by dividing an overlying layer of liver tissue (intrahepatic gallbladder). The fundus and inferior surface of the gallbladder are covered with peritoneum reflected from the liver. The gallbladder is 7 to 10 cm long, with an average volume of about 30 mL. With marked distention or acute obstruction, the viscus may contain up to 300 mL.

The gallbladder can be divided into four areas—fundus, body, infundibulum, and neck (Fig. 40-3). The fundus of the gallbladder begins at the anterior border of the liver and duodenum or transverse colon. The fundus usually projects 1 to 2 cm below the hepatic edge and is in contact with the anterior abdominal wall near the lateral border of the right rectus muscle. Indentation of the fundus accounts for the "phrygian cap" anomaly. The body of the gallbladder extends from the fundus into the tapered portion, or neck, which curves backward and upward toward the transverse fissure of the liver and terminates in the cystic duct. The neck usually has a gentle curve, the convexity of which may be enlarged to form the infundibulum, or Hartmann pouch. The neck occupies the deepest part of the gallbladder fossa and lies in the free portion of the hepatoduodenal ligament (see Fig. 40-2). The cystic duct lumen contains a thin mucosal septum, called the spiral valve of Heister (see Fig. 40-3). The valve may make catheterization of the cystic duct difficult but does not have true valvular function.

Vessels, Nerves, and Lymphatics

The arteries of the gallbladder are derived from the cystic branch of the hepatic artery.[3] The cystic artery arises from the right hepatic artery in 95% of cases, but it may arise from the left hepatic, common hepatic, gastroduodenal, or superior mesenteric arteries (Fig. 40-4). Double cystic arteries are present in 8% of cases, and an accessory cystic artery is present in 12% of cases. The course of the cystic artery varies greatly but is nearly always found within the hepatocystic triangle, the area bound by the cystic duct, common hepatic duct and liver margin. From its origin, it usually crosses behind the hepatic duct (84% of cases) but is sometimes anterior to that structure (16% of cases). The cystic artery proceeds to the neck of the gallbladder, where it divides into anterior and posterior divisions that supply the corresponding areas of the gallbladder. When the cystic

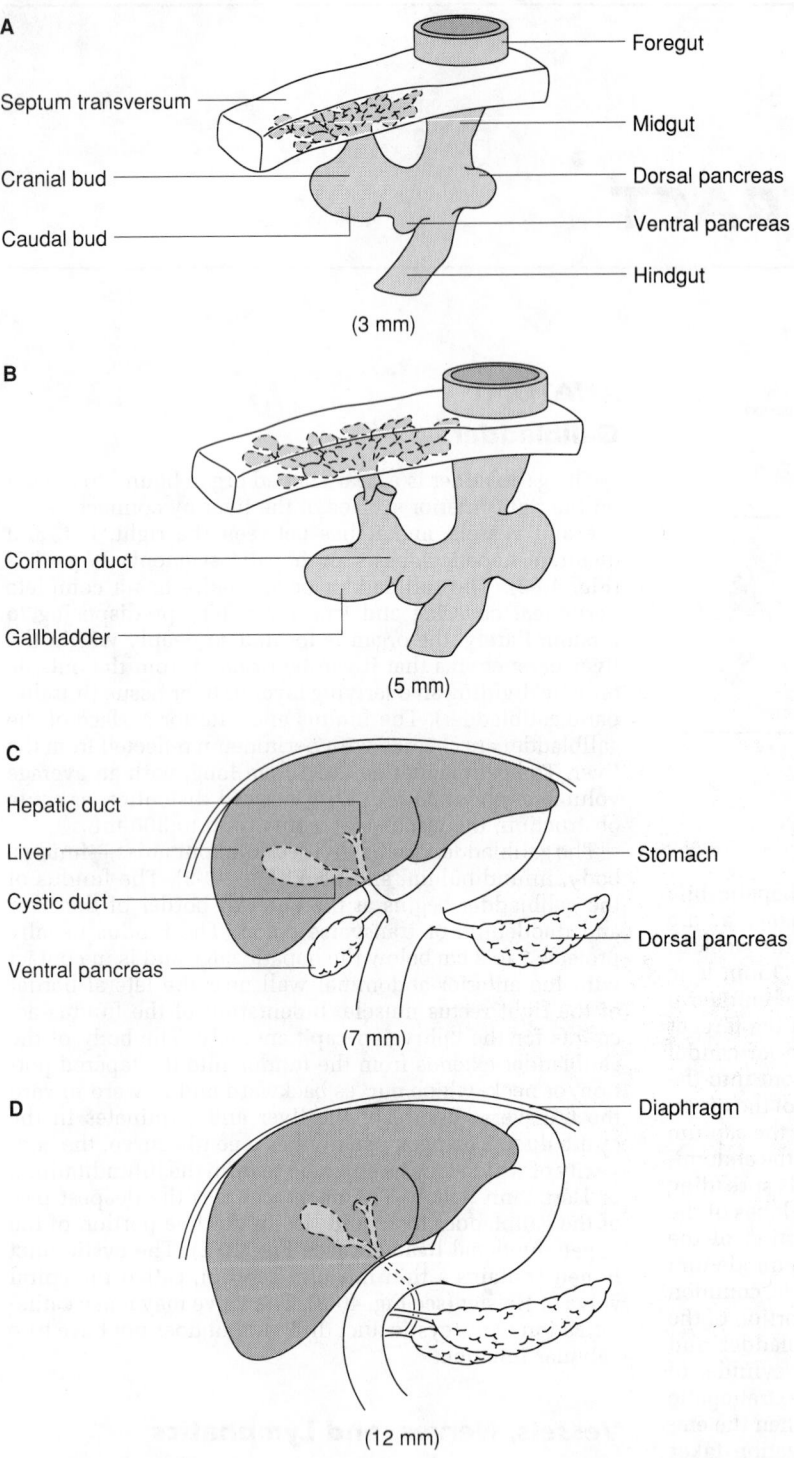

A

Septum transversum

Cranial bud

Caudal bud

Foregut

Midgut

Dorsal pancreas

Ventral pancreas

Hindgut

(3 mm)

B

Common duct

Gallbladder

(5 mm)

C

Hepatic duct

Liver

Cystic duct

Ventral pancreas

Stomach

Dorsal pancreas

(7 mm)

D

Diaphragm

(12 mm)

Figure 40-1. Sequence of the embryonic development of the biliary tract.

artery arises from the right hepatic artery, its course from its origin to the gallbladder is usually parallel and medial to the cystic duct. This relation is far from constant, however, and if the artery arises proximally from the right hepatic artery (33% of cases) or from the common hepatic artery, it may lie close to the common hepatic duct, which may be injured when the artery is clamped or ligated. When the cystic artery arises from the right hepatic artery close to the liver, the artery is related only to the upper part of the cystic duct (Fig. 40-5).

The cystic veins empty into the right branch of the portal vein and directly into the liver. Gallbladder lymphatics

drain into nodes at the neck of the gallbladder. Often, a visibly enlarged lymph node (cystic artery node or sentinel node) overlies the insertion of the cystic artery into the gallbladder wall. The nerves of the gallbladder are branches of the vagus and sympathetic nerves, which pass through the celiac plexus. The left (anterior) vagal trunk branches into hepatic and gastric components. The hepatic branch supplies fibers to the gallbladder, bile ducts, and liver. In addition to the well-described cholinergic effects of the vagus, numerous peptide-containing nerves exist in the vagi. These peptides include substance P, somatostatin, encephalins and vasoactive intestinal polypeptide

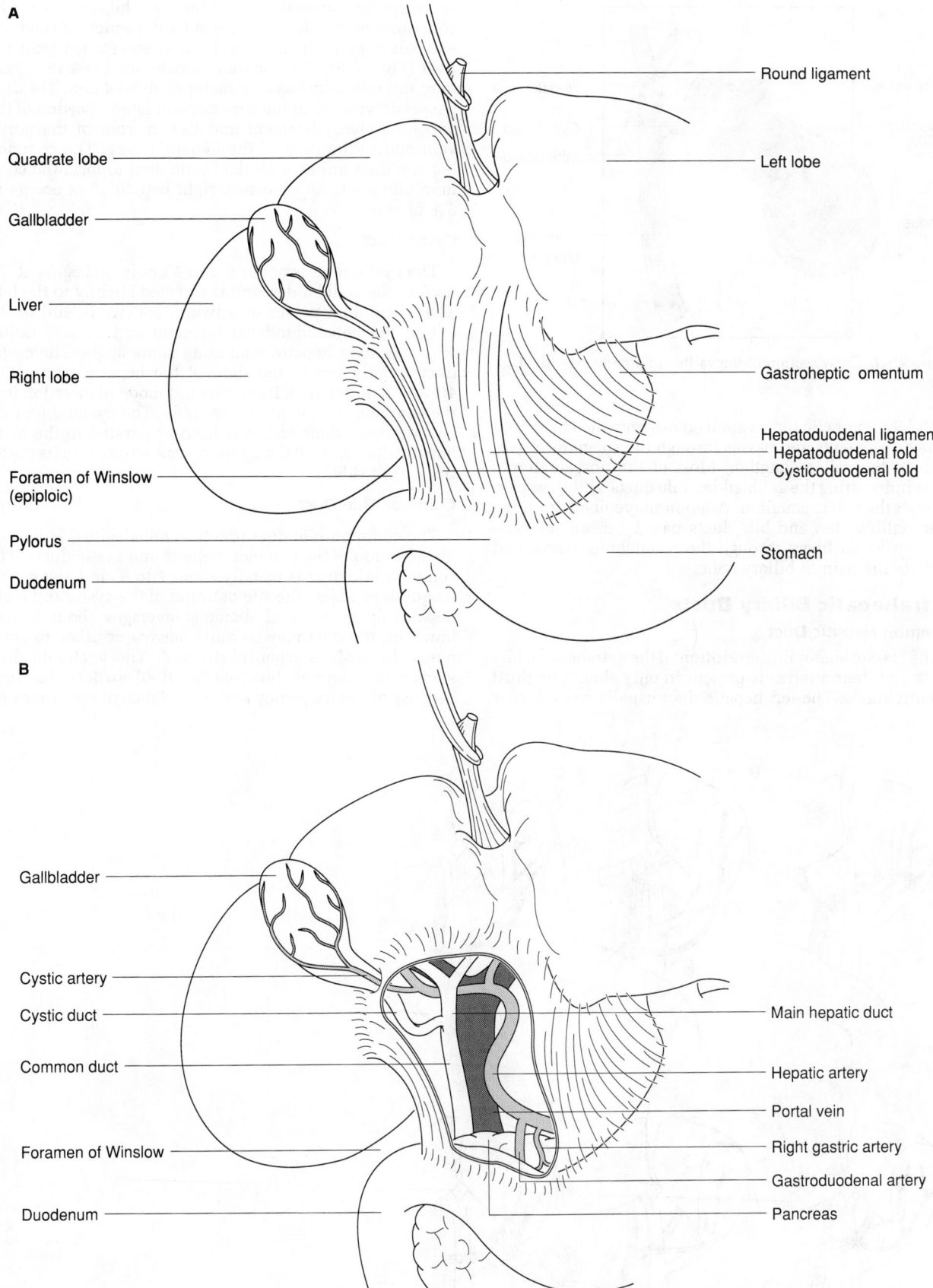

A

Quadrate lobe

Gallbladder

Liver

Right lobe

Foramen of Winslow
(epiploic)

Pylorus

Duodenum

Round ligament

Left lobe

Gastroheptic omentum

Hepatoduodenal ligament
Hepatoduodenal fold
Cysticoduodenal fold

Stomach

B

Gallbladder

Cystic artery

Cystic duct

Common duct

Foramen of Winslow

Duodenum

Main hepatic duct

Hepatic artery

Portal vein

Right gastric artery

Gastroduodenal artery

Pancreas

Figure 40-2. Anatomic relations of structures within the hepatoduodenal ligament.

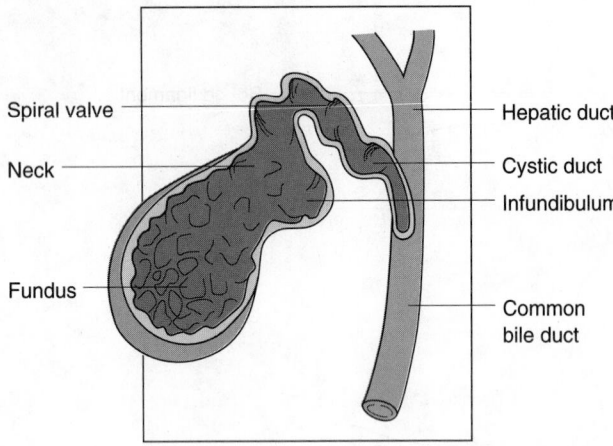

Figure 40-3. Cross section of the gallbladder and cystic duct.

(VIP).[4] Sympathetic innervation comes from the 7th to 10th thoracic segments and passes through the splanchnic ganglion to the celiac ganglion. Most of the postganglionic fibers innervating the gallbladder, bile ducts, and liver pass through the celiac ganglion. Afferent nerve fibers from the liver, gallbladder, and bile ducts pass by means of sympathic afferent fibers through the splanchnic nerves and mediate the pain of biliary colic.

Extrahepatic Biliary Ducts

Common Hepatic Duct

The classic anatomic description of the extrahepatic bile ducts and their arteries is present in only about one third of individuals. The left hepatic duct usually has a longer extrahepatic course than does the right hepatic duct. The common hepatic duct is formed by the union of the right and left hepatic ducts close to their emergence from the liver (Fig. 40-6). The common hepatic duct is 1 to 2.5 cm long and normally has a diameter of about 4 mm. The duct passes downward in the superior and lateral portion of the hepatoduodenal ligament and lies in front of the portal vein and to the right of the hepatic artery. The common hepatic duct unites with the cystic duct to form the common bile duct. An accessory right hepatic duct occurs in 5% of cases.

Cystic Duct

The cystic duct is about 0.5 to 4 cm long, begins at the neck of the gallbladder, and is directed slightly to the left. The cystic duct passes downward, backward, and to the left in the hepatoduodenal ligament and usually unites with the main hepatic duct at an acute angle. The cystic duct usually lies to the right of the hepatic artery (Fig. 40-7) and portal vein. Its course and mode of insertion into the common duct is highly variable. The cystic duct may be extremely short or run behind or parallel to the main hepatic duct and, after a spiral course, empty into its posterior or left side.

Common Bile Duct

The common bile duct (ductus choledochus) is formed by the union of the common hepatic and cystic ducts. The common bile duct is usually about 7 to 9 cm long, but its length depends on the site of union of the cystic and main hepatic ducts. Internal diameter averages about 5 mm; however, the duct may be quite narrow or dilate to enormous dimensions when obstructed. The anatomic divisions of the common duct (see Fig. 40-6) are described here because of the frequency and importance of operations on

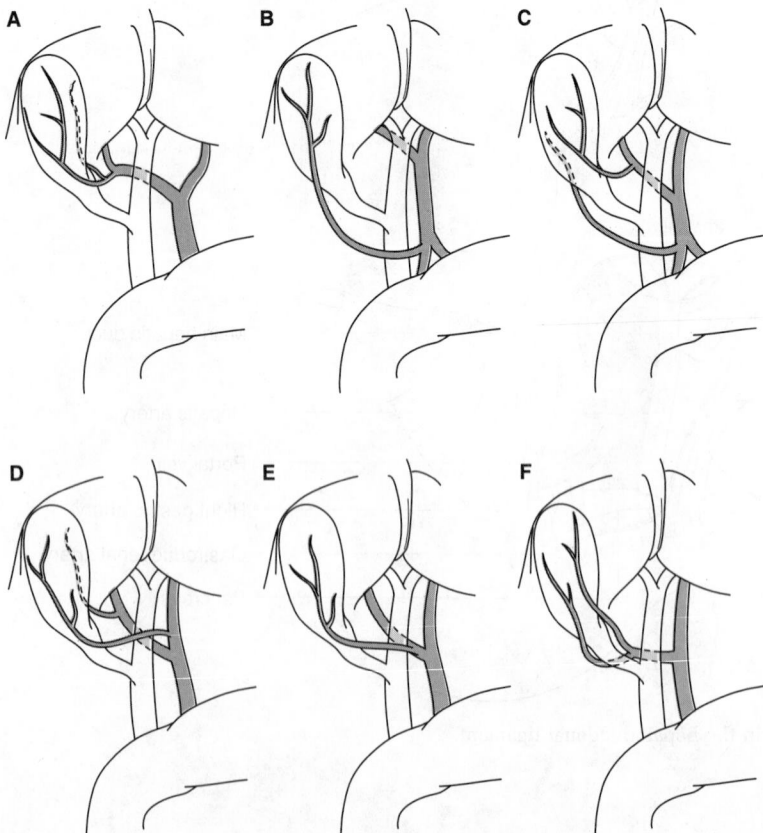

Figure 40-4. Normal and anomalous arterial supply to the gallbladder.

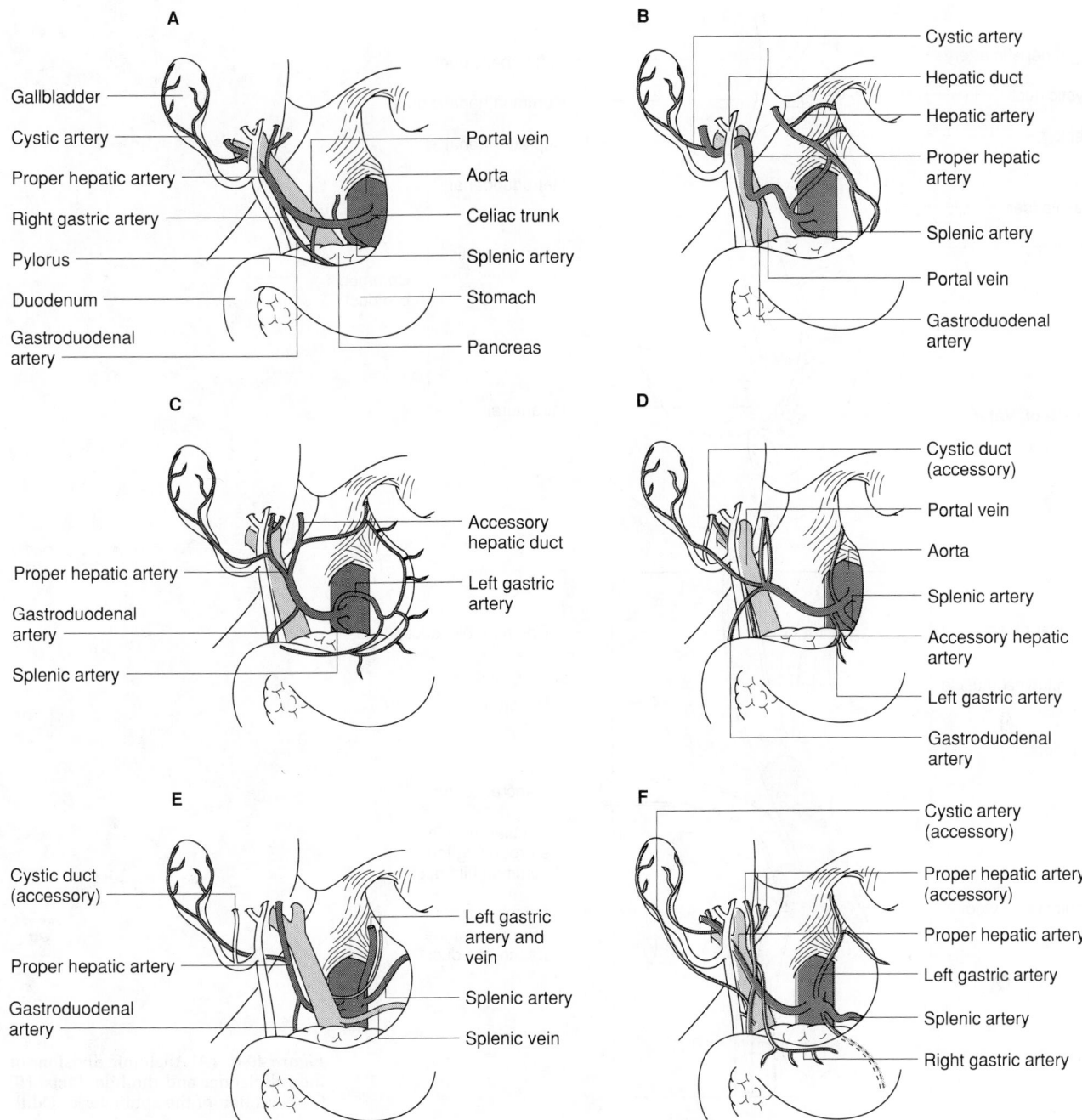

Figure 40-5. Variations in relations among the hepatic artery, portal vein, and bile ducts.

it. The supraduodenal portion passes downward and backward in the hepatoduodenal ligament in front of the epiploic foramen (foramen of Winslow) anterior and to the right of the portal vein. The hepatic artery and its gastroduodenal branch lie to the left of the supraduodenal portion of the duct. The retroduodenal portion lies behind and adherent to the first part of the duodenum, lateral to the portal vein, and in front of the vena cava. The pancreatic portion extends from the lower border of the first part of the duodenum to that point on the posteromedial wall of the second or descending part of the duodenum where the duct penetrates the intestine. This portion of the duct is either surrounded by the pancreas or runs in a groove in its posterior surface. The intramural portion of the common bile duct runs obliquely downward and laterally within the wall of the duodenum for 1 to 2 cm, opening

on a papilla of mucous membrane about 10 cm from the pylorus. The junction of the terminal common bile duct and pancreatic duct at the papilla takes one of three configurations that may be likened to a Y, V, or U. In about 70% of patients, there is a common channel of the bile duct and pancreatic ducts, thus a Y configuration (see Fig. 40-6B). In about 20%, the common channel is nonexistent (V configuration). In 10%, the two ducts enter the duodenum via separate openings (U configuration).

Vessels and Nerves

The arteries to the extrahepatic biliary ducts anastomose freely within the duct walls. The ductal arterial supply is derived primarily from the gastroduodenal and right hepatic arteries with major trunks running along the medial and lateral walls of the common duct at the 3- and 9-

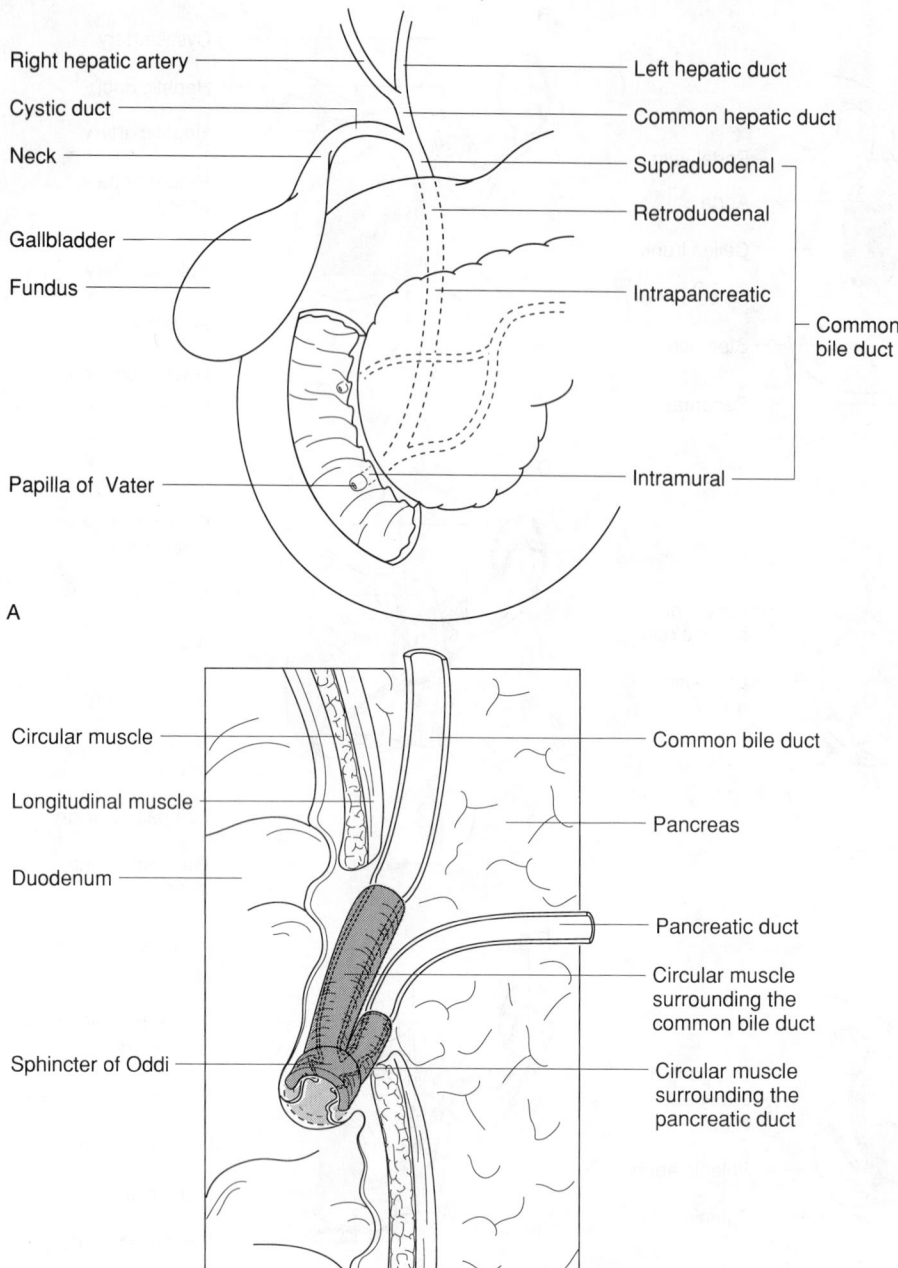

Figure 40-6. (*A*) Anatomic divisions of the gallbladder and the bile ducts. (*B*) Cross section of the sphincter of Oddi.

o'clock positions. The anterior surface of the common bile duct is covered by a plexus of thin-walled veins from which troublesome bleeding may occur while the duct is exposed. These veins usually can be pushed aside. The nerve supply to the common bile duct and sphincter of Oddi is the same as for the gallbladder. The density of neural fibers and ganglia increases near the sphincter of Oddi and includes several ganglionated plexuses connected to those of the gallbladder and duodenum.

HISTOLOGY AND ULTRASTRUCTURE
Gallbladder

The gallbladder wall consists of five layers.[2,5] The innermost layer is the epithelium, and the succeeding layers are the lamina propria, smooth muscle, perimuscular subserosal connective tissue, and serosa. There are no muscularis mucosa or submucosa in the gallbladder. Most cells in the mucosa are columnar cells, and their main function is absorption. These cells are aligned in a single row, with slightly eosinophilic cytoplasm, apical vacuoles, and basal or central nuclei.

The ultrastructure of the columnar cells features apical microvilli with filamentous rootlets. Vesicles found in these cells generally form from the intervillous cell membrane. The lateral cell membranes between cells are connected by junctional complexes that have complex interdigitations near the base. The intercellular spaces vary in size with absorptive activity of the mucosa; spaces are distended during water transport but otherwise are collapsed. The cytoplasmic structures consist of endoplasmic reticula, Golgi complexes, lysosomes, glycogen, mitochondria, mucous granules, and vesicles. The nucleus is rounded and sometimes contains a small nucleolus. The

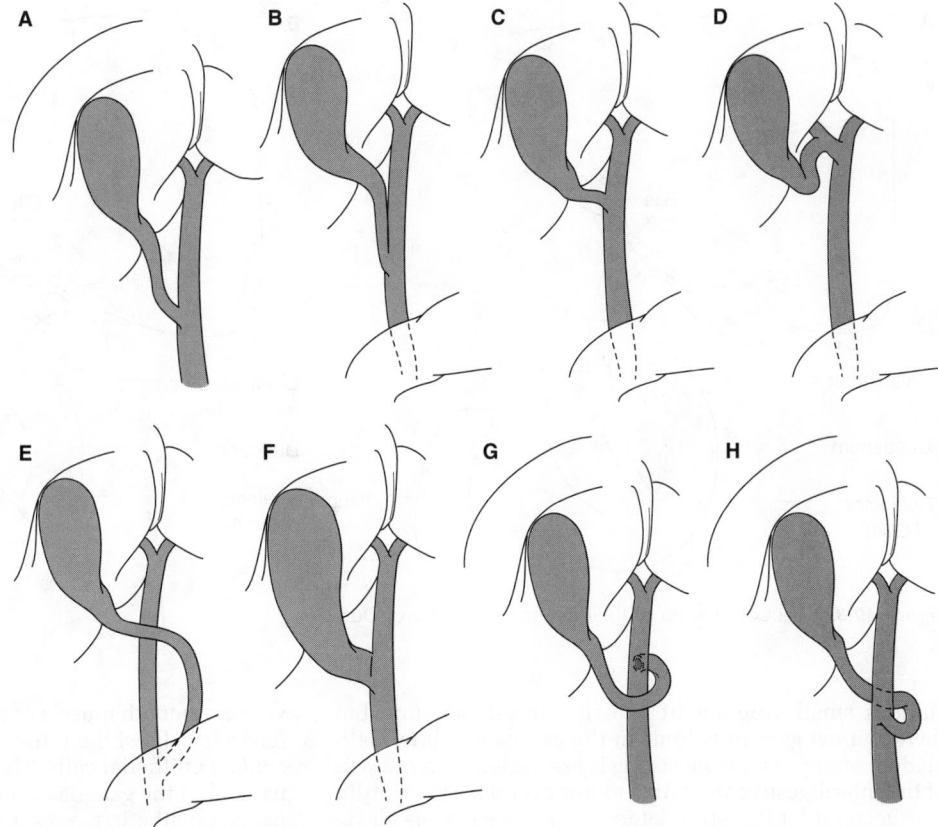

Figure 40-7. Variations in cystic duct anatomy.

mucosal histology changes depending on the part of the gallbladder. For example, the epithelial cells in the neck are tubuloalveolar and consist of cuboid or low columnar cells with clear cytoplasm and basal nuclei.

The lamina propria contains nerve fibers, vessels, lymphatics, elastic fibers, loose connective tissue, and occasional mast cells and macrophages. The muscle layer is a loose arrangement of circular, longitudinal, and oblique fibers without well-developed layers. Ganglia are found between smooth muscle bundles. The subserosa is composed of a loose arrangement of fibroblasts, elastic and collagen fibers, vessels, nerves, lymphatics, and adipocytes.

Rokitansky-Aschoff sinuses are invaginations of epithelium into the lamina propria, muscle, and subserosal connective tissue. These sinuses are present in about 40% of normal gallbladders and are present in abundance in almost all inflamed gallbladders. Ducts of Luschka are tiny bile ducts that drain directly from the liver into the body of the gallbladder. They are found in about 1% of normal gallbladders and have no relation to the Rokitansky-Aschoff sinuses or to cholecystitis but may lead to a bile leak after otherwise uncomplicated cholecystectomy.

Cystic Duct

The epithelium of the cystic duct is similar to that of the gallbladder. At the origin of the cystic duct is the spiral valve of Heister. This structure consists of bundles of transversely oriented smooth muscle that are thought to have a minor functional role during filling and emptying of the gallbladder.

Extrahepatic Bile Ducts

The extrahepatic bile ducts contain a columnar mucosa surrounded by a connective tissue layer. The surface is relatively flat, with basal nuclei and an absent or small nucleolus. The mucosa of the most distal segment of bile duct contains numerous mucus-secreting glands and is thrown into longitudinal folds called mucosal valvules. The lamina propria consists of collagen, elastic fibers, and vessels. Occasional lymphocytes are found, and pancreatic acini and ducts may be seen in the wall of the intrapancreatic portion of the distal common bile duct.

The bile duct wall is fibromuscular with smooth muscle cells scattered throughout the wall. Muscle fibers in the bile ducts are sparse and discontinuous. Muscle fibers that are present are usually longitudinal, although occasional circular fibers are observed. The distal common bile duct begins to develop a more substantial muscle layer in the intraduodenal portion of the duct, which becomes prominent at the sphincter of Oddi, where distinct bundles of longitudinal and circular fibers are clearly identified.

PHYSIOLOGY
Motor Function

As bile is secreted from the liver, it flows through the hepatic ducts into the common hepatic duct and continues through the common bile duct into the duodenum.[7,8] With an intact and contracted sphincter of Oddi, bile flow is directed into the gallbladder, where it is concentrated and stored (Fig. 40-8). In the postprandial state, about 70% of hepatic bile flows into the gallbladder before reaching the duodenum and entering the enterohepatic cycle. Patterns of gallbladder storage and emptying depend on a pressure gradient between the bile ducts and the gallbladder created by contraction of the sphincter. Peptide hormones and neural factors influence this gradient.[9] During the interdigestive phase, 90% of bile from the liver enters the gallbladder, while only a small fraction of the gallbladder bile enters the duodenum. In a bellows fashion, the gallbladder

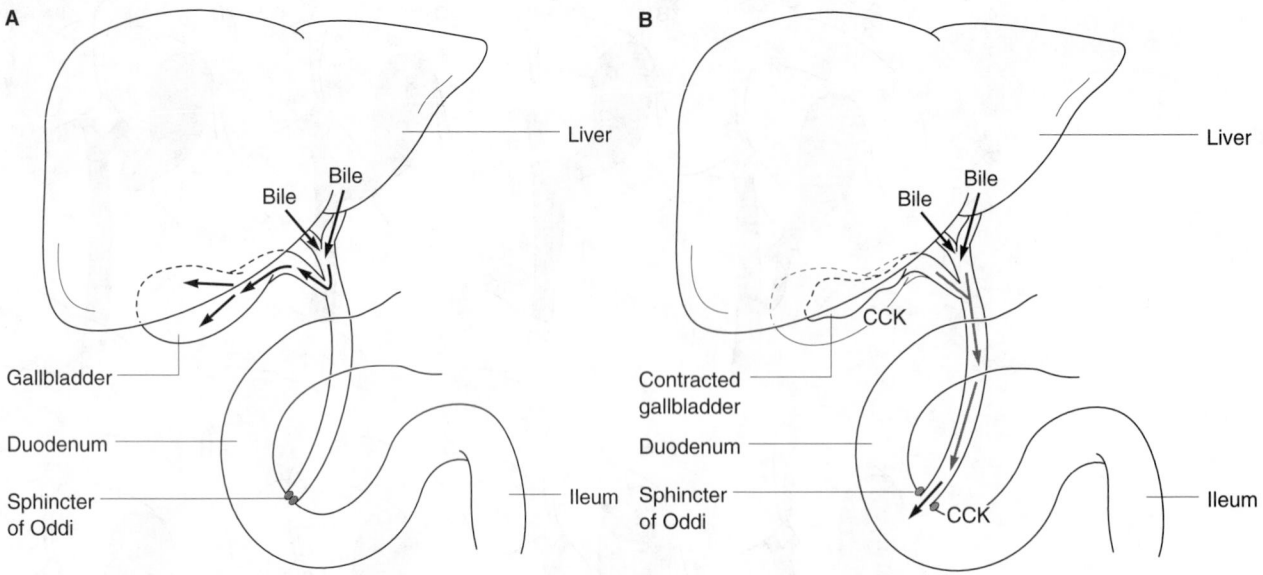

Figure 40-8. Effect of CCK on gallbladder and sphincter of Oddi.

empties small volumes of bile into the duodenum, but there is a net gain in volume in the gallbladder bile. Gallbladder emptying during fasting is associated with phase II of the interdigestive migrating motor complexes.[10] Motilin may account for this stimulatory effect since plasma elevations of motilin seem to correlate with the onset of phase II waves.[11] Following a meal, the gallbladder empties by a steady tonic contraction thought to be due to release of endogenous cholecystokinin (CCK) from the mucosa of the small intestine.[4]

The importance of these gallbladder motor events is speculative, but they have been invoked to explain cholesterol nucleation and gallstone formation. The bellows action of the gallbladder may reduce the vesicular phase (liquid crystals that lead to stone formation) and increase the micellar phase of stored bile. Periodic emptying during the interdigestive phase would thus remove the less dense vesicles, and alterations in the normal motor function would negate these favorable events and increase the risk of cholesterol stone formation.

Sphincter of Oddi

The sphincter of Oddi (see Fig. 40-6*B*) is about 4 to 6 mm in length. The sphincter's basal resting pressure is about 13 mmHg above the duodenal pressure.[6] The sphincter exhibits phasic contractions with a frequency of four per minute and a duration of 8 seconds. Pressure increases dramatically with phasic contractions, with an amplitude of 120 to 140 mm Hg. The regulation of bile flow is primarily controlled by the sphincter and not by the surrounding smooth muscle of the duodenum. Relaxation of the sphincter occurs with CCK stimulation, leading to diminished amplitude of phasic contractions and reduced basal pressure, allowing increased passive flow of bile into the duodenum. Parasympathetic stimulation also causes intermittent relaxation of the sphincter, and sympathetic splanchnic stimulation causes increased pressure.

Neurohormonal Regulation

The extrinsic nerves of the gallbladder consist of sympathetic fibers from the celiac ganglion and parasympathetic fibers from the vagus nerve.[12] The sympathetic fibers inner-

vate the smooth muscle of the blood vessels and the nonadrenergic cells of the intramural neural plexuses but do not contact epithelial cells. The parasympathetic fibers are visualized in the ganglia of the lamina propria. Traditionally, parasympathetic nerves were believed to control gallbladder contraction and relaxation of the sphincter of Oddi, whereas sympathetic fibers were believed to account for gallbladder relaxation and increased sphincter tone. These concepts have been modified to include a complex network of intrinsic nerves. The intrinsic nerves consist of cholinergic and peptidergic fibers, which are found in all layers of the gallbladder and terminate in proximity to smooth muscle cells, basement membrane of the epithelial cells, and blood vessels. Cholinergic and CCK-containing nerves contract the gallbladder, and VIP-positive nerves inhibit gallbladder contraction and dilate the gallbladder.[13,14] There are undoubtedly yet undiscovered neuropeptides and complex interactions between the various modulators involved in this regulation.

Motility of the gallbladder is an interactive process that involves direct neural control, neural stimulation with the release of adrenergic and cholinergic substances, neural stimulation with the release of peptides, and the direct effect of hormones and peptides on smooth muscle. Adrenergic stimulation usually causes relaxation because most E1-adrenergic receptors are inhibitory. Selective stimulation of the excitatory α-adrenergic receptors causes contraction. Sympathetic stimulation also causes increased net water absorption, probably through an α-adrenergic mechanism. The pylorocholecystic reflex is a cholinergic mechanism by which the gallbladder contracts in response to antral distention. The response to CCK is mediated both through cholinergic nerves and directly on smooth muscle fibers.

Afferent fibers transmit sensation of biliary discomfort to the right upper quadrant and to the right side of the back by way of the splanchnic system. The cause of biliary colic is unknown but is thought to be caused by increased pressure in the gallbladder secondary to a transient gallstone obstruction to outflow of bile from the gallbladder.

Hormonal and peptidergic receptors are located on the smooth muscle, vessels, nerves, and epithelium of the gallbladder. CCK stimulates gallbladder contraction[13] (see Fig. 40-8). CCK is localized in epithelial cells of the upper intesti-

Table 40-1. COMPARISON OF HEPATIC
AND GALLBLADDER BILE

	Hepatic Bile	Gallbladder Bile
Na (mEq/L)	140–159	220–340
K (mEq/L)	4–5	6–14
Ca (mEq/L)	2–5	5–32
Cl (mEq/L)	62–112	1–10
Bile salts (mEq/L)	3–55	290–340
Cholesterol (mg/dL)	60–70	350–930
Pigment (mg/dL)	50–170	
pH	7.2–7.7	5.6–7.4

(Davenport HW. Physiology of the digestive tract, ed 4. Chicago, Year Book, 1977)

nal tract, with the highest concentrations in the duodenum. CCK is released into the bloodstream by acid, fat, and amino acids in the duodenum. The four predominant molecular forms of CCK contain residues of 8, 33, 38 or 58 amino acids. The C-terminal octapeptide is the active portion of all the forms. CCK has a plasma half-life of 2.5 minutes and is metabolized by both the liver and the kidney. The degree of gallbladder contraction is directly related to the plasma concentration of CCK. The peptide acts directly on smooth muscle receptors of the gallbladder; optimal binding occurs at a pH of 5.5 and requires the presence of magnesium. CCK-stimulated gallbladder muscle contraction is calcium dependent and is also mediated by cholinergic vagal neurons. Gallbladder response to CCK stimulation is decreased after vagotomy or cholinergic blockade.

VIP inhibits contraction and causes gallbladder relaxation.[15] Somatostatin is a potent inhibitor of gallbladder contraction, whether mediated by CCK or vagal stimulation. Patients with somatostatinomas and those being treated with somatostatin analogues have a high incidence of gallstones, presumably due to somatostatin's potent inhibitory effect on gallbladder emptying in humans.[16]

The physiologic role of other hormones on gallbladder motor activity is unclear, but intravenous and pharmacologic doses have elicited various responses. Substance P causes contraction by a cholinergic mechanism. Enkephalin may abolish VIP-induced relaxation.[17] Norepinephrine results in gallbladder relaxation by means of a E1-adrenergic mechanism.[9,16]

Gallbladder afferent innervation is mediated by capsaicin-sensitive neurons. These neurons contain a number of neuropeptides, including substance P, neurokinin A, and calcitonin gene-related peptide.

MOTOR DYSFUNCTION
Gallbladder Dyskinesia

As the normal motility of the gallbladder and sphincter of Oddi have been characterized in the past decade, motor disorders have been described that can give rise to clinical syndromes. Motility abnormalities of the gallbladder and cystic duct present with symptoms suggesting gallstones. The most common presentation for patients with gallbladder motility disorders (chronic acalculous cholecystitis or gallbladder dyskinesia) is recurrent biliary-type pain. However, routine morphologic investigations of the biliary tree (by ultrasound or endoscopic retrograde cholangiopancreatography [ERCP]) display no evidence of gallstones or other anatomic abnormalities. Currently, the most specific test for diagnosing gallbladder dyskinesia is CCK-enhanced cholescintigraphy with assessment of gallbladder ejection

fraction. CCK is infused intravenously 15 to 30 minutes after injecting an analogue of 99m Tc imminodiacetic acid, and the ejection fraction of the isotope by the contracting gallbladder is calculated. An ejection fraction less than 35% is considered abnormal and cholecystectomy may be indicated.[18] A number of factors may lead to decreased gallbladder contraction such as a primary abnormality of gallbladder muscle, motor dysfunction secondary to chronic inflammation or lithogenic bile, suboptimal hormonal or neural stimulation or circulation of an inhibiting substance.[19]

Sphincter of Oddi Dysfunction

Abnormalities of the sphincter of Oddi may cause symptoms that are referable to the biliary tree or to the pancreas. Sphincter of Oddi dysfunction may arise de novo or lead to symptoms after cholecystectomy. Manometry of the sphincter of Oddi may be performed at the time of ERCP to characterize its basal pressure, the amplitude and frequency of contractions, and the direction of propagation of contractile waves.[4] Stenosis of the sphincter of Oddi is characterized by abnormally elevated basal pressure (higher than 40 mmHg), whereas dyskinesia is characterized by abnormalities of the other manometric parameters. Therapy for dysfunction of the sphincter of Oddi may be pharmacologic, using one of the newer prokinetic agents, or involve surgical or endoscopic division of the sphincter muscle.[20]

ABSORPTION

The gallbladder rapidly absorbs water and solutes from bile and concentrates the solute components 2- to 10-fold.[21] The changes in concentrations of solute components from hepatic bile to gallbladder bile are shown in Table 40-1 and Figure 40-9. The gallbladder has an active mucosa that can absorb water and solutes against significant concentration gradients. Water absorption is linked to the transport of ions. The two major mechanisms of absorption are active and passive. In passive absorption, sodium and chloride enter the gallbladder epithelial cells because of the electrochemical

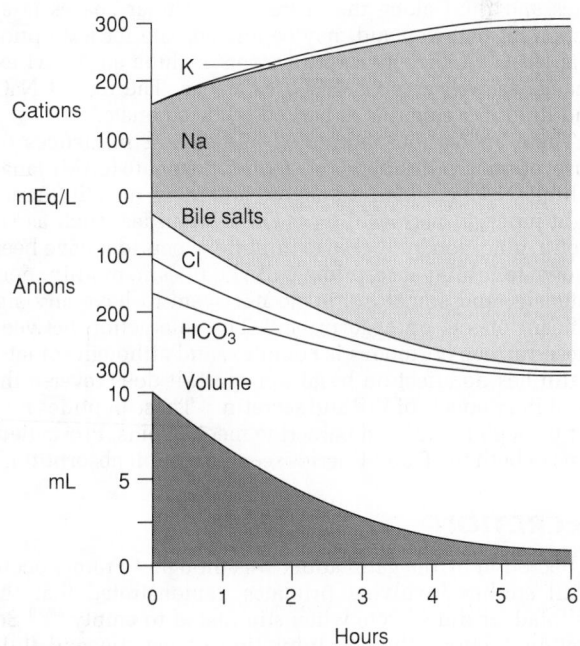

Figure 40-9. Changes in the volume and concentration of hepatic bile (*left*) to gallbladder bile (*right*).

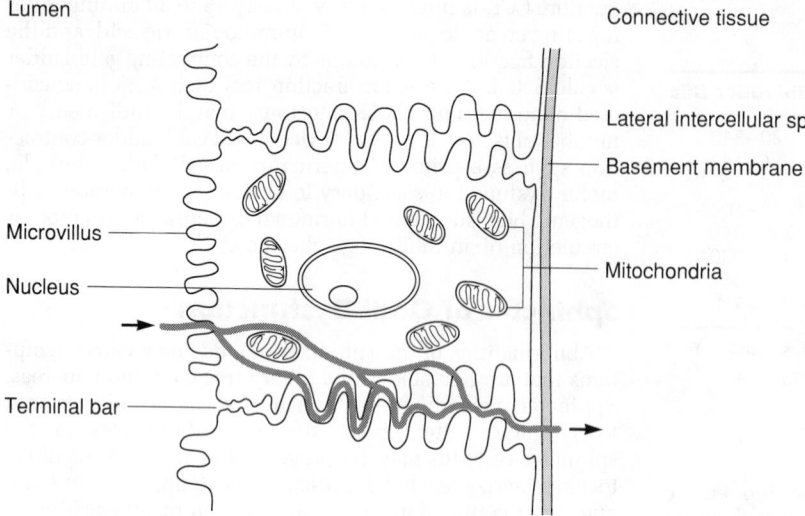

Figure 40-10. Cellular mechanisms of gallbladder mucosal absorption. The arrows indicate the route of water flow across the cell membrane and into the intercellular spaces. NaCl is pumped into the intercellular space, resulting in a hypertonic environment. As water enters, the space distends, and an isotonic solution enters the connective tissue space.

gradients. This results in an osmotic gradient, and water flows into the cell. Intracellular sodium is extruded across the basolateral membrane into the lateral intercellular spaces by active transport. The extrusion of sodium at the basolateral membrane may occur by electrogenic[22] or nonelectrogenic[23] mechanisms or both. Water enters the lateral intercellular space through the tight junctions at the mucosal surface in response to the solute concentration. Flow through the tight junctions into the lateral spaces is a passive mechanism. The transport of chloride is linked with sodium transport, and in experimental models, sodium absorption does not occur in the absence of chloride. This coupling between sodium and chloride probably occurs by an electrically neutral coupled mechanism and results in neutralization of any charge, preventing an electrochemical gradient.[24] The active transport of sodium against an electrochemical gradient is assisted by an Na^+-K^+-ATPase pump. Water moves with the passive and active transport of these solutes. The electrolyte and water transport therefore occurs not only across cells but also between cells (the intercellular spaces). The transport of electrolytes and fluid along the lateral intercellular spaces is an important pathway and may be a major site for absorption (Fig. 40-10). Other transport systems include an Na—H exchange as well as a Cl—HCO_3 exchange. The rate of NaCl and fluid movement is enhanced by bicarbonate.

There are various hormonal and neural influences on absorption. Cyclic adenosine monophosphate (cAMP) may inhibit NaCl-coupled transport and may also influence tight junction permeability.[25] Other peptides, such as secretin, glucagon, and gastric inhibitory peptide, have been shown to inhibit absorption. CCK, bombesin, motilin, neurotensin, and somatostatin do not seem to have any significant effects on absorption.[26] The interaction between these various hormones is complex, and although somatostatin has no effect on basal transport, it does reverse the inhibitory effects of VIP and secretin.[27] These peptides may act through neural and paracrine mechanisms. Prostaglandins of both the E and F series seem to inhibit absorption.[28]

SECRETION

Secretion by the gallbladder was thought to rarely occur until studies involving primates demonstrated that the gallbladder did secrete when stimulated to empty.[28,29] Secretion occurs either by inhibition of net ion and fluid absorption or with stimulation of a bicarbonate secretory mechanism. The mechanism of gallbladder secretion is poorly understood and may be related to elevations of cAMP or to exposure to prostaglandins and possibly certain peptides, such as VIP and secretin. The gallbladder epithelium also secretes mucin and nonmucin glycoproteins that may play an important role in the formation of gallstones.[30]

In experimental cholecystitis, substances such as morphine, loperamide, and enkephalin inhibit gallbladder secretion. This inhibition of secretion may contribute to the relief of symptoms associated with opiate treatment.

REFERENCES

1. Linder HH, Green RB. Embryology and surgical anatomy of the extrahepatic biliary tree. Surg Clin North Am 1964; 44:1273.
2. Frierson JF Jr. The gross anatomy and histology of the gallbladder, extrahepatic bile ducts, vaterian system and minor papilla. Am J Surg Pathol 1989;13:146.
3. Benson LA, Page RE. A practical reappraisal of the anatomy of the extrahepatic bile ducts and arteries. Br J Surg 1976;63:853.
4. Toouli J. Biliary tract. In: Kumar D, Wingate D, eds. An illustrated guide to gastrointestinal motility, ed 2. Edinburgh, Churchill Livingstone, 1993:393.
5. Gilloteaux J, Pomerants B, Kelly TR. Human gallbladder mucosa ultrastructure: evidence of intraepithelial nerve structures. Am J Anat 1989;184:321.
6. Carr-Locke DL, Gregg JA. Endoscopic manometry of pancreatic and biliary sphincter zones in man: basal results in healthy volunteers. Dig Dis Sci 1981;26:7.
7. Lanzini A, Northfield TC. Assessment of the motor functions of the gallbladder. J Hepatol 1989;9:383.
8. Lanzini A, Jazrawi RP, Northfield TC. Simultaneous quantitative measurements of absolute gallbladder storage and emptying during fasting and eating in humans. Gastroenterology 1987;92:852.
9. Banfield WJ. Physiology of the gallbladder. Gastroenterology 1975;69:770.
10. Svenberg T, Christofides ND, Fitzpatrick ML, et al. Interdigestive biliary output in man: relationship to fluctuations in plasma motilin and effect of atropine. Gut 1982;23:1024.
11. Svenberg T, Nilsson I, Samuelson K, et al. Studies on the causal relationship between gall-bladder emptying and motilin release in man. Acta Chir Scand 1984;520(Suppl):59.
12. Lundgren O, Svanvik J, Jivegard L. Enteric nervous system: II. Physiology and pathophysiology of the gallbladder. Dig Dis Sci 1989;34:284.
13. Bjorck S, Fahrenkrug J, Jivegard L, et al. Release of immunoreactive vasoactive intestinal polypeptide (VIP) from the gallbladder in response to vagus stimulation. Acta Physiol Scand 1986;128:639.

14. Lilja P, Fagan CJ, Wiener I, et al. Infusion of pure cholecystokinin in humans: correlation between plasma concentration of cholecystokinin and gallbladder size. Gastroenterology 1982; 83:256.
15. Jansson R, Svanvik J. Effects of intravenous vasoactive intestinal polypeptide (VIP) on gallbladder function in the cat. Gastroenterology 1978;75:47.
16. Fisher RS, Rock E, Levin G, et al. Effects of somatostatin on gallbladder emptying. Gastroenterology 1987;92:885.
17. Polack JM, Bloom SR, Sullivan SN, et al. Enkephalin-like immunoreactivity in the human gastrointestinal tract. Lancet 1977;1:972.
18. Sorensen MK, Fancher S, Lang MP, et al. Abnormal gallbladder nuclear ejection fraction predicts success of cholecystectomy in patients with biliary dyskinesia. Am J Surg 1993; 166:670.
19. Dodds WJ. Biliary tract motility and its relationship to clinical disorders. Am J Roentgenol 1990;155:247.
20. Geenen JE, Hogen WJ, Dodds WJ, et al. The efficacy of endoscopic sphincterotomy and post-cholecystectomy patients with Sphincter of Oddi dysfunction. N Engl J Med 1989; 320:82.
21. Wood JR, Svanvik J. Gall-bladder water and electrolyte transport and its regulation. Gut 1983;24:579.
22. Rose RC, Nahrwold DL. Electrolyte transport in Necturus gallbladder: the role of rheogenic Na transport. Am J Physiol 1980;238:6358.
23. Reuss L. Mechanisms of sodium and chloride transport by gallbladder epithelium. Fed Proc 1979;38:2733.
24. Duffey ME, Turnheim K, Frizzell RA, Schultz SG. Intracellular chloride activities in rabbit gallbladder: direct evidence for the role of the sodium-gradient in energizing "uphill" chloride transport. J Membr Biol 1978;42:229.
25. Duffey ME, Hainau B, Ho S, et al. Regulation of epithelial tight junction permeability by cAMP. Nature 1981;294:451.
26. Wood JR, Brennan LJ, Hormbrey JM, et al. Effects of regulatory peptides on gallbladder function. Scand J Gastroenterol 1982;17(suppl):528.
27. Wood JR, McLoughlin TA, Brennan LJ. VIP and secretin induced inhibition of gallbladder fluid absorption: reversal by somatostatin. Gastroenterology 1982;82:1213.
28. Wood JR, Saverymuttu SH, Heintze K. Gallbladder secretion. Gastroenterology 1977;73:629.
29. Leyssac P, Bukhave K, Frederiksen O. Inhibitory effect of prostaglandins on isosmotic fluid transport by rabbit gallbladder in vitro, and its modification by blockade of endogenous PGE-biosynthesis with indomethacin. Acta Physiol Scand 1974;92:496.
30. Lipsett PA, Hildreth J, Kaufman HS, et al. Human gallstones contain pronucleating non-mucin glycoproteins that are immunoglobulins. Ann Surg 1994;219:25.

SURGERY: SCIENTIFIC PRINCIPLES AND PRACTICE, Second Edition, edited by Lazar J. Greenfield, Michael W. Mulholland, Keith T. Oldham, Gerald B. Zelenock, and Keith D. Lillemoe. Lippincott–Raven Publishers, Philadelphia, © 1997.

CHAPTER 41

CALCULOUS BILIARY DISEASE

DAN I.N. GIURGIU AND JOEL J. ROSLYN

The first recognized case of cholelithiasis was reported more than 1500 years ago. For hundreds of years, people suffered from acute episodes of upper abdominal discomfort, probably as a consequence of gallstone disease, but their symptoms defied diagnosis and treatment. During the middle ages, a time when alchemists understood little about the process of gallstone formation, patients were advised to bathe in spas rich in magnesium sulfate to ameliorate their symptoms. We now know that such treatment may have been therapeutic because it stimulates gallbladder contraction and emptying. Few advances were made in the treatment of patients with biliary stone disease until the 1880s. In 1882, Carl Langenbach, a German surgeon, performed the first successful cholecystectomy. This event revolutionized the approach to cholelithiasis. Despite this clinical advance, little progress was made in our understanding of the pathogenesis of gallstone disease until the mid-1900s. During this period, physicians and scientists recognized the importance of increased concentrations of biliary cholesterol and alterations in hepatic biliary lipid metabolism as prerequisites for cholesterol stone formation. In more recent years, attention has focused on the role of altered gallbladder function in the pathogenesis of gallstones and the mechanisms by which changes in the physical properties of bile promote nucleation and stone formation.

Calculous disease of the biliary tract continues to be a major national and international health problem. The incidence of cholelithiasis varies widely throughout the world, as does the predominant type and actual location of gallstones. For more than a century, cholecystectomy had been the gold standard for the management of symptomatic gallstone disease. In the 1980s, a number of new and innovative techniques were developed for the nonoperative management of gallstones. The surgical management of cholelithiasis was challenged by the introduction of oral agents suitable for medical dissolution, reports of invasive techniques employing principles of contact dissolution, and biliary lithotripsy. For several years, this latter technology was popular among clinicians throughout the world. Subsequent developments have relegated this modality to a second-line intervention.

The management of gallstone disease has been revolutionized in recent years by the development of laparoscopic cholecystectomy and related procedures. This new technology continues to evolve. Its broad application to the management of biliary stone disease represents one of the greatest advances in surgery in this century, and parenthetically, one of its biggest challenges. Laparoscopy has rapidly become the preferred treatment for patients with symptomatic gallstone disease, including acute cholecystitis. In addition, this technology is now being extended to more complicated problems including common bile duct stone disease. Clinicians and hospital administrators continue to struggle with issues related to checking credentials, competency, as well as economic and legal issues. The next decade promises to be exciting in terms of defining the role of laparoscopic or minimally invasive surgery in treating patients with gallstone disease.

GALLSTONE CLASSIFICATION

Gallstones may be single or numerous, small or large, and they may differ in color, size, shape, and configuration. The composition of stones varies widely based on based on geography and form (Fig. 41-1). Nonetheless, the composition of stones in individual patients is uniform. There are essentially three types of gallstones—cholesterol, pigment, and mixed cholesterol and pigment stones. In the United States and most Western countries, about 10% of all stones are pure cholesterol, 15% are pigment, and the remaining 75% are mixed. In most Asian countries, patients tend to have pigment stones. Pigment stones are further classified as brown or black. These distinctions are important for understanding varyious causes but may have little influence for surgical decision making.

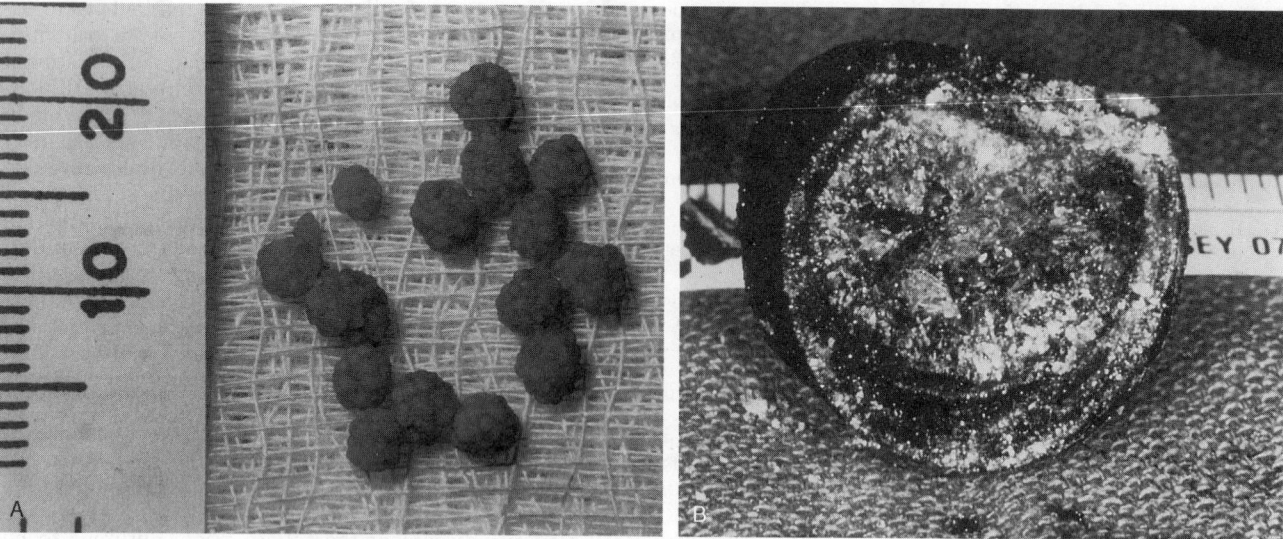

Figure 41-1. Gallstones from patients demonstrating multiple small cholesterol calculi (*A*) and single, large mixed stone (*B*).

Calculi may be found either in the gallbladder and extrahepatic biliary tract or in the intrahepatic ductal system. Although most Western patients with cholelithiasis have stones in the gallbladder, calculi are occasionally found in the intrahepatic or extrahepatic bile ducts. Stones situated in the extrahepatic biliary tract are classified as either primary or secondary, depending on the site of origin. Primary common duct stones form exclusively in the intrahepatic or extrahepatic bile ducts and are generally soft, smooth, and yellowish tan. These stones usually conform to the shape of the bile duct and rarely contain significant amounts of cholesterol. In contrast, secondary (or retained) stones form in the gallbladder and subsequently pass into the common bile duct, either through the cystic duct or a biliary fistula. These stones are chemically similar to coexisting stones in the gallbladder. Intrahepatic stone disease is a well recognized entity in the Orient and probably results from chronic biliary infection leading to stricture formation and stasis.

INCIDENCE

The incidence of biliary calculous disease varies widely throughout the world. In the United States, about 10% of the population has cholelithiasis. In addition to the 25 million people with documented gallstone disease, another 800,000 new cases are diagnosed each year. In other parts of the world, biliary stone disease is much less common. The 3% incidence of gallstones that has been reported in several African countries has been causally linked to genetic or dietary factors. The incidence of gallstone disease in the Far East is considerable, constitutes a medical-social problem of enormous magnitude, and is probably related to a number of demographic factors, including infestation with bacteria or parasites. Although cholesterol and mixed stones continue to be the predominant types found in the United States, pigment stones are being seen with increasing frequency in this country. Interestingly, the incidence of calcium bilirubinate stones is decreasing in the Far East while cholesterol stones are increasing. These trends are probably a consequence of changes in diet and environmental factors.

EPIDEMIOLOGY

Age

The physiologic explanation for the increasing incidence of gallstone disease in the elderly is unclear. The proportion of cholesterol present in bile and the cholesterol saturation index are significantly increased in elderly women compared with younger subjects. The increased incidence of gallstones observed in elderly men has been linked to changing androgen/estrogen ratios and the associated effects on biliary lipid metabolism and alterations in gallbladder motility. Ultrasonographic studies indicate that gallbladder sensitivity to cholecystokinin (CCK), the primary hormonal stimulus for gallbladder contraction, decreases with aging. Serum concentrations of pancreatic polypeptide increase with age. Experimental data suggest that this peptide affects postcontractile gallbladder filling. Further studies are needed to clarify the effects of these peptides and others on gallbladder contractility in the geriatric population.

Although gallstones are rarely found in healthy children and adolescents, they have been reported in young patients with hemolytic disorders, congenital anomalies, ileal disorders, and the short bowel syndrome, as well as in children maintained on long-term total parenteral nutrition (TPN). Epidemiologic studies have demonstrated a linear relation between increasing age and the prevalence of cholelithiasis (Table 41-1).

Hereditary and Ethnic Factors

Although certain population groups and individual families have been shown to have an inordinately high incidence of cholesterol gallstones, the role that heredity plays in the pathogenesis of biliary calculous disease remains uncertain. The realization that gallstone incidence in an ethnic population varies with geography suggests that environmental and perhaps dietary composition may be equally important as hereditary factors in determining propensity to develop stones. The Pima Indians of the southwestern United States have a high incidence of gallstones, which approaches 73% in women between the ages of 25 and 34 years. Numerous studies have attempted to define

Table 41-1. **GALLBLADDER DISEASE PREVALENCE BY AGE GROUP**

Age (y)	Percentage With Stones	
	Female	Male
10–39	5.0	1.5
40–49	12.0	4.4
50–59	15.8	6.2
60–69	25.4	9.9
70–79	28.9	15.2
80–89	30.9	17.9
90+	35.4	24.4

(Modified from Bateson MC. Gallbladder disease and cholecystectomy rates are independently variable. Lancet 1984;2:621)

the specific genetic defects that are responsible for the high degree of cholesterol saturation of bile that characterizes this population. Possible explanations for this phenomenon include an increase in hepatic biliary cholesterol secretion and a concomitant decrease in bile acid secretion. The low incidence of gallstones in people of East Africa may be secondary to hereditary and ethnic factors, although variations in dietary composition cannot be excluded as a causative factor.

Gender and Hormones

Gallstone disease is much more common in women than in men. The higher incidence of cholelithiasis in women persists until the seventh or eighth decades of life, when the incidence approaches 20% in both men and women (see Table 41-1). The propensity to form gallstones in women is likely due to hormonally mediated changes in biliary lipid metabolism and gallbladder motor function. Administering exogenous estrogens to premenopausal and postmenopausal women, or to men, significantly increases the incidence of cholesterol gallstones. Experimental studies suggest that estrogen decreases activity of the hepatic enzyme responsible for converting cholesterol to bile acids, resulting in a decrease in bile acid synthesis and secretion and an associated increase in cholesterol saturation of bile. Ultrasonographic studies demonstrate an increase in absolute and residual gallbladder volume after contraction during the second and third trimesters of pregnancy. Moreover, the rate of emptying and the percentage of initial volume emptied are also diminished during this stage of pregnancy. These effects, which are likely due to progesterone, result in incomplete gallbladder emptying and stasis of bile, factors thought to be important to the cascade of events resulting in cholesterol gallstones.

Obesity

Clinical evidence suggests a doubling or tripling in the incidence of cholelithiasis among morbidly obese patients compared with age-matched normal-weight subjects. Metabolic studies have indicated that obese patients secrete hepatic bile that has an increased concentration of cholesterol, therefore predisposing to a cholelithogenic state. Interestingly, rapid weight loss has also been associated with secretion of cholesterol-saturated bile and increased incidence of gallstones. Although the mechanisms for this association remain unclear, an alteration in the enterohepatic circulation of bile acids with a concomitant reduction in bile acid pool size probably accounts for the increased incidence of stones with surgical weight-reduction proce-

dures. The reported increased incidence of cholelithiasis in patients who undergo gastric restrictive procedures may also be due to decreased gallbladder emptying as a result of restricted oral intake.

Diabetes

Patients with diabetes mellitus have a two-fold increase in gallstone disease compared with nondiabetics. Limited information is available regarding the composition of these stones. The finding that gallbladder bile from diabetics tends to be supersaturated with cholesterol suggests that these stones are almost certainly composed of cholesterol. In addition to having supersaturated bile, diabetics also have been shown to have a reduced bile acid pool and altered gallbladder motor activity. Studies in a group of high-risk diabetics indicate that the degree of cholesterol saturation of bile actually increases during insulin treatment, predisposing patients to cholesterol precipitation and gallstone formation.

Cirrhosis

Although the influence of alcohol on gallstone formation remains poorly defined, autopsy studies suggest that the incidence of cholelithiasis is significantly increased in patients with alcoholic cirrhosis. This finding is due to an increased incidence of pigment gallstones. Specific alterations in bile acid metabolism have been proposed as critical to the pathogenesis of cirrhosis-induced pigment stones. The observation that cholesterol gallstones are infrequently seen in cirrhotic patients who undergo cholecystectomy is consistent with biliary lipid studies indicating that bile from patients with cirrhosis has a greater cholesterol solubilizing capacity than control bile.

Vagotomy

Early clinical studies suggested that truncal vagotomy, an important component of peptic ulcer surgery, was associated with a two-fold increase in the incidence of gallstones. It has long been presumed that the association between truncal vagotomy and cholelithiasis is secondary to alterations in gallbladder motor activity. Evidence for this hypothesis is provided by ultrasonographic and laboratory investigations demonstrating dilated gallbladders and increased intragallbladder pressure in response to CCK octapeptide after vagotomy and pyloroplasty. Nonetheless, experimental studies designed to prove that truncal vagotomy increases the incidence of gallstone formation have failed to confirm this hypothesis.

Total Parenteral Nutrition

One of the great advances in medicine, and particularly in gastrointestinal surgery, has been the introduction of TPN as a means of providing nutritional support for patients who are unable to eat. Early anecdotal reports suggested that the long-term administration of parenteral nutrition predisposed to acalculous and calculous cholecystitis. This observation subsequently was confirmed in a number of large clinical studies that demonstrated an increased risk of cholelithiasis in both children and adults maintained on long-term parenteral nutrition. Ultrasonographic studies have traced the development of gallstone disease in these patients from simple stasis to sludge and

Table 41-2. PREVALENCE OF SLUDGE AND GALLSTONES IN PATIENTS RECEIVING TOTAL PARENTERAL NUTRITION*

Time on TPN (d)	Sludge (%)
12	0
21	6
42	50
>42	100

* Study based on ultrasonography. Six of 14 sludge-positive patients developed gallstones.
(Modified from Messing B, Bories C, Kunstlinger F, et al. Does total parenteral nutrition induce gallbladder sludge formation and lithiasis? Gastroenterology 1983;84:1012)

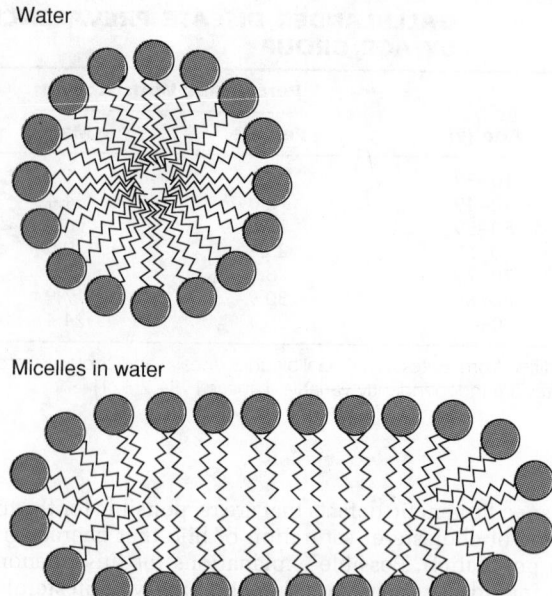

Figure 41-2. Schematic representation of the orientation of bile acid molecules as amphipathic units with hydrophobic ends pointed inward and hydrophilic ends pointed outward.

then to gallstone formation (Table 41-2). Preliminary studies suggest that most de novo stones in this setting are primarily composed of calcium bilirubinate. Although the pathogenesis of TPN-induced gallstone formation has not been defined, stasis of bile as a result of decreased gallbladder emptying appears to be a critical factor. Both experimental and clinical studies suggest that periodic, pharmacologically induced gallbladder emptying can alter these events and prevent gallstone formation in patients maintained on long-term TPN.

CHOLESTEROL GALLSTONES

The pathogenesis of cholesterol gallstones is multifactorial, and neither the liver nor the gallbladder alone has an exclusive etiologic role in the formation of calculi. Cholesterol calculi form as the result of a dynamic interaction between the liver and gallbladder, wherein factors present in cholesterol-saturated bile induce a series of alterations in gallbladder function that promote nucleation and stone growth.

Composition of Normal Bile

Bile is a solution secreted by the liver and is composed primarily of water, electrolytes, and organic solutes. This complex solution is isotonic with plasma and is essential for important physiologic functions, including cholesterol solubilization and digestive function. Bile salts, cholesterol, and phospholipids are the main solutes in bile and account for about 80% of the dry weight of bile. By definition, primary bile acids are synthesized from cholesterol in the liver. In humans, chenodeoxycholic and cholic acid (primary bile acids) are conjugated with taurine or glycine in the liver. Most of the cholesterol found in bile is synthesized de novo in the liver. Lecithin is the predominant phospholipid found in human bile and accounts for more than 90% of the phospholipid content.

Cholesterol Solubilization

Cholesterol is an organic molecule that is virtually insoluble in an aqueous medium such as bile. For many years, the formation of mixed-bile acid-lecithin-cholesterol micelles was thought to be critical in maintaining cholesterol in solution. Bile acids are amphipathic compounds that contain both hydrophilic polar groups (amino acids side chain) and hydrophobic nonpolar portions (Fig. 41-2). Although bile acids exist as individual ionized molecules in dilute solutions, increasing bile acid concentration is associated with aggregation of individual bile acid molecules into small clusters with outwardly oriented hydro-

philic polar ends and with the hydrophobic portions positioned inward. Incorporation of lecithin into the micelle induces swelling and facilitates incorporation of cholesterol into this matrix (Fig. 41-3). Although it is clear that this process occurs and that cholesterol is solubilized in micelles, the amount of cholesterol that ultimately is trans-

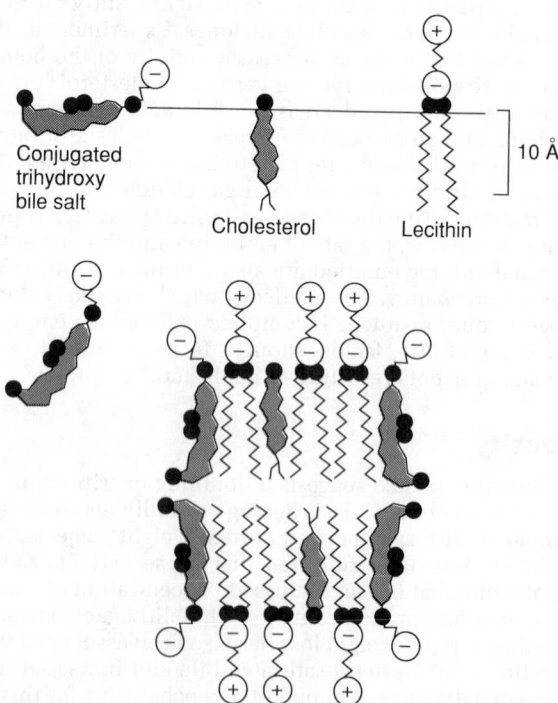

Figure 41-3. Bile acid–lecithin–cholesterol-mixed micelle. Polar ends of bile acids and lecithin are oriented outward, and hydrophobic, nonpolar portions make up the interior. Cholesterol is solubilized within the hydrophobic, nonpolar center.

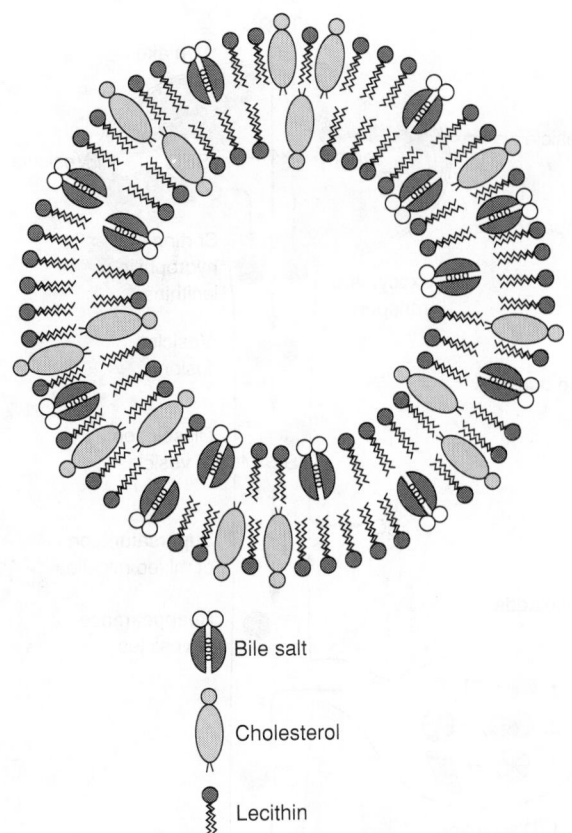

Figure 41-4. Unilamellar bile acid–lecithin–cholesterol vesicle. The amphipathic molecules of lecithin and bile acids form a lipid bilayer. Cholesterol is solubilized within the nonpolar portion of the bilayer.

ported in this manner rather than by vesicles is the source of considerable investigation. Nonetheless, the concept that the relation between cholesterol, phospholipids, and bile salts is an important determinant of cholesterol solubilization remains a basic principle of biliary physiology.

Several independent investigators have demonstrated that although some cholesterol is solubilized in mixed bile acid lecithin micelles, much of the biliary cholesterol normally present actually exists in a vesicular form. These vesicles solubilize greater quantities of cholesterol than micelles and are made up of lipid bilayers, similar to those normally found in cell membranes (Fig. 41-4). Up to 70% of the total amount of cholesterol normally found in human gallbladder bile is transported and solubilized in the vesicular form, with the remainder being transported in mixed micelles. The relative amounts of cholesterol transported in vesicles or micelles is related to the degree of bile concentration.

Cholesterol Saturation

Regardless of the mode of cholesterol transport, failure to solubilize all cholesterol present, either as a result of excessive quantity or alteration in the vehicle, is considered a critical step in the formation of gallstones. Theoretically, an increase in cholesterol concentration relative to bile acids can occur as a result of altered secretion of any of the three biliary lipid moities present in bile—cholesterol, bile acids, or lecithin. In 1968, Admirand and Small[1] first described the relation between cholesterol, phospholipids,

and bile salts in both health and during cholesterol gallstone formation. Their data have been displayed using triangular coordinates and have since been modified by others (Fig. 41-5).

It is generally accepted that the cholesterol content of bile exceeds its solubilizing capacity in patients with cholesterol gallstones. Cholesterol supersaturated bile can occur secondary to secretion of hepatic bile with either increased amounts of cholesterol or decreased amounts of bile acids. Although the former situation has been established as a cause of lithogenic bile in obese patients, decreased secretion of bile acids has been implicated as a causative factor of gallstone formation in patients with ileal disorders or ileal resection. Most people, even those without cholesterol gallstones, have bile that is nearly saturated with cholesterol. Moreover, during periods of starvation or fasting, normal people without gallstones secrete cholelithogenic bile. This finding suggests that factors other than cholesterol saturation of bile may play an important etiologic role in the pathogenesis of cholesterol gallstones. This concept is underscored by the finding that despite similar lithogenic indices, gallbladder bile from gallstone patients has decreased nucleation time compared with bile from patients without gallstones.

Nucleation and Mucus Secretion

Considerable evidence has been compiled indicating that aggregation of cholesterol–phospholipid vesicles is critical to nucleation and formation of cholesterol crystals. *Nucleation* refers to the process by which cholesterol

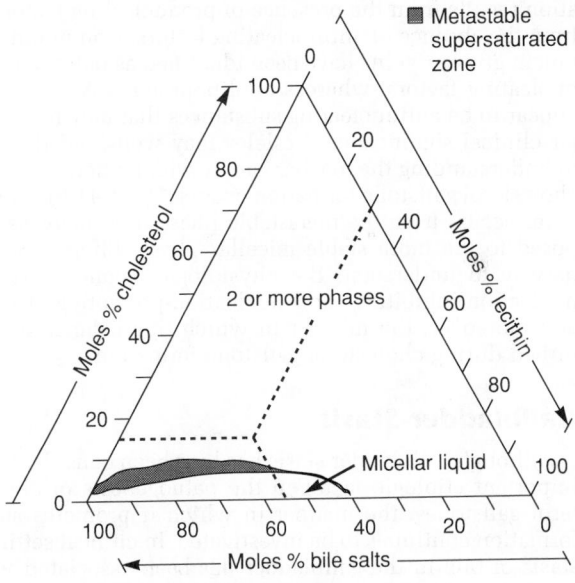

Figure 41-5. Tricoordinate phase diagram for determination of cholesterol saturation index. A given single point represents the relative molar ratios of bile salts, lecithin, and cholesterol. The range of concentrations found consistent with a clear, micellar solution (where cholesterol is fully solubilized) is limited to a small region in the lower left. The colored area directly above this region corresponds to a metastable zone in which bile initially appears clear but, with time, develops cholesterol crystals. All other regions represent bile solutions in which the cholesterol solubilization capacity is exceeded and rapid formation of cholesterol crystals occurs. (After Holzbach RT. Pathogenesis and medical treatment of gallstones. In: Slesinger MH, Fordtran JS, eds. Gastrointestinal diseases. Philadelphia, WB Saunders, 1989:1360)

monohydrate crystals form and agglomerate. Nucleation occurs more rapidly in gallbladder bile of patients with cholesterol gallstones compared with patients with saturated bile but no stones.

Experimental and clinical studies have suggested that cholesterol gallstone formation is associated with increased gallbladder mucus secretion.[2] Studies performed in the prairie dog animal model indicate that luminal factors present within cholesterol-saturated bile stimulate gallbladder mucus secretion. The observations that this activity occurs before cholesterol crystal formation and that human gallbladder mucin enhances in vitro nucleation of cholesterol crystals suggest that increased gallbladder mucus secretion may be a critical factor in the pathogenesis of cholesterol gallstones. This hypothesis is further supported by the observation that administering pharmacologic doses of aspirin to an animal model significantly inhibits mucus secretion and reduces the incidence of diet-induced cholesterol gallstones.

Nucleation time of gallbladder and hepatic bile correlates with nucleation time of vesicles as opposed to micelles. Similar relations between nucleation time and total protein and vesicular cholesterol concentration have been noted. Separation of vesicular and micellar fractions of cholesterol indicate that the nucleation of cholesterol crystals is significantly accelerated in the presence of bovine gallbladder mucin only in cholesterol-containing vesicles and not in mixed micelles. The physicochemical behavior of gallbladder mucin in bile is influenced by both mucin and electrolyte concentrations at the epithelial surface of the gallbladder, activities that have been shown to be altered in experimentally induced cholesterol gallstone formation. These data suggest that mucin may be the elusive nucleating factor. Debate continues as to whether nucleation results from the presence of pronucleating factors or from the absence of antinucleating factors. Nonmucin and mucin glycoproteins have been identified as potential pronucleating factors, whereas apolipoproteins A-I and A-II appear to be antinucleating substances that may have major clinical significance. Vesicles may well hold the link to understanding the mechanism by which nucleation and cholesterol gallstone formation occurs[3,4] (Fig. 41-6). Nucleation occurs from the metastable phase of vesicles as opposed to the more stable micellar phase. Efforts are underway to understand the physiologic balance between nucleation-inhibiting[5] and nucleation-promoting[6] factors and moreover, the manner in which this balance is disturbed during cholesterol gallstone formation.

Gallbladder Stasis

Although gallbladder stasis has long been considered an important etiologic factor in the pathogenesis of cholesterol gallstones, the manner in which it promotes stone formation continues to be investigated. In clinical settings, stasis of bile in the gallbladder has been associated with an increased incidence of cholelithiasis, including truncal vagotomy, pregnancy, and long-term administration of TPN. Experimental studies in diet-induced models of gallstone formation have suggested that specific defects in biliary motility, including decreased gallbladder contractility and increased cystic duct resistance, may result in impaired gallbladder emptying and biliary stasis. These findings have been confirmed in patients undergoing biliary scintigraphic studies in whom decreased motor response to CCK has been documented.

Early investigators suggested that a stagnant pool of bile in the gallbladder would result in a decrease in the amount of bile salts available for cholesterol solubilization and therefore predispose to saturation and crystal formation.

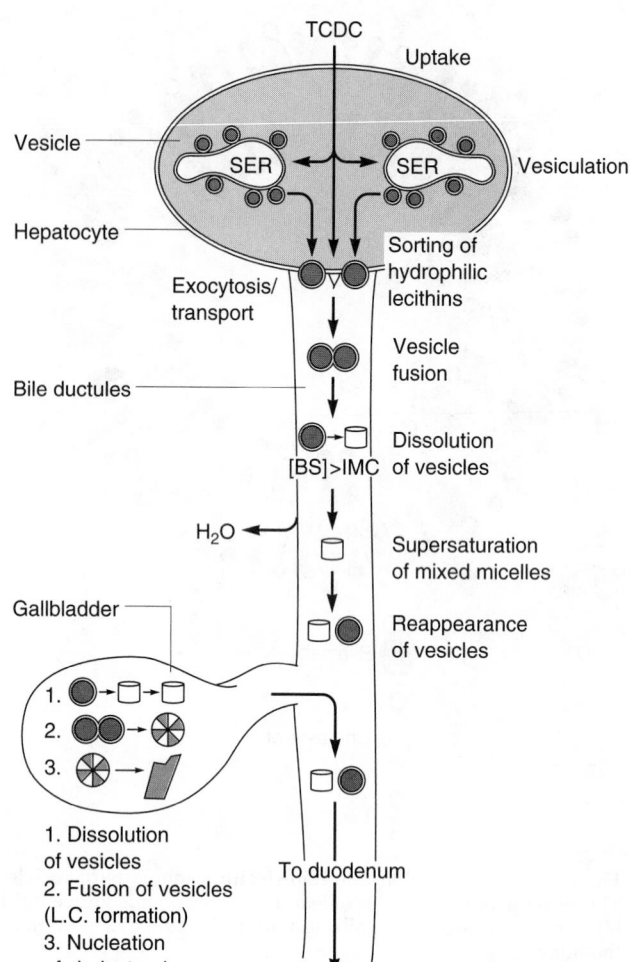

Figure 41-6. Schematic depicting the dynamic role of vesicles as vehicles for cholesterol in bile and how they relate to nucleation.

Stasis of bile in the gallbladder is thought to provide an ideal milieu for the precipitation of specific factors present in gallbladder bile. More recently, it has been proposed that alterations in gallbladder absorptive or secretory function may be a sequela of biliary stasis. The relation between gallbladder stasis and the concentration of nucleating or antinucleating factors continues to be examined as a possible critical factor in the cascade of events leading to stone formation (Fig. 41-7).

Biliary Calcium

Increased concentrations of calcium bilirubinate has long been recognized as an important etiologic factor in the formation of pigment gallstones. Recent studies have suggested that alterations in biliary calcium may be critical to the formation of cholesterol gallstones as well. For many years, it was believed that less than 30% of all cholesterol gallstones contained calcium. More recent studies indicate that the central matrix of almost all cholesterol gallstones contains some amount of calcium. In vitro studies show that the crystalline structures of calcium carbonate and cholesterol monohydrate are similar enough to support the growth of one crystal on the framework of the other. Laboratory and clinical studies suggest that cholesterol gallstone disease is characterized by increased gallbladder bile concentrations of total and ionized calcium. These find-

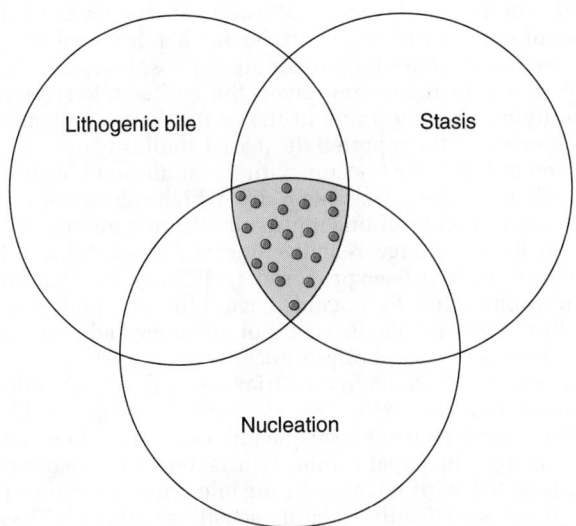

Figure 41-7. Gallstone pathogenesis is a multifactorial process that results from stasis of bile in the gallbladder in combination with a nucleation defect, all in the presence of cholesterol-saturated bile.

ings are of particular interest, given reports that calcium may promote fusion of vesicles and accelerate in vitro growth of cholesterol crystals. Moreover, elevated biliary calcium levels observed during gallstone formation may also play a role in modulating gallbladder absorptive function as discussed later in this chapter. The mechanism by which biliary calcium is increased remains unclear.

Altered Gallbladder Absorption

Although the primary function of the gallbladder is to concentrate bile by absorbing sodium and water during interdigestive periods, the manner in which this most fundamental activity is altered during gallstone formation has not been well defined. In vitro studies with diet-induced models of gallstone disease indicate that gallbladder fluid transport actually increases during the formation of experimentally induced cholesterol gallstones. Luminal factors present in cholesterol-saturated bile, specifically the ratio of phospholipids to bile salts, may influence gallbladder ion transport.

Calcium, another luminal factor, appears to be a key modulator of ion transport in the prairie dog model. Calcium, either via direct signaling or via intracellular mediators such as calmodulin and protein kinase C, may regulate absorptive and secretory responses observed at different stages of gallstone formation. Specific defects that occur in gallbladder epithelial ion transport during early stages of gallstone formation remain ill-defined but may involve alterations in calcium signaling in gallbladder epithelial cells. Recent in vitro studies have also demonstrated that gallbladder absorptive function is sensitive to hormonal factors, as evidenced by increased absorption of ions and water in response to octreotide, an analogue of somatostatin. The specific defects that occur in gallbladder epithelial ion transport during the early stages of stone formation remain obscure.

Biliary Prostaglandins

Data suggest that arachidonic metabolism is significantly altered during the formation of experimentally induced cholesterol gallstones. These changes in prostaglandin synthesis have been associated with mucus hypersecretion. Alterations in endogenous synthesis and release of prostanoids occur as a result of cholesterol feeding and have been linked with accumulation of gallbladder luminal fluid, a finding characteristic of patients with acute cholecystitis. Although several authors have suggested that altered concentrations of prostaglandins may affect gallbladder motor activity and absorptive function, these concepts have been challenged by at least one study, and it remains unclear whether the previously observed changes in prostaglandins are a cause or an effect of gallstones.

The traditional theory of cholesterol gallstone formation focused on the hepatic secretion of cholesterol-saturated bile. It is becoming increasingly apparent that the pathogenesis of cholesterol gallstones is multifactorial, and that a number of factors induce changes in hepatic metabolism and gallbladder function, which together result in a cascade of events leading to the formation of stones (Fig. 41-8).

PIGMENT GALLSTONES

Worldwide, pigment stones are the most common type of calculi found in the gallbladder. Epidemiologic studies have indicated that although cholesterol calculi account for most gallstones in the United States, pigment stones constitute about 30% of all gallbladder stones. Although the pathogenesis of cholesterol gallstones has been the subject of considerable investigation, there has been limited effort to study the mechanisms by which pigment gallstones form. A number of factors may explain this phenomenon, including the low incidence of pigment gallstones in the United States, lack of a suitable animal model, and the heterogeneous nature of pigment gallstones. Despite the diverse settings in which pigment gallstones are known to occur, the final common pathway in the pathogenesis of the various types of pigment calculi is altered solubilization of unconjugated bilirubin with precipitation of calcium bilirubinate and insoluble salts.

Classification

Pigment gallstones are characterized by their relatively high concentration of bilirubin (usually in excess of 40%) and their low cholesterol content. Most pigment gallstones are mixed stones and contain calcium bilirubinate as the main component. They have been further classified as either black or brown stones. Black-pigment stones are gen-

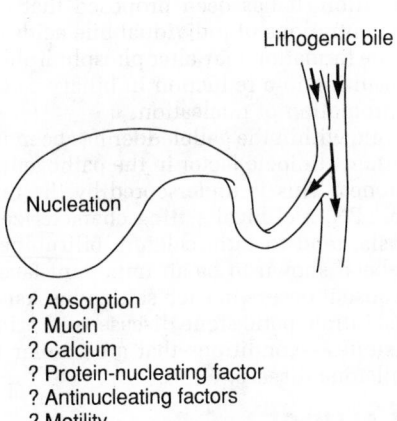

Figure 41-8. Proposed events that occur during cholesterol gallstone formation. A relation can be seen between hepatic metabolism and altered gallbladder physiology.

erally found in patients with hemolytic disorders or cirrhosis. These stones are typically tarry in appearance, are almost always located exclusively in the gallbladder, and are thought to occur as a result of alterations in biliary metabolism. In contrast, brown stones are the most common type found in Asian patients, are similar in composition to primary common bile duct stones, may be located throughout the intrahepatic or extrahepatic biliary tract, and are generally associated with infection.

Pathogenesis

Infection is thought to be a key factor in the pathogenesis of pigment gallstones.[7] Free unconjugated bilirubin produced by bacterial deconjugation is insoluble in water and combines with calcium in bile to produce a calcium bilirubinate matrix (which is well known as the predominant component of most pigment gallstones). Bacteria are found within the calcium bilirubinate–protein matrix of brown-pigment stones but are absent from either black-pigment or cholesterol gallstones. These findings are consistent with epidemiologic studies indicating that brown stones are found in patients living in areas where biliary infections are endemic, whereas black-pigment stones are typically found in patients with hemolytic disorders or cirrhosis.

The realization that pigment stones also occur in patients with hemolytic disorders or cirrhosis, during maintenance of long-term TPN, and after ileal resection suggests that biliary infection as a unified hypothesis cannot explain the pathogenesis of all pigment gallstones. The high incidence of pigment gallstones in patients with hemolytic disorders probably results from excessive loads of bilirubin presented to the liver for excretion. Two possible explanations for the high incidence of pigment gallstones in cirrhotics include hypersplenism leading to increased hemolysis and impaired hepatic conjugation of bilirubin. It has been proposed that unconjugated bilirubin may be secreted directly into hepatic bile where, in the presence of increased amounts of cholesterol, the bilirubin moiety is driven out of the micelle and is available for precipitation with calcium. The finding that endogenously synthesized β-glucuronidase is secreted in human bile suggests another possible factor in the pathogenesis of pigment gallstones. The presumed role of calcium in the pathogenesis of pigment gallstone formation has been substantiated by the finding that bile is supersaturated with calcium bilirubinate. In a manner similar to cholesterol solubilization, mixed micelles are thought to be an important factor in regulating calcium binding. Increased concentrations of biliary calcium in animals and humans with pigment gallstones have been correlated with specific changes in bile acid composition. It has been proposed that changes in relative concentrations of individual bile acids associated with gallstone formation may alter phospholipid–bile acid micelles, resulting in a reduction in biliary calcium solubility and promotion of nucleation.

Stasis of bile within the gallbladder has been implicated as an important etiologic factor in the pathogenesis of pigment gallstones. This is underscored by the finding that patients on TPN, a clinical setting characterized by gallbladder stasis, tend to form calcium bilirubinate stones. Sepsis has been shown to be an important facet of stone disease because it occurs in such settings as Asian cholangiohepatitis, intrahepatic stone disease, and primary common duct stones—conditions that are similar to brown-pigment gallstone disease.

BILIARY SLUDGE

The importance of biliary sludge as a precursor of cholesterol and pigment gallstones has recently been recognized.[8] Sludge, as determined ultrasonographically, is partly composed of calcium bilirubinate crystals and may be a consequence of biliary stasis. Biochemical analysis of sludge demonstrates large amounts of phospholipids. This is particularly interesting given the earlier observations identifying phospholipids in the central core of pigment gallstones and the reported decreased solubility of unconjugated bilirubin that occurs with the addition of lecithin. Nonetheless, the mechanism by which phospholipids alter the solubility of unconjugated bilirubin and contribute to biliary sludge remains unclear. Several possible explanations have been proposed, including direct binding of phospholipids to unconjugated bilirubin and phospholipid-induced displacement of unconjugated bilirubin from bile salt–phospholipid micelles.

Recent observations that ceftriaxone, a third-generation cephalosporin, reversibly leads to sludge in the gallbladder is of interest because ceftriaxone induces specific biochemical changes in hepatic bile. Ceftriaxone administration is associated with changes in organic anion excretion in the liver, specifically calcium-sensitive anions.[9] These changes in hepatic metabolism then presumably lead to an environment conducive to sludge formation in the gallbladder. Although stone formation per se has not been confirmed as a result of this drug, further studies examining the factors responsible for changes in ion flux may help elucidate the mechanism of altered absorption and its role in stone formation.

GALLSTONE DISEASE

The spectrum of clinical syndromes associated with cholelithiasis is as varied as the multiple causes associated with the pathogenesis and formation of cholesterol and noncholesterol gallstones. Studies suggest that about 50% of patients with gallstone disease are truly asymptomatic. Most patients with symptoms secondary to cholelithiasis complain of recurring right upper quandrant pain (biliary colic). Others will have symptoms consistent with acute cholecystitis, choledocholithiasis, or gallstone pancreatitis. The difficulty lies in identifying those patients at risk for developing these specific complications of gallstone disease. To date, this has not been possible. Recently completed, prospective longitudinal studies have attempted to trace the natural history of asymptomatic gallstones in well-defined populations. Although these studies suggest that only a small percentage of patients with asymptomatic stones develop serious complications, the data may not be representative of the general population. Of patients with cholelithiasis who are symptomatic, less than half ultimately undergo some type of biliary tract procedure. Less than 1% of all patients presenting with an initial complication of gallstones have a fatal outcome during that hospitalization.

Asymptomatic Stones

The optimal treatment for patients with asymptomatic gallstones has been debated for many years. Several relatively recent reports have suggested that the natural history of asymptomatic gallstones is benign and that early or prophylactic cholecystectomy is rarely indicated. In two such studies, data suggest that less than 10% of patients with asymptomatic gallstones will develop significant symptoms over a 5-year period. Some concerns have been raised regarding these data, and important questions remain unanswered.[10] An issue central to this controversy is the definition of what truly constitutes an asymptomatic patient. It is apparent that a significant number of patients with cholelithiasis do not have postprandial pain but instead have dyspepsia, vague epigastric discomfort, or even

enteric mucosal-to-mucosal anastomosis. A number of alternatives for elective repair of bile duct strictures exist. The choice of procedure is dictated by the location of the stricture, the history of previous unsuccessful attempts at repair, and the surgeon's personal preference. Simple excision of a bile duct stricture and end-to-end bile duct anastomosis or repair of the damaged duct can rarely be accomplished because of the invariable loss of duct length as a result of fibrosis associated with the injury. Similarly, anastomosis of the proximal bile duct to the duodenum as a choledochoduodenostomy is not suitable for most postcholecystectomy strictures because an adequate length of bile duct for creating a tension-free anastomosis to the duodenum usually cannot be obtained. Thus, in almost all cases, hepaticojejunostomy constructed to a Roux-en-Y limb of jejunum is the preferred procedure.

Many surgeons believe that a transanastomotic stent is helpful in almost all cases. In the early postoperative period, a stent is used to decompress the biliary tree and to provide access for cholangiography. If the injury involves the common bile duct or the common hepatic duct at least 2 cm distal to the hepatic duct bifurcation, and adequate proximal bile duct mucosa can be defined, the use of long-term biliary stents is not necessary. In these situations, the preoperatively placed percutaneous transhepatic catheter or operatively placed T-tube is used to decompress the biliary–enteric anastomosis for 4 to 6 weeks postoperatively. When adequate proximal bile duct is not available for a good mucosa-to-mucosa anastomosis, long-term stenting of the biliary–enteric anastomosis with Silastic transhepatic stent is recommended. For strictures involving the hepatic duct bifurcation, both the right and left main hepatic ducts should be individually stented.

An operative technique for biliary reconstruction with transhepatic stents employs the preoperatively placed percutaneous transhepatic catheters.[4,5] The porta hepatis is dissected, which usually involves separating adhesions of the duodenum and hepatic flexure of the colon to the Glisson capsule and the gallbladder fossa. Identification of the proximal biliary segment can be difficult and can be aided by the presence of the transhepatic biliary catheter. The bile duct is then divided at the lowest extent of the stricture and dissected proximally. A segment of the strictured duct should be resected and submitted for pathologic examination. The distal duct is then oversewn, and the bile duct proximal to the stricture is carefully dissected circumferentially in a cephalad direction for a distance not to exceed 5 mm. Excessive dissection should be avoided to prevent vascular compromise of this segment of duct, which will be used for the anastomosis. After mobilization and division of the bile duct, the biliary catheters protrude through the proximal end (Fig. 43-10A). A radiologic guide wire is then placed through these catheters. A series of progressively larger coudé catheters are then passed over the guide wire, dilating the system to allow the placement of a Silastic stent. The Silastic stents are 70 cm long and come in 12F to 22F sizes. Multiple side holes are present along 40% of the length of the stent. These side holes are left to reside within the intrahepatic biliary tree and the portion of the Roux-en-Y jejunal limb used for the biliary anastomosis. The end of the stent without the side holes exits through the hepatic parenchyma and is brought out through a stab wound in the upper anterior abdomen. After stent placement, a Roux-en-Y jejunal limb is prepared, and the anastomosis is then performed as an end-to-side hepaticojejunostomy (see Fig. 43-10B).

An alternative technique has been described for management of bile duct strictures involving the bifurcation and one or both of the hepatic ducts in which a side-to-side anastomosis of the left hepatic duct to the Roux-en-Y limb is constructed. A long opening along the anterior surface of the left hepatic duct is anastomosed to the side of the Roux-en-Y limb. Because it is possible to dissect the anterior surface of the left hepatic duct high up into the hepatic parenchyma, this procedure permits anastomosis to normal mucosa, even though there can be fibrosis and stricture at the bifurcation of the ducts and within the distal portion of the hepatic duct. This technique can avoid the need for postoperative stenting.

Results

Morbidity and Mortality

Repairs of bile duct strictures are performed primarily in major medical centers by experienced surgeons, yet these operations are still associated with significant morbidity and mortality. In 1982, a review of 38 series published since 1900, containing over 7643 procedures performed on 5586 patients, reported an overall operative mortality rate of 8.3%.[6] In the past decade, however, most series have reported mortality rates of less than 5%. Factors frequently associated with operative mortality include advanced age, coexistent disease, and a history of major biliary tract infection. The state of underlying liver disease, however, is the most important determinant of operative morbidity and mortality. In patients with advanced biliary cirrhosis and portal hypertension, operative mortality rates can approach 30%, with most deaths due to liver failure. Bile duct strictures located proximally are also associated with increased technical difficulty and thus also contribute to slightly increased risk.

Postoperative morbidity rates approach 20% to 30%. Complications may include the usual postoperative complications, such as hemorrhage, cardiopulmonary problems, urinary tract infection, and wound infection. Complications specific to the repair of bile duct strictures include anastomotic leaks at the site of the biliary–enteric anastomosis, cholangitis, and hepatic insufficiency from preexisting biliary cirrhosis. Most anastomotic leaks documented by postoperative cholangiography or by bilious drainage from intraoperatively placed drains can be successfully managed nonoperatively. Transhepatic stenting diverts biliary secretions externally in the face of a leak and is one of the major advantages of this technique.

Long-Term Results. Excellent long-term results can be achieved in 70% to 90% of patients who undergo repair of bile duct strictures (Table 43-1). The definition of satisfactory results in most series requires that patients have no symptoms, jaundice, or cholangitis. Length of follow-up is important in analyzing final results because recurrent strictures can occur up to 20 years after the initial procedure[2,3] (Fig. 43-11). About two thirds of restrictures are evident within 2 years, and 90% are seen within 7 years. The percentage of patients with good results is inversely related to the number of previous repairs. Other factors that favor a good outcome include young age at the time of stricture repair, use of a Roux-en-Y biliary–enteric anastomosis, absence of infection and hepatic fibrosis, and use of transhepatic stents.

Nonoperative Management

Operative management of bile duct strictures is technically difficult and continues to be associated with significant postoperative morbidity and mortality. Moreover, in all series, recurrent strictures develop in a proportion of patients. These factors, in addition to technical advances in the fields of therapeutic radiology and endoscopy, have

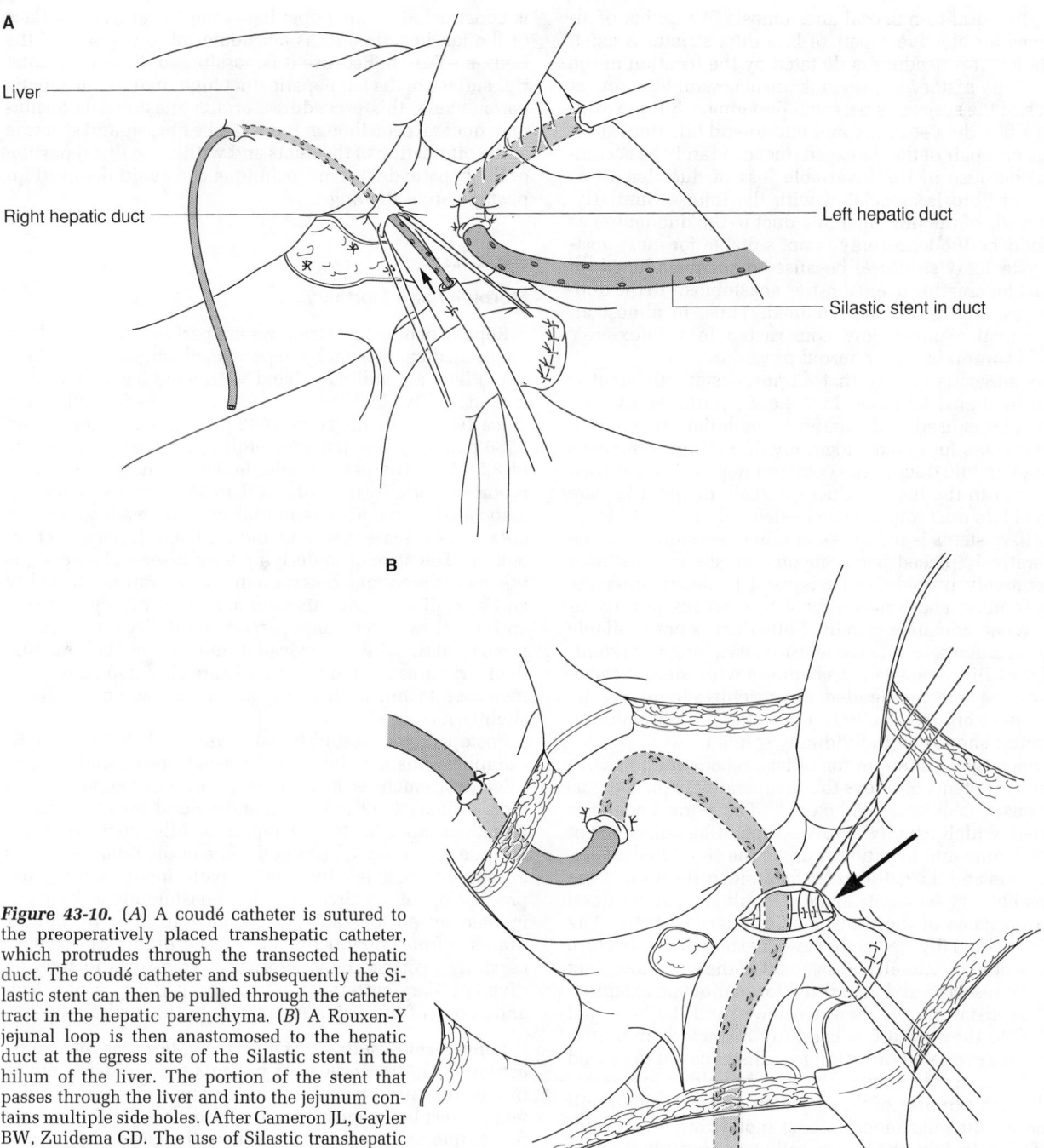

Figure 43-10. (*A*) A coudé catheter is sutured to the preoperatively placed transhepatic catheter, which protrudes through the transected hepatic duct. The coudé catheter and subsequently the Silastic stent can then be pulled through the catheter tract in the hepatic parenchyma. (*B*) A Rouxen-Y jejunal loop is then anastomosed to the hepatic duct at the egress site of the Silastic stent in the hilum of the liver. The portion of the stent that passes through the liver and into the jejunum contains multiple side holes. (After Cameron JL, Gayler BW, Zuidema GD. The use of Silastic transhepatic stents in benign and malignant strictures. Ann Surg 1978;188:552)

Table 43-1. **RESULTS OF SURGICAL MANAGEMENT OF BILE DUCT STRICTURES**

Investigators	Patients	Success (%)	Follow-Up (mo)
Pitt et al, 1982[2]	66	86	60
Pelligrini et al, 1984[3]	60	78	102
Genest, 1986	105	82	60
Innes, 1988	22	95	72
Pain, 1988	163	72	133
Pitt et al, 1989[5]	25	88	57
David et al, 1993[8]	35	83	50

led to the development of nonoperative techniques for management of bile duct strictures.

Percutaneous Balloon Dilation

The largest nonoperative experience in the management of benign bile duct strictures is using the percutaneous transhepatic route. The procedure in many cases can be performed with a combination of local anesthesia and intravenous sedation. In this technique, access to the proximal biliary tree is gained, and the stricture is traversed with a guide wire under fluoroscopic guidance. At this point, dilation of the stricture is performed using angioplasty-type balloon catheters, chosen on the basis of the location of the stricture and the diameter of the normal

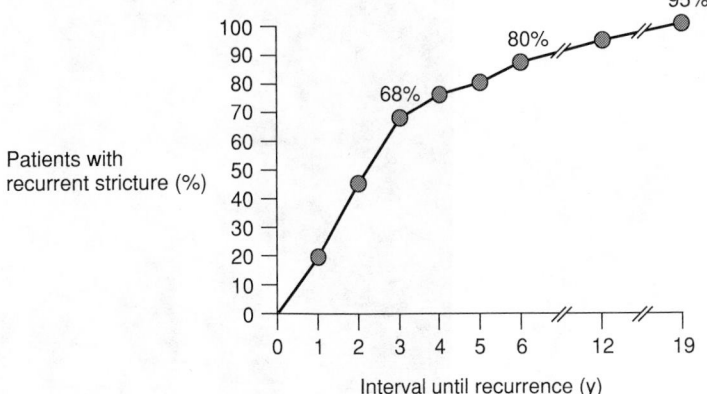

Figure 43-11. The cumulative percentage of recurrent strictures with respect to the time from the initial repair until the next repair. (After Pitt HA, Miyamoto T, Parapatis SK, et al. Factors influencing outcome in patients with postoperative biliary strictures. Am J Surg 1982;144:14)

duct (Fig. 43-12). After the procedure, a transhepatic stent is left in place across the stricture to allow access to the biliary tree for follow-up cholangiography, repeat dilation, and maintenance of a lumen during the healing process. In most series, numerous dilations are required.

The early results in a number of series have been encouraging (Table 43-2). In a multicenter review, 3-year follow-up showed a 67% patency rate for anastomotic and a 76% patency for iatrogenic primary bile duct strictures, yielding an overall 70% success rate.[7] Others have achieved successful dilation in 87.5% of patients with primary ductal strictures and in 72.5% of patients with biliary–enteric anastomotic strictures, with an overall success rate of 78%.[8]

Complications of balloon dilation are frequent. Cholangitis, hemobilia, and bile leaks can occur in up to 20% of patients. Bleeding, usually from the hepatic parenchyma, has been reported, with transfusions often necessary. Sepsis due to cholangitis can occur despite antibiotic prophylaxis. Sepsis and significant bleeding seldom occur in patients dilated by a T-tube tract, suggesting that much of the morbidity is the result of traversing the hepatic parenchyma by the large percutaneously placed catheters.

Endoscopic Balloon Dilation

The experience with endoscopic balloon dilation is more limited. This technique is technically possible only in patients with primary bile duct strictures or with strictures at a choledochoduodenal anastomosis. This technique begins with ERC and endoscopic sphincterotomy. The stricture is traversed retrograde with an atraumatic guide wire, and sequential balloon dilation is employed. Reevaluation with cholangiography is performed every 3 to 6 months. Redilation is performed as necessary. In most cases, an endoprosthesis is left in place after dilation for at least 6 months.

The reported experience with endoscopic dilation of benign bile duct strictures is shown in Table 43-3. The largest experience comes from the group in the Netherlands and is discussed under Comparative Data.[9] A similar experience was reported in the United States.[10] In this series, 18 of 25 strictures were postoperative in nature. Strictures were located at the cystic duct junction in 17 patients and in the distal bile duct in the remaining 8 patients. Twenty-two of 25 patients (88%) had significant clinical benefit from the therapy. Only two complications occurred in this series—one case each of pancreatitis and cholangitis.

Comparative Data

Comparison of results of nonoperative dilation with those of surgery have been difficult. Few centers have a significant experience with both operative and nonopera-

tive management. Furthermore, the definition of a successful procedure, the reporting of complications, and the length of follow-up have not been consistent in the literature. There are no prospective randomized studies to compare these techniques. However, two retrospective comparative studies exist. In the first study, a retrospective review of the results at the Johns Hopkins Hospital between 1979 and 1987 compared percutaneous balloon dilation and surgery in 43 patients with benign postoperative bile duct strictures.[5] Twenty-five patients underwent surgical repair with Roux-en-Y choledochojejunostomy or hepaticojejunostomy with postoperative transhepatic stenting for a mean of 13 ± 1.3 months. Twenty patients had percutaneous balloon dilation, a mean of 3.9 times, and were stented transhepatically for a mean of 13.3 ± 2 months. Three patients were managed with both surgery and balloon dilation. The two groups were similar with respect to multiple parameters that might have influenced outcome, including age, sex, associated medical problems, and presentation with either obstructive jaundice or biliary fistulas.

No patients died after any of the procedures. Procedure-related morbidity occurred in 20% of surgical patients and in 35% of the patients undergoing balloon dilation. For both groups, a successful outcome was defined as no evidence of cholangitis or jaundice requiring another procedure more than 12 months from the onset of treatment. A failed treatment was defined as the need for crossover to the other treatment modality, either operation or dilation, or late death from liver failure, biliary sepsis, or portal hypertension. A successful repair was achieved in 89% of the surgical patients and in only 52% of the balloon dilation patients (Fig. 43-13). The overall late mortality rate in this series was 10%. One late death occurred in the surgical group, whereas three late deaths followed balloon dilation (4% versus 15%, respectively). No deaths, however, were attributed to liver failure, biliary sepsis, or portal hypertension associated with the bile duct stricture.

To define further the relative benefits of the two procedures, total hospital stay and total procedural costs were determined. As expected, initial hospitalization was longer for surgery than for balloon dilation. When rehospitalization for further dilation, complications, or recurrences were considered, total hospital stay did not differ significantly between the two groups. Cost data paralleled hospitalization data and did not differ significantly between the groups. Thus, the authors concluded that until properly designed, randomized, prospective controlled trials can be performed, surgical repair for benign postoperative strictures appears to be associated with fewer problems and a greater success rate.

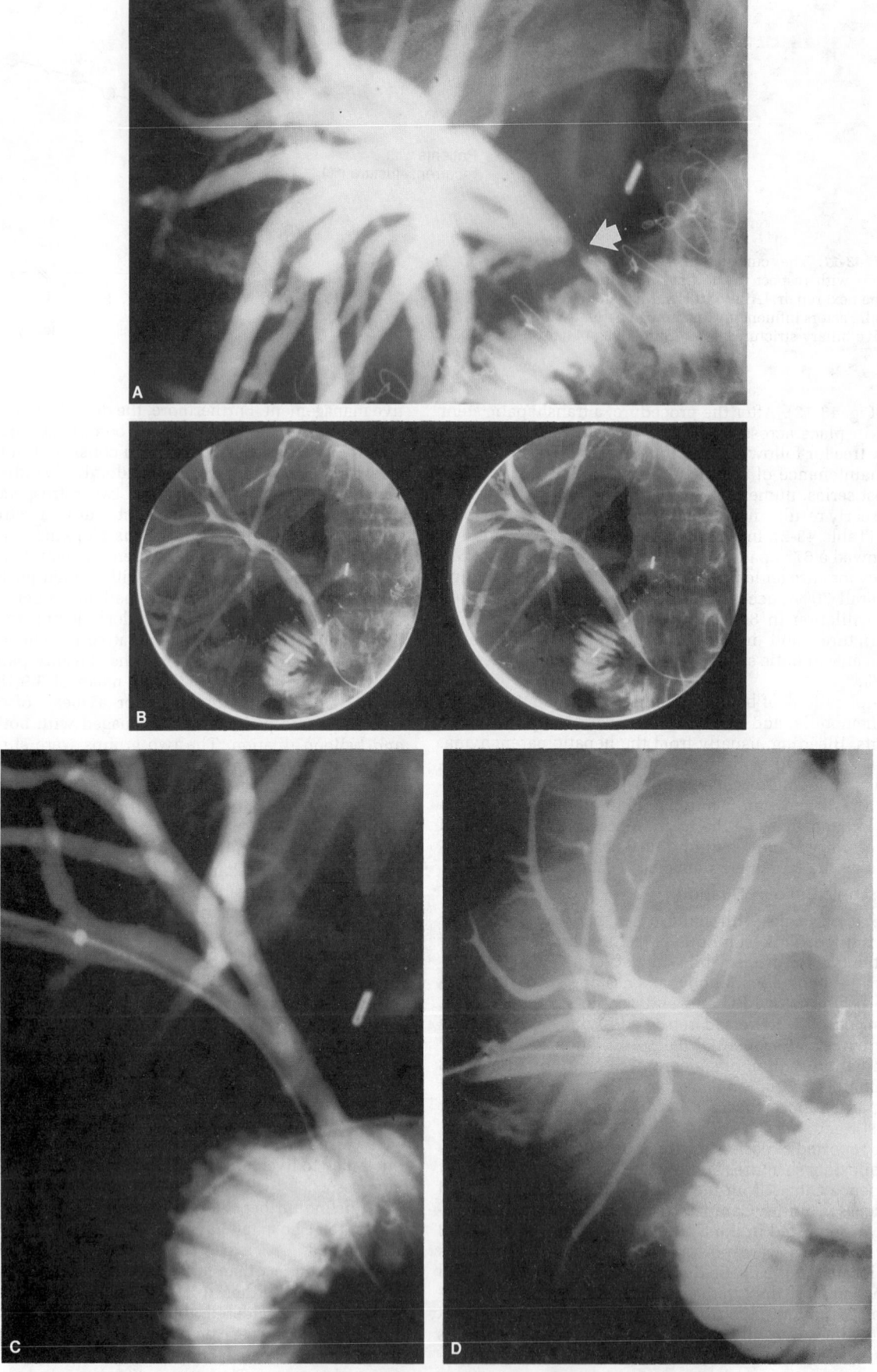

Figure 43-12. (*A*) Transhepatic cholangiogram demonstrating stricture (*arrow*) at a previous choledochojejunostomy. (*B*) Progressive dilation of the strictured anastomosis with an angioplasty balloon catheter. (*C*) Postdilation stenting of the anastomic stricture for prolonged periods. (*D*) Subsequent cholangiogram demonstrating resolution of the anastomotic stricture. (Pitt HA, Kaufman SL, Coleman J, et al. Benign postoperative biliary strictures: operate or dilate? Ann Surg 1989;210:417)

Table 43-2. RESULTS OF TRANSHEPATIC BALLOON DILATION OF BILE DUCT STRICTURES

Investigators	Patients	Success (%)	Follow-Up (mo)
Mueller et al, 1987[7]	61	70	36
Williams, 1987	64	78	28
Moore, 1987	18	83	33
Pitt et al, 1989[5]	20	55	59
Citron et al, 1991	28	93	38

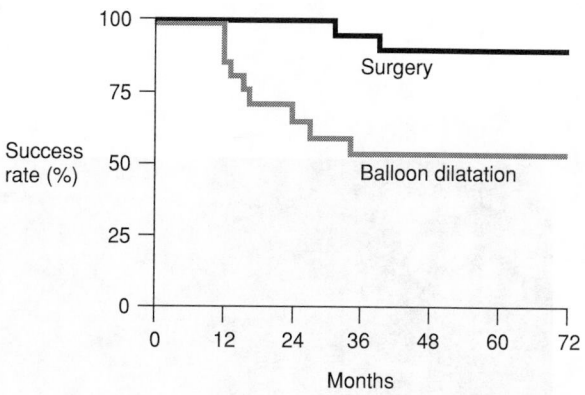

Figure 43-13. Actuarial success rates over 72 months for surgery (89%) and balloon dilation (52%). The difference is statistically significant ($P < .01$). (After Pitt HA, Kaufman SL, Coleman J, et al. Benign postoperative biliary strictures: operate or dilate? Ann Surg 1989;210:417)

In the second comparative study, the group from the Netherlands compared endoscopic versus surgical treatment of benign bile duct strictures.[9] Thirty-five patients were treated surgically, and 66 were treated by endoscopic stenting. Patient characteristics, initial injury, previous repairs, and the level of obstruction were comparable in both groups. Surgical therapy consisted of Roux-en-Y hepaticojejunostomy, and endoscopic therapy consisted of placement of endoprosthesis with trimonthly elective exchange for 1 year. Successful stent placement was accomplished in 94% of patients managed endoscopically. Six of the 66 endoscopic patients, however, underwent surgical reconstruction either for failed stent placement or for other reasons. Early complications occurred more frequently in the surgically treated group (26% versus 8%; $P < .03$). However, the only procedure-related death occurred in a patient who developed severe pancreatitis after endoscopic stent placement. Late complications, which included primarily episodes of cholangitis, occurred only in the endoscopic group (27%). The overall complication rates, therefore, were similar at 26% for surgical patients and 35% for endoscopic patients. The mean follow-up and definition of success were similar. After surgery, excellent results were observed in 83% of patients, with 6 patients developing a recurrent stricture at a mean of 40 months after the initial operation. After endoscopic stenting, excellent results were observed in 72% of patients, with 18% of patients developing restricture at a mean of 3 months after stent removal. The investigators concluded that endoscopic stenting should be considered for the initial attempt at definitive management in suitable patients in hopes of avoiding reoperation.

PRIMARY SCLEROSING CHOLANGITIS

Primary sclerosing cholangitis is an idiopathic disease characterized by intrahepatic and extrahepatic inflammatory strictures of the bile ducts that cannot be attributed to other specific causes. The cause of primary sclerosing cholangitis is unknown. Many experts consider primary sclerosing cholangitis to be an autoimmune reaction because it is associated with other autoimmune diseases, such as ulcerative colitis, retroperitoneal fibrosis, and Riedel thyroiditis (Table 43-4). It is likely that a number of

causes, including viral or bacterial infections, toxic drug reactions, and congenital anomalies, can all result in the same end-stage injury that is recognized as primary sclerosing cholangitis.

The usual clinical presentation of patients with primary sclerosing cholangitis involves intermittent jaundice, which begins insidiously in the fourth or fifth decade of life. Right upper quadrant pain, pruritus, fever, weight loss, and fatigue can also occur. The disease is characterized by cyclic remissions and exacerbations. Despite the nomenclature, acute cholangitis is uncommon without previous biliary manipulation or surgery. The diagnosis is suggested by clinical presentation associated with cholestatic liver function test abnormalities. The levels of bilirubin often fluctuate with respect to the remissions and exacerbations of the disease and the extent of hepatic injury. Alkaline phosphatase is usually elevated out of proportion to the serum bilirubin and is a more persistent finding. The diagnosis, however, usually is confirmed by cholangiography, which reveals multiple dilations and strictures (beading) of the intrahepatic and extrahepatic bile ducts (Fig. 43-14). ERC is the preferred procedure because of difficulties in cannulation of the intrahepatic ducts by the percutaneous transhepatic route because the ducts are usually nondilated and fibrotic. The disease should be followed closely by cholangiography and liver biopsy to pro-

Table 43-3. RESULTS OF ENDOSCOPIC BALLOON DILATION OF BILE DUCT STRICTURES

Foutsch, 1985	Patients	Success (%)	Follow-Up (mo)
Foutsch, 1985	9	55	6
Geenen et al, 1989[9]	25	88	48
David et al, 1993[8]	46	83	48

Table 43-4. DISEASES ASSOCIATED WITH PRIMARY SCLEROSING CHOLANGITIS

Disease	Frequency (%)
Ulcerative colitis	40–60
Pancreatitis	12–25
Diabetes mellitus	5–10
Retroperitoneal fibrosis	Rare
Riedel thyroiditis	Rare
Crohn's disease	Rare
Histiocytosis X	Rare
Sicca complex	Rare
Rheumatoid arthritis	Rare
Hypertrophic osteoarthropathy	Rare
Sarcoidosis	Rare
Angioimmunoblastic lymphadenopathy	Rare
Acquired immunodeficiency syndrome	Rare

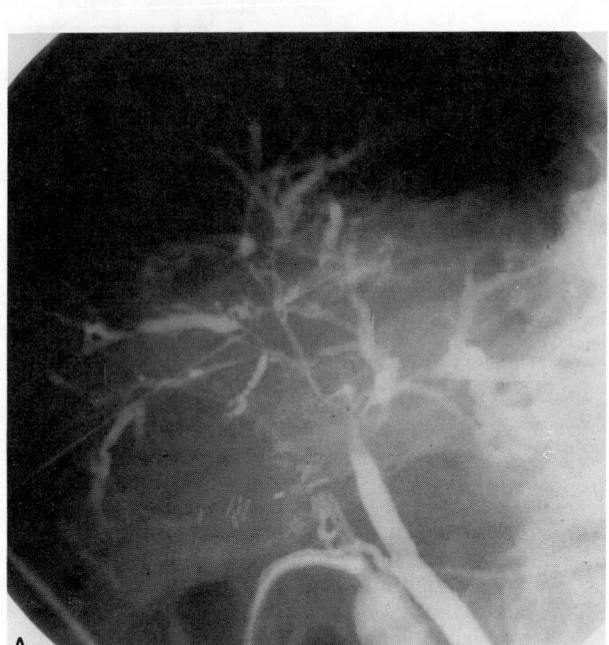
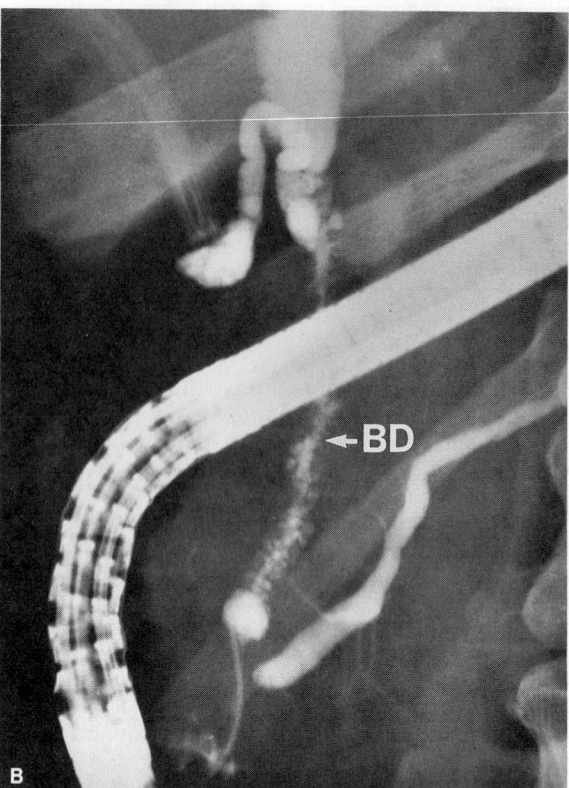

Figure 43-14. (*A*) Cholangiogram of a patient with primary sclerosing cholangitis. Multiple irregular strictures and dilation (beading) of intrahepatic bile ducts can be seen. (*B*) Endoscopic retrograde cholangiogram showing extensive involvement of extrahepatic bile duct (BD) with primary sclerosing cholangitis. (*B* from Lillemoe KD, Pitt HA, Cameron JL. Primary sclerosing cholangitis. Surg Clin North Am 1990;70:1390)

vide appropriate management before the development of biliary cirrhosis.

No known specific medical therapy is effective for primary sclerosing cholangitis. The most encouraging results, from a prospective, randomized, placebo-controlled trial, suggest that ursodeoxycholic acid significantly improves serum liver function tests and liver histologic appearance. Nonoperative dilation therapy (discussed earlier), by either the transhepatic or endoscopic route, has been used for dominant strictures. In a multicenter review of percutaneous balloon dilation, only 43% of patients with primary sclerosing cholangitis had successful long-term results.[7] The results of endoscopic dilation and stenting may be more favorable.

Because of the lack of effective medical therapy, an aggressive surgical approach is advocated for most symptomatic patients with primary sclerosing cholangitis. One surgical approach, in patients with a dominant stricture at the hepatic duct bifurcation, uses resection of the bifurcation and long-term transhepatic stenting with Silastic stents. This mode of therapy was reported in 31 patients.[11] Indications for operation included persistent jaundice in 29 patients and recurrent cholangitis in 2 patients. Five of the 31 patients had secondary biliary cirrhosis before surgery, with the remaining 26 having varying degrees of fibrosis without cirrhosis. The 1- and 5-year actuarial survival rates for patients with fibrosis were 92% and 71%, respectively whereas the actuarial survival rate at 1 and 5 years was 20% in patients with established biliary cirrhosis (Fig. 43-15). Four patients have undergone hepatic transplantation for progressive disease.

The other surgical option for treatment of primary sclerosing cholangitis is hepatic transplantation. In a review from the University of Pittsburgh of 55 consecutive hepatic transplantations for primary sclerosing cholangitis, the 1- and 2-year actuarial survival rates were 71% and 57%, respectively.[12] These rates were similar to those reported for hepatic transplantation for all patients during that time period. A more recent report from the University of Nebraska showed better results, with an actuarial survival rate of 88% at 4 years.

Resection of the hepatic duct bifurcation and long-term transanastomotic stenting in selected patients can preclude or delay the need for hepatic transplantation. Moreover, this operation does not eliminate or influence the results of hepatic transplantation. Resection of the hepatic bifurcation and long-term transhepatic stenting can be recommended for selected patients with primary sclerosing cholangitis with severe strictures at or distal to the hepatic duct bifurcation but without established biliary cirrhosis. In patients with biliary cirrhosis, hepatic transplantation is recommended.

BILE DUCT STRICTURES SECONDARY TO CHRONIC PANCREATITIS

Chronic pancreatitis is an uncommon cause of benign bile duct strictures, resulting in less than 10% of such cases. Transient partial obstruction of the distal common bile duct due to inflammation and edema frequently occurs in patients with acute pancreatitis. With chronic pancreatitis, however, the clinical problem is distal bile duct obstruction due to inflammation and parenchymal fibrosis of

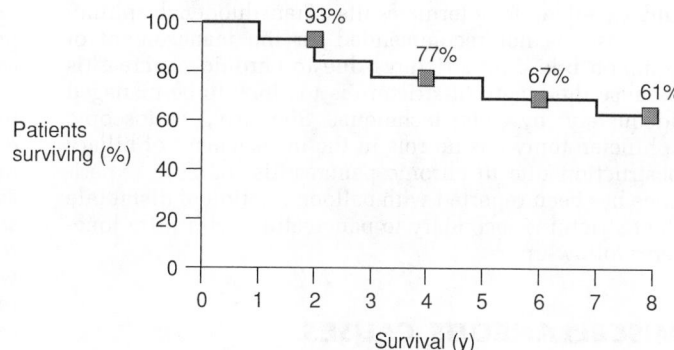

Figure 43-15. Actuarial survival rates among 31 noncirrhotic patients with primary sclerosing cholangitis who underwent resection of the hepatic bifurcation and long-term transhepatic stenting. (Lillemoe KD, Pitt HA, Cameron JL. Primary sclerosing cholangitis. Surg Clin North Am 1990; 70:1397)

the gland. These strictures classically involve the entire intrapancreatic segment of the common bile duct and are associated with dilation of the entire proximal biliary tree (Fig. 43-16). In most cases, the cause of the chronic pancreatitis is alcoholism. Often, advanced disease is present in that the incidence of pancreatic calcification, diabetes, and malabsorption is increased at the time of presentation with jaundice compared with patients with chronic pancreatitis without jaundice. Common bile duct strictures have been reported to occur in 3% to 29% of patients with chronic alcoholic pancreatitis. In a review of a number of clinical series, the overall incidence of common bile duct strictures in patients with chronic pancreatitis was 5.7%.[13] The exact

incidence of common bile duct strictures is not known, however, because cholangiography is not routinely performed in patients with chronic pancreatitis.

The clinical presentation of patients with common bile duct strictures secondary to chronic pancreatitis is variable. Some patients have no symptoms, with the diagnosis of bile duct strictures suggested only by abnormal liver function tests. The serum alkaline phosphatase appears to be the most sensitive laboratory finding and is elevated in over 80% of patients. Abdominal pain with or without jaundice is another common presentation. In some cases, the abdominal pain can be difficult to distinguish from the pain associated with chronic pancreatitis. Failure to recognize and address a bile duct stricture, however, can lead to ultimate failure of operative procedures performed for chronic pain in patients with chronic pancreatitis. Finally, the development of jaundice in patients with chronic pancreatitis must be differentiated from underlying periampullary malignancy.

The definitive evaluation of patients with a bile duct stricture due to chronic pancreatitis is cholangiography. Either endoscopic retrograde cholangiopancreatography (ERCP) or PTC can be useful. ERCP offers the advantage of demonstrating pancreatic ductal anatomy and possible abnormality, which is essential in optimal surgical management of chronic pancreatitis. Both techniques allow decompression of the obstructed biliary tree if necessary for cholangitis or severe jaundice. A long (usually 2 to 4 cm), smooth, gradual tapering of the common bile duct is most compatible with a benign stricture due to chronic pancreatitis (see Fig. 43-16).

The indications for surgical management of common bile duct strictures due to chronic pancreatitis are clear in patients with significant pain, jaundice, or cholangitis. Controversy exists, however, concerning the necessity of biliary decompression in patients with an asymptomatic elevation of serum alkaline phosphatase. In general, biliary bypass is indicated because changes from obstructive biliary cirrhosis have been observed in liver biopsy specimens obtained from patients with long-standing, functionally significant biliary obstruction due to chronic pancreatitis.[14,15]

Choledochoduodenostomy and Roux-en-Y choledochojejunostomy are acceptable methods of biliary bypass in patients with bile duct strictures due to chronic pancreatitis. Choledochoduodenostomy is preferred by many surgeons because it does not divert bile from the duodenum, is technically easier to perform, and leaves the jejunum intact for any associated procedures required for decompression of an obstructed gastrointestinal tract or pancreatic duct. The results of surgical management of distal bile duct structures due to chronic pancreatitis are usually excellent, with a low rate of perioperative complications

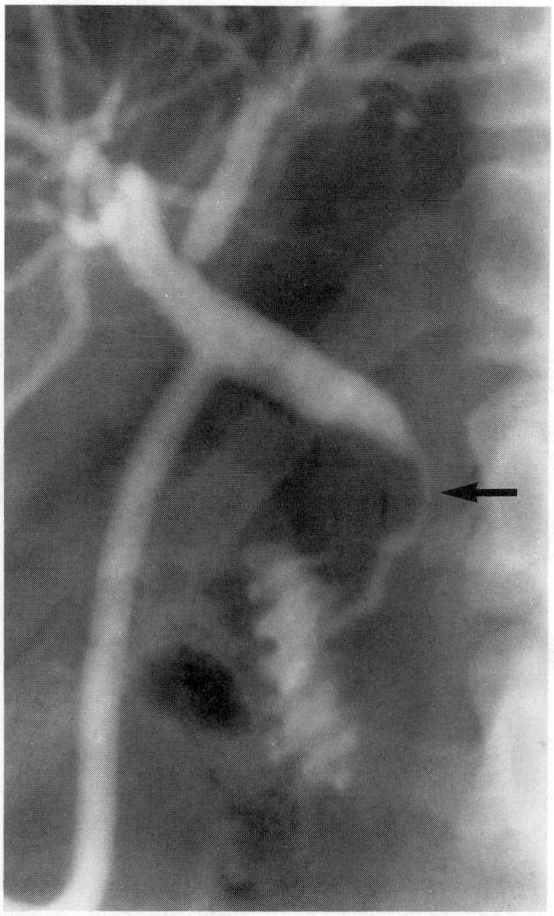

Figure 43-16. Cholangiogram of a patient with a long distal common bile duct stricture (*arrow*) due to chronic pancreatitis.

and excellent long-term results. Transduodenal sphincteroplasty is not recommended for the management of common bile duct strictures due to chronic pancreatitis because the length of stricture is too long to be managed adequately by this technique. Similarly, endoscopic sphincterotomy has no role in the management of biliary obstruction due to chronic pancreatitis. Limited experience has been reported with balloon dilation of distal bile duct strictures secondary to pancreatitis, with little long-term follow-up.

MISCELLANEOUS CAUSES OF BILE DUCT STRICTURES

Benign strictures of the bile duct can result from the chronic inflammation associated with gallstones in either the gallbladder or common bile duct. This is an uncommon cause of bile duct strictures and a rare complication of gallstone disease. Bile duct strictures due to cholelithiasis are usually associated with a narrowing at the level of the common hepatic duct caused by a stone impacted in the infundibulum of the gallbladder. The narrowing can be caused by two means. First, simple compression can occur from a large stone lying adjacent to the common hepatic duct. Second, chronic or acute inflammation arising from the gallbladder or cystic duct can extend to the contiguous bile duct, resulting in stricture formation. The biliary obstruction associated with either of these conditions is known as *Mirizzi syndrome*.

The clinical presentation of a bile duct stricture due to cholelithiasis is often associated with acute cholecystitis and hyperbilirubinemia. In some long-standing cases, these findings exist in the face of chronic gallbladder symptoms. If hyperbilirubinemia is present and urgent cholecystectomy is not indicated, ERCP or PTC can help to delineate the biliary anatomy preoperatively. Most cases that are associated with acute cholecystitis, however, are recognized at the time of cholecystectomy and operative cholangiography. When the duct compression is associated with acute inflammation, the common hepatic duct almost always returns to normal after the offending stone has been removed by cholecystectomy and the inflammatory process has resolved. Care must be taken during the dissection to avoid creation of a defect in the common hepatic duct. Rarely, after the acute episode has resolved, a well-established stricture presents months to years after the acute episode. In such cases, management by Roux-en-Y hepaticojejunostomy is appropriate.

Strictures due to choledocholithiasis are also rare. The presumed mechanism is erosion of the epithelium of the distal duct, creating inflammation with subsequent fibrosis and stricture. Because of the anatomic tapering of the common bile duct, nearly all stones are entrapped in the intrapancreatic portion of the duct and are often difficult to remove by the supraduodenal route.

Excessive intraoperative manipulation at the time of bile duct exploration with forceps, scoops, and catheters can often create additional trauma to an already friable distal duct. After the stone has been removed, the distal bile duct should be gently sized with a soft rubber catheter to be sure that no stricture exists. If a stricture persists after stone removal, it may not be recognized until the time of postoperative T-tube cholangiography. If recognized in the postoperative period, time should be allowed for resolution of inflammation before considering stricture repair. If a distal bile duct stricture does persist, a biliary–enteric anastomosis with either Roux-en-Y choledochojejunostomy or a choledochoduodenostomy is indicated. If the proximal duct is adequately dilated (more than 2 cm in diameter)

to allow a large choledochoduodenal anastomosis, this procedure is usually preferable because of its technical ease and excellent results.

Stenosis of the sphincter of Oddi, or papillitis, is a benign intrinsic obstruction of the outlet of the common bile duct, usually associated with inflammation, fibrosis, or muscular hypertrophy. Sphincter stenosis can result in any of three clinical conditions: (1) common bile duct obstruction due to fibrotic stenosis of the papilla, (2) recurrent pancreatitis, or (3) recurrent right upper quadrant pain without jaundice or pancreatitis. The pathogenesis of the inflammation of sphincter stenosis is unclear. In many cases, it is thought to be due to the trauma of the passage of multiple small stones from the common duct through the ampulla. This trauma results in inflammation, scarring, and stricture formation. Many patients with papillary stenosis have no gallstones. Other potential mechanisms include primary sphincter motility disorders and congenital anomalies. The clinical presentation is usually either jaundice or cholangitis. In some cases, an impacted common bile duct stone may be present. The diagnosis can be supported with cholangiography either by the percutaneous transhepatic or endoscopic route. This condition can be managed by sphincterotomy performed either endoscopically or operatively. If a cholecystectomy was performed previously, endoscopic papillotomy is the initial procedure of choice.

Cholangiohepatitis is an unusual infection of the biliary tree frequently associated with *Clonorchis sinensis* and other parasites. These infections are most commonly seen in natives of Asia. Most patients present with recurrent episodes of cholangitis. Cholangiography can demonstrate multiple strictures of both the intrahepatic and extrahepatic biliary tree, with the bile ducts filled with sludge and stones (Fig. 43-17). Surgical management consists of cholecystectomy and improved biliary drainage with either Roux-en-Y choledochojejunostomy or choledochoduodenostomy. Access to the biliary tree for postoperative management of intrahepatic stones or sludge should be maintained with either transhepatic biliary stents or a choledochojejunocutaneous or subcutaneous fis-

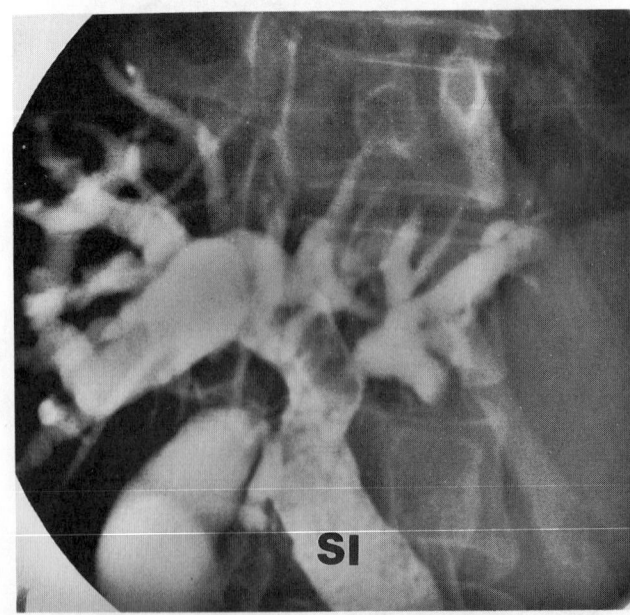

Figure 43-17. Cholangiogram of a patient with oriental cholangiohepatitis with diffuse bile duct dilation. The biliary tree is filled with sludge (Sl) and stones.

tula. No specific medical management is available for this condition.

Finally, rare causes of benign intrahepatic and extrahepatic bile duct strictures have been reported secondary to intrahepatic arterial infusion of 5-fluorouracil used in the treatment of hepatic metastases of colorectal carcinoma. The clinical picture closely resembles primary sclerosing cholangitis but usually can be managed by simple discontinuation of infusion and, in some cases, percutaneous transhepatic drainage. Surgery should be reserved for patients with persistent evidence of biliary obstruction. A similar cholangiographic appearance has been reported in patients with acquired immunodeficiency syndrome. The pathogenesis of this injury is believed to be viral in nature and related to cytomegalovirus infection. No experience in the surgical management of this condition has been reported.

REFERENCES

1. Branum G, Schmitt C, Baille J, et al. Management of major biliary complications after laparoscopic cholecystectomy. Ann Surg 1993;17:53.
2. Pitt HA, Miyamoto T, Parapatis SK, et al. Factors influencing outcome in patients with postoperative biliary strictures. Am J Surg 1982;144:14.
3. Pelligrini CA, Thomas MJ, Way LW. Recurrent biliary stricture: patterns of recurrent and outcome of surgical therapy. Am J Surg 1984;147:175.
4. Cameron JL, Gayler BW, Zuidema GD. The use of Silastic transhepatic stents in benign and malignant biliary strictures. Ann Surg 1978;188:552.
5. Pitt HA, Kaufman SL, Coleman J, et al. Benign postoperative biliary strictures: operate or dilate? Ann Surg 1989;210:417.
6. Warren KW, Christophi C, Armendari ZR. The evolution and current perspectives of the treatment of benign bile duct strictures: a review. Surg Gastroenterol 1982;1:141.
7. Mueller PR, van Sonnenberg E, Ferrucci Jr T, et al. Biliary stricture dilatation: multicenter review of clinical management in 73 patients. Radiology 1986;160:17.
8. Williams HF, Bender CE, May GR. Benign postoperative biliary strictures: dilatation with fluoroscopic guidance. Radiology 1987;163:629.
9. David PHP, Tanka AKF, Rauws EAJ, et al. Benign biliary strictures: Surgery or endoscopy? Ann Surg 1993;217:237.
10. Geenen DJ, Geenen JE, Hogan WJ, et al. Endoscopic therapy for benign bile duct strictures. Gastrointest Endosc 1989; 35:367.
11. Lillemoe KD, Pitt HA, Cameron JL. Primary sclerosing cholangitis. Surg Clin North Am 1990;70:1381.
12. Marsh JW Jr, Iwatsuki S, Makowka L, et al. Orthotopic liver transplantation for primary sclerosing cholangitis. Ann Surg 1988;207:21.
13. Stahl TJ, O'Connor A, Ansel M, et al. Partial biliary obstruction caused by chronic pancreatitis: an appraisal of indications for surgical biliary drainage. Ann Surg 1988;207:26.
14. Warshaw AL, Schapiro RH, Ferrucci JT Jr, et al. Persistent obstructive jaundice, cholangitis, and biliary cirrhosis due to common bile duct stenosis in chronic pancreatitis. Gastroenterology 1976;70:562.
15. Afroudakis A, Kaplowitz N. Liver histopathology in chronic bile duct stenosis due to chronic alcoholic pancreatitis. Hepatology 1981;1:65.

COLON, RECTUM, AND ANUS

SURGERY: SCIENTIFIC PRINCIPLES AND PRACTICE, Second Edition, edited by
Lazar J. Greenfield, Michael W. Mulholland, Keith T. Oldham, Gerald B. Zelenock,
and Keith D. Lillemoe. Lippincott–Raven Publishers, Philadelphia, © 1997.

CHAPTER 44

COLONIC ANATOMY AND PHYSIOLOGY

THOMAS A. MILLER

The major function of the gastrointestinal tract is to absorb water, nutrients, and other substances, such as electrolytes, minerals, and vitamins. To ensure that the ingested material is delivered to the appropriate site for absorption, an exquisitely developed muscular system exists within the wall of the gut. This system allows propulsion of luminal contents in a well-coordinated fashion and enables adequate mixing so that absorption can occur with optimal efficiency. Because the stomach, small intestine, and large bowel serve different functions in this absorptive process, motility patterns differ considerably among these three regions, even though fundamentally common mechanisms underlie the motor function of each section. The differing mechanisms that exist in these three anatomic regions relate to the different luminal contents to which they are exposed. For example, gastric contents are primarily in the form of suspended solid particles, whereas in the small intestine, they are more fluid. By the time luminal contents have reached the large intestine, they are semisolid to solid in composition. Thus, it is not surprising that much of the movement through the stomach and proximal small bowel is rapid, whereas throughout the distal small intestine, movement is much slower, and in the colon, propulsion is slow. Because of these differences in luminal content, it is appropriate that the main motor function of the stomach and proximal small bowel is one of mixing and rapid distal propulsion, while that of the distal small bowel is primarily mixing and slow distal propulsion. In contrast, the role of the colon is mixing, temporary storage, and very slow distal propulsion.

The mechanisms responsible for these different motility patterns are being unraveled, and much remains to be learned. In contrast to the stomach and small intestine, in which control systems modulating motility have been reasonably well defined, the organization and control of colonic motor activity requires much more elucidation.

ANATOMY OF THE COLON

General Considerations

The human colon has often been described as consisting of the appendix, cecum, ascending colon, transverse colon, descending colon, sigmoid colon, rectum, and anal canal. For the purposes of this chapter, the rectum and anal canal are not considered part of the colon. Further, the appendix, while arising from the cecum, has no obvious coordinating effect on colonic function, and thus is not considered a separate anatomic region. Defining the colon in this fashion, the total length averages 4.5 to 6 feet.

The various anatomic components of the colon are shown in Figure 44-1. The right colon has generally been designated as consisting of the cecum, the ascending colon, the hepatic flexure, and the proximal transverse colon. The left colon is comprised of the distal transverse colon, the splenic flexure, the descending colon, the sigmoid colon, and the rectosigmoid colon. Although the transverse and sigmoid colons are suspended in the peritoneal cavity by specific mesenteries, both the ascending and descending colonic segments are fixed to the retroperitoneum. The greatest diameter of the colon exists in the cecum, with the caliber of the lumen decreasing progressively from the cecum to the sigmoid.

Two major arterial systems supply the colon (Fig. 44-2). The right colon is predominantly supplied by the superior mesenteric artery. The major branches of this artery that perfuse the right colon include the ileocolic branch, which supplies the ileocecal junction; the right colic, which supplies the ascending colon; and the middle colic artery, which supplies the hepatic flexure and the transverse colon to its midpoint. The left colon is predominantly supplied by the inferior mesenteric artery, which derives its origin from the abdominal aorta. The distal transverse colon and the descending colon obtain their blood supply from the left colic branch of the inferior mesenteric artery, while the sigmoid colon obtains its blood supply from sigmoid branches. All along the colon, the colic arteries bifurcate and form vascular arcades so that the resultant marginal artery forms an anastomosis between the superior mesenteric artery and the inferior mesenteric artery. Considerable anatomic variation exists with respect to this arterial arcade, and a complete anastomosis is present in only 15% to 20% of people.

Accompanying the arteries perfusing the colon are corresponding veins (Fig. 44-3). The veins draining the right colon enter a major confluent vein, the superior mesenteric vein, while those draining the left colon form the inferior mesenteric vein. Both veins empty into the portal vein, which in turn drains into the liver. Lymphatic plexuses in both the submucosal and subserosal layers of the bowel drain into major lymphatic vessels and lymph nodes that accompany the veins and arteries (Fig. 44-4).

Similar to the small intestine, the colonic wall contains four layers: mucosa, submucosa, muscularis, and serosa (Fig. 44-5). The specific features of muscle fibers in the submucosa and the muscle bundles in the muscularis proper are discussed later. The neural elements that participate in colonic contractility and their anatomic location are described in a subsequent section.

Colonic Epithelium

The mucosal surface of the colon consists of a columnar epithelium, like that of the small intestine, but because the colon does not possess a physiologically important absorp-

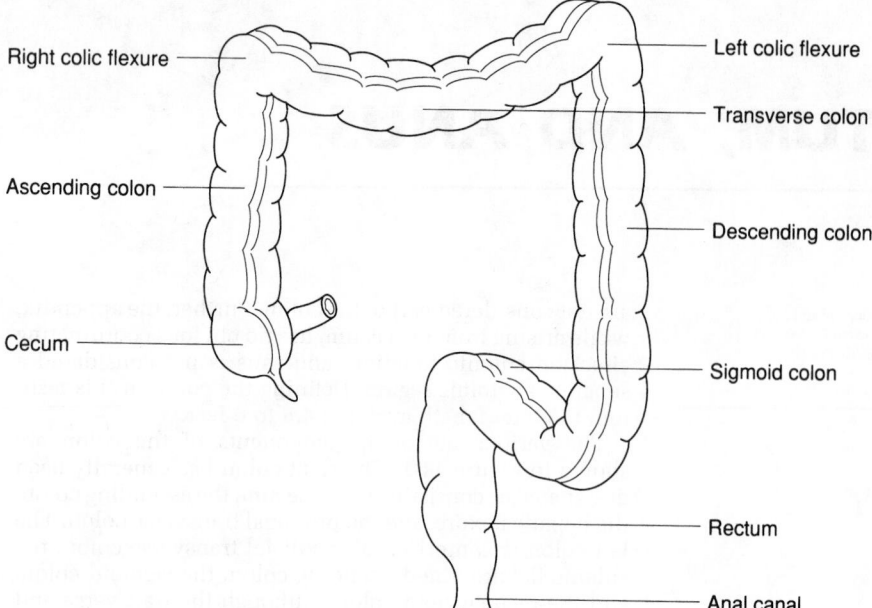

Figure 44-1. Anatomic components of the colon.

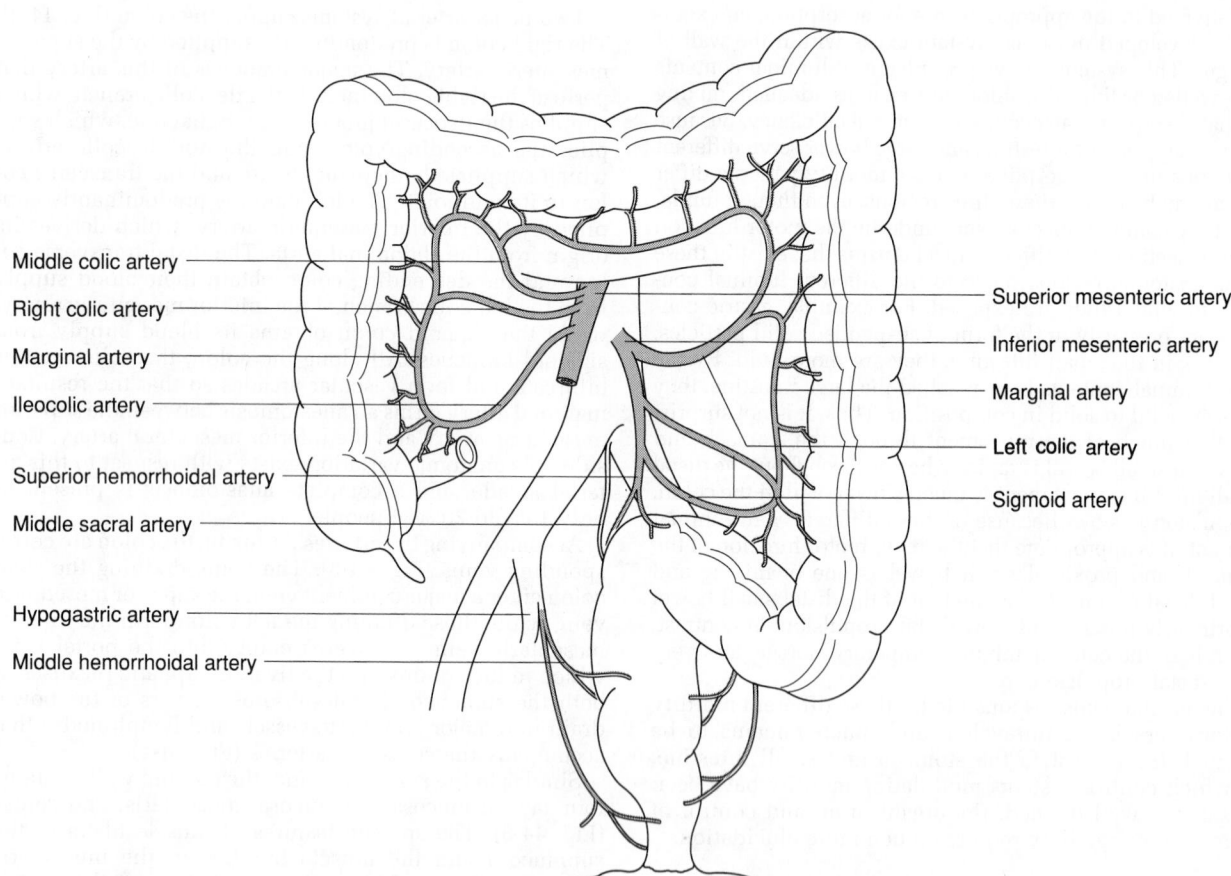

Figure 44-2. Arterial blood supply of the colon.

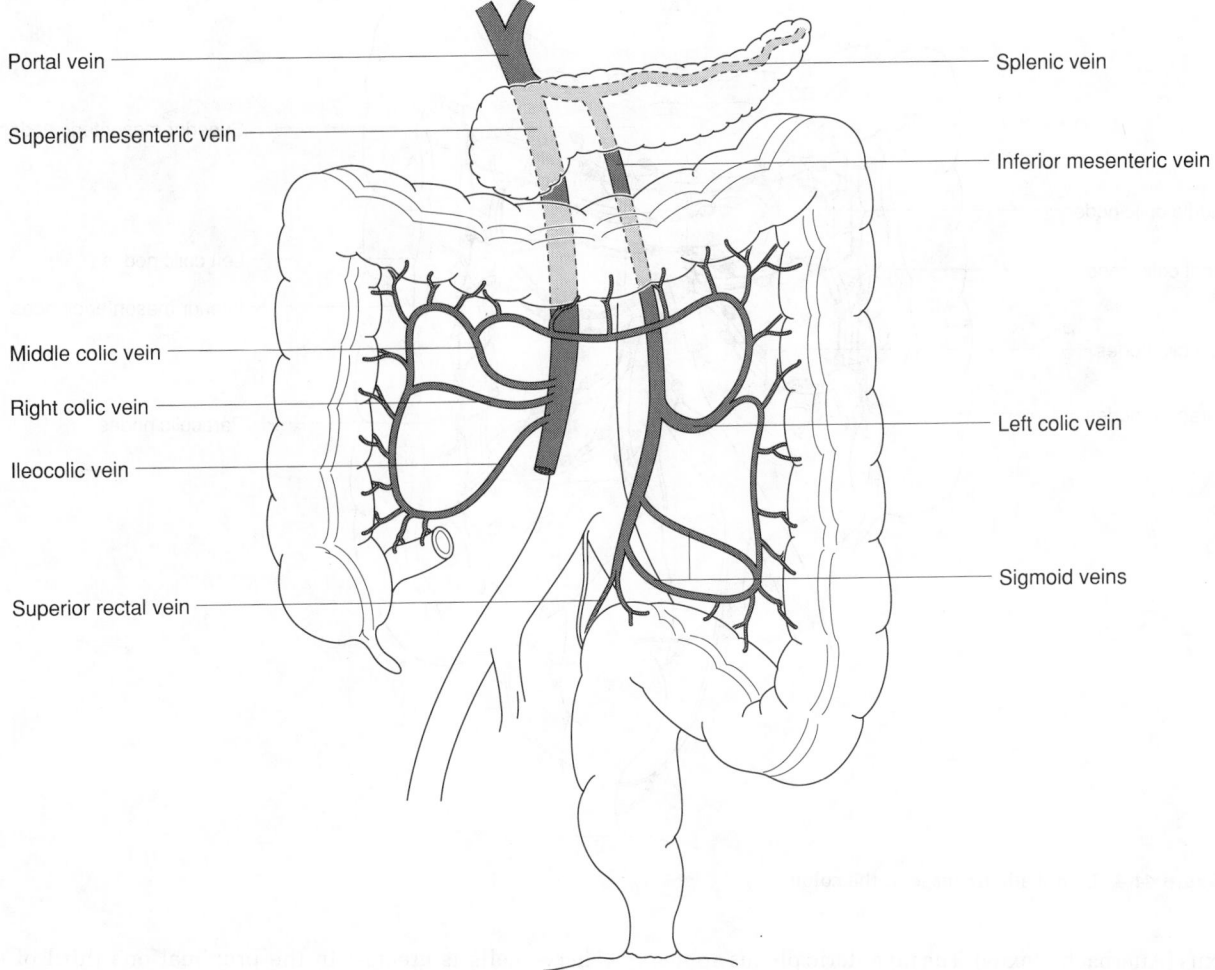

Figure 44-3. Venous drainage of the colon by the portal vein.

Portal vein

Superior mesenteric vein

Middle colic vein

Right colic vein

Ileocolic vein

Superior rectal vein

Splenic vein

Inferior mesenteric vein

Left colic vein

Sigmoid veins

tive role, the components of the colonic epithelium are less sophisticated. Thus, in the colon, villi are absent. In contrast to the small intestine, the mucosa is generally flat. All along the mucosal surface, the Lieberkühn crypts open into the colonic lumen. The epithelium of the lower portion of the crypts consists of undifferentiated mucus-secreting goblet cells, scattered endocrine cells, and columnar cells. The upper part of the crypts is composed of differentiated columnar cells, goblet cells, and fewer endocrine cells. The mucosa between the crypts is columnar in type.

Muscular Structure of the Colonic Wall

Like the stomach and small intestine, the musculature of the colon is smooth muscle and is arranged in three general layers. The innermost layer comprises the muscularis mucosa that resides below the epithelium as one moves from the intestinal lumen to the outer serosal lining. The muscularis mucosa has both an inner circular and outer longitudinal layer, but generally the two layers are fixed so that the muscle bundles are tightly interwoven. Surrounding the muscularis mucosa is a thick layer of circular smooth muscle that subtends the entire circumference of the colon. The anatomic structure of this circular smooth muscle is not unlike that found in the stomach and small intestine. An outer longitudinal muscle sur-

rounds the circular muscle. In contrast to the stomach and small intestine, in which bundles of the longitudinal muscle layer are uniformly distributed around the circumference of the bowel, the longitudinal muscle layer of the colon is grouped into three thick bands known as the *taeniae*. Although some longitudinal muscle is present between these taeniae, it is generally thin, with the bulk of the muscle mass residing in the taeniae. One taenia is located along the mesenteric insertion of the colon, while the other two are positioned about the same distance from one another. It is this configuration of the longitudinal muscle that gives rise to the sacculated appearance of the human colon, known as *haustration*. The three taeniae begin in the cecum and continue throughout the large bowel to the point where the sigmoid colon ends and the rectum begins. At this point, the three taeniae become more broad based and fuse so that the longitudinal muscle layer is distributed uniformly around the circumference of the rectum.

Neural Components

Similar to other regions of the gut, two groups of plexuses exist within the wall of the colon. The submucosal plexus (Meissner plexus) is located between the muscularis mucosa and the circular muscle layer of the muscularis propria. Sandwiched between the circular muscle and the outer longitudinal muscle is the myenteric

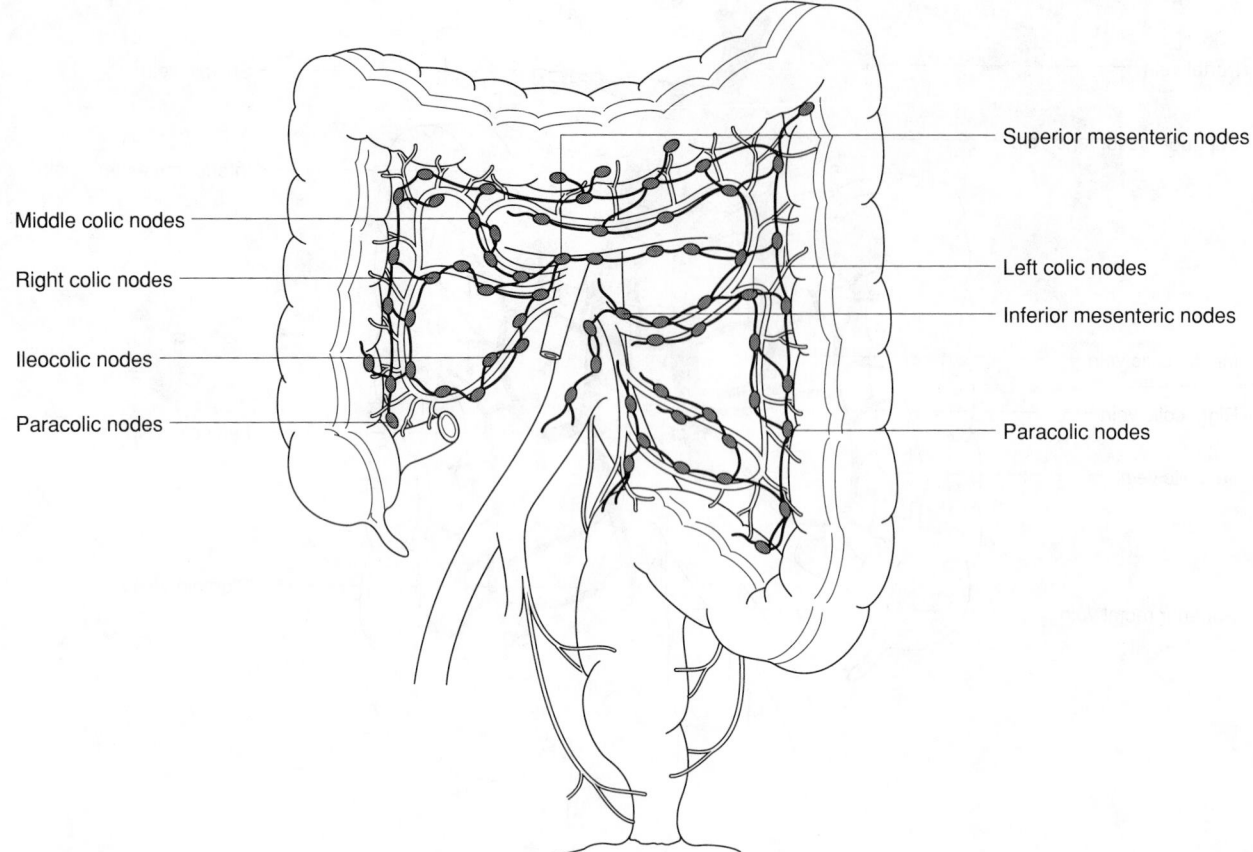

Figure 44-4. Lymphatic drainage of the colon.

plexus (Auerbach plexus). The myenteric plexus appears to be intimately involved with colonic motility. The plexus is composed of ganglia and clusters of nerve cell bodies that are linked together by bundles of nerve processes. Although the myenteric plexus is well developed throughout the entire length of the colon, the density of nerve cells is greatest in the proximal one third of the colon, similar to the density that exists throughout the small intestine. The physiologic significance of this organization remains to be defined, but it almost certainly contributes to the different motility patterns that exist throughout the large bowel.

PHYSIOLOGY OF COLONIC CONTRACTION

In contrast to the stomach and small intestine, in which the motility patterns in response to food and various neurohumoral stimuli have been reasonably well characterized, the patterns of colonic motor activity and the mechanisms responsible for its control are only partially understood. One explanation for this relates to the complexity of colonic motility when compared with other regions of the gut. Although the colon extends anatomically from the cecum to the junction of the sigmoid colon with the rectum, each region of the large bowel appears to have distinct motor activity independent of other regions. The ascending colon, for example, is primarily involved with mixing, stirring, and kneading the fecal material so that uniform exposure to the mucosal surface occurs, allowing adequate absorption of the liquid chyme that enters the colon during a 24-hour period. Thus, it is not surprising that propulsion of the fecal contents in a caudal direction occurs slowly from the colonic motor activity of the right colon. In contrast, the left colon is more of a storage reservoir for the semisolid to solid feces that exist within its lumen, and its contractile patterns are more concerned with forward movement of this fecal content distally and ultimate defecation. Only within the past decade has sub-

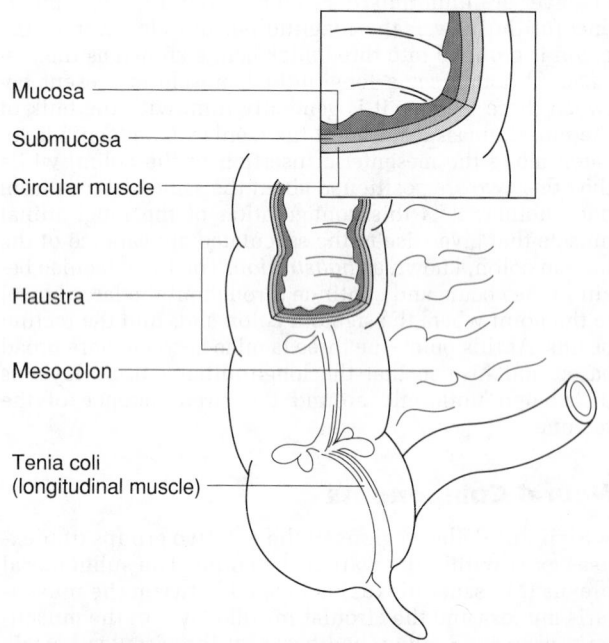

Figure 44-5. Layers of the colonic wall.

stantial progress been made in defining these patterns and how they interrelate with each other. Much of this progress has been possible because of the development of computer technology to elucidate the characteristics of these patterns and the mechanisms responsible for their control and modulation. Overall, the primary motor functions of the large bowel are concerned with mixing, storage, and slow distal propulsion.

To accomplish these goals, the human colon exhibits several different types of contractions.[1,2] One type, known as *individual phasic contractions,* initiates contractile patterns of both short and long duration. Short-duration contractions last less than 15 seconds, in contrast to the longer duration form, which last 40 to 60 seconds. Although both types of contraction can be recorded from circular muscle, most studies suggest that long-duration contractions arise primarily from the longitudinal muscle, while short-duration contractions emanate from circular muscle. The frequency of short-duration contractions in humans ranges from 2 to 13 per minute, while that of long-duration contractions ranges from 0.5 to 2 per minute. These contractions are primarily responsible for mixing colonic contents thoroughly to allow optimal absorption and then slowly propelling the semisolid to solid feces distally. The long-duration contractions appear to be especially important in enhancing this distal movement.

Underlying each of these phasic contractile patterns is a basic electrical pattern within smooth muscle cells that enables each cell to control its contractions as well as couple them with adjacent cells. For short-duration phasic contractions, periodic depolarizations of individual smooth muscle cells called *electric control activity* (ECA) appear to be important. ECA is a basic electrical rhythm or pacemaker activity of the large bowel and is characterized by slow waves similar to those identified in the stomach and small intestine. In contrast to the relative regular frequency and amplitude of these waves in more proximal gut regions, the amplitude and frequency of ECA in the colon are variable. Two frequency patterns have been identified in both animals and humans. The patterns include a low frequency range of 2 to 9 cycles per minute that is generally found in the ascending and sigmoid colon, and a higher frequency of 9 to 13 cycles per minute that is more commonly observed in the transverse and descending colon. Although the ECA appears to be present in circular smooth muscle, its existence in longitudinal muscle has been less certain. ECA is temperature and oxygen dependent and appears to be calcium dependent. The disorganized and variable colonic ECA is precisely what is needed to produce spatially disorganized short-duration contractions because the purpose of these contractions is mainly to mix and agitate the colonic contents. This disorganization of the ECA occurs not only along the length of the colon but also around its circumference.

The long-duration contractions appear to be controlled by a different electrical activity called the *contractile electrical complex.* This complex consists of intermittent bursts of electrical activity that oscillate at a frequency in the range of 25 to 40 cycles/min. The contractions resulting from these electrical bursts of activity are more powerful and sustained than those arising from the ECA, hence the designation long-duration phasic contractions. These contractions play an important role in mixing and enabling the nearly solid luminal contents to move back and forth. Further, because of their more profound nature, they enable movement of the fecal content to proceed in a slow but coordinated caudal fashion. Like the ECA, the contractile electrical complex responsible for long-duration contractions is calcium dependent and appears to require the

opening of voltage-sensitive calcium channels in the cell membrane.

In addition to these two types of phasic colonic contractions, the human colon also exhibits ultrapropulsive contractions called *giant migrating contractions.* They are of long duration and amplitude and propagate over a substantial length of the colon in contrast to the phasic contractions, which either do not propagate or propagate over short distances. The giant migrating contractions cause mass movements of colonic contents and the emptying of the area of the colon in which they occur. Under healthy conditions, they occur infrequently (ie, once or twice a day) and in the distal colon provide the force necessary to propel feces in a rapid fashion during the process of defecation. Little is known about the mechanisms responsible for the generation of giant migrating contractions. It is known, however, that their frequency can be profoundly increased during states of colonic inflammation. When this occurs, diarrhea can result, and considerable fluid and electrolytes can be lost in the fecal material because sufficient time was not allowed for absorption of these substances.

Because giant migrating contractions are infrequent in contrast to the short- and long-duration phasic contractions, the mean transit time through the whole length of the colon is prolonged compared with the rate of transit in the stomach or small intestine. In men, this transit time averages 33 hours; in women, it can be as long as 47 hours. This slow transit is fortunate because it allows defecation to occur at socially convenient times and under voluntary control.

NEUROHUMORAL CONTROL OF COLONIC MOTILITY

In addition to the inherent myogenic control of colonic motor function, both neural and humoral components play important roles in modulating colonic motility.[1,2] Three levels of neural control influence colonic contractions: the enteric, autonomic, and central nervous systems. The enteric nervous system plays an especially prominent role in the control of colonic motility. As previously discussed, the enteric nerves of the colon are organized into two major plexuses. The myenteric plexus (Auerbach plexus) is located between the longitudinal and circular muscles of the bowel wall; the submucosal plexus (Meissner plexus) is located between the muscularis mucosa and the circular muscle layer of the muscularis propria. In each plexus, the cell bodies of neurons are grouped into ganglia from which neurons project to the respective muscle groups that they supply. Motor neurons projecting to the circular and longitudinal muscle layers are of two types: excitatory and inhibitory. The neurotransmitter of the excitatory neurons is acetylcholine. The neurotransmitter for inhibitory motor neurons, often called *nonadrenergic noncholinergic* (NANC) *neurons,* remains uncertain. Putative neurotransmitters thought to play a role in NANC neuronal transmission include adenosine triphosphate, vasoactive intestinal polypeptide, and nitric oxide. Cholinergic excitatory neurons stimulate colonic muscle contraction, whereas the NANC inhibitory neurons inhibit them. Whether colonic contraction is stimulated or inhibited when activated simultaneously depends on the magnitude of the two neural inputs. In addition to modulating phasic contractions of slow and long duration, NANC inhibitory neurons are also thought to produce descending inhibition ahead of giant migrating contractions and thereby modulate defecation.

Peptidergic neurons have also been identified in the colonic wall using a variety of histochemical and immunocytochemical methods. Most of the transmitters for these neurons are peptides and include such diverse agents as somatostatin, substance P, opioids, calcitonin gene–related peptide, neuropeptide Y, vasoactive intestinal peptide, and gastrin-releasing peptide. Nonpeptide transmitters, such as γ-aminobutyric acid and serotonin, can also be functionally important. The physiologic role of these neurons as modulators of colonic motility remains undefined.

Also part of the enteric nervous system are various sensory neurons that perceive mechanical and chemical stimuli from the luminal contents. Their axons project both to motor neurons and to prevertebral ganglia and higher neural centers. Mediators of such sensory input appear to be substance P and calcitonin gene–related peptide. Their role in transmitting sensory information remains uncertain, but because they have been shown to synapse on the excitatory and inhibitory motor neurons, they probably play an important role in modulating spontaneous contractions.

As components of the autonomic nervous system, the vagus and the pelvic nerves are parasympathetic neural inputs, while the lumbar colonic, the splanchnic, and the hypogastric nerves comprise sympathetic components. Fibers from these nerves can affect a number of enteric ganglia and provide important pathways for input from the central nervous system to the colon and for reflex actions and modulation between different portions of the colon and between the colon and other organs. Norepinephrine is the primary neurotransmitter of sympathetic nerves in the colon and, through such neural transmission, regulates the release of acetylcholine at presynaptic terminals in the enteric ganglia. Parasympathetic neural transmission is mediated exclusively through acetylcholine.

The central nervous system primarily modulates colonic motor function under conditions of stress or during voluntary defecation. Such modulation is transmitted through the autonomic nerves (such as the vagus, pelvic, hypogastric, lumbar colonic, and splanchnic nerves) to the enteric ganglia. Through such autonomic neural control, the brain stimulates or inhibits colonic contractions by motor excitatory and inhibitory neurons.

In addition to the neurohumoral input just described, various peptides can modulate colonic motor activity under physiologic conditions. Substances such as cholecystokinin (CCK), gastrin, secretin, neurotensin, and pancreatic polypeptide are known to increase after eating. Experimentally, each of these peptides has been shown to stimulate or inhibit contraction of muscle strips. Whether postprandial concentrations of these peptides exhibit any significant effects on colonic motor activity remains to be determined but seems probable. Likewise, prostaglandins and motilin are powerful stimulants of intestinal smooth muscle and can be assayed radioimmunologically throughout the gut; whether they have a physiologic role, however, cannot be stated at this point. Many of the common laxatives that are used clinically to induce defecation have been assumed to stimulate colonic motor function. Studies in vitro, using various muscle strips, have failed to support this notion. On the other hand, bile acids, especially deoxycholic acid, appear to be direct stimulants of colonic motor activity, as has been assumed for decades. Finally, various drugs, such as erythromycin, cisapride, opioids, and serotonin antagonists, are known to alter colonic motor activity through a direct increase or decrease in the rate of transit. Exactly how these effects are mediated, though, remains undefined. Some of these drugs alter neural inputs to colonic motor cells, whereas others have direct effects on the cells themselves. Precise information regarding mechanism of action must await further investigation.

PHYSIOLOGIC ALTERATIONS IN COLONIC MOTILITY

Movements of the colon commonly occur soon after eating. In fact, in some people, this linkage is so well developed that the ingestion of certain foods almost guarantees that a bowel movement will soon follow. For others, the colonic response to eating is less predictable, and the extent and magnitude of the response is variable. The colonic response, when it occurs, affects both the frequency of the colonic contraction and the amplitude of pressures generated. The response is most marked in the sigmoid colon, but studies in which other regions have also been evaluated indicate that the whole length of the colon responds to eating in varying degrees.

Because original work examining the relation of eating to colonic function evoked this response after entry of food into the stomach, it was thought to have a gastric origin, and thus has been termed the *gastrocolic reflex*. Considerable debate exists concerning the actual role that the stomach plays in mediating this response. Disagreement is based on the observations that gastric distention does not commonly elicit the response: it begins somewhat slowly and persists after the stomach has normally emptied its contents, it can be demonstrated in patients who have previously been subjected to complete gastrectomy, and it can be elicited when food is placed directly into the duodenum. Whether the stomach initially triggers the response, and the duodenum and other portions of the proximal bowel sustain it, remains to be determined. There is little question, however, that the stomach is not necessary for the response to occur. Of further interest is the fact that different kinds of foods can modulate the intensity of the response. Thus, the ingestion of fat tends to increase colonic motility, while amino acids appear inhibitory. These findings suggest that mucosal chemoreceptors are responsible for its mediation.

Equally confusing is the mechanism by which chemoreceptive sensors effect changes in colonic motility. Evidence exists supporting a role for both neural and humoral pathways. Although data suggest that an intact cholinergic innervation is necessary to mediate the response, evidence also suggests that an adrenergic mechanism is involved. Further, whether the response is generated by direct neurogenic muscular contraction or a transient suspension of neurogenic inhibition remains to be clarified. Equally uncertain is the role that various hormones play in mediating this response. For example, gastrin, in physiologic doses, can increase colonic motor activity and initiate spike potentials in the human sigmoid and rectum. CCK appears to have similar stimulatory effects on colonic motor function. Thus, if hormones are involved in the colonic response to eating, it is conceivable that their release and subsequent colonic motor effects are modulated by various components of food as they pass through the gastrointestinal tract. Accordingly, gastrin release by food in the stomach could trigger the effect, whereas CCK release in the proximal bowel could sustain the effect.

Although a clear response in colonic motor function can be demonstrated after eating, the components responsible for this response and the mechanisms necessary for its transmission are far from understood. Multiple areas of the stomach and the bowel may evoke this response without one specific anatomic region being necessary for its generation. Equally likely is the possibility that both humoral substances and neural pathways are involved in modulating this response rather than one or the other.

COLONIC EPITHELIAL TRANSPORT

Compared with the small intestine, the epithelium of the colon is relatively impermeable and requires a considerably longer period of time to absorb the salt, water, and carbohydrate presented to it. Between 500 and 1500 g of a semiliquid material that can contain as much as 100 g of carbohydrate enter the colon on a daily basis. Most of this substance is absorbed, yielding a stool output that weighs about 200 g, indicating the effective absorptive capacity of the colonic mucosa. In fact, studies have shown that even larger amounts of carbohydrate and volumes of plasma-like solutions approaching 5 L can be effectively handled by the colon, when perfused at a steady rate into the cecum, without resulting in osmotic diarrhea. The reason for this efficient absorptive capacity, despite the relative impermeability of the colonic epithelium, relates to the close interrelation between epithelial transport and colonic motor activity.

To understand this relation, it must be remembered that transit through the large bowel takes about 10 times as long as that through the small intestine, usually requiring 2 or 3 days. Such slow passage provides optimal opportunity for the luminal contents to come into surface contact with the absorptive epithelium. Thus, sodium and water, which are extracted against high electrochemical and osmotic gradients, are efficiently absorbed. Further, the relatively static conditions of the colon allow the proliferation of vast numbers of anaerobic bacteria, which in turn break down carbohydrate to volatile fatty acids, which then are rapidly absorbed. Thus, the more rapid the colonic transit, the less efficient are these absorptive processes.

Although the mechanisms by which colonic motor patterns contribute to absorption are just becoming clearly understood, the various colonic contractile patterns have direct bearing on this process. Ringlike contractions, which move luminal contents in either antegrade or retrograde direction or which keep the contents stationary, enhance surface contact of the luminal slurry with enterocytes, optimizing conditions for absorption. Ringlike contractions, which are responsible for the haustration commonly seen on barium studies of the colon, also ensure that adequate mixing occurs and that the absorptive epithelium is brought into direct contact with luminal material, even that in the center of the lumen. Although the viscous nature of the colonic contents can make it difficult for substances in the center of the lumen to gain access to the absorptive epithelium, the haustral contractions enhance absorption by bringing the epithelial surface to the material in the colonic bulk. The net effect of this process is a highly efficient absorptive mechanism.

These mixing patterns also appear to stir the unstirred layer. This layer, which consists of a zone of water and mucus immediately adjacent to the epithelium, retards absorption; the thicker the layer, the greater is this retardation. By generating convection currents, the mixing patterns of the colon disrupt this layer and thereby enable more efficient surface contact between the luminal contents and the epithelial surface so that absorption can proceed without difficulty.[3] Evidence also exists indicating that the products of carbohydrate fermentation can stimulate salt and water absorption, presumably by influencing motor activity through various enteric neural reflexes. Further studies are needed, however, to define more clearly the nature of these reflexes and the precise conditions under which they occur.

In addition to the contractile patterns just described, more sustained contractions have been identified that develop in the left colon and result in the propulsion of the colonic contents into the rectum and toward the anus (Fig. 44-6). As discussed earlier, these giant migrating contractions produce mass movements and usually occur once or twice a day in humans.[4] Their primary purpose is to clear the colon of its contents. Although the stimuli for these contractions remain to be clarified, a variety of luminal substances appear to play important roles in their initiation. Fatty acids, bile acids, and various indigestible particles all have been shown to induce contractile patterns. In addition, luminal distention, various laxatives, and cholinergic stimulation have been shown to initiate contractile patterns. Under physiologic conditions, a balance appears to exist between mass movements that enable evacuation of waste materials on a regular basis and the slower mixing type of contractions that promote absorption of salt and water as well as bacterial proliferation for adequate carbohydrate salvage. When this balance is perturbed, as can occur with laxative abuse, derangements in bile acid production, excessive delivery of undigested particles to the colon, or disruption of the colon's normal bacterial flora by the inappropriate use of broad-spectrum antibiotics, excessive numbers of contractions of long duration can supervene, resulting in diarrhea.

DEFECATION

As already observed, giant migrating contractions produce mass movement in which undigested fecal content is propelled toward the rectum for eventual elimination from the body. The evacuation of these waste materials by

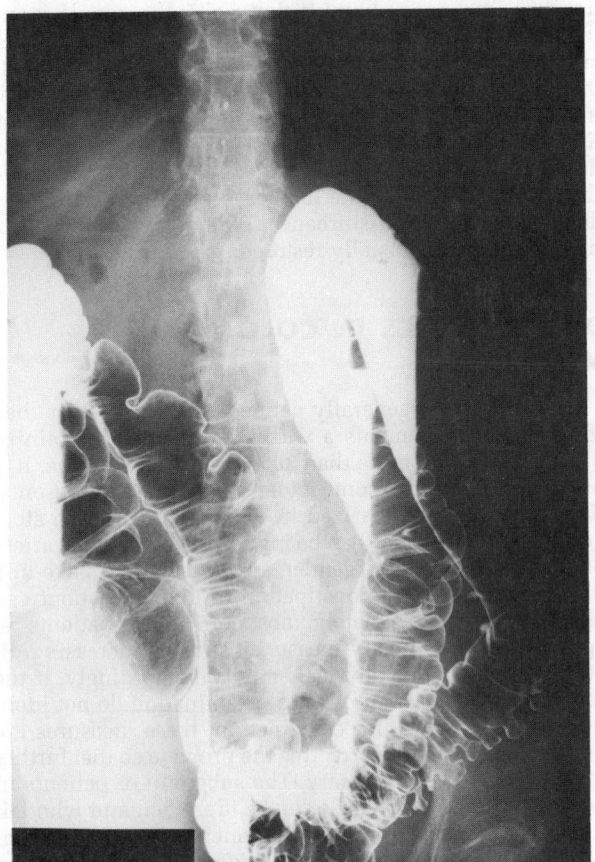

Figure 44-6. Air-contrast barium enema demonstrates extensive sigmoid diverticulosis without colonic narrowing. (Corman ML. Diverticular disease. In: Colon and rectal surgery. Philadelphia, JB Lippincott, 1989:670)

the rectum is known as defecation. The initiation of this response has been the subject of considerable study and appears to be elicited by mechanoreceptors that are located in the anorectal region. The exact location of these mechanoreceptors is still debated. Prevailing experimental opinion suggests that they reside in the mucosa, although some evidence indicates that the seromuscular layers are the site of origin.[5] Such receptors appear to be more numerous, or at least more sensitive, in the distal rectum than at more proximal locations. Balloon distention experiments involving the rectum have demonstrated that induction of sphincter relaxation is more effective as the balloon is moved more caudad. Clinical studies suggest that only the distal anorectal region is necessary for defecation to occur. A remnant of anorectal tissue about 6 cm from the anal–mucocutaneous junction can serve normal defecatory function when more proximal regions of the rectum are resected surgically.

Although it has generally been assumed that the rectal vault remains empty before the actual act of defecation, both clinical examination of the rectum, in which some stool is usually retrieved, and radiologic studies suggest that the rectum is commonly filled with fecal material in the absence of the urge to defecate. Exactly how changes in stool volume and coincident wall pressure excite the anorectal mechanoreceptors to initiate the act of defecation remains uncertain. Similarly, how relaxation of the anal sphincter initiates muscular movements in the distal colon to ensure that defecation proceeds smoothly and is sustained until complete evacuation has occurred requires further study.

The role that the nervous system plays in coordinating the defecatory process must also be considered. For defecation to occur, not only must the anal sphincter relax and the distal colon contract to move the fecal contents distally, but other ancillary processes must act to coordinate this process by raising the intraabdominal pressure. This involves a number of actions, including closure of the glottis, descent of the diaphragm, and contraction of the abdominal musculature. Injuries to the cerebral cortex and the spinal cord above the lumbosacral region can disturb defecation, but the disturbance is often transient, and in time, normalcy is usually restored.

DISTURBANCES IN COLONIC MOTILITY

Constipation is generally defined as having fewer than three bowel movements a week or excessively straining during defecation more than 20% to 25% of the time. It is usually a symptom of some underlying disease; representative causes are summarized in Table 44-1. Because stool volume and frequency can be influenced by a wide variety of factors (eg, age, diet, gender, and personality make-up), the precise causes of constipation in a given patient can remain elusive. Fortunately, most constipated patients respond to simple dietary measures, such as increasing dietary fiber intake or physical activity. Accordingly, if the underlying history and physical examination do not identify a specific cause for constipation, these measures are usually successful in correcting the problem so that further investigation is unnecessary. The subgroup of patients in whom no underlying cause can be identified and who fail to respond to these simple management strategies are generally considered to have *chronic idiopathic constipation*, which is usually categorized as colonic inertia, dysfunction of the pelvic floor, or normal transit constipation.[2]

Colonic inertia, or slow transit constipation, is primarily a disease of young women. Despite attempts at initiating

Table 44-1. CAUSES OF CONSTIPATION

FUNCTIONAL	MEDICATIONS
Slow transit	Narcotics
Pelvic floor dysfunction	Anticholinergics
Dietary	Antacids
Immobilization	Antihypertensives
Depression	Antidepressants
Irritable bowel syndrome	Iron
	Barium
NEUROLOGIC	
Central nervous system (stroke, Parkinson disease, Alzheimer disease)	**OBSTRUCTIVE**
	Tumor
	Diverticulitis
Spinal (multiple sclerosis, tumor, herniated disc, trauma, myelocele)	Inflammatory bowel disease
	Ischemic
	Volvulus
Nervi erigentes damage	Endometriosis
Aganglionosis (Hirschsprung disease, Chagas disease)	**SYSTEMIC**
	Scleroderma
ENDOCRINE	Uremia
Hypothyroidism	Amyloidosis
Hypercalcemia	Hypokalemia
Pheochromocytoma	
Diabetes	

bowel movements with fiber supplementation, large doses of laxatives, and enemas, sustained success is usually not forthcoming. The cause of this condition is totally unknown. Because of its predominance in young women, hormonal factors have been implicated, but never substantiated. A likely cause is some aberration in the neurochemical control of the colon, possibly within the enteric nerves. Abnormalities within the neural elements of the myenteric plexus of such patients have been demonstrated.[6] Such findings suggest that disturbances in neuromodulation of colonic motility play a role in this subset of patients. Other proposed possibilities include disturbances in colonic neurotransmission by humoral agents such as vasoactive intestinal peptide. In any event, the treatment of colonic inertia has proved difficult, and many patients have required subtotal colectomy to correct the severe constipation. Diagnosis of this condition is usually achieved by assessing colonic transit with various radioopaque markers. After ingestion of such markers, sequential abdominal films are taken to assess movement of markers in each segment of the colon. Total transit time in normal subjects averages about 35 hours. Total transit time in excess of 72 hours is clearly abnormal.

Evaluation of pelvic floor function can usually be accomplished with balloon expulsion, in which a rectally placed balloon is filled with 50 mL of water. If function of the pelvic floor is abnormal, evacuation of this balloon does not occur spontaneously, and additional weight may need to be added for facilitation of passage to occur. If pelvic floor dysfunction is suspected, it can be evaluated further with anorectal manometry, electromyography, and various scintigraphic evacuation studies. Depending on the information obtained with these studies, pharmacologic management or surgical intervention may be necessary.

If normal colonic transit and pelvic floor function are demonstrated in patients with constipation in whom no other discernible cause can be identified, normal transit constipation is a likely diagnosis. Because this entity is a variant of the irritable colon syndrome (see later), there is no role for surgery.

Similar to constipation, the mechanisms responsible for diarrhea are also poorly defined. Although disordered motility appears to play an important role, precise motility patterns differ depending on whether the diarrhea has an underlying osmotic, secretory, inflammatory, or idiopathic cause. Common opinion suggests that diarrhea occurs because of a hypermotile state, whereas hypomotility is responsible for constipation. Experimentally, data supporting these notions conflict. Although colonic transit time is decreased during diarrhea, a number of studies have indicated that overall motor activity of the colon is actually decreased rather than increased.[2] Evidence appears to suggest that loss of phasic activity with a consequent increase in colonic transit, enhancement in the number of large-amplitude migrating contractions, or both of these circumstances is the common motility disturbance in most diarrheal states. Disturbances in neural transmission can also be responsible for diarrhea, but with the exception of diabetic diarrhea, this appears to be a less common cause.

Various emotional states, such as anxiety and depression, can also influence colonic motor function. Both diarrhea and constipation have been described in patients afflicted with the same emotional disorder. Unfortunately, the few studies that have been conducted in an attempt to ascertain the effect of emotions on colonic motility have generally been poorly controlled, and the results from one laboratory have commonly contradicted those obtained from another. Further, what might be emotionally stressful to one person is of no consequence to another, so that standardization of emotional stress to determine its effect on colonic motility is difficult. The best that can be said is that emotional stress does appear to be linked with alterations in colonic motor function in some patients, but how such aberrations are mediated cannot yet be stated with any degree of certainty.

DIVERTICULOSIS OF THE COLON

Diverticulosis of the colon is a commonly encountered clinical problem that results from high intraluminal pressures that give rise to mucosal herniations through the colonic wall (Fig. 44-7; see Fig. 44-6). The initiating pressure head within the colonic lumen appears to be a consequence of disordered colonic motility. Several lines of evidence support this notion. These include the demonstration of thickened circular muscle adjacent to the diverticulum, with a concomitant narrowing of the luminal diameter; the observation that this thickening precedes the development of the diverticulum, often by many years; and the finding that intraluminal pressures in the region of the diverticulum are considerably more pronounced with pharmacologic stimulation by agents such as morphine when compared with pressure measurements in uninvolved regions of the colon. Why this thickening occurs is unknown. An interesting finding in patients with this disease has been an increased density in nerve tissue in the intramural ganglia in resected specimens. Whether this increase is the cause or consequence of the disease is uncertain. Despite the muscle thickening commonly encountered in diverticulosis, the myoelectric activity in patients with this disease is no different than that observed in control subjects.

Epidemiologically, considerable evidence links the muscular thickening and subsequent development of diverticulosis with the low-residue food that makes up a major portion of diets in industrialized countries. Exactly how such a diet initiates the muscular aberration is unknown. One possibility is that the low fecal volume resulting from this diet requires a greater propulsive force to initiate its movement caudad and subsequent evacuation through defecation. The muscular thickening may simply be a response to this diet to enable generation of this propulsive action. In support of this possibility is the clinical observa-

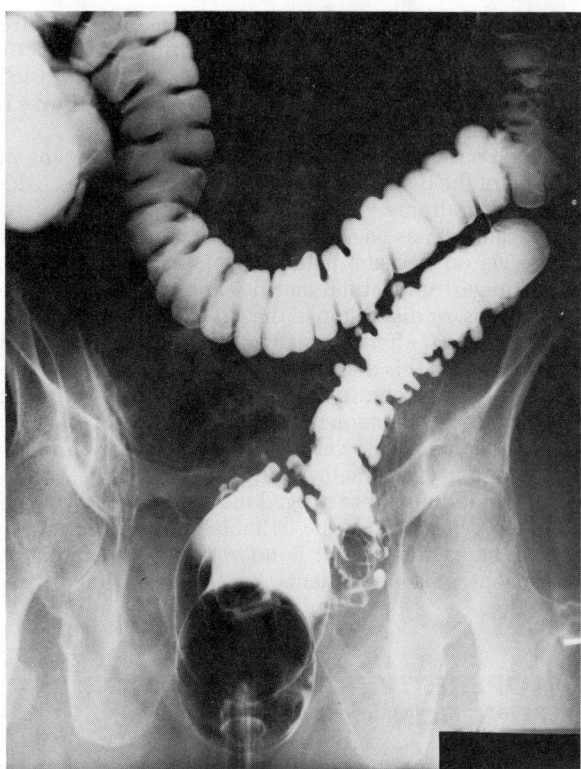

Figure 44-7. Extensive sigmoid diverticular disease with slight spasm but no stigmata of acute inflammation. (Corman, ML. Diverticular disease. In: Colon and rectal surgery. Philadelphia, JB Lippincott, 1989:670)

tion that patients with diverticular disease can often be managed effectively by increasing the fiber content and roughage in the diet to increase the stool volume. Whether actual complications of established diverticular disease can be prevented by bulking agents remains controversial.

IRRITABLE COLON SYNDROME

Numerous patients are examined by physicians each year with a symptom complex of abdominal pain, distention, and an abnormality in bowel function that can range from constipation to diarrhea. Often, no organic basis for this symptom complex can be identified. Such patients have been labeled as having psychosomatic bowel disease, functional bowel disorder, or more commonly, the irritable colon syndrome. Although a psychogenic basis for this disorder has generally been presumed, a significant number of patients with this symptom complex have no obvious psychological abnormality nor identifiable stress, depression, or anxiety. Equally problematic has been the difficulty in demonstrating clearcut motor abnormalities in patients with this syndrome.

In patients with diarrhea-predominant irritable colon syndrome, whole-gut transit times are usually shorter than normal, while in those with the constipation-predominant form, transit times are longer. Although abnormal colonic myoelectric activity has been postulated as an explanation for the altered motility in patients with the irritable colon syndrome, agreement on this issue has been by no means uniform. Further, some evidence exists that abnormal gut hormone secretion or sensitivity plays a role in this entity. Specifically, CCK has been demonstrated to increase colonic contractions and reproduce postprandial pain in patients with this syndrome, suggesting a role for this gastrointestinal peptide. Against a role for this agent is the observation that blockade of the CCK receptor responsible for colonic contraction did not alter the clinical course of patients with this syndrome.

Another observation suggests that visceral afferent innervation of the bowel is altered in patients with the irritable colon syndrome.[1] This hypothesis has considerable merit because it has been demonstrated that visceral afferent innervation mediates both visceral sensation and reflex changes in gastrointestinal motility and that sensations of pain, fullness, or distention of the gut can occur with alterations in visceral afferent mechanisms. Although individual patients with this disease vary greatly from one another in terms of their colonic motility patterns, groups of patients have been shown on manometric studies of the colon to experience pain at lower distending volumes and pressures than in asymptomatic control subjects. Whether one or a combination of these alleged disturbances is responsible for the symptoms of the irritable colon syndrome remains to be established. It is no wonder, therefore, that management of such patients has proved difficult and perplexing.

POSTOPERATIVE COLONIC MOTOR DYSFUNCTION

Gut motility can be severely altered after operations in the abdominal cavity.[7,8] This effect is related not only to the fact that an operation has been performed but also, more importantly, to what type of operation has been carried out. Postoperative ileus occurs because the abdomen has been entered during surgery and the intraabdominal contents have been handled. This handling may be merely moving various organs from one position to another or can involve dissection around or in the vicinity of a particular viscus to aid in performing the particular procedure. Regardless, a period of bowel inactivity almost always occurs that affects the colon.

Both neural and humoral agents, acting either alone or in combination, contribute to the functional intestinal aperistalsis after operation. Other factors that influence the length of ileus include medications administered preoperatively, anesthetic and analgesic agents employed, the extent to which the bowel is manipulated and handled, whether any concomitant dissection was carried out, and the metabolic status of the patient preoperatively as well as postoperatively. Abnormalities in potassium and calcium metabolism are known to alter intestinal motility, as does the protein status of the patient. Opioid compounds can profoundly alter the motor activity of the large bowel. Available data indicate that both meperidine and codeine depress contractile activity of the colon. The effect of morphine is controversial, but most data suggest that its effects on colonic contraction are not substantial or inconsistent.

As described earlier, operations on the stomach can alter colonic activity in response to a meal, but these changes appear to be short-lived. Thus, pyloroplasty, various degrees of subtotal gastrectomy, and even total gastrectomy can alter the response to eating for a short time, but perturbations appear to be transient. More important is the means by which gastrointestinal continuity is reestablished after an operation on the stomach, particularly if a portion of the stomach is resected. Thus, if a Billroth I operation is performed, no major alteration in intestinal motility usually occurs, but dumping can be a problem if a Billroth II procedure has been carried out. Even with this procedure, however, alterations in colonic activity

are uncommon. More important is biliary diversion performed to prevent reflux of bile acids into the stomach remnant after a distal gastric resection. In this circumstance, a Roux-en-Y procedure is usually performed, and bile acids are thus discharged into the small intestine more distally. Depending on the effects that such rerouting have on small bowel motility, bile acids may find egress into the proximal colon in higher concentrations than usual. This circumstance stimulates significant increases in colonic motility patterns so that diarrhea occurs. Treatment of this condition can involve dietary manipulation, administration of various pharmacologic agents to bind bile salts, and, when these are not effective, another surgical procedure to correct the egress of bile into the proximal bowel.

Although transsection of the intestine with reanastomosis would predictably alter motor function, studies in the small bowel in animals have shown that any decrease in the migrating motor complex appears to correct itself within several months. Similar myoelectric changes can be observed in the human small intestine after transsection and reanastomosis, but these appear to be of no clinical consequence because no significant perturbation in intestinal motility has been observed that can be quantified. Studies involving transsection of the colon with reanastomosis in animals are meager. The few studies that have been done have generated conflicting data, so extrapolation to the human situation is virtually impossible.

COLONIC PSEUDOOBSTRUCTION

Acute obstruction of the colon in the absence of any identifiable mechanical obstructing lesion is known as Ogilvie syndrome (Fig. 44-8). It denotes a clinical picture resembling that of a lesion obstructing flow along the

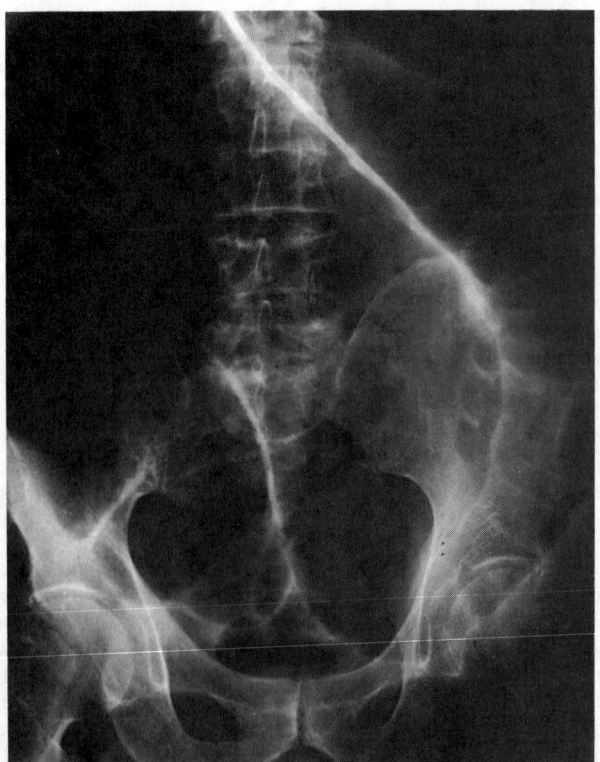

Figure 44-8. Pseudoobstruction of the colon (Ogilvie syndrome). (Corman ML. Miscellaneous colon and rectal conditions. In: Colon and rectal surgery. Philadelphia, JB Lippincott, 1989:977)

intestine even though no mechanical cause is present. The result of this circumstance is a failure of propulsive forces to overcome normal resistances to flow. Acute pseudoobstruction usually involves the proximal colon but can extend throughout the transverse colon and, rarely, the descending colon as well. The cause of this syndrome is unknown, but it almost always arises in critically ill or bedridden patients who have serious concomitant disease. The syndrome is occasionally seen in traumatized patients, particularly if a vertebral fracture involving the back is present. The hallmark of the disease is severe abdominal distention without marked pain or tenderness. Later in the disease, symptoms are not dissimilar to those of true mechanical obstruction. Roentgenographic films of the abdomen show marked gaseous distention of the colon that is typically localized to the right colon.

The role that various pharmacologic agents, such as analgesics, antibiotics, or cardiotropic drugs, play in initiating the disease or causing persistence remains unknown. Although laxative abuse has been implicated as a possible inciting factor in nursing home and bedridden patients, the evidence for this contention is not established.

The major problem with Ogilvie syndrome is the risk of cecal perforation. This risk is substantial, and the more prolonged the cecal distention, the greater this risk becomes. Although a considerable debate exists in the literature about the extent to which cecal dilation can occur before perforation becomes a likely possibility, some type of decompressive procedure should be considered when the cecum reaches 10 to 12 cm in diameter. Fiberoptic colonoscopy is the treatment of choice and is initially successful in 90% or more of patients. In the event that colonoscopy does not work or is not readily accessible, cecostomy is the accepted alternative therapy.

In contrast to acute pseudoobstruction, chronic pseudoobstruction is rare. It can result from a variety of etiologic possibilities, including visceral myopathy, visceral neuropathy such as Hirschsprung disease, connective tissue disorders, generalized nerve diseases, and various endocrine or metabolic disturbances. Drug-related pseudoobstruction is also a common cause of this entity. Because the more chronic forms of pseudoobstruction are not commonly managed by surgeons, they are not discussed further.

REFERENCES

1. Sarna SK. Colonic motor activity. Surg Clin North Am 1993; 73:1201.
2. McIntyre PB, Pemberton JH. Pathophysiology of colonic motility disorders. Surg Clin North Am 1993;73:1225.
3. Read NW. Colon: relationship between epithelial transport and motility. Pharmacology 1988;36(Suppl 1):120.
4. Karaus M, Sarna SK. Giant migrating contractions during defecation in the dog colon. Gastroenterology 1987;92:925.
5. Goligher JC, Highes ESR. Sensibility of the rectum and colon: its role in the mechanism of anal continence. Lancet 1951; 1:453.
6. Krichnamurthy S, Schuffler MD, Rohrmann CA, Pope CE II. Severe idiopathic constipation is associated with a distinctive abnormality of the colonic myenteric plexus. Gastroenterology 1985;88:26.
7. Becker JM. Normal peristalsis and abnormalities in intestinal motility. In: Miller TA, ed. Physiologic basis of modern surgical care. St Louis, CV Mosby, 1988:347.
8. Christensen J. Colonic motility. In: Schultz SS, Makhlouf GM, Rauner BR, eds. The gastrointestinal system: handbook of physiology, vol 1, sec 6. Bethesda MD, American Physiological Society, 1989:939.

SURGERY: SCIENTIFIC PRINCIPLES AND PRACTICE, Second Edition, edited by Lazar J. Greenfield, Michael W. Mulholland, Keith T. Oldham, Gerald B. Zelenock, and Keith D. Lillemoe. Lippincott–Raven Publishers, Philadelphia, © 1997.

CHAPTER 45

ULCERATIVE COLITIS

JAMES M. BECKER

Chronic ulcerative colitis is a diffuse inflammatory disease of unknown cause that affects the mucosa of the rectum and colon. This chronic disease features remissions and exacerbations characterized by rectal bleeding and diarrhea. Ulcerative colitis has no clearly identified cause or specific medical therapy, and it affects patients in their youth or early middle age. The disease has serious local and systemic long-term effects. Although medical therapy can affect the inflammatory process and control most symptomatic flares, it provides no definitive treatment for the disease. Total removal of the colon and rectum provides complete cure. Newer surgical alternatives have eliminated the need for a permanent ileostomy after definitive resection of the involved colon and rectum.

Although diarrheal illnesses have been described since the early writings of Hippocrates, it was not until 1875 that ulcerative colitis was more specifically characterized and distinguished by clinical and pathologic criteria from common infectious enteritis. With the description of regional enteritis in the 1930s by Crohn, separation of ulcerative colitis from Crohn's disease of the intestine appeared relatively straightforward. The two diseases appeared initially to have distinct pathologic features, and each affected a different organ system. During the past several decades, a marked overlap has been appreciated not only pathologically but also in anatomic distribution between the two conditions. In more than 10% of patients, a clear distinction cannot be made between the two. This distinction has become an extremely important factor because the surgical approaches to ulcerative colitis and Crohn's colitis are different.

Sigmoid colostomy was the first well-documented surgical procedure for inflammatory bowel disease. Not until 1940 did it become clear that definitive treatment required either total proctocolectomy or at least subtotal abdominal colectomy with ileostomy. The ostomy was associated with a high complication rate until Brooke and others proposed immediate maturation of the stoma in the 1950s. Proctocolectomy with the Brooke ileostomy emerged as the procedure of choice for ulcerative colitis. Numerous techniques have been proposed for the restoration of continence after colectomy. The continent ileostomy, or Kock pouch, was used in the 1970s with moderate success. This has been challenged in the past decade with the development of anal sphincter–sparing operations.

EPIDEMIOLOGY

Early studies of the epidemiology of chronic ulcerative colitis suffered from several important deficiencies. More recent studies have suggested that the incidence is about 6 per 100,000 per year, and that the prevalence is between 50 and 70 cases per 100,000 per year.[1] The incidence of ulcerative colitis is highest in developed or urban regions of the world and lowest in developing regions, although there are signs that the incidence rates of inflammatory bowel disease may be leveling off in the developed countries and starting to increase in the developing world. Ulcerative colitis is being reported with increasing frequency in Japan, India, Thailand, and other countries in Asia. Epidemiologic studies have also supported the earlier impression of a higher incidence of ulcerative colitis among Jews (two to four times the incidence versus non-Jews) and in whites (four times the incidence versus nonwhites). The patients are more commonly Western than Asian; in the Western population, they are much more often Northern European, Anglo-Saxon, or from the northern portion of Eastern Europe. Increasing incidence has also been observed in non-Jewish, black, and Hispanic populations.

Most cases of ulcerative colitis have their onset between the ages of 15 and 40 years, but the age range extends from infancy to very old age. Ulcerative colitis has its onset after age 60 years in about 3% to 5% of the cases. Throughout the age range, males and females are affected about equally. Clearcut familial patterns have been observed in ulcerative colitis. Ten to 25% of patients with ulcerative colitis have first-degree relatives with the disease. A number of families have been reported with up to eight members affected over several generations. Both Crohn's disease and ulcerative colitis can occur within the same family, but there appears to be an 80% to 90% concordance for the same disease category within sibships. Monozygous twins have a higher concordance for inflammatory bowel disease than dizygous twins. In addition, the HLA phenotypes AW24 and BW35 are associated with ulcerative colitis, particularly in Israeli Jews of European origin. The AW24 phenotype is increased in frequency in patients with early onset of chronic ulcerative colitis and moderate to severe disease. Geographic as well as racial differences influence the occurrence of the disease, and there is no conclusive evidence regarding the genetic versus the environmental determination of familial patterns.

CAUSE

The cause of ulcerative colitis remains unknown despite intensive work by many investigators. Most scientific attention has been devoted to infectious and immunologic hypotheses. Other avenues of investigation have included dietary, environmental, vascular, neuromotor, allergic, and psychogenic causes.

The investigation of bacterial and viral agents continues to be an area of active research, although there is considerable uncertainty as to the fundamental role that infectious agents play in the pathogenesis of ulcerative colitis. Whether the infectious agents are more likely to be triggers of disease or perpetuators of disease is of great controversy. To be a trigger, an infectious agent would have to act by initiation or reactivation. Agents could initiate an autoimmune response by altering antigens, affecting molecular immunity, or increasing immune responsiveness. The microbial agent might also trigger the pathologic response by increasing mucosal permeability or by stimulating epithelial injury or localized ischemia. The microbial agent could reactivate the inflammatory process directly, by secondary infection, or by the release of toxins. Evidence for microbial agents as triggers in inflammatory bowel disease is only indirect. Dysentery has been associated with flares of ulcerative colitis; in countries with high rates of dysentery, there appears to be an increased incidence of ulcerative colitis. Upper respiratory infections have been associated with apparent reactivation or flares of ulcerative colitis. The seasonal pattern observed in many patients with ulcerative colitis suggests a pattern of initiation and reactivation.

Other investigators have suggested that infectious agents may perpetuate the disease. The full clinical expression of ulcerative colitis requires an intact mucosal immune system and also depends on normal intestinal flora and their products. Thus, alterations in the disease may result from changes in intestinal flora. In addition, treatment interventions may affect disease activity by altering the flora and therefore the energetic or immunologic environment. As discussed later in this chapter, short-chain fatty acids are effective in treating diversion colitis and are natural products of the intestinal flora. Metronidazole may have an effect on ulcerative colitis by altering the flora. Finally, remissions of inflammatory bowel disease have been observed anecdotally in patients with acquired immunodeficiency syndrome.

Studies suggesting that particular pathogens, including *Chlamydia* sp, cytomegalovirus, and *Yersinia* sp, were primary agents in the pathogenesis of ulcerative colitis have not been substantiated by further work. *Clostridium difficile* toxin activity has been associated with relapses of ulcerative colitis but appears to be correlated better with prior antibiotic administration than with disease activity. Specific strains of *Escherichia coli* have been identified in patients with ulcerative colitis. A viral cause also appears unlikely because the disease cannot be transmitted, and viral particles have not been identified.

Speculation that chronic ulcerative colitis is an autoimmune disease has been considerable. A number of immunologic studies have supported this concept, and there is a great deal of interest in the role of cytokines and immunoregulatory molecules in the control of the immune response in patients with inflammatory bowel disease.[2] For example, many patients with ulcerative colitis have circulating antibodies to normal colonic epithelium that cross-react with specific enterobacterial lipopolysaccharide antigens. In addition, lymphocytes may be rendered cytotoxic to colonic epithelium by incubation with serum from patients with ulcerative colitis. Affected patients have also been found to have alterations of T- and B-lymphocyte activation and homing properties. Although total lymphocyte and T-lymphocyte counts are generally normal in ulcerative colitis patients, thymosine-dependent T-lymphocyte response may be abnormal, suggesting an immune-deficient state.

A number of investigators have argued that the immunologic events that have been observed in patients with ulcerative colitis are nonspecific epiphenomena and are not clinically useful disease markers. Little correlation exists between systemic immunity and clinical status of the patient. The changes are nonspecific, particularly those in regard to heat-shock proteins and lymphocyte function. The changes in the systemic immune system may simply reflect inflammation, rather than being specific for the disease. In contrast, many investigators believe that there is growing support for altered mucosal immunity in the pathogenesis of inflammatory bowel disease.

Cytokines may play a role in inflammatory bowel disease. Cytokines are proteins secreted by activated immunocytes that influence the activity, differentiation, or rate of proliferation of other cells. Cytokines exert activities by autocrine, paracrine, and endocrine effects. They have inflammatory as well as immunoregulatory activities. Cytokines may amplify the immune response by activating the proliferation or the chemotactic activity of effector cells or by stimulating mesenchymal cells to proliferate and increase production of eicosanoids, cytokines, and growth factors.

Specific activities of interleukins that are potentially relevant to inflammatory bowel disease have been identified. Most important of these may be interleukin-1 (IL-1), which activates T and B lymphocytes as well as macrophages and neutrophils. IL-1 stimulates production of eicosanoids, cytokines, growth factors, and destructive enzymes; increases adhesion of neutrophils and monocytes to endothelial cells; induces acute-phase response as well as fever, anorexia, and sleep; and stimulates collagen production and thus fibrosis. IL-1 has been shown to be elevated in ulcerative colitis as well as in experimental models of colitis. The increase in IL-1 levels appears to correlate with severity of disease. Alterations in IL-2, IL-6, IL-8, and interferon-γ have been identified in tissues from patients with ulcerative colitis. The production of interferon during inflammation could play a significant role in the differentiation of mature memory and effector cells within the intestine. Tumor necrosis factor may also be particularly important in the activation of mesenchymal cells but has not been fully evaluated in ulcerative colitis. Thus, it appears that cytokines are integrally involved in the pathogenesis of inflammatory bowel disease with both immunoregulatory and proinflammatory properties.

It has been proposed that ulcerative colitis represents an energy-deficient state of the colonic epithelium, with decreased levels of free coenzyme A and lower oxidation of butyrate to carbon dioxide in the colonic mucosal cells of patients with ulcerative colitis.[3] Based on this theory, it has been suggested that short-chain fatty acids might be therapeutically beneficial. Patients with diversion colitis (occurring after formation of a bypassed rectal segment) were found to have reduced short-chain fatty acid levels within the bypassed segments. Treatment with intraluminal instillation of an isotonic short-chain fatty acid solution resulted in complete endoscopic healing in all patients. Reoccurrence resulted when saline was substituted for the short-chain fatty acid solution.[4] Luminal short-chain fatty acids have also been shown to accelerate healing of surgical anastomoses and to increase regional blood flow and oxygen uptake. Although short-chain fatty acids may play a role in the pathogenesis and treatment of ulcerative colitis, this issue requires further study in the clinical setting.

Despite the imperfections and differences, the accumulated evidence, especially the presence of chronic ulcerative colitis in three or more members of a family spanning several generations, the increased frequency among first-degree relatives, and the increased concordance rates of inflammatory bowel disease in monozygous twins, strongly suggest a genetic influence. The genetic mechanisms involved are not known, although multiple gene alterations are likely. Genetic possibilities in ulcerative colitis include a polygenetic mode of inheritance, a specific form of somatic gene mutation in mesenchymal stem cells, the growth of a forbidden clone of cells whose mutant humoral products attack the colonic mucosa, and a rare additive major gene.[5] The identification of specific biologic markers of chronic ulcerative colitis would greatly facilitate genetic epidemiologic studies and further clarify the nature of the disorder. The study of the genetically modified transgenic rat model and the genetic deletion, or "knockout," animal model may provide important clues to the genetic nature of ulcerative colitis.

Further experimental and clinical work is necessary to evaluate the etiologic possibilities in ulcerative colitis. During the past decade, animal models of intestinal inflammation have substantially augmented our understanding of the pathogenesis of ulcerative colitis, particularly in the areas of inflammatory mediators and cytokine regulation, genetic susceptibility, and the influence of ubiquitous luminal bacterial constituents.[6–9] Inducible models, such as administration of acetic acid, trinitrobenzene sulfonic acid–ethanol, and indomethacin to rats, and feeding dextran sodium sulfate to mice, are inexpensive, easily accomplished, and reproducible, making these models the preferred routes for testing novel pharmaceutical agents. Submucosal injection of the bacterial cell wall with polymer peptidoglycan-polysaccharide[10] and intravenous administration of preformed immune complexes after rectal installation of formalin[11] elicit more immunologically and environmentally relevant inflammatory responses than the toxin-induced models, permitting more in-depth dissection of immunoregulatory mechanisms of acute and chronic intestinal inflammation. The cotton-top tamarin is unique in that it exhibits spontaneous colitis with associated adenocarcinoma of the colon.

Unprecedented advances in molecular biology provide techniques to overexpress or delete selected genes in rodents. In vivo overexpression (transgenic) or deletion (knockout) of genes encoding targeted cytokines, T-cell receptors, HLA molecules, and intracellular messengers by basic scientists outside of the inflammatory bowel disease field have unexpectedly created a whole new class of animal models of inflammatory bowel disease. Spontaneous intestinal inflammation in these genetically engineered rodents, in addition to the colitis that follows a spontaneous genetic mutation in C_3H/HeJ mice and restoration of T-lymphocyte subsets in immunocompromised hosts, now permit exciting new approaches to exploring mechanisms of chronic, spontaneous gastrointestinal inflammation.

PATHOLOGY

Ulcerative colitis, for the most part, is a disease confined to the mucosal and submucosal layers of the colonic wall. Ulcerative colitis is a continuous disease, with the rectum essentially always involved and the remainder of the colon diseased to a greater or lesser extent. Occasionally, with severe pancolitis, the terminal ileum shows secondary mild inflammation and dilation, a process that has been called *backwash ileitis*. On gross inspection, the colonic mucosa demonstrates healed granular superficial ulcers superimposed on a friable and thickened mucosa with increased vascularity. Patients may also demonstrate superficial fissures and small and regular pseudopolyps. This appearance is in contradistinction to the transmural inflammatory changes found in Crohn's disease of the colon, in which all layers of the colonic wall may be involved in a granulomatous inflammatory process (Table 45-1). In its earlier stage, the typical lesion consists of infiltration of round cells and polymorphonucleocytes into the crypts of Lieberkühn at the base of the mucosa, forming crypt abscesses. Light microscopy reveals poor staining and vacuolization of overlying epithelial cells. Swelling of mitochondria, widening of intercellular spaces, and broadening of the endoplasmic reticulum are observed by transmission electron microscopy. As the lesions progress, there is a coalescence of crypt abscesses and desquamation of overlying cells to form an ulcer. This cryptitis is associated with undermining of adjacent, relatively normal mucosa, which becomes edematous and assumes a polypoid con-

Table 45-1. PATHOLOGIC FEATURES OF CROHN'S DISEASE AND ULCERATIVE COLITIS

	Crohn's Disease	Ulcerative Colitis
Transmural inflammation	Yes	Uncommon
Granulomas	50%–75%	No
Fissures	Common	Rare
Submucosal thickening, fibrosis	Common	No
Submucosal inflammation	Common	Uncommon

figuration as it becomes isolated between adjacent ulcers. Collagen and a luxurious growth of granulation tissue occupy the areas of ulceration, which extend down to, but rarely through, the muscularis. Although ulcerative colitis is generally confined to the mucosa and submucosa, in the most severe forms of the disease, especially in toxic megacolon, the disease process may extend to the deeper muscular layers of the colon and even to the serosa. Rarely, crypt abscesses penetrate the muscularis propria, often extending along a blood vessel. In this situation, the colon may perforate, and there may be confusion about the diagnosis.

CLINICAL FEATURES

Ulcerative colitis usually presents with bloody diarrhea, abdominal pain, and fever. Sixty percent of patients present with a relatively mild attack that occurs as a segmental colitis involving the distal colon (80%) or as a pancolitis (20%). Five to 15% of patients with disease limited to the rectosigmoid area show eventual progression to involve most, if not all, of the length of the colon. Twenty-five percent of all patients present with a moderate attack in which bloody diarrhea is the major symptom. In a small number of patients (15%), ulcerative colitis has an acute and catastrophic fulminating course. These patients develop the relatively sudden onset of frequent bloody bowel movements, high fever, weight loss, and diffuse abdominal tenderness.

Physical findings are directly related to the duration and presentation of the disease. Weight loss and pallor are usually present. In the active phase, the abdomen in the region of the colon is tender to palpation. During acute attacks or in the fulminating form of the disease, there may be signs of an acute surgical abdomen accompanied by fever and decreased bowel sounds. In patients with toxic megacolon, abdominal distention may be identified. Examination of the integument, tongue, joints, and eyes is important because the presence of disease in these areas may suggest inflammatory bowel disease as a likely cause of the diarrheal illness.

Extraintestinal manifestations of ulcerative colitis are observed in a number of organ systems. The extracolonic manifestations of ulcerative colitis can be categorized as the *colitic group,* the *pathophysiologic group,* and the *miscellaneous group* of disorders. The activity of the colitic group of extracolonic manifestations parallels the activity of the underlying bowel disease, being present and most active when the colitis is active and subsiding when the colitis goes into remission. Included in this group are ocular lesions, including iritis or uveitis, which are seen in 0.5% to 3% of patients, conjunctivitis, episcleritis, keratitis, retinitis, and retrobulbar neuritis. With the exception of ulcerative panophthalmitis, ocular symptoms are closely related to disease activity and respond to therapy with steroids or other immunosuppressive agents.

Articular disorders, including peripheral joint disease, arthralgias, swelling, pain, and redness with migratory involvement, usually parallel the intensity of the colitis and respond to medical or surgical treatment. The joints of the lower extremities are most frequently involved. Overall, 15% to 20% of patients manifest endopathologic peripheral arthritis. Ankylosing spondylitis is seen in 1% to 6% of patients, and sacroiliitis is observed in 4% to 18% of patients. Both of these conditions can result in permanent fixation of the spine and should be treated aggressively. Bone involvement specific to the axial skeleton is less closely related to the inflammatory state of the colon and may precede clinical evidence of ulcerative colitis.

Lesions of the skin and oral cavity are frequently observed in patients with ulcerative colitis. Aphthous stomatitis and gingivitis and erythema nodosum are observed less frequently in ulcerative colitis than in Crohn's disease. In contrast, pyoderma gangrenosum is more frequently observed in ulcerative colitis (0.6%) than in Crohn's disease.

Liver and biliary tract disorders occur commonly in patients with chronic ulcerative colitis. Up to 80% of patients demonstrate histologic evidence of pericholangitis on liver biopsy, with hepatic involvement more common in patients with pancolitis. Between 50% and 90% of patients with ulcerative colitis have fatty infiltration of the liver. One to 10% of patients manifest chronic active hepatitis, and about 1% develop biliary cirrhosis. One of the most difficult complications, sclerosing cholangitis, is observed in 1% to 4% of patients with ulcerative colitis. Affected patients present with pruritus, alkaline phosphatase elevation, right upper quadrant pain and tenderness, and jaundice. The diagnosis is confirmed by endoscopic retrograde cholangiopancreatography or transhepatic cholangiography. Controversy surrounds the treatment of this disorder. Although some patients respond to colectomy, most show progression of their hepatic disease even after colon resection. Surgical drainage, internal stent placement, and antibiotics have all been reported to be of value in the treatment of symptomatic sclerosing cholangitis. Patients with progressive liver failure ultimately require orthotopic liver transplantation. Affected patients are also at greater risk of developing carcinoma of the bile duct, although this may also develop de novo in patients with ulcerative colitis.

Patients with ulcerative colitis are at slightly greater risk for the development of thromboembolic disease and vasculitis. Rarely, they develop renal disease, clubbing, bronchial and pulmonary abnormalities, and amyloidosis in association with their inflammatory bowel disease.

DIAGNOSIS

The diagnosis of acute ulcerative colitis is one of exclusion. There are no pathognomonic laboratory, radiographic, or histologic features. In all patients presenting with diarrhea or bloody diarrhea, an infectious cause must be excluded. Stool samples and biopsy specimens should be evaluated for *Campylobacter* sp, *Salmonella* sp, pathogenic *E coli, Aeromonas* sp, *Plesiomonas* sp, amebic colitis, and *C difficile.* Particularly important and difficult to exclude are pseudomembranous colitis, the proctocolitis seen increasingly in homosexual men, and traveler's diarrhea. It has become increasingly important to distinguish ulcerative colitis from granulomatous colitis. Major distinguishing clinical characteristics of Crohn's colitis and ulcerative colitis are shown in Table 45-2.

Flexible sigmoidoscopy is the first step in diagnosis because ulcerative colitis involves the distal colon and rectum in 90% to 95% of cases. Mild cases may only show a loss of normal vascular pattern, a granular texture, and microhemorrhages when the friable mucosa is touched or wiped (Color Fig. 45-1). In more advanced cases, when the disease is moderately active, the mucosa becomes more grossly pitted, and spontaneous bleeding is seen (Color Fig. 45-2). In severe cases, there is macroulceration with profuse bleeding and purulent exudate (Color Fig. 45-3). In advanced disease, areas of ulceration may surround areas of heaped-up granulation tissue and edematous mucosa, so-called pseudopolyps. The use of flexible sigmoidoscopy has improved diagnostic accuracy and patient acceptability. Colonoscopy may be useful in determining the extent and activity of the disease, particularly in patients in whom the diagnosis is unclear or cancer is suspected.

Table 45-2. DISTINGUISHING CHARACTERISTICS OF CROHN'S COLITIS AND ULCERATIVE COLITIS

Characteristics	Crohn's Colitis	Ulcerative Colitis
Location	Small bowel involvement	Colon only (rare backwash ileitis)
Anatomic distribution	Asymmetric distribution (skip lesions)	Contiguous involvement beginning distally
Rectal involvement	Rectal sparing common	Involved 90%
Gross bleeding	Absent 25%–30%	Universal
Perianal disease	≤75%	Rare, may be severe
Fistulization	Yes	No
Granulomas	50%–75%	No

Endoscopy can be useful in distinguishing between ulcerative colitis and Crohn's colitis (Table 45-3).

Barium enema examination of the colon is useful in most patients, although potentially dangerous in those with toxic megacolon. When ulcerative colitis develops, mucosal granularity and microhemorrhages produce a diffusely reticulated pattern, on which are superimposed countless punctate collections of contrast material lodged in microulcerations. A mild case of acute ulcerative colitis may be manifested by a diffusely granular appearance, which is best seen on air-contrast barium enema. In more advanced cases, the colon develops irregular margins with spiculated and undermining "collar-button" ulcers that can be well demonstrated on full-column barium enema. End-stage, or burned-out, ulcerative colitis is characterized by shortening of the colon, loss of normal redundancy in the sigmoid region and at the splenic and hepatic flexures, disappearance of the haustral pattern, a featureless mucosa, absence of discrete ulcerations, and narrowed caliber of the bowel. Chronic inflammation may lead to diffuse mucosal atrophy, leaving behind hypertrophic islands of inflamed mucosa and granulation tissue, which assume a polypoid shape and are called *pseudopolyps*. These pseudopolyps may carpet the colon, simulating the polyposis syndrome, or they may be discrete, as in the case of filiform pseudopolyposis.

A plain abdominal radiograph may be useful in patients with severe ulcerative colitis. An abdominal film may demonstrate colonic dilation, which has been called *toxic megacolon*, in 3% to 5% of patients (Fig. 45-1). Most frequently, this dilation is observed in the transverse colon. There may be free air within the peritoneal cavity from perforation of the diseased colon.

Table 45-3. ENDOSCOPIC FEATURES OF CROHN'S DISEASE AND ULCERATIVE COLITIS

Endoscopic Features	Crohn's Disease	Ulcerative Colitis
Mucosal involvement	Discontinuous	Contiguous
Discrete ulcers (aphthous ulcers)	Common	Rare
Surrounding mucosa	Relatively normal	Abnormal
Longitudinal ulcer	Common	Rare
Cobblestoning	In severe cases	No
Rectal involvement	Sparing common	Involved in 90%
Mucosal friability	Uncommon	Common
Vascular pattern	Normal	Distorted

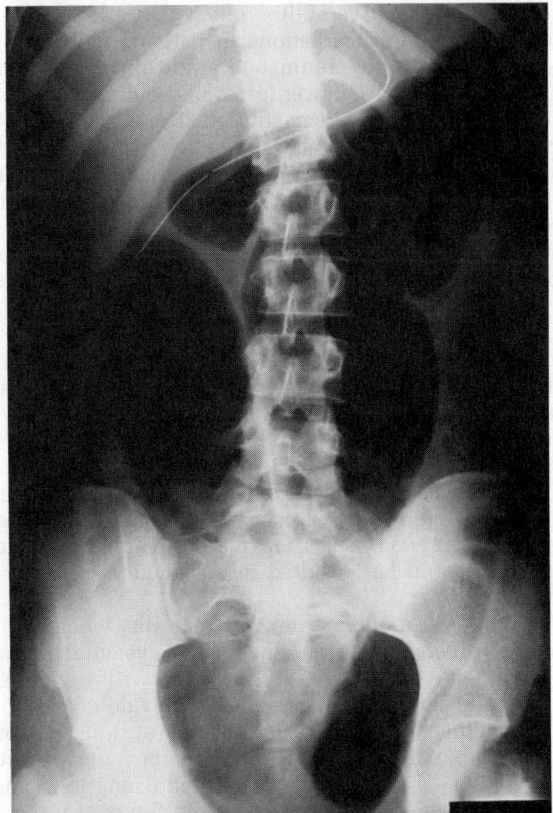

Figure 45-1. Colonic dilation, particularly of the transverse colon, in a patient with toxic megacolon.

MEDICAL MANAGEMENT

The principal categories of drug treatment for ulcerative colitis include symptomatic antidiarrheal and antispasmodic agents, sulfasalazine and its analogues, corticosteroids and adrenocorticotropic hormone (ACTH), immunosuppressive antimetabolites, and certain antibiotics.[12] Future therapy may also consist of soluble mediator blockade, immune mediator blockade, and oxygen radical scavengers. Once the diagnosis of ulcerative colitis has been clearly established, the decision regarding treatment depends on the severity of symptoms and on the severity and extent of disease as indicated by radiographic and endoscopic studies.

Sulfasalazine has been used in the management of the chronic phases of ulcerative colitis for the past 50 years. Sulfasalazine may exert its pharmacologic effect by inhibiting mucosal prostaglandin synthesis. The sulfasalazine molecule consists of 5-amino salicylic acid (5-ASA), linked by an azo bond to sulfapyridine. Evidence suggests that 5-ASA is the therapeutically active moiety, with the sulfapyridine acting as a vehicle for drug delivery to the lower gastrointestinal tract. Most of the drug's toxicity is attributable to the sulfapyridine. Reversible hypospermia and infertility are observed in male patients. About 25% to 30% of patients experience headaches, nausea, anorexia, and dyspepsia, and patients allergic to sulfa drugs develop fever and rash. Less common side effects include hemolysis and neutropenia, which are related to serum sulfapyridine levels. In some patients, sulfasalazine may actually cause exacerbation of the disease. Overall, sulfasalazine has been found to be effective in treating mild to moderate disease in 75% to 80% of patients. Sulfasalazine has not been of significant value in treating patients with severe acute ulcerative colitis, but it may play a role in controlling acute exacerbations in patients with chronic disease. In an effort to eliminate the side effects associated with the sulfa carrier, newer forms of the drug, such as 5-ASA and 4-ASA, have been studied. The basic concept is to prevent the active molecule from being absorbed in the proximal bowel. This may be accomplished by coating the tablet so that it dissolves only at an alkaline pH of 6 or 7, corresponding to the pH in the terminal ileum or colon. In all studies to date, these compounds have been shown to be as efficacious as sulfasalazine in treating acute ulcerative colitis as well as in preventing relapse.

The other common therapeutic modality for treatment of mild distal ulcerative colitis is the use of topical steroids. Steroid enemas are effective for patients with proctitis and proctosigmoiditis but have little value for patients with more extensive, left-sided disease or pancolitis. In an attempt to avoid systemic effects of steroid enemas, tixocortol pivalate was synthesized by adding a thiol ester group at position 21 on the hydrocortisone molecule. In trials, this agent has been useful for treating patients with left-sided colitis and has resulted in a reduction in systemic steroid side effects.

Patients with moderate ulcerative colitis, whether left-sided or universal, require some form of systemic therapy. These patients initially can be managed with topical steroid therapy and oral sulfasalazine. If they do not respond to this regimen, oral corticosteroids are introduced. Corticosteroids remain the mainstay of therapy during acute attacks. Between 40 and 60 mg of prednisone in a single daily dose is effective in most cases in terms of inducing remission. If the patient's clinical symptoms and sigmoidoscopic findings improve, the steroid dosage can be tapered after several weeks. Although maintenance steroids may be useful in controlling symptoms in patients with continuing activity, maintenance therapy with low-dose corticosteroids for patients with inactive disease has not been demonstrated to prevent relapse. Patients must be monitored carefully for the long-term adverse sequelae of corticosteroid use, including hypertension, hyperglycemia, cataracts, osteoporosis, and osteomalacia.

Some 10% to 20% of patients with ulcerative colitis have more severe clinical courses and require hospitalization. These patients need nutritional support, generally with intravenous hyperalimentation, and correction of anemia. Patients with more active disease or toxicity require parenteral steroids in the form of hydrocortisone. There has been controversy about whether intravenous ACTH plays any role in the treatment of severe ulcerative colitis. In general, ACTH appears to have a similar response rate to hydrocortisone, although it may be more effective in patients not previously treated with corticosteroids. The usual doses recommended are in the range of 300 mg/d of hydrocortisone or 40 IU/d of ACTH. Total parenteral nutrition plays no primary role in ameliorating the inflammatory response in ulcerative colitis but allows nutritional maintenance and repletion during the treatment phase. During an acute episode of severe colitis, narcotic pain medications and antidiarrheals should be avoided to prevent provocation of toxic megacolon. Once the patient has responded clinically, oral foods can be started, and the patient can begin receiving oral steroids as parenteral steroids are tapered.

A number of immunosuppressive agents have been used for the management of ulcerative colitis, including azathioprine and 6-mercaptopurine. Because these drugs do not produce a clinical response for several months, they have no role in treatment of acute flares of ulcerative colitis. Cyclosporine (C_sA), which has a more rapid onset of action, has been advocated for the treatment of severe, refractory acute ulcerative colitis. Both uncontrolled trials and one controlled study suggest that high-dose C_sA is efficacious for severe ulcerative colitis. There is, however, significant theoretic risk of irreversible C_sA-associated nephropathy after treatment of ulcerative colitis with high-dose C_sA. Severe infectious complications may also occur.[13]

Although widely prescribed for both ulcerative colitis and Crohn's disease, metronidazole and other antibiotics are of no proven value in the treatment of inflammatory bowel disease. In addition, the drugs have associated side effects. The major problem with metronidazole is patient intolerance secondary to side effects, such as the metallic taste and paresthesias.

SURGICAL CONSIDERATIONS

Nearly half of patients with chronic ulcerative colitis undergo surgery within the first 10 years of their illness, mainly because of the chronic nature of the disease and the tendency for relapse. In addition, occasional fulminant complications occur with ulcerative colitis, and a significant risk of malignant degeneration exists. The indications for surgery vary widely, and these differing indications have different implications for the timing of surgery and the choice of operative procedure. Indications for surgical intervention include (1) massive unrelenting hemorrhage, (2) toxic megacolon with impending or frank perforation, (3) fulminating acute ulcerative colitis that is unresponsive to steroid therapy, (4) obstruction from stricture, (5) suspicion or demonstration of colonic cancer, (6) systemic complications, and (7) intractability. An additional indication for surgery in children is failure to mature at an acceptable rate. For most patients with ulcerative colitis, a colectomy is performed when the disease enters an intractable, chronic phase and becomes a physical and social burden to the patient. With sphincter-sparing operations available for patients with ulcerative colitis, it has become critically important to avoid standard proctectomy whenever possible and to distinguish diagnostically patients with ulcerative colitis from those with Crohn's disease.

Indications for Surgery

Intractable Disease

A failure of medical management, reflected by chronic physical disability and physiologic dysfunction, is by far the most common indication for surgery in chronic ulcerative colitis.[14] This indication is also the hardest to define. Intractability can best be characterized as the severe and persistent impairment of a patient's quality of life, created by the underlying disease or by the treatment required for that disease. Elective operations for medically intractable ulcerative colitis include total proctocolectomy with Brooke ileostomy or continent ileostomy (Kock pouch), subtotal colectomy with ileostomy or ileorectal anastomosis, and colectomy with mucosal proctectomy and ileoanal anastomosis. In the past, when total proctocolectomy combined with ileostomy was the only definitive alternative, patients frequently delayed surgery for as long as possible, often to the point at which their life-styles and health were remarkably restricted. With the availability of newer surgical alternatives, patients and their physicians are electing surgery much earlier in the course of the disease. Criteria regarding timing of operation and indications for surgery are therefore undergoing considerable revision.

Extracolonic Disease

The relation between systemic extracolonic manifestations of ulcerative colitis and colectomy is not entirely clear. Except for extreme retardation of growth and development, extracolonic complications of ulcerative colitis rarely provide an independent indication for operation. Although the arthritis and skin lesions associated with chronic ulcerative colitis do respond to colectomy, ankylosing spondylitis and liver dysfunction or failure may not respond. Studies suggest that progression of sclerosing cholangitis appears to bear no relation to the presence or absence of the colon or to the degree of the inflammatory process within the diseased mucosa. A colitis-related extraintestinal manifestation that occasionally emerges as a potential surgical indication is progressively destructive pyoderma gangrenosum. In patients with active colitis (about half), colectomy tends to be followed by resolution of skin lesions. A rare but urgent extracolonic indication for colectomy is massive hemolytic anemia, usually Coombs test positive, that is unresponsive to steroid and immunosuppressive therapy. In this case, colectomy is generally accompanied by splenectomy. The most common extraintestinal indication for surgery in ulcerative colitis is retardation of growth and development in children and adolescents. Colectomy can be of dramatic benefit in children with ulcerative colitis.

Cancer Prophylaxis

Most authors agree that significant dysplasia or suspected cancer is a clear indication for colectomy.[15] Earlier studies suggested that the risk of cancer is relatively low for the first 10 years after the onset of ulcerative colitis (roughly 2% to 3%), and then begins to climb at a rate of 1% to 2% per year. Thus, by the time the patient has had the disease for 20 years, the risk of colon cancer may be as high as 20%. Many epidemiologists believe that earlier studies overestimated the risk of malignancy due to referral and ascertainment biases inherent in retrospective surveys from tertiary referral hospital centers.[16]

The question of timing of surgery for cancer prophylaxis remains controversial. In fact, there are few patients in whom this is the sole indication for operation. The role of rectal or colonic biopsy in directing the timing of colectomy also remains controversial. Several studies have demonstrated that more than 10% of patients have a more proximal colonic malignancy at the time that a random rectal biopsy shows severe dysplasia. Certainly, in a patient with long-standing colitis, unequivocal high-grade dysplasia in the absence of acute inflammation is an indication for colectomy. Some newer evidence suggests that even low-grade dysplasia, if it is unequivocal and unassociated with inflammation, should prompt colectomy.

The presence of carcinoma is not a contraindication to mucosal proctectomy with ileoanal anastomosis, unless the tumor is found to be of an advanced stage or is located within the rectum. If there is uncertainty about the stage of the tumor at the time of the initial operation, subtotal colectomy with ileostomy and Hartmann closure of the rectum can be performed. This operation would allow subsequent conversion to ileoanal anastomosis if the patient remains disease free.

Surgical Emergencies

Only 15% of patients with ulcerative colitis present initially with catastrophic illness. Several well-identified complications require urgent operation for survival of patients with ulcerative colitis. These include (1) massive, unrelenting hemorrhage; (2) toxic megacolon with impending or frank perforation; (3) fulminating acute ulcerative colitis that is unresponsive to steroid therapy; (4) acute colonic obstruction from stricture; and (5) suspicion or demonstration of colon cancer.

Acute perforation occurs infrequently, with the incidence directly related to both the severity of the initial attack and extent of the disease in the bowel. Although the overall incidence of perforation during a first attack is less than 4%, if the attack is severe, the incidence rises to about 10%. If the patient has pancolitis, the perforation rate is 15%; if the pancolitis is associated with a clinically severe attack, the perforation rate rises to nearly 20%. Perforation is the most lethal complication of acute colitis, with an associated mortality rate of 40% to 50%. Although free colon perforation occurs much more frequently in the presence of toxic megacolon than in its absence, it is important to remember that toxic megacolon is not a prerequisite for the development of perforation. In the presence of colonic perforation, the operation should be definitive without being overly aggressive. Abdominal colectomy with ileostomy and Hartmann closure of the rectum is the procedure of choice.

Obstructions caused by benign stricture formation occur in 11% of patients, with 34% of the strictures occurring in the rectum. Strictures are usually the result of submucosal fibrosis and occasionally mucosal hyperplasia. Although they do not usually cause acute obstruction, the lesions must be differentiated from carcinoma by biopsy or excision, and particular attention should be given to ruling out Crohn's disease. Strictures caused by carcinoma are less common than those caused by benign disease and are more prone to perforate.

Massive hemorrhage secondary to ulcerative colitis is rare, occurring in fewer than 1% of patients and accounting for about 10% of urgent colectomies performed for ulcerative colitis. Prompt surgical intervention is indicated after hemodynamic stabilization. Uncontrollable hemorrhage from the entire colorectal mucosa may be the one clear indication for emergency proctocolectomy. If possible, the rectum should be spared for later mucosal proctectomy with ileoanal anastomosis, realizing that about 12% of patients will have continued hemorrhage from the retained rectal segment.

Anorectal complications of ulcerative colitis are more common than generally appreciated, occasionally confusing the differential diagnosis between Crohn's colitis and ulcerative colitis. Most rectal symptoms occur within the first year of onset of symptoms and in part correlate with the severity of disease. Overall, up to 18% of patients with ulcerative colitis develop perirectal or ischiorectal abscesses and associated anal fistulas.

Acute toxic megacolon occurs in 6% to 13% of patients with ulcerative colitis. Initial treatment for toxic megacolon includes intravenous fluid and electrolyte resuscitation, nasogastric suction, broad-spectrum antibiotics to include anaerobic and aerobic gram-negative coverage, and total parenteral nutrition to improve nutritional status. Although the therapeutic role of steroids in toxic megacolon is controversial, most patients presenting with a severe attack of ulcerative colitis are already on steroid therapy and thus need stress doses of corticosteroids to prevent adrenal crisis. When toxic megacolon is promptly treated, subsequent surgery is not inevitable. Even among patients in whom prompt resolution has occurred, about half require surgery within a year, and most eventually require colectomy.

In the presence of acute toxic megacolon caused by ulcerative colitis, surgery can be associated with a high operative morbidity and mortality rate. Postoperative complications, including sepsis, wound infection, abscess, fistula, or delayed wound healing, have been reported in up to half of patients.[17] Postoperative mortality rates range between 11% and 16% and, for the subset of patients with perforation, 27% to 44%. The overall mortality rate after emergency surgery is 8.7%; the mortality rate is 6.1% for total abdominal colectomy and 14.7% for proctocolec-

A

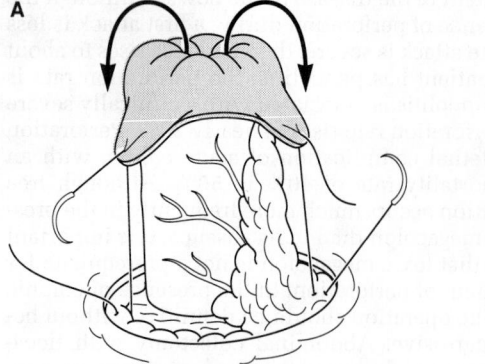

B

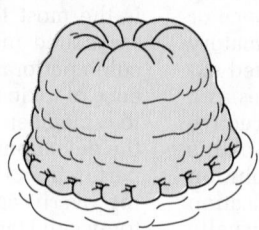

Figure 45-2. Construction of an end ileostomy. The terminal ileum is brought 5 cm through an abdominal wall defect, everted, and sutured to the more proximal ileal seromuscularis and then dermis to mature the ileostomy.

tomy. This observation suggests that more conservative surgery is appropriate in the acute setting. With the popularity of anal sphincter–sparing procedures, the surgeon should always weigh the possibility of the need for later surgery for restoration of continence. Specifically, leaving the rectum intact allows its use for subsequent mucosal proctectomy and ileoanal anastomosis.

Surgical Approaches

Because chronic ulcerative colitis is cured once the colon and rectum are removed, single-stage total proctocolectomy with ileostomy has historically been the procedure of choice for elective surgical treatment.[18] Despite the fact that this operation eliminates all diseased tissue and the risk of malignant transformation, it has remained controversial and poorly accepted by patients and their physicians. This reluctance is primarily because a permanent abdominal ileostomy is required after standard proctocolectomy. Although immediate maturation of the stoma (Fig. 45-2) eliminated many of the mechanical problems associated with ileostomy, patients receiving even the most carefully constructed ileostomies are incontinent of gas and stool and must wear an external collecting bag day and night. Several studies have demonstrated that, although 90% of patients with a Brooke ileostomy are able to adjust to the stoma, between 25% and 50% of patients with ileostomies complain of appliance-related problems.[19] These include skin irritation or excoriation, discomfort, leakage and odor, the financial burden of caring for an ileostomy with modern disposable stomal devices, and the time and effort that are required. Perhaps more important than these problems are the significant psychologic and social implications of a permanent ileostomy, particularly for young and physically active patients. It is for this reason that surgeons have long sought other alternatives to total proctocolectomy and ileostomy.

Proctocolectomy and Ileostomy

Until about 15 years ago, single-stage total proctocolectomy with ileostomy was the operation of choice when complications of ulcerative colitis were treated electively. Currently, proctocolectomy is the procedure of choice in relatively few patients with ulcerative colitis. The operation carries the advantages that it is curative, there is no anastomosis to heal, and it only requires a single operation. It provides the patient with a predictable functional result and eliminates the fear of anal incontinence.

The disadvantage of total proctocolectomy is that it results in permanent fecal incontinence. Patients require an external ileostomy device, which may need emptying four to eight times per day. Also, significant complications are

associated with the operation. A 20% overall morbidity rate is reported for elective, 30% for urgent, and 40% for emergency proctocolectomy. The risks are primarily hemorrhage, contamination, sepsis, and neural injury. Ten to 25% of patients require stoma revision. Ten to 20% have perineal wound problems after a standard abdominal perineal proctectomy. Fifteen to 20% of patients have bowel obstruction at some point in the postoperative period. Of major concern are bladder and sexual dysfunction associated with parasympathetic nerve injury. Impotence is reported to occur in to up 5% of male patients after proctectomy for benign disease.

Subtotal Colectomy

Subtotal colectomy, Brooke ileostomy, and Hartmann closure of the rectum, or ileorectal anastomosis (Fig. 45-3), have been employed in the surgical treatment of ulcerative colitis for decades. The operation eliminates an abdominal stoma if ileorectal anastomosis is performed and, because the pelvic autonomic nerves are not disturbed, impotence and bladder dysfunction are not a risk. As described earlier, subtotal colectomy with ileostomy is the procedure of choice in the emergency setting or if the diagnosis of

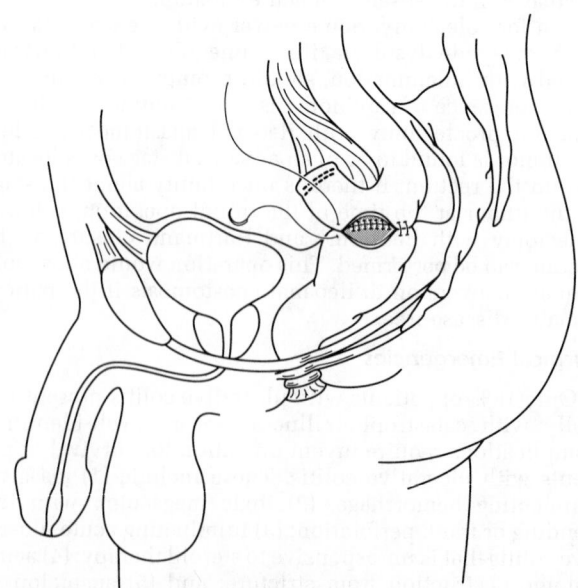

Figure 45-3. Ileorectal anastomosis after abdominal colectomy. This represents a nondefinitive operation for select patients with chronic ulcerative colitis.

ulcerative colitis, as opposed to Crohn's disease, cannot be clearly established. Although abdominal colectomy with ileorectal anastomosis is a less extensive procedure that usually leaves the patient with full continence, it has not gained wide popularity because it is not a curative operation. The inflammatory process persists in the retained rectum in essentially all patients, and there is an ongoing risk of malignancy that may be as high as 17% after 20 years.[20] At least 10% of patients require subsequent proctectomy for uncontrollable proctitis, and another 10% require proctectomy because of a poor functional result. Even in patients who do well, the stool frequency is high in the early postoperative period, eventually averaging four or five stools per 24 hours. The operation is also associated with a number of operative complications, including small bowel obstruction, which has been reported in 10% to 20% of patients. In addition, there is the potential for leakage of the anastomosis between the ileum and the disease-bearing rectum. The operation is clearly contraindicated in patients with anal sphincter dysfunction, severe rectal disease, rectal dysplasia, or frank cancer. Subtotal colectomy with ileorectal anastomosis is clearly a compromise operation. With the availability and success of the definitive mucosal proctectomy and ileoanal anastomosis, ileorectal anastomosis is applicable in few patients.

Continent Ileostomy

Kock first described the continent ileostomy, made entirely of terminal ileum and consisting of an intestinal pouch that serves as a reservoir for stool, with an ileal conduit connecting the pouch to a cutaneous stoma[21] (Fig. 45-4). The operation was modified several years later to include an intestinal nipple valve between the pouch and the stoma. For construction of the pouch and the valve, 45 to 50 cm of terminal ileum is used. The proximal 30 to 35 cm is formed into a pouch, and a nipple valve is constructed by intussuscepting the outflow tract from the pouch and then securing it with sutures or staples. The reservoir is sutured to the peritoneum and fascia, and the efferent limb is brought out through the abdominal wall as a flush stoma. Patients empty the pouch by passing a soft plastic tube through the valve by way of the stoma. The advantage of this operation is that it is a curative procedure because it is associated with total proctocolectomy. The

technique offers the patient a potentially new life-style by making the ileostomy continent and thereby avoiding an external appliance.

The continent ileostomy has been associated with a high complication rate.[22] Most of the complications are related to displacement of the nipple valve, producing fecal incontinence, and difficulty in intubating and emptying the pouch. Valve failure has been reported to occur in between 4% and 40% of patients. Ten to 20% of patients suffer bowel obstruction. The operation carries the same risk of bladder dysfunction, impotence, and perineal wound problems as standard proctocolectomy and ileostomy. Several syndromes of ileostomy dysfunction related to the Kock pouch have also been reported. These are variably described as stagnant loop syndrome, enteritis, nonspecific ileitis, and pouchitis. Clinical features include diarrhea, malabsorption of fat and vitamin B_{12}, proliferation of anaerobic bacteria, inflammation of the pouch, and incontinence. Patients may also develop fistulas between the pouch and the skin or other enteric organs. Crohn's disease is a clear contraindication to performing this operation. Despite these complications, patient satisfaction with the continent ileostomy is high.

Although the Kock ileostomy has advantages over the Brooke ileostomy, its high rate of mechanical, functional, and metabolic complications has limited its clinical usefulness. In centers that offer all surgical alternatives to patients with ulcerative colitis requiring colectomy, few Kock pouches are being constructed. The continent ileostomy may be useful in patients who have already undergone total proctocolectomy and ileostomy and, after careful counseling, are extremely desirous of an attempt at a continence-restoring procedure.

Ileoanal Anastomosis

Rather then ablating the entire rectum, anus, and anal sphincter, advantage can be taken of the fact that ulcerative colitis is a mucosal disease. The rectal mucosa can be selectively dissected out and removed down to the dentate line of the anus.[23] This preserves an intact rectal muscular cuff and anal sphincter apparatus. Continuity of the intestinal tract can be reestablished by extending the ileum into the pelvis endorectally, and circumferentially suturing it to the anus in an end-to-end fashion (Fig. 45-5). The potential

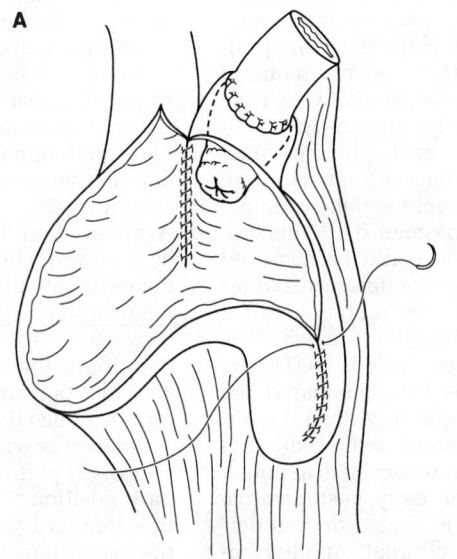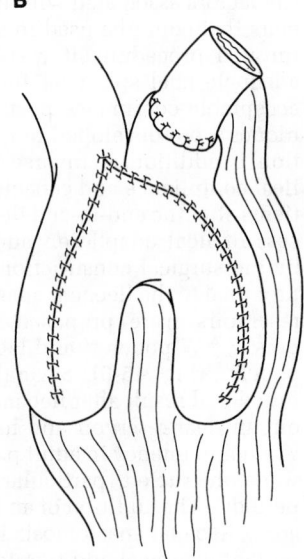

Figure 45-4. The continent ileostomy (Kock pouch) consists of an ileal reservoir and nipple valve constructed by intussuscepting the efferent limb and fixing it in place with sutures or staples. This provides a continent internal intestinal reservoir that the patient can drain by intubating the pouch through the flush cutaneous stoma several times throughout the day.

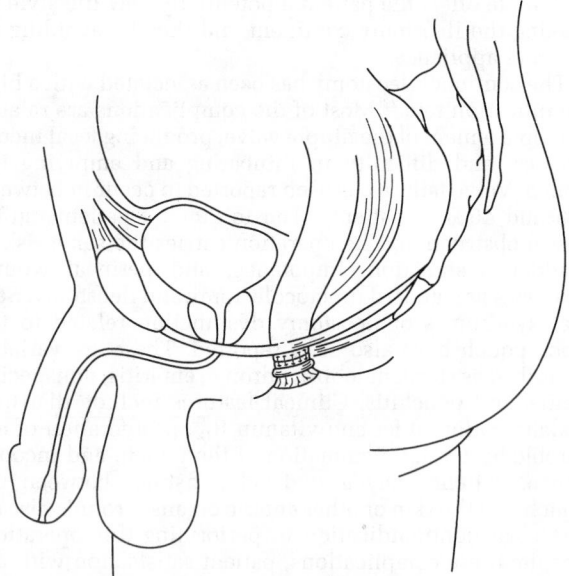

Figure 45-5. End-to-end ileoanal anastomosis after colectomy, mucosal proctectomy, and endorectal ileoanal pull-through.

advantages of this approach are that it eliminates all diseased tissue and is as definitive an operation as total proctocolectomy. Because the pelvic dissection is confined to the endorectal plane, it preserves parasympathetic innervation to the bladder and genitalia and eliminates the problem of urinary dysfunction or impotence. Because the abdominal perineal proctectomy is eliminated, it avoids a long-term draining perineal wound. A permanent abdominal stoma is unnecessary because of the ileoanal anastomosis. Finally, if performed carefully, it preserves the anorectal sphincter and maintains continence.

During the past 15 years, there has been increasing interest in the ileoanal pull-through procedure. This interest developed, in part, because other alternatives such as the Kock pouch were not as successful as originally hoped. In addition, important technical advances had been made. By the early 1980s, larger reports from various centers suggested that acceptable morbidity could be achieved. Although the functional result was encouraging, it was still variable and unpredictable. Attempts were made to identify factors associated with improved outcome and parameters that could be used in selecting patients for the pull-through procedure. It was found that patients required adequate anal sphincter function preoperatively to have acceptable continence postoperatively. Manometric techniques were developed to quantitate anal sphincter function. In addition, an inverse correlation was found between ileal compliance and capacity and stool frequencies in patients after the end-to-end ileoanal anastomosis.[24] This process of ileal adaptation and dilation could be hastened by the surgical construction of a ileal pouch or reservoir proximal to the ileoanal anastomosis. Several types of ileal reservoirs were proposed, including the J-pouch,[25] S-pouch,[26] W-pouch,[27] and lateral side-to-side isoperistaltic pouch[28] (Fig. 45-6). Several studies have compared the functional result after ileoanal anastomosis with and without an ileal reservoir and have demonstrated a reduction in stool frequency in adult patients in whom an ileal pouch was constructed, particularly in the early postoperative period.[29] The addition of an ileal pouch in children undergoing ileoanal anastomosis is not as clearcut. Another important technical addition to the operation is a temporary

diverting loop ileostomy. This allows fecal diversion during the early weeks of ileal pouch and ileoanal anastomotic healing, thereby reducing the incidence of pelvic sepsis and ileal pouch and ileoanal anastomotic dehiscence. Some surgeons have eliminated the loop ileostomy in good-risk patients.

Although it was thought initially that only patients who were young and had relatively quiescent disease were candidates for ileoanal anastomosis, the indications have been considerably liberalized during the past 10 years. Patients are not candidates if other medical problems or the severity of the colitis preclude a 4- to 6-hour operation. Although some series have reported that younger patients have a superior result when compared with older patients, others have not found this to be the case. Many surgeons are comfortable in offering ileoanal anastomosis to patients in their sixth decade if they are in relatively good health and have adequate anal sphincter function. Obesity significantly increases the technical difficulty of ileoanal anastomosis, but it is only a relative contraindication to the operation. Disease severity has not been found to be associated with enhanced operative morbidity, nor to correlate with subsequent functional results. Crohn's disease is an absolute contraindication to the operation. The most important criterion for electing ileoanal anastomosis is that the patient fully understand the physiology and technique of the operation and have realistic expectations about the outcome. If possible, all potential candidates for ileoanal anastomosis should be seen several weeks before the proposed surgery. Flexible sigmoidoscopic examination is performed to confirm the diagnosis and to assess the status of the inflammatory process of the rectal mucosa. Anorectal manometry is performed using either a pneumohydraulic perfused catheter system or solid-state transducers.[30,31] In patients with active disease of the rectum, steroid or sulfasalazine treatment is accelerated in the immediate preoperative period.

For most patients, the operation is performed in two stages. The first stage consists of abdominal colectomy, mucosal proctectomy, endorectal ileal pouch–anal anastomosis, and diverting loop ileostomy. During the second stage, performed at least 8 weeks after the initial operation, the loop ileostomy is closed. In patients in whom an emergency colectomy was required, the operation is staged. The first stage consists of abdominal colectomy, ileostomy, and Hartmann closure of the rectum. During the second stage, the rectal mucosa is dissected free, and the ileoanal anastomosis is performed with loop ileostomy. Finally, the loop ileostomy is closed. A group of patients who required prior abdominal colectomy followed by a staged mucosal proctectomy with ileal pouch–anal anastomosis was compared to matched patients who had undergone colectomy with ileoanal anastomosis at a single operative setting.[32,33] Previous abdominal colectomy was associated with a higher cumulative operative morbidity rate, prolonged hospital stay, increased costs, and a less optimal functional result. Aggressive and extended medical therapy, including cyclosporine, has been associated with an increased incidence of patients requiring staged subtotal colectomy with delayed ileoanal anastomosis. Therefore, patients with ulcerative colitis who have relative indications for urgent colectomy (bleeding, intractability, or toxic megacolon) should be given a full medical trial in an attempt to perform semielective surgery in a single stage.

Colectomy with mucosal proctectomy and ileoanal anastomosis is performed with the patient in a modified lithotomy position.[34,35] An abdominal colectomy is performed in a standard fashion through a midline incision. The entire rectal mucosal dissection is done transanally. A circumferential incision is made at the dentate line, and the

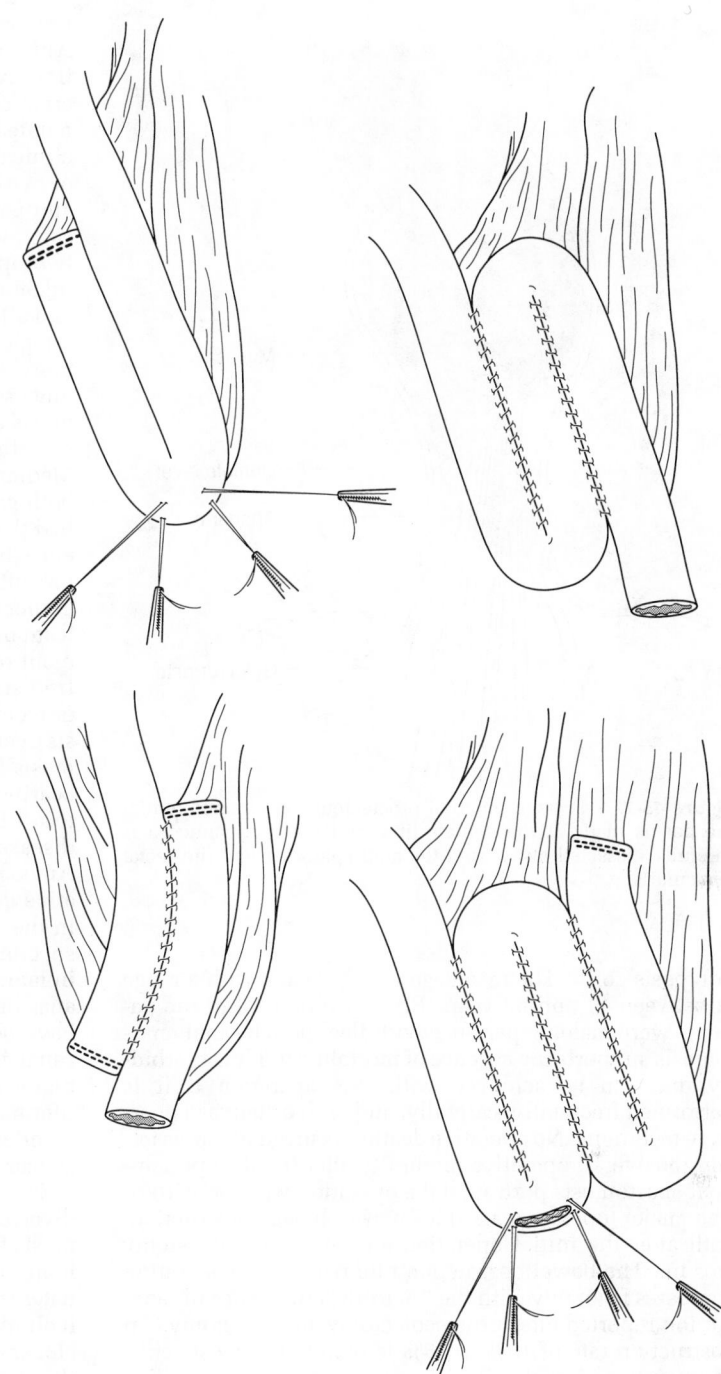

Figure 45-6. Ileal pouch configurations in patients undergoing ileal pouch–anal anastomosis.

rectal mucosa is carefully dissected away from the anal sphincter and then the rectal muscularis (Fig. 45-7).

With the mucosal dissection completed, the ileal pouch is constructed using suturing techniques or mechanical staplers (Fig. 45-8). The ileal pouch is extended into the pelvis endorectally, and its apex is opened and sutured circumferentially to the dentate line (Fig. 45-9). A loop ileostomy is then constructed 40 cm proximal to the pouch (Fig. 45-10).

Four weeks after the initial operation, standardized radiographic studies are performed to assess continence and the integrity of the ileal pouch and ileoanal anastomosis. Eight weeks after ileoanal anastomosis, anal manometry is repeated, and ileal pouch capacity is measured. The loop

ileostomy is then closed using a stapling technique, which has greatly simplified this operation (Fig. 45-11).

Poor stool consistency, increased stool frequency, and nocturnal leakage of stool are the most common postoperative complaints in patients after ileoanal anastomosis. In an effort to control stool output, patients have been placed on loperamide hydrochloride, a synthetic opioid antidiarrheal agent, and supplementary fiber in the form of psyllium hydrophilic mucilloid. In addition, patients are placed on a high-fiber diet.

The postoperative morbidity and functional results in most large series after ileoanal pull-through have been encouraging. Eighty-two percent of the patients in one series were operated on for ulcerative colitis and 18% for familial

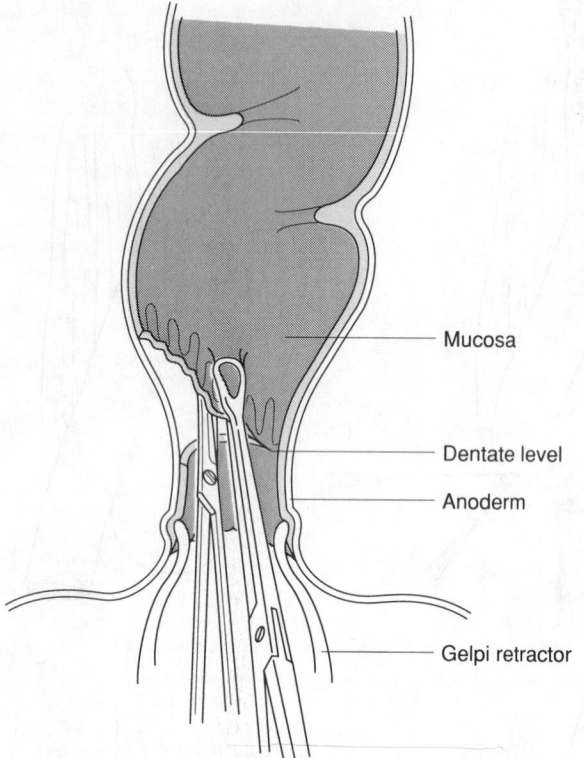

Mucosa

Dentate level

Anoderm

Gelpi retractor

Figure 45-7. Transanal mucosal proctectomy. A circumferential incision is made at the dentate line, and the rectal mucosa is carefully dissected away from the anal sphincter and the rectal muscularis.

polyposis coli.[36] The mean age was 35 years, with a range of between 11 and 67 years. Sixty-two percent of the patients were male. Experience with ileal pouch–anal anastomosis supports the absence of mortality and low morbidity that can be achieved with this operation if it is performed frequently, carefully, and with a standard operative technique. No operative deaths occurred in the series, and the overall operative morbidity after the ileal pouch–anal anastomosis portion of the operation was about 10%. The major operative morbidity was bowel obstruction, both after the initial operation and after loop ileostomy closure. The bowel obstruction rate requiring reoperation compares favorably with the 7% to 13% incidence of reoperation reported after proctocolectomy and ileostomy. An obstruction rate of 10% to 25% is reported in most series of patients undergoing ileal pouch–anal anastomosis (Fig. 45-12). Pelvic and wound infections have been reported to occur in 10% to 20% of patients undergoing ileoanal anastomosis, although the overall infection rate was reduced to about 5% in several more recent large series. A 5% to 10% failure rate necessitating conversion to permanent ileostomy has been reported in several series.

Although results with mucosal proctectomy and ileal pouch–anal anastomosis have been excellent, divergent points of view have arisen regarding the operative technique and its effect on anal physiology and functional result. A number of surgeons have advocated an alternative approach to conventional endoanal rectal mucosal resection that eliminates distal mucosal proctectomy.[37–39] Instead, the distal rectum is divided near the pelvic floor, leaving the anal canal largely intact. The ileal pouch is then stapled to the top of the anal canal. The rationale for this approach is that, by preserving the mucosa of the anal transition zone, the anatomic integrity of the anal canal is

preserved and the rate of fecal incontinence improved. Although several studies have suggested that patients have improved sensation and better functional results after preservation of the anal transition zone, this has not been documented by prospective study. A prospective, randomized, clinical trial compared ileal pouch–anal anastomosis with or without mucosectomy.[40] Thirty-two consecutive age- and gender-matched patients, under the care of one surgeon, were assigned prospectively and randomly to one of two operative groups. Patients were stratified for disease (ulcerative colitis and familial adenomatous polyposis), and all had preoperative and postoperative anorectal physiologic and manometric studies. Patients with mucosectomy were compared prospectively with those without mucosectomy, receiving a stapled ileoanal pouch anastomosis about 2 cm above the dentate line. A W-pouch and diverting loop ileostomy were performed in all patients. Median frequency of defecation for 24 hours was four in both groups. One patient, in the nonmucosectomy group, had the reservoir removed. There was no significant difference in nocturnal evacuations between the groups. All patients in both groups had excellent continence. The authors recommended full anorectal mucosectomy to eradicate mucosal disease totally and to prevent late development of colorectal cancer. A second prospective randomized study from Finland also demonstrated no functional or technical advantage of the stapled low rectal anastomosis over standard rectal mucosectomy with ileoanal anastomosis.[41] The obvious concern is that, by leaving disease-bearing mucosa in the anal canal, the patients are exposed to a lifelong risk of persistent or recurrent inflammatory disease as well the potential for malignant transformation. Among 50 patients treated with proctocolectomy for ulcerative colitis at the Mayo Clinic, 90% had disease present in the mucosa within 1 cm of the dentate line, where the specimens were carefully examined histologically.[42] This inflamed mucosa is left behind by ileal pouch–distal rectal anastomosis. In addition, dysplasia and adenocarcinoma have been described in the mucosa of the proximal anal canal in patients with ulcerative colitis. Until this technique is further evaluated, patients will require careful lifetime surveillance. Mucosectomy must be recommended in patients with rectal dysplasia, proximal rectal cancer, diffuse colonic dysplasia, and familial polyposis.[38]

Several reports have questioned the need for a proximal diverting ileostomy at the time of ileal pouch–anal anastomosis for ulcerative colitis.[43] The avoidance of a diverting loop ileostomy has several theoretic advantages: it eliminates the additional surgery needed to close the ileostomy, it eliminates the complications of ileostomy and ileostomy closure, and it may reduce diversion enteritis. A diverting ileostomy, however, reduces the risk of leakage from the ileal pouch or ileoanal anastomosis, a serious complication associated with significant morbidity and the potential for total loss of the ileal pouch. Only prospective, randomized, controlled trials will answer the question.

In large series of patients undergoing ileoanal anastomosis, the overall morbidity and mortality rates have been low.[44] The most frequent late complication in patients undergoing ileoanal anastomosis is ileal pouch dysfunction, or pouchitis, which has been reported to occur in 10% to 50% of patients undergoing this procedure for ulcerative colitis. Pouchitis is an incompletely defined and poorly understood clinical syndrome consisting of increased stool frequency, watery stools, cramping, urgency, nocturnal leakage of stool, arthralgia, malaise, and fever. The syndrome is similar to that found in patients with Kock continent ileostomy pouches. The cause of this condition is unknown; speculated causes include early Crohn's disease, bacterial overgrowth or bacterial dysbiosis, either pri-

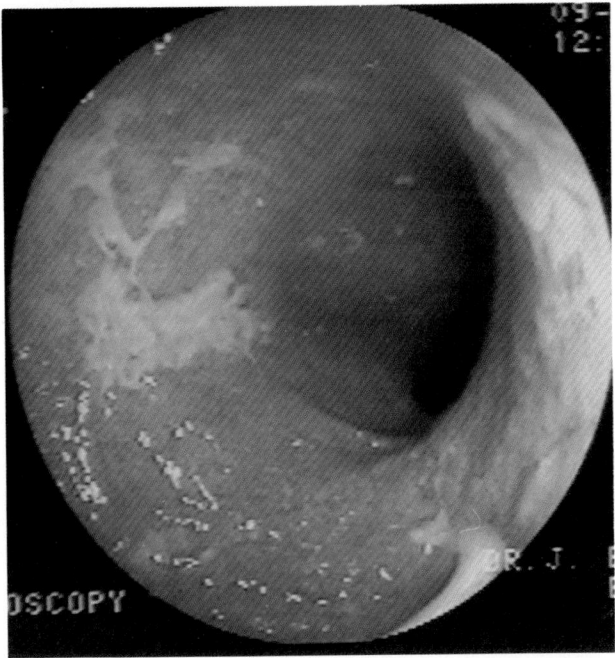

Color Figure 45-1. Endoscopic appearance of the rectum in a patient with mild ulcerative colitis, with mucosal granularity and loss of the normal vascular pattern.

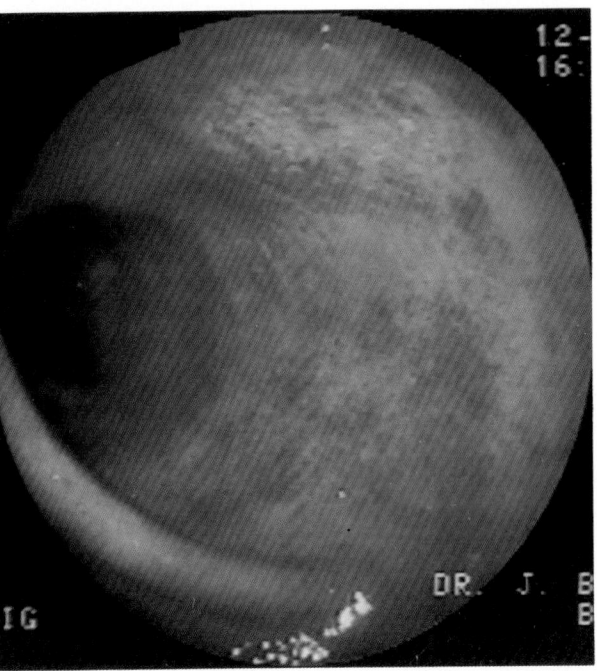

Color Figure 45-2. Endoscopic appearance of the rectum in a patient with moderate ulcerative colitis, with pitted mucosa and spontaneous hemorrhage.

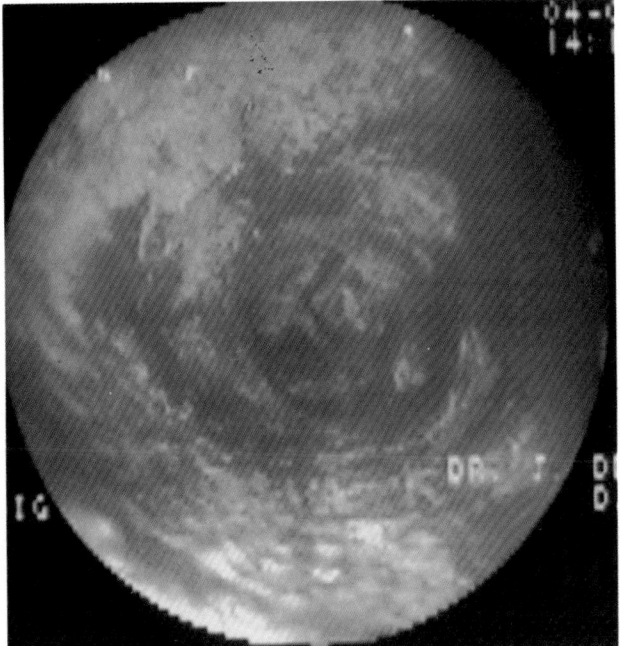

Color Figure 45-3. Endoscopic appearance of the rectum in a patient with severe ulcerative colitis, with frank ulceration, bleeding, and a purulent exudate.

mildly increased flatulence as the primary manifestation of their disease. Gallstone patients who complain of non-specific dyspeptic symptoms without biliary colic are less likely to have a satisfactory result from cholecystectomy. The fact that up to 70% of such patients derive significant benefit from cholecystectomy, however, suggests that these nonspecific symptoms are frequently due to biliary calculi. Thus, designating these patients as asymptomatic is inappropriate.

Insufficient data are available to accurately determine the natural history of patients with cholelithiasis. The role, therefore, of prophylactic management remains unclear. Medical dissolution with oral agents as a primary therapeutic modality for cholelithiasis has been disappointing, and these results, coupled with the cost of such treatment, suggest that this modality is probably not an appropriate means of dealing with asymptomatic stones. Similarly, there is little data to suggest any role for biliary lithotripsy or contact dissolution in the overall treatment of asymptomatic patients. Early cholecystectomy should be considered in any patient with asymptomatic gallstones who is particularly concerned about developing complications from biliary tract disease or in patients who have major risk factors and in whom operation is not contraindicated because of poor medical condition. For example, acute cholecystitis is a potentially life-threatening complication when it occurs in an immunosuppressed patient. For this reason, early cholecystectomy has been recommended in patients who have asymptomatic gallstones and who are undergoing laparotomy for other reasons or for major organ transplantation. The ease with which laparascopic cholecystectomy can be performed in most areas has led to some liberalization of indications for surgery in the asymptomatic patient. The wisdom and validity of this recommendation remains to be established.

Diagnosis

Abdominal Radiography

Although supine and upright abdominal radiographs are essential in the early evaluation of patients with an acute abdomen, their usefulness is limited in patients with cholelithiasis. Visualization of gallstones on plain abdominal radiographs is possible only in the 20% of patients whose stones are grossly calcified. Unusual clinical settings in which abdominal radiographs may be helpful in evaluating patients with biliary calculi include the identification of gas trapped in the center of a cholesterol gallstone during formation, air in the wall and lumen of the gallbladder as seen in emphysematous cholecystitis, air in the biliary tree as a result of a biliary enteric fistula, or the outlining of the gallbladder in patients with porcelain gallbladders or milk of calcium bile.

Oral Cholecystography

Traditionally, the oral cholecystogram has been the gold standard for the diagnostic evaluation of patients with calculous disease of the biliary tract (Fig. 41-9). This test is based on the excretion of halogen compounds by the liver into bile with gallbladder visualization after reabsorption of water and solutes, resulting in concentration of the dyes. Although the accuracy for oral cholecystography has been reported to be as high as 95%, several important conditions preclude satisfactory examination, including acute illness, poor patient compliance, inability to absorb the tablets as a result of emesis, malabsorption, or diarrhea, and jaundice or hepatic dysfunction.

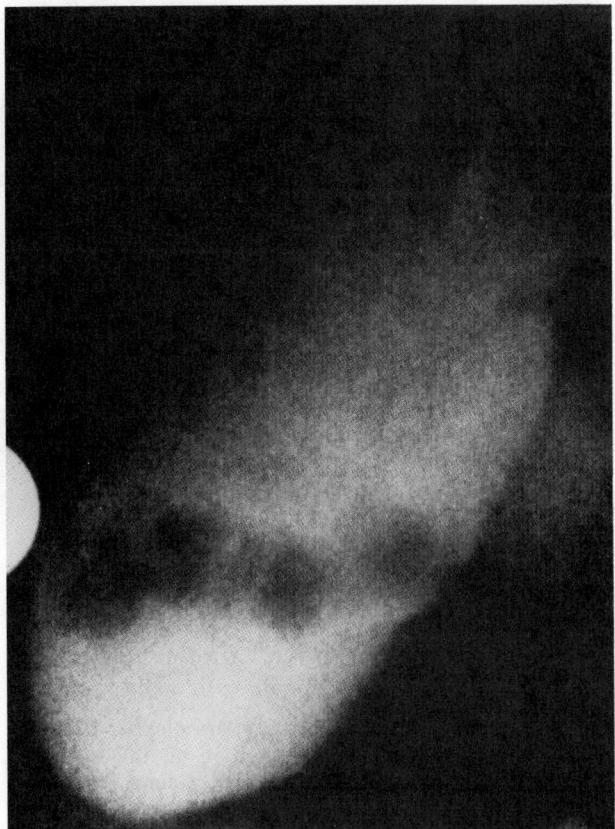

Figure 41-9. Oral cholecystogram demonstrating multiple radiolucent, free-floating stones in the gallbladder.

Abdominal Ultrasonography

Abdominal ultrasonography is the preferred test for evaluating patients with suspected cholelithiasis or cholecystitis (Fig. 41-10). Ultrasonography has several theoretical advantages over conventional oral cholecystography. These include absence of radiation exposure, independence of patient compliance, and no requirement for intact digestive and hepatic function. Although abdominal ultrasonography is most useful in identifying gallstones, it may also facilitate the diagnosis of cholecystitis. Most large series suggest that diagnostic accuracy and sensitivity for cholelithiasis exceeds 95%. Information derived from ultrasonography includes size and shape of the gallbladder, gallbladder wall thickness, and the presence of pericholecystic fluid collections. A sonographic Murphy sign has been described, in which the ultrasonography technician probes the point of maximal tenderness and correlates this with location of the gallbladder. Several studies have suggested that this sign has an 85% accuracy rate in patients with acute cholecystitis. Nonetheless, although abdominal ultrasonography is most helpful in identifying the presence or absence of gallstones, it is of limited use in distinguishing chronic from acute cholecystitis. In addition to identifying stones in the gallbladder or bile duct, abdominal ultrasonography provides important information regarding the anatomy of bile ducts, pancreas, and other structures in the area of examination.

Hepatobiliary Scintigraphy

Radionuclides, such as ^{99m}Tc−substituted iminodiacetic acid derivatives, can be used to provide a direct image of the gallbladder and biliary tract. These radionuclide

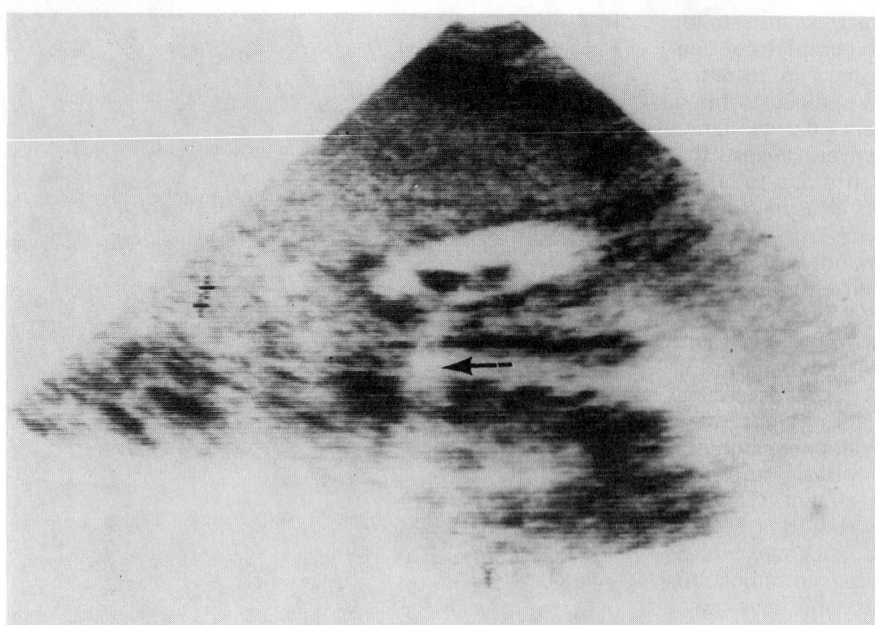

Figure 41-10. Abdominal ultrasonogram demonstrating echogenic foci within the gallbladder causing acoustic shadowing (*arrow*) typical of cholelithiasis.

agents, administered intravenously, are cleared from the blood by hepatocytes and excreted in an unconjugated form directly into the biliary ductular system. The newer generation of biliary scintigrams provides improved visualization with less radiation exposure for the patient, using isotopes with a relatively short half-life. Different analogues are available that may be preferable in patients with different degrees of jaundice. The varying usefulness of these agents is based on the rate of hepatocyte uptake, renal excretion, and transport from the hepatocyte into the biliary ducts.

Hepatobiliary scintigraphy provides information on the patency of bile ducts, including the cystic duct. The recognition that cystic duct obstruction is the sine qua non of acute cholecystitis provides the rationale for stating that a specific diagnosis of acute cholecystitis can be made with biliary scintigraphy. Cystic duct obstruction, and by implication cholecystitis, is diagnosed when normal imaging of the liver and common bile duct with prompt visualization of the duodenum is observed but with absence of label in the gallbladder. Failure to visualize the gallbladder after 60 minutes is diagnostic of cystic duct obstruction and highly suggestive of acute cholecystitis. No visualization of the cystic duct and gallbladder after 4 hours, even in patients with altered hepatic cellular function, is also highly suggestive of cholecystitis. Potential false-positive examinations can occur in patients receiving TPN or experiencing a prolonged fast. Caution should be exercised in interpreting a scan in which imaging of the liver is obtained without evidence of radionuclide in any portion of the extrahepatic biliary system. Although these findings may occasionally be observed in patients with complete extrahepatic obstruction secondary to either stones or tumor, this scenario is more frequently indicative of diffuse hepatic parenchymal disease. Most large series suggest that radionuclide scanning has a diagnostic accuracy and sensitivity for acute cholecystitis approaching 98%.

The diagnostic role of hepatobiliary scintigraphy in patients with acute right upper quadrant symptoms remains poorly defined. The diagnosis of acute cholecystitis is established based on clinical criteria, although it may be confirmed by biliary scintigraphy. Often, however, the information provided by the scan is superfluous. Most clini-

cians are suspicious of the diagnosis in an appropriate clinical setting and seek to document the presence or absence of gallstones. The presence of gallstones in a patient who has right upper quadrant tenderness, mild leukocytosis, and fever is sufficient to confirm the diagnosis of acute cholecystitis without performing a hepatobiliary scan. In patients with atypical symptoms in the presence of other possible confounding diagnoses, such as peptic ulcer disease, biliary scintigraphy may be particularly useful in establishing a precise diagnosis.

Biliary Drainage and Cholecystokinin Cholecystography

Occasionally, patients may present with what appear to be classic symptoms of biliary calculous disease, yet have no evidence of cholelithiasis on either oral cholecystography or abdominal ultrasonography. Although many of these patients have disorders unrelated to the biliary tract, a small percentage have either small stones that are undetectable by conventional modalities, cholesterolosis, or biliary dyskinesia. For these patients, duodenal drainage studies with examination of bile for cholesterol crystals, in conjunction with CCK cholecystography, have proved useful. After placement of a tube in the second portion of the duodenum (under fluoroscopic control), intravenous CCK is administered, and bile is collected. Gallbladder radiography or ultrasonography is used to evaluate gallbladder motility. Criteria for a positive study include reproduction of pain, absence of visible gallbladder contractions, and abnormal bile containing cholesterol or calcium bilirubinate crystals. Over 80% of patients with abnormal test results, either in terms of duodenal drainage studies or gallbladder motility, have significant improvement of their symptoms after cholecystectomy.

Common Clinical Features

Nonspecific Symptoms

Patients with cholelithiasis may complain of vague, poorly localized abdominal discomfort. Although the pain typically occurs postprandially, patients may be unable to specify the interval between the meal and pain. The discomfort is generally localized in the right upper quadrant, although a significant number of these patients complain of mid-epigastric pain. Other nonspecific complaints that may be present in gallstone patients include increased flatulence, eructations, or heartburn.

Biliary Colic

Biliary colic usually results from an impacted stone in the cystic duct or Hartmann pouch or from passage of a stone through this ductular structure. The term *colic* may be somewhat misleading in that the character of the pain is generally different from pain that occurs with intestinal or ureteral obstruction. In the latter settings, the patient typically describes an intermittent discomfort that is spasmodic and of relatively short duration. In contrast, biliary colic is characterized by a rapid increase in pain intensity, with a plateau of discomfort that lasts for several hours, followed by a gradual decrease in intensity (Fig. 41-11). Classically, the pain of biliary colic is situated in the right upper quadrant or middle epigastrium. The back discomfort that is frequently observed in patients with biliary colic is usually located in the inferomedial aspect of the right scapula, although pain may also occur in the right shoulder. Episodes of biliary colic typically occur postprandially and are often associated with nausea and emesis. These attacks are often precipitated by fatty meals, although most foods can also bring about gallbladder contractions and painful episodes.

Acute Cholecystitis

The clinical manifestations of biliary colic and acute cholecystitis may overlap, and clinical distinction is often difficult. Nonetheless, it is helpful to think of them as distinct entities. Similar to biliary colic, the initiating factor in the pathogenesis of acute cholecystitis is impaction of a stone either in the cystic duct or the pouch of Hartmann (Fig. 41-12). The onset and character of pain associated with acute cholecystitis is comparable to that observed in patients with biliary colic. Unlike biliary colic, however, in which the pain generally lasts for several minutes to hours, the pain of acute cholecystitis persists and may be unremitting for several days. With progression of the inflammatory process, the gallbladder may become more distended, ultimately resulting in inflammation of the contiguous parietal peritoneum. At this juncture, the patient typically complains of more localized right upper quadrant

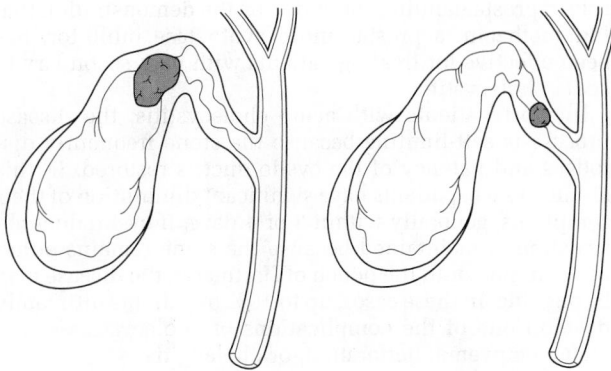

Figure 41-12. Acute cholecystitis occurs when a stone becomes lodged in the cystic duct or Hartmann pouch.

pain. This sometimes subtle alteration in the pattern of symptoms reflects the shift from visceral to parietal pain. Many patients have associated constitutional symptoms of anorexia, nausea, and vomiting. As a result of associated peritoneal irritation, the patient is reluctant to move and is most comfortable lying still. The classic physical finding of acute cholecystitis is a positive Murphy sign, which refers to inspiratory arrest during deep palpation in the right upper quadrant. There is a wide variation in the spectrum of complaints and physical findings in patients with acute cholecystitis, and often, only persistence of right upper quadrant pain and discomfort distinguishes this diagnosis from simple biliary colic. Laboratory data are helpful but frequently nonspecific. Most patients with uncomplicated acute cholecystitis have mild leukocytosis, ranging from 12,000 to 15,000/μL. Mild jaundice may be present in up to 20% of patients and is typically due to contiguous inflammation as opposed to bile duct obstruction.

Pathogenesis. Although acute cholecystitis is one of the more common abdominal emergencies, the specific events and factors responsible for its development remain unclear. Cholecystitis occurs in about 10% to 20% of patients with symptomatic gallstones. Obstruction of the cystic duct incites an inflammatory response in the gallbladder. The primary event in the development of acute cholecystitis is biochemical in nature, and bacterial infection plays a minor role in the genesis of the disease. A number of potential mediators of the inflammatory response have been identified, including bile acids, lithogenic bile, pancreatic juice, lysolecithin, phospholipase A, and prostaglandins. Each of these substances in experimental models is capable of inducing cellular injury and inflammation. Although early studies focused on the injurious roles of bile acids and pancreatic juice, more recent studies have examined the etiologic role of lysolecithin, phospholipase A, and prostaglandins. Lysolecithin originates from the hydrolysis of lecithin and is typically present in small amounts in normal bile. In patients with acute cholecystitis, the amount of lysolecithin relative to lecithin increases. Moreover, lysolecithin has been shown to alter cellular integrity and to induce changes typical of acute cholecystitis. Phospholipase A, an enzyme that catalyzes the conversion of lecithin to lysolecithin, is increased in the presence of biliary stasis. Perhaps the most intriguing group of mediators that have been proposed are prostaglandins. Prostaglandins have been shown to mediate inflammation in a variety of clinical settings, and some studies have suggested alterations in prostanoid metabolism during gallstone formation. Further evidence for an etiologic

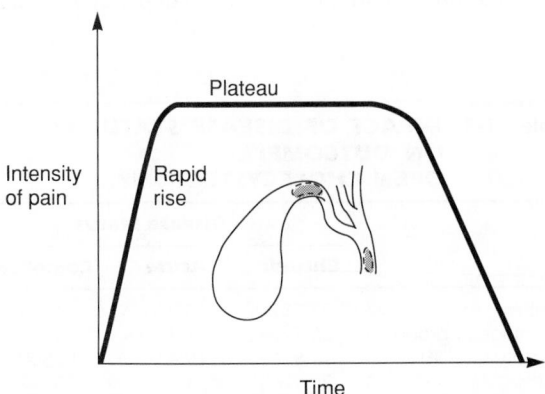

Figure 41-11. Diagram representing the chronologic pain intensity of biliary colic. Characteristically, the pain is of sudden onset, builds in intensity, and then remains steady for several hours. (After Schoenfield L. Manifestations of cholelithiasis. In: Diseases of the gallbladder and biliary system. New York, John Wiley & Sons, 1977:118)

role of prostaglandin is provided by the demonstration that indomethacin, a prostaglandin synthetase inhibitor, has been effective for treating patients with pain secondary to acute cholecystitis.

In most patients with acute cholecystitis, the disease process is self-limiting because the stone frequently dislodges and patency of the cystic duct is restored. In this circumstance, patients have significant diminution of their symptoms, generally within 3 or 4 days. If cystic duct obstruction is maintained because the stone remains either in the lumen or in the pouch of Hartmann, the disease may be ongoing. In these cases, up to 10% of patients ultimately develop one of the complications of cholecystitis—gangrene, empyema, perforation, or cholangitis.

Pathology. Obstruction of the cystic duct with a stone and the associated inflammatory response can cause significant edema of the gallbladder wall as a result of venous and lymphatic outflow obstruction. On gross examination, the gallbladder is typically distended with gallbladder wall thickening and obvious edema. At the time of laparotomy, the gallbladder may be surrounded by omentum or adherent to the duodenum and contiguous structures. Depending on the evolution of the disease, there may be gross evidence of ischemia, particularly in the least vascularized portion of the gallbladder, the fundus. Histologically, acute cholecystitis is manifested by mucosal and subserosal edema, hypervascularity, and infiltration of the submucosa with polymorphonuclear leukocytes. In addition to the changes typical of acute cholecystitis, most acutely diseased gallbladders also have evidence of chronic inflammation, with lymphocytic infiltration of the submucosal layer and flattening of the mucosa.

Bacteriology. In normal, healthy persons without gallstones, the incidence of positive bile cultures is essentially zero. In contrast, between 30% and 70% of patients with the clinical diagnosis of acute cholecystitis have positive bile cultures. Most of the bacteria cultured from these patients are of enteric origin, with the most common organism being *Escherichia coli.* Other bacteria typically found include species of *Enterobacter, Klebsiella,* and *Enterococcus.* The incidence of positive bile cultures is significantly higher in patients with acute cholecystitis (30% to 70%) compared with patients with chronic cholecystitis who are operated on for biliary colic (20% to 50%). The presence of bacteria in the bile of patients with acute cholecystitis is a source of significant morbidity and mortality. In most cases, the organisms leading to wound infection are identical to those found in the patient's bile. Prospective studies have demonstrated that the incidence of positive bile cultures increases significantly with age. The incidence of positive bile cultures in patients who undergo cholecystectomy is somewhere between 20% and 30% for those under 50 years of age and increases to over 50% for those 70 years of age or older.

Septic complications continue to be a source of significant morbidity after cholecystectomy, particularly when the indication for operation is acute cholecystitis. These septic complications can best be prevented by the judicious use of appropriate antimicrobial agents. The goal of antimicrobial therapy should be to establish adequate serum and tissue levels of antibiotic rather than to select an antibiotic that is excreted into the bile. Risk factors for the development of septic complications after cholecystectomy include patient age over 70 years, operation for acute cholecystitis, history of obstructive jaundice, and the presence of common duct stones with or without jaundice. Prospective studies have confirmed the benefit of prophylactic antibiotic therapy for these patients. Given the bacteriology that is typical of patients with uncomplicated cho-

lecystitis, appropriate antibiotic regimens should provide for adequate coverage of gram-negative aerobes. Anaerobic infections, such as *Clostridium perfringens*, are unusual but may be identified with intraoperative Gram stain. If a septic complication develops postoperatively, the choice of antibiotics should be based on operative cultures as well as cultures from the wound or intraabdominal fluid collections.

MANAGEMENT OF GALLSTONES
Cholecystectomy

The earliest attempts at surgical treatment for gallstone disease focused on cholecystostomy and stone removal. Surgeons realized, however, that this approach was associated with a significant risk of gallstone recurrence, approaching 50% to 80% within 5 years. In 1882, Carl Langenbuch performed the first successful cholecystectomy, and this procedure quickly became the procedure of choice for treating patients with cholelithiasis. For the last 100 years, open cholecystectomy has been the standard of care. The development of laparoscopic techniques for gallbladder removal has revolutionized the approach to patients with symptomatic gallstone disease. Over the past 5 years, laparoscopic cholecystectomy has supplanted open cholecystectomy as the treatment of choice in managing calculous biliary disease.

Open Cholecystectomy

Experience with open cholecystectomy is vast, spanning generations of surgeons and having been practiced in virtually every country throughout the world. Over time, this operation has proved to be safe and effective. In a collected series of about 20,000 patients who underwent cholecystectomy between 1946 and 1973 at 10 different institutions, from the United States and throughout the world, the overall mortality rate was 1.6%. This figure is comparable to a 1.7% mortality rate reported for more than 12,000 patients operated on for calculous biliary tract disease between 1932 and 1979 at a single US university center. In this latter group, the operative mortality rate for patients who underwent elective cholecystectomy was 0.1%.[11] More recently, a US population-based study examining the outcome of all open cholecystectomies performed in a 12-month period in two states reported an overall mortality rate of 0.17%, morbidity rate of 14.7%, and estimated incidence of bile duct injuries of 0.2%[12] (Table 41-3). In this study, morbidity and mortality were dependent on age as

Table 41-3. IMPACT OF DISEASE STATUS ON OUTCOME: OPEN CHOLECYSTECTOMY

	Disease Status		
	Chronic	Acute	Complicated
Number	27,892	13,246	1336
Percentage of group	65.7	31.2	3.1
Morbidity rate (%)	11.9	19.4*	25.2*
Deaths	29	34	8
Mortality rate (%)	0.10	0.26*	0.60*
Length of stay (d)	4.8	6.6*	8.6*
Cost ($)	5,881	9,043*	12,510*

* *P* <.0001 versus chronic cholecystitis.
(Roslyn JJ, Binns GS, Hughes FX, et al. Open cholecystectomy: a contemporary analysis of 42,474 patients. Ann Surg 1993;218:129)

Table 41-4. EFFECT OF AGE ON OUTCOME: OPEN CHOLECYSTECTOMY

	Age (y)	
	<65	>65
Number	30,059	12,415
Percentage of group	70.8	29.2
Morbidity rate (%)	10.2	25.7*
Deaths	9	62
Mortality rate (%)	0.3	0.50*
Length of stay (d)	4.7	7.3*
Cost ($)	5,980	9,728

* $P < .0001$ versus age <65 y.
(Roslyn JJ, Binns GS, Hughes FX, et al. Open cholecystectomy: a contemporary analysis of 42,474 patients. Ann Surg 1993;218:129)

Table 41-5. COMPLICATIONS OF LAPAROSCOPIC CHOLECYSTECTOMY IN 77,604 PATIENTS

Complication	Patients
Bile duct injury	459 (0.6%)
Vascular injury	193 (0.25%)
Bowel injury	109 (0.14%)
Mortality	33 (0.04%)

(Modified from Deziel DJ, Millikan KK, et al. Complications of laparoscopic cholecystectomy: a national survey of 4,292 hospitals and an analysis of 77,604 cases. Am J Surg 1993;165:9)

well as disease status (Table 41-4). These as well as other data reported from several US surgical centers have shown that open cholecystectomy can be performed with a mortality rate that approaches zero.[13] These rates of morbidity and mortality have become the standard against which newer operative treatment modalities must be compared. In elective situations, open cholecystectomy is being performed in most hospitals throughout the world on patients who are admitted the day of surgery with an overall stay of 2 to 4 days.

Laparoscopic Cholecystectomy

In 1988, anecdotal reports suggested that the gallbladder could be removed laparoscopically without the need for laparotomy. In recent years, laparoscopic cholecystectomy has become the treatment of choice rather than open cholecystectomy for managing calculous biliary disease. The indications for laparoscopic cholecystectomy are analagous to open cholecystectomy and include the presence of symptomatic gallstones. Occasionally, asymptomatic patients or individuals with atypical symptoms or complaints suggestive of biliary dyskinesia should be considered for gallbladder removal, either laparoscopically or using the open technique.

As experience with this technology has increased, recommendations regarding contraindications for it have evolved. Absolute contraindications include inability to perform laparascopic cholecystectomy because of inadequate training or equipment, poor candidate for general anesthesia, uncorrected coagulopathy, peritonitis, or suspected gallbladder carcinoma. Judgment should be exercised when considering laparoscopic cholecystectomy for patients with acute cholecystitis, morbid obesity, previous upper abdominal surgery, cirrhosis and portal hypertension, or pregnancy.

Despite early experiences that suggested a higher incidence of common bile duct injury using this technique, recent large-series reports from Canada,[14] Europe,[15] and the United States[16,17] confirm that laparoscopic cholecystectomy can be performed safely with overall morbidity rates ranging from 3% to 10%, and mortality rates between 0 and 0.1%. Injury to the bile ducts occurs in 0.2% to 0.6% of cases (Table 41-5).

There is a definite learning curve associated with performing laparoscopic cholecystectomy (Fig. 41-13). Bile duct injuries are most likely to occur during one's early operative experience with this procedure[18]. Recognizing this fact points to the need for especially close supervision by an experienced laparoscopic surgeon during the early training period. Widespread acceptance for this technique

is growing because of the obvious advantages of reduced hospital days, earlier return to normal activity, less pain, and better cosmesis. A 1992 National Institutes of Health consensus conference recognized the value of laparascopic cholecystectomy and recommended that efforts be made to make this procedure as safe and cost-effective as possible. Principles of performing laparascopic cholecystectomy have been well described and certain technical points differ from conventional open cholecystectomy (Fig. 41-14).

Delayed Versus Early Cholecystectomy

The issue of delayed versus early cholecystectomy in patients with acute cholecystitis has long been the focus of debate and controversy. Traditionally, the standard practice was to admit patients with acute cholecystitis to the hospital for intravenous therapy and antibiotics. As the inflammatory process resolved, these patients would be discharged with the plan to perform an elective cholecystectomy 6 to 10 weeks later. The rationale for this strategy was to allow resolution of the acute inflammatory process and to facilitate the operative procedure. This traditional approach of intense medical management was challenged by a number of reports that demonstrated significant advantages to early cholecystectomy. These studies indicated that morbidity and mortality were no different in patients who underwent early or delayed cholecystectomy and that early cholecystectomy was associated with reduced hospitalization, cost, and episodes of

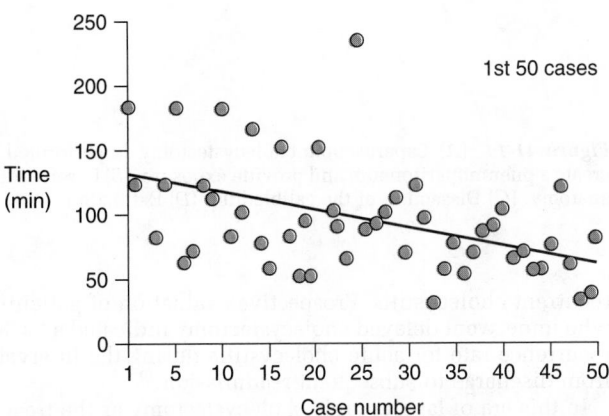

Figure 41-13. Data demonstrating the learning curve for performance of LC as reflected by time required. (Peters JH, Ellison EC, Innes JT, et al. Safety and efficacy of laparoscopic cholecystectomy: a prospective analysis of 100 initial patients. Ann Surg 1991;213:3)

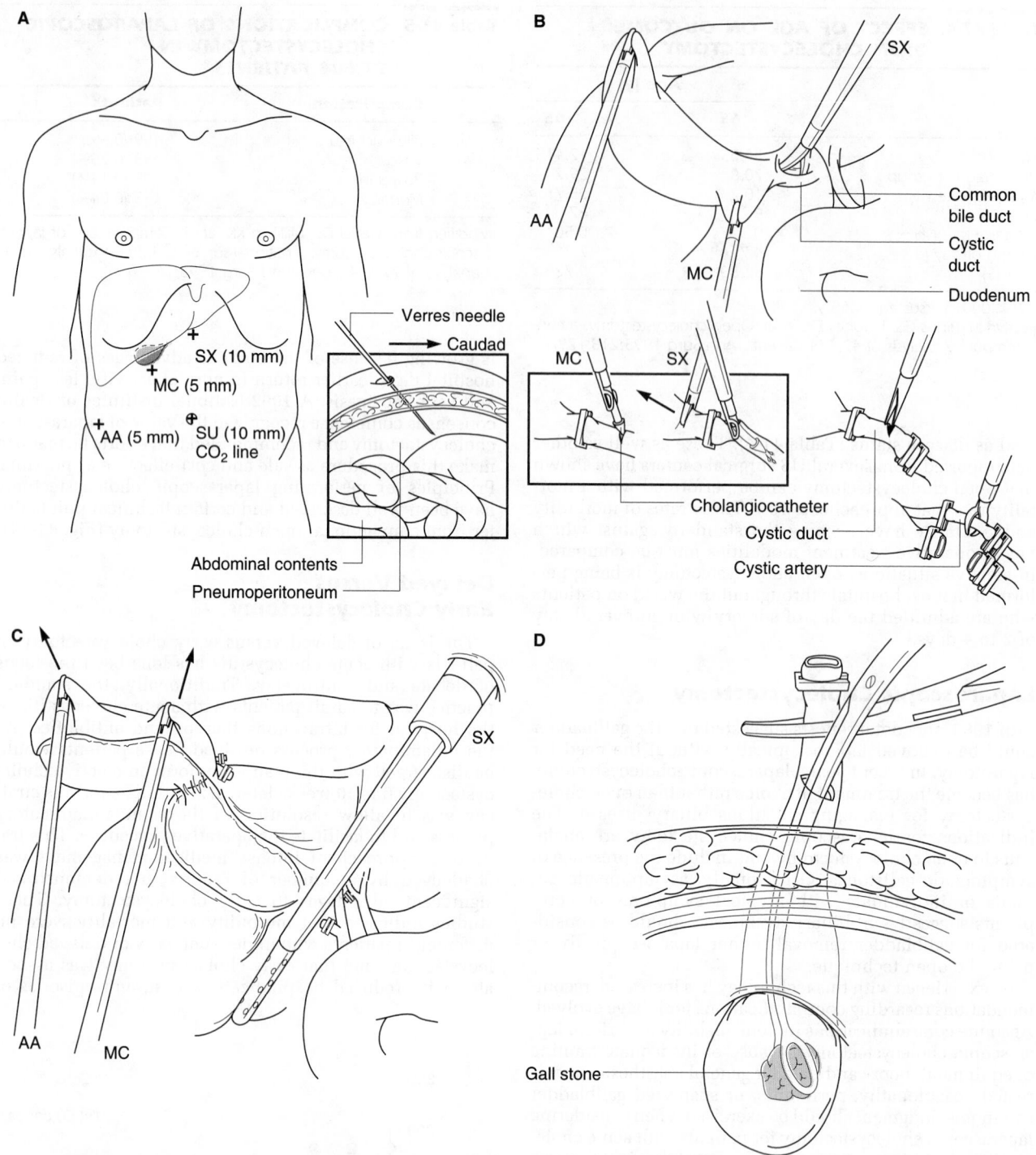

Figure 41-14. (*A*) Laparoscopic cholecystectomy is performed in a series of steps designed to create a pneumoperitoneum and provide exposure. (*B*) Careful identification of ductal and vascular anatomy. (*C*) Dissection of the gallbladder. (*D*) Extraction.

recurrent cholecystitis. Prospective evaluation of patients who underwent delayed cholecystectomy indicated a 24% recurrence rate for acute cholecystitis during the interval from discharge to subsequent readmission.[19]

In this era of laparoscopic cholecystectomy as the treatment of choice, the debate has shifted in favor of early rather than delayed intervention as morbidity and mortality appear to be the same or even less when the gallbladder is removed expeditiously in patients with acute cholecystitis. An initial attempt to laparoscopically remove the gall-

bladder should be considered, although both patient and physician should recognize that conversion to an open procedure may be required. Most series suggest that the rate of converting from elective laparoscopic cholecystectomy to open cholecystectomy approximates 3% to 5%, whereas in the setting of acute cholecystitis, the rate should be 20% to 30%. Performing laparoscopic cholecystectomy in the presence of acute inflammation can be challenging, and this procedure should only be undertaken by experienced laparoscopists. Surgeons should be cognizant of the following specific principles that may apply to safely performing laparascopic cholecystectomy in the setting of acute cholecystitis:

1. Exposure and retraction are essential.
2. Large, sharp forceps should be used for grasping.
3. The gallbladder should be decompressed.
4. Anatomy should be defined before the structures are divided.
5. Cholangiography should be considered.
6. Sufficient time should be allowed.
7. There is a low threshold for conversion to open cholecystectomy.

Role of Intraoperative Cholangiography

Common bile duct stones are found in about 8% to 12% of all patients who undergo cholecystectomy for symptomatic gallstone disease. An effective way to identify common duct calculi uses intraoperative cholangiography. In most instances, this is accomplished by the placing a small catheter through the cystic duct and instilling 10 to 20 mL of dye. A retrospective review of 4000 patients who underwent cholecystectomy during a 25-year period suggests that the decrease in unnecessary duct explorations resulting from routine intraoperative cholangiography is the single most important factor in reducing the overall mortality associated with cholecystectomy. Many arguments against the routine use of cholangiography relate to technical aspects of the procedure, wasted time and expense, and false-positive studies. The introduction of the movable C arm and fluoroscopic cholangiography has allowed the surgeon to definitively identify and evaluate the biliary ductal system in a matter of minutes and has greatly facilitated intraoperative evaluation.

Considerable discussion has focused on the role of intraoperative cholangiography in the performance of laparascopic cholecystectomy. Initial recommendations included routine intraoperative cholangiography to identify ductular anatomy and hopefully reduce the incidence of common bile duct injury. Current thought subscribes to using selective intraoperative cholangiography during laparascopic cholecystectomy, employing criteria that is analagous for open cholecystectomy. When anatomic structures are not clearly distinguishable during laparascopic cholecystectomy, intraoperative cholangiography is mandated to avoid serious injury to vital structures. Inability to perform intraoperative cholangiography under these circumstances represents an indication for conversion to an open procedure.

Medical Dissolution

Dissolution of existing gallstones with pharmacologic agents has long been a treatment goal. Confirmation of the hypothesis that altered hepatic secretion of cholesterol is a primary factor in the pathogenesis of cholesterol gallstones has prompted numerous attempts at gallstone dissolution by reducing bile lithogenicity. Years of intense investigation culminated in the identification and subsequent commercial release of chenodeoxycholic acid (CDCA). Data from the National Cooperative Gallstone Study, which included more than 900 patients, helped establish the rate and frequency of stone dissolution with CDCA.[20] Patients meeting criteria for selection were randomly assigned to receive high-dose CDCA, low-dose CDCA, or placebo. The rate of complete stone disappearance was only 13.5% in the high-dose CDCA group, and another 28% in this group had partial dissolution. In addition to this disappointingly

low success rate, other problems have been identified with the use of CDCA, including the need for at least 9 months of intense therapy and probably a lifetime of maintenance therapy to prevent recurrence of stones; the need to limit dietary cholesterol, especially among obese patients; potential toxicity and side effects; and high cost. As with any therapy that leaves the gallbladder in situ, gallstone recurrence is a major problem. Actuarial life-table analysis indicates that the risk of gallstone recurrence in patients who have undergone dissolution of gallstones with oral bile acid therapy is 12.5% after 1 year, 50% by 5 years, and 61% by 11 years. CDCA reportedly desaturates bile and dissolves cholesterol gallstones by a mechanism independent of simple expansion of bile salt pool size. CDCA is a specific inhibitor of HMG-CoA reductase, the rate limiting enzyme for cholesterol biosynthesis.

Ursodeoxycholic acid (UDCA) is now commercially available. Initial data suggest that this agent may be a better, safer, and more effective drug for gallstone dissolution than CDCA. Even with UDCA, however, the rate of complete dissolution only approaches 40%. It has been estimated that only 10% of all US patients with gallstones would be suitable candidates for medical dissolution therapy. The indications for the use of CDCA and UDCA are limited, particularly since the introduction of laparascopic cholecystectomy.

The mechanism by which UDCA affects desaturation and gallstone dissolution has not been completely elucidated. Although it was initially thought to affect cholesterol synthesis, UDCA now appears to act by modifying cholesterol absorption. In addition, there is evidence that UDCA may have a primary effect on cholesterol nucleation. In patients with cholesterol gallstones, the administration of low-dose UDCA significantly decreases the cholesterol saturation index and prolongs nucleation time. Furthermore, 3 months of treatment with UDCA significantly increased the serum concentration of apolipoprotein A-I, suggesting that this serum lipoprotein may play a role in the observed effects on nucleation time.

Medical dissolution of gallstones has been achieved only in cholesterol gallstones. Limited information is available on the dissolution of noncholesterol, calcium bilirubinate stones. A series of in vitro investigations, however, suggests that pigment gallstone material can be solubilized by a solvent system that contains a mucolytic agent, a chelating agent, and a strong detergent. Further research is clearly needed in the area of medical dissolution for both cholesterol and noncholesterol gallstones.

Contact Dissolution

Percutaneous transhepatic cholecystolitholysis (direct contact dissolution) has been recommended as a potential therapy for patients with symptomatic cholesterol gallstone disease.[21] The rationale for this technique is based on percutaneous transhepatic catheter placement in the gallbladder and infusion of an agent that has a high capacity for cholesterol dissolution. The procedure involves the percutaneous placement of a pigtail catheter through the liver and into the gallbladder, with rapid alternating infusion and aspiration of a specific agent that dissolves cholesterol (Fig. 41-15). This can be accomplished using local analgesia and fluoroscopic or ultrasonographic guidance. Preliminary studies suggest that this procedure can be done safely in carefully selected patients with a relatively high degree of success.

Methyl tert-butyl ether (MTBE) is an aliphatic ether, liquid at body temperature, that rapidly dissolves cholesterol. Preliminary animal and human studies suggested that this agent was as well tolerated as dimethyl ether and would

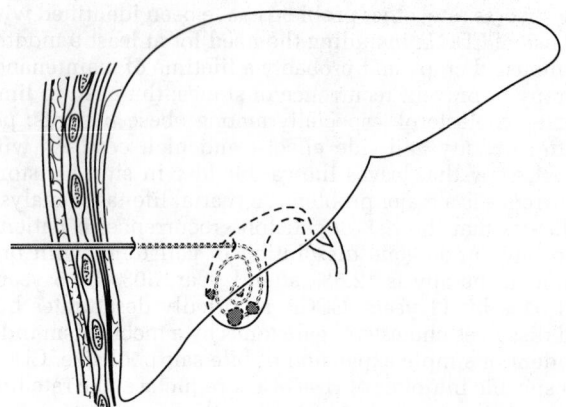

Figure 41-15. Schematic demonstration of the technique of percutaneous placement of pigtail catheter into the gallbladder. Methyl tert-butyl ether is infused and aspirated through the catheter.

be effective in dissolving cholesterol gallstones. MTBE has been used in only a small number of patients. Patient selection is of utmost importance, and potential candidates for MTBE dissolution include high-risk patients with symptomatic stones or those who refuse operation. For this modality to be effective, stones must be composed of cholesterol, and a patent cystic duct must be demonstrated by either oral cholecystography or biliary scintigraphy. Documented side effects include transient abdominal pain, nausea, emesis, duodenitis, sedation, and complications directly related to catheter placement. Stones have been documented to reoccur in about 10% of patients who have been followed for 36 months. Although experience with this procedure is limited, it has been estimated that 30% of patients have evidence of stone recurrence in 2 years, and 60% within 5 years. Although this modality may have specific indications, its application to the general population is limited.

Biliary Lithotripsy

In 1980, electrohydraulic shock wave lithotripsy (ESWL) was introduced as a treatment for patients with nephroureterolithiasis. This therapy has since been applied to more than 500,000 patients and has largely replaced open surgical procedures for the management of kidney stones. Although the inherent anatomic and physiologic differences between the genitourinary and biliary tracts prompted early concern about the efficacy and potential side effects of biliary lithotripsy, considerable experience has been gained with ESWL.[22]

The scientific principle underlying the use of this technology is based on the generation of high-energy shock waves within a water medium. These shock waves, composed of both high and low frequencies, can be generated by electromagnetically produced deflections of a membrane, underwater spark discharges, or piezoelectric crystals. These shock waves travel faster than the speed of sound and, when focused on a specific point, can cause fragmentation.

Potential advantages of biliary lithotripsy include shortened hospitalization, avoidance of surgical intervention and associated complications, and high rate of acceptance by patients. Based on preliminary trials, a number of selection criteria were established: history of biliary tract pain; one to three radiolucent gallbladder stones with diameters less than 30 mm; and a functioning gallbladder as demon-

strated by oral cholecystography. Patients who were specifically excluded from consideration for biliary lithotripsy included those with more than three stones, very large or calcified stones, a nonfunctioning gallbladder, or manifest complications of gallstone disease, such as cholecystitis, cholangitis, jaundice, or pancreatitis. Inclusion criteria may be broadened in the future. In a series of 62 patients of whom 60% were estimated to be noncandidates for lithotripsy using conventional criteria, complete stone clearance was achieved in about 60%.[23] Although this was a limited study, the authors suggested that selection criteria for patients undergoing biliary lithotripsy should be broadened. Applying present exclusion criteria, the suitability for ESWL was assessed in 100 consecutive patients who underwent cholecystectomy at a university center.[24] The results from this study suggested that only 19% of US patients undergoing cholecystectomy would be eligible for ESWL. This figure is similar to that reported in the European literature. In preliminary studies using lithotripsy combined with adjuvant and litholytic medications (usually UDCA), gallstone fragmentation has been achieved in virtually all selected patients. Fragment clearance occurred within 2 months in 30% of patients, within 4 months in 48%, and in 91% of patients between 12 and 18 months. These early results have been confirmed by subsequent reports, including a national cooperative study that consisted of more than 200 patients.[25] In patients who underwent ESWL for asymptomatic gallstone disease, 35% experienced transient biliary colic, 5% had cystic duct obstruction, and 2% had evidence of mild pancreatitis. Prior to 1989, ESWL appeared to be the most promising nonoperative modality for managing symptomatic gallstones. The widespread application of laparascopic cholecystectomy has caused this concept to be reevaluated.

Nonoperative Treatment for Gallstone Disease: Unresolved Issues

Medical dissolution, contact dissolution, and biliary lithotripsy have all been advocated as important adjuvant modalities for treating patients with gallstone disease. Their widespread application has been limited by various critical factors including recurrence rates, cost, need for careful patient selection, and perhaps most importantly by the emergence of laparascopic cholecystectomy. Technologic refinements will almost certainly improve the overall efficacy of these modalities. Nonetheless, it is doubtful that any will evolve as a major intervention now that stone disease can be cured in most patients with a relatively simple, minimally invasive procedure.

CHOLECYSTITIS IN SPECIFIC CLINICAL SETTINGS

Acalculous Cholecystitis

Acalculous cholecystitis is an unusual but potentially lethal complication of gallbladder disease. The cause of this clinical entity has not yet been determined. Most clinical and experimental studies suggest a multifactorial etiology that varies, depending on the clinical situation. Stasis of bile in the gallbladder has long been considered an important factor in the pathogenesis of this disorder. Biliary stasis can occur as a result of ampullary spasm secondary to the administration of narcotics, decreased gallbladder emptying during periods of prolonged fasting, or cystic duct occlusion secondary to edema. Moreover, altered viscosity of bile as a result of dehydration and multiple transfusions with an associated increase in pigment load has also been implicated as an important factor. The combination of biliary stasis and increased bile viscosity may lead to altered concentration of specific biliary lipids and other luminal factors that may predispose to irritation and inflammation of the gallbladder mucosa. In this manner, a cascade of events could be initiated with the release of specific biochemical mediators of the inflammatory response.

The estimated incidence of acute acalculous cholecystitis is about 3% of all surgical biliary tract cases treated in most large centers. Acalculous cholecystitis has been reported as a postoperative complication and in critically ill patients following trauma or burns. Most postoperative patients who develop acute acalculous cholecystitis have had an intraabdominal procedure 2 to 14 days before the onset of symptoms. Diagnosis of acalculous cholecystitis poses a considerable challenge to the clinician, especially when it occurs in intensive care unit patients. These patients typically have multiple medical and surgical problems, and as a result, the diagnosis may be delayed. Several studies suggest that the associated morbidity and mortality rates of acalculous cholecystitis, when it occurs in intensive care patients, is between 40% and 60%. The liberal use of ultrasound for early diagnosis and operative treatment may reduce the mortality associated with this disease; portable ultrasound is available in most institutions and can be brought to the bedside. Surgical treatment is warranted for all patients with acute acalculous cholecystitis. Cholecystectomy may be contraindicated because of the patient's unstable overall condition. Under these circumstances, a cholecystostomy, either through a minilaparotomy or percutaneously, is the procedure of choice. Percutaneous cholecystectomy can be safely performed by interventional radiologists in most centers. Although this procedure allows for the decompression and drainage of infected gallbladder bile, it obviously does not cure gangrenous cholecystitis.

Diabetes and Cholecystitis

For many years, it has been assumed that diabetics have an increased incidence of cholesterol gallstones and are more likely to develop acute cholecystitis with a greater incidence of postoperative complications. Anecdotal experience suggested that diabetics were more susceptible to septic complications, presumably due to some defect in immune function. Such a defect has yet to be identified. Nonetheless, the recommendation in many areas was that diabetics should be considered for early cholecystectomy regardless of severity or nature of symptoms. Given the large number of patients involved, the full implementation of this policy would have significant social and economic impact. In a recent prospective review of 175 diabetic and nondiabetic patients who underwent cholecystectomy, the incidence of gallbladder perforation, wound infection, and overall morbidity and mortality was not significantly different between the two groups.[26] These authors concluded that diabetes itself is not a significant risk factor for severe biliary tract disease. In addition, they recommended that decision making in diabetic cases should be based on criteria that apply to all patients, regardless of presence or absence of diabetes. This remains, however, a very controversial issue.

Cholecystitis in the Elderly

Considerable evidence indicates that gallstone disease is more virulent in the elderly than in the younger population. This contention is based on clinical observations demonstrating an increased incidence of choledocholithiasis, emphysematous cholecystitis, perforation of the gallbladder, and septic complications of cholecystitis in the elderly. Although some have proposed that these findings are secondary to differences in the evolution of the disease process, it is more likely that they represent the by-product of delayed diagnosis. Risk/benefit analyses suggest that elective cholecystectomy can be safely performed in elderly patients with minimal morbidity and mortality. Moreover, the reported five-fold increase in mortality when emergency cholecystectomy is performed in the elderly suggests that an aggressive attitude is warranted in the elderly patient with symptomatic gallstone disease. The two most common causes of death in older patients who undergo cholecystectomy are sepsis and cardiovascular disease. In a series of 88 elderly patients who underwent cholecystectomy, the overall mortality rate was 7%—nearly 10 times the rate for younger patients. The importance of timing of treatment in the elderly patient with acute cholecystitis is underscored by analysis of these data. Medical therapy, consisting of intravenous fluids and antibiotics, was attempted in 44% of these patients with cholecystitis. Emergency cholecystectomy became necessary in 97% of this subgroup because of failure to respond to conservative supportive treatment. The morbidity and mortality rates were 44% and 10% respectively in patients who required emergency cholecystectomy. In contrast, the morbidity and mortality rates were 22% and 2% in the group of patients who underwent semiurgent operations. Elderly patients with acute cholecystitis are best treated by timely diagnosis, early stabilization, and semiurgent cholecystectomy. Choledocholithiasis has been reported in 20% to 54% of elderly patients undergoing cholecystectomy. This figure is in contrast to the 8% to 12% rate of common duct stones reported in the general population. The increased incidence of common duct stones in the elderly probably reflects long-standing, untreated disease. The clinical impact of this increased incidence of choledocholithiasis in the elderly is underscored by the mortality rates for common duct exploration, which increase with age. The mortality rate associated with choledochotomy is 0.9% in patients younger than age 50 years and 7.6% to 29% in patients older than age 70 years.

Cirrhosis and Cholecystitis

Regardless of the type of gallstones present, several studies have demonstrated that cholecystectomy in cirrhotic patients is associated with significant rates of morbidity (50%) and mortality (10%). Difficulties encountered in cirrhotic patients who undergo cholecystectomy are due to associated portal hypertension, thrombocytopenia secondary to hypersplenism, and coagulopathy. Indications for cholecystectomy in a cirrhotic patient should be more restrictive than in the noncirrhotic patient. Operations should be undertaken only in patients who are truly symptomatic or who have developed one of the complications of gallstone disease, such as acute cholecystitis, perforation, fistula formation, or empyema of the gallbladder. Much of the bleeding encountered during cholecystectomy in the cirrhotic patient results from attempts to completely remove the gallbladder from its hepatic bed. It is acceptable to leave the posterior wall of the gallbladder in situ under these circumstances and to perform a partial cholecystectomy with cauterization of the remaining mucosa.

Total Parenteral Nutrition–Induced Gallbladder Disease

The reported incidence of asymptomatic and symptomatic gallstone disease in the subset of patients receiving long-term TPN (both children and adults) is between 40%

and 45%. The diagnosis of gallbladder disease in patients maintained on long-term TPN may not be readily apparent because of the complex underlying gastrointestinal disorders often present in these patients. This finding may contribute to the delay in diagnosing symptomatic biliary disease in this setting. One report indicated that 40% of patients with TPN-induced gallbladder disease required emergency cholecystectomy, and severe acute cholecystitis was present in more than 50%.[27] The reported morbidity and mortality rates associated with cholecystectomy were 54% and 11%, respectively. In this high-risk group, early cholecystectomy is indicated when stones first appear and should be considered in patients without stones who are committed to a long-term course of TPN and who are undergoing laparotomy for other reasons. Pharmacologic prophylaxis with periodic stimulated gallbladder contraction is practiced in some centers, and its clinical value should be further explored.

COMPLICATIONS OF CHOLECYSTITIS

Hydrops

Obstruction of the cystic duct by an impacted stone can result in hydrops, in which the gallbladder becomes filled with a clear or whitish mucoid material. Little is known about the pathophysiology of hydrops of the gallbladder except that the mucoid material probably results from altered gallbladder epithelial secretion. The gallbladder frequently becomes enlarged, and patients may present with signs and symptoms suggestive of acute cholecystitis, although occasionally, their only complaint is of a mass in the right upper quadrant. Cholecystectomy is the treatment of choice.

Emphysematous Cholecystitis

Emphysematous cholecystitis is an unusual but potentially lethal complication of cholecystitis and is manifested by the radiographic demonstration of gas within either the gallbladder lumen or wall. This entity accounts for about 1% of all cases of cholecystitis. Interestingly, stones are absent in about one third of patients with acute emphysematous cholecystitis. Emphysematous cholecystitis is more common in elderly men, and about 40% of all cases occur in diabetics. The radiographic demonstration of gas within the lumen of the gallbladder wall occurs as a result of gas-producing bacteria. The most common organisms cultured are *C perfringens*, although mixtures of this anaerobe with *E coli* and species of *Klebsiella* are also noted. The clinical course of patients with emphysematous cholecystitis is frequently characterized by rapid onset with severe abdominal pain, constitutional symptoms of nausea and vomiting, and evidence of severe sepsis. Common sequelae are gangrene (74%) and perforation of the gallbladder (21%). The potential for serious morbidity and mortality in patients with acute emphysematous cholecystitis is so great that emergent cholecystectomy is warranted when this diagnosis is suspected.

Empyema

Empyema of the gallbladder is a variant of acute cholecystitis. The pathogenesis of empyema is similar to acute uncomplicated cholecystitis, and the only significant difference is the presence of pus in the gallbladder lumen. These patients are often toxic, and emergent cholecystectomy is mandated.

Gallbladder Perforation

Perforation of the gallbladder occurs in about 3% to 10% of all patients with acute cholecystitis. This complication of biliary calculous disease has been traditionally classified into three types—type 1, acute free perforation with bile stained peritoneal fluid; type 2, subacute perforation with pericholecystic or right upper quadrant abscess formation; and type 3, chronic perforation with formation of either cholecystoenteric or cholecystocutaneous fistulas. Acute and subacute perforation of the gallbladder have been associated with underlying vascular, metabolic, or other disorders. Several authors have reported a 20% to 25% incidence of severe atherosclerotic heart disease or diabetes in patients with acute perforation of the gallbladder. The gallbladder fundus is the most common site of acute perforation. Anatomically, this area corresponds to the least vascularized portion of the gallbladder. In patients with subacute perforations or chronic perforations with fistula formation, repeated bouts of cholecystitis probably lead to scarring and fibrosis, with adherence of adjacent structures. Pressure necrosis and inflammation can develop around gallstones impacted in the wall of the gallbladder, with subsequent erosion of the stone through the gallbladder wall into contiguous organs. In most cases, this process occurs gradually so that protective adhesions between the gallbladder, omentum, and colon are formed and prevent diffuse contamination. In this setting, either a localized abscess or fistula results.

Although computed tomography (CT) may be an inferior modality for detecting gallstones, it is better than ultrasonography for detecting abscesses and free fluid that might be present in patients with either type 1 or 2 perforations. Barium upper gastrointestinal studies help define any fistulous communications among the stomach, duodenum, and gallbladder. Acute free perforation of the gallbladder is less common than the other types of perforation. The clinical suspicion of acute perforation of the gallbladder warrants prompt and aggressive treatment with fluid resuscitation, nasogastric decompression, intravenous administration of broad-spectrum antibiotics, and expeditious laparotomy. In a series of 51 patients with gallbladder perforation, the operative rates of morbidity (60%) and mortality (27%) were significantly greater in patients with acute free perforations than in those with type 2 or 3 perforations.[28]

Cholecystoenteric fistulas are the most common type of gallbladder perforation, accounting for about 40% of all reported cases. Depending on the size of the fistulous communication, a gallstone may pass through this tract. In most cases, the stone passes through the intestinal tract without symptoms. If a stone is large enough (greater than 2 cm in diameter), however, it may become lodged in a portion of the gastrointestinal tract and cause a mechanical small bowel obstruction. This condition, called *gallstone ileus*, is relatively rare and accounts for fewer than 5% of all cases of intestinal obstruction. The diagnosis of gallstone ileus may be suggested by the presence of intrahepatic biliary air on abdominal radiography. Patients with gallstone ileus are best treated as if they had mechanical small bowel obstruction, that is, with aggressive fluid resuscitation, broad-spectrum antibiotics, and early laparotomy. In most cases, the diagnosis is made at the time of laparotomy when a gallstone is palpated at the site of obstruction. Frequently, the stone is found in the terminal ileum. The primary goals at laparotomy are correction of the obstruction and removal of the offending stone. Since many of these patients are elderly and ill, cholecystectomy and take-down of the biliary enteric fistula may not be appropriate. Enterolithotomy alone, without cholecystectomy, has an associated mortality rate of 5% in contrast to the 15% mortality rate for patients who undergo both procedures at the same time.

CHOLEDOCHOLITHIASIS

Bile duct stones can be classified by stone composition, location in the biliary tract, time relation to cholecystectomy, and source. The most clinically useful and relevant system focuses on the source of bile duct stones as either primary or secondary. Primary common duct stones, also referred to as recurrent, are calculi that form de novo outside the gallbladder in either the intrahepatic or extrahepatic bile ducts. Secondary, or retained stones, form in the gallbladder and pass into the choledochus by the cystic duct or occasionally through a cholecystocholedochal fistula. The distinction between primary and secondary common duct stones has long been thought to have great therapeutic implications. Primary duct stones form as a result of biliary stasis and biliary infection; therefore, removing the stone without correcting the underlying abnormality may predispose to a high stone recurrence rate for patients with primary common duct stones. In contrast, secondary or retained stones can typically be removed without the need for a biliary bypass or drainage procedure. With the advent and widespread use of endoscopic sphincterotomy, many clinicians believe the issue of stone type is no longer of paramount importance in therapeutic decision making, since improved biliary drainage and stone removal can often be achieved without laparotomy.

Incidence

Although the definition of primary versus secondary stones seems straightforward, the criteria by which these stones are so designated continues to be an area of confusion. The incidence of bile duct stones in patients undergoing cholecystectomy for either acute or chronic cholecystitis is 8% to 15%. In addition, about 1% to 2% of all patients who undergo cholecystectomy have stones left in the bile duct that require further intervention. Depending on the criteria selected, the incidence of primary common bile duct stones in patients with documented choledocholithiasis varies widely. Criteria for primary common duct stones include previous cholecystectomy; at least a 2-year symptom-free period after cholecystectomy; the presence of soft, easily crushable, light-brown stones or sludge; and no evidence of a long cystic duct remnant or a biliary stricture resulting from prior surgery. Using these criteria, recurrent or primary bile duct stones probably account for 4% to 10% of all cases of choledocholithiasis.

Pathogenesis and Morphology of Common Bile Duct Stones

In general, retained common duct stones are biochemically similar to coexisting stones in the gallbladder. Almost all mixed or cholesterol stones found in the common bile duct are of gallbladder origin. Primary bile duct stones are exclusively of the pigment variety. They are classically described as earthy, soft, brown or yellowish tan, easily crushable, noncholesterol in nature, and conforming to the shape of the duct. Secondary bile duct stones, on the other hand, are similar in consistency to gallstones, are faceted, and often are cholesterol in nature. Primary stones lack a crystalline nidus and typically are associated with a variable amount of sludge or pasty concretions. In addition, the shape of primary common duct stones often conforms to that of the distal common bile duct. Biliary stasis has been implicated in the

pathogenesis of primary common duct stones. Early experimental evidence suggested that common duct stones formed in the presence of partial common bile duct obstruction. Ampullary stenosis and functional duct dilatation have been associated with an increased risk of primary common duct stone formation. Manometric studies indicate that aberrant patterns of sphincter of Oddi motility are present in patients with common duct stones. It remains to be determined, however, whether these findings are the cause or the effect of primary common duct stones. The presence of paravaterian diverticula of the duodenum has also been associated with an increased risk of choledocholithiasis.

Considerable evidence also links the presence of bacteria with formation of primary common duct stones. There is an increased incidence of positive bile cultures in patients with primary common duct stone disease. The obvious role of bacteria in Asian cholangiohepatitis suggests that the bacterial deconjugation of bilirubin by β-glucuronidase with the formation of insoluble bilirubin salts may play a critical role in primary common duct disease. Studies have identified bacterial microcolonies in the central matrix of common duct stones. Bacterial isolates in patients with brown-pigment common duct stones include the aerobic gram-negative rods *E coli* and *K pneumoniae* as well as anaerobes, including bacteroides and *Clostridium* sp. All these bacterial isolates possess β-glucuronidase activity at physiologic pH. This profile of biliary bacteria, with a predominance of aerobic organisms, is consistent with an ascending route of infection from the small intestine. The mechanism by which bacteria gain access to the common bile duct, as well as the relative contributions of stasis and abnormal biliary motility to the ultimate formation of primary common duct stones, remain to be investigated.

Natural History

The multifactorial origin of common duct stones, coupled with the heterogeneous settings in which they occur, has caused some difficulty in defining the natural history of choledocholithiasis. Stones may be present for years in the bile duct without causing any problems and may come to the attention of both patient and physician only when common duct obstruction occurs. When obstruction is sudden and complete, the patient frequently experiences biliary colic, bacteremia with chills, fever, leukocytosis, and the subsequent clinical development of jaundice. Although septic cholangitis may be the most dramatic manifestation of choledocholithiasis, a more gradual, progressive obstruction may also occur, with minimal symptomatology. When stones are in the bile duct but are not impacted, the symptom complex may be one of pruritus, with or without jaundice, transient elevation of alkaline phosphatase, and episodic abdominal or back discomfort. Small stones may enter the common bile duct from the gallbladder and actually pass into the duodenum without producing symptoms. Stones less than 3 mm in diameter rarely have clinical manifestations unless they accumulate simultaneously in the distal bile duct or become trapped in an abnormally narrowed bile duct or ampulla. As previously stated, stones that exceed the diameter of the ampulla may remain for years, causing minimal difficulty, or they may be associated with severe cholangitis. The uncertainties about the history of common duct stones suggest that the documentation of choledocholithiasis is an indication for stone removal. The best way to achieve this, however, is controversial.

Clinical Evaluation and Diagnosis

The critical factor in both the diagnostic evaluation and pathophysiology of common duct stone disease is obstruction of the common bile duct. Unlike malignant strictures,

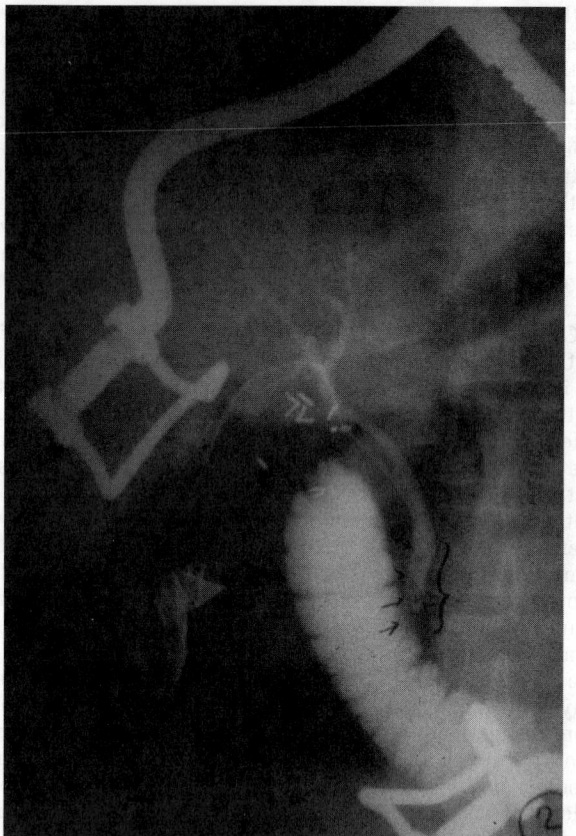

Figure 41-16. Intraoperative cholangiogram performed during OC demonstrating multiple, small, nonobstructing distal stones.

common duct obstruction from stone disease is typically characterized by incomplete obstruction, low levels of hyperbilirubinemia, and fluctuating symptoms of pain and jaundice. Although pain is unusual in patients with malignant strictures, it is present in more than 90% of patients with primary common duct stone disease and is frequently manifested by mid epigastric pain with radiation into the back. Charcot triad (jaundice, pain, and fever) is present in less than 25% of patients with choledocholithiasis. Laboratory evaluation provides important clinical information about the cause of jaundice. In the absence of significant obstruction, liver function tests may be normal. Serum alkaline phosphatase is the most sensitive indicator of ductal obstruction because this enzyme is released from the biliary ductal epithelium. Levels rise rapidly in response to duct obstruction. Serum glutamic oxaloacetic transaminase and serum glutamic pyruvic transaminase are released from injured hepatocytes, and although these levels may be elevated in patients with cholangitis, they are relatively normal in uncomplicated cases of choledocholithiasis.

While biochemical tests may provide evidence suggestive of extrahepatic biliary obstruction, further definition of biliary anatomy is generally useful in developing a management strategy. The first issue to resolve is whether there is intrahepatic or extrahepatic biliary dilatation or both. Ultrasonography has been shown to be a simple, safe, and accurate way to identify biliary dilatation. CT scans provide comparable information and also may identify mass lesions, such as tumors in the distal bile duct, periampullary region, or in the head of the pancreas. The presence of biliary dilatation in patients with known stone disease may suffice, and no further diagnostic evaluation may be necessary. It is often helpful, however, to further define

the biliary anatomy. This is particularly true in patients with primary common duct stones or in other settings in which the cause of the obstruction is unclear. Precise delineation of the intrahepatic and extrahepatic biliary tree and localization of anatomic abnormalities can best be achieved with either percutaneous transhepatic cholangiography or endoscopic retrograde cholangiopancreatography (ERCP). In patients with presumed primary common duct stone disease, ERCP offers certain advantages over percutaneous transhepatic cholangiography. ERCP provides visualization of the ampulla and periampullary region and allows for therapeutic intervention if sphincterotomy is indicated and feasible.

Clinical Syndromes

Management of Common Bile Duct Stones Found During Cholecystectomy

About 7% of patients who undergo elective cholecystectomy are found to have unsuspected common duct stones as documented by intraoperative cholangiography (Fig. 41-16). Complete stone removal is the goal for all common duct stones identified during cholecystectomy. The first step in the successful exploration of the common bile duct is to adequately dissect the choledochus. The bile duct should be dissected off its surrounding adventitia anteriorly for about 2 to 3 cm. In addition, mobilization of the duodenum (Kocher maneuver) is generally performed to

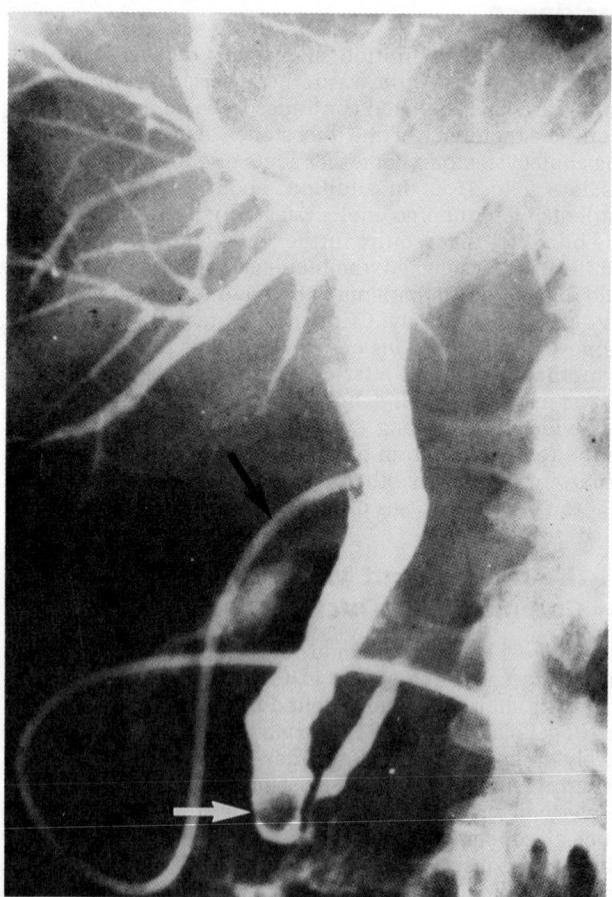

Figure 41-17. T-tube cholangiogram demonstrating retained gallstone in distal common bile duct (*white arrow*). The presence of a T tube (*black arrow*) and the size of the stone make this a favorable situation for radiologic extraction of stone.

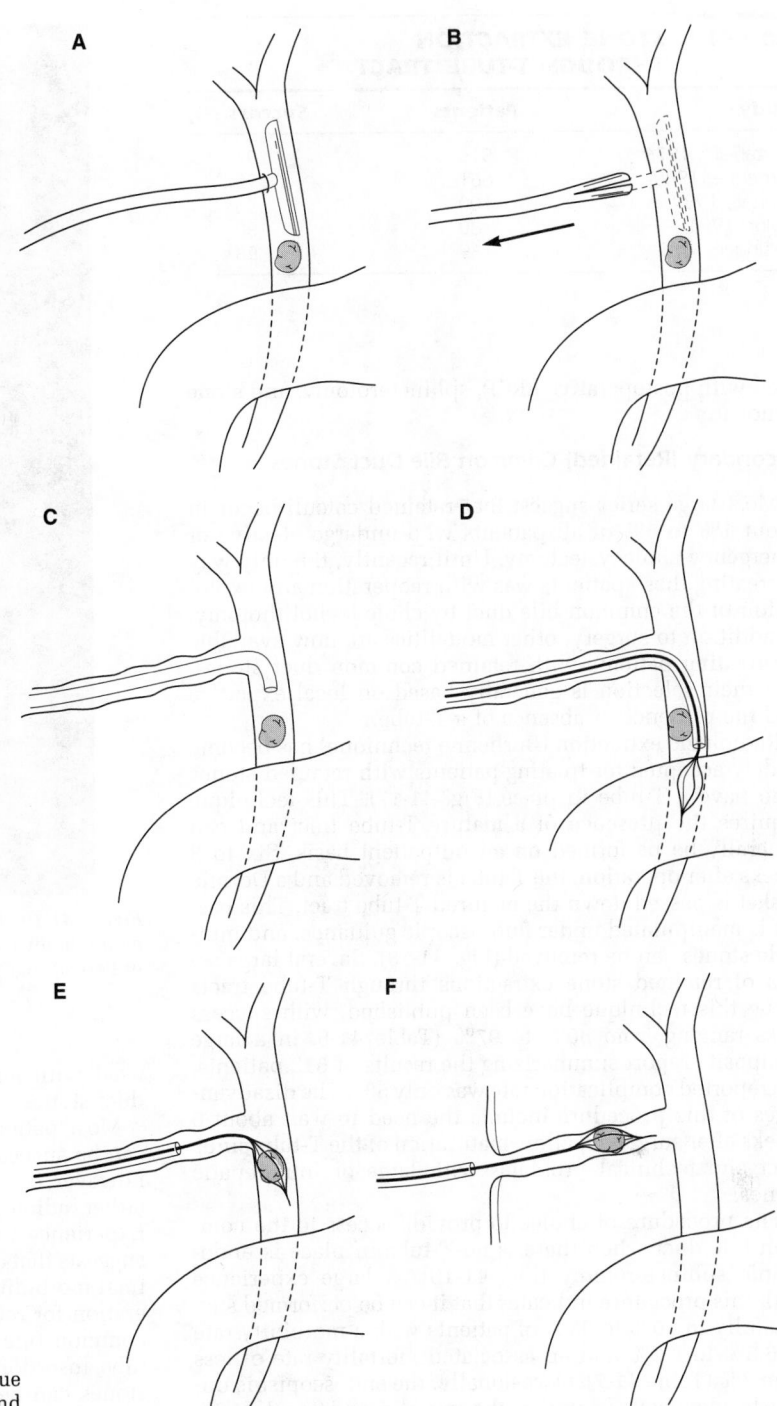

Figure 41-18. Illustration of Burhenne technique with placement of basket down matured tract and stone extraction.

facilitate guiding of instruments into the bile duct. Completion of the Kocher maneuver and adequate choledochotomy facilitates attempts at stone extraction with forceps, irrigation, or perhaps even by "milking" the duct. Choledochoscopy is a useful adjunct and improves the success rate of common bile duct exploration. In addition to visualizing stones, the choledochoscope often aids in their removal under direct vision with the use of endoscopic grasping forceps, baskets, or biliary balloons. Experience with completion cholangiography suggests that bile duct spasm can cause false-positive studies. For this reason, completion choledochoscopy is recommended to confirm that the duct has been cleared of all stones and associated debris.

Common bile duct stones found unexpectedly during a laparoscopic procedure present the surgeon with a different set of choices from that for stones found during an open procedure where one would invariably proceed to common duct exploration. Although converting to an open procedure for the purposes of common duct exploration is acceptable and should be considered based on the surgeon's experience and expertise, other options should also be entertained. Trancystic dilatation and exploration with stone removal is being performed more often and appears to be safe and effective. Laparascopic cholecystectomy is feasible for these cases, but experience is limited. Depending on the clinical situation, many surgeons may opt to complete the removal of the gallbladder and then pro-

Table 41-6. STONE EXTRACTION THROUGH T-TUBE TRACT

Study	Patients	Success (%)
Mazzariello, 1976	516	97
Burhenne, 1980	661	95
Caprine, 1980	100	96
Taylor, 1984	80	80
Geisinger, 1980	189	88

ceed with postoperative ERCP, sphincterotomy, and stone removal.

Secondary (Retained) Common Bile Duct Stones

Most large series suggest that retained calculi occur in about 1% to 5% of all patients who undergo elective or emergency cholecystectomy. Until recently, the only way of treating these patients was with reoperation and exploration of the common bile duct by choledocholithotomy. In addition to surgery, other modalities are now available for treating patients with retained common duct stones, and their selection is generally based on local expertise and the presence or absence of a T-tube.

Radiologic extraction (Burhenne technique) has become widely accepted for treating patients with retained stones who have a T-tube in place (Fig. 41-17). This technique requires the presence of a mature T-tube tract and can generally be performed on an outpatient basis. Six to 8 weeks after operation, the T-tube is removed and a Dormia basket is passed down the matured T-tube tract. This basket is manipulated under fluoroscopic guidance, and multiple stones can be removed (Fig. 41-18). Several large series of retained stone extractions through T-tube tracts using this technique have been published, with success rates ranging from 80% to 97% (Table 41-6). In a large composite report summarizing the results of 612 patients, the reported complication rate was only 5%. The disadvantages of this procedure include the need to wait about 6 weeks after surgery to allow maturation of the T-tube sinus tract and technical problems with large or intrahepatic stones.

The procedure of choice to provide access to the common bile duct when there is no T-tube in place is endoscopic sphincterotomy (Fig. 41-19). A large experience with this procedure indicates that it can be performed successfully in 80% to 95% of patients with a morbidity rate of 6.5% to 8.7% and an associated mortality rate of less than 2% (Table 41-7). Occasionally, the endoscopist is unable to adequately cannulate the ampulla, and transhepatic passage of a guide wire by the radiologist may facilitate this procedure. A multidisciplinary approach to retained common bile duct stones with a combination of radiologic and endoscopic technologies should be considered in such difficult cases.

The role of biliary lithotripsy has been evaluated in a multicenter trial involving 56 patients with bile duct stones. Stone fragmentation was successfully performed in 91% of patients, and clearance occurred in 79%. Although more experience must be gained with this new modality, ESWL may be a safe and effective adjunct to the treatment of bile duct stones in certain patients. A number of chemical solvents have been applied topically to dissolve bile duct stones. MTBE has been used successfully in the contact dissolution of gallbladder stones, but its role in the dissolution of bile duct stones has not been well defined. To date, monooctanoic acid is the only agent that has been

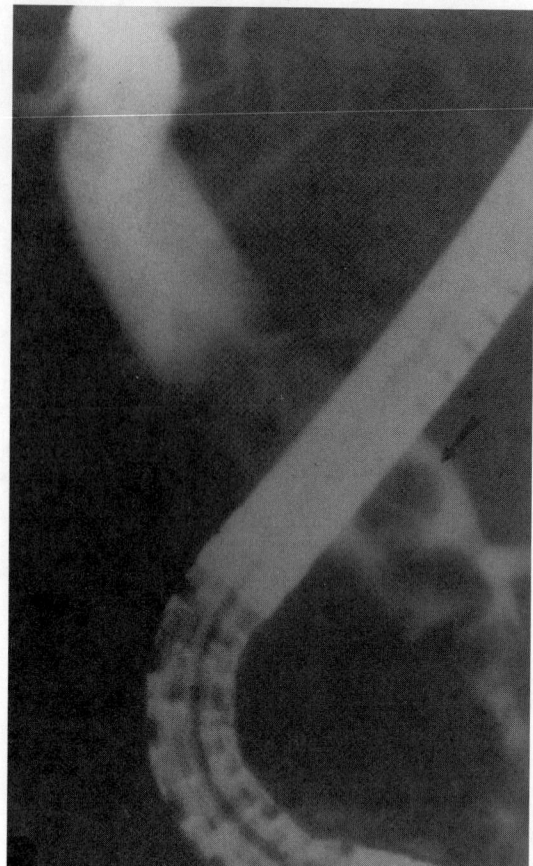

Figure 41-19. ERCP demonstrating multiple stones in distal common bile duct. Complete duct clearance was ultimately achieved in two sittings after endoscopic sphincterotomy.

used with any success to dissolve cholesterol common duct stones.

Most patients with retained common bile duct stones can be successfully treated nonoperatively. Occasionally, however, common bile duct stones may not be amenable to either radiologic extraction or endoscopic sphincterotomy. Experience with reoperation for retained bile duct stones suggests that operations can be performed safely with minimal morbidity and mortality. Most patients requiring operation for retained common duct stones should undergo common bile duct exploration, stone extraction, and T-tube insertion. Generally, when reoperation is required, stones can be adequately removed, so a drainage procedure, such as transduodenal sphincteroplasty or biliary enteric bypass, is not needed. If, however, patients have

Table 41-7. ENDOSCOPIC SPHINCTEROTOMY FOR BILE DUCT STONES

Study	Patients	Success (%)	Morbidity (%)	Mortality (%)
Viceconte, 1981	296	86	7	0.8
Leese, 1985	394	98	10	0.8
Safrany, 1977	265	92	10	1.2
Koch, 1977	267	95	7	0.8
Siegel, 1981	267	97	5	0.8
Escourrou, 1983	443	92	7	1.5
Wurbs, 1983	808	95	7	1.4

multiple stones or subsequently develop evidence of retained common bile duct stones after initial reexploration and require another reoperation, a biliary drainage procedure is advised.

Primary (Recurrent) Common Bile Duct Stones

Experience has demonstrated the efficacy of ERCP with endoscopic sphincterotomy for treating patients with primary common bile duct stones. Success of this procedure depends on the size of the stones, the number of stones involved, the degree of stenosis or narrowing of the distal bile duct, and the expertise of the endoscopist. Some patients may not be suitable candidates for endoscopic sphincterotomy because of the presence of a duodenal diverticulum adjacent to the ampulla of Vater. If sphincterotomy cannot be performed or is unsuccessful, an endoscopically placed catheter can be left in the bile duct for decompression. If the patient is a suitable operative risk and endoscopic sphincterotomy has not been possible or was technically unsatisfactory, operative exploration of the bile duct should be undertaken with the goal being removal of all stones. Stasis in the extrahepatic biliary system is presumed to be an important etiologic factor in the pathogenesis of primary bile duct stones. If one accepts this premise, simple stone removal without attention to improvement of biliary drainage is inadequate for the management of primary bile duct stones.

Optimal treatment of patients with primary common bile duct stones should achieve two goals—removal of stones and prevention of recurrences. Many of these patients have multiple stones in both the choledochus and intrahepatic ducts, and complete removal may not be feasible. Furthermore, it may be difficult to prevent stone recurrence. Therefore, the goal should be to select and perform a procedure that facilitates passage of any residual or recurrent stones into the small bowel and thereby reduces the likelihood of cholangitis, jaundice, or pancreatitis. The procedure selected should be simple and safe with minimal morbidity and mortality but should effectively minimize the need for a second operation or endoscopic procedure. The presence of primary common duct stones has been considered by most authors to be an absolute indication for formal drainage of the biliary tree with either choledochoduodenostomy, choledochojejunostomy, or transduodenal sphincteroplasty. The introduction of endoscopic techniques has added a new dimension to an already existing dilemma. The central question is no longer whether patients with primary common duct stones require a drainage procedure at the time of laparotomy, but rather whether they need an operation at all.

The observation that essentially all primary common duct stones are pigment stones has precluded the effective use of dissolution agents for treating these patients. The appropriate application of endoscopic sphincterotomy (papillotomy) in properly selected patients with primary common duct stones may achieve both stone removal and prevention of recurrence. After a successful papillotomy, stones frequently pass spontaneously into the duodenum or can be manually extracted using a variety of instruments and techniques. The realization that stones are often too large to pass or cannot be easily removed has prompted the evaluation of several experimental ancillary techniques to induce stone fragmentation and thereby facilitate either spontaneous passage or manual extraction. These new techniques include ultrasonic fragmentation and electrohydraulic laser lithotripsy.

When surgery is indicated for patients with primary common duct stones, the surgeon has three options—transduodenal sphincteroplasty, side-to-side choledochoduodenostomy, or Roux-en-Y choledochojejunostomy. Advocates of duodenal sphincteroplasty report minimal morbidity and

mortality associated with this procedure. A vast experience has been obtained with choledochoduodenostomy, which can be a satisfactory procedure for treating patients with primary common duct stones. Concern has been expressed about the accumulation of debris in the distal biliary tree, the so-called sump syndrome, although there is limited evidence to suggest that it occurs with any frequency. Occasionally, the duodenum may be scarred and mobilization difficult. In such instances, or if the bile duct is small or thin walled, a Roux-en-Y choledochojejunostomy is performed. This provides a satisfactory anastomosis and excellent biliary drainage to a defunctionalized limb.

REFERENCES

1. Admirand WH, Small DM. The physicochemical basis of cholesterol gallstone formation in man. J Clin Invest 1968; 47:1043.
2. Lee SP, La Mont JT, Carey MC. Role of gallbladder mucus hypersecretion in the evolution of cholesterol gallstones. J Clin Invest 1981;67:1712.
3. Halpern Z, Dudley MA, Kibe A, et al. Rapid vesicle formation and aggregation in abnormal human biles. Gastroenterology 1986; 90:875.
4. Harvey PRC, Somjen G, Gilat T, et al. Vesicular cholesterol in bile: relationship to protein concentration and nucleation time. Biochim Biophys Acta 1988;958:10.
5. Burnstein MJ, Ilson RG, Petrunka CN, et al. Evidence for a potent nucleating factor in the gallbladder bile of patients with cholesterol gallstones. Gastroenterology 1983;85:801.
6. Holzbach RT, Kibe A, Theil E, et al. Biliary proteins: unique inhibitors of cholesterol crystal nucleation in human gallbladder bile. J Clin Invest 1984;73:35.
7. Maki T. Pathogenesis of calcium bilirubinate gallstones: role of E. coli, β-glucuronidase and coagulation by inorganic ions, polyelectrolytes, and agitation. Ann Surg 1966;164:90.
8. Lee SP, Maher K, Nicholls IF. Origin and fate of biliary sludge. Gastroenterology 1988;94:170.
9. Kim YS, Kestell MF, Lee SP. Gallbladder sludge: lessons from ceftriaxone. J Gastroenterol Hepatol 1992;7:618.
10. Gracie WA, Ransohoff DF. The natural history of silent gallstones: the innocent gallstone is not a myth. N Engl J Med 1982;307:798.
11. Glenn F. Trends in surgical treatment of calculous disease of the biliary tract. Surg Gynecol Obstet 195;140:877.
12. Roslyn JJ, Binns GS, Hughes EF, et al. Open cholecystectomy: a contemporary analysis of 42,474 patients. Ann Surg 1993;218:129.
13. Ganey JB, Johnson PA Jr, Prillaman PE, et al. Cholecystectomy: clinical experience with a large series. Am J Surg 1986;151:352.
14. Barkun JS, Barkun AN, Meakins JL. Laparoscopic versus open cholecystectomy: the Canadien experience. Am J Surg 1993; 165:455.
15. Perissat J. Laparoscopic cholecystectomy: the European experience. Am J Surg 1993;165:444.
16. Gadacz TR. U.S. experience with laparoscopic cholecystectomy. Am J Surg 1993;165:450.
17. Deziel DJ, Millikan KW, Economou SG, et al. Complications of laparoscopic cholecystectomy: a national survey of 4,292 hospitals and an analysis of 77,604 cases. Am J Surg 1992; 165:9.
18. Southern Surgeons Club. A prospective analysis of 1518 laparoscopic cholecystectomies. N Eng J Med 1991;324:1073.
19. Norrby A, Herlin P, Holmin T, et al. Early or delayed cholecystectomy in acute cholecystitis? A clinical trial. Br J Surg 1983;70:163.
20. Schoenfield LT, Lachin JM, The Steering Committee, The National Cooperative Gallstone Study Group. Chenodiol (chenodeoxycholic acid) for dissolution of gallstones: the National Cooperative Gallstone Study: a controlled trial of efficacy and safety. Ann Intern Med 1981;95:257.
21. Thistle JL, May GR, Bender CE, et al. Dissolution of cholesterol gallbladder stones by methyl tert-butyl ether administered by percutaneous transhepatic catheter. N Engl J Med 1989;320:633.

22. Sackman M, Delius M, Sauerbruch T, et al. Shock-wave litho-tripsy of gallbladder gallstones. N Engl J Med 1988;318:393.

23. Dorzi A, Monson JRT, O'Morain C, et al. Extension of selection criteria for extracorporeal shockwave lithotripsy for gall-stones. BMJ 11989;299:302.

24. Magnuson TH, Lillemoe KD, Pitt HA. How many Americans will be eligible for biliary lithotripsy? Arch Surg 1980;124:1185.

25. Burnett D, Ertan A, Jones R, et al. Use of external shockwave lithotripsy and adjuvant ursodiol for treatment of radiducent gallstones: a national multicenter study. Dig Dis Sci 1989;34:1011.

26. Walsch DB, Eckhauser FE, Ramsburgh SR, et al. Risk associated with diabetes mellitus in patients undergoing gallbladder surgery. Surgery 1982;91:254.

27. Roslyn, JJ, Pitt HA, Mann LL, et al. Parenteral nutrition-induced gallbladder disease: a reason for early cholecystec-tomy. Am J Surg 1984;148:58.

28. Roslyn JJ, Thompson JE Jr, Darvin H, et al. Risk factors for gallbladder perforation. Am J Gastroenterol 1987;82:636.

SURGERY: SCIENTIFIC PRINCIPLES AND PRACTICE, Second Edition, edited by Lazar J. Greenfield, Michael W. Mulholland, Keith T. Oldham, Gerald B. Zelenock, and Keith D. Lillemoe. Lippincott–Raven Publishers, Philadelphia, © 1997.

CHAPTER 42

BILIARY NEOPLASMS

DAVID L. NAHRWOLD AND LILLIAN G. DAWES

Although cancers of the gallbladder and biliary tract are relatively uncommon, accounting for about 4260 deaths a year in the United States,[1] they continue to present a challenge to physicians. These tumors have been recognized since the 18th century, yet they continue to carry a grave prognosis. They are clinically silent until their late stages, and therefore, most are diagnosed only when they are surgically unresectable. Complete surgical resection has been the only proven cure, and unfortunately, good adjuvant therapy is yet to be realized. With improvements in diagnostic imaging, increased awareness of the disease, and the development of better chemotherapeutic or radiation treatments for these cancers, the future may hold more promise.

BENIGN TUMORS OF THE GALLBLADDER AND BILE DUCTS

Benign gallbladder and bile duct tumors are extremely rare. Overall, gallbladder tumors and pseudotumors occur more frequently than benign tumors of the bile ducts. The estimated incidence of benign gallbladder tumors in patients who have had cholecystectomies ranges from 0.5% to 3%. Benign bile duct tumors are much less common; only 4 (0.02%) were found in 20,000 consecutive patients who had biliary tract operations at the Mayo Clinic.[1]

Pathology

Benign Gallbladder Tumors

Benign tumors of the gallbladder most commonly present as polyps or polyploid lesions. Polyps can be pseudotumors or hyperplastic conditions (thought to result from inflammatory conditions), or adenomas, which are most likely premalignant lesions. Other benign tumors, such as adenomyosis, heterotopia, or tumors of the supporting tissues of the gallbladder, are rarely seen.

Pseudotumors

Cholesterolosis, or "strawberry gallbladder," is manifested by yellow spots visible on the surface of the mucosa. This proliferation of foamy macrophages filled with cholesterol in the lamina propria can also result in the formation of polyps, called *cholesterol polyps*. These polyps are thought to result from a disturbance in cholesterol metabolism. Other pseudotumors of the gallbladder are *inflammatory polyps,* which are composed of a vascular connective tissue stalk with a single layer of columnar epithelial cells and have a chronic inflammatory cell infiltrate. These lesions are not considered to be premalignant lesions and are thought to result from chronic inflammation.

Adenomas

Adenomas with hyperplasia of the epithelial layer of the gallbladder, like adenomas in other gastrointestinal tract organs, can be sessile or papillary. Papillary adenomas are sometimes called *papillomas,* and multiple papillomas are called *papillomatosis.* Carcinoma in situ has been reported in these lesions, and they are thought to be premalignant lesions. The cause of adenomas of the gallbladder is unknown. The role of gallstones in the formation of adenomas is also unknown; most are not associated with the presence of gallstones.

Adenomyosis

An adenomyoma of the gallbladder is a rare intramural mass or nodule. This lesion is characterized by proliferation of the mucosal epithelium and hypertrophy of the muscular layers of the gallbladder. Histologically, in addition to muscular hypertrophy, invagination of epithelial mucosa between muscle layers is evidenced by the presence of Rokitansky-Aschoff sinuses and Luschka crypts[2]; these histologic changes are also seen with chronic cholecystitis. Because most of these rare tumors have been reported to occur in the fundus, it has been postulated that a functional cystic duct obstruction or biliary dyskinesia is responsible for the muscular hypertrophy and the development of adenomyosis of the gallbladder. Nonetheless, the cause of this condition is unknown.

Other Benign Gallbladder Tumors

Other types of gallbladder tumors, such as heterotopic lesions or tumors of the supporting tissues of the gallbladder, have been reported and are extremely rare.[1] Heterotopia consists of nodules of ectopic tissue not normally seen in the gallbladder, such as intestinal, pancreatic, or gastric epithelium. Tumors of the supporting tissues, such as hemangiomas, lipomas, leiomyomas, or granular cell tumors, can also occur in the gallbladder.

Benign Bile Duct Tumors

Benign tumors of the extrahepatic bile ducts are extremely rare. Only 2 cases in 5200 biliary tract surgeries were reported in one series.[1] Papillomas or adenomas can occur in the extrahepatic bile ducts, as can multiple polyps or papillomatosis of the bile ducts. Isolated reports of these adenomatous lesions in association with adenocarcinoma suggest these may be premalignant lesions.[3] Tumors of the supporting tissues, such as fibromas, leiomyomas, angioleiomyomas, or carcinoids, are rarely found in the bile ducts.

Clinical Findings

Benign gallbladder tumors cause symptoms similar to those caused by cholelithiasis. Biliary symptoms, including right upper quadrant pain and discomfort, fatty food intolerance, nausea, vomiting, and an increase in flatulence, are common complaints in patients with symptomatic benign gallbladder tumors. Often, it is difficult to separate symptoms caused by these tumors from those caused by concomitant gallstones because many of these benign tumors are diagnosed as incidental findings at the time of cholecystectomy.

Benign tumors of the bile ducts present with symptoms relating to bile duct obstruction. Most often, these tumors are diagnosed during evaluation of jaundice or after treatment for biliary infection. The jaundice is often intermittent. Other patients have nonspecific symptoms, such as dyspepsia or elevated serum alkaline phosphatase levels.

Diagnosis and Treatment

Gallbladder tumors, when diagnosed preoperatively, can be visualized by ultrasound, oral cholecystography, or less commonly, computed tomography (CT). A filling defect that does not move with changes in position is probably a benign or malignant gallbladder polyp. Symptomatic patients who have a lesion in the gallbladder should have cholecystectomy. Because neither ultrasound nor cholecystography can distinguish benign from malignant lesions, all gallbladders that contain polypoid lesions should be removed.[4]

Ultrasound can also be used for initial evaluation of jaundice in a patient with a benign tumor of the bile duct, but unequivocal demonstration of these tumors requires either percutaneous transhepatic cholangiography or endoscopic retrograde cholangiography. Whenever tumors in the bile ducts are demonstrated, surgical excision is indicated to relieve intermittent jaundice and cholangitis. Excision of a benign tumor with reanastomosis of the bile duct is often possible. If so much duct is removed that a tension-free anastomosis cannot be done, reconstruction of the biliary tree with a biliary–enteric anastomosis is preferred, usually by choledochojejunostomy. Papillomatosis of the bile ducts is difficult to treat. When biliary papillomatosis is limited to one segment of the biliary tree, radical excision is preferable; however, hyperplastic lesions can extend throughout the biliary duct system. Re-

currence is frequent after curettage; therefore, resection should be performed whenever possible.[1]

GALLBLADDER CANCER

Gallbladder cancer was first described in 1777 and first successfully treated in 1890.[5] Surgical therapies ranging from simple cholecystectomy to hepatic resection have been recommended for the treatment of gallbladder cancer. Part of the difficulty in defining optimal treatment relates to the facts that gallbladder cancer continues to carry a poor prognosis and its rarity limits the institution of controlled, randomized trials.

Incidence

Gallbladder cancer accounts for 3% to 4% of all gastrointestinal tract tumors, and about 2% of all biliary tract procedures are done for gallbladder cancers. Gallbladder cancer has an incidence of about 2.5 per 100,000 population. About 6500 people die from gallbladder cancer each year.[5]

Gallbladder cancer is much more frequent in women, with a female/male ratio of 3:1. The disease is most commonly seen in elderly women, with the mean age of 65 years at diagnosis.[6] Southwest Native Americans, Alaskans, Mexicans, and Hispanics living in the United States have an estimated five or six times greater incidence of gallbladder cancer than the general population.[5] On the other hand, gallbladder cancer is much less common in blacks and is extremely rare in certain Bantu tribes, in whom cholelithiasis is also infrequent.

The association of gallstones with gallbladder cancer is well known (Fig. 42-1). Seventy to 90% of all patients with gallbladder cancer have gallstones, and about 0.4% of all patients with gallstones have gallbladder cancer.[5] The association of gallstones with cancer can be related to gallstone size; larger stones have a greater cancer risk. There is a 10-fold increase in the incidence of gallbladder cancer in patients who have gallstones that are larger than 3 cm in diameter.[7] It has been postulated that the larger gallstones have been present in the gallbladder for long periods of time, causing chronic irritation of the gallbladder wall, thus predisposing to the development of carcinoma. Experimental models of gallbladder cancer have supported the role of chronic cholelithiasis in promoting the develop-

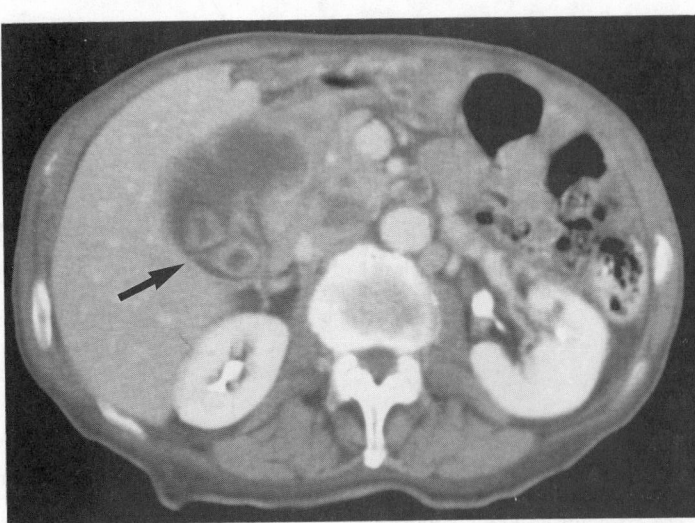

Figure 42-1. CT scan of a patient with gallbladder cancer. Gallstones (*arrow*) are seen in up to 90% of patients with gallbladder cancer. Also visible are the irregular gallbladder wall and the dilated gallbladder, which resulted from cystic duct obstruction due to tumor invasion.

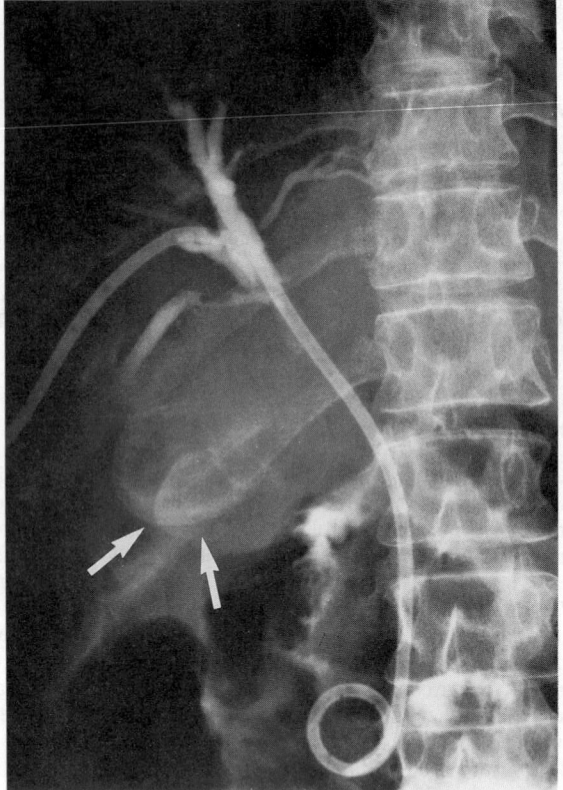

Figure 42-2. Gallbladder cancer often presents with stage V disease. This cholangiogram demonstrates a percutaneous stent placed through the transhepatic route to relieve biliary obstruction caused by an advanced gallbladder cancer. A porcelain gallbladder is present (*arrows*).

ment of gallbladder carcinoma. The presence of cholesterol pellets in the gallbladder increased the incidence of gallbladder carcinoma from 6% to 68% in hamsters fed the carcinogen dimethylnitrosamine.[5] The higher incidence of gallbladder cancer in chronic typhoid carriers is also thought to result from chronic irritation.

The potential risk of cancer in patients with gallstones gives rise to concern because asymptomatic gallstone patients are not treated by cholecystectomy. Epidemiologic studies on the 20-year risk of developing gallbladder carcinoma in patients with gallstones has been estimated to be in the range of 0.13% for the general population and up to 1.5% in high-risk populations (such as Native Americans).[5] It is evident that this small risk of developing gallbladder cancer in patients with gallstones even over the long-term does not warrant routine cholecystectomy in all patients with gallstones. There are, however, exceptions. Calcification of the wall of the gallbladder, the so-called porcelain gallbladder, is associated with a 25% to 60% incidence of gallbladder cancer. The presence of a porcelain gallbladder, therefore, should alert the physician to the high probability of a malignancy, and a cholecystectomy should be performed unless contraindicated for other reasons (Fig. 42-2).

Pathology

Eighty to 90% of gallbladder cancers are well-differentiated adenocarcinomas. Adenocarcinomas of the gallbladder can be subdivided into various types, including papillary, serous, colloid, or glandular carcinomas. A small percentage of gallbladder cancers are squamous cell in origin, but this type accounts for only about 5% of all gallbladder cancers. The remainder of gallbladder cancers, about 10%, are anaplastic neoplasms.

The mode of spread can be predicted by the lymphatic and venous drainage of the gallbladder. Venous drainage is into the venules that drain directly into the adjacent liver. The most common mode of spread of gallbladder cancer is through direct extension into the liver, particularly liver segments IV and V. The lymphatic drainage of the gallbladder is to the cystic duct lymph node, to periportal lymph nodes, and then to celiac and superior mesenteric lymph nodes. Spread to the cystic lymph node and other periportal lymph nodes is of diagnostic significance. These tumors also can spread into and around the cystic duct and can extend into the common bile duct, causing biliary obstruction. Thus, the first clinical symptom encountered is often jaundice (Fig. 42-3). Besides direct ex-

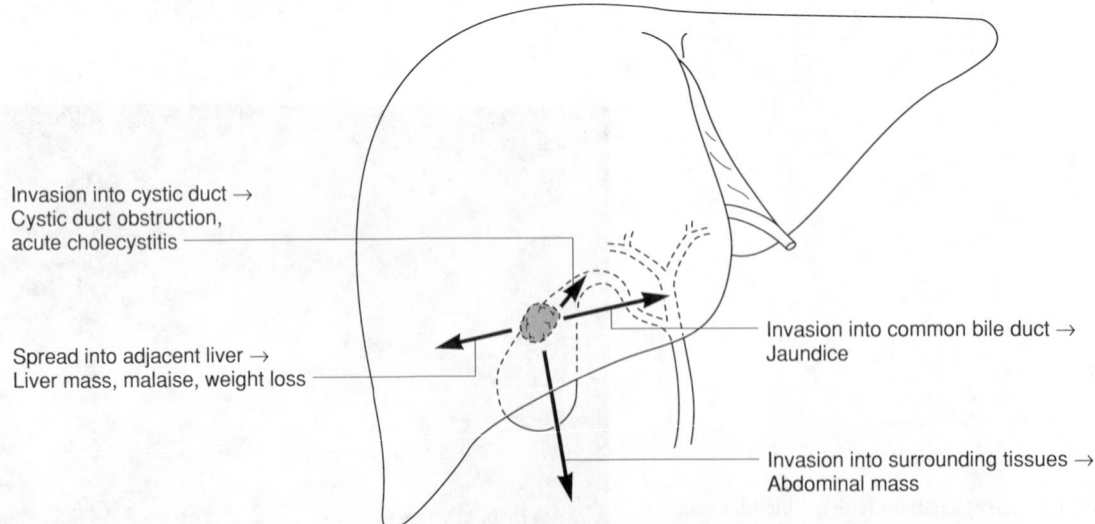

Invasion into cystic duct →
Cystic duct obstruction,
acute cholecystitis

Spread into adjacent liver →
Liver mass, malaise, weight loss

Invasion into common bile duct →
Jaundice

Invasion into surrounding tissues →
Abdominal mass

Figure 42-3. Tumor spread and presenting signs in gallbladder cancer. Gallbladder cancer commonly spreads by direct extension into surrounding tissues. This tumor extension results in the clinical presentations of jaundice, acute cholecystitis, abdominal mass, and weight loss.

Table 42-1. STAGING SYSTEM FOR GALLBLADDER CANCER

Stage	Extent of Tumor
I	Mucosa only
II	Muscularis and mucosa
III	Subserosa, muscularis, and mucosa
IV	Cystic lymph node involvement and layers of the gallbladder wall
V	Distant spread

tension and lymphatic spread of tumor, distant metastasis is possible but is less commonly seen.

A staging system has been developed that takes into consideration the lymphatic and venous drainage of the gallbladder.[8] This system is used to describe the extent of disease with gallbladder carcinoma and has been shown to be of prognostic value (Table 42-1). Stage I disease is limited to the mucosa of the gallbladder. Stage II includes involvement of the mucosa and the muscularis layers. In stage III, the subserosa is infiltrated by tumor. Stage IV includes involvement of all the layers of the gallbladder wall as well as cystic lymph node involvement. Stage V includes distant spread, either into the liver or adjacent organs. Unfortunately, most patients with gallbladder carcinoma present with stage V disease.

As outlined by the American Joint Committee on Cancer, a TNM classification is also being used to describe the extent of disease with gallbladder cancer. The primary tumor (T) is designated as T1 when it is confined to the mucosa (T1a) or to the muscle layer of the gallbladder (T1b). T2 tumors invade the perimuscular connective tissue, and T3 tumors perforate the serosa or invade into one adjacent organ (2-cm extension into the liver or less). T4 tumors have local extension into several adjacent organs, or they extend into the liver for more than 2 cm. The regional lymph node metastases are to cystic duct, pericholedochal, or hilar lymph nodes (N1) or to peripancreatic, periduodenal, periportal, celiac, or superior mesenteric lymph nodes (N2). Staging depends on the primary tumor, the regional lymph nodes, and metastatic disease (Table 42-2).

Diagnosis

The signs and symptoms of gallbladder cancer are similar to those of gallstones. For smaller tumors, it may be difficult to distinguish the symptoms of concomitant gallstones from those of gallbladder carcinoma. Right upper quadrant pain, discomfort, and dyspepsia can result from both. Patients with gallbladder cancer frequently have advanced disease and present with nonspecific signs of malaise, weight loss and anorexia, or obstructive jaundice (see Fig. 42-3). Occasionally, in the later stages of the disease, patients present with a mass in the right upper quadrant. Tumor invasion of the cystic duct causing cystic duct obstruction can result in the development of acute cholecystitis. Jaundice occurs when the tumor extends into the common bile duct. The diagnosis often is not made preoperatively but is made at the time of laparotomy for jaundice or acute cholecystitis. Tumors with the best prognosis are those found incidentally at the time of cholecystectomy for symptomatic gallstone disease. This emphasizes the importance of opening all gallbladders at the time of cholecystectomy so that any suspicious lesions can immediately be examined histologically.

Treatment

When gallbladder cancer is limited to the mucosa and submucosa, cholecystectomy is adequate treatment and has a good prognosis, with up to 100% 5-year survival rate. When the cancer involves the deeper layers of the gallbladder wall, the prognosis is more grim. A 64% 5-year survival rate was reported in patients who had carcinoma confined to the mucosa and submucosa, whereas none of the patient who had cancer involving all layers of the gallbladder wall survived longer than 2.5 years.[9] Even though these tumors were relatively localized at the time of cholecystectomy, cholecystectomy alone was not adequate therapy for long-term survival.

In hope of improving these survival rates and considering the lymphatic and venous drainage of the gallbladder, it has been recommended that gallbladder cancer be treated by cholecystectomy with a wide resection of the liver around the gallbladder bed (liver segments IV and V) and regional lymphadenectomy.[10] This procedure has been termed *radical cholecystectomy* or *extended cholecystectomy* and at times can also involve resection of the adjacent bile duct. In a retrospective review of this treatment, a prolongation of median survival was found, but the 5-year survival rate was not significantly improved.[11] When reoperation has been performed on patients with gallbladder cancer found incidentally at the time of cholecystectomy, residual disease has been found in the lymph nodes or adjacent liver, and resection of this residual disease may improve survival.

Others have advocated a more radical resection to include a hepatic resection with bile duct resection and sometimes a pancreaticoduodenectomy.[12] Reports of long-term survival with this aggressive approach need to be viewed in light of increased associated postoperative mortality. In other reports, hepatic lobectomy has not resulted in improvement, with only isolated cases of prolonged survival.[13] Given improved surgical technique and improved perioperative care, hepatic lobectomy, pancreaticoduodenectomy, or both may be indicated in a select group of patients.

For patients with invasive but resectable disease, a wedge resection of the liver with a 2- to 3-cm margin around the gallbladder, along with cholecystectomy and lymph node dissection, is recommended. The lymph node dissection should include all the lymph nodes and surrounding areolar tissue from the bifurcation of the common hepatic ducts to the distal common bile duct as well as the lymph nodes along the hepatic artery up to the celiac axis (Fig. 42-4). If the gallbladder cancer is near the cystic duct or if the bile duct is involved with tumor, a bile duct resection at the time of extended cholecystectomy is warranted.

For stage V disease, the goal of treatment is palliation. Because these patients frequently present with obstructive jaundice, a major goal of treatment is relief of jaundice and its attendant symptoms, such as pruritus and cholangitis.

Table 42-2. TNM CLASSIFICATION FOR STAGING OF CANCER OF THE GALLBLADDER

Stage	Stage Grouping
I	T1, N0, M0
II	T2, N0, M0
III	T1, T2 or T3, N0 or N1, M0
IVA	T4, N0 or N1, M0
IVB	Any T, N2, M0 or any T, any N, M1

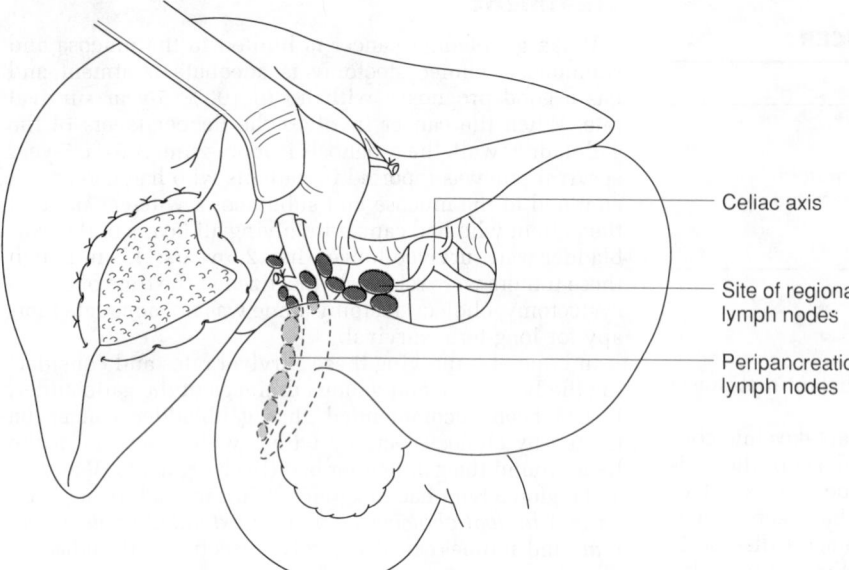

Celiac axis

Site of regional
lymph nodes

Peripancreatic
lymph nodes

Figure 42-4. Treatment for invasive gallbladder cancer is cholecystectomy and a wedge resection of the liver along with a regional lymphadenectomy. The wedge resection of the liver is illustrated along with the lymph node regions that drain the gallbladder and that should be removed during operation for gallbladder cancer.

Percutaneous, endoscopic, or operative drainage of the biliary tree can be performed. A biliary–enteric anastomosis (anastomosis of a loop of bowel to the biliary ducts proximal to the obstruction) can be performed for palliation when the diagnosis is determined operatively. When both the diagnosis and unresectability of the tumor are determined before operation, drainage of the biliary tree for palliation can be performed by stent placement, either endoscopically or by the transhepatic route.

Although radiation and chemotherapeutic regimens have been tried, none has been associated with a good response. The Eastern Cooperative Oncology Group reported on a randomized trial for three chemotherapy regimens for inoperable disease (5-fluorouracil [5-FU] alone, 5-FU and streptozocin, or 5-FU and methyl-CCNU); there was no difference in survival rates among groups, and only 5 of 53 patients with gallbladder cancer had objective response to treatment. The potential benefit of adjuvant radiotherapy is also difficult to evaluate because routine radiation doses have not been used, series are usually of fewer than 10 cases, and heterogeneous lesions are compared. Further investigation is needed to determine the exact roles of chemotherapy and radiation in the treatment of gallbladder carcinoma.

For symptomatic cholelithiasis, the treatment of choice is laparoscopic cholecystectomy. Laparoscopic removal of a gallbladder cancer is not recommended. Tumor implantation at the trocar sites has been observed when gallbladder cancer has been removed laparoscopically, and there is concern that the laparoscopic manipulation of the tumor can lead to tumor dissemination.[14] If gallbladder cancer is suspected, an open cholecystectomy and exploration is warranted. Laparoscopy has been used to stage gastrointestinal malignancies, and a staging laparoscopy may be appropriate before open operation if metastatic disease is suspected.

Prognosis

The prognosis of gallbladder cancer remains poor, with an average survival in the range of 6 months. Less than 5% of patients survive 5 years, because 90% of gallbladder cancer patients present with stage V disease. In 1947, a series of 36 patients was reported with a 5-year survival rate of 2.8%.[15] Since then, there has been no appreciable improvement in survival, with a 3% 5-year survival rate in a series of 71 patients reported in 1989.[16] Future efforts should be directed toward earlier detection of gallbladder cancer and better adjuvant therapy. Increased awareness of the potential for gallbladder cancer should lead to more routine examinations of the gallbladder in the operating room at the time of cholecystectomy so that the appropriate lymphatic dissection and wedge resection of the liver can be done in the hope of improving survival and cure rates for this disease.

CARCINOMA OF THE BILE DUCTS

Incidence

Cancer of the bile ducts is even less common than gallbladder carcinoma and is seen in 0.01% to 0.46% of all autopsies. Unlike gallbladder cancer, which is more frequent in females, males have a higher incidence of bile duct cancer. The average age range of diagnosis is between 50 and 70 years.[17,18]

Similar to gallbladder cancer, there is an association between bile duct cancer and gallstones. This association is, however, not as striking as for gallbladder cancer; only 25% to 57% of patients with bile duct cancer have gallstones. Biliary tract infection is associated with these tumors; for example, patients with *Clonorchis sinensis* infection and chronic typhoid carriers have a higher incidence of bile duct cancer than the general population. Congenital hepatic fibrosis and choledochal cysts are also associated with bile duct cancer. Patients with ulcerative colitis have a markedly increased incidence. This predisposition is independent of whether the patient has had adequate treatment, either medical or surgical, of their colonic disease. In addition, bile duct tumors in colitis patients tend to follow a more aggressive course.[19]

Staging

Bile duct cancer is classified according to its location within the ductal system. The tumors are generally divided into three major locations: upper third, middle third, and lower third[17,18] (Fig. 42-5). The most common location is

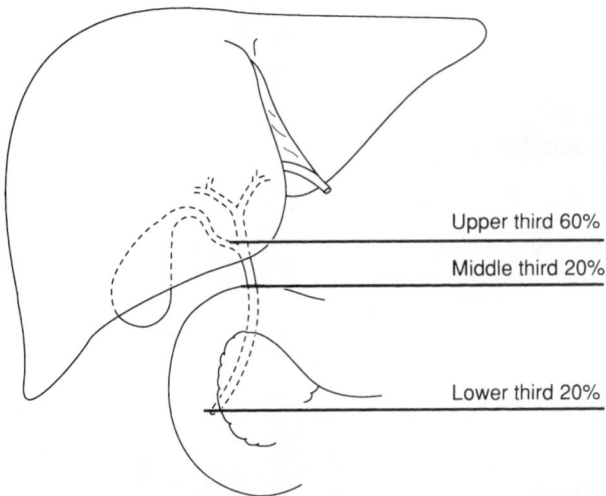

Figure 42-5. Distribution of bile duct cancers.

Upper third 60%

Middle third 20%

Lower third 20%

the upper third, where the confluence of the hepatic ducts is involved. Tumors in the upper third have been called *Klatzkin tumors,* after Gerald Klatzkin, who reported on 13 such patients with tumors at the bifurcation of the hepatic ducts. Middle-third tumors are located between the cystic duct and the upper border of the duodenum. Lower-third lesions are located between the upper border of the duodenum and up to but not including the Vater ampulla.

Staging for bile duct cancer can also be defined with a TNM classification as outlined by the American Joint Committee on Cancer. T refers to the primary tumor, with Tis as carcinoma in situ, and with T1 denoting tumor invasion into the mucosa (T1a) or into the muscle layer of the bile duct (T1b). T2 is used to designate tumors invading the perimuscular connective tissue. When the tumor invades adjacent structures, such as the liver, pancreas, or duodenum, the bile duct cancer is described as a T3 lesion. When present, lymph node metastases can be either N1, with metastasis in the cystic duct, pericholedochal, or hilar

lymph nodes, or N2, with metastases in the peripancreatic, periduodenal, celiac, or mesenteric lymph nodes. Stage I denotes T1 tumors, without lymph node or metastatic disease. Stage II is for T2 tumors without metastases. Stage III includes lymph node metastases with T1 or T2 primary tumors. Stage IV is for locally invasive disease, T3 tumors but no distant metastasis, and stage V indicates distant metastatic disease. The use of this classification in addition to site-specific information is recommended to promote more uniform description of extent of disease for these rare tumors.

Clinical Findings

Similar to gallbladder cancer, bile duct cancers spread by direct extension. With the close proximity of the bile ducts to the branches of the portal veins and hepatic arteries, these tumors are often unresectable because of vascular invasion, especially when they are located near the bifurcation into the right and left hepatic ducts. Jaundice is the most frequent presenting symptom, occurring in about 90% of patients. Abdominal pain (30% to 50%) and cholangitis (10% to 30%) are other common initial findings. Patients may present late with symptoms of weight loss, anorexia, pruritus, or anemia. These symptoms are seen with varying frequencies. Patients uniformly have elevated alkaline phosphatase levels, which may be the only clinical finding.

Diagnosis

Diagnosis is most often made during evaluation of jaundice. The evaluation begins with an ultrasound to detect ductal dilation. Ultrasound examination demonstrates intrahepatic ductal dilation and, depending on the site of the tumor, variable degrees of common bile duct dilation. Ultrasound or CT demonstrates intrahepatic biliary obstruction but rarely the tumor itself (Fig. 42-6A). When biliary obstruction is present, further visualization of the biliary tree is required, either through percutaneous transhepatic cholangiography (see Fig. 42-6B) or endoscopic retrograde cholangiopancreatography (ERCP). Percutane-

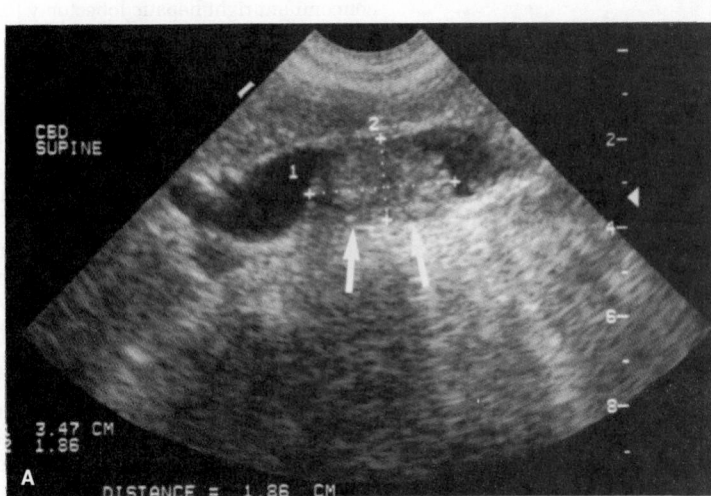

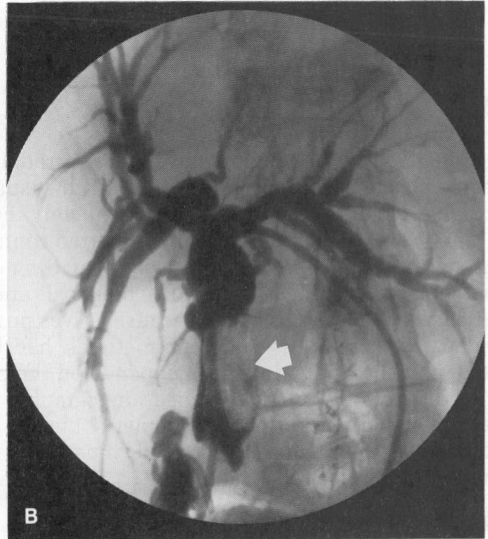

Figure 42-6. Ultrasound examination is useful in the initial evaluation of obstructive jaundice. (*A*) This ultrasound scan reveals an enlarged common bile duct with a filling defect (*arrows*) subsequently found to be a bile duct cancer. (*B*) A transhepatic cholangiogram further delineates the biliary tree and the location (*arrow*) of this obstructing tumor within the common bile duct.

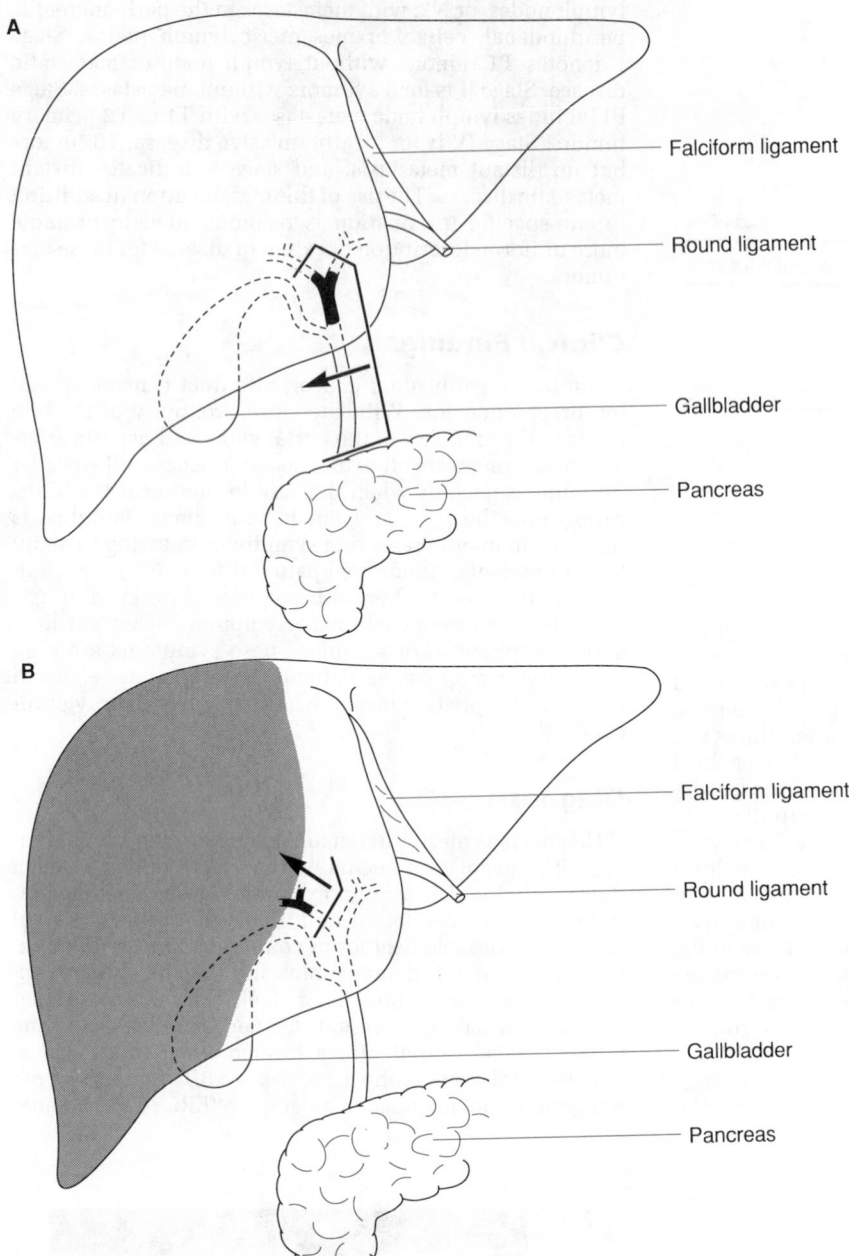

A

Falciform ligament

Round ligament

Gallbladder

Pancreas

B

Falciform ligament

Round ligament

Gallbladder

Pancreas

Figure 42-7. Surgical resection of hilar bile duct tumors in different locations. (*A*) Resection limited to extrahepatic bile ducts. (*B*) Resection of right bile duct with concomitant right hepatic lobectomy (*blue area*).

ous transhepatic cholangiography is preferred for more proximal lesions because ERCP can fail to visualize the proximal portion of the biliary tree adequately. For lower bile duct lesions, ERCP may be the preferred route of cholangiography. It has the advantages of providing opportunity to obtain brushings for cytologic diagnosis and having a lessened chance for bile leak because a liver puncture is avoided. Successful use of both methods has been reported, and the optimal method depends on the expertise of the institution. Selective celiac angiography helps to determine whether there is involvement of major adjacent vascular structures, such as the portal veins, to aid in determination of surgical resectability.

Surgical Therapy

Middle- and Lower-Third Bile Duct Tumors

For lesions of the middle and lower thirds of the bile duct, resection of the bile duct tumor with reanastomosis is the procedure of choice when possible. For small middle-third bile duct carcinomas, resection with reanastomosis of the common bile duct may be possible, but for larger lesions, reconstruction with a biliary–enteric anastomosis, usually a choledochojejunostomy (anastomosis of the common bile duct to the jejunum) is required. For lower-third lesions, the Whipple procedure (pancreaticoduodenectomy) is necessary. Overall, both middle- and lower-third lesions have a better prognosis than tumors in the hilum.

Hilar Tumors

Much debate centers around the extent of resection warranted for hilar bile duct carcinoma. Like gallbladder cancer, the prognosis for patients with hilar bile duct cancer is extremely poor, with mortality rates of 80% to 90% at 5 years. Poor survival reflects the fact that most of these tumors are unresectable at the time of diagnosis. Previous series reported up to a 25% surgical morbidity rate, and little improvement was made in survival when resection

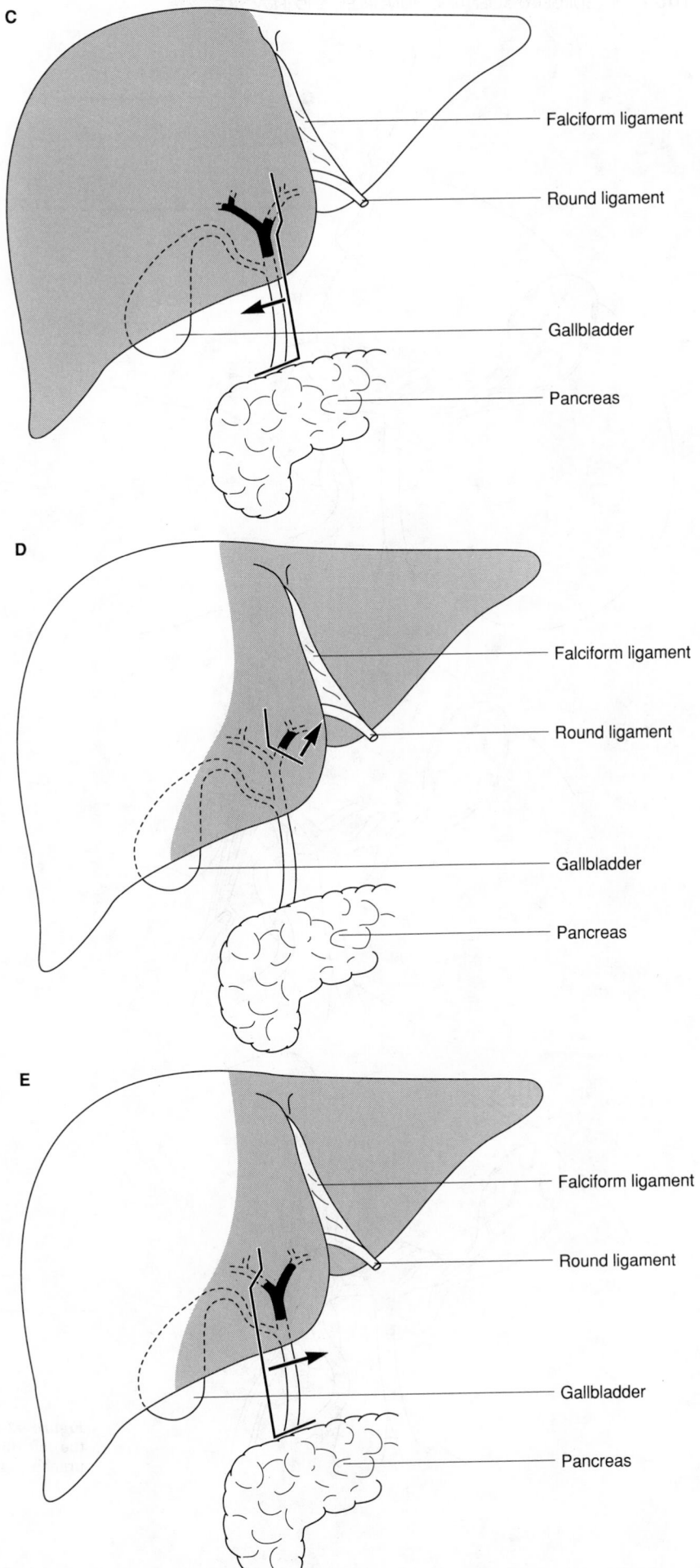

C — Falciform ligament

Round ligament

Gallbladder

Pancreas

D — Falciform ligament

Round ligament

Gallbladder

Pancreas

E — Falciform ligament

Round ligament

Gallbladder

Pancreas

Figure 42-7. *(Continued)* (*C*) Resection of ductal bifurcation combined with right hepatic trisegmentectomy (*blue area*). (*D*) Resection of left bile duct with concomitant left hepatic lobectomy (*blue area*). (*E*) Resection of duct bifurcation with left hepatic lobectomy (*blue area*).

A

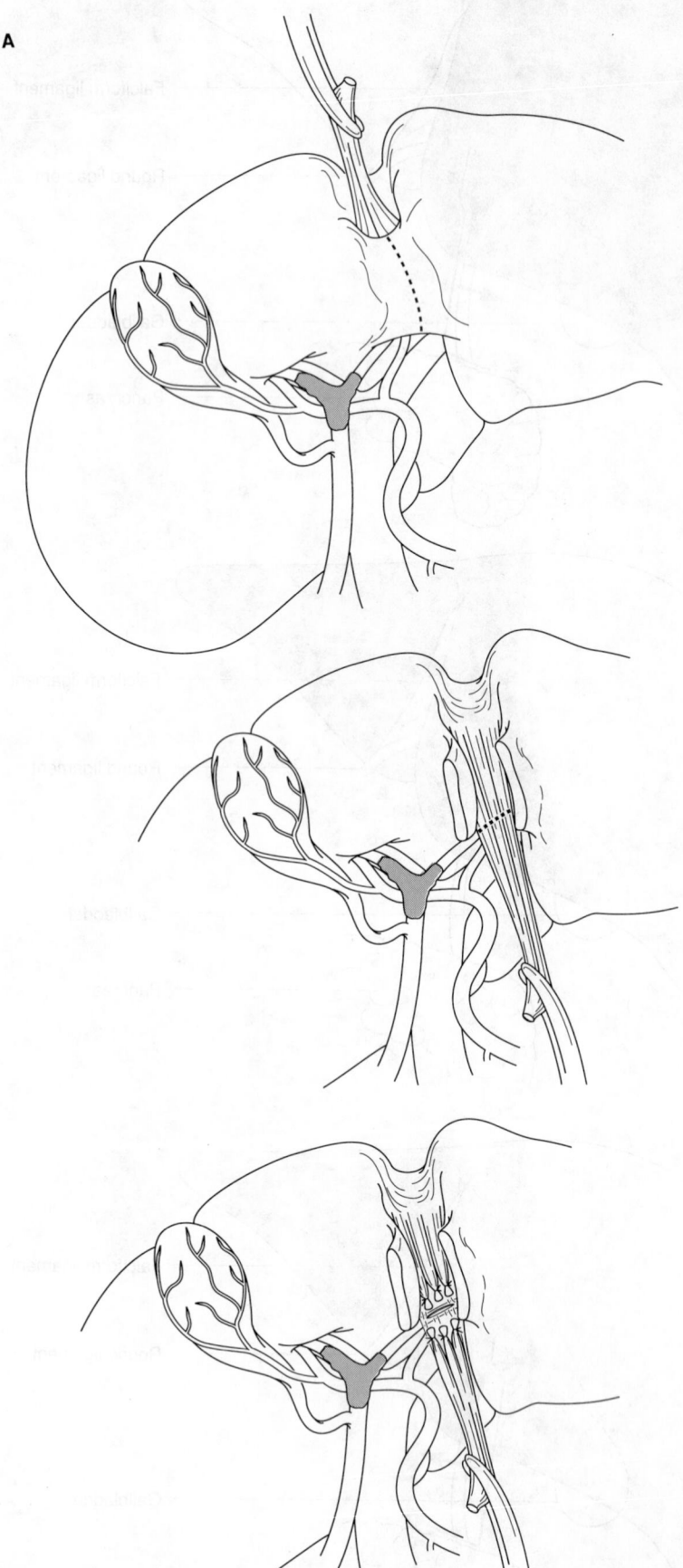

Figure 42-8. Surgical approach to biliary drainage for the left ductal system, illustrating round ligament approach to the left hepatic duct.

was compared with palliative procedures. Patients who underwent resection survived for only 11 to 33 months, compared with a 33-month median survival of patients with U-tube stenting and radiotherapy.[20,21] More recent series showed improvements in both surgical morbidity and survival rates after resection of hilar bile duct cancer. A 5-year survival rate of 21% for patients undergoing curative resection has been compared with a 6% 5-year survival rate after palliative stenting.[22] A 5-year survival rate of 30% and an operative mortality rate of only 4% for 25 patients who underwent resection for bile duct cancer have also been recorded, but those 25 patients represented only 17% of all patients who underwent exploration.[23] This latter finding is consistent with most series; most patients have hilar bile duct cancers that are unresectable at the time of diagnosis. In addition to being the only chance for cure, an improved quality of survival has also been reported for patients who undergo resection.

Unless contraindicated for other reasons, surgical exploration should be performed in all patients whose tumors are potentially resectable. Hepatic lobectomy is indicated for potential cure. Resection can include extended right hepatic lobectomy for lesions extending along the right hepatic ducts into the liver or invading the vascular supply to the right lobe. A left hepatic lobectomy or extended left hepatic lobectomy is performed for lesions extending into the left lobe of the liver (Fig. 42-7). Regardless of the surgical therapy, stenting of the biliary anastomosis is important because postoperative strictures and recurrent tumor are common, and long-term stents allow for cholangiographic follow-up and for dilation should strictures arise.

Aggressive surgical therapy with vascular reconstructions has been proposed to improve the dismal prognosis of more extensive disease. Hepatic transplantation has also been performed for these tumors, but the results are unfortunately hampered by a high rate of recurrence in the posttransplantation period, and thus hepatic transplantation is not a recommended treatment.[16]

Determination of Resectability

Hilar bile duct tumors are considered unresectable under the following conditions:

- There is metastatic disease, growth into surrounding structures, or peritoneal metastasis.
- There is extensive vascular invasion, that is, tumor invading the main portal vein or tumor involving both right and left portal veins or right and left hepatic arteries.
- There is tumor within the second-order biliary radicles of both hepatic lobes.

CT scans help to delineate the extent of local invasion. Cholangiography not only is the gold standard for diagnosis but also is helpful in determining resectability because if both the right and left biliary ducts have extension of tumor beyond the secondary biliary radicles, these tumors are unresectable. Angiography aids in determining the extent of vascular involvement. Surgical exploration should be considered for all good-risk patients whose tumors are potentially resectable.

Surgical Treatment of Unresectable Tumors

For the patients whose tumors are unresectable, surgical decompression of the biliary tree can be performed. Several methods can accomplish palliative surgical biliary drainage for hilar tumors. In the Longmire procedure, the lateral portion of the left lobe is transected, and the dilated left hepatic duct is identified and anastomosed to a loop of jejunum. This method is seldom used today because other surgical alternatives and percutaneous stenting are available. Another method of surgical decompression of the left ductal system is the round ligament approach.[24] In this approach, the bridge of tissue just beneath the ligamentum teres is opened to expose the dilated left hepatic duct. An anastomosis with a loop or Roux-en-Y limb of jejunum can then be made (Fig. 42-8). The right hepatic ductal system can also be approached from beneath the gallbladder bed, and a right hepaticojejunostomy is performed. U-tube stenting can also be established at the time of operation. A Silastic tube is placed through the abdominal wall, through the liver, across the tumor, out the bile duct, and through the abdominal wall. Because of problems with leakage around the site of exit from the common bile duct, a Roux-en-Y limb of jejunum is advocated to act as a conduit for this tube from the common duct to the abdominal wall when using a U-tube for biliary decom-

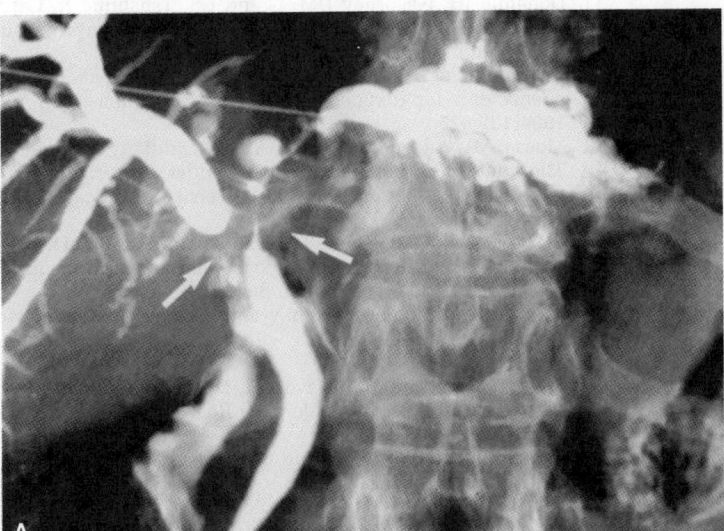
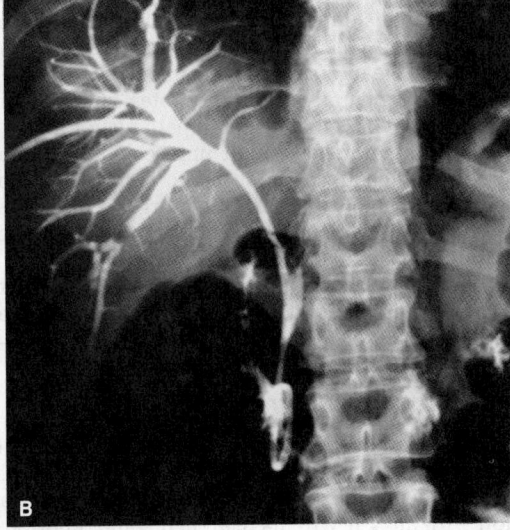

Figure 42-9. (*A*) Cholangiogram showing a hilar or Klatzkin tumor involving both the right and left ductal systems. (*B*) This tumor was unresectable, but successful palliation was accomplished with placement of a percutaneous stent through the right ductal system.

Table 42-3. ADVANTAGES AND DISADVANTAGES OF ENDOSCOPIC AND TRANSHEPATIC STENTING

	Endoprosthesis	External Stents
Placement	With endoscopic retrograde cholangiopancreatography and sphincterotomy	Percutaneous transhepatic approach
Electrolyte balance	No loss of fluid and electrolytes	External loss of fluid and electrolytes
Incidence of cholangitis	Less cholangitis and infection	Permits entry of bacteria from external sources
Care and comfort	Better patient comfort	Requires daily care
Access	Does not permit easy access	Easily exchanged; permits cholangiographic follow-up and placement of intracavitary radiotherapy

pression. Some surgeons prefer to have percutaneous stents placed preoperatively to serve as a guide for hilar ductal dissections and to facilitate the placement of operative stents.[18]

Nonsurgical Palliative Stenting

Improved palliation of patients with extensive unresectable disease is possible with nonsurgical percutaneous or endoscopic stenting. Stents can be placed across an obstructing, unresectable bile duct cancer either at the time of ERCP or by the percutaneous transhepatic approach (Fig. 42-9). Both types of stents have the potential complications of cholangitis, bleeding, or bile leakage along with recurrent obstruction from catheter occlusion. Endoprostheses have the advantages of improved patient comfort, no loss of electrolytes, and a reduced incidence of cholangitis and infection (Table 42-3). They are technically more difficult to place in proximal bile duct lesions, however, and they do not provide easy access for changing of the catheters or for repeat cholangiography. For proximal ductal lesions, the transhepatic approach is the technically preferred method. With external catheters, iridium (^{192}Ir) wires can be placed for the administration of intracavitary radiotherapy. Because percutaneous drains are used for palliation, drainage of one ductal system may be sufficient to relieve jaundice or pruritus or to treat cholangitis. Bilateral stent placements may be necessary for the control of biliary infection if an undrained segment is infected.

Palliative percutaneous or endoscopic stents can result in significant complications, such as cholangitis, bleeding, or bile leaks. The 30-day mortality rates for percutaneous or endoscopic stenting are also significant and range from 15% to 33%.[20] This high mortality may partially reflect the advanced stage of disease at the time of stenting. Similarly, 18% to 33% operative mortality rates have been reported for surgical bypass.[20] In general, patients with bile duct tumors who have metastatic or unresectable disease should have percutaneous or endoscopic stenting, avoiding the complications and discomfort of surgery. If tumors are explored for potential resectability and found intraoperatively to be unresectable, one of the surgical drainage or stenting procedures should be performed if possible. Patients with surgical bypass for palliation have less cholangitis and may have improved quality of life and survival.[20]

Adjuvant Therapy

Adjuvant radiotherapy has been proposed in an effort to improve the survival with bile duct carcinoma. External-beam irradiation, intraoperative irradiation, or local irradiation with an ^{192}Ir wire have all had some reported benefit. The number of cases is small, however, and further studies are needed to define the role of adjuvant radiotherapy. Treatment with postoperative radiotherapy may also re-

duce recurrence rates and prolong survival in patients with surgically resected tumors.[22] Various chemotherapeutic regimens have been tried, but no effective treatment for bile duct cancers has been developed.

REFERENCES

1. Nahrwold DL. Benign tumors and pseudo tumors of the biliary tract. In: Way LW, Pellegrini CA, eds. Surgery of the gallbladder and bile ducts. Philadelphia, WB Saunders, 1987:459.
2. Reubner BH, Montgomery CK. Pathology of the liver and biliary tract. New York, Wiley Medical, 1982:325.
3. Neumann RD, Livolsi VA, Rosenthall WS, Burrell M, Ball TJ. Adenocarcinoma in biliary papillomatosis. Gastroenterology 1976;70:779.
4. Majeski JA. Polyps of the gallbladder. J Surg Oncol 1986: 32:16.
5. Piehler JM, Crichlow RW. Primary cancer of the gallbladder: a collective review. Surg Gynecol Obstet 1978;147:929.
6. Morrow CE, Sutherland DE, Florack G, Eisenberg MM, Grage TB. Primary gallbladder carcinoma: significance of subserosal lesions and results of aggressive surgical treatment and adjuvant chemotherapy. Surgery 1983;94:709.
7. Diehl AK. Gallstone size and the risk of gallbladder cancer. JAMA 1983;250:2323.
8. Nevin JE, Moran TJ, Kay S, King R. Carcinoma of the gallbladder: staging, treatment and prognosis. Cancer 1976;37:141.
9. Bergdahl L. Gallbladder carcinoma first diagnosed at microscopic examination of gallbladders removed for presumed benign disease. Ann Surg 1980;191:19.
10. Glenn F, Hayes DM. The scope of radical surgery in the treatment of malignant tumors of the extrahepatic biliary tract. Surg Gynecol Obstet 1954;99:529.
11. Donahue JH, Nagorney DM, Grand CS, Tsushima K. Carcinoma of the gallbladder: does radical resection improve outcome? Arch Surg 1990;125:237.
12. Nakamura S, Mishiyam R, Yokoi Y, et al. Hepatopancreatoduodenectomy for advanced gallbladder carcinoma. Arch Surg 1994;129:625.
13. Moosa AR, Anagnost M, Hall AW, Moraldi A, Skinner DB. The continuing challenge of gallbladder cancer: survey of thirty years' experience at the University of Chicago. Am J Surg 1975;130:57.
14. Clair DG, Lautz DB, Brooks DC. Rapid development of umbilical metastases after laparoscopic cholecystectomy for unsuspected gallbladder carcinoma. Surgery 1993;113:355.
15. Sheinfeld W. Cholecystectomy and partial hepatectomy for carcinoma of the gallbladder with local liver extension. Surgery 1947;22:48.
16. Silk YN, Douglass HO, Nava HR, Driscoll DL, Tartarian G. Carcinoma of the gallbladder: the Roswell Park experience. Ann Surg 1889;210:751.
17. Tompkins RK. Treatment and prognosis in bile duct cancer. World J Surg 1988;12:109.
18. Langer JC, Langer B, Taylor BR, Zeldin R, Cummings B. Carcinoma of the extrahepatic bile duct: results of an aggressive surgical approach. Surgery 1985;98:752.
19. Akwari OE, van Heerden JA, Foulk WT. Cancer of the bile ducts associated with ulcerative colitis. Ann Surg 1975;181:303.

20. Ottow RT, August DA, Sugarbaker PH. Treatment of proximal biliary tract carcinoma: overview of techniques and results. Surgery 1985;97:251.
21. Terblanche J, Kahn D, Bornman PC, Werner D. The role of U-tube palliative treatment in the high bile duct carcinoma. Surgery 1988;103:624.
22. Cameron JL, Pitt HA, Zinner MJ, Kaufman SL, Coleman J. Management of proximal cholangiocarcinomas by surgical resection and radiotherapy. Am J Surg 1990;159:91.
23. Pinson CW, Rossi RL. Extended right hepatic lobectomy, left hepatic lobectomy and skeletonization resection for proximal bile duct cancer. World J Surg 1988;12:52.
24. Plumaged LH, Kelley CJ. Hepaticojejunostomy in benign and malignant high bile duct stricture: approaches to the left hepatic ducts. Br J Surg 1984;71:257.

SURGERY: SCIENTIFIC PRINCIPLES AND PRACTICE, Second Edition, edited by Lazar J. Greenfield, Michael W. Mulholland, Keith T. Oldham, Gerald B. Zelenock, and Keith D. Lillemoe. Lippincott–Raven Publishers, Philadelphia, © 1997.

CHAPTER 43

BILIARY STRICTURES AND SCLEROSING CHOLANGITIS

KEITH D. LILLEMOE

Benign strictures of the biliary tree are one of the most difficult challenges that a surgeon faces. Although numerous technologic developments have facilitated diagnosis and management, bile duct strictures remain a significant clinical problem. If unrecognized or managed improperly, life-threatening complications, such as biliary cirrhosis, portal hypertension, and cholangitis, can develop. To avoid these complications, virtually every patient with a bile duct stricture should undergo evaluation and treatment with the goal of relieving the obstruction to bile flow and its associated hepatic injury.

Benign bile duct strictures can have numerous causes:

Postoperative Strictures

Injury at primary biliary operations
    Laparoscopic cholecystectomy
    Open cholecystectomy
    Common bile duct exploration
Injury at other operative procedures
    Gastrectomy
    Hepatic resection
    Portacaval shunt
Stricture of a biliary–enteric anastomosis
Blunt or penetrating trauma

Strictures Due to Inflammatory Conditions

Chronic pancreatitis
Cholelithiasis and choledocholithiasis
Primary sclerosing cholangitis
Stenosis of the sphincter of Oddi
Duodenal ulcer
Crohn's disease
Viral infections
Toxic drugs

Most biliary strictures occur after primary operations on the gallbladder or biliary tree. With the introduction of laparoscopic cholecystectomy, bile duct injuries and associated strictures have been seen with an increased frequency. Operative injury to the bile ducts can also occur during nonbiliary operations on the gallbladder or biliary tree or as a result of external penetrating or blunt abdominal trauma. Inflammatory conditions and fibrosis due to chronic pancreatitis, gallstones within the gallbladder or the bile duct, stenosis of the sphincter of Oddi, or biliary tract infections can also cause benign bile duct strictures. Finally, primary sclerosing cholangitis, a rare disease of unknown cause, can result in multiple strictures of the intrahepatic and extrahepatic bile ducts. This chapter focuses primarily on postoperative bile duct strictures and primary sclerosing cholangitis.

POSTOPERATIVE BILE DUCT STRICTURES

Pathogenesis

Most benign bile duct strictures result from operations in or near the right upper quadrant. Over 80% of strictures occur after injury to the bile ducts during cholecystectomy. The exact incidence of bile duct injury is unknown, because many cases may go unreported in the literature. Data suggest that the incidence of bile duct injury during open cholecystectomy is 1 in 500 to 1000 cases. The incidence of bile duct injury during laparoscopic cholecystectomy is clearly higher. Although a wide range in the incidence of injury can be found in reported series, the most accurate data most likely come from surveys encompassing thousands of patients. These reports reflect the results from a large number of surgeons in both the community and teaching hospitals. The results of such series suggest an incidence of bile duct injury during laparoscopic cholecystectomy ranging from 0.3% to 0.6%.

A number of factors are associated with bile duct injury during either open or laparoscopic cholecystectomy, including acute or chronic inflammation, inadequate exposure, patient obesity, and failure to identify structures before clamping, ligating, or dividing them. More specific causes of bile duct injury also exist. Bleeding from the cystic or hepatic arteries can lead to bile duct injury during attempts to gain hemostasis. The generous application of Liga clips at either open or laparoscopic cholecystectomy to hilar areas not well visualized can result in placing a clip on or across a bile duct, with resultant injury (Fig. 43-1). Failure to recognize congenital anatomic anomalies of the bile ducts, such as insertion of the right hepatic duct into the cystic duct or a long common wall between the cystic duct and the common bile duct, can also lead to injury (Fig. 43-2). A number of technical factors are associated with laparoscopic cholecystectomy that can also increase the risk of bile duct injury when compared with the open procedure. These include the use of an end-viewing laparoscope, which alters the surgeon's perspective of the operative field. Excessive cephalad retraction of the gallbladder fundus can cause the cystic duct and common bile duct to become aligned in the same plane. This distortion often results in the classic laparoscopic injury, in which the common bile duct is mistaken for the cystic duct and clipped and divided[1] (Fig. 43-3). The role of intraoperative cholangiography in preventing bile duct injury during laparoscopic cholecystectomy is controversial. Based on a number of published series advocating either routine or selective cholangiography, it appears that cholangiography does not prevent bile duct injury. The procedure, however, can minimize the extent of injury. Finally, ample evidence exists to support the conclusion that the experience of the surgeon in performing laparoscopic cholecystectomy can be correlated with the risk of bile duct injury.

The importance of ischemia of the bile duct in the formation of postoperative strictures has been emphasized. Un-

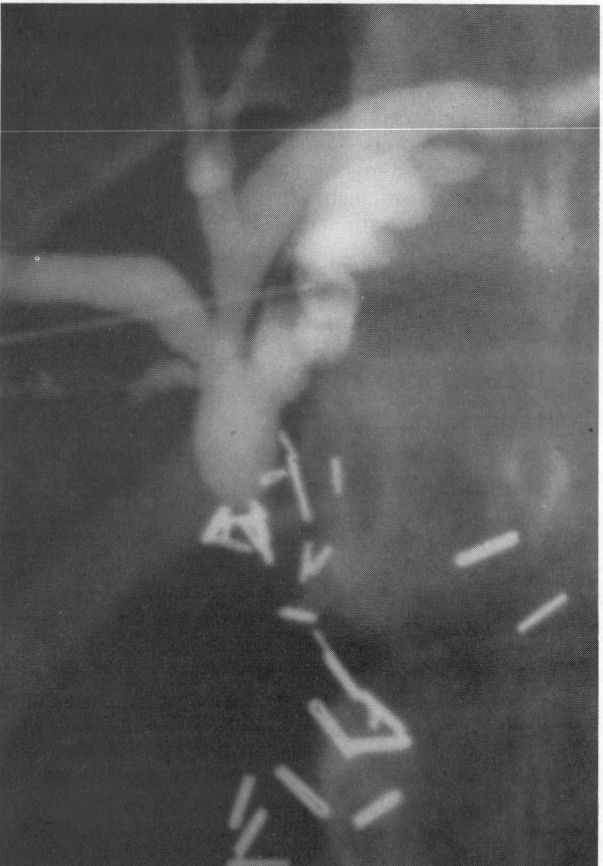

Figure 43-1. Percutaneous transhepatic cholangiogram in a patient with a bile duct stricture secondary to iatrogenic injury during cholecystectomy. Numerous surgical clips can be seen in the area of the stricture. (Lillemoe KD, Pitt HA, Cameron JL. Postoperative bile duct strictures. Surg Clin North Am 1990;70:1356)

necessary dissection around the bile duct during cholecystectomy or bile duct anastomosis can divide or injure the major arteries of the bile duct that run in the 3- and 9-o'clock positions (Fig. 43-4). Another important factor contributing to the formation of biliary strictures is the intense connective tissue response with fibrosis and scarring that can occur after bile duct injury. Experimental studies of bile duct ligation in a canine model have demonstrated immediate and sustained elevation of bile duct pressure and progressive increase in bile duct diameter. Histologic changes at 1 month after ligation have shown that the bile duct wall is thickened, with a reduction of mucosal folds and loss of surface microvilli, associated with a well-defined epithelial degeneration. Biochemical analysis of connective tissue response to ligation showed that collagen synthesis and Prolene hydroxylase activity is increased within 2 weeks in the obstructed bile duct and is sustained throughout the period of observation. Finally, a marked local inflammatory response can develop in the adjacent tissue in association with bile leakage, which occurs with many bile duct injuries. This inflammation can be further intensified in the face of infection. This inflammation results in fibrosis and scarring in the periductal tissue, further contributing to stricture formation. These factors can be of major importance in bile duct injuries during laparoscopic cholecystectomy, which are frequently associated with bile leaks.

After cholecystectomy and common bile duct exploration, the two most common operations associated with bile

duct injury are gastrectomy and hepatic resection. The most common situation resulting in bile duct injury during gastrectomy involves dissection of the pyloric region and the first portion of the duodenum in the face of inflammation from peptic ulcer disease. The injury occurs during mobilization of the duodenum either for creation of a Billroth I gastroduodenostomy or for closure of the duodenal stump. Biliary injury during liver resection is most likely to occur during dissection of the hepatic hilum.

In addition to iatrogenic bile duct injury occurring during cholecystectomy or other operations, bile duct strictures can also occur at biliary anastomoses. Such strictures can occur at a biliary–enteric anastomosis performed for reconstruction after resection for benign or malignant disease of the pancreaticobiliary system, or after end-to-end bile duct anastomosis performed for hepatic transplantation or for repair of traumatic injury. Ischemia of the anastomosis due to excessive skeletonization of the duct in preparation for the anastomosis is an important factor in many such strictures.

Unfortunately, the recurrence of bile duct strictures after an initial attempt at repair is not uncommon and can also account for a number of anastomotic strictures.[2,3] A number of other factors have been evaluated in patients who have developed a recurrent bile duct stricture, including the location of the stricture, the length of follow-up, the influence of previous operations, the type of operation performed, the type of sutures used, and the use and duration of postoperative stenting.[2] Previous attempts at repair and performance of a procedure other than choledochojejunostomy or hepaticojejunostomy and stricture location higher

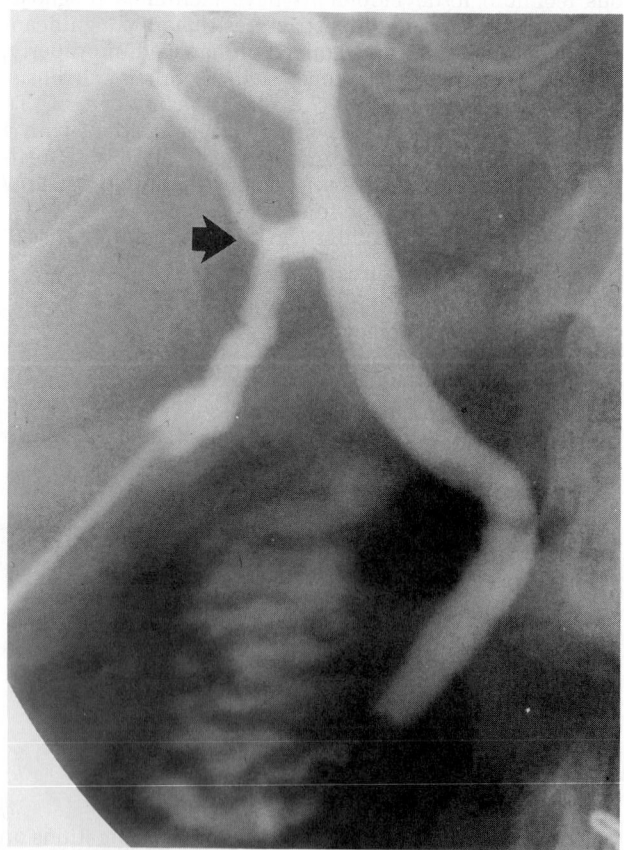

Figure 43-2. Operative cholangiogram demonstrating a right lobe segmental bile duct entering the cystic duct (*arrow*). Division of the cystic duct proximal to this insertion can result in a bile leak or obstruction of bile flow from a significant segment of the liver.

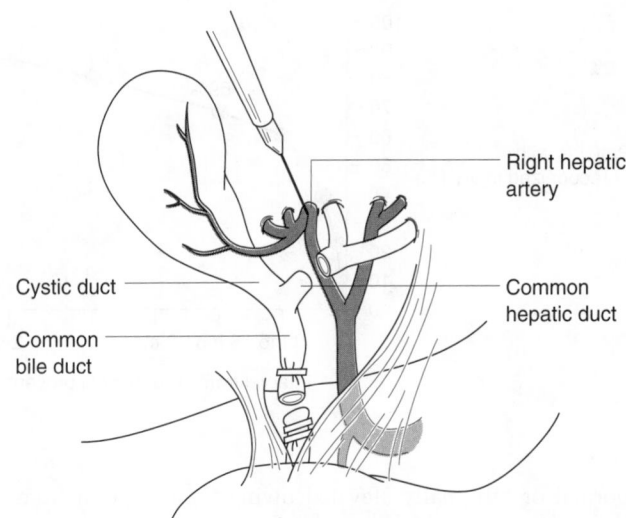

Figure 43-3. Classic laparoscopic bile duct injury. The common bile duct is mistaken for the cystic duct and transected. A variable extent of the extra-hepatic biliary tree is resected with the gallbladder. The right hepatic artery, in background, is also often injured. (After Branum G, Schmidt C, Baile J, et al. Management of major biliary complications after laparoscopic cholecystectomy. Ann Surg 1993; 217:532)

in the biliary tree appear to be associated with a higher incidence of recurrent stricture. The type of suture material used for repair does not influence the outcome. When postoperative biliary stents are used, a longer period of stenting appears to be favorable. Finally, long-term follow-up of a bile duct anastomosis is important because strictures can develop years after the original anastomosis.

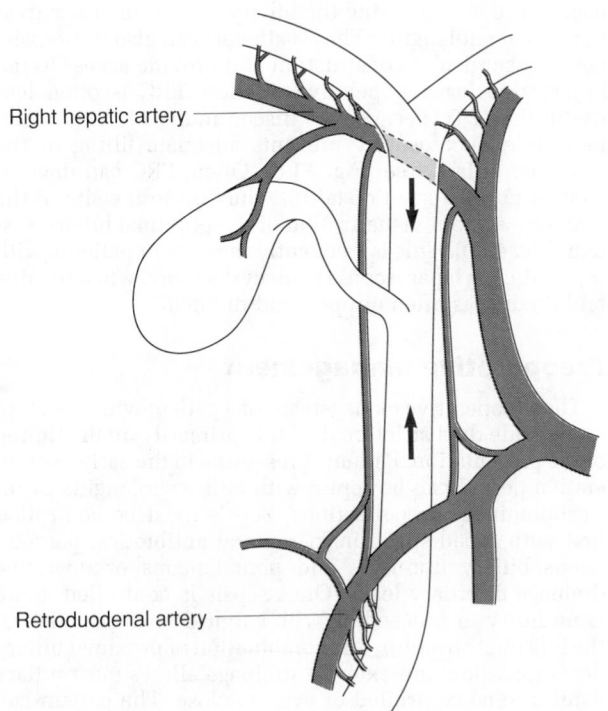

Figure 43-4. Diagrammatic view of the blood supply of the human bile duct. The blood supply to the bile ducts in the hilum of the liver (*above*) and to the intrapancreatic bile duct (*below*) from adjacent arteries is profuse. The supraduodenal bile duct blood supply is axial and tenuous, with 60% from below and 38% from above. The small main axial vessels (3- and 9-o'clock arteries) are vulnerable and easily damaged. (After Terblanche J, Allison HF, Northover JMA. An ischemic basis for biliary strictures. Surgery 1983;94:52)

Clinical Presentation

Most patients with benign postoperative bile duct strictures present early after their initial operation (Fig. 43-5). After open cholecystectomy, only about 10% of postoperative strictures are actually suspected within the first week, but nearly 70% are diagnosed within the first 6 months, and over 80% are diagnosed within 1 year of surgery.[2] In series reporting bile duct injuries during laparoscopic cholecystectomy, the injury is usually recognized either during the procedure or, more commonly, in the early postoperative period.

Patients suspected of having a postoperative bile duct stricture within days to weeks of initial operation usually present in one of two ways. One presentation is the progressive elevation of liver function tests, particularly total bilirubin and alkaline phosphatase levels. These changes can often be seen as early as the second or third postoperative day. The second mode of early presentation is with leakage of bile from the injured bile duct. This presentation appears to occur most often in patients presenting with bile duct injuries after laparoscopic cholecystectomy. Bilious drainage from operatively placed drains or through the wound after cholecystectomy is abnormal and represents some form of biliary injury. In patients without drains (including patients in whom the drains have been removed), the bile can leak freely into the peritoneal cavity, or it can loculate as a collection. Free accumulation of bile into the peritoneal cavity results in either biliary ascites or bile peritonitis. Similarly, a loculated bile collection can result in sterile biloma (Fig. 43-6) or in an infected subhepatic or subdiaphragmatic abscess.

Patients with postoperative bile duct strictures who present months to years after the initial operation frequently have evidence of cholangitis. The episodes of cholangitis are often mild and respond to antibiotic therapy. Repetitive episodes usually occur before the definitive diagnosis. Less commonly, patients may present with painless jaundice and no evidence of sepsis. Finally, patients with markedly delayed diagnoses may present with advanced biliary cirrhosis and its complications.

Laboratory Investigations

Liver function tests usually show evidence of cholestasis. The serum bilirubin can fluctuate; occasionally, it is normal. In patients with bile leakage, the bilirubin can be

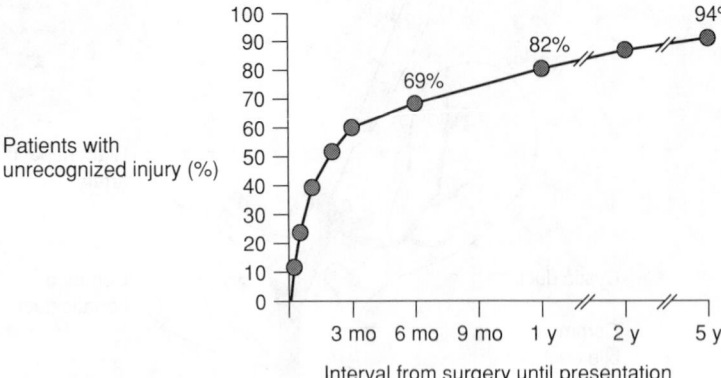

Figure 43-5. The cumulative percentage of patients developing symptoms is shown with respect to the time interval from the procedure during which the injury occurred until the presentation of the symptoms. (After Pitt HA, Miyamoto T, Parapatis SK, et al. Factors influencing outcome in patients with postoperative biliary strictures. Am J Surg 1982;144:14)

normal or minimally elevated owing to absorption from the peritoneal cavity. When elevated, serum bilirubin usually ranges from 2 to 6 mg/dL unless secondary biliary cirrhosis has developed. Serum alkaline phosphatase is usually elevated. Serum transaminase levels can be normal or minimally elevated except during episodes of cholangitis. If advanced liver disease exists, hepatic synthetic function can be impaired, with lowered serum albumin and a prolongation of prothrombin time. Serum electrolytes and complete blood count are typically normal unless there is associated biliary sepsis.

Radiologic Examinations

The imaging techniques of abdominal ultrasound and computed tomography (CT) play an important initial role in the evaluation of patients with benign postoperative biliary strictures. In patients who present in the early postoperative period with evidence of a bile leak or biliary sepsis, these studies are useful to rule out the presence of intraabdominal collections that might require drainage (see Fig. 43-6). CT and ultrasound are also important in the initial evaluation of the patient presenting with a bile duct stricture months to years after initial operation. Both studies can confirm biliary obstruction by demonstrating a dilated biliary tree. CT is especially useful in identifying the level of obstruction of the extrahepatic bile duct.

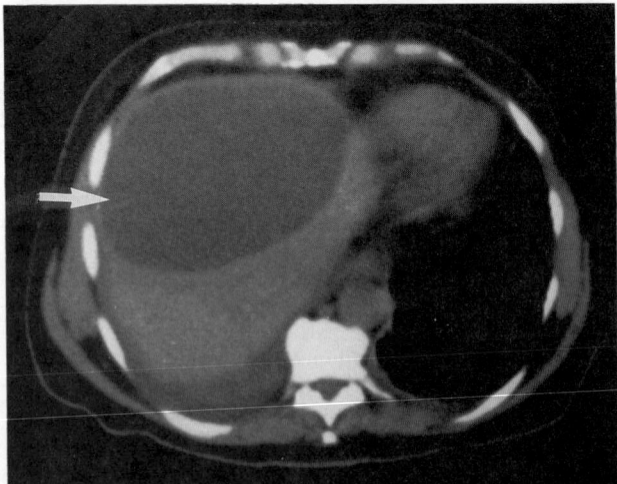

Figure 43-6. Large bile duct collection (biloma; *arrow*) occurring after bile duct injury. (Lillemoe KD, Pitt HA, Cameron JL. Postoperative bile duct strictures. Surg Clin North Am 1990;70:1362)

In patients suspected of having early postoperative bile duct injury, a radionucleotide biliary scan can confirm bile leakage. In patients with postoperative external bile fistula, injection of water-soluble contrast media through the drainage tract (sinography) can often define the site of leakage and the anatomy of the biliary tree. Sinography can also identify intraabdominal collections and facilitate nonoperative drainage.

The gold standard for evaluation of patients with bile duct strictures is cholangiography. Percutaneous transhepatic cholangiography (PTC) is generally more valuable than endoscopic retrograde cholangiography (ERC). PTC is more useful in that it defines the anatomy of the proximal biliary tree that is to be used in the surgical reconstruction (Fig. 43-7). Furthermore, PTC can be followed by placement of percutaneous transhepatic catheters, which can be useful in decompressing the biliary system to either treat or prevent cholangitis. These catheters can also be of assistance in surgical reconstruction and provide access to the biliary tree for nonoperative dilation. ERC is often less useful than PTC because the discontinuity of the extrahepatic bile duct usually prevents adequate filling of the proximal biliary tree (Fig. 43-8). Often, ERC can demonstrate a normal-sized distal bile duct up to the site of the stricture without visualization of the proximal biliary system (Fig. 43-9). This is frequently the case in patients with injury during laparoscopic cholecystectomy, when the distal bile duct is often clipped and divided.

Preoperative Management

The preoperative management of a patient with a postoperative bile duct stricture depends primarily on the timing of the presentation. Patients presenting in the early postoperative period can be septic with either cholangitis or intraabdominal bile collections. Sepsis must be controlled first with broad-spectrum parenteral antibiotics, percutaneous biliary drainage, and percutaneous or operative drainage of biliary leaks. Once sepsis is controlled, there is no hurry in proceeding with surgical reconstruction of the bile duct stricture. The combination of proximal biliary decompression and external drainage allows most biliary fistulas to be controlled or even to close. The patient can then be discharged home to allow several months to elapse for resolution of the inflammation in the periportal region and recovery of overall health status.

The management of a suspected bile duct injury after laparoscopic cholecystectomy presenting with a bile leak deserves special mention. Often, when bile leakage is suspected, the surgeon believes that urgent surgical exploration is necessary. Unfortunately, at laparotomy, the marked inflammation associated with bile spillage and the

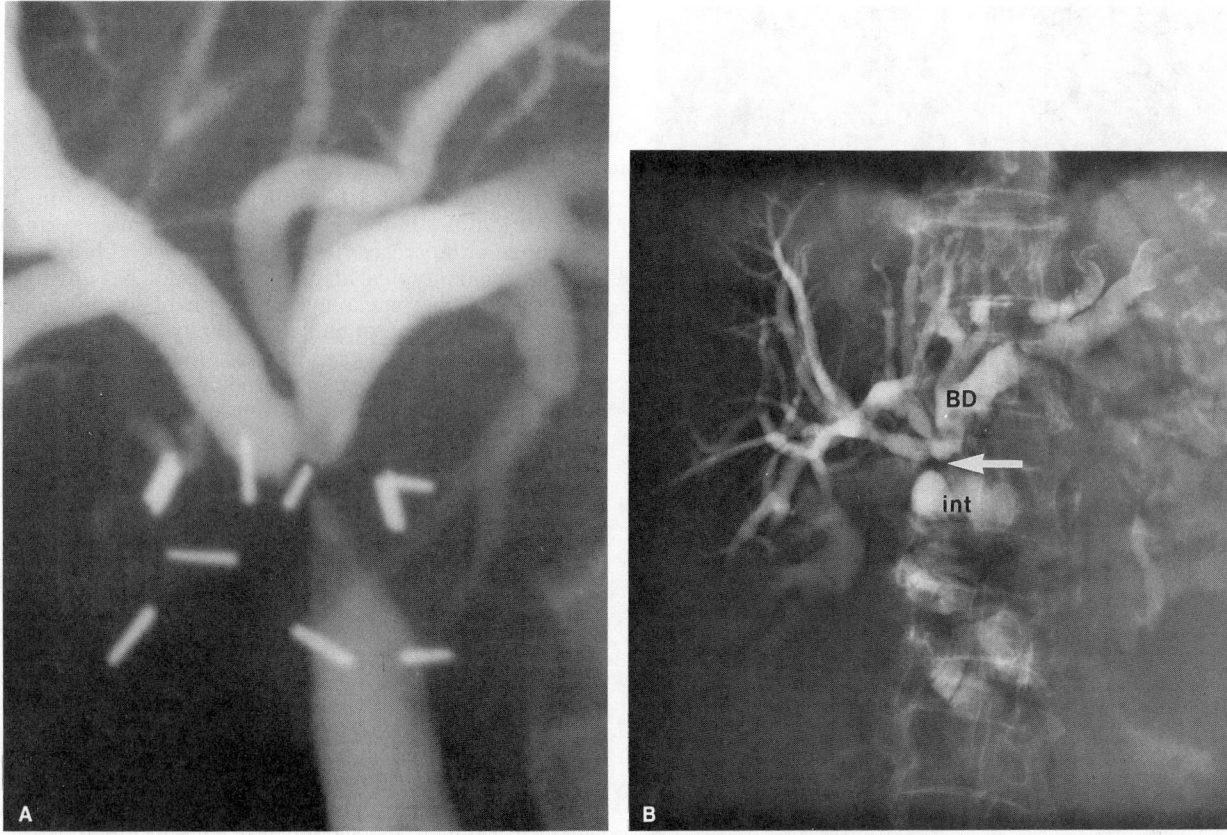

Figure 43-7. (*A*) Percutaneous transhepatic cholangiogram demonstrating bile duct stricture (*arrow*) at hepatic duct bifurcation with proximal duct dilation. (*B*) Percutaneous transhepatic cholangiogram demonstrating stricture at a hepaticojejunostomy anastomosis. BD, bile duct; int, intestine.

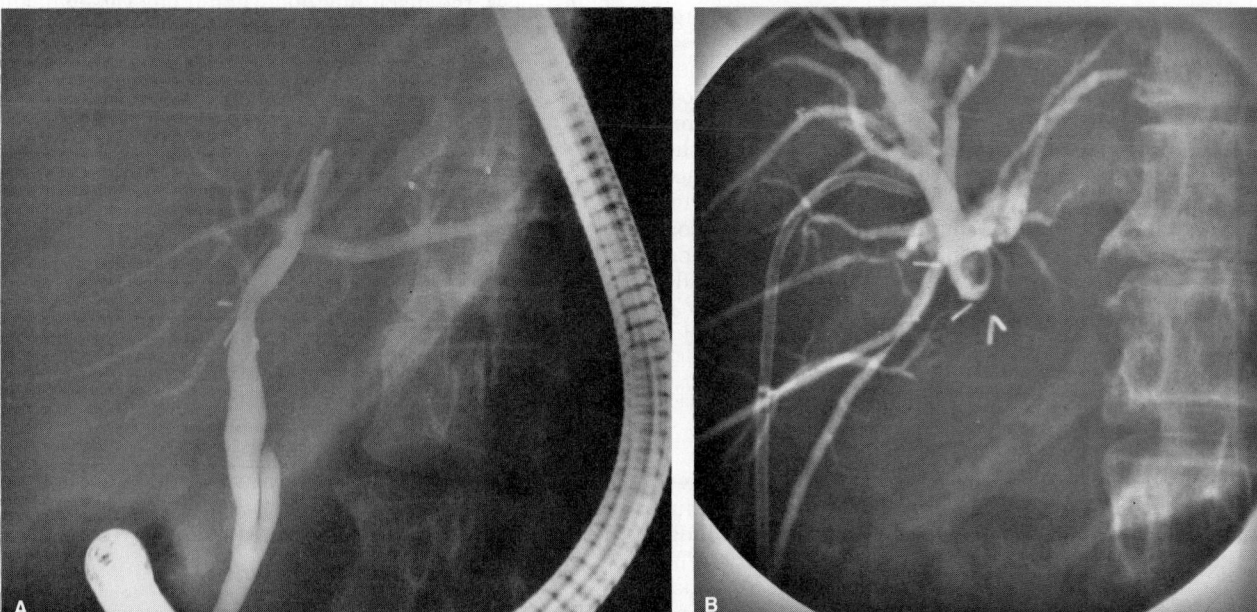

Figure 43-8. (*A*) Endoscopic retrograde cholangiogram showing a relatively normal biliary tree in a patient with a postoperative bile collection (see Fig. 43-6). (*B*) Percutaneous transhepatic cholangiogram of same patient, showing entire right hepatic posterior lobe segment obstructed as the result of ligation of the segmental duct. The patient had an unrecognized anatomic variant similar to that shown in Figure 43-2.

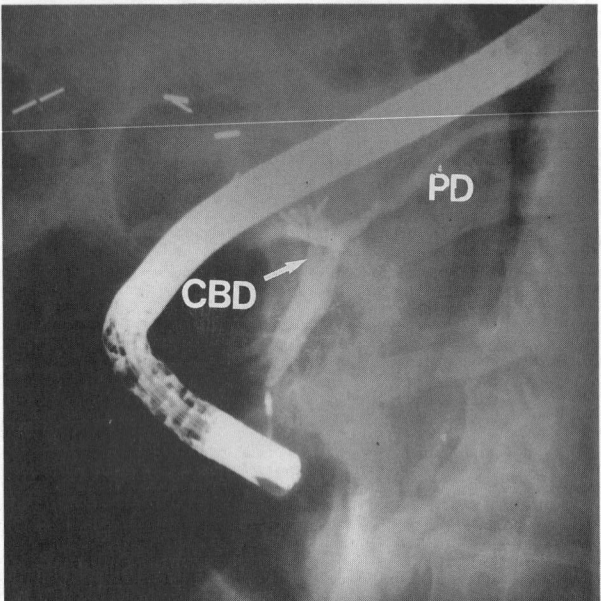

Figure 43-9. Endoscopic retrograde pancreaticocholangiogram showing filling of a normal pancreatic duct (PD). The common bile duct (CBD), however, does not fill beyond the large clip that appears to be placed across the duct. (Lillemoe KD, Pitt HA, Cameron JL. Postoperative bile duct strictures. Surg Clin North Am 1990;70:1363)

small decompressed biliary tree that appears retracted high into porta hepatis make recognition of the injury and repair virtually impossible. In such cases, every attempt should be made to define the biliary anatomy by preoperative cholangiography and to control the bile leak with either percutaneous or endoscopic stents. In many cases, early operative intervention is not required because the bile either can be drained percutaneously or simply is absorbed from the peritoneal cavity. Delayed reconstruction, aided by percutaneous biliary catheters, then allows optimal surgical results.

In patients who present with a biliary stricture remote from the initial operation, symptoms of cholangitis can necessitate urgent cholangiography and biliary decompression. Biliary drainage is best accomplished by the transhepatic method, although successful endoscopic stent placement can also be accomplished. Parenteral antibiotics and biliary drainage should be continued until sepsis is controlled. In patients who present with jaundice but without cholangitis, cholangiography should be performed to define the anatomy. Preoperative biliary decompression in patients without cholangitis has not been demonstrated to improve outcome.

Surgical Management

The goal of operative management of bile duct stricture is the establishment of bile flow into the proximal gastrointestinal tract in a manner that prevents cholangitis, sludge or stone formation, restricture, and biliary cirrhosis. This goal is best accomplished with a tension-free anastomosis between healthy tissues. A number of surgical alternatives exist for primary repair of bile duct strictures, including end-to-end repair, Roux-en-Y hepaticojejunostomy or choledochojejunostomy, choledochoduodenostomy, and mucosal grafting. The choice of repair depends on a number of factors, including the extent and location

of the strictures, the experience of the surgeon, and the timing of the repair.

Immediate Repair of Intraoperative Bile Duct Injury

In many cases, initial proper management of bile duct injury recognized at the time of cholecystectomy can avoid the development of a bile duct stricture. Unfortunately, recognition of a bile duct injury is uncommon during either open or laparoscopic cholecystectomy. If bile leakage is observed or atypical anatomy is encountered during laparoscopic cholecystectomy, early conversion to an open technique and prompt cholangiography are imperative. If a segmental or accessory duct less than 3 mm has been injured and cholangiography demonstrates segmental or subsegmental drainage of the injured ductal system, simple ligation of the injured duct is adequate. If the injured duct is 4 mm or larger, however, it is likely to drain multiple hepatic segments or the entire right or left lobe and thus requires operative repair.

If the injury involves the common hepatic duct or the common bile duct, repair should also be carried out at the time of injury. The aims of any repair should be to maintain ductal length and not to sacrifice tissue as well as to effect a repair that will not result in postoperative bile leakage. To accomplish these goals, all repairs at the time of initial operation should involve some sort of external drainage. If the injured segment of the bile duct is short (less than 1 cm), and the two ends can be opposed without tension, an end-to-end anastomosis can be performed with placement of a T-tube through a separate choledochotomy either above or below the anastomosis. Generous mobilization of the duodenum out of the retroperitoneum (Kocher maneuver) can be useful to help approximate the injured ends of the bile duct. An end-to-end repair, however, should be avoided if the ductal injury is near the hepatic duct bifurcation.

For proximal injuries or if the injured segment of bile duct is greater than 1 cm in length, an end-to-end bile duct anastomosis should be avoided because of the excessive tension that usually exists in these situations. In these circumstances, the distal bile duct should be oversewn, and the proximal bile duct should be débrided of injured tissue and anastomosed in an end-to-side fashion to a Roux-en-Y jejunal limb. The use of a Roux-en-Y jejunal limb is preferable to anastomosis to the duodenum because, in the latter case, an anastomotic leak results in a duodenal fistula.

The long-term results of immediate repair of common bile duct injuries is uncertain. Most injuries occur away from major centers, and therefore, even the successes are unlikely to be reported in the literature. In a Swedish report, early primary repair with end-to-end anastomosis resulted in good results in only 22% of patients. Anastomotic leak requiring reoperation occurred in 32% of patients, and late stricture occurred in another 37% of patients. In patients undergoing immediate repair with a biliary–enteric anastomosis, good results were seen in 54% of patients, with strictures occurring in only 12% of patients. Similar poor late results were observed in another series in which 29 of 36 patients with primary end-to-end repair developed postoperative strictures within 4 years.

Elective Repair of Established Strictures

Several principles are associated with successful repair of a biliary stricture: exposure of healthy proximal bile ducts that provide drainage of the entire liver; preparation of a suitable segment of intestine that can be brought to the area of the stricture without tension, most frequently a Roux-en-Y jejunal limb; and creation of a direct biliary–

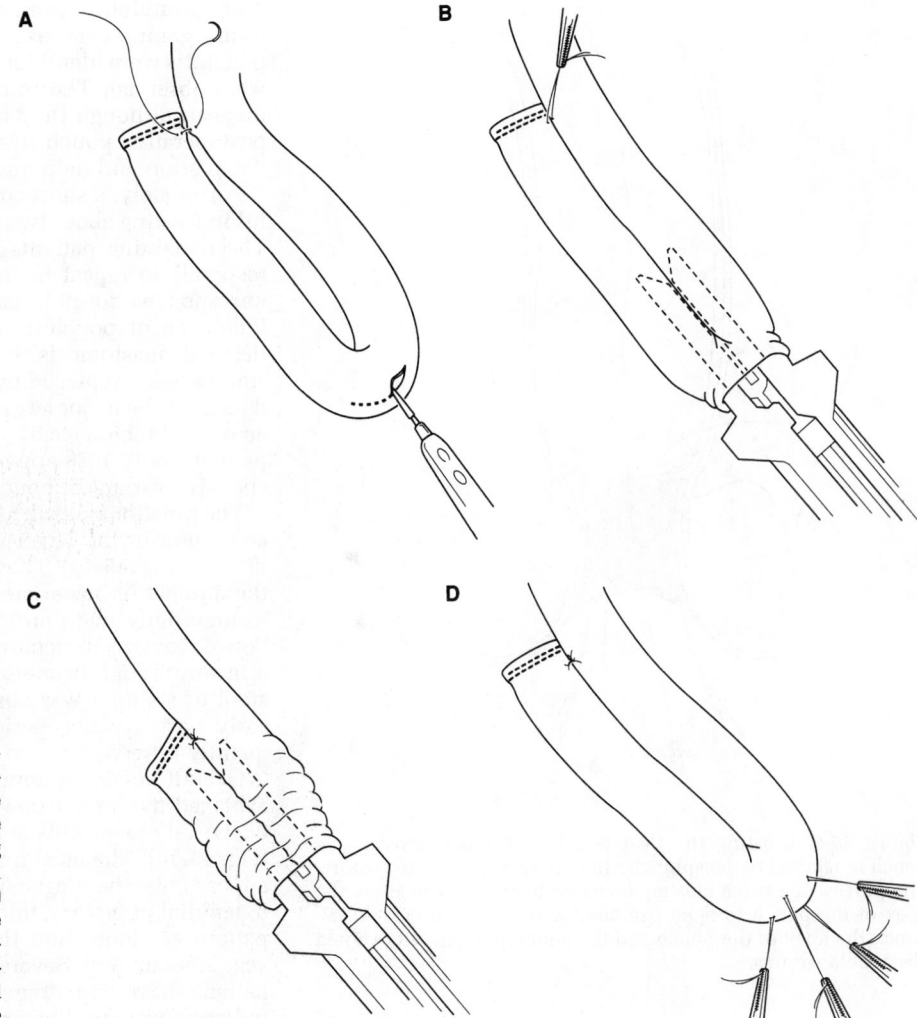

Figure 45-8. Ileal J-pouch construction. (*A*) Using electrocautery, an enterotomy is created at the apex of the 15-cm loop of terminal ileum. (*B*) The forks of an intestinal anastomosing stapler are pressed into the intestinal limbs, and the instrument is fired. (*C*) This is repeated once or twice while the limbs are telescoped onto the stapler, until a 15-cm side-to-side anastomosis is completed. (*D*) The apical enterotomy is closed with a simple pursestring stitch.

mary or secondary malabsorption, stasis, ischemia, and nutritional or immune deficiencies.[45] Investigators characterized axonal necrosis of enteric autonomic nerves in continent ileal pouches.[46] Axonal necrosis, an ultrastructural diagnosis, was previously demonstrated in samples of small intestine obtained from patients with Crohn's disease. These same findings were demonstrated in patients with pouchitis in association with the presence of mucosally invasive bacteria. This association suggested mechanistic similarities for the pathogenesis of Crohn's disease and pouchitis.

The role of stasis as an important etiologic factor in pouchitis is confused by the fact that stasis occurs to some degree in nearly all ileal pouches, and most authors fail to differentiate pouchitis from pouch dysfunction. Most available evidence suggests that stasis is not responsible for pouchitis directly. Nevertheless, the patient with poor pouch function must be identified accurately, and scintigraphic emptying studies perform this task well.[47] Although perturbation of the bacterial flora, a bacterial dysbiosis, may be responsible for pouchitis, no link has been found between a specific microbial pattern and pouchitis. Although a cause-and-effect relation is purely speculative, short-chain fatty acid concentrations are decreased in patients with pouchitis,[48,49] and low concentrations of butyric acid correlate with severe villous atrophy. Another possible cause of pouchitis is a relative deficit of gluta-

mine.[35] Based on these preliminary observations, nutritional repletion using either butyrate or glutamine may be an option for the prevention or management of pouchitis. Ischemia may likewise cause pouchitis.[50] Under conditions of hypoperfusion, xanthene oxidase activity may act as a potent source of oxygen-free radicals that cause tissue damage.

An important clinical clue is the observation that there is a significantly higher incidence of pouchitis in patients who exhibited extraintestinal manifestation of their inflammatory bowel disease before colectomy.[51] Pouchitis occurred in 40% of patients who exhibited extraintestinal manifestations, compared with a 20% incidence of pouchitis in those patients in whom extraintestinal manifestations were absent. This leads to the speculation that pouchitis may be a further manifestation of inflammatory bowel disease. A striking clinical observation has been the difference in frequency of pouchitis between patients operated on for ulcerative colitis and those operated on for familial polyposis coli. In one series of more than 400 patients evaluated over 10 years, no cases of pouchitis were observed in patients with familial polyposis, while a 19% observance was seen in chronic ulcerative colitis patients.

Pouchitis remains a clinically defined syndrome. Much of the controversy surrounding pouchitis revolves around the fact that no clear diagnostic criteria have been established. Clinical, endoscopic, and histologic criteria have

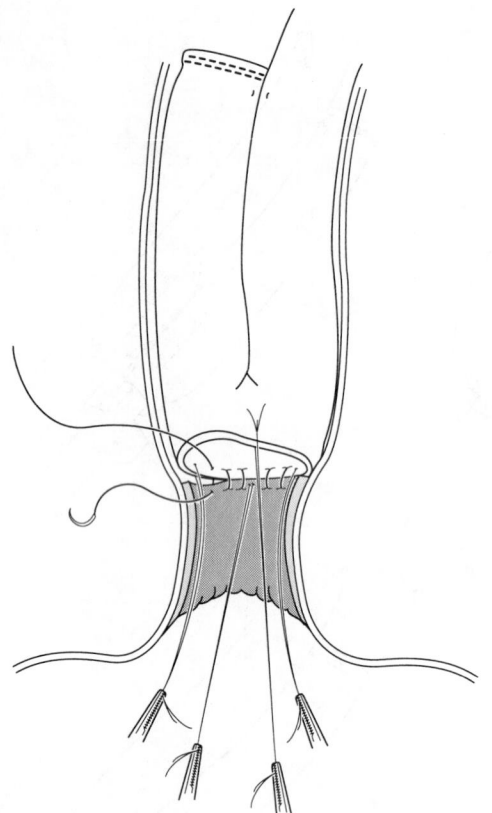

Figure 45-9. Creating the ileal pouch–anal anastomosis. The pouch is secured to the sphincter in each quadrant with a suture. The pursestring stitch closing the enterotomy is cut to allow the apex of the pouch to open. An anastomosis is then created between the apex of the pouch and the anoderm using interrupted absorbable sutures.

all been applied without clear controls or norms. Some authors have tried to base the diagnosis on endoscopic criteria. They have suggested that mild pouchitis is characterized by swelling, friability, and erythema of the mucosa. Superficial ulcers occur in moderate pouchitis, whereas severe pouchitis is characterized by diffuse erythema, copious exudate, and extensive superficial ulceration and even necrosis. The relations among endoscopic appearances, clinical symptoms, and histologic changes are unclear. Although investigators have shown a significant relation between the endoscopic and histologic features of acute inflammation, 24 of 46 patients with endoscopic abnormalities showed microscopically normal appearances.[52] Similarly, others have been unable to define morphologic abnormalities that distinguish patients with pouchitis from those without.[53]

Histologic assessment causes even further confusion. Chronic inflammatory changes are observed in essentially all ileal pouches, are thought to be an unavoidable response to fecal stasis, and are unrelated to clinical results in terms of stool frequency and incontinence.[35,52] Moreover, some degree of acute inflammation is present in up to two thirds of pouches, although more severe and extensive infiltrates with acute inflammatory cells are seen in association with symptomatic pouchitis. Investigators have attempted to quantify the presence and degree of inflammatory infiltrate in patients with pouchitis using white-cell scanning techniques.[34] They showed that in pouchitis there is a migration of neutrophils from the circulation to the inflamed ileal reservoir. By combining a positive in-

dium granulocyte scan and an increased 4-day fecal indium granulocyte excretion, all patients with severe pouchitis were identified. A number of false-positive scans were observed. The role of such scanning techniques is unclear, although they may help distinguish nonspecific postoperative pouch dysfunction from acute mucosal inflammation and help quantify the response to therapy.

Fortunately, a short course of metronidazole is successful in treating about two thirds of patients with pouchitis. The remaining patients have recurrent pouchitis, which responds to repeat metronidazole therapy, or a chronic, unresponsive form. It has been argued that, with the high incidence of pouchitis observed in some patients after ileoanal anastomosis, one disease (ulcerative colitis) is simply being replaced by another (pouchitis). Analysis of data from the major large clinical series, however, suggests an overall incidence of pouchitis of about 15%.[23] Of these patients, only 10% appear to develop a recurrent or unresponsive variant of pouchitis.

The functional result after ileoanal anastomosis has been consistent in the larger series with adequate late follow-up data (Fig. 45-13). These studies have demonstrated that the number of bowel movements was in the range of four to nine daily, with an average of six per day. Nocturnal bowel movements occurred one to two times nightly, with a mean of slightly more than one. Nocturnal seepage of stool or staining was observed in 20% of patients in the early postoperative period, but by 1 year, it was infrequently observed.

Overall, mean 24-hour and nocturnal stool frequencies averaged five or six bowel movements per 24 hours and 0.5 bowel movements at night in the late follow-up period (Fig. 45-14). The most important determinants of outcome appear to be the diagnosis of ulcerative colitis as opposed to familial polyposis, the preoperative stool frequency and pattern of stools, and the capacity of the ileal pouch 1 year after surgery. Several studies have demonstrated that patients have an extremely high level of satisfaction and performance after ileoanal anastomosis, particularly compared with those who have undergone conventional Brooke ileostomy.

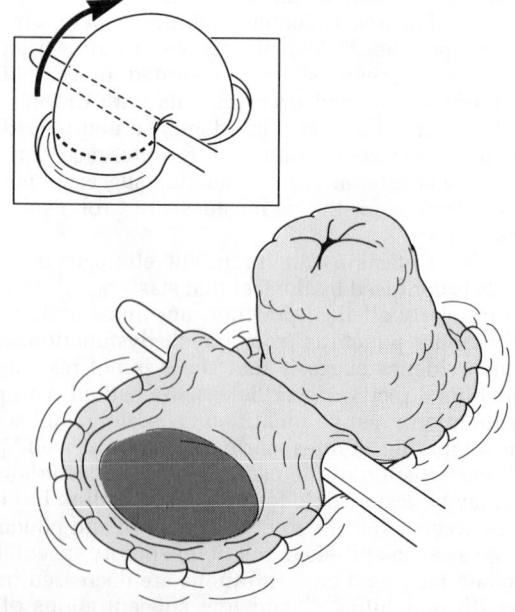

Figure 45-10. A loop ileostomy is constructed 40 cm proximal to the ileal pouch and is matured over a rod.

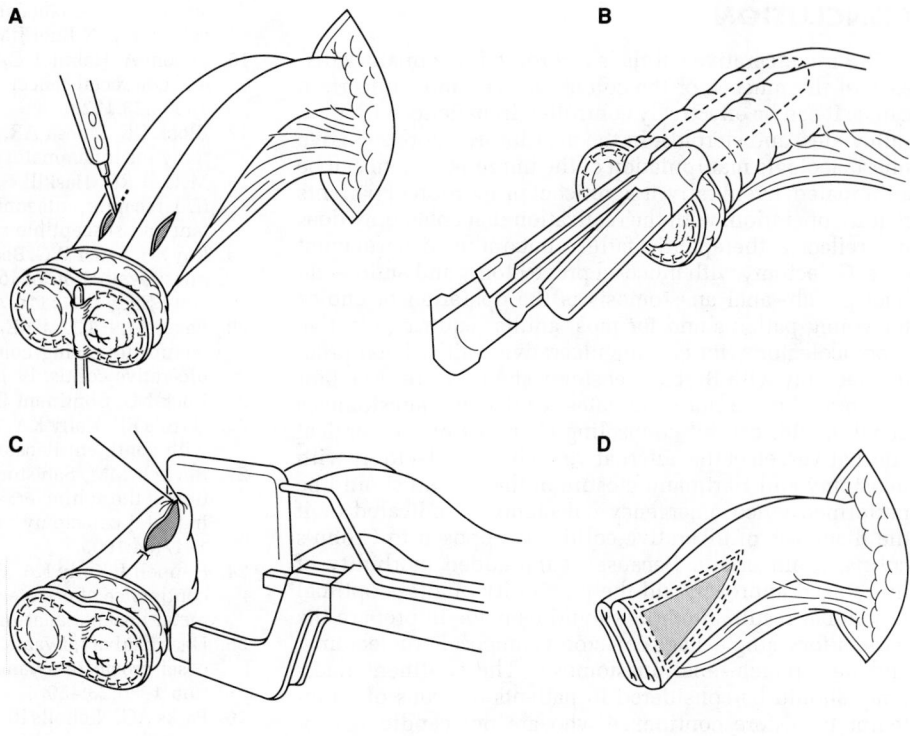

Figure 45-11. Closure of loop ileostomy. (*A*) A transverse elliptical incision is made around the stoma, and the limbs are dissected free. (*B*) The antimesenteric surfaces of the limb are tacked together, and the jaws of an anastomosing stapler are passed through enterotomies and down into the lumen of each of the intestinal limbs. The stapler is then fired to create a side-to-side anastomosis between the afferent and efferent ileal limbs. (*C*) A linear stapler is placed and fired below the former stoma and below the edges of the enterotomy. The stoma and distal limbs are amputated, and the stapler is released. (*D*) The anastomosis is dropped back into the peritoneal cavity, and the peritoneum, fascia, and skin are closed.

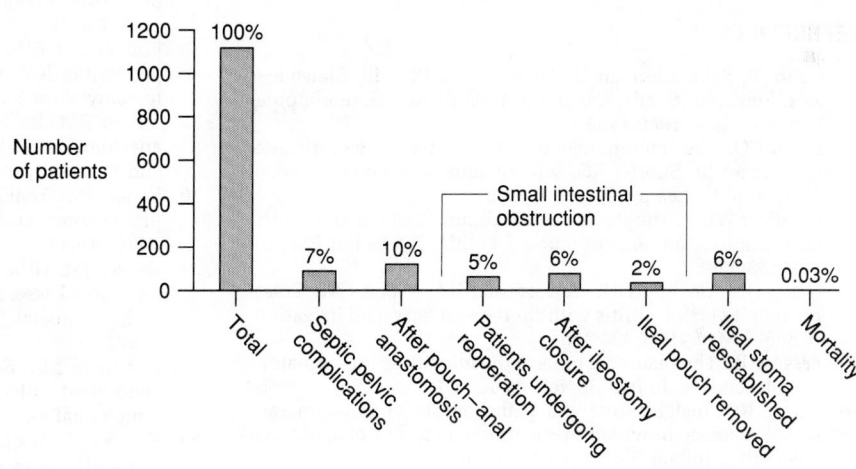

Figure 45-12. Operative morbidity after colectomy and ileoanal anastomosis in 12 clinical series.

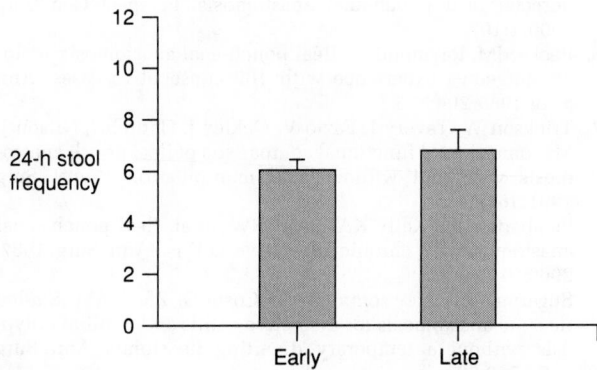

Figure 45-13. Early and late postoperative daily stool frequency in patients after colectomy and ileal pouch–anal anastomosis as reported in 12 clinical series.

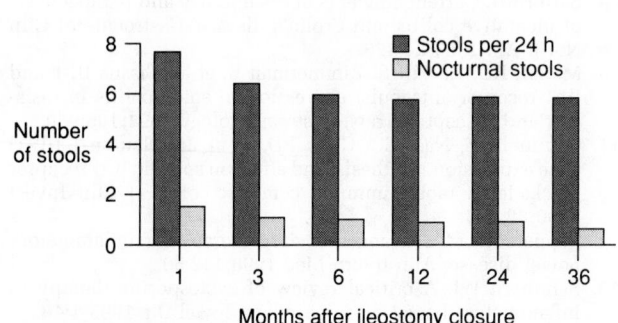

Figure 45-14. Twenty-four-hour and nocturnal stool frequencies after colectomy and ileoanal anastomosis in the author's series of patients.

CONCLUSION

Chronic ulcerative colitis is a chronic inflammatory disease of the mucosa of the colon and rectum of uncertain cause. It can be effectively controlled in patients with diet, salicylates, and steroids. In the near future, more selective pharmacologic manipulation of the immune system can be anticipated. Eventually, a significant proportion of patients require operation, with the realization that colectomy does not reflect a therapeutic failure but rather a permanent cure. Colectomy with mucosal proctectomy and endorectal ileal pouch–anal anastomosis is the operation of choice for young patients and for most adults requiring elective proctocolectomy for chronic ulcerative colitis. Total proctocolectomy with Brooke ileostomy should be reserved for patients who are not candidates for ileoanal anastomosis or who, after careful counseling about all of the surgical alternatives, elect that alternative. Subtotal colectomy with ileostomy and Hartmann closure of the rectum should be performed when emergency colectomy is indicated or if the diagnosis of ulcerative colitis, as opposed to Crohn's colitis, is uncertain. Because of the added morbidity of this staged approach and the possibility of a less optimal functional result, attempts should be made to prepare the patient for a single-stage colectomy, mucosal proctectomy, and ileal pouch–anal anastomosis. The continent ileostomy should be considered in patients desirous of an attempt to restore continence who are not candidates for ileoanal pull-through or in whom total proctocolectomy with ileostomy has already been performed.

REFERENCES

1. Cello JP, Schneiderman DJ. Ulcerative colitis. In: Sleisenger MH, Fordtran JS, eds. Gastrointestinal disease. Philadelphia, WB Saunders, 1989;1435.
2. Elson CO. The immunology of inflammatory bowel disease. In: Kirsner JB, Shorter RG, eds. Inflammatory bowel disease. Philadelphia, Lea & Febiger, 1988;97.
3. Roediger WEW. The starved colon: diminished mucosal nutrition, diminished absorption, and colitis. Dis Colon Rectum 1990;33:858.
4. Harig HM, Soergel HH, Koworowski RA, Wood CM. Treatment of diversion colitis with short chain fatty acid irrigation. N Engl J Med 1989;230:23.
5. Kirsner JB. The historical basis of the idiopathic inflammatory bowel diseases. Inflam Bowel Dis 1995;1:2.
6. Sartor RB. Insights into the pathogenesis of inflammatory bowel diseases provided by new rodent models of spontaneous colitis. Inflam Bowel Dis 1995;1:64.
7. Sartor RB. Animal models of intestinal inflammation: relevance to IBD. In: MacDermott RP, Stenson W, eds. Inflammatory bowel disease. New York: Elsevier, 1991;337.
8. Stenson WF. Animal models of inflammatory bowel disease. In: Tagran SR, ed. Inflammatory bowel disease: from bench to bedside. Baltimore: Williams & Wilkins, 1994;180.
9. Sartor RB. Current concepts of the etiology and pathogenesis of ulcerative colitis and Crohn's disease. Gastroenterol Clin North Am 1995;24:475.
10. McCall RD, Haskill S, Zimmerman E, et al. Tissue IL-1 and IL-1 receptor antagonist expression in enterocolitis in resistant and susceptible rats. Gastroenterology 1994;106:960.
11. Cominelli F, Nast CC, Clark BD, et al. Interleukin-1 (IL-1) gene expression, synthesis, and effect on specific IL-1 receptor blockade in rabbit immune complex colitis. J Clin Invest 1990;86:972.
12. Peppercorn M. Advances in drug therapy for inflammatory bowel disease. Ann Intern Med 1990;112:50.
13. Sandborn WJ. A critical review of cyclosporine therapy in inflammatory bowel disease. Inflam Bowel Dis 1995;1:48.
14. Sachar DB. Colectomy in ulcerative colitis: indications. In: Bayless TM, ed. Current management of inflammatory bowel disease. Philadelphia, BC Decker, 1989.
15. Collins RH, Feldman M, Fordtran JS. Colonic cancer, dysplasia, and surveillance in patients with ulcerative colitis: a critical review. N Engl J Med 1987;316:1654.
16. Ekbom A, Helmick C, Zack M, Adami H-O. Ulcerative colitis and colorectal cancer: a population based study. N Engl J Med 1990;323:1228.
17. Block GE, Moosa AR, Siminowitz D, et al. Emergency colectomy for inflammatory bowel disease. Surgery 1977;82:531.
18. McCall RD, Haskill S, Zimmerman E, et al. Tissue IL-1 and IL-1 receptor antagonist expression in enterocolitis in resistant and susceptible rats. Gastroenterology 1994;106:960.
19. Roy PH, Sauer WG, Beahrs OH, et al. Experiences with ileostomies: evaluation of long-term rehabilitation in 497 patients. Am J Surg 1970;119:77.
20. Baker WN, Glass RE, Ritchie JK, Aylett HS. Cancer of the rectum following colectomy and ileorectal anastomosis for ulcerative colitis. Br J Surg 1978;65:682.
21. Kock NG. Continent ileostomy. Prog Surg 1973;12:180.
22. Dozois RR, Kelly KA, Beart RW, Beahrs OH. Improved results with continent ileostomy. Ann Surg 1980;192:319.
23. Ravitch MM, Sabiston DL Jr. Anal ileostomy with preservation of the sphincter: a proposed operation in patients requiring total colectomy for benign lesions. Surg Gynecol Obstet 1947;84:1095.
24. Heppell J, Kelly KA, Phillips SF, et al. Physiologic aspects of continence after colectomy, mucosal proctectomy and endorectal ileoanal anastomosis. Ann Surg 1982;195:435.
25. Utsunomiya J, Iwama T, Imajo M, et al. Total colectomy, mucosal proctectomy and ileoanal-pull-through. Dis Colon Rectum 1980;23:459.
26. Parks AG, Nicholls RJ, Belliveau P. Proctocolectomy with ileal reservoir and anal anastomosis. Br J Surg 1980;67:533.
27. Nicholls RJ, Pezim ME. Restorative proctocolectomy with ileal reservoir for ulcerative colitis and familial adenomatous polyposis: a comparison of three reservoir designs. Br J Surg 1985;72:470.
28. Fonkalsrud EW. Endorectal ileoanal anastomosis with isoperistaltic ileal reservoir after colectomy and mucosal proctectomy. Ann Surg 1984;199:151.
29. Taylor BM, Beart RW Jr, Dozois RR, et al. Straight ileoanal anastomosis vs ileal pouch-anal anastomosis after colectomy and mucosal proctectomy. Arch Surg 1983;118:696.
30. Becker JM. Anal sphincter function after colectomy, mucosal proctectomy, and endorectal ileoanal pull-through. Arch Surg 1984;119:526.
31. Becker JM, Hillard AE, Mann FA, Kestenberg A, Nelson JA. Functional assessment after colectomy, mucosal proctectomy, and endorectal ileoanal pull-through. World J Surg 1985;9:589.
32. Zenilman ME, Soper NJ, Dunnegan D, Becker JM. Previous abdominal colectomy affects functional results after ileal pouch-anal anastomosis. World J Surg 1990;14:594.
33. Ferzoco SJ, Becker JM. Does aggressive medical therapy for acute ulcerative colitis result in a higher incidence of staged colectomy? Arch Surg 1993;129:420.
34. Becker JM, Parodi JE. Total colectomy with preservation of the anal sphincter. Surg Ann 1989;21:263.
35. Becker JM, Soper NJ. Colectomy, mucosal proctectomy, endorectal ileal pouch-anal anastomosis. Perspect Gen Surg 1990;1:107.
36. Becker JM, Raymond JL. Ileal pouch-anal anastomosis: a single surgeon's experience with 100 consecutive cases. Ann Surg 1986;204:375.
37. Trickson W, Tavery I, Fazio V, Oakley J, Church J, Nilson J. Manometric and functional comparison of ileal pouch anastomosis with and without anal manipulation. Am J Surg 1991;161:90.
38. Pemberton JH, Kelly KA, Beart RW, et al. Ileal pouch–anal anastomosis for chronic ulcerative colitis. Ann Surg 1987;206:504.
39. Sugarman HJ, Newsome HH, DeCosta G, Zfass AM. Sta-led ileoanal anastomosis for ulcerative colitis and familial polyposis without a temporary diverting ileostomy. Ann Surg 1991;213:606.
40. Seow-Choen T, Sunoda A, Nicholls RJ. Prospective randomized trial comparing anal function after hand sewn ileoanal anastomosis with mucosectomy versus stapled ileoanal anas-

tomosis without mucosectomy in restorative proctocolectomy. Br J Surg 1991;78:430.

41. Luukkonen P, Jarvinen H. Stapled vs hand-sutured ileoanal anastomosis in restorative proctocolectomy. Arch Surg 1993; 128:437.

42. Ambroze WL, Pemberton JH, Dozois R, Carpenter HA, O'Rourke JS, Ilstrup DM. The historical pattern and pathological involvement of the anal transition zone in patients with ulcerative colitis. Gastroenterology 1993;104:514.

43. Utsunomiya J, Iwama T, Imajo M, et al. Total colectomy, mucosal proctectomy and ileoanal-pull-through. Dis Colon Rectum 1980;23:459.

44. De Silva JH, Millard PR, Kettlewell M, Mortensen NJ, Prince C, Jewell DP. Mucosal characteristics of pelvic ileal pouches. Gut 1991;32:61.

45. Pemberton JH. The problem with pouchitis. Gastroenterology 1993;104:1209.

46. Dvorak AM, Onderdonk AB, McLeod RS, et al. Axonal necrosis of enteric autonomic nerves in continent ileal pouches. Ann Surg 1993;217:260.

47. O'Connell PR, Rankin DR, Weiland LH, Kelly KA. Enteric bacteriology, absorption, morphology and emptying after ileal pouch-anal anastomosis. Br J Surg 1986;73:9009.

48. Nasmyth DG, Godwin PG, Dixon MF, Williams NS, Johnston D. Ileal ecology after pouch-anal anastomosis or ileostomy: a study of mucosal morphology, fecal bacteriology, fecal volatile fatty acids, and their interrelationship. Gastroenterology 1989;96:817.

49. Wischmeyer P, Grotz RL, Pemberton JH, Phillips SF. Treatment of pouchitis after ileo-anal anastomosis with glutamine and butyric acid. (Abstract) Gastroenterology 1992:102:A947.

50. Levin KE, Pemberton JH, Phillips SF, Zinsmeister AR, Pezim ME. Role of oxygen free radicals in the etiology of pouchitis. Dis Colon Rectum 1992;35:452.

51. Becker JM, Dunnegan D. Ileal pouch function and dysfunction following ileal pouch-anal anastomosis. In: MacDermott RP, ed. Inflammatory bowel disease: current status and future approach. Amsterdam, Elsevier Science Publishers, 1988:689.

52. Moskowitz RL, Shepherd NA, Nicholls RJ. An assessment of inflammation in the reservoir after restorative proctocolectomy with ileoanal ileal reservoir. Int J Colorectal 1986;1:167.

53. Becker JM, Parodi JE. Total colectomy with preservation of the anal sphincter. Surg Ann 1989;21:263.

SURGERY: SCIENTIFIC PRINCIPLES AND PRACTICE, Second Edition, edited by Lazar J. Greenfield, Michael W. Mulholland, Keith T. Oldham, Gerald B. Zelenock, and Keith D. Lillemoe. Lippincott–Raven Publishers, Philadelphia, © 1997.

CHAPTER 46

COLONIC POLYPS AND POLYPOSIS SYNDROMES

C. RICHARD BOLAND AND R.S. BRESALIER

The gastrointestinal tract accounts for more neoplastic disease than any other organ system in the body. In North America, carcinomas of the colon and rectum have attracted the greatest interest because of their relatively high incidence and because appropriate intervention can dramatically modify their associated morbidity and mortality. The adenoma is the usual precursor of colorectal cancer, and early removal of adenomatous polyps can interrupt the natural history of the disease and prevent death. A variety of pathologic lesions can present as polyps within the colon, but the adenoma is the only lesion that is truly neoplastic and carries a risk for the development of cancer. During the past decade, understanding of the genetic events that lead to the development of colorectal polyps has advanced greatly, and progress in the clinical management of these lesions has been equally brisk. It is imperative that the biology, natural history, and clinical behavior of premalignant lesions in the colon, as well as the genetic basis of the polyposis syndromes, be well understood because these have important impact on patient treatment.

CLASSIFICATION OF COLORECTAL POLYPS

The term *polyp* (from the Greek *polypous,* a morbid excrescence) refers to a macroscopic protrusion of the colonic mucosa into the bowel lumen. This can result from abnormal growth of the mucosa or from a submucosal process that causes the mucosa to protrude into the lumen. Mucosal polyps can be *sessile,* protruding directly from the colonic wall, or *pedunculated,* extending from the mucosa through a fibrovascular stalk.

Mucosal polyps in the colon can be divided into *neoplastic,* with malignant potential, and *nonneoplastic,* with no malignant potential (Table 46-1). Neoplastic polyps include benign adenomatous polyps that may evolve to carcinoma, adenomatous polyps that contain foci of intramucosal carcinoma (carcinoma in situ), and adenomatous polyps in which carcinoma has penetrated the muscularis mucosae (invasive carcinoma). Sometimes a polyp is found in which carcinoma has completely obliterated the adenomatous tissue from which it arose (polypoid carcinoma). Nonneoplastic mucosal polyps include hyperplastic polyps, juvenile polyps, Peutz-Jeghers hamartomas, and a variety of inflammatory polyps, including those associated with idiopathic inflammatory bowel disease. Any submucosal lesion can expand to push the mucosa into the bowel lumen and thus appear as a polypoid lesion. Examples include lipomas, colitis cystica profunda, pneumatosis cystoides intestinalis, lymphoid aggre-

---

Table 46-1. CLASSIFICATION OF COLORECTAL POLYPS

MUCOSAL POLYPS

Neoplastic

BENIGN

Adenomatous polyps (dysplastic mucosa)
    Tubular
    Tubulovillous
    Villous

MALIGNANT

Carcinoma in situ
Invasive carcinoma
Polypoid carcinoma

Nonneoplastic

Hyperplastic polyps
Juvenile polyps
Peutz-Jeghers polyps
Inflammatory polyps
Normal epithelium

SUBMUCOSAL POLYPS

Lipomas
Leiomyomas
Colitis cystica profunda
Pneumatosis cystoides intestinalis
Lymphoid aggregates
Lymphoma (primary or secondary)
Carcinoids
Metastatic neoplasms

gates, primary or secondary lymphomas, carcinoid tumors, and other metastatic neoplasms.

NEOPLASTIC MUCOSAL POLYPS

Most colorectal cancers arise in preexisting adenomatous polyps. These are macroscopic neoplastic lesions consisting of dysplastic epithelium that has the potential to evolve to malignancy. Carcinomas of the colon and rectum do not arise de novo. The mucosal epithelium progresses through a series of molecular and cellular events that lead to altered proliferation, cellular accumulation, and glandular disarray, which becomes macroscopically evident in the form of the adenomatous polyp. Further genetic alterations result in the evolution to higher degrees of cellular atypia and glandular disorganization (dysplasia), which may evolve to carcinoma. This is known as the adenoma-to-carcinoma sequence.

Several pieces of evidence support the assumption that colorectal adenocarcinomas arise from adenomatous polyps. The descriptive epidemiology of colonic adenomas parallels that of carcinomas. Adenomas are rare in geographic regions with low colon cancer prevalence, and the distribution of adenomas in the colon parallels that of carcinomas. Adenomas often occur in anatomic proximity to colon cancers, and cancer risk is proportional to the number of adenomas present synchronously or metachronously in a patient. Cancer is often present in polyps removed endoscopically or surgically, and the risk of cancer is proportional to the degree of dysplasia or atypia in the polyp. Conversely, histologically evident residual adenomatous tissue may be found within carcinomas. Most important, results from several studies indicate that removal of adenomatous polyps during surveillance proctosigmoidoscopy decreases the risk of subsequent death from colorectal cancer.

Pathogenesis

Molecular Biology

Genetic changes that lead to the development of adenomas (and carcinomas) can be organized into three major classes: alterations in protooncogenes, loss of tumor-suppressor gene

activity, and abnormalities of genes involved in DNA repair (Fig. 46-1). Much of what is known about molecular genetic events that occur during the adenoma-to-carcinoma sequence has come from the study of familial colon cancer syndromes. It is now clear, however, that adenoma and carcinoma development is always associated with genetic changes. In familial adenomatous polyposis (FAP), hereditary nonpolyposis colorectal cancer (HNPCC), and other familial syndromes, genetic alterations are inherited in the germline. Environmental factors may contribute additional genetic mutations that lead to malignant transformation. "Sporadic" polyps and cancers are associated with multiple somatic mutations contributed by environmental insults.

Cellular protooncogenes are a group of evolutionarily conserved genes that play a role in signal transduction and normal regulation of cell growth. Inappropriate activation of these genes leads to abnormal transmission of growth regulatory messages from the cell surface to the nucleus, resulting in altered cellular proliferation. Mutations of the K-*ras* oncogene, for example, can be found in about 65% of sporadic colorectal neoplasms and appear to play a role in the transition from the early adenoma to more advanced stages of adenomatous change. Only 9% of small adenomas have *ras* gene mutations, whereas 58% of adenomas larger than 1 cm have altered K-*ras* genes. Although activation of *ras* alone is not sufficient for progression to carcinoma, understanding its role in stimulating proliferation may lead to development of antitumor therapies aimed at interrupting signals that lead to tumor cell growth.

Allelic losses of chromosome 5q occur early during carcinogenesis in the colon. Originally described in association with familial adenomatous polyposis coli (APC), mutations of the APC gene on chromosome 5 are found in more than 60% of sporadic adenomas.[1] APC acts as a tumor-suppressor gene, and abnormalities in APC may lead to disruption of normal cell–cell adhesion through interactions with the cellular adhesion molecule E-cadherin and cytoskeletal proteins called *catenins*.

Alterations in genes that help maintain DNA fidelity during replication are characteristic of patients with HNPCC.[2] Alterations in genes designated hMSH2, hMLH1, hPMS2 and possibly hPMS1 lead to the inability to repair base pair mismatches, and result in DNA replication errors (the

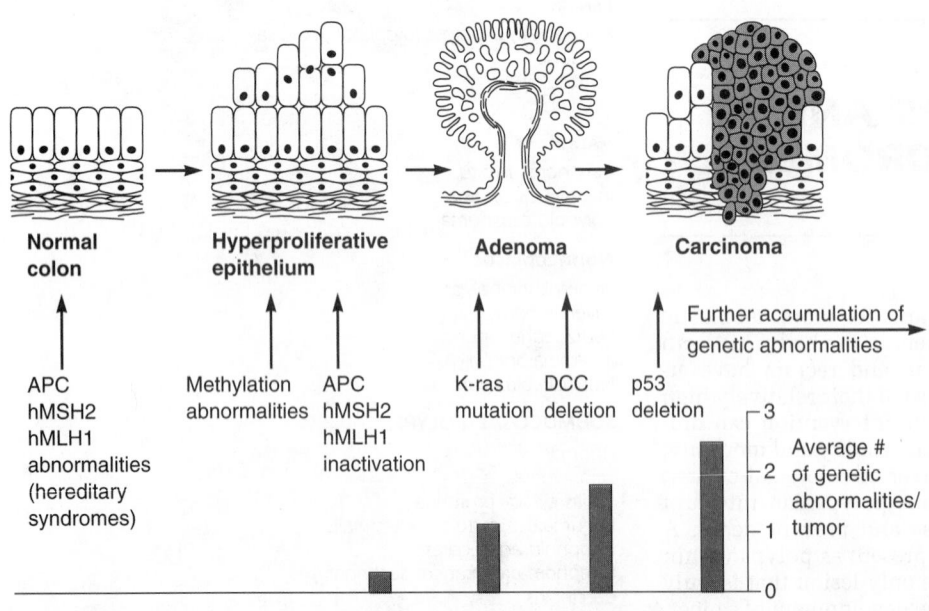

Normal colon → **Hyperproliferative epithelium** → **Adenoma** → **Carcinoma**

Further accumulation of genetic abnormalities

APC hMSH2 hMLH1 abnormalities (hereditary syndromes) / Methylation abnormalities / APC hMSH2 hMLH1 inactivation / K-ras mutation / DCC deletion / p53 deletion

Average # of genetic abnormalities/ tumor

Position in the adenoma-carcinoma sequence (above)

Figure 46-1. Molecular genetic events during the adenoma-to-carcinoma sequence. The progression to adenoma and carcinoma is associated with an accumulation of alterations in oncogenes (k-*ras*), tumor suppressor genes (APC, DCC, p53), and genes involved in maintaining the fidelity of DNA synthesis (DNA repair genes hMSH2, hMLH1). Alterations in APC, k-*ras*, and the DNA repair genes occur as early events in the development of adenomas, while deletion of DCC and p53 occur during the evolution from adenoma to carcinoma. The exact sequence of events is approximate. (Modified from Bresalier RS, Toribara NW. In: Eastwood GL, ed. Premalignant conditions of the gastrointestinal tract. New York, Elsevier 1991)

RER-positive phenotype) and increased susceptibility for the accumulation of cancer-causing mutations. Although this hypermutable phenotype is characteristic of HNPCC, similar alterations can be found in about 15% of sporadic colorectal cancers as well as in premalignant lesions.

Other genetic changes occur later in the adenoma-to-carcinoma sequence. Stepwise tumor progression is associated in more than 75% of cases with loss of the tumor-suppressor gene designated DCC (deleted in colorectal cancer) on chromosome 18q. This gene may be involved in maintaining normal cell–cell adhesive interactions, and its loss from a stage II (Dukes B) cancer is associated with a significantly worse prognosis. Deletions of chromosome 17p involve the p53 tumor-suppressor gene, whose product normally prevents cells with damaged DNA from progressing from G_1 to S phase in the cell cycle. Inactivation of the p53 gene mediates the conversion for adenoma to carcinoma.

Abnormal Proliferation

The development of adenomatous polyps is associated with abnormal cellular proliferation, a hallmark of neoplasia. In the normal colon, DNA synthesis and cellular proliferation occur only in the lower and middle regions of the crypt. Cells that have migrated to the upper crypt become terminally differentiated and can no longer divide. Disordered proliferation and aberrant crypt development are characteristic of adenomas. Abnormal proliferation can be detected throughout the crypt even in the grossly normal-appearing mucosa of some patients at especially high risk for adenoma development, such as those with FAP or HNPCC. This may be associated with alterations in biochemical markers of cellular proliferation, such as ornithine decarboxylase and protein kinase C. The initiating event for the adenoma, however, is thought to be inactivation of the APC tumor-suppressor gene, which has led to its designation as the "gatekeeper" for colorectal neoplasia.

Histopathology and Malignant Potential

Adenomatous polyps are characterized according to their physical characteristics, size, glandular structure, and degree of dysplasia. These characteristics have important implications for clinical management. Polyps may be sessile with a broad-based attachment to the colonic wall, or pedunculated, attached to the colonic wall by way of a fibrovascular stalk (Fig. 46-2). This typically determines the ability of the endoscopist to remove the polyp completely by snare polypectomy. Diminutive polyps measure 5 mm or less in diameter and have little likelihood of containing high-grade dysplasia or invasive carcinoma. Malignant potential increases with polyp size in all histologic groups of adenoma.

Adenomas are classified histologically according to their glandular structure. Aberrant (dysplastic) crypts and microadenomas may be the earliest lesions detected in the flat mucosa of at-risk patients. These enlarge and progress to macroscopic adenomatous polyps. Tubular adenomas are characterized by a complex network of branching adenomatous glands, whereas villous adenomas contain glands that extend straight down from the surface to the base of the polyp (Fig. 46-3). Often, both histologic types coexist in a mixed tubulovillous adenoma. The malignant potential of an adenomatous polyp correlates with its degree of villous architecture.

All adenomas by definition consist of dysplastic mucosa. The term *dysplasia* refers to abnormalities in crypt architecture (such as irregular branching or crowded "back-to-back" glands) and cytologic detail (enlarged pleiomorphic

and hyperchromatic nuclei with multiple mitoses and pseudostratification; Fig. 46-4). Dysplasia may be mild, moderate, or severe, depending on the degree of accumulation of these characteristics. Severe, or high-grade, dysplasia represents carcinoma in situ when the basement membrane is intact. Extension into the lamina propria denotes intramucosal carcinoma. Invasion into the muscularis mucosae defines invasive carcinoma and the malignant polyp. The degree of dysplasia often correlates with polyp size and extent of villous architecture.

Even though all adenocarcinomas of the colon and rectum arise in adenomatous polyps, not all polyps evolve into carcinoma. The malignant potential of adenomatous polyps is related to polyp size and histologic characteristics. Large polyps and those with a higher proportion of villous architecture are more likely to contain coincident carcinoma (Fig. 46-5). These features are interdependent, however, because large polyps are more likely to be villous and to contain higher degrees of dysplasia. Adenomas that measure 0.5 cm or less are most often tubular adenomas and rarely contain severe dysplasia or carcinoma (less than 0.5% in autopsy series). Likewise, only 1% to 2% of adenomatous polyps less than 1 cm contain carcinoma, but autopsy studies suggest that 40% of adenomas greater than 2 cm contain cancer. Data derived from examination of colonoscopic polypectomy specimens indicate similar trends but suggest a lower incidence of cancer-containing polyps.

Epidemiology

Prevalence

The descriptive epidemiology of adenomatous polyps of the colon and rectum parallels that of colorectal carcinoma with relation to geographic distribution, age prevalence, and genetic susceptibility. Like colorectal cancer, adenomas are common in Western countries like the United States, but their prevalence is low in areas of Asia, South America, and sub-Saharan Africa. Estimates of adenoma prevalence in the United States vary depending on the mode of data collection. Data from older studies were collected from autopsies and sometimes grouped all polyps together, whereas more recent studies have examined adenoma prevalence in the context of endoscopic screening. Studies using colonoscopy suggest an adenoma prevalence in patients without symptoms who are older than 50 years that ranges between 20% and 40%. Prevalence rates from autopsy studies are 50% higher. Based on autopsy studies, one half to two thirds of people older than 65 years may have colonic adenomas. Adenoma prevalence increases with age in all populations. Age-associated prevalence rates suggest that adenomas precede carcinomas in a given population by 5 to 10 years. Advancing age also correlates with multiplicity of polyps, polyp size, and higher degrees of dysplasia. In addition, 30% to 50% of patients with one adenoma have a synchronous adenoma elsewhere in the colon.[3]

Anatomic Distribution

Autopsy series and colonoscopic examination of patients who do not have symptoms suggest that although adenomas are uniformly distributed throughout the colon, clinically important larger adenomas have a distribution more similar to carcinoma, with a left-sided predominance.

Heredity

Heredity plays a role not only in the gastrointestinal polyposis syndromes and in HNPCC but also in development of sporadic adenomas. Sporadic or nonsyndromic

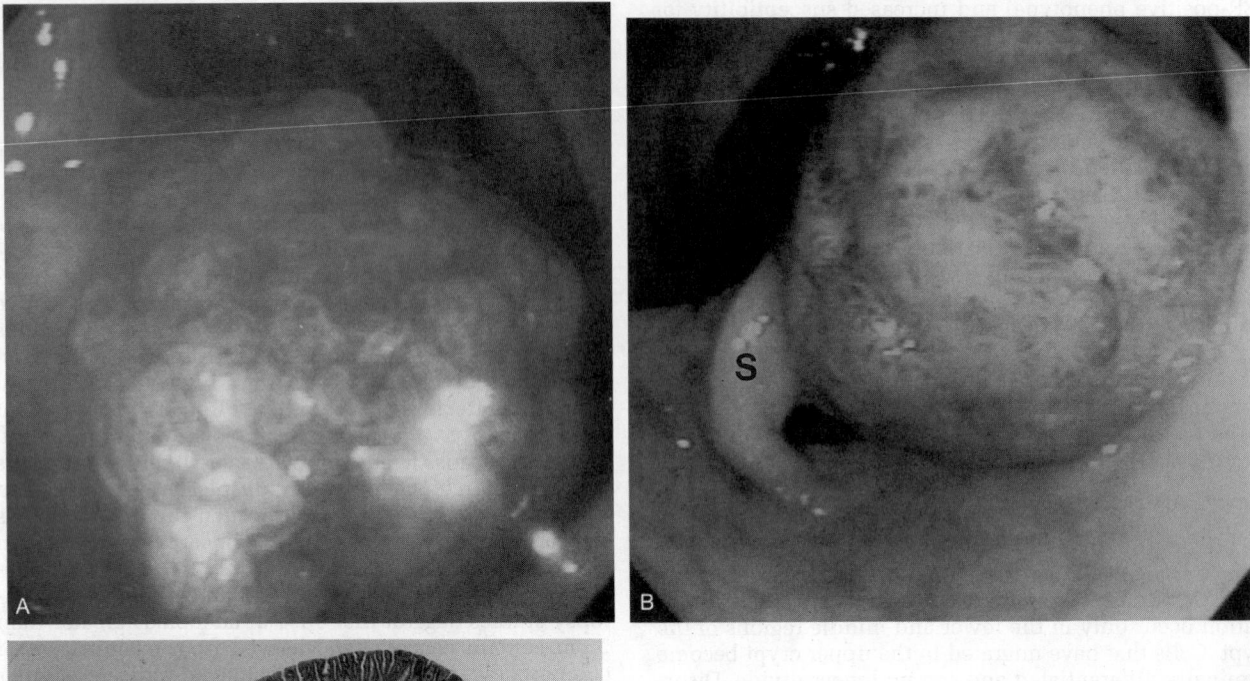

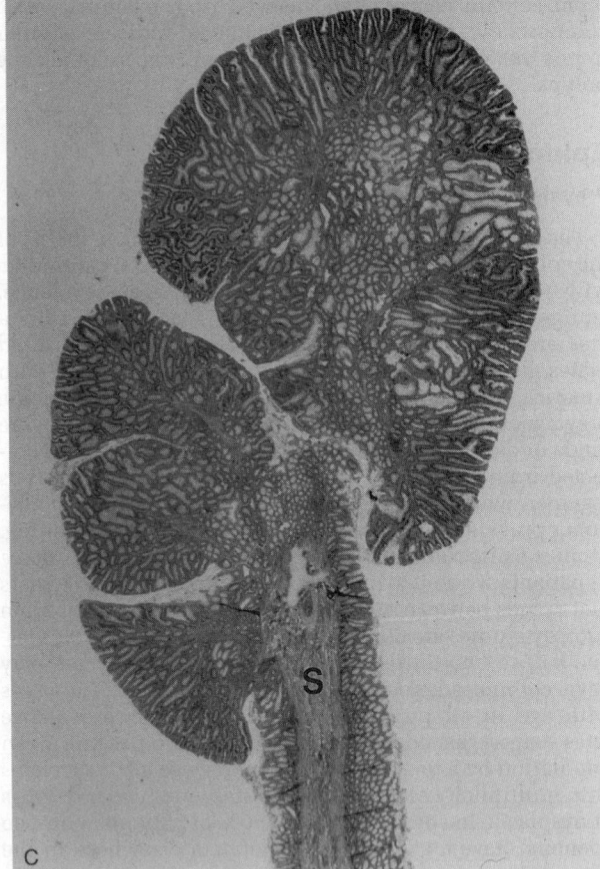

Figure 46-2. Mucosal polyps of the colon may be sessile and protrude directly from the colonic wall, or pedunculated, extending from the mucosa through a fibrovascular stalk. (*A*) Large sessile polyp seen at colonoscopy. The polyp has a broad-based attachment to the mucosa. (*B*) Large pedunculated polyp seen at colonoscopy. The polyp is attached to the mucosa through a distinct stalk (S). (*C*) Low-power photomicrograph of a pedunculated polyp (a tubular adenoma) cut in cross section to demonstrate its fibrovascular stalk (S).

adenomatous polyps and colon cancers represent 95% of colorectal neoplasms. Clinical studies, including case-control and prospective analyses, indicate a two- to three-fold increased risk for colon cancer among first-degree relatives of patients with a history of colonic adenoma or carcinoma. In some cases, it appears that common adenomas may be inherited with a susceptibility that is autosomal dominant but only partially penetrant. Therefore, it has been suggested that inheritance determines individual susceptibility to neoplasia, whereas environmental factors determine which susceptible people have adenomas and carcinomas of the colon.

Natural History

Although adenomas are a common occurrence in people older than 50 years, and most carcinomas arise in adenomatous polyps, relatively few adenomas progress into carcinoma. There is little precise data on what percentage of

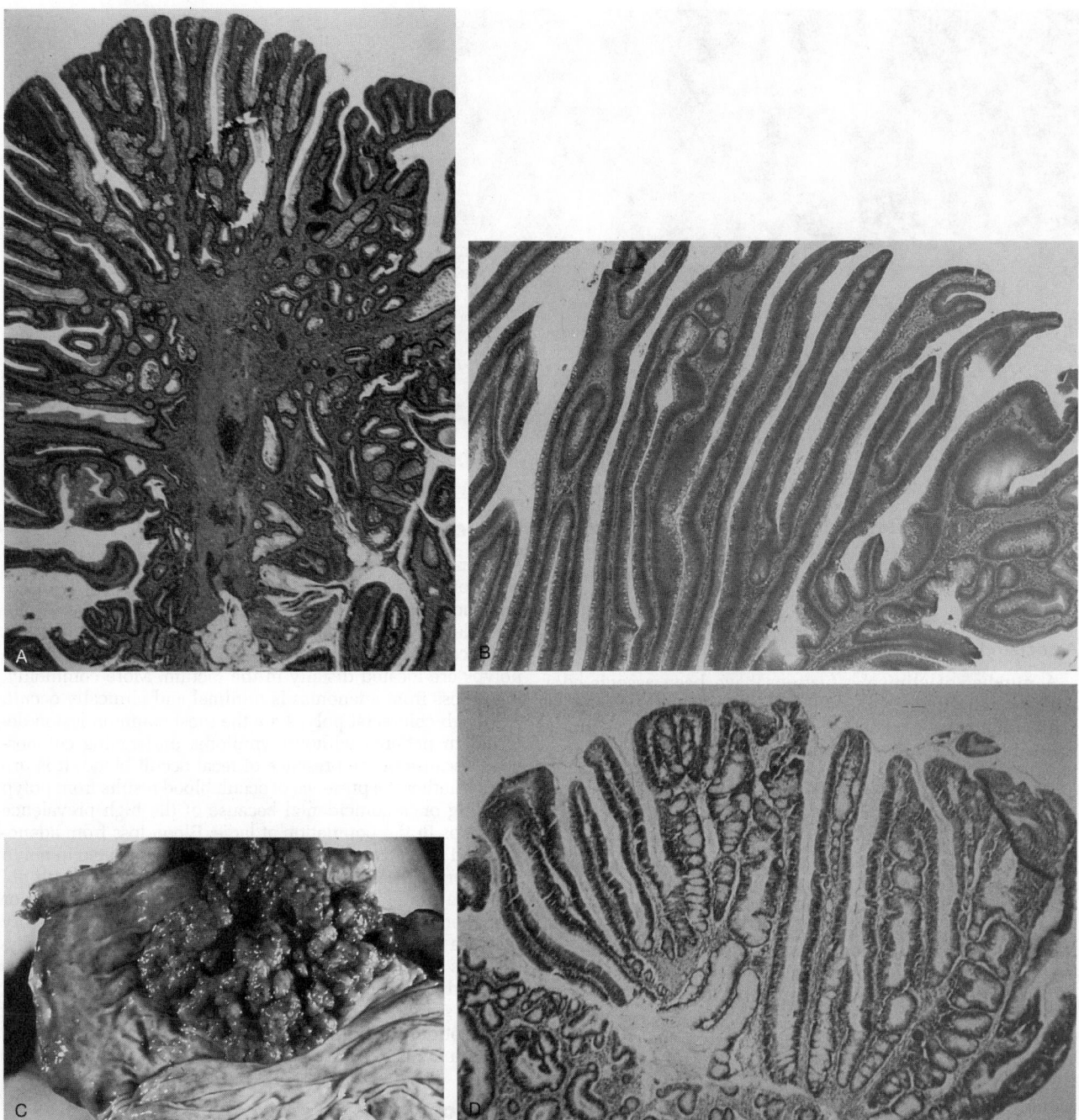

Figure 46-3. Histology of adenomatous polyps. (*A*) Tubular adenomas are characterized by a complex network of branching adenomatous glands (also see *C*). (*B*) Villous adenoma. This polyp consists of glands that extend straight down from the surface to the base of the polyp. This gives the appearance of finger-like projections, which may be suggested by the gross appearance of the polyp. (*C*) Surgical specimen demonstrating a large sessile polyp with finger-like fronds typical of a villous adenoma. (*D*) Tubulovillous adenoma. Many polyps contain both tubular and villous components on histologic examination.

adenomas evolve to carcinomas. In Norway, an example of a high-risk Western population, it has been estimated that 29% of the population older than 35 years of age have colorectal adenomas. The annual conversion rate from adenoma to carcinoma in this group (based on cancer incidence from multiple tumor registries) was calculated to be 0.25%. In other words, there is a 2.5% risk that colorectal cancer will develop in a polyp-bearing person within 10 years. The annual conversion rates to invasive cancer for people with adenomas larger than 1 cm, villous compo-

nents, and severe dysplasia were estimated to be 3%, 17%, and 37%, respectively, based on these inferences.

Both longitudinal follow-up of a small number of people with unresected adenomas and age distribution studies provide indirect evidence that the evolution from adenoma to carcinoma takes at least 5 to 10 years. Age prevalence data from the National Polyp Study, for example, suggest that it may take as long as 5 to 10 years for normal-appearing mucosa to develop into a macroscopically visible adenomatous polyp, and an additional 3 to 5 years for

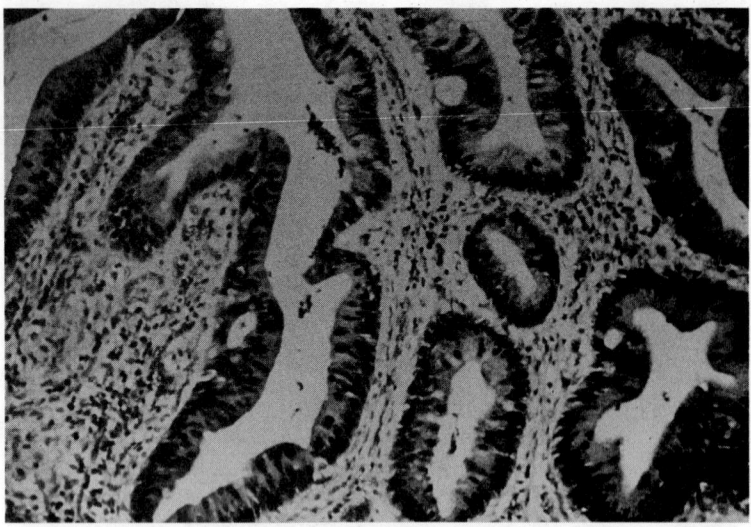

Figure 46-4. Moderate dysplasia. Dysplastic mucosa is characterized by crowded, irregular glands and cells with enlarged hyperchromatic nuclei of varied size and shape that do not line up uniformly on the basement membrane (pseudopallisading). Adenomas are composed of dysplastic mucosa, which may vary in degree of atypia. These changes precede the development of invasive carcinoma.

invasive carcinoma to develop. Case-control studies also support that the development of adenomas in the colon and the evolution to carcinoma occur slowly. Several studies have estimated that the protective effect of screening sigmoidoscopy may last at least 10 years.

Associated Disease States

A number of clinical situations have been associated with a greater than average risk of adenoma development, but the evidence in most cases is tenuous. Although adenomas and carcinomas develop frequently in patients who have undergone urinary diversion by way of ureterosigmoidoscopy, this is largely of historical interest. Nonetheless, patients who have had this procedure require periodic colonoscopic surveillance for adenoma and carcinoma development. An increased prevalence of colonic adenomas and carcinomas has been reported in patients with acromegaly, and patients with elevated gastrin levels have been reported to be at risk for neoplasia. Alleged associations between colorectal adenomas and a history of prior cholecystectomy, atherosclerosis, acrochordous (skin tags), and hyperplastic polyps remain unproved.

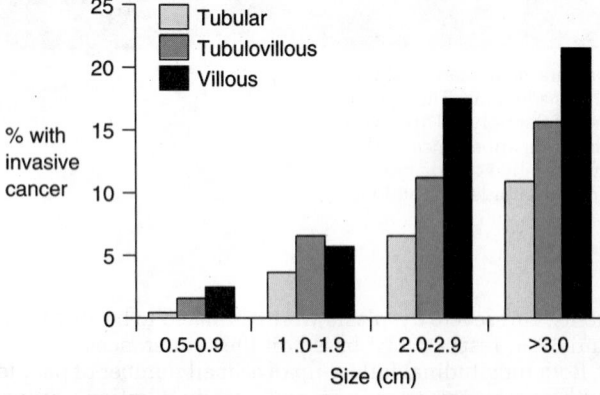

Figure 46-5. The relation of adenoma size and histology to malignant potential based on an analysis of 7000 endoscopically removed polyps. The incidence of polyp-associated carcinoma determined from examination of polypectomy specimens is lower than that derived from early autopsy studies. (Data derived from Shinya H, Wolff WI. Morphology, anatomic distribution, and cancer potential of colonic polyps. Ann Surg 1979;1990:675).

Clinical Features

Adenomatous polyps of the colon and rectum are highly prevalent in Western societies, but most patients with colonic adenomas do not have symptoms directly referable to these lesions. Overt bleeding manifesting as hematochezia may occur with larger polyps, which may be evident when polyps are located distally in the rectum. More commonly, blood loss from adenomas is minimal and clinically occult. Although colorectal polyps are the most common lesion detected in patients without symptoms undergoing colonoscopy because of the presence of fecal occult blood, it is unclear whether the presence of occult blood results from polyp bleeding or is coincidental because of the high prevalence of polyps in the population at large. Blood loss from adenomas and a positive fecal occult blood test are related to polyp size. Very large colonic polyps may be associated with obstructive symptoms, such as lower abdominal cramping or alterations in bowel habits, but this is unusual. Secretory diarrhea with accompanying hypokalemia and hypochlorhydria has been associated with very large villous adenomas of the distal colon and rectum. This is a rare syndrome, and the search for secretagogues such as vasoactive intestinal polypeptide or prostaglandins in patients with polyps and diarrhea is infrequently productive.

Adenomas Associated With Hereditary Nonpolyposis Colorectal Cancer and Its Variants

Hereditary nonpolyposis colorectal cancer (Lynch syndrome) is a disease of autosomal dominant inheritance in which cancers arise in discrete adenomas, but polyposis (ie, hundreds of polyps) does not occur. This entity is defined by the Amsterdam criteria: families must have least three relatives with colorectal cancer, one of whom is a first-degree relative of the other two. Colorectal cancer must involve at least two generations, and at least one cancer case must occur before 50 years of age. Adenomas and carcinomas arising in HNPCC occur at an early age (adenomas may occur in the 20s and 30s, with a mean age for carcinoma development of 40 to 45 years) and are often proximal in location and multiple. Some families with HNPCC (Lynch syndrome II, cancer family syndrome) are prone to cancers of the female genital tract (endometrium and ovary) and other sites in addition to colorectal neoplasms.

The frequency of HNPCC in the general population is

yet to be determined, but HNPCC may account for as much as 4% to 6% of colorectal cancer. A germline mutation in one of four genes that play a role in DNA mismatch repair—hMSH2 (human Mut S homologue 2), hMLH1 (human Mut L homologue 1), hPMS1 and hPMS2 (human postmeiotic segregation 1 and 2)—occurs in patients with HNPCC, leading to RERs. Precisely how RERs lead to adenoma and carcinoma development is unknown.

Turcot syndrome is characterized clinically by the concurrence of primary brain tumors and multiple colorectal adenomas. Evidence suggests that this can result from two distinct types of germline defects: mutation of the APC gene (ie, a variant of FAP) or mutation of a mismatch-repair gene (ie, a variant of HNPCC).

Diagnosis

Most colorectal adenomas are asymptomatic and are often detected in the setting of evaluation of unrelated colonic symptoms or occult blood in the stool. Similarly, adenomatous polyps are frequently detected as the result of screening patients without symptoms for colorectal neoplasia. Nevertheless, data strongly suggest that detection and removal of adenomatous polyps have an important impact on reducing colorectal cancer-related mortality.

Fecal Occult Blood Tests

Screening studies from both Scandinavia and the United States indicate that about 30% of patients without symptoms who are 50 years of age or older and who undergo colonoscopy for follow-up of a positive fecal occult blood test result have a polyp detected. Blood loss from polyps and positive fecal occult blood test results are related to polyp size. In one study that used rehydrated Hemoccult slides (rehydration results in greater sensitivity but also increases the number of false-positive tests), only 15% of polyps less than 1 cm were associated with a positive Hemoccult test, whereas 80% of polyps greater than 2 cm were positive. In another study, standard testing with Hemoccult cards detected 17% of adenomas less than 1 cm and 42% of adenomas greater than 1 cm in size. An immunochemical fecal occult blood test is promising, but not yet widely tested. It detected 36% of adenomas less than 1 cm and 76% of adenomas greater than 1 cm in a small group of patients. A prospective randomized study of fecal occult blood tests using rehydrated Hemoccult cards suggested that annual tests reduced colorectal cancer–related deaths by 33%. How much of this impact resulted from detection and removal of adenomas per se (as opposed to detection of early cancers) is unclear. Results from the National Polyp Study, however, strongly indicate that removal of index polyps detected by fecal occult blood test and other methods, together with subsequent colonoscopic surveillance, results in a lower than expected incidence of colon cancer compared with historical reference groups.

Sigmoidoscopy

The National Cancer Institute, the American Cancer Society, the American College of Physicians, the American Gastroenterological Association, and the World Health Organization Collaborating Center for Prevention of Colorectal Cancer all advocate screening sigmoidoscopy every 3 to 5 years in conjunction with yearly fecal occult blood tests beginning at 50 years of age. The benefit of sigmoidoscopy in interrupting the adenoma-to-carcinoma sequence is suggested by a number of studies. Investigators have compared the use of rigid sigmoidoscopy in 261 members of the Kaiser Permanente Medical Care Program who died of cancer of the rectum or distal colon versus that in 868 matched controls. Only 8.8% of those with cancer had

undergone screening sigmoidoscopy, compared with 24.2% of controls. The impact of sigmoidoscopy was limited to development of fatal colon cancer within reach of the sigmoidoscope and was long-standing (at least 10 years). Others have determined the long-term risk of colorectal cancer development after rigid sigmoidoscopy and polypectomy in 1618 patients with rectosigmoid adenomas. The overall risk of subsequent rectal cancer in these patients was similar to that in the general population, but subject analysis revealed that risk depended on histologic type, size, and number of adenomas removed.[4-6]

The 60-cm flexible sigmoidoscope has supplanted the rigid scope because it causes less discomfort to the patient, visualizes 2.5 times more surface area, and detects two to three times more adenomas. Flexible sigmoidoscopy can be learned by paramedical personnel and has been successfully used in screening programs by nurse-practitioners.

Other Screening Modalities

Given the high cost of repeated screening of average-risk patients who do not have symptoms for adenomas and carcinomas and the long natural history of the adenoma-to-carcinoma sequence, some have advocated the performance of a single air-contrast barium enema or colonoscopy at 50 years of age, with no further screening in patients without symptoms who have negative examinations. The appropriateness of this approach is unclear, however, and this alternative to yearly fecal occult blood tests plus periodic sigmoidoscopy has not gained wide acceptance.

Hydrocolonic sonography (instillation of water in the colon followed by extracorporeal ultrasound examination) has been suggested as a means of detecting large adenomas in the colon, but this test is insensitive and not an accepted screening tool. Detection of adenoma-associated antigens or mutated protooncogenes such as K-ras in stool is possible, but the effectiveness of such methods as a screening measure is doubtful.

Management of Adenomas

Index Polypectomy

Once detected, adenomas should be completely removed, preferably by endoscopic snare polypectomy (Fig. 46-6). Polypectomy is relatively safe and easily performed when adenomas are small or pedunculated but is more difficult when polyps are large or sessile. Potential complications include bleeding and perforation of the polypectomy site. Large sessile villous adenomas (ie, more than 2 cm) have a great potential for malignant degeneration. If such lesions cannot be completely removed by snare polypectomy, segmental surgical resection may be necessary. Diminutive polyps, on the other hand, carry little malignant potential. If they are too small for snare polypectomy, ablation with a hot biopsy forceps is a reasonable approach. Because 30% to 50% of patients with one adenoma have a synchronous adenoma elsewhere in the colon, the entire colon should be "cleared" by colonoscopy in polyp-bearing patients.

Follow-Up. Additional metachronous adenomas are likely to develop in the future in patients who have had adenomas removed. Colonoscopic surveillance studies have provided estimates of the frequency and time course of recurrence in these patients. Data from the National Polyp Study suggested a recurrence rate of 32% to 42% by 3 years after index polypectomy. A prospective colonoscopic analysis also demonstrated a cumulative recurrence rate at 3 years of 42%. Most adenomas detected at this 3-year interval were small tubular adenomas. Age greater

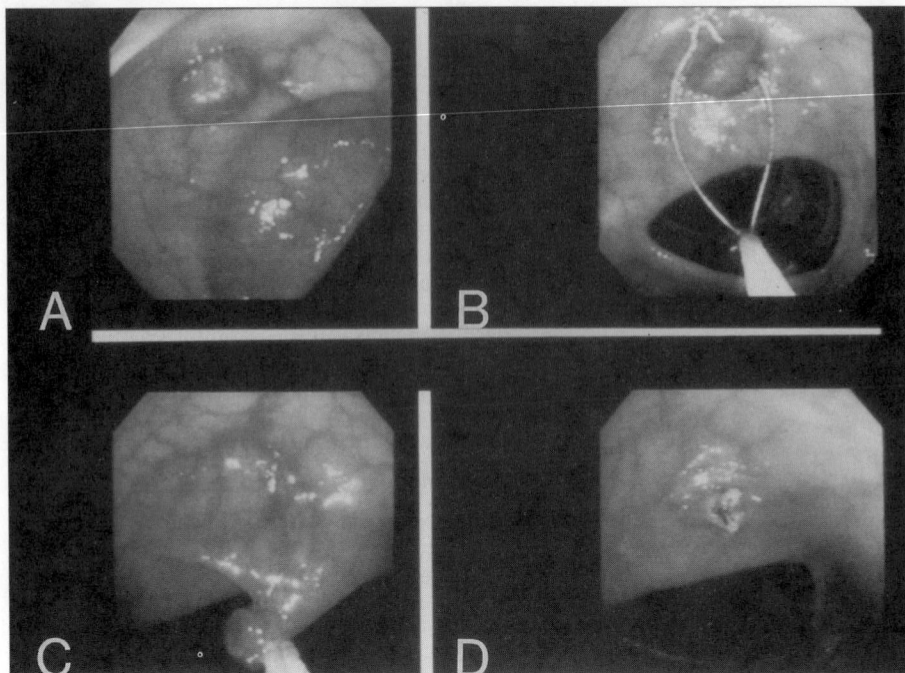

Figure 46-6. Endoscopic snare polypectomy. (*A*) A small colonic polyp. (*B*) The polypectomy snare is placed around the polyp. (*C*) The snare is closed around the base of the polyp, and the head of the polyp is gently pulled away from the wall and into the lumen. Current is applied to cut the stalk to cauterize the site. (*D*) The postpolypectomy site.

than 60 years, multiple adenomas at index polypectomy, and large size of the index adenoma predicted polyp recurrence in the National Polyp Study, but only multiplicity predicted recurrence of polyps with advanced pathologic features (greater than 1 cm, high-grade dysplasia or invasive cancer) at follow-up. The 3-year recurrence rate in patients with a known history of adenoma (42%) was higher than the incidence rate of de novo adenoma appearance during this period in patients who had no adenomas detected on index colonoscopy (16%).[7]

The high recurrence rate of adenomas after index polypectomy supports the use of postpolypectomy surveillance in those with known histories of adenoma. Colonoscopy is the preferred means of follow-up in these patients. Air-contrast barium enemas may detect most large polyps in the colon but may miss smaller lesions. The published sensitivity of air-contrast barium studies for detecting colorectal polyps is 85% to 95%, but data from the National Polyp Study suggest a substantially lower sensitivity rate, probably because of lack of detection of small polyps. Colonoscopy is the most accurate means of evaluating the colonic mucosa and allows biopsy and removal of suspicious lesions.

The National Polyp Study was organized in 1978 by the American Gastroenterological Association, the American Society of Gastrointestinal Endoscopy, and the American College of Gastroenterology as a long-term randomized prospective multicenter study to assess postpolypectomy surveillance. Data from the National Polyp Study indicate that repeat colonoscopy need not be performed at intervals less than every 3 years in patients whose index polyp demonstrates no evidence of high-grade dysplasia or carcinoma. Although patients undergoing postpolypectomy surveillance at both 1 and 3 years after index polypectomy had a greater number of polyps detected in this study compared with those undergoing colonoscopy at 3 years only, the percentage of patients whose adenomas had advanced pathologic features was similarly low in both groups (3.3%).

The National Polyp Study has demonstrated that colonoscopic polypectomy and surveillance result in a 76% to 90% reduction in colorectal cancer compared with histori-

cal reference groups. This and other studies have demonstrated, however, that in patients with no family history of colorectal cancer, most adenomas detected at interval follow-up are small tubular adenomas. In addition, when the index polyp is a small tubular adenoma, the risk of the subsequent development of a histologically important lesion is low. This is especially true of the diminutive polyp (ie, less than 6 mm in diameter). Given the high cost of repeated colonoscopies, this emphasizes the need to establish better who will most benefit from colonoscopic surveillance and who may require less rigorous follow-up.

Management of Malignant Polyps

Endoscopic polypectomy is adequate treatment for an adenomatous polyp that contains cancer if it can be demonstrated to be confined to the head of the polyp (ie, carcinoma in situ or intramucosal carcinoma; Fig. 46-7). The adequacy of simple polypectomy has been controversial in cases in which malignant cells have invaded the polyp stalk (Fig. 46-8), but most studies now indicate that polypectomy is adequate treatment provided that a margin of greater than 2 mm is present, the cancer is not poorly differentiated, and there is no vascular or lymphatic invasion. The presence of cancer at or near the margin is significantly associated with adverse outcome, even in the absence of other unfavorable parameters. On the other hand, in the absence of unfavorable histology and with a negative margin, the incidence of residual cancer is low (less than 1%). These criteria are more difficult to assess in sessile polyps. If an adequate margin cannot be demonstrated or negative histologic parameters are present, surgery is recommended to treat the possibility of regional lymph node metastases.

Primary Prevention of Adenoma Recurrence

Primary prevention relates to the ability to identify genetic, environmental, and biologic factors that cause cancer and to alter their effects. Laboratory, clinical, and epidemiologic

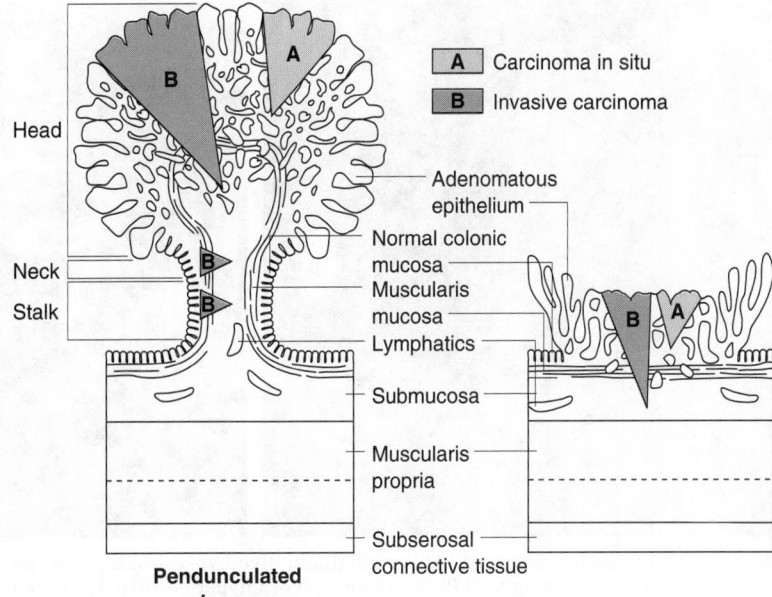

Figure 46-7. Diagrammatic representation of cancer-containing polyps. Pedunculated adenoma is described on the left and a sessile adenoma on the right. In carcinoma in situ, malignant cells are confined to the mucosa. These lesions are adequately treated by endoscopic polypectomy. Polypectomy is adequate treatment for invasive carcinoma only if there is a sufficient margin (perhaps 2 mm), if the carcinoma is not poorly differentiated, and if there is no evidence of venous or lymphatic invasion. (After Haggitt RC, Glotzbach RE, Soffen EE, et al. Prognostic factors in colorectal carcinomas arising in adenomas: implications for lesions removed by endoscopic polypectomy. Gastroenterology 1985;89:328)

evidence suggest that the regular use of nonsteroidal antiinflammatory drugs (NSAIDs), including aspirin, is associated with a decreased risk for colorectal cancer development. The number of colorectal adenomas discovered among regular NSAID users is lower than in nonusers in most observational studies. The only published randomized trial that assessed the effect of NSAIDs on colorectal cancer development in an average-risk population the Physicians Health Study) demonstrated a small but nonsignificant decrease in incident polyps among the aspirin group.[8] Therefore, although the data on NSAID use and primary prevention of adenomas are promising, they are insufficient to support a clinical recommendation for regular NSAID use to prevent polyp recurrence. Trials of antioxidant vitamins such as β-carotene and vitamins C and E have not convincingly demonstrated any effect on adenoma recurrence. Although supplemental calcium reduces proliferative activity in the mucosa of experimental animals and patients at high-risk for colorectal cancer development, clinical evidence for a reduction in polyp occurrence in average-risk patients has not been demonstrated.

NONNEOPLASTIC MUCOSAL POLYPS
Hyperplastic Polyps

Hyperplastic polyps are small, usually sessile lesions most frequently encountered in the distal colon and rectum (Fig. 46-9A). Although grossly indistinguishable from small adenomas, they carry no potential for malignant degeneration. Microscopically, hyperplastic polyps are characterized by a serrated epithelial pattern due to micropapillary luminal in-foldings of columnar absorptive cells and mature, frequently hyperdistended goblet cells (see Fig. 46-9B). Elongation and subsequent infolding of the epithelium may be due to an expanded, but otherwise normally located, replication zone in the crypt. The cytologic atypia found in adenomatous polyps is not seen in these lesions. Hyperplastic and adenomatous glands occasionally coexist in a polyp, and in some cases even share the same basement membrane. This is not strong evidence that adenomas derive from hyperplastic polyps. Abundant evidence documents the divergent growth and differentiation pat-

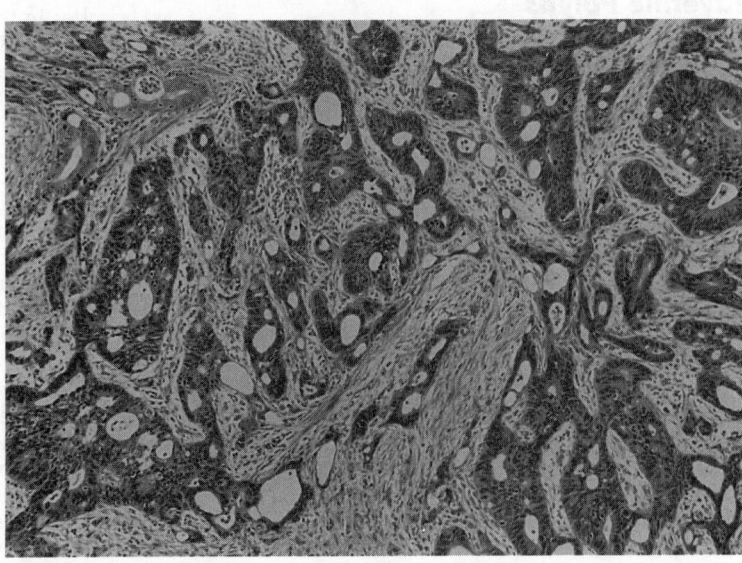

Figure 46-8. Invasive carcinoma in the stalk of an adenomatous polyp.

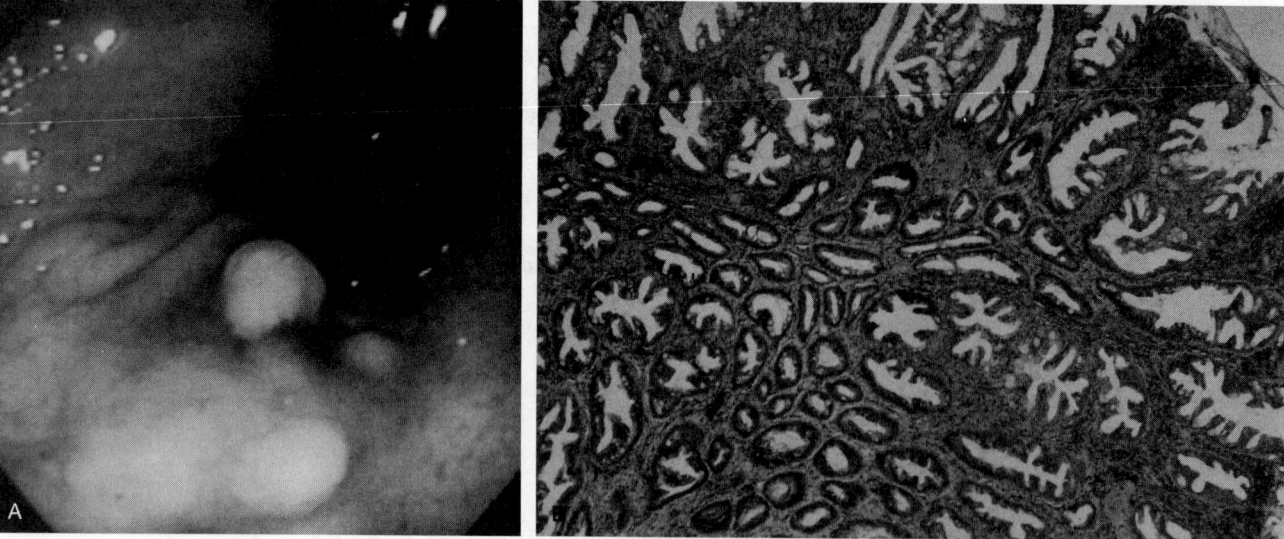

Figure 46-9. Hyperplastic polyps. (*A*) Several diminutive hyperplastic polyps seen in the rectum during flexible sigmoidoscopy. (*B*) Photomicrograph of a hyperplastic polyp characterized by elongated glands with papillary infoldings, which have a typical serrated epithelial pattern.

terns of hyperplastic polyps and adenomas. Another entity, the so-called mixed hyperplastic adenomatous polyp, exhibits the architectural, but not the cytologic, features of hyperplastic polyps. These lesions demonstrate the cytologic features of adenomas, and are considered adenoma variants (also called *serrated adenomas*).

Hyperplastic polyps are common age-related lesions found in about one third of the population older than 50 years. Although they often coexist with adenomas in polyp-bearing patients, there is no convincing evidence that hyperplastic polyps are harbingers of adenoma development. They are most common in the distal colon and rectum, and usually diminutive. Because hyperplastic polyps are asymptomatic and carry no malignant potential, no specific treatment is required for these lesions. If a hyperplastic polyp is the only lesion detected on index flexible sigmoidoscopy or colonoscopy, no further evaluation is indicated.

Juvenile Polyps

Juvenile polyps, also known as *retention polyps*, can occur sporadically or as part of a familial polyposis syndrome. These mucosal polyps consist of dilated cystic mucus-filled glands, abundant lamina propria, and inflammatory infiltrates. Seventy-five percent occur in children younger than 10 years of age, often appearing as single pedunculated cherry-red polyps with a smooth surface and contour. The exact prevalence of such lesions has not been determined, but they appear to be acquired lesions detected in about 2% of children who do not have symptoms. Juvenile polyps often present in the form of hematochezia because they are highly vascularized lesions. Rectal prolapse and autoamputation may occur with distal lesions, whereas intussusception may be precipitated by proximal juvenile polyps found in the context of familial syndromes. Individually, these polyps have no malignant potential, but symptomatic polyps should be removed to prevent further complications. Juvenile polyposis, on the other hand, is associated with an increased risk of early cancer development.

Inflammatory Polyps

Inflammatory mucosal polyps are common in the setting of idiopathic inflammatory bowel disease. Marked inflammation and ulceration coexist with granulation tissue in a distorted mucosal architecture that appears polypoid (Fig. 46-10*A*). Subsequent healing leads to residual islands of mucosa interspersed with denuded epithelium (the so-called pseudopolyps; see Fig. 46-10*B*). Severe chronic inflammation of any kind, including a variety of infectious diseases (tuberculosis, amebiasis, schistosomiasis, amebic colitis), may result in inflammatory polyps that resemble those found in the active stages of idiopathic inflammatory bowel disease.

SUBMUCOSAL POLYPS

Submucosal masses can expand to push the colonic mucosa into the bowel lumen and thus appear as polypoid lesions. Many submucosal lesions (eg, lipomas, leiomyomas) are clinically asymptomatic, and their significance lies in their differentiation from neoplastic lesions. Others are malignant lesions that require early detection, such as lymphomas and metastatic tumors. Many submucosal lesions are not detected on endoscopic mucosal biopsy because standard biopsy forceps do not reach beyond the mucosa. If a submucosal lesion is suspected, multiple biopsies of the same site sometimes provides tissue for diagnosis.

Lipomas are benign fatty tumors that occur throughout the gastrointestinal tract but are most commonly found in the cecum near the ileocecal valve (Fig. 46-11). They appear endoscopically as soft smooth polyps that are pliable and deformable. The overlying mucosa is intact but may be light yellow in appearance. These are benign lesions that have little clinical significance.

Isolated lymphoid nodules consisting of benign lymphoid tissue may appear as sessile smooth polyps of various size, with a predilection for the distal colon and rectum. These are usually asymptomatic. Diffuse nodular lymphoid hyperplasia also occurs in children as an incidental finding. These must be distinguished from primary or secondary lymphoma

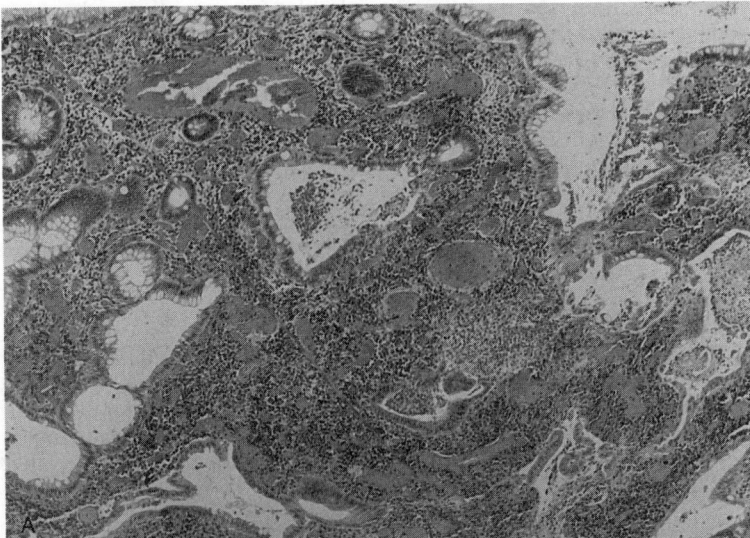
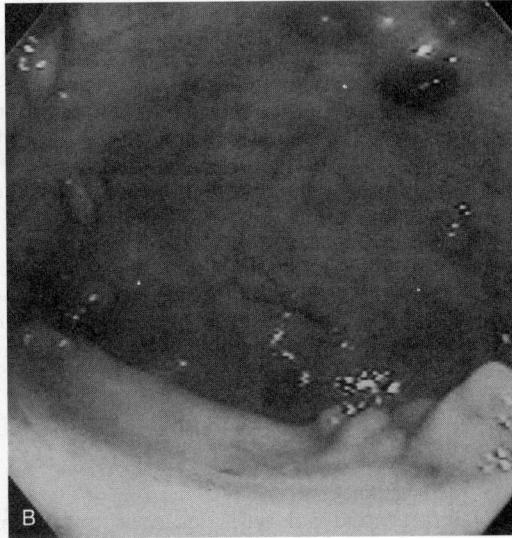

Figure 46-10. Inflammatory polyps. (*A*) Severe mucosal inflammation with inflammatory infiltrates and granulation tissue shown here microscopically can appear clinically with a polypoid configuration. (*B*) Resolution of inflammation can leave islands of intact mucosa among large areas of denuded epithelium, resulting in the presence of pseudopolyps.

of the large intestine, which may present as mucosal nodularity resembling the pseudopolyposis of inflammatory bowel disease.

Pneumatosis cystoides intestinalis has the appearance of multiple air-filled cysts within the submucosa. This may be an incidental finding in patients with chronic obstructive pulmonary disease, scleroderma, or asymptomatic pneumoperitoneum secondary to recent surgery or instrumentation, in which air or colonic gas diffuses into the cysts. These sometimes resolve with administration of oxygen. A far more virulent form of pneumatosis is associated with fulminant mucosal inflammation, ischemia, or necrotizing enterocolitis in children. These cysts are thought to result from mucosal invasion by gas-producing bacteria.

Colitis cystica profunda is a rare condition in which the intestinal wall is thickened by submucosal mucus-filled cysts of various size and an accumulation of fibroblasts in the lamina propria. This condition can present as an ulcerating or mass lesion in the rectosigmoid in association with the solitary rectal ulcer syndrome. Although the pathogenesis of this condition is unknown, it may result from the downward displacement of colonic glands during chronic inflammation and healing. The appearance of aberrant submucosal glandular epithelium and acellular mucous lakes should not be mistaken for colloid carcinoma because this lesion has no malignant potential.

Carcinoid tumors of the rectum appear as isolated, small, yellow-gray submucosal nodules. These are often inciden-

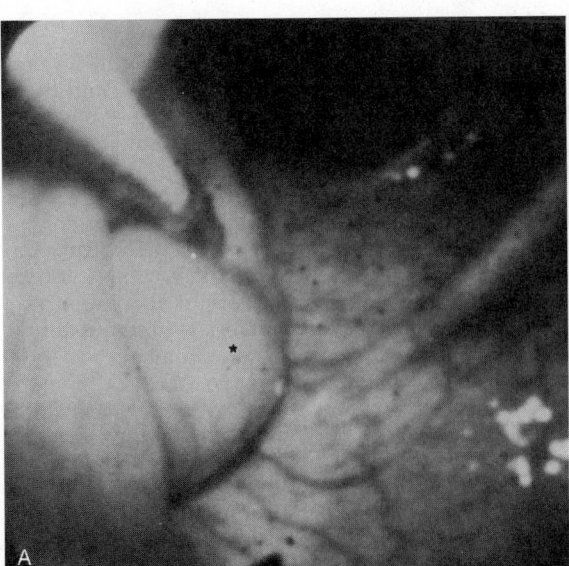
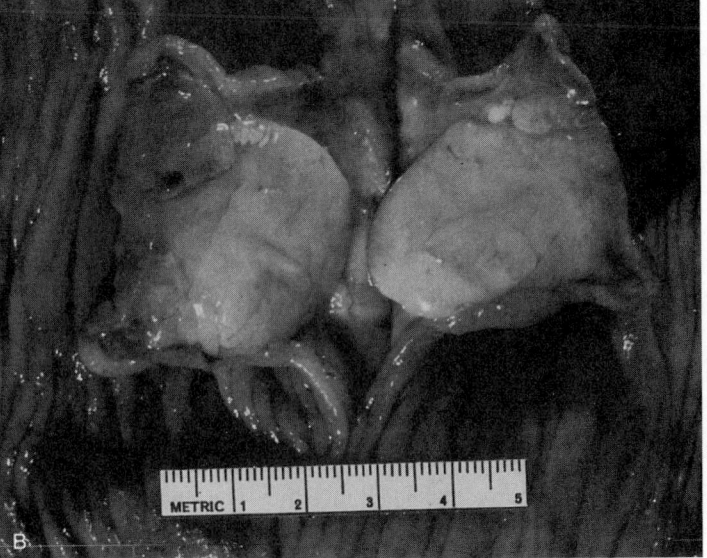

Figure 46-11. Submucosal lipoma. (*A*) Cecal lipoma seen at colonoscopy (*asterisk*). The submucosal fatty tissue causes protrusion of the mucosa into the lumen, which appears as a polyp. (*B*) Colectomy specimen demonstrating a large submucosal lipoma cut in cross section.

tal findings during sigmoidoscopy. Most are less than 1 cm and have low malignant potential. These are amenable to local excision. Lesions larger than 2 cm are more commonly malignant but seldom give rise to metastases. They should, however, be treated aggressively with complete excision. Rectal carcinoid tumors are usually asymptomatic but may present with hematochezia. They are not associated with the carcinoid syndrome. Carcinoid tumors in the proximal colon may be locally invasive or metastasize to the liver, liberating vasoactive peptides into the systemic circulation and producing the carcinoid syndrome.

Other lesions that can present as submucosal polyps include metastatic tumors, such as malignant melanoma, and benign lesions, such as leiomyomas, fibromas, lymphangiomas, hemangiomas, and endometriosis.

GASTROINTESTINAL POLYPOSIS SYNDROMES

Gastrointestinal polyposis indicates the presence of a systemic process that promotes the development of multiple polyps throughout the gastrointestinal tract. In some instances, the polyps are located predominantly in the colon; however, in many syndromes, polyps may be found in the stomach, small intestine, colon, and rectum. The classification of the polyposis syndromes has traditionally been based on the histologic characteristics of the polyps, but gradually an awareness of the genetic basis for the most important of these syndromes has permitted more precise diagnosis and individualized approaches to treatment.

Familial Adenomatous Polyposis

Familial adenomatous polyposis is an inherited disease characterized by the development of multiple adenomatous polyps throughout the colon and rectum (Fig. 46-12). The polyps first appear in adolescence, with median age of onset being about 16 years. The number of polyps in each patient is variable, and they increase in number and size with advancing age. The genetic basis for this disease is a germline mutation in the adenomatous polyposis coli (APC) gene located on chromosome 5q. In part, the age of onset, number of polyps, and age at which cancer develops are determined by the location of the mutation in the APC gene. More than 5000 polyps eventually develop in patients with the most severe types of mutations, and cancer develops in these patients at a mean age of 35 years. Additional factors not related to the mutation on the APC gene, some genetic and some environmental, also modify the clinical characteristics of the disease.[9,10]

Gastrointestinal Features

Polyps in the stomach and small intestine develop in about 90% of patients with FAP. The gastric polyps primarily consist of fundic gland hyperplasia, which is not a premalignant lesion. Occasionally, gastric adenomas are found, but stomach cancer is only rarely reported as a complication of FAP in North America, where the incidence of gastric cancer is low.

Small intestinal neoplasia is not rare in FAP, and principally occurs in the periampullary region of the duodenum. Duodenal adenomatous polyps, which typically appear later than the colonic lesions, may be multiple but tend not to carpet the proximal small intestine. The ampulla of Vater is a particular target for neoplastic development. With time, carcinoma develops in up to 5% of these patients, suggesting that this area requires surveillance. Adenomas and carcinomas occur in the jejunum and ileum, but these are rare. Polyps in the terminal ileum are more likely to represent lymphoid aggregates than adenomas and undergo biopsy for diagnostic purposes.

Classically, it has been stated that the natural history of FAP is for cancer to develop at a median age of 40 to 45 years. In fact, the development of cancer is variable, and again is based in part on the location of the germline mutation in the APC gene. Colon cancer is rare before 30 years of age, and cancer may not develop in patients with the attenuated form of FAP until they are in their 50s or 60s. Thus, the treatment of these patients relies increasingly on a genetic characterization of the disease.

Extraintestinal Features

Traditionally, patients with manifestations of FAP together with extraintestinal manifestations were considered to have Gardner syndrome. It is now appreciated that families with FAP all have extraintestinal manifestations and that there is no distinction between Gardner syndrome families and other FAP families. FAP is characterized by osteomas of the mandible, skull, and long bones and a variety of other benign soft tissue tumors, such as fibromas and lipomas (Fig. 46-13). Osteomas are commonly found in the skull and may be multiple. Some of these lesions have been reported to regress and later reappear. Osteomas may be found in the mandible, and radiographs of the mouth may reveal impacted or supernumerary teeth. Congenital hypertrophy of retinal pigmented epithelium (CHRPE) is present in some families with FAP, depending on the location of the mutation in the APC gene. CHRPE lesions may be seen in the general population but are small and usually single. Multiple, bilateral, and large CHRPE lesions are essentially diagnostic of FAP.

Malignant tumors are considered to be nearly inevitable consequences in the colon and may occur occasionally in the duodenum or (less commonly) elsewhere in the gastrointestinal tract. Patients with FAP are also at increased risk for brain tumors (particularly medulloblastomas), thyroid tumors, adrenal tumors, and benign and malignant tumors of the hepatobiliary tree. The occurrence of a malignant brain tumor in conjunction with intestinal polyposis was traditionally referred to as *Turcot syndrome*. Medulloblastomas are a rare complication of FAP, but there is a 99-fold increased risk of this tumor in FAP families. Interestingly, one of the index families initially reported by Turcot in 1959 did not have FAP but rather HNPCC, characterized by an excess of astrocytomas, such as glioblastoma multiforme.

Desmoid Tumors

When FAP is recognized, a colectomy should be performed long before the development of cancer, and there are strategies to reduce the likelihood of cancer development in the upper gastrointestinal tract. Desmoid tumors, however, later develop in 10% to 15% of patients with FAP, often as a complication of laparotomy but sometimes spontaneously. These are benign but aggressive tumors of mesenteric fibroblasts that can envelop and obstruct the gastrointestinal tract, arteries, veins, or ureters. In some instances, desmoid tumors virtually fill the abdominal cavity with tissue that makes additional abdominal exploration impossible. Desmoid tumors can be lethal.

Genetic Basis

Familial adenomatous polyposis occurs when a germline mutation in the APC gene inactivates the function of the APC gene product. In most instances, the genetic lesion creates a premature stop codon in the APC gene, which in turn leads to the translation of a truncated APC protein. The APC gene encodes for a large protein (311 kd) that binds to at least two other cytoskeletal elements—namely the catenins and E-cadherins. Depending on the location of the premature stop codon, the mutant protein is of variable

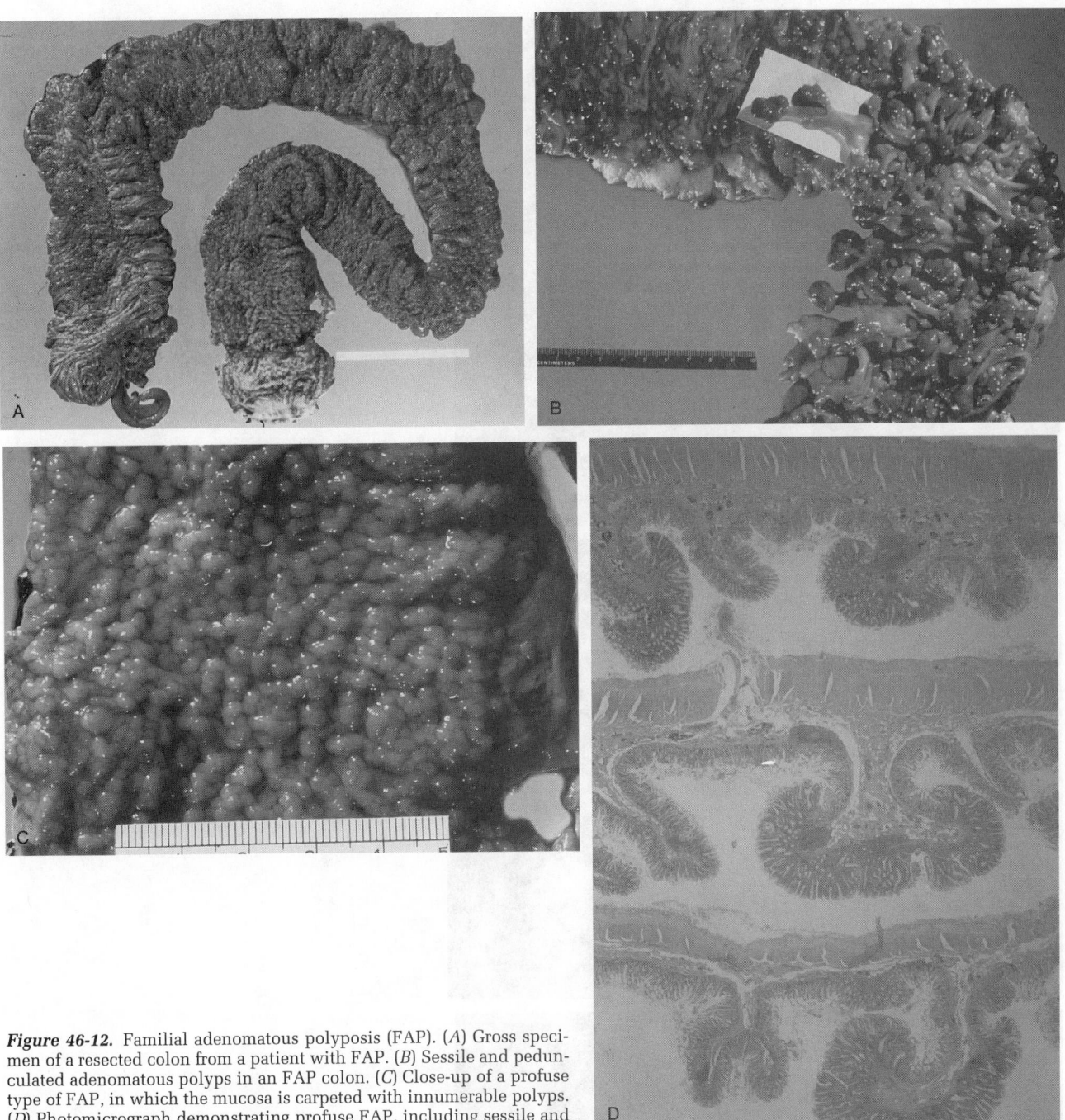

Figure 46-12. Familial adenomatous polyposis (FAP). (*A*) Gross specimen of a resected colon from a patient with FAP. (*B*) Sessile and pedunculated adenomatous polyps in an FAP colon. (*C*) Close-up of a profuse type of FAP, in which the mucosa is carpeted with innumerable polyps. (*D*) Photomicrograph demonstrating profuse FAP, including sessile and pedunculated adenomatous polyps.

length. The APC gene encodes 2844 codons (ie, one for each amino acid) and is broken into 15 translated exons. The structure of the APC gene is unique inasmuch as the exon makes up about 75% of the coding sequences of the gene. This long, open reading frame is unusually large, making it a natural target for the types of mutations that result in premature stop codons.[10]

The location of the germline mutation is of some clinical significance (Fig. 46-14). For example, mutations that occur at the 5′ end of the gene, particularly in the first three exons, encode for products that are intrinsically unstable and typically not detectable in tissues. This results in a clinically mild form of FAP called attenuated adenomatous polyposis coli. Families with this mutation have a smaller number of polyps, later onset of disease, and may

enter into their sixth or seventh decade having cancer. To complicate matters, however, family members with the same mutation may have variable manifestations of the disease. Indeed, some members who inherit this mutation have few polyps yet may pass on an increased risk of cancer to their progeny. In contrast, mutations that occur at the 5′ end of the 15th exon (in particular, in a brief segment between codons 1250 and 1464) develop a particularly virulent form of the disease with a larger number of polyps and an increased risk of colorectal cancer development at an early age (median age, 34 years). A large proportion of acquired mutations that occur in sporadic cancers also occur in this "hot spot," typically between codons 1309 and 1464. It appears that these mutations occur downstream (ie, toward the carboxyl terminus) in a portion of the APC

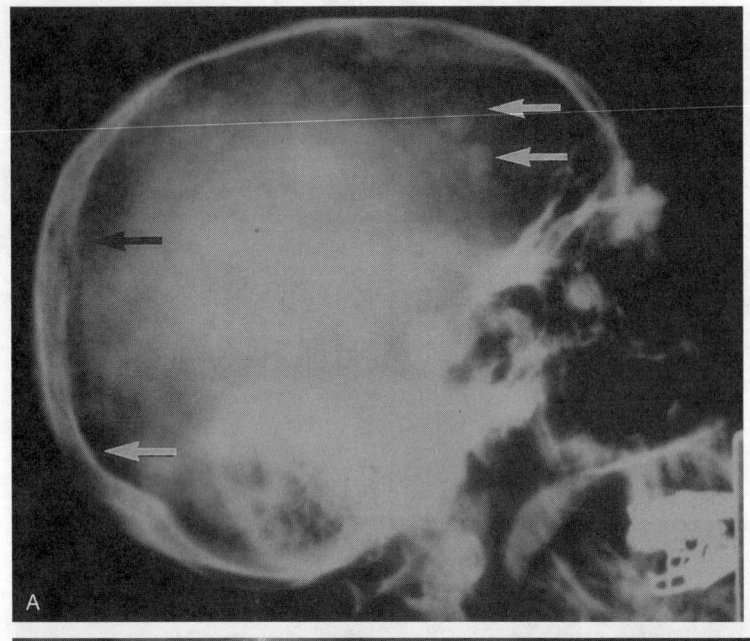

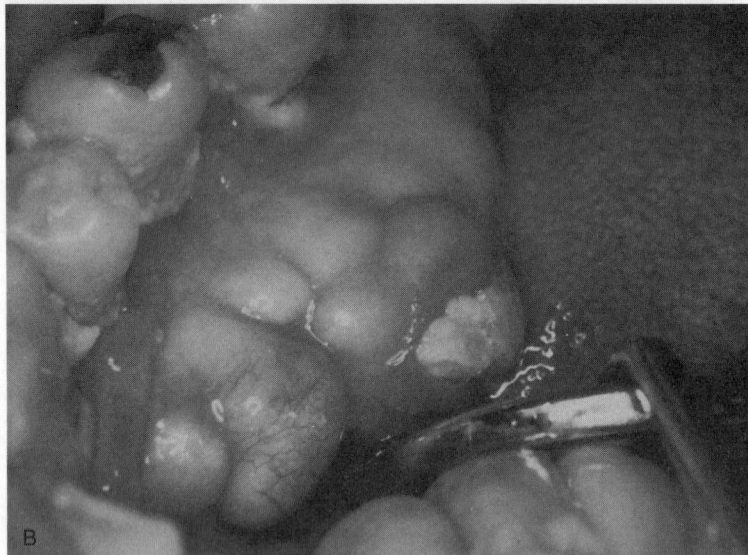

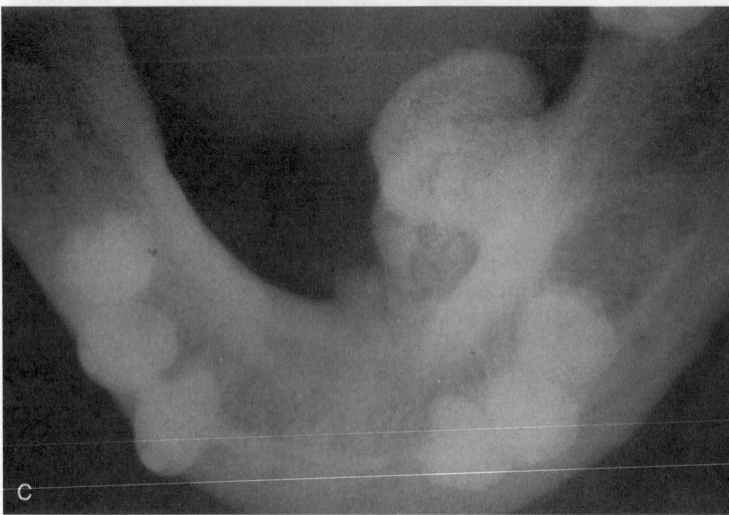

Figure 46-13. Extraintestinal manifestations of familial adenomatous polyposis (FAP). (*A*) Skull film demonstrating osteomas of the calvarium (*arrows*). (*B*) Photograph of the mandible demonstrating protuberant mandibular osteomas. (*C*) Mandibular radiograph demonstrating a large osteoma of the mandible. (*D*) Chest radiograph demonstrating multiple fibromas (*arrows*) in a patient with FAP. (*continues*)

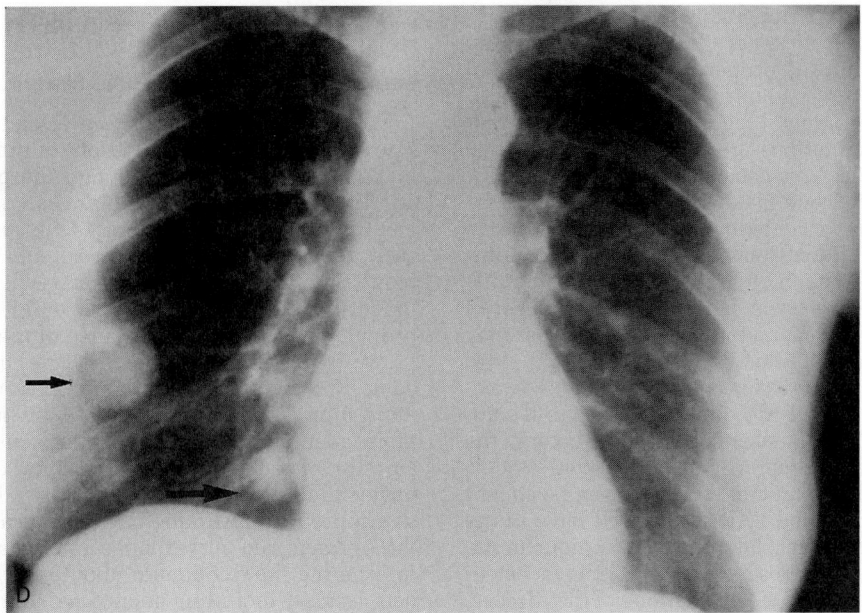

Figure 46-13. *(Continued)*

protein that associates with other cytoskeletal proteins. Thus, mutations in this region result in abnormal proteins that interfere with the wild-type protein and prevent normal cytoskeletal assembly. Mutant proteins that are truncated before this region are less capable of interfering with cytoskeletal assembly, and proteins that are truncated but nearly complete in length may be less deleterious to cellular function.

FAP families that have the CHRPE lesions usually have their mutations in exons 9 to 15, and this manifestation rarely occurs in families with mutations in any of the first 8 exons. Thus, detailed knowledge of the location of the germline mutation can help predict the expected clinical manifestations in these patients and can be used to guide therapy. Diagnostic screening tests that permit an estimation of the location of these mutations are available clinically.

Diagnosis

The clinical diagnosis of FAP is usually not problematic. When FAP is known in a family, the at-risk relatives should undergo surveillance sigmoidoscopy on an annual basis beginning in their middle teenage years. The entire colon is at risk of developing neoplasia, so sigmoidoscopy is sufficient to detect carriers of the abnormal gene. The appearance of a single adenoma in a teenager at risk for this disease greatly increases suspicion of the disease; however, the typical slow progression of the disease permits observation of these patients until multiple adenomas appear. After the first adenoma appears, diffuse adenoma development is typical during the next few years. The lesions must undergo biopsy to confirm that they are adenomas. No other disease produces multiple adenomatous polyps in young patients.

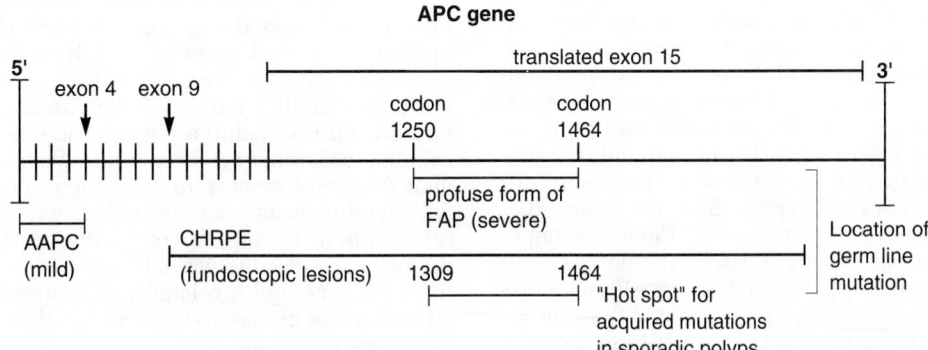

Figure 46-14. This scheme of the APC gene illustrates the genotype–phenotype correlations. Most of the mutations of the APC gene result in premature stop codons; therefore, the site of the mutation usually indicates the relative length of the mutant protein product. Mutations at the 5′ end of the gene produce AAPC, a milder form of the disease. The retinal lesions—CHRPE—occur when the mutations occur between exons 9 and 15. The portion of the APC gene that binds to other cytoskeletal elements in the cell (β-catenins) is represented in the 15th exon. Mutations in a hot spot immediately downstream from the β-catenin–binding site result in a more virulent, profuse form of familial adenomatous polyposis. This site is also the location of most of the acquired mutations in sporadic colorectal neoplasms.

The diagnosis of FAP is often made without prior suspicion in adults. In some instances, the disease had been present in relatives, but the proper diagnosis was not appreciated. About 25% of patients, however, have a germline lesion in the APC gene that is not present in either parent. These new mutations are more frequent in FAP than in some other diseases because the large size of the 15th exon of the APC gene makes it a suitable target for nucleotide insertions or deletions. These create frame shifts and subsequent downstream premature stop codons. In ambiguous cases—which often include attenuated disease, in which there are fewer polyps and later onset of disease (ie, attenuated adenomatous polyposis coli), it may be useful to confirm a suspected diagnosis with an in vitro truncated protein test. This test is about 60% to 80% sensitive in patients who have FAP, depending on the laboratory. Although the lack of sensitivity is a problem, the test is highly specific and reproducible. Therefore, once a positive test is found, the mutant APC gene can be sought in other relatives. Unrelated FAP families all have mutations in the APC gene, but most families have unique mutations. Although many families have CHRPE lesions, osteomas, or other extraintestinal manifestations of the disease, the appearance of these is sufficiently variable that they are a poor substitute for endoscopic examination or direct genetic testing.

In a family with FAP, each first-degree relative of an affected patient has a 50% likelihood of inheriting the mutated gene. By age 16, about half of affected patients have polyps. With each passing year, a negative sigmoidoscopic examination reduces further the likelihood that a patient carries the gene. Greater certainty can be obtained if the family's genetic lesion can be found and excluded in an at-risk family member.

Management

Surgery is the only reasonable management option in FAP, and the clinical decision involves the selection of the operation and its timing. The diagnosis of FAP is often made in adolescence, but there is typically a delay of 20 years or more from the appearance of the first adenomas until cancer develops. Thus, it is usually prudent to wait until the patient has reached full physical maturity before planning surgery.

The safest surgical approach is a total proctocolectomy with an ileoanal anastomosis. Any residual rectal mucosa that is left behind is at risk for the development of neoplasia. Even with careful endoscopic surveillance of the rectal segment, invasive carcinomas may develop.

Small adenomatous polyps of the rectum can spontaneously regress after a subtotal colectomy and ileorectal anastomosis, which underscores the reversible nature of the benign adenoma. It subsequently has been found that adenomas can regress in FAP in response to treatment with sulindac (Clinoril). Several reports have confirmed that even large numbers of polyps regress on 150 to 200 mg of sulindac twice per day.[11] Unfortunately, the polyps reappear when the drug is stopped, and there have been reports that cancer has developed despite treatment with sulindac. Medical treatment is therefore not a safe first-line treatment for FAP, but it may be of some benefit in patients who refuse operative intervention. Although there are no data to support this approach, sulindac may be a useful adjunct in patients with milder forms of FAP (ie, smaller numbers of polyps with relative rectal sparing) and in circumstances in which residual rectal tissue must be left behind. Sulindac does not appear to be effective in the management of upper gastrointestinal tract neoplasia. Furthermore, there is no evidence that sulindac plays any role in the management of sporadic adenomatous polyps or advanced colorectal neoplasia in any setting.

Management of Extracolonic Features

In addition to the risks of colorectal neoplasia, osteomas, lipomas, fibromas, and a variety of other lesions develop in patients with FAP. Although the osteomas, fibromas, and lipomas can degenerate into sarcomas, this is a sufficiently rare event that prophylactic surveillance and surgery are not indicated. Likewise, the CHRPE lesions do not require therapy. Gastric carcinoma is distinctly uncommon in North American populations, and it is not necessary to provide endoscopic surveillance of the stomach.

The two major management issues after removal of the colon and rectum are periampullary neoplasia and desmoid tumors. Ninety percent of FAP patients have one or more adenomas in the duodenum, usually close to the ampulla of Vater. These lesions should be excised for biopsy and destroyed by electrocautery, laser, or other ablative approaches. Although no data are available to indicate the optimal safe surveillance intervals, it seems prudent to examine the duodenum about every 2 years. Complex neoplasms—including adenomas with varying degrees of dysplasia—may require individualized management, including the use of biliary stents while performing extensive ablative therapy of the periampullary region. Surgical approaches may be required for advanced neoplasms (ie, carcinoma in situ or frank carcinoma), but therapeutic endoscopy remains the first option. Duodenotomy with local surgical excision is an option for these lesions.

Desmoid tumors are aggressive benign tumors of fibroblasts that can cause multiple clinical complications; they are a significant cause of morbidity and mortality in FAP. These tumors typically grow slowly and can surround or compress vascular structures, nerves, or the abdominal viscera. Surgical management is generally avoided unless simple local excision of an abdominal wall lesion is possible, and postoperative recurrences are common. Radiotherapy has been used to control the growth of some of these, but it is not always successful. There is no uniformly successful medical approach to this disease. A combination of sulindac plus tamoxifen may be tried for intraabdominal tumors, and has been successful in some patients. Cytotoxic chemotherapy with doxorubicin was successful in a patient whose tumor was refractory to other treatment.

Variants

A number of names have been attached to variations of FAP to emphasize the presence of particular extracolonic findings. The most prominent of these has been Gardner syndrome, which is the same as FAP because all Gardner syndrome families have mutations in the APC gene, and virtually all FAP families have the stigmata previously attributed to Gardner syndrome. A few families with prominent sebaceous cysts were once referred to as having Oldfield syndrome, and families with brain tumors have been referred to as having Turcot syndrome. All of these syndromes represent the variable expression of mutations in the APC gene and are largely of historical interest. The current mode of classifying FAP families is based on the APC gene mutation.

Peutz-Jeghers Syndrome

Peutz-Jeghers syndrome is an autosomal dominant familial syndrome characterized by multiple gastrointestinal polyps and characteristic skin pigmentation. The gene responsible for this disease has been neither identified nor mapped; carriers of the gene are predisposed to a number of early-onset cancers.

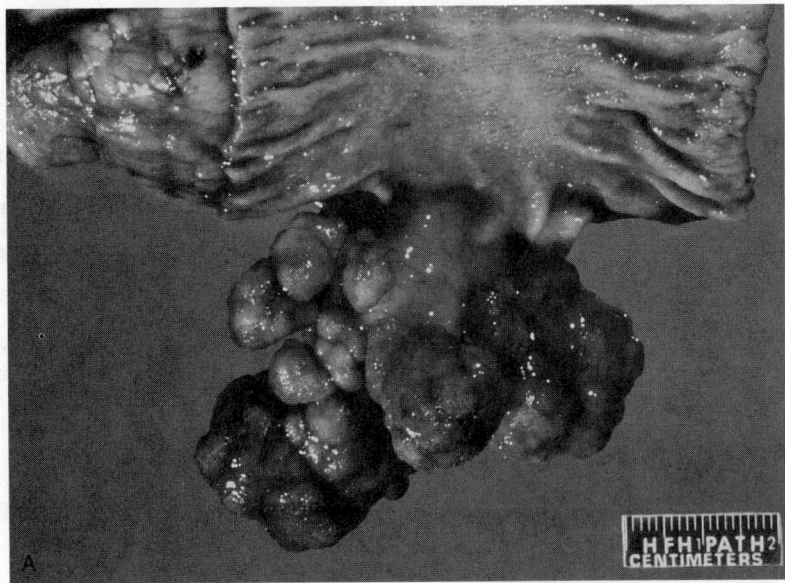

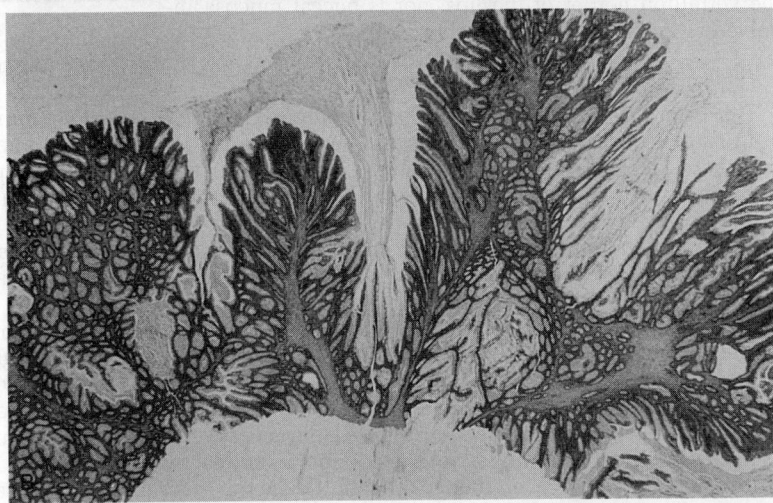

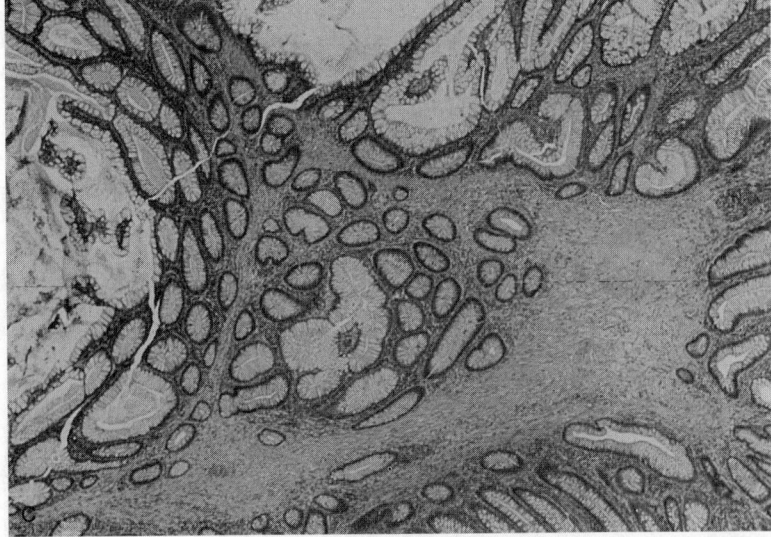

Figure 46-15. Peutz-Jeghers syndrome. (*A*) Gross specimen of a Peutz-Jeghers polyp, illustrating a large, multilobular lesion. (*B*) Low-power photomicrograph of a Peutz-Jeghers polyp of the colon, revealing the smooth muscle stroma covered by nonneoplastic colonic epithelium. (*C*) Higher-powered photomicrograph of the Peutz-Jeghers polyp indicates that the stroma contains arborizing bands of smooth muscle.

Gastrointestinal Features

The gastrointestinal polyps in Peutz-Jeghers syndrome are nonneoplastic hamartomas consisting of a supportive framework of smooth muscle tissue covered by somewhat hyperplastic epithelium (Fig. 46-15). These are distinctive from juvenile polyps and show no inflammatory cell infiltrate. Polyps may be found in the stomach, small intestine, or colon, and in each instance they have a distinctive appearance. Peutz-Jeghers polyps can usually be identified as such by the pathologist, and the characteristic cutaneous pigmentation makes this syndrome easily detected.

Skin Lesions

The cutaneous manifestations of Peutz-Jeghers syndrome may be found early in life and consists of dark, macular lesions on the mouth (both on the skin and in the buccal mucosa), nose, lips, hands, feet, genitalia, and anus. These lesions tend to become less obvious by the time of puberty. The cutaneous lesions of Peutz-Jeghers syndrome are present from birth, which does not occur with ordinary freckles. Moreover, ordinary freckles typically do not extend beyond the vermilion border of the lips, nor is buccal mucosa involved as occurs in Peutz-Jeghers syndrome.

Clinical Complications

The principal complication of Peutz-Jeghers syndrome is intestinal obstruction, which may occur in infancy or childhood. This complication is most prominent in the small intestine because of its narrower diameter. Gastrointestinal bleeding may also occur in this disease.

Cancer in the small intestine or colon can occur in Peutz-Jeghers syndrome; however, this is an uncommon complication.[12] It is thought that neoplasia may arise from foci of adenomatous epithelium that may be found in some Peutz-Jeghers polyps. The risk of cancer is such that prophylactic surgery is not recommended.

Patients with Peutz-Jeghers syndrome are at increased risk for cancers outside of the gastrointestinal tract as well. Cancer developed in about half of the patients in one large study, at a median age of about 50 years. Organs at risk include the gastrointestinal tract, gonads, breasts, pancreas, and biliary tree. Ovarian cysts and sex cord tumors are seen in 5% to 12% of female patients, and boys are at risk for endocrinologically active Sertoli cell testicular tumors that may produce feminizing features before puberty. No internal organ is at sufficiently high risk for cancer that a specific screening regimen or prophylactic surgery is indicated. The clinician should be aware of these risks, however, and should be particularly alert to gonadal tumors (which are otherwise rare) and breast cancer (for which screening should start at an early age, and bilateral disease should be suspected).

Management

The management of Peutz-Jeghers syndrome is limited to removal of polyps, using endoscopic techniques when possible. Surgery may be required for intussusception caused by small intestinal polyps. The risk of neoplastic development should be kept in mind, but these patients are not candidates for prophylactic removal of any section of the gastrointestinal tract. As mentioned earlier, gonadal neoplasms and breast cancer are potential complications that may require surgery.

Juvenile Polyposis

Juvenile polyps are pathologically characteristic lesions that can occur as solitary lesions or as part of a polyposis syndrome. Juvenile polyps are most commonly solitary lesions found in the rectums of children. The lesions may be large and are made up of an edematous, mildly inflamed lamina propria covered by normal colonic epithelium (Fig. 46-16). Multiple polyps may be found, which raises the suspicion for a familial juvenile polyposis syndrome. Three different syndromic presentations have been reported; it is not known, however, whether these are truly distinctive syndromes. They may consist of familial juvenile polyposis limited to the colon, familial juvenile polyposis throughout the gastrointestinal tract, and familial juvenile polyposis limited to the stomach. The genetic basis of this syndrome is not understood.

The manifestations of juvenile polyposis can vary but are largely limited to bleeding, interception, obstruction, or the passage of autoamputated lesions. Patients with familial juvenile polyposis are at some increased risk for the development of colorectal cancer. It has been suggested that the presence of mixed juvenile and adenomatous polyps indicates which lesions are premalignant. It is im-

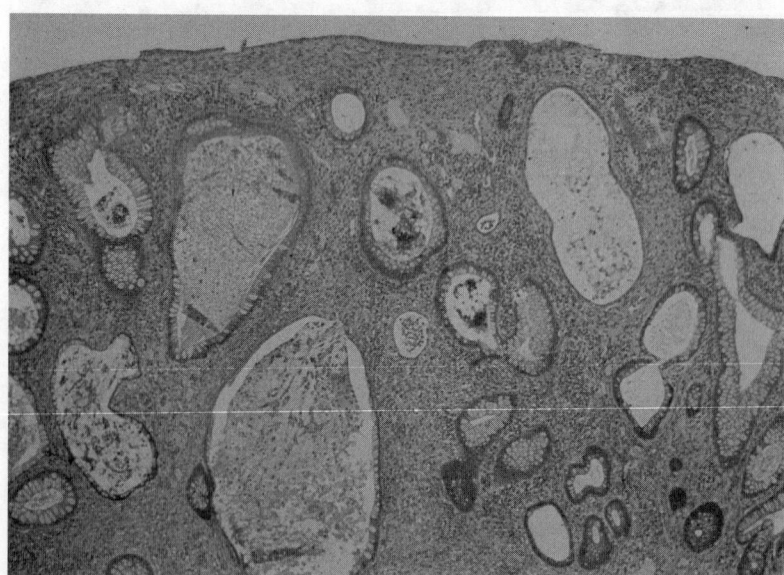

Figure 46-16. Photomicrograph of a juvenile polyp reveals an attenuated surface epithelium overlying an edematous lamina propria with fluid and mucus-filled cystic structures.

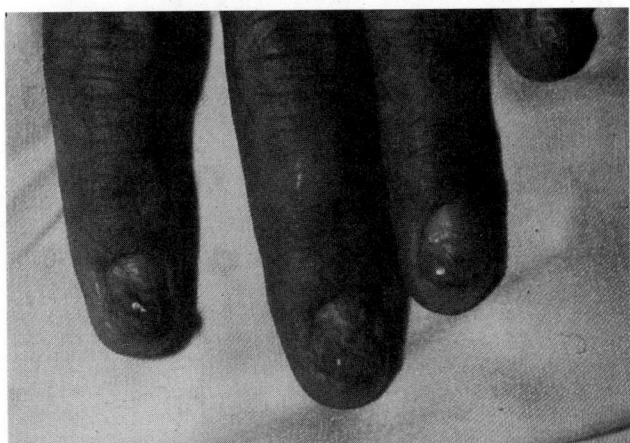

Figure 46-17. Cronkhite-Canada syndrome. Onycholysis and hyperpigmentation are characteristic cutaneous manifestations of Cronkhite-Canada syndrome, which is a nonfamilial, poorly understood, acquired condition consisting of multiple juvenile, inflammatory-type gastrointestinal polyps and characteristic cutaneous findings.

portant that the pathologist examine lesions carefully for the presence of adenomatous tissue in such polyps. When mixed lesions are found, patients in these families should be subjected to colonoscopic surveillance, perhaps as often as every 2 years.

Other Familial Polyposis Syndromes

A variety of other rare syndromes may give rise to multiple gastrointestinal polyps.[13] Cowden syndrome consists of multiple gastrointestinal hamartomas and may be complicated by multiple lesions of the face that arise from follicular epithelium and are pathologically trichilemmomas. Patients with multiple trichilemmomas should be considered for the diagnosis of Cowden syndrome. Gastrointestinal polyps, which are usually asymptomatic, may develop in these patients. The polyps include a variety of hamartomas, such as hyperplastic polyps and ganglioneuromas of the colon. Glycogenic acanthosis of the esophagus may also occur and usually is found incidentally as multiple, diminutive, flat polyps of the esophagus. These patients are at increased risk of development of breast cancer and of a variety of benign and malignant complications of the thyroid gland. No specific therapy need be directed toward the gastrointestinal tract.

Other diseases, such as neurofibromatosis (von Recklinghausen syndrome) and the basal cell nevus syndrome, may be associated with multiple gastrointestinal polyps; however, symptomatic complications of these polyps are uncommon.

Nonfamilial Gastrointestinal Polyposis Syndromes

Multiple gastrointestinal polyps are occasionally seen in nonfamilial syndromes. The Cronkhite-Canada syndrome is an acquired, nonfamilial syndrome characterized by cutaneous lesions (Fig. 46-17), chronic diarrhea, protein-losing enteropathy, and gastrointestinal polyps. The enter-

opathy may produce progressive inanition that results in death. The diarrhea is attributable to diffuse mucosal injury of the small intestine but may be complicated by bacterial overgrowth. Gastrointestinal polyps are present in most patients and occur in the stomach, small intestine, colon, and rectum. These polyps are pathologically similar to juvenile, retention-type polyps. The lamina propria is edematous and contains an inflammatory infiltrate. As has been reported in juvenile polyps, the lesions in this syndrome may contain adenomatous epithelium, and occasionally carcinomas have complicated this disease. A variety of medical and surgical measures have been used to treat this disease, and primary attention should be drawn to the treatment of the diarrhea and maintenance of the nutritional status. The cutaneous lesions consist of onycholysis, alopecia, and hyperpigmentation. In a number of cases, treatment of the bacterial overgrowth with antibiotics and maintenance of the nutritional status have resulted in complete resolution of the cutaneous features. Curiously, the cutaneous features may resolve despite persistence of the gastrointestinal polyps.

Other acquired lesions that may present with multiple gastrointestinal pseudopolyps include inflammatory pseudopolyps in the setting of inflammatory bowel disease, lymphoma, pneumatosis cystoides intestinalis, and multiple lipomas or hyperplastic polyps. None of these syndromes requires specific surgical treatment.

REFERENCES

1. Spirio L, Olschwang S, Groden J, et al. Alleles of the APC gene: an attenuated form of familial polyposis. Cell 1993; 755:951.
2. Burt RW. Hereditary polyposis syndromes and inheritance of adenomatous polyps. Semin Gastrointest Dis 1992;3:13.
3. Neugat AO, Jacobson JS, Ahsan H, et al. Incidence and recurrence rates of colorectal adenomas: a prospective study. Gastroenterology 1995;108:402.
4. Winawer SJ, Zauber AG, Ho MN, et al. Prevention of colorectal cancer by colonoscopic polypectomy. N Engl J Med 1993; 329:1977.
5. Cooper HS, Deppisch LM, Gourley WK, et al. Endoscopically removed malignant polyps: clinicopathologic correlations. Gastroenterology 1995;108:1657.
6. Atkin WS, Morson BC, Cuzick J. Long-term risk of colorectal cancer after excision of rectosigmoid adenomas. N Engl J Med 1992;326:658.
7. Winawer SJ, Zauber AG, O'Brien MJ, et al. Randomized comparison of surveillance intervals after colonoscopic removal of newly diagnosed adenomatous polyps. N Engl J Med 1993; 328:901.
8. Giavannucci E, Rimm EB, Stampfer MJ, et al. Aspirin use and the risk for colorectal cancer and adenoma in male health professionals. Ann Intern Med 1994;121:241.
9. Nagase H, Miyoshi Y, Horii A, et al. Correlation between the location of germ-line mutations in the APC gene and the number of colorectal polyps in familial adenomatous polyposis patients. Cancer Res 1992;52:4055.
10. Powell SM, Petersen GM, Krush AJ, et al. Molecular diagnosis of familial adenomatous polyposis. N Engl J Med 1993; 329:1982.
11. Giardiello FM, Hamilton SR, Krush AJ, et al. Treatment of colonic and rectal adenomas with sulindac in familial adenomatous polyposis. N Engl J Med 1993;328:1313.
12. Giardiello FM, Welsh SB, Hamilton SR, et al. Increased risk of cancer in the Peutz-Jeghers syndrome. N Engl J Med 1987;316:1511.
13. Marra G, Armelao F, Vecchio FM, Percesepe A, Anti M. Cowden's disease with extensive gastrointestinal polyposis. J Clin Gastroenterol 1994;18:42.

SURGERY: SCIENTIFIC PRINCIPLES AND PRACTICE, Second Edition, edited by Lazar J. Greenfield, Michael W. Mulholland, Keith T. Oldham, Gerald B. Zelenock, and Keith D. Lillemoe. Lippincott–Raven Publishers, Philadelphia, © 1997.

CHAPTER 47

COLORECTAL CANCER

ALFRED E. CHANG

Adenocarcinoma of the large intestine is the second most common malignancy in the United States, with more than 155,000 new cases diagnosed annually.[1] The only malignancy more prevalent than colorectal cancer is lung cancer. Colorectal carcinoma is the second leading cause of all cancer-related deaths. If diagnosed in its early stages, however, this malignancy is curable by surgical treatment with minimal morbidity and mortality.

Because of the potential for cure of early-stage disease, the definition of populations at risk and screening of asymptomatic patients are important considerations. Controlled clinical trials have demonstrated that the multidisciplinary approach to the treatment of localized colorectal cancer has improved the morbidity and mortality of this disease. For recurrent disease, various therapeutic approaches are reviewed. Other colorectal tumors, such as lymphomas, sarcomas, and carcinoid tumors, are distinct from adenocarcinoma and are discussed separately at the end of the chapter.

EPIDEMIOLOGY

Worldwide, colorectal cancer ties breast cancer as the third most frequent cancer, after gastric and lung cancers.[2] An important feature of colorectal cancer is its broad geographic variation in incidence, with the differences between population groups ranging as high as 30-fold (Fig. 47-1). These differences appear not to be the result solely of genetic factors, because populations migrating from low- to high-incidence regions experience an increase in the rate of colorectal cancer. Such data provide indirect evidence that environmental factors are involved in the pathogenesis of this disease. Industrialized countries have the highest incidences, and numerous studies have linked dietary factors to the development of colorectal cancer (see later). Evidence suggests that this disease may be responsive to dietary manipulations and therefore that its incidence may be reducible.

In the United States, the age-specific incidence of colorectal cancer rises steadily from the second to ninth decades. The rates of colon and rectal cancer are generally similar between men and women. Since the 1950s, there have been no dramatic changes in incidence trends, although there has been a slight upward drift in colon cancer incidence among people aged 55 years and older.[3] During the same period, there appears to be a favorable trend toward a lower mortality rate for rectal cancer.

In North America, there are no geographic regions with a substantially increased risk that would suggest the presence of an important carcinogenic agent, although urban populations and people of higher socioeconomic background tend to have higher incidences of colorectal cancers. In addition, there have been no consistent findings of high-risk occupations, and smoking does not play an etiologic role.

ETIOLOGY

Dietary Factors

Evidence from epidemiologic studies suggest that dietary factors play important causative and protective roles in the development of large bowel cancers. Fat intake has been the most consistently positive association and fiber intake the most consistently inverse association noted in the incidence of colorectal cancer.

In comparisons between countries, the rates of colon cancer are strongly associated with the intake of animal fat and meat[4] (Fig. 47-2). The associations between per capita consumption of total fat, saturated fat, and cholesterol and national incidence rates of colon cancer are strongly positive.[5] The proposed mechanism by which dietary fat may increase the risk for colonic cancer is its interaction with bile acids, discussed in more detail later.

The relation between fiber intake and colon cancer was

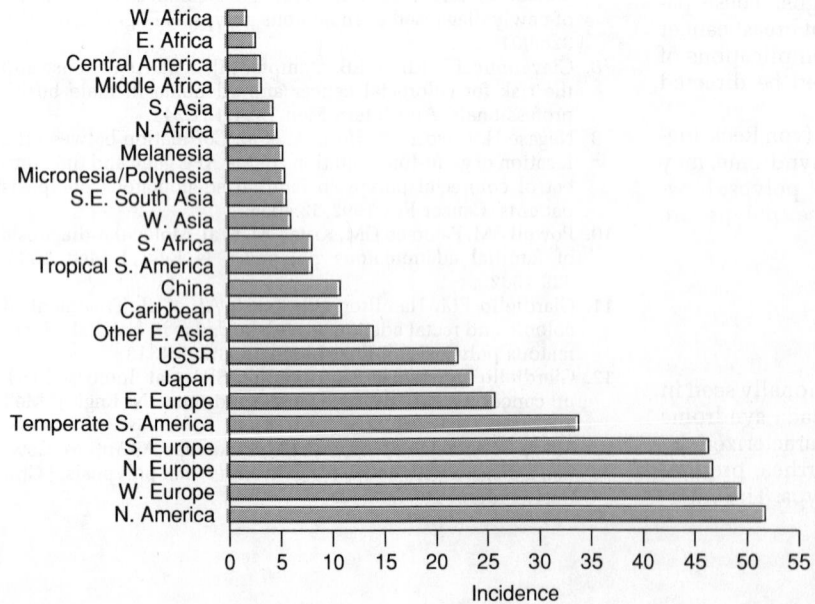

Figure 47-1. Incidence of colorectal cancer per 100,000 population in 23 geographic regions during 1980. (After Parkin DM, Laara E, Muir CS. Estimates of the worldwide frequency of sixteen major cancers in 1980. Int J Cancer 1988; 41:184)

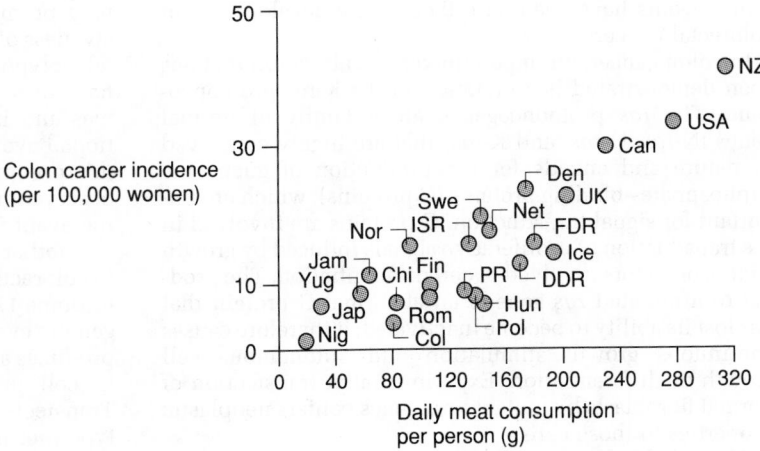

Figure 47-2. Correlation between meat intake and the incidence of colon cancer among women in 23 countries. (After Willett W. The search for the causes of breast and colon cancer. Nature 1989; 338:389)

initially noted by Burkitt,[6] who reported low rates of colon cancer in areas of Africa where fiber consumption and stool bulk were high. In general, epidemiologic studies have demonstrated that fiber intake is higher in nonindustrialized countries with lower incidences of colon cancer. However, countries with high fiber intake also tend to have lower intakes of fat and frequently have lower life expectancy, introducing confounding variables. The role of fiber was originally seen simply as the provision of bulk to dilute potential carcinogens and speed their transit through the colon. Data now suggest that this is an oversimplification and that the relation between fiber intake and colon cancer is more complex. Certain fibers can bind mutagens, reducing their contact with colonic epithelium; others can favorably change the fecal pH or participate in other complex interactions.

The difficulty in sorting out the association of fiber intake with colon cancer risk reflects the heterogeneous nature of fiber, the nondigestible component of carbohydrates. Fiber is derived from cereal products, vegetables, and fruit. Dietary fiber comprises a diverse collection of carbohydrates that are unlikely to have identical physiologic effects. Although the role of fiber in protecting against colorectal cancer is strong, the specific foods related to this effect are poorly defined.

Mutagenesis

Carcinogenesis in the colon and rectum has been described in terms of an initiation–promotion model based on experimental observations in laboratory animals. According to this model, the first step involves initiating factors that directly interact with cellular deoxyribonucleic acid (DNA) to induce mutations in the genome. Afterward, the process is driven by promotional factors, which are not mutagenic by themselves but enhance cellular proliferation of previously mutated cells. Although this concept represents an oversimplification of a complex, multistep process, it serves as a useful framework to understand data generated from animal models examining the pathogenesis of large bowel cancer. One can enhance or reduce tumorigenesis in experimental animals both by maneuvers that modify the generation of a mutagen (or carcinogen) and by those that alter promotional factors long after the administration of an initiating agent.

The human diet contains a myriad of naturally occurring mutagens or substances that can be metabolized into mutagens. A wide range of such substances are generated from interactions between the diet, microbial flora, and colonic

mucosal enzymes. There are also protective mechanisms present throughout the mucosa to detoxify these compounds. The action of carcinogens on DNA appears not to be an entirely random process. Mutagens typically alkylate DNA at specific carbon residues and cause nucleotide misreading during the next cycle of DNA replication. A mutation commonly seen early in colonic carcinogenesis results in activation of the *ras* protooncogene, one of several genetic events presumed to be involved in malignant transformation.[7] This mutational event may be involved in initiation or promotion of carcinogenesis. Because of the ubiquitous presence of mutagens in the gut, many strategies that aim to reduce colon cancer attempt to interfere with the interaction between mutagens and the target colonic cells.

From animal studies, the role of fat in the pathogenesis of colon cancer appears to be that of a promotional factor. With increasing fat intake, there is a significant increase in total fecal bile acid. Available data suggest that bile acids stimulate the generation of reactive oxygen metabolites that enhance the conversion of unsaturated fatty acids to compounds that promote cellular proliferation. Theoretically, this would facilitate the emergence of a mutated clone of neoplastic cells. Enhanced proliferation of these transformed cells can either compress the time required for carcinogenesis or, perhaps, make the process more efficient. An extension of this concept is the observation that increased dietary calcium has been associated with a decreased risk for colorectal cancer. Experimental data demonstrate that an increase in dietary calcium tends to inhibit colonic proliferative indices.

Molecular Genetics

The elucidation of the molecular events leading to the development of colorectal cancers has been aided by the observation that adenocarcinomas can arise from adenomas. There appears to be an orderly histologic progression of cellular transformation—from normal colonic epithelium, to small adenomas, to large adenomas, and then to carcinomas—which has allowed investigators to study the genetic alterations that may give rise to these changes. Cancers are believed to result from a series of genetic alterations leading to the progressive disordering of the normal mechanisms that control cell growth. There are at least three distinct mechanisms by which normal cell growth can be changed to a neoplastic pattern. These involve genetic alterations in oncogenes, tumor suppressor genes, and mismatch repair genes. Examples of all of these mutational events have been described in the development of colorectal cancers.

In colon cancer, an important genetic alteration that has been demonstrated is a mutation of the K-*ras* protooncogene. The *ras* protooncogenes are a family of normal genes (N-*ras*, H-*ras*, and K-*ras*) that are highly conserved in nature and encode for the production of guanosine triphosphate–binding proteins (G proteins), which are important for signal transduction. G proteins are involved in the transduction of proliferative signals induced by growth factors or factors involved in cell differentiation. The product of a mutated *ras* gene is an abnormal G protein that has lost its ability to become inactivated; it therefore causes continuous growth stimulation and autonomous cell growth or differentiation. Experimentally, transfection of normal fibroblasts by mutated *ras* genes confers neoplastic properties to those cells.

About half of colorectal carcinomas and a similar percentage of adenomas larger than 1 cm in diameter have been found to have the *ras* gene mutation.[7,8] By contrast, less than 10% of adenomas smaller than 1 cm have this mutation. The *ras* gene mutation may be the initiating event in some colorectal carcinomas or, alternatively, it may promote the clonal expansion of a mutated cell population. It appears that the *ras* gene mutation alone is not responsible for tumorigenesis. Other molecular events appear to be required in addition to *ras* gene mutations.

Loss of specific chromosomal regions (known as loss of heterozygosity, or LOH) is another genetic alteration that is associated with the development of colorectal neoplasms in a high percentage of cases. These chromosomal regions have been hypothesized to contain tumor suppressor (or growth suppressor) genes. The products of these genes normally regulate growth and differentiation in a negative fashion, and their loss promotes neoplastic development. One such gene, which is linked to familial adenomatous polyposis (FAP), has been mapped to the long arm of chromosome 5q and is referred to as the APC (adenomatosis polyposis coli) gene. The APC gene was identified in 1991.[9,10] It acts as a tumor suppressor gene, meaning that it normally functions to suppress cell growth. If the APC gene is mutated, this growth control is lost. The gene codes for a 300-kd protein that has recently been shown to bind to β-catenin, implying an important role in cell adhesion and possibly cytoskeleton function.[11,12] It is hypothesized that disruption of cell adhesion and cytoskeleton function can lead to loss of contact inhibition, which

may promote neoplastic transformation as well as invasiveness of cancer cells. Among patients without the familial polyposis syndrome, allelic losses of chromosome 5q have been observed in 20% to 50% of colorectal carcinomas and in 30% of adenomas. Furthermore, APC mutations have been identified in early adenomas and even in microscopic lesions thought to precede adenomas. This observation suggests that APC mutation may be an initiating event in colorectal carcinogenesis.

Another tumor suppressor gene thought to be important in colorectal tumorigenesis is the p53 gene located on chromosome 17p. Alteration in p53 is one of the most common genetic events seen in human malignancies. The p53 gene produces a DNA-binding phosphoprotein that is important in cell proliferation, differentiation, and cell survival. Transfection of human colon cancer cell lines with a wild-type (normal) p53 gene prevents expression of the malignant phenotype.[13] Allelic loss of p53 has been observed in over 75% of colorectal carcinomas; however, it is rarely observed in adenomas. This gene therefore appears to be associated with the transition from adenoma to carcinoma and may facilitate tumor progression.

Another common genetic alteration associated with colorectal tumors is an allelic loss of chromosome 18q. This is where the "deleted in colorectal carcinoma" gene, termed DCC, is located. Mutations in DCC are present in 47% of late adenomas and 73% of carcinomas but in less than 13% of early- and intermediate-stage adenomas.[14] This indicates that alterations of this gene occur later in tumorigenesis. The DCC protein shares significant homology with the family of neural cell adhesion molecules that regulate cell adhesion and recognition. The loss or mutation of the DCC gene may play a role in tumorigenesis by altering normal cell–cell or cell–matrix interactions that are important in cell growth and differentiation.[15]

The development of colorectal cancer is a multistep process wherein malignant carcinomas arise from benign adenomas. This progression has provided a framework for understanding the molecular events that occur during tumorigenesis. As already indicated, there are at least four defined genetic alterations associated with colorectal cancers: *ras* gene mutations, and allelic deletions of chromosomes 5q (APC), 17p (p53), and 18q (DCC). The development of colorectal cancer from adenomas appears to reflect an accumulation of these molecular events (Fig. 47-3). These are clearly not the only genetic alterations that can occur, because many other chromosome losses have been

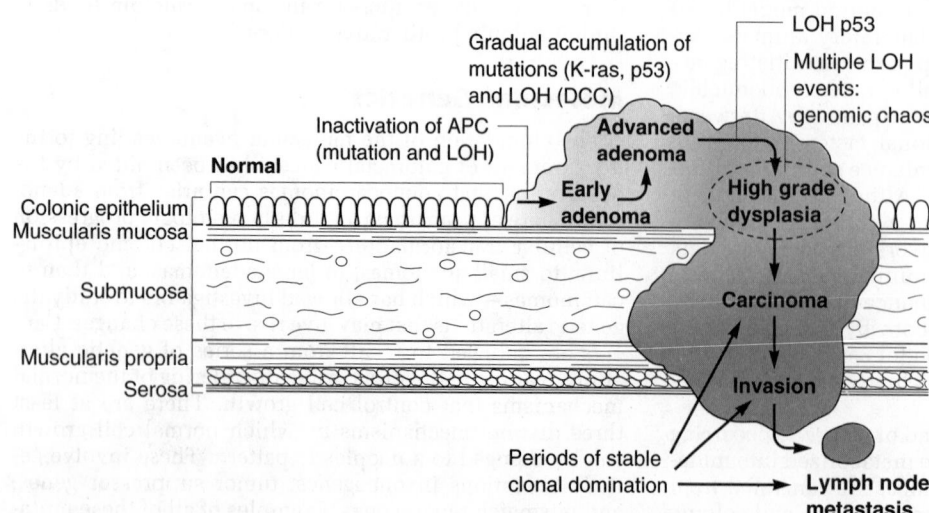

Figure 47-3. Model of genetic events mediating neoplastic progression of the colon. LOH, loss of heterozygosity. (After C.R. Boland, University of Michigan, Ann Arbor)

observed. In addition, a significant loss of methyl groups in DNA has been found to occur early in colorectal tumor development. Hypomethylation of DNA has been shown to contribute to the instability of the cell genome, which can enhance the rate at which genetic alterations, such as allelic losses, occur.

A new mechanism by which colorectal tumors arise was discovered by evaluating germline mutations in patients with hereditary nonpolyposis colorectal carcinoma (HNPCC). There is a highly conserved family of genes involved in DNA repair; their alteration disrupts the repair function and can lead to somatic mutations and genome instability, which can eventually give rise to cancer formation. These genes include *hMSH2*, located on chromosome 2p, and *hMLH1*, located on chromosome 3, and they belong to a family of genes known as mismatch repair genes. Mutations of *hMSH2* and *hMLH1* were found to be the underlying genetic defect in HNPCC.[16,17] It is estimated that between 5% to 10% of all colorectal carcinomas arise among kindreds with HNPCC. This genetic mutation may also play a role in the development of sporadic cancers, because 13% of such tumors have been found to exhibit it.

As genetic events are further defined in colorectal tumorigenesis, clinical applications may become evident. For instance, the identification of certain genetic alterations in tumor cells has prognostic significance (see Prognostic Factors). Specific germline genetic defects that can be assessed in peripheral blood cells may provide useful markers for identification of individuals at high risk for colorectal cancer (ie, persons with FAP or HNPCC). In the future, potential reversals of these genetic alterations may lead to new therapeutic strategies.

CLINICAL RISK FACTORS

Familial

Several familial polyposis syndromes (Table 47-1), which are characterized by the development of numerous adenomatous polyps, are associated with a high risk for large bowel cancers. The most significant of these syndromes is familial polyposis coli, or FAP. This syndrome is relatively rare in the United States, with an incidence of about 1 in 10,000 persons, and accounts for less than 1% of all colorectal cancers. People affected with this syndrome develop multiple adenomatous colonic polyps at a median age of 16 years, and increasing numbers of polyps are detected with increasing age. The disease is inherited as an autosomal dominant trait with essentially 100% penetrance. Unless proctocolectomy is performed in early adulthood, virtually all affected patients develop cancer by age 55. This syndrome represents the extreme end of the colon cancer spectrum and serves as a model of the adenoma-to-carcinoma sequence reviewed in the previous section. Adenomas appear first, and cancers develop later. It is important to identify these families so that family members can be examined frequently, because half of them go on to develop the syndrome. The variants of this syndrome, and those of other polyposis syndromes, are described in more detail in Chapter 46.

Two types of familial colon cancer syndromes have been described that are not associated with polyposis; they are broadly termed HNPCC.[18,19] The first is Lynch syndrome I, which is inherited as an autosomal dominant trait that produces multiple colon cancers two to three decades earlier than is typically seen. The cancers that develop have a predilection for the proximal colon. In 65% to 88% of cases, cancer develops in the proximal large intestine; in the general population, 20% to 30% that occur in that location. Lynch syndrome II, also called cancer family syndrome, is a closely related inherited disease that includes all the features seen in Lynch syndrome I but also is characterized by the early onset of carcinoma at other sites, including the endometrium, ovaries, and stomach. The Lynch syndromes are thought to be the most common forms of familial colon cancer and account for about 5% to 10% of all cases of colon cancer.

For most colorectal cancer patients with sporadic disease, there is evidence of an increased incidence in family members. Relatives of patients with sporadic colon cancer have a two- to three-fold increased risk of developing large bowel cancer compared with the general population. This association has not been characterized as a specific genetic disorder. More probably, familial factors may mediate differential susceptibility to environmental or dietary risks.

Inflammatory Bowel Disease

A strong association exists between inflammatory bowel disease and bowel cancer. For patients with ulcerative colitis, the incidence of malignancy is proportional to the extent of colonic involvement, age at onset, severity, and duration of disease. The duration of inflammatory bowel disease is a critical factor in predicting the likelihood of adenocarcinoma. About 3% of patients develop cancer during the first 10 years after the onset of colitis, and an additional 20% in each of the next two decades.[20] Treatment of cancers in patients with ulcerative colitis has a cure rate similar to that for noncolitic patients.[21]

Patients with Crohn's disease are also at increased risk for colon cancer as well as small bowel cancer. The risk of malignancy is lower than that reported for ulcerative colitis. As with ulcerative colitis, the cancers tend to occur at an earlier age than in patients without inflammatory bowel disease.

Polyps

Colorectal polyps can be divided into two broad categories: neoplastic and nonneoplastic. Nonneoplastic polyps include hyperplastic, inflammatory, juvenile, and hamartomatous polyps, none of which are precursors to colorectal cancer. Neoplastic polyps are adenomas and have

---

Table 47-1. CLINICAL RISK FACTORS FOR COLORECTAL CANCER

GENETIC

Polyposis syndromes
  Familial polyposis coli
  Gardner syndrome
  Turcot syndrome (CNS tumors)
  Oldfield syndrome (sebaceous cysts)
  Peutz-Jeghers syndrome (hamartomas)
Nonpolyposis syndromes
  Lynch syndrome I
  Lynch syndrome II (associated extracolonic cancers)
Preexisting disease
  Ulcerative colitis
  Crohn disease
  Prior colorectal cancer
  Neoplastic polyps
  Pelvic irradiation
  Breast or genital tract cancer

GENERAL

Age >40 y
Family history of colorectal cancer

Table 47-2. NEOPLASTIC COLORECTAL POLYPS

Type	Histologic Features	Incidence (%)	Invasive Malignancy (%)
Adenomatous (tubular adenoma)	Branching tubules embedded in lamina propria	75	5
Villous (villous adenoma)	Finger-like projections of epithelium over lamina propria	10	40
Intermediate (tubulovillous adenoma)	Mixture of adenomatous and villous patterns	15	22

the potential to develop into malignant cancers. The incidence of colorectal malignancy is two to five times higher in patients with adenomatous polyps than in those without them. Patients with multiple polyps are twice as likely to develop carcinoma as patients with a single polyp. Evidence suggests that there is a common inherited susceptibility toward both sporadic colonic adenomatous polyps and colorectal cancer.[22]

Adenomas can be divided into tubular adenomas (75% to 100% tubular components), tubulovillous adenomas (25% to 75% villous components), and villous adenomas (75% to 100% villous components). The most common type is tubular adenoma, or adenomatous polyp, which constitutes about 75% of neoplastic polyps[23] (Table 47-2). Tubulovillous adenomas account for 15% and pure villous adenomas for 10% of neoplastic polyps. All adenomas contain some degree of dysplasia or cellular atypia. This dysplasia can be graded from mild to severe. Carcinoma in situ and severe dysplasia have been grouped together under the classification of high-grade dysplasia. In carcinoma in situ, there is no invasion into the muscularis mucosa, as there is in invasive carcinoma (Fig. 47-4). The incidence of invasive malignancy differs markedly for the three types of adenomas and increases with the size of the adenoma. In general, malignancies are seen in 5% of adenomatous polyps, in 22% of tubulovillous adenomas, and in 40% of villous lesions. Although villous lesions are much less common, they are more likely to harbor a malignancy.

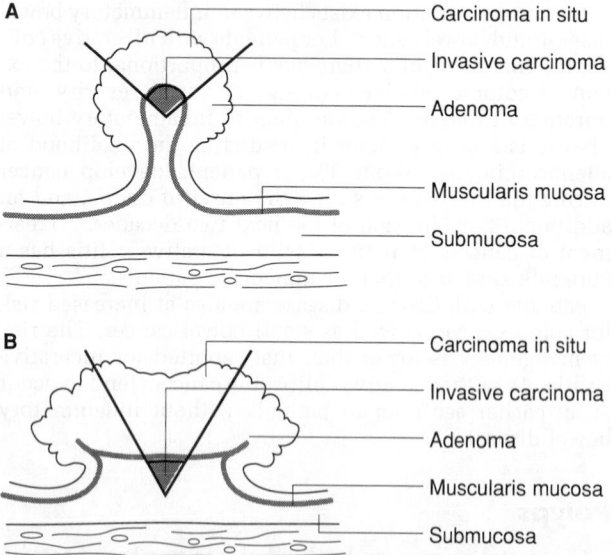

Figure 47-4. Anatomic distinction between carcinoma in situ and invasive malignancy in a pedunculated (*A*) or sessile (*B*) adenomatous polyp. In carcinoma in situ, there is no invasion into the muscularis mucosa.

Other Risk Factors

People older than 40 years of age have an increased risk for colorectal cancer, and this risk increases proportionally to the eighth decade. Patients who have received irradiation for gynecologic cancer have a two- to three-fold increased risk for development of colorectal cancer. Patients with previously resected colorectal cancer have a three-fold increased risk of developing a second primary large bowel cancer. Women with breast or genital tract cancer also have an increased risk for large bowel cancer.

DIAGNOSIS

Symptoms

The diagnosis of colorectal cancers can be made based on the evaluation of the symptomatic patient or through screening programs. The symptoms of colorectal cancer can be nonspecific, such as intermittent pain, bleeding, nausea, and vomiting. Bleeding may present as melena, which is more commonly associated with right colon cancers, or as gross red blood, associated with left colon and rectal cancers. Lesser amounts of bleeding may be detected as part of a fecal occult blood test. Patients with chronic blood loss may develop iron-deficiency anemia associated with fatigue.

Malignant obstruction can result in abdominal pain with nausea and vomiting. In the presence of obstruction, there may be a perforation either at the site of the tumor or through the proximal uninvolved intestine. For rectal tumors, compromise of the rectal reservoir can cause a change in bowel habits, such as constipation or a decreased stool caliber. For locally advanced rectal cancers, symptoms of tenesmus, urgency, and perineal pain can occur.

Diagnostic Tests

A broad range of diagnostic studies can be employed in the evaluation of a suspected large bowel cancer. The least expensive and potentially most informative study for rectal tumors is the digital examination. This permits the localization of distal rectal and anal neoplasms. In addition, stool can be obtained for evaluation of bleeding.

Rigid sigmoidoscopy with a 25-cm instrument is comparatively inexpensive but is limited by the length of intestine that can be examined and by patient compliance. Flexible fiberoptic sigmoidoscopy has gained more acceptance. Instruments measuring 35 and 65 cm are available, and an examination of the sigmoid colon and rectum can usually be performed after cleansing enemas. Patient acceptance is much higher than with rigid sigmoidoscopy.

The barium enema is the traditional study for the diagnosis of colonic polyps and cancers. The double-contrast technique using air insufflation is superior to the standard single-contrast barium enema to detect early polyps or cancers. The classic apple-core defect has been described for colonic cancers (Fig. 47-5). Proctosigmoidoscopy should

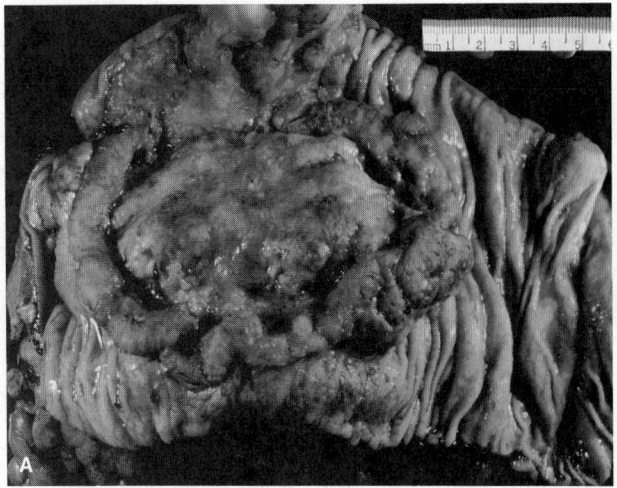
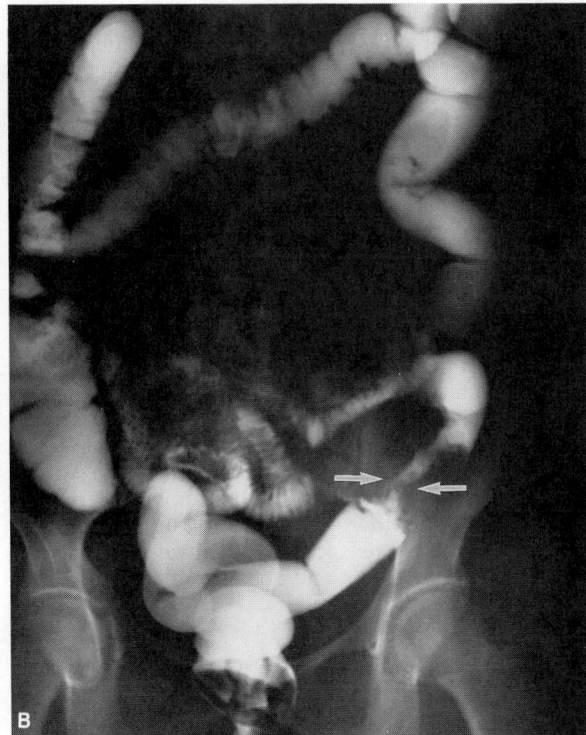

Figure 47-5. Surgical specimen with correlating barium enema examination of an invasive sigmoid carcinoma. (*A*) The tumor is a circumferential lesion. (*B*) The barium enema study demonstrates features of the apple-core defect (*arrows*).

also be performed to exclude rectal lesions, because visualization of the rectum is inadequate on barium enema. One advantage of barium enema over colonoscopy is the routine visualization of the right colon, which is not possible in 5% to 10% of colonoscopic examinations.

Colonoscopy with the 180-cm fiberoptic instrument is the most widely used diagnostic study to evaluate the colon. A valuable aspect of this procedure is the ability to obtain mucosal biopsy specimens and perform polypectomies. The incidence of severe complications that require surgical intervention (eg, hemorrhage, perforation) is 0.1% to 0.3%.

Increasingly, the diagnosis of colorectal cancer is made on the evaluation of a positive fecal occult blood test. The most commonly employed test to detect occult blood uses guaiac-impregnated paper slides that change color in the presence of peroxidase activity from hemoglobin. Several factors affect the utility of this test. First, not all colonic cancers or polyps are associated with bleeding, and even in those that are, bleeding is often intermittent in nature. Second, patients must be instructed to remain on low-peroxidase diets (no rare beef) before testing to avoid false-positive results. Third, certain medications, such as iron, cimetidine, antacids, and ascorbic acid, may interfere with the peroxidase reaction and may lead to a false-negative result. The experience with fecal occult blood testing in asymptomatic populations has shown that about 2.5% of tested patients are positive. Among those patients, only 10% to 15% have colorectal cancer.[24]

Screening

For screening purposes, asymptomatic patients can be divided into those in the high-risk category and the general population. People in the high-risk group were described previously. First-degree relatives of patients with known hereditary colon cancer syndromes should undergo colonoscopy by age 20 and regularly thereafter. Patients who have had adenomatous polyps removed should have

yearly colonoscopy until no further polyps are seen and then every 3 to 5 years thereafter. Patients with ulcerative colitis should have surveillance colonoscopy after 8 to 10 years of disease activity. Based on the findings, a subsequent surveillance program can be formulated.

In the asymptomatic general population, the efficacy of screening programs has been controversial. Testing for fecal occult blood is relatively inexpensive and simple, and it is the most commonly used screening test. In one prospective trial, more than 20,000 patients were randomly divided into two groups. Those in the first group were encouraged to undergo regular fecal occult blood testing, and those in the second group were advised to see a physician if colonic symptoms developed.[25] This study revealed that cancers diagnosed in the group that underwent screening were detected earlier than those diagnosed based on development of symptoms. Data regarding mortality from colorectal cancers were not available in this study. In a study of more than 46,000 participants, screening by fecal occult blood testing resulted in a statistically significant reduction of 33% in mortality rate from colorectal cancer.[26] In this study, asymptomatic individuals between the ages of 50 to 80 years were randomly assigned to screening once a year, to screening every 2 years, or to a control group. The 13-year cumulative mortality rate from colorectal cancer per 1000 participants was 5.88 in the annually screened group, 8.33 in the biennially screened group, and 8.83 in the control group. The reduced mortality rate in the annually screened group was associated with improved survival secondary to the detection of earlier stage cancers. The results of biennial fecal occult blood testing were not significantly different from those of the control group. This study was the first to demonstrate that screening by fecal occult blood testing can reduce the mortality rate from colorectal cancer. For the general population, the National Cancer Institute and the American Cancer Society advocate yearly fecal occult blood tests and flexible sigmoidoscopy every 3 to 5 years beginning at the age of 50 years.

Although these are reasonable guidelines, the cost-effectiveness of this program has yet to be ascertained.

STAGING
Pathology

Ninety to 95% of all large bowel cancers are adenocarcinomas, with the remaining histologic types being squamous cell carcinomas, adenosquamous carcinomas, lymphomas, sarcomas, and carcinoid tumors. Most colonic adenocarcinomas are moderately differentiated or well differentiated tumors. About 20% of adenocarcinomas are poorly differentiated or undifferentiated, and they are associated with a poorer prognosis. Another commonly described characteristic of adenocarcinomas is the relative amount of mucin that is produced. Ten to 20% of tumors are described as mucinous or colloid carcinomas based on abundant production of mucin. These tumors are associated with a poorer 5-year survival rate compared with nonmucinous tumors. Other histologic features associated with a poorer prognosis include blood vessel invasion, lymphatic vessel invasion, and absence of a lymphocytic response to the tumor.

Dukes Classification

The most important prognostic factor in colorectal cancer is the depth of invasion of the primary tumor. The first practical staging system to incorporate this observation was described by Dukes, who classified the depth of invasion of rectal tumors in stages from A to C. In his original classification, stage A indicated penetration through the muscularis propria but not through the intestinal wall (Fig. 47-6). Stage B represented penetration through the muscu-

laris propria into the perirectal fat. Stage C represented metastasis to lymph nodes regardless of the extent of intestinal wall penetration. This classification was strictly confined to rectal tumors lying beneath the peritoneal reflection, and therefore the concept of serosal involvement was not relevant.

Since Dukes' original description, various modifications of this system have been described to stage tumors in the rectum as well as throughout the colon. Because of these variations, the specific classification system used in a particular instance must be identified.

Modified Astler-Coller Staging System

One of the more commonly used staging systems is the modified Astler-Coller system (see Fig. 47-6). According to this system, stage A represents tumors that invade into the mucosa only. Stage B1 tumors invade into but not through the muscularis propria. Stage B2 lesions invade through the intestinal wall without adjacent organ involvement, whereas stage B3 tumors involve adjacent organs. Stage C tumors involve regional lymph nodes and are subgrouped into stages C1, C2, and C3, according to depth of intestinal wall penetration. Stage D represents evidence of distant organ involvement. In general, the 5-year survival rate for patients with stage D disease is less than 10%. Survival rates after curative resection for the other stages of colorectal cancer are summarized in Table 47-3. Overall, the 5-year survival rates for stages A, B, and C are 90%, 77%, and 47%, respectively. Additional studies have revealed that among Dukes stage C patients, the number of positive lymph nodes is a significant predictor of survival and should be incorporated into the staging of colorectal tumors[27] (Fig. 47-7).

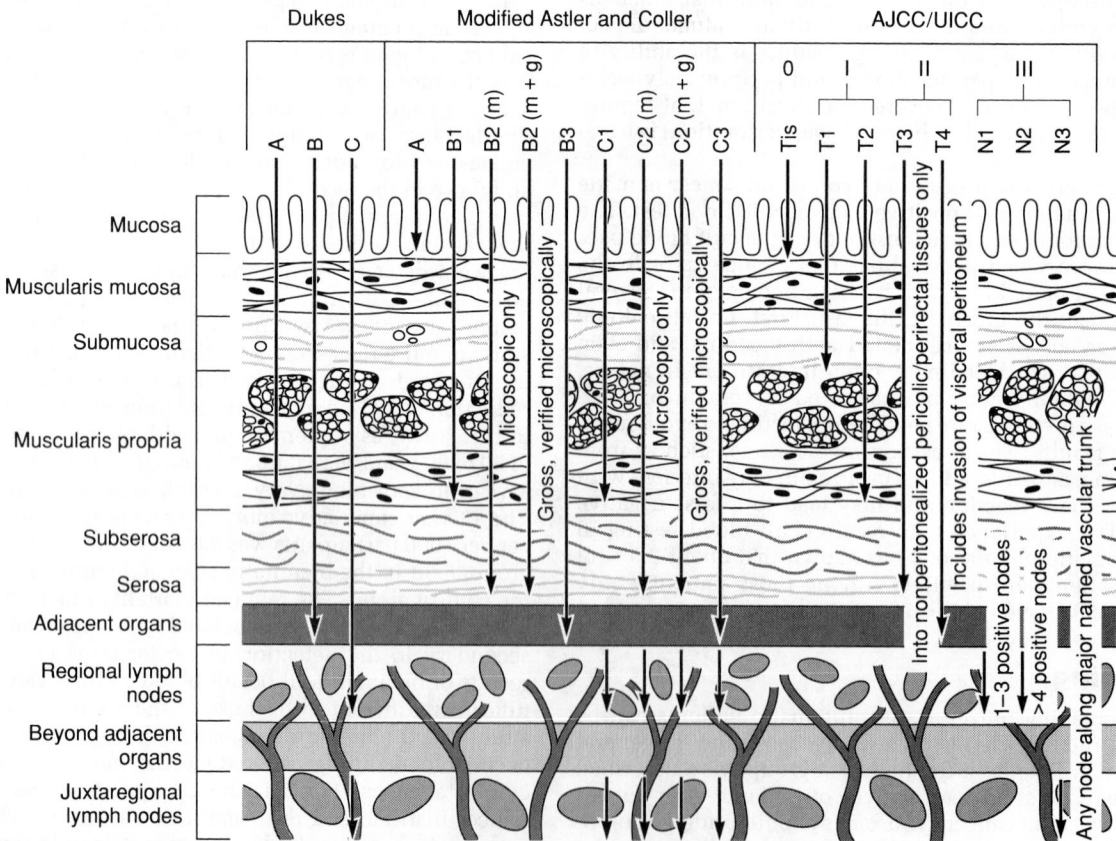

Figure 47-6. Schematic description of the staging systems with respect to depth of invasion.

Table 47-3. FIVE-YEAR SURVIVAL RATES OF PATIENTS WITH OPERABLE COLORECTAL CANCER

Investigators	Patients	5-Year Actuarial Survival Rate by Stage (%)								
		A	B	B1	B2	B3	C	C1	C2	C3
Corman et al, 1973[44]	244	98	79	—	—	—	42	—	—	—
Eisenberg et al, 1982[45]	1704	82	73	—	—	—	40	—	—	—
Pihl et al, 1980[46]*	615	88	78	—	—	—	60	—	—	—
Willett et al, 1984[47]*	533	90	—	75	70	64	—	63	45	38
Minsky et al, 1988[48]*	294	92	—	93	90	66	—	78	56	33
TOTAL	3390	MEAN 90	77				47			

* Restricted to colon cancers.

TNM Classification

The American Joint Committee on Cancer and the International Union Against Cancer (AJCC/UICC) have proposed an alternative staging system based on the extent of the primary tumor (T), regional node involvement (N), and metastasis (M). In contrast to the modified Astler-Coller system, this TNM system allows for carcinoma in situ (termed Tis) and stratifies according to number of positive nodes (see Fig. 47-6). Stage 0 consists of Tis tumors that do not metastasize; stage I are T1 and T2 tumors; stage II are T3 and T4 tumors; and stage III are any tumors with nodal involvement (N1 to N3). Stage IV includes any cancer with distant metastases. Equivalent Dukes and modified Astler-Coller stages according to the TNM classification are defined in Table 47-4. The TNM method has been generally adopted in the field of oncology as the universal colorectal cancer staging system.

Prognostic Factors

Although pathologic stage is the major determinant of prognosis, many clinical and pathologic features have been described to correlate with survival. Many of these factors are interrelated and may reflect the same characteristics. Table 47-5 summarizes some of the reported factors and how they have been associated with survival.

More recently, genetic markers have been identified that relate to prognosis. Tumor DNA content has been shown to be a significant prognostic factor. With the use of flow cytometry, tumors can be categorized as aneuploid (abnormal DNA content) or diploid (normal DNA content). Patients with aneuploid tumors have been reported to have higher recurrence rates and decreased survival rates than patients with diploid tumors.[28] By amplification of microsatellite markers, the allelic loss of chromosome 18q has been found to have significant prognostic effect in patients with node-negative colorectal cancer (ie, stage II tumors).[29] The DCC gene is located on 18q and is hypothesized to be a tumor suppressor gene in colorectal tumor formation (see Molecular Genetics). In a retrospective analysis, the 5-year survival rate among patients with stage II disease and no evidence of allelic loss of 18q was 93%. By contrast, stage II patients with allelic loss of 18q had a 5-year survival rate of 54%, which was similar to that of node-positive patients (ie, stage III). In the same study, the survival rate of stage III patients was not affected by the status of chromosome 18q. Genetic markers have an increasingly important role in the evaluation of patients with cancer.

Natural History

The natural progression of colorectal cancer can be categorized into three components: local invasion, lymphatic spread, and hematogenous spread. Studies described by

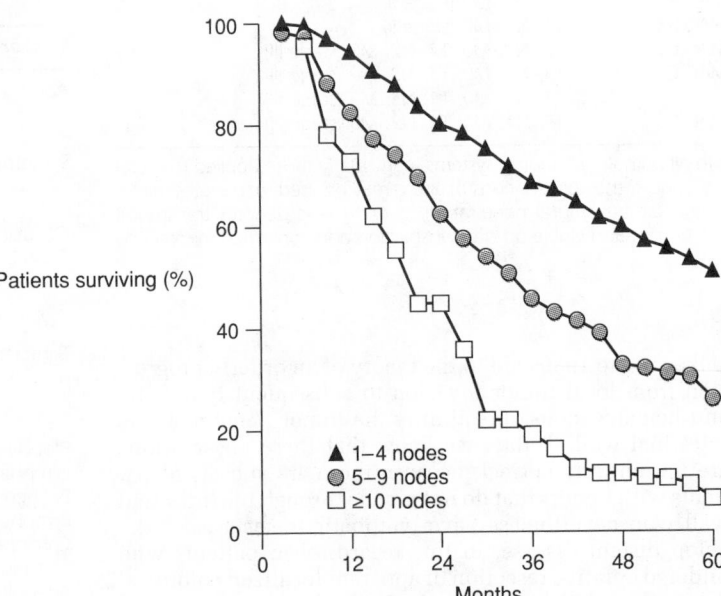

Figure 47-7. Survival of Dukes stage C patients according to the number of positive nodes.

Table 47-4. STAGING CLASSIFICATION OF COLORECTAL CANCER*

Stage	Description
TNM SYSTEM	
Primary Tumor	
Tx	Primary tumor cannot be assessed
T0	No evidence of tumor in resected specimen (prior polypectomy or fulguration)
Tis	Carcinoma in situ
T1	Invades into submucosa
T2	Invades into muscularis propria
T3/T4	Depends on whether serosa is present
SEROSA PRESENT	
T3	Invades through muscularis propria into subserosa
	Invades serosa (but not through)
	Invades pericolic fat within the leaves of the mesentery
T4	Invades through serosa into free peritoneal cavity, or through serosa into a contiguous organ
NO SEROSA (distal two thirds of rectum, posterior left or right colon)	
T3	Invades through muscularis propria
T4	Invades other organs (vagina, prostate, ureter, kidney)
Regional Lymph Node Involvement	
NX	Nodes cannot be assessed (eg, local excision only)
N0	No regional node metastases
N1	1–3 positive nodes
N2	4 or more positive nodes
N3	Central nodes positive
Distant Metastasis	
MX	Presence of distant metastases cannot be assessed
M0	No distant metastases
M1	Distant metastases present
DUKES STAGING SYSTEM CORRELATED WITH TNM	
Dukes A	T1, N0, M0 (stage I)
	T2, N0, M0 (stage I)
Dukes B	T3, N0, M0 (stage II)
	T4, N0, M0 (stage II)
Dukes C	T (any), N1, M0; T (any), N2, M0 (stage III)
Dukes D	T (any), N (any), M1 (stage IV)
MODIFIED ASTLER-COLLER (MAC) SYSTEM CORRELATED WITH TNM	
MAC A	T1, N0, M0 (stage I)
MAC B1	T2, N0, M0 (stage I)
MAC B2	T3, N0, M0 (stage II)
MAC B3	T4, N0, M0 (stage II)
MAC C1	T2, N1, M0; T2, N2, M0 (stage III)
MAC C2	T3, N1, M0; T3, N2, M0 (stage III)
	T4, N1, M0; T4, N2, M0 (stage III)
MAC C3	T4, N1, M0; T4, N2, M0 (stage III)

* In all pathologic staging systems, particularly those applied to rectal cancer, the abbreviations *m* and *g* may be used; *m* denotes microscopic transmural penetration; *g* or *m + g* denotes transmural penetration visible on gross inspection and confirmed microscopically.

Dukes in the 1930s led to the theory of an orderly progression from local tumor invasion to subsequent lymphatic and hematogenous spread after the tumor penetrated the intestinal wall. Today, we know that these observations are not entirely correct, because there are subsets of patients with tumors that do not invade through the intestinal wall who nevertheless have lymphatic metastases or develop distant disease. In this regard, even patients who undergo curative resection of apparent localized colorectal cancers should be viewed as harboring blood-borne metas-

tases. The risk of developing disseminated disease can be predicted by the depth of tumor invasion into the intestinal wall and the involvement of draining lymph nodes. Therapies designed to reduce the development of recurrent disease after surgical resection are discussed in later sections of this chapter.

Local growth of an adenocarcinoma is initially characterized by intramural expansion of the tumor into the bowel lumen. Subsequent lateral invasion into the intestinal wall usually progresses in a transverse direction rather than longitudinally, and thereby leads to circumferential involvement of the intestine. The incidence of lymphatic metastasis increases with extent of local invasion through the intestinal wall; however, 10% to 20% of patients with cancer limited to the intestinal wall are also found to have positive lymph nodes.

The liver is the most common site of hematogenous spread of colorectal cancer; liver metastasis occurs in about half of all cases.[30] The liver is the first capillary network exposed to tumor emboli traveling through the portal system and represents the major venous drainage of the colon and upper rectum. The liver can be the sole site of tumor metastasis, as evidenced by the success of resection of liver metastases for cure in selected patients. By contrast, the lower rectum has a dual drainage system, the portal system and the vena cava, by way of the middle and inferior hemorrhoidal veins, respectively. Some think that isolated lung metastases can develop from lower rectal tumors by travel of tumor emboli through the systemic venous drainage system. The lung is the second most common site of metastasis for colorectal tumors. Tumor involvement of other sites in the absence of liver and lung metastases is unusual. In certain circumstances, isolated bone metastases to the sacrum or vertebral bodies can arise from tumor embolism by portal–vertebral venous communications known as the Batson plexus.

Another potential mode of spread is by intraluminal or extraluminal exfoliation of tumor cells with subsequent implantation. Tumor implantation may occur during surgical resection with spillage of tumor cells, leading to recurrences in bowel anastomoses, abdominal incisions, or other intraabdominal sites. For tumors penetrating the in-

Table 47-5. PROGNOSTIC FACTORS FOR PRIMARY COLORECTAL CANCER

Factor	Association
Age	Patients <40 y old often present with more advanced stage disease
Symptoms	Symptomatic patients tend to have more advanced stage disease
Obstruction and perforation	Poorer prognosis when present
Location of primary	Rectosigmoid and rectal cancers have lower cure rates compared with cancers elsewhere in the colon
Tumor configuration	Exophytic tumors are associated with less advanced stage cancer compared with ulcerative tumors
Blood vessel invasion	Poorer prognosis when present
Lymphatic vessel invasion	Poorer prognosis when present
Perineural invasion	Poorer prognosis when present
Lymphocytic infiltration	Improved prognosis when present
Carcinoembryonic antigen study	Poorer prognosis when elevated before primary tumor resection
Aneuploidy	Poorer prognosis when present

testinal wall, shed tumor cells can implant intraperitoneally and cause peritoneal carcinomatosis.

A summary of the natural history of patients who present with colorectal cancer is depicted in Figure 47-8.[30] For every 100 patients initially evaluated, 30 have clinically evident distant spread, and the remaining 70 undergo resection for their localized disease. Among these 70 patients, 45 are cured and the remainder develop recurrent disease. Extrapolation of these figures to the approximately 155,000 patients diagnosed with colorectal cancer each year in the United States implies that 69,750 patients can be cured with surgical resection alone; the remaining 85,250 patients develop recurrent disease after resection or have disseminated tumor at the time of diagnosis.

TREATMENT OF PRIMARY COLORECTAL TUMORS
Neoplastic Polyps

With the availability of colonoscopy, endoscopic polypectomy has become the standard approach for the treatment of neoplastic polyps unless there are medical contraindications. The risk of this procedure is extremely low, with a complication rate of less than 1%. Almost all pedunculated polyps can be removed endoscopically with a snare. Sessile lesions can frequently be removed piecemeal but may require several sessions. A dilemma in treating colonic polyps occurs if a resected lesion contains a malignant focus. A decision must then be made about the need for a colectomy. If the lesion does not penetrate the muscularis mucosa, it should be considered an in situ malignancy that does not have the propensity to metastasize and, therefore, does not require further surgery. If the lesion penetrates the muscularis mucosa, it is an invasive cancer and may require surgery (see Fig. 47-2). In general, if there is evidence of invasion, colectomy with resection of paracolonic lymph nodes is indicated. In selected cases of pedunculated polyps, conservative management without colectomy may be undertaken if the lesion does not contain poorly differentiated tumor cells or evidence of vascular invasion and if a negative resection margin has been obtained at the level of the stalk. Lesions that are poorly differentiated or have evidence of vascular invasion, regardless of a negative surgical margin, should be treated by colectomy.

Large villous tumors of the rectum can pose a challenge. Total excision is required to accurately assess the presence of invasive cancer. Transanal excision with sphincteric muscle and mucosal approximation is preferred; however, other approaches, such as low anterior resection, coloanal procedures, or abdominoperineal resection, may have to be employed to totally excise extensive benign rectal lesions.

Invasive Colorectal Cancers
Surgery

Surgical options for colorectal cancer depend on the location of the primary tumor. These surgical procedures are summarized as follows:

Intraperitoneal colon and upper third of the rectum
Resection and anastomosis
Middle third of the rectum
Abdominoperineal resection
Low anterior resection
Abdominosacral resection
Coloanal resection
Local excision or fulguration
Primary radiation therapy
Lower third of the rectum
Abdominoperineal resection
Local excision or fulguration
Primary radiation therapy

Before surgical resection, evaluation for sites of metastatic disease is important. A careful physical examination determines the presence of hepatomegaly, ascites, or adenopathy. For rectal tumors, the distance of the tumor from the anal verge and its mobility are important in assessing resectability and type of operation required. Rectal ultra-

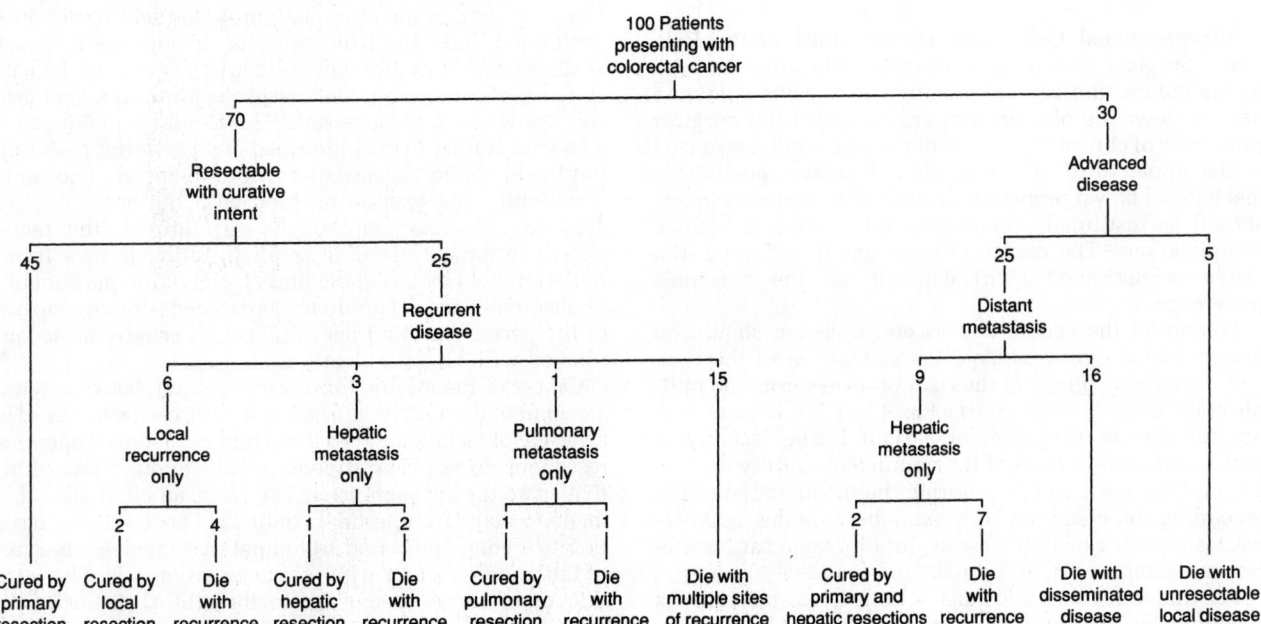

Figure 47-8. Algorithm depicting the natural history of patients with colorectal cancer.

sound can be helpful in assessing extent of local invasion and the presence of enlarged lymph nodes within the mesorectum. Laboratory studies should include a complete blood count, liver function studies, and a carcinoembryonic antigen (CEA) assay. Determination of a baseline CEA level can be useful in the subsequent follow-up of the patient (see later section). Abnormal liver function studies may indicate the need to perform an abdominal computed tomographic (CT) scan to assess the presence of liver metastases. It is not unreasonable to perform a preoperative abdominal CT scan in all patients with colorectal cancer. The presence of metastatic disease may alter the planned surgical procedure; that is, a low rectal cancer with evidence of hepatic metastases may be better palliated with fulguration than with abdominoperineal resection. A full colonoscopy or air-contrast barium enema should be performed to rule out other primary colorectal polyps or cancers.

The surgical goals in the resection of a primary colorectal cancer are to achieve an en bloc resection that encompasses an adequate amount of normal colon proximal and distal to the tumor, to obtain adequate lateral margins if the tumor is adherent to contiguous structures, and to remove regional lymph nodes. Accomplishment of these goals optimizes the chance of preventing locoregional recurrence of the disease. The extent of bowel resection has been the subject of numerous debates. From pathologic studies, tumor rarely extends intramurally more than 2 cm beyond the area of gross involvement. Traditionally, 5 cm of normal large intestine proximal and distal to the tumor has been advocated as a margin that is adequate to completely encompass intramural spread. The actual margin of intestine removed is often determined by the extent of the lymphadenectomy. The paracolic and intermediate draining lymph nodes should be removed as part of a curative resection (Fig. 47-9). Extensive resections of bowel along with more central or retroperitoneal lymph nodes are not indicated because they produce minimal additional oncologic benefit but substantially increase operative complications. At the time of surgical resection, a thorough investigation of the abdominal viscera, particularly the liver and peritoneal surfaces, should be performed. If evidence of disseminated disease is apparent, a less extensive resection of the primary lesion for palliation to avoid obstructive or bleeding complications may be indicated.

Intraperitoneal Colon and Upper Third of the Rectum. Surgical resections of cancers from different sites in the colorectum require attention to specific anatomic details. Resection plus primary anastomosis is the surgical procedure of choice for cancers of the colon and for cancers of the upper third of the rectum. Whenever possible, a mechanical bowel preparation, along with oral antibiotics, should be instituted preoperatively to reduce infectious complications. The choice of anastomotic technique (ie, staple versus hand-sewn) depends on the surgeon's preference.

Tumors of the cecum and ascending colon should be resected by a right hemicolectomy. Ligation of the ileocolic, the right colic, and the right branches from the middle colic artery is required (see Fig. 47-9). For hepatic flexure tumors, an extension of a right hemicolectomy is performed with ligation of the middle colic artery near its origin. Care must be taken during the mobilization of the ascending colon and hepatic flexure because the right ureter, testicular or ovarian vessels, inferior vena cava, superior mesenteric vein, and duodenum are close together.

For transverse colon lesions, a transverse colectomy is accomplished by proximal ligation of the middle colic artery (see Fig. 47-9). Cancer of the splenic flexure can be treated with a segmental resection in which the middle transverse colon is anastomosed to the middle descending colon. For this procedure, the left colic artery is divided and the middle colic artery is preserved. Mobilization of the splenic flexure requires care to avoid injury to the spleen.

A left hemicolectomy with removal of intestine from the middle transverse to the distal sigmoid colon can be used for descending colon tumors (see Fig. 47-9). High ligation of the inferior mesenteric artery is necessary in this operation. For sigmoid cancers, a segmental resection can be performed with ligation of the sigmoid artery near its origin. Rectosigmoid cancers and tumors confined to the upper third of the rectum are removed by an anterior resection. The upper third of the rectum is about 12 to 16 cm from the anal verge and is located above the peritoneal reflection (Fig. 47-10). The pelvic peritoneum is incised circumferentially around the rectum, and the intestine is mobilized from the presacral fascia. Laterally, the middle hemorrhoidal vessels are ligated, and anteriorly, the rectum is mobilized from the seminal vesicles and prostate or vagina. The mesenteric vessels are divided at the origin of the sigmoid artery or higher, at the origin of the inferior mesenteric artery, if further mobilization of the splenic flexure is required to obtain a tension-free anastomosis.

Middle and Lower Third of the Rectum. Cancers located in the lower third of the rectum, between the anorectal ring and 7 to 8 cm from the anal verge, are reliably treated by abdominoperineal resection (see Fig. 47-10). The procedure involves wide excision of the rectum to include the lateral attachments and pelvic mesocolon and establishment of a colostomy. The extent of surgery for an abdominoperineal resection is illustrated in Figure 47-11. With the patient in a modified lithotomy position, the abdominal and perineal procedures can be performed simultaneously by two teams or sequentially by one team. Alternatively, the abdominal procedure can be completed with the patient in the supine position, and the perineal portion completed afterward, with the patient turned in the lateral position. On opening of the abdomen, evidence of intraabdominal spread is ascertained. The discovery of extensive disseminated disease may eliminate the need for an abdominoperineal resection, because a local excision or fulguration to preserve anal function may be more appropriate for palliation. If an abdominoperineal resection is performed, ligation of the superior hemorrhoidal vessels at their origin from the left colic artery is required. Occasionally, if extensive nodal disease is present, higher arterial ligation may be necessary. The rectum is mobilized in a fashion similar to that described for an anterior resection, but the dissection is carried down to the pelvic floor muscles, which are excised en bloc with the anus. An end sigmoid colostomy is brought out through the rectus sheath. Efforts to exclude small intestine from a future radiation field by use of the uterus, omentum, peritoneum, or absorbable mesh should be considered. Primary closure of the perineal wound over drains can usually be accomplished without complications.

Cancer of the middle third of the rectum, between 8 and 12 cm from the anal verge (see Fig. 47-10), can be managed by a variety of techniques. For these tumors, abdominoperineal resections do not yield superior results to other procedures that spare the anal sphincter. Therefore, an effort should be made to maintain intestinal continuity. Low anterior resection is a commonly used technique that involves resection of the middle rectum with primary anastomosis. The introduction of the end-to-end anastomosis (EEA) stapler has increased the use of this sphincter-saving procedure (Fig. 47-12). If a transanal reconstruction with a stapler is contem-

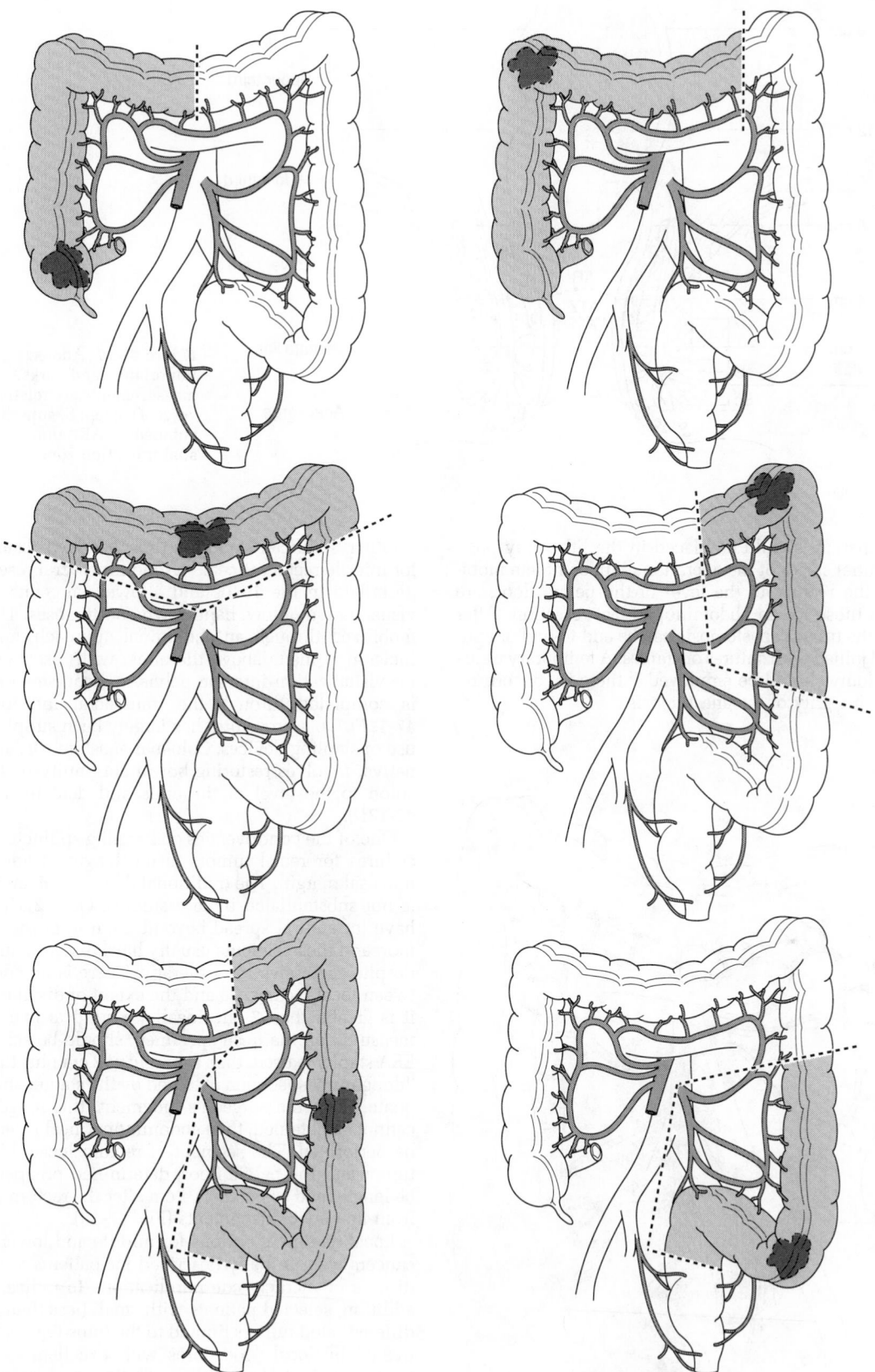

Figure 47-9. Segmental resections for cancers of the colon and upper third of the rectum.

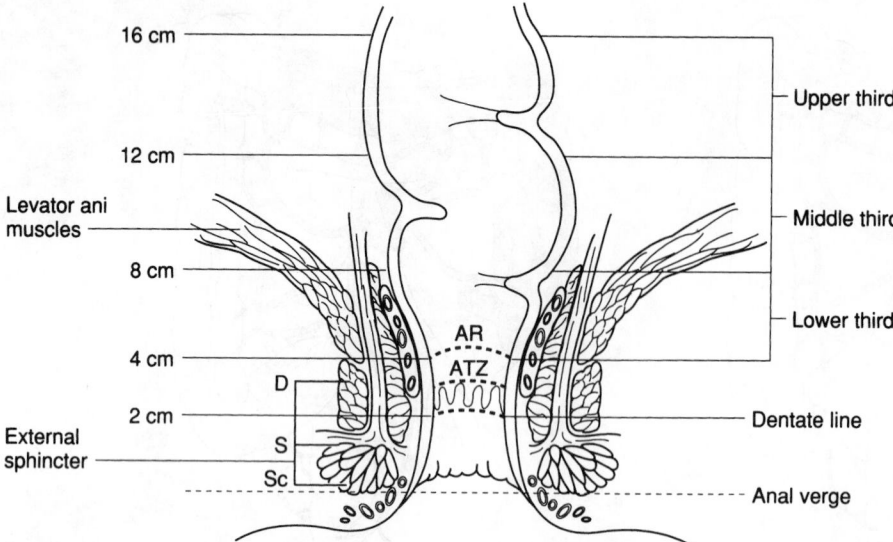

Figure 47-10. Anorectal anatomy with important landmarks. Approximate measurements are relative to the anal verge. D, deep; S, superficial; Sc, subcutaneous; AR, anorectal ring; ATZ, anal transition zone.

plated, the patient should be placed in the lithotomy position. The initial stages of the operation, with complete mobilization of the rectum to the level of the pelvic floor, are identical to those for an abdominoperineal resection. After removal of the tumor, anastomosis can be end-to-end or end-to-side, and joined with sutures or staples. A temporary transverse colostomy should be employed if there is concern regarding the integrity of the anastomosis.

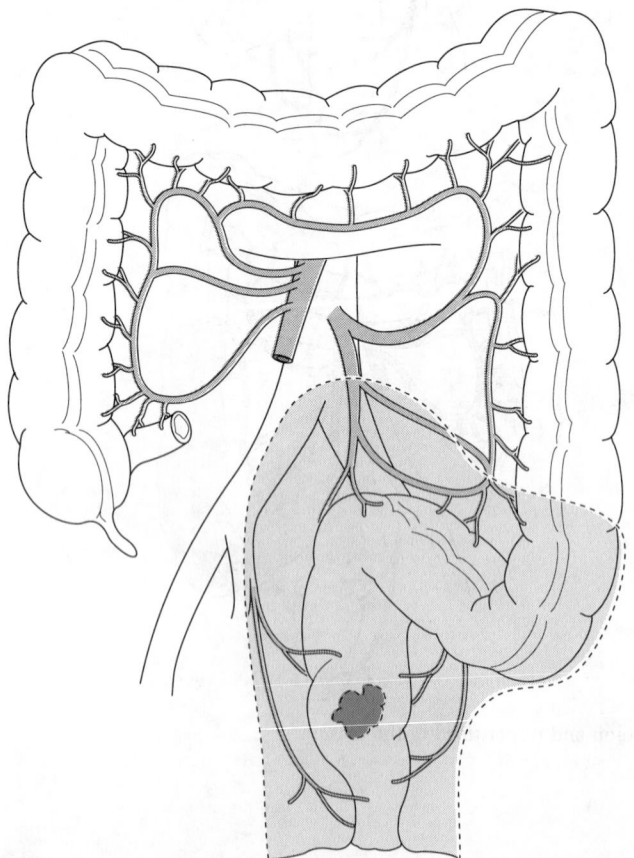

Figure 47-11. Extent of surgery in abdominoperineal resection.

Other sphincter-saving approaches have been described for middle rectal cancers.[31] Abdominosacral resections were described in the 1940s and allowed surgeons more direct visualization of low, hand-sewn anastomoses. The rectum is mobilized through an abdominal approach, and a second incision is made above the anus, with resection of coccyx for visualization into the pelvis. A hand-sewn anastomosis is completed through the transsacral incision (see Fig. 47-12E). This procedure has largely been supplanted by the use of stapling devices. Coloanal anastomosis, another alternative, involves restoring bowel continuity by bringing the colon to the level of the anus and dentate line (see Fig. 47-12D).

One of the controversies concerning sphincter-saving procedures for rectal tumors is the length of adequate distal mucosal margin. The traditional dictum of 5 cm for a margin is not substantiated by any studies. Only 2.5% of patients have intramural spread beyond 2 cm from the palpable tumor, and these patients usually have dissemination of tumor despite aggressive local therapy. There is no correlation between local recurrence and the extent of distal margin when it is greater than 2 cm. Ideally, a surgical margin of 3 cm, measured on the fresh specimen, should be achieved. If the EEA stapler is used, then a margin of 2 cm plus the additional "doughnut" specimen obtained by the stapler should be adequate. If, in the surgeon's judgment, this length of margin cannot be obtained, then abdominoperineal resection should be performed. The segment of rectum located between the tumor and the pelvic floor, determined preoperatively, can be lengthened as much as 4 cm after the rectum is mobilized from its pelvic attachments (Fig. 47-13).

Local treatment options for middle and lower third rectal cancers were initially described for patients with advanced disease or medical contraindications to radical surgery. In addition, selected patients with small (less than 3 cm), well-differentiated tumors limited to the intestinal wall have been treated by local procedures with excellent results. These treatments include excision, ablation, and irradiation. Full-thickness bowel wall excisions can be performed by a transanal route with primary closure of the defect. If negative surgical margins are achieved, then consideration of adjuvant chemotherapy and radiation should be recommended to optimize locoregional tumor control. If the surgical margins are positive, then a more definitive procedure should be performed (ie, low anterior resection or abdominoperineal resec-

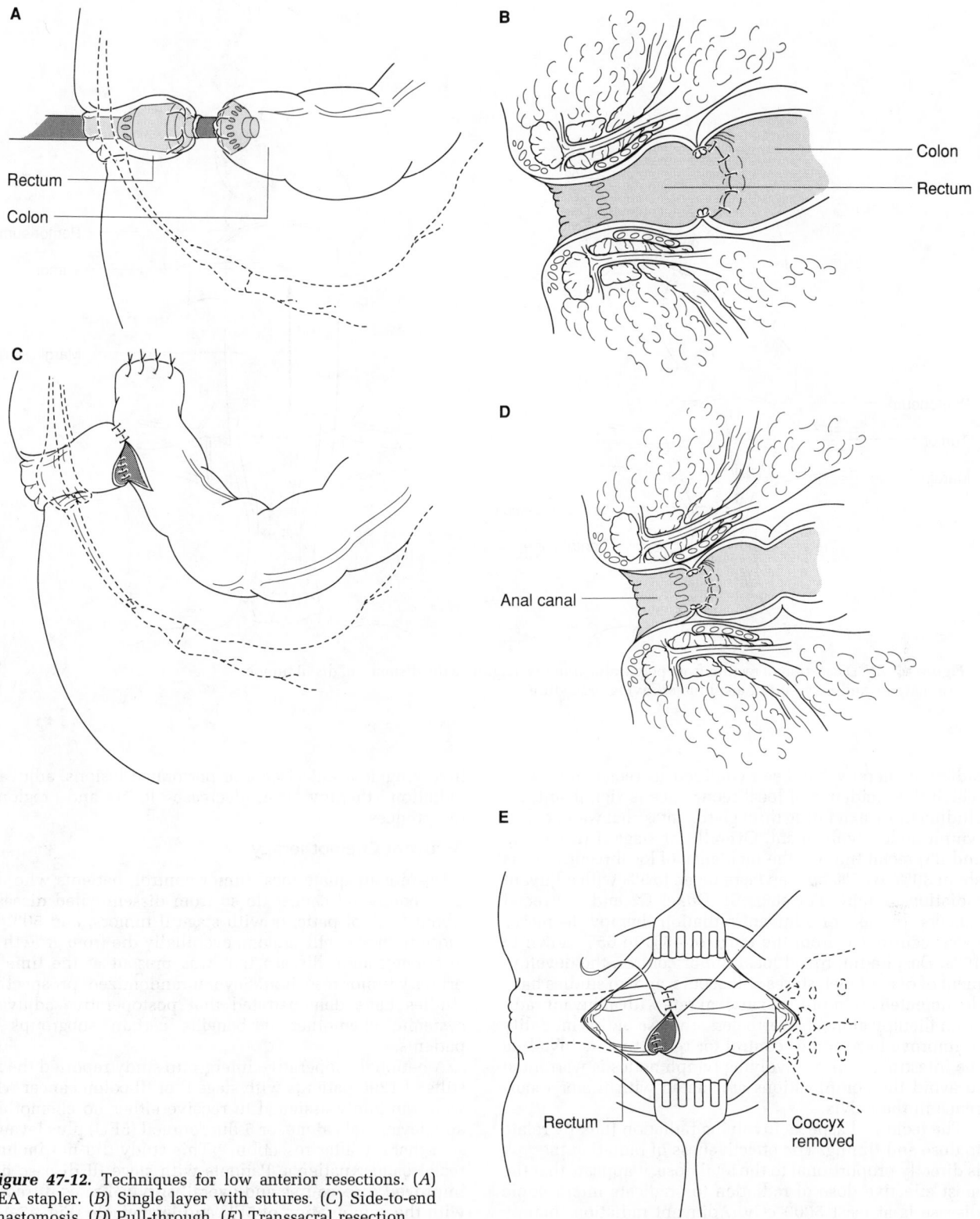

Figure 47-12. Techniques for low anterior resections. (*A*) EEA stapler. (*B*) Single layer with sutures. (*C*) Side-to-end anastomosis. (*D*) Pull-through. (*E*) Transsacral resection.

tion). Alternatively, posterior approaches have been described, with removal of the coccyx, proctotomy, and closure, or posterior division of the anal sphincter, proctotomy, and closure with reconstruction of the anal sphincter muscles. Ablation by transanal electrofulguration of the tumor in multiple stages has been reported to be an acceptable treatment in patients who are poor surgical candidates; however, this procedure cannot be employed for circumferential tumors.[32] Endocavitary irradiation as primary curative therapy to treat early cancers has been reported with some success. In locally advanced colorectal tumors, the neodymium:yttrium aluminum garnet laser has been found to be effective in palliating obstructive or bleeding lesions.

Adjuvant Radiation Therapy

Radiation therapy combined with surgical resection for colorectal cancer has been demonstrated to reduce the incidence of local tumor recurrence. In general, the use of

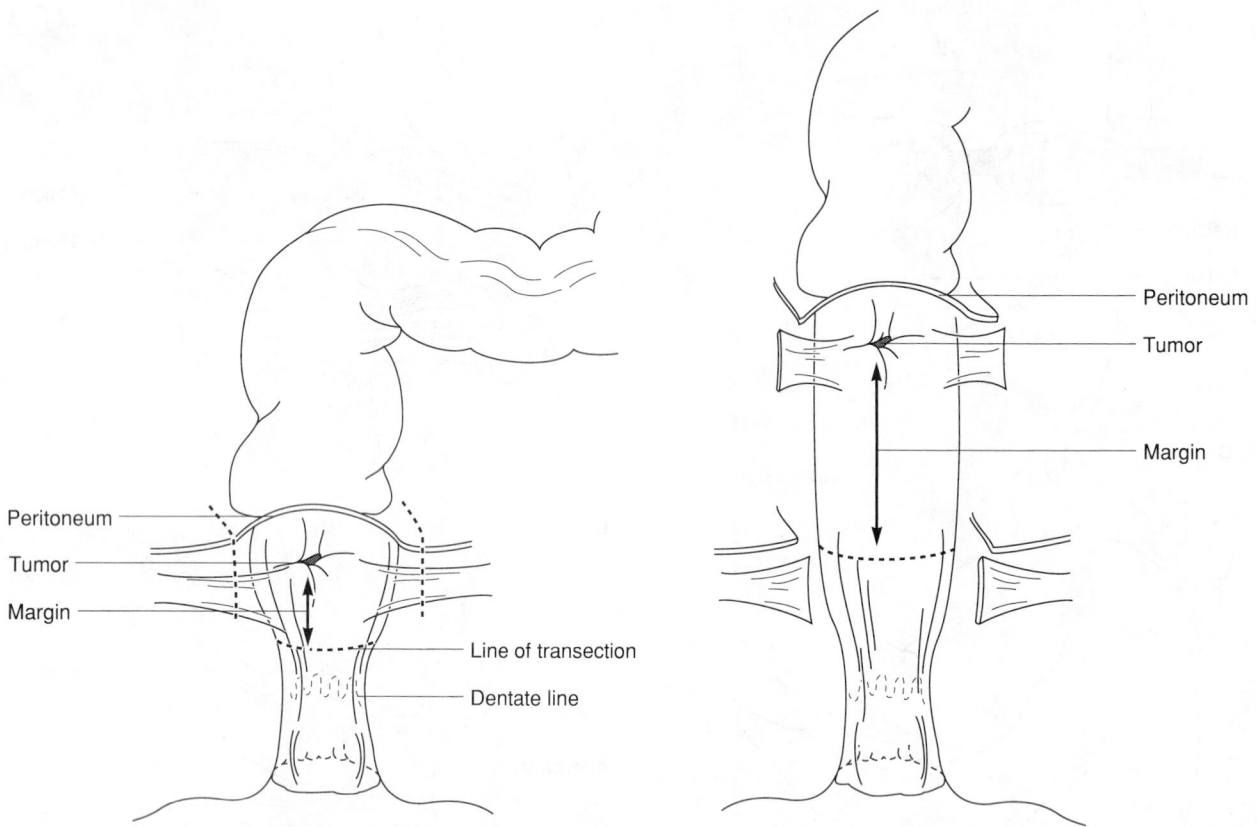

Figure 47-13. Dissection of rectum from pelvic attachments lengthens the distance of distal tumor-free margins and may permit a sphincter-saving procedure.

radiation therapy has been confined to rectal tumors in which the incidence of local recurrence is significant, including those extending through the intestinal wall or with lymph node involvement. Overall, for stage II (Dukes B2 and B3) rectal tumors, the incidence of local recurrence is about 30% to 35% but can be reduced to 5% with adjuvant radiation therapy. For stage III (Dukes C2 and C3) rectal cancers, the use of adjuvant radiation therapy decreases local recurrences from the range of 45% to 65% down to 10%. Despite improved local tumor control, the development of distant metastases still occurs, and no studies have documented an improved survival rate with adjuvant radiation therapy alone. Nevertheless, the use of this modality to improve local tumor control for rectal tumors invading the intestinal wall or involving lymph nodes is warranted to avoid the complications associated with tumor recurrence in the pelvis.

The technical aspects involving radiation therapy relate to dose and timing. The effectiveness of radiation therapy is directly proportional to the total dose. It appears that the most effective dose of radiation to eradicate microscopic disease is at least 5000 cGy. Adjuvant radiation therapy can be delivered preoperatively, postoperatively, or in combined sandwich approach, whereby small doses of preoperative treatment are followed by postoperative treatment to a high total cumulative dose. No studies clearly indicate that one approach is superior.

Less experience has been reported for adjuvant radiation therapy of resected colon cancer. Adjuvant radiation therapy for colon cancer is associated with special problems of toxicity because of the large amount of small intestine that may lie in the treatment field. Nevertheless, several reports indicate that in high-risk cases, such as tumors involving adjacent viscera or perforated lesions, adjuvant radiation therapy can decrease local and regional recurrences.

Adjuvant Chemotherapy

Despite adequate local tumor control, patients who die from colorectal cancer do so from disseminated disease. About 25% of patients with stage II tumors, and 50% of those with stage III tumors, eventually die from growth of micrometastatic disease that was present at the time of primary tumor resection. Several randomized, prospective studies have demonstrated that postoperative adjuvant systemic chemotherapy benefits certain subgroups of patients.

A national cooperative intergroup study reported the results of 1296 patients with stage II or III colon cancer who were randomly assigned to receive either no chemotherapy, levamisole alone, or 5-fluorouracil (5FU) plus levamisole therapy after resection.[33] This study did not include rectal cancer patients. Patients with stage III disease had improved disease-free and overall survival rates if treated with the combination of 5FU and levamisole (Fig. 47-14). The survival curve of patients treated with levamisole alone was similar to that of the control population. The results in patients with stage II tumors were equivocal and too preliminary to allow definitive conclusions.

In another study of 1166 patients with stage II and III colon cancers, the National Surgical Adjuvant Breast and Bowel Project (NSABP) reported an improved survival rate in patients randomly assigned to receive adjuvant chemotherapy (5FU, semustine, and vincristine), compared with those receiving no further treatment after resection.[34] In a follow-up study, the NSABP evaluated the efficacy of ther-

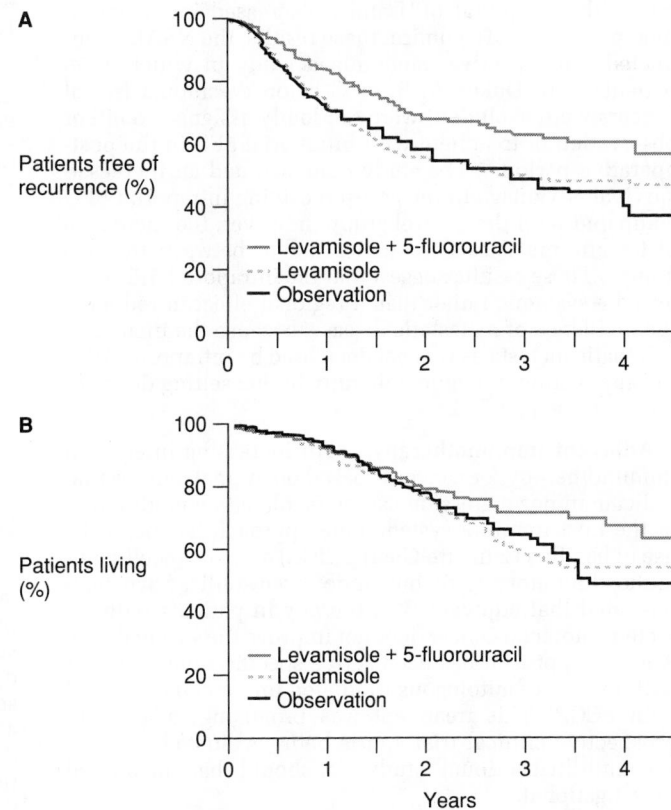

Figure 47-14. Improved disease-free and overall survival in patients with colon cancer who received adjuvant chemotherapy. (After Moertel CG, Fleming TR, MacDonald JS, et al. Levamisole and fluorouracil for adjuvant therapy of resected colon carcinoma. N Engl J Med 1990;322:352)

apy with 5FU, semustine, and vincristine versus 5FU plus leucovorin in stage II and III colon cancer patients.[35] Treatment with 5FU plus leucovorin resulted in significantly improved survival rates and appeared to be the better combination of drugs. Semustine, which has been reported to have a leukemogenic effect, is no longer administered in this setting. Based on an evaluation of prospective, randomized studies, the National Institutes of Health recommended that patients with stage III colon cancer be offered adjuvant chemotherapy as standard treatment to improve the survival rate.[36]

In colon cancer, local recurrence is infrequent; in rectal cancer, the use of adjuvant chemotherapy combined with radiation has proved effective in improving local control and increasing the survival rate. In rectal cancer, it is almost as important to prevent local failure and ensuing symptoms as it is to prevent death from distant failure. As noted in the previous section, radiation therapy is routinely recommended for patients with stage II or III rectal cancers. In a randomized, prospective study, 204 patients with stage II or III rectal cancers were randomly assigned to receive either postoperative radiation alone or radiation plus chemotherapy with 5FU and semustine.[37] The group that received chemotherapy had improved local tumor control and an increased overall survival rate (Fig 47-15). In another prospective study, semustine was found not to be an essential component for effective adjuvant therapy.[38] Based on these and other clinical studies, the National Institutes of Health has recommended that patients with stage II or III rectal cancers should receive postoperative chemotherapy and radiation as standard care.[36]

Other Adjuvant Therapies

Adjuvant Portal Vein Chemotherapy. The liver is the most common site of metastatic disease for colorectal cancer. Metastasis is established by tumor cells embolized into the portal vein. From anatomic studies, it is known that micrometastases to the liver are initially fed by portal blood flow. These observations form the rationale for the administration of adjuvant intraportal 5FU chemotherapy in an attempt to decrease the incidence of liver metastasis. In an initial study, 244 patients who had resections of Dukes A, B, or C colorectal tumors were randomly assigned to receive or not receive continuous intraportal 5FU with heparin immediately after surgery.[39] Patients with Dukes B and C tumors appeared to have an improved survival

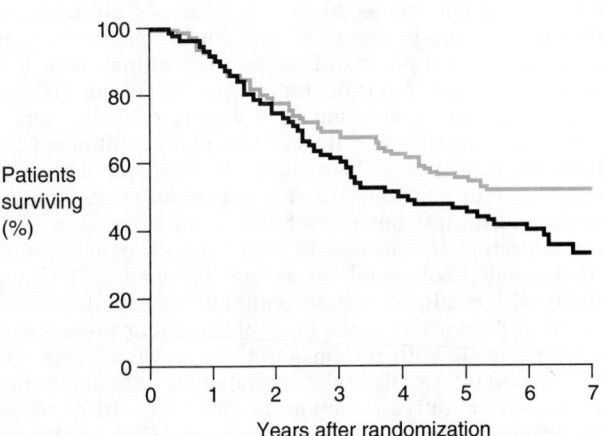

Figure 47-15. Improved overall survival in patients with stage II or III rectal cancer who received adjuvant chemotherapy plus radiation (*blue line*) versus radiation alone (*black line*) postoperatively (*P* = .025). (After Krook J, Moertel C, Gunderson L, et al. Effective surgical adjuvant therapy for high-risk rectal carcinoma. N Engl J Med 1991;324:709)

rate with intraportal 5FU and a decreased incidence of liver metastases. To confirm these results, the NSABP conducted a prospective, randomized study in which 1158 patients with Dukes A, B, or C colon carcinoma (rectal cancers were excluded) were randomly assigned to either observation or treatment with intraportal 5FU in the postoperative period.[40] The study demonstrated an increased survival advantage in the group receiving intraportal 5FU compared with the control group; however, the incidence of hepatic metastasis was not different between the two groups. These results suggest that the intraportal 5FU conferred a systemic rather than a regional effect in reducing the incidence of metastatic disease; because the incidence of hepatic metastasis was not decreased by intraportal 5FU, the application of regional therapy in this setting does not appear to be justified.

Adjuvant Immunotherapy. An increasing interest in immunotherapy for cancer is based on animal studies that indicate tumor regression can be mediated by modulation of the host immune system. One approach has been the use of bacillus Calmette-Guérin (BCG) as a nonspecific immunostimulatory agent, but randomized studies have demonstrated that adjuvant BCG therapy in patients with resected colorectal cancer does not improve the survival rate. Another approach has been active specific immunization with the use of autologous irradiated tumor cells admixed with BCG.[41] This treatment was promising in a small, prospective clinical trial and is being evaluated in a larger multiinstitutional study; it should be considered investigational.

TREATMENT OF RECURRENT COLORECTAL CANCER

A subset of patients with recurrent colorectal cancer can be cured. Therefore, a comprehensive follow-up program in patients who have undergone resection of their primary tumor is appropriate. Fifty percent of cancers that recur do so within 18 months of surgery, and 90% of recurrences are evident by 3 years. Therefore, careful follow-up should be performed during the 3-year period after primary tumor resection. Besides identifying recurrences, a careful follow-up program also identifies the 5% of patients who develop a metachronous primary tumor of the large intestine.

The CEA assay is a sensitive serologic test in the diagnosis of recurrent colorectal cancer. CEA is a glycoprotein that was originally described as a tumor-specific antigen derived from neoplasms of the gastrointestinal tract. It is now known that CEA is not tumor-specific because its concentration can be elevated by a variety of malignancies from different sites and by some benign conditions. CEA is an oncofetal antigen because it is also expressed by early embryonic or fetal cells. CEA is not useful as a screening or diagnostic test but is useful as a tumor marker. CEA concentration is elevated in over 90% of patients with disseminated colorectal cancer and in about 20% of patients with localized disease. Serum levels usually are elevated in proportion to the mass of the tumor present and often correlate with response to therapy. CEA levels provide useful information when elevated levels fall to normal levels after curative resection. In about two thirds of patients with recurrent disease, an increased CEA level is the first indicator of the tumor; therefore, serial CEA testing, combined with regular physical examinations, is one of the most useful means for detecting recurrent colorectal cancer. General guidelines for the follow-up of patients after colorectal resections for cancer are outlined in Table 47-6.

Table 47-6. GUIDELINES FOR FOLLOW-UP OF PATIENTS AFTER POTENTIALLY CURATIVE SURGERY

Procedure or Test	Frequency
History and physical examination	Every 6 mo for 3 y, then yearly
Carcinoembryonic antigen study	Every 6 mo for 3 y, then yearly
Fecal occult blood	Every 6 mo for 3 y, then yearly
Liver chemistries	Yearly*
Abdominal CT	Yearly*
Total colonoscopy	Yearly*
Chest radiograph	Yearly*

* After 5 years, if there is no evidence of recurrence, the procedure or test should be performed every 2 to 3 years for the remainder of the patient's life.

Hepatic Metastases

The liver is the most frequent site of blood-borne metastases from primary colorectal cancers. In a subgroup of patients, the liver is the only site of recurrent disease, and surgical excision of the metastases is the only curative option for these patients. Overall, surgical resection is associated with a 5-year survival rate of 25% to 30%[42] (Fig. 47-16). Patients eligible for hepatic resection of metastatic disease are those who have no evidence of extrahepatic tumor, no medical contraindications for surgery, and fewer than four lesions, and their lesions are amenable to resection with negative surgical margins.

Patients who have unresectable hepatic metastases that appear to be confined to that organ have been treated with regional chemotherapy through the hepatic artery (eg, 5FU, 5FU-deoxyribonucleoside [FUdR]). Several studies have demonstrated significantly higher tumor response rates with regional chemotherapy compared with systemic chemotherapy, but an improved survival rate with this therapy has not been demonstrated clearly in randomized trials.

Pulmonary Metastases

About 10% of all patients with colorectal cancer develop pulmonary metastases, usually in association with widespread metastatic disease. Because the colon is drained solely by the portal system, one would not expect metastases to the lung without evidence of tumor in the liver. In contrast, rectal cancers may spread through the portal or systemic venous systems and can theoretically give rise to isolated pulmonary metastases. In selected patients, particularly those with rectal cancers, resection of pulmonary recurrences can result in a 5-year survival rate of 20%.[43]

Local Recurrence

Local recurrence of colon cancer occurs in about 20% of cases, and the local lesion is the only site of recurrence in about one third of these cases. If the recurrent tumor is isolated to the suture line, resection of this recurrence can be curative. Locoregional failure occurs in 30% to 65% of patients with transmural or node-positive rectal cancers. Often, pelvic recurrences of rectal cancer after a low anterior or abdominoperineal resection are diffuse and associated with disseminated disease. If pelvic recurrences are localized, they should be resected if negative surgical margins can be achieved. Surgical procedures necessary to accomplish this include en bloc partial sacrectomy or total pelvic exenteration.

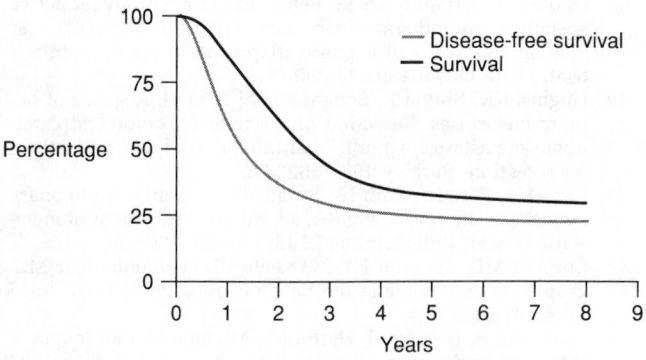

Figure 47-16. Disease-free and overall survival in patients who underwent hepatic resection for colorectal carcinoma metastases to the liver. (After Hughes KS, Simon R, Songhorabodi S, et al. Registry of hepatic metastases: resection of the liver for colorectal carcinoma metastases: a multiinstitutional study of indications for resection. Surgery 1988;103:278)

Disseminated Disease

Recurrent colorectal cancer is not usually localized to one site that is amenable to surgical resection. More commonly, colorectal cancer recurs in multiple sites. In these cases, systemic therapy may be considered. No studies have clearly documented that systemic therapies for disseminated colorectal cancer improve the survival rate; however, systemic treatment is commonly used for palliation.

The most commonly employed agent is 5FU, a fluoropyrimidine. As a single agent, 5FU has an objective response rate of 10% to 20%. Promising studies have shown that the antitumor activity of 5FU can be enhanced by folinic acid (leucovorin). The tumor response rates of this combination of drugs have been in the range of 30% to 40%. 5FU combined with leucovorin is the first-line regimen for treatment of disseminated colorectal cancer. Biologic agents alone have not been found to be active in disseminated colorectal cancer. Biologic therapy refers to cancer treatment mediated through the action of natural host mechanisms or the administration of natural mammalian substances. The biologic agent interferon-α has shown promising activity when combined with 5FU. Further studies to evaluate the efficacy of this combined therapy are needed.

OTHER COLORECTAL TUMORS
Carcinoid Tumors

Carcinoid tumors are neoplasms derived from cells that are capable of synthesizing a wide variety of hormones. Most gastrointestinal tract carcinoids occur in the ileum and the appendix. The rectum is the next most common site, and occasionally carcinoid tumors occur in the colon. Tumor size is an extremely important prognostic factor. About 60% of rectal carcinoids present as asymptomatic submucosal nodules measuring less than 2 cm in diameter. Transanal local excision suffices for definitive therapy, because small tumors rarely metastasize. Malignant potential is seen almost exclusively in tumors larger than 2 cm. More radical excisions of larger rectal lesions may be required for local control; however, the results of radical excisions for large rectal carcinoids are poor, because these tumors are prone to metastasize.

Lymphomas

Colorectal lymphomas are rare and account for less than 0.5% of all colorectal malignancies. In most cases, widespread dissemination of lymphoma is documented and underscores the concept that lymphoma of the gastrointestinal tract is a systemic disease with tumor cells present in other organ sites. Because this disease is highly responsive to chemotherapy and radiation, surgery is not the primary mode of therapy. If the clinical workup reveals a focal site of disease in the large intestine, surgical resection may be considered. Usually, for localized, low-grade colorectal lymphomas, radiation therapy is considered first-line therapy. For intermediate- and high-grade lymphomas, chemotherapy, combined with radiation therapy, should be the primary treatment modality. The role of surgery for colorectal lymphomas has been primarily for diagnostic and staging purposes and for the management of treatment-related complications (ie, perforation or bleeding).

Sarcomas

Colorectal sarcomas are extremely rare and account for less than 0.1% of all large bowel malignancies. The most common histologic sarcoma subtype is leiomyosarcoma. With these tumors, the most significant prognostic indicator is tumor grade. Patients with high-grade tumors do poorly. These tumors usually metastasize to the liver and peritoneal surfaces. If the tumors are clinically localized at initial presentation, a radical en bloc excision should be performed to obtain a margin of uninvolved normal tissue. Because of the rarity of this tumor, no studies have addressed whether adjuvant radiation therapy or chemotherapy is beneficial.

REFERENCES

1. Silverberg E, Boring CC, Squires TS. Cancer statistics 1990. CA 1990;40:9.
2. Parkin DM, Laara E, Muir CS. Estimates of the worldwide frequency of sixteen major cancers in 1980. Int J Cancer 1988;41:184.
3. Devesa SS, Silverman DT, Young JL, et al. Cancer incidence and mortality trends among whites in the United States, 1947–1984. J Natl Cancer Inst 1987;79:701.
4. Willett W. The search for the causes of breast and colon cancer. Nature 1989;338:389.
5. Willett WC, MacMahon B. Diet and cancer: an overview. N Engl J Med 1984;310:697.
6. Burkitt DP. Epidemiology of cancer of the colon and rectum. Cancer 1971;28:3.
7. Bos JL, Fearon ER, Hamilton SR, et al. Prevalence of *ras* gene mutations in human colorectal cancers. Nature 1987;327:293.
8. Fearon ER, Vogelstein B. A genetic model for colorectal tumorigenesis. Cell 1990;61:759.
9. Kinzler KW, Nilbert MC, Su L, et al. Identification of FAP locus genes from chromosome 5q21. Science 1991;253:661.
10. Groden J, Thliveris A, Samowitz W, et al. Identification and characterization of the familial adenomatous polyposis coli gene. Cell 1991;66:589.
11. Rubinfeld B, Souza B, Albert I, et al. Association of the APC gene product with beta-catenin. Science 1993;262:1731.
12. Su L, Vogelstein B, Kinzler K. Association of the APC tumor suppressor protein with catenins. Science 1993;262:1734.
13. Baker SJ, Markowitz S, Fearon ER, et al. Suppression of human colorectal carcinoma cell growth by wild-type p53. Science 1990;249:912.
14. Fearon ER, Cho KR, Nigro JM, et al. Identification of a chromosome 18q gene that is altered in colorectal cancers. Science 1990;247:49.
15. Fearon ER, Jones PA. Progressing toward a molecular description of colorectal cancer development. FASEB J 1992;6:2783.
16. Fishel R, Lescoe MK, Rao MRS, et al. The human mutator

gene homolog MSH2 and its association with hereditary non-polyposis colon cancer. Cell 1993;75:1027.

17. Papadopoulos N, Nicolaides NC, Wei Y, et al. Mutation of a mut L homolog in hereditary colon cancer. Science 1994; 263:1625.

18. Lynch HT, Harris RE, Bardawil WA, et al. Management of hereditary site-specific colon cancer. Arch Surg 1970; 112:170.

19. Boland CR, Troncale FJ. Familial colonic cancer without antecedent polyposis. Ann Intern Med 1984;100:700.

20. Devroede GJ, Taylor WF, Sauer WG, et al. Cancer risk and life expectancy of children with ulcerative colitis. N Engl J Med 1979;285:17.

21. Gyde SN, Prior P, Thompson H, et al. Survival of patients with colorectal cancer complicating ulcerative colitis. Gut 1984;25:228.

22. Cannon-Albright LA, Skolnick MH, Bishop T, et al. Common inheritance of susceptibility to colonic adenomatous polyps and associated colorectal cancers. N Engl J Med 1988;319:533.

23. Muto T, Bussey HJR, Morson BC. The evolution of cancer of the colon and rectum. Cancer 1975;36:2251.

24. Hardcastle JD, Armitage NC, Chamberlin J, et al. Fecal occult blood screening for colorectal cancer in the general population. Cancer 1986;58:397.

25. Hardcastle JD, Farrands PA, Balfour TW. Controlled trial of faecal occult blood testing in the detection of colorectal cancer. Lancet 1983;2:1.

26. Mandel JS, Bond JH, Church TR, et al. Reducing mortality from colorectal cancer by screening for fecal occult blood. N Engl J Med 1993;328:1365.

27. Wolmark N, Fisher B, Wieand HS. The prognostic value of the modifications of the Dukes' C class of colorectal cancer. Ann Surg 1986;203:115.

28. Kokal WA, Gardine RL, Sheibani K, et al. Tumor DNA content in resectable, primary colorectal carcinoma. Ann Surg 1989;209:188.

29. Jen J, Kim H, Piantadosi S, et al. Allelic loss of chromosome 18q and prognosis in colorectal cancer. N Engl J Med 1994;331:213.

30. August DA, Ottow RT, Sugarbaker PH. Clinical perspective of human colorectal cancer metastasis. Cancer Metastasis Rev 1984;3:303.

31. Yeatman TJ, Bland KI. Sphincter-saving procedures for distal carcinoma of the rectum. Ann Surg 1989;209:1.

32. Madden JL, Kandalft SI. Electrocoagulation as a primary curative method in the treatment of carcinoma of the rectum. Surg Gynecol Obstet 1983;157:164.

33. Moertel CG, Fleming TR, MacDonald JS, et al. Levamisole and fluorouracil for adjuvant therapy of resected colon carcinoma. N Engl J Med 1990;322:352.

34. Wolmark N, Fisher B, Rockette H, et al. Postoperative adjuvant chemotherapy or BCG for colon cancer: results from NSABP protocol C-01. J Natl Cancer Inst 1988;80:30.

35. Wolmark N, Rockette H, Fisher B, et al. The benefit of leucovorin-modulated fluorouracil as postoperative adjuvant therapy for primary colon cancer: results from National Surgical Adjuvant Breast and Bowel Project protocol C-03. J Clin Oncol 1993;11:1879.

36. Steele GD Jr, Augenlicht LH, Begg CB, et al. National Institutes of Health Consensus Development Conference statement: adjuvant therapy for patients with colon and rectal cancer. JAMA 1990;264:1444.

37. Krook JE, Moertel CG, Gunderson LL, et al. Effective surgical adjuvant therapy for high-risk rectal carcinoma. N Engl J Med 1991;324:709.

38. Gastrointestinal Tumor Study Group. Radiation therapy and fluorouracil with or without semustine for the treatment of patients with surgical adjuvant adenocarcinoma of the rectum. J Clin Oncol 1992;10:549.

39. Taylor I, Machin D, Mullee M, et al. A randomized controlled trial of adjuvant portal vein cytotoxic perfusion in colorectal cancer. Br J Surg 1985;72:359.

40. Wolmark N, Rockette H, Wickerham DL, et al. Adjuvant therapy of Dukes' A, B, and C adenocarcinoma of the colon with portal-vein fluorouracil hepatic infusion: preliminary results of National Surgical Adjuvant Breast and Bowel Project protocol C-02. J Clin Oncol 1990;8:1466.

41. Hoover HC, Brandhorst JS, Peters LC, et al. Adjuvant active specific immunotherapy for human colorectal cancer: 6.5-year median follow-up of a phase III prospectively randomized trial. J Clin Oncol 1993;11:390.

42. Hughes KK, Simon R, Songhorabodi S, et al. Registry of hepatic metastases. Resection of the liver for colorectal carcinoma metastases: a multi-institutional study of indications for resection. Surgery 1988;103:278.

43. Kern KA, Pass HI, Roth JA. Surgical treatment of pulmonary metastases. In: Rosenberg SA, ed. Surgical treatment of metastatic cancer. Philadelphia, JB Lippincott, 1987:69.

44. Corman ML, Swinton NW, O'Keefe DD, Veidenheimer MC. Colorectal carcinoma at the Lahey Clinic, 1962–1966. Am J Surg 1973;125:424.

45. Eisenberg B, Decosse JJ, Harford F, Michalek J. Carcinoma of the colon and rectum: the natural history reviewed in 1704 patients. Cancer 1982;49:1131.

46. Pihl E, Hughes ESR, McDermott FT, et al. Carcinoma of the colon: cancer-specific long-term survival—a series of 615 patients treated by one surgeon. Ann Surg 1980;192:114.

47. Willett CG, Tepper JE, Cohen AM, et al. Failure patterns following curative resection of colonic carcinoma. Ann Surg 1984;200:685.

48. Minsky BD, Mies C, Rich TA, et al. Potentially curative surgery of colon cancer: patterns of failure and survival. J Clin Oncol 1988;6:106.

SURGERY: SCIENTIFIC PRINCIPLES AND PRACTICE, Second Edition, edited by Lazar J. Greenfield, Michael W. Mulholland, Keith T. Oldham, Gerald B. Zelenock, and Keith D. Lillemoe. Lippincott–Raven Publishers, Philadelphia, © 1997.

CHAPTER 48
ANAL CANCER
SANTHAT NIVATVONGS

Anal cancers are uncommon, accounting for about 2% of large bowel cancers. The anal canal, which extends from the anorectal ring to the anal verge, is lined with several different kinds of epithelium, each of which is susceptible to neoplastic transformation. Below the dentate, or pectinate, line is squamous epithelium, and the epithelium above the dentate line is columnar. The change from squamous to columnar epithelium is not abrupt. For a distance of about 1 cm above the dentate line, there is a gradual transition where columnar, cuboidal, transitional, or even squamous epithelium can be found. This area of transition is often referred to as the *transitional* or *cloacogenic zone* (see Fig. 52-3 in Chap. 52). The anal canal above and below the dentate line has different routes of lymphatic drainage. In addition, when the same histologic type of neoplasm develops in these areas, for example, a squamous cell carcinoma, differences in biologic behavior are evident. For these reasons, carcinomas of the anal region should be classified in two categories in relation to the dentate line as recommended by the World Health Organization.[1] In this classification, the anal canal is arbitrarily divided into the area above the dentate line, known as the *anal canal,* and the area below the dentate line, known as the *anal margin.*

Unlike carcinoma of the rectum, staging for anal carcinoma does not work well. The Dukes system is irrelevant because part of the lymphatic drainage is in the inguinal region and is outside extent of the resection. The TNM system has also been tried without practical value.[2,3]

CARCINOMA OF THE ANAL MARGIN
Squamous Cell Carcinoma

Squamous cell carcinomas of the anal margin, in gross appearance, resemble those occurring in skin elsewhere in the body. They grow slowly and typically have rolled, everted edges with central ulceration. Any chronic un-healed or indurated ulceration in the anal area should be considered a squamous cell carcinoma until biopsy proves otherwise. Squamous carcinomas are usually well differentiated histologically, with well-developed patterns of keratinization (Fig. 48-1). Lymphatic spread from squamous carcinomas of the anal margin is mainly to inguinal lymph nodes. Despite their superficial location, most lesions are usually diagnosed late, with half of cases detected more than 24 months after onset of symptoms.[4] Examination of inguinal areas at regular intervals after excision of the primary lesion is indicated because subsequent metastasis to the groin lymph nodes is common.

Because squamous cell carcinomas of the anal margin are late to metastasize, a wide local excision can be performed as definitive surgical therapy.[5] If, on histologic examination, the carcinoma has invaded the underlying sphincter muscles, metastasis can occur proximally along the superior rectal nodes and laterally along the middle rectal nodes. An abdominoperineal resection is indicated.[6-8] In selected cases, radiotherapy in the form of radium implantation can be used with satisfactory results.[9] A radical groin nodal dissection should be performed only if metastasis to the inguinal lymph nodes is clinically suspected. Overall 5-year survival rates for squamous cell carcinoma of the anal margin vary from 35% to 82%, depending on different degrees of advancement of the disease.[6,10-12]

Basal Cell Carcinoma

Basal cell carcinoma of the anal margin is rare and occurs three times as frequently in men as in women. The lesions are characterized by central ulceration and irregular, raised edges. Basal cell carcinomas are usually superficial, are not fixed to deeper structures, and rarely metastasize. Al-though metastases are not common, inguinal lymphade-nopathy develops frequently from reactive inflammation. Almost one third of patients with basal cell carcinoma of the anal margin are misdiagnosed as having hemorrhoids, anal fistulas, or perianal eczema, causing delay in treat-ment.[13] The patient most frequently presents with com-plaints of mild discomfort, itching, or bleeding.

Local excision with a margin of normal tissue is the treatment of choice. Local recurrence after excision is com-mon, however, and occurs in almost one third of patients.[13] Reexcision is indicated. Abdominoperineal resection is re-served for large lesions and for uncontrollable local recur-rences. The 5-year survival rate in one series is 73%, but no patients died as the result of the basal cell carcinoma.[13]

Bowen Disease

Bowen disease of the perianal skin is a rare, slow-growing intraepidermal squamous cell carcinoma (carci-noma in situ; Fig. 47-2). The lesions appear as a discrete, scaly, or crusted plaque, sometimes exhibiting a moist sur-face. The patient may report itching, burning, or spotty bleeding. Although symptoms and gross appearance are suggestive, only a biopsy can confirm the diagnosis. Sig-nificantly, 70% to 80% of patients with Bowen disease have or eventually develop one or more primary internal malignancies or primary cancer of the skin with metasta-sis.[14] An essential part of the workup is, therefore, to ex-clude other primary malignancies. Wide local excision is the treatment of choice. Microscopic examination is indi-cated to confirm a clear resectional margin. Bowen disease can extend into the anal canal, requiring a wide excision of anoderm. In this circumstance, it may be necessary to use flaps to prevent postoperative anal stricture.

Perianal Paget Disease

Sir James Paget first described the disease that bears his name in relation to the nipple of the breast in women. Extramammary Paget disease can be found in the axilla and in the anogenital region, including the labia majora, penis, scrotum, groin, pubic area, perineum, perianal re-

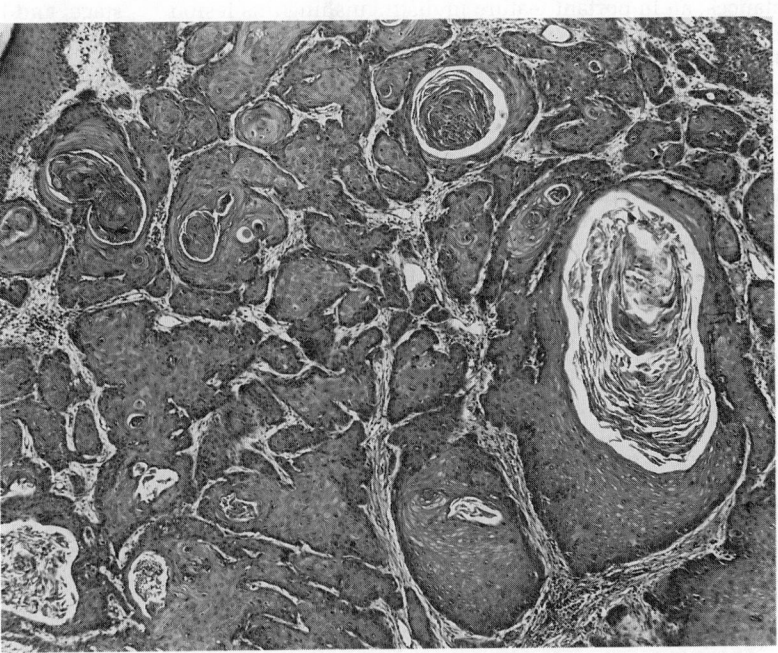

Figure 48-1. Photomicrograph of squamous cell carcinoma of the anal margin.

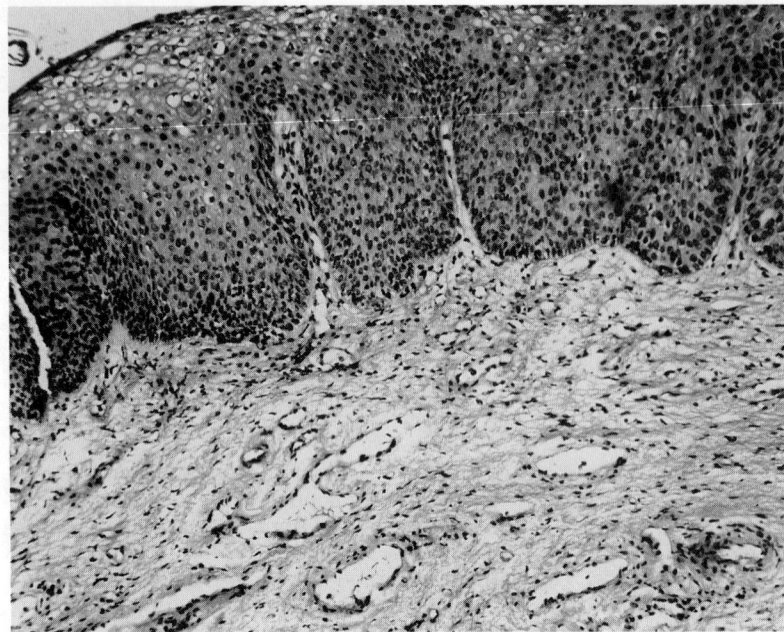

Figure 48-2. Bowen disease. Atypical epithelial cells involve the full thickness of the epidermis (carcinoma in situ).

gion, thigh, and buttock. Paget disease of the perianal area is a rare malignant neoplasm of the intraepidermal portion of apocrine glands with or without associated dermal involvement.[15,16] Paget disease has a long preinvasive phase, but if untreated, an invasive adenocarcinoma of the apocrine gland type develops. The disease is more common in women than men, with the highest incidence in the seventh decade.

Similar to Bowen disease, about 80% of patients with Paget disease are found already to have or subsequently to develop a second primary carcinoma, such as carcinoma of the breast or rectum. Intractable anal itching is usually present for many months. Macroscopically, the lesion appears as an erythematous, scaly, or eczematoid plaquelike lesion, similar to other benign perianal lesions, making clinical diagnosis difficult. A definite diagnosis is made by biopsy, which shows characteristic Paget cells—large, pale, vacuolated cells with hyperchromatic eccentric nuclei (Fig. 47-3). The cells invariably contain acid mucosubstances, an important feature in distinguishing this lesion from melanoma and Bowen disease. Wide local excision is the treatment of choice in the absence of invasive carcinoma. Because of the high incidence of local recurrence and residual tumor, it is vitally important to obtain an adequate resectional margin. Grossly, the extent of involvement is ill defined, and multiple punch biopsies may be required to determine the extent of involvement.[17] For more advanced lesions with underlying carcinoma, an abdominoperineal resection is indicated. Inguinal lymph node dissection is performed only if groin lymph nodes are clinically positive for metastasis. Because of the commonly delayed diagnosis (average, 4 years), about 25% of patients with perianal Paget disease have metastases when they seek treatment.[18,19] The sites of metastases, in order of frequency, are inguinal and pelvic lymph nodes, liver, bone, lung, brain, bladder, prostate, and adrenal gland. The prognosis is poor once metastasis has occurred.[18]

CARCINOMA OF THE ANAL CANAL
Adenocarcinoma

Adenocarcinomas of the lower rectum occasionally extend downward to involve the anal canal; therefore, it may not be possible to determine the origin of the lesion. One might also consider the rare possibility of secondary implantation of a carcinoma of the colon or rectum.

The ducts of the anal glands are lined by squamous epithelium close to their opening in the crypts, by transitional epithelium in the middle portion, and, in the depth of the gland, by mucin-secreting columnar epithelium. The histologic picture of these lesions may be one of adenocarcinoma, mucoepidermoid carcinoma, or basaloid or transitional cell carcinoma.[20] The most characteristic feature of anal duct carcinoma is its extramucosal origin. If a break occurs in the surface epithelium, as is often seen clinically, greater perianal involvement or deeper infiltration may be the only clue to the anal duct origin of these lesions.[21] Patients with anal ductal carcinoma usually present with complaints of pain, bleeding, and perianal mass.[22] Symptoms related to a mass in the anal canal are less common. Penetration beyond the anal canal can masquerade as perianal or ischioanal abscess or anal fistula. The diagnosis of ductal adenocarcinoma is usually made at an advanced stage, and the disease has frequently spread beyond hope for cure.

Adenocarcinomas developing in long-standing anal fistulas have occasionally been reported,[23] and it has been suggested that these carcinomas are due to chronic irritation of the epithelium around either the internal or the external openings of fistulas. Other investigators, however, believe that carcinomas in fistulas are ductal in origin.[20]

Local excision is reserved for selected patients with small carcinomas (not larger than 3 cm). Local excision is appropriate only for carcinomas that are limited to the submucosa, with well-differentiated histology. For most patients, an abdominoperineal resection is the treatment of choice. The roles of preoperative and postoperative radiotherapy have not been well defined.

Epidermoid Carcinoma

Squamous cell carcinoma, basaloid (cloacogenic) carcinoma, and mucoepidermoid carcinoma of the anal canal are histologic variants of epidermoid carcinoma. Because the responses of both tumors to treatment are similar to results observed with squamous cell carcinoma, most authors have grouped them with squamous cell carcinoma.[24]

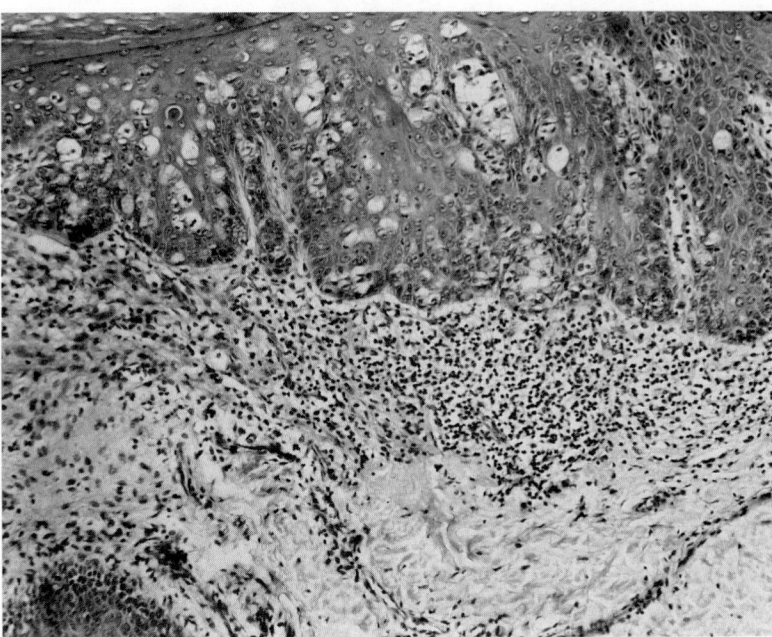

Figure 48-3. Perianal Paget disease. Paget cells are above the basal layer.

Squamous Cell Carcinoma

Squamous cell carcinoma arises from the cloacogenic area of epithelium. Squamous cancers are typically flat, ulcerating neoplasms that occur more frequently in women. The histologic picture resembles squamous cell carcinoma of the anal margin, except there is little or no keratin. Minor perianal problems, such as bleeding, occur in about half of patients. Other symptoms include rectal pain and anal mass. Almost one third of patients in most series had an initial incorrect diagnosis of benign or inflammatory disease.

Squamous cell carcinomas of the anal canal have been found to metastasize to superior rectal lymph nodes in about 40% of cases and to the inguinal nodes in about 33% of cases. The overall, corrected 5-year survival is about 50%.[25]

Basaloid (Cloacogenic) Carcinoma

Basaloid carcinoma is a variant of squamous cell carcinoma and, to some degree, resembles basal cell carcinomas of the skin. *Basaloid* refers to the histologic appearance of palisade nuclei seen in the periphery of clumps of cells that characterize this malignancy (Fig. 47-4). Histologically, these tumors are unlike typical skin basal cell carcinomas in that areas of eosinophilic necrosis exist within clumps of the neoplastic cells. Nuclear atypia and the presence of giant cells are characteristic, especially of the anaplastic variety. A female preponderance exists, and the average age of diagnosis is 60 years, with a range of 40 to 80 years. This type of carcinoma arises from the transitional zone above the dentate line, and the term *transitional cloacogenic carcinoma* is also used.[18,26] The clinical features are similar to those of squamous cell carcinomas of the anal canal.

As in squamous cell carcinomas of the anal canal, about half of patients already have regional lymph node involvement at operation.[2] The prognosis is related most closely to grading of the carcinoma. The 5-year survival rate is 90% for patients with well-differentiated lesions and 60% for those with moderately differentiated tumors. Patients with anaplastic lesions almost never live 5 years. The overall 5-year survival rate is about 50%.

Mucoepidermoid Carcinoma

Mucoepidermoid carcinoma is a variant of squamous cell carcinoma with the same histologic pattern except for the presence of mucin. Mucin staining varies in amount from lesion to lesion and within different areas of the same lesion. There is a slight female preponderance, and the average age of presentation is 55 years. The behavior and prognosis of these lesions are similar to those of squamous cell and basaloid carcinomas.

Treatment of Epidermoid Carcinoma

Local Excision. Local excision should be reserved for those early or well-differentiated lesions that involve only the submucosa but may also be considered for patients who are poor risks for extensive surgery. In general, the recurrence rate is high after local excision.[27]

Abdominoperineal Resection. In the past, abdominoperineal resection with wide excision of perineal tissue formed the basis of treatment.[7,8,28] In women, the posterior vaginal wall should also be excised because the incidence of invasion to the area is high (20%).[29] In one series, 43 patients were considered as having had curative resections, 17 had local or distal recurrent disease.[28]

The 5-year survival rate after an abdominoperineal resection is 30% to 70%, with an average of 50%.[2,3] Local recurrence rate after an abdominoperineal resection is 25% to 35%.[2,30] Such a high recurrence rate probably reflects the behavior of the carcinoma and the rich multiple pathways of the lymphatic network in the anorectum and the pelvis. To improve long-term survival and to save some patients from having a colostomy, use of abdominoperineal resection as the primary treatment for epidermoid carcinoma has been challenged by the use of combined-modality therapy.

Combination Therapy. Nigro[31] instituted a protocol consisting of preoperative irradiation and chemotherapy, with the intent of containing the disease to a more localized form for more effective removal by radical operation. Chemotherapy was added with the belief that it permitted the use of a more modest dose of irradiation. The treatment regimen is as follows:

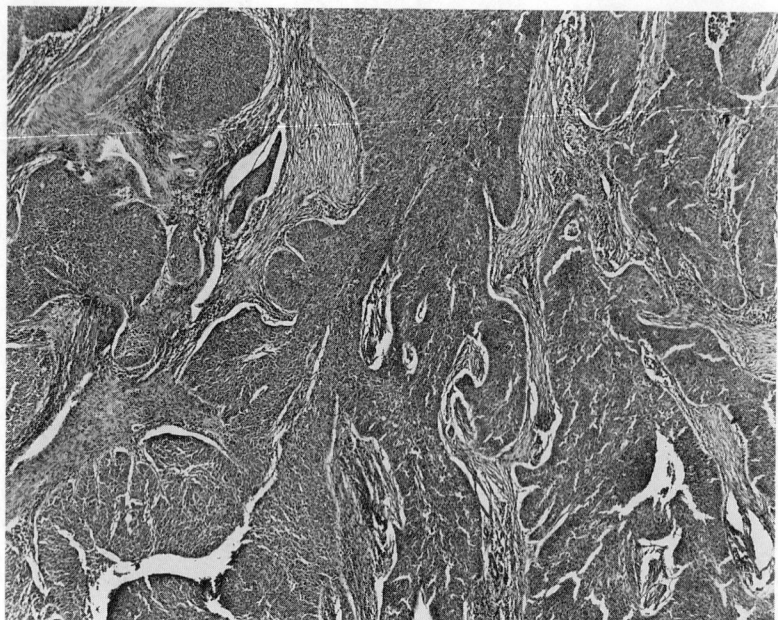

Figure 48-4. Basaloid (cloacogenic) carcinoma of the anal canal.

- External irradiation—30 Gy, to the primary tumor, pelvic, and inguinal nodes from day 1 to day 21 (2 Gy/d, 5 days a week)
- Systemic chemotherapy—5-fluorouracil at 1000 mg/m^2/24 h, as a continuous infusion for 4 days, starting on day 1 of radiotherapy and repeated on days 28 through 31
- Mitomycin C at 15 mg/m^2 intravenous bolus on day 1

If the lesion disappears grossly, and its microscopic absence is confirmed by biopsy, no further treatment is necessary. If residual cancer is present, and if there is no evidence of disseminated disease, abdominoperineal resection should be performed. Surgery is performed 4 to 6 weeks after completion of the irradiation. Of 104 patients evaluated for the effect of chemoradiotherapy, 97 had no gross tumor remaining in the anal canal. In 7 patients, gross tumor is present, although reduced in size. Eighty-two patients were alive and apparently free of disease from 2 to 11 years after therapy.[31] Other series show complete response rates in the range of 70% to 90%.[32] It appears that this combined regimen is at least as effective as the previous standard treatment with abdominoperineal resection, with a significant fraction of patients spared operation.

The combined chemoradiotherapy has become a popular and well-accepted form of therapy for epidermoid carcinoma of the anal canal. Controversy exists about relative importance of each of the components, and these uncertainties may help explain the numerous variations in dose scheduling that have been used and the departures from the original combination of 5-fluorouracil and mitomycin C that have been made, including the use of bleomycin and cisplatin.[25] Using chemoradiation, complete regression has been reported in the neighborhood of 90% in most series.[31,33–35] Chemoradiotherapy has become the standard treatment for epidermoid carcinoma of the anal canal. Abdominoperineal resection should be reserved for residual or recurrent disease after the chemoradiation or for the complications of radiotherapy.

Inguinal Node Dissection. Because of the high morbidity rate associated witH inguinal lymph node dissection, the risk of the added procedure outweighs the benefit, and

prophylactic groin dissection is not recommended.[28] The simultaneous appearance of inguinal metastasis is an ominous sign. In one series, only 2 of 14 patients with simultaneous nodal metastases survived 5 years.[14] In contrast, the subsequent appearance of inguinal metastasis has a better outlook. Fifteen of 20 such patients survived 5 years after the radical groin dissection. Elective irradiation of clinically normal inguinal nodes greatly reduces the risk of late node failure and carries little morbidity.[36] Only 1 of 38 such patients had a late recurrence in the inguinal area after undergoing combination chemotherapy and radiotherapy. In series in which the inguinal nodes are not treated electively, the late nodal recurrence rate is 15% to 25%.[2,37,38]

MALIGNANT MELANOMA

Melanoma, a rare malignant tumor of the anal canal, accounts for 0.5% to 1% of malignant neoplasms of the anal canal. The anal canal, nevertheless, represents the third most common site for melanomas, exceeded only by skin and eyes. Almost all anal melanomas arise from the epidermoid lining of the anal canal. Most melanomas occur adjacent to the dentate line, although a few reports have been made of these tumors arising in the rectum.

Rectal bleeding is the most common symptom. Melanoma is suspected when a deeply pigmented lesion is seen. Most tumors, however, are pigmented lightly or are non-pigmented, and they are often misdiagnosed as polyps or epidermoid carcinomas. In amelanotic malignant melanomas, tissue biopsy can be misinterpreted as an undifferentiated epidermoid carcinoma.

Anal canal melanomas have a marked tendency to spread submucosally into the rectum, but they rarely invade adjacent organs, probably because most patients die before this occurs. Lymphatic spread to the mesenteric nodes is seen in about one third of patients at the time of diagnosis; spread to the inguinal nodes is less common. Hematogenous spread to the liver and lung is early and rapid, accounting for most of the deaths.[39]

Melanomas of the anal canal are radioresistant and do not respond to chemotherapy or immunotherapy. The surgical approach to this malignant neoplasm is controversial.

There is no statistical difference in survival when patients treated by abdominoperineal resection are compared with those treated by wide local excision.[40-42] Both 5-year survival rates are about 15% to 17%. Tumor size and configuration do not affect the mean survival. In most cases, there is no clearcut choice of treatment, although abdominoperineal resection is more effective than wide local excision in preventing local recurrence.[42] For patients at low risk, an abdominoperineal resection is a reasonable treatment for removal of undetected mesenteric lymph node metastases.

REFERENCES

1. Jass JR, Sobin LH. Histologic typing of intestinal tumors. World Health Organization. Springer-Verlag, New York, 1989: 41.
2. Boman BM, Moertel CG, O'Connell MJ, et al. Carcinoma of the anal canal: a clinical and pathologic study of 188 cases. Cancer 1984;54:114.
3. Frost DB, Richards PC, Montague ED, Giacco GG, Martin RG. Epidermoid cancer of the anorectum. Cancer 1984;53:1285.
4. Moller C, Saksela E. Cancer of the anus and anal canal. Acta Chir Scand 1970;136:340.
5. Morson BC. The pathology and results of treatment of squamous cell carcinoma of the anal canal and anal margin. Proc R Soc Med 1960;53:416.
6. Greenall MJ, Quan SHQ, Stearns MW, Urmacher C, DeCosse JJ. Epidermoid cancer of the anal margin: pathologic features, treatment, and clinical results. Am J Surg 1985;149:95.
7. Beahrs OH, Wilson SM. Carcinoma of the anus. Am Surg 1976;184:422.
8. Quan SHQ. Anal and para-anal tumors. Surg Clin North Am 1978;58:591.
9. Papillon J. Radiation therapy in the management of epidermoid carcinoma of the anal region. Dis Colon Rectum 1974;17:181.
10. Shrout WH, Wang C, Dorson PJ, Block GE. Depth of invasion, location, and size of cancer of the anus dictate operative treatment. Cancer 1983;51:1291.
11. Brown DK, Oglesby AB, Scott DH, Dayton MT. Squamous cell carcinoma of the anus: a twenty-five year retrospective. Ann Surg 1988;54:337.
12. Pintor MP, Northover JMA, Nicholls RJ. Squamous cell carcinoma of the anus at one hospital from 1948 to 1984. Br J Surg 1989;76:806.
13. Nielsen OV, Jensen SL. Basal cell carcinoma of the anus: a clinical study of 34 cases. Br J Surg 1981;68:856.
14. Stearns MW Jr, Quan SHQ. Epidermoid carcinoma of the anorectum. Surg Gynecol Obstet 1970;131:953.
15. Rosai J. Ackerman's surgical pathology, ed 7. St Louis, CV Mosby, 1989:634.
16. Armitage NC, Jass JR, Richman PI, Thomson JPS, Philips RKS. Paget's disease of the anus: a clinicopathological study. Br J Surg 1989;76:60.
17. Beck DE, Fazio VW. Perianal Paget's disease. Dis Colon Rectum 1987;30:263.
18. Helwig EG, Graham JH. Anogenital (extramammary) Paget's disease: a clinicopathological study. Cancer 1963;16:387.
19. Grodsky L. Uncommon nonkeratinizing cancers of the anal canal and perianal region. NY State J Med 1965;65:894.
20. Nielsen OV, Koch E. Carcinoma of the anorectal region of extramucosal origin with special reference to the anal ducts. Acta Chir Scand 1973;139:299.
21. Hagihara P, Vazquez MD, Parker JC Jr, Griffin WO Jr. Carcinoma of anal ductal origin. Dis Colon Rectum 1976;19:694.
22. Abel ME, Chiu YSY, Russell TR, Volpe PA. Adenocarcinoma of the anal glands: results of a survey. Dis Colon Rectum 1993;36:383.
23. Thompson HR. Carcinoma of the anorectal region arising from the intramuscular and apocrine glands. Proc R Soc Med 1956;49:469.
24. Goldman S, Glimelius B, Pahlman L, Stahle E, Wilander E. Anal epidermoid carcinoma: a population-based clinico-pathological study of 164 patients. Int J Colorectal Dis 1988;3:109.
25. Gordon PH. Squamous cell carcinoma of the anal canal. Surg Clin North Am 1988;68:1391.
26. Grinvalsky HT, Helwig EG. Carcinoma of the anorectal junction. I. Histologic considerations. Cancer 1956;9:480.
27. Jensen SL, Hagen K, Harling H, Shokouh-Amiri MH, Nielsen OV. Long-term prognosis after radical treatment for squamous cell carcinoma of the anal canal and anal margin. Dis Colon Rectum 1988;31:273.
28. Welch JP, Malt RA. Appraisal of the treatment of carcinoma of the anus and anal canal. Surg Gynecol Obstet 1977;145:837.
29. Klotz RG Jr, Pamukcoglu T, Sonilliard DH. Transitional cloacogenic carcinoma of the anal canal. Cancer 1967;20:1727.
30. Greenall MJ, Quan SHQ, Urmacher C, DeCosse JJ. Treatment of epidermoid carcinoma of the anal canal. Surg Gynecol Obstet 1985;161:509.
31. Nigro ND. Multidisciplinary management of cancer of the anus. World J Surg 1987;11:446.
32. Deans GT, McAleer JJA, Spence RAJ. Malignant anal tumors. Br J Surg 1994;81:500.
33. Meeker WR Jr, Sickle-Santello BJ, Philpot G, et al. Combined chemotherapy, radiation and surgery for epithelial cancer of the anal canal. Cancer 1986;57:525.
34. Cummings BJ. Current management of epidermoid carcinoma of the anal canal. Gastroenterol Clin North Am 1987;16:125.
35. Flaur MS, John MJ, Mowry PA. Definitive combined modality therapy of carcinoma of the anus: a report of 30 cases including results of salvage therapy in patients with residual disease. Dis Colon Rectum 1987;30:495.
36. Cummings BJ, Thomas QM, Keane TJ. Primary radiation therapy in the treatment of anal canal carcinoma. Dis Colon Rectum 1982;25:778.
37. Stearns MW, Urmacher C, Sternborg SE, Woodruff J, Attiyeh FF. Cancer of the anal canal. Curr Prob Cancer 1980;4:1.
38. Papillon J, Montbarbon JF. Epidermoid carcinoma of the anal canal: a series of 276 cases. Dis Colon Rectum 1987;30:324.
39. Chiu YS, Unni KK, Beart RW Jr. Malignant melanoma of the anorectum. Dis Colon Rectum 1980;23:122.
40. Goldman S, Glimelius B, Pahlman L. Anorectal malignant melanoma in Sweden: report of 49 patients. Dis Colon Rectum 1990;33:874.
41. Antoniuk PM, Tjandra JJ, Webb BW, Petras RE, Milsom JW, Fazio VW. Anorectal malignant melanoma has poor prognosis. Int J Color Dis 1993;8:81.
42. Brady M, Kavolius J, Quan SHQ. Anorectal melanoma. Dis Colon Rectum 1994;37:P13.

SURGERY: SCIENTIFIC PRINCIPLES AND PRACTICE, Second Edition, edited by Lazar J. Greenfield, Michael W. Mulholland, Keith T. Oldham, Gerald B. Zelenock, and Keith D. Lillemoe. Lippincott–Raven Publishers, Philadelphia, © 1997.

CHAPTER 49

DIVERTICULAR DISEASE

GORDON L. TELFORD AND MARY F. OTTERSON

Diverticular disease of the colon includes both diverticulosis and diverticulitis. *Diverticulosis* refers to an abnormal state in which noninflamed diverticula are present with or without symptoms. *Diverticulitis* is present when one or more diverticula become inflamed. This inflammation can lead to perforation of the diverticulum with pericolic infection (*peridiverticulitis*) or abscess formation, free perforation with peritonitis, fistula formation, or obstruction.

Before 1940, diverticulosis of the colon was recognized infrequently. Retrospective reviews of colon radiographs and examinations of pathologic specimens from this period recorded an incidence of diverticulosis of 5% to 10%.[1] Diverticulosis has become much more commonly recognized in Western countries. The incidence depends on the age of the population studied, varying from less than 2% in patients younger than 30 years old to 30% to 50% in patients older than 50 years of age.[2] Although most patients with diverticulosis of the colon have no or only mild symptoms, complications of hemorrhage or infection occur in 15% to 30% of affected patients, and about 30% of these patients require operative treatment. Thus, colonic diverticular disease remains a major public health problem in the United States and a continuing challenge for general surgeons.

PATHOLOGIC ANATOMY

True diverticula involve all layers of the bowel wall: mucosa, submucosa, and muscularis externa. False diverticula involve only mucosa and submucosa that herniate through the muscularis externa. Most diverticula of the colon are false diverticula. True diverticula are rare. Most false diverticula emanate from weak points in the colonic wall where mesenteric blood vessels penetrate the circular muscle layer (Fig. 49-1). Diverticula also can occur along the antimesenteric border in the intertaenial area.[3]

Most colonic diverticula are found in the sigmoid colon, although they can be scattered throughout the intraabdominal colon.[1-3] In up to 65% of patients, diverticulosis is limited to the sigmoid colon. In about 35% of patients, at least one other area of the colon is involved. Only 1% to 4% of patients do not have involvement of the sigmoid colon.

PATHOPHYSIOLOGY

Diverticulosis has been described as a disease of Western industrialized civilization, although it may better be described as the disease of affluence and refined food products. As the people of Western nations have decreased their intake of dietary fiber, the incidence of diverticulosis has increased. Decrease in fiber is the most consistent factor associated with the high incidence of diverticulosis in Western populations.[4] In contrast, diverticulosis is rare in less affluent, nonindustrialized countries. Diverticulosis is also unusual in Japan, however, where the population continues to eat a diet high in fiber.

A perplexing problem is how a diet low in fiber results in the formation of diverticula. One hypothesis states that when circular muscular contractions occur in patients with small amounts of stool in their colons, which is the case in patients whose diets are low in fiber, the colonic lumen can be totally occluded. When two such contrac-

tions occur close together, the lumen of the intervening segment of colon is isolated from the remainder of the colon, and high pressure is generated in that segment. Theoretically, increased pressure results in the formation of diverticula by placing increased tension on the colonic wall. In some people, there also appears to be a decrease in tensile strength of the colon wall. Pressure–volume curves in patients with diverticulosis demonstrate decreased colon wall tension compared with controls. The combination of colonic segmentation and decreased wall tension may be more important than either factor in isolation.

CLINICAL PRESENTATION AND DIFFERENTIAL DIAGNOSES

Diverticulosis

Most patients with evidence of colonic diverticula on barium enema have no symptom or only mild symptoms. In patients with symptoms of abdominal pain and evidence of noninflamed diverticula on barium enema, the diverticula are not usually the cause of symptoms (Fig. 49-2). Noninflamed colonic diverticula are not a noted cause of pain or discomfort. A more plausible explanation for the pain that occurs in patients with diverticula is the excessive pressure exerted by segmentation of the colon. Although diverticulosis should be considered in the differential diagnosis of a patient with intermittent, mild to moderate lower abdominal pain, it is imperative that other causes of the pain be considered. Other diagnoses that should be eliminated include chronic constipation, diverticulitis, irritable bowel syndrome, and adenocarcinoma of the colon. If pain is severe and constant, a diagnosis of diverticulitis should be more seriously considered. Irritable bowel syndrome is thought by some to be a prediverticular condition and a diagnosis made by exclusion. In patients in whom barium enema does not demonstrate diverticula, a diagnosis of irritable bowel or chronic constipation should not be made until colonoscopy has definitively eliminated carcinoma.

Diverticulitis

The usual symptoms of diverticulitis include fever, lower abdominal pain, and lower abdominal tenderness. A lower abdominal mass, tachycardia, and an elevated white blood cell count with a left shift are frequently noted. Abdominal pain and tenderness can vary markedly, depending on the precise location of the inflammation and

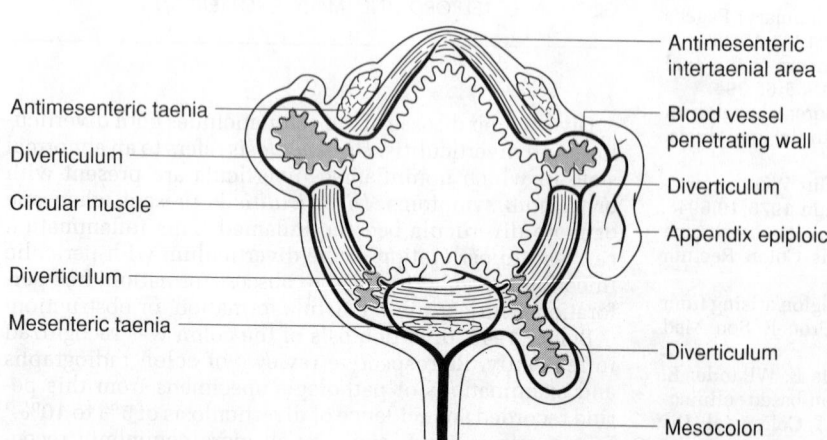

Antimesenteric taenia

Diverticulum

Circular muscle

Diverticulum

Mesenteric taenia

Antimesenteric intertaenial area

Blood vessel penetrating wall

Diverticulum

Appendix epiploica

Diverticulum

Mesocolon

Figure 49-1. Cross section of the colon illustrating the relation of diverticula to the blood vessels penetrating the circular muscle layer, the taeniae, and the appendices epiploicae.

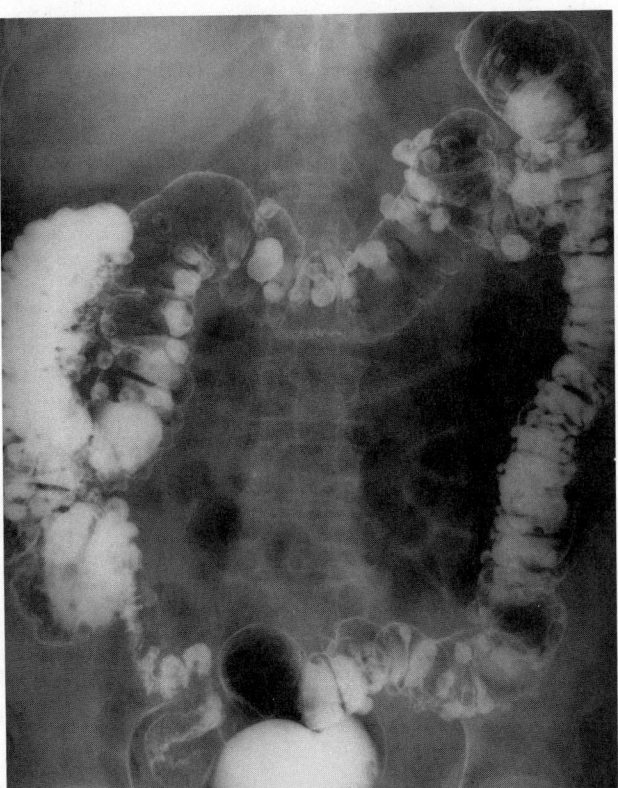

Figure 49-2. Barium enema showing multiple diverticula of the colon.

whether there is free perforation into the abdominal cavity. When there is free perforation and generalized peritonitis, it is often difficult to differentiate diverticulitis from other causes of perforated viscus. Suspicion of diverticular complications is heightened when the process is localized to the left lower quadrant and there is a palpable, tender mass. The differential diagnosis for diverticulitis without free perforation includes perforated colon cancer, acute appendicitis, perforated peptic ulcer, acute-onset ulcerative colitis, acute-onset Crohn's colitis, and ischemic colitis.

Perforated colon cancer is difficult to differentiate from diverticulitis. Both diseases frequently involve the sigmoid colon, and both can produce a tender, left lower quadrant mass. Patient histories are frequently similar because both diseases can cause vague, poorly defined lower abdominal pain. Although helpful, colonoscopy is not always diagnostic. The inflammation that results from the perforation can make colonoscopy difficult, and it may be impossible to see the involved area. Therefore, if a diagnosis of carcinoma cannot be eliminated preoperatively, a thorough examination must be performed intraoperatively. The patient's history is usually helpful in differentiating appendicitis from diverticulitis unless the diverticula are right sided in origin. Ulcerative colitis, Crohn's colitis, and ischemic colitis can be diagnosed by colonoscopy or flexible sigmoidoscopy. For ulcerative colitis or Crohn's disease, the patient's history usually includes a diagnosis of inflammatory bowel disease, but when the onset is acute, diverticulitis may be difficult to distinguish.

Hemorrhage

Hemorrhage can occur as a result of either diverticulosis or diverticulitis, although massive bleeding is more typically associated with diverticulosis (Fig. 49-3). It is im-

portant to distinguish hemorrhage as a complication of diverticulosis from colonic angiodysplasia.[5] Similar to diverticulosis, patients who bleed from angiodysplasia are usually asymptomatic before hemorrhage, and the blood loss can be massive. Carcinoma of the colon is seldom a cause of acute massive bleeding. Patients who develop massive bleeding secondary to inflammatory bowel disease usually have a history of colitis. Occasionally, a patient with colitis presents with a fulminant course and no history of the disease. Ischemic colitis is usually accompanied by a history of abdominal pain, diarrhea, and vascular occlusive disease. The differential diagnosis of lower gastrointestinal bleeding must always include the various causes of massive upper gastrointestinal bleeding.

Obstruction

Diverticulitis and its complications account for about 13% of cases of large bowel obstruction. Significant problems in evaluating patients with sigmoid colon obstruction are the relatively high incidence (7%) of carcinoma in patients with symptomatic sigmoid diverticular disease and the relative difficulty of making the diagnosis of carcinoma of the colon when a large phlegmonous mass is present.[6] Colonoscopy is helpful only when the endoscope can pass the area of obstruction and biopsy specimens can be obtained. A negative colonoscopy in a patient with obstruction and resultant inflammation and edema does not eliminate carcinoma.

DIAGNOSIS AND THERAPY

Diverticulosis

Patients with a combination of chronic, intermittent, lower abdominal pain and diverticula on barium enema should be treated symptomatically. The diverticula are not considered to be the cause of the pain, and surgical therapy is not indicated. Colectomy should be reserved for treatment of complications of diverticular disease.

Population studies have demonstrated that diverticula can be prevented by consuming a diet high in fiber, and such a diet has been widely prescribed for the treatment of symptomatic diverticulosis. No study, however, has shown that a diet high in fiber prevents the complications of diverticulosis. Likewise, the efficacy of fiber supplements or bulk laxatives to treat the pain associated with diverticula is controversial. Studies have demonstrated that an increase in dietary fiber can improve symptoms related to constipation. Vegetarians have a lower incidence of diverticulosis than nonvegetarians. Recommendations for increasing dietary fiber are probably worthwhile.

In over 70% of patients with diverticular hemorrhage, bleeding stops spontaneously, and 75% of these patients do not have recurrent bleeding. In the 25% of patients whose bleeding recurs, even if the bleeding is managed successfully by nonoperative means, segmental colectomy should be performed because most of these patients have subsequent hemorrhage. The management of diverticular hemorrhage is discussed in more detail in Chapter 50.

Reports suggest that angiodysplasia of the right colon is a more common cause of massive lower gastrointestinal bleeding than previously appreciated. In one series, half the patients with angiodysplasia had diverticula, which is not surprising because both diseases occur predominately in the elderly. All the bleeding angiodysplastic lesions were in the right colon, which explains why massive colonic hemorrhage tends to be right-sided in origin.

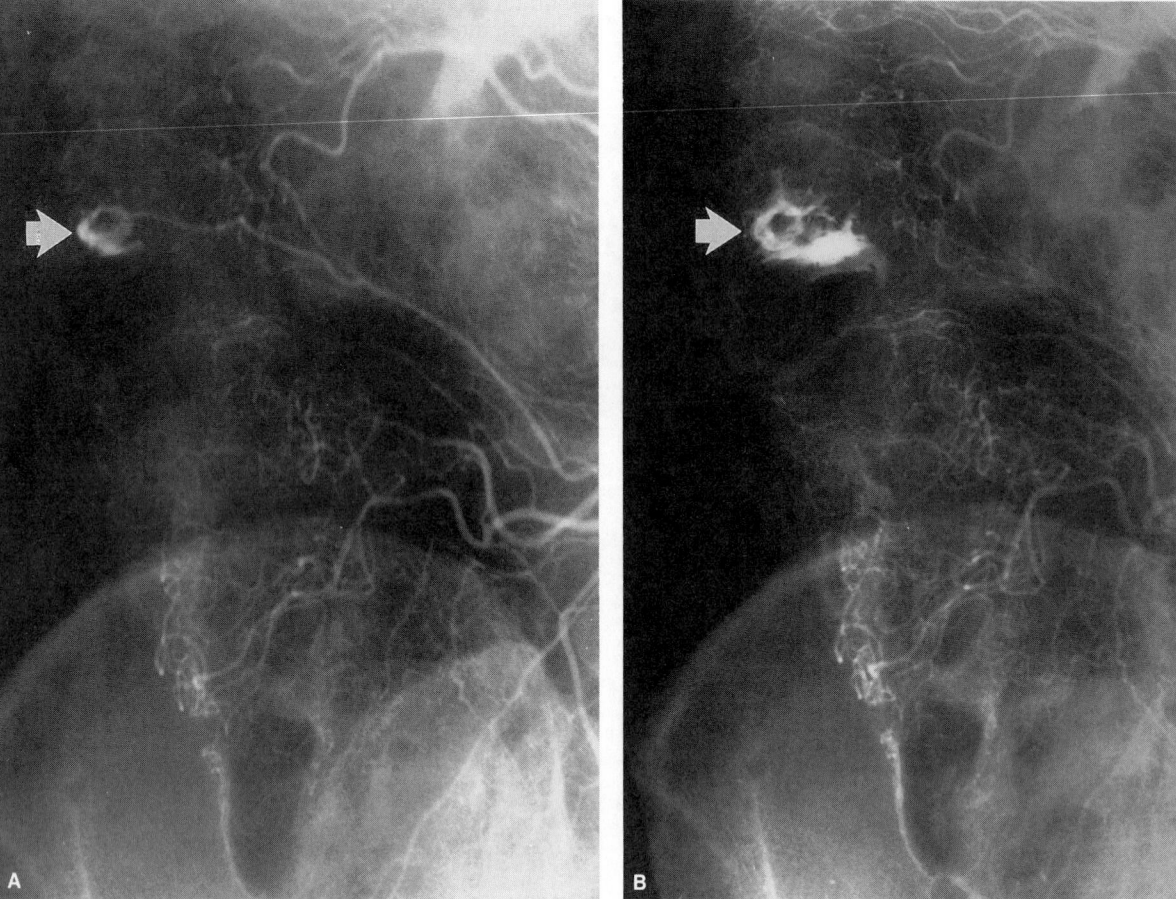

Figure 49-3. Superior mesenteric arteriogram from a patient with bleeding from a right colon diverticulum. (*A*) Early roentgenogram with contrast material outlining the diverticulum (*arrow*). (*B*) Late roentgenogram demonstrating overflow of contrast material into the colonic lumen.

Diverticulitis

Diverticulitis is a complication of diverticulosis. One theory is that diverticulitis occurs when impaction of feces in a single diverticulum causes obstruction of the neck of the diverticulum or abrasion of the thin-walled diverticulum, resulting in invasive infection. Another theory states that microperforation occurs as a result of increased intraluminal pressure, leading to spillage of colonic contents. Either event could result in infection of the surrounding pericolic tissues or free perforation. The process, once initiated, could result in a self-limiting infection without clinical symptoms or could cause progression to clinically significant infection, requiring hospitalization and surgical intervention. When the infection is progressive, other complications can occur.

Most patients with an acute episode of diverticulitis severe enough to require hospitalization can be treated with intravenous fluids, bowel rest, broad-spectrum antibiotics, and analgesics. Signs and symptoms of severe diverticulitis include fever, tachycardia, leukocytosis with left shift of the differential count, abdominal pain (usually in the left lower quadrant) severe enough to require analgesics, abdominal tenderness, and a lower abdominal mass.

If nausea, vomiting, or abdominal distention develops, nasogastric suction should be instituted. The patient should be reexamined frequently for signs of progression of disease. If, despite maximal therapy, the patient does not improve within 48 hours, complications of diverticulitis probably exist, and further therapy is necessary. Only about 20% of patients develop complications of diverticulitis with their first episode; this rises to 60% with recurrent episodes. Although a water-soluble contrast enema radiograph frequently provides the diagnosis of diverticulitis (Fig. 49-4), computed tomography (CT) has become the preferred diagnostic test in patients who do not improve within 49 hours, who are assumed to have a complication of diverticulitis (Fig. 49-5). CT is especially useful in delineating the complications of diverticulitis, including perforation and abscess formation.[7] In addition, at the time of CT scan, percutaneous drainage catheters can be placed if an abscess is identified. After CT drainage of an abscess, 50% to 90% of patients undergo a successful one-stage procedure of segmented colectomy and primary anastomosis.[8] If percutaneous drainage is not feasible or an abscess is not identified, surgical intervention is recommended.

At the time of exploratory laparotomy, if the disease is localized, a segmental colectomy should be performed. The distal extent of the resection should always extend to the proximal rectum to decrease the chance of recurrence. The proximal extent of resection should include the segment involved with the acute disease plus any additional colon with signs of chronic disease or many diverticula. With this approach, the recurrence rate after surgical resection is less than 10%. The only absolute contraindications to primary anastomosis are free perforation with generalized peritonitis, obstruction with unprepared bowel, and intraoperative conditions that do not warrant primary anastomosis, such as septic shock, ureteral injury, and

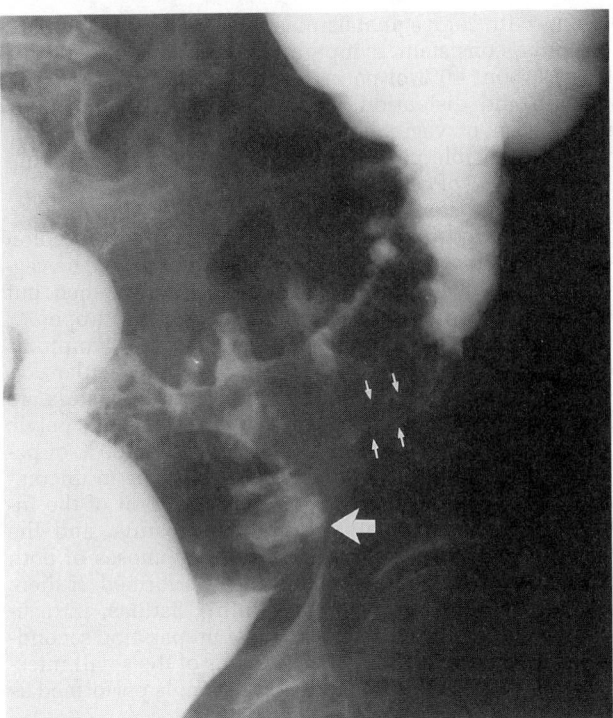

Figure 49-4. Barium enema examination of the sigmoid colon with signs of diverticulitis. There is persistent narrowing, intramural tracking (*small arrows*), and an abscess inferior to the sigmoid colon (*large arrow*).

other medical conditions that make a prolonged operation inadvisable. If resection is thought to be unsafe in the presence of a massive phlegmon or the patient is too unstable to undergo a resection, a diverting end colostomy with mucous fistula and drainage may be appropriate, with planned colonic resection at a later date after inflammation subsides. This approach is seldom necessary, however, and most patients can undergo resection of the diseased segment of bowel at the initial operation.

Most patients improve on a regimen of intravenous fluids, bowel rest, and broad-spectrum antibiotics, and emergency surgery is not necessary. Intravenous antibiotics should be continued for 7 to 10 days, and intravenous fluids and bowel rest should be continued until colonic

function has normalized. A contrast enema should be performed subsequently to confirm the presumed diagnosis and to evaluate the extent of disease. If there is minimal disease and no sign of obstruction, fistula formation, or abscess, the patient can be discharged and followed as an outpatient. If any of these complications are present, a segmental resection should be performed before discharging the patient. After a second episode of diverticulitis, a resection should be performed because the risk of further episodes of diverticulitis increases with each episode.

Obstruction

Patients who have experienced one or more episodes of diverticulitis can develop a fibrotic colonic stricture and large bowel obstruction. When obstruction is diagnosed, it is important to differentiate between diverticulitis and colon carcinoma or colonic volvulus. All patients should undergo sigmoidoscopy or colonoscopy so that biopsy specimens can be obtained of any masses. Water-soluble contrast radiographs of the colon should be obtained to define completeness of obstruction. The extent of the workup depends on the condition of the patient and the completeness of the obstruction. Patients with an incomplete obstruction should be given a thorough but rapid preoperative evaluation in an attempt to secure an exact diagnosis. Because patients with complete obstructions require urgent operation, it is not always feasible to complete all tests before surgery.

If the obstruction is partial, complete preoperative bowel preparation should be carried out, including oral antibiotics. Patients with high-grade colonic obstructions do not tolerate rapid bowel preparation with laxatives or polyethylene glycol. Such patients should be prepared slowly, with extra time allowed for completion of the bowel cleansing. Once bowel preparation is complete, the patient with incomplete obstruction can undergo one-stage resection and primary anastomosis. Unless colon carcinoma has been eliminated as a possible diagnosis, a cancer operation should be performed for this circumstance.

The patient with complete obstruction cannot undergo preoperative bowel preparation, and a one-stage operation is not be feasible. In this case, diverting colostomy should be performed as an urgent operation to relieve the obstruction. Resection of the diseased, obstructed segment of bowel can be performed during this operation or can be delayed until additional workup is complete. The workup to differentiate between carcinoma and diverticulitis

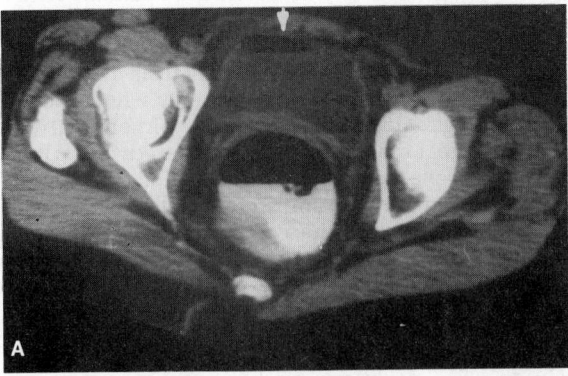
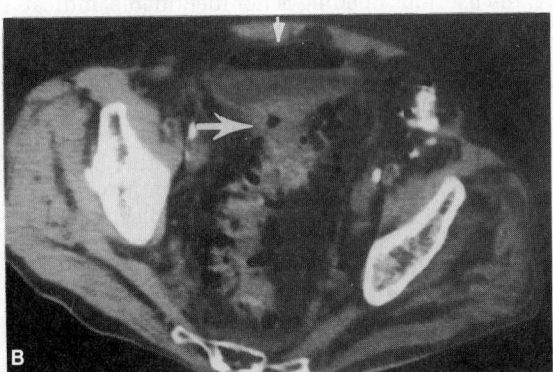

Figure 49-5. (*A*) CT scan demonstrating air in the urinary bladder (*arrow*) in the presence of a colovesical fistula secondary to diverticulitis. (*B*) Air in the urinary bladder (*small arrow*) in association with a paravesical inflammatory mass (*large arrow*). (Sarr MG, Fishman EK, Goldman SM. Enterovesical fistula. Surg Gynecol Obstet 1987;164:2)

should be completed after the patient has recovered from the initial surgery.

When the patient has recovered from the first operation, which usually takes at least 1 month, the next procedure is performed. Depending on the placement of the colostomy, the second operation can be resection of the colostomy and the diseased segment of colon and reestablishment of bowel continuity by colocolostomy. When the diseased segment of bowel was removed during the first operation, the secondary procedure can include colostomy closure.

Fistula Formation

Diverticular disease can also be complicated by the development of fistulas from the diseased colon to other viscera or to skin. Colovesical fistulas account for about half of fistulas due to diverticulitis. Most patients with colovesical fistulas present with urinary tract symptoms, including urgency, dysuria, pneumaturia, and fecaluria. Despite what in retrospect often appear to be obvious symptoms, the diagnosis of colovesical fistula can be difficult to establish conclusively. Recurrent urinary tract infections in an elderly man should increase suspicion. Barium enema usually demonstrates diverticula and occasionally shows sigmoid narrowing. Only rarely is the fistulous tract actually filled. Cystoscopy demonstrates hyperemia and inflammation consistent with chronic cystitis. Although these findings can be localized to some extent, indicating the presence of a fistulous communication, the fistulous opening is seldom seen. CT with intraluminal contrast material has emerged as the most sensitive test for the presence of a colovesical fistula. In addition, after the rectal administration of barium, the patient's urine sediment should be checked for barium by radiograph of a spun urine sample. The presence of barium in the urine is diagnostic of a colovesical fistula. In over 90% of patients, air is in the urinary bladder, and an indurated segment of sigmoid colon is observed adjacent to a locally thickened bladder wall.[9]

Most patients with colovesical fistulas are treated effectively with a one-stage procedure consisting of segmental colectomy and closure of the fistulous opening in the bladder. The proximal margin of resection should include the entire segment of thickened, contracted colon and any additional colon that is involved in the acute inflammation. As stated earlier, although it is not necessary to resect all the colon involved with diverticulosis, the resection should include sufficient colon to allow the anastomosis to be performed in an area of colon relatively free of diverticula. The distal resection margin should be the proximal rectum. If the fistulous opening is not identifiable, indicating that it is small in diameter, nothing needs to be done to identify the bladder fistula. Urinary catheter drainage for 7 to 10 days, followed by cystographic verification of closure of the fistula, is sufficient therapy. Depending on the severity of the related complications of diverticulitis (obstruction, inflammation, abscess, sepsis, other fistulas), it may occasionally be necessary to perform a two-stage procedure, the first stage being segmental colectomy and colostomy formation and the second stage consisting of closure of the colostomy. Either the one- or two-stage procedure can be done with low morbidity and mortality and with less than a 5% recurrence rate. The three-stage approach of diverting colostomy, then resection, and finally colostomy closure is not recommended because the inflammatory process and the fistula are not removed at the first operation, leaving potential sources of sepsis.

Although rare in the past, recent reports indicate an increase in the occurrence of colovaginal fistulas. Almost all patients with colovaginal fistulas have had hysterectomies. The only consistent symptom is feculent vaginal discharge. About 40% of patients have intermittent abdominal pain and distention. A mass may be felt on pelvic examination; on vaginal speculum examination, the fistula opening is visible in 85% of cases. The diagnosis is confirmed in 50% of cases by barium enema.

Unless other complications of diverticulitis are present, a one-stage procedure is appropriate. The involved colon is resected and a primary anastomosis performed. The vaginal defect is closed if this can be easily accomplished, but such a defect usually closes spontaneously if left open.

Diarrhea, abdominal pain, and constitutional symptoms are frequently observed in patients with diverticular coloenteric fistulas. The usual signs of coloenteric fistula are abdominal tenderness, abdominal distention, and pelvic mass. Barium enema is diagnostic in 40% to 100% of patients. The preferred operative management of an uncomplicated coloenteric fistula is en bloc resection of the involved segment of small intestine, the fistula, and the diseased segment of colon. Primary anastomoses of both the small intestine and colon are then performed. If there are complicating factors, such as other fistulas, intraabdominal abscess, or inadequate bowel preparation secondary to obstruction, primary anastomosis of the small intestine, combined with colostomy formation, is performed as the first stage of a two-stage procedure.

DIVERTICULITIS OF THE CECUM AND ASCENDING COLON

The actual incidence of right-sided diverticula is not known; estimates based on barium enema examinations are between 5% and 10%.[2] The incidence of true diverticula is higher in the cecum and ascending colon than in the remainder of the colon, but false diverticula still predominate. True diverticula tend to be solitary and to originate in the anterior cecum close to the ileocecal valve. They occur in only 1% to 2% of the population. Most are asymptomatic, and the diagnosis is usually made by pathologic examination.

When patients with right-sided diverticula develop diverticulitis, the symptom complex is similar to that in acute appendicitis, and misdiagnosis is frequent.[10,11] Patients with right-sided diverticulitis are generally younger than patients with left-sided disease and are older than most patients with appendicitis.[10] Patients with right-sided diverticulitis are usually in their late 30s or 40s; patients with left-sided diverticulitis are usually more than 50 years of age.[10] Patients with right-sided diverticulitis have a longer duration of illness than patients with appendicitis, infrequently vomit, and feel pain initially in the right lower quadrant rather than the middle abdomen. Despite these dissimilarities, misdiagnosis of acute appendicitis is made in over 60% of patients who are later found to have right-sided diverticulitis.[10,11] In only 20% of cases is the correct diagnosis made preoperatively. CT scanning may improve diagnosis of right-sided diverticulitis. CT findings include thickening of the colonic wall, extraluminal mass involving the cecum or ascending colon, and signs of pericolic inflammation. CT scanning is recommended in patients with atypical appendicitis who are elderly and in whom right-sided diverticulitis is being considered as a diagnosis. Barium enema examination is seldom helpful because many patients have a single diverticulum that is not visible on barium examination. Associated findings, such as compression of the colon, are nonspecific and usually nondiagnostic.

At the time of operation, it may be difficult to establish a diagnosis of diverticulitis of the cecum or ascending colon. Most series report a correct intraoperative diagnosis in fewer than 60% of cases.[10] The presence of an intact, normal appendix eliminates appendicitis as the diagnosis in almost all circumstances. Usually, a large inflammatory mass involves the cecum and ascending colon. In many cases, however, it is difficult to distinguish the mass from a perforated carcinoma, and a right hemicolectomy should be performed. If the resection can be accomplished without contamination of the peritoneal cavity and a mechanical bowel preparation had been accomplished preoperatively, a primary anastomosis is acceptable. If there is spillage of abscess contents or bowel preparation was not feasible, an end ileostomy and mucous fistula can be performed. When the only abnormality noted at laparotomy is an inflamed diverticulum, a few authors propose leaving the diverticulum in situ and treating the patient with broad-spectrum antibiotics. If this therapy is undertaken, an appendectomy should be performed to avoid confusion if right lower quadrant symptoms recur. Most patients treated in this manner do not develop recurrent diverticulitis.

If the diagnosis of right-sided diverticulitis is made before operation, the patient should be treated as with sigmoid diverticulitis. If improvement is noted with intravenous fluids, broad-spectrum antibiotics, bowel rest, and analgesics, therapy should be continued and further testing performed when the patient recovers. If the patient does not improve or deteriorates, laparotomy is recommended.

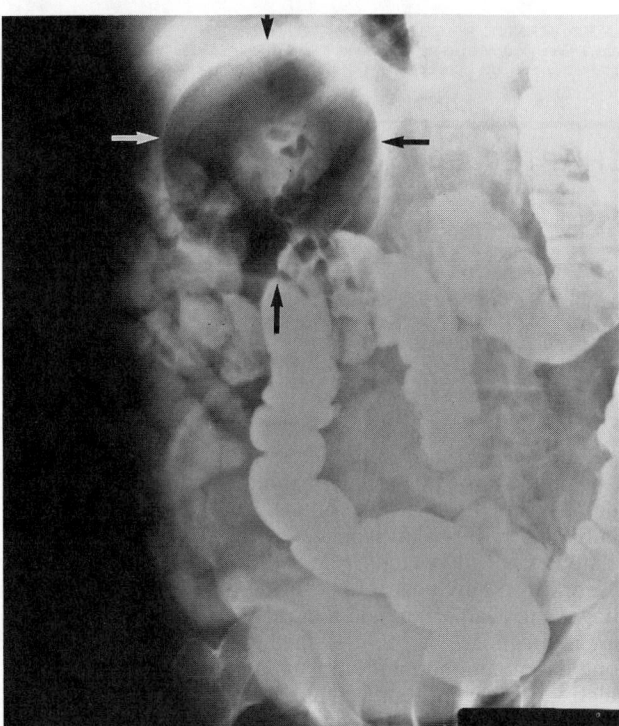

Figure 49-6. Postevacuation film of barium enema, demonstrating a giant colonic diverticulum (*arrows*) partially filled with barium. (McNutt R, Schmitt D, Schulte W. Giant colonic diverticula. Dis Colon 1988;31:625)

GIANT COLONIC DIVERTICULUM

Although uncommon, giant colonic diverticulum is a well-described clinical entity. Giant diverticula usually occur in the sigmoid colon, although they have been described in other areas of the left colon. Giant diverticula almost always arise from the antimesenteric border of the colon, unlike most left-sided diverticula, which develop where the vascular supply passes through the muscularis externa. Most are gas filled and therefore visible on plain abdominal radiographs. They range in size from 3 to 35 cm, with an average of 13.5 cm.

The pathogenesis of giant diverticula is not understood; they are assumed to be a complication of diverticulosis and not a separate entity. The most widely accepted explanation is that inflammation of a diverticulum causes narrowing of its neck and results in a ball-valve mechanism that entraps gases that pass into the diverticulum from the colon.

The predominant symptoms are abdominal pain, bloating, nausea, vomiting, and diarrhea. Physical findings include abdominal tenderness and a movable, lower abdominal mass. Perforation causes abdominal pain, leukocytosis, fever, and signs of localized or generalized peritonitis.

Although the diagnosis can be suspected based on plain radiographs of the abdomen, barium enema and CT scanning confirm the diagnosis. On barium enema, the diverticula fills with barium in 50% to 70% of cases, and frequently, other diverticula are demonstrated (Fig. 49-6). CT scanning of giant diverticula performed with intraluminal contrast usually demonstrates apposition of the colon and the giant diverticulum as well as the presence of barium in the diverticulum. On CT scan, wall thickness is variable and has not proved to be diagnostic.

Giant colonic diverticula are managed surgically. The patient should undergo standard mechanical bowel preparation, including oral antibiotics. The diverticulum, along with the adjacent colon, should be resected in continuity. Bowel continuity can usually be restored by end-to-end primary anastomosis.

REFERENCES

1. Spriggs EI, Marxer OA. Intestinal diverticula. Q J Med 1925;19:1.
2. Hughes LE. Postmortem survey of diverticular disease of the colon. Gut 1969;10:336.
3. Slack WW. The anatomy, pathology and some clinical features of diverticulitis of the colon. Br J Surg 1962;50:185.
4. Mendeloff AI. Thoughts on the epidemiology of diverticular disease. Clin Gastroenterol 1986;15:855.
5. Welch CE, Athanasoulis CA, Galdabini JJ. Hemorrhage from the large bowel with special reference to angiodysplasia and diverticular disease. World J Surg 1978;2:73.
6. Greenlee HB, Pienkos EJ, Vanderbilt PC, et al. Acute large bowel obstruction. Arch Surg 1974;108:470.
7. Labs JD, Sarr MG, Fishman EK, et al. Complications of acute diverticulitis of the colon: improved early diagnosis with computerized tomography. Am J Surg 1988;155:331.
8. Stabile BE, Puccio E, Van Sonnenberg E, Neff CC. Preoperative percutaneous drainage of diverticular abscesses. Am J Surg 1990;159:99.
9. Woods RJ, Lavery IC, Fazio VW, et al. Internal fistulas in diverticular disease. Dis Colon Rectum 1988;31:591.
10. Gouge TH, Coppa GF, Eng K, Ranson JH, Localio SA. Management of diverticulitis of the ascending colon: 10 years' experience. Am J Surg 1983;145:387.
11. Graham SM, Ballantyne GH. Cecal diverticulitis: a review of the American experience. Dis Colon Rectum 1987;30:821.

SURGERY: SCIENTIFIC PRINCIPLES AND PRACTICE, Second Edition, edited by
Lazar J. Greenfield, Michael W. Mulholland, Keith T. Oldham, Gerald B. Zelenock,
and Keith D. Lillemoe. Lippincott–Raven Publishers, Philadelphia, © 1997.

CHAPTER 50

ACUTE GASTROINTESTINAL HEMORRHAGE

RICHARD H. TURNAGE

Acute hemorrhage from the gastrointestinal (GI) tract is a common clinical problem encountered by a variety of medical and surgical disciplines. The morbidity and potential mortality risks associated with this condition necessitate that all physicians who care for these patients have a working knowledge of the principles of resuscitation, diagnostic evaluation, and therapeutic options. The differential diagnosis of acute GI hemorrhage encompasses a long list of common and unusual conditions. Fortunately, relatively few conditions comprise most causes commonly seen in practice. The initial evaluation and basic therapy for these patients are similar regardless of the underlying cause. Localizing the site of hemorrhage relative to the ligament of Treitz directs the evaluation and treatment. Sites of hemorrhage have been defined as within either the upper or lower GI tract based on the anatomic relation of the lesion to the ligament of Treitz. Hemorrhage from the esophagus, stomach, and duodenum accounts for about 80% of cases of GI hemorrhage, with nearly all of the remainder coming from the colon. The small intestine is the site of hemorrhage in about 1% of cases. The causes of overt upper and lower GI hemorrhage are listed in Tables 50-1 and 50-2, respectively.

CLINICAL PRESENTATION

A directed history and physical examination provides initial evidence of the site of hemorrhage. *Hematemesis,* the vomiting of blood, usually indicates a source of hemorrhage proximal to the ligament of Treitz. Aspiration of blood or "coffee grounds" from a nasogastric tube is also

Table 50-1. DIFFERENTIAL DIAGNOSIS OF ACUTE UPPER GASTROINTESTINAL HEMORRHAGE

Peptic ulcer disease
  Duodenal ulcer
  Gastric ulcer
Acute gastritis
  Stress gastritis
  Alcoholic gastritis
  Drug-induced gastritis
Gastroesophageal varices
Mallory-Weiss tear
Dieulafoy disease
Esophageal, gastric, or duodenal tumors
Aortoduodenal fistula
Esophagitis
Angiodysplasia
Hemobilia
Pancreatitis-induced pseudoaneurysm

Table 50-2. DIFFERENTIAL DIAGNOSIS OF ACUTE LOWER GASTROINTESTINAL HEMORRHAGE

Colonic diverticular disease
Colonic vascular ectasias
Small intestinal diverticular disease
  Meckel's diverticulum
  Pseudodiverticula
Inflammatory bowel disease
  Chronic ulcerative colitis
  Crohn's disease
Colonic neoplasms
Small intestinal neoplasms
Angiodysplasia
Aortoenteric fistula
Colitis
  Infectious
  Ischemic
  Radiation-induced
Internal hemorrhoidal disease

indicative of an upper GI source. *Melena,* the passage of black tarry stools, is usually associated with an upper GI source, but lower GI sources may also be associated with melena, particularly small intestinal and right colonic lesions. Melena is produced by the breakdown of blood by enteric bacteria and may be seen with as little as 50 mL of blood added to the alimentary tract. *Hematochezia* is the passage of bright red blood through the rectum and is most commonly associated with colonic lesions. Upper GI sources may produce hematochezia in cases of massive hemorrhage. The rate of bleeding in this instance is frequently associated with hemodynamic instability.

The clinical history may suggest the etiology of hemorrhage as well as determine the presence of prognostic factors. The onset of hemorrhage following several days of worsening epigastric or upper abdominal pain suggests peptic ulcer disease; whereas, hematemesis or melena following vomiting or retching suggests a Mallory-Weiss tear. Massive, painless upper GI hemorrhage in a patient with cirrhosis should suggest the diagnosis of variceal hemorrhage, although other etiologies including peptic ulcer disease must also be considered. Massive, painless lower GI hemorrhage in an elderly patient suggests bleeding from colonic diverticula.

The presence of cardiac, pulmonary, and renal disease significantly influences the patient's outcome. Medication use, especially nonsteroidal antiinflammatory agents (NSAIDs), aspirin, corticosteroids, and anticoagulants, should be reviewed. The use of NSAIDs is associated with a marked increase in the incidence of upper GI mucosal lesions and bleeding, particularly in the elderly.

A systematic physical examination should document the magnitude of the hemorrhage and the patient's ability to compensate. Massive hemorrhage is associated with signs and symptoms of shock, including cool, clammy, mottled skin, tachycardia, tachypnea, flat jugular veins, oliguria, and perhaps hypotension. These responses may be altered by the patient's age, concomitant medical problems, and medications. Physical examination should also document evidence of cirrhosis and portal hypertension (eg, ascites, spider angiomas, hepatosplenomegaly, palmar erythema, and large hemorrhoidal veins). A rectal examination can reveal the presence of bright red blood or melena.

Initial Evaluation and Resuscitation

As soon as a patient presents with GI hemorrhage, two large-bore intravenous lines should be placed in peripheral veins and intravascular volume resuscitation begun with an isotonic saline solution. Lactated Ringer solution is often preferred to 0.9% normal saline because the amount of sodium and chloride administered in lactated Ringer solution more closely approximates the electrolyte composition of the whole blood. Most patients stop bleeding spontaneously, and crystalloid volume resuscitation is all that is required. The massively bleeding patient should receive packed red blood cells to restore the intravascular volume and oxygen-carrying capacity. The decision to transfuse blood or blood products depends on the individual needs of the patient and the disease process encountered. The risks of the blood product (ie, infection and allergic reactions) must be carefully weighed against the risks of withholding transfusion (ie, anemia, decreased oxygen-carrying capacity, coagulopathy).

The propensity of the lesion to rebleed or to continue bleeding is an important factor in the decision to transfuse blood. Esophageal varices have a significant risk of recurrent or continued hemorrhage, and the transfusion of blood should be used earlier in the treatment of patients bleeding from this cause. Although most gastric and duodenal ulcers cease bleeding spontaneously, endoscopic findings of active hemorrhage or a visible vessel identify a lesion in which rebleeding or continued bleeding is likely. In contrast, the identification of patients with conditions associated with a low likelihood of continued hemorrhage or rebleeding (eg, Mallory-Weiss tears) should prompt crystalloid resuscitation in stable patients who appear to have stopped bleeding.

The hemodynamic reserve of a patient should also be carefully considered in the decision to use blood products. Compromised cardiac reserve, pulmonary disease, and vascular disease necessitate optimizing oxygen delivery, often with the use of blood products. In such patients, the risk of myocardial ischemia and infarction may be greater than the risk from the transfusion of blood products.

On presentation, blood is drawn for type and crossmatch, complete blood count with platelet count, electrolyte determination, liver function tests, and coagulation profiles. It is important to emphasize that on presentation, the hematocrit or hemoglobin level does not accurately reflect the magnitude of acute blood loss. Estimates of the severity of hemorrhage must be based on clinical parameters.

A nasogastric tube should be placed shortly after presentation and the presence of gastric blood determined. The absence of blood in bilious gastric fluid suggests a lower intestinal source. If no bilious fluid is obtained, esophagogastroduodenoscopy is necessary to exclude a duodenal source of hemorrhage. The unreliability of nasogastric aspiration for excluding an upper GI source of bleeding has been repeatedly confirmed; nearly 20% of patients with a clear nasogastric aspirate are bleeding from an upper GI source.[1] If hemorrhage has been significant, gastric lavage through a large-bore tube is used to clear the stomach of clot to facilitate endoscopy. Many patients stop bleeding before or during resuscitation and cleansing of retained blood from the stomach. Iced solutions are not recommended for gastric lavage because of the potential for systemic hypothermia with attendant adverse effects on coagulation, oxygen delivery, and hemodynamic stability.

Careful hemodynamic monitoring of these potentially critically ill patients is vital to successful management. Patients who are actively bleeding and those who have recently sustained significant hemorrhage should be admitted to an intensive care unit for close monitoring of hemodynamic parameters and for signs of continued or recurring hemorrhage. The presence of significant underlying illness, such as cardiac, renal, hepatic, or pulmonary insufficiency, necessitates invasive cardiac monitoring

with central cardiac and arterial catheters. The information gained from these devices allows cardiac performance to be optimized during intravascular volume replacement. Central venous catheterization should be performed only after initial volume resuscitation through peripheral sites. The placement of a urinary catheter and frequent monitoring of heart rate, blood pressure, gastric aspirate, and mentation are the minimum necessary to monitor all patients who have suffered GI hemorrhage. The importance of prompt, adequate resuscitation was first suggested by the observation that delayed or inadequate resuscitation was a significant factor contributing to the death of patients bleeding from peptic ulcer disease.[2]

Diagnostic Procedures

Despite well-described clinical scenarios for nearly all of the common causes of GI hemorrhage, none are adequately reliable to define the site and cause of hemorrhage. Therefore, invasive diagnostic approaches required. The first step in determining the etiology of bleeding is to place a nasogastric tube and examine the gastric aspirate. If blood is found in the stomach, an immediate esophagogastroduodenoscopy often defines the site of hemorrhage. In upper GI bleeding cases in which esophagogastroduodenoscopy is unsuccessful and in many cases of lower GI bleeding, other diagnostic methods are required to define the site and cause of hemorrhage and to appropriately begin to plan therapy. A general algorithm for evaluating acute upper and lower GI hemorrhage is presented in Figures 50-1 and 50-2, respectively.

Endoscopy

Esophagogastroscopy. The widespread availability of flexible endoscopy has revolutionized the diagnostic approach to patients suffering GI hemorrhage. Numerous studies have documented the unequivocal diagnostic superiority of endoscopy over contrast radiography in demonstrating sites of upper GI hemorrhage. The literature documents a diagnostic sensitivity of 70% to 85% and a high specificity (about 90%) for endoscopy in bleeding patients. Contrast radiography has been shown to correctly define the site of hemorrhage in less than 50% of all cases and is associated with at least a 30% error rate.[3] The consensus is that endoscopy demonstrates benefits that are not reflected in mortality statistics. The early definitive diagnosis of surgically correctable lesions in patients who rebleed facilitates operative planning and may prevent delays, a factor that is clearly associated with increased morbidity and mortality. Endoscopic identification of the source of hemorrhage may allow the clinician to estimate the risk of subsequent rebleeding or continued hemorrhage, and it facilitates long-term management. Endoscopy plays an important therapeutic role and has been shown to reduce the need for operative management as well as the risks of morbidity and mortality.

The timing of endoscopy is crucial. Proponents of early endoscopy (within 12 hours of admission) cite an increased likelihood of observing the suspected lesion bleeding. Less than 20% of lesions visualized 24 hours or more after hemorrhage have endoscopic signs of active or recent bleeding.[4] This can be important for patients with more than one disease process identified at endoscopy. When performed early, endoscopy is over 90% sensitive in demonstrating the site of hemorrhage. Factors that limit the diagnostic efficacy of endoscopy in actively bleeding patients are primarily related to impaired visibility, abnormal anatomy, and processes that simulate ulcers. The most common cause of diagnostic failure is blood retained in the stomach and duodenum, preventing adequate inspec-

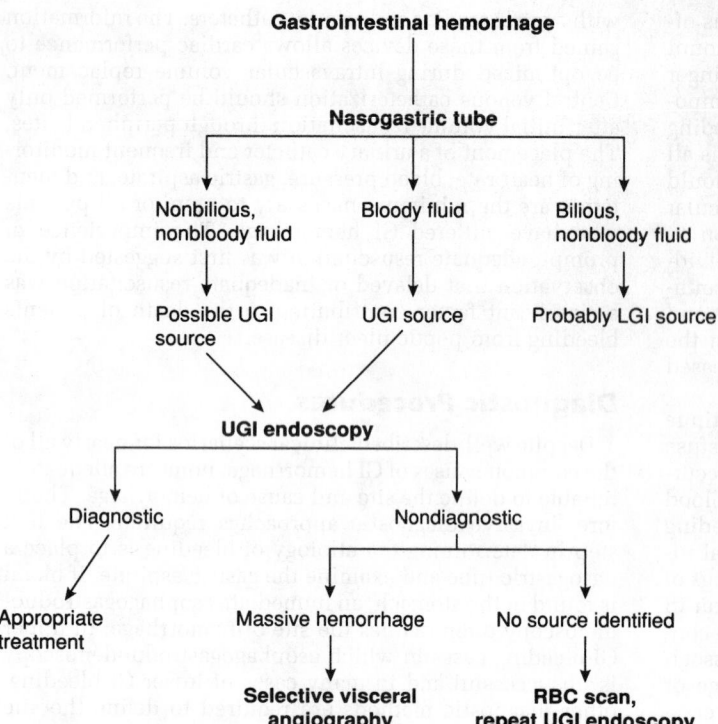

Figure 50-1. Diagnostic steps in the evaluation of acute upper gastrointestinal hemorrhage.

tion of mucosal surfaces. Pathologic changes, such as scarring of the duodenal bulb from chronic peptic ulcer disease, may prevent adequate inspection and lead to diagnostic failure. In addition, the endoscopist may be mislead by a number of factors that simulate an ulcer or occur concomitantly with the lesion responsible for the hemorrhage. Antacids adherent to the mucosa may simulate peptic ulcerations, particularly when mixed with blood. Nasogastric tube suction artifacts and endoscopic trauma may also mimic acute mucosal erosions.

Performing an emergent or urgent esophagogastroscopy in an actively bleeding or recently bleeding patient is associated with an increased incidence of complications related to the procedure. In one survey, the complication rate was 0.9%, about eight times higher than the 0.13% complication rate found in a survey of elective procedures.[1,5] Potential complications include aspiration, recurrent or increased hemorrhage, respiratory depression from sedatives, and perforation of the esophagus, stomach, or duodenum. The risks of endoscopy can be minimized by performing the procedure in the intensive care unit with adequate monitoring of the patient's respiratory and hemodynamic parameters. Endoscopy should be performed in a hemodynamically stable patient after volume resuscitation.

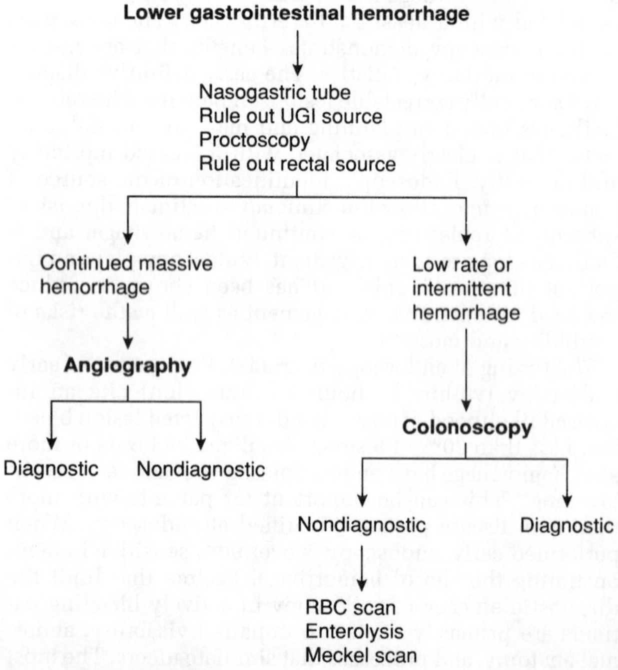

Colonoscopy. The frequent presence of asymptomatic colonic diverticulosis and vascular ectasia in the elderly makes it imperative to precisely determine the site of lower GI hemorrhage. In general, colonoscopy and selective visceral angiography are the most useful diagnostic procedures for determining the cause of lower GI hemorrhage. The best candidates for colonoscopy are patients who are minimally bleeding at the time of the study. Colonic lavage with polyethylene glycol solution clears the lumen of clot and stool, providing adequate visualization of the mucosa. The lavage solution can be administered orally or by an enteral feeding tube placed in the stomach or duodenum. As with esophagogastroduodenoscopy for upper GI hemorrhage, the diagnostic efficacy of colonoscopy decreases significantly as the length of time from the initial hemorrhage increases. Thus diagnostic studies should be performed expeditiously after the patient is resuscitated and stabilized. The appropriate use of colonoscopy requires a clinically stable patient who is not profusely bleeding. Massive hemorrhage or hemodynamic instability produce a situa-

Figure 50-2. Diagnostic steps in the evaluation of acute lower gastrointestinal hemorrhage.

tion in which diagnostic yield is minimal and the potential for complications is significant.

The colonoscopic diagnosis of vascular ectasia can be more difficult than angiographic diagnosis, especially in the presence of acute bleeding. Vascular ectasia may be mimicked by the vascular spiders, varices, and venous stars of chronic liver disease, telangiectasia associated with chronic renal failure, hereditary telangiectasia, vasculitic lesions, and focal hypervascularity of radiation, ulcerative colitis, Crohn's disease, and ischemic colitis. In addition, traumatic and suction artifacts produced during the examination may be confused with vascular ectasia. Furthermore, following significant bleeding and hypovolemia, blood flow is shunted away from the colonic mucosa, and vascular ectasia may not be evident in inadequately resuscitated patients.

Because hemorrhage associated with diverticular disease is often massive, colonoscopy may have limited efficacy in patients bleeding from this cause. In patients with diverticular bleeding, diverticula are readily identified; however, the precise site of hemorrhage can be difficult to discern. The presence of blood throughout the colon does not ensure a right-sided lesion because blood readily refluxes retrograde from the left colon to the right. Colonoscopy is valuable in excluding uncommon causes of acute colonic hemorrhage, such as colitis, polyps, and cancer.

Intraoperative Enteroscopy. Intraoperative endoscopy has been shown to be valuable in the rare patient without clear definition of the site of bleeding prior to laparotomy. The procedure can be performed without undue difficulty and may allow localization of the site of hemorrhage, thus limiting the extent of resection. Localization of Dieulafoy and angiodysplastic lesions in the stomach may allow precise resection or ligation. Transillumination of the intestine during intraoperative enteroscopy may demonstrate angiodysplastic lesions, and insufflation of the intestine may aid in the demonstration of small bowel diverticula. This procedure should be performed before committing patients to subtotal colectomy without clear documentation of the source of lower GI hemorrhage.

Selective Visceral Angiography

Selective visceral angiography is a useful and safe diagnostic tool in patients with severe upper and lower GI hemorrhage. Diagnostic angiography is primarily used for patients in whom endoscopy cannot be performed or has been unsuccessful in finding the source of hemorrhage. Successful angiographic identification of the source of hemorrhage mainly depends on the presence of active arterial bleeding at the time of the study. This requirement usually necessitates that the procedure be performed shortly after admission to the hospital. Extravasation of contrast is seen if the patient is bleeding at rates greater than 0.5 to 1 mL/min.[6] This figure, derived from animal studies, correlates with the loss of 4 to 5 units of blood per day in humans. Patients are likely to be bleeding at a rate that is angiographically detectable if they require continuous volume infusion to maintain hemodynamic stability. No studies compare the diagnostic accuracy of angiography and endoscopy for demonstrating sites of upper GI bleeding, and selective visceral angiography and endoscopy are complementary in evaluating an actively bleeding patient. In massively bleeding patients, endoscopic visualization is often severely limited, and selective mesenteric arteriography is often useful for demonstrating the site of bleeding (Fig. 50-3). Selective visceral angiography may be particular valuable in elucidating the etiology of lower GI hemorrhage. Angiography may detect vascular patterns diagnostic of vascular ectasia, or it may demonstrate extravasation of contrast into the lumen of the bowel as seen with hemorrhage from diverticula. Of greatest importance is the localization of the site of hemorrhage in those patients bleeding massively. Failure to visualize a bleeding point is usually due to the cessation of active bleeding at the time of angiography. The risks of angiography are primarily related to technical complications of the procedure (eg, arterial thrombosis and embolism) and to acute renal insufficiency from the intravascular contrast agent.

Radionuclide Scans

Abdominal scintigraphy with ^{99m}Tc sulfur colloid and ^{99m}Tc-labeled red blood cells may be useful for localizing intermittent bleeding or lesions with slow rates of hemor-

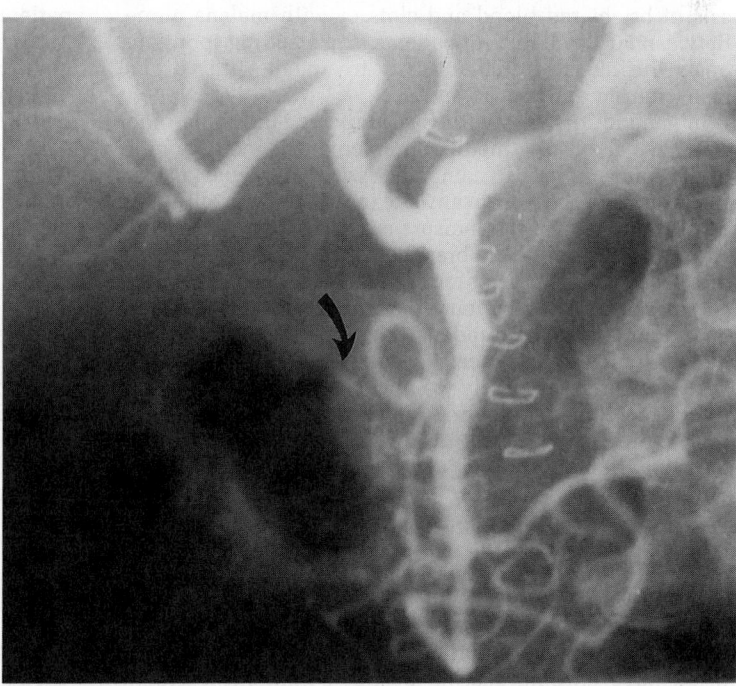

Figure 50-3. Selective celiac arteriography with injection into the common hepatic artery in a patient bleeding from a duodenal diverticulum. Extravasation of contrast from a branch of the gastroduodenal artery can be seen (*arrow*).

rhage. Abdominal scintigraphy done after the injection of radiolabeled erythrocytes detects bleeding at rates as low as 0.1 mL/min. ^{99m}Tc-labeled red blood cells are most commonly used because of their longer circulating half-life and less uptake by the liver and spleen than radiolabeled sulfur colloid. Because ^{99m}Tc sulfur colloid is rapidly cleared by the reticuloendothelial system (plasma disappearance half-time is 1.5 to 2.5 minutes), only actively bleeding sites are demonstrated. Furthermore, because the agent is avidly accumulated by Kupffer cells and other reticuloendothelial cells, bleeding at the hepatic and splenic flexures of the colon and duodenum may be obscured by isotope concentrations in the liver and spleen. Injection of radiolabeled red blood cells with scanning at 12 hours or longer may allow for the detection of slow or intermittent hemorrhage. Although nuclear scanning lacks the spatial resolution and diagnostic precision of angiography and endoscopy, it can be valuable for localizing the site of hemorrhage not apparent otherwise. This technique can be particularly valuable in evaluating intermittent lower GI hemorrhage in patients in whom endoscopy has been inconclusive. Precise localization of the site of hemorrhage may be obscured by the rapid distribution of isotope throughout the intestine by peristalsis or by accumulation in the right colon.

PEPTIC ULCER DISEASE

Peptic ulcer disease is the most common cause of acute upper GI hemorrhage, accounting for nearly 40% of cases in most series. About 15% to 20% of patients with peptic ulcer disease experience bleeding during the course of their disease, and bleeding is the initial manifestation in about 20%. Hemorrhage is the principal cause of death from peptic ulcer disease and has replaced intractable pain as the most frequent indication for surgery. Complications of peptic ulcer disease occur more commonly in older patients who often have medical problems that profoundly influence their morbidity and mortality.

Duodenal ulcers occur slightly more frequently than gastric ulcers. Penetration of the ulcer through the posterior wall of the duodenal bulb is associated with erosion into the gastroduodenal artery or one of its branches, resulting in brisk hemorrhage. Patients may present with hematemesis of bright red blood and clots or with melena alone. Between 80% and 90% of patients stop bleeding spontaneously during the initial stages of treatment with volume resuscitation and gastric lavage.

In general, patients with gastric ulcers tend to be older and have coexisting medical problems that increase morbidity and mortality compared with duodenal ulcers. Bleeding may occur from any site in the stomach, although ulcers occurring at the incisura are most common. At this site, involvement of the branches of the left gastric artery may result in brisk, if not torrential, hemorrhage. The clinical presentation of patients bleeding from gastric ulcers is similar to that of duodenal ulcers, with hematemesis, melena, and hematochezia. Hemorrhage complicating a gastric ulcer is less likely to subside spontaneously, more likely to rebleed following endoscopic hemostasis, and thus more likely to require operative intervention than bleeding due to duodenal ulcer.

An important risk factor for the development of GI hemorrhage and gastroduodenal ulcer formation is the use of NSAIDs. The stomach appears to be more susceptible than the duodenum to this injury. NSAID use has been associated with a continuum of mucosal injury, ranging from small acute mucosal hemorrhages to large chronic ulcers. It has been estimated that 10% to 15% of regular NSAID users have chronic gastric ulcers.[7] Symptoms correlate poorly with the degree of mucosal injury because as many as 20% of ulcers penetrating the muscularis are asymptomatic.[8] Case control and cohort studies have suggested that NSAIDs are associated with a relative risk of GI hemorrhage and ulceration ranging from about 2 to 9.1.[9] The risk of NSAID-associated complications is highest in the elderly. Patients with a prior history of peptic ulcer disease also appear to be at increased risk of NSAID-associated GI hemorrhage. Furthermore, a number of studies have documented significantly higher mortality rates among users of NSAIDs when compared with nonusers.[10]

The tremendous frequency with which NSAIDs are used by the elderly underscores the magnitude of this problem. The prudent use of these agents is an important responsibility of the prescribing physician. Those patients at increased risk of NSAID-induced hemorrhage should probably receive the prostaglandin E_1 analogue, misoprostol, which has been shown to prevent NSAID-induced gastric erosions and ulcers.[11] Histamine (H_2)-receptor blockers (ranitidine and cimetidine) are effective in preventing NSAID-induced duodenal ulcers, but appear to have little effect on the occurrence of gastric lesions.[8,12,13]

Attentive monitoring and aggressive resuscitation are important first steps in the successful treatment of patients bleeding from peptic ulcer disease. In those who stop bleeding spontaneously, treatment of the ulcer disease should be initiated, usually with cimetidine or ranitidine. Despite the lack of evidence that H_2-receptor antagonists reduce the rate of rebleeding, surgery, or death, the use of these agents is justified by their demonstrated ability to promote healing of peptic ulcers independent of the occurrence of GI hemorrhage.[14]

Endoscopic Treatment

Patients who continue to bleed or who have endoscopic findings suggestive of recurrent or continued hemorrhage are candidates for endoscopic therapy. A variety of endoscopic techniques are available to arrest hemorrhage from bleeding ulcers. All stop hemorrhage by inducing coagulation necrosis of the bleeding vessel and surrounding tissue using thermal or laser energy or by inducing thrombosis or sclerosis of the bleeding vessels. The precise method of treatment is less important than the correct selection of patients and the experience of the endoscopist.

Laser technology has been applied to the control of GI hemorrhage since 1974. Experience has accumulated with both argon and neodymium:yttrium aluminum garnet (Nd:YAG) lasers with more than 95% of centers using the Nd:YAG laser for photocoagulation. When directed into tissue, the absorbed light energy of the laser is converted into heat, which subsequently coagulates the tissue. The depth of tissue coagulation with the Nd:YAG laser is 1.7 mm, whereas that of the argon laser is 0.36 mm.[15] The low tissue penetration of the argon laser produces a technical disadvantage in the treatment of actively bleeding or larger vessels. Controlled trials and several uncontrolled clinical studies have examined the use of lasers in the treatment of acute GI hemorrhage with reports generally supporting the efficacy of lasers in controlling acute hemorrhage. In one randomized trial of 129 patients with nonvariceal bleeding, 100% initial hemostasis was achieved in the laser-treated group.[16] There were no differences in mortality or in the need for emergency surgery, but laser therapy significant reduced clinical rebleeding. It is significantly that in this study, nearly one third of the patients were excluded because of equipment failure or inability to gain adequate access to the lesion.[16] In another study of 138 patients with arterial bleeding, visible vessels, or other stigmata of recent hemorrhage, a significant reduction in the rebleeding rate, need for surgery, and mortality was achieved with laser photocoagulation.[17]

Thus, it appears that laser technology can be safely used to treat many causes of upper GI hemorrhage with reasonable effectiveness in inducing permanent hemostasis, but it is highly operator-dependent and can only be applied to favorably located lesions. Successful hemostasis depends on precisely identifying the bleeding vessel with an en face orientation to the lesion. Treatment with a tangential orientation to lesions is not possible, resulting in a significant 10% to 30% technical failure rate. The expense of this technology and the fact that laser units are not portable have encouraged the development and more frequent use of other methods of hemostasis.

Heater probes and monopolar and bipolar electrocoagulation probes control upper GI hemorrhage as effectively as the lasers, but lack many of its disadvantages. Monopolar probes apply high-frequency electrical current to the tissue, resulting in localized heating to 100°C and sealing of the bleeding vessel by coagulation necrosis of the surrounding tissue and vessel wall. To control bleeding, gentle pressure is applied to compress the vessel wall and occlude the lumen during coagulation. In uncontrolled trials, monopolar electrocoagulation probes have been shown to effectively arrest nonvariceal hemorrhage in 80% to 95% with about 12% of patients rebleeding and ultimately requiring operative treatment.[18] The depth of thermal injury is unpredictable with dry electrodes and varies with the amount of contact pressure and tissue adherence. Irrigating the tip of the electrode with water limits the area and depth of coagulation, prevents tissue adherence, and limits the risk of clot dislodgement. The risk of perforation is about 2%.

Multipolar electrocoagulation (bicap) probes consist of three equally spaced pairs of bipolar microelectrodes. This orientation of electrodes allows coagulation of tissue from tangential approaches and eliminates some of the disadvantages of the monopolar probe, such as the unpredictable depth of thermal injury, adherence of tissue, and clot dislodgement. Electrocoagulation is carried out circumferentially around a vessel, with a depth of tissue coagulation between 1 and 5 mm, depending on the power used and the pressure applied to the probe. This method of electrocoagulation appears promising, with randomized studies of actively bleeding patients demonstrating significant reductions in emergency operations, transfusion requirements, duration of hospital stay, and overall treatment cost.[19]

Direct thermal coagulation of a bleeding point can also be produced by applying a heater probe, consisting of an aluminum tip coated with Teflon. The tip is rapidly heated to 250°C by an inner coil. The tip can be irrigated with a water jet to prevent accumulation of debris and clot. Heat conducted from the probe produces tissue coagulation to a depth of 1 to 5 mm. En face and tangential applications are effective in achieving hemostasis as long as the bleeding vessel is precisely identified. Clinical experience with this technique has demonstrated excellent results, with an initial hemostatic efficacy that exceeds 90% and a reduction in the rebleeding rate.

The injection of sclerosants has been well described as a method of treating esophageal varices and has recently been popular for controlling nonvariceal bleeding sites. Sodium morrhuate and ethanolamine oleate are most commonly used to treat esophageal varices, whereas ethanol and polidocanol are most commonly used for nonvariceal sites. These agents act by thrombosing bleeding vessels and causing necrosis and subsequent fibrosis of surrounding tissue. Epinephrine has been used to arrest acute upper GI hemorrhage, presumably by causing temporary vasoconstriction and platelet aggregation in the bleeding vessel. Clinical experience with sclerosants has been similar to that obtained with electrocoagulation. In one large multicenter study of 332 actively bleeding patients or patients with stigmata of recent hemorrhage who underwent injection of 98% alcohol around the lesions, only 2 patients continued to bleed, 20 rebled, and 10 required emergency operative intervention.[20] Similar success has been achieved with polidocanol, either alone or with epinephrine.

A 1989 National Institutes of Health consensus statement concluded that the two most promising forms of endoscopic hemostatic therapy for treating bleeding gastroduodenal ulcers were the heater probe and multipolar electrocautery.[21] A metaanalysis of 25 randomized trials of endoscopic therapy for bleeding ulcers concluded that endoscopic treatment methods have a beneficial effect on survival by reducing the rate of recurrent hemorrhage. This analysis suggested that endoscopic therapy results in a relative reduction of 69% in recurrent bleeding, 62% in emergent surgery, and 30% in mortality rate, with the greatest benefit seen in actively bleeding ulcers and ulcers with nonbleeding visible vessels.[22] The effectiveness of early aggressive endoscopic diagnosis and treatment is further supported by a report of 562 patients bleeding from a variety of causes of whom only 2.5% required emergency operations to control hemorrhage.[23]

The successful use of endoscopic therapies has relegated operative procedures to a rescue role for those cases in which endoscopy is unsuccessful in arresting hemorrhage. To define which patients require prompt operative treatment, the following factors must be considered: the magnitude of the hemorrhage; the physiologic ability of the patient to withstand continued or recurrent hemorrhage; and the likelihood of recurrent or continued hemorrhage. Patients older than 60 years and those with significant concurrent medical problems should undergo operative intervention earlier during the course of the hemorrhage. These patients poorly tolerate continued hemorrhage, recurrent hypotension, and repeated transfusions. Delayed operative intervention has been strongly associated with increased mortality. Commonly accepted indications for operative management of bleeding peptic ulcers include the following: (1) massive hemorrhage unresponsive to resuscitation; (2) continued bleeding unresponsive to nonoperative measures; (3) recurrent hemorrhage following initial pharmacologic or endoscopic control; (4) two or more hospitalizations for ulcer hemorrhage; (5) a second coexisting indication for operation.

The type of operation depends on the pathology encountered. For bleeding gastric ulcers, the operation of choice is gastric resection (to include the ulcer in the resected specimen) with or without vagotomy, depending on the ulcer type (see Chap. 23 on gastric and stress ulcers). For patients bleeding from duodenal ulcers, truncal vagotomy, pyloroplasty, and oversewing of the bleeding vessel is the most widely used operation. Highly selective vagotomy with duodenotomy and oversewing of the bleeding vessel has also been recommended. Direct ligation of the bleeding vessel through the duodenotomy should incorporate the gastroduodenal artery proximal and distal to the ulcer as well as the transverse pancreatic artery (Fig. 50-4).

The mortality rate traditionally reported for acute GI hemorrhage is 10%, with a large number of deaths directly related to exsanguination. This figure has not changed significantly in the past 40 years. Advances in critical care and in endoscopy have been offset by an increasingly older and chronically ill population. Clinically important prognostic factors are listed in Table 50-3.

Age is a significant prognostic factor that influences out-

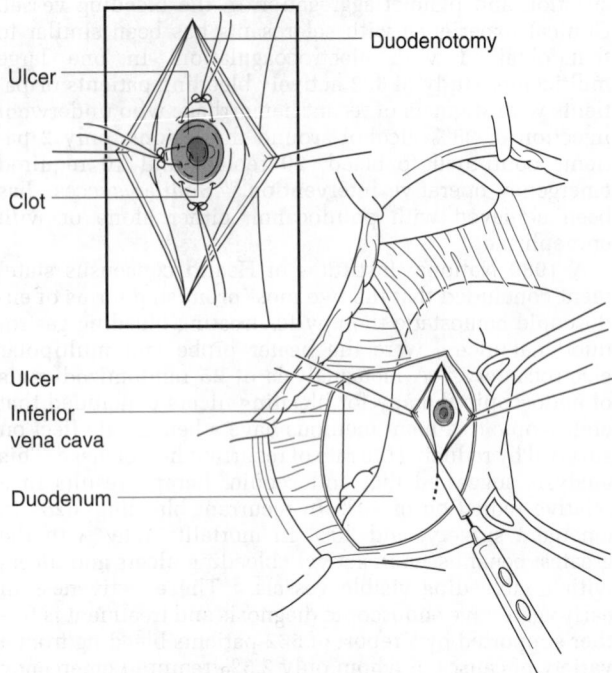

Figure 50-4. Diagram demonstrating the site of hemorrhage and method of ligation used for ulcers penetrating the posterior wall of the duodenal bulb. At this location, ulcers commonly erode into the gastroduodenal artery at the takeoff of the transverse pancreatic artery. Three-point ligation of these vessels (U-stitching) is important to prevent recurrent hemorrhage from the transverse pancreatic artery.

come in nearly every report. In a national survey of patients bleeding from a variety of upper GI sources, the mortality rate was 8.7% for patients younger than 60 years and 13.4% for those over 60.[1]

Concurrent chronic illness also markedly affects morbidity and mortality. Congestive heart failure, cardiac arrhythmias, central nervous system diseases, cirrhosis, cancer, pneumonia, chronic obstructive pulmonary disease, and renal disease have been associated with increased death rates among patients bleeding from upper GI sources. Patients who bleed while admitted to the hospital for other medical conditions were found to have a particularly high risk of dying. In one survey, the mortality rate for patients who bled while hospitalized for other conditions was 33%, whereas those presenting to the hospital with hemorrhage had a 7.1% mortality rate.[1]

Patients sustaining hemorrhagic shock are also at a high risk of dying. The mortality rate for these patients was 28% compared with 6% for those with blood pressures greater than 80 mmHg. The duration of hemorrhage and the volume of blood replacement have been directly related to mortality. The mortality rate for patients who bled more than 5 units of blood was 20%, whereas those requiring less than 5 units had a mortality rate of 5%.[1]

The appearance of the ulcer during endoscopy has also been correlated with the likelihood of persistent or recurrent hemorrhage and the necessity for operative intervention. A "visible vessel" in the base of an ulcer is associated with a 50% to 70% risk of rebleeding and increased mortality risks. Endoscopic findings of active bleeding, such as the spurting or streaming of blood from under a clot, also suggests a patient with a higher risk of requiring multiple units of blood and operative management and with increased morbidity and mortality.

STRESS GASTRITIS

Acute erosions of the gastric mucosa is a common phenomenon in critically ill patients. In early studies, esophagogastroduodenoscopy demonstrated evidence of stress gastritis in as many as 60% to 100% of critically ill patients. The incidence of overt hemorrhage is only about 10% to 20%, with just 2% to 5% of patients requiring transfusion. The incidence of stress gastritis appears to be have decreased since the 1970s when it was a frequently encountered problem in intensive care units. This reduction has been attributed to the widespread use of prophylactic gastric alkalinization and improved care and nutritional support of critically ill patients.

In general, stress gastritis is characterized by the appearance of multiple superficial gastric ulcerations within 12 to 14 hours of an acute injury. These lesions, initially localized to the fundus and body of the stomach, later involve the entire gastric surface. Patients at greatest risk include those with sepsis, major burns, or severe trauma. Patients with respiratory, hepatic, or renal insufficiency also appear to be at high risk of developing stress gastritis. In this setting, the disease appears to represent the gastric component of the multiorgan failure syndrome.

The pathogenesis of this disease is discussed in detail in Chapter 23. The primary defect is in the protective processes that maintain the integrity of the gastric mucosal barrier. Although some hydrogen ions are required for the development of stress gastritis, it is clear that the hypersecretion of acid is not the cause of mucosal injury. Altered gastric mucosal blood flow and impaired clearance of hydrogen ions from the mucosa appear to be of particular importance. Stress gastritis should be differentiated from the deep, often solitary ulcerations occurring in patients with severe central nervous system lesions (Cushing ulcers).

Overt bleeding is often heralded by the appearance of flecks of blood in the gastric aspirate. In general, hemorrhage is the only symptom that stress gastritis patients experience. The superficial nature of the lesions makes perforation unlikely.

GI hemorrhage in critically ill patients portends a very poor prognosis. In a study of 179 patients admitted to a medical intensive care unit, the mortality rate for patients who developed GI hemorrhage was 64% compared with 9.5% for those who did not bleed. Most deaths were attributed to coexisting organ failure.[24]

Several authors have suggested that certain populations are at greater risk for developing this complication than others. In a study of critically ill patients admitted to a

---

Table 50-3. PROGNOSTIC FACTORS FOR PATIENTS SUFFERING ACUTE UPPER GASTROINTESTINAL HEMORRHAGE

CLINICAL

Age over 60 y
Concurrent cardiac, pulmonary, hepatic, or renal disease
Massive hemorrhage
   Transfusion requirements (more than 5 units of blood)
   Hypotension
Continued hemorrhage
Bleeding gastroesophageal varices

ENDOSCOPIC

Visible vessel
Active hemorrhage with blood spurting or streaming from under a clot

medical intensive care unit, only respiratory failure and the presence of a coagulopathy appeared to significantly increase the risk of upper GI hemorrhage.[24] Similar results were obtained in a recent multicenter trial of 2252 patients. Patients requiring mechanical ventilation for more than 48 hours and those with a coagulopathy were significantly more likely to develop GI bleeding than patients without these factors.[25] Despite the identification of high-risk groups, in current clinical practice, most patients admitted to the intensive care unit receive prophylaxis.

Prophylactic therapy is directed toward preventing hemorrhage, primarily by neutralizing gastric acid, augmenting mucosal defenses, and removing or preventing of physiologic stress. Antacids and H_2-receptor antagonists appear to decrease the incidence of overt hemorrhage from stress gastritis with similar efficacy. Maintenance of an intragastric pH level greater than 3.5 to 4 has been associated with a reduced risk of hemorrhage. The frequent administration of antacids (up to every hour) can impose a significant burden on the nursing staff and thus makes H_2-receptor antagonists the the favored treatment. The addition of H_2-receptor antagonists to total parenteral nutrition solutions provides a simple and cost- effective way to administer these agents.

The alkalinization the gastric contents is associated with oral and fecal flora colonization of the stomach and may increase the risk of respiratory complications. Bacterial colonization of the stomach has been documented in 90% to 100% of critically ill patients being treated with antacids within 4 days of admission to the intensive care unit.[26] Colonization has been associated with an increased rate of nosocomial pneumonia, which can be reduced by using sucralfate as the prophylactic agent instead of antacids or cimetidine.[27] Several trials have shown that sucralfate is as effective as antacids or cimetidine in preventing overt hemorrhage from stress gastritis.[27]

In critically ill patients who experience overt hemorrhage, attention to blood replacement, intravascular volume restoration, and correction of coagulation defects are all important primary measures. Underlying sepsis must be sought and treated. Basic principles of resuscitation, as well as gastric lavage with saline, stop hemorrhage in more than 75% to 80% of patients. As soon as the patient is resuscitated, urgent endoscopy is indicated to determine the etiology of the hemorrhage. Many clinicians use antacids or H_2- receptor antagonists or both as first-line treatment of hemorrhage from stress gastritis. Several studies have suggested that antacid titration of gastric pH to greater than 5 stops active hemorrhage and prevents recurrent bleeding. Frequently, the doses required to arrest hemorrhage are much higher than those used for prophylaxis. H_2-receptor antagonists have also been used to arrest hemorrhage from stress gastritis.

Although endoscopic techniques have proved to be effective in arresting upper GI hemorrhage from peptic ulcer disease, there has been much less experience with this treatment for patients with stress gastritis. The high percentage of patients who stop bleeding spontaneously necessitate a large study population to prove efficacy of these techniques. In a series of 852 patients with a variety of causes of upper GI hemorrhage, endoscopic laser coagulation initially controlled bleeding in 92% of patients with acute gastric lesions, such as erosive gastritis or vascular malformations. The rebleeding rate in this series was 14%.[15]

Intraarterial infusion of vasopressin and transcatheter arterialembolization have also been used to successfully arrest hemorrhage from stress gastritis. Selective catheterization of the left gastric artery with continuous infusion of vasopressin, 0.2 to 0.4 IU/min, has been applied to arrest hemorrhage in patients not responding to more conserva-

tive methods. A randomized trial demonstrated initial control of bleeding in 80% of patients and permanent control in 67%.[28] Anecdotal experience with transcatheter embolization has also been reported. Hemorrhage from erosive gastritis is often diffuse, and the rich submucosal plexus of the stomach is so extensive that there is rarely one major artery supplying the area of hemorrhage, making embolization less likely to be effective. Embolization may be of greatest benefit in a small subset of high operative risk patients for whom other treatments have failed and a single bleeding site can be identified.

Less than 2% of patients bleeding from erosive gastritis ultimately require operative intervention to arrest hemorrhage. The dilemma facing the surgeon is that this patient poorly tolerates extensive procedures, yet lesser operations often fail to control hemorrhage. Regardless of the operation performed, mortality risk depends on the underlying illness, particularly in the presence of multiple organ failure. Mortality rates between 30% and 60% are commonly quoted, with as many as one fourth of deaths a direct result of continued hemorrhage.

A variety of surgical treatment options have been reported. These have included vagotomy and pyloroplasty with oversewing of bleeding sites, vagotomy and hemigastrectomy, total gastrectomy, and gastric devascularization. Most have been associated with similar mortality and rebleeding rates. The operative approach is best individualized to the patient's clinical status. In patients who are bleeding from relatively few discrete points, the combination of vagotomy, pyloroplasty, and oversewing of bleeding sites has been advocated as the procedure of choice. Rebleeding rates ranging from 25% to 61% have been reported.[29] Patients bleeding from diffuse disease should undergo more aggressive treatment. The combination of vagotomy, hemigastrectomy, and oversewing of bleeding points has been touted as more successful in these patients; however, rebleeding rates of 11% to 44% and operative mortality rates ranging from 33% to 63% have been associated with this procedure.[29] More extensive operations, such as near total gastrectomy or total gastrectomy are associated with significant mortality although they successfully stop hemorrhage.

GASTROESOPHAGEAL VARICES

Cirrhosis is a leading cause of death in the United States, and variceal hemorrhage is the common mode. About 30% of people with cirrhosis develop gastroesophageal varices, and of these patients, about 30% bleed as a result, usually within 1 to 2 years of diagnosis. Gastroesophageal varices are a significant cause of upper GI hemorrhage, accounting for about 20% of such cases. Patients with bleeding gastroesophageal varices tend to have much higher rebleeding rates, transfusion requirements, lengths of hospitalization, and risk of death than do patients bleeding from nonvariceal causes.[30]

Although the basic tenets of resuscitation for massive variceal hemorrhage are similar to those for any source of massive hemorrhage, intravenous volume resuscitation should be performed with fluids that have minimal sodium. The hyperaldosteronemic state of cirrhosis promotes sodium and water retention, with aggravation of ascites and peripheral edema. Accurate blood replacement is imperative because overtransfusion increases central venous pressure and worsens portal hypertension, thus exacerbating hemorrhage. Invasive cardiac monitoring with Swan-Ganz catheterization may be particularly useful for guiding volume replacement. Coagulation deficits should be aggressively corrected by administering fresh frozen plasma. Thrombocytopenia, secondary to hypersplenism or dilution, should be treated promptly with pooled platelet transfusions. Sedatives are best avoided or used sparingly because cirrhosis impairs the liver's ability to metabolize these drugs. Adequate prophylaxis for delirium tremens should be administered.

As with other sources of upper GI hemorrhage, early endoscopy is imperative for successful diagnosis and therapy (Fig. 50-5). The identification of varices alone is not adequate to incriminate them as the source of the hemorrhage. Up to half of patients with cirrhosis bleed from a source other than varices. Furthermore, endoscopy may identify factors associated with a heightened risk of variceal hemorrhage, including the size and number of varices as well as the presence of red, blue, or other colored spots on the varix. The presence of gastric and duodenal varices and portal hypertensive changes in the gastric mucosa (portal gastropathy) can also influence therapeutic decisions and prognosis.

Vasopressin has commonly been used early in the management of variceal hemorrhage. An initial dose of 20 IU IV over 20 minutes, followed by an infusion of 0.2 to 0.6 IU/min IV, is used. The infusion is continued for 48 to 72 hours or until bleeding ceases, at which time the agent is tapered. If bleeding continues during this therapy, other treatments are instituted (eg, sclerotherapy or balloon tamponade). Surprisingly, given the widespread acceptance of vasopressin for the early management of bleeding esophageal varices, there have been no controlled prospective trials demonstrating a clear beneficial effect on outcome. A metaanalysis of four controlled trials comparing vasopressin infusion with placebo or conventional therapy demonstrated a 52% success rate with vasopressin for the initial control of hemorrhage but a 45% rebleeding rate. Vasopressin demonstrated no beneficial influence on survival.[31]

The risks of vasopressin are related primarily to cardiovascular effects, especially systemic vasoconstriction. This effect is particularly significant in patients with coronary artery disease. Coronary artery vasoconstriction may induce myocardial ischemia and infarction. Systemic hypertension and cardiac arrhythmias have also been associated with vasopressin. The simultaneous administration of nitroglycerin ameliorates many of the adverse hemodynamic effects of vasopressin and may enhance the effectiveness of vasopressin in controlling variceal bleeding. Although vasopressin therapy alone is clearly not adequate to definitively treat bleeding esophageal varices, this treatment may provide initial control of hemorrhage, reducing transfusion requirements and providing time for adequate resuscitation before definitive treatment.

Another temporizing method used for massively bleeding patients is balloon tamponade. The instrument most commonly used is a gastric tube with esophageal and gastric balloons. A proximal esophageal tube for aspirating swallowed secretions is also available. Pressure from the inflated gastric and esophageal balloons tamponades bleeding varices, controlling hemorrhage in more than 80% of cases. On deflation of the balloons, however, hemorrhage recurs in 25% to 50% of patients, thus limiting this technique to a temporizing role.[32] The greatest value of these tubes is for arresting massive hemorrhage that has been unresponsive to other measures, allowing time for resuscitation before definitive treatment.

When used inappropriately, the tubes are associated with significant morbidity and mortality. Complications occur in 4% to 9% of patients, the most frequent being aspiration pneumonitis. Measures to prevent pulmonary complications include endotracheal intubation before tube insertion and the placement of an esophageal tube to remove swallowed salivary secretions. Other significant complications include esophageal rupture or necrosis and

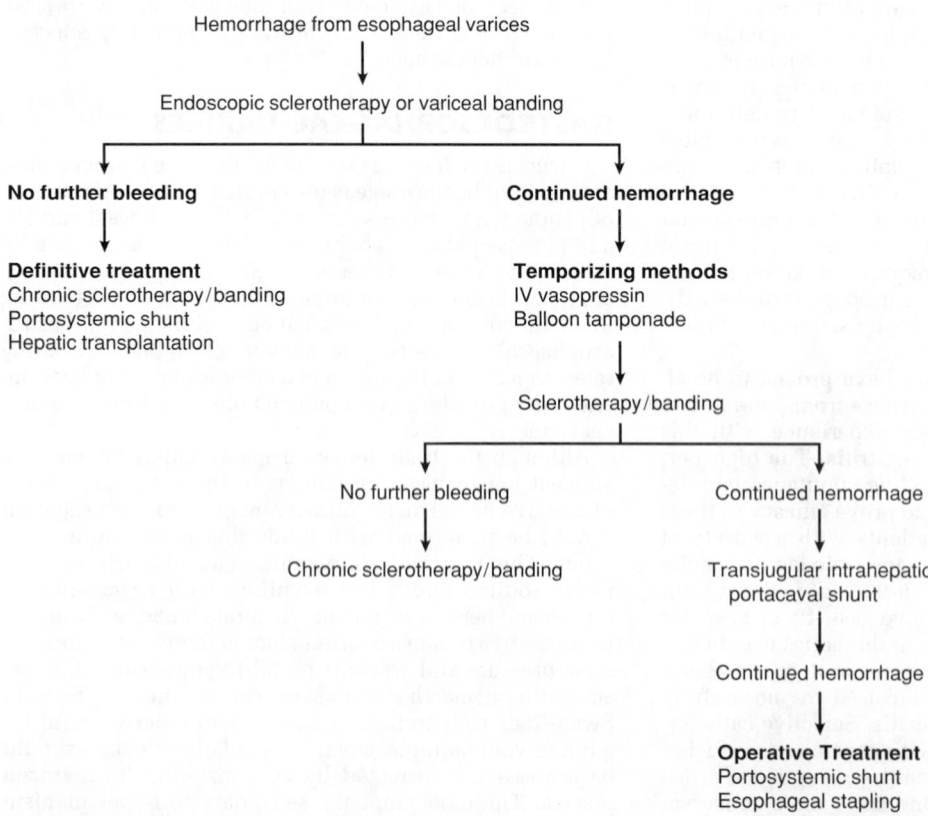

Figure 50-5. Therapeutic maneuvers in the management of acute hemorrhage from esophageal varices.

airway occlusion secondary to pharyngeal migration of the balloon.

A patient bleeding from esophageal varices should undergo urgent sclerotherapy or banding of varices at the time of the first emergency endoscopy. Endoscopic sclerotherapy has become the most widely used treatment for initial control of bleeding esophageal varices. Several controlled trials have confirmed that sclerotherapy arrests acute variceal hemorrhage in 90% to 95% of patients. A single treatment controls variceal bleeding in more than 70% of patients, and a second treatment increases the rate of control to between 90% and 95%. Sclerotherapy has been shown to be more effective than either balloon tamponade or vasopressin used alone. Patients who have stopped bleeding should undergo immediate sclerotherapy because the risk of recurrent hemorrhage is significant without the institution of definitive treatment. Continued or recurrent hemorrhage after sclerotherapy require temporary control with balloon tamponade and vasopressin, usually followed by urgent operative intervention.

Following control of the initial hemorrhage, sclerotherapy is repeated in 5 to 10 days and then at 1- to 3-week intervals until the varices have been obliterated. In general, this takes from three to five sclerotherapy sessions. During this period, prior to complete variceal obliteration, the risk of recurrent bleeding is at its highest. Chronic sclerotherapy appears to be at least as effective as portacaval or selective splenorenal shunt surgery in terms of preventing hemorrhage, ensuring survival, and preserving hepatic function. A metaanalysis of seven trials suggests that overall survival for patients with variceal bleeding was improved by sclerotherapy.[33]

Complications following sclerotherapy occur in 10% to 20% of patients and include local manifestations, such as perforation, stricture formation, and ulceration. Systemic complications, including fever and sepsis, have also been reported.

A more recent method of endoscopic control of variceal hemorrhage involves the mechanical ligation and strangulation of variceal channels by applying small, elastic O rings similar to those used for banding internal hemorrhoidal veins. In uncontrolled trials, variceal ligation was found to be comparable to endoscopic sclerotherapy in terms of controlling variceal hemorrhage and preventing recurrent bleeding; however, it caused substantially less morbidity, particularly esophageal ulceration and subsequent stricture formation.[34] Two randomized controlled trials comparing variceal ligation with sclerotherapy reported similar findings.[35,36]

Preliminary experience has been reported with nonoperative decompression of the portal venous system using a percutaneously created channel between a hepatic vein and the portal vein. This procedure, termed *transjugular intrahepatic portosystemic shunting*, uses expandable 8- to 10-mm metallic stents to maintain shunt patency. By supporting the shunt wall, the metallic stent prevents the elastic recoil of the hepatic parenchyma from occluding the shunt lumen and was associated with acute control of variceal hemorrhage in 29 of 30 patients in one large series.[37] For the most part, follow-up has been short with this procedure; however, shunt occlusion or stenosis appear to occur in a substantial number of patients when followed long-term. In one series of 96 patients who successfully underwent this procedure, shunt occlusion developed in 9 patients and shunt stenosis in 6 others. Many of these occluded shunts were successfully reopened with renewed patency. Shunt occlusion has been attributed to technical factors, intimal hyperplasia, and in situ thrombosis. In patients bleeding from esophageal varices, transjugular intrahepatic portosystemic shunting may be useful in the man-

agement of continued bleeding despite endoscopic treatment. This may be of particular value in place of an emergent portacaval shunt in a Child class C cirrhosis patient.

The operative management of bleeding esophageal varices is discussed in detail in Chapter 38.

MALLORY-WEISS TEARS

The Mallory-Weiss syndrome involves acute upper GI hemorrhage that occurs after retching or vomiting. These lesions account for about 5% to 15% of patients with upper GI bleeding. Mallory and Weiss described the presence of a laceration of the gastric cardia and postulated that violent emesis against an unrelaxed cardia was the mechanism of injury. Similar mucosal tears were produced in cadavers by forcing gastric contents against an occluded gastroesophageal junction. Other studies have demonstrated that vomiting raises intragastric pressure to levels capable of mucosal laceration.

The stereotypical patient with Mallory-Weiss syndrome is an alcoholic who begins to retch and vomit after an alcohol binge; however, endoscopy has identified significant numbers of patients with this who have no history of alcohol abuse. Initially, the vomitus is gastric contents without blood. Subsequently, the patient develops hematemesis and melena.

Initial management is similar to that for other sources of upper GI hemorrhage and includes volume resuscitation, gastric lavage, and decompression. Most patients with Mallory-Weiss tears stop bleeding spontaneously, either before treatment or after these early measures. Once bleeding has stopped, rebleeding is rare.

In patients who continue to bleed despite these maneuvers, nonoperative and operative therapeutic options are available. Nonoperative management, consisting of endoscopic electrocoagulation or injection therapy, has been successfully applied to these lesions. In cases not amenable to endoscopic therapy, operative management consists of oversewing the laceration through an anterior longitudinal gastrotomy in the middle third of the stomach. The mortality rate in recent series has been between 5% and 10%, with deaths related to associated diseases, most notably cirrhosis.

LOWER GASTROINTESTINAL HEMORRHAGE

The passage of maroon or bright red blood through the rectum suggests a source of hemorrhage distal to the ligament of Treitz. Although numerous potential causes of lower GI hemorrhage are possible (see Table 50-2), colonic diverticulosis and vascular ectasia of the colon are the most common. The relative frequency with which these conditions lead to lower GI hemorrhage is difficult to ascertain because both are common in the general population and are typically asymptomatic. Small bowel sources and other colonic pathology are relatively unusual causes of acute GI hemorrhage.

The first diagnostic step is gastric aspiration or esophagogastroduodenoscopy to rule out an upper GI source. As alluded to earlier, peptic ulcer disease is the most common cause of hematochezia and melena. Anoscopy and flexible or rigid sigmoidoscopy exclude sources of hemorrhage below the peritoneal reflection of the rectum, such as bleeding internal hemorrhoids.

The frequent presence of asymptomatic colonic diverticulosis and vascular ectasia in the elderly makes precise determination of the site of hemorrhage imperative. Recent improvements in outcome reflect more accurate preoperative localization of the bleeding source, permitting more directed and limited treatment. In general, colonoscopy and selective visceral angiography are the most useful diagnostic procedures for determining the site of lower GI hemorrhage. Because diagnostic efficacy decreases as the length of time from the initial hemorrhage increases, diagnostic studies should be performed expeditiously following resuscitation and stabilization of the patient. Colonoscopy may be of greatest value in patients who have stopped bleeding or who are bleeding at a slow rate, whereas selective visceral angiography is most valuable in patients who are actively bleeding at a rate that requires intravenous fluid and blood infusion to maintain hemodynamic stability. Abdominal scintigraphy following the infusion of ^{99m}Tc-labeled red blood cells may delineate the site of hemorrhage in those patients bleeding intermittently or at rates below those detectable by angiography. Preoperative localization of the site of hemorrhage is imperative to successfully treating these patients, and only rarely should laparotomy be performed without knowledge of the site of hemorrhage. In selected patients, intraoperative enteroscopy may be of value in defining the site of hemorrhage.

Colonic Diverticulosis

In Western society, the prevalence of colonic diverticula increases with age, and about 50% of people in their ninth decade of life are affected. About 20% of patients with diverticulosis have symptoms attributable to these lesions, but less than 5% experience hemorrhage.[38] Hemorrhage from diverticular disease is most often massive, associated with hematochezia and varying degrees of hemorrhagic shock. Classically, patients present with a sudden occurrence of mild lower abdominal discomfort, rectal urgency, and the subsequent passage of a large maroon or melenic stool. Because the colon can contain large volumes of blood, neither the volume nor the frequency of bloody stools is a reliable guide to the rate of hemorrhage. Despite the massive nature of hemorrhage, most patients with diverticular disease stop bleeding spontaneously (about 20% of patients suffer continued hemorrhage requiring urgent laparotomy). Fewer than 25% of patients suffer a second episode of diverticular hemorrhage, but most patients who do experience this subsequently have further bleeding.

Bleeding associated with diverticular disease comes from a perforated vasa recta located at the neck or apex of a diverticulum. The vasa recta penetrates the colonic wall from the serosa to the submucosa through obliquely oriented connective tissue septa. Protrusion of colonic mucosa through this connective tissue plane results in apposition of the diverticulum and the vasa recta. Eventual rupture of the arterial wall produces hemorrhage into the lumen of the bowel. Despite the well-known predilection of diverticular disease to the left colon, most bleeding comes from right-sided lesions.

The massive nature of the hemorrhage associated with diverticular disease limits the usefulness of colonoscopy. Rarely is a bleeding vessel seen within a diverticulum, and the presence of blood or clot within diverticula is of no diagnostic benefit. Selective mesenteric arteriography may demonstrate the luminal extravasation of contrast; however, in one study of patients bleeding from diverticulosis, angiographic localization was effective in less than 20% of patients.[39] Failure to visualize a bleeding point is usually due to cessation of active bleeding at the time of angiography.

Patients who stop bleeding should be treated expectantly because there is a relatively low risk of recurrent hemorrhage. About 10% of patients bleeding from colonic diverticula continue to bleed and ultimately require operative intervention. As with upper GI hemorrhage, the elderly and often infirm nature of the patients suffering diverticular hemorrhage necessitates prompt and accurate replacement of intravascular volume.

Nonoperative methods of arresting GI hemorrhage, including angiographic embolization and endoscopic electrocoagulation, have been reported. The end artery location of the vasa recta with limited collateral flow limits the usefulness of angiographic embolization because of a significant risk of colonic infarction. The rapid nature of the hemorrhage and the difficulty in defining the site of hemorrhage through the endoscope have prevented endoscopic treatments from being beneficial for bleeding diverticula.

Patients who continue to bleed from diverticular disease should undergo resection of the colon segment that contains the site of hemorrhage. If the bleeding diverticulum is located in the right colon, a right colectomy with ileotransverse colostomy is indicated. Subtotal colectomy for nonlocalized colonic hemorrhage rarely should occur. Subtotal colectomy is associated with greater perioperative morbidity rates than is segmental resection. In addition, postoperative diarrhea presents a significant problem to elderly patients. If the patient continues to bleed massively from the colon and all attempts at preoperative and intraoperative localization are unsuccessful, subtotal colectomy with ileoproctostomy may be required.

Colonic Vascular Ectasia

Vascular ectasias are believed to arise from the age-related degeneration of previously normal intestinal submucosal veins and overlying mucosal capillaries. These lesions are located most frequently in the cecum and ascending colon, although they may be found in the transverse and left colon or rectum in 20% to 30% of cases. Multiple lesions are common being present in 40% to 75% of all cases.[40] Endoscopically, these lesions appear as flat or slightly raised red lesions that are 2 to 10 mm wide. They may be round, stellate, or have sharply circumscribed fernlike margins. A prominent feeding vessel may be evident as well as a surrounding halo.

Microscopically, vascular ectasias consist of dilated, thin-walled vessels that appear to be ectatic veins, venules, and capillaries localized to the submucosa and mucosa. Concomitantly, a dilated submucosal vein is frequently found, and occasionally, an enlarged artery. It is believed that this variability of histologic patterns represents different stages of disease, with early changes being ectatic capillaries and venules and later lesions composed of arteriovenous communications.

The incidence of colonic vascular ectasias in the general population is difficult to determine because most patients who undergo evaluation are experiencing symptoms. Investigators have found colonic vascular ectasias in 2% to 6% of patients undergoing colonoscopy, depending on the indication for endoscopy.[40] In asymptomatic patients undergoing colonoscopic screening for neoplasms, the incidence of vascular ectasias was 0.93%.[40,41] These lesions may present with hematochezia, melena, occult blood loss, or iron deficiency anemia depending on the stage of the vascular malformation. Early lesions, histologically characterized by ectatic capillaries and venules, commonly present with low-grade recurrent bleeding and episodic hematochezia or melena. Most of these early lesions stop bleeding spontaneously and are rarely associated with life-threatening hemorrhage. Advanced lesions, histologically characterized as arteriovenous communications, may present with massive hemorrhage and hematochezia, progressing to hemorrhagic shock and death. Ten to 15% of patients present in this manner. Another 10% to 15% of patients present with occult intestinal blood loss, iron-deficiency anemia, and episodic heme-positive stools. Over 90% of patients stop bleeding spontaneously, thus allowing time for adequate evaluation before definitive treatment.

Vascular ectasias may be diagnosed by either colonoscopy or by selective mesenteric angiography. Colonoscopy has been reported to have a sensitivity of 80% in demonstrating vascular ectasias.[42] However, colonoscopic diagnosis of these lesions in actively bleeding patients may be confounded by the presence of various other incidental lesions, including traumatic and suction artifacts produced during the examination. In addition, after significant bleeding and hypovolemia, the shunting of blood flow away from the intestinal mucosa may obscure these lesions in inadequately resuscitated patients.

Selective mesenteric angiography may also demonstrate these lesions and compliment colonoscopy, particularly in patients who are massively bleeding or in whom colonoscopy was unrevealing or incomplete. Characteristic angiographic findings include the following:

1. A densely opacified and slowly emptying, dilated, tortuous vein. This finding is seen in 90% of patients and is best observed during the late venous phase of the angiogram.
2. A vascular tuft. This cluster of vessels, which empties slowly with opacification persisting into the venous phase, is seen in 66% to 75% of patients.
3. An early-filling vein. This is usually a segmental vein in the cecum or right colon, although at times, it may be the ileocolic vein. Early-filling veins can characteristically be visualized within 5 seconds after injecting them with contrast (Fig. 50-6). The extravasation of contrast material into the lumen of the bowel during angiography is seen in a minority of cases.

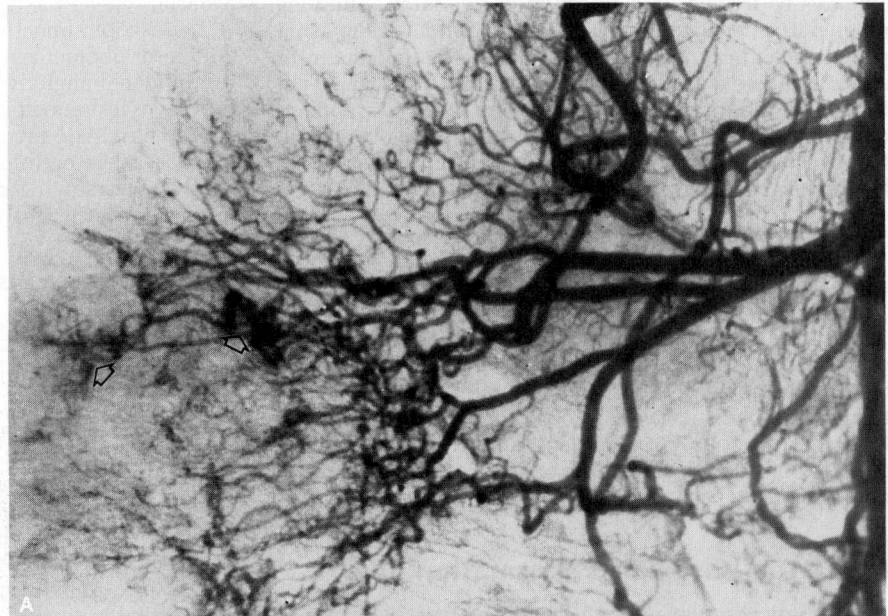

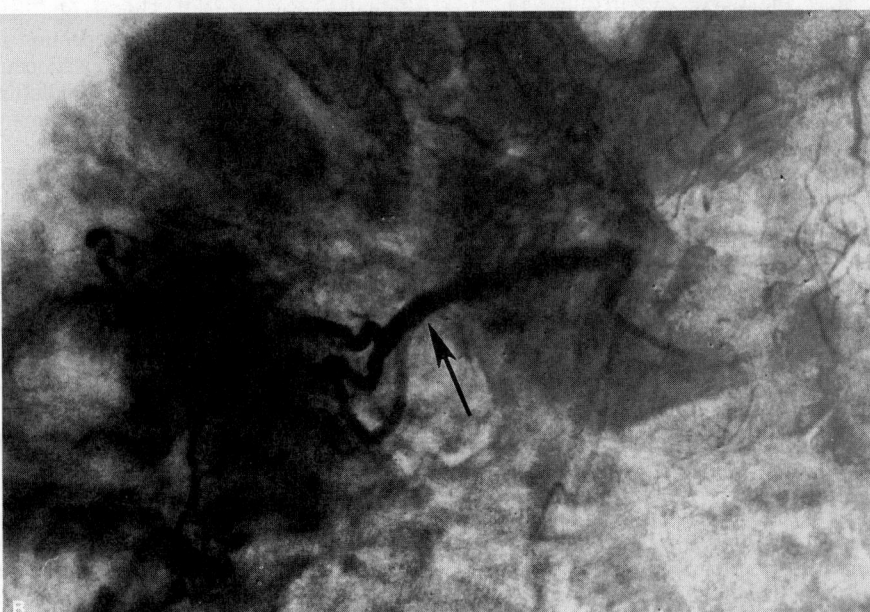

Figure 50-6. (*A*) Selective superior mesenteric arteriography demonstrating a vascular tuft (*arrows*) characteristic of vascular ectasia located within the right colon. (*B*) Selective superior mesenteric arteriography demonstrating early filling of the ileocolic vein (*arrow*) in a patient with vascular ectasia of the right colon.

The natural history of these lesions was revealed by the clinical course of 101 patients with colonic vascular ectasias.[42] Of the 15 asymptomatic individuals without a history of bleeding, none bled during a period of follow-up to 68 months (mean, 23 months). For 31 patients with overt bleeding or anemia who were treated only with blood transfusion, the rebleeding rate at 1 and 3 years was 26% and 46%, respectively. This suggests that the risk of bleeding for incidentally discovered lesions is minimal, whereas the risk for recurrent hemorrhage for most symptomatic patients is substantial and may increase with time.

Patients bleeding from colonic vascular ectasias can be treated with endoscopy. Nonrandomized investigations with vascular ectasias managed with monopolar electrocoagulation, endoscopic injection sclerotherapy, contact probes and lasers have been published with similar results. All methods appear to be effective for treating bleeding vascular ectasias and all are associated with procedure-related morbidity rates of 2% to 10%. Perforation has been reported in all of these experiences with rates of 2% to 3%.

Patients bleeding from vascular ectasias in whom endoscopic hemostatic methods are unsuccessful or unavailable can be treated with resection of the colon following preoperative localization of the bleeding site. For the usual patient bleeding from a vascular ectasia in the cecum or ascending colon, a right colectomy with ileotransverse colostomy is the treatment of choice. The value of preoperative localization of the bleeding site cannot be overstated, and every effort should be made to determine the site of hemorrhage prior to laparotomy.

UNUSUAL CAUSES OF ACUTE GASTROINTESTINAL HEMORRHAGE

As outlined in Tables 50-1 and 50-2, a wide variety of other pathologic processes may present with acute GI hemorrhage. Although these lesions generally comprise a relatively small percentage of the total number of cases of overt GI hemorrhage, they can present vexing problems to the clinician faced with a bleeding patient in whom the usual etiologies have been excluded.

Dieulafoy Vascular Malformation

Dieulafoy vascular malformation is an unusual cause of recurrent hematemesis, in which bleeding originates from an unusually large (1 to 3 mm diameter) artery running through the gastric submucosa for variable distances. Erosion of the gastric mucosa overlying the vessel results in necrosis of the arterial wall and brisk hemorrhage. The size of the mucosal defect is usually small (2 to 5 mm) and without evidence of chronic inflammation.

Painless hematemesis and melena are typical. Recurrent bleeding with spontaneous cessation are also common. In a collective review of 101 cases, the mean age of the patients was 52 years, and the lesion occurred twice as frequently in men as women. There was no significant association with alcohol abuse or antecedent symptoms.[43]

The diagnosis is most frequently made endoscopically by demonstrating arterial bleeding from a pinpoint mucosal defect. Occasionally, a small arterial vessel may be seen protruding from the gastric mucosa. Characteristically, the lesions are located within 6 cm of the esophagogastric junction along the lesser curvature.

Management consists of excising the gastric wall bearing the lesion through wedge resection of the proximal lesser curvature. Endoscopic electrocoagulation and ligation of the bleeding vessel have also been reported, although experience with this unusual lesion has been limited.

Angiodysplasia of the Stomach and Intestine

Angiodysplastic lesions may occur throughout the GI tract. They appear similar to colonic lesions being minute, flat or slightly raised red lesions with round or stellate shapes. Margins are characteristically sharp with a pale mucosal halo surrounding the lesion. The lesions are frequently multiple and are found most commonly in the stomach and duodenum, although esophageal and small intestinal involvement has also been described. A strong association with other chronic diseases, most notably chronic renal insufficiency and aortic stenosis, has also been well established.

Several factors may confound endoscopic diagnosis. The minute size and sessile nature of the lesions allow them to be concealed in inadequately distended gastric or duodenal folds. The lesions may be readily mistaken for submucosal hemorrhage associated with acute gastritis or trauma artifact from a nasogastric tube or the endoscope. The lesions may be demonstrated arteriographically and have many of the features described for colonic vascular ectasia.

Endoscopic injection of sclerosants, electrocoagulation, and laser photocoagulation have all been used to treat gastroduodenal angiodysplasia with good results. The multiplicity of lesions often necessitates several courses of therapy to eliminate recurring hemorrhage. Surgical resection of the gastric or intestinal wall containing the lesion as well as oversewing of the bleeding lesion have been reported to successfully control hemorrhage.

Aortoenteric Fistula

A communication between the aorta and the intestine may occur as a result of a variety of diseases, such as abdominal aortic aneurysm and infectious aortitis (primary aortoenteric fistula). Most of those encountered currently are due to the erosion of an aortic vascular prosthesis through the wall of the distal duodenum (secondary aortoenteric fistula). The incidence of aortoenteric fistula following aortic reconstructive surgery is about 1% with most of these fistulas arising from the proximal graft anastamosis. Secondary aortoenteric fistulas are believed to develop after prolonged contact of a prosthetic graft with a fixed segment of intestine, ultimately leading to erosion of the graft through the bowel wall. This results in a low-grade infection around the graft, and if the infection involves the suture line, dehiscence of the anastamosis occurs with massive hemorrhage. Bleeding may result from dehiscence of the anastamosis with bleeding into the bowel lumen, or it may occur from the edges of the eroded intestine.

The interval between aortic reconstructive surgery and the onset of GI hemorrhage may range from a few days to many years; the median interval is about 3 years.[44] Although aortoenteric fistula may present with an episode of severe and exsanguinating hemorrhage, it is more commonly intermittent and recurrent. Most patients have an initial episode (ie, herald bleed) that is followed in hours, days, or weeks by catastrophic hemorrhage. Patients may also complain of back or abdominal pain and less commonly have fever or signs of sepsis from infection around the graft.

The diagnosis of an aortoenteric fistula must be considered in any patient with an aortic prosthesis or an abdominal aortic aneurysm who presents with GI hemorrhage. Endoscopy should be urgently performed following the initial resuscitation to disclose evidence of an aortoenteric fistula or another cause of bleeding (eg, peptic ulcer disease with stigmata of recent hemorrhage). If endoscopy fails to demonstrate an aortoenteric fistula or other convincing source of bleeding and the patient is not massively bleeding, computed tomography may be helpful in detecting perigraft infection or other evidence of an aortoenteric fistula. In patients who are actively bleeding, exploratory laparotomy with exposure of the proximal graft should be undertaken. Identifying an aortoenteric fistula or erosion requires resection of the graft with extraanatomical bypass and repair of the duodenal wall.

Meckel's Diverticulum

Meckel's diverticulum is an unusual cause of acute GI hemorrhage, particularly in adults. About 25% of patients with symptomatic Meckel's diverticula present with hemorrhage.[45] In a series of 17 patients who bled from Meckel's diverticula, 11 experienced frank hemorrhage while 6 had chronic occult blood loss. The incidence of GI hemorrhage is greatest in the first decade of life and steadily decreases from that point. In one series, no patient older than 40 years of age and only one patient older than 31 years bled from a Meckel's diverticulum.[45] The pathogenesis of this bleeding involves the occurrence of ectopic gastric mucosa with peptic ulceration of adjacent bowel wall. Although these lesions may be demonstrated by enteroclysis, abdominal scintigraphy following the intravenous injection of radiolabeled technetium demonstrates the ectopic gastric mucosa and suggests the correct diagnosis. Treatment consists of resecting the diverticulum with a cuff of adjacent bowel. Diverticulectomy alone be associated with persistence of the ulcer and the possibility of recurrent hemorrhage.

Small Intestinal Diverticulum

Diverticular disease of the small intestine is another uncommon cause of either upper GI hemorrhage (duodenal) or lower GI hemorrhage (jejunoileal diverticula). The pathogenesis is similar to that of colonic diverticula with erosion of a vasa recta through the diverticular wall and the acute onset of hemorrhage. Depending on the location of the diverticulum, patients may present with either hematemesis, melena, or hematochezia. Hemorrhage from this source can be a vexing diagnostic problem because jejunoileal lesions are beyond the reach of the endoscope and bleeding from duodenal diverticula may be difficult to discern through it. Mesenteric angiography or intraoperative enteroscopy may localize the site of hemorrhage in actively bleeding patients. This is primarily because of the frequent occurrence of multiple lesions. Segmental resection of the involved intestine is the treatment of choice.

Inflammatory Bowel Disease

Rectal bleeding is found in nearly all patients with ulcerative colitis and in about 25% of patients with Crohn's disease; however, severe hemorrhage occurs in only 1% to 5% of patients. In general, bleeding from these lesions tends to be self-limiting, and resection of the site of hemorrhage is only rarely required. Hemorrhage occurring during the onset of fulminant ulcerative colitis can be treated with colectomy, retaining the rectum as a Hartmann pouch to allow subsequent performance of an ileoanal pull-through procedure.

REFERENCES

1. Gilbert DA, Silverstein FE, Tedesco FJ, et al. The national ASGE survey on upper GI bleeding. III. Endoscopy in upper GI bleeding. Gastrointest Endosc 1981;27:94.
2. Devitt JE, Brown FN, Beattie WG. Fatal bleeding ulcer. Ann Surg 1966;164:840.
3. Morris DW, Wevine GM, Soloway RD, et al. Prospective randomized study of diagnosis and outcome in acute upper GI bleeding: endoscopy versus conventional radiography. Am J Digest Dis 1975;20:1103.
4. Leinike JA, Schaffer RD, Hogan WJ, Green JE. Does timing affect the significance of diagnostic yield? Gastrointest Endosc 1976;22:228.
5. Silvis S, Nebel O, Rogers G, Sugawa C, Mandelstam P. Endoscopic complications: results of the 1974 American Society of GI Endoscopy survey. JAMA 1976;235:928.
6. Nusbaum M, Baum S. Radiographic demonstration of unknown sites of GI bleeding. Surg Forum 1963;14:374.
7. Hirschowitz BI, Lanas A. NSAID association with GI bleeding and peptic ulcer. AAS 1991;35:93.
8. Ehsanullah RSB, Page MD, Tildesley G, Wood JR. Prevention of gastroduodenal damage induced by non-steroidal anti-inflammatory drugs: controlled trial of ranitidine. BMJ 1988;297:1017.
9. Strom BL, Taragin MI, Carson JL. GI bleeding from the nonsteroidal anti-inflammatory drugs. AAS 1990;29:27.
10. Armstrong CP, Blower AL. Non-steroidal anti-inflammatory drugs and life threatening complications of peptic ulceration. Gut 1987;28:527.
11. Lanza FL, Fakouhi D, Rubin A, et al. A double-blind placebo-controlled comparison of the efficacy and safety of 50, 100, and 200 mcg of misoprostol qid in the prevention of ibuprofen-induced gastric and duodenal mucosal lesions and symptoms. Am J Gastroenterol 1989;84:633.
12. Robinson MG Griffin JW, Bowers J, et al. Effect of ranitidine on gastroduodenal mucosal damage induced by nonsteroidal antiinflammatory drugs. Dig Dis Sci 1989;34:424.
13. Roth SH, Bennett RE, Mitchell CS, Hartmean RJ. Cimetidine therapy in nonsteroidal anti-inflammatory drug gastropathy: double-blind long term evaluation. Arch Intern Med 1987;147:1798.
14. Collins R, Langman M. Treatment with histamine H2 antagonists in acute upper GI hemorrhage: implications of randomized trials. N Engl J Med 1985;313:660.
15. Keifhaber P, Keifhaber D, Huber F, Nath G. Endoscopic neodymium:YAG laser coagulation in GI hemorrhage. Endoscopy 1986;18:46.
16. Rutgeerts P, Van Trappen G, Broecbaert L, et al. Controlled trial of YAG laser treatment of upper digestive hemorrhage. Gastroenterology 1982;83:410.
17. Swain CP, Brown SG, Salmon PR, Kirkham JS, Northfield TC. Controlled trial of Nd:YAG laser in bleeding peptic ulcers. Gut 1983;24:A967.
18. Moreto M, Zaballa M, Ibanez S, Setien F, Figa M. Efficacy of monopolar electrocoagulation in the treatment of bleeding gastric ulcer. Endoscopy 1987;19:54.
19. Jessen K, Gilbert DA, Tytgat GNJ, Papp JP. Bipolar electrocoagulation in active UGI haemorrhage. Gastroenterology 1983;21:268.
20. Asaki S. Endoscopic haemostasis by local absolute alcohol injection for UGI tract bleeding: a multicentre study. In: Okabe H, Honda T, Ohshiba S, eds. Endoscopic surgery. New York, Elsevier, 1984:105.
21. Therapeutic endoscopy and bleeding ulcers: NIH consensus conference. JAMA 1989;262:1369.
22. Sacks HS, Chalmers TC, Blum AL, Berrier J, Pagano D. Endoscopic hemostasis: an effective therapy for bleeding peptic ulcers. JAMA 1990;264:494.
23. Sugawa C, Steffes CP, Nakamura R, et al. Upper GI bleeding in an urban hospital: etiology, recurrence and prognosis. Ann Surg 1990;212:521.
24. Schuster DP, Rowley H, Feinstein S, McGue MK, Zuckerman GR. Prospective evaluation of the risk of upper GI bleeding after admission to a medical intensive care unit. Am J Med 1984;76:623.
25. Cook DJ, Fuller HD, Guyatt GH, et al. Risk factors for GI bleeding in critically ill patients. N Engl J Med 1994;330:377.
26. DuMoulin GC, Paterson DG, Hedley-Whyte J, et al. Aspiration of gastric bacteria in antacid-treated patients: a frequent cause of postoperative colonisation of the airway. Lancet 1982;1:242.
27. Driks MR, Craven DE, Celli BR, et al. Nosocomial pneumonia

in intubated patients given sucralfate as compared with antacids or histamine type 2 blockers. N Engl J Med 1987;317:1376.

28. Athanasoulis CA. Medical progress: therapeutic applications of angiography. N Engl J Med 1980;302:1117.

29. Robert A, Kauffman GL Jr. Stress ulcers, erosions and gastric mucosal injury. In: Sleisenger MH, Fordtran JS, eds. GI disease: pathophysiology, diagnosis, management, ed 4. Philadelphia, WB Saunders, 1989:772.

30. Silverstein FE, Gilbert DA, Tedesco FJ, Buenger NK, Persing J. The national ASGE survey on upper GI varices. II. Clinical prognostic factors. Gastrointest Endosc 1981;27:80.

31. Grace ND. Variceal hemorrhage: pharmacologic approach. In: McDermott WV, Bothe A, eds. Surgery of the liver. Boston, Blackwell Scientific, 1988:303.

32. Hermann RE, Traul O. Experience with the Sengstaken-Blakemore tube: a prospective study. Gastroenterology 1971;61:291.

33. Terblanche J, Krige JE, Bornam PC. The treatment of esophageal varices. Annu Rev Med 1992;43:69.

34. Stiegmann GV, Goff JS, Sun JH, Davis D, Silas D. Technique and early clinical results of endoscopic variceal ligation (EVL). Surg Endosc 1989;3:73.

35. Stiegmann GV, Goff JS, Michaletz-Onody PA, et al. Endoscopic sclerotherapy as compared with endoscopic ligation for bleeding esophageal varices. N Engl J Med 1992;326:1527.

36. Laine L, El-Newihi HM, Migikovsky B, Sloane R, Carcia F. Endoscopic ligation compared with sclerotherapy for the treatment of bleeding esophageal varices. Ann Intern Med 1993:119:1.

37. LaBerge JM, Ring EJ, Gordon RL, et al. Creation of transjugular intrahepatic portosystemic shunts with the wallstent endoprosthesis: results in 100 patients. Radiology 1993;187:413.

38. McGuire HH, Haynes BW. Massive hemorrhage from diverticulosis of colon. Ann Surg 1972;175:847.

39. Boley SJ, DiBiase A, Brandt LJ, et al. Lower intestinal bleeding in the elderly. Am J Surg 1979;137:57.

40. Foutch PG. Angiodysplasia of the GI tract. Am J Gastroenterol. 1993;88:807.

41. Foutch PG, Rex DK, Lieberman DA. Prevalence of colonic angiodysplasia (AD) among healthy, asymptomatic people. Gastrointest Endosc 1993;39:A296.

42. Richter JM, Hedberg SE, Athanasoulis CA, et al. Angiodysplasia: clinical presentation and colonoscopic diagnosis. Dig Dis Sci 1984;29:481.

43. Veldhuyzen van Zanten SJO, Bartelsman JF, Schipper ME, Tytgat DN. Recurrent massive haematemesis from Dieulafoy vascular malformations: a review of 101 cases. Gut 1986; 27:213.

44. Nagy SW, Marshall JB. Aortoenteric fistulas. Postgrad Med 1993;93:211.

45. Mackey WC, Dineen P. A fifty year experience with Meckel's diverticulum. Surg Gynecol Obstet 1983;156:56.

CHAPTER 51

ANTIBIOTIC-ASSOCIATED COLITIS

F. ROBERT FEKETY

Mild diarrhea is a common side effect of antibiotic therapy; it is usually more of a nuisance than a serious problem. Most cases of diarrhea are of unknown cause but are thought to be related to alterations in the ecology of the fecal flora. Treated supportively, they resolve quickly after antibiotic administration is stopped. In marked contrast, about 10% to 20% of cases of antibiotic-associated diarrhea are complicated by a bacterial toxin–induced colitis, which is potentially serious. In these patients, the inflamed colonic mucosa is often covered with an adherent nodular exudate called a *pseudomembrane,* which consists of dead leukocytes, mucosal epithelial cells, mucus, and fibrin adherent to the inflamed mucosa. Visible pseudomembranes are not evident in all cases of antibiotic-associated colitis, especially early in the illness, but microscopic study of biopsy specimens of early lesions may reveal pseudomembranes as well as colitis. Any patient who experiences diarrhea within 6 weeks of receiving antibiotics, especially in the hospital, should be suspected of having pseudomembranous colitis (PMC), which is both serious and treatable. Many patients with PMC have mild diarrhea, especially early during the illness. Before the antibiotic era, PMC was most often found at autopsy or at the time of emergency colectomy.

Toxin-producing strains of *Clostridium difficile,* a component of the normal fecal flora, are the cause of almost all cases of antibiotic-associated colitis,[1] but rare cases have been attributed to toxigenic *Staphylococcus aureus, Salmonella* sp, *Clostridium perfringens* type C, *Plesiomonas shigelloides, Yersinia enterocolitica, Shigella* sp, *Campylobacter* sp, *Aeromonas* sp, cytomegalovirus, *Entamoeba histolytica,* and *Listeria monocytogenes.* Except for the *Staphylococcus* sp, pseudomembranes are only rarely detected in association with these organisms. Human immunodeficiency virus can also cause an intestinal inflammatory process that may be confused with *C difficile* colitis when it occurs in patients with acquired immunodeficiency syndrome who are receiving antimicrobial agents. Although there is no solid evidence that *C difficile* causes chronic inflammatory bowel diseases such as Crohn's colitis and chronic idiopathic ulcerative colitis, patients with these conditions are not immune to development of *C difficile* colitis, and when they do develop *C difficile* colitis, they may be mistakenly thought to have an acute exacerbation of the chronic disease.

PATHOLOGY

The key feature of antibiotic-associated colitis is an acute polymorphonuclear inflammation of the colonic mucosa and submucosa. Pseudomembranes may be absent in some patients with colitis; in addition, pseudomembranous plaques may be dislodged during processing of biopsy specimens. The inflammation usually affects only the epithelium and lamina propria, but necrosis and involvement of deeper tissues can occur in severe cases, and secondary infection may develop. Extensive transmural necrosis can result in toxic dilation of the colon, perforation, and peritonitis. The lesions of antibiotic-associated colitis can be found throughout the colon, but they are usually most prominent in the rectosigmoid; in about 10% of cases, lesions are restricted to the cecum or transverse colon.[2] In the latter circumstance, patients present with little or no diarrhea but with prominent abdominal pain, fever, and leukocytosis. The ileum is rarely involved in *C difficile* colitis but is often involved in staphylococcal enterocolitis. *C difficile*–associated diarrhea occurs at all ages but is most common in elderly adults and in debilitated patients. Antibiotic-associated colitis occurs but is surprisingly rare in infants and young children, up to half of whom harbor both the organism and its toxins in their stools. The reason for its rarity in this age group is not known; one proposed explanation is that receptors for the toxins on the colonic mucosal surfaces are sparse in infants. The disease can be difficult to diagnose in infants, especially when associated only with chronic diarrhea and hypoproteinemia. A therapeutic trial with vancomycin may be the only way to determine whether the presence of *C difficile* toxins in stools of infants with diarrhea is clinically meaningful.

PATHOGENESIS AND PREVENTION

C difficile is a spore-forming, gram-positive, obligate anaerobic bacillus present in the normal intestinal flora of 3% to 5% of healthy adults. The organism is ubiquitous in soil and water. Antibiotics promote acquisition and carriage by humans. Many studies have documented transmission in hospitals and nursing homes. *C difficile* can be found in the stools and environment of up to 15% to 20% of antibiotic-treated, hospitalized adults without diarrhea,[3,4] but diarrhea later devlops in as many as 30% of these patients. The organism is difficult to detect in stools using ordinary laboratory techniques, but a selective agar medium containing cycloserine, cefoxitin, and fructose has made this task easy. The addition of 0.2% highly purified sodium taurocholate increases the detectability of small numbers of spores in stools of asymptomatic carriers or from contaminated surfaces.

C difficile does not produce colitis by invasion of tissues; in fact, it is only rarely invasive. Colitis results from toxin production *within* the intestinal lumen, with the subsequent binding of these toxins to the mucosa.[4,5] The two most important toxins of *C difficile* are a 308-kd enterotoxin usually referred to as *toxin A* and a 270-kd toxin, referred to as *toxin B*.[5] Toxins A and B are closely related structurally and appear to share cellular mechanisms of action. The toxins attack mucosal cell membranes and microfilaments, producing depolymerization of actin, cytoplasmic contraction, hemorrhage, necrosis of epithelial cells, inflammation, chemoattraction of neutrophils, increased capillary permeability, and loss of protein and fluid into the intestinal lumen. Toxin B also interferes with mucosal integrity and protein synthesis in humans.[5] Other toxins produced by *C difficile* can increase intestinal myoelectric responses and peristalsis in the laboratory, but their clinical importance in the causation of diarrhea and cramping abdominal pain has not been established. Isolates that produce toxin A or B almost invariably produce the other toxin as well, but not necessarily to the same degree, which may account for some variation in the manifestations and severity of the illness.

Groups at high risk for PMC after treatment with antibiotics include elderly patients, patients undergoing abdominal surgery or cesarean section, those in intensive care units, and those with cancer, leukemia, uremia, burns, or colonic stasis. Even short-term antibiotic administration, such as for prophylaxis or treatment of minor infections, can precipitate PMC. The disease can follow oral, intramuscular, intravenous, or topical administration of antibiotics. The list of inciting or inducing antimicrobial agents is headed by penicillins and cephalosporins but includes practically every antimicrobial used in the treatment of infections in humans, including vancomycin and metronidazole (paradoxically, these two drugs are preferred in the treatment of PMC), antifungal agents, antiviral agents, and antineoplastic agents. Clindamycin is no longer the most common precipitating agent for PMC, because it is no longer used as often as it was a few decades ago. The pathogenetically important consequence of antimicrobial administration involves alterations of an unknown nature in the normal colonic flora that permit *C difficile* to proliferate and to produce large amounts of toxins within the intestinal lumen, with the subsequent development of *C difficile*–associated diarrhea. Not surprisingly, PMC may not begin until *after* antibiotics have been discontinued, especially if the *C difficile* isolate is susceptible to the

antimicrobial that was given or if the acquisition of the organism occurs *after* the antibiotics are discontinued. Despite clinical impressions to the contrary, the relative risks of different antimicrobial agents as inducers of PMC cannot be stated with confidence because antibiotic-specific attack rates in comparable groups of patients have not been determined.

Unusually high rates of PMC have been reported from numerous hospitals, and the organism can be transmitted nosocomially either by the hands of personnel who come into contact with patients who are carriers of the organism, especially if they have diarrhea, or by contact with contaminated surfaces.[3] Roommates of carriers are at increased risk of becoming colonized with the organism. *C difficile* colitis is increasing in frequency and is now the fourth most common nosocomial infection reported to the Centers for Disease Control and Prevention. *C difficile* diarrhea and colitis are more frequent than postoperative wound infections. Ironically, perioperative prophylactic antibiotics have decreased the frequency of postoperative wound infections but have increased the likelihood of developing antibiotic-associated colitis. Even short courses of antibiotics can facilitate the acquisition of *C difficile*. Person-to-person cross-infection by hand transmission is the primary way the organism is spread in hospitals, and careful handwashing and use of gloves while caring for patients with the disease and for asymptomatic carriers is important in preventing transmission.

Instruments inserted into the gastrointestinal tract should be thoroughly cleaned after use and disinfected with sodium hypochlorite (500 to 1600 ppm), alkaline glutaraldehyde, or ethylene oxide. Although vegetative forms of the organism are oxygen-sensitive and easily killed, spores are more resistant. Most experts believe that prophylaxis with oral vancomycin or metronidazole is not efficacious in prevention of antibiotic-associated colitis in high-risk patients. Although these agents do not reliably eradicate carriage of *C difficile*, they cause marked alteration in the colonization resistance of the fecal flora. Measures helpful in the prevention of *C difficile* colitis are summarized in Table 51-1.

In studies on immunization to toxins A and B using a hamster model, toxin A played a more important role in the pathogenesis of the disease than did toxin B, which does not bind to the intestinal mucosa of hamsters. Both toxins, however, bind to the colonic mucosa of humans.[5]

Table 51-1. PREVENTION OF *CLOSTRIDIUM DIFFICILE* COLITIS

GENERAL

Prudent use of antibiotics (narrow spectrum, short courses)
Handwashing between patients
Enteric isolation: single rooms, stool precautions, use of gloves
Immunization with *C difficile* toxoids (future)
Toxin adsorbents: cholestryramine, colestipol sucralfate (still experimental)

OUTBREAK SETTING

Education about the disease
Handwashing before and after each patient
Use of gloves for handling positive patients
Cohorting of affected patients
Treatment of fecal carriers with oral metronidazole, bacitracin, or vancomycin to reduce fecal shedding of *C difficile*
Disinfection of unit and fomites to kill spores and vegetative forms with 2% alkaline glutaraldehyde or hypochlorite solutions (1600 ppm)
Closure of unit (as a last resort)

Immunoglobulin G and neutralizing antibodies to toxin A and B have been detected in the sera of adults, but immunoglobulin G antibody titers do not correlate well with neutralizing antibodies in serum.[6] Whether these antibodies can offer protection against colitis in humans is not known. In one report, antibodies against C difficile antigens were found much more commonly in sera from young adults than in sera from elderly persons,[6] who are more susceptible to C difficile colitis. More immunologic studies with these toxins are needed, and it is hoped they will lead to development of toxoids effective in preventing the disease in humans.

The organisms of the normal intestinal flora that are important in suppressing colonization, overgrowth, and toxin production by C difficile have not been well delineated. Leading candidates are other Clostridium sp (including nontoxigenic isolates of C difficile), Bacteroides sp, Escherichia coli, and enterococci. Reports from the preantibiotic era of PMC suggested that dietary changes, malnutrition, hypoalbuminemia, anesthesia, surgery on the intestinal tract, colonic stasis, changes in bowel motility, uremia, cancer chemotherapy, and various medications may be important in precipitating the disease, probably by producing changes in the bowel flora similar to those produced by antibiotics.

CLINICAL MANIFESTATIONS

The severity of C difficile colitis varies widely. Not surprisingly, recognition of a severe or unusual case of the disease in a hospital often triggers a heightened awareness of the disease. With more frequent testing, recognition of many mild cases can create the illusion of an outbreak.

C difficile is responsible for only 10% to 20% of cases of antibiotic-associated diarrhea in hospitalized patients. The typical patient with C difficile colitis has profuse watery or mucoid, green, foul-smelling, liquid stools along with cramping abdominal pain beginning 3 to 9 days after starting antibiotics. There is wide variation in this pattern, and cases have been recognized only 1 day after starting antibiotic therapy. In about 20% of patients, diarrhea does not occur until up to 6 weeks *after* antibiotic therapy has been discontinued. The diarrheal stools often contain small amounts of blood but are rarely grossly bloody unless the patient has a coagulopathy. Hypovolemic shock, hypoproteinemia, edema, cecal perforation, toxic dilation of the colon, secondary sepsis, and hemorrhage are the most serious complications of severe PMC. Toxic dilation and perforation with PMC are surgical emergencies. If C difficile colitis goes unrecognized and untreated, the outcome can be fatal, and mortality rates of 10% to 20% have been reported in untreated elderly or chronically debilitated patients with PMC.

Some patients with antibiotic-associated colitis present with acute abdomens with localized abdominal pain, signs of peritonitis, and little or no diarrhea.[7] These patients may have disease restricted to the cecum and proximal colon, which may pursue a fulminant course. The clinical picture can be confused with Ogilvie syndrome or pseudoobstruction of the colon. Some patients with leukemia or granulocytopenia who are undergoing antibiotic therapy or antineoplastic chemotherapy develop ileocecitis (or typhlitis) caused by C difficile. This form of the disease may be triggered by cancer chemotherapy in the absence of antibiotic use.[8]

A severe form of the disease with little or no diarrhea is relatively frequent in women given prophylactic antibiotics for a cesarean section.[9] The altered colonic motility associated with pregnancy and surgical delivery, along with use of morphine or other opiates for postoperative

pain, contributes to development of toxic dilation of the colon without diarrhea. Unfortunately, stool studies for the presence of C difficile or its toxins usually take too long to be of much use in a patient who has an acute surgical abdomen. This atypical, nondiarrheal form of the illness is difficult to diagnose unless colonoscopy is performed or it is strongly suggested by a positive indium-33–labeled leukocyte scan or an abnormal computed tomographic (CT) scan of the abdomen.[10,11] CT scans may show distention and thickening of the wall of the colon along with pericolonic inflammation and peritonitis (Figs. 51-1 and 51-2). Concomitant toxic megacolon or ileus greatly interferes with effective antibiotic therapy of C difficile colitis using the preferred oral route, and many of these patients require emergency subtotal colectomies.

C difficile is an important cause of the ischemic enterocolitis that complicates Hirschsprung disease in infants and young children.[12] When such patients have signs of colitis, even if they have not received antibiotics, C difficile should be suspected and treatment with oral vancomycin begun promptly.

CLINICAL DIAGNOSIS

Patients with antibiotic-associated colitis usually have watery, mucoid, greenish, foul-smelling stools. They also have severe, crampy abdominal pain and tenderness, unexplained fever, and leukocytosis. High fever (39.4° to 40.5°C [103° to 105°F]), a peripheral leukocyte count of 35,000/μL to more than 50,000/μL, dehydration, electrolyte imbalance, and hypoalbuminemia not only are common with PMC but strongly indicate colitis rather than benign or simple diarrhea. The measures most useful in confirming the diagnosis of C difficile–associated diarrhea are summarized in Table 51-2.

The fecal leukocyte test is a simple, rapid screening measure that is sometimes useful in supporting the diagnosis of C difficile colitis. Polymorphonuclear leukocytes are found in stained smears of stools from about one third of patients with antibiotic-associated colitis. The finding in stained smears of three to five leukocytes in at least five high-dry fields suggests colitis and is strong evidence against the diagnosis of benign or simple antibiotic diar-

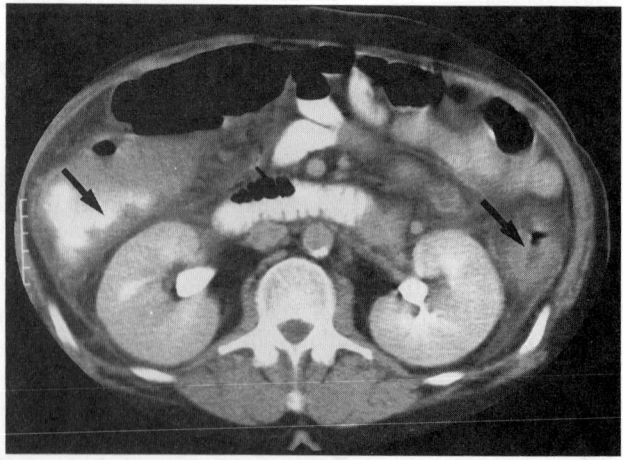

Figure 51-1. CT scan of abdomen in an elderly neurosurgical patient with fever and diarrhea postoperatively. Stools were positive for *Clostridium difficile* cytotoxin. The arrow at left indicates irregularly thickened cecal mucosa; the arrow at right indicates luminal narrowing, mucosal thickening, and edema of the descending colon.

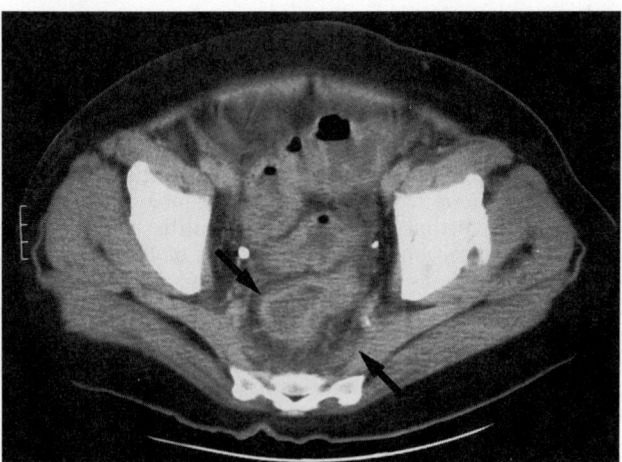

Figure 51-2. CT scan of another level of a patient with pseudomembraneous colitis. The arrow at left points to thickening of the rectal mucosa; the arrow at right indicates edema and inflammation in the perirectal soft tissues.

staphylococci first began to be troublesome in hospitals, *S aureus* was thought to be the cause of pseudomembranous enterocolitis. The clinical features of staphylococcal enterocolitis are similar to those of *C difficile* colitis, except that the former often involved the distal ileum, which is uncommon with *C difficile* colitis. Vancomycin was effective in treating staphylococcal PMC. In retrospect, some experts believe this form of the disease to have been caused by *C difficile*, which was not recognized to play a role in this disease process until 1977 to 1978.[1,4] So-called staphylococcal enterocolitis seemed to disappear after the introduction of penicillinase-resistant penicillins and cephalosporins in the early 1960s, and PMC remained an uncommon disease until the early 1970s, when clusters of cases related to the use of clindamycin were first recognized.

In the differential diagnosis of patients with nonspecific colitis associated with antibiotic use beginning outside the hospital, it is important also to consider Crohn's disease, idiopathic ulcerative colitis, ischemic colitis, gold-induced colitis, chemical colitis, and infection with other intestinal pathogens, such as *S aureus, C perfringens* type C (enteritis necroticans), *Salmonella* sp, *Edwardsiella* sp, *Shigella* sp, *E coli* (especially the 0157:H7 serotype if the colitis is hemorrhagic), and *P shigelloides*. Other organisms that can cause diarrhea, usually without colitis, include enterotoxigenic *E coli, Bacillus cereus, E histolytica, Campylobacter* sp, *Yersinia* sp, *Strongyloides* sp, cytomegalovirus, *Listeria* sp, *Aeromonas* sp, *Vibrios* sp, and possibly other Enterobacteriaceae genera, *Pseudomonas* sp, and *Candida* sp. When a patient develops diarrhea *after* admission to the hospital and after antibiotics have been administered, stool cultures for these conventional pathogens are probably not indicated unless tests for *C difficile* are negative.

rhea, but it is not specific for *C difficile* (Fig. 51-3). A negative test for fecal leukocytes does not rule out the diagnosis of colitis. Viewed in this way, many consider examination for fecal leukocytes a good first step in the workup of patients with antibiotic-associated diarrhea. Clostridia rarely predominate in stained smears of feces from patients with PMC, but gram-positive cocci resembling staphylococci occasionally are abundant; when they are, the diagnosis of staphylococcal enterocolitis is suggested.

Early in the antibiotic era, when penicillinase-producing

Table 51-2. DIAGNOSING *CLOSTRIDIUM DIFFICILE* COLITIS

Test	Comments
LABORATORY TESTS ON FECES	
Test for fecal leukocytes	A simple screening test but sensitivity only 30%–50%. A positive test rules out benign or simple antibiotic diarrhea
Stool culture for *C difficile*	Results delayed. Not diagnostic, since 10%–25% of patients in hospitals may carry the organism, and only 75% of isolates produce toxins
Tests for the presence of fecal toxins	
Cytopathic effect of toxin B in tissue cultures	Gold standard laboratory test, but some cell lines are not as sensitive as others, so false-negative results may occur. Time-consuming, expensive, and not widely available. Requires antitoxin neutralization for specificity
ELISA tests for toxins A or B	Rapid, widely available, relatively inexpensive. Sensitivity varies and may be only fair (75%–85%). If cut point is chosen to minimize false-negative results, false-positive results become a problem
Latex agglutination for *C difficile*	Rapid and inexpensive. Detects glutamate dehydrogenase (neither a toxin nor specific for *C. difficile*). Many false-positive and false-negative results
RADIOLOGIC STUDIES	
Plain film of the abdomen	Nonspecific and useful only when colitis is far-advanced or complications such as toxic megacolon or perforation are present.
Barium enema	Nonspecific findings. May precipitate perforation or megacolon
Computed tomography	Safe, but expensive, and not highly specific. Can be useful, especially when patients present with an acute abdomen without diarrhea. May demonstrate unsuspected pseudomembranous colitis
Radionuclide scan (indium-labeled white blood cells)	May detect inflammation, but does not diagnose cause
PROCEDURES	
Flexible sigmoidoscopy	Most rapid way to make the diagnosis. Expensive. Misses about 10% of cases (those with only minor or proximal colonic lesions). Biopsy of minor or nonspecific lesions increases yield.
Colonoscopy	Rapid and most sensitive way to make the diagnosis. Expensive and may be hazardous in impending perforation

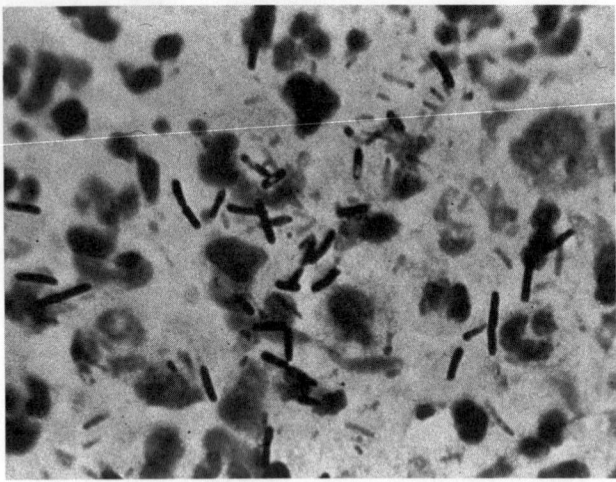

Figure 51-3. Giemsa-stained smear of feces from patient with *Clostridium difficile* colitis. The important finding is that many leukocytes are present. Although organisms resembling clostridia are also numerous, this is often not the case.

The diagnosis of PMC is most rapidly and certainly established by flexible sigmoidoscopy or colonoscopy, which can detect inflammation and pseudomembranes. Endoscopy, however, is expensive, uncomfortable for a sick patient, not always possible, and it can precipitate perforation or toxic megacolon, especially if air insufflation is used. Proctoscopy can be helpful in this situation. Endoscopy can detect friability, hemorrhage, edema, ulcers, colitis, and nodular or diffuse pseudomembranous lesions. Four types of pseudomembranous lesions have been recognized: (1) large, adherent pseudomembranes; (2) small (2- to 8-mm) nodular or plaquelike elevated lesions; (3) small, faint, flat, circular or ringlike whitish yellow lesions on an erythematous background; and (4) pseudomembranes that are seen microscopically in biopsy specimens of inflamed mucosa. The first three types of lesions can be seen in Figure 51-4. Microscopically, the lesions often appear to erupt from the mucosal surface and are called *volcano* or *summit* lesions. The characteristic nodules and plaques are essentially diagnostic and are usually most numerous in the distal colon, sigmoid, and rectum. Up to 10% of patients with PMC have lesions restricted to the cecum or proximal colon. The diagnosis may not be possible in these patients unless full colonoscopy or CT scanning is performed. Right-sided disease should be suspected when patients with antibiotic-associated diarrhea and toxin-positive stools have no visible lesions during sigmoidoscopy. A staphylococcal cause in humans should be suspected when there is involvement primarily of the right side of the colon and cecum and when tests for *C difficile* are negative. In these patients, oral vancomycin is the preferred treatment. *C difficile* has been reported to involve the distal ileum after colectomy, but otherwise this is rare.

Plain abdominal radiographs can suggest ileus, edema, ascites, perforation, or toxic dilation of the colon, and air-contrast barium enema studies can show thumbprinting, the accordion sign, and other signs of PMC. These findings are not specific, however, and are often absent early. More important, barium studies can precipitate toxic megacolon, perforation, or other complications and are best avoided.

LABORATORY DIAGNOSIS

The tests most useful for diagnosing *C difficile* colitis include stool cultures for the organism and tests on stools for the presence of *C difficile* toxins. A search for fecal leukocytes is a simple and useful screening test because a positive test indicates mucosal inflammation and excludes the benign form of antibiotic diarrhea; however, no more than a third of patients with *C difficile* colitis have positive fecal leukocyte test results.

About 85% of adults with antibiotic-associated diarrhea and cultures positive for *C difficile* have colitis. The isolation of *C difficile* from stools of a patient with diarrhea does not prove that the patient has colitis caused by *C difficile* because about 25% of isolates of *C difficile* obtained from humans are nontoxigenic and nonpathogenic. In addition, at least 3% of healthy adults are asymptomatic carriers of toxigenic isolates of *C difficile*. In hospitals in which PMC is frequent, 15% to 30% of asymptomatic adult patients treated with antibiotics have been found to carry the organism. Nevertheless, a positive culture can be useful in making management decisions, because it increases the likelihood that the patient has toxin-positive stools.

Demonstration of the presence of either toxin A (the enterotoxin) or toxin B (the cytotoxin) in stools of adults with diarrhea is helpful but does not prove that the patient has colitis. Some adults (and many colonized infants) have the toxin in stools and yet have no symptoms. Cell culture evidence for cytotoxicity by cytotoxin B is the most reliable laboratory aid in the diagnosis of PMC. This test is the gold standard used to evaluate all newer tests, but it is expensive, takes at least 24 hours, and is not readily available in most hospitals. At least 95% of adults with antibiotic-associated diarrhea and toxin B–positive stools have colitis. Toxin B tests are often sent out to a reference laboratory, so it should be remembered that this toxin is heat and acid labile and can easily be inactivated during storage, transport, or processing. When proctosigmoidoscopy is performed on patients with strongly positive toxin B titers and is normal, it is likely that these patients have colitis at a proximal site, such as the cecum, or mild, nonspecific colitis without pseudomembranes. Enzyme-linked immunosorbent assay (ELISA) tests on stools to detect toxin A (or B) are much more easily, inexpensively, and rapidly performed (2 to 3 hours) than the cytotoxin test for toxin B in many hospital clinical laboratories. When toxin B is present, toxin A is present, and vice versa, with rare

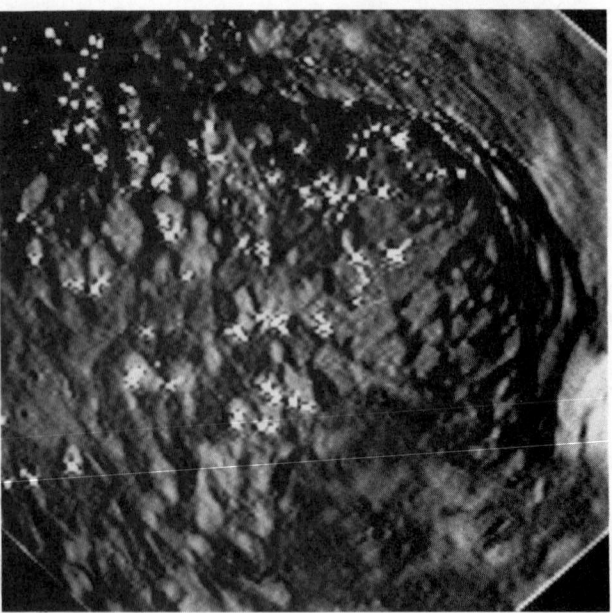

Figure 51-4. Sigmoidoscopic appearance of lesions typical of *Clostridium difficile* pseudomembraneous colitis.

exceptions. The results can be obtained in just a few hours using the ELISA test for toxin A. ELISA has become the preferred alternative to the cytotoxin B test. The endpoint chosen for reading ELISA tests is somewhat arbitrary and is a compromise between minimizing false-negative results and not increasing the frequency of false-positive results. Toxin A tests manufactured by different companies do not always agree with one another. As usually employed, sensitivity ranges from 75% to 90%, with about 5% to 10% false-positive results.[13] The clinician should keep the possibility of a false-negative or false-positive result in mind when basing management decisions on ELISA tests for the toxins. Consequently, experts recommend that at least two different tests be performed on stools from patients suspected of having PMC. A latex agglutination test is available that detects an antigen (glutamate dehydrogenase) of *C difficile* that is of no pathogenetic significance and that is produced by several other species of organisms found in the intestinal tract; the result is that the test also suffers from a lack of sensitivity and specificity. When the ELISA test for toxin A is negative, it can be helpful to repeat it or to perform another test for *C difficile*–associated diarrhea, such as culture, toxin B test in cell cultures, the latex agglutination test, or endoscopy. Use of the polymerase chain reaction to probe for and detect gene sequences of toxin A or B of *C difficile* in feces of patients suspected of having PMC has become possible. Although not yet commercially available, the test is rapid, sensitive, and specific, and in the future it may become the preferred test for confirming the diagnosis of PMC.[14]

TREATMENT OF *CLOSTRIDIUM DIFFICILE* COLITIS

Antibiotics

Oral therapy with antimicrobial agents is always preferred for antibiotic-associated colitis, since it is far more reliable than parenteral therapy.[15] Because susceptibility tests on *C difficile* isolates are rarely performed as a guide to the treatment of individual patients, treatment is empiric and based on published data from studies with large numbers of isolates. *C difficile* is usually susceptible to vancomycin, metronidazole, and bacitracin. Empiric therapy should begin while awaiting results of tests designed to implicate *C difficile* if the patient is elderly, debilitated, severely ill, or likely to have a severe form of the disease. Empiric therapy is designed to correct fluid and electrolyte imbalances and to prevent hypoproteinemia, edema, toxic colonic dilation, colonic perforation, and other complications. Either vancomycin or metronidazole is preferred as specific therapy. *C difficile* isolates are always susceptible to vancomycin and are usually susceptible to metronidazole (97% of the time), and most isolates are susceptible to bacitracin and teicoplanin. The latter antibiotic, which is similar to vancomycin, has been popular in Europe but is not available in the United States. Most isolates are susceptible to bacitracin, rifampin, or teicoplanin. The minimal inhibitory concentrations of these antimicrobial agents for most isolates of *C difficile* are about 5 mg/L or less. *C difficile* are susceptible at concentrations found in stools when therapy is administered orally unless the drug does not reach the colonic lumen because of ileus. Metronidazole is usually undetectable in stools when given orally, presumably because it is converted into the antibacterially active derivative by susceptible bacteria and is also absorbed so well systemically that no active drug is found in the lumen of the gut.

Not all patients with antibiotic-associated colitis need treatment with specific antimicrobial agents. When pa-

tients have only mild or moderate illness, it may be sufficient to discontinue the precipitating antibiotic and to give supportive therapy with fluid and electrolyte replacement. If the patient improves within a few days, supportive therapy may be continued, and diarrhea usually subsides completely within 7 to 10 days. If not, specific antibiotic therapy should be given, usually for another 7 to 10 days. To facilitate return of the normal fecal flora and colonization resistance, many experts believe the duration of treatment with vancomycin or metronidazole should be brief rather than long (usually no longer than 10 to 14 days). If the inducing antibiotic must be continued, specific oral antimicrobial treatment with vancomycin or metronidazole should be started promptly, even if the symptoms of colitis are mild. Discontinuation of the inducing antibiotic after recognition of colitis is not essential if specific therapy for PMC is given. The antibacterial effects of vancomycin on *C difficile* in vitro are not antagonized by other antimicrobial agents; thus, vancomycin or metronidazole can suppress the disease despite continuation of therapy with antimicrobial agents. Nonetheless, it is a good idea to change to another appropriate antimicrobial regimen for treating the original infection when possible.

Vancomycin

The efficacy of vancomycin has been so well documented that this drug must be considered the most reliable treatment for PMC. No isolates of *C difficile* are resistant to vancomycin, and it is also the drug of choice for oral therapy of staphylococcal enterocolitis. Metronidazole, bacitracin, and teicoplanin are alternatives for treating mild or moderately severe illness or when vancomycin is not tolerated. Because of problems associated with the emergence of vancomycin-resistant enterococci and coagulase-negative staphylococci in hospitals, most experts recommend that vancomycin or teicoplanin not be used for the treatment of *C difficile* diarrhea or colitis unless diarrhea or colitis is severe or the patient is critically ill.

C difficile isolates are almost always susceptible to vancomycin at concentrations of less than 5 mg/L, and few isolates have been identified that require more than 16 mg/L. Because vancomycin is poorly absorbed into the systemic circulation when given orally at a dosage of 125 to 500 mg four times a day, concentrations far exceeding 16 mg/L, the maximal concentration required for inhibition of *C difficile*, are easily achieved in stool. Indeed, when a dose of 500 mg is given orally four times a day, stool concentrations average 2000 mg/L or more. The higher dose is usually reserved for patients with impending ileus or who are severely ill. Even patients with profuse diarrhea achieve adequate concentrations of vancomycin in stools with these regimens. Although small amounts of vancomycin can be absorbed systemically, toxic serum concentrations have never been reported with oral therapy, even when the patient has renal failure. Systemic side effects are rare or nonexistent with use of oral vancomycin, even in patients with inflamed colonic mucosa. Good antibacterial activity within colonic tissues does not appear necessary for the management of PMC; instead, cessation of toxin production within the lumen or at the mucosal surface seems sufficient. *C difficile* colitis should be viewed as a colonic intoxication rather than as an infection. Patients treated with oral vancomycin usually show improvement in fever, diarrhea, abdominal cramps, and malaise in 48 to 72 hours, and toxin titers in stools begin to decline shortly after treatment is begun.[16] Diarrhea and fever may require 1 to 2 weeks to resolve, especially if the patient is severely ill or has extensive lesions, or if treatment was delayed. Treatment should continue for at least 7 days but is rarely needed for more than 14 days. Some investigators believe that therapy should be continued until toxins are no longer detectable in stools, but routine tests to detect the toxins in stools of patients who are doing well are generally believed unnecessary. Stool cultures often remain positive for *C difficile* after successful treatment, usually without negative consequences for the patient. Because there is no reliable treatment for the asymptomatic carrier state, routine cultures for detecting *C difficile* in stools of asymptomatic patients to anticipate and prevent relapses are unnecessary except for epidemiologic purposes.

In a randomized study of treatment of *C difficile*–associated diarrhea with vancomycin, no statistically or clinically significant differences were found in the overall clinical or bacteriologic responses of patients treated with oral vancomycin in dosages of 125 or 500 mg every 6 hours.[16] For treatment of infants and children with antibiotic-associated colitis, a dose of 500 mg/1.73 m^2 every 6 hours orally has been recommended. Because the diagnosis of *C difficile* colitis is extremely difficult to establish in infants, a therapeutic trial with vancomycin is sometimes used to confirm the diagnosis in infants with protracted diarrhea after antibiotic therapy.

Vancomycin is the drug of choice for oral therapy of staphylococcal enterocolitis, which may be suspected when Gram-stained smears of stools show a preponderance of gram-positive cocci and leukocytes, or when tests for *C difficile* are negative despite the presence of colitis. A vancomycin dosage of 500 mg four times a day is preferred in this setting. Because of concerns that parenteral or oral use of vancomycin could encourage the outgrowth of vancomycin-resistant enterococci and staphylococci, investigators recommend that metronidazole be used preferentially for the oral therapy of *C difficile* colitis unless the patient has failed therapy, is pregnant, is a child, is unable to tolerate metronidazole, or is severely ill.

Metronidazole

Metronidazole, an inexpensive antimicrobial, is usually active against *C difficile* and is effective in the treatment of most patients with antibiotic-associated colitis, even though stool concentrations of the drug after oral administration are often undetectable. In a randomized comparative study of treatment of *C difficile* diarrhea or colitis in adult men, oral metronidazole was associated with a cure rate (within 7 days) of 92%, whereas the cure rate was 100% with oral vancomycin.[17] Although this difference was not statistically significant, patients who failed metronidazole therapy and were switched to vancomycin then responded. Metronidazole has a metallic taste but is well tolerated, is significantly less expensive than vancomycin, and is associated with the same rate of posttreatment carriage, relapse, and side effects as vancomycin. The usual oral dose of metronidazole for *C difficile* colitis is 500 to 750 mg three times daily or 250 mg four times daily for 7 to 10 days.

Metronidazole has a number of potentially serious side effects and is not recommended for use in pregnant women or children. In addition, metronidazole is not approved in the United States by the Food and Drug Administration for the treatment of *C difficile* colitis or diarrhea. Although metronidazole has the advantage of not encouraging the emergence of vancomycin-resistant enterococci or staphylococci, it is not useful in the treatment of rare patients with staphylococcal enterocolitis.

Other Antimicrobials

Several investigators have reported successful treatment with oral bacitracin, and there is little doubt that bacitracin can be an effective alternative to vancomycin and metronidazole. The most common dosage in these studies was 25,000 IU (about 500 mg) four times a day for 7 to 19 days. The response to bacitracin was slower and less certain than with vancomycin; furthermore, stool carriage rates and toxin titers declined less rapidly and less often than with vancomycin. Some patients experienced a relapse after bacitracin therapy and were then treated successfully with vancomycin. Most isolates of *C difficile* are susceptible to bacitracin, but some require more than 20 IU/mL (about 1000 mg/L) for inhibition, which is an extremely high concentration, probably indicating resistance. Bacitracin is a useful alternative to vancomycin or metronidazole but is often not readily available; it is not a primary treatment for the disease.[18]

Rifampin is active in vitro against *C difficile* isolates but should not be used for treatment of *C difficile* colitis except in combination with some other active drug because of the high rate of development of resistance when given alone. Rifampin has been used orally along with vancomycin, with apparent success in an uncontrolled study for treatment of recurrent colitis.[19] Rifampin achieves high concentrations intracellularly, but there is no good evidence for synergism with vancomycin against *C difficile*.

Anion Exchange–Binding Resins

Cholestyramine and colestipol are anion exchange–binding resins that were used in treatment of PMC before the cause of the disease was known. Cholestyramine binds toxin B (and possibly also toxin A) as its presumed mechanism of beneficial action in PMC. Cholestyramine can also bind vancomycin, so the simultaneous use of cholestyramine and low doses of vancomycin should be avoided. Cholestyramine *may* prevent the development of diarrhea and other symptoms during an episode of *C difficile* diarrhea without adversely affecting the normal fecal flora. The agent has no demonstrable inhibitory effects on *C difficile*. Because many patients with colitis respond slowly or not at all to cholestyramine and often require a change to oral treatment with specific antibiotics, cholestyramine is usually reserved for patients with mild illness or with recurrent or relapsing *C difficile* colitis. The usual oral dose of cholestyramine for treatment of PMC in adults is 4 g three or four times a day. Obstipation is the most serious side effect of anion-binding resins.

Antidiarrheal Agents

Antiperistaltic agents, such as loperamide or diphenoxylate with atropine (Lomotil), are best avoided in patients with antibiotic-associated colitis.[20] Although these agents provide relief of symptoms, they may do this by causing pooling of fluid within the intestinal lumen. Diphenoxylate with atropine is especially dangerous in infants because of this effect and other side effects. The conditions of some patients worsen after administration of antiperistaltic drugs; the drugs may improve diarrhea but promote more severe damage to the colon because of pooling of toxin-containing fluid within the bowel lumen, with toxic dilation of the colon a possible result. The antiperistaltic effects of morphine and related opiates given to postoperative patients for relief of pain may also decrease the signs of diarrhea that would alert one to the possibility of PMC and may thus predispose to severe colitis and toxic megacolon.

Treatment of Patients Unable to Take Oral Therapy

Patients who are unable to take vancomycin or metronidazole orally can be given it through a nasogastric tube along with intermittent clamping. Patients with ileus or obstruction may not achieve adequate concentrations of vancomycin within the colonic lumen, where it is needed to stop toxin production. These patients pose a formidable therapeutic problem and, not surprisingly, have a relatively high death rate. Most investigators believe there is no reliable parenteral regimen for treatment of PMC. Most patients treated parenterally with vancomycin have little or none of it in their stool unless they are bleeding from colonic lesions. Although metronidazole given intravenously is excreted by way of the hepatobiliary route, the drug may be completely reabsorbed from the small intestine unless the transit time is rapid. Thus, patients with colitis treated intravenously with vancomycin or metronidazole may not achieve therapeutic concentrations within the bowel lumen, where it is most needed.[21,22] Reliance on intravenous antibiotics for treatment of colitis, to the exclusion of oral or intraluminal therapy, is not recommended. Evidence suggests that metronidazole given intravenously is beneficial in some patients, either because of leakage of the drug across the mucosa into the lumen, because of increased permeability or bleeding, or even because of transport of the active metabolite across the mucosa into the colon. The physician should not rely on these possibilities; other alternatives exist.

When parenteral therapy for PMC is unavoidable (as in patients with paralytic ileus and severe colitis), some authorities recommend treatment with both intravenous metronidazole and intravenous vancomycin, supplemented by vancomycin given by means of a nasogastric tube with intermittent clamping, an ileostomy or colostomy, an enema, or a catheter passed to the cecum colonoscopically. Passage of a long intestinal tube nasogastrically to the distal ileum or through the ileocecal valve into the cecum under fluoroscopic control may be possible in some patients, permitting perfusion of the colon from above and under low pressure with vancomycin-containing solutions. A vancomycin concentration of 500 to 1000 mg/L can be used as a perfusate. Oral metronidazole has no role in this setting because the drug usually is completely absorbed systemically from the small intestine, and little or none reaches the colonic lumen even if the mucosa is hyperpermeable.

Surgical Measures

Patients with PMC can deteriorate rapidly and develop life-threatening fulminant colitis, toxic megacolon, or perforation. Urgent subtotal colectomy is necessary to deal with these life-threatening emergencies. A colostomy or ileostomy can be a good way to facilitate instillation of vancomycin or metronidazole into the colonic lumen of patients with ileus or obstruction. C difficile–associated diarrhea may occur in the small bowel after colostomy, and PMC may be the cause of early colostomy dysfunction that goes unsuspected until mucosal plaques become apparent on the everted bowel at the colostomy opening.[23]

Treatment of Patients With Relapse or Recurrence of Colitis

Most patients with C difficile colitis do not suffer multiple recurrences, but another episode of colitis has been observed up to 8 weeks after apparent resolution of the disease in 10% to 20% of patients treated with vancomycin, metronidazole, or bacitracin. Recurrences occur at about the same rate after all forms of specific antimicrobial treatment and usually respond promptly to repeated therapy with vancomycin, metronidazole, or bacitracin. Recurrences may be caused by germination of spores persisting

in the colon (relapse) or by acquisition by the permissive colon of organisms from environmental or human contacts (reinfection). Persistence is more common than reinfection, but management is the same in either case. Unfortunately, the C difficile carrier state cannot be reliably eradicated with antimicrobial agents in the hope of preventing recurrences.

Although most patients with PMC have one recurrence at most, some unfortunate patients experience multiple episodes. It is not unusual for patients to have 5 to 10 intermittent episodes of diarrhea and colitis during a 6- to 24-month period. Although no entirely satisfactory way to prevent these episodes is known, anecdotal observations and experiences support management with either short (7 to 10 days) or long (4 to 6 weeks) courses of therapy with oral vancomycin, metronidazole, or bacitracin. Sometimes, drug therapy is followed by gradual tapering of the dose, with or without cholestyramine therapy, for a period of weeks after antibiotic therapy has been completed. Oral vancomycin plus rifampin has been used empirically for treatment and prevention of multiple relapses, with apparent success.[19] None of these regimens was proved to be better than the others in well-controlled studies. Five children with chronic relapsing C difficile colitis were treated successfully with specific antibiotics plus intravenous γ-globulin at a dose of 400 mg every 3 weeks based on the theory that they may have defective immune responses to the toxins.[24]

Theoretically, the best way to prevent relapses is by restoration of the normal fecal flora. Patients with multiple relapses have been treated with enemas containing feces obtained from healthy people or by the oral or rectal administration of a nontoxigenic isolate of C difficile or a mixture of pure cultures of organisms isolated from stools, in the hope of suppressing C difficile or its toxins. Direct attempts at recolonization of the colon include orally administered yogurt or other Lactobacillus sp preparations, such as lactobacillus GG,[25] or by the oral administration of a nonpathogenic yeast, Saccharomyces boulardii. Results with S boulardii have been especially promising. In 1994, investigators reported the results of a double-blind, placebo-controlled intervention study in patients with recurrent C difficile diarrhea and colitis.[26] Patients received treatment with live yeast, S boulardii (1 g/d), or placebo for 4 weeks in combination with standard oral antibiotic therapy given for 10 days. There were no side effects with the yeast other than thirst and mild constipation. The efficacy of S boulardii was significant: its recurrence rate was 34.6%, compared with 64.7% on placebo. The yeast was not of significant benefit in preventing a recurrence of colitis in patients experiencing their first attack of the disease (recurrence rate was 19.3% with the yeast, compared with 24.2% on placebo). Unfortunately, although the yeast is available in Europe, it is not yet available in the United States. The mechanism of the benefit of S boulardii has not been established.

REFERENCES

1. Bartlett JG. Antibiotic-associated pseudomembranous colitis. Rev Infect Dis 1979;1:530.
2. Tedesco FJ, Corless JK, Brownstein RE. Rectal sparing in antibiotic-associated pseudomembranous colitis: a prospective study. Gastroenterology 1982;83:1259.
3. Fekety R, Kim K-H, Brown D, et al. Epidemiology of antibiotic-associated colitis: isolation of Clostridium difficile from the hospital environment. Am J Med 1981;70:906.
4. Rifkin GD, Fekety R, Silva J, et al. Antibiotic-induced colitis: implication of a toxin neutralized by Clostridium sordellii antitoxin. Lancet 1977;2:1103.
5. Mitty RD, LaMont JT. Clostridium difficile diarrhea: pathogen-

esis, epidemiology and treatment. Gastroenterologist 1994; 2:61.

6. Bacon AE, Fekety R. Immunoglobulin G directed against toxins A and B of *Clostridium difficile* in the general population and patients with antibiotic-associated diarrhea. Diagn Microbiol Infect Dis 1994;18:205.

7. Drapkin MS, Worthington MG, Chang TW, Razvi SA. *Clostridium difficile* colitis mimicking acute peritonitis. Arch Surg 1985;120:1321.

8. Cudmore MA, Silva J, Fekety R, et al. *Clostridium difficile* colitis associated with cancer chemotherapy. Arch Intern Med 1982;142:333.

9. Arsura EL, Fazio RA, Wickremesinghe PC. Pseudomembranous colitis following prophylactic antibiotic use in primary caesarean section. Am J Obstet Gynecol 1985;151:87.

10. Yankes JR, Baker ME, Cooper C, Gorbatt J. CT appearance of focal pseudomembranous colitis. J Comput Assist Tomogr 1988;12:394.

11. Brunner D, Feifarek, C, McNeely D, Haney P. CT of pseudomembranous colitis. Gastrointest Radiol 1984;9:73.

12. Brearly S, Armstrong GR, Nairn R, et al. Pseudomembranous colitis: a lethal complication of Hirschsprung's disease unrelated to antibiotic usage. J Pediatr Surg 1987;22:257.

13. Brazier JS. Role of the laboratory in investigations of *C. difficile* diarrhea. Clin Infect Dis 1993;16(Suppl 4):S228.

14. Kuhl SJ, Tang YJ, Navarro L, et al. Diagnosis and monitoring of *Clostridium difficile* infections with the polymerase chain reaction. Clin Infect Dis 1993;16(Suppl 4):S234.

15. Fekety R, Shah AB. Diagnosis and treatment of *Clostridium difficile* colitis. JAMA 1993;269:71.

16. Fekety FR, Silva J, Kauffman C, Buggy B, Deery H. Treatment of antibiotic-associated *Clostridium difficile* colitis with oral vancomycin: comparison of two dosage regimens. Am J Med 1989;86:15.

17. Teasley PG, Gerding,DN, Olson MM, et al. Prospective randomized trial of metronidazole versus vancomycin for *Clostridium difficile*–associated diarrhea and colitis. Lancet 1993;2:1043.

18. Dudley MN, McLaughlin JC, Carrington G, et al. Oral bacitracin vs vancomycin therapy for *Clostridium difficile*–induced diarrhea: a randomized double-blind trial. Arch Intern Med 1986;146:1101.

19. Buggy BP, Fekety R, Silva J. Therapy of relapsing *Clostridium difficile*–associated diarrhea and colitis with the combination of vancomycin and rifampin. J Clin Gastroenterol 1987;9:155.

20. Novak E, Lee JG, Seckman E, et al. Unfavorable effect of atropine-diphenoxylate (Lomotil) therapy in lincomycin caused diarrhea. JAMA 1976;235:1451.

21. Guzman R, Kirkpatrick J, Forward K, Lim F. Failure of parenteral metronidazole in treatment of pseudomembranous colitis. J Infect Dis 1988;158:1146.

22. Oliva SL, Guglielmo BJ, Jacobs R, Pons VG. Failure of intravenous vancomycin and intravenous metronidazole to prevent or treat antibiotic-associated pseudomembranous colitis. J Infect Dis 1989;159:1154.

23. Stein HD, Sirota RA, Yudis M, et al. Pseudomembranous colitis as a cause of early colostomy dysfunction. J Clin Gastroenterol 1994;18:165.

24. Leung DY, Kelly CP, Boguniewicz M, et al. Treatment with intravenously administered gamma globulin of chronic relapsing colitis induced by *Clostridium difficile* toxin. J Pediatr 1991;118:633.

25. Gorbach SL, Chang TW, Golden B. Successful treatment of relapsing *Clostridium difficile* colitis with lactobacillus GG. Lancet 1987;2:1519.

26. McFarland LV, Surawicz CM, Greenberg RN, et al. A randomized placebo-controlled trial of *Saccharomyces boulardii* in combination with standard antibiotic for *Clostridium difficile* disease. JAMA 1994;271:1913.

SURGERY: SCIENTIFIC PRINCIPLES AND PRACTICE, Second Edition, edited by Lazar J. Greenfield, Michael W. Mulholland, Keith T. Oldham, Gerald B. Zelenock, and Keith D. Lillemoe. Lippincott-Raven Publishers, Philadelphia, © 1997.

CHAPTER 52

ANORECTAL DISORDERS

SANTHAT NIVATVONGS

ANATOMY OF THE RECTUM AND ANAL CANAL

The Rectum

The rectum extends from the level of the promontory of the sacrum to the level of the levator ani muscle and varies in length from 12 to 15 cm. The rectum differs from the colon in that the outer layer is covered circumferentially by longitudinal muscle rather than the three taeniae bands. The rectum has two or three lateral curves that form submucosal folds in the lumen, known as the valves of Houston. The posterior part of the rectum is devoid of peritoneum and is covered with the endopelvic fascia. The presacral fascia is a strong, endopelvic fascia that covers the entire anterior surface of the sacrum and also covers the underlying vessels and nerves. At about the level of S-4, the presacral fascia runs forward and downward, and attaches to the rectum.[1] This is referred to as rectosacral fascia (Fig. 52-1). It is necessary to cut this fascia for full mobilization of the rectum, as in abdominoperineal resection or low anterior resection. Peritoneum covers the upper two thirds of the rectum anteriorly, and the upper one third of the rectum is covered by peritoneum laterally. The lower third of the rectum is entirely devoid of peritoneum. In general, the anterior peritoneal reflection is about 6 to 8 cm from the anal verge. The extraperitoneal portion of the rectum is covered by the endopelvic fascia, which, on the anterior surface, is called Denonvilliers fascia. The lateral endopelvic fascia is thicker and is called the lateral rectal stalks, which also require division for full mobilization of the rectum.

Anal Canal

The anal canal, about 4 cm in length, is the terminal portion of the large bowel that passes through the levator ani muscle and opens to the anal verge. The muscular wall of the anal canal, as a continuation of the circular muscular layer of the rectum, is thickened and forms the internal sphincter. The anal canal is wrapped by the external sphincter muscle and the puborectal muscle, which are arranged in three U-shaped loops.[2] The top loop is formed by the puborectal muscle, which originates from the pubis. The intermediate loop is the superficial external sphincter muscle; the origin of this loop, at the tip of the coccyx, is known as the anococcygeal ligament. The basal loop is composed of the subcutaneous portion of the external sphincter muscle (Fig. 52-2).

The upper portion of the anal canal, where the internal sphincter muscle becomes thickened and the puborectal muscle wraps around (felt on digital examination of the lateral and posterior quadrants), is called the anorectal ring. From the level of the anorectal ring distally and between the internal and external sphincter muscles, the longitudinal muscle coat of the rectum is joined by fibers of the levator ani and puborectal muscles to form the conjoined longitudinal muscle (Fig. 52-3). These muscle fibers

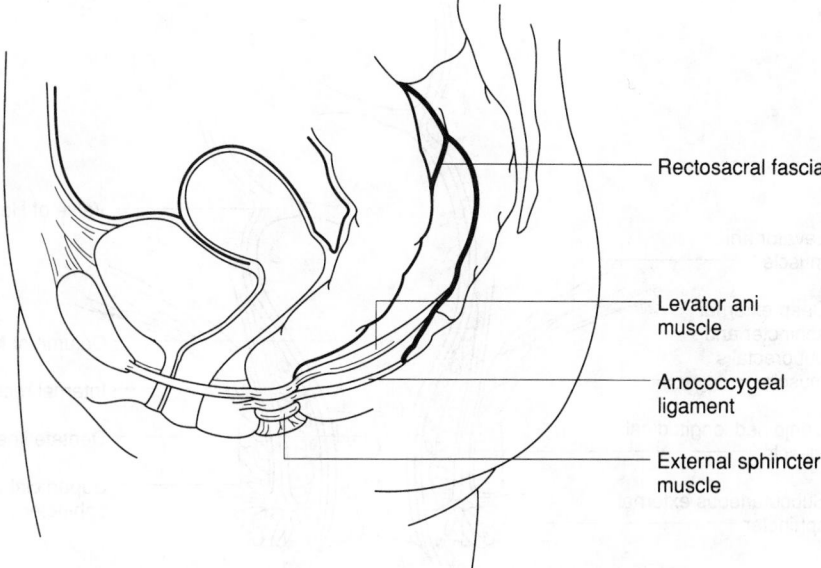

Figure 52-1. Fascial attachments of the rectum.

may traverse the lower portion of the distal external sphincter to insert in the perianal skin, causing wrinkling of the anal verge. This wrinkling is referred to as corrugator cutis ani.

At about the midpoint of the anal canal, 2 cm from the anal verge, there is an undulating demarcation called the dentate or pectinate line. Longitudinal folds of the mucosa above the dentate line are known as the columns of Morgagni. For a distance of about 1 cm above the dentate line, the epithelial lining may be columnar, transitional, or stratified squamous epithelium; this area is referred to as the transitional or cloacogenic zone. The area above the transitional zone is lined by columnar epithelium, and the area below the dentate line is lined by squamous epithelium (see Fig. 52-3). This is also the area where the internal hemorrhoidal plexus lies.

Pelvic Floor Muscles

The pelvic floor muscles consist of the levator ani muscle and the iliococcygeal muscle. The levator ani muscle is a broad, thin muscle that forms the floor of the pelvic cavity and is innervated by the fourth sacral nerve. This muscle has traditionally been considered to consist of three muscles—the iliococcygeal, the pubococcygeal, and the puborectal. Studies suggest that it consists only of the iliococcygeal and pubococcygeal muscles, and that the puborectal muscle is actually a part of the deep portion of the external sphincter.[3,4]

The iliococcygeal muscle arises from the ischial spine and posterior part of the obturator fascia, passes downward, backward, and medially, and becomes inserted on the last two segments of the sacrum and the anococcygeal

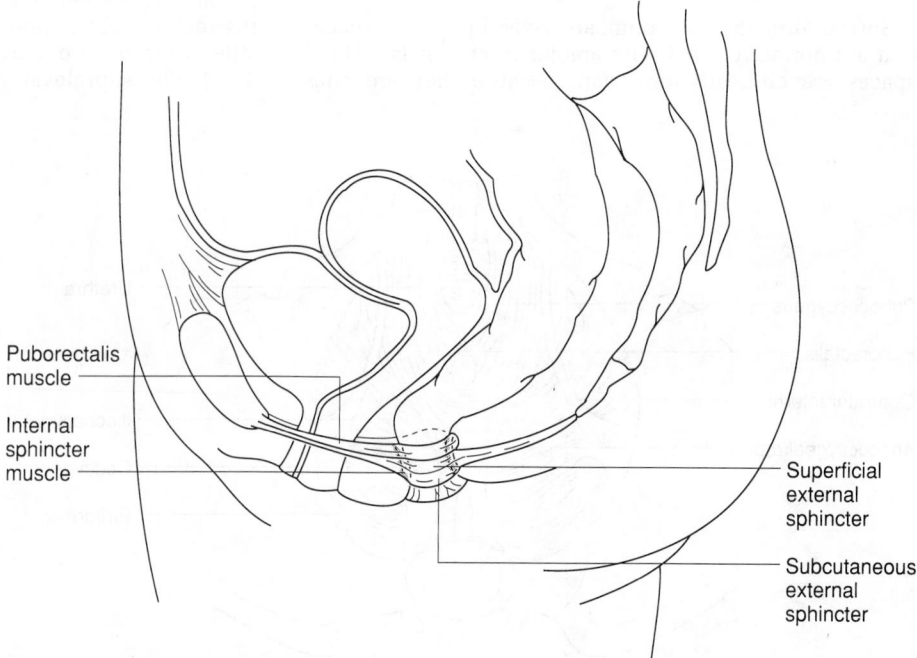

Figure 52-2. Arrangement of the external sphincter muscles.

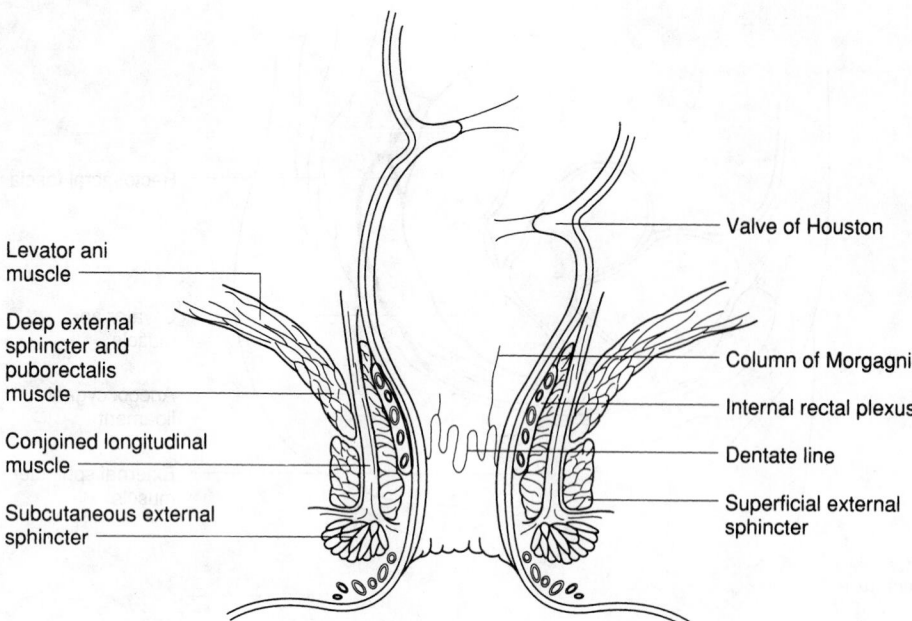

Levator ani
muscle

Deep external
sphincter and
puborectalis
muscle

Conjoined longitudinal
muscle

Subcutaneous external
sphincter

Valve of Houston

Column of Morgagni

Internal rectal plexus

Dentate line

Superficial external
sphincter

Figure 52-3. Anatomy of the anal canal.

raphe (Fig. 52-4). The pubococcygeal muscle arises from the anterior half of the obturator fascia and the back of the pubis. The fibers of the pubococcygeal muscle are directed backward, downward, and medially, where they decussate with fibers of the opposite side. The line of decussation is called the anococcygeal raphe (see Fig. 52-4). Some fibers that lie more posteriorly are attached directly to the tip of the coccyx and the last segment of the sacrum. This muscle also sends fibers to share in the formation of the conjoined longitudinal muscle. The puborectal and levator ani muscles have a reciprocal action: as one contracts, the other relaxes. During defecation, there is puborectal relaxation accompanied by levator ani contraction, which widens the hiatus and elevates the lower rectum and anal canal. When a person is in the upright position, the levator ani muscle supports the viscera.

Perianal and Perirectal Spaces

Surrounding the anorectum are several potential spaces that are normally filled with areolar tissues or fat. These spaces are clinically important because they are sites where abscesses can form. The perianal space immediately surrounds the anus. Laterally, the perianal space is contiguous with the subcutaneous fat of the buttocks. Medially, it is bound by the anoderm to the level of the dentate line. The ischioanal space is a triangular-shaped region below the levator ani muscle, bound medially by the external sphincter muscle, laterally by the ischium, and inferiorly by the transverse septum of the ischiorectal fossa (Fig. 52-5). The ischioanal space on each side is filled with fat and contains the inferior rectal vessels and lymphatics. The deep postanal space connects the ischioanal space on each side posteriorly and lies between the levator ani muscle above and the anococcygeal ligament below (Fig. 52-6). The deep postanal space is an important pathway in the formation of abscess; spread from one ischiorectal fossa to the other may result in a so-called horseshoe abscess. The intersphincteric space lies between the internal and external sphincter muscles. It is continuous with the perianal space below and extends above into the wall of the rectum. The supralevator spaces are situated on each side of the rectum above the levator ani muscle (see Fig. 52-5). The supralevator spaces communicate posteriorly

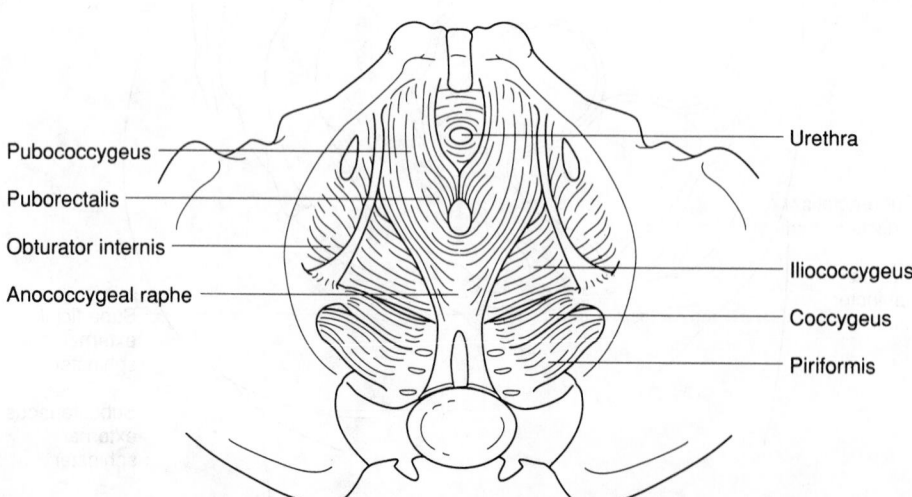

Pubococcygeus

Puborectalis

Obturator internis

Anococcygeal raphe

Urethra

Iliococcygeus

Coccygeus

Piriformis

Figure 52-4. Muscles of the pelvic floor.

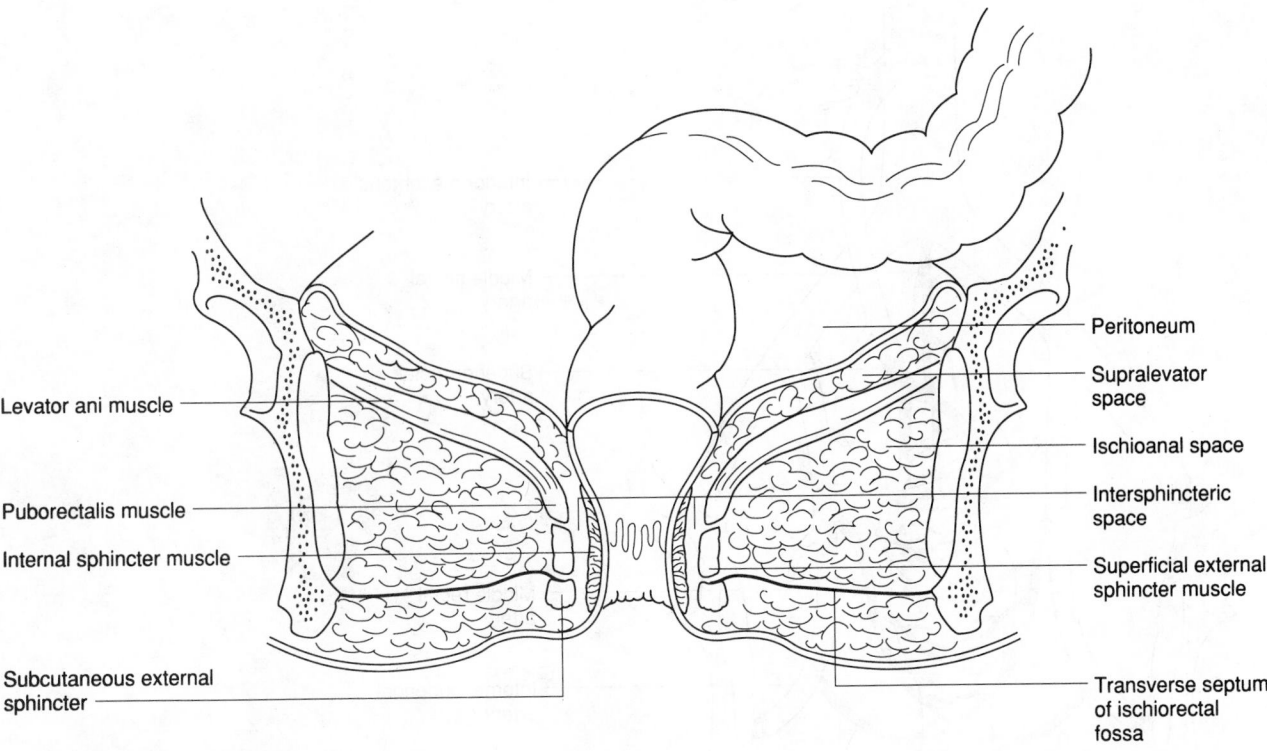

Figure 52-5. Anatomy of the perianorectal spaces (anteroposterior view).

and may allow spread of infection cephalad into the retroperitoneum (see Fig. 52-6).

Arterial Supply of the Rectum and Anal Canal

The superior rectal (hemorrhoidal) artery is the continuation of the inferior mesenteric artery and descends posterior to the rectum, where it bifurcates to supply the rectum and the upper portion of the anal canal (Fig. 52-7). The middle rectal (hemorrhoidal) arteries arise from the internal iliac artery on each side and enter the lower portion of the rectum anterolaterally at the level of the levator ani muscle; the middle rectal vessels do not enter the rectum by means of the lateral stalks, as previously believed. The middle rectal arteries anastomose with the branches of the superior rectal artery. The inferior rectal arteries (hemorrhoidal) arise from the internal pudendal artery, a branch of the internal iliac artery, and traverse the ischioanal fossa on each side to supply the anal sphincter muscles. There is no evidence of anastomosis between the superior and inferior rectal arteries. The middle sacral artery provides an insignificant amount of blood supply to the rectum. It arises posteriorly, just above the bifurcation of the aorta,

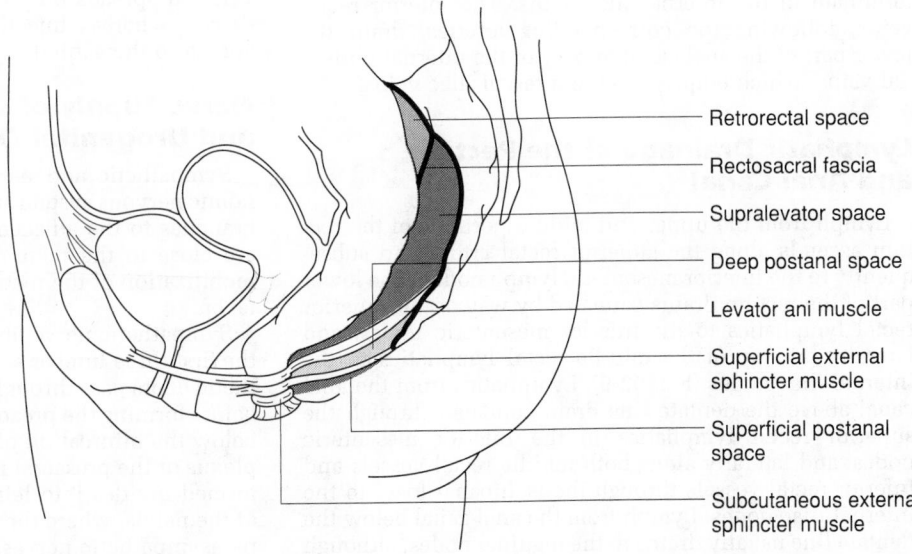

Figure 52-6. Anatomy of the perianorectal spaces (lateral view).

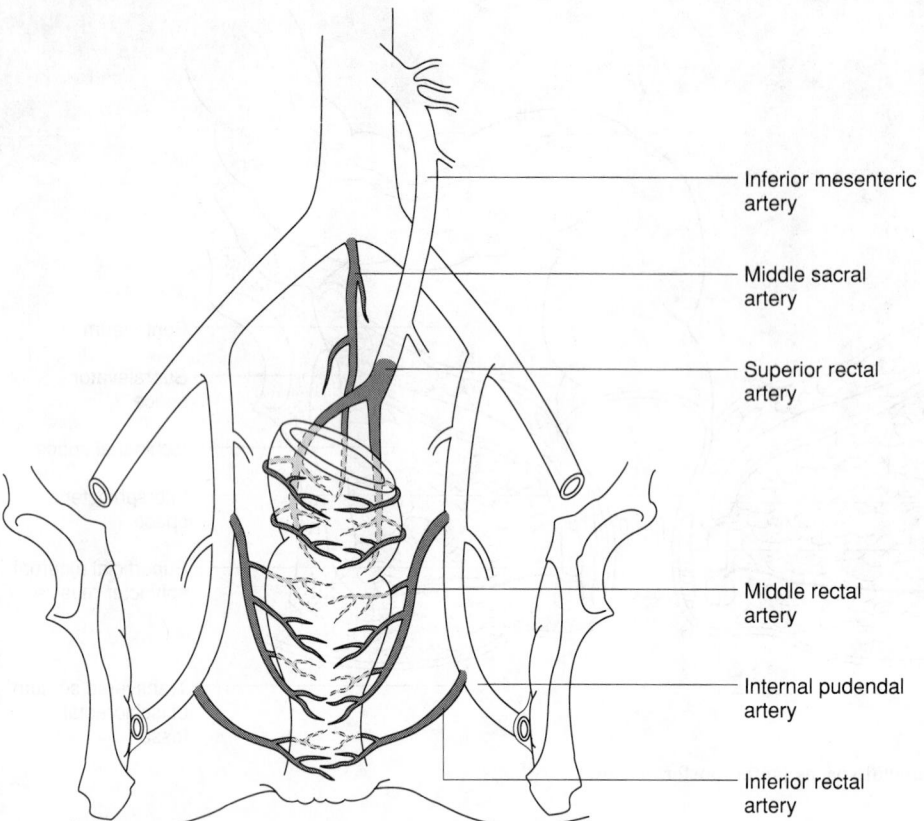

- Inferior mesenteric artery
- Middle sacral artery
- Superior rectal artery
- Middle rectal artery
- Internal pudendal artery
- Inferior rectal artery

Figure 52-7. Arterial supply of the rectum and anal canal.

and descends over the lumbar vertebra, sacrum, and coccyx.

Venous Drainage of the Rectum and Anal Canal

The return of blood from the rectum and anal canal occurs by two systems—portal and systemic (Fig. 52-8). The superior rectal (hemorrhoidal) vein drains the rectum and upper part of the anal canal into the portal system through the inferior mesenteric vein. The middle rectal veins drain the lower part of the rectum and the upper part of the anal canal; they accompany the middle rectal arteries and terminate in the internal iliac veins. The inferior rectal veins, following the corresponding arteries, drain the lower part of the anal canal by way of the internal pudendal veins, which empty into the internal iliac veins.

Lymphatic Drainage of the Rectum and Anal Canal

Lymph from the upper and middle portions of the rectum ascends along the superior rectal artery and subsequently to the inferior mesenteric lymph nodes. The lower part of the rectum drains cephalad by way of the superior rectal lymphatics to the inferior mesenteric nodes, and laterally by way of the middle rectal lymphatics to the internal iliac nodes (Fig. 52-9). Lymphatics from the anal canal above the dentate line drain cephalad through the superior rectal lymphatics to the inferior mesenteric nodes, and laterally along both middle rectal vessels and inferior rectal vessels through the ischioanal fossa to the internal iliac nodes. Lymph from the anal canal below the dentate line usually drains to the inguinal nodes, although

it can also drain to the superior rectal lymph nodes or along the inferior rectal lymphatics to the ischioanal fossa, if obstruction occurs in the primary drainage (Fig. 52-10). Retrograde lymphatic spread of carcinoma of the rectum and anal canal occurs only when there has been extensive involvement of perirectal structures, serosal surfaces, veins, and perineural lymphatic and proximal lymphatic channels.

Studies of the lymphatic drainage of the anorectum in women have shown that when dye is injected 5 cm above the anal verge, it spreads to the posterior vaginal wall, uterus, cervix, broad ligament, fallopian tubes, ovaries, and cul-de-sac. When dye is injected 10 cm above the anal verge, it spreads only to the broad ligament and the cul-de-sac, whereas injection at the 15-cm level shows no spread to the genital organs.[5]

Nerve Supply of the Rectum and Urogenital Organs

Sympathetic and parasympathetic nerves of the autonomic nervous system supply the anorectum and also send branches to the adjacent urogenital organs. Nerve trunks are close to the rectum and are prone to injury during mobilization of the rectum unless specific precautions are taken.

Sympathetic nerve fibers to the rectum are derived from the first three lumbar segments of the spinal cord. Sympathetic fibers pass through ganglionated sympathetic chains before forming the preaortic plexus. Preaortic fibers extend below the bifurcation of the aorta to form the hypogastric plexus or the presacral nerve (Fig. 52-11). The plexus thus formed divides into left and right branches on each side of the pelvis, where they are joined by the branches of the parasympathetic nerves.

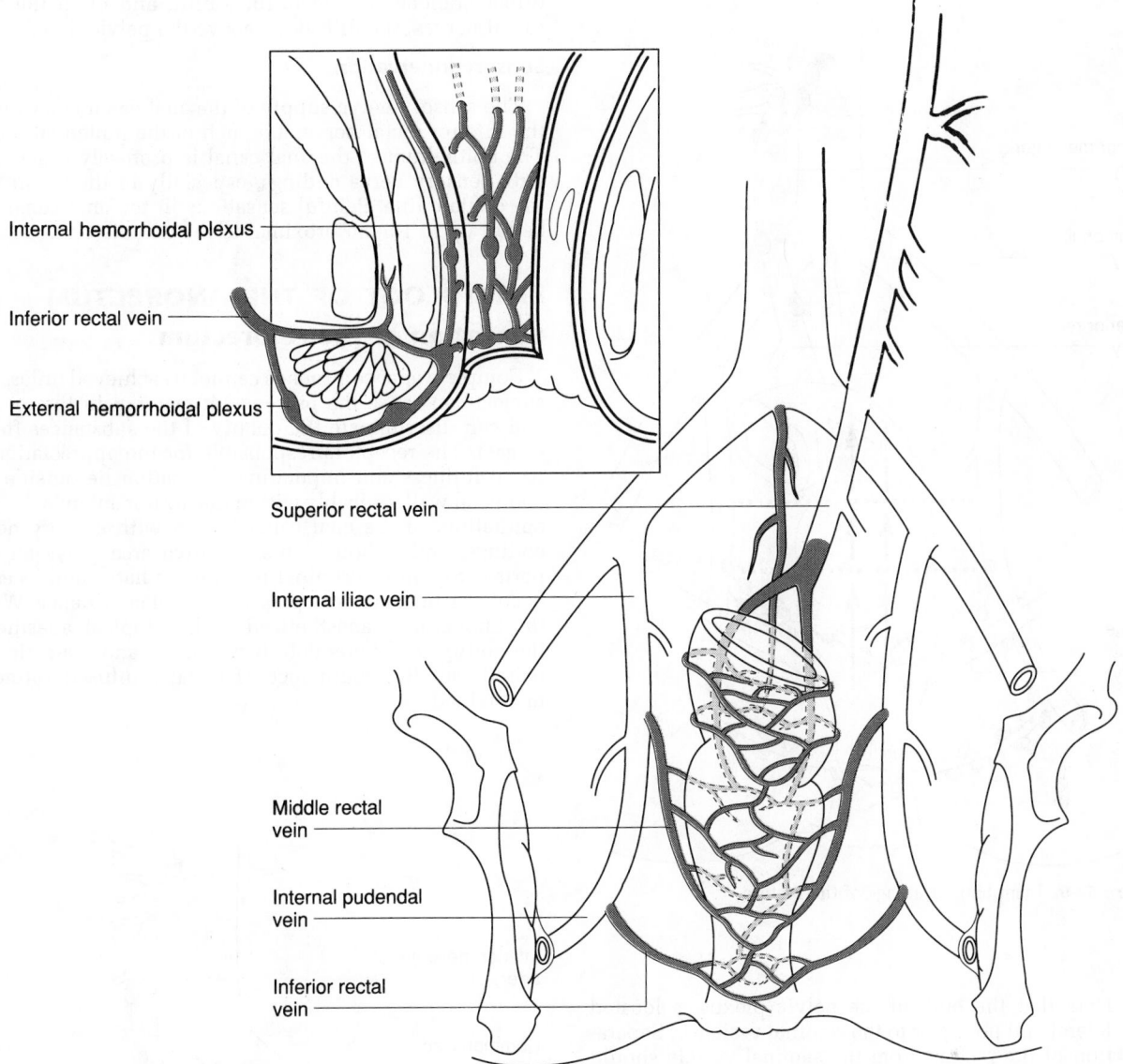

Internal hemorrhoidal plexus

Inferior rectal vein

External hemorrhoidal plexus

Superior rectal vein

Internal iliac vein

Middle rectal vein

Internal pudendal vein

Inferior rectal vein

Figure 52-8. Venous drainage of the rectum and anal canal.

The pelvic parasympathetic nerve supply is from the nervi erigentes, which originate from the second, third, and fourth sacral nerve roots. The fibers pass inward and forward to join the sympathetic nerve fibers to form the pelvic plexus (see Fig. 52-11). From the pelvic plexuses, both types of nerve fibers are distributed to urinary and genital organs.

In women, the sympathetic nerve fibers from the hypogastric plexus are directed toward the uterosacral ligament close to the rectum. In men, the nerve fibers from the hypogastric plexus pass immediately adjacent to the anterolateral wall of the rectum in the retroperitoneal tissue.

The pelvic plexus gives rise to the periprostatic plexus, an important subdivision that is essential to sexual function in men. The periprostatic plexus distributes fibers to the prostate, seminal vesicles, corpora cavernosum, terminal part of the vas deferens, prostatic and membranous urethra, ejaculatory ducts, and bulbourethral glands. Both parasympathetic and sympathetic nervous systems are involved in erection. Nerve impulses from the parasympathetic nerves, which lead to erection, produce vasodilation and increase blood flow in the cavernous spaces of the

penis. Activity of the sympathetic system adds to vascular engorgement and sustained erection. Moreover, sympathetic activity causes contraction of the ejaculatory ducts, seminal vesicles, and prostate, with subsequent expulsion of semen into the posterior urethra. Depending on which nerves have been damaged, deficiencies may include incomplete erection, lack of ejaculation, retrograde ejaculation, or total impotence.[6]

The following precautions can be exercised during operations on the pelvic colon to avoid nerve injuries:

1. When mobilizing the rectosigmoid colon and the upper rectum for nonmalignant disease, dissect close to the bowel wall posteriorly and do not disturb the retroperitoneal tissue, to avoid injury to the hypogastric plexus.
2. Cut the peritoneum on each side close to the rectum and brush off the retroperitoneal tissue laterally to avoid injury to the left and right branches of the hypogastric plexus.
3. Divide the lateral stalks close to the rectum to avoid injury to the nervi erigentes and the pelvic plexus.

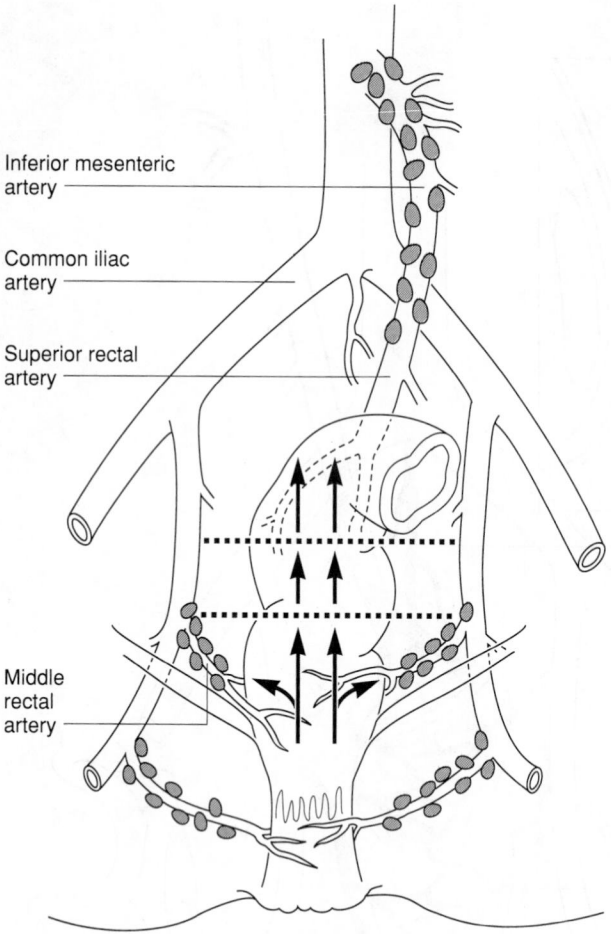

Figure 52-9. Lymphatic drainage of the rectum.

4. Note that the bulk of the pelvic plexus is located lateral and posterior to the seminal vesicles.[7] Separation of the rectum from the seminal vesicle should start at the midline. This is carried laterally to the edge of the seminal vesicle, then curves inferiorly to avoid injury to the neurovascular bundle.

The pudendal nerve arises from the sacral plexus (S-2 to S-4). It leaves the pelvis through the greater sciatic foramen, crosses the ischial spine, and then continues in the pudendal canal toward the ischial tuberosity in the lateral wall of the ischioanal fossa on each side. Three of its important branches are the inferior rectal, perineal, and dorsal nerves of the penis or clitoris. The pudendal nerve is anatomically protected from injury during mobilization of the rectum. Sensory stimuli from the penis and clitoris are mediated by a branch of the pudendal nerve and thus are preserved after proctectomy.

Nerve Supply of the Anal Canal

Motor Innervation

The internal sphincter is supplied by both sympathetic and parasympathetic nerves. The sympathetic and parasympathetic nerves are inhibitory to the internal anal sphincter. The external sphincter is supplied by the inferior rectal branch of the internal pudendal nerve and the perineal branch of the fourth sacral nerve. The levator ani is supplied not only by the pudendal nerve but also by

direct branches of the third, fourth, and often the fifth sacral nerves, the fifth lying above the pelvic floor.

Sensory Innervation

The sensory nerve supply of the anal canal comes from the inferior rectal nerve, a branch of the pudendal nerve. The epithelium of the anal canal is profusely innervated with sensory nerve endings, especially in the vicinity of the dentate line. Painful sensations in the anal canal can be felt up to 1.5 cm proximal to the dentate line.

PHYSIOLOGY OF THE ANORECTUM

Sensation of the Anorectum

Complete anal continence cannot be achieved unless the subject can sense the presence of material in the rectum and can discriminate the quality of the substances (feces or gas). The receptors responsible for the appreciation of rectal fullness and impending evacuation lie outside the anorectal wall, probably within the levator ani muscle. The epithelium of the anal canal is rich with sensory nerve endings, and although this sensitive area plays an important role in discriminating between flatus and feces, it is not a critical factor in preserving anal continence. When the anoderm is anesthetized with a topical anesthetic, the ability to differentiate between air and water is impaired, but the continence of rectally infused saline is maintained.[8]

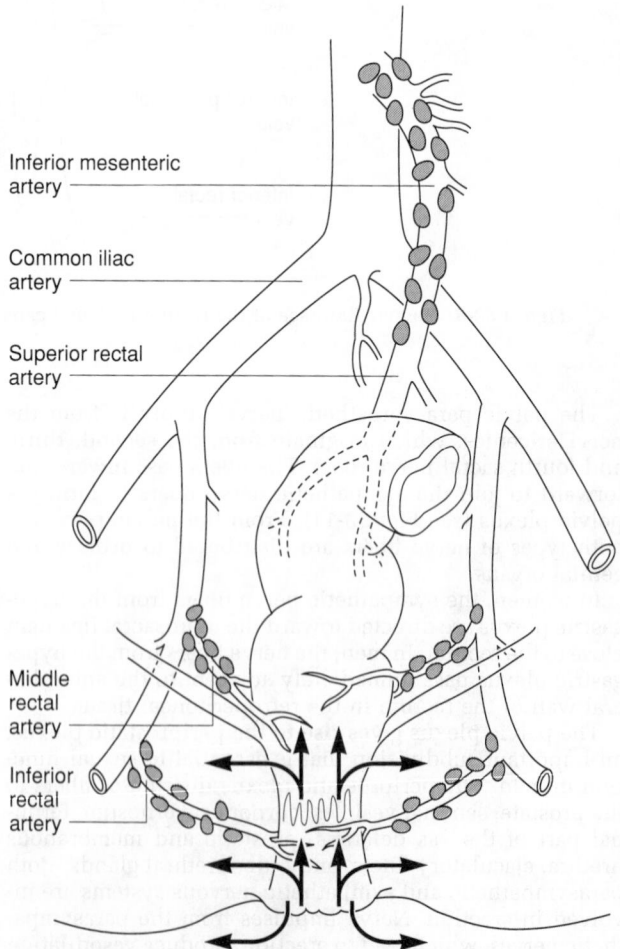

Figure 52-10. Lymphatic drainage of the anal canal.

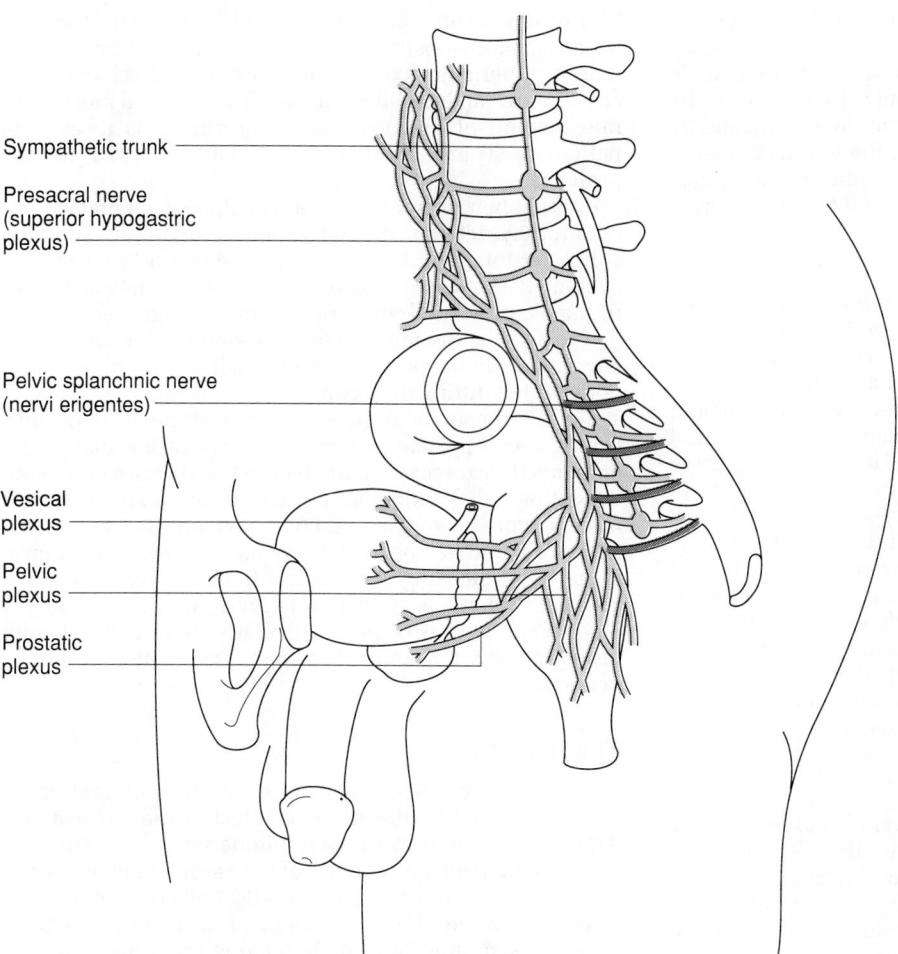

Sympathetic trunk

Presacral nerve
(superior hypogastric
plexus)

Pelvic splanchnic nerve
(nervi erigentes)

Vesical
plexus

Pelvic
plexus

Prostatic
plexus

Figure 52-11. Sympathetic and para-sympathetic nerve supply of the rectum.

Mechanism of Anal Continence

Stool can accumulate in the rectum for a variable period of time before the urge to defecate is experienced. The ability of the rectum to retain stool is known as reservoir continence. Continence is favored by the influence of pelvic muscles on rectal shape. The anal canal is pulled forward by the puborectal muscle, which, as a U-shaped sling, creates an angle of 80 to 90 degrees to the rectum. This anorectal angle, maintained by the continuous tonic activity of the puborectal muscle, is effective in preventing stool in the rectum from entering the anal canal. Although it has been postulated that the mucosa of the anterior wall of the lower rectum is pressed firmly into the anal canal, creating a flap valve effect, recent studies have suggested that continence is maintained by sphincteric action rather than such a valvular mechanism. In the upper part of the anal canal, there are usually three submucosal anal cushions, which may contribute to the mechanism of anal closure and cause high pressure in the anal canal.

The internal sphincter, because it is innervated by the autonomic nervous system, is not subject to voluntary control. This powerful muscle exists in a continuously tonic state and is responsible for maintaining closure of the resting anal canal. The high-pressure zone of the anal canal at rest is due to the actions of the internal sphincter. The external sphincter contributes to anal pressure only when a bolus of stool is present within the anal canal. The increase in pressure during voluntary contraction (squeeze pressure) is due exclusively to the activity of the external sphincter. The high resting pressure in the anal canal acts as a barrier to prevent leakage of mucus and gas.

When the rectum is distended, the internal sphincter relaxes (rectoanal reflex). This relaxation allows the rectal content to move down to the anal canal. In contrast, the external sphincter contracts when the rectum is distended. Reflex contraction of the external sphincter prevents rectal content from leaking through the anus. A marked distention of the rectum, however, inhibits external sphincter contraction, and the voluntary act of straining also inhibits the external sphincter and the pelvic floor muscles. Although volitional contraction of the external sphincter can be sustained only for short periods, it is the most important mechanism of voluntary continence.

Defecation

Defecation, the act of evacuating fecal material from the rectum, is a complex process that involves both a reflex response and voluntary performance. When a fecal bolus enters the rectum, the stretch receptors, believed to reside within the muscles of the pelvic floor, register a sensation and an urge to defecate. Distention of the rectum causes a reflex relaxation of the internal sphincter and contraction of the external sphincter and puborectal muscle, allowing the rectal content to make contact with the anal canal. This contact allows the sensory epithelium of the anal canal to sense and discriminate the nature of the material. If rectal distention is maintained, the rectal musculature adapts to decrease the rectal pressure, the accommodation response. The act of defecation proceeds with the subject assuming the squatting or sitting position to straighten out the angle between the rectum and the anal canal. Expulsion of the feces is accomplished by contraction of the rectum and by increased intraabdominal pressure by the Valsalva maneuver. After defecation is completed, voluntary sphincters contract actively, and the normal postural tone is restored.

HEMORRHOIDS

In the upper anal canal there are cushions of submucosal tissue that are composed of connective tissue containing venules and smooth muscle fibers. There are usually three cushions—left lateral, right anterior, and right posterior. This anatomic arrangement is remarkably constant and bears no relation, as previously thought, to the terminal branches of the superior rectal vein. The function of these cushions is to aid in anal continence. During the act of defecation, when they become engorged with blood, they cushion the anal canal and support the anal canal lining. The anal cushions are supported by muscles that arise partly from the internal sphincter and partly from the conjoined longitudinal muscles. *Hemorrhoid* is the pathologic term used to describe the downward displacement of the anal cushion causing dilatation of the contained venules.[9,10] Hence, hemorrhoids develop when the supporting tissues of the anal cushion deteriorate.[11]

Classification

External hemorrhoids are dilated venules of the inferior hemorrhoidal plexus located below the dentate line. Thrombosed external hemorrhoids are intravascular clots in the venules of the external hemorrhoids. Internal hemorrhoids are the anal cushions located above the dentate line that have become prolapsed. The appearance and symptoms of internal hemorrhoids depend on the severity. For practical purposes, internal hemorrhoids are graded according to the degree of prolapse.

> *First degree:* The anal cushions slide down beyond the dentate line on straining.
> *Second degree:* The anal cushions prolapse through the anus on straining but reduce spontaneously.
> *Third degree:* The anal cushions prolapse through the anus on straining or exertion and require manual replacement into the anal canal.
> *Fourth degree:* The prolapse is not manually reducible.

Clinical Manifestations

The most common complaints of burning, itching, swelling, and pain usually are not from hemorrhoids but result from pruritus ani, anal abrasion, anal fissure, thrombosed external hemorrhoids, or prolapsed anal papilla. The most common manifestation of hemorrhoids is painless, bright red rectal bleeding associated with bowel movement. In severe hemorrhoids, the patient commonly describes the bleeding episode as blood dripping into the toilet bowl. A feeling of incomplete evacuation is also common. In chronic prolapse, exposed rectal mucosa often causes perianal irritation and mucus staining on the underwear. Congestion of external hemorrhoids or skin tags can cause discomfort or pain. Symptoms are aggravated by constipation and diarrhea.

Examination

Definitive diagnosis of hemorrhoids is made by examination. An enema administered shortly before examination will make a complete inspection easier and more thorough.

The examination can be performed in the left lateral or prone jackknife position. Anal skin tags, an external fistula opening, perianal excoriation from anal discharge, and anal fissure can be easily detected. The best and most accurate method of diagnosis for hemorrhoids is to ask the patient to sit and strain on the toilet and watch for the prolapse.

Internal hemorrhoids cannot be palpated. Digital examination may detect anal stenosis or an anal scar. The anal sphincter tone and sphincter squeeze can be subjectively evaluated. A mass in the anal canal can be detected, and, in males, prostatic hypertrophy can be diagnosed.

Anoscopy is the ideal method to examine the anal canal. For patients in the prone jackknife position, the table should not be tilted during the examination. The patient is asked to strain to estimate the degree of prolapse of the hemorrhoids. During anoscopy, one must exclude a coexisting anal fissure or fistula. Proctoscopy should be used in all cases to rule out coexisting rectal abnormalities, particularly carcinoma and inflammatory bowel disease, both of which can cause symptoms similar to hemorrhoidal complaints. In young patients, if the rectal bleeding is obviously from the hemorrhoids, a complete colonic examination is not indicated. In patients older than 50 years of age, particularly those with a family history of cancer, a complete colonic examination should be performed.

Treatment

According to modern concepts, prolapse of anal cushions is initiated by the shearing effect of the passage of a large, hard stool or by the precipitous act of defecation, as in urgent diarrhea. If prolapse of the vascular cushions can be prevented or if the congesting effect of a tight anal canal can be abolished, the anal cushions return to their normal state and symptoms are ameliorated without necessitating removal of the cushions themselves. Therefore, the rationale of giving bulk in the diet is to eliminate straining at defecation. A high-fiber diet usually reduces symptoms of hemorrhoids and is ideal for first- and second-degree hemorrhoids.

Rubber Band Ligation

Rubber band ligation is suitable for second-degree and first-degree hemorrhoids that do not respond to bulk-forming agents, and it is suitable for some third-degree hemorrhoids. The procedure may be performed in the office with the patient prepared with an enema. Aspirin, nonsteroidal antiinflammatory drugs, and anticoagulants must be discontinued at least 1 week before and for 2 weeks after the procedure. The procedure is performed through an anoscope. The band should be placed on the rectal mucosa just above the internal hemorrhoid (Fig. 52-12). Usually, one hemorrhoid is ligated per session, with additional ligation performed 4 to 6 weeks later; ligation of two or three hemorrhoids at one setting has been practiced with good results.

Rubber band ligation is not painless. The patient should be warned of anal discomfort or even pain, usually from anal sphincter spasm. Warm sitz baths reduce the pain, and an appropriate analgesic should be prescribed. A bulk-forming agent should be taken for at least 6 to 8 weeks. Immediate severe or progressive pain is an indication of misplaced rubber band ligation, too close to the dentate line, and requires immediate removal of the rubber band. There has been concern about the safety of rubber band ligation because of reports of deaths due to acute perianal sepsis. Symptoms of delayed anal pain, urinary retention, and fever are clues to the development of perianal infection. Prompt and aggressive treatment should include anti-

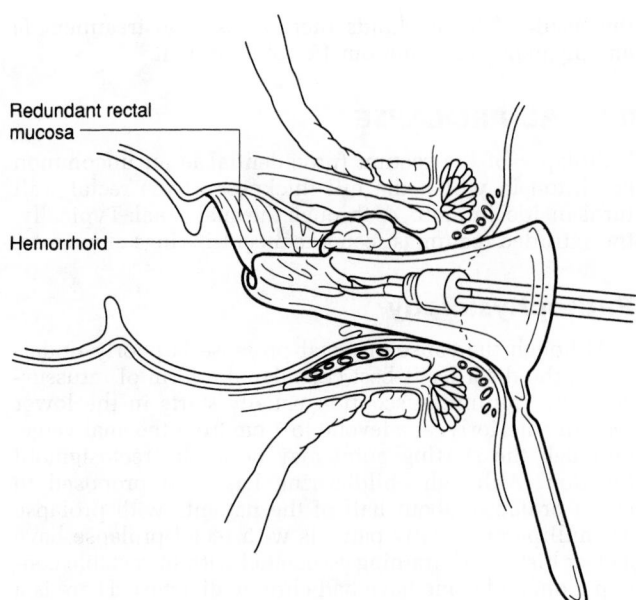

Figure 52-12. Rubber band ligation of an internal hemorrhoid.

biotics, drainage of abscesses, and excision of necrotic tissues. Severe infection after rubber band ligation is rare. Because of these potentially severe complications, rubber band ligation should not be performed in patients with immune deficiencies.

Infrared Photocoagulation

Infrared photocoagulation is a relatively new technique that coagulates tissue protein or evaporates water in the cells, depending on the intensity and duration of application. An infrared probe is applied just proximal to the internal hemorrhoids through an anoscope. Infrared photocoagulation results for first- and second-degree hemorrhoids are comparable to those of rubber band ligation. Pain and complications occur infrequently. A regular electrocautery unit with a flat or ball tip works as well or even better.

Hemorrhoidectomy

Hemorrhoidectomy should be considered when the hemorrhoids are severely prolapsed through the anus, requiring manual replacement, or when hemorrhoids are complicated by associated pathology, such as ulceration, fissures, fistulas, large hypertrophied anal papillae, or extensive skin tags. In most cases, hemorrhoidectomy can be performed using local anesthesia with mild sedation. In muscular or obese individuals, general or regional block anesthesia may be preferable. The procedure is performed with the patient in the prone jackknife position. The cheeks of the buttocks are taped apart. An elliptic excision starts at the perianal skin, includes external and internal hemorrhoids, and ends at the anorectal ring. The mucosa and submucosa are dissected off of the underlying internal sphincter muscle (Fig. 52-13). Unless there is an associated anal stenosis or chronic anal fissure, internal sphincterotomy is not performed. The entire wound is closed with running absorbable sutures. The largest and the most redundant hemorrhoid should be excised first. No packing is placed in the anal canal.

Urinary retention is a common complication of hemorrhoidectomy, unless intravenous fluids are restricted during the procedure and minimized for the next 6 to 8

hours.[12] Warm sitz baths are started the next morning, as is bran or psyllium seed. A mild laxative is given the following night. Lasers have also been used for hemorrhoidectomy. The public demand for laser hemorrhoidectomy is great because of the belief that laser hemorrhoidectomy is less painful and has better results than conventional hemorrhoidectomy; there has been no evidence for such claims.[13]

MANAGEMENT OF SPECIAL SITUATIONS

Thrombosed External Hemorrhoids

Thrombosis is a fairly common complication of hemorrhoidal disease. Most patients give no history of straining or physical exertion and do not have histories of hemorrhoidal disease. The complication develops with an abrupt onset of anal mass and pain that peaks within 48 hours. Usually, the pain becomes minimal after the fourth day.

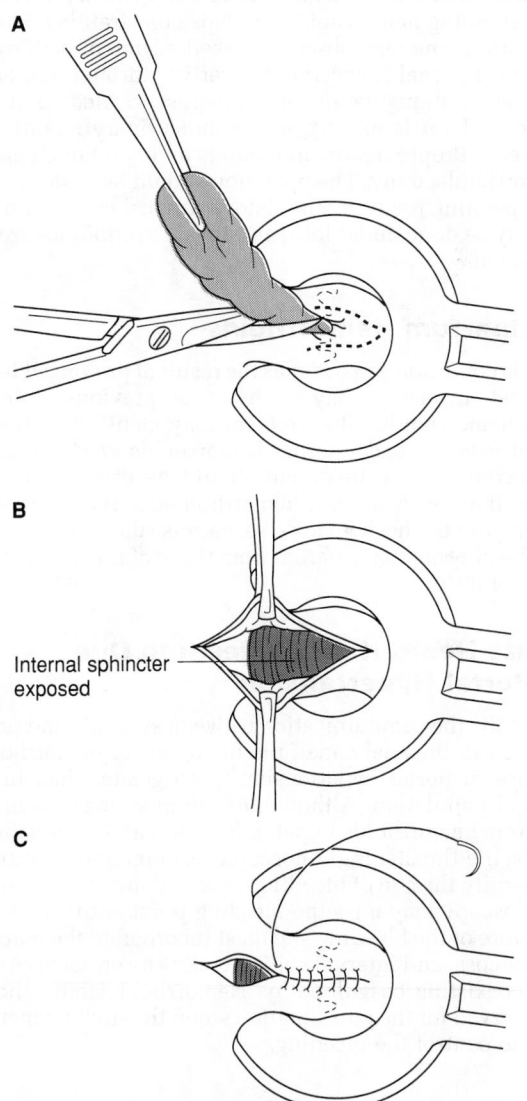

Figure 52-13. Technique of interanal closed hemorrhoidectomy. (*A*) Exposure of hemorrhoid with elliptic excision starting at perianal skin and extending to anorectal ring. (*B*) Submucosal hemorrhoidal plexus dissected from the internal sphincter, anoderm, and mucosa. (*C*) Wound closed with a running suture.

Occasionally, the skin overlying the hematoma becomes necrotic, causing bleeding and discharge or infection, which causes further necrosis and more pain. Treatment should be aimed at relief of severe pain, prevention of recurrent clot, and prevention of residual skin tags. If the patient is examined during severe pain, excision of the clot should be performed. Conversely, if the pain is already subsiding and the clot is starting to shrink, thrombosis may be managed conservatively with warm sitz baths for comfort, proper anal hygiene, and bulk-producing agents such as bran or psyllium seed. The entire clot must be removed if operation is chosen. The procedure can often be performed with the use of local anesthesia, and the wound can be left open without packing. Relief of pain is usually immediate. Postoperative care is simple and is aimed at keeping the wound clean with warm sitz baths or washing. An analgesic drug may be required during the first 24 hours.

Strangulated Hemorrhoids

Strangulation results from prolapsed third-degree hemorrhoids that have become irreducible. History reveals a long-standing hemorrhoidal prolapse on straining. On examination, one may observe marked edema of both external and internal hemorrhoids everting through the anus. Untreated, strangulation may progress to ulceration and necrosis. Pain is usually severe and urinary retention is common. Proper treatment requires an urgent or emergent hemorrhoidectomy. The operation should be performed in the operating room or ambulatory surgical center and can usually be done under local anesthesia. Antibiotics are not indicated.

Postpartum Hemorrhoids

This condition can occur as the result of prolonged labor. The patient may or may not have had previous problems with hemorrhoids. The problem may manifest as thrombosed external and internal hemorrhoids or strangulated hemorrhoids. The treatment should be directed accordingly. If an excision or a hemorrhoidectomy is indicated, one should not hesitate to do so, because the complications and healing are not different from those of the nonpostpartum condition.

Acute Hemorrhoidal Bleeding Due to Portal Hypertension

Despite the communication between systemic and portal systems in the anal canal, the incidence of hemorrhoidal disease in portal hypertension is no greater than in the normal population. Although uncommon, massive bleeding from hemorrhoids in patients with portal hypertension can be life-threatening. Anoscopic examination is essential to identify the site of bleeding; proctoscopy or flexible sigmoidoscopy may miss the bleeding point entirely.

Suture of the bleeding site must incorporate the mucosa, submucosa, and internal sphincter. It is essential to correct any coexisting coagulopathy. Hemorrhoidectomy should be reserved for the rare situation when the stick-tie method fails to control the bleeding.

Hemorrhoids in Inflammatory Bowel Disease

Hemorrhoidal problems in inflammatory bowel disease are uncommon. Most anal problems are the result of diarrhea causing perianal irritation and swelling, rather than the result of hemorrhoids themselves. The treatment is anal hygiene and symptomatic relief of pain.

RECTAL PROLAPSE

Prolapse of the rectum (procidentia) is an uncommon condition in which the full thickness of the rectal wall turns inside out, into, or through the anal canal. Typically, the extruded rectum is seen as concentric rings of mucosa.

Pathophysiology

Although the cause of rectal prolapse is poorly understood, the disorder is best considered a form of intussusception. The intussusception usually starts in the lower rectum anteriorly, at a level 6 to 7 cm from the anal verge, although the starting point may be at the rectosigmoid junction. Although childbearing has been proposed to cause prolapse, about half of the patients with prolapse are nulliparous. Many patients with rectal prolapse have a clear history of straining associated with intractable constipation, and some have had chronic diarrhea. There is a high incidence of rectal prolapse in patients affected by mental retardation.

Studies of anorectal function and defecation dynamics in patients with rectal prolapse reveal that these patients have impaired resting and voluntary sphincter activity, decreased functional rectal capacity, and impaired continence. A failure of normal relaxation of the external sphincter and pelvic floor musculature during defecation attempts is also seen.

Anatomic Abnormalities

Prolapse of the rectum predominates in females, with a female/male ratio of 5:1 or 6:1. Several anatomic defects or abnormalities are consistently demonstrated in patients with chronic rectal prolapse:

- Abnormally deep rectovaginal or rectovesical pouch
- Lax and atonic musculature of the pelvic floor
- Lack of normal fixation of the rectum and an elongated mesorectum
- Redundant rectosigmoid and sigmoid colon
- Lax and atonic sphincters

These defects are most likely the effect of long-standing prolapse rather than the cause.

Classification

Rectal prolapse is classified in the following manner[14]:

- Incomplete (partial) rectal prolapse: prolapse of rectal mucosa only
- Complete rectal prolapse (involving all layers)
    First degree—occult prolapse
    Second degree—prolapse to, but not through, the anus
    Third degree—protrusion through the anus for a variable distance

Clinical Manifestations

One of the early symptoms of rectal prolapse is anorectal discomfort during defecation. Difficulty in initiating bowel movements and the feeling of incomplete evacuation are common. Some patients require digital evacuation of the stool in the rectum. In many patients, the prolapse causes obstruction that leads to chronic constipation. In an overt prolapse, initially the protrusion occurs only during or after defecation. As the problem becomes more pronounced, the protrusion may be precipitated by coughing, exertion, or walking. In patients with grade I (occult) and grade II prolapse, perineal pressure, difficult with defecation, and incomplete evacuation may be the only complaints. Fecal and urinary incontinence are associated symptoms in prolapse of long duration.

Diagnosis

Diagnosis of rectal prolapse is easy if the prolapse has come through the anus. Typically, the protrusion has circumferential mucosal folds. When the prolapse remains in the rectum or anal canal (occult prolapse), the diagnosis is difficult. Redness of the rectal mucosa, especially anteriorly at 6 to 7 cm from the anal verge, provides a clue. In grade II prolapse, in which the protrusion is to but not through the anus, the rectal prolapse is often confused with prolapsed hemorrhoids.

Evaluation

Although not useful for the diagnosis of rectal prolapse, barium enema is indicated in certain patients to rule out an associated lesion, particularly in patients who have had recent constipation. Total colonoscopy is an acceptable alternative to barium enema. Anal manometry is helpful for the evaluation of patients with incontinence and for follow-up of anal sphincteric function after the repair. Defecating proctogram is useful to confirm the diagnosis of grade I and grade II rectal prolapse if an intussusception can be demonstrated.

Complications

Complications due to rectal prolapse are rare. Ulceration from chronic trauma to the prolapsed rectum is frequent but rarely severe. Strangulation is uncommon. Spontaneous rupture of the prolapsed rectum with evisceration of small bowel through the anus is even more rare.

Treatment

The modern concept of repair of rectal prolapse involves removal of the intussusception and measures to prevent intussusception from recurring. Most methods of repair are by the transabdominal approach, although in most elderly or unfit patients a transperineal approach is more appropriate.

The rectal sling operation, a method introduced by Ripstein, is the technique used most often for rectal prolapse in the United States. The operation consists of the construction of a sling of Teflon or Marlex that wraps the fully mobilized rectum anteriorly and attaches to the presacral fascia (Fig. 52-14A). In a large series with long-term follow-up reported from the Lahey Clinic, the operative death rate was 0.7%. Complications included hemorrhage from presacral veins in 8%, stricture at the site of the sling in 2%, and recurrence in 10%. Men had higher rates of recurrence than women (24% versus 8%), suggesting difficulty in mobilizing the rectum in the narrow male pelvis.[15]

The Ivalon sponge wrap operation has been more popular in the United Kingdom. The Ivalon sponge is formed from a polyvinyl alcohol that creates a fibrotic reaction to enhance adhesion of the rectum to the sacrum. Unlike the Ripstein procedure, the sponge, which is sewn to the sacrum, wraps the rectum posteriorly but not circumferentially (see Fig. 52-14B). A purported advantage of the posterior wrapping over the anterior wrapping is its freedom

from obstruction of the rectum. One of the most concerning complications of using the Ivalon sponge is pelvic sepsis, which has been reported to occur in 2.6% to 16% of patients.

Recurrence rates of 2% to 16% with follow-up periods of 3 to 10 years have been reported. The use of Marlex mesh instead of Ivalon sponge has been reported with excellent results, with no recurrences in a 2-year follow-up of 86 patients.[16]

Anterior resection of the rectum, in a manner that removes all redundant colonic loops, has also been reported as a treatment for rectal prolapse. A complete mobilization of the rectum to the level of the levator ani muscle is essential. A suitable length of rectum and sigmoid colon is resected, and a primary anastomosis is performed. In a series of 123 patients, the recurrence rate was 8.9% with a mean follow-up of 10 years. The mortality rate was 0.7% and the overall morbidity rate was 29%.[17]

Transabdominal rectosigmoid resection and rectopexy is a composite surgical procedure with a full mobilization of the rectum to the level of the pelvic floor musculature. The redundant sigmoid and the rectum are resected with primary anastomosis. The endorectal tissue and peritoneum on each side of the mid-rectum are then sutured to the presacral fascia (Fig. 52-15). The recurrence rate has been reported to be 6% to 9% with a 3- to 4-year follow-up.[18] Transabdominal rectosigmoid resection and rectopexy has become the preferred choice of the abdominal approaches.

Perineal rectosigmoidectomy is a transperineal approach in which the prolapsed rectum and redundant sigmoid colon are excised endorectally. The prolapse has to protrude at least 3 cm through the anus. The operation is performed with the patient in the lithotomy (Fig. 52-16) or prone jackknife position. The operation is well tolerated by patients, and the postoperative pain is minimal. Several recent series report a recurrence rate of about 10% with a relatively short-term follow-up.[19,20] Perineal rectosigmoidectomy is an excellent choice for patients with the prolapse extruded at least 3 cm, particularly elderly patients.

The modified Delorme procedure is another transperineal approach. This technique is used for rectal prolapse that comes down to but not through the anus, or for overt prolapse that protrudes less than 3 cm through the anus. The procedure is conducted with the patient in the prone jackknife position. The submucosa from the dentate line is stripped circumferentially with the use of electrocautery. This is continued proximally until it is taut. At this point, the submucosal tube is transected anally. The proximal cut end is then brought down and anastomosed to the dentate line. The denuded rectal wall is incorporated into the stitches to eliminate the dead space. Eight such stitches are required with additional interrupted simple stitches in between (Fig. 52-17). Similar to perineal rectosigmoidectomy, it is well tolerated by patients and causes little postoperative pain. The recurrence rate is about 10% at 3 years' follow-up.[21,22]

Incontinence in Rectal Prolapse

By the time rectal prolapse is diagnosed, half of the patients already have anal incontinence. Loss of continence is not caused solely by prolonged protrusion, with mechanical stretching of the sphincter. Incontinence in rectal prolapse is caused by damage to the pudendal nerve that supplies the sphincter muscles, probably from prolonged stretching.[23] About 50% of patients with fecal incontinence from rectal prolapse improve after repair of the prolapse. Because the return of continence takes as long as 6

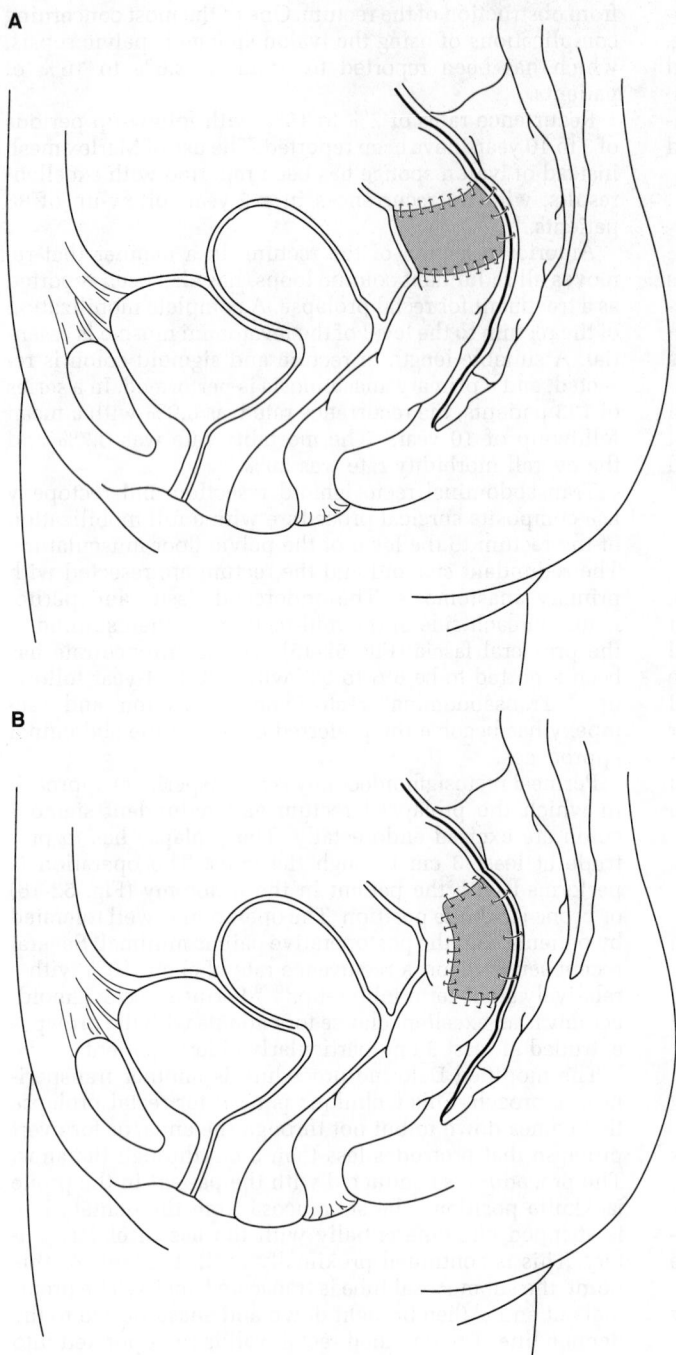

Figure 52-14. (*A*) Teflon sling repair (Ripstein repair). The Teflon mesh is wrapped around the rectum anteriorly and sutured to the rectum. (*B*) Ivalon sponge repair. The Ivalon sponge is sutured to the presacral fascia, then wrapped around the rectum posteriorly.

to 12 months, operative treatment for incontinence should be postponed for a year.

ANAL FISSURE

Definition

Anal fissure is an ulcer in the lower portion of the anal canal. Fissures can be classified as acute or chronic and further subdivided as either primary or secondary. A primary fissure occurs without association with other local or systemic diseases. Secondary fissure develops in association with other systemic diseases, such as Crohn's disease, leukemia, aplastic anemia, or agranulocytosis.

Pathophysiology

Most tears of the anal canal can be traced to the passage of a large, hard stool or explosive diarrhea; trauma to the anus; or tearing during vaginal delivery. In men, almost all of the fissures are located in the posterior midline, whereas 10% of fissures in women are in the anterior midline. Numerous studies on anal sphincteric function reveal that the resting anal pressure (internal sphincter) in patients with anal fissure is significantly higher than normal, whereas the squeeze pressure (external sphincter) is not different from normal. The studies also show that the high anal pressure is caused by an increased tone of the internal sphincter muscle and not by internal sphincter muscle spasm, because the

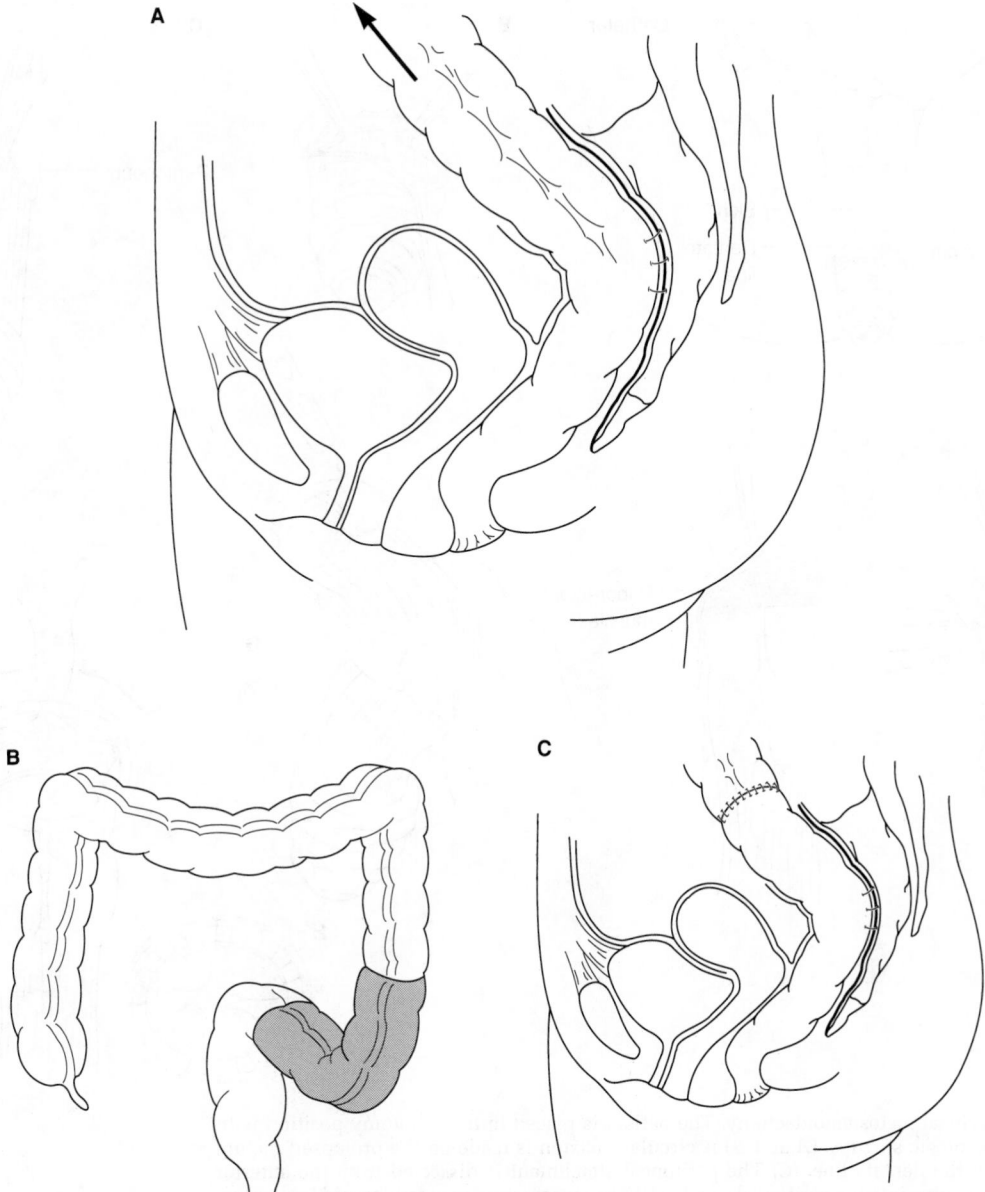

Figure 52-15. Transabdominal proctopexy. (*A*) After full mobilization of the rectum, the endorectal fascia and peritoneum on each side is sutured to presacral fascia, below the promontory of the sacrum. (*B*) Resection of redundant rectosigmoid colon. (*C*) Completed colonic anastomosis.

inhibitory reflex remains normal in these patients. Increased pressure is not caused by external sphincter muscle because, during squeeze, the anal pressure increases normally. An abnormal internal anal sphincter reflex in response to rectal distention has been reported. It was characterized by an overshoot contraction immediately after a normal relaxation. The most recent study suggests that the unhealed ulcer is caused by reduced anodermal blood flow as the result of increased anal pressure.[24] These reports suggest that reflexively stimulated internal sphincter muscle plays a role in the pathogenesis of anal fissure and that surgical approaches should be directed to the internal, rather than external, anal sphincter.

Clinical Manifestations

Anal pain, particularly during and after bowel movement, is the most prominent symptom. The pain is described as burning, throbbing, or dull aching. In acute anal fissure, the pain can be severe and incapacitating and may last for many hours. If there is fever, fissure may mimic an anorectal abscess, especially intersphincteric abscess. Bleeding is common and, as a rule, stains the toilet paper upon wiping. Constipation is a common association, because the pain may cause patients to be reluctant to have a bowel movement.

Diagnosis

Although pain and bleeding are typical of anal fissure, the diagnosis is confirmed by examination. When performed gently, inspection of the anus by spreading the buttocks will reveal the fissure in most cases. On digital examination, the fissure can be appreciated as a small fibrotic defect. Digital examination can also detect tightness of the anal canal, another clue indicating an anal fissure. A small anoscope is useful to visualize the fissure. Proctos-

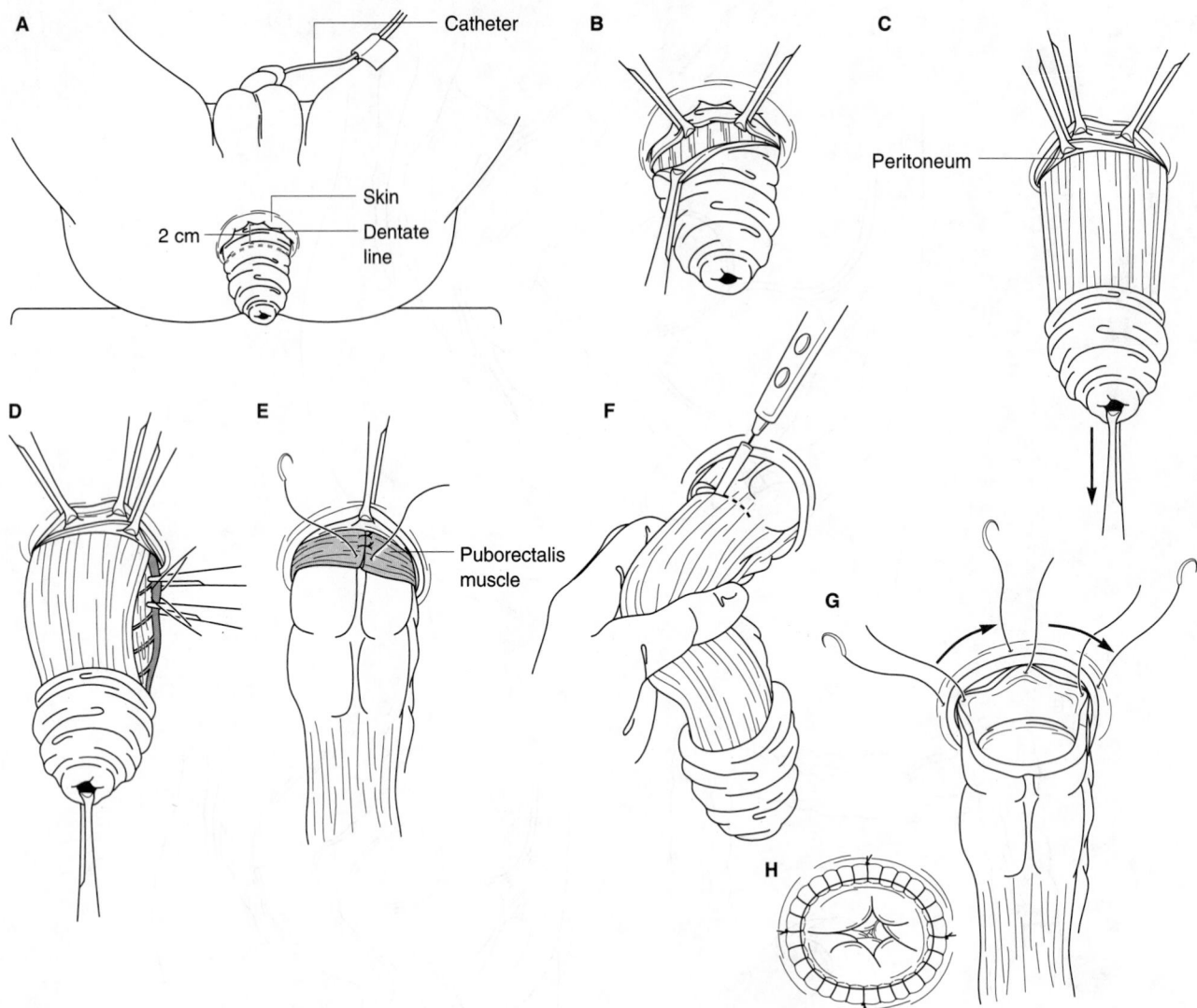

Figure 52-16. Perineal rectosigmoidectomy. The patient is placed in the lithotomy position with both legs in gynecologic stirrups. (*A* and *B*) A circular incision is made on the prolapsed rectum 2 cm proximal to the dentate line. (*C*) The peritoneal attachment is dissected from the anterior rectal wall, thus opening into the peritoneal cavity. (*D*) The mesorectum or mesosigmoid is clamped and divided laterally and posteriorly. (*E*) The previously opened peritoneum is sutured to the anterior wall of the rectum or sigmoid colon as high as possible. This is followed by approximation of the puborectalis (optional). (*F*) The anterior wall of the protruding rectum is cut 1 cm distal to the anal verge. (*G*) Stay sutures of 3-0 synthetic absorbable material are placed in four quadrants. (*H*) Anastomosis with running stitches.

copy or flexible sigmoidoscopy should be done to exclude any associated abnormalities of the anal canal and rectum, especially inflammatory bowel disease. Occasionally, the examination must be performed under general anesthesia because of severe pain.

Management

Initial treatment of acute anal fissure is pain relief, with proper anal hygiene and warm sitz baths to relax the anal canal. Of equal importance are bulk-forming agents, such as bran or psyllium seed, to relieve constipation. Application of a topical anesthetic jelly directly to the fissure before bowel movement is helpful. Acute anal fissure should heal within 6 weeks. Surgery is not usually required unless the fissure is an exacerbation of a chronic anal fissure.

Chronic anal fissure is usually deep, exposing the internal anal sphincter. Occasionally, chronic anal fissure has a triad of fissure, sentinel skin tag, and hypertrophied anal papilla. The sentinel tag is the fibrotic or edematous skin adjacent to the fissure. Chronic anal fissure is unlikely to heal with conservative management, and if the pain persists, surgery should be considered.

Lateral internal sphincterotomy has become the treatment of choice for chronic anal fissure.[25] The procedure can be performed under local, regional, or general anesthesia. Most patients can return home on the same day of the surgery.

In the closed method, the left or right lateral quadrant of the anal canal is exposed with an anal speculum. The speculum is gently and gradually opened to its maximum. The stretched internal sphincter can be easily felt, like a bow string. A knife blade is passed through the skin at

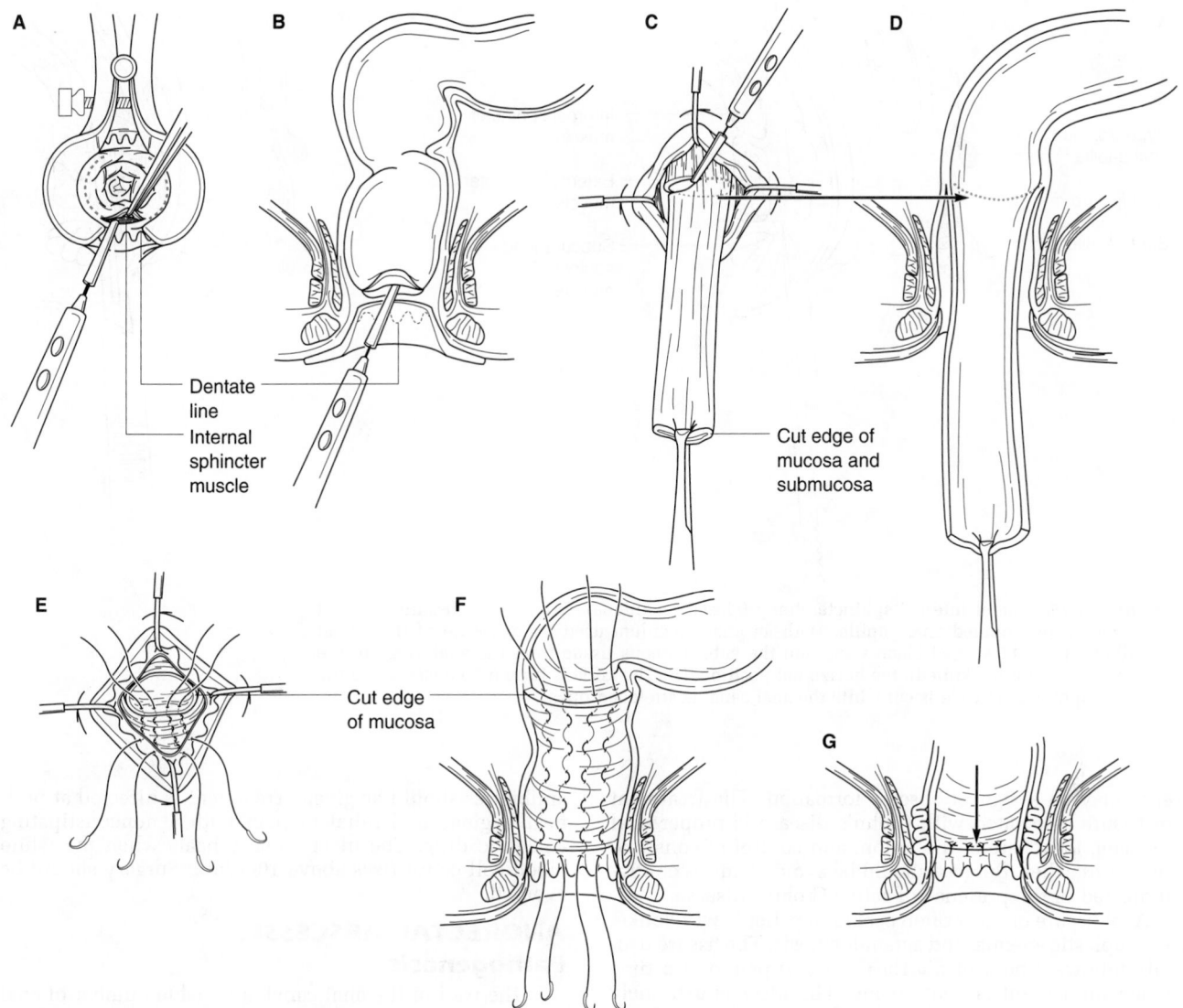

Figure 52-17. Modified Delorme procedure. Patient is placed in the prone position. (*A* and *B*) With a Pratt speculum used for exposure, a circumferential incision is made 1 cm proximal to the dentate line. The submucosa is dissected from the underlying internal sphincter. At the level of the anorectal ring, the Pratt speculum is replaced by Gelpi retractors placed at a right angle to the dentate line. (*C* and *D*) Proximal to the anorectal ring, the dissection continues in the mucosal plane until the mucosa resists being pulled down. The mucosal tube is then cut. (*E* and *F*) With 3-0 synthetic absorbable sutures, the mucosa at the upper cut end is brought down to the mucosa at the lower cut end, taking along the denuded anorectal wall. Eight such sutures are placed all around. (*G*) At completion of the anastomosis, the anorectum is plicated.

the lateral border of the internal sphincter muscle, in the subcutaneous plane, with the blade in the horizontal position. The knife blade is then advanced to the level of the dentate line. At this point, the blade is turned 90 degrees, with the cutting edge on the muscle. The internal sphincter muscle is then cut to its full thickness by gentle pressure on the blade while it is withdrawn. The stab wound is left open (Fig. 52-18). The fissure in the posterior or anterior midline is left undisturbed, but the redundant skin or the hypertrophied anal papilla can be excised as appropriate.

With the open technique, the skin and subcutaneous tissue from the dentate line to the anal verge are incised; an anal speculum is used to expose the left or right lateral quadrant. The internal sphincter muscle is identified and incised to its full thickness. The wound is closed with running sutures (Fig. 52-19).

Fissurectomy with anoplasty using a skin flap to cover the wound is suitable for cases in which there are markedly redundant skin tags around the fissure. A triangular skin flap with the apex at the fissure and the wide base at the perianal skin is created. Internal sphincterotomy is performed in the bed of the fissure from the dentate line to its lateral border. If preferred, the fissure can be excised. The full-thickness flap is then slid to cover the wound and is closed with running sutures (Fig. 52-20).

Secondary Anal Fissure

Fissures or ulcers in Crohn's disease are larger and deeper than primary anal fissures. The skin around the ulcer is edematous, macerated, and erythematous. As a rule, pain is not as severe as that associated with idiopathic primary fissure; severe pain from a fissure in Crohn's dis-

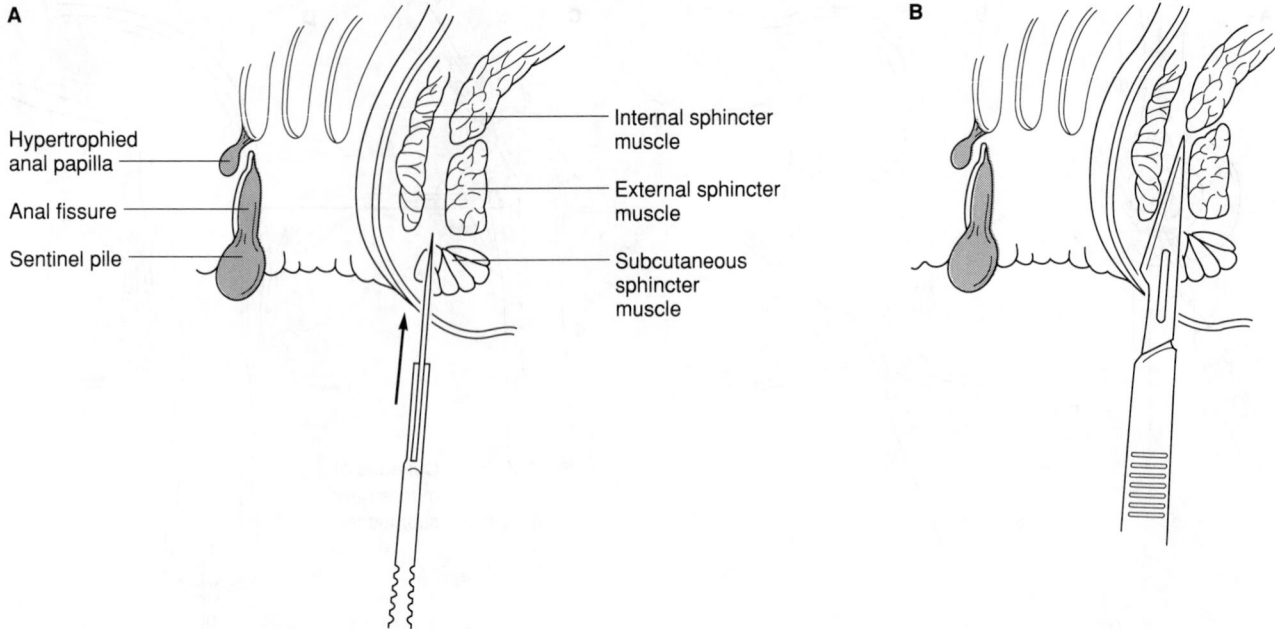

Figure 52-18. Lateral internal sphincterotomy (closed technique). (*A*) Triad of fissure, sentinel pile, and hypertrophied anal papilla. With an anal speculum used for exposure of the lateral quadrant, a no. 11 scalpel blade stabs into the subcutaneous tissue from the anal verge to the dentate line, with the knife in the horizontal position. (*B*) The knife is turned 90 degrees and the internal sphincter muscle is cut while the anal canal is stretched open.

ease may be a sign of abscess formation. The treatment of fissure associated with Crohn's disease is proper anal hygiene, local care of the lesion, and control of constipation or diarrhea. Surgery should be avoided and is contraindicated in the presence of active Crohn's disease.

Anal fissure or ulcer often occurs in patients with leukemia, aplastic anemia, and agranulocytosis. The fissure usually follows a bout of diarrhea or constipation at a time when the patient is neutropenic. The ulcer is extremely painful, usually superficial, and often necrotic at its base. Fever or septicemia is common; if present, broad-spectrum

antibiotics should be given. Treatment is directed at perineal hygiene and relief of pain with a nonconstipating analgesic drug. The ulcer usually heals when the white blood cell count rises above 1000/mL. Surgery should be avoided.

ANORECTAL ABSCESSES
Pathogenesis

In the wall of the anal canal, a variable number of anal glands (4 to 10) lined by stratified columnar epithelium have direct openings into the anal crypts at the dentate

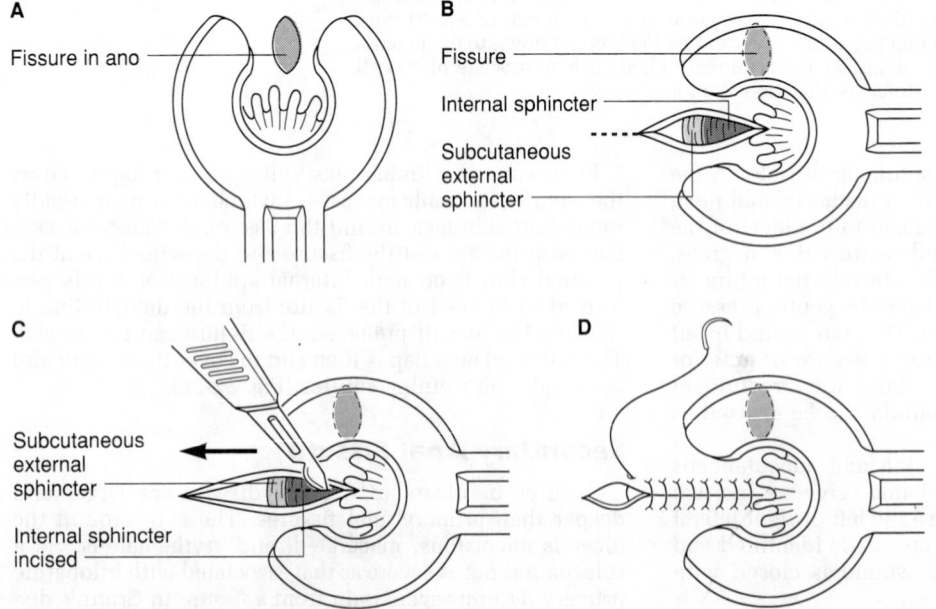

Figure 52-19. Lateral internal sphincterotomy (open method). (*A*) The fissure in the midline is left alone. (*B*) With a speculum used to expose the left lateral quadrant, an incision is made through the subcutaneous tissue to expose both the subcutaneous external sphincter and the internal sphincter. (*C*) The internal sphincter is incised to its full thickness; care is taken not to cut the external sphincter. (*D*) The wound is closed.

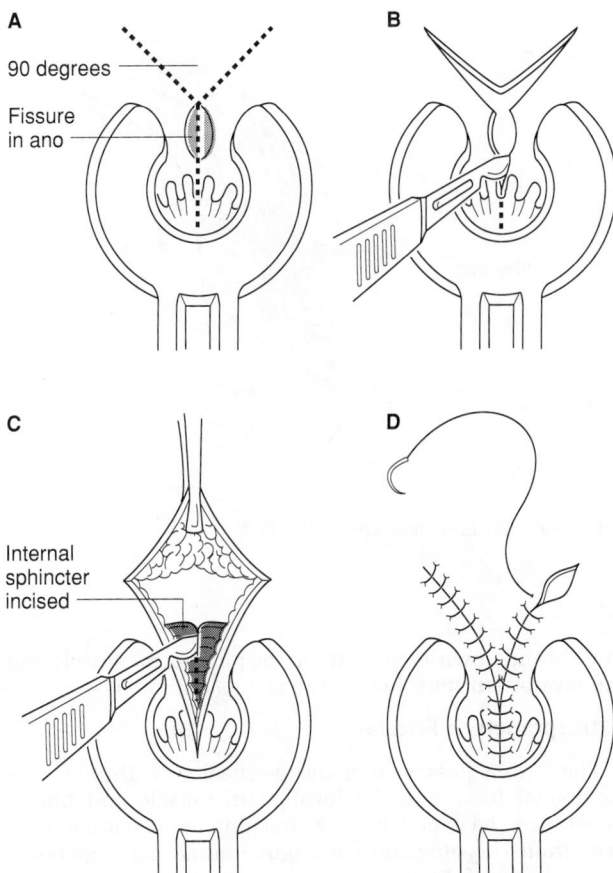

Figure 52-20. Internal sphincterotomy with V-Y anoplasty. (*A*) The skin flap is outlined, with the apex at the fissure, at a right angle. (*B*) A full-thickness skin flap is created. (*C*) Internal sphincterotomy is made through the fissure, in its full thickness to the dentate line. (*D*) The skin flap is advanced to cover the wound and is sutured.

line. Infection of the anal glands is the most common origin of perianal abscesses. Because the anal glands lie between the internal and external sphincter muscles, an intersphincteric abscess is formed. The infection may then spread to different spaces (Fig. 52-21). The locations of abscesses, in order of frequency, are perianal, ischioanal, intersphincteric, and supralevator.

Clinical Manifestations

The initial symptom of most anorectal abscesses is severe pain in the anal region. The pain is throbbing or dully aching in character and is aggravated by walking, straining, coughing, and sneezing. Depending on the location of the abscess, a swollen mass may be felt. Fever or even septicemia may be present. In some patients, urinary retention occurs.

Management

Like an abscess in any other part of the body, an anorectal abscess must be drained as soon as possible. In general, antibiotics are not necessary after the abscess is adequately drained, but in patients with immune deficiencies and in those with prostheses or cardiac valvular abnormalities, appropriate antibiotics should be instituted.

Perianal abscesses are the most superficial and the easi-

est to treat. The abscess is usually small and can be drained under local anesthesia. A cruciate incision is made on the most prominent part of the skin and subcutaneous tissue overlying the abscess cavity. Redundant skin edges are excised to prevent premature closure of the abscess. No packing is necessary.

An ischioanal abscess causes a diffuse swelling of the ischioanal fossa. The drainage is the same as in perianal abscess. Bilateral ischioanal or horseshoe abscess has its origin in the deep postanal space, with spreads to both sides of the ischioanal space. A horseshoe abscess should be drained through the deep postanal space. A longitudinal incision is made in the skin between the tip of the coccyx and the anus to expose the anococcygeal ligament. The anococcygeal ligament is incised along its fibers, and the deep postanal space is entered. After the abscess cavity is drained and irrigated, a counter-drainage incision is made on one or both limbs of the ischioanal space. No packing is needed.

Unlike perianal and ischioanal abscesses, there are no apparent signs of swelling or induration in the perianal area in intersphincteric abscesses. The diagnosis is suspected when anorectal pain is so severe that rectal examination is impossible. A deep-seated tenderness is present when circumanal pressure is applied. Most intersphincteric abscesses are located in the posterior quadrant. An indurated or bulging mass can be felt in the anal wall above the dentate line and can extend into the rectum to a variable distance. Intersphincteric abscesses are drained by incising the anal canal lining and incising through the internal sphincter muscle. The abscess cavity is curetted and irrigated with saline solution until clean. No packing is placed. Postoperative care consists of warm sitz baths for comfort. A bulk-producing agent is started the next day.

Supralevator abscess is uncommon and can be difficult to diagnose. Because of its proximity to the abdominal cavity, a supralevator abscess can mimic acute intraabdominal conditions. Digital examination reveals an indurated or bulging tender mass on either side of the lower rectum or posteriorly above the level of the anorectal ring. The supralevator abscess may arise in one of three ways: through upward extension of an intersphincteric abscess, by upward extension of an ischioanal abscess, or from intraabdominal processes such as diverticular abscess, appendiceal abscess, or abscess from Crohn's disease. It is essential to determine the origin of the abscess before treatment. If the abscess is secondary to upward extension of an intersphincteric abscess, it should be drained into the rectum. If such an abscess is drained through the ischioanal fossa, a complicated suprasphincteric fistula can be formed. If a supralevator abscess arises from the upward extension of an ischiorectal abscess, it should be drained through the ischioanal fossa. Attempts at draining this kind of abscess into the rectum may result in an extrasphincteric fistula. If the abscess is secondary to an intraabdominal disease, the primary disease is treated and the supralevator abscess is drained into the rectum, through the ischioanal fossa, or through the abdominal wall.

FISTULA-IN-ANO

Fistula-in-ano is a chronic form of perianal abscess that is spontaneously or surgically drained but in which the abscess cavity does not heal completely, becoming instead an inflammatory track with a primary opening (internal opening) in the anal crypt at the dentate line and a secondary opening (external opening) in the perianal skin.

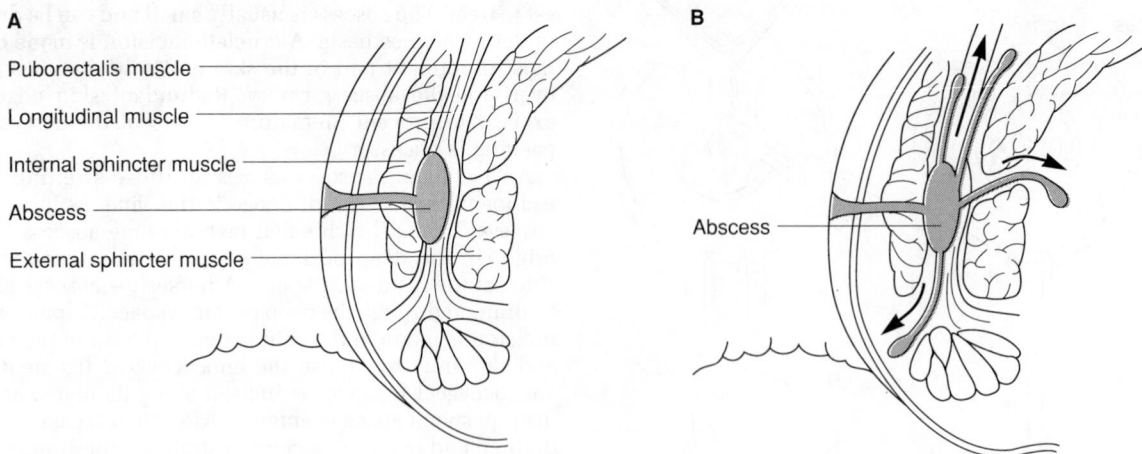

Figure 52-21. Pathways of infection start in the intersphincteric space (*A*) and then spread to perianal spaces, forming perianal abscesses (*B*).

Classification

There are four main forms of fistula-in-ano, based on the relation of the fistula to the sphincter muscles[26] (Fig. 52-22).

Intersphincteric Fistula

The fistulous track is in the intersphincteric plane. The external opening is usually in the perianal skin close to the anal verge.

Transsphincteric Fistula

The fistula starts in the intersphincteric plane or in the deep postanal space. The fistulous track traverses the external sphincter, with the external opening at the ischioanal fossa. Horseshoe fistulas are in this category.

Suprasphincteric Fistula

The fistula starts in the intersphincteric plane in the mid–anal canal and then passes upward to a point above the puborectal muscle. The fistula passes laterally over this muscle and downward between the puborectal muscle and the levator ani muscle into the ischioanal fossa.

Extrasphincteric Fistula

The fistula passes from the perineal skin through the ischioanal fossa and the levator ani muscle and finally penetrates the rectal wall. Extrasphincteric fistulas may arise from a cryptoglandular origin, trauma, a foreign body, or a pelvic abscess.

Clinical Manifestations

Most patients have a previous history of anorectal abscess subsequently associated with intermittent drainage. Recurrence of a perianal abscess suggests the presence of a fistula-in-ano. The external opening is usually visible as a red elevation of granulation tissue with purulent or serosanguineous drainage on compression. In the simple or superficial fistula, the track can be palpated as an indurated cord. Deeper fistulas usually are not palpable.

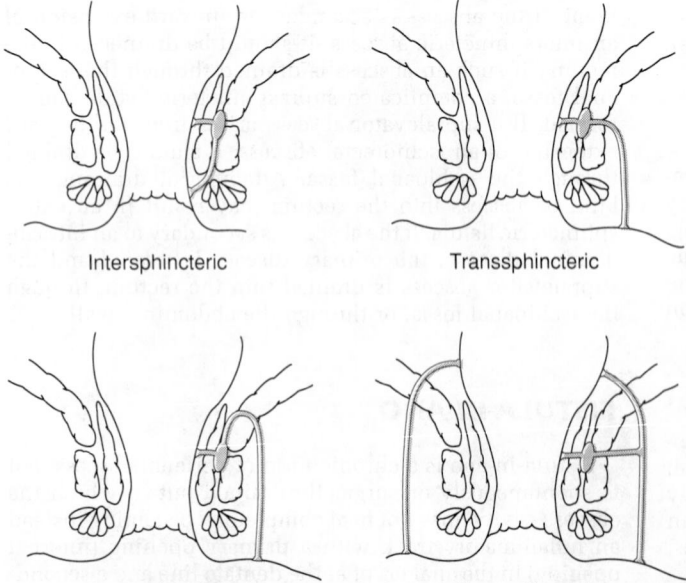

Intersphincteric   Transsphincteric

Suprasphincteric   Extrasphincteric

Figure 52-22. The four main anatomic types of fistula.

Anoscopy should be done to identify the internal opening. Proctoscopy or flexible sigmoidoscopy is performed to rule out other lesions and inflammatory bowel disease. A fistula probe can be introduced into the fistulous track to determine its direction, although it is not always possible to pass the probe through the internal opening.

Several disorders must be considered in the differential diagnosis of a fistula-in-ano. Hidradenitis suppurativa is differentiated by the presence of multiple perianal skin openings. A pilonidal sinus with perianal extension and infected perianal sebaceous cysts must be considered. It is important to exclude fistulas associated with ulcerative colitis and Crohn's disease. Diverticulitis of the sigmoid colon, with perforation and fistulization to the perineum, rarely occurs. Low rectal and anal canal carcinomas may present as a fistula in the perineum.

Management

The principles of fistula surgery include unroofing the fistula, eliminating the primary opening (infective source), and establishing adequate drainage.[27] Failure to open the entire track may lead to recurrence. In most fistulas, the treatment of choice involves opening the entire fistulous track, with a guide in place. Granulation tissues are curetted and the edges of the wound marsupialized. Fistulectomy, the excision of the fistulous track, has no advantages over fistulotomy. Horseshoe fistula, an uncommon form of fistula-in-ano, is a direct extension of an intersphincteric abscess and usually starts in the deep postanal space. Radical unroofing results in a large wound and is not necessary. Incision of the deep postanal space combined with excision of the lateral tracks is the procedure of choice.

In young patients, transection of the internal and external sphincter muscle in the posterior half, when performed in the course of a fistulotomy, does not always jeopardize anal continence. In older patients and in women, however, transection of the external sphincter muscle, particularly in the anterior half, risks incontinence. When sphincter transection appears likely, some authors recommend the use of a seton. A seton is a suture, usually silk, that is drawn through a fistula. Setons are used to tie around the muscles covering the fistula to create fibrosis, and to cut the muscles. The seton is threaded through the fistulous track and tied over the muscles. In the second stage (average interval, 6 to 8 weeks), fistulotomy is performed. Incontinence after the proper use of a seton is uncommon, even when the fistula is deep.

Anal Fistula Associated With Crohn's Disease

Fistulas associated with Crohn's disease are often asymptomatic. They resemble the ordinary fistulas seen in patients without Crohn's disease in that there is an indurated opening in the skin that exudes pus and a palpable track passing toward the anal canal. The fistulas can be simple and superficial, complex with multiple tracks, or deep with the origin in the upper anal canal or lower rectum.

The most important part of treatment is adequate and aggressive medical therapy, including medications for active Crohn's disease.[28] Metronidazole has been found to be useful in some patients. Surgery is indicated only for those fistulas associated with an abscess.

PILONIDAL SINUS

Most authors now accept the fact that pilonidal sinuses are caused by infection of the hair follicle in the sacrococcygeal area. Reports that pilonidal sinus occurs in unusual positions such as the umbilicus, healed amputation stumps, and interdigital clefts all support the acquired etiology of this disease. Pilonidal sinuses are more likely to occur in the hirsute patient.

Clinical Manifestations

The average patient with pilonidal disease is a hirsute, moderately obese man in his second or third decade. Pilonidal disease is rare in people under age 15, rises sharply to peak between 16 and 20 years, and remains high until age 25, when the incidence declines quickly. Pilonidal disease may present as an acute abscess at the sacrococcygeal area that ruptures spontaneously, leaving unhealed sinuses with chronic drainage. When sinuses develop, pain is usually minimal.

Diagnosis

A painful and fluctuant mass is the most common presentation of the acute process. In its earliest stage, only cellulitis may be present, whereas in the chronic state the diagnosis is confirmed by the sinus opening in the intergluteal fold, about 5 cm above the anus. Most sinus tracks run cephalad (93%); the rest run caudad (7%) and may be confused with fistula-in-ano or suppurative hidradenitis. On careful examination, one can always find a pit or pits in the midline, representing infected hair follicles. The differential diagnoses include furuncles of the skin, anal fistula, syphilitic or tuberculous granulomas, and osteomyelitis with multiple draining sinuses in the skin. Actinomycosis in the sacral region has been described as virtually indistinguishable from pilonidal disease.

Treatment

Drainage of a pilonidal abscess can almost always be done under local anesthesia. A longitudinal incision is made lateral to the midline in the coccygeal area. The incision is deepened into the subcutaneous tissue, entering the abscess cavity. All the hairs in the abscess cavity, if present, must be removed, and the wound is lightly packed with fine gauze. The patient is instructed to clean the wound at least once a day and to apply light packing. An antibiotic is not usually indicated.

Conservative excision of chronic pilonidal sinuses consists of minimal excision of midline pits or sinuses, with the abscess cavity thoroughly cleaned of hairs and debris. The cavity may be packed and permitted to heal by second intention. In a follow-up of 149 patients for a mean of 3.5 years, the cure rate was 84%.[29] The advantage of this technique is the minimal surgery and wound involved. Healing is rapid, and usually the wounds are completely closed within 3 weeks. This is the technique of choice for most primary pilonidal sinuses with or without abscess.

A variation of this approach consists of opening the sinus track in the midline. The debris and granulation tissues are curetted. The fibrous edges of the track are sutured to the edges of the wound all around. This technique minimizes the size and depth of the wound and also prevents the wound from premature closure. Wounds treated in this way require about 6 weeks to heal.

Excision of pilonidal sinuses with primary closure of the wound is simple but has a high recurrence rate. Primary closure is appealing because of complete wound healing within 7 to 10 days. To avoid recurrence or breakdown of the midline wound, the anatomy of the natal crease needs to be altered. Z-plasty can achieve this goal. Excision of pilonidal sinuses with primary Z-plasty fills out and flattens the natal crease, directs the hair-points away from the midline, largely prevents maceration, reduces suction effects in the soft tissues of the buttocks, and minimizes friction between adjacent surfaces. The excision is carried down to the subcutaneous tissue. The limbs of the Z are cut to form a 30-degree angle with the long axis of the wound. Full-thickness flaps are raised, and the flaps are transposed and sutured. A closed-suction drain is placed under the full-thickness flaps. Z-plasty avoids the midline wound, which is the main cause of slow healing and recurrences. Because of the rather extensive dissection compared with the conservative excision outlined above, Z-plasty should be reserved for recurrent pilonidal sinuses.

Postoperative Care

The postoperative care is as important as the operation. The wound should be washed in the bathtub or shower at least once a day. If the cavity is large, it should be packed with fine gauze. If it is small, it should be swabbed to remove any foreign body, especially hair, at least once a day. The patient should return for follow-up at 1- to 2-week intervals until the wound is completely healed.

Pilonidal Sinus Complicated by Carcinoma

Carcinoma arising from chronic pilonidal sinus is rare; 32 cases had been reported in the world literature up to 1981.[30] Most of the lesions are well-differentiated squamous cell carcinomas. The appearance of the wound should alert one to suspect carcinoma. There is usually an ulcer with a friable, bleeding, and fungating margin. Wide excision is the treatment of choice. When inguinal node metastasis is present, the prognosis is poor; review of the literature shows a 5-year survival rate of 51%. Inguinal node metastasis occurs in 14% of patients at the time of diagnosis.[30]

RECTOVAGINAL FISTULA

A rectovaginal fistula is a communication between the anterior wall of the anal canal or rectum and the posterior wall of the vagina. Causes of rectovaginal fistula include the following:

- Congenital maldevelopment
- Trauma
   Obstetric
   Operative
   Blunt and penetrating injury
   Foreign body
- Infection of anal canal or vaginal septum
- Pelvic irradiation
- Neoplasm

Rectovaginal fistulas are considered low if a repair can be done from a perineal approach and high if repair can be accomplished only transabdominally (Fig. 52-23).

Rectovaginal fistulas can be classified as simple or complex, based on location, size, and cause:

Simple
Low to mid-vaginal septum
2.5 cm or less in diameter
Traumatic or infectious cause

Complex
High vaginal septum
2.5 cm or more in diameter
Inflammatory bowel disease, irradiation, neoplastic cause

Symptoms of rectovaginal fistulas depend on location, size, and cause. In low or small fistulas, the most common complaint is passage of gas per vagina. In large fistulas, symptoms include vaginal discharge with fecal odor, passage of flatus and stool per vagina, and vaginitis. Some patients have fecal incontinence as well.

Definitive diagnosis is made by examination. In low fistula, digital examination of the anal canal reveals scar and a defect in the anterior wall. Bimanual examination with one finger in the rectum and a finger of the other hand in the vagina is also helpful. Anoscopy can also detect the opening in the anal canal. Middle and high fistulas require proctoscopy. If the fistula cannot be seen, a tampon is placed in the vaginal canal and 100 mL of diluted methylene blue is instilled into the anorectum. After a time, the tampon is removed and checked for evidence of blue staining. Barium enema is usually not helpful but may be indicated in certain patients with inflammatory bowel disease or previous irradiation.

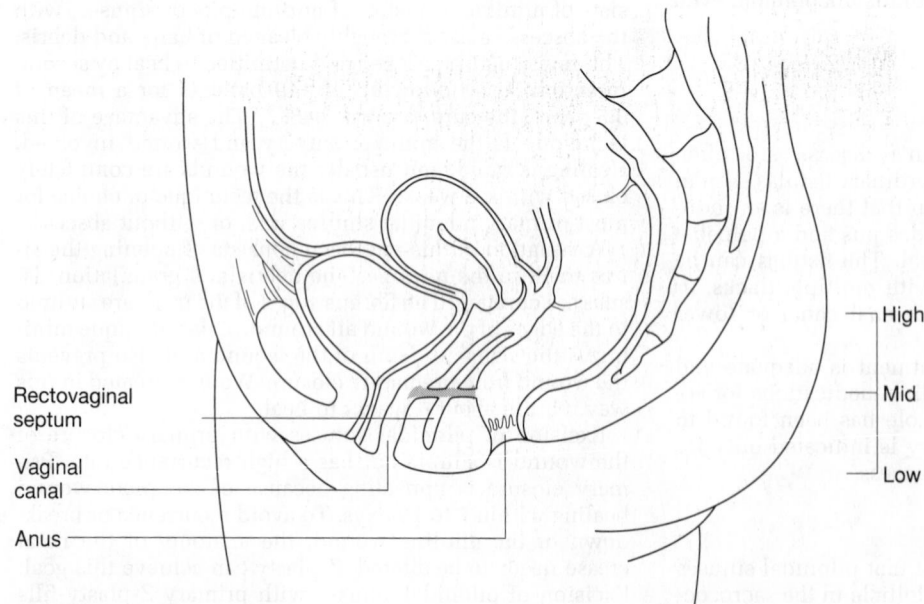

Rectovaginal septum

Vaginal canal

Anus

High

Mid

Low

Figure 52-23. Rectovaginal fistula classified by location. Fistulas are low when at or just cephalad to the dentate line, high when near the cervix, and mid when located in between.

Spontaneous or nonoperative healing of a rectovaginal fistula depends primarily on its cause and, to a lesser extent, on its size. About one half of small rectovaginal fistulas secondary to obstetric trauma heal spontaneously.

Removal of a foreign body is often followed by healing. Similarly, proper treatment of an infectious process may allow the fistula to heal. Fistula due to Crohn's disease or irradiation rarely heals spontaneously. For a low, simple fistula and some mid-rectovaginal fistulas, endorectal advancement of an anorectal flap technique gives the best results. The rectal flap, which consists of mucosa, submucosa, internal sphincter, and the circular muscle of the lower rectum, is outlined lateral and distal to the fistula. It is important to base the flap at least 4 cm cephalad to the fistula, and the base should be about twice the length of the flap to ensure adequate blood supply. After the flap is raised from the apex to the base, the underlying fistula and the excess flap are excised. The cut edges of the internal sphincter and the circular muscle of the lower rectum are approximated, thus obliterating the opening of the fistula in the anal canal. The opening in the vagina is left open for drainage. The anorectal flap is then advanced over the repaired area and sutured (Fig. 52-24). If the rectovaginal fistula is associated with incontinence resulting from injury to the external sphincter, a sphincteroplasty is also performed. In this technique, the ends of the transected muscle are identified and mobilized. The fistula is excised, and the muscle ends are then overlapped and sutured. The results of endorectal advancement flap for treatment of simple rectovaginal fistula are good, with 83% of treated patients achieving primary healing of the fistula.[31] It is important to wait, usually 3 to 6 months, until the inflammation has subsided before considering a surgical repair.

High fistulas and some mid-rectovaginal fistulas require a transabdominal approach. Simple fistulas with healthy surrounding tissues can be repaired by mobilization of the rectovaginal septum, division of the fistula, and layer closure of the rectal defect without bowel resection. If the local tissues are damaged by irradiation, infection, or inflammatory diseases, an extended low anterior resection should be performed. Although most simple rectovaginal fistulas do not require a diverting colostomy, complex rectovaginal fistulas are best managed by a preliminary colostomy. However, the tissues should be allowed to recover before definitive repair takes place. For elderly or unfit patients, for most radiation-induced fistulas, and for rectovaginal fistulas associated with Crohn's disease, a permanent colostomy may be the procedure of choice.

ANAL INCONTINENCE

The term *anal incontinence* covers a broad spectrum of anorectal functional impairment, ranging from simple involuntary passage of flatus to complete loss of sphincteric tone with involuntary passage of formed stool.

Anal incontinence results when there is loss or disturbance of normal anorectal anatomy or physiology. A contracted rectum, poor rectal compliance, or a resection of the rectum with loss of normal rectal reservoir function may result in incontinence. A neurologic problem may disturb anorectal sensation, which provides awareness of the presence of stool in the anorectum. More than half of the patients with long-standing rectal prolapse have anal incontinence, presumably from stretching of the pudendal nerve, which causes dysfunction of the sphincter muscles. A large volume of diarrheal stool emptying rapidly into the anorectum may overcome the continent mechanism, even in healthy persons. Direct mechanical injuries to the sphincter muscles include obstetric tear, fistulotomy, hemorrhoidectomy, internal sphincterotomy, anal stretching, and perianal trauma.

Examination of the patient starts with observation of any fecal materials in the undergarments and the degree of perianal skin excoriation. Gaping or laxity of the anus may be obvious, indicating neurogenic dysfunction of the sphincteric muscles. Abnormal perineal descent, in which the downward movement of the anus on straining is more than 2 cm below the plane of ischial tuberosities, may indicate damage to the levator ani muscle. A scar or defect in the anal region may indicate surgical injuries to the sphincter muscle. Digital examination can accurately sense the tone of the internal sphincter muscle, and voluntary squeezing of the anal canal can estimate the function of the external sphincter muscle, especially the puborectal muscle. Flexible sigmoidoscopy should always be performed. A barium enema or total colonoscopy is usually indicated. Anal manometry is useful to evaluate the status of the internal and external sphincteric muscles and may also be helpful in evaluating the results of operation.

Regulation of bowel habit, particularly decreasing the bowel movement to once a day or once every other day, usually improves the condition. A high-fiber diet makes the stool formed and bulky and makes it easier for patients to evacuate and empty the rectum. Antidiarrheal drugs may be prescribed judiciously.

Biofeedback is used in the treatment of anal incontinence to retrain the anorectum to be aware of the sensation of rectal fullness and to retrain contraction of the sphincteric muscles. Biofeedback training helps 50% to 100% of patients with various causes of anal incontinence.[32-34] The most common system consists of a triple-balloon catheter attached to a pressure transducer. With the patient watching the rectal manometer tracings, the balloon is inflated, and the patient is coached to contract the sphincter muscle to elevate the sphincter tracing. Several sessions may be required before the patient is aware of the sensation in the rectum and can specifically contract the anal sphincter. Eventually, the patient can learn to contract the sphincter muscle without the instrument. A small, portable anorectal biofeedback system can be used to practice at home.

Operative treatment is reserved for patients resistant to conservative management. Sphincteroplasty is most suitable for incontinence secondary to obstetric injury or injury secondary to anorectal surgery. The procedure involves a curved incision in the perianal skin where the sphincter muscle has been transected. The sphincter muscle, including the puborectal muscle, is mobilized enough so that it can be wrapped over itself with modest tension (Fig. 52-25). This operation is successful in about 80% of patients.[35]

Postanal intersphincteric sphincteroplasty was designed for incontinence caused by prolapse of the rectum and for certain cases of idiopathic incontinence. The approach is through the intersphincteric plane posteriorly. The levator ani muscle is approximated to restore the anorectal angle to normal. The puborectal muscle and the external sphincter muscles are also tightened with sutures. The procedure also lengthens the anal canal to a significant degree. The success rate of this operation varies from 70% to 90%.[36-38]

Gracilis muscle transposition functions as a substitute anal sphincter. The procedure is suitable for cases in which there is significant loss of the anal sphincter muscle mass or when other techniques have failed. The gracilis muscle from the thigh is mobilized and detached from its insertion at the tibial tuberosity. The gracilis is then tunneled through the perineum and encircles the anal canal to replace the anal sphincter muscle. The results of this operation vary from good to total failure.[39,40] Gluteal

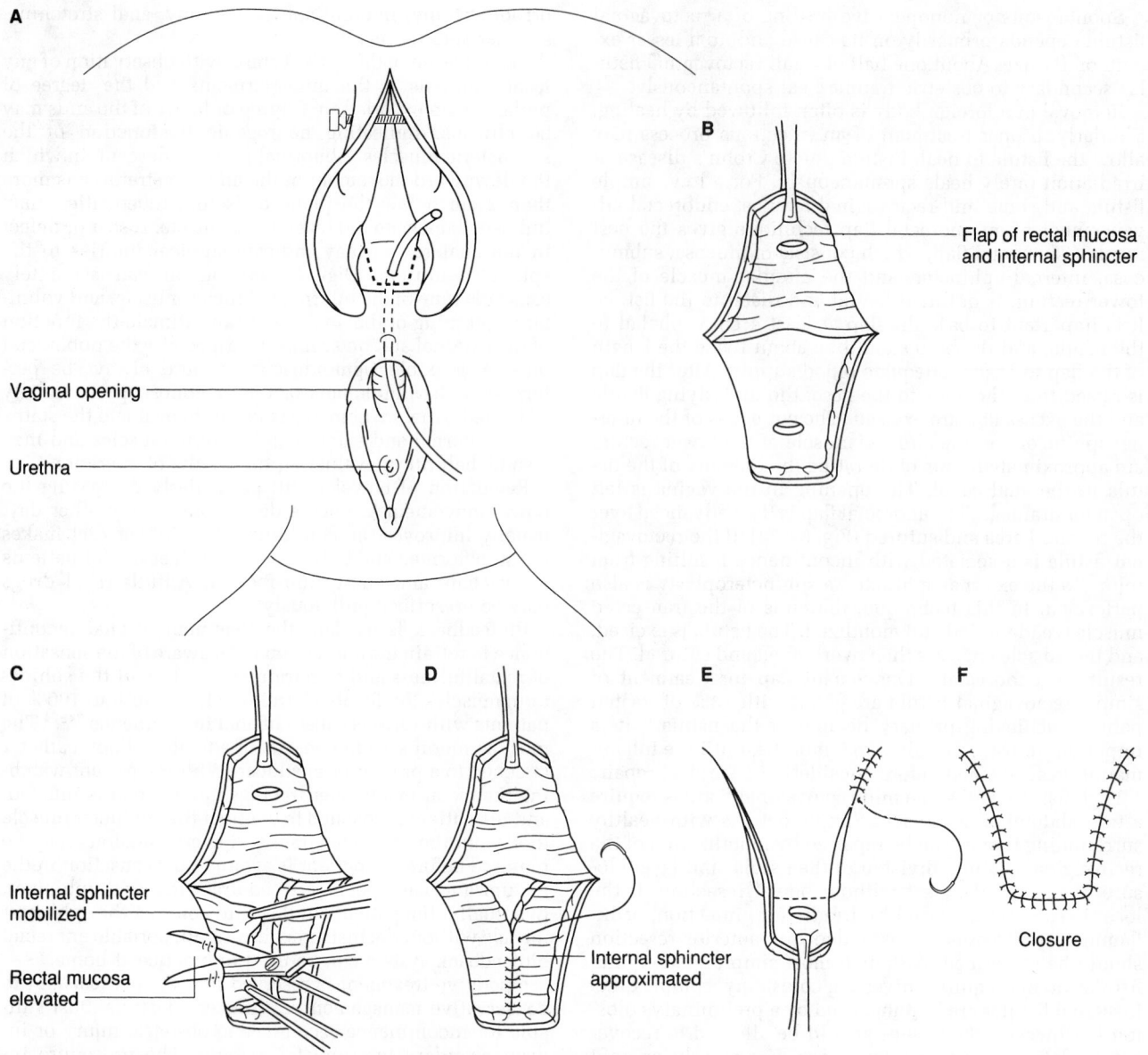

A

Vaginal opening

Urethra

B

Flap of rectal mucosa
and internal sphincter

C

Internal sphincter
mobilized

Rectal mucosa
elevated

D

Internal sphincter
approximated

E

F

Closure

Figure 52-24. Endorectal advancement of anorectal flap. (*A*) Exposure is gained by an anal speculum, and the fistula is identified. Outline of endorectal flap, extending proximally to 7 cm from the anal verge. (*B*) The full-thickness flap is created to include the internal sphincter muscle. (*C*) Lateral mobilization is made on each side in the submucosal plane. (*D*) Anorectal wall on each side is approximated. (*E* and *F*) The endorectal flap is pulled down to cover the wound and sutured. The fistula is excised. The aperture in the vagina is not sutured but is left open for drainage.

muscle transposition can also be performed in a similar fashion.[41]

For patients who are incapacitated from complete fecal incontinence, and whose chances of success from anal sphincter repair are slim, a permanent end-sigmoid colostomy is the best choice. Artificial and electrically stimulated neoanal sphincters have been tried, but both are still in their experimental stage.[42,43] Their applications to clinical use in the future may be possible in selected cases.

SEXUALLY TRANSMITTED DISEASES OF THE ANORECTUM

Anal Condylomata Acuminata

Anal condylomata acuminata are caused by human papilloma virus (HPV), primarily HPV-6 and HPV-11. In most patients, the warts involve the perianal skin, anal verge, and anoderm. Occasionally, the lesions also involve the mucosa of the upper anal canal and the lower rectum. The extent of the disease varies from a few small warts to an extensive mass occluding the anus. The diagnosis is usually obvious by the characteristic papillary appearance. Anoscopic examination is essential to detect intraanal involvement. Because most cases are transmitted by sexual contact, other coexisting venereal diseases, especially gonorrhea and syphilis, should be excluded.

Small perianal warts can be destroyed by applying podophyllin solution or bichloracetic acid. Both podophyllin and bichloracetic acid are caustic; therefore, the uninvolved skin should be protected with petroleum jelly before these agents are applied so that caustic injury can be prevented. Extensive warts in the perianal area, or in the anal canal, are best treated by excision with a small iris scissors, followed by electrocoagulation of the bases.

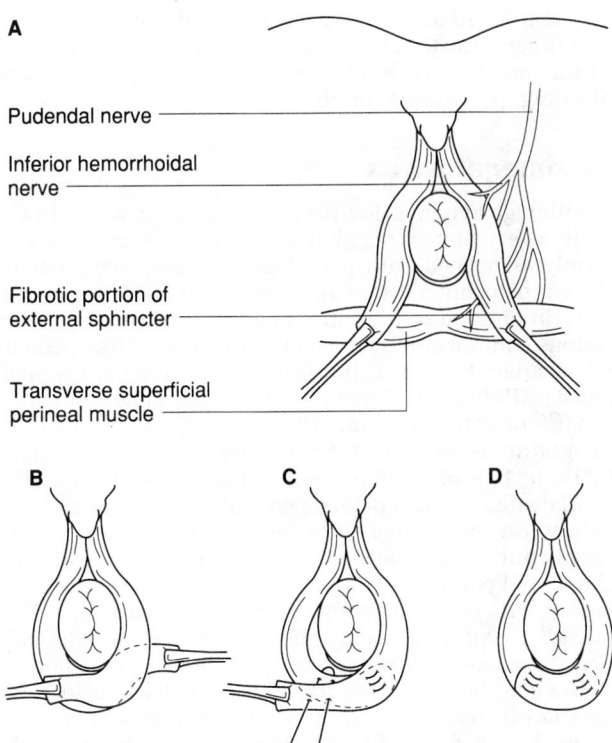

Figure 52-25. Wrap-around anal sphincteroplasty.

Pudendal nerve

Inferior hemorrhoidal nerve

Fibrotic portion of external sphincter

Transverse superficial perineal muscle

Frequent postoperative follow-up is necessary because the recurrence rate is as high as 65%. The follow-up should be done at 2 to 4 weeks, until at least 3 months have passed with no disease recurrence. Immunotherapy (with the use of autogenous wart tissue vaccine) in conjunction with excision of the lesions has been found to be effective, but the role of immune mechanisms in recurrent wart formation has yet to be determined.

Malignant transformation of condylomata acuminata is rare and is usually associated with long-standing disease. The microscopic picture includes squamous dysplasia with proliferation and disorganization of epidermal cells, individual cell keratinization, keratin pearl formation, an increased number of normal and abnormal mitoses, and, most important, invasion into the underlying tissue. Treatment of anal condylomata acuminata with invasive carcinoma should follow the treatment of squamous cell carcinoma of the anal margin and epidermoid carcinoma of the anal canal (see Chap. 48).

Buschke-Löwenstein tumor or giant condyloma acuminatum was once believed to be a malignant transformation of a large condyloma acuminatum. Although no universal agreement has been reached, there is a growing consensus that this entity probably represents a verrucous carcinoma.[44] Verrucous carcinoma is a slow-growing, aggressive, essentially nonmetastasizing variant of a well-differentiated squamous cell carcinoma. Its clinical course is one of relentless progression and expansion of the neoplasm causing extensive erosion and pressure necrosis of the surrounding tissues. It may invade the ischioanal fossa, perirectal tissues, and even the pelvic cavity. The treatment is determined by the extent of the lesion and varies from a wide local excision to an abdominoperineal resection.

Gonococcal Proctitis

Patients with gonococcal proctitis are generally asymptomatic but may have mild anal burning, pain, discharge, or bleeding in the acute phase. Proctoscopic examination reveals hyperemic and edematous anorectal mucosa with purulent discharge in the anal crypts at the dentate line. In the chronic phase, the anorectum may appear normal. Diagnosis is confirmed by observing *Neisseria gonorrhoeae* on stained smears of the discharge and by plating the exudate immediately onto Thayer-Martin culture medium. In the United States, antimicrobial resistance in the gonococcus continues to evolve, and coinfection with *Chlamydia trachomatis* is a serious problem. Chlamydial infection may be documented in up to 45% of gonorrhea cases when adequate chlamydial cultures are performed.

Amoxicillin, 3 g, ampicillin, 3.5 g orally, aqueous procaine penicillin G (APPG), 4.8 million IU intramuscularly, and ceftriaxone, 250 mg intramuscularly, are the drugs of choice. Amoxicillin, ampicillin, and penicillin (but not ceftriaxone) are accompanied by probenecid, 1 g by mouth. APPG may be less desirable because of associated pain and toxicity. Tetracycline hydrochloride, 500 mg by mouth four times daily for 7 days, or doxycycline, 100 mg by mouth twice daily for 7 days, is included to treat coexisting chlamydial infection. For patients in whom tetracycline is contraindicated or not tolerated, erythromycin base or stearate, 500 mg by mouth four times daily for 7 days, or erythromycin ethylsuccinate, 800 mg by mouth four times daily for 7 days, may be used. For those allergic to penicillin, one may use spectinomycin, 2 g intramuscularly, tetracycline, 500 mg orally four times daily for 7 days, or doxycycline, 100 mg by mouth twice daily for 7 days.

All patients treated for gonorrhea should have a serologic test for syphilis. Patients with incubating syphilis (seronegative, without clinical signs of syphilis) are likely to be cured by all the above regimens except spectinomycin used alone. Patients with gonorrhea who have documented syphilis or are established sex partners of syphilis patients should be treated for syphilis as well as for gonorrhea.

Follow-up cultures should be obtained from the anorectum 3 to 7 days after completion of treatment. If gonorrhea persists after treatment with one of the nonspectinomycin regimens, patients should be treated with spectinomycin, 2 g intramuscularly, or with ceftriaxone, 250 mg intramuscularly. Recurrent gonococcal infections after treatment with recommended schedules are commonly caused by reinfection rather than treatment failure and indicate a need for improved sex partner tracing and patient education. Because antimicrobial resistance is a cause of treatment failure, all posttreatment isolates should be tested for antimicrobial susceptibility.

Chlamydial Proctitis

Chlamydia trachomatis is the most common cause of sexually transmitted disease in the United States, affecting 4 million Americans each year. Although most chlamydial infections affect the urethra, anorectal involvement among male homosexuals is common. Proctoscopy reveals a picture of nonspecific proctitis with friable, granular, and edematous mucosa. Immunofluorescent microscopy provides an accurate and rapid diagnosis. The specimen should be collected by swabbing the anorectal mucosa.

Treatment includes tetracycline hydrochloride, 500 mg by mouth four times daily for 7 days, or doxycycline, 100 mg by mouth twice daily for 7 days. For patients in whom tetracyclines are contraindicated, erythromycin base or stearate, 500 mg by mouth four times daily for 7 days, or erythromycin ethylsuccinate, 800 mg by mouth four times daily for 7 days, may be used. When taken as directed, the tetracycline and erythromycin regimens listed above are highly effective (over 95% cure rate). Therefore, posttreatment *C trachomatis* test-of-cure cultures may be omitted if laboratory resources are limited. Although cultures may not become positive until 3 to 6 weeks after treatment, when they are positive, patients should be retreated with one of the above regimens, and any interim sex partners should also be contacted.

Two new drugs have been approved by the FDA for the treatment of *Chlamydia*—azithromycin, 1 g orally in a single dose, and ofloxacin, 300 mg orally two times a day for 7 days. A substantial advantage of azithromycin, in comparison with all other therapies, is that a single dose is effective; this antimicrobial may prove most useful for situations in which compliance with a 7-day regimen of another antimicrobial cannot be ensured. In view of the high efficacy of tetracycline and doxycycline, cost should also be considered when selecting a treatment regimen.[45]

Herpes Simplex Viral Proctitis

Anorectal herpes is caused by herpesvirus hominis type II, the same organism implicated in genital herpes. The usually severe anorectal pain is associated with fever, inguinal adenopathy, tenesmus, constipation, anorectal discharge, and bleeding. Neurologic symptoms in the distribution of the sacral roots are noted in some patients. These may include urinary retention, dyspareunia, and impotence. Examination reveals erythematous areas with small groups of vesicles that rupture and become ulcerated. Proctoscopic examination may reveal a nonspecific proctitis.[46,47]

The diagnosis can be made by staining the exudate with the Papanicolaou or Giemsa method. A finding of multinucleated giant cells is diagnostic. One may also use immunofluorescence or immunoperoxidase staining of lesion scrapings to detect the herpes simplex virus (HSV) antigens. Both techniques are rapid and useful when positive but are less sensitive than viral isolation in tissue culture from the vesicles or ulcers.

For the first episode, acyclovir, 200 mg by mouth five times daily for 7 to 10 days, is effective if initiated within 6 days of the onset of lesions. This treatment shortens the median duration of first-episode eruptions by 3 to 5 days and may reduce systemic symptoms in primary episodes. For patients with severe symptoms or complications that necessitate hospitalization, acyclovir, 5 mg/kg intravenously every 8 hours for 5 to 7 days, is recommended. This treatment shortens the median course of first episodes by about 7 days. Topical acyclovir ointment has a marginal benefit in decreasing virus shedding but has no significant effect on symptoms or healing time.

For recurrent anorectal herpes, because benefit may be minimal, treatment should be limited to those patients who typically have severe symptoms and who are able to begin therapy at the beginning of the prodrome or within 2 days of the onset of lesions. Acyclovir, 200 mg orally five times a day for 5 days, is used. It shortens the mean clinical course by about 1 day. Intravenous and topical acyclovir are not indicated for recurrences.

ANORECTAL DISEASES IN PATIENTS WITH AIDS AND HIV POSITIVITY

Kaposi Sarcoma

Kaposi sarcoma, normally a rare tumor of the skin, is the most common malignant tumor in AIDS patients. Most Kaposi sarcoma tumors of the colon and rectum are asymptomatic, but bleeding, diarrhea, and obstruction may occur. The lesion has a characteristic red, round, submucosal nodule with central umbilication. A deep biopsy is re-

quired to yield an accurate result. The diagnosis is useful as a prognostication because there is no effective medical treatment. Surgery is indicated only to control massive bleeding, perforation, or obstruction.

Cytomegalovirus

Although cytomegalovirus (CMV) has been found in virtually every human organ system, its presence is not uniformly associated with pathologic changes. Symptomatic CMV proctocolitis occurs in at least 10% of AIDS patients. CMV in immunocompromised patients, however, leads to serious complications. In about 50% of the AIDS patients who harbor the virus, the infection is serious. Disseminated CMV has been identified at postmortem examination in 90% of patients with AIDS, with 30% having CMV in the gastrointestinal tract. CMV enteroproctocolitis occurs in 5% to 10% of AIDS patients but is responsible for 70% of all deaths in AIDS patients who undergo major abdominal surgery on an emergency basis.[48,49] Symptoms of CMV enterocolitis are diarrhea, fever, right lower quadrant abdominal pain, and weight loss. Not uncommon are coinfection with one or more opportunistic agents such as *Salmonella*, *Shigella*, *Campylobacter*, *Clostridium difficile*, *Cryptosporidium*, *Microsporida*, *Entamoeba*, and *Giardia*.

The morphologic hallmarks of CMV enteroproctocolitis are sharply demarcated areas of shallow ulcers, frequently covered with fibrin. Biopsy gives an accurate diagnosis. The pathognomonic histopathologic features include large basophilic intranuclear CMV inclusions. The problems that most commonly necessitate emergency or urgent surgical intervention are bleeding and perforation of the CMV ulcers. These complications occur in 60% to 100% of emergency exploratory celiotomies performed in AIDS patients. Medical treatment consists of ganciclovir.[49]

Lymphoma

There is an increased incidence of non-Hodgkin's lymphoma in patients with HIV positivity and AIDS. In the United States, about 3% of AIDS cases present with lymphoma. When the gastrointestinal tract is the primary site, the stomach is affected more than the colon. Identification of anorectal lymphoma is difficult because the disease is extraluminal in most cases. Most patients are brought to the operating room with perianal abscesses as a preoperative diagnosis.[49] The diagnosis relies on microscopic identification of B-cell immunoblastic configuration of extranodular lymphoma. A consideration in the treatment of AIDS-related lymphoma is that radiation and chemotherapy may actually accelerate the demise of the patient through further immunosuppression. It is worthwhile, in patients with resectable tumors, to excise the lesion.[50]

Anal Carcinoma in HIV-Positive Patients

Recent studies show a remarkable increase in anal carcinoma in both men and women in the United States, rising at an annual rate of 2%.[51] Three populations have emerged as being potentially at risk for anal carcinoma: women with a history of sexual activity and, in particular, women with a history of cervical carcinoma; men with a history of anal-receptive intercourse; and HIV-positive men and women. Squamous cell carcinoma of the anus and squamous cell carcinoma of the cervix are histologically similar, and it is now widely accepted that their pathogenesis is similar, with oncogenic HPV as the cause. HPV-16 and HPV-18 are most strongly associated with invasive squamous cell carcinoma of the cervix. The mechanism by which HPV contributes to the development of anogenital squamous cell carcinoma is not fully understood. HPV proteins may have a role in this process. HPV establishes itself in the basal cell layer of the epithelium. This area contains the only dividing cells of the epithelium, and it is from this area that the remainder of the epithelium is derived. It has been shown that the likely anal carcinoma precursor, high-grade anal intraepithelial neoplasia, is also associated primarily with HPV-16. A recent study showed that anal HPV infection is found in 54% of men with AIDS or the AIDS-related complex.[51]

Groups at high risk for developing anal carcinoma should have a proctosigmoidoscopic and anoscopic examination. The application of 3% acetic acid will help to identify areas of abnormal epithelium for biopsies. High-grade intraepithelial dysplasia should be treated with local excision or electrocoagulation. Low-grade dysplasia can be followed periodically.[51] Invasive carcinoma should be treated with the standard regimen of combined chemoradiation. In patients with AIDS, invasive squamous cell carcinoma of the anus has a poor prognosis, and the moribund condition of these patients usually precludes effective treatment.

Anorectal Ulcers in HIV-Positive Patients

The anal-receptive male has an increased proclivity for various viral, bacterial, and parasitic diseases of the anorectum. In a review of 160 seropositive patients, 33% had anal and rectal symptomatology. Anal ulcers are common among HIV-positive patients. About half of the anal ulcers are idiopathic.[52] Most ulcers are in the posterior midline of the anus, somewhat closer to the dentate line than the ordinary anal fissure. Idiopathic ulcers in HIV-positive patients are extremely erosive, dissecting along the submucosal and intersphincteric planes and many times skeletonizing the internal sphincter muscle. These erosions create pockets in which stool and pus collect, causing severe pain, especially on defecation.

Examination of the anorectum under general anesthesia is usually necessary. Biopsy specimens should be taken and sent for viral culture and dark-field examination if indicated. If lymphoma is suspected, the tissue should be sent for typing. Pocketing of the ulcers should be corrected by division of a portion of the internal sphincter muscle along with débridement. In patients with intolerable pain from anal ulcers, a sigmoid colostomy gives symptomatic relief. Specific ulcers in HIV-positive patients are usually from syphilis, tuberculosis, HSV, cytomegalovirus, and other bacterial infections.

REFERENCES

1. Crapp AR, Cuthbertson AM. William Waldeyer and the rectosacral fascia. Surg Gynecol Obstet 1974;138:252.
2. Shafik A. A new concept of the anatomy of the anal sphincter mechanism and the physiology of defecation. The external anal sphincter: a triple-loop system. Invest Urol 1975;12:412.
3. Oh C, Kark AE. Anatomy of the external sphincter. Br J Surg 1972;59:717.
4. Shafik A. A new concept of the anatomy of the anal sphincter mechanism and the physiology of defecation. II. Anatomy of the levator ani muscle with special reference to puborectalis. Invest Urol 1975;13:175.
5. Block IR, Enquist IF. Lymphatic studies pertaining to local spread of carcinoma of the rectum in females. Surg Gynecol Obstet 1961;112:41.
6. Bauer JJ, Gelernt IM, Salky B, et al. Sexual dysfunction following proctectomy for benign diseases of the colon and rectum. Ann Surg 1983;197:363.
7. Walsh PC, Schlegel PN. Radical pelvic surgery with preservation of sexual function. Ann Surg 1988;208:391.
8. Cherry DA, Rothenberger DA. Pelvic floor physiology. Surg Clin North Am 1988;68:1217.
9. Thomson WHF. The nature of hemorrhoids. Br J Surg 1975;62:542.
10. Loder PB, Kamm MA, Nicholls RJ, Phillips RKS. Hemorrhoids: pathology, pathophysiology and etiology. Br J Surg 1994;81:946.
11. Bernstein WC. What are hemorrhoids and what is their relationship to the portal venous system? Dis Colon Rectum 1983;26:829.
12. Buls JG, Goldberg SM. Modern management of hemorrhoids. Surg Clin North Am 1978;58:469.
13. Leff EI. Hemorrhoidectomy—laser vs. nonlaser: outpatient surgical experience. Dis Colon Rectum 1992;35:743.
14. Beahrs OH, Theuerkauf FJ Jr, Hill JR. Procidentia: surgical treatment. Dis Colon Rectum 1972;15:337.
15. Roberts PL, Schoetz DJ Jr, Coller JA, Veidenheimer MC. Ripstein procedure: the Lahey Clinic experience: 1963–1985. Arch Surg 1988;123:554.
16. Keighley MR, Fielding JW, Alexander-Williams J. Results of Marlex mesh abdominal rectopexy for rectal prolapse in 100 consecutive patients. Br J Surg 1983;70:229.
17. Wolff BG, Dietzen C. Abdominal resectional procedures for rectal prolapse. Semin Colon Rectal Surg 1991;2:184.
18. Gemlo BT, Madoff RD. Suture rectopexy with colon resection for rectal prolapse. Semin Colon Rectal Surg 1991;2:193.
19. Williams JG, Rothenberger DA, Madoff RD, Goldberg SM. Treatment of rectal prolapse in the elderly by perineal rectosigmoidectomy. Dis Colon Rectum 1992;35:830.
20. Finlay IG, Aitchison M. Perineal excision of the rectum for prolapse in the elderly. Br J Surg 1991;78:687.
21. Uhlig BE, Sullivan ES. The modified Delorme operation: its place in surgical treatment of massive rectal prolapse. Dis Colon Rectum 1979;22:513.
22. Nivatvongs S. Rectal prolapse: techniques of transperineal repair. Perspect Colon Rectal Surg 1991;4:101.
23. Parks AG, Swash M, Urich H. Sphincter denervation in anorectal incontinence and rectal prolapse. Gut 1977;18:656.
24. Schouten WR, Briel JW, Auwerda JJA. Relationship between anal pressure and anodermal blood flow. Dis Colon Rectum 1994;37:664.
25. Gordon PH, Vasilevsky CA. Lateral internal sphincterotomy: rationale, technique and anesthesia. Can J Surg 1985;28:28.
26. Parks AG, Gordon PH, Hardcastle JE. A classification of fistula-in-ano. Br J Surg 1976;63:1.
27. Vasilevsky CA, Gordon PH. Results of treatment of fistula-in-ano. Dis Colon Rectum 1985;28:225.
28. Allan A, Keighley MRB. Management of perianal Crohn's disease. World J Surg 1988;12:198.
29. Bascom J. Pilonidal disease: long-term results of follicle removal. Dis Colon Rectum 1983;26:800.
30. Pilipshen SJ, Gray G, Goldsmith E, Dinem P. Carcinoma arising in pilonidal sinuses. Am Surg 1981;193:506.
31. Lowry AC, Thorson AG, Rothenberger DA, et al. Repair of simple rectovaginal fistula: influence of previous repairs. Dis Colon Rectum 1988;31:676.
32. Lowry AC, Jensen LL. Biofeedback for fecal incontinence. Perspect Colon Rectal Surg 1992;5:210.
33. Miner PB, Donnelly TC, Read NW. Investigation of mode of action of biofeedback in treatment of fecal incontinence. Dig Dis Sci 1990;35:1291.
34. MacLeod JH. Management of anal incontinence by biofeedback. Gastroenterology 1987;93:291.
35. Fang DT, Nivatvongs S, Vermeulen FD, et al. Overlapping sphincteroplasty for acquired anal incontinence. Dis Colon Rectum 1984;27:720.
36. Henry MM, Simson JN. Results of postanal repair: a retrospective study. Br J Surg 1985;72(Suppl):S17.
37. Keighley MRB. Postanal repair: how I do it. Int J Colorectal Dis 1987;2:236.
38. Womack NR, Morrison JF, Williams NS. Prospective study of the effects of postanal repair in neurogenic fecal incontinence. Br J Surg 1988;75:48.

39. Corman ML. Gracilis muscle transposition for anal incontinence: late results. Br J Surg 1985;72(Suppl):S21.

40. Yoshioka K, Keighley MRB. Clinical and manometric assessment of gracilis muscle transplant for fecal incontinence. Dis Colon Rectum 1988;31:767.

41. Pearl RK, Prasad ML, Nelson RL, Orsay CP, Abcarian H. Bilateral gluteus maximus transposition for anal incontinence. Dis Colon Rectum 1991;34:478.

42. George BD, Williams NS. Electrically stimulated gracilis neoanal sphincter. Semin Colon Rectal Surg 1992;3:104.

43. Christiansen J. The artificial anal sphincter. Semin Colon Rectal Surg 1992;3:98.

44. Gordon PH. Condyloma acuminatum. In: Gordon PH, Nivatvongs S, eds. Principles and practice of surgery for the colon, rectum, and anus. St Louis, Quality Medical Publishing, 1992:311.

45. Minnesota Department of Health. Disease control newsletter, vol 22, 1994:1.

46. Jacobs E. Sexually transmitted diseases of the anorectum and intestine. Perspect Colon Rectal Surg 1989;2:27.

47. Milsom JW. Herpes simplex infections of the anorectum. Semin Colon Rectal Surg 1992;3:222.

48. Soderlund C, Brett GA, Engstrom L, et al. Surgical treatment of cytomegalovirus enterocolitis in severe human immunodeficiency virus infection: report of eight cases. Dis Colon Rectum 1994;37:63.

49. Wexner SD. AIDS: what the colorectal surgeon needs to know. Perspect Colon Rectal Surg 1989;2:19.

50. Williams RA, Wilson SE. Surgical intervention in AIDS. Am Coll Surg Bull 1990;75:13.

51. Palefsky JM. Rising incidence of anal cancer in HIV-positive patients: implications for the colorectal surgeon. Perspect Colon Rectal Surg 1994;7:115.

52. Gottesman L. Treatment of anorectal ulcers in the HIV-positive patient. Perspect Colon Rectal Surg 1991;4:19.

HERNIA, MESENTERY, AND RETROPERITONEUM

SURGERY: SCIENTIFIC PRINCIPLES AND PRACTICE, Second Edition, edited by Lazar J. Greenfield, Michael W. Mulholland, Keith T. Oldham, Gerald B. Zelenock, and Keith D. Lillemoe. Lippincott–Raven Publishers, Philadelphia, © 1997.

CHAPTER 53

INGUINAL ANATOMY AND ABDOMINAL WALL HERNIAS

JAMES A. KNOL AND FREDERIC E. ECKHAUSER

The surgical treatment of hernia dates from the first century BC with the writings of Celsus, who described herniorrhaphy as performed by Heliodorus.[1] Hernia repair is one of a group of operations that are basic to general surgery. Nevertheless, controversy can arise over the optimal approach and technical details of repairing almost any hernia. The approach considered to be correct is often the one engendered by the surgeon's training and may be a matter of tradition. The recent advent of laparoscopic hernia repair has generated considerable dispute among surgeons. The study of gross anatomy has been predominant in contributing to the understanding of hernias and their peculiar defects. The contributions of the physiologist, biochemist, and even the molecular biologist are only recently having an impact on the science of hernias and their repair. The effect of mechanical stresses on tissue and the processes of wound healing are being elucidated at all levels. Nevertheless, hernia repair is still more art than science and remains mainly based on empiricism.

Hernias play a significant role in surgical disease. An estimated 5% of the population is affected by a spontaneously occurring hernia during their lifetime. Many people also develop a secondary hernia, most frequently in the area of a previous incision or other operatively induced injury to the abdominal wall. Worldwide, hernia is the most common cause of intestinal obstruction and is the third most common cause in the United States. Disabilities associated with hernias and hernia repair are not inconsequential. In the case of large abdominal wall hernias and particularly large incisional hernias, multiple recurrences are not uncommon. The hernias of the abdominal wall are listed in Table 53-1.

INGUINAL ANATOMY

Anterior Abdominal Wall

The anterior abdominal wall consists of a group of lateral sheet-like muscles and paired, longitudinally oriented flat muscles on either side of the midline. The lateral muscula-ture of the abdominal wall consists of three layers, each of which has fascicles running at an oblique angle to the others. Each muscle inserts into an aponeurosis, a flat broad tendon of dense directional connective tissue. The aponeurosis inserts into the midline linea alba, a decussation of the tendon fibers from the contralateral abdomen, and into other bony and connective tissue structures, depending on the direction of the fascicles. Medially, the musculature consists of the longitudinally oriented, paired paramidline rectus abdominis muscles. The rectus abdominis muscles originate on the ribs superiorly and on the pubis inferiorly, and they insert into one to four transversely oriented tendinous bands that are variably spaced along the length of the muscle.

Running lateral to the rectus abdominis muscles is a longitudinal, slightly curved depression, the linea semilunaris, where the muscular fibers are transformed to aponeurotic fibers for each of the lateral muscle layers. The most superficial of the lateral muscles is the external oblique muscle, which originates on the lower eight ribs, with obliquely and inferiorly directed fascicles inserting into its aponeurosis (Fig. 53-1). The internal oblique muscle lies deep to the external oblique muscle. Its obliquely and superiorly oriented fascicles arise from the iliopsoas fascia deep to the lateral portion of the inguinal ligament, the anterior two thirds of the iliac crest, and the lumbodorsal fascia. It inserts into its aponeurosis and into the lower ribs and cartilages superiorly. The transversus abdominis muscle is the innermost of the lateral abdominal wall musculature, and its fascicles are generally transversely oriented. It originates from the iliopsoas fascia deep to the lateral inguinal ligament and from the iliac crest, the lumbodorsal fascia, and the lower costal cartilages. It inserts principally into its aponeurosis.

Table 53-1. HERNIAS OF THE ABDOMINAL WALL

INGUINAL ABDOMINAL WALL

Indirect inguinal
Direct inguinal
Femoral

ANTERIOR ABDOMINAL WALL

Umbilical
Epigastric
Spigelian
Supravesical

PELVIC

Obturator
Sciatic
Perineal

LUMBAR

Superior lumbar triangle (Grynfelt)
Inferior lumbar triangle (Petit)

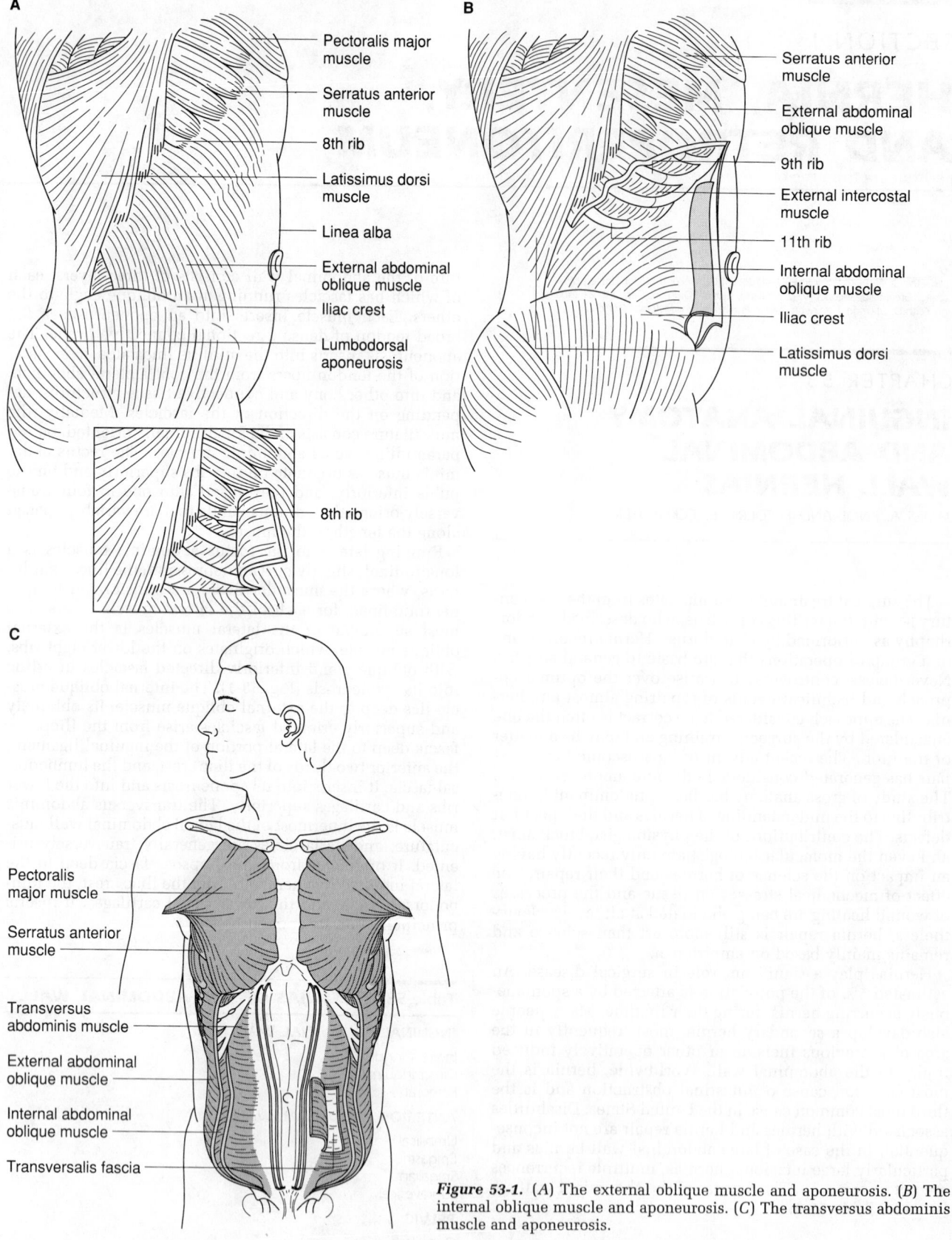

Figure 53-1. (*A*) The external oblique muscle and aponeurosis. (*B*) The internal oblique muscle and aponeurosis. (*C*) The transversus abdominis muscle and aponeurosis.

Each of these muscles is ensheathed within a fascia, a thin transparent layer of connective tissue intimately attached to the muscle and its aponeurosis. Two of these fasciae are frequently referred to as the innominate fascia, which overlies the external oblique muscle, and the transversalis fascia, which lies on the deep side of the transversus muscle and extends to form an essentially complete fascial envelope of the abdominal cavity. Separating the peritoneum from the transversalis fascia is a variable layer of preperitoneal fat.

The semicircular line is defined by the lower edge of the posterior sheath about 3 to 6 cm below the level of the umbilicus, and its convexity is directed superiorly. Above the semicircular line, the internal oblique aponeurosis splits into posterior and anterior laminae. The posterior lamina joins with the transversus abdominis aponeurosis to form the posterior rectus sheath. The anterior lamina fuses with the external oblique aponeurosis to form the anterior rectus sheath. Below the semicircular line, the internal oblique and transversus abdominis aponeuroses fuse to form an internal lamina of the anterior sheath, with

the external oblique aponeurosis forming the external lamina of the anterior sheath. Below the semicircular line, the rectus muscles are nearly fused in the midline, and their posterior surface is covered with transversalis fascia. There is an intricate and criss-crossing pattern of these fibers from the different aponeurotic layers, particularly as they decussate at the midline[2] (Fig. 53-2).

Posterolateral (Lumbar) Abdominal Wall

The posterolateral abdominal wall is composed of three layers of muscles, comprising a total of eight muscles. The deep muscles include the quadratus lumborum muscle, the psoas major muscle, and the transversus abdominis muscle. The quadratus lumborum originates from the iliac crest and the iliolumbar ligament between iliac crest and 5th lumbar transverse process and inserts on the 12th rib. The psoas muscle arises from vertebrae T-12 through L-5 and passes downward under the inguinal ligament to in-

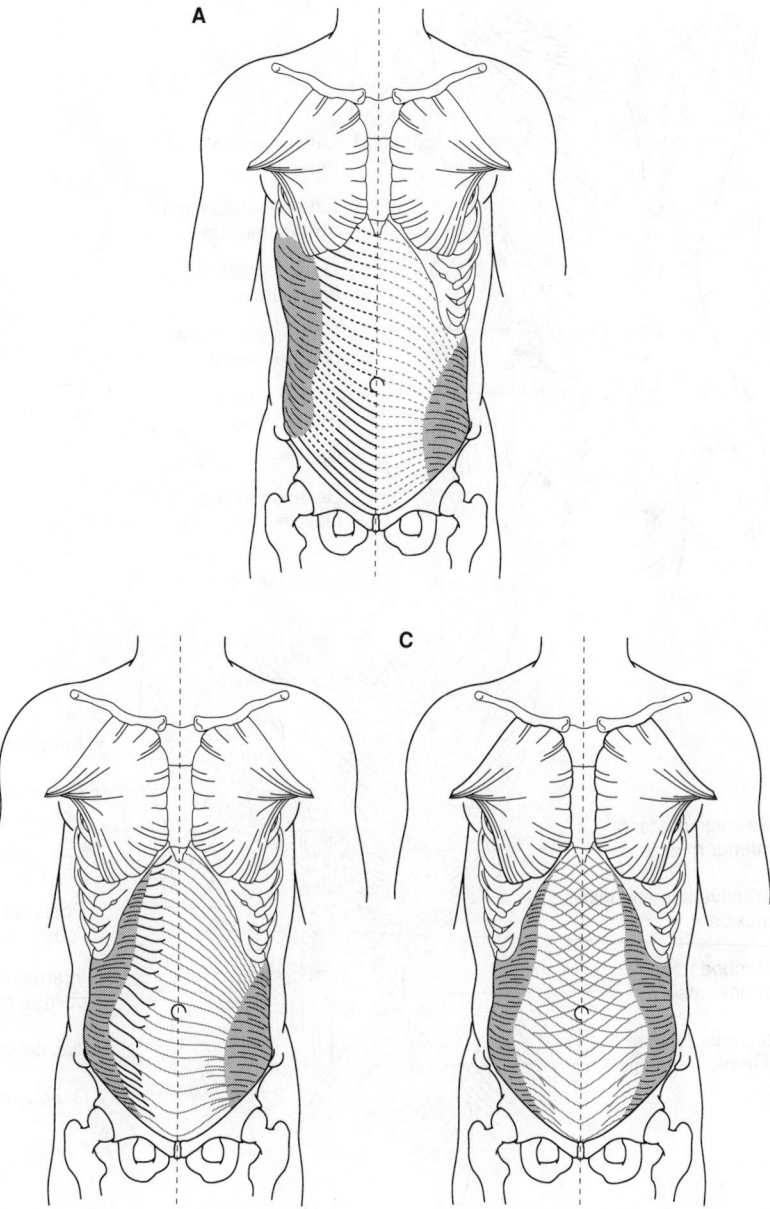

Figure 53-2. Pattern of the crossing of the aponeurotic fascicles of the abdominal wall musculature. (*A*) Fascicles from right external oblique and anterior lamina of left internal oblique. (*B*) Fascicles from right transversus abdominis and posterior lamina of left internal oblique. (*C*) Fascicles between right and left transversus abdominis.

sert on the lesser trochanter of the femur. The transversus abdominis has been described above. Defects in this muscle give rise to lumbar hernias.

The middle level of musculature includes the sacrospinalis, internal oblique, and serratus posterior inferior muscles. The latter muscle arises from the lumbodorsal fascia and runs anteriorly to insert onto the four lowest ribs. The sacrospinalis muscle runs along the spinous processes the entire length of the spine. The internal oblique muscle is described in the preceding section.

The superficial muscles include the external oblique muscle, described in connection with the anterior abdominal wall, and the latissimus dorsi muscle. The latter originates on the posterior third of the iliac crest, the spinous processes of the sacral and lumbar vertebrae, and the lumbodorsal fascia. From a broad origin, the muscle converges on a tendon inserting into the intertubercular groove of the humerus.

Spontaneously occurring lumbar hernias appear principally in two anatomic regions, the superior lumbar triangle (of Grynfelt-Lesshaft) and the inferior lumbar triangle (of Petit; Fig. 53-3). The superior lumbar triangle is larger and more constant than the inferior lumbar triangle and is the more common site of a spontaneous lumbar hernia. This space is bounded above by the 12th rib, the posterior lumbocostal ligament, and the serratus posterior inferior muscle; inferiorly by the superior border of the internal oblique muscle; and posteriorly by the lateral border of the sacrospinalis muscle. The floor of the superior lumbar triangle is transversus abdominis muscle, and the roof is the latissimus dorsi muscle. The inferior lumbar triangle is bordered posteriorly by the latissimus dorsi muscle, anteriorly by the external oblique muscle, and inferiorly by the iliac crest.

Inguinal Region

Complete familiarity with the normal anatomy of the inguinal region is required to understanding inguinal and femoral hernias and their repairs. A comprehensive trea-

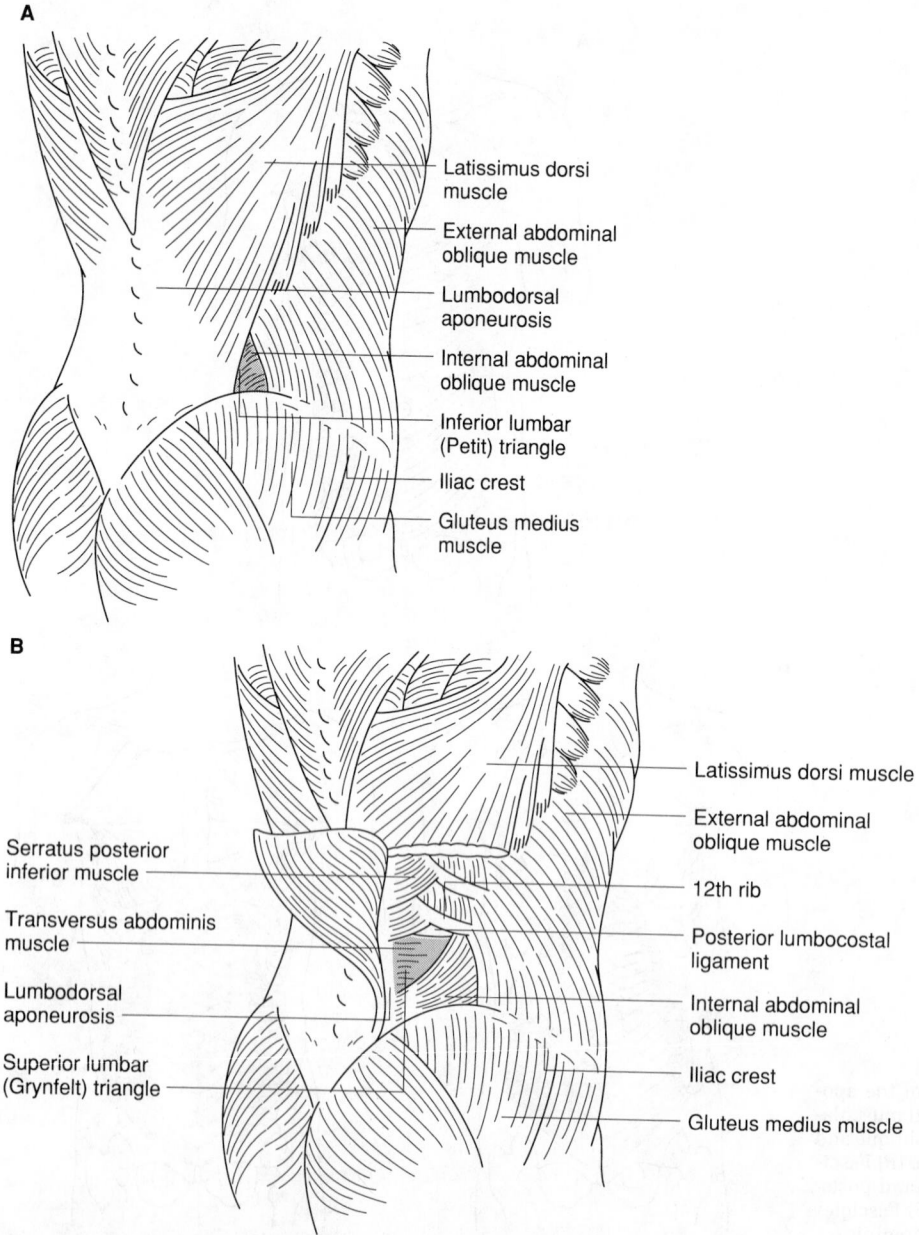

Figure 53-3. The lumbar abdominal wall with the inferior lumbar triangle (*A*) and the superior lumbar triangle (*B*).

tise on the anatomy of this region is not given here but can be found in the writings of Skandalakis and coworkers[1] and of McVay.[3]

Within the skin and subcutaneous tissues in the region superior to the inguinal crease, lie the superficial circumflex iliac, superficial epigastric, and external pudendal arteries, with their accompanying veins. They arise from the proximal femoral artery and course superiorly. These vessels are routinely encountered in the operative approach to the inguinal region.

The external oblique muscle and aponeurosis, with its inferiorly and medially directed fascicles, and the overlying innominate fascia lie deep to the subcutaneum. The inguinal ligament (Poupart) is the inferior edge of the external oblique aponeurosis and extends from the anterior superior iliac spine to the pubic tubercle, turning under itself posteriorly and then superiorly to form a shelving edge (Fig. 53-4). Medially, the inguinal ligament turns under even further to form the lacunar ligament, as part of its insertion on the pubis, and the reflected inguinal ligament, consisting of aponeurotic fibers coursing medially and superiorly toward the linea alba. The superficial inguinal ring is a triangular opening in the external oblique aponeurosis, with its apex superiorly and positioned slightly above and lateral to the pubic tubercle, through which the cord exits the inguinal canal.

The internal oblique muscle originates on the iliopsoas muscle fascia and forms an aponeurosis medially. This contributes to the rectus sheath, which exists only as an anterior rectus sheath in the inferior abdominal wall. Although the fascicles of the internal oblique generally run obliquely upward in the upper abdomen, they run almost transversely in the inguinal region. The lowermost fibers form a muscular arch, which runs slightly superiorly to the arch of the underlying transversus abdominis muscle. These fibers lie immediately superior to the cord in the inguinal canal. Infrequently, they turn inferiorly to form an aponeurosis that fuses with that of the transversus abdominis muscle and forms a true conjoint tendon. Strictly speaking, none of the foregoing structures plays a role in the anatomy of inguinal or femoral hernias.

The transversus abdominis muscle is the most important layer of the abdominal wall for preventing inguinal hernia. The muscle originates on the iliopsoas fascia laterally. Although its fascicles usually are oriented transversely, in the inguinal region they course obliquely downward. Here, the predominantly aponeurotic fibers of the transversus abdominis muscle form an arch that inserts inferiorly on the pectineal (Cooper) ligament and medially forms part of the internal lamina of the (anterior) rectus sheath. The transversalis fascia is the connective tissue layer that lines the musculature of the abdominal cavity. The transversalis fascia, where it is a component of the inguinal floor, tends to be somewhat more dense than where it lies internal to muscle bundles. Fascia as a structure is distinct from aponeurosis, and the usual character of the transversalis fascia in the inguinal floor is a rather thin, not particularly strong, clear layer between muscle and the preperitoneal fat.

The conjoined tendon is commonly alluded to in descriptions of inguinal hernia repairs. The conjoined tendon is the fusion of the aponeuroses of the internal oblique and transversus muscles where they insert on the pubic tubercle and superior pubic ramus. This structure is actually present in only 3% of persons. The structures, which in combination are usually designated the conjoined tendon, include the transversus abdominis aponeurosis, the lateral edge of the rectus sheath, and the transversalis fascia. Skandalakis and coworkers[1] suggest the term *conjoined area* as a substitute term to denote the area of the medial structures that is used in repairing an inguinal hernia.

Structures that are lateroinferior to the area of inguinal and femoral hernias and are used in hernia repairs are the pectineal (Cooper) ligament, the iliopubic tract, and the femoral sheath. The pectineal ligament is a constant ligamentous structure running along the superior aspect of the superior pubic ramus. In addition to periosteum, its components include fibers that originate from the pectineus muscle, the insertion of the lacunar ligament, and the insertion of the transversus abdominis aponeurosis. The iliopubic tract is an aponeurotic band formed from the most inferior part of the transversus abdominis muscle and aponeurosis. It passes anterior to the femoral vessels and extends from the anterior superior iliac spine and iliopsoas fascia laterally to the iliopectineal arch just lateral to the femoral vessels, and then to the superior pubic ramus medially. The iliopubic tract forms the anterior margin of the femoral sheath and the inferior margin of the internal ring. Although closely associated with the inguinal ligament, the iliopubic tract is a separate structure and part of the deep aponeurotic layer (Fig. 53-5). The iliopectineal arch is a thickening of the iliacus fascia where the muscle exits the pelvis. The fascia arches anteriorly, lateral to the external iliac vessels, to join other fibers from the inguinal ligament, from a portion of the origin of the internal oblique and transversus abdominis muscles, and from part of the lateral attachment of the iliopubic tract. The external iliac vessels pass posterior to the inguinal ligament and iliopubic tract and anterior to the pectineal ligament to enter the femoral sheath. The femoral sheath is composed of transversalis, pectineus, psoas, and iliacus fasciae, to form three compartments. The most medial compartment consists of the femoral canal, through which a femoral hernia might pass. The lateral boundary of the femoral canal is the femoral vein, and the medial margin is transversus abdominis aponeurosis insertion and transversalis fascia. The femoral canal contains lymphatic channels and lymph nodes.

Two defined regions in the inguinal area are the inguinal canal and Hesselbach triangle. The inguinal canal is the course of the spermatic cord or round ligament through

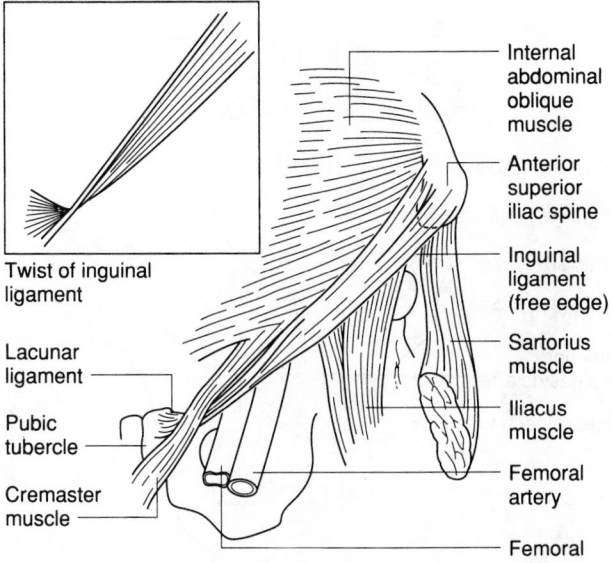

Figure 53-4. The anatomy of the inguinal ligament. The 180-degree twist of the external oblique aponeurosis forms a shelving edge in the lower portion of the ligament.

Labels in figure:
- Twist of inguinal ligament
- Lacunar ligament
- Pubic tubercle
- Cremaster muscle
- Internal abdominal oblique muscle
- Anterior superior iliac spine
- Inguinal ligament (free edge)
- Sartorius muscle
- Iliacus muscle
- Femoral artery
- Femoral vein

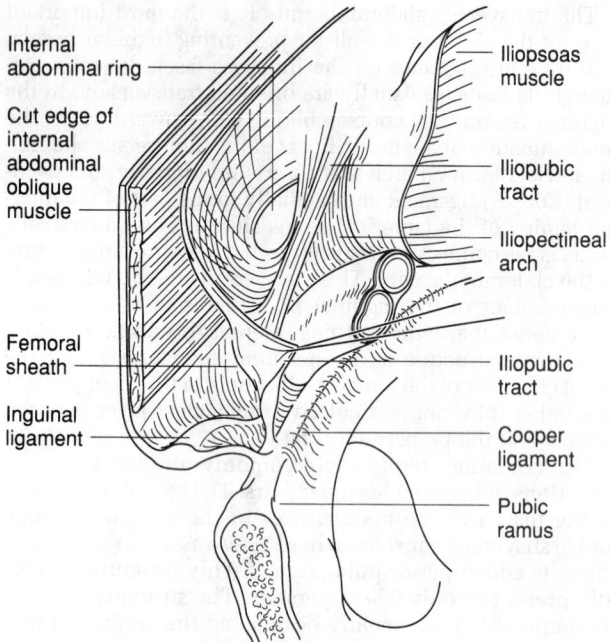

Figure 53-5. The deep aponeurotic layer at the groin.

the abdominal wall. The internal inguinal ring is bounded by the arch of the internal oblique and transversus abdominis muscles superiorly and medially and the iliopubic tract laterally and inferiorly. The ring is surrounded by transversalis fascia. The floor of the inguinal canal consists of transversus abdominis aponeurosis and transversalis fascia in three fourths of persons and of transversalis fascia alone in the remainder. The superficial ring was described earlier in this section. The roof of the canal is the external oblique aponeurosis, and the inferior margin is the inguinal ligament. The term Hesselbach triangle refers to the margins of the floor of the inguinal canal (Fig. 53-6). The laterosuperior side consists of the inferior epigastric vessels and the lateroinferior side is the inguinal ligament. The medial side is the lateral edge of the rectus sheath.

The spermatic cord has as its core the ductus deferens and the testicular artery and vein, which are enclosed within the internal spermatic fascia, an extension of the transversalis fascia onto the cord. An indirect hernia sac, when present, is found within the internal spermatic fascia. The cremaster muscle is an extension of the internal oblique muscle onto the cord and is invested in the cremasteric fascia. The cord is enclosed in the internal spermatic fascia and cremaster muscle and its fascia throughout the inguinal canal. On exiting the canal at the superficial inguinal ring, the innominate fascia extends onto the cord as the external spermatic fascia. In females, the cremaster muscle is represented by few muscle fibers, and the fasciae are present but less developed over the round ligament.

Arising anteriorly from the external iliac artery, immediately before its entrance into the femoral sheath, the inferior epigastric artery, with its accompanying vein, runs obliquely medially and upward in the preperitoneal fat, posterior to transversalis fascia and close to the inferior margin of the internal inguinal ring. Inguinal hernias arising superior to the inferior epigastric vessels are indirect inguinal hernias, whereas those arising inferior to these vessels are direct inguinal hernias. The external spermatic artery arises from the inferior epigastric artery just inferior

to the internal inguinal ring and runs along the spermatic cord to supply the cremaster muscle.

The iliohypogastric and ilioinguinal nerves are motor and sensory nerves to the muscles and skin of the inguinal region. They originate principally from the 1st lumbar nerve root but may have contributions from the 12th thoracic root. The nerves penetrate the transversus abdominis muscle at a point above the middle of the iliac crest, lie beneath the internal oblique muscle up to a point just medial and superior to the anterior superior iliac spine, and then penetrate the internal oblique muscle to lie beneath the external oblique aponeurosis. The iliohypogastric nerve may give off an inguinal branch that joins the ilioinguinal nerve. The main nerve runs on the anterior surface of the internal oblique muscle and aponeurosis medially, superior to the internal ring and lowest internal oblique fibers, to penetrate the superficial layer of the rectus sheath and innervate the suprapubic skin. The ilioinguinal nerve runs anterior to the spermatic cord in the inguinal canal and, at the superficial inguinal ring, branches into the sensory supply to the pubic region and the upper scrotum or labium majus pudendi. The genital branch of the genitofemoral nerve, which arises from lumbar roots one and two, perforates the transversalis fascia and transversus abdominis aponeurosis usually just inferior to the internal ring. It courses along the posterior surface of the spermatic cord and supplies motor fibers to the cremaster muscle. At the superficial inguinal ring, it divides to provide sensory innervation to the scrotum and medial aspect of the upper thigh.

An understanding of the inguinal anatomy as viewed from the superior-posterior, or internal, aspect is crucial for repairing inguinal and femoral hernias using the preperitoneal and laparoscopic methods[4] (Fig. 53-7). Vessels and nerves that are not exposed to injury by the anterior approach to the inguinal region are at risk from the internal approach because they are superficial, although covered with a variable layer of adipose and a thin layer of membranous connective tissue, and are somewhat unpredictable in position. From the intraperitoneal approach, the medial umbilical ligament is the landmark for the lateral extent of the bladder, and the lateral umbilical ligament identifies

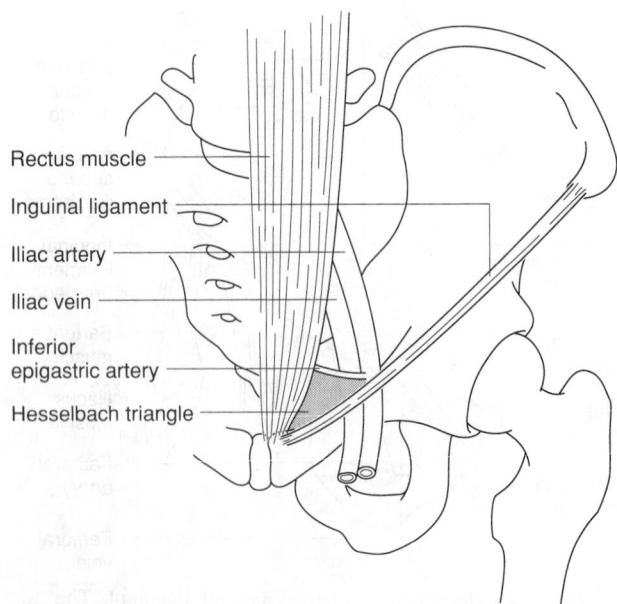

Figure 53-6. Hesselbach triangle.

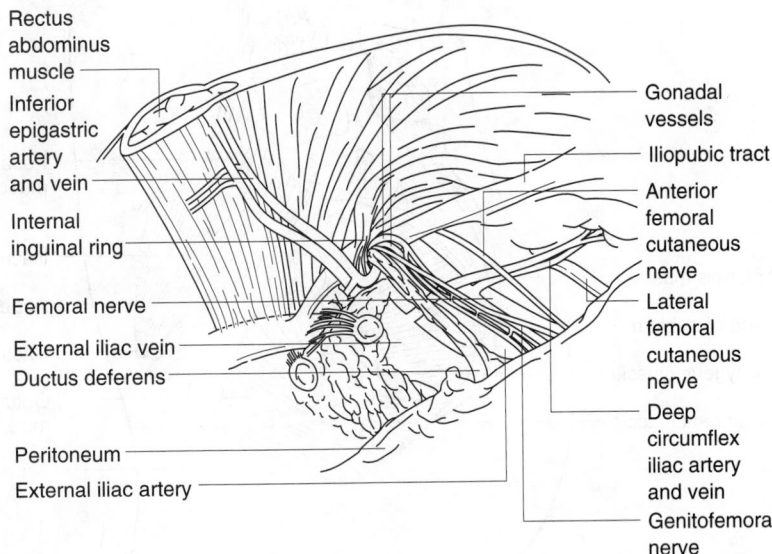

Figure 53-7. Anatomy of the inguinal region from the internal aspect, as seen with the laparoscopic approach.

the inferior epigastric vessels. In the preperitoneal space, the internal inguinal ring lies at the apex of a triangle in men formed medially by the ductus deferens and laterally by the testicular vessels. At the base of the triangle, under a layer of membranous connective tissue are the external iliac vessels. This triangle has been called the "triangle of doom," referring to the consequences of injuring the external iliac vessels during laparoscopic surgery, particularly the placement of staples, in this area.

Connective tissue structures that can be discerned from the internal approach are the pubic tubercle, the lacunar ligament, the pectineal (Cooper) ligament, the iliopubic tract, the lateral border of the rectus abdominis muscle, and the transversus abdominis muscular arch.

Blood vessels in this region include the deep circumflex iliac artery and vein, which arise from the external iliac vessels just cranial to the iliopubic tract and run laterally posterior to the iliopubic tract; the inferior epigastric artery and veins, which arise from the external iliac vessels usually cranial to the iliopubic tract and immediately turn inferiorly before curving superiorly along the anterior abdominal wall; and, in half or more of patients, an aberrant obturator artery arises from the external iliac artery near the internal ring, crosses the femoral ring and the pectineal (Cooper) ligament, and exits through the obturator ring. Other aberrant vessels are occasionally present within this surgical field.

Nerves that course through this region frequently do not have precise locations in reference to the other structures. The genital branch of the genitofemoral nerve usually lies on and runs parallel to the external iliac artery. The femoral branch of the genitofemoral nerve passes on the surface of the iliacus muscle lateral to the external iliac vessels to pass through the iliopubic tract just lateral to the internal inguinal ring. The lateral femoral cutaneous nerve usually runs on the iliacus muscle to pass posterior to the deep circumflex iliac vessels and enter the thigh posterior to the iliopubic tract and inguinal ligament just medial to the anterior superior iliac spine. However, there are frequently unnamed nerves that run between the femoral branch of the genitofemoral nerve and the lateral femoral cutaneous nerve, or combinations of these nerves, which penetrate the iliopubic tract lateral to the internal inguinal ring. The femoral nerve courses in the groove between iliacus and psoas muscles just lateral to the external iliac artery, runs

posterior to the deep circumflex vessels, iliopubic tract and inguinal ligament to enter the thigh. The lateral area between the iliopubic tract and the gonadal vessels has been named the "triangle of pain."

PELVIC ANATOMY

The pelvic anatomy pertinent to hernias consists of the musculoaponeurotic structures of the pelvis and the apertures through which structures pass from inside to outside the pelvis. The obturator internus muscle arises from the margins of the obturator foramen and the obturator membrane (Fig. 53-8). The muscle fascicles converge and exit the pelvis at the lesser sciatic foramen and insert by means of a tendon on the medial surface of the greater trochanter of the femur. The obturator vessels and nerve pass through the obturator canal, which is superior in the obturator foramen. The obturator canal is 2 to 4 cm long and runs obliquely from the pelvis to enter the medial thigh between the pectineal, long adductor, and external obturator muscles (see Fig. 53-9). The piriformis muscle arises from the anterior surface of the second through fourth sacral vertebrae and somewhat from the sacrotuberous ligament, and its fibers converge to form a tendon that exits the pelvis through the greater sciatic foramen (see Fig. 53-8). Above and below the tendon, in the greater sciatic foramen, are the suprapiriform and infrapiriform foramens (Fig. 53-10). Through the former pass the superior gluteal vessels and nerves. The sciatic nerve, perineal nerves, and pelvic vessels pass through the infrapiriform foramen. A dense parietal pelvic fascia, continuous with the endopelvic fascia, overlies the obturator internus and piriformis muscles and fuses with the sheaths of the vessels and nerves exiting through the foramens. The particularly dense lower margin of the parietal pelvic fascia, extending from the posterior surface of the pubis to the ischial spine, is called the linea terminalis, from which the levator ani muscles arise.

The pelvic diaphragm suspends the pelvic organs, closes the outlet of the pelvis, and provides a component of the muscles of fecal continence (Fig. 53-11). Adhering to the undersurface of the pelvic diaphragm anteriorly and attached to the inferior ramus of the pubis is the urogenital diaphragm, a thickened fascia-like structure. The lateral portion of the levator ani muscle arises from the posterolateral body of the pubis and the linea terminalis and forms, with its counterpart

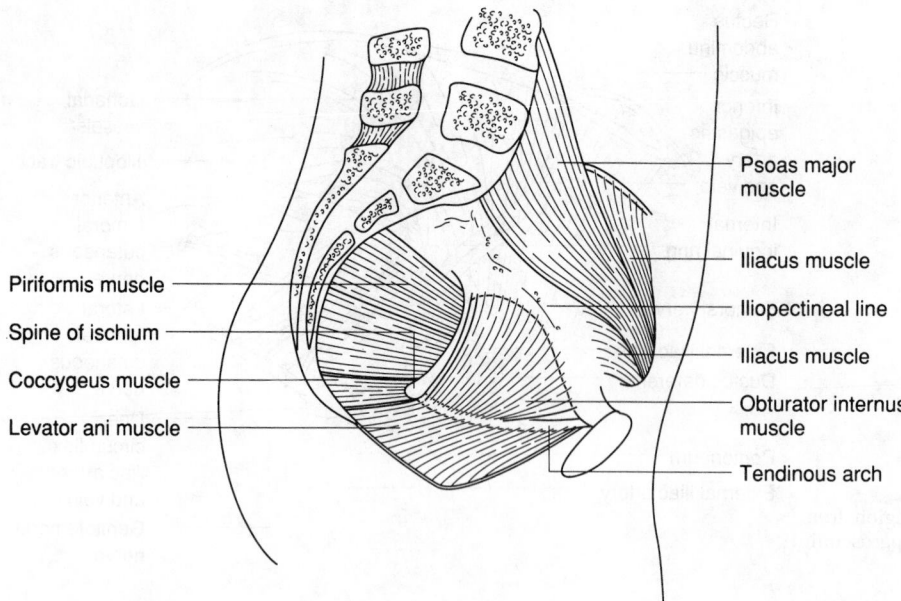

Psoas major muscle

Iliacus muscle

Iliopectineal line

Iliacus muscle

Obturator internus muscle

Tendinous arch

Piriformis muscle

Spine of ischium

Coccygeus muscle

Levator ani muscle

Figure 53-8. Musculature of the pelvis.

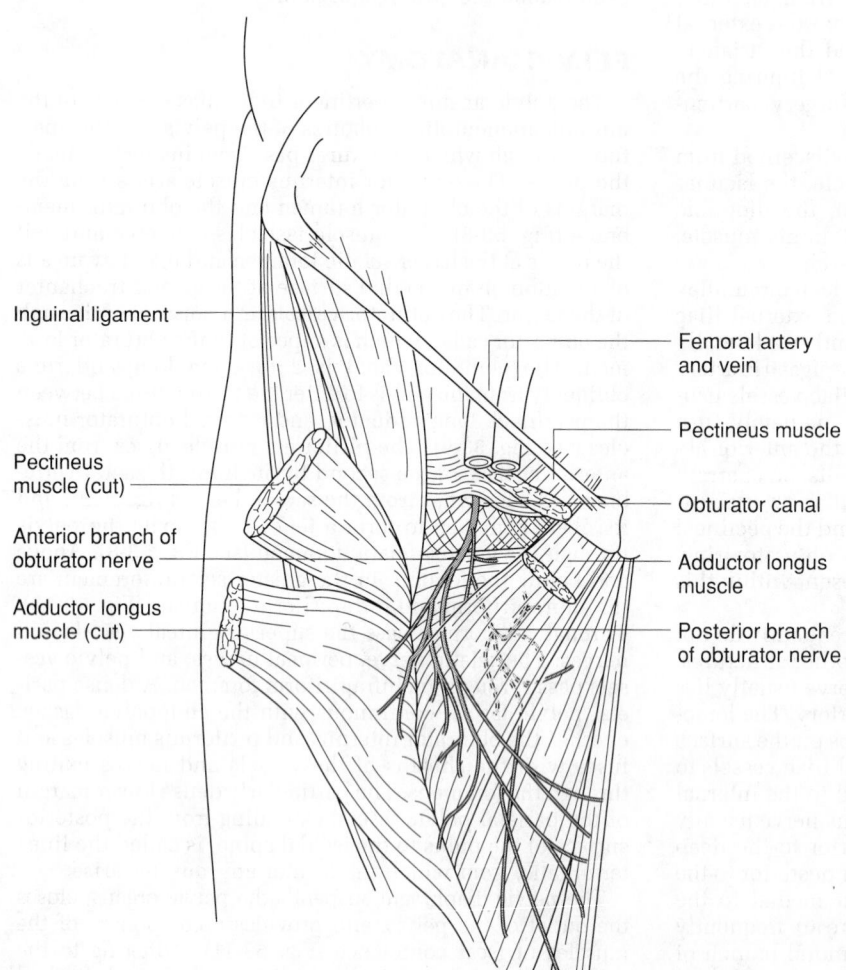

Inguinal ligament

Pectineus muscle (cut)

Anterior branch of obturator nerve

Adductor longus muscle (cut)

Femoral artery and vein

Pectineus muscle

Obturator canal

Adductor longus muscle

Posterior branch of obturator nerve

Figure 53-9. External relations of the obturator canal.

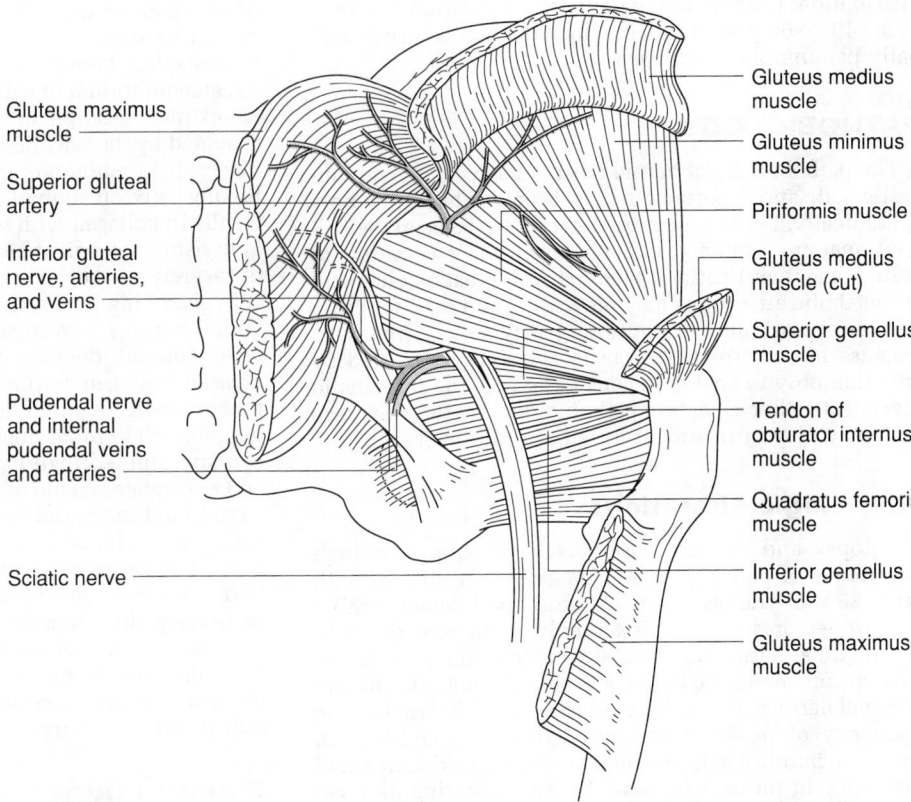

Figure 53-10. External relations of the sciatic foramens.

from the opposite side, the anococcygeal raphe. The pubococcygeal portion of the levator ani muscle originates from a more medial portion of the body of the pubis, runs posteriorly, and joins the longitudinal layer of the rectal wall near the perineum. The coccygeus muscle originates from the spine of the ischium, the sacrospinous ligament and the coccyx. The fascia that lines the pelvis and is continuous with the transversalis fascia is called the endopelvic fascia, which wraps around the viscera exiting through the pelvic diaphragm and so resists herniation along these organs.

EPIDEMIOLOGY

Hernias are commonly occurring processes, although there are no hard data on incidence. Estimates are that spontaneous abdominal hernias occur in 5% of the world's population over a lifetime, but based on US population statistics and operative rates, the prevalence may be as high as 10%. Inguinal hernias, the most common, occur five times as often as other types hernia types and constitute 80% of the total. Umbilical hernias constitute about 14% of hernias, femoral hernias about 5%, and other types are rare. The incidence of incisional hernias follows the frequency of abdominal surgery and is high in countries such as the United States, where about 115,000 incisional hernia repairs are done per year. There is a male prevalence in inguinal hernias of about 7:1 (male to female), whereas there is a female dominance in femoral and umbilical hernia of 1.8:1 and 1.7:1 (female to male), respectively. Incisional hernias also predominate in females by 2:1. For inguinal hernia, which occurs at all age levels, frequency increases with age. Umbilical hernia has a bimodal age

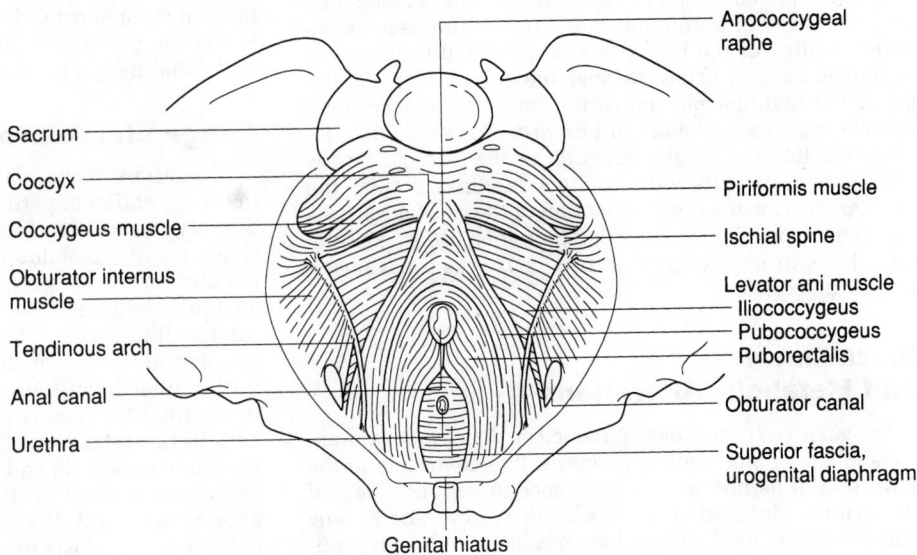

Figure 53-11. Pelvic diaphragm.

distribution, peaking in the pediatric population and then in the 40- to 60-year group, in which the hernias are principally paraumbilical hernias.

PATHOBIOLOGY

The pathobiology of hernia has not been extensively investigated, and information has been forthcoming only sporadically. For the most part, hernias have been considered anatomic deficits, either congenital or acquired or both. Some investigations have suggested that biochemical or metabolic alterations may play a role and that, for groin hernias at least, altered physiology may also be involved. Because most hernias have been successfully treated by attention only to anatomic considerations, the impetus to investigate other aspects of pathobiology and the relevance they may play in treatment have been minimal.

Physiologic Alterations

Autopsy and surgical observers have reported a high prevalence of patent processus vaginalis in infants, with up to 25% of youngsters in late childhood demonstrating a continued presence of this anomaly. In the past, the indirect inguinal hernia has been attributed to the presence of a patent processus vaginalis, and most, if not all, indirect inguinal hernias were consigned to a congenital cause. The frequency of patent processus vaginalis in children in whom no hernia can be demonstrated and the documented frequency of indirect inguinal hernia appearing de novo in the elderly suggest that indirect inguinal hernia cannot be attributed to a patent processus vaginalis alone. Animal studies have confirmed that inguinal herniation occurs infrequently despite patency of the processus vaginalis.

Investigations of how the internal inguinal ring responds to increases in intraabdominal pressure, such as during cough or Valsalva maneuver, have demonstrated a valve- or shutter-like effect at the ring in what is considered its normal state. Despite the presence of patent processus vaginalis, tensing of the abdominal wall normally closes the internal inguinal ring down to a slit through which intestine cannot protrude. In cases of indirect inguinal hernia, there is a deficient shutter function of the internal inguinal ring, and the ring constricts little, if at all. In such cases, the bowel has ready access to the patent process vaginalis, with the increase in intraabdominal pressure providing the impetus to force abdominal contents through the internal ring into the patent processus vaginalis.

In rats, traumatic injury to the internal ring is associated with the onset of herniation into a patent processus vaginalis. Healing of the injury is associated with reversal of the bowel's ability to pass through the internal ring. Paralysis of the inguinal portion of the transversus abdominis muscle is also associated with herniation. Despite the observation that the shutter function of the internal ring is deficient in patients with indirect inguinal hernia, the mechanism causing the dysfunction of the shutter remains a matter of speculation. For other types of hernias, possible alterations in physiology that may cause them have been largely unexplored.

Biochemical and Metabolic Alterations

Several investigators have provided evidence that there are metabolic and biochemical processes that contribute to the formation of hernias and to recurrence of hernias. Some of this evidence is based on the biochemistry of wound healing and of collagen formation and maintenance. Although tendinous, aponeurotic, and mature scar tissues have been regarded as stable, nearly inert tissues, increasing evidence suggests that these tissues are usually in a state of homeostasis, an equilibrium of collagen formation and collagenolysis. An extreme example of the metabolic activity of collagen is provided by the now rare disease called lathyrism, in which ingested ϵ1-aminopropionitrile prevents covalent cross-linking between and within forming collagen molecules and results in collagen with reduced tensile strength. Clinically, lathyrism causes giant hernias and other disorders as a result of severely weakened collagen.

In searching for biochemical factors associated with inguinal hernias, investigators have reported decreased collagen content, decreased wet weight of collagen, and decreased collagen formation in rectus sheath biopsies of patients with inguinal hernia as compared to patients undergoing abdominal operations for other conditions. Others have studied inguinal floor tissues from the ipsilateral and contralateral side of patients with inguinal hernia and have found increased rates of both collagen synthesis and catabolism, almost 10 times that in dense coherent collagen. They proposed that the primary process in inguinal hernia was collagenolysis, with the increased synthesis a secondary phenomenon. During the past decade, few data have been forthcoming to further elucidate the role of collagen metabolism on hernia formation. The nature and significance of altered collagen metabolism in hernia formation remains obscure.

Chronic Injury

Chronic trauma in the form of overstretching of musculoaponeurotic structures is likely to be a significant factor in spontaneously occurring hernias. Although minimal experimental data exist to support this contention, various forms of clinical evidence are suggestive. Direct inguinal hernias occur with unusual frequency in athletically competing young adults compared with their sedentary counterparts. Moreover, chronically increased intraabdominal pressure is frequently associated with the onset of hernias. Thus, hernias may first become evident in patients with chronic cough from chronic obstructive pulmonary disease, obstructive uropathy, massive ascites, massive splenomegaly, pregnancy, and with obstipation from colorectal cancer. Finally, although the experience is anecdotal, patients frequently relate a specific episode of muscular straining during which a sudden discomfort occurred, followed by hernia symptoms of discomfort or bulge. In cases of incisional hernias, chronic tension on the scar at the musculoaponeurotic level during the scar remodeling phase can result in a thin scar that poorly resists stresses. Incisional hernia may occur months to years later.

Congenital Anatomic Variants

Alterations in anatomic structures have been implicated in the formation of particular hernias. Although it does not directly result in the formation of a hernia, the consequent weakness of the abdominal wall becomes less resistant to the chronic stresses imposed in some individuals, so that anatomic structural weakness together with other factors can result in hernia. The absence of transversus abdominis aponeurotic fibers in the lateral portion or the whole of the inguinal floor (in up to 25% of persons) may predispose to inguinal hernias. A pattern of single decussation of fibers in the formation of the linea alba may predispose a person to epigastric and paraumbilical hernias.[2] Anatomic variations in the transition of the transversus abdominis aponeurosis and the posterior lamina of the internal oblique aponeurosis from posterior to anterior at the junction of the semilunar and semicircular lines may predispose a patient to spigelian hernia.

The umbilical hernia is an example of the failure of usual developmental progression. Although a defect always exists at the umbilicus at birth, this defect closes in most individuals. In a small percentage, the defect remains open in infancy as a hernia but closes eventually, and in the remainder the defect continues as a hernia. There is a genetic predisposition for umbilical hernias.

DIAGNOSTIC CONSIDERATIONS

The history and physical examination are the modalities almost exclusively used for diagnosing and delineating hernias. Questions should be directed toward the presence of a bulge, the conditions under which the bulge appears, and whether the bulge ever disappears and under which conditions. Also of importance are pain or discomfort associated with a particular area, especially in the area of a bulge, and the relation of that discomfort to certain activities, particularly those that increase intraabdominal pressures. A search for a precipitating event in the onset of the symptoms is of interest but is seldom of major benefit in establishing a diagnosis. Any bowel complaints should be sought, particularly symptoms of intermittent bowel obstruction such as distention, bloating, vomiting, and intermittent diarrhea and constipation. Inquiry should be made into previous hernias and the results of any previous repairs, the intake of any medications that might retard healing such as steroid or antineoplastic drugs, and any familial predisposition to hernias or known connective tissue defects such as Marfan syndrome. The review of systems should include those factors that might lead to increased intraabdominal pressure and so precipitate hernia emergence or make recurrence more likely. These factors include obstructive uropathy, rectal and left-sided colon cancers, chronic obstructive pulmonary disease or chronic cough, constipation, and ascites.

A complete physical examination should include general examination of the abdomen and rectal area, as well as testing of stool for occult blood. Examination for suspected groin (inguinal or femoral), obturator, sacral, or perineal hernias is best initiated with the patient in a standing position where the abdominal contents exert maximal gravity-induced pressure at the sites of potential hernias. Additional intraabdominal pressure is then best obtained by Valsalva maneuver, which can be sustained longer than pressures generated by cough. Palpation is directed toward a bulge that enlarges or appears with the Valsalva maneuver. Evaluation of the abdominal wall defect is usually not possible or necessary with inguinal and pelvic hernias. An attempt should be made to reduce gently any palpable bulge. If it is not clear whether a palpable mass is reducible or is a hernia, placing the patient in the recumbent position often permits reduction of the hernia without immediate reemergence. Resumption of the standing position should then allow confirmation by reappearance of the bulge.

Examination for inguinal hernia in the male is best accomplished by invagination of the index finger into the skin of the scrotum to follow the ductus deferens to the superficial ring. The tip of the index finger is better left at or just within the superficial ring when palpating for a bulge or impulse. If the fingertip lies far within the inguinal canal at the time of Valsalva, the bulging outward of the floor of the canal can easily be mistaken for hernia, especially as the fingertip is squeezed between internal and external oblique aponeuroses. In females, the inguinal region is examined by palpation directly over the area of the superficial inguinal ring. If no bulge is found, performing the Valsalva maneuver while pressure is applied over the

internal inguinal ring may elicit tenderness when an indirect inguinal hernia is present. For either sex, differentiating between indirect and direct inguinal hernia at physical examination is imprecise and of little meaning to the surgeon, because the operative approach is likely to be the same for either. A large superficial inguinal ring does not signify an inguinal hernia.

Femoral hernia should be sought at the femoral triangle medial to the femoral artery and inferior to the inguinal ligament. Obturator hernia infrequently presents with a palpable bulge in the proximal thigh just anterior to the origin of the adductor muscles of the thigh. Sciatic hernias may present with a bulge in the medial gluteal area, lateral to the sacrum. Perineal hernias present with a bulge lateral to the vagina or anus.

Ventral hernias are often best initially evaluated with the patient in the supine position. Valsalva or straight leg raises nearly always demonstrate the presence of an abdominal wall defect and a bulge. Difficulties in evaluation may arise in those patients with significant adipose tissue in the subcutaneous layer of the abdominal wall and in patients with an interparietal hernia. Particular discomfort with pressure over the area of suspected hernia with Valsalva maneuver should increase suspicion of hernia in these cases but is not diagnostic. The reducibility of the hernia, the size of the defect, and the proportion of abdominal contents chronically outside the confines of the abdominal cavity are important factors. Previous scars and any changes in the overlying skin are also meaningful.

When a question remains regarding the presence of a hernia or the differentiation from a mass overlying the abdominal or pelvic wall, radiographic studies may sometimes provide additional information. Plain radiographs of the abdomen taken in views tangential to the abdominal wall in the area of the suspected hernia defect may depict gas-containing bowel outside the confines of the abdominal wall. Likewise, barium contrast studies of the gastrointestinal tract may demonstrate bowel emerging from a defect in the abdominal wall. A problem with these studies is that the abdominal and pelvic wall cannot be accurately visualized.

Ultrasound may allow delineation of hernias with acceptable identification of the abdominal wall structures and of gas or fluid in most cases. Computed tomography (CT) usually delineates abdominal and pelvic wall structures, and often identifies wall defects. Gas, fluid collections, and contrast within bowel outside the confines of the abdominal or pelvic walls are frequently demonstrable with CT, particularly if Valsalva and special maneuvers are incorporated by the radiographer. Herniography, using nonionic medium iohexol as contrast in the peritoneal cavity, usually demonstrates both the presence and site of origin for inguinal and pelvic hernias.[5] The technique has not been widely practiced but may be useful in persons with groin or pelvic pain in the absence of findings by physical examination.

Differential diagnosis of inguinal hernia includes hydrocele, lipoma or other tumor, spermatocele, varicocele, undescended testis, or metastasis from testicular neoplasm. Femoral hernia must be differentiated from lymphadenopathy, lipoma, aneurysm or pseudoaneurysm of the femoral artery, lymphocele, hematoma, or the presentation of a psoas abscess. Incisional and recurrent hernias can be confused with cysts or seromas, neoplastic masses, and abscesses.

CLINICAL MANIFESTATIONS
Uncomplicated Hernias

The predominant symptoms associated with uncomplicated hernias are a dull ache and a bulge. The ache may be more or less intense, and is occasionally described as

1218 SURGERY: SCIENTIFIC PRINCIPLES AND PRACTICE

a burning or a pain. It is usually exacerbated by activity and may become particularly intense with coughing and sneezing but is often relieved by recumbency. Any bulge is usually reported by the patient to be more prominent when active and ambulating or with any maneuver that increases intraabdominal pressure and to be decreased or nonexistent in the recumbent position. Occasionally, neuralgia develops in the distribution of a sensory nerve lying at the site of the hernia, such as the ilioinguinal nerve for inguinal hernia or the obturator nerve for obturator hernia. Infrequently, a hernia may be totally asymptomatic and discovered in the course of a physical examination.

Complications of Hernias

The major complications of hernias are incarceration, bowel obstruction, and bowel strangulation. Bowel obstruction or strangulation are estimated to occur with about 5% of hernias. A complication is more likely to occur with a large-volume hernia sac relative to the hernia defect diameter and in hernias in which the bowel has access to the hernia sac. The presence of bowel incarceration greatly increases the risk for bowel obstruction and strangulation.

Incarceration

Incarceration denotes the condition in which viscera are contained within a hernia sac and cannot be disgorged from the sac. Conditions under which incarceration occurs include the following: (1) adhesion formation between a portion of the interior of the sac and the viscus; (2) adhesion formation between the neck of the sac at several sites, such that viscera within the sac cannot then exit; and (3) development of edema in hernia contents or contortion and adhesion between viscera within the sac so that exit of the contents is difficult. Patients with an incarcerated hernia may be asymptomatic except for the presence of a bulge. Pain associated with an incarcerated hernia is indicative of strangulation.

Attempting to reduce an apparently incarcerated asymptomatic hernia is relatively safe, as long as excessive force is not applied. With gentle kneading, many apparently unreducible hernias are found to reduce. An incarcerated hernia with associated discomfort or signs of bowel obstruction is best treated with urgent hernia repair. In some cases, gentle attempts at reducing a symptomatic, seemingly incarcerated hernia may be without consequence. Reduction of the symptomatic hernia may result in the reduction of gangrenous bowel into the peritoneal cavity. Reduction of bowel with necrotic areas eventuates in bowel perforation and peritonitis with associated 10% to 30% mortality rates and high levels of morbidity. Vigorous attempts at reduction may result in reduction en masse, in which the viscera remain within the peritoneal sac after reduction, with the entire sac and its contained viscera forced through the abdominal wall defect into the preperitoneal layer. Reduction en masse usually occurs when a small fibrous neck traps the enclosed viscera. It is associated with a high risk for continued entrapment or progression to obstruction or strangulation.

Obstruction

Worldwide, hernias are the leading cause of intestinal obstruction. The obstruction is almost exclusively small intestinal. Only rarely is the colon, or even more rarely the stomach, the site of obstruction. In the United States, where abdominal operations are frequent, hernia is the third most common cause of bowel obstruction after intraabdominal adhesions and abdominal cancer. In any patient with a suspected bowel obstruction, it is mandatory to assess for the presence of hernia. If it is responsible for the bowel obstruction, it is also mandatory to repair the hernia as well as relieve the bowel obstruction.

In most cases, if the bowel obstruction can be attributed to the hernia, the primary operative attack can focus on the hernia. Assessing bowel viability is possible without laparotomy in most cases, and releasing adhesions holding the bowel within the sac is more easily accomplished through direct entry into the hernia sac. Inguinal, femoral, umbilical, and incisional hernias predominate in causing hernia-induced bowel obstruction, and these hernias are usually best approached directly. Pelvic and lumbar hernias, as well as internal hernias, may be occult sources of bowel obstruction and are also usually best repaired from an intraabdominal approach. Reducing the herniated and incarcerated bowel may be difficult from the intraabdominal approach, necessitating a counter-incision over the external presentation of the hernia.

Strangulation

Strangulation implies compromise of the blood supply to a viscus, which, in the case of hernia, is usually a segment of small bowel. Strangulation may be of acute onset with torsion of the contents of the hernia occluding the arterial inflow and venous outflow from a segment of bowel. A less acute onset may arise from bowel obstruction, venous outflow obstruction, or even lymphatic obstruction. In this subacute onset, increasing edema in the mesentery gradually occludes venous outflow, with increasingly rapid accumulation of interstitial fluid to the point of exceeding arteriolar pressure and subsequent ischemia.

In almost all cases of strangulation, there is concomitant bowel obstruction. The exception is the Richter hernia, in which the herniated lateral wall of the viscus may strangulate without obstruction (Fig. 53-12). Most patients who develop a strangulated hernia have a known hernia, and incarceration may be present for some time before strangulation. In up to 40% of cases, particularly with femoral hernia, the episode of strangulation may occur within a few days of the first indication of the hernia.[6] Pain usually accompanies strangulation but may be inconspicuous in those with diabetic neuropathy and in the elderly. Strangulation is a concern whenever bowel obstruction is due to hernia, and urgent operation is indicated. Strangulation is associated with a mortality rate of about 10% and major morbidity.[6]

The operative approach for potentially strangulated bowel within a hernia is generally identical to that for the hernia itself. Care must be exercised with necrotic bowel to prevent disruption of the bowel wall and spillage of bowel contents. Dissection must be carried out to access viable bowel proximal and distal to the strangulated bowel,

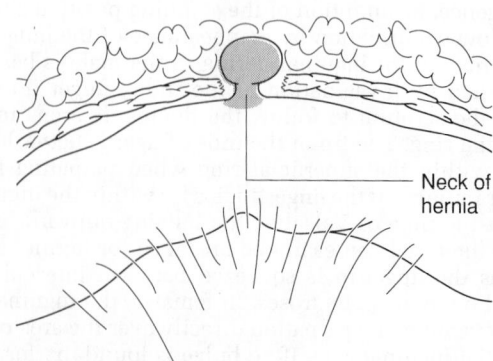

Neck of hernia

Figure 53-12. Richter hernia.

after which bowel resection can be carried out through the same incision used to repair the hernia. For hernias approached from within the abdomen, traction on the strangulated bowel within the hernia must be avoided to prevent bowel rupture and spillage of contents. Frequently, a counter-incision over the external aspect of the hernia and dissection of the bowel from the sac using an external approach is safest.

TREATMENT

The indications for hernia repair must be individualized to each patient and situation. In general, the presence of a hernia can be considered an adequate indication for hernia repair. Certainly, the presence of complications due to the hernia necessitates correcting those complications and usually repairing the hernia. As with any treatment, the benefits of operative repair must be weighed against the natural history of the disease, the extent to which the treatment can correct the problem, the possibility of treatment-related injury, and the interference of concomitant disease with the treatment results.

With few exceptions, the natural history of abdominal wall hernia is that the size of the defect and the sac enlarges over time, and that such enlargement increases the difficulty of adequate repair and the chances of recurrence of the hernia. How the risk of a major complication relates to the length of time that a hernia is present has not been rigorously demonstrated. Nevertheless, such complications are more likely to occur in a patient the longer the exposure to a hernia and the larger the sac relative to the hernia defect. In addition, major complications necessitate an emergent operation with attendant high mortality and morbidity in relation to elective repair. Therefore, if an operative hernia repair is to be done, it is better done sooner than later, assuming adequate preoperative preparation.

Expectant treatment is appropriate for umbilical hernias less than 3 cm in diameter and for small epigastric hernias in children under 2 to 4 years old, provided the hernia is not enlarging and is not incarcerated. These two types of hernias have been observed to disappear in these young children. Although some have advocated strapping to maintain such hernias in a reduced position to permit closure, no well-controlled data exist to support the use of strapping. The age beyond which operative repair becomes necessary has not been defined, but there is little evidence that spontaneous closure occurs except rarely in children older than 6 years or in those with enlarging hernias.

Nonoperative therapy is appropriate in patients for whom the risk of mortality and morbidity due to concomitant disease is greater for operative repair of their hernia than for potential complications from the hernia. The mortality rate for repair of most hernias is 1% or less. For those patients with coexisting medical illness, however, mortality and morbidity are much increased for emergent operation due to a hernia complication than for the elective repair of the identical hernia. Using a corset or binder may be appropriate in the patient with an easily reducible ventral or lumbar hernia who is a poor candidate for hernia repair. These devices are contraindicated for the patient with an incarcerated hernia or a hernia with a narrow neck relative to the sac. The use of a truss, an external support device using a system of straps to exert regional pressure over the hernia defect, should generally be avoided. Trusses do not consistently maintain a hernia in the reduced state, and they put an unreduced hernia in greater jeopardy of strangulation. The pressure exerted induces edema by decreasing lymphatic and venous flow out of the herniated bowel. Trusses may also injure the skin overlying the hernia. Most patients for whom trusses are prescribed would be better served by and suffer less morbidity from an appropriate hernia repair.

Principles of Treatment

Hernia repair is directed first at the sac and its contents, and second at the defect in the delimiting structure, usually the abdominal wall. Although the procedure is occasionally challenging, particularly in reducing incarcerated visceral contents, there are few controversial areas in the handling of the sac. To prevent entering and subsequently entrapping visceral contents within a peritoneal sac as a type of internal hernia, the sac with a narrow neck should be closed at its neck after evacuating the visceral contents, and the excess sac should be excised. A sac with a broad entrance, having a similar diameter to that of the sac, need not be excised or closed. Later incarceration of bowel contents within its confines is not a risk, and it needs only to be reduced beneath the abdominal wall repair.

The sliding hernia is a special case in terms of handling the sac. In this hernia, the visceral peritoneum covering a portion of a retroperitoneal organ makes up a portion of the sac, requiring that the retroperitoneal organ also be included in the herniated tissues (Fig. 53-13). For sliding hernias, the means of closing and excising the narrow-necked sac must avoid injury to the sliding organ or its blood supply. Various techniques have been devised to handle the sliding hernia, but the best results have followed the simplest procedures. Reperitonealization of the sliding viscus is unnecessary, and simple closure of the peritoneum after excising grossly redundant portions is sufficient. The essential element in repairing the sliding hernia is a satisfactory repair of the abdominal wall defect.

Effective repair of the abdominal wall defect is the sine qua non of hernia repair, and controversy continues about how best to accomplish this goal in repairing a range of hernia types. In general, the principles of wound closure apply (ie, the direct apposition of strong musculoaponeurotic structures without tension). Closure under no tension whatsoever is rarely achieved, so the goal must be to minimize the tension at the closure. How much tension is too much has not been scientifically demonstrated. Contrary

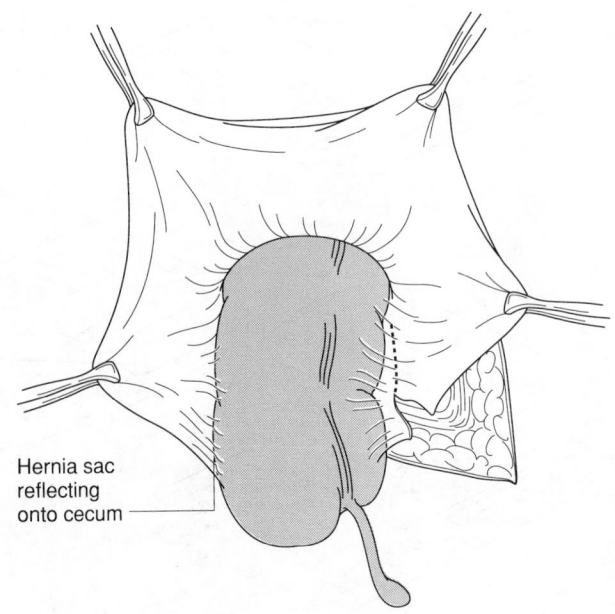

Figure 53-13. Sliding hernia (right indirect inguinal).

to conditions in primary wound closure, hernias are frequently associated with a long-standing tissue deficit in which abdominal wall is either actually missing as a result of tissue necrosis or gradual attenuation or is effectively missing because of chronic retraction and scarring. Additionally, the musculoaponeurotic tissues at the margins of the hernia defect may be attenuated or, especially with incisional hernias, fenestrated from previous closure methods. Various techniques have been advocated to overcome these more adverse conditions associated with closure of hernia wounds.

One technique is the use of a relaxing incision, which is an incision in an aponeurosis that overlies dense muscle, with the relaxing incision oriented roughly parallel to but separated from the area of hernia or wound closure by at least several centimeters. The relaxing incision allows the aponeurotic structure to slide over the underlying muscle to allow closure of the hernia defect under decreased tension. The underlying muscle with its intact underlying transversalis fascia prevents herniation at the site of the relaxing incision.

Another technique is the use of musculoaponeurotic or aponeurotic flaps that are rotated or folded over and then sutured to the musculoaponeurotic structures at the margin of the hernia defect. Use of such flaps requires that the blood supply to the dislocated tissue be maintained. Although a nonvascularized aponeurosis initially performs satisfactorily for a repair, over time the collagen is resorbed and the hernia is likely to recur. When using flaps, it is also necessary to leave adequate supporting structures in the area from which the flap has been derived.

Much more commonly used than flaps are nonviable free grafts. Some grafts consist of collagen, including autologous fascia lata and homograft aponeurotic structures. The grafts more frequently consist of prosthetic materials, including polypropylene mesh, expanded polytetrafluoro-

ethylene sheet, and tantalum wire mesh. For large defects, such grafts are almost essential to allow closure. Collagen grafts have proved unsatisfactory in many applications; far from being inert, the nonvascularized collagen graft is resorbed and recurrent hernia often develops.

Plastic meshes or sheets are chosen for most applications. Ideal characteristics for these grafts are strength, flexibility, durability, ease of tailoring, lack of stimulation of inflammatory response, and promotion of fibroblastic response and ingrowth. An important consideration in placement of such grafts is the method of fixation to the musculoaponeurotic structures at the margin of the defect. Underlaying the material with suturing or a sandwich technique, achieved by folding the graft over the margin or using two layers of graft, appears to allow less recurrence of hernia at the margins than does the overlay technique (Fig. 53-14).

Complications of Operative Treatment

Many complications can occur with operations on the abdomen. Complications specific to hernia repairs include injury to motor or sensory nerves, which leads to muscular atrophy in the distribution of those nerves and may predispose the patient to recurrent hernia at the initial or an adjacent site. Sensory nerve injury may lead to disabling symptoms from neuromas, myofascial type pain, or reflex sympathetic dystrophy. Severe symptoms due to sensory nerve entrapment or injury are common in inguinal hernia repairs.

Vascular injuries may occur to viscera for which the blood supply courses through the region of the hernia repair, resulting in ischemia or necrosis. In some cases, recognition of injury to visceral blood supply is delayed and

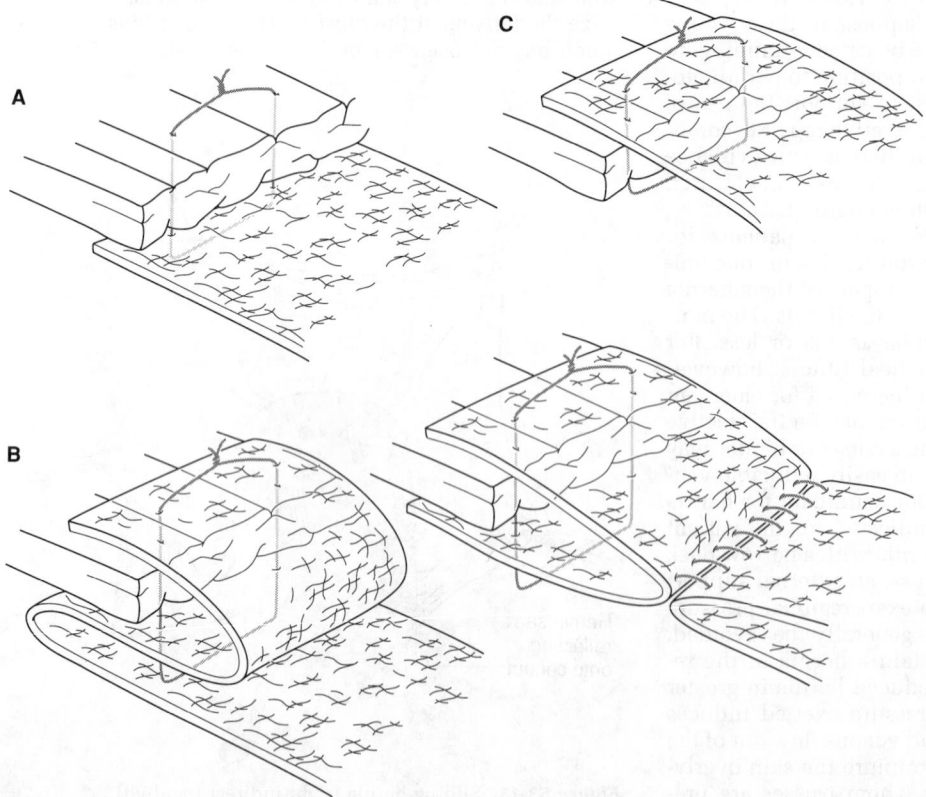

Figure 53-14. Various techniques for suturing prosthesis to the abdominal wall. (*A*) Underlay. (*B*) Sandwich. (*C*) Overlay.

results in gangrene and its sequelae. The particular vessels at risk with hernia repairs are given in the discussions of the various hernias. Injury can occur to nearby organs that are not visible but are separated from the repair by little distance and tissue. Injuries to the bladder and the femoral vein can occur with groin hernia repairs. Injury to bowel can occur during repair if the bowel is inadequately dissected from the hernia margins.

Hernia recurrence is the bane of the surgeon because it is a sign that the applied treatment has failed. Hernia recurrence rates after primary groin hernia repair should be infrequent but varied in several large series from less than 1% to almost 9%.[7] The prevalence of recurrent hernia may be higher after repair of recurrent groin hernia, but several researchers have been able to achieve less than a 3% rate of second recurrence. On the other hand, the recurrence rate after incisional hernia repair may exceed 30%.

Factors responsible for hernia recurrence include those relevant to incisional hernia—closure under excessive tension, failure to exclude adjacent musculoaponeurotic defects and to identify and use an adequately strong musculoaponeurotic margin, and wound infection. Other factors in hernia recurrence generally relate to inadequate collagen formation in the wound, including protein and vitamin malnutrition and the concomitant therapeutic administration of corticosteroids or antimetabolites. Finally, a chronically high intraabdominal pressure, the causes of which include obstructive uropathy, chronic coughing, ascites, and chronic straining at stool, is associated with an increased rate of hernia recurrence.

Preoperative and Postoperative Care

Before hernia repair, the factors that may have contributed to the development of the hernia must be investigated. Contributing elements must first be nullified or alleviated as much as possible. Increased intraabdominal pressure due to obstructive uropathy or ascites should be reversed before repairing the hernia. Partially obstructing rectal cancer as a cause of increased intraabdominal pressure should be evaluated by history and stool occult blood testing. Screening sigmoidoscopy for those over 40 years old was recommended in the past, but it is not cost-effective and is no longer recommended routinely. Chronic cough should be treated to the extent possible.

Open wounds in the region of the hernia should be allowed to heal if at all possible before repair, and must be healed before the use of a nonabsorbable prosthesis as part of the repair. Large chronic granulating wounds are best closed by split-thickness skin grafting. Chronic corticosteroid administration should be at as low a level as possible, and antimetabolites should be discontinued.

Anesthetic Considerations

Most primary repairs of groin hernias can be performed on an outpatient basis under local anesthesia. Most methods of local anesthesia for groin hernia incorporate a combination of ilioinguinal-iliohypogastric nerve block, field block, and direct infiltration. Procedures less likely to be satisfactorily completed under local anesthesia are those that require more than 90 minutes to complete, those associated with extensive intraperitoneal dissection (eg, scrotal hernia), or those performed for recurrent inguinal hernia. Spinal, epidural, and general anesthesia, alone or in combination, are effective for groin hernias and can be used for outpatient surgery under appropriate conditions.

Small anterior abdominal wall hernias can be repaired under local anesthesia. Epidural or spinal anesthetic may also be useful for anterior abdominal wall hernias where the hernia lies in the middle or lower abdomen and little intraperitoneal dissection is likely. The immediate availability of general anesthesia is recommended for incisional hernias and epigastric hernias, in which a much more extensive repair may be required because of multiple defects or when there is a need to dissect extensive intraabdominal adhesions. The patient must therefore be considered a candidate for general anesthesia and evaluated as such before the elective repair of anterior abdominal wall hernias.

General anesthesia, alone or as an adjunct, is necessary for all patients with hernias requiring an intraabdominal approach (including the laparoscopic approach) or extensive intraperitoneal dissection (eg, a large incarcerated hernia) and for those patients with large hernias in which the hernia contents have lost right of domain. These patients also require hospitalization postoperatively because postoperative ileus is likely.

Patients With Massive Hernias

In massive hernias, a large proportion of the abdominal contents reside within the hernia on a permanent basis, whether or not they are incarcerated, and they are said to have lost the right of domain within the abdominal cavity. The abdominal wall is chronically contracted, and the acute replacement of the hernia contents within the abdominal cavity at the time of repair can be accomplished only by markedly increasing intraabdominal pressure. Reduction of hernia contents results in the following: (1) acutely increased inspiratory pressures, due to forcibly elevated diaphragms; (2) decreased venous return; (3) sometimes, renal insufficiency due to vena cava and renal vein compression; and (4) increased tension on the hernia repair. In addition to right of domain issues, chronic traction on the mesentery in these massive hernias has often resulted in chronic congestion and edema of the bowel wall, further increasing the difficulty of reduction. In some cases of massive hernia, the skin stretched over the hernia thins and even ulcerates. Moreover, dependency of a large sac often leads to lymphedema, dermatoses, and occasionally cellulitis of the overlying skin.

The repair of massive hernias almost always requires the use of prosthetic material. Therefore, skin ulceration, dermatoses, and cellulitis must be treated before hernia repair. Occasionally, the patient must be placed at bed rest for a few days preoperatively to decrease the dependent pressure of the hernia contents on the skin.

Progressive pneumoperitoneum has been recommended for repairing these massive hernias.[8] Progressive pneumoperitoneum involves injecting 500 to 1500 mL of air every 1 to 3 days for 14 to 21 days before hernia repair. Putative benefits include physiologic acclimation to increased intraabdominal pressures and the elevation of the diaphragms, stretching of the abdominal wall to increase the volume of the abdominal cavity before replacement of hernia contents, and reduction of adhesions in the hernia. No study has sufficiently compared the physiologic and result parameters between groups who were treated with and without progressive preoperative pneumoperitoneum. Whether increased intraabdominal pressure does much more than stretch the hernia sac and overlying skin is open to question.

TYPES OF HERNIAS
Spontaneously Occurring Hernias
Inguinal and Femoral Hernias

Inguinal hernias are the most commonly occurring nonincisional hernias. Because the anatomy of femoral and inguinal hernias is similar, these two are often discussed together (see the earlier discussion of their anatomy, epidemiology, and diagnosis). Inguinal hernias are divided into indirect and direct hernias. The anatomic landmark distinguishing them is the inferior epigastric blood vessels, although the actual difference is in the mechanism of formation (Fig. 53-15). Indirect inguinal hernias occur through the internal inguinal ring in a protrusion of peritoneum along the spermatic cord lying within the internal spermatic fascia. These hernias arise in some cases from incomplete closure of the processus vaginalis, the tongue of peritoneum that descends with the testis in fetal life. Large, indirect inguinal hernias descend into the scrotum along the spermatic cord. In contrast, direct inguinal hernias occur through the floor of the inguinal canal, separate from the spermatic cord. Direct inguinal hernias occur because of a breakdown of the transversus abdominis aponeurosis and transversalis fascia and tend to occur in individuals who engage in activities requiring intense abdominal wall muscle tension. Simultaneous ipsilateral indirect and direct inguinal hernias are known as pantaloon hernias. Femoral hernias occur into the femoral canal.

Since Bassini described the inguinal hernia repair that bears his name in 1884, the repair of inguinal and femoral hernias has been guided primarily by attempts to restore the anatomy of the inguinal region. A review of the many operative methods that have been recommended and used to repair inguinal hernias is beyond the scope of this text. Nevertheless, principles that apply to repair of hernias in this region are illustrated by discussion of commonly used repairs. First, all repairs of indirect and femoral hernias require the following procedures: (1) identification of the hernia sac; (2) evacuation of the sac; and (3) identification of any sliding component, whether from bladder, cecum, sigmoid colon, appendix, or ovary. In some cases of femoral hernia, difficulty in achieving reduction of the incarcerated bowel may require an infrainguinal ligament counterincision or division of the inguinal ligament. The direct hernia sac is generally broad-based compared to its length and infrequently requires ligation and excision; it most frequently is reduced beneath the inguinal floor closure. The second principle is a secure closure of the defect and the assurance of a strong tissue plane at the inguinal floor or at the opening of the femoral canal for femoral hernias.

The portion of the inguinal hernia repair that has given rise to the more important technical differences is the provision of a strong inguinal floor, often referred to as reconstruction of the inguinal floor. The inguinal floor is the site of direct inguinal hernias, but the superior portion of the floor is also attenuated or destroyed by the enlargement of the internal inguinal ring in medium to large indirect inguinal hernias.

The Bassini repair is an inguinal hernia repair used worldwide and has been a standard against which other repairs are judged. The repair as described initially divided the inguinal floor structures (ie, the transversus abdominis aponeurosis and transversalis fascia) and apposed the medial portions of these two structures and the lateral edge of the rectus sheath (ie, the conjoint area structures) to the shelving edge of the inguinal (Poupart) ligament. A common practice in the United States has been to approximate these structures by imbrication without dividing the inguinal floor. The Shouldice (Canadian Bassini) repair is similar but approximates these same structures in an overlapping fashion with two rows of running sutures (Fig. 53-16). The Bassini repair has been criticized because it does not precisely restore the anatomy of the inguinal floor, since anatomically, the transversus abdominis aponeurosis and transversalis fascia insert into the pectineal ligament and not the inguinal ligament. A femoral hernia cannot be repaired by an unmodified Bassini repair because the orifice to the femoral canal lies deep to the inguinal ligament.

Cooper ligament repair, of which McVay has been a strong proponent, divides and excises the central attenuated portion of the inguinal floor in its standard implementation. It repairs the inguinal floor by approximation of the conjoint area structures and the transversus abdominis aponeurosis and transversalis fascia to the pectineal (Cooper) ligament between the pubic tubercle and the femoral vein (Fig. 53-17). More laterally, the transversus abdominis muscle and aponeurosis and transversalis fascia are approximated to the iliopubic tract and femoral sheath up to the internal ring. This repair is also appropriate for femoral hernias.

The relaxing incision is important for repairs of direct and large indirect inguinal hernias to prevent excessive tension in the closure (see Fig. 53-17). Failure to make a relaxing incision has been implicated in a greater incidence of recurrence for these repairs. The relaxing incision

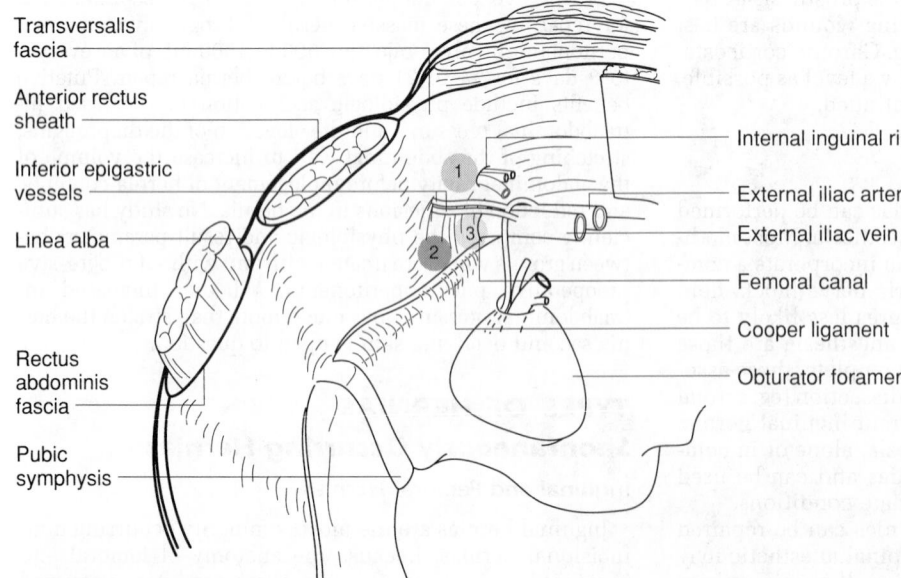

Transversalis fascia

Anterior rectus sheath

Inferior epigastric vessels

Linea alba

Rectus abdominis fascia

Pubic symphysis

Internal inguinal ring

External iliac artery

External iliac vein

Femoral canal

Cooper ligament

Obturator foramen

Figure 53-15. Posterior view of the inguinal region. (1) Site of indirect inguinal hernia, along the spermatic cord. (2) Site of direct inguinal hernia, through the inguinal floor. (3) Site of femoral hernia, the internal orifice of the femoral canal.

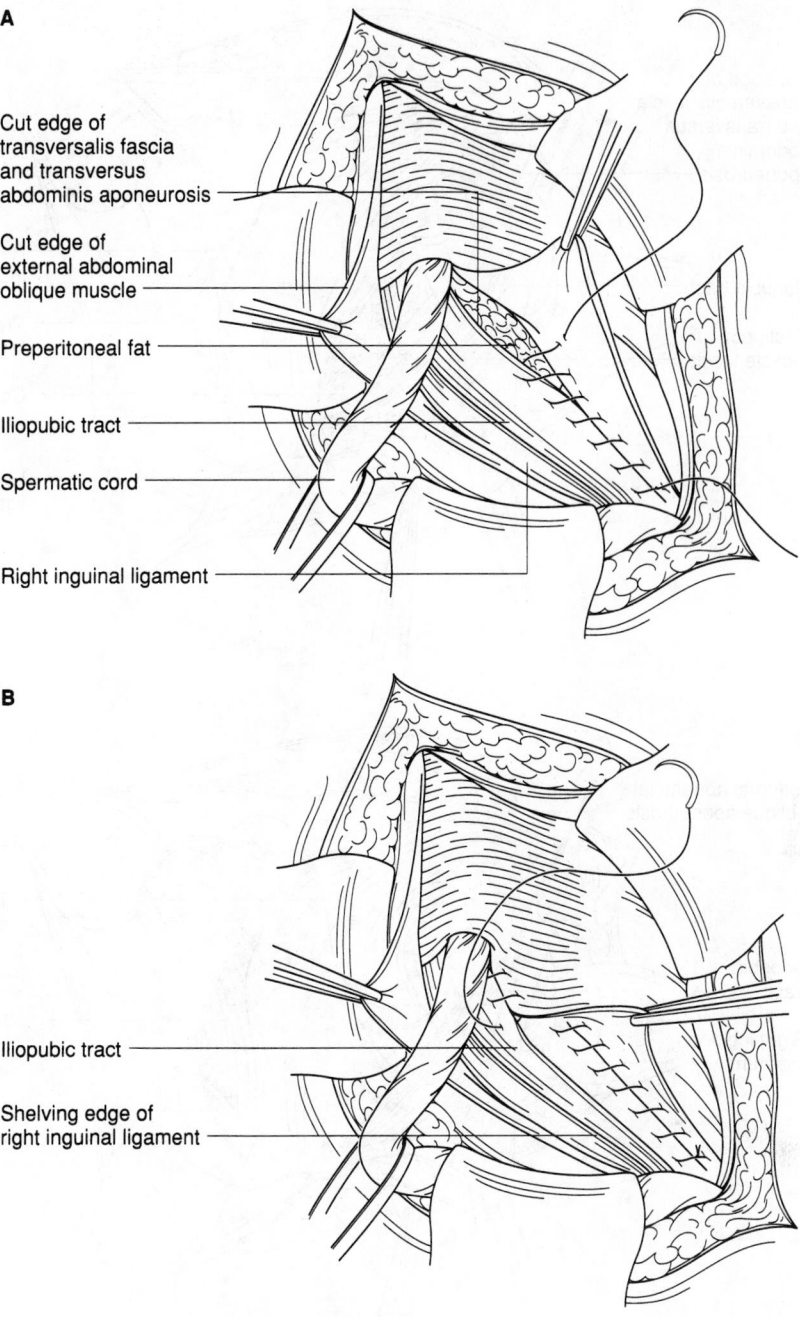

A

Cut edge of
transversalis fascia
and transversus
abdominis aponeurosis

Cut edge of
external abdominal
oblique muscle

Preperitoneal fat

Iliopubic tract

Spermatic cord

Right inguinal ligament

B

Iliopubic tract

Shelving edge of
right inguinal ligament

Figure 53-16. Shouldice inguinal hernia repair. (A) The first of the suture lines approximates the lateral cut edge of transversus abdominis aponeurosis and transversalis fascia to the undersurface of these same structures near the edge of the rectus abdominis muscle. (B) The second suture line joins the medial cut edge of the inguinal floor to the iliopubic tract and shelving edge of the inguinal ligament. Two additional suture lines, approximating progressively more superficial medial to lateral musculoaponeurotic structures, are frequently omitted.

is made in the internal lamina of the anterior rectus sheath in a craniocaudad direction extending from 1 to 2 cm above the pubis to a level approximately opposite the internal inguinal ring. The resulting defect is covered posteriorly by the body of the rectus muscle and anteriorly by the anterior leaf of the rectus sheath, preventing herniation at that site.

The polypropylene mesh repair is becoming widely used as a standard repair for all primary direct and large indirect inguinal hernias. The mesh incites the formation of scar tissue to further increase tensile strength beyond that provided by the mesh alone. Prosthetic materials, including tantalum wire and polypropylene meshes, have been used for many years for large or recurrent inguinal and femoral hernias. In recurrent or large hernias, a deficit of strong tissue may preclude a low-tension repair using adjacent endogenous tissues, in which case prosthetic tissue has

been used as a substitute. For primary hernia repairs using mesh in the most frequently used method (popularized by Lichtenstein), the mesh is laid over the undisturbed inguinal floor, posterior to the spermatic cord, and sutured to the shelving edge of the inguinal ligament, the pubis, and the internal oblique fascia (Fig. 53-18). Two tails fashioned in the upper portion of the mesh are slighty wrapped and sutured on either side of the spermatic cord as it exits the internal inguinal ring. Results reported for inguinal hernias primarily repaired with mesh have been excellent. Improvement over traditional methods for primary repair has not been demonstrated, however, and the slight risk of infection of the prosthetic material must be considered.

The preperitoneal approach to groin hernia repair is advocated most frequently for the recurrent inguinal or femoral hernia but is also applicable to primary hernia repair. This approach uses a more or less transverse incision

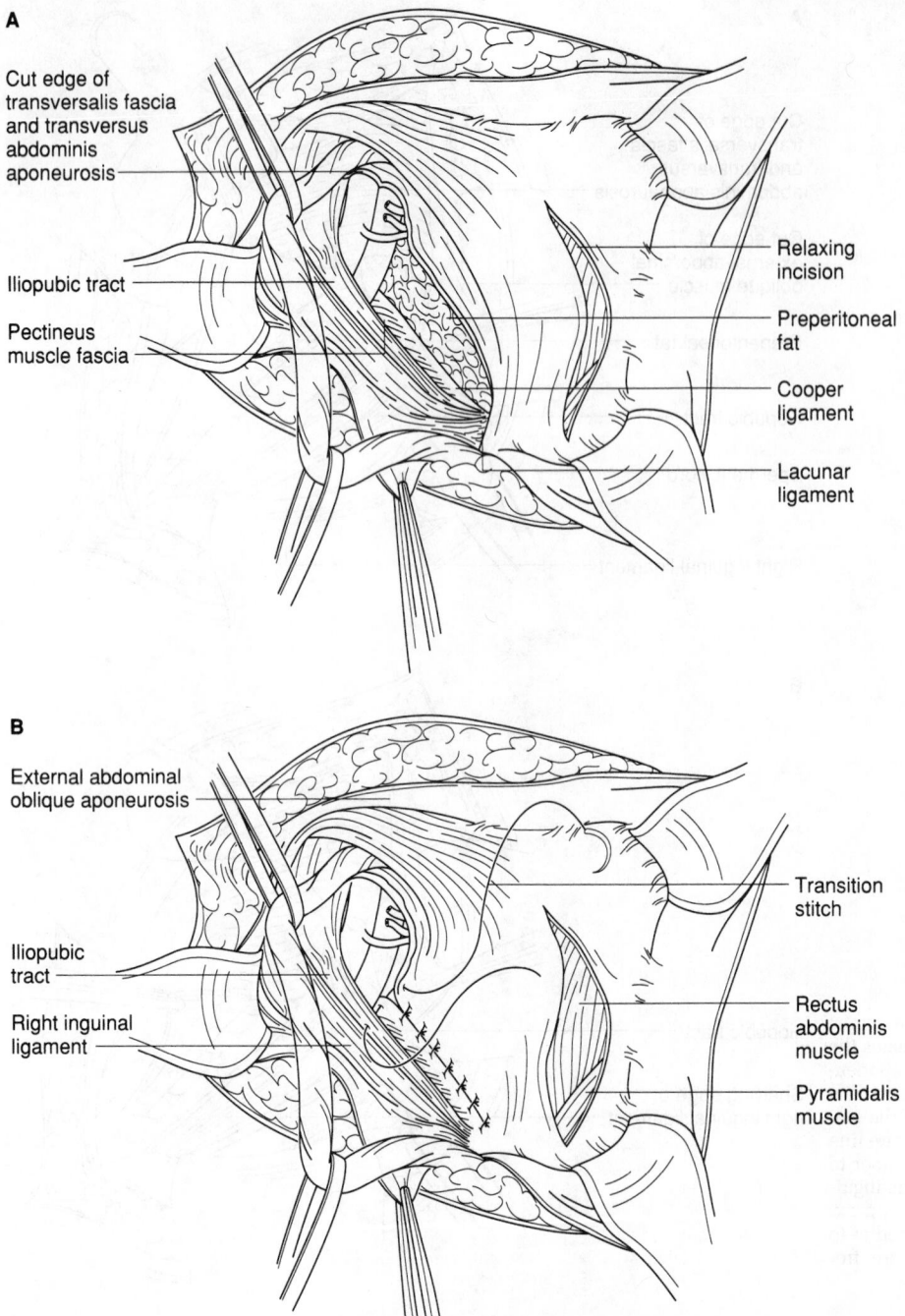

A

Cut edge of
transversalis fascia
and transversus
abdominis
aponeurosis

Iliopubic tract

Pectineus
muscle fascia

Relaxing
incision

Preperitoneal
fat

Cooper
ligament

Lacunar
ligament

B

External abdominal
oblique aponeurosis

Iliopubic
tract

Right inguinal
ligament

Transition
stitch

Rectus
abdominis
muscle

Pyramidalis
muscle

Figure 53-17. Cooper ligament repair. (*A*) Anatomy with the attenuated inguinal floor excised and the relaxing incision made. (*B*) Approximation of the conjoined structures medially to the Cooper ligament laterally, with placement of the transition stitch through conjoined structures, Cooper ligament, pectineus muscle fascia, and iliopubic tract. The internal ring is closed by approximation of transversalis fascia and transversis abdominis muscle medially to iliopubic tract laterally.

placed only a little more superior than that used for the anterior approaches to inguinal and femoral hernias discussed previously. The musculoaponeurotic structures of the abdominal wall are divided down to the preperitoneal fat plane, which is deep to the transversalis fascia. The preperitoneal fat and underlying peritoneum are pushed posteriorly to expose the inguinal floor, internal inguinal ring, and femoral canal orifice from the posterior surface. A Cooper ligament repair is then accomplished from this posterior preperitoneal approach. A relaxing incision is strongly recommended. Mesh can also be placed from this approach when indicated.

Femoral hernia repair requires the interposition of a musculoaponeurotic structure medial to the femoral vein to close

the inlet to the femoral canal. Apposition of the lacunar ligament and shelving edge of the inguinal ligament to the pectineal ligament has been suggested by some surgeons but is accomplished only with high tension on the apposed edges and is liable to recurrence. The anterior or posterior (preperitoneal) approaches using the pectineal ligament and iliopubic tract are the most widely recommended.

The approach to bilateral groin hernias is based on the extent of the hernia defect. For hernias that require inguinal floor reconstruction (all direct and moderate to large indirect inguinal hernias, all femoral hernias), simultaneous repair of bilateral hernias results in recurrence of one or both of the hernias twice as frequently as if the hernias were repaired sequentially. For repairs requiring only

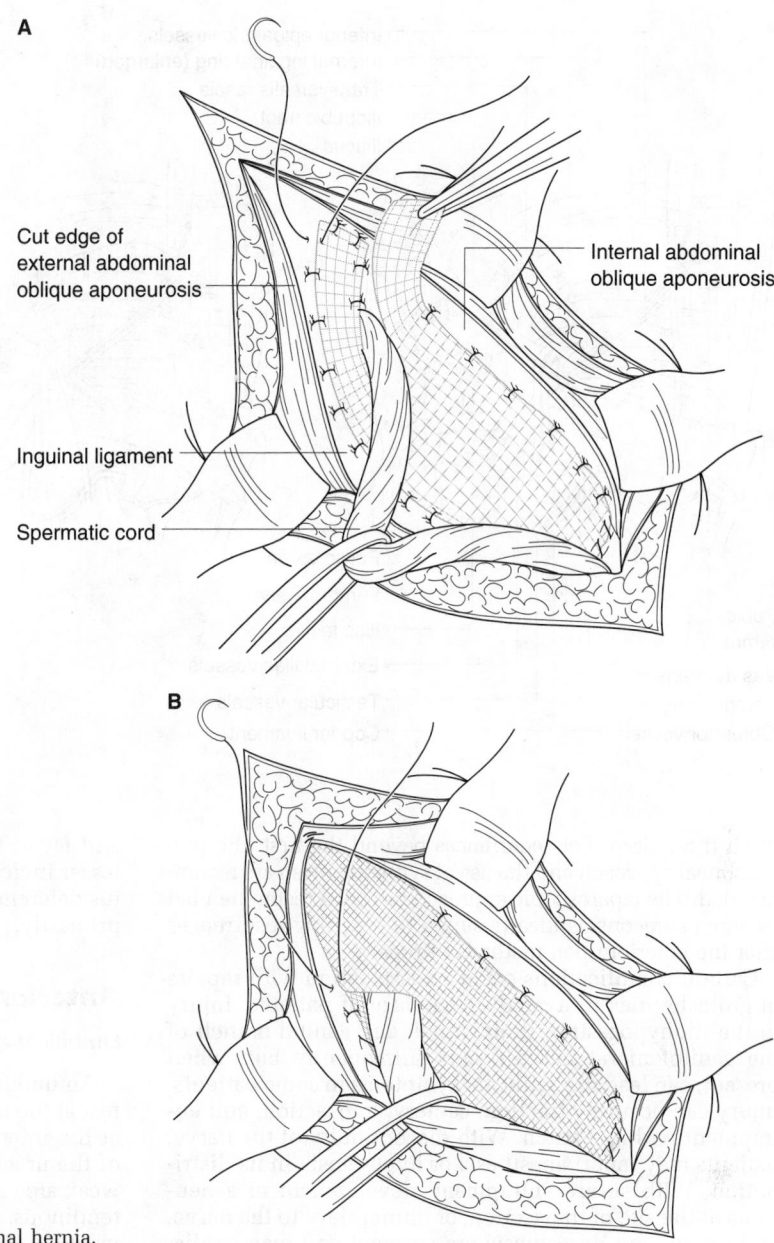

Figure 53-18. Placement of mesh in repair of inguinal hernia.

tightening of the internal ring in addition to excision and closure of the sac, simultaneous bilateral hernia repair does not lead to an increased recurrence rate, such as in the pediatric age group in which bilateral simultaneous inguinal hernia repair is routine. Determination of the need for floor reconstruction in older juveniles and adults can usually be made only at operation, and therefore, repair of bilateral groin hernias is better done with two separate operations separated by 4 to 6 weeks.

The laparoscopic approach to repairing groin hernias has only recently been developed. The most common laparoscopic approach is transabdominal, wherein the peritoneum in the inguinal area is opened, and the repair is performed in the preperitoneum. The second most common method is an entirely preperitoneal approach. After reducing visceral contents out of the hernia, the repair is performed by placing a sheet of prosthetic mesh over the internal aspect of the inguinal floor and internal ring area (Fig 53-19). Several variations in method have been advocated, but no laparoscopic method has the long-term fol-

low up data to show it is equal or superior to the open methods of groin hernia repair.

Repair of recurrent inguinal or, much less commonly, femoral hernia requires judgment based on experience. Some recurrences after direct inguinal hernia repairs are due to indirect inguinal hernias, which presumably were not evident at the time of the initial repair. The most common site of recurrence after inguinal floor reconstruction is medial at the pubic tubercle. The anterior approach to recurrent inguinal or femoral hernia, particularly at the first recurrence, is frequently satisfactory. In many cases, no relaxing incision was made at the initial repair, and, with care, an entirely adequate repair can be performed using one of the techniques discussed above. If a deficit of aponeurotic tissue exists, methods using polypropylene mesh as an overlay, or preferably as an underlay, and tailored around the spermatic cord have proved highly successful. The preperitoneal approach also has many advantages, including avoidance of the inevitable scar encountered with the anterior approach, excellent assessment of the defect, and the ease of placing synthetic

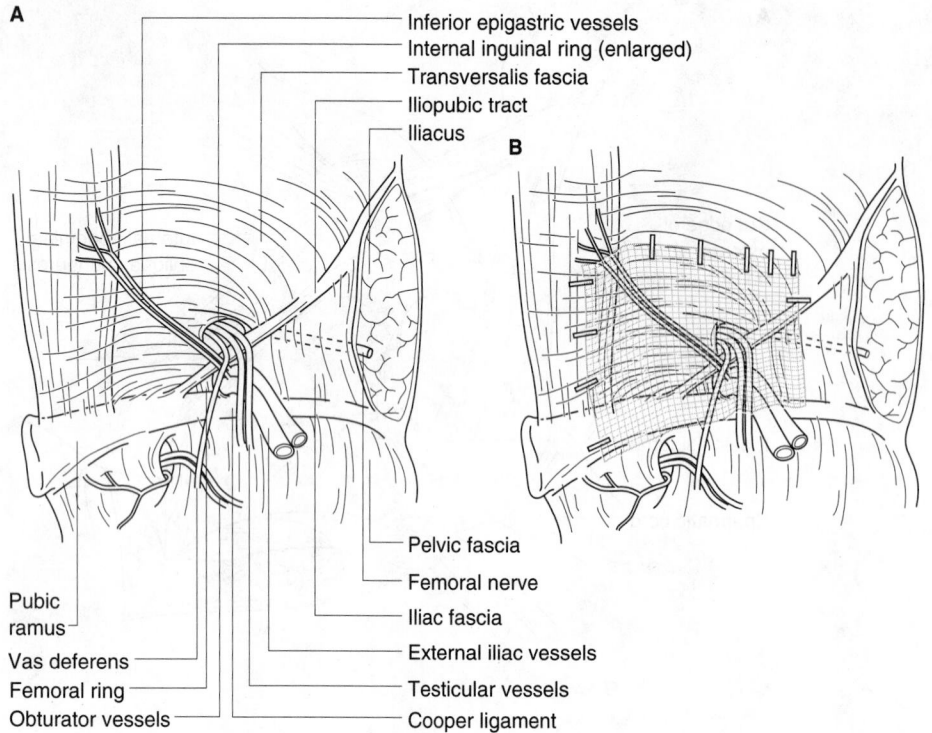

A

- Inferior epigastric vessels
- Internal inguinal ring (enlarged)
- Transversalis fascia
- Iliopubic tract
- Iliacus

B

- Pelvic fascia
- Femoral nerve
- Iliac fascia
- External iliac vessels
- Testicular vessels
- Cooper ligament

Pubic ramus
Vas deferens
Femoral ring
Obturator vessels

Figure 53-19. Placement of mesh internally in the inguinal region in laparoscopic repair of right groin hernia.

mesh if required. For recurrences beyond the first, the preperitoneal approach and the use of synthetic mesh are recommended. The laparoscopic approach has been recommended by some surgeons as ideally suited to repairing recurrences after the anterior open methods of repair.

Certain complications occur in association with repairs of groin hernias in a small percentage of patients. Injury to the iliohypogastric, ilioinguinal, and genital branch of the genitofemoral nerve occurs infrequently but, when present, can lead to significant symptoms in some patients. Injury can occur by traction, cautery, transection, and entrapment within a stitch. With discontinuity of the nerve, patients may report anesthesia or hypesthesia in its distribution. With suture entrapment, development of a neuroma at the site of transection, or blunt injury to the nerve, groin pain, and dysesthesia are frequent and may be disabling in some patients. Carefully dissecting and identifying the nerves during both the dissection and reconstruction stages of the hernia repair are necessary to avoid such injuries. Avoiding these nerves is much more difficult in repairs of recurrent groin hernias. Observed division of a nerve should be treated by ligation. Pain due to nerve entrapment or injury is usually most effectively treated by neurectomy of a portion of the involved nerve or nerves in their course proximal to their distribution in the groin. Appropriate nerve blocks are useful in diagnosis of the specific nerves involved and as an indicator of the utility of a neurectomy.[9] Nerve injuries can occur after laparoscopic hernia repair, most frequently to the lateral femoral cutaneous nerve but also to the ilioinguinal nerve. Most laparoscopic nerve injuries are from staples placed lateral to the gonadal vessels and posterior to the iliopubic tract.

Injury to the testicular artery to the testis during inguinal or femoral herniorrhaphy may occasionally result in ischemic necrosis or atrophy of the testis. Usually, unless there is dissection into the scrotum as with a concomitant hydrocelectomy, the testis can usually survive on collateral circulation. Division of the entire spermatic cord frequently results in postoperative testicular swelling, tenderness,

and fever, but spontaneous resolution is the rule, with a lesser incidence of testicular atrophy. Division of the ductus deferens, unless intentionally done, should be repaired primarily.

Anterior Abdominal Wall Hernias

Umbilical and Paraumbilical Hernias

An umbilical hernia results from an abdominal wall defect at the umbilicus. The round ligament usually attaches at the inferior rim of the umbilicus along with remnants of the urachus and the umbilical arteries, thus creating a weak area in the fascia superiorly. In addition, the lowest tendinous intersection of the rectus abdominis muscle usually inserts into the linea alba at a level just above that of the umbilicus.[2]

Umbilical hernia in children is usually considered to be congenital. About 10% of umbilical hernias in adults are thought to be the result of a congenital defect carried into adulthood. Most adult umbilical hernias are acquired and are called paraumbilical hernias. These typically occur in multiparous females. Other patients with increased intraabdominal pressure, particularly with concomitant chronic abdominal distention as from ascites, are also at increased risk for developing paraumbilical hernia. With vigorous contraction of the rectus muscle at parturition, significant stress is placed on the lowest tendinous intersection. This stress is transmitted to an overstretched linea alba at the superior aspect of the umbilicus, resulting in paraumbilical hernia. Chronic abdominal distention also can weaken the linea alba. Finally, 80% of paraumbilical hernias occur in patients with a single midline aponeurotic decussation (occurring in 30% of the population) as compared with 20% in those with a triple midline aponeurotic decussation[2] (Fig. 53-20). Umbilical and paraumbilical hernias vary from small to extremely large. Incarceration is frequent in the large hernias, which typically have a small neck. An umbilical hernia can be especially danger-

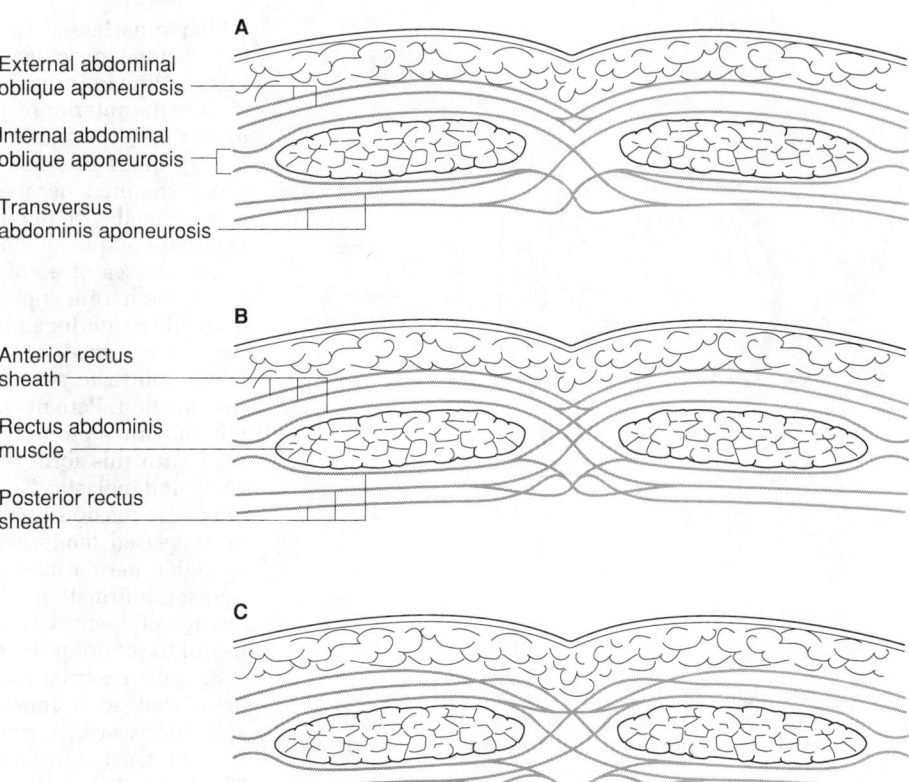

External abdominal
oblique aponeurosis

Internal abdominal
oblique aponeurosis

Transversus
abdominis aponeurosis

Anterior rectus
sheath

Rectus abdominis
muscle

Posterior rectus
sheath

Figure 53-20. Patterns of midline decussation of the aponeuroses. (*A*) Single anterior and single posterior lines of decussation. (*B*) Single anterior and triple posterior lines of decussation. (*C*) Triple anterior and posterior lines of decussation. (After Askar O. Surgical anatomy of the aponeurotic expansions of the anterior abdominal wall. Ann R Coll Surg Engl 1977;59:313)

ous in an elderly patient or in any adult patient with an altered sensorium, since the usual manifestations of strangulation may not be apparent.

Indications for operation in adults include symptoms, incarceration, large hernia relative to the neck, and trophic changes in the overlying skin. Among adults with associated ascites, repair is advocated to avoid potentially serious complications. Discoloration or ulceration of overlying skin or a rapid increase in the size of the hernia heralds impending rupture. Spontaneous rupture of the hernia in these patients can be catastrophic and is frequently associated with mortality rates approaching 30%.[10] By comparison, elective umbilical hernia repair can be performed safely in patients with ascites with acceptable mortality and morbidity.[11]

Most elective umbilical hernia repairs can be performed on an outpatient basis using local, regional, or general anesthesia. The umbilicus should be preserved except in unusual circumstances such as the patient with multiple recurrences. The defect is usually approached using a curved infraumbilical incision. A small hernia sac can be isolated by blunt dissection, using a curved hemostat, and then carefully divided at the fascial level, leaving a remnant of sac attached to the overlying skin. In large hernias, direct entry into the sac facilitates reduction of bowel and identification of the aponeurotic defect. The musculoaponeurotic margin surrounding the hernia defect should be cleared of fat and peritoneum for about 1 cm in all directions to facilitate closure, but injury to the aponeurotic structures should be avoided. The surgeon should palpate the undersurface of the linea alba to check for an unsuspected epigastric hernia.

With approximation of or substitution for aponeurotic structures, the goal is to avoid excess tension. The hernia defect in paraumbilical hernias tends toward the transverse, and defects of 3 cm or less can usually be closed transversely without much tension. Larger defects should use prosthetic mesh to avoid excess tension. Relaxing incisions in the lateral anterior rectus sheath relieve tension poorly at the umbilicus because of the tendinous insertion in the rectus abdominis muscles at this level. Imbrication or overlapping of the fascial edges has been suggested for repairing umbilical and paraumbilical hernia but has no experimental or clinical support and cannot be recommended. These methods only increase the tension at the repair.

Epigastric Hernias

Hernias occurring in the midline of the abdomen are collectively referred to as hernias of the linea alba. Those occurring above the level of the umbilicus are called epigastric hernias. Infraumbilical linea alba hernias are rare. Estimates of prevalence of epigastric hernias range from less than 1% to as high as 5% of the population. Epigastric hernias are two to three times more common in men than in women and usually present in patients 20 to 50 years of age, although cases have been reported in infants.

The cause of epigastric hernias is a combination of stress on the linea alba and a congenital variation in the structure of the linea alba. Nearly all epigastric hernias occur in cases of only a single midline decussation of aponeurotic fibers[2] (see Fig. 53-20). Distention of the abdominal wall, moreover, results in the separation of the decussating aponeurotic fibers in a transversely oriented rhomboid pattern. Vertically oriented aponeurotic fibers extending from the anterior diaphragm to the linea alba midway between xiphoid and umbilicus have also been demonstrated (Fig. 53-21). Vigorous diaphragmatic contraction can thereby exert a disruptive force on the predisposed linea alba to produce an epigastric hernia at this midpoint, which is the most common location.

Epigastric hernias are usually small, but they vary con-

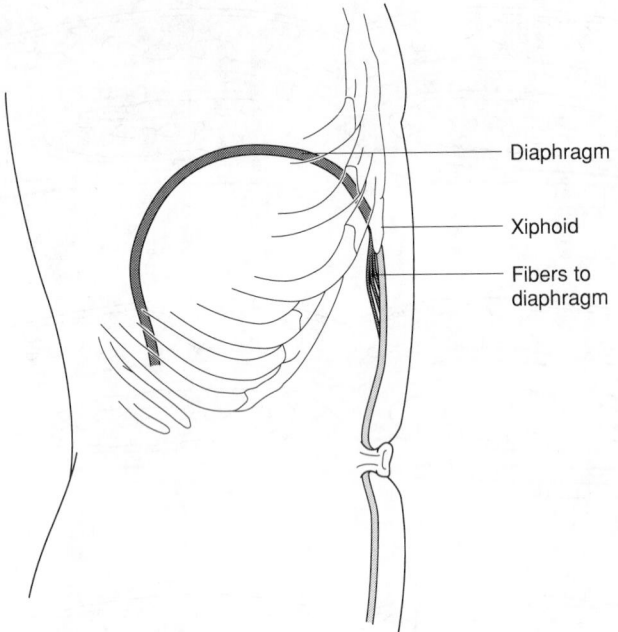

Figure 53-21. Aponeurotic fibers to the midline from the diaphragm. (After Askar O. Surgical anatomy of the aponeurotic expansions of the anterior abdominal wall. Ann R Coll Surg Engl 1977;59:313)

siderably in size. Most of these defects occur in the midline. The small defects contain only preperitoneal fat with no sac. With increasing size, fat in the falciform ligament and eventually a peritoneal sac and abdominal viscera may be contained within the hernia. The preperitoneal fat in small defects is usually incarcerated. Multiple defects may be present in up to 20% of patients.

The diagnosis of an epigastric hernia can usually be made by the presence of a painful midline abdominal mass. In general, small hernia defects are associated with the most pain, with decreasing pain as the defect enlarges. Infrequently, especially in obese individuals, an abdominal wall mass may not be palpable. In such situations, a history of pain exacerbated by exertion and relieved by reclining may help to support the diagnosis. The differential diagnosis includes subcutaneous or fascial abdominal wall tumors.

Congenital epigastric hernias may disappear spontaneously, and expectant therapy is acceptable for patients up to 5 or 6 years old if they are asymptomatic. Surgery is recommended for all adult patients with symptoms or with a hernia defect greater than 1.5 to 2 cm in diameter. Because more than one linea alba defect may be present, exposing the entire linea alba from xiphoid to the umbilicus is recommended. Methods of repair depend on the size of the defects, but anatomic and physiologic principles relating to the midline aponeurosis should be observed. Converting the entire epigastric midline to an incision that is then closed has been recommended. For small defects, simple closure with obliquely placed suture after reduction or removal of preperitoneal fat from the defect has been recommended. Recurrent epigastric hernias in up to 10% of cases have been reported with the latter method, most likely as the result of additional undetected and unrepaired weaknesses in the epigastric midline.

Spigelian Hernias

A spigelian hernia is an unusual abdominal wall defect; fewer than 400 cases have been reported in the world literature.[12] This hernia occurs through the linea semilunaris, which runs lateral to the rectus abdominis muscle and between the muscular fibers of the internal oblique muscle and the line of insertion of the external oblique aponeurosis into the anterior rectus sheath. Spigelian hernias almost exclusively occur inferior to the linea semicircularis (Fig. 53-22). Such a hernia in the suprapubic area would be a direct inguinal hernia. This hernia is almost uniformly interparietal with the hernia sac dissecting posterior to the external oblique aponeurosis (Fig. 53-23).

The causes of a spigelian hernia are unclear. In most cases, the hernia appears to be acquired and is associated with other anterior abdominal wall hernias. Most spigelian hernias are small (1 to 2 cm in diameter) and develop in the fourth to seventh decades of life. There is no sex predilection. Patients usually present with localized pain without much prominence of a bulge. Incarceration is common with this form of hernia because the fascial ring is small and inelastic. The pain is generally exacerbated with muscular tension in the abdominal wall, and there may be increased tenderness during Valsalva. Palpation of a spigelian hernia may be difficult, especially in obese patients. Confirmation of the diagnosis is frequently difficult outside of operative exploration. Ultrasound or CT can be useful to pinpoint the fascial defect and herniating tissue.

Spigelian hernias should be repaired because of the risks associated with incarceration. The operative repair is straightforward. A transverse incision over the bulge or defect is carried through the external oblique aponeurosis. The sac, when present, is opened and dissected to the neck of the hernia, abdominal contents are returned to the abdominal cavity, and the sac is excised at its neck. If necessary for reduction of contents, the rectus sheath can be opened and the rectus muscle retracted medially. Care should be exercised for the inferior epigastric vessels that lie inferomedially. Preperitoneal fat is removed from the defect, which is then closed transversely by simple suture closure of the transversus abdominis and internal oblique muscles (Fig. 53-24). Recurrence is rare, but multiple defects may be present at the time of initial repair.

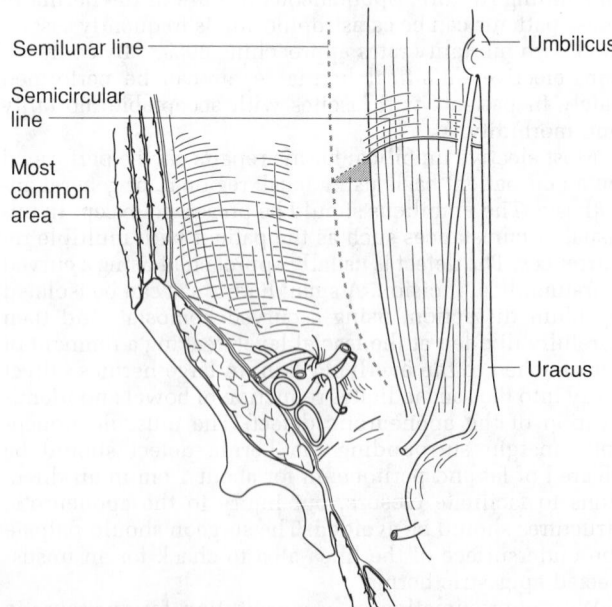

Figure 53-22. The posterior aspect of the anterior abdominal wall indicating the semilunar (spigelian) line and the most common site of spigelian hernia.

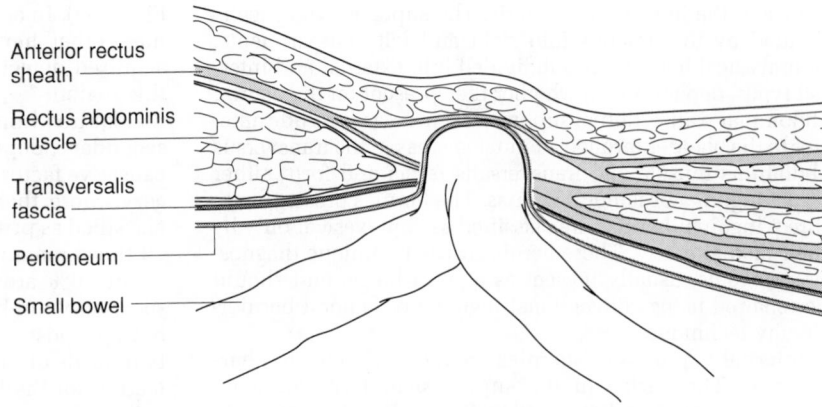

Figure 53-23. Schematic cross section of a spigelian hernia.

Interparietal Hernias

Interparietal or interstitial hernias are rare abdominal wall defects in which the hernia sac lies between layers of the abdominal wall. Fewer than 600 cases of primary interparietal hernia have been reported in the world literature. These hernias include the preperitoneal hernia, a term that refers to an internal hernia in which the sac lies between the peritoneum and the transversalis fascia, and those hernias in which a portion or the entirety of the herniated structures are loculated between layers of the fasciomusculoaponeurotic portion of the abdominal wall. Spontaneous interparietal hernias occur almost exclusively in the inguinal region and are much more common in males. Interparietal hernias are predominantly right-sided, and nearly 70% occur in patients with an ectopic or maldescended testicle.[12] Congenital factors as well as mechanical factors are invoked in the causes of these hernias.

A correct preoperative diagnosis of interparietal hernia is rarely made. Most patients with complicated interparietal hernias present with bowel obstruction. The presence of a tender mass above and lateral to the internal inguinal ring may provide a clue to the diagnosis. The finding of a maldescended testicle may help to establish the diagnosis.

Because the presentation is usually bowel obstruction, most of these hernias are discovered from within the abdominal cavity. If a preperitoneal hernia is encountered, the neck should be divided and ligated after reducing the sac contents into the abdomen.

An interparietal hernia sac should be managed in a similar fashion, but the internal inguinal ring should be treated as an indirect inguinal hernia. If a maldescended testicle is encountered, particularly in an adult, it should be removed and the internal inguinal ring should be closed. The area should be carefully inspected to rule out the presence of an associated inguinal or femoral hernia. If encountered, these defects can be managed at the same time using conventional preperitoneal repair techniques.

Supravesical Hernias

Supravesical hernias are uncommon abdominal wall hernias that are rarely encountered in clinical practice. The classification of these hernias can be confusing, but the common starting point is the supravesical space. This space is bounded inferiorly by the transverse fold of the urinary bladder, laterally by the umbilical ligaments (obliterated umbilical arteries), and superiorly by a gradual fusion of the vesical fascia with transversalis fascia somewhere between the umbi-

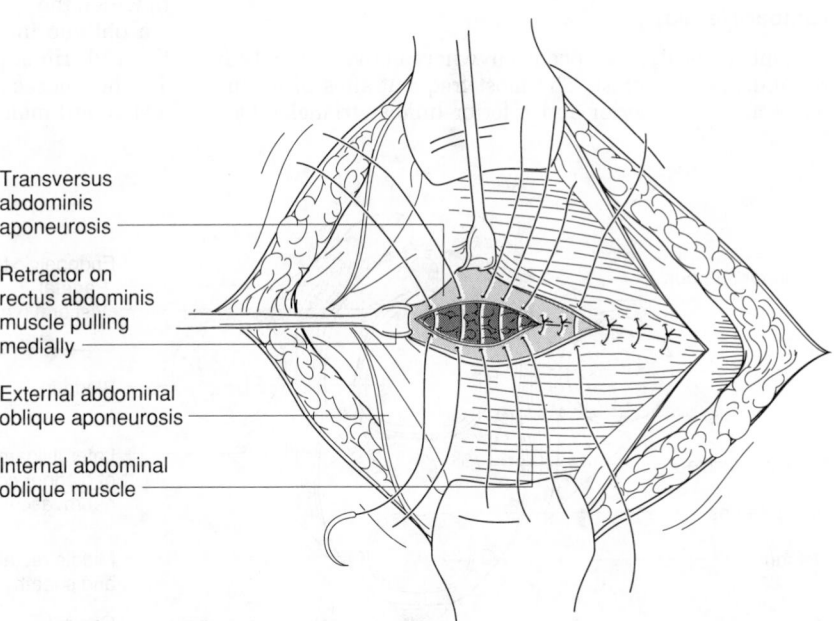

Figure 53-24. Repair of a spigelian hernia.

licus and the linea semicircularis. The supravesical space is divided by the urachus into right and left compartments. Supravesical hernias are subdivided into external and internal types, depending on whether they present on the ventral abdominal wall. External supravesical hernias protrude anterior to the bladder through attenuated areas in the transversus abdominis muscle and transversalis fascia and form either direct inguinal or femoral hernias. The hernias presenting as direct inguinal hernias are classified as supravesical only by their medial defect. These hernias cause no unique diagnostic problems, usually present as a groin bulge, and should be repaired using conventional inguinal or femoral herniorrhaphy techniques.

Internal supravesical hernias are more difficult to characterize. They arise in the supravesical fossa and, according to a system developed by Skandalakis and coworkers,[13] are classified by whether they course in front of, beside, or behind the bladder. Figure 53-25 illustrates the anatomic landmarks used to characterize the various spaces around the bladder. To understand the possible pathways of the various internal supravesical hernias, one must have a thorough knowledge of the retropubic and retrovesical spaces in both males and females. The most common type is the anterior retropubic hernia in the space of Retzius.[14]

Internal supravesical hernias are extremely rare, and fewer than 70 cases have been reported in the world literature. These hernias are more common in men, and most cases present later in life. Internal supravesical hernias are thought to be developmental defects in the lower abdominal fasciae that become exaggerated with aging or with factors that chronically increase intraabdominal pressure. Bowel symptoms predominate, but urinary tract complaints are present in up to 30% of patients. In many patients, symptoms are vague and nonspecific. There is no place for expectant treatment of these patients because of the risk of bowel strangulation. A transperitoneal approach through a lower midline incision is recommended. Once the diagnosis has been correctly established, the hernia can usually be reduced without difficulty. Nonviable intestine may be encountered in up to 15% of patients, necessitating bowel resection. The neck of the sac should be divided and closed to prevent possible hernia recurrence.

Lumbar and Pelvic Hernias

Lumbar Hernias

Lumbar hernias can occur anywhere between the 12th rib and the iliac crest. The most frequent sites of occurrence are the superior and inferior lumbar triangles (see Fig. 53-3). In addition to superior and inferior lumbar hernias, other herniations can occur through congenital or acquired defects in the musculoaponeurotic structures in this region.

Acquired lumbar hernias may be classified as primary or secondary, depending on whether there is an identifiable causative factor, such as infection, trauma, or previous surgery. More than half of the reported lumbar hernias are classified as primary (spontaneous or acquired atraumatic). Of those remaining, 25% are secondary or traumatic, and about 20% are congenital.[15] It is likely that many more secondary lumbar hernias occur but go unreported or have been purposely excluded from the reported series. Roughly two thirds of lumbar hernias occur in males, with a predilection for the left side.

Symptoms vary from a vague sense of discomfort associated with appreciation of a bulge in the lumbar area to severe, localized pain and a tender nodule that may be attributable to herniation of retroperitoneal fat through a lumbofascial defect with subsequent incarceration. The presence of a mass in the lumbar region is usually sufficient to establish the diagnosis. Incarceration should be suspected in any patient with a nonreducible mass or signs of bowel obstruction. Strangulation occurs in about 10% of cases and seems to be more common in patients with primary or atraumatic forms of lumbar hernia. The differential diagnosis of a mass occurring in the lumbar region includes lumbar hernia, abscess, hematoma, benign or malignant soft tissue tumors of fatty, connective tissue or muscle origin, solid and cystic renal tumors including hydronephrosis, and panniculitis associated with other rheumatoid manifestations. An appropriate systems review combined with radiologic studies such as intravenous pyelography, ultrasound, or CT helps to establish a correct diagnosis in most cases.

The natural history of lumbar hernias is gradual progression in size. Larger hernias are far more difficult to repair than smaller defects. Therefore, most authorities recommend that all lumbar hernias should be repaired unless the patient is a prohibitive operative risk. Weight reduction should be encouraged in all patients with large hernias before operation.

Optimal exposure of any lumbar hernia defect is best achieved by placing the patient in a lateral decubitus position on the operating table with the kidney rest elevated to widen the space between the 12th rib and the iliac crest. An oblique incision is used extending from the level of the 12th rib superiorly to the iliac crest anteroinferiorly. The hernia sac and contents are dissected and handled in a standard manner. Reconstruction of the hernia defect is

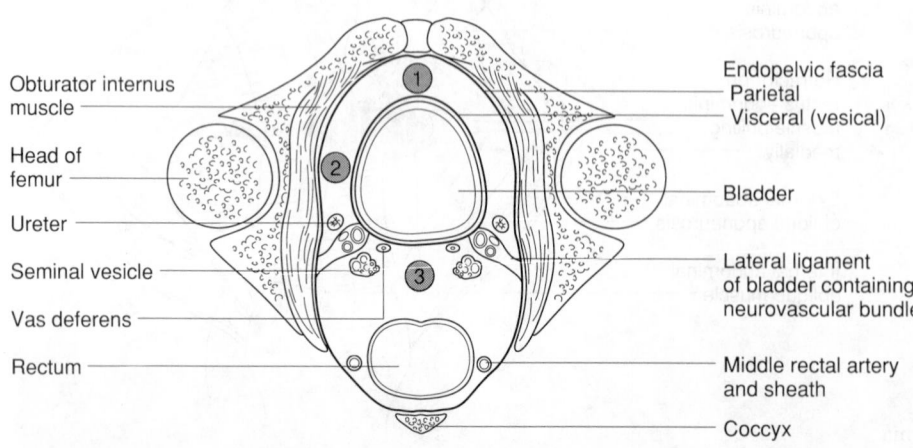

Obturator internus muscle
Head of femur
Ureter
Seminal vesicle
Vas deferens
Rectum

Endopelvic fascia
— Parietal
— Visceral (vesical)
Bladder
Lateral ligament of bladder containing neurovascular bundle
Middle rectal artery and sheath
Coccyx

Figure 53-25. Anatomic relations in supravesical hernia. (1) Site of anterior internal supravescial hernia. (2) Site of lateral internal supravesical hernia. (3) Site of posterior internal supravesical hernia.

the challenging aspect of the operation. The many techniques include using autologous tissue or prosthetic materials. One technique for repairing lower lumbar hernias includes a layered closure of the hernia defect using multiple layers and flaps from adjacent musculoaponeurotic structures (Fig. 53-26). Other more complicated procedures require the use of flaps or autologous graft. Because of the paucity of these hernias, no procedure has achieved a clear precedence by virtue of its successes. Large lumbar defects are the more troublesome but can usually be managed successfully with grafts of prosthetic material.

Obturator Hernias

An obturator hernia is a hernia that occurs through the obturator canal, accompanied by the obturator vessels and the obturator nerve. The vessels lie lateral to the sac in about half the cases. This hernia is an anterior pelvic hernia. It occurs rarely, although somewhat more frequently than sciatic or perineal hernia. Most obturator hernias occur in older women and are predominantly right-sided.

Obturator hernias are acquired lesions that are thought to result from progressive laxity of the pelvic floor associated with multiparity and increasing age. Obturator hernias begin with protrusion of preperitoneal fat into the pelvic orifice of the obturator canal. With progression, a sac of peritoneum begins to invaginate into the obturator canal. The final stage is associated with herniation of an organ, usually ileum, through the canal. Usually the herniated loop of intestine reduces spontaneously and symptoms tend to be intermittent. Repeated herniation leads to scarring and eventual incarceration with possible strangulation.

Symptoms are frequently intermittent but tend to be acute and become increasingly severe with incarceration of the hernia. Intestinal symptoms predominate, but dysesthesia or pain in the medial thigh with occasional radiation to the hip joint is often present. Dysesthesia results from compression of either division of the obturator nerve. Relief of the pain on flexion of the thigh and exacerbation on extension, adduction, or medial rotation are characteristic. Although the hernia is never externally visible, in a small

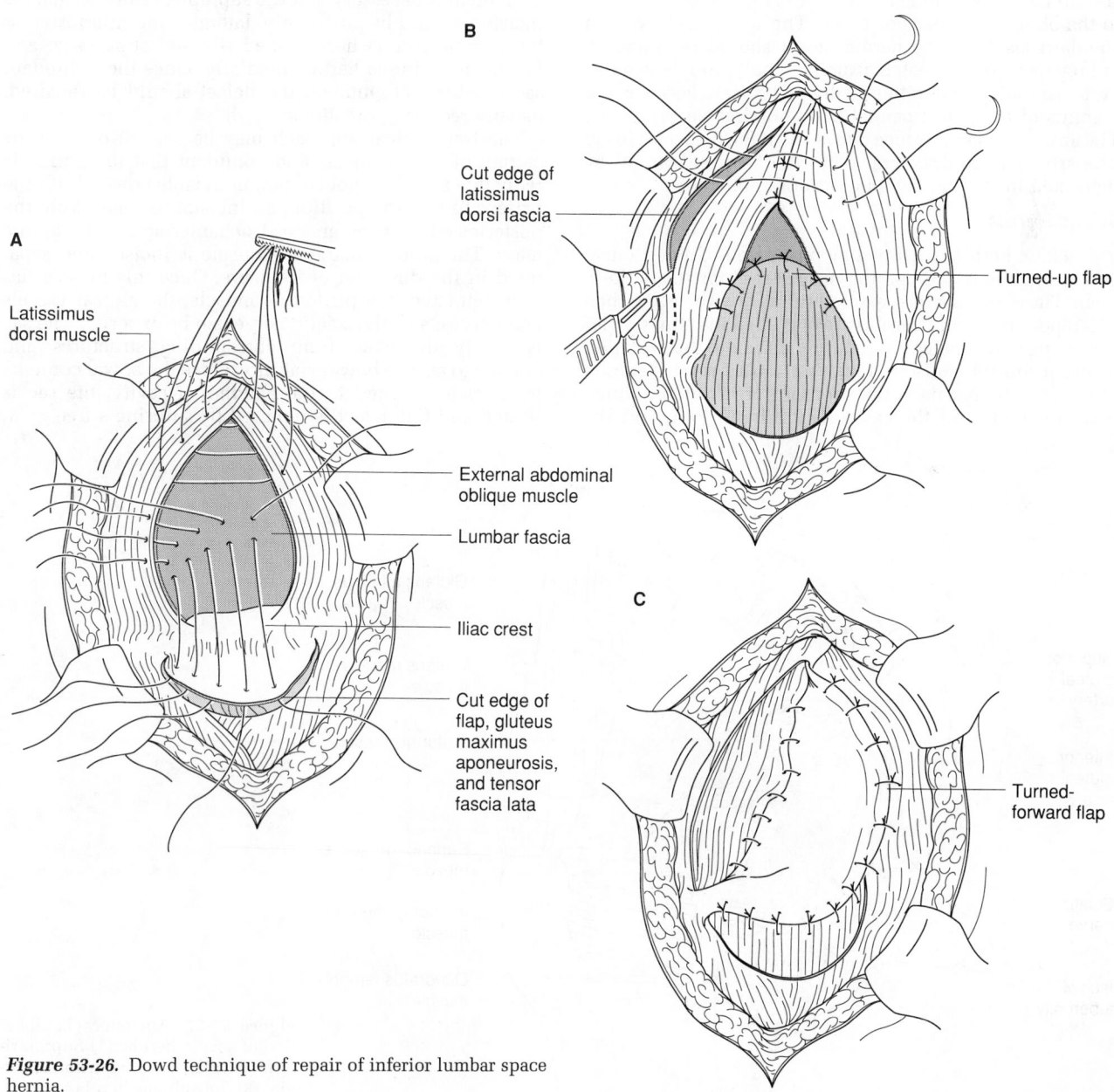

Figure 53-26. Dowd technique of repair of inferior lumbar space hernia.

percentage of patients, a mass can be palpated in the upper, medial thigh. This can best be appreciated with the thigh flexed, externally rotated, and abducted. The mass or defect can be palpated on vaginal examination.

A correct preoperative diagnosis of an obturator hernia is made in about one third of patients presenting with intestinal obstruction. Plain radiography is rarely helpful except to show evidence of partial or complete bowel obstruction. When in doubt, the diagnosis of an obturator hernia can usually be confirmed with either ultrasound or CT.

Treatment is operative. There is no place for expectant therapy, especially in a patient with pain and paresthesias along the inner aspect of the thigh or with clinical or radiographic evidence of bowel obstruction. Many surgical approaches have been promoted, but the transabdominal approach should be used because it has several advantages. It best confirms the diagnosis and exposes the obturator canal orifice, vessels, and nerve, also permitting bowel resection when required. Adhesions of contents within the hernia are uncommon, and the hernia can usually be reduced with gentle traction. If the hernia defect needs to be widened to reduce the contents, the obturator membrane should be incised along its inferior margin to avoid injury to the obturator vessels or nerve. The sac is dealt with in standard fashion. The hernia defect should be repaired, but repair requires a patch, usually of polypropylene mesh or expanded polytetrafluoroethylene sheet, because the margins of the defect cannot be approximated primarily. The anticipated recurrence rate is low if the defect is closed properly. The contralateral obturator foramen should be inspected to ensure that a defect does not exist.

Sciatic Hernias

A sciatic hernia is defined by protrusion of a peritoneal sac and contents through the major or minor sciatic foramen. These hernias are extremely rare, with fewer than 100 reported. Sciatic hernias are classified into three types according to where they exit the pelvis and to their relation to the piriformis muscle (Fig. 53-27). The most common type of sciatic hernia is the suprapiriform variant, which constitutes 60% of the cases. The infrapiriform and the

subspinous (lesser sciatic) variants occur in 30% and 10% of cases, respectively.[16]

Symptoms of a sciatic hernia are variable. Many patients present with an uncomfortable or slowly enlarging mass in the gluteal or infragluteal area. Occasionally, bowel sounds can be auscultated over the mass, indicating the presence of bowel in the hernia sac. Obstructive symptoms may predominate if bowel becomes incarcerated. Classic sciatica may occur. Sciatic nerve involvement is usually due to compression and may present as either motor or sensory dysfunction. Ureteral obstruction may also occur because of its inclusion with the herniated tissues. When the clinical diagnosis is in doubt, ultrasound or CT may be useful

The treatment of sciatic hernia is surgical. Transperitoneal and transgluteal approaches have been described. Occasionally, a combined approach is required. The transperitoneal approach is preferred if bowel obstruction or strangulation is suspected. The hernia contents can usually be reduced with gentle traction. If enlargement of the hernia neck becomes necessary to reduce the contents, care must be taken to avoid injuring the adjacent vessels and nerve. Visualization of these structures and incision away from them is necessary. For the suprapiriformis hernia, the incision should be posteriorly, laterally and inferiorly; for the infrapiriformis hernia, medially and superiorly; and for the subspinous hernia, medially. Once the redundant sac has been amputated, the defect should be repaired, usually requiring prosthetic mesh.

The transgluteal approach may be used if one can be certain of the diagnosis and confident that the hernia is reducible and does not contain nonviable bowel. With the patient in a prone position, an incision is made from the posterior edge of the greater trochanter across the hernia mass. The gluteus maximus muscle is incised and separated in the direction of its fibers. Once this muscle has been retracted, the piriformis muscle, the gluteal vessels and nerves, and the sciatic nerve can be exposed. The sac is gently dissected from surrounding structures and opened to ensure bowel viability. Once the bowel contents have been returned to the abdominal cavity, the sac is ligated and the defect is repaired by suturing a free graft,

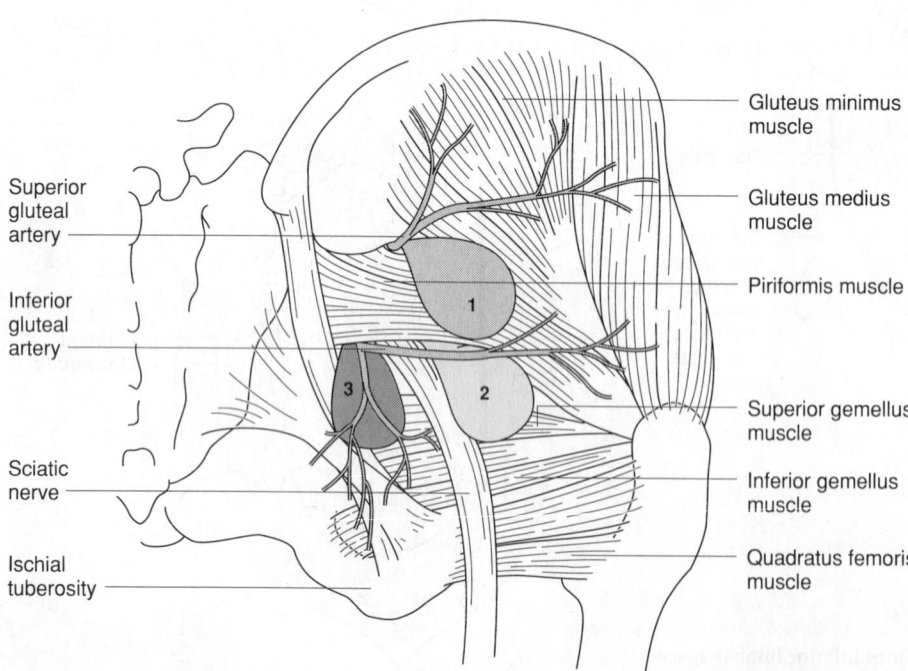

Figure 53-27. Anatomic classification of sciatic hernia. (1) Suprapiriform hernia. (2) Infrapiriform hernia. (3) Subspinous hernia.

usually prosthetic mesh, to close the particular defect (Fig. 53-28). Alternatively, autologous fascia or prosthetic mesh can be used to close the defect between the piriformis muscle and the iliac or ischial bone.

Perineal Hernias

A perineal hernia is a protrusion of tissues through the muscles and fasciae of the pelvic diaphragm. These hernias are categorized as primary, having no discernible cause, or as secondary, occurring after trauma or surgery to the pelvic floor. Primary perineal hernias are rare, with about 100 cases reported. They are more common in older, multiparous women. The cause of primary perineal hernia is thought to be related to progressive attenuation of the pelvic floor associated with multiple pregnancies.

Perineal hernias can occur through multiple sites in the pelvic diaphragm. Anterior and posterior perineal hernias are distinguished by their location relative to the transverse perineal muscles (Fig. 53-29). Anterior hernias occur only in females and are classified as labial, pudendal, or vaginolabial depending on their site of presentation. Posterior hernias may protrude directly through the pelvic floor and present between the rectum and the ischial tuberosity. They are more frequent in females.

Symptoms are usually related to protrusion of a perineal mass that makes it difficult for the patient to sit down. Bowel symptoms may supervene if colon or small intestine becomes incarcerated in the hernia defect. The diagnosis can usually be established by the history of a recurring or persistent bulge in the perineum and confirmed by physical examination. Bimanual rectal or vaginal examination may help to clarify the diagnosis. In addition to perineal hernia, the differential diagnosis of a perineal mass includes abscess, soft tissue tumors such as lipomas or fibromas, rectal prolapse, rectoceles and cystoceles, and vaginal polyps.

The treatment of perineal hernia is surgical repair. The transabdominal approach is preferred because a better closure can be performed and because the viability of any incarcerated bowel can be assessed. The patient is placed in the Trendelenburg position to elevate the bowel from the pelvis. Once identified, the sac contents are withdrawn into the abdomen and the sac itself is everted and amputated at the fascial level. If the fascial defect is small, direct closure with nonabsorbable suture may be sufficient. If the opening is patulous, prosthetic mesh should be used to close the defect.

Internal Hernias

Internal hernias are defects in peritoneum through which bowel and occasionally other viscera pass. In contrast to the abdominal wall hernia, no musculoaponeurotic defects are involved in these hernias. In the case of trans-

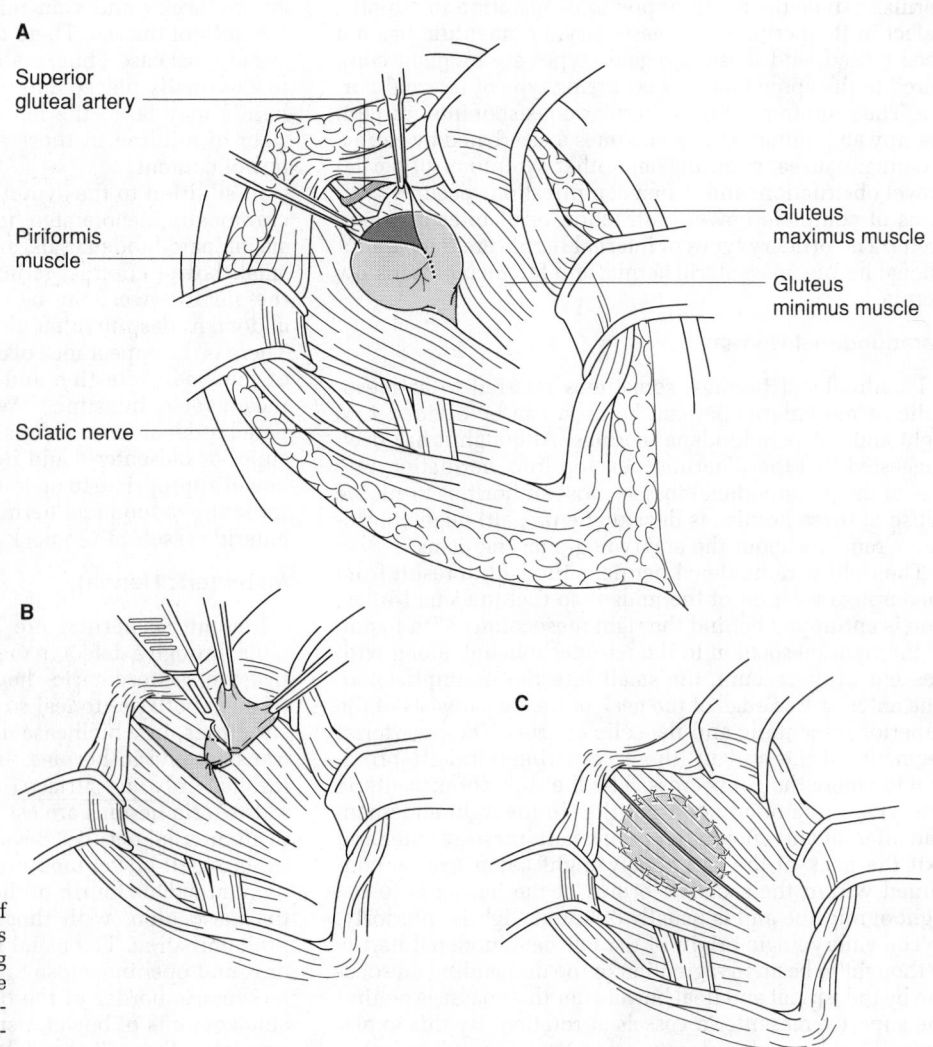

Figure 53-28. Transgluteal repair of sciatic hernia. (*A*) Gluteus maximus separated; sac opened; and ring around neck of sac incised to reduce contents. (*B*) Neck of sac ligated; excess sac excised. (*C*) Mesh prosthesis used to close defect.

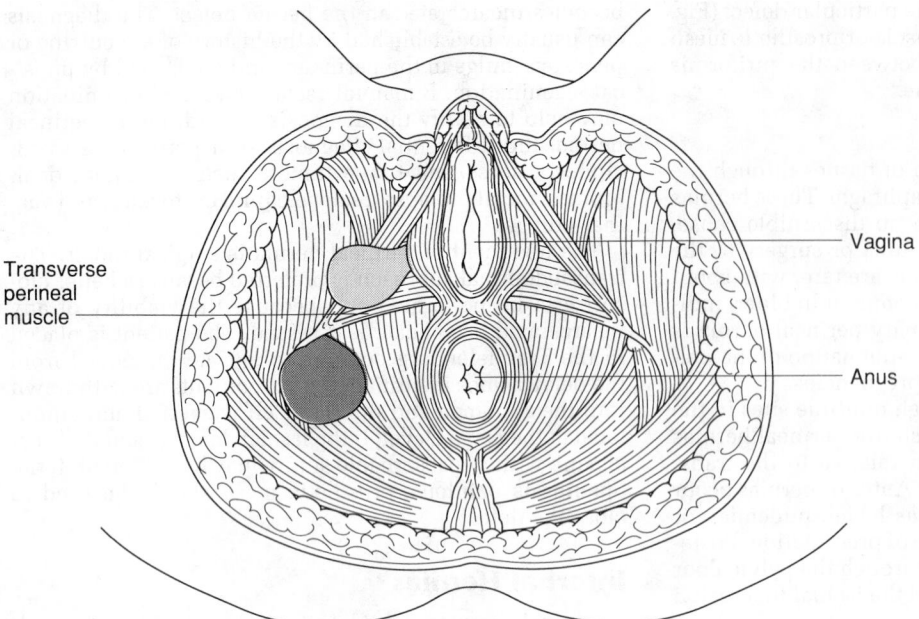

Figure 53-29. Perineal hernia. Transverse perineal muscles distinguish anterior from posterior perineal hernias.

mesenteric hernias, the designation false hernia is sometimes applied, since no peritoneal sac is present. Internal hernias can be the result of previous operation in which a defect in the peritoneum, mesentery, or omentum has not been closed, and these iatrogenic types are frequent compared to the spontaneously occurring type of internal hernia. The symptoms of these hernias consist of intermittent, crampy abdominal pain, sometimes exacerbated by eating; bloating; nausea, vomiting, and other symptoms of partial bowel obstruction; and, when complications occur, symptoms of complete bowel obstruction or of intestinal gangrene. The primary types of internal hernia are the paraduodenal hernia, mesenteric hernia, and foramen of Winslow hernia.

Paraduodenal Hernias

Paraduodenal hernias, sometimes referred to as mesocolic or mesentericoparietal hernias, can be divided into right and left paraduodenal hernias. Although it has been suggested that these hernias develop from herniation into one of the paraduodenal fossae, most authorities think the cause of these hernias is developmental, although controversy remains about the embryologic mechanisms.

The right paraduodenal hernia is thought to result from incomplete rotation of the midgut so that the small intestine is entrapped behind the right mesocolon. With fusion of the right mesocolon to the retroperitoneum, along with descent of the cecum, the small intestine is imprisoned. The anterior free edge of the neck of the sac consists of the superior mesenteric and ileocolic arteries. The prearterial segments of the midgut (those occurring normally proximal to where the gut is crossed by the superior mesenteric artery) are in a nonrotated position in the right abdomen, and afferent and efferent loops of small intestine enter and exit the neck of the sac. Rarely, right colon can be contained within the sac. The orifice of the hernia is to the right of midline and is usually oriented slightly inferiorly.

The embryologic origin of the left paraduodenal hernia is thought to be an invagination of the descending mesocolon by the jejunal and ileal bowel after their passage behind the superior mesenteric vessels at rotation. By this explanation, the vascular structures of the descending colon resist invagination and, after fusion of the descending mesocolon over the entrapped small bowel, the inferior mesenteric artery and vein remain as the anterior margin of the neck of the sac. There is no intestine seen entering the sac in most cases, but small bowel exits the sac to progress to a normally placed and rotated cecum. The orifice of the hernia may be to the left of midline or displaced to the right of midline in those hernias with larger amounts of bowel content.

In addition to the symptoms common to many types of chronically incarcerated hernias, the preoperative diagnosis of paraduodenal hernia can be suspected based on small bowel contrast radiography, in which a portion of the small bowel may be confined within an area of the abdomen despite alterations in the patient's position. There is the appearance of a constant clumping of a portion of the small intestine and a delay in transit through the incarcerated intestine.[17] With any approach to the right paraduodenal hernia, considerations include avoiding the superior mesenteric and ileocolic vessels and placing the bowel appropriate to operations for malrotation. Similarly, for left paraduodenal hernia, attention to the inferior mesenteric vessels at the neck of the sac must be maintained.

Mesenteric Hernias

Mesenteric hernias are protrusions of peritoneal contents through a defect in the mesentery, omentum, or broad ligament. Mesenteric hernias occur more commonly through both peritoneal surfaces of one of these sheet-like structures, in which case no sac exists and they are called transmesenteric hernias. In addition, they may herniate through only one surface (intramesenteric) and have a sac. Mesenteric hernias are estimated to constitute about 10% of all internal hernias. Seventy percent of the defects occur in the small bowel mesentery, mainly in that of the terminal ileum. One fourth of the defects have been reported in the mesocolon, with those in the transverse mesocolon predominating. The usual finding is a 2-cm diameter oval or round opening, close to but not directly adjacent to the mesenteric border of the bowel, with firm margins. Variable amounts of bowel, usually small intestine, are found herniated through the defect at operation. These defects have been found in all age groups, with no sex predilection. Repair requires reduction of bowel and closure of the defect.

Foramen of Winslow Hernias

Hernia through the foramen of Winslow is rare, with fewer than 200 cases reported. In more than half of these, the cecum is involved as a portion or the whole of the herniated viscera. In such cases, the cecum is untethered in the right lower quadrant. Ascending colon and terminal ileum may accompany the cecum through the foramen of Winslow. The classic presentation includes epigastric pain eased by flexion of the trunk, a tympanitic epigastric mass, and no previous abdominal surgery. Abdominal radiography frequently reveals a collection of gas or feces in the epigastrium with the stomach displaced anteriorly and to the left. Reduction of the herniated bowel may require approach through the gastrocolic ligament into the lesser space, occasionally requiring colotomy or enterotomy to decompress the bowel first. In the case of the mobile cecum, cecopexy is recommended. Closure of the foramen can be accomplished with a small reflected flap of peritoneum, but the need for such a closure is unknown.

Incisional Hernias

Repairing an incisional hernia can be difficult. Incisional hernias can be small (less than 1 cm) or large, with nearly the entire abdominal contents contained within the hernia. Several factors make these hernias particularly challenging. First, incisional hernias are often related to a postoperative wound infection, in which case associated fasciitis or muscle necrosis may have resulted in loss of tissue. Second, a previous abdominal wall closure under tension or with a technique that resulted in tension on particular sutures may have led to a multifenestrated region of the musculoaponeurotic abdominal wall near or slightly back from its margin (Fig. 53-30). Third, chronic retraction of the abdominal muscle results in a larger defect. Fourth, a

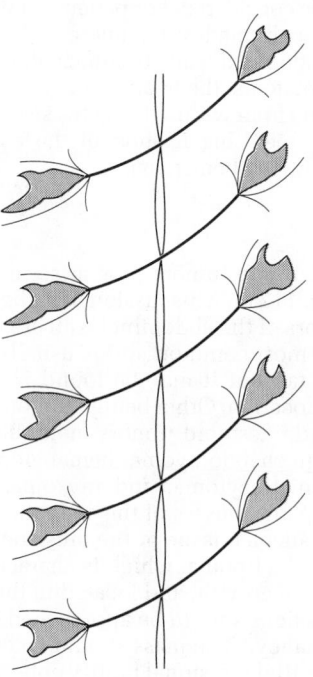

Figure 53-30. Buttonhole defects occurring at sites of suturing of the abdominal wall.

large potential space remains anterior to the abdominal wall closure; postoperative fluid accumulation in this space contributes to the wound infection rate of about 5%. Also, extensive adhesions are often associated with incarcerated herniated bowel in the larger hernias. During lysis of adhesions, the bowel is sometimes entered, increasing the risk of wound infection. Finally, in patients in whom a significant portion of the abdominal contents lie within the hernia, returning the contents to the abdominal cavity can result in respiratory embarrassment by forcible elevation of the diaphragms and cardiovascular problems by limiting venous return through compression of the inferior vena cava.

A high recurrence rate accompanies repair of incisional hernias. Three factors are responsible for most recurrences: (1) wound infection; (2) insufficient dissection and exposure of the true musculoaponeurotic edge and failure to exclude adjacent musculoaponeurotic defects; and (3) closure under excess tension. Elements contributing to infection were discussed earlier in this chapter. The other two factors contributing to recurrence are predominantly technical and largely avoidable. Adequate dissection of the margins, clearing of peritoneum and fat overlying the musculoaponeurotic edges, and identification of buttonhole defects formed from previous suture closure are required to achieve direct apposition and continuity of musculoaponeurotic structures.

Tension at the repair should be avoided. Simple primary closure of incisional hernias larger than 3 to 4 cm in least diameter is likely to result in recurrence because of the excess tension. The use of relaxing incisions decreases tension and may be particularly useful in midline hernias, in which the relaxing incision is made parallel to the midline in the lateral portion of the anterior rectus sheath. Although an increased subcutaneous space is created by the prefascial dissection needed to make the relaxing incision, a primary musculoaponeurotic closure can be achieved, avoiding the use of prosthetic mesh. Closure of the defect with a musculoaponeurotic flap also avoids the use of prosthetic mesh but is a rarely used technique.

Prosthetic materials are frequently needed to close large incisional hernias (see the earlier discussion of graft materials). Unless the risk of inoculation of organisms is low, permanent graft materials should be avoided. Infected permanent graft infrequently heals completely. More often, persistent sinus tracts, intermittent subcutaneous infections, and occasionally, enterocutaneous or colocutaneous fistulas result from infected graft. For open or infected wounds, polyglycolic acid mesh is recommended when there is risk of evisceration. Granulation tissue forms well over this mesh, allowing skin grafting, and the mesh itself resorbs beginning at about 3 weeks, leaving no permanent foreign body as a persistent locus of infection. For open or infected wounds without risk of evisceration, split-thickness skin graft on clean or granulating tissue achieves closure. Over weeks to months, an areolar tissue plane develops between bowel and the skin. Once complete skin closure is achieved and the loosening of the skin over the bowel occurs, reoperation can be performed using primary repair or placement of permanent prosthetic material, as indicated.

ABDOMINAL WALL

The abdominal wall is a lattice of criss-crossing muscles. This supports, confines, and protects the abdominal visceral contents. The abdominal wall permits variation in intraabdominal pressure for defecation, micturition, vomiting, and coughing. It assists in respiration as accessory musculature, allows erect posture by serving as a muscular counter to the paraspinous muscles, and allows lateral and forward bending. The anatomy of the abdominal wall is unique in that the greater part of most of the muscles insert only into an aponeurosis or tendon that is not attached to bone or cartilage.

The directions of the muscles, the areas of overlap and lack of overlap, and the functions of the aponeuroses and tendons are important in understanding incisions, formation and repair of hernias, as well as reconstruction of the abdominal wall after trauma or tumor excision. Three sets of lateral muscles arise from the ribs, spine, and pelvic skeleton, each oriented at an angle to the next. These insert into broad central aponeuroses, which insert into the midline tendon (linea alba). The combined force vector of the lateral musculature is in a lateral direction. The aponeuroses of the lateral muscles ensheathe the vertically oriented rectus abdominis muscles, which arise on the ribs superiorly and on the pubis inferiorly, and insert into one to four transversely oriented tendinous bands variably spaced along the length of the muscle. These tendinous bands are fused to the anterior but not to the posterior rectus sheath.

The blood supply, venous drainage, lymphatic drainage, and innervation of the abdominal wall principally run obliquely downward from posterior to anterior, essentially extensions of the intercostal blood and lymphatic vessels and nerves onto the abdominal wall. Several centimeters of decussation occur across the midline for these supporting elements. The superior epigastric and inferior epigastric arteries and veins form an anastomosing vascular supply and drainage coursing vertically within the rectus abdominis muscle. Nonmidline incisions that do not run parallel to the nerves necessarily sever them. The result is a loss in skin sensation and motor innervation to abdominal musculature, which may cause muscular atrophy. Maintaining arterial supply to the abdominal wall requires care, particularly to avoid multiple incisions not running parallel to the course of the arteries.

Rectus Sheath Hematomas

Rectus sheath hematoma results from arterial or venous bleeding into the rectus sheath, most commonly from arterial bleeding. The rectus sheath superior to the semicircular line (4 to 6 cm below the level of the umbilicus) is essentially a flattened tube with nondistensible walls. Dissection of blood along the length of the sheath is limited anteriorly by the tendinous insertions of the rectus muscle into the sheath. Bleeding into the sheath occurs only when intravascular pressure exceeds intrasheath pressure. In the upper sheath, only arterial bleeding continues to the point of symptomatic distention of the rectus sheath. The resulting hematoma continues to cause symptoms by exerting pressure on the sheath and only slowly resolves, sometimes with resultant rebleeding. Most reported rectus sheath hematomas occur in the lower abdomen.[18] Below the semicircular line, the posterior aspect of the rectus is enclosed only by a thin layer of muscular fascia and preperitoneal fat, and a much larger hematoma can accumulate before causing distressing symptoms, with frequent extension into the perivesical fat and into the retroperitoneum. Venous bleeding is occasionally responsible for hematomas below the level of the semicircular line.

Rectus sheath hematomas predominate in women by about 3 to 1. The mean age of incidence is in the late fifth decade, but the hematomas occur in ages ranging from 20 to 80 years. In younger patients, there is no gender predominance, but there is a difference in cause, with pregnancy the most frequent cause in young women and trauma or muscular exertion the most common causes in young men.

Spontaneous formation of rectus hematoma is rare but can occur with vasculitis, arteriovenous malformations, a severe coagulopathy, or the administration of anticoagulants. The usual cause is trauma, most commonly stab wounds through the epigastric artery, such as needle injuries when suturing the abdominal wall or when performing paracentesis; vigorous contraction or stretching of the rectus abdominis muscle causing tears of the muscle with arteriolar or arterial bleeding; or, occasionally, blunt trauma to the abdominal wall. Events as trivial as sneezing, coughing, or twisting to the side have initiated rectus hematoma. Predisposing factors include the use of anticoagulants, old age, hypertension, and arteriosclerosis.

Abdominal pain is almost always described at presentation. The pain is often described as severe and usually is exacerbated by movements that require muscular contraction of the abdominal wall. On examination, there is tenderness over the rectus sheath, often voluntary guarding, and often a diffuse mass sensation in the area of tenderness. Contraction of the rectus muscles exacerbates the pain and the tenderness. Peritoneal signs are absent. Ecchymosis may occur but usually appears several days after the onset of pain. In cases where the hematoma dissects or originates inferiorly and expands into the paravesical and preperitoneal space, the hematocrit may fall significantly; however, hemodynamic instability is distinctly unusual.

In half or more of reported cases, the diagnosis is not made before operative exploration because the findings are misleading or the diagnosis is not considered. In most cases, the diagnosis can be made securely on clinical grounds. When it is unclear whether the source of pain is intraabdominal or abdominal wall, ultrasound and particularly CT can delineate the hematoma and localize it to the abdominal wall in almost all cases.

Treatment must take into consideration the cause, if known, and whether the hematoma is stable or progressive. Coagulopathies should be corrected when possible, although continuation of anticoagulation in selected patients has been reported without adverse sequelae. In trauma, concomitant injuries must be considered. For patients in whom the hematoma is stable, pain medication and avoidance of muscular stress on the abdominal wall are sufficient. For patients with progressive hematoma, the treatment of choice is evacuation of the hematoma from within the rectus sheath and hemostasis, sometimes requiring ligation of the epigastric vessels above and below the hematoma.

Tumors

Various soft tissue tumors may arise in the abdominal wall (see Chap. 112 for a discussion of malignant soft tissue tumors). Tumors of the abdominal wall are usually benign. Lipoma is the most common and is usually located in the subcutaneous fat, but it may be found in a subfascial or preperitoneal location. Other benign tumors of the abdominal wall include desmoid tumors, neurofibroma, nodular fasciitis, benign rhabdomyoma, hemangioma, lymphangioma, fibrous histiocytoma, and myxoma. These tumors present as palpable masses of the abdominal wall, involving the subcutaneous tissue or the muscular or fascial layers. Except for the lipoma, which is characteristically soft, stable in terms of growth, and located in the subcutaneous tissue, these lesions should be approached with the suspicion of malignancy. The mass should be evaluated by CT scans and an initial incisional biopsy obtained in a manner consistent with possible need for future surgery for sarcoma. Once histologic diagnosis has been ascertained, excision is the treatment of choice for these benign lesions and is straightforward except in the case of desmoid tumor, which tends to recur.

Desmoid Tumors

Desmoid tumors are fibromatous tumors that may resemble low-grade fibrosarcoma but never metastasize. The tumor often infiltrates adjacent muscle and has a high incidence of recurrence despite seemingly adequate gross resection. The tumors are usually categorized by location—extraabdominal, abdominal, or mesenteric.

Desmoid tumors are rare, occurring in 2 to 4 persons per 1 million population. There are four peaks in the age distribution of desmoid tumor.[19,20] The highest frequency is during peak fertility years (27.2 ± 4.4 years); desmoids in this group are 1.8 times more frequently found in women, and 92% of tumors are abdominal. The juvenile group (4.5 ± 3.5 years) is composed mostly of females, with abdominal tumors constituting 23% of this group. In the middle-age group (43.9 ± 6.9 years), there is a nearly 1:1 ratio by sex, and 72% of tumors are abdominal. The old-age group (68.1 ± 4.4 years) demonstrates equal distribution between extraabdominal and abdominal sites and between sexes.

The histologic features of desmoid are characterized by well-differentiated fibroblasts, few or absent mitoses, and lack of cytologic features of malignancy.[20] Collagen is usually abundant, and the central portions may be nearly acellular. The presence of sarcolemmic giant cells is distinctive. No pseudocapsule is found. Evidence of a muscle cell component to these tumors is demonstrated by characteristics of myofibroblasts in 30% of cells and by findings of positivity for both desmin and muscle actin on immunohistochemistry. The pattern of growth is infiltration into adjacent muscle, including the bladder, and into adjacent periosteum, but it rarely involves fixation to the peritoneum or penetration of underlying bowel. Invasion of skin has never been reported.

Three biologic characteristics have been observed in patients with desmoid tumors. First, abdominal wall desmoid tumors are associated with previous operation at the tumor site in one third of cases.[20] This relation to operative or other penetrating trauma is not reported in extraabdominal desmoid tumors. Second, half the patients with desmoid tumors, and nearly all those with Gardner syndrome who develop desmoid tumors, have bone malformations. These malformations include cortical thickening, exostosis, cystic areas of translucency, and compact islands in the femur. This finding has prompted genetic analysis suggesting that an autosomal dominant genetic factor is important in the formation of these tumors. Finally, the tumors exhibit evidence of hormonal responsiveness, with significantly higher growth rates in hormonally active women than in men or postmenopausal women. Positive estrogen receptor assays have been found in a high percentage of tumors in some studies.

The most frequent presenting symptom is a nontender palpable abdominal wall mass.[25] There is no predilection for any given portion of the abdominal wall. The median diameter of the tumor at the time of diagnosis is 10 cm.[21] Diagnostic imaging is best carried out by CT or magnetic resonance (MR) imaging, which delineates the extent of involvement of the layers of the abdominal wall and potential intraperitoneal extension.[25]

Initial treatment of abdominal wall desmoid tumors is surgical, though controversy remains about the role of adjuvant radiotherapy. Because the margins of the tumor are not easily determined and because the tumor often infiltrates muscle and periosteum, limited margins around the gross tumor frequently result in microscopic tumor at the

margin. Recurrence rates for abdominal desmoid tumors vary from 9% to 40%, and recurrence is frequent with inadequate margins.[21,22] A 5-cm margin of resection is considered adequate, with mono bloc resection of rib cage, pubic or iliac bone, or involved portions of organs such as bladder to achieve those margins.[21] Reconstruction of abdominal wall with polypropylene mesh is necessary in most cases. Musculofascial rotational grafts with split-thickness skin grafting is necessary in some cases for soft tissue reconstruction. In patients in whom adequate margins of resection are achieved, there is no evidence for benefit from adjuvant radiotherapy. Second and third resections after recurrence have been associated with no higher rate of recurrence than primary resection.[20]

Radiotherapy alone has achieved local control in desmoid tumor in as many as 100% of tumors treated primarily and in 75% of recurrent tumors.[23] Radiation doses of at least 60 Gy are considered necessary for consistent control.[24] Few abdominal wall tumors so treated have been reported, since the required radiation dose risks major damage to adjacent bowel. The role of primary radiation treatment of the abdominal wall desmoid is, therefore, a limited one.

Other therapies for desmoid tumors have been used for recurrent tumor, including tamoxifen, indomethacin, sulindac, and varied antineoplastic chemotherapeutic regimens. No consistent results and no controlled trials have been reported for any of these agents.

MESENTERY
Anatomy

The mesentery develops embryologically as a dorsal structure providing access for vasculature, lymphatics, and nerves. Between the 6th and 12th weeks of development, when the intestine is principally extracoelomic, intestinal rotation occurs in a counterclockwise direction about the superior mesenteric artery. With return of the intestine to the coelomic cavity at about the 12th week, the mesentery in the area of duodenum, pancreas, ascending colon, and descending colon disappears into a retroperitoneal fusion. Malrotation of the intestine and the accompanying alterations are discussed in Chapter 103.

The mesentery consists of the small bowel mesentery, the transverse mesocolon, and the sigmoid mesocolon. The small bowel mesentery extends from above, where it is in the midline anteroinferior to the third portion of the duodenum, diagonally downward to the right, almost to the pelvic brim in the right lower quadrant. The transverse mesocolon extends transversely across the abdomen anterior to the lower second portion of the duodenum, the lower margin of the head, body, and sometimes the tail of the pancreas, and, on the left, anterior to the left kidney. The sigmoid mesocolon has a base anterior to the left pelvic brim, the left common iliac vessels, and the left ureter.

At the base of the small bowel mesentery lies the ileocolic artery and vein, which are branches of the respective superior mesenteric vessels and which supply vasculature to the right colon and terminal ileum. The more proximal small bowel receives its vasculature by way of major trunks that divide into arcades and then anastomose with corresponding arcades from the next most proximal and distal trunk. From these arcades, vasa rectae course directly to the mesenteric margin of the bowel. In some cases, secondary arcades are formed. Occasionally, there is no anastomosing arcade between adjacent trunks. The major vasculature in the transverse mesocolon is the middle colic artery, usually the second or third branch of the superior mesenteric artery, and the corresponding vein, which joins with the right gastroepiploic vein to form the gastrocolic trunk, a high tributary into the superior mesenteric vein. In some cases, a supplementary transverse colic artery courses to the left of the middle colic vessels, with a direct origin off the superior mesenteric artery. The sigmoid mesocolon contains sigmoid arteries, branches of the inferior mesenteric artery, and the sigmoid veins, tributaries of the inferior mesenteric vein. Lymphatic drainage channels in the mesenteries accompany the course of the arterial supply and drain into the cisterna chyli. Sympathetic and parasympathetic innervation also accompany the arterial vessels.

Inflammatory Diseases of the Mesentery

Acute Mesenteric Lymphadenitis

Acute mesenteric lymphadenitis is a clinical syndrome of acute and marked right lower quadrant abdominal pain associated with mesenteric lymphatic enlargement and a normal appendix. Acute mesenteric lymphadenitis is the most common final diagnosis in patients operated on for presumed acute appendicitis in whom a normal appendix is found.[25] This clinical syndrome was designated *nonspecific acute lymphadenitis* in the 1950s. Although nonspecific acute lymphadenitis was once considered a distinct clinical entity without known cause, increasingly specific infectious agents have been discovered to account for the lymphadenitis and other clinical aspects of the syndrome.

Acute mesenteric lymphadenitis is a disease of the young, generally occurring in persons under 20 years old, and with equal incidence by gender. Some investigators have suggested its frequency is increased in the spring and autumn. It has also been associated with concurrent or preexisting rhinopharyngitis.

Although the designation acute mesenteric lymphadenitis suggests an entity with a single cause, several infectious and other specific causative factors have been identified. There are many conditions in which mesenteric lymphadenitis may be found. Many have been associated with a clinical syndrome and operative gross findings equivalent to those attributed to acute mesenteric lymphadenitis. *Yersinia enterocolitica,* in particular, and *Yersinia pseudotuberculosis* have both been associated with a pseudoappendicitis syndrome in children over 5 years old.[26] Culture and histologic evaluation of lymph nodes found at operation, stool culture, and antibody titers are necessary to identify causal agents in many of the cases that might have been previously categorized as nonspecific acute mesenteric lymphadenitis.[26]

The pseudoappendicitis syndrome, in which mesenteric lymphadenitis is encountered as the major finding during laparotomy, usually presents with pain as the initial symptom, beginning in the middle to upper abdomen and descending, in most cases, toward the right lower quadrant. Rebound tenderness and muscular rigidity are usually absent. Abdominal tenderness may shift to the left with the patient in the left lateral decubitus position. Nausea, vomiting, diarrhea, or constipation may be present. Body temperature and white blood cell count are normal to elevated.

Generally, the diagnosis of a normal appendix and mesenteric lymphadenitis is made at operation for suspected appendicitis. Because some of the etiologic processes responsible for acute mesenteric lymphadenitis may require treatment or have prognostic implications, nodal histology and culture should be obtained, examination of the terminal ileum recorded, and consideration given to stool culture and serologic titers for potential microbial agents. Differentiation between acute mesenteric lymphadenitis and acute appendicitis has been reported by using ultrasonography with a graded compression technique.

Treatment and prognosis for acute mesenteric lymphadenitis are wholly dependent on its cause. The course of disease with infectious agents such as *Yersinia enterocolitica* is self-limited in most cases and resolves before a definitive diagnosis is obtained. Yersinial infection may also require treatment with appropriate antibiotics and may be associated with recurrent pain.[28] Other infectious agents such as tuberculosis require treatment in all cases. With Crohn disease, no specific treatment is necessarily indicated.

Mesenteric Panniculitis

Mesenteric panniculitis is an inflammatory process of the adipose tissue of the mesentery. The condition has been referred to by various names, including *retractile mesenteritis, isolated lipodystrophy, retroperitoneal xanthogranuloma, sclerosing lipogranulomatosis,* and *lipogranuloma of the mesentery.* Although there is some variation in the abnormal picture, the inflammatory conditions of the mesentery are usually grouped as mesenteric panniculitis. Because the condition is rarely encountered, its presentation is usually confusing and leads to suspicion of some more serious abnormal condition.

Mesenteric panniculitis occurs most often in the fifth decade of life, but it has occurred in persons between the ages of 7 and 82 years.[29,30] The disease occurs predominantly in males, with a male-to-female ratio of 2 to 1. The small bowel mesentery is the most frequent site of mesenteric panniculitis, but the mesocolon may also be involved or be the sole site.[30] In collected series, 20% to 30% of patients developing mesenteric panniculitis have had previous abdominal surgery. Other concomitant and abnormal abdominal processes have been present in 22% to 67% of patients when mesenteric panniculitis was diagnosed.

The etiology and pathogenesis of mesenteric panniculitis are unknown. The coexistence of other abnormal abdominal processes or previous abdominal operations cannot explain most cases. Bacterial infection has only infrequently been demonstrated in association with the inflammatory process.[29] The clinical presentation makes it unlikely to be a variant of Weber-Christian disease. Other hypothetical causes include trauma, drugs, and allergic reactions.

Grossly, the disease is characterized by a thickened, hard, rubbery or nodular mesentery or by multiple mesenteric masses of similar consistency.[29] The process most often involves the root of the small bowel mesentery and often encompasses the mesenteric vessels. In advanced cases, vascular obstruction (usually venous) or lymphatic obstruction have been reported. The mesocolon and, infrequently, the omentum may be involved. Irregular areas of discoloration, ranging from gray to reddish brown to pale yellow areas suggesting fat necrosis, are scattered throughout the mesentery. In some patients, there may be foreshortening and scarring of the mesentery with distortion of the bowel. Microscopic findings include abnormal fat cells with foamy cytoplasm and infiltration by mononuclear inflammatory cells. Lipid-laden macrophages are invariably present. Foreign-body giant cells, fatty necrosis, calcification, and collagenous replacement are present in some patients, especially in more advanced cases.

Symptoms occurring in patients with mesenteric panniculitis include abdominal pain (70%), vomiting (30%), and abdominal mass or swelling (16%).[29] Other complaints have been anorexia, weight loss, constipation, diarrhea, and rectal bleeding. Physical examination reveals an abdominal mass in 50% to 65% of patients.[30] Abdominal tenderness, abdominal distention, fever, and signs of peritoneal irritation are present in a small number of patients.

Laboratory studies may disclose an elevated erythrocyte sedimentation rate. Except for leukocytosis in a few patients, other biochemical or hematologic alterations are unusual. Small and large bowel barium contrast studies often reveal extrinsic displacement of intestinal loops, dilated loops of small bowel, and a spiculated or serrated mucosal surface characteristic of an extrinsic inflammatory mass.[31] With involvement of the colon, there may be poor distensibility of the colon, with narrowing or even the appearance of an obstructing lesion. Recent reports of the CT characteristics of mesenteric panniculitis suggest that CT may permit diagnosis without the need for laparotomy.[32] Laparotomy for operative evaluation and biopsy of the mass remains necessary for definitive diagnosis.

Mesenteric panniculitis requires treatment only infrequently. Resection or bypass is usually necessary only for bowel obstruction. Mesentery resection, bypass, or proximal diversion is indicated in fewer than 15% of patients with disease involving the small bowel. The prognosis in mesenteric panniculitis is good. Lethal disease has been described in only 2 of the more than 120 patients reported in the literature. Abdominal pain continues or recurs in about 25% of patients after diagnosis by laparotomy. Although there have been several lymphomas reported in conjunction with mesenteric panniculitis, the relation between the two remains unclear.

Neoplasms of the Mesentery

Primary tumors of the mesentery are rare. They may be classified as cystic or solid. Cystic neoplasms of the mesentery occur more frequently than do solid neoplasms. Not all cysts of the mesentery are neoplastic.

Cystic Tumors of the Mesentery

The incidence of cystic neoplasms of the mesentery is difficult to estimate because of failure of histologic classification in almost all reported series of mesenteric cystic lesions. Cystic lymphangioma, a benign tumor, predominates, but rare malignant neoplasms including lymphangioendothelioma and cystic leiomyosarcoma have been reported.

Cystic Lymphangiomas. Twenty-nine percent of mesenteric cysts fulfill histologic criteria for cystic lymphangioma.[34] These benign neoplasms are found predominantly in children and young adults, with a mean age of 10 years, most occurring in the first decade of life, with none found after 40 years. Occurrence in males is 2 or 3 times higher than in females.[33,34] Grossly, cystic lymphangioma is indistinguishable from mesenteric cyst. Cystic lymphangioma is usually multilocular, containing clear fluid, with occasional hemorrhagic, calcified, or shaggy fibrinous areas on the lining. Light microscopy reveals a lining of endothelial cells, the presence of foam cells, and a wall containing small lymphatic spaces, lymphoid tissue, and smooth muscle. By contrast, simple mesenteric cysts have cuboidal or columnar lining cells, or lack lining, and do not include lymphatic elements or smooth muscle in the wall. Ultrastructurally, the lining cells in cystic lymphangioma resemble those of lymphatic channels.

About 90% of patients present with symptoms, which is true of mesenteric cysts in general in the pediatric and adolescent age groups. Symptoms may include abdominal pain, fever, and emesis. Half of patients have ascites, and about one quarter have an abdominal mass.

Solid Tumors of the Mesentery

Primary solid tumors of the mesentery are extremely rare, with fewer than 200 reported in the literature in English. Most neoplasms involving the mesentery are metastatic from bowel or other primary malignancies or a manifestation of lymphoma. Because of the rarity of solid tumors of the mesentery, most reports are of individual tumors. A broad range of cell types are represented in the mesentery, and corresponding tumors for most of these cell types have been reported. If lymphoma and mesothelioma are excluded, two thirds of solid mesenteric tumors are benign, and occurrence is equal by gender. The age at presentation ranges from a few months to 90 years or older.[33]

Mesotheliomas. A tumor that does not arise from the mesentery per se, mesothelioma is a tumor of the peritoneum. Mesothelial tumors of the peritoneum include benign mesothelioma, divided into adenomatoid and localized fibrous mesothelioma; borderline mesothelioma, composed of multicystic and well-differentiated papillary mesothelioma; and malignant mesothelioma, which is categorized into epithelial, fibrosarcomatous, and mixed-type mesothelioma.[35] Although peritoneal malignant mesothelioma is the most common of these, it is rare, with an estimated annual incidence of one to two cases per 1 million persons.[36] Only 10% to 20% of all mesotheliomas arise on the peritoneum, with most arising in the pleura. Peritoneal malignant mesothelioma occurs predominantly in adult males but also occurs rarely in children with equal sex incidence. The incidence of malignant mesothelioma is greatest late in the fifth decade of life, benign mesothelioma early in the fourth decade, and cystic mesothelioma late in the third decade. The nonmalignant types are more common in women.[37] The link with heavy asbestos exposure 20 to 40 years before is now well established.

The clinical presentation of peritoneal malignant mesothelioma is usually abdominal pain, which may be migratory rather than limited to a specific region of the abdomen. Abdominal distention and complaints associated with partial bowel obstruction are also frequent. Physical examination may reveal ascites or an abdominal mass. Similar findings are usual for cystic mesothelioma. Laboratory tests are generally not helpful in the diagnosis. Cytology of ascitic fluid may be positive for malignant cells in cases of malignant mesothelioma, but the diagnosis of mesothelioma cannot be confidently made cytologically. CT scans frequently demonstrate tumor masses and ascites but are not specific for mesothelioma. Laparotomy or laparoscopy for multiple biopsies is required in almost all cases to make the diagnosis.

The gross appearance of peritoneal malignant mesothelioma is not specific and may often easily be mistaken for carcinomatosis from other cancers. Findings at laparotomy or autopsy include tumor nodules on visceral and parietal peritoneum, diffuse thickening of the peritoneum, adhesions and agglutination of the abdominal contents, and encasement of the liver and spleen. Local invasion into bowel or other adjacent structures occurs in one third of cases of malignant mesothelioma of the peritoneum, and lymphatic metastases in about one half. Microscopically, malignant mesothelioma exhibits epithelial, mesenchymal, or mixed patterns, and usually more than one pattern is seen in an individual case. The differentiation from carcinoma can be difficult, even with special histochemical staining techniques. Ultrastructural examination may establish the mesothelial character of the cells by demonstrating cytoplasmic tonofilaments and microvilli and glycogen-like granules in the cytoplasm.

A multicystic mass attached to the peritoneal surface is typical for cystic mesothelioma.[37] Invasion and metastasis have not been described for cystic mesothelioma. Cystic mesothelioma exhibits small cysts lined by a single layer of flattened to cuboidal mesothelial-like cells, with frequent papillary clusters of a few cells within the cyst lumens.

Peritoneal malignant mesothelioma is treated with combination therapy. Surgical therapy by itself is not curative but is directed toward debulking and treatment of intestinal obstruction. Multidrug chemotherapy, usually including doxorubicin as one of the agents, administered systemically and sometimes as intraperitoneal chemotherapy, has shown activity. Whole abdomen radiotherapy has been used in treatment, but its effectiveness in the limited doses possible remains unknown.

The prognosis for patients with peritoneal malignant mesothelioma is dismal, with median survival of about 1 year after presentation.[36] Treatment appears to prolong survival in some patients compared to historic controls. Death usually results from progressive bowel obstruction. Prognosis for patients with cystic mesothelioma is good.

Desmoid Tumors. The desmoid tumor is the most common tumor of the mesentery. The histologic features, biologic characteristics, and treatment are similar to those of the abdominal wall desmoid, discussed earlier. Mesenteric desmoid tumors constitute 8% of all desmoid tumors and are about one sixth as frequent as abdominal wall desmoid tumors.[38] The relation of these tumors to Gardner syndrome is notable (see Chapter 46). Close to one third of patients with colonic polyposis and Gardner syndrome exhibit desmoid tumors. Bone malformations occur with a significantly higher incidence in association with both desmoid tumors and Gardner syndrome. It has been postulated that the genes for desmoid syndrome and Gardner syndrome, both also autosomal dominant, affect expression of mesenchymal structural components and, though not the same, are closely related.[20] Abnormalities in chromosome 5, which contains the familial adenomatous polyposis gene, have been reported in some desmoid tumors in those with and without Gardner syndrome.[39]

Lipomatous Tumors. Tumors of fat-cell derivation constitute about 22% of reported cases of mesenteric solid tumors, 70% of which are benign lipomas.[34] Liposarcomas exhibit spread by peritoneal implantation but have not been reported to disseminate by embolic metastases.

Stromal Tumors. These tumors were previously referred to as *smooth muscle tumors,* although histochemical studies reveal no true smooth muscle. They constitute about 10% of solid mesenteric tumors. The malignant variant is more commonly found than the benign. Malignancy in stromal tumors is more likely where smaller, rounded cellularity is seen and where mitoses are easily found. The malignant tumors more frequently metastasize by peritoneal implants, but hematogenous metastases do occur, not uncommonly to the liver.

Vascular Tumors. About 7% of solid mesenteric tumors are vascular in origin. Hemangiopericytoma, a malignant tumor, is the most common. Almost as commonly reported are hemangiomas.

Neurofibromas. Neurogenous cell-origin tumors make up about 6% of solid mesenteric tumors. Tumors of this cell type in the mesentery are almost exclusively benign neurofibromas.

Other Tumors. Other cell types that present as mesenteric tumors are teratomas (germ-cell origin) and mesenchymomas or hamartomas (mixed-element tumors).[33]

Clinical Elements

For both cystic and solid primary neoplasms of mesentery, symptoms relate primarily to the size and position of the tumor. Symptoms are frequently absent until the tumor reaches such size that partial bowel obstruction occurs. The most common symptom is abdominal pain, usually cramping and intermittent. Other symptoms, in order of decreasing frequency, are nausea, vomiting, distention, constipation, and diarrhea. Complications associated with the tumor may lead to the specific symptoms associated with such complications.

A palpable abdominal mass is the most frequent physical finding and relates to the size of the tumor. Solid neoplasms are palpable in 70% to 82% of patients and cystic neoplasms in 25% to 62% of patients at diagnosis. Characteristic of mesenteric masses is mobility on palpation in the transverse but not in the craniocaudad axis of the body. A less common abdominal finding is the presence of ascites.[34] Complications of mesenteric neoplasms include bowel obstruction, volvulus of bowel around the tumor with intestinal infarction and peritonitis, torsion of the tumor, hemorrhage into the tumor with rapid enlargement and occasionally anemia, and rupture with cystic tumors.

Diagnostic studies, for the most part, yield nonspecific results. Laboratory studies are likely to be normal. Plain abdominal radiography may depict displacement of bowel gas and occasionally presence of calcium (in a teratoma). Gastrointestinal contrast studies, in the absence of bowel complications from the neoplasm, reveal only displacement of intestinal loops or extrinsic compression of bowel. Ultrasound, CT, and MR imaging yield the greatest amount of information about mesenteric neoplasms. Sonography delineates the internal structure of cystic structures better than CT scans.[40] MR imaging can more precisely locate the tumor because of its multiplanar reconstruction capabilities. No modality can differentiate solid primary from secondary or metastatic tumor or even from inflammatory lesions with any certainty. Likewise, malignant cystic lesions cannot be reliably distinguished from benign.

Treatment for mesenteric neoplastic lesions is complete excision. Suspected malignant lesions should be resected with as wide a margin as the surgeon judges acceptable. How extensive such margins need be remains an open question. The small intestine frequently requires resection of malignant tumors because of encroachment on the vascular supply or close approximation or involvement of the bowel. Even the benign tumors may require bowel resection for complete excision. About 75% of patients with mesenteric cystic lymphangiomas require small intestinal resection to permit complete excision of this cystic neoplasm.[33,34] The neoplasms of the mesentery have a tendency to recur with less than complete excision. Because of the extreme rarity of malignant mesenteric tumors, the role of chemotherapy, radiotherapy, or other potential therapies is unknown.

Mesenteric Cysts

Mesenteric cysts are uncommon, occurring in about 1 in 100,000 general hospital admissions and 1 in 4000 to 34,000 pediatric hospital admissions.[39] Neoplastic mesenteric cysts were discussed earlier. The most commonly occurring nonneoplastic mesenteric cysts can be referred to as *mesothelial cysts.* Such cysts occur predominantly in adults, with a mean age of 45 years, are about twice as commonly found in women as in men,[34] and are located in the small bowel mesentery in about 60% of cases and in the large-bowel mesentery in 40%.[41] Mesothelial cysts are multiloculated in about 5% of cases and occasionally multiple cysts are present. The pathobiology in formation of these cysts remains a matter of speculation. Histologic features are a lining of cuboidal or columnar cells or an absent lining, a wall containing no lymphatic elements or smooth muscle (but occasionally calcium), and ultrastructurally, a mesothelial type of lining cell. These cysts may contain chyle if located in the mesentery of the proximal bowel, but they more often contain clear fluid when located in the distal small bowel or colonic mesentery.

Symptoms and potential complications parallel those found with neoplastic cysts (see earlier discussion) and correlate with size of the cyst. Diagnostic imaging is best accomplished with ultrasonography, CT, or MR imaging.[40] Enucleation of the cyst is the treatment of choice and is usually easily accomplished because the mesenteric blood vessels and bowel only infrequently adhere closely to the cyst wall. Internal drainage of the cyst into the peritoneal cavity after excision of the major portion of the wall is an acceptable alternative. Marsupialization is a poor alternative because of the not infrequent need for a second operation to close a draining sinus. Simple aspiration has a high rate of cyst recurrence and is a poor alternative as well. Although the incidence of malignant change is low, the cyst wall should be examined for rough, friable, papillary projections that suggest malignancy.

OMENTUM
Anatomy

The omenta are broad, thin structures covered on both surfaces with peritoneum and extending from the stomach to other organs. The greater omentum develops from the dorsal mesogastrium. Subsequent to the rotations and fusions of the gastrointestinal tract during intrauterine development, the greater omentum descends from the greater curvature of the stomach anterior to the transverse colon and much of the small bowel. It folds back on itself to fuse to the serosal layer of the transverse colon and mesocolon and to a variable extent to the serosal layer of the cranial portions of the ascending and descending colon. The anterior and posterior layers of greater omentum fuse so that no actual lesser sac exists between the two layers. The portion of greater omentum extending from the greater curvature of the stomach to the transverse colon is called the *gastrocolic ligament*. The greater omentum contains mainly adipose and vascular tissues.

The lesser omentum extends from the lesser curvature of the stomach to the inferior and medial aspect of the liver at the level of the hilum and extends superiorly anterior to left margin of the caudate lobe. The lesser omentum usually has a portion nearly devoid of adipose tissue superior to the stomach that is designated the *pars flaccida*. Structures coursing through the lesser omentum are the anterior and posterior vagus nerves to the stomach, the vagus nerves to the liver and gallbladder, the right gastric artery, the ramifications of the left gastric artery, and the left hepatic artery in persons in whom it arises from the left gastric artery. Posterior to the lesser omentum is the right superior portion of the lesser sac.

The greater omentum is called the "policeman" of the abdomen because it is often found encompassing an area of intraabdominal inflammation. Its adherence to inflammation in such cases, however, is passive and results from random movement and its mobility within the abdominal cavity. Nevertheless, adherence to areas of inflammation can effectively seal or wall off leaks from a viscus and isolate other causes of peritoneal inflammation. The greater omentum may also serve as a depot of significant volumes of adipose tissue. The lesser omentum serves principally as a supporting structure.

Omental Torsion

Torsion of the omentum is an infrequently occurring condition in which twisting of the omentum causes ischemia with associated pain. Unremitting torsion may result

in ischemic necrosis of the compromised portion of omentum. Torsion of the omentum is classified as primary, in which no identified coexisting condition is assigned causation, and secondary, occurring in association with adhesions of the free end of the omentum. The torsion may be unipolar, in which the free end of omentum undergoes torsion, or bipolar, in which the omentum is twisted between its base and an adhesion to the free end. Primary torsion occurs in males more often than in females by a ratio of 3 to 2 and occurs more often in the third and fourth decades, although it is reported for all age groups. Secondary torsion is much more common than primary torsion. Secondary omental torsion often occurs with the neck of a hernia serving as the attachment point, with bipolar torsion occurring to the intraabdominal portion of omentum. Less frequently, a unipolar torsion of the omentum transpires within the hernia sac. Inflammatory or postoperative adhesions may also serve as an attachment point in secondary torsion.

Primary torsion occurs most frequently in the right portion of the greater omentum, and it has been postulated that the greater weight and freedom of the right omentum predispose it to torsion when compared to the other portions of the omentum.[42] The gross pathologic findings with omental torsion are congestion, thrombosis of omental veins, areas of hemorrhage, and occasionally frank necrosis.

The usual clinical presentation is that of a patient with a single episode of acute abdominal pain of sudden onset, unremitting, and ranging from mild to severe in intensity. The pain localizes to the right lower quadrant in about 80% of patients. Nausea and vomiting are also frequent symptoms. A low-grade fever may be present. Abdominal tenderness, guarding, and mild rebound tenderness, usually in the right lower quadrant, are frequent, and an abdominal mass is palpable in half of patients.[42] Leukocytosis occurs in one half to two thirds of cases. Preoperative diagnosis is uncommon. The usual preoperative diagnosis is acute appendicitis, or, less often, acute cholecystitis. At laparotomy, free serosanguinous intraabdominal fluid is often present. Omental torsion should be suspected when the appendix is normal in combination with the above constellation of symptoms and findings. Treatment consists of excising the involved portion of omentum.

Omental Cysts

Omental cysts are rare, with an incidence of one fourth to one third that of mesenteric cysts.[43] These cysts are pathobiologically the same as described above for mesenteric cysts. Diagnostic methods are similar. Localization to the omentum may be difficult preoperatively but may be suggested by a greater mobility, particularly in the longitudinal axis, than in mesenteric cysts. Treatment is excision or enucleation, either of which is usually accomplished without difficulty. As with mesenteric cysts, after removal but before closing the abdomen, the cyst interior must be examined for papillary projections suggesting possible malignancy.

Omental Neoplasms

Primary omental neoplasms are rare, with fewer than 500 cases reported. The classification of primary mesenteric tumors is applicable to primary omental tumors. The distribution of types of tumors is different for the omentum than for the mesentery. Almost all omental neoplasms are metastases, usually from an intraabdominal primary malignancy. Benign cystic neoplasms, principally cystic lymphangioma, are the predominant primary tumors, but the true incidence is uncertain.

Most of the solid primary omental tumors are reported

in small numbers, so that epidemiologic information is sparse or suspect. Based on collected series, these tumors are found at all ages but most frequently in the fifth and sixth decades. A slight predominance for females has been suggested. Omental neoplasms may be divided into a group of exclusively benign small tumors found incidentally at laparotomy, and a group of larger tumors in patients operated on for symptoms attributable to the omental mass.[44] Of the latter group, slightly more than half are malignant. Leiomyoma is the most common type of benign solid omental neoplasm, and hemangiopericytoma, an extremely rare vascular tumor, is the single most common malignant tumor.

The clinical presentation of the symptomatic omental tumor is one of abdominal pain, abdominal distention, a sense of weight in the abdomen, and less frequently, weakness and weight loss, diarrhea, and nausea and vomiting. A palpable mass is usually present and is often mobile. The site from which the mass arises may not be apparent, especially with larger masses. The solid or cystic nature of the mass may be detected by abdominal ultrasound and CT scans, but its origin in the omentum is usually not detectable by preoperative studies. Abdominal roentgenograms and gastrointestinal contrast studies usually are nonspecific, revealing only displacement of bowel.

At operation, a solid mass encountered within the omentum must always precipitate a search for a primary tumor from which it may have metastasized. If the mass is judged a primary tumor, it should be totally excised with margins, because malignant primary omental tumors are sarcomas. Peritoneal and liver metastases occur more frequently than lung metastases from solid omental malignant tumors and should be sought. The benign tumors are almost always easily excised, but the malignant tumor may defy resection.[44] Prognosis for patients with benign omental tumors is excellent, but for those with primary malignancies, the outlook is poor. The results of chemotherapy, radiotherapy, and combination therapy for these malignant tumors are unknown.

RETROPERITONEUM

Anatomy

The retroperitoneum is that portion of the torso posterior to the peritoneal cavity. The retroperitoneum is contiguous with the soft tissues laterally, anteriorly (preperitoneum), and inferiorly that lie between the peritoneum and the abdominal wall musculature, and with the mesentery. There exist potential communications with the mediastinum and with the perineum and lower extremities in the planes along structures passing into or from the abdomen as defined by the musculoskeletal boundaries. Organs encompassed by or lying within the retroperitoneum include the adrenals, kidneys, ureters, bladder, pancreas, duodenum in its second through fourth portions, ascending and descending colon, upper two thirds of the rectum, upper vagina, ovaries, seminal vesicles, a portion of the vas deferens, the abdominal aorta and iliac arteries, the abdominal inferior vena cava and the iliac veins, and the major accompanying lymphatics including the cisterna chyli. The esophagus, upper stomach, liver, and spleen also have an interface with the retroperitoneum. Most of the blood supply, the venous drainage (with the exception of the liver), and the lymphatic drainage of the body below the diaphragms and thoracic dermatomes courses through the retroperitoneum.

The retroperitoneum can be divided into the lumbar fossa and the iliac fossa. The lumbar fossa extends from the 12th rib and thoracic vertebra to the sacral promontory and iliac crest and is bounded posteriorly by the fasciae of the quadratus lumborum and psoas muscles. The iliac fossa extends from the iliac crest to the margins of the pelvis and to the deep aspect of the lateral half of the inguinal ligament, with the iliac muscle fascia forming the floor.

Retroperitoneal Abscess

The significance of the retroperitoneum in considering abscess formation is that there are few anatomically delimiting structures within the retroperitoneum. As a consequence, an inflammatory process involving the retroperitoneum can spread widely. The muscle fasciae forming the posterior limits of the retroperitoneum generally confine abscesses in this region to the retroperitoneal space or to the subfascial space. The Gerota fascia (renal fascia) constitutes the single (bilateral) limiting structure of major consequence within the retroperitoneal tissues, separating the perirenal fat from the remainder of the retroperitoneum, although there is also a tendency for spread of infection to be limited at the periaortic tissue. Abscesses most commonly found in the retroperitoneum include perinephric abscess, lateral extension of pelvic abscess, abscess associated with perforated cecum, ileum, or duodenum, extension from retroperitoneal appendicitis, and abscess associated with acute pancreatitis. Necrotizing pancreatitis frequently extends into the right and left paracolic gutter, the base of the transverse mesocolon, and occasionally extends into the small bowel mesentery, the perivesical space, and the scrotum or femoral triangle. Subfascial abscesses most commonly are due to Pott disease (tuberculosis of the spine) and frequently erode into or anterior to the psoas muscle. Subfascial abscess may extend inferiorly to the iliac fossa and beneath the inguinal ligament. From there, the abscess may extend in various directions—to the femoral triangle in the groin, along the profunda femoris artery to the medial thigh, posteriorly along the sciatic nerve to the gluteal region, or posteriorly to the lumbar region.

The origin of a retroperitoneal abscess may be difficult to pinpoint, even at the time of operation. CT scanning is the best study for evaluating the retroperitoneum, but identifying the precise origin of the inflammatory process may be impossible. Similarly, at operation, the surgeon must be prepared to expose the retroperitoneum widely if the origin of the abscess is to be located.

Limited drainage, whether by operation or by sonographic-directed or CT-directed percutaneous drainage, may be satisfactory where the abscess is localized but is insufficient in instances of more widespread retroperitoneal abscess. Similarly, a retroperitoneal surgical approach to retroperitoneal abscess is suitable for localized purulence, but the transabdominal approach is appropriate for more extensive abscesses. Abscesses are often multiple and separated by uninvolved areas of retroperitoneum.

Chylous Ascites

Chylous ascites is the accumulation within the peritoneal cavity of chyle, a lymphatic fluid with a high lipid content. Usually, the chylous ascites is milky white, but the fat content of such fluid varies with the ingestion of fat. Ascitic fluid that is whitish and turbid may not be chylous ascites but may be of a similar character due to cellular breakdown as with bacterial peritonitis or neoplasm. Chylous fluid usually has a lipid content greater than plasma and a protein content more than half that of plasma. Microscopic fat is usually present. Although there are exceptions, the ratio of neutral fat to total lipid is almost always higher than that of plasma. Only lymph drainage from the intestine and possibly the liver contains the requisite level of fat to be the source of chylous fluid.

The physiology of intestinal lipid absorption is relevant to an understanding of the formation and treatment of chylous ascites. Triglycerides require hydrolysis to monoglycerides and fatty acids in the intestinal lumen before they can be absorbed. Micelles, formed in the intestinal lumen from monoglycerides, fatty acids, and cholesterol, in combination with bile salts, come into contact with the brush border of the intestinal mucosal cells, and the lipids enter the cell by passive diffusion, where rapid esterification occurs. Fatty acids larger than 12 carbons, which constitute about two thirds of dietary fat, are reesterified into triglycerides, coated with a layer of protein, cholesterol, and phospholipid to form chylomicrons, and secreted into the lacteals (intestinal wall lymph ducts). Access to the circulation is by way of the mesenteric lymphatics that enter the cisterna chyli, which in turn becomes the thoracic duct. Short- and medium-chain fatty acids (those containing 12 or fewer carbons) are transported within the intestinal mucosal cell directly into the portal venous system as free fatty acids and do not enter the lymph in significant proportion.

The cisterna chyli lies at the anterior surface of the first and second lumbar vertebrae, slightly to the right of the aorta.[45] Right and left lumbar, descending thoracic, intestinal, and liver lymphatics join the cisterna, which ascends to become the thoracic duct at about the T-12 to L-1 vertebral body junction. The thoracic duct ascends in the right posterior mediastinum until the T-5 to T-4 region. It then crosses to the left and ascends in the left retropleural space to join the venous system at the junction of the left subclavian and internal jugular veins. Normal lymph flow in the thoracic duct is estimated to be less than 1.5 L/d, mostly originating from the intestine and liver.

Chylous ascites may result from injury to a major lymphatic duct or to the cisterna. Experimental studies suggest that for lymphatic leakage to persist, widespread occlusion of lymphatic and lymphaticovenous collaterals within the abdomen must also be present. Similarly, except in nephrotic syndrome and cirrhosis, spontaneously occurring chylous ascites occurs only with extensive occlusion of retroperitoneal lymphatics. Malignancy is the predominant cause (88%) of spontaneous chylous ascites in adults, with lymphoma the most common malignancy.[46] In the pediatric age group, chylous ascites is two times more frequent in infants than in older children and is only infrequently due to malignant causes, with 40% of cases resulting from idiopathic and congenital causes.[47]

Diagnostic studies must include not only documentation of the lymphatic origins of the abdominal fluid but also an attempt to delineate the cause of the chylous ascites. Paracentesis and analysis of chylous fluid typically reveal elevated triglycerides, protein, and leukocyte levels, with a predominance of lymphocytes. The turbidity and milkiness of the fluid may vary and reflect both chylomicron size and triglyceride level. Unfortunately, cytology is seldom positive despite the presence of malignancy.[46] Lymphangiography or lymphoscintigraphy may define the site of lymphatic leak for patients in whom the leak is from the cisterna or retroperitoneal lymphatics but not when from mesenteric and hepatic lymphatics. Lymphangiography is of moderate usefulness in documenting retroperitoneal neoplastic processes giving rise to the chylous ascites. Of noninvasive studies, CT is the test of choice, with a high diagnostic yield in nontraumatic chylous ascites in adults. Frequently, laparotomy with node biopsy is required for histology and typing in cases suspected to be cancer, particularly for lymphoma, in which CT-guided needle aspiration biopsy cannot delineate nodal architecture.

The symptoms associated with chylous ascites include abdominal distention in almost all patients; abdominal pain, anorexia, weight loss, and edema in about half of patients; and weakness, nausea, dyspnea, weight gain, lymphadenopathy, early satiety, fever, or night sweats in a smaller number of patients. Physical examination yields findings of ascites in most patients. About half the patients have pleural effusion or peripheral edema. Other signs, in decreasing frequency, include palpable lymphadenopathy, caput medusae, cachexia, abdominal mass, hernia, cystocele or rectocele, and, in about 10% of patients, abdominal tenderness.[46]

Treatments for chylous ascites have been directed toward decreasing lymph and triglyceride accumulation. Successful resolution of chylous ascites has been achieved using a fat-restricted diet with added medium-chain triglycerides in an attempt to reduce the lymphatic transport of triglycerides and perhaps intestinal lymph flow. Although there have been reports of success using such dietary manipulation, many failures have also been reported. Cessation of all oral intake with administration of total parenteral nutrition has been effective in patients with nonneoplastic causes for the chylous ascites.[47]

In most patients with chylous ascites, treatment is likely to be successful only when directed toward the underlying cause. For patients with lymphoma, therapy effective against the lymphoma is likely to eliminate chylous ascites. Similar results are achieved with therapy directed toward the tuberculous and parasitic causes of chylous ascites. Radiotherapy and chemotherapy may provide temporary relief from chylous ascites in patients with solid neoplasms, but when the neoplasm is not cured by such treatment, the chylous ascites almost always recurs. Surgical attack on the source of the ascites may be curative when a specific site of leak can be identified or other cause can be eliminated, but it is likely to fail under other circumstances.

Removing the ascites may be required to relieve dyspnea, pleural effusion formation, or pain from progressive abdominal distention. Diuretics, salt restriction, and bed rest does little to relieve pain. Paracentesis is usually only transiently effective. Although a single paracentesis is associated with low risk of complications, repeated paracenteses for chylous ascites have considerable morbidity. Removing the ascitic fluid with automatic venous reinfusion using LeVeen or Denver peritoneovenous shunts has been temporarily successful, but patency of such shunts for longer than a few months is rare with chylous ascites. For traumatic or postsurgical causes, in which spontaneous resolution of the lymphatic leak is likely, peritoneovenous shunting has had reported success despite minimal success in other settings.

The prognosis for patients with chylous ascites is much better in infants and children than in adults, principally because of the different causes of the condition. A mortality rate of 21% is reported among infants and children.[47] Proper nutritional support has been advocated to further decrease mortality in infants and children. By contrast, a mortality rate of 88% has been reported in adults.[46] Patients with chylous ascites with associated neoplasm typically have a grave prognosis.

Retroperitoneal Fibrosis

Retroperitoneal fibrosis is a rare condition, occurring about once in every 30,000 hospital admissions.[48] This condition, in which fibrosis develops in the retroperitoneal space, is significant because the process generally encompasses the ureters and eventually causes hydronephrosis and kidney damage. Retroperitoneal fibrosis may also obstruct the extrahepatic bile duct and occasionally causes inferior vena caval or iliac vein obstruction. It may also be associated with retroperitoneal malignancy. Retroperitoneal fibrosis occurs most commonly in the fifth and sixth decades, with only 5% of cases occurring before age 20 years and 5% after age 70 years. It is twice as common in males than females.

The pathobiology of retroperitoneal fibrosis remains to be delineated. In fully two thirds of cases, retroperitoneal fibrosis is idiopathic. An autoimmune process has been suggested as the potential cause. Evidence includes fibrosis extending beyond the retroperitoneum, reports of concomitance with other entities considered autoimmune in cause, reports of coexisting systemic vasculitis, and the frequent response to corticosteroids. A reaction to a substance in the atherosclerotic aorta has also been proposed based on the similar fibrosis that is associated with 5% to 23% of abdominal aortic aneurysms.[48] These possible causes for idiopathic retroperitoneal fibrosis await confirmation.

About 12% of cases of retroperitoneal fibrosis have been associated with the use of methysergide, a serotonin antagonist used for vascular and migraine headache, and in this subgroup females outnumber males 2 to 1. The mechanism by which fibrosis is induced in association with methysergide is unknown. In most cases in which the retroperitoneal fibrosis is discovered early, discontinuing the methysergide has resulted in disappearance of radiologic findings of fibrosis. Other drugs have been implicated as causative agents for retroperitoneal fibrosis but with little supporting data.

Primary or metastatic malignancy in the retroperitoneum is found in 8% of patients with retroperitoneal fibrosis. There is equal prevalence by gender, and patient ages have ranged from the second through the seventh decade. Sarcomas are the most common primary tumors, but non-Hodgkin and Hodgkin lymphomas and ureteral cancer have also been found. Metastases have originated from cancer of the stomach, breast, colon, carcinoid, pancreas, prostate, ovary, and cervix.[49] The focus of tumor may be small but may induce desmoplasia that is grossly indistinguishable from the benign variants of retroperitoneal fibrosis.

Grossly, retroperitoneal fibrosis presents as a grayish white, rubbery, and dense thickening in the retroperitoneum, usually several centimeters thick and encompassing all retroperitoneal structures. The usual location is along the lower abdominal aorta, often including the bifurcation, but the fibrosis has extended to the mediastinum, rarely into the pelvis,[48] and as a localized epigastric or paranephric mass.[50] Microscopically, a spectrum occurs that in early stages is marked by islands of adipose cells surrounded by cellular areas composed of mature plasma cells, small round lymphocytes, eosinophils, and fibroblasts. Less inflammatory-appearing areas may reveal capillary proliferation, more fibroblasts, and collagen formation. Other (late) areas show fibrosis, with few cells, most of which are distorted mature plasma cells. Differentiation from sclerosing lymphoma is assisted by identifying mature plasma cells in benign retroperitoneal fibrosis by methyl green–pyronine staining.

Ninety percent of patients present with dull, noncolicky pain in the back, flank, or abdomen. Other symptoms include weight loss, nonspecific gastrointestinal complaints, and uncommonly, lower extremity edema, malaise, and dysuria. Physical signs, found in less than 10% of patients, include palpable abdominal mass, hypertension, fever, and oliguria or anuria. Laboratory studies may be normal in 25% of patients, but 55% have an elevated blood urea nitrogen and 6% have pyuria.

Diagnosis is most commonly suggested by intravenous pyelography. The combination of medial deviation of the ureter, hydroureteronephrosis, and extrinsic ureteral compression are highly suggestive of retroperitoneal fibrosis. CT or MR imaging is indicated when retroperitoneal fibrosis is suspected to more completely delineate the extent of disease. Either method can define the level of ureteral involvement and depict the mass appearance of the fibrotic process.[51] Patients may have decreased renal function, contraindicating intravascular contrast agents and thereby compromising visualization of ureters and great vessels by CT scanning. Because MR imaging requires no contrast and may differentiate malignant from nonmalignant retroperitoneal fibrosis,[52] it may be the diagnostic study best suited to this disease. Exploratory laparotomy with multiple deep biopsies of the retroperitoneal process is an essential part of diagnosis, since foci of carcinoma, when present, may be sparse within the predominantly sclerotic reaction.

Treatment for retroperitoneal fibrosis must identify and deal with potential causative agents, relieve the ureteral obstruction, and reverse the inflammatory fibrotic process. Methysergide, if used, should be discontinued. Renal obstruction may need to be relieved acutely, either by retrograde ureteral stents or by percutaneous nephrostomy tubes. With significant renal compromise, associated electrolyte and fluid imbalances and hypertension must be addressed, and dialysis is occasionally required. Long-term resolution of ureteral obstruction most frequently has been accomplished by operative freeing of the ureters from the fibrosis and displacing them laterally or within the peritoneal cavity. Although renal function is improved in over 90% of cases so treated, in as many as one third of patients, ureteral obstruction recurs on the ipsilateral or contralateral side.[48] Postoperative morbidity, including ureteral leaks, is not inconsequential.[53] Some researchers recommend an initial 2- to 3-week trial of corticosteroids before any operation and report resolution of ureteral obstruction in a high percentage of patients so treated, with response occurring within 7 to 10 days.[53] Failure after this brief course of steroids is an indication for operative treatment. Regressions as a response to tamoxifen administration and to aggressive immunosuppressive therapy have been reported.[54,55]

Prognosis for patients with nonmalignant retroperitoneal fibrosis is good. Survival rates of 86% to 100% for several years have been reported.[48] Extension of the fibrosis to the mediastinum or porta hepatis is associated with significantly poorer prognosis. Survival in most cases of malignant retroperitoneal fibrosis is only a few months.

Retroperitoneal Neoplasms

Tumors and cysts of the retroperitoneum may be similar to those rare tumors and cysts occurring in the mesentery and omentum. Much more frequently, tumors of the retroperitoneum are those of the structures that lie in the retroperitoneum, such as the pancreas, kidneys, ureters, adrenals, and neural crest tissues. Metastatic tumor is not uncommon because the retroperitoneum contains major lymphatic channels. In general, tumors in the retroperitoneum are asymptomatic until they have achieved a large size, unless they secrete substances that are active in the body and cause early symptoms. Surgical resection of retroperitoneal tumors is often compromised by the proximity or involvement of multiple important structures.

REFERENCES

1. Skandalakis JE, Gray SW, Skandalakis LJ, et al. Surgical anatomy of the inguinal area. World J Surg 1989;13:490.
2. Askar OM. Aponeurotic hernias: recent observations upon

paraumbilical and epigastric hernias. Surg Clin North Am 1984;64:315.

3. McVay CB. Abdominal wall. In: McVay CB. Anson and McVay surgical anatomy. Philadelphia, WB Saunders, 1984:484.

4. Brick WG, Colborn GL, Gadacz TR, et al. Crucial anatomic lessons for laparoscopic herniorrhaphy. Am Surg 1995; 61:172.

5. Gullmo 8F. Herniography. World J Surg 1989;13:560.

6. McEntee GP, O'Carroll A, Mooney B, et al. Timing of strangulation in adult hernias. Br J Surg 1989;76:725.

7. Stoppa RE. The treatment of complicated groin and incisional hernias. World J Surg 1989;13:545.

8. Raynor RW, Del Guiercio LRM. Update on the use of preoperative pneumoperitoneum prior to the repair of large hernias of the abdominal wall. Surg Gynecol Obstet 1985;161:367.

9. Starling JR, Harms BA. Diagnosis and treatment of genitofemoral and ilioinguinal neuralgia. World J Surg 1989;13:586.

10. Lemmer JH, Strodel WE, Knol JA, et al. Management of spontaneous umbilical hernia disruption in the cirrhotic patient. Ann Surg 1983;198:30.

11. O'Hara ET, Asghar O, Patek AJ Jr, et al. Management of umbilical hernia associated with hepatic cirrhosis and ascites. Ann Surg 1973;181:85.

12. Schumpelick V, Zinner M, eds. Atlas of hernia surgery. Philadelphia, BC Decker, 1990:223.

13. Skandalakis JE, Gray SW, Burns WB, et al. Internal and external supravesical hernia. Am Surg 1976;42:142.

14. Skandalakis JE, Gray SW. Supravesical hernia. In: Nyhus LM, Condon RE, eds. Hernia, ed 2. Philadelphia, JB Lippincott, 1974:395.

15. Dowd CN. Congenital lumbar hernia at the triangle of Petit. Ann Surg 1907;45:245.

16. Watson LF. Hernia, ed 3. St Louis, CV Mosby, 1948:476.

17. Berardi RS. Paraduodenal hernias. Surg Gynecol Obstet 1981; 152:99.

18. Zainea GG, Jordan F. Rectus sheath hematomas: their pathogenesis, diagnosis, and management. Am Surg 1988;54:630.

19. Kiel KD, Suit HD. Radiation therapy in the treatment of aggressive fibromatoses (desmoid tumors). Cancer 1984;54:2051.

20. Reitamo JJ, Scheinin TM, Hayry P. The desmoid syndrome. New aspects in the cause, pathogenesis and treatment of the desmoid tumor. Am J Surg 1986;151:230.

21. Shiu MH, Weinstein L, Hajdu SI, et al. Malignant soft-tissue tumors of the anterior abdominal wall. Am J Surg 1989; 158:446.

22. Easter DW, Halasz NA. Recent trends in the management of desmoid tumors: summary of 19 cases and review of the literature. Ann Surg 1989;210:765.

23. Miralbell R, Suit HD, Phil D, et al. Fibromatoses: from postsurgical surveillance to combined surgery and radiation therapy. Int J Radiat Oncol Biol Phys 1990;18;535.

24. Bataini JP, Belloir C, Mazabraud A, et al. Desmoid tumors in adults: the role of radiotherapy in their management. Am J Surg 1988;155:754.

25. Gilmore OJA, Browett JP, Griffin PH, et al. Appendicitis and mimicking conditions: a prospective study. Lancet 1975; 2:421.

26. Tertti R, Vuento R, Mikkola P, et al. Clinical manifestations of *Yersinia pseudotuberculosis* infection in children. Eur J Clin Microbiol Infect Dis 1989;8:587.

27. Puylaert JBCM. Mesenteric adenitis and acute terminal ileitis: US evaluation using graded compression. Radiology 1986; 161:691.

28. Saibo A. The *Yersinia enterocolitica* infection in acute abdominal surgery. Ann Surg 1983;198:760.

29. Durst AL, Freund H, Rosenmann E, et al. Mesenteric pan-

niculitis: review of the literature and presentation of cases. Surgery 1977;81:203.

30. Adachi Y, Mori M, Enjoji M, et al. Mesenteric panniculitis of the colon: review of the literature and report of two cases. Dis Colon Rectum 1987;30:962.

31. Monahan DW, Poston WK, Brown GJ. Mesenteric panniculitis. South Med J 1989;82:782.

32. Kopecky KK, Lappas JC, Baker MK, et al. Mesenteric panniculitis: CT appearance. Gastrointest Radiol 1988;13:273.

33. Gonzalez-Crussi F, Sotelo-Avila C, DeMello DE. Primary peritoneal, omental, and mesenteric tumors in childhood. Semin Diagn Pathol 1986;3:122.

34. Takiff H, Calabria R, Yin L, et al. Mesenteric cysts and intraabdominal cystic lymphangiomas. Arch Surg 1985;120:1266.

35. Hutchinson R, Sokhi GS. Multicystic peritoneal mesothelioma: not a benign condition. Eur J Surg 1992;158:451.

36. Plaus WJ. Peritoneal mesothelioma. Arch Surg 1988;123:763.

37. Katsube Y, Mukai K, Silverberg SG. Cystic mesothelioma of the peritoneum: a report of five cases and review of the literature. Cancer 1982;50:1615.

38. Hayry P, Scheinin TM. The desmoid (Reitamo) syndrome: etiology, manifestations, pathogenesis, and treatment. Curr Probl Surg 1988;25:225.

39. Bridge JA, Sreekantaiah C, Mouron B, et al. Clonal chromosomal abnormalities in desmoid tumors. Cancer 1992;69:430.

40. Ros PR, Olmsted WW, Moser RP Jr, et al. Mesenteric and omental cysts: histologic classification with imaging correlation. Radiology 1987;164:327.

41. Kurtz RJ, Heimann TM, Beck AR, et al. Mesenteric and retroperitoneal cysts. Ann Surg 1986;203:109.

42. Brady SC, Kliman MR. Torsion of the greater omentum or appendices epiploicae. Can J Surg 1979;22:79.

43. Walker AR, Putnam TC. Omental, mesenteric, and retroperitoneal cysts: a clinical study of 33 new cases. Ann Surg 1973;178:13.

44. Stout AP, Hendry J, Purdie FJ. Primary solid tumors of the great omentum. Cancer 1963;16:231.

45. Heyl A, Veen HF. Iatrogenic chylous ascites: operative or conservative approach. Neth J Surg 1989;41:5.

46. Press OW, Press NO, Kaufman SD. Evaluation and management of chylous ascites. Ann Intern Med 1982;96:358.

47. Unger SW, Chandler JG. Chylous ascites in infants and children. Surgery 1983;93:455.

48. Buff DD, Bogin MB, Faltz LL. Retroperitoneal fibrosis: a report of selected cases and a review of the literature. NY State J Med 1989;89:511.

49. Usher SM, Brendler H, Ciavarra VA. Retroperitoneal fibrosis secondary to metastatic neoplasm. Urology 1977;9:191.

50. Osborne BM, Butler JJ, Bloustein P, et al. Idiopathic retroperitoneal fibrosis (sclerosing retroperitonitis). Hum Pathol 1987;18:735.

51. Mulligan SA, Holley HC, Koehler RE, et al. CT and MR imaging in the evaluation of retroperitoneal fibrosis. J Comput Assist Tomogr 1989;13:277.

52. Arrive L, Hricak H, Tavares NJ, et al. Malignant versus nonmalignant retroperitoneal fibrosis: differentiation with MR imaging. Radiology 1989;172:139.

53. Higgens PM, Bennett-Jones DN, Naish PF, et al. Nonoperative management of retroperitoneal fibrosis. Br J Surg 1988;75:573.

54. Clark CP, Vanderpool D, Preskitt JT. The response of retroperitoneal fibrosis to tamoxifen. Surgery 1991;109:502.

55. McDougal WS, MacDonell RC Jr. Treatment of idiopathic retroperitoneal fibrosis by immunosuppression. J Urol 1991; 145:112.

56. Manten H, Barkin JS, Rogers AI. Chylous ascites. Postgrad Med 1982;71:79.

57. Koep L, Zuidema GD. The clinical significance of retroperitoneal fibrosis. Surgery 1977;81:250.

SURGERY: SCIENTIFIC PRINCIPLES AND PRACTICE, Second Edition, edited by
Lazar J. Greenfield, Michael W. Mulholland, Keith T. Oldham, Gerald B. Zelenock,
and Keith D. Lillemoe. Lippincott–Raven Publishers, Philadelphia, © 1997.

CHAPTER 54

ACUTE ABDOMEN AND APPENDIX

CARSON D. LIU AND DAVID W. MCFADDEN

ACUTE ABDOMEN

Nearly everyone has experienced sudden abdominal pain at some time in their life. Whether self-limited, as in gastroenteritis, or imminently life-threatening, as in perforated peptic ulcer or colon cancer, the physical and psychosocial impacts may be overwhelming. About 250,000 people miss work each day because of digestive or abdominal problems. In the United States, abdominal pain accounts for more hospital admissions than any other disease category.[1] However, the term *acute abdomen* applies to only a small number of these. It implies a pathophysiologic process that has a sudden onset and may be corrected by surgical manipulation.

Symptoms are the subjective manifestations of a disturbance in function and represent pathophysiologic states rather than specific diseases.[2] In the gastrointestinal tract, numerous alterations in physiologic function can be implicated. These include changes in secretion, absorption, motility, synthesis, digestion, and transport. The resultant symptoms can include abdominal (or extraabdominal) pain, dysphagia or odynophagia, anorexia, weight loss, nausea and vomiting, bloating or distention, constipation, flatulence, and diarrhea.[3] Signs of disease are the objective demonstrations of a pathologic process. These include tenderness, rigidity, masses, altered bowel sounds, bleeding, malnutrition, jaundice, and stigmata of hepatic dysfunction.[2,4]

The case history remains one of the most useful tools in the diagnosis of digestive diseases.[5] The surgical consultant should thoroughly review every detail of the illness with the patient. The art of physical examination is also of great importance in the diagnosis of abdominal pain. Combining the elicited symptoms from a complete history and the signs from a comprehensive physical examination allows the surgeon to establish a differential diagnosis. It is important to formulate a thorough but cost-effective diagnostic evaluation that may require blood tests, radiographs, and histologic confirmation.[6]

Pain

Pain, from the Latin *poena*, meaning punishment, penalty, or torment, is the singular sensory experience that humans use to identify disease within themselves. It is one of the greatest motivational drives known to man.[7] Most diseases of the abdominal viscera are associated with pain sometime during their course (Fig. 54-1). A brief review of abdominal embryology and pain physiology will assist the clinician in evaluating the patient with acute or chronic abdominal pain.

The gastrointestinal tract consists of a foregut, midgut, and hindgut. Each segment has its own blood supply and innervation and retains these relations throughout development and into adulthood. The foregut extends from the oropharynx to the duodenum at the level of the entrance of the common bile duct. It includes the pancreas, liver, biliary tree, and spleen. The midgut is composed of the distal duodenum, jejunum, ileum, appendix, ascending colon, and proximal two thirds of the transverse colon. The hindgut consists of the remainder of the colon and rectum down to the cloacal bulge, which constitutes the interface between the surface ectoderm and endoderm of the cloaca, corresponding to the dentate line.[2,6]

The peritoneum is a continuous visceral and parietal layer. Although both layers are mesodermally derived, they develop separately and have separate nerve supplies. This is important for diagnostic reasons. The visceral layer (ie, the layer surrounding all intraabdominal organs) is supplied by autonomic nerves (sympathetic and parasympathetic), and the parietal peritoneum is supplied by somatic innervation (spinal nerves).[1] The pathways relaying the sensation of pain differ for each layer. They also differ in quality. Visceral pain is characteristically dull, crampy, deep, or aching, and it may involve sweating and nausea. Parietal pain is sharp, severe, and persistent.[6] Visceral organs have very little pain sensation, but stretching of the mesentery and stimulation of the parietal peritoneum cause severe pain.

Normal embryologic development of the abdominal viscera proceeds with bilateral autonomic innervation, resulting in visceral pain that is usually perceived as arising from the midline. The location of pain in the midline is determined by the embryologic origin of the involved viscus. Epigastric pain is typical of foregut origin. Periumbilical pain signifies pain emanating from the midgut. Hypogastric or lower abdominal midline pain indicates a hindgut origin. Pelvic pain is more typical of disease originating in structures derived from the cloaca.[2]

For abdominal pain to be recognized by the patient, nociceptors, or pain receptors, must be noxiously stimulated. Two types of neuronal fibers are involved. A-δ fibers are rapid transmitters and give rise to sharp, well-localized pain sensations. These fibers are distributed to muscle and skin and are involved with somatic pain transmission through spinal nerves. C fibers are slow transmitters. They generate the sensation of dull, poorly localized pain that is gradual in its onset and of long duration.[6] These fibers are located intramurally in hollow viscera and in the capsule of solid organs. They are found in muscle, periosteum, and the parietal peritoneum and are involved in visceral pain transmission through the autonomic nervous system.[2]

Different neural pathways are responsible for pain mediation, depending on whether the source of the pain is the parietal peritoneum or the visceral peritoneum. The anterior and lateral abdominal walls are supplied by nerves arising from spinal segments T-7 to L-1. The posterior abdominal wall is innervated from spinal segments L-2 to L-5. Pain arising from the abdominal wall is relayed to the spinal cord through the spinal nerves. Because these pain fibers enter the spinal cord ipsilaterally, pain is perceived as originating from that side. Also, such pain localizes to the area of the abdomen from which it originates. In contrast, pain arising from intraabdominal viscera is perceived to arise in the midline because sensory input from such viscera enters the spinal cord on both sides.

Abdominal pain can be divided into three categories: visceral, somatic, and referred. The aforementioned intramural sensory receptors of the abdominal organs are responsible for visceral pain. Some destructive stimuli to the abdominal viscera are painless. For example, almost all abdominal organs are insensitive to pinching, burning, stabbing, cutting, and electrical and thermal stimulation. The same is true for the application of acid and alkali to normal mucosa.[6]

The four general classes of visceral stimulation that result in abdominal pain are the following:

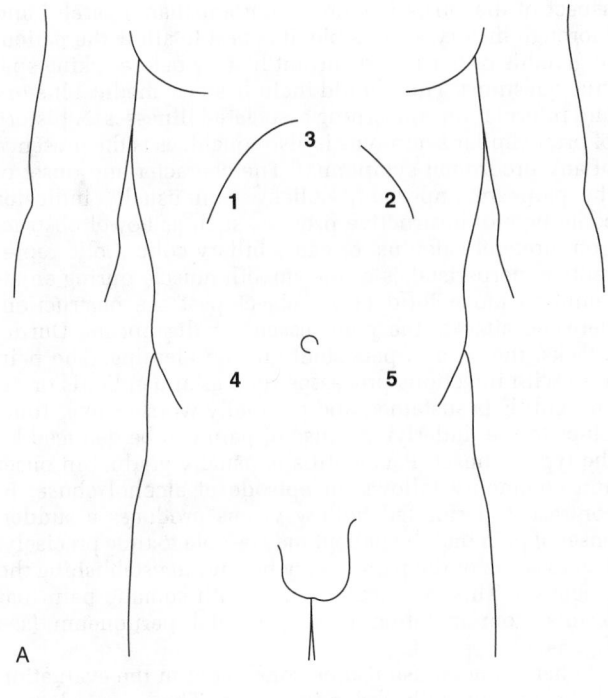

A

Figure 54-1. Abdominal pain map.

B

RIGHT UPPER QUADRANT PAIN (1)

Cholecystitis
Choledocholithiasis
Retrocecal appendicitis
Pancreatitis
Subdiaphragmatic abscess
Hepatic abscess
Hepatitis (A, B, C)
Peptic ulcer
Hepatic metastasis
Choledochocyst
Hepatic vein obstruction
 (Budd-Chiari syndrome)
Herpes zoster
Pneumonia
Hepatomegaly from congestive
 heart failure
Myocardial ischemia
Pericarditis
Pleuritis
Empyema
Pulmonary infarction

LEFT UPPER QUADRANT PAIN (2)

Splenomegaly
Splenic infarction
Splenic artery aneurysm
Splenic rupture (from blunt
 trauma)
Fractured ribs
Gastritis
Peptic ulcer disease
Pancreatitis
Herpes zoster
Pneumonia
Myocardial ischemia
Pericarditis
Pleuritis
Empyema
Pulmonary infarction

EPIGASTRIC PAIN (3)

Pancreatitis
Gastritis
Peptic ulcer disease
Cholecystitis
Reflux esophagitis
Myocardial ischemia
Pericarditis

RIGHT LOWER QUADRANT PAIN (4)

Appendicitis
Ruptured peptic ulcer (Valentino
 syndrome)
Cholecystitis
Intestinal obstruction
Diverticulitis
Crohn's disease
Leaking abdominal aortic
 aneurysm
Ectopic pregnancy
Ovarian cyst
Salpingitis
Ovarian torsion
Endometriosis
Mittelschmerz
Renal calculi
Psoas abscess
Seminal vesiculitis
Abdominal wall hematoma

LEFT LOWER QUADRANT PAIN (5)

Diverticulitis
Appendicitis
Colon cancer
Intestinal obstruction
Splenomegaly
Gastritis
Inflammatory bowel disease
Leaking abdominal aortic
 aneurysm
Ectopic pregnancy
Ovarian cyst
Salpingitis
Ovarian torsion
Endometriosis
Mittelschmerz
Renal calculi
Psoas abscess
Seminal vesiculitis
Abdominal wall hematoma

DIFFUSE PAIN

Early appendicitis
Peritonitis
Gastroenteritis
Pancreatitis
Mesenteric thrombosis
Abdominal aortic aneurysm
Intussusception
Colitis
Intestinal obstruction
Inflammatory bowel disease
Leukemia
Sickle cell crisis
Mesenteric adenitis
Metabolic, toxic and bacterial
 causes

- Stretching and contraction
- Traction, compression, and torsion
- Stretch alone
- Certain chemicals

The mediating receptors for these responses are located intramurally in hollow organs, on serosal structures such as the visceral peritoneum and capsule of solid organs, within the mesentery (especially associated with large mesenteric vessels and ligaments), and within the mucosa. These receptors are polymodal (responsive to both mechanical and chemical stimuli). Mucosal receptors respond primarily to chemical stimulation.[6] The major forces

that evoke visceral pain arise from geometric forces (such as stretching and distention) that result in increased wall tension. Other factors responsible for visceral pain include ischemia and inflammation.[1] Visceral pain almost always heralds intraabdominal disease but may not indicate the need for surgical therapy. When visceral pain is superseded by somatic pain, the need for surgical intervention becomes likely.[8]

Somatic or visceral pain arises from irritation of the parietal peritoneum. Mediated mainly by spinal nerve fibers that supply the abdominal wall, somatic pain is localized and perceived as arising from one of the four quadrants of the abdominal wall. In contrast to visceral pain, in which geometric changes are responsible for the stimulation of nerve endings, somatic pain arises as a response to acute changes in pH or temperature, as seen in bacterial or chemical inflammation.[6,7] In addition, somatic pain is felt in response to sudden increases in pressure, as with a surgical incision. Somatic pain is perceived as sharp and pricking and is usually constant. In many clinical situations it is probable that the perception of pain results from multiple stimuli. The pain of pancreatic cancer probably arises from the combination of serosal stretch, vascular and mesenteric compression, and direct neural infiltration. The sensitivities of visceral receptors are also affected by circumstances. Pressure on or chemical application to normal gastric mucosa is usually painless, but if the mucosa is inflamed, these same stimuli are quite painful.[6]

Referred pain is felt in an area of the body other than the site of its origin and is one of the characteristic qualities of abdominal pain. Referred pain usually arises from a deep structure, is superficial at its distant presenting location, and often is sharp, localized, and persistent at the distant site. It occurs secondary to the existence of shared central pathways for afferent neurons arising from different sites.[8] Two associated features of referred pain are skin hyperalgesia and increased muscle tone of the abdominal wall. A classic example is the ruptured spleen that results in irritation of the left hemidiaphragm, which is innervated by the same cervical nerves. In this setting, referred pain is perceived as arising in the left shoulder (Kehr sign), which is also supplied by those nerve roots. A knowledge of referred pain and its patterns may be of diagnostic assistance when other evidence of disease is lacking or absent (Table 54-1).

Acute Abdominal Pain

Acute abdominal pain is loosely defined as pain present for less than 8 hours. The key to the management of patients with acute abdominal pain is early diagnosis. No

---

Table 54-1. POSSIBLE ORIGINS FOR REFERRED PAIN

RIGHT SHOULDER

Diaphragm
Gallbladder
Liver capsule
Right-sided pneumoperitoneum

RIGHT SCAPULA

Ballbladder
Biliary tree

GROIN OR GENITALIA

Kidney
Ureter
Aorta or iliac artery

BACK—MIDLINE

Pancreas
Duodenum
Aorta

LEFT SHOULDER

Diaphragm
Spleen
Tail of pancreas
Stomach
Splenic flexure (colon)
Left-sided pneumoperitoneum

LEFT SCAPULA

Spleen
Tail of pancreas

---

aspect of diagnosis is more important than a careful and thorough history. If possible, it is best to allow the patient to give his or her entire current history before asking specific questions. This should include a past medical history and information concerning associated illnesses. A history of prior similar symptoms is also sought, as is the presence of any prodromal symptoms.[8] The character and onset of the pain are important. Colicky pain usually indicates some type of obstructive process, such as bowel obstruction, ureteral calculus, or acute biliary colic. Colic represents hyperperistalsis of the smooth muscle during an attempt to move fluid or an object past the obstruction. Between attacks, the pain lessens or disappears. During attacks, the pain is persistent and unrelenting. The pain seen with infectious processes such as appendicitis or diverticulitis is sustained and gradually worsens over time. Clues to the underlying cause of pain can be deduced by the type of onset. Pancreatitis is usually gradual in onset and commonly follows an episode of alcohol abuse. In contrast, a perforated hollow viscus produces a sudden onset of pain that the patient may be able to time precisely. The location of the pain is very helpful in establishing the diagnosis. This is especially true with somatic pain that results from irritation of the parietal peritoneum (see Fig. 54-1).

Other factors must also be considered in the evaluation of the patient with abdominal pain. These include any previous history of intraabdominal disease, previous abdominal surgery, and current medications. Familial or concomitant diseases in family members should also be sought. A woman's precise menstrual history should be obtained because this may be the sole clue to the presence of gynecologic pathology.[9]

The first and most important step in the physical examination of the patient with an acute abdomen is careful observation of the patient's body habitus and facial expression. Unwillingness to change body position suggests an underlying peritonitis. Hip flexion with the knees drawn up to maintain comfort suggests abdominal wall and possibly peritoneal irritation.[8] Restriction of diaphragmatic excursion with respiration, as noted by shallow breathing and the use of accessory respiratory muscles, is also consistent with peritoneal irritation. In contrast, colicky pain is often manifested by intense movement in an effort to alleviate pain, followed by restful intervals between colicky periods. Inspection of the abdomen for hernial bulges, masses, distention, or areas of inflammation should be performed. Careful auscultation of the abdominal cavity for the presence or absence and quality of bowel sounds is performed. The presence and location of bruits should be noted. A careful auscultation of the chest, particularly in the diaphragmatic area, should be undertaken to document diaphragmatic movement and to search for a basilar pneumonia that may simulate an acute abdominal condition. Gentle palpation of all quadrants of the abdomen should be performed last. Gentle, rather superficial, palpation of the abdomen should be performed initially, proceeding from the quadrant with the least symptomatology to the most painful area. Peritoneal signs or masses, suggested by the superficial examination, may then be confirmed by a deeper, still gentle palpation. Classic rebound tenderness is fraught with examiner error; a percussion test is kinder and more specific.[2] Having the patient cough, laugh, or maximally distend the abdomen may localize the disease, especially in children.[10] Patients in pain who were previously examined by an unskilled physician are often quite sensitized to the manipulations that are used to elicit rebound. Therefore, a skilled examiner must use other diversions to confirm peritonitis. The so-called stethoscope test, which consists of using a stethoscope to depress and release the abdomen, is useful. Similarly, shaking the pelvis from side to side may elicit true rebound tenderness. Hyperesthesia is uncommonly present but is defined as skin that is exquisitely sensitive to gentle touch. Hyperesthesia exists because the dermatome is supplied by the same nerve roots as an area of parietal peritoneum.

Many laboratory tests offer useful information in the evaluation of patients with an acute abdominal condition. Minimally, a complete blood count, urinalysis, serum amylase, and, for women with lower abdominal pain, a β-human chorionic gonadotropin, or pregnancy test, should be requested. Serum electrolytes, blood urea nitrogen, creatinine, and glucose are useful in determining the patient's hydration status, renal function, and basic metabolic state. Liver chemistries are helpful in patients with upper abdominal pain or stigmata of liver disease. In general, laboratory tests should not be performed unless their results will alter the need for additional tests or therapy.[11] Frequently, at the time of venipuncture, an intravenous cannula can be inserted and used for hydration or administration of medication.

Four radiologic views of the chest and abdomen are essential in patients with abdominal pain and no obvious diagnosis.[12] The physician must be aware of the stress of a trip to the radiology suite on the patient and of the time involved and must therefore ensure stability of the patient's hemodynamic status before this endeavor takes place. An upright and supine film of the abdomen and an upright and lateral radiograph of the chest are then performed. Although only 10% of patients with an acute abdomen have abnormalities on screening roentgenography, radiographs are still suggested in patients unless a clear-cut diagnosis is established.[13] Pneumoperitoneum, gas–fluid levels, fecaliths, gallstones, ascites, and obliteration of the psoas shadows are all helpful diagnostic findings that can be seen on the four screening films.[14] Contrast gastrointestinal studies, ultrasonography, computed tomography (CT) scans, and arteriography may be suggested or required given the specific findings and clinical suspicions of the evaluating physician.[15,16]

No laboratory or radiologic maneuver should be performed unless its result will alter the need for additional tests or treatment. If the patient appears to have appendicitis and an operation is planned, it serves no purpose to obtain an abdominal series to look for a fecalith. Also, test results should not duplicate previous tests. Gallstones delineated by ultrasound do not require additional radiologic examinations. A balance should be sought, taking into consideration cost, yield, morbidity, and accuracy. Finally, one must resist the "Mount Everest" syndrome,[17] wherein a test is performed because the facilities exist for its performance.

Numerous surgical causes exist for the patient presenting with acute abdominal pain. These are covered individually in the chapters dealing with specific organ systems. A review of nearly 1200 patients presenting for emergency evaluation of abdominal pain affords some interesting findings.[18] The most common diagnosis was nonspecific abdominal pain, occurring in 35% of patients. Appendicitis (17%), intestinal obstruction (15%), urologic problems (6%), and gallstones (5%) were the leading surgical causes. The largest number of admissions consisted of patients 10 to 29 years of age (31%) and patients 60 to 79 years of age (29%). Surgical procedures were required in 47% of patients. The increased proportion of elderly patients in this study mirrors the rise in the elderly population. Large series of elderly patients presenting with acute abdominal pain have found the leading diagnoses to be cholelithiasis, nonspecific pain, malignancy, incarcerated hernia, ileus, and gastroduodenal ulcer.[7] The presence of comorbid processes, especially cardiovascular disease, stresses the need for rapid diagnosis and timely operative surgery if appropriate.[19]

Gynecologic Causes of the Acute Abdomen

Organ systems other than those classically associated with the alimentary tract must also be considered. Gynecologic causes of acute abdominal pain include pelvic inflammatory disease (PID), ectopic pregnancy, tuboovarian cysts, torsion, hemorrhage or abscess, and mittelschmerz.[9] PID must be considered in virtually every woman of reproductive age with lower abdominal pain. It includes tuboovarian abscess with or without rupture. Whereas PID is usually appreciated bilaterally, an abscess is unilateral in over 70% of cases. Acute pain is reported in 90% of patients, fever and chills in 50%, fever in 60%, and leukocytosis in 68%.[9] Pelvic examination usually reveals extreme pelvic tenderness and increased pain on cervical motion.[20] Peritoneal signs in the upper abdomen suggest leakage or rupture of a pelvic abscess, usually requiring surgical intervention. Differentiation of PID from acute appendicitis is particularly difficult, especially in women of childbearing age, and the rate of false-positive explorations approaches 40%. Table 54-2 outlines a few of the salient differences.

Ectopic pregnancy occurs once in 200 conceptions, leading to 50,000 cases per year in the United States. Risk factors include prior salpingitis, tubal ligation, prior tubal repair, presence of an intrauterine device, and prior ectopic pregnancy. Pain and abnormal uterine bleeding are seen in 97% and 86% of patients, respectively.[21] Human chorionic gonadotropin (hCG) testing and culdocentesis are essential for diagnosis.

Hemorrhage from functional ovarian cysts can also simulate an acute surgical abdomen. Symptoms typically begin at or around the time of ovulation. Pain is classically severe, abrupt in onset, and often bilateral. Pregnancy testing by serum hCG should distinguish this process from ectopic pregnancy. Operation is rarely required to treat hemorrhage associated with rupture of a follicular ovarian cyst. Adnexal torsion presents with lower abdominal, lateralized pain that may be colicky. As with other pelvic conditions, ultrasonography and laparoscopy are helpful tools in diagnosis and management.[11]

Urologic Causes of the Acute Abdomen

Urologic conditions that may simulate an acute surgical abdominal condition include renal, perirenal, or bladder infections; obstructions of the ureter, renal pelvis, or bladder; and acute intrascrotal events. Uncomplicated pyelone-

Table 54-2. APPENDICITIS DIFFERENTIATED FROM PELVIC INFLAMMATORY DISEASE (PID)

Finding	Appendicitis	PID
Nausea and vomiting	+++	+
Menstrual cycle	No preference	60% in first 14 d
History of venereal disease	+	+++
Mean duration of symptoms	32 h	65 h
Cervical motion or adnexal tenderness	+	+++
Guarding or tenderness	Right lower quadrant	Bilateral

phritis is rarely a diagnostic problem and does not often present as an acute abdominal event. In contrast, renal and perirenal abscesses may present acutely and may mimic appendicitis, diverticulitis, or cholecystitis. An intravenous pyelogram (IVP) is abnormal in most cases, as is urinalysis. Acute ureteral or renal pelvis obstruction is the most common condition to be confused with nonurologic causes of the acute abdomen. Urinalysis, plain abdominal radiography, and IVP are usually confirmatory.[22]

Acute testicular torsion and other intrascrotal events present with prominent abdominal pain in 25% to 50% of cases. A careful examination of the scrotum usually reveals an elevated testicle on the affected side, along with profound tenderness.[22]

The Acute Abdomen in Specific Conditions

Nonsurgical conditions that simulate the acute abdomen include a number of pulmonary, cardiac, neurologic, metabolic, toxic, infectious, and hematologic problems, as described in Table 54-3. The differential diagnosis of acute abdominal pain in the pediatric patient is outlined in Table 54-4. In the first few years of life, congenital abnormalities are the most common source of abdominal symptoms of surgical importance.[23] Histories are difficult to obtain, and the physical examination in the newborn or infant can be extremely misleading in that no discernible tenderness may be present. Plain abdominal films should be used more liberally in the pediatric population. In older children, the history and physical findings are more easily elicited, and diagnosis is generally more clear. Certain features in children should be mentioned. Anorexia is often absent in children with appendicitis or other intraabdominal inflammatory conditions.[10] The sigmoid colon is often redundant in children. If it is adjacent to an inflamed appendix, diarrheal symptoms may predominate, leading to a

Table 54-3. NONSURGICAL CAUSES OF THE ACUTE ABDOMEN

METABOLIC

Diabetic ketoacidosis
Porphyria
Adrenal insufficiency
Uremia
Hypercalcemia

TOXIC

Insect bites
Venoms (scorpion, snake)
Lead poisoning
Drugs

MISCELLANEOUS

Hemolytic crises
Rectus sheath hematoma

NEUROGENIC

Herpes zoster
Abdominal epilepsy
Spinal cord tumor, infection
Nerve root compression

CARDIOPULMONARY

Pneumonia
Myocardial infarction
Myocarditis
Empyema
Costochondritis

Table 54-4. DIFFERENTIAL DIAGNOSIS OF THE ACUTE ABDOMEN IN THE PEDIATRIC POPULATION

Infants	Children	Adolescents
Viral enteritis	Meckel's diverticulitis	Pelvic inflammatory
Intussusception	Cystitis	disease
Pyelonephritis	Viral enteritis	Viral enteritis
Gastroesophageal	Appendicitis	Mittelschmerz
reflux	Crohn's disease	Crohn's disease
Bacterial enterocolitis	Bacterial	Pancreatitis
Pneumonitis	enterocolitis	Pneumonia
Appendicitis	Trauma (child	Hematocolpos
Pyloric stenosis	abuse)	Bacterial enterocolitis
Testicular torsion	Pneumonitis	Psychosomatic illness
Mesenteric cysts	Pancreatitis	Peptic ulcer
Ruptured tumors	Ruptured tumors	Poisoning
Pancreatitis	Poisoning	Trauma
Meckel's diverticulitis	Pyelonephritis	Ectopic pregnancy
Hirschsprung disease		Pregnancy
Strangulated hernia		Cholelithiasis
Poisoning		
Trauma (child abuse)		

false diagnosis of gastroenteritis. In children, microscopic hematuria and pyuria are often seen with appendicitis, whereas leukocytosis is less common.[23]

Acute abdominal conditions after cardiac surgery occur in only 1% of patients. However, abdominal complications are responsible for 7% to 10% of the total postoperative mortality rate for cardiac surgery because of their associated 25% to 60% mortality rate. Gastrointestinal bleeding, acute cholecystitis, mesenteric ischemia, pancreatitis, and acute colitis are the diagnoses most commonly reported.[24]

Immunocompromised patients constitute a heterogeneous group that includes those receiving allografts, chemotherapy, or immunosuppressive drugs for autoimmune disorders, and individuals with the acquired immunodeficiency syndrome (AIDS).[25-28] Each of these groups has specific abdominal complications that must be appreciated and suspected by the evaluating physician (Table 54-5).

Acute, nonspecific abdominal pain is a frequent final diagnosis. It accounts for up to 43% of patients with abdominal pain presenting for emergency evaluation.[29] One retrospective study found this to be the 6th and 10th most common cause of hospital admission for women and men, respectively.[18] A long-term study found that 77% of these patients remained healthy and symptom-free at 5 years' follow-up, 7% had been readmitted (one third of whom had acute appendicitis), and the rest had diagnosed recurrences of acute nonspecific abdominal pain. Malignancy was found in only 1 of 230 patients, or 4% of patients over the age of 50 years.[29]

Abdominal wall pain is a diagnosis to be considered in patients with acute abdominal pain. Causes to be evaluated include iatrogenic peripheral nerve injuries, hernia, myofascial pain syndromes, the rib tip syndrome, abdominal pain of spinal origin, and spontaneous rectus sheath hematomas.[30]

Each year about 10,000 new spinal cord injury patients are added to the nearly 200,000 paraplegics residing in the United States. Acute abdominal conditions are common but difficult to diagnose in these patients. One excellent review of 21 such patients found that the interval between the spinal cord injury and hospitalization for the acute abdominal complaint averaged 15 years. The average patient was 43 years old. Diseases most commonly seen were acute cholecystitis (36%), perforated peptic ulcer (14%),

Table 54-5. ACUTE ABDOMINAL PAIN ASSOCIATIONS IN THE IMMUNOCOMPROMISED PATIENT

CYTOMEGALOVIRUS INFECTION

Interstitial pneumonitis
Mononucleosis
Pancreatitis
Hepatitis
Cholecystitis
Gastrointestinal ulceration

PANCREATITIS

Steroids
Azathioprine
Cytomegalovirus
Pentamidine

HEPATITIS

Hepatitis A, B, and C
Cytomegalovirus
Epstein-Barr virus

CHOLECYSTITIS

Cytomegalovirus
Acalculous cholecystitis
Campylobacter

HEPATOSPLENIC ABSCESS

Fungal
Mycobacterial
Protozoal
Splenic rupture

BOWEL PERFORATION

Lymphoma, leukemia (especially after chemotherapy)
Cytomegalovirus
Colon ulcers
Kaposi sarcoma
Pseudomembranous colitis
Mycobacteria
Iatrogenic

ACUTE GRAFT-VERSUS-HOST DISEASE
PSEUDOACUTE ABDOMEN
FECAL IMPACTION
STANDARD ABDOMINAL PROCESSES

Appendicitis
Cholecystitis
Diverticulitis
Bowel obstruction
Ulcer disease
Pelvic inflammatory disease
Perirectal abscess
Urinary tract infection
Lymphadenitis

NEUTROPENIC ENTEROCOLITIS

and renal disease (9%). Physical examination was frequently not helpful. Leukocytosis was seen in 57%, and radiologic studies (plain radiographs, CT scans, oral cholecystograms, sonograms, and barium studies) led to the correct diagnosis in 77% of cases. The overall mortality rate was 10%, and there was a 38% operative morbidity rate.[31]

Acute abdominal pain in the patient on oral anticoagulation is another difficult clinical situation. In a recent review of 51 patients with this presentation from the literature,[32] nausea and vomiting were seen in 78%, fever occurred in 29%, and decreased bowel sounds were present in 76% of patients. The most common diagnosis was intramural hematoma of the bowel (86% of all patients). Most hematomas (67%) were found in the jejunum; the

next most common site was the ileum (28%). Other diagnoses reported were bowel infarction in 6% of patients, volvulus in 4%, and miscellaneous causes in 6%. The overall mortality rate was 14%. The challenge for the surgeon is to differentiate patients with intramural hematoma from the minority of patients who will require surgery. Laparotomy or laparoscopy is recommended for patients who fail to improve or who worsen over a 24- to 36-hour observation period.

APPENDIX

Appendectomy is the most common surgical procedure performed on an emergency basis in Western medicine.[33] Appendicitis significantly affects productivity because it reduces the work force by virtue of its impact on a relatively young, healthy segment of the population. The negative appendectomy rate is about 22% to 26% in broad-based reviews. The perforation rate is as low as 3.6% in a subset of young males, but it is significantly higher in the elderly population.[34] Some authors have advocated a norm using a negative appendectomy rate of 15% while attempting to maintain the perforation rate below 15%.[35] Acceptance of a higher negative appendectomy rate allows for a lower rate of perforation. A perforated appendix requiring antibiotic therapy is the major cause of prolonged hospital stays with appendicitis. The most common causes of abdominal pain when a negative appendectomy is done are gynecologic in nature. Appendicitis is difficult to diagnose in the elderly (older than 60 years) and the very young (younger than 3 years) because of other abdominal pathologies that mimic appendicitis and because of the lack of specific symptoms. Decreased dietary fiber, decreased water intake, familial history, or infection may predispose the patient to develop appendicitis.[36] The morbidity rate is about 15% to 20% in most reports of appendicitis, with wound infection from a gangrenous or perforated appendix being the most common complication. Perioperative antibiotic therapy has greatly improved the morbidity rate of appendicitis, but perforation of the appendix is not prevented by antibiotics; nor has the incidence of perforation been reduced in the United States in recent years.

History

In 1889, Fitz described the sequence of appendiceal inflammation, perforation, abscess formation, and peritonitis.[37,38] Since the initial descriptions of the pathophysiology of appendicitis, appendectomy has remained one of the most common abdominal surgeries performed on an urgent basis. In addition to acute appendicitis, carcinoid tumors, and neuromas of the appendix,[39,40] mucoceles caused by epithelial tumors with appendiceal distention[41] and a variety of other appendiceal abnormalities have been described. By far the most common etiology of appendicitis is luminal obstruction resulting in inflammation and eventual suppuration.

Anatomists have questioned the purpose of the appendix since its initial description. Leonardo da Vinci considered the appendix to serve and protect the cecum from rupture by too great an accumulation of "superfluous wind" because it had the ability to dilate and contract.[38,42] Current belief is that the appendix is a vestigial organ with no function in humans. Phylogenetic studies have shown a progressive development of the appendix in anthropoid apes as the primate scale is ascended.[38] In carnivores such as the dog, wolf, tiger, and lion, the appendix is absent. In herbivores, a long and well-developed cecum is observed. In omnivores, which include apes, wombats, and man, a portion of the cecum is smaller in diameter with a prominent lymphoid aggregation susceptible to inflammation or atrophy.[38] The presence of lymphoid aggregates has led to the hypothesis that the appendix has a role in immune surveillance of the gut. Others postulate an exocrine function to assist in the digestion of plants. In a 24-hour period, the adult human appendix produces a maximum of 2 mL of fluid containing mucin, amylase, and proteolytic enzymes. It is implausible that this volume aids substantially in the digestion of plant material presented to the colon. A pressure gradient normally exists along the long axis of the appendix with 10 mmHg of intraluminal pressure at the distal tip and 5 mmHg at the base, thus prohibiting the entrance of food material into the lumen of the appendix. Lymphoid nodules with substantial populations of both B cells and T cells are found in the lamina propria of the appendix, differentiating it from the colon.[43] The lymphoid aggregates have morphologic features similar to those of the Peyer patches of the gut-associated lymphoid tissue.[33] Some hypothesize that the appendix is not a vestigial organ but may have a function similar to that of the thymus or bursa of Fabricius.[38] The role of the appendix remains controversial, but its unique lymphoid aggregations and its location differentiate it from the colon or cecum.

Anatomy

The appendix develops from the cecal diverticulum of the fetus. At 6 weeks' gestation, the cecal primordium begins as a conical outpouching along the antimesenteric border of the caudal limb of the midgut loop. The appendix is delineated during the fifth month of gestation when the apex of the cecal outpouching does not enlarge as rapidly as the rest of the cecum. Variable positions of the appendix occur when the cecum and appendix are displaced downward into the right iliac fossa as the proximal colon enlarges. During colonic elongation, the appendix localizes either posterior to the cecum (retrocecal) or posterior to the colon (retrocolic), or it may descend over the brim of the pelvis (pelvic or descending). About 64% of the population have the appendix located retrocecally, and 31% have the appendix located over the pelvic brim.[44] The appendix elongates by birth, and the cecal wall enlarges unequally after birth, causing the appendix to be located

posteromedially. Delayed diagnosis of appendicitis has been attributed to unusual anatomic positions. Gangrene and perforation of the appendix have been reported in 69% of patients who had either a delayed presentation of symptoms or diagnosis when the appendix was located in the true pelvis, behind the ileum or ileocolic mesentery, or retrocolic or retroperitoneal.

The appendiceal length varies from 2 to 20 cm and averages 9 cm. Children have longer appendices that might atrophy during adulthood. The three taeniae coli of the ascending colon consolidate at the base of the appendix with the anterior taenia serving as a landmark when traced along the anterior cecum. The appendix is connected to the lower aspect of the ileal mesentery by the mesoappendix. The main appendicular artery is a branch of the ileocolic artery that courses behind the ileum, through the mesoappendix, and along the appendiceal wall until it reaches the tip of the organ. The appendicular artery courses along the free border of the mesoappendix until it reaches the distal appendix, at which time it lies along the wall of the appendix (Fig. 54-2). During acute inflammation, the appendicular artery becomes susceptible to thrombosis as the appendix becomes enlarged.

The lymphatics draining the appendix include vessels from the body and tip of the appendix that drain posteriorly into the upper and lower ileocolic nodes. The lymph vessels from the base of the appendix drain to the anterior ileocolic lymph nodes. The lymph nodes along the ileocolic chain may be hyperplastic during appendicitis.

The neural innervation of the appendix is from the autonomic nervous system, without any direct innervation from pain fibers. The absence of pain fibers as with other viscera, explains the lack of localized symptoms until an inflamed appendix irritates the peritoneum. The sympathetic nerve supply originates from the superior mesenteric plexus, whereas the parasympathetic innervation arises from the vagus nerve. The submucosal plexus and the myenteric plexus are spread irregularly through the appendix on histologic examination.[38]

The orifice of the appendix opens to the cecum with a semilunar mucosal fold forming a valve. In the adult, the lumen may be partially or entirely obliterated, but the average luminal width is between 0.5 and 1 cm. The base of the appendix is normally located at about the level of the

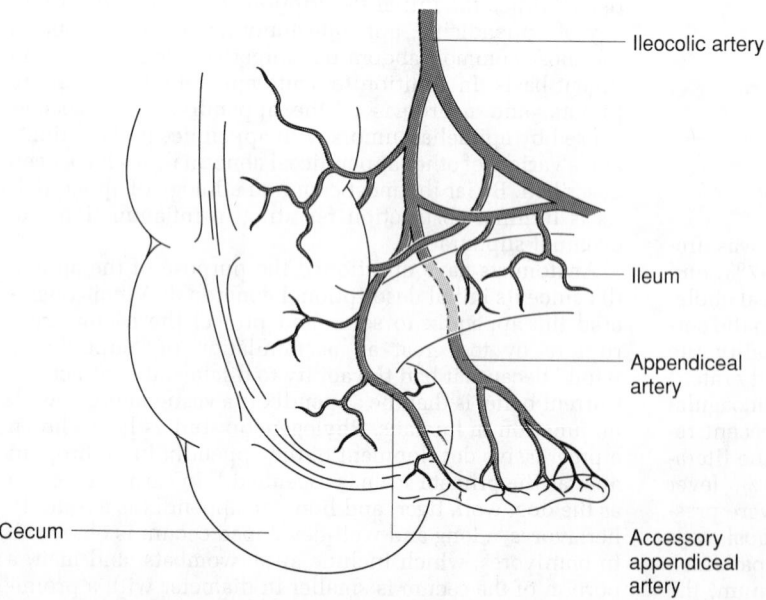

Figure 54-2. Anatomy of and blood supply to the appendix.

S-1 vertebral body, at the McBurney point. The serosa covers the entire appendix, with longitudinal muscle fibers forming an almost complete layer immediately beneath this. At the base, the longitudinal muscles form rudimentary taeniae continuous with the taeniae coli of the colon. A layer of circular muscle forms a thicker inner layer. The submucosa contains lymphoid tissue that may hypertrophy and obstruct the lumen during acute appendicitis. Finally, the appendix is lined throughout by a mucosal luminal surface. The mucosa has features similar to those of the colon, but lymphoid tissue is concentrated more densely, resembling the ileum.

The subepithelial layer contains neurosecretory cells that increase in number in older patients. With the use of lead staining, few neurosecretory cells are visualized in appendices of children up to the age of 9 years. As the age of the patient increases, more neurosecretory cells are observed in the submucosa.[46] This finding correlates with an age-related increase in the number of carcinoid tumors as the number of neurosecretory cells increases.

Pathophysiology

The most common cause of appendicitis is obstruction of the appendiceal lumen. In young children and young adults, the most common cause of luminal obstruction is lymphoid hyperplasia from the submucosal follicles, which are abundant. The pathogenesis is controversial and likely multifactorial, but dehydration and viral infections have been hypothesized as causes of lymphoid hyperplasia. In older adults, fecaliths are one cause of luminal obstruction that may be visible on abdominal radiographs including the right lower quadrant or the pelvic area. Luminal obstruction of the appendix causes an increase in mucus production. Bacteria are trapped in the distal appendix in relatively high concentrations because of the relation to the right side of the colon. Bacterial overgrowth from stasis and luminal obstruction causes eventual dilatation of the appendix. As the appendix enlarges, venous and lymphatic flow are compromised, causing further dilatation of the appendix. Venous hypertension and luminal distention contribute to increased appendiceal wall tension according to the Laplace law, wherein wall tension is proportional to the thickness of the wall divided by the radius squared. With increasing wall tension, blood flow is eventually compromised and diminishes most acutely to the distal appendix (flow = pressure/resistance). The decrease in arterial blood flow may cause vessel thrombosis with necrosis of the appendiceal wall (Fig. 54-3). When full-thickness necrosis occurs, perforation of the appendix takes place, and its fecal and suppurative contents are released into the abdominal cavity. Peritoneal irritation occurs, with appendiceal abscess formation or generalized peritonitis occurring if the enteric spill is large.

Lymphoid hyperplasia has a peak incidence during the teenage years, correlating well with the higher incidence of acute appendicitis at this age. Gastroenteritis involving infectious agents such as *Shigella* and *Salmonella* is associated with lymphoid follicle hyperplasia and acute appendicitis. Other systemic diseases such as upper respiratory infections, infectious mononucleosis, and measles have been shown to cause a generalized lymphoid hyperplasia in the appendix. Lymphoid hyperplasia accounts for 60% of acute appendicitis and occurs mainly in the young.

In adults, fecalith formation accounts for about 30% of acute appendicitis. The formation of an appendiceal fecalith begins with the random entrapment of vegetable fiber, with deposition of mucus causing eventual concretion of the mucus entrapment. Multiple layers of concretions

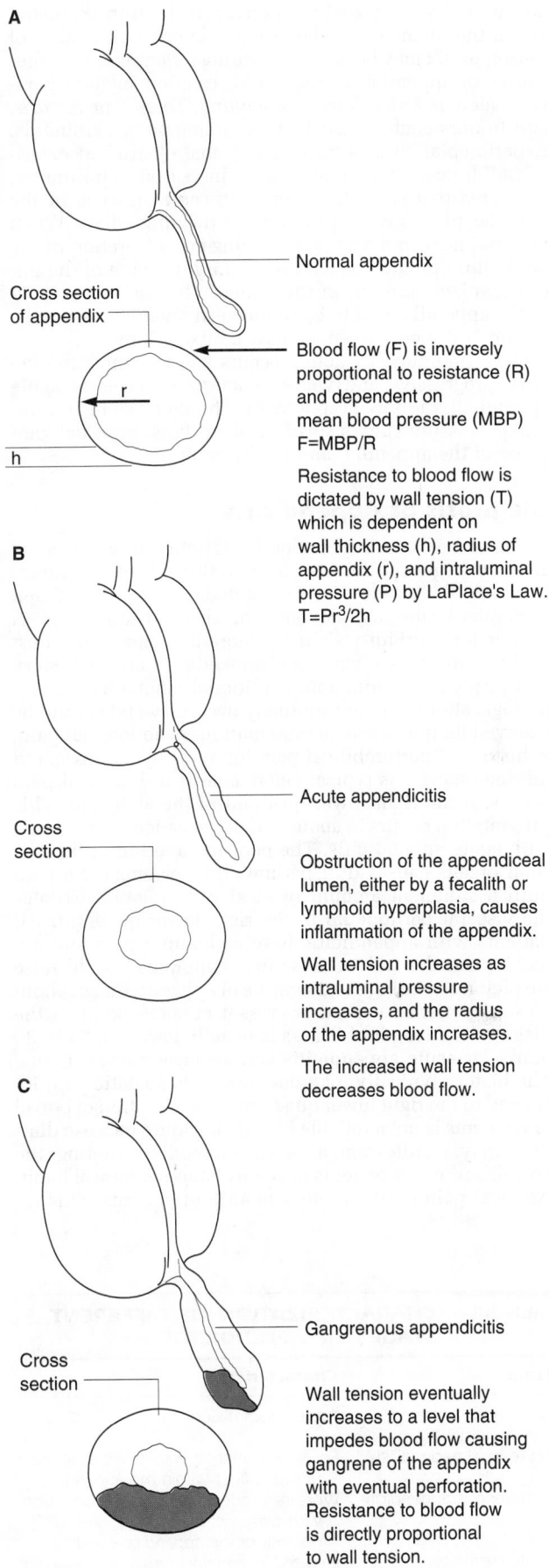

Figure 54-3. Pathophysiologic stages of appendicitis.

are formed with a gradual increase in fecalith diameter. When the diameter reaches 1 cm or more, obstruction of the appendix may occur with ensuing inflammation. Other causes of appendiceal luminal obstruction include parasites such as *Enterobius vermicularis*, *Taenia*, or *Ascaris*, and tumors such as cecal adenocarcinoma or carcinoids. Experimental studies have shown that obstructed exteriorized human appendices have increased intraluminal pressures that can exceed the perfusion pressure in the vascular plexus within the wall of the appendix.[47] When mucosal ischemia occurs, sloughing and ulceration of the epithelium progresses with secondary invasion of the microorganisms present in the lumen. The bacteria present in the appendix tend to be commensal organisms from the cecum and therefore encompass a mixed flora.

Once luminal obstruction occurs and inflammation begins, progressive and well-characterized stages of acute appendicitis follow (Table 54-6). The increase in intraluminal pressure causes stasis of blood flow, eventual gangrene of the appendix, and finally rupture.

Diagnosis of Appendicitis

The aim of reducing appendiceal rupture is achieved by an early diagnosis. Because the mortality rate of appendicitis is low (0.6% when nonperforated, less than 5% when perforated), the consequence of delayed diagnosis is greater for morbidity than for mortality rates. The most useful tools in the diagnosis of appendicitis are the history and physical examination. Additional laboratory and radiologic studies are not routinely necessary and should be reserved for questionable presentations of abdominal pain. A history of periumbilical pain followed by anorexia and minimal nausea is typical before emesis or localized pain occurs in the right lower quadrant of the abdomen. This presentation occurs in about half of the patients presenting with acute appendicitis. The poor innervation of the visceral organs causes dull periumbilical or epigastric pain until a sufficient amount of local inflammation irritates the visceral peritoneum in the right lower quadrant. All patients with appendicitis have abdominal pain and anorexia, and the lack of these two symptoms should raise suspicion regarding the diagnosis of appendicitis. In about 90% of patients, nausea is present at some point in the history. The length of illness is usually less than 24 to 36 hours for acute appendicitis and averages several hours. The history typically includes crescendo somatic pain localized to the right lower quadrant. The alteration of bowel movements is not a reliable historical feature because diarrhea may result from a pelvic appendix irritating the bowel, and many patients have no changes in bowel habit. Atypical pain occurs in 40% to 45% of patients. This in-

cludes patients who present with localized right lower quadrant pain immediately and those with diffuse periumbilical pain. These patients tend to be elderly or those who are taking antibiotics that mask the symptoms.

The physical examination will generally distinguish appendicitis from other abdominal pathologies. Right lower quadrant pain on palpation is typically present and involves guarding with peritoneal irritation upon percussion. Simple movement of the bed usually elicits right lower quadrant pain. Other physical signs associated with appendicitis include the initiation of pain in the right lower quadrant during palpation of the left lower quadrant (Rovsing sign), increased pain with coughing (Dunphy sign), pain on internal rotation of the hip (obturator sign), and pain during extension of the right hip (iliopsoas sign). All result from parietal peritoneal inflammation and somatic pain. The iliopsoas sign is typical of a retrocecal appendix, whereas the obturator sign suggests a pelvic appendix. During a rectal examination or pelvic examination, focal tenderness is elicited more on the right side, but palpation of a tender mass is indicative of a pelvic abscess.

Laboratory and Radiologic Diagnosis

The cost-effectiveness of various tests has come under great scrutiny. When the history and physical examination are definitive, no other investigation is required. The review that follows is applicable to patients when the diagnosis is not initially clear. After the history and physical examination, a white blood cell (WBC) count with a peripheral smear is helpful. About two thirds of patients with appendicitis present with an elevated WBC count (more than 10,000 WBC/mL), whereas fever is absent in most cases. Elderly patients with appendicitis tend to have normal WBC counts, but fewer than 4% to 5% will have a normal differential count of WBCs. Almost 95% of patients with acute appendicitis present with a predominance of polymorphonuclear leukocytes and relative lymphopenia. A urinalysis is commonly obtained in the emergency room when the diagnosis of appendicitis is entertained. In one study, an abnormal urinalysis was discovered in 48% of patients with acute appendicitis before appendectomy. This remained abnormal in 12% on postoperative day 6.[48] Hematuria, pyuria, and proteinuria are frequently found in patients with acute appendicitis. These findings should not necessarily lead the surgeon away from the initial diagnosis suspected from the history and physical examination.

Radiologic examinations should be used in questionable cases. Abdominal radiographs are rarely useful in children, but in adults, fecaliths may occasionally be visualized along with a paucity of gas in the right lower quadrant of the abdomen (Fig. 54-4). A perforated or gangrenous appendix may exhibit extraluminal gas on radiographs, but this occurs in only 1% of cases. Loss of the right psoas shadow usually represents late appendicitis with retroperitoneal inflammation.

Ultrasonography

Recent developments in the technique and interpretation of ultrasonography have made this a valuable adjunct to physical examination in young women and in patients with atypical symptoms. Graded abdominal compression is used to displace the cecum and ascending colon, exposing retrocecal and pelvic locations. A typical target appearance identifies the appendix by characteristic reflecting properties of wall elements (Fig. 54-5). Findings associated with appendicitis include wall thickening beyond the normal 8 to 10 mm, luminal distention, and a lack of compressibility. The visualized appendix usually

---

Table 54-6. CHARACTERIZATION OF DIFFERENT STAGES OF APPENDICITIS

Stage	Characteristics
Acute nonperforated appendicitis	Acute inflammation
Acute focal appendicitis	Focal inflammation with localized abscess of mixed flora within the appendix
Gangrenous appendicitis	Worsening edema with arterial occlusion with persistent infection causing necrosis of the appendiceal wall
Acute perforated appendicitis	Elevated intraluminal pressure leading to perforation through the gangrenous portion of the appendix

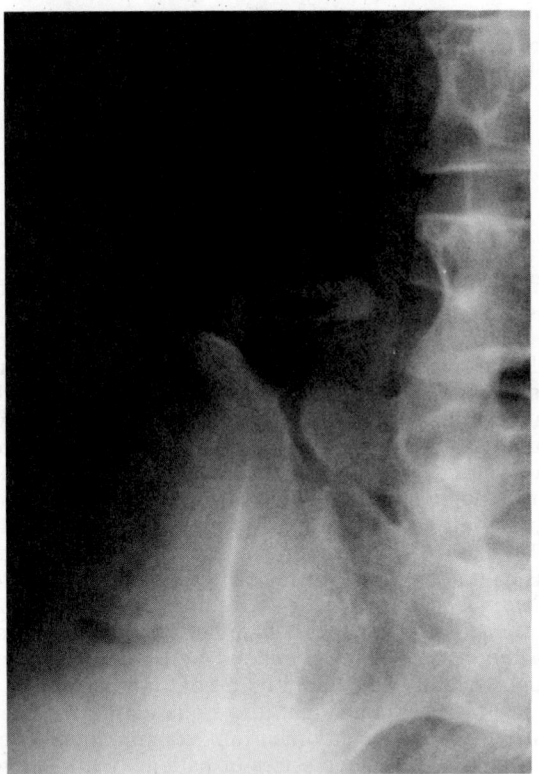

Figure 54-4. Appendicolith as seen on abdominal radiograph.

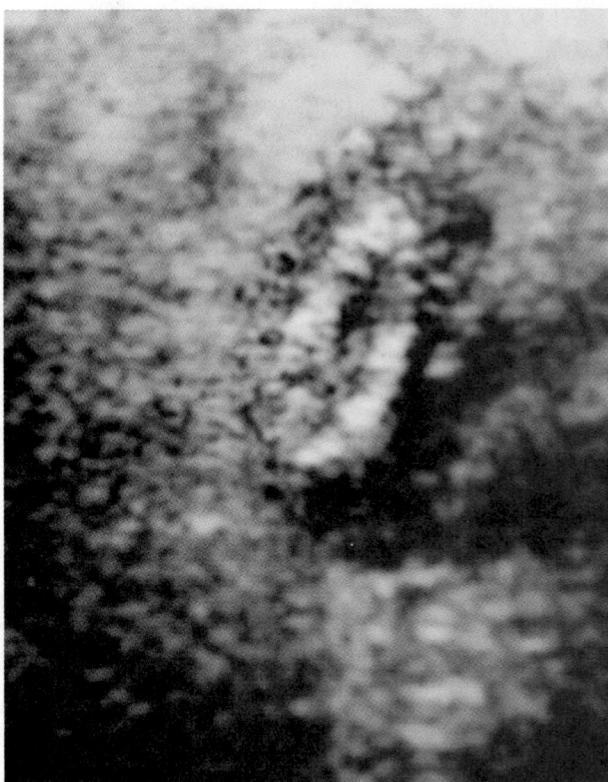

Figure 54-5. Target appearance of an acutely inflamed appendix as seen on ultrasound scan.

coincides with the site of localized pain and tenderness. Advanced appendicitis is indicated sonographically by asymmetric wall thickening, abscess formation, associated free intraperitoneal fluid, surrounding tissue edema, and decreased local tenderness to compression. Marked wall thickening without distention is present in Crohn's disease of the appendix, often in association with ileal or cecal disease. Rare findings, such as appendiceal neoplasms and mucoceles, may also be well visualized. Ultrasonography is critically operator dependent, and care must be taken to avoid overinterpreting a technically inadequate examination. With this caveat, the sensitivity of ultrasound in the diagnosis of appendicitis from several centers has been reported in excess of 80%, with a specificity of 90%.

Computed Tomography

Recent refinements in resolution to the 0.5- to 1-cm range have improved the accuracy of CT imaging in detecting the nature and extent of abdominal disease. This has been most useful in patients presenting with obscure inflammatory processes of the abdomen in whom the diagnosis of appendicitis is not foremost. In the specific evaluation of atypical patients for possible appendicitis, the CT examination should be considered only if ultrasound is unavailable or unrevealing for technical reasons, most commonly in cases of gaseous abdominal distention. The risks of radiation exposure must be considered, particularly in young, potentially pregnant women.

The normal appendix may be difficult to locate on CT examinations not specifically focused on this question. Variability of appendiceal location, surrounding fat, and scan quality may require extra scans at finer intervals (Fig. 54-6). Appendicoliths are seen in one fourth of all people as a ringlike or homogeneous calcific density on CT. This sensitivity is much higher than that of plain abdominal radiographs. Specific CT findings of appendicitis become

more prominent with advanced disease. They include a distended, thick-walled, edematous appendix seen as a target structure, inflammatory streaking of surrounding fat, and the presence of an appendicolith (Fig. 54-7). Early appendicitis may be impossible to distinguish from the normal appendix, but this is true of all modalities, including direct visual inspection. CT findings suggestive of appendicitis include a pericecal phlegmon or abscess, and

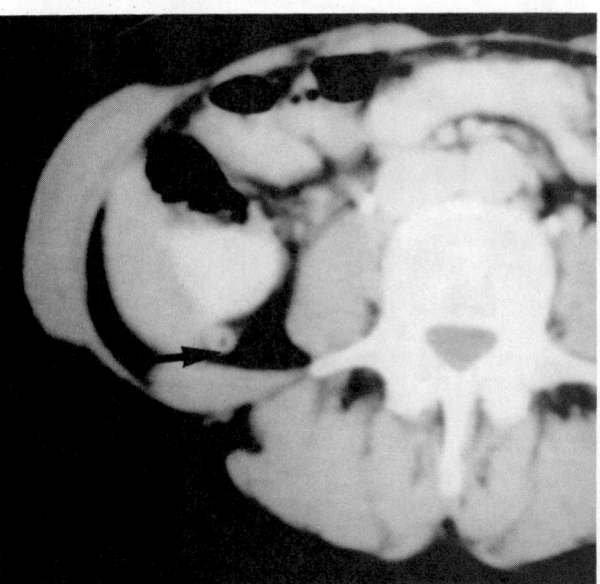

Figure 54-6. CT appearance of a normal appendix (*arrow*).

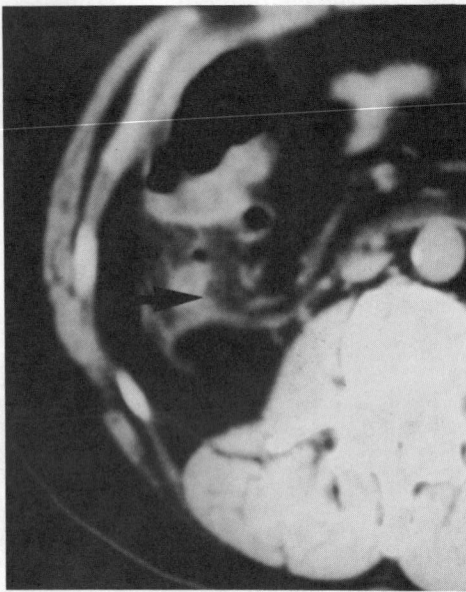

Figure 54-7. CT appearance of early acute appendicitis with edema and loss of water–fat interface.

small amounts of right lower quadrant intraabdominal free air that signal perforation (Fig. 54-8). Other processes, such as cecal diverticulitis and perforated cecal carcinoma, may create a similar appearance. In the patient presenting with an appendiceal mass, CT is useful in planning nonoperative management. A phlegmon responsive to antibiotic treatment can be distinguished from abscesses that may require drainage. Nonappendiceal causes of lower abdominal pain can frequently be defined. A 90% sensitivity for detecting intraabdominal inflammation has been reported for CT scanning, and in 80% of these patients a specific diagnosis can be made.

Barium Contrast Studies

Historically, single-contrast barium enema in the unprepared patient has been used for the diagnosis of atypical appendicitis. This remains a simple, safe, and readily available test that has strong proponents. Generally, however, ultrasound and CT examinations are preferred. A barium study allows for the following:

- Assessment of luminal patency of the appendix
- Examination of the colonic wall for mass effects or secondary effects of appendicitis
- Diagnosis of right colonic or terminal ileal mucosal disease that may simulate appendicitis

When barium contrast fills the appendix, appendicitis is unlikely but not impossible. Up to 10% to 20% of normal appendices do not fill during barium study. Partial filling of the appendix with appendicitis at the tip and appendicitis that develops without luminal obstruction are potential causes of a false-negative study. Some information can be gleaned from such studies, however, because even with luminal patency the mucosal defect usually leads to irregularity that can be outlined by barium. Cecal indentation by an inflammatory appendiceal mass or extravasation of barium from a site of perforation may also be evident (Figs. 54-9 and 54-10). Right colon mucosal changes due to infectious colitis *(Yersinia enterocolitica; Salmonella, Shigella,* or *Campylobacter* sp; or the toxigenic effects of *Escherichia coli* 0157:H7), idiopathic inflammatory bowel disease, or cecal neoplasms may be defined by a barium study, although severe, toxic colitis is a contraindication to any contrast study. Not all right lower quadrant inflammatory conditions are detected on barium examination, however. For example, in a large series of patients with equivocal presentations, 40% of barium studies were also equivocal. Barium enema complements ultrasound and CT examinations in defining mucosal lesions of the cecum and appendix. It should be considered in settings of chronic or recurrent abdominal pain. It should be used for acute appendicitis when the diagnosis is suspected but unclear and when both CT and ultrasound are not helpful.

Treatment

Laparoscopy

If the diagnosis of appendicitis is unclear, laparoscopy may be very helpful to rule out appendicitis while also examining for gynecologic pathologies. Recent series reported a confirmation of acute appendicitis in 59% of pa-

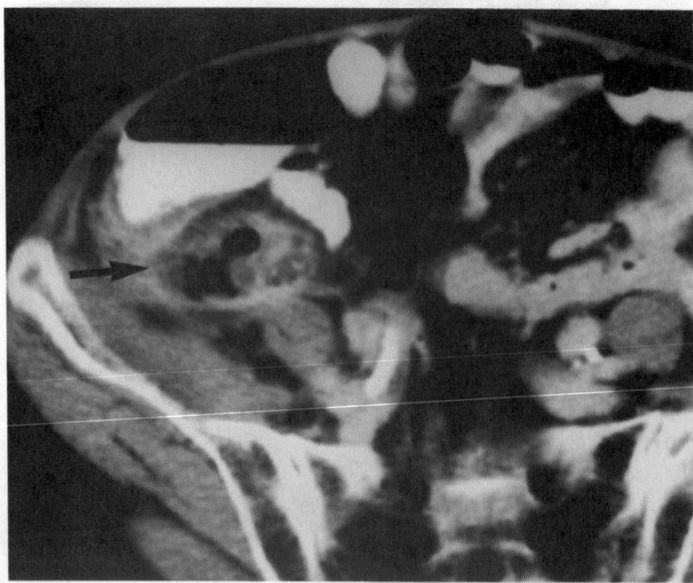

Figure 54-8. CT appearance of appendicitis with perforation and abscess formation.

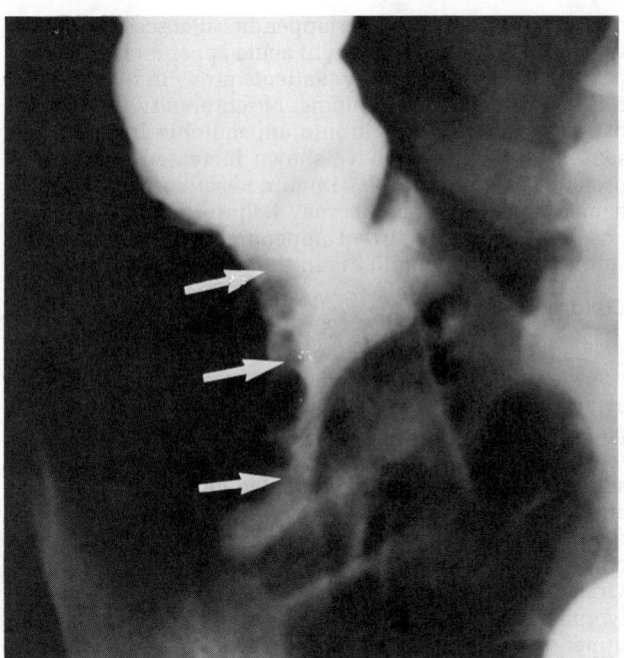

Figure 54-9. Barium enema showing an appendiceal mass indenting the cecum.

tients who presented with right lower quadrant symptoms, whereas 35% of females with a diagnosis of suspected appendicitis had gynecologic pathology noted by laparoscopy.[48] Some have advocated diagnostic laparoscopy in all females presenting with symptoms of acute appendicitis to reduce unnecessary appendectomy. Laparoscopy can be either diagnostic or therapeutic for acute appendicitis. Each approach has its advocates.[49] The benefits of laparoscopic appendectomy include decreased postoperative pain, a better cosmetic outcome, and a more rapid return to full activities. Some of the disadvantages of laparoscopic appendectomy include a slightly increased operative time, possibly increased cost, and increased postoperative emesis.[50]

Laparotomy

The standard management of appendicitis remains open appendectomy by way of a limited right lower quadrant incision. Before the induction of anesthesia, the surgeon should note the point of maximal tenderness. While the patient is under anesthesia, masses should be palpated if possible. The McBurney point (at the junction of the middle and lateral thirds of a line drawn from the umbilicus to the right anterosuperior iliac spine) does not universally mark the tip of the appendix, and palpation without the patient guarding may be useful in placing the incision. In general, an inferior incision below the maximal tender area will help in rotating the cecum into the wound. Various skin incisions have been described to give maximal exposure. The McBurney incision is the classical oblique appendectomy incision through the McBurney point to the lateral edge of the rectus sheath. Alternatively, a skin line or transverse incision placed 1 to 2 cm medial to the anterosuperior iliac spine is used. All are generally performed with a muscle-splitting technique through all layers lateral to the rectus abdominis muscle as entrance into the abdomen is gained.

A low horizontal skin incision also improves the postoperative appearance in young patients. The incision is continued through the superficial fascia until the external oblique muscle aponeurosis is exposed. The fibers of the aponeurosis are opened sharply, and the muscle fibers themselves are bluntly separated, as are the fibers of the internal oblique and transversus abdominis muscles. The peritoneum is incised, and cultures can be obtained to help direct antibiotic therapy postoperatively for ruptured appendices. The base of the appendix always lies at the confluence of all three taeniae. The cecum is mobilized into the wound, and the appendix is mobilized into the wound as adhesions are bluntly dissected. Ligation of the mesoappendix is usually performed from the distal tip to the base of the appendix. In some difficult cases involving a long appendix, reversing the ligation of the mesoappendix can facilitate appendectomy. The appendiceal stump is usually cauterized to prevent mucocele formation. The appendiceal stump may be inverted with a pursestring suture in the cecum or by placing a Z-stitch. Copious irrigation with saline should be performed in cases of perforated appendicitis to prevent formation of a pelvic or subhepatic abscess. The peritoneum and muscular fasciae are usually closed with a running absorbable suture. The skin can be closed in nonperforated cases of appendicitis, and delayed primary closure is routine in cases of ruptured appendicitis.

If a normal appendix is encountered during appendectomy, the terminal ileum and pelvic structures (ie, ovaries, fallopian tubes, uterus) need to be visualized to rule out other surgically treatable problems. Meckel's diverticulum may exist in the terminal ileum of the young, whereas Crohn's disease of the terminal ileum may be discovered in any age group. If a normal appendix is seen, but Crohn's disease affects the terminal ileum, an appendectomy is still warranted and will not affect the rate of fistula formation.[51]

Nonoperative Treatment

If a distinct mass in the right iliac fossa is palpated at presentation and the patient has no systemic manifestations such as fever or clinical peritonitis, a nonoperative approach can be undertaken.[38] This approach was popularized before modern antibiotics became available. It is safe

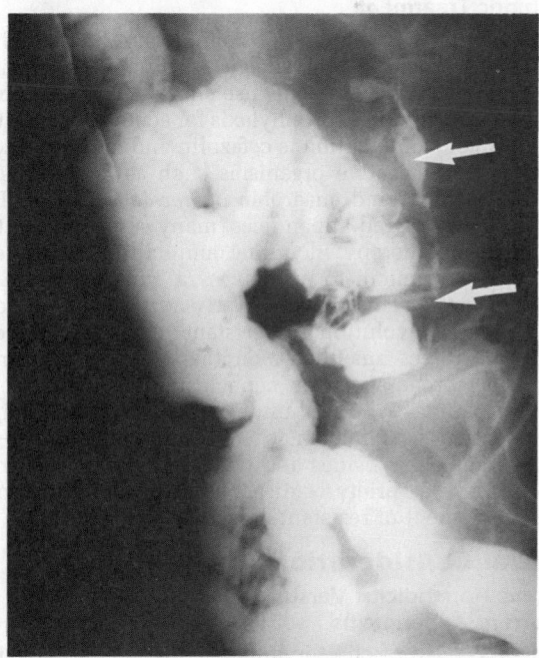

Figure 54-10. Barium enema showing a retrocecal appendix with perforation and extravasation of barium.

to remove the appendix with antibiotic coverage in virtually any patient. However, this is periodically a useful approach in the nontoxic patient with a clear diagnosis of an appendiceal abscess. The patient is fasted with this approach while intravenous fluids are administered. Broad-spectrum antibiotics are given to cover enteric organisms while the pulse is closely followed, because tachycardia is one of the first signs that conservative therapy is not benefiting the patient. Increasing pain, progressive tachycardia, and failure to respond after 24 to 48 hours require operative intervention. Periappendiceal abscesses usually resolve in 10 to 14 days without appendectomy or drainage. With modern-day CT, patients with well-formed periappendiceal abscesses can undergo CT-guided placement of pigtail drainage catheters to help resolve the abscess more rapidly, rather than depending on the abscess to drain internally into the cecum. If the abscess is palpable, it is often best to externally drain it percutaneously, although this remains an issue that demands clinical judgment. Limitations of percutaneous drainage include the inadequacy of draining multiloculated abscesses, inaccessible locations, and the possible need for general anesthesia in young patients. This approach is virtually always followed by an interval appendectomy. If symptoms of pain and abscess persist after a catheter drainage procedure, formal surgical drainage with appendectomy may be warranted and is safe.

Interval Appendectomy

Most surgeons wait about 6 weeks to 3 months after the nonoperative treatment of a perforated appendix to perform an interval appendectomy. Technical difficulties during interval appendectomy range from severe to minimal, depending on the nature of the initial abscess. The primary benefit, however, is that the operation is conducted in the absence of frank purulence. No adequate prospective trials have been performed examining the necessity for interval appendectomy after appendiceal rupture, but it remains standard practice. Prospective studies in children have shown that percutaneous catheter drainage is beneficial, but it has not been reported whether recurrence of appendicitis is a common entity after appendiceal rupture.

Antibiotic Treatment

The patient with appendicitis should not be rushed to the operating room without adequate hydration and antibiotic treatment. Most surgeons use short-course (less than 24 hours) antimicrobial prophylaxis for acute appendicitis. One common combination is cefazolin and metronidazole to cover gram-negative organisms such as *E coli*, gram-positive bacteria, and anaerobic *Bacteroides fragilis*. For presumably ruptured appendices, many surgeons use triple antibiotic therapy including ampicillin, metronidazole, and gentamicin to encompass a wide spectrum of enteric bacteria. This may be overly aggressive and contribute to the evolution of resistant organisms. Recent studies have recommended monotherapy with a second-generation, broad-spectrum cephalosporin such as cefotetan for patients who will undergo surgery as the definitive treatment.[52] Cefotetan is economical and effective, whereas aminoglycosides and other more potent antimicrobials have a variety of disadvantages, including cost, the development of resistant organisms, and toxicity.

Special Considerations
Chronic Appendicitis Versus Recurrent Appendicitis

The existence of chronic appendicitis is controversial. Various authors have described chronic right lower quadrant pain or recurrence of mild symptoms.[38] Some patients may have symptoms of periappendiceal abscess, cecal diverticular disease, or recurrent acute appendicitis that appear to indicate chronicity. Patients prone to recurrent fecaliths may have symptoms of chronicity, but these patients do not have chronic appendicitis in the truest sense. Recent studies have shown increased numbers of protein gene product 9.5 immunoreactive nerves in inflamed appendices.[53] This may help to definitively diagnose chronically recurrent appendicitis as well as more subtle cases of appendicitis in the future.

Children

The diagnosis of appendicitis is difficult in young children for the obvious reasons that an accurate history of symptoms is not provided by the patient and abdominal pain from other causes is common. In early childhood, nausea, vomiting, and abdominal tenderness are frequent signs of extraabdominal disease. Meningitis, otitis media, and pneumonia should be specifically excluded. Older children have different diagnostic alternatives to appendicitis. The vomiting and voluminous diarrhea common in viral gastroenteritis are rare in appendicitis. Mesenteric lymphadenitis is usually associated with an antecedent upper respiratory tract viral prodrome, as in Henoch-Schönlein purpura. The latter classically has the associated findings of purpuric skin lesions, arthritis, and nephritis. Intussusception is most common in children younger than 2 or 3 years of age before appendicitis becomes common. Vomiting and episodic abdominal pain that is not localized suggest the diagnosis of intussusception in this age group. Together with findings of an elongated tender abdominal mass and guaiac-positive stool, the diagnosis of intussusception can be clear on the basis of history and physical examination. Primary peritonitis is not rare in children, particularly prepubertal females. It is almost invariably mistaken for acute appendicitis. Typhlitis, acute cecal inflammation, must be considered in the neutropenic patient with progressive right abdominal tenderness. This focal form of neutropenic colitis may be associated with pneumatosis intestinalis of the cecal wall, and this finding helps differentiate the disease from appendicitis. In the profoundly neutropenic patient with right lower quadrant tenderness, the mainstay of treatment is systemic antibiotic administration until the neutropenia is resolved. Surgical exploration is associated with extraordinary mortality in these patients.

Younger children who cannot give histories tend to present to the emergency department multiple times and eventually are given the diagnosis of appendicitis when gangrene or perforation occurs.[54] In most contemporary reviews of childhood appendicitis, the perforation rate is about 50%. In one study, 34% of children (54 of 158 patients) with appendicitis during the first 3 years of life presented with an appendiceal mass. For this subgroup of very young children, complication rates may be reduced and hospital stays shortened if the appendiceal mass is managed nonoperatively.[55]

Congenital Abnormalities. Rare reports of congenital appendiceal abnormalities have been published. These include agenesis and differing degrees of hypoplasia as described by Collins.[38,56] Other congenital abnormalities totaling about 100 cases include appendix multiplex and horseshoe anomalies of the appendix. The classification of appendix multiplex[57] involves Wallbridge's type A anomaly (a single-based appendix with varying degrees of partial appendiceal duplication arising from a single cecum); a type B anomaly (consisting of two distinct appendixes arising from a single cecum); and a type C anomaly (containing a double cecum, each with its own separate appendix and associated with genitourinary or other hindgut abnormalities).[38]

Elderly Pateints

Elderly patients with appendicitis have higher morbidity and mortality rates than the rest of the population because of the delay in presentation of symptoms and the delay in diagnosis. A higher incidence of perforated appendicitis occurs in the elderly, but unlike young children, the elderly have much less reserve when challenged with peritonitis. These patients may have fewer complaints of pain compared with young adults, and the pain may be described as a dull right lower quadrant pain. Furthermore, localization to the right lower quadrant is delayed, and an elevation in the WBC count may be nonexistent. Over 30% of elderly patients have a ruptured appendix at time of surgery. Elderly patients tend to have more medical problems, which causes a delay in the definitive treatment of appendectomy. As a result, more elderly patients die from ruptured appendices because of a delay in surgery or the absence of surgery. The elderly may have a mortality rate in excess of 5% from a perforated appendix, in contrast to a mortality rate of less than 1% in other patients. When a patient older than 60 years of age undergoes an appendectomy, inspection for a coexistent right-sided colon carcinoma should be routine during laparotomy.

Pregnancy

Anatomic and physiologic changes alter the presentation of appendicitis during the second and third trimesters of pregnancy. Abdominal pain, nausea, and vomiting are all common in early pregnancy. Nausea and vomiting may be difficult to distinguish from symptoms due to the pregnancy; however, localizing right lower quadrant tenderness is still a reliable sign of acute appendicitis. After the fifth month of gestation, the appendiceal position—and therefore the site of pain—is shifted superiorly above the right iliac crest, and the appendix tip is rotated medially by the gravid uterus (Fig. 54-11). Abdominal tenderness becomes less localized as distention of the abdomen lifts the peritoneum away from the appendix and cecum. Nevertheless, tenderness remains the most important clinical finding. Fever is less common, and leukocytosis is difficult to interpret given that this is a normal feature of pregnancy. The clinical diagnosis of appendicitis is more difficult at this stage, and ultrasound may be helpful in distinguishing obstetric pathology from appendicitis. If peritoneal signs supervene in late pregnancy, this usually signifies perforation and may have grave consequences. Perforation has been associated with a fetal mortality rate of over 30% and a maternal mortality rate of 1% to 2%. Simple acute appendicitis has a negligible maternal mortality rate, and the risk of fetal loss is about 10%. Urgent exploration should be undertaken once the diagnosis of appendicitis has been made. There is no role for nonoperative management in this setting. A negative laparotomy rate of 15% to 40% resulting from an aggressive approach to this disease is appropriate. Appendicitis remains the most frequent nonobstetric indication for laparotomy during pregnancy.

AIDS Patients

Although patients with AIDS are more susceptible to cytomegalovirus-related bowel perforations, there is no evidence that they have a higher rate of acute suppurative appendicitis.[38] Predictably, however, morbidity and mortality rates are higher for this group of patients, and the diagnosis of acute appendicitis is more difficult because opportunistic infectious agents causing enterocolitis may mimic the disease. Some AIDS patients have presented with primary Kaposi sarcoma of the appendix,[58] which elicits symptoms similar to those of acute appendicitis. When pathology reports after an apparently routine appendectomy show rare opportunistic infections, a workup for AIDS should be entertained.

Incidental Appendectomy

Incidental appendectomy refers to the prophylactic removal of the normal appendix during laparotomy for another condition. The decision to resect the appendix dur-

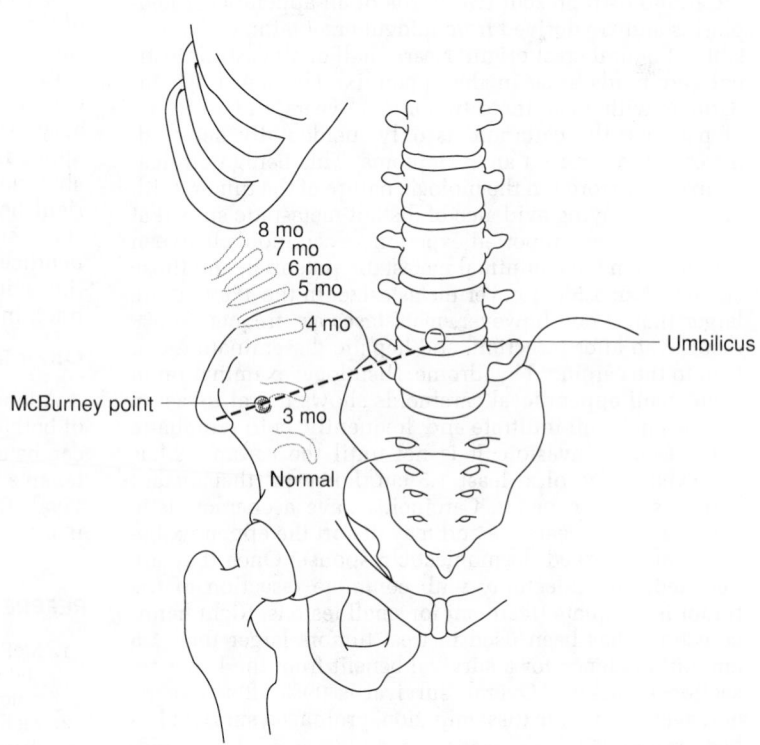

Figure 54-11. Location and orientation of the appendix in pregnancy.

ing another abdominal operation depends on the risk-to-benefit ratio. It requires clinical judgment and remains controversial. Even though removal of the appendix is the most common urgent operation in the Western Hemisphere, most of the population will live a full life with a normal appendix. It is estimated that 100 to 115 incidental appendectomies must be performed, without complications or death, to prevent one needed appendectomy in the elderly. Some suggest that incidental appendectomies can be safely performed in patients younger than 60 years of age. Incidental appendectomies are controversial in a child or an adult, but they are clearly not indicated in the elderly. The argument in favor of incidental appendectomy is that it is cost-effective in terms of reducing the morbidity of an additional surgery, reducing hospitalization, and eliminating possible perforation in the future.

Several studies have looked at incidental appendectomies in the adult population. In trauma patients undergoing laparotomy, incidental appendectomy does not affect overall complication rates. Other patients undergoing laparotomy for the staging of Hodgkin disease have an increase in wound infection rates. In patients older than 50 years of age undergoing cholecystectomy, a significant increase in morbidity was observed in those who had incidental appendectomy. The deficiency in all past studies of this issue is the lack of blinded long-term trials to assess the true cost and benefit. Although appendectomies can be safely performed, the subjection of patients to even a small unnecessary risk is difficult to justify in a litigious society.[59] At present, individual judgment regarding specific patients remains necessary in this area.

Neoplasms of the Appendix

Neoplasms of the appendix are rare, occurring in 1.08% to 1.3% of all appendectomy specimens.[60] Carcinoid tumors are the most common, followed in frequency by benign and malignant mucoceles.

Carcinoids

Carcinoids represent two thirds of all appendiceal neoplasms and are derived from midgut argentaffin cells, possibly of neural crest origin. Nearly half of all gastrointestinal carcinoids arise in the appendix. The mean age for patients with a carcinoid tumor is 41 years. In two thirds of patients, the carcinoid is only incidentally detected, never having caused any symptoms. This benign clinical course is mirrored in the biologic nature of the tumor, with only 0.5% having evidence of distant metastatic spread at resection. In one reported experience, carcinoids between 1.5 and 2 cm have minimal metastatic potential, and those smaller than 1.5 cm never metastasize. In the 1% that are larger than 2 cm, however, metastases are frequent; 80% recur even after resection, and hepatic dissemination can lead to the carcinoid syndrome. Histologic examination of even small appendiceal carcinoids shows mural invasion by the small cell infiltrate and, frequently, both lymphatic and vascular invasion. It is not until the carcinoid has achieved a size of at least 1.5 cm, however, that distant spread seems to occur. Carcinoids have a characteristic firm, yellow appearance and may distort the appendix because of a marked desmoplastic response. Once they are detected, appendectomy with complete resection of the tumor is adequate treatment for small lesions. Right hemicolectomy has been used to treat tumors larger than 1.5 cm, but evidence for a survival benefit from the larger resection is lacking. Overall survival is 99% after 5 years, and even with wide dissemination, prolonged survival has been reported.

Mucinous Cystadenoma and Cystadenocarcinoma

Mucoceles of the appendix include both benign and malignant disease. Both benign cystadenomas and malignant cystadenocarcinomas are characterized by an obstructed, mucin-filled appendix displacing the cecum. Plain abdominal radiographs and barium studies may show a right lower quadrant mass effect and calcification in the mucocele wall. Contents are near water density on CT scan and show little echogenicity by ultrasound. Calcification is more sensitively detected by these two techniques. In benign cystadenomas, the neoplastic, mucus-secreting mucosa of the appendix does not have invasive or metastatic potential. Most lesions are small and asymptomatic. Appendectomy is curative, even in patients with a ruptured cystadenoma that results in mucinous ascites. In contrast, neoplastic mucosa from a cystadenocarcinoma has, by definition, invaded the appendiceal wall and possibly other peritoneal sites. Mucin secretion from peritoneal tumor implants is the cause of pseudomyxoma peritonei. This differs from simple mucinous ascites by having cellular tumor elements present in the mucin, and it is a serious complication of cyst rupture before or during surgical treatment. Inflammatory changes associated with peritoneal tumor implants are a cause of recurrent intestinal obstruction, adhesion formation, and fistulas. Most of these patients are symptomatic, and wide resection of the primary disease, together with debulking of peritoneal implants, is indicated. Indolent progression of metastases commonly results in prolonged survival rates (50% at 5 years). During this time, patients may require repeated laparotomies for complications of the disease. No effective adjuvant treatment has been described.

Adenocarcinoma

Adenocarcinoma of the appendix is exceedingly rare. Analysis of the reported world literature suggests that these tumors occur in older patients and develop at the base of the appendix. Early occlusion of the lumen with development of appendicitis is the most common presentation. The diagnosis is not made preoperatively and is rarely considered during surgery because the appearance of the tumor may mimic perforated appendicitis with an inflammatory mass. Up to one half of patients have metastatic disease at diagnosis, and the peritoneum is the most common site of spread. Survival is proportional to tumor stage. Dukes stage A disease may be treated simply with appendectomy if all disease can be removed with reasonable margins. Dukes stage B and C lesions require formal right hemicolectomy for disease control that is, stage for stage, similar to that of colon carcinoma after 5 years. Appendiceal adenocarcinoma also appears to have an association with secondary tumors, often of the gastrointestinal tract, in up to 35% of patients.

Other Rare Neoplasms

Adenocarcinoids are rare tumors with histologic features of both carcinoids and adenocarcinomas that, if localized, can be treated by appendectomy. High-grade or locally extensive lesions require hemicolectomy for reasonable survival. Lymphomas and metastatic carcinomas of the appendix have also been described.

REFERENCES

1. McFadden DW, Zinner MJ. Approach to the patient with acute abdomen and fever of abdominal origin. Philadelphia, JB Lippincott, 1991.
2. McFadden DW, Zinner MJ. Manifestations of gastrointestinal disease. New York, McGraw-Hill, 1994.

3. Hiatt JR. Management of the acute abdomen. Postgrad Med 1990;87:38.
4. Eastwood GL, Avanduk C. Manual of gastroenterology: diagnosis and therapy. Boston, Little, Brown, 1989.
5. Spiro HM. Gastrointestinal consultation. Chicago, Year Book Medical Publishers, 1990.
6. Klein KB, Mellinkoff SM. Approach to the patient with abdominal pain. Philadelphia, JB Lippincott, 1991.
7. McFadden DW, Zinner MJ. Gastroduodenal disease in the elderly. Surg Clin North Am 1994;74:113.
8. Cutler BS, Dodson TF, Silva WE, Salm TJV. Manual of clinical problems in surgery. Boston, Little, Brown, 1984.
9. Burnett LS. Gynecologic causes of the acute abdomen. Surg Clin North Am 1988;68:385.
10. Nesblett WW, Pietsch JB. Acute abdominal conditions in children and adolescents. Surg Clin North Am 1988;68:415.
11. Paterson-Brown S, Vipond MN. Modern aids to clinical decision-making in the acute abdomen. Br J Surg 1990;77:93.
12. Levine MS. Plain film diagnosis of the acute abdomen. Emerg Med Clin North Am 1985;3:541.
13. Eisenberg RL, Heineken P. Evaluation of plain abdominal radiographs in the diagnosis of abdominal pain. Ann Surg 1983;197:464.
14. Roh JJ, Thompson JS. Value of pneumoperitoneum in the diagnosis of visceral perforation. Am J Surg 1983;146:830.
15. Schaff MI, Tarr RW. Computed tomography and magnetic resonance imaging of the acute abdomen. Surg Clin North Am 1988;68:23.
16. Balthazar EJ, Chako AC. Computerized tomography in acute gastrointestinal disorders. Am J Gastroenterol 1990;85:1445.
17. Pickleman J. Abdominal pain. St Louis, CV Mosby, 1987.
18. Irvin TT. Abdominal pain: a surgical audit of 1190 emergency admissions. Br J Surg 1989;76:1121.
19. Schamburek RD, Farrar JT. Disorders of the digestive system in the elderly. N Engl J Med 1990;322:438.
20. Sweet RL, Gibbs RS. Infectious diseases of the female reproductive tract. Baltimore, Williams & Wilkens, 1990.
21. Weckstein LN. Current perspective on ectopic pregnancy. Obstet Gynecol Surg 1985;40:259.
22. Koch MO, McDougal WS. Urologic causes of the acute abdomen. Surg Clin North Am 1988;68:399.
23. Hatch EI. The acute abdomen in children. Pediatr Clin North Am 1985;32:1151.
24. Rosemurgy AS, McAllister E, Karl RC. The acute surgical abdomen after cardiac surgery involving extracorporeal circulation. Ann Surg 1988;207:323.
25. Glenn J, Funkhouser WK, Bloom L, et al. Acute illnesses necessitating urgent abdominal surgery in neutropenic cancer patients. Surgery 1989;105:778.
26. Stellato TA, Shek RR. Gastrointestinal emergencies in the oncology patient. Semin Oncol 1989;16:521.
27. Villar HG, Warneke JA, Nora B, et al. Role of surgical treatment in the management of complications of the gastrointestinal tract in patients with leukemia. Surg Gynecol Obstet 1987;165:217.
28. Wade DS, Nava HR. Neutropenic colitis. Cancer 1992;69:17.
29. Jess P, Bjerregaard B, Brynitz S, et al. Prognosis of acute nonspecific abdominal pain. Am J Surg 1982;144:338.
30. Gallegos NC, Hobsley M. Abdominal wall pain: an alternative diagnosis. Br J Surg 1990;77:1167.
31. Neumayer LA, Bull DA, Mohr JD, et al. The acutely affected abdomen in paraplegic spinal cord patients. Ann Surg 1990;212:561.
32. Euhus DM, Hiatt JR. Management of the acute abdomen complicating oral anticoagulation therapy. Am Surg 1990;56:581.
33. Tsuji M, Puri P, Reen DJ. Characterization of the local inflammatory response in appendicitis. J Pediatr Gastroenterol Nutr 1993;16:43.
34. Agafonoff S, Hawke I, Khadra M, et al. The influence of age and gender on normal appendicectomy rates. Aust N Z J Surg 1987;57:843.
35. Silverman VA. Appendectomy in a large metropolitan hospital: retrospective analysis of 1,013 cases. Am J Surg 1981;142:615.
36. Nelson M, Barker DJ, Winter PD. Dietary fibre and acute appendicitis: a case-control study. Human Nutrition—Applied Nutrition 1984;38:126.
37. Bett W. A short history of some common diseases. London, Oxford University Press, 1934.
38. Williams R. Pathology of the appendix and its surgical treatment. London, Chapman & Hall, 1994.
39. Masson P. Carcinoids (argentaffin cell tumours) and nerve hyperplasia of the appendicular mucosa. Am J Pathol 1928;4:181.
40. Michalany J, Galindo W. Classification of neuromas of the appendix. Beitr Pathol 1973;150:213.
41. Higa E, Rosai J, Pizzimbono CA, Wise L. Mucosal hyperplasia, mucinous cystadenoma and mucinous cystadenocarcinoma of the appendix: a re-evaluation of appendiceal "mucocele." Cancer 1973;32:1525.
42. McMurrich JP. The organs of digestion, from Leonardo da Vinci—the anatomist. Baltimore, Williams & Wilkins, 1930.
43. Bjerke K, Brandtzaeg P, Rgonum TO. Distribution of immunoglobulin cells is different in normal appendix and colon mucosa. Gut 1986;27:667.
44. Moore KL. The developing human: clinically oriented anatomy. Philadelphia, WB Saunders, 1982.
45. Poole GV. Anatomic basis for delayed diagnosis of appendicitis. South Med J 1990;83:771.
46. Dhillon AP, Williams RA, Rode J. Age, site and distribution of subepithelial neurosecretory cells in the appendix. Pathology 1992;24:56.
47. Wangensteen OH, Dennis C. Experimental proof of the obstructive origin of appendicitis in man. Ann Surg 1939;110:629.
48. Cox MR, McCall JL, Padbury RT, Wilson TG, Wattchow DA, Toouli J. Laparoscopic surgery in women with a clinical diagnosis of acute appendicitis. Med J Aust 1995;162:130.
49. Connor TJ, Garcha IS, Ramshaw BJ, et al. Diagnostic laparoscopy for suspected appendicitis. Am Surg 1995;61:187.
50. Ortega AE, Hunter JG, Peters JH, Swanstrom LL, Schirmer B. A prospective, randomized comparison of laparoscopic appendectomy with open appendectomy: Laparoscopic Appendectomy Study Group. Am J Surg 1995;169:208.
51. McCue J, Coppen M, Rasbridge S, Lock M. Crohn's disease of the appendix. Ann R Coll Surg Engl 1988;70:300.
52. Hopkins JA, Wilson SE, Bobey DG. Adjunctive antimicrobial therapy for complicated appendicitis: bacterial overkill by combination therapy. World J Surg 1994;18:933.
53. Sebastiano PD, Fink T, Weihe E, et al. Changes of protein gene product 9.5 (PGP 9.5) immunoreactive nerves in inflamed appendix. Dig Dis Sci 1995;40:366.
54. Stone HH, Sanders SL, Martin JD. Perforated appendicitis in children. Surgery 1971;69:673.
55. Puri P, Boyd E, Guiney E, O'Donnell B. Appendix mass in the very young child. J Pediatr Surg 1981;16:55.
56. Collins DC. Agenesis of the vermiform appendix. Am J Surg 1951;82:689.
57. Wallbridge PH. Double appendix. Br J Surg 1963;50:346.
58. Ravalli S, Vincent RA, Beaton HI. Acute appendicitis secondary to Kaposi's sarcoma in the acquired immunodeficiency syndrome. N Y State J Med 1991;91:401.
59. Fisher KS, Ross DS. Guidelines for therapeutic decision in incidental appendicectomy. Surg Gynecol Obstet 1990;171:95.
60. Lyss AP. Appendiceal malignancies. Semin Oncol 1988;15:129.

SURGERY: SCIENTIFIC PRINCIPLES AND PRACTICE, Second Edition, edited by
Lazar J. Greenfield, Michael W. Mulholland, Keith T. Oldham, Gerald B. Zelenock,
and Keith D. Lillemoe. Lippincott–Raven Publishers, Philadelphia, © 1997.

CHAPTER 55

SPLEEN

ANTHONY A. MEYER

The spleen has a complex physiologic role, as evidenced by its multiple functions. The normal spleen has three principal functions. It serves an important role as an organ of red blood cell (RBC) maintenance by altering or destroying abnormal RBCs, and it even produces new RBCs in specific circumstances. The spleen is also an immune organ, participating in both specific and nonspecific inflammatory responses. Lastly, the spleen acts as a capacitor and occasionally as a reservoir of cellular blood elements. This may be of physiologic consequence in humans with disorders affecting the splenic circulation. Disorders of the spleen are usually the result of acquired processes that lead to one or more manifestations of splenic dysfunction.

Primary diseases that affect the spleen are typically the result of abnormalities of the cells that populate the spleen, predominantly lymphoid cells and macrophages. Secondary disorders of the spleen generally involve altered physiologic function.

It is important for surgeons to understand the pathophysiology of both primary and related disease processes as they pertain to the spleen; this is the basis for a rational surgical approach to the pathologic splenic conditions reviewed here. Specific issues that relate to the management of the traumatized spleen are addressed in Chapter 11, which discusses the larger subject of trauma.

SPLENIC ANATOMY

Embryology

The spleen arises during the fifth week of gestation from mesenchymal tissue in the dorsal mesogastrium between the pancreas and stomach. Incomplete fusion of this mesenchymal anlage during embryogenesis can result in the formation of accessory spleens between the stomach and pancreas. These accessory spleens are found in about 20% of normal patients and can be identified at celiotomy or on technetium sulfur colloid scan, although not all accessory spleens are apparent with use of this latter technique.

When the abdomen is fully developed, the spleen resides in the left upper quadrant posterior to the stomach, as shown in Figure 55-1. It is an elliptic, lobulated solid organ with a convex surface that abuts the diaphragm and a concave surface that faces the stomach and tail of the pancreas. The spleen lies anterior and medial to the 9th, 10th, and 11th ribs. A normal spleen is shown in Figure 55-2. The normal adult spleen generally weighs between 125 and 175 g. It measures about 15 cm along its cranial–caudal axis and 8 cm along its smaller elliptic axis, and it is 2 to 3 cm thick. The spleen most often has lobulations on the anterior or ventral edge, closest to the hilum. Splenic parenchymal tissue is enveloped by an outer capsule, which is fibrous but quite thin. This capsule can be stripped easily from the splenic substance; this may result in continuous oozing of blood from the exposed surface. This is an important technical concern for the operating surgeon. The relation of the spleen to adjacent organs is illustrated in

Figure 55-3. The concave surface of the spleen lies along the greater curvature of the stomach and the tail of the pancreas.

The blood supply enters the concave splenic substance at the splenic hilum. The convex surface of the spleen is bounded by the peritoneal surface of the diaphragm. Caudad to the spleen are the attachments to the colon and left kidney. There may be lateral attachments of the spleen to the diaphragmatic peritoneal surface, but these are often absent unless infection or some other pathologic process has occurred in that area. The concave surface of the spleen has an ellipsoid area of peritoneal attachment to its surface. These peritoneal attachments surround the central portion of the splenic hilum where the blood vessels and lymphatics enter the parenchyma. The anterior peritoneum extends onto the anterior surface of the pancreas.

Blood Supply

The blood flow to the spleen accounts for as much as 5% of cardiac output. Because of this blood flow, the spleen may function as a reservoir, providing intravascular volume expansion if needed. The spleen is principally perfused by the splenic artery, a primary branch of the celiac axis. The splenic artery is a tortuous vessel that passes posterior and superior to the pancreas. It may become calcified or aneurysmal with certain pathologic states. The splenic artery does not give rise to significant secondary branches until it enters the splenic hilum. The splenic artery separates into two or three branches that penetrate the splenic parenchyma. There is no consistent segmental arterial anatomy, and arterial collaterals exist, which prevent standardized anatomic partial splenectomy based on blood supply.[1] Typically, one to three arterial branches from the left gastroepiploic artery form the vasa brevia or short gastric vessels. These enter the spleen superior to the splenic artery but are within the same hilar area invested by the peritoneum. These short gastric arteries are usually sufficient for splenic survival if the splenic artery must be sacrificed. The short gastric arteries are accompanied by veins that may penetrate the splenic substance itself or that may join with other vascular branches at the splenic hilum. It is these veins that provide collateral systemic–portal venous drainage, which can be exploited to provide selective decompression of distal esophageal or gastric varices.

The splenic vein arises from a confluence of secondary and tertiary veins draining the splenic hilum, generally originating within 1 to 2 cm of the splenic substance. The individual branches are arrayed linearly from cephalad to caudad. The splenic vein passes posterior and inferior to the pancreas, joining the inferior mesenteric vein and eventually the superior mesenteric vein to form the portal vein. These vascular relations are shown in Figure 55-4.

Histology

Splenic structure is directly related to the spleen's normal function and to its altered roles in disease. It is classically divided into red pulp, an area predominantly populated with erythrocytes, and white pulp, an area characterized by a predominance of lymphocytes and macrophages. The volume of the spleen is about 75% to 85% red pulp and 20% white pulp.[1] Unlike any other solid organ, the spleen has no discrete compartments, lobes, or segments. The fibrous splenic skeleton consists of collagen trabeculae that have a random, incomplete framework extending from the hilum to the capsule. Blood vessels penetrate the substance of the spleen within these trabeculae.

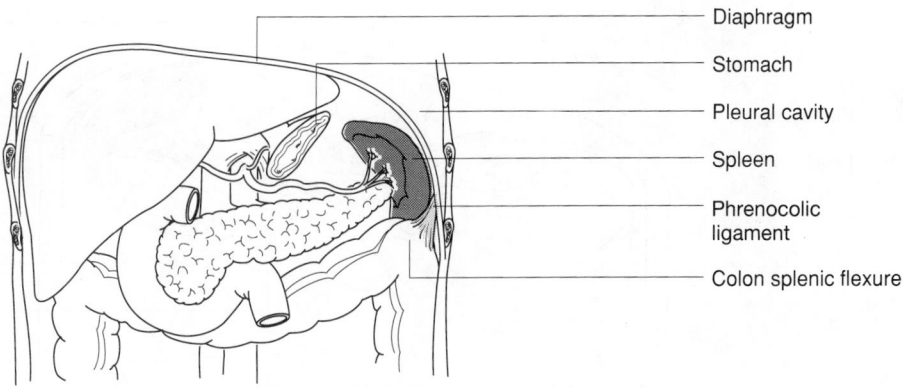

Diaphragm

Stomach

Pleural cavity

Spleen

Phrenocolic ligament

Colon splenic flexure

Visceral surface of spleen

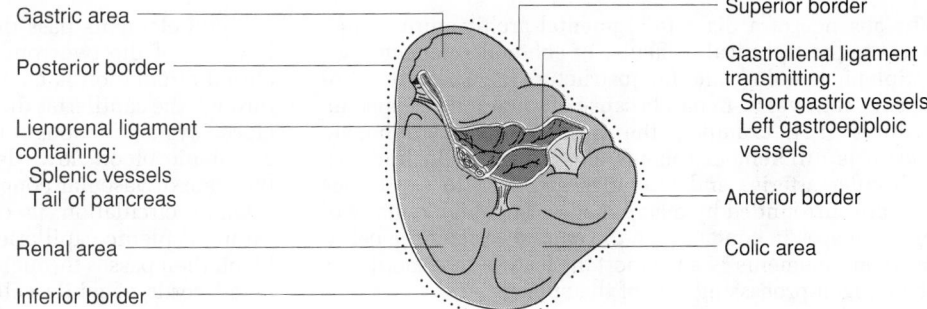

Gastric area

Posterior border

Lienorenal ligament containing:
  Splenic vessels
  Tail of pancreas

Renal area

Inferior border

Superior border

Gastrolienal ligament transmitting:
  Short gastric vessels
  Left gastroepiploic vessels

Anterior border

Colic area

Figure 55-1. Anatomic relation of the spleen to the liver, diaphragm, pancreas, colon, and kidney. The stomach is sectioned to illustrate the anatomic relation in situ.

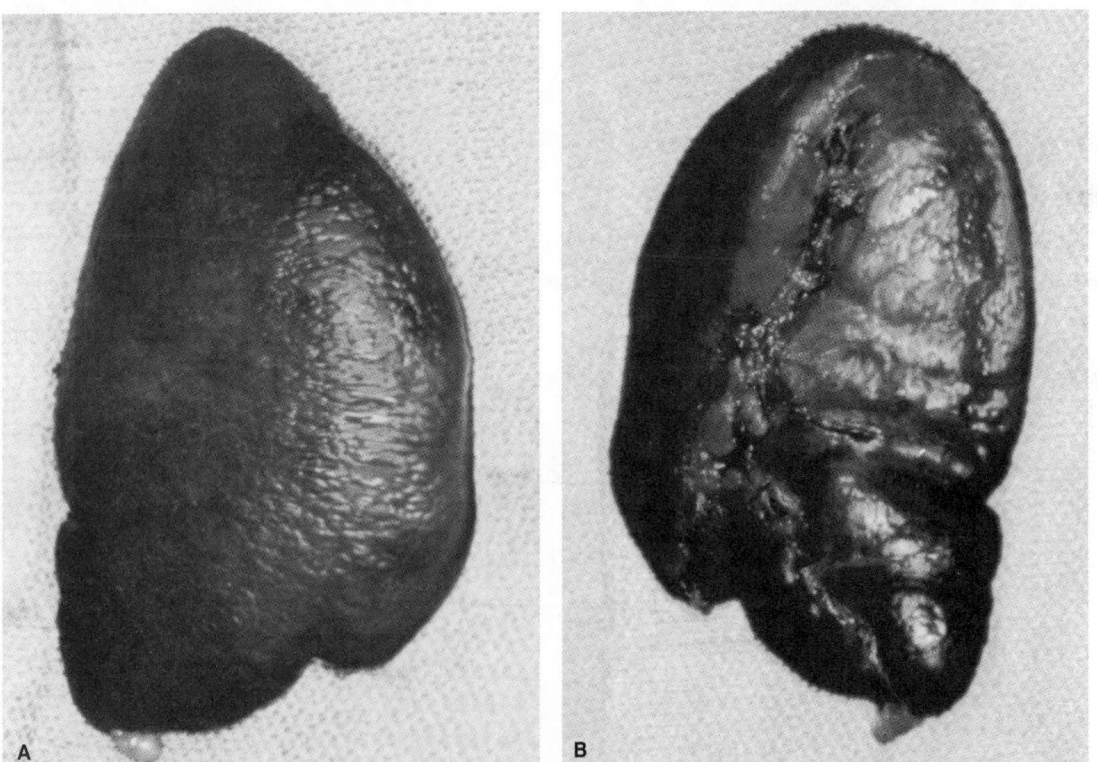

A   B

Figure 55-2. (A) The lateral or diaphragmatic surface of the spleen, showing the lobulated edge and the glistening capsule. (B) The hilar surface of the spleen, showing the ligatures on the cephalad short gastric vessels and the caudal hilar vessels.

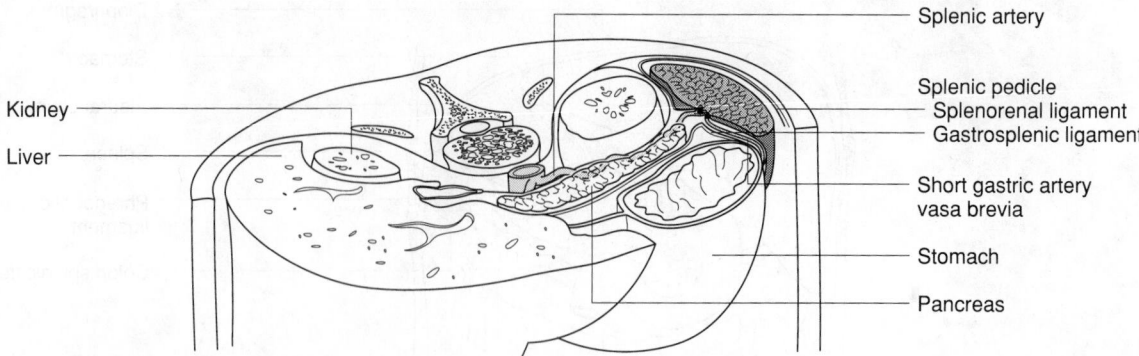

Figure 55-3. The relations of the spleen to the abdominal and retroperitoneal viscera are seen in a cross section of the left-facing torso.

The absence of a discrete segmental architecture contributes to the technical difficulty of subtotal splenectomy.

Splenic histology and microstructure have been the subject of controversy, in part because of some species-specific features. For example, the periarteriolar lymphocyte sheath is different in rodents and humans.[2] In humans, trabecular arteries and arterioles give rise to capillaries that are surrounded by macrophages. This high density of macrophages in contact with the capillaries and the cellular blood elements is an important feature that facilitates the antigen-processing role of the spleen.

Blood elements pass through splenic capillaries to follow one of the two routes depicted in Figure 55-5. The closed circulation is characterized by blood cells passing through the capillaries directly into venous sinusoids. This closed system is thought to account for about 10% to 20% of splenic blood flow, depending on the individual and the state of vascular congestion of the spleen.

Open circulation is characterized by blood passing through splenic capillaries into the splenic red pulp. The blood then passes through lakes of RBCs with loosely organized cords of white cells. The RBCs then move slowly

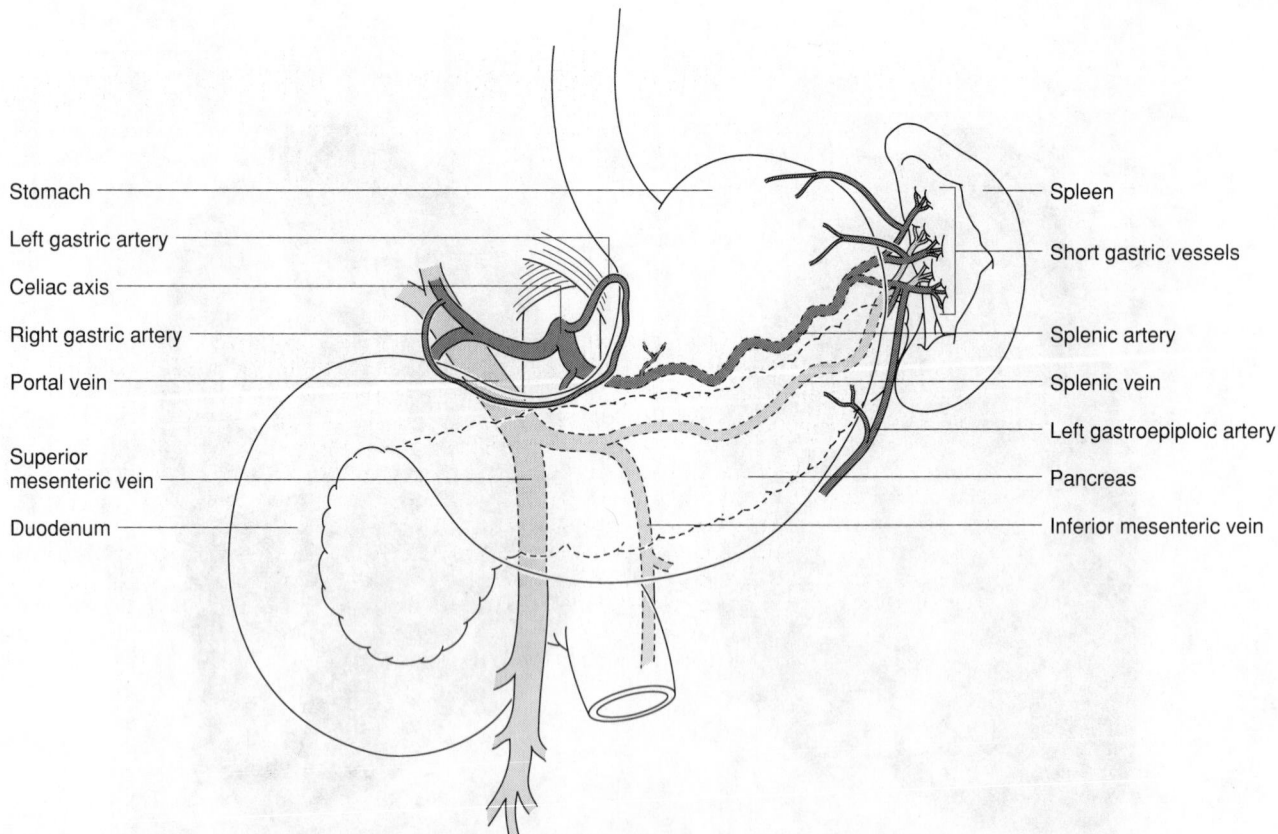

Figure 55-4. The arterial blood flow to the spleen is derived from the splenic artery, the left gastroepiploic artery, and the short gastric arteries (vasa brevia). The venous drainage into the portal vein is also shown.

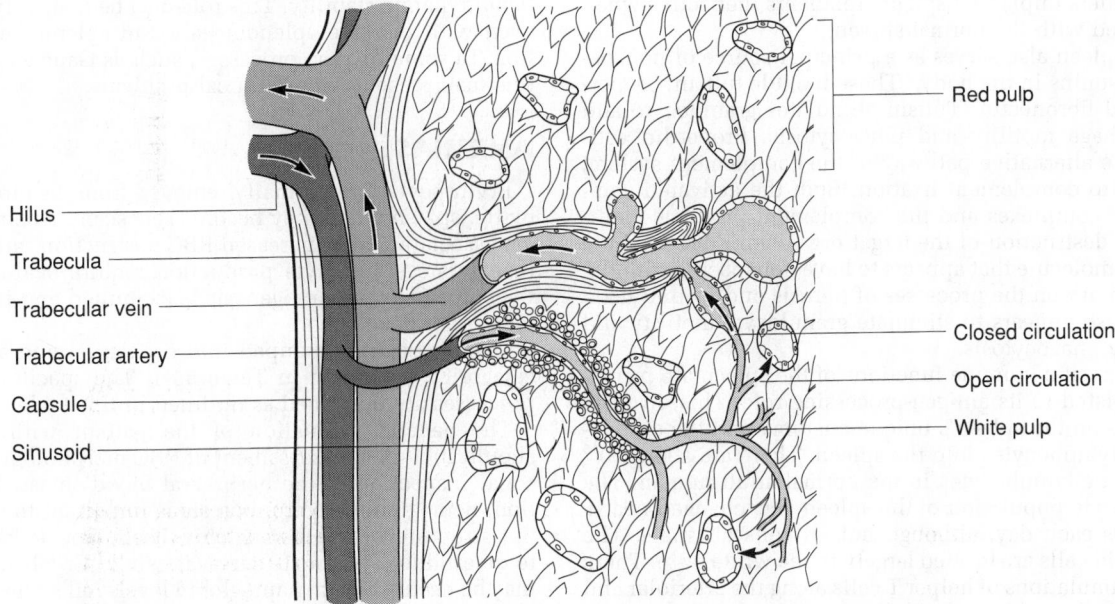

Hilus
Trabecula
Trabecular vein
Trabecular artery
Capsule
Sinusoid

Red pulp
Closed circulation
Open circulation
White pulp

Figure 55-5. The splenic microanatomy is shown with depictions of both the open and closed circulations.

into the sinusoids, which in turn empty into the trabecular veins. Eighty to 90% of splenic blood flow is processed through this open system.

Impairment of splenic blood supply can occur by several mechanisms. Torsion, which is rotation of the spleen on its vascular pedicle, is one such occurrence that is uncommon. The patient usually presents with pain, and the diagnosis is made by establishing that the spleen is anatomically present but nonfunctional. Ultrasonography or computed tomography (CT) demonstrates the former, whereas the lack of splenic function is demonstrable by the absence of technetium sulfur colloid extraction from plasma or the lack of splenic blood flow on arteriography.

Vascular abnormalities can lead to primary splenic problems. These can be secondary to events such as thrombosis of the splenic vein or aneurysmal abnormalities of the splenic artery. They can occur secondary to acute pancreatitis or other local inflammatory events. Splenic vein thrombosis can lead to regionalized portal hypertension with gastric and sometimes distal esophageal varices. Massive upper gastrointestinal bleeding can result from this. If this is a possible cause of upper gastrointestinal hemorrhage, it is essential that the diagnosis be established, because management consists of straightforward splenectomy with predictable success. If this hemorrhage is presumed secondary to cirrhosis-induced portal hypertension, and treatment is based on this mistaken assumption, considerable morbidity may result. Arteriography with venous phase studies is important in the elective surgical evaluation of bleeding esophageal varices. The presence of distal esophageal varices should not be taken to exclude splenic vein thrombosis as the underlying cause of bleeding.

SPLENIC PHYSIOLOGY

Knowledge of splenic physiology is critical when considering the secondary role of the spleen in systemic diseases and when identifying appropriate surgical involvement.

Erythrocyte Maintenance

One of the principal roles of the spleen is to maintain functional erythrocyte mass. The spleen serves this role in erythrocyte maintenance by repairing RBCs that have become damaged during general circulation. Erythrocytes that cannot be repaired by removal of membrane defects are destroyed in the red pulp. The spleen can even remove malarial parasites from infected RBCs.

The degree of RBC destruction in the spleen can be approximated by the presence of markers of RBC remnants. These include Howell-Jolly bodies, which are nuclear remnants; Heinz bodies, which are denatured hemoglobin deposits; and Pappenheimer bodies, which are iron granules from hemoglobin degradation.

Erythrocyte maintenance in the spleen can even include extramedullary hematopoiesis. This is common during fetal development but is generally not seen after birth. In cases of greatly accelerated erythrocyte destruction, hematopoiesis in both the liver and spleen can occur.

Exaggerated erythrocyte destruction can lead to problems in the spleen. This is described in detail in the sections on anemias and hemoglobinopathies. Congestion of the spleen with hemoglobin S (sickle) erythrocytes can lead to splenic congestion and segmental infarcts. In most children with sickle cell disease, the spleen is infarcted and atrophic by the age of 5 years.

Immune Function

Immune function in the spleen consists of two basic components: nonspecific and specific immune responses. Nonspecific immune function is largely characterized by removal of particulate matter by the macrophages. The spleen contains 25% of the fixed tissue macrophage population in the body. Furthermore, it is more efficient than the liver at removing incompletely opsonized bacteria. The liver is most effective at removing bacteria with a high density of surface opsonins. The unique splenic open microcirculation system accounts for the removal of these poorly opsonized bacteria. Alteration of the microcirculation renders implanted splenic remnants ineffective when compared with the normal spleen.

The spleen also serves as a principal source of nonspecific opsonins in the body.[3] These include tuftsin, properdin, and fibronectin. Tuftsin stimulates granulocyte and macrophage motility and phagocytosis. Properdin activates the alternative pathway of the complement system, leading to complement fixation. Both the activated complement complexes and the complement products facilitate the destruction of the target organism. Fibronectin is a macromolecule that appears to have nonspecific stimulatory activity on the processes of fibrosis and wound healing. It also appears to stimulate granulocyte motility and possibly phagocytosis.

The specific immune functions of the spleen are principally related to its antigen-processing role. This, in turn, depends on the spleen's unique anatomy and the circulation of lymphocytes into the spleen. There are about 10^{10} circulating lymphocytes in the normal adult human. The lymphocyte population of the spleen is exchanged nearly 50 times each day, although not all cells circulate. The lymphoid cells are located largely in the white pulp. There are accumulations of helper T cells along the arteriolar and capillary sheaths. Plasma cells are most easily identified along arteries and arterioles. They are also present in follicles throughout the spleen. These follicles may have marginal sinuses populated predominantly by helper T cells, but they are not as well described in humans as in rodents.

Antigen passing through the circulation comes into contact first with macrophages and helper T cells in the area of the arterioles and capillaries. How the spleen participates further in antigen processing depends on whether a humoral or cellular response develops to the antigen. T-cell populations respond to antigenic stimuli with synthesis of cytokines. Activated T cells recirculate in the body to modulate this response. Some antigens are transmitted to antibody-synthesizing cells by macrophages and helper T cells. These pass through the perivascular tissues into the follicles and corona sections of the spleen. Here, they come into contact with dendritic macrophages and helper T cells that stimulate and control immunoglobulin synthesis. The spleen is the largest producer of IgM in humans; therefore, splenectomy yields substantial decreases in IgM synthesis. This may recover spontaneously over several years. Splenectomy also decreases the helper T cell/suppressor cell ratio as measured by CD4/CD8 with fluorescent activated cell-sorting techniques. These changes are known to suppress many aspects of host resistance to infection.

Contributions to the specific and nonspecific components of the immune system are an important part of normal splenic function. Their absence due to splenic malfunction or splenectomy can lead to significant impairment of immune function.

Vascular Capacity

The spleen also serves as an intravascular reservoir. This is usually a limited role in humans, because the human spleen is relatively small and does not have well-preserved contractile properties. Effective incorporation of splenic blood into the circulating blood volume occurs by vasoconstriction of the splenic artery and with diminution of the splenic blood pool by increased venous outflow. This contribution to the intravascular volume is relatively small considering the limited size of the organ.

In disease states, the splenic volume can be substantial. Portal hypertension or other causes of hypersplenism can lead to massive splenomegaly, in which considerable blood volume is pooled in the spleen. In such patients, splenic surgery or injury may have a significant effect on

hemodynamic stability. This role may be relatively minor, even with massive splenomegaly and splenic sequestration. In some disease processes, such as Gaucher disease, this may present major clinical problems.

ANEMIAS

Erythrocytes are normally removed from the circulation by the spleen when they become senescent. Anemias that are associated with increased RBC destruction rather than inadequate erythrocyte production require evaluation of the spleen as the pathogenesis is examined and the treatment plan developed.

Anemias can be grouped into congenital and acquired categories, as shown in Table 55-1. The specific disease processes are described as outlined in this table.

The general evaluation of the patient with anemia should include an assessment of RBC morphology by personal inspection of the peripheral blood smear. In addition, hemoglobin electrophoresis is important to examine the structure of the hemoglobin itself. Specialized tests to determine erythrocyte survival using ^{51}Cr-labeled RBCs may be useful. Serum haptoglobin levels reflect hemolysis. The total bilirubin level in plasma reflects hemoglobin turnover, but this is generally determined by the efficacy of hepatocyte bilirubin conjugation and is therefore of limited clinical use in the anemic patient. Infants with hemolytic anemias have reliably elevated plasma levels of unconjugated bilirubin, but this is less predictable in adults.

Congenital Anemias

Congenital anemias involve abnormalities of erythrocyte structure, of metabolism, or of the hemoglobin itself.

Erythrocyte Structure Abnormalities

Hereditary spherocytosis is the most common of the congenital hemolytic anemias related to an abnormality in erythrocyte structure. The hemoglobin molecule itself is

---

Table 55-1. CLASSIFICATION OF ANEMIAS

CONGENITAL

Erythrocyte Structure Abnormalities

Hereditary spherocytosis
Hereditary elliptocytosis
Hereditary pyropoikilocytosis
Hereditary xerocytosis
Hereditary hydrocytosis

Erythrocyte Metabolism Abnormalities

Glucose-6-phosphate dehydrogenase
Pyruvate kinase deficiency

Hemoglobinopathies

Sickle cell disease
Thalassemia
   Major
   Minor

ACQUIRED

Autoimmune Hemolytic Anemia

Primary
Secondary
   Warm antibody
   Cold antibody

Aplastic

Neutropenia
Chemotherapy

normal. Affected RBCs have a deficiency of spectrin, an essential component of the cell membrane that contributes to both durability and deformability. Spectrin deficiency in the erythrocyte membrane is associated with increased permeability to sodium, leading to increased intracellular volume and loss of the normal, biconcave, discoid erythrocyte morphology. The characteristic diagnostic feature of affected erythrocytes is increased osmotic fragility because of already maximal intracellular volumes. Spherocytes placed in hypotonic sodium lyse rapidly because of this feature of the disease. The resulting spherical erythrocytes are rigid and do not pass normally through the splenic microvasculature. Splenic sequestration and accelerated erythrocyte destruction result.

The precise incidence of hereditary spherocytosis is unclear. It is an autosomal dominant trait associated with a positive family history in about three quarters of patients, the remainder presumably being spontaneous new mutations. The severity of the anemia with hereditary spherocytosis is variable and is loosely correlated with the amount of spectrin present in the erythrocytes.

Patients have varying degrees of symptoms related to hereditary spherocytosis, although the severity is usually reasonably constant within families. Patients with mild cases may have acute exacerbations induced by concurrent viral infections, which may cause further erythrocyte destruction and may precipitate an anemic crisis. Splenomegaly is expected, generally by 1 year of age. Jaundice may occur and may present as neonatal jaundice. Pigment gallstones develop in untreated patients and may be found by 5 years of age.

Hereditary spherocytosis requires splenectomy at some time. If the disease process is not severe, it is best to wait until the patient is at least 6 to 8 years of age. This decreases the risk of overwhelming postsplenectomy sepsis in later years. Indications for earlier operation include aplastic crisis, severe anemia, growth failure, and possibly gallstones. Splenectomy does nothing to correct the spectrin deficiency, but it leads to relatively normal RBC survival by eliminating the site of erythrocyte consumption. Affected RBCs remain as spherocytes after splenectomy but function relatively normally from the standpoint of gas exchange.

Gallstones with bilirubin pigment are expected in patients with hemolytic anemias as a consequence of constant hemolysis. The natural history of asymptomatic gallstones in this circumstance is not clear. In general, cholecystectomy is recommended at the time of splenectomy when hemolytic anemia and cholelithiasis coexist. Because splenectomy does not correct the physiologic cause of the anemia, additional gallstones form if the gallbladder is left in situ.

Hereditary elliptocytosis is also an abnormality of RBC membrane structure that is associated with decreased levels of spectrin. This is an autosomal dominant trait that is relatively common, affecting about 1 in 2000 persons. The consequences of this abnormality are elliptic erythrocytes. Like spherocytes, these abnormal RBCs may have an increase in the rate of spontaneous destruction, leading to hemolytic anemia.

The relative severity of the hereditary elliptocytosis determines the need for splenectomy. Most patients have few elliptocytes on smear and do not need treatment, whereas those with symptoms of severe anemia require splenectomy. As with hereditary spherocytosis, splenectomy does not alter the fundamental erythrocyte abnormality, but it does help to prolong RBC survival by removing the organ of erythrocyte destruction. In general, splenectomy is indicated for severe hemolytic anemia.

Hereditary pyropoikilocytosis is a rare recessive variant of hereditary spherocytosis seen in the African American population. In contrast to elliptocytosis, hereditary pyropoikilocytosis causes predictably severe anemia and excessive erythrocyte destruction. In some patients, the severity of the hemolytic anemia decreases during childhood. In other patients, the anemia persists and may require early splenectomy.

Hereditary hydrocytosis is a rare hemolytic anemia associated with abnormalities in the RBC membrane transport of sodium and potassium. These abnormalities lead to decreased levels of hemoglobin and larger intracellular volumes in the erythrocytes. This in turn leads to increased osmotic fragility and accelerated RBC destruction. Splenectomy is often useful in treating patients with hydrocytosis because it prolongs RBC survival. It does not eliminate the cause of the increased osmotic fragility. Persistent hemolysis results, although the relative rate of hemolysis decreases.

Hereditary xerocytosis is a cellular abnormality that leads to intracellular water loss with resulting increases in the amount of hemoglobin per unit volume of RBCs. These erythrocytes have an elevated mean corpuscular hemoglobin content. The cause of the intracellular dehydration appears to be excessive loss of intracellular potassium, followed by passive water loss through the cell membrane. Increased erythrocyte destruction associated with hereditary xerocytosis is generally modest, and the anemias are often of limited clinical significance. Therefore, splenectomy is not often indicated.

Erythrocyte Metabolism Abnormalities

Glucose-6-phosphate dehydrogenase (G6PD) deficiency and pyruvate kinase deficiency are the two principal erythrocyte metabolism abnormalities that lead to hemolytic anemia. G6PD deficiency is caused by one of several X-linked genetic abnormalities and is present in up to 200 million people worldwide. It is most common in the African American, Mediterranean, African, and Middle Eastern populations. Generally, it is not clinically apparent; hemolytic anemia occurs in most patients only after the consumption of certain medications or exposure to specific chemicals. A partial list of oxidizing agents known to induce acute hemolytic anemia in patients with G6PD deficiency follows:

- Acetylsalicylic acid (high dose)
- Phenacetin
- Nitrofurantoin
- Sulfamethoxazole
- Doxorubicin
- Nalidixic acid
- Acetanilid
- Primaquine
- Phenazopyridine
- Methylene blue
- Niridazole
- Furazolidone
- Fava beans

The diagnosis is established by measurement of erythrocyte G6PD levels. Affected individuals have activity levels less than 10% of normal.

Splenectomy is rarely indicated in patients with G6PD deficiency. Management generally consists of simply avoiding exposure to precipitating agents. Vitamin E and desferrioxamine may be useful, presumably because of their antioxidant activities, but their roles are unclear.

Pyruvate kinase deficiency is an enzymatic deficiency transmitted as an autosomal recessive trait. Pyruvate kinase is important in adenosine triphosphate synthesis, and its deficiency is associated with diminished erythrocyte survival. The severity of the anemia associated with pyruvate kinase deficiency can be variable. Patients with disease severe enough to require blood transfusions may benefit from splenectomy. Although splenic sequestration of erythrocytes is not characteristic of pyruvate kinase deficiency, RBC survival is enhanced by empiric splenectomy. This is generally reserved for children older than 5 to 6 years of age with severe anemia or an ongoing transfusion requirement.

Hemoglobinopathies

Sickle cell disease and thalassemia are the principal hemoglobinopathies that cause clinically important disease. Sickle cell anemia is largely restricted to people of African descent. Hemoglobin S (HgbS) results when the substitution of valine for glutamic acid in the sixth position of the β-chain of normal hemoglobin A (HgbA) occurs. About 0.5% of African Americans are homozygous for HgbS, whereas 8% are heterozygous for HgbS. Clinical symptoms are directly dependent on the amount of HgbS present, and this can be variable. Factors that can influence this are the presence of other hemoglobins, such as fetal hemoglobin (HgbF) and hemoglobin associated with thalassemia (HgbC). The physiologic result of HgbS is that rigid, sickle-shaped erythrocytes occur when oxygen saturation diminishes. These altered RBCs lack the normal ability to deform with microvascular passage, leading to capillary occlusion and shortened RBC survival.

Patients who are homozygous for HgbS usually have small sequential splenic infarcts as a result of microvascular occlusion, and the spleen is usually small, fibrotic, and dysfunctional by the age of 5 years. Splenectomy is sometimes appropriate if autosplenectomy does not occur. Occasionally, acute splenic infarction leads to significant pain and precipitates a sickle cell crisis, for which splenectomy may be beneficial. Rarely, patients with HgbS disease develop acute and massive splenic erythrocyte sequestration with splenomegaly that may require urgent splenectomy. Other elective operations are generally performed after planned blood transfusion to reduce the HgbS fraction to less than 40%, thereby reducing the risk of a sickle cell crisis.

The thalassemias are a group of some 30 disorders of hemoglobin synthesis characterized by the formation or inappropriate production of hemoglobin chains, generally α or β chains. β-Thalassemia is characterized by a deficiency of the β chain and a corresponding excess of α chains, whereas α-thalassemia results from α-chain deficiency and β-chain excess. Thalassemia minor is heterozygous β-thalassemia and is generally accompanied by mild clinical disease. Thalassemia major (Cooley anemia) is homozygous β-thalassemia and is a severe clinical anemia. Clinical severity of the resulting anemia depends on the amount of abnormal hemoglobin present. Some forms of thalassemia with major hemoglobin chain deficiencies are incompatible with life. Patients with the more common thalassemia minor variants may have little or no symptomatology.

Thalassemia patients may develop significant splenomegaly and hypersplenism, resulting in sequestration of platelets and white cells. Splenectomy can significantly improve these specific problems; therefore, they are considered operative indications. Transfusion is the mainstay of medical therapy.

Acquired Anemias

Autoimmune Hemolytic Anemia

Autoimmune hemolytic anemia results from acute RBC destruction secondary to complement fixation of antibodies bound to the surface of the erythrocyte. Autoimmune hemolytic anemias are usually associated with medications that induce antibody synthesis. Numerous drugs have been implicated in this process; these include antibiotics such as β-lactams and aminoglycosides, quinidine, phenacetin, and multiple sulfur-containing drugs. Other events that can trigger autoimmune hemolytic anemia include viral infections, malignancies, and both chronic and acute inflammatory processes.

Many acute hemolytic anemias resolve spontaneously with removal of the etiologic agent, but treatment may be required if hemolysis is severe or persistent. Empiric glucocorticoid therapy is generally the first line of treatment, and the effect is thought to reside in the inhibition of the endogenous inflammatory response. Patients with persistent symptoms often benefit from splenectomy, even in the absence of demonstrable increases in erythrocyte sequestration in the spleen. As many as 75% of these patients have significant improvement in the anemia after splenectomy.

The diagnosis of an autoimmune hemolytic anemia is usually established by a positive direct Coombs test. This is a bioassay that yields hemolysis when complement is added to a preparation of the patient's erythrocytes. These cells already have antibody bound to their surface. This is in contrast to the indirect Coombs test, which detects other substances bound to the RBC surface by adding exogenous immunoglobulin and then reacting with complement components.

Autoimmune hemolytic anemias are classified as those associated with warm antibody or cold antibody. Warm-antibody autoimmune hemolytic anemias are more common and are usually the result of IgG antibodies to the erythrocyte. They are associated with RBC destruction in the spleen. Splenectomy is beneficial for about half of these patients.

Autoimmune hemolytic anemias associated with cold antibodies are all IgM related. These bind at temperatures below 28°F and produce symptoms only in patients exposed to low temperatures. The antibody-coated RBCs in these patients are usually destroyed in the liver. About half of these anemias are associated with *Mycoplasma* infection. Chronic anemia symptoms are more common in cold-antibody anemias than in warm-antibody anemias.

A primary autoimmune hemolytic anemia is one in which there is no demonstrable association with medication, infection, tumor, or other disease. The diagnosis is made by a positive direct Coombs test. The severity and duration of these primary anemias are variable, and treatment is based on the magnitude of the clinical findings. Patients who have minimal symptoms may not require splenectomy. Patients who are stable can be observed for a short time to see if the anemia improves.

Aplastic Anemia

Aplastic anemia is an acute disease process with total or near-total failure of production of erythrocytes and other bone marrow–derived cells. It is most commonly associated with drug reactions and occasionally is associated with infections or other unknown causes. Splenectomy may be useful in some patients with RBC aplasia, although the mechanism is unclear and a physiologic basis for a good result is not obvious. Routine splenectomy for aplastic anemia cannot be recommended.

Primary neutropenia is a selective anemia in which the spleen has an undetermined contribution, and splenectomy is not usually indicated.

Anemias may be induced before bone marrow transplant. Splenectomy has been used as part of the preparation for, or in conjunction with, bone marrow transplantation in some centers. With the development of recombinant growth factors for myeloid precursors, the necessity for splenectomy in this situation may change.

IMMUNE (IDIOPATHIC) THROMBOCYTOPENIC PURPURA

Immune thrombocytopenic purpura has traditionally been called idiopathic thrombocytopenic purpura (ITP). Identification of circulating antibodies to platelet antigens in these patients and the good response to empiric immunosuppressive therapy led to the hypothesis that ITP is an autoimmune phenomenon. Further study has indicated that the presence of circulating antiplatelet antibodies is not specifically diagnostic of ITP. These antibodies are present in many normal individuals and do not specifically correlate with thrombocytopenia in patients with ITP.[4] The precise amount of antiplatelet antibody is difficult to detect because of varied binding affinities between antibody and platelet antigen. In addition, these are generally IgG antibodies without complement receptors (FC), which makes detection more difficult. Another important reason for the absence of a simple diagnostic algorithm for ITP is that it is a syndrome that results from many etiologies. These include both congenital and acquired disorders, with both immune and nonimmune causes, and are summarized in Table 55-2.[5]

ITP is classically diagnosed by clinical symptoms, including petechiae, gingival bleeding, and soft tissue ecchymoses. Initial blood examination identifies a low circulating platelet count, often below 50,000/μL. Bone marrow aspirate or core biopsy demonstrates normal or increased levels of megakaryocytes. If antiplatelet antibody is present and no other cause for thrombocytopenia is identified, the diagnosis of ITP is made. ITP occurs most commonly in young women, but it is not limited to this group. Subgroups of patients, including those with human immuno-

deficiency virus infection and acquired immunodeficiency syndrome, have been found to have an increased risk of ITP.

On physical examination, patients with ITP may have persistent clinical evidence of bleeding but generally do not have significant abdominal findings. The spleen is not enlarged. The presence of a palpable spleen in the patient with apparent ITP should lead one to search for another cause of splenomegaly and thrombocytopenia.

The initial treatment of ITP consists of systemic glucocorticoids, generally prednisone, 1 to 2 mg/kg/d. About 60% to 80% of patients with acute ITP respond to this therapy. The dose is reduced during the next several weeks with monitoring of the platelet count. Patients with thrombocytopenia from causes other than ITP usually continue to have normal or near-normal platelet counts. Patients whose platelet counts begin to drop after cessation of steroids are generally considered to have chronic ITP and become candidates for splenectomy.

ITP in children requires a different management strategy. In over 90% of children younger than 10 years of age, ITP resolves spontaneously and requires no specific therapy. Splenectomy in children should be reserved for those who have important consequences of abnormal bleeding, such as intracranial hemorrhage.

The mechanism by which glucocorticoids improve the platelet count appears to be an increase in platelet production.[6] Corticosteroids do not suppress the levels of antiplatelet antibody or limit the rate of peripheral destruction of platelets. This increase in platelet production diminishes as the corticosteroid dose is tapered, or even if it is continued at high levels for long periods.

Splenectomy remains the principal treatment for ITP. As noted earlier, the platelet count rises to adequate levels in about 80% of patients who undergo the procedure.[7] Ninety percent of patients who have had good responses to corticosteroids have improved platelet counts after splenectomy. Of patients who do not respond to corticosteroids, about 60% respond to splenectomy.[8,9] Splenectomy is effective because of its ability to remove a site of platelet destruction. Because the spleen is the site of most platelet sequestration in ITP, splenectomy should eliminate this source of platelet consumption. Furthermore, splenectomy removes a significant source of antiplatelet IgG production.

The timing of splenectomy for ITP is controversial. Because the potential causes of thrombocytopenia are numerous, the diagnosis of ITP generally requires some time to determine whether the thrombocytopenia recurs after corticosteroid treatment.

Additional tests may be required to eliminate other possibilities. In general, there is no benefit to delay once the diagnosis of chronic ITP is made. When it is apparent that the thrombocytopenia is not a self-limited problem, splenectomy should be performed at the earliest convenience. This limits some of the adverse effects of chronic steroid therapy and also limits the associated immune suppression.

Patients in whom the thrombocytopenia does not respond to splenectomy may require other forms of therapy. If corticosteroid therapy is continued, the dosage is usually lower than that used before splenectomy. Other medical regimens have included general immunosuppressive drugs such as vincristine, danazol, azathioprine, and cyclophosphamide.[5,6] Generally, males have more incomplete or adverse responses to splenectomy, but data on this are unclear.

It is important to closely evaluate low platelet counts in the absence of clinical symptoms. Some patients have aggregation of platelets in the standard EDTA anticoagulant solutions in most blood tubes, yielding a falsely low

Table 55-2. CLASSIFICATION OF CAUSES OF IMMUNE THROMBOCYTOPENIC PURPURA

CONGENITAL
Immune
Drug induced
Autoimmune neonatal thrombocytopenia
Maternal antibody–induced neonatal thrombocytopenia
Infection

Nonimmune
Drug induced
Erythroblastosis hemangioma
Infection
Giant cavernous hemangioma

ACQUIRED
Immune
Drug induced
Sepsis
Posttransfusion purpura
Allergic reaction
Acute or chronic autoimmune thrombocytopenia

Nonimmune
Drug induced
Disseminated intravascular coagulation
Thrombotic thrombocytopenic purpura
Acquired immunodeficiency syndrome

(Adapted from Koller CA. Immune thrombocytopenic purpura. Med Clin North Am 1980;64:761)

platelet count that is persistent from test to test. In these patients, blood should be gathered in a heparin tube, thus avoiding similar platelet aggregation.

THROMBOTIC THROMBOCYTOPENIC PURPURA

Thrombotic thrombocytopenic purpura (TTP) is a relatively rare syndrome with no definitive diagnostic test or clinical characteristic. The principal clinical features of TTP are thrombocytopenic purpura, fever, a microangiopathic hemolytic anemia, mental status changes with possible peripheral neuropathy, and renal dysfunction. About half of the patients diagnosed as having TTP have all five of these clinical characteristics.

The pathogenesis of the disease is unknown. It is thought to result from the loss of an inhibitory mechanism for platelet aggregation.[10] This results in multiple focal areas of thrombosis and tissue infarction, often involving the brain. It is possible that a circulating substance that binds platelets is responsible, but this has not been specifically identified despite extensive effort. TTP is associated with a number of different clinical events. Among these are medication reactions, new infections, and inflammatory or autoimmune diseases. It is difficult to identify common characteristics among these patients.

The treatment of TTP is generally focused on removal of the plasma constituents that lead to platelet aggregation. Plasmapheresis is particularly effective and has decreased the 1-year mortality rate of 50% to 80% to about 10%. Splenectomy was initially proposed for TTP but has been shown to have little benefit and instead is associated with a considerable risk of postsplenectomy sepsis. The high mortality associated with splenectomy for TTP was not seen when patients were treated with plasmapheresis preoperatively. The role of splenectomy in TTP remains unclear, and plasmapheresis remains the principal treatment. Splenectomy may be considered if plasmapheresis is ineffective.

Hemolytic uremic syndrome is a disease of children that is associated with systemic vasculitis. Like patients with TTP, children with hemolytic uremic syndrome have a constellation of clinical problems, including thrombocytopenia, renal failure, microangiopathic hemolytic anemia, and mental status changes. The pathogenic mechanisms are unclear. About half the children have been found to have enteric *Escherichia coli* 0157:H7, which may be pathogenic because of renotoxin production. The incidence of hemolytic uremic syndrome seems to be increasing in the United States, although the reasons are unknown.[11] The disease is most severe if the peripheral blood polymorphonuclear neutrophil count is above $15,000/\mu L$ and the patient has bloody diarrhea or a short prodrome. Treatment generally consists of nonspecific supportive care. Splenectomy is rarely indicated in these patients, and its role is not established.

POSTSPLENECTOMY SEPSIS

Postsplenectomy sepsis (PSS) refers to the increased risk of systemic infection in patients who have undergone splenectomy. This includes an increased risk of routine bacterial infections and, more important, an increased risk of overwhelming systemic sepsis, predominantly associated with gram-positive encapsulated bacteria such as streptococcal organisms. The increase in conventional bacterial infections is difficult to quantify and probably results from some limitation of general immune function that is associated with splenectomy. The increased incidence of imme-

diate postoperative infection is more closely associated with transfusion, rather than the choice of splenectomy versus splenic preservation.[12] The risk of overwhelming infection from poorly opsonized bacteria is due to a decrease in the specific immune response to particular bacterial antigens and to a reduced capacity to clear bacteria from the blood.

The increased incidence of overwhelming infection after splenectomy was described by King and Schumacker in 1952.[13] Multiple subsequent studies have confirmed this increased risk and further refined the ability to identify it. The mortality rate from PSS is about 50%.[14,15] The incidence of PSS in children is as high as 4% during a follow-up of nearly 10 years and ranges from 0.3% to 1.8% in adults during an 8-year follow-up. The highest incidence of PSS is in those who had splenectomy for associated malignancies or those who had an incidental splenectomy during other surgical procedures in adulthood. In children, the patients most at risk for PSS are those who had splenectomy for either congenital or acquired anemias. It is important to remember that any patient who has undergone splenectomy or who has hyposplenism is at risk for PSS.

The clinical course of overwhelming PSS commonly has no identifiable event. Typically, there is no prodromal infection. The most common causative organisms are *Streptococcus pneumoniae, Haemophilus influenzae,* and *Neisseria meningitidis.* Other less common encapsulated organisms have also been identified. In addition, organisms without classic polysaccharide cell walls can occasionally produce overwhelming infection in postsplenectomy patients.

Clinically, patients develop symptoms of sepsis, including hypotension, coagulopathy, and multiple organ failure. Patients can also develop Friderichsen-Waterhouse syndrome, with adrenocortical hemorrhage. This may be independent of the specific organism identified, but blood cultures are usually positive. Furthermore, the bacterial count in the blood is considerably higher than in nonsplenectomized patients with similar infections. This syndrome is generally not associated with decreased plasma cortisol levels.

The identification of PSS has greatly changed the approach to management of splenic injuries and diseases. Routine removal of the spleen because of injury or involvement in other primary diseases has been carefully reexamined. Splenic preservation after trauma or incidental injury is now the preferred method of treatment. After splenic injury, splenectomy is reserved for patients in whom splenic repair or nonoperative management is unsuccessful.

Splenic autotransplantation has been proposed as an alternative means of splenic preservation in patients whose spleens are too severely injured for in situ repair. Splenic autotransplantation has been attempted with several methods. The most common technique involves placement of a fragmented or surgically harvested spleen into an omental pouch. Persistence of these implants can be documented by periodic liver–spleen scans postoperatively. In animal and human models, the transplanted tissue does not appear to have normal splenic function. There are increased numbers of abnormal erythrocytes circulating in the peripheral blood of patients who have had autotransplants when compared with those who have had subtotal splenectomy. Morphologically, the splenic transplants have abnormal architecture and abnormal blood supply. Most important, splenic autotransplants have a diminished ability to protect against PSS when compared with a normal spleen.[8,14,16]

It is possible that the altered blood supply causes splenic autotransplants to function in a manner different from that of the intact spleen during bacterial antigen processing and clearance. In the intact spleen with normal blood flow, the bacterial antigens pass through the splenic arterioles into the periarterial or lymphatic sheaths.[17] This allows for exposure of the antigens to macrophages and helper T cells, with subsequent migration of the antigen into the germinal centers, where antibody production can be maximized. This unique blood flow enhances the clearance of poorly opsonized encapsulated bacteria. This does not occur in autotransplants, in which the blood flow characteristics along the path of these immune cells in the normal spleen are lost.[18] Because of this, antigen processing is greatly reduced and bacterial clearance is impaired.[19] Preservation of part of the spleen in the normal position with normal blood supply is probably an essential mechanism to preserve splenic function and prevent overwhelming PSS.

The management of PSS is nonspecific and includes supportive care and administration of broad-spectrum systemic antibiotics. Prevention is the goal, with efforts focused on partial splenectomy when possible and vaccination when total splenectomy is necessary. Immunizations are discussed in the section of this chapter that includes the technical aspects of splenectomy.

HYPERSPLENISM

Hypersplenism is not a specific disease but rather a physiologic state characterized by splenomegaly, a decrease in circulating levels of some blood cells or platelets, bone marrow hypertrophy in response to the decrease in circulating blood elements, and some degree of improvement by splenectomy. Most hypersplenism is secondary to some other disease process, but primary hypersplenism does occur. Primary hypersplenism usually develops in women. The diagnosis depends on identification of the physiologic state without an apparent etiology. A diagnosis of primary hypersplenism can be made only after a thorough search for other physiologic abnormalities. The presence of splenic enlargement alone is insufficient evidence for the diagnosis of hypersplenism.

Splenectomy is indicated for patients with true primary hypersplenism. These patients rarely respond to glucocorticoid therapy, and prolonged courses of steroids are not indicated. Such therapy results in additional risks with no benefit to the patient.

Disease processes associated with secondary hypersplenism include the following:

Increased venous pressure
- Portal hypertension
- Splenic vein thrombosis
- Severe congestive heart failure

Malignancy
- Leukemias (especially chronic)
- Lymphoma

Chronic inflammatory diseases
- Felty syndrome
- Systemic lupus erythematosus
- Sarcoidosis

Metabolic abnormalities
- Amyloidosis
- Gaucher disease
- Niemann-Pick disease

Infection
- Mononucleosis
- Bacterial endocarditis
- Parasites
- Fungus

Other
- Myelofibrosis with myeloid metaplasia
- Polycythemia vera

Although these individual disease processes are variable, the general mechanism by which they generate hypersplenism is increased blood sequestration in the spleen. This may result from venous outflow obstruction caused by anatomic occlusion, such as splenic vein thrombosis, or from increased splenic venous pressure, as with portal hypertension. Venous congestion can also occur secondary to a variety of inflammatory diseases and metabolic disorders.

Regardless of the underlying cause, patients with hypersplenism have the physiologic state of blood pooling within the spleen. The decision about the need for splenectomy is based on the magnitude of the symptoms related to hypersplenism and the relative risk of the operation. Although Eichner defines hypersplenism as the time at which the "spleen is more harmful than beneficial,"[20] this does not take into account the late risks of splenectomy. When considering splenectomy for hypersplenism, one should consider both the operative risks and the early and late postoperative outcomes.

Several specific disease processes that are associated with hypersplenism are discussed in this section.

Portal Hypertension

Portal hypertension results in congestion of the spleen secondary to elevated venous pressure in both the short gastric veins and the splenic vein. This is associated with collateral vein formation, including the usually avascular attachments to the colon and diaphragm.

Patients with hypersplenism from portal hypertension usually present with thrombocytopenia as the primary manifestation. The role of splenectomy in such patients is controversial. Although splenectomy may transiently increase the number of platelets in the peripheral circulation, it generally does not improve survival. At the time of surgery, these patients have considerable risk for massive bleeding and subsequent complications related to hepatic dysfunction. These latter complications include ascites, coagulopathy, and wound complications. The severity of the underlying liver disease is the determining factor for this group of patients. Some believe that splenectomy is contraindicated in patients with portal hypertension.[21] Indeed, the perioperative risks are considerably greater than normal. This should be considered as a last option, and even then it should be realized that the operative and perioperative morbidity and mortality are high.

Splenic Vein Thrombosis

Splenic vein thrombosis is often discovered when bleeding gastric varices develop in a patient with a history of chronic pancreatitis. Lankisch[22] reports a 95% likelihood of splenic vein thrombosis if splenomegaly and esophageal and gastric varices are present in a patient with acute or chronic pancreatitis. It is important in this circumstance to establish the cause of bleeding and patency of the splenic vein, because clinical management is dictated entirely by these data. Splenic vein thrombosis is best managed by splenectomy, and improvement in the hypersplenism is predictable.[23]

Gaucher Disease

Patients with several metabolic abnormalities associated with hypersplenism may benefit from splenectomy. Gaucher disease is among these. Gaucher disease is an autosomal recessive metabolic disorder characterized by deficiency of the enzyme β-glucocerebrosidase. This abnormality is most common among Ashkenazi Jews and leads to an accumulation of glucocerebroside in macrophages throughout the body.

The severity of the disease is directly correlated with the relative deficiency of glucocerebrosidase. The most quiescent form is identified in adults. The spleen can become very large, resulting in significant hypersplenism. Patients with juvenile forms of the disease have many more diverse and severe symptoms, with especially debilitating neurologic dysfunction. These patients generally do not survive to adulthood, so the need for splenectomy in their management is usually not an issue.

In adult patients with Gaucher disease, hypersplenism is often a considerable problem. Pain and incapacitating abdominal distention may occur from massive splenomegaly. These patients are at increased risk for overwhelming PSS; partial splenectomy to preserve some splenic tissue has been recommended. It is unclear whether partial splenectomy is beneficial in these patients. Generally, adults with hypersplenism secondary to Gaucher disease require splenectomy.

Felty Syndrome

Felty syndrome is a systemic inflammatory disease characterized by the clinical triad of severe rheumatoid arthritis, splenomegaly, and decreased numbers of circulating granulocytes. These patients also have an increased incidence of leg ulcers. The granulocytopenia is believed secondary to the development of circulating antibodies to granulocytes. Patients are at increased risk for systemic infection because of the granulocyte deficiency. It has been difficult to identify the relation between the severe rheumatoid arthritis and the antigranulocyte antibody.

Patients who have severe granulocytopenia, unremitting leg ulcers, and evidence of systemic infection are the best candidates for splenectomy. Some improvement generally occurs in the clinical symptoms after removal of the spleen, but no evidence indicates that splenectomy is of therapeutic benefit for rheumatoid arthritis.

Systemic Lupus Erythematosus

Systemic lupus erythematosus is another chronic inflammatory disease process; it is characterized by the development of antibodies to DNA. Patients often have a positive direct Coombs test, although they do not have a clinically significant degree of hemolysis. Hypersplenism occurs in these patients, but the pathogenesis is not known. Splenectomy is reserved for those who have clinically significant hypersplenism.

Sarcoidosis

Sarcoidosis is a disease of overproduction of immune proteins. The splenic macrophages and reticular tissue can accumulate sarcoid protein, resulting in hypersplenism. The indications for splenectomy in sarcoidosis are related to the severity of the hypersplenism.

Infection

Systemic infections of many types can lead to hypersplenism secondary to acute and chronic inflammatory changes in the spleen itself. Patients with sepsis may develop splenomegaly with engorgement of macrophages and lymphoid cells in the parenchyma itself. This increase in noncirculating lymphoid cells may be the response of increased immunoglobulin synthesis, as well as increased trapping of activated macrophages. In certain parasitic infections, clearing of parasites from the RBCs in the splenic red pulp may be enhanced. In most types of bacterial or fungal infection, splenomegaly or hypersplenism is incidental. In most of these instances, the hypersplenism resolves with appropriate therapy, and splenectomy is not indicated. Infectious mononucleosis is associated with viral infection and often results in splenomegaly and occasionally hypersplenism. As in other situations where infection-related causes of hypersplenism are found, splenectomy is not generally indicated. In these circumstances, spontaneous acute rupture of the pathologic spleen or rupture that is secondary to trauma may require surgical intervention. Splenic salvage may be difficult in such situations, but it has been described.

Malignancies

The role of the spleen in malignant disease is discussed elsewhere. Hypersplenism can occur secondary to a variety of malignancies, but it is most commonly associated with chronic leukemoid or lymphocytic leukemias. The chronic leukemias and lymphomas lead to sequestration of cellular blood elements in the spleen, and splenomegaly with hypersplenism is a notable occurrence in these disease processes. Because the underlying disease is often subclinical and requires only limited chemotherapy with an excellent long-term prognosis, these patients usually benefit from splenectomy, with considerable postoperative improvement. Hypersplenism with thrombocytopenia is the usual problem, and this almost invariably improves after splenectomy.

Other

Several other disease processes may lead to hypersplenism. The two most common are myelofibrosis with myeloid metaplasia and polycythemia vera. For these as well as other diseases in which secondary hypersplenism occurs, splenectomy should be considered empirically. The operative indications depend on the underlying disease process, the magnitude of the hypersplenism-induced symptoms, and the individual operative risk.

Myelofibrosis With Myeloid Metaplasia

Myelofibrosis with myeloid metaplasia is a variable process that has characteristics of both primary inflammatory and malignant disease. The diagnosis is made by the finding of increased megakaryocytes in the bone marrow with concomitant fibroblast proliferation.[24] Patients usually develop extramedullary hematopoiesis in the spleen and liver. The degree of myelofibrosis is related to the severity of the hypersplenism. Patients with this disease may have associated problems, such as essential thrombocytosis, polycythemia vera, and chronic myelogenous leukemia. The precise pathogenesis of the process is unclear, and a considerable number of these patients eventually develop leukemia.

The spleen has both desirable and problematic characteristics associated with this disease process. It is the site of the extramedullary hematopoiesis that is a compensatory effort to preserve normal cell counts within the circulation. The spleen also sequesters large numbers of cells. Because of this sequestration, spleen size may be considerable. The patient may develop symptoms of abdominal pain and distention. Gastric emptying may be abnormal because of the splenic size alone. Patients with myelofibrosis and myeloid metaplasia have some of the largest spleens encountered in clinical medicine.

Treatment of this syndrome is generally nonoperative. Initially, treatment with glucocorticoids is undertaken as a means to control splenic sequestration and maintain adequate circulating blood cell counts. Splenectomy is considered when hypersplenism is severe and refractory to this approach.[8] Unfortunately, splenectomy has limited benefit and considerable potential for postoperative problems. Splenectomy does not improve survival from the disease, but it does alleviate some of its symptoms.[25] Patients develop larger platelets and thrombocytosis and may be hypercoagulable after splenectomy. Portal vein thrombosis has been described after splenectomy for myelofibrosis and myeloid metaplasia. Aspirin used at or immediately after splenectomy may attenuate the hypercoagulable state.

Long-term consequences of progressive myeloid metaplasia are difficult to determine. About 25% of patients with this problem develop acute myelogenous leukemia. This may be a variant form of leukemia because it is typically unresponsive to chemotherapy.

Polycythemia Vera

Polycythemia vera is a disease process characterized by uncontrolled production of RBCs and their precursors. Other blood cell lines may also be included, but uncontrolled erythrocyte production is the hallmark of the disorder. Extramedullary hematopoiesis is uniform, and 75% of these patients have a palpable spleen, whereas nearly half have hepatomegaly. Splenectomy has little or no role in patients with hypersplenism from polycythemia vera because it is ineffective. Generally, intermittent phlebotomy to remove excess erythrocytes is the best therapy.

MISCELLANEOUS DISEASES OF THE SPLEEN

Hyposplenism

Hyposplenism is the condition in which the peripheral blood has elements suggestive of an asplenic state, despite the anatomic presence of a spleen. This is described in patients with sickle cell disease, inflammatory bowel disease, collagen vascular diseases, and other autoimmune processes. The spleen in a patient with hyposplenism may be any size—small, normal, or enlarged.

The classic peripheral blood smear findings of hyposplenism include Howell-Jolly bodies and spur cells (acanthocytes). These findings in the presence of a spleen are diagnostic of hyposplenism. Hyposplenism is associated with an increased risk for systemic infection, including PSS. Failure of the erythrocyte maintenance mechanisms of the spleen appears to be associated with abnormalities of the specific and nonspecific immune functions of the spleen as well.

Neoplastic Disease

As the largest single lymphoid organ in the body, the spleen becomes involved with many lymphoid malignancies. It is also secondarily affected by malignancies in other parts of the body. Another possibility is that of metastatic deposition of solid tumors from nonlymphoid sources into the spleen. Despite the high blood flow through the spleen and a microanatomy designed to trap circulating cells, the spleen is a relatively rare site of solid tumor metastatic disease compared with the liver. This may be the result of effective local defenses that destroy abnormal cells. Another mechanism of splenic involvement with malignant disease is the rare primary nonlymphoid tumor that arises in the spleen. Any of these scenarios may result in abnormal splenic function.

Primary Tumors of the Spleen

Hemangiomas are the most common primary nonlymphoid tumors of the spleen. These usually present as a single lesion and may be large by the time of diagnosis. Multiple lesions also occur. Hemangiomas of the spleen are often associated with hemangiomas of other organs, especially the liver. The primary risks of splenic hemangiomas are rupture and platelet sequestration. Clinically significant coagulopathies have been associated with large hemangiomas of the spleen.

Although hemangiomas are benign tumors, a tissue diagnosis cannot be made until the spleen has been removed. It is unclear whether partial splenectomy has a role in the management of these lesions because of the possible risk of recurrence in the remaining splenic tissue. In general, the entire spleen is removed.

Hamartomas can develop in any tissue, including the spleen. The histopathology is variable, although the origin is uniformly from the white pulp. These lesions are usually discovered as incidental findings during evaluations for unrelated reasons. Both cystic and solid hamartomas are described. Generally, hamartomas have no specific clinical consequences, unless they are related simply to the size and the mass effect. Differentiation of a splenic hamartoma from other lesions may be difficult or impossible based on imaging evaluation alone. Splenectomy is usually performed as a diagnostic maneuver.

Lymphangiomas of the spleen are cystic lesions that generally do not cause primary symptoms but may lead to secondary splenic abnormalities, such as hypersplenism. Splenic lymphangiomas are usually associated with liver lymphangiomas and have involvement in multiple areas of the body. Lung, skin, and bone involvement is often associated with lymphangiomas of the spleen. As with other splenic lesions, the specific disease process is usually identified at the time of splenectomy.[26]

Angiosarcoma is an extremely rare malignant disorder of the spleen. It is uncommon without similar tumors in other organs, concurrent angiosarcoma of the liver being the most frequent. Splenectomy is done for diagnosis and generally provides the only therapy required. At the time of operation, other areas of angiosarcoma involvement can be identified. Additional therapy is dictated by the extent of disease at other sites of involvement.

Hodgkin's Disease

Hodgkin's disease is the result of a malignant lymphoid neoplasm. Its relatively unusual characteristics consist of a localized origin and limited regional spread. Systemic dissemination of Hodgkin's disease is a relatively late occurrence. Hodgkin's disease is pathologically defined by the presence of giant, multinucleated Sternberg-Reed cells in the abnormal lymphoid tissue.

The cellular classification of Hodgkin's disease from the Rye, New York, conference includes lymphocyte predominance, nodular sclerosis, mixed cellularity, and lymphocyte depletion. Many new attempts at classification based on morphology and cell-surface immunologic characteristics have been undertaken. Current molecular biology techniques offer the potential for new means of classification, but these are still being developed. It is unclear whether any new system will supplant the Rye classification system.

The exact cell of origin of Hodgkin's disease varies among individuals. It is also unclear whether the cell type is consistent from patient to patient. Macrophages and T cells are both reported as the cell of origin of Hodgkin's disease. Hodgkin's disease can develop in any lymphoid tissue. In about 10% of patients, the spleen is the primary site. The role of staging splenectomy in Hodgkin's disease has decreased significantly. Staging laparotomy to assess the pathologic extent of Hodgkin's disease is no longer routine; however, this issue is controversial.

In the past, up to 42% of patients with Hodgkin's disease had a change in staging at laparotomy. With the development of more sophisticated imaging techniques, the value of staging laparotomy is less clear.[27] Some institutions continue to perform staging laparotomy, whereas others avoid it totally. The spleen is positive for Hodgkin's disease in 30% of patients with the disease.[28]

The decision to proceed with staging laparotomy depends on the clinical stage of the disease. Table 55-3 provides the Ann Arbor classification for clinical staging. The histopathologic criteria for different types of Hodgkin's disease are also important. Placement of the disease into these subcategories permits a much improved prognostic effort.

If staging laparotomy is elected, specific tissues require sampling.[28,29] Classically, a thorough abdominal exploration is performed, followed by sampling of lymphoid tissue. Needle liver biopsies and wedge biopsies of the liver are performed in both lobes, usually using the anterior edge of the relevant lobe. Splenectomy is considered standard. Careful search is made for perihilar lymph nodes. Sampling of lymph nodes is then performed, including all large lymph nodes. Representative nodes from several areas are also taken if no specific large nodes are identified. The areas that require sampling are the bilateral iliac regions and the periaortic, portahepatic, and celiac node areas. These biopsies are summarized in Figure 55-6. These areas are all marked with nonmagnetic radiopaque clips. This permits targeting of radiotherapy through CT or magnetic resonance imaging after review of the permanent pathology. Each lymph node and its origin are identified on the specimen, and the tissues are sent separately for pathologic evaluation. Bone marrow biopsies or aspiration should be performed at that time, if they have not already been done. There is some debate as to whether an appendectomy should be performed at laparotomy.

Few complications result from a planned staging laparotomy with splenectomy, and the operative mortality rate should be under 1%. There may be late morbidity related to the development of secondary malignancies, especially acute myelogenous leukemia. The question of whether splenectomy increases the risk for this is unanswered. This is one reason why staging laparotomy and splenectomy are debated in the management of Hodgkin's disease.

Non-Hodgkin's Lymphoma

Unlike Hodgkin's disease, other lymphomas are generally systemic diseases at the time of diagnosis. Primary disease limited to the spleen is rare. Lymphomas are classified according to their aggressiveness and by morphologic appearance of the tumor cells:

Low-Grade Aggressiveness

- Small lymphocytic
- Follicular small cleaved cell
- Follicular mixed cell

Intermediate-Grade Aggressiveness

- Follicular large cell
- Diffuse small cell
- Diffuse mixed cell
- Diffuse large cell

High-Grade Aggressiveness

- Lymphoblastic
- Small noncleaved cell
- Immunoblastic

These categories are stratified for biologic behavior on the basis of histology. The lymphomas may also be staged with the Ann Arbor classification system as used for patients with Hodgkin's disease. Distinctions between different stages are less clear, and the system's ability to predict outcome is much less accurate in patients who have non-Hodgkin's lymphoma.

Splenectomy has a limited role in the management of lymphoma. The clinical ability to identify lymphomatous involvement of the spleen is poor. One third of spleens that are involved with tumor are of normal size. Furthermore, only one third of the spleens in patients with lymphoma have tumors identified in them. In general, operative intervention for splenic lymphoma is restricted to patients who have symptomatic disease related to their spleen or patients in whom the lymphoma is not identified until the spleen is removed for diagnostic purposes.

Hairy Cell Leukemia

Hairy cell leukemia is a lymphocytic leukemia characterized by abnormal B cells in 90% of cases and abnormal T cells in the other 10%. It is initially diagnosed morphologically by the ruffled leukocyte cell membranes seen on light and electron microscopy. The diagnosis is enhanced by selective staining for tartrate-resistant acid phosphatase, which is present in about 90% of patients with hairy cell leukemia. These hairy cells are seen predominantly in the red pulp. The spleen in patients with hairy cell leukemia is enlarged and has white surface deposits that resemble sugar coating (Fig. 55-7).

Clinically, patients with hairy cell leukemia have splenomegaly and pancytopenia. Hairy cell leukemia is more common in men and most often occurs after age 50. The pancytopenias are the result of sequestration of all blood elements in the spleen, as well as marrow replacement by leukemic cells and diminished production of blood cellular components. Hairy cell leukemia is seen with coexistent malignancies in more than 10% of patients; it also has an increased incidence of coexisting infections.

The role of splenectomy in hairy cell leukemia is controversial. Splenectomy for symptomatic hypersplenism is beneficial in over 80% of patients. It improves all cell counts and lessens the risks of hemorrhage. Splenectomy is associated with improved survival, possibly because of avoidance of the complications of pancytopenia. Medical therapy with α-interferon is being evaluated, but the long-term outcome compared with splenectomy is not known.

Table 55-3. ANN ARBOR STAGING SYSTEM FOR HODGKIN'S DISEASE

STAGE

Stage I	Single lymph node region or extralymphoid site
Stage II	Two or more lymph node areas or one extralymphoid site with one lymph node area; but all are on one side of the diaphragm
Stage III	Multiple lymph node sites on both sides of the diaphragm. With localized extralymphoid sites, this is IIIE; with splenic involvement, IIIS; and with both, IIIES
Stage IV	Diffuse involvement of extralymphoid organs, with or without adenopathy

CLINICAL MODIFIERS

A	No systemic symptoms
B	Temperature above 38°C, night sweats, or weight loss

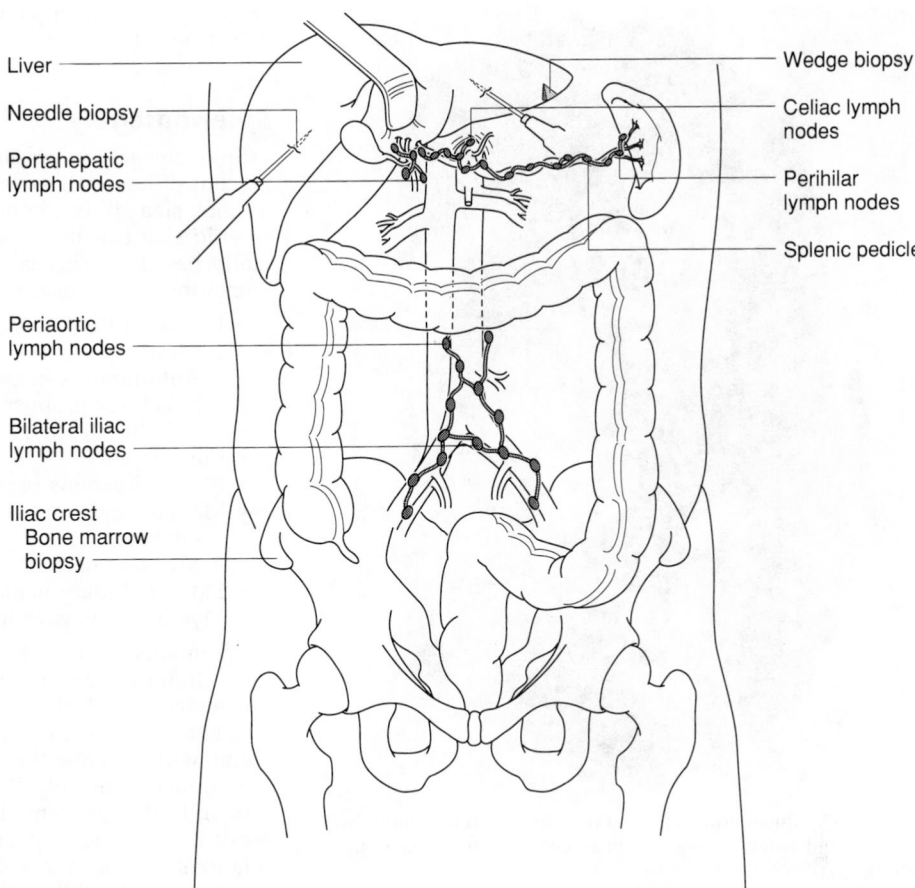

Liver

Needle biopsy

Portahepatic lymph nodes

Wedge biopsy

Celiac lymph nodes

Perihilar lymph nodes

Splenic pedicle

Periaortic lymph nodes

Bilateral iliac lymph nodes

Iliac crest
Bone marrow biopsy

Figure 55-6. The tissues to be removed or to undergo biopsy in a staging laparotomy for Hodgkin's disease. Splenectomy, liver biopsy, and lymph node sampling in the specific sites are shown. Bone marrow biopsy can be done if necessary.

Chronic Myelogenous Leukemia

Chronic myelogenous leukemia (CML) is seen most often in the third and fourth decades of life and is slightly more common in men than in women. It is associated with the Philadelphia chromosome, which is a 22/9 gene translocation. This Philadelphia chromosome is present in 90% of patients with CML.

Most patients with CML (80%) progress to acute myelogenous leukemia; this is characterized by a blast crisis. This usually occurs 1 to 4 years after the diagnosis of chronic myelogenous leukemia is established. Splenectomy is performed for symptoms of splenomegaly or exaggerated splenic sequestration of cellular elements. Splenectomy does not have an effect on the survival of patients with CML.

Chronic Lymphocytic Leukemia

Chronic lymphocytic leukemia is a B-cell leukemia that is predominantly a disease of the elderly. It is more common in men than in women. Clinically, it presents as adenopathy and splenomegaly with exaggerated peripheral lymphocyte counts. Characteristically, 20% or more of patients develop a second malignancy, and a considerable number develop acute hemolytic anemia. Treatment of chronic lymphocytic leukemia involves different forms of chemotherapy and occasionally corticosteroids. Radiation therapy has been used to control large spleens, but splenectomy remains the principal management strategy. Splenectomy results in a considerable decrease in the peripheral lymphocyte count in more than 80% of patients. Transfusion requirements are decreased after splenectomy because of prolonged RBC survival and better primary cellular pro-

duction. The spleen may have areas of acute infarction, as shown in Figure 55-8.

Patients with chronic lymphocytic leukemia generally die from complications related to infection or bleeding if they do not develop lethal secondary malignancies.

Treatment of Hematologic Malignancies

Patients who undergo bone marrow transplantation for leukemia or lymphoma may need splenectomy before transplantation. It is generally performed several weeks before the bone marrow transplant to allow the patient time to recover from the operation.

Splenic Cysts

True splenic cysts are uncommon. They can be either congenital or acquired. The latter usually occur after traumatic injury. Pseudocysts of the spleen may result from pancreatitis. These pseudocysts arise from the pancreas but present with some or all of the cyst within the splenic parenchyma. Pseudocysts and posttraumatic acquired cysts often resolve spontaneously and can be successfully treated by simple aspiration. Splenectomy is considered if the cyst persists or becomes symptomatic, regardless of etiology.

Some splenic cysts are secondary to parasitic or nonparasitic infections, particularly from hydatid disease. As with other echinococcal infections, primary attention is directed at killing all of the parasites. The residual cyst can be surgically addressed if it presents a problem after nonoperative treatment of the infection.

Nonparasitic cysts of the spleen are rare, and patients

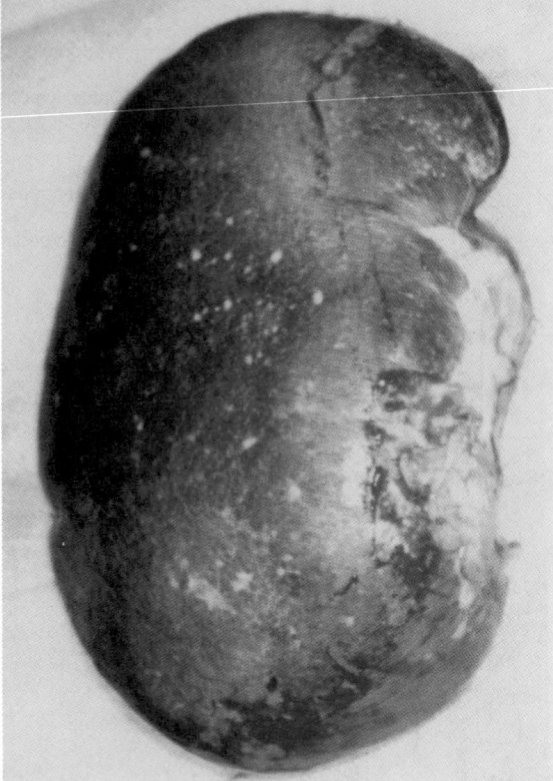

Figure 55-7. Spleen from a patient with hairy cell leukemia. Note the whitened anterior edge of the spleen and the white "sugar-coating" spots on the surface.

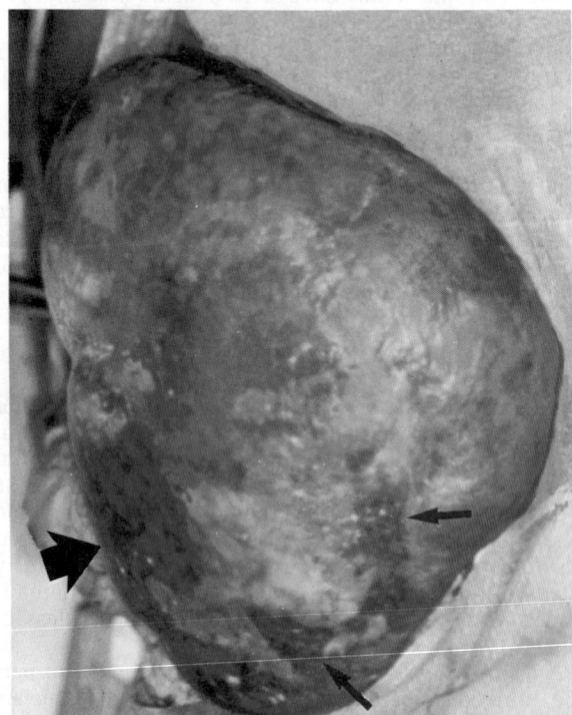

Figure 55-8. A massively enlarged, 2.2-kg spleen from a patient with chronic lymphocytic leukemia. Superficial areas of infarction are indicated by thin arrows and splenic infarction by the thick arrow.

usually present with pain. The presence of a parenchymal defect on CT usually results in splenectomy to rule out other causes. A schematic example is seen in Figure 55-9.

Splenomegaly

Splenomegaly is present in about 3% of patients. Five percent of hospitalized patients have palpable spleens of normal size. It is unclear how accurate assessment of splenic size can be, because these assessments are normally based on clinical studies without objective documentation. The causes of splenomegaly are as follows:

- Increased RBC destruction
- Inflammatory processes
    Autoimmune hemolytic anemia
    Infectious problems
- Metabolic disorders
- Congestion
- Elevated venous pressure
- Malignancy
    Leukemia
    Myelofibrosis
- Extramedullary hematopoiesis
- Myelofibrosis with myeloid metaplasia

Splenomegaly is not itself an indication for splenectomy. In most patients, splenomegaly is transient and has no deleterious effects. The finding of splenomegaly should lead to evaluation, including a complete blood and platelet count with examination of the peripheral blood smear. Additionally, the spleen should be imaged to evaluate its size and other abnormalities. CT is the best means of assessing splenic size, parenchymal abnormalities, and the relations to other intraabdominal structures. Liver–spleen scans assess the ability of the spleen to take up particulate matter but are relatively insensitive. In addition, they suffer from the operator-dependent nature of the study. After diagnostic evaluation, the surgeon should participate in evaluating the cause of splenomegaly and planning treatment.

SURGICAL MANAGEMENT OF SPLENIC PATHOLOGY

The surgical management of splenic disease is based on the type of disease, the severity of disease, the goals of surgery, and the relative risks and benefits of surgery.[29]

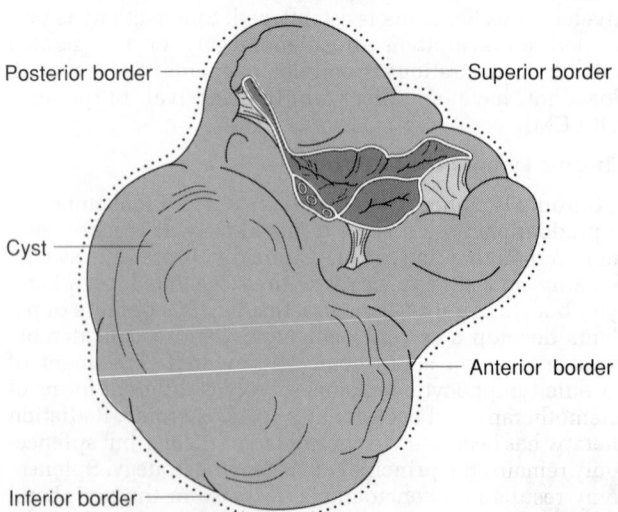

Figure 55-9. The visceral surface of a spleen with a true congenital splenic cyst.

These factors relate to the underlying disease process as well as to other individual medical problems. In general, nonoperative management of splenic pathology should be used when it is superior to or as effective as surgical therapy.[30] Splenic surgery should not be avoided or delayed when appropriate indications exist. A list of the most common diseases for which splenectomy should be considered follows.

Thrombocytopenia
- ITP
- TTP

Malignancy
- Hairy cell leukemia
- Hodgkin's disease
- Non-Hodgkin's lymphoma
- Other primary splenic tumors
- Metastatic or locally invasive tumor

Anemia
- Autoimmune hemolytic anemia
- Hereditary hemolytic anemia
- Medullary fibrosis with myeloid metaplasia

Hypersplenism
- Primary hypersplenism
- Other causes of hypersplenism

Miscellaneous
- Leukopenias
- Metabolic disorders
- Gaucher disease
- Granulomatous disease
- Cysts
- Abscesses
- Idiopathic splenomegaly

Trauma

Partial splenectomy has been advocated for some diseases in which splenic involvement is limited. In such circumstances, preservation of a small segment of the spleen must not allow recurrence of the original problem. Because the technical hazards of partial splenectomy are significant, and because the functional preservation of splenic tissue is somewhat problematic, the reliance on partial splenectomy is limited. It remains an experimental procedure for primary or secondary diseases of the spleen, with the important exception of trauma.

Splenic salvage techniques are used routinely in the management of splenic trauma. This is an accepted, standard procedure for the minimally injured spleen or when partial resection is possible.[31] Increasingly, isolated splenic trauma seen on abdominal CT scan after injury is managed nonoperatively. This is associated with a good outcome in most series of hemodynamically stable patients. Decisions regarding nonoperative versus operative treatment should be based on clinical parameters, because grading of splenic injury by CT does not correlate with the need for splenectomy.[32,33] The goal of splenic preservation is to decrease the incidence of overwhelming PSS in patients who might otherwise have been rendered asplenic. Most problems discussed in this review are those in which the entire spleen is involved in the disease process. Total splenectomy is almost always the choice when dealing with nontraumatic problems involving the spleen. Techniques for both splenectomy and splenorrhaphy are discussed in this chapter.

Techniques for Splenectomy

The spleen is generally approached through one of two exposures. The first involves an upper midline incision that extends along the xiphoid process. This permits ade-

quate mobilization of the spleen and its hilum, and allows predictable control of the vascular supply to the spleen. The other commonly used approach for splenectomy is the left subcostal incision. This incision is placed below the left costal margin from the midline and is extended laterally to the anterior axillary line, if necessary. This is carried down through the rectus abdominis muscle and peritoneum, exposing the intraperitoneal spleen below the costal margin. This approach permits direct access to the spleen and makes control of its lower and lateral attachments easier. Access to the upper attachments of the spleen may be slightly more difficult when compared with the midline approach. The choice between these two incisions depends on the surgeon's preference and may be based on the size of the spleen and the need to explore the rest of the abdomen. There are no objective data that favor either incision.

After entry into the peritoneum, abdominal exploration is routine. Adequate exposure of the left upper quadrant, regardless of the incision, is best accomplished with a firm retractor, either hand-held or fixed. Packs are used to hold the colon away from the inferior edge of the spleen and the stomach medially away from the medial aspect of the spleen. The left lateral segment of the liver is mobilized by dividing the triangular ligaments; it is then folded and retracted to the left with the stomach. The spleen is inspected visually and then carefully palpated to estimate its size and the degree of attachment to the diaphragm and surrounding structures. The lesser sac can be opened for examination and ligation of the splenic vessels, if necessary. Accessory spleens are sought along the cephalad and caudal edges of the pancreas behind the stomach. The area of the gastrohepatic ligament is another potential area for an accessory spleen. The greater omentum and the splenic hilum must be examined as well. Accessory spleens are present in about 20% of individuals. It is unclear how much these accessory spleens function, but total splenectomy should include a thorough search for and excision of any accessory spleens.

The blood vessels to the spleen are examined either through the lesser sac or at the splenic hilum, the latter being more common. Evidence of significant portal hypertension or thrombosis may be useful in selecting the ap-

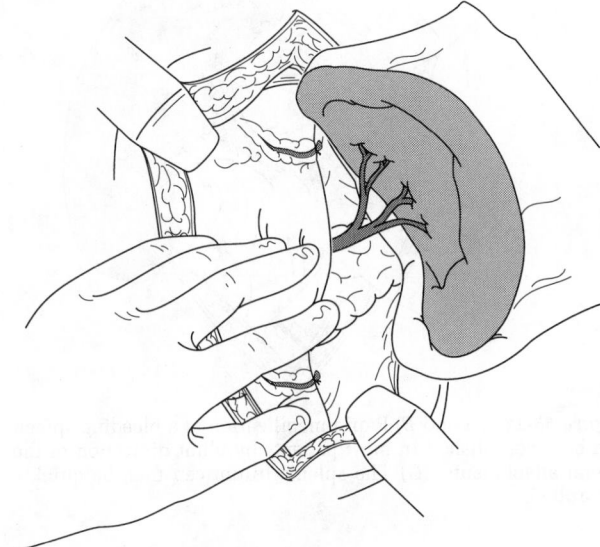

Figure 55-10. Lateral mobilization permits the spleen to reach the surface of a midline wound despite the presence of intact hilar vessels.

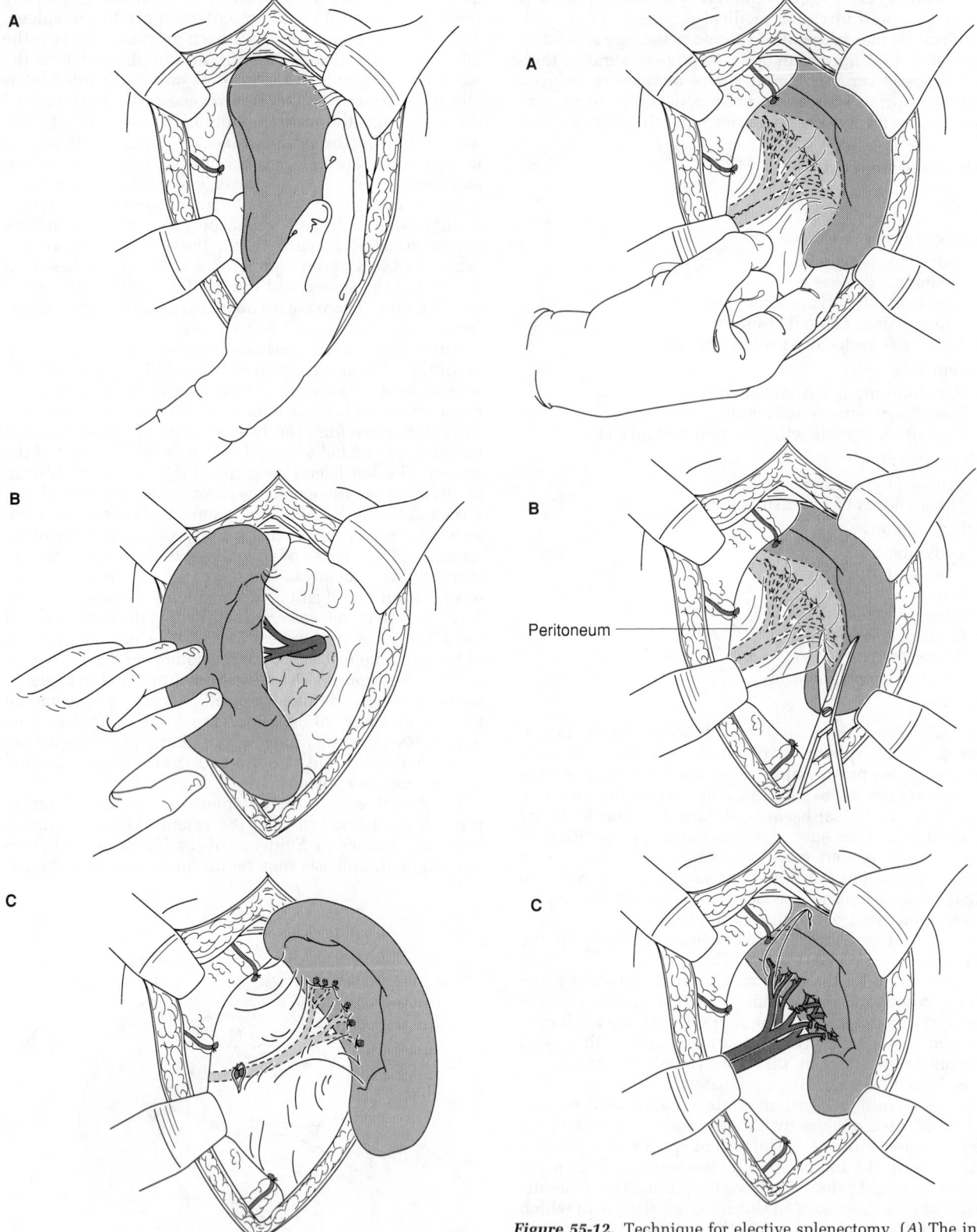

Figure 55-11. (*A* and *B*) Rapid mobilization of a bleeding spleen can be accomplished in most patients by blunt dissection of the lateral attachments. (*C*) The splenic hilum can then be quickly controlled.

Figure 55-12. Technique for elective splenectomy. (*A*) The inferior pole is reflected laterally by the assistant's fingers, exposing the lower edge of the hilar peritoneal envelope. (*B*) The hilar peritoneum is opened, here shown progressing from inferior to superior. (*C*) Individual vessels are identified and suture ligated.

proach to splenectomy. Large spleens with a dilated splenic vasculature may be removed safely and more easily after ligation of the splenic artery, remote from the splenic hilum. This usually can be accomplished through the lesser sac, identifying the splenic artery cephalad to the pancreas.

The sequence in which the splenic attachments are taken down varies among surgeons. Some alter their approach depending on the anatomy of the individual patient. The short gastric vessels (vasa brevia) can be ligated and divided as the initial step. The lateral and lower attachments to the spleen can be taken first. Regardless of the technique, it is best to proceed in an orderly fashion with good visualization. Mobilization to facilitate the dissection can usually be performed without injury to the spleen or tearing the major hilar vessels.

The posterior peritoneal attachments can generally be divided by direct visualization with scissors or electrocautery between the jaws of a right-angle clamp. Once these posterior attachments have been divided, the spleen can be readily brought into the abdominal wound. Mobilization of the spleen is shown in Figure 55-10. In this figure, the spleen, which is still attached by its pedicle, is lying in the midline incision. If the spleen is ruptured or otherwise abnormal, rapid mobilization can be accomplished by delivering the spleen into the wound by hand, as in Figure 55-11.

The spleen can be removed from either the cranial or caudal pole. For example, after division of the lienocolic attachments to the inferior surface, the peritoneal envelope is opened. The lower pole is reflected laterally, revealing the caudad edge of the hilar peritoneum (Fig. 55-12A). The peritoneum can be divided by cautery or scissors (see Fig. 55-12B). This peritoneal division is carried up to the hilum, where identification of the splenic vessels is made. The individual splenic vessels are carefully dissected and divided between ties or clamps. The proximal ends of the vessels are usually suture ligated with 3-0 silk (see Fig. 55-12C). After dissection and ligation of the splenic artery and vein, additional attachments can be divided between clamps along the superior aspect of the peritoneal attachments to the greater curvature of the stomach.

There are usually two or three vascular attachments of the upper greater curvature of the stomach to the spleen. These short gastric vessels are clamped and suture ligated. Any remaining attachments of the spleen are divided, and the organ can be removed and sent for pathology. If there is any question of malignant disease, it is best to have the pathologist present in the operating room to take the specimen for touch preparations or specific immunologic staining techniques to identify lymphocyte subpopulations.

Massive bleeding during splenectomy is encountered when the splenic vessels are perforated during dissection

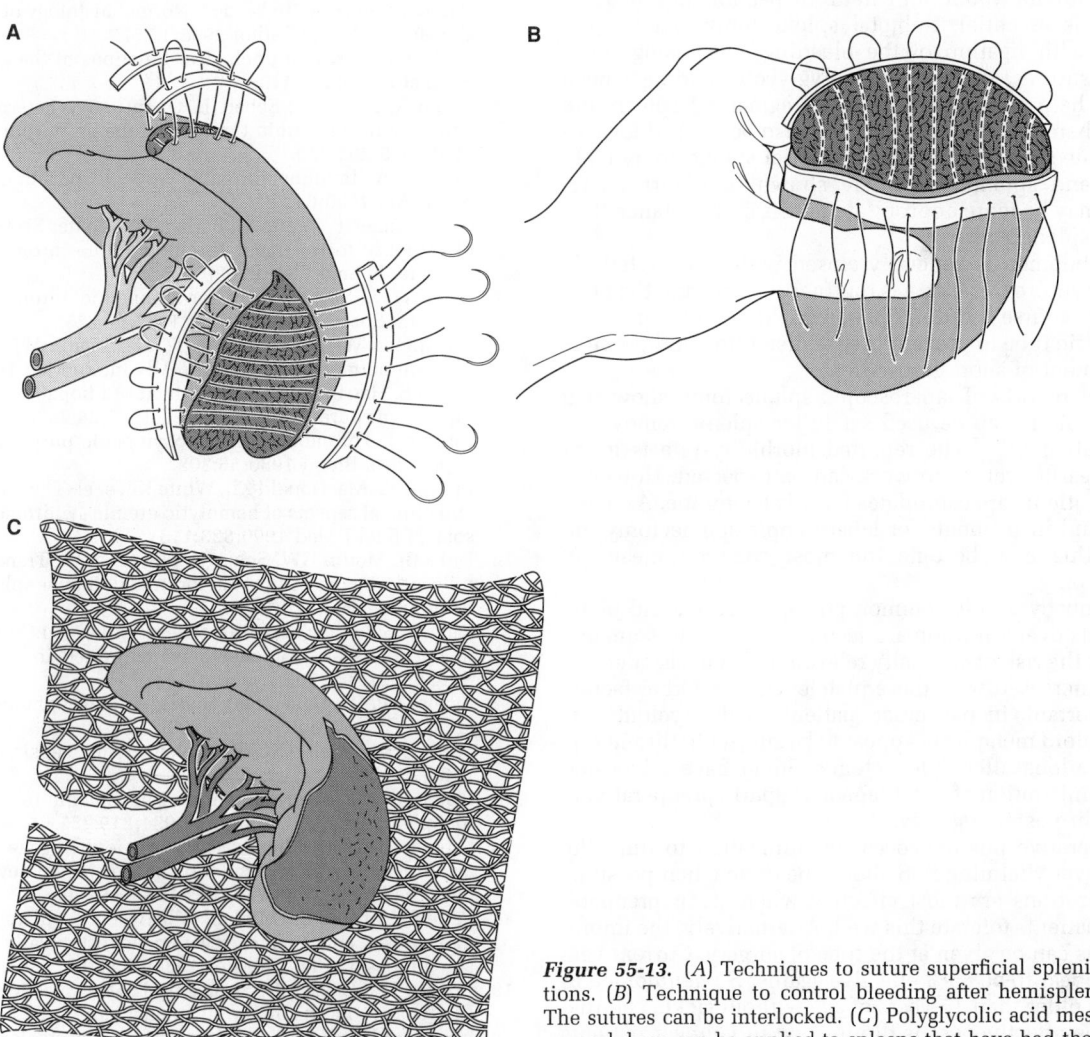

Figure 55-13. (*A*) Techniques to suture superficial splenic lacerations. (*B*) Technique to control bleeding after hemisplenectomy. The sutures can be interlocked. (*C*) Polyglycolic acid mesh sheets or mesh bags can be applied to spleens that have had the capsule stripped away.

of the hilum. This occasionally occurs because of traction on the splenic or hilar vessels during dissection. It is best not to blindly place a clamp on the hilum of the spleen. The tail of the pancreas is usually in the immediate area, and pancreatic injury may result in pseudocyst or fistula formation. If significant bleeding occurs, it is better to reach down and occlude the vessels between the thumb and the finger while the vessels are dissected. Massive bleeding can also occur from lateral attachments or accessory vessels if portal hypertension is present. In general, this should be anticipated before the procedure is begun, and all attachments should be divided and tied carefully.

Bleeding from the short gastric vessels can occur late postoperatively from dislodgment of a tie or transection without ligature. It is important to carefully inspect the short gastric vessels on the greater curvature of the stomach and the splenic hilum after the spleen has been removed.

Generally, drains are not used for elective splenectomy. These have been associated with increased complications, particularly infection. If a drain is necessary, a closed-suction drain should be used. Measurement of the amylase content of any drained fluid is done the first postoperative day. If this is negligible and output volume is small, the drain can be removed. Persistent, large-volume drainage or drainage fluid with a high amylase content warrants leaving the drain in place until the area can be investigated by either sonography or CT.

Partial splenectomy and splenorrhaphy are accomplished by use of the same principles. Mobilization of the spleen into the wound for careful inspection and repair of injuries is essential. Subtotal splenectomy can be performed with ligation of the bleeding edge using interlocking sutures. Mesh bags of polyglycolic acid have been used to help apply pressure to a fragmented spleen and control hemorrhage. Staplers have also been used for partial splenectomy.[34] Examples of partial splenectomy techniques and splenic repair are shown in Figure 55-13. Drains may be more appropriate in this circumstance than in total splenectomy.

The abdomen is generally closed with interrupted absorbable sutures. The skin is routinely closed, and the postoperative course is ordinarily benign. Many surgeons use a nasogastric tube to prevent gastric distention and possible dislodgment of short gastric ties.

Recent reports of laparoscopic splenectomy show that this technique can be used safely for splenic removal in some patients.[35-37] The reported morbidity rate is lower and an earlier return to work can be expected. However, not all patients are candidates for this technique. As experience and instruments for laparoscopic splenectomy improve, this may become the most common means of splenectomy.

Thrombocytosis is common postoperatively, and platelet counts over 1 million are seen fairly often. It is unclear whether the risk of clinically relevant thrombosis or embolism is increased with these platelet counts. Other factors are important. In particular, patients with myelofibrosis and myeloid metaplasia appear to be subject to thrombotic complications after splenectomy. Some have advocated the administration of subcutaneous heparin preoperatively or aspirin postoperatively.

Preoperative pneumococcal immunization to limit the risk of overwhelming PSS should be done when possible. Immunizations are most effective when given preoperatively; patients tolerate this well. Alternatively, the immunizations can be given at the time of surgery. Current vaccines appear to be 85% effective against *S pneumoniae* in patients older than 15 years of age without sickle cell disease. The effectiveness is diminished in younger patients or if the patient has sickle cell disease or other hematologic

disorders.[38] Regardless of the immunization status, prophylactic penicillin should be considered in all children, all patients with sickle cell disease, and all patients who have underlying hematologic diseases.[39]

The role of booster or secondary immunizations is unclear. These are associated with local and systemic side effects such as fever, chills, and other symptoms.

Apparent acceleration of atherosclerosis has been described after splenectomy. This is believed to be secondary to the increased number of circulating platelets or possibly other immune mechanisms that involve the atherosclerotic process.

Additionally, the question of an increased incidence of malignancy after splenectomy has been raised. This is a difficult issue to address, and no consensus exists.

The incidence of complications after splenectomy is as high as 17% among patients with primary hematologic disorders.[26] A 1% mortality rate has been described in similar patients. The most common complication in these patients was bleeding, which occurred in 4%. Significant postoperative bleeding was most common in patients with very large spleens, including 30% of patients with spleens larger than 2 kg.

REFERENCES

1. Skandalakis PN, Colborn GL, Skandalakis LJ, Richardson DD, Mitchell WE Jr, Skandalakis JE. The surgical anatomy of the spleen. Surg Clin North Am 1993;73:747.
2. Van Krieken JHJM, te Velde J. Normal histology of the human spleen. Am J Surg Pathol 1988;12:777.
3. Lockwood CM. Immunological functions of the spleen. Clin Haematol 1983;12:449.
4. Dixon R, Rosse W, Ebbert L. Quantitative determination of antibody in idiopathic thrombocytopenic purpura. N Engl J Med 1975;292:230.
5. Koller CA. Immune thrombocytopenic purpura. Med Clin North Am 1980;64:761.
6. Gernsheimer T, Stratton J, Ballem PJ, Slichter SJ. Mechanisms of response to treatment in autoimmune thrombocytopenic purpura. N Engl J Med 1989;320:974.
7. Coon WW. Splenectomy for idiopathic thrombocytopenic purpura. Surg Gynecol Obstet 1987;64:225.
8. Harrington WJ Jr, Harrington TJ, Harrington WJ. Is splenectomy an outmoded procedure? Adv Intern Med 1990;35:415.
9. Ahn YS, Harrington WJ. Treatment of idiopathic thrombocytopenic purpura. Annu Rev Med 1977;28:299.
10. Cuttner J. Thrombotic thrombocytopenic purpura: a 10-year experience. Blood 1980;56:302.
11. Martin DL, MacDonald KL, White KE, et al. The epidemiology and clinical aspects of hemolytic uremic syndrome in Minnesota. N Engl J Med 1990;323:1161.
12. Duke BJ, Modin GW, Schecter WP, Horn JK. Transfusion significantly increases the risk for infection after splenic injury. Arch Surg 1993;128:1125.
13. King H, Schumacker HB Jr. Splenic studies. 1. Susceptibility to infections after splenectomy performed in infancy. Ann Surg 1952;136:239.
14. Evans D. Post-splenectomy sepsis ten years or more after operation. J Clin Pathol 1985;38:309.
15. Shaw JHF, Print CG. Postsplenectomy sepsis. Br J Surg 1989;76:1074.
16. Pisters PW, Pachter HL. Autologous splenic transplantation for splenic trauma. Ann Surg 1994;219:225.
17. Groom AC. The Microvascular Society Eugene M. Landis award lecture. Microcirculation of the spleen: new concepts, new challenge. Microvasc Res 1987;34:269.
18. Felle P, Harding B. Differences between the histology of normal spleen and that of regenerated ectopically implanted splenic tissue. Eur Surg Res 1988;20:220.
19. Cooney DR, Dearth JC, Swanson SE, Dewanjee MK, Telander RL. Relative merits of partial splenectomy, splenic reimplantation, and immunization in preventing postsplenectomy infection. Surgery 1979;86:561.

20. Eichner ER. Splenic function: normal, too much and too little. Am J Med 1979;66:311.
21. El-Khishen MA, Henderson JM, Milikan WJ, et al. Splenectomy is contraindicated for thrombocytopenia secondary to portal hypertension. Surg Gynecol Obstet 1985;160:233.
22. Lankisch PG. The spleen in inflammatory pancreatic disease. Gastroenterology 1990;98:509.
23. Bradley EL III. The natural history of splenic vein thrombosis due to chronic pancreatitis: indications for surgery. Int J Pancreatol 1987;2:87.
24. Groopman JE. The pathogenesis of myelofibrosis in myeloproliferative disorders. Ann Intern Med 1980;92:857.
25. Wilson RE, Rosenthal DS, Moloney WC, et al. Splenectomy for myeloproliferative disorders. World J Surg 1985;9:431.
26. Rolfes RJ, Ros PR. The spleen: an integrated imaging approach. Crit Rev Diagn Imaging 1990;30:41.
27. Rosenberg SA. Laparotomy and splenectomy in Hodgkin's disease: a reappraisal after 20 years. Scand J Haematol 1985;34:289.
28. Taylor MA, Kaplan HS, Nelsen TS. Staging laparotomy with splenectomy for Hodgkin's disease: the Stanford experience. World J Surg 1985;9:449.
29. Johansson T, Bostrom H, Sjodahl R, Ihse I. Splenectomy for haematological diseases. Acta Chir Scand 1990;156:83.
30. Munser G, Lazar G, Hocking W, Busuttil W. Splenectomy for hematologic disease: the UCLA experience with 306 patients. Ann Surg 1984;200:40.
31. Lucas CE. Splenic trauma: choice of management. Ann Surg 1991;213:98.
32. Kohn JS, Clark DE, Isler RJ, Pope CF. Is computed tomographic grading of splenic injury useful in the nonsurgical management of blunt trauma? J Trauma 1994;37:870.
33. Becker CD, Spring P, Glattli A, Schweizer W. Blunt splenic trauma in adults: can CT findings be used to determine the need for surgery? AJR Am J Roentgenol 1994;162:343.
34. Uranus S, Kronberger L, Kraft-Kine J. Partial splenic resection using the TA-stapler. Am J Surg 1994;168:49.
35. Carroll BJ, Phillips EH, Semel CJ, et al. Laparoscopic splenectomy. Surg Endosc 1992;6:183.
36. Delaitre B, Maignien B. Laparoscopic splenectomy: technical aspects. Surg Endosc 1992;6:305.
37. Taddeo F, Sessa R, Sessa E, Minelli S. Video laparoscopic treatment of spleen injuries: report of two cases. Surg Endosc 1994;8:910.
38. Bolan G, Broome CV, Facklam RR, Plikaytis BD, Fraser DW, Schlech WF III. Pneumococcal vaccine efficacy in selected populations in the United States. Ann Intern Med 1986;104:1.
39. Barrett DJ. Human immune responses to polysaccharide antigens: an analysis of bacterial polysaccharide vaccines in infants. Adv Pediatr 1985;32:139.

SURGICAL ENDOCRINOLOGY

SURGERY: SCIENTIFIC PRINCIPLES AND PRACTICE, Second Edition, edited by
Lazar J. Greenfield, Michael W. Mulholland, Keith T. Oldham, Gerald B. Zelenock,
and Keith D. Lillemoe. Lippincott–Raven Publishers, Philadelphia, © 1997.

CHAPTER 56

THYROID GLAND

NORMAN W. THOMPSON

ANATOMY

Embryology

The thyroid gland originates from the primitive alimentary tract and is predominantly of endodermal origin. It arises as a midline diverticulum from the floor of the pharynx in the region of the foramen cecum at about the third gestational week and becomes recognizable about 1 month after conception. The main body of the thyroid descends into the neck from this origin as a hollow cylinder of epithelial cells that becomes consolidated as it migrates caudally. It then develops into a bilobed solid organ. The original attachment to the buccal cavity at the foramen cecum is the thyroglossal duct, which ruptures and is resorbed during the sixth week of gestation. The distal end of the duct may be retained as the pyramidal lobe of the adult thyroid. The median thyroid anlage develops into the lateral thyroid lobes and their isthmus, which covers the upper two or three tracheal rings.

As the lateral lobes develop, follicles are noted. By the time the embryo is 60 mm long, colloid is found within them. Thyroid glandular function develops by the third month, when iodine trapping occurs and thyroid hormones are first secreted. During formation of lateral lobes, the ultimobranchial fourth pharyngeal pouches give rise to the calcitonin-producing C cells that migrate from the neural crest to this location. These coalesce and enter the lateral and posterior upper two thirds of the thyroid lobes, where they are distributed among follicles. Their concentration is limited to the upper and middle portions of the gland, particularly in their posterior and medial aspects. In some vertebrates, the C cells from the fourth and fifth pharyngeal pouches form ultimobranchial bodies that remain as separate calcitonin-secreting organs. The C cells of the human thyroid are the only nonendodermal component of the adult gland.

The most common developmental malformations requiring surgical intervention are thyroglossal duct cysts and fistulas. Less common is the lingual thyroid gland, which is usually associated with agenesis of other thyroid tissues. Thyroglossal cysts usually occur at or near the midline, from the base of the tongue to the suprasternal notch. About 75% are found just inferior to the hyoid bone. They are most often noted in infancy or early childhood, although they can be found at any age. They are equally distributed between the sexes and can be identified by their elevation in the neck when the tongue is protruded. Choking and dysphagia can occur, but it is usually a mass or infection of the cyst that leads to medical evaluation. Frequently, spontaneous rupture or surgical drainage (in infection) results in a chronically draining fistula. Sinuses or cysts may be lined by columnar, cuboidal, or even squamous epithelium, but the wall usually contains some thyroid tissue. As a result, cysts may be the origin of thyroid cancer, which is usually papillary in type. All thyroglossal duct cysts should be excised because of the potential for infection.

The basic principle of the operation is to excise the entire cyst as well as the thyroglossal tract up to its origin at the foramen cecum. Because the tract so frequently passes through the center of the hyoid bone, removal of its central portion is crucial to success. Recurrence results from failure to excise the entire tract to the base of the tongue. Excision of a portion of the hyoid bone requires no repair and incurs no disability. This approach nearly eliminates the problem of recurrence. When papillary carcinoma arises in a thyroglossal duct or cyst, total excision of the cyst and tract may be sufficient. When lymph node metastases are already present, total thyroidectomy must be considered with regional excision of all involved nodes. Such procedures are then followed by radioactive iodine (^{131}I) scintiscanning and treatment with radioactive iodine if residual disease is found.

Lingual thyroids represent failure of the median thyroid anlage to descend normally. This tissue is often the only thyroid tissue present. When there is airway obstruction, interference with swallowing, or hemorrhage, surgical excision may be required. Most lingual thyroid glands can be decreased in size by suppressing thyroid-stimulating hormone (TSH) with exogenous thyroid hormone administration. Treatment with ^{131}I followed by thyroid hormone replacement therapy is another alternative to surgical excision. Because thyroid replacement therapy is well accepted by patients, excision and transplantation of lingual thyroid tissue is rarely performed.

Ectopic thyroid tissue is found in other locations within the central compartment of the neck. Remnants can be found even in the anterior mediastinum. More often, a nodule of thyroid tissue below the lower poles of the thyroid represents sequestered thyroid nodules usually associated with multinodular goiters. Thyroid nodules in the carotid sheath or lateral neck represent metastases of well-differentiated thyroid carcinoma. The concept that normal thyroid tissue could appear in the lateral neck (*lateral aberrant thyroid*) as an embryologic accident has been abandoned. A small primary thyroid carcinoma is found within the ipsilateral thyroid lobe even when it appears to be normal on gross examination. This is usually a follicular variant of papillary carcinoma and may have few of the cytologic features typical of carcinoma metastatic to lymph nodes.

Anatomic Relations

In geographic regions where dietary iodine is abundant, the normal adult thyroid gland weighs between 14 and 20 g, but it is larger in regions with iodine deficiency. The thyroid lobe lies adjacent to the thyroid cartilage and is situated anterolateral to the larynx and trachea, which are united anteriorly just below the cricoid cartilage by an isthmus. Thus, the thyroid partially surrounds the upper trachea, and the lateral posterior portion of the lobe may expand behind the upper trachea. The pyramidal process or distal remnant of the thyroglossal duct is present in about half of all adults and varies from a small vestige to a well-defined structure extending to the hyoid bone. Although found more often on the left side of the isthmus, it may be found in the midline or on the right side. It may be enlarged and nodular in patients with multinodular goiters, lymphocytic thyroiditis, or Graves disease. The anterior portion of the thyroid gland is covered by the infrahyoid muscles and their fasciae. Posterolaterally, the lobes are bounded by the carotid sheaths.

The thyroid gland lies in the visceral compartment of the neck and is invested by a thin layer of connective tissue derived from pretracheal fascia. Above the isthmus, this fascia forms the anterior suspensory ligament of the thyroid. It envelops the pyramidal process as well as the group of lymphatics referred to as *Delphian lymph nodes*. This fascia should not be confused with the true capsule of the thyroid gland, which is an integral part of the gland and cannot be separated from the parenchyma without sharp dissection. The pretracheal fasciae is referred to as the *thyroid sheath* and varies in consistency and completeness among individuals. Posteromedially, it is usually condensed and firmly attaches the gland to the upper two or three tracheal rings and the cricoid cartilage. This posteromedial suspensory ligament is referred to as the *ligament of Berry* and is surgically important because of its relation to the recurrent laryngeal nerve[1] (RLN; Fig. 56-1).

The RLN usually lies just lateral to the ligament before entering the larynx, but in about 25% of patients the nerve is surrounded by the ligament before its entrance into the larynx. The sheath is also important because of its relation to the parathyroid glands and the branches of the inferior thyroid artery. As the thyroid sheath envelops the lateral posterior portion of each lobe, it frequently covers the superior parathyroid gland before continuing laterally to form a portion of the carotid sheath. As a result, the superior parathyroid gland may lie between the sheath and the thyroid capsule, within the sheath, posterior to the sheath in a potentially open plane, or occasionally anterior to the sheath. The inferior parathyroid gland likewise may be within the sheath, particularly when the gland is adherent to the lower pole of the thyroid. By dissecting the sheath from the thyroid capsule, the parathyroid gland can usually be identified and preserved during thyroid resection. The inferior thyroid artery branches ramify on the thyroid gland between the sheath and the capsule. They are best identified before clamping after the sheath has been lifted from the capsule.

The thyroid gland is a vascular organ supplied by four main arteries: two superior and two inferior. The superior thyroid artery usually arises as the first anterior branch of the external carotid artery just above the bifurcation of the common carotid artery. It descends medially on the surface of the inferior pharyngeal constrictor muscle to divide into an anterior and posterior branch at the apex of the thyroid lobe on its anteromedial surface. Its relation to the external branch of the superior laryngeal nerve is important during thyroid lobectomy. The inferior thyroid arteries usually arise from the thyrocervical trunks a few centimeters from their origin in the subclavian artery and ascend behind the carotid sheath before passing downward and medial to enter the thyroid gland at its middle portion. There are no arteries directly entering the lower poles from below, with the exception of a thyroidea ima artery that may replace

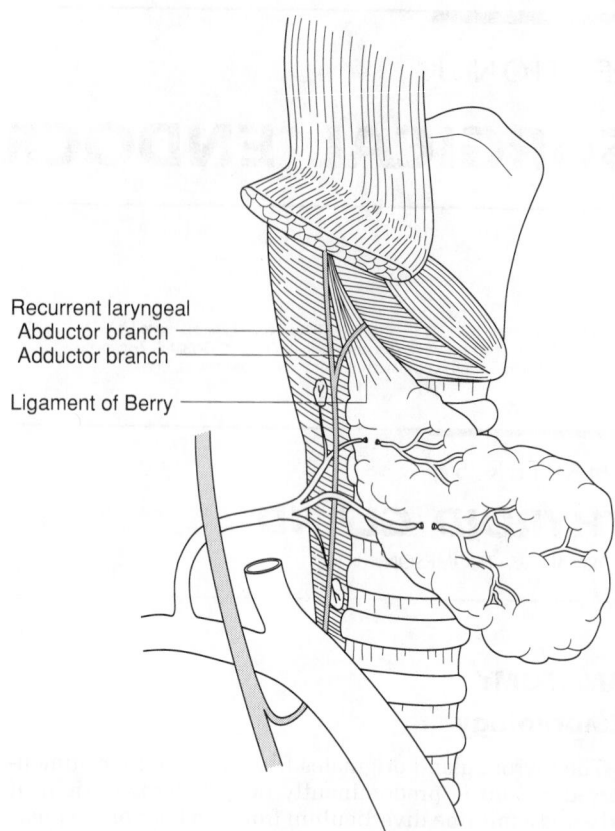

Figure 56-1. The ligament of Berry is carefully transected after full mobilization of the lobe and visualization of the distal recurrent laryngeal nerve. Fine clamps are used because small branches of the inferior thyroid artery frequently run in the ligament.

Recurrent laryngeal
Abductor branch
Adductor branch
Ligament of Berry

an absent inferior artery. Thyroidea ima arteries arise from either the innominate artery or the aorta in 1% to 4% of individuals, entering the lower surface of the isthmus after coursing on the trachea. Occasionally, an ima artery may enter the lower pole on the right side.

The relation of the inferior thyroid artery to the RLN has important surgical implications. The inferior artery may pass over, under, or between RLN branches in its course to the larynx. With the exception of a nonrecurrent laryngeal nerve arising from the vagus nerve, there is always a crossing. The inferior thyroid artery is also the principal blood supply to both superior and inferior parathyroid glands in most individuals. Although there may be a rich anastomosis between the superior and inferior thyroid arteries, the end artery supplying each parathyroid gland arises from an inferior thyroid artery or one of its branches in more than 80% of individuals.

The venous drainage of the thyroid gland is from three pairs of principal veins that freely anastomose on the gland's surface. The superior veins course with the superior arteries and empty into the internal jugular vein at the level of the carotid bifurcation. The middle thyroid veins are inconsistent but are present in about 50% of individuals. They arise from the anterolateral surface of the thyroid in its middle portion and drain directly into the internal jugular veins. The middle vein, when present, must be divided and ligated when mobilization of the thyroid lobe is performed. The inferior thyroid veins typically form two trunks, which descend from the lower pole of the gland and drain into their respective innominate and brachiocephalic veins. The veins from both sides may join in the midline and form a plexus in front of the trachea, which drains into the left innominate vein. The inferior veins most often follow the course of the thyrothymic ligament, which connects the lower pole of the thyroid to the cervical tongue of the thymus gland.

The lymphatic drainage of the thyroid gland is an important consideration in the surgical treatment of thyroid carcinoma. The thyroid gland is richly endowed with lymphatics, and the flow may drain in many directions from the gland. Intraglandular channels are found beneath the capsule and communicate through the isthmus to the opposite lobe. In addition, they drain into perithyroidal channels and lymph nodes. The regional nodes include the paraglandular or capsular nodes; the pretracheal lymph nodes superior to the isthmus; the paratracheal nodes; the RLN chain; the anterosuperior mediastinal nodes; the upper, middle, and lower jugular nodes; and the retropharyngeal and esophageal nodes. Lateral cervical nodes within the posterior triangle may also be involved in patients with more advanced thyroid cancers. Lymph nodes within the submaxillary triangle are infrequently involved with metastases from thyroid carcinomas. Dissections of involved lymph nodes are performed commonly for thyroid cancers. Patients with papillary carcinomas often have clinically apparent nodal metastases, and about 90% of children and adolescents with papillary carcinoma have lymph node involvement. Medullary carcinoma also has a predilection for lymphatic spread, and most patients with palpable primary tumors have lymph node metastases at the time of operation. In these cases, the central compartment nodes must be routinely dissected, including excision of all lymph nodes from the level of the hyoid bone above to the innominate artery below and lateral to the jugular vein.

The anatomic relations of greatest importance during thyroidectomy are those of the RLN, the superior laryngeal nerve, and the parathyroid glands to the thyroid gland. Injury to the RLN results in paralysis of the vocal cord on the ipsilateral side. The cord either may remain in a paramedial position or may be abducted, lateral to the midline. When the paralyzed cord is approximated by the functioning contralateral cord, the patient may have a normal but weakened voice. Shortness of breath may occur in some individuals because the airway is decreased in size. When the vocal cord is paralyzed in an abducted position, closure is prevented, and a severely impaired voice and ineffective cough result. Bilateral cord palsies can result in either a complete loss of voice or an airway obstruction requiring emergency intubation or tracheostomy. If both vocal cords are paralyzed in an abducted position, airway obstruction may not develop for months or until contraction of the cords gradually causes them to approach the midline. In these cases, upper respiratory infection may necessitate an emergency procedure to restore an airway. Bilateral permanent RLN injury during surgery is always disastrous but can be avoided in nearly all patients. Knowledge of the possible courses of the RLNs and familiarity with the surgical techniques designed to avoid their injury are essential elements in the strategy for thyroidectomy.

The right RLN arises from the vagus nerve at its crossing with the first portion of the subclavian artery (Fig. 56-2). It then passes around the posterior aspect of the artery before ascending lateral to the trachea, eventually entering the larynx posterior to the thyroid gland at the level of the cricothyroid articulation. The right RLN usually courses about 1 to 2 cm lateral to the tracheoesophageal groove at the level of the lower thyroid pole. At the level of the inferior thyroid artery, the nerve is closer to the trachea. The nerve may divide into one or more branches here, although its bifurcation is more likely to occur as the nerve

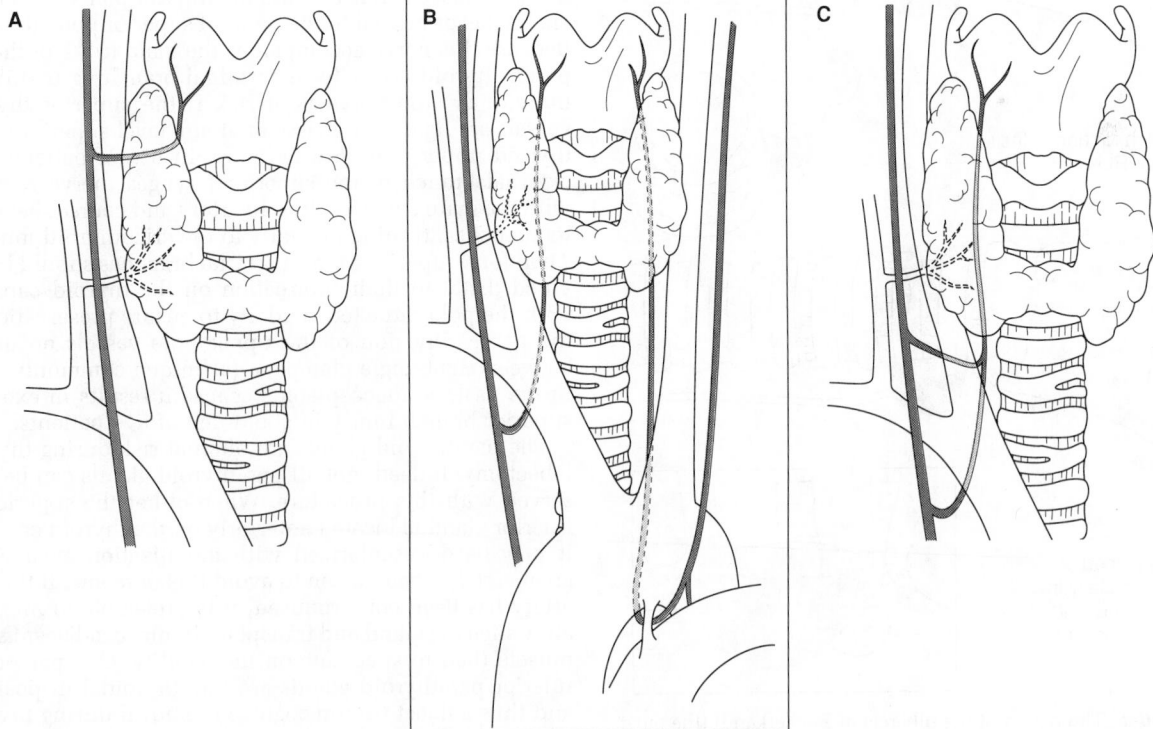

Figure 56-2. Anomalous variations in the course of the right recurrent laryngeal nerve. (*A*) Nonrecurrent nerve from vagus. (*B*) Normal course of right recurrent laryngeal nerve. (*C*) Rare nonrecurrent nerve and recurrent laryngeal nerve joining to form the common distal nerve.

enters the larynx. The RLN junction with the inferior thyroid artery is often considered the most vulnerable location in thyroidectomy because of the many nerve–artery relations at their crossing; one study reported 28 variations.

The relation is unpredictable because the nerve may be anterior or posterior to the main arterial trunk or between one or more arterial branches. Thus, many surgeons prefer to identify the RLN below the inferior thyroid artery level and trace its course to the nerve junction. Others consider the RLN to be most vulnerable in the area superior to the junction with the artery and proximal to the ligament of Berry. There, the RLN frequently branches and may actually traverse the ligament. In this area, the nerve cannot be identified until the most lateral posterior extension of the thyroid lobe has been rotated medially. This extension of thyroid tissue is called the *tubercle of Zuckerkandl* (Fig. 56-3). The terminal segment of the RLN invariably courses directly under this lateral posterior extension of thyroid tissue. The attachment of the ligament of Berry to the trachea and cricoid cartilage is intimately related to the recurrent nerve, and in 25% of patients the nerve traverses the ligament (Fig. 56-4). Successful surgery requires knowledge of the anatomy as well as technical precision. Identification of the RLN before division of the ligament of Berry may reduce the risk of surgical injury to the nerves.

With this approach, even a nonrecurrent right laryngeal nerve arising directly from the vagus nerve can be readily identified before entry into the larynx. A nonrecurrent right laryngeal nerve is found in 0.5% to 1% of individuals. In addition, about 0.2% of patients have both a recurrent and a nonrecurrent laryngeal nerve, with union at or below the inferior thyroid artery and formation of a single distal trunk (see Fig. 56-2). Although it may not be necessary to visualize the distal course of every RLN as the ligament is dissected, it is prudent to do so. If done routinely, permanent nerve injury can be avoided in almost all cases.

The left RLN arises from the vagus nerve as it courses over the arch of the aorta. It passes inferior and medial to the aorta and ascends to the larynx, often in the tracheal esophageal groove. There are many variations in its relation to the inferior thyroid artery, but nonrecurrent left laryngeal nerves are extremely rare and have been reported only in patients with situs inversus. Another anatomic variation of surgical importance is when an RLN is found on the anterior lateral aspect of the trachea, at or even below the lower pole of the thyroid. Such a medial course is virtually always found on the left. No vertical structure on the trachea near the inferior thyroid pole should be divided until it is absolutely identified.

The superior laryngeal nerve arises from the vagus nerve at the base of the skull and descends along the internal carotid artery to the level of the hyoid cornu, where it divides into two branches. The larger, or internal, branch is a sensory nerve and penetrates the thyrohyoid membrane before innervating the larynx. The smaller external branch lies on the lateral surface of the inferior pharyngeal constrictor muscle and usually descends just medial to the superior thyroid artery as it enters the cricothyroid muscle. During thyroid lobectomy, the external branch is usually not seen because it is beneath the inferior pharyngeal muscle fasciae or medial to the point of superior pole division. Because this nerve accompanies the main trunk of the superior thyroid artery to its terminal branching in 15% of individuals, the nerve is at risk if the superior thyroid vessels are ligated en masse or at any level superior to the thyroid upper pole. Furthermore, in 6% of patients, the external branch of the superior laryngeal nerve remains with the main superior thyroid artery and courses between its branches, turning medially to the cricothyroid muscle. Therefore, superior thyroid arterial branches should be divided distal to their bifurcation on the thyroid capsule, with the pole retracted caudally to ensure preservation of the nerve. Division of the upper pole vessels en masse between right-angle clamps, a technique commonly used in the past, is unacceptable because it results in external superior branch injury in about one of five patients.

The parathyroid glands are often at risk during thyroid lobectomy. Indeed, not all parathyroid glands can be preserved with this procedure. When either the superior or inferior gland is located anteriorly on the thyroid capsule, it may be devascularized with mobilization even when great care has been taken to avoid this outcome. If the end artery has been compromised, it is preferable to immediately slice the gland and transplant it into an adjacent strap muscle than to speculate on its viability. One percent of inferior parathyroid glands are intrathyroidal in position and thus subject to unrecognized removal during thyroid lobectomy. If these glands are recognized intraoperatively by the surgeon, they can still be salvaged by local transplantation into striated muscle. Although inadvertent parathyroidectomy may occur in patients with large goiters

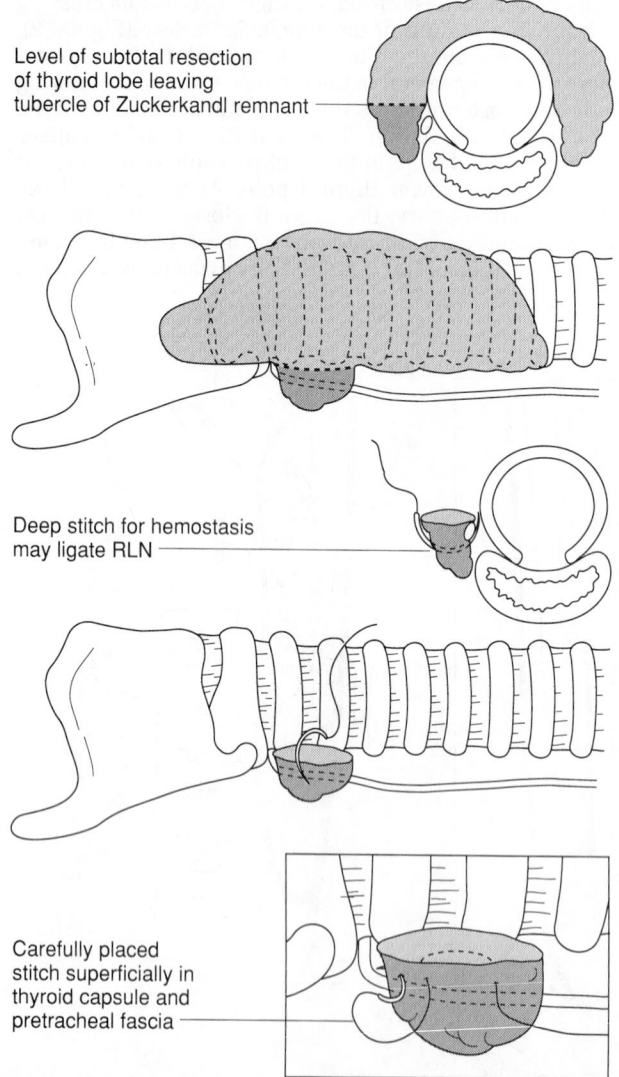

Level of subtotal resection of thyroid lobe leaving tubercle of Zuckerkandl remnant

Deep stitch for hemostasis may ligate RLN

Carefully placed stitch superficially in thyroid capsule and pretracheal fascia

Figure 56-3. The region of the tubercle of Zuckerkandl (the most posterior extent of the thyroid lobe) and the distal course of the recurrent laryngeal nerve (RLN). The relation of the RLN to the remaining remnant of thyroid and the mechanism for possible RLN injury are shown.

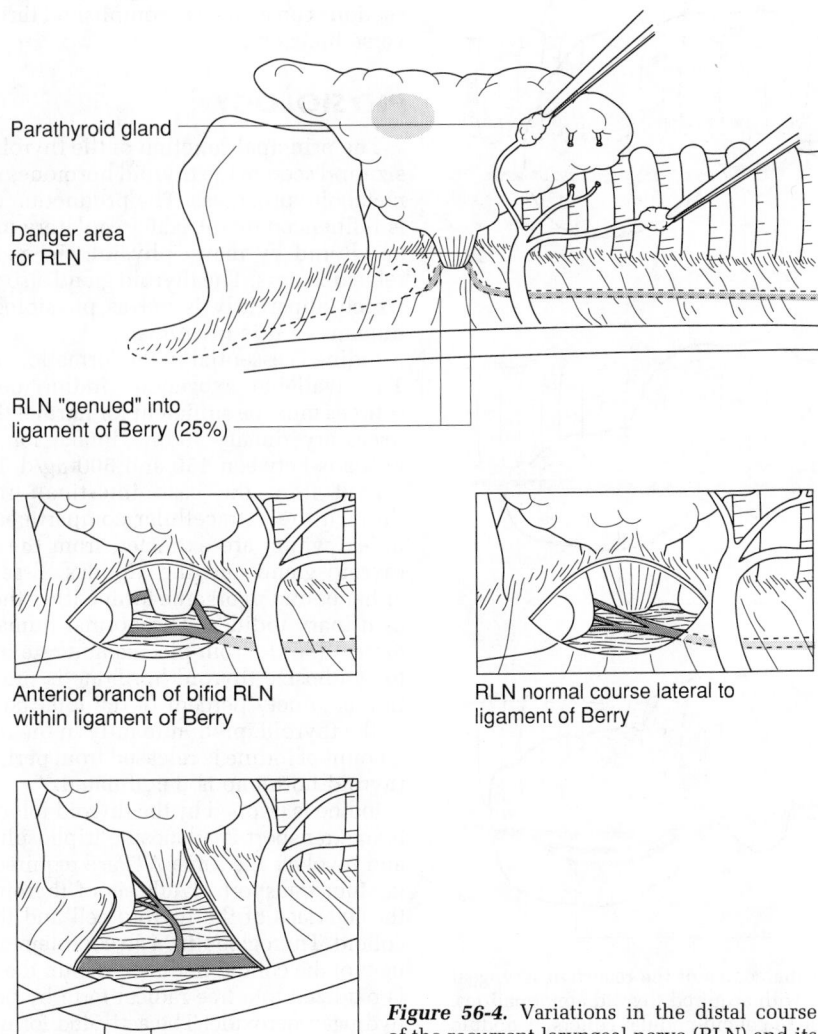

Parathyroid gland

Danger area for RLN

RLN "genued" into ligament of Berry (25%)

Anterior branch of bifid RLN within ligament of Berry

RLN normal course lateral to ligament of Berry

Non-RLN arising from vagus (1%) on right side

Figure 56-4. Variations in the distal course of the recurrent laryngeal nerve (RLN) and its relation to the posterior (Berry) ligament of the thyroid gland. This is the region where the nerve is most at risk during thyroidectomy.

or metastases to lymph nodes, the most common cause of hypoparathyroidism after thyroidectomy is injury to the blood supply of the parathyroid glands.

The principal blood supply to both parathyroid glands is the inferior thyroid artery. Parathyroid glands invariably have a single end artery supplying them, and if the main trunk of the inferior thyroid artery is ligated during thyroidectomy, there is no collateral blood supply to maintain their viability. It is preferable to divide only the branches of the inferior thyroid artery medial to those that supply either of the parathyroid glands. This requires individual clamping of smaller vessels under the thyroid sheath, since these vessels penetrate the thyroid capsule. This technique is essential to prevent permanent hypoparathyroidism during total thyroidectomy. Ligation of the main trunk of the inferior thyroid artery was commonly used for bilateral subtotal thyroidectomy in the past. It did not routinely cause hypoparathyroidism only because enough collateral blood supply was maintained to reach the end artery to one or more parathyroid glands. Ligation of the main trunk of the inferior thyroid artery must be avoided.

Abnormal changes within the thyroid gland or the surrounding lymph nodes may cause anatomic alterations that complicate thyroidectomy. For example, patients with diffuse goiters related to Hashimoto or Graves disease may have parathyroid glands in a position more anterior than usual. As a result, all four glands may require careful dissection from the thyroid capsule in a medial to lateral direction to avoid devascularization, even in a subtotal thyroidectomy. In patients with nodular goiters, particularly when there is a substernal extension, the RLNs may be deviated and stretched over the anterolateral surface of the goiter at the thoracic inlet. In addition, an occasional nodule may develop within the tubercle of Zuckerkandl. As a result, the RLN may be found either on the surface of the lobe or posterior to it. These variations should always be considered during thyroid lobectomy of an abnormal gland (Fig. 56-5). A detailed knowledge of the embryology and anatomic variations can help avoid surgical complications of RLN and external laryngeal nerve injury. Hypoparathyroidism can be minimized or totally avoided by the careful surgeon.

Generally, the surgical approach to the thyroid is through a transverse skin line incision 2 to 3 cm above the clavicles. Its length is determined by the size of the thyroid gland. The technique for the performance of a total thyroidectomy is shown in Figures 56-6 through 56-10. Skin flaps including the subcutaneum and platysma muscle are developed cranially to the level of the notch of the thyroid

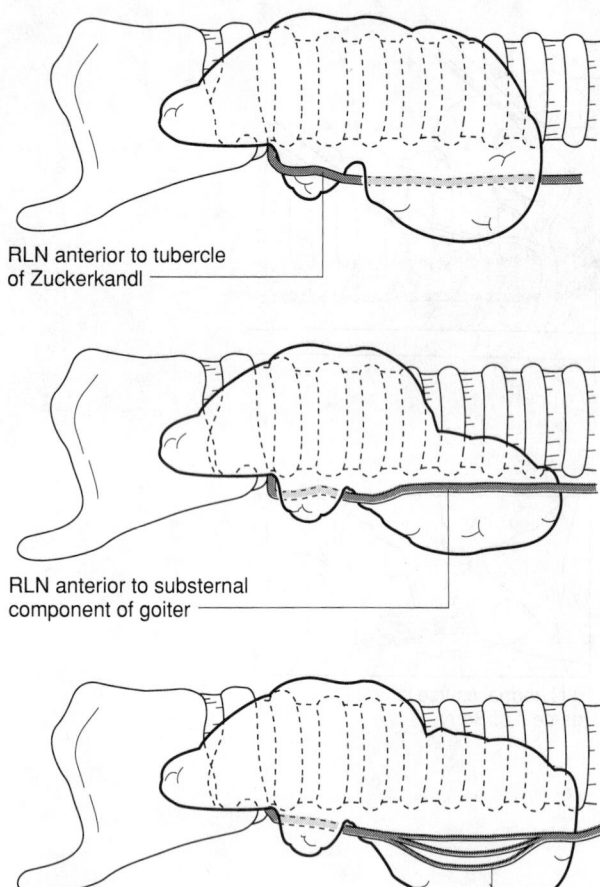

RLN anterior to tubercle
of Zuckerkandl

RLN anterior to substernal
component of goiter

RLN palsy from stretching
by large goiter

Figure 56-5. Variations in the course of the recurrent laryngeal nerve (RLN) are associated with acquired thyroid abnormalities. This is most commonly due to colloid nodular goiters. A nodule of thyroid may grow and enlarge under the distal RLN in the region of the most posterior extent of the thyroid (tubercle of Zuckerkandl), placing the nerve anterior to a lobule of thyroid tissue and vulnerable to injury. A substernal extension of thyroid may descend under the RLN rather than anterior to it and, when stretched out over the substernal extension, may cause RLN palsy.

cartilage and caudally to the suprasternal notch. The infrahyoid muscles are separated in the midline and retracted laterally without transection. Occasionally, patients with large goiters require division of the strap muscles. Retractors expose the superior thyroid vessels when the lateral upper pole is sufficiently mobilized and the avascular space between the upper thyroid lobe and the cricothyroid muscle is entered. With caudal retraction, these vessels are easily visualized, as is the ectopically located external branch of the superior laryngeal nerve.[2]

Mobilization of the upper pole is facilitated by dividing the anterior suspensory muscle over the larynx before entering the avascular space. Once the upper pole is freed, division of the middle thyroid vein allows medial retraction of the thyroid lobe, after which even large substernal goiters can be gently dissected from within the thoracic inlet or mediastinum. Regional lymph node dissections are readily accomplished by extending the incision bilaterally and elevating the upper flap to the level of the hyoid bone. Vertical incisions for lymph node dissections are unnecessary and are cosmetically less desirable than extended transverse incisions. Extensive modified bilateral neck dissections can also be accomplished through extended transverse incisions.

PHYSIOLOGY

The principal function of the thyroid gland is to synthesize and secrete the thyroid hormones necessary for normal metabolic processes. The production of thyroid hormones is influenced by intricate regulatory mechanisms and may be altered by many physiologic, pathologic, and drug-related factors. The thyroid gland also produces calcitonin, which apparently is not as physiologically important in humans as it is in animals.

Iodine is essential in the formation of thyroid hormones. The available exogenous iodine derived from dietary sources must be sufficient for normal thyroid function. The necessary dietary iodine intake for normal physiologic needs is between 150 and 500 μg/d. Iodine is rapidly absorbed from the gastrointestinal tract and distributed through the extracellular compartment in the form of iodides, which are extracted from the plasma by both the thyroid gland and the kidneys. Essentially all iodine is either bound in organic form within the thyroid or excreted as urinary iodides. The normal human thyroid is able to extract iodide from plasma at a rate of 2 μg/h. The ability to synthesize thyroid hormone is present only in thyroid tissue. Ninety percent of the total body iodine is present in the thyroid, predominantly in the organic form. A small amount of iodine is released from peripheral tissues, where thyroid hormone is deiodinated.[3,4]

Iodine is trapped by the thyroid follicular cell. Transmembrane transport is adenosine triphosphate (ATP) dependent and involves the same ATPase required for sodium and potassium transport. Synthesis of thyroid hormone occurs at the interface of the thyroid cell and the thyroglobulin-rich colloid. Thyroglobulin, a glycoprotein, is the primary constituent of the colloid nodules. Within the follicular cell, iodine is oxidized to a free radical form by peroxidases, including hydrogen peroxide. The activated form of iodine attaches to the amino acid tyrosine, forming either monoiodotyrosine or diiodotyrosine. This important organification of iodine is inhibited by reducing substances such as propylthiouracil (PTU). The iodotyrosines then combine with each other in a reaction that involves tyrosine side-chain cleavage and oxidation. If monoiodotyrosine and diiodotyrosine couple, the result is triiodotyrosine (T_3), whereas the union of two diiodotyrosines results in thyroxine (T_4). These newly formed thyroid hormones are stored in the thyroglobulin, which is located centrally within a cluster of thyroid cells. This storage material is the colloid of the thyroid follicle. Thyroid hormone remains stored until its release is initiated by TSH. TSH-stimulated follicular cells form pseudopodia that encircle portions of the thyroglobulin colloid with cell membrane, forming vesicles that fuse with enzymes containing lysosomes. Initially, the enzymes induce thyroglobulin hydrolysis, during which disulfide double bonds within the thyroglobulin are reduced. Glutathione supplies the hydrogen ion for this reduction, and this reaction is facilitated by the transhydrogenase enzyme. Proteases complete this process by cleaving T_4 and T_3 from the thyroglobulin and releasing them into the circulation. The thyroglobulin molecule is normally too large to be transported across the follicular cell membrane, although small quantities may enter the plasma. In general, large quantities of thyroglobulin enter the circulation only after acute injury to the thyroid follicle in conditions such as subacute thyroiditis or radiation. Nevertheless, many patients with goiter and even some with normal thyroid glands may have detectable levels of plasma thyroglobulin. Measurement of serum thyroglobulin levels can detect persistent or recurrent differentiated thyroid cancers.[5–7]

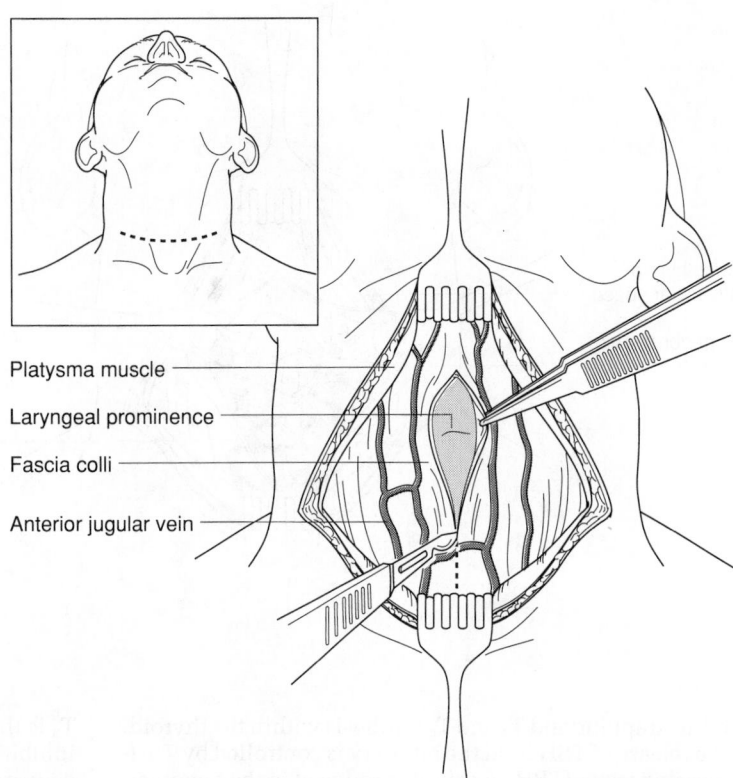

Platysma muscle

Laryngeal prominence

Fascia colli

Anterior jugular vein

Figure 56-6. The curvilinear cervical incision for thyroidectomy is placed in a skin crease or Langer line two fingerbreadths above the clavicles. After skin–platysmal muscle flaps have been developed from the thyroid cartilage notch to the sternal notch, the strap muscles are split in the midline and reflected off the involved thyroid lobe.

The thyroid gland is the only endogenous source of T_4, whereas most T_3 is produced by the peripheral conversion of T_4. Under normal circumstances, only about 20% of T_3 is secreted directly from the thyroid gland. Peripheral T_4 conversion results from 5'-monodeiodinase cleavage of 5'-iodine from the outer ring of T_4. This reaction takes place in the liver, muscles, kidney, and anterior pituitary. In some thyroid diseases (eg, Graves disease and toxic nodular goiter), the proportion of T_3 secreted directly by the thyroid gland may be markedly increased. Some T_4 is converted to reverse T_3 by removal of the 5'-iodine from the inner ring of T_4. Unlike T_3, the reverse compound has no metabolic activity.

Once thyroid hormones are released into the circulation, they are bound to thyroid-binding globulin (TBG; 85%), albumin (10%), and transthyretin (prealbumin; 15%). These binding proteins allow the thyroid hormones to remain soluble in plasma, contributing to systemic distribution to various target-cell populations. A limited amount of thyroid hormone circulates freely in the plasma in metabolically active form (free T_4, free T_3). Pregnancy and the use of oral contraceptives alter the serum-binding protein levels and hence the total T_4 and T_3 levels, but they do not affect the free T_4 or T_3 concentrations.

TSH, a glycoprotein secreted by the pituitary gland, regulates not only the release of thyroid hormone but also

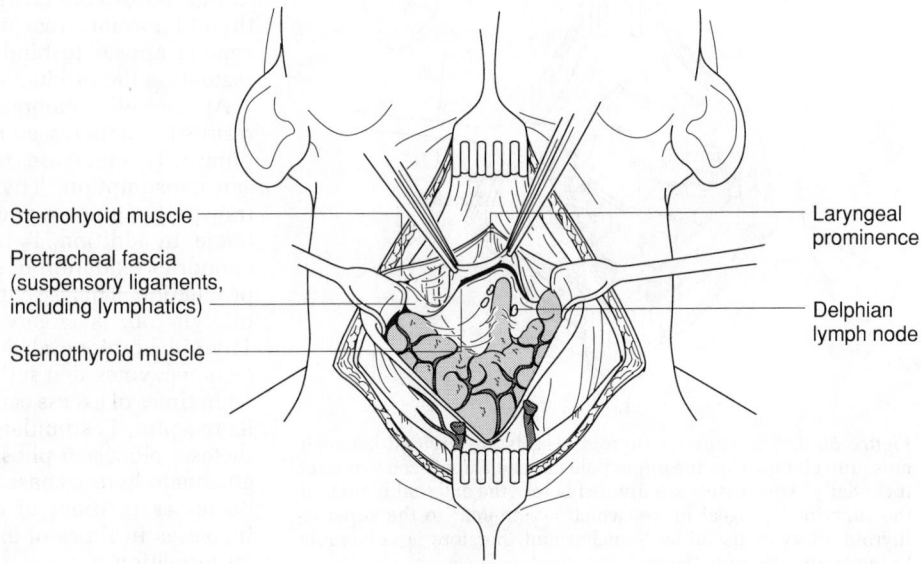

Sternohyoid muscle

Pretracheal fascia (suspensory ligaments, including lymphatics)

Sternothyroid muscle

Laryngeal prominence

Delphian lymph node

Figure 56-7. The anterior suspensory ligament, from the laryngeal prominence or notch of the thyroid cartilage, is exposed, as are the medial borders of the upper thyroid lobes. A pyramidal lobe can be present on either side and may extend to the hyoid bone.

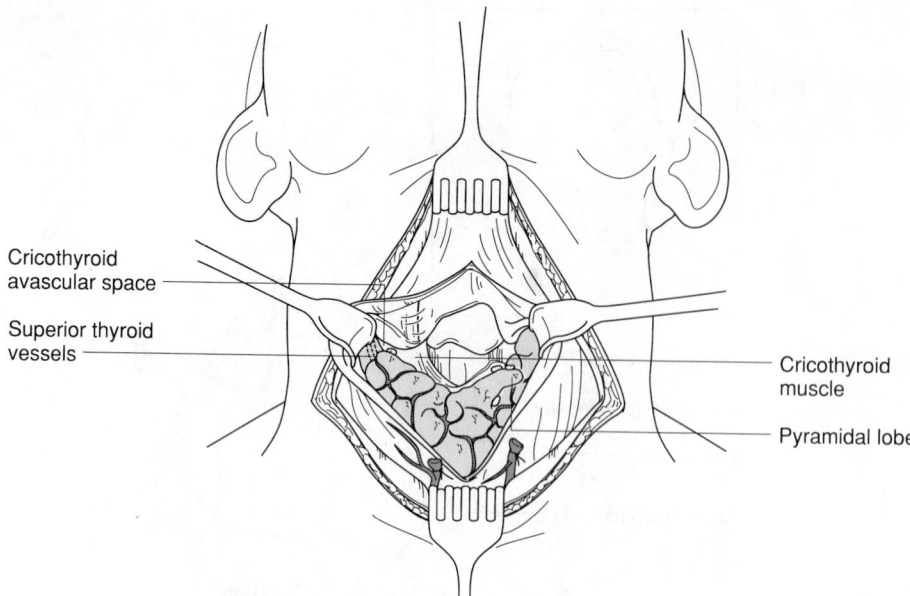

Cricothyroid avascular space

Superior thyroid vessels

Cricothyroid muscle

Pyramidal lobe

Figure 56-8. The pretracheal fascia and any pyramidal lobe or thyroglossal tract are divided from the level of the hyoid and reflected caudally to the cricoid. This includes any prelaryngeal (Delphian) lymph nodes. Reflection of the anterior suspensory ligament allows entrance into the avascular space between the upper pole of the thyroid gland and the larynx.

iodine trapping and T_4 and T_3 synthesis within the thyroid. The release of TSH from the pituitary is controlled by TSH-releasing factor (TRH), a peptide produced in the hypothalamus and transferred to the pituitary by way of the portovenous circulation. T_3 and T_4 inhibit the action of TRH on the anterior pituitary, decreasing the secretion of TSH.

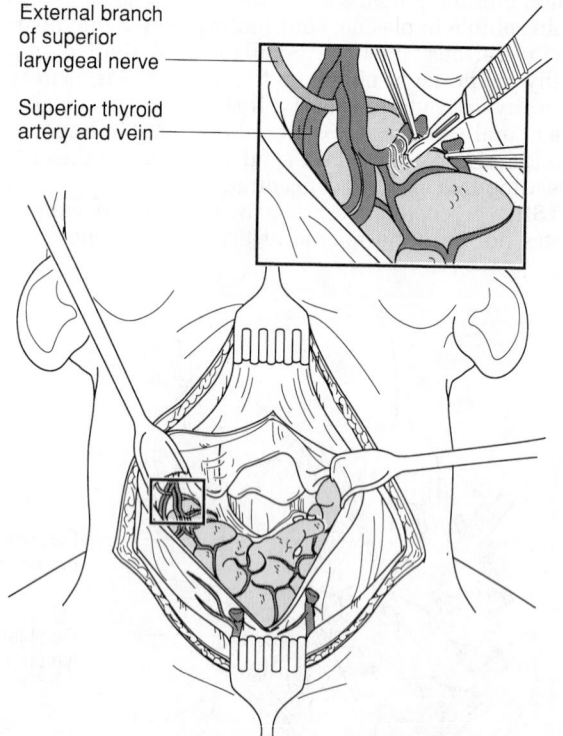

External branch of superior laryngeal nerve

Superior thyroid artery and vein

Figure 56-9. The superior thyroid vessels are divided between mosquito clamps after the upper pole has been mobilized to retract it caudally. The vessels are divided below the external branch of the superior laryngeal nerve, which is adherent to the superior thyroid artery or its initial branches and therefore is vulnerable to injury in 20% of patients.

T_3 is thought to play a greater role than T_4 in this feedback inhibition of TSH secretion because the pituitary readily converts T_4 to T_3. The amount of available iodine also influences the intrathyroidal regulation of thyroid hormone secretion. Large amounts of ingested iodine, or iodine administered as contrast media, may decrease iodine trapping and hence hormone synthesis. When there is iodine depletion or deprivation, a compensatory increase in iodine trapping occurs. These reciprocal regulatory changes in iodine trapping function to maintain a constant thyroid hormone pool.

The effect of thyroid hormone at the cellular level depends on the binding of T_3 with a specific intracellular receptor. Free thyroid hormone traverses the cell membrane by diffusion. After adherence to a high-affinity intracellular binding protein, it migrates to the nuclear membrane, which it traverses by active transport. There, T_3 binds to a nuclear receptor, which in turn regulates transcription and translation and protein synthesis.[8] The thyroid hormone receptor is part of a family that includes steroids, estrogen, and vitamin D, each with different affinities but shared characteristics.[9] Thus far, two different thyroid hormone receptors have been identified. These receptors appear to bind to different DNA segments, thus regulating the production of different gene products.

At the cell membrane, an excess of thyroid hormone results in an increased number of ATP-dependent sodium pumps. This increases resting energy expenditure and oxygen consumption. Thyroid hormone also facilitates the transport of glucose and amino acids across the cell membrane. In addition, T_3-induced energy derived from mitochondrial oxidation of substrate results in increased ATP production. This essential process, called oxidative phosphorylation, is largely regulated by thyroid hormone.[10] Thyroid hormone also increases the production of lipogenic enzymes that induce the production and storage of fat in times of excess carbohydrate ingestion. Coupled with its receptor, T_3 stimulates the production of fatty acid synthetase, glucose-6-phosphate dehydrogenase, 6-phosphogluconate hydrogenase, and related enzymes. Because T_3 decreases in times of caloric deprivation or illness and increases in times of excess, T_3 may either limit or favor fat formation.

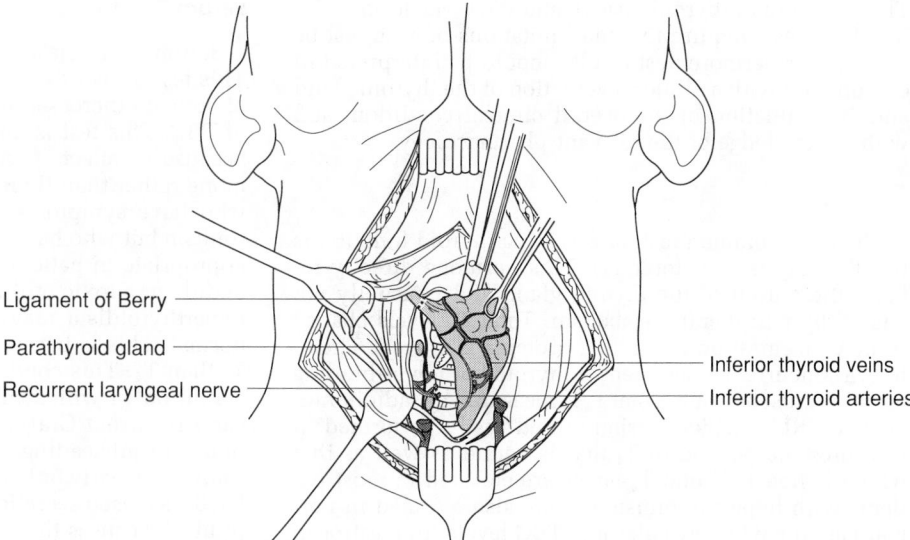

Figure 56-10. The distal branches of the inferior thyroid artery are divided when a total lobectomy is performed. Any parathyroid glands on the thyroid capsule are gently teased away from the capsule, medial to lateral, preserving the end artery to the gland. The lobe is retracted medially.

Ligament of Berry
Parathyroid gland
Recurrent laryngeal nerve
Inferior thyroid veins
Inferior thyroid arteries

Heat production (thermogenesis regulation) is another important function of thyroid hormone. Whenever substrates are oxidized, energy is released. The energy is either captured and stored as ATP or used to generate heat. At the cell membrane, the activity of the increased number of sodium pumps stimulated by T_3 requires energy and results in heat generation. In the nucleus, thyroid hormones induce the production of new proteins. Each of these steps requires energy and results in heat production. Similarly, mitochondrial oxidative phosphorylation is a heat-generating process.

Pharmacologic Factors and Treatment

A number of substances interfere with the normal production of thyroid hormone by blocking one of the relevant enzymatic steps. Chronic ingestion of these blocking agents in a normal individual can result in hypothyroidism and secondary goiter formation as a result of increased TSH secretion. On the other hand, some drugs are useful in the treatment of hyperthyroidism. Iodine was the first effective drug to be used in the treatment of thyrotoxicosis. When given in large enough doses, it can acutely block the organification and coupling steps and prevent the release of thyroid hormone. Iodine also inhibits the enzymatic reduction of the double bonds in thyroglobulin. This in turn prevents thyroglobulin mobilization and thyroid hormone release. Furthermore, iodine in large doses probably inhibits the ability of TSH to stimulate cyclic AMP release at the follicular cell membrane.

Commonly used antithyroid drugs are PTU, methimazole (Tapazole), and carbimazole. Although carbimazole is widely used in Great Britain, only PTU and methimazole are commonly used in the United States. PTU interferes with the incorporation of iodine into the tyrosine residues of thyroglobulin by inhibiting the peroxidase enzymes, thus preventing oxidation of iodide to iodine. It also inhibits the peripheral deiodination of T_4 to T_3. Although both PTU and methimazole are thionamides, methimazole does not have this peripheral effect. Thus, PTU is the preferred drug for patients with thyroid storm. PTU has a plasma half-life of 2 to 3 hours after a standard 100-mg dose is administered. A dose of 500 mg may yield effective levels for 6 to 8 hours. Methimazole, when given in standard doses of 10 to 25 mg, has a plasma half-life of 6 to 13

hours. Therefore, patients given PTU for long-term therapy require at least three daily doses for effective inhibition of thyroid synthesis. Methimazole, however, is effective when given only once or twice daily. Both drugs are associated with undesirable side effects that range from annoying to life-threatening. About 3% of patients taking PTU demonstrate at least one side effect during the first 3 months of therapy, whereas the prevalence with methimazole is about 7%. The most common of these side effects is a skin rash. The most serious side effect of these drugs is agranulocytosis, which has a reported prevalence of 0.12% with methimazole and 0.44% with PTU. Some studies suggest an incidence as low as 1 in 500 patients. This dangerous complication is irreversible and is always a consideration when treating patients. In addition to long-term therapy of thyrotoxicosis with the thionamides, short-term preoperative preparation for 5 to 6 weeks is routine. These drugs are effective in the treatment of thyrotoxicosis during pregnancy, but because of unrestricted placental passage, they inhibit the production of thyroid hormone in the fetus and result in a secondary rise in TSH and the subsequent development of a fetal goiter. Therefore, if treatment is necessary during pregnancy, minimal doses of antithyroid drugs should be used to reduce the risk of fetal hypothyroidism and goiter.

During the past two decades, β-adrenergic antagonists have been used in the treatment of hyperthyroidism. Propranolol is the most widely used of these drugs. However, β-blockade does not alter thyroid function per se. Rather, its effect is to provide symptomatic relief of hyperthyroidism because of interference with the action of thyroid hormones at the cellular level. These drugs alleviate the symptoms of hyperthyroidism within 1 or 2 days when administered orally and within as little as 1 hour when given intravenously. Propranolol inhibits the conversion of T_4 to T_3. Many hyperthyroid patients are prepared for operation with propranolol alone, but because of its relatively short action and the 5- to 7-day half-life of T_4, the drug must be continued for up to 1 week postoperatively if thyroid storm is to be avoided.

Laboratory Tests of Thyroid Function

A large number of laboratory tests are available to assess thyroid function either directly or indirectly. No single test is sufficient to evaluate thyroid function in all patients.

The spectrum of thyroid disease and the variable sensitivity of the tests require that the limitations of each test be known. Furthermore, test results should be interpreted in conjunction with a clinical evaluation of the thyroid gland and an evaluation of the overall clinical condition, and with a knowledge of the relevant pharmacology.

T_4 Assay

The most common test for assessing thyroid function is the T_4 assay (serum total T_4). This hormone directly reflects the output of the thyroid gland and is usually not altered by peripheral metabolism. Total T_4 levels change if the concentration of binding proteins is altered. Therefore, a concurrent assessment of thyroid hormone–binding proteins must be done. Total T_4 is measured by radioimmunoassay (RIA), which is simply and easily performed. It measures the portion of T_4 that is bound as well as that which is free T_4. Total T_4 levels are elevated in most patients with hyperthyroidism but are also elevated in normal patients who have elevated TBG levels from estrogen use, pregnancy, congenital TBG excess, and other disorders. In patients with hypothyroidism, total T_4 levels are decreased. T_4 levels are also reduced in individuals taking anabolic steroids and in those with nephrotic syndrome and inherited TBG deficiency. The latter conditions are associated with low levels of thyroid hormone–binding proteins. These patients may have normal thyroid function if their free T_4 levels are normal.

T_3 Resin Uptake Test

The T_3 resin uptake test is used to measure thyroid hormone–binding proteins and is not a measurement of either total T_3 or free T_3 concentrations. In this assay, a binding resin is used rather than antibody (T_4 test), and radiolabeled T_3 is used rather than labeled T_4. The radiolabeled T_3 binds either to binding protein or to the resin. If there are fewer sites left on the binding protein because of occupation by excess thyroid hormone, then more of the labeled T_3 binds to the resin, giving a high reading. The T_3 resin uptake is low if there are more binding sites on the protein because of excess TBG, and it is low in patients with hypothyroidism who have less hormone to occupy available protein-binding sites. When the levels of both total T_4 and T_3 resin uptake are similarly abnormal, a true thyroid hormone production abnormality is present. In clinically significant hypothyroidism, both total T_4 and T_3 resin uptake are decreased. During pregnancy and in women who are taking oral contraceptives, total T_4 levels are elevated and T_3 resin uptake is decreased because of excess TBG.

Free T_4 Index

The free T_4 index is a calculation obtained by multiplying the total T_4 by the T_3 resin uptake. When the total T_4 is high because of increased binding protein, the T_3 resin uptake is low and the free T_4 index is normal. The information provided by this calculation is similar to but not as precise as that derived from the free T_4 test. The free T_4 index should not be confused with the free T_4 test.

Free T_4

Free T_4 (serum free thyroxine) concentration can also be measured by RIA. The test has proved to be sensitive and accurate. In borderline cases of hyperthyroidism, an elevated level of free T_4 confirms the diagnosis. This test is a direct measurement of the biologically available T_4 in the circulation.

Serum Total T_3

Serum total T_3 is another test that uses an RIA technique. This test measures both protein-bound and free T_3; levels of both are increased in patients who have elevated levels of TBG. This test is not appropriate for general screening because it reflects peripheral metabolism of thyroid hormone rather than thyroid function. It is useful in patients who have symptoms and findings suggesting hyperthyroidism but who have a normal T_4. The test is particularly appropriate in patients suspected of having either a toxic nodule or a toxic multinodular goiter. In both conditions, hyperthyroidism may be present although the free T_4 is normal. This is because such nodules often secrete more T_3 than T_4. This condition is called T_3 toxicosis. Another condition in which more T_3 than T_4 may be secreted is early recurrent Graves disease. Total T_3 level determinations are misleading in evaluating patients for hypothyroidism. In early or borderline hypothyroidism, the stimulated increased secretion of TSH (low T_4 level reaching the pituitary) causes the thyroid to preferentially produce T_3, resulting in normal serum levels until the disease is severe.

Serum TSH

Until recently, the TSH RIA was not sensitive enough to demonstrate low levels of TSH. More sensitive techniques have increased the value of TSH measurement for assessing thyroid function. With the development of TSH monoclonal antibodies in the mid-1980s, immunometric assays (IMAs) first became commercially available. IMAs use two TSH antibodies, one monoclonal antibody bound in excess to a solid phase, and a second, labeled TSH antibody of either monoclonal or polyclonal origin. In an IMA, the solid-phase TSH antibody extracts TSH molecules out of the serum sample. The second TSH antibody is labeled with a signal (an isotope, enzyme, fluorophor, or chemiluminescent molecule) and binds to the solid phase, but only if a TSH molecule of serum origin forms a bridge between the two TSH antibodies. After the reaction has reached equilibrium, the unbound assay constituents are washed away so that the label bound to the solid phase is proportional to the serum TSH concentration. The type of label used determines the nomenclature of the new IMAs. An immunoradiometric assay uses ^{125}I; immunoenzymetric assay uses an enzyme; immunofluorometric assay uses a fluorophor; and immunochemiluminometric assay uses a chemiluminescent molecule.[11] The remarkable improvements in assay sensitivity achieved with the introduction of TSH IMA technology required the invention of descriptive terms such as *sensitive, ultrasensitive,* and *supersensitive.* A TSH IMA should be designated as sensitive only if it can distinguish between the depressed serum TSH values typical of hyperthyroidism and the euthyroid levels with a 99% statistical confidence level.

A generational classification has also been developed based on the concept that each generation represents a 10-fold improvement in functional assay performance. The commonly used TSH RIA (or first-generation TSH assay) displays functional assay sensitivity limits between 1 and 2 mIU/L. Most TSH IMAs have a functional sensitivity in the range of 0.1 to 0.2 mIU/L; these are considered second-generation assays. Third-generation TSH IMAs display an additional 10-fold improvement in functional sensitivity, with an assay limit of 0.01 to 0.02 mIU/L. Use of third-generation TSH IMAs is limited, whereas almost all major laboratories in the United States use TSH IMAs rather than the old TSH immunoradioassay (IRA). The only assays that have been shown to exhibit third-generation functional performance are the immunochemiluminometric assays. Because many commercially used IMAs only marginally meet second-generation standards, it is important for the clinician to be aware of the type of assay available and its sensitivity. Serum TSH measurements provide the most sensitive and accurate method for assessing peripheral thyroid hormone action in healthy ambulatory patients. The normal range for serum TSH values varies about 10-fold from 0.4 to 4.5 mIU/L. Any value within this range is generally considered to reflect a clinically euthyroid state. Serum TSH values that are persistently above or below this broad normal range are considered to be a reflection of an abnormal thyroid status. The TSH IMA has now established itself as a first-line test.[12]

Because major acute medical or psychiatric illnesses are capable of producing transient abnormalities in serum TSH secretion, these applications apply only to ambulatory and otherwise well patient populations. The finding of a normal serum TSH value in ambulatory populations virtually excludes the diagnosis of thyroid dysfunction. The test may be used to screen ambulatory patients at risk for primary thyroid dysfunction, such as those with autoimmune diseases that affect organ systems (eg, myasthenia gravis, pernicious anemia, rheumatoid arthritis, systemic lupus erythematosus), those with a family history of autoimmune thyroid disease, and the elderly. In each group, the prevalence of autoimmune thyroid disease appears to be significantly increased. TSH measurement is also ideally suited for optimizing thyroid hormone replacement therapy because it provides the most precise endpoint for determining the adequacy of peripheral thyroid hormone action. A minimum of 4 to 8 weeks between oral T_4 dosage adjustments is required to achieve a new stable serum TSH level. Another use is to optimize thyroid hormone levels for suppressive therapy of both benign and malignant growths.

Comparison of TSH suppression using older tests and recent, more sensitive assays shows that TSH suppression is a relative and not an absolute phenomenon. The differences reported in clinical responses to thyroid hormone suppressive therapy in the past may reflect the degree to which TSH levels were suppressed. The minimal criterion for adequate TSH suppression is to provide the least amount of T_4 therapy required to reduce basal serum TSH values below 0.1 mIU/L. Suppression of TSH to this level is used to treat patients who have or are presumed to have TSH-dependent differentiated thyroid cancer.

TRH Test

The thyrotropin-releasing hormone stimulation test (TRH test) determines the functional status of the pituitary TSH secretory mechanism. It also determines the presence of autonomous thyroid function in a patient with a functioning thyroid nodule that may not have produced clinical hyperthyroidism. It may also determine whether TSH secretion is blunted in patients with pituitary tumors. Although the TRH test was formerly used to evaluate patients with possible but borderline hyperthyroidism, the sensitive TSH assay has replaced it in this situation. The test is performed by administering 500 μg of TRH intravenously, assaying TSH after 30 and 60 minutes, and comparing these measurements with previously obtained baseline TSH levels. Normally, the TSH level rises at least 6 μIU/mL from the baseline level.

Serum Antibodies

Serum thyroid antibodies are designated as antimicrosomal and antithyroglobulin. In autoimmune diseases of the thyroid (eg, Graves and Hashimoto disease), their levels are frequently measured. About 80% of patients with Hashimoto thyroiditis have detectable autoantibodies. The antimicrosomal antibody test is the more useful of the two because the results are much more frequently positive and unequivocal. Antithyroglobulin antibody levels are often normal in patients with autoimmune disease of the thyroid gland. The presence of these antibodies does not determine the functional status of the thyroid, but they are a clue to the underlying disease. Most patients with Graves disease have detectable thyroid-stimulating immunoglobulins not usually found in other hyperthyroid conditions. Immunoglobulin determinations are not necessary in the usual patient with Graves disease. They are useful in evaluating patients who have apparent Graves ophthalmopathy but who are otherwise euthyroid and have no goiter. In this disorder, elevated levels of thyroid-stimulating immunoglobulins confirm the diagnosis.

Serum Thyroglobulin Assay

Thyroglobulin is not usually released into the circulation in large quantities, but it can be present when there is a destructive process within the thyroid gland (eg, thyroiditis, radiation injury, Graves disease, multinodular goiter). The most common use of the thyroglobulin assay is to follow up patients with differentiated thyroid carcinoma. It is not a diagnostic test for cancer in patients with untreated thyroid tumors, but it is useful in assessing the adequacy of therapy and in monitoring the patient for recurrent or metastatic disease. This is especially true after total thyroidectomy or subtotal resection and ablation of the thyroid remnant with radioactive iodine.[6]

Measurement of serum thyroglobulin levels complements the use of ^{131}I scintiscanning in the detection of residual local or metastatic disease.[13] In some institutions, it has replaced repeated ^{131}I scanning once a negative scan has been obtained. Several recent studies support the use of serum thyroglobulin levels for detecting tumor recurrence, even when the patient has had only a thyroid lobectomy, provided that the patient's TSH is suppressed with thyroid hormone. In one study, serum thyroglobulin levels lower than 10 μg/L were shown to confirm the absence of tumor recurrence in patients after lobectomy as well as after total thyroidectomy.[7] In this study, the specificity was 100% and the sensitivity 80% in patients with lobectomy alone. Despite the presence of residual normal thyroid tissue, measurement of serum thyroglobulin levels can exclude the presence of significant metastases in most patients after lobectomy for thyroid cancer. In another postoperative study, 429 patients with well-differentiated thyroid cancer received thyroid hormone suppression therapy, and 61 were found to have metastases. Forty were detected by thyroglobulin increases, whereas 21 metastases were nonfunctioning and were detected by other diagnostic procedures.[5] Thyroglobulin measurements by either IRA or immunoradiometric assay techniques were found to be equally satisfactory. Of the patients with high thyroglobulin levels, 92% had metastases and 8% had large thyroid remnants. Levels were high in 80% of the patients with metastases. More important is the fact that thyroglobulin levels were high in 76% of the patients with metastases that were unable to take up radioiodine. In most cases, a high thyroglobulin level, even after a negative thyroid scan, indicates metastatic disease.

THYROID IMAGING

Imaging modalities that are useful in the appraisal of thyroid disorders include ultrasonography, radiologic fluorescent scanning, single photon emission computed tomography, positron emission tomography, radiologic transmission computed tomography (CT), magnetic resonance (MR) imaging, and radioisotope scintiscanning. Of these, radionuclide imaging and ultrasonography have proved most useful. CT and MR imaging are useful in certain circumstances.

Radionuclide Imaging

Radionuclide imaging plays an important role in the evaluation of the thyroid gland. It is unique in that the mechanism by which the gland is visualized depends on its function. All of the other imaging modalities depend on the physical characteristics of the thyroid gland, such as the pattern of sound reflection, the absorption of x-rays, and the density of protons. Many radionuclides have been used, but only three are routinely used for thyroid imaging. These are technetium-99m pertechnetate (^{99m}Tc), iodine-123 (^{123}I), and iodine-131 (^{131}I). ^{99m}Tc is the radionuclide most commonly available for thyroid imaging. The pertechnetate molecules are trapped by the thyroid by use of an active transport mechanism similar to iodine; however, they are not organified and stored in the colloid. Although ^{99m}Tc itself has a half-life of only 6 hours, it is generated from ^{99}Mo, a product of nuclear fission with a half-life of 67 hours. The ^{99m}Tc generator requires only weekly replacement of ^{99}Mo and is a practical and inexpensive source of ^{99m}Tc. This isotope emits γ-rays of 140 keV, and other forms of radiation are negligible. After intravenous injection, ^{99m}Tc is rapidly trapped in the thyroid gland. Within 20 minutes, 0.3% to 3% is extracted from plasma, but it remains in the thyroid only transiently. The photon energy of 140 keV is optimal for scintigraphy with available gamma cameras. A thyroid study after intravenous ^{99m}Tc can be completed in less than 1 hour. The amount of radiation exposure with ^{99m}Tc is minimal (absorbed thyroid dose, 0.01 to 0.035 Gy) and is far less than that with ^{131}I. A normal scan image displays uniformly accumulated tracer in both lobes on anteroposterior and oblique views.

^{123}I is trapped and organified by the thyroid gland, allowing a more complete assessment of thyroid function. Because ^{123}I is produced in a cyclotron and has a relatively short half-life (13.2 hours), it is not readily available, must be delivered daily, and is expensive. ^{123}I emits x-rays of 159 keV with a negligible emission of β-particles and γ-rays. After oral administration, it is absorbed in the stomach and trapped by the thyroid within 4 hours. Its uptake reaches a plateau of about 5% to 30%, and these peak levels last for at least 24 hours. Traditionally, images are obtained at 4 and 24 hours, both of which are inconvenient times for the patient, requiring a long wait and a return the next day. Nevertheless, iodine uptake provides useful information about thyroid function. Routine imaging uses either ^{99m}Tc or ^{123}I. Imaging with ^{99m}Tc frequently provides enough information to serve as an acceptable alternative to ^{123}I. For cases in which assessment of both organification and trapping is necessary, ^{123}I testing can be done later.

^{131}I has generally the same biologic behavior as ^{123}I, but it has a high proportion of β-radiation and a long half-life (8.1 days), resulting in a much higher level of radiation to the patient. Its primary γ-radiation at 364 keV is suboptimal for imaging with available scintillation cameras, and the resulting images are inferior to those from other isotopes. However, it is the tracer of choice in the search for functioning metastatic thyroid tumors. Its half-life allows imaging at 24, 48, and 78 hours, and the delineation of metastases is improved because of almost complete background uptake clearance. The benefits of ^{131}I outweigh all disadvantages for this specific clinical indication. It is important as a therapeutic agent in the treatment of patients with hyperthyroidism and functioning metastatic thyroid carcinoma because of the destructive effects of its β-radiation.[14]

Ultrasound

Diagnostic ultrasonography is a simple, safe, and noninvasive imaging technique that offers an effective method for differentiating solid and cystic thyroid lesions. With the availability of high-frequency real-time imaging, dramatic improvements in visualization of the thyroid gland have been realized. High-resolution imaging can be obtained with either a 7.5- or a 10-MHz transducer. The high-resolution small parts scanner is capable of detecting a 3-mm thyroid nodule. It is sensitive enough that a new concern has been the demonstration of nonpalpable thyroid lesions of uncertain clinical importance.

Ultrasound examination provides anatomic information about the thyroid gland. Specific nodules are usually described as cystic, mixed cystic, solid, or pure solid. A recent review of 16 clinical reports showed that 69% of the nodules studied were solid, 19% were cystic, and 12% were mixed. Patients coming to operation with solid lesions showed the highest prevalence of carcinoma (21%). Twelve percent of mixed lesions also proved to be malignant. The finding of a pure cystic lesion did not exclude the presence of carcinoma, although cystic carcinoma was rare. In 30 other series that identified 2300 thyroid cysts, 229 patients underwent operation. Twenty-one of these patients had carcinomas (1% of the total, 10% of those selected for operation). Although ultrasonography can readily identify cystic thyroid lesions, this is also easily accomplished by fine-needle aspiration (FNA). In clinics, where this procedure is commonly performed, ultrasound examination of the thyroid is rarely necessary.

Computed Tomography and Magnetic Resonance Imaging

Contrast-enhanced CT scans and MR images can demonstrate thyroid abnormalities as well as the relation of the gland to contiguous anatomic structures. They can also demonstrate subclinical cervical lymphadenopathy. Patients with elevated calcitonin levels after a total thyroidectomy for medullary carcinoma are candidates for CT or MR imaging. Neither study can differentiate benign from malignant thyroid lesions or, for that matter, metastatic from benign lymph nodes. Their use in other thyroid problems should be considered only after a radionuclide scan has been obtained if needed because the iodine contained in the contrast materials blocks the uptake of radionuclides for a period of 6 weeks or more. We use CT and MR only to evaluate substernal goiter.

Approach to Thyroid Imaging

Radioisotope scanning measures the functional activity of the thyroid gland and maps its correlation with physical findings. For routine scanning, ^{131}I has been replaced by either ^{123}I or ^{99m}Tc. Because of the lower radiation exposure, cost, and ease of use, ^{99m}Tc is preferentially used. Both of these isotopes can identify nonfunctioning (or cold) nodules, which are areas of decreased activity compared with the surrounding thyroid tissue. The differential diagnosis of a solitary nonfunctioning nodule includes carcinoma, colloid nodule, nonfunctioning adenoma, and cyst. The prevalence of carcinoma ranges from 5% to 20% in cold nodules, and such lesions require further evaluation. If the scan detects other nonfunctioning areas in addition to the palpable nodule, the gland is at low risk for carcinoma because most patients with this finding have a multinodular goiter.

Another important benefit of nuclide scanning is the demonstration of functioning, or hot, nodules, seen as areas of increased activity. A solitary discrete area of increased activity is most often found in a young patient with an otherwise normal thyroid gland. Multiple hot spots are typically found in an older patient with a multinodular goiter. In patients with solitary or multiple functioning nodules, their TSH dependence must be considered. With rare exceptions, hot nodules are not malignant. A functioning solitary nodule that is independent of TSH is considered an autonomous nodule and can be the cause of hyperthyroidism. A functioning TSH-dependent nodule invariably represents regional hypertrophy of otherwise normal tissue because of degenerative processes in the surrounding thyroid gland. TSH dependence is established by a follow-up isotope scan after a 5-day course of orally administered T_3. This suppression scan shows persistent activity in the autonomous nodule but almost no uptake in the hypertrophic or reactive nodule. The prevalence of functioning nodules among all solitary nodules varies between 4% and 15%.

Because of the important information that can be obtained from radioisotope scanning, many endocrinologists routinely obtain either a ^{99m}Tc scan or an ^{123}I iodine scan as part of the initial evaluation of the patient with a solitary nodule. The possibility of carcinoma is an extremely important consideration in a patient with a solitary nonfunctional nodule in one lobe of an otherwise normal thyroid gland. In the midwestern United States, the prevalence of cancer in such nodules has been found to be 35% to 45%. It is higher in younger individuals. The presence of a cold nodule is insufficient information to determine a treatment plan. Although nearly all carcinomas are cold, most cold nodules are benign. FNA cytology is considered the most reliable evaluation for the diagnosis of thyroid nodules that are nonfunctional or hypofunctional by nuclide scan (see later discussion).

FUNCTIONAL DISORDERS

Hyperthyroidism

Hyperthyroidism (or thyrotoxicosis) is associated with clinical manifestations related to an excess of thyroid hormone. Although there are many causes, three are of primary concern to the surgeon. Graves disease, or toxic diffuse goiter, is most common, accounting for more than 80% of all patients with hyperthyroidism. The other two relevant causes of hyperthyroidism are toxic nodular goiter and a single toxic nodule. Common causes that rarely require surgery are postpartum thyroiditis, iodine-induced hyperthyroidism (jodbasedow syndrome), self-administered or iatrogenic hyperthyroidism, struma ovarii, functioning metastatic carcinoma, and several rare forms of thyroiditis.[15] Graves disease, toxic nodular goiter, and the autonomously functioning toxic nodule are considered here.

Graves Disease

Graves disease is an autoimmune disease with clinical manifestations that result from thyroid-stimulating immunoglobulins and other tissue-specific antibodies. These antibodies bind to the TSH receptors on the follicular cell and stimulate thyroid function. Other antibodies appear to be related to clinical manifestations as diverse as exophthalmos and pretibial myxedema, although the precise mechanisms are unknown. Hereditary factors, female gender, and emotional trauma have been implicated in the pathogenesis of Graves disease. Among families with Graves disease, the simultaneous presence of Hashimoto thyroiditis or another autoimmune thyroid disease is more common. The incidence of Graves disease is six to seven times higher in females than in males.

Clinical Manifestations. The clinical manifestations of Graves disease include thyrotoxicosis, diffuse goiter, exophthalmos, and, infrequently, pretibial myxedema. Not all patients develop this classic picture. The systemic manifestations of hyperthyroidism include heat intolerance, thirst, increased appetite, weight loss, sweating, palpitations, and tremor. These symptoms develop most commonly in young patients, but the disease can have its onset at any age. Exophthalmos is not a feature of hyperthyroidism but rather a variable manifestation of Graves disease, appearing before other symptoms, during the active phase of the disease, after definitive treatment of the disease, not at all, or in patients who never develop a goiter or hyperthyroidism. About one third of patients develop ocular manifestations and the signs and symptoms of thyrotoxicosis simultaneously. The ocular findings of Graves disease include exophthalmos with proptosis, spasms of the upper lid, lid retraction, and supraorbital and infraorbital swelling. Extrinsic ocular muscle weakness is present in about 40% of patients and is particularly apparent with upward gaze. Severe eye disease is characterized by venous congestion and edema.

The initial manifestation of Graves disease in older patients may be atrial fibrillation or myocardial dysfunction (eg, angina pectoris or congestive heart failure). These patients may not have obvious goiters, and if ocular signs are absent, the diagnosis may be overlooked. With or without ocular findings, the thyroid gland may be diffusely enlarged, symmetric, and smooth, which is characteristic, but it may also be irregular.

Diagnosis. In about 3% of patients, the thyroid is normal in size. In addition to elevated T_4 or T_3 levels, or both, the uptake of radioiodine by the thyroid is markedly elevated, with up to 90% of the dose concentrated within the gland after 24 hours. Diffuse, increased uptake of ^{131}I within a symmetrically enlarged gland is diagnostic and differentiates Graves disease from other causes of thyrotoxicosis, such as Hashimoto thyroiditis or toxic nodular goiter. As a result, some endocrinologists routinely obtain a ^{131}I scan even when the diagnosis of Graves disease is relatively secure clinically.

Medical Treatment. The treatment of Graves disease must be individualized on the basis of age, general health, severity of disease, gland size, and the patient's preference. The three appropriate treatment approaches include therapy with thionamide drugs, radioactive iodine, and thyroidectomy. All are safe and predictably successful, and their roles are complementary. Because there are good alternatives, patients should be well informed of the relative merits and disadvantages of each approach. During the past several decades, the indications for operation have dramatically narrowed, particularly in the United States, where a resurgence in the use of antithyroid drugs has occurred along with a liberalization in the use of ^{131}I.[16] At the same time, there has been greater concern about the potential surgical complications associated with thyroidectomy for Graves disease. Nevertheless, thyroidectomy remains an important alternative for selected patients with Graves disease.

Antithyroid drugs are the initial therapy in most patients with Graves disease, either as definitive therapy or in preparation for ^{131}I or surgical ablation. Because of the high failure rate of long-term treatment (6 to 24 months) with thionamides, the use of these drugs as definitive treatment had decreased until recently. Improved results and evidence that these drugs may have a direct effect on the basic immunologic cause of the disease have recently been reported and have prompted a reevaluation. Decreased plasma levels of immunoglobulins and antithyroid antibodies have shown no prognostic value.

The major risk of prolonged thionamide therapy is a small but important 0.5% incidence of agranulocytosis. Other major drawbacks include the long duration of treatment and the possibility of recurrence when the drug is stopped. Even after 1 year of treatment, the rate of recurrence in the following year is as high as 43%. Five years after treatment, only 25% of patients remain in remission. Unlike other definitive treatments, thionamide treatment does not result in hypothyroidism if an appropriate dosage of the drug is given. The improved results of some recent series appear to be based on improved patient selection rather than any other factor. Patients with a small or normal-sized gland have a remission rate of 75% or greater. When the goiter is large, the success rate is less than 30%. Patients with high T_3 levels or a high T_3/T_4 ratio also appear to fare less well. Although human leukocyte antigen typing was once considered a significant prognostic factor for pharmacologic selection, recent evidence does not support this concept.

Finally, there is increasing evidence that children and young adults are unlikely to remain in remission even after long-term thionamide therapy. Despite this evidence, most children and young adults in the United States are treated with either PTU or methimazole for extended periods of time, particularly if the gland is not greatly enlarged. For those whose therapy fails, surgical or possibly ^{131}I treatment is required.

For more than 45 years, ^{131}I has been used to treat patients with Graves disease. It is a definitive treatment with predictable and lasting results in most patients, and it has few, if any, serious side effects. [131]I treatment delivers 0.06 to 100 Gy to the thyroid gland and is ablative in its effect. Hypothyroidism is a nearly inevitable result of effective therapy, although it may take years to become clinically apparent. About 70% of patients treated with ^{131}I are hypothyroid within 10 years of treatment. After a therapeutic dose of ^{131}I, several months or more are needed before the hyperthyroidism is controlled. Subsequently, patients must be monitored closely to determine when or if thyroid replacement therapy is required. Although attempts have been made to use low-dose ^{131}I therapy to treat Graves disease, a dose adequate to control hyperthyroidism results eventually in hypothyroidism. Most patients are treated successfully by one dose, but because of rapid ^{131}I turnover or other reasons, a small percentage may require a second or even a third dose. The risk of recurrence of hyperthyroidism after an initial response is less than 5%. Despite the theoretic risks of chromosomal damage and oncogenesis, there are no data for either risk after 40 years of study. Nevertheless, this approach remains a concern in the treatment of children because of the limited experience and possibility of cumulative effects. An increased incidence of parathyroid adenomas may occur among patients receiving ^{131}I therapy.

Most adult patients in the United States are treated with ^{131}I as definitive therapy for Graves disease. Exceptions are women in the childbearing years, patients with concomitant thyroid nodules, those with extremely large glands, and, increasingly, those who are opposed to ^{131}I therapy. The resistance to ^{131}I therapy appears to be emotional rather than based on any evidence of long-term adverse effects of [131]I.

Surgical Treatment. Thyroidectomy for Graves disease offers rapid and permanent treatment. Preparation for operation with medical therapy can be accomplished within 6 weeks with the use of a thionamide and, if necessary, within 1 week with the use of β-adrenergic blocking agents. After hospitalization for 2 or 3 days and 2 to 3 weeks of recuperation, the patient is cured and can resume full activity. Thyroidectomy for Graves disease is a safe procedure with a minimal risk of either vocal cord paralysis or permanent hypoparathyroidism in the well-prepared patient. These risks range from 0.4% for RLN injury to less than 1% for permanent hypoparathyroidism. Thyroid crisis or mortality from operation is almost nonexistent. Although the extent of resection of thyroid tissue is still controversial, acceptable resections are highly successful in that they reliably provide a cure with only a small chance of recurrent hyperthyroidism. Recent large series show a recurrence of 3.2% with subtotal resections and no recurrence with total thyroidectomy.[15,17–19] Some patients with Graves disease have concomitant thyroid nodules; when malignant, this carcinoma is also definitively treated along with Graves disease.

Thyroidectomy has been advocated for the patient who is noncompliant and incapable of long-term management with thionamide drugs. Thyroidectomy has also been advocated for the patient with ophthalmopathy because of the possibility that progressive eye disease is more likely to be controlled after total ablation of the thyroid. Ocular disease is likewise controlled in most patients after ^{131}I ablation. There is no clear evidence that total thyroidectomy offers a significant advantage in the treatment of eye disease, although several small series have shown excellent results. Overall costs of these medical and surgical options appear to be similar.

Preoperative preparation of the hyperthyroid patient is essential to avoid intraoperative or postoperative thyroid storm. This complication is avoidable, and its incidence is zero in nearly all recent large series. Thionamide drugs administered for a period of 4 to 8 weeks preoperatively or until the patient is euthyroid, with or without the addition of β-adrenergic blocking agents or iodine, are considered the safest preparatory regimen. PTU, 200 to 400 mg/d, and methimazole, 30 to 60 mg/d, are most commonly used in the United States. In most patients, propranolol is given in doses ranging from 40 to 460 mg at the initiation of thionamide therapy to afford immediate symptomatic relief. Although propranolol usually controls the symptoms and signs of hyperthyroidism that are attributable to the peripheral effects of T_3 and T_4, the drug has no effect on either the synthesis or the release of thyroid hormones. The initial dose of β-blocking agent may be decreased after several weeks or when the thionamide drugs have become effective.

Iodine is administered for 2 weeks before the operation in addition to thionamide to decrease the vascularity of the gland, to make the gland firmer, and to simplify resection. Iodine is given as saturated potassium iodide (50 mg per drop), usually 1 drop three times daily, or as Lugol solution (iodine plus potassium iodide, 6 mg of iodine per drop), 5 to 10 drops three times daily. During the past decade, the routine use of iodine was found to be unnecessary because propranolol was equally effective in decreasing thyroid gland vascularity.

Propranolol alone or in combination with iodine has been widely used by many as preparation for operation and has been found to be safe.[15] Generally, thionamides are used in elective situations because of the additional safety provided. In patients intolerant to thionamides, propranolol alone can be administered for 1 to 2 weeks or until the clinical manifestations of hyperthyroidism are eliminated. These patients must receive a propranolol dose on the morning of operation, at 6-hour intervals in the immediate postoperative period, and for 5 or 6 days postoperatively to avoid thyroid storm. In the patient resistant to high doses of propranolol, the addition of iodine for 2 weeks before operation can be effective. This combination should be successful in patients with severe thyrotoxicosis who are still tachycardiac even after 500 mg/d or more of propranolol. The longer-acting β-adrenergic antagonists such as nadolol (Corgard) and atenolol (Tenormin) have been used with excellent clinical results. These drugs can be given only once daily for 7 to 10 days and on the morning of operation. The disadvantage of using only β-blockade in a preoperative preparation is the need for close monitoring during the perioperative period. A particular advantage of this approach is its use in patients who have had significant adverse reactions to thionamides, particularly bone marrow suppression.

The appropriate extent of thyroidectomy for Graves disease is controversial. The traditional approach is a bilateral subtotal thyroidectomy, leaving a remnant of 2 to 4 g of viable thyroid tissue on either side. A second approach is a total lobectomy on one side, leaving a larger remnant on the contralateral side. In both approaches, the goal is to ensure permanent euthyroidism by leaving a thyroid remnant sufficient to prevent hypothyroidism but not so large as to allow for recurrent hyperthyroidism. The appropriate remnant size cannot be determined because the two objectives of the procedure are mutually exclusive. Although leaving a 6- to 8-g remnant does lead to a high percentage of euthyroidism (70%), 3% to 4% of patients remain hyperthyroid, and an additional 25% to 30% become hypothyroid. Although many surgeons and physicians consider hypothyroidism an acceptable result in the definitive treatment of Graves disease, recurrent hyperthyroidism is unacceptable, particularly in the patient who has refused ^{131}I. Because manipulating the remnant size does not produce euthyroidism in any predictable way, a third alternative is to perform total thyroidectomy. This procedure has the advantage of completely eliminating recurrences but does so with the disadvantage that all patients require lifelong thyroid replacement. Because total thyroidectomy offers the least chance of recurrence and progressive eye involvement, it has gained increasing favor in the management of Graves disease. Reports from a number of centers have shown that there is little or no increased risk of either RLN injury or permanent hypoparathyroidism when a total or near-total thyroidectomy is performed by an experienced thyroid surgeon.[19] Bilateral subtotal thyroidectomy and total thyroidectomy have proved to be equally safe if the nerve is positively identified and traced to its entrance into the larynx. With care taken to preserve the blood supply to the parathyroid glands, the incidence of hypoparathyroidism after total thyroidectomy for either benign or malignant disease is about 1% or less.

Determining the extent of thyroidectomy for Graves disease requires a balance between the risks and benefits of subtotal versus total thyroidectomy. This decision is arrived at by each surgeon during preoperative discussions with the patient and is guided by surgical judgments based on the findings at operation. There are three guiding principles in determining the procedure to be performed. First, permanent hypoparathyroidism is a serious and lifelong complication. It should be avoided by modifying the operation if anatomic factors related to the parathyroid glands make it necessary. Second, recurrent hyperthyroidism represents operative failure and usually requires ^{131}I for treatment, negating the primary reason for which thyroidectomy is usually selected. Therefore, any thyroid remnant left to ensure preservation of parathyroid tissue should be as small as possible. Third, hypothyroidism should not be considered a complication or an important factor in determining remnant size, but rather an expected and eas-

ily treated sequela of the definitive treatment of Graves disease in many patients.

Over the past two decades, we have performed either a total or near-total thyroidectomy in most patients with Graves disease. Most of these patients were children, young adults, or women in the childbearing years; patients with recurrence after long-term thionamide drug therapy; and those opposed to the use of ^{131}I. No patients developed RLN palsy, permanent hypoparathyroidism, or recurrence of the disease. All patients with total or near-total thyroidectomy require levothyroxine replacement therapy after operation and have been euthyroid as determined by annual testing. No patient had difficulty complying with this therapy. Most patients had total thyroidectomies, unless both parathyroid glands were not considered viable after the initial total lobectomy and isthmectomy. In these cases, a small posterior thyroid remnant was left on the contralateral side when either or both parathyroid glands were adherent to the thyroid capsule. In no case was more than 1 or 2 g of thyroid parenchyma left in situ. Alternatively, a few adult patients willing to accept the small risk of recurrence and the possible need for ^{131}I or a second operation underwent total lobectomy, isthmectomy, and subtotal lobectomy, leaving a 6- to 8-g remnant. This operation, like bilateral subtotal thyroidectomy with a 3- to 4-g remnant on each side, is associated with a 3% to 5% recurrence rate and a 30% to 40% incidence of hypothyroidism. These patients require careful lifelong follow-up for either recurrence or the late development of hypothyroidism.

Toxic Multinodular Goiter

Hyperthyroidism in the patient with a multinodular goiter usually develops in women older than 50 years of age, but it is seen occasionally in younger patients. Most patients have had a nontoxic nodular goiter for many years. Eventually, enough nodules become autonomous so that hyperthyroidism develops insidiously. In some patients, the hyperthyroidism is so mild that it is not suspected until the patient is placed on thyroid suppression therapy because of the enlarging goiter. Even low doses of thyroid can then cause overt hyperthyroidism. It can also be precipitated or exacerbated by iodides in medications or after the administration of contrast media done for many radiologic procedures (jodbasedow phenomenon). Older patients may present with toxic multinodular goiters and cardiac findings such as atrial fibrillation, tachycardia, congestive heart failure, or unexplained or accelerated angina. Unexplained weight loss, anxiety, and insomnia may also develop. Masked hyperthyroidism occurs when the goiter has been overlooked and the manifestations of thyrotoxicosis are unrecognized.

The preferred treatment for most patients with toxic multinodular goiters is thyroidectomy after adequate preparation renders the patient euthyroid. ^{131}I may be an alternative in selected poor-risk patients with goiters that are not causing airway compression. Although ^{131}I can be used to treat the hyperthyroidism, large (greater than 50 mCi) and often repeated doses of ^{131}I may be required. ^{131}I does not significantly reduce the goiter size and may, because of radiation-induced thyroiditis, cause acute enlargement. This may be hazardous in the patient with some degree of preexisting airway compression. Any airway symptoms, particularly in patients with substernal goiters, should be considered strong contraindications to the use of ^{131}I.

Standard surgical treatment of toxic nodular goiter has consisted of bilateral subtotal thyroidectomy. Remnant size is not as important as the excision of all autonomous nodules. Because thyroid replacement or suppression is used routinely to prevent recurrence of goiter when a subtotal resection is done, the risk of hypothyroidism is not a consideration in determining remnant size. Recurrent hyperthyroidism after adequate resection of a toxic nodular goiter does not occur. Alternative procedures are total lobectomy, isthmectomy and contralateral subtotal lobectomy, or total thyroidectomy. Total lobectomy on the dominant side is easier and safer to perform than subtotal resection of the lobe, provided that the parathyroid glands can be identified and preserved. Permanent hypoparathyroidism should be avoidable in essentially all patients. Caution must be taken with the RLNs, which may be displaced from their normal locations by the abnormal growth of nodules, particularly in the region of the tubercle of Zuckerkandl. The nerve may be found on the lateral surface of the thyroid rather than posterior to the gland, and on occasion it may be stretched out over a large nodule that has descended substernally. Recognition of these possibilities prevents inadvertent nerve injury in patients with large multinodular goiters.

Solitary Toxic Nodule

Patients with autonomous functioning nodules causing thyrotoxicosis are usually younger than those with toxic multinodular goiters. The peak incidence occurs during the fifth decade, and women are much more commonly affected. Autonomously functioning nodules causing hyperthyroidism are invariably at least 3 cm in diameter. Smaller solitary hot nodules are not usually associated with hyperthyroidism. The natural history of these nodules is that they enlarge, develop central necrosis, and become cold. Only about 20% of all autonomous hot nodules eventually enlarge to the point at which clinical hyperthyroidism develops.

Thyroiditis

There are three types of thyroiditis that can cause thyroid abnormalities of surgical significance. The most common is chronic lymphocytic thyroiditis, an autoimmune disease that can occur in any age group. Subacute thyroiditis is much less common and is believed to be caused by a viral infection. It occurs most often in young women and usually resolves spontaneously in weeks or months. Occasionally, the disease causes unilateral thyroid enlargement that simulates malignancy. The rarest form of thyroiditis is Riedel struma, which can mimic a diffuse thyroid carcinoma because of the fibrotic infiltrative process that results. The surgical implications of each of these diseases are considered in the following section.

Hashimoto Disease

Struma lymphomatosa, chronic lymphocytic thyroiditis, and Hashimoto disease are synonymous terms referring to a relatively common cause of diffuse goiter. Although it can occur in any age group, it is most common in middle-aged women. The prevalence in autopsy studies has been about 2%, but the estimated clinical prevalence in women is nearly 5% and has been steadily increasing. It is considered an autoimmune disease, and most patients have high levels of circulating antimicrosomal and antithyroglobulin antibodies. Both humoral and cell-mediated immunity are involved in the resulting inflammatory response. The tendency of Hashimoto disease and Graves disease to occur in members of the same family is well recognized and suggests a genetic predisposition to these diseases. Environmental factors also appear to play a significant role, because Hashimoto disease occurs more commonly in geographic areas where the dietary intake of iodine is high. It is also common in patients who received radiation in infancy or childhood.

Hashimoto thyroiditis results in defective hormone synthesis characterized by a lack of organification of trapped iodine. The reduced functional capacity of the thyroid increases TSH secretion, and a goiter develops. Because of the associated fibrosis and the thyroid gland lobulations, palpation of the gland may suggest a nodular goiter or a neoplasm. Abnormal findings include small follicles depleted of thyroglobulin, varying degrees of fibrosis, and diffuse lymphocytic infiltration with germinal centers. Although a goiter is characteristic, some patients may have a smaller than normal but firm and rubbery thyroid gland. Hashimoto disease is the most common cause of spontaneous hypothyroidism in adults, but many patients may have the disease for years with normal thyroid function. Rarely, the disease may cause mild thyrotoxicosis (hashitoxicosis), especially during the acute phase of the disease when there may be an excessive release of thyroid hormone. This phase is usually self-limiting and can be managed symptomatically with antithyroid drugs or propranolol. Transient hyperthyroidism is seen most commonly in young women several months after pregnancy.

The usual clinical manifestations are those of a diffuse and slowly progressive goiter. The goiter is usually asymptomatic unless accompanied by local pressure symptoms or the insidious onset of mild hypothyroidism. The gland is usually firm and rubbery with a somewhat lobulated surface that may be asymmetric, simulating a neoplasm or adenomatous goiter. The clinical and laboratory findings, particularly an elevated antimicrosomal antibody titer, are usually sufficiently characteristic to establish the diagnosis. Treatment with thyroid hormone (0.15 mg of levothyroxine daily) usually results in regression of the goiter. Despite TSH suppression therapy, the goiter may continue to enlarge and cause compression or a significant cosmetic deformity. In these situations, partial thyroidectomy may be indicated. Furthermore, Hashimoto thyroiditis may coexist with an adenomatous goiter or a solitary nodule within the diffusely enlarged or normal-sized gland. Thyroidectomy may be indicated for treatment of a solitary nodule, particularly if it is cold, suspicious, definitely malignant, or solid and if FNA biopsy is indeterminate.

An increased incidence of papillary carcinoma in patients with Hashimoto disease has not been substantiated by recent findings. Nevertheless, well-differentiated carcinoma does occur in glands involved with thyroiditis. Even if the diagnosis of Hashimoto disease has been made, a suspicious nodule should be evaluated as if the underlying thyroiditis did not exist. There is a relation between Hashimoto disease and the occurrence of thyroid lymphoma. In one experience, 80% of thyroid lymphomas seen during the past 20 years developed in glands that showed evidence of Hashimoto disease.[20] Nevertheless, the incidence of lymphoma is so low that prophylactic thyroidectomy to prevent its occurrence is not indicated. Any rapid enlargement of a thyroid gland involved with Hashimoto thyroiditis should be carefully evaluated. FNA cytology should be performed if lymphoma is suspected.

Subacute Thyroiditis

Granulomatous, de Quervain, and subacute thyroiditis are terms that refer to a disease that usually occurs in young women within weeks of an upper respiratory or other viral infection. There may be systemic manifestations such as weakness, depression, easy fatigability, neck pain in the region of the thyroid, or referred pain to the ear or angle of the jaw. The thyroid is usually tender to palpation, and the diagnosis often can be made without laboratory studies or biopsy. The disease is usually self-limited for a few weeks, during which time symptomatic relief can be achieved with salicylates or possibly corticosteroids. In some patients, the disease may persist for several months or longer. Recovery is usually associated with restoration of normal thyroid function. In unusual patients, the disease may be confined to one lobe and may result in a firm, slightly tender mass suggesting carcinoma. Lobectomy may be indicated to rule out the presence of malignancy. Total thyroidectomy may be considered for persistent painful thyroiditis after months of steroid therapy have failed to alleviate the disease.

Riedel Struma

Goiter with a woody or fibrous component involving the adjacent strap muscles and carotid sheaths is referred to as Riedel struma. Its identity as a separate entity has been debated because of its rarity; fewer than 100 new cases have been reported during the last 25 years. The causes of Riedel struma are not known, but it is associated with other types of fibrotic processes such as retroperitoneal fibrosis, sclerosing cholangitis, and fibrosing mediastinitis. The process involves both lobes of the thyroid and the isthmus. The infiltrating fibrotic process involves the strap muscles and may extend to the carotid sheath and other surrounding organs as well. Clinically, it resembles an infiltrative undifferentiated thyroid carcinoma or lymphoma and cannot be differentiated without biopsy.

Although considered self-limited, the process may be associated with considerable morbidity as a result of localized pain and compression of adjacent tissues. Airway compression is best treated by open biopsy and excision of the isthmus and as much of the fibrotic process as possible without endangering the RLNs. Occasionally, tracheostomy may be required. Because the histopathology can be mimicked by some types of lymphoma, careful immunohistochemical staining should be performed before the diagnosis of Riedel struma is established. In patients who do not require urgent decompression of the airway, treatment with steroids may prove beneficial. Although nonsteroidal antiestrogens have been used with success in the treatment of other fibrotic processes, such as desmoid tumors and retroperitoneal fibrosis, their value in the treatment of Riedel struma remains to be proved.

SOLITARY THYROID NODULE

The thyroid nodule continues to be a major source of concern to both physicians and surgeons evaluating patients with thyroid problems. In the United States, the most common indication for a thyroid operation is a solitary nodule with the possibility of malignancy. In the past, all solitary thyroid nodules that failed to respond to TSH suppression were removed. However, a more cost-effective and accurate assessment should be made before choosing surgical excision, further observation, or thyroid hormone suppression. Selective management is emphasized because of the relatively high frequency of benign nodules.

The prevalence of thyroid nodules in the adult population ranges from 4% to 8%. Almost all are colloid nodules or follicular adenomas. In several recent surveys in the United States, 4% of adults between 30 and 60 years of age were found to have one or more palpable thyroid nodules.[21] Thus, about 9,000,000 American adults have thyroid nodules, and an additional 250,000 people are thought to develop new nodules each year. In contrast, the National Cancer Institute estimates that only 11,300 new cases of thyroid cancer were diagnosed in 1979.[22] About 1025 people die as a result of thyroid cancer each year. Worldwide, the annual incidence of thyroid carcinoma ranges from about 4 to 7 per 100,000 people. It is apparent from these figures that the process of selecting patients for surgery is of great practical importance. Many individuals with nodules are not considered surgical candidates. This group includes many patients who, after careful evaluation, are found to have small multinodular goiters rather than single nodules.

Diagnostic Studies

The history and physical examination are still the most important considerations for patients with thyroid nodules. In many patients, an asymptomatic nodule is first discovered during a routine physical examination. Often, these patients are unaware of any thyroid enlargement or symptoms, even after the nodule has been identified. Nearly half of asymptomatic nodules are discovered by patients themselves. The relation between irradiation exposure during infancy or childhood and thyroid carcinoma is well known, and many patients with this exposure present themselves for a thyroid evaluation. This relation should always be specifically sought when taking the history. A history of low-dose radiation exposure is a strong factor favoring a more aggressive approach to a thyroid nodule. In the past, nearly one in five patients with thyroid carcinoma younger than 30 years of age was found to have such a history. Other important considerations are the use of thyroid hormones and any change in the nodule during treatment. Growth of a nodule in a patient taking suppressive doses of thyroid hormone suggests that the nodule is autonomous and may be malignant.

A careful examination of the neck can often determine whether a nodule is likely to be thyroid carcinoma. Large, firm lymph nodes in the lower third of the neck are often present, particularly in children and in young adults with papillary carcinoma. Lymphadenopathy in association with an ipsilateral thyroid nodule should always be considered the result of malignancy until proved otherwise. Obvious fixation of a nodule to surrounding structures implies malignancy. The palpable consistency of a solitary nodule is not always helpful. Some malignancies are soft or cystic, whereas an occasional benign nodule may be hard and calcified. A firm nodule with an irregular outline should raise the question of malignancy. Hoarseness without RLN palsy may occur with either benign or malignant nodules. On the other hand, paralysis of the RLN on the side of a thyroid nodule always suggests a carcinoma.

An evaluation of the entire thyroid gland is important. A careful search is made for evidence of Hashimoto disease, diffuse enlargement, and other nodules. The presence of other nodules, the absence of adenopathy, normal vocal cord function, and no history of irradiation reduce the probability of malignancy. Before a management plan is recommended, further diagnostic evaluation is needed.

Imaging Studies

Thyroid scintiscans are often used to supplement the findings of a physical examination. In most cases, the results of scintigraphy are not decisive in determining the treatment of thyroid nodules. A nodule is usually at least 1 cm or more in diameter before it is seen on a thyroid scan. The scintiscan, regardless of the isotope administered, usually fails to delineate a nodule that cannot be palpated on physical examination unless it is substernal in location. Many patients are referred for surgical treatment after a thyroid scan has demonstrated a cold nodule. Most cold thyroid nodules are benign. It is only when a nodule is hyperfunctioning (hot) that the isotope scan becomes specific. Only rarely is a warm or hot nodule a well-differentiated thyroid carcinoma. Because only 5% of all solitary nodules are hot, the overall specificity of thyroid scintiscans is low. Nevertheless, thyroid scans are the most common screening study obtained in patients with a thyroid nodule. Therefore, their limitations should be understood by surgeons treating patients with thyroid nodules.

^{99m}Tc is the preferred agent for routine imaging of the thyroid gland. When a nodule is hot with ^{99m}Tc, the possibility of malignancy, particularly papillary carcinoma, is low but not totally excluded. ^{123}I is necessary to assess the functional activity of a nodule. Thyroid function studies probably should be done in all patients with large nodules, although most patients prove to be euthyroid. When a previous scintiscan has demonstrated a hyperfunctioning nodule, thyroid function studies may detect excessive thyroid hormone production. A hot nodule larger than 3 cm may cause thyrotoxicosis, whereas lesions smaller than this rarely do so. Functional nodules are excised for the treatment of hyperthyroidism rather than for the suspicion of malignancy. Whether the routine use of scintigraphy can be justified for the purpose of identifying hot nodules that would otherwise remain unrecognized is controversial. A scintiscan may be of value when the thyroid gland cannot be completely palpated because of its substernal extension or because of a patient's thick and muscular neck. In these circumstances, a scan may outline the lower extent of the thyroid gland and also delineate cold and hot nodules that would otherwise escape detection.

Ultrasonography has been widely used during the past 20 years to supplement the scintiscan and the physical examination of the thyroid. In many centers, radiologists report that ultrasonographic diagnosis is accurate in 95% of patients in identifying cysts and complex and solid nodules. Since the adoption of FNA, sonography has been virtually abandoned in the evaluation of the palpable thyroid nodule. Although sonography can identify thyroid lesions as small as 3 mm in diameter, it cannot differentiate between benign and malignant lesions on the basis of any specific characteristics.

Needle Biopsy

Needle biopsy techniques used extensively in Scandinavia for more than 30 years have gained wide acceptance and enthusiastic advocates in the United States during the past 10 years. An early theoretic concern about needle biopsy was the fear of implanting thyroid carcinoma in the needle tract when using a large needle. During a 25-year period in which more than 20,000 FNA biopsies of palpable thyroid nodules were performed at the Karolinska Hospital, implantation of thyroid cancer did not occur.[23] The possibility of implantation of malignant cells is not a deterrent to FNA cytologic techniques, and there are virtually no complications when FNA is performed properly. The technique of aspiration biopsy has been described.[22,23] The technique is applicable to any palpable thyroid nodule, regardless of size. The results in large series show that false-negative diagnoses were made in less than 10% of patients and false-positive diagnoses were made in less than 2%. When interpreted by a skilled cytologist, this technique is highly accurate and is considered the preferred method of selecting patients for surgery. Nearly 80% of patients with thyroid nodules were spared surgical exploration as a result of such studies, as noted in one report.[22] Because of the risk of false-negative diagnoses (10%), advocates of this technique emphasize the importance of clinical judgment in addition to the cytologic study in selecting operative candidates. Worldwide experience during the last decade was similar to the Swedish experience in that false-positive cytologic diagnoses of thyroid cancer were rare. As a diagnostic method, this technique closely parallels histopathologic standards of accuracy. In most cases, FNA cytology biopsy enables the pathologist to distinguish nonneoplastic from neoplastic nodules and to identify the type of malignant tumor. Papillary, medullary, and anaplastic carcinoma all have a typical cytologic appearance. Cytologic studies cannot differentiate malignant from benign follicular or Hürthle cell neoplasms. A definitive diagnosis depends on histologic examination of the entire excised tumor. The introduction of FNA cytology has dramatically reduced the number of diagnostic surgical operations for benign lesions in centers where it has been extensively used. In most Scandinavian hospitals, FNA is routinely performed before operative intervention is considered. At one time in the United States, a major factor limiting the use of FNA was a shortage of pathologists experienced in the interpretation of thyroid cytology. This is no longer the case.

FNA cytology is used to evaluate most solitary nodules of the thyroid. In patients with thyroid nodules and a history of previous head and neck radiation, operation is generally recommended regardless of the cytologic findings. In these patients, both benign and malignant lesions may develop, and the chances of sampling error are considerable. As a result, a negative biopsy does not reliably rule out carcinoma. In other patients in whom the clinical evaluation detects obvious signs of cancer, an FNA may not be necessary. The cytologic evaluation can be used to determine the specific cell type of the tumor. When cytologic studies are positive for papillary or medullary neoplasms of the thyroid, a definitive operation may be planned and carried out without the necessity of frozen section confirmation.

In addition to cytologic evaluation with FNA, this technique is useful in the diagnosis of cystic lesions of the thyroid. In cases in which the nodule is found to be a cyst, the fluid is aspirated and the physical examination is repeated. If a nodule is still present, a specific FNA cytology test is carried out on the solid component. When nothing is palpable after aspiration, an operation can be avoided if the cyst does not recur. Cysts larger than 4 cm invariably recur despite repeated aspirations and usually require surgical excision to be eradicated. Most cysts smaller than 4 cm with no solid component can be eliminated, but it may require three or four aspirations to achieve this permanently. About 15% of all patients referred with nodules actually have a cyst. Not all cysts should be considered harmless, because about 10% are malignant. These are usually papillary carcinomas in patients between 20 and 40 years of age. If a cyst does not completely disappear with aspiration, repeated FNA cytologic examination of any residual solid component is necessary.

FNA cytology and cyst aspiration have contributed significantly to the evaluation of the patient with a thyroid nodule. In addition to the careful history and physical examination, FNA has become the most important diagnostic technique for selecting patients for operation. Twenty years ago, the incidence of carcinoma in patients with thyroid nodules selected for operation, after evaluation with routine scintigraphy and a trial of suppression, was about 30%.[21] In the last decade, with the routine use of FNA, the incidence of carcinoma in nodules excised because of the suspicion of carcinoma has been close to 50%.[23]

Thyroid Suppression

It has been suggested that TSH suppression by the administration of thyroid hormone causes 50% of benign thyroid nodules to decrease in size or disappear. As a result, thyroid suppression has been used frequently, both as a diagnostic maneuver and as therapy for thyroid nodules. An occasional nodule may regress within 6 weeks with or without treatment. Most are not solid nodules but rather hemorrhagic cysts that develop acutely. These should be observed for a reasonable time (6 weeks) or aspirated if painful. Most nodules that disappear with thyroid hormone treatment are actually lobulations of the gland or diffuse enlargement of a lobe associated with either Hashimoto disease or a colloid goiter. Although an occasional discrete nodule larger than 1 to 2 cm decreases in size or even disappears, this occurs in less than 5% of solitary, noncystic thyroid nodules. A well-differentiated thyroid cancer may decrease in size after TSH suppression. If diagnostic suppression is routinely used, strict criteria for the selection of patients for thyroidectomy must be used. Unless the lesion resolves completely, carcinoma cannot be ruled out with certainty.

With the increasing use of FNA in the diagnosis of benign thyroid disease, thyroid suppression is best used for therapeutic reasons such as preventing further enlargement of a nodule or preventing the development of new nodules.[24-26]

Operative Treatment

Total extracapsular thyroid lobectomy and isthmectomy is the procedure of choice when a decision has been made to surgically remove a thyroid nodule. The entire lobe with the isthmus is submitted for frozen-section pathologic examination if FNA has not already resulted in a definitive diagnosis of carcinoma. When a nodule is located in the isthmus, it may be excised with a margin of normal thyroid tissue on both sides for the biopsy. In performing total lobectomy, both parathyroid glands are carefully preserved with their blood supply by either dissecting them from the surface of the thyroid gland or completely avoiding them if they are not in the immediate proximity of the thyroid capsule. This is done in the event that total thyroidectomy is necessary if either the frozen or permanent histologic sections confirm the presence of thyroid carcinoma.

Total lobectomy offers the best opportunity for accurate histologic diagnosis and is associated with the lowest incidence of complications when the need for reoperation is considered. In one experience, 800 consecutive cases of total unilateral lobectomy were performed for benign or malignant nodules suspected of being cancerous, and no permanent RLN palsies occurred.[27] Primary total lobectomy is safer than a partial lobectomy followed by resection of the residual lobe after a delayed diagnosis of malignancy. Reoperation to complete a lobectomy after an interval of several days or weeks is associated with a greater risk to both the RLN and the parathyroids on the ipsilateral side. Furthermore, the possibility of implanting carcinoma cells is increased by subtotal lobectomy.

Although there is controversy as to whether a total lobectomy and isthmectomy or a total thyroidectomy is the best definitive operation for a unilateral papillary carcinoma, a subtotal lobectomy is universally considered an inadequate operation.[28] A definitive cancer operation can be accomplished with one procedure in 80% of cases when a skilled thyroid pathologist is available for frozen-section interpretation. Therefore, it is crucial that a frozen-section diagnosis be made whenever open surgical biopsy of a thyroid nodule is performed so that a definitive operation can be selected. In patients with well-encapsulated follicular and Hürthle cell tumors, this procedure may not be possible until multiple sections through the capsule have been taken during permanent section study. As a result, a definitive operation may not always be possible in one stage in this group of patients. For those situations in which a firm diagnosis has not already been established, a lobectomy or biopsy should not be done without the aid of a competent pathologist familiar with the histopathology of thyroid lesions on frozen sections. When the diagnosis of carcinoma has been established preoperatively by FNA, the surgeon may determine what definitive thyroid operation is required, which may be modified by the gross findings at operation.[20,23]

THYROID CARCINOMA

Thyroid cancer is not one disease but rather a spectrum of neoplasms ranging in virulence from the most indolent visceral carcinoma to the most lethal. Fortunately, papillary carcinoma, which is the most common, is usually associated with an excellent prognosis, particularly in patients younger than 40 years of age. Seventy to 80% of the 11,000 new patients with thyroid carcinoma diagnosed annually in the United States have papillary carcinoma. The incidence of clinically apparent thyroid carcinoma has increased by nearly 50%. The reasons for this are not entirely clear but include such factors as dietary iodine abundance, radiation exposure, environmental mutagens, and improved diagnostic methods. This increase has not occurred in all types of thyroid neoplasms—it has been limited to papillary carcinoma. Most patients with thyroid carcinomas have solitary thyroid nodules. Selecting the patients with thyroid nodules who should undergo operation is based on clinical judgment and FNA. Factors strongly favoring operative intervention are solitary nodules in individuals younger than 20 years of age or older than 60 years of age, a history of irradiation, and suspicious aspiration cytology and growth while the patient was on thyroid suppression. Aspiration cytology has become the most important technique for the selection of operative candidates.

Classification

Thyroid carcinomas are classified as papillary, follicular, Hürthle cell, medullary, and anaplastic. Lymphomas also occur as primary neoplasms arising from the thyroid gland. The thyroid gland is also a site for metastatic carcinoma on rare occasions. Conventionally, only papillary and follicular carcinomas are considered differentiated. Although some classifications have included Hürthle cell carcinomas as a subtype of follicular neoplasms, they are considered separate because these tumors are incapable of concentrating iodine and do not respond to TSH. Although similar to follicular carcinomas in angioinvasive characteristics, pure Hürthle cell malignancies frequently invade lymphatics as well, a feature usually found only in advanced follicular carcinomas. Both papillary and follicular cancers may induce a Hürthle cell reaction around and within some tumors. These cells are not neoplastic but reactionary, and the biologic behavior of the tumor is not altered because of their appearance. Such neoplasms are classified as either papillary or follicular and not as Hürthle cell or mixed tumors. The term papillary carcinoma includes all thyroid neoplasms with characteristic cytologic findings, as well as those with easily recognized papillary configurations. The tumor may form well-defined follicles and show no pattern of papillae whatsoever. Previously, some authors classified these tumors as mixed papillary–follicular carcinomas, but they are now more appropriately designated as follicular variants of papillary carcinoma. Their biologic behavior is similar to that of other papillary carcinomas. With the use of cytologic criteria, carcinomas previously diagnosed as follicular can be identified as papillary and correctly classified with consistency. These tumors have the same propensity to spread to the lymph nodes that the more easily recognized papillary carcinomas demonstrate. They rarely metastasize to bone, a frequent site for metastatic follicular carcinoma.[20]

Several subtypes of papillary carcinoma are unpredictable in their biologic behavior and frequently prove aggressive and unresponsive to conventional therapy. These include the insular, columnar, and tall cell carcinomas. They are more likely to occur in older patients, and their prognosis, regardless of therapy, must be considered guarded. Because none of these variants retain the ability to concentrate iodine, they are functionally undifferentiated neoplasms. Fortunately, these types are rare and constitute less than 1% of papillary carcinomas. When recognized, they should be treated aggressively by total thyroidectomy and resection of all involved lymphatics. Treatment of these carcinomas with other techniques has been uniformly unsuccessful. Evidence suggests that nearly all anaplastic or undifferentiated (giant or spindle cell) carcinomas arise from follicular or papillary carcinomas that are often long-standing. Even when most of the neoplasm appears differentiated on pathologic study, it is classified on the basis of the most aggressive cell type recognized. This is particularly important for prognostic purposes.

The management of differentiated thyroid carcinoma remains controversial, especially in relation to the optimal management of papillary carcinoma and, to some degree, the treatment of follicular carcinoma when clinically confined to the thyroid gland.

Papillary Carcinoma

Papillary carcinomas are divided into three groups based on size and local extent of the primary tumor: minimal, intrathyroidal, and extrathyroidal (invasion through the true thyroid capsule). These categories are clinically useful as determinants of prognosis. Minimal thyroid carcinoma refers to those papillary carcinomas that are less than 1 cm in diameter and not associated with any clinically apparent lymph node metastases. In contrast to clinically significant papillary carcinomas, these are common and are found in 2% to 13% of adult thyroid glands serially sectioned after autopsy studies of individuals who died from other causes. Most of these microscopic carcinomas are a few millimeters in diameter, but they may be associated with microscopic cervical lymph node metastases. They may be misinterpreted as clinically significant cancer reported by a pathologist after a lobectomy or subtotal thyroidectomy for otherwise benign thyroid disease. In most cases, no further surgical treatment is required. For tumors between 0.5 and 1 cm, a total lobectomy and isthmectomy is satisfactory treatment.[27,29]

If a lesion of this size was excised as part of a subtotal lobectomy, the surgeon needs to decide whether the remaining lobe should be removed at a second operation. This decision can be individualized on the basis of a number of factors, including the age of the patient, whether there is an adequate margin of normal thyroid tissue surrounding the resected tumor, whether there is a history of previous head or neck irradiation, or whether there are multiple tumor sites. In general, excision of the remaining thyroid tissue to complete a total lobectomy is favored in patients with evidence of tumor multicentricity, a history of head and neck irradiation, or a borderline tissue margin. Minimal papillary carcinoma in association with a benign thyroid nodule or neoplasm should create no significant problem in subsequent management, provided that the surgeon performs a total lobectomy and isthmectomy for any nodule that is considered possibly malignant and involves one lobe of the thyroid.

Most clinically significant papillary carcinomas are 1 to 4 cm in diameter and are contained within the thyroid capsule. Multicentricity is relatively common and can be found on gross sectioning of the thyroid gland in 20% to 30% of cases. Furthermore, after serial sectioning of the entire thyroid gland in patients with papillary carcinoma, microscopic foci are found in 70% to 80%. Differentiating multicentricity from intraglandular lymphatic dissemination may be impossible, but this does not appear to be clinically important. Cervical lymph node metastases in the central compartment, anterior mediastinum, or lateral cervical lymph nodes lateral to the carotid sheath are found in about 30% of all patients with papillary carcinoma. The presence of lymph node metastases does not correlate as closely to the size of the tumor as it does to the age of the patient. The younger the patient, the greater the likelihood of metastatic lymph node involvement. Nearly all patients younger than 15 years of age have metastases to lymph nodes.

The presence or absence of lymph node metastases in patients with intrathyroidal primary papillary carcinomas does not appear to have an appreciable effect on long-term survival of the patient if distant metastases are not present at the time of initial treatment. Extension of a primary papillary carcinoma through the thyroid capsule, even when there are no lymphatic metastases, is a poor prognostic sign, indicating biologic aggressiveness of the tumor. Tumors as small as 1 cm in diameter may on occasion invade the capsule into the RLN or other surrounding structures. This feature of the primary tumor must be taken into consideration when determining definitive treatment of the neoplasm.

Multivariate analysis has been used during the past decade to define the risk factors for cancer recurrence and death due to differentiated thyroid cancer. This was first done in 1979 by Cady and others from the Lahey Clinic with a patient cohort of 30 years.[30,31] They created a simplified clinical scoring system that placed patients into risk groups with greatly different prognoses. The scale, referred to as the AMES clinical scoring system, was based on Age, distant Metastases, Extent of the primary tumor, and Size of the primary tumor. It was possible to separate nearly 90% of all patients at low risk of death from the group that was at high risk of death from differentiated thyroid cancers.

A similar scale was developed at the Mayo Clinic after four statistically significant factors were identified and after multiple regression analysis of variables affecting outcome was used for patients with papillary carcinoma. The Mayo Clinic scoring scale, referred to as the AGES clinical scoring system, was based on the Age of the patient, the Grade of the tumor, and the Extent and Size of the primary tumor.[32] Both of these systems are commonly used to determine the prognosis and report the results of patients treated for thyroid carcinoma.[33] Of the factors determining low risk, age is the most important. Men younger than 40 years of age and women younger than 50 years of age have a low risk of death from differentiated thyroid malignancies if no distant metastases are present at the time of initial treatment. Papillary carcinomas larger than 4 cm or with extension of the primary tumor through the capsule are associated with increased risk.

DNA ploidy has also been evaluated in a number of studies. Patients with papillary carcinoma who died of disease within 12 years were shown to have increased nuclear DNA values (aneuploidy), whereas patients who were alive at least 10 years after diagnosis had diploid DNA levels.[34] Other studies have failed to confirm these results. In an evaluation of DNA measurements using flow cytometry techniques on archival tissues from follicular neoplasms at the Mayo Clinic, the DNA ploidy did not differentiate between benign and malignant neoplasms. Although some groups are using DNA analysis to assist in therapeutic decisions in patients with thyroid carcinoma, the overall value of this information remains to be determined. DNA analysis appears to be more useful in prognosis than in therapeutic decision making.

The surgical resection of papillary carcinoma is the cornerstone of treatment. The extent of resectional therapy of clinically significant papillary carcinoma remains controversial. There is general agreement that the minimal operation for such tumors is a total lobectomy and isthmectomy. If a history of previous head or neck irradiation is confirmed, total or near-total thyroidectomy should be performed because of the high incidence of multifocal neoplasms. Another factor associated with a less favorable prognosis is invasion of the neoplasm through the thyroid capsule. Total or near-total thyroidectomy is indicated in this circumstance as well. In children with papillary carcinoma, the disease usually is not discovered until multiple cervical metastases are already present. In patients 15 years of age or younger, more than 90% have cervical metastases and 20% have pulmonary metastases when the diagnosis is initially made. Bilateral thyroid lobe involvement and anterior mediastinal lymph node involvement are common. In addition to total thyroidectomy, nearly all children require regional or modified neck dissections as well as routine excision of the anterior mediastinal lymph nodes through the cervical incision. A sternal splitting incision is rarely, if ever, necessary to excise involved lymph nodes in patients with papillary carcinoma. The modified neck dissection for jugular and posterior cervical lymph node involvement preserves the jugular vein, sternocleidomastoid muscle, and spinal accessory nerve. All grossly involved lymph nodes are excised, but no effort is made to do this en bloc. Usually, this can be accomplished through an extended transverse collar incision. Vertical incisions, which can cause disfiguring scars, should be avoided.

Some surgeons favor total lobectomy and isthmectomy for papillary carcinomas in low-risk patients.[28,35] Others recommend that thyroidectomy be performed for all patients with papillary carcinomas larger than 1 cm in diameter.[27,36–40] Recurrent nerve injury and hypoparathyroidism are rare. The advantage of scanning for residual cervical or distant metastases without the use of ablative doses of ^{131}I outweighs any potential risks of the procedure. Furthermore, total thyroidectomy eliminates local cervical recurrence in patients in whom all gross tumor was completely excised at the initial operation. Occult pulmonary metastases can be detected and treated with ^{131}I within 6 weeks of operation.[41] Regardless of the extent of the resection, all patients with papillary carcinoma are eventually given thyroid replacement therapy sufficient to suppress TSH. There is no additional medication burden attached to total thyroidectomy. When follow-up scintiscans show no residual uptake after total thyroidectomy, it is possible to assure patients that recurrence is unlikely. This cannot be done if residual normal thyroid tissue remains, unless it is first ablated with large doses of [131]I.

Many surgeons advocate total lobectomy and isthmectomy for the adult patient with unilateral papillary carcinoma confined to the thyroid gland. This procedure decreases the potential risk to the contralateral RLN and to the parathyroid glands. For low-risk patients, surgeons with little experience can perform total lobectomy and isthmectomy. Although most patients do well, 7% develop local recurrence after lobectomy, and half of these patients die from recurrent disease, although this may not occur for 15 to 25 years after operation.[42]

During the last two decades, there has been marked improvement in the technique and performance of this procedure. In centers where total thyroidectomy is done frequently, the complication rates compare favorably with those for lobectomy and near-total thyroidectomy. In most series, the incidence of permanent hypoparathyroidism is about 1%. This occurs primarily in patients who have had bilateral extensive disease.[36,37,40,43,44] Unfortunately, no randomized studies of similarly staged papillary carcinomas demonstrate that total thyroidectomy is superior to lobectomy and isthmectomy or to near-total thyroidectomy in reducing long-term morbidity and mortality. Several retrospective studies do show that total thyroidectomy and the use of ^{131}I when indicated are advantageous and reduce mortality during long-term follow-up. The extent of thyroidectomy for papillary carcinoma must be determined and is based on the surgeon's training, experience, and preference. In addition, the risk factors must be taken into consideration. Total thyroidectomy is advocated for papillary carcinoma because the operation eliminates possible remnant recurrence due to intraglandular lymphatic spread or multicentricity, facilitates the use of postoperative ^{131}I to detect and treat occult or obvious metastases, and avoids the necessity of therapeutic ^{131}I to ablate normal thyroid tissue.

Follicular Carcinoma

Follicular carcinomas can be classified as those with macroinvasion and those with microinvasion of either the capsule or tumor vessels. Other terms used to describe these two groups are high-grade angioinvasive and low-grade encapsulated follicular carcinomas. Follicular carcinoma has steadily decreased in incidence during the time that dietary iodine has increased. This type of carcinoma accounted for 20% to 40% of patients with thyroid carcinoma when endemic goiter was common in the Great Lakes region of the United States. In some geographic areas of the world where goiter remains endemic and iodine deficiency is still prevalent, follicular carcinoma may be even more common than papillary carcinoma. Follicular carcinoma accounts for about 10% of all new carcinomas.[45] Most patients being treated are those with minimal invasion of the capsule or vessels within the neoplasms. Such tumors are seldom diagnosed definitively by either needle aspiration cytology or frozen-section diagnosis at the time of lobectomy. Most often, the diagnosis is made after study of permanent sections. If the pathologist is fortunate enough to make a section through an area showing definitive features of capsular or angioinvasion at the time of frozen section, the diagnosis can be established immediately. Microinvasive encapsulated follicular carcinomas are rarely associated with metastatic lymph nodes, and distant metastases involving bone are also rare at the time of diagnosis.

Angioinvasive follicular carcinomas are usually large and often show invasion of perithyroidal and lateral neck veins at the time of diagnosis. They may already have metastasized to distant sites, most often to bone. The tumor thrombus within a perithyroidal vein may extend into the jugular or great veins of the mediastinum or the right atrium. These tumors can be readily diagnosed by the surgeon at the time of operation because the perithyroidal veins are usually white and enlarged. The tumor thrombus within the vein can be detected by gentle palpation. The primary tumor in these cases may extend into the contralateral lobe or through the thyroid capsule into surrounding structures, such as the trachea or RLN. Multivariate analysis scoring systems have been used to determine prognosis. The age factor has again been shown to be significant. Most patients younger than 40 years of age do well, but patients older than 50 years of age have a guarded prognosis.[28,32,33,46,47]

Follicular carcinomas of the thyroid are treated by total thyroidectomy. Lymphatic dissections are not usually required because only about 5% of all patients have lymphatic involvement.[36,37,40,45,47–49] The most effective therapy for bone or pulmonary metastases is radioactive iodine. The controversy in the surgical management of follicular carcinoma is whether patients with low-grade encapsulated neoplasms diagnosed by permanent section evaluation after total lobectomy should be treated with total thyroidectomy. If no distant metastases are present, recurrence in the contralateral lobe or elsewhere is extremely rare. Multicentricity and intraglandular spread through the lymphatics are not significant factors in encapsulated follicular carcinomas. Because of the difficulty in the intraoperative diagnosis of follicular carcinoma when encapsulated and the high incidence of microscopic carcinoma in follicular neoplasms larger than 4 cm, a total thyroidectomy is recommended. About 80% of follicular neoplasms 4 cm or larger are judged malignant after permanent section study. In patients with smaller follicular neoplasms that are found to be malignant as determined by microinvasion of the capsule, completion thyroidectomy is usually not done; instead, the patients are observed closely after performance of a ^{99m}Tc bone scan to rule out occult bone metastases. The recurrence rate in this small group of patients is low. Other patients with follicular carcinoma treated by total thyroidectomy require a ^{131}I scan 6 weeks after their operative procedure.

Medullary Carcinoma

Medullary carcinoma of the thyroid (MCT) accounts for only about 7% of all malignant tumors of the thyroid. Nevertheless, an intense interest developed in this tumor because of its hereditary occurrence in 20% to 30% of all cases and its secretion of a biologic marker (calcitonin) that allows detection of its presence when the tumor is too small to palpate. Furthermore, the cells of origin (parafollicular or C cells) are derived from the neural crest and can produce peptide and amine hormones. MCT has been found to be a more aggressive tumor than either papillary or follicular carcinoma, particularly in younger patients. It metastasizes at an early age to perithyroidal lymph nodes and eventually may involve multiple distant sites, including the liver, lung, and bones. Although the 10-year survival rate is only 50%, the tumor growth rate in individual patients has shown great variability. Early detection and appropriate surgical treatment are important and have improved the cure rate in familial cases.

MCT appears in three clinical settings. First, as a sporadic tumor, it is usually detected as a thyroid nodule in one lobe of the gland, although detection may not occur until a large neck mass or metastatic lymph nodes become apparent. Patients with sporadic disease are nearly always 30 years of age or older when the disease occurs. Second, MCT occurs as a component of the multiple endocrine neoplasia (MEN IIa) syndrome with or without adrenal medullary disease (pheochromocytomas) or hyperparathyroidism. A family history of thyroid carcinoma with or without pheochromocytoma is invariably present. MCT in the MEN IIa syndrome is always bilateral and multicentric and arises from C-cell hyperplasia. MCT usually does not develop before age 12 and is almost always clinically apparent before age 30. Third, MCT is found as a component of the MEN IIb syndrome with or without bilateral adrenal medullary disease and always with the facies and autonomic nervous system dysplasia expressed as a ganglioneuromatosis from the lips to the anus. These patients often have a marfanoid habitus and skeletal deformities as well. The MEN IIb syndrome occurs as a sporadic mutation, but its familial occurrence is more common because patients are surviving long enough to reproduce. MCT or its precursor, C-cell hyperplasia, develops by age 2 in MEN IIb and is also always bilateral and multicentric. As a result of its early appearance and late detection, the disease is usually more advanced when treatment is instituted. Nevertheless, the biologic behavior of MCT in patients with the MEN IIb syndrome is considered more aggressive than that of tumors occurring sporadically or in patients with MEN IIa disease.

The minimal treatment of MCT is total thyroidectomy.[50] In patients with tumors that occur sporadically, this allows for excision of any intraglandular lymphatic spread and careful immunohistopathologic study (C-cell hyperplasia) of the contralateral lobe. If no changes are found, the otherwise obligatory evaluation of other family members may be avoided, although this point is debatable because C-cell hyperplasia may not always be easily detected. Sporadic MCT usually presents as a solitary nodule in the upper half of the lateral lobe on either side. Metastatic lymph nodes may be detected, although the primary tumor is occult. The diagnosis is made most often by FNA cytology before operation.

The cellular characteristics of MCT are readily identified by FNA cytology. A basal serum calcitonin assay should be obtained along with a pentagastrin-stimulated determination of plasma calcitonin levels.[51] The level of calcitonin is of some predictive value in estimating the amount of tumor present and whether metastatic lymph nodes are likely to be involved. Even when the history is negative for MEN IIa and there are no physical findings of MEN IIb, plasma catecholamine levels should be determined, particularly if the patient is hypertensive before thyroidectomy. An added benefit of preoperative FNA examination and measurement of plasma calcitonin levels is that the patient can be informed preoperatively of the need for total thyroidectomy and possible neck dissection. Furthermore, a thallium scintiscan should be considered preoperatively because some MCT tumors and their metastases concentrate this substance sufficiently and can thus be readily visualized. When the primary tumor is well visualized with thallium, this agent can be used postoperatively to search for occult metastases if the calcitonin level remains or becomes elevated.

Most patients with sporadic disease have lymph node metastases when diagnosed, and a central compartment dissection sparing the parathyroid glands is indicated. If lateral lymph nodes are involved, a modified neck dissection should be done. Occasionally, capsular invasion of the lymph nodes with involvement of contiguous structures requires a formal radical dissection. Patients with the MEN II syndromes must be evaluated for possible pheochromocytomas before the treatment of MCT. Operations for pheochromocytoma should always take precedence over any neck procedures. Total thyroidectomy is essential in patients with MEN IIa disease. This must be a complete bilateral extracapsular excision because C cells are embryologically concentrated in the region of the posterior and middle to upper thyroid lobes.

Failure to remove all thyroid tissue inevitably leads to recurrent disease. For this reason, some surgeons routinely obtain a ^{131}I scintiscan postoperatively to determine whether the thyroidectomy is complete. If it is not complete, an ablative dose of ^{131}I is given to destroy any remaining thyroid tissue possibly containing C cells. At the time of exploration for the MEN IIa syndrome, only enlarged parathyroid glands should be excised in patients with hyperparathyroidism (usually only one or two). Although many MEN IIa patients have one or even two enlarged parathyroid glands, only about 20% of patients with this disease become hypercalcemic. Despite the fact that the normal-sized glands are usually hyperplastic microscopically, recurrence after less than a subtotal parathyroidectomy is extremely rare. On the other hand, near-total parathyroidectomy often results in permanent hypoparathyroidism and should be avoided. On the basis of the biologic behavior of hyperparathyroidism in this syndrome, total parathyroidectomy and autotransplantation have little value.[52]

If the MCT is discovered by calcitonin screening and no tumor is palpable, central compartment lymph nodes may be tumor free. Nevertheless, even normal-sized nodes should be sampled for frozen-section examination to determine whether a complete and thorough central compartment dissection is required. Lateral lymph node involvement is treated by modified neck dissection, which may be bilateral and performed in one or two stages.

Patients with the MEN IIb disease require total thyroidectomy as soon as the syndrome is recognized, preferably by the age of 2 years. In familial cases, the characteristic findings are sufficient to justify operation even without calcitonin testing. If the diagnosis is not made until adolescence or later, both central compartment involvement and lateral node involvement require neck dissection for definitive treatment.[53] Older patients may have liver or bone involvement, which prevents any curative operative attempts.

When the lateral lymph nodes are involved with MCT, a biochemical cure as determined by calcitonin testing is most unlikely. As a result, a formal radical neck dissection is considered by many to be futile. Nevertheless, this is appropriate if the procedure is required to excise all areas of gross disease because of lymph node invasion of local tissues. Controversy remains as to whether this should be done if no clinical disease is present after total thyroidectomy and central compartment dissection, and if the postoperative calcitonin level remains elevated.[54] A meticulous radical neck dissection is favored by some surgeons, and biochemical cure has been achieved in some of these patients.[55] Others advocate regional excision of any palpable nodes as they develop, or regional excision based on positive thallium scans when the disease is limited to the lateral neck or anterior mediastinum. One of the causes of failure of radical neck dissection based entirely on an elevated calcitonin level is that the MCT may already have spread hematogenously to involve the liver, lungs, or bone and may still be clinically occult. Because of this possibility, selective venous sampling for calcitonin may rule out systemic disease before any neck dissections are performed.[56]

Germline missense mutations within the coding region of the *ret* protooncogene were identified in patients with MEN IIa and familial medullary thyroid cancer in 1993.[57,58] Subsequent studies confirmed that point mutations in the *ret* protooncogene occurred in nearly all families studied and that specific point mutations could be related to the variable phenotypic expressions, such as hyperparathyroidism and pheochromocytomas, that occur in some families.[59] Discovery of the involved gene in MEN IIa and familial medullary thyroid cancer has subsequently allowed a DNA-based strategy for direct mutation detection and diagnosis. A variety of DNA-based techniques to identify *ret* mutations have been developed, including direct sequencing, single stranded conformational polymorphisms (SSCP), restriction enzyme analysis, and denaturing gradient gel electrophoresis (DGGE).[60-62] The latter technique has proved highly sensitive in detecting all nucleotide variations in *ret* exons 10 and 11, including the 35 potential MEN IIa and familial medullary thyroid cancer mutations. Because direct mutation detection is highly sensitive and specific, screening needs to be performed only once to establish genetic susceptibility and determine the possible need for a total thyroidectomy without other biochemical testing. This avoids repeated examinations and biochemical studies and the need to rely on an elevated calcitonin level before recommending

a total thyroidectomy. It is also considered prudent to obtain a mutational analysis in patients with sporadic MCT to rule out germline changes in the *ret* protooncogene. It is estimated that 10% to 20% of patients with MCT that is considered sporadic actually have MEN IIa. All family members at risk for having MEN IIa should have mutational analysis performed as early as possible, preferably before 5 years of age. For those with negative studies, no further testing is indicated. Prophylactic total thyroidectomy is recommended for patients shown to have proven mutations consistent with MEN IIa. This should be performed before the age of 10 years, when MCT begins to develop from C-cell hyperplasia in MEN IIa patients. Preoperative testing with pentagastrin and calcium stimulation for calcitonin elevation is no longer used in these patients. Postoperative biochemical testing for pheochromocytomas, hypercalcemia, and calcitonin remains useful. Sampling of central compartment lymph nodes probably should be performed, even in young patients without any palpable intrathyroidal tumor. However, it seems likely that most patients with prophylactic operations will not require central compartment lymph node dissection or parathyroidectomy, except when a clearly enlarged gland is encountered.[62] Our approach is to perform total thyroidectomy at 5 years of age in MEN IIa patients and before 2 years of age in MEN IIb patients because MCT develops in that group at a very early age. Mutational analysis is already revolutionizing the management of MEN IIa and familial medullary thyroid cancer families and eventually should have a major impact on the morbidity and mortality from the MCT component of these syndromes.

Hürthle Cell Carcinoma

Hürthle cell neoplasms are relatively uncommon and account for 3% to 5% of all thyroid carcinomas. These tumors were previously classified as a variant of follicular carcinoma but are now considered separately because of their different biologic behavior. These lesions do not have the ability to take up iodine or to synthesize thyroid hormones, characteristics that truly differentiate them from follicular carcinoma. Nevertheless, they are probably derived from follicular cells, because with immunohistochemical staining, thyroglobulin is often found. Although follicular carcinoma metastasizes to the lymph nodes infrequently, and does so only in patients with advanced disease, Hürthle cell carcinoma infiltrates lymphatics early and metastasizes to the lymph nodes in a significant number of cases. It also metastasizes hematogenously, most often to the bone and lung. With the use of FNA cytology, more patients with Hürthle cell neoplasms are encountered at an early stage. Because it is impossible to differentiate benign from malignant Hürthle cell neoplasms on the basis of cytology alone, any nodule composed entirely of Hürthle cells is considered an indication for lobectomy and more definitive evaluation of the neoplasm and its capsule.[23]

Controversy about the treatment of Hürthle cell neoplasms centers on the well-differentiated tumors without traditional microscopic findings of malignancy. A definitive diagnosis of Hürthle cell adenoma is not always possible because some lesions are associated with lymph node or distant metastases. In one study, total thyroidectomy was advised for true Hürthle cell neoplasms.[27] Many patients with Hürthle cell nodules as a reaction to Hashimoto disease and patients with colloid nodular goiter were excluded from consideration. Subsequently, excellent long-term results were reported after lobectomy and isthmectomy for Hürthle cell adenomas. Total thyroidectomy is unnecessary when a diagnosis of adenoma can be made. As pathologists became more interested in this particular tumor, it became apparent that a reliable diagnosis of adenoma can be made in many cases. The recommendation for lobectomy and isthmectomy alone rather than total thyroidectomy appears to be valid when a pathologist can find no evidence of capsular invasion or angioinvasion after extensive study of permanent sections. On the other hand, Hürthle cell carcinomas verified by standard histopathologic criteria are best treated by total thyroidectomy because of their propensity to spread by lymphatic as well as hematogenous dissemination.

There is no satisfactory adjunctive therapy for this neoplasm because it does not take up radioactive iodine, it is radioresistant, and it does not respond to chemotherapy. Local and regional recurrences are common after inadequate surgical therapy. Total thyroidectomy has markedly decreased the incidence of local recurrence. If the lymphatics are involved, a central compartment dissection on the ipsilateral side is indicated. If lateral nodes are involved, a modified radical neck dissection to clear all nodes is essential. Because of the high incidence of capsular invasion or angioinvasion with lesions greater than 4 cm, total thyroidectomy is advised, as it is for follicular neoplasms of that size. Permanent sections have shown that a minimum of 80% of neoplasms of this size show histopathologic evidence of invasion.

Anaplastic Carcinoma

Undifferentiated or anaplastic thyroid carcinoma has decreased in incidence during the past few decades and parallels the decrease in follicular carcinoma in iodine-rich geographic areas. Most anaplastic carcinomas of the spindle or giant cell type arise in differentiated thyroid cancers that have been present for a long period. Although most are follicular carcinomas, the tumor clearly can arise in patients with papillary carcinoma, Hürthle cell carcinoma, and, rarely, medullary carcinoma. The improved treatment of differentiated carcinoma may also be a factor in the decreasing incidence of this neoplasm. At one time in the midwestern United States, the incidence of anaplastic carcinoma was considerably higher, constituting about 20% of all thyroid carcinomas encountered. In recent decades, the incidence of anaplastic carcinoma has fallen to less than 2% of all thyroid carcinomas. It usually occurs in older patients with long-standing goiters. Careful microscopic evaluation of specimens removed and studied has shown that about 80% of these arose in differentiated carcinomas.

Pathologic classification based on ultrastructural evaluation and immunohistochemical staining has improved determination of the carcinoma's incidence. At one time, small cell carcinomas constituted nearly half of all anaplastic thyroid carcinomas, and most if not all of these were found to be lymphomas or MCT. Small cell thyroid carcinoma is now rare. Because of the much improved prognosis for thyroid lymphoma as compared with anaplastic carcinoma, it is important to make this differentiation.[20] A surgeon should never accept the diagnosis of small cell anaplastic carcinoma until all appropriate studies have been performed to rule out lymphoma or MCT.

It is fortunate that anaplastic carcinomas have become infrequent because the giant and spindle cell varieties are among the most rapidly lethal malignancies known. Most are too far advanced for adequate operative treatment when first diagnosed. The diagnosis can usually be made or suspected by physical findings and FNA cytology. In some patients without airway obstruction, no operative intervention is indicated because of poor prognosis. In other patients, establishing an airway by debulking and tracheostomy is all that can be done. If an early anaplastic thyroid cancer is confined within the thyroid, a total thyroidectomy offers the only possibility of cure, and such cases have been reported with long-term survival. Operative therapy has been followed by external radiation to the neck and mediastinum, but its value and necessity in these infrequent cases are unknown.

RADIOACTIVE IODINE

Radioactive iodine is used only in patients who have differentiated thyroid carcinomas. It is of no value in the treatment and follow-up of patients with Hürthle cell or medullary carcinomas. Many papillary carcinomas are capable of taking up radioactive iodine. Most papillary carcinomas in patients younger than 50 years of age do so, provided that the patient has had a total thyroidectomy and there is no normal thyroid tissue to compete for the ^{131}I. About 20% of all papillary carcinomas do not trap sufficient iodine for imaging. Most occur in patients older than 60 years of age. Patients with the tall cell variant of papillary carcinoma, insular carcinoma, or clear cell carcinoma do not produce an image with ^{131}I. Nearly all metastatic follicular carcinomas retain the ability to trap ^{131}I sufficiently for imaging and therapy. Even well-differentiated papillary and follicular carcinomas cannot compete successfully for ^{131}I with normal thyroid tissue. Unless all tissue has been removed or subsequently ablated with an initial dose of ^{131}I, many metastases cannot be detected.

^{131}I scintiscanning is performed 6 weeks after total thyroidectomy, during which time no thyroid hormone is administered. TSH levels are measured and are usually markedly elevated during the latter part of the 6-week interval. Two to 5 mCi of ^{131}I is administered for a standard metastatic thyroid scan.[14] If a localized uptake of radioactive iodine indicates metastatic disease, a therapeutic dose of ^{131}I is administered. When a ^{131}I scan is positive for lymph node disease, a decision must be made as to whether these metastases should be surgically excised or treated with ^{131}I. Surgical excision of lymph node metastases identified by ^{131}I scanning is generally recommended if they are palpable. In some patients, palpable lymph nodes appear within the latter 2 weeks as a result of TSH stimulation. This usually implies a good prognosis because these tumors depend greatly on TSH stimulation. When no lymph nodes are palpable and a ^{131}I scan shows disease in the lateral neck, a therapeutic dose, usually in the range of 150 to 180 mCi, is given. For patients with evidence of metastases in the lungs, the initial ^{131}I dose should be at least 180 mCi and more often 200 mCi, depending on the size of the individual.[63] In patients with no uptake outside of the central compartment, the use of ^{131}I is individualized. If there is uptake of up to 1% to 2% of radioactive iodine in the region of the ligament of Berry, this may represent a few thyroid cells left at the time of total thyroidectomy, and no therapeutic dose is administered. If the primary tumor was extensive and possibly shaved from the trachea or RLN, a therapeutic dose is administered to ensure that all malignant cells have been eradicated. Therapeutic doses of ^{131}I are administered only to those patients in whom residual carcinoma or metastatic carcinoma is strongly suspected.[64]

The therapeutic administration of ^{131}I requires 2 or 3 days of hospitalization, after which replacement doses of levothyroxine are administered. For patients who require no ^{131}I, levothyroxine is started immediately and given for life. The dose usually ranges from 150 to 200 $\mu g/d$. After a therapeutic dose of radioactive iodine, a follow-up scan is done within 1 year; if negative, no further ^{131}I is administered. If evidence of residual disease remains, a second dose, usually around 200 mCi, is administered. A follow-up scan is again obtained during the subsequent year. Rarely, three or four doses may be required for extensive metastatic disease in the lungs before the disease can be arrested. In some patients, particularly those with pulmonary metastases that are readily apparent on chest roentgenogram or CT scan, cure of the disease may not be possible with radioactive iodine. When the disease can be detected only by ^{131}I after a total thyroidectomy, eradication of all pulmonary metastases is often possible. This experience has emphasized the need for early detection and therapeutic [131]I. Pulmonary metastases can be effectively eradicated with timely treatment.[41,65,66] The most common site for distant metastatic follicular carcinoma is bone. Although these metastases are more resistant to ^{131}I therapy, the uptake can be intense, and effective palliation can be achieved for long periods. Most patients with follicular carcinomas treated with ^{131}I survive for 5 years or longer. Several patients with bone metastases have survived for up to 15 years after ^{131}I therapy. The overall mortality rate for distant metastatic disease in patients with differentiated cancer is about 75% after 5 years. With treatment consisting of total thyroidectomy and ^{131}I, this has been reduced to 25%.[65]

The long-term survival rate of patients in the good-risk category with differentiated carcinomas of the thyroid has been 90% or higher. Before the use of total thyroidectomy and ^{131}I, the overall mortality rate for all papillary carcinomas was about 12% at the end of 10 years. This has improved to a 98% survival rate during the past two decades. The 10-year survival rate for follicular carcinoma, which formerly was about 70%, has also improved to over 90%.[27,39,47] Nevertheless, patients with angioinvasive follicular carcinoma, particularly with distant metastases, are rarely, if ever, cured with therapy; they usually die from their disease. Patients with variants of papillary carcinoma, such as tall cell carcinoma, have a mortality rate of 30% to 40% at the end of 5 years, as do some patients with extensive papillary carcinoma incapable of concentrating radioactive iodine.

REFERENCES

1. Hollinshead WH. Visceral structures of the neck. In: Anatomy for surgeons, vol 1. The head and neck. New York, Harper & Row, 1968:567.
2. Thompson NW, Olsen WR, Hoffman GL. The continuing development of the technique of thyroidectomy. Surgery 1973;73:913.
3. Bergman DA. Thyroid physiology and immunology. Otolaryngol Clin North Am 1990;23:231.
4. Tong W. Thyroid hormone synthesis and releasing. In: Werner SC, Ingbar SH, eds. The thyroid: a fundamental and clinical text, ed 3. New York, Harper & Row, 1971:24.
5. Girelli ME, Busuardo B, Amerio R, et al. Serum thyroglobulin levels in patients with well-differentiated thyroid cancer during suppressive therapy: study on 429 patients. Eur J Nucl Med 1985;10:252.
6. Van Herle AJ, Uller RP. Elevated serum thyroglobulin: a marker of metastases in differentiated thyroid carcinoma. J Clin Invest 1975;56:272.
7. Harney RD, Matheson NA, Grabowski PS, Rogers AB. Measurement of serum thyroglobulin is of value in detecting tumor recurrence following treatment of differentiated thyroid carcinoma by lobectomy. Br J Surg 1990;77:324.
8. Oppenheimer J. Thyroid action at the nuclear level. Ann Intern Med 1985;102:374.
9. Evans R. The steroid and thyroid hormone receptor superfamily. Science 1988;240:889.
10. Sterling K. Thyroid hormone action at the cell level. N Engl J Med 1979;300:117.
11. Spencer CA, LoPresti JS, Patel A, et al. Applications of a new chemiluminometric TSH assay to subnormal measurement. J Clin Endocrinol Metab 1990;70:453.
12. Spencer CA, Nicoloff JT. Serum TSH measurement: a 1990 status report. Thyroid Today 1990;13:1.
13. Ramanna L, Waxman AD, Brachman MB, et al. Correlation of thyroglobulin measurements and radioiodine scans in the follow-up of patients with differentiated thyroid cancer. Cancer 1985;55:1525.
14. Beierwaltes WH. The treatment of thyroid carcinoma with radioactive iodine. Semin Nucl Med 1978;8:79.
15. Lennquist S, Smeds S. The hypermetabolic syndrome: hyperthyroidism. In: Friesen SR, Thompson NW, eds. Surgical endocrinology: clinical syndromes, ed 2. Philadelphia, JB Lippincott, 1990:127.
16. Wartofsky L, Glinoer D, Solomon B, et al. Differences and similarities in the diagnosis and treatment of Graves disease in Europe, Japan and the United States. Thyroid 1991;1:129.
17. Lazarus JH, Wade SH. The role of surgery in the management of thyrotoxicosis. In: Johnston I, Thompson NW, eds. Endocrine surgery. London, Butterworths, 1983:1.
18. Falk SA. The management of hyperthyroidism, a surgeon's perspective. Otolaryngol Clin North Am 1990;23:361.
19. Perzik SL. Total thyroidectomy in the management of Graves disease: a review of 282 cases. Am J Surg 1976;132:480.
20. Lloyd RV. The thyroid. In: Lloyd R, ed. Endocrine pathology. New York, Springer-Verlag, 1990:37.
21. Hoffman GL, Thompson NW, Heffron C. The solitary thyroid nodule: a reassessment. Arch Surg 1972;105:379.
22. Miller JM, Hamburger JI, Sini S. Diagnosis of thyroid nodules. JAMA 1979;241:481.
23. Lowhagen T, Granberg PO, Lundell G. Aspiration biopsy cytology (ABC) in nodules of the thyroid gland suspected to be malignant. Surg Clin North Am 1979;59:3.
24. Cheung PSY, Lee JMH, Boey JH. Thyroxine suppressive therapy of benign solitary thyroid nodules: a perspective study. World J Surg 1989;13:818.
25. Spiliotis JD, Chalmoukis A, Androulakis JA, et al. Thyroxine suppressive therapy of benign solitary thyroid nodules: some problems. World J Surg 1991;15:304.
26. Gharib H, James EM, Charbeueau JW, et al. Suppressive therapy with levothyroxine for solitary thyroid nodules: a double-blind controlled clinical study. N Engl J Med 1987;317:70.
27. Thompson NW, Nishiyama RH, Harness JK. Thyroid carcinoma: current controversies. Curr Probl Surg 1978;15:1.
28. Rossi RL, Cady B, Silverman ML, et al. Current results of conservative surgery for differentiated thyroid carcinoma. World J Surg 1986;10:612.
29. Thompson NW. The resection therapy of carcinoma of the thyroid. Surg Rounds 1984:100.
30. Cady B, Rossi R. An expanded view of risk-group definition in undifferentiated thyroid carcinoma. Surgery 1988;104:947.
31. Cady B, Sedgwick CE, Meissner WA, et al. Risk factor analysis in differentiated thyroid cancer. Cancer 1979;43:811.
32. Hay ID. Prognostic factors in thyroid carcinoma. Thyroid Today 1989;12:1.
33. Byar DP, Green SB, Sor P, et al. A prognostic index for thyroid carcinoma: a study of the EORTC Thyroid Cancer Cooperative Group. Eur J Cancer 1979;15:1033.
34. Cohn K, Backdahl M, Forsslund BM, et al. Prognostic value of nuclear DNA content in papillary thyroid carcinoma. World J Surg 1988;12:559.
35. McConahey WM, Hay ID, Woolner LB, et al. Papillary thyroid cancer treated at the Mayo Clinic through 1970: initial manifestations, pathologic findings, therapy and outcome. Mayo Clin Proc 1986;61:978.
36. Clark OH. Total thyroidectomy: the treatment of choice for patients with differentiated thyroid cancer. Ann Surg 1982;196:361.
37. Lennquist S. Surgical strategy in thyroid carcinoma: a clinical review. Acta Chir Scand 1986;152:321.
38. Lennquist S, Persliden J, Smeds S. The value of intraoperative scintigraphy as a routine procedure in thyroid carcinoma. World J Surg 1988;12:586.
39. Mazzaferri LE, Young RL. Papillary thyroid carcinoma: a 10 year follow-up report of the impact of therapy in 567 patients. Am J Med 1981;70:511.

40. Reeve TS, Delbridge L. Thyroid cancers of follicular cell origin: the place of radical or limited surgery. Prog Surg 1988; 19:113.

41. Casare D, Zorat PL, Bushnardo B, Girelli ME. Pulmonary metastases from differentiated thyroid carcinoma detected only by radionuclide imaging. Br J Radiol 1981;54:362.

42. Tollefson HR, DeCosse JJ. Papillary carcinoma of the thyroid: recurrence in the thyroid gland after initial surgical treatment. Am J Surg 1963;106:728.

43. Attie JN, Khafif RA. Preservation of parathyroid glands during total thyroidectomy. Am J Surg 1975;130:399.

44. Calabro S, Auguste LJ, Attie JN. Morbidity of completion thyroidectomy for initially misdiagnosed thyroid carcinoma. Head Neck Surg 1988;10:235.

45. Harness JK, Thompson NW, McLeod MK, Eckhauser FE, Lloyd RV. Follicular carcinoma of the thyroid gland: trends and treatment. Surgery 1984;96:972.

46. Donohue JH, Goldfien SD, Miller TR, et al. Do the prognoses of papillary and follicular thyroid carcinoma differ? Am J Surg 1984;148:168.

47. Young RL, Mazzaferri EL, Rahea J, et al. Pure follicular thyroid cancer: impact of treatment in 214 patients. J Nucl Med 1980;21:733.

48. Thompson NW, Nishiyama RH, Harness JK. Thyroid carcinoma: current controversies. Curr Probl Surg 1978;15:1.

49. Yamashita T, Fujimoto Y, Kodama T, et al. When is total thyroidectomy indicated as a treatment of follicular carcinoma? World J Surg 1988;12:539.

50. Thompson NW. Surgery for medullary thyroid carcinoma. In: Fee WE Jr, Goepfert H, Johns ME, Strong EW, Ward PH, eds. Head and neck cancer. Philadelphia, BC Decker, 1990:2.

51. Wells SA, Bayin SB, Linehan WM, et al. Provocative agents and the diagnosis of medullary carcinoma of the thyroid gland. Ann Surg 1978;188:139.

52. Allo MD, Thompson NW. Hyperparathyroidism as a part of the MEN I and MEN II syndromes. In: Kaplan EL, ed. Surgery of the thyroid and parathyroid glands: clinical surgery international. New York, Churchill Livingstone, 1983:177.

53. Norton JA, Froome LC, Farrell RE, Wells SA Jr. Multiple endocrine neoplasia type IIb. Surg Clin North Am 1979;59:109.

54. Block MA, Jackson CE, Tashijian AH. Management of occult medullary carcinoma of the thyroid evidenced only by serum calcitonin level elevations after apparently adequate neck operations. Arch Surg 1987;113:368.

55. Tisell LE, Hansson G, Jansson S, Salander H. Reoperation in the treatment of asymptomatic metastasizing medullary carcinoma of the thyroid. Surgery 1986;99:60.

56. Mrad B, Gardet P, Roche A, et al. Value of venous catheterization and calcitonin studies in the treatment and management of clinically inapparent medullary thyroid carcinoma. Cancer 1989;63:133.

57. Mulligan LM, Kwok JB, Healey CS, et al. Germ-line mutations of the ret proto-oncogene in multiple endocrine neoplasia type 2a. Nature 1993;363:458.

58. Doris-Keller H, Dou S, Chi D, et al. Mutations in the ret proto-oncogene are associated with MEN IIa and FMTC. Hum Mol Genet 1993;7:851.

59. Mulligan LM, Eng C, Healey CS, et al. Specific mutations of the ret proto-oncogene are related to disease phenotype in MEN IIa and FMTC. Nat Genet 1994;6:70.

60. Wells SA, Chi DD, Toshima K, et al. Predictive DNA testing and prophylactic thyroidectomy in patients at risk for multiple endocrine neoplasia type IIa. Ann Surg 1994;220:237.

61. Decker RA, Peacock ML, Borst MJ, et al: Progress in genetic screening of multiple endocrine neoplasia type IIa: is calcitonin testing obsolete? Surgery 1995;118:256.

62. Decker DA, Geiger JD, Cox CE, et al. Prophylactic surgery for MEN IIa following genetic diagnosis: is parathyroid transplantation indicated? World J Surg 1996 (in press).

63. Beierwaltes WH, Nishiyama RH, Thompson NW. Survival time and cure in papillary and follicular thyroid carcinoma with distant metastases. J Nucl Med 1982;23:561.

64. Goolden AWG. The indication for ablating normal thyroid tissue with ^{131}I in differentiated thyroid carcinoma. Clin Endocrinol 1985;23:81.

65. Harness JK, Thompson NW, Sisson JC, Beierwaltes WH. Differentiated thyroid carcinoma: treatment of distant metastases. Arch Surg 1974;108:410.

66. Leeper RD. The effect of ^{131}I therapy on survival in patients with metastatic papillary or follicular thyroid carcinoma. J Clin Endocrinol Metab 1973;6:1143.

SURGERY: SCIENTIFIC PRINCIPLES AND PRACTICE, Second Edition, edited by Lazar J. Greenfield, Michael W. Mulholland, Keith T. Oldham, Gerald B. Zelenock, and Keith D. Lillemoe. Lippincott–Raven Publishers, Philadelphia, © 1997.

CHAPTER 57

PARATHYROID GLANDS

GERARD M. DOHERTY AND SAMUEL A. WELLS, JR

ANATOMY

Typically, four parathyroid glands exist—two superior and two inferior[1] (Fig. 57-1). The normal parathyroids are flat, ovoid, and red-brown to yellow. They measure 5 to 7 mm × 3 to 4 mm × 0.5 to 2 mm and weigh between 30 and 50 mg each. The lower glands are usually larger than the upper. The superior glands are most often embedded in the fat on the posterior surface of the upper thyroid lobe near the site where the recurrent laryngeal nerve enters the larynx. The inferior glands are usually more ventral and lie close to or within that portion of the thymus gland that extends from the inferior pole of the thyroid gland into the chest. Although this anatomy is fairly consistent, substantial variations from the norm can occur, and it is essential that the surgeon have a thorough understanding of these anatomic variations before beginning a neck exploration for hyperparathyroidism.

Variations in parathyroid anatomy are primarily caused by differences in patterns of embryogenesis. During the fourth and fifth weeks of fetal development, the embryo develops a series of four pharyngeal pouches (Fig. 57-2). The superior parathyroid actually arises from the fourth pharyngeal pouch in conjunction with the lateral thyroid, and the inferior gland arises from the third pouch along with the thymus. The derivatives of each pouch then migrate together so that the superior parathyroid usually remains in close association with the upper pole of the thyroid, although it may occasionally be loosely attached by a long vascular pedicle, migrating caudally along the esophagus into the posterior mediastinum. Occasionally, a gland may be totally embedded in the thyroid parenchyma. The inferior parathyroid descends with the thymus, but this migration may be extremely variable. Inferior glands can be found anywhere from the pharynx to the mediastinum. Regardless of their location, they usually adhere to the thymus or are within the thyrothymic ligament. Supernumerary glands can be identified in up to 15% of patients, most often in association with the thymus. Autopsy studies suggest that four parathyroid glands are virtually always present.

The arterial supply to both the superior and inferior parathyroids is usually from the inferior thyroid artery, although it may arise from the superior thyroid or thyroid ima arteries or from the rich anastomosis of vessels supplying the larynx, trachea, and esophagus. It has been suggested that a mediastinal parathyroid gland that descended during embryonic development usually receives its blood supply from either the internal mammary artery

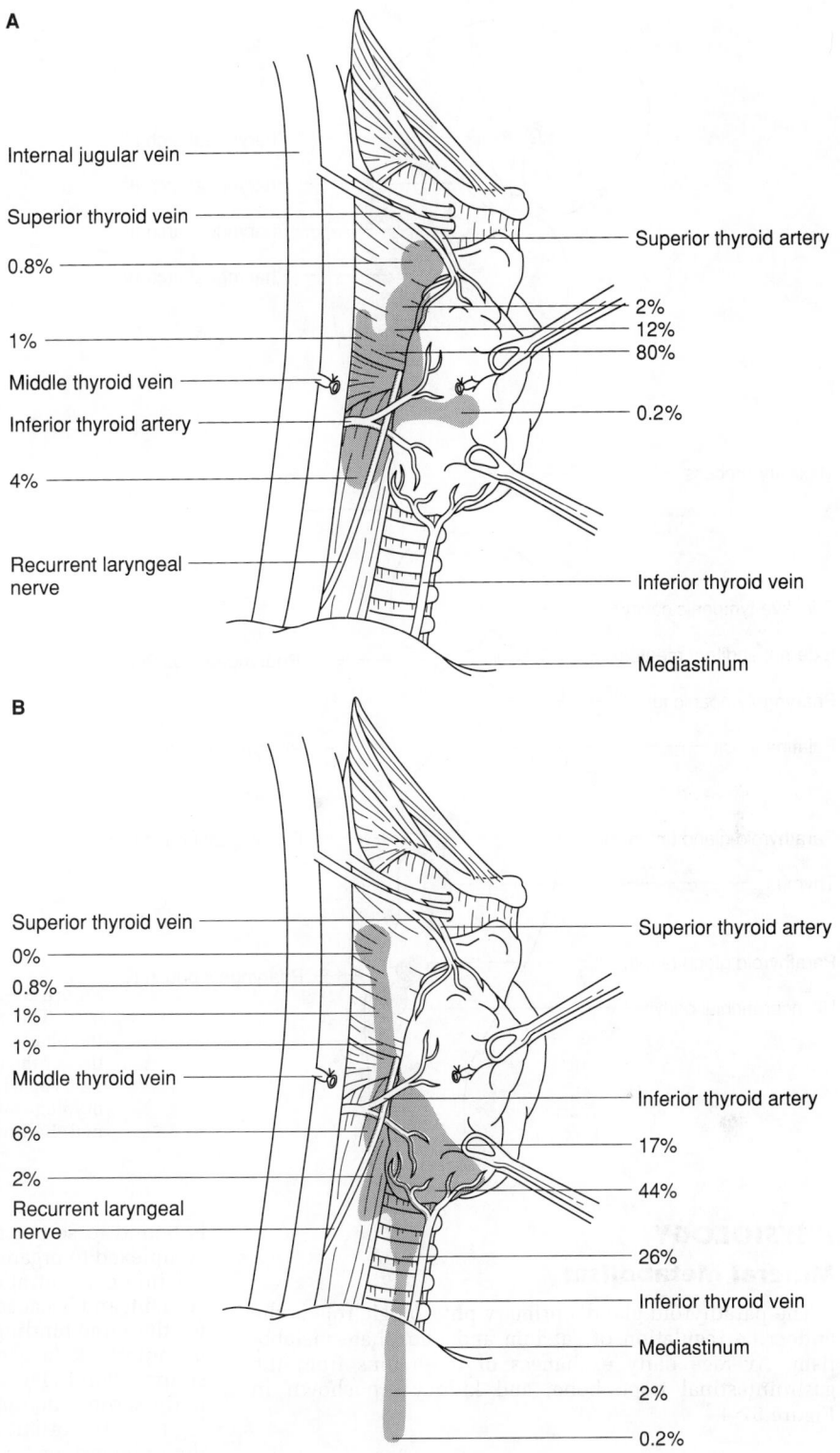

A

Internal jugular vein

Superior thyroid vein

0.8%

1%

Middle thyroid vein

Inferior thyroid artery

4%

Recurrent laryngeal
nerve

Superior thyroid artery

2%
12%
80%

0.2%

Inferior thyroid vein

Mediastinum

B

Superior thyroid vein
0%
0.8%
1%
1%
Middle thyroid vein

6%
2%
Recurrent laryngeal
nerve

Superior thyroid artery

Inferior thyroid artery

17%

44%

26%

Inferior thyroid vein

Mediastinum

2%

0.2%

Figure 57-1. Location of the superior (*A*) and inferior (*B*) parathyroid glands from 503 autopsy studies. The more common locations are indicated by the shaded areas. The numbers represent the percentage of glands found at each location. Typically, the glands were found posterolateral to the thyroid and above or below the junction of the inferior thyroid artery with the recurrent laryngeal nerve. (After Akerstrom G, Malmaers J, Bergstrom R. Surgical anatomy of human parathyroid glands. Surgery 1984;95:14)

or small arteries within the thymus. In adults, however, an enlarged parathyroid gland that migrates into the mediastinum usually carries with it the corresponding branch of the inferior thyroid artery. The inferior, middle, and superior thyroid veins, which drain the parathyroid glands, empty into the internal jugular vein or the innominate vein.

Histologically, the normal adult parathyroid is about half parenchyma and half stroma, including fat cells (Fig. 57-3). In children, the gland is almost entirely composed of parenchymal chief cells. Beginning at puberty, adipocytes appear, and with age, they occupy an increasing proportion of the gland. Also with increasing age, acidophilic, mitochondria-rich oxyphil cells are present in increasing numbers and are intermixed with the glycogen-laden, polygonal, water-clear cells. The functional significance of the various cell types remains unclear, although the water-clear cells and oxyphil cells are probably derived from the chief cell and secrete parathyroid hormone (PTH).

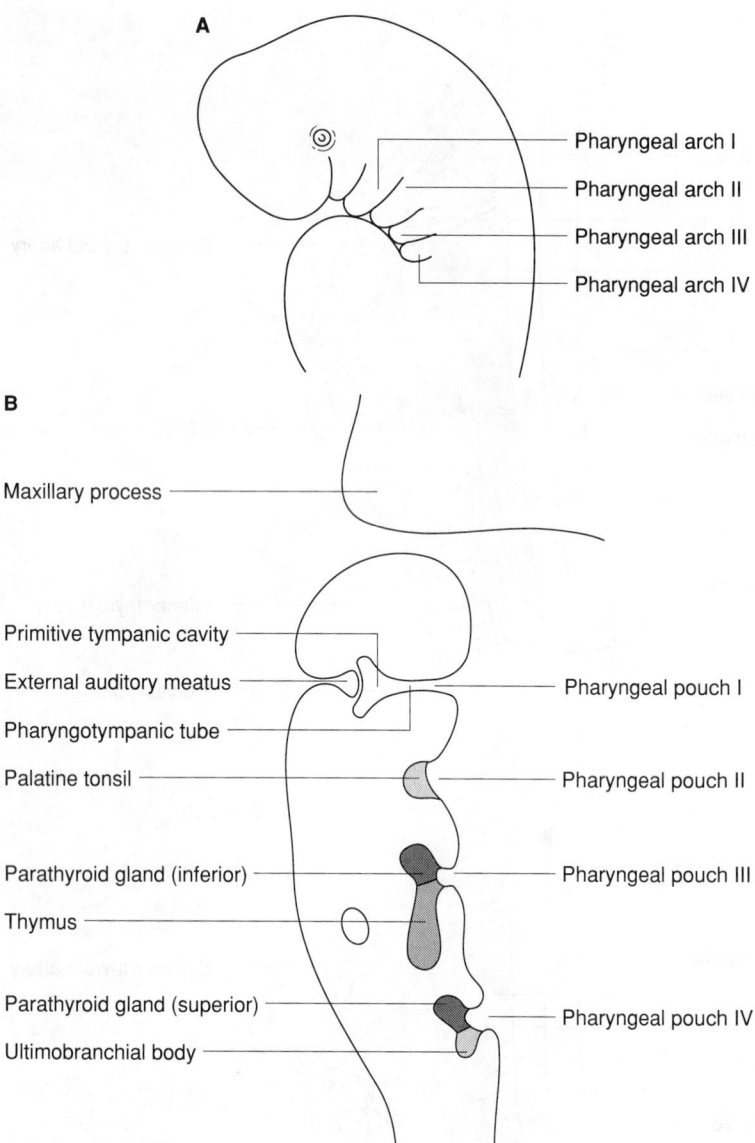

A

- Pharyngeal arch I
- Pharyngeal arch II
- Pharyngeal arch III
- Pharyngeal arch IV

B

Maxillary process

Primitive tympanic cavity

External auditory meatus — Pharyngeal pouch I

Pharyngotympanic tube

Palatine tonsil — Pharyngeal pouch II

Parathyroid gland (inferior) — Pharyngeal pouch III

Thymus

Parathyroid gland (superior) — Pharyngeal pouch IV

Ultimobranchial body

Figure 57-2. (*A*) Pharyngeal arches in a 5-week embryo. The corresponding pouches extend from within the pharynx into each arch. (*B*) Schematic representation of the differentiating epithelium of the respective pharyngeal pouches. (After Langman J. Medical embryology and human development: normal and abnormal. Baltimore, Williams & Wilkins, 1975:262)

PHYSIOLOGY

Mineral Metabolism

The parathyroid gland's primary physiologic role is the endocrine regulation of calcium and phosphate metabolism. Average daily exchanges of these ions from the gastrointestinal tract, bone, and kidney are shown in Figure 57-4.

Calcium

Calcium ion plays a critical role in all biologic systems. It participates in enzymatic reactions and is a mediator in hormone metabolism. Calcium is intimately involved in the physiology of neurotransmission, muscle contraction, and blood coagulation. It is the major cation in bone and teeth. It represents about 2% of the average body weight, and almost all calcium is contained in the skeleton. The normal range of serum calcium is 9 to 10.5 mg/dL (4.5 to 5.2 mEq/L), and daily variation in the normal person is generally less than 10%. About half of the total serum calcium is in an ionized, biologically active form; 40%

is bound to serum protein, mainly albumin; and 10% is complexed to organic ions such as citrate. The total serum calcium concentration is a function of the serum protein content, and because hydrogen ion competes with calcium for the same binding sites on albumin, the body fluid pH is important. In general, for every 1-g/dL change in the serum albumin level, there is a direct, 0.8-mg/dL alteration in the serum calcium concentration. Almost all the physiologically important activity of calcium is represented by the unbound, or free, fraction.

Calcium is absorbed in its inorganic form from the duodenum and proximal jejunum. Percentage absorption is precisely regulated based on body calcium status. The calcium in the extracellular fluid is constantly being exchanged with that in the intracellular fluid, the exchangeable bone, and the glomerular filtrate. Calcium reabsorption by the kidney is closely related to that of sodium, and about 99% of the filtered load is reabsorbed under normal conditions.

Phosphate

Phosphate anion is also an integral component of most biologic systems. It is critical to the pathways of glycolysis and is the functional group for a number of high-energy

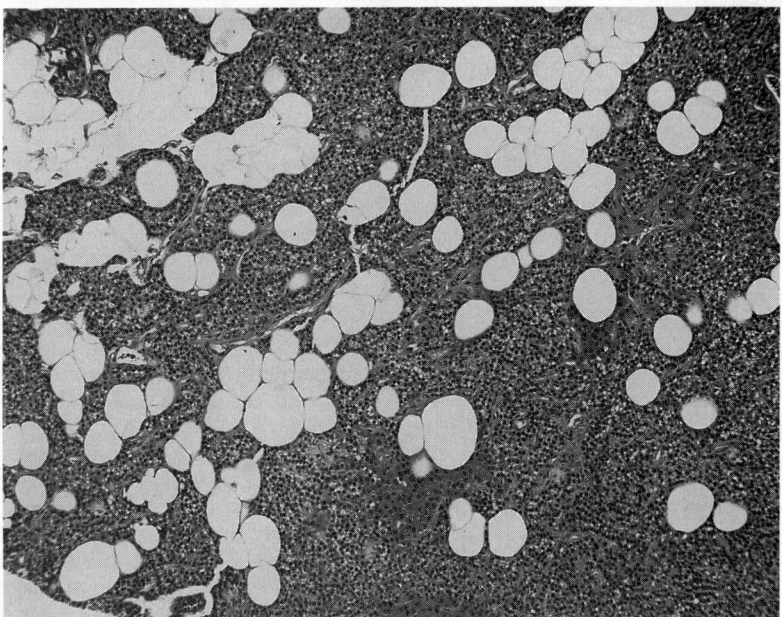

Figure 57-3. A normal adult parathyroid is composed of about half parenchyma and half fat (×150).

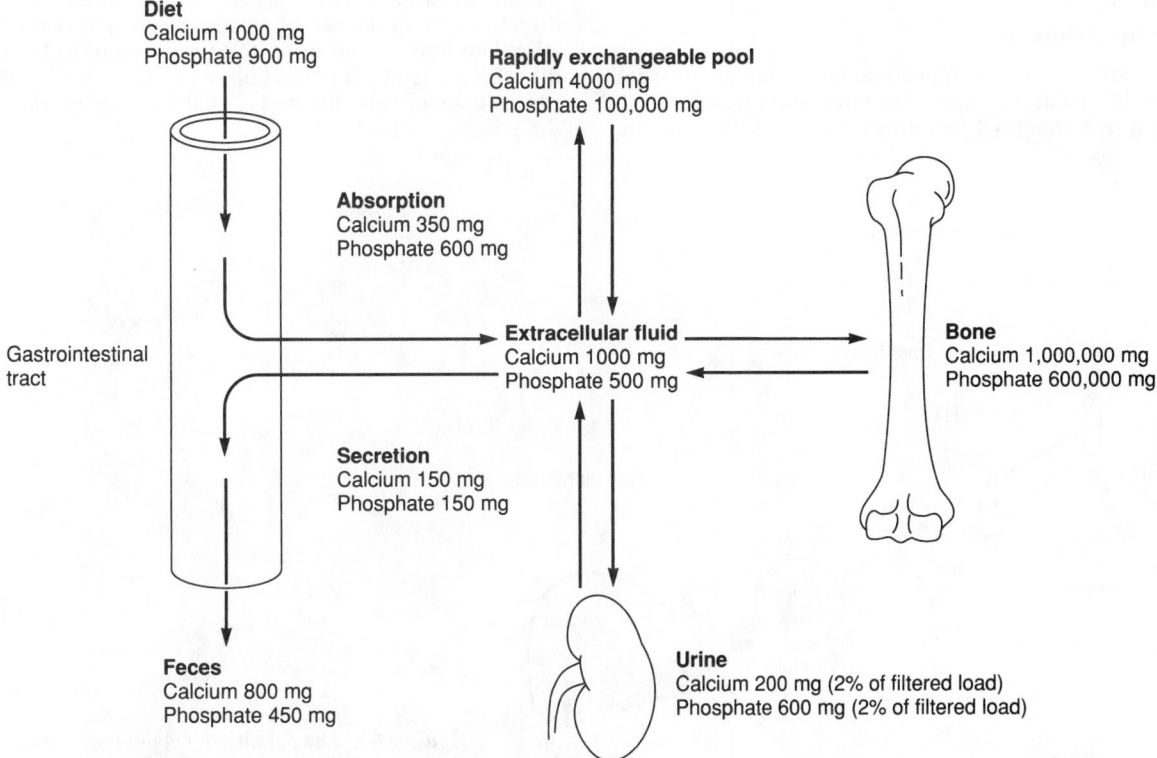

Figure 57-4. Average daily calcium and phosphate turnover in humans. (After Aurbach GD, Marx SJ, Spiegel AM, et al: Parathyroid hormone, calcitonin, and the calciferols. In: Textbook of endocrinology, ed 7. Philadelphia, WB Saunders, 1985:1144)

Table 57-1. HORMONAL REGULATION OF CALCIUM AND PHOSPHATE METABOLISM

	Parathyroid Hormone	Vitamin D	Calcitonin
Gastrointestinal tract	No direct effect	Stimulates calcium and phosphate absorption	No direct effect
Skeleton	Stimulates calcium and phosphate resorption	Stimulates calcium and phosphate transport	Inhibits calcium and phosphate resorption
Kidneys	Stimulates calcium resorption Inhibits phosphate resorption	No direct effect	Inhibits calcium and phosphate resorption

transfer compounds, including adenosine triphosphate. It is also the major anion in crystalline bone. Normal plasma phosphate ranges from 2.5 to 4.3 mg/dL, and the level varies inversely with that of the serum calcium. The relation is such that the product of plasma calcium and phosphate is constant and ranges between 30 and 40 mg/dL. When it increases above this level, there is a potential for calcium phosphate complex precipitation in body tissues.

In contrast to calcium, the percentage of phosphate absorbed from the diet is relatively constant, and excretion usually provides the major mechanisms for regulating phosphate balance (see Fig. 57-4). Also unlike calcium, the readily exchangeable soft tissue stores of phosphate, such as those in muscle, are large.

Regulation of Calcium and Phosphate Metabolism

The maintenance of calcium and phosphate homeostasis depends on major contributions from three organ systems—the gastrointestinal tract, the skeleton, and the kidneys—with minor contributions from the skin and liver.[2] The primary hormonal regulators of this metabolism are PTH, vitamin D, and calcitonin. The actions of each of these hormones on the organs are summarized in Table 57-1.

Parathyroid Hormone

Parathyroid hormone appears to be the single most important hormonal regulator of calcium and phosphate metabolism in humans. It has direct effects on the skeleton and kidney and indirect effects on the intestine, mediated through vitamin D. In target tissues, PTH binds first to membrane receptors, activating adenyl cyclase to generate cyclic adenosine monophosphate (cAMP), which in turn regulates other intracellular enzymes.

In bone, the effects of PTH are complex, stimulating both resorption and new bone formation. In its simplest form, however, sustained elevations stimulate osteoclasts and inhibit osteoblasts. Osteocytes, in the matrix of cortical bone, may also act to reabsorb matrix in response to PTH, a process referred to as *osteocytic osteolysis*. Calcium and phosphate mobilization in response to PTH occurs in two phases. Initially, mineral is mobilized from areas of rapid equilibrium. This is followed by a more sustained release mediated by newly synthesized lysosomal and hydrolytic enzymes. In the kidney, PTH increases the reabsorption of extracellular fluid calcium at any given concentration, although excess secretion, because of the hypercalcemia, increases the net daily amount of urinary calcium excretion. Reabsorption in the proximal tubule and Henle loop is linked with sodium transport such that factors that alter sodium transport concomitantly alter calcium reabsorption. In contrast, reabsorption in the distal nephron is independent of sodium and directly influenced by PTH. PTH also increases phosphate excretion. This is accompanied by enhanced bicarbonate secretion. PTH probably has no direct effects on the gastrointestinal tract, although it does stimulate hydroxylation of 25-hydroxyvitamin D to 1,25-dihydroxyvitamin D in the kidney. This activated metabolite enhances calcium and phosphate absorption from the gut.

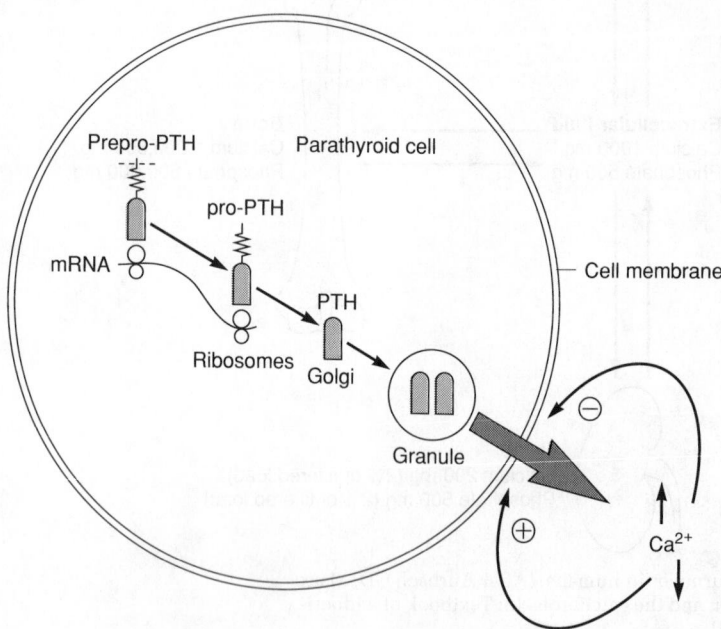

Figure 57-5. The parathyroid gland produces a precursor (prepro-PTH) that is sequentially cleaved to pro-PTH and PTH. PTH secretion is controlled by the extracellular fluid volume. (After Klee GG, Kao PC, Heath H. Hypercalcemia. Endocrinol Metab Clin North Am 1988;17)

PTH is synthesized initially as a precursor, prepropara-thyroid hormone, that is sequentially cleaved in the para-thyroid gland to proparathyroid hormone and then to PTH (Fig. 57-5). Secretion of this 84–amino acid molecule is controlled by a negative feedback loop with extracellular fluid calcium. Most PTH is secreted in this form and then cleaved in the liver into N- and C-terminal fragments. The N terminus contains most of the biologic activity and is rapidly degraded by the liver, whereas the inactive C termi-nus is slowly metabolized by the kidney.

Vitamin D

Vitamin D has two major sites of action. It increases intestinal absorption of calcium and phosphate. In addi-tion, in the skeleton, it promotes mineralization and en-hances PTH-mediated mobilization of calcium and phos-phate. It probably has no direct effect on the kidney.

Vitamin D_3, or cholecalciferol, is produced normally by the action of sunlight on 7-dehydrocholesterol in the skin (Fig. 57-6). It is then hydroxylated in the liver (25 position) and kidney (1 position) to form the active 1,25-dihydroxyvitamin D_3 (calcitriol). Vitamin D_2 is normally present in yeast and fungi but not in humans. It represents the major pharmacologic source of vitamin D. Pharmaceu-tical preparations include vitamin D_2 (ergocalciferol), 25-hydroxycholecalciferol (calcifediol), and 1,25-dihydroxy-cholecalciferol (calcitriol). 1-Hydroxycholecalciferol and dihydrotachysterol are synthetic preparations that re-quire only 25-hydroxylation for activity and so are useful for supplementation in renal failure patients who lack the 1-hydroxylase.

Calcitonin

Calcitonin is a 32–amino acid protein produced by the parafollicular C (calcitonin) cells of the thyroid. These C cells are embryologically derived from the neural crest and, in lower animals, are found in the ultimobranchial bodies, which are glandular structures derived from the lowest branchial pouch. In humans, these structures are incorporated into the superior and lateral aspects of the thyroid lobes.

Total thyroidectomy, with removal of all the C cells, is well tolerated, and it has been concluded that calcitonin is not essential for the normal control of calcium metabo-lism in adult humans. It does inhibit bone resorption and can produce hypocalcemia in experimental animals. It also increases urinary calcium and phosphate excretion. These effects appear to be mediated primarily through cyclic adenosine monophosphate. Several secretogogues for cal-citonin have been identified, including catecholamines, gastrin, and cholecystokinin, but the most potent appear to be calcium and pentagastrin.

Mineral Homeostasis

Under normal conditions, serum calcium and phosphate levels vary minimally over the course of the day. Regula-tion occurs primarily through PTH but also through a se-ries of feedback loops involving vitamin D and calcitonin (Fig. 57-7). A fall in serum ionized calcium increases PTH secretion and stimulates production of 1,25-$(OH)_2D_3$. Con-

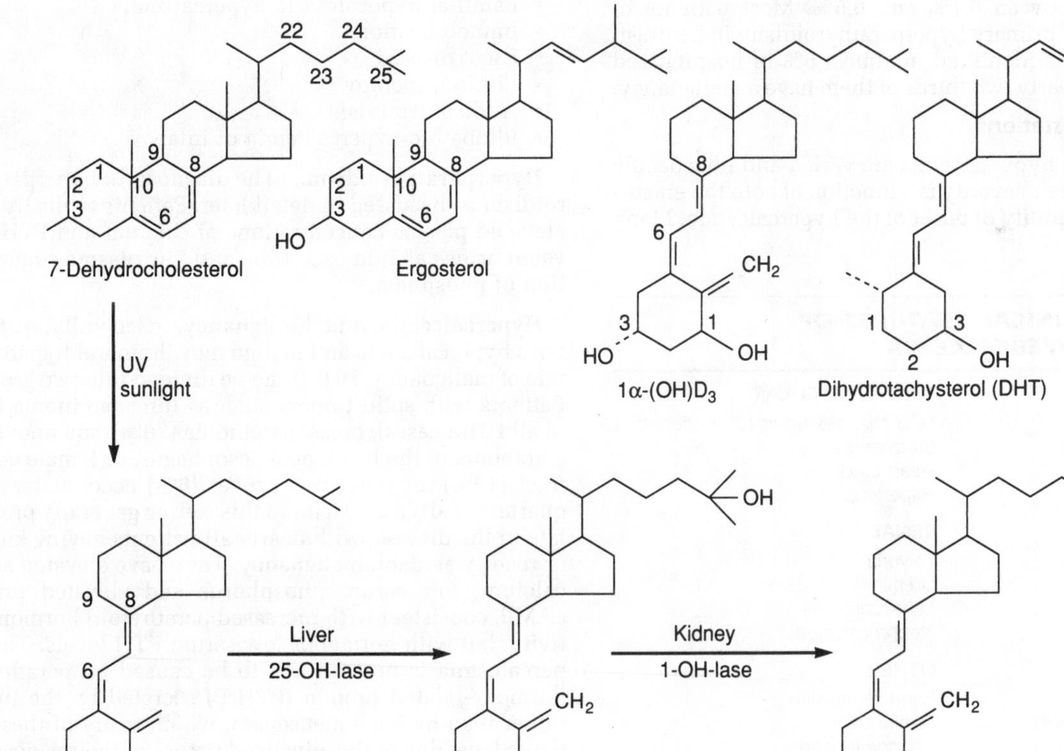

Figure 57-6. Synthesis of vitamin D_3. Ergosterol, $1\alpha\gamma$-(OH)D_3, and dihydrotachysterol are syn-thetic vitamin D preparations. (After Klee GG, Kao PC, Heath H. Hypercalcemia. Endocrinol Metab Clin North Am 1988;17:573)

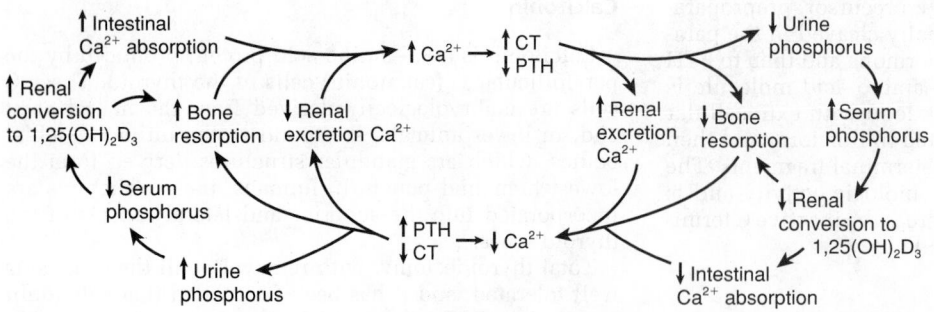

Figure 57-7. Feedback loops involved in the regulation of serum calcium and phosphorus. PTH, parathyroid hormone; CT, calcitonin.

versely, increases in serum calcium inhibit PTH secretion and the formation of active calciferol.

PATHOPHYSIOLOGY

Diseases of the parathyroid glands present almost exclusively as disorders of calcium metabolism. Hypercalcemia is the most common manifestation, and in the patient who presents with an elevated serum calcium level, the differential diagnosis can often be complex. A thorough understanding of both hypercalcemia and hypocalcemia is essential for the successful treatment of patients undergoing parathyroid surgery. Primary disorders of plasma phosphate are not usually related to surgical disease and are not discussed in detail here.

Hypercalcemia

Hypercalcemia is a relatively common clinical problem.[3] In the general population and in hospital outpatients, the incidence is between 0.1% and 0.5%. Most patients in this group have primary hyperparathyroidism. In contrast, hypercalcemia is identified in almost 5% of hospitalized patients, and nearly two thirds of them have a malignancy.

Clinical Manifestations

Symptoms of hypercalcemia are varied and nonspecific (Table 57-2). Their severity is a function of both the magnitude and the rapidity of onset of the hypercalcemia. Many of the manifestations are subtle and are evident only in retrospect, after the patient has been successfully treated for the cause of the elevated calcium. Specific symptoms and diagnostic tests are addressed in more detail in the discussion of hyperparathyroidism.

Differential Diagnosis

Although the diagnosis of primary hyperparathyroidism can, after appropriate investigation, be established with confidence in most patients, all causes of hypercalcemia must be considered and excluded. The multiple causes of hypercalcemia include the following:

- Hyperparathyroidism
- Malignancy
- Vitamin A or D intoxication
- Thiazide diuretics
- Hyperthyroidism
- Milk–alkali syndrome
- Sarcoidosis and other granulomatous diseases
- Familial hypocalciuric hypercalcemia
- Immobilization
- Paget disease
- Lithium therapy
- Addisonian crisis
- Idiopathic hypercalcemia of infancy

Hyperparathyroidism. The diagnosis of hyperparathyroidism is discussed in detail later. Patients typically have elevated plasma concentrations of calcium and PTH, elevated urine calcium excretion, and low plasma concentration of phosphate.

Hypercalcemia and Malignancy. Generally, patients with hypercalcemia and malignancy (humoral hypercalcemia of malignancy, HHM) can be divided into two groups.[4] Patients with solid tumors such as lung carcinoma (25% of all HHM cases), breast carcinoma (20%), squamous cell carcinoma of the head, neck, esophagus, or female genital tract (19%), or renal cell cancer (8%) account for three quarters of all cases. HHM in this setting generally presents late in the disease, with nearly all patients having known, or readily evident, malignancy. They have elevated serum calcium, low serum phosphorus and elevated urinary cAMP, consistent with increased parathyroid hormone activity, but with normal or low serum PTH levels. The hypercalcemia is now known to be caused by parathyroid hormone-related protein (PTHrP) secreted by the tumor, rather than by bone metastases, which many of these patients have due to the advanced nature of their cancers. In the second group, accounting for one quarter of cases, are patients with hematologic malignancies, such as multiple myeloma, certain lymphomas and leukemias, as well as a subset of the patients with breast cancer. These patients have elevated serum calcium levels, but in contrast to most patients with solid tumors and HHM, have elevated serum level of phosphate and low urinary cAMP. These patients

---

Table 57-2. CLINICAL FEATURES OF HYPERCALCEMIA

NEUROLOGIC	CARDIOVASCULAR
Lethargy	ECG changes (short QT, widened T)
Confusion	Bradycardia
Coma	Heart block
Headache	Hypertension
Depression	
Paranoia	**RENAL**
Muscle weakness	Polyuria
Hyporeflexia	Uremia
Incontinence	Renal colic
Memory loss	Nephrocalcinosis
Hearing loss	
Ataxia	**OTHER**
	Band keratopathy
GASTROINTESTINAL	Conjunctivitis
Constipation	Change in vision
Anorexia	Pruritus
Nausea and vomiting	Thrombosis
Polydipsia	Myalgia
Weight loss	
Pancreatitis	
Peptic ulcer	
Abdominal pain	

always have lytic bony lesions, and histologically demonstrate increased osteoclast bone resorption adjacent to tumor cells. Formerly, an osteoclast-activating factor was implicated as a bone-resorption–stimulating lymphokine secreted locally in and around the bone metastases. This osteoclast-activating activity is now thought to be an effect of other known cytokines, mainly interleukin-1β (IL-1β) and tumor necrosis factor-β (lymphotoxin). These cytokines promote local net bone resorption and thus produce hypercalcemia and hyperphosphatemia.

Vitamin D and Vitamin A Intoxication. When administered in excess, vitamins A and D can produce hypercalcemia. Affected patients tend to have normal or elevated serum phosphate levels associated with a low PTH level. Metastatic calcification may occur.

Thiazide Diuretics. Thiazides may increase serum calcium to a mild degree, primarily through hemoconcentration. Serum phosphate may also be depressed. It often takes several weeks for the hypercalcemia to resolve after the medication is discontinued.

Hyperthyroidism. Hyperthyroidism is associated with increased bone resorption. Often, the plasma PTH is low, and a history of other thyrotoxic symptoms can be elicited. The hypercalcemia usually resolves as the patient becomes euthyroid.

Milk–Alkali Syndrome. Typically, the milk–alkali syndrome occurs in patients with peptic ulcers who consume large quantities of milk and absorbable antacids. Usually, there is some degree of renal failure. PTH levels are low. This syndrome has become much less common with the increased use of nonabsorbable antacids and H$_2$-receptor antagonists.

Sarcoidosis and Other Granulomatous Diseases. These syndromes are associated with hypersensitivity to vitamin D. Apparently, the granulomas can convert the inactive vitamin D to its active form. These patients have elevated plasma globulins and low PTH levels. Large doses of cortisone for 10 days usually reduces the hypercalcemia. Biopsy of lymph nodes or the liver may confirm the diagnosis.

Familial Hypocalciuric Hypercalcemic Hyperparathyroidism. This disease is a generally asymptomatic, autosomal dominant condition characterized by mild to moderate hypercalcemia, hypocalciuria, and normal or only slightly elevated parathyroid hormone levels. It develops in people heterozygous for a mutation in the calcium-sensing receptor.[5] The mutation causes an increase in the set-point for extracellular calcium concentration; thus the "normal" calcium for these individuals is higher than in the normal population. No treatment is necessary, although people with this disease should receive genetic counseling. Neonatal severe hyperparathyroidism, which may be fatal, develops in children homozygous for mutations in this receptor. Treatment for neonates with this disease is controversial, but most benefit from early surgical management.[6]

Immobilization. Immobilization produces hypercalcemia by increasing the ratio of bone resorption to formation. These patients can usually be distinguished by history, although on laboratory evaluation, they have elevated serum levels of calcium and phosphate and a decreased serum concentration of PTH. Often, hypercalciuria exists, which may lead to the development of renal stones. Treatment is early mobilization and forced diuresis.

Other Causes. A variety of other diseases may produce hypercalcemia. For example, Paget disease (osteitis deformans) typically causes mild elevations in serum calcium. It can be diagnosed on the basis of the characteristic radiographic lesion. Adrenal insufficiency may be associated with hypercalcemia, although the symptoms are typically those of the primary abnormality. Lithium therapy appears to produce hypercalcemia by altering the parathyroid set-point for inhibition by calcium. Idiopathic hypercalcemia of infancy is a rare disorder that is probably the result of hypersensitivity to vitamin D. It occurs in infants with mental retardation and is satisfactorily treated with glucocorticoids. Other causes include aluminum-induced renal osteomalacia and a host of analytic errors related to improper specimen collection with prolonged tourniquet times, tube contamination, and instrument drift.

Medical Treatment

Although the choice of therapy is tailored to the cause of the hypercalcemia, several general measures can prove effective.[7]

For the patient with mild hypercalcemia, a decrease in dietary calcium is indicated. A reduction in intake of milk and other dairy products is suggested along with discontinuing thiazide diuretics and vitamin D preparations. Mobilization prevents bone demineralization and should be encouraged.

Patients with more marked hypercalcemia or severe symptoms should be admitted to the hospital for treatment with careful observation and monitoring. In the patient with severe hyperparathyroidism, although the definitive therapy is surgical, it is unwise to proceed with neck exploration until the calcium has been reduced to near normal. The mainstay of therapy is intravenous hydration, preferably with normal saline in sufficient quantities to maintain the urine output above 100 mL/h. These patients are often dehydrated before therapy, and fluid can be administered intravenously at a rate of 200 mL/h. Caution must be exercised in older patients who might have marginal cardiac reserve. This therapy exploits the kidney's parallel handling of calcium and sodium. The diuretic furosemide also increases sodium and calcium excretion but should not be used until the patient is well hydrated.

The endpoints of therapy are a decrease in the serum calcium and a reduction of symptoms. Saline diuresis is usually effective when the hypercalcemia results from hyperparathyroidism or from a benign cause. In contrast, the hypercalcemia of malignancy may produce severe symptoms associated with extremely high serum calcium levels that are difficult to control. In this setting, a variety of other measures may be considered (Table 57-3). Some of the agents used to treat hypercalcemia have significant toxicity and require close patient monitoring during treatment. Calcitonin is a fairly weak hypocalcemic agent, but it acts rapidly and appears to have less toxicity than many of the other drugs. Salmon calcitonin appears to be the most potent preparation. Glucocorticoids may be particularly efficacious in patients with sarcoidosis and other granulomatous diseases. Mithramycin has proved useful in patients with hypercalcemia of malignancy, but it has a cumulative toxicity (thrombocytopenia, hepatotoxicity, and nephrotoxicity). Biphosphonates appear to directly inhibit osteoclast activity. Disodium etidronate is the agent most commonly used. It is given intravenously and is particularly efficacious, although long-term use may be associated with significant osteomalacia. Prostaglandin synthetase inhibitors were initially considered useful, but their efficacy has proved to be limited. Intravenous phosphates and chelating agents have largely been abandoned because of their severe toxicity; however, oral phosphates may be beneficial in cases requiring prolonged therapy. Gallium nitrate is a promising agent for the potent inhibition of bone re-

---

Table 57-3. TREATMENT OF HYPERCALCEMIA

THERAPY OF PRIMARY DISEASE

Tumor resection (hypercalcemia of malignancy)
Parathyroidectomy (primary hyperparathyroidism)

EXPANSION OF EXTRACELLULAR VOLUME

Saline infusion

ENHANCEMENT OF URINARY CALCIUM EXCRETION

Extracellular volume expansion
Loop diuretics (furosemide and ethacrynic acid)

INHIBITION OF BONE RESORPTION

Calcitonin
Glucocorticoids
Plicamycin (Mithramycin)
Bisphosphonates
Gallium nitrate

REDUCTION OF INTESTINAL CALCIUM ABSORPTION

Low-calcium diet
Glucocorticoids

OTHER

Dialysis
Mobilization
Oral phosphate
Estrogens or progestogens (postmenopausal women with primary
    hyperparathyroidism)
Chloroquine (sarcoidosis)

(Modified from Attie MF. Treatment of hypercalcemia. Endocrinol
    Metab Clin North Am 1989;18:802)

---

sorption; however, it can have severe nephrotoxicity, and the clinical experience with its use is still limited. Amifostine (WR-2721) was initially considered useful for hypercalcemia, but further experience has demonstrated that its effects are limited and transient.

Hypocalcemia

Hypocalcemia can occur as a consequence of various acquired and hereditary diseases.[8] Generally, these disorders produce a deficiency or a defect in the action of either PTH or vitamin D. It is most commonly a significant clinical problem after neck operation for thyroid disease. Vitamin D deficiency is associated with compensatory PTH excess. The end result is rickets in children or osteomalacia in adults.

Clinical Features

The major signs and symptoms of hypocalcemia are a direct consequence of the reduction in plasma-ionized calcium, which increases neuromuscular excitability (Table 57-4). The earliest clinical manifestations are numbness and tingling in the circumoral area, fingers, and toes. Mental symptoms are also common. Patients become anxious, depressed, and occasionally confused. Tetany may develop, characterized by carpopedal spasm, tonic–clonic convulsions, and laryngeal stridor. The magnitude of symptoms at any given plasma concentration of ionized calcium varies from patient to patient. On physical examination, contraction of the facial muscles is elicited by tapping anterior to the facial nerve (Chvostek sign), although this sign may be positive in 10% of normal patients. Trousseau sign is elicited by occluding blood flow to the forearm for 3 minutes. The development of carpal spasm indicates hypocalcemia, although the test is unpleasant and clinically impractical.

Differential Diagnosis

The causes of hypocalcemia include the following:

- Hypoparathyroidism
- Vitamin D deficiency
- Pseudohypoparathyroidism
- Hypomagnesemia
- Malabsorption
- Pancreatitis
- Hypoalbuminemia
- Chelation of calcium
- Osteoblastic metastases
- Toxic shock syndrome
- Hyperphosphatemia

The most common cause of hypocalcemia by far is excision of or damage to the parathyroid glands during thyroid surgery.

Postoperative Hypoparathyroidism. Postoperative hypoparathyroidism commonly develops after total thyroidectomy for malignancy. Most patients undergoing operation on the thyroid experience some alteration in serum calcium, although they often are asymptomatic, and the low calcium probably represents contusion or temporary alteration of the blood supply to the parathyroids. The hypocalcemia is usually transient and is not treated unless significant symptoms develop. Occasionally, in patients with preoperative hyperparathyroidism and significant bone disease, as evidenced by either radiographic changes or an elevation of the serum alkaline phosphatase level, there is a marked skeletal calcium deposition and symptomatic hypocalcemia, so-called bone hunger. The plasma calcium usually reaches its nadir at 48 to 72 hours after surgery and then slowly returns to normal over 2 to 3 days. Occasionally, these patients may require calcium and vitamin D therapy for weeks or months after parathyroidectomy.

Idiopathic Hypoparathyroidism. A less common cause of hypoparathyroidism is idiopathic lack of function. It occurs in both sporadic and familial forms. In some

---

Table 57-4. CLINICAL FEATURES OF HYPOCALCEMIA

NEUROLOGIC

Circumoral parethesia
Light-headedness
Depression
Anxiety
Confusion
Chvostek sign
Trousseau sign
Irritability
Laryngeal spasm
Seizures

MUSCULOSKELETAL

Tetany
Cramps
Involuntary twitching
Osteomalacia

CARDIOVASCULAR

ECG changes (prolonged QT interval, T-wave peaking)
Arrhythmia
Tachycardia, hypotension

OTHER

Lenticular cataracts

cases, it develops as part of a polyglandular disorder and is thought to have an autoimmune basis. DiGeorge syndrome is a congenital disorder involving the branchial pouches that produces agenesis of the thymus and parathyroids. Hypoparathyroidism may also develop in newborns as a result of prenatal suppression of the fetal parathyroids by the hypercalcemic mother. It is also common in otherwise normal but premature infants.

Vitamin D Deficiency. Vitamin D deficiency may occur as a result of dietary deficiency or lack of exposure to the sun. Likewise, renal disease produces a decrease in the 1-hydroxylase activity necessary for formation of active vitamin D_3. The result is a decrease in calcium absorption and an increased secretion of PTH by the stimulated parathyroid glands. Osteomalacia, abnormal fractures, and the deformities of rickets may result.

Pseudohypoparathyroidism. Pseudohypoparathyroidism is a familial disease characterized by rotund appearance, shortening of the extremities, and sometimes mental deficiency. The defect does not lie in PTH secretion; in fact, most patients have elevated plasma levels of PTH with evidence of increased bone resorption. Rather, the kidney is unresponsive to the hormone, and as a consequence, the patients develop hypocalcemia and hyperphosphatemia. The deficit appears to lie in the renal adenyl cyclase system.

Hypomagnesemia. This unusual deficit may result from chronic alcoholism, malabsorption, parenteral nutrition, or increased renal clearance during therapy with aminoglycosides. The deficit appears to block the physical response to PTH as well as its release from the parathyroid gland.

Other Causes. In short gut syndrome, after extensive small-bowel resection or bypass, vitamin D and calcium may be absorbed in insufficient quantities. In pancreatitis, the massive soft tissue destruction and saponification that occur with hemorrhagic disease may sequester significant amounts of calcium in the retroperitoneum. There also appears to be some undefined systemic factor that contributes to the hypocalcemia in these patients. Hypoalbuminemia causes a reduction in the total plasma calcium level, although the ionized calcium remains in the normal range, and patients are asymptomatic. Circulatory substances, such as the citrate used to anticoagulate banked blood and radiographic contrast media, may bind to or chelate calcium. In patients with osteoblastic metastases, particularly associated with prostate carcinoma, hypocalcemia has been attributed to increased calcium flux into the lesions. Toxic shock syndrome is sometimes associated with hypocalcemia, but the mechanism has not been defined. Acute hyperphosphatemia, as a consequence of exogenous administration of phosphate or during the cytolytic chemotherapy of highly responsive tumors, such as Burkitt lymphoma and acute lymphoblastic leukemia, may produce symptomatic hypocalcemia associated with soft tissue calcification.

Medical Treatment

Treatment of hypocalcemia can be summarized as follows:

Symptomatic hypocalcemia: calcium gluconate or chloride
Symptomatic tetany—diphenylhydantoin
Correction of hypomagnesemia—magnesium chloride
Vitamin D supplementation
Ergocalciferol
Calcifediol (liver disease)
Calcitriol (renal disease)
Long-term therapy
  Calcium carbonate
  Low phosphate, oxalate diet
  Parathyroid grafting (immunosuppressed)

For acute symptomatic hypocalcemia, calcium should be administered intravenously. Calcium gluconate is less irritating to the veins, and the calcium release is slower, without the risk of overcorrection. Usually 20 to 30 mL of 10% solution is infused over a 15- to 20-minute period, and then 50 to 100 mL is administered over the next 12 hours in adults. Bicarbonate precipitates any calcium infused through the same intravenous line. Serum magnesium should always be measured, and hypomagnesemia should be corrected if present. In patients with convulsions from advanced tetany, intravenous calcium chloride therapy may prove useful, but symptoms should never be allowed to progress to this point.

Long-term therapy is gauged on the basis of symptoms. In the postoperative patient, the continued stimulus of mild hypocalcemia to any remaining parathyroid tissue may prove useful. Concomitant therapy with calcium and vitamin D is effective in a timely fashion. A starting dose of 1 g/d oral calcium carbonate is usually well-tolerated. Vitamin D can be administered as calcitriol, a synthetic vitamin D analogue. Most adults respond to a dose of 0.5 to 2.0 μg/d; reduced dosages may be necessary for patients with renal dysfunction.

A low phosphate and oxalate diet may also prove useful. Synthetic PTH is not yet available in sufficient quantities to make its use practical, and parathyroid allotransplantation is successful but requires immunosuppression therapy.

Hyperparathyroidism

Definitions

As with other endocrine tumors, parathyroid neoplasms are recognized not because of physical enlargement but because of the peripheral effects of excess hormone. Although the distinction is somewhat artificial, primary hyperparathyroidism develops spontaneously without apparent cause but possibly in response to exogenous stimuli. When the normal control of serum calcium is disturbed and there is increased autonomous production of PTH, the state is referred to as *primary hyperparathyroidism*. This category includes both benign single- and multiple-gland enlargements and the much rarer parathyroid carcinoma. In some cases, the disease is familial. In contrast, *secondary hyperparathyroidism* occurs when there is a defect in mineral homeostasis that leads to a compensatory increase in parathyroid function. This occurs most commonly in response to renal disease but may also develop as a consequence of the hypocalcemia associated with some diseases of the gastrointestinal tract, bone, or other endocrine organs. Occasionally, with prolonged secondary stimulation, the hyperfunctioning glands are no longer physiologically responsive to an increased ionized calcium. This rare, relatively autonomous state is referred to as *tertiary hyperparathyroidism* and develops most commonly after renal transplantation when the defect in calcium homeostasis is corrected.

Incidence

The advent in the 1970s of widespread screening of serum calcium as part of automated multichannel analysis has considerably altered our understanding of hyperparathyroidism. Before that time, primary hyperparathyroidism was thought to be a relatively rare condition. Most

Table 57-5. AGE- AND GENDER-SPECIFIC INCIDENCE OF PRIMARY HYPERPARATHYROIDISM

Age (y)	New Cases per 100,000	
	Men	Women
<39	5	8
40–50	26	104
>60	92	189
Total	18	56

(After Heath H III, Hodgson SF, Kennedy MA. Primary hyperthyroidism: incidence, morbidity, and potential economic impact in a community. N Engl J Med 1980;302:189)

patients presented with symptoms of disease, usually renal stones or bony manifestations. Today, as a result of screening, most patients are asymptomatic or only have vague symptoms or signs that can be related to hyperparathyroidism.[9] Occasionally, patients recognize that they had symptoms only after their well-being improves following parathyroidectomy. Incidence varies both with age and gender (Table 57-5), but hyperparathyroidism is believed to develop in about 50 to 100 people per 100,000 in the general population, with about 50,000 new cases occurring annually in the United States.[10] Marked variations have been noted worldwide; the reasons for these differences remain unclear.

Etiology

The cause of primary hyperparathyroidism is not known. Although the sequence of progression from secondary to tertiary disease in response to chronic stimulation has logical appeal, it is difficult to draw parallels with primary disease. As discussed later, most patients with primary hyperparathyroidism have disease of a single gland rather than multiple glands, unlike what might be predicted if an external stimulus were operative. Hyperparathyroidism is most common in postmenopausal women, the population group with the highest incidence of osteoporosis and the most significant alterations in cal-

cium and phosphate metabolism. Loss of renal function with aging is associated with elevations in PTH and decreases in phosphate clearance. It has been suggested but not demonstrated that a renal calcium leak, if sufficient, might result in a chronic calcium deficit, stimulating the parathyroids.

Genetic studies of parathyroid adenomas have described a new oncogene (*PRAD1*), which may be one step in the path to neoplasia in these tumors. Ongoing research indicates that overexpression of the normal *PRAD1* gene, also known as cyclin D1, allows progression of the cell cycle from the G1 phase to the S phase, thus promoting cellular growth and division. *PRAD1* is overexpressed in only a subset of parathyroid adenomas; further research may reveal other genetic alterations that contribute to the neoplastic growth.[11]

Hyperparathyroidism occurs in several familial forms. It is a major component of the multiple endocrine neoplasia (MEN) syndromes types I and IIa (discussed later). The parathyroid disease of these syndromes is multiglandular and transmitted in an autosomal dominant fashion. The genetic basis for MEN I is under intense investigation and appears to be due to a mutation of a tumor suppressor gene in the proximal long arm of chromosome 11. Several studies have demonstrated that in many MEN I tumors, including hyperplastic parathyroid tumors, there are deletions of this region of the chromosome, suggesting loss of a gene involved in growth regulation or tumor suppression.[12]

The genetic defect responsible for MEN IIa was recently identified after a detailed and systematic search.[13,14] The *RET* protooncogene was identified as the site of point mutations resulting in the substitutions of extracellular cysteine residues in this receptor tyrosine kinase. Further studies of these mutations may shed light on the variable penetrance of the parathyroid disease in MEN IIa.

Pathology

Single- Versus Multiple-Gland Disease. Although pathologic studies can readily distinguish parathyroid glands from other tissue, beyond this capacity, they may not prove useful. As discussed later, intraoperative decisions frequently depend on recognizing disease of one or more

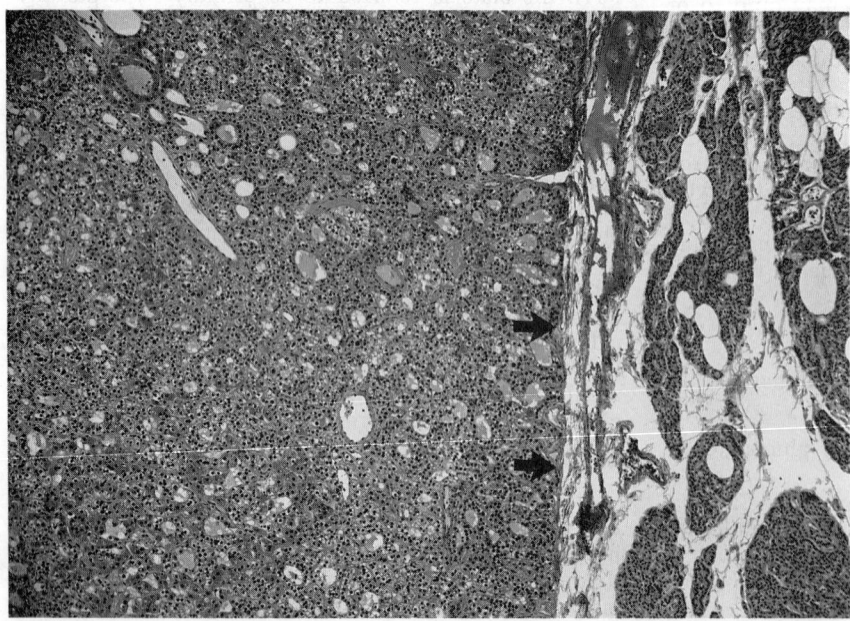

Figure 57-8. Classic histologic findings in parathyroid adenoma with a single focus of proliferating chief cells and a compressed rim of normal surrounding parathyroid (*arrows*) composed of half stroma and half fat (×90).

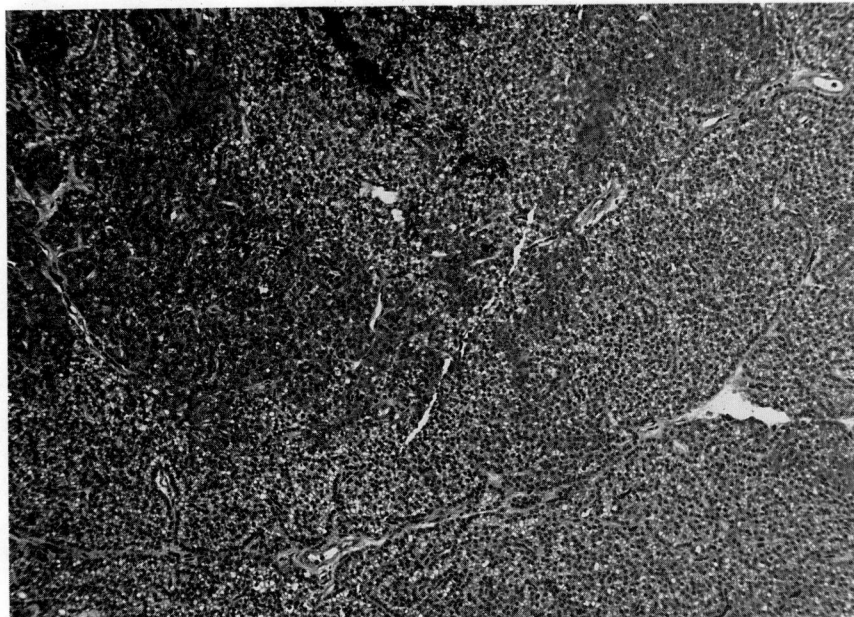

Figure 57-9. Classic findings in parathyroid hyperplasia with diffuse proliferation of cells and without any remaining normal gland (×150).

parathyroid glands, and in this regard, the histologic description of adenoma or hyperplasia may be totally unreliable in primary hyperparathyroidism.

Microscopically, the cell most commonly involved in primary hyperparathyroidism is the chief cell.[15] Less frequently, the oxyphil cell is the predominant cell type. Diseased glands typically have an increase in the proportion of stromal cells and a reduction in the proportion of stromal fat. Single diseased glands, or adenomas, have been classically described with a predominance of chief cells centering in a single focus, with a compressed rim of surrounding normal tissue (Fig. 57-8). In contrast, parathyroid hyperplasia has been characterized as a diffuse proliferation of clear cells in multiple glands, with little remaining normal tissue (Fig. 57-9). These criteria have proved to be totally unreliable. Patients with multiple-gland disease may have one gland that appears to be an adenoma and another that appears diffusely involved or even histologically normal with gross enlargement. Other methods of determining normal glands, including intracellular fat staining, measurements of glandular density, and flow cytometric analysis of cellular DNA content have all been used with some reported success, although none provides unequivocal differentiation between normal and abnormal glands.

By far the most reliable index of abnormality is the determination of gland size by visual inspection. The incidence of single- and multiple-gland enlargement in 100 consecutive patients with hyperparathyroidism is shown in Table 57-6. Treatment based on the visual assessment and judgment of the experienced surgeon has proved to be the best basis for intraoperative decisions. This requires that all four parathyroid glands be evaluated at the time of operation.

Carcinoma. Parathyroid carcinoma is a rare entity, and the histologic diagnosis can prove to be exceedingly difficult. The surgeon may suspect the diagnosis when dense invasion and scarring are encountered, although this may be secondary to some other inflammatory disease in the neck. Pathologic criteria include marked mitotic activity, dense fibrous stroma, and evidence of local invasion into the capsule or surrounding vessels. Malignant-appearing tumors, however, may pursue an apparently benign clinical course; the converse is less frequently true. An aneuploid pattern by flow cytometric analysis of tumor DNA content may help to distinguish carcinoma from atypical adenoma in borderline cases.[16] The only reliable criteria of malignancy are metastases, most commonly to the lymph nodes, lung, or liver, and true local invasion.

Systemic Effects

The use of automated technology for determining serum calcium has changed not only the estimated incidence of hyperparathyroidism but also the usual mode of presentation.[9] Before screening, three fourths of patients presented with renal disease, particularly nephrolithiasis, one third to one half had skeletal manifestations, and rare patients had both. Most recent series suggest that a least half of patients are diagnosed without renal or osseous disease, and many are asymptomatic (Table 57-7). Manifestations of the disease are protean but generally nonspecific and may be difficult to elicit in the history. A significant proportion of patients present without a readily quantifiable index of disease severity. This has created some controversy about the need for surgery in the asymptomatic and particularly elderly or high-risk patient.

The earliest complaints are often the vague symptoms of hypercalcemia as discussed previously. They vary with the magnitude of plasma calcium elevation and include muscle weakness, anorexia, nausea, constipation, poly-

Table 57-6. GLAND ENLARGEMENT IN 100 PATIENTS WITH PRIMARY HYPERPARATHYROIDISM

Enlarged Glands	Patients
1	65
2	15
3	10
4	10

(Wells SA Jr, Leight GS, Ross AJ. Primary hyperparathyroidism. Curr Probl Surg 1980;17:400)

Table 57-7. CLINICAL CHARACTERISTICS OF PATIENTS WITH PRIMARY HYPERPARATHYROIDISM

Characteristics*	Percentage of Population
Urolithiasis	4
Hypercalciuria (>250 mg/d)	22
Emotional disorder	20
Osteoporosis	12
Diminished renal function	14
Hyperparathyroid bone disease	8
Peptic ulcer disease	8
No problems related to hyperparathyroidism	51

* Listed are problems generally accepted as potentially caused or aggravated by hypercalcemia or hyperparathyroidism
(After Heath H III, Hodgson SF, Kennedy MA. Primary hyperthyroidism: incidence, morbidity, and potential economic impact in a community. N Engl J Med 1980;302:189)

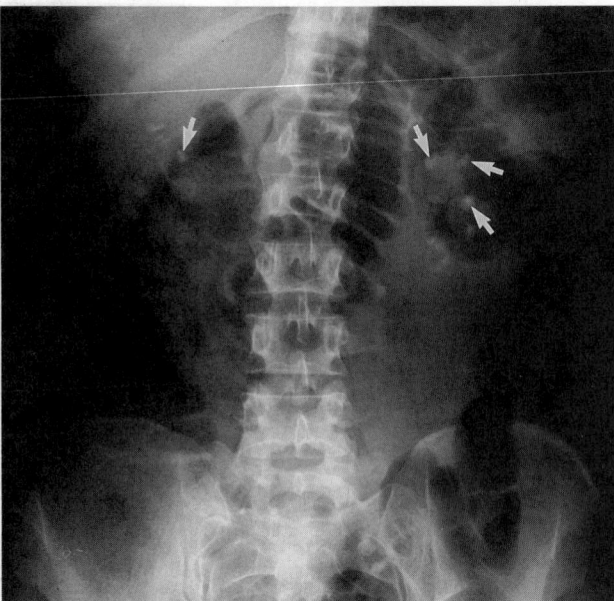

Figure 57-10. Abdominal film demonstrating nephrocalcinosis, or diffuse calcification of the renal parenchyma (*arrows*).

uria, and polydipsia. These nonspecific symptoms may or may not cause the patient to seek medical attention.[17] Some symptomatic patients have evidence of chronic disease involving the kidney or skeleton. Usually, only one of these systems is significantly involved in any individual patient. The most frequent symptoms in patients evaluated at the time of diagnosis in a large clinic are shown in Table 57-7. The treatment of hyperparathyroidism is designed to eliminate or halt the progression of the complications of the disease. Symptomatic patients can be divided into two groups. Members of the first group develop renal manifestations, have a slower onset of symptoms, and generally have lower serum calcium concentrations. Patients in the second group have a more rapid onset of symptoms, higher serum calcium levels, and significant bone disease. More recently, a third group has been recognized. These are the asymptomatic patients, characterized by the least active disease. No recognizable histologic or physiologic characteristics allow separation of patients with renal disease from those with bone disease.

Renal Manifestations. Renal complications develop because the hypercalcemia leads to increased urinary calcium excretion and because PTH increases the excretion of phosphate and produces urinary alkalosis. Both these events predispose to stone formation. Urinary stones may be treated surgically or with lithotripsy, and subsequent definitive treatment of the hyperparathyroidism reduces the rate of reformation. Nephrolithiasis develops in about 30% of patients. Of patients who present for the first time with renal colic, 5% to 10% are found to have primary hyperparathyroidism. Nephrocalcinosis (Fig. 57-10). represents calcification of the renal parenchyma and occurs in 5% to 10% of patients with hyperparathyroidism. It causes more significant renal damage than nephrolithiasis. In general, the more severe the renal damage, the less likely it is that nephrocalcinosis will improve after parathyroidectomy.

The increased incidence of hypertension in hyperparathyroidism correlates with the degree of renal impairment. This may be the most significant cause of morbidity in these patients, and although improvements in hypertension have been demonstrated in some patients after parathyroidectomy, there is no clear correlation between the two conditions.

Skeletal Manifestations. Parathyroid bone disease in its most classic and severe form, osteitis fibrosa cystica, is

seldom seen; however, 5% to 15% of patients present with significant symptoms of skeletal disease. Most commonly, these include bone pain and pathologic fractures.

Bone changes are often demonstrable with detailed plain radiographs of the hands (Fig. 57-11). Characteristically, subperiosteal resorption is evident on the radial aspect of

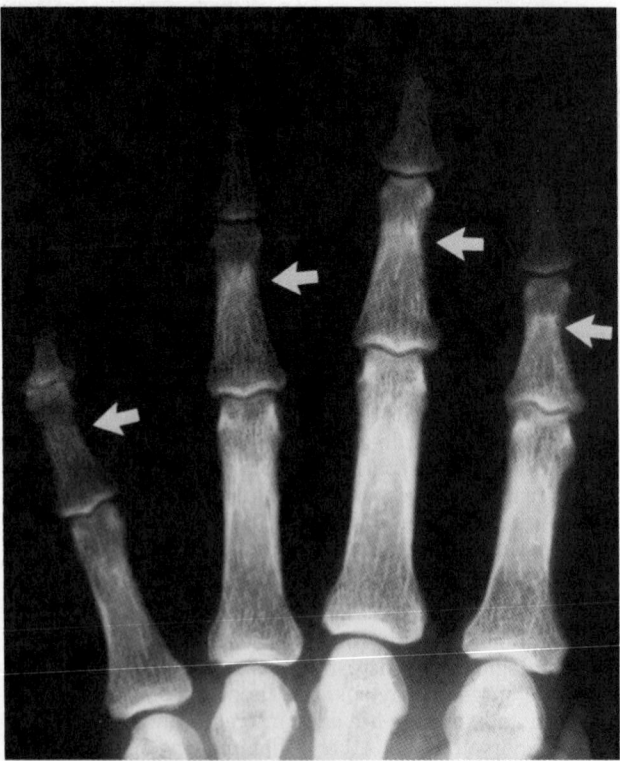

Figure 57-11. Magnification radiograph of the fingers in hyperparathyroidism, demonstrating subperiosteal cortical resorption (*arrows*), typically most visible on the radial aspect of the middle phalanges.

the middle phalanx of the second or third finger. There may be tufting of the distal phalanges, producing clubbing on physical examination. Other findings that typically involve the skull and long bones include bone cysts, "brown" tumors (ie, localized proliferations of osteoclasts), and diffuse demineralization or granularity.

More subtle bone loss can be detected using iliac crest bone biopsy or photon-beam densitometry. The significance of mild derangements detectable only with such sophisticated technology has been questioned, and further studies are needed to determine the postoperative outcome of the bone disease in patients with these presumably early manifestations of hyperparathyroidism.

Gastrointestinal Manifestations. Hypercalcemia is clearly associated with nonspecific gastrointestinal complaints, including nausea, vomiting, constipation, and anorexia, but attempts to demonstrate a definite relation between hyperparathyroidism and either peptic ulcer disease or pancreatitis remain unconvincing. Hypercalcemia stimulates increased gastric acid secretion experimentally and clinically and has been associated with pancreatitis. Therefore, a theoretic rationale for the complex of hyperparathyroidism and gastrointestinal complaints does exist. There also appears to be a slight increase in the incidence of cholelithiasis in patients with hyperparathyroidism, presumably as a result of the higher concentrations of calcium in bile.

Neuromuscular Manifestations. Neurologic and muscular complaints are those of hypercalcemia in general. Fatigability and proximal muscle weakness are among the most debilitating. Atrophy of type II muscle fibers, consistent with a neuropathic and not a myopathic cause, has been demonstrated. Sensory complaints include dysesthesia, reduced vibratory sense, and stocking-glove sensory deficits.

Psychologic Manifestations. The emotional disturbances of hyperparathyroidism are often subtle and difficult to quantitate. As with other forms of hypercalcemia, they range from depression or anxiety to psychosis and coma. Patients undergoing parathyroidectomy frequently experience a sense of well-being and relief of fatigue and dullness postoperatively, although they may have had no noticeable complaints preoperatively.

Other Manifestations. A variety of signs and symptoms of soft tissue calcification have also been described. Nonspecific arthralgia, particularly involving the proximal interphalangeal joints of the hands, is characteristic. There is an increased incidence of chondrocalcinosis. Pruritus, vascular and cardiac calcification, and band keratopathy of the cornea have all been noted. Several reports have suggested an increased incidence of malignancy, but these remain unsubstantiated.

Diagnostic Investigations

Of the various clinical manifestations, only the skeletal changes of hyperparathyroidism are pathognomonic. Usually, the evaluation focuses on the differential diagnosis of an elevated serum calcium concentration, and the diagnosis is essentially one of exclusion, ruling out other causes of hypercalcemia.

Physical Findings. Except in patients with the classic deformities of advanced bone disease, the physical examination is seldom helpful. Diseased parathyroids are infrequently palpable, except in patients with parathyroid carcinoma. A mass in the anterior neck in a patient with primary hyperparathyroidism is more commonly a thyroid nodule.

Calcium. Hypercalcemia is the single most important diagnostic finding; however, particularly in early or mild cases, serial analysis may show fluctuations in and out of the normal range. Coexistent hypoalbuminemia and acidosis may produce an apparently normal total serum calcium, even though the ionized fraction is actually elevated. Although cumbersome, methodology is available for determining serum-ionized calcium concentrations and may be helpful in the differential diagnosis of hypercalcemia.

Parathyroid Hormone. In the United States, PTH measurement has become an important method for establishing the diagnosis of hyperparathyroidism. Because of the heterogeneity of the various circulating forms of PTH, the initial clinical experience with radioimmunoassays gave conflicting and often confusing results. The methodology continues to be refined, and most current assays are sufficiently sensitive, specific, and reliable to recommend wide clinical use. Middle-region and two-site assays, as opposed to amino-terminal, carboxy-terminal, and intact hormone assays, appear to be the most dependable. The demonstration of an elevated plasma PTH concentration alone does not establish the diagnosis of hyperparathyroidism. In the setting of an inappropriately elevated serum calcium level, however, this finding is virtually diagnostic (Fig. 57-12).

Phosphate. Parathyroid hormone increases renal phosphate excretion and, in about half of patients, produces hypophosphatemia. In the presence of renal disease, however, the serum phosphate levels may be normal or significantly elevated.

Bicarbonate. Parathyroid hormone also increases bicarbonate excretion such that patients may develop a hyperchloremic metabolic acidosis. It has been suggested that the finding of an elevated serum chloride/phosphate ratio may be helpful in the differential diagnosis of hypercalcemia. A ratio greater than 30 is considered highly suggestive of hyperparathyroidism.

Magnesium. Hypomagnesemia develops in 5% to 10% of patients. After parathyroidectomy, if there is both hypocalcemia and hypomagnesemia, it may be difficult to correct the calcium until the serum magnesium has been corrected.

Other Diagnostic Tests. A variety of special diagnostic tests are now available. None are more specific than the measurements of serum concentrations of calcium and PTH, although they may be useful in equivocal cases. For example, 24-hour urinary calcium excretion is usually elevated in patients with hyperparathyroidism, although the finding is not specific for this disease. This test is helpful in identifying patients with familial hypercalcemic hypocalciuric hyperparathyroidism. Measurements of tubular reabsorption of phosphate less than 30% suggest primary hyperparathyroidism. Urinary cAMP is generated specifically as a consequence of PTH activation of renal tubular adenyl cyclase. Increased urinary concentrations are identified in most patients with primary hyperparathyroidism. This test has been used as a rapid way to assess surgical procedures intraoperatively.

Localization

Because of the ectopic location of some glands, the difficulty in differentiating single-gland from multiple-gland disease, and the fact that even the experienced endocrine surgeon occasionally has difficulty identifying an abnormal gland, attempts have been made to localize enlarged glands preoperatively. In the hands of an experienced surgeon, however, the cure rate for hyperparathyroidism at the initial operation approaches 95%. There is no evidence

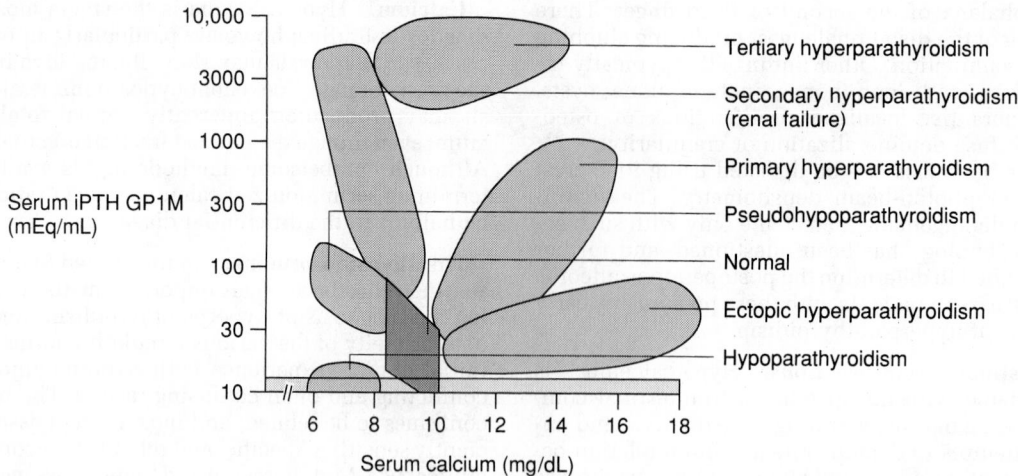

Figure 57-12. Relation between serum immunoreactive parathyroid hormone (iPTH) and serum calcium in patients with hypoparathyroidism, pseudohypoparathyroidism, ectopic hyperparathyroidism, and primary, secondary, and tertiary hyperparathyroidism. GP1M, guinea pig antiserum 1M. (After Clark OH, Way LW. Thyroid and parathyroid. In: Current surgical diagnosis and treatment, ed 8. Norwalk, CT, Appleton & Lange, 1989:249)

that preoperative localization reduces either the duration of an initial operation or the incidence of complications, and most surgeons feel that these techniques should be reserved for the patient undergoing reoperation after a failed initial procedure. A recent National Institutes of Health (NIH) Consensus Development Conference concluded that, "Preoperative localization in patients without prior neck operation is rarely indicated and not proven to be cost-effective."[18] This is particularly the case for the more invasive techniques, such as arteriography and venography, which have specific complications.

High-resolution real-time ultrasonography, CT scanning, magnetic resonance (MR) imaging, thallium–technetium subtraction scanning, and sestamibi scanning all appear to have comparable sensitivities of 50% to 60%. They may be less successful when employed at centers without significant experience in their use. Ultrasound is a more operator-dependent technique and is limited to the evaluation of the neck. It is a rapid and relatively inexpensive technique that permits confirmation by sonographically directed fine-needle aspiration for cytologic confirmation and immunoassay for PTH.

CT scanning is more expensive but less operator dependent than ultrasound. It clearly is superior in identifying deeper structures and for examining the retrosternal mediastinum. MR imaging is considerably more expensive than CT and has not been shown to be superior.

Thallium–technetium subtraction scanning depends on nonselective uptake of thallium by both the thyroid and parathyroid glands, whereas technetium is taken up only by the thyroid. The technetium scan is subtracted from the thallium scan, leaving only the parathyroid image. Despite its conceptual appeal, this method is less sensitive than the other diagnostic tests. Sestamibi is a radionuclide imaging agent originally developed for cardiac imaging. It also images parathyroid tissue on delayed scans and has been used recently for noninvasive parathyroid imaging. The single nuclide nature and short half-life, high-energy profile of this technique provides advantages in lateral, oblique, and three-dimensional imaging compared to technetium–thallium scanning. The sensitivity of sestamibi is still significantly lower than exploration by an experienced surgeon, however, and the appropriate use of the test appears to be limited to persistent or recurrent disease.

Treatment

Indications for Surgery. Recent reports have suggested that estrogen therapy, by reducing bone turnover and plasma calcium, may be useful in postmenopausal women with mild hyperparathyroidism. Generally, however, the only practical therapeutic option is surgery. Nephrolithiasis, bone disease, and neuromuscular symptoms all respond well to surgical intervention. In contrast, surgery in patients with renal failure, hypertension, and psychiatric complaints is not so uniformly successful, although it benefits some patients and is usually indicated in all patients but those at highest risk. The question of what to do with the large group of patients who have apparently asymptomatic disease requires particular discussion.

Management of Asymptomatic Hyperparathyroidism. An increasing proportion of patients with the diagnosis of hyperparathyroidism are asymptomatic. The appropriate treatment for these patients remains controversial. Although little evidence indicates that patients with asymptomatic mild disease eventually develop irreversible complications, such as renal failure, the natural history of the disease remains incompletely defined. Many of the manifestations of this disease may go unrecognized until they are corrected surgically. Still unanswered is the question of to what degree asymptomatic disease may contribute to generalized osteopenia in this predominantly postmenopausal female population.

One study followed a group of 142 asymptomatic patients without operation.[19] At the end of the 10-year study, over 20% of the patients had required surgery for an increase in serum calcium to greater than 11 mg/dL or for specific complications attributable to the disease. Another 20% were lost to or declined follow-up. The remaining patients either died of unrelated causes or had persistent asymptomatic disease. The authors concluded that, because of the large percentage (about 40%) of patients who either required operation or were lost to follow-up, they could not reliably recommend conservative management.

In October 1990, an NIH Consensus Development Conference reviewed the available evidence regarding the management of asymptomatic primary hyperparathyroidism.[18] The panel agreed that operation is the indicated treatment for all patients with symptoms, however, they recognized a subgroup of patients who have no symptoms attributable to hyperparathyroidism. Their conclusions included several indications for surgical intervention in asymptomatic patients:

- Markedly elevated serum calcium
- History of an episode of life-threatening hypercalcemia
- Reduced creatinine clearance
- Presence of one or more kidney stones detected by abdominal radiograph
- Markedly elevated 24-hour urinary calcium excretion
- Substantially reduced bone mass as determined by direct measurement

They mandated close (every 6 months) follow-up for those patients not treated by operation. In addition, surgery was agreed on for those patients for whom medical surveillance was neither desirable nor suitable. Such cases exist when a patient requests surgery, consistent follow-up is unlikely, coexistent illness complicates management, or the patient is young (<50 year old).

This remains an area of considerable controversy, and resolution of this question requires a randomized, controlled trial. The complication rate of operation by an experienced surgeon is less than 3%. Within a short period, the financial cost of medical follow-up exceeds that of treatment by operation. Based on these considerations and the uncertainty regarding the natural history of untreated disease, almost all patients should undergo operation and those who do not must be closely followed.

Principles of Surgical Correction. Although neck exploration for hyperparathyroidism may be straightforward, it sometimes becomes an arduous procedure requiring considerable patience because of the variability in both the location and the number of diseased glands. Persistent hyperparathyroidism and the necessity for reexploration can usually be avoided by a meticulous initial procedure. Reoperation is predictably more difficult than the initial operation, and the risks of damage to the recurrent laryngeal nerves and hypoparathyroidism are greater during reoperation.

It is essential that the surgeon be confident of the preoperative diagnosis and prospectively discuss the procedure with the patient. The potential complications of damage either to the recurrent laryngeal nerve or superior laryngeal nerve and the development of hypocalcemia require discussion. Likewise, the possibility of an unsuccessful initial operation needs to be explained, and the patient should recognize that reexploration, including median sternotomy, may be required.

The patient is explored under general anesthesia with a roll beneath the thoracic spine and with the neck extended. The neck is opened through a transverse incision two fingerbreadths above the sternal notch, and the platysma is similarly divided. Superior and inferior flaps are developed. The strap muscles are separated in the midline and retracted laterally; division is unnecessary. One lobe of the thyroid is chosen and rotated medially. Important landmarks include the tracheoesophageal groove, the recurrent laryngeal nerve, the inferior and superior thyroid arteries, and the middle thyroid vein (Fig. 57-13). In most patients, the nerve lies in the tracheoesophageal groove or just laterally. Occasionally, it may be more anterior. Uncommonly, it may originate directly from the vagus without passing around the right subclavian artery. Both these variations make the recurrent nerve more susceptible to injury. The external branch of the superior laryngeal nerve, which innervates the cricothyroid muscle, usually lies medial to the superior thyroid vessels and should be carefully preserved.

Although in the past some have advocated unilateral exploration if a single enlarged gland and one normal gland are identified on the first side explored, most surgeons now agree that all four glands need to be identified at the initial exploration because of the possibility of multiple-gland disease. Supernumerary glands may be present and should be sought at the initial procedure. Although frozen section has not been helpful in differentiating diseased and normal glands, it is essential for confirming the presence or absence of parathyroid tissue. Small, thin biopsy specimens are sharply incised from each gland with extreme care taken to avoid damaging their delicate blood supply.

The upper glands are usually located far dorsally on the surface of the thyroid lobe at the level of the upper two thirds of the gland. The lower glands are less constant and may be located anywhere from well above the thyroid to the anterior mediastinum. The lower glands are most commonly in the region where the thyrothymic ligament at-

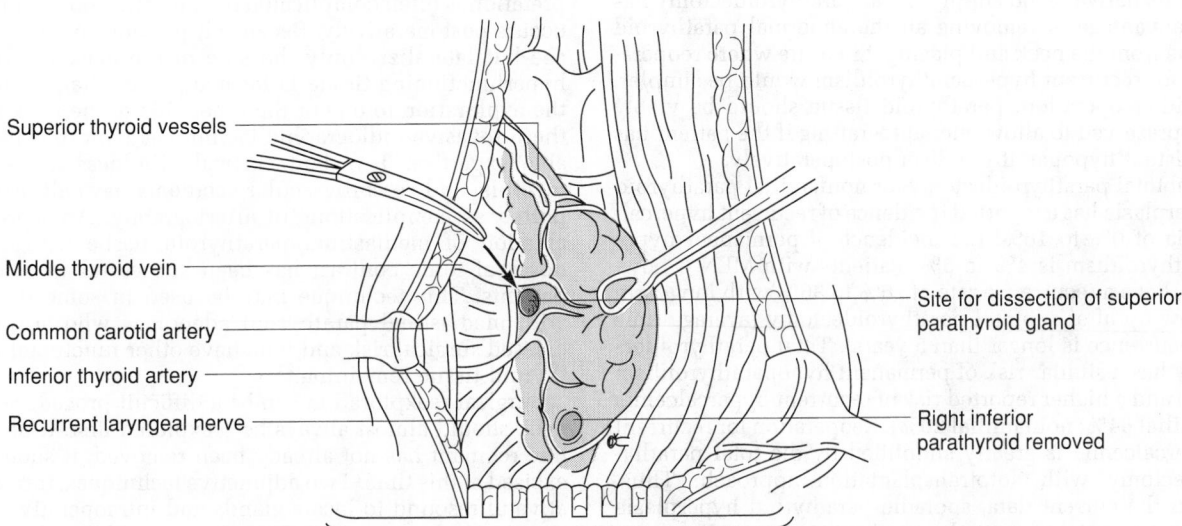

Figure 57-13. Lateral view of the right side of the neck after rotation of the thyroid lobe, emphasizing the important anatomic landmarks.

taches to the lower pole of the thyroid lobe. If the inferior glands cannot be localized, the thymic pedicle should be carefully examined and mobilized. Because of their common embryologic origin, the inferior gland is frequently associated with the thymic remnant. Parathyroid glands within the mediastinum sometimes can be removed by mobilizing the thymus through the cervical incision. If this is unsuccessful in identifying the parathyroid gland, the thyroid lobe on the side of the missing gland is mobilized and palpated. Intraoperative ultrasound examination may identify an intrathyroidal parathyroid gland. As a last resort, blind excision of the lobe may be indicated.

If after meticulous exploration of all these areas, three or four parathyroid glands have been identified, none of which is enlarged, most surgeons would favor terminating the operation.

Extent of Resection. The operative procedure performed is based on the number of enlarged glands identified. In many instances, the pathologist cannot reliably distinguish diseased from normal glands based on frozen section, and this remains a decision based on the surgeon's experience and judgment. Traditionally, single-gland disease has been treated by simple excision, whereas any combination of two- or three-gland enlargement is treated by resecting the diseased tissue and leaving the normal glands in place. The question of whether two- or three-gland enlargement implies the presence of disease in all glands (hyperplasia) has not been resolved. If one gland is large and the remaining three are normal in size, resection of the single parathyroid cures virtually all patients. Of 76 patients with two- or three-gland disease treated by excising the large glands and leaving the normal glands, only 8 (10.5%) had recurrent hypercalcemia, which tended to be mild (follow-up 12 to 140 months postoperatively). This approach seems satisfactory in most patients.[20]

Treating patients with four-gland disease has been more difficult. In many of these patients, the disease occurs as a component of one of the familial syndromes, particularly MEN I. Patients with four-gland parathyroid hyperplasia can be treated by subtotal parathyroidectomy (removing three and a half glands) or by total parathyroidectomy with autotransplantation of some parathyroid tissue into the nondominant forearm. Both operations depend on meticulous identification of all parathyroid tissue for adequate results. The putative advantage of the subtotal parathyroidectomy is that it leaves the remaining parathyroid tissue with its native blood supply. Total parathyroidectomy has the advantage of removing all the abnormal parathyroid tissue from the neck and placing it in a site where reoperation for recurrent hyperparathyroidism would be simpler. In either operation, parathyroid tissue should be viably cryopreserved to allow later autografting if the patient has persistent hypoparathyroidism postoperatively.

Subtotal parathyroidectomy for nonfamilial parathyroid hyperplasia has a reported incidence of recurrent hypercalcemia of 0% to 16%; the incidence of permanent hypoparathyroidism is 4% to 5%. Patients with MEN I, however, have a recurrence rate of 26% to 36% with long term follow-up after subtotal parathyroidectomy (average time to recurrence is longer than 5 years). Total parathyroidectomy has a similar risk of permanent hypoparathyroidism (5%) and a higher reported risk of recurrent hypercalcemia (familial 64%; nonfamilial 20%). Reoperation for recurrent hypercalcemia is greatly simplified by the total parathyroidectomy with autotransplantation approach. Thus, given the current data, sporadic parathyroid hyperplasia can be acceptably treated by either operation. However, the substantial risk of recurrent hypercalcemia following either operation makes the total parathyroidectomy with autotransplantation option preferable for patients with familial disease.

Technique of Parathyroid Autotransplantation. Total parathyroidectomy is performed, and a parathyroid is sliced into 15 to 20 pieces and autografted into a forearm muscle bed. The sites are marked with silk sutures. This location permits easy subsequent access under local anesthesia if the patient develops recurrent hypercalcemia. Function of the autograft is documented by normocalcemia, with the autograft as the only source of PTH, and by measuring higher concentrations of hormone in the antecubital vein draining the graft bed compared with that in the opposite arm. Lack of function is unusual; hypoparathyroidism develops in about 5% of patients. Glands should also be viably frozen in dimethyl sulfoxide and serum. If in the postoperative period it becomes clear that the patient is aparathyroid, the cryopreserved tissue can be reimplanted under local anesthesia.

Special Situations

Persistent or Recurrent Hyperparathyroidism. Persistent hyperparathyroidism occurs in less than 5% of patients after exploration by an experienced surgeon. Most commonly, it is the result of a single diseased gland still remaining in the neck or in the mediastinum. Recurrent disease develops after an interval of normocalcemia and may be the result of regrowth of diseased tissue, implantation from a tumor broken at the initial procedure, or even recurrent parathyroid carcinoma.

When evaluating these patients, it is essential to document that the initial diagnosis was indeed correct. Familial hypocalciuric hypercalcemia should be ruled out by measuring urinary calcium excretion.

Reviewing the original operative notes and pathology reports may provide clues to the position of missed glands. The locations of parathyroid tumors not found at the initial operation but identified on subsequent exploration in one large series are shown in Figure 57-14.

It is generally agreed that localization studies do have a place in the management of recurrent disease. Noninvasive methods are used first, and if these are unsuccessful in identifying the diseased gland, selective angiography and venous sampling for PTH are used. Selective angiography appears to be the most accurate technique, successfully localizing 50% to 80% of parathyroid glands that cannot be detected by any other modality. Venous sampling may also be helpful in some patients, although interpretation is often complicated by the collateralization that occurs postoperatively. Because it provides no direct image but lateralizes only the side of the neck where the hyperfunctioning tissue is located, it may help to direct the exploration to one or the other side of the neck. Both these invasive radiographic techniques require considerable expertise. Transient cortical blindness, transverse myelitis, and cerebrovascular accidents have all been reported as complications of arteriography. Angiographic ablation of mediastinal parathyroid tissue using large doses of ionic contrast has been successful in selected patients. This technique may be used in some patients with mediastinal parathyroid adenomas who are at increased surgical risk and who have other functional parathyroid tissue remaining.[21]

Surgical reexploration can be a difficult procedure. The neck should almost always be reexplored first. If the thymic remnant has not already been removed, it should be excised at this time. Two adjunctive techniques, intraoperative ultrasound to locate glands and intraoperative measurement of urinary cAMP to document the adequacy of resection, may be useful in patients undergoing operation for persistent disease.

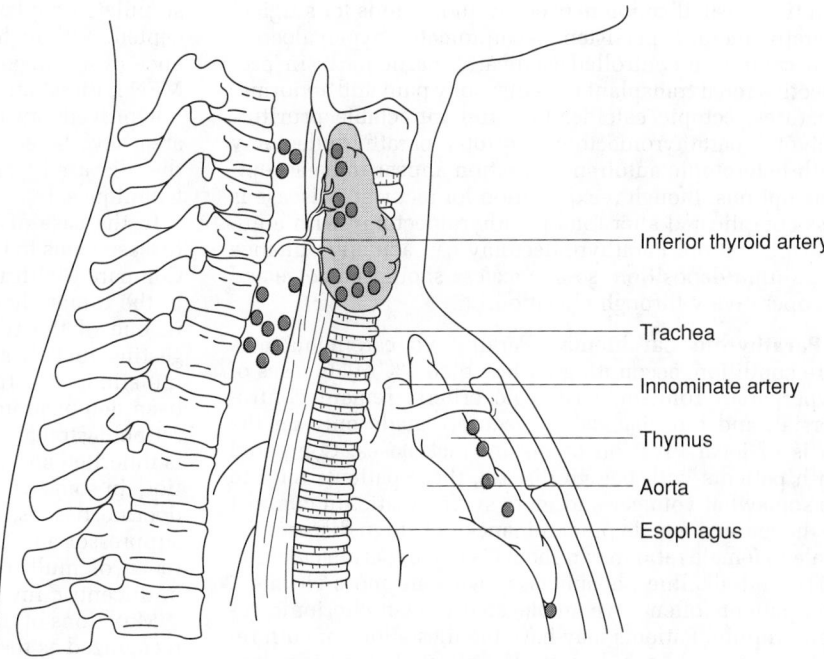

Inferior thyroid artery

Trachea

Innominate artery

Thymus

Aorta

Esophagus

Figure 57-14. Location of the parathyroid tumors missed on initial exploration but identified on subsequent operation. (After Brennan MF, Doppman JL, Marx SJ, et al. Reoperative parathyroid surgery for persistent hyperparathyroidism. Surgery 1978;83:669)

If the gland is not identified in the neck using the maneuvers described, the mediastinum is examined. Median sternotomy and exploration is necessary in only 1% to 2% of patients with hyperparathyroidism. Usually, a vertical incision is made from the center of the cervical incision to the xiphoid, and the sternum is divided. Successful transcervical mediastinal exploration is sometimes possible using the Cooper thymectomy retractor, a substernal retractor that permits more extensive mediastinal exploration and thymectomy through a cervical incision.[22] Any remaining thymic tissue is first isolated and examined. Inferior parathyroids most commonly migrate into the anterior mediastinum. If this exploration is negative, the area posterior and lateral to the trachea is then explored. Superior parathyroids may be found as far posterior as the esophagus and as far superior as the pharynx.

Surgical reexploration is successful in experienced hands in 60% to 80% of cases. There is an increased incidence of complications. Unilateral recurrent nerve injury occurs in 5% to 10% of patients and permanent hypoparathyroidism in 10% to 20% of patients postoperatively. Cryopreservation of excised tissue is an important component of the management of these patients, as it allows later autotransplantation if the patient becomes hypoparathyroid postoperatively. The risks of these complications are clearly outweighed by the clinical improvement in patients with advanced disease. Reoperation in asymptomatic patients with mild disease is controversial.

Hypercalcemic Crisis.   Occasionally, patients with hyperparathyroidism may become acutely hypercalcemic with severe symptoms. The pathogenesis appears to involve a vicious cycle of uncontrolled PTH secretion followed by hypercalcemia and secondary polyuria, dehydration, and reduced renal function, which exacerbates the hypercalcemia. Patients typically develop serum calcium concentrations in the range of 16 to 20 mg/dL, and the syndrome is manifested by rapidly developing muscle weakness, nausea and vomiting, lethargy, fatigue, and even coma. If the diagnosis of hyperparathyroidism is in question, ultrasound or CT scan may help to identify the enlarged gland.

Definitive treatment involves resecting the diseased parathyroid tissue, which is almost always curative. Generally, however, it is safer to lower the serum calcium level before operation.

Hyperparathyroidism in Pregnancy.   Hyperparathyroidism in pregnancy is a rare disorder that not only causes hypercalcemia in the mother but is associated with increased morbidity and mortality rates in the fetus. Even the newborn is at risk for the development of neonatal tetany. The risk of fetal complications is higher if the hyperparathyroidism is left untreated. The mother should undergo operation in the second trimester.

Neonatal Hyperparathyroidism.   Neonatal hyperparathyroidism occurs in infants who are homozygous for a mutation of the calcium-sensing receptor and is characterized by hypotonia, poor feeding, constipation, and respiratory distress.[6] Each parent of these children is affected by familial hypocalciuric hypercalcemia. The 1-year survival rate in children with symptoms is less than 50%, and patients without symptoms appear to have significant bone disease. Total parathyroidectomy with autotransplantation is the treatment of choice.[23]

Secondary Hyperparathyroidism.   Secondary hyperparathyroidism develops as a consequence of chronic renal failure. Phosphate retention and hyperphosphatemia reduce the serum calcium levels. This effect is aggravated by the reduction in 1-hydroxylase activity in the kidney, necessary for the activation of vitamin D_3. The secondary increase in PTH levels to compensate for these hypocalcemic effects is exacerbated by aluminum accumulation in bone. This aluminum, present both in the dialysate water and in phosphate-binding medications, contributes to the osteomalacia (renal osteodystrophy) that develops in all these patients after several years of dialysis. Therapy includes controlling the hyperphosphatemia by dietary restriction and phosphate-binding gels, calcium supplementation orally and in the dialysate bath, correction of acidosis, administration of vitamin D sterol, and reduction in aluminum intake in both the dialysate and the diet. Therapy should be initiated carefully because metastatic soft tissue calcification may occur. Indications for surgical therapy include persistent, symptomatic hypercalcemia that cannot be controlled medically, particularly in prospective renal transplant patients; bony pain and abnormal fractures; ectopic calcification; and intractable pruritus. Subtotal parathyroidectomy or total parathyroidectomy with heterotopic autotransplantation appear to be acceptable options, though reexploration for recurrent disease is less complicated after total parathyroidectomy with autotransplantation. Parathyroidectomy can actually enhance aluminum deposition, so any excess should be corrected preoperatively through chelation.

Parathyroid Carcinoma. Parathyroid carcinoma is a rare condition, accounting for less than 1% of all cases of hyperparathyroidism. Histologic criteria remain controversial, and the diagnosis is securely made only on the basis of local invasion or distant metastases. Compared with patients with benign disease, these patients tend to be somewhat younger and more symptomatic. In contrast to the marked female predominance in benign disease, the male to female ratio in carcinoma is equal. Serum calcium, PTH, and alkaline phosphatase levels are more elevated, and patients often have an elevated human chorionic gonadotrophin. Patients may have manifestations of both renal disease and bone disease. The affected gland is palpable in almost half of patients.

Initial treatment should include radical resection of the involved gland, the ipsilateral thyroid lobe, and the regional lymph nodes. Neither chemotherapy nor radiation therapy have shown any benefit. If the disease recurs, resection should be attempted because, if untreated, these patients usually succumb to uncontrolled hypercalcemia. The long-term prognosis is poor, and the opportunity for survival depends on complete initial resection.[24]

Multiple Endocrine Neoplasia

Although these familial disorders are typically characterized by a predisposition to the development of tumors of multiple endocrine organs, the parathyroid is characteristically involved in two of these conditions. These disorders are all inherited in an autosomal dominant fashion, and the tumors tend to be multicentric. The tumors may be benign or malignant and may occur metachronously or synchronously. MEN I is characterized by the concurrence of parathyroid hyperplasia, pancreatic islet cell tumors, and pituitary adenomas. MEN IIa consists of medullary thyroid carcinoma (MTC), pheochromocytoma, and parathyroid hyperplasia. MEN IIb includes MTC, pheochromocytoma, mucosal neuromas, and a distinctive marfanoid habitus. Together, these syndromes encompass much of the spectrum of endocrine neoplasia.

Pathogenesis

A unifying hypothesis for the MEN syndromes was offered by Pearse based on both embryologic and cytochemical studies.[25] He suggested that these tumors arise in cells that embryologically derive from the neural crest and are characterized by amine precursor uptake and decarboxylase activity (APUD cells). According to this theory, some defect in the development of the neural crest might explain the development of multicentric tumors in multiple organs. Although this could account for the development of MTC, pheochromocytomas, pituitary tumors, and the widespread nervous system hypertrophy of MEN IIb, the endocrine cells of the parathyroid and pancreas do not appear to be of neural crest origin. Subsequent attempts to develop another unifying hypothesis, whereby a tumor in one organ secretes endocrine products, which secondarily stimulate neoplasia in the other glands, have not been accepted. Although some evidence has suggested the presence of a mitogenic factor in the serum of patients with MEN I, direct attempts to define the pathophysiology have not proved rewarding. As a result, investigators in this area have taken a different approach, attempting to map the diseased gene through modern molecular genetic techniques.

In the case of MEN I, such methods have mapped the disease locus to the proximal long arm of chromosome 11. Compared with the normal cells of these patients, many of the tumors have demonstrated deletions in this region in one of the two normally present chromosomes, suggesting that these tumors may result from two separate mutations at a tumor suppressor gene, a model that has been demonstrated in other inherited neoplasms, such as retinoblastoma. According to this model, the first mutation is inherited and is unmasked only when the second mutation, in some cases a deletion, develops in susceptible endocrine tissues, resulting in complete loss of the tumor suppressor and the development of neoplasia. The occurrence of multiple second mutations would explain the multicentric involvement characteristic of these diseases.

Mutations of the *RET* protooncogene have recently been recognized as the cause of MEN IIa. Genetic testing is now available to identify affected family members, and to provide the opportunity for early treatment of medullary thyroid cancer in affected individuals.

Clinical Features and Management

Characteristically, MEN I develops in the third and fourth decades, and there is no gender predilection.[26] The gene is transmitted with nearly complete penetrance, and autopsy studies suggest that all three organs are affected in over 90% of patients. The phenotype varies, however, with over 90% of patients having hyperparathyroidism, but evidence of islet cell neoplasms (30% to 80%) and pituitary tumors (15% to 50%) is less common.

Parathyroid Disease. Hypercalcemia secondary to hyperparathyroidism is usually the first biochemical abnormality detected in MEN I and represents the best screening study for members of affected kindreds until direct genetic screening is available. Many of these patients are asymptomatic and have relatively mild hypercalcemia. When symptoms do develop, they typically involve the urinary tract rather than the skeleton.

Typically, these patients have four-gland disease, which may be particularly difficult to manage. These patients are best treated with total parathyroidectomy and heterotopic autotransplantation (as noted earlier).

Pancreatic Tumors. Patients with pancreatic tumors develop multicentric and diffuse hyperplasia of the pancreatic islets, which may occur in areas distant from any grossly evident tumor. In the absence of symptomatic disease, no solid evidence shows that screening for these tumors in affected kindred is of any benefit. In patients with hyperparathyroidism, the measurement of serum gastrin is helpful because gastrinomas are the most common islet cell lesion. Some evidence indicates that measuring serum concentrations of pancreatic polypeptide may provide a general screening measure for a variety of islet cell tumors.

Patients with gastrinomas typically develop a severe ulcer diathesis (Zollinger-Ellison syndrome) associated with secretory diarrhea. Serum gastrin levels are usually markedly elevated (above 100 pg/mL), although in patients with equivocal elevations (250 to 1000 pg/mL), provocative testing with secretin (2 μm/kg) may be useful. An absolute serum gastrin increase of 200 pg/mL is diagnostic.

Pancreatic tumors are typically multicentric and frequently malignant. In contrast to sporadic gastrinomas, biochemical cure of the gastrinoma is almost never possible, although exploration can reduce the need for antisecretory medications, and may reduce the risk of liver metastasis. H_2-receptor antagonists are often effective in controlling acid secretion, although very high doses may be necessary; the malignant disease is often indolent. In patients whose acid secretion is not controlled by H_2 blockers, omeprazole may be useful. Parietal cell vagotomy in this setting can reduce the amount of medications needed. Most surgeons now use total gastrectomy only as a last resort.

Insulinoma is the next most common pancreatic neoplasm. These tumors are usually small and multicentric. Patients present with a history of sweating, dizziness, confusion, and syncope consistent with neuroglycopenia and are relieved by consuming carbohydrates. The diagnosis is verified by documenting fasting hypoglycemia associated with inappropriately elevated plasma insulin levels. It appears that rapid calcium infusion is the most sensitive provocative test (Fig. 57-15). Preoperative tumor localization is usually achieved using a combination of CT scanning and arteriography along with transhepatic portal venous sampling for plasma insulin measurements to detect a gradient from specific pancreatic venous tributaries.

Because there is only limited medical therapy for insulinoma, these patients are treated operatively. Lesions in the tail of the gland can be enucleated if they are small, however distal pancreatectomy carries little morbidity. Tumors of the head can usually be enucleated, thereby avoiding pancreaticoduodenectomy. In patients with malignant disease, metastases may respond to streptozocin. Diazoxide, verapamil, or octreotide may successfully reduce insulin secretion and control symptoms. A complex carbohydrate diet can also help to stabilize serum glucose levels in the hyperinsulinemic patient.

Other islet cell lesions occur only rarely in association with MEN I.

Pituitary Adenomas. Prolactin-secreting tumors occur most commonly in this setting, although occasional patients develop Cushing disease or acromegaly. Symptoms may result from compression of the optic chiasm, which produces bitemporal hemianopsia, or from prolactin excess, which produces amenorrhea and galactorrhea in females and hypogonadism in males.

Bromocriptine inhibits prolactin secretion and shrinks many prolactinomas. Refractory tumors and those producing other hormones can be managed by pituitary ablation or radiation.

Other Tumors. MEN I is associated much less frequently with adrenocortical tumors and benign thyroid adenomas. Lipomas and carcinoid tumors may also occur.

Clinical Features

Like MEN I, the MEN II syndromes are inherited in an autosomal dominant fashion with complete penetrance but variable phenotype. Bilateral MTC occurs in every affected patient. More frequently than the other syndromes, MEN IIb may arise as a new mutation that can be transmitted to subsequent generations.

Medullary Thyroid Carcinoma. Medullary thyroid carcinoma accounts for about 10% of all thyroid malignancies, and 20% of cases occur in the familial setting of MEN IIa, MEN IIb, or familial non-MEN MTC. It is usually the first tumor that develops in these patients and typically appears in the second or third decade. Tumors are virtually always bilateral and develop in multiple areas of the middle and upper portions of the thyroid lobe (Fig. 57-16). Occasionally, in young people, a diffuse proliferation of parafollicular C cells, termed *C-cell hyperplasia,* is present without frankly invasive carcinoma. This finding is highly

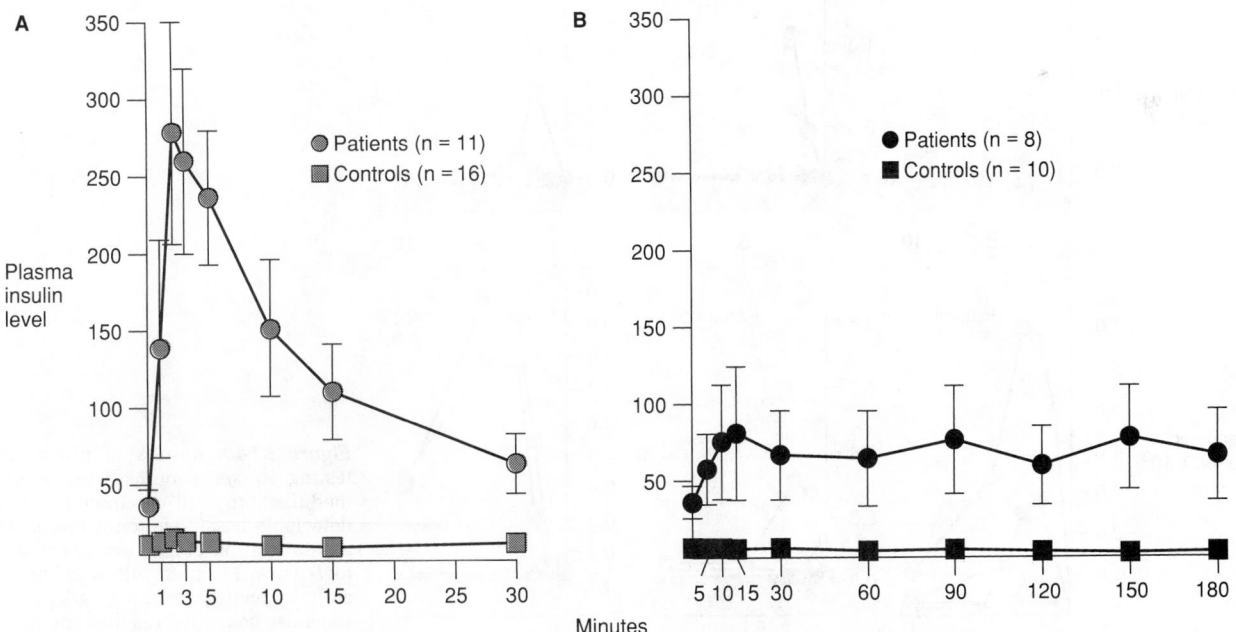

Figure 57-15. Provocative testing for insulinoma by rapid (2 mg/kg over 1 minute; *A*) or long (12 mg/kg over 3 hours; *B*) calcium infusion. Patients with insulinoma had a pronounced and rapid increase in plasma insulin levels when compared with normal controls. Effects of rapid calcium infusion were considerably more pronounced. (After Brunt LM, Veldhuis JD, Dilley WG, et al. Stimulation of insulin secretion by a rapid intravenous calcium infusion in patients with beta cell neoplasms of the pancreas. J Clin Endocrinol Metab 1986;62:210)

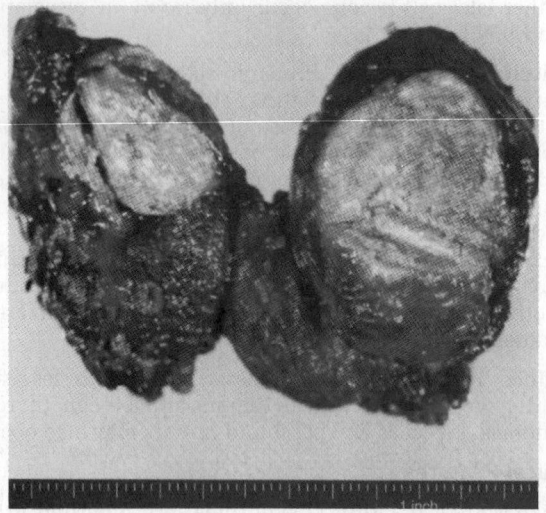

Figure 57-16. Primary medullary thyroid carcinoma from a total thyroidectomy specimen. The tumors are bilateral and centered in the upper pole.

suggestive of one of the familial MTC syndromes. Patients typically present with a neck mass and may have hoarseness, dysphagia, or palpable cervical adenopathy. Medullary thyroid carcinoma may produce a variety of hormones, including calcitonin, adrenocorticotrophic hormone, prostaglandin, and serotonin. The hypercalcitoninemia is often asymptomatic, although these patients can develop severe diarrhea.

By detecting minimal elevations of plasma calcitonin in patients, it is possible to diagnose MTC at a clinically occult stage.[27] Basal plasma calcitonin levels in normal subjects are in the range of 30 to 100 pg/mL. An increase to levels of 150 to 200 pg/mL occurs, however, after the administration of the potent secretagogues calcium and pentagastrin. Patients with MTC have striking increases (greater than 1000 pg/mL) in plasma calcitonin levels after provocative testing, which allows them to be readily identified. Patients with occult disease may have only minimally elevated basal calcitonin levels, which increase in response to secretagogues. The combined infusion of calcium and pentagastrin was the most effective screening test for familial MTC before genetic testing became available (Fig. 57-17). By provocative testing in kindred members at risk for disease, MTC was diagnosed at a preclinical stage, and a greater percentage of these patients were cured by surgical therapy. With genetic testing now available, early treatment of medullary thyroid cancer is possible for all affected people and will hopefully increase the number of people cured of this cancer.

Postoperatively, the presence of residual MTC can be readily detected by provocative testing. Recent reports have suggested that meticulous reoperation in patients with recurrent or persistently elevated plasma calcitonin levels postoperatively, including on occasion mediastinal dissection, can normalize elevated plasma calcitonin levels and apparently cure many of these patients.[28] In the patient with unresectable metastases, there are few therapeutic options. Neither radiation nor chemotherapy have significant benefit.

The clinical course of patients with the MEN type II syndromes is determined primarily by the status of their

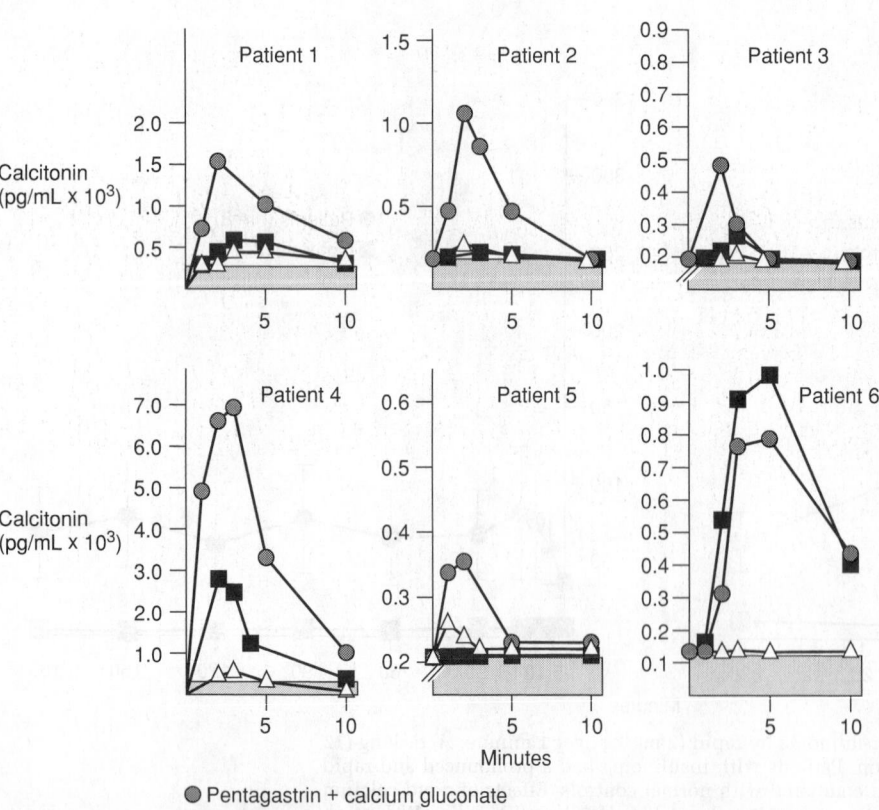

Figure 57-17. Results of provocative testing in six patients with familial medullary thyroid carcinoma and undetectable basal calcitonin levels. The administration of calcium gluconate, 2 mg/kg over 1 minute, followed immediately by pentagastrin, 0.5 μg/kg over 5 seconds, generally resulted in higher peak calcitonin levels than with either calcium gluconate or pentagastrin alone. (After Wells SA Jr, Baylin SB, Linehan WM, et al. Provocative agents and the diagnosis of medullary carcinoma of the thyroid gland. Ann Surg 1978;188:139)

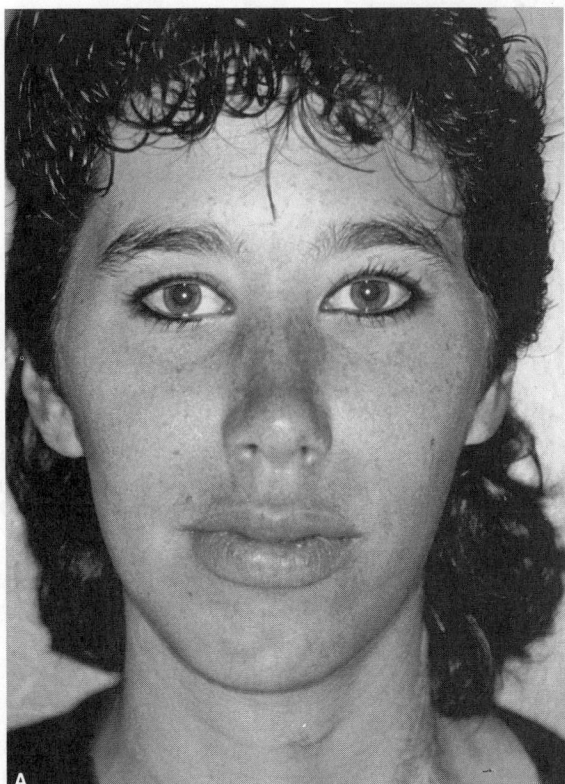
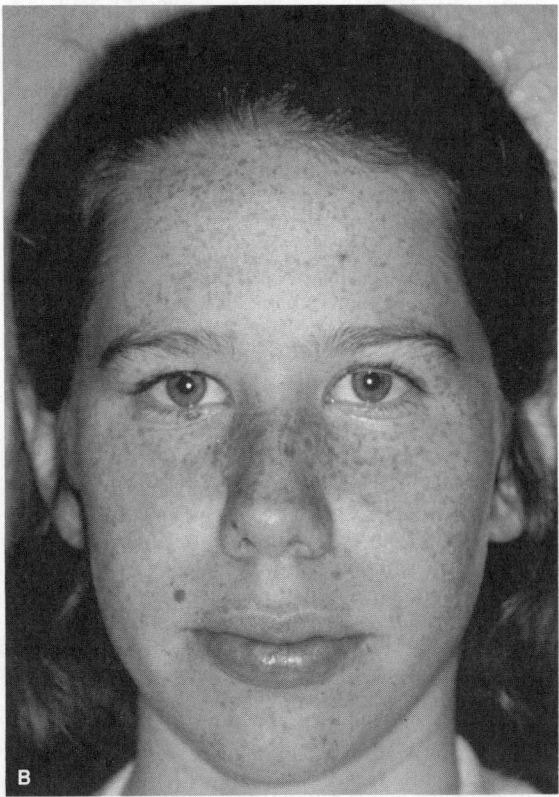
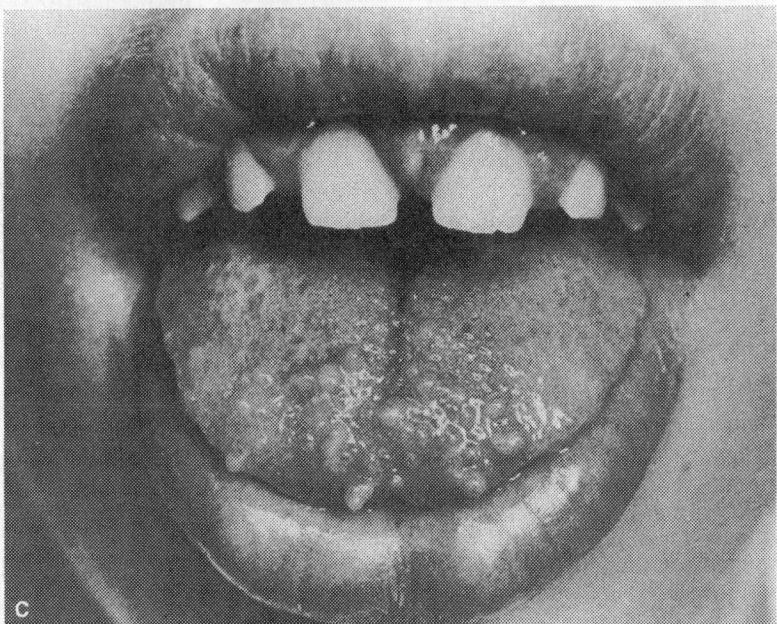

Figure 57-18. (*A* and *B*) Characteristic appearance of patients with
MEN 2b, demonstrating thick lips.
(*C*) Multiple mucosal neuromas on
the tongue of a patient with MEN 2b.
(Norton JA, Froome LC, Farrell FE,
et al. Multiple endocrine neoplasia
type 2b: the most aggressive form of
medullary thyroid carcinoma. Surg
Clin North Am 1979;59:109)

MTC. In the setting of MEN IIa, the tumors are often indolent with prolonged survival even in the presence of metastatic disease. By contrast, the tumors in patients with
MEN IIb occur at an earlier age and are generally more
aggressive neoplasms. Patients may succumb to the disease
at a young age. As a consequence of this aggressiveness,
the number of kindred with the disease is typically small,
and usually only a few generations are affected.

Pheochromocytomas. Pheochromocytomas are usually diagnosed during the initial screening or follow-up of
patients already diagnosed with MTC. They typically
appear in the second or third decade of life, and about 80%
are bilateral. Usually, they are benign but multicentric, and
they almost always arise in the adrenal medulla. Patients
with MEN IIa or IIb may first develop hyperplasia of the
adrenal medulla, grossly characterized by thickening of
the medullary tissue in both adrenal glands.

Pheochromocytomas may be asymptomatic, but most
commonly, patients develop pounding frontal headaches,
episodic diaphoresis, palpitations, or anxiety. Hypertension also occurs and is often episodic.

The diagnosis is made by measuring urinary excretion
of catecholamines and their metabolites. The best test is a
24-hour urine collection for total catecholamines, epinephrine, norepinephrine, metanephrine, and vanillylmandelic

acid. Patients with MEN IIa or IIb and MTC should be evaluated for pheochromocytoma before thyroidectomy. If the patient is found to have both lesions, adrenalectomy should be performed first, followed by neck exploration in 1 to 2 weeks. If urinary excretion rates are equivocal, CT scan of the abdomen can identify lesions 1 cm or larger in size, and sometimes hyperplasia is recognized. A relatively new technique for localization uses ^{131}I-metaiodobenzylguanidine scintigraphy. This agent, which is similar to norepinephrine, is taken up and stored in neurotransmitter vesicles. Normal glands are not visualized, whereas about 90% of pheochromocytomas can be seen. This test is particularly useful in identifying extraadrenal lesions. MR imaging is also sensitive for pheochromocytomas and has the advantage of differentiating pheochromocytoma from benign adenoma based on T2-weighted imaging characteristics.

Preoperatively, patients are hospitalized for α-adrenergic blockade with phenoxybenzamine. β-Adrenergic blockade with propranolol may be necessary if tachyarrhythmia subsequently develops, but it should not be initiated until after α-adrenergic blockade because of the risk of unopposed vasoconstriction. Intraoperative hypertension is controlled with a vasodilator, such as sodium nitroprusside or phentolamine. Patients are explored through the abdomen, with either a bilateral subcostal incision or a laparoscope, so that both adrenal glands, the sympathetic chain, and the organ of Zuckerkandl can all be examined. Bilateral pheochromocytomas are treated by bilateral adrenalectomy. In the patient with MEN II or IIb and a unilateral pheochromocytoma, only the diseased adrenal gland is removed. About 30% of patients treated in this manner eventually develop a tumor in the opposite gland. In the remaining patients, this approach avoids the necessity of glucocorticoid and mineralocorticoid replacement and the risks of addisonian crisis. After unilateral adrenalectomy, patients are carefully screened at 6-month or 1-year intervals.

Parathyroid Disease. Hyperparathyroidism develops in about one third of patients with MEN IIa, although it is usually asymptomatic. Occasionally, patients develop nephrolithiasis. Bone disease is unusual. Frequently, enlarged parathyroid glands are found at operation for MTC, although the patient is still normocalcemic. Multiglandular chief cell hyperplasia is the predominant histologic finding in MEN IIa. Parathyroid disease rarely develops in MEN IIb.

Total parathyroidectomy and heterotopic autotransplantation are performed in hypercalcemic patients with MEN IIa. In normocalcemic MEN IIa patients undergoing thyroidectomy for MTC, a total parathyroidectomy with heterotopic autotransplantation is performed at the same operation to ensure that the complete thyroidectomy does not compromise the parathyroid blood supply and to avoid reoperation in the neck for subsequent hyperparathyroidism. Evidence suggests that these patients are more easily treated, with a lower incidence of recurrent hyperparathyroidism than is seen in patients with MEN I.

Nonendocrine Manifestations of MEN IIb. In addition to MTC and pheochromocytoma, patients with MEN IIb develop marked abnormalities of the nervous and musculoskeletal systems. The classic phenotype is characterized by the presence of thick lips and a thin marfanoid habitus (Fig. 57-18A and B). There is a high incidence of associated skeletal abnormalities, including kyphosis, pectus excavatum, pes planus or cavus, and congenital dislocation of the hip. There is also evidence of diffuse autonomic nervous hypertrophy. Mucosal neuromas appear on the tongue (see Fig. 57-18C), eyelids, lips, and pharynx. Slit-lamp examination may reveal hypertrophied corneal nerves. Ganglioneuromatosis develops in the submucosal and myenteric plexuses of the gastrointestinal tract. Constipation is common, and radiographic findings may suggest megacolon or Hirschsprung disease.

REFERENCES

1. Akerstrom G, Malmaeus J, Bergstrom R. Surgical anatomy of human parathyroid glands. Surg 1984;95:14.
2. Mallette LE. Regulation of blood calcium in humans. Endocrinol Metabol Clin N Amer 1989;18:601.
3. Nussbaum SR. Pathophysiology and management of severe hypercalcemia. Endocrinol Metab Clin North Am 1993;22:343.
4. Strewler GJ, Nissenson RA. Hypercalcemia in malignancy. West J Med 1990;153:635.
5. Pollak MR, Brown EM, Chou Y-HW, et al. Mutations in the human Ca-sensing receptor gene cause familial hypocalciuric hypercalcemia and neonatal severe hyperparathyroidism. Cell 1993;75:1297.
6. Pollak MR, Chou Y-HW, Marx SJ, et al. Familial hypocalciuric hypercalcemia and neonatal severe hyperparathyroidism: effects of mutant gene dosage on phenotype. J Clin Invest 1994;93:1108.
7. Bilezikian JP. Management of acute hypercalcemia. N Engl J Med 1992;326:1196.
8. Tohme MF, Bilezikian JP. Hypocalcemic emergencies. Endocrinol Metab Clin North Am 1993;22:363.
9. Heath H. Clinical spectrum of primary hyperparathyroidism: evolution with changes in medical practice and technology. J Bone Miner Res 1991;6(Suppl 2):S63.
10. Heath H, Hodgson SF, Kennedy MA. Primary hyperparathyroidism: incidence, morbidity and potential economic impact in a community. N Engl J Med 1980;302:189.
11. Arnold A. Molecular mechanisms of parathyroid neoplasia. Endocrinol Metab Clin North Am 1994;23:93.
12. Larsson C, Friedman E. Localization and identification of the multiple endocrine neoplasia type 1 disease gene. Endocrinol Metab Clin North Am 1994;23:67.
13. Mulligan LM, Kwok JBJ, Healey CS, et al. Germ-line mutation of the RET proto-oncogene in multiple endocrine neoplasia type 2A. Nature 1993;363:458.
14. Donis-Keller H, Dou S, Chi D, et al. Mutations in the RET proto-oncogene are associated with MEN 2A and FMTC. Hum Mol Genet 1993;2:851.
15. Roth SI. Recent advances in parathyroid gland pathology. Am J Med 1994;50:612.
16. Levin KE, Chew KL, Ljung B-M, et al. Deoxyribonucleic acid cytometry helps identify parathyroid carcinomas. J Clin Endocrinol Metab 1994;67:779.
17. Wells SA, Leight GF, Ross A. Primary hyperparathyroidism. Curr Probl Surg 1980;17:398.
18. Potts JT Jr, Ackerman IP, Barker CF, et al. Diagnosis and management of asymptomatic primary hyperparathyroidism: consensus development conference statement. Ann Intern Med 1991;114:593.
19. Scholz DA, Purnell DC. Asymptomatic primary hyperparathyroidism: 10 year prospective study. Mayo Clin Proc 1981;56:473.
20. Wells SA, Leight GS, Hensley M, et al. Hyperparathyroidism associated with the enlargement of two or three parathyroid glands. Ann Surg 1994;202:523.
21. Doherty GM, Doppman JL, Miller DL, et al. Results of a multidisciplinary strategy for management of mediastinal parathyroid adenoma as a cause of persistent primary hyperparathyroidism. Ann Surg 1992;215:101.
22. Wells SA, Cooper JD. Closed mediastinal exploration in patients With persistent hyperparathyroidism. Ann Surg 1991;214:555.
23. Key LL, Thorne M, Pitzer B, et al. Management of neonatal hyperparathyroidism with parathyroidectomy and autotransplantation. J Pediatr 1990;116:923.
24. Wang C, Gaz RD. Natural history of parathyroid carcinoma. Diagnosis, treatment, and results. Am J Surg 1985;149:522.
25. Pearse AGE. Common cytochemical and ultrastructural char-

APUD series) and their relevance to the thyroid and ultimobranchial C-cells and calcitonin. Proc R Soc Lond B Biol Soc 1968;170:71.

26. Skogseid B, Rastad J, Oberg K. Multiple endocrine neoplasia type 1: Clinical features and screening. Endocrinol Metab Clin North Am 1994;23:1.
27. Cance WG, Wells SAJ. Multiple endocrine neoplasia type IIa. Curr Probl Surg 1985;22:1.
28. Moley JF, Wells SA, Dilley WG, et al. Reoperation for recurrent or persistent medullary thyroid cancer. Surgery 1993; 114:1090.

SURGERY: SCIENTIFIC PRINCIPLES AND PRACTICE, Second Edition, edited by Lazar J. Greenfield, Michael W. Mulholland, Keith T. Oldham, Gerald B. Zelenock, and Keith D. Lillemoe. Lippincott–Raven Publishers, Philadelphia, © 1997.

CHAPTER 58

ADRENAL GLANDS

H.H. NEWSOME, JR.

ANATOMY
Total Gland

The adrenal glands are paired structures located on each side of the body superior to the kidneys. They are flat and triangular structures, each weighing about 5 g. Three sets of adrenal arteries predominate—the *superior adrenal artery* is a branch of the inferior phrenic artery; the *middle adrenal artery* originates from the aorta on each side; and the *inferior adrenal artery* arises from each renal artery. Although some small random veins handle some effluent, most drainage is through a single, well-defined central vein, which empties into the renal vein on the left and into the vena cava on the right. Blood flow within the gland is predominantly from the cortex through the medulla into the central medullary venous system, forming the large adrenal vein. The adrenal gland is composed of two distinct regions. The outer, bright yellow, lipid-laden cortex gives the gland its characteristic external appearance. Sandwiched between the layers of the cortex is the thin, dark gray medulla. These features and relations are shown in Figure 58-1.[1]

Adrenal Cortex
Embryology

The cortex is mesodermal in origin. It arises near the gonads on the adrenogenital ridge at about the fifth week of gestation. This location explains the bits of cortical tissue (adrenal rests) found in various sites, such as the ovaries, spermatic cords, and testes. Histologically, fetal zonation of the cortex disappears shortly after birth.

Microscopy

The fully developed cortex is organized into three distinct zones. The *zona glomerulosa* is found just under the fibrous, outer capsule of the gland and contains ovoid clusters of cells. This thin, indistinct layer is the site of production of the mineralocorticoid, aldosterone. The middle layer, the *zona fasciculata,* is composed of cells in linear patterns arranged at right angles to the surface of the gland. The cells are full of lipid and are the source of the carbohy-drate-active steroid, cortisol, and the adrenal sex steroids. The internal layer, the *zona reticularis,* lies adjacent to the medulla, and the cells are arranged in a more random, sheetlike pattern. The cells of the inner zone are lipid replete. They secrete cortisol, androgens, and estrogens, and they maintain cholesterol stores as a precursor for steroidogenesis. A schematic representation of these zones is shown in Figure 58-2.

Adrenal Medulla
Embryology

The medulla is ectodermal in origin and is derived specifically from the neural crest. It is first seen in the 10-mm embryo and insinuates itself into the cluster of adrenocortical cells. The early cells from the neural crest are grouped into the *chromocell* system and the *neuronal system.* Both elements are represented in the population of adrenal medulla cells and explain the development of two distinct tumors—pheochromocytomas and neuroblastomas.

Microscopy

With light microscopy, the medullary cells appear as homogenous sheets with nestlike or cordlike orientation and abundant cytoplasm. Their large nuclei are characterized by variation in size and shape and by the occasional presence of abnormal forms. Of clinical significance is their content of catecholamines and other substances, such as neuron-specific enolase and chromogranin. These substances help to identify tumors arising from the neural elements.

On electron microscopy, abundant secretory granules can be seen in the cytoplasm of medullary cells. Their presence is in contrast to the adrenocortical cells, in which a similar abundance of smooth endoplasmic reticulum, mitochondria, and Golgi complexes are seen, but few secretory granules are present. The medullary secretory granules containing epinephrine are slightly smaller than those containing norepinephrine and are more electron dense, with a loose-fitting membrane. The granules are carried to the periphery of the cell, where catecholamines and other contents are released by exocytosis into the surrounding milieu.

PHYSIOLOGY
Adrenocortical Secretion

Although the control of secretion of the major categories of corticosteroid products differs somewhat, the early steroidogenic pathway is common to all steroids (Fig. 58-3). Generally, however, cholesterol is converted to $\delta 5$-pregnenolone, progesterone, 17-OH progesterone, and then either to the adrenal androgens or cortisol. Progesterone is converted to aldosterone by a different pathway. The amount of 17-ketosteroids (adrenal androgens) produced is 25 to 30 mg/d; 15 to 20 mg/d of the 17-hydroxysteroids (cortisol) is produced and 75 to 125 μg/d of aldosterone. As mentioned, aldosterone is produced primarily in zona glomerulosa, whereas the 17-ketosteroids and 17-OH corticosteroids are produced in the zonae fasciculata and reticularis. The outer zone and the latter two inner zones are under separate regulatory mechanisms.

Control of Cortisol Secretion

The proximate stimulator of cortisol production is the peptide hormone, adrenocorticotropic hormone (ACTH). It originates from the anterior pituitary gland and is regulated by corticotropin-releasing hormone (CRH). CRH is stored in the anterior hypothalamus and, on stimulation,

A

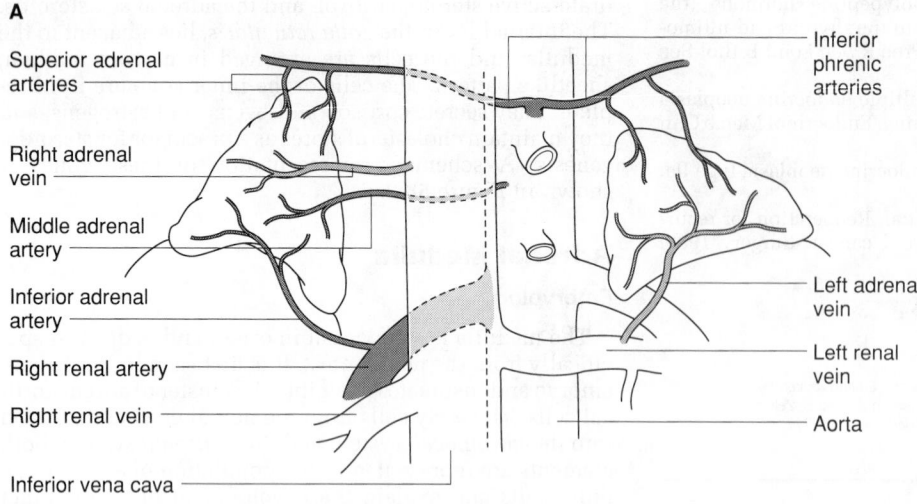

B

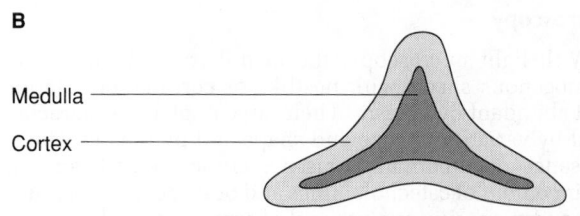

Figure 58-1. (*A*) The arterial and venous anatomy of the right and left adrenal glands. (*B*) Division of the gland into the outer cortex and inner medulla.

is released into the pituitary portal system where it reaches the anterior pituitary gland and releases ACTH. The stimulation of CRH is controlled by various neural influences. From the diurnal variation in CRH secretion, it is probable that intrinsic central nervous system influences are present. The increased cortisol production during fear or other emotional stress is another indicator of central nervous system regulation. On the other hand, the striking increase of cortisol secretion during pain and physical trauma attests to the importance of peripheral sensory pathways in stimulating cortisol production.

Release of CRH is under negative-feedback inhibition by cortisol. Although there is some evidence of a short-loop feedback of ACTH on CRH, both the slow and fast feedback by cortisol on the pituitary release mechanism are clinically noteworthy. Under normal circumstances, the set-point for negative-feedback inhibition of ACTH secretion is in the physiologic range of plasma cortisol concentrations. That is, a plasma cortisol concentration in the high-normal range of 15 to 20 μg/dL of plasma results in suppressed ACTH secretion and a consequent lowering of cortisol secretion by the adrenal cortex. Evidence also suggests that the fast feedback suppression, effected by acutely rising plasma cortisol concentrations, can suppress both CRH release and the response of ACTH to the stimulus of CRH. Considering the short half-life of plasma ACTH (measured in minutes) and its rapid onset of action compared with the longer plasma half-life of steroids and their slower onset of action, it is remarkable that this system can accomplish such fine homeostatic adjustment of plasma cortisol within a fairly narrow range. The feedback relations are shown in Figure 58-4.

Clinically important examples of the slow feedback mechanism occur during chronic exogenous steroid administration for steroid-dependent diseases or during endogenous steroid excess from adrenocortical tumors. Under either circumstance, the pituitary adrenal axis is suppressed not only during the period of steroid excess

but also for weeks and months after the steroid excess is corrected. The secretion of adrenal androgens, which are converted peripherally to estrogens, is basically controlled by the same mechanisms as cortisol secretion. This is distinct from the estrogens and androgens secreted by the gonads, which are regulated by a completely different set of pituitary peptides.

Control of Aldosterone Secretion

The primary proximate control of aldosterone secretion is by the octapeptide, angiotensin II. The production of circulating angiotensin II begins with the action of a peptidase enzyme, renin, which is produced predominately in the juxtaglomerular apparatus of the kidney, where it acts locally and where it is released into the system circulation. Both locally and when released, renin cleaves angiotensin I, a decapeptide derived from a large hepatic protein serving as renin substrate. Angiotensin I undergoes enzymatic cleavage in the lung to angiotensin II, which is the biologically active form of the peptide. Conversion of angiotensin I to angiotensin II is about 90% complete with one passage through the lung. The carboxypeptidase that is responsible for this cleavage is known as angiotensin-converting enzyme.

The rate of renin secretion is controlled by changes in the afferent arteriolar pressure in the renal cortex as well as by changes in sodium content in the renal tubule. These changes are sensed by the juxtaglomerular apparatus and by the macula densa. In general, a decrease in arterial pressure or in the sodium content of the renal tubule results in an increase in renin and angiotensin II production, with a subsequent increase in aldosterone secretion. Conversely, a sodium load, overhydration, or assumption of the supine position normally results in a decrease in renin and angiotensin production and a subsequent fall in aldosterone secretion.

At least two other factors influence aldosterone secretion. Aldosterone secretion is directly related to the serum

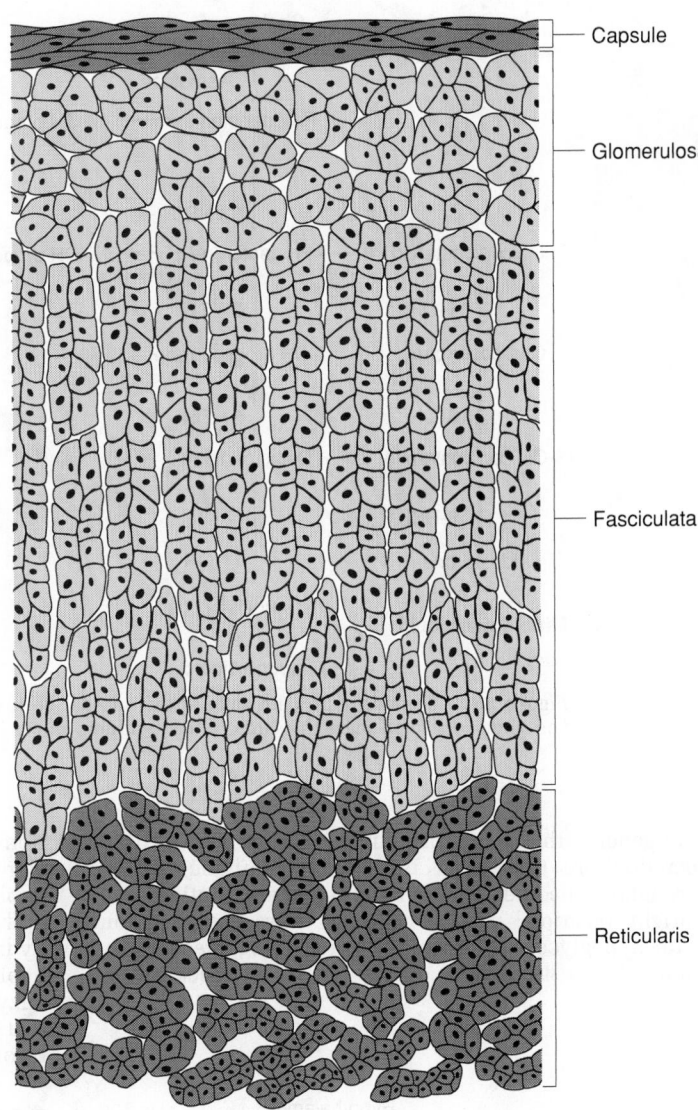

Capsule

Glomerulosa

Fasciculata

Reticularis

Medulla

Figure 58-2. Schematic representation of the microscopic anatomy of the adrenal cortex.

potassium concentration. In view of aldosterone's ability to promote potassium excretion in the urine, it is not surprising that an increase in serum potassium directly stimulates aldosterone production, whereas a decrease in serum potassium has the opposite effect. Because of its early point of action in the steroidogenic pathway, ACTH also increases aldosterone secretion, although it is much less potent in this regard than in its stimulation of cortisol. The stimulatory effects of potassium and ACTH on aldosterone secretion can be overcome by angiotensin II stimulation. These concepts are summarized in Figure 58-5.

Adrenomedullary Secretion

In reviewing the control of medullary secretion, it is useful to think of the adrenal medulla as a sympathetic ganglion. Instead of innervating postganglionic cells, the preganglionic sympathetic fibers innervate the secretory chromaffin cells. Stimulation of these cells increases the tyrosine hydroxylase activity and also moves the secretory granules to the surface of the cell, where exocytosis results in a discharge of the secretory product. The metabolic pathway in the medulla that culminates in catecholamine

production is as follows. Tyrosine is converted to dihydroxyphenylalanine and then to dopamine as the immediate precursor to norepinephrine. Norepinephrine is converted to epinephrine. The various compound structures and enzyme names are shown in Figure 58-6. A portion of the released norepinephrine and epinephrine is taken up again by the chromaffin cells, and part is released into the systemic circulation. In the systemic circulation, the catecholamines can undergo neuronal uptake and subsequent degradation, enzymatic degradation by other sites, or excretion in the urine. The catecholamines taken up by neurons are metabolized predominately by monoamine oxidase, and they eventually yield vanillylmandelic acid (VMA). The enzyme, carboxy-o-methyl transferase, is responsible for the extraneuronal inactivation. The major metabolic product of this enzyme is normetanephrine for norepinephrine or metanephrine for epinephrine. Another fraction of the circulating catecholamines binds to tissue receptors for epinephrine and norepinephrine, and biologic effects are achieved. A small fraction is also excreted in the urine as free epinephrine and norepinephrine, which provides a useful way to diagnose pheochromocytomas.

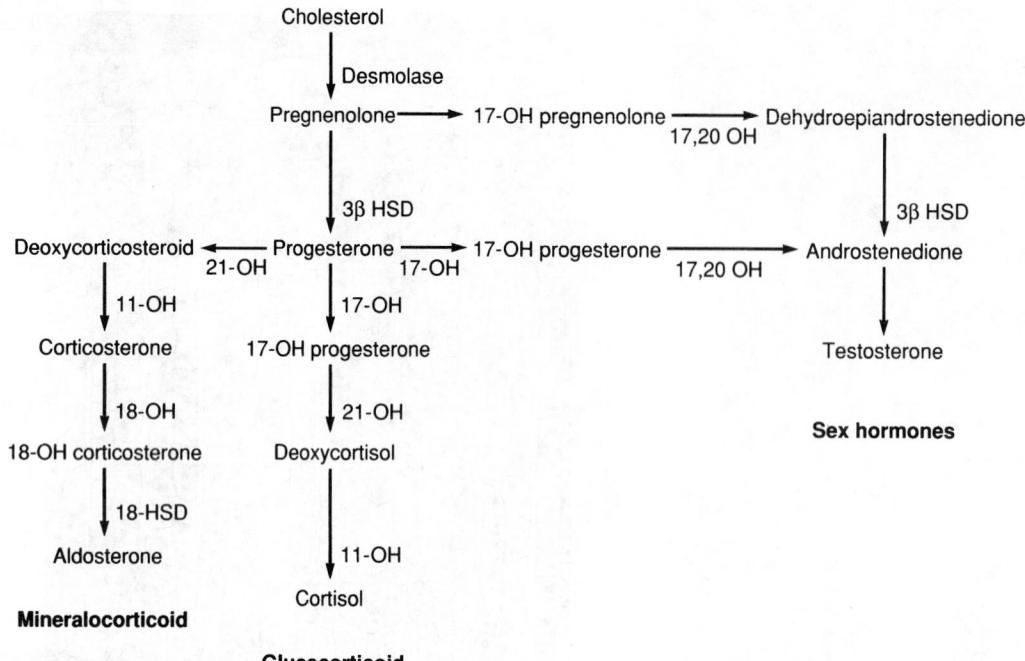

Figure 58-3. Steroidogenic pathways of the adrenal cortex. Sex hormones, mineralocorticoids, and glucocorticoids share the same initial synthetic steps.

In general, the factors that stimulate adrenal medullary secretion are those that increase sympathetic activity throughout the body. These include the assumption of an upright position, pain, emotional stress, hypotension, cold, hypoglycemia, and many others. Two mechanisms diminish the stimulatory effects. One is feedback inhibi-

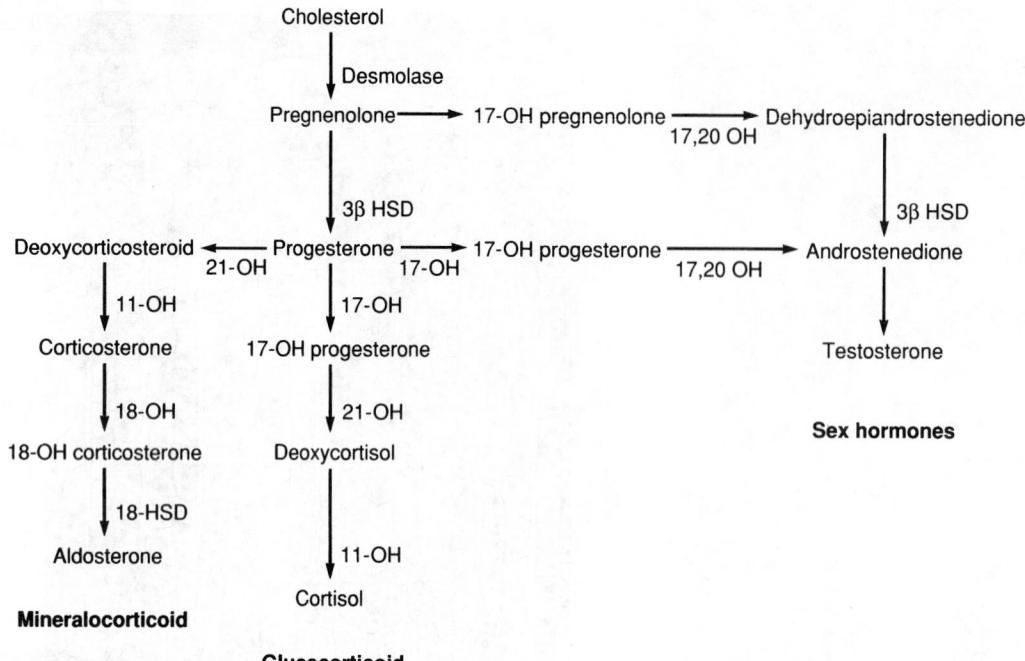

Figure 58-4. The feedback relations between the adrenal gland, the hypothalamus, and the anterior pituitary.

tion by norepinephrine on the presynaptic, preganglionic α_2-receptors. Stimulation of these receptors by norepinephrine decreases the release of acetylcholine. The second feedback mechanism is the suppression of tyrosine hydroxylase activity by high concentrations of norepinephrine. Because tyrosine hydroxylase is the rate-limiting enzyme in the synthetic pathway, increasing levels of the end product, norepinephrine, limit its own production through the effects on this short, negative-feedback loop.

PATHOPHYSIOLOGY

For the surgeon concerned with the adrenal gland, functional pathology is heavily weighted toward tumor formation. Some of the other entities, however, such as steroidogenic enzymatic defects in congenital adrenal hyperplasia, are important and are considered here. In general, hormonal overproduction is the characteristic underlying problem. Before considering the clinical impact of these states, it is necessary to examine the effects of steroids and catecholamines on peripheral tissues.

Steroids

After secretion into the blood, most steroid molecules are bound to specific plasma proteins and are present only to a limited degree in unbound, or free, form. Except in unusual situations in which there is an excess of steroid-binding proteins, increased total circulating hormone accurately reflects increased secretion. This is usually seen with stress states, functioning tumors, or congenital adrenal hyperplasia.

The circulating unbound steroid molecules pass freely through the cellular membrane of the target cell, where they bind with a specific cytosolic receptor. After the receptor transforms, the receptor–steroid complex is translocated into the nucleus. In the nucleus, this complex directs new messenger RNA production and thus results in new biologic behavior of the target cell. The general schema

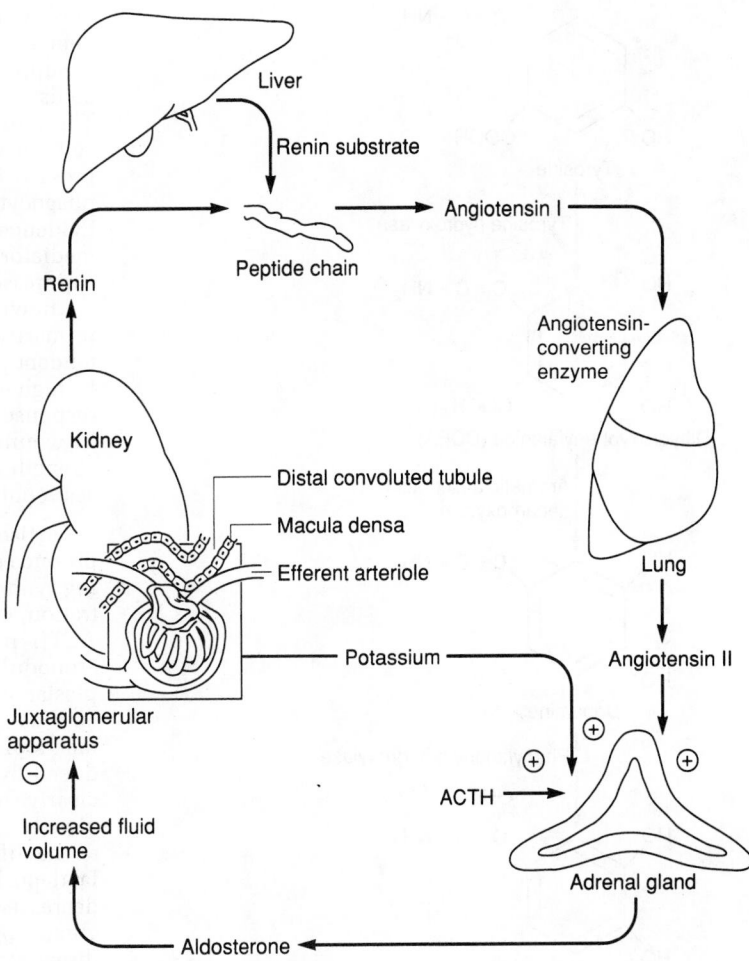

Figure 58-5. The relations of renin, angiotensin I, angiotensin II, and their anatomic sites of production and enzymatic conversion.

of cytosolic receptor and nuclear signal transduction is common to all steroids. It is the distribution of receptors, specific for each of the steroids, among various cell populations that determines the differential effects of steroids among tissues. Cortisol, which is the key endogenous hormone for carbohydrate-active effects, has receptors in almost all tissues of the body. Androgenic and estrogenic receptors are somewhat more restricted in their distribution, with key cell populations in such organs as breast, prostate, and external genitalia, although effects of sex steroids can be demonstrated in some other cells, such as hepatocytes. The mineralocorticoids, such as aldosterone and deoxycorticosterone, have receptors with an even more limited distribution to target tissues, such as the renal tubule, salivary glands, and colonic mucosa.

Cortisol

Normal Effects. Of the many systemic effects of the glucocorticoids, most are probably related to their effect on intermediary metabolism. In this regard, perhaps the most important action is the effect of steroids on protein breakdown. A direct proteolytic effect of steroids has been suggested by several lines of evidence. The glucocorticoids release branched-chain and other amino acids from muscle. This release provides substrate for gluconeogenesis and is one of the several mechanisms by which steroids produce an increase in this process. The steroid-induced release of amino acids from muscle occurs even in the absence of insulin and is not simply an antiinsulin effect. In addition to the direct proteolytic effect on muscle, ste-

roids accentuate the release of lactate from muscle. Both the lactate from muscle and the glycerol from fat cells released under the influence of epinephrine are additional precursors for gluconeogenesis. The glucocorticoids also have a direct effect on several of the gluconeogenetic hepatic enzymes, all of which promote hyperglycemia. Gluconeogenesis is one of the two primary mechanisms whereby glucocorticoids promote hyperglycemia. On the other side of the equation, glucocorticoids effect a decrease in glucose use by peripheral tissues. There appears to be an inhibition of glucose transport into fat cells. Second, glucocorticoids appear to decrease insulin binding by insulin-sensitive tissues. Together, the decrease in peripheral use of glucose and the increased production of glucose primarily by gluconeogenesis explain the tendency toward hyperglycemia produced by glucocorticoids. The final aspect of glucocorticoid influence on substrate use is the apparent accentuation of lipolysis by these steroids. Both serum triglycerides and free fatty acids are increased. Such an effect is obviously countered by that of insulin on adipocytes. It is believed that the truncal obesity seen in steroid excess is related to the predominance of the lipogenic effect of insulin on these truncal adipocytes over the lipolytic effect of glucocorticoids. The opposite relation may hold true for the receptors in fat of the extremities and would explain the comparatively scant fat in these areas with steroid excess.

Glucocorticoids have effects specific to particular systems, including the gastrointestinal tract, the cardiovascular system, kidneys, and bone, and to specific processes,

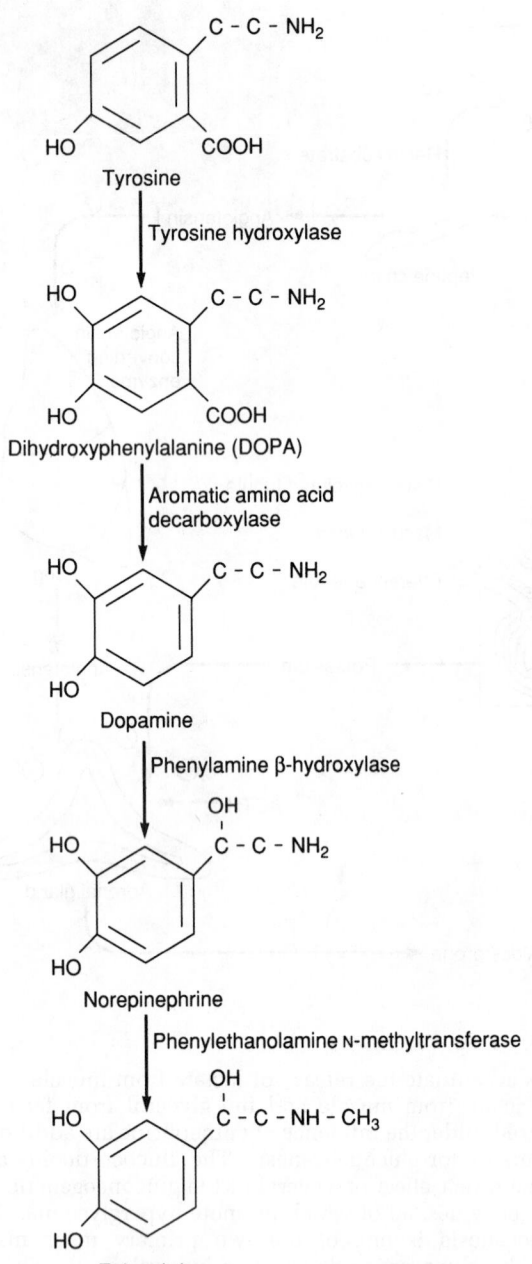

Figure 58-6. The enzymatic and structural relations on which the adrenal medullary synthesis of catecholomines depends.

including the inflammatory response, immune function, and wound healing. The most notable effect in the gastrointestinal tract is a decrease in the rate of mucosal cell replication. In addition, decreased mucosal and pancreatic prostaglandin synthesis occurs. This may have important implications for the cytoprotective mechanisms in the stomach and for maintaining pancreatic acinar integrity in the face of various insults. In the cardiovascular system, glucocorticoids appear to produce an increased chronotropic and inotropic effect on the heart along with an increased peripheral vascular resistance. Receptors in the distal renal tubules respond to glucocorticoids by inducing increased tubular resorption of sodium. These are a different class of receptors from those mediating the more potent actions of aldosterone. In bone, there is a clear decrease in the rate of bone formation. This is probably secondary to

delay in osteoblast development, resulting in qualitatively deficient protein constituents of the extracellular matrix.

Suppression of the inflammatory response by glucocorticoids is a particularly germane issue for surgical patients. The most obvious effect is the decrease of mononuclear cells in wounds. The function of these cells is also suppressed in terms of deficient chemotaxis and inadequate phagocytosis. Consequently, bacterial activity increases. Evidence is also accumulating that production of soluble mediators, important in the inflammatory process, may be suppressed in response to excess steroids.

Known steroidal effects on immune function are seen primarily in the behavior of cellular elements. There is a tendency to leukocytosis, eosinophilia, and lymphopenia. In higher ranges of steroid excess, there is a diminished response of lymphocytes to antigen stimulation. Finally, in wound healing, steroid-induced reductions in tensile strength are clearly demonstrable along with suppressed scar contraction and delayed epithelialization.

Cortisol Excess.   The varied causes of cortisol excess produce clinical features that are collectively called *Cushing syndrome*.[2] These include exogenous steroid administration, Cushing disease (pituitary ACTH excess), ectopic ACTH production, adrenal adenoma or carcinoma, micronodular pigmented hyperplasia, macronodular hyperplasia, and steroid-dependent adrenal hyperplasia. These entities are reviewed later in this chapter. Although treatments of these modalities differ, the clinical picture produced by the various causes is virtually the same and is clearly related to the cortisol actions mentioned previously. The peculiar fat distribution is probably related to the differential insulin and steroid receptors in various fat depositions in the body. Hyperglycemia is related to the decreased peripheral use of glucose as well as to increased gluconeogenesis. Muscle-wasting is primarily the result of direct steroidal effects on proteolysis. Abdominal striae and tendency to poor wound healing can be related to suppression of both scar contraction and inflammatory response. Increased susceptibility to infection is also related to immunosuppression. The apparent increases in incidence of peptic ulcer disease and acute pancreatitis are related to the effects on the gastrointestinal tract. Sodium retention and the effects on the cardiovascular system contribute to hypertension. Osteoporosis and perhaps growth retardation in children are related in part to the steroidal effects on bone growth. Although the primary manifestations of adrenal disorders in children are those of sexual ambiguity and virilization, as described later, the delay in growth is a particularly notable feature in children with glucocorticoid excess. Some of the extensive effects of cortisol are outlined in Table 58-1.

Androgens and Estrogens

Quantitatively, the major adrenal androgens are dehydroepiandrosterone, androstenedione, and testosterone. Androstenedione is the principal androgen converted in peripheral tissues to estrogens, and testosterone is the most potent masculinizing steroid on a per-weight basis.

Normal Effects.   In adults, androgens have the obvious effect of deepening the voice, producing a male hair distribution, coarsening the skin, toughening and darkening facial hair, and promoting protein deposition in muscles. Estrogens have virtually opposite effects. Androgens in the fetus stimulate wolffian duct development and elongate the genital tubercle. They promote midline migration of the labial folds and a fusion of these folds to form the scrotum. To complete the transformation, the urethral opening migrates to the tip of the phallus. All these events are androgen-dependent. Since the ovary in the normal

Table 58-1. SYSTEMIC EFFECTS OF CORTISOL

Function	Normal Amounts	Excessive Amounts
Metabolic		
Protein	Proteolysis	Muscle wasting
Glucose	Gluconeogenesis	Hyperglycemia
Fat	Low-use peripheral lipolysis	Limb thinness
	Central lipogenesis	Truncal obesity
Gastrointestinal	Mucosal cells	Ulceration
	Prostaglandin	Pancreatitis(?)
Cardiovascular	Chronotropic, inotropic	Hypertension
	Vascular resistance	
Renal	Sodium resorption	Hypertension
Bone	Osteoblastic development	Osteoporosis
Inflammatory and immune	Circulating cells	Infection
	Soluble mediators	
	Antigen processing	
Wound healing	Fibroblasts	Striae
	Epithelial cells	Dehiscence

female fetus does not secrete androgens, the genital tubercle, labial folds, and urethral opening all remain in the normal female position in this circumstance. Excess androgen in the male fetus manifests itself only after birth, when masculinization and precocious puberty are in evidence. Excess androgen in the female fetus causes neonatal virilization, as is seen with congenital adrenal hyperplasia.

Excess Sex Steroids. In both the child and adult, excess androgen or estrogen production by the adrenal gland almost always arises from carcinoma. Androgen excess in the female, in addition to producing the masculinizing features already mentioned, results in clitoral hypertrophy and, in the adult, menstrual cessation. Androgen excesses are difficult to detect in adult men, but in children precocious puberty occurs. In the rare adrenal carcinoma producing estrogen, menstrual irregularities may be the only clinical manifestation in the female, whereas the male may experience disturbing loss of libido, enlarged breast tissue, and female distribution of hair.

Enzymatic defects in the steroidogenic pathway can produce the syndrome known as *congenital adrenal hyperplasia*.[3] This syndrome presents predominantly in the neonatal period with sexual ambiguity. These enzymatic defects result in a lowered cortisol secretion, with consequent increased ACTH production and stimulation in the early steroidogenic pathway (Fig. 58-7). The specific enzyme defects present determine which clinical form the syndrome takes. The most common form is 21-hydroxylase deficiency. Both this defect and the 11β-hydroxylase deficiency result in excess androgen production in utero and masculinization with ambiguous genitalia in the female newborn. Masculinizing effects in the male may not be detected until precocious puberty is obvious. About 40% of patients with 21-hydroxylase deficiency have saltwasting or sodium loss by urine, which, in males, may result in earlier detection than in those without saltwasting. In the 11β-hydroxylase deficiency, there may also be hypertension because of excess secretion of deoxycorticosterone. In the 17-hydroxylase deficiency, hypertension caused by excess secretion of deoxycorticosterone and corticosterone occurs, and the testes may not secrete androgens, which may result in ambiguous female genitalia. In the female, ovarian failure to secrete estrogen prevents the appearance of secondary sex characteristics at the time of puberty. The 3-hydroxysteroid dehydrogenase deficiency is similar to the 21-hydroxylase deficiency, especially with

regard to the salt-wasting variety, in that both mineralocorticoid and glucocorticoid synthesis may be decreased. In both the 21-hydroxylase deficiency and the 3-hydroxysteroid dehydrogenase deficiency, mild forms may not become obvious until later in childhood, when precocious puberty may draw attention to the excess androgen secretion.

Aldosterone

Normal Effects. Aldosterone is the primary mineralocorticoid in humans. It influences sodium, potassium, and hydrogen ion transport. Receptors for aldosterone are found in the parotid gland and colonic mucosa, but the principal site of action is the distal renal tubule. Aldosterone increases tubular sodium resorption and decreases sodium excretion and potassium resorption with kaliuresis. Aldosterone also increases secretion of hydrogen ion into the urine. Under normal conditions, aldosterone secretion is controlled by total body sodium and potassium content and is relatively constant around a physiologic set-point regardless of variations in intake. Excess sodium intake suppresses renin secretion, angiotensin formation, and aldosterone secretion. The deficit in aldosterone results in increased urinary sodium loss and excretion of the administered sodium load. Conversely, a negative sodium balance stimulates renin, angiotensin, and aldosterone secretion, with resorption of sodium from the urine. This results in conservation of sodium and prevention of further negative sodium balance. Aldosterone control also affords some protection from excess serum potassium levels in

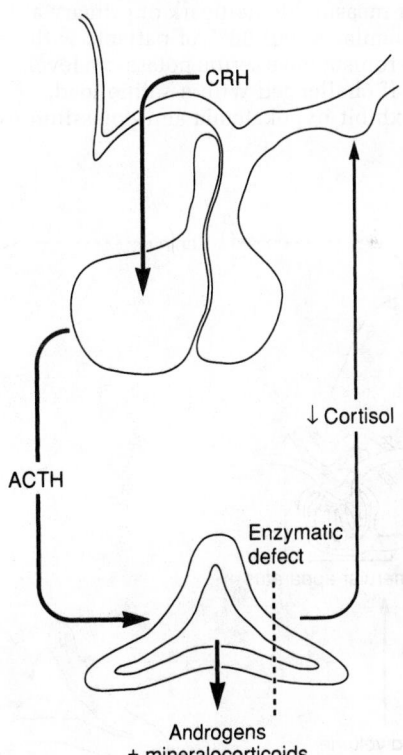

Figure 58-7. A variety of heritable enzymatic defects block the adrenal production of cortisol. This results in the loss of negative feedback to the hypothalamus with continued stimulation and excess production of androgens and possibly mineralocorticoids. The result is the congenital adrenal hyperplasia syndrome. The most common enzymatic deficiencies are 21-hydroxylase, 11β-hydroxylase and 3β-hydroxysteroid dehydrogenase (see Fig. 58-3).

that hyperkalemia stimulates aldosterone secretion, which in turn promotes renal potassium loss and helps lower serum potassium levels.

Aldosterone Excess. Primary hyperaldosteronism occurs with certain abnormal adrenal entities, in which secretion is not only excessive but autonomous; that is, it does not suppress by the usual mechanisms. These adrenal entities are adenoma, primary hyperplasia of the zona glomerulosa, and adrenal carcinoma producing aldosterone.[4] The rarity of adenomas that produce deoxycorticosterone precludes further mention here. Causes of secondary hyperaldosteronism are related to increased renin secretion, such as renal artery stenosis, congestive heart failure, and renal salt-wasting. Juxtaglomerular hyperplasia (Bartter syndrome) is a rare, nonhypertensive form of secondary hyperaldosteronism. These secondary, mainly nonsurgical, forms are not discussed here.

Primary hyperaldosteronism is characterized by mineralocorticoid hypersecretion, which promotes positive sodium balance secondary to stimulation of sodium resorption in the renal tubule.[5] The autonomy of aldosterone secretion prevents suppression by the excess total body sodium and expanded fluid compartments. This positive sodium balance results in an excess volume of 2 to 3 L of saline before a new steady state of expanded extracellular fluid volume is reached. This new steady state is attributed to an escape phenomenon whereby a certain volume of positive sodium balance is tolerated, after which additional sodium intake is promptly excreted. Thus, normal fluid homeostasis is preserved. With the expanded extracellular volume or positive sodium balance of primary aldosteronism, renin secretion and angiotensin formation are suppressed (Fig. 58-8).

Another measurable hallmark of primary aldosteronism is hypokalemia. About 80% of patients with primary hyperaldosteronism have serum potassium levels of 3.5 mEq/L or less. If challenged with a saline load, up to 95% of patients exhibit hypokalemia and potassium excretion of

Table 58-2. EFFECTS OF ALDOSTERONE SECRETION

Tubular Action	Normal Amounts	Excessive Amounts
Increased resorption of sodium	Protects against low-volume states	Hypertension Positive sodium balance Hyporeninemia
Decreased resorption of potassium	Protects against hyperkalemia	Hypokalemia Metabolic alkalosis Hyperglycemia Nocturia, polyuria Muscle weakness

more than 40 to 60 mEq/d in the urine because of an accentuated exchange of sodium for potassium in the renal tubule. In addition to hypernatremia and hypokalemia, metabolic alkalosis, due primarily to loss of hydrogen ions in the urine, is common. The increased tubular resorption of sodium, leading to the positive sodium balance, promotes hypertension. Hypokalemic nephropathy eventually leads to polyuria and nocturia. The hypokalemia further affects muscles by promoting weakness and paralysis. Hypokalemia also reduces β-cell insulin release, resulting in hypoinsulinemia and hyperglycemia. A summary of these events is given in Table 58-2.

Catecholamines

Normal Effects. The two major catecholamines, norepinephrine and epinephrine, mediate their effects through cellular membrane receptors. These receptors are found on many cell types, but their initial characterization was accomplished using smooth muscle. α-Receptors were found to be those that mediate contraction of smooth muscle, and β-receptors regulate relaxation. These were later characterized further into β_1- and β_2-receptors and α_1- and α_2-receptors. Several examples of β_1-receptor stimulation include increased inotropic and chronotropic responses in cardiac muscle, lipolytic effects in adipocytes, and a decrease in peripheral glucose use by most cells. Effects of β_2-receptors include relaxation of smooth muscle, especially that of the bronchus. Isoproterenol and epinephrine are well-known β-agonists. Effects of α_1-receptors are predominately contraction of smooth muscle in peripheral vascular beds and in the uterus. α_2-Receptors mediate platelet aggregation and, on presynaptic neuronal terminals, suppress the release of norepinephrine or acetylcholine. Both epinephrine and norepinephrine may have α-receptor effects, but the specific effects seem to depend both on the concentration of the catecholamines to which the receptors are exposed and the distribution of the various types of receptors within the tissues. For example, norepinephrine may have a β_2-receptor effect at high concentrations, whereas epinephrine exerts this effect at relatively low concentrations. On the other hand, white blood cells have a predominance of β-receptors and show little response to norepinephrine even at higher concentrations. Additional mechanisms modulate catecholamine effects. As the concentration of catecholamines increases, the receptor population decreases. This phenomenon is known as *down-regulation* and explains the relative insensitivity of a given tissue to catecholamines upon exposure to high concentrations (tachyphylaxis). With *up-regulation*, the number of receptors increase during the use of receptor antagonists or in the relative absence of catecholamines. This explains the increased sensitivity to catecholamines

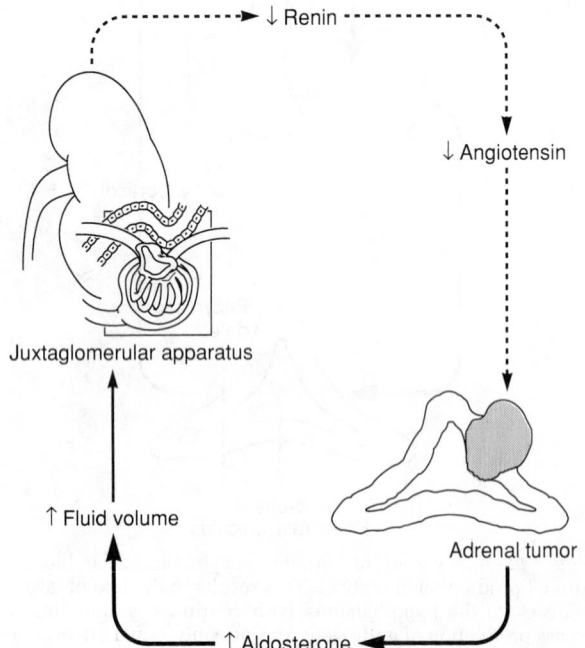

Figure 58-8. The physiologic consequences of primary hyperaldosteronism. The effects on the renin-angiotensin axis and intravascular volume are emphasized.

after surgical sympathectomy, for example. Another modulating mechanism is a change in adenyl cyclase activity as a postreceptor phenomenon. An excess of circulating thyroxine increases adenyl cyclase activity, which in turn increases cyclic adenosine monophosphate (cAMP) concentrations to amplify catecholamine activity. Thus, for a given α- or β-receptor number, sympathetic effects are amplified during a period of thyroxine excess.

Because of the wide distribution of catecholamine receptors, the effects achieved by catecholamines are predictably varied. The effects of catecholamines differ from those of steroids in at least two major ways. The onset of catecholamine action occurs within 1 or 2 minutes, as compared with 60 to 90 minutes for steroids. This difference reflects the quick mediation by membrane catecholamine receptors, whose changes are translated to the cAMP system. This contrasts with the slower mediation by cytosolic steroid receptors, which must be transported to the nucleus where changes are expressed through DNA and RNA synthesis. In part because of catecholamine's short plasma half-life, its effects tend to be short-lived. As mentioned, this rapid clearance is due to a combination of neuronal reuptake and the ubiquitous presence of the degradative catecholamine enzymes.

Catecholamine Excess. Pheochromocytomas are tumors primarily of the adrenal medulla.[6,7] They are classified as functioning when they produce catecholamines, always autonomously and usually in great excess. Although some of these tumors produce only epinephrine or norepinephrine, most produce the two catecholamines in combination. The predictable clinical effects of this endogenous catecholamine outpouring include hypertension, tachycardia, nervousness, and sweating (Table 58-3). Dopamine is also produced in variable amounts, with clinical consequences that are unclear.

The secretory effects of these tumors tend to fall into three patterns. Patients may have sustained hypertension without episodic increases in blood pressure or any other signs of markedly excessive secretion. Patients may be predominately normotensive with superimposed episodes of increased secretion manifested by tachycardia, hypertension, or flushing. Finally, patients may present with a combination of the two patterns, with sustained baseline hypertension and superimposed attacks of episodic hypertension. The episodes are best explained by changes in local blood flow since it is well documented that the tumors are not functionally innervated. A surge in blood flow in these tumors can wash out sinusoids rich in the catecholamines, producing a spike in circulating catecholamine concentrations. For patients with minimal clinical symptoms, it appears that released catecholamines are also taken up locally by the tumor and metabolized to their

inactive products. For this reason, a large tumor may be relatively asymptomatic because its active products are metabolized mainly on site. This yields inactive metabolites, and few, if any, active products reach the systemic circulation. Diagnostic sensitivity can therefore be improved by measuring both the metabolites and the catecholamines in the urine. As implied, some pheochromocytomas apparently do not secrete active substances of any kind; these are termed *nonfunctioning*.

DIAGNOSTIC INVESTIGATIONS

Patients with functioning adrenal lesions usually come to the attention of the health care delivery system by virtue of an incidental finding such as hypertension or hypokalemia; changes in appearance, such as redistribution of fat or abdominal striae; or with other symptoms, such as palpitations or muscular weakness. The various symptoms and findings specific for the types of functioning adrenal tumors were outlined previously. Both functioning and nonfunctioning adrenal tumors come to the attention of physicians as incidental findings on radiologic scan as well as through the use of modern imaging techniques, including computed tomographic (CT) scans, ultrasound, and magnetic resonance (MR) imaging of the abdomen. Therapeutic approaches to both functioning and nonfunctioning adrenal tumors are discussed in a subsequent section. Laboratory investigations used to determine the presence and type of functioning adrenal tumors and techniques used to determine their location are reviewed next.

Functional Assessment

The first diagnostic step in determining the functional state of an adrenal gland or lesion is to screen the urine or plasma for secretory products. The impetus for the screening is usually the presence of clinical findings or symptoms that suggest one of the various types of hyperfunctioning adrenal lesions, or it may simply be an incidental finding on an imaging test. Once hypersecretion is demonstrated, the specific type of pathology producing the syndrome must be determined with the aid of functional tests that manipulate the feedback mechanisms involved. In addition, relevant scanning and imaging tests can distinguish among the various types of lesions.

Hypercortisolism (Cushing Syndrome)

Screening Procedures. The simplest screening procedure for Cushing syndrome is the determination of plasma cortisol concentrations, preferably on multiple venous samplings. The sensitivity and specificity of this screening test is about 80% to 90%. The specificity can be increased by obtaining plasma samples at 8:00 AM and 6:00 PM. Diurnal variation of plasma cortisol is lost both in adrenal tumor formation and in the hypercortisolism of pituitary origin (Cushing disease). The measurement of 17-OH corticosteroids in the urine is perhaps more sensitive than cortisol measurements in plasma, but urine collection is more complicated than plasma sampling. Measurement of urinary free cortisol is perhaps the most sensitive screening method of all. In equivocal cases, the low-dose dexamethasone suppression test can be used. Dexamethasone, by negative feedback, suppresses the hypothalamic–pituitary secretion of ACTH and consequently lowers both plasma cortisol and urinary 17-OH corticosteroid excretion. Administration of 2 mg of dexamethasone suppresses plasma cortisol and urinary 17-OH corticosteroid by at least half when compared with control values taken with a normal pituitary–adrenal axis. In Cushing disease, with

Table 58-3. CATECHOLAMINE EFFECTS

Receptor Class	Normal Amounts	Excessive Amounts
β_1	Chronotropic, inotropic	Tachycardia
	Sweat glands	Sweating
	Decreased glucose use	Hyperglycemia
β_2	Smooth muscle relaxation	Hypotension
α_1	Smooth muscle contraction	Hypertension
	Gluconeogenesis	
	Glycogenolysis	Hyperglycemia
	Suppressed insulin effects	
α_2	Smooth muscle contraction	Pallor
	Platelet aggregation	

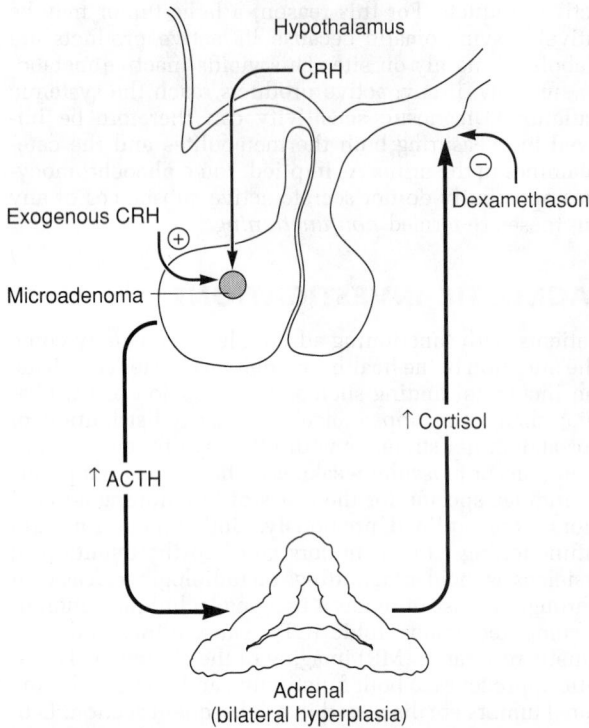

Figure 58-9. Cushing disease results from autonomous pituitary ACTH release. Dexamethasone does not suppress 17-OH corticosteroid production in patients with Cushing disease.

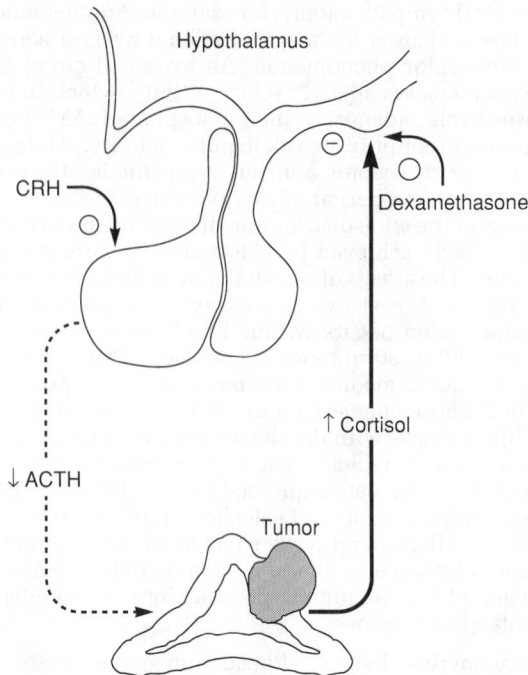

Figure 58-10. With a primary adrenal tumor producing hypercortisolism, pituitary ACTH is already maximally suppressed and dexamethasone produces no further decrease in output.

the set-point of ACTH secretion higher than normal, low-dose dexamethasone is insufficient to suppress ACTH.

Determining the Cause. Once hypersecretion of cortisol has been established, confirmation of specific abnormalities is undertaken by manipulating the negative feedback loop for steroids on the hypothalamic–pituitary unit. High-dose dexamethasone is used for this. The classic version of the test consists of 2 mg of dexamethasone administered every 6 hours for 24 hours. Measurement of 24-hour 17-OH corticosteroid excretion is obtained for baseline values on the day before dexamethasone administration. This is then repeated on the day of dexamethasone administration. A normal response to overnight suppression is to lower the 17-OH corticosteroid excretion by more than half. In the case of Cushing disease, the hypothalamic steroid receptors that allow negative feedback are intact but are set at a higher point. In this case, the 17-OH corticosteroid secretion does decrease significantly after high-dose dexamethasone administration. The schema for Cushing disease is shown in Figure 58-9. On the other hand, adrenal tumors, other causes of ectopic production of ACTH, and most cases of nodular hyperplasia do not respond to dexamethasone suppression with a decrease in steroid secretion. With an adrenal tumor, pituitary ACTH is already suppressed; therefore, dexamethasone cannot suppress it further (Fig. 58-10). With ectopic ACTH secretion, the tissue producing ACTH has no receptors for steroids, and negative feedback cannot be achieved. It is not clear why some cases of micronodular adrenal hyperplasia can be suppressed by dexamethasone. Because the classic dexamethasone suppression test uses cumbersome urinary measurements, an overnight test has been devised that uses a previous-day 8:00 AM plasma cortisol determination for control values and another sample taken at 8:00 the morning after the dexamethasone administration. The sensitiv-

ity and specificity of this simplified test are comparable to the classic form.

Potentially, the most helpful new test uses CRH to release ACTH and consequently to stimulate cortisol secretion. A standard dose of CRH is 1 μg/kg, or a maximum of 100 μg. The CRH is administered intravenously, and serial blood samples are obtained for about 3 hours after administration. The normal pituitary adrenal axis responds by a moderate increase in ACTH and cortisol. With Cushing disease, the ACTH and cortisol rise are accentuated. The overlap in results with this test for normal subjects and those with Cushing disease is not great. With adrenal autonomous production of cortisol (adrenal tumors or nodular hyperplasia) and with ectopic ACTH production, there is virtually no response to CRH. The diagnostic steps for Cushing syndrome are listed in Table 58-4.

Table 58-4. STEPS IN THE DIAGNOSIS OF CUSHING SYNDROME

SCREENING TESTS
Plasma cortisol—random and diurnal
Urinary 17-OH corticosteroids
Urinary free cortisol
Overnight low-dose dexamethasone

DETERMINING THE CAUSE
Standard dexamethasone suppression
  Positive—pituitary cause
  Negative—adrenal or ectopic cause
Corticotropin-releasing hormone stimulation
  Accentuated—pituitary cause
  No response—adrenal or ectopic cause
Petrosal sinus sampling
  Lateralizing—pituitary cause
  Nonlateralizing—adrenal or ectopic cause

Sex Steroid Excess

In adults, evidence of androgen excess is clinically apparent only in females. Although an ovarian source of androgen production must be sought in females, the predominant adrenal lesion is a cortical carcinoma. Male adults who become feminine are at high risk for having an adrenocortical carcinoma. In children, precocious puberty in males or virilization in females should point to the possibility of adrenal carcinoma. The differential diagnosis in children should include nonclassic or late 21-OH deficiency, 11β-OH deficiency, and primary ovarian tumors. The screening test for an adrenal source of excessive sex steroids is measurement of urinary 17-ketosteroids. This is abnormally high in patients with an adrenal source. In the feminine male, urinary estrogens should be measured. The dexamethasone suppression test in children is a useful means to determine whether one is dealing with the autonomous secretion of 17-ketosteroids by a tumor or whether the suppressible steroid secretion suggests an enzymatic defect in the steroidogenic pathway.

Congenital adrenal hyperplasia is usually brought to the physician's attention because of ambiguous genitalia in the female at birth. About 90% of these cases involve 21-OH deficiency. Male patients may be recognized early since about two thirds of these cases have salt-wasting. In either sex, it is an important diagnosis to make early. In the female, there is the question of gender assignment. Usually, the assignment is female, regardless of genotype, and an early operation should be planned. The objectives are to correct the clitoral hypertrophy, to create an adequate vagina and introitus, and to perform whatever cosmetic revision of the labia is required. In either male or female, prompt treatment of the salt-wasting may be life-saving. The diagnostic measurement of choice in the case of 21-OH deficiency is that of 17-OH progesterone, whereas 11-deoxycortisol is the major steroid produced for 11β-hydroxylase deficiency. Any enzymatic defect can be detected by evaluating for excess of proximal intermediates (see Fig. 58-3).

Hyperaldosteronism

For practical purposes, the best screening test in the hypertensive population for primary aldosteronism is the measurement of serum potassium levels. Since the prevalence of primary aldosteronism in the hypertensive population is less than 1 in 200 patients, it is not feasible to engage in more specific measurements in a screening program. When obtained with the patient in the fasting state and without any form of exercise or prolonged venostasis, the diagnostic sensitivity of this test for hypokalemia is close to 90%. Urinary potassium excretion above 30 mEq/24 h is confirmatory, especially when the serum potassium level is below 3.5 mEq/L. When there is borderline hypokalemia, salt supplementation at about 200 mEq/d can further improve the sensitivity of the screening test. Because there are so many other causes of hypertension and hypokalemia, the specificity of this test for hypokalemia is low, and further studies are required.

Determinations of urinary or plasma aldosterone and plasma renin are primary considerations in making a diagnosis of hyperaldosteronism. Taking 20 mg/24 h as the upper limit of normal, the sensitivity of a 24-hour urinary aldosterone measurement is up to 80%. When combined with a 3-day salt-supplemented diet, the sensitivity is increased to 95%. Measurement of plasma renin is also a reliable screening test for hyperaldosteronism. When plasma renin remains low when an upright position is assumed and during negative sodium balance, the likelihood of autonomous production of aldosterone is increased.

To confirm the diagnosis of primary aldosteronism, measurements must be made under special conditions that manipulate feedback control. The starting premise is that with primary aldosteronism, aldosterone values should be higher than in patients with other forms of hypertension, and these values cannot be lowered by various maneuvers that normally suppress aldosterone secretion. The infusion of 2000 mL of normal saline over a 4-hour period normally suppresses plasma aldosterone to less than 10 ng/dL, but in primary aldosteronism, it fails to suppress. The few false-positive results encountered with this test are typically associated with increased plasma renin activity, such as with renal artery stenosis. The captopril test takes advantage of the fact that this agent blocks the conversion of angiotensin I to angiotensin II. The test is therefore similar in concept to the saline infusion test, except that angiotensin II levels are lowered by pharmacologic means rather than by volume expansion. Another outpatient test calculates the integrated plasma aldosterone concentrations over a 24-hour period. It is unclear whether this test has advantages over the others mentioned. In the equivocal case, the patient should be brought into the hospital for dietary control and prolonged observation. The patient can be subjected to a period of volume expansion to test the autonomous nature of the aldosterone hypersecretion. Alternatively, treatment with sodium restriction and diuretics tests whether suppression of renin activity is fixed. These considerations can be reviewed by referring to Figures 58-5 and 58-8.

The problem of differentiating aldosterone-producing adenomas from hyperplasia of the zona glomerulosa remains. Because surgery is usually not effective in the latter situation, the differentiation is an important one. Although interest has been centered on localization procedures, several maneuvers can distinguish the two conditions. The first takes advantage of postural stimulation. Aldosterone and renin are measured at 8:00 AM after 2 hours in the recumbent position and again 2 to 4 hours later after quiet ambulation. With adenomas, plasma renin remains suppressed even on standing, and the plasma aldosterone tends to be lower on the second sampling because of decreasing ACTH levels as the morning progresses. Plasma renin activity is not as suppressed in patients with hyperplasia. The upright position produces postural response, which is a small increase in plasma renin activity, and plasma aldosterone consequently increases.

The second test is more promising and involves measuring an aldosterone precursor, 18-hydroxycorticosterone. For some unknown reason, this steroid is increased in patients with adenomas but remains in the normal range in those with hyperplasia. The 18-hydroxycorticosterone levels are above 100 μg/dL in virtually all patients with aldosterone-producing adenomas. An interesting subtype of primary adrenal hyperplasia is that which can be cured by surgery. These patients characteristically have elevated plasma 18-hydroxycorticosterone levels. Therefore, even if a patient with primary aldosteronism does not lateralize on CT or venous sampling, surgery may be curative in the presence of elevated 18-hydroxycorticosterone. Localization to distinguish aldosteronomas from hyperplasia is covered in the subsequent section. Table 58-5 provides a summary of screening and confirmation tests.

Catecholamines

In a patient suspected of having a pheochromocytoma, the most efficient and sensitive means of screening is to measure the catecholamines or their metabolic products in the urine. The normal person excretes less than 100 μg/d of the catecholamines, norepinephrine and epinephrine. Because of some overlap in values, specificity can be im-

---

Table 58-5. STEPS IN THE DIAGNOSIS OF ALDOSTERONISM

SCREENING TESTS

Serum potassium concentration—low
Urinary potassium excretion—high
Urinary aldosterone excretion—high
Plasma renin—low
Oral sodium loading

CONFIRMING TESTS

Plasma and urinary aldosterone
   Saline infusion
   Captopril
   Integrated plasma values
Plasma renin
   Negative sodium balance

TUMOR VERSUS HYPERPLASIA

Upright posture—plasma aldosterone and renin levels
   Tumor—remain suppressed
   Hyperplasia—slight rise
18-OH-corticosterone—high with tumor

---

proved by using a normal range of up to 250 μg/d. Although 24-hour samples can reduce the possible episodic variations in catecholamine excretion, shorter sampling periods can be useful, especially if corrected for creatinine excretion. In general, creatinine also should be measured in all 24-hour samples to check for completeness of collection. Because of their stability and relative freedom from substances interfering with their measurement, the metanephrines are preferred by some centers. A value of greater than 1 mg/24 h is usually considered positive. Measurement of either the urinary catecholamines or the metanephrines usually yields a 95% detection sensitivity. A combination of the two is reported to have a greater than 98% sensitivity. The measurement of VMA can also be added for a virtual 100% sensitivity in the patient with an actively secreting pheochromocytoma. As mentioned, the clinical pattern in patients with pheochromocytoma is either sustained hypertension; sustained hypertension with episodes of increased blood pressure, tachycardia, or flushing; or, rarely, mostly normotensive, with infrequent and unpredictable episodes of hypertension. Timing of the collection is critical in patients who have only episodic hypersecretion. Urine collection should be started immediately after a suspected attack of hypertension.

With the advent of sensitive radioimmunoassays and high-pressure liquid chromatography for determining catecholamine levels in plasma, attention has turned to the use of these measurements. Fluctuations in plasma catecholamine concentrations are much greater than those in urinary excretion, even in normal subjects. As the upper limits of normal plasma values are increased to account for fluctuations, the specificity is improved but at the sacrifice of sensitivity. Conversely, by lowering upper limits of normal to 750 pg/mL for norepinephrine or 110 pg/mL for epinephrine (supine position), the sensitivity is raised to about 90%. The specificity is low in this circumstance, however, because of the overlap of normal spikes in catecholamine concentrations with those concentrations produced by minimally secreting pheochromocytomas. In spite of these shortcomings, plasma values are useful in other contexts. Measuring catecholamines in the plasma has made possible the clonidine suppression test. In patients without pheochromocytoma, clonidine suppresses high basal plasma concentrations into the normal range, whereas concentrations in patients with pheochromocy-

toma are not suppressed. Another use of plasma catecholamine measurement is in examining the ratio of 3,4-dihydroxyphenoglycol (DHPG) to norepinephrine in plasma. DHPG is released from the chromaffin cell and adrenergic neurons to a much greater extent than norepinephrine in pheochromocytoma patients compared with patients who have essential hypertension. A rare but important use of plasma catecholamine determinations is in patients who have elevated catecholamine levels on several occasions but negative CT scans. In this case, superior and inferior vena cava sampling with measurement of the plasma catecholamines at various points along the vessels can pinpoint the location of the tumor by showing a step-up in the catecholamine concentrations. The various urinary and plasma tests for determining the presence of a pheochromocytoma are as follows:

- Urinary excretion
- Catecholamines
   Metanephrine, normetanephrine
   VMA
- Plasma epinephrine, norepinephrine
- Clonidine suppression test
- DHPG/norepinephrine ratio

In addition to the proper timing of urinary samples, several events, substances, and emotional states influence plasma and urinary catecholamine levels. Some of these are well-known events, whereas others relate to interfering substances that can falsely alter the assays, cause specific interferences with the assays, or affect catecholamine metabolism:

Endogenous Release

- Pain
- Hypotension
- Hypoglycemia
- Psychic distress
- Drug withdrawal
- Surgery

Interfering Drugs

- Catecholamines: calcium-channel blockers, captopril, α-agonists, β-blockers, α-blockers, methenamine mandelate
- VMA or metanephrine: clofibrate, nalidixic acid, methylglucamine
- Both catecholamines and metabolites: labetalol, levodopa, tricyclic antidepressants, phenothiazines, methyldopa, monoamine oxidase inhibitors

Localization Studies

Nonscintigraphic Studies

Although ultrasonography is the least expensive of the imaging procedures and is also able to distinguish solid from cystic lesions, its value is limited by the relative inaccessibility of the adrenal gland and by the small size of some of the adrenal lesions to be examined.

CT is the technique most commonly used to examine patients in whom adrenal abnormalities are suspected.[8] In addition, because of the widespread use of abdominal CT, this method most often discovers the unsuspected adrenal tumors. CT reliably detects adrenal tumors greater than 1 cm in diameter (Fig. 58-11). The sensitivity of CT for tumors that are 1 cm in diameter is about 80%, and it reaches 100% for tumors that are 3 to 4 cm. Although CT is noninvasive and reasonably sensitive, it is nonspecific. CT distinguishes cystic from solid adrenal abnormalities but does not distinguish functioning from nonfunctioning tumors,

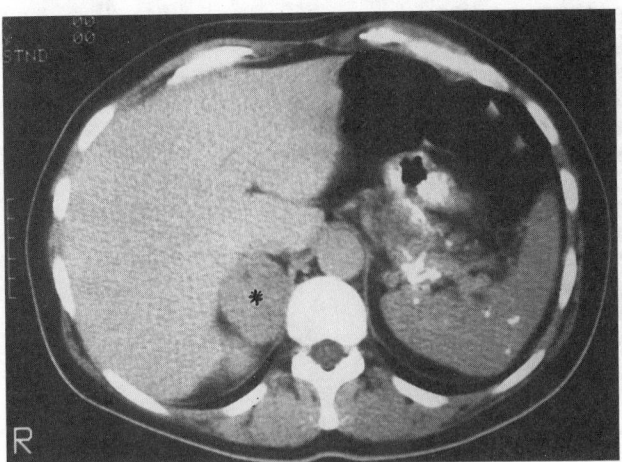

Figure 58-11. Abdominal CT scan showing right adrenal tumor (*asterisk*).

nor benign from malignant tumors, with any degree of reliability.

MR imaging has maintained a certain usefulness even after retrenchment from early optimistic predictions. It is more expensive and requires greater patient cooperation than CT, but it has greater versatility than CT because of the use of T1- and T2-weighted images. The relatively fast scanning time for the T1-weighted images provides an increased sensitivity for identifying adrenal lesions in comparison with the T2 sequences, which are more subject to motion artifact. In some cases, the T2-weighted images can provide a differential diagnosis of adrenal lesions. The T2-weighted images may distinguish such entities as metastatic or primary carcinoma and pheochromocytoma from adenomas, lipomas, myelolipomas, and cysts. On the T2-weighted images, carcinomas generally have increased signal intensity, whereas the fat-laden adenomas and hyperplasia show decreased intensity. T2-weighted images can provide adrenal/liver signal ratios that are higher for pheochromocytomas than for cortical adenomas or carcinomas. In a sense, MR imaging is complementary to CT in that the latter can better detect the lesion whereas the former can distinguish one type of lesion from the other. In addition, MR imaging is probably better than CT for distinguishing anatomic relations and extent of involvement of surrounding tissues by carcinomas. A T1-weighted MR image of a pelvic pheochromocytoma is shown in Figure 58-12*A*. The same tumor is shown by CT scan in Figure 58-12*B*.

Scintigraphic Imaging

Two radiopharmaceuticals have proved useful in imaging the adrenal gland. Adrenocortical lesions can be imaged by ^{131}I-6 β-iodomethyl-19-norcholesterol (NP-59), which is taken up as cholesterol in the adrenocortical steroidogenic pathway. The other agent is ^{131}I-methaiodobenzylguanidine (MIBG), a norepinephrine analogue. It indicates norepinephrine accumulation in storage vesicles and can detect sympathoadrenal tumors at any site in the body. NP-59 can accurately localize the adrenal cortex and any functioning tumors. NP-59 can distinguish adrenocortical hyperplasia from functioning adenomas or carcinomas. With the use of dexamethasone suppression, some cases of primary macronodular or micronodular adrenal hyperplasia, which do not suppress, can be distinguished from adrenal hyperplasia of pituitary origin, which does suppress. NP-59 has also been reported to distinguish unilat-

eral aldosterone-producing tumors from bilateral hyperplasia of the zona glomerulosa in patients with primary hyperaldosteronism. Finally, in patients with incidentally discovered nonfunctioning adrenal tumors, NP-59 can separate adenomas, which accumulate the agent, from carcinomas, either primary or metastatic, which do not. MIBG is a useful agent in localizing pheochromocytomas throughout the body, especially when the tumors are multiple, extraadrenal, recurrent, or metastatic.

Invasive Localization Techniques

Arteriography, venography, and selective venous sampling became less popular as experience with the imaging techniques listed previously increased. Specific sampling of adrenal venous blood in primary aldosteronism and vena cava sampling in occult pheochromocytomas are still occasionally useful techniques. In addition to the disadvantages inherent in invasive procedures using intravascular contrast agents, arteriography is specifically dangerous in the study of patients with pheochromocytomas. The injection can cause a sudden rise in catecholamines and precipitate a hypertensive crisis. The same phenomenon has been reported with adrenal phlebography in pheochromocytomas, but the more common complication with this technique is disruption and bleeding of the adrenal venous system.

Localization Overview

In general, CT is the first choice for imaging because of its noninvasive nature, its ease in performance, and its sensitivity. In nonfunctioning tumors, some additional information can be derived concerning the nature of the lesion by using MR imaging. NP-59 scintigraphy is particularly useful in cases of Cushing syndrome and in hyperaldosteronism, and MIBG may be required in cases of pheochromocytoma in which multiple, extraadrenal, recurrent, or metastatic pheochromocytomas are suspected. Vena cava sampling of catecholamines may also be helpful in these patients. Finally, adrenal venous sampling is usually reserved for questionable cases of primary aldosteronism. A summary of these considerations is shown in Table 58-6.

TREATMENT

Treatment of adrenal tumors is primarily surgical removal. The following secions describe the open, standard techniques, but in the next few years laparoscopic techniques will play a greater role.[9] Although pharmaceutical agents are useful in preparing the patient for surgery or in palliating the patient with recurrent adrenal carcinoma, no agents render definitive therapy for adrenal tumors. Congenital adrenal hyperplasia is the only primary, hyperfunctioning adrenal syndrome that is amenable to medical therapy for definitive treatment.

Adrenal Hypercortisolism

Nonoperative Treatment

Functioning benign lesions of the adrenal cortex that are not ACTH dependent, such as adenomas or macronodular hyperplasia, respond to metyrapone and aminoglutethimide, which inhibit enzymes in the adrenal steroidogenic pathway. Both agents can effect a decrease in the production of cortisol when there is no increase in ACTH secondary to feedback stimulation by lowered cortisol levels. These drugs are not satisfactory long-term agents because of their high incidence of drug reactions, patient noncompliance, and continued growth of the lesions. They may

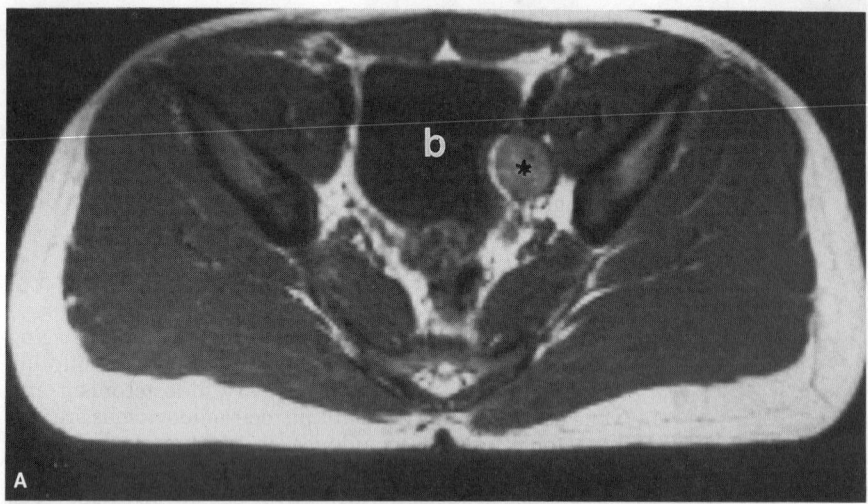

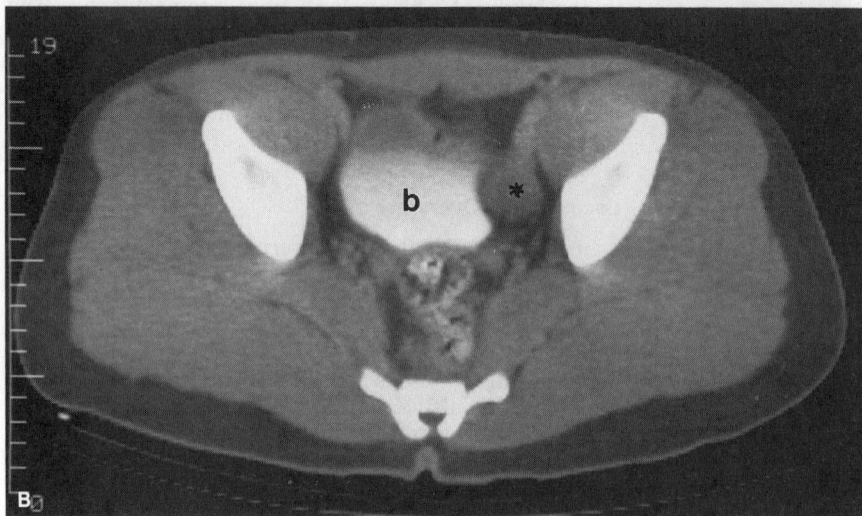

Figure 58-12. (*A*) T1−weighted MR image of a left pelvic pheochromocytoma (*asterisk*) compressing the bladder (b). (*B*) CT scan of the pelvis showing the left pelvic pheochromocytoma with bladder distortion (*asterisk*) as depicted in *A* (b).

Table 58-6. USE OF LOCALIZATION PROCEDURES

Procedure	Characteristics
RADIOGRAPHIC SCANS	
CT	Good first test; sensitive but not very specific
MR	Can identify some types of pathology and defines anatomy well; competes with scintigraphy in nonfunctioning tumors; lower sensitivity than CT; expensive
SCINTIGRAPHIC SCANS	
NP-59	Adrenocortical imaging can distinguish unilateral from bilateral disease in most instances; dexamethasone can add specificity, potential for identifying carcinomas in nonfunctioning tumors
MIBG	Adrenal medulla imaging can supplement CT scan when extraadrenal, recurrent, or metastatic pheochromocytomas are suspected
INVASIVE STUDIES	
Adrenal venous sampling	Greatest use in distinguishing adenoma from hyperplasia in primary aldosteronism; technically demanding; adrenal venography can cause hemorrhage
Vena cava sampling	Largely replaced by MIBG in search for extraadrenal pheochromocytomas
Arteriography	Can be dangerous with pheochromocytomas; largely replaced by noninvasive scanning

be useful in patients whose surgery must be delayed. Although malignant, functioning, adrenocortical lesions should be debulked whenever possible, several chemotherapy agents offer adjunct therapy. The most noteworthy is mitotane (o,p,-DDD).[10] This is a cytolytic agent that has a 30% to 70% response rate in terms of decreasing steroid output. Unfortunately, patient survival is not affected. External irradiation and chemotherapy have not been effective for these malignant tumors.

As mentioned, nonoperative treatment is definitive therapy for congenital adrenal hyperplasia. Usually, 5 mg/d of cortisone acetate is sufficient in infants and is gradually increased to 25 to 35 mg/d in adults. For the salt-losing variety, intravenous steroid administration occasionally is required on an acute basis until the salt-losing tendency is brought under control by cortisone treatment. If a mineralocorticoid is required, oral 9α-fludrocortisone (Florinef) can be given in a dosage of 0.1 to 0.2 mg/d for an infant. In the occasional noncompliant patient, deoxycorticosterone pivalate can be given in a dosage of 12.5 to 25 mg/mo intramuscularly.

Operative Treatment

Indication for operation in the patient with a unilateral functioning adrenal tumor is clear. In the patient with a nonfunctioning adrenal tumor, the need for surgery is related to the size of the tumor and its rate of growth.[11] There is consensus that a tumor larger than 6 cm should be removed. Some recommend that the acceptable size limit be 3 cm, especially when MR imaging suggests carcinoma or when functional studies suggest activity. When nonoperative therapy is elected, the patient should receive an adrenal scan 1, 3, and 6 months after the initial scan and yearly thereafter to assess growth of the lesion. If the tumor has grown, surgical removal is indicated. In bilateral functioning adrenocortical lesions, assessment of the pituitary–adrenal axis by dexamethasone suppression test and CRH stimulation must be done. If the pituitary is not implicated as the source of the hypercortisolism, bilateral adrenalectomy is indicated. In the case of nonfunctioning bilateral adrenal disease, the probability of metastasis to the adrenal gland is high. Image-guided needle biopsy may be the diagnostic approach of choice in that situation.

Preoperative preparation for adrenalectomy is straightforward. Other than the considerations of or preparation with enzyme inhibitors mentioned previously, the only specific issue is that of steroid replacement. It is best to treat patients prophylactically if there is any question about preexisting adrenal suppression or the possibility of adrenalectomy. At the start of the operation, 100 mg of hydrocortisone is administered intravenously and repeated in 4 hours.

The surgical approach is determined by the lateral position and size of the lesion. For small unilateral lesions, such as adenomas, a posterior approach through the bed of the 12th or 11th rib is preferred. An alternative extraperitoneal approach is through the flank, with the patient in the lateral decubitus position. The bilateral posterior approach is usually reserved for small, hyperplastic glands, such as in micronodular hyperplasia or hyperplasia of Cushing disease, in which pituitary treatment has failed. With transabdominal surgery, either unilateral subcostal or bilateral rooftop incisions are used for large adrenal tumors or macronodular hyperplasia, respectively. If the lesion proves to be a carcinoma growing into surrounding tissues, a thoracoabdominal approach may be necessary.

By far the most serious intraoperative complications are avulsion of the right adrenal gland from the inferior vena cava or a direct tear in the vena cava. The posterior approach is particularly hazardous in this regard because it is difficult to extricate a large tumor through the small posterior aperture. In addition, large tumors may be carcinomas, and the transabdominal approach allows for wide resection of lymph node-bearing areas and perhaps partial removal of attached surrounding structures. Other potential complications dependent on the incision include pneumothorax for the posterior approach and pancreatitis for the left abdominal approach.

The postoperative course involves tapering the exogenous steroid doses to maintenance levels in the case of bilateral adrenalectomy or to cessation in the case of unilateral adrenal removal. One simple regimen involves administering 100 mg of hydrocortisone intravenously every 6 hours during the first 48 hours. Some prefer alternating doses of intramuscular cortisone acetate in the event that intravenous access is lost. Provided that no intervening complications arise, the doses can be halved every 48 to 72 hours. In patients who have been exposed preoperatively to glucocorticoid excess, the maintenance dose may be as high as 100 mg/d for several months. Both high doses and normal maintenance of 35 to 50 mg/d can be given in the form of oral cortisone acetate as long as reliable alimentation and absorption have been achieved. It may be difficult to achieve normal maintenance dosages of 35 to 50 mg/d in many patients with Cushing syndrome without developing symptoms of steroid withdrawal. Also, the pituitary–adrenal axis remains suppressed for 6 to 12 months after operation, and even patients with normal contralateral adrenal glands cannot be taken off steroid replacement until after that time. Complications in the postoperative period include wound infection, pancreatitis, and thromboembolism. The latter complication has led some surgeons to prefer the preoperative placement of lower-extremity compression devices and their maintenance through the postoperative period. An alternative method is the use of low-dose heparin.

Hyperaldosteronism

Nonoperative Treatment

The only pharmaceutical agent that has practical benefit in this syndrome is spironolactone. This drug inhibits the sodium–potassium exchange in the distal tubule, normalizes serum potassium, and if tolerated for a period of time, can lower the blood pressure. Oral potassium chloride supplementation helps to correct the concomitant hypokalemia. Because of gynecomastia and other side effects, long-term spironolactone is problematic in some patients. Large doses of up 3 to 4 g/d may be required.

Operative Treatment

Primary aldosteronism due to an adrenal adenoma is best treated by surgically removing the adenoma. On the other hand, when the syndrome arises from adrenal hyperplasia, surgical removal of the adrenal gland is seldom curative. It is therefore essential that every effort be made to distinguish the two causes. Surgery is indicated only for adenomas or for those forms of hyperplasia that, on dynamic testing, behave as adenomas.

The important preoperative preparation is that of potassium replenishment. Correction of hypokalemia may be materially aided by the short-term use of spironolactone. Since the tumors are generally small and rarely malignant and hyperplasia is minimal, the unilateral or bilateral posterior approach is preferred. If bilateral adrenalectomy is anticipated, hydrocortisone should be administered as detailed above. Because these adenomas may be particularly small, it is necessary in some cases to thoroughly mobilize the adrenal gland and to examine it with bidigital palpation to assure an adequate examination. Pneumothorax and vena cava bleeding may occur as in other adrenalectomies, but the tissues are not as friable as those in chronic hypercortisolism. In addition, the lack of truncal obesity contributes to the comparative ease of surgery in primary hyperaldosteronism. Postoperatively, the patient usually experiences an uneventful recovery. Because of hyporeninemia, the remaining zona glomerulosa is usually temporarily suppressed, and a relative hypoaldosteronism may follow removal of an adenoma. Clinically, this is manifested by low blood pressure and hyperkalemia, which usually respond to the administration of a mineralocorticoid, such as fludrocortisone. Of course, bilateral adrenalectomy necessitates exogenous cortisol administration, which can usually be tapered to maintenance levels during the normal postoperative recovery period of 5 to 10 days.

Pheochromocytoma

Nonoperative Treatment

Nonoperative treatment of pheochromocytoma is generally unsatisfactory and entails pharmacologic blockade of the effects of catecholamines. Phenoxybenzamine and prazosin are two preferred agents that block the α-adrenergic effects of the catecholamines. The use of β-adrenergic blockers, such as labetalol, may be required in those patients with obvious β-adrenergic effects, such as resting pulse rates above 100 beats/min.

Operative Treatment

Because of the potential for wide swings in blood pressure and other effects of chronic catecholamine secretion, such as high blood glucose or cardiomyopathy, careful preoperative preparation is required in patients with these tumors.[12] It is customary to institute α-adrenergic blockade 2 to 3 weeks before anticipated surgery. This controls the blood pressure for cardiovascular reasons and allows restoration of a decreased blood volume. It is the consensus that preoperative preparation in this manner makes the intraoperative treatment of the patient much more safe. In patients who require β-adrenergic blockade, it is essential to first establish good α-adrenergic blockade. These patients are especially prone to cardiac failure induced by β-adrenergic blockade because of the cardiomyopathy that may preexist. β-Adrenergic blockade in the cardiomyopathic patient, with failure to first reduce the afterload by α-adrenergic blockade, can precipitate cardiac failure. Many surgeons prefer having a pulmonary artery catheter in place before and during surgery because of the potential cardiovascular instability. Preoperative sedation appears to be important. The use of rectal thiopental sodium (Pentothal) or diazepam is efficacious, especially in children.

In the operating room, several preinduction maneuvers should be carried out. Although pulmonary artery monitoring is considered optional, it is essential that intraarterial blood pressure monitoring be done. With catecholamine excess, the peripheral pulse may disappear, and auditory monitoring of the blood pressure is impossible. A large array of pharmaceutical agents should be immediately available. These include agents that lower blood pressure, such as phentolamine (Regitine) or nitroprusside; β-adrenergic blockers, such as esmolol; antiarrhythmic agents, such as lidocaine; and blood-pressure support agents, such as norepinephrine, to counteract possible postoperative hypotension. Opinions vary as to the preferred anesthetic agents, but the principle of smooth induction is universally held. Most important are an anesthesiologist who has had experience with these tumors and an anesthetic regimen that is familiar to the user.

It is customary to approach these tumors by the transabdominal route, usually through a generous bilateral, subcostal rooftop incision. The rationale for this approach includes the significant incidence of bilateral, extraadrenal tumors and malignant tumors. As more experience is gained with imaging techniques, including MIBG, it may be possible to localize adrenal tumors exclusively to one side with sufficient accuracy so that a posterior approach in these situations would be justified. The two major technical principles in operation for these tumors are to minimize the manipulation of the tumor and to isolate and ligate the adrenal vein as soon as possible in the sequence of dissection. It is during the period of tumor manipulation that the anesthesiologist must be most alert in counteracting arrhythmia and high blood pressure with the agents noted. Once the tumor is removed, the blood pressure may fall precipitously. This can be counteracted immediately by instituting an α-adrenergic agonist, such as norepinephrine. A preexisting low blood volume may also contribute to hypotension, and transfusion of one or two units of blood may be considered. Conversely, failure to bring the blood pressure down at least to normal on removal of a pheochromocytoma should raise suspicion of a second pheochromocytoma or of metastases. A thorough intraabdominal search along the vertebral bodies, aorta, contralateral adrenal gland, and urinary bladder should be done before closure.

Postoperatively, once the hypotension is corrected, the patient usually has an uneventful recovery. When all functioning pheochromocytomas have been removed, normalization of blood pressure is achieved in virtually 100% of patients.

Nonfunctioning Adrenal Tumors

As mentioned previously, the indications for surgery in these tumors are a diameter greater than 6 cm, growth of the smaller tumors during a period of observation, or questions of functional status. Because carcinomas smaller than 6 cm have been reported, some clinicians prefer to remove any tumors larger than 3 cm. The principles of surgical approach are much the same as those for functioning tumors. Tumors larger than 5 to 6 cm are probably best approached by the flank or transabdominal routes. Smaller tumors with a low index of suspicion for malignancy can easily be removed through the posterior approach.

OUTCOMES

The prognosis for patients with benign functioning adrenal tumors is generally excellent. For patients with Cushing syndrome caused by benign lesions, such as pituitary adenomas, adrenal adenomas, or macronodular hyperplasia, the cure rate approximates 100%. This is in marked contrast to untreated Cushing syndrome patients, who have historically suffered a 50% 5-year mortality rate. The same good prognosis is true for treated adrenal adenomas secreting aldosterone or benign pheochromocytomas producing catecholamines. A notable exception in the benign diseases is hyperplasia of the zona glomerulosa, in which, for some unknown reason, surgical removal of the adrenal glands usually does not cure the hypertension. The prognosis for adrenocortical carcinoma is not good. The overall 5-year survival rate is 20% to 25% for these malignancies. When there is localized disease at the time of surgery, the 5-year survival may be higher, in the 40% to 50% range. The true prognosis in childhood is not clear, but the data suggest a 2-year survival rate of about 20%. In some instances, these early tumors were removed without benefit of exogenous steroid therapy. The precise 5-year survival rate of malignant pheochromocytomas is difficult to determine because of the rarity of these tumors and the propensity of the metastases to appear many years later. Also, some of these patients live a long time with their disease. Patients with previous pheochromocytomas should therefore be followed periodically for many years because of the possibility of late-appearing metastases. The follow-up regimen can be better determined when more useful criteria for distinguishing benign from malignant tumors are developed. The mitotic index and the determination of ploidy on the flow cytometer may help in this regard.

REFERENCES

1. Silverman ML, Lee AK. Anatomy and pathology of the adrenal glands. Urol Clin North Am 1989;16:417.
2. Perry RR, Nieman LK, Cutler GB, et al. Primary adrenal causes of Cushing's syndrome: diagnosis and surgical management. Ann Surg 1989;210:59.
3. New MI. Basic and clinical aspects of congenital adrenal hyperplasia. J Steroid Biochem 1987;27:1.
4. Merrell RC. Aldosterone-producing tumors (Conn's syndrome). Semin Surg Oncol 1990;6:66.
5. Gordon RD. Primary aldosteronism: a new understanding. Med J Aust 1993;158:729.
6. Sheps SG, Jiang NS, Klee GC, et al. Recent developments in the diagnosis and treatment of pheochromocytoma. Mayo Clin Proc 1990;65:88.
7. Bravo EL, Gifford RW. Pheochromocytoma. Endocrinol Metab Clin North Am 1993;22:329.

8. Lamki LM, Haynie TP. Role of adrenal imaging in surgical management. J Surg Oncol 1990;43:139.

9. Suzuki K, Kageyama S, Ueda D. Laparoscopic adrenalectomy: clinical experience with 12 cases. J Urol 1993;150:1099.

10. Wooten MD, King DK. Adrenal cortical carcinoma. Cancer 1993;72:3145.

11. Gajraj H, Young AE. Adrenal incidentaloma. Br J Surg 1993; 80:422.

12. Pullerits J, Ein S, Balfe JW. Anaesthesia for phaeochromocytoma. Can J Anaesth 1988;35:526.

SURGERY: SCIENTIFIC PRINCIPLES AND PRACTICE, Second Edition, edited by Lazar J. Greenfield, Michael W. Mulholland, Keith T. Oldham, Gerald B. Zelenock, and Keith D. Lillemoe. Lippincott–Raven Publishers, Philadelphia, © 1997.

CHAPTER 59

PITUITARY GLAND

WILLIAM F. CHANDLER AND RICARDO V. LLOYD

The pituitary gland, or hypophysis, is a remarkably complex way-station in the connection between the brain and a wide range of organs throughout the body. The hypothalamus of the brain is the principal integrating organ for regulating the body's internal environment, and the pituitary is its major link with the organs outside the nervous system. The pituitary has been called the master gland; even with advances in modern neuroendocrinology, it remains worthy of that description.

EMBRYOLOGY, ANATOMY, AND PHYSIOLOGY

To appreciate the gross and microscopic anatomy of this small but complex gland, it is important to briefly review the embryologic development of the hypophysis. By the fourth week, an evagination in the roof of the stomodeal depression develops and is lined by the ectodermal cells of the cavity destined to become the pharynx (Fig. 59-1). This depression is known as the Rathke pouch. At the same time, a depression in the floor of the diencephalon develops and is called the infundibular process. This too is lined with ectodermal cells. These are cells of the future diencephalic portion of the brain and are, therefore, more

similar to central nervous system tissue. Over weeks, these two structures grow to meet each other—the infundibular process forming the neurohypophysis (pars neuralis) and the Rathke pouch forming the adenohypophysis (pars distalis). In lower animals, an intermediary lobe (pars intermedia) is also formed, but in humans this is present only as a minor cleft. As the adenohypophysis enlarges, its upper portion (pars tuberalis) partially surrounds the stalk connecting the pituitary to the brain. Eventually, the connection between the adenohypophysis and the oral cavity disappears, but occasionally it leaves ectopic remnants of nonfunctioning pituitary cells, which are known as pharyngeal pituitary tissue, along its path.

In an adult, the hypophysis is 6×9×12 mm and weighs about 0.6 g. It enlarges during pregnancy and weighs up to 1 g in multiparous women. The adenohypophysis constitutes 80% of the gland and contains the pars distalis, the pars tuberalis, and the remnant of the pars intermedia. The pars distalis is the major functional portion of the adenohypophysis, and in this chapter, it is considered synonymous with the adenohypophysis or anterior pituitary. The neurohypophysis, or posterior pituitary, is small and, according to its embryological development, should be considered virtually an extension of the hypothalamus of the brain.

Figure 59-2A shows that the combined neurohypophysis and adenohypophysis are connected to the base of the brain by a common stalk. The stalk blends into the median eminence of the hypothalamus and serves to transport both hormone-enriched portal blood to the adenohypophysis and nerve fibers to the neurohypophysis. The optic chiasm lies directly above the pituitary, just anterior to the stalk; thus, it is vulnerable to compression by a pituitary tumor. The supraoptic and paraventricular nuclei of the hypothalamus are depicted in Figure 59-2A, because they are the principal locations of cell bodies with axons headed for the neurohypophysis.

Figure 59-2B shows that the median eminence is the location in which blood destined for the adenohypophysis picks up its hormonal contribution from axons originating in various nuclei of the hypothalamus. Blood enters this region primarily from the superior hypophyseal artery and goes into gomitoli, which are small capillary plexes capable of picking up hormones within the median eminence. This blood is then transported by the portal system to influence secretory cells in the adenohypophysis. These cells in turn secrete hormones into the general circulation to stimulate end organs. This system involves the transport of the following:

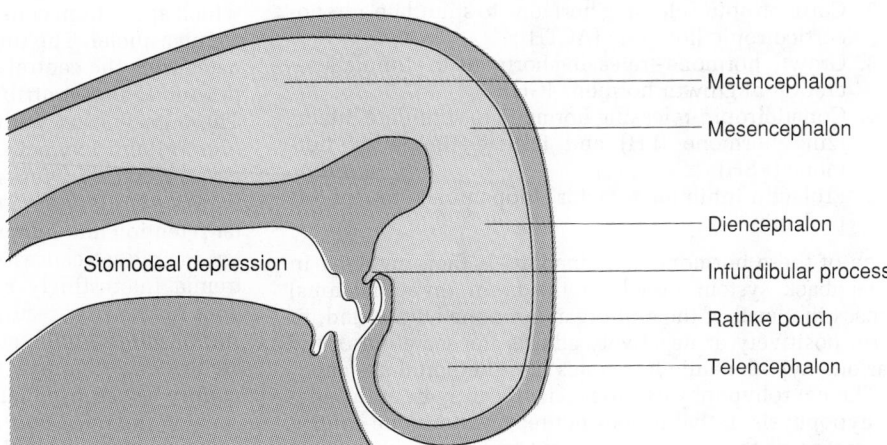

Figure 59-1. Diagram of 4-week embryo demonstrating how the Rathke pouch meets the infundibular process to form the anterior and posterior pituitary, respectively.

Stomodeal depression

Metencephalon

Mesencephalon

Diencephalon

Infundibular process

Rathke pouch

Telencephalon

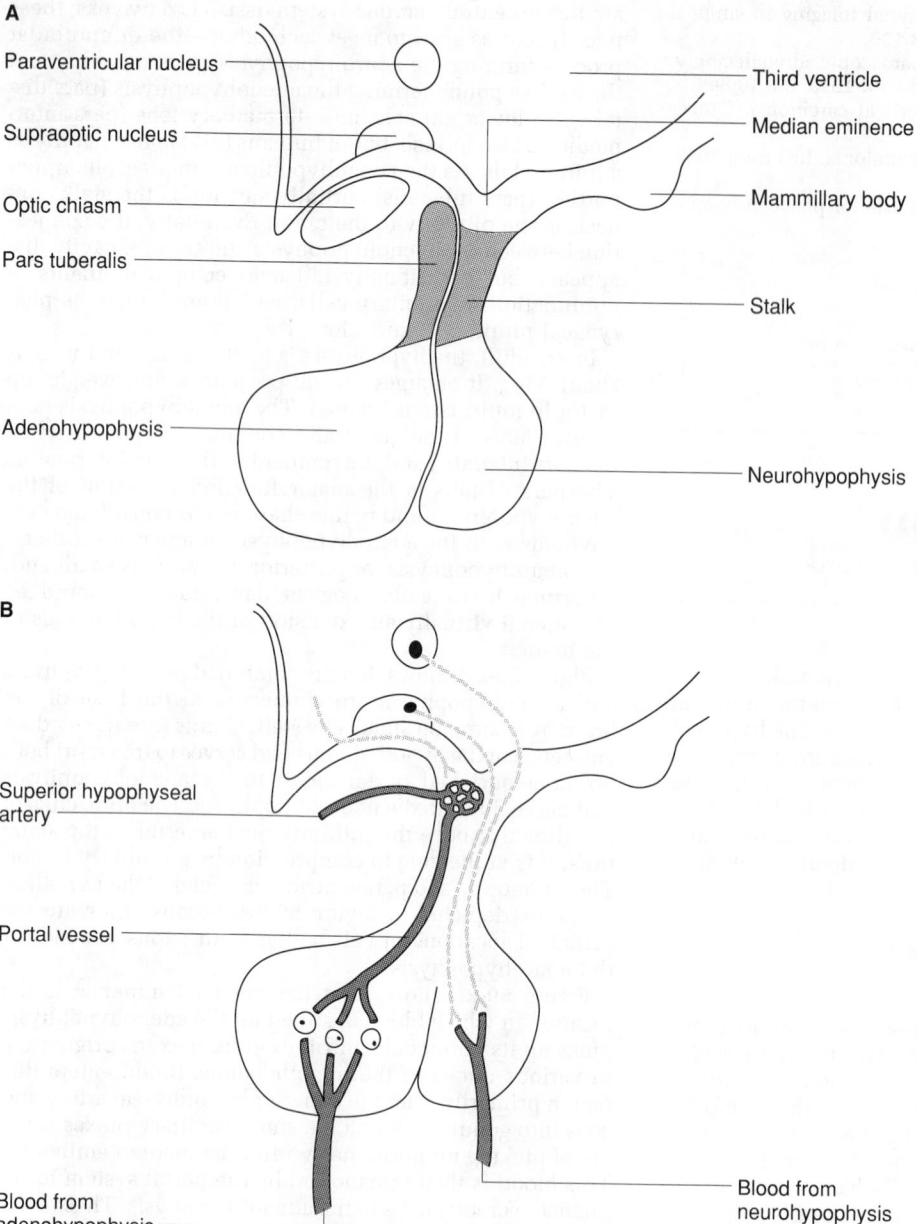

Figure 59-2. (*A*) Schematic diagram of pituitary and floor of the third ventricle as seen in midline sagittal view. Anterior is to the left. (*B*) Diagram on same schematic drawing of physiology of hormone release. The adenohypophysis receives releasing hormones through a portal venous system, and the neurohypophysis receives hormones directly from hypothalamic nuclei by means of neurons.

1. Thyrotropin-releasing hormone (TRH) to stimulate the secretion of thyroid-stimulating hormone (TSH)
2. Corticotropin-releasing hormone to stimulate adrenocorticotropic hormone (ACTH)
3. Growth hormone–releasing hormone to stimulate secretion of growth hormone (GH)
4. Gonadotropin-releasing hormone to stimulate luteinizing hormone (LH) and follicle-stimulating hormone (FSH)
5. Prolactin-inhibitory factor (dopamine) to inhibit prolactin

Each of these hormone combinations is then involved in a feedback system in which the brain (hypothalamus) senses the level of the end-organ hormone output and, in turn, positively or negatively adjusts the secretion of the various hypothalamic hormones into the portal system.

The neurohypophysis differs significantly from the adenohypophysis in that it does not receive hormone control by means of the portal system but by direct transport of hormones through nerve fibers. The principal input into the neurohypophysis is the supraopticohypophyseal tract, which arises from cells within the supraoptic and paraventricular nuclei. The tuberohypophyseal tract, which originates from the central and posterior portions of the hypothalamus, also contributes input to the neurohypophysis. These tracts carry both antidiuretic hormone (ADH; vasopressin) and oxytocin. ADH is secreted into the general circulation and causes the kidneys to absorb free water. Excess ADH (syndrome of inappropriate ADH) causes water retention and hyponatremia, and ADH shortage (diabetes insipidus) causes excess loss of water and hypernatremia. Interestingly, surgical loss of the neurohypophysis does not usually result in diabetes insipidus, because the stalk itself can still secrete ADH into the circulation. The feedback mechanism to the brain for release of ADH is mainly serum osmolarity, with hyperosmolar conditions causing the release of ADH and retention of water. Blood volume also controls the release of ADH; thus, hemorrhage causes water retention. Oxytocin functions only during pregnancy and causes both uterine contractions and milk let-down within the breasts.

The gross surgical anatomy of the pituitary is also critical to the surgeon, because the pituitary is closely surrounded by a number of important structures. Figure 59-3A illustrates the coronal cross section of the anatomy of the pituitary as seen from the front. The pituitary sits within the bony confines of the sella turcica (Turkish saddle) and is bordered laterally by the cavernous sinuses (venous), inferiorly and anteriorly by the sphenoid sinus (air), posteriorly by the dorsum sella, and superiorly by the membranous diaphragma sella. The cavernous sinuses each contain the siphon region of the internal carotid artery and portions of the cranial nerves III, IV, V, and VI, all within a venous plexus. The optic chiasm lies immediately above the diaphragma sella. Directly below the anterior and inferior portions of the sella is the aerated sphenoid sinus. This is sufficiently large in 97% of patients to allow a transnasal, transsphenoidal surgical approach to the pituitary (see Fig. 59-3B).

METHODS OF CELL ANALYSIS

Pituitary adenomas have been classified historically as acidophilic, basophilic, and chromophobic. Adenomas may show a variable staining pattern with conventional hematoxylin–eosin dyes, so it is difficult to classify adenomas based on these stains. For example, prolactinomas and sparsely granulated growth hormone adenomas may be acidophilic or chromophobic after hematoxylin–eosin staining (Table 59-1). Immunohistochemistry, ultrastructural studies, and in situ hybridization analyses for specific hormones are the most reliable methods of classifying pituitary adenomas today.

Other conventional stains that help in the analysis of pituitary adenomas include the reticulin stain, which helps to distinguish between pituitary hyperplasia and adenomas. The normal reticulin pattern is retained in hyperplasia and is similar to the normal pituitary but becomes disrupted in neoplasms. The periodic acid–Schiff reaction stains carbohydrates in ACTH-producing adenomas as well as in TSH- and FSH/LH-producing tumors.

Ultrastructural analysis of pituitary adenomas provides a great deal of information about the size and type of secretory granules, cellular synthetic activity, and unique features of specific adenoma subtypes. For example, misplaced exocytosis is seen in prolactin-producing tumors, type I microfilaments are present in ACTH-producing tumors, and abundant mitochondria are characteristic of oncocytic null cell adenomas. The unique honeycomb pattern of the Golgi complex is a distinct morphologic feature of FSH/LH-producing adenomas in women.[1] Because there is a great deal of pleomorphism and size variation in secretory granules, immunohistochemical studies at the light and ultrastructural levels are more reliable in classifying adenomas than the ultrastructural, morphologic appearance of secretory granules.

Immunohistochemical staining of pituitary adenomas with specific antibodies is a reliable method for classifying

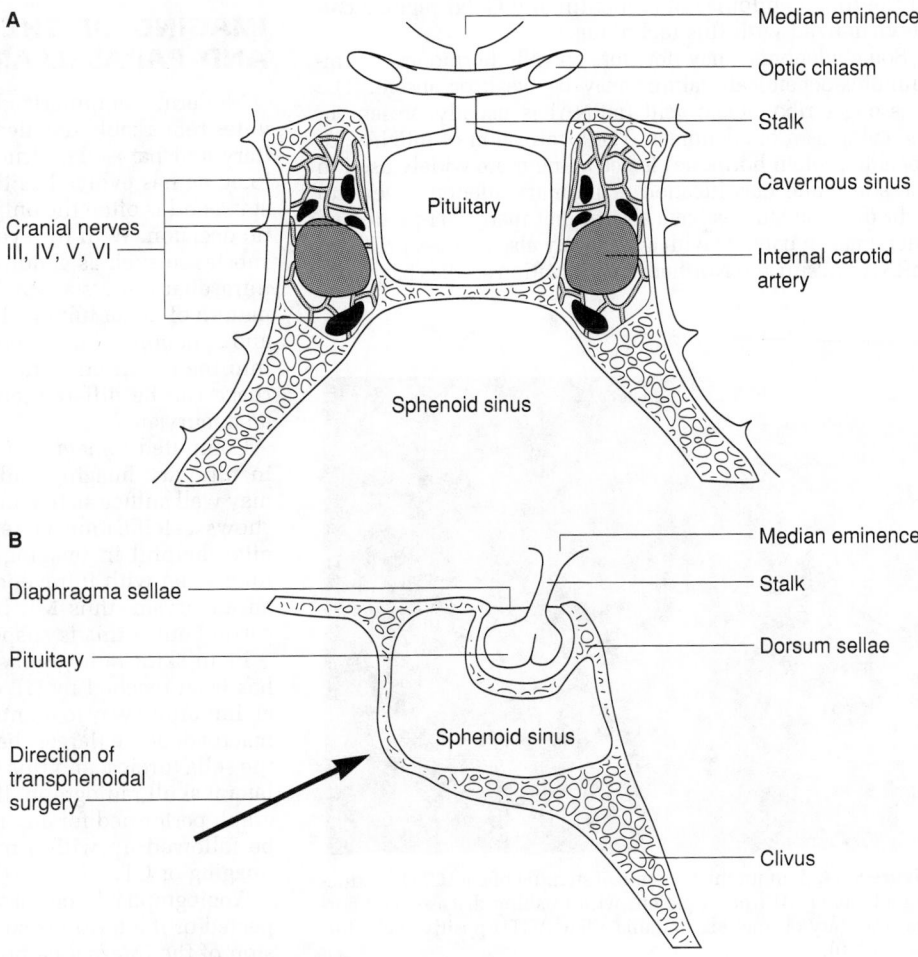

Figure 59-3. (*A*) Mid-pituitary coronal view of parasellar region. The sphenoid sinus is below and the cavernous sinuses are lateral. (*B*) Midsagittal view of pituitary and surrounding bony structures. Note the approach for transsphenoidal surgery. Anterior is to the left.

Table 59-1. FUNCTIONAL PITUITARY ADENOMAS: PATHOLOGIC FINDINGS

Adenoma Type	Incidence (%)	Staining*	Immunoreactivity	Ultrastructure
PRL-secreting				
Sparsely granulated	28	C	PRL	Few SG 150–500 nm misplaced exocytosis
Densely granulated	1	A	PRL	SG 400–1200 nm
GH-secreting				
Sparsely granulated	5	C–A	GH	SG 300–600 nm, fibrous bodies
Densely granulated	5	A	GH	SG 100–250 nm
Mixed GH cell–PRL cell	5	A–C	GH, PRL	Variable pattern
Mixed GH cell–PRL cell	1	A	GH, PRL	SG 150–450 nm and 350–1000 nm
ACTH-secreting	10	B	ACTH	SG 250–700 nm
				Prominent type I microfilaments
Gonadotroph cell adenoma	7–10	C–B	FSH, LH	SG 50–150 nm
				Distinct female pattern of honeycomb
				Golgi region
Thyrotroph cell adenoma	1	C–B	TSH	SG 50–250 nm

ACTH, adrenocorticotropic hormone; FSH, follicle-stimulating hormone; GH, growth hormone; LH, luteinizing
   hormone; PRL, prolactin; SG, secretory granules; TSH, thyroid-stimulating hormone.
* Conventional hematoxylin–eosin staining: A, acidophil; B, basophil; C, chromophobe.

adenomas according to the hormones that are being produced (Fig. 59-4). Highly purified polyclonal and monoclonal antibodies against prolactin, GH, ACTH, FSH-β, LH-β, and TSH-β, are available for immunohistochemical staining. Many studies with these antibodies have revealed that some pituitary tumors are composed of several cell types, which produce various hormones.[1] Ultrastructural immunohistochemistry provides another degree of refinement for classifying and studying adenomas, because the exact site of storage of the hormones in secretary granules and the subcellular sites of production and processing in the rough endoplasmic reticulin and Golgi regions can be visualized with this technique.

Some adenomas may not store specific hormones, so immunohistochemical staining may be weak or absent. The messenger ribonucleic acid (mRNA) is usually present in the cytoplasm of adenomas. The localization of mRNAs for specific protein hormones is becoming more widely used in the study and classification of pituitary adenomas. In situ hybridization studies have shown that many GH-producing adenomas in patients with acromegaly also express prolactin mRNA.[2] In situ and Northern hybridization studies have contributed to the understanding of adenoma subtypes. For example, clinically silent GH adenomas express GH mRNA, although the protein that is produced does not cause acromegaly. Other studies have shown that null-cell adenomas, which constitute up to 25% of pituitary neoplasms, commonly express the mRNA for gonadotropic hormones.

Although a great deal of information about the cell biology of pituitary adenomas has been gained through various methods of cell analysis, there are many gaps in our knowledge about the biology of these neoplasms.

IMAGING OF THE PITUITARY AND PARASELLAR REGION

Modern, computerized imaging technology now provides remarkably detailed multiplanar images of the pituitary and parasellar structures. Magnetic resonance (MR) imaging has evolved as the first choice for diagnostic imaging and is often the only test needed to reach a therapeutic decision. With intravenous infusion of a paramagnetic substance such as gadolinium, MR imaging demonstrates intrasellar tumors as small as 5 mm and shows the growth pattern of larger tumors. It reveals the extent of suprasellar and sphenoid sinus extension, as well as lateral extension into the cavernous sinuses (Fig. 59-5). Cysts and hemorrhage can be differentiated, as can blood flowing within an aneurysm.

Computed tomographic (CT) scanning also has a place in pituitary imaging and, if MR imaging is unavailable, may well suffice as the only mode of imaging. CT scanning shows calcification better than MR imaging and thus is often helpful in imaging a craniopharyngioma. CT scanning, even with intravenous contrast, cannot differentiate an aneurysm, thus MR imaging or angiography must be carried out if this is suspected.

Plain skull radiographs are not needed if the diagnosis has been reached by CT or MR imaging, but they remain an important way to identify incidental lesions. A pituitary macroadenoma (larger than 10 mm) causes enlargement of the sella turcica, and this can easily be observed on a plain lateral skull radiograph. If this finding is noted on a radiograph performed for any reason, such as trauma, it should be followed up with a more detailed study, such as MR imaging or CT.

Angiography is performed only if an aneurysm is suspected or if a lesion is so large that occlusion or compression of the internal carotid artery is in question.

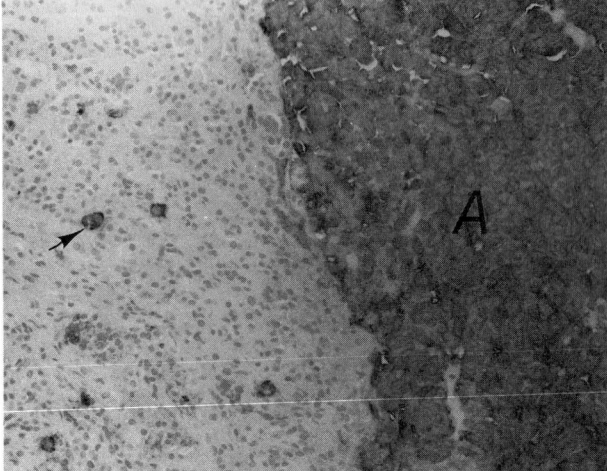

Figure 59-4. Immunohistochemical staining of an ACTH-producing adenoma (*A*) from a patient with Cushing disease. The normal pituitary on the left contains a few ACTH-positive cells (*arrow;* ×250).

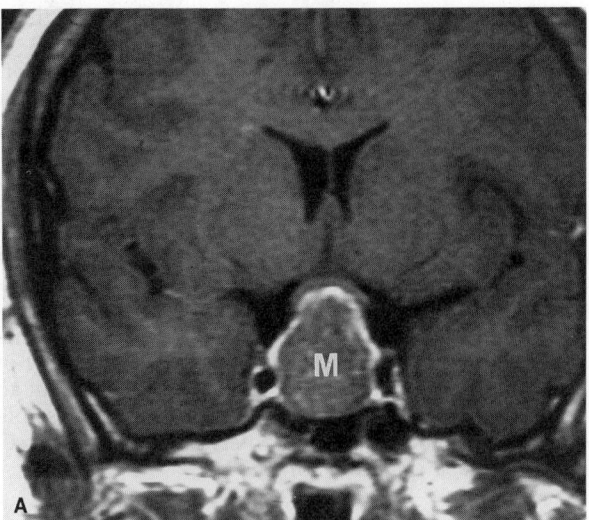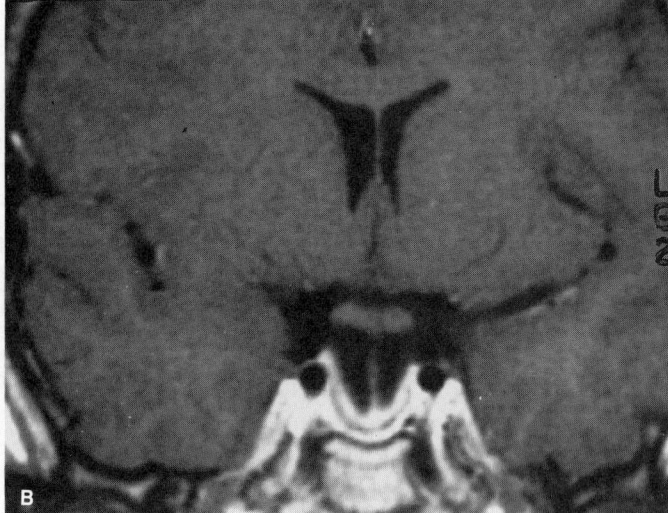

Figure 59-5. (*A*) Mid-pituitary coronal MR scan showing a pituitary macroadenoma (M). (*B*) Post-operative MR scan demonstrating gross total resection of tumor with cerebrospinal fluid in the sella.

CLINICAL AND ENDOCRINE EVALUATION

General Clinical Signs and Symptoms

Patients with pituitary lesions may present with symptoms and signs related to a mass effect on the pituitary and its surrounding structures, hypersecretion of hormones by the lesion itself, or a combination of both. Tumors or other mass lesions are generally larger than 1 cm before they produce symptoms related to compression. As a lesion enlarges, it may cause loss of function of the pituitary, usually manifested by a decrease in hormone secretion from the adenohypophysis. This may result in a loss of TSH and subsequent hypothyroidism. A decrease in ACTH results in Addison disease, and a decrease in LH and FSH causes amenorrhea. A decline in GH is noted only in children with a loss of normal growth progress. The one exception to this pattern is that generalized pituitary compression may cause a rise in prolactin, because the prolactin inhibitory factor (dopamine) from the hypothalamus may be compromised by the compression. Generalized compression from within the sella rarely results in loss of ADH from the neurohypophysis and subsequent diabetes insipidus. Lesions that originate in the region of the pituitary stalk, however, often present with early signs of diabetes insipidus. Symptoms related to loss of pituitary function are usually insidious in onset, with the exception of a sudden hemorrhage within the sella, or so-called pituitary apoplexy. Such hemorrhages are usually associated with the presence of a pituitary adenoma.

When mass lesions in the region of the pituitary enlarge, they may also compress or invade nearby structures, causing symptoms unrelated to endocrine function. As tumors or other lesions grow laterally from the sella, they encounter the various contents of the cavernous sinuses. These include the third, fourth, sixth, and first two divisions of the fifth cranial nerves, as well as the internal carotid artery. Compression of cranial nerves III, IV, or VI causes diplopia, and compression of cranial nerve V causes ipsilateral facial numbness. Invasion or constriction of the carotid may result in carotid occlusion, which in rare cases may result in cerebral infarction. Growth of a tumor in the relatively unrestricted upward direction is much more

common and often compresses the optic chiasm with resultant loss of vision, typically a bitemporal hemianopsia. Extensive upward intracranial growth may compress the hypothalamus or the third ventricle, causing hydrocephalus. Rarely, intracranial extension results in cortical irritation and associated seizures. Downward growth of tumors into the sphenoid sinus is common but causes no clinical symptoms or signs.

The syndromes associated with hypersecretion of pituitary hormones are discussed at length later in this chapter. They include Cushing disease (ACTH), acromegaly (GH), hyperprolactinemia (prolactin), and Nelson syndrome (ACTH after adrenalectomy). Rare cases of TSH-secreting adenomas have been documented. Traditionally, pituitary adenomas have been divided into nonfunctioning and functioning tumors, but it has been clear through immunohistochemical studies of the tumors that many nonfunctioning tumors are, in fact, endocrinologically active. Although these secreted hormones may not cause clinical symptoms or signs, they may serve as a marker for the presence of the tumor before and after treatment.

General Endocrine Evaluation

The extent of the endocrine evaluation of a patient with a pituitary lesion depends on the urgency of the situation (eg, if vision is impaired) and whether a hypersecretion state is suspected. If time permits, a careful evaluation of the endocrine status is warranted, including testing of pituitary reserve. Although this is most critical after treatment, it is ideal to have complete pretreatment evaluation for comparison. Pituitary endocrine evaluation should include baseline values for prolactin, GH, LH, FSH, testosterone (male), estrogen (female), cortisol, ACTH, electrolytes, glucose, and thyroid function tests, including TSH. Because baseline values may not reflect the ability of the pituitary to respond to stress, it is also important to test the reserve capacity of the pituitary. The most efficient way to test this is with insulin-induced hypoglycemia combined with TRH. Assuming the patient does not have a contraindication to transient hypoglycemia (ie, ischemic heart disease, cerebrovascular disease, or seizure disorder), insulin is given in a dosage of 0.10 to 0.15 IU/kg, such that the serum glucose falls below 40 mg/dL. In the patient with normal pituitary function, this causes a rise in cortisol to above 20 μg/dL and a rise in GH to above 10 ng/mL. In patients with compromised ACTH or GH production, a response is not noted. The administration of TRH should normally cause a rise in both TSH and prolactin. If indicated, gonadotropin-releasing hormone may be administered to increase the gonadotropins, LH and FSH.

If urgent surgical decompression is indicated, the previously mentioned baseline values are obtained, and the patient is prepared for surgery with sufficient hydrocortisone to cover the possibility of inadequate cortisol reserve. Careful postoperative evaluation is then carried out to determine if long-term replacement therapy is needed. It should be stressed that if the patient receives postoperative radiation therapy, the status of the pituitary should be checked periodically over the following years because pituitary function may slowly decline after radiation exposure.

If diabetes insipidus is suspected, urine-specific gravity and serum sodium should be checked, and fluid intake and output should be carefully evaluated.

Cushing Disease

Although the diagnosis of hypercortisolism (Cushing syndrome) is often reached after physical examination by an astute physician, sometimes the physical manifestations are not obvious. Often, the precise diagnosis as to the cause of hypercortisolism is difficult to ascertain, even with detailed endocrine and imaging tests. The findings of Cushing syndrome often include central obesity, hypertension, hirsutism, fatigue, easy bruisability, stria, moonlike facies, dorsal fat pad, and often depression or other mental changes. Less common abnormalities include headache, osteoporosis, diabetes mellitus, galactorrhea, periplural edema, and amenorrhea. Often, a patient presents without the classic cushingoid appearance and only complains of severe fatigue or depression.

The cause of hypercortisolism is an ACTH-secreting pituitary adenoma (Cushing disease) in up to 80% of cases, with the remainder due either to an adrenocortical tumor or to an ectopic neoplasm secreting ACTH or corticotropin-releasing factor. Pituitary-dependent hypercortisolism is much more common in women (80%), and an ectopic etiology more common in men (80%). Thus, if an adult man presents with rapid onset of Cushing syndrome, particularly with weight loss, an ectopic neoplasm must be strongly considered. It should also be kept in mind that increased cortisol levels may be due to primary depression, alcoholism, obesity, or drugs such as estrogens and phenytoin.

Because up to 60% of patients with pituitary etiologies have nondiagnostic imaging studies, the diagnosis often relies completely on endocrine testing.[3] Multiple measurements of cortisol and ACTH to evaluate the diurnal pattern are important but often misleading. They are mainly of value when clearly elevated. Urinary free cortisol excretion over 24 hours is an extremely important measurement. It is not elevated with obesity or medications, but it is elevated with depression or alcoholism. If the overnight dexamethasone screening test (1 mg at 10:00 PM) yields an 8:00 AM serum cortisol level of less than 5 μg/dL, then hypercortisolism is rarely present. Generally, patients with a pituitary etiology of hypercortisolism do not show suppression with the low-dosage dexamethasone test (0.5 mg every 6 hours for eight doses) but do with the higher dosage (2 mg every 6 hours for eight doses). Patients with adrenal or ectopic etiologies classically do not experience suppres-

sion with either dose. There are exceptions to both of these tests (Fig. 59-6).

When metyrapone is given, a rise in serum 11-deoxycortisol (or urinary 17-hydroxycortisol) is seen in normal or pituitary etiology patients. Unfortunately, a positive response does not absolutely rule out an adrenal or ectopic source of hypercortisolism. Perhaps the most specific diagnostic test is transfemoral catheterization with simultaneous measurements of ACTH levels in both inferior petrosal sinuses and a concurrent determination of the peripheral blood level. This approach has produced specific information about the existence of an ACTH-secreting pituitary tumor and even the laterality of the tumor. Along with this intensive endocrine workup, appropriate CT scanning of the adrenal glands and thorax should be carried out to look for adrenal or lung tumors. The additional possible etiology consists of simple hyperplasia of the pituitary secreting increased quantities of ACTH.

Acromegaly

As with Cushing syndrome, the diagnosis of acromegaly may be reached clinically when patients present with advanced stages of the disease. The obvious enlargement of facial features and acral enlargement may be subtle and the presenting symptoms may be nonspecific headaches, fatigue, arthralgias, decreased libido, or amenorrhea. Patients often have hypertension, diabetes mellitus, and the early onset of atherosclerotic cardiovascular disease. It is critical that this disease be diagnosed and treated, because the mortality rate is 50% greater than normal per decade beyond the age of 40 years. With rare exceptions, the cause of acromegaly is a GH-secreting pituitary adenoma. As with other functioning adenomas, the tumors may be small or large and invasive. Patients with larger tumors may, of course, present with visual loss. Rarely, elevated GH levels are secondary to GH-releasing hormone produced by an ectopic tumor.

The endocrine diagnosis rests largely on serum GH levels because 90% of patients have levels higher than 10 ng/mL. Normally, GH in a resting, nonstressed patient is less than 5 ng/mL, but both normal and acromegalic patients may have levels between 5 and 10 ng/mL. Somatomedin C, or insulin-like growth factor I, which mediates the effect of GH on peripheral tissues, should also be measured in all circumstances where GH excess is suspected. When acromegaly is apparent, but consistently elevated GH levels are not obtained, the glucose suppression test is the most useful diagnostic procedure. In normal patients, 1 to 2 hours after the oral administration of 100 g of glucose, the GH level falls well below 5 ng/mL. This suppression is not seen with GH-secreting adenomas, and often a paradoxical rise in GH is observed (Fig. 59-7).

Hyperprolactinemia

Because 60% to 70% of prolactin-secreting pituitary adenomas are microadenomas, most patients present with endocrine symptoms as opposed to local mass effects. Hyperprolactinemia in women usually causes amenorrhea and often galactorrhea and thus, in young women, provides a reason to seek medical evaluation early in the growth of the tumor. In men, this early warning sign is not available, and they almost invariably present with macroadenomas usually associated with loss of libido, infertility, or loss of vision. It should be kept in mind that the finding of amenorrhea or galactorrhea associated with an elevated prolactin level does not always indicate the presence of a pituitary tumor. Table 59-2 lists the other possible causes of hyperprolactinemia. Most important among these are

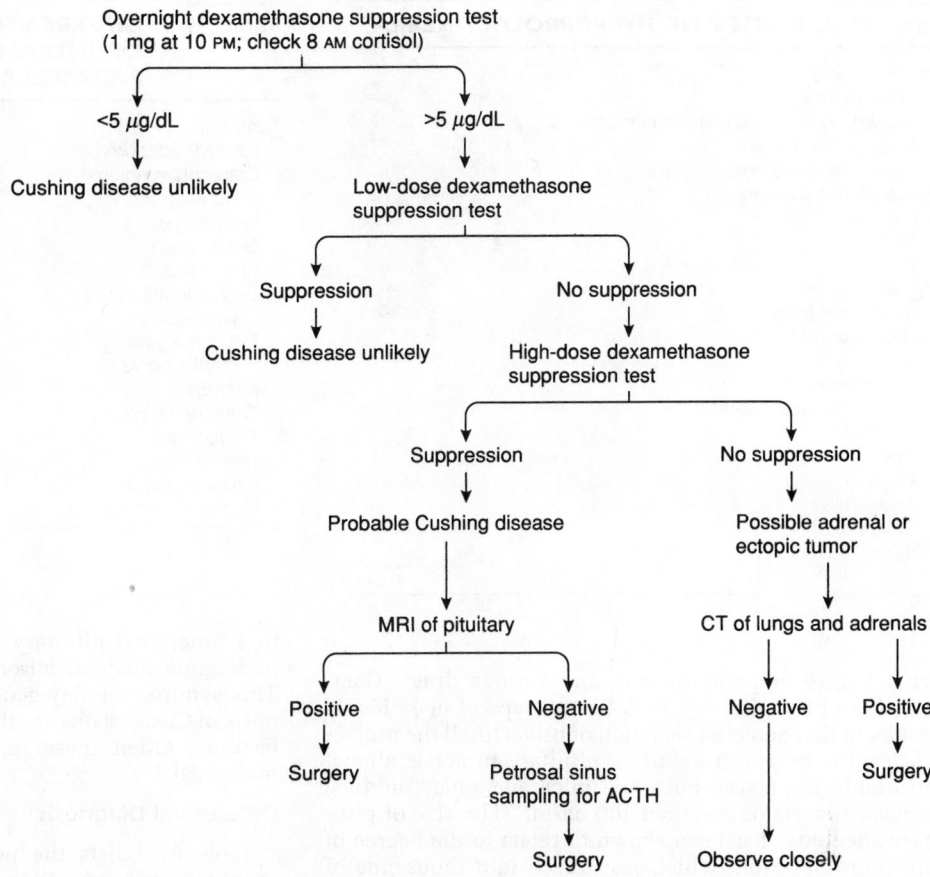

Figure 59-6. Workup and treatment of Cushing disease.

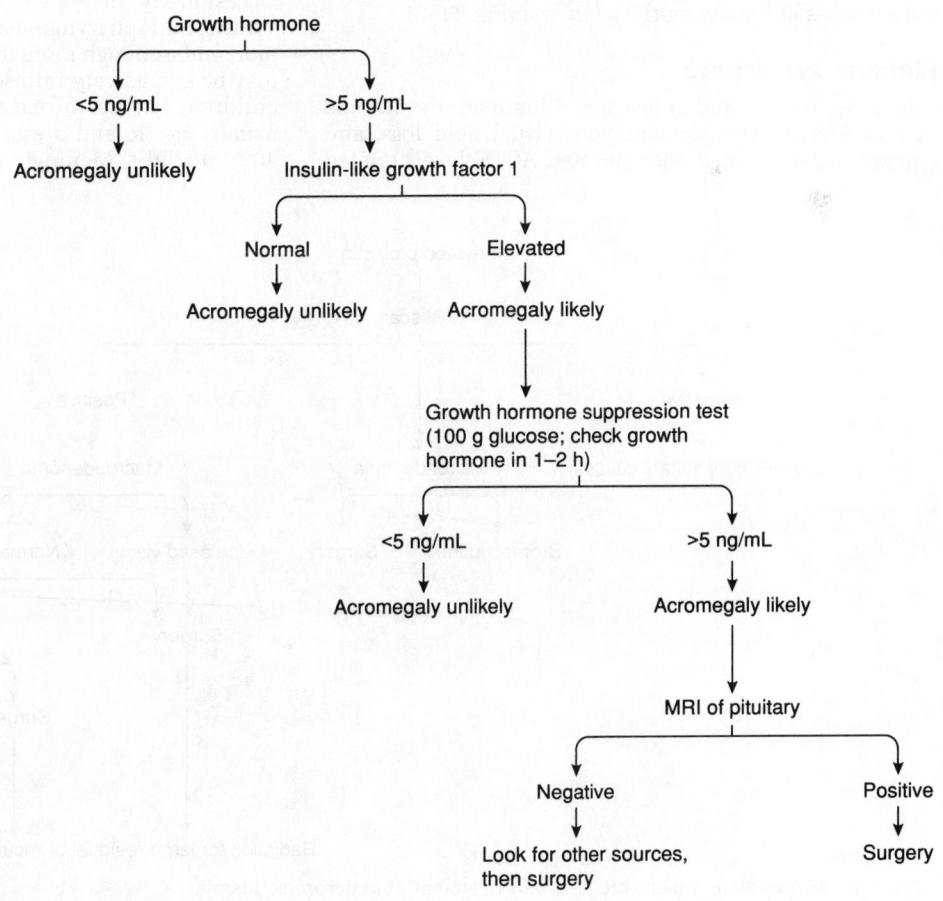

Figure 59-7. Workup and treatment of acromegaly.

Table 59-2. CAUSES OF HYPERPROLACTINEMIA

Pituitary disease
  Prolactinoma
  Growth hormone–secreting adenoma
  Pituitary stalk section
  Empty sella syndrome
Hypothalamic disease
  Tumors
  Sarcoidosis
  Radiation
Hypothyroidism
Chronic renal failure
Hepatic disease
Drugs
Phenothiazines
  Tricyclic antidepressants
  Estrogen
  Opiates
  Reserpine
  Verapamil
  Others
Pregnancy
Stress

Table 59-3. DIFFERENTIAL DIAGNOSES OF INTRASELLAR AND PARASELLAR LESIONS

Tumors	Cysts
Pituitary adenoma	Rathke cleft cyst
Craniopharyngioma	Pituitary cyst
Meningioma	Inflammatory and granulomatous
Lymphoma	lesions
Germinoma	Bacterial abscess
Chordoma	Sarcoidosis
Granular cell tumor	Eosinophilic granuloma
(choristoma)	(histiocytosis X)
Neuroma (arising from	Tuberculosis
cranial nerve V)	Mycoses
Metastatic	Granulomatous hypophysitis
Optic nerve glioma	Aneurysm
Epidermoid	Hamartoma
Dermoid	Empty sella syndrome
Infundibuloma	Pituitary apoplexy
Hypothalamic glioma	

renal failure, hypothyroidism, and various drugs. Compression of the pituitary stalk by any type of mass lesion results in the increased secretion of prolactin. If the prolactin level is over 150 ng/mL, a pituitary tumor is almost invariably the cause, but often microadenomas produce prolactin levels of less than 100 ng/mL. The size of pituitary adenomas has been shown to relate to the degree of prolactin elevation, which may reach into thousands of nanograms per milliliter. There are no reliable provocative tests to differentiate prolactinomas from other causes of hyperprolactinemia, so the diagnosis relies on ruling out other causes and imaging the adenoma (Fig. 59-8).

Nelson Syndrome

In 1958, Nelson and colleagues[4] identified a syndrome of progressive hyperpigmentation, visual field loss, and amenorrhea associated with elevated ACTH levels related to a functional pituitary adenoma in a patient who had undergone bilateral adrenalectomy for hypercortisolism. This syndrome today generally represents a missed diagnosis of Cushing disease that has been treated with adrenalectomy. Often these tumors are aggressive or frankly malignant.

Differential Diagnosis

Table 59-3 lists the possible lesions that may occur within the sella or in the parasellar region. Pituitary adenomas head the list, because they are the most common lesion in this region and constitute 8% to 10% of all brain tumors. Occasionally, they are cystic and confused with other lesions. Craniopharyngiomas are the next most common tumor, and although more often suprasellar in location, they may be exclusively intrasellar. They are more common in children, but up to one third occur in adults. They are usually cystic and are calcified in 70% of children and 40% of adults. Meningiomas are also more commonly su-

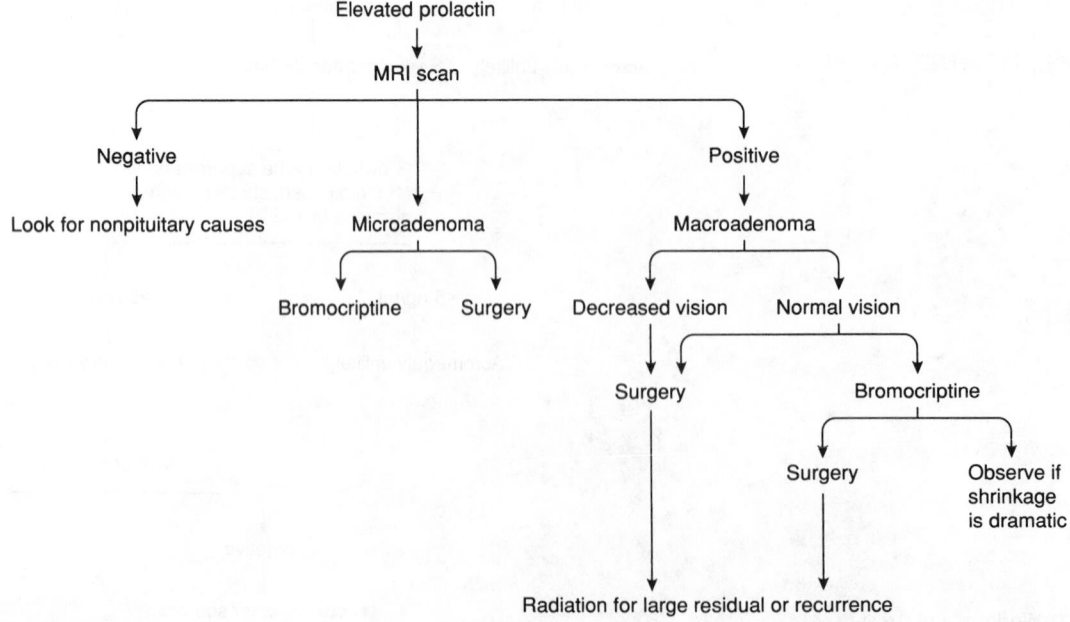

Figure 59-8. Diagnostic tests and treatment of hyperprolactinemia.

prasellar and enhance strongly on CT and MR imaging. Germinomas, or so-called ectopic pinealomas, generally involve the pituitary stalk and often causes diabetes insipidus. It is a general principle that if a patient presents with diabetes insipidus, one should think of a lesion other than a pituitary adenoma. Metastatic malignancies, commonly from lung and breast primary tumors, may be found in the pituitary, with 70% residing in the posterior pituitary. Optic nerve gliomas and hypothalamic gliomas may occasionally be confused with pituitary adenomas, as can the rare granular cell tumor (choristoma). Dermoids and epidermoids may occur intrasellarly, and fifth nerve neuromas may compress the sella.

Rathke cysts are benign congenital remnants that occur within the sella and can cause loss of pituitary function by local compression. These can be confused on imaging studies with cystic adenomas or craniopharyngiomas, and require biopsy and surgical decompression.

Inflammatory and granulomatous processes should also be kept in mind, including bacterial abscesses within the sella. Sarcoidosis may involve the pituitary or its stalk, as can the granulomas associated with histiocytosis X. Hamartomas may involve the pituitary stalk and hypothalamus and are impossible to differentiate from invasive gliomas on imaging studies.

Aneurysms, usually from the internal carotid arteries, but occasionally from the basilar artery, may appear within the sella and must be ruled out preoperatively with MR imaging or angiography.

The empty-sella syndrome is generally an anatomic variation that rarely causes symptoms. Patients with headaches or head trauma may undergo a skull radiograph or CT scan, and an enlarged sella may be found. With high-resolution CT or MR scanning, usually the elongated stalk is seen to reach the sellar floor, thus ruling out a cystic lesion. A contrast cisternogram may be used to visualize cerebrospinal fluid within the sella if necessary.

Pituitary apoplexy occurs symptomatically only rarely but may cause a profound and emergent situation. Infarction and hemorrhage, usually in a pituitary adenoma, causes sudden intrasellar expansion with severe headache and rapid loss of pituitary function, resulting in hypotension. There may also be sudden loss of vision and the development of cranial nerve palsies. Treatment in severe cases involves the administration of steroids and surgical decompression of the sella.

TREATMENT AND RESULTS

The treatment of primary pituitary adenomas is generally surgical, although certain exceptions exist. Even with modern imaging techniques, the unequivocal diagnosis of an adenoma is not reached until tissue is obtained. As seen in Table 59-3, the list of possible parasellar lesions is extensive, and it is not within the scope of this chapter to delineate the specific treatment for each lesion. Along with surgical removal or decompression of pituitary adenomas, additional treatment in the form of radiation or medical therapy is often indicated. In addition to treatment directed at the primary lesion, it is critical to thoroughly assess pituitary function before and after treatment to decide if hormone replacement is indicated.

More than 95% of pituitary adenomas can be approached by the transsphenoidal route. This is usually accomplished through a sublabial incision and a transseptal approach to the sphenoid. Once the sphenoid sinus has been entered, the operating microscope is brought in, the anterior wall of the sella is carefully drilled away, and the dura surrounding the pituitary is identified. The dura is opened and, if a macroadenoma is present, the tumor is usually seen directly beneath the dura. If a microadenoma is present, the surgeon must carefully dissect around and often through the pituitary to identify the small tumor.

Contraindications to this approach, and therefore indications for a craniotomy, include the following: (1) massive suprasellar extension; (2) extensive lateral intracranial extension; and (3) the rare dumbbell-shaped tumor with a tight construction at the level of the diaphragma sella. If a craniotomy is necessary, a right subfrontal approach to the optic nerve and chiasm is required, and the tumor is removed in a piecemeal fashion using the operating microscope and microinstruments.

Nonfunctioning Adenomas

Because patients with nonfunctioning adenomas usually present with the effects of a mass lesion, these tumors are rarely microadenomas. Although these can be either exclusively intrasellar in location or have extensive intracranial involvement, these tumors are almost all approached currently via the transsphenoidal route.

There are three goals of surgery for nonfunctioning macroadenomas: (1) establishment of a diagnosis; (2) decompression of surrounding structures; and (3) gross total removal of tumor tissue if possible. The first goal is usually accomplished easily, and although most tumors turn out to be adenomas, surprise findings are not unusual. Decompression is also usually accomplished readily because most tumors are soft and easily removed. Less than 5% of adenomas are so fibrous that decompression is difficult. Evidence for adequate decompression is provided by the consistent finding that 75% to 80% of patients with visual field losses show recovery after transsphenoidal tumor removal.[5] The third goal, that of total tumor resection, is much more difficult to accomplish with macroadenomas. It has been demonstrated that most macroadenomas (88% to 94%) invade at least the dura mater, and many have gross invasion of surrounding structures. This invasion makes complete surgical resection impossible and, therefore, these patients need to be followed indefinitely with high-quality imaging to monitor tumor progression or recurrence. Whereas it was once common practice to provide postoperative radiation to all macroadenomas, most neurosurgeons are content to watch for progression with high-resolution imaging and reserve local radiation for that indication. There is currently no medical treatment for nonfunctional adenomas.

Cushing Disease

Once it has been established that the cause of a patient's hypercortisolism is a pituitary lesion, the treatment of choice is transsphenoidal exploration of the pituitary. Because only 40% of such patients have positive imaging studies, many of these patients require careful and systematic exploration of the sellar contents by an experienced pituitary surgeon.[3] Microadenomas secreting ACTH may be very small and are often located deep within the gland itself. If a tumor is not evident on opening the dura and examining all surfaces of the pituitary, then incisions must be made into the gland and an internal exploration carried out. These microadenomas are usually in one lateral aspect of the pituitary gland, and the initial choice of which side to explore may be guided by the results of the preoperative petrosal sinus sampling for ACTH levels as described earlier. If no tumor is identified, then a decision must be made as to whether to resect all or a portion of the gland. If the endocrine evidence is convincing for a pituitary origin and the patient has no desire to have children, then total hypophysectomy is warranted. If the petrosal sinus sampling clearly indicates laterality of the ACTH secretion, then an appropriate hemiresection of the gland is carried out. Macroadenomas are treated with maximum tumor resection but, of course, are more difficult situations in which to accomplish endocrine remission. Obviously, patients with adrenal or ectopic lesions are treated by resection of tumors in these locations. Microadenomas are the source of ACTH secretion in about 75% of patients.[3,6,7] The postoperative remission rate in these patients is 88% to 96%, and the long-term recurrence rate appears to be no more than 5%. Therefore, selective microsurgical tumor resection in patients with microadenomas is clearly the current treatment of choice.

Some 10% to 20% of patients who undergo exploration have macroadenomas, and the postoperative remission rates in these patients have been reported to be from 33% to 61%.[3,6-9] Most of these patients require postoperative radiation therapy, which leads to remissions in some of the surgical failures. Those that fail to remit with both surgery and radiation require either a surgical adrenalectomy or medical suppression of adrenal function. In a small percentage of patients who have undergone adrenalectomy, the pituitary tumors continue to grow and secrete ACTH, thus producing Nelson syndrome.

Acromegaly

Like Cushing disease, acromegaly is a condition that ultimately threatens the life of the patient. For this reason, it must be treated aggressively, even at the expense of normal pituitary function. Over the past two decades a variety of medical, surgical, and radiation therapies have evolved that have proved effective at lowering GH levels. No single treatment is uniformly effective, and often a combination of treatments is necessary. The goals of treatment are to lower the circulating GH or somatomedin C levels to a normal range and to reduce the size of the mass lesion that is causing compression-related symptoms.

Unfortunately, only 20% to 34% of GH-secreting tumors are microadenomas, making microsurgical tumor resection less effective than in Cushing disease. When a microadenoma is selectively removed transsphenoidally, endocrine remission may be expected in 80% to 88% of cases.[10] When a macroadenoma is resected, immediate postoperative remission is reported in 30% to 68% of cases.[11] The rate of remission is inversely related to higher preoperative GH levels and larger invasive tumors. Preoperative treatment of macroadenomas with a somatostatin analogue may improve postoperative remission rates.[12]

Radiation therapy has proven moderately effective both as a primary mode of treatment and in conjunction with partial surgical resection. Proton-beam heavy-particle therapy has been reported in 510 patients, 428 of which were observed for between 1 and 20 years.[13] Analysis of these patients revealed that there is a progressive fall in GH levels beginning immediately after treatment and continuing for up to 20 years. After 2 years, 47.5% of patients have GH levels below 10 ng/mL; at 4, 10, and 20 years, the rate is 65%, 87.5%, and 97.5%, respectively. If a GH level of less than 5 ng/mL is considered a cure, this level is achieved in 75% of patients at 10 years and 92.5% of patients at 20 years. Conventional radiation therapy provides comparable results (10-year posttreatment levels below 10 ng/mL in 81% and below 5 ng/mL in 69%).

Bromocriptine, a dopamine receptor agonist, has been demonstrated to lower GH levels in 71% of 126 patients.[11] Unfortunately, GH levels of less than 10 ng/mL were achieved in only 14% of patients in this study. A clinical response was achieved in up to 95% of acromegalic patients, and reduced somatomedin C levels were found in

some patients with persistently elevated GH levels. Bromocriptine does not appear to be an effective primary treatment for acromegaly but may help to control GH and somatomedin C levels as an adjuvant therapy.

A somatostatin analogue has recently been used on an experimental basis and has been demonstrated to significantly reduce GH and somatomedin C levels in most patients. This treatment provides only minimal tumor shrinkage, and GH levels rise again immediately after cessation of the drug. This drug may prove to be useful in preoperative treatment or in surgical failures.[12] The recurrence of GH-secreting tumors appears to be only 4% after successful surgery and less than 1% after radiation.[14]

Given the variety of treatment modalities, a rational therapeutic approach is to resect tumors surgically when possible and to provide radiation therapy to those in whom a remission cannot be achieved. Somatostatin analogue is potentially useful as an adjuvant therapy in selected patients.

Prolactinomas

Prolactin-secreting adenomas are the most common functioning pituitary tumors but remain the most controversial with regard to treatment. The controversy exists because, unlike ACTH- or GH-secreting adenomas, there is reasonably effective medical treatment available in the form of dopamine agonists. The treatment options include medical therapy, usually with bromocriptine, transsphenoidal surgical resection, radiation therapy, or in some cases, no treatment. Because different considerations are involved with different sized tumors, the treatments are discussed according to size.

Macroadenomas

The goal in treating a patient with a large, prolactin-secreting adenoma is to decompress the optic pathways if involved and to reduce the prolactin levels to normal concentrations. Surgery is effective in improving vision in 80% of cases, but vision has also been reported to improve in patients treated with bromocriptine. The success of surgery in reducing prolactin levels to normal has generally been disappointing. The uniform finding of various investigators has been that the likelihood of normalizing prolactin levels is greatly reduced if the initial concentration is greater than 200 ng/mL or if the macroadenoma is larger than 10 mm.

Treatment of patients with macroadenomas using bromocriptine reduces prolactin levels significantly in almost all instances, and reductions to normal ranges are reported in over 46%.[14] In 90% of patients, the size of the tumor is decreased to some degree, and in many, the reduction is dramatic. It is also true, with rare exception, that the tumor returns to its original size once bromocriptine is stopped. It is recognized that up to 25% of patients with macroadenomas have an increase in tumor size during pregnancy, whereas this is true in less than 1% of microadenomas.[14]

It has been shown with a mixture of prolactin and nonfunctioning tumors that the recurrence rate is 21% 10 years after radiation plus surgery, 29% with radiation alone, and 91% with only surgery.[15] These data demonstrate the effectiveness of radiation therapy and the lack of effectiveness of surgery alone. The treating physician's obligation is to discuss in detail the treatment options with the patient and to decide on a specific course of action. A transsphenoidal debulking of the tumor is recommended, with remission achieved in up to 30% of patients. Usually, bromocriptine is used for 3 to 4 weeks preoperatively to reduce the size of the tumor. If a large invasive tumor is encountered, postoperative radiation therapy is recommended. If remission is not achieved but the tumor is grossly removed, then bromocriptine alone is used postoperatively. Surgery is particularly recommended if subsequent pregnancy is desired, because expansion of the tumor during pregnancy (off bromocriptine) is likely to occur, possibly jeopardizing vision. Careful follow-up with CT or MR imaging is required for the lifetime of the patient, because rapid tumor growth may occur. The recurrence rate of macroadenomas is from 25% to 75% within 5 years,[15] so adjunctive therapy is clearly indicated if the postoperative prolactin level begins to rise.

Microadenomas

The surgical treatment of prolactin-secreting microadenomas results in postoperative remission in a much higher percentage of patients. Two large series report remission in 77%[16] and 72%[17] of patients. In the latter report, 88% were in remission with prolactin levels below 100 ng/mL, and only 50% had prolactin levels above 100 ng/mL. The incidence of new postoperative hypogonadism was only 1%. Others[18] reported an immediate postoperative remission rate of 81% without bromocriptine pretreatment but only a 33% rate with pretreatment. These data suggest that bromocriptine induces fibrosis within the tumor and that the lower remission rate is related to this fibrosis. Primary medical treatment is safe and effective but may lower the chance of long-term surgical cure by causing fibrosis. As in macroadenomas, long-term continued therapy is indicated, because prolactin levels rapidly rise with cessation of dopamine agonists. Pregnancy is of less risk to the patient with a microadenoma because tumor expansion and visual loss are rare.

The recurrence rate in patients initially in remission after microsurgical tumor removal has been somewhat disappointing compared with other functioning tumors. Recurrences have uniformly been found to be higher in patients with postoperative prolactin levels in the upper end of the normal range. Recurrence rates of 17% to 50% over 5 years have been reported. Radiation therapy does not play a role in the treatment of microadenomas unless they recur in an aggressive manner.

The approach to prolactin-secreting microadenomas that can be seen on imaging studies is to carefully explain the medical and surgical options to the patient. Surgery is offered as a primary option because it allows the possibility of long-term remission without continued medical therapy. In the final analysis, patients must make an educated choice between primary medical or surgical treatment.

There are few objective data about surgical exploration of patients with presumed microadenomas. Unlike patients with Cushing disease or acromegaly, most patients with hyperprolactinemia and normasa l imaging studies have not been explored. Once other causes of hyperprolactinemia have been ruled out, dopamine agonists are generally tried to lower prolactin levels. These patients need to be carefully followed with imaging studies and prolactin levels. The incidence of subsequent development of obvious adenomas is unknown, but it appears to be as low as 5%.

REFERENCES

1. Kovacs K, Horvath E. Tumors of the pituitary gland. In: Hartmann WH, ed. Atlas of tumor pathology, series 2, fascicle 21. Washington, DC, Armed Forces Institute of Pathology, 1986:192.
2. Lloyd RV, Cano M, Chandler WF, et al. Human growth hormone and prolactin secreting pituitary adenomas analyzed by in situ hybridization. Am J Pathol 1989;134:605.
3. Chandler WF, Schteingart DE, Lloyd RV, et al. Surgical treatment of Cushing's disease. J Neurosurg 1987;66:204.
4. Nelson DH, Meakin JW, Dealy JB, et al. ACTH-producing tumor of the pituitary gland. N Engl J Med 1958;259:161.
5. Ebersold MJ, Quast LM, Laws ER, et al. Long-term results in transsphenoidal removal of nonfunctioning pituitary adenomas. J Neurosurg 1986;64:713.
6. Boggan JE, Tyrrell JB, Wilson CB. Transsphenoidal microsurgical management of Cushing's disease. J Neurosurg 1983;59:195.
7. Hardy J. Cushing's disease: 50 years later. Can J Neurol Sci 1982;9:375.
8. Kuwayama A, Kageyama N. Current management of Cushing's disease: part II. Contemp Neurosurg 1985;7:1.
9. Salassa RM, Laws ER, Carpenter PC, Northcutt RC. Cushing's disease: 50 years later. Trans Am Clin Climatol Assoc 1982;94:122.
10. Tindall GT, Tindall SC. Transsphenoidal surgery for acromegaly: long-term results in 50 patients. In: Black PM, Zervas NT, Ridgeway EC, et al, eds. Secretory tumors of the pituitary gland. New York, Raven Press, 1984:175.
11. Besser GM, Wass JAH. The medical management of acromegaly. In: Black PM, Zervas NT, Ridgeway EC, et al JB, eds. Secretory tumors of the pituitary gland. New York, Raven Press, 1984:155.
12. Barkan AL, Lloyd RV, Chandler WF, et al. Preoperative treatment of acromegaly with long-acting somatostatin: shrinkage of invasive pituitary macroadenomas and improved surgical remission rate. J Clin Endocrinol Metab 1988;67:1040.
13. Kliman B, Kjellberg RN, Swisher B, Butler W. Proton beam therapy of acromegaly: a 20 year experience. In: Black PM, Zervas NT, Ridgeway EC, et al, eds. Secretory tumors of the pituitary gland. New York, Raven Press, 1984:191.
14. Thorner MO, Evans WS, Vance ML. Medical management of prolactinomas: I. In: Black PM, Servas NT, Ridgeway EC, et al, eds. Secretory tumors of the pituitary gland. New York, Raven Press, 1984:53.
15. Sheline GE, Grossman A, Jones AE, et al. Radiation therapy for prolactinomas. In: Black PM, Zervas NI, Ridgeway EC, et al, eds. Secretory tumors of the pituitary gland. New York, Raven Press, 1984:93.
16. Hardy J. Transsphenoidal microsurgery of prolactinomas. In: Black PM, Zervas NT, Ridgeway EC, et al, eds. Secretory tumors of the pituitary gland. New York, Raven Press, 1984:73.
17. Randall RV, Laws ER, Abboud CF, et al. Transsphenoidal microsurgical treatment of prolactin-producing pituitary adenomas. Mayo Clin Proc 1983;58:108.
18. Landolt AM, Keller PJ, Froesch ER, et al. Bromocriptine: does it jeopardize the result of later surgery for prolactinomas? Lancet 1982;1:657.

SURGERY: SCIENTIFIC PRINCIPLES AND PRACTICE, Second Edition, edited by Lazar J. Greenfield, Michael W. Mulholland, Keith T. Oldham, Gerald B. Zelenock, and Keith D. Lillemoe. Lippincott–Raven Publishers, Philadelphia, © 1997.

CHAPTER 60

BREAST

DAVID A. AUGUST AND VERNON K. SONDAK

Diseases of the breast are among the disorders most commonly evaluated by general surgeons. Breast disease is an area in which the practicing surgeon may play the role of gatekeeper and primary care physician. Clinical and laboratory advances have had a major impact on the evaluation, treatment, and outcome of patients with benign and malignant breast disorders. This chapter presents a practical clinical approach to the care of patients with breast problems and a rational scientific basis for this approach.

Table 60-1. RESULTS OF OPERATIONS FOR BREAST CANCER IN THE 19th CENTURY

Series	Number	Local Recurrence Rate (%)
Cases collected before 1890	1305	65
Halsted radical mastectomy	50	6

(Adapted from Kinne W. Primary treatment of breast cancer. In: Harris JR, Hellman S, Henderson IC, Kinne DW, eds. Breast diseases. Philadelphia, JB Lippincott, 1987:260)

HISTORICAL PERSPECTIVE

Study of the Edwin Smith Surgical Papyrus (circa 1600 BC) reveals ancient Egyptian references to both benign breast diseases and breast cancer. Hippocrates discussed the treatment of breast cancer and suggested that in cases of deep-seated cancer, it was preferable not to treat the patient; he believed treatment hastened death. Galen described surgery for superficial breast cancers and emphasized the importance of purging and bleeding to allow the escape of "black bile." With the Renaissance in the 16th century came a renewed interest in breast diseases. The role of surgery for treatment of breast cancer was explored in a more systematic fashion.[1] Before 1890, however, the outlook for patients with breast cancer remained dismal. Local recurrence rates after breast cancer surgery averaged 65% and cure was rare (Table 60-1). In 1894, Halsted described the radical mastectomy.[2] This operation achieved a dramatic reduction in the incidence of local recurrence after surgery to 6%, and even cured some women.

In the past century, modest improvements have been made in breast cancer control and cure. It would be a mistake to conclude, however, that patients are not better off today than a century ago. Improved diagnostic tools and a better understanding of breast physiology and endocrinology have refined the evaluation and treatment of breast diseases. Since Halsted, insights into the modes of spread of breast cancer and the recognition of breast cancer as a systemic disease have revolutionized treatment. Surgically, less can be better. Improvement in breast cancer survival for selected patients has been realized through the use of systemic chemotherapy and hormonal agents. Recent discoveries suggest that further advances are imminent. Discovery of the BRCA-1 gene responsible for many instances of familial breast cancer, the elucidation of new prognostic factors, improved understanding of mechanisms of intracellular signaling, and clinical trials investigating carcinoma in situ and breast cancer chemoprevention promise improved care in the near future.

These advances have already resulted in major changes in clinical practice. As recently as 25 years ago, more than half of breast cancer patients in the United States underwent radical mastectomy. In 1981, however, this figure was only 4%; modified radical mastectomy had become the surgical procedure of choice[3] (Table 60-2). Equally striking transformations have occurred since 1981. By 1986, breast-conserving surgery for primary operable breast cancer was used for about one third of patients nationally, and in some regions of the United States, more than 40% of women were treated without the use of mastectomy.[4] There have also been marked increases in the use of radiotherapy, chemotherapy, hormone therapy, and breast reconstruction to treat breast cancer.[5,6] It is now rare for a patient not to receive multimodality therapy. It is likely that similar dramatic changes will occur during the next decade.

ANATOMY AND EMBRYOLOGY

Embryology and Development

The first manifestation of breast development in utero is the appearance of the milk line during the fifth week of gestation. This ridge of tissue runs from the base of the upper limb to the base of the lower limb. Over several weeks, all but the thoracic portion of this ridge regresses. From the seventh week of gestation to birth, the mammary anlage on the chest wall develops into an epithelial bud with 15 to 20 ducts, and the nipple develops its circular smooth muscle fibers. After birth, in utero exposure to maternal hormones may stimulate the neonatal breast to produce colostrum ("witch's milk"). This is generally expressible the first week after birth and may persist for as long as 1 month. From this point, aside from minor development of the ductal system, the breast is quiescent until puberty.

Failure of proper regression of the milk line leads to the most common congenital breast anomaly—accessory breast tissue. In the adult, accessory breast tissue can be found anywhere along the milk line, from axilla to groin. Most frequently, an accessory nipple (polythelia) is encountered; this anomaly is present in roughly 2% of the adult population and is seen in both sexes. Actual accessory breast tissue, separate from the main breast mound, is most commonly found in the axilla. Complete accessory breasts, possessing both breast tissue and a nipple (Fig. 60-1), are rare. Abnormal regression of the milk line can lead to underdevelopment of the breasts (hypoplasia). Complete absence of the breast (amastia) is usually associated with hypoplasia of the ipsilateral pectoralis musculature and chest wall (Poland syndrome).

At puberty, the female breast undergoes a series of changes that culminate in the adult appearance. As described by Tanner, these changes begin at about 10 years of age with elevation of the nipple (Fig. 60-2, Tanner stage I). Subsequently, the breast mound begins to appear (about age 11, Tanner stage II), followed by breast enlargement and increased areolar size and pigmentation (about age 12, stage III), projection outward of the areolar mound (about age 13, stage IV), and ultimately, regression of the areolar mound to form the final adult contour (about age 15, stage V). This sequence of developmental events is thought to be initiated by the high levels of unopposed estrogen present soon after menarche. During the next 1 to 2 years, ovulatory cycles replace the earlier anovulatory cycles. The resulting secretion of progesterone by the corpus luteum allows the later phases of breast maturation to occur. Both estrogen and progesterone are required for full development of the female breast.

Adult Anatomy

The breast sits on the anterior chest wall. In the adult female, it extends from the sternocostal junction medially to the mid-axillary line laterally and from the second to

Table 60-2. CHANGES IN BREAST CANCER SURGERY, 1972–1986

Year	Patients Undergoing Procedure (%)		
	Breast Conservation	Mastectomy	Radical Mastectomy
1972[3]	—	~40	~60
1976[3]	3	69	29
1981[3]	7	89	4
1985–1986[4]	33	66	<1

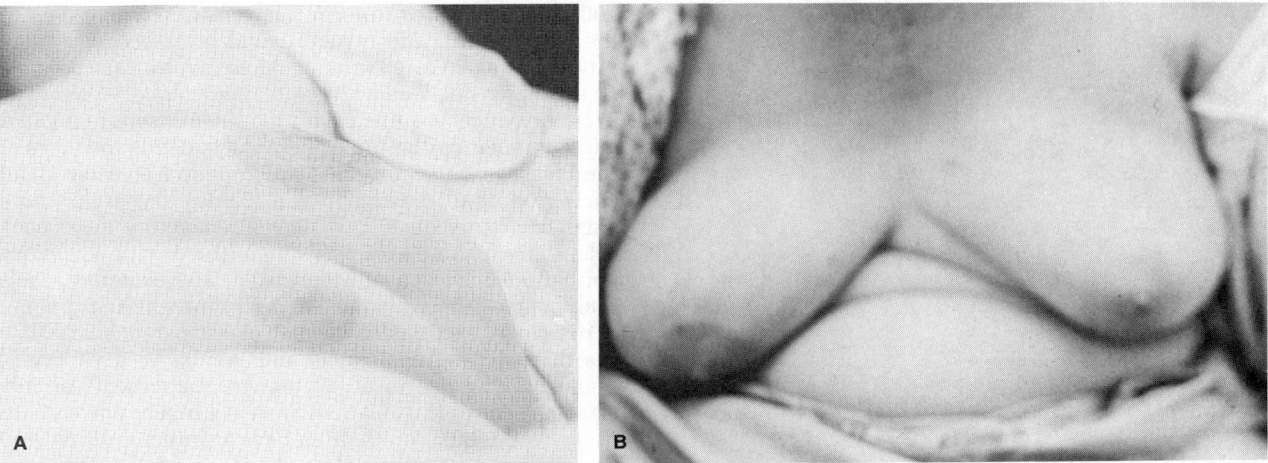

Figure 60-1. (*A*) Accessory breast and nipple directly inferior to the normal left breast in a 65-year-old woman. (*B*) When the woman is seated or standing, the accessory breast is hidden by the normal breast.

the sixth ribs in the midclavicular line (Fig. 60-3). The normal breast has a teardrop shape, resulting from an extension of breast tissue into the axilla, the axillary tail of Spence. The location of the nipple–areola complex is variable in the center of the breast mound.

The areola is a relatively flat area of pigmented skin that is usually well demarcated from the surrounding breast skin. Its surface is noteworthy for the presence of Montgomery tubercles. These numerous small protuberances are the openings of sebaceous glands that lubricate the nipple during lactation. Beneath the skin of the areola is a compact layer of circular smooth muscle; there are similar muscle fibers in the nipple. These are responsible for nipple erection. The entire breast, particularly the nipple, is richly supplied with sensory nerves.

The arterial supply to the medial and central breast comes from perforating branches off the internal mammary artery. The lateral thoracic artery, branches of the thoracodorsal and subscapular arteries, and perforating branches of the intercostal arteries nourish the lateral breast. The venous anatomy of the breast is noteworthy for a plexus of veins that begins in the subareolar region and ultimately drains into the intercostal, internal mammary, and axillary veins.

Lymphatic Drainage

The lymphatic anatomy of the breast is of interest to the surgeon because of the tendency of breast cancer to involve the regional lymph nodes. Thin-walled, valveless lymphatic vessels in the skin convey lymph to deep lymphatic channels in the subcutaneous fat and within the breast parenchyma. Studies using radioactive tracers demonstrate that at least 97% of lymphatic flow from the breast is into the axilla; the remainder courses to the internal mammary nodes.[7] These studies also show that lymph flowing into the internal mammary chain is not restricted in origin to the medial half and subareolar region of the breast, as was thought, but can originate in any quadrant of the breast.

In the axilla, lymphatic vessels terminate in lymph nodes embedded within the axillary fat pad. Isolated lymph nodes can also be found between the pectoralis major and minor muscles (Rotter nodes) and within or alongside the lateral edge of the breast (intramammary nodes). The axillary lymph nodes are found within an area bordered laterally by the latissimus dorsi muscle, superiorly by the axillary vein, and medially by the chest wall. Although the axilla extends inferiorly to the junction of

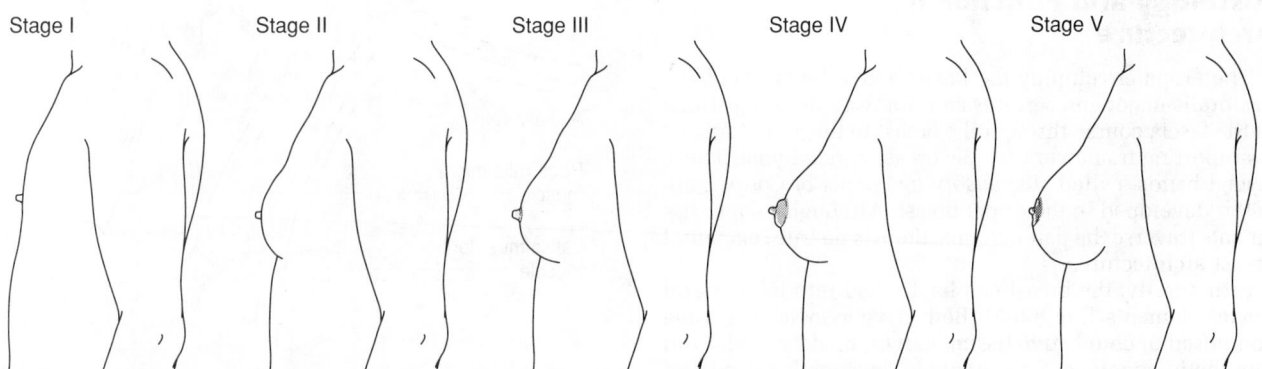

Figure 60-2. Developmental stages of the female breast beginning at the onset of puberty, as described by Tanner. Stage I, preadolescent elevation of the nipple without apparent glandular tissue. Stage II, appearance of the breast mound. Stage III, enlargement of the breast with increased areolar size and pigmentation. Stage IV, outward projection of the areola. Stage V, regression of the areola, establishing the normal adult contour.

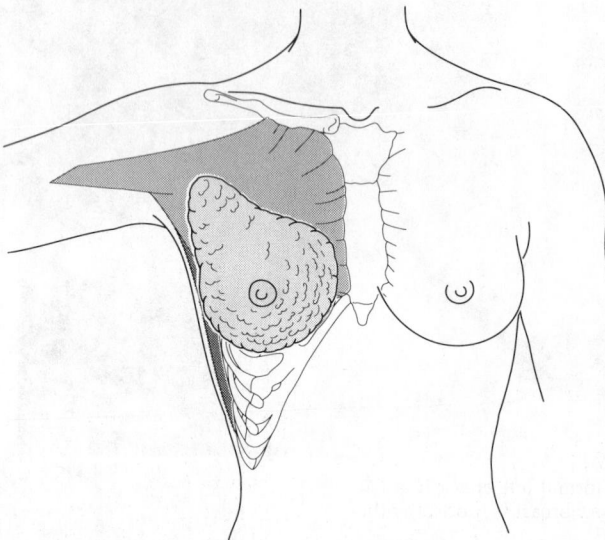

Figure 60-3. The adult female breast. The upper and medial two thirds of the breast lie on the pectoralis major muscle, and the lower, lateral third sits on the serratus anterior muscle.

the serratus anterior and latissimus dorsi muscles, nodes draining the breast are rarely found this far caudally. The floor of the axilla is formed by the subscapularis muscle. Also within the axillary fat pad are the intercostobrachial nerve (a sensory nerve supplying the underarm skin), the long thoracic nerve of Bell (a motor nerve to the serratus anterior and subscapularis muscles), and the thoracodorsal nerve (a motor nerve to the latissimus dorsi) adjacent to its accompanying artery and veins. Small arteries directly off the axillary artery and a variable number of venous tributaries of the axillary vein form the vascular supply for the axilla.

The lymph nodes within the axilla are divided into three levels based on their relation to the pectoralis minor muscle (Fig. 60-4). Level I encompasses the lymph nodes lateral to the lateral border of the pectoralis minor muscle; this subgroup contains most of the axillary nodes. The lymph nodes lying directly beneath the pectoralis minor muscle are classified as level II. Those lying medial to the medial border of the pectoralis minor and extending up to the apex of the axilla are level III nodes.

Histology and Functional Architecture

The fascia enveloping the breast abuts the fascia of the pectoralis major and serratus anterior muscles. Projections of the fascia course through the breast to the skin, forming a supporting framework for the breast parenchyma. These fascial bands, called *suspensory ligaments of Cooper,* are better developed in the upper breast. Although Cooper ligaments traverse the parenchyma, there is no true segmental breast architecture.

Structurally, the breast can be divided into lobular and ductal elements (Fig. 60-5). Both have associated stroma composed of connective tissue, nerves, blood vessels, and lymphatic channels. The *lobule* is the functional unit of the breast. Within a lobule, the terminal elongated tubular ducts are referred to as *alveoli.* The walls of the alveolar ducts consist of an inner layer of low columnar glandular cells overlying a stratum of myoepithelial cells; a prominent basement membrane surrounds these layers. Ten to

100 alveoli coalesce to form a larger duct, which defines the lobular unit. The myoepithelial layer becomes more prominent as 20 to 40 lobular ducts join to form progressively larger ducts and ultimately an *excretory duct.* The excretory ducts are lined with a double layer of cuboidal and columnar epithelium. These ducts define the lobes of the breast, each of which is a compound alveolar gland composed of all the alveoli and lobules that drain into a single excretory duct. The 10 to 20 excretory ducts each dilate into a short *excretory sinus* (lined with squamous epithelium) just beneath the areola. The excretory ducts then course perpendicularly to exit through the nipple.

Histologic sections of normal breast parenchyma slice the three-dimensional ducts and lobules in a variety of planes, giving rise to an asymmetric pattern of variably sized structures (Fig. 60-6A). Seen at a higher power, both ductal and lobular epithelium have a similar multilayered appearance, with cuboidal basal cells and flat surface cells (see Fig. 60-6B). The stromal components differ in appearance between the ducts and lobules, however. Lobules contain no elastic tissue. Connective tissue surrounding ducts appears histologically as a cuff of loose stroma, within which the ductal lymphatics are found. The lobular connective tissue is more vascular and cellular. Between lobules, the connective tissue is dense, although it may be heavily infiltrated by fat in the larger breast.

Anatomy of the Male Breast

Before puberty, the development of the male breast parallels that of the female breast. At puberty, however, the paucity of estrogen and progesterone precludes maturation of the lobular elements. The result is a rudimentary breast possessing ductal structures and a nipple–areola complex.

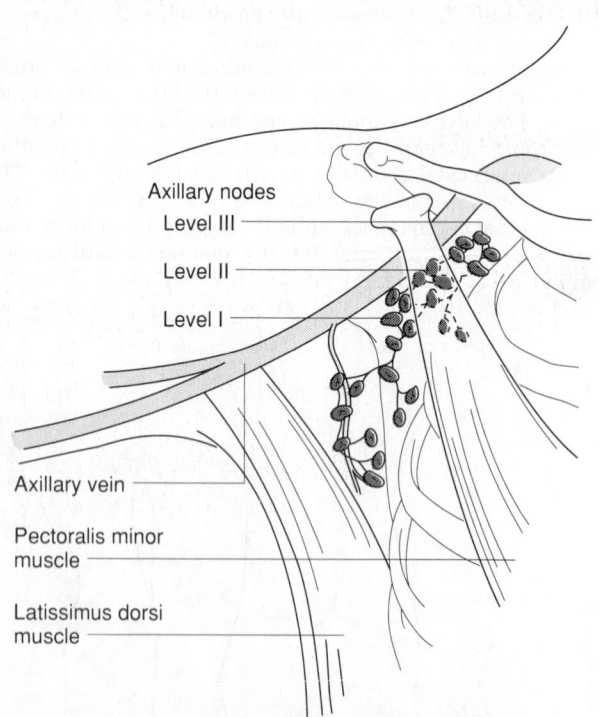

Figure 60-4. Anatomic classification of axillary lymph nodes into three levels based on their relation to the pectoralis minor muscle. Level I nodes are lateral to the edge of the muscle, level II nodes lie beneath the muscle, and level III nodes are medial to the muscle. Rotter nodes (*not shown*) are found between the pectoralis major and minor muscles, anterior to the axillary space.

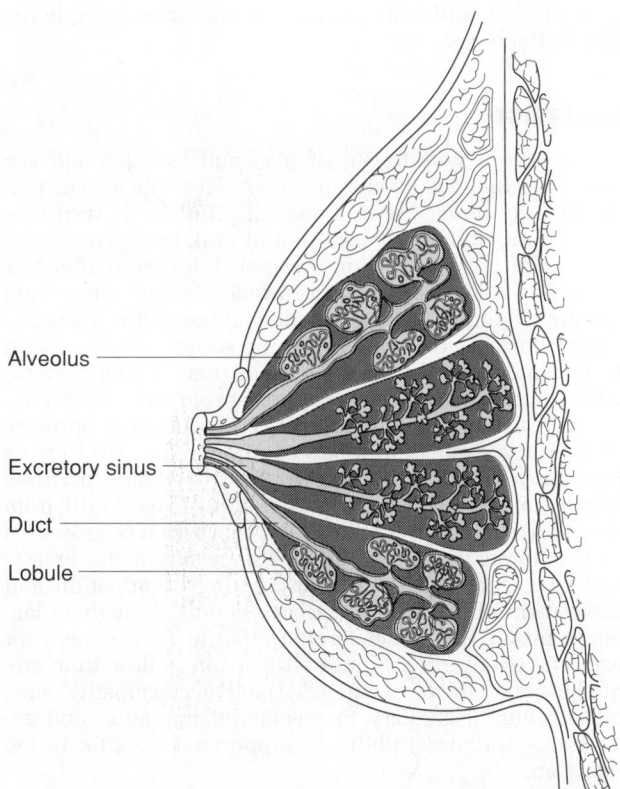

Figure 60-5. The basic functional unit of the breast is the lobule. Each lobule contains 10 to 100 elongated terminal ducts called *alveoli*. Ducts draining 20 to 40 lobules coalesce to form larger ducts, and ultimately an excretory duct. Each excretory duct dilates just beneath the nipple to form an excretory sinus. Ten to 20 excretory ducts drain the entire breast.

Because the in utero development of the male and female breast is similar, anomalies of breast development, such as aplasia and supernumerary nipples, are seen with equal frequency in both sexes. Palpable breast tissue (gynecomastia) may be found in male patients of all postpubertal ages.

PHYSIOLOGY
Cell Regulation

Breast growth, development, and function are orchestrated by a variety of hormones and growth factors, including estrogens, progestins, prolactin, oxytocin, corticosteroids, thyroid hormone, and growth hormone.[8] Binding of these substances to specific cellular receptors triggers their effects. Polypeptide hormone receptors are found on the cell-surface membrane; steroid hormones bind to intracellular receptors. Although estrogen, progesterone, and prolactin are the primary hormones acting on the breast, other hormones and growth factors are also important. Insulin and growth hormone are required for mammary epithelial cell division. Cortisol and insulin play a permissive role, allowing prolactin to differentiate alveolar cells into milk-secreting cells. Normal breast epithelial cells also exhibit membrane receptors for insulin-like growth factor and epidermal growth factor. The in vivo role of these substances is unclear, but in vitro, they have been reported to stimulate a variety of metabolic activities, including cell proliferation.[9]

Estrogens play a central role in breast development, growth, and differentiation.[9] Lipid-soluble, estrogens gain entry to the normal and malignant breast cell by diffusing through the cell membrane. Once within the cell, estrogens bind to the estrogen receptor (ER). Both normal and malignant breast cells contain ER, but the low levels of ER in normal breast tissue and in some breast cancers results in their testing ER-negative in clinical assays. The estrogen–ER complex binds with nuclear chromatin and, by poorly understood processes, influences transcription of messenger RNA (mRNA). This mRNA is ultimately translated into proteins (estrogen-induced translation products), such as the progesterone receptor (PR), and perhaps growth factors (insulin-like growth factor and transforming growth factor β) that can alter and regulate breast cell growth and metabolism. Similar mechanisms likely mediate the effect of other hormones and growth factors. Compounds such as tamoxifen work at least in part by preventing the binding of hormones and growth factors to their target receptors.

Menstruation

Mammary tissue is a target organ of pituitary trophic factors and circulating hormones. Cyclic changes associated with the menstrual cycle have a profound influence

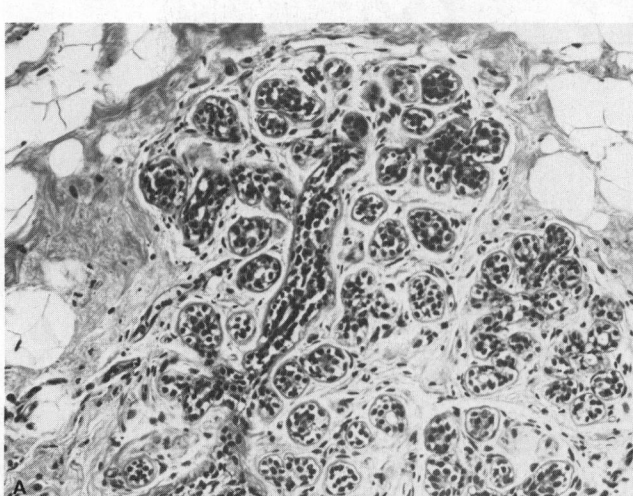
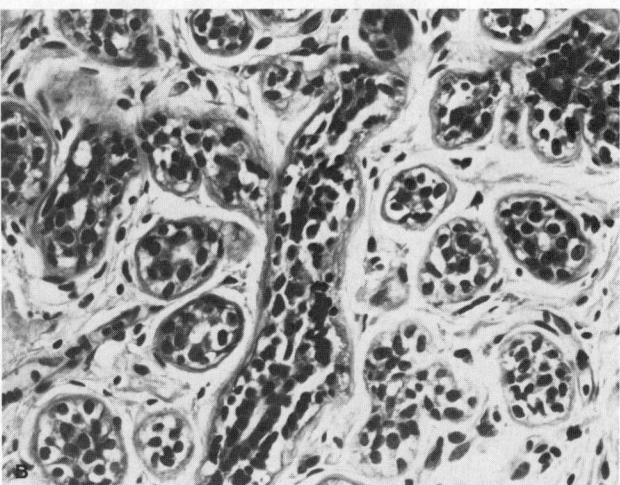

Figure 60-6. (*A*) Histologic section of normal breast tissue, showing sections of ducts and lobules in a variety of planes. (*B*) At higher magnification, the elastin surrounding the ductal elements and the cellularity and vascularity of the lobular elements are evident.

on female breast morphology and physiology (Fig. 60-7). The resting histology of the breast was discussed earlier. Breast engorgement and tenderness are at a minimum 5 to 7 days after menstruation. At this point in the cycle, breast palpation is most sensitive for detecting masses and most comfortable for the patient. Even during this interval of relative quiescence, increasing graafian follicle secretion of estrogen in response to pituitary elaboration of follicle-stimulating hormone--luteinizing hormone stimulates breast epithelial proliferation; mitoses may be observed in breast epithelial cells during this proliferative phase. As the luteal phase of the cycle is entered, progesterone levels rise. Mammary ductal dilation and differentiation of alveolar epithelial cells into secretory cells result. Continued estrogen stimulation increases blood flow to the breast. These ductal, secretory, and vascular events and associated interlobular edema cause the breast swelling, engorgement, and tenderness associated with the premenstrual phase. At the onset of menstruation, the rapid decline in circulating sex hormone levels leads to breast involution, and the cycle begins anew. Because the degree of proliferation and involution varies from cycle to cycle and between different areas of the breast, all cycling women have some breast nodularity.

Pregnancy

During pregnancy, marked ductular, lobular, and alveolar growth occurs under the influence of estrogen, progesterone, placental lactogen, prolactin, and chorionic gonadotropin. These changes prepare the breasts for milk production at parturition. Early in the first trimester, ductular sprouting and lobular formation proceed under estrogenic influence. Later in the first trimester, noticeable breast enlargement ensues, along with dilation of superficial veins and increased pigmentation of the nipple–areola complex. During the second trimester, lobular events predominate under the influence of progestins. Colostrum collects within the lobular alveoli. By parturition, the combined effects of vascular engorgement, epithelial

proliferation, and colostrum accumulation may triple the size of the breast.

Lactation

The abrupt withdrawal of placental lactogen and sex hormones that occurs with delivery leaves the breasts predominantly under the influence of pituitary-derived prolactin. Production and secretion of milk by alveolar cells results. Initially, colostrum is secreted, followed after 4 or 5 days by milk rich in lipid, protein, carbohydrate, and immunoglobulin. Milk production and secretion are maintained during lactation by ongoing secretion of prolactin by the anterior pituitary; the nursing infant's tactile stimulation of the nipple–areola complex prompts this pituitary activity. Oxytocin elaboration by the posterior pituitary also results from nipple–areola stimulation. By causing breast myoepithelial cells to contract, oxytocin increases intramammary ductal pressures, helping to eject milk from the lobules into the lactiferous ducts, where it is accessible to the nursing infant. Throughout lactation, the breasts remain engorged and nodular, making examination and assessment difficult. The presence of milk throughout lactation makes the ductal lumina a fertile environment for bacterial overgrowth should obstruction to flow from any of the major ducts occur. Obstructive mastopathy most often occurs secondary to areolar inflammation and accounts for the susceptibility to suppurative mastitis during lactation.

Postlactational Involution

Postlactational involution of the breast occurs during the 3 months after cessation of nursing. Regression of the extralobular stroma is the primary feature of this period, but there is also glandular and ductal atrophy. The breast gradually returns to its nulliparous state, but this process is not complete because some glandular hypertrophy persists indefinitely.

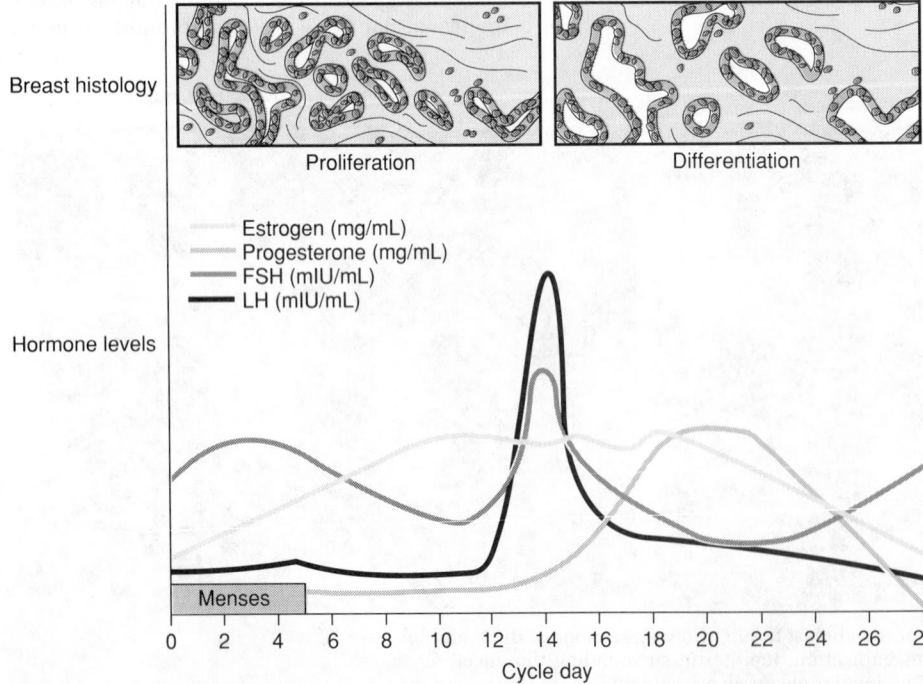

Figure 60-7. The effect of cyclic hormonal changes on the breast. FSH, follicle-stimulating hormone; LH, luteinizing hormone.

Menopause

In contrast to the events that occur when lactation ceases, the mammary involution that occurs with menopause involves actual loss of glandular tissue. Although some lobules always remain, the postmenopausal breast ultimately consists largely of fat, connective tissue, and mammary ducts. Fat replacement of lobular elements helps to maintain the breast contour; the breasts may become ptotic if lobular volume is not replaced with adipose tissue.

BREAST EXAMINATION

The breast examination is an opportunity to detect breast problems and to identify risk factors for the development of breast malignancy. It can reassure patients with normal examinations. If abnormalities are detected, it facilitates formulation of a diagnostic strategy that the patient can understand and support. This encounter may also be used to educate and encourage patients to participate actively in a screening program. The superficial location of the breast on the chest wall permits patient involvement in breast disease detection by breast self-examination (BSE). Without adequate education and training, however, BSE can be a source of anxiety and frustration for patients. Involving women in all aspects of their own breast care forges a strong partnership between physician and patient that can assist both parties.

Patient History

Most patients seek medical attention because of either breast-related tenderness or a lump. Others are referred for evaluation after mammographic detection of a nonpalpable lesion. The breast history should stress the nature of the presenting complaint and assessment of cancer risk factors. It is important to elicit symptoms such as pain, tenderness, and nipple discharge. The nature, duration, and relation of these symptoms to the menstrual cycle (or exogenous hormone intake) is important. Complaints of pain, tenderness, or nodularity that vary with the menstrual cycle are suggestive of a benign cause. Cancers are often asymptomatic. Patients should be questioned about findings at BSE.

A history of prior breast problems may suggest the diagnosis. The timing and nature of any previous breast problems and operations should be clarified. Details of the histologic findings from prior biopsies may be important; pathology reports, slides, or cell blocks should be obtained for review. For example, a past biopsy that revealed proliferative changes, lobular carcinoma in situ (LCIS), or papillomatosis suggests that the patient is at higher risk for development of invasive breast cancer. A history of breast cancer also confers increased risk for development of a new breast cancer (for more details, refer to Epidemiology and Risk Factors). Alternatively, knowledge of a previous breast cyst or abscess would raise suspicion for a recurrence of the condition.

A family history of breast cancer is among the most significant predictors of breast cancer risk. It is helpful to know not only the relation of the family member to the patient but also the age at which the cancer was diagnosed and if one or both breasts were involved. Bilateral breast cancer in a premenopausal first-degree relative implies as much as a 50% chance of breast cancer developing in the patient.[10] Family histories that reveal combinations of multiple first-degree relatives, multiple generations, or multiple occurrences of bilateral or premenopausal breast cancer strongly suggest the possibility of the presence of a genetic predisposition to breast cancer (familial breast cancer). Women belonging to families in which the autosomal dominant gene BRCA-1 (or breast cancer gene 1) is present have a 50% chance of inheriting this gene from their mother or father. Those women who inherit the gene have more than a 50% chance of development of invasive breast cancer by 50 years of age and a lifetime risk that approaches 85%. Clearly, women from such families must be evaluated and counseled appropriately.[11,12] In some, but not all, breast cancer families, men are also at increased risk for the development of breast cancer.

Other factors that should be addressed during an initial evaluation include menstrual history, reproductive history, and radiation exposure. Although hormone use has not been conclusively linked with an increased breast cancer risk, estrogens may alter the texture of the breast on examination and influence the development or regression of benign breast diseases; any prior or current use of hormones should be recorded.

Physical Examination

Physical examination of the breast is easiest during the week after menses, when tenderness and engorgement are at a minimum. Palpation of the supraclavicular and anterior and posterior cervical lymph node chains initiates the examination. Next, with the patient fully disrobed from the waist up, the breasts are inspected and compared (Fig. 60-8). Minor size differences (up to 10%) are common and of no significance. Careful observation for skin changes, dimpling, or nipple abnormalities is important. Subtle abnormalities in the lower quadrants may be accentuated by having the patient raise her arms above her head and by pectoral muscle contraction; these maneuvers should be a routine part of every breast examination. While the patient remains in the upright seated position, bimanual palpation of the breasts is carried out. Palpation of the axillae, including lymph nodes and the mammary tissue in the axillary tail, is best carried out in the sitting position. The number, size, consistency, and mobility of any palpable lymph nodes should be recorded.

Palpation of the breast is also performed with the patient supine. Placement of the patient's ipsilateral hand behind the head pulls the lateral quadrants and tail of the breast onto the chest wall, permitting palpation of the entire breast by compression against the thoracic cage. Palpation should proceed in an orderly fashion to ensure that the whole breast is examined. Subtly thickened areas may be compared with the contralateral breast to help assess their significance. Discrete or dominant nodules and thickenings should be described by their location (clock face position and distance from nipple), consistency, borders, and size; tender areas should also be recorded. Breast palpation is completed by gently squeezing the nipple–areola complex to detect subareolar masses and latent nipple discharge. If a discharge is evident, careful investigation of its duct of origin is important. The character of the discharge is significant. Milky, serous, or green-brown discharges are almost always benign in origin. Although bloody discharge most often results from an intraductal papilloma, it may mark an underlying cancer and should be evaluated further.

The routine breast examination should end with a discussion of the elements of BSE. BSE is best carried out just after menstruation is complete (monthly in nonmenstruating women) and should include observation in a mirror as well as palpation both upright in the shower and supine in bed. For the patient, emphasis should be placed on detecting changes and differences rather than on interpretation of self-examination findings.

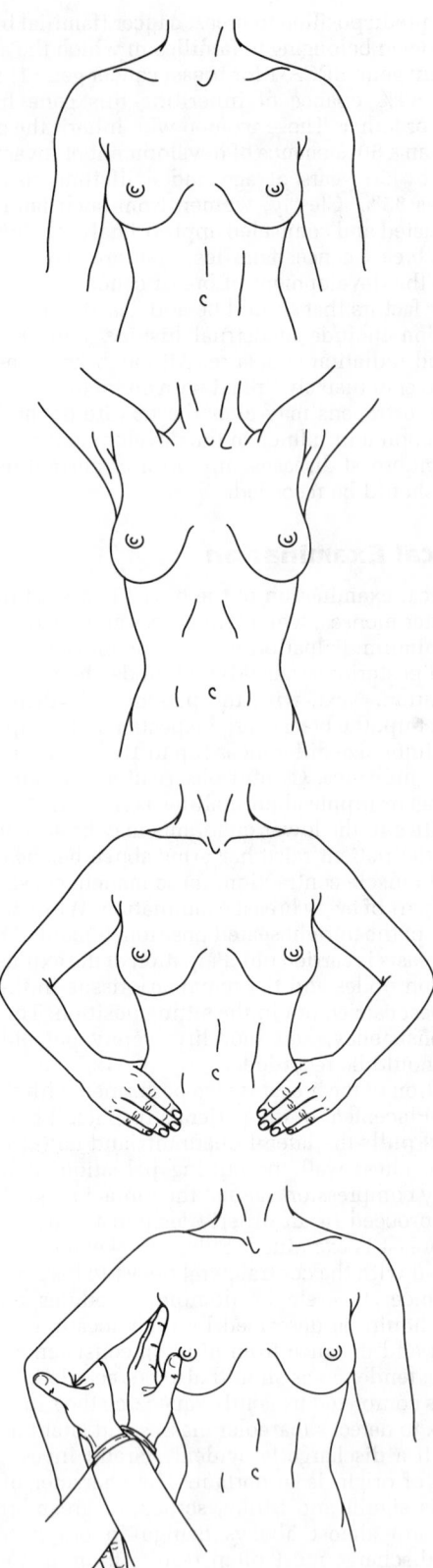

Figure 60-8. Positions for proper breast examination.

Imaging

Mammography, ultrasonography, and ductography are the proven breast imaging methods. Studies suggest that magnetic resonance (MR) imaging and positron emission tomography (PET) scanning may soon join the aforementioned as important clinical tools. Imaging methods are complements to, not substitutes for, a thorough history and physical examination. Only when these studies are used in concert with a thorough clinical examination is optimal screening and diagnostic specificity and sensitivity achieved.

Mammography was developed early in the 20th century. It did not become a widely used technique, however, until the findings of the Health Insurance Plan of New York and the Breast Cancer Detection Demonstration Project studies of screening mammography were disseminated.[13-15] These and other investigations demonstrated that 10% to 50% of cancers detected mammographically are not palpable. Conversely, palpation recognizes 10% to 20% of tumors not detectable mammographically.

The low level of radiation exposure associated with mammograms performed using dedicated equipment in certified centers (about 1 mGy to the glandular tissue per study) ensures that mammography is safe in women of screening age. The incidence of breast cancer begins to rise sharply at 40 years of age, and the sensitivity of mammograms increases with age as the dense parenchymal tissue of young women is progressively replaced by fatty tissue. Routine screening mammography has been shown to decrease breast cancer–related mortality in women without symptoms who are older than 50 years of age.[13-17] Although studies have questioned the benefit of screening mammography in women aged 40 to 50 years,[17,18] there are no well-performed prospective, randomized trials that definitively assess the ability of mammography in this age group to reduce breast cancer mortality. Some investigators have reported that excess biopsies and psychological, economic, and social costs result from the routine use of screening mammograms in women younger than 50 years of age.[17,19] Others believe, however, that women in this age group do benefit from regular, high-quality screening mammography.[20] The American Cancer Society recommends that mammographic screening begin at about age 40 (Table 60-3). The Board of Scientific Counselors of the National Cancer Institute has taken a noncommittal approach, suggesting, "For those women under 50, the National Cancer Institute will provide a summary of existing evidence and data and suggests these be discussed with each woman's physician or health care provider."[20]

Mammography also plays an important role in the evaluation of symptomatic breast disorders. Mammography may help establish a diagnosis in a woman presenting with a palpable mass or other clinical abnormality (Fig. 60-9). Additionally, mammography should be performed before biopsy in all women older than 30 years to detect synchronous, nonpalpable ipsilateral or contralateral disease.

Two mammography techniques are commonly em-

Table 60-3. AMERICAN CANCER SOCIETY RECOMMENDATIONS FOR ROUTINE MAMMOGRAPHIC SCREENING OF ASYMPTOMATIC WOMEN

Age (y)	Recommendation
40–49	Mammogram every 1–2 y
50+	Mammogram yearly

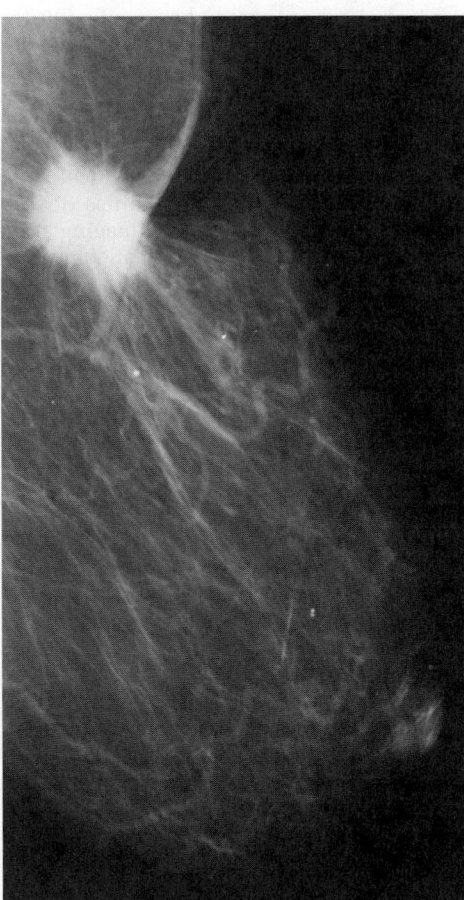

Figure 60-9. Left mediolateral mammogram revealing a 3.5-cm spiculated mass in the upper outer quadrant with associated skin thickening and retraction. Excisional biopsy demonstrated infiltrating ductal carcinoma. (Courtesy of Debra Ikeda, MD; from the Division of Breast Imaging, University of Michigan Medical School, Ann Arbor)

ployed. Film screen mammography is similar to usual radiographic methods, yielding black and white radiographs that are viewed on a light box. Xeroradiography uses an electrostatic detector plate coated with selenium, which distributes electric charge on its surface in a manner proportional to the amount of radiation reaching the plate. The resultant electrostatic image is converted to a blue-on-white photocopy image. Although each method has strengths and limitations, they are equally effective at detecting breast cancer. Film screen imaging involves a somewhat lower radiation dose. No matter which method is used, mammograms should be performed using dedicated, modern equipment and exacting technique, and they should be interpreted by a radiologist knowledgeable in breast imaging.

Although sensitive, mammography is not specific. Only about 25% of nonpalpable lesions detected mammographically are found to be malignant at biopsy. A spiculated density with ill-defined margins on a mammogram is almost certainly malignant (see Fig. 60-9). More commonly, features are seen that are suggestive but not diagnostic of cancer. These include clustered microcalcifications (Fig. 60-10), asymmetric density, ductal asymmetry, distortion of normal breast architecture, and skin or nipple distortion.

Ductography may be used in the evaluation of nipple discharge. A blunt-tipped small-caliber needle is inserted into the draining duct, a small volume of water-soluble contrast is injected, and orthogonal images are obtained. Filling defects generally represent intraductal papillomas (Fig. 60-11), but the findings are rarely specific enough to eliminate the need for histologic diagnosis.

Ultrasonography uses high-resolution, 1- to 10-MHz acoustic waves to image the breast. The most useful feature of ultrasound is its ability to distinguish between cystic and solid masses (Fig. 60-12). It is not an effective screening test for cancer. It cannot detect microcalcifications or small lesions. In selected situations, ultrasonography may help to confirm the diagnosis of a cyst or support a clinical impression of fibroadenoma. Doppler ultrasound is under investigation to determine whether differences in blood flow may be detected and used noninvasively to differentiate between benign and malignant masses in the breast and the axilla. Results to date have been mixed,[21,22] but improvements to the color Doppler technique are being studied.[23]

PET is a technique that produces images reflective of cellular biochemical activities, providing a functional as opposed to an anatomic view of tissues. Through the use of the tracer 2-[F-18]-fluoro-2-deoxy-D-glucose (FDG), PET allows preferential imaging of cells (such as primary and metastatic breast cancers) that have an abnormally high rate of glycolysis. PET has been used to image primary breast tumors, as a noninvasive method for staging axillary lymph nodes, and to detect metastatic disease.[24-26] Although resolution is limited (generally to lesions more than

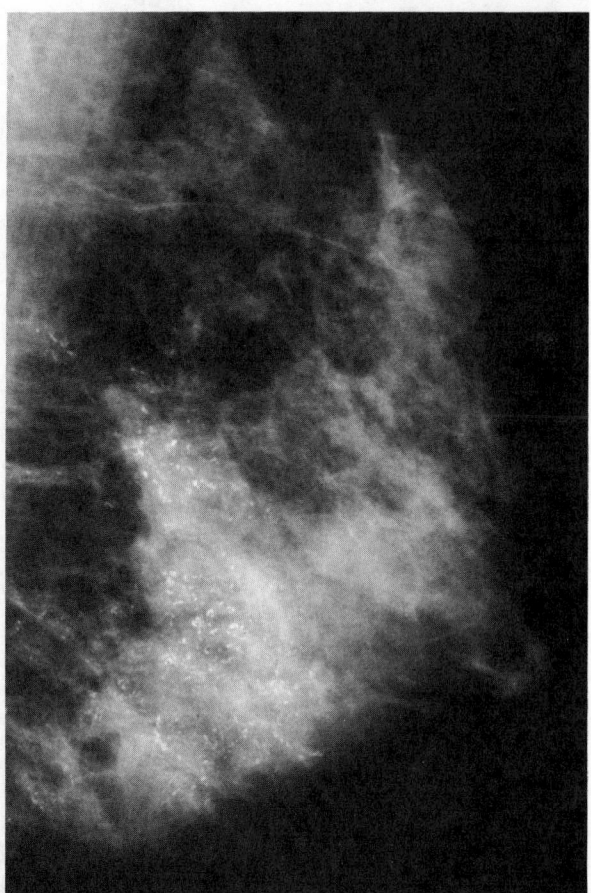

Figure 60-10. Left mediolateral oblique mammogram showing extensive irregular and branching microcalcifications throughout the lower breast. Biopsy demonstrated extensive ductal carcinoma in situ. (Courtesy of Debra Ikeda, MD; from the Division of Breast Imaging, University of Michigan Medical School, Ann Arbor)

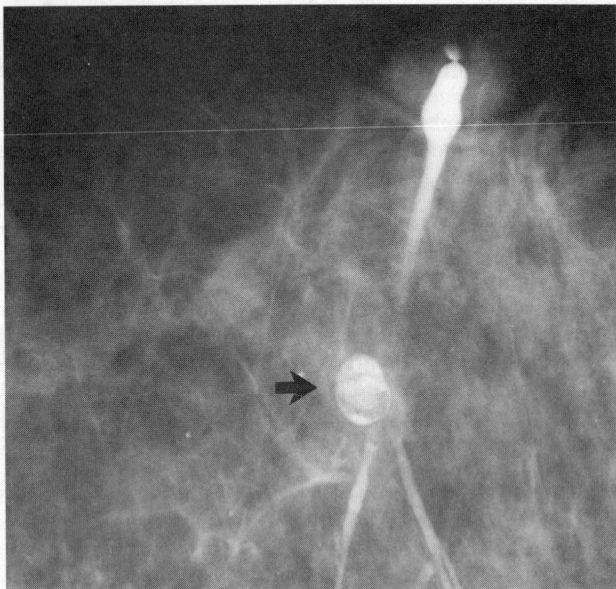

Figure 60-11. Magnification craniocaudal view obtained after duct injection (ductogram) showing focal ductal dilation with an associated filling defect (*arrow*). Biopsy revealed an intraductal papilloma. (Courtesy of Debra Ikeda, MD; from the Division of Breast Imaging, University of Michigan Medical School, Ann Arbor)

1 cm), the technique appears to be specific (90% or better positive predictive value). We have found PET with FDG to be particularly helpful in distinguishing radiation changes from recurrent disease, particularly in the axilla and the region of the brachial plexus.

Interest in MR imaging of the breast is high.[27] Dedicated breast MR machines and MR biopsy localization techniques are being developed. With the use of suitable enhancing agents (eg, gadolinium) and imaging and analysis methods designed to detect early enhancement (less than 10 to 60 seconds), excellent sensitivity and adequate specificity have been obtained. Although further improvement of the method and reduction of the cost are necessary before breast MR imaging becomes a useful and widely available addition to the breast imaging armamentarium, these developments are likely in the next 5 years.[23,28]

EVALUATION OF BREAST MASSES

Although an increasing number of breast abnormalities are detected by screening mammography, most breast cancers still present as a palpable mass.[29] A comprehensive approach to the evaluation of a palpable breast mass is outlined in Figure 60-13. A recent review also offers an excellent overview of this topic.[30]

In postmenopausal women, the replacement of glandular tissue by fat, the absence of hormone-related functional changes, and the high incidence of cancer make evaluation of breast masses relatively straightforward. After obtaining

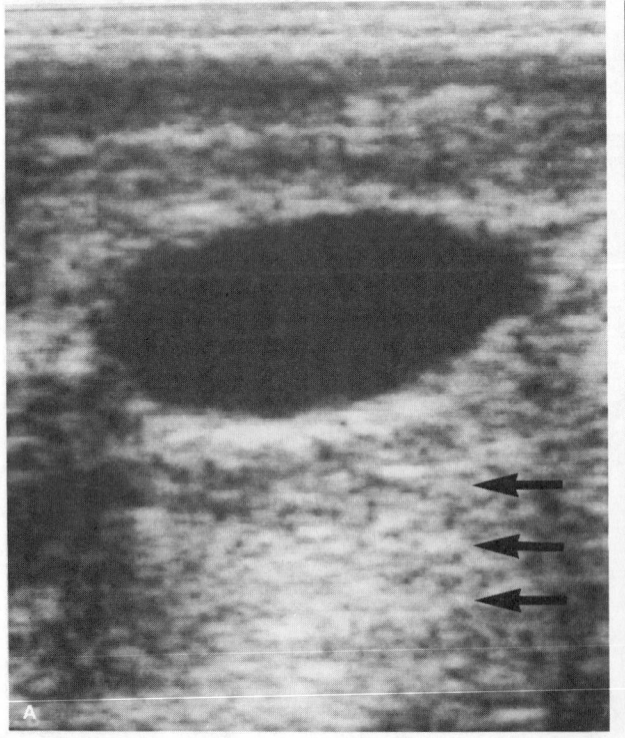
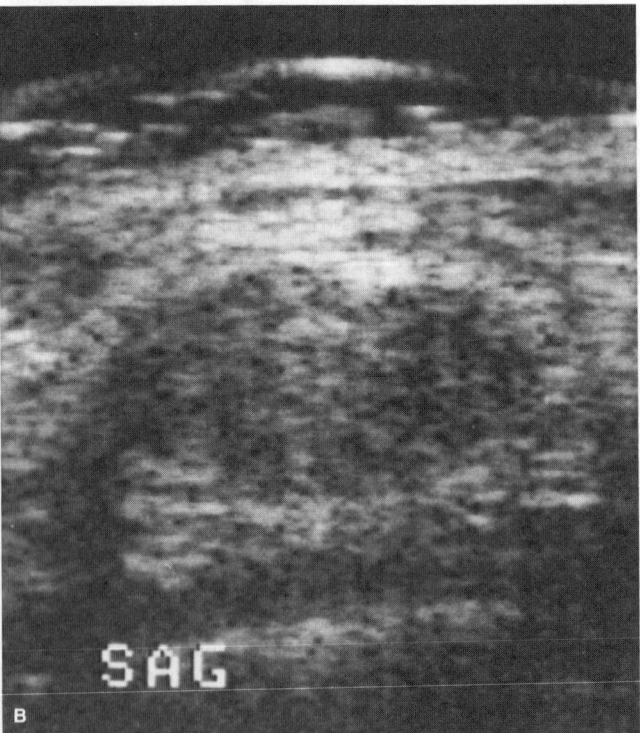

Figure 60-12. (*A*) Real-time ultrasound using a 7.5-MHz transducer showing a simple cyst. The mass is anechoic, is smooth-walled, and has enhanced through transmission of sound (*arrows*). (*B*) In contrast, this ultrasound of a fibroadenoma reveals a well-demarcated hypoechoic mass with only minimal through transmission. (Courtesy of Debra Ikeda, MD; from the Division of Breast Imaging, University of Michigan Medical School, Ann Arbor)

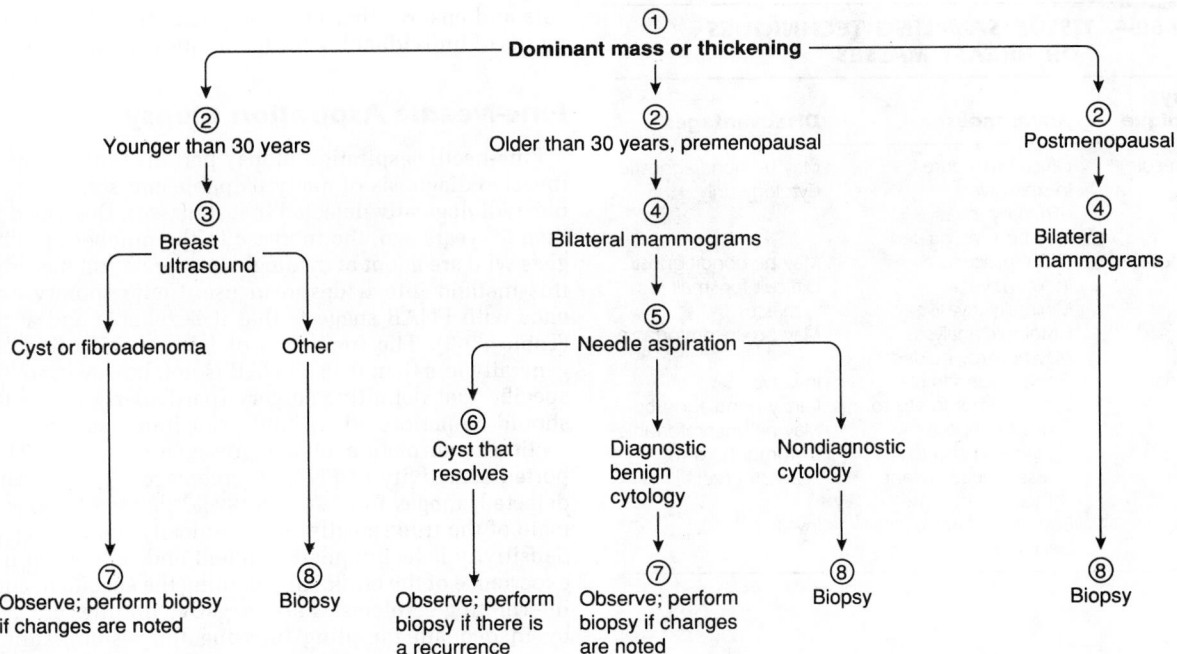

Figure 60-13. Algorithm for evaluation of a discrete breast mass.

(1) A *dominant mass* is a discrete area of breast parenchyma that is distinct in density or consistency from surrounding tissue in three dimensions. A *thickening* is a region of breast tissue that is not discrete but that is clearly distinguishable from the patient's other breast tissue. Recognition of a dominant mass or thickening may be aided by examining the corresponding location in the opposite breast; if the findings are symmetric, further evaluation may not be required.

(2) Age and menopausal status determine the workup of a dominant mass or thickening. Only 2% of breast cancers occur before the age of 30 years, whereas 70% are diagnosed after 50 years of age. In a young woman, if other factors corroborate an impression of a benign mass, observation may be warranted. All lesions in women older than 30 years (whether premenopausal or postmenopausal) must be assumed to be cancer until proved otherwise. In the presence of known major risk factors for breast cancer, evaluation in any woman should follow the algorithm for postmenopausal women, regardless of age.

(3) In women younger than 30 years, an ultrasound scan that corroborates a clinical impression of a simple cyst or fibroadenoma supports observation. Breast ultrasound is indicated after 30 years of age only when confirmation of a mammographic impression of a simple cyst is needed. The accuracy of breast ultrasound is not sufficient to allow its use to avoid the need for biopsy in women older than 30 years.

(4) The sensitivity and specificity of mammography for detecting malignant lesions improve with increasing age. Additionally, although the radiation exposure risk is low at any age, the risk decreases with age. Mammograms are rarely helpful before 30 years of age.

(5) Fine-needle aspiration is useful in premenopausal women older than 30 years. Aspiration may resolve a simple cyst or establish an unequivocally benign tissue diagnosis, obviating the need for further evaluation. If a lesion that is not a simple cyst is to be observed, the cytology must be both diagnostic and benign. Equivocal cytologic readings (eg, acellular, blood only, normal fat and mammary cells) require further workup (generally formal biopsy).

(6) Simple cysts that resolve completely after aspiration of nonbloody fluid may be observed. If they do not recur after aspiration, they may be assumed to be benign. A recurrent or enlarging cyst should undergo biopsy.

(7) Observation must be active, not passive. Reevaluation should occur in 2 to 3 months if it is elected to follow a discrete mass, and it should be repeated at least once thereafter. In women younger than 30 years, a decision to observe can be made if a clinical impression of benignity is substantiated by ultrasound or aspirate findings. In premenopausal women older than 30 years, a decision to observe should be made only with more stringent corroborative evidence—namely, a normal or benign-appearing mammogram *and* an aspirate that reveals either a simple cyst or unequivocally benign cytology. In postmenopausal women, tissue diagnosis of a discrete mass or thickening is mandatory. If observation is to be sensitive and useful, the baseline findings (location, size, consistency, tenderness) must be completely and accurately recorded and available for review by the same examiner at subsequent visits.

(8) *Biopsy* refers to a definitive tissue diagnosis made from unequivocally diagnostic fine-needle cytology or definitive histology from a sample obtained with a core-needle, incisional, or excisional biopsy.

Table 60-4. TISSUE SAMPLING TECHNIQUES FOR BREAST MASSES

Biopsy Technique	Advantages	Disadvantages
Fine needle	Office procedure Inexpensive Minimally invasive May be x-ray guided	May be nondiagnostic Cytology only
Core needle	Office procedure Inexpensive Minimally invasive Histologic analysis May be x-ray guided	May be nondiagnostic Difficult for small masses May be uncomfortable
Incisional	Good tissue sample Leaves tumor in situ to assist lumpectomy planning and to assess neoadjuvant therapy response	Invasive Rarely nondiagnostic May be uncomfortable (tumor hard to anesthetize)
Excisional	Best tissue sample Definitive	Invasive

bilateral mammograms to screen for concurrent, clinically unappreciated lesions, biopsy of the palpable mass is usually indicated. An adequate biopsy requires either cytologic analysis of diagnostic cells obtained by fine-needle aspiration biopsy (FNAB), or histologic examination of a tissue sample obtained by core-needle, incisional, or excisional biopsy.

For women younger than 30 years of age who are without major breast cancer risk factors, a well-circumscribed discrete breast mass suggests the presence of a simple cyst, fibroadenoma, or fibrocystic changes. Breast ultrasound can confirm the diagnosis of a simple cyst or, if a homogeneous, well-demarcated solid lesion is seen, support a diagnosis of fibroadenoma. Either lesion may be followed safely in a young patient, but a presumed fibroadenoma should be excised if it enlarges or changes in consistency. Cysts may be aspirated if they are large or symptomatic; they should be excised if they recur after aspiration. Even in a young woman, a dominant mass not typical of a cyst or fibroadenoma should undergo biopsy. In a study of 951 breast biopsies performed in young women, none of 178 patients younger than 21 years was found to have breast cancer, but 1.3% of biopsies in women aged 21 to 25 years and 4.0% in women aged 26 to 30 years were positive for malignancy.[31] These data indicate the importance of diagnostic vigilance, even in younger women.

The presence of functional, cycling glandular tissue in premenopausal women, combined with a progressively increasing incidence of cancer beyond the age of 30 years, makes evaluation of breast masses between age 30 and menopause problematic. Bilateral mammograms should be obtained to look for concurrent nonpalpable disease before undertaking a definitive diagnostic procedure.

The gold standard for breast mass diagnosis is excisional biopsy with formal pathologic analysis. Smaller tissue specimens (including cytologic specimens), however, are often diagnostic and may be easier to obtain (Table 60-4). Aspiration cytology can often distinguish between benign and cancerous lesions without the need to resort to more invasive diagnostic methods. Whatever tissue sampling method is chosen, only biopsy (examination of cells or tissue) and not physical examination or mammography can establish a definitive diagnosis and avoid delay in treatment. A positive biopsy rate of 20% to 30% is accept-

able and ensures that few if any cancers are missed. The merits of individual biopsy techniques are discussed next.

Fine-Needle Aspiration Biopsy

Fine-needle aspiration biopsy permits rapid, minimally invasive diagnosis of many palpable and some nonpalpable, radiologically detected breast masses. Described more than 50 years ago, the increase in the number of pathologists who are adept at cytologic interpretation has brought this method into widespread use. Contemporary experience with FNAB suggests that it is reliable and accurate (Table 60-5). The incidence of false-positive findings is generally less than 0.5%. FNAB is not, however, so highly specific that definitive surgery (particularly mastectomy) should be performed without prior intraoperative frozen-section confirmation of the presence of cancer. The reported sensitivity of FNAB (percentage of actual cancers detected) ranges from 70% to 99%[32]; 85% is a good estimate of the true sensitivity in clinically relevant settings. Sensitivity is technique-dependent and influenced by the experience of the clinician obtaining the specimen and the interpreting cytologist. False-negative findings are caused by inadequate sampling (missing the lesion), improper processing of the specimen, or inability of the cytologist to make a definite diagnosis. A diagnostic FNAB reveals cells that show a specific benign entity or that are unequivocally malignant. A finding of normal epithelial or fat cells may mean that the aspiration needle missed the intended target; these findings should be interpreted as nondiagnostic. Readings such as acellular, atypical, or suspicious are also nondiagnostic. Nondiagnostic aspirates mandate surgical biopsy and should not be relied on to guide definitive therapy.

FNAB of a solid lesion is carried out with a 20- or 21-gauge needle on a 10- or 20-mL syringe (Fig. 60-14). With the needle positioned in the lesion, short bursts of suction are applied to the syringe. A number of passes are made into the mass, and the needle is removed from the breast only after suction is released, to avoid aspirating the specimen from the needle up into the syringe barrel. The sample is extruded onto a glass slide, stabilized with aerosolized fixative, stained, and examined. Immunohistochemical hormone receptor assays can be performed if the sample is specially processed.

Table 60-5. SENSITIVITY, SPECIFICITY, AND ACCURACY OF FINE-NEEDLE ASPIRATION BIOPSY OF BREAST MASSES

Investigator	Sensitivity (%)	Specificity (%)	Accuracy (%)
Rimsten, 1975	84	99	95
Kline, 1979	89	98	97
Gardecki, 1980	87	95	90
Strawbridge, 1981	70	96	87
Bell, 1983	73	98	92
Abele, 1983	95	97	96
Wanebo, 1984	90	95	92
Norton, 1984	84	83	84
Ulanow, 1984	85	87	86
Frable, 1984	89	97	94
Lannin, 1985	87	100	96

(Adapted from Lanin DR, Silverman JF, Pories WJ, Walker C. Cost-effectiveness of fine-needle biopsy of the breast. Ann Surg 1985; 203:474)

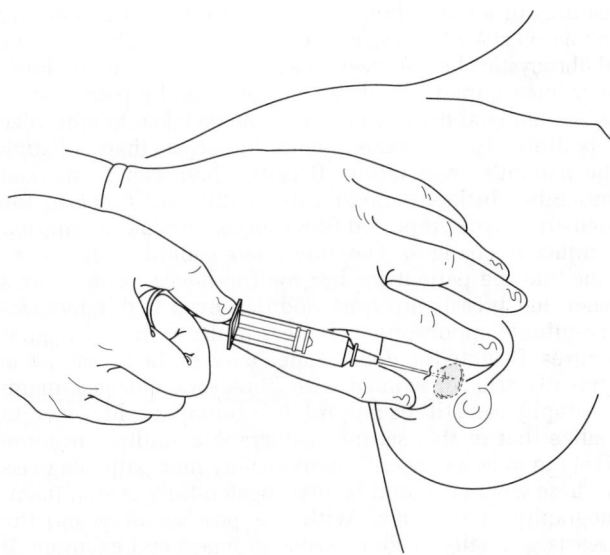

Figure 60-14. Technique of fine-needle aspiration biopsy of a breast mass.

Radiographically guided FNAB has been used to offer minimally invasive diagnosis of nonpalpable breast lesions detected mammographically. The technique is effective, especially for mass lesions (as opposed to microcalcifications). Mammograms are used to guide the aspirating needle into the suspicious lesion and to verify that the sampling was performed with the needle tip in proper position. Accuracy is comparable to that achieved with FNAB of palpable lesions.[33] As with FNAB of palpable lesions, however, nondiagnostic aspirates need to be followed up by surgical biopsy.

Core-Needle Biopsy

Core-needle biopsy, with a Tru-Cut or similar needle, is a helpful tissue sampling method for palpable masses.[34] Local anesthesia is used for the 2-mm incision through which the biopsy needle is introduced. The operator must stabilize the lesion with the nondominant hand to ensure that the needle traverses the palpable abnormality. A 1×10-mm tissue sample is obtained for histologic analysis, which, although inadequate for cytosol hormone receptor determination, is sufficient for immunohistochemical assay. There is also increasing experience with mammographically guided core needle biopsy of nonpalpable lesions.[28] Often, biopsies are performed more easily on such lesions using FNAB. If histology is desired, however, only core-needle biopsy accomplishes this without formal operation. The FNAB caveats about inadequate or nondiagnostic samples also apply to core-needle specimens. In particular, when a finding of normal or nondiagnostic breast tissue suggests that the lesion was not adequately sampled, a surgical biopsy should be performed.

Incisional and Excisional Biopsy

Incisional biopsy involves removal of a portion of a mass. Excisional biopsy, the removal of an entire mass, permits optimal diagnostic evaluation. Incisional biopsy should be reserved for those lesions too large (generally larger than 3 cm) to permit complete excision without causing unacceptable aesthetic sequelae.

When cancer is strongly suspected, prebiopsy evaluation by a medical oncologist or radiation oncologist allows eval-

uation of the primary tumor and facilitates subsequent treatment planning. Incisions paralleling the areolar border are generally preferable cosmetically (Fig. 60-15); they should be placed so as not to complicate a subsequent definitive operation if cancer is diagnosed. The incision should generally be made directly over the mass to avoid unnecessary contamination of normal tissue; an incision at the areolar border should not be used to tunnel to a peripherally located mass. Use of electrocautery at the edges of the specimen should be avoided to limit coagulation artifact, which may impair pathologic interpretation. Almost all breast biopsies can be performed in an outpatient setting using local anesthesia. For larger or deeper lesions, in anxious patients, or when a wire localization technique is used, supplemental intravenous sedation is helpful. Inadequate anesthesia traumatizes the patient, erodes the therapeutic relationship, and prevents a thorough and meticulous procedure. Orientation sutures are placed in the excised tissue so that positive margins can be precisely located by the pathologist. The fresh specimen is never placed in formalin; it should be placed in an empty container on ice so that the pathologist can prepare a portion of unfixed tumor for hormone receptor analysis. Frozen sections are rarely helpful and use tissue that might be better saved for detailed histopathologic or receptor analysis. After hemostasis is achieved, only the skin need be closed. Sutures within the breast parenchyma to close the dead space act as a nidus for wound infection and distort the surrounding breast architecture, yielding a poorer aesthetic result. The fibrin that quickly fills the dead space restores the normal contour of the breast.

Breast biopsy, when carried out properly, is an atraumatic procedure. The complication rate, however, is as high as 5% to 10%, primarily from minor wound infections and hematoma formation.

Wire Localization Biopsy

Nonpalpable lesions detected mammographically comprise an increasing proportion of biopsy cases. These lesions must be localized radiographically.[35,36] The technique is as described earlier, with a few additions. Immediately before operation, a localizing wire is inserted in proximity to the abnormality using orthogonal mammo-

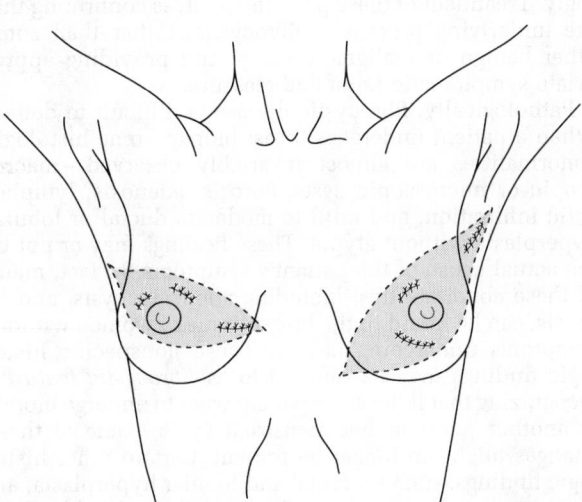

Figure 60-15. Orientation of incisions for surgical biopsy of the breast, shown in relation to potential mastectomy incisions (*shaded areas*).

graphic images (Fig. 60-16). The surgeon must review (preferably with the mammographer) the mammograms to formulate an operative approach. Whenever possible, the incision should be made perpendicular to the path of the wire to facilitate locating the wire and tracing it to the lesion. The excised specimen must undergo radiography before completion of the procedure to confirm that the target lesion (mass or microcalcifications) was adequately sampled or removed (see Fig. 60-16E). Only rarely is the target lesion missed, necessitating excision of additional breast tissue. About 25% of wire localization biopsies reveal malignancy.[35,36]

BENIGN BREAST DISORDERS

Most women who present to a surgeon for evaluation of a breast problem do not have cancer. Many clinicians, however, are uncomfortable caring for these patients. This is exacerbated by the confusing lexicon applied to benign breast disorders. This section provides a standard terminology and approach to benign breast disorders and addresses their clinical presentation as well as histologic findings.

Fibrocystic Disease

Many of the changes commonly referred to as *fibrocystic disease* are not diseases at all. Rather, they are the manifestations of breast tissue response (orderly or disorderly) to cyclic hormonal stimulation. Various terms for these changes have been proposed, including the pathologically inappropriate *chronic cystic mastitis* and the precise but overwhelming *aberrations of normal development and involution.* None of these has successfully competed with the well-entrenched term *fibrocystic disease.*

If the established terminology is to be retained, it should be modified to reflect clinical reality. When a patient is seen on examination to have nodular (lumpy) or tender breasts, she may or may not have associated symptoms. If she does not have symptoms or has minimal symptoms, the patient is referred to as having *fibrocystic changes.* Treatment beyond reassurance is unnecessary.

Clinically, patients with moderate or severe symptoms seeking relief of symptoms can legitimately be said to have fibrocystic *disease.* Patients with fibrocystic disease are subclassified as having mastodynia (breast pain), a breast mass, or a nipple discharge, and they are treated accordingly. Treatment of these patients involves confirming that the underlying process is fibrocystic, rather than some other benign or malignant entity, and providing appropriate symptomatic relief and reassurance.

Pathologically, fibrocystic disease is difficult to define. When a patient undergoes breast biopsy, some histologic abnormalities are almost invariably observed—macroscopic or microscopic cysts, fibrosis, adenosis, lymphocytic infiltration, and mild to moderate ductal or lobular hyperplasia without atypia. These findings may or not be the actual cause of the patient's symptoms. In fact, many of these abnormalities, including adenosis, cysts, and fibrosis, can be found in the breast tissue of women without symptoms undergoing biopsy. These nonspecific histologic findings may be referred to as *fibrocystic features,* recognizing that if the same patient were to undergo biopsy at another point in her menstrual cycle, some of these changes might no longer be present. Certain other histologic findings, such as ductal and lobular hyperplasia, are clearcut pathologic entities. These findings should not be dismissed as fibrocystic but rather specifically addressed, particularly in terms of subsequent cancer risk (see later).

When defined in this manner, the finding of fibrocystic features in a breast biopsy specimen does not confer any increased risk of breast cancer development. The presence of fibrocystic changes even in a symptomless patient, however, may impair breast cancer detection by palpation or by mammography. Several steps can be taken to minimize this difficulty, but none is more important than enlisting the patient's cooperation. Because there can be marked variability in breast nodularity at different times in the menstrual cycle, repeated BSE is necessary to discern truly significant changes. The physician should endeavor to schedule the patient for her routine breast examinations when her breasts are least nodular, even if this requires last-minute appointment changes in the event of irregular menses. Despite the dense appearance of the breast tissue typically seen in women with fibrocystic changes, mammography can still be helpful. It is important, however, to realize that in this setting radiographic studies are more likely to miss a cancer. Therefore, any new palpable mass in these women should be investigated fully even if mammography is negative. With the passage of years, the breasts generally become easier to image and examine. If all the above measures are taken, mastectomy should *never* be necessary solely because of breast nodularity impairing examination and screening.

Epidemiology and Risk Factors

Virtually every woman of reproductive age has occasional cyclic breast discomfort. Defining the incidence of benign breast disorders clinically, therefore, is problematic. Pathologic classification is equally untenable. The nature and severity of histologic abnormalities do not correlate well with the intensity of a patient's complaints. Indeed, histologically abnormal breast tissue can be found in nearly all women of reproductive age. Although this lack of pathologic correlation has led some investigators to call benign breast problems "nondisease,"[8] this view trivializes the legitimate discomfort of some patients.

Whatever the terminology, it is clear that benign breast disorders, particularly those pronounced enough to lead to biopsy, have a different set of risk factors and age distribution than breast cancer. The risk factors for benign breast disease include:

- Early menarche
- Late menopause
- Small breast size
- Normal or low body weight
- History of cyclic breast discomfort
- Irregular menses
- History of spontaneous abortions
- Premenopausal status

Most benign breast problems are encountered in menstruating women, with a steadily declining incidence after menopause. Mastodynia is frequently encountered in young women (late teens and 20s), with another peak in incidence in the years before menopause. Postmenopausal women have relatively few benign breast complaints, although users of replacement estrogen may experience some symptoms. Oral contraceptive use in premenopausal women, in contrast, has been shown to decrease the incidence of benign breast disease; this is particularly true with high-progesterone formulations.

Clinical Evaluation

For both patient and physician faced with any breast problem, differentiation between benign or malignant is the most important issue. Once it has been established that the patient does not have cancer, definition of the precise

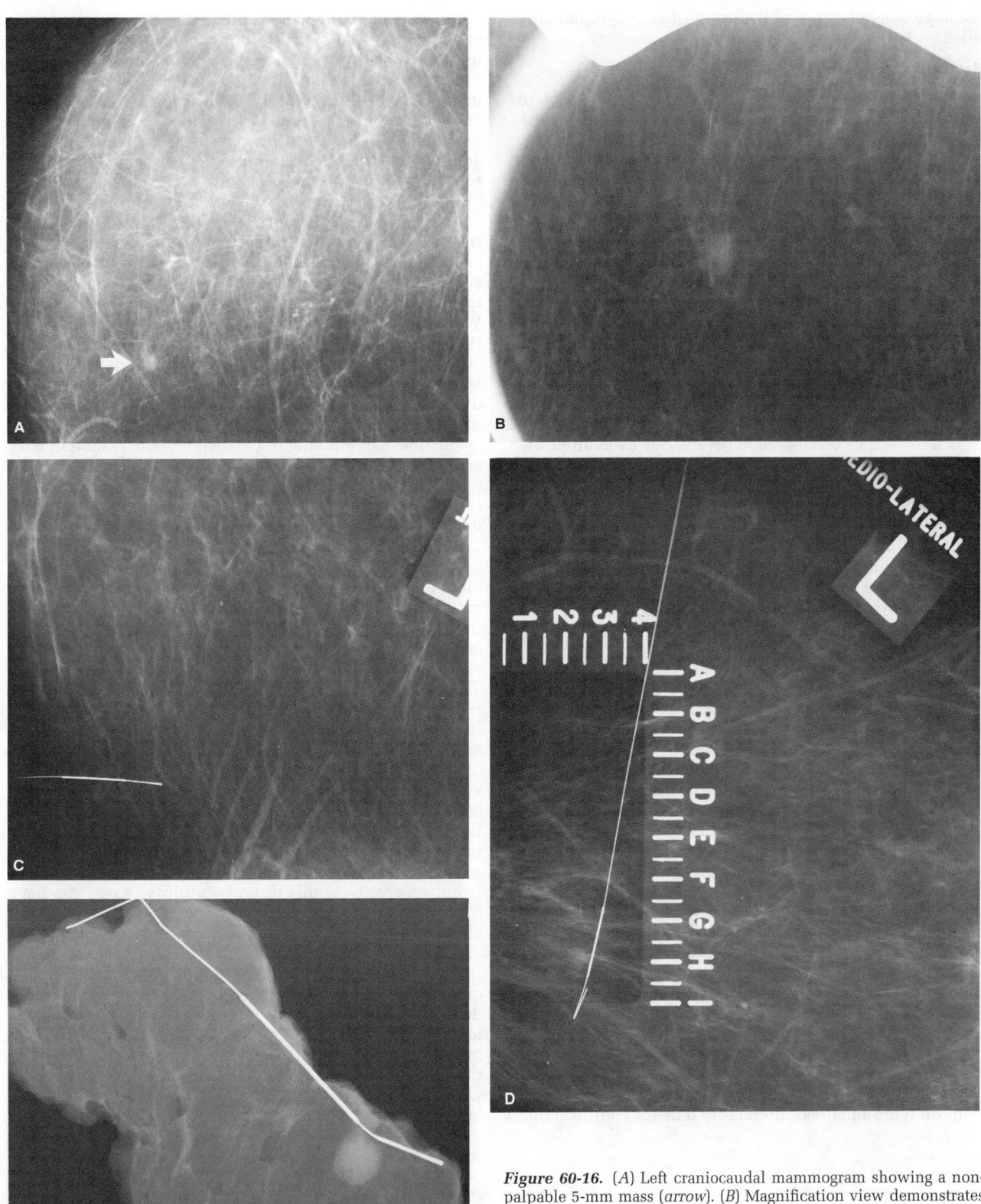

Figure 60-16. (*A*) Left craniocaudal mammogram showing a non-palpable 5-mm mass (*arrow*). (*B*) Magnification view demonstrates spiculated borders, suspicious for malignancy. (*C*) Magnification view after placement of a localization wire; the reinforced portion of the wire is just superior to the mass. (*D*) Orthogonal view. (*E*) Specimen radiograph containing the wire and the suspicious mass. Histologic evaluation revealed invasive ductal carcinoma. (Courtesy of Debra Ikeda, MD; from the Division of Breast Imaging, University of Michigan Medical School, Ann Arbor)

histology is less important than provision of symptomatic relief.

Mastodynia

One of the most common presenting complaints of women with benign breast disease is mastodynia (also referred to as *mastalgia*), which may be either cyclic (waxing or waning with the menstrual cycle) or continuous. Breast pain, especially cyclic mastodynia, is rarely associated with breast malignancy. Specific causes for the pain should be sought in all cases, however. The relation of the pain to the menstrual cycle should be ascertained. Cyclic mastodynia is most severe just before the menstrual period and least severe or absent in the days immediately after menstruation. It may be referred to the axilla, the undersurface of the upper arm, or the scapula. Pain that is unrelated to the menstrual cycle may be caused by an acute or subacute infection or a single, large cyst. Once physical examination and mammography, when appropriate, have ruled out a mass lesion, most patients require no treatment beyond reassurance. Mastodynia that begins as cyclic but progresses to become constant and severe, however, often signifies disease requiring more specific therapy.

Physical examination should confirm that the origin of the pain is the breast. Costochondritis of the upper ribs may be perceived by the patient as breast pain (Tietze syndrome). Reproduction of the pain by palpation of the affected rib allows the diagnosis of costochondritis to be made. This is a self-limiting condition; nonsteroidal anti-inflammatory drugs may be used if the pain is severe. In rare instances, pain of cardiac or cervical nerve root origin can be referred to the breast.

In most cases of mastodynia, breast examination reveals tender, nodular breasts, suggesting a diagnosis of fibrocystic disease. The examiner must determine whether a dominant mass, distinct from the surrounding breast tissue, is present. Such a mass could represent a cyst or confluent area of fibrocystic changes, either of which could be the cause of the patient's pain, or a cancer that likely is not the cause of the pain but an incidental finding. The evaluation of a dominant mass is described later.

After all appropriate steps to rule out the presence of a malignancy have been taken, an important element of the treatment of mastodynia is reassuring the patient that she does not have breast cancer. Patients should not be told that there is nothing wrong. Rather, they should counseled about their disorder, its causes, and its unrelatedness to subsequent cancer development. For most patients, occasional nonprescription analgesics are the only drug therapy required. Prescription analgesics, particularly narcotics, should not be used. Symptoms severe enough to prompt consideration of using such drugs mandate fuller evaluation and more specific therapy.

The relation of methylxanthines, particularly caffeine, to mastodynia and breast nodularity remains controversial.

Some women do, however, experience diminution of their symptoms and subjective improvement in breast nodularity by limiting or eliminating caffeine intake. We advise mastodynia patients to eliminate caffeinated beverages as much as possible for a period of 2 or 3 months. At the end of that time, the patient is in a good position to judge whether there has been an improvement in her pain. In addition to caffeine abstention, patients should be urged to stop smoking because nicotine is purported to worsen mastodynia, in addition to its other health risks.

A variety of medications have been advocated for the treatment of mastodynia (Table 60-6). Unfortunately, because of the subjective nature of the disease and its propensity to be better tolerated by the patient with reassurance, the exact benefit of most of these interventions is unclear. Vitamin E (α-tocopherol) has been touted as beneficial; however, clinical data do not support the use of this or other vitamins for this condition. In the United Kingdom, evening primrose oil has been used to treat cyclic mastodynia. This naturally occurring substance is a rich source of essential fatty acids. The hypothesis that women with cyclic mastodynia might be deficient in essential fatty acids led to its clinical use. This hypothesis must still be considered unproved, but studies have shown response rates comparable to those associated with caffeine abstinence. Noncyclic mastodynia does not appear to respond to evening primrose oil.

The use of hormonal agents to treat mastodynia has been more extensively tested. Danazol, a weak androgen, is the most effective drug available for treatment of mastodynia related to fibrocystic disease. Unfortunately, the androgenic side effects of danazol are troublesome enough to restrict its use to the most problematic cases of mastodynia. These undesirable effects include amenorrhea, body fat redistribution, hirsutism, acne, weight gain, and deepening of the voice. At high doses (more than 600 mg/d), these side effects are nearly universal, but even at lower doses (200 mg/d or less), many women report at least some adverse effects. Long-term danazol administration has been associated with liver function abnormalities as well. For those few patients with severe symptoms in whom lesser measures fail, a starting dose of 100 mg/d is used. Treatment must begin during the menses to be sure the patient is not pregnant. At this dose, two thirds of patients have some degree of interference with their menstrual cycles. If after 2 months, relief is incomplete and side effects are absent or minimal, the dose of danazol can be increased. If the side effects have been excessive and pain relief adequate, the dose can be decreased to 100 mg every other day. Although hepatic toxicity is unlikely, liver function tests should be checked after 2 months and again after 6 months. After 6 months of therapy, danazol is discontinued. About half of patients need no further therapy. In patients whose pain recurs and who are willing to resume taking the drug, low maintenance doses of danazol, 100

Table 60-6. DRUGS USED FOR THE TREATMENT OF MASTODYNIA

Drug	Mode of Action	Level of Benefit	Side Effects and Disadvantages
Danazol	Androgen	Very effective	Irregular menses, virilization
Evening primrose oil	Provides essential fatty acids	Effective for cyclic pain	Not widely available, expensive
Oral contraceptives	Stable hormonal cycles	Effective for cyclic pain	Contraceptive, bloating, weight gain, mood changes
Bromocriptine	Prolactin inhibitor	Effective for cyclic pain	Nausea, vomiting, headache
Tamoxifen	Antiestrogen	May be effective	Hot flashes, irregular menses, possible carcinogen
α-Tocopherol (vitamin E)	Vitamin	Ineffective (placebo)	Ineffective, expensive

mg every other day, may be employed, with surveillance of liver function tests every 6 months. Virtually all danazol-related side effects are reversible on discontinuing the drug.

Other hormonal agents have been investigated for the management of mastodynia. In young women, oral contraceptives have a variable effect on mastodynia. Some women experience relief of breast pain and nodularity, whereas others experience worsening of their symptoms. Not infrequently, the effect of oral contraceptives is dependent on the formulation of the pill. A trial-and-error search for the optimal preparation may be necessary.

In double-blind studies, mastodynia patients treated with the antiestrogen tamoxifen experienced significantly greater pain relief than did controls. Uncertainty about the long-term effects of tamoxifen, however, argue against the use of this agent for mastodynia. Other drugs that may play a role in the treatment of cyclic mastodynia include bromocriptine (a suppressor of prolactin secretion) and the luteinizing hormone–releasing hormone agonist goserelin (Zoladex). Mastectomy is almost never indicated for the sole purpose of relieving mastodynia, and it is not always successful even when performed.

Not infrequently, mastodynia is encountered in the fourth and fifth decades of life as ovarian estrogen production becomes more irregular in the years preceding menopause. In carefully selected patients who are approaching menopause, mastodynia and concomitant menstrual irregularities may be treated with exogenous replacement estrogen and progesterone initiated before the onset of hot flashes or complete amenorrhea. Generally, however, such patients can be treated with the reassurance that menopause will eventually resolve their pain. Mastodynia is not a contraindication to estrogen replacement therapy after menopause, although patients may experience a recrudescence of their symptoms.

Breast Mass

Specific benign disorders, such as fibroadenoma, that may present as a mass are described in the next section. A detailed approach to the evaluation of breast masses is presented elsewhere. Nevertheless, certain aspects of fibrocystic changes presenting as a mass warrant discussion.

A palpable breast mass may be a cyst. Cysts can either be aspirated with a fine needle or, in selected cases, observed to see if they will resolve. Persistent or enlarging cysts should be aspirated. If cyst fluid is obtained and the lesion disappears, the only subsequent management required is observation for recurrence. Cytologic evaluation of cyst fluid is not routinely indicated; the yield is low, and the nature of cyst fluid can make cytologic analysis of specimens from benign cysts misleading. If aspiration yields no fluid, the mass must be presumed to be a solid lesion, and cytologic examination of the aspirate should be carried out (see Fine-Needle Aspiration Biopsy). Bloody cyst fluid or a palpable mass that persists after aspiration of fluid suggests the possibility of cancer within a cyst. Excisional biopsy is mandated in such cases to exclude malignancy. Any palpable cyst that recurs after complete aspiration should likewise be excised.

At times, fibrocystic changes may present as a palpable mass in the absence of a macroscopic cyst. In most of these cases, physical examination reveals a palpable area of asymmetry rather than a true dominant mass. Reexamination at a different point in the menstrual cycle (optimally just after the end of menses) may reveal regression of the area, indicating that the patient may be safely observed. In postmenopausal women, even an area of asymmetric thickening should be viewed with suspicion because fi-

brocystic changes are rare unless the patient is taking exogenous estrogen.

Nipple Discharge

At one time or another, many women notice a nipple discharge. The physician must distinguish between normal physiology and a benign or malignant pathologic process. The most common physiologic basis for nipple discharge is lactation. Milk may continue to be secreted intermittently for as long as 2 years after breastfeeding has stopped, particularly with breast stimulation. Vigorous squeezing or stimulation of the breast can sometimes express secretions even years after lactation in multiparous women, and occasionally in women who have never been pregnant. This may occur during BSE, part of which involves squeezing the nipples. Generally, such nonspontaneous discharges are of little consequence, and patients can be safely reassured. Reevaluation is indicated if the discharge becomes spontaneous or blood tinged.

If physiologic nipple discharge has been excluded, the discharge should be characterized by its appearance. In the relatively rare case of a subareolar infection presenting as a discharge, the fluid is purulent and the nipple erythematous and tender. Antibiotics and drainage cure this problem. A milky white discharge, usually bilateral, that is not related to lactation or breast stimulation is termed *galactorrhea*. The presence of bilateral galactorrhea should prompt an evaluation for an underlying endocrinopathy causing increased prolactin secretion by the pituitary (hyperprolactinemia). Classically, this is associated with amenorrhea, but galactorrhea may be the only sign of hyperprolactinemia. The elevated prolactin level may be due to a prolactin-secreting pituitary adenoma, or it may be secondary to medication, such as phenothiazines, metoclopramide, oral contraceptives, α-methyl-DOPA, reserpine, or tricyclic antidepressants. An elevated prolactin level in a patient with galactorrhea who is not taking any causative medications should prompt a search for a pituitary microadenoma. Rarely, thyroid dysfunction can lead to hyperprolactinemia and galactorrhea; the presence of symptoms compatible with hyperthyroidism or hypothyroidism calls for evaluation of thyroid function along with the prolactin level. Galactorrhea that occurs without an underlying endocrinopathy may be safely followed.

Nipple discharges associated with fibrocystic changes are generally green, yellow, or brown. Intraductal papillomas and cancer lead to bloody or blood-tinged serous discharges. The brownish discharge of fibrocystic disease can be easily confused with old blood. Either a guaiac test or the even simpler expedient of dabbing the discharge with a gauze pad and examining the stain can differentiate the two.

A bloody or blood-tinged discharge must be evaluated promptly to exclude carcinoma. An underlying mass is not always present when breast cancer presents as a bloody discharge. Cytologic examination of the discharge is sometimes employed, but false-negative and false-positive results are common. An occasional pregnant patient may have blood-tinged discharge late in her pregnancy; this generally resolves within a few months of pregnancy and requires no further evaluation.

If the discharge is expressible at the time the patient is seen, a contrast ductogram may be obtained. Because of the discomfort associated with the performance of a ductogram, its use is largely reserved for bloody discharges, when the likelihood of a lesion being identified is highest. If a subareolar lesion is found, it is resected by either a partial or total subareolar duct excision, depending on whether the patient plans future breastfeeding. A fine lacrimal probe is inserted into the discharging duct at the time of surgery as a guide to the extent of resection and the path of the ductal system (Fig. 60-17). Nonbloody discharges due to fibrocystic changes in the underlying breast are managed surgically only if they are severe or unrelenting; the operative approach to duct excision is the same.

Specific Entities

The preceding discussion focused on fibrocystic changes; however, a number of benign entities should be recognized and treated as unique disorders. For some of these, the clinical presentation alone is sufficiently characteristic to allow for

diagnosis; others require a complete evaluation, including mammography and biopsy.

Fibroadenoma

Fibroadenoma represents the most common breast tumor in adolescents and young women but is also frequently encountered in older women. It generally presents as a palpable breast mass and must be differentiated from cancer. Multiple fibroadenomas are encountered in 10% to 15% of cases. Typically, fibroadenoma presents as a painless, slow-growing mass found incidentally on BSE. Often, the mass grows to a size of several centimeters and

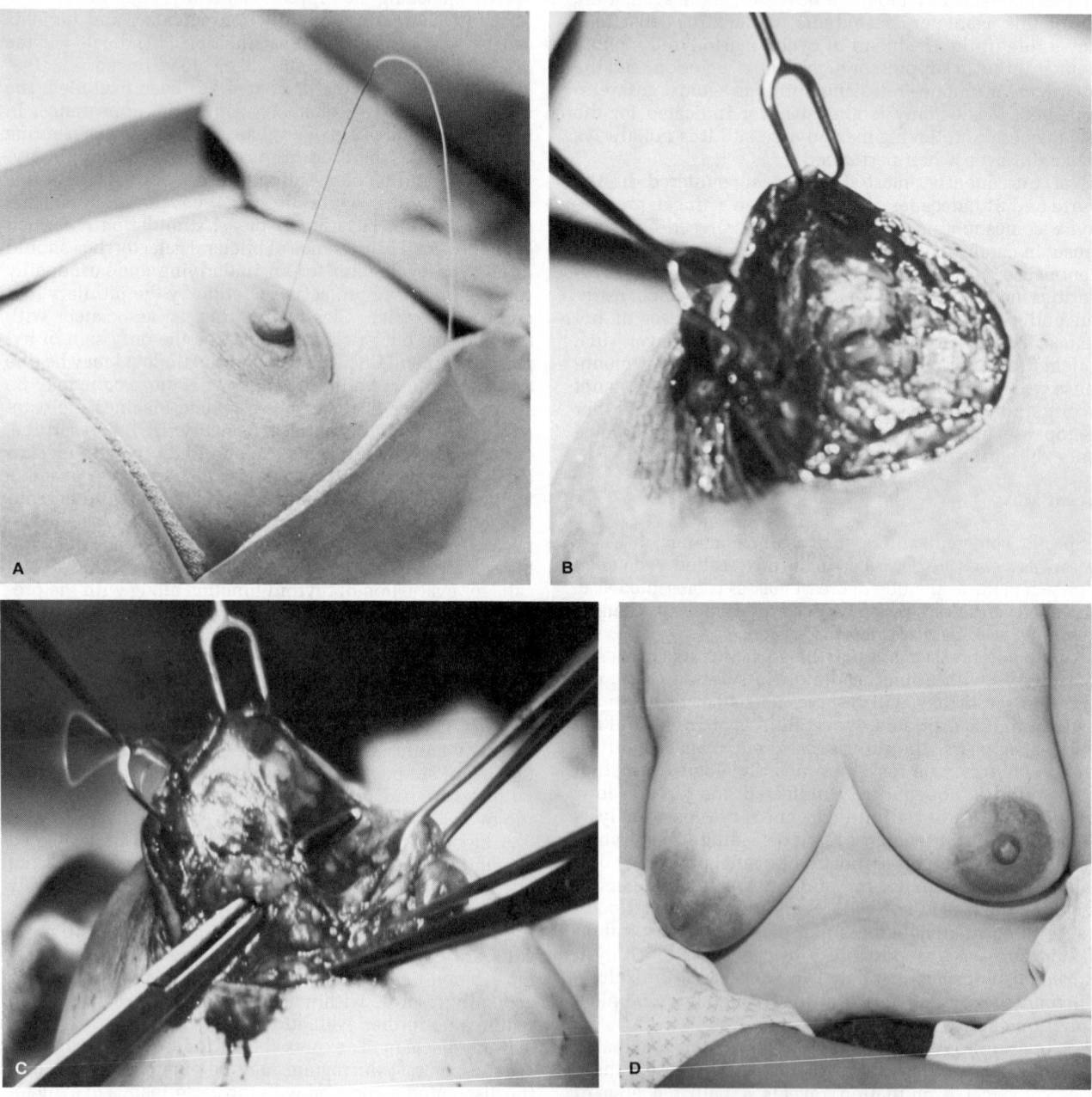

Figure 60-17. Subareolar duct excision for management of nipple discharge. (*A*) A probe is placed into the duct from which the discharge is emanating. An incision is then made along the areolar edge encompassing half of the circumference of the areola. (*B*) The nipple–areolar complex is elevated from the underlying subareolar tissue, leaving a small amount of subcutaneous fat. (*C*) The duct containing the probe is isolated. The subareolar tissue is excised in toto. A preoperative ductogram may assist in determining the depth of excision. The incision is closed using fine (5-0) absorbable suture for the subcuticular layer. (*D*) Postoperative result.

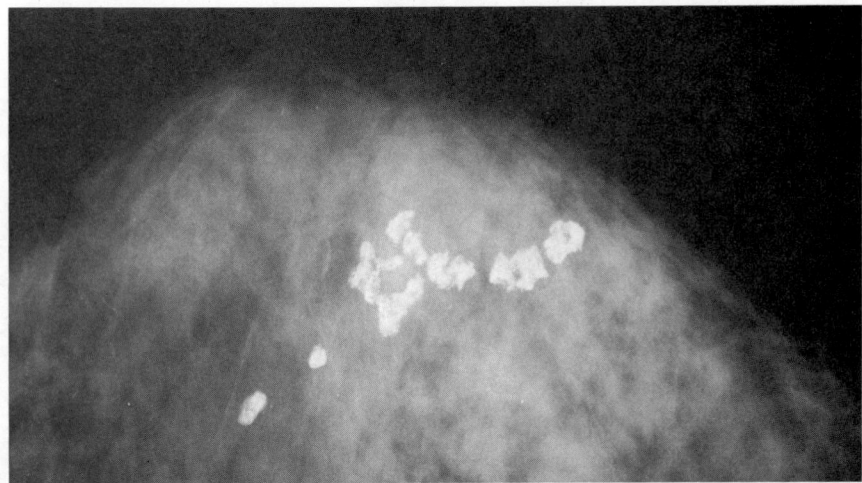

Figure 60-18. Mammographic appearance of a degenerating fibroadenoma displaying a characteristic pattern of dense, popcorn-like calcifications. (Courtesy of Debra Ikeda, MD; from the Division of Breast Imaging, University of Michigan Medical School, Ann Arbor)

remains stable thereafter. Although uncommon, variation in size with the menstrual cycle can occur. Lesions that have been stable for years may enlarge rapidly during pregnancy, suggesting that fibroadenomas are responsive to hormonal stimuli, at least in some cases.

Palpation of a fibroadenoma usually reveals a well-circumscribed, oval or round mobile mass with a firm, rubbery texture. In older women, degenerating fibroadenomas may be small and rock-hard on palpation. In any patient, an indistinct border or fixation to the surrounding breast tissue or skin suggests malignancy rather than fibroadenoma.

Because the mammographic appearance of a fibroadenoma is rarely characteristic, mammography plays little role in diagnosing this lesion. If the lesion has undergone degeneration, the resultant characteristic calcifications can allow for a specific radiologic diagnosis (Fig. 60-18). Ultrasonography can differentiate a solid mass from a cyst. Additionally, the ultrasonic appearance of a well-marginated, homogenous mass may be sufficiently characteristic to permit diagnosis of a fibroadenoma.

On gross inspection, fibroadenomas are well-encapsulated, rubbery, and white. The cut surface is glistening white and has irregular clefts distributed over it. Darker brown coloration suggests the possibility of phyllodes tumor (cystosarcoma phyllodes) rather than fibroadenoma. Microscopically, the derivation of fibroadenomas from lobular elements of the breast is obvious (Fig. 60-19). The hallmark of this lesion is the presence of stromal tissue, similar to the normal lobular stroma, combined with epithelium-lined, ductlike structures. There is no elastic tissue present in a fibroadenoma; such tissue is a feature of ductal elements.

Excisional biopsy is not necessary for every fibroadenoma. Women younger than 30 years of age with a characteristic physical examination and ultrasonographic appearance of fibroadenoma may be given the option of observation, with removal performed only if the lesion enlarges or changes in character. Above that age, a cytologic diagnosis of fibroadenoma should be made by FNAB if the lesion is to be observed. Excision is indicated if the cytology is not diagnostic or if the mass is changing. Many women prefer excisional biopsy even of a stable fibroadenoma to avoid repeat examinations and the attendant anxiety. Generally, fibroadenomas are thought not to be premalignant lesions, nor to indicate any increased risk for the development of breast cancer.[37] Recently, however, a large case-control study reported an increased risk of breast cancer development in women with a family history of breast

cancer plus the combination of fibroadenoma and associated fibrocystic or proliferative changes in the adjacent breast.[38] This study also showed that most women with simple fibroadenomas and no family history of breast cancer were not at increased risk.

Fibroadenomas larger than 5 cm in greatest diameter are called *giant fibroadenomas.* They frequently grow rapidly to attain that size. Rapid growth of a giant fibroadenoma may occasionally produce venous engorgement and a clinical appearance worrisome for inflammatory cancer. These unusual lesions occur at the extremes of reproductive age—just after menarche and just before menopause. In the younger age group, the rapid enlargement of normal breast tissue at the same time can mask the presence of a giant fibroadenoma, and patients sometimes present with breast asymmetry rather than a palpable mass. Giant fibroadenomas must be differentiated from the benign and malignant phyllodes tumors. The treatment of giant fibroadenomas at any age is complete excision without

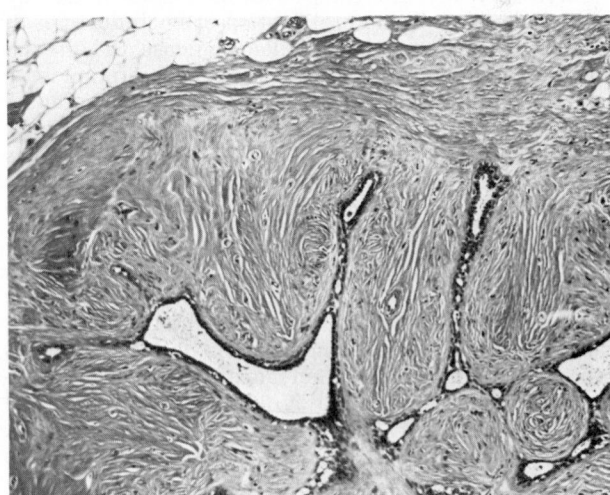

Figure 60-19. The histologic appearance of a typical fibroadenoma. This is a long-standing fibroadenoma excised from a middle-aged woman, demonstrating hyalinizing fibrosis of the stroma. This is in contrast to the loose, pale, fibrous stroma often present in younger fibroadenomas. No elastic tissue is present. (Courtesy of Harold Oberman, MD, Department of Pathology, University of Michigan Medical School, Ann Arbor)

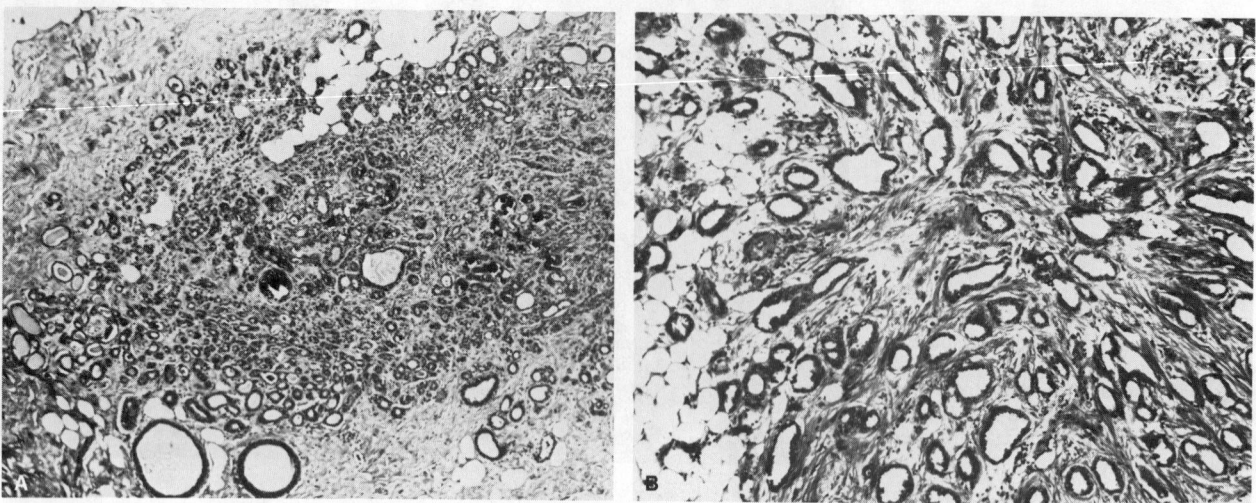

Figure 60-20. The histologic appearance of sclerosing adenosis (*A*) and invasive ductal cancer (*B*) can be similar and cause diagnostic uncertainty, especially on frozen-section examination. Sclerosing adenosis is characterized by its circumscription, the presence of bigger ducts near the periphery, and the presence of two layers in the duct lining (an inner epithelium and an outer myoepithelium). Cytologically, nuclear atypia is not generally seen in sclerosing adenosis. (Courtesy of Harold Oberman, MD, Department of Pathology, University of Michigan Medical School, Ann Arbor)

mastectomy. Recurrence is rare provided the lesion is completely excised.

Sclerosing Adenosis

Sclerosing adenosis is a histologic subtype of fibrocystic change that is not associated with an increased risk of cancer development. It is, however, one of the benign breast processes most likely to be confused radiologically and histologically with cancer. It may present as a palpable mass or as mastodynia. More commonly, it is detected on routine mammography as clustered microcalcifications without an associated palpable lesion. In these cases, wire localization and excision are required to establish a diagnosis.

Microscopically, sclerosing adenosis is characterized by intralobular fibrosis and proliferation of small ductules. If the fibrous component is particularly intense, the orientation of lobules and epithelial cells may be lost, mimicking carcinoma. Differentiating sclerosing adenosis from cancer on frozen-section examination can be particularly difficult and should not be attempted (Fig. 60-20). Pathologic clues to the benignity of sclerosing adenosis can be found in the regularity of the nuclei and the absence of mitoses.

Radial Scar

Radial scars, also called *radial sclerosing lesions,* are another benign entity that may easily be confused with cancer. A radial scar appears as a stellate, irregular mass lesion on mammography, often indistinguishable by radiographic criteria from cancer (Fig. 60-21). On sectioning, the gross appearance may be identical to cancer—an irregular, gray-white, hard lesion. Microscopically, the core of the radial scar is composed of fibroelastic tissue with entrapped glandular elements. Radiating from the central core, ducts with varying degrees of epithelial hyperplasia and cystic dilation can be seen. Surrounding areas of fibrocystic features, including sclerosing adenosis, are common. These associated changes probably account for any symptoms associated with the presence of the radial scar, which may well represent one point on the spectrum of

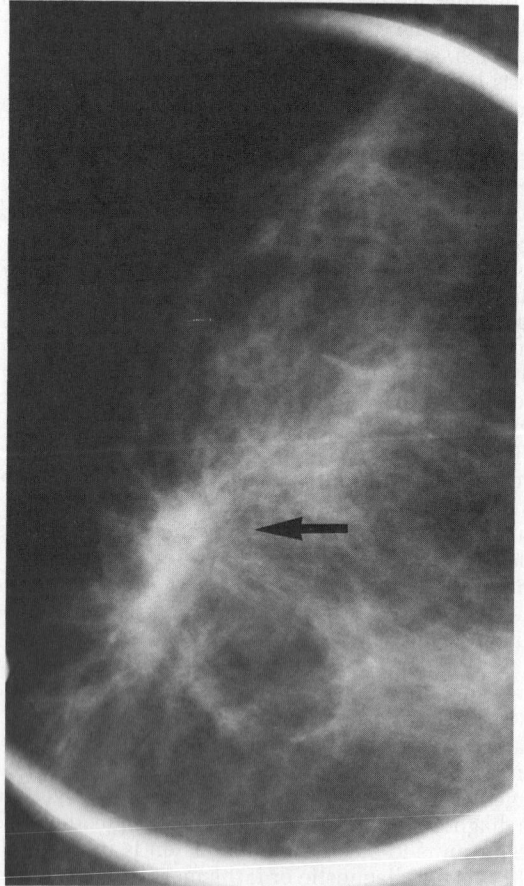

Figure 60-21. The radiographic appearance of a radial scar can be virtually indistinguishable from that of cancer. This mammogram displays a spiculated mass (*arrow*) that was not palpable. Wire localization biopsy yielded the diagnosis of radial scar without evidence of malignancy. (Courtesy of Debra Ikeda, MD; from the Division of Breast Imaging, University of Michigan Medical School, Ann Arbor)

fibrocystic change. This lesion is not associated with an increased cancer risk.

Fat Necrosis

Traumatic injury to the fatty tissue in the breast can incite an inflammatory response leading to fat necrosis. In only about half of cases, however, is a traumatic event recalled. This raises the possibility that other processes can induce the type of inflammation that culminates in the formation of this lesion. Fat necrosis can be confused with carcinoma; the attendant fibrosis simulates a mass and may cause skin dimpling and retraction. Therefore, these signs cannot be considered pathognomonic for malignancy. Microscopically, the presence of fat-laden macrophages and, later, of foreign-body giant cells are characteristic. No specific treatment is required.

Periductal Mastitis (Mammary Duct Ectasia)

Periductal mastitis, also called *plasma cell mastitis* or *mammary duct ectasia*, is an uncommon benign disorder characterized by the presence of dilated mammary ducts with inspissated secretions and marked periductal inflammation. Mammary duct ectasia appears to be a part of this disease complex rather than a separate entity. The presenting symptoms are noncyclic mastodynia associated with nipple retraction or discharge. In severe cases, subareolar abscesses form and can burrow through the skin at the areolar border to form mammary duct fistulas.

The pathogenesis of this condition is obscure. Younger women (early to middle 30s) tend to present with inflammatory and infectious processes, such as recurrent subareolar abscesses, whereas perimenopausal and postmenopausal women are more likely to present with nipple discharge, sterile subareolar masses, or nipple retraction. Many women with this disorder offer a history of difficulty breastfeeding. Periductal mastitis is probably a final common pathway that results from obstructed milk ducts. This obstruction may result from nipple abnormalities such as congenital inversion, from periductal fibrosis as part of fibrocystic disease, or from primary periductal inflammation.

For older women who present with the typical thick, white, creamy nipple discharge, reassurance may be the only treatment needed. If the discharge is bloody or if the presentation is one of spontaneous nipple retraction, differentiation from malignancy is required. When subareolar abscesses or mammary duct fistulas complicate the condition, treatment must be aimed at removing the affected duct complex. Antibiotic therapy alone rarely suffices. Simple cases can be treated with incision and drainage of the abscess since the pathologic process frequently begins in only one duct. Curative treatment of more advanced cases usually requires subareolar duct excision, often with open packing and postoperative antibiotics.

Other Causes of Mastitis and Abscess

Inflammatory and infectious processes involving the breast are relatively uncommon. Whenever mastitis or breast infection is suspected clinically, the possibility of an inflammatory carcinoma must be entertained (discussed later). Any inflammatory process that does not respond completely and promptly to antibiotics or drainage should be subjected to biopsy to rule out cancer. It also is sound practice to perform a biopsy of the abscess wall whenever open surgical drainage is performed.

Lactation and periductal mastitis are risk factors for development of breast infections. Infection complicates breastfeeding in fewer than 1 in 100 women, but these lactational infections still account for 80% of all breast infections. Presumably gaining access through the skin of the irritated nipple of the nursing woman, *Staphylococcus aureus* is by far the most common pathogen in this setting. The milk-filled breast, with its dilated ducts, provides an ideal milieu for the progressive growth of bacteria. Nursing women are most vulnerable to infection either in the first month of breastfeeding, when the skin of the nipples is most easily damaged, or much later, when the child has teeth that may traumatize the nipples.

Many breast infections begin as cellulitis, without abscess formation. If recognized at this stage, antibiotic treatment is usually successful. When an actual abscess is suspected, percutaneous aspiration can establish the diagnosis and allow for bacterial culture and sensitivity testing. Although some have tried nonoperative management of breast abscesses, open surgical drainage is the most prudent and effective treatment. In the United States, most lactating women in whom infections develop cease breastfeeding; lactation may be suppressed by bromocriptine, ice, and sometimes binding. There is, however, no absolute indication to cease nursing because of a breast infection. Nursing is often difficult for several days on the affected side; the breast should be mechanically emptied and the infant fed from the other breast until nursing can recommence.

Nonlactational infections other than those associated with periductal mastitis are rare and should always raise the specter of inflammatory cancer. Chronic breast infections can occur from some unusual pathogens, however. Actinomycosis can cause chronic, relapsing breast infections as an isolated process or as part of a systemic infection. Tuberculosis and syphilis are other rare causes of chronic, nonlactational breast infections.

Acute, noninfectious mastitis can be seen secondary to a variety of inflammatory processes, such as systemic lupus erythematosus. On rare occasions, acute mastitis complicates fibrocystic changes in the breast. In these cases, the source of the inflammation is presumed to be a spontaneously or traumatically ruptured benign cyst.

Galactocele

A galactocele is a breast cyst that is filled with milk rather than the usual cyst fluid. It is seen in women who are or who were recently lactating and likely represents a dilated, obstructed breast duct. It may also occur in postpartum women who do not breastfeed. The history of recent pregnancy and the character of the cyst fluid allow differentiation of a galactocele from periductal mastitis, wherein the fluid is more viscid and may be purulent. Mammography may reveal an interesting fat–fluid level as the milk within the cyst separates and the cream rises to the top (Fig. 60-22). Aspiration is the only treatment necessary. Although recurrences develop occasionally, repeated aspiration usually cures the condition.

Mondor Disease

Thrombophlebitis of one of the superficial veins of the breast can lead to a palpable, cordlike mass in the breast. This condition, referred to as *Mondor disease,* is identical to superficial thrombophlebitis elsewhere. Most cases have no identifiable cause, but strenuous exercise can sometimes bring on the condition. Vein ligation or coagulation during a breast biopsy can also be causative. Patients with Mondor disease may complain of burning breast pain. Physical examination reveals a characteristic cordlike mass in the superficial subcutaneous tissue of the breast. Most commonly, the affected vein is in the lower, outer quadrant. Skin retraction and dimpling may be present, particularly when the arms are raised.

Because of the skin changes and the palpable mass, Mondor disease is sometimes mistaken for cancer. When there is doubt, mammography can be helpful in confirming the diagnosis. Mondor disease is both benign and self-

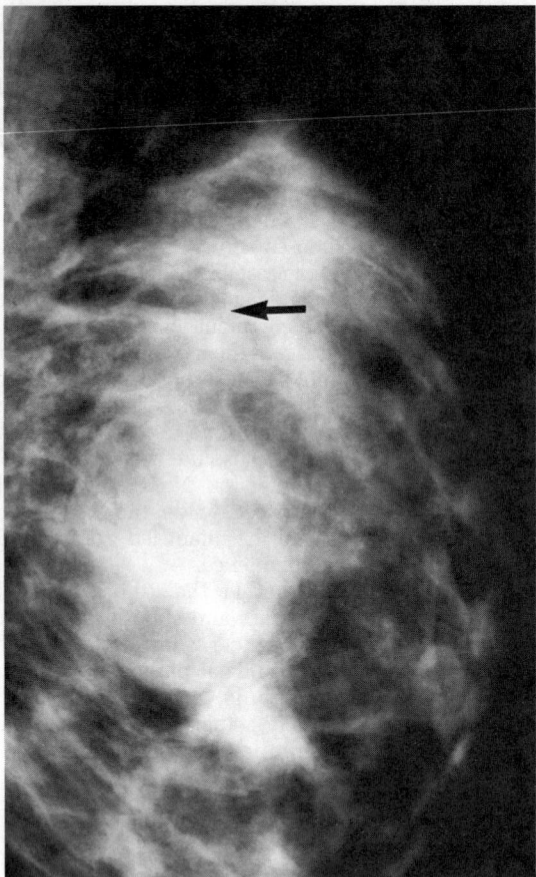

Figure 60-22. The diagnosis of a galactocele can be made with certainty when mammography reveals the characteristic fat–fluid level caused by separation of the lipid elements of milk within the cyst. Aspiration of milky fluid can also confirm the diagnosis and is usually the only treatment necessary. (Courtesy of Debra Ikeda, MD; from the Division of Breast Imaging, University of Michigan Medical School, Ann Arbor)

limited, so no specific treatment is required. Nonsteroidal antiinflammatory drugs often provide relief of symptoms, and recurrence is uncommon.

Intraductal Papilloma

Intraductal papilloma represents the most common cause of a bloody nipple discharge, although in about half of cases, the discharge is serous. Because the average size of an intraductal papilloma is 3 to 4 mm, they are rarely palpable.

Ductography may demonstrate the lesion, or it may be found after subareolar duct excision performed to treat the discharge. The lesion is usually solitary and generally is found within a few centimeters of the nipple. Characteristically, these lesions have a long, slender stalk and are vulnerable to torsion as they grow larger; this may be the source of the bloody discharge. Subareolar excision of the affected duct is curative. Data suggest that there is no increased incidence of breast cancer in women with solitary intraductal papillomas.

Rarely, patients are encountered with diffuse papillomatosis. In these patients, papillomas occur in multiple ducts, often bilaterally. The individual papillomas are usually larger and more distant from the nipple than are isolated papillomas. Serous rather than bloody discharge is characteristic of this condition. Unlike isolated papillo-

mas, diffuse papillomatosis is associated with an increased risk of breast cancer. The exact magnitude of this risk is unknown, but it has been reported that invasive cancer eventually develops in up to 40% of women with this condition. A high rate of recurrence of the nipple discharge is to be expected after excision unless the entire involved portion of the ductal system is removed.

Disorders of the Nipple

Diseases specifically involving the nipple are unusual. Their importance lies largely in the need to differentiate them from malignant processes that may involve the nipple secondarily. Nipple retraction is a common sign of breast carcinoma, and malignancy needs to be excluded whenever nipple retraction develops in an adult. Congenital nipple inversion is not infrequent, however, and is of no clinical significance. The condition may occur unilaterally or bilaterally. Women with congenitally inverted nipples may have difficulty with breastfeeding. Acquired nipple retraction can result from any process, benign or malignant, that leads to fibrosis and contraction of breast parenchyma. The most common benign cause of nipple retraction is periductal mastitis; this can usually be differentiated from malignancy clinically and mammographically. Fat necrosis and Mondor disease are benign causes of breast skin retraction. In the unusual cases when these disease processes are subareolar, nipple retraction can also occur.

Eczema and other erosive skin lesions involving the nipple are rare and must be differentiated from Paget disease and its associated malignancy (discussed later). Every eczematoid rash involving the nipple must be suspected of representing Paget disease, and biopsy should be performed if necessary to rule out this condition. When eczema involves the nipple, there is usually but not invariably evidence of eczema elsewhere. Eczema of the nipple is usually bilateral, symmetric, and limited to the nipple–areola complex. In contrast, Paget disease is most often unilateral, asymmetrically involves the nipple, and in advanced cases may completely obliterate the nipple and involve adjacent skin.

Repeated traumatic irritation and breastfeeding can cause erosive lesions of the nipple. The former condition is common in male and female runners and cyclists because of the friction of clothing on the nipple. It is usually easily recognized and may be prevented by use of appropriate protective clothing (such as a well-padded jogger's bra), adhesive strips, or petroleum jelly to minimize friction during exercise. The cracked, irritated nipples of the lactating breast are likewise easily recognized. Good hygiene, including cleansing the nipples of dried secretions with warm water, is vital to prevention of infection. Antibiotic or antifungal creams are used only if infection is established. These creams should be wiped off the nipple before breastfeeding and reapplied after cleansing the nipple. If only one breast is involved, temporarily nursing from only the unaffected side is prudent.

Adenomas and polyps of the nipple can occur and may be mistaken for Paget disease. Biopsy is appropriate if the diagnosis is in doubt; partial resections of the nipple can usually be performed with satisfactory cosmetic results and complete excision of the offending lesion.

A variety of subcutaneous cysts can afflict the nipple, including sebaceous cysts and retention cysts involving Montgomery glands. These are usually easily recognized as benign and treated with conservative local excision. If a cyst has become infected, secondary closure of the wound may be necessary.

BREAST CANCER

Epidemiology and Risk Factors

Cancer of the breast is an extremely common malignancy in Western societies. Until recently, it was the leading cause of cancer deaths among American women, a dubious distinction now held by lung cancer. Annually, breast cancer develops in about 182,000 American women (and 1400 men) and about 46,000 breast cancer deaths occur.[39] The incidence and mortality figures for the United States are about five times higher than the comparable figures in many Asian and African countries. Breast cancer mortality rates in this country have remained largely unchanged since the 1930s. The absolute incidence of breast cancer has slightly increased during this time, however, suggesting some decrease in the case-fatality rate.

Identifying patients at increased risk of development of breast cancer serves two purposes. Recognition of high-risk patients improves understanding of the factors involved in breast cancer development. It also allows planning of preventive and diagnostic strategies. Clinicians, however, must have a clear understanding of the significance of risk factors and how they should be used.

The absolute risk of development of a disease is the incidence of that disease over a lifetime. The relative risk of development of a disease is assessed by comparing the incidence rate of individuals possessing a given characteristic to the incidence rate of individuals in whom that characteristic is not present. Two points about this bear mentioning. First, relative risk is not assessed compared with the "average" person because if the characteristic of interest is common in the population as a whole, the average person may have that characteristic. Second, in most epidemiologic studies from which relative risk ratios are calculated, subjects are followed up for a limited time, not for their entire lives. Because the risk of development of breast cancer does not remain constant over a woman's entire life, direct extrapolation from relative risk data to absolute lifetime risk is inappropriate.

Many factors are associated with an increased risk of development of breast cancer (Table 60-7). The foremost risk factor for breast cancer is female gender. Men account for fewer than 1 in 130 breast cancer patients. Virtually all

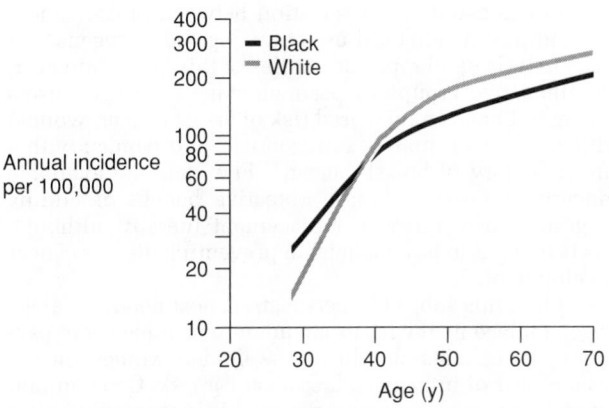

Figure 60-23. Age-specific incidence curves for breast cancer in white and black women in the United States, 1969 to 1971. The incidence curve rises sharply after 30 years of age and continues to climb thereafter, although the rate of rise lessens after menopause. Black women have a higher incidence of premenopausal, but not postmenopausal, breast cancer. (After Schottenfeld D, Epidemiology of breast cancer. In: Harness JK, Oberman HA, Lichter AS, Adler DD, Cody RL, eds. Breast cancer: collaborative management. Chelsea, MI, Lewis, 1988:55)

women are at risk of development of breast cancer. It has been estimated that, if the annual incidence and mortality rates remain unchanged, breast cancer will develop in as many as 1 in 8 women (12.2%) in her lifetime, and 3.6% of all women will die of the disease.[40] In actuality, breast cancer develops in about 7% of women (1 in 14) who reach 70 years of age. The risk of development of breast cancer is strongly age related. It is exceedingly rare in women under the age of 25, but the incidence increases steadily with age until menopause, at which time it rises further, albeit at a slower rate (Fig. 60-23). Premenopausal breast cancer is more likely to develop in black women than white women; this increased incidence does not persist after menopause. Black women are also more likely than whites to die of breast cancer.[41]

The internal hormonal milieu plays a decisive role in the pathogenesis of breast cancer. Greater exposure to uninterrupted hormonal (menstrual) cycles, as may be seen in nulliparous women or in those having early menarche or late menopause, fosters the development of breast cancer. Women who give birth to a child before 30 years of age are at decreased risk of development of breast cancer compared with those who give birth for the first time after age 30 or who never bear children. This protective effect is age-related because women who give birth before age 20 are at even lower risk. There is a suggestion that a second child born before age 25 conveys additional benefit.

A trend toward increased breast cancer risk with earlier menarche has been shown, with the relative risk being about 1.5 if the onset of menses is before 12 years of age. Late menopause (after age 55) is also a risk factor, with a relative risk of about two times that of earlier cessation of menses. Women who undergo oophorectomy before age 35 and do not take replacement estrogens have a two-thirds reduction in their breast cancer risk (relative risk, 0.3). Replacement estrogen therapy eliminates the beneficial effect of oophorectomy.

Exogenous hormone therapy has been extensively studied as a risk factor for breast cancer. Most investigations of oral contraceptive use do not demonstrate an associated increased risk of breast cancer development. Studies of estrogen replacement therapy for postmenopausal women have yielded equivocal results. Most contemporary studies

---

Table 60-7. BREAST CANCER RISK FACTORS

DEMOGRAPHIC FACTORS

Age more than 30 y
Female gender (130:1 female/male ratio)

GREATLY INCREASED RISK

Known carrier of breast cancer susceptibility gene
Strong family history—two or more first-degree relatives with bilateral or premenopausal breast cancer
Atypical ductal or lobular hyperplasia or lobular carcinoma in situ
Ductal carcinoma in situ, risk limited to ipsilateral breast

MODERATELY INCREASED RISK

Family history—one or more relatives with breast cancer, not bilateral or premenopausal
Menstrual history—menarche before age 12 y, menopause after age 55 y
Parity—nulliparity or first live birth after age 30 y
Radiation—exposure to low-dose ionizing radiation in childhood or adolescence
Previous breast cancer—low-grade, node-negative, or receptor-positive; lobular histology
Other cancers—colon or endometrial cancer
Diet—high-fat or high-calorie diet

fail to demonstrate an association between breast cancer risk and postmenopausal use of conjugated estrogens.[42] A metaanalysis of all reported studies of this topic, however, identified two groups of postmenopausal estrogen users who might have an increased risk of breast cancer: women with 15 years or more of estrogen use, and women with a family history of breast cancer.[43] Few data are available concerning possible breast-protective benefit of adding progesterone to estrogen replacement therapy, although this is thought to be beneficial in preventing uterine cancer development.

To place this subject in perspective, postmenopausal estrogen replacement with its attendant physiologic and psychological benefits should not be denied women on the basis of fear of increasing breast cancer risk. Concomitant progesterone replacement is reasonable in women who are at risk of development of endometrial cancer, that is, those who still have their uteri. When a diagnosis of breast cancer is made, however, hormonal therapy for contraception or postmenopausal replacement should be discontinued. This is the practice for all breast cancers, including receptor-negative tumors, because even these tumors may be influenced subtly by exogenous hormones. Any subsequent use of estrogen replacement therapy by women with an established diagnosis of breast cancer is generally avoided, although this is clearly a controversial area that needs further study.[44]

Most women with fibrocystic changes are not at increased risk of development of breast cancer. The 3% to 6% who are found at breast biopsy to have atypical epithelial hyperplasia (whether lobular or ductal), however, have a relative risk of breast cancer that is about 5 times that of women who do not have this finding. Women who have atypical hyperplasia and one or more close female relatives with breast cancer are at even greater risk of breast cancer development[37] (relative risk, 6 to 8; Fig. 60-24).

Breast cancer is a common disease in women; thus, a family history of a female relative with breast cancer is also common. Nevertheless, the history of one or more close relatives (sister, daughter, mother, maternal grand-

mother, or maternal aunt) having breast cancer is definitely associated with an increased risk of development of breast cancer. The risk increases further if the relative had bilateral breast cancer or was diagnosed with cancer while premenopausal. Women with a strongly positive family history (defined as two or more close relatives with bilateral, premenopausal breast cancer) have an absolute lifetime breast cancer incidence of 50% or greater. This incidence is sufficiently great that genetic screening (if available) and preventive measures, such as prophylactic mastectomies, should be considered (see later discussion).

A woman who has been treated for breast cancer in one breast is not immune to development of a second primary tumor in the opposite breast. Estimates of the magnitude of the risk vary, in part because it can occasionally be difficult to discriminate a second primary tumor from a metastasis of the original cancer. The annual risk of development of a second breast cancer may be as high as 1% per year. Overall, the absolute lifetime risk of development of a second carcinoma approaches 10%. This risk varies based on several identifiable patient and tumor characteristics. The younger the age at original diagnosis, the greater the likelihood of development of a second cancer. For a second primary tumor to develop, of course, the patient must survive her first cancer. Indeed, good-prognosis first primary tumors (eg, those that are small, node-negative, or histologically low grade) are associated with a higher risk of metachronous bilaterality. Other factors associated with bilateral breast cancer include family history of breast cancer, multicentric first tumor, and lobular histology of the first tumor. Patients with invasive lobular cancer have synchronous cancers in the other breast in as many as 3% of cases; with time, contralateral breast cancer develops in up to 30% of patients. LCIS is associated with a long-term risk of development of invasive cancer that is bilateral, even if the LCIS is found in only one breast. No matter what the histologic type of cancer, however, the recognition that breast cancer patients remain at risk for development of a second primary tumor mandates careful lifelong clinical and radiologic observation of the opposite breast.

Other breast cancer risk factors have been identified through epidemiologic studies.[45] Exposure to ionizing radiation at a young age (such as thymic irradiation, chest fluoroscopy, or mantle irradiation for Hodgkin disease) leads to a clearcut increase in breast cancer incidence later in life. The latency period is 10 to 30 years.[46,47] Dietary factors have also been linked to breast cancer development. Cross-cultural studies demonstrate that women from low-risk countries, such as parts of Asia and Africa, acquire the same high risk of breast cancer as their American counterparts when they move to this country and adopt a Western diet. The high fat content of the American diet in comparison to that of low-risk countries appears to be the source of this increased risk. Cancers associated with high-fat diets, namely endometrial cancer and colon cancer, are also more common in women who have had breast cancer, and vice versa. Obese postmenopausal women appear to be at increased risk for breast cancer, with a relative risk of about 2. Part of this risk may relate to hormonal influences of obesity. Increased body fat stores can lead to higher circulating levels of estrogen by peripheral conversion of steroids within the lipocytes. Furthermore, childhood obesity has been correlated with early menarche.

Despite the wealth of known risk factors, women who possess no identifiable risk factors account for most breast cancer patients. On an individual basis, no woman can be assumed not to have breast cancer solely on the basis of a favorable risk profile. More specifically, any woman older than 25 years of age with a palpable mass or abnormal

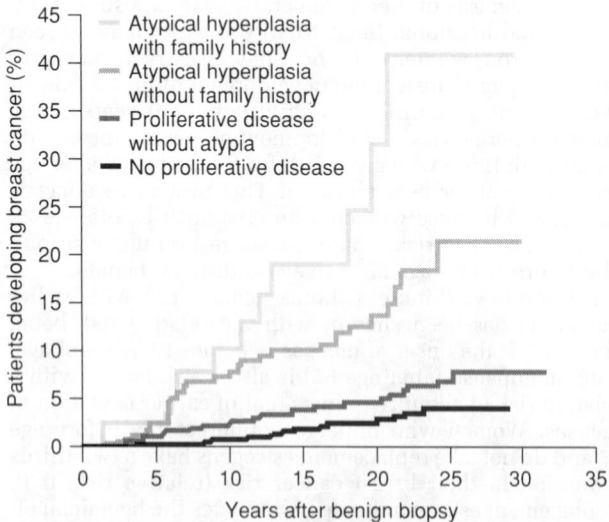

Figure 60-24. Cumulative risk of developing invasive breast cancer after a biopsy for benign breast disease. Women with proliferative disease with atypia (atypical ductal or lobular hyperplasia) are at significantly increased risk for developing invasive breast cancer. This is particularly true if a family history of breast cancer is present. (After Page DL, Dupont WD. Anatomic markers of human premalignancy and risk of breast cancer. Cancer 1990;66:1326)

mammogram, regardless of the presence or absence of any risk factors, should be considered at risk.

Inherited Breast Cancer Syndromes

It has long been recognized that women with a family history of breast cancer are at increased risk for development of the disease. Early epidemiologic studies comparing families of breast cancer patients with the general population consistently identified a two-fold to three-fold increase in risk conferred by a positive family history.[48,49] Because this degree of risk is similar in magnitude to that associated with other factors previously mentioned, it was difficult to implicate genetic (as opposed to environmental) causes conclusively. To investigate the issue further, Anderson and colleagues[10,50] developed a set of breast cancer pedigrees enriched for the presence of a family history of breast cancer, and compared them with control groups of patients with cancer who also had family histories of malignancy. Analysis of this database highlighted the significance of bilaterality of cancer, early age at onset of breast cancer, and the relationship of affected family members (first-degree versus other). Recognition that women who were the first-degree relatives of premenopausal patients with bilateral breast cancer had an approximate 50% risk of development of cancer helped confirm a genetic (indeed, autosomal dominant) basis for the increased risk seen in some families.

This work and similar studies also laid a foundation for the identification of a number of specific hereditary breast cancer syndromes. Understanding of these syndromes is important for a number of reasons. First, recognition of a family history consistent with the presence of such a syndrome can help assess the risk to an individual patient under evaluation and initiate counseling and screening of other potentially involved family members. As many as 11% of women younger than 50 years diagnosed at one referral center had family histories consistent with a hereditary form of breast cancer,[51] forming a significant group for which counseling and intervention should be considered. Second, recognition of cancer syndromes has facilitated study of genetic alterations common to many cancers and helped identify etiologic genetic events in the pathogenesis of many types of cancer.[52] Third, families with inherited predisposition to breast cancer have been an important resource for the identification of specific gene alterations that contribute to development of the disease. Finally, it is likely that the specific gene alterations identified in familial cancers also are present, through somatic mutation, in at least some sporadic breast cancers.

Four inherited syndromes appear to be particularly important in breast cancer. The Li-Fraumeni syndrome has an autosomal dominant mode of inheritance.[53] It is attributed to mutations in the p53 tumor-suppressor gene, a gene that codes for a protein that serves as a G_1 to S-phase checkpoint regulator of the cell cycle.[54] Affected patients suffer from excess occurrences of multiple types of cancer, including breast cancer and sarcomas (see Chap. 113). Initially, this syndrome was detected as an elevated risk of breast cancer in mothers of children with sarcomas.[55,56] Breast cancer is common in woman with Li-Fraumeni syndrome and is frequently premenopausal (77%) and bilateral 25%.[53]

More recently, a mutation has been characterized on the short arm of chromosome 2 in a gene associated with DNA repair. Predisposition to a wide range of malignancies, including breast and colon cancer, is associated with abnormalities at this locus.[57] Its relative contribution to breast cancer incidence remains to be determined.

The most exciting developments in inherited suscepti-

bility to breast cancer relate to the identification and cloning of the BRCA-1 gene,[58,59] which was initially localized to the long arm of chromosome 17 by linkage analysis.[60] Germline abnormalities in BRCA-1 may be responsible for as many as 5% of all breast cancers in the United States.[11,12] The gene is characterized by autosomal dominant inheritance with a high degree of penetrance. Breast cancer develops by 50 years of age in almost 60% of women who inherit the gene, and the lifetime risk approaches 85%. BRCA-1 can be inherited from a father as well as a mother. Because male carriers of the gene do not appear to be at increased risk for development of breast cancer, tracking of the gene through a family history requires careful questioning. BRCA-1 also confers at least a 10% lifetime risk for development of ovarian cancer. Family histories that reveal multiple young women with breast cancer associated with ovarian cancer should raise suspicion for the presence of BRCA-1.

Another breast cancer susceptibility gene, dubbed BRCA-2, has been localized by linkage analysis to a small region of chromosome 13q12-13.[61] BRCA-2 apparently confers a high risk of early-onset female breast cancer. Similar to BRCA-1, lifetime breast cancer risk approaches 90% in carriers of BRCA-2. The risk of ovarian cancer associated with BRCA-2 appears much lower than that associated with BRCA-1. Unlike BRCA-1, BRCA-2 may have an associated increased risk of male breast cancer.

Treatment of women suspected of having familial breast cancer syndromes is difficult.[11] The potential benefits of screening and counseling in these families are great. Identification of other family members at risk can facilitate aggressive screening. The only accepted method of prevention is bilateral mastectomy, but even this is not of proven value because small remnants of breast tissue that are invariably left behind may still pose a significant risk. Chemoprevention trials underway may also offer hope. Clearly, when women at risk experience their first breast cancer, bilateral mastectomy should be considered as a treatment option. Bilateral oophorectomy in BRCA-1 families should also be discussed. There are multiple potential pitfalls, however, in caring for patients and families suspected of harboring familial cancer syndromes. Mastectomy and oophorectomy are aggressive measures, and there are no long-term follow-up studies that accurately define their efficacy as prophylactic procedures.[12] Major confidentiality issues arise when undertaking genetic counseling for inherited cancer syndromes, particularly because of the interaction of family dynamics with complex medical and risk assessment issues. Information obtained during screening and counseling may affect insurability. With syndromes such as BRCA-1 and Li-Fraumeni that especially affect younger people, it is difficult to determine at what age counseling and intervention should begin. For example, should young males at risk for carrying and transmitting BRCA-1 (but perhaps at little or no personal risk) be informed before adolescence, only when considering marriage, or not at all? These and similar issues must be dealt with knowledgeably and thoughtfully. Multidisciplinary approaches that include geneticists, genetic counselors, psychosocial and family support professionals, and clinicians familiar with diagnosis and treatment of breast cancer are likely to be most effective.

Pathology

Every breast biopsy should be processed and analyzed so that, if a malignancy is found, the following features can be determined:

- Tumor size
- Hormone receptor status
- Status of excision margins
- Histologic type
- Status of pathologic prognostic features (eg, nuclear grade, angiolymphatic invasion, host lymphocytic response)

It is ultimately the surgeon's responsibility to ensure that the pathologist provides all histologic information necessary to formulate a proper treatment plan for the patient.

On receiving a breast biopsy specimen, the pathologist should first orient it and then ink the margins (Fig. 60-25). Next, the lesion should be bisected along the longest axis of the palpable tumor, and the length and width of the tumor should be measured. If the tumor is large enough, a portion should be removed and either submitted immediately for ER and PR determination or frozen for subsequent assay. If the pathologist deems the tumor too small to undergo cytosol receptor radioimmunoassay (about 1 g of tumor is required), immunohistochemical receptor determinations should be performed.

Invasive Carcinoma

Once a diagnosis of malignancy has been made, the single most important prognostic feature is the presence or absence of invasion through the basement membrane. Invasive carcinoma is potentially capable of regional and distant metastasis. Even tiny invasive cancers on occasion lead to the death of the patient. Theoretically, noninvasive

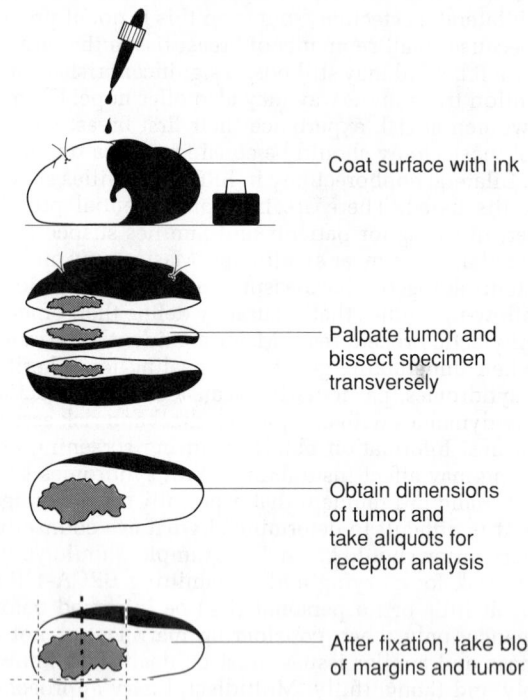

Coat surface with ink

Palpate tumor and bissect specimen transversely

Obtain dimensions of tumor and take aliquots for receptor analysis

After fixation, take blocks of margins and tumor

Figure 60-25. Every breast biopsy should be processed so that full analysis of tumor size and histologic type, margins, and hormone receptor status can be performed. The recommended pathologic procedure is illustrated here. The surgeon should place marking sutures in the operating room to orient the specimen for the pathologist. The pathologist begins by inking the specimen to facilitate subsequent microscopic identification of excision margins. The sample is then transected, and a portion is removed and processed separately for hormone receptor analysis. Only then is the remaining specimen placed into fixative. Breast biopsy specimens should not be sent to the pathologist in formalin or other fixatives.

cancers cannot metastasize and should be 100% curable by local therapy. Admittedly, this ideal is not actually reached because a tiny focus of invasion in an otherwise entirely noninvasive tumor might be missed by even the most diligent pathologist. Pure noninvasive breast cancers demand different management strategies and are discussed, along with details of their pathologic appearance, in a later section.

Invasive Ductal Carcinoma. Although the breast is composed of both lobular and ductal elements, most breast cancer arises within the ductal elements. Invasive ductal carcinoma (also called *infiltrating ductal carcinoma*) accounts for 70% to 80% of all cases of breast cancer. On gross inspection, the cut surface of an invasive ductal cancer is usually grayish white with irregular, spiculated edges. The lesion is hard and feels gritty when cut with a knife blade. Tiny calcifications may be evident within the tumor mass. Cystic changes within an invasive ductal cancer are uncommon, but areas of hemorrhage or necrosis may liquefy.

Although there is no single microscopic feature specific for infiltrating ductal carcinoma, it can be recognized histologically as an invasive adenocarcinoma involving the ductal elements (see Fig. 60-20B). The malignant ductal cells are often dispersed within a fibrous stroma, leading to the appellation *scirrhous carcinoma.* At times, the fibrous reaction is so great that malignant cells are lined up in strands a single cell wide. This pattern, however, is at least as commonly encountered with invasive lobular cancers (Fig. 60-26). When mixed histologies are encountered, the clinical behavior parallels that of the invasive ductal element, not the other subtype. Hence, these mixed tumors are considered together with pure invasive ductal carcinoma for prognostic purposes. In many cases, areas of in situ ductal carcinoma are seen; these may be within the tumor or adjacent to it. The presence of an in situ component does not adversely affect prognosis, although it may jeopardize attempts at breast conservation (see later). Invasion of nerves, blood vessels, and lymphatic channels in the breast parenchyma at the edges of a lesion may be seen; these findings generally carry a poorer prognosis. Invasive ductal carcinomas vary widely in their degree of differentiation and nuclear atypia.

Variants of Invasive Ductal Carcinoma. A number of less common types of breast cancer arise from the ductal epithelium and are hence best classified as variants of invasive ductal carcinoma. There are distinct histologic criteria for classifying these lesions; these criteria must be met throughout the entire tumor. Prognostically, histologically pure examples of these variant tumors are associated with a better long-term survival than type ordinaire invasive ductal cancer.

Medullary carcinoma is one of the more common variants, accounting for about 6% of all invasive breast cancers. These tumors can grow to a large size within the breast (5 to 10 cm) and are characteristically well circumscribed. On gross inspection, the tumors have a softer, more fleshy consistency than typical invasive ductal cancers, and they do not have the same gritty feel when sectioned. Histologically, the preeminent feature is a marked lymphocytic infiltrate without extensive fibrous reaction. The tumor cells are large, with pleomorphic nuclei, prominent nucleoli, and numerous mitoses. If not recognized as a medullary variant, the frequent mitoses and high degree of nuclear atypia can lead to the lesion being classified as a high-grade invasive ductal cancer, with a poorer prognosis. Conversely, common invasive ductal cancers sometimes have a moderate to marked lymphocytic infiltrate. These cancers do not have the more favorable prognosis of med-

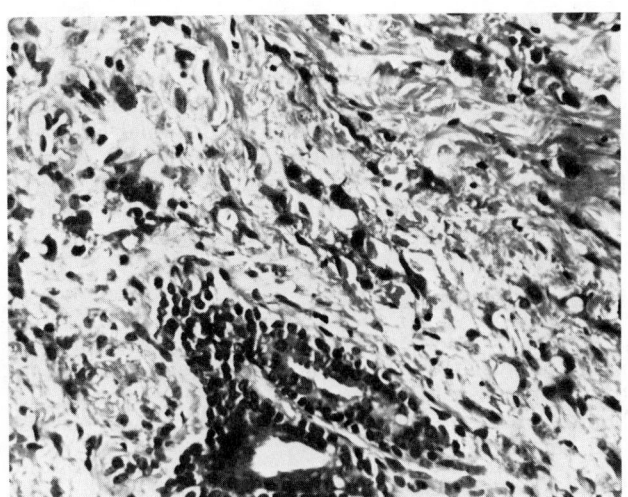

Figure 60-26. Histologic appearance of invasive lobular carcinoma. This may be contrasted with the appearance of invasive ductal carcinoma in Figure 60-20*B*. Invasive lobular carcinoma is characterized by cords of tumor containing single cells (Indian file). These cancer cells often surround normal ducts. Frequently, little atypia is seen. (Courtesy of Harold Oberman, MD, Department of Pathology, University of Michigan Medical School, Ann Arbor)

ullary carcinoma and are sometimes referred to as *atypical medullary cancers.* The more favorable prognosis of medullary carcinoma is observed even in the presence of axillary lymph node involvement. Medullary cancers are ER- and PR-negative in more than 90% of cases.

Tubular carcinoma is a well-differentiated form of ductal carcinoma that accounts for about 2% of all breast cancers. It is characteristically small; in one series, tubular cancers constituted 8% of breast cancers smaller than 1 cm. These lesions are typically found on screening mammography while still nonpalpable. On gross inspection, tubular carcinomas often appear much like ordinary invasive ductal cancers. The tumor is firm, and the cut surface is grayish white with irregular borders. Microscopically, the tumor is recognized by the presence of small tubules that resemble normal breast ductules. These tubular elements must constitute at least 75% of the invasive cancer for the tumor to be considered a pure tubular carcinoma. An intraductal (in situ) component is present in most cases, and calcifications are frequently detected within this portion of the tumor. The stroma is noteworthy for the presence of elastic tissue, sometimes in prominent amounts. Sclerosing adenosis can be mistaken for tubular carcinoma in some cases, particularly on frozen-section examination. Close inspection of the cytologic detail and of the pattern of dispersion of the glandular elements usually permits separation of these two entities.

Mucinous carcinoma, also referred to as *colloid carcinoma,* is encountered in 1% to 2% of breast cancer cases. Areas of mucinous differentiation are also seen in otherwise typical invasive ductal cancers. This tumor is often recognizable on gross inspection by virtue of its soft, gelatinous feel and moist, glistening, cut surface. It is usually well circumscribed. Microscopically, the hallmark of this variant is the presence of extracellular mucin secreted around tumor cells. This pattern should be seen in all cases of pure mucinous carcinoma. An intraductal component of similar-appearing tumor cells is a frequent feature. At times, the mucin production by the tumor is so profuse that actual malignant cells are rare, and many microscopic fields may have none at all. Interestingly, mucin accumula-

tion within tumor cells is not a feature of this cancer, although mucin can be detected in the tumor cells on electron microscopy.

Secretory carcinoma is one of the rarest breast cancer variants, but it is the most common form of breast cancer in children and adolescents. For this reason, it has also been called *juvenile carcinoma.* The term *secretory carcinoma* is preferred, however, because this tumor has been reported in patients in their eighth decade of life. The first report of secretory carcinoma detailed the cases of seven children aged 3 to 15 years, but subsequent series have put the mean age of patients with this variant at about 25 years. Little is distinctive about the clinical presentation or gross appearance of secretory carcinomas, other than their predilection for a younger age group. The tumors are usually encapsulated, rubbery, mobile, and slow-growing. When they arise in women in their teens and 20s, they can easily be mistaken for fibroadenomas. On histologic examination, the tumor exhibits a characteristic lobulated pattern composed of expanded ducts containing numerous small, secretion-filled glands (Fig. 60-27). The glandular secretion stains for mucin and with the periodic acid–Schiff reagent. Occasionally, a noninvasive component of secretory carcinoma surrounds the main tumor mass.

Invasive Lobular Carcinoma. Cancer arises from the lobular elements of the breast less frequently than from the ducts. The reasons for this are unknown. Recent series classify about 10% of breast cancers as lobular in histology. The clinical features, epidemiology, and risk factors associated with lobular carcinoma are similar in many respects to those for ductal carcinoma. Several unique features of lobular carcinoma are recognized, however. Lobular cancers do not form microcalcifications, so this radiologic hallmark of breast cancer is usually absent. They also tend to be extensively infiltrative, often without a distinct tumor mass. Hence, mammographic detection of lobular cancer may be difficult.

Almost every series has stressed a higher incidence of bilateral cancer in patients with invasive lobular cancer. The contralateral breast may be involved either synchronously (about 3% of patients) or metachronously (20% to

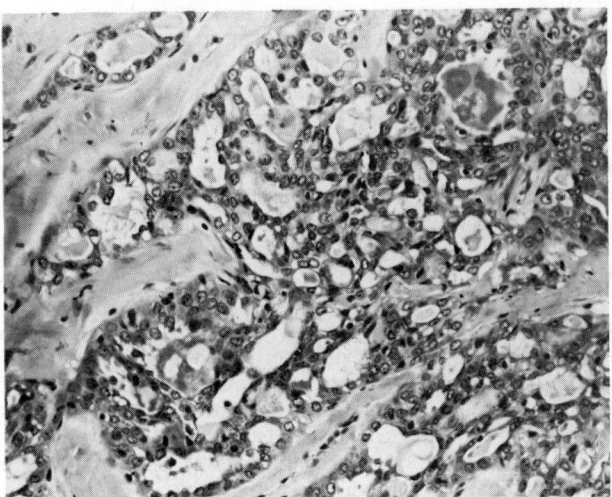

Figure 60-27. Histologic appearance of secretory carcinoma. Secretory carcinoma is characterized by its well-differentiated appearance. Both intracytoplasmic vacuolization and intraluminal secretions can be seen. (Courtesy of Harold Oberman, MD, Department of Pathology, University of Michigan Medical School, Ann Arbor)

30% of patients). About half of contralateral breast tumors are of lobular histology, a much greater percentage than in the general pool of invasive breast cancers.

Invasive lobular cancers are more common in women who were previously diagnosed as having LCIS. Women who undergo breast biopsy showing LCIS and who have no further treatment have about a 30% lifetime risk of development of invasive cancer. Fifty to 60% of these subsequent cancers are lobular; the remainder are ductal. On gross inspection, lobular cancers usually have indistinct margins. Indeed, there may be no visible abnormality in some lobular cancers, and an area of induration may be the only clue to the presence of the cancer. If a tumor mass is found, it is often tan and rubbery. Microscopically, the presence of sheets of tumor cells growing in a concentric fashion around normal, uninvolved ducts is diagnostic of invasive lobular cancer (see Fig. 60-26). This classic pattern, however, is not present in all cases or may occur in a portion of a tumor that is otherwise typical in appearance for an invasive ductal cancer. Mixed lobular and ductal cancers are generally categorized as ductal lesions. Other histologic characteristics of lobular carcinoma include the presence of small, uniform tumor cells, often dispersed in a line through a dense fibrous stroma. Most small cell breast cancers are in fact lobular carcinomas; increased recognition of this fact is probably the main reason for the greater proportion of cases diagnosed as lobular in more recent series. Occasionally, larger, signet-ring cells are seen. This pattern is associated with a poorer prognosis.

Other Histologic Types of Breast Cancer

A number of other variant histologies of breast cancer constitute fewer than 2% of all breast cancers.

Metaplastic carcinomas are breast adenocarcinomas that take on the appearance of a nonglandular tumor. The two common types of metaplasia are squamous and pseudosarcomatous; both may occur in the same lesion. Medullary carcinomas seem particularly prone to exhibit squamous metaplasia. When pseudosarcomatous metaplasia is present, elements resembling cartilage, bone, or undifferentiated spindle cells can be seen. Although these tumors have also been referred to as *carcinosarcomas,* this terminology should be restricted to tumors that are actually composed of separately derived epithelial and mesenchymal elements. Metaplastic carcinomas generally have a prognosis similar to the identical nonmetaplastic type; however, extensive metaplasia, particularly pseudosarcomatous metaplasia, confers a poorer prognosis.

Pure *squamous carcinomas* do occur in the breast, but these lesions are extremely uncommon and must always be differentiated from adenocarcinomas with extensive squamous metaplasia. Histologic, immunocytochemical, and ultrastructural examination of squamous cancers document the presence of substantial amounts of keratin. This tumor type appears to have a slightly worse prognosis than invasive ductal cancer.

Cancers arising from the sweat gland elements of the breast are termed *apocrine carcinomas.* Apocrine cancers are often seen in a setting of apocrine metaplasia elsewhere in the breast, although apocrine metaplasia is not widely regarded as a precancerous lesion. Like so many other variants, pure apocrine cancers must be distinguished from invasive ductal cancers with some apocrine features. Little is known about the outcome of patients with pure apocrine cancers.

Adenoid cystic carcinomas of the breast are identical in appearance to those arising in salivary glands. These tumors have a favorable prognosis; long-term survival has been reported even in cases left untreated for many years. When recurrence or metastases do occur, it is usually after a prolonged disease-free interval. This lesion has also been reported in the male breast. The tumors are almost always well circumscribed, and larger lesions frequently undergo cystic degeneration. Microscopically, the tumors are characterized by a mixed appearance of glandular (adenoid) and stromal (cystic or cylindromatous) elements. The proportion of glandular and stromal elements may vary greatly within the tumor, making it difficult to establish the diagnosis on small samples such as FNAB specimens.

Breast Cancer Biology

The past two decades have seen dramatic breakthroughs in our understanding of the biology of breast cancer. Continuing progress in the realms of cellular and molecular biology promise further improvements in tumor therapy and cancer prevention.

Cellular and Molecular Biology

Although the precise steps in breast carcinogenesis are not fully understood, a large body of clinical, histologic, cellular, and molecular evidence has developed to clarify the process. Clinicopathologic data strongly implicate a multistep continuum of change from normal breast epithelium to carcinoma in situ to invasive breast cancer. Wellings,[62] by classifying proliferative breast lesions on the basis of their site of origin and degree of hyperplasia, highlighted a morphologic spectrum extending from mild lobular changes with normal-appearing epithelial cells, through the development of hyperplasia and atypia, to carcinoma in situ, and finally to invasive cancer. Precursor lesions (ductal or lobular hyperplasia, ductal or lobular hyperplasia with atypia) that are seen before the development of carcinoma in situ share many of the cytologic features of carcinoma in situ.[63] Both precursor lesions and carcinoma in situ are associated with an increased risk for development of invasive carcinoma. In a seminal study, Dupont and Page[64] reported clinical outcomes in 3303 women who underwent breast biopsy with a median follow-up of 17 years. The relative risk of subsequent development of invasive breast cancer increased with position of the biopsy in the histologic continuum, ranging from 1.0 (nonproliferative, benign histology) to 1.9 (simple hyperplasia) to 5.3 (hyperplasia with atypia; see Fig. 60-24). The concept of precursor lesions progressing to frank carcinoma is further supported by the fact that LCIS, a precursor lesion late in the continuum, but still short of invasive cancer, on average occurs at a younger age than invasive breast cancer, about 45 years versus 55 years of age.[65] These data show the following:

1. There is a morphologic continuum that can be traced from normal breast epithelium through atypical hyperplasia to carcinoma in situ and finally invasive cancer.
2. The presence of a precursor lesion confers a significantly increased risk of subsequent development of invasive cancer.
3. Precursor lesions, on average, predate the appearance of invasive cancer.

Notwithstanding this evidence, one cannot assume that precursor lesions always directly progress and develop into cancer. It may only be concluded that proliferative lesions are associated with the development of cancer. This association may in fact represent the progression of precursor lesions to carcinoma, or it may be a consequence of a field effect, whereby the entire breast is under the influence of hormonal, genetic, and environmental factors that promote the independent development of both precursor lesions and frank carcinoma. It seems more likely, however, that these histopathologic findings are a consequence of progressive alterations in breast epithelial biology. With this uncertainty in mind, invasive cancer-associated lesions (atypical hyperplasia and carcinoma in situ) are best referred to as *precursor lesions,* recognizing the strength of the association without postulating a cause-and-effect relation.

Estrogens play a crucial role in breast carcinogenesis. These hormones are also a major mediator of primary and metastatic breast cancer growth in humans.[5] The ER mediates estrogen-induced effects in breast tissue.[66] ER expression is low in normal breast epithelium and is overexpressed relative to normal in many breast cancers; this may represent a remnant of a normal mechanism of mammary proliferation in neoplastic growth.[8] Hormone-receptor complexes are able to activate genes involved in mammary proliferation. Estrogen induces global transcription in the human-derived hormone-responsive MCF-7 cell line and induces expression of a variety of proteins with collagenolytic and protease activity thought relevant to invasive activity.[8] Clinically, the importance of various estrogen-related factors, such as age at menarche and menopause, parity, effects of oophorectomy, and exogenous hormone use, in relation to breast cancer risk highlights the central role of sex hormones in breast carcinogenesis. These relations are supported by observations made in animal models of breast carcinogenesis. Best characterized is the rat model of DMBA-induced breast.[67] In this model, presence of immature terminal end buds, estrogen, and the DMBA carcinogen are all necessary to induce cancers.

Considerable interest has focused on the role of transforming growth factors (TGF-α and TGF-β). TGF-α expression is induced by estradiol in MCF-7 cells and independently stimulates growth of MCF-7 cells. Seventy percent of human breast cancer cell lines with varying ER status contained TGF-α mRNA in one study.[68] Normal breast epithelial cells rapidly proliferating in culture also produce TGF-α.[69] TGF-β has been implicated as a growth-inhibitory polypeptide in human breast cancer cell lines. Its expression may be induced by antiestrogens.[70] Growth factor expression and dependence differ between normal and transformed breast epithelial cells. Growth factor production and sensitivity clearly change during breast carcinogenesis.

Genetic alterations are observed in many primary breast cancers. The c-*myc* protooncogene is amplified in many primary breast tumors.[71-74] Overexpression of the HER-2/*neu* protooncogene is observed in up to 40% of primary breast cancers.[75] Although some studies have implicated overexpression as a marker of unfavorable prognosis in node-positive breast cancer, others have not. HER-2/*neu* overexpression may be an early step in the development of a distinct histologic type of carcinoma in the breast.[75,76] It may also be an early marker of the development invasive potential in breast cancer precursor lesions. Protooncogenes c-H-*ras*, c-K-*ras*, and c-N-*ras* may also be overexpressed in breast cancers. In benign breast biopsy tissue, oncogene expression increases with the degree of proliferation and atypia.[77] In total, these findings imply that alterations in oncogene amplification and expression correlate with histologic markers of breast carcinogenesis and biologic behavior. This evidence supports the concept of a continuum of changes leading from normal to transformed mammary epithelium.

Tumor cell heterogeneity within a given breast cancer is often prominent. This is evidenced by cell-to-cell differences in histologic and biochemical markers of differentiation (tumor-associated antigens, hormone receptor expression, and hormone dependency) and cytogenetic, DNA ploidy, gene expression, and proliferation characteristics. This heterogeneity may have a profound influence on the clinical behavior of breast cancers and their responses to therapy.[78] Under investigation are the relations between the characteristics of individual cells and their invasive and metastatic potential and sensitivity to chemotherapy and radiotherapy. In this regard, the observation that the multidrug-resistance gene may also influence the invasive potential of cancer cells is particularly intriguing.[79]

Biology of Breast Cancer Dissemination

In 1907, Halsted stated, "Breast cancer in the broad sense is a local affliction, and there comes to the surgeon an encouragement to greater endeavor with the cognition that . . . the metastatic involvements are almost invariably by process of lymphatic permeation and not embolic by way of the blood."[80] This statement embodied Halsted's paradigm of the biology of breast cancer dissemination. He believed that breast cancer spread in an orderly, predictable, centrifugal fashion. Starting first as a local tumor, Halsted postulated the cancer sequentially permeated draining lymphatics, spread to contiguous regional lymph nodes, and only then spread by further lymphatic permeation to distant sites. As proof of this theory, he could point to the success of the radical mastectomy in reliably establishing local control and sometimes curing breast cancer (see Table 60-1). Because the radical mastectomy included wide excision of the lymphatic drainage routes of the breast (within which Halsted mistakenly included the pectoralis muscles), Halsted believed it got beyond the front of lymphatic permeation and achieved complete tumor extirpation. Because of its success, the Halsted radical mastectomy was broadly accepted; so too was the associated medical paradigm. This pathobiologic concept taken to its logical conclusion led to description of the extended radical mastectomy, which added en bloc resection of internal mammary lymph nodes to the Halsted mastectomy.[81]

Haagensen and Stout, strong proponents of radical mastectomy, were the first to question its application to all cases of breast cancer.[82] Subsequently, studies carried out by the National Surgical Adjuvant Breast Project (NSABP) and others led to rejection of the Halsted paradigm of breast cancer dissemination. In 1971, NSABP protocol B-04 was initiated. One aspect of the B-04 study compared radical mastectomy, total mastectomy (without lymph node dissection), and total mastectomy with radiotherapy to the chest wall and regional lymph nodes in patients with clinically negative axillary nodes. At 10-year follow-up, there were no differences in survival rate between the treatment groups.[83] Treatment of clinically normal axillary lymph nodes by resection (radical mastectomy) or with radiotherapy did not offer any survival advantage over local therapy without treatment of regional nodes (total mastectomy). These findings were not consistent with the Halsted hypothesis. They were compatible, however, with an alternative view (Fig. 60-28). It is now recognized that breast cancer dissemination is not orderly and predictable; it is capricious. Hematogenous spread is the primary mode of metastasis. Blood-borne spread may occur in the absence of nodal involvement. Furthermore, although breast cancer metastasis becomes more likely as a tumor enlarges and develops more cellular heterogeneity, hematogenous metastasis can occur at any time. Treatment of draining lymph nodes does not improve breast cancer survival because most patients with nodal metastases already have distant disease. The distant disease is not affected by locoregional therapy. Regional lymph node metastases are a marker of tumor dissemination and not necessarily an intermediate step in the process of distant metastasis.

Subsequent clinical trials have confirmed the validity of this new paradigm of breast cancer spread. There has been a concomitant change in the clinical approach to breast cancer

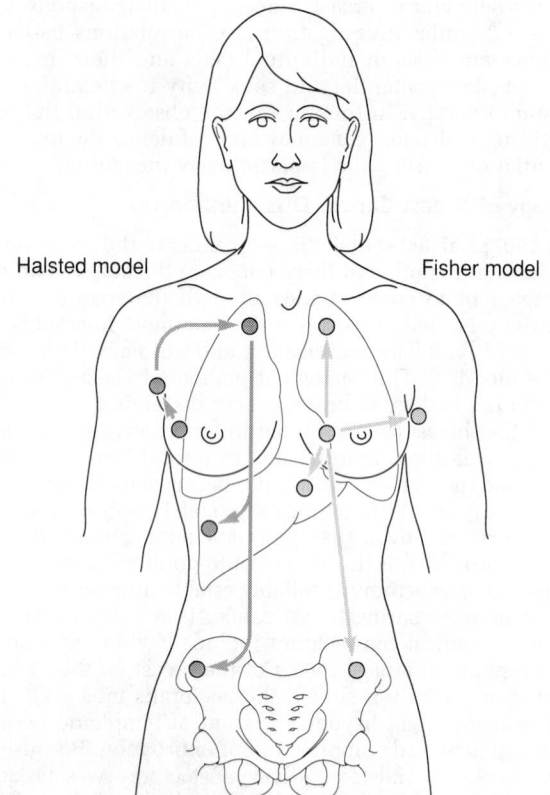

Halsted model   Fisher model

Figure 60-28. Halsted conceptualized an orderly spread of breast cancer from the primary tumor to the regional lymph nodes, and *then* distantly. Current thinking, as articulated by Fisher, recognizes that distant metastases may occur hematogenously, independent of nodal involvement.

treatment. First, it is now recognized that the efficacy of locoregional treatments should be measured solely by their success at controlling locoregional disease. More radical therapies directed at the chest wall and draining lymph nodes do not improve overall survival. Second, axillary dissection for clinically node-negative patients has been relegated to the status of a staging procedure. Presently, axillary node status is a reliable prognostic factor to help determine the need for adjuvant chemotherapy. Therefore, axillary lymph node dissection (ALND) is indicated as a staging procedure in most patients. If newer prognostic factors that are assessable noninvasively become available and can replace nodal status as a predictor of relapse, staging axillary dissection may become an anachronism. Third, because a breast cancer can disseminate at any time during its development, earliest detection and prevention rather than more aggressive surgery are the best strategies for reducing breast cancer morbidity and mortality. Fourth, the new paradigm justifies the aggressive use of adjuvant systemic treatment in patients at high risk for systemic disease, such as those with positive nodes or other pathologic indicators of poorer prognosis. It is the presence or absence of micrometastatic systemic disease, not local tumor, that determines ultimate survival. These four precepts form the basis of current clinical standards: use of breast-conserving therapy, use of axillary dissection as a staging technique, emphasis on breast cancer screening, and expanding application of adjuvant chemotherapy and hormonal therapy.

Staging

Breast cancer staging permits meaningful prognostic and therapeutic distinctions to be made. TNM staging permits grouping of breast tumors into clearly identifiable prognos-

tic categories. These groupings delineate treatment approaches; they identify those patients likely to benefit from adjuvant chemotherapy and radiotherapy and those patients in whom surgery plays only a secondary role.

Knowledge of breast cancer staging must also include familiarity with a well-defined process by which the relevant information is obtained to permit classification of patients, formulation of treatment plans, and accurate determination of prognosis. Precise staging is imperative if patients with breast cancer are to be treated appropriately. The importance of a thorough and complete physical examination with accurate recording of the findings cannot be overstated. Additionally, treating physicians must collaborate with pathologists to develop a standardized format for reporting pathology results that includes information on all relevant aspects of tumor size, tumor histology, extent of nodal involvement, resection margins, receptor status, tumor grade, and other prognostic factors. Finally, accurate staging requires appropriate radiologic evaluation, individualized for each patient according to signs, symptoms, and likelihood of the presence of metastatic disease.

American Joint Committee on Cancer Breast Cancer Staging Schema

TNM staging simplifies accurate description and classification of breast cancers. The American Joint Committee on Cancer (AJCC) staging schema, based on TNM criteria, separates patients with breast cancer into different prognosis and treatment categories. These groupings help to identify those patients likely to benefit from adjuvant chemotherapy and radiotherapy and those patients in whom surgery should not play a primary role in treatment.

The AJCC schema for staging breast cancer is summarized in Table 60-8.[84] The schema is based on clinical data, including tumor size, tumor extension, and nodal status determined by clinical examination and operation. If information is obtained from pathologic examination of biopsy or operative material, this should be specified. Ipsilateral supraclavicular lymph node involvement, previously classified as regional disease, is now recognized as equivalent to distant metastasis. This staging system effectively distinguishes prognostic groups (Table 60-9). The discrimination offered by the AJCC breast cancer staging schema has led to its wide acceptance.

Clinical Staging

Clinical staging begins with notation of the size and mobility of the primary tumor and lymph nodes. Clinically enlarged axillary nodes are found to contain tumor in only 75% of cases when examined histologically; similarly, the clinically normal axilla contains microscopic lymph node metastases 20% to 40% of the time.[85]

Because of their prognostic and therapeutic significance, a number of distinctive clinical patterns must be recognized if staging is to be accurate. The term *locally advanced breast cancer* (LABC) defines a group of patients who have an especially poor prognosis. Even in the absence of detectable metastatic disease, almost all of these patients have micrometastases present at the time of initial presentation. These patients have stage IIIb tumors in the AJCC schema; some patients with stage IIIa disease also share this particularly poor prognosis. The clinical features of breast cancer that identify this subset of patients (Table 60-10) are called *grave signs* and include edema of the skin of the breast, skin ulceration (not just dimpling), fixation of the tumor to the chest wall (not just to the pectoralis muscles), axillary nodes larger than 2.5 cm in diameter, and fixed axillary nodes.[86] An even poorer prognosis is associated with the presence of extensive breast edema

Table 60-8. TNM CLASSIFICATION FOR STAGING OF CANCER OF THE BREAST

TNM DEFINITIONS

Primary Tumor

TX	Primary tumor cannot be assessed
T0	No evidence of primary tumor
Tis	Carcinoma in situ
T1	Tumor 2 cm or less in greatest dimension
T2	Tumor more than 2 cm but not more than 5 cm in greatest dimension
T3	Tumor more than 5 cm in greatest dimension
T4	Tumor of any size with direct extension into chest wall (not including pectoral muscles) or skin edema or skin ulceration or satellite skin nodules confined to the same breast or inflammatory carcinoma

Regional Lymph Node Involvement

NX	Regional lymph nodes cannot be assessed
N0	No regional lymph node involvement
N1	Metastasis to movable ipsilateral axillary lymph node(s)
N2	Metastasis to ipsilateral axillary lymph node(s) fixed to one another or to other structures
N3	Metastasis to ipsilateral internal mammary lymph nodes

Distant Metastasis

MX	Presence of distant metastasis cannot be assessed
M0	No distant metastasis
M1	Distant metastasis present (including ipsilateral supraclavicular lymph nodes)

STAGE GROUPING

Stage 0	Tis, N0, M0
Stage I	T1, N0, M0
Stage IIA	T0–1, N1, M0
	T2, N0, M0
Stage IIB	T2, N1, M0
	T3, N0, M0
Stage IIIA	T0–2, N2, M0
	T3, N1–2, M0
Stage IIIB	T4, N1–2, M0
	Any T, N3, M0
Stage IV	Any T, any N, M1

Beahrs OH, Henson DE, Huller RVP, Kennedy RJ. Manual for staging of cancer, ed 4. Philadelphia, JB Lippincott, 1992:149)

involving more than one third of the skin, satellite tumor nodules in the ipsilateral breast, or the presence of arm edema.

The category of LABC includes patients with *inflammatory breast cancer*. The stigmata of this clinical syndrome include breast warmth, tenderness, erythema, and edema. The edema often results in an orange-peel appearance of the overlying skin (*peau d'orange*; Fig. 60-29). An underlying mass or palpable axillary lymph nodes may or may not

Table 60-9. APPROXIMATE 5-YEAR BREAST CANCER SURVIVAL RATE BY AJCC STAGE

Stage	5-Year Survival Rate (%)
I	90
II	75
III	50
IV	15

(Beahrs OH, Henson DE, Mutter RVP, Kennedy RJ. Manual for staging of cancer, ed 4. Philadelphia, JB Lippincott, 1992:149)

Table 60-10. RESULTS OF RADICAL MASTECTOMY IN THE PRESENCE OF SIGNS OF LOCALLY ADVANCED BREAST CANCER

Clinical Feature	Local Recurrence (%)	5-Year Disease-Free Survival Rate (%)
GRAVE SIGNS		
Edema of less than one third of skin of breast	32	23
Skin ulceration	14	36
Solid fixation to chest wall beyond pectoralis muscles	40	5
Axillary lymph node larger than 2.5 cm	13	38
Fixed axillary nodes	13	13
OTHER SIGNS		
Edema of more than one third of skin of breast	61	0
Satellite tumor nodules in breast	57	0
Inflammatory carcinoma	60	0
Edema of arm	50	0

(Haagensen CD. Diseases of the breast, ed 3. Philadelphia, WB Saunders, 1986:851)

be present. The histologic hallmark of inflammatory breast cancer is dermal lymphatic invasion demonstrable on skin biopsy, although the clinical syndrome (with its attendant poor prognosis) may be present in the absence of this finding. The signs of inflammatory breast cancer must not be mistaken as indicators of a benign infectious or inflammatory process; prompt mammography and biopsy of the skin and any palpable or radiographic breast lesions are mandatory. The importance of recognizing any of the signs of LABC relates to the dismal outcomes associated with surgical therapy in these patients. Treatment of patients with LABC generally involves initial chemotherapy, with surgery and radiotherapy deferred for subsequent consolidation of local tumor control.

The Surgeon's Role in Pathologic Staging

Accurate pathologic staging requires forethought to ensure that appropriate tissues are acquired and sent to the pathology laboratory in a condition that permits complete

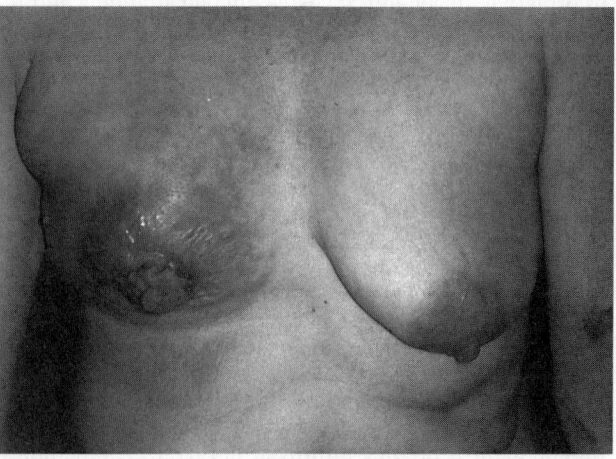

Figure 60-29. Appearance of locally advanced (inflammatory) breast cancer, showing erythema, edema, and skin involvement.

analysis. What is appropriate may vary from patient to patient. For example, knowledge of the pathologic status of the axilla may be irrelevant in a woman with known metastatic disease undergoing a mastectomy solely to achieve local control.

Pathologic staging begins with the initial biopsy. Adherence to a biopsy protocol as described previously (see Fig. 60-25) ensures that all relevant staging information is obtained. The primary surgical procedure for the treatment of a breast cancer should be planned so that all necessary staging data not previously acquired are obtained. Unless previously secured, fresh tumor needs to be obtained for hormone receptor analysis. A period of warm ischemia as short as 30 minutes may cause underestimation of ER levels.

The need to remove axillary nodes must be determined preoperatively. In most cases of invasive cancer, the prognostic and therapeutic information gained is compelling enough to recommend an axillary dissection. Axillary lymph node metastases will be found in about one third of clinically negative axillae, but only if a proper axillary dissection is performed. Removal of only level I nodes or "sampling" of axillary lymph nodes in a haphazard fashion increases the risk of injury to major axillary neurovascular structures and may understage up to 25% of women.[85] Proper staging of axillary lymph nodes should include en bloc removal and examination of level I and level II nodes. When conducted for staging, ALND should not include removal of level III axillary nodes; in fewer than 2% of cases are metastases present in level III nodes when the level I and level II nodes are negative.[85] Removal of level III nodes, however, does increase the incidence of postoperative arm lymphedema almost five-fold. ALND is performed with therapeutic intent when there is palpable disease in the axilla. Therapeutic axillary lymph node dissection should include removal of level I, II, and III nodes as needed to clear all evident gross disease.

The breast and axillary specimens should be processed by the pathologist according to a standardized protocol. Depending on the institution, the prognostic factors to be analyzed may include tumor size, margins, number and extent of involved nodes, histology, grade, invasiveness, proliferative activity, hormone receptor status, tumor protein expression, and oncogene amplification.

Pathologic Staging and Prognostic Factors

The TNM criteria for pathologic staging are of prognostic significance. Tumor size and axillary node status are highly significant predictors of outcome (Table 60-11). Standard histologic characteristics of the tumor are also informative. In general, invasive ductal carcinoma and invasive lobular carcinoma confer a somewhat worse prognosis than their variants. Tumor grade, the presence of angiolymphatic invasion, and the degree of host response (sinus histiocytosis in the draining nodes or lymphocytic infiltration of the tumor) also have prognostic significance. Unfortunately, all are subject to observer variability.[87,88] Race is also a predictor of outcome in the United States. Black women fare worse, even if all other variables taken into account.[89] Although all of these factors have statistical prognostic significance, their roles in choosing therapies for individual patients (except tumor size and node status) are still to be determined.

Emphasis has been placed on factors that can be assessed objectively and quantitatively to predict outcome. There is no doubt that hormone receptor status correlates with disease-free and overall survival.[90] ER and PR positivity independently predict improved survival. The standard quantitative radioimmune hormone receptor assay requires about 1 g of unfixed tumor and may underestimate

Table 60-11. FACTORS PROGNOSTIC FOR OUTCOME AFTER THERAPY FOR PRIMARY OPERABLE BREAST CANCER

Factor	Effect on Prognosis
Size	↓ with increasing tumor size
Axillary lymph nodes	↓ with increasing number of involved nodes; ↓ with more extensive involvement (gross worse than microscopic)
Hormone receptors	↑ with estrogen or progesterone receptor positivity
Histology	↑ with most variants of invasive ductal or lobular histologies
Grade	↓ with higher grade (cellular or nuclear dedifferentiation)
Angiolymphatic invasion	↓ if present
Proliferative activity	↓ with increased proliferation (as measured by thymidine incorporation or flow cytometry)
Tumor ploidy	↓ with increasing aneuploidy
Tumor angiogenesis	↓ with increasing angiogenic activity
Cathepsin D	?↓ with increasing tumor elaboration of cathepsin D
Oncogene amplification	?↓ with increasing amplification of HER-2/neu oncogene
p53 Protein accumulation	↓ with increasing immunocytochemically detected p53

↑, Improved prognosis; ↓, worse prognosis; ?, suggested by some studies but not others.

receptor levels if the tissue homogenate contains nontumor cells or if the specimen has been subjected to warm ischemia. Newer immunohistochemical methods of assessing ER status use monoclonal antibodies specific for the receptor. These methods are attractive because they may be used on small tissue specimens or even cytologic samples and can be applied to paraffin-embedded, formalin-fixed specimens. Although these immunohistochemical methods correlate with radioimmunoassays, they do not permit precise quantitation. When adequate fresh tissue is available, quantitative receptor assay is preferred.

Other quantitative tumor characteristics have been suggested as prognostic indicators. These include S-phase analysis, ploidy index, tumor-stimulated angiogenesis, cathepsin D expression, oncogene amplification, and p53 protein expression.[87,88] None of these newer factors has a proven clinical role. Demonstration of the utility of a prognostic factor is a two-step process. First, a putative factor must be shown to discriminate, independently of other known factors, between groups of patients with a better and poorer prognosis. Furthermore, the difference in prognosis between the groups must be great enough clinically so as to warrant potentially different therapeutic approaches. Second, it must be demonstrated in clinical trials that an intervention in the poorer prognosis group or withholding of treatment in the better prognosis group improves clinical outcomes. In breast cancer, only some prognostic factors meet these two criteria: tumor size, axillary lymph node status, presence of metastatic disease, and ER status.

Increased tumor cell proliferative activity is associated with a higher probability of cancer recurrence and patient death. The *thymidine-labeling index* is the percentage of cells (assessed autoradiographically) that, when incubated with tritiated thymidine, incorporate this labeled nucleotide. It is a measure of the proportion of cells in the DNA synthetic phase (S phase) of the cell cycle and reflects tumor cell proliferative activity. Flow cytometry is another means of assessing proliferative activity (S-phase analysis), and also analyzes the degree of tumor aneuploidy. Patients whose tumors are aneuploid, as opposed to diploid, have a worse prognosis. Immunohistochemical demonstration of active angiogenesis in the region of a primary breast tumor correlates with increased metastatic potential and poorer prognosis.[91,92] Cathepsin D, a protease secreted in excess by breast cancer cells in comparison with normal breast epithelial cells, has been reported to be an independent prognostic factor.[93,94] Patients with high tumor levels of cathepsin D have a poor prognosis, independent of nodal status or tumor size. It has further been suggested that oncogene analysis in breast cancers may predict outcome. Amplification of the HER/*neu* oncogene is associated with a poorer prognosis in some studies[95,96] but not others.[75] Finally, accumulation of immunohistochemically detected p53 protein within breast cancer cells has been postulated as an independent marker of poorer prognosis.[97]

Diagnostic Imaging and Clinical Laboratory Adjuncts for Staging

The use of clinical laboratory and radiologic studies in women with stage I or II breast cancer should be limited and focused (Table 60-12). Bilateral mammography is required in all women to search for concurrent ipsilateral and contralateral breast disease, which may be present in up to 10% of patients. In the absence of palpable or radiographic abnormality, further evaluation of the opposite breast is generally not indicated. Some surgeons have advocated mirror-image biopsy of the contralateral breast, especially when lobular carcinoma is the presenting diagnosis; this approach has fallen out of favor because of the low yield of invasive cancers in women with negative physical examinations and negative mammograms of the opposite breast.[98]

A complete blood count, liver function tests, and a standard chest radiograph complete the routine preoperative investigations. Further studies should be ordered only as symptoms and the initial screening tests indicate. A radionuclide bone scan is an extremely low yield test in symptomless, node-negative patients and should not routinely be performed.[99] Similarly, hepatic imaging by CT, ultrasound, or radionuclide scan is not necessary unless specific symptoms or blood work raise the possibility of liver metastases. For locally advanced tumors (stage III), or postoperatively when the pathologic staging indicates a poor prognosis (eg, multiple positive nodes), the higher likelihood of metastases indicates a radionuclide bone scan and a CT scan of the chest and liver to detect occult metastases and to establish a baseline for future follow-up. In contrast, patients with noninvasive cancers (ductal carcinoma in situ [DCIS] or LCIS) are at virtually zero risk of having metastatic disease and should not be subjected to *any* scans or radiographs for the purpose of ruling out metastases.

Treatment Planning

The nomenclature that describes procedures used to manage primary breast cancer is confusing. Terms such as *excision*, *wide local excision*, *tylectomy*, *partial mastectomy*, and *segmentectomy* are rarely precisely defined. Before discussing an approach to planning treatment for breast cancer, it will be helpful to first define some terms.

Terminology

Biopsy refers to procedures intended to obtain tissue for diagnostic and prognostic purposes. Biopsy procedures include FNAB, core-needle biopsy, and incisional or excisional surgical biopsies (see previous discussion). *Breast conservation* describes treatments undertaken to gain locoregional control of breast cancers in a manner that preserves an aesthetically acceptable breast. Breast conservation generally combines surgical excision of the palpable or radiographically evident tumor with radiotherapy to the remainder of that breast. If a breast-conserving approach is taken, the tumor excision should be performed with the intent of removing all gross and microscopic tumor to achieve negative margins. The term *lumpectomy* is used to connote such a procedure (even if there is really no palpable lump). The specimen removed during a lumpectomy may include an entire quadrant of the breast or merely a few milligrams of tissue, depending on the size of the tumor and its pattern of infiltration. As defined here, lumpectomy is a cancer operation performed according to the principles of en bloc tumor resection with sufficient margins to ensure removal of all tumor and without contamination of surrounding, normal tissues. *Reexcision lumpectomy* refers to a lumpectomy undertaken after a previous procedure (biopsy or lumpectomy) during which the cancer was not completely removed.

Total mastectomy is an operation that removes all breast tissue, including the nipple–areola complex. *Subcutaneous mastectomy* is a procedure that removes the bulk of the breast tissue but preserves the nipple–areola complex. Because this operation leaves breast tissue behind, it is neither an effective prophylactic nor cancer treatment procedure. *Axillary lymph node dissection* refers to the removal of level I and level II axillary lymph nodes en bloc with the axillary fat pad. ALND as defined here is the most appropriate staging procedure for assessing the presence of lymph node metastases. *Therapeutic ALND*, performed to remove nodes known to contain tumor, may be more extensive, depending on the location of the metastases within the axilla. *Radical mastectomy* involves en bloc excision of the breast, overlying skin, the pectoralis major and minor muscles, and level I, II, and III axillary nodes, sacrificing the long thoracic and thoracodorsal nerves. The combination of a total mastectomy with an en bloc ALND is called a *modified radical mastectomy* (MRM). This procedure conserves the pectoralis major muscle and its innervation from the medial pectoral nerve. MRM has been variously modified either to spare or remove the pectoralis minor muscle; common practice is to preserve it unless additional exposure for safe axillary dissection is needed. During MRM or ALND, most surgeons identify and preserve the long thoracic and thoracodorsal nerves. The intercostobrachial nerve, which traverses the axillary fat pad, is often sacrificed because the sensory deficit that results is rarely troublesome. The muscle- and nerve-preserving features of MRM as compared with radical mastectomy are associated with less chest wall and axillary deformity, a

Table 60-12. CLINICAL AND RADIOLOGIC STUDIES USEFUL FOR STAGING BREAST CANCER

Study	Indications
Complete blood count, liver function tests	Routine
Chest radiograph	Routine
Bilateral mammogram	Routine
Bone scan	Suggestive symptoms, locally advanced primary, abnormal alkaline phosphatase
CT of liver	Suggestive symptoms, abnormal liver function tests

reduced incidence of arm edema, and essentially normal arm and shoulder function.

Procedures designed to alleviate breast and chest wall deformities resulting from breast cancer surgery are referred to as *breast reconstruction*. These procedures are designed to provide attractive and symmetric breasts that meet patient expectations without compromising oncologic objectives. Breast reconstruction may be either *immediate* (performed at the time of mastectomy) or *delayed*.

Approaches to Locoregional Control of Breast Cancer

The scientific basis of locoregional treatment strategies for stage I and stage II breast cancer was established by a series of studies conducted during the 1970s and 1980s. Two NSABP protocols were particularly influential and are illustrative. NSABP protocol B-04 involved 1765 patients with primary operable breast cancer treated at 34 institutions between 1971 and 1974.[83] Women with clinically negative axillae were randomized to receive either radical mastectomy, total mastectomy followed by radiation to the chest wall and regional lymph nodes, or total mastectomy alone with removal of axillary nodes only if they subsequently turned clinically suspicious. Women with clinically positive nodes were randomized to receive either radical mastectomy or total mastectomy followed by locoregional radiotherapy. In clinically node-negative patients, there were no significant differences at 10 years in disease-free or overall survival rate between the three groups. Similarly, no significant differences were found in the two clinically node-positive groups (Table 60-13).

These results showed that total mastectomy with delayed node dissection only for nodes that subsequently turn positive, total mastectomy with locoregional radiotherapy, and radical mastectomy are clinically equivalent. Radical mastectomy, because of its attendant disfigurement and disability, has no role in the treatment of primary operable breast cancer; lesser procedures are equally effective with less morbidity. Furthermore, the finding that delay of axillary node dissection until there is clinical evidence of disease does not influence overall survival emphasized that the role of axillary dissection in clinically

node-negative patients is solely for staging. Removal of clinically negative nodes has no therapeutic benefit if regional recurrences are detected and treated promptly. ALND is indicated only when the staging information acquired will influence subsequent therapeutic choices.

NSABP study B-06 investigated the role of lumpectomy and radiotherapy in the treatment of stage I and II breast cancer.[100] During 8 years, 1843 women with tumors less than 4 cm in largest dimension, no fixation to underlying muscle or chest wall, no skin involvement, and no distant disease were randomly assigned to receive either MRM, lumpectomy with ALND, or lumpectomy, ALND, and breast irradiation. Pathologically negative margins on the lumpectomy specimen were required; patients with positive margins underwent mastectomy but were analyzed within their group of initial randomization. Patients with and without clinical axillary node involvement were enrolled in the study.

The results of the study were definitive. MRM offered no advantage over the other treatments when analyzed by disease-free or overall survival rate in either node-negative or node-positive patients (Table 60-14). Breast irradiation after lumpectomy reduced the likelihood of in-breast tumor recurrence from 39% to 10% but did not affect overall survival when compared with lumpectomy alone. This study demonstrated the equivalence of breast-conserving therapy (lumpectomy with or without breast irradiation) to more extensive procedures in the treatment of stage I and II breast cancer. In most instances, patient preference should be the key factor in choosing between mastectomy and breast conservation. Because the addition of breast irradiation to lumpectomy improved local control but not overall survival, radiotherapy may be used in a somewhat selective fashion. For example, an elderly woman with a small tumor who lives at a great distance from a radiotherapy facility could be managed with lumpectomy alone and careful follow-up. The average patient has a sufficiently high risk of in-breast recurrence after lumpectomy alone, however, to justify the routine use of postlumpectomy radiotherapy in cases of invasive cancer.

NSABP studies B-04 and B-06 and similar studies provide the scientific basis for simplifying and humanizing breast cancer treatment without compromising medical outcomes. They provide a firm foundation for the use of breast-conserving and less-than-radical mastectomy options.

The formulation of a treatment plan for a woman with newly diagnosed primary operable (stage I or II) breast cancer may be simplified by separately considering four issues—local control, regional control, adjuvant therapy for occult metastatic disease, and function and cosmesis (Table 60-15).

Local Control. NSABP protocols B-04 and B-06 established that, in most situations, total mastectomy and lumpectomy with breast irradiation are equally effective at preventing local tumor recurrence. With either therapy, local control is achieved in about 90% of patients. The presence of larger tumors (even 5 cm or larger) or clinically positive axillary nodes does not preclude achieving local control with breast conservation. A few factors, however, predict a higher likelihood of local failure after lumpectomy and radiotherapy. Residual gross or microscopic tumor after lumpectomy is one factor; this may be unavoidable if the cancer is large, insidiously infiltrative, or multifocal. Carcinoma in situ composing more than 25% of the tumor mass or present beyond the margins of the invasive tumor (*extensive intraductal component*) is associated with a higher incidence of local recurrence, particularly if the noninvasive component extends to the excision margin.[101] Thus, total mastectomy may be a better choice

---

Table 60-13. RESULTS OF NSABP PROTOCOL B-04 COMPARING RADICAL MASTECTOMY AND TOTAL MASTECTOMY WITH OR WITHOUT REGIONAL IRRADIATION FOR PRIMARY OPERABLE BREAST CANCER

	Survival Rate (%)			
	Disease-Free		Overall	
	5 y	10 y	5 y	10 y
NODE-NEGATIVE				
Radical mastectomy	60	47	75	58
Total mastectomy	56	42	74	54
Total mastectomy and regional irradiation	65	48	75	59
NODE-POSITIVE				
Radical mastectomy	45	29	62	38
Total mastectomy and regional irradiation	40	25	58	39

(Adapted from Fisher B, Redmond C, Fisher ER, et al. Ten-year results of a randomized clinical trial comparing radical mastectomy and total mastectomy with or without radiation. N Engl J Med 1985; 312:674)

Table 60-14. RESULTS OF NSABP PROTOCOL B-06 COMPARING TOTAL MASTECTOMY AND LUMPECTOMY WITH OR WITHOUT BREAST IRRADIATION FOR PRIMARY OPERABLE BREAST CANCER

	Disease-Free Survival Rate in Breast, 8 y* (%)	Disease-Free Survival Rate, 8 y† (%)	Overall Survival Rate, 8 y (%)
NODE-NEGATIVE			
Total mastectomy	—	75	88
Lumpectomy	63	68	87
Lumpectomy and irradiation	88	77	88
NODE-POSITIVE			
Total mastectomy	—	54	60
Lumpectomy	57	55	60
Lumpectomy and irradiation	94	59	68

* Proportion of women without an in-breast recurrence after breast conservation.

† Reoccurrence of tumor in the same breast after lumpectomy does not count against disease-free survival, because patients who underwent total mastectomy were not at risk for another ipsilateral occurrence of in-breast tumor.

(Adapted from Fisher B, Redmond C, Poisson R, et al. Eight-year results of a randomized clinical trial comparing total mastectomy and lumpectomy with or without irradiation in the treatment of breast cancer. N Engl J Med 1989;320:822)

if an extensive intraductal component is present and cannot be cleared with a negative margin reexcision or if lumpectomy cannot achieve negative margins on the invasive tumor.[102]

Regional Control. Treatments to establish regional control focus on the axilla. Clinically troublesome internal mammary node recurrences are rare, and prophylactic treatment does not improve survival; treatment of supraclavicular nodes is really an issue of distant, not regional, disease control. As demonstrated by NSABP protocol B-04, prophylactic treatment of the axilla with either radiotherapy or ALND does not improve survival, but ALND is often indicated for staging. There is no doubt, however, that therapeutic ALND or irradiation is indicated in the presence of known regional lymph node metastases.

Adjuvant Therapy. The indications for postoperative adjuvant therapy are addressed subsequently. In general, clinical and pathologic staging play crucial roles in the formulation of adjuvant treatment strategies. Staging measures critical to this decision-making process, such as ALND, should be incorporated into the primary therapy.

Function and Cosmesis. The objective of breast conservation is preservation of a breast that is aesthetically and functionally acceptable to the patient. A number of factors may contraindicate lumpectomy and radiotherapy even when it is oncologically equivalent to total mastectomy. The breast that remains after lumpectomy may be unacceptably small or distorted if the tumor is large relative to the breast size. If lumpectomy for a centrally located tumor requires nipple–areola excision, the result may be aesthetically unacceptable to some women. Radiotherapy requires roughly 6 weeks of daily treatments at an accredited facility, and this may be difficult for homebound or otherwise

encumbered patients. Despite these caveats, breast conservation is an excellent option for most women with primary operable breast cancer. In all instances when mastectomy is indicated or chosen, the option of breast reconstruction should be considered. Because many breast reconstruction procedures are performed at the time of mastectomy, this alternative must be considered early in treatment planning.

Treatment-Planning Process

The initial evaluation and treatment planning for patients with breast cancer is an interdisciplinary endeavor. The decisions to be made often require the expertise of surgical, medical, and radiation oncologists, reconstructive surgeons, radiologists, and pathologists. Additionally, breast cancer places psychosocial stresses on patients and their families. Although physicians must be attuned to these issues, nurse specialists and social workers can play a critical role in counseling patients and assisting them to deal with the bewildering array of facts, options, uncertainties, and fears they must confront. For these reasons, some centers have comprehensive programs for the evaluation, treatment, and support of women with benign and malignant breast diseases.[103]

This approach may be realized through a multidisciplinary unit attended by general, oncologic, and plastic surgeons, gynecologists, medical oncologists, radiation oncologists, radiologists, a psychiatrist, an epidemiologist, clinical nurse specialists, social workers, protocol coordinators, a data manager, and tumor registry and quality assurance representatives.[104] In this setting, patients can routinely receive multidisciplinary evaluations. An associated patient care conference permits interactive treatment planning, facilitation of care plans, coordinated follow-up, and support of clinical and basic research. Data support the clinical, financial, and patient satisfaction advantages of multidisciplinary breast care centers.[104–106]

Surgery for Primary Operable Breast Cancer

Surgery for treatment of primary operable breast cancer should establish local tumor control and acquire all relevant staging information. The role of the primary operation in staging was discussed previously. Surgery remains the most important method for the establishment of local control. When mastectomy is performed, failure to remove all tumor is likely to lead to local recurrence, even if systemic adjuvants are used. Similarly, breast conservation is more likely to be successful if all known tumor is surgically

Table 60-15. TREATMENT OPTIONS FOR PRIMARY OPERABLE BREAST CANCER

Objective	Options
Local control	Lumpectomy
	Lumpectomy with breast irradiation
	Mastectomy
Regional control	Axillary lymph node dissection
	Regional irradiation
Control of occult micrometastatic disease	Chemotherapy
	Hormone therapy
Improved function and cosmesis	Breast-conserving therapy
	Reconstruction (immediate or delayed)

removed before initiation of radiotherapy. The pain, hygienic problems, and emotional anguish that persistent or recurrent breast and chest wall disease can cause emphasize the importance of local control. With proper patient selection, local control generally can be achieved with either mastectomy or breast-conserving therapy.

Breast-Conserving Procedures

A breast-conserving procedure is suitable for all women with primary operable breast cancer, unless a specific contraindication exists (Table 60-16). Relative contraindications include size or location of the tumor such that the aesthetic result would not be acceptable to the patient, presence of factors that may interfere with posttreatment surveillance of the breast, multifocal tumor, presence of diffuse microcalcifications, specific contraindications to radiotherapy (discussed later), and patient preference for mastectomy. A breast-conserving operation is almost always followed by radiotherapy to the entire breast to reduce the local tumor recurrence rate from about 40% to 10%. The indications for axillary dissection were previously discussed; ALND frequently accompanies breast-conserving therapy.

The technique of lumpectomy has been well described.[107] The incision should be made directly over the tumor (see Fig. 60-15). In the case of a reexcision lumpectomy, an ellipse of skin encompassing the previous biopsy incision is removed en bloc with the specimen. The previous biopsy site should preferably not be entered. Reexcision lumpectomy may be more difficult after an excisional biopsy if there is no remaining palpable mass to guide the dissection. During lumpectomy, electrocautery is avoided until the specimen is removed to prevent cautery artifact at the margins. Orientation sutures are placed in the speci-

men. Placement of radioopaque clips in the lumpectomy bed facilitates subsequent radiotherapy planning. After securing hemostasis, the wound is closed without deep sutures or drains so that the cavity can fill with fibrin; as the fibrin organizes, the normal breast contour and consistency are restored. When ALND is performed as part of a breast-conserving procedure, it should be done through a separate incision, using fresh instruments, so that tumor cells are not spread to the axilla.

Complications of lumpectomy, including infection, hematoma, and poor cosmetic result, occur in 5% to 10% of cases.

Mastectomy

The indications for mastectomy have changed dramatically during the past 10 years. Total mastectomy is an appropriate means of establishing local control for any stage 0, I, or II breast cancer. It is the indicated treatment when the patient prefers mastectomy over other options or when breast-conserving therapy is contraindicated (see Table 60-16). Mastectomy may also play an important role in local control of stage III and stage IV breast cancer when used in conjunction with radiation and chemohormonal therapy. Mastectomy should not be the primary treatment in these settings.

MRM is performed when total mastectomy is the appropriate method of establishing local control and when ALND is indicated for staging or therapeutic reasons. As originally described by Patey and Dyson,[108] MRM includes division of the pectoralis minor muscle at the coracoid process to expose the axillary space and permit thorough removal of the highest (level III) lymph nodes. Many surgeons modify this technique by leaving the pectoralis minor muscle intact and limiting the dissection to level I and II nodes. This approach avoids injury to the medial and lateral pectoral nerves (avoiding pectoral atrophy) and reduces the incidence of post-ALND lymphedema while still adequately staging the axillary nodes.

The technique described here is that of MRM with preservation of the pectoralis minor muscle and of the medial pectoral, long thoracic, and thoracodorsal nerves. Long-acting muscle relaxants are avoided as part of the anesthetic management so that the relevant nerves can be stimulated during the dissection to facilitate positive identification. The skin incision is elliptic, encompassing the biopsy incision and the nipple–areola complex with at least 2-cm margins, and should be oriented to achieve optimal cosmesis and to facilitate subsequent reconstruction. Skin flaps are raised to encompass the entire breast (Fig. 60-30A). There is no plane that separates the breast from the dermis and subcutaneous fat. Proper flap thickness removes as much of the breast as possible while preserving adequate blood supply to the skin. Even the creation of flaps of minimal depth to ensure skin viability often results in some breast tissue being left behind; this is unavoidable.[109,110] Care must be taken while raising the flaps not to enter tissue planes contaminated by a recent biopsy. Next, the breast is elevated off the pectoralis major muscle; in the absence of gross involvement (in which case a portion of underlying muscle should be included in the resection), the pectoralis fascia may be preserved to facilitate reconstruction. For total mastectomy without ALND, dissection is concluded just beyond the lateral border of the pectoralis minor muscle. For MRM, the axillary portion of the procedure commences. The dissection is carried along the lateral border of the pectoralis minor muscle, with care taken to identify and preserve the medial pectoral nerve. The inferior border of the axillary vein is cleared from the medial edge of the pectoralis minor muscle laterally to the thoracodorsal vein. The dissection should not extend

---

Table 60-16. MASTECTOMY VERSUS BREAST-CONSERVING THERAPY FOR PRIMARY OPERABLE BREAST CANCER

FACTORS FAVORING BREAST-CONSERVING THERAPY

Patient preference for breast conservation
Tumor size and location in breast favorable for good aesthetic result
Unifocal tumor
Small or absent intraductal component of tumor
Postlumpectomy breast anticipated easy to follow by physical examination and mammography
Patient inability to tolerate general anesthesia

FACTORS FAVORING MASTECTOMY

Patient preference for mastectomy
Tumor size and location in relation to breast not favorable for good aesthetic result with breast conservation
Multifocal tumor
Extensive intraductal component of tumor
Inability to closely observe patient postoperatively
Inability to achieve negative margins on lumpectomy
Contraindication to radiotherapy (eg, prior chest irradiation, pregnancy, severe pulmonary disease, patient inability to keep appointments)

FACTORS IRRELEVANT TO CHOICE

Size of tumor (if it can be totally excised with acceptable aesthetic result)
Breast size (if tumor can be totally excised with acceptable aesthetic result)
Node status
Tumor histology
Anticipated need for adjuvant chemotherapy
Patient age

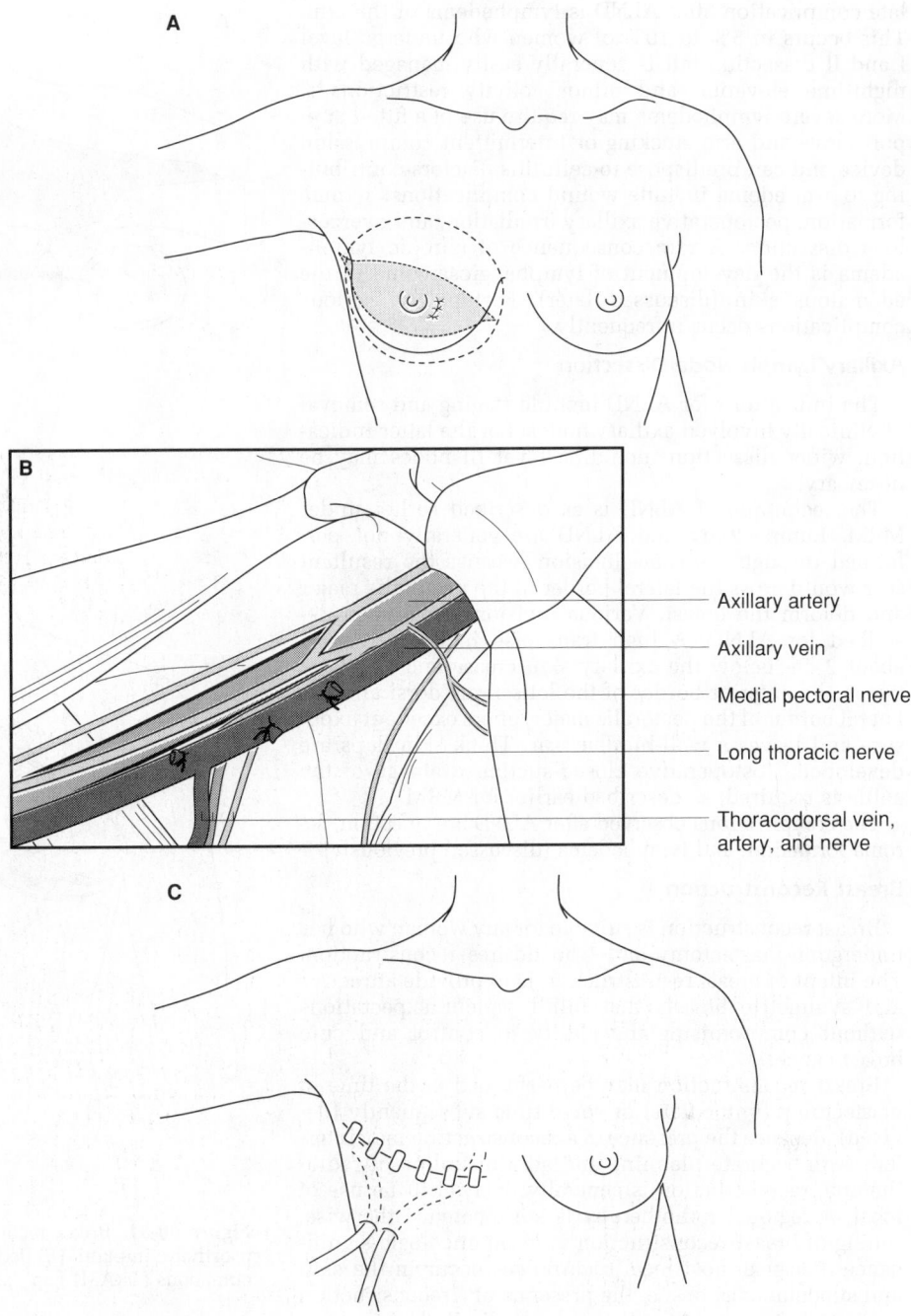

A

B

Axillary artery

Axillary vein

Medial pectoral nerve

Long thoracic nerve

Thoracodorsal vein, artery, and nerve

C

Figure 60-30. Technique of modified radical mastectomy.

cephalad to the vein to avoid injury to the axillary artery and brachial plexus and to reduce the incidence of postsurgical arm edema. Dissection along the thoracodorsal vein reveals the thoracodorsal artery and nerve (see Fig. 60-30*B*); care must be taken to protect these structures because latissimus function depends on an intact nerve. Furthermore, some reconstruction options depend on the presence of an intact neurovascular bundle. The long thoracic nerve is identified by carrying the dissection posteriorly along the chest wall; it must be carefully protected as it is dissected inferiorly until it enters the serratus anterior muscle. The intercostobrachial nerve may be divided or preserved. The specimen is then transected inferiorly and elevated off the subscapularis muscle to finish the dissection. The wound is closed over two suction drains, one on the chest wall and one in the axilla, both of which are brought through the skin lateral and inferior to the incision

(see Fig. 60-30*C*). They should remain in place until drainage is less than 30 to 40 mL/d from each (generally not more than 21 days). Dry sterile dressings are applied—these should not be pressure bandages so that vascular compromise of the flaps is avoided.

Early complications occur after MRM in up to 10% of cases. Wound infections involving the axillary portion of the operation can be particularly troublesome. Necrosis of the skin flaps with tissue loss can occur. Seromas can form under the skin flaps or in the axilla. These are best prevented by limiting formal rehabilitation exercises until after the drains are removed and leaving the drains in for up to 4 weeks, if necessary, until output has decreased below 30 to 40 mL/d. Seromas can be treated initially by simple aspiration. Reinsertion of a closed-suction drain under sterile conditions is generally required if the seroma recurs after two or three aspirations. The most common late complication after ALND is lymphedema of the arm. This occurs in 5% to 10% of women who undergo level I and II dissection but is generally easily managed with nighttime elevation and minor activity restrictions.[111] More severe lymphedema may require use of a fitted support glove and arm stocking or intermittent compression device and can predispose to cellulitis. Factors contributing to arm edema include wound complications, seroma formation, postoperative axillary irradiation, and overzealous dissection. A rare consequence of chronic lymphedema is the development of lymphangiosarcoma in the edematous skin (discussed later). Fortunately, serious complications occur infrequently.

Axillary Lymph Node Dissection

The indications for ALND include staging and removal of clinically involved axillary nodes. For the latter indication, wider dissection including level III nodes may be necessary.

The technique of ALND is as described earlier under MRM. Lumpectomy and ALND are generally not performed through the same incision because the resultant scar would cross the lateral border of the pectoralis major and deform the breast. Various incisions have been described for ALND. A high transverse incision, located about 2 cm below the axillary skin crease and lying between the anterior border of the latissimus dorsi and the lateral border of the pectoralis major, offers excellent exposure and leaves a well-hidden scar. Thick skin flaps are developed. Postoperative closed-suction drainage of the axilla is required, as described earlier for MRM.

The complications observed after ALND are infection, seroma formation, and lymphedema (discussed previously).

Breast Reconstruction

Breast reconstruction is suitable for any woman who has undergone mastectomy and who desires reconstruction. The intent of breast reconstruction is to provide attractive and symmetric breasts that fulfill patient expectations without compromising the ability to control and cure breast cancer.

Breast reconstruction may be performed at the time of mastectomy (immediate) or some time subsequently (delayed). Because the presence of a reconstruction may interfere with accurate planning and administration of radiotherapy, reconstruction is generally delayed if the use of local or regional radiotherapy is anticipated. Otherwise, timing of breast reconstruction is of no oncologic significance. Because most local recurrences occur in the skin and subcutaneous tissue, the presence of a reconstruction will not interfere with detection.[112] Similarly, a reconstruction does not complicate the administration of chemotherapy. There is rarely a medical indication to delay reconstruction. The recent trend is toward immediate reconstruction because of its convenience (one admission, one anesthetic, one recuperation) and psychosocial benefits.[113,114] Postponement is warranted when the need for radiotherapy is uncertain, the risk of complications that may delay adjuvant chemotherapy is high, or a patient is uncertain about her wishes regarding reconstruction.

Decisions pertaining to breast reconstruction should involve the reconstructive surgeon, radiation oncologist, medical oncologist, and psychosocial support staff. Patients should be informed early in the breast cancer evaluation process of possible reconstruction options.

Breast reconstruction techniques use either autogenous tissue or synthetic prostheses to recreate a breast mound[115] (Fig. 60-31). Generally, the use of autogenous tissue requires a more extensive operative procedure. Because this tissue is vascularized, long-term changes such as con-

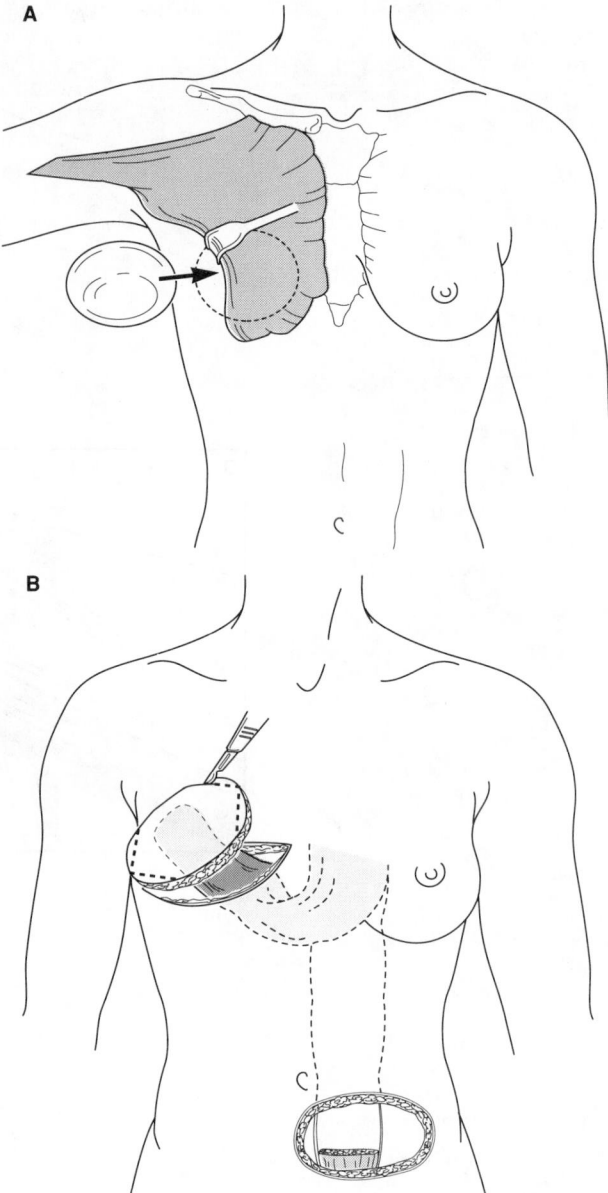

Figure 60-31. Breast reconstruction techniques. (*A*) Subpectoral prosthetic implant. (*B*) Pedicle transverse rectus abdominis myocutaneous (TRAM) flap.

tracture or fibrosis are uncommon. Autogenous tissue is ideal for use in previously irradiated fields or to manage skin and muscle defects caused by prior therapies.[116,117]

Prosthetic reconstruction is usually accomplished by the subpectoral placement of a saline- or silicon gel–filled implant. Controversy over long-term side effects associated with the use of silicon gel implants has caused most reconstructive surgeons to use only saline-filled prostheses.[118] Available data suggest that risks attributable to silicone gel prostheses (particularly autoimmune mediated disorders) are minimal.[119] Maintenance of an effective subpectoral pocket for an implant requires preservation of the pectoralis fascia and the medial pectoral nerve during mastectomy. Lack of adequate skin often limits the size of the prosthesis that may be implanted during an immediate reconstruction. To alleviate this problem, a subpectoral tissue expander can be placed at the time of mastectomy. Using an attached subcutaneous port, the expander is gradually inflated with saline for 6 to 12 weeks to stretch the overlying skin. When the subpectoral pocket is of sufficient size, it is a relatively simple procedure to remove the expander and replace it with a permanent prosthesis.

The transverse rectus abdominus myocutaneous (TRAM) flap is the autogenous reconstruction of choice.[116,117] Using the rectus abdominus muscle and abdominal wall pannus for bulk and an overlying skin island for skin replacement, the flap is either rotated on a superiorly based pedicle or transferred as a free flap with anastomosis of the thoraco-dorsal vessels to the inferior epigastric pedicle mobilized with the TRAM. TRAM flaps offer a soft mound with breastlike consistency. Because they are vascularized, they are resistant to the long-term changes, such as capsular contracture, that can complicate prosthetic reconstructions. The TRAM operation is complex and time-consuming. If the flap undergoes necrosis, a large soft-tissue defect may result; this devastating complication is fortunately rarely encountered. Because of its long-term stability and excellent aesthetic characteristics, the TRAM flap is often the procedure of choice for breast reconstruction. Complication rates are lower than those associated with prosthetic reconstruction.[6] The magnitude of the operation has not dissuaded some from favoring TRAM reconstruction even for bilateral, immediate procedures.[116] Other choices for autogenous breast reconstruction are the latissimus dorsi myocutaneous flap, the greater omentum pedicle flap covered with a skin graft, and the gluteus maximus free flap.

Whatever the method for restoring the breast mound, breast reconstruction often involves a second, delayed procedure. This operation may include reconstruction of a nipple–areola complex and modification of either the reconstructed or the contralateral breast to establish symmetry. Tissue sources for nipple–areola reconstruction include local skin, a portion of the contralateral nipple–areola complex, or pigmented skin from the upper inner thigh or the labia minora.[115]

Complications of breast reconstruction include infection, tissue loss, and poor cosmetic result. Flap loss due to vascular compromise may be particularly problematic with autogenous reconstruction. Conversely, prosthetic reconstructions are more prone to change over time. These changes may result in slippage of the implant or capsular contraction. In general, breast reconstruction, when carefully planned and executed, achieves a high degree of patient satisfaction.

Radiotherapy for Primary Operable Breast Cancer

Keynes[120] was among the first to recognize the possible complementary effects of radiotherapy and surgery on breast cancer; he began trials of breast-conserving cancer therapy in London in 1924. It is now well documented that the combination of surgical excision without mastectomy and breast irradiation to control subclinical residual tumor achieves local control, survival, and cure of breast cancer comparable to mastectomy in most circumstances. Long-term follow-up of patients treated in this fashion has established breast conservation as perhaps the preeminent mode of treatment of primary operable breast cancer. Radiotherapy may also be used after mastectomy to consolidate locoregional control.

Radiotherapy After Lumpectomy

Breast conservation usually involves the combined use of lumpectomy and radiotherapy to achieve local control of breast cancer. A number of specific contraindications to breast irradiation may preclude breast-conserving therapy.

The presence of tumor in two or more widely separated locations within the breast prevents delivery of a radiation boost to both excision sites and suggests the presence of occult multifocal disease. Prior lung, chest wall, or breast irradiation can make field-matching difficult and prevent delivery of uniformly adequate radiation doses. Pregnancy is an absolute contraindication to radiotherapy. If breast conservation is considered in this setting, either termination of pregnancy or delay of irradiation (which, if longer than 8 to 12 weeks, can be detrimental) is required; mastectomy is a safe alternative. Inability to achieve negative lumpectomy margins, especially when an extensive intraductal component is associated with the primary tumor, has been repeatedly incriminated in a higher incidence of in-breast tumor recurrence after lumpectomy and radiotherapy and thus is a relative contraindication to breast conservation.[101,102] Finally, because the two approaches are therapeutically equivalent, patient preference for mastectomy over breast conservation should be accommodated.

Any technique used for postlumpectomy irradiation of the breast must adequately cover the volume at risk, deliver a homogeneous dose throughout the target tissues, avoid overlapping or inadequate apposition of fields, and minimize the dose reaching the heart and lungs.[121] This may be accomplished using a three-field technique, with tangential medial and lateral beams for the breast and an en face anterior beam for the regional nodes (Fig. 60-32). The entire breast should be treated to a total dose of 4500 to 5000 cGy, using 180- to 200-cGy fractions daily, 5 days per week for 5 weeks. The controversy over the need for a radiation boost to the site of the primary tumor remains unresolved. If a boost is chosen, it may be administered using electrons, photons if greater penetration is required, or interstitial iridium-192 implants. The electron-beam technique, using about 1600 cGy over 8 days, is usually simplest and well tolerated. The issue of regional node irradiation has not been settled. Because most data suggest that therapy directed at regional nodes does not affect overall survival, even though it may improve regional control, regional irradiation is not routinely indicated. Treatment of high-risk nodal areas is reasonable, however, and the indications are as noted later for postmastectomy radiotherapy.

Complications resulting from breast irradiation are uncommon if both the lumpectomy and the radiotherapy portions of the technique are performed correctly. Acute complications of radiotherapy include fatigue, breast edema, and skin erythema (which may evolve to moist desquamation); these are almost always self-limiting and resolve over weeks (fatigue) to months (erythema) or years (edema). The most common long-term problems are rib fractures and minor arm edema, each of which occurs about 5% of the time. Other complications are rare. Radiation pneumonitis can be problematic in patients with preexisting pulmonary disease, and irradiation of the heart can cause pericarditis and accelerated coronary artery atherosclerosis. Brachial plexopathy secondary to radiotherapy can be difficult to distinguish from recurrent carcinoma in or around the plexus.

Radiotherapy After Mastectomy

It is well established that radiation to the chest wall and regional lymphatics after mastectomy decreases the incidence of locoregional failure.[122] Although it has been assumed that this does not translate into a survival benefit, recent data have readdressed this issue and suggest that adjuvant radiotherapy may in fact have a small, favorable impact on survival.[123] Further studies are needed.[124] For now, the established role of postmastectomy irradiation is to prevent the potentially disastrous sequelae of locoregional treatment failure in patients at substantial risk of

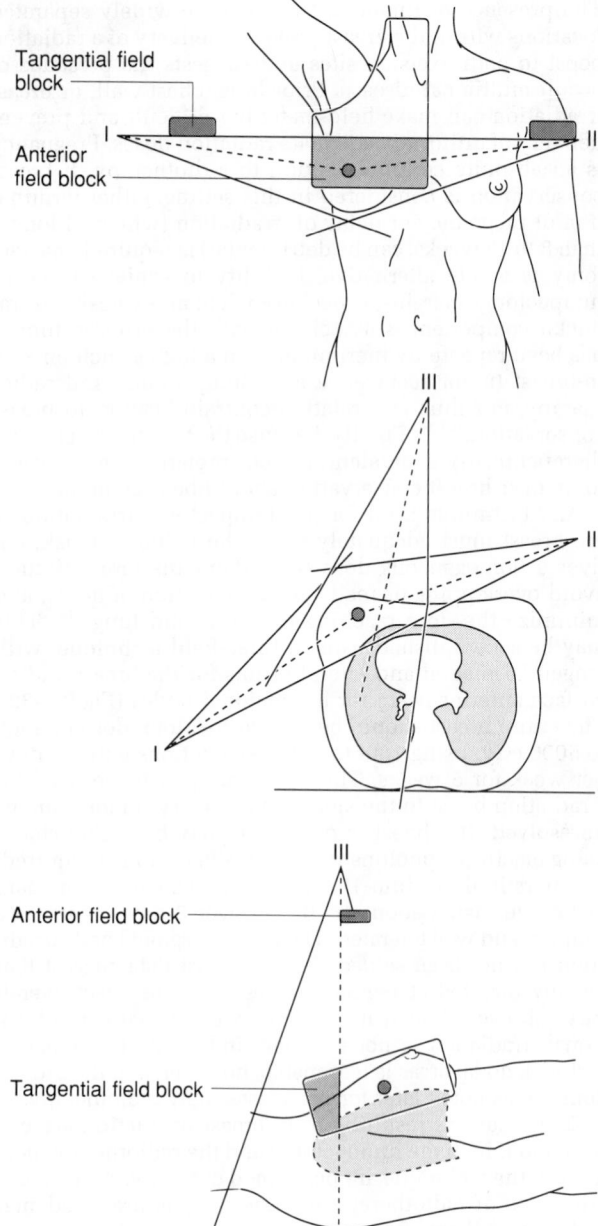

Figure 60-32. Technique of radiotherapy after lumpectomy.

developing recurrent locoregional disease. Such at-risk patients include those with multiple (four or more) involved axillary nodes, extracapsular extension of nodal tumor, or locally advanced primary tumors. Because the incidence of arm edema approaches 35% to 50% in women who undergo ALND plus axillary irradiation, this combination should be avoided whenever possible.

Adjuvant Systemic Therapy

The treatment of clinically localized breast cancer is no longer the sole province of the surgeon. Most breast cancer patients receive therapy in addition to their primary surgery. This adjuvant treatment may include radiotherapy, hormonal manipulation, and chemotherapy. Systemic therapy is administered to eradicate microscopic metastatic foci before they become clinically evident. Every patient with surgically resectable breast cancer should be evaluated for possible adjuvant systemic treatment.

Rationale

The recognition that microscopic foci of metastatic disease are present in many breast cancer patients at the time of surgery led to the development of strategies aimed at improving cure rates by adding systemic treatment before metastases become clinically evident. The probability that micrometastatic disease is present in a given patient varies greatly and depends on a number of factors. All women with invasive breast cancer are at some risk of having micrometastatic disease and hence dying of breast cancer. The precise indications for treatment of subgroups of breast cancer patients with adjuvant therapy are still evolving as understanding of adjuvant regimens and prognostic factors improves (Table 60-17).

The rationale for adjuvant treatment of occult systemic disease is strengthened by acceptance of a theory of cancer behavior known as the *Goldie-Coldman hypothesis.*[125] This theory proposes that malignant cells are likely to acquire spontaneous resistance to cytotoxic drugs as they progressively grow and divide, even without any exposure to those drugs (Fig. 60-33). Therefore, the sooner cytotoxic drugs are administered, the less likely there are to be tumor cells resistant to those drugs. Although this hypothesis has never been proved in humans, it is accepted throughout the oncologic community. The practical import of the Goldie-Coldman hypothesis is to suggest that a chemotherapy regimen that cannot cure a patient with advanced malignancy might well cure that same patient with micrometastatic disease.

Table 60-17. CURRENT RECOMMENDATIONS FOR ADJUVANT THERAPY IN STAGE I AND II BREAST CANCER

Tumor	Premenopausal Patient		Postmenopausal Patient	
	ER-Positive	ER-Negative	ER-Positive	ER-Negative
<1 cm, negative nodes	NT	NT	NT	NT
≥1 cm, negative nodes	Tam ± chemo	Chemo	Tam	Chemo
Positive nodes	Chemo	Chemo	Tam	Chemo

ER, estrogen receptor; PR, progesterone receptor; NT, no treatment indicated outside of a clinical study; Tam, treatment with tamoxifen for at least 5 years indicated; chemo, chemotherapy may be indicated for some patients in addition to or instead of tamoxifen; Chemo, chemotherapy is indicated.

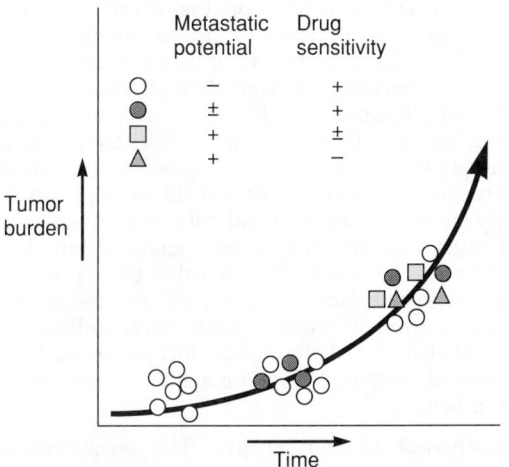

Figure 60-33. The kinetics of breast cancer growth, illustrating the development of metastatic potential and spontaneous resistance to cytotoxic drugs. Mammography can detect nonpalpable breast cancers before they have developed the ability to metastasize. Adjuvant chemotherapy, administered after surgical removal of a palpable cancer, allows treatment of a minimal tumor burden that may not yet have developed chemoresistance. Clinically evident metastatic disease, by virtue of the bulk of tumor and its inherent resistance, is rarely if ever curable by chemotherapy.

Another rationale for adjuvant administration of systemic therapy derives from the fact that the kinetics of cell kill by chemotherapeutic agents is logarithmic in nature.[126] This means that a given dose of drug kills a fixed proportion of susceptible tumor cells, not a fixed number. Hence, the same dose of chemotherapy required to decrease tumor burden from 10^8 to 10^6 cytoreduces a tumor from 10^5 to 10^3 tumor cells (a residuum that may be too small to allow regrowth). Therefore, a given total dose of chemotherapy administered to a patient with a smaller tumor burden is more likely to be curative.

These concepts form the foundation for modern adjuvant chemotherapy of breast cancer. After 30 years of investigation, many questions about indications for adjuvant therapy and optimal treatment regimens remain. Recommendations based on today's knowledge may be obsolete tomorrow.

Adjuvant Hormonal Therapy

Advanced breast cancer often responds to hormonal manipulation, which is generally well tolerated. Although hormonal therapy alters the growth rate of breast cancer cells, it may not entirely eradicate them.

One of the attractions of hormonal therapy is the availability of hormone receptor assays that serve as markers for response. In advanced breast cancer, patients whose tumors are positive for both ER and PR at a level of at least 10 fmol/mg have the highest likelihood of response to hormonal intervention (60% to 70%). Patients in whom only one of the two receptors is positive are somewhat less likely to respond. For those patients whose tumors lack both types of receptors, response rates to hormone therapy are low, but not zero. There has been increased interest in the possible use of adjuvant hormonal therapy in patients with hormone receptor–negative tumors; but strong support for this approach is not yet available.

Hormonal interventions may be either ablative or additive. Ablative measures include oophorectomy or ovarian irradiation, adrenalectomy or hypophysectomy, and antiestrogenic drugs, such as tamoxifen. Additive measures generally involve pharmacologic doses of female sex hormones, either estrogens or progestins, although corticosteroids and testosterone derivatives can be used. The choice for an individual patient is based on side-effect profiles; there is little difference in effectiveness among the options. Tamoxifen is by far the most commonly used hormonal intervention for both adjuvant and advanced disease treatment because of its ease of administration and minimal toxicity.

Adjuvant oophorectomy and ovarian irradiation were first investigated in trials initiated in the 1950s and 1960s. At that time, ER and PR determinations were unavailable. Hence, these studies generally included all premenopausal or perimenopausal women. In retrospect, it would be expected that at least half of these women were ER- and PR-negative and thus unlikely to benefit from hormonal therapy. None of these studies showed a clearcut survival advantage for women treated with ovarian ablation, although in some studies, a prolongation in disease-free survival was observed.

Despite availability of hormone receptor assays, studies of adjuvant hormonal therapy with tamoxifen have yielded similar results. Adjuvant tamoxifen leads to a prolonged disease-free interval in postmenopausal, ER-positive women with histologically positive lymph nodes and in premenopausal and postmenopausal, ER-positive women with negative lymph nodes. The National Cancer Institute (NCI) 1985 Consensus Conference on breast cancer adjuvant therapy recommended adjuvant tamoxifen as the treatment of choice for postmenopausal, ER-positive women with positive nodes[127] (see Table 60-17).

Many questions about the role of adjuvant tamoxifen remain unsettled. Available data suggest long-term tamoxifen use for 5 years is better than shorter regimens. Longer treatment does not seem to offer additional benefit.[127a] Whether adjuvant tamoxifen improves overall survival remains to be determined. Metaanalysis performed by pooling the results of many published trials suggests that there may indeed be a survival advantage associated with the use of adjuvant tamoxifen in postmenopausal women, on the order of 6%.[128]

Another contested issue involves the combination of tamoxifen with chemotherapy. Immunohistochemical studies have shown that even strongly ER-positive tumors contain some ER-negative cells. Thus, combination of tamoxifen with chemotherapy could be additive. Although initial fears that the cytostatic effect of tamoxifen might diminish the effectiveness of cytotoxic agents, which selectively kill rapidly dividing cells, have not been borne out, no conclusive survival advantage has yet been shown for combined tamoxifen and chemotherapy regimens over tamoxifen or chemotherapy alone.

Adjuvant Cytotoxic Chemotherapy

Breast cancer is considered relatively sensitive to chemotherapy. The cyclophosphamide, methotrexate, and 5-fluorouracil (CMF) regimen leads to objective responses in more than half of premenopausal women with metastatic breast cancer. Other active regimens for these patients include CMF plus vincristine and prednisone (CMFVP) and doxorubicin-containing regimens, such as Adriamycin plus cyclophosphamide (AC) and cyclophosphamide, Adriamycin, and 5-fluorouracil (CAF). These regimens also have activity in postmenopausal women, albeit to a slightly lesser degree.

Premenopausal, Node-Positive Patients. CMF and CMFVP were among the first regimens to be tested for adjuvant chemotherapy of premenopausal patients with positive lymph nodes. Numerous studies confirm that these women have both longer disease-free survival and longer overall survival when treated with adjuvant CMF or CMFVP after "curative" surgery. The 1985 NCI Consensus Conference on breast cancer adjuvant therapy listed adjuvant chemotherapy with CMF or a similar regimen as the treatment of choice for premenopausal, node-positive women regardless of receptor status[127] (see Table 16-17). The results obtained in Milan were among the first to demonstrate this survival benefit[129] (Table 60-18).

Postmenopausal, Node-Positive Patients. In the initial Milan trial, postmenopausal patients treated with CMF had an improved disease-free survival rate, but there was no significant difference in overall survival rate (see Table 16-18). Other randomized, controlled trials of adjuvant chemotherapy in postmenopausal women have demonstrated similar results. Because the use of adjuvant tamoxifen in postmenopausal, node-positive, ER-positive women achieves similar results, and because tamoxifen is generally much less toxic than chemotherapy, the 1985 NCI Consensus Conference proposed adjuvant tamoxifen as the treatment of choice for such women. The NCI Conference also concluded that these women should not receive chemotherapy on a routine basis, although they advised further clinical trials.[127] This approach was further supported when a metaanalysis of all available randomized studies showed a survival benefit for adjuvant tamoxifen therapy in postmenopausal patients.[128]

Premenopausal and Postmenopausal, Node-Negative Patients. When many of the early studies of adjuvant chemotherapy were conducted, node-negative patients were excluded from participation. The risk for distant metastases was considered too low to justify the anticipated toxicity. The success of adjuvant chemotherapy in node-positive patients, combined with the recognition that 30% or more of node-negative breast cancer patients suffer recurrence of their disease, led to new studies specifically addressing node-negative patients.

Several trials of adjuvant chemotherapy with CMF or related regimens have been conducted in node-negative patients. Most studies attempted to define high-risk subgroups of node-negative patients by including only those with large or hormone receptor–negative tumors. The early results of all these trials have been similar: the disease-free survival rate is definitely improved with adjuvant chemotherapy. These studies are generally not mature

enough to draw definitive conclusions about the overall survival rate. The findings of several of these trials impressed the NCI sufficiently to issue a clinical alert, urging clinicians to consider adjuvant chemotherapy or hormonal therapy for all patients with tumors large enough to have hormone receptor levels measured.[130] There was much debate about the advisability and possible prematurity of these recommendations. The benefit of adjuvant chemotherapy in increasing survival rate in node-negative patients must still be considered uncertain, but it is supported by available data[128] (see Table 60-17). Ideally, the role of prognostic factors (eg, tumor size, receptor status, oncogene amplification, and proliferative indices) to identify those at high risk should be further defined to allow treatment of only those node-negative women who truly stand to benefit.[131]

Neoadjuvant Chemotherapy. The term *neoadjuvant chemotherapy* refers to preoperative use of cytotoxic drugs. Several rationales exist for such an approach. The first and most compelling is in patients with large, technically unresectable tumors for which preoperative chemotherapy might cause sufficient shrinkage to allow resection. Even for resectable tumors, it might be advantageous to begin systemic chemotherapy as soon as a diagnosis of cancer is made rather than delay it until convalescence from surgery is complete.

The efficacy of preoperative chemotherapy for resectable breast cancer is under investigation in a novel trial by the NSABP (Protocol B-18). In this trial, women with breast cancer diagnosed by needle biopsy are randomized to receive four cycles of chemotherapy with doxorubicin and cyclophosphamide either before or after surgery. Tamoxifen is added to the treatment regimen for all women older than 50 years. This trial is particularly innovative because it treats all women similarly regardless of hormone receptor or nodal status. Indeed, that is the only way such a trial can be conducted because half of these patients will not have had hormone receptor assays or ALND before systemic treatment commences. The design of this trial tests many of the fundamental principles of adjuvant therapy described previously; its results are eagerly awaited and could potentially change many long-held ideas about breast cancer treatment.

Duration, Dose Intensity, and Coordination With Other Modalities. Data suggest that a relatively short duration of high-dose chemotherapy administered soon after surgery is ideal. Trials using CMF failed to show any advantage for 2 years of treatment over 1 year. Many protocols specify treatment for only 6 to 9 months. This is in marked contrast to tamoxifen, which seems most appropriately used for 5 years.[127a,128] The optimal duration, regimen, and dose of drugs is still a matter of debate.

The widespread use of breast-conserving procedures employing postoperative radiotherapy requires consideration of the problem of coordinating chemotherapy and radiation. Three options exist: radiation may be given before, during, or after chemotherapy. The former option is least attractive because it forces an additional 6- to 8-week delay before systemic therapy begins. This seems unwise given the desire to initiate systemic treatment as close to the time of diagnosis as possible. With longer-duration chemotherapy regimens, such as CMF given for 9 to 12 months, radiation is usually integrated into the chemotherapy schedule. Typically, one or two initial cycles of chemotherapy are given, with radiation delivered concurrent with the next two cycles. Some clinicians withhold methotrexate during radiation because of possible increased skin toxicity. At the conclusion of radiotherapy, chemotherapy resumes as before until completion of the prescribed dose. Prospective

Table 60-18. TEN-YEAR DISEASE-FREE AND OVERALL SURVIVAL RATES WITH AND WITHOUT ADJUVANT CHEMOTHERAPY AFTER DEFINITIVE SURGERY FOR NODE-POSITIVE PRIMARY OPERABLE BREAST CANCER

| | Survival Rate (%) | | | |
| | Disease-Free | | Overall (%) | |
Patients	Obs	CMF	Obs	CMF
Premenopausal	31	48*	45	59*
Postmenopausal	32	38	50	52
ALL	31	43*	47	55

Obs, observation alone after surgery; CMF, 1 year of adjuvant chemotherapy with cyclophosphamide, methotrexate, and 5-fluorouracil.
* P < .05 compared with observation alone.
(Bonadonna G, Rossi A, Valagussa P. Adjuvant CMF chemotherapy in operable breast cancer: ten years later. World J Surg 1985;9:707)

studies have shown that full amounts of chemotherapy can be given along with radiotherapy when proper attention is paid to technique.

Doxorubicin is associated with a marked radiation-potentiating effect and is best avoided during radiotherapy. Fortunately, most doxorubicin-containing regimens are of short duration, on the order of 4 to 6 months. Hence, radiotherapy can be safely deferred until the entire course of chemotherapy is completed. Longer periods of treatment are often used for locally advanced breast cancer, and it may not be appropriate to defer chest wall irradiation in these patients for a year or more. Typically, in these patients, chemotherapy is given first to assess response. Surgery or radiotherpay is then carried out, with chemotherapy resuming as soon as possible postoperatively and continuing during radiotherapy. Doxorubicin is withheld from chemotherapy cycles given during the radiotherapy.

Counseling and Support

The psychosocial and functional stresses experienced by women during the evaluation, treatment, and recuperation phases of breast cancer are substantial. The patient may confront issues relating to mortality, illness, disability, sexuality, body image, spousal adjustment, family relationships, and fear of recurrence. Changes in the approach to breast cancer care during the past 20 years have eased some of these psychosocial dilemmas but have complicated others. Fear of disfigurement and loss of sexual identity have been replaced in part by confusion over the bewildering array of treatment options available. Two-stage procedures (biopsy followed by later definitive operation) and outpatient evaluation have substituted the anxiety caused by delay of diagnosis and therapy for the fear and uncertainty that once accompanied one-stage procedures. The long-term consequences of breast cancer and its therapy are such that even women who are cured remain breast cancer patients for the rest of their lives.[132-134]

Fortunately, the past 20 years have witnessed a greater appreciation of these psychosocial issues. From the outset, forthrightness on the part of the physician is crucial to establish a mature and open relationship with the patient. As soon as a diagnosis of cancer is suspected, it is appropriate to involve nurses, social workers, previously treated breast cancer patients, and other counseling resources to reassure and support the patient. Early consultations with medical and radiation oncologists and reconstructive surgeons can help explain various treatment options. Postoperatively, a variety of resources are available. Aggressive physical therapy can limit the duration of disability and help to involve the patient in her own care. Reach to Recovery and similar self-help groups can have an enormous impact on practical and psychosocial aspects of breast cancer survivorship. Local groups sponsored by the American Cancer Society or area hospitals provide educational, physical, and emotional sustenance. Optimal care of the breast cancer patient requires knowledge and use of all these resources.

Follow-Up Procedures

Because the unpredictable nature of breast cancer permits metastatic disease to appear even decades after primary therapy, and because the risk of development of a contralateral breast malignancy is lifelong, follow-up of "curatively" treated patients must continue indefinitely. Of patients who are going to relapse, 50% to 75% do so within 2 years, and more than 85% relapse within 5 years. More than 70% of the recurrences are distant, but anywhere from 10% to 30% of recurrences are local. Bone and lung or pleura are the most common initial sites of distant relapse (50% and 25%, respectively). Thus, follow-up should be directed toward surveillance of the locoregional area, the skeleton, and the thoracic cavity, and it should be especially intensive for the first 2 to 5 years after treatment. The risk of development of a contralateral breast cancer has been estimated to be 0.5% to 1% per year. The risk is increased in women whose first breast cancer is diagnosed before the age of 50 years, in patients with a positive family history (first-degree relative), in patients with multicentric first tumors, and in patients whose first carcinoma was of the invasive lobular histology.

A follow-up regimen is outlined in Table 60-19. If breast-conserving therapy is undertaken, a baseline mammogram should be obtained 2 to 4 months after completion of radiotherapy. Annual mammography thereafter, commencing on the anniversary of the initial diagnosis, is indicated. For patients at high risk for recurrent disease, it is appropriate to obtain a baseline radionuclide bone scan after completion of primary therapy. The high incidence of false-positive findings and the often symptomatic nature of bone metastases suggest that bone scans not be used routinely thereafter but only to evaluate clinically suspected bony metastases. An attempt should be made to corroborate bone scan abnormalities with plain film findings.

Management of Locally Advanced Breast Cancer

Certain patients whose tumors appear localized and technically resectable are poor candidates for surgery because of their prohibitive incidence of locoregional recurrence and dismal long-term prognosis (see Table 60-10). The locoregional extent of disease is usually much greater than appreciated, and almost all these patients have subclinical micrometastatic disease at the time of presenta-

Table 60-19. **ROUTINE FOLLOW-UP STUDIES IN THE CURATIVELY TREATED BREAST CANCER PATIENT**

Study	Year 1	Year 2	Years 3–5	After Year 5
	Intervals Between Follow-Up Studies			
Physical examination	4 mo	4 mo	6 mo	12 mo
Chest radiograph	Baseline only	As needed	As needed	As needed
Mammogram	12 mo*	12 mo*	12 mo	12 mo
Bone scan	Baseline only†	As needed	As needed	As needed

* Ipsilateral mammogram obtained 6 months and 1 year after breast-conserving therapy; contralateral breast imaged yearly.
† Baseline study obtained only in high-risk patients, and then subsequently as signs or symptoms indicate.

tion. These patients have stage III disease and are referred to as having LABC. Proper treatment of these women requires recognition of the clinical signs of LABC. In these patients, primary surgical therapy alone is of little benefit.[135]

Experience with radiotherapy of these tumors to doses greater than 6000 cGy demonstrated that local control could be achieved at rates comparable to those seen with surgery alone.[136] Combination of surgery with either preoperative or postoperative radiotherapy reduced the incidence of locoregional recurrences to the 10% to 20% range, but distant failure remained a frequent, lethal occurrence, with 5-year disease-free survival rates of less than 30%.[137] One recent approach to the treatment of LABC has been the use of neoadjuvant therapy.[135] Treatment is initiated with combined chemohormonal therapy and continues until maximal clinical response is achieved. Patients are then restaged clinically, radiographically, and pathologically, including repeat breast biopsy. Patients with a complete pathologic response (no tumor in the rebiopsy specimen) receive breast irradiation to consolidate local control. If residual tumor is found, patients undergo MRM and postoperative radiotherapy. Neoadjuvant therapy offers the theoretic advantage of administering systemic treatment immediately to deal with the occult metastatic disease that is invariably present and ultimately determines outcome. It also affords the opportunity to observe tumor response to chemotherapy and may allow some patients to avoid mastectomy. Experience with a similar protocol demonstrated a response rate of over 90%, with about 30% complete pathologic responses and improved relapse-free survival.[138] Neoadjuvant therapy does not complicate subsequent surgical procedures.

These results highlight the diagnostic and adjuvant role of surgery in the treatment of patients with LABC. Aggressive systemic therapy offers the best hope of disease control in these women.

Management of Recurrent Disease

Despite potentially curative resection, at least 20% of node-negative and 60% of node-positive breast cancer patients have a recurrence of their disease at some time after surgery. Almost all women who suffer a recurrence of breast cancer ultimately die of the disease. Breast cancer recurrences can be divided into three broad categories—local, involving the breast or chest wall; regional, involving the first draining lymph nodes (axillary or internal mammary); and distant, involving secondary node groups and distant sites. The surgeon caring for breast cancer patients must be familiar with each of these possibilities and have a working knowledge of the management options available for each type of disease recurrence.

Local Recurrence After Mastectomy

Recurrence on the chest wall after mastectomy is ominous. The incidence of chest wall recurrence as the first site of treatment failure was investigated in 1392 patients treated with mastectomy.[139] Of these, 917 were found to have negative axillary nodes and had no further therapy besides mastectomy; the remainder had positive nodes and received adjuvant systemic therapy. No patients received postoperative chest wall irradiation. Overall, 6.5% of node-negative and 8.8% of node-positive women undergoing mastectomy for breast cancer had chest wall recurrence as their initial site of failure. These investigators did not break down subsequent outcome based on whether the first recurrence was in the chest wall, regional nodes (including supraclavicular nodes), or both. After locoregional recurrence in their series, distant metastatic disease developed

within 2 years in about 30% of initially node-negative and about 70% of initially node-positive patients. By 10 years after locoregional recurrence, most (about 60%) of initially node-negative and almost all (more than 90%) of initially node-positive patients had evidence of metastatic disease.

Treatment options for local recurrence are limited. For patients with solitary local recurrences not fixed to the chest wall, wide resection may be possible. Such lesions are rare, however, and most chest wall recurrences are not amenable to excision. Radical resections, including parts of the chest wall in continuity, have been reported by some researchers. Given the high likelihood of metastatic disease developing within a few years, this seems overly aggressive for most cases. Patients with local recurrence who have not had prior chest wall irradiation should receive radiotherapy. The radiation field should include the entire chest wall as well as the supraclavicular and internal mammary nodes. Spot radiation of only the site or sites of recurrence should be avoided. Such "postage stamp" fields often result in out-of-field recurrences, and the patchwork of treated areas makes subsequent definitive radiotherapy impossible. A full course of at least 4500 to 5000 cGy should be delivered to the entire chest wall, with consideration given to a boost dose to any sites of gross tumor.

Far more difficult to manage are chest wall recurrences after radiotherapy has been administered. Such lesions may involve multiple, confluent areas of chest wall skin in a so-called en cuirrasse pattern (Fig. 60-34). Additional radiotherapy is usually impossible using standard techniques without exceeding the tolerance of adjacent normal tissues, such as heart, lung, and brachial plexus. Innovative approaches to this difficult condition have included electron-beam irradiation, which penetrates only 7 to 10 mm into the dermis, sparing underlying vital structures. Sufficient additional radiation can sometimes be given to achieve local control without prohibitive skin toxicity.

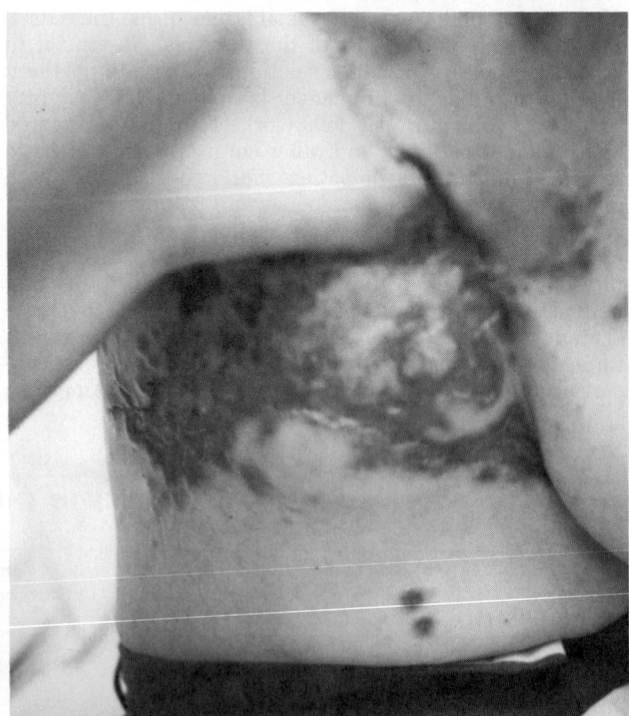

Figure 60-34. Chest wall recurrence of breast cancer after modified radical mastectomy. Multiple plaque-like areas of tumor are present and are beginning to coalesce over the chest wall (en cuirrasse pattern).

Topical hyperthermia, wherein the chest wall is heated to raise tumor temperature to 41°C or hotter, can be used in conjunction with additional radiotherapy. Although supported by experimental data, combined hyperthermia and radiation of locally recurrent breast cancer has not yet been proved superior to radiotherapy alone.[140]

Experience with systemic chemotherapy as primary treatment for chest wall recurrence has been disappointing. It may be that postsurgical scarring and obliteration of vascularity, further exacerbated by chest wall irradiation, limits penetration of blood-borne drug into the tumor. Interestingly, experimental protocols involving high-dose chemotherapy combined with autologous bone marrow replacement for patients with advanced breast cancer report a high rate of chest wall failure, even if all other disease sites have regressed.

Because postmastectomy local recurrence is often rapidly followed by metastatic disease, it is logical to postulate a role for adjuvant systemic therapy once local measures have achieved control of chest wall disease. Few data are available relevant to this approach. Certain subgroups of patients who suffer chest wall recurrence appear to have a worse prognosis, namely those whose original tumor had metastasized to the regional nodes, those who have a short interval between mastectomy and recurrence, and those with multiple rather than solitary chest wall nodules. Such patients should be seen in consultation by a medical oncologist and considered for adjuvant chemotherapy.

Local Recurrence After Breast-Conserving Surgery

In contrast to the dismal prognosis associated with postmastectomy local recurrence stands the more favorable prognosis for women with in-breast recurrence after breast-conserving therapy. As previously stated, NSABP protocol B-06 demonstrated that overall survival rates were equal in the lumpectomy alone and lumpectomy plus radiation groups despite the three-fold higher in-breast recurrence rate in nonirradiated patients.[100] Two reasons may account for the lack of impact of in-breast recurrence on survival. First, total mastectomy is an excellent salvage operation for most women suffering recurrence. Second, in-breast recurrences can usually be detected early with conscientious physical examinations and regular mammography. Recent data, however, suggest that an in-breast recurrence after breast conservation is a prognostic factor. Women with an in-breast recurrence have a higher likelihood of development of systemic disease than do women who remain disease-free in the breast. It should not be concluded, however, that the local recurrence is the cause of the poorer prognosis. In fact, those women would have had a poorer prognosis even if they presciently underwent mastectomy for original treatment of their breast cancers. The in-breast recurrence, thus, may be thought of as a post hoc prognostic indicator.[141]

In-breast recurrences and their morbidity can be minimized in several ways. Some recurrences can be prevented by strict adherence to good technique (negative margins on the lumpectomy and meticulous radiotherapy). Early detection of recurrences through careful follow-up facilitates therapy. Total mastectomy is usually the treatment of choice when this problem occurs despite good technique.

Regional Nodal Recurrence

With properly conceived and executed local or regional therapy, regional node recurrence, defined as recurrence in the first draining node groups, should be rare. Less than 3% of patients have recurrence of disease in the axilla after ALND. Despite the fact that the internal mammary nodes are rarely treated, less than 1% of patients have internal mammary node recurrence as their first site of disease failure. Supraclavicular and cervical lymph node metastases are not truly regional recurrences because neither node group primarily drains the breast. In patients with positive axillary nodes, however, the supraclavicular nodes are the next lymphatic site at risk for tumor spread. Progressive disease in Rotter (interpectoral) nodes may present as an apparent solitary chest wall recurrence, when in fact it represents a regional recurrence. In patients who have had radiotherapy to the supraclavicular or axillary areas, recurrence in these locations may be difficult to differentiate from postirradiation changes. Either may present as a brachial plexopathy, with pain, muscle-wasting, and progressive hand and arm weakness. Magnetic resonance imaging, and more recently positron emission tomographic scanning, have proved helpful in discriminating between recurrence and radiation injury.

Regional recurrences after inadequate node dissection can sometimes be salvaged by a more radical dissection. Most commonly, however, regional and supraclavicular–cervical nodal disease is treated with radiotherapy to the entire involved node basin. Nodal recurrences in previously irradiated fields are generally treated with systemic therapy, usually with poor results. Data suggest that the prognosis of patients with nodal recurrences is similar to that of patients with postmastectomy chest wall recurrences, namely a high incidence of early development of metastatic disease and few long-term survivors.

Management of Metastatic Disease

Distant metastatic disease from breast cancer is almost never amenable to surgical salvage, and the prospect for cure by any means is near zero. Nonetheless, rare patients with biopsy-proven metastatic disease can have dramatically long survival with good quality of life. For most patients with metastatic breast cancer, treatment should be considered palliative; that is, it should relieve symptoms and improve quality of life without adding excessive toxicity. Three main treatment options are widely used—systemic chemotherapy, hormonal manipulation, and localized radiotherapy (Table 60-20). The choice of therapy is

Table 60-20. OPTIONS FOR THE TREATMENT OF METASTATIC BREAST CANCER

CHEMOTHERAPY

Doxorubicin
Cyclophosphamide
Methotrexate
5-Fluorouracil
Vincristine
Vinblastine
Cisplatin
Paclitaxel

RADIOTHERAPY

Localized radiotherapy to discrete, symptomatic sites of disease or weight-bearing bone metastases
Whole-brain radiotherapy for intracranial metastases

HORMONE THERAPY

Surgical ablation
  Oophorectomy
  Adrenalectomy
  Hypophysectomy
Diethylstilbestrol (estrogen)
Tamoxifen
Megestrol acetate
Fluoxymesterone
Prednisone

based on the site, hormonal sensitivity, and aggressiveness of the metastatic disease and on the age, overall state of health, and menstrual status of the patient. Still under active investigation is very-high-dose systemic chemotherapy with bone marrow transplantation, one modality that may offer improved survival compared with standard-dose regimes.[142]

Chemotherapy

Chemotherapy for metastatic breast cancer is more likely to be employed for young women, those with ER-negative tumors, those with visceral organ involvement, and those with rapidly advancing or life-threatening disease. Properly administered, systemic chemotherapy can provide palliation with acceptable toxicity. The most active single agent for the treatment of breast cancer is doxorubicin; other commonly used drugs include cyclophosphamide, methotrexate, vincristine, paclitaxel (Taxol), and 5-fluorouracil. Less frequently used drugs with known activity include cisplatin, thiotepa, mitoxantrone, and mitomycin C. The new agents docetaxel (Taxotere) and vinorelbine (Navelbine) have been documented to have significant activity in metastatic breast cancer.

Generally, combinations of agents are used in treating metastatic breast cancer. The CMF regimen leads to complete and partial remissions in more than half of premenopausal women with metastatic breast cancer. Regimens with similar activity include CAF and other doxorubicin-containing regimens. All of these regimens are slightly less active in postmenopausal women. Response rates are highest in women who have not received prior treatment for metastatic disease. Prior adjuvant chemotherapy is not consistently associated with a poorer response to chemotherapy, particularly if a long interval has elapsed between adjuvant therapy and the development of metastases.

It is believed that a dose–response relation exists for most cytotoxic agents, and therefore higher doses of chemotherapy may be more likely to lead to tumor regression. Colony-stimulating factors may minimize or reverse the myelosuppression of cytotoxic chemotherapy and permit dose escalation with increased tumor kill. An alternative approach to bypass the dose-limiting effects of myelosuppression is autologous bone marrow transplantation. After administration of lethal doses of chemotherapy, the patient is rescued from the deadly myelosuppressive effects of the chemotherapy by reinfusion of previously harvested autologous marrow. The toxicity of marrow transplantation regimens is formidable, and treatment-related death rates of 3% to 10% or more have been reported. Response rates are high, but the duration of response is often short. Active investigation of this modality is ongoing, with the goal of determining whether this treatment actually offers the possibility of cure to a subset of patients.[142]

Hormonal Therapy

Endocrine therapy is appropriate as first-line treatment for nearly all women with ER-positive metastatic breast cancer. Because clinical response to hormonal therapy may take 6 to 8 weeks, chemotherapy is preferred for those patients with rapidly progressing disease. ER-negative tumors are only infrequently treated with hormonal therapy because the response rate is under 10%.

Tamoxifen is the agent of choice for first-line hormonal therapy of metastatic breast cancer. Both premenopausal and postmenopausal patients can receive this agent, and side effects are minimal. The usual dose is 10 mg orally twice a day, and there is little evidence to suggest that higher doses provide significant additional benefit. Its main toxicities are hot flashes, fluid retention, and mood changes; less common but more serious are thromboembolic events and cataract formation. Animal studies have suggested a carcinogenic effect of tamoxifen, with increased numbers of uterine and hepatic tumors in experimental models. An apparent increase in uterine cancer has been seen in humans, but the incidence is low and certainly should not limit the use of this drug in patients with advanced disease. Megestrol acetate (Megace), a progestational agent, is effective second-line therapy in women whose metastases remain non–life-threatening after initial response to tamoxifen. Patients who do not respond at all to tamoxifen usually do not respond to alternative hormonal interventions. The main side effects of megestrol acetate are depression and weight gain. Premenopausal women with metastatic breast cancer can also be treated by oophorectomy. This is associated with a response rate similar to tamoxifen but without the need to take a pill twice a day. Oophorectomy is generally reserved for selected women whose disease responded to tamoxifen and megestrol acetate but subsequently progressed. In the future, follicle-stimulating hormone–luteinizing hormone agonists may play a role in breast cancer treatment by selectively interfering with the stimulus to ovarian secretion, causing a reversible "medical castration," obviating the need for oophorectomy.

A third-line choice for postmenopausal or oophorectomized premenopausal women is surgical or medical adrenalectomy to eliminate this extraovarian source of sex hormones. Once commonly used, bilateral surgical adrenalectomy is now of historical import only. Aminoglutethimide is the drug most commonly used to cause reversible adrenal blockade; hydrocortisone is administered concurrently to prevent symptoms of steroid deficiency.

Radiotherapy

Radiotherapy has a limited but important role in the palliative treatment of metastatic breast cancer. Its use in treating local and regional recurrences has already been described. Radiation is effective in relieving pain from bony metastases and preventing pathologic fractures in asymptomatic weight-bearing bones involved with metastatic disease. Most commonly, asymptomatic metastases in the vertebral bodies, pelvis, or femur are treated to prevent disabling fractures. Severe pain from bone metastases too widespread to be amenable to external-beam irradiation can be effectively palliated by the oral administration of strontium-89, a radioactive bone-avid isotope. Localized radiotherapy to symptomatic sites can also be combined with endocrine manipulations or cytotoxic chemotherapy in patients with widespread disease. Central nervous system metastases to the brain, spinal cord, or meninges are best palliated by radiation to the neuraxis.

Mastectomy

A small percentage of breast cancer patients have metastatic disease at the time of initial presentation. In these patients, removing the primary breast tumor does not affect overall outcome. If left without adequate treatment, however, the breast tumor can pose a major local control problem and cause intractable cosmetic, hygienic, and pain-management problems. Total mastectomy is occasionally indicated solely to obtain local control in these patients. The term *toilet mastectomy* has been applied in this setting; obviously, this is not a term well-accepted by patients. ALND should not accompany mastectomy in these patients unless grossly enlarged axillary nodes are contributing to the patient's locoregional control problem.

Noninvasive Breast Carcinoma

Noninvasive (in situ) cancer is defined as a neoplastic entity confined entirely within its epithelium of origin and without invasion through the basement membrane. Noninvasive cancer has no access to lymphatic or vascular elements and hence cannot metastasize. Before the advent of routine screening mammography, in situ breast cancer was a rarely encountered curiosity. It either was found incidentally during biopsy of a benign lesion or presented as a palpable tumor mass, and it virtually always was treated by mastectomy. Mammography now enables detection of microscopic noninvasive cancers, and such lesions constitute an increasing percentage of breast cancer cases. Combined with the increasing use of breast-conserving procedures for invasive breast cancer, clinicians have been forced into a dramatic rethinking of the clinical approach to noninvasive breast cancer.

Like invasive breast cancer, noninvasive cancer arises either from the ductal or lobular elements. Unlike their invasive counterparts, the clinical presentation and behavior of DCIS and LCIS differ markedly (Table 60-21).

Ductal Carcinoma in Situ

Ductal carcinoma in situ has traditionally been referred to as *intraductal carcinoma*. This latter name, although technically accurate, has spawned considerable confusion and limits appreciation of the difference between invasive and noninvasive ductal cancers. For this reason, the former term is preferred. Invasive breast cancer can have a significant intraductal (ie, noninvasive) component, either within or adjacent to the main tumor mass; the term DCIS excludes tumors with any microscopic evidence of invasion beyond the basement membrane.

Clinical Presentation.   Before the widespread adoption of screening mammography, the few patients seen with symptomatic DCIS presented with a palpable mass. Today, a palpable mass of pure DCIS is decidedly unusual. The use of routine screening mammography, coupled with wire-localization biopsy of nonpalpable abnormalities, has led to a marked increase in the number of patients diagnosed with nonpalpable DCIS. Generally, clustered microcalcifications are the mammographic hallmark of DCIS, but such calcifications can also be seen with invasive breast cancer. There is no radiographic finding specific for DCIS, but as many as 60% of nonpalpable cancers detected mammographically are of this type. Purely noninvasive breast cancer can also present as erosion of the nipple. This is termed *Paget disease*, although this presentation may be associated with invasive cancer as well (see later). The age distribution of DCIS does not differ significantly from that of invasive ductal cancer. The proportion of breast cancers diagnosed as DCIS is a function of the extent to which

screening mammography is used in the population. In many series, 10% to 20% of new cancers are DCIS.[104] The epidemiology and risk factors for DCIS appear to parallel those of invasive ductal cancer. About 5% of male breast cancers are DCIS; these may present with a bloody nipple discharge.

Pathology.   If a palpable mass of DCIS is present, it may be grossly indistinguishable from an invasive ductal cancer. On sectioning the mass, necrotic areas of cancer cells may be seen extruding from the cut surface (so-called comedo necrosis). Areas of nonpalpable DCIS may be recognized if there are associated calcifications; cutting through such areas often has a characteristic gritty feel. The microscopic hallmark of DCIS is the presence of cancer cells confined within the lumina of the ducts, with no evidence of invasion through the basement membrane (Fig. 60-35). Several microscopic patterns of DCIS are recognized, any or all of which may coexist in the same tumor. The most common types are comedo, cribriform, and papillary.

Prognosis.   The prognosis for all types of DCIS is uniformly good. Lymph node metastases occur in less than 1% of cases; presumably, an area of microinvasive cancer was not sampled in the biopsy or in the pathology specimen. Although the prognostic importance of noninvasive breast cancer lies in its propensity to develop into invasive malignancy, the natural history of DCIS is still not entirely characterized. In a unique study, 25 cases of DCIS were found on re-review of some 10,000 breast biopsy specimens originally reported as benign.[143] Because the noninvasive malignancy was not initially recognized, these patients did not undergo any treatment after the biopsy. Ten patients in this group had long-term data available, with an average follow-up of more than 21 years. Seven of the 10 had invasive breast cancer after a mean of 9.7 years; 3 remained disease-free until death. The lack of follow-up on the other 15 patients precluded making an absolute estimate of the risk of invasive cancer development for the entire group.

Two facts about microscopic DCIS have become clear. First, not every woman who undergoes complete excision of a focus of DCIS develops invasive ductal cancer. Various series suggest that invasive breast cancer never develops after excisional biopsy alone in 50% or more of patients. Second, when a subsequent invasive cancer does occur, it is almost always of the invasive ductal type and located in the same quadrant of the breast as the initial DCIS. The latent period before the development of invasive cancer usually exceeds 5 years.

Management.   Appropriate management of DCIS hinges on understanding the natural history of the disease and the wishes of the patient. Radical or modified radical mastectomy is clearly inappropriate for a disease with virtually no ability to spread to the regional lymphatics. Total mastectomy is associated with a nearly 100% cure rate for this condition.

Although total mastectomy remains the gold standard for treatment of DCIS, there is increasing experience with breast-conserving therapy. Unfortunately, no clinical trials are available that directly compare breast conservation to mastectomy for DCIS. Therefore, breast conservation should be offered with the understanding that a recurrence could be in the form of invasive cancer, with the attendant worse prognosis. NSABP protocol B-17 randomly assigned 818 women to receive either lumpectomy alone or lumpectomy followed by breast irradiation for breast-conserving treatment of DCIS.[144] Localized tumor and histologically tumor-free lumpectomy margins were required for enrollment in the study. The incidence of adverse events, de-

Table 60-21. CLINICAL FEATURES OF DUCTAL CARCINOMA IN SITU VERSUS LOBULAR CARCINOMA IN SITU

	Ductal	Lobular
Age distribution	<50% Premenopausal (same as invasive ductal cancer)	75% Premenopausal
Palpable mass	Rare	Never
Radiographic findings	Microcalcifications	Usually none
Node involvement	<1%	None
Subsequent cancer risk	Invasive ductal cancer	Invasive ductal or lobular cancer
	Same breast	Either breast
	Same quadrant	Any quadrant

(Modified from Harris JR, Hellman S, Henderson IC, Kinne DW, eds. Breast diseases. Philadelphia, JB Lippincott, 1987:365)

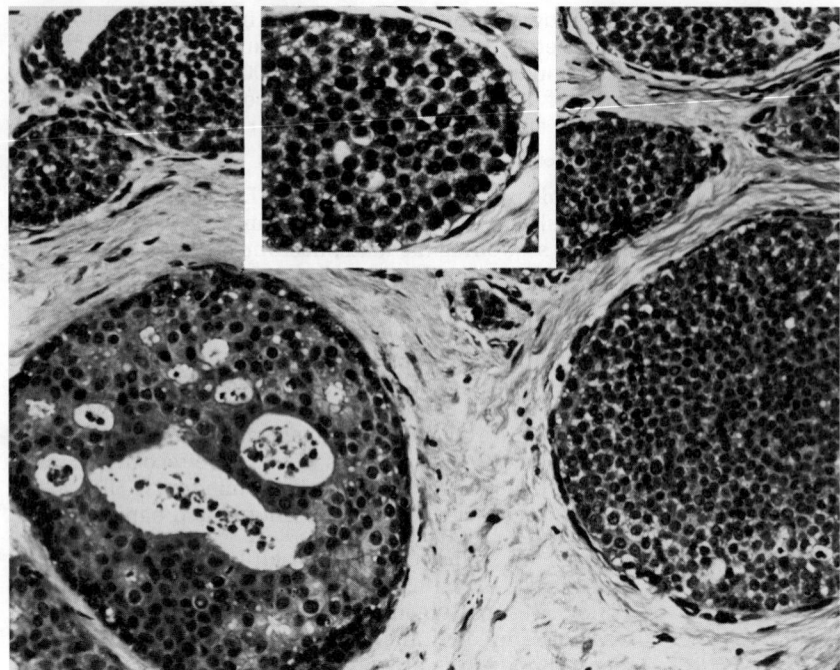

Figure 60-35. Histologic appearance of ductal carcinoma in situ (*left*) and lobular carcinoma in situ (*right*) found side by side in a single breast biopsy specimen. The lobular type is characterized by the minimal cohesion of the cells and the cellular uniformity (*inset*); it lacks the bridges of cells seen in ductal carcinoma in situ. (Courtesy of Harold Oberman, MD, Department of Pathology, University of Michigan Medical School, Ann Arbor)

fined as subsequent discovery of an ipsilateral or contralateral breast cancer (whether in situ or invasive), regional or distant metastasis, development of a second primary (nonbreast) cancer, or noncancer death, was compared between the two groups. The 5-year event-free survival rate (median follow-up, 43 months) was significantly better in women who received radiotherapy than in those who did not (Table 60-22). The improvement was attributable to a reduction in the occurrence of ipsilateral breast cancers. Furthermore, whereas 50% of the ipsilateral recurrences in the nonirradiated group were invasive cancers, only 29% of the recurrences in women receiving radiotherapy were invasive.

These data strongly suggest that when breast conservation is chosen for treatment of DCIS, the combination of lumpectomy with radiotherapy should be employed. Most striking is the apparent ability of breast irradiation to reduce the incidence of subsequent development of invasive breast cancer. Breast conservation may be offered to DCIS patients in whom the entire tumor can be surgically re-

moved with negative histologic margins and in whom the remaining breast tissue can be reliably assessed clinically and radiographically. DCIS may be multifocal and may spread along the ducts throughout any and all quadrants of the breast. Hence, inability to excise areas of DCIS with a negative histologic margin may represent a contraindication to breast conservation. The presence of extensive microcalcifications throughout the breast may be another contraindication to breast conservation. These calcifications may represent further areas of DCIS. Even if they do not, their presence could impair mammographic detection of a recurrence. NSABP study B-24, in progress, is designed to address whether breast-conserving therapy can be extended to some women with these apparent contraindications.

Two cautionary notes about breast conserving therapy for DCIS are important. First, the NSABP B-17 data, which are the best data available, are derived from patients with relatively short-term follow-up. Second, the 84% event-free survival rate observed in NSABP B-17 for patients undergoing lumpectomy and radiotherapy is worse than that achievable with simple mastectomy. Thus, breast conservation for DCIS commits patients to more careful long-term follow-up and likely subjects them to additional subsequent treatment to deal with recurrences. Although it is unlikely that the poorer event-free survival rate associated with breast conservation will translate into a poorer overall survival rate, this has never been demonstrated in a clinical trial. Close follow-up for all women undergoing breast conservation for DCIS is mandatory.

Lobular Carcinoma In Situ

Lobular carcinoma in situ accounts for about one third of noninvasive breast cancers. Studies of its natural history have led to a rethinking of the meaning of carcinoma in situ. The available evidence suggests that LCIS is not so much a committed predecessor of invasive lobular cancer as a marker of susceptibility of the breasts to malignant change. All the lobular and ductal elements of both breasts are marked "at risk" by the presence of LCIS anywhere in either breast. The pervasive nature of this risk, combined

---

Table 60-22. RESULTS OF NSABP PROTOCOL B-17 COMPARING LUMPECTOMY WITH AND WITHOUT BREAST IRRADIATION FOR DUCTAL CARCINOMA IN SITU

	Annual Incidence (%) of First Event	
Type of Event	Lumpectomy	Lumpectomy and Irradiation
Ipsilateral breast cancer		
Noninvasive	2.6	1.5
Invasive	2.6	0.6
Other	1.5	1.7
TOTAL	6.7	3.8

(Adapted from Fisher B, Constantino J, Redmond C, et al. Lumpectomy compared with lumpectomy and radiation therapy for the treatment of intraductal breast cancer. N Engl J Med 1993;328:1581)

with the lack of clinical signs and symptoms, makes the care of women with this problem a challenge.

Clinical Presentation. LCIS is almost always an incidental finding. There are usually no signs or symptoms associated with its presence. Unlike DCIS, which can occasionally be manifest as a clinically apparent mass, LCIS is virtually never palpable. The clustered calcifications typical of DCIS are usually absent in LCIS, so there are few mammographic clues to its presence. In one series of 50 LCIS patients whose lesions were found after biopsy of a mammographic abnormality, calcifications were found histologically within the LCIS in only 4 (8%). In the remaining 46 cases, a coexistent benign lesion was responsible for the radiographically detected lesion that led to biopsy, and the LCIS was discovered incidentally.[145]

LCIS patients are significantly younger than patients with invasive breast cancer. Three-fourths of affected patients are premenopausal. LCIS is an infrequent finding in women older than 75 years. When the opposite breast is sampled at the time of diagnosis, contralateral LCIS is found in 30% to 50% of cases. Because LCIS has few associated signs and symptoms, the frequency with which bilaterality is detected is related to the diligence with which it is sought. Series in which bilateral mastectomies were performed on all patients with LCIS report the highest rates of bilaterality. Because there is no known added significance to the finding of bilateral as opposed to unilateral LCIS, routine use of contralateral breast biopsies is not indicated.

Pathology. LCIS is not recognizable on gross inspection. It is often found in conjunction with other clinically more apparent lesions that led to performance of the breast biopsy. Because fibroadenomas are benign lesions of lobular origin, in the infrequent case in which malignancy occurs within a fibroadenoma, it is most commonly LCIS. It is believed that the LCIS is a coincidental finding in these cases and is not a result of malignant degeneration of the fibroadenoma. Microscopically, LCIS is characterized by a proliferation of cancer cells in the acini and terminal ductules of the breast lobules, without invasion through the basement membrane (see Fig. 60-35). The lobules may become distended by progressive proliferation of malignant cells. The tumor cells are characteristically large, poorly cohesive, and have small, round nuclei with infrequent mitoses. Considerable pleomorphism can be manifest, however, and more anaplastic variants of LCIS are sometimes seen. LCIS must be differentiated from atypical lobular hyperplasia. This distinction can at times be difficult and is usually based on the degree of atypia and the percentage of the lobule involved with the malignant change (75% is a common cutoff for a diagnosis of LCIS). Because patients with atypical lobular hyperplasia have an increased risk for invasive cancer development similar to that in LCIS patients, most authorities regard these two lesions as part of a spectrum of lobular neoplasia.

Prognosis. The prognosis of LCIS is solely related to the subsequent development of invasive carcinoma[146] (Table 60-23). Invasive cancer develops in about one third of patients with biopsy-demonstrated LCIS; half of these cancers occur in the index breast and half in the contralateral breast. The subsequent breast cancers can be either lobular or ductal in histology.

Management. In the confusion about how best to treat patients with LCIS, one fact seems clear: both breasts are at equal risk, so both breasts should be treated the same. Resection of all areas of LCIS with breast conservation is generally not possible because of the multifocality of the disease. In any event, this would not diminish the risk for

Table 60-23. DEVELOPMENT OF INVASIVE CANCER AFTER UNTREATED LOBULAR CARCINOMA IN SITU*

Status at Follow-Up†	Patients	Percentage of Total	Percentage of Patients With Follow-Up
Known invasive cancer	32	32	38
Never developed invasive cancer	52	53	62
Lost to follow-up	15	15	—
TOTAL	99	100	—

* Ninety-nine patients were retrospectively identified as having biopsy-demonstrated lobular carcinoma in situ but received no further treatment.
† Median follow-up was 25 years.
(Rosen PP, Lieberman PH, Braun DW, et al. Lobular carcinoma in situ of the breast. Am J Surg Pathol 1978; 2:225)

breast cancer development in the normal breast tissue that remained. Accordingly, the two available treatment options are observation of both breasts to detect subsequent cancer development or bilateral, total mastectomies. Ultimately, it is the well-informed patient who must make the final decision.

Bilateral, total mastectomies, usually offered with immediate reconstruction, obviate the need for long-term follow-up. This is an appropriate choice for patients who cannot or prefer not to adhere to a follow-up regimen that includes annual mammography, twice-yearly physical examinations, and monthly self-examination. Bilateral mastectomies may also be preferable for LCIS patients with family histories of breast cancer, who are at higher risk of development of invasive cancer. The magnitude of the risk that accompanies a diagnosis of LCIS is insufficient justification to many women for bilateral mastectomies. Informed, motivated patients often choose careful follow-up rather than bilateral mastectomies. Before doing so, the patient should be fully aware of the observation schedule. It is critical to emphasize that LCIS conveys a lifetime risk. Observation is not prevention and is successful only if careful follow-up detects subsequent cancers at an early and potentially curable stage. Whether nonsurgical means of preventing breast cancer development will be applicable to the population of LCIS patients is a matter of intensive investigation (see later).

Prophylactic Mastectomy for the High-Risk Patient

The only treatment available that can reliably prevent breast cancer from developing is total mastectomy. The risk of cancer development is rarely so great as to justify prophylactic removal of a clinically normal breast. In those few situations in which it merits consideration, however, prophylactic mastectomy may be not only life-saving but also life-affirming. The anxiety associated with the risk of breast cancer development, particularly if relatives have died of metastatic disease, can be a major motivating factor to undergo prophylactic mastectomy. When properly performed along with breast reconstruction, the surgery may be associated with great relief and a marked improvement in quality of life.

Appropriately considered for prophylactic mastectomy are patients at high risk of development of breast cancer by virtue of strong family histories of the disease, patients with known primary breast cancer with a high propensity for contralateral occurrence, and patients with histologic markers conferring a high risk for subsequent invasive cancer development.

Indications

Three considerations enter into the decision-making process for prophylactic mastectomy: (1) the risk of invasive breast cancer development, (2) the ability to observe the patient, and (3) the anxiety level about cancer development. Each of these factors must be assessed in every patient considered for prophylactic surgery. The presence of a markedly increased risk for the development of invasive breast cancer is the sine qua non; anxious or difficult-to-follow women who are not at increased risk for breast cancer are not candidates for prophylactic mastectomy.

Several situations are associated with a sufficiently high risk of development of invasive cancer such that prophylactic mastectomy warrants consideration (Table 60-24). Women with two or more close relatives who have had bilateral or premenopausal breast cancer are at high risk of development of breast cancer. This risk may exceed 50% over the lifetime of the patient. Some patients may come from families with clear genetic predisposition for development of breast cancer secondary to the presence of BRCA-1 and BRCA-2 or other well-characterized cancer syndromes; in the near future, availability of genetic testing may select the women of these families who are most appropriate candidates for prophylactic surgery. Other women with lesser family histories may also be at increased risk for development of breast cancer compared with the general population, but generally, this risk is not great enough to warrant consideration of prophylactic mastectomy.

The presence of biopsy-proven LCIS is associated with an increased risk of development of invasive cancer in both breasts. Invasive cancer develops in about 30% of women with LCIS in their lifetimes. Patients with LCIS and a family history of breast cancer may be at even higher risk. Bilateral mastectomies as prophylaxis against subsequent invasive cancer are appropriate for some women with LCIS.

Women who have one breast cancer may be at increased risk of development of a contralateral breast primary. No patient should undergo surgical therapy for breast cancer without first having bilateral mammography and careful examination of the opposite breast. If these simple measures to detect synchronous invasive cancer are performed, there is no compelling evidence to support routine use of contralateral biopsy or mastectomy, even in patients with invasive or noninvasive lobular cancer.[98] Accordingly, patients with unilateral breast cancer in the absence of some other specific factor placing them at high risk are not generally candidates for prophylactic contralateral mastectomy.

Table 60-24. CRITERIA FOR CONSIDERATION OF PROPHYLACTIC MASTECTOMY

ONE OF THE FOLLOWING

Strong family history of breast cancer
Lobular carcinoma in situ
Atypical hyperplasia and a family history of breast cancer

PLUS ANY ONE OF THE FOLLOWING

High anxiety about cancer development
Limited access to follow-up
Difficult to follow clinically or radiographically
Patient preference for prophylactic surgery

The only established alternative to bilateral mastectomies for high-risk women is close observation with frequent physical examinations and screening mammography. Hence, an individual patient's access to and suitability for long-term follow-up must be considered in the decision-making process for prophylactic surgery. The dense, glandular breasts of young women can be difficult to image mammographically, impeding early breast cancer detection. Similarly, pronounced fibrocystic changes may limit the ability of physical examination to detect a small breast cancer. Not all patients have access to the full spectrum of resources necessary for appropriate follow-up. Finally, some women are ill-suited to the psychosocial burden of a lifetime of close medical follow-up and are unlikely to comply. All these considerations, coupled with the patient's level of anxiety about cancer development, need to be assessed before deciding how to treat a woman at high risk of development of breast cancer. It must be re-emphasized that although considerations of follow-up and anxiety level are important, by themselves these are not indications for prophylactic mastectomy. They are relevant only within the context of a high-risk patient.

Choice of Operation

Total mastectomy is an operation designed to remove all breast tissue, including the nipple–areola complex. It is the only procedure appropriate for breast cancer prophylaxis. Simultaneous removal of axillary lymph nodes is not indicated; ALND in this situation is unnecessary and potentially morbid. Subcutaneous mastectomy, wherein the nipple–areola complex is preserved, leaves breast tissue behind. Although this operation may somewhat reduce the overall cancer risk, after subcutaneous mastectomy women remain at risk for cancer development in the remaining breast tissue and need follow-up examinations and mammography just as if they had not had surgery. Cases of breast cancer developing after subcutaneous mastectomy have been reported in the literature.[147]

Unfortunately, not even total mastectomy can invariably remove all breast tissue. Particularly if thick skin flaps are created, as much as 1% to 2% of breast tissue may remain. A few cases of breast cancer arising within the skin flaps after total mastectomy have been described. Although such cases are extremely uncommon, they serve to emphasize the fact that a total mastectomy for prophylaxis should be performed with just as much attention to technique as the same operation done for known breast cancer. Concessions should not be made in the name of an improved cosmetic result.

Reconstruction

A high percentage of women who undergo prophylactic mastectomies have reconstructions performed. Reconstruction should be encouraged because it permits patients to make informed decisions about surgery with less fear of deformity. To this end, every patient considering prophylactic breast surgery should have the opportunity to meet a reconstructive surgeon before the procedure. She should be able to review the entire range of immediate and delayed reconstruction possibilities, including photographs of reconstructed patients. Although it is a major operative undertaking, bilateral prophylactic mastectomies with immediate, bilateral TRAM flap reconstructions is a safe and effective option for most women.[116] Because of the convenience and psychosocial advantages of immediate reconstruction, this option may well be the procedure of choice for women choosing prophylactic surgery. At times, the opportunity to meet and speak with women who have already undergone postmastectomy reconstruction is invaluable to the patient. The patient's needs and desires should take precedence in deciding among reconstruction options.

Prospects for Nonsurgical Prevention of Breast Cancer

Prevention strategies for breast cancer are still in their infancy, and none is available to replace surgery. Experimental data, however, demonstrate that tamoxifen can prevent breast carcinogenesis in susceptible animals.[148] Even more intriguing, studies in surgically treated breast cancer show a lower incidence of contralateral breast cancer in women receiving adjuvant tamoxifen compared with placebo.[128,149,150] Some studies, however, suggest that tamoxifen-treated women have an increased incidence of thromboembolic events and may be at increased risk of development of uterine cancer.[128,151] More investigation needs to be carried out before tamoxifen can be advocated as a chemopreventive agent for breast cancer. In this regard, two major randomized trials are underway—one in the United States and one in the United Kingdom—to evaluate tamoxifen for cancer prevention in women at high risk for breast cancer development, including those with LCIS. Also undergoing evaluation as a potential breast cancer chemopreventive agent is the retinoid compound fenretinide (4-hydroxyphenylretinide, also called 4-HPR).

Cystosarcoma Phyllodes and Sarcomas of the Breast

Mesenchymal tumors arising in the breast are rare. Their recognition is important, however, because the natural history and treatment of breast sarcomas differ markedly from those for breast carcinomas. Mesenchymal breast tumors are best stratified into two groups—the phyllodes tumors, which are unique to the breast, and those soft tissue sarcomas of the breast that can also occur elsewhere in the body. These latter tumors may arise de novo within the breast or may be encountered after previous treatment for breast carcinoma.

Cystosarcoma Phyllodes (Phyllodes Tumor)

Johannes Müller named and provided the first description of cystosarcoma phyllodes in 1838. In retrospect, the name *cystosarcoma phyllodes* was a poor choice. The term *sarcoma* implies a malignancy, but cystosarcoma phyllodes may behave in a completely benign fashion. Because of this, many pathologists have proposed dropping the word *cystosarcoma* from the name or reserving its use for only malignant tumors. The name *phyllodes tumor* has been advanced as a generic label for both benign and malignant variants.

Clinical Presentation. Phyllodes tumor presents as a painless breast mass. The patient may have a history of sudden enlargement of a previously stable nodule. The mass may attain huge size, with prominent vascularity and thinning of the overlying skin. Even with large tumors, skin fixation, edema, and axillary node involvement rarely occur. Phyllodes tumor is encountered most commonly in women aged 30 to 40 years, but it can occur at any age. Because phyllodes tumor arises from the lobular elements of the breast, it is essentially nonexistent in males. Mammography usually shows a well-circumscribed lesion indistinguishable from a fibroadenoma. One or more borders may be indistinct radiologically, suggesting the presence of a malignant lesion. Rarely, areas of cystic degeneration are seen within an otherwise solid mass, allowing a specific mammographic diagnosis to be made. Ultrasonography generally cannot differentiate phyllodes tumor from fibroadenoma.

Pathology. On gross inspection, most phyllodes tumors are well circumscribed and often have a distinctive brownish color. The cut surface is soft, slimy, and occasionally cystic. A characteristic leaflike pattern, from which the name *phyllodes* is derived, may be evident. Microscopically, the tumor is composed of both stromal and epithelial elements. Fibroadenomas, which are also composed of the same two elements, differ from phyllodes tumors in that they have a much less cellular stroma and lack the nuclear atypia and mitotic figures. Phyllodes tumor is almost always distinguishable from fibroadenoma on histologic grounds.

The differentiation of benign from malignant phyllodes tumors may be more difficult. Malignant changes can occur focally within an otherwise benign-appearing lesion and must be carefully sought. Even lesions thought to be clearly benign occasionally manifest malignant behavior, but several criteria are generally predictive of outcome. These include the number of mitoses per high-power field, the character of the tumor margin (infiltrating versus pushing), the degree of cellular atypia, the presence or absence of stromal overgrowth, and increased stromal cellularity (Fig. 60-36). About one fourth of all phyllodes tumors are histologically malignant by these criteria, but metastatic disease develops in only a fraction of these patients.

Management. The optimal treatment for a benign or malignant phyllodes tumor is wide excision with a margin of normal breast tissue. This margin must be histologically free of involvement because even benign lesions can recur after incomplete excision. If this can be done leaving an adequate cosmetic appearance, mastectomy is not necessary. Total mastectomy is reserved for large lesions in small-breasted women or recurrences after previous local excision that are not amenable to repeat local excision. ALND is not performed in the absence of biopsy-proven nodal involvement, even for malignant phyllodes tumors, because axillary node metastases are uncommon.

Other Sarcomas of the Breast

Any histologic subtype of sarcoma can arise within the mesenchymal elements of the breast. Most commonly, however, breast sarcomas arise from the fibrous stroma of the breast. These tumors lack the biphasic (stromal and epithelial) appearance of malignant phyllodes tumor and have been called *stromal sarcomas* or *monomorphic sarcomas* to emphasize this difference. Angiosarcomas also appear to have a propensity to occur in the breast, for unknown reasons. Males as well as females may be affected by primary (nonphyllodes) breast sarcomas.

The principles of sarcoma therapy applied elsewhere in the body govern the workup and management of nonphyllodes breast sarcomas. Axillary node involvement is rare. Wide local excision is the key to preventing local recurrence; total or radical mastectomy is indicated only if necessary to excise the tumor adequately (Fig. 60-37). Postoperative radiotherapy is employed for high-grade sarcomas or if the adequacy of excision is questionable. ALND is reserved for biopsy-proven nodal metastases. Adjuvant chemotherapy after complete surgical resection has not been proved to be of benefit for breast sarcomas.[152]

Sarcomas Arising After Treatment of Breast Cancer

Radiation-induced sarcomas may arise in either the bone or the soft tissue of the chest wall after mastectomy and postoperative radiotherapy and must be differentiated from chest wall recurrence of the original breast cancer.

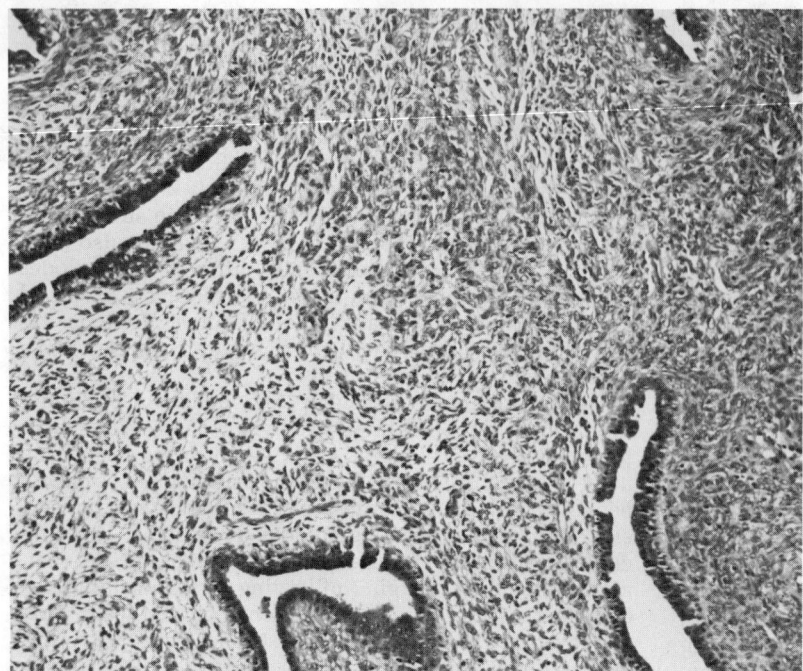

Figure 60-36. Histologic appearance of malignant phyllodes tumor (so-called cystosarcoma phyllodes). Phyllodes tumors are characterized by their exaggerated intracanalicular pattern of ductal elements and their stromal cellularity. Malignant lesions, such as the one pictured here, manifest hypercellularity at their margins, cellular atypia, and exaggerated stromal overgrowth. (Courtesy of Harold Oberman, MD, Department of Pathology, University of Michigan Medical School, Ann Arbor)

The long duration between treatment of the original cancer and presentation of the sarcoma (averaging about 10 years) may be a clue to the nature of the lesion, but biopsy is always necessary to establish the diagnosis. Treatment options are limited by the high doses of radiation previously given to the area. The overall outlook is worse than for standard soft tissue or bone sarcomas. Few patients survive 5 years. Patients have been described in whom postirradiation sarcomas developed in the breast after lumpectomy and radiotherapy[153]; although some of these patients may be saved with total mastectomy, most will succumb to metastatic disease.

An even worse prognosis is associated with lymphangiosarcoma, which generally develops in the setting of lymphedema. Originally described in postmastectomy patients,

it is now recognized that long-standing lymphedema of any kind predisposes to the development of lymphangiosarcoma. Most of these tumors develop in patients with massive lymphedema, usually as a result of the combination of a complete axillary dissection (including level III nodes) and axillary irradiation. A single, discrete tumor is rarely encountered. Rather, the multiple purplish red nodules may easily be mistaken for bacterial cellulitis. Postmastectomy lymphangiosarcomas are virtually always high-grade lesions; they usually spread rapidly to involve most of the arm as well as the shoulder and chest wall. Pulmonary metastases are common by the time the lesion is diagnosed (Fig. 60-38). Most patients die of disease within 2 years.

For patients without pulmonary metastases, forequarter (interscapulothoracic) amputation provides the best chance

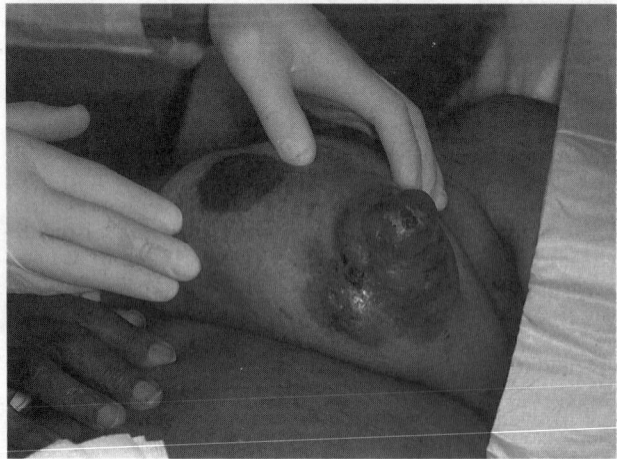

Figure 60-37. Large, low-grade sarcoma involving the skin of the left breast. This lesion was ulcerated and bled easily, requiring electrocautery. Removing the lesion with histologically negative margins required total mastectomy. There was no clinical evidence of axillary node involvement, and node dissection was not performed.

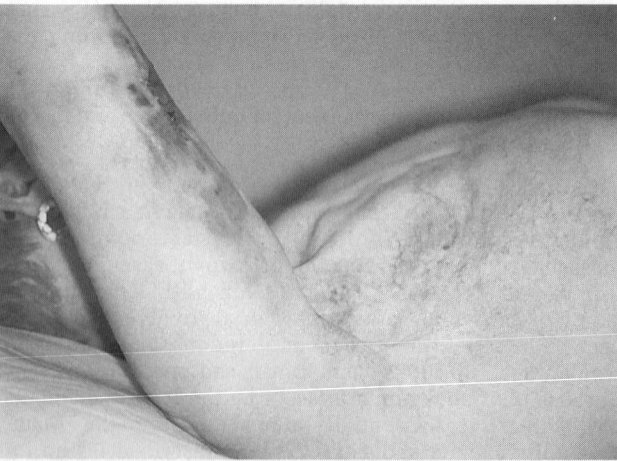

Figure 60-38. High-grade lymphangiosarcoma arising on the right arm 21 years after radical mastectomy and chest wall irradiation for breast cancer. The patient presented with pulmonary metastases at the time of diagnosis. This patient did not have significant lymphedema subsequent to her mastectomy.

for local control. Given the nearly uniform development of disseminated disease within a short time after diagnosis, however, less radical surgery combined with regional or systemic chemotherapy seems more appropriate for most patients. Avoidance of level III node dissections and of the combination of ALND and axillary irradiation should minimize the likelihood of massive lymphedema and nearly eliminate the occurrence of this tumor.

Paget Disease of the Nipple

Paget disease is characterized by a weeping, eczematoid lesion of the nipple (Fig. 60-39). There is often accompanying edema and inflammation. Biopsy of the nipple reveals malignant cells within the milk ducts. The lesion is invariably associated with an underlying invasive or in situ ductal carcinoma. The underlying cancer can be detected mammographically in some cases.[154] The prognosis of Paget disease is that of the underlying cancer. Standard treatment is mastectomy, with ALND only if invasive carcinoma is present. There is limited experience with wide nipple–areola complex excision followed by radiotherapy. This may be appropriate in some cases.[155]

Breast Cancer During Pregnancy and Lactation

Breast cancer that occurs during pregnancy or lactation poses unique therapeutic and ethical challenges for both the patient and the physician.[156] Up to 4% of breast cancers occur during pregnancy or within a year thereafter. In fact, data suggest that the effect of pregnancy on breast cancer risk is biphasic. Although the long-term and net effect of pregnancy is to reduce breast cancer risk, there seems to be a short-term excess of breast cancer cases during the 10 to 15 years after a first pregnancy as compared with nulliparous controls.[157] Diagnosis of breast cancer in the pregnant or lactating woman may be difficult and is frequently delayed because of the breast engorgement, tenderness, and nodularity associated with these states. Early reports stressed the dismal outcomes that seemed to be attached to a diagnosis of breast cancer during pregnancy or lactation, but more recent studies indicate that, stage

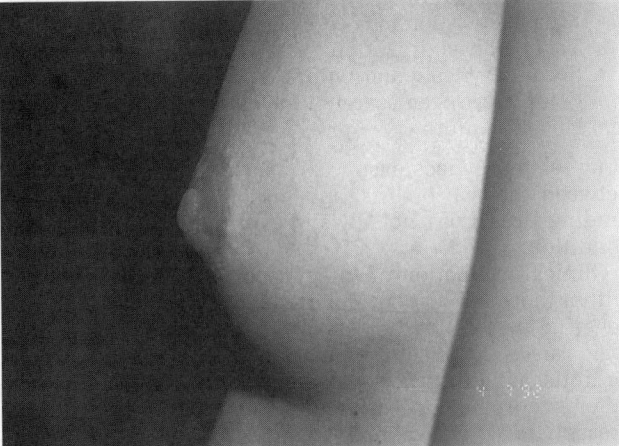

Figure 60-39. Paget disease of the nipple. An eczematoid reaction involves most of the papilla and the lower half of the areola. There was no evidence of invasive cancer on examination or mammography. The patient was treated with excision of the nipple–areolar complex and postoperative irradiation. She is without evidence of recurrence or metastasis.

for stage, the prognosis does not differ from that for groups of similar, nonpregnant women. Overall, however, pregnant and lactating women tend to have a worse prognosis because of the relatively high incidence of poor prognostic factors (particularly negative hormone receptors and positive axillary nodes) and perhaps because of delay in diagnosis.

Therapy of breast cancer during lactation involves cessation of breastfeeding and treatment as indicated for nonlactating patients. Pregnancy makes the treatment choices more problematic. Termination of pregnancy and suppression of lactation in and of themselves are not therapeutic, although they may simplify therapy. Radiotherapy is contraindicated with a fetus in utero because it is impossible to deliver tumoricidal doses without potentially dangerous fetal exposure. If breast conservation is to be considered, the pregnancy must be terminated or the radiotherapy delayed until after delivery. Mastectomy is generally safe during pregnancy and lactation with careful anesthetic management. Adjuvant chemotherapy or hormonal therapy is rarely given to pregnant or lactating women because of the risks of fetal exposure. Adjuvant therapy may be delayed, or if the risk of recurrence is low, omitted completely. There are no known direct effects of breast cancer on the fetus; no incidents of transplacental metastasis of breast cancer have been reported. Similarly, there is no demonstrated risk to the mother of subsequent pregnancy, although delay of such for 3 to 5 years is prudent because this is the period of highest risk for recurrence.

Occult Breast Cancer Presenting as Axillary Metastases

Breast cancer may present with enlarged axillary lymph nodes as the first sign of disease. On rare occasions, careful physical examination and mammography fail to detect a primary tumor in the breast even after lymph node biopsy reveals metastatic adenocarcinoma. This raises two important questions: What is the likelihood that an undetectable breast cancer is present? How should subsequent evaluation and treatment proceed?

The workup should focus on careful pathologic examination of the nodal tissue, looking for clues to the origin of the tumor, and a brief search for other primary tumors. If these endeavors are unrevealing, an occult breast primary tumor may be assumed.[158] Pathologic examination should include hormone receptor assay and special stains and electron microscopy to rule out lymphoma, melanoma, apocrine tumors, and other unusual primary tumors. Careful breast examination and mammography are mandatory. A complete physical examination should include careful skin and thyroid assessment and testing for fecal occult blood. Laboratory and radiographic investigation, in the absence of suggestive physical findings, should be limited to a complete blood count, liver function tests, carcinoembryonic antigen determination, and chest radiograph.

Historically, women with adenocarcinoma in the axillary lymph nodes and no known primary tumor have been treated with mastectomy, presuming an underlying subclinical breast primary. Indeed, careful sectioning of the breast reveals cancer in 55% to 100% of these patients.[159] In all cases, a complete axillary dissection should be performed because about two thirds of patients have cancer in nodes other than the one that underwent biopsy.[159,160] Regarding therapy of the breast itself, researchers variously recommend mastectomy or breast conservation. Proponents of the former argue that mastectomy establishes a firm primary tumor diagnosis in most cases, establishes locoregional control, and cures a significant number of women. Supporters of the latter suggest that since the primary tumor is likely to be in the breast and is probably small, radiotherapy should effectively treat the patient while conserving the breast. Limited experience with the latter approach prevents definitive appraisal of its efficacy, but it does appear promising.[159,160] Adjuvant therapy is recommended for all patients as for any other primary operable stage II breast cancer. The 5-year survival rate in patients with occult primary tumors and axillary metastases is about 60%, not significantly different than for women with known primary tumors and axillary metastases.

BREAST DISEASES OF EXTRAMAMMARY ORIGIN

A variety of problems may arise in the nonglandular portions of the breast. Additionally, derangements of hormonal regulation elsewhere in the body can manifest themselves through their effects on the breast as an endocrine target organ. It is important to recognize these problems as extraglandular in origin so that evaluation and treatment proceeds along lines appropriate for their true causes.

Diseases of the skin overlying the breast should be treated as such, and not as breast disorders. For example, the concept of wide local excision and regional node dissection for a melanoma arising in the skin of the breast must be differentiated from that of lumpectomy and ALND for a primary breast cancer. For melanoma and other malignancies arising in the region of the breast, mastectomy is inappropriate unless required to obtain adequate margins.

A variety of neoplasms of mesenchymal origin may arise in the breast. Included are any of the histologic benign and malignant varieties of soft tissue tumors. Fibromatosis (desmoid tumors), fat necrosis, foreign-body reactions, sarcoidosis, lymphoma, and various infections (including those of mycobacterial origin) have also been described. Superficial thrombophlebitis of the thoracoepigastric vein (Mondor disease) was mentioned earlier. Because the breast is responsive to hormonal influences, endocrine abnormalities may produce mammary sequelae. Most common is galactorrhea resulting from abnormal elaboration of prolactin secondary to a pituitary adenoma, a thyroid disorder, or medications. Measurement of a serum prolactin level is appropriate in women who have not lactated within the prior year with onset of new, bilateral galactorrhea. Gynecomastia may relate to abnormalities of estrogen metabolism seen accompanying cirrhosis, feminizing tumors, and genetic defects. Postmenopausal women who present with signs and symptoms of new-onset fibrocystic changes should be evaluated for the possible presence of a hormone-producing ovarian neoplasm.

MALE BREAST DISEASES

The absence of estrogen and progesterone in the normal postpubertal male precludes the maturation of breast tissue. Before puberty, however, the development of the male breast is similar to that of the female breast. Because the lobular elements depend on female hormones for development, the adult male breast remains a rudimentary structure possessing ductal elements and a nipple–areola complex. Along with the lack of cyclic hormone changes, this accounts for the low incidence of both benign and malignant disorders in the male breast. Derangements of the normal male hormonal milieu can be associated with a much higher incidence of breast disease. Most commonly, males present to a surgeon for evaluation of enlargement of one or both breasts and, much less commonly, for treatment of breast cancer.

Gynecomastia

Gynecomastia is defined as palpable enlargement of the male breast. Nonspecific breast enlargement from fat deposition in obese patients must be differentiated from true gynecomastia; in the latter case, there is a distinct disk of breast tissue palpable immediately beneath the nipple–areola complex. Gynecomastia may occur as a consequence of physiologic situations wherein the normal hormonal milieu of the male is perturbed. Transplacental hormonal stimulation can lead to breast enlargement and even milk production (colostrum) in both males and females in the first month of life. At the onset of puberty, the estrogen/testosterone ratio may be high in some males, and this can persist for several years. Asymptomatic gynecomastia is a surprisingly common finding in adolescent males, probably because of this relative imbalance. One study demonstrated a 39% incidence of gynecomastia between ages 11 and 14, declining to 14% by age 16.[161] In elderly men, declining serum levels of testosterone in the presence of physiologic estrogen levels may be associated with gynecomastia. The precise role estrogen plays in physiologic gynecomastia is unclear because asymptomatic breast enlargement may be found even when hormonal imbalances cannot be implicated.

Pathologic causes of estrogen excess or testosterone deficiency are also associated with gynecomastia. In many cases of gynecomastia, no cause is found. Clinically significant gynecomastia has been associated with use of a number of drugs as well as with other causes:

- Idiopathic
- Drug-induced
  Androgens
  Cimetidine
  Cyproterone
  Digoxin
  Griseofulvin
  Isoniazid
  Marijuana
  Metoclopramide
  α-Methyl-DOPA
  Reserpine
  Spironolactone
  Tricyclic antidepressants
- Klinefelter syndrome (XXY chromosomal abnormality)
- Testicular feminization
- Secondary testicular failure
- Ectopic estrogen secretion
- Hepatic failure

Drug-related gynecomastia is often unilateral or unequal between the two breasts, and discontinuation of the offending drug does not always lead to resolution of the condition.

Clinical evaluation of the gynecomastia patient begins with a thorough history and systems review aimed at uncovering underlying hormonal, pharmacologic, or pathologic causes. Physical examination may reveal stigmata of an underlying disorder, such as liver dysfunction, Klinefelter syndrome, or a testicular tumor. Palpation of the breast tissue is critical both to verify the presence of gynecomastia and to exclude the possibility of cancer. Benign gynecomastia feels disk-shaped or spheric, firm, and rubbery. The breast tissue is symmetric and centered directly below the nipple. Irregularly-shaped masses, or those not immediately below the nipple–areola complex, must be suspected of malignancy. Mammography is feasible in males as well as females and should be employed in any patient in whom malignancy is suspected. Testicular ultrasound is not used routinely if the testes are normal to palpation. Liver function tests can help to exclude some causes of gynecomastia. A formal endocrine evaluation is not indicated for gynecomastia unless some other sign of hormonal imbalance is found on routine examination. FNAB cytology has proved disappointing in excluding malignancy in gynecomastia; equivocal or atypical findings are common in histologically benign cases.

Treatment of gynecomastia involves correction or elimination of the underlying cause, if any, combined with reassuring the patient about the benignity of the condition. For most patients, particularly older males with bilateral disease, exclusion of malignancy is all that is required. Younger males, especially those with unilateral breast enlargement, may be bothered by the presence of gynecomastia and desire excision. Although hormonal agents have been used with anecdotal success, this seems excessive for patients who require only reassurance, and inadequate and overly noxious for those who are troubled by their appearance.

The standard surgical treatment of gynecomastia consists of a subcutaneous mastectomy performed under local anesthesia. General anesthesia or hospitalization are rarely required. An incision circumscribing 180 degrees of the areola is combined with short, transverse extensions. The entire nipple is raised as a skin flap, with a generous amount of subcutaneous fat and a small amount of breast tissue left adherent to prevent nipple sloughing or inversion. Wider skin flaps are raised as needed in all directions to encompass the entirety of the enlarged breast tissue, which is then dissected off the underlying pectoralis major muscle. The skin is closed with a subcuticular suture and adhesive strips. A small-caliber, closed-suction drain may be employed and removed within 24 to 48 hours.

Male Breast Cancer

Fewer than 1% of all cases of breast cancer occur in men. Male breast cancer patients often present at a more advanced stage than their female counterparts. This is attributable both to delay in presentation (10 to 18 months in some series) and to the smaller amount of breast tissue, which permits early invasion into the chest wall. The mean age at diagnosis, about 60 to 65 years, is higher in men than in women. Few clearcut risk factors have been identified for breast cancer in males. The presence of gynecomastia is not associated with subsequent development of cancer, yet protracted hyperestrogenemic states, which are associated with gynecomastia, are linked to breast cancer development. Klinefelter syndrome patients are markedly hyperestrogenemic; the incidence of breast cancer in males with this condition approaches 6%. Schistosomiasis has been associated with an increase in the frequency of male breast cancer; this parasitic infestation leads to chronic liver failure and hyperestrogenemia. In Egypt, where schistosomiasis is endemic, male breast cancer is more common than prostate cancer. Chronic liver disease from other causes theoretically should carry with it a similar increased risk of development of male breast cancer, but most patients with severe hepatic dysfunction do not survive long enough for this increased risk to be manifest. Long-term estrogen therapy in males is another potential risk factor for development of male breast cancer. Several well-documented cases exist of primary breast cancer developing in males taking exogenous estrogen.

Radiation to the chest wall, particularly in childhood or adolescence, is associated with a higher risk of development of breast cancer. The magnitude of this risk appears

to be similar to that seen in females receiving radiation at the same time of life. A family history of breast cancer has been reported in some patients with male breast cancer. The significance of a family history of female breast cancer is difficult to interpret given the prevalence of this disease. Female relatives of male breast cancer patients do not appear to have a higher breast cancer rate than would be expected in the general population. It will be of interest to see whether any cases of male breast cancer can be attributed to the presence of the newly isolated breast cancer susceptibility gene BRCA-1 or to similar genetic abnormalities. The BRCA-2 gene does appear to confer an increased risk of breast cancer development in male as well as female carriers.[61]

Because the normal male breast does not have lobular elements, male breast cancer is almost always ductal in origin. Only a few confirmed cases of invasive lobular cancer or LCIS have been reported in genetically normal males without a history of hormone use.[162,163] All other histologic types of breast cancer seen in women can be seen in men. Both inflammatory breast cancer and Paget disease have been reported. About 80% of male breast cancers are ER-positive, a higher percentage than in women.

The most common presentation of male breast cancer is a hard, painless breast lump. Bloody nipple discharge and skin ulceration are more common than in female patients. In contrast to gynecomastia, male breast cancer is usually hard, asymmetric, fixed to the skin or chest wall, and frequently associated with axillary adenopathy. Mammography can be useful in establishing a diagnosis of malignancy in questionable cases. Even if the mammogram does not reveal cancer, biopsy of a breast mass should be performed if indicated clinically. Male patients who have had cancer in one breast can be followed up with mammography of the contralateral breast to detect a second primary tumor. Mammographic detection of nonpalpable breast cancer in a clinically normal opposite breast has been reported.

The scant amount of breast tissue in males mandates a different surgical approach to breast cancer than in females. Early involvement of skin and muscle is common. In these cases, radical mastectomy with split-thickness skin grafting may be necessary. Most tumors, however, may be treated by modified radical mastectomy; en bloc excision of underlying pectoralis major without complete removal of the muscle may be required. Although postoperative radiotherapy improves local control, survival has not been shown to be affected.

Metastases to the axillary nodes are frequent in male breast cancer, occurring in about 55% of cases. Survival of male patients with node-positive breast cancer is poor (Table 60-25). Therefore, adjuvant systemic chemotherapy has been advocated. The limited number of patients has precluded the performance of large, randomized studies of adjuvant therapy. Nonetheless, nonrandomized data suggest that node-positive male patients benefit from adju-

Table 60-25. BREAST CANCER IN MALES: 5- AND 10-YEAR OVERALL SURVIVAL RATES

Patients	Survival Rate (%)	
	5 y	10 y
Node-negative	79	62
Node-positive	28	4
ALL	49	35

(Crichlow RW. Carcinoma of the male breast. Surg Gynecol Obstet 1972;134:1011)

vant chemotherapy in a fashion analogous to their female counterparts.

When metastatic disease develops in a male breast cancer patient, endocrine manipulations are the first line of therapy. Between 50% and 80% of patients respond to hormone therapy. As in women, ER-positive tumors are far more likely to regress with hormonal therapy than ER-negative tumors. Available treatments include orchiectomy, pharmacologic doses of estrogen (diethylstilbestrol), tamoxifen, progestational agents, antiandrogens, and adrenalectomy. Tamoxifen is the most convenient and best tolerated of these agents. For patients who are ER-negative, who fail first-line hormone therapy without ever responding, or who have major visceral disease (usually liver involvement), combination chemotherapy is the treatment of choice. Active agents are the same as for female breast cancer; response rates to commonly employed chemotherapy regimens are essentially the same as in women.

Other Breast Diseases

Diseases of the male breast other than gynecomastia and cancer are rare. Because lobular elements are absent in normal males, pathologic processes arising from these elements (such as fibroadenomas or LCIS) are essentially unheard of except in patients who are on long-term estrogen therapy or who have Klinefelter syndrome. Other lesions, such as ductal ectasia, do occur, although at a much reduced frequency compared with women. Principles of treatment parallel those of the same lesions in women.

REFERENCES

1. Wagner FB Jr. History of breast disease and its treatment. In: Bland KI, Copeland EM, eds. The breast: comprehensive management of benign and malignant diseases. Philadelphia, WB Saunders, 1991:1.
2. Halsted WS. The results of operations for cure of cancer of the breast performed at the Johns Hopkins Hospital from June 1889 to January 1894. Johns Hopkins Hosp Bull 1894–1895;4:297.
3. Wilson RE, Donegan WL, Mettlin C, et al. The 1982 national survey of carcinoma of the breast in the United States by the American College of Surgeons. Surg Gynecol Obstet 1984;159:309.
4. Farrow DC, Hunt WC, Samet JM. Geographic variation in the treatment of localized breast cancer. N Engl J Med 1992;326:1097.
5. Harris JR, Lippman ME, Veronesi U, Willett W. Breast cancer (parts I, II, and III). N Engl J Med 1992;327:319.
6. August DA, Wilkins EG, Rea T. Breast reconstruction in older women. Surgery 1994;115:663.
7. Hultborn KA, Larsen LG, Rahgnult I. The lymph drainage from the breast to the axillary and parasternal lymph nodes: studies with the aid of colloidal ¹⁹⁸Au. Acta Radiol 1955;43:52.
8. Dickson RB, Lippman ME. Control of human breast cancer by estrogen, growth factors, and oncogenes. In: Lippman ME, Dickson RB, eds. Breast cancer: cellular and molecular biology. Boston, Kluwer, 1988:119.
9. Dickson RB, Lippman ME. Growth regulation of normal and malignant breast epithelium. In: Bland KI, Copeland EM, eds. The breast: comprehensive management of benign and malignant diseases. Philadelphia, WB Saunders, 1991:363.
10. Anderson DE, Williams WR. Familial cancer: implications for healthy relatives. In: Chaganti RSK, German J, eds. Genetics in clinical oncology. New York, Oxford University, 1985:241.
11. Biesecker BB, Boehnke M, Calzone K, et al. Genetic counseling for families with inherited susceptibility to breast and ovarian cancer. JAMA 1993;269:1970.
12. King M-C, Rowell S, Love SM. Inherited breast and ovarian cancer. What are the risks? What are the choices? JAMA 1993;269:1975.
13. Baker LH. The Breast Cancer Detection Demonstration Project: 5 year summary report. Cancer 1982;32:194.
14. Habbema JD, van Oortmarssen GJ, van Putten, et al. Age specific reduction in breast cancer mortality by screening: an analysis of the results of the Health Insurance Plan of Greater New York. J Natl Cancer Inst 1986;77:317.
15. Feig SA. Decreased breast cancer mortality through mammographic screening: results of clinical trials. Radiology 1988;167:659.
16. Tabar L, Fagerber CJG, Gad A, et al. Reduction in mortality from breast cancer after mass screening with mammography: randomized trial from the breast cancer screening working group of the Swedish National Board of Health and Welfare. Lancet 1985;1:829.
17. Kerlikowske K, Grady D, Rubin SM, et al. Efficacy of screening mammography: a meta-analysis. JAMA 1995;273:149.
18. Miller AB, Baines CJ, To T, et al. Canadian national breast screening study: breast cancer detection and death rates among women aged 40 to 49 years. Can Med Assoc J 1992;147:1459.
19. Davis DL, Love SM. Mammographic screening. (Editorial) JAMA 1994;271:152.
20. Kaluzny AD, Rimer B, Harris R. The National Cancer Institute and guideline development: lessons from the breast cancer screening controversy. (Commentary) J Natl Cancer Inst 1994;86:901.
21. Adler DD, Hyde DL, Ikeda DM. Quantitative sonographic parameters as a means of distinguishing breast cancers from benign solid breast masses. J Ultrasound Med 1991;10:505.
22. Dixon JM, Walsh J, Patterson D, Chetty U. Colour Doppler ultrasonography studies of benign and malignant breast lesions. Br J Surg 1992;79:259.
23. Greenstein S, Troupin RH. Nonmammographic imaging of the breast: current issues and future prospects. Semin Roentgenol 1993;28:231.
24. Wahl RL, Cody RL, Hutchins G, Mudgett E. Primary and metastatic breast carcinoma: initial clinical evaluation with the radiolabeled glucose analogue of 2-[F-18]-fluoro-2-deoxy-D-glucose. Radiology 1991;179:765.
25. Tse NY, Hoh CK, Hawkins RA, et al. The application of positron emission tomographic imaging with fluorodeoxyglucose to the evaluation of breast disease. Ann Surg 1992;216:27.
26. Nieweg OE, Kim EE, Wong W-H, et al. Positron emission tomography with fluorine-18-deoxyglucose in the detection and staging of breast cancer. Cancer 1993;71:3920.
27. Harms SE, Flamig DP. MR imaging of the breast. J Magn Reson Imaging 1993;3:277.
28. D'Orsi CJ, Adler DD, Ikeda DM, et al. Breast imaging. Radiology 1994;190:936.
29. Rosato FE, Rosenberg AL. Examination techniques: role of the physician and patient in evaluating breast diseases. In: Bland KI, Copeland EM, eds. The breast: comprehensive management of benign and malignant diseases. Philadelphia, WB Saunders, 1991:409.
30. Donegan WL. Evaluation of a palpable breast mass. N Engl J Med 1992;327:937.
31. Ferguson CM, Powell RW. Breast masses in young women. Arch Surg 1989;124:1338.
32. Layfield LJ, Glasgow BJ, Cramer H. Fine-needle aspiration in the management of breast masses. Pathol Annu 1989;24:23.
33. Helvie MA, Baker DE, Adler DD, et al. Radiographically guided fine-needle aspiration of nonpalpable breast lesions. Radiology 1990;174:657.
34. Cady B. How to perform breast biopsies. Surg Oncol Clin North Am 1995;4:47.
35. Campbell ID, Royle GT, Coddington R, et al. Technique and results of localization biopsy in a breast screening programme. Br J Surg 1991;78:1113.
36. Sailors DM, Crabtree JD, Land RL, Rose WB, Burns RP, Barker DE. Needle localization for nonpalpable breast lesions. Am Surg 1994;60:186.
37. Consensus Statement. Is "fibrocystic disease" of the breast precancerous? Arch Pathol Lab Med 1986;110:171.
38. Dupont WD, Page DL, Parl FF, et al. Long-term risk of breast cancer in women with fibroadenoma. N Engl J Med 1994;331:10.

39. Wingo PA, Tong T, Bolden S. Cancer statistics, 1995. CA 1995;45:8.
40. Miller BA, Feuer EJ, Hankey BF. The significance of the rising incidence of breast cancer in the United States. In: DeVita VT, Hellman S, Rosenberg SA, eds. Important advances in oncology 1994. Philadelphia, JB Lippincott, 1994:193.
41. Eley JW, Hill HA, Chen VW, et al. Racial differences in survival from breast cancer: results of the National Cancer Institute black/white cancer survival study. JAMA 1994;272:947.
42. Colditz GA, Stampfer MJ, Willett WC, et al. Prospective study of estrogen replacement therapy and risk of breast cancer in postmenopausal women. JAMA 1990;264:2648.
43. Steinberg KK, Thacker SB, Smith SJ, et al. A meta-analysis of the effect of estrogen replacement therapy on the risk of breast cancer. JAMA 1991;265:1985.
44. Cobleigh MA, Berris RF, Bush T, et al. Estrogen replacement therapy in breast cancer survivors: a time for change. JAMA 1994;272:540.
45. Kelsey JL, Berkowitz GS. Breast cancer epidemiology. Cancer Res 1988;48:5615.
46. Hildreth NG, Shore RE, Dvoretsky PM. The risk of breast cancer after irradiation of the thymus. N Engl J Med 1989;321:1281.
47. Miller AB, Howe GR, Sherman GJ, et al. Mortality from breast cancer after irradiation during fluoroscopic examinations in patients being treated for tuberculosis. N Engl J Med 1989;321:1285.
48. Slattery ML, Kerber RA. A comprehensive evaluation of family history and breast cancer risk: the Utah population database. JAMA 1993;270:1563.
49. Garber JE. Familial aspects of breast cancer. In: Harris JR, Hellman S, Henderson IC, Kinne DW, eds. Breast diseases. Philadelphia, JB Lippincott, 1991:142.
50. Anderson DE, Badzioch MD. Risk of familial breast cancer. Cancer 1985;56:383.
51. Lynch HT, Guirgis HA, Brodkey F, et al. Genetic heterogeneity and familial carcinoma of the breast. Surg Gynecol Obstet 1976;142:693.
52. Garber JE, Goldstein AM, Kantor AF, Dreyfus MG, Fraumeni JF Jr, Li FP. Follow-up study of 24 families with Li-Fraumeni syndrome. Cancer Res 1991;51:6094.
53. Li FP, Fraumeni JF Jr, Mulvihill JJ, et al. A cancer family syndrome in 24 kindreds. Cancer Res 1988;48:5358.
54. Glebov OK, McKenzie KE, White CA, Sukumar S. Frequent p53 gene mutations and novel alleles in familial breast cancer. Cancer Res 1994;54:3703.
55. Birch JM, Hartley AL, Marsden HB, et al. Excess risk of breast cancer in mothers of children with soft tissue sarcomas. Br J Cancer 1984;49:325.
56. Hartley AL, Birch JM, Marsden HB, et al. Breast cancer risk in mothers of children with osteosarcoma and chondrosarcoma. Br J Cancer 1986;54:819.
57. Vasen HFA. Inherited forms of colorectal, breast, and ovarian cancer: guidelines for surveillance. Surg Oncol Clin North Am 1994;3:501.
58. Miki Y, Swensen J, Shattuck-Eidens D, et al. A strong candidate for the breast and ovarian cancer susceptibility gene BRCA1. Science 1994;266:66.
59. Futreal PA, Liu Q, Shattuck-Eidens D, et al. BRCA1 mutations in primary breast and ovarian carcinomas. Science 1994;266:120.
60. Hall JM, Lee MK, Newman B, et al. Linkage of early-onset familial breast cancer to chromosome 17q21. Science 1990;250:1684.
61. Wooster R, Neuhausen SL, Mangion J, et al. Localization of a breast cancer susceptibility gene, BRCA2, to chromosome 13q12. Science 1994;265:2088.
62. Wellings SR. Development of human breast cancer. Adv Cancer Res 1980;31:287.
63. Page DL, Dupont WD, Rogers LW, et al. Atypical hyperplastic lesions of the female breast: a long term follow-up study. Cancer 1985;55:2698.
64. Dupont WD, Page DL. Risk factors for breast cancer in women with proliferative breast disease. N Engl J Med 1985;312:146.
65. Rosen PP, Lieberman PH, Braun DW, et al. Lobular carci-
66. Strobl JS, Thompson EB. Mechanisms of steroid hormone action. In: Auricchio F, ed. Sex steroid receptors. Field Educational Halia Acta Medica, Rome, 1985:9.
67. Russo J, Russo I. Biological and molecular bases of mammary carcinogenesis. Lab Invest 1987;57:112.
68. Bates SE, Valverius E, Salomon D, et al. Expression and estrogen regulation of transforming growth factor α (TGFα) mRNA in human breast cancer. Proceedings of the Annual Meeting of the American Association for Cancer Research, Atlanta, GA 1987;28:240.
69. Kobrin MS, Samosondar J, Kudlow JE. Transforming growth factor-α secreted by untransformed bovine anterior pituitary cells in culture. J Biol Chem 1986;261:14414.
70. Knabbe C, Lippman ME, Wakefield L, et al. Evidence that TGFβ is a hormonally regulated negative growth factor in human breast cancer. Cell 1987;48:417.
71. Escot C, Theillet C, Lidereau R, et al. Genetic alterations of the c-myc proto-oncogene (myc) in human primary breast carcinomas. Proc Natl Acad Sci USA 1986;83:4834.
72. Cline MJ, Battifora H, Yokota J. Proto-oncogene abnormalities in human breast cancer: correlations with anatomic features and clinical course of disease. J Clin Oncol 1987;5:999.
73. Bonilla M, Ramirez M, Lopez-Cueto J, Gariglio P. In vivo amplification and rearrangement of c-myc oncogene in human breast tumors. J Natl Cancer Inst 1988;80:665.
74. Guerin M, Barrois M, Terrier MJ, et al. Overexpression of either c-myc or c-erbB-2/neu protooncogenes in human breast carcinomas: correlation with poor prognosis. Oncogene 1988;3:21.
75. van de Vijver MJ, Peterse JL, Moot WJ, et al. Neu-protein in overexpression in breast cancer: association with comedo-type ductal carcinoma in situ and limited prognostic value in stage II breast cancer. N Engl J Med 1988;319:1239.
76. Maguire HC, Hellman ME, Greene MI, Yeh I. Expression of c-erb-2 in in situ and in adjacent invasive ductal adenocarcinomas of the female breast. Pathobiology 1992;60:117.
77. Whittaker JL, Walker RA, Varley JM. Differential expression of cellular oncogenes in benign and malignant human breast tissue. Int J Cancer 1986;38:651.
78. Muss HB, Thor AD, Berry DA, et al. c-erbB-2 expression and response to adjuvant therapy in women with node positive early breast cancer. N Engl J Med 1994;330:1260.
79. Weinstein RS, Jakate SM, Dominguez JM, et al. Relationship of the expression of the multidrug resistance gene product (p-glycoprotein) in human colon carcinoma to local tumor aggressiveness and lymph node metastasis. Cancer Res 1991;51:2720.
80. Halsted WS. The results of radical operations for the cure of cancer of the breast. Ann Surg 1907;46:1.
81. Urban JA, Baker HW. Radical mastectomy in continuity with en bloc resection of the internal mammary lymph node chain. Cancer 1952;5:992.
82. Haagensen CD, Stout AP. Carcinoma of the breast. II. Criteria of operability. Ann Surg 1943;118:859.
83. Fisher B, Redmond C, Fisher ER, et al. Ten-year results of a randomized clinical trial comparing radical mastectomy and total mastectomy with or without radiation. N Engl J Med 1985;312:674.
84. Beahrs OH, Henson DE, Hutter RVP, Kennedy RJ. Breast. In: Manual for staging of cancer, ed 4. Philadelphia, JB Lippincott, 1992:149.
85. Chevinsky AH, Ferrara J, James AG, Minton JP, Young D, Farrar WB. Prospective evaluation of clinical and pathologic detection of axillary metastases in patients with breast carcinoma. Surgery 1990;108:612.
86. Haagensen CD. Clinical classification of the stage of advancement of breast carcinoma. In: Diseases of the breast. Philadelphia, WB Saunders, 1986:851.
87. McGuire WL, Clark GM. Prognostic factors and treatment decisions in axillary-node–negative breast cancer. N Engl J Med 1992;326:1756.
88. Elledge RM, McGuire WL, Osborne CK. Prognostic factors in breast cancer. Semin Oncol 1992;19:244.
89. Coates RJ, Clark WS, Eley JW, Greenberg RS, Huguley CM

noma in-situ of the breast: detailed analysis of 99 patients with average follow-up of 24 years. Am J Surg Pathol 1978;2:225.

Jr, Brown RL. Race, nutritional status, and survival from breast cancer. J Natl Cancer Inst 1990;82:1684.

90. McGuire WL, Clark GM, Dressler LG, Owens MA. Role of steroid hormone receptors as prognostic factors in primary breast cancer. Natl Cancer Inst Monogr 1986;1:19.

91. Weidner N, Semple JP, Welch WR, Folkman J. Tumor angiogenesis and metastasis: correlation in invasive breast carcinoma. N Engl J Med 1991;324:1.

92. Gasparini G, Weidner N, Bevilacqua P, et al. Tumor microvessel density, p53 expression, tumor size, and peritumoral lymphatic vessel invasion are relevant prognostic markers in node-negative breast carcinoma. J Clin Oncol 1994;12:454.

93. Spyratos F, Maudelonde T, Brouillet J-P, et al. Cathepsin D: an independent prognostic factor for metastasis of breast cancer. Lancet 1989;2:1115.

94. Kute TE, Shao Z-M, Sugg NK, Long RT, Russell GB, Case LD. Cathepsin-D as a prognostic indicator for node-negative breast cancer patients using both immunoassays and enzymatic assays. Cancer Res 1992;52:5198.

95. Slamon DJ, Clark GM, Wong SG, et al. Human breast cancer: correlation of relapse and survival with amplification of the HER-2/*neu* oncogene. Science 1987;235:177.

96. McCann AH, Dervan PA, O'Regan M, et al. Prognostic significance of c-*erbB*-2 and estrogen receptor status in human breast cancer. Cancer Res 1991;51:3296.

97. Thor AD, Moore DH II, Edgerton SM, et al. Accumulation of p53 tumor suppressor gene protein: an independent marker of prognosis in breast cancers. J Natl Cancer Inst 1992;84:845.

98. Smith BL, Bertagnolli M, Klein BB, et al. Evaluation of the contralateral breast: the role of biopsy at the time of treatment of primary breast cancer. Ann Surg 1992;216:17.

99. Yeh KA, Fortunato L, Ridge JA, Hoffman JP, Eisenberg BL, Sigurdson ER. Routine bone scanning in patients with T1 and T2 breast cancer: a waste of money. Ann Surg Oncol 1995;2:319.

100. Fisher B, Redmond, Poisson R, et al. Eight-year results of a randomized clinical trial comparing total mastectomy and lumpectomy with or without irradiation in the treatment of breast cancer. N Engl J Med 1989;320:822.

101. Schnitt SJ, Abner A, Gelman R, et al. The relationship between microscopic margins of resection and the risk of local recurrence in patients with breast cancer treated with breast-conserving surgery and radiation therapy. Cancer 1994; 74:1746.

102. Spivack B, Khanna MM, Tafra L, et al. Margin status and local recurrence after breast-conserving surgery. Arch Surg 1994;129:952.

103. Harness JK. Organizing for collaborative management: what are the options? In: Harness JK, Oberman HA, Lichter AS, Adler DD, Cody RL, eds. Breast cancer: collaborative management. Chelsea, MI, Lewis, 1988.

104. August DA, Carpenter LC, Harness JK, et al. The benefits of a multidisciplinary approach to breast care. J Surg Oncol 1993;53:161.

105. August DA, Middleton S. The financial feasibility of a multidisciplinary approach to breast care. (Abstract) 15th Annual San Antonio Breast Cancer Symposium, 1992.

106. August DA, Ehrlich D, Carpenter LC. Patient evaluation of care within a multidisciplinary breast care center. Quality Management in Health Care 1995;3:1.

107. Margolese R, Poisson R, Shibata H, et al. The technique of segmental mastectomy (lumpectomy) and axillary dissection: syllabus from the National Surgical Adjuvant Breast Project workshops. Surgery 1987;102:828.

108. Patey DH, Dyson WH. The prognosis of carcinoma of the breast in relation to the type of operation performed. Br J Cancer 1948;2:7.

109. Barton FE Jr. Breast cancer, preventive mastectomy and breast reconstruction. In: Selected readings in plastic surgery. 1988:1.

110. Goldman LD, Goldwyn RM. Some anatomical considerations of subcutaneous mastectomy. Plast Reconstr Surg 1973; 51:501.

111. Hoe AL, Iven D, Royle GT, Taylor I. Incidence of arm swelling following axillary clearance for breast cancer. Br J Surg 1992;79:261.

112. Slavin SA, Love SM, Goldwyn RM. Recurrent breast cancer following immediate reconstruction with myocutaneous flaps. Plastic Reconstr Surg 1994;93:1191.

113. Stevens LA, McGrath MH, Drus RG, et al. The psychological impact of immediate breast reconstruction for women with early breast cancer. Plast Reconstr Surg 1984;73:619.

114. Wellisch DK, Schain WS, Noone RB, et al. Psychological correlates of immediate versus delayed reconstruction of the breast. Plast Reconstr Surg 1985;76:713.

115. Vasconez LO, Lejour M, Gamboa-Bobadilla M. Breast reconstruction. Philadelphia, JB Lippincott, 1991.

116. Wilkins EG, August DA, Chang AE, Smith DJ. Immediate, bilateral transverse rectus abdominis musculocutaneous (TRAM) flap reconstruction after mastectomy. Am Surg 1993;59:519.

117. Wilkins EG, August DA, Kuzon WM, Chang AE, Smith DJ. Immediate transverse rectus abdominis myocutaneous flap reconstruction following mastectomy. J Am Coll Surg 1995;180:177.

118. Angell M. Do breast implants cause systemic disease? Science in the courtroom. N Engl J Med 1994;330:1748.

119. Gabriel SE, O'Fallon WM, Kurland LT, Beard CM, Woods JE, Melton LJ. Risk of connective-tissue diseases and other disorders after breast implantation. N Engl J Med 1994; 330:1697.

120. Keynes G. Conservative treatment of cancer of the breast. Br J Med 1937;2:643.

121. Harris JR, Hellman S. Conservative surgery and radiotherapy. In: Harris JR, Hellman S, Henderson IC, Kinne DW, eds. Breast diseases. Philadelphia, JB Lippincott, 1987:299.

122. Lichter AS. Is radiation therapy in conjunction with mastectomy indicated for the treatment of operable breast cancer? Cancer Invest 1987;5:243.

123. Cuzick J, Stewart H, Rutqvist L, et al. Cause-specific mortality in long-term survivors of breast cancer who participated in trials of radiotherapy. J Clin Oncol 1994;12:447.

124. Pierce LJ, Lichter AS. Postmastectomy radiotherapy: more than locoregional control. (Editorial) J Clin Oncol 1994; 12:444.

125. Goldie JH, Coldman AJ. A mathematic model for relating the drug sensitivity of tumors to their spontaneous mutation rate. Cancer Treat Rep 1979;63:1727.

126. Skipper HE, Schabel FM, Mellett LB, et al. Implications of biochemical, cytokinetic, pharmacologic, and toxicologic relationships in the design of optimal therapeutic schedules. Cancer Chemother Rep 1970;54:431.

127. Consensus Development Conference Report. Adjuvant chemotherapy for breast cancer. JAMA 1985;254:3461.

127a. Fisher B, Dingam J, Wieand S, Wolmark N, Wickerham DL, contributing investigators. Duration of tamoxifen (TAM) therapy for primary breast cancer: 5 versus 10 years (NSABPB-14). Proc Am Soc Clin Oncol 1996;15:113.

128. Early Breast Cancer Trialists' Collaborative Group. Systemic treatment of early breast cancer by hormonal, cytotoxic, or immune therapy: 133 randomised trials involving 31 000 recurrences and 24 000 deaths among 75,000 women. Lancet 1992;339;1.

129. Bonnadonna G, Valagussa P, Rossi A, et al. Ten-year experience with CMF-based adjuvant chemotherapy in resectable breast cancer. Breast Cancer Res Treat 1985;5:95.

130. Clinical Alert from the National Cancer Institute, May 18, 1988. Breast Cancer Res Treat 1988;12:3.

131. NIH consensus conference. Treatment of early-stage breast cancer. JAMA 1991;265:391.

132. Vinokur AD, Threatt BA, Caplan RD, Zimmerman BL. Physical and psychosocial functioning and adjustment to breast cancer: long-term follow-up of a screening population. Cancer 1989;63:394.

133. Vinokur AD, Threatt BA, Vinokur-Kaplan D, Satariano WA. The process of recovery from breast cancer for younger and older patients: changes during the first year. Cancer 1990; 65:1242.

134. Vinokur AD, Vinokur-Kaplan D. "In sickness and in health": patterns of social support and undermining in older married couples. J Aging Health 1990;2:215.

135. Sorace RA, Bagley CS, Lichter AS, et al. The management of nonmetastatic locally advanced breast cancer using primary induction chemotherapy with hormonal synchronization followed by radiation therapy with or without debulking surgery. World J Surg 1985;9:775.

136. Baclesse F. Five-year results in 431 breast cancers treated solely by roentgen rays. Ann Surg 1965;161:103.

137. Bedwinek J, Rao DV, Perez C, et al. Stage III and localized stage IV breast cancer: irradiation alone vs. irradiation plus surgery. Int J Radiat Oncol Biol Phys 1982;8:31.

138. Weber BL, Merajver SD, August DA, et al. High response rate and breast conservation in locally advanced breast cancer (LABC) using combined modality therapy with hormonal synchronization. (Abstract) Proc Am Soc Clin Oncol 1992;11:75.

139. Crowe JP Jr, Gordon NH, Antunez AR, et al. Local-regional breast cancer recurrence following mastectomy. Arch Surg 1991;126:429.

140. van der Zee J, van Rhoon GC, Wike-Hooley, et al. Thermal enhancement of radiotherapy in breast carcinoma. In: Overgaard J, ed. Hyperthermic oncology 1984, vol 4. London, Taylor & Francis, 1985:387.

141. DiPaola RS, Orel, SG, Fowble BL. Ipsilateral breast tumor recurrence following conservative surgery and radiation therapy. Oncology 1994;8:59.

142. Bezwoda WR, Seymour L, Dansey RD. High-dose chemotherapy with hematopoietic rescue as primary treatment for metastatic breast cancer: a randomized trial. J Clin Oncol 1995;13:2483.

143. Betsill WL, Rosen PP, Lieberman PH, et al. Intraductal carcinoma: long-term follow-up after treatment by biopsy alone. JAMA 1978;239:1863.

144. Fisher B, Constantino J, Redmond C, et al. Lumpectomy compared with lumpectomy and radiation therapy for the treatment of intraductal breast cancer. N Engl J Med 1993;328:1581.

145. Beahrs O, Shapiro S, Smart C. Report of the working group to review the National Cancer Institute–American Cancer Society Breast Cancer Detection Demonstration Projects. J Natl Cancer Inst 1979;62:240.

146. Rosen PP, Lieberman PH, Braun DW, et al. Lobular carcinoma *in situ* of the breast. Am J Surg Pathol 1978;2:225.

147. Goodnight JE Jr, Quagliana JM, Morton DL. Failure of subcutaneous mastectomy to prevent the development of breast cancer. J Surg Oncol 1984;26:198.

148. Jordan VC, Lababidi MK, Langan-Fahey S. Suppression of mouse mammary tumorigenesis by long-term tamoxifen therapy. J Natl Cancer Inst 1991;83:492.

149. Fisher B, Constantino J, Redmond C, et al. A randomized clinical trial evaluating tamoxifen in the treatment of patients with node-negative breast cancer who have estrogen-receptor–positive tumors. N Engl J Med 1989;320:479.

150. Rutqvist LE, Cedermark B, Glas U, et al. Contralateral primary tumors in breast cancer patients in a randomized trial of adjuvant tamoxifen therapy. J Natl Cancer Inst 1991;83:1299.

151. Davidson NE. Tamoxifen: panacea or pandora's box? (Editorial) N Engl J Med 1992;326:885.

152. Glenn J, Kinsella T, Glatstein E, et al. A randomized, prospective trial of adjuvant chemotherapy in adults with soft tissue sarcomas of the head and neck, breast, and trunk. Cancer 1985;55:1206.

153. Edeiken S, Russo DP, Knecht J, et al. Angiosarcoma after tylectomy and radiation therapy for carcinoma of the breast. Cancer 1992;70:644.

154. Ikeda DM, Helvie MA, Frank TS, et al. Paget disease of the nipple: radiologic-pathologic correlation. Radiology 1993;189:89.

155. Osteen RT. Paget disease of the nipple. In: Harris JR, Hellman S, Henderson IC, Kinne DW, eds. Breast diseases. Philadelphia, JB Lippincott, 1991:797.

156. Gallenberg MM, Loprinzi CL. Breast cancer and pregnancy. Semin Oncol 1989;16:369.

157. Lambe M, Hsieh C-C, Trichopoulos D, Ekbom A, Pavia M, Adami H-O. Transient increase in the risk of breast cancer after giving birth. N Engl J Med 1994;331:5.

158. Baron PL, Moore MP, Kinne DW, et al. Occult breast cancer presenting with axillary metastases: updated management. Arch Surg 1990;125:210.

159. Merson M, Andreola S, Galimberti V, Bufalino R, Marchini S, Veronesi U. Breast carcinoma presenting as axillary metastases without evidence of a primary tumor. Cancer 1992;70:504.

160. Moore MP, Yahalom J. Occult primary tumor with axillary metastases. In: Harris JR, Hellman S, Henderson IC, Kinne DW, eds. Breast diseases. Philadelphia, JB Lippincott, 1991:817.

161. Nydick M, Bustos J, Dale JH, Rawson RW. Gynecomastia in adolescent boys. JAMA 1961;178:449.

162. Nance KV, Reddick RL. In situ and infiltrating lobular carcinoma of the male breast. Hum Pathol 1989;20:1220.

163. Michaels BM, Nunn CR, Roses DF. Lobular carcinoma of the male breast. Surgery 1994;115:402.

SURGERY: SCIENTIFIC PRINCIPLES AND PRACTICE, Second Edition, edited by
Lazar J. Greenfield, Michael W. Mulholland, Keith T. Oldham, Gerald B. Zelenock,
and Keith D. Lillemoe. Lippincott–Raven Publishers, Philadelphia. © 1997.

CHAPTER 61

LUNG NEOPLASMS

VALERIE W. RUSCH

Primary and metastatic lung neoplasms are the most common diseases treated by thoracic surgeons. The clinical management of lung neoplasms, especially primary lung cancer, has evolved considerably during the past 20 years. Significant advances have been made in our understanding of the natural history of lung cancer and in the methods of selecting patients for surgical resection. The roles of both extended and limited pulmonary resection have been defined. Multimodality therapy has become increasingly important and requires that surgeons be able to identify patients for adjuvant treatment and understand how to integrate surgical resection with radiotherapy and chemotherapy. Molecular genetic techniques have begun to reveal the fundamental biology of lung cancer and hold hope of newer, more effective treatments. This chapter emphasizes current information about tumor biology, multimodality therapy, and the rationale for surgical intervention in both primary and metastatic lung neoplasms.

LUNG CANCER

Incidence and Epidemiology

The incidence of lung cancer has risen steadily since the 1930s. More than 170,000 new cases occur annually in the United States, making lung cancer the second most common malignancy and the most common cause of cancer-related deaths in both men and women. Although men still account for two thirds of the cases, there has been a dramatic increase of the disease in women because of their increased cigarette smoking during the past 50 years. At least 40 carcinogens have been identified among the constituents of cigarette smoke, including the α-emitters polonium-210 and lead-210, benzo[a]pyrene, and several nitrosamines.[1] The relative importance of each of these carcinogens and the exact mechanisms by which they initiate or promote lung cancer are still undefined. The level of exposure to carcinogens (ie, the number of pack-years smoked) influences the risk of developing lung cancer, yet only about 20% of smokers ever develop lung cancer. Moreover, some people without known exposure to tobacco smoke or other carcinogens develop lung cancer. This suggests that a genetic predisposition to lung cancer exists.[2] Epidemiologic studies indicate an increased familial risk of lung cancer, most likely associated with a mendelian codominant inheritance of an autosomal gene, par-

ticularly in people who develop lung cancer before they are 50 years of age. This putative genetic abnormality is unidentified and needs to be investigated through genetic linkage studies.[3]

People who develop lung cancer may have genetic abnormalities that limit their ability to detoxify the carcinogens in tobacco smoke. Abnormalities of the cytochrome P450 enzyme system, which transforms the polycyclic aromatic hydrocarbon procarcinogens in cigarette smoke into potent carcinogens, are thought to be important determinants of individual susceptibility to lung cancer. These include abnormalities in expression of the CYP1A1, CYP2D6, and GSTM1 genes, all of which affect the metabolism of tobacco-related carcinogens.[4]

Environmental carcinogens are also risk factors for lung cancer and may interact synergistically with cigarette smoke. This is particularly true of asbestos; it has been estimated that smokers exposed to asbestos have a 92-fold greater risk of lung cancer than the general population of nonsmokers.[5] Occupational carcinogens associated with an increased risk of lung cancer include arsenic, chromium, nickel, copper, beryllium, vinyl chloride, and benzene. Uranium mining has been associated with an increased risk of lung cancer, particularly small cell lung cancer, that is independent of smoking. Radon, an inert gas released during the decay of uranium-238, is ubiquitous in indoor and outdoor air and is a potentially important cause of lung cancer in the general population. Well-insulated homes trap radon that would ordinarily be dispersed into the atmosphere, creating potentially hazardous levels of exposure.[2]

Pathologic Classification

Carcinomas of the lung are divided into two major categories—small cell and non–small cell lung cancers. About 80% of lung cancers are non–small cell lung cancers, whereas 20% are small cell lung cancers. The two types differ by their histology and clinical behavior, but frequent admixtures of small cell and non–small cell in individual tumors suggest a common origin for all lung cancers. The possibility of this common origin is supported by the in vitro finding that c-myc or N-myc amplified small cell lung cancer cell lines undergo transition toward the non–small cell phenotype after insertion of an activated ras gene.[6] Non–small cell lung cancers are subdivided into squamous cell cancers, adenocarcinomas, and large cell cancers. The criteria for the histologic classification of lung tumors are shown in Tables 61-1 and 61-2.

Most squamous cell tumors arise centrally, in the mainstem, lobar, or segmental bronchi, but one third occur in the small bronchi of lung tissue. In contrast, adenocarcinomas arise peripherally in the pulmonary parenchyma. During the past 20 years, there has been a gradual shift in the incidence of non–small cell types, with adenocarcinomas overtaking squamous cell cancers as the most common type. The reasons for this trend are unknown. The frequency of histologic cell types seen in two large lung can-

Table 61-1. HISTOLOGIC CLASSIFICATION OF LUNG TUMORS

WHO*	WPL-LCSG†
	01 Carcinoma in situ
1. Squamous cell carcinoma (epidermoid carcinoma)	10 Squamous cell carcinoma
	11 Well-differentiated
Variant:	12 Moderately differentiated
a. Spindle cell (squamous carcinoma)	13 Poorly differentiated
2. Small cell carcinoma	20 Small cell
a. Oat cell carcinoma	21 Lymphocyte-like or oat cell
b. Intermediate cell type	22 Intermediate
c. Combined oat cell carcinoma	
3. Adenocarcinoma	30 Adenocarcinoma
a. Acinar adenocarcinoma	31 Well-differentiated
b. Papillary adenocarcinoma	32 Moderately differentiated
	33 Poorly differentiated
c. Bronchioloalveolar carcinoma	34 Bronchiolar or alveolar
d. Solid carcinoma with mucus formation	
4. Large cell carcinoma	40 Large cell undifferentiated
Variants:	41 Giant cell
a. Giant cell carcinoma	
b. Clear cell carcinoma	
5. Adenosquamous carcinoma	50 Poorly differentiated carcinoma
6. Carcinoid	60 Bimulticomponent or multidifferentiated
	70 Carcinoid
7. Bronchial gland carcinoma	
a. Adenoid cystic	
b. Mucoepidermoid carcinoma	
c. Others	
8. Others	80 Bronchial gland tumors
	81 Adenoid cystic
	82 Mucoepidermoid
	83 Mixed tumors

* World Health Organization. Adapted from: Histological typing of lung tumours. Tumori 1981;67:253.
† Working Party for the Study of Lung Cancer. Modified by Lung Cancer Study Group, National Cancer Institute.

cer screening programs is shown in Table 61-3. Large cell cancers remain the least common form of non–small cell lung cancer, especially because immunohistochemistry and electron microscopy allow many of these to be classified as poorly differentiated forms of either squamous cell or adenocarcinoma. Bronchioloalveolar carcinoma, a subtype of adenocarcinoma, is characterized histologically by the growth of malignant cells along the walls of alveoli without destruction of the normal pulmonary architecture. Despite this uniform histologic appearance, bronchioloalveolar carcinomas have varying biologic behaviors. They can present either as indolent, well-circumscribed, small, peripheral pulmonary nodules or as aggressive tumors with diffuse pneumonic involvement. Bronchioloalveolar carcinoma is more likely to be multifocal than are the other types of non–small cell lung cancer. Early-stage squamous cell cancers, adenocarcinomas, and large cell cancers differ somewhat in their clinical behavior, but up to 45% of non–small cell lung tumors show more than one of the three cell types, again suggesting a common origin for all lung cancers.[7]

Small cell lung cancers are part of the larger family of neuroendocrine tumors that arise in many different areas of the body. In the lung and bronchial tree, neuroendocrine

Table 61-2. HISTOLOGIC CRITERIA USED FOR DIAGNOSING COMMON LUNG NEOPLASMS*

SQUAMOUS CELL CARCINOMA

Keratin formation, keratin pearl formation, intercellular junctions (bridges, processes) located between adjacent cells. These junctions are referred to as *prickles* or *spines*.

ADENOCARCINOMA

Definite gland formation or the presence of mucus production in a solid tumor, as determined by a mucosubstance special stain (eg, PAS-D, mucicarmine)

UNDIFFERENTIATED LARGE CELL CARCINOMA

Large cells with vesicular nuclei and prominent eosinophilic nucleoli; no evidence of squamous or glandular differentiation; negative for mucin stain

MULTICOMPONENT TUMOR (MIXED SQUAMOUS CELL AND ADENOCARCINOMA)

Tumors composed of more than one histologic type according to criteria as defined above

* Developed by the pathology section of the Lung Cancer Study Group.

tumors include a spectrum ranging from the well-differentiated, indolent, typical carcinoid tumor, to the more aggressive, atypical carcinoid tumor, to large cell neuroendocrine carcinomas, and finally to small cell cancer. Light microscopy permits the distinction between two subtypes of small cell lung cancer: oat cell carcinoma, a tumor composed of small round uniform cells; and intermediate small cell cancer, a tumor composed of less regular, polygonal cells. These two categories are characterized respectively in small cell lung cancer cell lines as *classic* and *variant* subtypes. Classic cell lines express a panel of four biomarkers, including L-dopa decarboxylase, neuron-specific enolase, creatine kinase, and bombesin-like immunoreactivity. Variant cell lines express creatine kinase and low amounts of neuron-specific enolase but not the other two markers. Variant cell lines also reveal amplification and expression of the oncogene c-*myc*, whereas classic cell lines do not. The variant cell line or intermediate form of small cell cancer is associated with a more malignant clinical course.

Biology

Relatively little is known about the genetic events involved in lung tumorigenesis. Multiple chromosomal abnormalities are present and vary even within histologically

Table 61-3. FREQUENCY OF HISTOLOGIC CELL TYPES FROM TWO LARGE SCREENING PROJECTS*

Cell Type	Memorial Sloan-Kettering (%)	Mayo Clinic (%)	
		Prevalence	Incidence
Adenocarcinoma	45	27	24
Squamous cell carcinoma	33	43	30
Undifferentiated carcinoma			
Small cell	16	13	26
Large cell	6	17	19

* Based on results from 20,000 screened patients.
(Petts SB Jr, Wernly JA, Akl BF. Lung Cancer: current concepts and controversies. West J Med 1986;J145:52).

similar tumors. One of the most prominent cytogenetic changes is deletion of material from the short arm of chromosome 3 (3p14-23).[8] This occurs in all small cell and in many non−small cell cancers. The critical gene residing in this region has not yet been identified but is presumably a tumor suppressor gene.

Other frequent abnormalities include deletion of the short arms of chromosomes 1, 9, 13, and 17 and polysomy of chromosome 7. In the case of chromosomes 13 and 17, genetic loss has been localized to known tumor suppressor genes, the retinoblastoma (Rb) and the p53 genes, respectively. Other deletions, rearrangements (usually nonreciprocal translocations), and polysomies are also common.[9] Unlike some hematologic malignancies, which are characterized by a single predominant chromosomal abnormality, karyotypes in non−small cell lung cancer are complex, even in early-stage tumors. Of course, not all of these chromosomal abnormalities necessarily reflect genetic changes that are biologically important.

At the molecular level, lung cancers, like other solid tumors, are characterized by the activation of oncogenes, the expression of growth factor loops, and the inactivation of tumor suppressor genes. The most frequently activated oncogene in non−small cell lung cancer is K-ras. Other members of the ras gene family, N-ras and H-ras, are rarely activated. The ras family of oncogenes becomes activated through point mutations of codon 12, 13, or 61. About one third of lung adenocarcinomas harbor a point mutation in codon 12 of the K-ras oncogene. This abnormality occurs less frequently in bronchioloalveolar carcinoma, a biologically indolent form of adenocarcinoma, and is not seen in tumors of pure squamous or small cell histology.

K-ras point mutations are linked to smoking. Occupational exposure to asbestos may increase the risk of K-ras mutations. In contrast, simultaneous exposure to tobacco smoke and to high levels of radioactivity, such as occurs in uranium miners, does not lead to the development of lung cancers with K-ras point mutations. These people more typically develop small cell lung cancers, which are characterized primarily by mutations in the tumor suppressor gene p53.

The presence of K-ras point mutations defines a subgroup of patients with lung adenocarcinoma in whom the disease-free and overall survival rates are short.[10] The correlation between K-ras point mutations and survival has been sufficiently consistent in retrospective studies that it may be appropriate to incorporate this molecular abnormality as a stratification factor in prospective clinical trials.

Growth factors and their receptors appear to play a role in lung tumorigenesis through autocrine or paracrine loops. For example, the epidermal growth factor receptor (EGFR) and one of its ligands, transforming growth factor-alpha (TGF-α) are thought to function as an autocrine loop in non−small cell lung cancer, analogous to the well-characterized autocrine loop of gastrin-releasing peptide and its receptor in small cell lung cancer cell lines. Several immunohistochemical studies of EGFR and of TGF-α suggest that these are overexpressed in primary tumors. Enhanced expression at the RNA level is also reported in selected non−small cell lung cancer cell lines. One study examined the differential expression of EGFR and of its ligands TGF-α, epidermal growth factor (EGF), and amphiregulin (AR) at the RNA level by Northern analysis and at the protein level by immunohistochemistry in primary non−small cell lung cancers and paired samples of benign lung tissue. EGF expression was not seen in either tumor or benign lung tissue. Overexpression of EGFR was found in 45% of tumors; while overexpression of TGF-α was seen in 61% of tumors, and decreased expression of AR was seen in 63% of tumors. Differential expression of EGFR, TGF-α, and AR was not influenced by cell type and tumor stage and did not correlate with disease-free or overall survival.[11] Thus, differential expression of EGFR and of some of its ligands is a common event in non−small cell lung cancers and may participate in initial tumor growth without necessarily influencing tumor progression.

Other studies, primarily in non−small cell lung cancer cell lines, have reported overexpression of the platelet-derived growth factor and of its receptor and of the HER2/neu receptor protein.[12] The clinical importance of the altered expression of these growth factors and their receptors needs to be defined.

The p53 tumor suppressor gene, which is frequently altered in human solid tumors, is either mutated or overexpressed in over half of non−small cell lung cancers. Structural and immunohistochemical abnormalities of p53 were investigated by in a tumor bank of paired non−small cell lung cancers and benign lung tissue developed by the Lung Cancer Study Group (LCSG).[13] Of the 85 patients studied, 64% showed p53 overexpression, and 51% had mutant p53 sequences in exons 5 to 8. However, the concordance rate between overexpression and mutation was only 67%, suggesting that several mechanisms contribute to p53 overexpression. In this clinically well-defined cohort of patients for whom follow-up data were available, p53 overexpression but not mutation was associated with a significantly worse overall survival rate.

Similar to K-ras point-mutations, p53 structural and immunohistochemical abnormalities are linked to smoking. However, only 10% or less of non−small cell lung cancers are found to contain both p53 abnormalities and K-ras mutations.

The type of p53 mutations are both carcinogen and tumor specific. Most mutations are missense rather than nonsense mutations and occur in highly conserved regions of the gene, usually in CpG dinucleotides. Lung cancers are characterized by G:C to T:A transversions in the nontranscribed DNA strand. Even aerodigestive tract tumors, which share a common cause in exposure to tobacco, manifest different patterns of p53 mutations.

Mutations of p53 in primary lung tumors are reported to be conserved in metastases developing from that tumor. Thus, the type of p53 mutation might discriminate between a new tumor, a second primary tumor, or a metastasis.

Another tumor suppressor gene commonly inactivated in non−small cell lung cancer is the Rb susceptibility gene. The Rb gene is inactivated in about one third of primary non−small cell lung cancers of all histologic types. No clear correlation has been established between Rb inactivation and survival in patients with early-stage non−small cell lung cancer.[14]

Several molecular genetic abnormalities linked to tumor progression are reported in primary non−small cell lung cancers. These abnormalities include lack of expression of the A- and H-related blood group antigens and expression of the protein encoded by bcl-2, which is known to be involved in apoptosis (programmed cell death).[15]

The carcinogenesis models suggest that clinical tumors develop as a result of multiple steps, including the activation of oncogenes and the inactivation of tumor suppressor genes. At least three abnormalities known to occur frequently in overt tumors (ie, deletion of the short arm of chromosome 3, abnormal expression of the p53 gene, and overexpression of the EGFR) have also been found in dysplastic bronchial epithelium. These are likely early steps involved in lung tumorigenesis. The precise sequence of these and other molecular steps leading to the transformation of normal bronchial epithelial cells to metaplasia, dysplasia, carcinoma in situ, or invasive and metastatic cancer remains to be determined.

Primary tumors, even when histologically similar, manifest disparate cellular abnormalities, which affect cell function at the cell surface (eg, EGFR and its ligands), within the cytoplasm (eg, K-*ras*), and ultimately within the nucleus (eg, Rb and p53). Some genetic changes may affect only tumor initiation or growth, whereas others may affect tumor progression (metastasis) or may act at several stages in lung tumorigenesis. As already mentioned, primary tumors with p53 mutations or overexpression rarely show K-*ras* point mutations or inactivation of Rb. This suggests that different cellular pathways may lead to clinically similar outcomes. For instance, EGFR activation leads to activation of the *ras* pathway or may induce transcription by activation of a group of proteins (the Stat proteins) through tyrosine phosphorylation. Conversely, p53 may promote cell proliferation by transactivating the EGFR promoter in the nucleus. Understanding the interplay between genetic changes in non–small cell lung cancers will provide insights into mechanisms of tumor growth and progression and will ultimately identify potential targets for cancer therapy.

NON–SMALL CELL LUNG CANCER

Non–small cell lung cancer is the most common lung neoplasm. Unfortunately, the mortality rate for this disease continues to rise in direct proportion to its incidence. This reflects the fact that only about 30% of patients are candidates for surgical resection. About 50% of patients present with disseminated disease, and another 20% present with disease that is too advanced locally to allow surgical resection. Modest improvements have occurred in the chemotherapy for non–small cell lung cancer, but none substantial enough to produce a significant impact on the overall mortality of this disease. Surgical resection remains the only curative form of treatment, and few patients are candidates for this approach.

Table 61-4. TNM CLASSIFICATION FOR STAGING SYSTEM OF NON–SMALL CELL LUNG CANCER

TNM DEFINITIONS

Primary Tumor

TX Tumor proved by the presence of malignant cells in bronchopulmonary secretions but not visualized roentgenographically or bronchoscopically, or any tumor that cannot be assessed as in a retreatment staging

T0 No evidence of primary tumor

Tis Carcinoma in situ

T1* A tumor that is 3 cm or less in greatest dimension, surrounded by lung or visceral pleura, and without evidence of invasion proximal to a lobar bronchus at bronchoscopy

T2 A tumor more than 3 cm in greatest dimension, or a tumor of any size that either invades the visceral pleura or has associated atelectasis or obstructive pneumonitis extending to the hilar region. At bronchoscopy, the proximal extent of demonstrable tumor must be within a lobar bronchus or at least 2 cm distal to the carina. Any associated atelectasis or obstructive pneumonitis must involve less than an entire lung

T3 A tumor of any size with direct extension into the chest wall (including superior sulcus tumors), diaphragm, or the mediastinal pleura or pericarcium without involving the heart, great vessels, trachea, esophagus, or vertebral body, or a tumor in the main bronchus within 2 cm of the carina without involving the carina

T4† A tumor of any size with invasion of the mediastinum or involving the heart, great vessels, trachea, esophagus, vertebral body, or carina or presence of malignant pleural effusion

Regional Lymph Node Involvement

N0 No demonstrable metastasis to regional lymph nodes

N1 Metastasis to lymph nodes in the peribronchial or the ipsilateral hilar region, or both, including direct extension

N2 Metastasis to ipsilateral mediastinal lymph nodes and subcarinal lymph nodes

N3 Metastasis to contralateral mediastinal lymph nodes, contralateral hilar lymph nodes, ipsilateral or contralateral scalene lymph nodes, or supraclavicular lymph nodes

Distant Metastasis

M0 No (known) distant metastasis

M1 Distant metastasis present—specify sites

STAGE GROUPING

Occult carcinoma	TX, N0, M0
Stage 0	Tis, carcinoma in situ
Stage I	T1, N0, M0
	T2, N0, M0
Stage II	T1, N1, M0
	T2, N1, M0
Stage IIIa	T3, N0, M0
	T3, N1, M0
	T1–3, N2, M0
Stage IIIb	Any T, N3, M0
	T4, any N, M0
Stage IV	Any T, any N, M1

* The uncommon superficial tumor of any size with its invasive component limited to the bronchial wall that may extend proximal to the main bronchus is classified as T1.

† Most pleural effusions associated with lung cancer are due to tumor. There are, however, some few patients in whom cytopathologic examination of pleural fluid (on more than one specimen) is negative for tumor and in whom the fluid is nonbloody and is not an exudate. In cases in which these elements and clinical judgment dictate that the effusion is not related to the tumor, the patient should be staged T1, T2, or T3, excluding effusion as a staging element.

Non−small cell lung cancer is classified into four stages. The staging system and the descriptors for each TNM stage are outlined in Table 61-4. In 1986, this system replaced the original American Joint Committee on Cancer staging system that had been in use since 1977. The current TNM system is internationally accepted, reconciles differences between the original staging system and a previous radiation oncology staging system, and incorporates information acquired during the past 15 years about factors affecting long-term survival. Specifically, it recognizes the negative effect of hilar nodal involvement on survival by shifting T1, N1 tumors from stage I to stage II; and it recognizes that stage III tumors encompass a broad spectrum of disease by subdividing them into stages IIIa and IIIb. Distant metastatic disease has been moved out of stage III and designated as stage IV in the new system. It is important to be aware of these changes because lung cancer survival rates published before 1986 may differ from current survival figures simply by virtue of use of the older staging system rather than because of true alterations in outcome.

Clinical Presentation and Diagnosis

Early-stage non−small cell lung cancers can cause hemoptysis, atelectasis, or postobstructive pneumonia if they are located centrally, or they can cause pain if they are located peripherally and extend into the chest wall, spine, or brachial plexus. However, most patients are referred to the surgeon because of an asymptomatic nodule or mass on a chest radiograph. Old chest radiographs are helpful in this situation. If the lesion has not grown in the past 2 years, it is more likely to be benign. Radiographic characteristics, such as a smooth contour, dense homogeneous calcification, or "popcorn" calcification, suggest diseases other than lung cancer (Fig. 61-1). Tissue diagnosis can be established by bronchoscopy for centrally located lesions or by percutaneous needle aspiration for peripheral

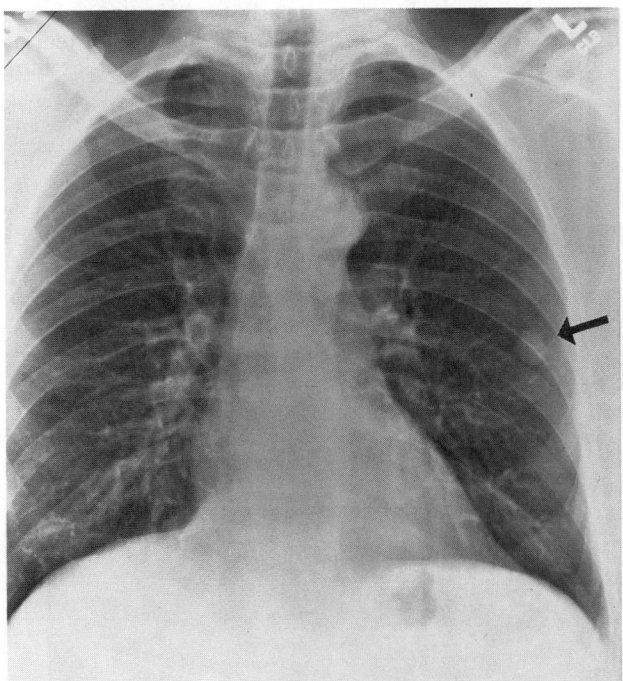

Figure 61-1. Smooth, well-circumscribed, left mid-lung field nodule (*arrow*) that did not change on serial chest radiographs during a 2-year period. This is most likely a benign pulmonary nodule, perhaps a hamartoma.

masses. Exploratory thoracotomy without a preoperative diagnosis is acceptable if the history and radiographic findings strongly suggest the possibility of lung cancer or if attempts to obtain a tissue diagnosis have failed and there is no evidence of distant disease. An algorithm for the management of solitary pulmonary nodules is shown in Figure 61-2.

Selection of Treatment

Selection of treatment for patients with non−small cell lung cancer is based on the stage of the disease at diagnosis and on the patient's overall medical condition. Stage IV disease is treated primarily with chemotherapy. Stage IIIb disease is treated with radiotherapy or combined chemoradiotherapy. Outside of well-controlled clinical trials using multimodality therapy for specific subsets of patients, surgical resection has no role in stage IIIb disease. In contrast, surgical resection is the treatment of choice for stages I and II. The most controversial area is the management of stage IIIa disease, for which surgical resection is occasionally the primary treatment but which is treated more often by a combination of chemotherapy, surgical resection, and radiotherapy.

The aims of the initial evaluation of a patient with non−small cell lung cancer are to determine whether distant metastatic disease is present and to assess the extent of intrathoracic disease. Common metastatic sites include the brain, supraclavicular nodes, contralateral lung, bone, liver, and adrenal glands. A thorough history and physical examination, combined with a plain chest radiograph and baseline laboratory data (complete blood count and serum sodium, calcium, alkaline phosphatase, and lactate dehydrogenase levels), may suggest the presence of metastatic disease. Abnormal findings are then investigated further by selected radionuclide, computed tomographic (CT), or magnetic resonance imaging scans and by needle aspiration biopsy or open biopsy, if necessary, to prove the extent of disease.

If the initial clinical evaluation does not suggest the presence of distant disease, the extent of further evaluation by various scans is controversial. Some physicians always perform a complete metastatic work-up with CT scans of the chest and abdomen, a CT or magnetic resonance imaging scan of the brain, and a bone scan. CT scanning of the chest and abdomen has become standard, as much to evaluate the extent of the primary tumor and the status of the mediastinal lymph nodes as to detect metastases in the ipsilateral or contralateral lung, liver, or adrenals. Additional scans in asymptomatic patients may detect the 5% to 10% of metastases that are occult, but these scans are not clearly cost-effective in patients with clinical stage I or II tumors who have no clinical indications of disease.

If there is no clinical evidence of extrathoracic disease, it is important to determine whether mediastinal nodal metastases (N2 or N3 disease) are present. This is accomplished by a combination of CT scanning and mediastinoscopy.[16] Mediastinal nodes 1 cm or less in diameter on CT scan are almost always benign. Mediastinal nodes larger than 1.5 cm are often malignant but are also sometimes enlarged because of underlying pulmonary disease or postobstructive pneumonia. Peripheral tumors without associated mediastinal adenopathy on CT scan have a 10% or less chance of nodal metastases and do not require mediastinoscopy (Fig. 61-3). In contrast, more centrally located tumors, or tumors with mediastinal adenopathy discovered by CT scan, warrant mediastinoscopy (Fig. 61-4). Most tumors can be adequately staged by cervical mediastinoscopy, which allows access to the

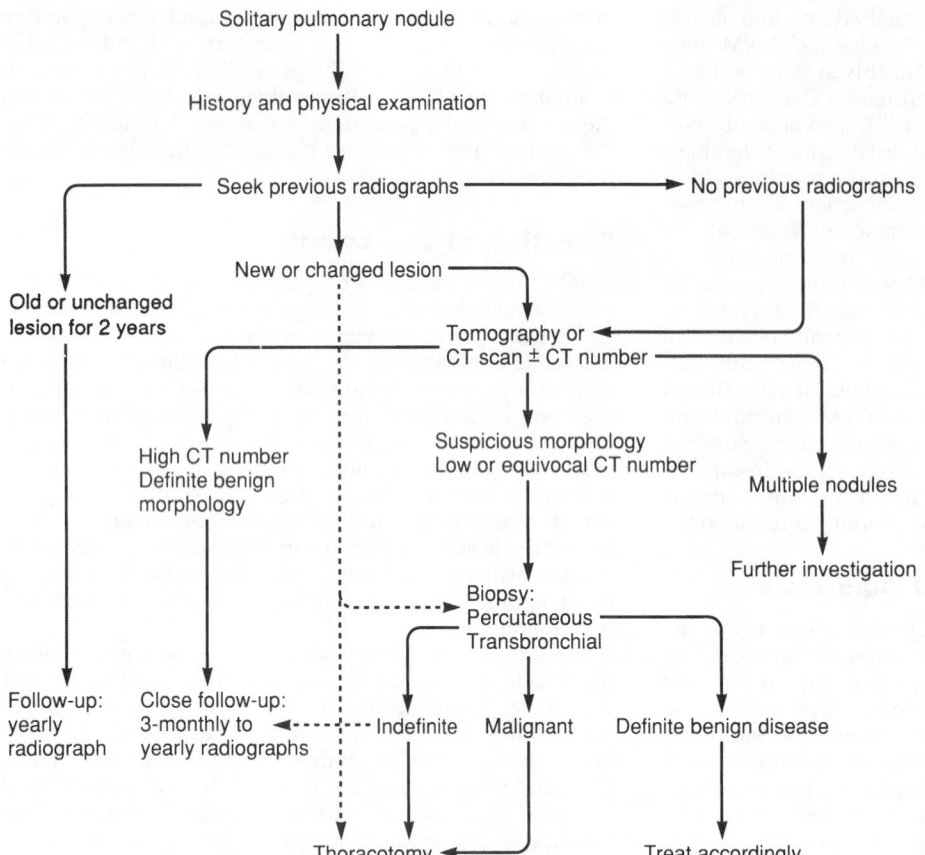

Figure 61-2. Algorithm for decision making in patients who present with solitary pulmonary nodules.

left and right paratracheal nodes, the right tracheobronchial angle nodes, and the subcarinal nodes. However, left upper lobe tumors drain both to the left paratracheal and tracheobronchial nodes and to the subaortic nodes. Complete mediastinal nodal staging requires either a combined cervical and parasternal approach or an extended cervical mediastinoscopy, whereby biopsy is performed on the subaortic nodes by passing the mediastinoscope over the aortic arch between the innominate and left carotid arteries. In the hands of experienced surgeons, mediastinoscopy carries virtually no mortality and minimal morbidity and fails to diagnose only the 10% of involved mediastinal nodes that are not technically accessible by this approach. Thus, mediastinos-

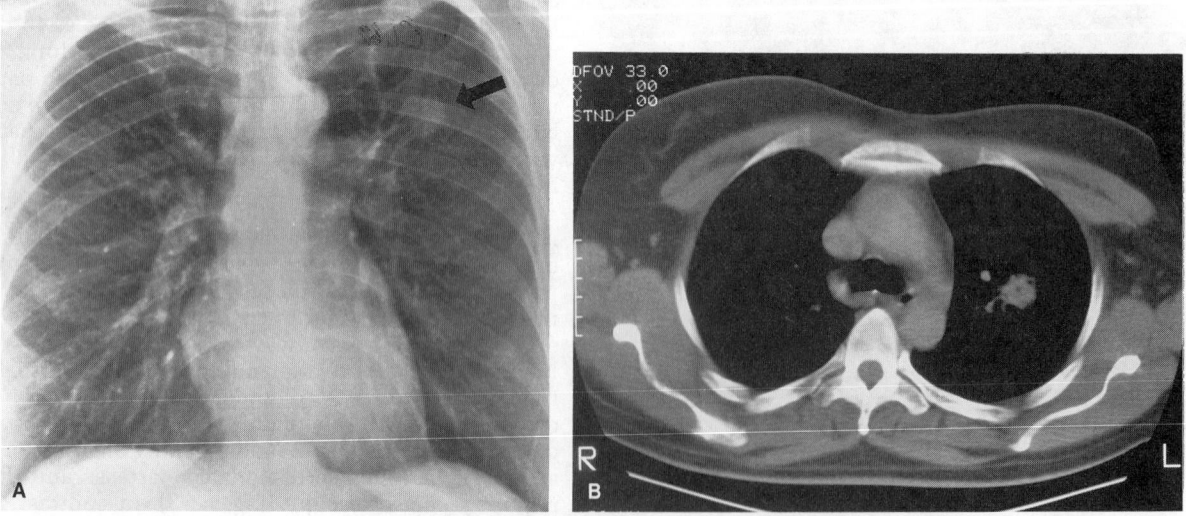

Figure 61-3. Solitary, irregular, left upper lobe mass (*arrow*) diagnosed incidentally on a routine chest radiograph in a 50-year-old nonsmoking woman. Chest CT scan confirmed the presence of the mass but did not demonstrate any mediastinal adenopathy. At exploratory thoracotomy, the patient had a T1, N0 adenocarcinoma.

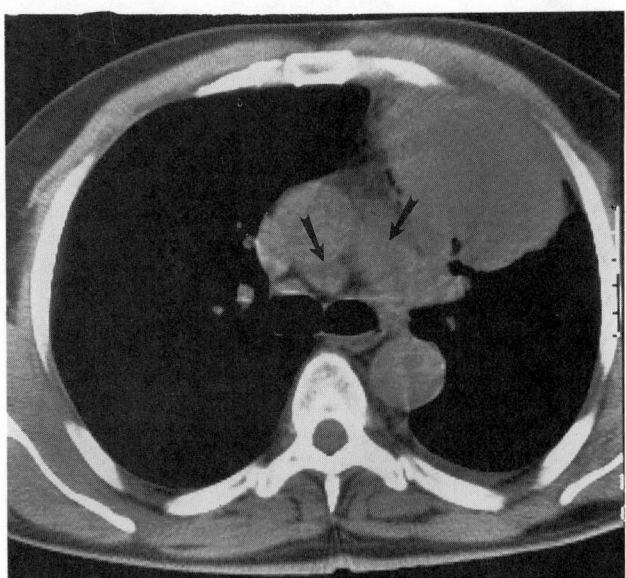

Figure 61-4. CT scan of a patient with a huge left upper lobe squamous cell cancer. Mediastinal adenopathy was observed on CT scan in the aortopulmonary window and in the pretracheal regions (*arrows*). Mediastinoscopy demonstrated enlarged but benign lymph nodes.

copy is crucial to avoiding a thoracotomy in patients with unresectable disease.

Patients with early-stage non–small cell lung cancer must also be evaluated to determine whether their pulmonary function and overall medical condition permit pulmonary resection. Because lung cancer patients are predominantly smokers older than 40 years of age, underlying coronary disease is common and is often a source of perioperative morbidity or mortality. The patient's cardiac status should be rigorously assessed if the history, physical examination, or baseline electrocardiogram suggests any cardiac dysfunction. Pulmonary function tests are obtained to determine the patient's ability to tolerate pulmonary resection. The details of pulmonary function testing as they relate to the risk of pulmonary resection are well covered in standard thoracic surgical texts and are not discussed in depth here. The forced expiratory volume in 1 second (FEV_1) is the most useful single parameter because most lung cancer patients have chronic obstructive pulmonary disease. In general, pulmonary resection can be tolerated if the postresection FEV_1 is 800 mL/s or greater. Patients who have an initial FEV_1 of 2 L/s or more can usually tolerate any form of pulmonary resection, including a pneumonectomy. Patients whose FEV_1 is less than 2 L/s should have a ventilation–perfusion lung scan performed to determine how much the area of planned pulmonary resection contributes to overall lung function. Sometimes, it contains primarily nonfunctional lung, particularly if the tumor is centrally located. Lung cancer patients may also have restrictive or interstitial lung disease because of occupational exposure to carcinogenic chemicals or dusts. This can be diagnosed by alterations in the total lung capacity, the vital capacity, and the diffusion capacity. Baseline arterial blood gases mainly identify patients whose risk is high because of CO_2 retention (ie, P_{CO_2} greater than 50 mmHg). Hypoxemia may simply reflect the presence of a shunt or ventilation–perfusion mismatch caused by the tumor and is not usually helpful in selecting patients for pulmonary resection. Measure-

ments of parameters such as the diffusion capacity are not routine in many pulmonary function laboratories, however. Unless the laboratory is specifically aware of what parameters need to be measured, a seriously incomplete evaluation may be performed. It is important for the surgeon to understand which tests need to be ordered and to know how to interpret them.

Patients who are smoking actively at the time of diagnosis should quit smoking for at least 2 weeks before surgery. Patients are placed on intensive bronchodilator therapy and are treated with appropriate antibiotics if they have chronic bronchitis. These measures greatly reduce the risk of postoperative atelectasis or pneumonia.

Surgical Resection of Stage I and II Disease

Stage I and II non–small cell lung cancers are best treated by surgical resection. The goals of pulmonary resection in patients with lung cancer are to remove the primary tumor completely and to stage it definitively. The details of surgical techniques and of perioperative care are amply described in standard thoracic surgical texts and are not discussed here. The extent of pulmonary resection is dictated by the location and the size of the primary tumor and by whether there is involvement of the adjacent bronchopulmonary nodes. Depending on these factors, a pneumonectomy, lobectomy, or bilobectomy is the appropriate operation and should provide microscopically negative vascular and bronchial margins. Several retrospective series suggest that limited resections, wedge resection, or segmentectomy, rather than lobectomy, may be adequate for some early-stage (T1, N0) tumors. However, a prospective randomized trial by the North American LCSG has shown that limited resection is associated with a higher rate of local recurrence and poorer survival than lobectomy in patients with T1, N0 tumors, especially adenocarcinomas.[17]

Tumors with direct extension into the chest wall, diaphragm, or pericardium should undergo resection of the adjacent involved structure en bloc with the pulmonary resection. Reconstruction is performed as necessary (Fig. 61-5). On the other hand, tumors that have extensive endobronchial disease without involvement of the surrounding vascular or lymphatic structures can sometimes be completely removed by a lobectomy with segmental resection of the bronchus (sleeve resection), thereby preserving lung function.

Clinical staging of mediastinal nodes is inaccurate and should not be substituted for careful intraoperative staging performed by mediastinal nodal sampling or mediastinal lymph node dissection. Meticulous pathologic staging provides accurate prognostic information and allows appropriate decisions to be made regarding the use of postoperative adjuvant therapy. Complete en bloc mediastinal lymph node dissection is advocated by some groups as the most accurate means of staging. For right-sided tumors, this involves en bloc removal of the entire subcarinal packet of nodes and en bloc removal of all the paratracheal lymph nodes located between the trachea posteriorly, the superior vena cava anteriorly, the innominate artery superiorly, and the tracheobronchial angle inferiorly. For left-sided tumors, the dissection includes en bloc removal of the subcarinal nodes and of the subaortic and periaortic nodes. If technically accessible, the left tracheobronchial angle nodes are also removed. Whether this extensive dissection results in more accurate staging than simply sampling lymph nodes from each one of these areas remains controversial. No matter which method is chosen, each

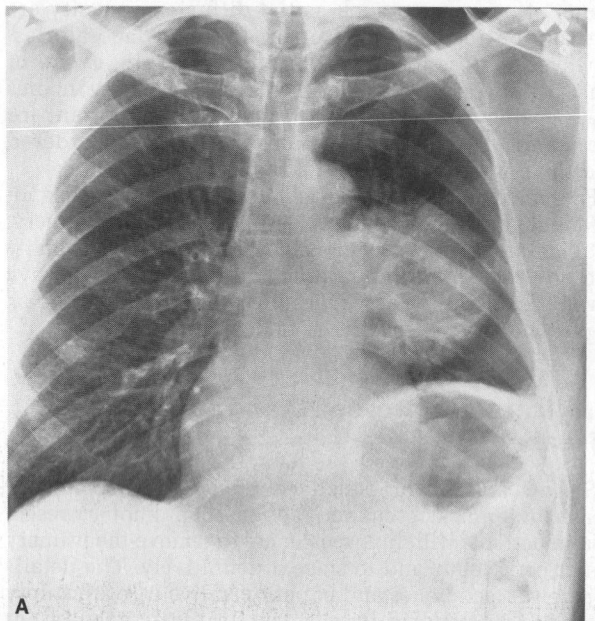

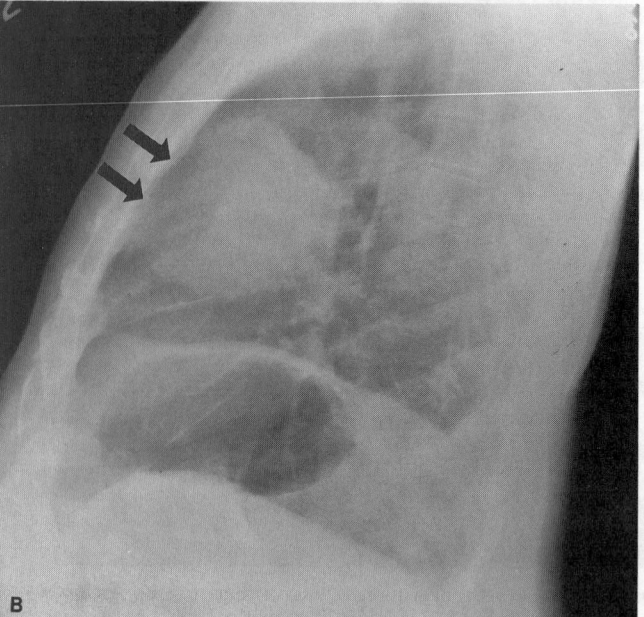

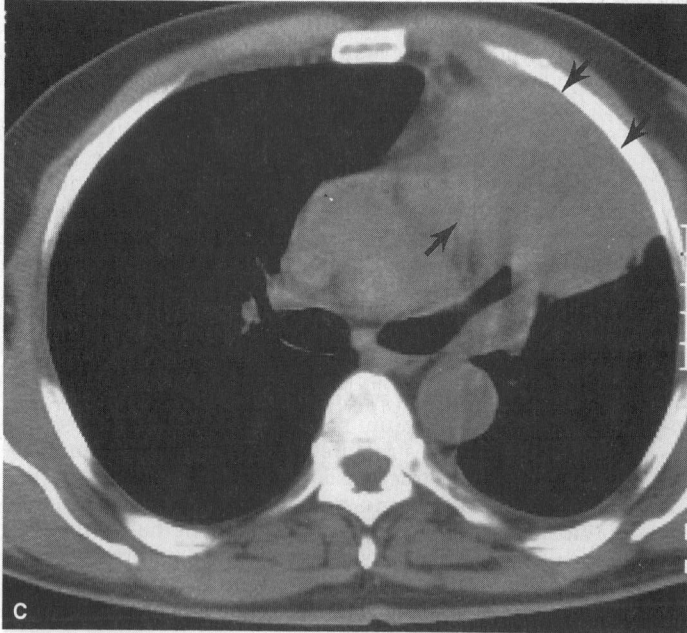

Figure 61-5. Imaging studies from the same patient as in Figure 61-4. (*A*) Posteroanterior chest radiograph shows an elevated left hemidiaphragm suggestive of phrenic nerve involvement by the mass. (*B*) Lateral chest radiograph shows extension of the mass to the anterior chest wall (*arrow*). (*C*) CT scan suggests both pericardial and chest wall involvement (*arrows*). At thoracotomy, the patient had involvement of the chest wall, phrenic nerve, and pericardium. All were resected en bloc with the tumor.

lymph node group must be identified by the surgeon and submitted appropriately labeled to the pathologist. Standard nomenclature and numbering systems are available in lymph node maps designed for this purpose. The lymph node map of Naruke (Fig. 61-6) is gradually being supplanted by the lymph node map developed by the American Thoracic Society and modified by the LCSG (Fig. 61-7). The latter map has more precise anatomic definitions of the location of lymph nodes and allows correlation of CT scan findings with surgical findings.

Survival

The long-term survival after surgical resection for non–small cell lung cancer is linked to the pathologic stage of disease. The overall 5-year survival rates are shown in Table 61-5. They range from 60% to 80% for stage I tumors, from 40% to 50% for stage II tumors, and from 20% to 30% for stage IIIa tumors. Nodal involvement has the strongest

adverse influence on survival. This is well illustrated by the differences in survival among subsets of stage IIIa tumors. Large peripheral tumors that extend directly into the chest wall but have no nodal involvement (T3, N0) are associated with a 40% to 50% 5-year survival rate after complete resection, whereas only a 15% survival rate is seen when hilar or mediastinal nodes are involved. The status of the primary tumor has a lesser but still important effect on survival. Within stage I, for instance, T1, N0 tumors have an 80% 5-year survival rate, substantially better than the 60% 5-year survival rate of T2, N0 tumors.

Several series suggest that histology also has an impact on survival. In stage I or II non–small cell lung cancer, the North American LCSG consistently observed a better disease-free and overall survival for squamous cell cancer than for nonsquamous tumors. The influence of histology has not been reported in all series and is not seen in stage III and IV tumors. However, T and N status and histology

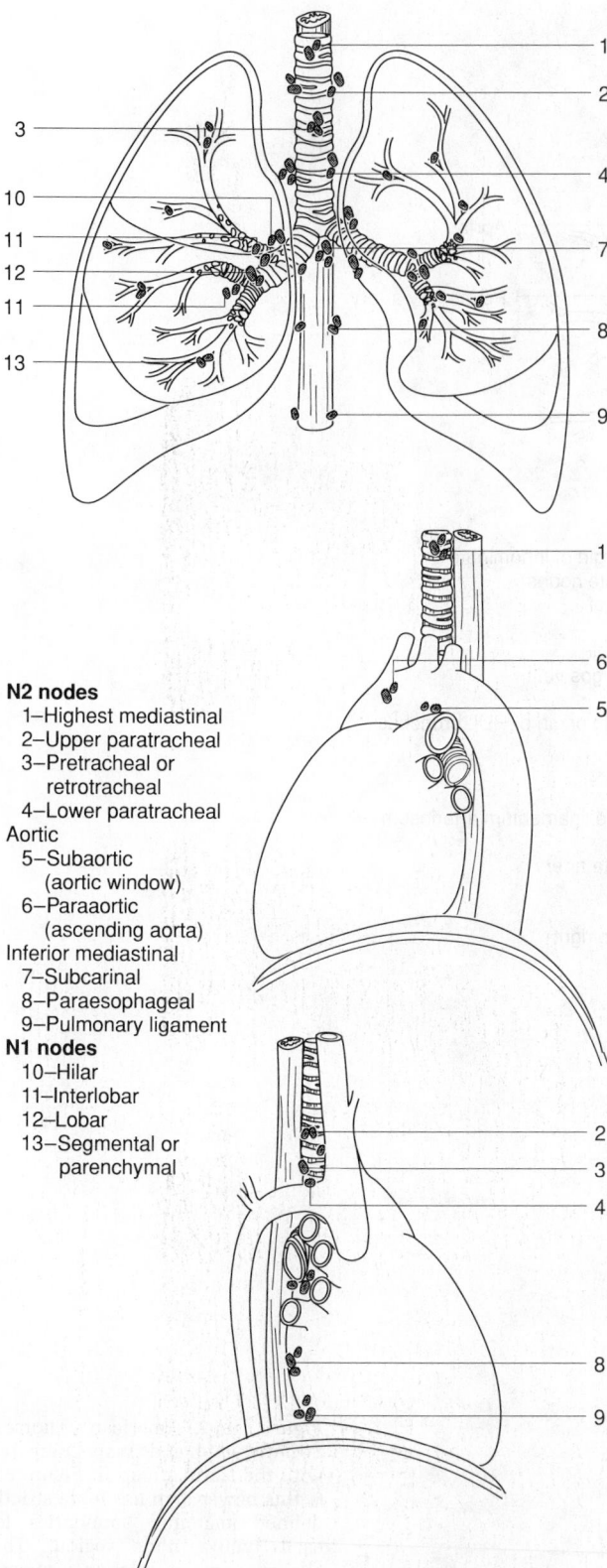

N2 nodes
1—Highest mediastinal
2—Upper paratracheal
3—Pretracheal or
   retrotracheal
4—Lower paratracheal
Aortic
5—Subaortic
   (aortic window)
6—Paraaortic
   (ascending aorta)
Inferior mediastinal
7—Subcarinal
8—Paraesophageal
9—Pulmonary ligament
N1 nodes
10—Hilar
11—Interlobar
12—Lobar
13—Segmental or
   parenchymal

Figure 61-6. Naruke lymph node map. (After Manual for staging of cancer, ed 3. Philadelphia, JB Lippincott, 1988:115)

provide only a crude estimate of outcome. Within a given TNM category and histology, it is still impossible to discern which patients will experience relapse. A better understanding of lung cancer biology is needed to define which patients are truly at risk for recurrence.

Patterns of Recurrence

The predominant sites of relapse for all stages of non–small cell lung cancer after surgical resection are distant metastases. Whether the original tumor was stage I or III, the risk of metastatic disease is remarkably consistent at 70% to 80%. Local recurrence is more common with squamous cell carcinomas than with tumors of nonsquamous histology. For all stages of disease, the brain is the single most common site of relapse. Brain metastases also occur more frequently in nonsquamous tumors. Other common metastatic sites include bone, ipsilateral or contralateral lung, liver, and the adrenal glands.

Up to 80% of recurrences develop in the first 2 years after operation, and virtually all recurrences related to the original primary tumor occur within 5 years after operation. No more than half of patients with stage II and III disease survive long term, so it is difficult to gauge what happens to this patient group beyond 5 years. Most stage I patients, however, particularly those with T1, N0 tumors, do enjoy long-term survival. As a result, they experience patterns of disease not seen in the remainder of the lung cancer population. The North American LCSG followed 907 patients with T1, N0 tumors for a minimum of 5 years after operation.[18] Recurrences of the original primary tumor were rare after 5 years, but after that time, the occurrence rate of new pulmonary cancers increased. Patients also faced consistent risk of new nonpulmonary primary cancers during the first 5 years after operation and thereafter. New nonpulmonary malignancies developed in a wide variety of sites, but breast, colon, and prostate cancers were the most common.

This emphasizes the importance of long-term follow-up after resection of early-stage non–small cell lung cancer. Most thoracic oncologists see their lung cancer patients every 3 months during the first 2 years after operation, then every 6 months until 5 years after operation, and annually thereafter. There is no single way to detect recurrence, so follow-up includes a combination of history, physical examination, serial chest radiographs, and screening blood tests, including a complete blood count and chemistry profile.

Adjuvant Therapy

The substantial risk of recurrent disease after resection of early-stage non–small cell lung cancer has engendered efforts to improve survival rates by the addition of adjuvant therapy. Retrospective single institution studies suggest that postoperative adjuvant therapy is beneficial. The major prospective randomized trials of adjuvant therapy in resected non–small cell lung cancer were performed by the North American LCSG, a multidisciplinary clinical cooperative research group funded by the National Cancer Institute. The results of these trials show that adjuvant therapy can alter the patterns of relapse and improve disease-free but not overall survival.

In stage I disease, few patients relapse, and there is no specific means of identifying those who will. Therefore, if adjuvant treatment is used in this group, it must be relatively nontoxic. In the early 1970s, a single-institution, nonrandomized study suggested that immunotherapy with intrapleural bacillus Calmette-Guérin (BCG) might improve survival after resection of stage I lung cancer. This prompted a large prospective randomized trial by the LCSG comparing intrapleural BCG to placebo in patients with resected stage I non–small cell lung cancer. Treatment was well tolerated, but no survival advantage was observed in the group of patients treated with BCG.[19]

Several retrospective series suggested that mediastinal irradiation might improve survival after resection of stage

A

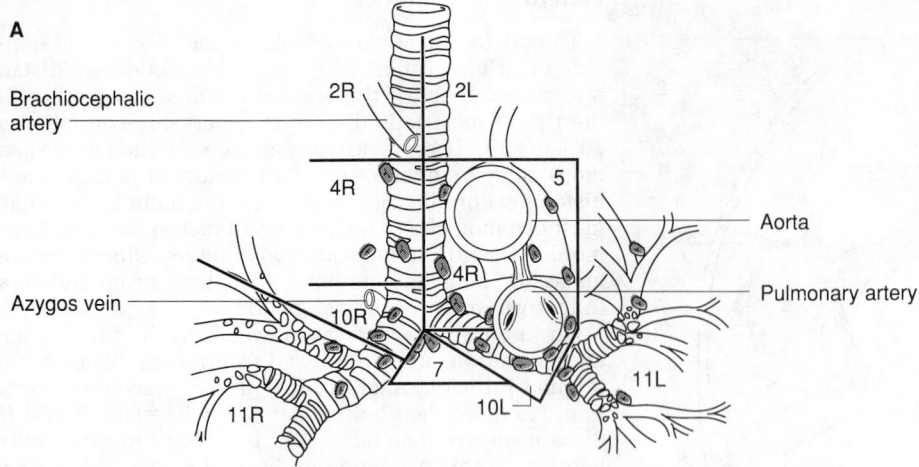

N2 nodes
Superior mediastinal nodes

2 [2R–*Right upper paratracheal:* Between intersection of caudal margin of innominate
   artery with trachea and the apex of the lung (suprainnominate nodes)
   2L–*Left upper paratracheal:* Between top of aortic arch and apex of
   the lung (supraaortic nodes)

4 [4R–*Right lower paratracheal:* Between intersection of caudal margin
   of innominate artery with trachea and cephalic border of azygos vein
   4L–*Left lower paratracheal:* Between top of aortic arch and carina

10 [10R–*Right tracheobronchial:* From cephalic border of azygos vein to origin of RUL bronchus
   10L–*Left tracheobronchial:* Between carina and LUL bronchus
      (medial to ligamentum arteriosum)

Aortic nodes

[5–*Aortopulmonary:* Subaortic and paraaortic nodes; lateral to the ligamentum arteriosum
   (proximal to first branch of left PA)
   6–*Anterior mediastinal:* Anterior to ascending aorta or innominate artery

Inferior mediastinal nodes

[7–*Subcarinal:* Caudal to carina of the trachea
   8–*Paraesophageal:* Dorsal to posterior wall of the trachea and to right
      or left of the midline of the esophagus
   9–*Pulmonary ligament:* Within the pulmonary ligament

N1 nodes

[11–*Interlobar*
   12–*Lobar*
   13–*Segmental*
   14–*Subsegmental*

B

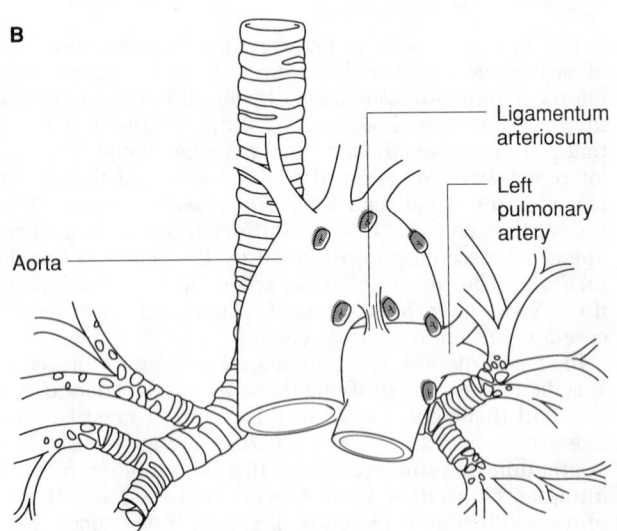

Figure 61-7. American Thoracic Society lymph node map. Compared with the Naruke map in Figure 61-6, this newer map has more strictly defined anatomic boundaries for each lymph node region. This allows easy correlation between findings at operation and findings on the chest CT scan. (After Am Rev Resp Dis 1983;127:659)

Table 61-5. **NEW STAGE DATA BASE: CUMULATIVE PERCENTAGE SURVIVING 5 YEARS AND MEDIAN SURVIVAL BY CLINICAL AND SURGICAL TNM SUBSETS**

TNM Subset	Clinical			Surgical		
	Patients	Patients Surviving (%)	Median Survival (mo)	Patients	Patients Surviving (%)	Median Survival (mo)
T1, N0, M0	591	61.9	60+	429	68.5	60+
T2, N0, M0	1012	35.8	26	436	59.0	60+
T1, N1, M0	19	33.6	20	67	54.1	60+
T2, N1, M0	176	22.7	17	250	40.0	29
T3, N0, M0	221	7.6	8	57	44.2	26
T3, N1, M0	71	7.7	8	29	17.6	16
Any N2, M0	497	4.9	11	168	28.8	22
Any M1	1166	1.7	6	—	—	—
Total	3753			1436		

II and especially stage IIIa tumors. In many communities, postoperative radiotherapy became the standard of care in this setting. Because patients with squamous cell tumors have the highest risk of local recurrence, they are the most likely to benefit from adjuvant radiotherapy. The LCSG conducted a trial comparing mediastinal irradiation to no treatment after complete resection of stage II and III squamous cell carcinomas.[20] Radiotherapy did not improve survival but was remarkably effective in preventing local recurrence.

Patients with nonsquamous tumors are especially prone to distant metastases and therefore constitute the ideal target group for adjuvant chemotherapy. The LCSG evaluated the benefit of adjuvant CAP (cyclophosphamide [Cytoxan], doxorubicin [Adriamycin], and cisplatin) chemotherapy in three separate randomized trials. In the first trial, patients with completely resected stage II and III adenocarcinomas and large cell cancers were randomized to receive postoperative CAP chemotherapy versus immunotherapy.[21] Disease-free survival was better in the chemotherapy group, but there was no difference in overall survival between the two groups. In the second trial, chemoradiotherapy was superior to radiotherapy alone in patients with incompletely resected stage IIIa adenocarcinoma or large cell carcinoma. Unfortunately, these modest benefits were not seen in a third trial that compared adjuvant CAP chemotherapy to no treatment after complete resection of early-stage (T2, N0 and T1, N1) lung cancer.[22]

Radiotherapy is still often given to patients after resection of stage IIIa tumors but with the understanding that it serves mainly to prevent local recurrence. Adjuvant chemotherapy for stage II or III completely resected tumors is not widely accepted because of its failure to improve overall survival in clinical trials.

Treatment of Stage IIIa Disease

Role of Surgical Resection

Stage IIIa non–small cell lung cancer includes a heterogenous group of tumors with widely varying survival rates after surgical resection. T3, N0 tumors involving the chest wall, pericardium, diaphragm, or main-stem bronchi are the most favorable stage IIIa tumor subsets. Complete resection is associated with a 5-year survival rate of 25% to 40% and is considered the standard treatment of these tumors.[23,24] Exclusion of the presence of N2 mediastinal nodal disease by mediastinoscopy is mandatory before thoracotomy because less than 10% of patients with T3, N2 tumors are cured by surgical resection alone.[25]

The most controversial and complex part of the treatment of stage IIIa non–small cell lung cancer is the management of patients with N2 disease. Reported 5-year survival rates after resection for N2 disease are usually 20% to 30% but range from 0% to 40%. This variation reflects the extent of mediastinal nodal involvement, the T status of the primary tumor, and the ability to perform a complete resection. With respect to mediastinal nodal involvement, adverse prognostic factors include the presence of extracapsular nodal disease, multiple levels of involved lymph nodes, and the presence of superior mediastinal nodal metastases.

Many reported series present an inappropriately optimistic view of the benefit of surgical resection for N2 disease because they focus on highly selected groups of patients. The experience reported by Martini and Flehinger[26] places surgical resection for N2 disease in perspective because it examines the outcome of treatment of all patients with N2 disease, not just a small subset. From 1974 to 1981, 1598 patients were seen with non–small cell lung cancer, of whom 706 had mediastinal nodal metastases. Only 151 patients, or 21% of all patients with N2 disease, had technically complete resections of the primary tumor and all accessible mediastinal lymph nodes. The survival rate of these 151 patients was 29% at 5 years. Moreover, the subset of 33 patients who had clinical N2 disease (mediastinal nodal involvement extensive enough to be visible on chest radiograph or at bronchoscopy) had only an 8% survival rate at 3 years. Thus, only 16.7% of all patients really benefited in the long term from surgical resection. Outcome was also influenced by the T status of the primary tumor, with T2 or T3 tumors faring significantly worse than T1 tumors. These results have been corroborated by the experience of several other groups (Table 61-6). Most surgeons consider resecting only those patients who have a T1 or T2 primary tumor and single-level, intranodal N2 disease.

Two randomized clinical trials challenge the concept of surgical resection as primary treatment for any patients with N2 disease. Rosell and colleagues[27] randomized 60 patients with stage IIIa non–small cell lung cancer (16 of whom did not have N2 disease) to undergo surgical resection or to receive three cycles of cisplatin-based chemotherapy followed by surgical resection. The median survival was significantly longer (26 versus 8 months) in the patients receiving preoperative chemotherapy than in patients going directly to surgical resection. A similar study from the M. D. Anderson Cancer Center confirms these results.[28] Both trials were stopped early because of the highly significant differences between the two study arms. These two studies suggest that it may be appropriate to

Table 61-6. RESULTS OF PHASE III TRIALS COMPARING RADIOTHERAPY ALONE TO SEQUENTIAL CHEMORADIOTHERAPY FOR STAGE III NON–SMALL CELL LUNG CANCER

Investigators	Patients	Chemotherapy	Radiotherapy (Gy)	Group	Survival	
					Median (mo)	2-y (%)
van Houtte et al, 1984[64]	59	CDDP and VP-16	55(C)	CT-RT	11	—
				RT	11	—
Dillman et al, 1990[32]	180	CDDP and Vbl	60(C)	CT-RT	13.8	26
				RT	9.7	13
Mattson et al, 1988[65]	228	CAP	55(S)	CT-RT	11.0	19
				RT	10.4	17
Morton et al, 1988[66]	121	MACC	60(C)	CT-RT	10.5	23
				RT	9.7	12
Trovo et al, 1990[67]	111	CAMP	4500(C)	CT-RT	11.7	15
				RT	10	15
Le Chevalier et al, 1991[68]	353	VCPC	65(C)	CT-RT	12	21
				RT	10	14

CDDP, cisplatin; VP-16, etoposide; CAP, cyclophosphamide, doxorubicin, cisplatin; MACC, methotrexate, doxorubicin, cyclophosphamide, lomustine; CAMP, cyclophosphamide, doxorubicin, methotrexate, procarbazine; Vbl, vinblastine; (C), continuous course; (S), split course.

consider all patients with N2 disease diagnosed at mediastinoscopy for induction chemotherapy. Unfortunately, because pretreatment mediastinoscopy was not mandated in either trial, some patients who did not have N2 disease were included. The results of these trials are not universally accepted because of the small numbers of patients enrolled, the lack of systematic pretreatment staging, and the unusually poor survival of patients in the control arms.

Rationale for Neoadjuvant Therapy

Although a few patients with minimal N2 disease benefit from surgical resection as their primary form of treatment, most patients have more extensive nodal involvement and are not surgical candidates. Until the 1980s, the standard treatment for such patients was radiotherapy. The survival rates after radiation are harder to interpret than after surgical resection because most series include a mixture of stage IIIa and IIIb patients and do not define the precise extent of nodal involvement. Sequential trials by the Radiation Therapy Oncology Group showed that high-dose, continuous irradiation yields the best chance of local control.[29] Distant metastatic disease, however, is the dominant form of relapse after radiotherapy, just as it is after surgical resection. The poor long-term survival after irradiation or surgical resection and the risk of distant metastatic disease prompted investigation of multimodality therapy for stage III non–small cell lung cancer.

Early Trials of Neoadjuvant Therapy

The concept of preoperative therapy followed by surgical resection (*neoadjuvant* therapy) dates back to 1955 when Bromley[30] used an average dose of 47 Gy to treat 66 patients before surgical resection. At operation, no viable tumor was found in 29 of 62 (47%) patients, but 10 patients died of complications in the first month, and only 2 patients were alive 5 years after operation. At the time, the natural history of non–small cell lung cancer was not as well understood, the methods of staging not as accurate, and the importance of distant metastases not fully recognized. Effective chemotherapy did not exist, and it was hoped that an approach that increased resectability might lead to better long-term survival. Thus, early neoadjuvant trials focused on using preoperative irradiation.

Several subsequent studies further explored this approach.[31] All these trials were flawed by a lack of pretreatment staging, by the use of widely varying amounts of radiation, and by excessively long intervals between irradiation and surgical resection. Nonetheless, it was apparent that aggressive local treatment did not improve long-term survival even though radiation could sterilize tumor in a significant number of patients. Fifty to 80% of patients developed distant metastases during or shortly after treatment, emphasizing the need for systemic therapy in stage III non–small cell lung cancer.

Recent Neoadjuvant Therapy Trials

Chemotherapy is now the primary treatment for most patients with stage IIIa (N2) disease, with surgical resection, radiotherapy, or both being added to optimize control of locoregional disease. Many neoadjuvant therapy trials have been performed. Most are phase II studies, designed to test the feasibility of this treatment. It is difficult to assess whether one neoadjuvant regimen is superior to others because of wide variations in the types of induction therapy and the eligibility criteria among trials. The initial neoadjuvant trials using induction chemotherapy were developed in the early 1980s when less information about the natural history of stage III lung cancer was available. Therefore, they included a heterogeneous patient population. A better understanding of the natural history of early-stage lung cancer and the use of the new International Staging System in 1986 have allowed recent trials to focus on more uniform patient populations and have made it easier to interpret trial results.

Although many different treatment regimens have been used in neoadjuvant trials, they can be grouped into two major categories: (1) chemoradiotherapy without surgical resection and (2) chemotherapy or chemoradiotherapy followed by surgical resection.

Trials of Chemoradiotherapy Without Surgical Resection. The feasibility of combined chemoradiotherapy without surgical resection for stage III non–small cell lung cancer was shown in several phase II trials. Several phase III randomized trials have compared radiotherapy alone with combined chemoradiotherapy. These trials cannot be equated with trials of neoadjuvant therapy that include surgical resection because patients entered on nonsurgical trials are staged clinically without the benefit of mediastinoscopy. Therefore, nonsurgical trials include mixtures of stage IIIa and IIIb cancers and may even include some patients who have earlier-stage disease but are thought erroneously to be stage III because of mediastinal adenopathy on CT scan.

Three different strategies have been investigated for combining chemotherapy and radiotherapy. The concept of alternating chemotherapy and radiotherapy has been explored in phase II trials but has not been tested in randomized trials. Phase III trials comparing radiotherapy to chemoradiotherapy have used either sequential treatment with induction chemotherapy followed by radiotherapy or concurrent chemoradiotherapy. Both of these approaches have theoretic advantages. Sequential treatment potentially allows more intensive chemotherapy and higher-dose irradiation, whereas concurrent chemoradiotherapy potentially allows both radiosensitization and effective systemic therapy, provided the combined toxicity is tolerable.

The results of phase III trials comparing radiotherapy alone to sequential chemoradiotherapy are outlined in Table 61-6. These trials confirmed the feasibility of combined-modality treatment, and some found modest treatment advantages (eg, better control of systemic disease). The trial conducted by the Cancer and Leukemia Group B (CALGB) showed a significant improvement in overall survival for the chemoradiotherapy arm.[32] An intergroup trial by the Radiation Therapy Oncology Group and Eastern Cooperative Oncology Group confirms the results of the CALGB trial. This three-arm randomized study compared standard fractionation radiotherapy, hyperfractionated radiotherapy, and sequential chemoradiotherapy as given in the CALGB trial. Preliminary results found that patients in the chemoradiotherapy arm experienced a better survival than those receiving either form of radiotherapy alone.[33]

At least four randomized trials comparing radiotherapy to concurrent chemoradiotherapy have been reported (Table 61-7). Two of these, the trial by the European Organization for Research and Treatment of Cancer and the trial by the LCSG, have shown a benefit for the combined modality arm. The European trial demonstrated improved overall survival for patients who received daily cisplatin and concurrent radiotherapy.[34] As mentioned previously the LCSG trial, performed in patients who had earlier-stage disease (ie, positive surgical margin, or the highest mediastinal node positive after surgical resection) found an improved, recurrence-free survival in the chemoradiotherapy arm. The benefit in overall survival was lost after the third year of follow-up.[35]

The varying results among phase III trials comparing radiotherapy to chemoradiotherapy may be related to several factors, including differences in total radiation dose and method of administration (split versus continuous course); differences in chemotherapy dose, especially with respect to cisplatin; and differences in patient selection based on staging criteria. Taken as a whole, the results of multiple phase II and III trails show that combined chemoradiotherapy can be administered safely to patients with stage III non–small cell lung cancer and leads to a modest but real survival benefit compared with radiotherapy alone.

Neoadjuvant Trials That Include Surgical Resection. These trials have also used two different treatment strategies: induction chemotherapy alone or concurrent chemoradiotherapy before surgical resection. The rationale for chemotherapy alone as induction treatment is that it potentially allows greater dose intensity as well as the use of some drugs, such as mitomycin, that cannot be administered in conjunction with radiation. Proponents of this approach also believe that chemotherapy provides as effective induction treatment as combined chemoradiotherapy and that separating the two modalities allows the use of irradiation postoperatively when a higher total dose can be given. Proponents of concurrent preoperative chemoradiotherapy believe that this approach provides adequate systemic treatment of micrometastatic disease and more effective control of bulky primary and mediastinal tumors.

Neoadjuvant Trials Using Chemotherapy Alone Before Surgical Resection. Several small phase II trials have demonstrated the feasibility of combining induction chemotherapy with subsequent pulmonary resection in patients with initially unresectable stage III non–small cell lung cancers. As mentioned previously, Martini and colleagues[26] retrospectively identified a large group of patients with clinical N2 disease who did not benefit from surgical resection as their primary form of treatment. In 1984, they initiated a trial of high-dose cisplatin-based chemotherapy followed by surgical resection for these patients. Induction therapy included vinblastine, mitomycin, and cisplatin (MVP regimen). Postoperative irradiation was given to patients who had persistent mediastinal nodal tumor at thoracotomy, and all patients received two additional cycles of postoperative chemotherapy. From 1984 to 1991, 136 patients were treated in this manner.[36] The overall response rate to induction chemotherapy was 77% (105 of 136 patients), and the complete resection rate was 65% (89 of 136 patients). There was no histologic evidence

Table 61-7. RESULTS OF PHASE III TRIALS COMPARING RADIOTHERAPY TO CONCURRENT CHEMORADIOTHERAPY FOR STAGE III NON–SMALL CELL LUNG CANCER

Investigators	Patients	Chemotherapy	Radiotherapy (Gy)	Group	Survival Median (mo)	2-y (%)
Ansari et al, 1991[69]	200	CDDP days 1, 22, 43	60	CRT	9	5
			60	RT	10	9
Trovo et al, 1991[70]	180	Daily CDDP	60(C)	RT	ND	—
			45(C)	CRT	ND	—
Schaake-Koning et al, 1992[34]	334	Weekly CDDP	55(S)	CRT	—	19
		Daily CDDP		CRT	—	26
				CRT	—	13
Sadeghi et al, 1991[71]	154	CAP	40(S)	CRT	~20	~40
			40(S)	RT	~14	~35

CDDP, cisplatin; CAP, cyclophosphamide, doxorubicin, cisplatin; (C), continuous course; (S), split course; ND, no difference; CRT, concurrent chemoradiotherapy; RT, radiotherapy.

of tumor in the resected specimens of 19 patients, for a complete pathologic response rate of 21% (19 of 89 patients). The overall survival rate for all 136 patients at 5 years was 17%, with a median survival of 19 months, a distinct improvement over the historical survival rate of 8% at 3 years for this group of patients. There were seven treatment-related deaths (5%), five of which were postoperative deaths.

Two other groups, the Toronto group and the LCSG, performed trials designed to corroborate this experience. Similar response and resectability rates were seen, but the treatment-related mortality rate was higher, in the range of 15%.[37,38] These three studies demonstrate that neoadjuvant therapy with MVP is feasible and effective. The low mortality rate in the Memorial trial reflects careful patient selection and management by physicians experienced in the use of this regimen. As usual, it is difficult to reproduce the results of a single-institution trial in a multiinstitutional setting. Enthusiasm for the MVP regimen in the oncology community at large has been tempered by the perceived risk of mitomycin-induced pulmonary toxicity, especially postoperative adult respiratory distress syndrome, and the side effects of high-dose cisplatin. Many oncologists believe that similar results can be achieved with less toxic regimens. Analysis of the Memorial experience identified 12 patients (8.8%) thought to have mitomycin-related pulmonary toxicity. This appeared to be dose-related, occurring only in patients who had received a total dose of 24 mg/m[2], and these patients responded to treatment with corticosteroids.

Neoadjuvant Trials Using Combined Chemoradiotherapy Before Surgical Resection. Most neoadjuvant trials used both chemotherapy and radiotherapy as induction treatment. Trials of this design have been reported by the LCSG, the Rush-Presbyterian group, and the CALGB (Table 61-8). The most recent and largest phase II neoadjuvant trial using concurrent chemoradiotherapy was performed by the Southwest Oncology Group (SWOG). This study enrolled both stage IIIa (N2) and IIIb patients, including patients with N3 disease, and mandated pathologic documentation of initial tumor stage. The induction therapy was two cycles of cisplatin and etoposide (VP-16) with 4500 cGy of fully concurrent radiation. For the 126 eligible patients entered in study, the response rate to induction therapy was 59%, and the resectability rates were 85% for patients with stage IIIa (N2) and 80% for patients with stage IIIb tumors. The 2-year survival rate was 37% for

stage IIIa (N2) and 39% for stage IIIb patients, considerably better than historical experience for these same groups of patients.[39]

Two notable differences between the SWOG trial and earlier neoadjuvant trials were the use of higher-dose continuous radiation (ie, 4500 cGy, as opposed to 3000 cGy continuous or 4000 cGy split-course irradiation) and the fully concurrent manner in which the chemotherapy and radiotherapy were administered. The use of radiation doses *above* 4500 cGy with concurrent cisplatin-based chemotherapy was explored in two small single institution trials.[40,41] Both found prohibitive treatment-related morbidity and mortality related to postoperative adult respiratory distress syndrome and bronchial stump leaks.

Is There an Optimal Neoadjuvant Regimen? Concurrent chemoradiotherapy has been the most common induction treatment for unresectable stage III non–small cell lung cancers, but caution should be exercised in drawing conclusions from the numerous reported neoadjuvant trials. There are considerable differences among these trials with respect to eligibility criteria, accuracy of pretreatment staging, and induction regimens. Some trials (eg, the LCSG and SWOG trials) included both stage IIIa (N2) and IIIb (T4 and N3) tumors, while some trials (eg, the Rush-Presbyterian trials) intentionally included both tumors that were stage IIIa but not N2 (T3 N0-1) and a few stage IIIb (T4) tumors, and other trials (eg, the Memorial Sloan-Kettering trial) included stage IIIa (N2) tumors but no stage IIIb tumors. The inclusion of these different tumor stages accounts in part for the differences in response, resectability, and survival rates. In addition, the staging of patients before induction therapy was primarily clinical in early neoadjuvant trials. Greater experience with this form of treatment, the use of the new International Staging System, and a growing appreciation of the heterogeneity of stage III disease have led to the use of more stringent staging in recent studies, such as the SWOG trial.

The criteria for taking patients to thoracotomy after induction treatment also vary among these trials. Some trials, particularly the early ones, offered patients surgical resection only if they had a radiographic response to induction therapy. Other trials mandated thoracotomy in all patients unless they had evidence of progressive disease. Therefore, the resectability rates are not comparable among various trials. Both the Rush-Presbyterian and the SWOG trials have shown that there can be a discrepancy between radiographic and pathologic response and that resectability is

Table 61-8. RESULTS OF REPRESENTATIVE NEOADJUVANT TRIALS FOR STAGE III NON–SMALL CELL LUNG CANCER USING INDUCATION CHEMORADIOTHERAPY FOLLOWED BY SURGICAL RESECTION

Study	Patients at Eligible Stage	Chemotherapy	Radiotherapy cGy	Survival Median (mo)	Survival 2y (%)
LCSG, 1987	IIIA, IIIB: 39	CAP × 3	3000 (S), 10 fractions	11	8
Rush-Presbyterian, 1989[72]	IIIA: 85 (including 19 N0)	CDDP (60 mg/m[2]) + 5-FU ± VP-16 × 4	4000 cGy (S), 20 fractions	21.8	40 (3-y)
LCSG, 1991[73]	IIIA, IIIB: 85	CDDP (75 mg/m[2]) + 5-FU × 2	3000 cGy (C), 15 fractions	13	~20
CALGB, 1992[74]	IIIA: 41 (including 8 N0-1)	CDDP (100 mg/m[2]) + Vbl + 5-FU × 2	3000 cGy (C), 15 fractions	15.5	~30
SWOG, 1993[39]	IIIA, IIIB: 126	CDDP (50 mg/m[2] days 1 and 8) + VP-16 × 2	4500 cGy (C), 30 fractions	13 (IIIa) 17 (IIIb)	37 (IIIa) 39 (IIIb)

LCSG, Lung Cancer Study Group; CALGB, Cancer and Leukemia Group B; SWOG, Southwest Oncology Group; CDDP, cisplatin; Vbl, vinblastine; 5-FU, 5 fluorouracil; CAP, cyclophosphamide, doxorubicin, cisplatin; VP-16, etoposide; (C), continuous course; (S), split course.

not necessarily linked to radiographic response. The response, resectability, and survival rates are not uniformly reported. In some cases, the resectability rates are reported as a percentage of the patients who had a radiographic response, and only the survival rate of patients who had a resection is emphasized. In reality, these rates should be reported as percentages of the total number of patients entered in a study. The use of a smaller denominator falsely suggests better results.

Taken as a whole, trials of neoadjuvant therapy have demonstrated the feasibility of combined-modality treatment in stage III non–small cell lung cancer. The resectability and survival rates of these locally advanced tumors appear to be at least 50% higher than they were historically with surgical treatment alone. Induction regimens that use high-dose cisplatin (greater than 100 mg/m²) or high-dose radiation (4000 cGy or greater) appear to produce higher response rates. Radiation doses of 5500 cGy or higher, however, have been associated with a prohibitive risk of postoperative adult respiratory distress syndrome and bronchial stump leak, especially in patients undergoing pneumonectomy. In the Memorial Sloan-Kettering experience, induction therapy with chemotherapy alone has been as effective as concurrent chemoradiotherapy, but unfortunately, the MVP regimen has been associated with greater toxicity and lower response rates in the multiinstitutional setting. Thus, regimens that use standard-dose cisplatin (100 mg/m² in single or divided dose) with a synergistic agent such as etoposide and moderate doses of concurrent radiation (40 or 45 Gy) are effective and may be more easily administered to the general population of lung cancer patients.

For patients with stage III non–small cell lung cancer who are not candidates for surgical resection (ie, medically inoperable), chemoradiotherapy has superseded radiotherapy alone as standard care. Whether sequential chemoradiotherapy is superior to concurrent therapy remains to be seen in future clinical trials. For patients who can tolerate an operation, the most urgent question is whether neoadjuvant therapy followed by surgical resection is superior to chemotherapy and higher-dose radiotherapy. This is the subject of a prospective randomized multiinstitutional trial. In all completed trials, the major form of relapse has been distant metastatic disease, underscoring the need for new and more effective forms of systemic treatment.

NEUROENDOCRINE TUMORS

Neuroendocrine tumors of the lung share a common histogenesis but manifest varying clinical behavior, ranging from indolent (typical carcinoid) to rapidly growing and aggressive (small cell lung cancer).

Carcinoid Tumors

Carcinoid tumors arise from the neuroendocrine stem cells of the bronchial epithelium and are classified as either typical or atypical. Typical carcinoids consist microscopically of uniform round cells with small nuclei and fine granular chromatin (Fig. 61-8). Mitoses and lymph node metastases are infrequent. Atypical carcinoids are more pleomorphic and may have areas of increased cellularity with disorganization of the architecture and tumor necrosis. Mitoses are present within the context of a recognizable carcinoid pattern. Lymph nodes metastases occur in about half the patients.[42]

About 40% of carcinoids are located centrally and may be diagnosed by bronchoscopy. At bronchoscopy, they appear as pink or purple friable endobronchial masses covered by intact epithelium (Fig. 61-9). The remainder of carcinoid tumors are seen as well-circumscribed nodules on chest radiographs. Typical carcinoids occur more frequently in the central or lobar airways than do atypical carcinoids. About half of all patients present with symptoms, which include hemoptysis, postobstructive pneumonitis, and dyspnea. The carcinoid syndrome is rarely associated with bronchial carcinoids and occurs primarily in the 2% of patients who have metastatic disease, particularly liver metastases. Other endocrinopathies occur rarely, including Cushing syndrome, inappropriate antidiuretic hormone secretion, and hypoglycemia.[43]

Standard treatment of bronchial carcinoids is complete surgical resection with mediastinal lymph node sampling or dissection. Lobectomy is required in about 50% of patients. Lesser resections (segmentectomy, sleeve resection) are adequate for complete resection in about 20% of patients. Endoscopic resection is invariably associated with local recurrence and should be used only as a palliative maneuver in patients whose general medical conditions preclude thoracotomy and pulmonary resection.[43]

The long-term survival rate after surgical resection exceeds 90% in patients with typical carcinoids even when hilar or mediastinal nodal metastases are present. In contrast, patients with atypical carcinoids have a 60% 5-year survival rate after complete resection. Outcome is more closely linked to histology than the tumor size, location, or nodal involvement. Recurrence is more frequent with tumors greater than 3 cm in size and in patients who present with lymph node metastases.[44]

Large Cell Neuroendocrine Carcinomas

Large cell neuroendocrine carcinoma is characterized by a neuroendocrine appearance on light microscopy but with large cells, a low nuclear/cytoplasmic ratio, a high mitotic rate, and necrosis.[45] Large clinical series of patients with this entity have not yet been reported, but a series of 23 patients suggests that this is a smoking-related tumor often associated with a poor prognosis despite complete resection. Initial experience does not suggest that these tumors are either chemotherapy or radiotherapy responsive.[46] Management of large cell neuroendocrine carcinoma is identical to that of non–small cell lung cancer.

Small Cell Lung Cancer and the Role of Surgery

Small cell lung cancers grow rapidly and disseminate widely by the time of diagnosis. They are rarely the domain of the surgeon. In contrast to non–small cell tumors, they are notably responsive to chemotherapy. Over two thirds of all patients initially experience a complete or partial response to chemotherapy. In most cases, these responses are not durable, and the overall 5-year survival rate remains in the range of 10%. Improvements in multimodality therapy with chemoradiation, however, have led to a better outcome in patients with early-stage (limited) disease, with reported 4-year survival rates as high as 30%.

The staging system for small cell lung cancer was developed by the Veterans Administration Lung Cancer Staging Group and divides patients into those with limited and those with extensive disease. This distinction is based on what can be encompassed by a tolerable radiotherapy portal. Limited disease is defined as a tumor confined to one hemithorax and its regional lymph nodes, including the ipsilateral, mediastinal, and supraclavicular nodes and the contralateral hilar nodes. Ipsilateral pleural effusions, left recurrent laryngeal nerve involvement, and superior vena

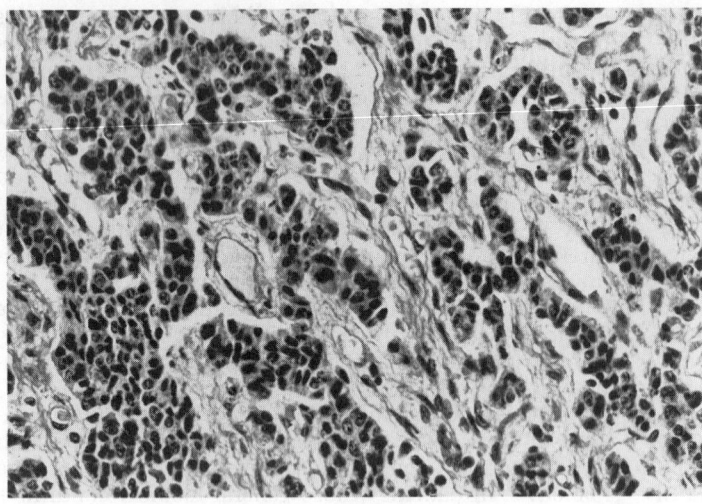

Figure 61-8. Photomicrograph of a typical carcinoid with interlacing cords and masses of uniform cells. Vascular stroma is apparent.

cava obstruction are considered limited diseases, whereas pericardial disease and bilateral pulmonary involvement are considered extensive diseases. With improvements in the treatment of small cell lung cancer during the past decade, it has become evident that this staging system is inadequate. A review by the SWOG of prognostic variables in its 2580-patient small cell lung cancer data base found that the two-stage system should be extended into a four-stage system using serum lactate dehydrogenase level, age, and pleural effusion as additional staging criteria.[47]

Even these changes in the staging system would not address the specific subset of small cell cancer patients seen by the surgeon. Fewer than 10% of all small cell cancer patients are candidates for possible pulmonary resection. They have peripheral tumors with no nodal involvement or only hilar nodal involvement, which would be classified as T1–2, N0–1 tumors in the non–small cell lung cancer staging system. Such tumors are often diagnosed at exploratory thoracotomy for an asymptomatic coin lesion. Several retrospective series have demonstrated a 50% 5-year survival rate after resection of T1, N0 or T2, N0 small cell lung cancers. For completely resected T1–2, N1 tumors, the 5-year survival rate approximates 30%.[48] Because of the propensity for small cell cancers to disseminate, adjuvant chemotherapy has traditionally been given to patients after surgical resection, even though, by virtue of the small numbers of patients available, there are no prospective randomized trials to demonstrate whether this is of benefit.[49] Relapse in the primary site, which is a problem for most patients with limited-stage small cell lung cancer, is distinctly uncommon after complete resection of these early tumors. The role of surgical resection for patients with mediastinal nodal involvement (N2 disease) is less clear and should probably be confined to well-controlled clinical trials.

With the increasing use of percutaneous needle aspiration for the diagnosis of coin lesions, many patients with early-stage small cell lung cancer are diagnosed preoperatively. Once identified, such patients should be evaluated in conjunction with a medical oncologist. Surgical resection should be considered after distant disease has been excluded by a metastatic evaluation that includes a bone scan and CT scans of the chest, abdomen, and brain. Some oncologists also perform bone marrow biopsies. Because the role of surgical resection in patients with N2 disease remains questionable, mediastinal nodal disease should be excluded by mediastinoscopy. This should be performed separately from thoracotomy because it can be difficult for the pathologist to diagnose small cell cancer on a frozen section. In the absence of better data, adjuvant postoperative chemotherapy is considered standard treatment. If surgical resection has been complete, radiation is not given because there is no evidence that it improves either local control or long-term survival.

BRONCHIAL ADENOMAS

Bronchial adenomas constitute about 1% of all lung neoplasms and no more than 2% of tumors for which surgical resection is performed. The term *adenoma* is misleading because these tumors constitute a group of tumors that can be of either low- or high-grade malignancy. This group includes cystic carcinoma, mucoepidermoid carcinoma, and mucous gland adenoma—the only truly benign tumor.

The presenting signs and symptoms of these tumors depend on their location. Peripheral tumors are asymptomatic, generally presenting as a nodule on routine chest radiograph. Proximally located tumors present with

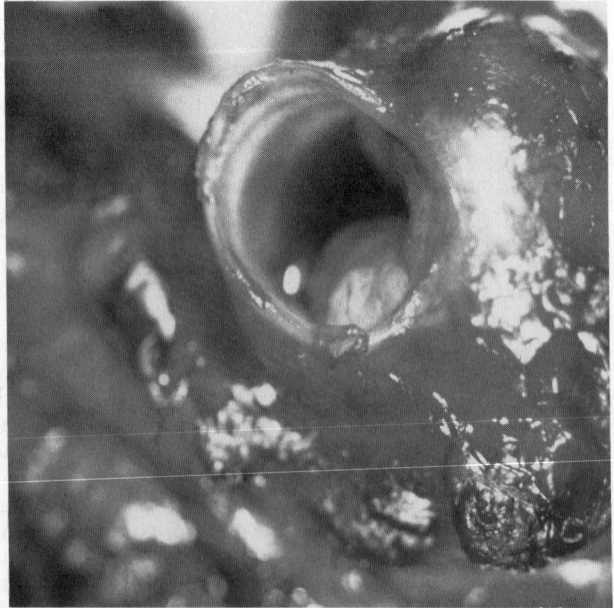

Figure 61-9. Bronchoscopic view of a carcinoid tumor.

hemoptysis or signs of airway obstruction, including cough, recurrent infection, wheezing, or stridor. Because of the slow growth of these tumors, signs and symptoms may develop over a period of years. Incompletely obstructing tumors frequently masquerade as asthma for prolonged periods of time.

Peripheral tumors are diagnosed by percutaneous needle aspiration biopsy or at the time of thoracotomy. Tumors in major airways are diagnosed by bronchoscopy. Other studies, such as CT scans, are rarely required to make the diagnosis but may be of value in planning therapy.

Because most of these tumors do not metastasize, complete excision, preserving as much pulmonary tissue as possible, is the goal. Whenever possible, sleeve resections of main bronchi are employed to preserve pulmonary tissue.

Adenoid Cystic Carcinoma

Adenoid cystic carcinomas are slowly growing malignant tumors that arise from the submucosal glands of the trachea and main bronchi (Fig. 61-10). They have also been called cylindromas, adenoid cystic basal cell carcinomas, adenomyoepitheliomas, and pseudoadenomatous basal cell carcinomas. Adenoid cystic carcinomas behave much like the major and minor salivary gland tumors of the same name, to which they are microscopically identical. An important aspect of their clinical behavior is that they tend to spread in the submucosal plane along the perineural lymphatics, well beyond the obvious endoluminal component of the tumor.

Whenever possible, total excision by tracheal resection or tracheobronchial resection is the treatment of choice.[50] This is not always possible because of the extensive submucosal spread of tumor. In such cases, palliative resec-

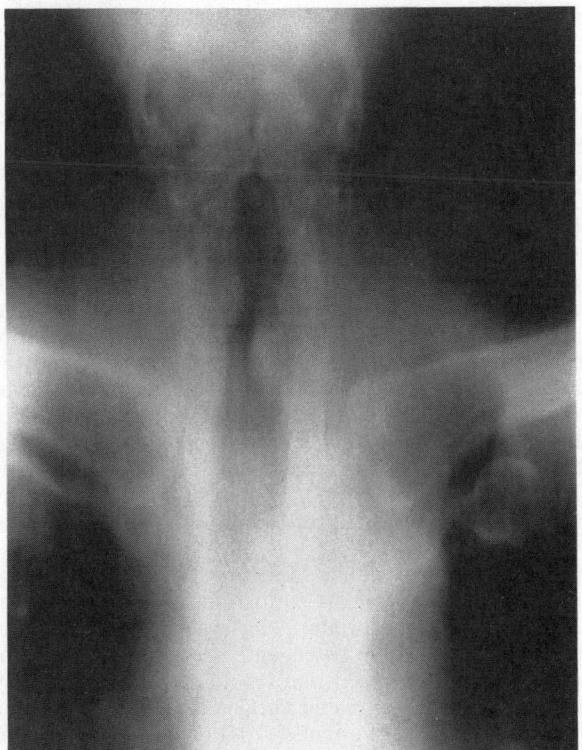

Figure 61-10. Tracheogram demonstrating the high airway obstruction of an adenoid cystic carcinoma of the upper trachea.

tion may be necessary. Postoperative radiotherapy is indicated because these tumors are radiation sensitive.

When no surgical resection is feasible because of the extent of the lesion, a palliative treatment option is endoscopic laser removal followed by radiotherapy (both brachytherapy and external-beam irradiation).

When complete surgical resection is possible, the prognosis is excellent. However, because of the slow-growing nature of the tumor and its responsiveness to radiotherapy, prolonged survival is possible even with incomplete resection or palliative measures. Patients frequently live 10 years or more with persisting disease, including pulmonary metastases. In such cases, repeated efforts at palliation are indicated.

Mucoepidermoid Carcinoma

Mucoepidermoid carcinomas are rare bronchial tumors, accounting for no more than 2% of all bronchial adenomas. Mucoepidermoid carcinomas present in patients of all ages.

Mucoepidermoid carcinomas may be of low- or high-grade malignancy and have the same microscopic appearance as mucoepidermoid tumors of salivary gland origin. These tumors also arise in the glandular submucosa, presenting as submucosal lesions. Low-grade tumors have a large proportion of mucous cells, whereas high-grade tumors have a large proportion of squamous cells.

The principles of treatment of mucoepidermoid tumors are similar to those of carcinoid tumors. The more malignant variety must be treated as bronchogenic carcinoma. The outlook for these tumors depends on the grade of malignancy and the stage of the disease. High-grade tumors have the same prognosis as bronchogenic carcinoma. Complete surgical resection is the mainstay of treatment. Mucoepidermoid tumors are too rare to permit the evaluation of combined-modality therapy for the more aggressive high-grade tumors.[51]

Mucous Gland Adenoma

Mucous gland adenomas are rare submucosal tumors that arise from mucous glands and are also known as bronchial cysts and papillary cystadenomas. Because of their totally benign behavior, they can usually be treated by endoscopic excision. Thoracotomy and surgical resection are indicated only if the distal lung has been destroyed by chronic infection or if endoscopic removal is technically contraindicated or incomplete.

BENIGN TUMORS OF THE LUNG

The lung is composed of epithelial, mesodermal, and endodermal cells. Benign tumors may arise from any of these cells. They may present as endobronchial lesions or peripheral nodules. Endobronchial tumors present with signs and symptoms related to airway obstruction or bleeding. Tumors arising in peripheral airways or in association with pulmonary parenchyma usually present as undiagnosed asymptomatic solitary pulmonary nodules. The many types of benign lung tumors are listed in Table 61-9.

Hamartoma

The most frequently occurring benign tumors are hamartomas. A hamartoma consists of an unusual arrangement of normally occurring cells. In the lung, the most frequent component is cartilage. A hamartoma usually presents as a solitary pulmonary nodule with an extremely slow growth pattern. Classically, the radiographic appearance is a well-

Table 61-9. TYPES OF BENIGN LUNG TUMORS CLASSIFIED ACCORDING TO THEIR CELLULAR ORIGIN

EPITHELIAL
Polyps
Papilloma

MESENCHYMAL
Nerve
Granular cell myoblastoma
Neurilemoma
Neurofibroma
Chemodectoma
Muscle
Leiomyoma
Others
Lipoma
Chondroma
Plasma cell granuloma
Teratoma

ENDOTHELIAL
Sclerosing hemangioma
Glomus tumor
Arteriovenous malformation

circumscribed nodule that may contain popcorn calcification. If previous chest radiographs are available, these tumors are found to have been present for many years. Their growth pattern is variable but generally slow.

The diagnosis of these lesions can be made by CT scan if appropriate calcification is demonstrated. Needle aspiration is frequently diagnostic of a cartilaginous benign lesion.

Controversy exists regarding whether these lesions should be excised for pathologic diagnosis. Certainly, they do not require excision unless they are proximal and cause symptoms related to endobronchial obstruction or unless carcinoma cannot be ruled out. If transthoracic needle aspiration biopsy confirms the nature of these hamartomas, many surgeons elect to follow patients with annual chest radiographs rather than surgical excision. Occasionally, significant growth during follow-up necessitates excision.

Arteriovenous Malformations

Arteriovenous malformations are the result of direct connection between branches of the pulmonary artery and pulmonary vein. They are congenital and frequently present as symptomatic pulmonary nodules. Most occur in the lower lobes, and they are occasionally identified by an enlarged draining pulmonary vein running from the lesion to the mediastinum. If associated with Osler-Weber-Rendu disease, the arteriovenous malformations are multiple. The lesions are usually not recognized until at least the second decade of life. Often, they enlarge progressively in response to increasing flow.

Symptoms include dyspnea (due to arteriovenous shunting and hypoxemia), parenchymal hemorrhage, hemoptysis, and neurologic sequelae related to emboli. Up to half of patients have significant mortality or morbidity related to the disease.

Until 1978, surgery was the only method of treatment and required either local excision, segmentectomy, lobectomy, or in extreme cases, pneumonectomy. Other successful treatment techniques include embolotherapy using percutaneous catheters, embolization coils, or balloons.

Because of the frequent multiplicity of the lesions, embolotherapy is now the treatment of choice.

Other Benign Tumors

Other benign tumors may present as endobronchial lesions (commonly fibromas, lipomas, chondromas, and granular cell myoblastomas). These tumors may be removed endoscopically, but frequently they also require surgical excision when the diagnosis is in doubt or when incomplete excision has occurred endoscopically. Peripheral tumors often are removed for diagnosis.

OTHER MALIGNANT TUMORS OF THE LUNG

As with benign tumors, malignant tumors arising from epithelial, mesodermal, or endodermal cell lines can occur in the lung. Sarcomas arising from soft tissue or large vessels and carcinosarcomas are treated in a similar fashion to sarcomas occurring elsewhere. Primary pulmonary lymphomas usually are excised for confirmatory diagnosis. Other rare tumors include primary melanomas of the bronchus, malignant teratomas, and pulmonary blastomas. Treatment of these tumors primarily involves complete surgical resection. Radiotherapy and chemotherapy do not have well-defined roles in the treatment of any of these tumors but are occasionally used in particular situations.

SURGICAL RESECTION OF PULMONARY METASTASES
Historical Background

Pulmonary resection for metastatic disease was initially reported in the European literature by Divis in 1927.[52] The first such resection in North America was performed by Barney and Churchill[53] in 1939. A solitary mass removed by lobectomy proved to be a metastasis from renal cell carcinoma. The patient subsequently had a nephrectomy for the primary tumor and survived disease-free for more than 20 years.

From 1940 to the mid-1960s, pulmonary metastasectomy was performed infrequently and only in highly selected patients. At Memorial Sloan-Kettering Cancer Center, 25 patients with pulmonary metastases were treated surgically from 1940 to 1965. Operation was not considered unless the patient had a long disease-free interval after the resection of the primary tumor and had three or fewer lesions confined to one lung. From 1941 to 1962, the Mayo Clinic performed 221 pulmonary resections on 205 patients for metastatic disease.[54] Multiple nodules were not considered a contraindication to resection, but it was thought that bilateral disease was associated with a poor prognosis and should not be resected. The indications for pulmonary metastasectomy were restricted, and although not explicitly stated, the large number of operations performed may reflect the high volume of cases seen at the Mayo Clinic rather than the common use of surgical resection.

In the 1970s, experience from several institutions suggested that more liberal indications for pulmonary metastasectomy were appropriate. A striking example was the treatment of metastatic osteogenic sarcoma at Memorial Sloan-Kettering Cancer Center. From 1940 to 1965, only 5 such patients were treated surgically. During the same period, only 24 of 145 patients (17%) survived 5 years after resection of their primary tumors, and 118 of these patients (81%) died of pulmonary metastases. This experience prompted a more aggressive approach to the management of pulmonary metastases. Starting in 1965, a consecutive series of 22 patients with osteogenic sarcoma underwent pulmonary metastasectomy. Patients were considered for operation even if they had bilateral metastases or required multiple thoracotomies to remove all gross tumor. A total of 59 thoracotomies were performed in these 22 patients, with an overall 5-year survival rate of 32%. The dramatic improvement in survival compared with historical experience strongly supported the aggressive use of pulmonary metastasectomy in these patients.[55]

During the past 25 years, surgical resection has become a widely accepted treatment for pulmonary metastases; however, some of the criteria for patient selection remain controversial. In addition, advances in chemotherapy have changed the indications for surgical resection. For some cancers, pulmonary metastasectomy is performed to prolong life expectancy, whereas in others, it serves mainly to restage disease or to provide adjuvant treatment after initial chemotherapy. The role of pulmonary metastasectomy will undoubtedly continue to evolve as improvements in systemic treatment occur. This review provides a perspective on the approach to the surgical management of pulmonary metastases.

Clinical Presentation and Diagnosis

Metastases are asymptomatic 85% of the time and are usually detected on a routine chest radiograph. Patients who have resection of a primary tumor known to be prone to subsequent pulmonary metastases should have a chest radiograph as part of their routine follow-up care. On a chest radiograph, metastases usually present as well-circumscribed, spherical solid masses with well-defined borders (Fig. 61-11). Cavitation is occasionally seen in large lesions that have central necrosis.

Metastases to the lung usually arise in the pulmonary parenchyma. Endobronchial metastases are uncommon and occur most frequently with renal cell, colon, and breast cancers. More often, endobronchial disease represents extension of contiguous parenchymal disease. The extent of endobronchial tumor can affect the approach to

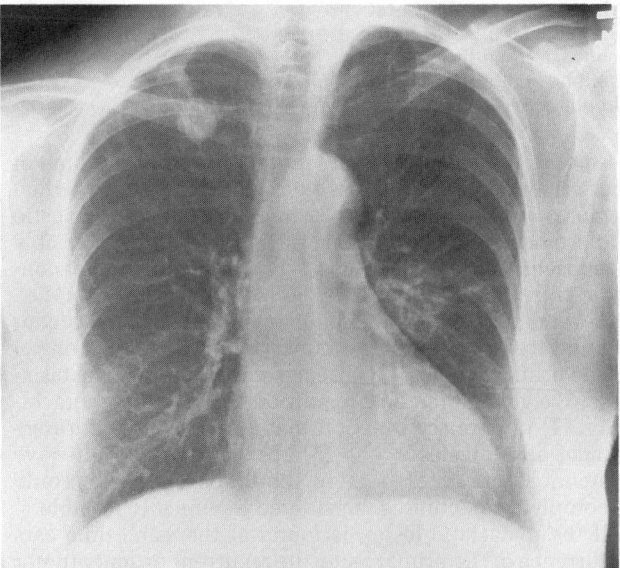

Figure 61-11. Chest radiograph of a patient with bilateral pulmonary metastases from endometrial cancer. The right upper lobe mass is well circumscribed and has the radiographic appearance typical of a metastasis.

surgical resection. For that reason, bronchoscopy should be performed before thoracotomy for centrally located pulmonary metastases.[56]

Hilar or mediastinal nodal involvement sometimes accompanies pulmonary metastases. The determinants of nodal involvement and the prognostic and therapeutic implications remain poorly understood. Lymphangitic spread can occur with or without concomitant pulmonary nodules. This occurs most frequently in breast cancer and produces a characteristic radiographic appearance of diffusely increased interstitial markings and a clinical presentation of severe dyspnea out of proportion to the radiographic findings.

When pulmonary metastases are thought to be present on a chest radiograph, a CT scan should be done to determine their number, location, size, and potential resectability. Plain chest radiographs detect only lesions of at least 9 mm in size. New lesions of this size seen on chest radiograph in a patient already treated for a malignancy have a 90% chance of being malignant.

Even a CT scan underestimates the number of pulmonary metastases. In a study correlating radiologic and surgical findings, only 73% of 237 nodules were identified preoperatively by CT scan (Fig. 61-12). Of the lesions not detected by CT scan, 87% were metastatic tumors, 8% were benign, and 4% were new primary bronchogenic carcinomas of the lung.[57]

Patients who present with multiple pulmonary nodules in the setting of a previously treated malignancy rarely pose a diagnostic dilemma. Patients who present with solitary pulmonary nodules are more problematic. Generally, a solitary lesion is more likely to be a metastasis if the primary tumor was a sarcoma or a melanoma. If the primary tumor originated in the head, neck, or breast, it is more likely to be a new primary lung cancer. It has an equal chance of being metastatic or a new primary if the initial tumor was of gastrointestinal or genitourinary origin. Percutaneous fine-needle aspiration biopsy usually yields a tissue diagnosis, but the necessity of a biopsy in the case of a solitary lesion is questionable. If the patient fits the selection criteria for resection, a biopsy of the lesion may best be done as an excisional biopsy. Because the findings on needle biopsy do not alter the recommendations for excision of a solitary lesion, this procedure should be done only if the patient is not an operative candidate, if an alternative method of treatment is indicated, or if the patient requests knowing the diagnosis before consenting to surgery.

Criteria for Surgical Resection

The disease-free interval, the number of metastatic nodules, and the tumor doubling time have been used as criteria for the surgical resection of pulmonary metastases. Each of these factors remains controversial with respect to its impact on long-term outcome.

The disease-free interval is defined as the time from the resection of the primary tumor to the diagnosis of metastases. The length of the disease-free interval is thought to confer prognostic significance and varies greatly among published reports. Examples of this are shown in Table 61-10.

The number of metastatic nodules resected has also been considered predictive of survival. In sarcomas, some have reported that the presence of four nodules is a significant breakpoint in survival; however, the significance of the number of nodules varies among reported series. Most consider the completeness of resection the best predictor of survival. Obviously, when a shower of numerous, tiny (1-

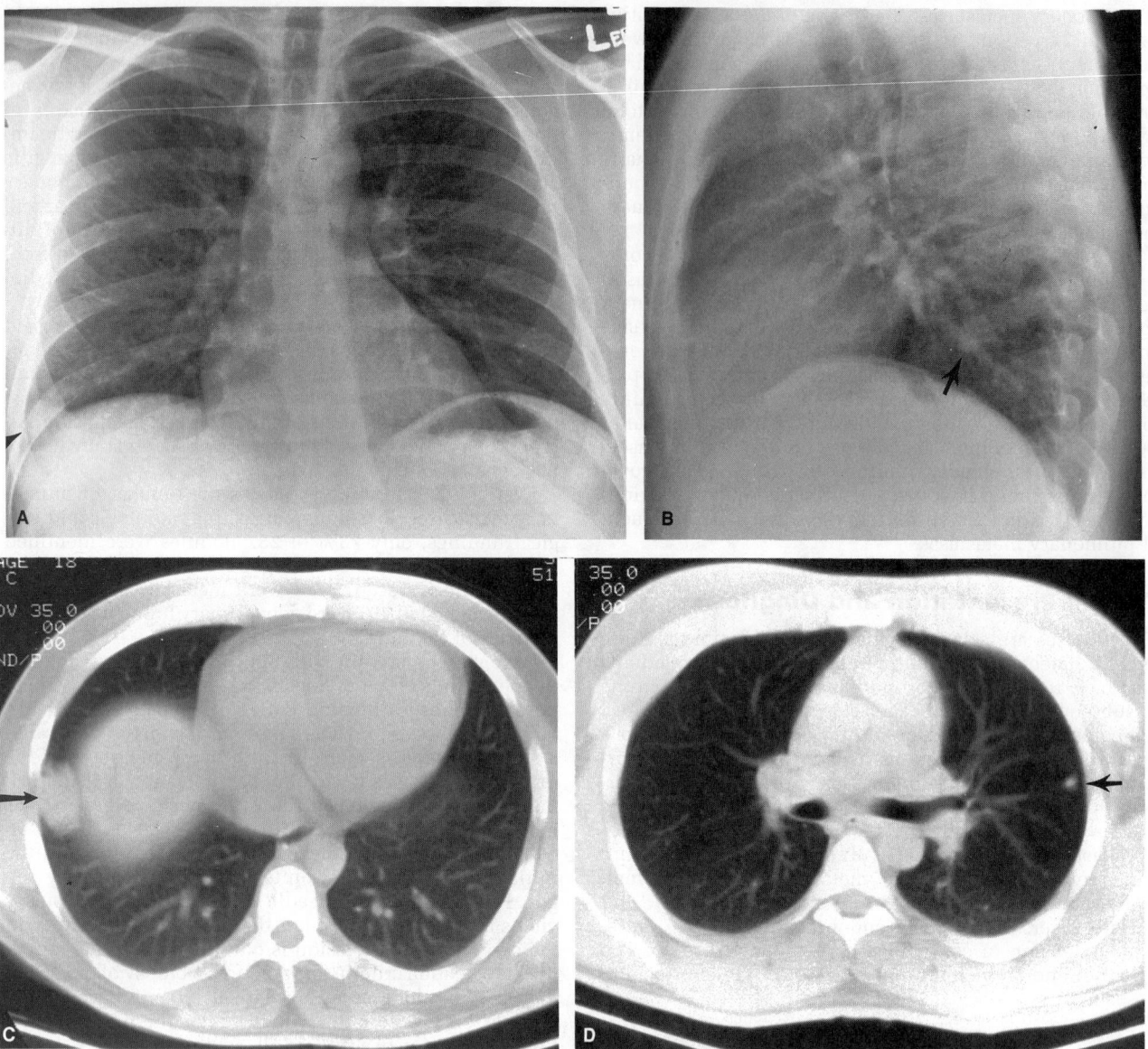

Figure 61-12. Imaging studies from a patient with metastatic embryonal rhabdomyosarcoma. Chest radiographs show a right lower lobe mass (*arrow in A*) that is best seen on the lateral view (*arrow in B*). CT scan confirmed the presence of this mass (*arrow in C*) and showed an additional left upper lobe nodule (*arrow in D*). At surgical exploration, however, the patient had multiple bilateral pulmonary metastases that measured less than 5 mm and therefore could not be seen on CT scan.

to 2-mm) lesions is encountered, complete resection is not possible.

Tumor doubling time is a measure of the aggressiveness of tumor growth. The importance of this was first recognized by Joseph,[58] who found 40 days to be the significant time with respect to long-term survival. They reported a

Table 61-10. SELECTED SERIES SHOWING A SIGNIFICANT IMPACT OF DISEASE-FREE INTERVAL ON OVERALL SURVIVAL

Investigators	Patients	Disease-Free Interval
Creagan et al, 1979[75]	112	>1 y
Morrow et al, 1980[76]	167	>5 y
Takita et al, 1981[77]	234	>7 mo
Putnam et al, 1984[78]	67	>1 y
van de Wal et al, 1986[79]	80	>1–5 y
Depadt G et al, 1985[80]	68	>2 y

44-month median survival with a tumor doubling time of more than 40 days, and less than half that survival when tumor doubling times were 20 to 40 days. The prognostic importance of tumor doubling time, however, was variable in subsequent reports (Table 61-11), and many do not consider this a criterion for surgical resection.

Several guidelines must be met before a patient is considered for resection of pulmonary metastases: (1) control of the primary tumor, (2) absence of extrathoracic metastases, (3) a general medical condition that permits thoracotomy, (4) pulmonary function that allows complete resection of all metastases, and (5) absence of more effective systemic treatment. Resection should be undertaken only if complete resection is considered technically feasible.[59]

If the metastatic lesion is found at the same time as a recurrence of the primary site, the recurrent primary tumor should be treated before the metastatic disease is treated to prevent further seeding of the metastatic site. When the primary tumor and the metastasis are diagnosed simultaneously, lung resection may precede the surgery for the

Table 61-11. SELECTED SERIES REPORTING THAT TUMOR DOUBLING TIME SIGNIFICANTLY INFLUENCES OVERALL SURVIVAL

Investigators	Patients	Tumor Doubling Time (d)
Ramming, 1980[81]	91	>40
Takita et al, 1981[77]	234	>45
Putnam & Roth, 1990[82]	67	>20
van de Wal et al, 1986[79]	80	>136

primary disease if doubt exists about whether the pulmonary disease can be completely resected and immediate subsequent resection of the primary tumor is planned.

When a patient meets the criteria for resection of one or more pulmonary metastases, consideration must be given to the natural history of the tumor and to whether effective systemic therapy is available. Experience in breast cancer, testicular cancer, and osteogenic sarcoma illustrate this point. In contrast to sarcomas, in which metastatic disease is usually confined to the lungs, pulmonary metastases from breast cancer signal the development of widely disseminated disease. Because effective systemic therapy is available for breast cancer, surgical resection of pulmonary metastases is rarely indicated.[60]

In germ cell cancer, the advent of effective chemotherapy radically altered the management of pulmonary metastases and rendered an incurable disease curable. Chemotherapy is now the primary form of treatment. Surgical resection is reserved for patients who have gross residual disease after the initial chemotherapy and whose serum tumor markers (β-human chorionic gonadotropin and α-fetoprotein) have fallen to normal levels. Persistent elevation of tumor markers signifies residual active tumor and is an indication for continuing chemotherapy. Negative tumor markers in the presence of gross disease on chest radiograph or CT scan usually signify residual benign teratoma. Removal of teratoma is performed to prevent its degeneration to a more malignant form of germ cell tumor and to avoid the potential complications of local tumor growth. Thus, surgical resection plays a strictly adjuvant role in the treatment of malignant germ cell tumors.[61]

The development of more effective chemotherapy regimens for sarcomas, especially osteogenic sarcomas, has also altered the management of pulmonary metastases in this disease. Surgical resection is part of a multimodality treatment approach, but the manner in which chemotherapy and resection should be combined is less clear than in germ cell cancer. The timing of an operation in relation to chemotherapy depends on the number, size, and location of pulmonary metastases at diagnosis and on whether the patient has received any previous chemotherapy. Often, surgical resection is sandwiched between several cycles of chemotherapy, with the aim of controlling both gross and micrometastatic disease. This approach allows assessment of the sensitivity of the patient's tumor to chemotherapy and determines the advisability of continuing the regimen postoperatively. The thoracic surgeon should collaborate with the medical oncologist in planning a multidisciplinary treatment program for the patient with pulmonary metastases from sarcoma.

Preoperative Evaluation

The preoperative evaluation of the patient undergoing resection of pulmonary metastases is similar to that of the patient undergoing removal of a primary lung cancer. Pul-

monary function is assessed by pulmonary function tests, arterial blood gases, and, if necessary, ventilation–perfusion lung scanning to ensure that the patient has sufficient reserve to tolerate complete resection of the metastases. Patients who received chemotherapy may have a substantial reduction in their pulmonary function. This is particularly true of patients treated with bleomycin and mitomycin, which can markedly diminish the diffusion capacity and can occasionally and unpredictably cause an adult respiratory distress–type syndrome postoperatively. Maintaining patients on 35% or less inspired oxygen intraoperatively is thought to help prevent this complication.

Attention should be given to smoking cessation just as it is for lung cancer patients because patients who smoke actively up to the time of operation are at risk for postoperative atelectasis or pneumonia.

It is also important to assess the patient's general medical condition and cardiovascular status. Older patients may have underlying coronary artery disease that requires preoperative treatment and additional perioperative monitoring. Patients who previously received chemotherapy, especially doxorubicin, may have impaired cardiac function. A preoperative radionuclide (MUGA) scan or echocardiogram should be performed to determine the left ventricular ejection fraction and to assess whether intraoperative hemodynamic monitoring is necessary. Other drugs, such as cisplatin, can impair renal or neurologic function and may influence perioperative management.

In patients who recently received chemotherapy, the timing of surgery should be planned in conjunction with the medical oncologist so that the operation is not performed when the patient is neutropenic or thrombocytopenic. Resumption of chemotherapy postoperatively should also be a joint decision between surgeon and medical oncologist so that it does not compromise wound healing.

Surgical Technique

The surgical approach to resection of pulmonary metastatic lesions follows two guidelines—complete resection of the disease and maximal sparing of functioning lung tissue. Wedge resections should be done whenever possible. These can be carried out with staples, electrocautery, or laser. A lobectomy or pneumonectomy is performed only when wedge resection will not provide a complete resection.

Unilateral disease is approached by a standard anterolateral or posterolateral thoracotomy incision. Patients with bi-

Table 61-12. SITES OF PRIMARY TUMOR IN PATIENTS UNDERGOING RESECTION OF PULMONARY METASTASES AT MEMORIAL SLOAN-KETTERING CANCER CENTER, 1960–1990

Site	Patients
Colon or rectum	111
Testes	102
Kidney	65
Melanoma	64
Breast	60
Head or neck	65
Uterus	14
Bladder	13
Cervix	9
Lung	3
Other	10
TOTAL	516

Table 61-13. RESULTS OF PULMONARY RESECTIONS FOR METASTASES AT MEMORIAL SLOAN-KETTERING CANCER CENTER

	Patients	Median Survival
RENAL CELL CANCER*		
No evidence of disease	12	81 mo
Alive with disease	10	39 mo
Dead of disease	41	22 mo
HEAD AND NECK CANCERS†		
Epidermoid	40	44 mo
Salivary gland	20	20 y
Thyroid	5	10 y
COLON CANCER‡		
Dukes A	10	58 mo
Dukes B	25	47 mo
Dukes C	33	33 mo

* 1960–1990; 65 patients.
† 1960–1990; 64 patients.
‡ 1965–1988; 111 patients.

lateral pulmonary metastases should have simultaneous resection of the bilateral lesions if technically feasible. This can be accomplished by a median sternotomy or a clamshell incision (bilateral anterior thoracotomy with transverse sternotomy).[62] A clamshell incision provides better exposure to the posterior aspects of the lungs, particularly the left lower lobe, which is difficult to access by a median sternotomy.[63] Bilateral pulmonary nodules may require sequential posterolateral thoracotomies if they are centrally located and good exposure of the hilar vessels is needed.

Results

Surgical resection remains the mainstay of treatment for pulmonary metastases from many solid tumors that cannot be treated effectively with chemotherapy. These include colon cancer, renal cell cancer, melanoma, some head and neck tumors, and endometrial cancer. The frequency of primary tumor sites in patients with pulmonary metastases is illustrated in Table 61-12.

Experiences with resection of pulmonary metastases from renal cell cancer, from head and neck cancer, and from colon cancer are summarized in Table 61-13. These results again demonstrate that complete resection of metastatic disease is associated with prolonged survival in carefully selected patients. The surgical removal of pulmonary metastases is widely accepted, but its role has evolved as more effective chemotherapy has become available for some cancers. It is important that the surgeon understand the indications for operation, the potential side effects of initial chemotherapy, and the ways in which surgical resection should be integrated into the overall treatment plan for these patients.

REFERENCES

1. Winters TH, Di Franza JR. Radioactivity in cigarette smoking. N Engl J Med 1982;306:364.
2. Bonney GE. Interactions of genes, environment, and life-style in lung cancer development. J Natl Cancer Inst 1990;82:1236.
3. Sellers TA, Bailey-Wilson JE, Elston RC, et al. Evidence for Mendelian inheritance in the pathogenesis of lung cancer. J Natl Cancer Inst 1990;82:1272.
4. Czerwinski M, McLemore TL, Gelboin HV, Gonzalez FJ. Quantification of CYP2B7, CYP4B1, and CYPOR messenger RNAs in normal human lung and lung tumors. Cancer Res 1994;54:1085.
5. Selikoff IJ, Hammond EC, Churg J. Asbestos exposure, smoking, and neoplasia. JAMA 1968;204:106.
6. Falco JP, Baylin SB, Lupu R, et al. v-ras^H Induces non-small cell phenotype, with associated growth factors and receptors, in a small cell lung cancer cell line. J Clin Invest 1990;85:1740.
7. Roggli VL, Vollmer RT, Greenberg SD, McGavran MH. Lung cancer heterogeneity: a blinded and randomized study of 100 consecutive cases. Hum Pathol 1985;16:569.
8. Kok K, Osinga J, Carritt B, et al. Deletion of a DNA sequence at the chromosomal region 3p21 in all major types of lung cancer. Nature 1987;330:578.
9. Miura I, Siegfried JM, Resau J, Keller SM, Zhou J-Y, Testa JR. Chromosome alterations in 21 non–small cell lung carcinomas. Genes Chrom Cancer 1990;2:328.
10. Rodenhuis S, Slebos RJC. Clinical significance of ras oncogene activation in human lung cancer. Cancer Res 1992;52:2665s.
11. Rusch V, Baselga J, Cordon-Cardo C, et al. Differential expression of the epidermal growth factor receptor and its ligands in primary non–small cell lung cancers and adjacent benign lung. Cancer Res 1993;53:2379.
12. Derynck R, Goeddel DV, Ullrich A, et al. Synthesis of messenger RNAs for transforming growth factors α and β and the epidermal growth factor receptor by human tumors. Cancer Res 1987;47:707.
13. Carbone DP, Mitsudomi T, Chiba I, et al. p53 immunostaining positivity is associated with reduced survival and is imperfectly correlated with gene mutations in resected non–small cell lung cancer: a preliminary report of LCSG 871. Chest 1994;106:3775.
14. Reissmann PT, Koga H, Takahashi R, et al. Inactivation of the retinoblastoma susceptibility gene in non-small-cell lung cancer. Oncogene 1993;8:1913.
15. Miyake M, Taki T, Hitomi S, Hakomori S-I. Correlation of expression of H/Le^y/Le^b antigens with survival in patients with carcinoma of the lung. N Engl J Med 1992;327:14.
16. Patterson GA, Ginsberg RJ, Poon PY, Cooper JD. A prospective evaluation of magnetic resonance imaging, computed tomography, and mediastinoscopy in the preoperative assessment of mediastinal node status in bronchogenic carcinoma. J Thorac Cardiovasc Surg 1987;94:679.
17. Ginsberg RJ, Rubinstein L, the Lung Cancer Study Group. Randomized trial of lobectomy versus limited resection for T1N0 non–small cell lung cancer. Ann Thorac Surg 1995;60:615.
18. Thomas P, Rubinstein L, the Lung Cancer Study Group. Cancer recurrence after resection: T1 N0 non–small cell lung cancer. Ann Thorac Surg 1990;49:242.
19. Mountain CF, Gail MH. Surgical adjuvant intrapleural BCG treatment for stage I non–small cell lung cancer: preliminary report of the National Cancer Institute Lung Cancer Study Group. J Thorac Cardiovasc Surg 1981;82:649.
20. The Lung Cancer Study Group. Effects of postoperative mediastinal radiation on completely resected stage II and stage III epidermoid cancer of the lung. N Engl J Med 1986;315:1377.
21. Holmes EC, Gail M, the Lung Cancer Study Group. Surgical adjuvant therapy for stage II and stage III adenocarcinoma and large-cell undifferentiated carcinoma. J Clin Oncol 1986;4:710.
22. Feld R, Rubinstein L, Thomas PA, the Lung Cancer Study Group. Adjuvant chemotherapy with cyclophosphamide, doxorubicin, and cisplatin in patients with completely resected stage I non-small-cell lung cancer. J Natl Cancer Inst 1993;85:299.
23. McCaughan BC, Martini N, Bains MS, McCormack PM. Chest wall invasion in carcinoma of the lung: therapeutic and prognostic implications. J Thorac Cardiovasc Surg 1985;89:836.
24. Martini N, Yellin A, Ginsberg RJ, et al. Management of non–small cell lung cancer with direct mediastinal involvement. Ann Thorac Surg 1994;58:1447.
25. Mehran RJ, Deslauriers J, Piraus M, Beaulieu M. Survival related to nodal status after sleeve resection for lung cancer. J Thorac Cardiovasc Surg 1994;107:576.
26. Martini N, Flehinger BJ. The role of surgery in N2 lung cancer. Surg Clin North Am 1987;67:1037.
27. Rosell R, Gómez-Codina J, Camps C, et al. A randomized trial

comparing preoperative chemotherapy plus surgery with surgery alone in patients with non–small-cell lung cancer. N Engl J Med 1994;330:153.

28. Roth JA, Fossella F, Komaki R, et al. A randomized trial comparing perioperative chemotherapy and surgery with surgery alone in resectable stage IIIA non–small-cell lung cancer. J Natl Cancer Inst 1994;86:673.
29. Perez CA, Pajak TF, Rubin P, et al. Long-term observations of the patterns of failure in patients with unresectable non–oat cell carcinoma of the lung treated with definitive radiotherapy: report by the Radiation Therapy Oncology Group. Cancer 1987;59:1874.
30. Bromley LL, Szur L. Combined radiotherapy and resection for carcinoma of the bronchus: experiences with 66 patients. Lancet 1955;2:937.
31. Payne DG. Pre-operative radiation therapy in non–small cell lung cancer of the lung. Lung Cancer 1991;7:47.
32. Dillman RO, Seagren SL, Propert KJ, et al. A randomized trial of induction chemotherapy plus high-dose radiation versus radiation alone in stage III non–small cell lung cancer. N Engl J Med 1990;323:940.
33. Sause W, Scott C, Taylor S, et al. RTOG 8808 ECOG 4588, preliminary analysis of a phase III trial in regionally advanced unresectable non–small cell lung cancer. Proc ASCO (Abstract) 1994;13:325.
34. Schaake-Koning C, van den Bogaert W, Dalesio O, et al. Effects of concomitant cisplatin and radiotherapy on inoperable non–small cell lung cancer. N Engl J Med 1992;326:524.
35. Sadeghi A, Payne D, Rubinstein L, Lad T, the Lung Cancer Study Group. Combined modality treatment for resected advanced non–small cell lung cancer: local control and local recurrence. Int J Radiat Oncol Biol Phys 1988;15:89.
36. Martini N, Kris MG, Flehinger BJ, et al. Preoperative chemotherapy for stage IIIa (N2) lung cancer: the Sloan-Kettering experience with 136 patients. Ann Thorac Surg 1993;55:1365.
37. Burkes RL, Ginsberg RJ, Shepherd FA, et al. Induction chemotherapy with mitomycin, vindesine, and cisplatin for stage III unresectable non–small cell lung cancer: results of the Toronto phase II trial. J Clin Oncol 1992;10:580.
38. Wagner H Jr, Lad T, Piantadosi S, the Lung Cancer Study Group. Randomized phase II evaluation of preoperative radiation therapy and preoperative chemotherapy with mitomycin-C, vinblastine, and cisplatin in patients with technically unresectable stage IIIA and IIIB non–small cell cancer of the lung. (Abstract) Lung Cancer 1991;7(Suppl):157.
39. Albain KS, Rusch VW, Crowley JJ, et al. Concurrent cisplatin/etoposide plus chest radiotherapy followed by surgery for stages IIIA (N2) and IIIB non–small cell lung cancer: mature results of Southwest Oncology Group Phase II study 8805. J Clin Oncol 1995;13:1880.
40. Yashar J, Weitberg AB, Glicksman AS, Posner MR, Feng W, Wanebo HJ. Preoperative chemotherapy and radiation therapy for stage IIIa carcinoma of the lung. Ann Thorac Surg 1992;53:445.
41. Fowler WC, Langer CJ, Curran WJ Jr, Keller SM. Postoperative complications after combined neoadjuvant treatment of lung cancer. Ann Thorac Surg 1993;55:986.
42. Arrigoni MG, Woolner LB, Bernatz PE. Atypical carcinoid tumors of the lung. J Thorac Cardiovasc Surg 1972;64:413.
43. McCaughan BC, Martini N, Bains MS. Bronchial carcinoids: review of 124 cases. J Thorac Cardiovasc Surg 1985;89:8.
44. Martini N, Zaman MB, Bains MS, et al. Treatment and prognosis in bronchial carcinoids involving regional lymph nodes. J Thorac Cardiovasc Surg 1994;107:1.
45. Travis WD, Linnoila I, Tsokos MG, et al. Neuroendocrine tumors of the lung with proposed criteria for large-cell neuroendocrine carcinoma: an ultrastructural, immunohistochemical, and flow cytometric study of 35 cases. Am J Surg Pathol 1991;15:529.
46. Lequaglie C, Patriarca C, Cataldo I, Muscolino G, Preda F, Ravasi G. Prognosis of resected well-differentiated neuroendocrine carcinoma of the lung. Chest 1991;100:1053.
47. Albain KS, Crowley JJ, LeBlanc M, Livingston RB. Determinants of improved outcome in small-cell lung cancer: an analysis of the 2,580-patient Southwest Oncology Group data base. J Clin Oncol 1990;8:1563.
48. Shah SS, Thompson J, Goldstraw P. Results of operation without adjuvant therapy in treatment of small cell lung cancer. Ann Thorac Surg 1992;54:498.
49. Shepherd FA, Evans WK, Feld R, et al. Adjuvant chemotherapy following surgical resection for small-cell carcinoma of the lung. J Clin Oncol 1988;6:832.
50. Chin HW, DeMeester T, Chin RY, Boman B. Endobronchial adenoid cystic carcinoma. Chest 1991;100:1464.
51. Heitmiller RF, Mathisen DJ, Ferry JA, Mark EJ, Grillo HC. Mucoepidermoid lung tumors. Ann Thorac Surg 1989;47:394.
52. Divis G. Einbertrag zur Operativen, Behandlung der Lungengeschuuilste. Acta Chir Scand 1927;62:329.
53. Barney JD, Churchill ED. Adenocarcinoma of the kidney with metastases to the lung cured by nephrectomy and lobectomy. J Urol 1939;42:269.
54. Thomford NR, Woolner LB, Clagett OT. The surgical treatment of metastatic tumors in the lungs. J Thorac Cardiovasc Surg 1965;49:357.
55. Martini N, Huvos AG, Miké V, Marcove RC, Beattie EJ Jr. Multiple pulmonary resections in the treatment of osteogenic sarcoma. Ann Thorac Surg 1971;12:271.
56. Mountain CF, McMurtrey MJ, Hermes KE. Surgery for pulmonary metastasis: a 20-year experience. Ann Thorac Surg 1984;38:323.
57. McCormack PM, Ginsberg KB, Bains MS, et al. Accuracy of lung imaging in metastases with implications for the role of thoracoscopy. Ann Thorac Surg 1993;56:863.
58. Joseph WL. Criteria for resection of sarcoma metastatic to the lung. Cancer Chemother Rep 1974;58:285.
59. Rusch VW. Pulmonary metastectomy: current indications. Chest 1995;107:3225.
60. Lanza LA, Natarajan G, Roth JA, Putnam JB Jr. Long-term survival after resection of pulmonary metastases from carcinoma of the breast. Ann Thorac Surg 1992;54:244.
61. Toner GC, Panicek DM, Heelan RT, et al. Adjunctive surgery after chemotherapy for nonseminomatous germ cell tumors: recommendations for patient selection. J Clin Oncol 1990;8:1683.
62. Roth JA, Pass HI, Wesley MN, White D, Putnam JB, Siepp C. Comparison of median sternotomy and thoracotomy for resection of pulmonary metastases in patients with adult soft-tissue sarcomas. Ann Thorac Surg 1986;42:134.
63. Bains MS, Ginsberg RJ, Jones WG, et al. The clamshell incision: an improved approach to bilateral pulmonary and mediastinal tumor. Ann Thorac Surg 1994;58:30.
64. van Houtte P, Klastersky J, Nguyen H, et al. Comparative randomized study of chest radiotherapy preceded or not by chemotherapy with cisplatin, etoposide, and vindesine for the treatment of NSCLC. (Abstract) Proc Am Assoc Cancer Res 1984;25:785.
65. Mattson K, Holsti LR, Holsti P, et al. Inoperable non–small cell lung cancer: radiation with or without chemotherapy. Eur J Cancer Clin Oncol 1988;24:477.
66. Morton RF, Jett JR, McGinnis WL, et al. Thoracic radiation therapy alone compared with combined chemoradiotherapy for locally unresectable non–small cell lung cancer: a randomized, phase III trial. Ann Intern Med 1991;115:681.
67. Trovo MG, Minatel E, Veronesi A, et al. Combined radiotherapy and chemotherapy versus radiotherapy alone in locally advanced epidermoid bronchogenic carcinoma: a randomized study. Cancer 1990;65:400.
68. Le Chevalier T, Arrigada R, Quoix E, et al. Radiotherapy alone versus combined chemotherapy and radiotherapy in nonresectable non–small cell lung cancer: first analysis of a randomized trial in 353 patients. J Natl Cancer Inst 1991;83:417.
69. Ansari R, Tokars R, Fisher W, et al. A phase III study of thoracic irradiation with or without concomitant cisplatin in locoregional unresectable non–small cell lung cancer (NSCLC): a Hoosier Oncology Group (HOG) protocol. (Abstract) Proc Am Soc Clin Oncol 1991;10:A823.
70. Trovo MG, Minatel E, Franchin G, et al. Radiotherapy (RT) versus RT enhanced by cisplatin (DDP) in stage III non–small cell lung cancer (NSCLC): randomzied cooperative study. (Abstract) Lung Cancer 1991;7:590.
71. Sadeghi A, Payne D, Rubenstein L, the Lung Cancer Study Goup. Combined modality treatment for resected advanced non–small cell lung cancer: local control and local recurrence. Int J Radiat Oncol Biol Phys 1991;15:89.
72. Faber LP, Kittle CF, Warren WH, et al. Preoperative chemo-

therapy and irradiation for stage III non–small cell lung cancer. Ann Thorac Surg 1989;47:669.

73. Weiden PL, Piantadosi S. Preoperative chemotherapy (cisplatin and fluorouracil) and radiation therapy in stage III non–small cell lung cancer: a phase II study of the Lung Cancer Study Group. J Natl Cancer Inst 1991;83:266.

74. Stauss GM, Herndon JE, Sherman DD, et al. Neoadjuvant chemotherapy and radiotherapy followed by surgery in stage IIIA non–small cell carcinoma of the lung: report of a Cancer and Leukemia Group B phase II study. J Clin Oncol 1992;10:1237.

75. Creagan ET, Fleming TR, Edmonson JH, et al. Pulmonary resection for metastatic nonosteogenic sarcoma. Cancer 1979; 44:1908.

76. Morrow CE, Vassilopoulos PP, Grage TB. Surgical resection for metastatic neoplasms of the lung: experience of the University of Minnesota hospitals. Cancer 1980;45:2981.

77. Takita H, Edgerton F, Karakousis C, et al. Surgical management of metastases to the lung. Surg Gynecol Obstet 1981;152:191.

78. Putnam JB Jr, Roth JA, Wesley MN, et al. Analysis of prognostic factors in patients undergoing resection of pulmonary metastases from soft tissue sarcomas. J Thorac Cardiovasc Surg 1984;87:260.

79. van de Wal HJ, Verhagen A, Lecluyse A, et al. Surgery of pulmonary metastases. Thorac Cardiovasc Surg 1986;34:153.

80. Depadt G, Delacrois R, Mauretta J, et al. Surgical treatment of pulmonary metastasis: problems and prospects. In: Hellman K, Eccles SA, eds. Proceedings. Philadelphia, Taylor and Francis, 1985;5.

81. Ramming KP. Surgery for pulmonary metastases. Surg Clin North Am 1980;60:814.

82. Putnam JB Jr, Roth JA. Prognostic indicators in patients with pulmonary metastases. Semin Surg Oncol 1990;6:291.

SURGERY: SCIENTIFIC PRINCIPLES AND PRACTICE, Second Edition, edited by Lazar J. Greenfield, Michael W. Mulholland, Keith T. Oldham, Gerald B. Zelenock, and Keith D. Lillemoe. Lippincott–Raven Publishers, Philadelphia, © 1997.

CHAPTER 62

CHEST WALL, PLEURA, MEDIASTINUM, AND NONNEOPLASTIC LUNG DISEASE

MARK D. IANNETTONI AND MARK B. ORRINGER

ANATOMY

Respiration

The thoracic cage is a dynamic, continuously active combination of skeletal, muscular, and articulating tissues, the primary function of which is to provide movement to generate ventilation of the lungs. The thoracic cage also protects the thoracic viscera and supports the upper extremities. As active, coordinated muscle contractions occur during inspiration, intrathoracic, intrapleural, and intrapulmonic pressures fall, and atmospheric air is drawn into the lungs. Expiration is mainly a passive event that occurs as the expanded thoracic dimensions of inspiration return to baseline levels.

During inspiration, the body of the sternum is elevated outward and forward by motion of the ribs at their vertebral articulations. The first through fourth ribs and cartilages are relatively short and immobile, whereas the fifth through seventh are the longest and most flexible. Synchronous contraction of the intercostal muscles in inspiration,

with some assistance from the scalene muscles, elevates the thoracic cage as a unit and results in an increase in both the anteroposterior and lateral dimensions of the chest. Finally, as the muscular diaphragm contracts and flattens during inspiration, the superoinferior dimension of the chest also increases.

The primary muscles of inspiration are the diaphragm, which contributes 75% to 80% of ventilation during quiet respiration, and the intercostal muscles (especially the external intercostal and the anterior portions of the internal intercostal), which are responsible for 20% to 25% of respiratory movement. The accessory muscles of respiration (ie, the sternocleidomastoid muscles, serratus, levators of the ribs, trapezius, pectoral, latissimus dorsi) come into play in cases of respiratory distress.

At the end of quiet inspiration, when contraction of the inspiratory muscles has expanded the rib cage maximally against atmospheric pressure, elastic recoil of the lungs and rib cage results in a rise of intrapulmonic pressure that forces air out of the lungs until intrapulmonic pressure equals atmospheric pressure. Vigorous expiration that occurs, for example, with straining or shouting, is facilitated by contraction of the abdominal wall musculature that forces abdominal viscera against the diaphragm.

Skeletal Support

The bony chest wall is made up of the sternum, 10 pairs of ribs and their costal cartilages, 2 pairs of ribs without cartilages, and 12 thoracic vertebrae and their intervertebral disks (Fig. 62-1). These bony elements surround the thoracic cavity, which extends from the thoracic inlet above to the outlet below. The boundaries of the thoracic inlet are the manubrium of the sternum anteriorly, the first ribs laterally, and the first thoracic vertebra posteriorly. The anterior border of the thoracic inlet is 2 to 3 cm below its posterior border. The endothoracic (Sibson) fascia makes up the roof of the thoracic inlet and extends into the base of the neck with the parietal pleura, which is just beneath it. The thoracic outlet is bounded by the xiphoid process anteriorly, the fused 7th through 10th costal cartilages anterolaterally, and portions of the 11th and 12th ribs and the 12th thoracic vertebra posteriorly, and it is separated from the abdomen by the diaphragm. The outlet is higher anteriorly than it is posteriorly, and it is lowest in the mid-axillary line laterally.

The sternum is 15 to 20 cm in length and consists of three sections—the manubrium, the body (gladiolus), and the xiphoid process. Wider in its upper half (5 cm) than in its lower half (2.5 to 3 cm), the manubrium articulates along its upper border with the clavicles and laterally with the cartilages of the first and upper halves of the second ribs. The junction of the manubrium and body of the sternum—the sternal angle or angle of Louis—corresponds to the second interspace laterally and the top of the fourth thoracic vertebral body posteriorly. The body of the sternum, somewhat more than twice the length of the manubrium, articulates with the lower half of the second costal cartilages and the cartilages of the third through seventh ribs. The lower end of the body of the sternum articulates with the xiphoid process and is at the lateral level of the 10th or 11th thoracic vertebrae. The xiphoid cartilage has a variable length and ends in the rectus sheath. Although the lateral aspects of the sternum are covered by the sternal origins of the pectoralis major muscles, the midline is virtually subcutaneous and therefore readily accessible for a median sternotomy incision.

Developmentally, the ribs are initially entirely cartilaginous and extend horizontally from their respective vertebral bodies to the sternum. With embryonic growth, the

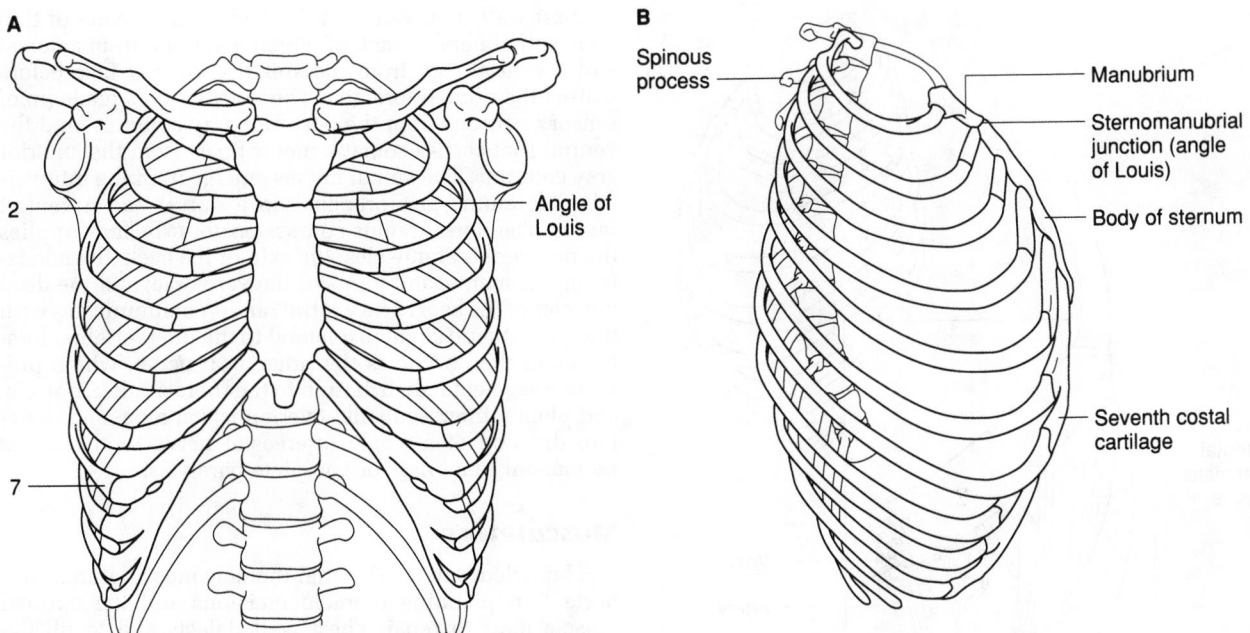

Figure 62-1. Skeletal support of the thorax. Anterior (*A*) and lateral (*B*) views. Note the anterior cartilaginous component of the upper 10 ribs, the fused costal cartilages of ribs 7 through 10, the location of the sternomanubrial junction (angle of Louis) at the level of the second rib, and the oblique course of the ribs laterally from posterior to anterior.

vertebral ends of the ribs migrate cephalad, so that the heads of the ribs, particularly ribs two through nine, eventually come to articulate with both their vertebral body and the one immediately above. As ossification occurs, the unossified anterior end remains as cartilage. Each rib extends backward from the vertebrae and then turns forward toward the sternum at the angle of the rib. The upper seven pairs of true ribs articulate with the sternum at their respective sternocostal junction. The lower five pairs of false ribs do not articulate directly with the sternum. The cartilages of ribs 8, 9, and 10 each articulate with the cartilage of the rib above, and ribs 11 and 12 terminate in cartilaginous tips that end in the muscle of the abdominal wall. The fused cartilages of ribs 7 through 10 make up the common costal arch. This anatomic relation has great significance to the thoracic surgeon. A chest wall infection that involves the upper anterior ribs may be eradicated by complete excision of the entire avascular costal cartilage, whereas infections involving a portion of the 7th through 10th costal cartilages often require complete excision of the entire costal arch for resolution.

The ribs gradually increase in length from the first through the seventh, which is the longest, and then progressively shorten to the 12th. Each rib has a *head,* usually with facets, which articulates with its vertebral body and the one above (Fig. 62-2). The 2.5-cm-long *neck* has a tubercle with an articular cartilage that meets a facet on the transverse process of the respective vertebral body, thereby forming the costotransverse joint. The *shaft* of the rib begins at the *angle,* which is usually the lateral margin of the erector spinae muscles. The costal groove along the inferior aspect of each rib contains the intercostal vessels and nerves. Therefore, when placing pericostal sutures to reapproximate the ribs after a thoracotomy, or when performing a thoracentesis or chest tube insertion, the undersurface of the rib should be avoided to prevent untoward bleeding from a lacerated intercostal artery or neuralgia from an injured intercostal nerve. The junction of the ribs with their respective cartilages is marked by a palpable elevation, the costochondral junction.

Each intercostal space is made up of three layers of muscle and their respective deep fascia (Fig. 62-3). The external intercostal muscle courses obliquely forward and downward from the lower border of the rib above to the upper border of the rib below and extends from the tubercle of the rib posteriorly to the start of the costal cartilage in front. Beneath this is the internal intercostal muscle, which courses in an opposite direction, downward and backward. The neurovascular bundle—the intercostal vein, artery, and nerve (from above downward)—is located deep to the second muscle layer within the endothoracic fascia, just superficial to the parietal pleura. The next layer, the innermost intercostal muscle, is less well developed and is unimportant from a clinical standpoint. The

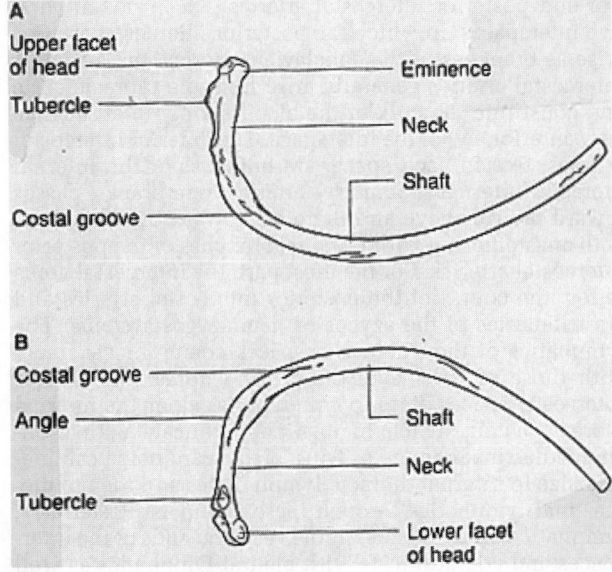

Figure 62-2. Anatomy of the rib as viewed from above (*A*) and below (*B*).

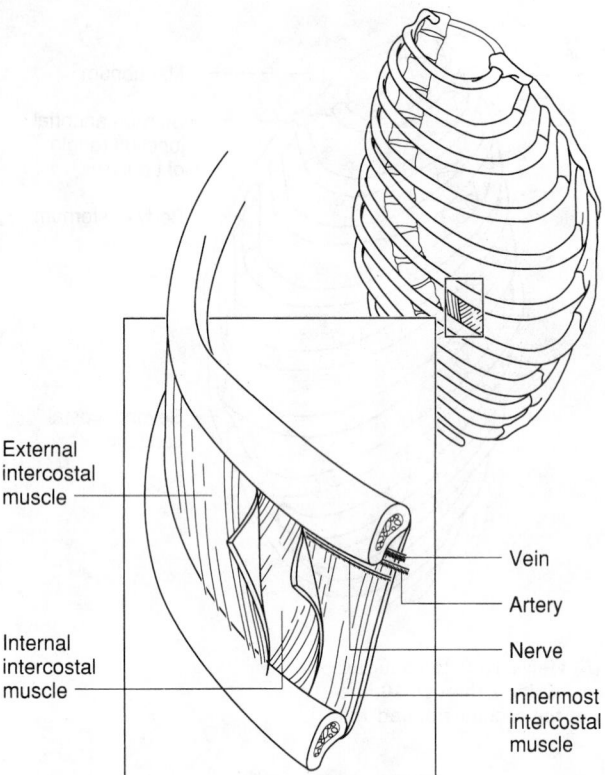

Figure 62-3. Anatomy of the intercostal space. The major intercostal muscles are the external and internal. The neurovascular bundle courses in the costal groove along the inferior aspect of the rib.

endothoracic fascia is a fibroareolar layer of varying depth beneath the innermost intercostal layer. It is the site at which a subpleural dissection is carried out, separating the parietal pleura from the chest wall.

Blood Supply, Venous Drainage, and Lymphatics

Each intercostal space receives blood supply from anterior and posterior intercostal arteries. Except for the first two interspaces, in which the posterior intercostal arteries arise as branches of the subclavian arteries, the posterior intercostal arteries generally arise from the thoracic aorta and constitute the bulk of the blood supply to all but the very anterior end of the interspace. The anterior intercostal arteries, two in each space, are branches of the internal thoracic (internal mammary) arteries; one branch passes toward the rib above and the other toward the rib below, both anastomosing with terminal branches of the posterior intercostal arteries. For the most part, the intercostal veins follow the course of the posterior intercostal arteries and are tributaries of the azygos or hemiazygos systems. The lymphatics of the intercostal spaces communicate freely with those of the mediastinum. The upper four or five intercostal spaces drain to lymph nodes along the internal thoracic chain, which in turn communicate with bronchomediastinal channels. Thus, breast carcinoma can metastasize to internal thoracic lymph nodes and then to mediastinal lymphatics through these channels. Posteriorly, lymphatics drain to nodes at the vertebral ends of the interspaces and communicate with pleural lymphatics as well as with the thoracic duct above and the cisterna chyli below.

Chest wall innervation is derived from 12 pairs of thoracic spinal nerves, each of which is formed from a dorsal and a ventral root from the spinal cord that fuse before exiting the normal foramen. The dorsal root is made up of sensory neurons from the posterior gray columns, and the ventral root carries somatic motor fibers from the anterior gray columns. The spinal nerves emerge from the intervertebral foramina and branch into a dorsal and a ventral ramus. The dorsal ramus courses posteriorly and supplies the paravertebral muscles; the skin of the back; the periosteum, ligaments, and joints of the vertebrae; and the deep muscles of the back. The ventral ramus communicates with the sympathetic chain just lateral to the intervertebral foramen and then becomes the intercostal nerve, which provides a segmental distribution to the thoracic skin, muscle, and pleura. Intersegmental overlap is common, and therefore division of a single intercostal nerve rarely causes permanent numbness or complete paralysis.

Musculature

A knowledge of the external thoracic musculature is important in planning thoracic incisions and the optimal muscle flaps to repair chest wall defects and to fill the pleural space as treatment of chronic empyemas or complications of previous pulmonary resection (Fig. 62-4). The *sternocleidomastoid muscle* arises from the manubrium medially and the medial third of the clavicle laterally; it inserts on the mastoid bone at the base of the skull. The *pectoralis major muscle* arises from the medial clavicle, the sternum, the anterior ribs, and the external oblique fascia and inserts on the greater tubercle of the humerus at the bicipital groove. Its lower margins form the anterior fold of the axilla. Its predominant blood supply is the pectoral branch of the thoracoacromial artery, which arises from the axillary artery medial to the proximal border of the pectoralis minor and can be found reliably emerging from the clavipectoral fascia about 2 cm medial and 2 cm caudal to the coracoid process of the scapula. Innervation of the pectoralis major is from the medial and lateral pectoral nerves, which are named from the cord of the brachial plexus from which they arise and not from their anatomic position. The functions of the pectoralis major are adduction and medial rotation of the arm. This muscle can be mobilized on its vascular pedicle to permit repair of anterior thoracic defects, particularly those of the upper three fourths of the sternum, and as a musculocutaneous flap after ablative head and neck operations.

The *pectoralis minor muscle*, deep to the pectoralis major, arises from the second through fifth ribs and inserts on the coracoid process of the scapula. It is also supplied by the medial and lateral pectoral nerves and functions to depress and rotate the shoulders downward.

The *serratus anterior muscle* originates from the upper eight ribs anteriorly and passes upward and laterally, attaching on the anterior surface of the medial aspect of the scapula. This muscle holds the scapula against the chest wall, particularly when adducting and elevating the arms above the horizontal plane. The long thoracic nerve, which passes inferiorly in the mid-axillary line, just beneath the anterior border of the latissimus dorsi muscle, provides innervation to the serratus anterior, and injury to this nerve results in a winged scapula, an annoying and cosmetically unsightly protrusion of the scapula from the posterior thorax.

On the posterior thorax, the *trapezius muscles* provide the margins of the neck and the upper shoulders. Each arises from the nuchal line of the occipital bone, the ligamentum nuchae of the neck, and the spines of the seventh cervical and all the thoracic vertebrae. The fibers of trape-

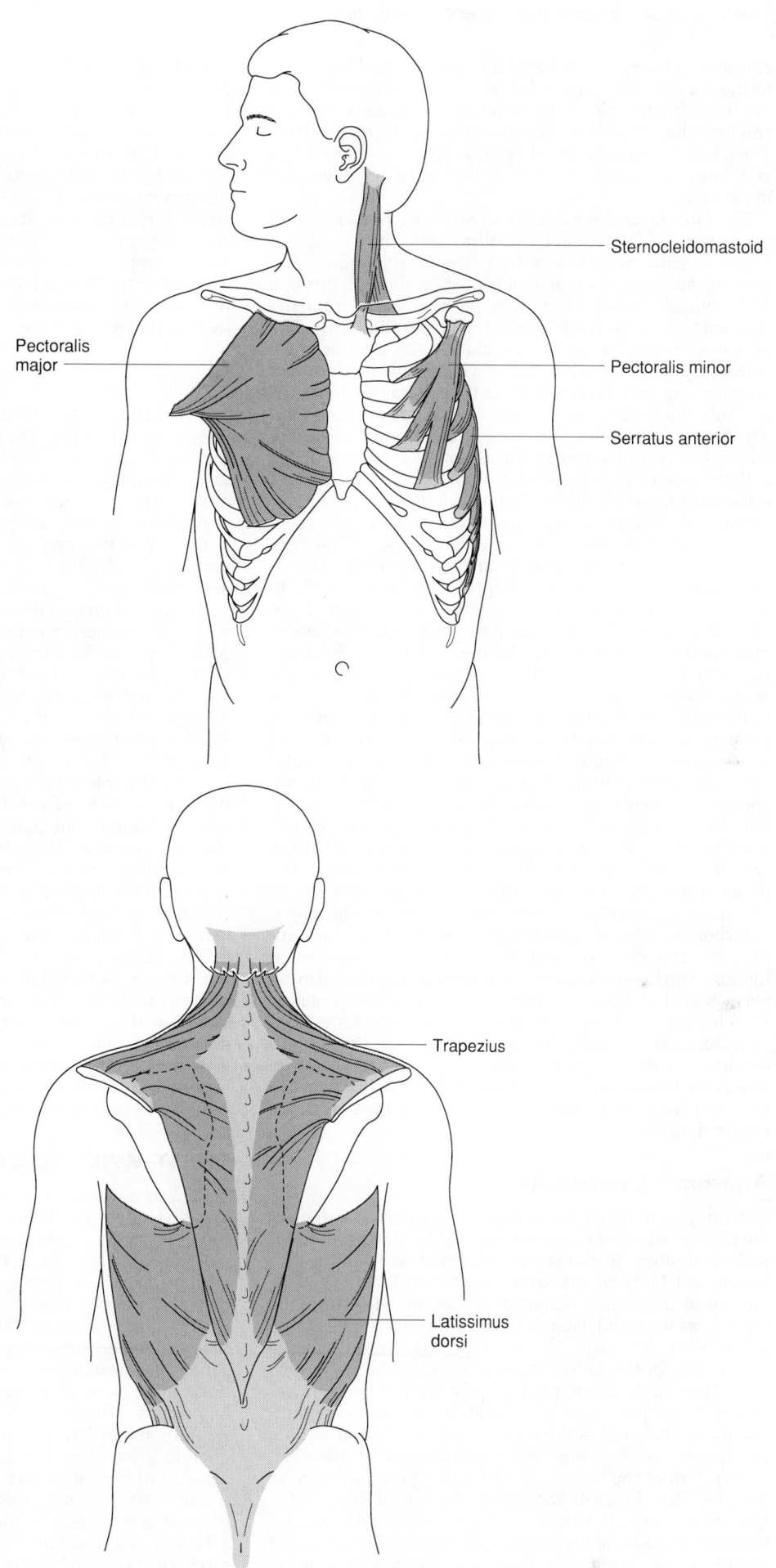

Sternocleidomastoid

Pectoralis major

Pectoralis minor

Serratus anterior

Trapezius

Latissimus dorsi

Figure 62-4. Thoracic musculature. (*A*) Anterior view. (*B*) Posterior view.

zius sweep laterally and insert on the spine and acromion of the scapula and on the lateral clavicle. Innervation of the trapezius muscles is from the spinal accessory nerves and branches of the third and fourth cervical spinal nerves. The trapezius muscles stabilize the scapulae and shoulders and are important in the wide range of shoulder movements.

The *latissimus dorsi muscle* covers a triangular area of the lower and lateral back extending from the sacrum up to the seventh thoracic vertebrae. The muscle arises from a broad aponeurosis that is attached to the 7th through 12th thoracic vertebral spinous processes and from the aponeuroses of the lumbodorsal fascia and iliac crest. The upper border of the muscle attaches to the inferior angle of the scapula by muscle bundles. The muscle then courses laterally and inserts on the lesser tubercle of the humerus and into the intertubercular groove. The major blood supply of the latissimus dorsi is the thoracodorsal artery, which is a continuation of the subscapular branch of the axillary artery. The thoracodorsal artery has a fairly constant course, reaching the latissimus along its upper border about 2 cm from the lateral edge of the muscle and 8 to 10 cm from the humeral insertion of the muscle. The constancy of this vascular pedicle and the size of the latissimus, which permits great mobility, allow this muscle to be used for reconstruction of almost any portion of the chest wall, pleural cavity, and head and neck. The latissimus dorsi muscle is invested by the dorsal superficial fascia, which connects to the thick skin of the back by dense septa. Because latissimus muscle provides blood supply to its overlying skin through multiple perforating arteries, the muscle is ideally suited as a carrier for its overlying skin and subcutaneous tissue as a combined musculocutaneous flap. Innervation of latissimus dorsi is by the thoracodorsal nerve of the posterior cord of the brachial plexus, which carries fibers from C-6, C-7, and C-8. The latissimus dorsi functions to extend, adduct, and internally rotate the arm. It also pulls the shoulder downward and posteriorly. Beneath the trapezius and latissimus dorsi muscle layers is a layer of muscles (levator scapulae, rhomboid major, and rhomboid minor muscles) that function to elevate, adduct, and retract the scapula. These muscles are innervated by the dorsal scapular nerve; the levator scapulae also receive branches from C-4 and C-5. The serratus posterior muscle, which arises from the aponeuroses of the ligamentum nuchae and the spinous processes of the seventh cervical vertebrae as well as the first three thoracic vertebrae, attaches to the upper edges of the first three to five ribs and is also regarded as an accessory muscle of inspiration.

Anatomic Landmarks

A number of topographic thoracic anatomic landmarks are particularly useful in assessing and localizing intrathoracic pathology. For example, the junction of the manubrium and body of the sternum (the angle of Louis) is located at the upper margin of the second rib. On plane anteroposterior and lateral chest radiographs, this angle aligns with the carina in the mid-mediastinum and the upper edge of the fourth thoracic vertebral body posteriorly. The nipple in men is typically located at the lower border of the pectoralis major muscle, lateral to the midclavicular line, and in the fourth intercostal space. Nipple location in women is more variable because of the variation in size of the breast. The *triangle of auscultation* on the posterior thorax is formed by the lateral edge of the trapezius muscle, the upper border of latissimus dorsi, and the medial border of the scapula. Because of the absence of significant overlying chest wall musculature at this point,

auscultation of underlying respiratory sounds is most clear in this area. Both subclavian veins cross the first rib anterior to the attachment of the serratus anterior muscle on the scalene tubercle of the first rib. These vessels are therefore localized for subclavian puncture just lateral to the angle formed by the clavicle and the first rib. Because the diaphragm can ascend to the level of the fourth intercostal space during deep expiration, particularly if the patient is crouching forward, any penetrating wound of the thorax from the nipple line downward may have entered the peritoneal cavity. The junction of the body and the xiphoid process of the sternum is roughly at the level of the 10th to 11th thoracic vertebrae.

Pleura

Embryologically, the lungs begin as diverticula of the foregut and grow into the thoracic cavity, thereby displacing the pleural sac. A portion of the pleural sac is applied to the lung buds as the visceral pleura, whereas the part of the pleural sac that is applied to the chest wall becomes the parietal pleura. The parietal and visceral pleurae join at the root of the lung and at the pulmonary ligament. The parietal pleura is subdivided into its costal, mediastinal, and diaphragmatic portions, designated by the adjacent structures. Topographic relations of the pleura to the chest wall are remarkably constant (Fig. 62-5). Superiorly, the pleura extends into the base of the neck. Anteriorly, the pleurae meet just behind the angle of Louis. The right pleural edge continues downward near the midline and then diverges laterally at the sixth or seventh costal cartilage. The left pleura is generally displaced laterally by the heart from the fourth through the sixth interspaces. The lowest extent of the pleura occurs laterally in the mid-clavicular line, at the level of the 11th rib. The pleural edge then follows a horizontal course along the 12th rib to the 12th thoracic vertebra. Thus, flank approaches to the kidneys or adrenal glands over the 11th or 12th ribs can result in entry into the pleural cavity and the need for a chest tube.

The lower edge of the lung does not extend as far inferiorly as the inferior extent of the pleura. Superiorly, the cupola of the pleura is characteristically located behind the inferior and medial borders of the scalenus anterior muscle and is therefore vulnerable to damage during operations in this vicinity (eg, scalene node biopsy, anterior scalenotomy for thoracic outlet syndrome, or subclavian vein puncture). The cupola of the pleura is also crossed superficially in the neck by both the phrenic and vagus nerves that are descending into the thorax.

CHEST WALL TUMORS

Tumors of the chest wall are relatively uncommon, constituting only 1% to 2% of all tumors in the body. Although reported series of chest wall tumors frequently exclude patients with soft tissue tumors and focus only on those with primary bone tumors, it has become increasingly evident that the soft tissues are an important origin of chest wall tumors and in fact account for half of these tumors that are treated surgically.[1] Although it is common to regard a chest wall mass as a primary tumor on initial evaluation, about 57% of resected chest wall tumors prove to be primary, whereas 43% are metastatic from other sites.[2] Solitary metastatic tumors to the chest wall most frequently arise from the genitourinary tract, the thyroid gland, and the colon. Renal cell and thyroid cancers have a predilection to metastasize to the sternum, where they occasionally present as pulsatile masses.

Overall, 60% of chest wall tumors are malignant, most arising either from bone or cartilage. Primary tumors of the

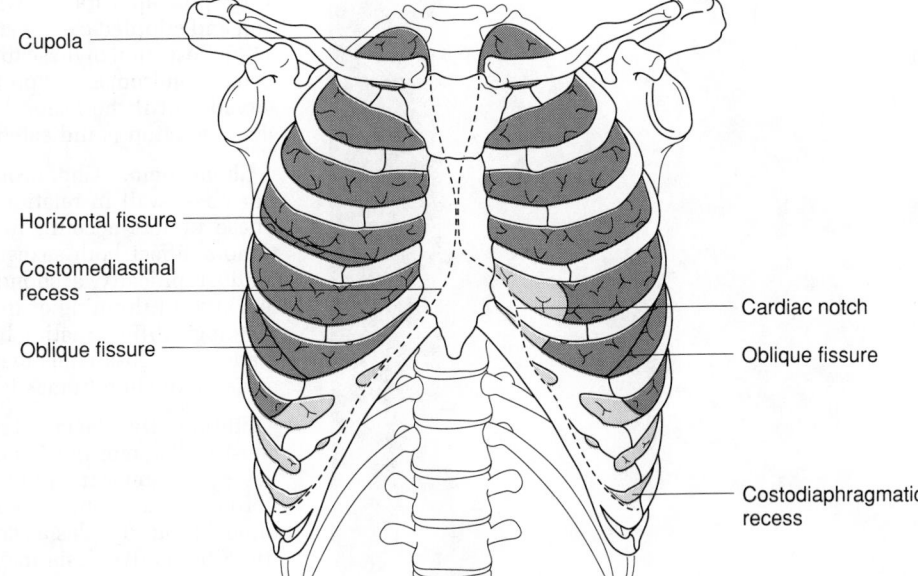

Figure 62-5. Topographic relations of the pleura to the chest wall. Laterally, the pleura extends to the level of the 11th to 12th ribs. The anterior reflection of the mediastinal and costal pleurae forms the costo-mediastinal recess, whereas the reflections of the costal and diaphragmatic pleurae form the costo-diaphragmatic recess.

ribs are more common than those of the sternum. Soft tissue sarcomas are the next most common chest wall malignancies, followed by multiple myeloma, Ewing sarcoma, and a variety of tumors, including malignant fibrous histiocytoma, synovial sarcoma, liposarcoma, rhabdomyosarcoma, undifferentiated sarcoma, and malignant hemangioendothelioma. Benign primary chest wall tumors include osteochondromas, chondromas, desmoid tumors, fibrous dysplasia, lipomas, fibromas, and neurilemomas.

Presentation

Only 20% of chest wall tumors are asymptomatic, typically detected initially on a routine chest radiograph. In contrast, 80% of these tumors present as an enlarging mass that is painful in 50% to 60% of patients. Fever, leukocytosis, and eosinophilia may be present, depending on the tumor type. Certain histologic tumors predominate in specific age groups, although chest wall tumors can occur at any age. In assessing the patient, the location of the tumor may have direct implications on the type of operation required for its resection. Posterior thoracic tumors may involve the spine and require a combined neurosurgical and thoracosurgical approach. Tumors low on the chest wall may involve the diaphragm and necessitate partial diaphragmatic resection and reconstruction. High anterior chest wall tumors may require resection of the adjacent clavicle and dissection of the mass away from the great vessels of the neck.

Preoperative Evaluation

Standard posteroanterior and lateral chest radiographs assist in localizing the mass, determining the presence of rib destruction, identifying associated pulmonary disease such as lung metastases, and defining the presence of a pleural effusion that would merit thoracentesis and cytologic evaluation.

Although computed tomography (CT) is of little value in determining bone destruction because of the oblique course of the ribs, which are imaged at right angles to the long axis of the body, CT is of great value in demonstrating the relation between the mass and contiguous structures,

defining the dimensions and consistency of the tumor, revealing the presence of synchronous metastases to the lungs, assessing the mediastinum for adenopathy, and demonstrating any associated pleural tumor or fluid. CT scanning should include both chest and abdominal views so that the kidneys can be assessed as a potential source of a primary tumor and hepatic metastases can be excluded.

For chest wall tumors located near the axilla, angiography may be helpful in defining involvement of the axillary artery. When the need for a muscle flap from a previously irradiated field is anticipated, angiography may be useful in defining the integrity of the vascular pedicle. Because 43% of chest wall tumors are due to metastatic disease, a bone scan should be performed in all patients with tumors of the chest wall, ribs, or sternum to rule out other sites of metastatic disease that might preclude resection. In most cases, excision of chest wall tumors does not involve a major pulmonary resection. Baseline pulmonary function testing and determination of arterial blood gases is helpful in assessing the relative operative risk of patients in whom removal of a major portion of the lung is anticipated.

A thorough physical examination of the patient with a chest wall tumor is important in identifying an unsuspected primary site of the tumor. The thyroid gland should be carefully palpated, breast and abdominal masses excluded, and urine and stool examined for occult blood.

Diagnosis

Controversy surrounds the need or desirability of a preoperative biopsy of chest wall tumors. Historically, the emphasis has been placed on regarding all new chest wall tumors as malignant and treating them directly with wide excision. The difficulty in differentiating histologically a low-grade chondrosarcoma from a high-grade chondroma is notorious. Therefore, an initial nonexcisional biopsy was discouraged because of the concern about local recurrence of the tumor after incomplete resection. A clear change in this earlier philosophy is evolving for several reasons. With the advent of multimodality therapy for some chest wall tumors, the most efficacious ordering of chemotherapy, radiotherapy, or surgery has been based on tumor histology. In a large experience from Memorial

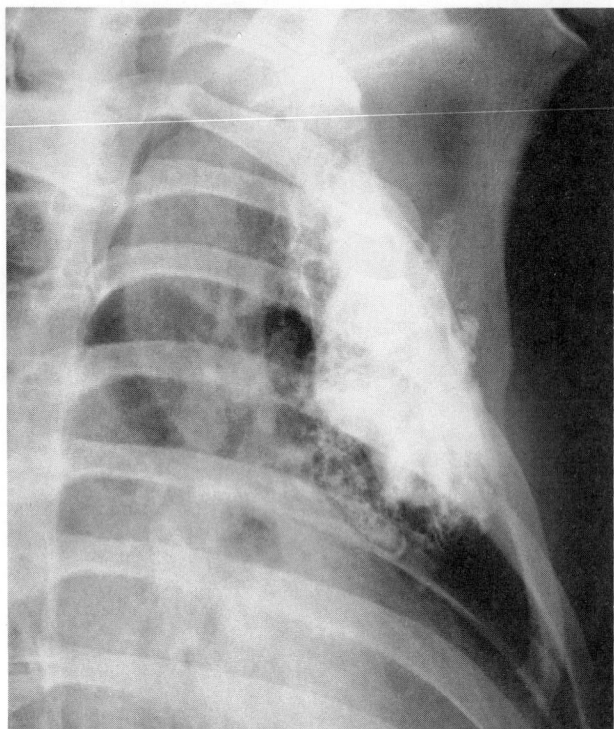

Figure 62-6. Osteochondroma of left second rib. The stippled calcification within the tumor and the intact cortex of the rib are characteristic.

Sloan-Kettering Cancer Center, patients with osteogenic sarcoma, plasmacytomas, and Ewing sarcoma had improved survival rates with combined multimodality treatment, and resection was the best primary treatment for chondrosarcoma.[3,4] Although it was earlier argued that the precise histologic diagnosis of chest wall tumors was often extremely difficult, the availability of electron microscopy and immunohistochemical techniques now permits greater diagnostic accuracy. Further, neither an increased incidence of local recurrence nor decreased survival after properly performed preoperative biopsies has been documented. Therefore, biopsy of a chest wall mass through an incision that is amenable to excision when skin flaps are raised at a later date is now recommended. Multiple core-needle biopsies, not fine-needle aspirations, may provide sufficient diagnostic tissue without the need for a larger operative biopsy. The tissue obtained at biopsy should be submitted for permanent histopathologic assessment, immunohistochemical studies, and electron microscopic study. Appropriate treatment planning based on available adjuvant therapy can then be undertaken with the knowledge of the tumor's histology.

Primary Tumors of the Ribs and Sternum

Benign Rib Tumors

Osteochondroma. Only 10% of rib tumors are benign, and osteochondromas, the most common benign bone tumor, account for half of these.[1] The tumor occurs more frequently in men, with a male/female ratio of 3:1. Osteochondromas begin in childhood and grow until completion of skeletal maturity. They are frequently asymptomatic, and the development of pain may signify malignant degeneration. Osteochondromas have a characteristic ra-

diographic appearance, with a peripheral rim of calcification and stippled calcification within the tumor mass (Fig. 62-6). Resection of these tumors in adults is recommended. Osteochondromas in prepubertal children may be observed, but if the lesion becomes painful or increases in size, resection is indicated.

Chondroma. Chondromas typically arise on the anterior chest wall in relation to the costochondral junction. These tumors account for 15% of benign thoracic cage tumors, affect both sexes equally, and occur at any age. Radiographically, a chondroma presents as an expansile lesion with thinning of the overlying cortex. Because the histologic differentiation between a chondroma and a low-grade chondrosarcoma may be exceedingly difficult, wide excision of chondromas is recommended.

Fibrous Dysplasia. This abnormality presents as a chest wall tumor but is not neoplastic. Fibrous dysplasia is a cystic abnormality of the rib that is characterized by fibrous replacement of the medullary cavity of the rib. Most often, fibrous dysplasia occurs as a solitary bone abnormality. Fibrous dysplasia may also occur as part of Albright syndrome (multiple bone cysts, pigmented skin, and precocious puberty in girls). Fibrous dysplasia most often involves the posterolateral ribs, affects both sexes equally, and produces a characteristic radiographic appearance of an expansile rib lesion with thinning of the overlying cortex and a central ground-glass appearance (Fig. 62-7). Asymptomatic lesions may be followed in children because cessation of growth is common at the onset of puberty. Enlarging or painful lesions should be resected locally.

Histiocytosis X. Like fibrous dysplasia, histiocytosis X is a nonneoplastic condition of the ribs. In this case, the

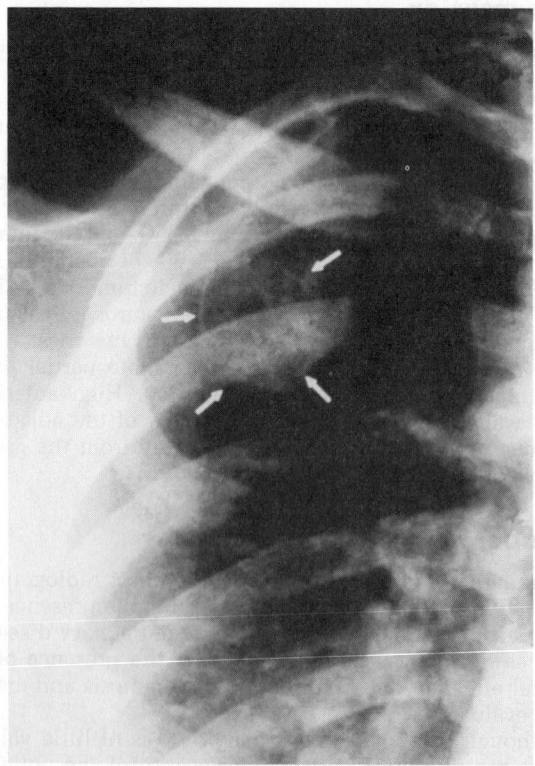

Figure 62-7. Fibrous dysplasia of the rib. Note the characteristic expansion and thinning of the cortex (*arrows*) and the central ground-glass appearance.

rib abnormality is part of a spectrum of reticuloendothelial diseases that include eosinophilic granuloma, Letterer-Siwe disease, and Hand-Schüller-Christian disease. The bone abnormalities of histiocytosis X most often involve the skull, but 10% to 20% of patients have rib abnormalities that are similar for all three forms of the disease. Radiographically, histiocytosis X causes an expansile rib lesion that is associated with periosteal new bone formation and irregular cortical destruction. The characteristic histology of histiocytosis X involves infiltration of the marrow and bone by eosinophils and histiocytes. In eosinophilic granuloma, there is only involvement of bone, either solitary or at multiple sites. Diagnostic excisional biopsy may be required and cures the lesion if it is solitary. If there are multiple bone lesions, low-dose radiotherapy in the range of 300 to 600 cGy to each area of involvement may be beneficial. Hand-Schüller-Christian disease and Letterer-Siwe disease are systemic conditions that are characteristically associated with fever, malaise, weight loss, lymphadenopathy, and splenomegaly. Hematologic assessment may demonstrate leukocytosis, eosinophilia, and anemia. These conditions tend to be more protracted and necessitate corticosteroids and chemotherapy. Eosinophilic granuloma tends to occur in young to middle-aged adults. Letterer-Siwe disease usually occurs in infants, and Hand-Schüller-Christian disease appears in children.

Malignant Rib Tumors

Chondrosarcoma. Chondrosarcoma is the most common primary chest wall malignancy, typically occurring as a solitary lesion and affecting the first four ribs. These tumors generally occur in patients older than 40 years of age and present as an anterior chest wall mass (Fig. 62-8). Seventy-five percent arise anteriorly from the costal cartilage, either at the costochondral or sternochondral junctions. Twenty-five percent arise posteriorly from the cartilaginous articulations with the head of the rib. The typical clinical presentation is that of a slowly growing chest mass that has been painful for months. There is a characteristic radiographic appearance of a lobulated mass in the medullary portion of the rib with poorly defined margins and associated cortical destruction. Mottled calcification is typical. Chondrosarcomas tend to grow slowly and to recur locally if they are inadequately excised. A report of the results of treatment in 88 patients with chest

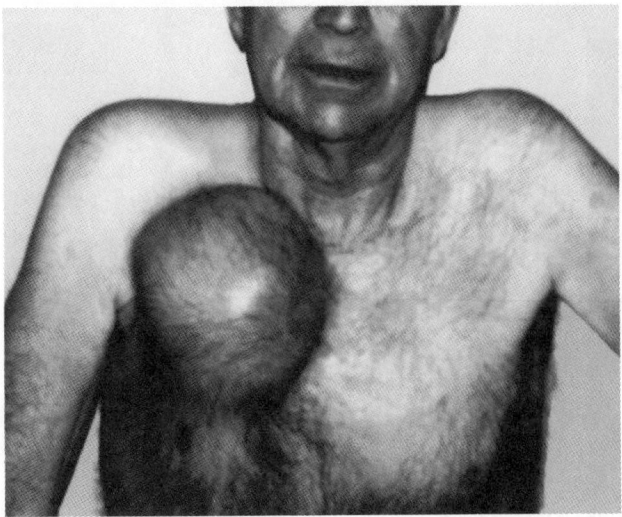

Figure 62-8. Large chondrosarcoma arising from the right anterior third costochondral junction.

wall chondrosarcomas documented an overall 5-year survival rate of 64% and a median survival of 184 months.[3] The major predictors of survival were metastatic disease at the time of presentation, age greater than 50 years, and complete resection. Sex, tumor grade, and tumor size had no significant impact on survival. Metastasis to lymph nodes, lung, bone, and other distant sites is well documented. Chondrosarcomas should be resected with at least a 4- to 5-cm margin of normal tissue on all sides, and with such wide resection, 10-year rates survival of nearly 97% have been reported.[5]

Ewing Sarcoma. Ewing sarcoma of the rib accounts for about 10% of all primary malignancies of the bony thorax. These tumors have a predilection for children and adolescents and affect boys twice as often as girls. The tumors characteristically present as a painful soft tissue swelling of the chest wall with an associated pleural effusion. One of the hallmarks of this chest wall tumor is systemic symptoms of fever, fatigue, malaise, and weight loss with laboratory studies showing a leukocytosis and elevated sedimentation rate. Nearly half of these patients have hematogenous metastasis to the lungs or central nervous system at the time of presentation. Radiographically, Ewing sarcoma demonstrates both lytic and blastic areas of bone destruction. Elevation of the periosteum and multiple layers of subperiosteal new bone formation produce an onion skin appearance of the overlying bone. This finding may occur with other bone tumors. Because of the radiographic appearance and associated fever and leukocytosis, Ewing sarcoma may be easily confused with osteomyelitis. The unique histology of Ewing sarcoma includes broad sheets of small polyhedral cells that have a pale cytoplasm and small hyperchromatic nuclei. Differentiation from lymphoma can be difficult and may necessitate evaluation with light microscopy, special stains, and electron microscopy. One of the distinguishing features of Ewing sarcoma is its sensitivity to radiotherapy, which until recently was the treatment of choice. Surgery also appears to have an important role in the treatment of this tumor. Although resection combined with radiotherapy may be appropriate for localized lesions, tumors that are greater than 10 cm in diameter or associated with appreciable soft tissue infiltration have a demonstrated poor prognosis, and in this latter group, multimodality therapy has been applied. Combination therapy using doxorubicin (Adriamycin), cyclophosphamide, and vincristine with localized radiotherapy and resection is being evaluated with encouraging results; reported 3-year disease-free survival rates approach 50%.[6] A report of a 40-year experience with Ewing sarcoma indicates that patients pretreated with chemotherapy followed by local resection have 5- and 10-year survival rates of 48%, and only the development of distant metastasis has a significant impact on survival.[5]

Osteogenic Sarcoma. Osteogenic sarcoma of the rib is far less common than that in the extremity and accounts for only 6% of primary bony chest wall malignancies. This tumor occurs most commonly in teenagers and young adults and presents as a painful mass fixed to the underlying rib. The characteristic radiographic "sunburst" is due to the typical calcification at right angles to the involved cortex that occurs with osteogenic sarcoma. These tend to be large, lobulated tumors that destroy cortical bone and extend into soft tissues. Vascular invasion and pulmonary metastases are common. Wide excision of the involved bone and adjacent soft tissues has been the mainstay of treatment; radiotherapy has essentially no role in the treatment of these tumors. The prognosis is generally poor, with a 5-year survival rate of only 20%. Multimodality therapy is used for osteogenic sarcoma with encouraging results; some investigators have reported a 90% disease-free survival rate with a preoperative chemotherapy regimen that includes vincristine, methotrexate, doxorubicin, bleomycin, dactinomycin, and cyclophosphamide.[7,8]

Plasmacytoma. This tumor accounts for nearly one third of all chest wall tumors. Although isolated, solitary plasmacytomas do occur, as a rule, this condition is indicative of systemic multiple myeloma, and patients without other manifestations of the systemic disease generally develop it with longer observation. Radiographically, these tumors typically present as osteolytic, "punched-out" rib defects. There is frequently an associated soft tissue component greater than that seen with other chest wall tumors (Fig. 62-9). Plasmacytoma of the chest wall is more common in men and typically occurs in the fifth through seventh decades of life. The common presenting symptom is pain, and as indicated earlier, although there may be an appreciable soft tissue component within the thorax, there may be no palpable mass on physical examination. Systemic signs and symptoms include fever, malaise, anemia, and an elevated sedimentation rate. Eighty-five percent of these patients have abnormal serum protein electrophoresis, and 50% have hypercalcemia and Bence Jones protein in the urine. The diagnosis of plasmacytoma of the chest wall can be made with a biopsy of the lytic lesion showing the characteristic plasma cells. These tumors are sensitive to alkylating agents (melphalan) in combination with prednisone, and local radiotherapy also provides an excellent response. Because in most cases chest wall plasmacytomas are part of a systemic disease, wide excision and chest wall reconstruction is difficult to justify. In the rare case of a solitary plasma cell tumor, however, resection may be curative when systemic disease can not be demonstrated by immunoelectrophoresis or imaging studies for lytic lesions. The reported 5-year survival rate after resection of chest wall plasmacytoma usually includes patients who have developed amyloidosis or multiple myeloma and ranges from 20% to 40%.[9]

Tumors of the Sternum and Clavicles

Fifteen percent of all primary chest wall bone tumors arise in the sternum, and more than 95% of these are malignant.[9] Most are chondrosarcomas, plasmacytomas, malignant lymphomas, and osteogenic sarcomas. Carcinomas of the breast, thyroid, and kidney frequently metastasize to the sternum. Clavicular tumors account for less than 1% of all primary bone tumors, and more than 90% are malignant. More than two thirds of these are either plasmacytomas or Ewing sarcoma and are therefore radiosensitive. Metastatic disease affects the clavicles more frequently than primary malignancy. The treatment of sternal and clavicular tumors is wide resection of the entire involved bone with a 4-cm margin.

Soft Tissue Sarcomas

Soft tissue sarcomas account for about 20% of malignant chest wall tumors. The most common histologic types include fibrosarcoma, leiomyosarcoma, liposarcoma, synovial sarcoma, neurofibrosarcoma, and malignant fibrous histiocytoma. Sarcomas are typically surrounded by a pseudocapsule of compressed normal tissue that is inevitably invaded by the tumor. Sarcomas have an aggressive biologic behavior and tend to metastasize, particularly to the lungs, within 2 years of diagnosis. Even with adequate excision, the incidence of local recurrence is about 10%, and studies are investigating the use of multimodality therapy, including postoperative radiotherapy and chemotherapy with doxorubicin and cyclophosphamide.

Malignant fibrous histiocytoma is an aggressive tumor that characteristically spreads locally along fascial planes and muscle fibers and therefore has a high incidence of local recurrence after resection. This tumor occurs most often between the ages of 50 and 70 years, and two thirds occur in men. Some evidence suggests that these tumors may be radiation induced, with several reported cases arising in areas of the chest wall previously irradiated for breast cancer, Hodgkin disease, and myeloma.[10] Because these tumors are resistant to both radiation and chemotherapy, wide resection is the treatment of choice, and the 5-year survival rate is about 38%. Postoperative radiotherapy is indicated if the margins of resection are inadequate.[11]

Rhabdomyosarcoma is basically a tumor of children and young adults that presents as a rapidly enlarging nonpainful chest mass. With its rapid growth rate, associated tumor necrosis and hemorrhage are common. Advances using multimodality therapy have greatly altered the prognosis of this disease. When wide resection of the tumor is followed by irradiation and multidrug chemotherapy (pri-

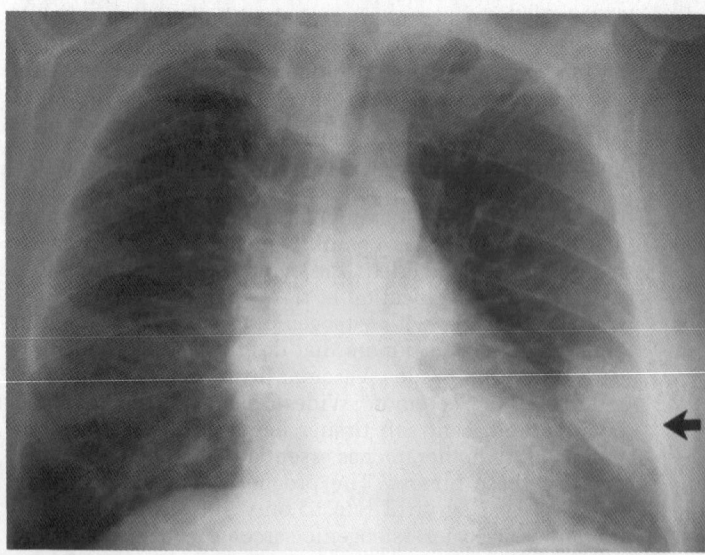

Figure 62-9. Plasmacytoma of the left seventh rib, showing characteristic cortical destruction and relatively large soft tissue component projecting into the chest.

marily with doxorubicin, cyclophosphamide, dactino-mycin, and vincristine), a 5-year survival rate of 70% can be achieved.

Chest Wall Resection

Using available methods of chest wall resection and reconstruction, operative mortality rates range from 1% to 4.5%.[1] The morbidity associated with these operations is remarkably low and includes pulmonary insufficiency, wound infection, bleeding, and ischemic necrosis of the rotated flap. Positioning of the patient for a chest wall resection and reconstruction is determined by the location of the chest tumor as well as the need for a muscle flap rotation for reconstruction. Most chest wall tumors are approached with the patient in a lateral decubitus position, as for a posterolateral thoracotomy; sternal tumors are resected with the patient in the supine position. A double-lumen endotracheal tube is helpful in the assessment of involvement of the contiguous lung, allowing either separation of adhesions or en bloc resection of pulmonary parenchyma when required. An old scar from a previous incisional biopsy should be excised with the specimen, and the skin incision must be planned accordingly. It is important to determine which muscle flaps will be used for reconstruction before making the incision because division of a potential muscle flap may limit the amount of tissue available for reconstruction. Skin and subcutaneous tissue are elevated superiorly to at least one intercostal space above the upper extent of the tumor. The overlying chest wall musculature is then incised to that interspace, which is then entered, allowing an initial exploration of the undersurface of the rib cage and the inward extent of the tumor. An adequate resection of a primary chest wall tumor involves a margin of 4 cm in all directions, which may translate to one or two ribs above and below the palpable limits of the mass. Each rib to be removed is divided anteriorly and posteriorly, identifying, ligating, and dividing each respective intercostal neurovascular bundle with absorbable suture. Musculature overlying the mass is divided with electrocautery and is left attached to the rib segment to be removed so as to avoid violation of the pseudocapsule of the tumor. The lower skin and subcutaneous flap are elevated, and again, an appropriate interspace is selected for incision well below the palpable margin of the tumor. The lower interspace incision is made, and the segment of chest wall to be resected is thereby freed. Assessment of involvement of contiguous structures (pleura, lung, and diaphragm) is then made, and the surgical stapler is used to divide adherent lung with the tumor mass rather than attempting to divide adhesions that may contain tumor. Resection of adherent diaphragm also may be required. When resecting a chest wall tumor, a wide margin of resection, rather than conservation of tissue for reconstruction, should be the most important consideration. Particularly when operating for a chest wall sarcoma, chest wall musculature overlying the tumor should not be separated from it because entry into the pseudocapsule compromises the margin and sets the stage for local tumor recurrence. In contrast, metastatic tumors to the chest wall and primary rib tumors frequently have relatively little involvement of adjacent soft tissue so that preservation of the overlying muscle is acceptable. A rib involved by tumor should be resected completely from its cartilaginous articulations at either end. Ribs above and below the tumor are resected to achieve an adequate margin and need not be removed in their entirety.

Chest Wall Reconstruction

Techniques

During the past decade, considerable progress has been made in techniques for providing both skeletal and soft tissue replacement after chest wall resection. Before that time, segments of chest wall that were invaded by lung cancer were resected en bloc with the diseased portion of lung, or wide resection of chest wall tumors was carried out without any method of bony reconstruction. The overlying skin and residual chest wall musculature were simply closed over the skeletal defect, accepting the functional loss and poor cosmetic result of the subsequent lung hernia. Reports have established the feasibility and value of providing immediate chest wall support after removal of appreciable segments of the chest wall. Providing a firm, stable replacement for the lost skeletal support of the chest wall has some obvious advantages:

- Preventing paradoxical movement of the underlying lung with respiration and therefore permitting a more vigorous cough and respiratory function
- Achieving a more acceptable cosmetic result in a patient who is young and vigorous and may have a relatively long life expectancy; and finally
- Providing protection for the underlying intrathoracic organs

A variety of factors influence the need for and type of skeletal reconstruction. Full-thickness skeletal defects of the chest wall that are less than 5 cm in diameter generally require no reconstruction. Posterior thoracic defects smaller than 10 cm, particularly those involving the upper ribs, are covered by the overlying scapula and do not require reconstruction. Replacement of the bony thorax is used most frequently in anterior and anterolateral chest wall defects. A variety of prosthetic material is available for stabilization of the chest, including Marlex mesh, Prolene mesh, and 2-mm-thick polytetrafluoroethylene (Gore-Tex) patch. Each of these materials has its proponents, and all have provided satisfactory results. Another popular variation is the Marlex methyl methacrylate sandwich (Fig. 62-10). This technique involves cutting two pieces of Marlex mesh several centimeters larger than the chest wall defect. A thin, 3- to 4-mm layer of methyl methacrylate is spread over one layer of the mesh to a size that is 1 to 2 cm smaller than the chest wall defect on all sides. An optional small sheet of steel mesh can then be added to prevent fragmentation of the methyl methacrylate, followed by the second Marlex layer. As the methyl methacrylate begins to harden, it is molded to the contour of the chest in the region of the defect. The prosthesis is then anchored carefully in place using heavy 0 or 1-0 nonabsorbable sutures placed either through adjacent sternum or around the edges of the cut rib as figure-of-eight or horizontal mattress sutures. The edges of the prosthesis are further anchored to adjacent soft tissue with a running whipstitch of 2-0 suture. The muscle and skin are then closed over the prosthesis.

When using prosthetic patch material that is not impregnated with methyl methacrylate, the material is stretched tightly in all directions to enhance early chest wall stability. Marlex, a single-stitch knit, is rigid in only one direction, whereas Prolene, a double-stitch knit, is rigid in all directions. When Marlex is used for chest wall reconstruction, drainage of the space beneath the overlying muscle and skin is achieved by means of a chest tube because serous fluid passes through the interstices of the mesh and into the chest. Gore-Tex soft tissue patch is a solid sheet through which neither air nor fluid can pass. A chest cathe-

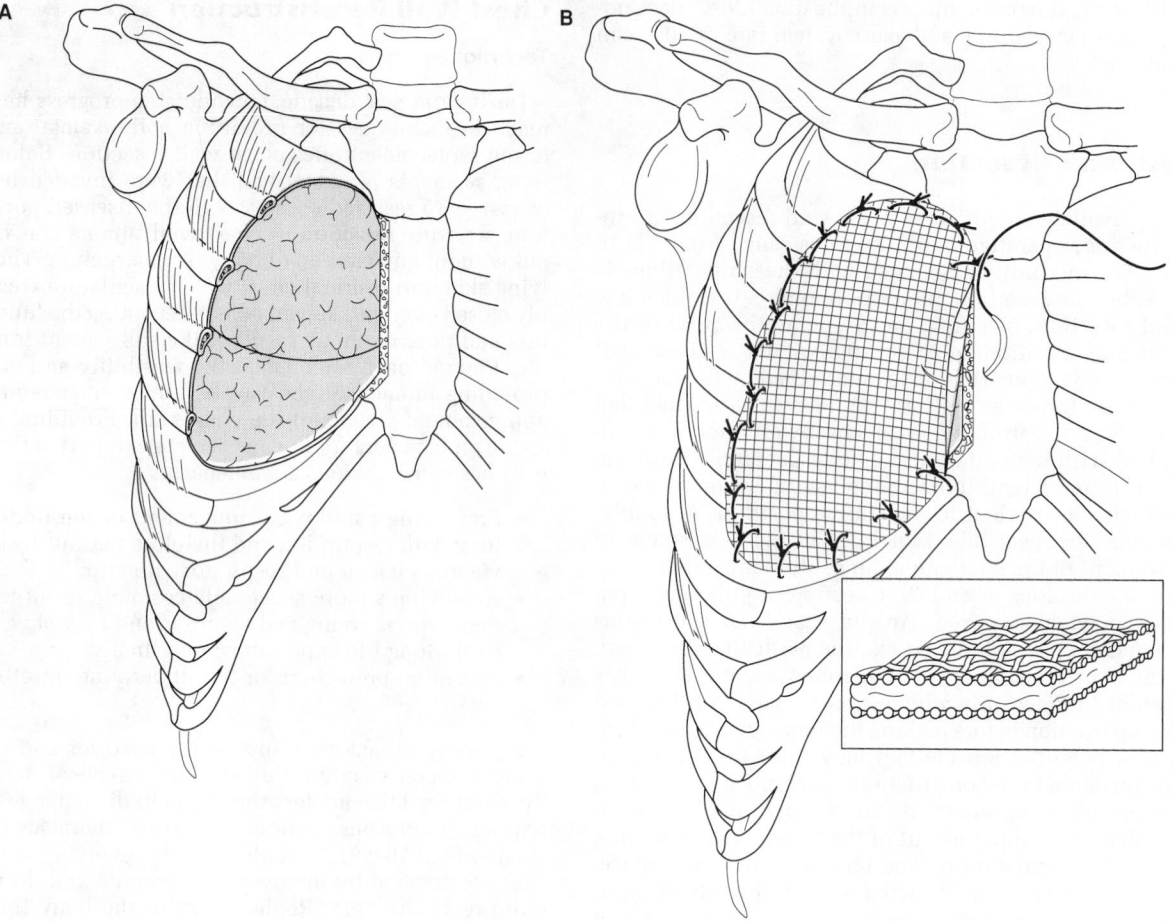

Figure 62-10. Marlex methyl methacrylate sandwich technique for chest wall reconstruction. (*A*) Upper anterior chest wall defect resulting from resection of ribs two to five and a portion of sternum. (*B*) Marlex methyl methacrylate prosthesis being sutured in place. Heavy, nonabsorbable sutures either encircling the ribs or passed through the sternum are used to anchor the prosthesis in place. (*Inset*) Detail of prosthesis showing sandwich of hardened methyl methacrylate between two sheets or Marlex.

ter to evacuate the pleural space as well as a drain to evacuate serous fluid from beneath the overlying skin and muscle flap are therefore needed when Gore-Tex is used.

At times, reconstruction of both the soft tissue of the chest wall and of skeletal support is required. For example, large areas of osteoradionecrosis of the skin and underlying anterior chest wall requires wide, full-thickness excision back to healthy tissue and replacement not only of skeletal support but also of soft tissue coverage. Similarly, wide excision of previous biopsy or drain sites and of adjacent overlying muscle is required when treating chest wall sarcomas, and care must be taken not to violate the pseudocapsule of the tumor. The resulting full-thickness chest wall defect requires soft tissue coverage as well as replacement of the ribs.

If relatively little skin and subcutaneous tissue have been resected, even if the underlying chest wall muscle has been removed with the chest en bloc, the skin and subcutaneous tissue can be closed over the prosthetic patch material with an acceptable cosmetic and functional result. This is particularly true in patients who have relatively thick layers of subcutaneous tissue. In fact, particularly in elderly women with large, pendulous breasts, the breast tissue alone can be used to cover full-thickness defects resulting from wide excision of areas of osteoradionecrosis (Fig. 62-11). The operation may not be cosmetically

appealing, but for patients who have suffered with chronic nonhealing chest wall ulcers, the procedure provides an acceptable and gratifying result. Furthermore, because such wounds are invariably contaminated, the potential for infection after placement of prosthetic material exists, and this complication can be managed only by removal of the entire prosthetic foreign body.

For relatively small chest wall defects that do not require skeletal reconstruction, and for those situations in which it is desirable not to use prosthetic material, full-thickness chest wall defects can be managed by transposition of a variety of muscle and myocutaneous flaps. When there are no available muscle flaps for coverage, the omentum can be used to cover prosthetic material and then skin grafted at a later date. This situation is rare given the vast array of muscle flaps available.[12]

Muscle Flaps for Chest Wall Reconstruction

Latissimus Dorsi. Because of its size (the largest flat muscle of the thorax), its mobile thoracodorsal vascular pedicle, and its blood supply to the overlying skin, the latissimus dorsi muscle can be elevated and rotated either alone or with its overlying skin to cover the lateral and central back as well as the entire anterior chest (Fig. 62-12). Thus, an island of skin about 10 × 16 cm can be

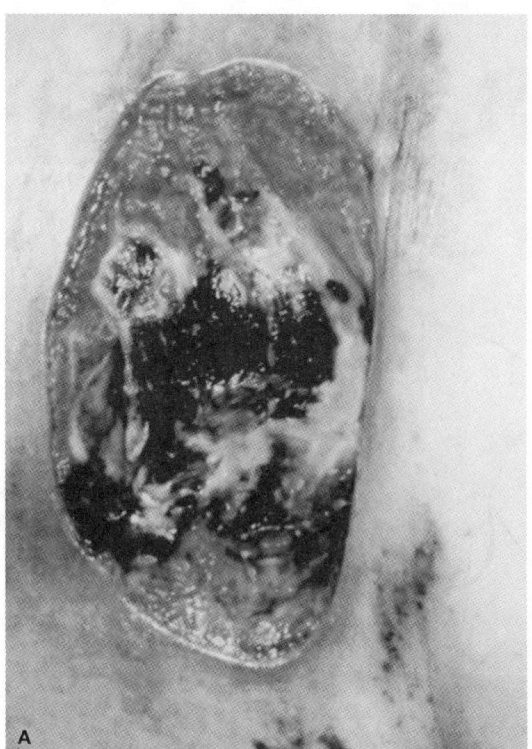
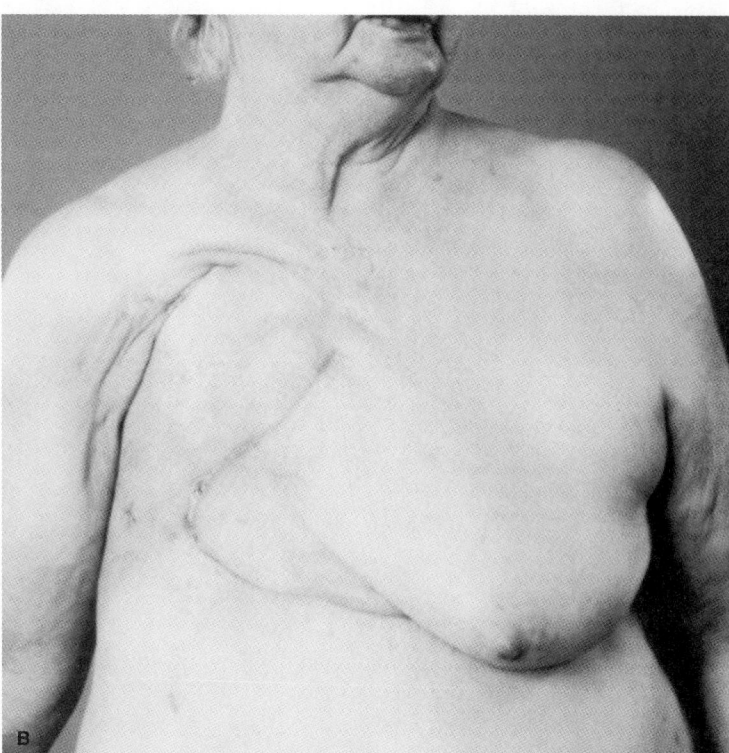

Figure 62-11. Operation for chest wall reconstruction. (*A*) A 7 × 8-cm ulcerated chest wall lesion resulted from osteoradionecrosis after a right radical mastectomy and radiation therapy for breast cancer. The ulcer overlies a portion of the sternum adjacent to the left breast. (*B*) After a full-thickness chest wall resection of the type illustrated in Figure 63-10*A*, coverage of the resulting defect has been achieved by mobilizing the left breast medially.

transposed from the posterior thorax to the anterior chest wall.

Pectoralis Major. The pectoralis major muscle, the second largest flat muscle of the chest wall, is particularly useful for anterior chest wall defects, especially those involving the upper three fourths of the sternum. Like the latissimus dorsi muscle, the pectoralis muscle provides blood supply to its overlying skin, which permits its use as a musculocutaneous flap and allows transfer of skin for reconstruction after head and neck cancer surgery. It is also useful for rotating inward into the chest to fill the thoracic cavity when there is a need to obliterate an infected pleural space. Bilateral pectoralis flaps can be used for repair of sternal defects left after débridement of an infected median sternotomy. Division of the humeral attachments of the muscle permits its transposition medially without undue tension on its thoracoacromial neurovascular bundle (Fig. 62-13). The pectoralis major flap generally does not reach sufficiently inferiorly to permit coverage of lower-third sternal defects. When the defect involves the entire length of the sternum, addition of a rectus abdominis muscle flap is required.

Rectus Abdominis. The mobilized rectus abdominis muscle, based on the internal mammary artery, is most useful for repair of low sternal anterior chest wall defects (Fig. 62-14). The inferior epigastric vessels are divided as the muscle is mobilized inferiorly, permitting its rotation upward onto the chest wall. When using the rectus abdominis to repair a median sternotomy defect after cardiac surgery, a preoperative angiogram is useful to document patency of the internal thoracic artery. The transverse rectus abdominis flap is a musculocutaneous flap in which a large ellipse of lower abdominal skin is based on one rectus muscle and the intact superior epigastric vessels. This flap is useful for coverage of anterior chest and inferior axilla defects.

Other Muscle Flaps. The external oblique muscle, based on the lower thoracic intercostal vessels, can be used to close defects of the lower chest wall and upper abdomen. The serratus anterior muscle, based on its thoracodorsal vascular pedicle, may be used to close anterior thoracic defects and to fill intrathoracic cavities. Refinements in microsurgical technique have permitted the application of free flap techniques to some chest wall defects. For example, tensor fascia lata muscle with fascia lata and overlying skin have been transferred as a free flap based on the lateral femoral circumflex vessels to cover chest wall defects.

PLEURA

Anatomy

The pleural space is a closed serous sac. The pleura consists of two parts, the parietal pleura, which is applied to the thoracic wall, and the visceral pleura, which covers the surface of the lung and is intimately applied to it. Each of these pleural surfaces is lined by a mesothelial layer that secretes a small amount of lubricating fluid.

The parietal pleura has four subdivisions: (1) the costal, against the ribs and intercostal muscles; (2) the diaphragmatic, covering the thoracic surface of the diaphragm; (3) the mediastinal, investing the mediastinum; and (4) the cervical, at the apex of the pleural space. Parts of the parietal pleura are in contact as potential spaces in the costodiaphragmatic sinus and the costomediastinal sinus (see Fig. 62-5), except in deep inspiration. At both pulmonary hila,

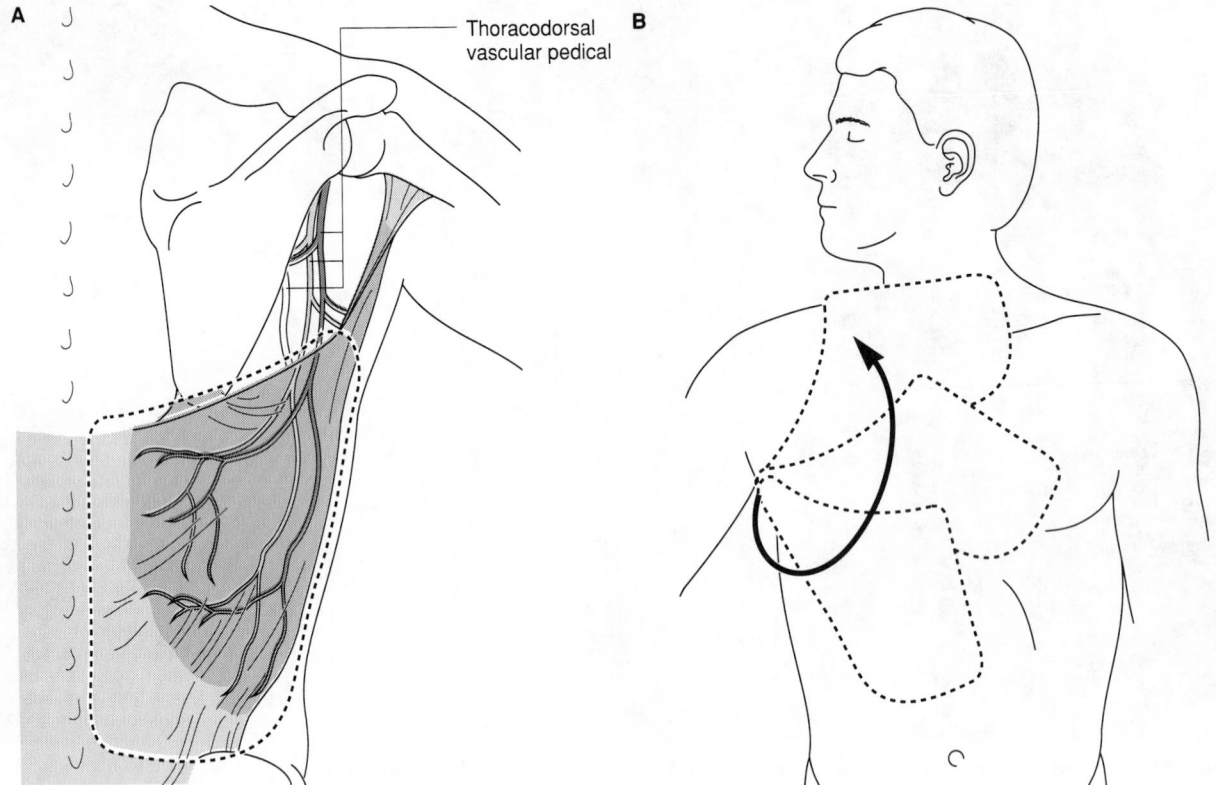

Figure 62-12. Latissimus dorsi muscle rotation flap for chest wall reconstruction. (*A*) Posterior view showing detachment of the origins of the muscle. The dominant blood supply, the thoracodorsal artery, is preserved. (*B*) Anterior view showing the extent to which the mobilized muscle reaches.

the mediastinal pleura reflects onto the lung and becomes the visceral pleura. The anterior and posterior reflections of the pleura from the inferior aspect of the root of the lung to the diaphragmatic surface form the inferior pulmonary ligament. The parietal pleura receives its arterial supply from the intercostal, internal mammary, superior phrenic, and anterior mediastinal arteries, and the venous drainage corresponds to these arteries. The visceral pleura, conversely, is supplied by tributaries of the bronchial and pulmonary arteries; venous drainage is into the pulmonary, not bronchial, veins. The central portion of the diaphragmatic pleura and the mediastinal pleura are innervated by the phrenic nerves, whereas the intercostal nerves innervate the costal and peripheral diaphragmatic pleurae. The parietal pleura is much more sensitive to contact than the visceral pleura.

An extensive network of lymphatics in the connective tissue beneath the pleural mesothelial cells drains the pleura. The lymphatics of the visceral pleura coalesce with the superficial efferent lymphatics of the lung and form a subpleural lymphatic plexus that drains to mediastinal, intercostal, and substernal, phrenic, and anterior and posterior mediastinal lymph nodes. There is also communication at the apex of the chest between cervical and costal pleural lymphatics and axillary lymph nodes. The parietal and visceral pleural lymphatics drain into the right lymphatic duct, whereas those on the left drain into the left thoracic duct. Abnormalities of the pleura include effusions, empyema, pneumothorax, chylothorax, and tumors.

Pleural Effusions

A pleural effusion is a sign of systemic or pleural disease. The typical symptoms are pleuritic chest pain and dyspnea. Large effusions that prevent contact between the vis-

ceral and parietal pleura during respiration are seldom associated with pleuritic chest pain. Tumors involving the parietal pleura generally produce constant dull pain. Large pleural effusions interfere with expansion of the lung and produce dyspnea, shortness of breath, and atelectasis.

Because of the hydrostatic and colloid osmotic pressure across the pleura, pleural fluid normally flows from the parietal pleura into the pleural space and then to the visceral pleura, where it is absorbed. About 5000 to 10,000 mL of fluid crosses the pleural space each day. The small amount of pleural fluid ordinarily present in the pleural space has a low protein content of about 1.5 g/dL. Lymphatic drainage removes between 150 and 500 mL of fluid from the pleural space each day. Pleural fluid may accumulate in the chest if there is (1) increased hydrostatic pressure (eg, congestive heart failure); (2) increased capillary permeability (eg, pneumonia); (3) decreased plasma colloid oncotic pressure (eg, hypoalbuminemia); (4) increased negative intrapleural pressure (eg, in atelectasis); and (5) impaired drainage of the pleural space by lymphatics obstructed by tumor.

Pleural effusions are traditionally characterized as either *transudates* or *exudates*. The causes of transudative and exudative pleural effusions are shown in Table 62-1. Transudates are the result of abnormal formation or absorption of pleural fluid and do not indicate primary pulmonary pathology, in contrast to exudates, which result from diseased pleura or pleural lymphatics. When the pleura is diseased by infection, pulmonary embolism, or tumor, increased capillary permeability for protein occurs. Pleural lymphatics obstructed by tumor cannot absorb pleural fluid at a normal rate. When a pleural effusion is diagnosed as transudate, additional diagnostic studies are unneces-

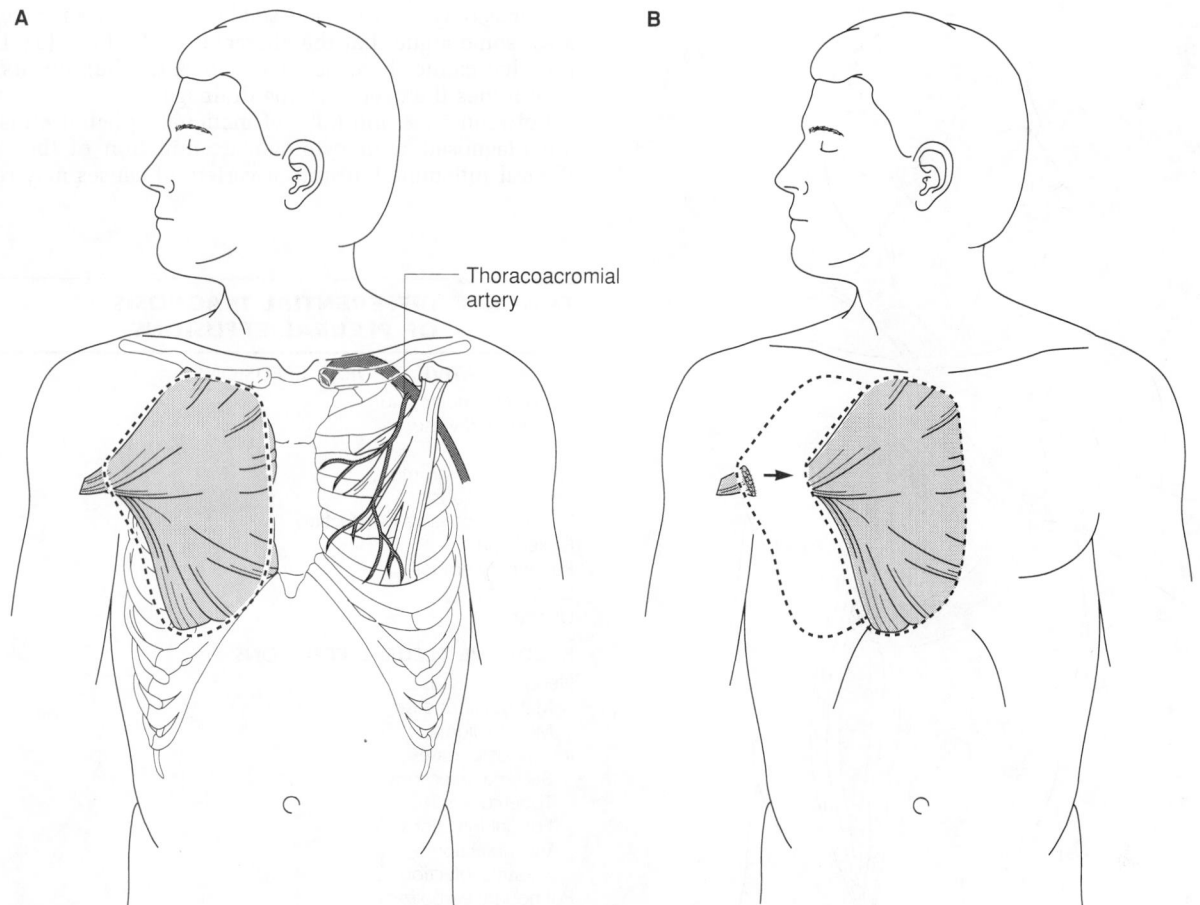

A

B

Thoracoacromial
artery

Figure 62-13. Pectoralis major muscle rotation flap. (*A*) Mobilization of the flap by detaching the clavicular, sternal, and chest wall origins as well as the insertion of the muscle on the greater tubercle of the humerus. The dominant blood supply, the thoracoacromial artery, which arises from the axillary artery medial to the proximal border of the pectoralis minor muscle is shown on the left side, where the pectoralis major muscle has been removed. (*B*) Medial transposition of the muscle flap, preserving the thoracoacromial neurovascular bundle.

sary, and treatment is directed at the systemic cause. Conversely, when an effusion is found to be an exudate, further diagnosis to identify the exact nature of pleural or lymphatic disease is indicated.

It was thought in the past that pleural effusions with a protein content of more than 3 g/dL or a specific gravity od greater than 1.016 were exudates. It is now known that long-standing transudates can have high protein content, simulating exudates and leading to an error in characterization of the effusion in 10% of cases. Light[13] used simultaneous determinations of pleural fluid and serum protein and lactic acid dehydrogenase to differentiate transudates from exudates. From a clinical standpoint, the differentiation is important because 43% of pleural exudates are due to malignant disease, whereas 83% of transudates are the result of congestive heart failure.

On the standard upright chest radiograph, blunting of either costophrenic angle is indicative of the accumulation of between 250 to 400 mL of fluid. Lateral decubitus films that allow fluid to shift to the dependent portion of the thoracic cavity help differentiate fluid in the costophrenic angle from pleural thickening and fibrosis, which do not change configuration with a shift in the patient's position. Accumulation of pleural fluid between the lung and the diaphragm is called a *subpulmonic effusion* and gives the false impression of an elevated hemidiaphragm. When pleural fluid is trapped within a fissure of the lung, its

spheric contour may result in a masslike pseudotumor. The CT scan is an extremely sensitive indicator of the presence of a pleural effusion. In 70% of patients with large pleural effusions that fill one hemothorax, the underlying cause is a pleural malignancy, but massive effusions may also be the result of tuberculosis, empyema, or transudates from congestive heart failure or cirrhosis.[14]

Physical and Chemical Characteristics of Effusions

Transudates are characteristically straw-colored, clear, and odorless, with a white blood cell count of less than 1000/μL. Because most exudates contain white blood cells, they are usually cloudy. Parapneumonic effusions, pulmonary infarctions, pancreatitis, and early tuberculosis are associated with effusions that contain a predominance of neutrophils. Conversely, in tuberculosis, lymphoma, or malignancy, lymphocytes tend to predominate in the pleural effusion. Thick, viscous creamy pleural fluid may suggest either an empyema or a chylothorax. On centrifugation of this fluid, the supernatant is clear in empyema fluid but remains milky with a chylous effusion. A bloody pleural effusion occurring in a patient with no history of trauma or pulmonary infarction is indicative of neoplasm in 90% of cases. Because a red blood cell count as low as 5000 to 10,000/μL can cause a pleural effusion to be red, the finding of blood-tinged pleural fluid per se has little diagnostic value and is often the result of local needle trauma from

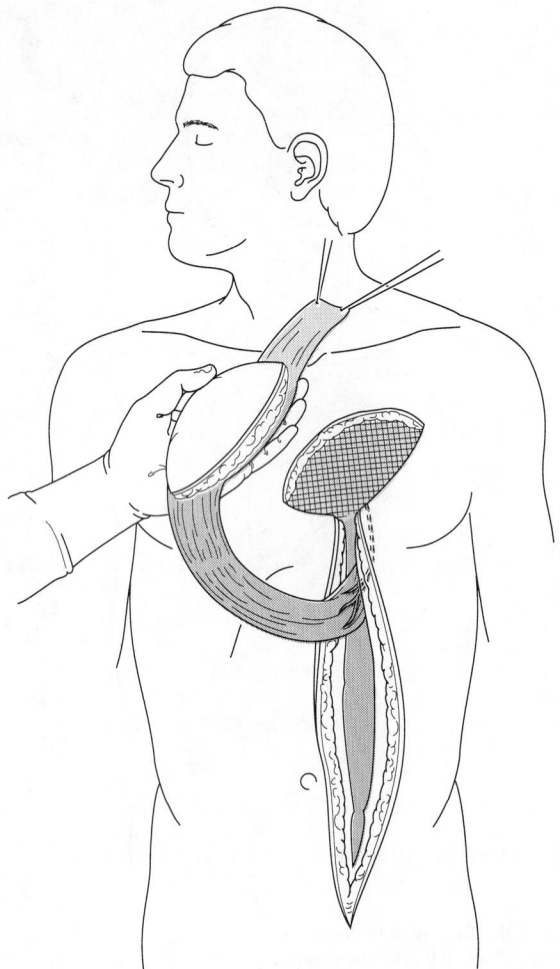

Figure 62-14. Rectus abdominis muscle rotation flap. Shown is the mobilization of the rectus abdominis muscle, which is based on the superior epigastric artery (the continuation of the internal thoracic artery), and rotation of the muscle and overlying skin to fill an anterior chest wall defect.

the thoracentesis. Cloudy or foul-smelling pleural effusions that are likely due to infection should always be cultured and Gram stained. Effusions due to tuberculosis are notoriously difficult to diagnose because the acid-fast bacilli rarely are identified on staining and are cultured in only 30% of cases.

Pleural effusions, particularly on the left, are not uncommon in patients with acute pancreatitis or a chronic pancreatic pseudocyst that results in a pancreaticopleural fistula, and therefore the finding of a pleural fluid amylase level that is several times greater than that in the serum may be diagnostic of the source of the fluid. At times, particularly in an edentulous patient who does not have sufficient oral bacteria to cause serious mediastinitis or empyema, an occult esophageal perforation may present as an unexplained pleural effusion. Salivary amylase can be differentiated from pancreatic amylase by laboratory studies. A pleural fluid glucose level lower than that in the serum is characteristic of empyema, tuberculosis, rheumatoid arthritis, and neoplasms. It has been suggested that the pH of pleural fluid in patients with acute bacterial pneumonia and an associated parapneumonic effusion is an important indicator of the need for chest tube drainage; an effusion with a pH of 7.2 or less has a high likelihood of becoming contaminated with bacteria and requiring tube

thoracostomy.[15,16] As discussed later, this is a controversial area; some argue that the character of the fluid (eg, thick pus that cannot be evacuated with a needle), not its pH, determines the need for tube drainage.[17]

Between 50% and 60% of malignant pleural effusions are diagnosed with cytologic examination of the fluid. Pleural inflammation from a variety of causes may result

---

Table 62-1. DIFFERENTIAL DIAGNOSIS OF PLEURAL EFFUSIONS

TRANSUDATIVE PLEURAL EFFUSIONS

Congestive heart failure
Pericardial disease
Cirrhosis
Nephrotic syndrome
Peritoneal dialysis
Superior vena cava obstruction
Myxedema
Pulmonary emboli
Sarcoidosis
Urinothorax

EXUDATIVE PLEURAL EFFUSIONS

Neoplastic diseases
  Metastatic disease
  Mesothelioma
Infectious diseases
  Bacterial infections
  Tuberculosis
  Fungal infections
  Viral infections
  Parasitic infections
Pulmonary embolization
Gastrointestinal disease
  Esophageal perforation
  Pancreatic disease
  Intraabdominal abscess
  Diaphragmatic hernia
  Postabdominal surgery
  Endoscopic variceal sclerotherapy
Collagen vascular diseases
  Rheumatoid pleuritis
  Systemic lupus erythematosus
  Drug-induced lupus erythematosus
  Immunoblastic lymphadenopathy
  Sjögren syndrome
  Wegener granulomatosis
  Churg-Strauss syndrome
Postcardiac injury syndrome
Asbestos exposure
Sarcoidosis
Uremia
Meigs syndrome
Yellow nail syndrome
Drug-induced pleural disease
  Nitrofurantoin
  Dantrolene
  Methysergide
  Bromocriptine
  Procarbazine
  Amiodarone
Trapped lung
Radiotherapy
Electrical burns
Urinary tract obstruction
Iatrogenic injury
Ovarian hyperstimulation syndrome
Chylothorax
Hemothorax

(Data from Light RW. The physiology of pleural fluid production and benign pleural effusion. In: Shields TW, ed. General thoracic surgery, ed 4. Malvern, PA, Williams & Wilkins, 1994:676)

in reactive changes in the mesothelial pleural cells that may erroneously be interpreted as neoplasm on cytologic evaluation. Because mesothelial cells may be confused with lymphocytes on cytologic assessment, the cytologic diagnosis of pleural effusion due to lymphoma is notoriously unreliable. Needle biopsy of the pleura in patients with tuberculous pleuritis and pleural effusion is extremely useful in diagnosing the disease; granulomas or mycobacteria are identified on histologic assessment in as many as 80% of patients. Although cultures of pleural fluid in patients with tuberculosis are positive in fewer than 30% of cases, pleural biopsy cultures are positive in over 75%. Pleural biopsy identifies the presence of tumor in about half of patients with malignant effusion, and therefore the diagnostic yield is increased to at least 80% by combining cytologic assessment of the pleural fluid with needle biopsy of the pleura.[18]

At times, the cause of a pleural effusion may be unexplained after extensive chemical and cytologic evaluations of the fluid and needle biopsy of associated thickened pleura. Although a diagnostic thoracotomy can be performed to rule out the presence of such treatable conditions as lymphoma or tuberculosis, pleuroscopy is an effective alternative that is associated with less morbidity.[19] Pleuroscopy is performed with the patient under general anesthesia and using a double-lumen endotracheal tube to permit single-lung ventilation. The patient is positioned with the affected side up. Fluid is evacuated from the chest with either a needle or trocar, and the lung on the affected side is collapsed by selective ventilation. Through a limited interspace incision, the thoracoscope (which may be a sterile, rigid bronchoscope or esophagoscope) is introduced and used to inspect the pleural surfaces of the lung, the chest wall, and the diaphragm. Biopsy forceps are used to obtain appropriate specimens for culture and histologic evaluation. The thoracoscope is withdrawn, air is evacuated from the chest, and the wound is closed. If there has been no resulting air leak from biopsy of the visceral pleura, no chest tube may be necessary, and the procedure can be performed on an outpatient basis. Thoracoscopy has been used to determine the cause of pleural effusions because the conventional methods of thoracentesis or pleural biopsy are effective in only 60% of cases. Thoracoscopy has a reported diagnostic yield of greater then 90% for malignant effusions and leads to a diagnosis in up to 75% of cases when other methods have failed.[20]

Treatment of Malignant Pleural Effusions

Although most pleural effusions due to nonneoplastic disease respond to treatment of the underlying cause and, if asymptomatic, require thoracentesis only for diagnostic purposes, those due to malignant disease often present a therapeutic challenge that warrants interventional treatment. Effusions originating from a neoplasm within the mediastinum or obstruction of lymphatics by tumor may respond to either appropriate chemotherapy or radiotherapy. In patients with large malignant effusions adversely affecting cardiorespiratory dynamics, a thoracentesis may provide gratifying palliation. The thoracentesis should be performed using a plastic catheter rather than a needle to minimize the incidence of injury to the lung and a resulting pneumothorax that may require chest tube insertion. When a thoracentesis is needed, the effusion should be tapped dry, so that it can be determined on subsequent chest radiograph if the lung expands fully or if it has become trapped down by tumor, fibrosis, or a proteinaceous layer. As is the case with all pleural space problems, whether due to air (pneumothorax), effusion, or pus (empyema), successful resolution requires the apposition of visceral and parietal pleural surfaces. If after evacuation of a large amount of fluid from the pleural cavity, a follow-up chest radiograph shows failure of the lung to reexpand, fluid probably will once again accumulate within the pleural dead space. If a chest tube has been used to evacuate the fluid, and the lung fails to expand on subsequent chest radiographs obtained during the next 1 to 2 days, the chest tube should be removed before the pleural space becomes infected, and either an alternative form of therapy should be initiated or a decision made to use repeated thoracentesis as necessary. Repeated thoracentesis may give gratifying relief of symptoms in patients with malignant effusions, but rapid accumulation of fluid within several days suggests the need for alternative therapy.

If after thoracentesis in a patient with a malignant effusion, the lung expands well, but the effusion eventually recurs, chemical pleurodesis, which produces an inflammatory pleuritis with obliteration of the pleural space, may be highly effective. Chemical pleurodesis is performed through a small (24F to 28F) chest catheter inserted through a low lateral interspace. Although a variety of agents, such as radioactive isotopes (^{198}Au or $Cr^{34} PO^4$), nitrogen mustard, quinacrine, and talc have been used in the past to achieve chemical pleurodesis, talc and bleomycin are the most popular agents used. Complete evacuation of fluid and expansion of the lung should be verified with a chest radiograph before instilling the sclerosing agent intrapleurally. Intrapleural tetracycline was used in the past to achieve chemical pleurodesis in patients with recurrent malignant pleural effusions, but it is no longer available commercially for this purpose. Talc and bleomycin are the most popular agents used for chemical pleurodesis. When performing bleomycin pleurodesis, 240 mg of bleomycin in 50 to 100 mL of normal saline is instilled into the previously placed chest tube, which is flushed with an additional 20 mL of saline. The chest tube is then clamped, and the patient is placed in both lateral decubitus positions, supine, and prone for 30 minutes in each position to ensure complete dispersion of the bleomycin throughout the pleural cavity. The chest tube is then unclamped, connected to suction, and removed when the pleural space is obliterated on chest radiograph and chest tube drainage is less than 100 mL/d. Bleomycin pleurodesis successfully manages 50% to 60% of malignant pleural effusions. The use of pharmaceutical talc for pleurodesis has been shown to be significantly less expensive and more effective in the management of pleural effusions, especially when introduced thoracoscopically.[21,22] Thoracoscopic pleurodesis requires operative intervention and one-lung ventilation but can be achieved through a single chest tube port using the thoracoscope for simultaneous suction, inspection, and biopsy. Loculations can be separated with the thoracoscope, and then insufflation of 5 g of pharmaceutical talc can either be done through the same port or an additional one. A chest tube is inserted, the lung is reexpanded, and pleural symphysis is achieved. Alternatively, after adequate evacuation of the effusion with a chest tube, a slurry of 5 g of talc can be combined with 50 to 100 mL of normal saline and instilled through the tube into the pleural cavity. Positioning is similar to that described for bleomycin. Instillation of talc through a chest tube is not as effective as talc delivered thoracoscopically, but the former method obviates the need for an operative procedure under general anesthesia.

Rarely, a patient who has undergone thoracoscopic pleurodesis still requires further intervention for a persistent malignant pleural effusion that has failed other forms of therapy. In this case, pleurectomy may be an option. This operation generally requires a thoracotomy and involves removal of as much of the diseased visceral and parietal pleura as is possible, so that expansion of the lung and symphysis between the two pleural surfaces can occur. This treatment is most appropriate in patients with metastatic carcinoma of the breast and occasionally in those with carcinoma of the lung. As anticipated, intraoperative blood loss for pleurectomy may be excessive, and complication rates greater than 20% and mortality rates between 10% and 20% have been reported.[23] Reported experience with partial pleurectomy using thoracoscopy has compared favorably with that done through an open procedure and has been associated with a mortality rate of about 10%.[24] In another series, there were no deaths, and no significant complications, and the average length of hospitalization was 5 days.[25] A valved subcutaneous pleuroperitoneal shunt operated by manual compression has been used to treat refractory malignant pleural effusions without the need for a thoracotomy. Active patient involvement is needed because manipulation of the shunt is required for pumping and clearing the reservoir. Therefore, only patients with good preoperative status are candidates.[26,27] Problems with occlusion of the shunt are common, and there has not been tremendous enthusiasm for this approach.

Thoracic Empyema

The accumulation of pus in the pleural space is referred to as *thoracic* or *pleural empyema,* or *empyema thoracis.* Empyemas may be characterized as acute or chronic, localized or diffuse, or unilateral or bilateral. Pus is the fluid product of inflammation and contains leukocytes and the debris of dead cells and tissues. In general, empyema fluid has a white-cell count greater than 15,000 cells/μL, a protein level greater than 2.5 to 3 mg/dL, and a specific gravity greater than 1.018.[28] Pleural fluid with a pH less than 7, a glucose level less than 40 mg/dL, and a lactate dehydrogenase (LDH) level greater than 1000 IU/L, in addition to gram-positive staining, is defined as an empyema. These physical characteristics alone, however, are not as important in establishing the need for tube drainage as the gross characteristics of the fluid, which should be too thick or viscous to be aspirated adequately with a thoracentesis needle.

Using the American Thoracic Society 1962 classification, there are three phases in the natural history of empyema:

1. The acute or exudative phase, in which sterile pleural fluid forms as a response to inflammation. This fluid has a low viscosity, low white-cell count, low LDH level, and a normal glucose level and pH. The visceral and parietal pleura are not fused.
2. The transitional or fibrinopurulent phase, in which the fluid becomes more turbid as the number of white blood cells within it increases. A fibrinous peel develops on both pleural surfaces, eventually limiting expansion of the lung. Pleural fluid pH and glucose levels begin to fall, and the LDH level increases.
3. The chronic or organizing phase, in which there is an ingrowth of capillaries and fibroblasts into the fibrous pleural peel. The pleural fluid in this phase is characteristically viscous and consists of 75% sediment when placed in a test tube and allowed to settle. This phase typically occurs 4 to 6 weeks after the onset of the process and defines the empyema as being in the chronic phase. The pleural fluid in the chronic phase typically has a pH less than 7 and a sugar level below 40 mg/dL.

At least half of empyemas are secondary to pneumonia (Table 62-2). Twenty-five percent occur as a result of com

Table 62-2. CAUSES OF EMPYEMA

Cause	Frequency (%)
Pyogenic pneumonia	50
Postsurgical	25
Subphrenic abscess extension	10
Posttraumatic	3–5
Lung abscess rupture	1–3
Generalized sepsis	1–3
Pulmonary tuberculosis	1
Pulmonary mycotic infection	1
Spontaneous pneumothorax	<1
Parasitic infection	<1
Retained tracheobronchial foreign body	<1

(Modified from Miller JI Jr. Infections of the pleura. In: Shields TW, ed. General thoracic surgery, ed 3. Philadelphia, Lea & Febiger, 1989:634)

plications of esophageal, pulmonary, or mediastinal surgery, and about 10% arise as extensions from subphrenic abscesses. Before the antibiotic era, *Streptococcus* sp and *Pneumococcus* sp were the organisms most frequently cultured from empyemas. *Staphylococcus aureus* became the most common organism between 1955 and 1965 and remains the most frequent causative organism in children younger than 2 years of age. Gram-negative organisms (eg, *Pseudomonas* sp, *Klebsiella pneumoniae, Escherichia coli, Aerobacter aerogenes, Proteus* sp, and *Salmonella* sp) are frequently found. With the availability of anaerobic culture techniques, these organisms, particularly *Bacteroides fragilis,* have been recovered with increasing frequency.

Patients with empyema present with pleuritic chest pain and a feeling of heaviness or discomfort on the affected side. Fever, cough with purulent sputum production, and shortness of breath are common. On physical examination there are decreased breath sounds and dullness to percussion on the affected side. Complications of empyema in the chronic phase include empyema necessitatis, in which the intrathoracic infection works its way through the chest wall and presents at the surface of the skin as a draining sinus, costochondritis and osteomyelitis of the ribs, bronchopleural fistula, mediastinal or pericardial infection, and disseminated infection such as a brain or renal abscess.

The standard posteroanterior and lateral chest radiographs are among the most important diagnostic modalities. The finding of pneumonia with a large pleural effusion or complete opacification of one hemothorax is common. Air–fluid levels or multiple loculations may also be seen. With large effusions, the trachea and mediastinum may be shifted to the contralateral side. Most parapneumonic empyemas are posterior and lateral and extend to the diaphragm (Fig. 62-15). The aerated lung can be seen anteriorly. The differentiation between a lung abscess and empyema can be difficult and may require additional diagnostic studies, such as bronchoscopy, bronchography, or a CT scan. The CT scan is helpful in demonstrating the extent of the empyema and areas of loculation. The most important test in diagnosing an empyema is a thoracentesis in which pus is recovered from the pleural cavity. This fluid should be sent for Gram stain, culture and sensitivity testing, and analysis of pH, white-cell count with differential, sugar, protein, and LDH. Thin, watery parapneumonic effusions that are infected may be treated with repeated thoracentesis and appropriate antibiotic therapy, although it has been suggested that pleural fluid with a pH below 7, a sugar content less than 40 mg/dL, and an LDH level higher than 1000 IU/dL is indicative of empyema requiring drainage.

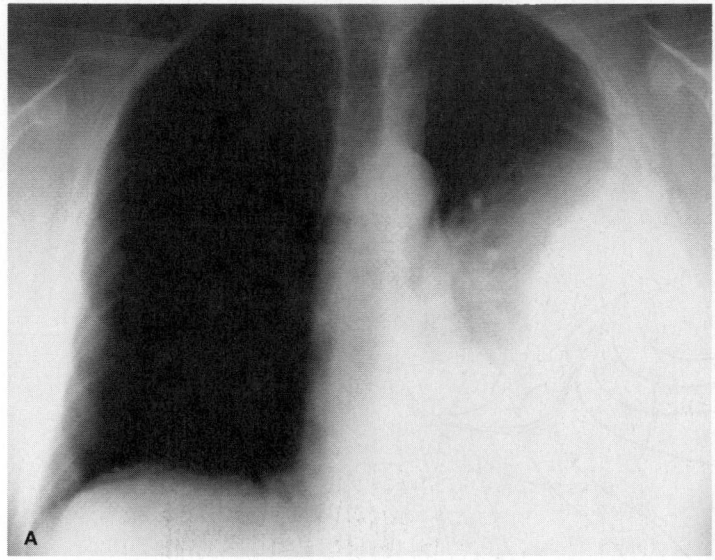
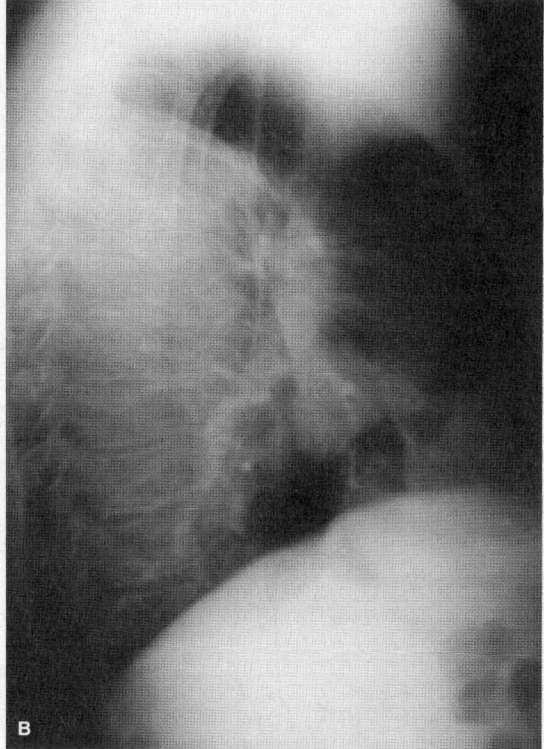

Figure 62-15. Typical parapneumonic empyema presenting as a lateral fluid collection extending to the diaphragm. Posteroanterior view (*A*) and lateral view (*B*), which localizes the collection of fluid to the posterior chest. This empyema was treated with a rib resection and drainage.

In the past, when thick pus was obtained on aspiration of pleural fluid, the plastic catheter used to perform the thoracentesis was taped to the skin and the patient taken to the radiology department for an empyemagram. Sixty to 90 mL of pus was aspirated from the chest and replaced with an equal volume of Dionosil Oily. This contrast material fell to the most dependent position of the empyema cavity. Upright posteroanterior and lateral chest radiographs defined the inferior extent of the cavity. Cross-table lateral radiographs in the right and left lateral decubitus positions demonstrated the medial and lateral extent. With these landmarks identified on the chest radiograph, it was possible to count down over the appropriate rib to determine the most dependent position for subsequent tube drainage of the empyema. Dionosil is no longer available commercially, however, and CT has replaced the empyemagram for localizing and defining the extent of empyemas. The same principles of dependent drainage apply, however, and the cavity should be localized with a needle in the operating room before open drainage. The patient who develops a spontaneous empyema should undergo bronchoscopy to rule out endobronchial obstruction by tumor or foreign body that may interfere with subsequent reexpansion of the lung.

When gross pus is recovered from the chest during thoracentesis, tube drainage is indicated. Although dependent drainage of the empyema cavity with a large-bore, 36F chest tube may result in satisfactory resolution of the process, particularly in cases of parapneumonic empyemas, chest tube drainage alone is frequently inadequate in other situations.[17] For example, postoperative empyemas, such as those after pulmonary resection or esophageal operations, and empyemas occurring in immunosuppressed patients are more effectively treated by rib resection and drainage. Proper rib resection requires accurate dependent positioning of a large-bore, end-hole drainage tube into the empyema cavity and is facilitated by localizing the most dependent point with chest radiographs and a chest CT scan. The procedure is usually performed with the patient

under general anesthesia. After aspirating pus from the appropriate low interspace overlying the empyema, a 5-cm segment of the adjacent rib is resected, and the exposed intercostal neurovascular bundle is divided to minimize intercostal neuralgia caused by later pressure by the empyema tube. The underlying thickened pleura is incised, gross pus is evacuated, loculations are disrupted, and using the operative suction, vigorous irrigation and aspiration of the empyema cavity are carried out before insertion of a large-bore (46F) empyema drainage tube. The end of the tube is intentionally low in the cavity to ensure adequate drainage. No side holes are cut in the tube because the ingrowth of granulation tissue into the side holes may make subsequent tube removal for cleansing difficult. The tube is sutured to the skin and connected to underwater seal and suction, which are maintained for 7 to 10 days in an effort to pull the lung against the chest wall and help obliterate the empyema cavity. At the end of this period, the patient is taken to the radiology department, where the chest tube is disconnected from underwater suction and left open to air as a repeat chest radiograph is obtained. If the lung does not fall away from the chest wall, the empyema tube is cut off at the skin and secured in place. During the ensuing 4 weeks, the tube is periodically removed and the empyema cavity irrigated as gradual contraction of the cavity occurs, and the tube is gradually shortened and eventually withdrawn. If reexpansion of the lung does not occur after 6 to 8 weeks of drainage, either a thoracotomy with decortication or marsupialization of the empyema cavity (Eloesser flap construction; Fig. 62-16) is performed.

Decortication is indicated if the patient's general condition is relatively good and the lung has failed to expand after drainage of the empyema. Decortication of the lung involves removing the fibrous rind or peel that has formed on the pleural surface overlying the lung. The procedure is aimed at freeing the trapped lung, thereby allowing reexpansion and obliteration of the pleural space. The opera-

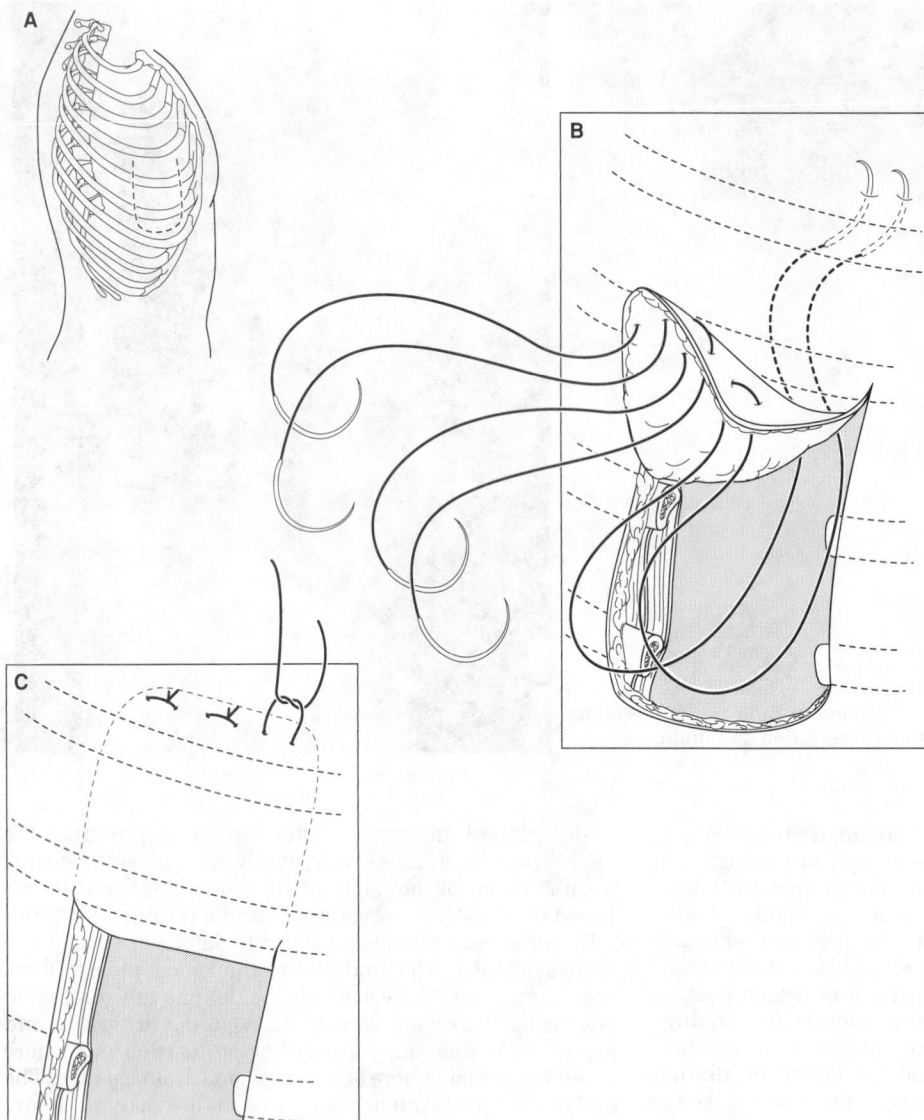

Figure 62-16. Marsupialization of empyema cavity (Eloesser flap). (*A*) U-shaped skin and subcutaneous flap is fashioned over two ribs that overlie the dependent portion of the empyema cavity. (*B*) Five-centimeter segments of the two ribs are resected, and the neurovascular bundles of these two interspaces are ligated and divided. Mattress sutures of nonabsorbable material (eg, polypropylene) are placed through the end of the flap and then through the upper chest wall. (*C*) As the sutures are tightened, the flap is drawn into the chest, resulting in an epithelium-lined cavity that drains freely without the need for an indwelling tube.

tion is performed through a standard posterolateral thoracotomy, and the vascularity of the inflammatory adhesions encountered may result in significant intraoperative blood loss. Patients with a persistent pleural space after decortication can be treated with a limited thoracoplasty (collapse of the chest wall) or muscle flap rotation to obliterate the cavity.[29] An algorithm for the management of parapneumonic or nonoperative empyema is shown in Figure 62-17.

Spontaneous Pneumothorax

Tuberculosis was thought to be the cause of spontaneous pneumothorax until the early 1930s, when it was first appreciated that in most patients with this condition there is no infectious cause. In fact, spontaneous pneumothorax occurs most often in young, otherwise healthy people who rupture a subpleural bleb that in 90% of cases is located either at the apex of the upper lobe or the superior segment of the lower lobe. Spontaneous pneumothorax has an incidence of 6 to 15 cases per 100,000 population, and the condition affects men three to four times more commonly than women. Spontaneous pneumothorax is more com-

mon in tall, asthenic patients who have long, narrow chests. There is a predilection for patients in the 20- to 30-year age range. The right lung seems to be more commonly involved.

Although it might be reasoned that spontaneous pneumothorax occurs when the patient is engaged in forceful activity requiring a vigorous Valsalva maneuver, this is not the case, and most episodes begin when the patient is sedentary. The presenting symptoms are characteristic and include chest pain and shortness of breath in 95% of patients. Ten percent of patients complain of associated cough. Although the precise cause of pneumothorax is unknown, associated conditions include a history of smoking, meconium staining at birth in neonates who develop pneumothorax, and occasionally abnormalities of the first or second ribs. Pneumothorax may complicate the course of malignancy involving the lung, chronic obstructive pulmonary disease, cystic fibrosis, penetrating chest trauma, tracheobronchial disruption, or esophageal perforation. Catamenial pneumothorax is a variety of spontaneous pneumothoraces that occur in temporal relation to menstruation.[30] Originally thought to be the result of air entering the peritoneal cavity through the female genital tract

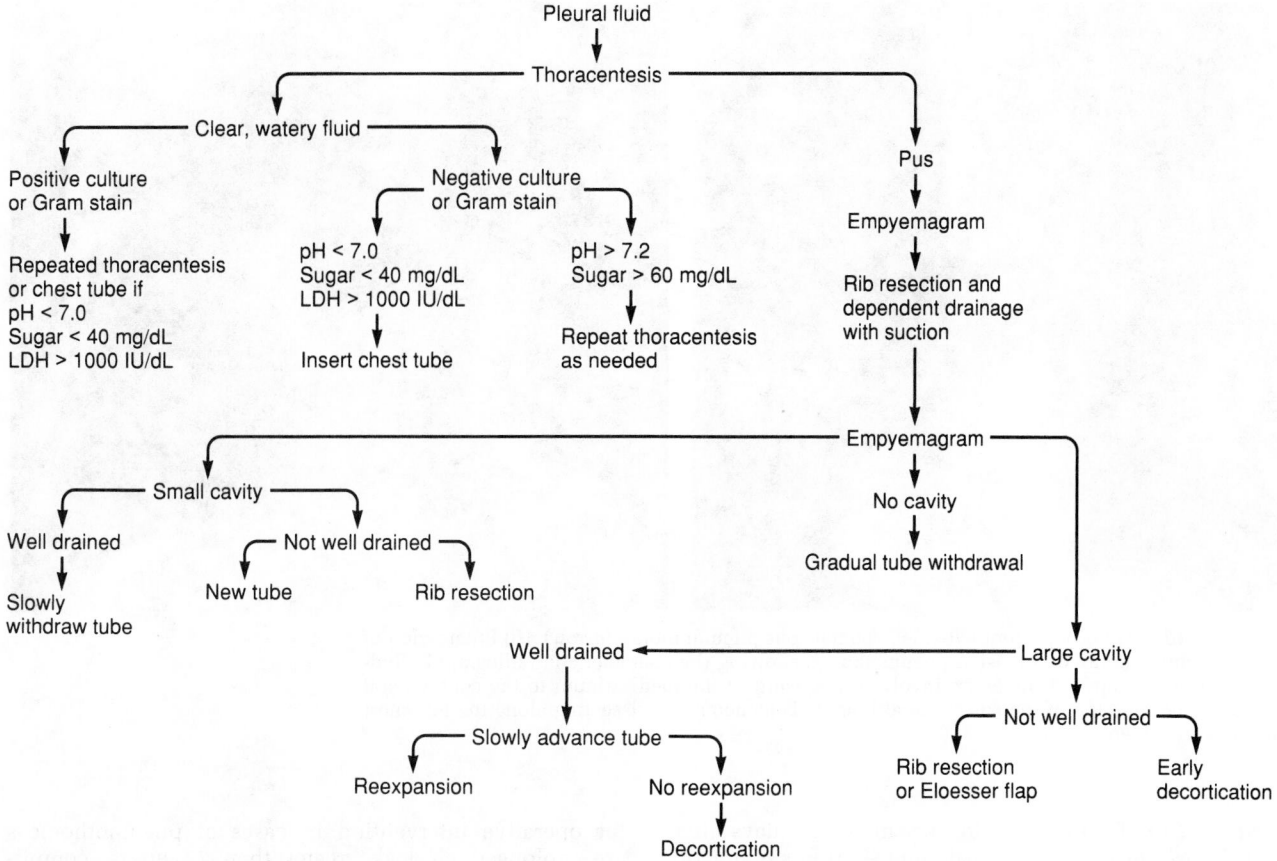

Figure 62-17. Management of empyema. (After Miller JI Jr. Infections of the pleura. In: Shields TW, ed. General thoracic surgery, ed 3. Philadelphia, Lea & Febiger, 1989:637)

and then passing into the chest through tiny transdiaphragmatic channels, catamenial pneumothorax is now believed to be the result of endometrial implants on the lung that create a defect on the visceral pleura during menstruation.

About half of patients who sustain an initial spontaneous pneumothorax have a subsequent recurrence, and after the second pneumothorax, three fourths recur.[31] Complications of spontaneous pneumothorax include tension pneumothorax, hemopneumothorax, persistent air leak, pneumomediastinum, and subcutaneous emphysema. Tension pneumothorax occurs in only 2% to 3% of patients and results from a tangential tear in the visceral pleura that permits air to enter the pleural space during inspiration but closes during exhalation. The resulting increased pressure within the pleural cavity causes shift of the mediastinum to the contralateral side with compression of the uninvolved lung, diminished venous return to the heart, and eventual decreased cardiac output (Fig. 62-18). This condition is incompatible with life and is readily apparent in a young patient presenting with marked respiratory distress; decreased breath sounds over one hemothorax, which is hyperresonant to percussion; and shift of the trachea toward the contralateral side. When the diagnosis is suspected, prompt and decisive action is indicated, and time should not be taken to await the return of a chest radiograph. Rather, a large-bore, 14-gauge needle should be inserted into the second interspace anteriorly. The characteristic hiss of air under pressure is heard as pressure within the pleural cavity is relieved. The patient's condition improves dramatically because a simple pneumothorax is far better tolerated physiologically and can be treated by placement of a chest tube. About 20% of patients with

spontaneous pneumothorax have associated pleural effusion. In 5% of patients, frank hemothorax occurs from bleeding in the torn adhesions between the visceral and parietal pleura. The bleeding is typically on the chest wall side of the adhesion and may stop if chest tube drainage achieves complete reexpansion of the lung against the chest wall. Thoracotomy for control of the bleeding may be required.

In 95% of patients, placement of an apical chest tube results in cessation of the air leak within 12 to 24 hours. A persistent air leak after 72 hours generally warrants surgical intervention if the patient's condition permits. If air from the ruptured pulmonary bleb dissects in a retrograde fashion in the interstitial planes along the bronchi or pulmonary vasculature, pneumomediastinum may be seen on the chest radiograph. This is seldom significant, except in infants in whom compression of the great vessels may occur. Rarely, an occasional patient presents with bilateral simultaneous pneumothorax. About 10% of patients who develop a pneumothorax on one side ultimately have a pneumothorax on the other side, and pleurodesis is recommended in any patient who develops a pneumothorax on one side after having had the same problem on the other. Patients who develop subcutaneous emphysema after placement of a chest tube for spontaneous pneumothorax do not have satisfactory decompression of the air leak and require repositioning of the tube or correction of malfunctioning drainage equipment.

Spontaneous pneumothorax occurring in young, otherwise healthy patients is often remarkably well tolerated, even when the lung is virtually collapsed, so long as tension does not develop. It is not uncommon for college-

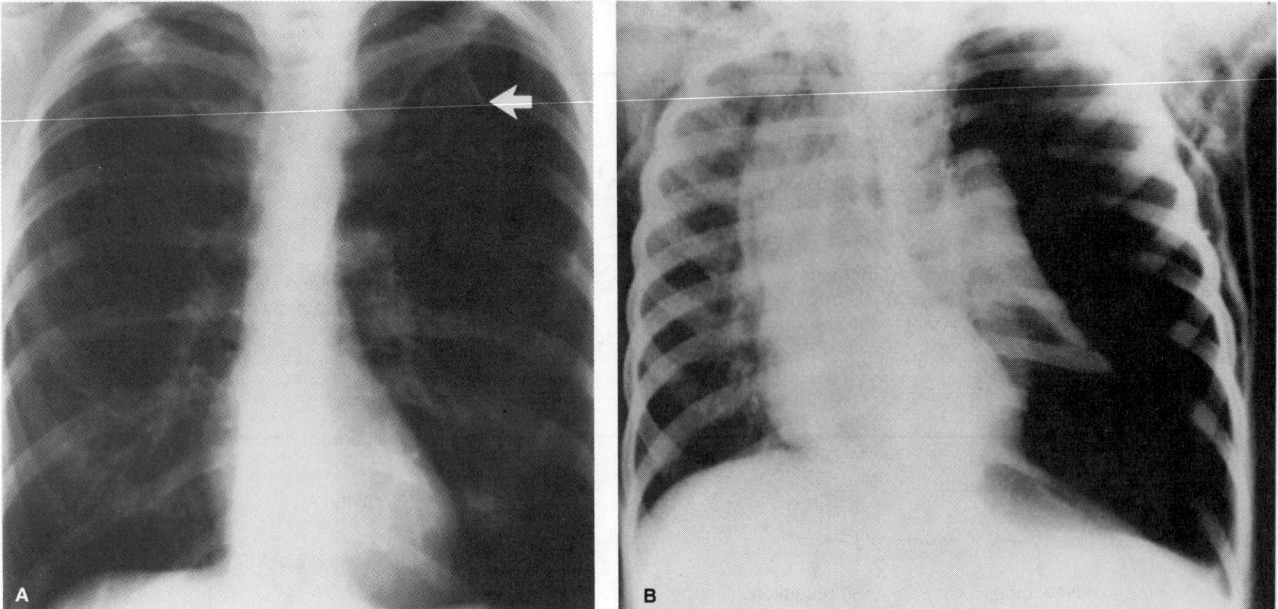

Figure 62-18. (*A*) Forty percent left-sided spontaneous pneumothorax (*arrow*). (*B*) Progression of simple pneumothorax to a tension pneumothorax, showing the characteristic radiographic findings—virtual collapse of the entire involved lung, shift of the mediastinum to the contralateral side, and compression of the contralateral lung. Subcutaneous air dissecting along the left chest wall is also evident.

aged patients, for example, to present several days after their initial episode of chest pain and shortness of breath, now without symptoms, but with a chest radiograph showing a 30% to 40% or larger pneumothorax. It is not unreasonable to follow such patients with a repeat chest radiograph for 1 or 2 days on an outpatient basis and then at 1- to 2-week intervals because air is absorbed from the pleural cavity at a rate of about 1% per day, and gradual resolution of the process occurs if the bleb has sealed. Patients who do not have symptoms from the pneumothorax are best treated with an apically placed chest tube because most pulmonary blebs responsible for the development of a spontaneous pneumothorax are located at the apex of the chest. The apical chest tube is most easily inserted behind the pectoralis major muscle fold just below the axillary hairline. In this location, there are no large extrathoracic muscles to traverse, and the scar that remains after removal of the tube is more cosmetically acceptable than when the tube is inserted in the mid-clavicular line anteriorly.

As indicated previously, in most patients with spontaneous pneumothorax, spontaneous resolution or successful treatment with a chest tube is achieved. Indications for operative intervention include (1) a history of a previous pneumothorax; (2) continued air leak or failure of a properly placed chest tube to result in reexpansion of the lung after 3 to 5 days; (3) massive air leak with inability to reexpand the lung within 24 hours; (4) bilateral pneumothoraces occurring either simultaneously or at different times; (5) patient occupation for which recurrent pneumothorax would constitute a major threat to life (eg, airline pilot, diver); (6) residence in a remote area; and (7) demonstrable large pulmonary bullae. Thoracostomy tube drainage is the treatment of choice for an initial pneumothorax.[32] In a randomized study evaluating tube thoracostomy versus immediate thoracoscopic stapling of blebs, there was no benefit with respect to decreased length of stay, cost, or long-term outcome in patients who had early thoracoscopic intervention compared with those who underwent initial tube thoracotomy. The recommendations

for operative intervention in cases of pneumothoraces are prolonged air leak greater then 72 hours, complicated pneumothorax, recurrent pneumothorax, or bilateral pneumothoraces.[19]

The operative treatment of pneumothorax has been achieved through a variety of incisions, including an anterior thoracotomy, lateral thoracotomy, median sternotomy, and transaxillary minithoracotomy. Thoracoscopy has been used successfully in the treatment of pneumothorax and is appealing because of the limited thoracic incision it requires. Through three 1-inch incisions, ports are placed that allow entry into the thoracic cavity after one-lung anesthesia has been established (Fig. 62-19). Bleb ex-

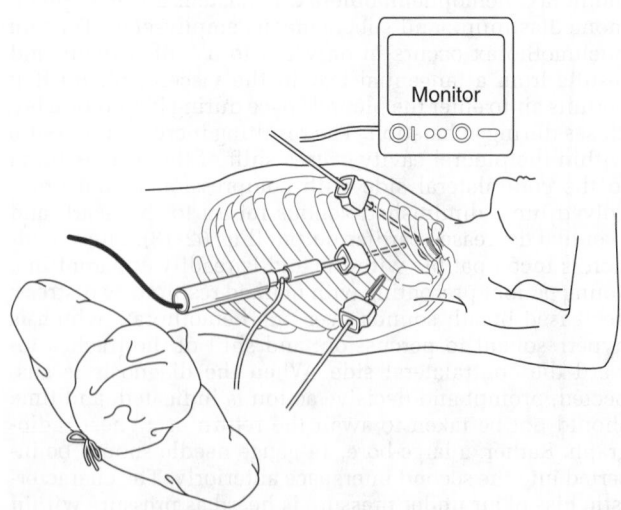

Figure 62-19. Positioning and instrumentation for thoracoscopy procedures. (After Daniel TM, Wyatt DA. Pneumothorax and bullous disease. In: Kaiser LR, Daniel TM, eds. Thoracoscopic surgery. Boston, Little, Brown, 1993:85)

cision and pleurodesis are readily performed with this approach. The theoretic advantages of thoracoscopy—decreased postoperative pain, decreased hospitalization and decreased expense—have not been realized, but there does not seem to be a significant difference in this regard between thoracoscopic bleb resection and open bleb resection and pleurodesis.[33] Parietal pleurectomy has been advocated by some as the operative approach of choice for recurrent spontaneous pneumothorax. After stripping away the parietal pleura and draining the chest, the visceral pleura adheres to the chest wall, preventing recurrence of the pneumothorax. We do *not* favor this approach, nor do most thoracic surgeons. Not only is this a more extensive operation than is required for this condition, but if there should be a subsequent need to reenter the chest (eg, to treat a later lung tumor), it is technically much more difficult. Because spontaneous pneumothorax is most often due to a pulmonary bleb involving the visceral pleura, the most appropriate surgical approach appears to be directed at the lung rather than the chest wall. We prefer a transaxillary minithoracotomy, entering the third intercostal space through an 8- to 10-cm curvilinear incision placed 1 to 2 cm below the axillary hairline and extending from the anterior border of latissimus dorsi behind to the posterior edge of the pectoralis major muscle anteriorly (Fig. 62-20). Care is taken to avoid the long thoracic nerve that courses along the chest wall just beneath the anterior edge of the latissimus dorsi muscle. After entering the chest, the apex of the lung is inspected, and in most cases, tiny pulmonary blebs can be identified in this location. After stapling the blebs with the surgical stapling device, a mechanical pleurodesis is carried out by vigorous gauze abrasion of the parietal and visceral pleural surfaces that are accessible through the incision. A single 28F apical chest tube is inserted and can usually be removed within 48 hours. Recurrent pneumothorax occurs in less than 1% of patients after this procedure. Although the transaxillary minithoracotomy is adequate in most young, otherwise healthy patients with spontaneous pneumothoraces, patients with other underlying pulmonary pathology, such

as chronic obstructive pulmonary disease with obvious blebs at locations other than the apex, or catamenial pneumothorax in which there may be multiple endometrial implants along the diaphragmatic surface of the lung, should be approached through a more traditional posterolateral thoracotomy.

Chylothorax

The thoracic duct is a posterior mediastinal structure that may have variable anatomy (Fig. 62-21). The duct originates from the confluence of the cisterna chyli at variable levels from the 10th thoracic to the 3rd lumbar vertebrae. The cisterna chyli is about 3 to 4 cm long and 2 to 3 cm in diameter and is located to the right side of the abdominal aorta. From the cisterna chyli, a single thoracic duct enters the posterior mediastinum through the aortic hiatus at the level of T-10 to T-12 and to the right of the aorta. Above the diaphragm, the duct courses cephalad along the anterior surface of the vertebral column posterior to the esophagus and between the aorta and azygos vein. At about the level of T-4 to T-5, the duct crosses to the left of the spine under the aortic arch and then continues along the left side of the esophagus and into the neck behind the left subclavian artery. In the neck, the duct is always located anterior to the vertebral artery and vein, thyrocervical trunk, and phrenic nerve and medial to the scalenus anticus muscle. The thoracic duct drains into the venous system at the confluence of the left subclavian and internal jugular veins. Within the chest, the thoracic duct has numerous lymphaticovenous anastomoses with the azygos, intercostal, and lumbar veins. It is for this reason that the duct can be ligated at any point in the chest or neck without serious consequences. Forty percent of patients have two or more thoracic ducts.

Knowledge of thoracic duct anatomy is important in understanding why injury to the thoracic duct and subsequent leak of chyle into the pleural space (chylothorax) can occur after penetrating or blunt trauma, hyperextension injuries to the spine, forceful vomiting, violent coughing,

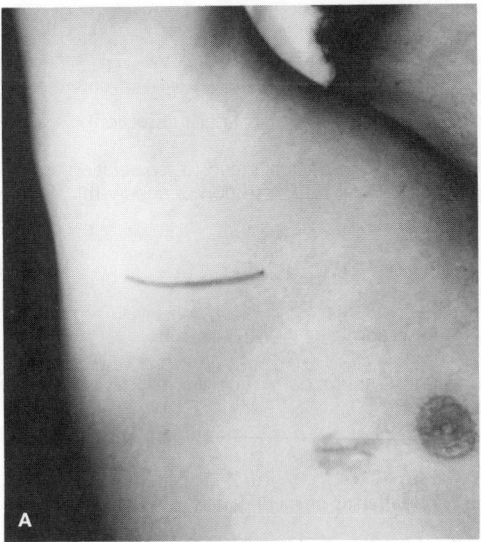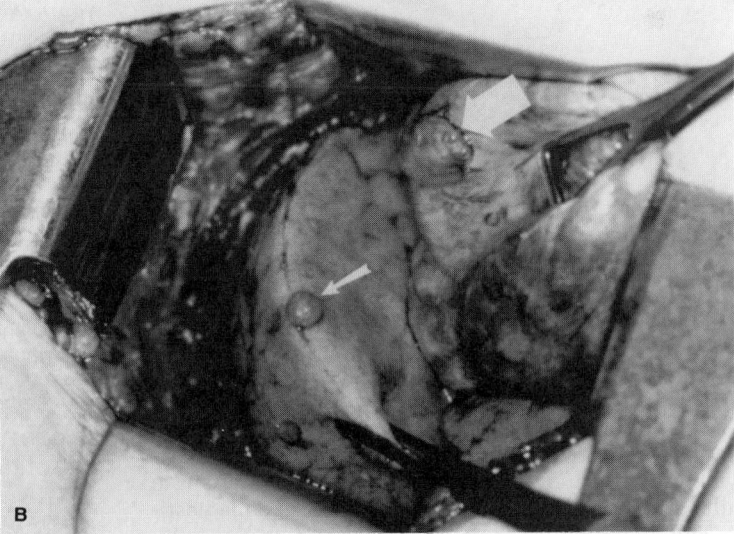

Figure 62-20. Transaxillary mini-thoracotomy used for resection of apical blebs and pleurodesis for spontaneous pneumothorax. (*A*) The patient is in the left lateral decubitus position with his arm suspended from the ether screen. The 8- to 10-cm incision beneath the axillary hair line extends from the edge of the latissimus dorsi behind to the pectoralis major muscle anteriorly. A scar from a previous chest tube is seen adjacent to the nipple. (*B*) Typical subpleural blebs demonstrated through incision shown in *A*. The large arrow marks right upper lobe bleb; the small arrow marks bleb in superior segment of right lower lobe.

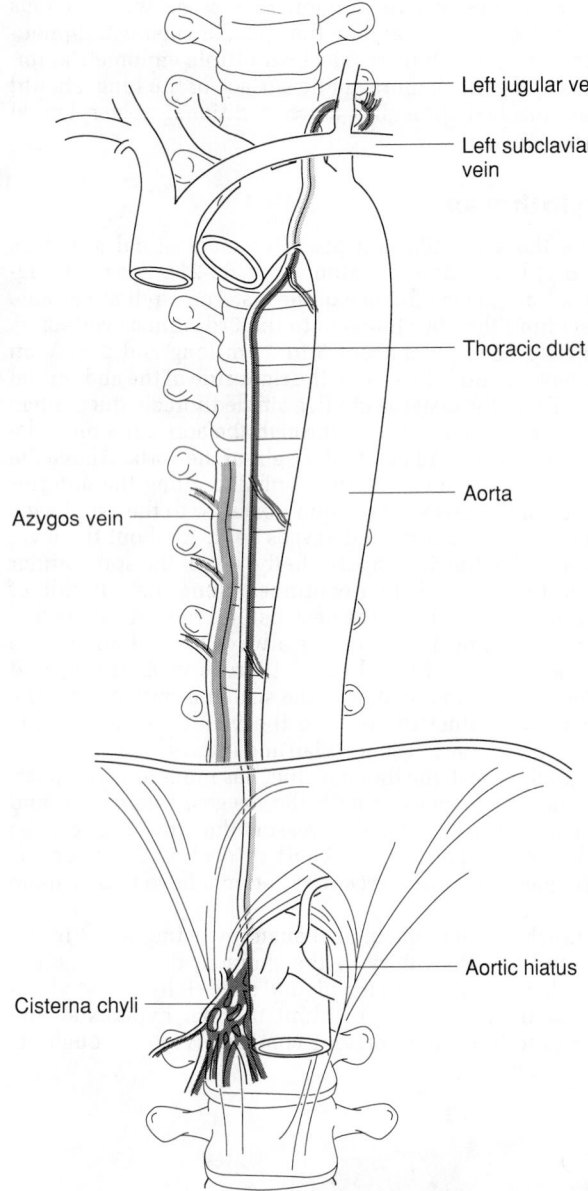

Figure 62-21. Course of the thoracic duct.

and in association with posterior mediastinal tumors. Iatrogenic thoracic duct injury can occur during operations in the left thorax involving the aortic arch or esophagus, where the duct passes from the right side of the spine to the left side to ascend into the neck. Similarly, operations on cervical or abdominal lymph nodes or the lungs can result in a chylothorax.

When the thoracic duct is injured, chyle accumulates in the posterior mediastinum until the mediastinal pleura eventually ruptures into one or both chests, resulting in a chylothorax. Accumulation of chyle in the pleural space results in compression of the ipsilateral lung and mediastinum and may produce chest discomfort and dyspnea. Although the diagnosis of chylothorax is generally apparent when the characteristic opalescent, milky pleural fluid is obtained on a thoracentesis performed to evaluate a pleural effusion, in the first several days after a major thoracic or abdominal operation, when the patient has had no oral intake and therefore has little fat within the lymph, the pleural fluid may appear clear or serosanguineous, and the diagnosis of a chylothorax may be delayed.

Differentiation between chylous and nonchylous effusions is facilitated by a knowledge of the physical and biochemical properties of chyle. Thoracic duct lymph contains 0.4 to 6 g of fat/100 mL, depending on dietary intake, and from 2.2 to 5.9 g of protein/100 mL, about half the concentration of plasma protein.[34] The albumin/globulin ratio is 3:1. Ninety-five percent of thoracic duct lymph originates in the liver or intestinal lymphatics, the latter of which absorb 60% to 70% of ingested fat, which is transported to the bloodstream through the thoracic duct. Chyle has a lymphocyte count between 400 and 6800/μL. Typically, chyle has a specific gravity of 1.012 to 1.025 and is alkaline, odorless, sterile, and bacteriostatic. The diagnosis of a chylothorax in a patient who is eating may be made by staining the pleural fluid with Sudan red, which stains the fat globules. A cholesterol/triglyceride ratio of less than 1 is characteristic of a chylous effusion, whereas nonchylous effusions typically have a ratio of greater than 1. Pleural fluid that has a triglyceride level of less than 50 mL/dL has less than a 5% chance of being chylous, whereas fluid with a triglyceride level of greater than 110 mL/dL has a 99% chance of being chyle.[34] To establish a diagnosis of chylothorax, lipoprotein analysis of pleural fluid to verify the presence of chylomicrons may be required. Most often, particularly in postoperative patients, the diagnosis of chylothorax is seldom subtle or difficult to make once milky fluid has been identified. Injuries to the thoracic duct below the T-5 to T-6 level usually result in a right-sided chylothorax, whereas those above this level usually cause left-sided chylous effusions.

Chylothorax has a variety of causes (Table 62-3). Half of

Table 62-3. CAUSES OF CHYLOTHORAX

CONGENITAL

Thoracic duct atresia
Thoracic duct fistula
Birth trauma

TRAUMA

Blunt
Penetrating
Surgical
   Cervical (lymph node biopsy or radical neck dissection)
   Thoracic
      Aortic operations (patent ductus arteriosus, coarctation repair, operations for vascular ring, resection of aneurysm)
      Pulmonary resection
      Esophagectomy
      Mediastinal tumor excision
      Sympathectomy
   Abdominal
      Lymph node dissection
      Sympathectomy
Diagnostic procedures (translumbar aortogram, subclavian vein catheterization)

TUMORS

INFECTIONS

Granulomatous lymphadenitis or mediastinitis
Filariasis

OTHER

Vena cava or subclavian vein thrombosis
Pulmonary lymphangiomyomatosis

(Modified from DeMeester TR, Lafontaine E. The pleura. In: Sabiston DC Jr, Spencer FC, eds. Surgery of the chest, ed 5. Philadelphia, WB Saunders, 1990:456)

chylothoraces in adults are due to tumors, and three fourths of these are the result of lymphomas. The treatment of postoperative chylothorax is controversial. Chylothorax unassociated with trauma to the thoracic duct may at times respond to nonoperative therapy, such as intravenous hyperalimentation (to diminish output from the fistula), chemical pleurodesis, and mediastinal irradiation. Postoperative chylothorax, conversely, may pose more of a therapeutic dilemma because loss of large amounts of chyle from a chest tube can result in substantial fluid shifts, electrolyte imbalance, loss of serum protein and albumin, and decrease in peripheral lymphocytes with subsequent altered immune response. Particularly after an esophagectomy in a patient with chronic esophageal obstruction, loss of protein-rich chyle for a prolonged period is simply not well tolerated and may be associated with a mortality rate in excess of 30%.[35] Particularly after a major thoracic operation, if prolonged or excessive serosanguineous chest tube drainage suggests the possibility of a thoracic duct injury, the administration of 60 to 90 mL/h of cream by mouth or nasogastric feeding tube for 3 to 6 hours results in an obvious change in the character of the drainage to the typical milky fluid of chyle. At times, conservative management of postoperative chylothorax with chest tube drainage, low-residue enteral feedings, or intravenous hyperalimentation and correction of fluid and electrolyte imbalance may be successful and has been advocated for up to 14 days. We do not recommend this approach. Particularly in the patient who has undergone an esophagectomy, if chest tube drainage exceeds 250 to 300 mL for two consecutive 8-hour shifts 3 or 4 days after establishing a diagnosis of chylothorax and initiating the standard measures described earlier, cream should be administered either through a previously placed jejunostomy tube or a nasogastric tube at a rate of 60 to 90 mL/h for 4 to 6 consecutive hours to ensure an active flow of chyle from the chest tube at the time of operation. A transthoracic approach to the injured thoracic duct, usually on the same side as the pleural drainage, is most effective. A double-lumen endotracheal tube permits one-lung anesthesia and ventilation of the contralateral side during visualization of the site of injury to the thoracic duct, which is ligated and suture ligated above and below this point. Because of the abundance of alternative collateral pathways for lymphatic drainage in the chest, such thoracic duct ligation has no adverse consequences. Thoracoscopic drainage and thoracic duct occlusion, either by direct ligation for clip application at the level of the aortic hiatus, has been reported.[36] Alternatively, transabdominal thoracic duct ligation at the aortic hiatus is an effective option, but one that may be difficult in a patient who has undergone an esophageal resection with mobilization of the stomach through the diaphragmatic hiatus in the original esophageal bed, making access to the aortic hiatus difficult. Although there is a natural tendency to treat postoperative chylothoraces conservatively for as long as possible, delay in definitive therapy may result in serious and irreparable volume, electrolyte, protein, lymphocyte, and vitamin depletion that can be lethal. At times, an aggressive approach to control the chyle fistula is live-saving. Surgical intervention in patients with postoperative iatrogenic chylothorax is usually successful because there is a well-localized thoracic duct injury that can be identified, isolated, and controlled. In contrast, chylothorax due to obstruction of mediastinal lymphatics by tumor is frequently the result of diffuse oozing of chyle from multiple sites within the mediastinum, and therefore precise identification of the source of the chyle leak is difficult, and operative intervention is seldom rewarding.

Tumors of the Pleura

Benign tumors of the pleura are exceedingly rare and include lipomas, endotheliomas, and angiomas. They characteristically arise from the subpleural tissues of the chest wall and are resected when they present as an asymptomatic mass on chest radiograph. Cysts of the pleura occur predominantly at the pleuropericardial reflection. They originate from the parietal pleura and present as a characteristic rounded mass adjacent to the right-sided heart border on chest radiograph. Although, in the past, these pericardial cysts were resected for diagnostic purposes, the advent of the CT scan has allowed determination of the cystic nature of these lesions and CT-guided transthoracic aspiration for cytologic assessment of the fluid. Periodic follow-up with chest radiographs is an acceptable approach in most cases.

Mesothelioma is by far the most common primary tumor of the pleura. Epidemiologically, there is a strong relation between asbestos exposure and the development of mesothelioma.[37] The exact relation between asbestos exposure and mesothelioma remains unclear. A history of asbestos exposure is not always obtainable in patients who have mesothelioma; the reported relation varies between 0% and 80%.[38] Although 6% to 7% of deaths in asbestos workers are the result of either pleural or peritoneal mesothelioma, 20% of deaths are the result of bronchogenic carcinoma, the incidence of which is also markedly increased in patients with asbestos exposure. There are two types of asbestos fibers based on crystalline structure—serpentine (chrysolite) and amphibole. Included within amphibole are amosite, tremolite, crocidolite, and anthophyllite. The most harmful of these latter fibers is crocidolite, or blue asbestos.

Mesotheliomas are typically divided into the diffuse and localized types. Diffuse mesothelioma is virtually always malignant. Although the localized form of mesothelioma is often benign, many of the localized tumors are malignant. The histologic evaluation of mesotheliomas is notoriously difficult, and an understanding of the embryology of the pleura explains this. The pleura forms from two lamellae, which originate from mesoderm. The parietal lamella fuses with the ectoderm and forms the somatopleura. The visceral lamella fuses with the endoderm and forms the splanchnopleura. Therefore, all three germ cell layers are represented in the formation of the pleura, and mesotheliomas may be composed of varying degrees of epithelial and mesenchymal elements.

Localized Benign Mesothelioma

Benign pleural mesotheliomas characteristically arise from the visceral pleura of the lung as a pedunculated tumor on a stalk.[38] These tumors sometimes arise from the mediastinal, diaphragmatic, or parietal pleura and can occur within the lung parenchyma, mimicking a bronchogenic tumor. They vary in size from small lesions of several centimeters to massive lesions that fill the hemithorax. Benign mesotheliomas may be associated with a bloody pleural effusion that does *not* represent nonresectable malignant disease, one of the few instances in which a lung mass with a bloody pleural effusion is not synonymous with incurability.

Most benign mesotheliomas present as asymptomatic tumors discovered on a routine chest radiograph. Chest pain, cough, shortness of breath, and a pleural effusion may also occur. One peculiar characteristic of this tumor is the association with hypertrophic pulmonary osteoarthropathy in about 20% of patients, most often with tumors larger than 7 cm in size. Dramatic hypoglycemia that is eliminated by removal of the tumor may also occur with benign mesothelioma.

Most of these tumors are diagnosed when the patient undergoes a thoracotomy for diagnosis of a chest mass discovered on chest radiograph. The typical gross appearance of a cauliflower mass arising from the lung surface generally allows the surgeon to make the diagnosis. The tumor is removed by applying a surgical stapler across lung parenchyma at least 1 cm from the site of origin of the stalk of the tumor. Recurrence is rare, and when it happens, transition to the malignant form of the tumor should be suspected.

Localized Malignant Mesothelioma

Patients with localized malignant mesothelioma, unlike their counterparts with the benign form of the disease, typically have symptoms of chest pain, cough, dyspnea, and fever. Pulmonary osteoarthropathy is unusual with a localized malignant tumor. Wide local excision is again the treatment of choice, and the diagnosis of malignancy is established histologically. Because seeding of the adjacent pleura can occur during resection of these tumors and result in subsequent recurrence, careful handling of the tumors during resection is important. Postoperative radiotherapy and chemotherapy has been used in patients who have undergone incomplete resections. With incomplete resection, median survival is only 7 months.

Diffuse Malignant Mesothelioma

This form of mesothelioma arises from any pleural surface and grows in a characteristic spreading fashion along the pleural surfaces, including the interlobar fissures. The entire lung ultimately is enveloped and compressed by a thick rind of tumor. Diffuse mesothelioma most often begins in the lower aspects of the pleural cavity. The tumor often extends through the diaphragm and into the peritoneal cavity as well as into the ribs and chest wall. Involvement of regional lymph nodes and hematogenous spread to liver, lung, brain, and adrenal glands is common. Histologically, malignant mesotheliomas have both fibrous (sarcomatous) and epithelial (papillary) components. The epithelial components resemble adenocarcinoma and typically form papillary fronds projecting into dilated cystic spaces on histologic evaluation. Some tumors may show a preponderance of sarcomatous elements, whereas the mixed variety of mesothelioma contains both epithelial and sarcomatous elements. Because mesotheliomas do not typically produce mucin, periodic acid–Schiff stain for mucin may be helpful in the histochemical differentiation from adenocarcinoma. Immunohistochemistry and electron microscopy may also be necessary to establish the diagnosis. Malignant mesotheliomas have the greatest incidence in the sixth and seventh decades of life, but one quarter of patients are younger than 50 years of age. Men are affected more commonly than woman, at a ratio of 2:1 to 5:1. The characteristic presenting symptoms are chest pain, dyspnea, cough, and weight loss. Chest radiographs demonstrate pleural effusions in more than 75% of patients. The chest CT scan, which is perhaps the best study for evaluating the pleura, is extremely helpful in documenting the extent of the tumor. Irregular and nodular pleural thickening with contraction of the involved hemithorax is common, as are pleural plaques, often calcified, in the opposite chest. There may be extension into the chest wall with rib and soft tissue involvement.

The diagnosis of malignant mesothelioma can be difficult. Cytologic evaluation of the pleural fluid may be nondiagnostic; needle biopsy of the thickened pleura has a much greater diagnostic yield. Thoracoscopy and biopsy or a small diagnostic thoracotomy and biopsy may be required. Butchart and associates[39] proposed the most frequently used classification for the staging of malignant mesothelioma:

Stage I—involvement of ipsilateral pleura and lung
Stage II—involvement of chest wall, mediastinum, pericardium, or contralateral pleura
Stage III—involvement of chest and abdomen, or lymph nodes outside the chest
Stage IV—distant hematogenous metastases

In an attempt to achieve more accurate and unified staging, Rusch and Ginsberg[40] proposed the TNM system adopted by the Union Internationale Contre le Cancer (Table 62-4). The treatment of diffuse malignant mesothelioma is discouragingly ineffective; survival after diagnosis rarely is longer than 2 years and averages between 10 and 14 months.[41] Evidence suggests that patients with the epithelial type of mesothelioma have a limited but significantly better survival when treated with combination chemotherapy and radiotherapy followed by radical

---

Table 62-4. TNM CLASSIFICATION FOR STAGING OF MESOTHELIOMA

TNM DEFINITIONS

Primary Tumor

Tx	Primary tumor cannot be assessed
T0	No evidence of primary tumor
T1	Primary tumor limited to ipsilateral parietal, or visceral pleura, or both
T2	Tumor invades any of the following: ipsilateral lung, endothoracic fascia, diaphragm, pericardium
T3	Tumor invades any of the following: ipsilateral chest wall muscle, ribs, mediastinal organs or tissues
T4	Tumor extends to any of the following: contralateral pleura or lung by direct extension, peritoneum or intraabdominal organs by direct extension, cervical tissues

Regional Lymph Node Involvement

Nx	Regional lymph nodes cannot be assessed
N0	No regional lymph node metastases
N1	Metastases in ipsilateral bronchopulmonary or hilar lymph nodes
N2	Metastases in ipsilateral mediastinal lymph nodes
N3	Metastases in contralateral mediastinal, internal mammary, supraclavicular, or scalene lymph nodes

Distant Metastasis

Mx	Presence of distant metastases cannot be assessed
M0	No known distant metastasis
M1	Distant metastasis present

STAGING GROUPING*

Stage I	T1, N0, M0
	T2, N0, M0
Stage II	T1, N1, M0
	T2, N1, M0
Stage III	T3, N0, M0
	T3, N1, M0
	T1, N2, M0
	T2, N2, M0
	T3, N2, M0
Stage IV	Any T, N3, M0
	T4, any N, M0
	Any T, any N, M1

* Staging solely on clinical measures is designated cTNM. Staging that can be done in clinical pathologic information is designated as pTNM. Clinical and pathologic groups are identical.
(Adapted from Rusch VW, Ginsberg RJ. New concepts in the staging of mesotheliomas. In: Deslaurier J, Lacquet LK, eds. Thoracic surgery. St Louis, CV Mosby, 1990:340)

pleuropneumonectomy.[42,43] As with other neoplasms, the presence of lymph node metastases significantly impacts on survival. As many as 25% of patients with malignant mesothelioma have involvement of mediastinal lymph nodes at the time of surgery. Therefore, as with other malignancies, precise staging of the tumors is extremely important in defining outcome studies. In selected patients with stage I disease, a radical pleuropneumonectomy sometimes is effective. The morbidity and mortality from this operation are high, and long-term survival is rare. Some have advocated pleurectomy followed by postoperative brachytherapy through implanted radiation catheters, but brachytherapy has not been associated with significantly prolonged survival in these patients. Primary radiotherapy has also been used as treatment for mesothelioma. Combination chemotherapy using either single-agent or combination protocols with cisplatin and doxorubicin also has proponents, but the prognosis with this tumor remains dismal.

Pleural Metastases

The pleura is frequently involved with metastatic disease. In men, the most common primary sites are lung and lymphoma, which account for 70% of malignant effusions. In women, cancers involving the breast, genital tract, and lung account for more than 70% of malignant effusions.[44]

MEDIASTINUM

The mediastinum is the central portion of the chest and extends from the thoracic inlet above to the diaphragm below. It is bounded anteriorly by the sternum, laterally by the mediastinal pleura, and posteriorly by the vertebral bodies. To assist in the localization of mediastinal abnormalities, the mediastinum is traditionally divided into superior, anterior, middle, and posterior compartments (Fig. 62-22). If on a lateral chest radiograph, a line is drawn

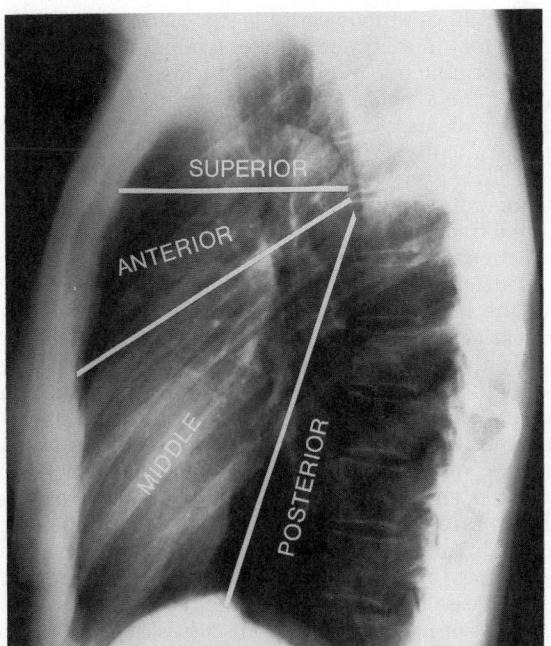

Figure 62-22. Compartments of the mediastinum. The superior and inferior mediastinum are separated by a line drawn from the sternomanubrial junction anteriorly on a lateral chest radiograph to the lower edge of the fourth vertebral body posteriorly. The inferior mediastinum is divided into anterior, middle, and posterior compartments by the pericardium.

from the lower end of the manubrium to the lower edge of the body of the fourth thoracic vertebral body, the superior mediastinum is the area above that line. The pericardial sac and its contents divide the inferior mediastinum into its anterior, middle, and posterior compartments. The contents of the mediastinum and its compartments are as follows:

Superior Mediastinum
Thymus gland
Aortic arch and great vessels
Upper trachea
Upper esophagus

Anterior Mediastinum
Thymus gland
Lymph nodes

Middle Mediastinum
Pericardium
Heart
Tracheal bifurcation
Main-stem bronchi
Subcarinal and peribronchial lymph nodes
Ascending aorta

Posterior Mediastinum
Esophagus
Descending aorta
Nerves (sympathetic, parasympathetic, and intercostal)

CT has permitted visualization of mediastinal structures that in the past were obscured on the standard posteroanterior chest radiograph by the sternum, spine, and cardiac silhouette (Fig. 62-23).

Infection

Acute Mediastinitis

Acute infection of the mediastinum, regardless of the cause, is associated with great morbidity and mortality. Although acute mediastinitis can follow cardiac operations in which the mediastinum has been opened or penetrating wounds of the chest or tracheobronchial tree, the most common cause of acute suppurative mediastinitis is an esophageal perforation, which can have a wide variety of causes. The causes, clinical presentation, diagnosis, and treatment of esophageal perforations are reviewed in Chapter 19. Infection after a median sternotomy for cardiac surgery is a serious complication, especially if the patient has prosthetic aortic graft material at the base of the wound. Mediastinitis in this setting is typically heralded by sternal instability, drainage from the wound, and fever. Various approaches have been used to treat postoperative sternal wound infections. These range from simple débridement and sternal reapproximation to staged reconstruction and the use of muscle flap rotation into the sternal wound edges. We favor thorough sternal and mediastinal débridement and one-stage reconstruction with a rotated muscle flap or omentum to fill the retrosternal space, unless the space is relatively small and obliteration can be achieved with suction drains. Regardless of the technique used, it is important to obliterate the retrosternal space to prevent reaccumulation of infection. Adequate débridement of all exposed cartilage from the sternum and ribs is critical because cartilage is avascular, does not heal, and promotes formation of a chronic draining wound sinus. If the sternum is clearly devascularized, it is necessary to remove completely all necrotic bone and cartilage and to then fill the anterior mediastinal space with a muscle flap, which also aids with chest wall stability. A vascularized muscle or omental pedicle should be used to ensure resolution of the infectious process. Space obliter-

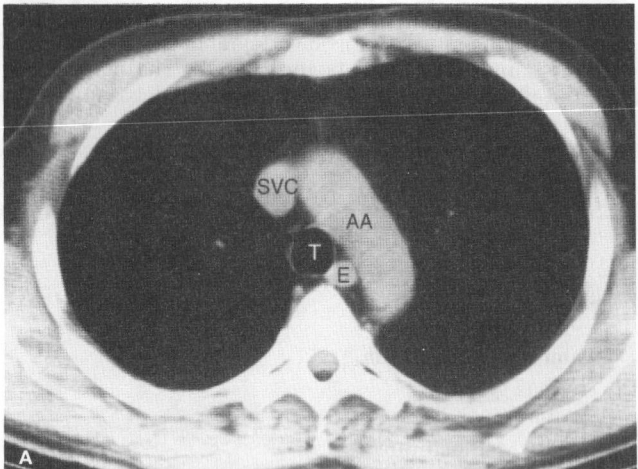

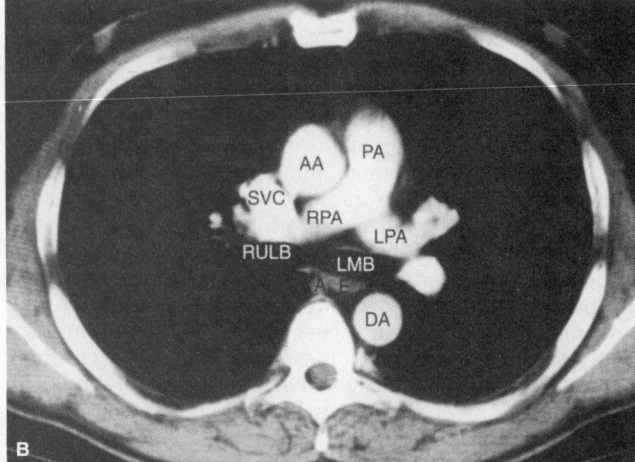

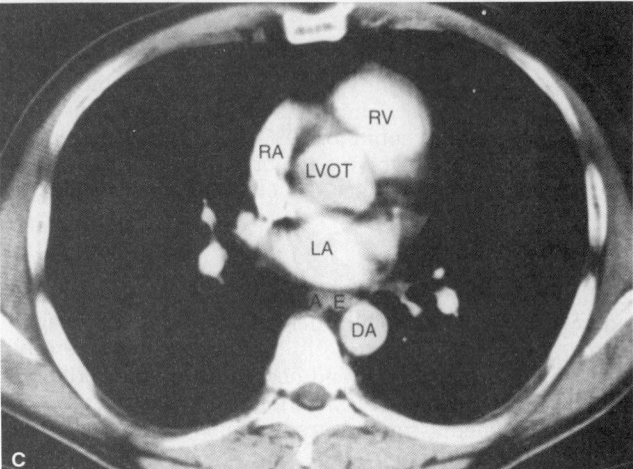

Figure 62-23. Normal mediastinal anatomy as shown with CT scans. (*A*) Scan at level of the aortic arch and mid trachea. T, trachea; E, esophagus; AA, aortic arch; SVC, superior vena cava. (*B*) Scan at level of carina. RULB, right upper lobe bronchus; LMB, left main-stem bronchus; AA, ascending aorta; DA, descending aorta; A, azygos vein; E, esophagus; SVC, superior vena cava; PA, main pulmonary artery; LPA and RPA, left and right pulmonary arteries. (*C*) Scan at the level of the left atrium. LA, left atrium; RA, right atrium; LVOT, left ventricular outflow tract; RV, right ventricle; A, azygos vein; E, esophagus; DA, descending aorta.

ation with an omental flap and reapproximation of the sternum may be performed if the wound is not grossly contaminated and intraoperative Gram stain is negative. This approach may have a long-term advantage because more than half of patients who require sternal débridement and flap interposition without reapproximation of the bone have chronic postoperative pain after reconstruction.[45,46] If a grossly infected wound is encountered or there has been a failed attempt at sternal reconstruction, however, the patient is left with either draining sternal wound sinuses or an open sternotomy incision. Sternal débridement and rotation of pectoralis major and rectus abdominis muscle flaps as described previously fills the chest wall defect with vascularized healthy tissue that usually achieves resolution of the infectious problem.

Descending Necrotizing Mediastinitis

Descending necrotizing mediastinitis is a lethal form of acute mediastinitis in which infection arising from the oropharynx spreads to the mediastinum.[47] This form of mediastinitis typically develops as a complication of oropharyngeal infection (eg, odontogenic, peritonsillar, or retropharyngeal abscesses, Ludwig angina, or infection after a pharyngeal perforation). Although transcervical drainage is generally adequate treatment for acute mediastinitis resulting from a cervical esophageal perforation, this approach does *not* provide adequate drainage in the patient with descending necrotizing mediastinitis, and the resulting mortality rate for this condition approaches 40%. Although the standard chest radiograph may demonstrate

typical findings of mediastinitis, the CT scan is the most valuable tool in this condition for evaluating the presence of a gas-forming infection within the mediastinum and for following the adequacy of surgical drainage.

These patients are ill with fever, pleuritic chest pain, dysphagia, and varying degrees of airway obstruction resulting from dissection of large amounts of air and acute inflammation within the mediastinal fascial planes. They require a tracheostomy to ensure an adequate airway during treatment of the acute mediastinitis. If only the superior mediastinum is involved and the infection remains above the level of the fourth thoracic vertebra, standard transcervical mediastinal drainage may be adequate. This is rarely the case, however. Most of these patients have extensive mediastinitis, which requires a combination of transcervical and subxiphoid or transthoracic drainage. Broad-spectrum aerobic and anaerobic antibiotic coverage should be instituted immediately when the diagnosis is considered, and culture-specific antibiotics should be used as the culture reports return. The highly lethal nature of this fulminant infection cannot be overemphasized, and patients may experience exsanguination from erosion of the great vessels of the neck and mediastinum, aspiration, cranial nerve paralysis, brain abscesses, and necrotizing fasciitis. Recognition of the fact that one is dealing with more than localized upper mediastinal infection of the type commonly associated with acute esophageal perforations is critical. Aggressive drainage of the mediastinum using the cervical, subxiphoid, or transthoracic route is virtually the only means of salvaging these patients.

Chronic Granulomatous Mediastinitis

Granulomatous infections of the chest frequently involve paratracheal (right more than left) and subcarinal mediastinal lymph nodes. In the past, tuberculosis was the most common cause of mediastinal granulomatous infection; histoplasmosis is now the leading etiologic agent.[48] The granulomatous reaction within the mediastinal lymph node may incite an intense surrounding inflammatory response that produces mediastinal fibrosis, which can cause compression of the superior vena cava (SVC), esophagus, trachea, or airways. Resection of large, acutely inflamed mediastinal lymph nodes involved with histoplasmosis has been recommended to minimize the late sequelae of this disease. In cases of vena cava obstruction due to mediastinal fibrosis, vascular reconstruction using either a spiral vein graft or a Gore-Tex graft may be required if symptoms are severe. Another potential complication of mediastinal granulomatous disease is necrosis of the adjacent esophageal and tracheobronchial walls with the development of a bronchoesophageal fistula. This complication requires a transthoracic approach, identification and division of the fistulous opening, closure of both the tracheal and esophageal openings, and interposition of a flap of viable adjacent pleura or mediastinal fat to prevent reformation of the fistula.

Mediastinal Tumors and Cysts

Although mediastinal tumors can arise primarily, secondary metastases to mediastinal lymph nodes and direct invasion of the mediastinum by tracheobronchial, esophageal, or other malignancies are common. The differential diagnosis of a mediastinal mass includes neoplasms as well as congenital cysts, which are not neoplastic. Therefore, most reported series of mediastinal tumors include both congenital and neoplastic processes. Neurogenic tumors are most common and account for 21% of mediastinal masses, followed by thymomas (20%), cysts (20%), and lymphomas (12%).[49] The locations of tumors in the various mediastinal compartments are as follows:

Anterior Mediastinum

Thymoma
Teratoma
Carcinoma
Lymphangioma
Hemangioma
Lipoma

Superior Mediastinum

Thymoma
Lymphoma
Thyroid adenoma
Parathyroid adenoma

Posterior Mediastinum

Neurogenic tumor
Enteric cyst

Middle Mediastinum

Pericardial cyst
Bronchogenic cyst
Lymphoma

Mediastinal masses cause symptoms (chest pain, cough, or dyspnea) in nearly two thirds of adult patients. Nearly half of symptomatic mediastinal tumors are malignant, whereas 95% of asymptomatic mediastinal masses discovered on routine chest radiograph are benign. Children have a higher incidence of malignancy of mediastinal tumors than adults.

Patients with mediastinal masses and evidence of involvement of adjacent structures are more likely to have malignant disease. For example, hoarseness is indicative of recurrent laryngeal nerve invasion, Horner syndrome signifies invasion of the stellate ganglion, SVC syndrome or tracheal compression suggests mediastinal infiltration by tumor, and back pain may be indicative of chest wall invasion with intercostal nerve involvement.

A variety of radiographic studies are of help in assessing the patient with a mediastinal mass. The standard posteroanterior and lateral chest radiograph assists in localization of the mass. Fluoroscopy, barium esophagogram, and laminography have also been of value. These latter studies have all but been replaced by contrast-enhanced CT magnetic resonance (MR) imaging, and which provide the most information about the exact location of the mediastinal mass, its vascularity, relation to adjacent mediastinal structures, and consistency (ie, cystic, solid, or fat). Aortography is at times needed to differentiate a mediastinal tumor from an aneurysm. Fine-needle aspiration or core-needle biopsy of mediastinal masses under CT scan or fluoroscopic guidance may provide enough tissue for cytologic or pathologic diagnosis, which is useful in planning treatment. Using the flexible fiberoptic bronchoscope and fluoroscopic guidance, a transbronchial needle aspiration of subcarinal or paratracheal lymphadenopathy may establish a diagnosis while avoiding a major operation.[50] Mediastinoscopy, which requires general anesthesia, involves passage of a rigid endoscope through a low cervical incision along the anterior trachea into the mid-mediastinum. This procedure provides access to paratracheal and subcarinal lymph nodes for the purpose of biopsy but is inappropriate for the assessment of an anterior mediastinal mass. Because the mediastinoscope follows the course of the trachea into the mid-mediastinum, it cannot be angled forward sufficiently to reach the anterior mediastinum. In patients thought to have an unresectable anterior mediastinal or anterior hilar tumor (eg, lymphoma or metastatic carcinoma), a limited anterior second or third interspace parasternal (Chamberlain) approach can be used. Diagnosis of the paratracheal, superior mediastinal, and hilar regions can also be obtained through a transaxillary, third interspace minithoracotomy, displacing the apex of the lung downward. When these modalities fail, one-lung anesthesia and the use of thoracoscope-directed biopsy is appropriate in most patients who require diagnosis before complete excision. For most newly diagnosed mediastinal masses, unless there is strong evidence to suggest unresectability, excisional biopsy is the standard approach.

Neurogenic Tumors

Neurogenic tumors, the most common mediastinal tumors, typically occur in a paravertebral location in the posterior mediastinum, where they arise from the intercostal nerves or sympathetic nerve trunks. Their classic appearance on a standard posteroanterior and lateral chest radiograph is that of a rounded paravertebral mass (Fig. 62-24). The spectrum of neurogenic tumors includes neurilemoma, neurofibroma, neurosarcoma, ganglioneuroma, neuroblastoma, paraganglioma, and pheochromocytoma. In adults, most neurogenic tumors are benign; in children, they tend to be malignant. Because of their neural crest origin, some neurogenic tumors have hormonal activity. Elevated vasoactive intestinal polypeptide levels have been reported with ganglioneuromas and neurofibromas, whereas elevated urinary vanillylmandelic acid levels occur with ganglioneuromas. Therefore, just as is the case with pheochromocytomas, neurogenic mediastinal tumors may produce hypertension, flushing, diaphoresis, diarrhea, and abdominal distention.

Mediastinal neurofibromas arise from the nerve sheaths

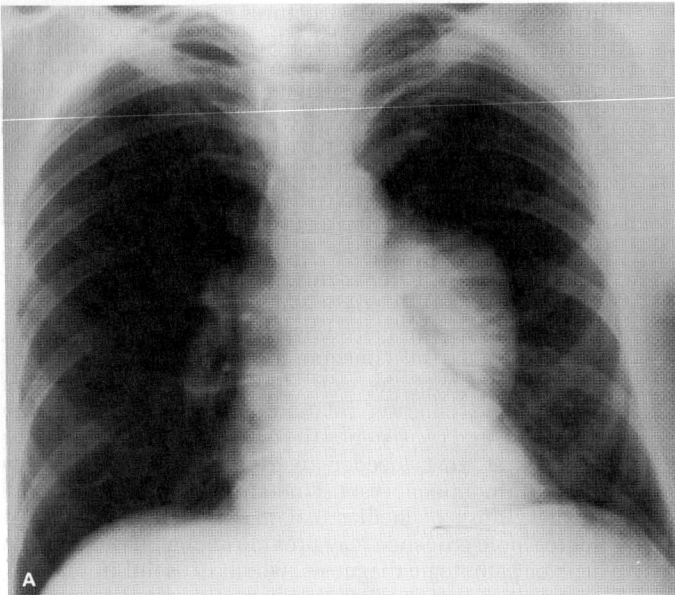

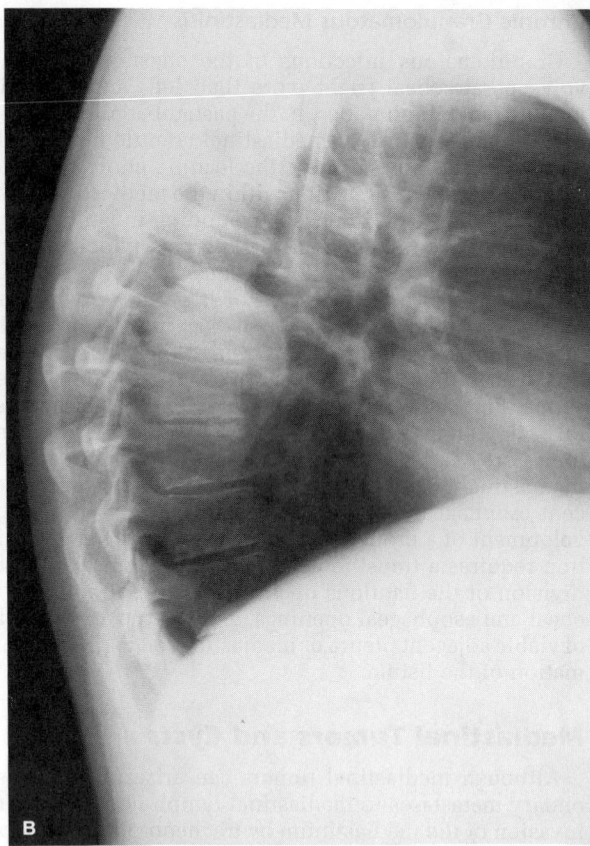

Figure 62-24. Posteroanterior (*A*) and lateral (*B*) chest roentgenograms showing a mediastinal neurofibroma that appears as a typically rounded posterior mediastinal paravertebral mass.

and fibers and occur in patients with von Recklinghausen disease. Ganglioneuromas arise from the sympathetic chain, contain ganglion cells, and are the most common neurogenic tumor in children. The biologic behavior of these tumors varies considerably. One type of ganglioneuroma, the ganglioneuroblastoma, is associated with an 85% 5-year survival rate if it is completely excised.[51] At the other extreme are the neuroblastomas, which are highly aggressive and malignant tumors that require multimodality therapy combining resection, radiation, and chemotherapy. Neuroblastomas in children may be associated with a neurologic syndrome that includes cerebellar ataxia, opsoclonus, and polymyoclonia; these neurologic changes often regress when the tumor is resected. The cellular DNA content of the tumor has been used as a predictor of response to chemotherapy and as a prognostic indicator in children with neuroblastomas[52] (see Chap. 105).

Because of a low but well-documented incidence of malignant degeneration of neurogenic tumors in adults, resection of suspected neurogenic tumors is recommended both for diagnostic and therapeutic purposes. A major preoperative concern in the patient with a neurogenic tumor is whether there is an intraspinous extension of the tumor through the intervertebral foramen (Fig. 62-25). A tumor with both an intraspinous and intrathoracic component is termed a *dumbbell* neurogenic tumor and has the potential for intraoperative disaster if it is not recognized and planned for preoperatively. Ten percent of patients with neurogenic mediastinal tumors have an intraspinous component of their lesion. This should be suspected in any patient with a posterior mediastinal tumor who presents with either radicular pain, vertebral body pedicle erosion, or enlargement of an intervertebral foramen on spinal radiographs or CT scan. In such situations, either a myelogram or magnetic resonance imaging scan of the spine is

indicated to determine if there is an intraspinous component of the tumor. Patients with an asymptomatic posterior mediastinal tumor that is suspected on the basis of chest radiograph and CT scan to be a neurogenic tumor require only a routine preoperative assessment before thoracotomy. Those in whom an intraspinous component

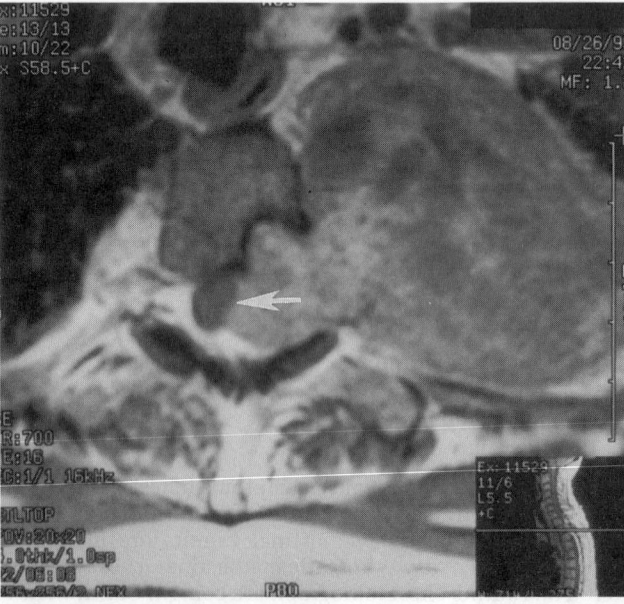

Figure 62-25. MR image demonstrating intraspinous and intrathoracic components of a dumbbell neurogenic tumor. Arrow indicates the intraspinous component compressing the spinal cord.

of the tumor has been demonstrated require a combined neurosurgical–thoracosurgical approach. If such a dumbbell tumor is inadvertently amputated during resection of the intrathoracic component of the tumor, allowing the remainder of the tumor to retract into the spinal canal, subsequent intraspinous bleeding may result in paraplegia or death. Therefore, when dealing with a dumbbell neurogenic tumor, the intraspinous component should be resected first and then the intrathoracic component. This is achieved in one operation by extending the posterior laminectomy neurosurgical incision into a posterior thoracotomy in the appropriate interspace.[53]

Pheochromocytoma

Pheochromocytomas are hormonally active tumors of the sympathetic nervous system. They are termed *chromaffin* tumors because of their affinity for chromic salts on staining. Chromaffin tissue is of neural crest origin and occurs in the adrenal medulla, in the sympathetic ganglia, in the paraganglia along the sympathetic chain and the organ of Zuckerkandl, in small nests scattered along the aorta, in walls of blood vessels, and in the heart, prostate, and ovary. Any of these aberrant collections of chromaffin tissue can give rise to pheochromocytomas. Paragangliomas (chemodectomas) of the parasympathetic nervous system do not contain chromaffin and, unlike pheochromocytomas, usually do not produce hormones. These tumors typically occur in carotid body, glomus jugulare, aorticopulmonary glomus, vagal body, and ciliary glomus chemoreceptor tissues.

Ninety percent of pheochromocytomas occur in the adrenal gland, where they produce excessive catecholamines, predominantly norepinephrine. Ten percent of pheochromocytomas occur in an extraadrenal location, and fewer than 2% of all pheochromocytomas occur in the chest. This latter figure may prove to be falsely low because more mediastinal pheochromocytomas are diagnosed using the relatively newly developed radiopharmaceutical ^{131}I-metaiodobenzylguanidine (131-MIBG), which for the first time has permitted scintigraphic localization of pheochromocytomas.[54] Using the 131-MIBG scan in combination with contrast-enhanced CT, a growing number of cardiac pheochromocytomas are reported.[55]

Intrathoracic pheochromocytomas present both diagnostic and therapeutic challenges. These relatively rare tumors most often are localized to the posterior mediastinum, as is the case with most thoracic neurogenic tumors. In this latter location, where they arise from the paravertebral sympathetic ganglia, they are readily resectable, as are most posterior mediastinal neurogenic tumors. Conversely, when preoperative scanning localizes these tumors to the mid-mediastinum, the surgeon is basically dealing with a cardiac tumor that is arising from either the coronary paraganglia or the visceral autonomic paraganglia of the atria (Fig. 62-26). Unlike pheochromocytomas of the abdomen or posterior chest, these tumors do not shell out from adjacent tissue. They frequently require resection of involved myocardium or coronary vessels with pericardial patching or coronary artery bypass grafting, and therefore cardiopulmonary bypass must be available for their removal.

Teratoma

Teratomas are composed of cells that arise from more than one embryonic germ cell layer. Totipotential cells of the ovary, testis, and embryonic rests that can differentiate into any of the three primary germ cells layers give rise to teratomas. Mediastinal teratomas typically occur as dermoid cysts in the anterior mediastinum, frequently growing to large size and containing hair and teeth. Most terato-

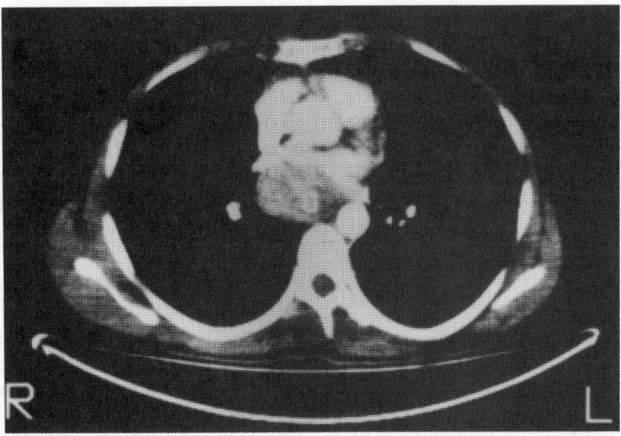

Figure 62-26. CT scan showing cardiac pheochromocytoma (cursor) originating from the posterior aspect of the left atrium. The patient was a 19-year-old woman with hypertension and elevated urinary catecholamines. Her tumor was localized to the posterior mediastinum with an MIBG scan and more precisely defined with this contrast-enhanced CT scan, showing the vascular cardiac tumor.

mas are benign, and the 10% to 20% that are malignant are frequently associated with elevated α-fetoprotein and carcinoembryonic antigens. When a malignant teratoma is suspected preoperatively, serum tumor marker levels should be obtained and a needle biopsy performed to establish a tissue diagnosis. Multidrug chemotherapy, based primarily on cisplatin, is then instituted, and when the tumor markers fall to a normal range, wide resection of the tumor is carried out. Although most teratomas are benign and can be resected through a median sternotomy, their large size and the surrounding inflammatory response that they induce may complicate the resection.[56]

Thymoma

Thymic tumors occur more frequently in adults than in children. Rarely, infants with marked thymic enlargement due to hyperplasia require emergent thymectomy to relieve their cardiorespiratory embarrassment. This approach is now thought to be preferable to radiotherapy, which was used in the past, but which is associated with a definite increased risk of malignancy in the field of radiation.

The relation between the thymus gland and myasthenia gravis has been appreciated for many years. Myasthenia gravis is generally regarded as an immunologic disorder in which serum antibodies form against acetylcholine receptors in the muscle.[57,58] The thymus gland has been postulated to be the source of the acetylcholine receptor–like antigen. Some 10% to 20% of patients with myasthenia gravis have thymomas, and 60% have thymic hyperplasia. Nearly 75% of patients with thymomas develop myasthenia gravis within 10 years. Thymoma has been associated with other conditions besides myasthenia gravis, specifically, red blood cell aplasia, Cushing syndrome, hypogammaglobulinemia, and collagen vascular disease.

Thymectomy is generally most beneficial in young women with myasthenia gravis who have no thymomas and a short duration of their disease. Most neurologists still use anticholinesterase drugs (pyridostigmine and neostigmine), immunosuppressants (azathioprine, antilymphocyte serum, antithymocyte serum), and occasionally steroids as the primary treatment for myasthenia gravis. Any patient who has a thymoma should undergo a thymectomy both to establish the diagnosis of the mediastinal mass and to prevent potential spread of the tumor. One quarter of thymomas are malignant. Traditional teaching has held that the diagnosis of malignant thymoma is extremely difficult on the basis of histologic criteria, the most important determinant of malignancy being the surgeon's assessment of invasion by the tumor of adjacent tissues such as pleura, blood vessels, pericardium, or lung. The Masaoka staging system for thymoma combines both operative findings and histologic evaluation to guide therapy[59] (Table 62-5).

A variety of techniques for removing the thymus have been proposed and include a transcervical approach and either a partial or full median sternotomy (Fig. 62-27). Although a normal-size thymus gland can be resected either transcervically or through a partial upper sternal split, a thymoma requires a full sternotomy. Malignant thymomas seldom metastasize widely, but local recurrence due to droplet seeding of the pleura during resection is well described. It is therefore important that these tumors are resected completely and with avoidance of tumor spill. Adherent pericardium, pleura, or lung should be resected with malignant thymomas, which should then be treated with postoperative mediastinal radiotherapy. A 10-year survival rate of 87% has been reported for encapsulated thymoma, 62% for locally invasive, and 40% if there is pleural seeding.[60] A report from Memorial Sloan-Kettering Cancer Center indicates that patients with completely resected malignant thymomas have an 80% 5-year and a 70% 10-year survival rate, compared with 70% and 28% 5- and 10-year survival rates, respectively, for partial resection, or 38% and 24% rates for biopsy only. With the addition of chemotherapy and radiotherapy for patients with stage II or greater disease, survival was markedly improved by the addition of neoadjuvant radiation and chemotherapy.[61]

Miscellaneous Tumors

Mediastinal lymph node involvement by lymphoma may present as an anterior mediastinal mass on chest radiograph. Because the accurate diagnosis of lymphoma by cytology of tissue obtained from fine-needle aspiration is notoriously difficult unless there is associated adenopathy at other sites that are more amenable to biopsy, biopsy of mediastinal lymph nodes may be required to obtain adequate diagnostic specimens. Either mediastinoscopy (for paratracheal or subcarinal adenopathy), or an anterior mediastinotomy through a parasternal second or third interspace incision (Chamberlain) approach is used. Radical resection or debulking of mediastinal lymphoma is inappropriate therapy because these tumors are more responsive to combined radiation and chemotherapy.

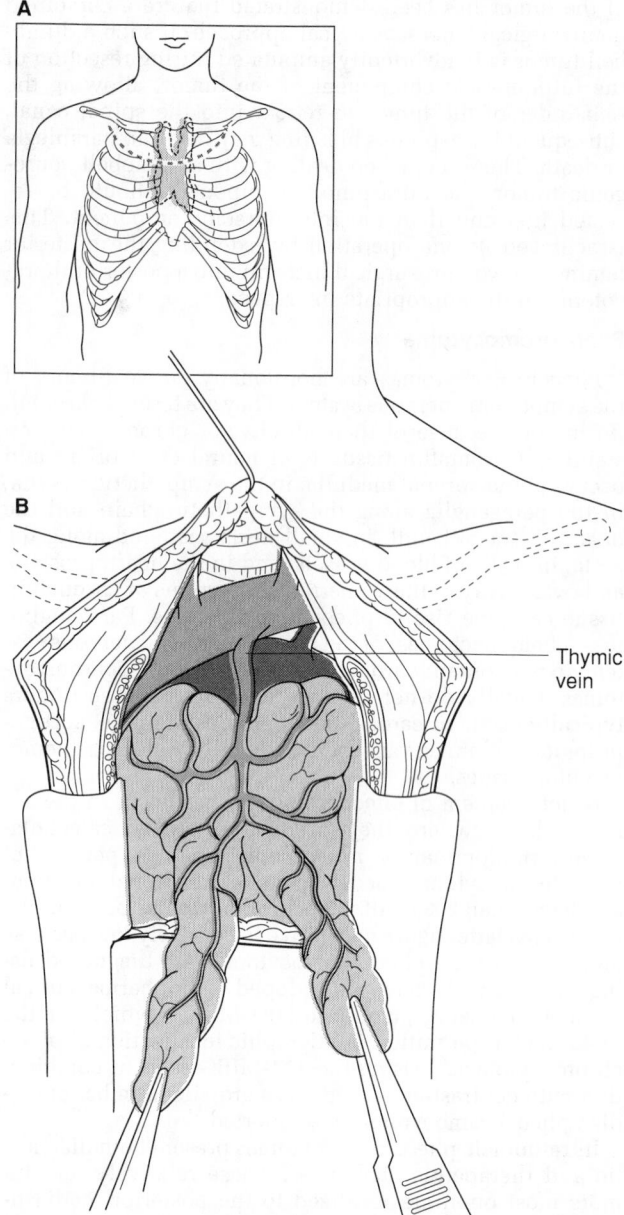

Figure 62-27. Technique of thymectomy. (*A*) Skin incision for partial sternotomy used to resect either a normal-sized thymus gland or one containing a small tumor. The incision placed over the sternomanubrial junction avoids a cervical scar and is more cosmetically appealing. After raising a skin and subcutaneous flap, the upper sternum is divided. (*B*) After the cervical extensions of the thymus gland are mobilized downward, the thymic vein is identified, ligated, and divided where it joins the innominate vein.

Table 62-5. MASAOKA STAGING SYSTEM FOR THYMOMA

Stage	Definition
I	Macroscopically, completely encapsulated; microscopically, no capsular invasion
IIA	Macroscopic invasion in surrounding fatty tissues or mediastinal pleura
IIB	Microscopic invasion into the capsule
III	Macroscopic invasion into a neighboring organ, such as pericardium, great vessels, or lung
IVA	Pleural or pericardial dissemination
IVB	Hematogenous or lymphogenous metastases

(Adapted from Masaoka A, Monden Y, Nakahara K, et al. Follow-up study of thymomas with special references to their clinical stages. Cancer 1981:48,2485)

Large goiters of the thyroid gland may grow retrosternally into the superior mediastinum. Although these substernal goiters present as an anterior superior mediastinal mass on chest radiograph, their resection rarely requires a sternal split, and they can virtually all be resected through a standard transcervical approach. Because tracheomalacia may result from prolonged pressure on the trachea by the enlarged thyroid, prolonged ventilatory assistance may be required postoperatively. Ectopic mediastinal thyroid tissue may present as a thyroid adenoma. These tumors characteristically present as asymptomatic mediastinal masses. Ten percent of parathyroid adenomas are located within

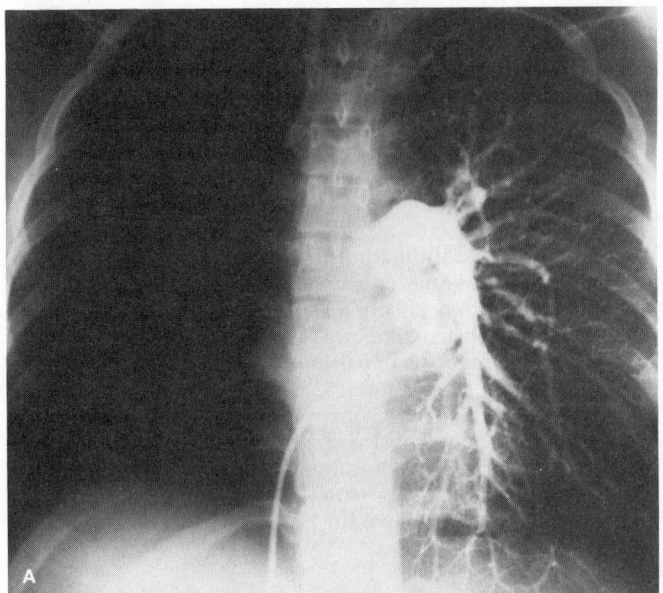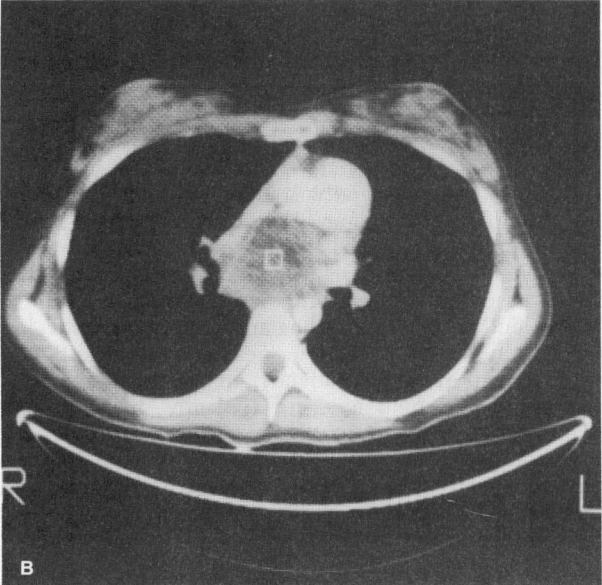

Figure 62-28. Bronchogenic cyst causing pulmonary artery compression. (*A*) Pulmonary angiogram in a 30-year-old woman presenting with acute shortness of breath. The right pulmonary artery is cut off by an extrinsic mediastinal mass. (*B*) CT tomography shows the mass to be cystic (*cursor*), and the right pulmonary artery draped over it. This proved to be a bronchogenic cyst.

the anterosuperior mediastinum and may require a variety of studies for diagnosis and localization (eg, venous angiography with sequential parathyroid hormone assays and CT, thallium, and technetium scanning). Less common mesenchymal tumors of the mediastinum include fibrosarcomas and liposarcomas, fibrous histiocytomas, leiomyosarcomas, and mesotheliomas. Mediastinal tumors of the vascular and lymphatic systems (hemangiomas, hemangiopericytomas, and lymphangiomas) are extremely rare and usually occur in the anterior mediastinum.

Mediastinal Cysts

Mediastinal cysts are classified as bronchogenic, enteric (duplication), or pericardial. Bronchogenic cysts originate from the primordial respiratory tissues of the ventral foregut and are generally found in proximity to the trachea, main-stem bronchi, or posterior carina. They have a ciliated respiratory epithelial lining. Although usually asymptomatic in adults and presenting as a smooth mediastinal mass near the carina, these cysts can attain large size and cause compression of adjacent structures (Fig. 62-28). Enteric (duplication or enterogenous) cysts arise from the dorsal foregut from which the alimentary tract evolves and are therefore located in proximity to the esophagus in the posterior mediastinum, occasionally being found intramurally within the wall of the esophagus (Fig. 62-29). Functioning gastric epithelium that lines some of these cysts may result in ulceration and bleeding. Technetium scanning has been used to localize gastric mucosa within the mediastinum. Enterogenous cysts are often associated with vertebral body abnormalities and spinal cord attachments.

Almost 75% of pericardial cysts occur in the right cardiophrenic angle, either in continuity with the pericardial space or separately as a pericardial developmental abnormality. They rarely cause symptoms and are most often detected on a chest radiograph obtained for other reasons. In the past, resection of these masses was recommended to establish a tissue diagnosis; the CT scan now usually can identify the cystic nature of the lesion, making the need for resection less compelling. Percutaneous CT-guided needle aspiration of

pericardial cysts has been recommended, and the fluid obtained is evaluated cytologically.

Mediastinal Emphysema (Pneumomediastinum)

Entry of air into the mediastinum may occur from the tracheobronchial tree, the neck, or the abdomen. Both penetrating wounds of the mediastinum as well as blunt chest trauma may be responsible for mediastinal emphysema. Compression injuries of the thorax may cause a marked

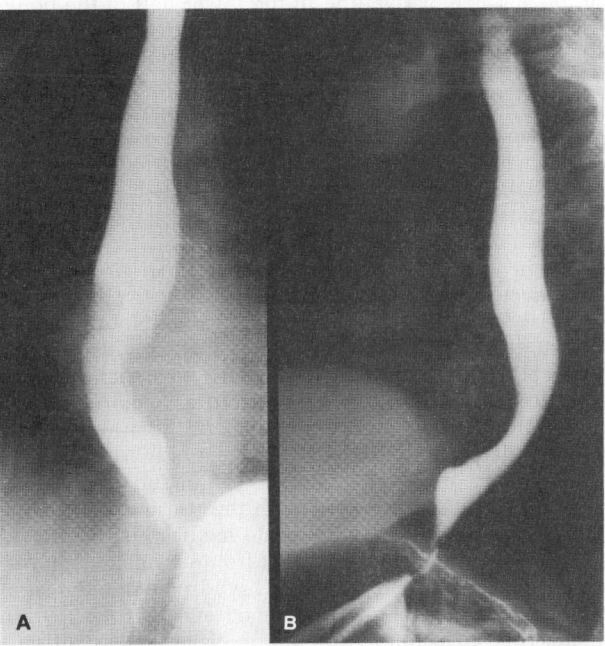

Figure 62-29. Barium esophagogram, posteroanterior (*A*) and lateral (*B*) views, showing an intramural esophageal duplication cyst.

rise in intrathoracic pressure, rupture of peripheral alveoli, and the initiation of dissection of air in the interstitial planes of the lung toward the hilum and then into the mediastinum. A forceful sneeze or bout of asthma can produce mediastinal emphysema in the same way (spontaneous mediastinal emphysema).

Mediastinal emphysema may have a dramatic clinical presentation but is usually not life-threatening. Patients often complain of retrosternal discomfort and have subcutaneous crepitus at the base of the neck. As air continues to dissect upward from the mediastinum into the subcutaneous tissue planes, cervical, fascial, thoracic, truncal, scrotal, and extremity swelling and crepitus can develop. Air within the periorbital tissues may cause sufficient swelling to prevent the patient from opening the eyelids. A precordial crunch is heard typically during systole (Hamman sign) on auscultation over the anterior chest. Air is seen in the mediastinal tissue planes, along the pericardium, and in the soft tissues of the neck, chest, and upper abdomen on chest radiographs. Rarely in adults, tension pneumomediastinum may interfere with venous return to the heart and result in cardiovascular collapse. Most often, spontaneous mediastinal emphysema is self-limiting and requires little treatment other than sedation and supplemental oxygen. If an associated pneumothorax is identified, a tube thoracostomy should be performed. If the patient is distressed by the inability to open the eyes, 5-mm decompressing incisions made in the skin folds of the eyelids or neck using local anesthesia permit the subcutaneous air to be milked out by gentle pressure, allowing the patient to open the eyes.

Superior Vena Cava Syndrome

Superior vena cava syndrome is due to obstruction of the SVC and presents clinically as facial and upper extremity edema, distention of the veins of the head, neck, arms, and upper thorax, and a dusky rubor of these areas suggesting cyanosis. Patients complain of periorbital swelling, a full feeling in their head, and a roaring in the ears aggravated by lying supine or bending. Although congestive heart failure, cirrhosis, and constrictive pericarditis may be included in the differential diagnosis, these conditions are excluded by the absence of swelling in the lower half of the body. Seventy-five percent of patients with SVC syndrome have malignant disease within the mediastinum compressing the SVC, most often bronchogenic carcinoma involving the right upper lobe. SVC obstruction can also result from lymphoma and metastatic carcinoma within the mediastinum. Twenty-five percent of patients with SVC syndrome have a benign cause for this problem, such as mediastinal granulomatous disease, idiopathic mediastinal fibrosis, goiter, or bronchogenic cysts.

Despite the rather characteristic clinical presentation that leaves little doubt as to the diagnosis, many physicians still feel compelled to obtain a venogram. Not only does this study add little information to that provided by the physical examination, but it may also be associated with considerable morbidity if injected contrast material extravasates into the subcutaneous tissues of the arm when an injection is performed in the presence of marked venous hypertension. The venogram for evaluation of SVC obstruction has been replaced with the use of MR imaging and angiography, which delineate mediastinal structures as well as vascular impingement from extrinsic compression.[62] In most patients with SVC syndrome due to malignant disease, cure is not possible because of the extent of mediastinal invasion by the tumor. Nevertheless, a tissue diagnosis is important because it may alter therapy. Therefore, sputa should be collected for cytologic evaluation. A

central lung mass identified on CT scan may be diagnosed with bronchoscopy and biopsy or transthoracic fine-needle aspiration biopsy. Mediastinoscopy has also been used in patients with SVC syndrome, although there are two concerns with the use of this procedure in this setting. First, mediastinal venous hypertension *may* be responsible for bleeding complications. Second, SVC obstruction may produce submucosal edema of the tracheobronchial tree that can precipitate acute airway obstruction when aggravated by endotracheal intubation that is required for general anesthesia in these patients. Both radiotherapy and chemotherapy are often effective in providing rapid and acute relief of SVC obstruction due to malignant disease. Because of the poor prognosis of patients with SVC obstruction due to malignant disease, surgical therapy is seldom indicated. Most patients with SVC obstruction due to benign disease gradually develop chest wall and mediastinal venous collaterals, so that their symptoms improve with time. In rare cases, autogenous or prosthetic vein graft replacement or bypass is used to relieve the SVC obstruction.

TRACHEA
Primary Tumors

Primary tumors of the trachea (excluding the larynx and main bronchi) are uncommon; the most frequent types are squamous cell carcinoma, adenoid cystic carcinoma (cylindroma), and carcinoid adenoma.[63,64] Even rarer are the reported chondrosarcoma, carcinosarcoma, pseudosarcoma, spindle-cell sarcoma, adenosquamous carcinoma, squamous papilloma, fibroma, hemangioma, chondroma, chondroblastoma, granular cell myoblastoma, and leukemia. Tracheal tumors produce stridor, cough, dyspnea, hemoptysis, and recurrent pneumonia. Squamous carcinoma of the trachea can occur in either an exophytic or ulcerative form, and mediastinal or pulmonary metastases are present in one third of patients at the time of diagnosis. Adenoid cystic carcinomas were formerly termed cylindromas, but because these are *not* benign tumors, this designation is incorrect. These tumors characteristically spread within the tracheal wall for a distance that is greater than that evidenced on gross inspection, and therefore frozen-section confirmation of adequate margins is important at the time of operation. The goal of resection is to remove gross tumor only, however, because frozen-section diagnosis is frequently positive for microscopic tumor, which may run throughout the airway. Regional lymph node involvement is also common. Because adenoid cystic carcinoma is a radiosensitive tumor, even when resection margins are positive and regional lymph node spread is present, long-term survival may be achieved with postoperative radiotherapy.

Secondary Tumors

Carcinomas of the esophagus, lung, thyroid, and larynx may all involve the trachea. Contiguity of the posterior membranous trachea with the cervical and upper thoracic esophagus accounts for involvement by esophageal carcinomas. It is for this reason that all patients with cancers involving the upper and mid-esophagus to the level of the carina should undergo preoperative bronchoscopy to rule out tracheobronchial invasion. Again, because of the proximity of the trachea and esophagus, particularly at the point at which the left main-stem bronchus originates from the carina and passes in front of the esophagus, tracheoesophageal fistulas in this area may occur. Bronchogenic carcinoma may extend up the major bronchi and involve the trachea. In most cases, involvement of the trachea by esophageal or lung cancers represents surgically incurable disease. Thyroid carcinoma, particularly the follicular or papillary forms, may invade the trachea and sometimes is amenable to radical resection. Tracheal stomal recurrences after laryngectomy for carcinoma occasionally can be resected with gratifying long-term results, provided that the disease is localized.

Extrinsic Compression

Large goiters that descend retrosternally and cause chronic compression of the trachea in the thoracic inlet and superior mediastinum may be associated with appreciable chondromalacia and respiratory distress after their removal and require a temporary tracheostomy. Congenital vascular rings, aneurysms of the innominate artery, or an anomalous subclavian artery passing behind the trachea and esophagus may also produce tracheal compression.

Inflammatory Stenosis

Tracheal strictures may follow the healing of endotracheal tuberculosis, severe diphtheria, and sclerosing mediastinitis, now attributed to histoplasmosis. Tracheal lacerations or disruptions from blunt trauma are generally well managed by obtaining control of the airway, evaluating the extent of the injury bronchoscopically, and primary repair.[65] At times, stenosis at the site of the injury may require later tracheal resection and reconstruction.

Cooper and Grillo[66] identified the role of cuffed endotracheal and tracheostomy tubes in the subsequent development of tracheal injury and postintubation strictures. It is now recognized that postintubation tracheal damage can be manifested as glottic edema, vocal cord granulomas, erosion of the arytenoid cartilages, granulation tissue at the site of tracheostomy, distortion of the tracheal cartilage at the point of tracheostomy, tracheomalacia or stenosis at the site of the endotracheal balloon, or granulation tissue at the site of erosion by the tip of the endotracheal or tracheostomy tube[67] (Fig. 62-30). Largely because of the work of Grillo and his associates, the development of high-volume, low-pressure cuffs for endotracheal and tracheostomy tubes was encouraged. Nevertheless, it is important to emphasize that hyperinflated high-volume cuffs can still produce tracheal injury, and careful monitoring of cuff pressures to prevent overinflation and tracheal ischemia is still mandatory. The possibility of postintubation tracheal trauma should be considered in any patient who develops signs of upper airway compromise within the first few months after extubation. The patient with a severe postintubation tracheal stenosis may be relatively symptomless if sedentary while convalescing from a major operation or illness, and the airway problem does not manifest itself until the patient is more active after discharge from the hospital.

Diagnosis of Tracheal Pathology

Abnormalities of the tracheal air column are often evident on a standard chest radiograph or lateral films of the neck. Tracheal laminograms provide the best assessment of the length of tracheal involvement relative to the vocal cords and carina and are thus invaluable in planning operative intervention (Fig. 62-31). The standard CT of the chest is useful for assessing mediastinal involvement by tracheal tumors but has little value in evaluation of benign tracheal stenosis. The efficiency of spiral or helical CT scanning in delineating tracheal and bronchial pathology has been demonstrated[68] (Fig. 62-32).

As a rule, bronchoscopic evaluation of tracheal stenoses

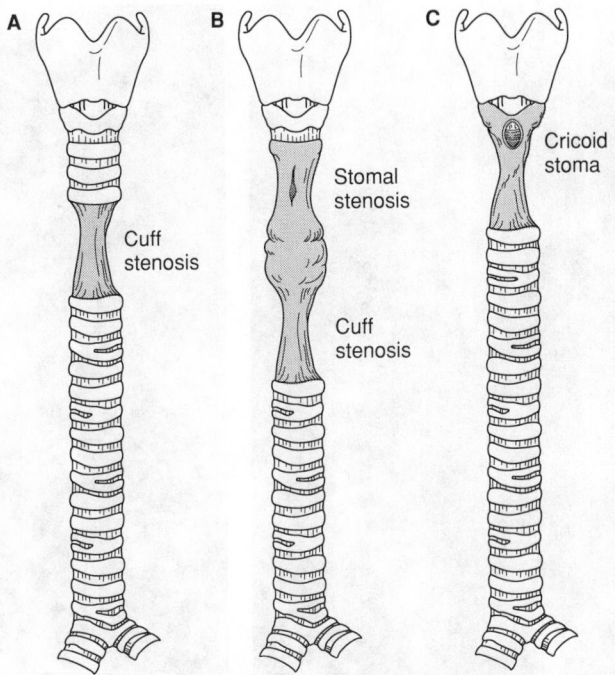

Figure 62-30. Postintubation tracheal injuries. (*A*) Stenosis at site of endotracheal tube cuff. Pressure necrosis by the cuff typically results in a circumferential injury and stenosis. (*B*) Injuries due to tracheostomy tubes include stenosis at the level of the stoma and cuff stenosis (generally lower than with an endotracheal tube). The segment between the two injuries may be malacic. (*C*) Subglottic stenosis resulting from either too high a tracheostomy or erosion of the tracheostomy tube through the cricoid cartilage.

should be carried out with equipment and facilities available for definitive tracheal resection because instrumentation of a critical tracheal stenosis may precipitate local edema and complete airway obstruction. Granulation tissue occurring at the site of a tracheostomy stoma or the tip of a tracheostomy tube may be excised with biopsy forceps through the rigid bronchoscope. Respiratory distress resulting from an obstructing tracheal tumor may be relieved by coring out the tumor through the rigid bronchoscope, thereby converting the required tracheal surgery to an elective procedure.

Treatment of Obstructing Tracheal Lesions

Because primary tracheal tumors are rare, and at least one third are incurable when initially seen because of mediastinal invasion or pulmonary metastases, few surgeons have a large experience with resectional therapy. Resection should be reserved for patients with localized, potentially curable lesions. Perelman and Koroleva[64] have reported on 75 sleeve or carinal resections for primary tracheal tumors with a 5-year survival of 13% for squamous cell and 66% for adenoid cystic carcinoma. Patients with benign tracheal obstruction are best treated with tracheal resection and reconstruction using techniques that have been well described and established by Grillo and Mathisen.[69]

The adult trachea averages 11 cm in length from the inferior border of the cricoid cartilage to the carina. The vocal cords are located 1.5 to 2 cm above the inferior border of the cricoid cartilage. Most lesions involving the upper half of the trachea are approached through an anterior collar incision, which may be extended downward as a T,

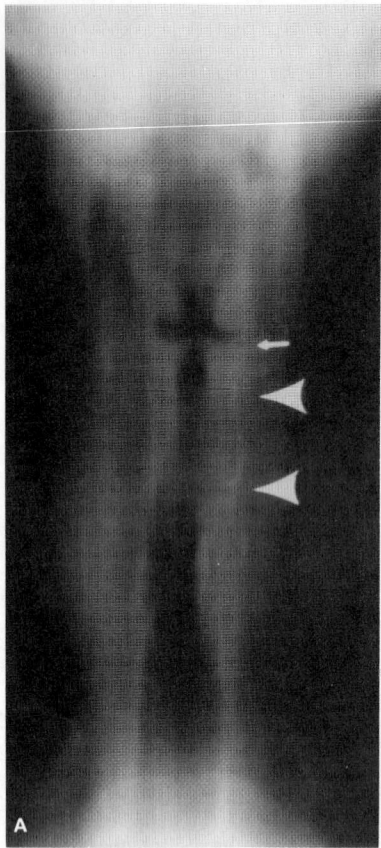
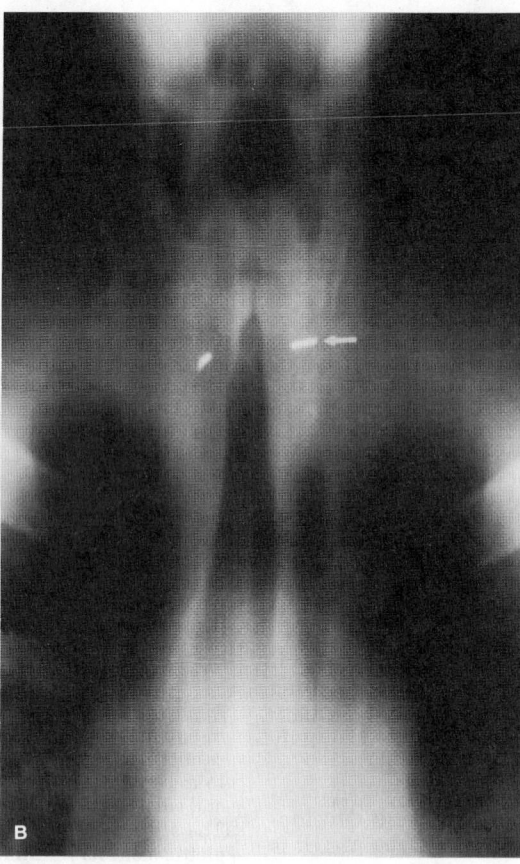

Figure 62-31. Tracheal laminograms. (*A*) This 7-cm-long subglottic stenosis (*between large arrows*) begins just below vocal cords (*small arrow*). (*B*) Postoperative view after resection and primary anastomosis. Silver clips (*arrow*) mark the level of the anastomosis.

using a partial upper sternal split if necessary. Lesions of the lower half of the trachea are approached through a right fourth interspace posterolateral thoracotomy. Because the blood supply of the trachea enters laterally, mobilization of the trachea for a sleeve resection and anastomosis is carried out in the pretracheal plane and posteriorly between the membranous trachea and esophagus to avoid

devascularization of the trachea. Flexion of the cervical spine allows resection of 4.5 cm of trachea with a primary reanastomosis. When approaching lesions of the lower trachea through a right thoracotomy, mobilizing the hilum of the lung and freeing its carinal attachments allow resection of a 3-cm length of lower trachea. Additional length for reconstruction can be obtained by cervical flexion. Grillo and associates[70] have reported good or satisfactory results in 93% of 273 patients so operated on, with a 1.8% mortality.

Tracheoinnominate Artery Fistula

A tracheostomy tube may erode into the innominate artery, producing life-threatening hemorrhage. This is more common in young women with long, gracile necks whose intrathoracic trachea may be elevated into the operative field by extension of the neck during tracheostomy. Once the patient's neck is placed into a more neutral position, the tracheostomy stoma descends into the thoracic inlet, and the tube may come into apposition with the overlying innominate artery (Fig. 62-33). Alternatively, a tracheostomy or endotracheal tube cuff may erode through the tracheal wall and into the adjacent innominate artery. An impending tracheoinnominate artery erosion may be heralded by the return of bright-red blood on suctioning of the indwelling tracheal tube. The diagnosis may be confirmed by temporarily deflating the tracheal cuff with resulting major hemorrhage. This may be controlled in the acute situation by overinflation of the tracheal cuff against the adjacent innominate artery or by digital compression of the innominate artery against the sternum by the finger inserted through the tracheostomy stoma (see Fig. 62-33). Finger pressure is then maintained as the patient is trans-

Figure 62-32. Helical CT reconstruction demonstrating a long tracheal stenosis (*arrow*) just below the level of the thoracic inlet. This method of imaging allows greater detail when compared with tomograms.

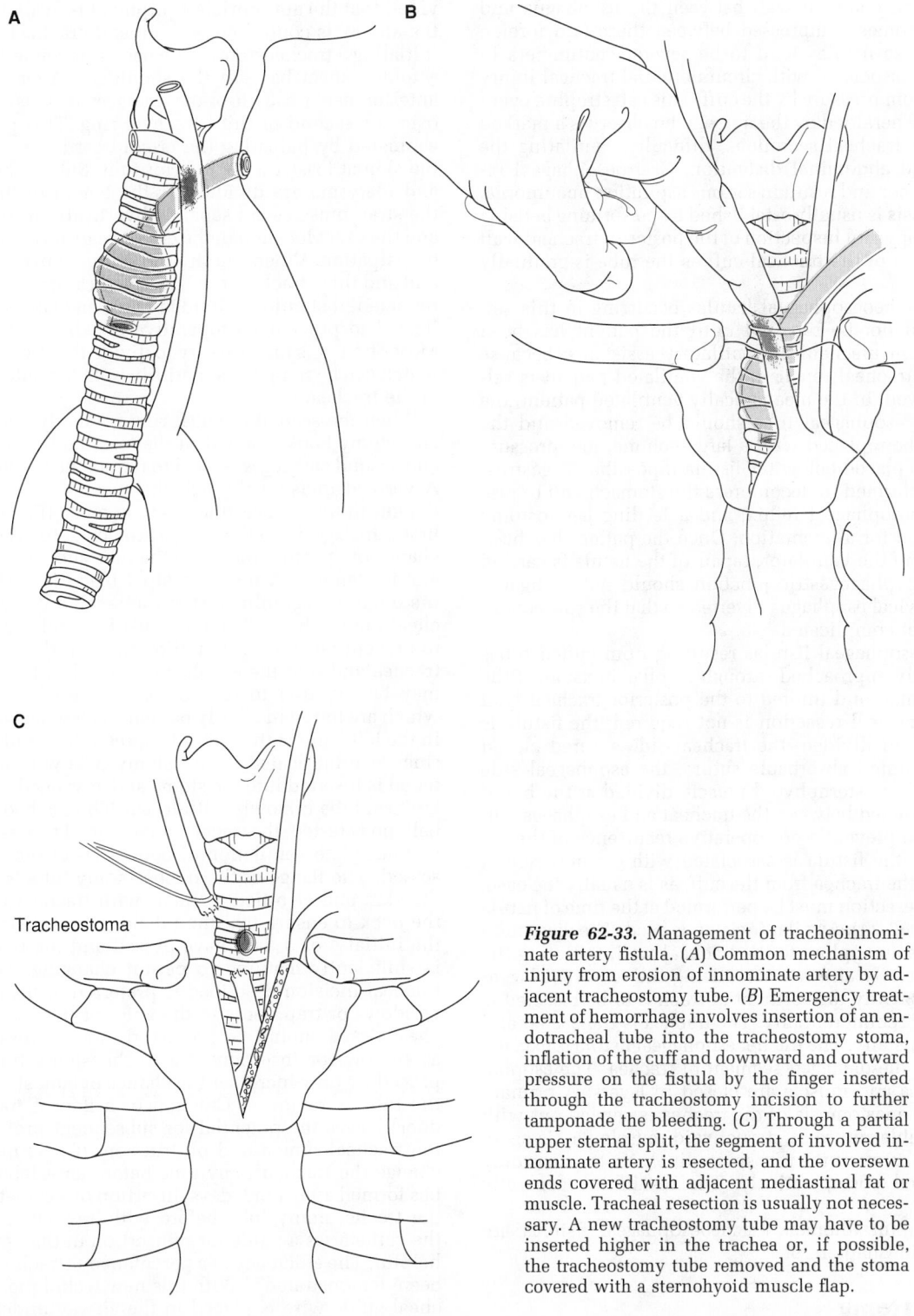

A

B

C

Tracheostoma

Figure 62-33. Management of tracheoinnominate artery fistula. (*A*) Common mechanism of injury from erosion of innominate artery by adjacent tracheostomy tube. (*B*) Emergency treatment of hemorrhage involves insertion of an endotracheal tube into the tracheostomy stoma, inflation of the cuff and downward and outward pressure on the fistula by the finger inserted through the tracheostomy incision to further tamponade the bleeding. (*C*) Through a partial upper sternal split, the segment of involved innominate artery is resected, and the oversewn ends covered with adjacent mediastinal fat or muscle. Tracheal resection is usually not necessary. A new tracheostomy tube may have to be inserted higher in the trachea or, if possible, the tracheostomy tube removed and the stoma covered with a sternohyoid muscle flap.

ferred to the operating room. Because of the local inflammation and inevitable contamination of the wound, resection of the involved segment of the innominate artery, oversewing both ends with nonabsorbable suture and covering the suture lines with adjacent mediastinal or thymic fat or muscle, rather than attempting arterial reconstruction, is advised. The incidence of serious neurologic sequelae from acute interruption of the innominate artery flow is low in the young population. If a low tracheostomy stoma is in fact identified at the time of innominate artery

division, muscle flap closure of the stoma should be done and a higher new stoma created. No tracheal resection is required for a tracheoinnominate artery fistula.

Acquired Tracheoesophageal Fistula

A patient requiring prolonged mechanical ventilation may develop a tracheoesophageal fistula as a result of erosion at the site of the cuffed tracheal tube.[71] This is more common when there is an indwelling esophageal feeding tube and the common wall between the esophagus and trachea becomes compressed between these two foreign bodies. These fistulas tend to be several centimeters in length and associated with circumferential tracheal injury resulting from pressure by the cuff. This catastrophic event is generally heralded by the nurse, who observes a marked increase in tracheal secretions, difficulty ventilating the patient, and abdominal distention. Gastroesophageal reflux may occur and result in serious aspiration pneumonia. The diagnosis is usually established by performing bedside bronchoscopy and inspection of the posterior tracheal wall in the region of the tracheal cuff as the tube is gradually withdrawn.

Acute tracheoesophageal fistulas occurring in this setting should not be repaired until the patient has been weaned from mechanical ventilatory assistance because successful tracheal repair in the ventilated patient is seldom achieved. In the mechanically ventilated patient, the indwelling esophageal tube should be removed and the tracheal tube replaced with a large-volume, low-pressure cuffed tube placed below the fistula if possible. A gastrostomy is performed to decompress the stomach and to prevent gastroesophageal reflux, and a feeding jejunostomy is performed for alimentation. Once the patient has been weaned from the ventilator, repair of the fistula is carried out. The esophagogastric junction should not be ligated nor the cervical esophagus diverted so that the subsequent repair is not complicated.

Tracheoesophageal fistulas resulting from cuffed tubes are generally approached through a collar incision. If the fistula is small and limited to the posterior tracheal wall so that a tracheal resection is not required, the fistula is identified and divided, the tracheal side sutured closed with interrupted absorbable suture, the esophageal side closed, and the sternohyoid muscle divided at the hyoid bone and rotated between the tracheal and esophageal suture lines to prevent a postoperative recurrence of the fistula. When the fistula is associated with circumferential damage to the trachea from the cuff, as is usually the case, a tracheal resection must be performed at the time of fistula repair (Fig. 62-34). A collar incision is used. The dissection is kept closely applied to the tracheal wall, reflecting the thyroid laterally and not visualizing the recurrent laryngeal nerves. Only the segment of trachea to be resected is dissected circumferentially. The trachea is transected and intubated distally. The tracheoesophageal fistula is excised along with the damaged segment of trachea. The esophageal mucosa and muscle are closed in layers. A primary end-to-end anastomosis of the trachea is carried out with 4-0 absorbable suture. A sternohyoid muscle flap is again interposed between the two suture lines. No tracheostomy tube is used postoperatively. The results are generally excellent.

Acquired intrathoracic tracheoesophageal fistulas are discussed in Chapter 19.

Tracheostomy

As a general rule, tracheostomy should not be performed as an emergency. Whenever possible, an adequate airway should be restored with either an endotracheal tube or a rigid ventilating bronchoscope so that a more complete evaluation of the problem and an unrushed, more controlled, elective tracheostomy can be performed. Undertaking a tracheostomy without adequate initial airway control or proper equipment—including surgical instruments, tracheostomy tubes, lighting, and suction—may be a prelude to disaster.[72]

A tracheostomy may be performed either at the bedside or in the operating room almost with equal facility, provided that the appropriate equipment is available. Ideally, the airway is controlled with an endotracheal tube before initiating a tracheostomy. The neck is extended by placing a folded sheet beneath the shoulders. After draping the anterior neck, a 3- to 4-cm transverse incision is made over the second or third tracheal ring. This point can be estimated by palpating the cricoid cartilage and incising the skin at least 1.5 cm inferior to it. Subcutaneous tissue and platysma are divided for the length of the incision, the strap muscles are separated vertically in the midline, and the exact location of the cricoid cartilage is ascertained by palpation. When the thyroid isthmus overlies the second and third tracheal cartilages and cannot be adequately retracted, it should be divided between clamps and suture ligated to prevent postoperative bleeding complications. Most often, it is unnecessary to divide the thyroid isthmus, which can be retracted superiorly from the anterior surface of the trachea.

When the second tracheal ring is clearly defined, a tracheostomy hook inserted in the midline between the first and second cartilages is used to retract the trachea upward. A vertical incision through the second, third, and often the fourth tracheal cartilage is then made (Fig. 62-35). The first cartilage is deliberately protected to minimize the chance of upward erosion by the tube and subsequent subglottic stenosis. A no. 11 scalpel blade is used to incise the trachea, beginning just at the level of entry of the tracheal hook. The knife blade must be carefully controlled to prevent posterior penetration through the membranous trachea and into the esophagus behind it. Heavy scissors may be required to divide calcified tracheal cartilages, which are found in elderly patients. A tracheal dilator held in the left hand is then used to spread the divided tracheal rings as a lubricated tracheostomy tube with the cuff deflated is inserted into the stoma and advanced as the endotracheal tube is slowly withdrawn. The tracheostomy tube balloon is tested, the trachea is suctioned through the tube, and adequate ventilation of both sides of the chest is assessed. The flange of the tracheostomy tube is sutured to the skin and also tied in place with tracheal ties around the neck to ensure that the tube does not dislodge before the initial 4 or 5 days have passed and the tracheostomy is sufficiently matured to permit changing. The vertical tracheal incision described is preferred to the creation of windows or trap doors in the anterior tracheal wall. Tracheal tissue should be preserved, not cut away to make a window for insertion of a tracheostomy tube. Such a procedure only increases the chance of later stenosis when the tube is removed. Creation of a flap of trachea (trap door) leaves the potential for subsequent protrusion into the tracheal lumen and obstruction. If it is necessary to change the tracheostomy tube before an established tract has formed after 4 or 5 days, insertion of a catheter through the tracheostomy tube before withdrawing it and using the catheter as a guide for reinsertion of the new tube are helpful. The efficiency of a percutaneous tracheostomy has been demonstrated.[73] With this new technique, a transtracheal guide wire is placed in the airway under bronchoscopic guidance, and progressive dilation of the tracheal opening and insertion of a tracheostomy tube performed without the need for an open procedure. Long-term complications of this new technique are as yet unknown, but the immediate results appear as good as standard operative tracheostomy, and percutaneous tracheostomy has the advantage of being a much simpler procedure that is readily performed at the bed side.

Cricothyroidotomy

Cricothyroidotomy is an alternative to the standard tracheostomy, but because it is performed nearer the vocal cords, there is the potential for an increased inci-

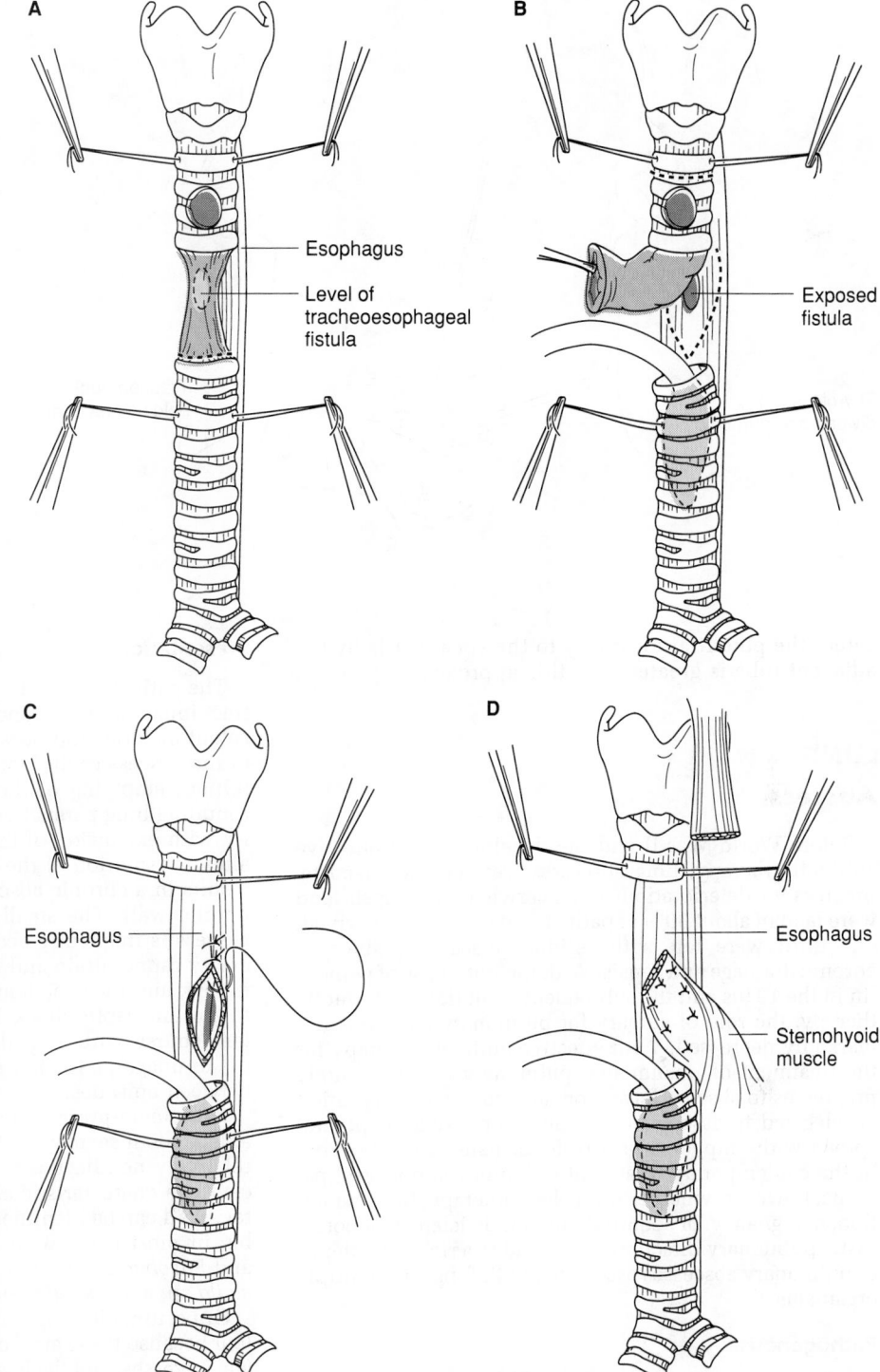

Figure 62-34. Management of post-intubation tracheoesophageal fistula. (*A*) Only the length of damaged trachea to be resected (usually including the tracheostomy stoma) is circumferentially mobilized above and below the fistula to avoid devascularizing the remaining trachea. Stay sutures secure the trachea above and below this segment. (*B*) The trachea is transected, the distal trachea intubated across the field, and the fistula identified by elevating the damaged tracheal segment. (*C*) The stenotic tracheal segment is resected and closure of the esophageal fistula begun, being certain to invert the mucosa. A two-layered closure is completed. (*D*) After interposing the mobilized sternohyoid muscle and suturing it over the esophageal closure, an end-to-end tracheal anastomosis is performed.

dence of subglottic tracheal stenosis. As with a standard tracheostomy, cricothyroidotomy is best performed after securing control of the airway with an endotracheal tube. With the surgeon standing at the patient's right side, the thyroid cartilage is stabilized between the thumb and middle finger with the left hand while the cricothyroid space is identified by palpation with the left index finger (Fig. 62-36). A 1.5-cm transverse incision is made over this area, a hemostat is used to spread and dissect bluntly to the cricothyroid membrane, and a no. 11 scalpel blade is used to puncture the membrane. The opening in the cricothyroid membrane is enlarged with a tracheal dilator as the endotracheal tube is withdrawn, and a cuffed tracheostomy tube is inserted into the trachea and tied in place. The trapezoid-shaped cricothyroid space averages 0.9 × 3 cm and generally accommodates an 8-mm tracheostomy tube. The advantage of this approach is that the thyroid isthmus and blood vessels encountered in the lower neck are avoided with a cricothyroidotomy. As indi-

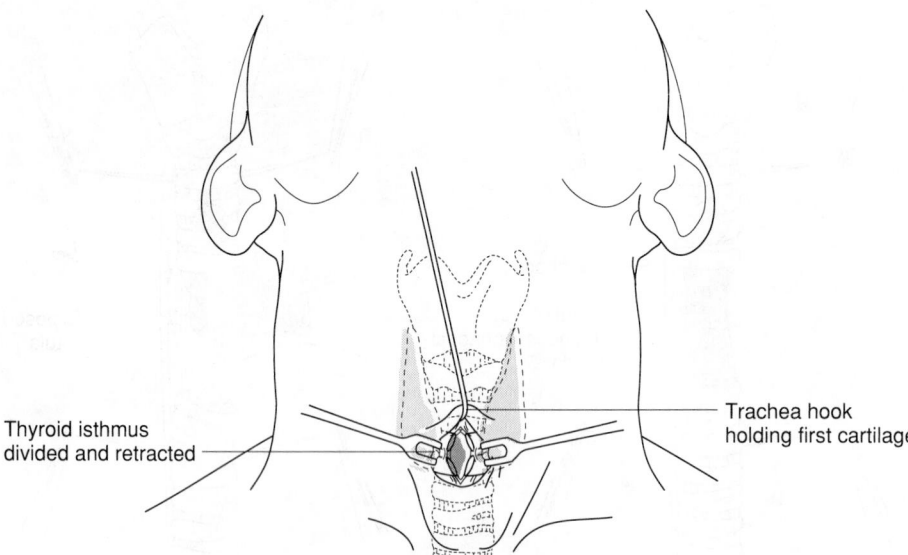

Thyroid isthmus
divided and retracted

Trachea hook
holding first cartilage

Figure 62-35. Standard tracheostomy using a vertical incision through the second and third tracheal rings.

cated, the potential for injury to the vocal cords by the adjacent tube is greater with this approach.

LUNG

Abscess

Before World War II and the development of effective antibiotic therapy, lung abscesses were characterized by progressive deterioration and overwhelming sepsis and were fatal in about 30% of patients. Of those who survived, one third were left with residual disease manifest as chronic drainage and sepsis. With the initial use of penicillin in the 1940s and the subsequent evolution of antibiotic therapy, the role of surgery for pulmonary abscesses has markedly decreased. With effective antibiotic therapy for the treatment of pneumonia, pulmonary infection rarely progresses to abscess formation, and surgical intervention is relegated to associated complications, such as pleural spread with empyema or a residual parenchymal cavity. In the contemporary treatment of immunosuppressed patients, however, whether from chemotherapy, transplantation, malignancy, or acquired immunodeficiency, opportunistic pulmonary infections have lead to a rising incidence of pulmonary abscesses associated with fungal or multiple organisms.

Pathogenesis

The common cause of most lung abscesses is aspiration of infected material or a compromised neurologic state. Pulmonary abscesses are associated with anaerobic infections in patients who have poor oral hygiene, carious teeth, or gingival disease. This aspirated material becomes lodged in the bronchial tree, an area of local necrosis results, and suppurative cavity infection rapidly ensues. These areas of infarction are frequently found in the posterior segment of the upper lobe or in the superior segment of the lower lobe because of the dependent drainage of the infected material aspirated. Liquefaction necrosis from anaerobic organisms rarely allows identification of the causative agent because the culture techniques are inappropriate or because antibiotic therapy is initiated before cultures are obtained.

Presentation

The patients typically present with an upper respiratory tract infection, fever, and sepsis with expectoration of purulent material and possibly hemoptysis. Communication of the abscess cavity with the bronchial tree allows intermittent emptying of the cavity and aeration of the surrounding lung parenchyma. Complete collapse of the cavity with expansion of the lung obliterates the cavity and allows resolution of the abscess. A poorly drained cavity results in a chronic abscess with the formation of a thick fibrotic wall. The small bronchiolar fistula draining the abscess is frequently occluded by edema or debris. If the cavity cannot drain and remains internalized, rupture can follow, and these patients may present with pyopneumothorax and septic shock. Patients may have a chronic indolent course with episodes of productive sputum during the drainage phase and a relatively nonproductive cough between episodes.

Radiologic presentation demonstrates consolidation in a dependent segment of the lung and in the early phase is relatively nondiagnostic. With bronchial drainage of the cavity, a characteristic air–fluid level and the thick cavitary wall can be identified (Fig. 62-37). Isolates are anaerobic in most cases with *Bacteroides, Peptostreptococcus,* and *Fusobacterium* sp. Aerobes tend to be *S aureus, Klebsiella* sp, and *Pseudomonas* sp.

Opportunistic lung infections are a more difficult problem because these are frequently multiple rather than single abscesses, and the host is immunocompromised. Bacterial infections in these patients most commonly include *S aureus* and *Pseudomonas, Proteus,* and *Klebsiella* sp as well as fungal organisms such as *Aspergillus* and *Mucor* sp.

Treatment

The initial treatment for any pulmonary abscess consists of antibiotic therapy and adequate drainage. Penicillins or clindamycin have been shown to be most effective, and after adequate initial response with intravenous administration, oral antibiotics appear effective. As mentioned, identification of the etiologic organism to direct them is problematic, but the effort should not be neglected. Adequate drainage is achieved with both pulmonary physiotherapy and postural drainage. Bronchoscopy is consid-

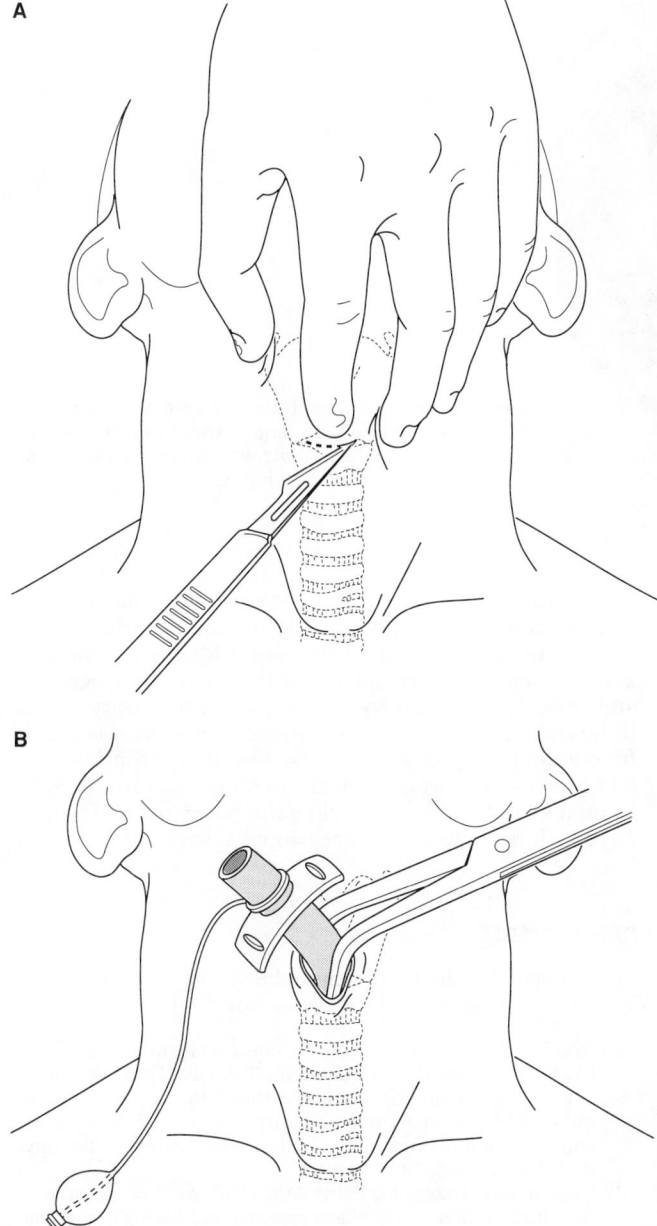

Figure 62-36. Cricothyroidotomy. (*A*) Identification of the cricothyroid membrane by palpation and incising the membrane transversely. (*B*) Insertion of a tracheostomy tube through the cricothyroid membrane, which is spread with a tracheal dilator.

ered standard to determine whether an endobronchial lesion, foreign body, or extrinsic pathology is the cause of inadequate drainage. When inadequate drainage is found, endobronchial drainage should be established with rigid bronchoscopy. It is imperative, however, that appropriate contralateral airway protection be provided to prevent operative drainage into the opposite lung. Operative treatment is required in less than 10% of patients. Indications include overwhelming sepsis, an abscess larger than 6 cm in diameter, bronchopleural fistula, life-threatening hemoptysis, and empyema.[74] In the chronic stage, surgical treatment is indicated for patients without resolution, or for a cavity that has been persistent for longer than 5 weeks. In these cases, pulmonary resection is recommended. The mortality from pulmonary resection is increased because of the underlying diseases in many of these patients.

External drainage with rib resection is occasionally required for uncontrolled disease; however, reports of CT-guided percutaneous drainage with irrigation of the cavity through the catheter suggest that this is a reasonable alternative.[75] A similar option using placement of expandable metal stents to drain a pulmonary abscess has been described.[76] The contemporary mortality rate from pyogenic pulmonary abscess related to community-acquired pneumonia is about 5%. Mortality is substantially higher, however, with nosocomial infection and immunologically compromised hosts.[77]

Bronchiectasis

Bronchiectasis results from infection of the distal bronchi, most commonly in the basilar segments, with dilation and destruction of the bronchial walls. This results in fibrosis, poor drainage, and further destruction of the lung and airways. Bronchiectasis can be either congenital or acquired, although the bronchial injury is always a progressive degenerative process. The most common causes of congenital bronchiectasis include cystic fibrosis, congenital cystic bronchiectasis, α_1-antitrypsin deficiency, Kartagener syndrome, and occasionally intralobar bronchopulmonary sequestration. Acquired bronchiectasis can result from virtually any cause of chronic airway obstruction. This leads to distal infection with retained purulent bronchial secretions, mucous plugs, and further injury to the distal conducting airways. This cycle leads to dilation of the distal small airways, mucous and fluid collection, and further tissue destruction with airway collapse.[78]

Pathogenesis

Bronchiectasis is traditionally divided into three groups based on gross pathologic features:

Cylindric—characterized by dilated bronchi of regular configuration

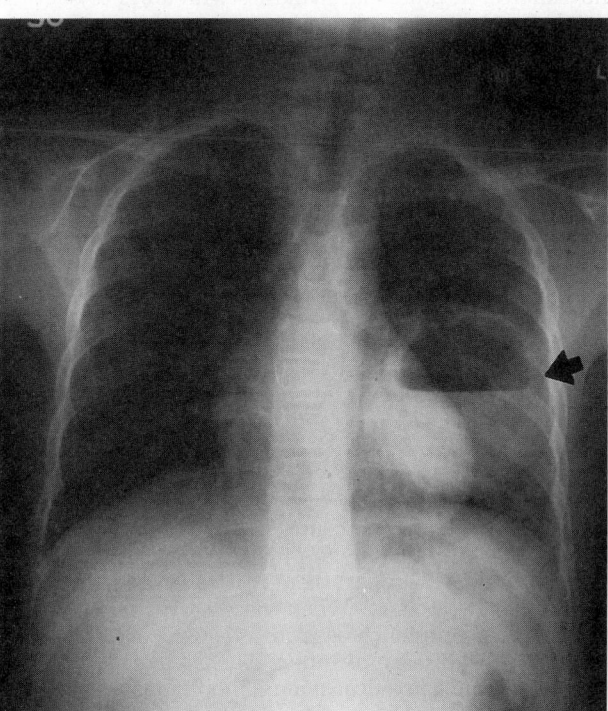

Figure 62-37. Chest roentgenogram showing a large abscess of the left lung with an air–fluid level (*arrow*).

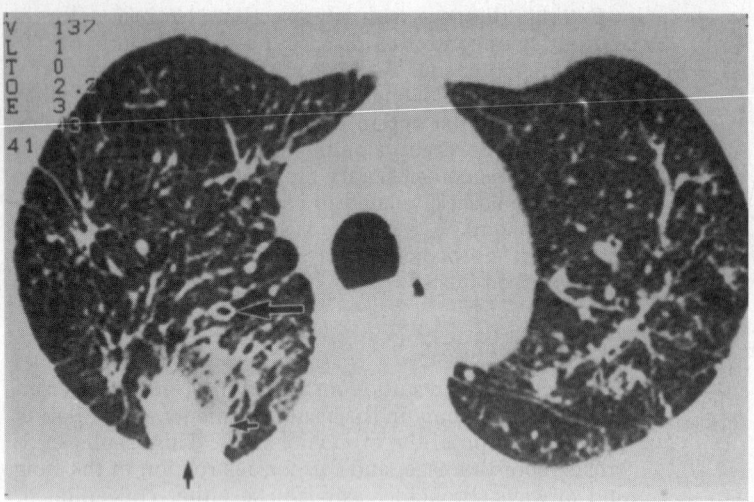

Figure 62-38. High-resolution CT scan of chest revealing bronchiectasis. The large arrow indicates the dilated airway. The small arrow indicates areas of undrained secretions and collapse.

Varicose—characterized by greater dilation and irregularity

Saccular or cystic—characterized by aneurysmal-type dilation in the periphery; the bronchi are frequently filled with fluid collections

In virtually all instances, these effects are more marked in distal bronchi because there is less structural support, whereas the proximal bronchi have a more complex skeleton, including cartilage, which is resistant to dilation.

Diagnosis

Patients are usually characterized by chronic productive cough with recurrent pulmonary infections. Foul-smelling sputum, fever, and hemoptysis and common. Hemoptysis results from increased bronchial collateral circulation intimately associated with tissue destruction in the bronchial tree and occurs in about half the patients who have acquired chronic bronchiectasis. The chest radiograph may show increased bronchial markings with areas of overinflation; however, plain chest films are usually not diagnostic. Previously, bronchography was recommended to delineate the tracheal bronchial tree. With the advent of high-resolution CT scanning, however, bronchography has become obsolete (Fig. 62-38). High-resolution CT scanning and dynamic CT scanning are the optimal means for evaluation of lung parenchyma, allowing visualization of the small airways, dilated bronchioles, and mucus- or fluid-filled cysts. Exhalation CT scanning can also give information about air trapping.[79] Bronchoscopy is the standard means to determine whether the disease is due to intrinsically abnormal airways or to other endobronchial pathology such as a foreign body, neoplastic process, or extrinsic compression. Bronchoscopy also facilitates the process of obtaining appropriate cultures and establishing drainage of a diseased segment.

Treatment

Treatment for bronchiectasis is largely supportive. It consists of antibiotics to control infection and aggressive pulmonary physiotherapy to promote drainage of the diseased segments.[80] Surgical therapy is reserved for failures of medical treatment. When necessary, parenchyma-sparing procedures such as segmentectomy are preferred; however, the disease is often extensive and requires lobectomy from a practical standpoint. Preoperative ventilation–perfusion scans are helpful to delineate areas of nonfunctioning parenchyma that can be resected with little physiologic cost. Anesthesiologists must carefully manage the remaining lung to prevent spillage of purulent secretions into areas of physiologic importance. Surgery in these patients may also be necessary for life-threatening hemoptysis, which is not controlled with arteriography and embolization. Surgery is infrequently necessary; when indicated, it must be individualized to preserve as much functioning parenchyma as possible. In appropriate circumstances, however, surgical resection can provide substantial symptomatic relief, slow the progression of parenchymal lung injury, and occasionally save the patient's life.

REFERENCES

1. Pairolero PC. Chest wall tumors. In: Shields TW, ed. General thoracic surgery, ed 4. Malvern, PA, Williams & Wilkins, 1994:579.
2. Pass HI. Primary and metastatic chest wall tumors. In: Roth JA, Ruckdeschel JC, Weisenburger TH, eds. Thoracic oncology. Philadelphia, WB Saunders, 1989:546.
3. Fulton BM, Wessner-Dunlap S, Karpeh M, et al. Primary bony and cartilaginous sarcomas of chest wall: results of therapy. Ann Thorac Surg 1992;54:226.
4. Karpeh BM, Ukoha O, Bains MS, et al. Medical tumors of the chest wall: solitary plasmacytoma and Ewing's sarcoma. J Thorac Cardiovasc Surg 1993;105:89.
5. McAfee MK, Pairolero RC, Bergstralh EJ, et al. Chondrosarcoma of the chest wall: factors affecting survival. Ann Thorac Surg 1985;40:535.
6. Ryan MB, McMurtrey MJ, Roth JA. Current management of chest-wall tumors. Surg Clin North Am 1989;69:1061.
7. Rosen G, Caparros B, Huvos AC, et al. Preoperative chemotherapy for osteogenic sarcoma: selection of postoperative adjuvant chemotherapy based upon the response of the primary tumor to preoperative chemotherapy. Cancer 1982;49:1221.
8. Raymond AK, Chawla SP, Carrasco CH, et al. Osteosarcoma chemotherapy effect: a prognostic factor. Semin Diagn Pathol 1987;4:212.
9. Dahlin DC, Unni KK. Bone tumors: general aspects and data on 8,542 cases. Springfield, IL, Charles C Thomas, 1986.
10. Venn GE, Gellister J, DaCosta PE, Goldstraw P. Malignant fibrous histiocytoma in thoracic surgical practice. J Thorac Cardiovasc Surg 1986;91:234.
11. Wallner KE, Nori D, Burt M, et al. Adjuvant brachytherapy for treatment of chest wall sarcomas. J Thorac Cardiovasc Surg 1991;101:888.
12. Seyfer AE, Graeber GM, Wind GG. Atlas of chest wall reconstruction. Rockville, MD, Aspen Systems, 1986.
13. Light RW. Parapneumonic effusions and infections of the pleural space. In: Light RW, ed. Pleural diseases, ed 2. Philadelphia, Lea & Febiger, 1990:130.

14. Kennedy L, Sahn SA. Noninvasive evaluation of the patient with a pleural effusion. Surg Clin North Am 1994;4:451.

15. Broaddus VC, Light RW. What is the origin of pleural transudates and exudates? Chest 1992;102:658.

16. Houston MC. Pleural fluid pH: diagnostic, therapeutic, and prognostic value. Am J Surg 1987;154:333.

17. Lemmer JH, Botham MJ, Orringer MB. Modern management of adult thoracic empyema. J Thorac Cardiovasc Surg 1985;90:849.

18. Prakash VBS, Reiman HM. Comparison of needle biopsy with cytologic analysis for the evaluation of pleural effusion: analysis of 414 cases. Mayo Clin Proc 1985;60:158.

19. Kaiser LR. Pleural masses and effusions. In: Kaiser LR, Daniel TM, eds. Thoracoscopic surgery. Boston: Little, Brown, 1993:59.

20. Kohman LJ. Thoracoscopy for the evaluation and treatment of pleural space disease. Surg Clin North Am 1993;4:467.

21. LoCicero J. Thoracoscopic management of malignant pleural effusion. Ann Thorac Surg 1993;56:641.

22. Hartman DL, Gaither JM, Kesler KA, Mylet DM, Brown JW, Mathur PN. Comparison of insufflated talc under thoracoscopic guidance with standard tetracycline and bleomycin pleurodesis for control of malignant pleural effusions. J Thorac Cardiovasc Surg 1993;105:743.

23. Martini N, Bains MS, Beattie EJ, Jr. Indications for pleurectomy in malignant effusion. Cancer 1975;35:734.

24. Harvey JC, Erdman CB, Beattie EJ, Jr. Early experience with videothoracoscopic hydrodissection pleurectomy in the treatment of malignant pleural effusion. J Surg Oncol 1995;59:243.

25. Waller DA, Morritt GN, Forty J. Video-assisted thoracoscopic pleurectomy in the management of malignant pleural effusion. Chest 1995;107:454.

26. Reich H, Beattie EJ, Harvey JC. Pleuroperitoneal shunt for malignant pleural effusions: a one-year experience. Semin Surg Oncol 1993;9:160.

27. Tsang V, Fernando HC, Goldstraw P. Pleuroperitoneal shunt for recurrent malignant pleural effusions. Thorax 1990; 45:369.

28. le Roux BT, Mohlala ML, Odel JA, et al. Suppurative diseases of the lung and pleural space. I. Empyema thoracis and lung abscess. Curr Probl Surg 1986;6:23.

29. Miller JI, Mansour KA, Nahai F, et al. Single-stage complete muscle flap closure of the postpneumonectomy empyema space: a new method and possible solution to a disturbing complication. Ann Thorac Surg 1984;38:227.

30. Lillington GA, Mitchell SP, Wood GA. Catamenial pneumothorax. JAMA 1972;219:1328.

31. Gaensler EA. Parietal pleurectomy for recurrent spontaneous pneumothorax. Surg Gynecol Obstet 1956;102:293.

32. Cole FH, Cole FH, Khandekar A, Maxwell JM, Pate JW, Walker WA. Video-assisted thoracic surgery: primary therapy for spontaneous pneumothorax? Ann Thorac Surg 1995;60:931.

33. Waller DA, Forty J, Morritt GN. Video-assisted thoracoscopic surgery versus thoracotomy for spontaneous pneumothorax. Ann Thorac Surg 1994;58:372.

34. Robinson CLH. The management of chylothorax (collective review). Ann Thorac Surg 1985;39:90.

35. Ferguson MK, Little AG, Skinner DB. Current concepts in the management of postoperative chylothorax. Ann Thorac Surg 1985;40:542.

36. Shirai T, Amano J, Takabe K. Thoracoscopic diagnosis and treatment of chylothorax after pneumonectomy. Ann Thorac Surg 1991;52:307.

37. Rusch VW. Diffuse malignant mesothelioma. In: Shields TW, ed. General thoracic surgery, ed 4. Philadelphia, Lea & Febiger, 1994:731.

38. Antman KH, Pass HI, Delaney T, et al. Benign and malignant mesothelioma. In: DeVita V, Hellman S, Rosenberg SA, eds. Principles and practices of oncology ed 2. Philadelphia, JB Lippincott, 1993:1399.

39. Butchart EG, Ashcroft T, Barnsley, et al. Pleuropneumonectomy in the management of diffuse malignant mesothelioma of the pleura: experience with 29 patients. Thorax 1976;31:15.

40. Rusch VW, Ginsberg RJ. New concepts in the staging of mesotheliomas. In: Deslaurier J, Lacquet LK, eds. Thoracic surgery. St Louis, CV Mosby, 1990:340.

41. Lau MR, Gregor A, Hodson ME, et al. Malignant mesothelioma of the pleura: a study of 52 treated and 64 untreated patients. Thorax 1984;39:255.

42. Sugarbaker DJ, Jaklitsch MT, Liptay MJ. Mesothelioma and radical multimodality therapy: who benefits? Chest 1995; 107:345S.

43. Sugarbaker DJ, Strauss GM, Lynch TJ, et al. Node status has prognostic significance in the multimodality therapy of diffuse, malignant mesothelioma. J Clin Oncol 1993;11:1172.

44. Johnson WW. The malignant pleural effusion: a review of cytopathologic diagnoses of 584 specimens from 472 consecutive patients. Cancer 1985;56:905.

45. Ringelman PR, Vander Kolk CA, Cameron D, Baumgartner WA, Manson PN. Long-term results of flap reconstruction in median sternotomy wound infections. Plast Reconstr Surg 1994;93:1208.

46. Scully HE, Leclerc Y, Martin RD, et al. Comparison between antibiotic irrigation and mobilization of pectoral muscle flaps in treatment of deep sternal infections. J Thorac Cardiovasc Surg 1985;90:523.

47. Wheatley MJ, Stirling MC, Kirsh MM, et al. Descending necrotizing mediastinitis: transcervical drainage is not enough. Ann Thorac Surg 1990;49:780.

48. Garrett HE Jr, Roger CL. Surgical intervention in histoplasmosis: collective review. Ann Thorac Surg 1986;42:711.

49. Davis RD Jr, Oldham HN Jr, Sabiston DC Jr. The mediastinum. In: Sabiston DC Jr, Spencer FC, eds. Surgery of the chest, ed 6. Philadelphia, WB Saunders, 1995:582.

50. Wang KP. Staging of bronchogenic carcinoma by bronchoscopy. Chest 1994;106:588.

51. Adam A, Hochholzer L. Ganglioneuroblastoma of the posterior mediastinum: a clinicopathologic review of 80 cases. Cancer 1981;47:373.

52. Look AT, Hayes FA, Nitschke R, et al. Cellular DNA content as a predictor of response to chemotherapy in infants with unresectable neuroblastoma. N Engl J Med 1984;311:321.

53. Grillo HC, Ojemann RG, Scannell G, et al. Combined approach to "dumbbell" intrathoracic and intraspinal neurogenic tumors. Ann Thorac Surg 1983;36:402.

54. Shapiro B, Orringer MB, Gross MD. Mediastinal paragangliomas and pheochromocytomas. In: Shields TW, eds. Mediastinal surgery. Philadelphia, Lea & Febiger, 1991:254.

55. Sisson JC, Shapiro B, Beierwaltes WH, et al. Locating pheochromocytomas by scintigraphy using 131-I metaiodobenzylguanidine. Cancer 1984;34:86.

56. Dulmet EM, Macchiarini P, Suc B, Verley JM. Germ cell tumors of the mediastinum: a 30-year experience. Cancer 1993;72:1894.

57. Sanders DB, Scoppetta C. The treatment of patients with myasthenia gravis. Neurol Clin 1994;12:343.

58. Richman DP, Agius MA. Myasthenia gravis: pathogenesis and treatment. Semin Neurol 1994;14:106.

59. Wilkins EW Jr, Grillo HC, Scannell JG, et al. Role of staging in prognosis and management of thymoma. Ann Thorac Surg 1991;51:888.

60. Maggi G, Casadio C, Cavallo A, et al. Thymoma: results of 241 operated cases. Ann Thorac Surg 1991;51:152.

61. Blumberg D, Port JL, Weksler B, et al. Thymoma: a multivariate analysis of factors predicting survival. Ann Thorac Surg 1995;60:908.

62. Khimji T, Zeiss J. MRI versus CT and US in the evaluation of a patient presenting with superior vena cava syndrome: case report. Clin Imag 1992;16:269.

63. Grillo HC, Mathisen DJ. Primary tracheal tumors: treatment and results. Ann Thorac Surg 1990;49:69.

64. Perelman MI, Koroleva NS. Primary tumors of the trachea. In: Grillo HC, Eschapasse H, eds. International trends in general thoracic surgery, vol 2. Philadelphia, WB Saunders, 1987:91.

65. Mathisen DJ, Grillo HC. Laryngotracheal trauma. Ann Thorac Surg 1987;43:254.

66. Cooper JD, Grillo HC. The evolution of tracheal injury due to ventilatory assistance through cuffed tubes: a pathologic study. Ann Surg 1969;169:343.

67. Grillo HC. Surgical treatment of postintubation tracheal injuries. J Thorac Cardiovasc Surg 1979;78:860.

68. Whyte RI, Quint LE, Kazerooni EA, Cascade PN, Iannettoni MD, Orringer MB. Helical CT in the evaluation of tracheal stenosis. Ann Thorac Surg 1995;60:27.

69. Grillo HC, Mathisen DJ. Surgical management of tracheal strictures. Surg Clin North Am 1988;68:511.

70. Grillo HC, Zannini P, Michelassi F. Complications of tracheal reconstruction. J Thorac Cardiovasc Surg 1986;91:322.

71. Mathisen DJ, Grillo HC, Wain JC, Hilgenberg AD. Management of acquired non-malignant tracheoesophageal fistula. Ann Thorac Surg 1991;52:759.

72. Orringer MB. Endotracheal intubation and tracheostomy: indications, techniques, and complications. Surg Clin North Am 1980;60:1447.

73. Ciaglia P, Firshing R, et al. Elective percutaneous dilational tracheostomy. Chest 1985;87:715.

74. Wiedemann HP, Rice TW. Lung abscess and empyema. Semin Thorac Cardiovasc Surg 1995;7:119.

75. Ha HK, Kang MW, Park JM, Yang WJ, Shinn KS, Bahk YW. Lung abscess: percutaneous catheter therapy. Acta Radiol 1993;34:362.

76. Okuda Y, Sawada S, Kobayashi M, Tanigawa N, Senda T, Morioka N. Percutaneous internal fistulization of a lung abscess after incomplete external drainage. Cardiovasc Intervent Radiol 1994;17:339.

77. Mori T, Ebe T, Takahashi M, Isonuma H, Ikemoto H, Oguri T. Lung abscess: analysis of 66 cases from 1979 to 1991. Ann Intern Med 1993;32:278.

78. Nicotra MB. Bronchiectasis. Semin Respir Infect 1994;9:31.

79. Webb WR. High-resolution computed tomography of obstructive lung disease. Radiol Clin North Am 1994;32:745.

80. Barker AF. Bronchiectasis. Semin Thorac Cardiovasc Surg 1995;7:112.

SURGERY: SCIENTIFIC PRINCIPLES AND PRACTICE, Second Edition, edited by
Lazar J. Greenfield, Michael W. Mulholland, Keith T. Oldham, Gerald B. Zelenock,
and Keith D. Lillemoe. Lippincott–Raven Publishers, Philadelphia, © 1997.

CHAPTER 63

CONGENITAL HEART DISEASE AND CARDIAC TUMORS

RALPH S. MOSCA, FLAVIAN M. LUPINETTI,
AND EDWARD L. BOVE

ATRIAL SEPTAL DEFECT

The formation of the atrial and ventricular septa occurs between the third and sixth weeks of fetal development. After the fusion of the paired heart tubes into a single tube folded on itself, the distal portion of the tube causes an indentation in the roof of the common atrium. Near this portion of the roof, the septum primum arises and extends in a crescentic formation toward the atrioventricular (AV) junction. The gap remaining between the septum primum and the developing tissues of the AV junction is named the *ostium primum*. Before the septum primum fuses completely with the endocardial cushions, a series of fenestrations appears in the septum primum that coalesce into the ostium secundum. During this coalescence, the septum secundum grows downward from the roof of the atrium, parallel and to the right of the septum primum. The septum primum does not fuse but creates an oblique pathway, called the *foramen ovale*, from the right atrium to the left. After birth, the increase in left atrial pressure usually closes this pathway, resulting in complete separation of the atria. Probe patency of foramen ovale is commonly observed in normal individuals.[1]

An *atrial septal defect* (ASD) is a hole in the atrial septum (Fig. 63-1). ASDs are most commonly located in the central aspect of the septum and are referred to as *ostium secundum* or *fossa ovalis defects*. Ostium secundum defects account for more than 80% of all atrial septal defects. These defects may range from a simple patent foramen ovale to complete absence of the septum primum. In the latter condition, the inferior vena caval orifice may appear to connect directly with the left atrium. In 5% to 10% of patients, the defect occurs along the remnant of the right horn of the sinus venosus and is referred to as a *sinus venosus ASD*. Most often, this occurs adjacent to the superior vena cava and is associated with partial anomalous pulmonary venous return. The superior vena cava orifice appears to straddle the ASD, its posterior wall being continuous with the left atrium itself. Defects in the AV septum are commonly referred to as *ostium primum ASDs*. This actually represents a more complex form of atrial defect and is more properly referred to as the incomplete

form of *AV septal defect* (AVSD). These are associated with abnormal mitral valve morphology. Coronary sinus defects occur when the coronary sinus is partially or completely unroofed in the left atrium. These defects result from deficiency in the remnant of the left horn of the sinus venosus and allow communication between right and left atria through the defect in the wall of the coronary sinus. One or more of the above types of ASDs may coexist.

Anomalies of pulmonary venous connection may be seen with ASDs, most commonly those of the sinus venosus type.[2] In this condition, the pulmonary veins from the right upper and middle lobes enter the superior vena cava near the cavoatrial junction. Uncommonly, some or all of the right pulmonary veins may enter the right atrium directly, with or without an associated ASD. In a rare condition known as the *scimitar syndrome*, the right pulmonary vein courses inferiorly along the pericardial border and enters the heart in the region of the junction between the right atrium and the inferior vena cava. An ASD is frequently present. Scimitar syndrome is usually associated with a hypoplastic right lung that is supplied by an anomalous systemic artery originating from the abdominal aorta.

ASDs result in increased pulmonary blood flow secondary to left-to-right shunting through the defect. The flow of blood is directed from the left atrium to the right atrium because of the greater diastolic compliance and lower diastolic pressures in the right ventricle. When pulmonary flow is twice that of the systemic circulation (Qp/Qs ratio higher than 2), symptoms generally occur. Lesser degrees of shunting may be asymptomatic and remain so until late in life. The most common symptoms are fatigue, shortness of breath, and recurrent respiratory infections. Atrial dysrhythmias are common in adulthood. *Paradoxical embolism*, a term applied to systemic emboli that arise from the peripheral veins, is a rare complication of ASD. These emboli, which would normally go to the lungs, instead pass through the ASD to the systemic circulation.

Classic physical findings with large ASDs consist of a normal first heart sound and wide, fixed splitting of the second heart sound. This results from the relatively fixed left-to-right shunt throughout all phases of the cardiac cycle. A soft ejection flow murmur across the pulmonary valve occurs as a result of the increased volume of flow. Additionally, a diastolic flow murmur may be audible across the tricuspid valve. A prominent right ventricular lift and increased intensity of the pulmonary component of the second sound may occur with pulmonary hypertension. Chest radiograph demonstrates cardiomegaly with enlargement of the right atrium, right ventricle, and pulmonary artery. The left atrium does not enlarge. The pulmonary vascular markings are increased. The electrocardiogram (ECG) shows right axis deviation and an incomplete right bundle-branch block pattern. When right bundle-branch block is associated with a leftward or superior axis, an AVSD should be strongly suspected. Two-dimensional (2D) echocardiography is used to visualize the defect as well as any associated anomalies of pulmonary venous return. Right ventricular volume overload with a flat or

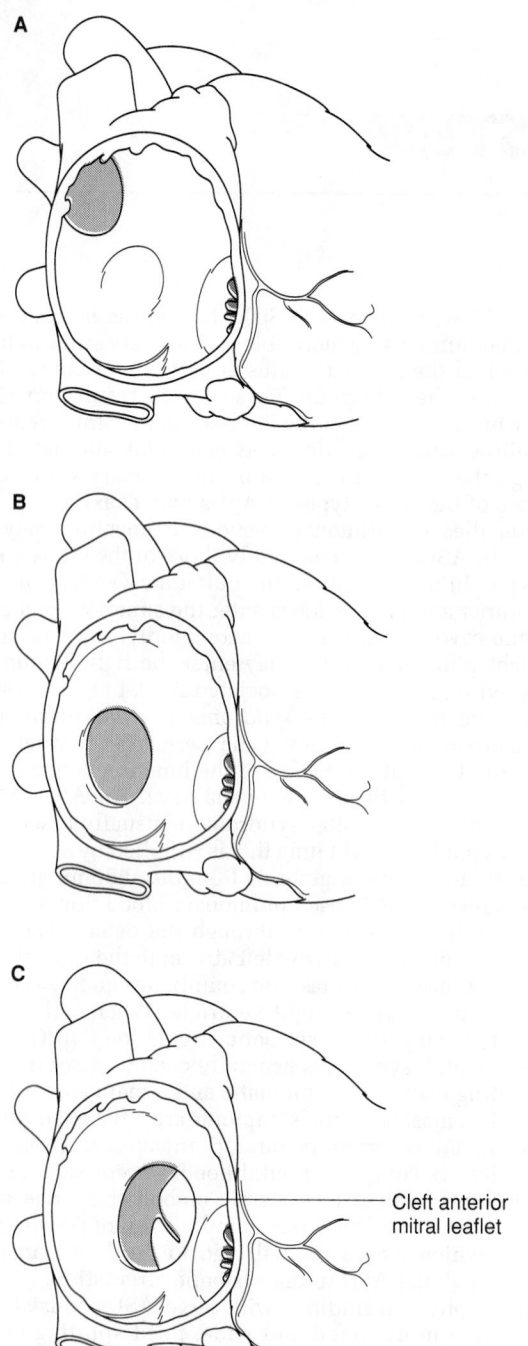

Figure 63-1. The anatomy of atrial septal defects. In the sinus venosus type (*A*), the right upper and middle pulmonary veins frequently drain to the superior vena cava or right atrium. (*B*) Secundum defects generally occur as isolated lesions. (*C*) Primum defects are part of a more complex lesion and are best considered as incomplete atrioventricular septal defects.

Cleft anterior mitral leaflet

reversed septal motion is evidence of a significant volume of left-to-right shunting. Cardiac catheterization is rarely used today in isolated cases of ASD when 2D Doppler echocardiography in addition to the other noninvasive evaluations demonstrate the classic findings. Cardiac catheterization may be important in assessing the quantity of left-to-right shunting and the degree of pulmonary hypertension in patients in whom the pulmonary vascular resistance is thought to be elevated. Although rare, the chronic

left-to-right shunt from an ASD may produce pulmonary vascular occlusive disease later in life. When the Qp/Qs ratio is less than 1.5 and the pulmonary to systemic vascular resistance (Rp/Rs) ratio exceeds 0.7, advanced pulmonary occlusive disease may be present. An absolute pulmonary vascular resistance in excess of 10 to 12 Woods units/m² indicates inoperability.[3]

Any ASD with a significant left-to-right shunt producing volume overload should be closed surgically. This occurs with a Qp/Qs ratio of approximately 1.5 or greater. The degree of left-to-right shunting tends to increase with advanced age as left ventricular dysfunction causes decreasing left ventricular compliance. Congestive heart failure (CHF), supraventricular dysrhythmias, and pulmonary hypertension occur with increasing frequency by the third to fourth decade of life in patients with large untreated ASDs. Even smaller defects may be associated with paradoxical embolism, particularly during pregnancy. Elective repair is advised before school age in patients with moderate to large ASDs.

ASDs can be readily repaired using standard techniques of cardiopulmonary bypass through a midline sternotomy approach. Alternatively, a right thoracotomy or bilateral submammary incision can be used for cosmetic reasons. The heart and venous return are carefully inspected to examine for anomalies of pulmonary venous connection or the presence of a left superior vena cava. Direct superior and inferior vena cava cannulation is used, and the core temperature is lowered to 32°C. Aortic cross-clamping with elective myocardial arrest using an infusion of cold cardioplegic solution is then performed. Alternatively, the aorta is left unclamped, and the heart is electively fibrillated to prevent the ejection of air during exposure of the ASD. A right atriotomy is made, and the atrial septum is carefully inspected. Closure of ostium secundum defects is accomplished either by direct suture or by the insertion of a patch. Care must be taken to accurately identify all edges of the ASD, particularly in cases where the entire septum primum is absent. In these situations, the eustachian valve may be mistaken for the lower rim of the ASD and used in the repair, inadvertently diverting inferior vena cava blood in the left atrium. Sinus venosus ASDs associated with partial anomalous pulmonary venous connection are repaired by inserting a patch, redirecting the pulmonary veins behind the patch to the left atrium. Care must be taken not to obstruct the pulmonary veins or superior vena cava. Generally, the superior vena cava is dilated and provides ample room for inserting the patch. In some situations, one or more pulmonary veins may enter the superior vena cava far superiorly. When the abnormally connecting pulmonary vein represents part or all of the right upper lobe only, it may be best not to incorporate this vein in the repair to avoid creating an obstruction to venous return. The resultant left-to-right shunt generally has a Qp/Qs ratio of less than 1.5 and should not cause problems later in life.

First performed in 1976,[4] transcatheter closure of ASDs using the umbrella device is increasing in popularity. Initial devices were hampered by arm fracture and have been replaced by the Bard clamshell occluder.[5] These devices will likely play an increasing role in the future treatment of ASDs.

The results for ASD closure are excellent, and the hospital mortality rate approaches zero. Morbidity is minimal and convalescence is generally uncomplicated. Uncommonly, atrial arrhythmias or significant left atrial hypertension may occur soon after repair. The latter is due to the noncompliant small left atrial chamber and generally resolves rapidly.

VENTRICULAR SEPTAL DEFECT

The ventricular septum forms in part from the endocardial cushions and in part by the relatively greater growth of the ventricles compared to the interventricular foramen. The spiral septation of the embryologic great arteries also contributes to septal formation. Ventricular septal defect (VSD) is a common anomaly and ranks behind only bicuspid aortic valve in the frequency of congenital heart defects. VSDs account for 20% to 25% of all cardiac lesions and are present in 2 of every 1000 live-born infants. Although VSDs may occur in any portion of the ventricular septum, certain typical locations tend to predominate (Fig. 63-2). Most defects are single and are located high in the ventricular septum, just beneath the aortic valve. When the defects abut the tricuspid valve annulus, as is usually the case, they are termed *perimembranous VSDs*, referring to their involvement of the membranous septum. The typical VSD, representing about 80% of all defects, is perimembranous and located in the infundibular septum, which is the portion of the septum separating right and left ventricular outflow tracts. Defects located high in the infundibular septum, immediately beneath the pulmonary valve, are referred to as *supracristal, infundibular,* or *subarterial VSDs.* These defects account for about 5% to 10% of all VSDs. The infundibular septum may be extremely deficient or virtually absent in these defects, with little or no

muscle separating the aortic and pulmonary valves. In about 5% of VSDs, the defect lies in the inlet septum beneath the septal leaflet of the tricuspid valve. These perimembranous inlet defects are also referred to as *atrioventricular canal-type defects.* The remaining VSDs are composed entirely of muscular edges and are most commonly located in the apical muscular portion of the ventricular septum. These defects are often multiple and may be associated with additional perimembranous VSDs.

Associated lesions are common with VSDs, and the defect itself is often a part of a more complex lesion. Prolapse of the aortic valve with aortic insufficiency may be caused by the VSD itself. This is more common with subpulmonic or supracristal defects. VSDs may be associated with left heart obstructive lesions, such as aortic stenosis, mitral stenosis, and coarctation.

Isolated VSDs result in left-to-right shunting with increased pulmonary blood flow. The hemodynamics and symptoms in patients with isolated VSDs depend on the size of the defect and the magnitude of the shunt. As the normally elevated pulmonary vascular resistance of the neonate falls during the first few weeks of life, the degree of left-to-right shunting increases, resulting in signs and symptoms of CHF. This generally occurs after the first 4 to 6 weeks of life in patients with large VSDs. Large or nonrestrictive VSDs are present when the defect size approximates

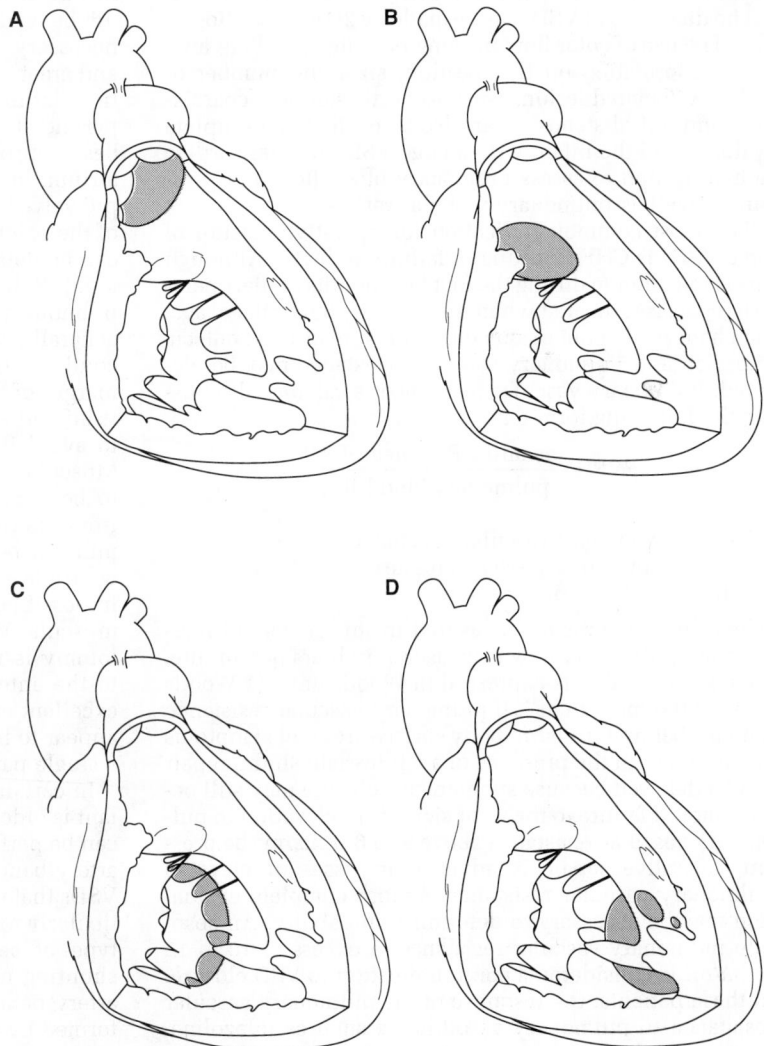

Figure 63-2. The anatomy of ventricular septal defects (VSDs) as seen through the right ventricle. (*A*) Subarterial VSDs, or high type, are generally bordered superiorly by the pulmonary valve annulus. (*B*) Perimembranous VSDs are the most common, extending from the membranous septum into the infundibular septum. (*C*) Inlet defects are located predominantly beneath the septal leaflet of the tricuspid valve. (*D*) Muscular VSDs are situated away from the valves, toward the cardiac apex.

the size of the aortic annulus, resulting in systemic or near systemic right ventricular pressure and a Qp/Qs ratio generally in excess of 2.5 or 3. Moderate VSDs are restrictive in size, with right ventricular pressure generally at about half systemic levels or less. The Qp/Qs ratio is 1.5 to 2.5. With small ventricular defects, right ventricular pressure remains normal and the Qp/Qs ratio is less than 1.5.

Large VSDs generally present at about 6 weeks to 2 months of age, a time when the normally elevated pulmonary vascular resistance falls, allowing an increase in the left-to-right shunt. CHF is manifested by tachypnea, tachycardia, diaphoresis with poor feeding, and inadequate weight gain. About half of all VSDs discovered in infancy undergo spontaneous closure. Although this is less likely with nonrestrictive defects, all VSDs are initially managed medically with the administration of digoxin and diuretics to control symptoms of CHF. The increased pulmonary blood flow and pressure seen with moderate and large VSDs may lead to a gradual increase in pulmonary arterial resistance and the development of pulmonary vascular occlusive disease. Advanced changes of pulmonary vascular disease generally do not occur until 2 years of age in patients with isolated large VSDs. Histologically, these changes have been classified by Heath and Edwards.[6] Grade 1 changes consist of medial hypertrophy alone, with grade 2 changes involving intimal proliferation. Grades 1 and 2 are considered reversible. More advanced findings consist of intimal fibrosis (grade 3) and progressive dilatation lesions, including arteriolar necrosis (grades 4 to 6). These advanced changes are not reversible.

The diagnosis of VSD may be made by 2D echocardiography. The use of color flow imaging provides excellent anatomic information on the location, size, and number of VSDs. Associated lesions, such as aortic stenosis, coarctation, and mitral stenosis, can also be evaluated. Complete evaluation of the infant with a large VSD includes cardiac catheterization to assess pulmonary blood flow and pressure as well as pulmonary vascular resistance.

The most common indication for operative closure of large VSDs is CHF resulting in failure to thrive. Although this is uncommon during the first few months of life, operative repair is indicated when it occurs. By 6 months of age, the chances of spontaneous defect closure of large defects diminish and pulmonary vascular resistance may be elevated. Pulmonary vascular resistance is calculated by using the following formula:

$$PVR = \frac{\text{mean PAP} - \text{mean LAP}}{\text{pulmonary blood flow}}$$

where:
PVR = pulmonary vascular resistance
PAP = pulmonary artery pressure
LAP = left arterial pressure

When the pressures are measured in millimeters of mercury and pulmonary flow is measured in liters per minute, the resulting value is expressed in Woods units (1 Woods unit = 80 dynes·s/cm^5). If pulmonary vascular resistance remains below 4 units/m^2 body surface area and symptoms are minimal, in the presence of a left-to-right shunt, repair can be deferred because spontaneous closure may still occur. Should failure to thrive or significant elevation in pulmonary vascular resistance above 4 to 6 units/m^2 be present, operative repair is advised. In cases of elevated pulmonary vascular resistance, a more complete evaluation may be necessary to determine operability. An absolute pulmonary vascular resistance in excess of 10 to 12 units/m^2 is considered a contraindication to VSD closure. In these patients, the response of the pulmonary vascular resistance to pulmonary vasodilators such as tolazoline, isoproterenol, or oxygen may be used to assess whether

the resistance remains fixed. The response to exercise may be helpful in older children. In favorable situations, pulmonary vascular resistance falls, associated with an increase in the Qp/Qs ratio, indicating that operation remains advisable. If the Qp/Qs ratio remains less than 1.5 with a pulmonary to systemic resistance ratio in excess of 0.6 to 0.7, operation is contraindicated. When this occurs, patients begin to develop right-to-left shunting, particularly with exercise, and the signs and symptoms of CHF are no longer apparent. VSD closure in these patients prevents the compensatory right-to-left shunting that is necessary to maintain cardiac output as pulmonary vascular resistance increases or systemic vascular resistance falls. Moderate defects that do not result in significant pulmonary artery hypertension or elevation in pulmonary resistance can continue to be observed if symptoms are minimal. Even in these situations, surgical closure is indicated by 3 to 5 years of age, because spontaneous defect closure is highly unlikely beyond that time.

In most cases, the surgical treatment of VSDs consists of primary repair using cardiopulmonary bypass. Most infants can be treated using deep hypothermia with low-flow bypass at systemic temperatures of 20° to 25°C. Cold cardioplegic solution is used to protect the heart. In some instances, a period of deep hypothermia and circulatory arrest may be used to facilitate exposure.[7] Perimembranous VSDs may be adequately exposed and closed using the right atrial approach. Retraction on the leaflets of the tricuspid valve allows exposure of the margins of the defect. In rare situations, the superior margin of the defect may not be well visualized, and a right ventriculotomy may be necessary. The defect is closed with a patch in all cases, and great care must be taken to avoid injuring the conduction tissue that lies along the posterior and inferior rim of perimembranous infundibular defects. Inlet VSDs are also best approached through the tricuspid valve and right atrium. In some situations, the arrangement of the tricuspid valve tensor apparatus may impair accurate placement of the patch. In these cases, the base of the tricuspid valve can be detached 1 to 2 mm away from its annular attachment. Subpulmonary VSDs are best exposed through the pulmonary artery or right ventricle. Because these defects generally do not extend to the perimembranous region, the conduction tissue is remote from its edge. The superior margin of the defect is composed of the pulmonary valve itself and suturing must be done to the base of the leaflets to avoid injuring both the aortic and pulmonary valves. Muscular VSDs present a special problem and may need to be approached from the left ventricle. When viewed from the right ventricular side, these defects often appear multiple because the coarse trabeculations within the right ventricle make delineating the edges of the VSD nearly impossible. This is particularly true of anterior and apical muscular VSDs. In these situations, an apical left ventriculotomy is made. The incision is carefully placed lateral to the anterior descending coronary artery and provides excellent exposure of the muscular septum. Defects often appear to be single from this view and can be closed with a single patch of prosthetic material.[8]

In certain situations, repair is best delayed until the infant is older and palliation with pulmonary artery banding can be performed. Although rarely used today, pulmonary artery banding may be indicated with complex muscular VSDs that require left ventriculotomy in small infants, particularly for those patients with the so-called Swiss cheese type of septum, in whom elimination of all residual shunting may be impossible. Removal of the pulmonary artery band and closure of the defects can then be performed by age 2 or 3 years.

The results for closure of isolated VSD are excellent,

even in infants. The hospital mortality rate approaches zero for uncomplicated defects. Young age, VSD location, and elevated pulmonary vascular resistance are no longer considered important risk factors. Major associated lesions may still adversely affect outcome. Although elevations in pulmonary vascular resistance do not increase operative mortality, late survival may be substantially reduced.

AORTIC STENOSIS

Obstruction to left ventricular outflow can occur at multiple levels (Fig. 63-3). The most common level of obstruction is due to valvar aortic stenosis, although the obstruction may be located in the subvalvar or supravalvular areas as well. Valvar aortic stenosis is secondary to various abnormalities of aortic valve development, most commonly a bicuspid aortic valve with fusion of the commissures. A bicuspid aortic valve is estimated to occur in about 2% of the population. Less commonly, variable degrees of fusion along the commissures of a tricuspid valve may be found. In neonates, significant aortic stenosis is most often due to unicommissural valve. The most common lesions associated with aortic stenosis are coarctation of the aorta, VSD, and mitral stenosis. Although valvar aortic stenosis may present at any age, most patients are diagnosed in childhood with the finding of an asymptomatic murmur. In infancy, CHF may develop, but symptoms are distinctly uncommon beyond that age until adulthood is reached. Although rare in childhood, angina may occur when myocardial blood flow cannot adequately perfuse the hypertrophied and hypertensive ventricular muscle. In the neonate, angina may present as periodic episodes of inconsolable crying. The third classic symptom of aortic stenosis, syncope, results from an inability of the left ventricle to in-crease cardiac output through the fixed valve orifice on demand, as occurs during exercise.

The physical findings in patients with aortic stenosis include a reduced pulse volume, precordial thrill, and an ejection systolic murmur at the cardiac base that radiates into the neck. The presence of a systolic ejection click signifies that the stenosis is valvar. Severe stenosis may be accompanied by a fourth heart sound as well as paradoxical splitting of the second sound. Physical findings are notoriously unreliable in predicting the severity of the lesion. The chest radiograph is rarely helpful and is often normal. There may be prominence of the left ventricular apex and a dilated ascending aorta. The ECG usually shows left ventricular hypertrophy, but may also be normal. In addition, 2D echocardiography is extremely useful in determining the site and severity of the lesion. The left ventricular outflow tract gradient can be estimated with Doppler techniques, which show good correlation with cardiac catheterization.

The neonate presenting with critical aortic stenosis and CHF requires urgent operative intervention. Many of these patients have severe low cardiac output and metabolic acidosis. These conditions may be improved by endotracheal intubation and inotropic support. An infusion of prostaglandin maintains the patency of or opens the ductus arteriosus and allows increased systemic blood flow. Although symptoms are rare in children older than infants, operation is indicated when any of the classic triad of heart failure, angina, or syncope occur in association with a left ventricular outflow tract gradient of at least 50 mmHg. Even in the absence of symptoms, a gradient in excess of 75 mmHg is considered severe. Patients with aortic valve gradients between 50 and 75 mmHg present a difficult dilemma. In the absence of symptoms, these patients should be care-

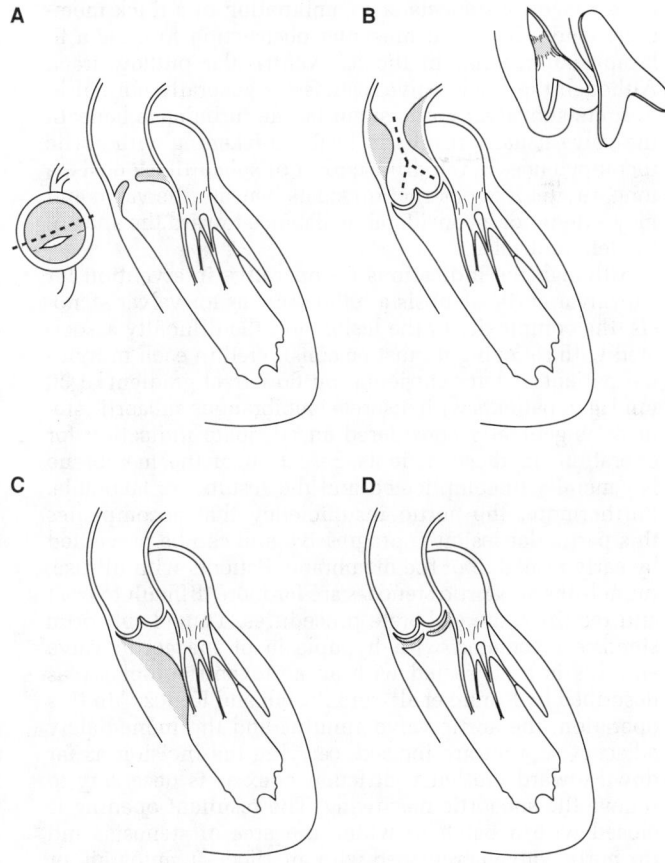

Figure 63-3. The anatomy of the types of congenital aortic stenosis. (*A*) Valvar aortic stenosis. (*B*) Supravalvular aortic stenosis and its repair (*inset*). (*C*) Tunnel-type subvalvar aortic stenosis. (*D*) Membranous subvalvar aortic stenosis.

fully observed. An ECG that demonstrates left ventricular strain or ischemia, at rest or with exercise, is considered an indication for operation.

Relief of valvar aortic stenosis in infants and children is generally accomplished using standard techniques of cardiopulmonary bypass with direct exposure of the aortic valve. Incision of fused commissures to within 1 to 2 mm of the valve annulus can then be done. Careful assessment of valve morphology is essential to avoid dividing a false raphe and producing leaflet prolapse and severe aortic regurgitation. Increasingly, reports indicate that balloon dilation of the aortic valve is effective in reducing the gradient without producing regurgitation, even in the neonate. For the older child, balloon dilatation is the procedure of choice, with operation reserved for the more complex lesions and those with annular hypoplasia. For the neonate, the large catheters required for dilatation have been associated with significant femoral arterial complications. The preferred approach is via the umbilical[9] or carotid[10] arteries. Alternatively, transventricular dilation through the left ventricular apex has proved effective with or without normothermic cardiopulmonary bypass to support the circulation. This technique avoids the myocardial ischemia produced by aortic cross-clamping. Although satisfactory relief of the gradient is generally accomplished, it is usually impossible to abolish the entire obstruction completely. A bicuspid aortic valve may be intrinsically stenotic when the total length of its free edges is less than the circumference of the aorta.[11] The goal of treating critical aortic stenosis in the neonate is to relieve the aortic obstruction without creating significant aortic insufficiency.

Subvalvar aortic stenosis occurs beneath the aortic valve and may be discrete or diffuse. In the discrete type, a fibrous membrane is located immediately beneath the aortic valve leaflets. Anteriorly, the membrane is attached to the septum and posteriorly to the anterior leaflet of the mitral valve in the region of aortic–mitral continuity. Often, discrete subaortic stenosis is a combination of a thick membrane and a localized muscular obstruction forming a fibromuscular collar in the left ventricular outflow tract. Although the aortic valve leaflets are generally normal in discrete subvalvar aortic stenosis, the turbulence beneath the valve usually results in leaflet thickening with aortic incompetence. In the diffuse form of subaortic stenosis, a long, tunnel-like obstruction exists beneath the valve and may extend for a considerable distance toward the apex of the left ventricle.

Although the indications for operative intervention for subvalvar aortic stenosis are the same as for valvar stenosis, the complexity of the lesion and the difficulty associated with relieving it must be considered in each individual patient. A left ventricular outflow tract gradient of 30 mmHg in patients with discrete membranous subaortic stenosis is generally considered an adequate indication for operation. In these patients, resection of the membrane is generally uncomplicated and the results are favorable. Furthermore, the aortic insufficiency that accompanies this particular lesion is progressive and can be prevented by early resection of the membrane. Patients with diffuse, tunnel-like subaortic stenoses are far more difficult to treat and require more elaborate procedures. Tunnel subaortic stenosis associated with hypoplasia of the aortic valve annulus is best treated with an aortoventriculoplasty as described by Konno et al[12] and Rastan and Koncz.[13] In this operation, the aortic valve annulus and the immediately adjacent septum are incised, carrying the incision as far down toward the left ventricular apex as is necessary to relieve the subaortic narrowing. The resultant opening is closed with a patch to widen the area of stenosis, and the aortic valve is replaced with an allograft, autograft, or

prosthesis. When the aortic valve annulus is adequate, the septal incision is confined to the immediate subvalvar area, and a patch is used to widen the left ventricular outflow tract without replacing the aortic valve.

Supravalvar aortic stenosis is an obstruction beginning distal to the aortic valve; it also exists in either a discrete or diffuse form. The discrete form is localized to the immediate supravalvar area just above the aortic valve commissures. This produces an hourglass deformity of the ascending aorta. The intraluminal thickening results in adherence of the three leaflets of the aortic valve to the area of obstruction, partially obstructing coronary flow in diastole ("cusp tuck"). This intramural thickening and fibrosis may extend into the orifices of the coronaries themselves, further impairing coronary blood flow. Although the disease presents most commonly in the discrete or localized form, some patients have diffuse vascular abnormalities, with thickening of the aortic wall extending further distally into the aortic arch and its branches.

The signs and symptoms of supravalvar aortic stenosis are similar to other forms of left ventricular outflow tract narrowing. Occasionally, supravalvar aortic stenosis may be associated with Williams syndrome, a constellation of elfin facies, mental retardation, and hypercalcemia. Diagnosis is established with cardiac catheterization and angiography. This is necessary to accurately define the extent of obstruction as well as any associated anomalies. The most common associated condition is peripheral pulmonary artery stenosis, which may be diffuse and severe.

Operation is indicated for patients with supravalvar aortic stenosis with outflow tract gradients higher than 50 mmHg. At operation, a patch is placed across the area of obstruction along the ascending aorta, extending it deep into the noncoronary sinus of Valsalva. On occasion, it may be advisable to insert an upside-down, Y-shaped patch with one limb of the Y extending into the noncoronary sinus of Valsalva and the other into the right coronary sinus to augment the narrowed supravalvar area in two places. In addition, the intramural tissue is generally resected by partial endarterectomy.

The results of surgery for the localized form of supravalvar aortic stenosis are generally good, with low operative mortality and excellent long-term survival. Obstruction is generally well relieved. The diffuse form of the disease is more difficult to treat and recurrence more likely to occur. When diffuse severe supravalvar pulmonary stenosis coexists, operative repair is far more hazardous and long-term results are poor.

TETRALOGY OF FALLOT

Tetralogy of Fallot is the most common congenital heart defect that results in cyanosis. In this condition, anterior displacement of the infundibular septum results in hypoplasia of the right ventricular outflow tract and pulmonary valve annulus. A large malalignment VSD with overriding of the aorta results. Right ventricular hypertrophy occurs secondary to the outflow tract obstruction. These are the four components of the tetralogy (Fig. 63-4). The anatomic hallmark of this condition is the anterior displacement of the infundibular septum, along with its leftward extension. The infundibular septum inserts anterior to the anterior extension of the septal band, rather than between its anterior and posterior extensions. The pulmonary valve itself is stenotic in most cases and often bicuspid in nature. The annulus of the pulmonary valve may be hypoplastic as is frequently the case when the infundibular stenosis is severe. Abnormalities of pulmonary artery development are also common, with diffuse mild hypoplasia predominating. A branch pulmonary artery stenosis, more fre-

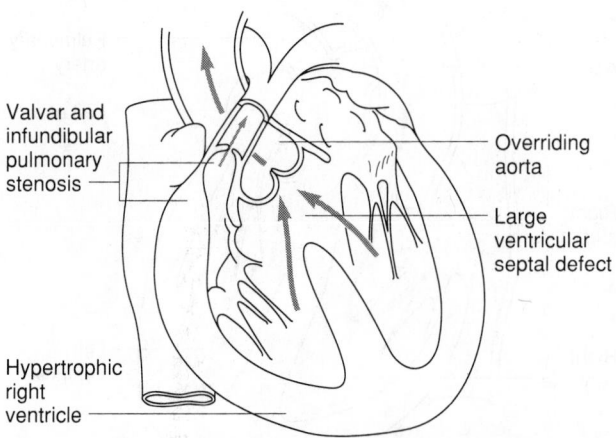

Figure 63-4. The four anatomic features of the tetralogy of Fallot. The primary morphologic abnormality, anterior and superior displacement of the infundibular septum, results in the malalignment ventricular septal defect, overriding of the aortic valve, and obstruction of right ventricular outflow. The right ventricular hypertrophy is a secondary occurrence.

quently of the left pulmonary artery at the region of the insertion of the ligamentum arteriosum, may also be seen. Absence of a unilateral pulmonary artery is rarely found. When pulmonary valvar atresia accompanies the tetralogy of Fallot, pulmonary blood flow is then supplied by multiple aortopulmonary collaterals with or without a patent ductus arteriosus (PDA). These vessels generally originate from the upper descending thoracic aorta and traverse the mediastinum to reach the hilum of each lung. They join the true intralobar pulmonary arteries in the lung and are indistinguishable from these vessels histologically. In most patients, hemodynamically significant stenoses occur between the aortic origin and the intrapulmonary vessels. The VSD in tetralogy of Fallot is nonrestrictive. The defect is cradled between the anterior and posterior limbs of the septal band and most commonly extends to the annulus of the tricuspid valve and involves the membranous septum. The aortic arch may be on the right, crossing over the right main-stem bronchus in 25% of patients with tetralogy of Fallot. The coronary arteries are usually normal, but in about 3% to 5% of patients, the anterior descending coronary originates from the right sinus of Valsalva and crosses over the right ventricular outflow tract to reach the interventricular groove. Other uncommon associated anomalies include absence of the pulmonary valve, multiple VSDs, and complete atrioventricular canal defect.

Patients with tetralogy of Fallot present with cyanosis, the severity of which depends on the degree of right ventricular outflow tract obstruction. Frequently, cyanosis is mild at birth and may be undetected for weeks or even months. Patients with severe hypoplasia of the pulmonary outflow tract and annulus, as well as those with pulmonary atresia, present with important cyanosis at birth or soon thereafter. Closure of the ductus arteriosus may unmask the cyanosis. In a few patients, the outflow tract obstruction may be so mild that patients initially present with large VSDs with left-to-right shunting and CHF.

When the right ventricular outflow tract obstruction is predominantly located in the infundibulum and is muscular in nature, patients may be subject to cyanotic spells. These episodes are most commonly seen in tetralogy but occur in patients with other forms of cyanotic defects as well. The spells are characterized by aggravation of the patient's cyanosis, labored breathing, and a fall in arterial

blood pressure. These events may be triggered by anything that reduces systemic vascular resistance, from vigorous physical exertion to a warm bath or a fever. Other factors that can increase the right-to-left shunt and exacerbate the degree of cyanosis include hyperpnea, the Valsalva maneuver, tachycardia, and dehydration. Although most episodes resolve spontaneously in a few minutes, they may lead to seizures or death. Immediate treatment is directed toward relieving the hypoxia and reducing the right ventricular obstruction. Supplemental oxygen, sedation with morphine, and beta blockade may help in this regard. The occurrence of cyanotic spells is an indication for surgical intervention.

Physical examination in patients with tetralogy of Fallot generally reveals some degree of cyanosis. There may be clubbing of the fingers and toes in older patients. The precordium is generally quiet, without thrill, and the second sound may appear to be single because of the soft pulmonic component. A mid-intensity systolic ejection murmur is present, which may decrease in intensity with increasing degrees of outflow tract obstruction. Continuous murmurs may be audible over the back secondary to collaterals. CHF is rare and generally occurs only in the presence of large systemic to pulmonary collaterals or in the later stages of the disease with associated ventricular failure or aortic incompetence. Chest radiography may demonstrate the classic boot-shaped heart with a concave pulmonary outflow tract and an upward-tipped apex secondary to right ventricular hypertrophy. The heart size is generally normal, and the pulmonary vascular markings are decreased. There may be a right aortic arch. 2D echocardiography demonstrates the position and nature of the VSD, defines the nature of the outflow tract obstruction, and often can visualize the branch pulmonary arteries and proximal coronary arteries. For these reasons echocardiography is often the only procedure required before surgery. Cardiac catheterization is occasionally necessary to accurately outline the anatomy of the pulmonary arteries and the presence of important coronary abnormalities.

The most common indications for operative intervention include increasing cyanosis and the occurrence of cyanotic spells. Although spells may be treated by propranolol, more definitive surgical intervention is generally indicated. Important considerations for determining the type and timing of surgical repair include size and distribution of the pulmonary arteries, coronary artery abnormalities, and the presence of right ventricle to pulmonary artery discontinuity. Although complete repair during infancy can be accomplished in most patients, certain anatomic features dictate that two-stage repair with preliminary shunting is optimal. Severe pulmonary artery hypoplasia represents an absolute contraindication to repair in infancy. In the past, patients with pulmonary atresia and multifocal pulmonary blood flow from aortopulmonary collaterals have been treated with preliminary shunting, ligation of collaterals, and unifocalization of nonconfluent branch pulmonary arteries. However, many of these patients were unable to undergo complete repair. For this reason, many centers now favor the early establishment of continuity between the right ventricle and the pulmonary artery. This promotes uniform central pulmonary artery growth and allows the interventional cardiologist access to the branch pulmonary arteries for dilatation, coil occlusion, and stenting. A team approach is often necessary to optimize the pulmonary vasculature for complete repair. The presence of an anomalous anterior coronary artery from the right coronary artery may limit the surgeon's ability to relieve pulmonary valvar hypoplasia using a transannular patch, and a conduit may be necessary. Although this can be done in infancy, repair may be best deferred until a larger conduit can be inserted. Conversely, when the pulmonary valve annulus is of adequate size and the infundibular stenosis is localized, repair can then be accomplished in the neonate or infant, avoiding ventriculotomy entirely.

When necessary, palliation is best accomplished with a modified Blalock-Taussig shunt.[14] The modified form consists of positioning a Gore-Tex conduit between the undivided subclavian artery and ipsilateral pulmonary artery. Generally, a 4- or 5-mm shunt is used through a right thoracotomy. Patency rates are excellent; however, there is a small but real risk of pulmonary artery distortion.

Complete repair consists of VSD closure and relief of right ventricular outflow tract obstruction. The VSD is closed transatrially, often avoiding a ventriculotomy. Traction on the anterior and septal leaflets of the tricuspid valve generally affords excellent exposure, even in neonates. Relief of right ventricular outflow tract obstruction can involve division and resection of hypertrophic musculature, pulmonary valve commissurotomy, and patch enlargement of the outflow tract, extending it across the annulus when necessary. Muscle resection can often be avoided entirely, particularly in neonates. The outflow tract is enlarged beginning with incision of the anterior limb of the septal band, division of the hypertrophied parietal extensions of the infundibular septum, and relief of any other obstructing muscle bundles to the level of the moderator band. Pulmonary valve annular size can be assessed intraoperatively, and the prediction made about the postoperative right ventricle/left ventricle pressure ratio. If this ratio is less than 0.75, the annulus is left intact. If the outflow tract is judged to be deficient, pulmonary valve commissurotomy or a limited transannular patch may be needed. Only in cases of severe tubular infundibular stenosis is an extended right ventriculotomy warranted. The pulmonary valve regurgitation that results is well tolerated in the absence of tricuspid regurgitation, severe right ventricular dysfunction, significant residual VSD, or outflow tract obstruction. It is imperative to be certain that residual branch pulmonary artery stenosis of either the right or left pulmonary artery is not present; otherwise, important outflow tract obstruction will remain distal to the outflow patch. In special circumstances, the insertion of a pulmonary valve prosthesis, generally a cryopreserved homograft, is indicated. These circumstances include severe pulmonary artery hypoplasia, absent pulmonary valve syndrome with aneurysmal pulmonary arteries in infancy, surgically inaccessible distal pulmonary artery stenosis, and unilateral absence of a pulmonary artery. Pulmonary regurgitation in these situations is poorly tolerated. The operative mortality rate is between 2% and 5%. Results for patients with tetralogy of Fallot and pulmonary atresia are less optimal, particularly in the presence of multiple aortopulmonary collaterals. The long-term results of repair avoiding an extended ventriculotomy are likely to be excellent because the incidence of late right ventricular dysfunction and dysrhythmias is surely reduced.[15]

TRANSPOSITION OF THE GREAT ARTERIES

Transposition of the great arteries (TGA) is a congenital cardiac anomaly in which the aorta arises from the right ventricle and the pulmonary artery originates from the left ventricle (ventriculoarterial discordance; Fig. 63-5). In the form of transposition considered here, the connections between the atria and sventricles are normal (concordant). TGA is a relatively common cardiac anomaly and is the most common form of congenital heart disease presenting

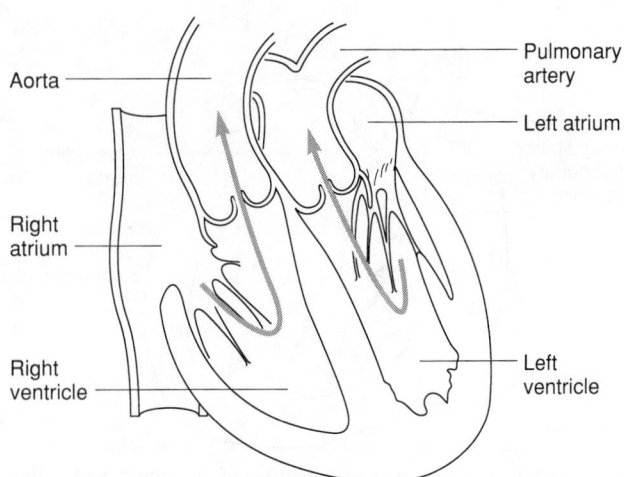

Figure 63-5. The anatomy of the most common type of transposition of the great arteries. The ascending aorta is usually located anterior and to the right of the pulmonary artery.

as cyanosis in the first week of life. The degree of cyanosis depends on the amount of mixing between the pulmonary and systemic circulations. In TGA, oxygenated pulmonary venous blood is returned to the lungs and desaturated systemic blood to the body, because the two circulations exist in parallel. To sustain life, some mixing of these two circulations must occur to allow oxygenated blood to reach the systemic circulation and the desaturated blood to reach the lungs. Mixing may occur at a number of levels, but it occurs most commonly at the atrial level through an ASD or patent foramen ovale. Often, a VSD or PDA serves as an additional site for cardiac mixing. In TGA, no fixed shunt can occur in one direction without an equal amount of blood passing in the other direction; otherwise, one circulation would eventually empty into the other. Therefore, the amount of desaturated blood reaching the lungs (effective pulmonary blood flow) must equal the amount of saturated blood reaching the aorta (effective systemic blood flow).

The newborn with TGA is noticeably cyanotic within hours of birth. As the ductus arteriosus closes, particularly in the face of a restrictive ASD, severe cyanosis occurs and may result in a metabolic acidosis. In the presence of a large VSD, cyanosis may be mild and go undetected for the first few weeks of life. When significant pulmonary stenosis is present, cyanosis may be profound even with adequate mixing. In these cases, cyanosis is also caused by a decrease in absolute pulmonary blood flow.

The physical findings in the neonate with TGA and intact ventricular septum are often unimpressive. Apart from cyanosis, there may be no other abnormal clinical findings. The ECG is normal at birth, demonstrating the typical pattern of right ventricular dominance. Although the classic chest radiographic appearance of an egg on its side may be seen, this finding is often obscured by an enlarged thymic shadow. Echocardiography clearly demonstrates the abnormal ventriculoarterial connection by demonstrating that the posterior great vessel arising from the left ventricle is a pulmonary artery that bifurcates soon after its origin. The anterior great vessel is the aorta and arises from the right ventricle. Associated lesions, including VSD, left ventricular outflow tract obstruction, and coarctation of the aorta, may also be diagnosed. Although used less frequently, cardiac catheterization may be helpful to confirm the basic anatomy, discern associated lesions, define the coronary anatomy, and improve cardiac mixing using a balloon atrial septostomy.

The infant with TGA and severe cyanosis requires prompt diagnosis and treatment to improve mixing and to increase the arterial oxygen saturation. This is best done either by early surgical repair or by balloon atrial septostomy, a technique developed by William Rashkind in 1966.[16] The procedure involves inserting a balloon-tipped catheter across the foramen ovale into the left atrium. The catheter is inflated and forcibly withdrawn, tearing the septum primum and enlarging the ASD. An immediate increase in mixing generally occurs, with a substantial increase in arterial oxygen saturation. In some situations, even the presence of an adequate atrial communication does not ensure adequate mixing, and the infant may remain severely cyanotic. This may be due to associated left ventricular outflow tract obstruction or a failure of the elevated neonatal pulmonary vascular resistance to fall toward normal levels. In the latter situation, the compliance of both circulations remains about equal, and no mixing occurs across the ASD. An infusion of prostaglandin may help by increasing mixing at the great vessel level through the PDA and by decreasing pulmonary vascular resistance. Often, this infusion may then be weaned within the next few days as pulmonary vascular resistance decreases.

Definitive surgical treatment of patients with TGA has changed dramatically in the past decade with the advent of the arterial switch procedure. Before this procedure, repair of patients with TGA was generally delayed until at least 6 months of age. Historically, palliative procedures were often necessary to improve the systemic saturation of these patients before definitive repair. If balloon atrial septostomy failed to adequately enlarge the ASD, a Blalock-Hanlon septectomy was performed. Rarely used today, this operation provides a method of surgically enlarging the ASD without cardiopulmonary bypass. In patients with large VSDs, significant CHF and pulmonary hypertension are present early in life. The main pulmonary artery may be banded to reduce distal pulmonary artery pressure and prevent the development of pulmonary vascular occlusive disease. About 25% of patients with hemodynamically large VSDs may develop changes of pulmonary vascular disease by 3 months of age; therefore, early reduction of pulmonary artery pressure is essential. Adjustment and

positioning of the pulmonary artery band are critical for proper palliation. Too tight a band results in unacceptable cyanosis, whereas too loose a band does not adequately reduce distal pulmonary arterial pressure. Migration of the pulmonary artery band distally may result in branch pulmonary artery stenosis with excessive flow to one lung and diminished or absent flow to the other. If the band is placed too proximal, pulmonary valve function may be impaired and the valve distorted. For these reasons, pulmonary artery banding for uncomplicated cases of TGA is avoided. In those cases of transposition with severe left ventricular outflow tract obstruction, total pulmonary flow is reduced and systemic to pulmonary artery shunting is indicated. A classic or modified Blalock-Taussig shunt is used to increase pulmonary blood flow and allows postponement of definitive repair until a later age.

Until recently, definitive repair was achieved by redirecting venous inflow at the atrial level. First successfully performed by Senning in 1959, the operation was simplified by Mustard in 1964[17] (Fig. 63-6). In both techniques, the atrial septum is repositioned such that superior and inferior vena cava blood drains to the mitral valve and then to the left ventricle and pulmonary artery. Pulmonary venous blood drains on the other side of the partition to the tricuspid valve and right ventricle. The right ventricle then ejects the oxygenated blood to the systemic circulation. The Mustard operation uses a large patch of pericardium or prosthetic material to create the intraatrial baffle. In the Senning procedure, the patient's atrial tissue is used and little or no foreign material is necessary. Although physiologic repair at the atrial level has achieved a low operative mortality rate (less than 5%) even in infants, a number of late problems have occurred. Obstruction to vena cava inflow, particularly at the superior vena cava-right atrial junction, still occurs in about 5% of patients and may be considerably more common when the procedure is done in the infant. Additionally, pulmonary venous obstruction may occur and is often difficult to repair. Perhaps because of the complex atrial suture lines, atrial dysrhythmias are common and occur in more than half of patients observed long term. In addition, pacemakers may be necessary for troubling bradyarrhythmias in as many as 10% of these patients.

The most serious long-term complication of repair by

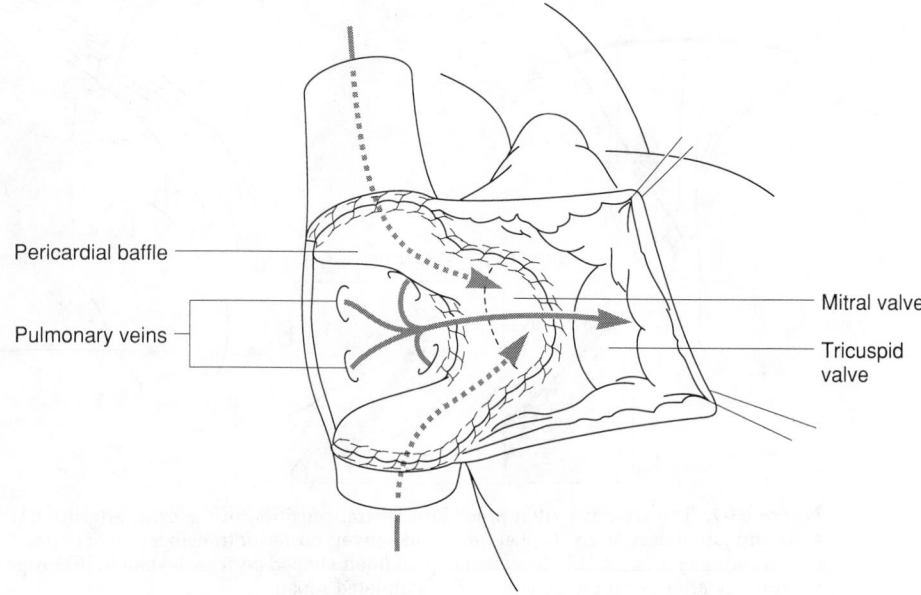

Figure 63-6. The Mustard operation for transposition of the great arteries. In this procedure, the atrial septum is excised and replaced with a pericardial baffle, redirecting pulmonary venous blood over the baffle to the tricuspid valve. Superior and inferior vena caval blood then drains to the mitral valve.

Pericardial baffle — Pulmonary veins — Mitral valve — Tricuspid valve

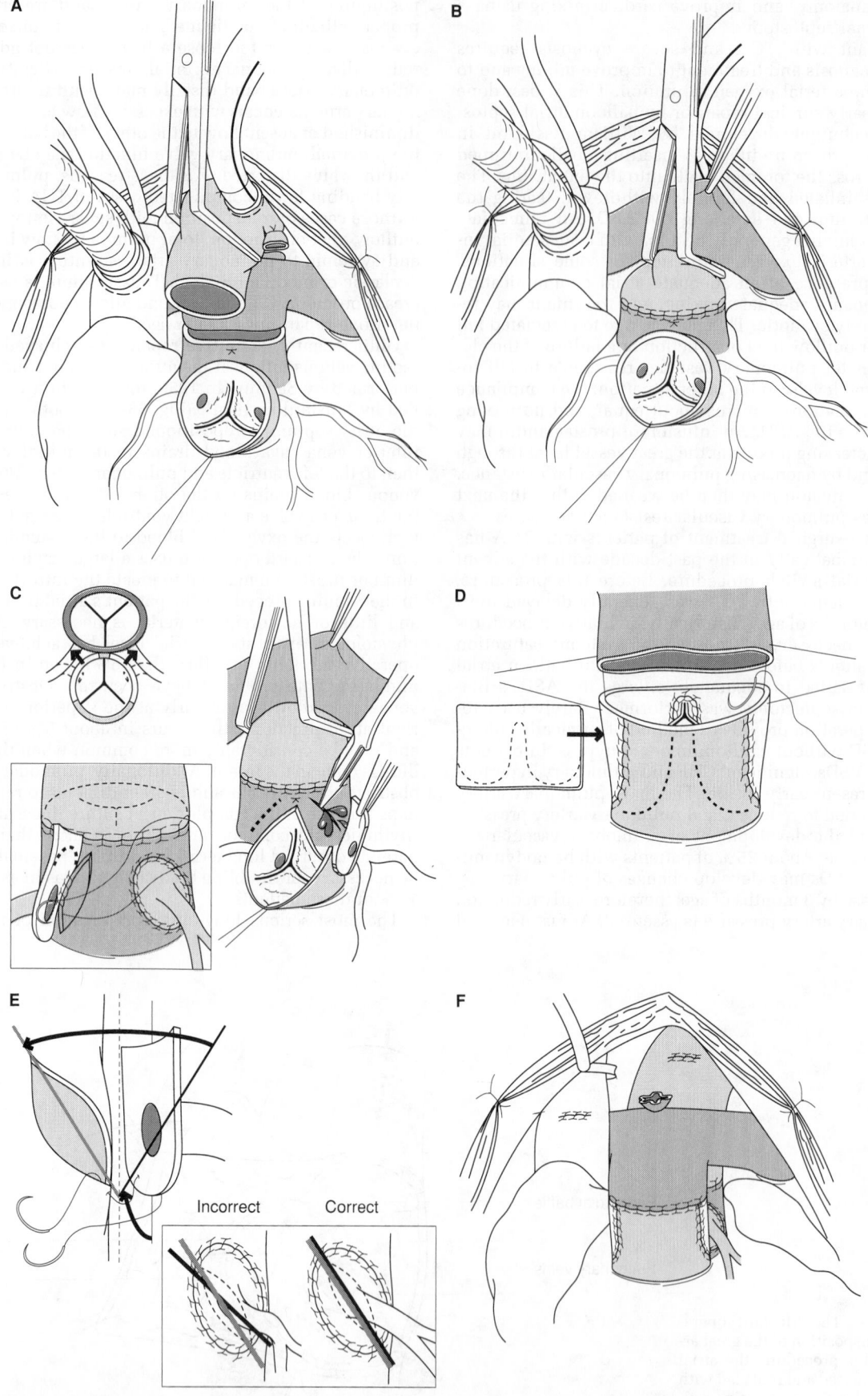

Figure 63-7. The arterial switch procedure for transposition of the great arteries. (*A*) Division of aorta and pulmonary artery. (*B*) LeCompte maneuver; posterior translocation of aorta. (*C*) Mobilization of coronary arteries. (*D*) Placement of pantaloon-shaped pericardial patch. (*E*) Proper alignment of coronary arteries on the neoaorta. (*F*) Completed repair.

either the Senning or Mustard technique has been right ventricular dysfunction. Right ventricular failure with an enlarged, poorly contractile chamber and secondary tricuspid regurgitation have been found in a significant number of these patients with long-term follow-up studies. The true incidence of significant right ventricular failure in these patients remains difficult to define and is clearly influenced by an earlier era of operation with different methods of myocardial protection and surgical technique. The fact that many of these infants had their definitive repair performed after many months of significant cyanosis may also have influenced right ventricular function.

These long-term complications of atrial repair prompted a reexamination of direct arterial repair for transposing the great arteries. The "arterial switch" procedure was first successfully performed by Jatene in 1977 and has become the optimal surgical procedure for infants with this condition.[18] Current techniques have reduced the operative mortality to levels comparable to that of atrial repair. Additionally, because operation is performed early in life, this approach has virtually eliminated the interim morbidity and mortality associated with postponing surgery until at least 6 months of age. The operative technique involves transecting both great vessels with direct reanastomosis to reestablish ventriculoarterial concordance (Fig. 63-7). Additionally, the coronary arteries are removed from the anterior aorta and relocated to the posterior great vessel (neoaorta). The extensive experience gained with this procedure has confirmed that any variant of coronary artery anatomy can be successfully repaired, although clearly, certain unusual forms impose a higher risk. Because most patients with TGA have intact ventricular septa, left ventricular pressure falls early in life as pulmonary vascular resistance decreases. In this situation, it is essential that the arterial repair be performed within the first 2 to 3 weeks of life, while the left ventricle is still able to meet systemic workloads. Patients presenting later can have the left ventricle retrained with a preliminary pulmonary artery banding and aortopulmonary shunt followed by the definitive arterial repair. Although patients with large VSDs do not require early repair because of decreased left ventricular pressure, experience has indicated that even in this subgroup, the operation must be performed within the first month of life, before secondary complications such as pulmonary hypertension, CHF, or infection develop.

Patients with fixed left ventricular outflow tract obstruction are not candidates for the arterial repair, because correction would result in systemic ventricular outflow tract obstruction. Most of these patients also have large VSDs. Palliation early in life with systemic to pulmonary artery shunting is preferred, and definitive repair is then postponed until age 3 to 5 years. At that time, the Rastelli procedure is performed by redirecting left ventricular blood through the VSD and to the anterior aorta by placing an intraventricular patch (Fig. 63-8). The pulmonary artery is ligated, and right ventricle to distal pulmonary artery continuity is reestablished with a valve-bearing conduit.

DOUBLE-OUTLET RIGHT VENTRICLE

Double-outlet ventricle includes a variety of malformations in which, by 50% or more, both great arteries arise from one ventricle. Although double-outlet left ventricles occur, a far more common anomaly is the double-outlet right ventricle (DORV). A VSD is usually present in DORV, and there may other defects, including discordant ventriculoarterial connections, valvar or subvalvar stenosis of the pulmonary, or aortic outflow and single ventricle.

The physiologic consequences of DORV vary, depending on the associated defects. The three most critical factors determining the net effects on the circulation are the size of the VSD, the presence or absence of pulmonary stenosis, and the presence and degree of left-sided obstruction. As a result, DORV may clinically resemble an isolated VSD, tetralogy of Fallot, or TGA.

The size and location of the VSD are important considerations in planning operative management. The VSD may be primarily directed toward the aorta, toward the pulmonary artery, equally toward both arteries (doubly committed), or remote from both great vessels (noncommitted). The location of the VSD affects the direction of flow of oxygenated blood and thus affects the degree of cyanosis. VSDs in DORV seldom undergo spontaneous closure. This is fortunate, because closure would result in severe hemodynamic decompensation or death.

If the VSD is large and nonrestrictive, it can be closed with a tunnel-like patch that directs left ventricular flow into the aorta. A restrictive VSD must be enlarged to avoid creating subaortic stenosis. For patients with DORV and pulmonary stenosis, repair requires right ventricular outflow tract reconstruction with a patch or a valved allograft conduit, as well as patch closure of the VSD.

DORV with transposition-type physiology may be treated by a variety of methods, depending on the specific anatomic details. With one approach, the VSD is patched to baffle left ventricular output into the pulmonary artery,

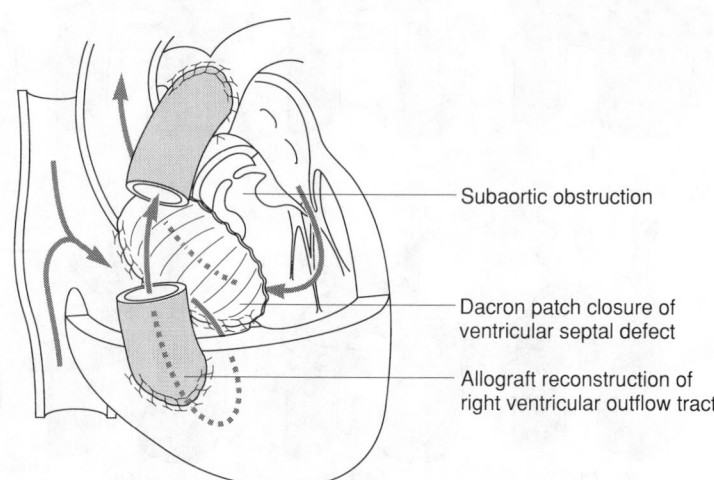

Figure 63-8. The Rastelli procedure for transposition of the great arteries with ventricular septal defect and pulmonary stenosis. A prosthetic patch is placed within the right ventricle, directing left ventricular blood through the defect to the aorta. The main pulmonary artery is ligated, and right ventricular blood then passes through a conduit to the distal pulmonary arteries.

- Subaortic obstruction
- Dacron patch closure of ventricular septal defect
- Allograft reconstruction of right ventricular outflow tract

and an atrial (Senning or Mustard) or arterial type of correction is then performed. A second approach requires constructing an intraventricular patch that connects the left ventricle to both great vessels, dividing the pulmonary artery at its origin, and inserting a conduit from the right ventricle to the distal pulmonary artery. In the Damus-Kaye-Stanzel operation, patch closure of the VSD and division of the pulmonary artery are performed. The proximal pulmonary artery is then anastomosed to the side of the ascending aorta. An extracardiac conduit is then placed from the right ventricle to the distal pulmonary artery. This approach may be particularly advantageous when the VSD is far removed from the aortic valve, making a direct connection impossible.

TRUNCUS ARTERIOSUS

Truncus arteriosus is a rare anomaly that accounts for 0.4% to 4% of all cases of congenital heart disease. A single arterial vessel arises from the heart, overriding the ventricular septum and giving rise to the systemic, coronary, and pulmonary circulations. Two classification schemes have been proposed—one by Collett and Edwards[19] in 1949 and the other by Van Praagh and Van Praagh[20] in 1965 (Fig. 63-9). The Collett and Edwards classification focused on the origin of the pulmonary arteries from the common arterial trunk as follows:

Type I: Common arterial trunk gives rise to a main pulmonary artery and the aorta.
Type II: Right and left pulmonary arteries arise directly and in close proximity from the posterior wall of the truncus.
Type III: Right and left pulmonary arteries arise from more widely separate orifices on the posterior truncal wall.
Type IV: Branch pulmonary arteries are absent. Pulmonary blood flow is derived from aortopulmonary collaterals.

The following system offered by Van Praagh and Van Praagh, a somewhat more surgically oriented scheme, is based on the presence or absence of a VSD, the degree of formation of the aorticopulmonary septum, and the status of the aortic arch:

Type A—with a VSD
Type B—without a VSD
1. The aorticopulmonary septum is partially developed (partially separate main pulmonary artery).
2. The aorticopulmonary septum is absent (no main pulmonary artery segment) both branch pulmonary arteries arise from the common trunk.
3. Absence of either branch pulmonary artery.
4. Hypoplasia, coarctation, atresia, or absence of the aortic isthmus in association with a large PDA.

Persistent truncus arteriosus occurs as a result of the failed development of the aorticopulmonary septum and subpulmonary infundibulum (conal septum). Normal septation leads to both pulmonary and systemic outflow tracts, the division of the semilunar valves, and aorta and pulmonary arteries. Failure of septation results in a VSD (absence of the infundibular septum), a single semilunar valve, and a single arterial trunk.

Most cases are associated with a ventricular septal defect reminiscent of the VSD associated with tetralogy of Fallot. Unlike the VSD in this tetralogy, the superior margin of the defect is formed by the truncal valve.

The truncal valve leaflets are often dysmorphic, being thickened, fleshy, and often restricted in their motion. Leaflet number is highly variable with about 65% being tricuspid, 25% quadricuspid, and 9% bicuspid. As a result of these abnormally developed valve leaflets, about half of the patients present with some degree of truncal valve regurgitation. Truncal valve stenosis can be seen alone or in combination with regurgitation and is present in about one third of cases of truncus arteriosus. Significant obstruction is predicted by gradients of greater than 30 mmHg in the presence of normal cardiac output.

The pulmonary arteries are usually of normal size, and most often arise from the left posterolateral aspect of the truncal artery, often in close proximity to the truncal valve and ostium of the left coronary artery.

Associated lesions include patent foramen ovale, atrial septal defect (10%), persistent left superior vena cava

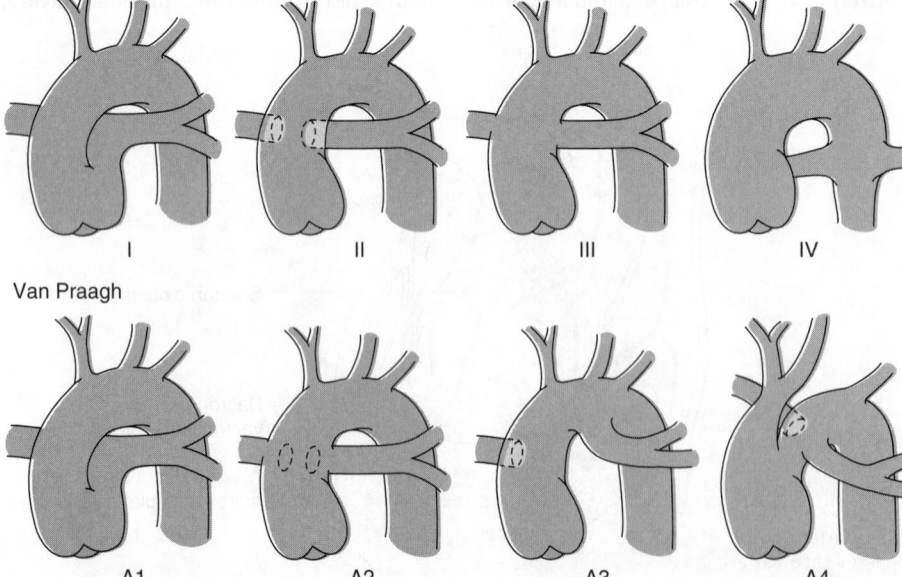

Figure 63-9. Truncus arteriosus: Classification schemes as described by Collett and Edwards and by Van-Praagh and VanPraagh. (Hernanz-Schulman M, Fellows KE. Persistent truncus arteriosus: pathologic, diagnostic, and therapeutic considerations. Semin Roentgenol 1985; 20:121)

(10%), and mitral valve anomalies (5%). Interrupted aortic arch (usually type B) occurs about 20% of the time, and a right aortic arch coexists in 25% to 35% of cases. Coronary artery abnormalities are common (50%) and can lead to coronary arterial injury during repair. Noncardiac anomalies are present in about 20% of cases and may contribute to death. In particular, the DiGeorge syndrome is often associated with truncus arteriosus, and screening of these infants is routine.

The anatomy of truncus arteriosus results in obligatory mixing of the systemic and pulmonary venous blood at the level of the VSD and truncal valve producing arterial saturations of 85% to 90%. The systemic arterial saturation depends on the volume of pulmonary blood flow which in turn is determined by the pulmonary vascular resistance (PVR). As the PVR begins to fall, pulmonary overcirculation ensues leading to pulmonary congestion. This nonrestrictive left-to-right shunt may lead to the early development of irreversible pulmonary vascular obstructive disease.

The presence of truncal valve abnormalities poses further hemodynamic burdens. Truncal valve regurgitation leads to ventricular dilatation and low diastolic coronary perfusion pressures and can result in myocardial ischemia. Truncal valve stenosis promotes ventricular hypertrophy, increases myocardial oxygen demand, and limits coronary and systemic perfusion, especially with the large volume run-off into the pulmonary vascular bed.

Neonates with truncus arteriosus present with signs of CHF and collapsing peripheral pulses. Chest radiography shows marked cardiomegaly, pulmonary plethora, often with minimal thymus shadow, and a right aortic arch. The ECG most often depicts biventricular hypertrophy. Echocardiography is the diagnostic procedure of choice and can demonstrate the truncal vessel, the structure and function of the truncal valve, associated lesions such as interrupted aortic arch, and often the pulmonary artery anatomy. Cardiac catheterization is reserved for cases in which the anatomy is unclear or further information is needed about the status of the truncal valve and for those in whom the status of the pulmonary vasculature is unclear (ie, infants older than 3 months at diagnosis).

The natural history of patients born with truncus arteriosus is early demise. More than 80% of patients succumb by 1 year. Early death is due to CHF. Survivors may do well for a period of time until the development of pulmonary vascular obstructive disease and Eisenmenger syndrome.

The ultimate treatment of truncus arteriosus is surgical therapy. Medical treatment is directed toward controlling CHF by fluid restriction, diuretics, digitalis, and afterload reduction. The onset of tachypnea can be used as a marker to identify declining pulmonary vascular resistance and the optimal timing for repair. Complete repair entails separating the pulmonary arteries from the truncus, repairing the resulting defect in the aorta, closing the ventricular septal defect, and restoring the right ventricular outflow tract continuity using an extra cardiac conduit. Severe truncal valve regurgitation requires truncal valve replacement, which is best done using a small cryopreserved allograft. An associated interrupted aortic arch is repaired by constructing a primary end-to-end anastomosis of the distal ascending aorta with proximal augmentation if necessary.

The results of truncus arteriosus repair have improved greatly over the last two decades. Before the importance of early operation to avoid irreversible pulmonary vascular disease was appreciated, most institutions repaired patients at an average age of 2 to 5 years. Most patients had pulmonary vascular disease, and mortality rates ranged from 25% to 88%. Ebert showed that repair in the first 6 months of life was not only possible but preferable, and he reported a mortality rate of 9%. Recent reports demonstrate improving results with mortality rates for complicated neonatal repairs, ranging from 11% to 20%.[21,22] The presence of aortic arch interruption, severe truncal valve regurgitation, coronary artery anomalies, and age older than 3 months are generally considered important risk factors. Primary repair promptly after presentation is the standard therapy for truncus arteriosus.

CORONARY ARTERY ANOMALIES

Anomalies of coronary artery anatomy are divided into three categories based on their functional significance. Those abnormalities that are of no functional significance are usually detected as incidental findings on cardiac catheterization and occur in about 3 of 1000 patients; however, such coronary artery anomalies may have a somewhat higher than expected frequency of atherosclerotic stenosis. The most common example of this type of finding is the origin of the circumflex coronary artery from the right coronary sinus or as a branch of the right coronary artery.

The second type of coronary anomaly has no intrinsic physiologic effects but because of its presence in patients with other cardiac defects, this type of anomaly alters the surgical management. A common example is an abnormal course of the left anterior descending coronary artery in a patient with tetralogy of Fallot. This abnormal course occurs in 3% to 5% of patients with tetralogy and may prevent a right ventricular incision that might otherwise be performed as part of the operative repair.

The most important types of coronary artery anomalies are those that produce significant adverse effects on the myocardium. Coronary arteriovenous fistula is the most common major anomaly of the coronary circulation. In these defects, the coronary arteries arise normally from the aorta but connect with (in descending order of frequency) the right ventricle, the right atrium (including the coronary sinus or the superior vena cava), the pulmonary artery, the left atrium, the left ventricle, or bronchial veins. This produces a left-to-right shunt, which may result in symptoms of CHF. Angina, endocarditis, myocardial infarction, and, in infants, failure to thrive are other presenting manifestations.[23] The diagnosis can be established by cardiac catheterization or by echocardiography and Doppler ultrasound. Intraoperative echocardiographic and Doppler studies may help to localize the fistula.

The natural history of coronary artery fistulas has not been well defined. In light of the possible increase in size and possible predilection to develop subacute bacterial endocarditis or rupture, however, most investigators recommend obliterating the fistula unless the shunt is insignificant (Qp/Qs less than 1.3/1). Rare fistulas that are discrete and easily located can be closed without cardiopulmonary bypass. More commonly, operation requires opening the recipient cardiac chamber on bypass to identify and securely close all fistulous communications. Furthermore, obliterating the fistula may compromise coronary flow distal to the fistula, and coronary bypass may need to be performed to prevent myocardial ischemia.

The second most frequent clinically important coronary artery anomaly is origin of a coronary artery from the pulmonary artery. This abnormality is more frequently observed in the left coronary artery than in the right. The magnitude of physiologic derangement varies with the extent of collateral formation between the abnormal coronary and the normal vessels. In the postnatal period, as pulmonary vascular resistance falls, a decrease in the perfusion pressure in the distribution of the abnormal artery may result in a steal of blood from the normal coronary circulation into the low-pressure pulmonary artery. If collaterals from the right coronary artery are good and myocardial perfusion remains adequate, this may not present until later in life when the diagnosis is established as part of an evaluation for a cardiac murmur. When there are poor collaterals from the opposite coronary vessel, however, the resulting steal may have profound effects in the neonatal period because of myocardial ischemia. This may manifest itself by irritability, difficulty in feeding, ECG evidence of ischemia and infarction, and evidence of ischemic mitral regurgitation. Typically, symptoms first occur at about 6 weeks to 3 months of life. This anomaly usually requires angiography to establish the anatomic diagnosis, although echocardiography can often describe the origin and course of the coronary arteries. Surgical correction should be performed promptly when this condition is identified. The operative treatment used has varied with the age of the patient and the specifics of the coronary anatomy. When collaterals are extensive, simple ligation of the anomalous vessel at its origin has been used to eliminate the steal into the pulmonary circulation without impairing myocardial perfusion. Although this approach may be life-saving, particularly in the symptomatic infant, it results in a one–coronary artery system, leaving left coronary flow dependent on collaterals from the right. This situation often results in chronic ischemia later in life. Attempts at restoring a normal arterial supply with coronary artery bypass using a saphenous vein, internal mammary artery, or subclavian artery have been successful. Bypass operations may be technically difficult in the diminutive vessels of the infant, and long-term patency is suboptimal, particularly when saphenous vein is used. The optimal surgical approach is to construct a direct connection between the aorta and the anomalous coronary, either by direct implantation or by the creation of tunnel in the pulmonary artery. This technique has proved successful in neonates and has excellent long-term results.[24]

A potentially dangerous abnormality exists when the left main coronary artery arises from the right coronary sinus and passes between the pulmonary artery and the aorta. Fatal complications may also occur when the right coronary artery arises from the left coronary sinus and passes between the great arteries, particularly when the right coronary is dominant. The precise pathophysiologic sequence by which these abnormalities cause death is the subject of debate. This condition often causes sudden death during vigorous physical exertion in young, healthy individuals. It has therefore been suggested that an increase in aortic and pulmonary artery pressure causes extrinsic compression of the coronary artery (the vascular vise). Others have observed that the orifice of these anomalous arteries is elliptical and have hypothesized that the increase in aortic diameter with increased cardiac output causes coronary obstruction by further narrowing the orifice. Regardless of the precise physiologic events, diagnosis of this abnormality is an indication for operative treatment. Typically, coronary artery bypass with the internal mammary artery can be performed with a low operative risk.

PATENT DUCTUS ARTERIOSUS

Normally, pulmonary vascular resistance declines and pulmonary blood flow increases proportionately after birth. The resultant increase in arterial oxygen tension stimulates the closure of the ductus arteriosus. This may fail to occur because of other cardiac or pulmonary conditions associated with abnormally low arterial oxygen or may be an isolated lesion. Isolated PDA is most frequently observed in premature infants. These patients typically are in respiratory distress, but it may be difficult to determine

whether this is attributable to the PDA or to an immature pulmonary bed.

Indomethacin administration can cause the ductus to close. Indomethacin works by inhibiting cyclooxygenase and diminishing endogenous prostaglandins that contribute to ductal patency. Part of the effect of indomethacin may also be attributed to an increase in norepinephrine release, which in turn causes the richly innervated ductus to constrict. Indomethacin may adversely affect kidney and platelet function and is contraindicated in patients with sepsis, coagulopathy, intracranial hemorrhage, and hepatic dysfunction. The efficacy of indomethacin is variable in babies weighing more than 1 kg. Operative closure can be done safely in even the smallest neonates. Prophylactic surgical closure of the ductus arteriosus in extremely premature babies has been shown to reduce the risk of necrotizing enterocolitis.[25] The improvement in pulmonary function is often dramatic and may permit ventilator-dependent patients to be rapidly extubated.

In older children, a PDA usually presents as an asymptomatic murmur—the classic "machinery" murmur—with or without a hyperdynamic precordium. Pharmacologic closure of the ductus is rarely successful beyond the neonatal period, and surgical closure is required. Operation is indicated for isolated PDA in virtually all cases to prevent eventual development of pulmonary vascular changes and congestive failure. Even the small ductus that is hemodynamically insignificant should be closed to prevent the complications of endocarditis, which may be a consequence of abnormally turbulent blood flow in this area.

In virtually all infants and most older children, ductus closure is accomplished by ligation through a left thoracotomy. Some surgeons prefer to divide the ductus in patients in whom it can be safely accomplished. In premature infants, closure can be accomplished with vascular hemoclips through a minithoracotomy. Careful definition of the anatomy—most importantly, the recurrent laryngeal nerve—permits accomplishing this procedure with an extremely low risk of complications. The mortality rate of the operation approaches zero.

Recent advances include thoracoscopic ligation and transcatheter closure. Transcatheter closure using the techniques of the Rashkind double umbrella is possible in older infants and children.[26] Small PDAs can also be closed using coils. Although initial results have been encouraging, further follow-up is necessary to judge the results compared with the gold standard of surgical closure. Finally, thoracoscopic closure of PDAs has reached the clinical arena. Advances in pediatric fiberoptics and the improved smaller thoracoscopic equipment have made closure possible with acceptable initial results.[27]

The rare adult with a PDA can pose difficult technical problems. Pulmonary artery pressures in these cases may be markedly elevated, and an aneurysm of the ductus may occur. The ductus in older individuals is highly susceptible to calcification, which may make simple ligation hazardous. In other patients, recurrent episodes of endocarditis or endarteritis may make the ductal tissue extremely friable. Safe operative division in some cases requires cardiopulmonary bypass with suture closure from within the pulmonary artery.

ATRIOVENTRICULAR SEPTAL DEFECT

Defects in the embryologic development of the endocardial cushions may result in a variety of morphologic abnormalities in the AV valves and the atrial and ventricular septa. These anomalies range from the ostium primum ASD to the complete AVSD (or AV canal defect), with a spectrum of intermediate forms. PDA and tetralogy of Fallot are occasionally seen in association with these defects. A high percentage of patients with abnormalities of the AV structures have Down syndrome.

Complete AVSD is an anomaly in which there is a common AV orifice rather than separate mitral and tricuspid orifices, accompanied by a deficiency of the endocardial cushion tissue resulting in an ASD and an inlet type of VSD. AVSDs are classified per Rastelli into the following three types according to the morphology of the anterior leaflet of the common AV valve:

Type A: The anterior bridging leaflet is divided and attached to the septum by multiple chordae.
Type B: The anterior bridging leaflet is attached to a papillary muscle in the right ventricle
Type C: The anterior bridging leaflet is free-floating, with no attachments except to the valve annulus.

Despite the extreme degrees of abnormal supporting structures that are commonly found, the valves themselves are almost always competent.

AVSD is rarely diagnosed in the neonatal period, because the pulmonary vascular resistance remains elevated for longer than usual. The occasional patient with significant AV valve insufficiency may present as a newborn. Usually in the first 6 to 12 months of life, excessive pulmonary blood flow produces severe congestive failure, manifested by dyspnea, poor feeding, and delayed growth. Patients who present beyond age 2 or 3 years often have Eisenmenger syndrome with irreversible pulmonary vascular disease.

Physical examination of patients with AVSDs demonstrates increased precordial activity and fixed splitting of the second heart sound. The chest radiograph in these individuals shows increased pulmonary vascularity and cardiomegaly. The ECG shows right ventricular or biventricular hypertrophy.

Echocardiography provides excellent assessment of the anatomy in AVSDs and defines the presence or absence of valvular insufficiency. Echocardiography also provides important information about the relative sizes of the ventricles. Hypoplasia of one ventricle may dictate an alteration in the operative approach. Despite the proven value of echocardiography as a sole diagnostic modality for AVSD, many groups continue to recommend catheterization before operative intervention, primarily to evaluate pulmonary artery resistance especially in patients with Down syndrome who are older than 6 months. If the pulmonary artery resistance is high, it is important to remeasure it while the child is breathing 100% oxygen. If the pulmonary resistance falls, it implies that much of the elevated resistance is dynamic and can be managed in the perioperative period by vigorous ventilation and supplemental oxygen. Markedly elevated pulmonary resistance (more than 8 to 10 Wood units) that does not respond to oxygen administration may in some cases contraindicate repair.

Operative treatment is almost always necessary as soon as symptoms are observed to prevent further clinical deterioration. Even in the absence of symptoms, operation is best performed before 6 months of age. Pulmonary artery banding, which permits delaying the repair until the child is larger, is no longer used today. This approach exposes the child to the risks of two operations, and the overall mortality exceeds that of primary repair in infancy.

Correcting AVSDs requires patch closure of both septal defects, with reattachment of the valve apparatus to the newly constructed septa. Separate atrial and ventricular patches or a single patch for both chambers can be used.[28] During closure of the ventricular defect, the surgeon must carefully avoid injury to the conduction system, which

passes along the posterior and inferior rim of the ventricular septum.

The success of the operation is highly dependent on the status of the pulmonary vascular resistance and the surgeon's ability to maintain competence of the mitral and tricuspid valves. Because the mitral valve usually has three component leaflets, much debate has focused on whether this valve should be made into a two-leaflet structure at operation by approximating the "cleft" between the two septal leaflets with sutures. Many surgeons believe this separation is not a true cleft that should be closed, but is rather a commissure in a three-leaflet valve that should be preserved. Others believe mitral competence is best preserved by closing this cleft, making this valve a two-leaflet structure. When important insufficiency is present, the location of the regurgitation must be precisely determined at operation to perform an accurate valvuloplasty.

The immediate operative results are good, especially if the patient is treated before the development of pulmonary vascular disease. Patients with severe preoperative valvar regurgitation, those with significant associated defects, and those with pulmonary vascular disease do not fare as well. Late reoperation sometimes is necessary because of problems with the mitral or tricuspid valve, but should be rare if initial operative management is carried out precisely.

COARCTATION OF THE AORTA

Coarctation of the aorta (COA) is a narrowing that most commonly occurs in the upper descending aorta just distal to the left subclavian artery. COA is thought to occur when this area contains ectopic tissue from the ductus arteriosus. As the ductus undergoes normal involution and closure, this ectopic tissue also constricts, leaving a luminal narrowing. Coarctations vary in the degree of luminal stenosis and the length of aorta affected. Typically, there is a shelflike projection of aortic media and intima at the area of tightest obstruction. COA may be associated with tubular hypoplasia of the more proximal aortic arch. Coarctation is associated with Turner syndrome.

A prominent feature of COA is extensive development of collateral arteries. These collaterals, which typically involve the internal mammary arteries and the intercostal arteries, produce many of the classic findings of COA. Extensive flow through the collaterals causes pulsations under the ribs and near the scapula, bruits that may be heard diffusely over the chest wall, and rib notching as seen on chest radiograph.

The most common cardiac anomaly found in association with COA is a bicuspid aortic valve, which may or may not be of clinical importance. VSDs and severe aortic stenosis may be seen as well, particularly in highly symptomatic neonates.

In the newborn period, COA may present with profound CHF. The precordium is typically hyperdynamic, and a harsh murmur is audible over the left chest and back. Femoral pulses are diminished or undetectable. The onset of symptoms may coincide with closure of the ductus. Before ductal closure, differential cyanosis (pink upper body and cyanotic lower body) provides evidence that the lower body is dependent on ductal flow. Rib notching is not seen in this early period, although cardiomegaly is observed radiographically.

Older children are almost always asymptomatic. These patients are usually diagnosed because of upper extremity hypertension with diminished or absent lower extremity pulses. The chest film generally shows rib notching and the typical 3 shadow in the aortic knob. Asymmetry of the rib notching may suggest anomalous origin or stenosis of a subclavian artery. Adults presenting with COA may have developed severe hypertension as well as congestive failure. No single cause of hypertension in COA has been defined. Mechanical obstruction to ventricular ejection is one component leading to elevated arterial pressure. Hypoperfusion of the kidneys with resulting activation of the renin–angiotensin–aldosterone axis probably contributes to some degree. Abnormal aortic compliance, variable capacity of collateral vessels, and abnormal setting of baroreceptors have also been implicated in the pathogenesis of hypertension.

Many patients with COA can be diagnosed on physical examination alone. Echocardiography frequently can provide excellent demonstration of the anatomy and estimate the pressure gradient. Aortography with pressure measurement can be used when the diagnosis is unclear and permits definition of other possible cardiac anomalies. In adolescents and adults, the aortogram may be particularly useful to the surgeon in demonstrating the presence or absence of collaterals, because this may influence the operative management.

In the neonate with COA and CHF, operative repair is performed as a life-saving measure. In older children, COA should be repaired to prevent the long-term sequelae of hypertension, heart failure, endocarditis, aortic rupture, and intracranial vascular lesions. Patients with COA and severe hypertension should undergo operation as early as possible. The earlier the operation is performed, the more likely the patient is to become normotensive.

The surgical technique varies with the patient's age and particular anatomy.[29] Resection of the coarctation segment with direct end-to-end anastomosis is preferred in those cases where the anatomy demonstrates that a direct anastomosis can be achieved without excessive tension. This method of repair has the benefit of removing all diseased tissue, particularly residual ductal tissue, which may contract and cause further narrowing if left behind. Absorbable sutures can be used to perform the reconstruction in the hope that growth of the aorta will not be compromised. The subclavian flap angioplasty is an alternative technique used to enlarge the narrowed portion of the aorta with viable arterial wall. The affected portion of the aorta is opened longitudinally and augmented with the adjacent subclavian artery. Blood flow to the left arm is subsequently provided by collateral vessels. Although growth and function of the arm almost always remain normal, long-term studies have demonstrated slight limb-length discrepancy in some patients. Less commonly, reconstruction with a patch or an end-to-end interposition graft is performed. Many surgeons believe that patch reconstruction carries a high risk of aneurysm formation. These aneurysms occur not on the patched side of the aorta but on the opposite wall.

One of the major intraoperative concerns during COA repair is the problem with interrupting distal aortic blood flow, particularly to the spinal cord. The risk of paraplegia after this operation is low but is elevated in the absence of large collaterals. It is often advisable to place a femoral artery catheter to monitor lower body arterial pressure during the operative repair. If inadequate distal perfusion pressure is found, some method of providing additional lower body flow should be performed. We prefer partial cardiac bypass using either the femoral artery or distal thoracic aorta for arterial supply and the femoral vein or left atrium for venous return. This maintains blood flow to the spinal cord, kidneys, and other organs and assists in managing overall hemodynamics during aortic clamping and unclamping. Newborns with coarctation and large VSDs have a particularly high risk of hemodynamic instability. These patients are best treated by simultaneous VSD closure in addition to coarctation repair with a median

sternotomy and a short period of hypothermic circulatory arrest.

The treatment of patients after COA repair often focuses on controlling hypertension. This hypertension may be observed regardless of the degree of anatomic obstruction relief, and the blood pressure may exceed preoperative levels. The pathogenesis of this so-called paradoxical hypertension is thought to be related to stimulation of sympathetic nerve fibers in the aortic wall. An infusion of sodium nitroprusside or intermittent administration of propranolol is usually effective in keeping arterial pressure within an acceptable range.[30]

Abdominal discomfort during this time may be a symptom of mesenteric arteritis. This problem is thought to result from restored pulsatile flow to the visceral vessels, resulting in spasm and potential intestinal ischemia. This complication, which can be fatal, is almost completely preventable by proper control of blood pressure. In addition, it is advisable to strictly forbid oral intake until bowel function returns.

Some reports have described balloon dilatation as an effective therapy for COA, although false aneurysms, dissection, and inadequate dilatation have been problems with this technique and may complicate a subsequent operation. Balloon dilatation appears to have a more promising application to the 7% to 10% of recurrent coarctations after initial surgical repair. In these cases, the additional aortic wall mass from scarring and adhesions may make this technique safer. The long-term results of coarctation repair are generally good with the optimal technique in infants and children being resection with primary end-to-end anastomosis.

UNIVENTRICULAR HEART

A univentricular heart is a congenital anomaly characterized by the presence of only one ventricular chamber connected to the atria. To be classified as a ventricle, a chamber must receive at least half of an inlet valve. In the most common form of univentricular heart, both the mitral and tricuspid valves connect to a morphologic left ventricle (double-inlet left ventricle), which ejects blood through a hypoplastic outlet chamber and then to the aorta. The outlet chamber cannot be considered a ventricle, regardless of its size, because it does not receive an inlet valve. Univentricular hearts are frequently associated with malpositions of the great vessels and varying degrees of obstruction to pulmonary blood flow. In double-inlet left ventricle, the aorta is usually anterior and to the left of the pulmonary artery.

Infants with univentricular hearts have variable presentations, depending on the status of the pulmonary blood flow.[31] When pulmonary flow is excessive, cyanosis may be mild and the dominant feature is CHF. Pulmonary stenosis decreases pulmonary blood flow, and the degree of cyanosis is therefore increased. Associated lesions may further complicate the picture, such as coarctation of the aorta, subaortic stenosis, or a restrictive ASD. Patients with moderate pulmonary stenosis may achieve a well-balanced circulation with acceptable systemic oxygenation and normal pulmonary artery pressure. These patients may be symptom-free well into adolescence. Most patients, however, require intervention early in life to reduce pulmonary blood flow if excessive or to increase this flow in the presence of severe pulmonary stenosis. Pulmonary vascular obstructive disease develops early when pulmonary blood flow is excessive. With the possible exception of patients with well-balanced pulmonary and systemic blood flow, the prognosis for patients with unoperated univentricular hearts is poor. More than half of these patients die early of CHF or dysrhythmias.

In the presence of excessive pulmonary blood flow and pulmonary hypertension, operation should be performed early in life to control pulmonary blood flow and to prevent the development of pulmonary vascular occlusive disease. Options include pulmonary artery banding or division of the main pulmonary artery in conjunction with a controlled aortopulmonary shunt. Pulmonary artery banding is a less complicated procedure; however, it is often difficult to accurately adjust the pulmonary flow, and too proximal or too distal a band can lead to pulmonary artery distortion, further complicating later operations. Another option is division of the main pulmonary artery, side-to-side anastomosis with the native aorta, and a modified Blalock-Taussig shunt (modified Damus-Kaye-Stanzel procedure). This procedure more accurately limits the pulmonary blood flow and eliminates the possibility of subaortic obstruction which can occur when the systemic blood flow depends on egress through a bulboventricular foramen. Pulmonary stenosis may be palliated by a systemic-to-pulmonary artery shunt procedure. We prefer a modified Blalock-Taussig shunt with a right thoracotomy in most patients. This procedure increases systemic saturation with minimal risk of causing excessive pulmonary blood flow or pulmonary artery distortion. In infants older than 4 to 6 months, a Hemifontan connection, in which the superior vena caval flow is directed into the pulmonary arteries, can be used to increase effective pulmonary blood flow. This procedure maximizes pulmonary flow without providing volume overload to the single ventricle. It is most commonly used as part of a complete atriopulmonary connection, often as a preliminary first stage.

The goal of surgical correction for patients with univentricular hearts involves total diversion of all vena caval blood directly into the pulmonary arteries; this is called the Fontan procedure.[32] This procedure was first successfully performed in a patient with tricuspid atresia but has since evolved as an excellent way to establish physiologic repair for patients with more complex forms of univentricular heart. Although many modifications of the technique have been made, the best approach involves direct anastomosis of the right atrium and superior vena cava to the pulmonary artery without the use of a valve. Systemic and pulmonary venous blood flow is divided in the atrium by using a prosthetic patch (ie, lateral tunnel technique). All pulmonary venous flow then empties into the ventricular chamber through the AV valves, while superior and inferior vena caval blood drains through the atriopulmonary anastomosis (Fig. 63-10). For the Fontan procedure to be performed with a low operative mortality and an acceptable functional result, certain criteria must be met. Normal pulmonary artery pressure (below 20 mmHg) and pulmonary vascular resistance (less than 2 Woods units) are the most important prerequisites. Additionally, it is essential that ventricular function and atrioventricular valve function are normal. Many of the criteria originally proposed, including normal cardiac rhythm, right atrial hypertrophy, normal systemic venous return, and age older than 4 years, have little or no importance. Although the Fontan procedure cannot be considered a truly corrective operation, it offers benefits that cannot be equaled by any of the other palliative procedures. The major advantages include restoration of normal systemic oxygen saturation and reduction of ventricular volume overload. These benefits may well protect against later ventricular failure and the complications associated with long-standing cyanosis. The addition of a fixed orifice right-

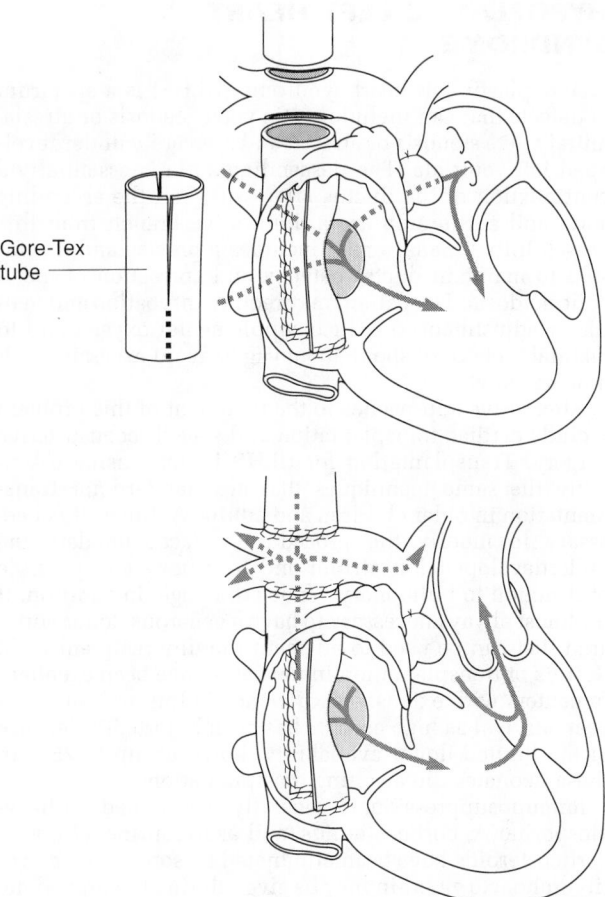

Figure 63-10. Total cavopulmonary connection for univentricular heart. The internal orifices of the superior and inferior vena cavas are connected in the right atrium with a patch cut from a Gore-Tex tube. The superior vena cava is divided just above its junction, with the right atrium and both ends anastomosed to the right pulmonary artery. The main pulmonary artery is ligated.

to-left shunt (ie, fenestrated Fontan), which preserves systemic output in the face of transient elevations in pulmonary vascular resistance, may help to reduce early postoperative morbidity.[33]

Ventricular septation procedures have also been successfully performed in patients with univentricular hearts. The subset of patients with double-inlet left ventricles, anterior and leftward aortas, a nonrestrictive outlet foramen, and mild or no pulmonary stenosis are best suited for septation. This anatomy allows placement of a relatively direct and straight prosthetic patch in the ventricle that separates the pulmonary and systemic circulations. The septation procedure has been associated with a relatively high morbidity, primarily related to complete heart block, thus reducing its overall effectiveness. A few centers have continued to apply this procedure in carefully selected patients.

The operative risk for the Fontan procedure when all preoperative risk factors are within acceptable limits is 5% to 10%. Although the operation may be used in patients who do not meet one or more of these criteria, the risk may increase substantially. Survivors are significantly improved, and most function in New York Heart Association class I or II. Although long-term results are encouraging, late complications may be seen. Continued surveillance for arrhythmias, CHF, protein-losing enteropathy, and hepatic dysfunction remain important.

HYPOPLASTIC LEFT HEART SYNDROME

Hypoplastic left heart syndrome (HLHS) is a spectrum of defects that can include aortic valve stenosis or atresia, mitral valve stenosis or atresia, and a severely underdeveloped left ventricle. The descending aorta is essentially a continuation of the ductus arteriosus, and the ascending aorta and aortic arch are a diminutive branch from this vessel. Initial management includes a prostaglandin infusion to maintain ductal patency and correction of metabolic acidosis. The patient may require intubation and ventilator adjustment to reduce supplemental oxygen and to maintain a PCO_2 of about 40 mmHg to avoid excessive pulmonary flow.

Alternative approaches to the treatment of this problem include cardiac transplantation and staged reconstructive surgery. Transplantation for HLHS is done using essentially the same techniques that are standard for transplantation in older children and adults. At times, it is necessary to modify the procedure to accommodate the underdeveloped left atrium and to relieve any possible obstruction to pulmonary venous drainage. In addition, it is almost always necessary to have a generous donor aortic arch that can be used to augment the tiny recipient arch. Results of transplantation in neonates have been excellent in centers with extensive experience in this area, and a 2-year survival as high as 70% has been reported.[34] Because of the limited donor availability, however, up to 25% of these neonates die awaiting transplantation.

Immunosuppression is generally maintained with cyclosporine A, corticosteroids, and azathioprine, although corticosteroids have been eliminated by some groups. Antilymphocyte globulin may be given during the immediate postoperative period and during treatment of rejection. Myocardial biopsies are done infrequently because of difficulty with access. Although transplantation remains a viable option, it is plagued by problems of infection, acute rejection, and the possibility of graft atherosclerosis.

Even if transplantation could be performed with perfect results, the limited supply of donor hearts necessitates reconstruction for a large number of babies with HLHS. The operation developed by Norwood and colleagues for first-stage palliation of this defect has permitted excellent growth and development[35] (Fig. 63-11). The Norwood procedure converts the pulmonary artery into the main outlet for what is to be a functional single ventricle. The aortic arch is augmented with a large piece of allograft artery and anastomosed to the pulmonary root. The distal pulmonary arteries are separated from their origin and are supplied with blood through a systemic–pulmonary artery shunt. Critical elements of this operation include excising the interatrial septum, extending the arch augmentation beyond the ductus arteriosus, preserving coronary artery perfusion, and creating an appropriately sized aortopulmonary shunt. Postoperatively, careful ventilator management is mandatory to help adjust pulmonary vascular resistance and maintain the proper balance of pulmonary and systemic blood flow. Subsequent reconstructive management of HLHS includes a bidirectional superior vena cava–pulmonary artery anastomosis at about 6 months to 1 year of age, followed by completion of a modified Fontan reconstruction at about 18 months. In the latter operation, inferior vena caval blood is routed to the pulmonary artery, thus providing a physiologic repair by diverting all systemic venous return directly to the lungs.

Survival after first-stage reconstruction for HLHS exceeds 80% in experienced centers.[36] The use of an intermediate procedure in which the superior vena cava is transected and anastomosed to the undivided pulmonary artery is anticipated to improve late survival and reduce the risk of the Fontan procedure. Again, the bidirectional Glenn procedure or Hemifontan operation relieves the volume load on the ventricle while improving effective pulmonary blood flow. Although the reconstructive route entails three separate operations, when the results for primary transplantation include patients who die while waiting for donor organs, the replacement and reconstructive approaches have similar short-term results.

PRIMARY NEOPLASMS OF THE HEART AND PERICARDIUM

Primary tumors of the heart and pericardium are extremely rare. Metastatic lesions are 20 to 30 times more common. Of primary cardiac tumors, benign lesions predominate over malignant ones by a 3:1 ratio. The presentation of cardiac tumors may include congestive failure, angina, syncope, pulmonary hypertension, pulmonary or systemic emboli, arrhythmias, hemolysis, and a variety of systemic manifestations that may create a puzzling clinical picture.

Initial diagnostic studies in patients with cardiac neoplasms are rarely specific. An occasional tumor may calcify, facilitating roentgenographic diagnosis. ECG may show nonspecific chamber enlargement or rhythm disturbances. The diagnosis of these tumors has been greatly advanced in recent years by 2D echocardiography, although distinguishing a tumor from thrombus may be difficult. Cardiac catheterization and angiography may be unable to identify the tumor by negative-contrast images. Furthermore, transseptal puncture to identify the most common cardiac tumors, located in the left atrium, may be hazardous because of the risk of systemic embolism.

The most common primary cardiac neoplasm is the myxoma. This may present in patients of either sex, of any age, and in any cardiac chamber. Familial predilections to myxomas exist. Although some pathologists have argued that myxomas are really organized thrombi, most believe they are true neoplasms. Over 75% of myxomas arise in the left atrium, and 5% are multiple. Myxomas are most commonly attached to the fossa ovalis and are said to never arise from the cardiac valves. Myxomas are yellow-brown to pale gray gelatinous masses of up to 15 cm in diameter. They rarely extend deeper than the endocardium. Malignant degeneration is not thought to occur in myxomas, although their ability to recur after inadequate resection and their occasional multiplicity may create a suspicion of malignant behavior.

Because they commonly arise in the left atrium, these lesions may present with symptoms typical of mitral valve disease, including murmurs, atrial arrhythmias, systemic emboli, and CHF. One striking symptom that should arouse suspicion of a myxoma is dyspnea that varies dramatically with posture, especially dyspnea that is aggravated by an upright position.

All myxomas should be resected because of their potential for causing CHF and stroke. At operation, the myxoma should be completely excised, including its base on the atrial septum. Often, a small patch is required to close the remaining atrial septal defect. A careful inspection of all cardiac chambers for possible undiagnosed tumors is a mandatory part of this procedure. The operative mortality rate approaches zero, and the long-term outlook is generally completely benign.

Rhabdomyoma is the most common cardiac tumor in infancy and childhood, usually presenting before the age of 1 year. Most are located in the left or right ventricle and often protrude into the ventricular lumen, where they may

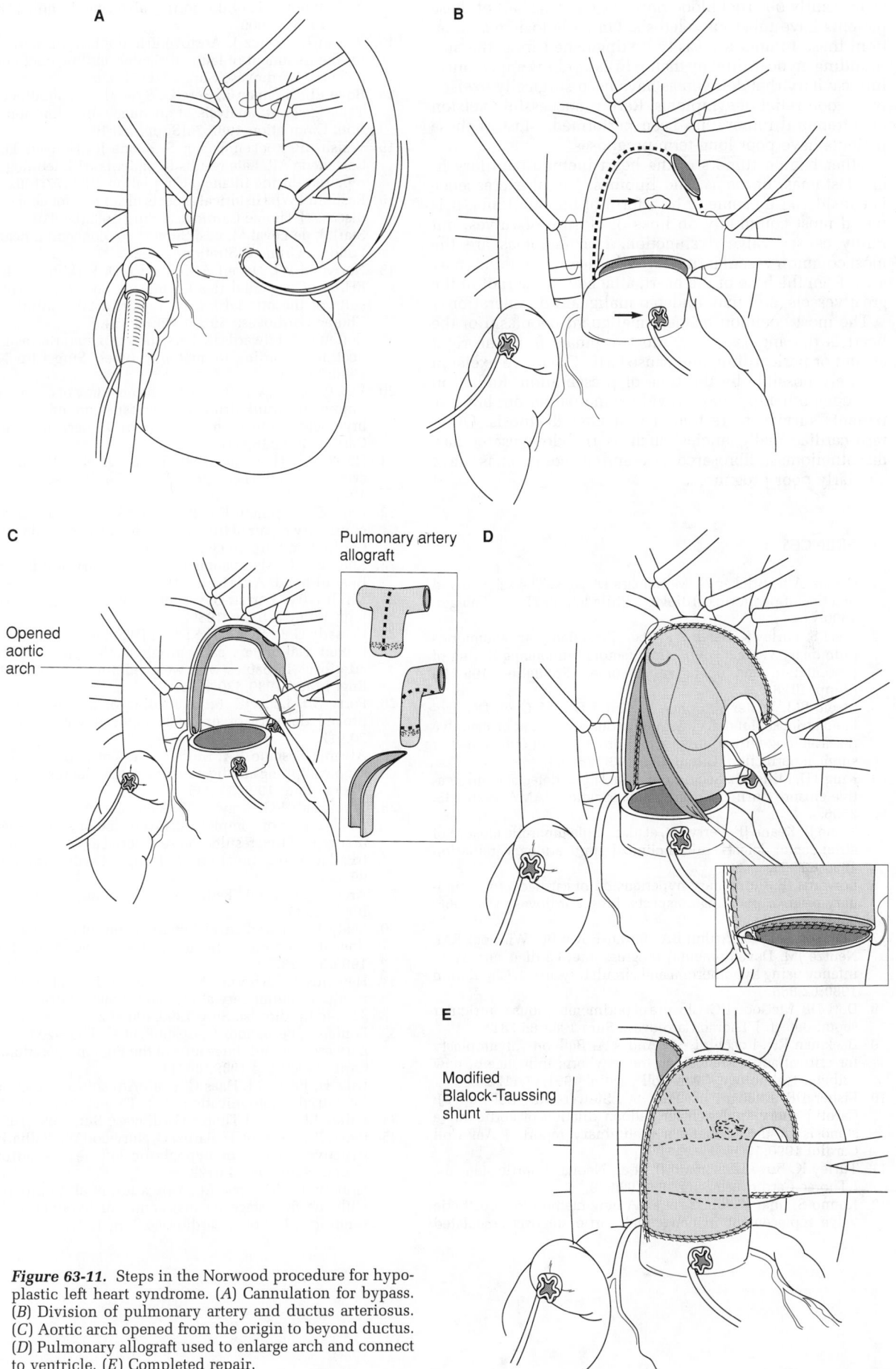

Figure 63-11. Steps in the Norwood procedure for hypoplastic left heart syndrome. (*A*) Cannulation for bypass. (*B*) Division of pulmonary artery and ductus arteriosus. (*C*) Aortic arch opened from the origin to beyond ductus. (*D*) Pulmonary allograft used to enlarge arch and connect to ventricle. (*E*) Completed repair.

significantly obstruct blood flow. As many as half of these patients have tuberous sclerosis. On pathologic examination, these tumors are easily distinguished from the surrounding myocardium by their whitish yellow appearance. Intracavitary rhabdomyomas have been surgically excised with good relief of symptoms. Rarely, successful excision of intramural tumors has been performed. Most of these patients have poor long-term prognoses.

Other benign tumors of the heart include papillary fibroelastomas, fibromas, and lipomas. Lambl excrescence is considered by some to be a form of fibroelastoma. It is found most commonly on lines of closure of valves, but rarely causes valve dysfunction. Hemangiomas are the most common vascular tumors of the heart. Teratomas may arise from the base of the heart, attached to the root of the great vessels, and may undergo malignant degeneration.

The most common primary malignant neoplasm of the heart is the angiosarcoma. Most originate from the right atrium or pericardium and cause CHF. Operative excision is rarely possible by the time of presentation. Radiation and chemotherapy may provide some palliation, but few patients survive more than a year after diagnosis. Other rare cardiac malignancies, such as rhabdomyosarcomas, mesotheliomas, fibrosarcomas, and osteosarcomas have similarly poor prognoses.

REFERENCES

1. Garson A Jr, Bricker JT, McNamara DG, eds. The science and practice of pediatric cardiology. Philadelphia, Lea & Febiger, 1990.
2. Yee ES, Turley K, Hsieh WR, Ebert PA. Infant total anomalous pulmonary venous connection: factors influencing timing of presentation and operative outcome. Circulation 1987;76 (Suppl III):83.
3. Steele PM, Fuster V, Cohen M, Ritter DG, McGoon DC. Isolated atrial septal defect with pulmonary vascular obstructive disease: long-term follow-up and prediction of outcome after surgical correction. Circulation 1987;76:1037.
4. King TD, Mills NL. Secundum atrial septal defects: nonoperative closure during cardiac catheterization. JAMA 1976;235:2506.
5. Rome JJ, Keane JF, Perry SB, et al. Double umbrella closure of atrial septal defects: initial clinical applications. Circulation 1990;82:751.
6. Edwards JE. Pulmonary hypertension of cardiac and pulmonary origins: pathologic aspects. Prog Cardiovasc Dis 1966;9:205.
7. Clarkson PM, MacArthur BA, Barratt-Boyes BG, Whitlock RM, Neutze JM. Developmental progress after cardiac surgery in infancy using hypothermia and circulatory arrest. Circulation 1980;62:855.
8. Doty DB, McGoon DC. Closure of perimembranous ventricular septal defect. J Thorac Cardiovasc Surg 1983;85:781.
9. Beekman RH, Rocchini AP, Andes A. Balloon valvuloplasty for critical aortic stenosis in the newborn: influence of new catheter technology. J Am Coll Cardiol 1991;17:1172.
10. Fisher DR, Ettedgui JA, Park SC, Siewers RD, DelNido PJ: Carotid artery approach for balloon dilation of aortic valve stenosis in the neonate: a preliminary report. J Am Coll Cardiol 1990;15:1633.
11. Turley K, Bove EL, Amato JJ, et al. Neonatal aortic stenosis. J Thorac Cardiovasc Surg 1990;99:679.
12. Konno S, Imai Y, Iida Y, et al. A new method for prosthetic valve replacement in congenital aortic stenosis associated with hypoplasia of the aortic valve ring. J Thorac Cardiovasc Surg 1975;70:909.
13. Rastan H, Koncz J. Aortoventriculoplasty: a new technique for the treatment of left ventricular outflow tract obstruction. J Thorac Cardiovasc Surg 1976;71:920.
14. Bove EL, Kohman L, Sereika S, et al. The modified Blalock-Taussig shunt: analysis of adequacy and duration of palliation. Circulation 1987;76(Suppl III):19.
15. Walsh EP, Rockenmacher S, Keane JF, Hougen TJ, Lock JE, Castaneda AR. Late results in patients with tetralogy of Fallot repaired during infancy. Circulation 1988;77:1062.
16. Rashkind WJ. Historical aspects of surgery for congenital heart disease. J Thorac Cardiovasc Surg 1982;84:619.
17. Stark J, de Leval M, eds. Surgery for congenital heart defects. London, Grune & Stratton, 1983.
18. Norwood WI, Dobell AR, Freed MD, Kirklin JW, Blackstone EH, the Congenital Heart Surgeons Society. Intermediate results of the arterial switch repair: a 20-institution study. J Thorac Cardiovasc Surg 1988;96:854.
19. Collett RW, Edwards JE. Persistent truncus arteriosus: a classification according to anatomic types. Surg Clin North Am 1949;29:1245.
20. Van Praagh R, Van Praagh S. The anatomy of common aortico-pulmonary trunk (truncus arteriosus communis) and its embryologic implications: a study of 57 necropsy cases. Am J Cardiol 1965;16:406.
21. Hanley FL, Heinemann MK, Jonas RA, et al. Repair of truncus arteriosus in the neonate. J Thorac Cardiovasc Surg 1993;105:1047.
22. Bove EL, Lupinetti FM, Pridjian AK, et al. Results of a policy of primary repair of truncus arteriosus in the neonate. J Thorac Cardiovasc Surg 1993;105:1057.
23. Roberts WC. Major anomalies of coronary arterial origin seen in adulthood. Am Heart J 1986;111:941.
24. Kirklin JW, Barratt-Boyes BG. Cardiac surgery. New York, John Wiley & Sons, 1986.
25. Cassady G, Crouse DT, Kirklin JW, et al. A randomized, controlled trial of very early prophylactic ligation of the ductus arteriosus in babies who weighed 1000 g or less at birth. N Engl J Med 1989;320:1511.
26. Perry SB, Lock JE. Front loading of double umbrellas: Improved delivery of umbrella devices. Am J Cardiol 1992;70:917.
27. Alvarez-Tostado RA, Millan MA, Tovar LA, et al. Thoracoscopic clipping and ligation of a patent ductus arteriosus. Ann Thorac Surg 1994;57:755.
28. Weintraub RG, Brawn WJ, Venables AW, Mee RBB. Two-patch repair of complete atrioventricular septal defect in the first year of life: results and sequential assessment of atrioventricular valve function. J Thorac Cardiovasc Surg 1990;99:320.
29. Arciniegas E, ed. Pediatric cardiac surgery. Chicago, Year Book, 1985.
30. Sealy WC. Paradoxical hypertension after repair of coarctation of the aorta: a review of its causes. Ann Thorac Surg 1990;50:323.
31. Hawkins JA, Thorne JK, Boucek MM, et al. Early and late results in pulmonary atresia and intact ventricular septum. J Thorac Cardiovasc Surg 1990;100:492.
32. Fontan F, Fernandez G, Costa F, et al. The size of the pulmonary arteries and the results of the Fontan operation. J Thorac Cardiovasc Surg 1989;98:711.
33. Laks H, Pearl JM, Haas G, et.al. Advantages of an adjustable interatrial communication. Ann Thorac Surg 1991;52:1089.
34. Bailey LL, et al. J Thorac Cardiovasc Surg 1993;105:805.
35. Pigott JD, Murphy JD, Barber G, Norwood WI. Palliative reconstructive surgery for hypoplastic left heart syndrome. Ann Thorac Surg 1988;45:122.
36. Iannettoni MD, Bove EL, Mosca RS, et al. Improving results with the first stage reconstruction of hypoplastic left heart syndrome. J Thorac Cardiovasc Surg 1994;107:934.

SURGERY: SCIENTIFIC PRINCIPLES AND PRACTICE, Second Edition, edited by Lazar J. Greenfield, Michael W. Mulholland, Keith T. Oldham, Gerald B. Zelenock, and Keith D. Lillemoe. Lippincott–Raven Publishers, Philadelphia, © 1997.

CHAPTER 64

VALVULAR HEART DISEASE

O. WAYNE ISOM AND TODD K. ROSENGART

The introduction of the pump oxygenator by Gibbons in 1953 transformed the landscape of potential cardiac operations by allowing open heart surgery. Various valvular operations were introduced by such pioneers as Bahnson, Harken, McGoon, Lillehei, and others, but results, especially for valvular insufficiency, were often suboptimal. Then, in 1963, the Starr-Edwards ball-valve prosthesis, named for the surgeon and mechanical engineer responsible for its development, ushered in the newest era of valvular surgery. Since then, many modifications and different forms of prosthetic heart valves have been developed. Today, more than 10,000 operations for valve repair or replacement are performed in the United States each year, although the ideal prosthetic valve has yet to be designed. In a sense, these limitations attest to the true elegance in form and function of the native human heart valve.

ANATOMY AND PATHOLOGY

The proper function of the heart, a biologic pump, is entirely dependent on the proper functioning of the heart valves. The two sets of valves, the atrioventricular (AV) and semilunar valves, that bridge the pressure gradients between the atria and ventricles, and the ventricles and the peripheral circulations, respectively, are well designed for this task. Each valve goes through at least 2.6 billion cycles of opening and closing in the course of a normal lifetime.

The tricuspid valve, guarding the right AV orifice, and the mitral, or bicuspid, valve, guarding the left AV orifice, are so named because of the number of their leaflets. Each is a fibrous structure lined by endocardium. The leaflets, or cusps, of the valves are continuous with the anuli fibrosi at the base of the heart and continuous with each other at lines of attachment called commissures. The chordae tendineae tether the free edges of the leaflets to the intra-

ventricular papillary muscles, thus preventing reflux during ventricular contraction.

The tricuspid valve consists of a large anterior leaflet, attached to the anterior wall of the heart, a posterior leaflet at the right margin of the heart, and a septal leaflet attached to the interventricular septum (Fig. 64-1). The large anterior papillary muscle sends chordae to anterior and posterior leaflets. A variable posterior papillary muscle and a prominent septal, or conus, papillary muscle may send chordae to the posterior and septal leaflets.

The mitral valve consists of a large anterior (aortic) leaflet and a smaller posterior (mural) leaflet, which are in continuity with the posterior wall of the aorta and the posterior wall of the heart at the AV groove, respectively. Large anterior and posterior papillary muscles send chordae to each leaflet.

The identical semilunar valves, the aortic and pulmonary, guard the outlets of the two ventricles. They are so named because of the shape of the three valvules, or cusps, they comprise. The valvulae are attached at their base to the annulus and are attached to each other at the commissures. The thin, free margins of the valvulae are divided into two lunulae by a thickening at the midpoint, known as the nodulus of Arantius. The three nodules coapt with their opposite members in diastole, thereby sealing the central orifice of the valve. Distal to the valve proper are the sinuses of Valsalva, gentle dilations of the aortic and pulmonary roots that may play a role in maximizing blood flow and minimizing turbulence. In the aortic root, the left and right coronary arteries normally arise at the base of the left and right aortic leaflets, respectively. The third, noncoronary cusp is located posteromedially. The aortic valve bears important anatomic relations to the mitral valve, the interventricular septum, and the conduction system (Fig. 64-2).

Aortic valvular stenosis is the most common type of valvular lesion, followed by mitral stenosis. In a recent review of valvular operations, 80% of excised valves were stenotic, and 14% were purely regurgitant (Table 64-1). Multivalvular replacement was required in 22% of cases in this report.

Rheumatic heart disease remains the most common cause of heart valve dysfunction and the most common cause of multivalvular disease, despite current medical treatment of streptococcal infections. The mitral valve is most commonly affected, followed by the aortic and the pulmonic valves. It is uncommon to have significant rheumatic valvular disease without mitral valve involvement. Rheumatic heart disease is by far the most common cause of mitral stenosis (Table 64-2) and was responsible for 48%

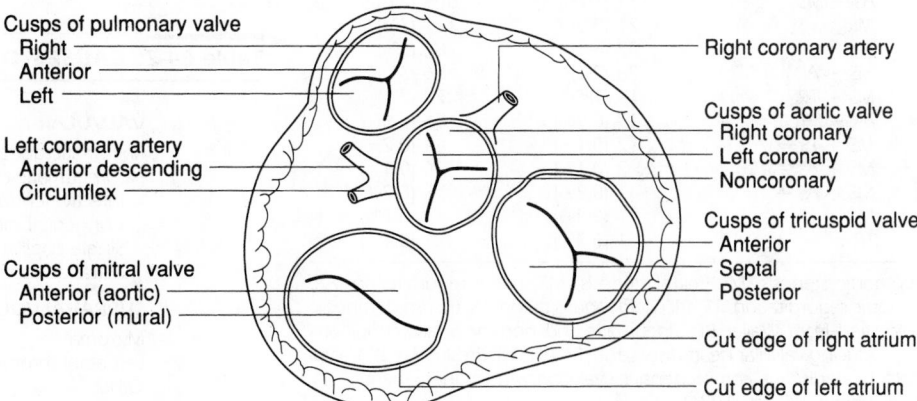

Figure 64-1. Cross-sectional representation of the normal anatomic relations of the semilunar (aortic and pulmonary) and atrioventricular (mitral and tricuspid) valves.

Cusps of pulmonary valve
Right
Anterior
Left

Left coronary artery
Anterior descending
Circumflex

Cusps of mitral valve
Anterior (aortic)
Posterior (mural)

Right coronary artery

Cusps of aortic valve
Right coronary
Left coronary
Noncoronary

Cusps of tricuspid valve
Anterior
Septal
Posterior

Cut edge of right atrium

Cut edge of left atrium

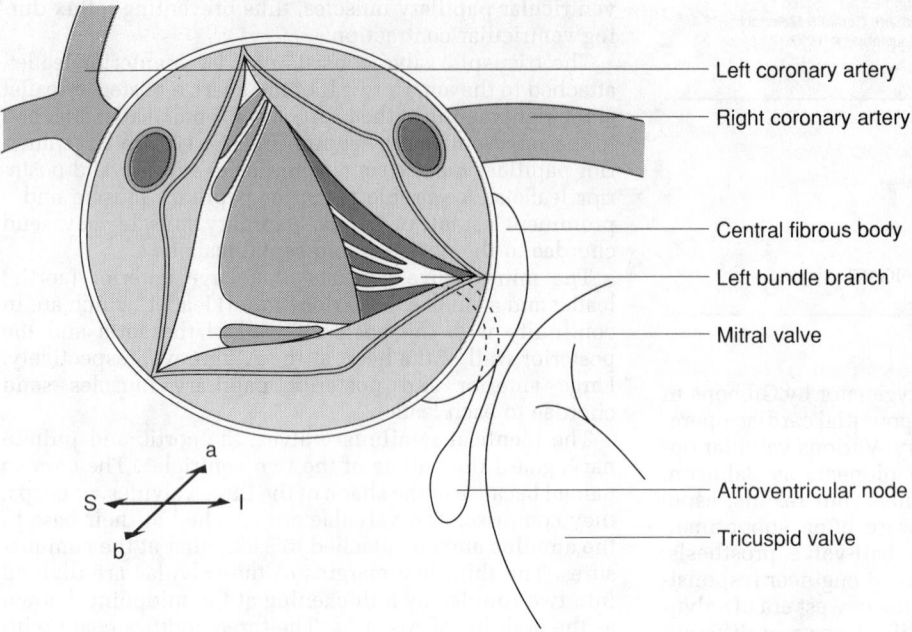

Left coronary artery

Right coronary artery

Central fibrous body

Left bundle branch

Mitral valve

Atrioventricular node

Tricuspid valve

Figure 64-2. Schematic diagram of the anatomic relations of the aortic valve showing the mitral valve posterolaterally and the septum medially. (After Wilcox BR, Anderson RN. Surgical anatomy of the heart. New York, Raven Press, 1985)

of pure mitral regurgitant lesions in Robert's review of 1010 necropsy cases of mitral valve disease.[1] Multivalvular disease was present in 41% of patients with mitral valve disease in this series. Tricuspid insufficiency in rheumatic heart disease is almost always a functional complication of left-sided disease, usually mitral stenosis, rather than primary rheumatic involvement of the tricuspid valve. Only 5% of rheumatic heart disease patients have significant stenosis of the tricuspid valve.

Although stenosis is predominant, rheumatic heart disease produces both stenotic and regurgitant lesions. Pure mitral stenosis is seen in 25% of patients with rheumatic heart disease, whereas 40% have both mitral stenosis and insufficiency. The pathologic anatomy of rheumatic valvular stenosis usually involves a combination of fusion of the valve commissures and cusps, producing the so-called fish-mouth deformity, and fusion and shortening of the

chordae tendineae. Leaflet cusp shortening caused by fibrosis can lead to valvular insufficiency. Shortening, fibrosis, and fusion of the chordae tendineae or the papillary muscles can also be responsible for regurgitation.

Degenerative processes are another common cause of heart valve dysfunction. Myxomatous changes, characteristically becoming clinically prominent in the third or fourth decade of life, most often affect the mitral valve, resulting in mitral valve prolapse or frank insufficiency. Jeresaty[2] reported that myxomatous degeneration is responsible for 62% of isolated mitral regurgitation (MR). Less commonly, floppy aortic valve leaflets can result in aortic insufficiency (AI), or both valves can be affected together.

Mitral annular calcification is an extremely common degenerative finding in older patients that uncommonly produces valvular dysfunction. Severe mitral annular calcification can create an unpliable annulus that does not properly contract with systole and may infrequently be responsible for MR. Mitral annular calcification with extension into the mitral or aortic leaflet substance can lead to mitral or aortic stenosis.

Valvular calcification produces immobile, heavily calcified leaflets that neither open nor close properly. Calcification thereby creates a predominantly stenotic lesion

Table 64-1. RELATIVE FREQUENCY OF VALVULAR LESIONS

Lesion	Patients	Valves
AS	491 (35%)	491 (28%)
MS	404 (23%)	404 (28%)
AS + MS	254 (18%)	508 (29%)
MR	121 (8%)	121 (7%)
AR	82 (6%)	82 (5%)
MS + AR	28 (2%)	56 (3%)
MS + TR	14 (1%)	28 (2%)
AR + MR	13 (0.9%)	26 (2%)
MS + TS	2 (0.1%)	4 (0.2%)
MS + AS + TS	2 (0.1%)	6 (0.4%)
MS + AS + TR	1 (0.3%)	3 (0.2%)
MR + TR	1 (0.3%)	2 (0.1%)
TR	1 (0.3%)	1 (0.1%)

AS, aortic stenosis; MS, mitral stenosis; MR, mitral regurgitation; AR, aortic regurgitation; TR, tricuspid regurgitation; TS, tricuspid stenosis. (Modified from Waller BF. Rheumatic and non-rheumatic conditions producing valvular heart disease. In: Frankl WS, Brest AN, eds. Valvular heart disease: comprehensive evaluation and management. Philadelphia, FA Davis, 1986)

Table 64-2. CAUSES OF MITRAL STENOSIS

VALVULAR

Rheumatic disease
Nonrheumatic disease
    Infective endocarditis
    Congenital mitral stenosis
    Single papillary muscle (parachute valve)
    Mitral annular calcification

SUPRAVALVULAR

Myxoma
Left atrial thrombus
Other

Table 64-3. CAUSES OF LEFT VENTRICULAR OUTFLOW TRACT OBSTRUCTION

VALVULAR (AORTIC STENOSIS)

Acquired
  Rheumatic disease
  Degenerative (fibrocalcific) disease
    Tricuspid valve
    Congenital bicuspid valve
  Infective endocarditis
  Other
Congenital
  Tricuspid valve with commissural
    fusion
  Unicuspid unicommissural valve
  Hypoplastic annulus

SUPRAVALVULAR

Membranous
Hourglass
Hypoplastic

SUBVALVULAR

Hypertrophic cardiomyopathy
Discrete (membranous) subaortic stenosis
Tunnel subaortic stenosis

---

with some degree of valvular insufficiency. The calcified trileaflet aortic valve is responsible for aortic stenosis in 90% of patients over the age of 65 years.[3] Turbulent flow caused by a congenitally bicuspid valve probably accelerates this normal wear-and-tear phenomenon of calcific degeneration and stenosis. The peak clinical occurrence of bicuspid valve stenosis is in the fifth and sixth decades of life. The bicuspid valve is initially somewhat regurgitant but becomes more stenotic as it progressively calcifies. Fenoglio and associates[4] found that 46% of patients over the age of 50 years and 73% of patients over the age of 70 years with a bicuspid valve had some degree of stenosis. In one operative series, 56% of aortic stenosis was related

to a bicuspid valve, 17% to rheumatic heart disease, predominantly with associated mitral disease, and 12% to calcified, trileaflet valves. Other causes of aortic stenosis are far less common (Table 64-3).

The bicuspid aortic valve is the most common manifestation of congenital valvular disease. As much as 1% to 2% of the population is estimated to have a bicuspid aortic valve. Commissural fusion of a tricuspid semilunar valve ranks second. Other, less common forms of congenital valvular disease frequently cause severe dysfunction before adulthood.

Endocarditis usually affects valves with congenital or acquired impairment and is typically a left-sided lesion, reflecting the normal distribution of preexisting valvular disease. Acute endocarditis is increasingly affecting normal valves and is more likely to result in significant valve dysfunction. Endocarditis is the ranking cause of fatal AI in the adult population. Endocarditic destruction of the valve or supporting structures can render the valve incompetent. Healed endocarditis can lead to leaflet fibrosis, producing a stenotic lesion. Uncommonly, large vegetations can interfere with normal valvular coaptation and produce insufficiency or functional obstruction.

AI and mitral insufficiency can also be produced by disease distinct from the valve itself (Tables 64-4 and 64-5). Aortic root dilation, whether from dissection, Marfan disease, cystic medial necrosis, or other causes, prevents normal coaptation of the aortic valve leaflets and can produce acute or chronic AI. Less commonly, trauma or dissection can lead to loss of the commissural support for the valve leaflets.

The nonvalvular causes of MR are far greater than those

Table 64-4. ETIOLOGY OF AORTIC INSUFFICIENCY

	Pathology		
Cause	**Leaflet**	**Aortic Root**	**Loss of Commissural Support**
COMMON			
Rheumatic disease	+	−	−
Congenital disease	+	−	±
Endocarditis	+	−	±
LESS COMMON			
Syphilis	±	+	−
Connective tissue disease (eg, Marfan syndrome)	+	+	−
Aortic dissection	−	+	+
UNCOMMON			
Trauma	+	+	+
Hypertension	±	±	±
Inflammatory disease (ankylosing spondylitis, Reiter syndrome)	+	+	−

(Modified from Greenberg BH. Acquired aortic valve disease. In: Greenberg BH, Murphy E, eds. Valvular heart disease. Littleton, MA, PSG Publishing, 1987:157)

Table 64-5. CAUSES OF MITRAL REGURGITATION

DISORDERS OF THE MITRAL VALVE LEAFLETS

Loss of contracture of valvular tissue
  Rheumatic fever
  Endocarditis
  Systemic lupus erythematosus
Congenital
  Cleft leaflet (isolated)
  Endocardial cushion defect
Connective tissue disorders
Other

DISORDERS OF THE MITRAL ANNULUS

Calcification
Dilatation
Destruction

DISORDERS OF THE CHORADAE TENDINEAE

Rupture of the chordae tendineae
  Endocarditis
  Myocardial infarction
  Connective tissue disorder
  Other
Thickening or fusion of the chordae tendinae
Elongation of the chordae tendineae

DISORDERS OF THE PAPILLARY MUSCLES

Dysfunction of rupture of papillary muscle
  Ischemia or infarction
  Endocarditis
  Inflammatory disorder
Malalignment
  Left ventricular dilatation
  Hypertrophic cardiomyopathy
  Infiltrative cardiomyopathy
Other

(Modified from Silverman ME, Hurst JW. The mitral complex: clues to its afflictions. Cardiovasc Clin North Am 1973;5:35)

of AI because the mitral valve apparatus is far more complex. MR can be caused by dysfunction at any level of the mitral valve apparatus, including the left ventricle proper. Chordal rupture caused by endocarditis, myxomatous degeneration, rheumatic heart disease, or acute left ventricular (LV) dilation can result in acute, severe MR and rapid cardiac decompensation. LV dysfunction can produce MR through inadequate contraction of the annulus during systole. Marked LV dilation can stretch the mitral annulus to the point at which leaflet coaptation is not possible at all. LV dilation, even segmental dyskinesis, can also be responsible for MR by creating malalignment of the papillary muscles and their respective chordae, leading to improper leaflet coaptation.

The papillary muscles are perfused by terminal branches of the coronary arteries and are thus highly susceptible to ischemia or even infarction. In fact, some degree of ischemia-related MR is seen in as many as 30% of coronary bypass patients. The posterior papillary muscle is more commonly involved, being supplied by branches of the posterior descending artery only, whereas the lateral (anterior) papillary muscle receives a dual supply from branches of the left anterior descending and circumflex marginal arteries. MR is usually transient, being related to ischemia only, but it can be severe and irreversible if associated with papillary necrosis.

Tricuspid regurgitation is the predominant form of right-sided valvular dysfunction but is most often secondary to left-sided disease. Tricuspid regurgitation is most often caused by right ventricular dilation, which in turn is caused by pulmonary hypertension from left-sided valvular lesions or left-sided heart failure. Mitral stenosis is the valvular lesion most often responsible for creating secondary tricuspid regurgitation. Other, less common causes of tricuspid and pulmonic valvular diseases are listed in Table 64-6.

PATHOPHYSIOLOGY

Valvular dysfunction produces two forms of stress on the heart—volume overload and pressure overload. Both represent increased cardiac afterload (ie, increased systolic wall stress). Tremendous cardiac reserves normally exist in the patient with valvular heart disease. Because of various compensatory mechanisms, the patient with valvular disease can persist in an asymptomatic, well-compensated state until severe valvular and ventricular dysfunction have developed. In contrast, the patient developing acute valvular dysfunction without a period of gradual adaptation can rapidly succumb to severe heart failure.

Chamber enlargement, shifts along the Frank-Starling curve (Fig. 64-3), myocardial hypertrophy, and increased adrenergic stimulation are among the mechanisms that allow the heart to adapt to valvular dysfunction that develops gradually. Increased diastolic filling of the ventricle increases myocardial sarcomere length, or preload. This allows optimal overlap between myofilaments at 2.2 μm. Hemodynamically, this results in improved ventricular ejection as a function of ventricular filling; this is demonstrated as a shift along the length-active tension relation, or Frank-Starling curve (see Fig. 64-3).

The Laplace law (see Appendix 64-1) predicts that wall stress increases with increasing ventricular radius, or preload, but is inversely related to wall thickness. Therefore, ventricular hypertrophy, another compensatory mechanism, acts to decrease wall stress. Cardiac myocytes do not replicate after the neonatal period; increases in myocardial mass are produced by myocyte hypertrophy, not hyperplasia. Hypertrophy, in turn, requires the derepression of myocyte DNA. Stress imposed by increased preload or afterload, depletion of myocyte adenosine triphosphate (ATP), accumulation of cell degeneration products caused by wear and tear, and humoral stimuli such as thyroid hormone have been implicated as stimulating agents.

CONGESTIVE HEART FAILURE

Heart failure is the common endpoint in the natural history of most forms of valvular dysfunction and is associated with failure of the compensation mechanisms described earlier. Precisely defined, heart failure signifies an inability of the heart to pump blood at a level adequate for the metabolic demands of the body. In patients with valvular dysfunction, heart failure can initially be caused by abnormal hemodynamic loads in the face of normal myocardial function. Heart failure must therefore be distinguished from myocardial failure, in which myocardial contractile properties have deteriorated. Acute AI, for example, imposes a sudden imbalance in forward cardiac flow with essentially intact myocardial function.

Heart failure must also be distinguished from a systemic congested state, caused by such peripheral factors as abnormal fluid retention, and from circulatory failure, the state of inadequate systemic perfusion secondary to heart failure or such other causes as blood loss or abnormalities in systemic vascular resistance. High output failure describes a state of failure with abnormally high systemic flow, a hyperdynamic circulation, as can be seen with thyrotoxicosis. The far more prevalent low output failure is characterized by decreased systemic flow and systemic vasoconstriction.

Heart failure can be further categorized by specific mechanisms and manifestations. Two basic classifications are backward failure, first proposed in 1832 by Hope, and forward failure, suggested by Mackenzie some 80 years later. Backward failure refers to blood accumulation and pressure increases upstream from the failing ventricle, represented by pulmonary edema in the face of LV failure or systemic venous congestion in the setting of right-sided heart failure. *Forward failure* refers to the inadequate delivery of blood into the circulation caused by the diminished pumping function of the heart. Mental confusion,

---

Table 64-6. CAUSES OF RIGHT-SIDED VALVULAR DYSFUNCTION

TRICUSPID VALVE	PULMONIC VALVE
Regurgitation	Regurgitation
RV or annular dilatation	Annular dilatation
RV infarct	Pulmonary hypertension
RV hypertension	Marfan syndrome
RV failure	Other
Marfan syndrome	Congenital defects
Congenital	Endocarditis
Ebstein anomaly	Carcinoid heart disease
AV canal	Iatrogenic or other
Rheumatic heart disease	Stenosis
Tricuspid valve prolapse	Congenital pulmonic stenosis
Papillary muscle	Rheumatic heart disease
dysfunction	Carcinoid heart disease
Infective endocarditis	Cardiac tumors
Carcinoid heart disease	Other
Right atrial myxoma	
Endomyocardial fibrosis	
Other	
Stenosis	
Rheumatic disease	
Congenital tricuspid atresia	
Right atrial tumors	
Carcinoid heart disease	
Constrictive pericarditis	
Other	

AV, atrioventricular; RV, right ventricular.

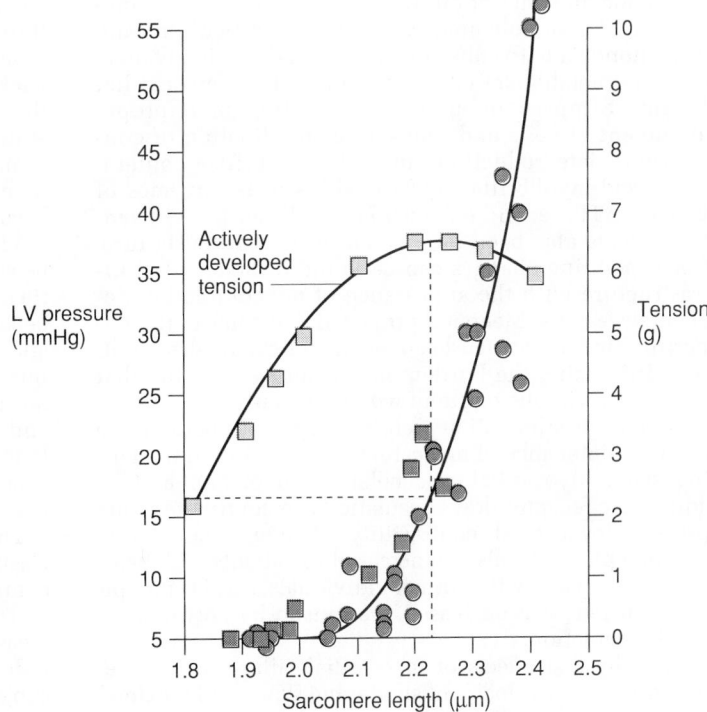

Figure 64-3. Frank-Starling relation describing ventricular contractility as a function of left ventricular (LV) end-diastolic volume. Data are derived from animal studies. The upper curve represents myocardial tension development as a function of sarcomere length; the lower curve represents resting ventricular pressure as a function of sarcomere length. (After Spotnitz JH, Sonnenblick EH, Spiro D. Relationship of ultrastructure to function in the intact heart: sarcomere structure relative to pressure-volume curves of the intact left ventricles of dog and cat. Circ Res 1966;18:57)

weakness, and sodium and water retention are manifestations of forward failure secondary to hypoperfusion of the brain, skeletal muscle, and kidneys, respectively. Although these two hemodynamic states can be separated in theory, they are almost invariably present together in the clinical setting.

Systolic and diastolic dysfunction both contribute to the clinical picture of heart failure. Systolic failure is more familiar and refers to the pump failure described earlier. Diastolic failure is a relatively newer concept, referring to the impaired ability of the ventricle to fill properly, and is probably related to abnormal ventricular relaxation properties and chamber stiffness. Diastolic failure is reflected in decreased ventricular compliance and elevation of ventricular end-diastolic pressure at a given level of filling. Venous congestion in the circulation upstream from the failing ventricle, either pulmonary or systemic, is the result. Inadequate filling of the ventricle in diastole further leads to inadequate systolic function because of inadequate preload (see earlier).

Heart failure most commonly refers to left-sided heart failure, with *forward* and *backward* failure referring to systemic hypoperfusion and pulmonary congestion, respectively. Less commonly, isolated right-sided heart failure can predominate, with isolated systemic venous congestion (backward failure) and decreased flow to the left side of the heart (forward failure). A mixed clinical picture is again most typical.

The principle of ventricular interdependence describes the interaction between left- and right-sided heart function, and the progression observed between failure of one side of the heart and failure of the other. Several mechanisms can play a part. Mechanical constraints are imposed by one ventricle on the other as the expansion of one chamber within the single pericardial sac limits the proper filling of the other. Systemic hemodynamic changes such as hypervolemia affect both sides of the heart equally. Biochemical alterations such as myocardial levels of catechol-

amines and actomyosin ATPase activity can spread from one ventricle to the other.

Myocardial Failure

Although the exact cause of myocardial fatigue has not yet been determined, studies of intact and isolated heart muscle provide some insight into this phenomenon. Myocardial hypertrophy is associated with increased production of mitochondria and increased myofibrillar mass, presumably to meet the increased contractile energy demands of the stressed myocytes (Fig. 64-4). Decreased or inadequate myocardial energy function, or an inadequate ratio of mitochondrial mass to myofibrillar mass, can contribute to myocardial failure. Calcium uptake and redistribution within the cell are critical to nor-

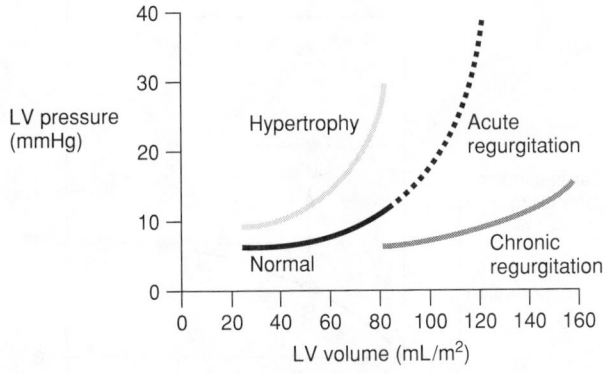

Figure 64-4. Schematic representation of the pathophysiology of compensatory hypertrophy of the heart in valvular heart disease and the peripheral sequelae of congestive failure. LV, left ventricular. (After Meerson FZ, Katz AM, eds. The failing heart: adaptation and deadaptation. New York, Raven Press, 1983)

mal myocyte contraction. Damage to, or improper function of, the sarcolemma, sarcoplasmic reticulum, and mitochondria with subsequent abnormalities in myocyte calcium metabolism can also contribute to myocardial fatigue. Slippage of myocytes (resulting in improper alignment of cells and ineffective coordination of contraction), late reductions in cell myofibrillar content, decreased myofibrillar ATPase, shifts in isoenzymes of myosin ATPase, and exhaustion of cellular protein synthesis have also been implicated in myocardial failure. Corresponding changes can be found in myocardial ultrastructure with the appearance of noncontractile, degenerative cells. Meerson[5] proposed that some of the hypertrophied myocytes become necrotic and drop out, thus increasing the burden on remaining cells in what becomes a vicious circle of worsening failure.

Adrenergic stimulation probably plays an important role in the maintenance of myocardial contractility in the failing state. Myocardial catecholamine depletion and β-adrenergic receptor down-regulation can contribute to depressed myocardial contractility. Although circulating norepinephrine levels are increased in patients with heart failure compared with normal individuals, cardiac norepinephrine release is decreased, presumably because of myocardial depletion.

The physical effects of myocardial failure include reduced maximal velocity of shortening (V_{max}) and maximal isometric tension. These changes are demonstrated in depressed length-active tension curves (ie, an increased end-diastolic volume is required to generate the same level of tension). This represents a rightward shift of the Frank-Starling curve (Fig. A in 64-5). Baseline ejection fractions are reduced and rise subnormally with elevation in end-diastolic volume. LV end-diastolic pressure (LVEDP) increases proportionally with increases in LV end-diastolic volume (LVEDV), based on the compliance of the ventricle. In turn, compliance can be modified by ventricular hypertrophy or dilation (see Fig. 64-4). The increased LVEDP is transmitted back across the mitral valve orifice as increased left atrial (LA) pressures.

Peripheral Manifestations

The clinical presentation of congestive heart failure is dominated by its peripheral sequelae. As described earlier, pulmonary congestion caused by the damming up of blood behind the ineffectively contracting ventricle is one of the leading manifestations of heart failure. Elevated LA pres-

sures associated with ventricular failure are transmitted through the pulmonary venous system. The increased pulmonary hydrostatic pressure overwhelms the counterbalancing osmotic pressure gradient. Edema fluid escapes into the interstitial space from the pulmonary capillaries, resulting in the signs and symptoms of pulmonary congestion. Pulmonary edema, the most extreme form of pulmonary congestion, is associated with transalveolar accumulation of edema fluid.

Vital capacity is reduced with pulmonary congestion because air in the lungs is replaced by interstitial and intraalveolar fluid, as well as engorged vessels. The lungs become stiffer as intraparenchymal fluid decreases compliance. The work of breathing increases because increased intrapleural pressures must be generated to expand collapsed airways and stiffer lungs. Tidal volume decreases and respiratory frequency increases to compensate. Ventilation and perfusion mismatches result in increased dead space to tidal volume ratios, an increased alveolar-arterial gradient, and even hypoxemia.

The patient's first symptom of this process is breathlessness, or dyspnea. Dyspnea is probably caused by a complex interaction of various intrapulmonary, chest wall, and skeletal stretch receptors as well as chemoreceptors measuring blood gas levels. An inappropriate length-to-tension relation in skeletal muscles, suggesting that the subject is getting inadequate breath per tension generated by these muscles, is probably central to the pathophysiology of dyspnea. Skeletal muscle fatigue caused by forward cardiac failure and increased work of breathing can heighten this sensation.

Orthopnea and paroxysmal nocturnal dyspnea are specific forms of dyspnea caused by redistribution of blood from the abdomen and lower extremities to the central vascular compartment during recumbency. The failing ventricle inadequately ejects this increased central blood flow, leading to increased levels of ventricular end-diastolic pressure and to pulmonary congestion. Orthopnea can occur at any time of recumbency; paroxysmal nocturnal dyspnea is specifically related to sleep-time changes in physiology, probably including decreased adrenergic stimulation of the ventricle and depression of respiratory drive. Orthopnea develops within minutes of assuming recumbency, resolves quickly, and is characteristically relieved by the patient sleeping on additional pillows—the basis of the term *two-pillow orthopnea*. Paroxysmal nocturnal dyspnea can last for 30 minutes or longer.

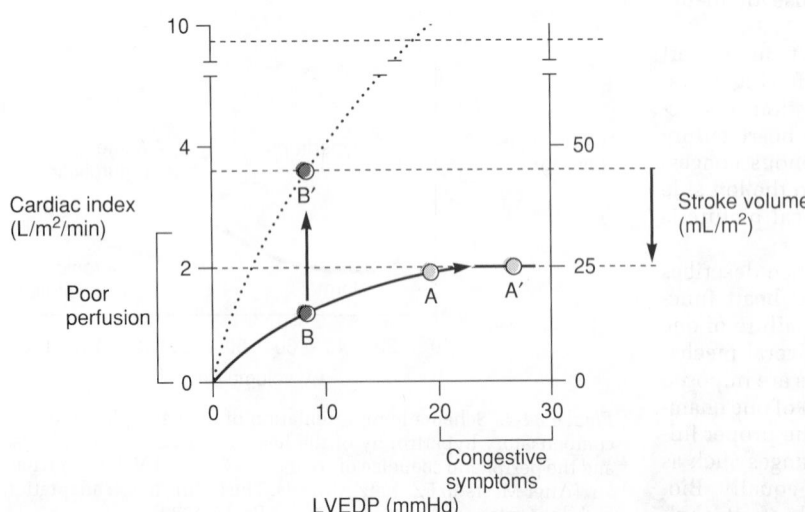

Figure 64-5. Diagram demonstrating the relation between left ventricular end-diastolic pressure (LVEDP) and cardiac index (*left ordinate*) or stroke volume (*right ordinate*) in a normal heart (*dotted line*) and a failing heart (*solid line*). Congestive symptoms can be expected with LVEDP above 20 mmHg, and inadequate systemic perfusion with cardiac index below 2.2 L/m²/min. In the failing heart, increases along the flat portion of the Frank-Starling curve (A to A') produce increases in LVEDP and congestive symptoms without improving perfusion. Improved myocardial function (B to B') allows greater cardiac ejection and systemic perfusion at a given LVEDP. Ventricular filling (LVEDP) can thereby be maintained at levels below the threshold of congestive symptoms. (After Hall RJC, Julian DG. Diseases of the cardiac valves. New York, Churchill Livingstone, 1984:487)

Transalveolar diapedesis of red cells can produce blood-tinged or pink sputum in patients with congestion. Chronic bronchitis due to an edematous bronchial mucosa can also produce blood-tinged sputum. Frank hemoptysis can occur with greater elevations of pressure. Rarely, pulmonary apoplexy with profuse bleeding results from rupture of a thin-walled bronchial vein. This is most characteristic of early mitral stenosis. It is rarely life threatening.

With prolonged periods of pulmonary congestion, reactive constriction develops in pulmonary arterioles, followed by obliterative changes in the microcirculation. These changes are initially beneficial, preventing pulmonary congestion and increased capillary pressures by reducing pulmonary flow. Eventually, fixed pulmonary hypertension results.

Heart failure also has a significant peripheral effect on the kidney and on the various neurohumoral mechanisms regulating salt and water balance. Decreased renal blood flow and glomerular filtration rates cause increased sodium and water retention through direct renal hydrodynamics. Low renal perfusion, low sodium load presented to the macula densa, and increased β-adrenergic stimulation of the juxtaglomerular complex also activate the renin-angiotensin-aldosterone axis in patients with low-output states. Elevated plasma levels of renin are commonly found in patients with congestive failure. Angiotensin II, a potent vasoconstrictor, acts along with the increased adrenergic tone to raise peripheral vascular resistance in patients with failure, exacerbating the effects of low flow on the kidney. Aldosterone further increases sodium and water retention.

Resetting of the LA stretch receptors and increased renal efferent sympathetic activity lead to elevation of arginine vasopressin (antidiuretic hormone; ADH), which is produced in the pituitary, to levels about twice normal in patients with failure. Vasopressin is a potent vasoconstrictor and acts like angiotensin II in this regard. ADH also increases water reabsorption in the distal renal tubule. Decreased levels of atrial natriuretic factor can also contribute to water and salt retention.

Expansion of the extracellular fluid volume caused by these neurohormonal perturbations becomes manifest as peripheral edema when fluid accumulation exceeds 5 L. Ascites represents fluid accumulation in the abdominal cavity that is caused by increased back-pressure in the veins draining the peritoneum and abdominal viscera. Increased capillary permeability and hypoalbuminemia caused by liver failure and protein-losing enteropathy associated with failure can also contribute to ascites. Hydrothorax, usually symmetric, is caused by similar mechanisms. If unilateral, hydrothorax is characteristically found on the right. Massive generalized edema, termed anasarca,

is a severe and late manifestation of extracellular fluid accumulation.

Elevated systemic venous pressure that causes tissue congestion and edema can lead to end-organ failure. Hepatomegaly can develop before the onset of peripheral edema, especially with right-sided failure. Acute hepatic congestion with rapid increases in liver size can cause tenderness because of stretching of the Glisson capsule. Impaired hepatic function can be associated with increases in transaminases, bilirubin, and alkaline phosphatase. Bilirubin and serum glutamic-oxaloacetic transaminase levels higher than 10 times normal can be seen. Cardiac cirrhosis, with central necrosis and extensive fibrosis, can develop with long-standing hepatic congestion, along with hypoalbuminemia, prolongation of prothrombin times, and frank jaundice. Hepatic hypoglycemia and liver failure are uncommon late findings.

PATHOPHYSIOLOGY OF SPECIFIC VALVULAR DYSFUNCTION

Although congestive heart failure is the common endpoint for all forms of valvular heart disease, each form of valvular dysfunction imposes a hemodynamic burden on the heart in a unique fashion. Each lesion must therefore be considered separately.

Mitral Stenosis

The normal adult mitral valve orifice size is 4 to 6 cm². Reduction of orifice size to 2 cm² represents mild mitral stenosis; this is the point at which a transvalvular pressure gradient first appears (Fig. 64-6). At an orifice area of 1 cm², considered critical mitral stenosis, the transvalvular gradient required to maintain normal resting cardiac output is 20 mmHg. Assuming a low-normal LVEDP of 5 mmHg, this represents an LA pressure of 25 mmHg. Transmitted back through the pulmonary veins to the pulmonary alveolar capillary network, this increased pressure leads to the signs and symptoms of pulmonary congestion (see earlier discussion).

The transvalvular gradient associated with mitral stenosis can be severely exacerbated by any increases in cardiac output and transmitral flow. The law of Poiseuille (see Appendix) predicts that increased flow across a point of fixed resistance results in an increase in the pressure gradient that is equal to the square of the change in flow. Any increase in cardiac output therefore results in a disproportionate increase in transmitral gradient, LA pressure, and pulmonary congestion. Furthermore, at a given level of

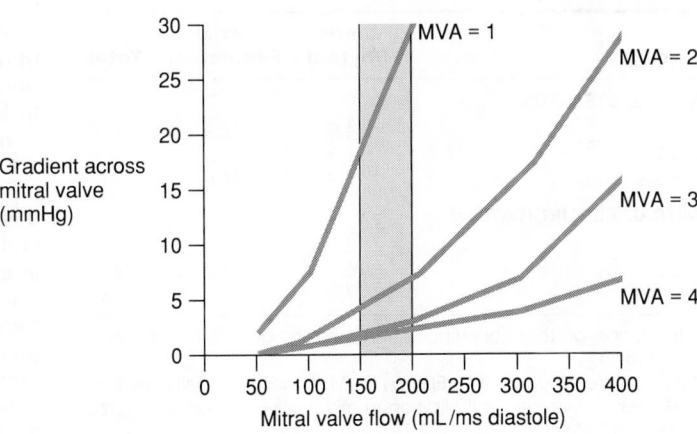

Figure 64-6. Mitral valve gradient as a function of mitral valve flow. The blue area represents normal transvalvular flow. The gradient increases exponentially with decreases in mitral valve area (MVA). (After Dalen JE. Valvular heart disease, ed 2. Boston, Little, Brown, 1987:53)

cardiac output, any increase in heart rate decreases the diastolic filling time available for flow across the stenotic valve. This also results in increased flow per unit time and an increase in the transvalvular gradient. The pathophysiology of dyspnea on exertion is related to these mechanisms.

Effective atrial contraction associated with sinus rhythm helps to counter increases in LA pressures. Normal atrial contraction augments diastolic filling of the ventricle by up to 30% in mitral stenosis patients. This increases ventricular preload and allows for more effective myocardial contraction (see Fig. 64-3). Mean LA pressure needed to maintain a given level of ventricular function is thus lowered. Loss of this atrial kick, as with the onset of atrial fibrillation, results in a 20% decrease in cardiac output. The increase in heart rate usually associated with the onset of atrial fibrillation leads to further deleterious increases in transvalvular gradient, as described earlier.

The onset of atrial fibrillation correlates with increased age and LA dilation. LA dilation is associated with fibrosis and disorganization of atrial fibers, leading to disparate atrial conduction times and refractory periods. These factors serve as fertile ground for the ectopic foci and reentrant circuits that ultimately degenerate into supraventricular tachycardias and atrial fibrillation. In one study, only 3% of patients with LA diameters less than 40 mm were in atrial fibrillation, compared with 80% of patients with diameters greater than 45 mm and older than 40 years of age.

Mural thrombi and thromboembolism are serious sequelae of mitral stenosis that are directly related to the presence of atrial fibrillation (Table 64-7). One fourth of all mitral stenosis deaths before the era of surgical correction were due to this cause. Half of all emboli appear to enter the cerebral circulation. Emboli can go to the coronaries, resulting in ischemia or myocardial infarction; to the kidneys, resulting in hematuria or hypertension; to the splanchnic circulation; or to the periphery. Multiple or recurrent emboli occur in 25% of cases. Rarely, a large pedunculated thrombus obstructs the valve orifice, leading to hemodynamic collapse and sudden death. The risk of embolism has also been directly related to age and inversely related to cardiac output. Eighty percent of patients suffering from thromboembolism are in atrial fibrillation; conversely, embolism or stroke can be the first symptom of mitral stenosis in 12% of patients.[6]

Table 64-7. ASSOCIATION OF THROMBOEMBOLISM WITH ATRIAL FIBRILLATION AND AGE IN PATIENTS WITH MITRAL VALVE DISEASE*

Age (y)	Sinus Rhythm	Atrial Fibrillation	Total
MITRAL STENOSIS			
≤35	4.5	27.5	9.0
>35	11.3	32.3	23.9
Total	7.9	31.5	19.0
MITRAL REGURGITATION			
≤35	3.7	15.8	8.6
>35	16.7	25.0	23.2
Total	7.6	22.2	16.7

* Incidence of thromboembolism in percentage of total patients studied.
(Modified from Coulshed N, Epstein EJ, McKindrich CS, Galloway RW, Walker, E. Systemic embolisation in mitral valve disease. Br Heart J 1970;32:26)

Mitral stenosis is the most sparing of the left-sided valvular lesions in terms of ventricular function. The pathophysiology, signs, and symptoms of mitral stenosis are mostly related to pressure buildup and stasis upstream from the point of valvular obstruction. LVEDP is normal or even below normal in about 85% of patients. The cardiac output is normal in two thirds of patients. When cardiac output is reduced, it is usually due to decreased preload because of slow filling through the stenotic valve rather than to depressed myocardial contractility. In longstanding mitral stenosis, pulmonary artery (PA) pressure can exceed systemic pressure. At PA pressures greater than 70 mmHg, impedance to right heart outflow frequently results in right-sided heart failure, with right ventricular dilation, tricuspid insufficiency, and even pulmonic insufficiency. Further decreases in left heart preload result, and low cardiac output syndrome develops.

Aortic Stenosis

The normal aortic valve orifice measures from 2.6 to 3.5 cm². The aortic valve becomes a point of fixed resistance in the LV outflow tract at an orifice area of 1 cm². Gradual pressure loading of the ventricle caused by increasing valvular obstruction leads to myocardial sarcomere replication and LV hypertrophy (see earlier). LV systolic pressures thereby increase commensurately with increasing valvular stenosis. Adequate cardiac output and normal systemic pressures are maintained until late in the course of aortic stenosis but at the expense of ventricular systolic pressures 50% to 100% greater than normal. LV systolic pressures over 300 mmHg can develop, and hypertrophy can result in hearts weighing up to 500 to 700 g. Eventually, myocardial hypertrophy leads to significantly decreased ventricular compliance, increased LVEDP, and pulmonary congestion.

Effective atrial contraction allows volume loading of the noncompliant ventricle without causing significant elevation of the mean LA pressure, similar to the role played by the atrium in patients with mitral stenosis. Lower LA mean pressures allow the pulmonary circulation to remain decompressed despite relatively high LVEDP. The onset of atrial fibrillation or AV dissociation can consequently be poorly tolerated, as in mitral stenosis patients.

Inadequate myocardial perfusion, especially in the subendocardial region, is another negative outcome of LV hypertrophy. Angina pectoris develops in two thirds of patients with severe aortic stenosis, although one half of these patients also have significant coronary disease. Ischemia can develop for several reasons. Aortic stenosis often results in significant increases in systolic ejection pressures, which are generated over a longer systolic ejection phase. Myocardial oxygen demand is thereby increased, which lowers the threshold for ischemia. Coronary perfusion occurs predominantly in diastole, and the increases in intramyocardial pressure and LVEDP mentioned earlier present resistance to coronary flow. The absolute increase in LV mass associated with aortic stenosis can further act to outstrip coronary supply.

Syncope, which is observed in 25% of symptomatic aortic stenosis patients, is probably due to limitations in cardiac output and decreased cerebral perfusion. Periods of systemic vasodilation can lead to dramatic decreases in arterial pressure when a fixed cardiac output is present. These periods can exacerbate syncopal episodes in the patient with severe aortic stenosis. Tachycardia can also be poorly tolerated because prolonged ejection times are required to maintain adequate flow through the stenotic valve. Eventually, as maximal LV hypertrophy is achieved, an adequate pressure gradient across the stenotic aortic orifice can no longer be maintained, and LV failure ensues. A persistent cycle of increases in LVEDP and LVEDV, increasing ventricular systolic dysfunction, and worsening heart and pulmonary failure follows. Right-sided heart failure develops as pulmonary hypertension causes an increase in right-sided heart afterload. Death occurs in 10% to 20% of patients, usually secondary to congestive heart failure. Sudden death, possibly secondary to arrhythmia, is responsible for mortality in most of the remainder.

LV dilation can also cause mitral annular enlargement and concomitant MR, which results in further deterioration in forward ventricular ejection. High LV systolic pressures associated with aortic stenosis can significantly worsen MR. Severe decompensation can follow in these cases.

Aortic Insufficiency

Aortic insufficiency produces a volume-loading strain on the left ventricle, unlike the pressure-loading strain of aortic stenosis. Increased diastolic loading of the ventricle comes from regurgitant flow through the aortic root. The volume-loaded ventricle empties more efficiently and completely than normal, as dictated by the principles of the Frank-Starling curve. This volume-related enhancement of contractility is the predominant compensatory mechanism in patients with AI.

With increased diastolic loading of the ventricle and with LV chamber enlargement, the law of Laplace predicts that LV wall tension increases proportionally with the increase in LV radius. This increased ventricular afterload represents increased LV work, and myocardial oxygen consumption rises. Increased wall tension produces a compensatory increase in LV wall thickness, as mentioned earlier. The law of Laplace further dictates that this decreases wall stress and, consequently, decreases myocardial oxygen demands. Maintenance of a normal LV wall thickness to volume ratio therefore allows a normal amount of noncontractile systolic work to be performed in patients with AI. The amount of subendocardial ischemia and angina produced is consequently far less than that seen in aortic stenosis patients.

The sum effect of volume enlargement and wall thickening is the dramatically enlarged heart, known as cor bovinum. AI can produce ventricles weighing as much as 1 kg—the greatest increase in ventricular mass produced by any of the valvular lesions. LV compliance remains relatively low until late in the course of AI, despite the degree of ventricular hypertrophy present, and LVEDP remains low. This has been attributed to slippage of the myocardial sarcomeres, which replicate in parallel in patients with AI, unlike the sarcomere replication in series associated with aortic stenosis.

LV chamber enlargement and hypertrophy allow for greatly increased stroke volumes and cardiac outputs in patients with severe, chronic AI. Cardiac outputs can increase to 30 L/min, 20 L of which possibly returns to the heart as regurgitant flow. Diastolic retrograde flow into the LV results in aortic root decompression and sometimes dramatic decreases in systemic diastolic pressures. Gradual myocardial decompensation often progresses in patients with AI before the onset of symptoms. Limitations in cardiac output produce symptoms of fatigue and weakness only when stroke volume plateaus with end-stage disease. At this point, any additional regurgitant flow cannot be ejected. LVEDP rises, net forward flow decreases, and cardiac failure ensues.

Acute AI, as might be seen with aortic dissection, results in relatively small regurgitant fractions compared with chronic AI because inadequate time is available for the

evolution of chamber enlargement and other compensatory mechanisms. LVEDP rises rapidly because of backward flow into a small, noncompliant ventricle. Rapid equalization of systemic and ventricular pressures can result. The dramatic elevation in LVEDP is transmitted back to the pulmonary circulation and can produce fulminant pulmonary congestion. Fortunately, high diastolic LV pressures often cause mitral preclosure, thereby protecting the pulmonary circuit. Significant increases in LVEDP and ventricular wall tension can produce dramatic myocardial ischemia. Low cardiac output syndrome or frank cardiovascular collapse, with tachycardia, peripheral vasoconstriction, and systemic hypotension, is not uncommon.

Mitral Regurgitation

Maximal cardiac ejection is achieved in patients with AI predominantly through adaptive shifts of loading conditions along the Frank-Starling curve. In patients with MR, adaptation is further aided through the mechanism of afterload reduction. In fact, the primary pathophysiologic feature of MR is systolic unloading of the LV into the low-pressure left atrium.

As left ventricular pressure rises with the onset of systole, chamber pressure exceeds LA pressure well before it reaches aortic root pressure. Consequently, as much as one half of LV volume can be ejected through the incompetent mitral valve before the aortic valve has even opened. Reflow of the regurgitant volume from the atrium to the left ventricle during diastole produces a volume-loaded state similar to that seen with AI. Contractility improves, as predicted by the Frank-Starling curve, in an equivalent fashion. Systolic unloading, which is not found with AI, allows enhanced emptying of the LV during systole, and ejection fractions are characteristically supranormal. As with AI, only a small portion of the ejected fraction results in net forward flow. Because of these mechanisms, end-systolic volumes are usually smaller in patients with MR compared with AI, and a given level of end-systolic volume can represent greater dysfunction. Furthermore, normal ejection fractions and fractional shortening ratios in MR patients can actually reflect severe LV dysfunction. Ventricular function is therefore a key index of disease progression in patients with MR.

Myocardial ischemia is uncommon in patients with MR because afterload reduction into the left atrium yields increased ejection fractions and stroke volumes with only slight increases in oxygen consumption.[7] Diastolic overloading of the LV increases LV radius and wall tension as described by the law of Laplace, but afterload unloading into the low-pressure atrial chamber through the mitral pop-off valve yields a net decrease in systolic wall tension and systolic work.[8] The volume-loaded LV also hypertrophies, increasing LV wall thickness and further decreasing wall stress. The constant ratio of LV mass to end-diastolic volume allows maintenance of normal levels of noncontractile work, analogous to the compensatory mechanism found in patients with AI.

The left atrium responds to the MR along a spectrum of adaptations that is the chief determinant of symptoms in patients with MR.[8] A high-compliance chamber with a large, low-pressure capacitance is characteristic of chronic MR. A low-compliance, small, hypertrophied atrium at relatively high pressure is the characteristic response to acute MR. In the low-compliance system, or in end-stage MR, the capacitance of the left atrium is often exceeded. Back-pressures transmitted to the pulmonary system result in the characteristic stigma of pulmonary congestion. The chronically dilated or high-compliance LA is thinned and fibrotic, and atrial fibrillation is common. Sinus rhythm is common in acute MR.

Eventually, as the left atrium and mitral orifice size grow and regurgitant flow increases, maximal systolic ejection is reached. More diastolic filling of the ventricle is met by fixed forward ejection, and end-diastolic volume increases. This leads to a further increase in mitral orifice size, more mitral insufficiency, and a self-perpetuating cycle of left-sided heart dilation and low-output failure. As Edwards and Burchell stated, "Mitral regurgitation begets more mitral regurgitation."[9] As with other forms of end-stage valvular disease, pulmonary hypertension, pulmonary vascular hypertrophy, right ventricular hypertrophy, and right ventricular dysfunction develop as well.

In acute MR, adaptation is not possible, and fulminant cardiac decompensation often ensues. LVEDP rises rapidly as the noncompliant, small-capacitance LV is subjected to sudden, severe increases in diastolic filling. The relatively thin-walled ventricle is subjected to the oxygen demands of a high-stress system. Similar compliance restrictions in the left atrium lead to ventricularization of this chamber with pressures up to 40 to 70 mmHg. Pulmonary edema and right-sided heart failure are frequent sequelae.

Other Valvular Dysfunction

The pathophysiology of right-sided valvular dysfunction is analogous to that of left-sided disease. Symptoms in patients with tricuspid regurgitation are usually related to the primary, left-sided pathology. Systemic venous hypertension can produce hepatic congestion and dysfunction with ascites, jaundice, and other stigmata of cirrhosis. Peripheral edema or abdominal swelling can be prominent.

Tricuspid stenosis with a tricuspid valve gradient as small as 5 mmHg can elevate right atrial pressures enough to cause similar symptoms of systemic venous hypertension. Anasarca can be a late finding. Dyspnea from isolated tricuspid stenosis or tricuspid regurgitation is uncommon and suggests other problems. As with mitral stenosis, restrictive tricuspid valve flow in patients with tricuspid stenosis or limited net forward flow in patients with severe tricuspid regurgitation can produce symptoms of low cardiac output. Left-sided pressures and flow rates, upstream from the restrictive lesion, are normal or even decreased.

The pathophysiology of multivalvular disease, most commonly seen with rheumatic heart disease, is obviously more complex than that of single lesions. The upstream lesion is often responsible for producing the more proximal lesion, as with mitral stenosis and tricuspid regurgitation, or aortic stenosis and MR. Alternatively, combined valvular dysfunction can be part of the same disease process, as with AI and MR in Marfan syndrome. The upstream lesion often masks the effects of the distal lesion and makes accurate diagnosis more difficult. For example, significant mitral stenosis may not permit enough upstream flow to allow the pathologic changes of AI to develop. Mitral stenosis associated with aortic stenosis inhibits the LV hypertrophy and elevation of the transaortic gradient normally produced by isolated aortic stenosis. Conversely, AI and MR can act synergistically. Reflux from the aortic root all the way to the pulmonary circulation can cause severe dysfunction with these dual lesions. Accurate diagnosis of multiple lesions is consequently essential in formulating appropriate treatment strategies.

DIAGNOSIS

The initial assessment of patients with valvular heart disease still depends on a careful history and physical examination, despite the recent introduction of advanced diagnostic techniques. A careful history and physical examination reveals important information regarding the kind of valvular disease present, and it also provides some estimate of the severity, duration, and prognosis of the dysfunction. This is supplemented by data obtained from the chest roentgenogram and 12-lead electrocardiogram (ECG); M-mode, two-dimensional (2D), and color Doppler echocardiography; the flow-directed PA catheter; and, ultimately, cardiac catheterization. Some now advocate surgical intervention without catheterization as the reliability of noninvasive procedures improves.

Physical Examination

Cardiac examination must include careful palpation and auscultation, with provocative maneuvers as appropriate. Phonocardiography can supplement this examination but is infrequently used. Examination of the peripheral arterial pulses, inspection of the jugular venous pattern, and a thorough search for systemic findings such as edema, ascites, or jaundice must be conducted.

Pulsus parvus et tardus, a late-peaking, low-pulse pressure impulse, is the classic change found in the carotid pulse of patients with critical aortic stenosis. This is usually a late finding, because a normotensive or even hypertensive state is maintained until severe dysfunction has developed. The classic mid-systolic murmur of aortic stenosis is produced by turbulent, high-velocity flow across the narrowed aortic valve. This murmur is heard best at the base of the heart and usually radiates to both carotid arteries. Radiation of a high-pitched component to the cardiac apex with an intervening quiet area, known as the Gallavardin phenomenon, can mimic MR. A sustained, forceful, nondisplaced apical impulse (PMI) should be palpable, produced by prolonged ventricular ejection through the stenotic valve. High-grade lesions can also produce palpable vibrations known as thrills in the aortic auscultation area and a carotid shudder due to transmission of the turbulent aortic flow.

AI characteristically produces a hyperdynamic circulation with marked increases in systemic arterial pulse pressure. This hyperdynamic response produces a wide variety of signs, such as the Corrigan water-hammer pulse, Musset sign (head bobbing in time with heart beat), or Quincke sign (capillary pulsations in fingertips detected with light compression). The PMI is displaced laterally and is bounding. Cardiac auscultatory findings include a high-pitched, decrescendo diastolic murmur that is best heard in expiration at the left sternal border with the patient leaning forward. The Austin Flint murmur, an apical, mid to late diastolic rumble, represents turbulence between forward mitral flow and regurgitant aortic flow. Acute AI may produce only a short diastolic murmur because rapid equalization of aortic and ventricular diastolic pressures limits the amount of regurgitant flow. Conversely, peripheral signs of low cardiac output, such as cold, vasoconstricted extremities, can be pronounced.

MR, like AI, produces a hyperdynamic circulation with a brisk, laterally displaced PMI. Unlike AI, the peripheral findings of MR are otherwise unremarkable. The cardiac auscultatory findings of MR include a widely split S_2 due to early aortic valve closure. The holosystolic murmur of MR is a constant, blowing murmur heard best at the apex and usually radiating to the axilla. Regurgitation through a single leaflet can confusingly direct the murmur to the base of the heart, to the back, or even to the head. A diastolic murmur caused by high diastolic reflow across the mitral valve can also be present. There is little beat-to-beat variation of the MR murmur, as may be seen with aortic stenosis, and no increase in the murmur with inspiration, as seen in tricuspid regurgitation. The mid to late systolic click murmur of mitral valve prolapse is more variable than the murmur of MR and can be distinguished by several provocative maneuvers (Table 64-8).

Mitral stenosis produces few peripheral signs on physical examination but many cardiac findings. The PMI is nondisplaced and may be decreased in intensity. An opening snap and accentuated S_1, a diastolic rumble at the apex, and presystolic accentuation of the diastolic murmur may be heard on auscultation. The opening snap is produced by abrupt tensing of the fibrotic mitral valve. Both the opening snap and the first heart sound are decreased as the valve becomes increasingly calcified and immobile. Presystolic accentuation is caused by the increased flow associated with atrial contraction and is therefore usually lost with the onset of atrial fibrillation. Rales are associated with the onset of pulmonary congestion. Late signs of pulmonary hypertension may include an increased P_2, the Graham Steell murmur of pulmonary regurgitation, and further signs of right-sided heart failure.

Tricuspid regurgitation can be associated with a pulsatile liver, ascites, edema, right ventricular heave, and jugular venous distention with bounding *v* waves (*c-v* waves). The pansystolic murmur of tricuspid regurgitation is localized more to the left lower sternal border and tends to increase with inspiration (Carvallo sign) compared with the other systolic murmurs.

The cardiac findings of tricuspid stenosis are frequently masked by associated mitral stenosis. The examiner may notice a diastolic murmur heard best at the left lower sternal border that increases with inspiration. Conversely, the findings of marked jugular venous distention with a prominent *a* wave, ascites, or anasarca in the presence of clear lung fields are highly suggestive of tricuspid stenosis.

Electrocardiogram

The 12-lead ECG is useful in assessing the rhythm disturbances and the specific chamber enlargement that can be associated with valvular disease. More often, the data obtained are nonspecific indicators of overall cardiac function. Vectorcardiography, which determines axis orientation as a function of time, yields additional information but is infrequently used.

Increased QRS voltage associated with LV hypertrophy is a common finding associated with valvular heart disease. An LV strain pattern of sinus tachycardia depression, usually in the lateral leads, is often present. About 85% of patients with significant aortic stenosis have this finding, but systemic hypertension, AI, or other conditions can also cause hypertrophy. LA enlargement with a hypertrophic pattern can also be observed in up to 80% of patients with aortic stenosis. Left axis deviation secondary

to ventricular chamber enlargement can be seen in patients with AI.

Disease of the mitral and tricuspid valves is predominantly reflected in the electrocardiographic activity of the atria. Atrial ectopic activity and atrial fibrillation are common. Mitral stenosis produces a pattern of LA enlargement in 90% of cases; MR produces similar changes. Signs of right ventricular hypertrophy are present in 15% of patients with MR and in 50% of patients with PA systolic pressures exceeding 70 mmHg. In addition, 50% of patients with MR show signs of LV hypertrophy.

IMAGING TECHNIQUES
Chest Roentgenogram

The routine posteroanterior and lateral chest roentgenograms provide relatively nonspecific information about cardiac chamber enlargement and pulmonary congestion that may help in assessing the physiologic impact of valvular heart disease. The ready availability and low expense of the chest radiograph make it a useful means of observing the patient with valvular heart disease despite the introduction of more precise means of cardiac imaging, such as echocardiography. Other specific data can be obtained from the chest radiograph as well. Aortic stenosis is unlikely to be found in a patient older than 40 years of age in the absence of aortic root calcification. Kerley B lines, dense short horizontal lines at the costophrenic angles seen with interstitial edema, usually correlate with pulmonary wedge pressures greater than 20 mmHg and are an important physiologic correlate of valvular disease.

Echocardiography

Cardiac echocardiography has revolutionized the diagnosis of valvular heart disease. M-mode and 2D echocardiography allow real-time assessment of chamber size, wall thickness, and valve appearance and motion. Doppler echo with color Doppler overlay on the 2D image now provides bedside physiologic data regarding blood flow across stenotic or regurgitant valves. The introduction of transesophageal echocardiography should make continuous, real-time evaluation of morphologic parameters readily available in the unstable patient.

The practice of cardiac echocardiography rests on the principle that air, blood, and tissue reflect sound waves with different efficiency. The echo transducer transmits sound waves at a frequency usually between 1 and 7 MHz and receives reflected signals from the targeted structure. These reflected signals are then used to construct an image of the structure being scanned. M-mode echocardiography constructs an ice-pick image as a function of time at the

Table 64-8. PROVOCATIVE MANEUVERS IN PHYSICAL DIAGNOSIS OF VALVULAR DISEASE

Maneuver	Hypertrophic Cardiomyopathy	Aortic Stenosis	Mitral Regurgitation	Mitral Prolapse
Valsalva	+	−	−	±
Standing	+	+/0	−	+
Handgrip	−	−/0	+	−
Squatting	−	−/0	+	−
Amyl nitrite	++	+	−	+
Isoproterenol	++	+	−	+

(Modified from Paraskos JA. Combined valvular disease. In: Dalen JE, Alpert JS, eds. Valvular heart disease. Boston, Little, Brown, 1981)

one point at which the transducer is aimed. The 2D transducer uses a phased array to produce an echo image, usually 30 degrees in circumference. The 2D image suffers somewhat in sharpness compared with the M-mode image, and chamber dimensional measurements are consequently obtained from the M-mode image. Other limitations of echo imaging include interference with ultrasound transmission by air in overlying lung, motion artifact, and the limited number of viewing windows. Calcium and prosthetic valves are extremely echo dense relative to normal tissue, producing bright, contrasting images that are also hard to image. In general, 70% to 80% of echo studies are considered technically adequate.

Quantification of mitral stenosis is perhaps the valvular analysis most amenable to 2D imaging. Direct measurement of orifice size correlates exceptionally well with catheterization data. Decreased range of mitral valve excursion on the M-mode study (E-F slope), thickened leaflets, and decreased diastolic leaflet separation also yield useful information. Accurate LA sizing provides important diagnostic and therapeutic data for mitral disease. Conversely, LA thrombus is often sought in mitral stenosis patients but is not reliably revealed. The causes of MR, such as a ruptured chorda or flail leaflet, can be visualized, but quantification of MR depends on Doppler analysis.

Echocardiographic assessment of the aortic valve also yields data regarding orifice size and pathology. Abnormalities such as a bicuspid valve can usually be detected. Leaflet thickening and orifice narrowing are characteristic of aortic stenosis. AI can be suggested by diastolic fluttering of the mitral or aortic leaflet. Important prognostic data regarding LV diameters can also be accurately followed.

Doppler echocardiography uses basic Doppler principles to measure the velocity of red blood cells in a targeted area. The two most commonly used formats are the continuous-wave Doppler and the gated, or pulsed, Doppler. Continuous-wave Doppler samples all sound waves returned along the course of the transducer beam. Instantaneous mean velocity and direction of blood flow are determined from the frequency shift of the returning signal. Pulsed Doppler samples blood velocity at a specific point along the beam course, known as the sample volume. Continuous-wave Doppler suffers in that it cannot indicate where along the Doppler path the blood velocities are being reported. The chief disadvantage of pulsed Doppler is a phenomenon known as aliasing, which makes it difficult to accurately measure high-speed blood velocities. Continuous-wave Doppler is therefore most useful for measuring high-speed blood flow, such as that found in aortic stenosis; pulsed Doppler is used to assess flow at a specific point.

Modification of the Bernoulli principle relating velocity change to pressure drop across points of fixed resistance allows quantification of pressure gradients across stenotic valve orifices. The pressure drop across a stenotic valve can be approximated as $P = 4v^2$. Close correlation with subsequent catheterization data has been good. Velocity and pressure drop are underestimated if the pulse beam is not within 20 degrees of parallel to the blood jet.

Assessment of regurgitant flow is less accurate. Qualitative determination of the severity of regurgitant flow can be made with pulsed Doppler by measuring how far the high-flow jet extends from the incompetent valve. The detection of high-speed jets characteristic of periprosthetic leaks is possible with an accuracy of up to 94%. Doppler techniques are especially applicable for the assessment of tricuspid regurgitation because of the technical limitations of other studies.

Cardiac Catheterization

The first cardiac catheterization of a living human being is a classic story in the annals of pioneering medical discovery. It was reported by the discoverer, Forssmann, in 1929; he was 25 years old. He exposed a vein in his own left arm, introduced a ureteral catheter into the antecubital vein, and then walked to the radiology department, where he was able to document positioning of the catheter in the right atrium of his own heart. Forssmann reported that "there was a considerable distance between the operating rooms and the x-ray unit . . . while the probe was lying within my heart, but I was not aware of any unpleasantness."[10]

Cardiac catheterization, now performed with a mortality and significant morbidity rate of about 0.1% each, yields the most accurate functional data of all diagnostic studies and remains the diagnostic gold standard. A wide range of intracardiac pressures and hemodynamic parameters can be obtained by cardiac catheterization (Table 64-9). Access to the left side of the heart can be obtained by way of percutaneous introduction of catheters through the femoral (Judkins) or brachial (Sones) arteries. About 5% of severely stenotic aortic valves cannot be crossed with this retrograde approach. In these instances, a catheter can be passed from the venous circulation across the atrial septum to the left side of the heart. This technique is also useful in the presence of severe MR, when pulmonary capillary wedge pressure does not adequately estimate LVEDP, and in the presence of a tilting-disc aortic valve prosthesis.

Left and right atrial pressure waveforms, obtained by appropriately positioned catheters, normally contain two major positive components, the a and v waves (Fig. 64-7). The a wave corresponds to atrial systole, whereas the v wave is inscribed during ventricular systole, as the atrium fills with the venous return. The x descent follows the a wave as atrial pressure declines, only to be interrupted by the c wave, caused by closure and upward movement of the AV valve toward the atrial chamber. The x descent continues after the c wave, as blood slowly begins to refill the emptied atrial chamber. The v wave represents the upturn in this filling phase as atrial capacitance is reached. The y descent after the v peak corresponds with ventricular

Table 64-9. NORMAL CARDIAC HEMODYNAMIC PRESSURES AND VALUES

	Systolic	End-Diastolic	Mean
PRESSURE (mmHg)			
Right atrium			0–8
Right ventricle	15–30	0–8	
Pulmonary artery	15–30	3–12	9–16
Pulmonary artery wedge/ left atrium			1–10
Left ventricle	100–140	3–12	
Aorta	100–140	60–90	70–105
CARDIAC OUTPUT INDEX (L/min/m²)		2.6–4.2	
RESISTANCE (dynes·s/cm⁵)			
Pulmonary		20–130	
Systemic		700–1600	

(Modified from Grossman W, Barry WH. Cardiac catheterization. In: Braunwald E, ed. Heart disease: a textbook of cardiovascular medicine. Philadelphia, WB Saunders, 1988:287)

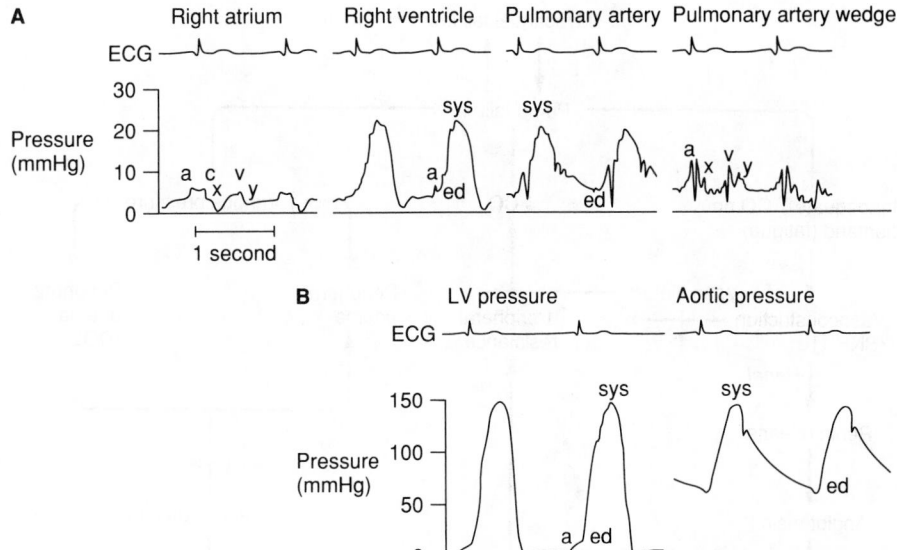

Figure 64-7. Normal pressure tracings from the right (*A*) and left (*B*) sides of the heart. (After Grossman W, Barry WH. Cardiac catheterization. In: Braunwald E, ed. Heart disease: a textbook of cardiovascular medicine, ed 3. Philadelphia, WB Saunders, 1988:250)

relaxation. The AV valve opens, and atrial blood empties during ventricular diastole into the ventricular chamber.

Atrial and ventricular pressures are normally about equal during diastole because of the low resistance to flow across the normal AV valve. The PA diastolic or pulmonary capillary wedge pressure, usually obtained with a flow-directed catheter, is normally an adequate reflection of LA pressure, and therefore LVEDP. The end-diastolic PA pressure and the mean PA wedge pressure are about equal in a low-resistance pulmonary circuit. Mean PA pressure is always higher than mean wedge pressure, because the systolic PA pressure is not transmitted to the wedged catheter position.

The various valvular lesions produce a spectrum of abnormalities of pressure gradients and waveforms. In patients with AI, the peripheral pulse pressure is widened because of reflow into the ventricle. The *a* wave in the PA or LA pressure trace is greatly increased in mitral stenosis as a result of atrial contraction against the stenotic mitral valve. Similar changes are seen in right atrial tracings in tricuspid stenosis. Ventricular stiffness caused by hypertrophy, especially in aortic stenosis, is also reflected in large *a* waves as the atrium contracts against the relatively high resistance of the hypertrophied ventricle. MR or tricuspid regurgitation produces a large *c-v* wave as diastolic atrial filling is augmented by flow back across the mitral valve during ventricular systole.

Pressure gradients across stenotic valves are determined by the measurement of pressures in the chamber above and below the lesion being examined (Fig. 64-8). Pressures can be measured by pullback of the catheter from one chamber to the next or, more accurately, by simultaneous pressure measurements with catheters placed in each chamber. Valve cross-sectional areas are determined by the Gorlin equations (see Appendix 64-1). These equations are derived from the basic hydrodynamic equation, flow = pressure ÷ resistance. A constant that is specific for each valve corrects for resistance to flow caused by blood viscosity and turbulence, predicted by the Poiseuille and Reynold equations, respectively. Flow is derived from cardiac output divided by the specific flow time across the valve being measured. Cardiac output, in turn, is calculated by the Fick principle, using indicator dilution curves, thermodilution techniques, or the classic oxygen method. High cardiac output or mixed regurgitant disease is a source of

error in these calculations. Real-time echocardiographic determinations may be superior in this regard.

Regurgitant lesions are graded qualitatively on a 1+ to 4+ scale, based on contrast injections made upstream from the lesion in question; for example, an aortic root injection is used to assess AI. Regurgitation of scale 1+ corresponds to a regurgitant fraction of about 20%, 2+ about 20% to 40%, 3+ between 40% and 60%, and 4+ greater than 60%. Fractions exceeding 30% to 40% (2+ or greater) are considered hemodynamically significant. The most troublesome lesion in this regard is tricuspid regurgitation, because no direct access to the right ventricle is technically feasible except across the valve itself. Artifactual tricuspid regurgitation can be caused by the catheter crossing the valve or by ventricular ectopic activity induced by right ventricular injections.

Radionuclide Angiography

Radionuclide cineangiography yields visual and numeric data regarding cardiac function and valvular disease. Combined with with technetium-99m, it yields accurate measurements of cardiac ejection fractions and is espe-

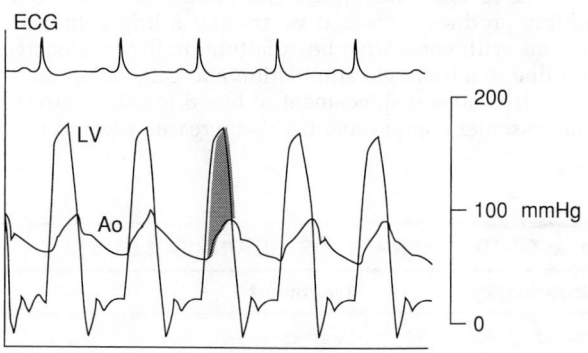

Figure 64-8. Left ventricular (LV) and aortic (Ao) pressure tracings in a patient with aortic stenosis. Peak-to-peak systolic gradient is approximately 80 mmHg. Mean aortic valve pressure gradient (*blue area*) is approximately 70 mmHg. (After Grossman W. Resistance to blood flow by stenotic valves. In: Cardiac catheterization and angiography. Philadelphia, Lea & Febiger, 1974:92)

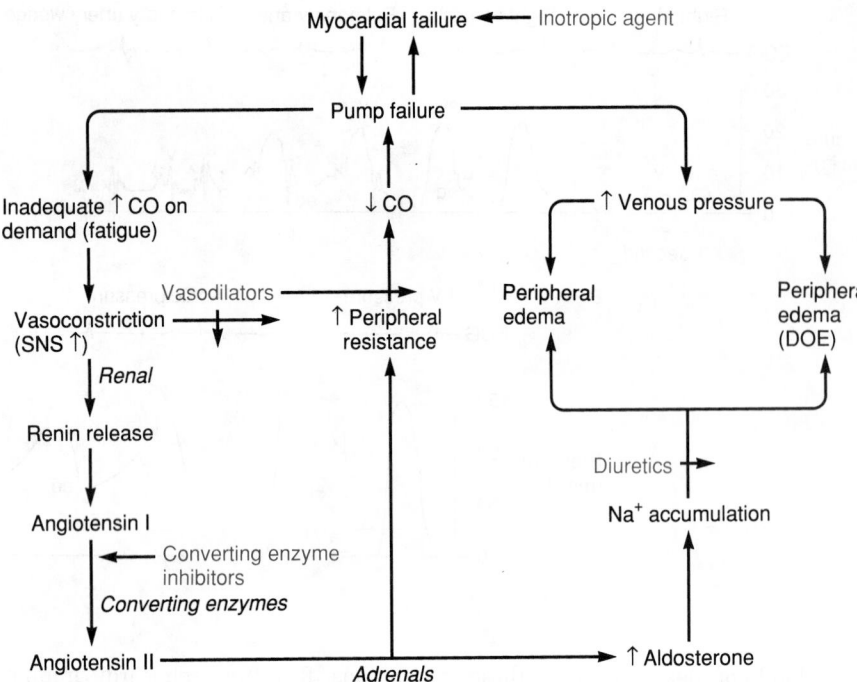

Figure 64-9. Schematic diagram of the pathophysiology of heart failure and the point of action of the three major therapeutic agents—diuretics, inotropic agents, and vasodilators. (After Schlant RC, Sonnenblick EH. Pathophysiology of heart failure. In: Hurst JW. The heart, ed 6. New York, McGraw-Hill, 1986:336)

cially useful in measuring forward flow in patients with regurgitation. Serial determination of ventricular function with radionuclide cineangiography is now a mainstay in the long-term follow-up of many valvular heart disease patients.

MEDICAL MANAGEMENT

The medical management of the patient with significant cardiac valvular dysfunction requires an understanding of the pathophysiology of valvular heart disease and the treatment of congestive heart failure (Fig. 64-9). Enhancement of cardiac function in patients with congestive failure secondary to valvular dysfunction is directed toward optimizing the three primary determinants of ventricular function—preload, afterload, and myocardial contractility (Table 64-10). Specific considerations vary, depending on which form of valvular dysfunction is being treated.

Congestive Heart Failure

Increased total body water and increased intravascular volume produce increased ventricular filling volumes in patients with congestive heart failure. Both venoconstriction due to adrenergic stimulation and catecholamine release also cause displacement of blood into the intrathoracic vascular compartment. This increased preload is, on

the one hand, beneficial, shifting ventricular contractility rightward on the Frank-Starling curve. On the other hand, increased ventricular distention represents an unwanted increase in ventricular afterload with consequent increases in myocardial oxygen consumption and deleterious effects on contractility. Because the ventricle is often operating on the flat portion of the Frank-Starling curve in patients with significant dysfunction (see A in Fig. 64-5), excessive elevation of preload increases pulmonary congestion and lowers the patient's functional capabilities without significantly improving cardiac output. Preload is effectively lowered with diuretics, such as furosemide, and venodilator agents, such as nitroglycerine. Excessive reduction in preload robs the ventricle of filling volumes needed to maintain effective contraction. The balance between beneficial decreases in afterload with improvement in pulmonary congestion, versus deleterious decreases in preload, cannot be discerned a priori. Careful clinical and hemodynamic monitoring of the patient after implementation of therapy is required.

A similar balance is struck in using arterial vasodilators to reduce afterload. Afterload reduction in the failing heart results in a substantial improvement in ventricular fiber shortening and an increase in stroke volume compared with the effects seen in the normal heart. The decrease in systemic vascular resistance induced by vasodilator agents is thereby often offset by an increase in cardiac output, and blood pressure remains stable or decreases only slightly. Afterload reduction is therefore most effective in patients with increased systemic vascular resistance, depressed cardiac output, and increased filling pressures. Excessive use of afterload reducers can result in significant hypotension.

Afterload reduction can be accomplished with such agents as nitroprusside, a rapidly acting intravenous agent, or hydralazine, an oral arterial vasodilator. The angiotensin-converting enzyme inhibitors, represented by captopril and enalapril, are another class of afterload reducing drugs that act primarily by inhibiting the vasoconstrictor angiotensin II. They are effective regardless of circulating renin levels.

Table 64-10. THERAPY OF HEART FAILURE

Abnormality	Treatment
Preload	Diuretics
	Venous dilators
Afterload	Arterial vasodilators
	Angiotensin-converting enzyme inhibitors
Contractility	Positive inotropic agents

(Schlant RC, Sonnenblick EH. Pathophysiology of heart failure. In: Hurst JW, ed. The heart, ed 6. New York, McGraw-Hill, 1986:319)

The quintessential and oldest positive cardiac inotropes are the digitalis glycosides, discovered over 200 years ago. Digitalis increases the rate of rise of intraventricular pressure during isovolumetric systole through a direct effect on Na^+-K^+-ATPase and the myocyte sodium pump. Adequate digitalis levels for patients in normal sinus rhythm appear to be between 1.5 and 2 ng/mL. The ventricular function curve is shifted upward and to the left (see B in Fig. 64-5), producing more stroke work at any given level of filling. Because the failing myocardium is working on a decreased length–active tension curve, the relative augmentation of contractility is greater in the failing heart than in the normal heart. Improvement in cardiac function allows decreased ventricular filling and creates a greater cardiac reserve because the ventricle is able to function at a lower point on the Frank-Starling curve. Decreased levels of LVEDP lead to decreased pulmonary congestion and symptomatic improvement. Increases in cardiac output can result in diuresis and decreased heart rate as sympathetic tone is diminished. Although digitalis can cause improvement in the functional class of the patient, there is no evidence that administration of this agent prolongs survival or retards the long-term course of myocardial dysfunction.

Several other positive inotropes share similar hemodynamic effects with digitalis, varying only by their mode of action. Dopamine is an endogenous catecholamine that is the immediate precursor in the biosynthesis of norepinephrine. Dopamine stimulates myocardial contractility by direct action on myocardial β_1-receptors and by indirect release of norepinephrine from sympathetic nerve terminals. Dopamine interacts with vasodilating dopamine$_1$ receptors in the coronary, renal, mesenteric, and cerebral vascular beds, producing decreases in systemic and renal vascular resistance at low (1 to 3 μg/kg/min) doses. Larger doses of dopamine cause vasoconstriction that overrides this dopaminergic effect, probably through interaction with serotonin and β_1 receptors. As with other agents that increase myocardial contractility, dopamine causes an increase in myocardial oxygen consumption, a deleterious effect that must be balanced with its ability to increase contractility.

Dobutamine, a synthetic sympathetamine with clinical β_1 and β_2 activity, addresses several side effects of dopamine that can be deleterious in selected circumstances. Dobutamine usually causes less of an increase in heart rate and decreases systemic vascular resistance in comparison with dopamine. This tends to cause a smaller relative increase or even a decrease in myocardial oxygen consumption. Dobutamine is generally the drug of choice for heart failure in the normotensive or hypertensive patient.

A new class of agents, represented by amrinone, works through inhibition of phosphodiesterase F-III. These agents, which increase intracellular levels of cyclic AMP, combine positive inotropic and vasodilator effects. Because these agents work through a cell pathway entirely separate from that of the sympathetamines, they can be particularly effective when sympathetic mechanisms have already been saturated with other compounds. The long half-life of amrinone may be a relative disadvantage.

Specific Considerations

Aortic Stenosis

The ventricle of patients with aortic stenosis can be significantly noncompliant, leading to large changes in LVEDP with small volume changes. Incremental adjustment of the volume status of these patients may be required to avoid dramatic changes in LVEDP, leading either to pul-

monary edema if excessively increased or to vascular collapse with inadequate ventricular filling. Negative inotropic agents should be avoided. Significant hemodynamic compromise associated with atrial fibrillation may require pharmacologic or electrical cardioversion.

Aortic Insufficiency

Peripheral vasodilators are the keystone to pharmacologic treatment of AI, producing a pressure gradient favoring blood flow to the periphery. Vasoconstricting agents such as norepinephrine bitartrate (Levophed) are contraindicated because they tend to increase afterload and exacerbate AI. Use of the intraaortic balloon pump is strictly contraindicated, because balloon inflation during diastole severely exacerbates AI. Valve replacement is often the only effective treatment for cardiac decompensation associated with acute-onset AI.

Mitral Stenosis

The primary effects of mitral stenosis are related to the pulmonary circulation; thus, treatment of pulmonary congestive changes is central to the medical management of mitral stenosis. Symptoms of dyspnea and pulmonary fluid overload can be dramatically improved with sodium restriction and diuresis. As mentioned earlier, dehydration must be cautiously avoided. Excessive loss of atrial preload can reduce the needed pressure gradient across the mitral valve, resulting in inadequate LV filling and vascular collapse.

Control of ventricular rate is also important in the medical management of mitral stenosis. The frequent occurrence of atrial fibrillation can be controlled with digitalis or with calcium-channel blockers or β-blockers. Maintenance of sinus rhythm appears to improve prognosis, although it is unclear whether this is a reflection of the associated complications of thromboembolism or relates to the underlying status of cardiac function. Antiarrhythmic therapy may therefore be indicated for frequent premature atrial contractions, often the harbinger of atrial fibrillation. Cardioversion may be indicated for atrial fibrillation, especially if significant hemodynamic compromise develops. Atrial fibrillation of recent onset (less than 6 months) and with an atrium less than 55 mm in diameter is less likely to be recurrent after cardioversion than long-standing atrial fibrillation in a dilated atrium.

Mitral Regurgitation

A multimodality approach is best suited to the medical management of MR. Ventricular preload reduction with diuretics or nitrates should serve to improve pulmonary congestion. Preload and afterload reduction with vasodilators should reduce the degree of MR by decreasing the LV–LA gradient and the mitral valve orifice size.[11] Improved LV emptying with decreased wall tension and decreased end-systolic volume should result. Positive inotropes can also be used to decrease the regurgitant orifice size by improving myocardial contractility. In the setting of acute, severe MR, aggressive afterload reduction with nitroprusside and balloon counterpulsation can be effective temporizing measures before operation.

Tricuspid Disease

Tricuspid stenosis and tricuspid regurgitation are most effectively treated with aggressive diuresis, applying the same cautions as indicated earlier. Correction of the primary left-sided disease can significantly improve the physiologic effects of secondary tricuspid regurgitation. In fact, total excision of the tricuspid valve can be well tolerated in the presence of normal right ventricular systolic pressures.

SURGICAL MANAGEMENT

Indications

The timing of surgical intervention remains an important and often controversial issue in caring for patients with valvular disease. Surgical indications generally include deterioration in ventricular function or functional class. If operative intervention is delayed inappropriately, postoperative ventricular function and functional class may fail to improve, and operative risks are significantly increased.

Timing of surgery is perhaps most critical for patients with AI or MR because symptoms may not develop until after irreversible myocardial dysfunction has occurred. Mean survival after development of symptoms in AI is only 4 years if angina is present and 2 years if congestive failure is present.[12] Thus, operative intervention is usually indicated for any functional class II patient with AI or MR. Others advocate operative repair of severe AI, as indicated by a diastolic blood pressure less than 50 mmHg, even in the asymptomatic patient.

Even with these criteria, functional improvement can be significantly reduced for patients undergoing aortic valve replacement for AI compared with those in the same preoperative class with aortic stenosis, because of the delayed onset of symptoms with AI. Fortunately, the availability of radionuclide cineangiography to determine LV ejection fractions and echocardiography to measure LV dimensions has greatly facilitated the accurate follow-up of ventricular function in these patients. Proposed operative criteria for AI that suggest ventricular decompensation include an end-systolic LV diameter larger than 55 mm (Fig. 64-10) and fractional shortening less than 30%, ejection fraction below 50%, and increases in LVEDV.[13,14] Similar criteria have been established for the timing of operation in MR patients.[15]

Operative intervention is usually advocated for critical mitral stenosis (mitral valve orifice less than 1 cm^2/m^2) or for any patient with symptoms. Systemic emboli, especially if recurrent, are also an indication for operation. Other parameters include a mean mitral valve gradient of 12 to 15 mmHg and an end-diastolic gradient of 8 to 10 mmHg. The onset of atrial fibrillation has also been suggested as an operative indication because prolonged atrial fibrillation seems to worsen the prognosis for patients with mitral stenosis. Some researchers do not recommend operation in the absence of symptoms, since a certain proportion of patients with mitral stenosis stabilize and little risk of irreversible myocardial dysfunction is incurred. Early operation does not appear to improve long-term survival in asymptomatic patients. Conversely, the 5-year survival rate for functional class III patients is only 62%, and it drops to 15% for class IV patients.[16]

Timing of surgery for aortic stenosis is somewhat less controversial. Operation is usually indicated for any symptoms, including emboli, a transvalvular gradient greater than or equal to 50 mmHg, and a calculated valve area less than or equal to 0.4 cm^2/m^2. Mean survival after the onset of angina is about 5 years; with syncope, it is 3 years, and with heart failure, 2 years (Fig. 64-11). Symptomatic patients with significant uncorrected aortic stenosis have 25% 1-year and 50% 2-year mortality rates.[17] Half of these deaths are sudden.

As mentioned earlier, functional tricuspid regurgitation most often improves with correction of left-sided disease. Duran and associates[18] reported a 100% late persistence of tricuspid regurgitation in the presence of significant pulmonary hypertension, compared with a 0% incidence without pulmonary hypertension. Furthermore, tricuspid regurgitation remained in 47% of pa-

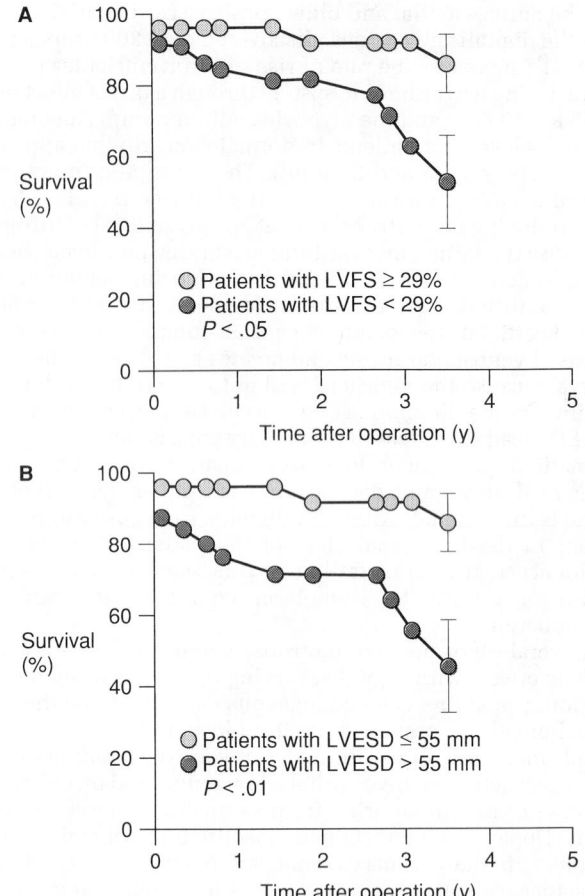

Figure 64-10. Survival after operation for aortic regurgitation as a function of left ventricular fractional shortening (LVFS; *A*) and left ventricular end-systolic diameter (LVESD; *B*). There is improved early and late survival with improved ventricular function. (After Bonow RO, Rosing DR, Kent KM, Epstein SE. Timing of operation for chronic aortic regurgitation. Am J Cardiol 1982;50:325)

tients undergoing mitral valve replacement with associated organic disease of the tricuspid valve, compared with no late tricuspid regurgitation in the absence of organic tricuspid disease. A tricuspid valve gradient of 5 mmHg or more is an indication for operative correction of tricuspid stenosis.

Surgical Options

Balloon valvuloplasty is a recently popularized approach to valvular disease that can be an advantageous alternative to open heart surgery in selected circumstances. Initial and intermediate-term results for selected cases of mitral stenosis have been encouraging.[19] Patients suitable for balloon valvuloplasty must have limited valvular and subvalvular calcification and fibrosis. This determination is made from a standardized echocardiographic scoring system.[20]

In contrast, percutaneous aortic balloon valvuloplasty suffers from a relatively high complication and recurrence rate.[21] Open heart surgery, with aortic valve replacement, therefore remains the primary option for most patients with critical aortic stenosis, although balloon aortic valvuloplasty has been advocated as a bridging technique in critically ill patients.[22]

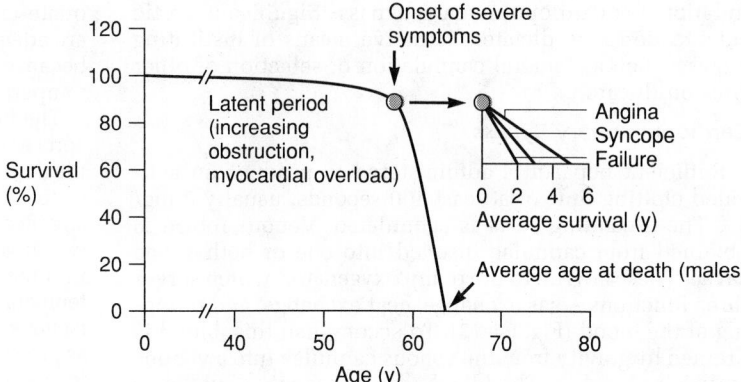

Figure 64-11. Natural history of aortic stenosis without operative intervention. (After Ross J Jr, Braunwald E. Aortic stenosis. Circulation 1968;38[Suppl 5]:61)

Mitral commissurotomy for mitral stenosis can be performed in 70% to 90% of patients but may be limited by extensive calcification, leaflet stiffness, chordal fusion, or associated MR, in that order.[23] Commissurotomy carries up to a 20% chance of reoperation within 5 years and a 60% chance at 10 years[24] but avoids the potential morbidity of a valve prosthesis during that time. Mitral valve repair for MR, which is applicable in most cases, depending on patient population, carries a 6% reoperation rate at 5 years for nonrheumatic disease, although 23% of repairs for rheumatic disease require reoperation at 5 years.[25] Aortic valve repair is not usually possible in the presence of calcific disease. Tricuspid valve annuloplasty (Fig. 64-12) is the preferred treatment for significant secondary tricuspid regurgitation, with valve replacement reserved for severe or primary disease.

Preoperative Care

Careful preoperative preparation of the patient about to undergo heart valve replacement can have important consequences in terms of eventual patient morbidity and mortality. Screening for occult infectious processes is critical to prevent contamination of the valvular prosthesis and prosthetic valve endocarditis. Dental abscesses should be treated before operation if the patient's cardiac status permits. Bleeding parameters and potential for coagulopathy should be assessed because of the need for intraoperative heparinization and postoperative anticoagulation. Gastrointestinal tract bleeding, in particular, should be thoroughly evaluated before valve replacement. Aspirin and other agents that can alter coagulation should be discontinued 1 week before surgery. Patients with significant respiratory compromise should be considered for preoperative pulmonary care. Cigarette smoking should be discontinued. Attention should be directed toward improving the nutritional status of the patient, if possible.

Preoperative enhancement of cardiac function can significantly improve operative survival. The concept of optimizing a patient may have originated with such preoperative treatment of patients with mitral stenosis, in whom prolonged periods of congestive failure may have contributed to significant accumulations of edema fluid. Operative survival correlates with preoperative functional class; therefore, treatment of congestive failure in the preoperative period and upgrading of functional class can have significant effects on the outcome of operation (see later discussion).

Surgical Technique

Operative technique at the outset of the procedure is similar whether valve repair or replacement is to be performed. A median sternotomy is almost always used and allows best access to the heart, although excellent exposure to the mitral valve can be obtained by way of a thoracotomy incision. After opening the pericardium, the surgeon can palpate the tricuspid valve and assess tricuspid regurgitation through a pursestring incision in the right atrial appendage. The aorta is assessed for calcification before can-

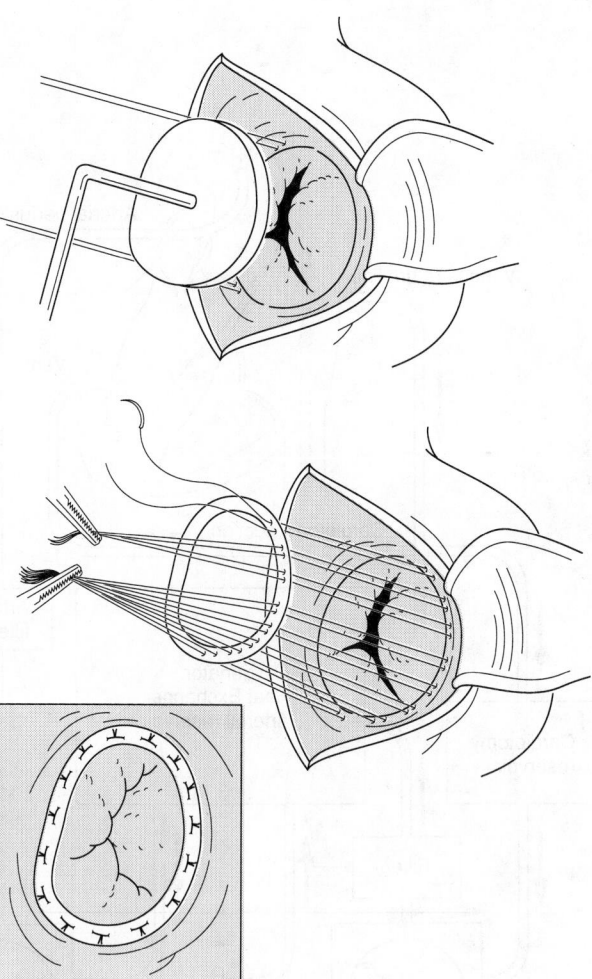

Figure 64-12. Carpentier tricuspid ring annuloplasty. Disproportionate intervals between sutures in the annulus compared with the ring allow pursestring suturing of the dilated annulus. (After Carpentier A, Deloche A, Hanania G, et al. Surgical management of acquired tricuspid valve disease. J Thorac Cardiovasc Surg 1974;67:53)

nulation for cardiopulmonary bypass. Significant aortic calcification may dictate alternative means of instituting bypass, such as femoral cannulation or selection of other sites on the arch.

Cardiopulmonary Bypass

Sufficient heparin is administered to produce an activated clotting time of at least 400 seconds, usually 3 mg/kg. The ascending aorta is cannulated. Venous return is obtained from cannulae inserted into one or both venae cavae. These are run to the pump oxygenator, which serves three functions—gas exchange, heat exchange, and pumping of the blood (Fig. 64-13). To accomplish this, blood is drained by gravity from the venous cannulae into a venous reservoir chamber. The blood passes through a bubble or membrane oxygenator that provides for gas exchange, and a heat exchanger that can rapidly warm or cool the blood. Finally, the blood is pumped back into the body, usually with a DeBakey-type roller pump or Bio-Medicus centrifugal pump. The pump oxygenator also contains various filters and other mechanisms to prevent introduction of air or thrombi into the arterial circuit.

Once bypass is appropriately initiated, the blood is usually cooled to 25° to 27°C. At this temperature, metabolic rates are such that flow rates of 1.6 L/m²/min provide ade-

quate circulation. Similarly, hematocrits of 20% to 25% are adequate and provide optimal rheologic characteristics because of increased blood viscosity at these lower temperatures.

The heart is then arrested by crossclamping the ascending aorta and injecting about 1000 mL of a cold potassium cardioplegic solution (potassium concentration, 30 to 35 mEq/L at 4° to 6°C) into the aortic root. Injections in the presence of significant AI require opening of the aortic root and direct cannulation of the coronary ostia to prevent reflux of injectate into the left ventricle and ventricular distention. Myocardial temperatures are usually maintained at 10° to 20°C, with reinjections of cold cardioplegic solution about every 20 minutes as protection during the ischemic crossclamp period. A topical iced slush or iced saline solution can also be used to help prevent rewarming due to operating room lights and the warmer blood flowing through the aorta and abdominal viscera below. Various protective agents, such as calcium-channel blockers, free-radical scavengers, and Krebs cycle precursors, can be added to the cardioplegic solution to help improve myocardial protection.

Mitral Valve Repair

After the heart is cooled and arrested, a longitudinal LA incision is made and appropriate retraction applied (Fig. 64-14). Some authors advocate oversewing the LA append-

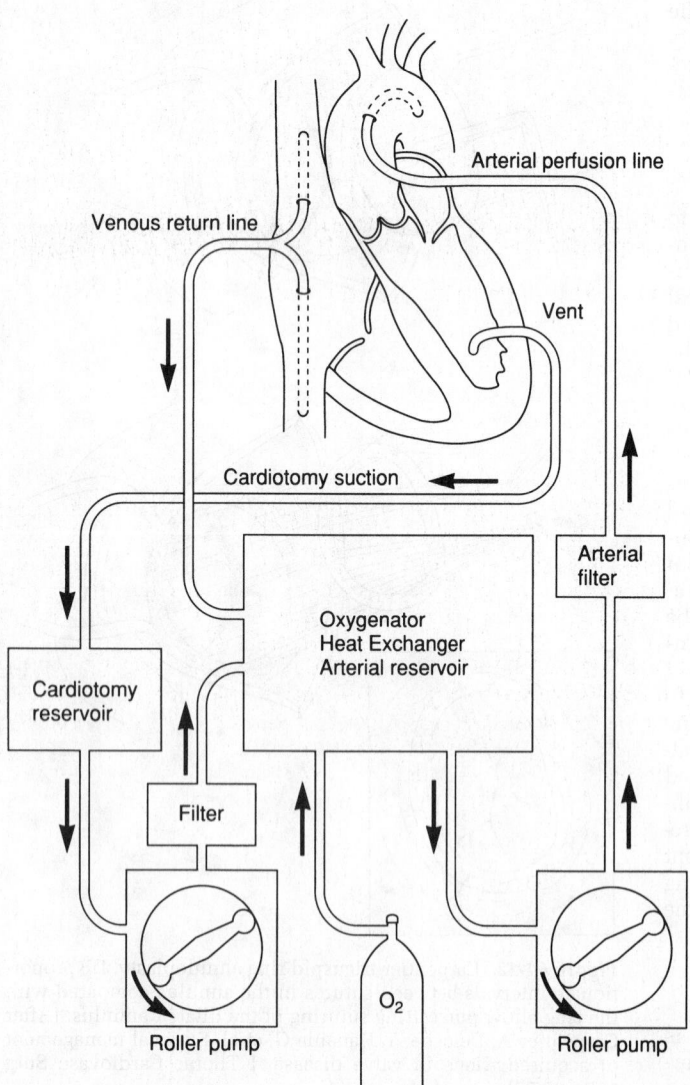

Figure 64-13. Schematic depiction of the main components of the pump oxygenator (heart–lung machine). (After Callaghan JC, Wartak J. Open heart surgery: theory and practice. New York, Praeger Press, 1986)

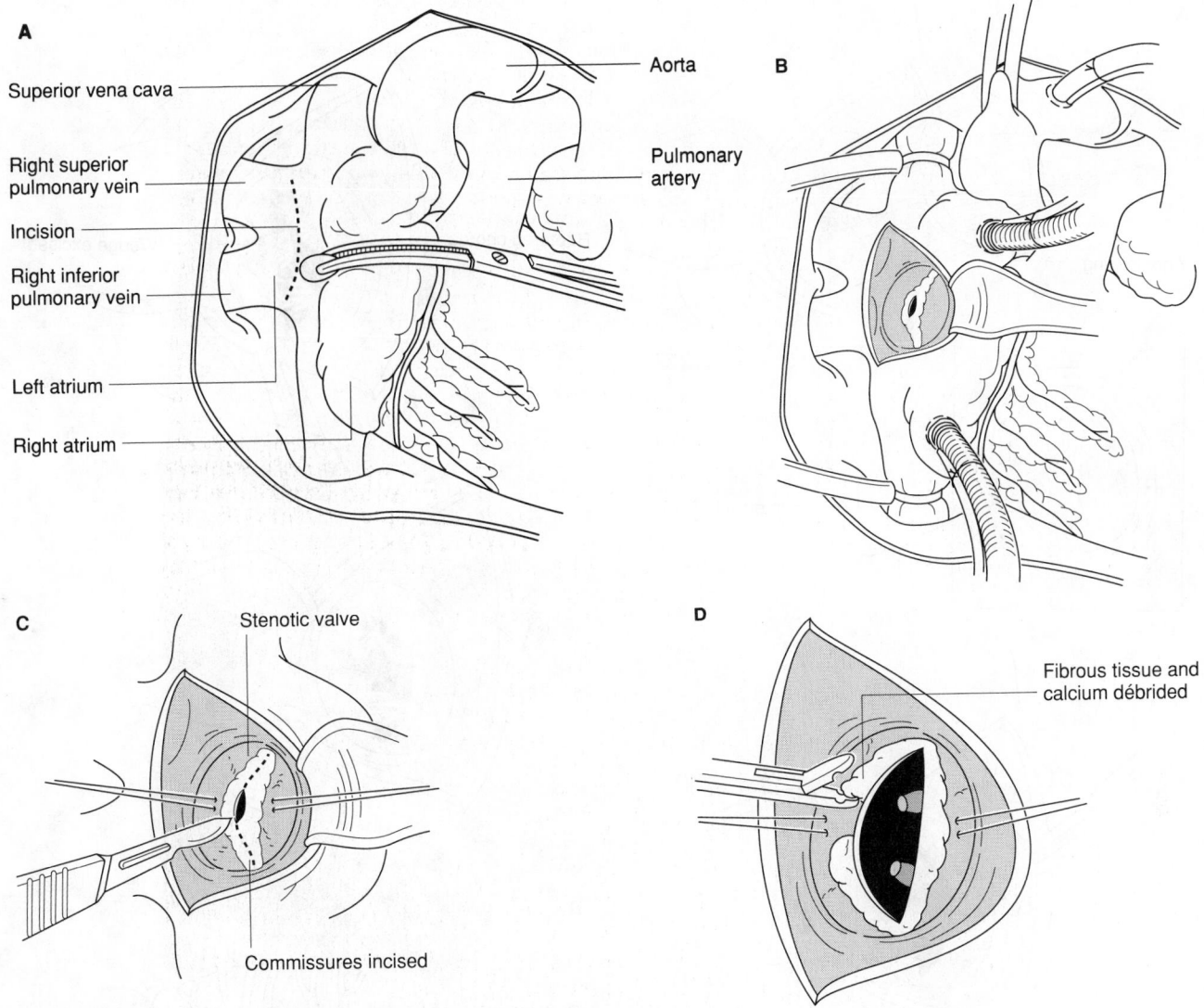

Figure 64-14. Mitral valve repair for stenotic disease. (*A* and *B*) Left atrial incision. (*C*) Mitral commissurotomy showing incision of fused commissures. (*D*) Débridement of excessive calcium.

age, especially in the presence of LA thrombus. In performing a mitral commissurotomy, the surgeon divides the fused commissures to a point a few millimeters from the valve annulus, ensuring that attachments to the chordae tendineae are left intact to prevent iatrogenic mitral insufficiency (see Fig. 64-14*C*). Fused chordae or even the papillary muscle can occasionally be split to improve valve mobility. Shortened secondary chordae to the mural leaflet can be divided. Curettage of excessive calcium can be undertaken, but posterior perforations must be carefully avoided (see Fig. 64-14*D*).

Mitral reconstruction for insufficiency may involve mitral annuloplasty, with plication of an enlarged annulus usually onto a semirigid, C-shaped ring (Fig. 64-15*A*), or mitral reconstruction by various other techniques, as described by Carpentier (see Fig. 64-15*B* through *D*). These may consist of quadrantic segmental resection of an enlarged mural leaflet, shortening of elongated chordae, or transposition of mural leaflet chordae to the aortic (anterior) leaflet. The most common repair performed for mitral regurgitation is posterior leaflet resection.[26]

Recent evidence has suggested that placement of a rigid annuloplasty ring can precipitate systolic anterior motion of the anterior mitral valve leaflet and left ventricular outflow tract obstruction. Placement of a flexible ring, or total avoidance of ring placement anteriorly, seems to alleviate this problem and allows improved LV function.

Valve Replacement

Mitral valve replacement begins with excising the diseased valve some 3 to 4 mm from the annulus (Fig. 64-16*A*). Heavily calcified valves can present difficulties in excision. Preservation of the posterior leaflet or at least some of the chordae to the posterior annulus is used by many surgeons, especially for nonrheumatic MR. This can improve postoperative LV function and help prevent posterior LV rupture, a grave complication of valve replacement.[27] Partial valvular preservation can be particularly attractive when the use of a tissue bioprosthesis is contemplated, because there is less risk of residual valvular tissue interfering with prosthetic function, as can occur with mechanical valves. Otherwise, most surgeons divide the chordae at their junction with the papillary muscles or divide the papillary heads.

After valve removal and appropriate débridement of calcium to allow passage of sutures into relatively compliant

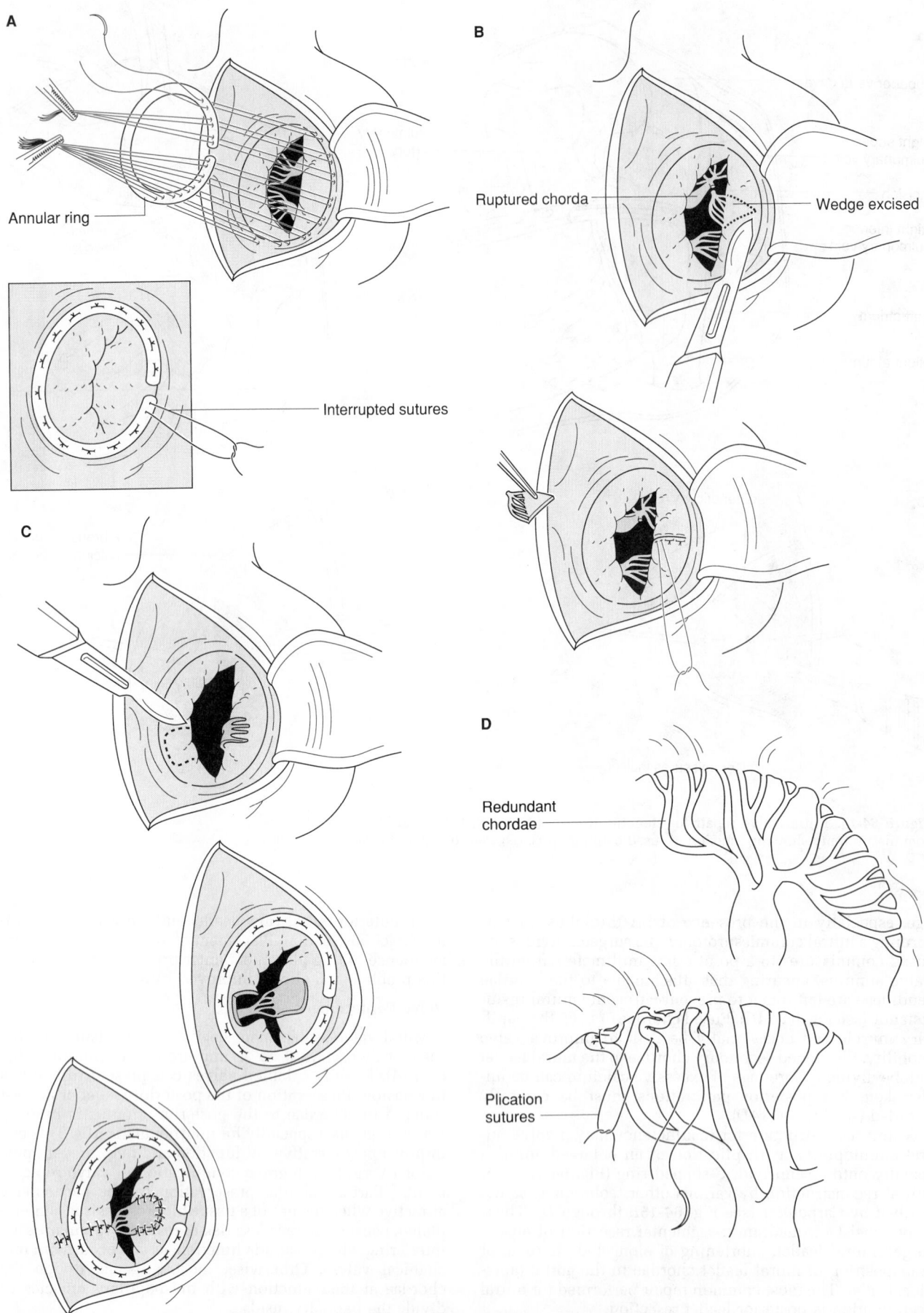

Figure 64-15. Mitral valve repair for regurgitant disease. (*A*) Annuloplasty. (*B*) Leaflet resection. (*C*) Chordal transposition. (*D*) Chordal plication. (After Galloway AC, Colvin SB, Baumann FG, et al. Current concepts of mitral valve reconstruction for mitral insufficiency. Circulation 1988;78:1087)

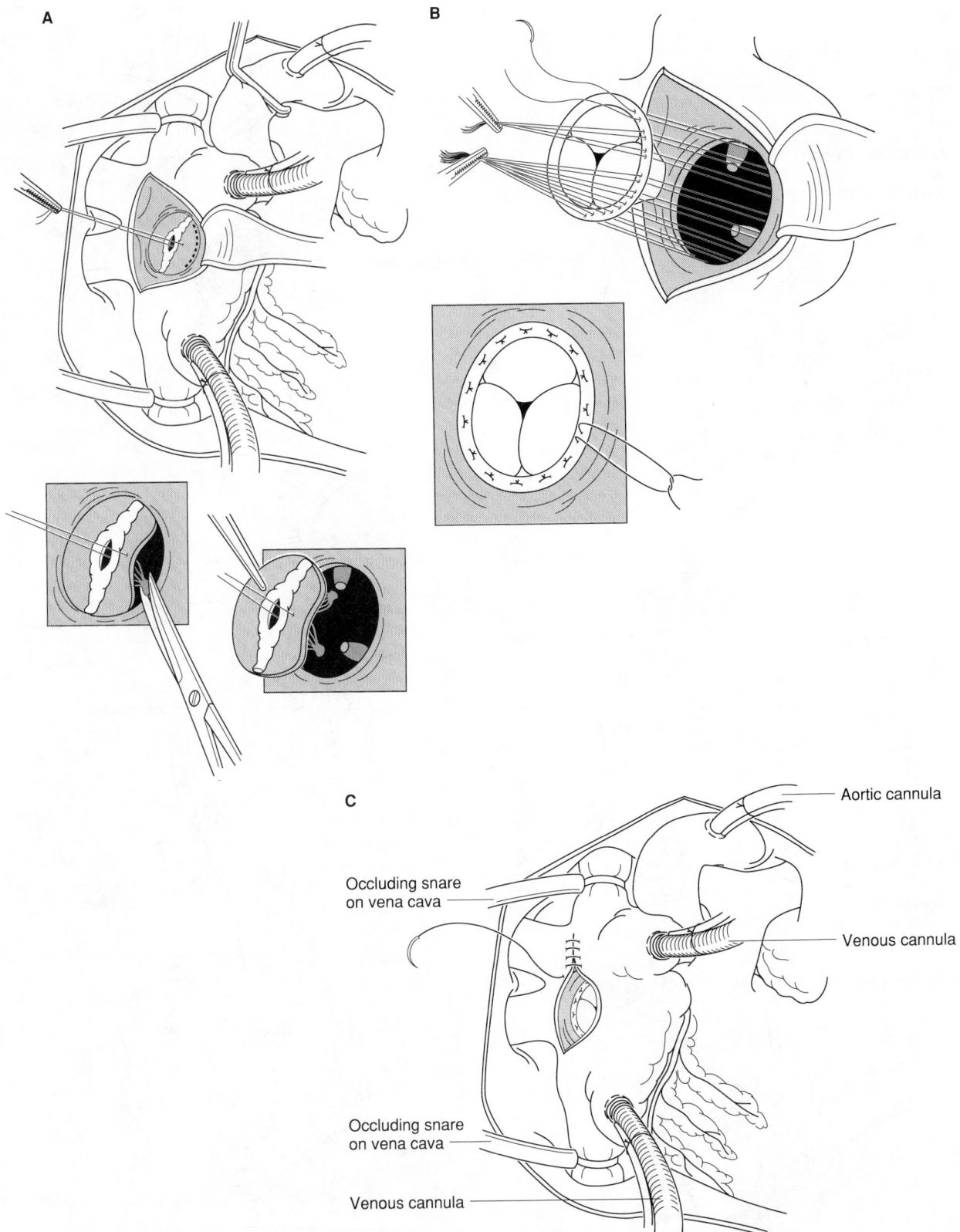

Figure 64-16. Mitral valve replacement. (*A*) Excision of diseased valve. (*B*) Suturing appropriately sized prosthesis. (*C*) Atriotomy closure.

tissue, the valve orifice is sized with a plastic sizer. Valve sizes of at least 29 mm allow reasonable flow in most patients. The prosthesis is usually sewn to the annulus with interrupted horizontal mattress sutures of nonabsorbable material, which are buttressed with small Dacron pledgets (see Fig. 64-16*B*). Sutures placed too deep can injure the

circumflex artery in the AV groove posterolaterally, the aortic leaflet mechanism anteriorly, or the AV node medially. The valve is lowered into place and the sutures tied down, ensuring that the valve annulus is seated properly to avoid the possibility of paravalvular leaks. It is important that the valve not be too big for the ventricular

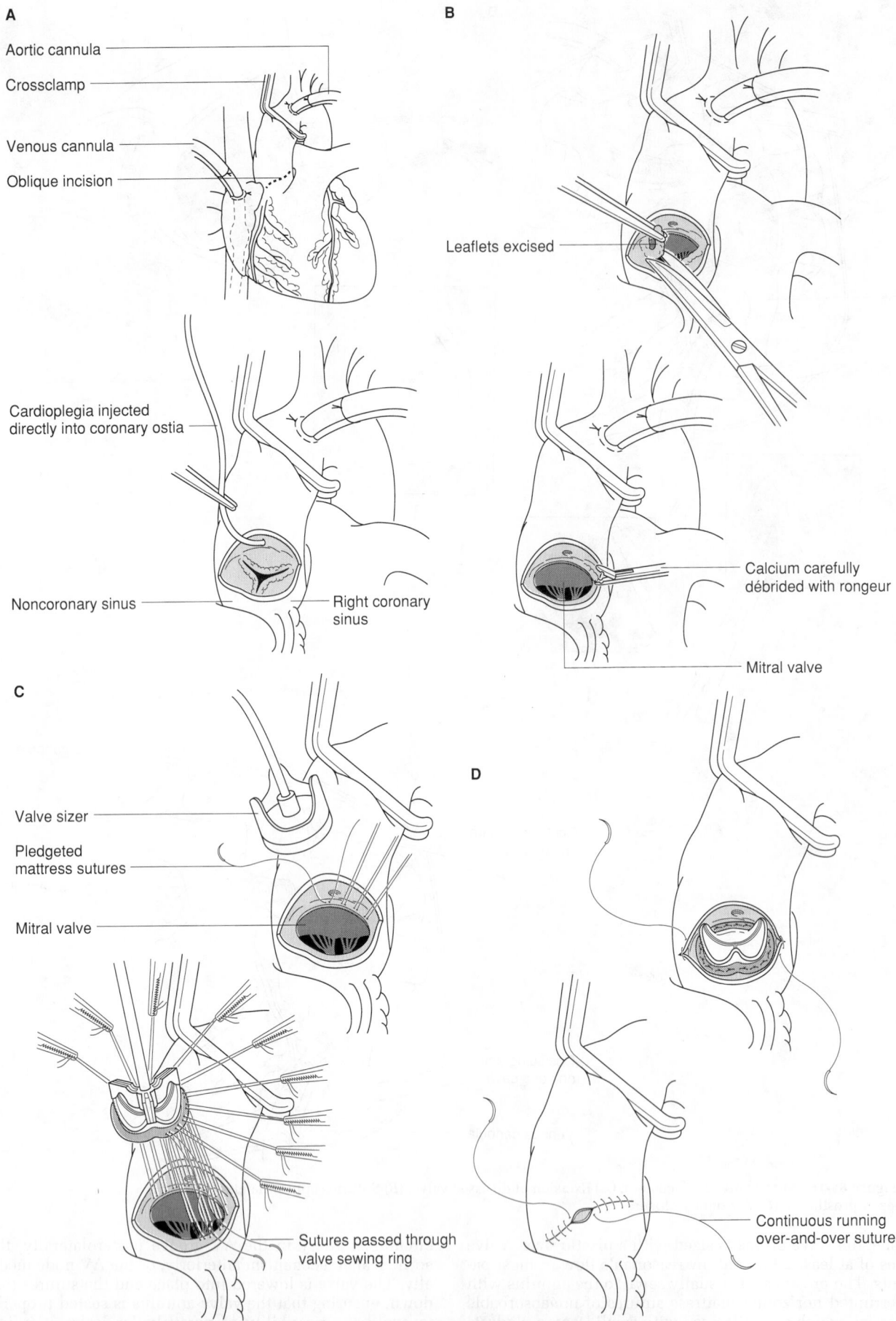

A

Aortic cannula

Crossclamp

Venous cannula

Oblique incision

Cardioplegia injected
directly into coronary ostia

Noncoronary sinus

Right coronary
sinus

B

Leaflets excised

Calcium carefully
débrided with rongeur

Mitral valve

C

Valve sizer

Pledgeted
mattress sutures

Mitral valve

Sutures passed through
valve sewing ring

D

Continuous running
over-and-over suture

Figure 64-17. Aortic valve replacement. (*A*) Aortotomy below crossclamp and aortic cannula. (*B*) Excision of heavily calcified valve. (*C*) Suturing of valve prosthesis. (*D*) Closure of aortotomy.

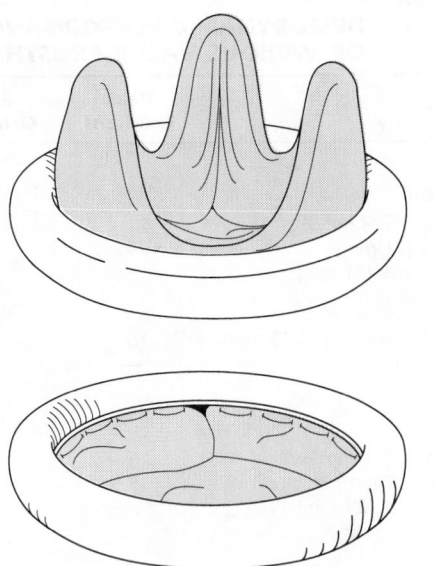

Figure 64-18. Carpentier-Edwards porcine bioprosthetic valve.

chamber, because this can contribute to outflow tract obstruction, AV groove or posterior wall rupture, or prosthetic dysfunction.

Aortic valve replacement is performed in a similar fashion (Fig. 64-17). After a transverse aortotomy has been made, the aortic valve is excised, making sure that stray chunks of calcium are carefully removed. The valve is usually excised at the level of attachment to the annulus, but care must be taken with heavily calcified valves to prevent perforations of the aortic wall. The valve orifice is appropriately sized and the valve sewn into place in a manner analogous to the process described earlier.

At this point, the blood is rewarmed, and the aortotomy or atriotomy incisions are oversewn. These closures are usually not completed until after the critical maneuver of de-airing. Failure to evacuate air from the left side of the heart can result in the serious complication of arterial air embolism, most notably cerebral embolism. Although various de-airing techniques are used, most involve electrically fibrillating the heart, filling the left heart chambers by momentarily decreasing the flow through the pump, and allowing air to escape through a venting site placed in some superior position. These maneuvers are assisted by placing the patient in a steep Trendelenburg position, massaging the heart, vigorously ventilating the lungs, and removing or partially removing the aortic crossclamp. A needle is often used to aspirate any residual air from the left ventricle. A small venting catheter can be placed across the valve prosthesis to further improve ventricular de-airing.

After these maneuvers, closure of the aortotomy or atriotomy incisions is completed (see Figs. 64-16*C* and 64-17*D*). Protamine is given to neutralize the remaining heparin dose, and atrial and ventricular epicardial pacing wires are placed in the event that they are needed for transient bradycardia or heart block.

Prosthetic Valves

The ideal prosthetic heart valve should be durable, non-thrombogenic, resistant to infection, and technically easy to insert; it should have optimal hydraulic function; and it should be subjectively acceptable to the patient.[28] The wide variety of prosthetic heart valves available clearly suggests that the ideal valve has not yet been developed. The tissue bioprosthetic valve and the mechanical valve trade off between strengths in low thrombogenicity and durability, respectively.

Most bioprosthetic valves are porcine heterografts that are fixed in glutaraldehyde (Fig. 64-18). Homograft aortic valves, derived from human cadavers and cryopreserved, have historically been of restricted clinical utility because of limited availability, high cost, and the greater degree of technical expertise required for implantation. The use of homografts has been repopularized, and they remain an important option for aortic valve replacement, especially in the young and in patients with endocarditis. The potentially increased durability of homografts due to improved preservation techniques and the adoption of a modified, less demanding surgical technique in which the homograft valve is implanted as a unit with the aortic root have contributed to this resurgence. The benefits of homograft insertion in terms of low incidences of endocarditis and thromboembolism and the consequent ability to avoid anticoagulation are additional advantages.

The original mechanical valves were of the ball-in-cage design (Starr-Edwards). These valves underwent several modifications to improve thrombogenicity and hydraulic function and are still in use (Fig. 64-19). These valves are by definition the most durable of the mechanical valves

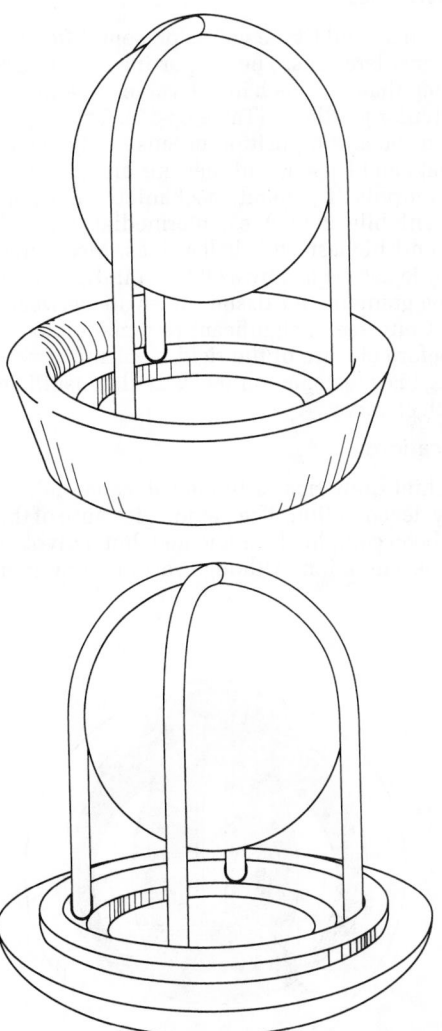

Figure 64-19. Starr-Edwards aortic (*top*) and mitral (*bottom*) ball valves.

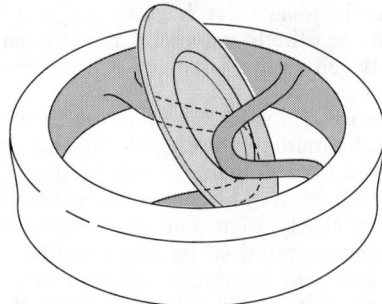

Figure 64-20. Björk-Shiley tilting-disc valve.

because they have been in the longest clinical use. The next and current generation of mechanical valves consists of modified versions of the tilting-disk valve, represented by the original Björk-Shiley valve (Fig. 64-20). Specific models of the convexoconcave Björk-Shiley valve suffered a 0.17% rate of strut fracture, sometimes associated with catastrophic valve failure, and they are not presently available in the United States. Recent modifications of the tilting-disk valve (St Jude) use a pivoting bileaflet mechanism made of Pyrolite carbon that eliminates the need for retaining struts (Fig. 64-21).

Hemodynamics

Mechanical and tissue valves present different hemodynamic considerations. The supporting ring in tissue valves is bulkier than in mechanical valves, leading to greater transvalvular gradients (Table 64-11). These gradients are higher in the aortic position because of the smaller valve sizes that can be used, and they are higher with increased cardiac outputs. In general, mechanical valve gradients are lowest with bileaflet valves, intermediate with tilting-disk valves, and highest with ball valves. Mean gradients for the St Jude can be as low as 0 to 5 mmHg, whereas corresponding gradients for tissue valves are between 6 and 23 mmHg. Conversely, significant retrograde blood flow can occur before closure of the rigid mechanical valve leaflet, resulting in a greater amount of valvular insufficiency with mechanical valves.

Complications

The chief drawback of tissue valves is their propensity for early degeneration. The pathologic cause of this process has not been completely elucidated, but it involves gradual calcific degeneration. Although various antimineralization

Table 64-11. HEMODYNAMIC PERFORMANCE OF VARIOUS VALVE PROSTHESES

Valve	Peak Gradient	Effective Orifice Area
AORTIC		
Mechanical		
Starr-Edwards (23 mm AV)	21	1.2
Björk-Shiley (21 mm)	24	1.3
St Jude Medical (21 mm)	6	1.7
Biologic		
Carpentier-Edwards (21–23 mm)	16	1.5–1.7
Hancock (21 mm)	—	1.3
MITRAL		
Mechanical		
Starr-Edwards (27 mm AV)	5	1.4
Björk-Shiley (29 mm)	5.5	1.9
St Jude Medical (29 mm)	2.5	2.8
Biologic		
Carpentier-Edwards (27–29 mm)	6	2.4
Hancock (modified) (27 mm)	8	1.8

AV, atrioventricular.
(Modified from Jamieson WRE. Bioprostheses are superior to mechanical prostheses. Z Kardiol 1986;75[Suppl 2]:258)

strategies, including alterations in fixation pressures and use of sodium dodecyl sulfate, are being investigated to decrease calcification, none have yet achieved clinical relevance. Degeneration of the tissue valves usually involves gradual leaflet calcification and thickening, leading to stenosis or insufficiency. Sudden and catastrophic tissue valve failure can occur as the result of leaflet tear or separation. Emergency replacement may be required in these instances. Valves at highest risk for degeneration are those exposed to high mechanical stresses and those in patients with accelerated calcium metabolism. Thus, children and young adults (younger than 35 years of age), patients with chronic renal failure, and those with high cardiac indices are at increased risk for valve failure. The mean durability of the porcine tissue valves is about 13 years (Fig. 64-22). Freedom from structural degeneration in one recent survey was 71% at 10 years and 31% at 15 years.[29]

Mechanical prosthetic valves such as the tilting-disk valve enjoy failure-free rates with anticoagulation of about

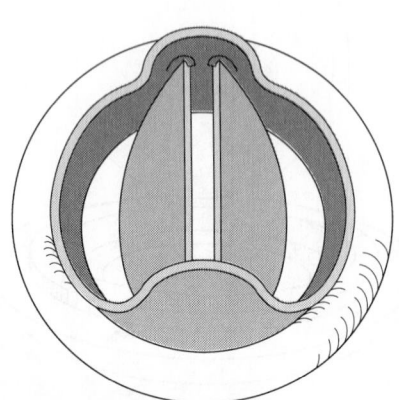

Figure 64-21. St Jude bileaflet valve.

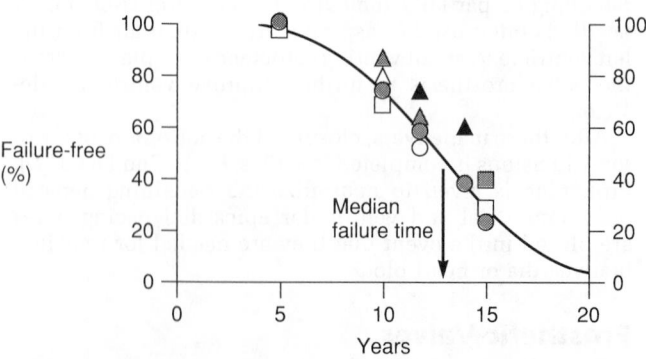

Figure 64-22. Representation of failure-free rates in tissue heterograft valves based on a compilation of published series with experience beyond 10 years. Median failure time is about 13 years. (After Starr A, Grunkemeier GL. The expected lifetime of porcine valves. Ann Thorac Surg 1989;48:317)

98% per year. Mechanical valve dysfunction is predominantly due to valve thrombosis, although rare failures include strut fracture, ball variance, and even ball or leaflet escape. Catastrophic failure is somewhat more common with the low-profile valve than with the ball valve. Thrombotic occlusion of the tilting-disk leaflet leaves it in a half-open, half-closed position, leading to severe stenosis and insufficiency. The mortality rate for thrombotic occlusion is between 33% and 100%, with an operative mortality rate of about 10%.

Auscultation remains one of the most effective means of screening for prosthetic valve dysfunction. Any diminution of prosthetic heart valve sounds can represent tissue ingrowth or thrombus formation. Any new or changed murmurs should also raise the suspicion of valvular dysfunction, although dysfunction can occur without any change in auscultatory findings. Further diagnostic evaluation can include fluoroscopic examination of mechanical valve leaflet motion, echo and Doppler echo studies, and even cardiac catheterization. Kontos and associates[30] reported that cardiac echo and fluoroscopy yield a prohibitive rate of false-negative results, with catheterization demonstrating 100% accuracy.

Treatment of prosthetic valvular dysfunction may require urgent or emergent operation and valve replacement. Less commonly, open thrombectomy is possible. Intraaortic balloon counterpulsation can be an effective measure for stabilizing the patient with prosthetic mitral insufficiency, and pharmacologic support should also be instituted, based on the type of prosthetic dysfunction involved. Some studies suggest a role for fibrinolytic therapy for the treatment of acute thrombotic occlusion of prosthetic valves, especially the tricuspid valve, with success rates of up to 75% reported.[31]

Hemolysis is another potential complication of mechanical valves most likely to occur with a prosthesis in the aortic position, with small valve sizes, or in the presence of a periprosthetic leak, especially in the mitral position. Hemolysis can be great enough to produce clinically apparent jaundice and require transfusion, but this usually resolves with time. Valve replacement may be required, especially if a periprosthetic leak exists. Other potential complications of valve replacement include endocarditis, atrial and ventricular arrhythmias, coronary ostial obstruction (aortic valve), LV rupture and AV groove tear (mitral valve), postpericardiotomy syndrome, and ventricular outflow tract obstruction.

On the basis of these relative advantages and disadvantages, mechanical valves are recommended for most patients. Tissue valves are generally preferred if there is a contraindication to anticoagulation, if life expectancy is less than 10 years, if future pregnancy is anticipated, or if there are technical considerations at the time of operation, such as a heavily calcified annulus, that favor tissue valve implantation. Tissue valves are almost exclusively used for tricuspid valve replacement because of thrombotic complications associated with the use of mechanical valves in this position.

Postoperative Care

The postoperative course of patients after valve surgery is in many ways similar to that of any patient undergoing operation, with similar neuroendocrine responses to the stress of surgery. The use of cardiopulmonary bypass superimposes additional metabolic changes, affecting almost every organ system. The speed of recovery is often influenced by the preoperative status of the particular organ system, the length of cardiopulmonary bypass, and postop-

erative cardiac function. Fortunately, cardiac hemodynamics can be expected to approach normal in most patients with the correction of valvular pathology.

The ultimate goal in terms of cardiac performance after valve surgery is maintenance of a cardiac output sufficient for nominal systemic perfusion. Qualitative assessment of cardiac function can be made by noting the mental status of the patient, as well as the color and temperature of the patient's extremities. Urine output is often high immediately after bypass but is subsequently a good indicator of organ perfusion. Conversely, systemic blood pressure is a poor indicator of hemodynamic function. Blood pressure is often elevated in the postoperative period as a result of elevated levels of catecholamines and other endogenous pressor agents. The PA thermodilution catheter allows direct quantification of cardiac index, which should be greater than 2 L/min/m^2. The mixed venous gas is a physiologic index of adequate perfusion; PvO_2 should be greater than 30 mmHg. Effective treatment of low cardiac output can consist of volume resuscitation to increase preload, the administration of positive inotropic agents, or the use of vasodilators to decrease afterload (Fig. 64-23).

Pulmonary dysfunction is common after bypass. Clinically significant effects are normally seen through the first 3 days, with 7 to 10 days required for complete reversal of pulmonary compromise. Tachypnea, increased alveolar-arterial oxygen gradients, and decreased functional residual capacity are observed. An increase in lung water, increased airway closure rate, and decreased pulmonary compliance are also found. Interstitial water accumulation may figure prominently in these changes and is directly related to pump time, the type of oxygenator used, and other technical considerations. Complement activation and leukocyte aggregation in the pulmonary microcirculation have been implicated as well. Preoperative pulmonary status is another independent risk factor for prolonged postoperative dysfunction. Therapy consists of diuresis, pulmonary toilet, and ventilatory support until appropriate extubation parameters are met.

Moderate to severe renal dysfunction can occur in 7% of patients, with transient azotemia in an additional 20%.[32] Preoperative LV function, renal function, age, prolonged cardiopulmonary bypass, and prolonged postoperative low-output state are significant risk factors. Renal failure carries a 65% to 85% mortality rate, which can be lowered by the early implementation of hemodialysis or peritoneal dialysis. Use of agents such as furosemide and mannitol to promote diuresis can be of additional benefit.

The risk of transient deterioration in intellectual ability or neurologic complication is 7% to 25%, with a smaller incidence of permanent or fixed focal defects.[33] Platelet, thrombin, calcium, cholesterol, and air microemboli have been implicated. Microemboli or periods of systemic hypotension appear to result in ischemia in central nervous system watershed zones, and infarcts have been documented in these vascular border zones. Age, preexistent neurologic dysfunction, and total cardiopulmonary bypass time are independent risk factors. Asymptomatic carotid bruits do not impose an additional risk. Neurologic defects can most often be expected to clear in hours to days. Treatment is supportive, because no specific therapy has clearly been documented to be effective.

Metabolic perturbations after cardiopulmonary bypass include a metabolic acidosis for the first several hours postoperatively, resulting from the washout of regions that were poorly perfused during hypothermia. Hypothermia usually resolves in the first 6 hours after operation. Sodium and water retention normally seen in surgical patients is exacerbated by bypass, with 5% increases in weight being average. Physiologic diuresis is usually assisted by the ad-

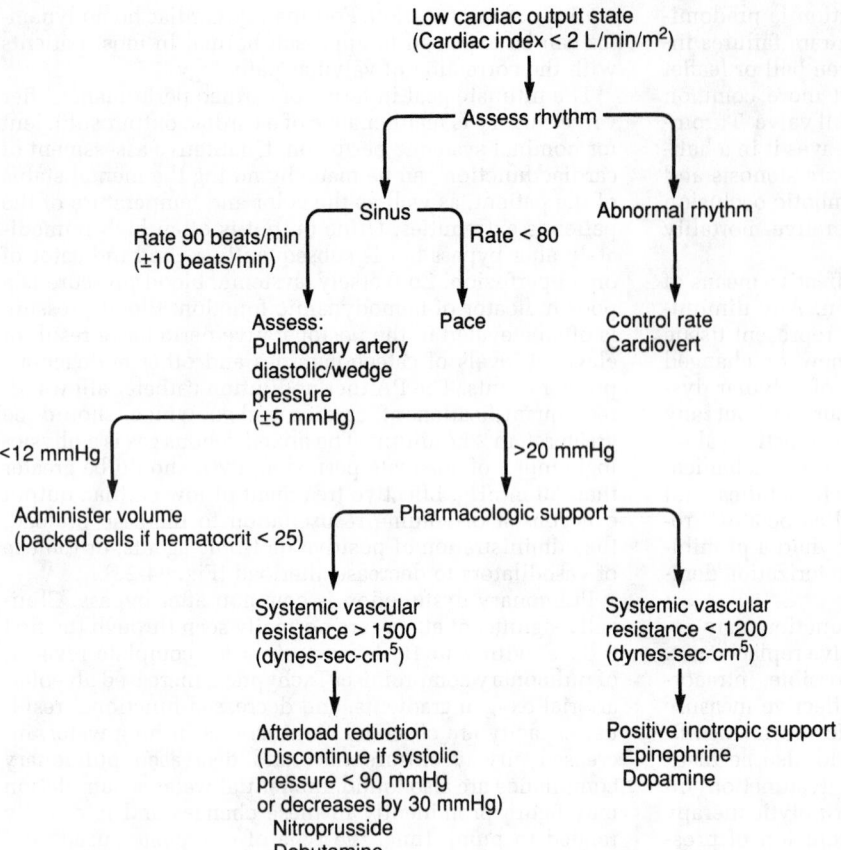

Figure 64-23. Suggested algorithm for treatment of postoperative low cardiac output syndrome. Indicated pressures vary depending on ventricular compliance and other factors.

ministration of exogenous diuretic agents. Hyperthermia and leukocytosis are also exacerbated after cardiopulmonary bypass and are not useful as guides to infection. Anemia, thrombocytopenia, and depletion of clotting factors can lead to immediate or delayed risks of bleeding and cardiac tamponade. Tamponade can also result from postpericardiotomy syndrome.

Mediastinitis occurs in 1.4% of patients after valve replacement and carries a mortality rate of up to 12.5% in the absence of other complications.[34] Unexplained fever and leukocytosis, especially in the setting of chest pain, tenderness, or an unstable sternum, should raise the suspicion of mediastinitis. Early use of muscle flaps can improve survival.

Jaundice, acalculous cholecystitis, pancreatitis, gastrointestinal bleeding, peptic ulcer disease, intestinal ischemia, and other acute abdominal complications can also occur with increased frequency and are present in almost 1% of patients after open heart surgery.[35] The pathophysiology of these complications can in part be related to poor organ perfusion during nonpulsatile cardiopulmonary bypass.

Surgical Results

Mortality

The overall operative mortality rate for valve replacement ranges from 5% to 12%. A study from the University of Toronto of almost 2500 patients demonstrated a 5.3% mortality rate for aortic valve replacement and a 6.6% mortality rate for mitral valve replacement.[36] The increased mortality for mitral replacement may reflect technical con-

siderations of the operation or the increased risk of correcting MR compared with AI (see later discussion). Independent risk factors for operation in this series were emergent surgery, previous valve surgery, coronary artery disease, and age. The type of mitral lesion was a univariant predictor of outcome in the Toronto report, with a 2.7% mortality rate for mitral stenosis, an 8.7% rate for MR, and a 10.1% mortality rate for mixed lesions. Others report no significant differences in operative mortality between operations for MR and mitral stenosis or between operations for AI and aortic stenosis when controlled for ventricular function. In the Toronto study, decreased LV function was an independent risk factor for mitral valve surgery only (Fig. 64-24). Other authors observe that significant deterioration in LV function or functional class approximately doubles the risk of aortic[37] or mitral valve replacement.[38] Blackstone and colleagues[39] reported that functional class IV patients suffered almost three times the operative mortality as class I patients.

The presence of ischemic MR or concomitant coronary disease in the Toronto group raised the mortality rate to 16% in patients undergoing mitral replacement, similar to results reported by others.[40] Reoperation more than doubles operative risk, as does double-valve replacement.[41] The presence of significant tricuspid regurgitation also doubled operative risk in the report from Toronto, but others report no increased risk of combined mitral operation and tricuspid valvuloplasty. Age was only a limited risk factor in the absence of other disability. Even in patients older than 80 years of age, valve surgery can be performed with a mortality rate as low as 4%.[42]

The operative mortality rate for mitral valve repair has

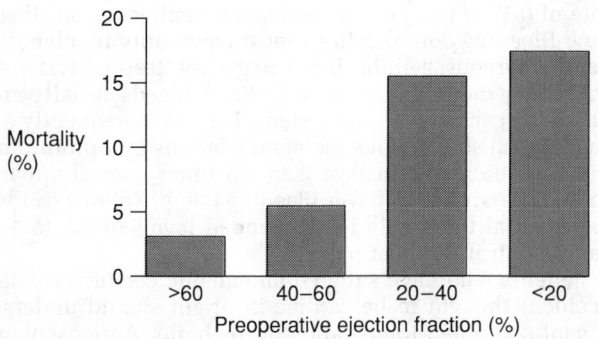

Figure 64-24. Bar graph of operative mortality after mitral valve replacement as a function of preoperative ejection fraction. (After Christakis GT, Weisel RD, David TE, et al. Predictors of operative survival after valve replacement. Circulation 1988;78[Suppl 1]:630)

generally been reported to be less than 5%—significantly lower than that for replacement.[26] However, similarly decreased mortality has recently been reported for mitral valve replacement when performed with preservation of posterior leaflet-chordae-papillary muscle continuity.[43]

Hemodynamic Results

Left ventricular chamber size, wall thickness, and LV mass decrease after valve replacement for aortic stenosis or AI.[44] Significant decreases in LV volume and wall stress can be detected by 7 to 10 days after operation in patients undergoing valve replacement for AI. Ejection fraction improves more in patients undergoing correction of aortic stenosis compared with those undergoing correction of AI. Diminished LV performance immediately after operation in patients with AI may be attributed to inadequate filling of the high-capacitance, volume-adapted ventricle, or it may be related to the relatively greater improvement in afterload associated with correction of aortic stenosis compared with correction of AI. Differences in underlying preoperative LV function can also play a role.

Correction of AI or MR relieves the ventricle of the afterload mismatch and increased wall stress associated with excessive diastolic volume loading. The resistance against which the ventricle is pumping is unchanged after correction of AI. The increase in ejection fraction after correction of AI indicates a decrease in net systolic afterload. Conversely, correction of MR forces the ventricle to pump against increased resistance because of the removal of the mitral pop-off mechanism of afterload reduction into the low-pressure left atrium. Ventricular afterload and systolic work are accordingly increased. In patients with good LV function, the ejection fraction decreases, but to levels that are still acceptable. LV hypertrophy eventually resolves, indicating an overall decrease in wall stress. In MR patients with significantly worsened LV function preoperatively, ejection fraction also decreases after mitral valve replacement, but to unacceptably low levels. LV hypertrophy does not resolve in these cases. LV dilation and functional deterioration are late results.

Functional Results

Excellent functional improvement can generally be expected for all valvular heart disease patients after successful operation. Karp and associates[45] reported that 75% of functional class III or IV patients improved to functional class I or II after mitral valve replacement for MR. O'Toole and colleagues[37] reported that all of their patients undergoing aortic valve replacement improved to or remained

functional class I or II. The most significant limitations on functional improvement are imposed by preoperative ventricular function and the function and durability of the prosthetic valve implanted. Thus, Barnhorst and associates[38] reported a 58% versus a 94% 5-year survival rate in patients undergoing aortic valve replacement with or without evidence of LV dysfunction, respectively. Although the 5-year survival rate for functional class II patients with mitral stenosis is 90% to 95%, this declines to 50% for functional class IV patients. Others report similar correlations between preoperative functional class or LV function and long-term survival and functional improvement for both aortic (see Fig. 64-14) and mitral valve replacement.[15] Complication-free survival rates for patients undergoing mitral valve repair appear to exceed those for replacement, although data from a prospective randomized trial comparing the two techniques are not available.[46]

ANTICOAGULATION

Anticoagulation in patients with native valve disease or in patients with prosthetic valves is indicated when the risk of thromboembolism associated with these conditions exceeds the morbidity of hemorrhagic complications caused by anticoagulant therapy (Table 64-12). A second caveat of anticoagulant therapy is that lower rates of thromboembolism must be demonstrated with treatment.

Indications

Data from several large studies allow stratification of the relative risk of thromboembolism for specific valvular disease. Rheumatic heart disease carries the highest risk of thromboembolism of any form of valvular heart disease. Mitral rheumatic disease patients have a 20% risk of developing clinically significant emboli, at an approximate rate

Table 64-12. ANTICOAGULANT RECOMMENDATIONS

Indication	Recommended Prothrombin Time Elevation With Warfarin Administration
PROSTHETIC HEART VALVES	
Mechanical	1.5–2
Bioprosthetic	1.3–1.5 (3 months postoperatively)
NATIVE VALVE DISEASE	
Rheumatic mitral valve	
Previous embolism	1.5–2 (1.3–1.5 after 1 y)
Atrial fibrillation	1.3–1.5
Dilated left atrium	
(>55 mm in diameter)	1.3–1.5
Aortic valve disease	No treatment*
Mitral valve prolapse	No treatment*
Mitral annular calcification	No treatment*
Infective endocarditis	No treatment*
ATRIAL FIBRILLATION	
Previous embolism	1.5–2 (1.3–1.5 after 1 y)
Mitral valve disease	1.3–1.5
Cardiomyopathy	
Dilated	1.3–1.5
Hypertrophic	1.3–1.5
Thyrotoxicosis	1.3–1.5†
Lone atrial fibrillation	No treatment*
Cardioversion	1.3–1.5†

* Unless other indications exist.

† Maintain therapy for 2 to 4 weeks after conversion to sinus rhythm.

of 1.5% to 4.7% per year and with a 10% to 15% mortality rate without treatment.[47] Patients with mitral valve disease and atrial fibrillation have as great as four to seven times the risk of thromboembolism compared with mitral valve disease patients in normal sinus rhythm (see Table 64-7). More specifically, patients in atrial fibrillation with mitral stenosis have about a 50% greater risk of thromboembolism than patients with MR—31.5% versus 22%, respectively.[48] In the same study, thromboemboli occurred in only 8% of patients in sinus rhythm with mitral stenosis or MR. Patients suffering a single embolic event have a 30% to 65% chance of suffering recurrent episodes; more than half of these occur within 6 months. Patients with large atria (diameter larger than 55 mm) are at increased risk for developing atrial fibrillation and therefore may be candidates for anticoagulation on that basis. Finally, advanced age and decreased cardiac index are also risk factors for thromboembolism. Anticoagulant therapy is therefore recommended for patients with atrial fibrillation and systemic emboli, atrial fibrillation and mitral valve disease, and atrial fibrillation with associated cardiomyopathy.[49]

Valvular lesions other than mitral valve disease carry a relatively low risk of embolism. Calcific emboli do not appear to be prevented by warfarin therapy. Anticoagulation is therefore not indicated for mitral valve prolapse, mitral annular calcification, or aortic valve disease without other risk factors. Emboli associated with endocarditis are usually not thrombotic in nature, and anticoagulation is not indicated for endocarditis unless other indications exist (eg, prosthetic valve endocarditis).

Reliable data from randomized trials of anticoagulant therapy in patients with prosthetic heart valves are sporadic, but some specific recommendations are available (see Table 64-12). Initial experiences with the Starr-Edwards ball valve showed an average embolic risk of 6% per year, ranging up to a 30% risk over the course of one study in which anticoagulants were not used. Anticoagulant therapy reduces this risk by three- to six-fold. The new generation of low-profile tilting-disk valves, although thought to have lower thrombosis potential, still demonstrates thromboembolic rates without anticoagulation of up to 3% per year. Bioprosthetic tissue valves have a low potential for thromboembolism, on the order of 2% per year. Half of all tissue valve thromboembolic episodes occur in the first 12 weeks after surgery. Lifelong anticoagulation is therefore recommended for all patients with mechanical valves, and an initial 3-month period of anticoagulation is recommended for patients with bioprosthetic valves to cover the early period of neointimal deposition. Antiplatelet therapy with either aspirin or dipyridamole (Persantine) may be an effective alternative treatment to lower thromboembolic risk, but the data conflict. These agents may be useful as an adjunct to warfarin in cases in which single-drug therapy is ineffective in preventing embolic complications.

Summarizing all prosthetic valve data, Edmunds[50] concluded that the cumulative risk of thromboembolism for mechanical valves with anticoagulation and prosthetic valves without anticoagulation was about equal at 2% per year. Anticoagulated patients with mechanical valves assume the added risk of bleeding complications, but 10% of patients with tissue valves in the aortic position, and up to 40% to 60% of patients with bioprosthetic mitral valves, eventually require warfarin anticoagulation, thus partially negating the benefit of the tissue prosthesis.

Complications

Data derived from patients with prosthetic valves who are on warfarin therapy suggest a uniform risk of major bleeding episodes of 1% to 2% per year, with a mortality rate of 0.17% per year for patients on anticoagulant therapy. Bleeding complications most commonly involve the central nervous, genitourinary, or gastrointestinal systems, including the retroperitoneum. Fatal bleeds usually involve the central nervous system. Trauma is frequently an inciting cause. Previous recommendations that prothrombin time be maintained at 2 to 2.5 times control appear to be excessive, and fewer bleeding complications can be expected at the newly recommended levels of 1.3 to 1.5 times control for most patients.[49,51]

Patients who have suffered an embolic cerebrovascular accident thought to be cardiac in origin should undergo urgent computed tomography of the brain. Anticoagulant therapy should be instituted immediately if the scan is negative. If a large or hemorrhagic infarct is observed, therapy should be postponed for 1 week.

Few studies address the management of patients requiring interruption of anticoagulation because of bleeding complications or because major surgery is planned. The authors believe that anticoagulation should be reversed by withholding warfarin several days before operation and allowing prothrombin time to decrease to about 14 to 15 seconds. Therapy should be resumed 1 to 2 days postoperatively in low-risk patients. High-risk patients should be switched to heparin preoperatively once the prothrombin time reaches subtherapeutic levels. The heparin can be discontinued immediately before operation and resumed as soon as 12 hours postoperatively if operative bleeding is not a problem. Rapid reversal of anticoagulation should be made with fresh frozen plasma transfusions, if necessary. Vitamin K administration makes subsequent warfarin therapy more difficult and should be avoided. The benefits of aspirin use through the perioperative period remain unconfirmed.

Contraindications

Anticoagulant therapy is specifically contraindicated in any patient with a predisposition for bleeding complications, from either systemic disease (eg, active ulcer disease) or coagulopathy; in those likely to incur trauma through occupation or pastime; in those likely to be poorly compliant; and in those with a desire for future pregnancy.

Anticoagulation in the pregnant patient is a significant problem. Warfarin is a small molecule that readily crosses the placental barrier. The immature fetal liver is susceptible to the effects of warfarin, and a protracted hypocoagulable state develops. Fetal clotting factors can take 2 to 3 weeks to return to normal after cessation of warfarin therapy. Warfarin is also a known fetal teratogen, especially with use during the first trimester. A fetal loss rate over 30% and a rate of premature labor over 50% have been reported with warfarin use during pregnancy.[52] Use of warfarin late in pregnancy can produce fetal neurologic complications as a result of intracranial hemorrhage. The trauma of delivery is a significant problem in this regard. Heparin is not transferred across the placental barrier but can produce fetal loss through placental hemorrhage.

Conversely, the pregnant woman is in a hypercoagulable state, with elevated levels of clotting factors and decreased fibrinolytic activity. Cessation of anticoagulation during pregnancy can lead to an incidence of cerebral events as high as 25%. Antiplatelet agents are not as toxic to the fetus as warfarin but do not confer adequate protection to the mother.

The best solution to this problem is the use of a bioprosthesis in patients wishing to become pregnant, with use of antiplatelet agents during pregnancy. If an unforeseen pregnancy develops in a patient with a mechanical valve, an alternating regimen of heparin and Coumadin has been recommended, which minimizes the deleterious effects of each agent. Subcutaneous heparin is substituted for warfarin as soon as pregnancy is diagnosed and continued to week 12. Oral anticoagulants are continued to week 37, when subcutaneous heparin is again substituted.

ENDOCARDITIS

Prosthetic heart valves and diseased native valves are at increased risk for the development of endocarditis, although infection of normal valves is occurring with increasing frequency. Of all patients with endocarditis in one recent study, 24% had rheumatic heart disease, 23% had congenital deformities, and 32% had normal valves.[53] Endocarditis is most commonly left sided, reflecting the normal distribution of valvular heart disease; right-sided endocarditis, often associated with intravenous drug abuse, usually affects normal or congenitally deformed valves. Hypertrophic cardiomyopathy, mitral valve prolapse associated with a murmur, and mitral annular calcification are also predisposing causes of endocarditis.

Pathology

Endocarditis of diseased valves can be precipitated by any transient bacteremia. Endocarditis can develop in a normal valve when a focus of a relatively virulent organism is established, such as *Staphylococcus aureus* osteomyelitis, or it can be incurred in any immunocompromised patient. Endocarditis in burn patients, or from infected long-arm lines or pacemaker pockets, characteristically affects nondiseased valves.

Endocarditis involving previously diseased valves characteristically runs an indolent, subacute course, whereas involvement of normal heart valves usually presents as an acute, often fulminant process. *Streptococcus viridans,* followed by *Enterococcus,* other streptococcal species, and *Staphylococcus,* in that order, are most often responsible for the subacute form of endocarditis.[53] *S aureus* is the organism most commonly responsible for acute endocarditis and involves normal valves in 40% to 60% of cases. *S aureus* is also the most common cause of infection in intravenous drug abusers.

Fungal and gram-negative rod infections are usually seen in patients with prosthetic valves, in intravenous drug abusers, or in immunocompromised patients. Normal valves are commonly involved, especially the tricuspid valve. Patients already on antimicrobial therapy for bacterial endocarditis can also become suprainfected with fungi or gram-negative rods.

The mitral valve is the customary site of native valve endocarditis in most series. Abscess formation is the most common perivalvular complication, occurring in 20% of cases, and it is most often caused by *S aureus* infections. Perivalvular spread is most common for aortic valve endocarditis. Other complications of endocarditic infection include leaflet tears and chordal rupture producing valvular insufficiency, aortic mycotic aneurysm, conduction defects, sinus of Valsalva aneurysms, intrapericardial rupture with pyogenic pericarditis, and valve thrombosis. Bulky fungal vegetations can produce functional valvular stenosis.

Prosthetic valve endocarditis, constituting 15% to 30% of all cases of endocarditis, can develop as an early form (less than 2 months postoperatively), usually related to extracardiac contamination from sources such as skin infections, or as a late form, usually related to bacteremic seeding of the valve. Prosthetic endocarditis is reported to occur in 1% to 2% of implants. In contrast to native valve endocarditis, the aortic valve is the most common site of prosthetic valve infections. *Staphylococcus epidermidis, S aureus,* and gram-negative rods are most often seen in the early form of prosthetic endocarditis, and streptococcal, staphylococcal, and gram-negative rod infections are seen in the late form. Overall, *S aureus* infections are more common in patients with prosthetic valves than in patients with native valve disease.

Presentation

The patient with endocarditis characteristically presents with fever, chills, or sweats. Fever is almost always present, unless the patient is elderly or debilitated. Septic emboli occur in about 30% of patients and produce a great variety of symptoms. Emboli most commonly involve the spleen, producing abdominal pain, but renal emboli can produce hematuria, middle cerebral artery emboli can cause hemiplegia, and coronary emboli can lead to myocardial infarction. Septic emboli from tricuspid valve infections can produce bilateral patchy pulmonary infiltrates with secondary pulmonary infarcts and abscesses. The classic physical stigmata of subacute endocarditis, such as Osler nodes, Janeway lesions, and Roth spots, are much less commonly seen today, probably because of the relatively early application of antimicrobial therapy.

Although most patients with endocarditis develop a murmur at some point in the course of their disease, almost one third have no murmur at the time of presentation. Furthermore, many patients have preexistent murmurs due to native valve disease or to the presence of a prosthetic valve. Only half of patients with prosthetic valves develop an altered murmur. Changing murmurs are usually found only with acute endocarditis and correspond with tissue destruction.

Blood cultures remain the mainstay of diagnosis, which is accurate in over 90% of cases. Most effective blood culturing calls for three to six sets of cultures obtained within 24 hours. Previous antibiotic treatment, intramyocardial abscess, or fungal infections can yield false-negative results. Two-dimensional echocardiography is a useful diagnostic adjunct, but small lesions (less than 3 mm) may be undetected. Vegetations that are detected by echo have been associated with an increased incidence of complications. Vegetations can persist despite sterilization of the lesion. Overall, echocardiography is accurate in 55% to 80% of cases.

Management

The mainstay of treatment for bacterial endocarditis is appropriate antibiotic prophylaxis (Table 64-13). Medical therapy for established endocarditis consists of intravenous administration of appropriate antibiotics at bactericidal levels for a period of 4 to 6 weeks. This is effective in 50% to 80% of cases, depending on the organism involved. An increased risk of medical failure is predicted by increased age, staphylococcal infections, and the development of heart failure. Medical therapy can be expected to sterilize one third to two thirds of prosthetic valve infections, and most authors recommend an initial trial of antibiotic therapy for prosthetic valve endocarditis. Antibiotic treatment of heterograft infections may be relatively more successful than that of mechanical valve infections, although earlier reports that heterografts are more resistant to infection than mechanical valves have not been confirmed.

Continued medical therapy of valvular endocarditis in the face of cardiac deterioration carries an 80% to 90% mortality rate. The mortality rate with early prosthetic valve infections with *Staphylococcus* or gram-negative rods is as high as 85%, whereas late *S viridans* infections result in far lower mortal-

Table 64-13. PROPHYLAXIS FOR BACTERIAL ENDOCARDITIS

CARDIOVASCULAR CONDITIONS AT RISK FOR ENDOCARDITIS	ANTIBIOTIC PROPHYLAXIS†
Conditions With Highest Risk Prosthetic heart valves Previous endocarditis **Conditions With Medium Risk** Acquired valvular disease Congenital heart disease (excluding most cases of secundum atrial septal defect and ligated patent ductus arteriosus) Intravenous drug abusers Hypertrophic cardiomyopathy Mitral valve prolapse with murmur **Conditions With Lowest Risk** High-risk or penicillin-allergic patients Transvenous pacemakers Mitral valve prolapse without murmur Indwelling central venous or intracardiac catheters	**Dental Procedures and Upper Respiratory Tract** For most patients 　Penicillin V, 2 g 1 hour before procedure 　Penicillin, 1 g 6 hours after initial dose Penicillin-allergic patients 　Erythromycin, 1 g orally 1 hour before procedure 　Erythromycin, 500 mg 6 hours after initial dose High-risk patients 　Ampicillin, 1–2 g *plus* 　Gentamicin, 1.5 mg/kg IM or IV given 30 minutes before procedure 　Penicillin V, 1 g orally 6 hours after initial dose 　Vancomycin, 1 g IV over 60 minutes, begun 60 minutes before procedure; no repeat dose is necessary
PROCEDURES THAT MAY CAUSE BACTEREMIAS Dental care with bleeding Surgery or instrumentation* 　Maxillofacial 　Upper gastrointestinal (endoscopy with biopsy) 　Genitourinary tract surgery 　Biliary 　Lower gastrointestinal Septic abortion of peripartum infection Manipulation or drainage of abscesses Débridement of burns	**Gastrointestinal and Genitourinary Tract Instrumentation or Surgery** For most patients 　Ampicillin, 2 g IM or IV *plus* 　Gentamicin, 1.5 mg/kg IM or IV given 30 minutes before procedure 　Repeat once 8 hours later Penicillin-allergic patients 　Vancomycin, 1 g IV over 60 minutes *plus* 　Gentamicin, 1.5 mg/kg IM or IV, given 60 minutes before procedure 　Repeat once 8–12 hours later For minor procedures or low-risk patients 　Amoxicillin, 3 g 1 hour before procedure 　Amoxicillin, 1.5 g 6 hours after initial dose

* Prophylaxis possibly indicated for liver biopsy, upper endoscopy without biopsy, oral intubation, barium enema, vaginal delivery, or uterine manipulations.
† 1985 American Heart Association recommendations.
(Modified from Byrd RC, Cheitlin MD. Endocarditis. In: Greenberg BH, Murphy E, eds. Valvular heart disease. Littleton, MA, PSG Publishing, 1987:234)

ity rates. The chief cause of death from endocarditis is congestive heart failure from AI. Congestive failure was the indication for operation in 56% of patients in a recent study, with emboli second at 42%.[54] Consequently, the development of a new AI murmur warrants careful consideration of surgical intervention, especially if accompanied by hemodynamic compromise. Other surgical indications include failure of antimicrobial therapy, as evidenced by persistently positive

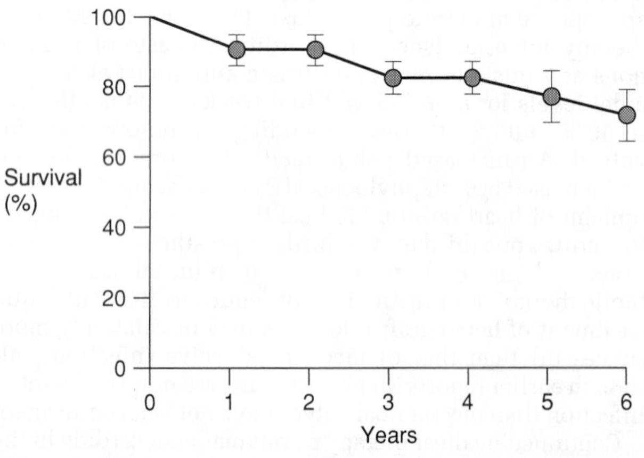

blood cultures, valvular insufficiency, perivalvular abscess, and pericarditis. Surgical intervention is often advocated for fungal and gram-negative rod infections because of the low cure rates associated with medical therapy. Others advocate delaying surgery to give a specified time course of antibiotics.

Surgical intervention is most often required for aortic valve endocarditis because of the high incidence of associated complications. Excision of the diseased valve, débridement of perivalvular abscesses, and valve replacement are the usual treatment. Surgical treatment of tricuspid disease can be performed without valve replacement, although valve replacement is probably preferable in this position as well.

Valve replacement in the hemodynamically stable patient results in an initially favorable outcome in 80% to 95% of cases. A valve reinfection rate of 1% to 13% can be expected. Late mortality rates between 20% and 60% have been reported and are greater for native mitral versus aortic disease and for early versus late prosthetic infections. David and associates[55] reported on 62 patients undergoing operation for active endocarditis, with a 0% operative mortality rate for native valve endocarditis and a 12.5% rate for prosthetic valve endocarditis. The 5-year survival rate was 86% ± 8% after operation for native valve endocarditis and 67% ± 11% for prosthetic valve endocarditis (Fig. 64-25).

Figure 64-25. Actuarial survival of all patients with active infective endocarditis. (After David TE, Bos J, Christakis GT, Brogman PR, Wong D, Feindel CM. Heart valve operations in patients with active infective endocarditis. Ann Thorac Surg 1990;49:704)

REFERENCES

1. Roberts WC. Morphologic features of the normal and abnormal mitral valve. Am J Cardiol 1983;51:1005.
2. Jeresaty RM. Mitral valve prolapse. New York, Raven Press, 1979.

3. Roberts WC, Perloff JK, Constantino T. Severe valvular aortic stenosis in patients over 65 years of age: a clinicopathologic study. Am J Cardiol 1971;27:497.

4. Fenoglio JJ Jr, McAllister HA Jr, DeCastro CM, Davia JE, Cheitlin MD. Congenital bicuspid aortic valve after age 20. Am J Cardiol 1977;39:164.

5. Meerson FZ. The myocardium in hyperfunction, hypertrophy, and heart failure. Circ Res 1969;25(Suppl II):1.

6. Wood P. An appreciation of mitral stenosis: a review. BMJ 1954;105I:1113.

7. Ross J Jr. Afterload mismatch in aortic and mitral valve disease: implications for surgical therapy. J Am Coll Cardiol 1985;5:811.

8. Braunwald E. Mitral regurgitation: physiologic, clinical, and surgical correlations. N Engl J Med 1969;281:425.

9. Edwards JE, Burchell HB. Pathologic anatomy of mitral insufficiency. Mayo Clin Proc 1958;33:497.

10. Forssmann W. Die Sondierung des rechten Herzens. Klin Wochenschr 1929;8:2085.

11. Yoran C, Yellin EL, Becker RM, Gabbay S, Frater RWM, Sonnenblick EH. Dynamic aspects of acute mitral regurgitation: effects of ventricular volume, pressure and contractility on the effective regurgitant orifice area. Circulation 1979;60:170.

12. Fischl SJ, Gorlin R, Herman MW. Cardiac shape and function in aortic valvular disease: physiologic and clinical implications. Am J Cardiol 1977;39:170.

13. Henry WL, Bonow RO, Rosing DR, Epstein SE. Observations on the optimum time for operative intervention for aortic regurgitation. Circulation 1980;61:484.

14. Levine HJ. Left ventricular function after correction of chronic aortic regurgitation. Circulation 1988;78:1319.

15. Schuler G, Peterson KL, Johnson AD, et al. Temporal response of left ventricular performance to mitral valve surgery. Circulation 1979;59:1218.

16. Olesen KH. The natural history of 271 patients with mitral stenosis under medical treatment. Br Heart J 1962;24:349.

17. Chizner MA, Pearle DL, deLeon AC Jr. The natural history of aortic stenosis in adults. Am Heart J 1980;99:419.

18. Duran CMG, Pomar JL, Colman T, Figueroa A, Revuelta JM, Ubago JL. Is tricuspid valve repair necessary? J Thorac Cardiovasc Surg 1980;80:849.

19. Turi ZG, Reyes VP, Raju BS, et al. Percutaneous balloon valvuloplasty versus surgical closed commissurotomy for mitral stenosis: a prospective, randomized trial. Circulation 1991;83:1179.

20. Tuzcu EM, Block PC, Palacios IF. Comparison of early versus late experience with percutaneous mitral balloon valvuloplasty. J Am Coll Cardiol 1991;17:1121.

21. Palacios I, Block PC, Brandi S, et al. Percutaneous balloon valvotomy for patients with severe mitral stenosis. Circulation 1987;75:778.

22. Smedira NG, Ports TA, Merrick SH, Rankin JS. Balloon aortic valvuloplasty as a bridge to aortic valve replacement in critically ill patients. Ann Thorac Surg 1993;55:914.

23. Smith WN, Neutze JM, Barratt-Boyes BG, Lower JB. Open mitral valvotomy: effect of preoperative factors on results. J Thorac Cardiovasc Surg 1981;82:738.

24. Heger JJ, Wann LS, Weyman AE, Dillon JC, Feigenbaum H. Long term changes in mitral valve area after successful mitral commissurotomy. Circulation 1979;59:443.

25. Galloway AC, Colvin SB, Baumann FG, et al. A comparison of mitral valve reconstruction with mitral valve replacement: intermediate-term results. Ann Thorac Surg 1989;47:655.

26. Cohn LH, Couper GS, Arlaki SF, et al. Long term results of mitral valve reconstruction for regurgitation of the myxomatous mitral valve. J Thorac Cardiovasc Surg 1994;107:143.

27. Lillehei CW, Levy MJ, Bonnabeau RCJ. Mitral valve replacement with preservation of papillary muscles and chordae tendineae. J Thorac Cardiovasc Surg 1964;47:532.

28. McClung JA, Stein JH, Ambrose JA, Herman MV, Reed GE. Prosthetic heart valves: a review. Prog Cardiovasc Dis 1983;26:237.

29. Starr A, Grunkemeier GL. The expected lifetime of porcine valves. Ann Thorac Surg 1989;48:317.

30. Kontos GJ, Schaff HV, Orszulak TA, Puga FJ, Pluth JR, Danielson GK. Thrombotic obstruction of disc valves: clinical recognition and surgical management. Ann Thorac Surg 1989;48:60.

31. Graver LM, Gelber PH, Denis TH. The risks and benefits of thrombolytic therapy in acute aortic and mitral prosthetic valve dysfunction: report of a case and review of the literature. Ann Thorac Surg 1988;46:85.

32. Abel RM, Buckley MJ, Austen G, et al. Etiology, incidence and prognosis of renal failure following cardiac operations: results of a prospective analysis of 500 consecutive patients. J Thorac Cardiovasc Surg 1976;71:323.

33. Branthwaite MA. Prevention of neurological damage during open-heart surgery. Thorax 1975;30:258.

34. Cheung EH, Craver JM, Jones EL, Murphy DA, Hatcher CR Jr, Guyton RA. Mediastinitis after cardiac valve operations: impact upon survival. J Thorac Cardiovasc Surg 1985;90:517.

35. Lawhorne TW, Davis WL, Smith GW. General surgical complications after cardiac surgery. Am J Surg 1978;136:254.

36. Christakis GT, Weisel RD, David TE, et al. Predictors of operative survival after valve replacement. Circulation 1988;78(Suppl I):25.

37. O'Toole JD, Geiser EA, Reddy S, Curtiss EI, Landfair RM. Effect of preoperative ejection fraction on survival and hemodynamic improvement following aortic valve replacement. Circulation 1978;58:1175.

38. Barnhorst DA, Oxman HA, Connolly DC, et al. Long-term followup of isolated replacement of the aortic or mitral valve with Starr-Edwards prosthesis. Am J Cardiol 1975;35:228.

39. Blackstone EH, Kirklin JW. Death and other time-related events after valve replacement. Circulation 1985;72:753.

40. Salomon NW, Stinson EB, Griepp RB, Shumway NE. Patient-related risk factors as predictors of results following isolated mitral valve replacement. Ann Thorac Surg 1977;24:519.

41. Isom OW, Spencer FC, Glassman E, et al. Long-term results in 1375 patients undergoing valve replacement with the Starr-Edwards cloth-covered steel ball prosthesis. Ann Surg 1977;86:310.

42. Rich MW, Sandza JG, Kleiger RE, Connors JP. Cardiac operations in patients over 80 years of age. J Thorac Cardiovasc Surg 1985;90:56.

43. Cohn LH, Couper ES, Kinchla NM, et al. Decreased operative risk of surgical treatment of mitral regurgitation with or without coronary artery disease. J Am Coll Cardiol 1990;16:1575.

44. Bonow RO. Left ventricular structure and function in aortic valve disease. Circulation 1989;79:966.

45. Karp RB, Cyrus RJ, Blackstone EH, Kirklin JW, Kouchoukos NT, Pacifico AD. The Björk-Shiley valve: intermediate-term follow-up. J Thorac Cardiovasc Surg 1981;81:602.

46. Akins CW, Hilgenberg AD, Buckley MJ, et al. Mitral valve reconstruction versus reoperation for degenerative or ischemic mitral regurgitation. Ann Thorac Surg 1994;S8668.

47. Nielson GH, Gales EG, Hossack KF. Thromboembolic complications of mitral valve disease. Aust NZ J Med 1978;8:3372.

48. Coulshed N, Epstein EJ, McKindrich CS, Galloway RW, Walker E. Systemic embolisation in mitral valve disease. Br Heart J 1970;32:26.

49. Levine HJ, Pauker SJ, Salzman EW. Antithrombotic therapy in valvular heart disease. Chest 1986;86(Suppl):365.

50. Edmunds LH Jr. Thromboembolic complications of current cardiac valvular prostheses. Ann Thorac Surg 1981;34:96.

51. Stein PD, Kantrowitz A. Antithrombotic therapy in mechanical and biological prosthetic heart valves and saphenous vein bypass grafts. Chest 1989;95(Suppl):107.

52. Sareli P, England MJ, Berk MR, et al. Maternal and fetal sequelae of anticoagulation during pregnancy in patients with mechanical heart valve prostheses. Am J Cardiol 1989;63:1462.

53. Bayliss R, Clark C, Oakley CM, et al. Incidence, mortality, and prevention of infective endocarditis. J R Coll Physicians Lond 1986;20:15.

54. Aslamaci S, Dimitri WR, Williams BT. Operative considerations in active native valve infective endocarditis. J Cardiovasc Surg 1989;30:328.

55. David TE, Bos J, Christakis GT, Brofman PR, Wong D, Feindel CM. Heart valve operations in patients with active infective endocarditis. Ann Thorac Surg 1990;49:701.

APPENDIX
PERTINENT FORMULAS
Laplace Law

$$CWS = \frac{(Pb)}{h}\left(1 - \frac{b^2}{2a^2} - \frac{h}{2b} + \frac{h}{8a^2}\right)$$

where:
CWS = circumferential wall stress in dynes/cm^2 × 10^3;
P = left ventricular pressure in dynes/cm^2; a and b
= major and minor semiaxes, respectively, in cm;
h = left ventricular wall thickness in cm

Gorlin Equation for Calculated Valve Areas*

$$P_1 - P_2 = \frac{F2}{k(\text{valve area})}$$

where:
P_1 and P_2 = pressure proximal and distal, respectively,
to stenotic valve in mmHg; k = correction constant
specific for each valve; F = flow across the valve in
mL/s; valve area is measured in cm^2

Modified Bernoulli Equation

$$P_1 - P_2 = 4(V_2^2 - V_1^2)$$

where:
P_1 and P_2 = pressure proximal and distal, respectively,
to stenotic valve in mmHg; V_2 and V_1 = blood velocity
distal and proximal, respectively, to valve in m/s

Modified Fick Equation

$$Q = \frac{V_{O_2}}{C(a - v)_{O_2}}$$

where:
Q = cardiac output; V_{O_2} = oxygen consumption;
$C(a - v)_{O_2}$ = arterial − mixed venous oxygen content
difference

Poiseuille Equation

$$Q = (\Delta P)r^4/8\rho l$$

and since

$$R = \Delta P/Q$$

then

$$R = 8l/\rho r^4$$

where:
Q = laminar flow; r = tube radius; l = tube length;
ρ = fluid viscosity; R = resistance

Reynold Equation

$$R_e - \frac{VD\rho}{\mu}$$

---

* Modified to express pressure drop as a function of flow.

where:
R_e = Reynold number (flow exceeding this number
becomes turbulent); V = average flow velocity;
D = tube diameter; ρ = fluid density; μ = fluid
viscosity

SURGERY: SCIENTIFIC PRINCIPLES AND PRACTICE, Second Edition, edited by
Lazar J. Greenfield, Michael W. Mulholland, Keith T. Oldham, Gerald B. Zelenock,
and Keith D. Lillemoe. Lippincott–Raven Publishers, Philadelphia, © 1997.

CHAPTER 65

ISCHEMIC HEART DISEASE
GLENN J.R. WHITMAN AND VERDI J. DISESA

CORONARY CIRCULATION
Coronary Arteries

The right and left coronary arteries originate from the
aorta just above the aortic valve cusps (Fig. 65-1). The
positions of the two arteries within the sinuses of Valsalva
designate the right and left coronary cusps. The third aortic
valve cusp is referred to as the *noncoronary cusp.*

The left main coronary artery travels posterolaterally to
the left behind the pulmonary artery and divides (usually
within 10 mm) into two main branches, the left anterior
descending (LAD) coronary artery and the left circumflex
coronary artery.

The LAD coronary artery emerges from behind the pulmonary artery to course anteriorly within the interventricular groove down to the cardiac apex, sometimes wrapping
around it onto the posterior interventricular groove. The
initial tributaries of the LAD are usually the first diagonal,
which takes off at an acute angle and runs over the anterolateral surface of the left ventricle, and the first septal perforator, which emerges at a right angle from the LAD and
penetrates the interventricular septum. The continuation
of the LAD may give off several more diagonal and septal
branches. This pattern of arborization means that the LAD
is responsible for nourishing the anterior, anterolateral,
septal, and apical walls of the left ventricle.

The circumflex coronary artery descends posteriorly
from the left main coronary and runs within the posterior
atrioventricular groove. In about 80% to 85% of patients,
it terminates with branches to the posterolateral wall of
the left ventricle. In the remainder of cases, it extends to
the crux of the heart and gives off the posterior descending
artery (PDA), which runs in the posterior interventricular
groove. The usual branches of the circumflex are referred
to as *obtuse marginal branches* because they cover myocardium where, as seen in the left anterior oblique (LAO)
projection, the heart's lateral wall and posterior wall form
an angle greater than 90 degrees.

The right coronary artery descends in the right atrioventricular groove to the crux, where in 80% to 85% of cases
it gives off the PDA, occasionally continuing and terminating as posterior left ventricular branches. The right ventricular free wall is fed by acute marginal branches from the
right coronary artery, which feed the heart where (as seen
in the LAO projection) it forms an angle of less than 90
degrees as it turns onto the diaphragm.

The artery responsible for supplying the PDA (ie, the
right coronary or left circumflex artery) determines
whether the coronary circulation is termed *right dominant*

A

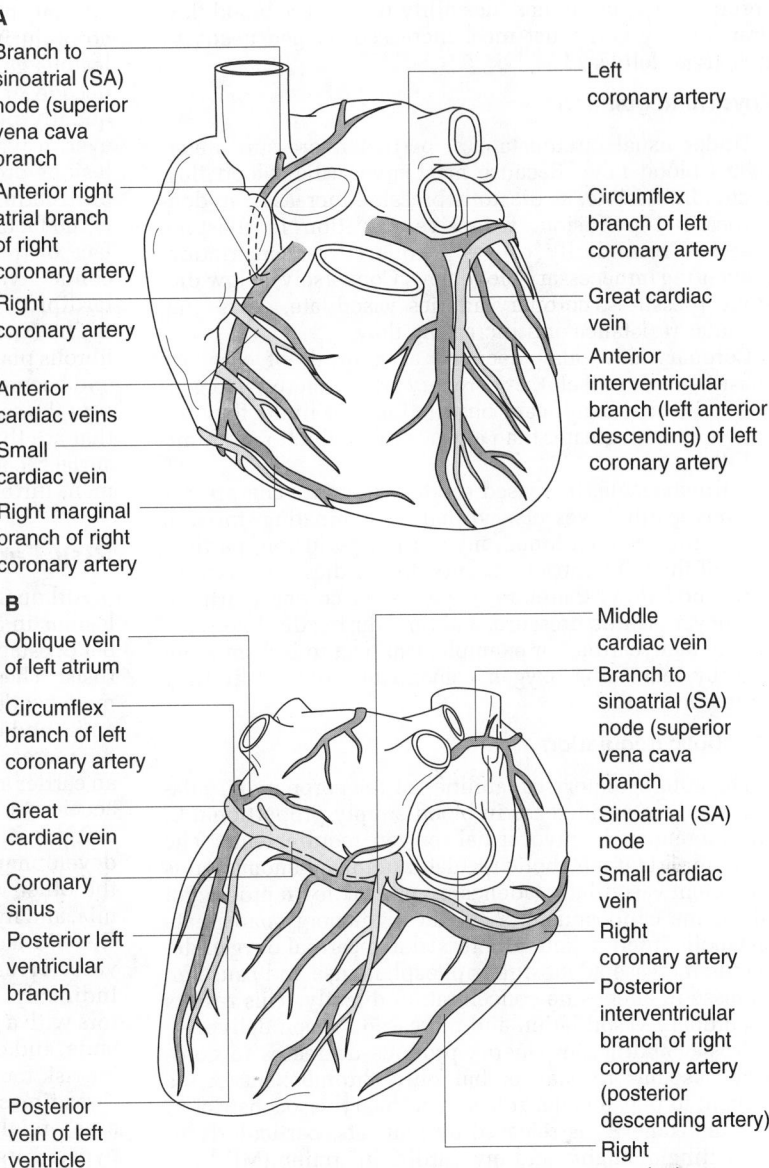

Branch to sinoatrial (SA) node (superior vena cava branch

Anterior right atrial branch of right coronary artery

Right coronary artery

Anterior cardiac veins

Small cardiac vein

Right marginal branch of right coronary artery

Left coronary artery

Circumflex branch of left coronary artery

Great cardiac vein

Anterior interventricular branch (left anterior descending) of left coronary artery

B

Oblique vein of left atrium

Circumflex branch of left coronary artery

Great cardiac vein

Coronary sinus

Posterior left ventricular branch

Posterior vein of left ventricle

Middle cardiac vein

Branch to sinoatrial (SA) node (superior vena cava branch

Sinoatrial (SA) node

Small cardiac vein

Right coronary artery

Posterior interventricular branch of right coronary artery (posterior descending artery)

Right marginal artery

Figure 65-1. Cardiac anatomy depicting the coronary arteries and cardiac veins. The origin of the left main coronary artery is left lateral and somewhat posterior with respect to the aorta, coursing behind the pulmonary artery and then dividing into the left anterior descending and circumflex coronary arteries. The right coronary artery comes off almost directly anterior, running in the atrioventricular groove. The great, middle, and small cardiac veins all come together at the level of the coronary sinus, which lies in the left inferior atrioventricular groove and empties into the right atrium.

or *left dominant*. The PDA gives off the atrioventricular nodal artery, and its occlusion can result in heart block.

Coronary Veins

The following three venous systems drain the coronary circulation:

1. The coronary sinus, located in the posterior atrioventricular groove, receives blood from the great, middle, and small cardiac veins as well as the posterior veins of the left ventricle. It empties into the right atrium. The great cardiac vein ascends along the LAD in the interventricular groove and then turns posteriorly to follow the circumflex coronary artery to empty into the coronary sinus. The middle cardiac vein returns from the apex along the posterior interventricular groove. The small cardiac vein follows the right coronary artery, both emptying at the level of the crux into the coronary sinus.
2. The thebesian veins are tiny venous orifices that drain

the myocardium by emptying directly into any of the four chambers of the heart.
3. The anterior cardiac veins drain the right ventricular coronary system, traversing the right ventricular free wall and crossing the atrioventricular groove to empty directly into the right atrium or a correlating vein at its base.

Coronary Blood Flow

Perfusion of any organ provides oxygen and nutrients to support function. Every minute, the heart uses about 8 to 10 mL of oxygen per 100 g of myocardium. Given the fact that myocardial blood flow is 70 to 90 mL/min/100 g and oxygen delivery is about 14 to 18 mL/min, myocardial oxygen extraction is high, and coronary sinus oxygen content is only 4 to 6 mL oxygen/100 mL blood. This corresponds to a P_{O_2} of about 20 mmHg and a hemoglobin saturation of about 30%. Therefore, even at rest, the heart extracts oxygen maximally, and increased oxygen demand cannot be met by increased oxygen extraction. Rather, the coronary circulation has the ability to increase blood flow dramatically and must meet increased oxygen needs by increased delivery.[1]

Physical Regulation

Under usual circumstances, perfusion pressure determines blood flow. Because most myocardial blood flow occurs in diastole, as diastolic pressure increases, so does myocardial perfusion. Excessive elevation in diastolic pressure secondarily causes coronary vasoconstriction, preventing unnecessary blood flow. Conversely, at low diastolic pressures, coronary arteries vasodilate, decreasing vascular resistance and increasing flow.

Coronary flow may decrease as a result of coronary spasm, intramural clot, or coronary atherosclerosis. In general, clinically significant obstruction that limits flow occurs only with greater than a two thirds reduction in luminal diameter.

During systole, increased cavitary pressure compresses intramyocardial vessels, virtually eliminating forward flow. Thus, as mentioned, myocardial perfusion, particularly of the left ventricle, occurs during diastole. Myocardial blood flow, therefore, depends on coronary arterial patency, diastolic pressure, and time during diastole. That is why tachycardia, for example, can lead to ischemia not only by increasing oxygen demand but also by limiting perfusion time.

Metabolic Regulation

The autoregulatory capabilities of the coronary circulation produce an increase in blood supply proportional to any increment in myocardial oxygen requirements. The most important metabolic regulator of this phenomenon is the potent vasodilator, adenosine, a breakdown product of adenosine triphosphate, a crucial high-energy phosphate metabolic intermediate.[2] Increased myocardial oxygen demands increase adenosine triphosphate use and cause an increase in adenosine concentration directly. This results in coronary vasodilation and increased oxygen delivery.

Prostaglandins, in general, produce decreases in coronary vascular resistance, but only thromboxane A_2 is thought to play a major role as a coronary vasoconstrictor. Thromboxane A_2 is released by platelets, particularly in the setting of angina and myocardial infarction (MI).[3]

Stimulation of cardiac sympathetic nerves directly vasoconstricts coronary arteries. This effect is usually overwhelmed by the autoregulatory vasodilatory response to increased myocardial oxygen demand caused by sympathetic stimulation. Although acetylcholine, which is released by parasympathetic or vagal stimulation, produces coronary vasodilation directly, it lowers heart rate and decreases contractility, resulting in diminished oxygen requirements and vasoconstriction.

CORONARY ATHEROSCLEROSIS

The Lesion

Although atherosclerotic plaques are not uniform within a patient or throughout a population, there are certain common identifiable characteristics. In all cases, atherosclerosis produces a mixture of proliferation of smooth muscle, formation by these cells of tissue matrix consisting of collagen, elastin, and proteoglycans, and accumulation of intracellular and extracellular lipid. The lesions characteristically occur within the intima, the innermost wall of the artery, and follow a progression from the benign "fatty-streak" lesion to the complicated plaque.

As early as childhood, fatty-streak lesions consisting of lipid-laden macrophages and smooth muscle cells line the arterial intima (Fig. 65-2). This process may occur in the aorta during the first decade of life, but coronary arterial lesions generally do not appear until the second or third decade of life. Fatty streaks are nonobstructive and frequently progress no further. In populations at risk, however, a whitish fibrous plaque may then develop. These lesions protrude into the arterial lumen and may become obstructing. Subintimal smooth muscle cell proliferation is the factor most responsible for this protrusion. The surface of the lesion is fibrous, the result of the buildup of connective tissue matrix and intracellular and extracellular lipid.

The advanced, complicated lesion results from an aging fibrous plaque. The necrotic core of the plaque may enlarge and become calcified. Hemorrhage into the plaque can disrupt the smooth, fibrous surface, with resulting ulcerations that are thrombogenic. Organization of clot on the plaque surface causes increased protrusion into the arterial lumen, further decreasing flow.

Risk Factors

Although the characteristics, locations, and severity of lesions in each person can vary, there appear to be a number of established risk factors that predispose to atherosclerosis.[4] These include advanced age, genetic predisposition, male gender, hypertension, diabetes mellitus, hyperlipidemia, and cigarette smoking. The presence of one risk factor increases the likelihood of developing the disease at an earlier age, and the presence of more than one risk factor accelerates the process even further.

Aging appears to have a complex association with the development of atherosclerotic coronary disease; many of the other risk factors, such as hypertension, hyperglycemia, and hyperlipidemia, are associated with aging as well. Genetic factors play a major role, with direct effects on vascular endothelial biology and arterial wall structure. Indirectly, genetic factors predispose patients to risk factors with a genetic basis, such as hypertension, hyperlipidemia, and diabetes. Male gender is a well-documented major risk for the development of coronary disease. Men are three times more likely than women to have coronary disease, and the development of angina, MI, or treatment with bypass surgery occurs 10 years earlier in affected men than women.

Hypertension

Although the mechanism is uncertain, high blood pressure exerts a profound influence on the development of ischemic heart disease. It has been suggested that the increase in heart stress at particular times may alter the vascular endothelium, predisposing to fatty deposition and plaque development. The risk for coronary artery disease increases with increasing blood pressure; in middle-aged men with blood pressures higher than 160/95 mmHg, the incidence of coronary disease is five times greater than in normotensive men. Control of hypertension decreases this risk, with the greatest benefit seen in patients whose diastolic blood pressure exceeds 105 mmHg before treatment.

Diabetes Mellitus

A clear association is seen between diabetes mellitus and atherosclerosis. In both insulin-dependent and non–insulin-dependent diabetic patients, the risk of coronary artery disease is at least doubled, and the risk is even higher in patients with juvenile-onset diabetes and in diabetic women. Unfortunately, although hyperglycemia and atherosclerosis are strongly linked, rigorous control of elevated blood glucose concentrations by insulin does not appear to affect coronary mortality.

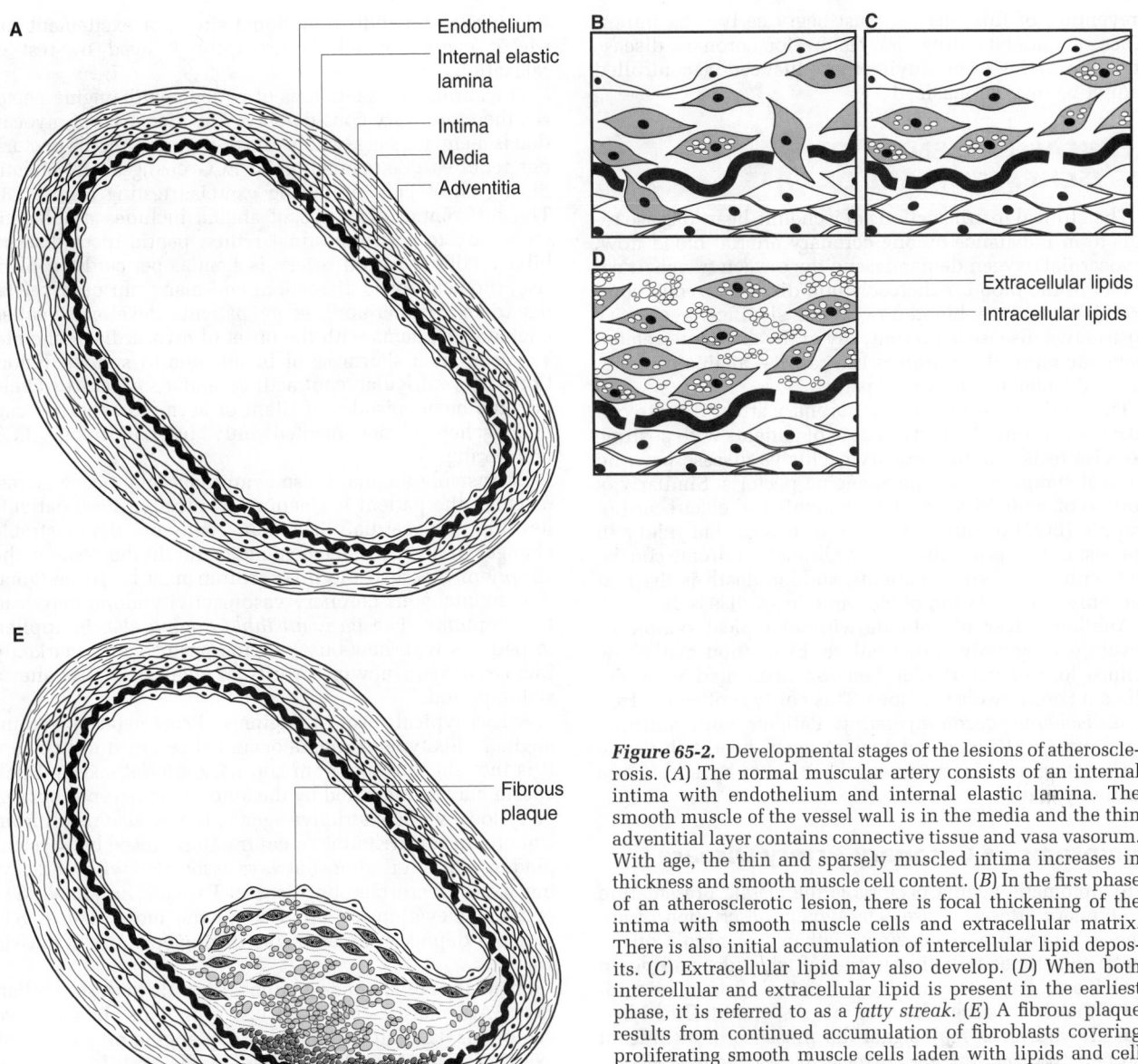

Figure 65-2. Developmental stages of the lesions of atherosclerosis. (*A*) The normal muscular artery consists of an internal intima with endothelium and internal elastic lamina. The smooth muscle of the vessel wall is in the media and the thin adventitial layer contains connective tissue and vasa vasorum. With age, the thin and sparsely muscled intima increases in thickness and smooth muscle cell content. (*B*) In the first phase of an atherosclerotic lesion, there is focal thickening of the intima with smooth muscle cells and extracellular matrix. There is also initial accumulation of intercellular lipid deposits. (*C*) Extracellular lipid may also develop. (*D*) When both intercellular and extracellular lipid is present in the earliest phase, it is referred to as a *fatty streak.* (*E*) A fibrous plaque results from continued accumulation of fibroblasts covering proliferating smooth muscle cells laden with lipids and cell debris. The lesion becomes more complex as continuing cell degeneration leads to ingress of blood constituents and calcification. (After Glomset JA, Ross R. Atherosclerosis and the arterial smooth muscle cells. Science 1973;180:1332)

Hyperlipidemia

Both hypercholesterolemia and hypertriglyceridemia are important risk factors for coronary artery disease. The Lipid Research Clinics Trial[5] demonstrated a direct association between plasma lipoproteins, cholesterol level, and morbidity and mortality from coronary artery disease. Furthermore, treated patients decreased their risk in direct proportion to the degree of cholesterol lowering. Hypertriglyceridemia appears to affect the incidence of coronary artery disease specifically in patients with familial combined hyperlipidemia, while accentuating the risk in diabetics and smokers.

High-density lipoproteins (HDL) contain about 20% of total plasma cholesterol. HDL level is inversely proportional to the risk of developing coronary artery disease. HDL is about 25% higher in women than in men, is raised by exercise and estrogens, and is decreased by androgens and cigarette smoking. High HDL levels offer some protection against the development of coronary artery disease.

Cigarette Smoking

Cigarette smoking is one of the most important risk factors for coronary artery disease, not simply because its acceleration of the disease is so evident but because its cessation so clearly decreases the risk. In men who smoke one pack of cigarettes per day, the death rate from coronary artery disease is 70% higher and the incidence of the disease three to five times greater than in nonsmokers. Cigarette smoking appears to potentiate other risk factors, such as hypertension and diabetes mellitus. Patients with these risk factors who also smoke experience a severe increase in coronary artery disease mortality.

Prevention

Angina pectoris and MI are late manifestations of coronary artery disease. Because atherosclerosis, as evidenced by fatty streaks and early complicated lesions, has been found in men as early as the second decade of life, primary prevention of this disease must begin early. The importance of understanding risk factors for coronary disease and eliminating or modifying those that can be controlled cannot be overemphasized.

CLINICAL PRESENTATION OF ISCHEMIC HEART DISEASE

The clinical manifestations of ischemic heart disease result from imbalance among coronary arterial blood flow, myocardial oxygen demands, and the oxygen transport capacity of the blood. Atherosclerotic disease directly compromises coronary blood flow. When significant coronary obstructive disease is present, any of the three interrelated ischemic clinical syndromes can result—angina pectoris, MI, and ischemic cardiomyopathy.

The clinical presentation of coronary artery disease can take many forms. As many as 25% of patients with positive exercise tests due to coronary occlusive disease have no clinical symptoms of typical angina pectoris. Similarly, a portion of acute MIs are silent; patients had electrocardiographic (ECG) or other evidence of myocardial injury in the past but no prior history of a clinical syndrome consistent with MI. In some patients, sudden death is the first and only manifestation of ischemic heart disease.

Another subset of patients without typical symptoms develops progressive heart failure. Evaluation may show diffuse loss of ventricular function associated with significant coronary obstructions. This entity is often referred to as *ischemic cardiomyopathy*. Patients with multiple symptomatic MIs who end up with severe heart failure due to loss of ventricular muscle can be said to have ischemic cardiomyopathy.

Symptoms of Coronary Artery Disease

Symptomatic angina pectoris is the classic presentation of coronary artery disease. The typical description of angina is a pressure or heaviness felt in the middle of the chest, sometimes radiating to the left shoulder and down the left arm. Patients typically clench their fists in the middle of the chest as they describe this discomfort. Other, less typical syndromes may signal the presence of significant coronary obstruction and myocardial ischemia. Patients may complain of abdominal pain, nausea, or belching. Other symptoms include back pain or pain in one or both shoulders, jaw pain, or hand heaviness or numbness. Stable angina pectoris is brought on by reproducible increases in myocardial demand for oxygen. Patients report that cer-

tain levels of activity, emotional stress, or excitement can trigger angina, which is promptly relieved by rest or relaxation.

The clinical presentations of patients with angina pectoris, therefore, vary considerably. The diagnosis of myocardial ischemia is suggested by the presence of angina pectoris but requires documentation of ECG changes of ischemia during chest pain or during exercise testing (Fig. 65-3). The differential diagnosis of angina includes esophagitis secondary to gastrointestinal reflux, peptic ulcer disease, biliary colic, visceral artery ischemia, pericarditis, pleurisy, thoracic aortic dissection, and many musculoskeletal disorders. Furthermore, some patients develop so-called angina equivalents with the onset of myocardial ischemia. These include shortness of breath due to sudden reductions in ventricular contractility and compliance. Other patients have episodes of silent or asymptomatic myocardial ischemia, documented only by continuous ECG monitoring.

In unstable angina, these symptoms may occur at rest or when the patient is sleeping. Typically, these patients develop myocardial ischemia without demonstrable changes in myocardial oxygen demand. In these cases, the *supply* of blood to the myocardium may be so marginal that spontaneous coronary vasoreactivity alone may lead to symptoms. The term *unstable angina* also is applied to patients with new-onset angina pectoris or a markedly increased frequency or severity of angina pectoris after a stable period.

A less typical form of angina is Prinzmetal or variant angina. This type of angina occurs at rest or during sleep. It is thought to result from coronary arterial spasm. Such spasm may be mediated by the autonomic nervous system or by local vasoconstrictive agents. It may also result from smooth muscle irritation or contraction caused by adjacent plaques. Spasm is almost always associated with underlying fixed atherosclerotic disease. Patients may have ST-segment elevation, as opposed to the more typical ST-segment depression that occurs during episodes of classic angina.

Physicians often grade angina according to the Canadian Heart Association scheme. Class I patients do not have symptoms. Class II patients develop angina on significant exertion. Class III patients have angina at mild exertion, and class IV patients develop symptoms at rest. A similar classification from the New York Heart Association is used to describe the severity of heart failure. Patients in New York Heart Association class I have no symptoms of heart failure; class II patients develop symptoms at significant

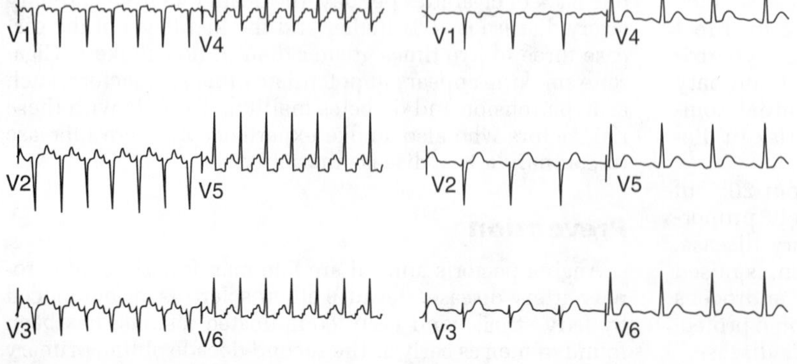

Figure 65-3. ECG from a 60-year-old man during an exercise test showing the standard precordial leads, V_1 through V_6. During exercise (*A*) ST segment depression and ischemia are seen in leads V_4 through V_6, which resolve after the exercise was stopped (*B*). (After Wagner GS. Ischemia due to increased myocardial demand. In: Marriott's practical electrocardiography, ed 9. Baltimore, Williams & Wilkins, 1994)

exertion; class III at mild exertion, such as normal daily activities; and class IV at rest.

Physical Examination

Usually, there are no detectable signs of coronary artery disease on physical examination, but there may be evidence of associated conditions. Patients may have clinical evidence of peripheral vascular disease with loss of pulses or presence of bruits in the carotid arteries, abdomen, or femoral arteries. Other signs, such as ocular xanthomas or hypertensive retinal changes, may provide corroborative evidence in patients at risk for coronary disease.

Diagnostic Studies

Laboratory studies may be useful for detecting cardiac risk factors, such as diabetes mellitus, hyperlipidemia, or hyperthyroidism. Anemia in the presence of subcritical or borderline coronary obstructions may precipitate angina due to myocardial ischemia from the reduced oxygen-carrying capacity of blood.

The ECG examination is frequently normal but may reveal evidence of old MI. Typically, these changes include Q waves or loss of R-wave progression in the precordial leads. Chronic ST-segment and T-wave changes may be suggestive of underlying coronary disease but are not specific.

Stress testing may be useful for detecting the presence of coronary disease or assessing the functional significance of coronary lesions. In the standard test, a patient undergoes graded exercise on a treadmill with ECG monitoring. If the patient develops signs or symptoms of angina pectoris associated with typical ischemic ECG changes, this is considered a positive test. The most diagnostic ECG changes are downward sloping ST-segment depressions. The accuracy of the test is reduced when the patient has underlying ECG abnormalities. Specificity may be improved if the test is combined with administration of thallium. Thallium is a radioactive isotope that is distributed intracellularly like potassium. When injected during exercise, if a patient develops coronary ischemia, the involved area of myocardium fails to take up thallium, and a defect is present on a myocardial scan. As the patient recovers from exercise and the ischemia is relieved, the previous defect fills in. In patients who cannot exercise, thallium imaging can be done after administration of dipyridamole. Dipyridamole is a coronary vasodilator that may reveal areas of relative underperfusion, leading to a thallium defect on scanning as with exercise testing. In patients in whom it is thought to be unsafe to exercise or give dipyridamole, a rest–rest thallium myocardial scan may reveal evidence of borderline regional myocardial perfusion. In this test, patients are scanned early after injection with thallium and again several hours later. A defect present on the early scan that fills in later is considered a sign of significant coronary obstruction. A defect that never fills in on thallium scanning is a sign of irreversibly scarred, nonviable myocardium.

Coronary arteriography, which is an invasive diagnostic procedure, is the only way to make the definitive diagnosis of significant coronary obstruction. Coronary arteriography is indicated in patients with atypical presentations and borderline or normal stress tests in whom there is a need to make a definitive diagnosis of coronary artery disease. Patients with classic anginal symptoms and ECG changes in whom the diagnosis of coronary disease is in little doubt should have coronary angiography only if they are refractory to medical therapy or candidates for revascularization. Regardless of symptoms, patients suspected of having severe coronary artery disease, such as left main stenosis or severe proximal three-vessel coronary disease, should have coronary arteriography to document their condition because of the survival benefits that accrue with revascularization. Other indications for diagnostic coronary arteriography include patients with other cardiac disease, such as valvular heart disease, in whom valve surgery is planned but in whom there is a risk of concomitant coronary disease. Examples include patients with aortic stenosis who have angina as part of their presentation. Patients with valvular heart disease who do not have angina but do have risk factors for coronary disease should also have angiography before surgery. These include men older than 45 to 50 years with one or more risk factors for coronary disease.

Medical Management

The medical management of coronary artery disease includes the identification and reduction of controllable risk factors. Obviously, patients can do little about a genetic predisposition for the development of coronary obstructions. Control of risk factors by weight reduction, smoking cessation, blood pressure control, and limitation of dietary fats is sensible. Patients with hyperthyroidism or anemia, which may exacerbate anginal symptoms, should have these underlying conditions corrected.

The goal of all therapy for angina pectoris is to decrease the imbalance between the myocardial oxygen supply and demand. Most of the medications that are useful in angina pectoris have a greater effect on reducing myocardial oxygen demand than on increasing supply. *Nitroglycerin*, one of the most commonly used agents, primarily dilates venous capacitance blood vessels, but at higher doses, it may also cause systemic arterial dilation. Although nitrate compounds do not appear to increase coronary blood flow in the normal heart, these drugs may result in some dilation of the coronary arterioles, with improvement in coronary collateral blood flow in patients with extensive atherosclerotic obstructive disease. The primary benefit of nitrates, however, appears to be the reduction of myocardial oxygen demand by reducing ventricular work. This is the result of a reduction in systemic vascular resistance and dilation of venous capacitance vessels, which lowers ventricular filling pressures, ventricular wall stress or tension, and contractile work.

β-Adrenergic blocking agents also reduce myocardial oxygen demand by decreasing both cardiac contractility and heart rate. These agents may also reduce blood pressure and systemic vascular resistance, further reducing the work of the heart. *Calcium-channel blocking agents*, such as nifedipine and diltiazem, have more complex cardiac and vascular effects that include a reduction in ventricular contractility, variable degrees of vasodilation, and possibly a direct protection of myocytes when these cells become hypoxic. Calcium-channel blocking agents may be particularly effective in patients with a component of coronary vasospastic disease.

ACUTE MYOCARDIAL INFARCTION

Acute MI is the direct result of interruption of blood supply to the myocardium. It is not the result of increased myocardial oxygen demand, but rather of loss of oxygen supply. It usually occurs after coronary artery thrombosis at the site of a significant stenosis over a complicated plaque. The clot may form as a result of plaque rupture or hemorrhage that incites thrombus formation, or it may be secondary to coronary spasm, further reducing luminal diameter, markedly decreasing flow, and leading to thrombosis. Although the acute event associated with MI is acute thrombosis, studies using cardiac catheterization have shown that about 20% to 30% of culprit coronary arteries are patent again within a few days of infarction. This is more common in nontransmural than transmural MIs.[6]

One major determinant of prognosis after acute MI is the amount of ventricular myocardium that undergoes necrosis. For post-MI patients with ejection fractions of more than 50%, the 3-year survival is nearly 90%, but when ejection fraction falls to less than 37%, the 3-year survival rate is only 50% (Fig. 65-4). Loss of 25% of ventricular myocardium leads to symptomatic cardiac dysfunction, whereas the acute loss of more than 40% is frequently associated with cardiogenic shock and death. Efforts to treat patients who are experiencing MI are therefore focused on decreasing myocardial loss by improving flow to the area at risk as quickly as possible. Interestingly, collateral blood supply, although unable to meet myocardial oxygen requirements completely, may supply enough flow to limit markedly the amount of myocardium lost. Thus, although well-developed collaterals may not prevent demand-induced angina, they may significantly diminish the loss of myocardium after an acute coronary occlusion.

Presentation

Pain is the most common presenting complaint in patients with MI. It is deep and visceral and frequently described as heavy or crushing. However, pain is by no means universally present, and 20% to 25% of patients (most often diabetic and elderly patients) do not have symptoms. The combination of substernal chest pain lasting for more than 20 to 30 minutes and diaphoresis is strongly suggestive of MI. Interestingly, anterior MIs (usually involving the LAD) result in sympathetic hyperactivity with tachycardia and hypertension, whereas inferior MIs (involving the right coronary artery) frequently have parasympathetic activity with bradycardia and hypotension.

Diagnosis

The classic ECG picture of an acute MI is the development of Q waves and elevated, coved ST segments in leads reflecting the affected area (Fig. 65-5). Clinicians frequently characterize MIs by the associated ECG changes. Transmural infarctions usually cause Q waves, whereas subendocardial or nontransmural infarctions are characterized by transient ST-segment changes with evolving T-wave inversion but without the development of Q waves.

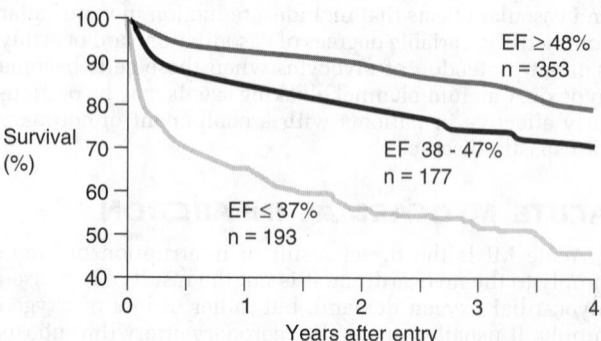

Figure 65-4. Survival of patients in the Multicenter Investigation on Limitation of Infarct Size (MILIS). Probability of survival is reduced in patients with poor ejection fraction (EF) at the time of admission for a myocardial infarction. (After Braunwald E. Circulation 1987;76[Suppl II]:406)

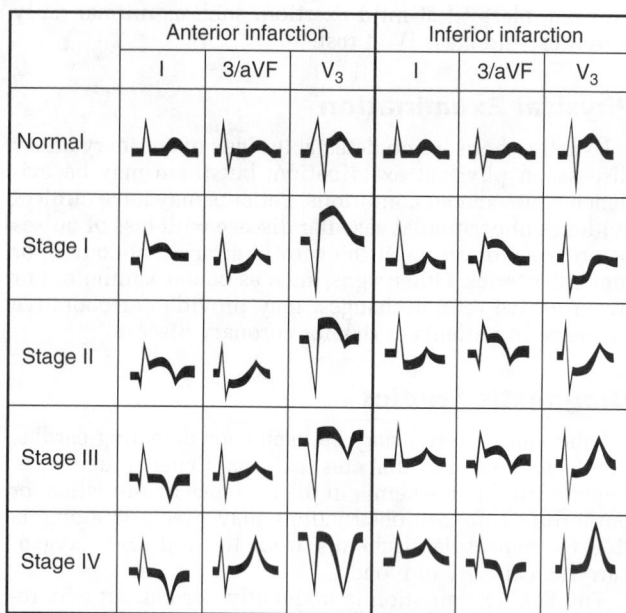

Figure 65-5. The pattern of evolution of the ECG in acute myocardial infarction. In the first stage, acute ST elevations are present in leads reflecting the affected area of myocardium. There are reciprocal ST depressions in leads away from the site of the infarct. Stage 2 T-wave inversion begins, which deepens in stage 3. ST segment elevations are no longer present. A Q wave may develop early, but by stage 4, Q waves are present and persistent T-wave inversions, which may be deep, are seen. (After Marriott HJL. Myocardial infarction. In: Practical electrocardiography, ed 7. Baltimore, Williams & Wilkins, 1983:379).

MIs are frequently referred to by these ECG changes and are called either Q-wave (transmural) or non–Q-wave (nontransmural or subendocardial) infarctions.

After MI, enzymes are released by necrotic myocytes in large enough quantities to be detected in serum. As a result, enzyme elevations have become the sine qua non of the diagnosis of MI. In particular, serum levels of creatine kinase, a cardiac enzyme involved with high-energy phosphate metabolism, are increased after myocardial cell death and rise substantially within 8 to 24 hours, returning to normal within 1 to 2 days. Creatine kinase has several tissue-specific isoenzymes; the isoenzyme found specifically in cardiac tissue is denoted as CK-MB. Because creatine kinase is found in brain (CK-BB) and muscle (CK-MM) and can rise significantly after stroke, surgery, cardiac catheterization, or simply an intramuscular injection, it is crucial to measure the specific isoenzyme CK-MB when ruling out MI. Characteristic CK-MB elevations occur in 95% of patients with clinically proven MI.

Management

During the early phase of MI, it may not be clear whether the patient has unstable preinfarction angina or whether the patient's symptoms indicate a process leading to irreversible myocardial injury. The ECG may be unrevealing, and cardiac isoenzymes may be unavailable. In this situation, oxygen should be administered, heart rhythm should be monitored, and lidocaine should be given to prevent ventricular fibrillation if warning arrhythmias occur. *Early evolving MI* is the term used to describe patients who are within 4 to 6 hours of the onset of continued chest pain. This group is important to recognize because ischemic myocardium may still be salvaged before irreversible necrosis.

Initial treatment should be to control pain, most frequently with intravenous morphine. Decreasing anxiety and pain may have a significant therapeutic effect, decreasing myocardial oxygen demand and limiting infarct size. Intravenous nitroglycerin, begun at a low dose of 0.2 μg/kg/min, to prevent the side effects of hypotension and headache may diminish infarct size, decrease sudden death, and lower the incidence of congestive heart failure.[7] The use of β-blockers is not uniformly agreed on, although they too have been shown to limit infarct size and decrease early mortality.[8] Hypotension and bradyarrhythmias occur more frequently with administration of β-blockers than with intravenous nitroglycerin. Their use in patients with acute MI who have increased sympathetic tone, however, is probably a safe and beneficial practice. Unlike β-blockers, calcium-channel blockers have little benefit in the acute MI setting.[9]

Thrombolytic agents convert plasminogen to plasmin, a powerful thrombolysin. It was hypothesized that administration of thrombolytic agents would lead to dissolution of coronary thrombosis, reversing the process that leads to MI. In the late 1970s, a European trial of one thrombolysin, streptokinase, revealed a significant benefit if the drug was given within 12 hours of acute MI.[10] Thrombolytic trials in the 1980s involving thousands of patients established the benefit of this approach, showing that thrombolysis reopens acutely occluded coronary arteries in most cases, restoring flow and reducing mortality.[11]

Although initial thrombolytic trials involved intracoronary administration of the drugs, the cumbersome necessity for emergency cardiac catheterization led to investigations of systemic intravenous administration, allowing virtually immediate therapy in the acute MI setting. Three intravenous thrombolytic agents are approved by the Food and Drug Administration: streptokinase, recombinant tissue-type plasminogen activator (rTPA), and anisoylated plasminogen streptokinase activator complex (APSAC). The most widely used is streptokinase, which has been effective in several large trials[12] and is inexpensive. APSAC was developed to enable treating physicians to give intravenous therapy as a bolus over a few minutes with maintenance of effect for a few hours, rather than requiring a continuous intravenous infusion, as is necessary with streptokinase and rTPA. However, results are not significantly better than with the other two drugs, APSAC is more expensive, and its prolonged half-life and thrombolytic effect can be a significant drawback rather than a benefit. rtPA is produced by recombinant DNA techniques and is significantly more expensive than streptokinase. Although it generates less of a systemic fibrinolytic effect than either streptokinase or APSAC, it produces higher patency rates.[13]

Systemic intravenous thrombolytic therapy unquestionably decreases morbidity and mortality after MI. The earlier the treatment, the greater the impact, with the greatest benefit accruing in patients treated within 1 to 2 hours of the onset of symptoms.[14] Furthermore, decreased morbidity secondary to a reduction in arrhythmias and ventricular power failure appears to benefit patients treated with thrombolytic therapy as well. Heparin and antiplatelet drugs such as aspirin produce an added benefit when combined with thrombolytic therapy, particularly in the case of rTPA, which has a short half-life and produces little antithrombin effect because it does not generate excessive fibrin degradation products.

Complications of thrombolytic therapy include allergic reactions in patients exposed to streptococci or streptokinase in the previous year, with reactions occurring in less than 2% of patients. Hemorrhage is a major problem with all lytic agents, commonly occurring at a site of vascular access. Stroke occurs in less than 1% of patients but may be catastrophic due to its hemorrhagic nature. Bleeding complications and strokes occur most frequently in elderly, female, hypertensive, and small patients.

Mechanical Intervention

The use of thrombolytic therapy with early recanalization of the culprit vessel responsible for the MI has had tremendous impact on the treatment and prognosis of patients experiencing acute MI. The issue then becomes whether anything more need be done acutely, considering that despite reperfusion, significant residual stenoses remain. The Thrombolysis in Myocardial Infarction phase 2 trial compared elective catheterization and percutaneous transluminal coronary angioplasty (PTCA) within the first 2 days of lytic therapy for MI to cardiac catheterization and PTCA only if ischemia developed later in the hospital course.[15] The more invasive approach failed to provide a benefit with respect to early or late mortality and, in fact, increased the patient's risk significantly. As a result of this and other trials, cardiac catheterization and PTCA should be withheld in most patients who have no symptoms after thrombolytic therapy for an acute MI. A more invasive approach is justified in patients who exhibit residual ischemia during their hospital stay either during convalescence or at a predischarge exercise stress test. PTCA may be appropriate, but if cardiac catheterization shows multivessel coronary artery disease or anatomy more suitable for bypass than PTCA, surgery should be carried out. Patients operated on within 30 days of acute MI have excellent early and long-term results.[16]

Indications for Surgery

Postinfarction Angina. Chest pain recurs in 10% to 15% of patients after acute MI, a frequency that increases dramatically if thrombolytic therapy is used. In that situation, the incidence of angina after MI may be as high as 30% to 35%. Postinfarction angina is an indication that myocardial cells are ischemic and often occurs when a patient is at rest. This generally indicates residual myocardial tissue at risk for infarct extension, which is a complication that can and should be avoided. After MI, the mortality rate may increase by 15% to as much as 40% if infarct extension occurs.[17] In fact, infarct extension may be the most powerful predictor of mortality after MI, as seen by an increase in the average 1-year mortality from about 18% to 65% if infarct extension occurs. Thus, postinfarction angina is an indication for cardiac catheterization, with mechanical intervention, such as PTCA or coronary bypass surgery, if indicated. This is particularly relevant because the mortality rate from coronary bypass surgery after MI is extremely low, less than 4% in most advanced centers.[16]

Cardiogenic Shock. The occurrence of cardiogenic shock after MI is uncommon. In the multicenter investigation for the limitation of infarct size, only 60 of 845 patients with acute MI developed cardiogenic shock.[18] That group had a 65% mortality rate, whereas in the group that did not develop shock, the mortality rate was only 4%. Infarct extension occurred in 23% of the shock group as opposed to 7% of the nonshock group. More important, in 50% of patients, shock developed more than 24 hours after admission. Evaluation of these patients revealed that age greater than 65 years, ejection fraction less than 35% on admission, a large MI as evaluated by the magnitude of the CK-MB leak, a history of diabetes mellitus, and a history of previous MI were all risk factors that predicted the development of shock. When three of these risk factors were present, the in-hospital mortality rate was 18%; with all five risk factors, the in-hospital mortality rate was 55%.[18]

Animal studies have shown that even in the face of prolonged regional myocardial ischemia, intervention with emergency revascularization may decrease the amount of damage sustained by the myocardium. These studies have focused on ways to decrease energy expenditure during early reperfusion as well as ways to tailor the initial reperfusate in an effort to decrease cell swelling, provide intermediary cellular metabolic substrates, and decrease oxidant injury. In this way, myocardium damaged by an ischemic insult can be drastically reduced.[19] This has led to a prospective study[20] evaluating the effect on mortality of emergency coronary bypass surgery in patients in cardiogenic shock after MI. In 80 consecutive patients in cardiogenic shock on vasopressors with intraaortic balloon pumps after MI, emergency coronary bypass was performed. If surgery occurred within 18 hours of onset of shock, the mortality rate was 7%; if surgery occurred after 18 hours, the mortality rate was 31%. This represents a definite improvement on the results of medical therapy (65% mortality) for this severe complication of MI. In those centers capable of performing surgery of this kind, it may be the ideal approach to patients in shock after MI. These results, which have not been duplicated by other institutions, must be viewed as preliminary.

Ventricular Septal Defect. Ventricular septal defects occur in about 2% of patients after MI. In general, this complication occurs at a time when the myocardium is at its weakest, about 3 to 5 days after MI. It occurs more commonly in anterior than posterior MIs and has a mortality rate with medical treatment of more than 90%. At greatest risk for the development of this complication are elderly hypertensive women with transmural infarction. Clinically, patients develop hypotension with congestive heart failure. Emergency cardiac catheterization reveals an oxygen step-up in the right ventricle, indicating a left-to-right shunt. Medical therapy involves decreasing afterload as much as possible, invariably using an intraaortic balloon pump as well as vasodilator therapy if possible. Preload is optimized, and surgery should be performed immediately. Previous approaches involved the stabilization of patients for a prolonged period in hopes that the infarcted area of myocardium would become firmer and hold sutures better. During the 3 weeks that were generally given for this process, however, patients frequently developed irreversible multiorgan system failure from shock and sepsis. Early operation before complications occur appears to carry a much better survival rate. Surgical opinion now favors early intervention for this complication.[21]

Acute Mitral Regurgitation. Papillary muscle rupture with acute mitral regurgitation occurs infrequently and is seen in less than 2% of patients. As with ventricular septal defect, it is seen between the third and fifth days when infarcted myocardium is at its weakest. Posteroinferior MIs lead to this complication more frequently than anterior infarctions, almost certainly because the circumflex and PDA distribution are the most crucial blood supplies to the papillary muscles. Clinically, this complication can present with signs and symptoms similar to a ventricular septal defect. There is the development of a new murmur and symptoms of congestive heart failure with hypotension. The pulmonary capillary wedge pressure tracing, however, shows prominent V waves, and there is no right ventricular oxygen step-up. Immediate medical therapy involves decreasing afterload with an intraaortic balloon pump. Surgery, although at increased risk, leads to a better survival than continued medical therapy, decreasing mor-

tality from more than 90% to less than 50%. Evidence has shown that if total mitral valve excision can be avoided by saving all or part of the subvalvular mitral apparatus, the mortality rate can be decreased even further from 20% with mitral valve replacement to 5% if the mitral valve apparatus is preserved with either repair or replacement. Long-term survival is also improved. In one series,[22] the 4-year survival rate was 89% in the group undergoing conservation of the mitral apparatus, as opposed to 59% in the group that had mitral valve replacement with total excision of the native valve.

Free Wall Rupture. Ventricular free wall rupture after MI occurs also at a time when the myocardium is at its weakest, in the period between the 3rd and 6th days after infarction. The incidence is not well known, but the medical mortality rate is exceedingly high (more than 90%). The benefits of surgical intervention are undocumented. A variety of case reports cite the dramatic rescue of some patients, but circumstances must be ideal. The free wall rupture must be small and contained, allowing time for diagnosis and operative intervention. Most commonly, free wall rupture leads to death. In some cases, it is contained and may go unrecognized until the development of a pseudoaneurysm, which is diagnosed at a later date.

MECHANICAL REVASCULARIZATION USING PERCUTANEOUS TRANSLUMINAL CORONARY ANGIOPLASTY

Percutaneous transluminal coronary angioplasty is a cardiac catheterization technique designed to reduce the degree of myocardial obstruction with improvement in regional coronary blood flow. In the mid-1970s, Gruentzig and Hoff designed a balloon dilation catheter for use in the coronary arteries and initiated this important treatment option for patients with ischemic heart disease. PTCA is performed in a standard cardiac catheterization laboratory. The technique is similar to coronary angiography. Under fluoroscopic guidance, a catheter is directed into the coronary artery to be treated. A guide wire is then placed across the obstructing lesion. A balloon catheter is then passed over the guide wire and the balloon positioned in the midportion of the obstructing lesion. Under fluoroscopic control, the balloon is inflated to a pressure of 4 to 10 atmospheres for 20 to 60 seconds, reducing the degree of coronary obstruction. Balloon inflation may be repeated several times. It is unclear whether the beneficial effect of this treatment is compression or fracture of the plaque or fracture of the more pliable part of the coronary vessel circumference. After withdrawing the balloon catheter, repeat coronary angiography is undertaken immediately to assess the degree of dilation and to look for dilation-related complications, such as arterial dissection or acute thrombosis. Since the first successful coronary angioplasty was reported in 1977, the number of PTCA procedures has increased dramatically to more than 200,000 cases per year in the United States.

Indications

The indications for PTCA are the same as for coronary artery bypass surgery, the main alternative revascularization technique. Patients with intractable symptoms and those with proximal coronary stenoses that place a large amount of myocardium at risk are potential candidates for angioplasty. The ideal lesion for angioplasty is a symmetric focal stenosis in an epicardial vessel. Long, asymmetric stenoses or those that are adjacent to bends in the artery or branch points are less likely to lead to a successful result. In general, PTCA is contraindicated if there is significant disease in the left main coronary artery, if the target coronary artery is less then 2 mm in luminal diameter, if there are multiple significant obstructive lesions in the same artery, or if there are complex obstructive lesions, such as those involving or straddling arterial bifurcations.

Complications

The primary risk of angioplasty is dissection of the coronary vessel with acute closure. This occurs in about 3% of cases and usually requires emergency coronary bypass surgery.[23] MI may result but can be aborted by immediate surgical revascularization. Other risks are similar to those of coronary angiography and include cerebral vascular accident and local arterial trauma. Improvements in balloon catheter design and fabrication have enhanced the success rate of PTCA and have allowed more extensive dilations in patients with multivessel or complex coronary artery disease. Also under development are atherectomy catheters, which incorporate tiny rotating blades for lysis of atheromatous plaque, and laser-tip catheters that vaporize intraluminal obstructions. Newer investigational devices also include coronary stents. These small, implantable, cylindric devices are designed to maintain patency of diseased arteries when more conventional balloon angioplasty is ineffective.

Results

Successful primary dilation of favorable coronary arterial obstructive lesions occurs in more than 90% of PTCA attempts, with an immediate complication rate of about 3%. The most significant long-term problem with PTCA is the high incidence of restenosis. Restenosis is probably the result of postdilation proliferation of intimal and smooth muscle cells in response to the angioplasty. Restenosis rates of between 20% and 40% within the first 4 to 6 months after PTCA have been reported in patients with initially successful dilation for simple lesions.[24] Restenosis rates as high as 60% have been reported for patients with complex lesions that required multiple dilations. Although redilation of recurrent stenotic lesions can be carried out successfully, many of these patients ultimately require bypass grafting.

CORONARY ARTERY BYPASS SURGERY

Coronary artery bypass grafting (CABG) is among the most commonly applied major surgical operations in the United States, with more than 250,000 procedures performed yearly. The goals of coronary artery bypass surgery are identical to the goals of medical treatment and PTCA— to treat ischemic heart disease by relieving the imbalance of myocardial oxygen supply and demand. The indications for coronary bypass surgery versus medical treatment or PTCA for an individual patient may be controversial. Choosing the optimal therapy for a given patient necessitates weighing variables, such as the pattern of the coronary artery obstructions, ventricular function, symptom severity, initial response to medical therapy, and presence of noncardiac diseases. Patients require individual evaluation to determine the potential short- and long-term benefits of surgical revascularization versus medical or less invasive angioplasty treatment.[25]

Indications

Patients are referred to as having *single-, double-,* or *triple-vessel disease* if there are significant atherosclerotic narrowings of one, two, or all three of the major arteries (ie, LAD, circumflex, and right coronary artery). In general, data from clinical trials and retrospective studies suggest that as the number of diseased major coronary arterial segments increases, the survival benefit of surgical therapy over medical therapy alone becomes greater (Table 65-1). This observation in general terms has been borne out by the three major prospective randomized coronary bypass studies, the Coronary Artery Surgery Study (CASS)[26], Veterans Administration Cooperative Study[27], and European reports[28] (see later). In patients with stable angina, the presence of severe proximal triple-vessel disease, especially in those with impaired left ventricular function, generally is an indication for surgical revascularization.

Another well-accepted indication for CABG is the presence of significant stenosis of the left main coronary artery. Both the Veterans Administration Cooperative Study[29] and the CASS study[26] provide overwhelming evidence for improved survival with surgical treatment of patients with left main artery disease. Most cardiologists and cardiac surgeons also believe there is a surgical benefit in patients with normal or depressed left ventricular function and two-vessel disease associated with a high-grade proximal LAD obstruction.[28] On the other hand, the need for surgery in patients with single- or double-vessel disease, without disabling symptoms or LAD involvement, has not been clearly established.[30]

Above all, the most common indication for CABG continues to be the relief of disabling angina refractory to medical therapy. Bypass surgery reduces or eliminates angina in more than 90% of patients, and those patients with the most severe anginal syndromes derive the greatest benefit. The randomized studies[26-29] have provided strong evidence that CABG is more effective than medical treatment for relieving angina, improving physical work capacity, and improving the overall quality of life. Finally, patients with silent ischemia (ie, patients without symptoms with significant atherosclerotic disease and myocardial ischemia demonstrated by ECG changes, exercise stress testing, and coronary angiography) have shown improved survival after CABG.

Patients with unstable angina are a heterogeneous group. In general, the occurrence of unstable (or crescendo) angina suggests that the patient is at risk for MI and death. These patients require aggressive medical therapy, including nitrates, β-adrenergic blockers, and calcium antago-

---

Table 65-1. INDICATIONS FOR CORONARY BYPASS SURGERY

ANATOMY

Left main coronary artery disease
Triple-vessel disease involving the proximal left anterior descending coronary artery with normal or diminished ejection fraction
Double-vessel disease involving the proximal left anterior descending coronary artery with normal or diminished ejection fraction

SYMPTOMS

Unstable (crescendo) angina
Post—myocardial infarction angina
Acute coronary occlusion after percutaneous transluminal coronary angioplasty
Symptoms unsuccessfully controlled with medical therapy
Controlled symptoms, but with unacceptable life-style

nists, as well as heparin anticoagulation to forestall coronary arterial thrombosis. If the patient continues to experience unstable or rest angina despite maximal medical treatment, urgent coronary angiography is indicated in preparation for PTCA or surgery.[31] Collective outcome data from several series of patients with unstable angina who underwent surgical revascularization demonstrated increased rates of perioperative MI, postoperative low cardiac output, and death as compared with patients who underwent CABG for chronic stable angina. Nonetheless, patients with unstable angina had *late* outcomes after CABG similar to patients with chronic stable angina: relief of angina was excellent, the late MI rate was low, and, most important, long-term survival was similar.

Although there does not appear to be an unequivocal role for CABG in the setting of acute MI, the development of recurrent angina early after infarction has become an accepted indication for operative intervention. These patients are at risk for infarct extension or for a second infarction. Even mild postinfarction angina mandates an aggressive response with coronary angiography and consideration of revascularization (see earlier).

As mentioned, emergency CABG is necessary in the about 3% of patients who develop coronary occlusive complications during PTCA. Most of these occlusions result from coronary dissections proximal or distal to the site of dilation. Emergency CABG is indicated as soon as it is apparent that an acute coronary occlusion has occurred, an event heralded by the onset of chest pain, ECG changes, and often hemodynamic instability. It is usually possible to verify the presence and nature of the acute coronary occlusion by immediate repeat coronary angiography, allowing for confirmation of the diagnosis.

Most patients in the process of an evolving MI have some attenuation of the ischemic injury and greater hemodynamic stability if intraaortic balloon counterpulsation is established promptly in the catheterization laboratory before transport to the operating room. If the patient develops severe hemodynamic instability despite balloon pump support, portable cardiopulmonary bypass perfusion with femoral arterial and venous cannulation may allow sufficient stabilization to transport the patient to the operating room. In general, these patients should be placed on cardiopulmonary bypass as quickly as possible to initiate cardioplegic arrest and myocardial cooling and to prevent further extension of the infarction.

Surgical Technique

In coronary artery surgery, the diseased coronary artery is bypassed by creation of an alternative conduit for delivery of blood beyond the coronary stenosis. Grafts are constructed by making an end-to-side anastomosis to the coronary artery distal to the obstruction. The proximal end of a vein graft is usually sutured end-to-side to the ascending aorta. When the aorta is diseased, the origin of the innominate artery is sometimes used. The most commonly used vein graft is the greater saphenous vein, although lesser saphenous vein is sometimes employed. The cephalic vein from the arm may be used, but its long-term patency is extremely poor.

Use of arterial grafts has increased. The most commonly used arterial graft is the left internal mammary artery (IMA). This artery is used most often as a pedicle graft, retaining its origin at the subclavian artery. The distal end is anastomosed end-to-side to the coronary artery. The most commonly grafted artery using the left IMA is the left anterior descending coronary artery. When multiple arterial grafts are desired, the right IMA can be used either as a pedicle graft or as a free graft, with the proximal anas-

tomosis made on the ascending aorta. More limited use has been made of the gastroepiploic artery, the radial artery, and the inferior epigastric artery. The main benefit of these arterial grafts is improved long-term patency. The actuarial probability of vein graft patency at 10 years is 50%. In contrast, the probability that the left IMA will be patent at 10 years is 90% to 95%. There is also evidence that early mortality is improved when at least one mammary artery graft is used.

To construct accurate anastomoses in a quiet, bloodless field, cardiopulmonary bypass must be employed for coronary bypass surgery (Fig. 65-6). With the patient on bypass and the heart empty, the distal ascending aorta is cross-clamped, and potassium cardioplegia solution is injected into the aortic root, causing nearly instantaneous cardiac arrest. The cardioplegic solution at a temperature of 4 to 10C induces rapid myocardial cooling along with cardiac arrest in diastole. In addition, many surgeons apply cold saline directly to the surface of the heart, either intermittently or continuously, to maintain the myocardial temperature from 10 to 15C during aortic cross-clamping. The most important components of cardioplegia are cold temperature and potassium (usually 15 to 20 mEq/L), which causes depolarization of the myocardial membrane and arrest of the heart in diastole. Myocardial temperatures of 10 to 15C decrease the metabolic rate of the heart by 80%, and arrest lowers the metabolic rate to as little as 5% of the normothermic, working heart.

A number of cardioplegia solutions are available, although the ones most commonly used are based on a dilute blood solution with potassium and often other additives. Some techniques employ initial warm induction of arrest followed by cold cardioplegia. A warm dose of cardioplegia before removing the cross-clamp has been advocated. This may be particularly useful in patients who suffered significant preoperative ischemic insults. Warm cardioplegia reperfusion supplies oxygen and substrates while maintaining diastolic arrest with its attendant decreases in metabolic demand. Some surgeons prefer to do the entire operation with the patient and the heart warm while cardioplegia is administered continuously.[32] Cardioplegia is more commonly administered antegrade by injection of the solution into the aortic root proximal to the cross-clamp. It has been shown that the retrograde administration of cardioplegia through placement of a cannula in the coronary sinus can lead to enhanced myocardial protection because significant coronary stenoses can prevent the homogenous delivery of cardioplegia, a problem obviated by the retrograde approach.[33] The combination of antegrade and retrograde cardioplegia may be optimal in some cases. The retrograde cardioplegia technique is often applied to patients who previously underwent CABG in an effort to avoid the complication of atheromatous emboli from diseased bypass grafts.[34] Retrograde cardioplegia is also helpful in the presence of significant aortic insufficiency.

CABG is performed with the aid of optical magnification. Monofilament sutures are used by most surgeons, with specific techniques varying from a single continuous running anastomosis to multiple interrupted sutures. In addition to individual vein or mammary artery graft anastomoses to specific arterial branches, two or more distal anastomoses can be constructed from a single vein or mammary artery. These sequential grafts are especially favored when multiple distal sites are planned for anastomosis or when there is a shortage of suitable conduit material.

When the distal anastomoses are completed, the aortic clamp is released. After initiating reperfusion, the heart often develops ventricular fibrillation but usually is cardioverted with a single direct-current electrical shock. By placing a partially occluding clamp on the ascending aorta,

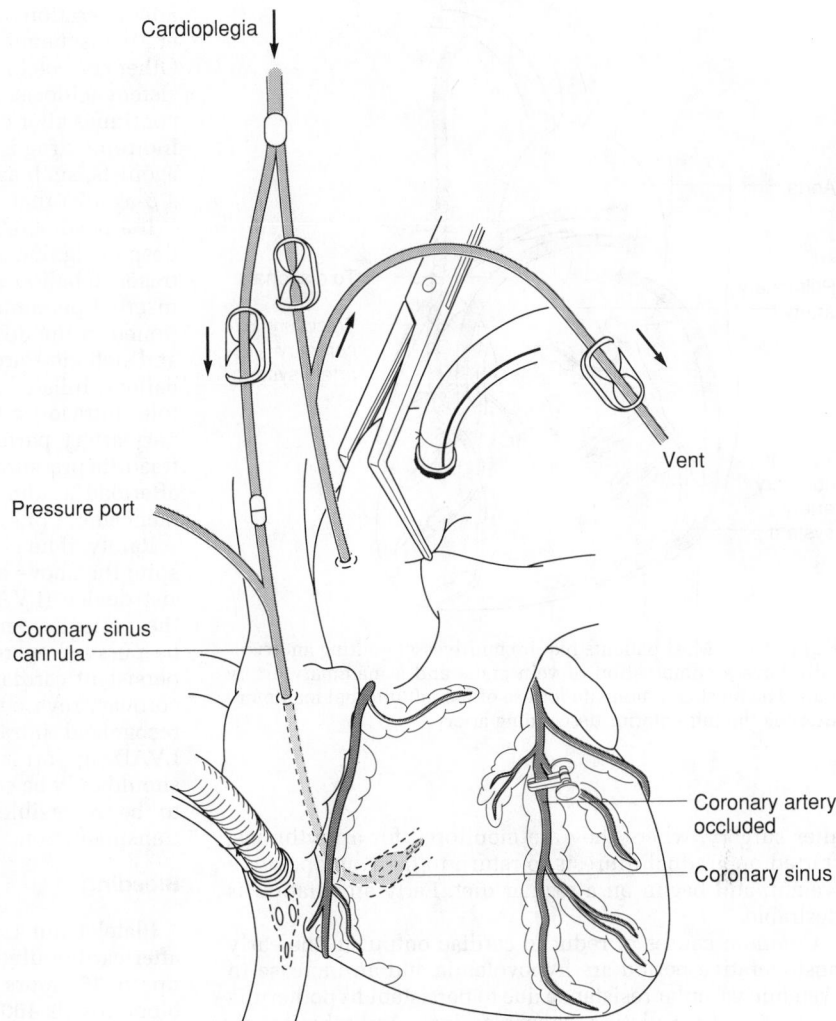

Figure 65-6. Cardiac instrumentation for retrograde cardioplegic administration through the coronary sinus. A catheter with an occlusive balloon tip has been placed within the coronary sinus through the right atrium. The cardioplegic solution can be administered by means of the coronary sinus or the aortic root (antegrade). There is a pressure-measuring side port on the coronary sinus catheter that can be used to prevent overdistention of the coronary venous system. (After Partington MT, et al. Studies of retrograde cardioplegia I. J Thorac Cardiovasc Surg 1989;97:613)

the proximal aortosaphenous vein graft anastomoses can be constructed as myocardial perfusion is maintained through the native circulation and the newly constructed mammary anastomoses (Fig. 65-7). In some cases, especially in reoperation, the proximal anastomoses are made during ischemic time with the cross-clamp still in place, obviating the need for the partial occluding clamp, which can be difficult to place and can cause atherosclerotic embolism in the presence of old grafts.

When performing CABG, if there are diffuse atherosclerotic changes, or if the site chosen for a distal anastomosis is heavily diseased, the surgeon may need to perform an endarterectomy to allow for a more reliable graft-to-artery anastomosis. There are conflicting data regarding the safety and efficacy of coronary endarterectomy because endarterectomy sites are more prone to early thrombosis and reocclusion. Endarterectomy of the distal right coronary artery, which is the most common site of endarterectomy, appears to be safe and well tolerated, in part because the right coronary artery is often already nearly totally occluded. Data regarding the long-term comparative value of endarterectomy on the LAD coronary artery versus grafting alone are not available. Endarterectomy is reserved for patients with such severe distal disease that it is necessary for distal flow. Because patients with diffuse distal disease are already prone to poor outcome, it has proved difficult to demonstrate a beneficial effect from coronary endarterectomy.

Postoperative Management

Postoperative cardiac surgical management is based on hemodynamic monitoring in an intensive care unit setting. Arterial blood pressure, central venous pressure, pulmonary capillary wedge pressure, cardiac output, and urine output all provide valuable information regarding the adequacy of arterial circulation, tissue perfusion, and organ function and should be followed closely. In addition, arterial blood gases, complete blood counts, electrolytes, and ECG should be evaluated at regular intervals. A chest radiograph should be taken on arrival in the intensive care unit and checked for position of the endotracheal tube, nasogastric tube, chest tubes, and Swan-Ganz catheter. Also, pleural effusion, pneumothorax, and mediastinal widening should be ruled out, and a follow-up chest film should be taken 8 to 12 hours later. Mediastinal and chest tube drainage should be recorded hourly. Shed blood can be autotransfused to minimize the use of banked blood products. Patients should be weighed to assist in fluid management. All patients develop a capillary leak syndrome after cardiopulmonary bypass and fluid accumulation, and a marked increase in total body sodium and weight gain of 5 to 10 kg are typical. After extubation, which normally occurs between 4 and 12 hours postoperatively, pulmonary toilet should be vigorous. Most CABG patients can be transferred to a step-down unit on the day

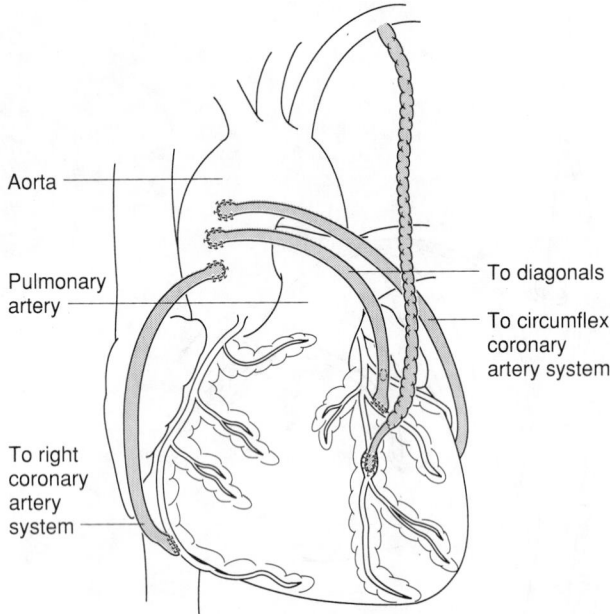

Figure 65-7. Most patients require multivessel grafting and typically have a combination of vein grafts and a mammary artery graft. The most common site for use of the left internal mammary artery is the left anterior descending artery.

after surgery, where they are monitored for arrhythmias, started on gradual diuresis to return to their preoperative weight, and begun on a regular diet. Early ambulation is desirable.

Common causes of reduced cardiac output in the early postoperative period are hypovolemia and an increase in systemic vascular resistance due to persistent hypothermia or increased circulating catecholamines. Arrhythmias, either bradycardia from resolving hypothermia, heart block thought secondary to transient but persistent cardioplegia effect, or supraventricular tachyarrhythmias, primarily atrial fibrillation, can also contribute to low cardiac output. Management is more often directed at correcting such alterations than at increasing ventricular contractility. Patients are vigorously rewarmed, given adequate crystalloid or colloid solution to optimize cardiac filling pressures, and often treated with a vasodilator agent such as sodium nitroprusside to maintain mean blood pressure between 65 to 75 mmHg in an effort to reduce systemic vascular resistance. Arrhythmias should be treated and bradycardia managed with atrial or atrioventricular pacing.

Low Cardiac Output

Causes of low cardiac output are summarized as follows:

- Inadequate preload
- Excessive afterload
- Poor ventricular contractility
    Perioperative ischemia
    Poor myocardial preservation
- Arrhythmia
- Severe acidosis
- Tension pneumothorax
- Tamponade

If the calculated cardiac index is less than 2 L/min/m² despite optimization of heart rhythm, preload (cardiac filling pressures), and afterload (systemic vascular resistance), an inotropic agent may be indicated to enhance contractility. Poor ventricular contractility immediately

after operation may be secondary to stunning from intraoperative ischemia or preoperative ventricular dysfunction. Other correctable factors, such as poor oxygenation or persistent acidosis, may be responsible. If low cardiac output continues after correction of acidosis and oxygenation, an inotropic drug is used. Appropriate first selections are β_1-agonists, such as dopamine, dobutamine, or epinephrine, a β-agonist that also has α-agonist activity.

If a postoperative patient remains in cardiogenic shock despite significant inotropic support, placement of an intraaortic balloon pump may be necessary. The balloon is inserted percutaneously into the femoral artery and positioned in the descending thoracic aorta. Balloon inflation and deflation are timed using the ECG signals, with the balloon inflated during diastole and deflated during systole. Intraaortic balloon counterpulsation increases coronary artery perfusion because balloon inflation raises intraaortic pressure during diastole and maximally decreases afterload as the balloon is actively deflated at the commencement of systole.

Rarely, if hemodynamic instability and shock persist despite the above aggressive measures, a left ventricular assist device (LVAD) should be considered. The cause of the patient's persistent low cardiac output state should be pursued aggressively before use of an LVAD because persistent cardiac dysfunction may be due to inadequate coronary revascularization, early graft occlusion, or an unrecognized intracardiac or valvular mechanical defect. LVAD support is extremely labor intensive and costly and should only be considered if myocardial failure is thought to be reversible or if the patient is a candidate for transplantation.

Bleeding

Platelet function and blood clotting factors are altered after cardiopulmonary bypass and may not normalize for up to 36 hours postoperatively. Average postoperative blood loss is 400 to 800 mL, and much of this shed blood can be reinfused. Continued bleeding at a rate greater than 200 mL/h for 4 hours or more postoperatively is considered excessive, and in these cases, specific abnormalities in coagulation should be corrected aggressively. It is simple and safe to give additional protamine to reverse residual heparin activity, but transfusion of platelets, fresh-frozen plasma, or cryoprecipitate should be considered only if coagulation studies indicate their need. Reexploration is required if bleeding continues after correction of coagulopathy.

Tamponade

Cardiac tamponade is a potentially lethal cause of low cardiac output early after operation. Clinical features include a decreasing output in the presence of a narrowed pulse pressure, rising cardiac filling pressures, pulsus paradoxus, a widened mediastinal silhouette on chest film, and decreased urine output. These classic signs may be absent or equivocal. Sudden cessation of excessive bleeding should make the physician alert to the possibility of tamponade. Transesophageal echocardiography can establish this diagnosis immediately and can assess ventricular function as well as preload, an extremely useful parameter in treating the patient in shock.

Late cardiac tamponade can occur up to several weeks after operation and can be caused by hemopericardium or a transudative pericardial effusion. Presenting symptoms may be obvious but frequently are subtle and include lethargy, mild respiratory distress, nonspecific chest discomfort, fluid retention, and hepatomegaly. The diagnosis is made by echocardiography, and the tamponade nearly always is managed successfully with either percutaneous or operative drainage.

Infection

The major wound complications after coronary artery surgery are sternal infection, dehiscence, and mediastinitis, problems that occur in 0.5% to 2% of patients. The wound infection rate is somewhat higher in patients who undergo bilateral mammary artery grafting, especially if they are elderly and diabetic. *Staphylococcus* sp is the responsible organism in most cases, and in an increasing number of these patients, the bacteria are methicillin resistant. Risk factors associated with postoperative wound infections are a preoperative hospital stay of longer than 2 days, chronic obstructive pulmonary disease with prolonged ventilator support, the use of bilateral IMA grafts, and low cardiac output.

Sternal dehiscence and mediastinitis may occur even in the absence of an apparent superficial wound infection or drainage. Helpful clinical features of these initially occult infections are fever, elevated white blood cell count, and sternal tenderness or instability. Once the diagnosis is made, however, immediate mediastinal reexploration and aggressive débridement of infected bone and cartilage are necessary because mediastinitis with sepsis can lead to a rapid deterioration of the patient. Primary reclosure of the wound is sometimes possible, but it is often necessary to use pectoral or rectus muscle flaps for wound closure not only to bring in a good blood supply but also to fill the void left by the débrided sternum.

Stroke

Cerebral vascular accident, or stroke, can be a devastating complication after bypass surgery. Stroke is usually due to atherosclerotic emboli that probably originate from the aorta and are loosened by cannulation, cross-clamping, or construction of the proximal anastomoses. Underlying cerebral vascular disease in conjunction with alterations in cerebral blood flow patterns due to cardiopulmonary bypass may also play a role. Strokes occur in 1% to 2% of low-risk patients after bypass surgery but in up to 10% of the elderly. The need to evaluate the extracranial cerebral circulation before bypass surgery is controversial. No data suggest that the investigation of asymptomatic carotid bruits and subsequent endarterectomy, if significant stenosis is found, reduce the incidence of stroke after bypass operation. In general, only symptomatic carotid stenoses should be addressed before bypass surgery. The timing of endarterectomy and CABG and whether they should be performed sequentially or as a combined procedure are also controversial. If the carotid disease is asymptomatic, factors affecting the timing of coronary surgery usually take precedence.

Postpericardiotomy Syndrome

Postpericardiotomy syndrome is a delayed pericardial inflammatory reaction characterized by fever, anterior chest pain, and a pericardial friction rub. It occurs in up to 30% of postoperative cardiac surgery patients. The syndrome is associated with the development of pericardial effusions, which rarely lead to cardiac tamponade. In addition, postpericardiotomy syndrome can result in mediastinal fibrosis and premature graft closure. Treatment with nonsteroidal antiinflammatory agents for 2 or more weeks usually eliminates the symptoms of postpericardiotomy syndrome, but corticosteroids may be required in patients with recurring episodes.

Risk Factors for Operative Mortality

The assessment and analysis of risk factors for operative mortality after coronary bypass surgery is an important component of the preoperative evaluation of patients with coronary disease (Table 65-2). Furthermore, as an increasing number of interested parties scrutinize the results of bypass surgery, preoperative risk stratification is crucial. Among the many factors that affect outcome after CABG are the patient's state of general health and the potential for complete revascularization. Incomplete revascularization due either to severe distal coronary artery disease or to inadequate conduits for bypass grafting is associated with a higher operative mortality and uncertain long-term outcome. Likewise, patients with concurrent medical problems, such as cerebrovascular, pulmonary, or renal insufficiency, are much more likely to sustain additional complications during CABG with a higher operative risk.[35]

Poor ventricular function is among the most important factors increasing the mortality risk of bypass surgery. Operative risk also is increased when the patient requires additional operative intervention, such as valve repair or replacement. Furthermore, when ventricular function is not improved by bypass grafting or when mitral valve replacement or ventricular reconstruction is required because of complications of previous infarction, long-term outlook is noticeably worsened.

Several reports have documented increased morbidity and mortality in elderly patients undergoing CABG. In the CASS study, the operative mortality rate in patients 70 years or older was nearly 8%, compared with an overall estimated mortality rate of about 3% in better-risk, younger patients. An important observation made of elderly patients is that this increased mortality is due to postoperative complications, such as stroke, respiratory failure, renal failure, or sepsis, and not cardiac failure. Although age is an incremental risk factor for early death after coronary bypass surgery, it is not a contraindication to surgery.[36]

The influence of the patient's gender on surgical outcome is less clear, despite several reports suggesting a higher operative risk for women. In many of these studies, women undergoing CABG were older with a higher incidence of unstable angina, preoperative congestive heart failure, hypertension, and diabetes. Some reports have attributed the increased risk of bypass surgery for women to their smaller physical stature, with a correspondingly smaller coronary arterial bed and its technical limitations. Probably, the higher risk for women is due to increased risk factors, such as advanced age and severity of the anginal syndrome.[37]

Other factors that increase operative risk include renal insufficiency, diabetes mellitus, peripheral vascular dis-

Table 65-2. PREDICTION OF THE RISK FOR OPERATIVE MORTALITY*

	Low	Medium	High
Age	60 y	75 y	75 y
Gender	Male	Female	Female
Diabetes	No	Yes	Yes
Unstable angina	Yes	No	Yes
Ejection fraction	65%	35%	25%
Three-vessel disease	Yes	Yes	Yes
Operative incidence	First	First	Redo
Predicted mortality rate	0.8%	3.4%	12%

* Based on The Society of Thoracic Surgery National Cardiac Database Risk Stratification Algorithm.

ease, cerebral vascular disease, respiratory insufficiency, and obesity. Most of these conditions are also associated with premature or accelerated atherosclerosis and a high incidence of generalized cardiovascular disease due to hypertension, hyperlipidemia, and abnormal carbohydrate metabolism. Patients with end-stage renal disease have an increased operative morbidity, often as a result of bleeding and infection. Mortality is also increased. Patients with a functioning kidney transplant have better outcomes than patients requiring chronic hemodialysis.

Reoperative CABG has become increasingly more frequent during the past several years and accounts for an increasing proportion of all CABG procedures carried out in the United States. Reoperative surgery has a higher operative mortality than primary bypass procedures. This is due to the technical difficulty of the procedure, which results from pericardial adhesions and scar formation, as well as the fact that patients who undergo reoperation are older, have more advanced coronary disease, and are more likely to be incompletely revascularized.[38]

Long-Term Outcomes

Controlled clinical trials have shown that surgical revascularization provides significant relief of anginal symptoms. Most series show initial elimination of angina in about 90% of patients, with about 70% of patients remaining free of cardiac events for 1 to 3 years. In one report, 67% of surviving patients were free of angina at 20 years after surgery. Reoperation improved survival in patients with recurrent symptoms.[39]

Several studies suggest that CABG may enhance ventricular function both in the immediate postoperative period and late after surgery. Nonetheless, controversy persists over the long-term functional effects of bypass surgery, especially on systolic function, with some reports even suggesting deterioration of ventricular performance. In a few controlled clinical trials, functional improvement has been documented both at rest and with exercise 8 months postoperatively. In addition, in one study, improvement in left ventricular ejection fraction was demonstrated and could be attributed to improved contractility in myocardial regions in which there had been demonstrable ischemia during exercise before surgery. Clinical improvement after coronary bypass surgery, including cessation of angina, stabilization of ventricular function, and, most important, enhanced survival, depends on short- and long-term graft patency. In a follow-up study that included postoperative coronary angiography, 82% of patients with at least one graft patent at 1-year coronary angiogram were alive 12 years after surgery, compared with only 42% of the patients who had no patent grafts 1 year after operation. Vein graft occlusion within the first few months of surgery is almost certainly due to poor blood flow, poor coronary arterial runoff, injury to the graft during preparation, or faulty surgical technique. Vein graft stenosis or graft failure within the first few years is associated with intimal hyperplasia, a process that is demonstrable angiographically in up to 75% of vein grafts after 1 year.

The overall occlusion rates for saphenous vein grafts are 5% to 20% during the first postoperative year, and 2% to 4% annually for the next 4 years, reaching 22% to 30% at 5 years and 50% at 10 years.

Use of the IMA graft has become increasingly favored because it greatly improves late patency. Patency rates for IMA grafts are 95% at 1 year, 94% at 8 years, and 85% or better at 10 years. This improved IMA graft patency has been reported for both pedicle and free IMA grafts. Excellent late IMA graft patency clearly correlates with increased patient survival, reduced symptom recurrence,

and fewer reoperations. In a study from the Cleveland Clinic, where IMA grafts have been used extensively, 10-year survival rates in patients with saphenous vein grafts for single-, double-, and triple-vessel disease were 88%, 79.5%, and 71%, respectively, compared with 93.4%, 90%, and 82.6% in a comparable group of patients who had IMA grafts to the LAD.

About 90% of primary post-CABG patients survive 5 years, 80% survive 10 years, and about 58% survive 15 years. Use of the IMA graft improves long-term survival to 89% at 10 years. Long-term surgical survival for all patients in the three major clinical trials was 58% at 11 years in the Veterans Administration study,[27] 71% at 12 years in the European study,[28] and 87% at 8 years in the CASS study.[26] At 5 years, 10% of the surgically treated patients in the CASS study had died. One quarter of these deaths were sudden coronary death, 47% were not sudden but of cardiac cause, and 28% were noncardiac deaths. In the European trial, there was a 92% 5-year surgical survival rate in patients with stable angina and good left ventricular function; this decreased to 71% at 12 years. Medical therapy in a matched group of patients resulted in 83% survival at 5 years and 67% at 12 years. The difference between medical and surgical therapy at 12 years is still significant, but of less magnitude, possibly owing to the fact that patients received only saphenous vein grafts. Better long-term survival should result from mammary grafting, which is universally performed.

About one in seven patients who had vein grafts required reoperation after 15 years, twice the reoperation rate of patients who received at least one mammary artery bypass. As reviewed earlier, patients who undergo reoperation have at least double the operative risk of primary elective CABG patients because the operation is technically more difficult, the patients' average age is higher, and atherosclerotic disease is more advanced. In addition, long-term results after reoperation are poorer because of these factors and because revascularization may not be as complete. Symptom relief is usually of shorter duration.

PRINCIPLES DERIVED FROM COOPERATIVE STUDIES

Although the clearest indication for mechanical intervention such as PTCA or CABG is unstable angina on maximal medical therapy, improvement in long-term survival in certain anatomic patterns of coronary disease provides another indication for bypass surgery. The three prospective, randomized trials comparing coronary bypass to medical therapy were carried out in the 1970s. Both surgical and medical management of coronary artery disease have improved dramatically since that time. For example, IMA use was negligible during the time period of these studies, as was the use of PTCA and platelet-inhibiting drugs. Regardless, important principles derived by these studies still shape the clinical approach to coronary artery disease.

Veterans Administration Cooperative Study

The Veterans Administration Cooperative Study[27] randomly assigned 686 male patients (average age, 50 years) to initial medical versus surgical therapy. All patients had medically stable angina, single-vessel disease or worse, and an ejection fraction of greater than 30%. Despite a much higher operative mortality rate than was acceptable even at that time, the study revealed a tremendous benefit derived from surgery for patients with left main artery disease.[29] In these patients, the 3-year survival rate was 93%

in the surgery group versus 68% in the medical group. Furthermore, patients with a history of hypertension, previous MI, abnormal resting ECG, and increasingly severe symptoms (high clinical risk), as well as patients with three-vessel disease and decreased left ventricular function (high anatomic risk), fared significantly better with surgery.

European Coronary Surgery Study

The European Coronary Surgery Study[28] examined only men younger than 65 years with mild to moderate angina who had normal left ventricular function and at least two-vessel disease. At 8 years follow-up, surgery improved survival in the population as a whole (89% versus 80%), in patients with three-vessel disease (92% versus 77%), and in patients with two-vessel disease involving the proximal LAD (90% versus 79%). There was no benefit to immediate surgery in single-vessel disease, even if it involved the proximal LAD (but the IMA was not used).

Coronary Artery Surgery Study

The CASS was a prospective, randomized study[26,40] carried out between 1975 and 1979 in the United States in men and women younger than 65 years who had symptoms no more severe than mild angina. At 10 years follow-up, the group as a whole derived no benefit from surgery. In patients with ejection fractions between 30% and 50%, however, surgery conferred an increased survival (79% versus 61%). Furthermore, in the observational studies that were part of this project, surgery provided a survival advantage in all patients with three-vessel disease, but patients who had the severest anatomic disease with the worst ventricular function benefitted the most. Although it appears that surgery provides the greatest benefit to those with left ventricular dysfunction, congestive heart failure is a major determinant of *poor* surgical outcome. When heart failure, not angina, is the predominant symptom, surgery leads to a poor result. Pulmonary rales, diuretic and digitalis use, and an enlarged heart are predictors of increased operative risk.[41] Nonetheless, in patients with significant angina, although left ventricular dysfunction increases surgical risk and decreases long-term survival, bypass surgery bestows the greatest benefit in terms of improved long-term survival.

TRANSPLANTATION VERSUS HIGH-RISK CORONARY BYPASS SURGERY

Patients with severely impaired ventricular function may be referred for bypass surgery when severe associated coronary obstructions are detected. Often, there is uncertainty about whether the patient who is at severely increased risk because of ventricular dysfunction is a candidate for bypass surgery, or whether transplantation should be pursued. In patients with ischemic but viable myocardium, ventricular function may improve after bypass surgery once adequate blood flow is restored. The term *hibernating myocardium* has been used to describe ventricular dysfunction secondary to inadequate coronary flow even in the absence of ECG changes or anginal symptoms.[42] *Ischemic cardiomyopathy* implies irreversible myocardial dysfunction associated with extensive myocyte necrosis and infarction. Surgical revascularization improves the contractile function of hibernating muscle, whereas there is little functional benefit derived from revascularization in ischemic cardiomyopathy with extensively scarred or infarcted myocardium.

In deciding whether to recommend transplantation or bypass surgery to a patient at high risk owing to severely depressed left ventricular function, it is therefore important to determine the viability of the myocardium. Anginal symptoms suggestive of reversible ischemia are often a useful measure of myocardial viability that would benefit from revascularization, and patients whose only symptom is heart failure should be approached with caution. Myocardial viability may better be assessed with positron emission tomography scans, but these are not widely available. Some cardiologists and surgeons find it useful to perform thallium scanning either with exercise, dipyridamole, or at rest to assess myocardial viability. Muscle that takes up thallium (early or late) is presumed to be viable. Radionuclide scanning provides data to estimate the potential for improved ventricular function with revascularization in patients with coronary obstructive disease and significant left ventricular dysfunction because it can identify poorly functioning but viable ischemic areas. A thallium defect with exercise or even at rest that subsequently fills on the delayed images is evidence that viable myocardium is present despite poor function. In a patient with these findings, especially if angina is present, surgery rather than transplantation is generally indicated if there is operable coronary disease. Postoperative outcome in these patients is acceptable and usually associated with improved left ventricular function. In patients with congestive heart failure and no evidence of reversible ischemia, bypass surgery is of high risk and low benefit, and transplantation should be considered.

REFERENCES

1. Messer JV, Wagman RJ, Levine HJ, Neill WA, Krasnow N, Gorlin R. Patterns of myocardial oxygen extraction during rest and exercise. J Clin Invest 1962;41:725.
2. Berne RM. The role of adenosine in the regulation of coronary blood flow. Circ Res 1980;47:807.
3. Robertson RM, Robertson D, Roberts LJ, et al. Thromboxane A_2 in vasotonic angina pectoris. N Engl J Med 1981;304:998.
4. McGill H. Risk factors for atherosclerosis. Adv Exp Med Biol 1977;104:273.
5. The Lipid Research Clinics Program. The Lipid Research Clinics Coronary Primary Prevention Trial results. II. The relationship of reduction in incidence of coronary heart disease to cholesterol lowering. JAMA 1984;251:365.
6. DeWood MA, Spores J, Notske R, et al. Prevalence of total coronary occlusion during the early hours of transmural myocardial infarction. N Engl J Med 198;303:897.
7. Flaherty JT, Becker LC, Bulkley BH, et al. A randomized prospective trial of intravenous nitroglycerin in patients with acute myocardial infarction. Circulation 1976;54:766.
8. Herlitz J, Elmfeldt D, Hjalmarson A, et al. Effect of metoprolol on indirect signs of the size and severity of acute myocardial infarction. Am J Cardiol 1983;51:1282.
9. Yusuf S, Held P, Fuberg C. Update of effects of calcium antagonists in myocardial infarction or angina in light of the second Danish verapamil infarction trial (DAVIT-II) and other recent studies. Am J Cardiol 1991;67:1295.
10. European Cooperative Study Group for Streptokinase Treatment in Acute Myocardial Infarction. Streptokinase in acute myocardial infarction. N Engl J Med 1979;301:797.
11. Fry ETA, Sobel BE. Coronary thrombosis. In: Zipes DP, Rowlands DJ, eds. Progress in cardiology, vol 2. Philadelphia, Lea & Febiger, 1990:199.
12. Yusuf S, Collins R, Peto R, et al. Intravenous and intracoronary fibrinolytic therapy in acute myocardial infarction: overview of results on mortality, reinfarction and side effects from 33 randomized control trials. Eur Heart J 1985;6:556.
13. White HD, Rivers JT, Maslowski AH, et al. Effect of intravenous streptokinase as compared with that of tissue plasminogen activator on left ventricular function after first myocardial infarction. N Engl J Med 1989;320:817.

14. Tiefenbrunn AJ, Sobel BE. The impact of coronary thrombolysis on myocardial infarction. Fibrinolysis 1989;3:1.

15. TIMI Study Group. Comparison of invasive and conservative strategies after treatment with intravenous tissue plasminogen activator in acute myocardial infarction: results of the Thrombolysis in Myocardial Infarction (TIMI) phase II trial. N Engl J Med 1989;320:618.

16. Naunheim KS, Kessler KA, Kanter KR, et al. Coronary artery bypass for recent infarction: predictors of mortality. Circulation 1988;78(Suppl I):I-122.

17. Maisel AS, Ahnve S, Gilpin E, et al. Prognosis after extension of myocardial infarct: the role of W wave on non-Q wave infarction. Circulation 1985;71:211.

18. Hands ME, Rutherford JD, Muller JE, et al. The in-hospital development of cardiogenic shock after myocardial infarction: incidence, predictors of occurrence, outcome and prognosis factors. JACC 1989;14:40.

19. Allen BS, Okamoto F, Buckberg GD, et al. Studies of controlled reperfusion after ischemia. XIII. Reperfusion conditions: critical importance of total ventricular decompression during regional reperfusion. J Thorac Cardiovasc Surg 1986;92:605.

20. Allen BS, Rosenkranz E, Buckberg GD, et al. Studies on prolonged acute regional ischemia. IV. Myocardial infarction with left ventricular failure. J Thorac Cardiovasc Surg 1989;98:691.

21. Daggett WM, Buckely MR, Akins CW, et al. Improved results of surgical management of postinfarction ventricular septal rupture. Ann Surg 1982;196:269.

22. David TE, Ho WL. The effect of preservation of chordae tendineae on mitral valve replacement for postinfarction mitral regurgitation. Circulation 1986;74(Suppl I):116.

23. Green MA, Gray LA Jr, Slater AD, Ganzel BL, Mavroudis C. Emergency aortocoronary bypass after failed angioplasty. Ann Thorac Surg 1991;51:194.

24. King SB III, Talley JD. Coronary arteriography and percutaneous transluminal coronary angioplasty: changing patterns of use and results. Circulation 1989;79(Suppl I):19.

25. Nwasokwa ON, Koss JR, Friedman GH, Grunwald AM, Bodenheimer MM. Bypass surgery for chronic stable angina: predictors of survival benefit and strategy for patient selection. Ann Intern Med 1991;114:1035.

26. Myers WO, Martshfield WI, Gersh BJ, et al. Medical versus early surgical therapy in patients with triple-vessel disease and mild angina pectoris: a CASS registry study of survival. Ann Thorac Surg 1987;44:471.

27. Detre KM, Takaro, T, Hultgren H, Peduzzi P, and the Study Participants. Long-term mortality and morbidity results of the Veterans Administration randomized trial of coronary artery bypass surgery. Circulation 1985;72(Suppl V):84.

28. Varnauskas E, and the European Coronary Surgery Study Group. Twelve-year follow-up of survival in the randomized European Coronary Surgery Study. N Engl J Med 1988;319:332.

29. Takaro T, Pifarre R, Fish R. Left main coronary artery disease. Prog Cardiovasc Dis 1985;28:229.

30. Akins CW. Controversies in myocardial revascularization: coronary artery surgery for single-vessel disease. Semin Thorac Cardiovasc Surg 1994;6:109.

31. Hammermeister KE, Morrison DA. Coronary bypass surgery for stable angina and unstable angina pectoris. Cardiol Clin 1991;9:133.

32. Gundry SR, Wang N, Bann D, et al. Retrograde continuous warm blood cardioplegia: maintenance of myocardial homeostasis in humans. Ann Thorac Surg 1993;55:358.

33. Noyez L, van Son JA, van der Werf T, et al. Retrograde versus antegrade delivery of cardioplegic solution in myocardial revascularization: a clinical trial in patients with three-vessel coronary disease who underwent myocardial revascularization with extensive use of the internal mammary artery. J Thorac Cardiovasc Surg 1993;105:854.

34. Rosengart TK, Krieger K, Lang SJ, et al. Reoperative coronary artery surgery: improved preservation of myocardial function with retrograde cardioplegia. Circulation 1993; 88(Suppl II):330.

35. Grover FL, Johnson RR, Marshall G, et al. Factors predictive of operative mortality among coronary artery bypass subsets. Ann Thorac Surg 1993;56:1296.

36. Smith JM, Rath R, Feldman DJ, Schreiber JT. Coronary artery bypass grafting in the elderly: changing trends and results. J Cardiovasc Surg 1992;33:468.

37. Barbir M, Lazem F, Ilsley C, et al. Coronary artery surgery in women compared with men: analysis of coronary risk factors and in-hospital mortality in a single centre. Br Heart J 1994;71:408.

38. Lytle BW, Loop FD, Taylor PC, et al. The effect of coronary reoperation on the survival of patients with stenoses in saphenous vein bypass grafts to coronary arteries. J Thorac Cardiovasc Surg 1993;105:605.

39. Lawrie GM, Morris GC Jr, Earle N. Long-term results of coronary bypass surgery: analysis of 1698 patients followed 15 to 20 years. Ann Surg 1991;213:355.

40. Myers WO, Schaff HV, Gersh BJ, et al. Improved survival of surgically treated patients with triple vessel coronary disease and severe angina pectoris. J Thorac Cardiovasc Surg 1989;98:487.

41. Nwasokwa ON, Koss Jr, Friedman GH, et al. Bypass surgery for chronic stable angina: predictors of survival benefit and strategy for patient selection. Ann Intern Med 1991;114:1035.

42. Braunwald E, Rutherford JD. Reversible ischemic left ventricular dysfunction: evidence for the hibernating myocardium. J Am Coll Cardiol 1986;8:1467.

SURGERY: SCIENTIFIC PRINCIPLES AND PRACTICE, Second Edition, edited by Lazar J. Greenfield, Michael W. Mulholland, Keith T. Oldham, Gerald B. Zelenock, and Keith D. Lillemoe. Lippincott–Raven Publishers, Philadelphia, © 1997.

CHAPTER 66

MECHANICAL CIRCULATORY SUPPORT

JOHN S. SAPIRSTEIN AND WILLIAM S. PIERCE

Mechanical circulatory support is indicated when the heart can no longer safely meet the perfusion requirements of the body. Severe cardiac dysfunction may be the result of an acute event such as a myocardial infarction, or it may be due to a more chronic process such as idiopathic cardiomyopathy. Return of cardiac function might reasonably be expected, or the decompensation could be the final stage of irreversible heart failure. A variety of devices, ranging from the widely available intraaortic balloon pump (IABP) to the sophisticated permanent total artificial heart (TAH), are used to treat patients with failing hearts. The appropriate support system is always that device that can provide the best potential results in the simplest possible manner.

INTRAAORTIC BALLOON PUMP

In the 1950s, Sarnoff and colleagues[1] proposed that myocardial oxygen consumption is a function of ventricular wall tension, rather than external factors such as stroke volume. The time during which wall tension developed also was considered a determinant of oxygen consumption. Thus, the *tension–time index* (TTI), the area under the arterial pressure trace, came to reflect the heart muscle's consumption of oxygen. Harken suggested in 1958 that decreasing the TTI would effectively support the failing heart, and his group[2] described a device that lowered the TTI by withdrawing blood from the arterial tree just before ventricular systole, returning it to the circulation during diastole. Limitations to this early counterpulsating device included a fairly high degree of hemolysis. In 1962, Moulopoulos and associates[3] described a catheter-mounted balloon that produced hemodynamic effects similar to the Harken pump, but without an extracorporeal circuit. They passed the balloon into the aorta and inflated it during ventricular diastole, thereby augmenting diastolic blood flow. Deflation just before ejection effectively decreased the heart's afterload and thus the work during systole. Kantrowitz and colleagues[4] reported the first clinical use of the IABP in 1968 and predicted rapidly expanding uses for this intervention. The indications for the IABP have grown, fostered by the availability in 1980 of percutaneous insertion techniques that allow the device's timely application without a formal surgical procedure.

IABP systems have become increasingly sophisticated (Fig. 66-1), but salutary effects still rest predominantly on modification of the heart's oxygen supply–demand equilibrium. Deflation of the intraaortic balloon just before ven-

tricular ejection presumably increases aortic compliance, resulting in a lower ventricular afterload (Fig. 66-2). Such a reduction decreases myocardial oxygen demand, manifested by a lower TTI or, using more rigorous descriptors of cardiac energetics, a smaller pressure–volume area.[5] Inflation of the balloon during diastole conversely increases the aortic root pressure, and the increased pressure gradient between the intraventricular cavity and the coronary orifices (the diastolic pressure–time index) augments coronary perfusion and oxygen supply. Benefits of the IABP as an adjunct to coronary vessel reperfusion strategies (described later) derive from the mechanics of increased intraluminal flow and pressure.

Indications
Myocardial Infarction

The first clinical application of the IABP was in cardiogenic shock secondary to acute myocardial infarction.[4] The combination of hypotension (systolic blood pressure less

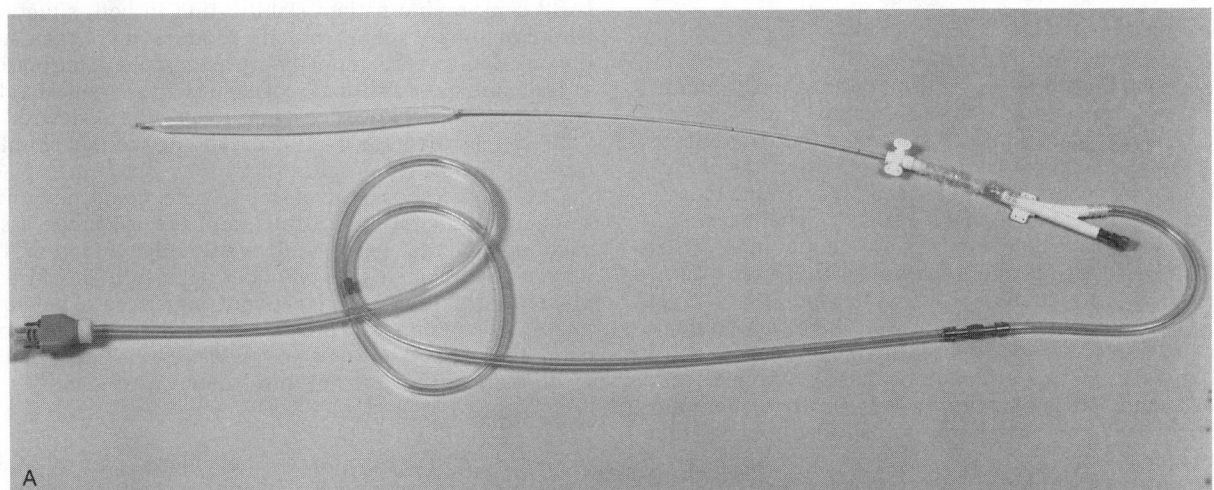

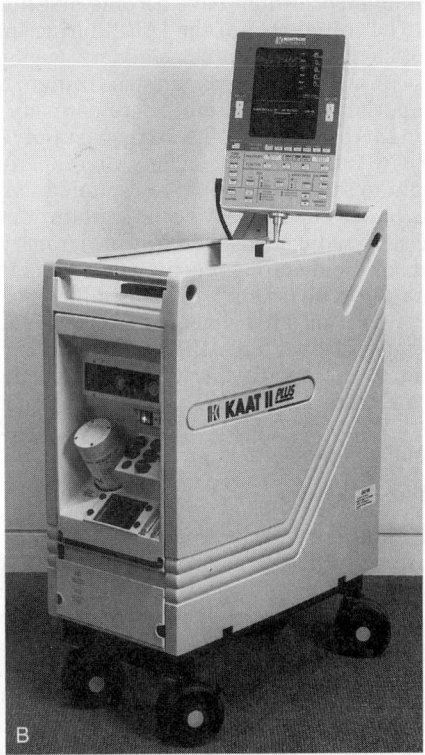

Figure 66-1. Intraaortic balloon pump. (*A*) Catheter-mounted balloon is typically passed into the thoracic aorta through a percutaneous insertion in the groin. (*B*) Drive console for the intraaortic balloon pump. (Courtesy of D. Frank, Arrow International, Reading, PA)

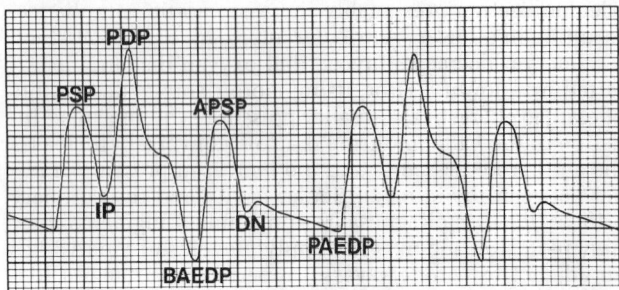

Figure 66-2. Aortic pressure tracing during intraaortic balloon pump support. Balloon counterpulsation is occurring after every other heartbeat (1:2 counterpulsation). With correct timing, balloon inflation (IP) begins immediately after aortic valve closure, signaled by the dicrotic notch (DN). Compared with unassisted ejection, the pump augments diastolic blood flow by increasing peak aortic pressure during diastole (PDP). Balloon deflation before systole decreases ventricular afterload, with lower aortic end-diastolic pressure (BAEDP versus PAEDP) and lower peak systolic pressure (APSP versus PSP). (Courtesy of St Jude Medical, Inc., Cardiac Assist Division, Minneapolis)

than 90 mmHg) and hypoperfusion (altered mental status, decreased urine output, cool and clammy skin) is the hallmark of cardiogenic shock, a syndrome that complicates about 8% of all myocardial infarctions.[6] Extension of myocardial injury occurs beyond the acutely infarcted muscle, and early animal studies in the 1970s documented significant diminution of the volume of myocardial injury when the IABP was used after coronary vessel occlusion.[7,8] Clinically, however, infarction size was not reduced with the IABP,[9] nor were outcomes improved. Emergent coronary artery bypass grafting in the setting of cardiogenic shock after myocardial infarction dramatically improves survival,[10] and some studies have shown better outcomes when IABP support is instituted before such revascularization.[11,12]

Nonsurgical techniques for reestablishing perfusion to ischemic myocardium have become first-line standards of care. The initial role of the IABP during thrombolysis or percutaneous transluminal coronary angioplasty (PTCA) was to provide hemodynamic stabilization, much as it was a temporizing intervention before coronary artery bypass grafting. Ameliorating the oxygen supply–demand balance with the IABP immediately after reperfusion was also thought to salvage more of the "stunned" myocardium. In 1991, however, the TAMI study group reported that the IABP also reduced reocclusion of coronary vessels after thrombolytic therapy for acute myocardial infarction.[13] Ishihara and coworkers[14] found similar results when the IABP was used after emergent PTCA, and experimental work suggests that the IABP can increase the rate of thrombolysis.[15] These and other findings have given some support for prophylactic use of the IABP during PTCA,[16] although whether clinical outcomes are ultimately improved by such a strategy remains unproved.

Cardiac Surgery

Low-output syndrome results from ventricular dysfunction occurring after a technically adequate cardiac surgical procedure. Most often, this entity first manifests as the inability to wean a patient from cardiopulmonary bypass (CPB). Contributing factors appear to include inadequate myocardial preservation during the procedure, long bypass periods (greater than 2 hours), and poor ventricular function before the operation. In patients for whom pharmacologic therapy is insufficient, mechanical support with the IABP has been proved effective. Between 3% and 10% of adult cardiac surgery patients require the IABP, with 50% to 90% of these devices being placed intraoperatively.[17–21] Initially, hospital mortality rates for these patients approached 65%,[21] but recent published series demonstrate mortality rates between 32%[19] and 44%.[18] These latter figures include the older, more hemodynamically compromised patients who routinely undergo cardiac procedures; considerably better survival rates with IABP use can be expected in younger patients with less extensive cardiac disease. The 5-year survival rate is 42%.[18] Postcardiotomy support remains the principal indication for IABP in the surgical patient.

Ventricular septal rupture and acute mitral regurgitation are surgical emergencies that can occur after acute myocardial infarction. Ischemia involving the posteromedial papillary muscle is the most common cause of acute mitral regurgitation, although nonischemic causes include chorda tendinae rupture and endocarditis; pulmonary edema is a frequent finding. Ventricular septal rupture usually develops within 1 week of the myocardial infarction, and it is characterized by a large left-to-right shunt. An IABP can provide patient stabilization in both situations before definitive surgical repair. Modulating oxygen supply and demand theoretically prevents rapid deterioration of ischemic myocardium associated with the mitral valve apparatus, while lowering ventricular afterload with an IABP can decrease the fraction of left heart output shunted into the low-pressure right heart.

Cardiogenic shock can develop from nonischemic insults such as viral myocarditis, and the IABP can assist such an injured heart until ventricular function improves.[22] If adequate recovery does not return, heart transplantation of the IABP-dependent patient is a potential option. Our group and others have had good experience using the IABP as a first-step, short-term bridging device when a donor organ is not immediately available.[23]

Noncardiac Surgery

Noncardiac surgery places the elderly patient at increased risk for myocardial infarction, and indices have been developed to quantify that risk. Prophylactic placement of an IABP in noncardiac surgical patients has been reported sporadically, and analyses support the judicious application of this approach in selected patients.[24,25] The physician must weigh any added margin of safety against potential morbidity associated with IABP use. This type of aggressive perioperative management has not gained widespread acceptance, but it should probably be used more widely.

Septic Shock

The pathophysiology of septic shock is markedly more complex than the cardiogenic form, and the merits of using IABP support in this clinical situation have been debated. In vivo studies have shown the hemodynamic benefit of counterpulsation in septicemia.[26,27] Limited clinical experience suggests that IABP may improve outcomes in septic patients.[28] Nonetheless, evidence that IABP support is beneficial during septic shock remains anecdotal, and it is not considered standard therapy.

Technique of Insertion and Operation

The percutaneous Seldinger method of insertion is most often employed. The common femoral artery is customarily entered, with skin puncture made about 3 cm below the inguinal ligament. This anatomic site permits adequate hemostasis with direct compression on catheter removal, and it limits distal limb ischemia associated with cannulation of the smaller superficial femoral artery. After passage of the flexible guide wire, the soft tissue tract and vessel are progressively dilated until an appropriately sized sheath can be inserted. Sheathless IABP catheters are available. Next, the furled catheter (standard size, 9.5F, 40-mL balloon) is passed proximally until its tip rests in the thoracic aorta just distal to the left subclavian artery, a point roughly at the level of the left second intercostal space. Fluoroscopic guidance can aid the procedure, and a standard chest radiograph is mandatory to confirm correct positioning. Direct, surgical placement is sometimes necessary (eg, in obese patients), in which case the catheter can be inserted through either a pursestring suture in the vessel or an anastomosed prosthetic graft. Alternative access sites, such as the axillary artery, are occasionally employed. The balloon catheter can also be placed directly into the aorta during thoracic surgical procedures.

Counterpulsation can be timed from either the electrocardiogram or the arterial pressure trace. The goal is to achieve balloon inflation immediately after aortic valve closure and deflation just before ventricular ejection. Anticoagulation protocols vary among institutions, but typically heparin or low-molecular-weight dextran is used. Meticulous wound management is needed to prevent local and systemic infection, and patients are uniformly confined to bed rest. Weaning of IABP support generally involves the gradual increase of the heartbeat/counterpulsation ratio. Back-bleeding at catheter removal decreases the likelihood of distal ischemic events. Removal may require a surgical procedure, particularly if the catheter had been placed surgically; formal embolectomy is usually performed in this situation.

Complications

Predictably, most complications of the IABP are vascular in nature. Overall complication rates have been reported between 12% and 30%.[29-32] Ischemia distal to the catheter insertion site is the most common complication, occurring in 9% to 25% of recipients; experience suggests that between about 40% and 80% of these patients require surgical intervention to treat the ischemic episode. Other, less common complications include infection and localized hematoma; vessel perforation with extensive hemorrhage; aortic dissection from catheter passage below the intima; pseudoaneurysm formation at the vessel puncture site; peripheral nerve damage; and lymphatic disruption with fistula formation. Balloon position can occlude major branches of the aorta and, depending on the extent of pre-existing vascular disease, can cause ischemia of the tissues supplied by these vessels. Examples of this scenario are intestinal "angina" from occlusion of the mesenteric vessels and upper extremity symptoms when the balloon impinges on the left subclavian artery. Cardiac function worsens if the catheter tip traverses the aortic valve. Rare events, such as catheter fracture and entrapment of the balloon, have been documented. The relatively small volumes of balloon gas used usually imply minimal sequelae in the rare event of intraluminal balloon rupture. The high solubility of carbon dioxide in blood offers an advantage to using this gas instead of helium in the IABP.

EXTRACORPOREAL MEMBRANE OXYGENATION AND VENTRICULAR ASSIST DEVICES

The first description of an IABP documented an effect with counterpulsation only if a threshold blood pressure (40 mmHg) existed. The IABP augments native heart func-

tion. If the left ventricle cannot produce a significant baseline systemic pressure—because of profound cardiogenic shock, physical injury to the heart, or severe dysrhythmias—IABP support is ineffective. In such situations, more elaborate measures for supporting the circulation may be beneficial. Circulatory support beyond the IABP most often involves application of a ventricular assist device (VAD). Clinical scenarios leading to device use are varied. In the acute, or temporary, setting, native heart function is expected to recover quickly; the cardiac surgical patient with postcardiotomy cardiogenic shock (PCCS) typifies this situation. More chronic support (ie, for weeks or months) may be necessary for the deteriorating transplantation candidate with end-stage heart failure for whom a donor organ is not available. The demand for donor hearts, however, far outstrips the supply. Thus, permanently implanted circulatory support systems could be extremely helpful for the thousands of cardiomyopathic patients with absolute or relative contraindications to allografting. Some available devices are appropriate for short-term applications in the acutely failing heart, while others are used exclusively for more chronic bridging to cardiac transplantation. Intensive work is also underway to design permanent implanted VADs.

Extracorporeal Membrane Oxygenation

Cardiopulmonary bypass has been used in the operating room for more than three decades. Successful CPB, however, is generally limited to a maximum duration of between 4 and 6 hours. Modifications to the CPB circuit, particularly the inclusion of membrane oxygenators, led to the development in the 1970s of extracorporeal membrane oxygenation (ECMO). Designed initially to treat pulmonary dysfunction,[33] ECMO uses either a venovenous or venoarterial bypass circuit; typical circuits involve cannulation of the common carotid or common femoral artery along with the internal jugular vein, a femoral vein, or both. Effective balloon counterpulsation has been difficult to achieve in children owing to the high elasticity of their aortas, and IABPs appropriately sized for very small patients are not widely available. These reasons, together with the relatively high incidence of primary pulmonary disease in children, have made ECMO an effective intervention for children.[34,35] There has been renewed interest in using ECMO in adults with cardiogenic shock unresponsive to IABP.[36,37] Experimental work also suggests a synergism when ECMO and IABP are combined in the acute management of myocardial infarction.[38] Although initial results are encouraging, the future potential of ECMO is unclear. ECMO may cause hematologic changes that deserve consideration. A whole-body inflammatory response occurs in response to circulatory bypass. For example, complement activation through the alternative pathway is an event well documented during both hemodialysis[39] and CPB.[40] Circulating C3a and C5a lead to neutrophil adherence, aggregation, and activation; activated neutrophils in turn release free radicals, proteases, and arachidonic acid metabolites that, among other things, attack cellular membranes. Although any mechanical circulatory support device with blood–artificial surface interfaces can conceivably promote these reactions, the likelihood appears higher in ECMO given the obligatory blood–oxygenator surface interactions. Moreover, the complexity of ECMO mandates continuous intensive care unit monitoring, often with the patient pharmacologically paralyzed, and the circuit requires high levels of anticoagulation. Thus, the VAD systems described next probably have broader clinical applications when IABP support is deemed insufficient.

Ventricular Assist Devices

During the past 20 years, many types of VADs have been designed, tested, and, less frequently, marketed. Some devices can only be applied to the left ventricle, whereas others are appropriate for both left- and right-sided use. Delivered flow has been pulsatile and nonpulsatile in character. This discussion is limited to devices available in the United States and to newer systems still under development that show the most promise of routine clinical use in the near future. Although certain devices are better suited than others for particular situations, all systems share the common attribute of being indicated only for patients with severe, refractory cardiac dysfunction. During the 1960s and 1970s, most of the recipients fulfilling this requirement were in cardiogenic shock secondary to acute myocardial infarction. In general, the results of such interventions were poor. More recently, the predominant indications for VADs have consisted mainly of PCCS and bridge to cardiac transplantation.[41] Our application of circulatory support beyond the IABP has been exclusively for bridge to transplantation.

General inclusion criteria for VAD implantation are listed in Table 66-1. Left ventricular assistance is the most common type of support employed. Isolated right heart failure in adults is rare. Right ventricular failure, when present, usually becomes evident after mechanical support of the failing left ventricle is initiated. The improved left-sided hemodynamics may unmask concomitant right heart dysfunction, or left ventricular decompression may actually precipitate right ventricular failure[42], in part because of the static and dynamic interactions, or cross-talk, between ventricles. If right ventricular failure does develop (see Table 66-1), pharmacologic support with inotropic agents and pulmonary vasculature dilators (isoproterenol, prostaglandin E_1, and nitric oxide) can be tried. Persistent dysfunction may require the addition of a right VAD.

Implantation of a VAD usually requires the use of CPB. Major complications of the devices include perioperative bleeding, infection, thromboembolism, and hemolysis. Hemolysis results from the physical trauma to erythrocytes caused by the mechanical pumps. High rates of hemolysis can lead to organ system injury and anemia. The risk for bleeding depends in part on the anticoagulation requirements of the specific device. Excessive bleeding may require transfusion of blood products, predisposing the patient to infection with blood-borne pathogens. Of particular concern for the bridge to transplantation patient is transmission of cytomegalovirus, infection with which can severely complicate posttransplantation management. Exposure to foreign antigens also makes subsequent location of an antigenically acceptable organ more difficult. Similarly, preexisting infection in a transplant recipient

Table 66-1. CHARACTERIZATION OF VENTRICULAR FAILURE

LEFT VENTRICULAR FAILURE

Cardiac index <1.8 L/min/m²
Left atrial pressure >20 mmHg
Peak systolic aortic pressure <90 mmHg
Scant urine output
Poor tissue perfusion

RIGHT VENTRICULAR FAILURE

Cardiac index <1.8 L/min/m²
Right atrial pressure >20 mmHg
Left atrial pressure <15 mmHg

about to receive induction immunosuppression is very dangerous. Patients who require mechanical circulatory support are at increased risk for infection for several reasons. At the time of device placement, these patients are hemodynamically unstable, a condition that compromises the immune response. The implanted components of the systems serve as a large, potential nidus for infection. Additionally, all available systems employ percutaneous elements that amplify the risk of developing foreign-body infections.

Nonpulsatile Devices

The efficacy of supporting the circulation for short periods of time with nonpulsatile blood flow is demonstrated by the more than 300,000 cardiac procedures performed each year with CPB. There are three general types of nonpulsatile VADs: roller-head pumps, centrifugal pumps, and axial flow pumps. These devices are not actuated in a phasic manner; rather, their pumps operate in a continuous, unidirectional fashion. Consequently, the pumps are, from a design standpoint, mechanically simple. The continuous, high-speed nature of these systems, however, tends to result in substantial blood trauma. An empiric law of fluid mechanics, the "no-slip" condition, requires that blood immediately adjacent to a pump surface be stationary; the rate of change of the blood's velocity on moving away from the stationary surface is called the *shear rate.* Stress on the blood and all of the elements suspended within it is directly proportional to the shear rate. Shear rates and the resulting shear stresses are created by all types of pumps, but the shearing caused by nonpulsatile pumps is particularly high. The stress imposed on erythrocytes can lead to membrane instability and hemolysis with release of free hemoglobin into the bloodstream. If the body's ability to scavenge hemoglobin (predominantly through haptoglobin-binding sites) is overwhelmed, plasma-free hemoglobin levels rise. Hemoglobin casts form in the renal tubules when plasma-free hemoglobin levels approach 40 mg/dL, and acute renal failure can then develop. Hemolysis also contributes to hepatic insufficiency, coagulopathies, and anemia. A relatively high degree of hemolysis has been documented in nonpulsatile pumps.[43]

Shear stresses also have profound effects on platelets and the clotting cascades. Shearing can elicit changes in the expression and functionality of platelet membrane glycoproteins,[44] inducing the binding of von Willebrand factor and fibrinogen. These events are critical to the activation and aggregation of platelets and the formation of platelet thrombi. Shearing also causes platelet fragmentation, exposing more cellular surface on which catalytic amplification of the clotting cascade can occur.[45] Nonpulsatile pumps have a tendency to cause thrombus formation and the subsequent risk of embolic events, in part because of the high shear stresses. Thrombus formation and relatively high levels of hemolysis, as well as some unique operational constraints mentioned later, have limited nonpulsatile ventricular support to short-term use (ie, lasting several days to a week). Nonpulsatile pumps, therefore, appear not to be the optimal choice for bridging to transplantation. Nonetheless, they are well suited to the temporary support of patients with PCCS.

Roller-Head Pumps. Most CPB machines incorporate roller-head pumps to deliver flow. Roller-heads compress the circuit's flexible tubing, thereby generating flow in a peristaltic fashion. Given the general familiarity with the set-up, it is not surprising that roller-head pumps have been employed outside of the operating room as VADs.[46] The primary advantage of a roller-head VAD is the fact that every institution performing cardiac surgery can conceivably use this relatively inexpensive support strategy. These pumps were not designed for protracted use in a single patient, and limitations to extended VAD application arise. As the pump head compresses the tubing, a jet of blood created within the narrow gap of the lumen creates high shear stresses. Prolonged exposure to repetitive compression also leads to fatigue deformation and spallation of the circuit's flexible tubing, and thus the physical integrity of the circuit must be carefully monitored. Vigilance is also mandatory because outflow obstruction can produce pressure overload and catastrophic tubing disruption. Conversely, an inlet cannula obstruction may result in air aspiration from around the cannulation site, leading to air embolism.

Centrifugal Pumps.   The goal of minimizing the risks associated with roller-head pumps while still keeping ventricular support simple and inexpensive has led to increasing use of so-called centrifugal pumps. Drawing on Bernoulli's theorem, these devices generate dynamic pressure from kinetic energy imparted to blood by a spinning chamber. The developed pressure gradient within the circuit then creates nonpulsatile blood flow. Two centrifugal pumps have been used extensively in the United States. The Bio-Medicus Bio-Pump (Medtronic Bio-Medicus, Inc, Eden Prairie, MN) contains rotating cones within the blood-spinning chamber. The Sarns centrifugal pump (Sarns/3M Health Care, Inc, Ann Arbor, MI), shown in Figure 66-3, relies on a familiar impeller mechanism to deliver energy to the blood. An axle and bearings support these blood-contacting elements. Reusable consoles spin the pumping chambers through the technique of magnetic coupling. Seals are designed to prevent the leakage of blood out of the pump heads.

Data from the voluntary registry of mechanical circulatory support show that, between 1983 and 1993, centrifugal pumps were the most commonly applied support devices (other than IABPs), constituting about half of all device use.[41] Most of the patients were being treated for PCCS, and 26% of these patients were discharged from the hospital. Nearly half of the patients were reported to have had excessive bleeding. This complication is not wholly unexpected given the anticoagulation regimens that usually are followed. In one center's experience, more than one quarter of patients with a Sarns device required reoperation or extensive blood transfusions as a result of bleeding.[47] To decrease the amount of anticoagulation necessary, pumps bonded with heparin are now available. The efficacy of such surface coatings is unclear.

Seal disruption, sometimes precipitating abrupt device failure, does occur in centrifugal pumps, and the development of seal-free pumps is underway.[48] Technical considerations like seal leakage and thrombus formation have limited the typical duration of support with centrifugal pumps to between 2 and 8 days, depending on the indication. Their low cost and ease of use, however, make these devices the mainstays of therapy for PCCS unresponsive to IABP.

Axial Flow Pumps.   Longer-term circulatory support with centrifugal pumps will not soon be practical, in part because the physical size of a complete system prevents, or at best severely limits, patient mobility. Consequently, several groups are developing small, implantable axial flow blood pumps (Fig. 66-4). These pumps deliver nonpulsatile blood flow in much the same way that a ship's propeller moves water.[49-51] Most of the systems are being designed to provide circulatory support lasting up to several months. The projects are all in the in vitro and early animal studies stages, meaning that clinical availability lies many years in the future. Beyond the considerable engineering challenges that remain to be solved, most notably the long-term maintenance of pump bearings, the potentially deleterious effects from long-term nonpulsatile blood flow need to be thoroughly evaluated. Only scant data have addressed the physiologic implications of chronically attenuating the circulation's pulsatility.[52]

Pulsatile Devices

Pulsatile VADs contain blood-pumping chambers that are completely isolated from their actuating mechanisms. As a result, the need for biocompatible seals and bearings

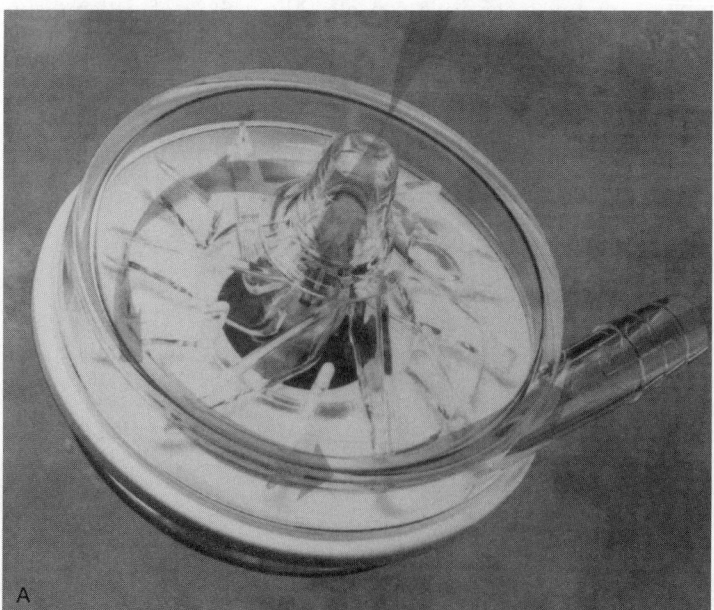
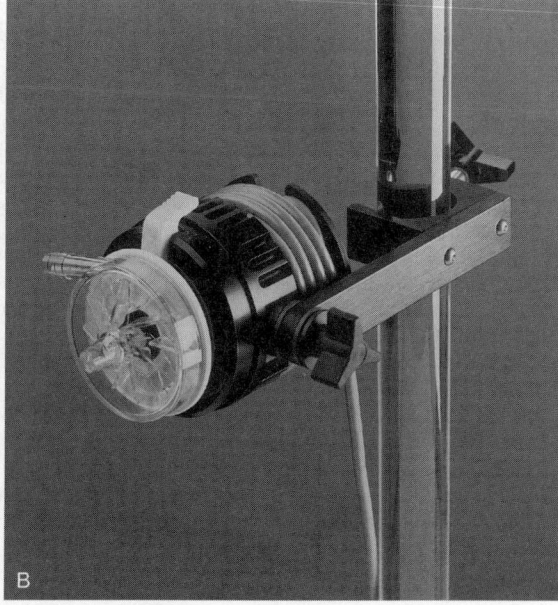

Figure 66-3. Sarns centrifugal blood pump. (*A*) Spinning impeller draws blood into pump through central port and ejects blood through tangential outlet port. (*B*) Disposable pump is driven by magnetic coupling to the reusable motor housing. (Courtesy of L. Tuttle, Sarns/3M Health Care, Ann Arbor)

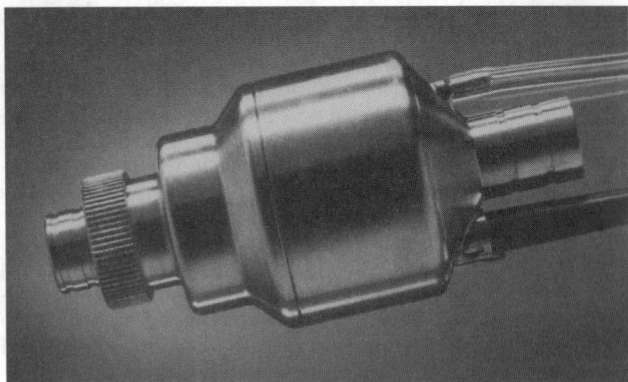

Figure 66-4. Nimbus AxiPump. This prototype of the axial flow blood pump has a 14-mm diameter and can generate flow up to 10 L/min. (Courtesy of K. C. Butler, Nimbus, Inc, Rancho Cordova, (CA)

is greatly reduced, and the systems are better suited for longer-term pumping. For this reason, pulsatile VADs are particularly advantageous when bridging a patient until heart transplantation. The issue of nonphysiologic blood flow is also less important with the pulsatile pumps.

Pierce-Donachy Ventricular Assist Device. The Pierce-Donachy VAD (Thoratec Laboratories Corp, Berkeley, CA) has been used throughout the United States and abroad in extensive clinical trials. The VAD (Fig. 66-5) is based on a seamless, 70-mL polyurethane blood sac that fits within a rigid polycarbonate case. An attached drive console withdraws and injects air into the case, causing the sac to fill or empty. The device lies in a paracorporeal position over the patient's upper abdomen, with the atrial or ventricular apex inlet cannula and the aortic or pulmonary arterial outlet cannula exiting the body through subcutaneous tunnels. The cannulas are fabricated from wire-reinforced polyurethane, and arterial graft material permits a standard end-to-side arterial anastomosis. Tilting disk prosthetic valves ensure unidirectional blood flow. A magnetic switch in the pump detects a completely filled sac, prompting the initiation of pump ejection with an air pulse. Alternatively, the pump can be run in synchrony with the native heart rhythm by means of the electrocardiogram signal. Fixed-rate pumping, independent of sac filling or heartbeat, is also possible. Left, right, or biventricular support is available with this type of device, and the implantation generally, but not always, is made during CPB. In cases in which atrial pressures are high enough to diminish the chances for air embolism, atrial inlet cannulation can be performed without CPB. The presence of prosthetic valves mandates systemic anticoagulation, usually sodium warfarin in a dose sufficient to raise the prothrombin time 1.5 to 2 times the control value.

The Pierce-Donachy VAD has been used to manage acute myocardial infarction, PCCS, and as a bridge to transplantation. Our use of the device during the past two decades has evolved to the point that we now implant it almost exclusively for the latter indication. As a bridging device, the Pierce-Donachy VAD offers survival statistics after transplantation that match those of nonsupported patients.[53]

Abiomed BVS 5000. The Abiomed BVS 5000 (Abiomed, Inc, Danvers, MA) is a commercially available extracorporeal pneumatic device. The system is designed for temporary situations in which the return of native heart function is anticipated, and PCCS is its predominant indi-

cation. The device can be applied to the left, the right, or both ventricles, although the bilateral configuration has been used in about 60% of supported PCCS patients.[54] Each disposable pump consists of two 100-mL, flexible chambers—one filling and one pumping—fabricated from polyurethane. The pumping chamber has polyurethane trileaflet valves at its inlet and outlet. The filling chamber continuously drains blood by gravity from the patient's atrium (Fig. 66-6), and it empties passively into the pumping chamber when the pressure gradient permits valve opening. Air pulses from a separate drive console compress the pumping chamber to effect asynchronous ventricular ejection whenever stroke volume reaches 80 mL. In a prospective, multicenter clinical trial, 29% of selected PCCS patients were ultimately weaned from their devices and then discharged from the hospital.[54] Complication rates for these extremely ill patients were high; excessive bleeding developed in three quarters of all PCCS recipients, and more than half of patients developed acute renal failure. However, 89% of discharged patients were leading functionally normal lives at 1-year follow-up, demonstrating the efficacy of this system, and it is now available for routine use in treating PCCS.

HeartMate 1000 IP. The HeartMate 1000 IP (Thermo Cardiosystems, Inc, Woburn, MA) is indicated for left ventricular support as a bridge to transplantation (Fig. 66-7), and a system appropriate for chronic, long-term use is under development (see later). The blood-contacting surfaces of this pump consist of sintered titanium microspheres and a textured polyurethane diaphragm. These surfaces promote the formation of a biologically active pseudoneointima shortly after exposure to blood.[55] Additionally, porcine xenograft valves are used at the inlet and outlet positions, and therefore the requirement for systemic anticoagulation is greatly reduced or obviated. The diaphragm is bonded to a rigid pusher-plate that moves back and forth with air pulses delivered from a drive unit; as the pusher-plate moves, blood alternately enters and leaves the pump through attached cannulas. The pump is placed intraperitoneally in the left upper quadrant, with the left ventricular apex inflow and aortic outflow cannulas traversing the patient's diaphragm. A percutaneous air line connects the pump to its drive console. About 68% of patients supported during clinical trials subsequently underwent car-

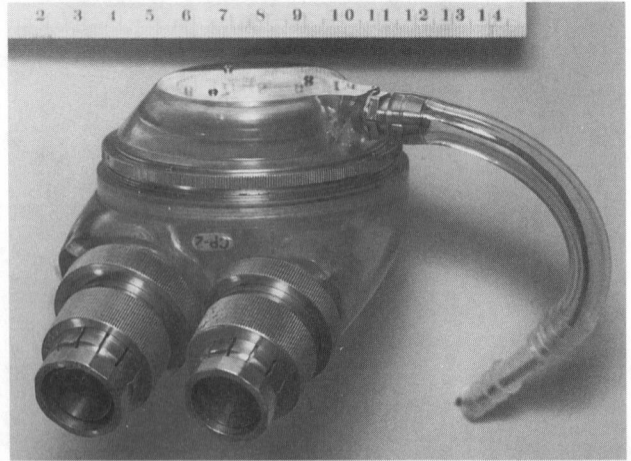

Figure 66-5. Pierce-Donachy ventricular assist device. This paracorporeal device contains a flexible, 70-mL blood sac. A magnetic switch in the case detects a filled sac, causing pump ejection, with a pulse of air delivered from the attached drive console (not shown).

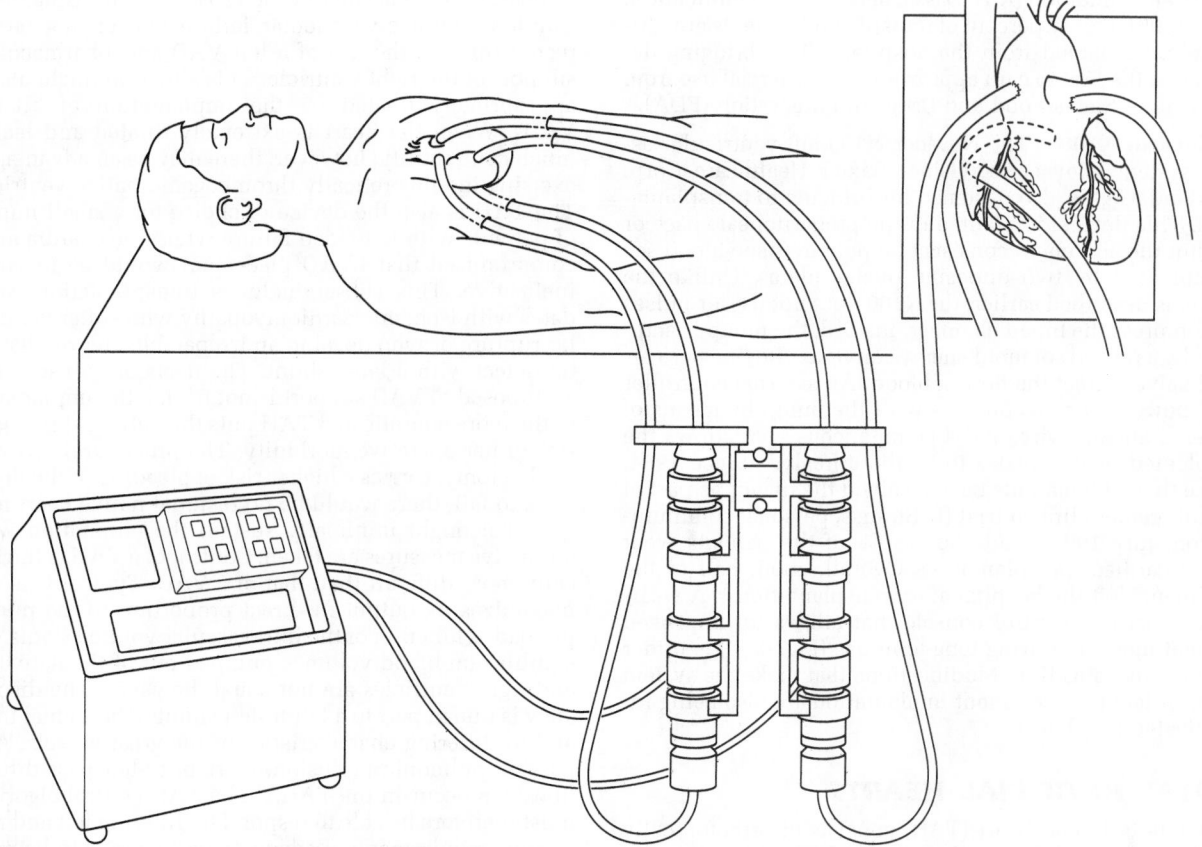

Figure 66-6. Abiomed BVS 5000 with atrial pump inflow.

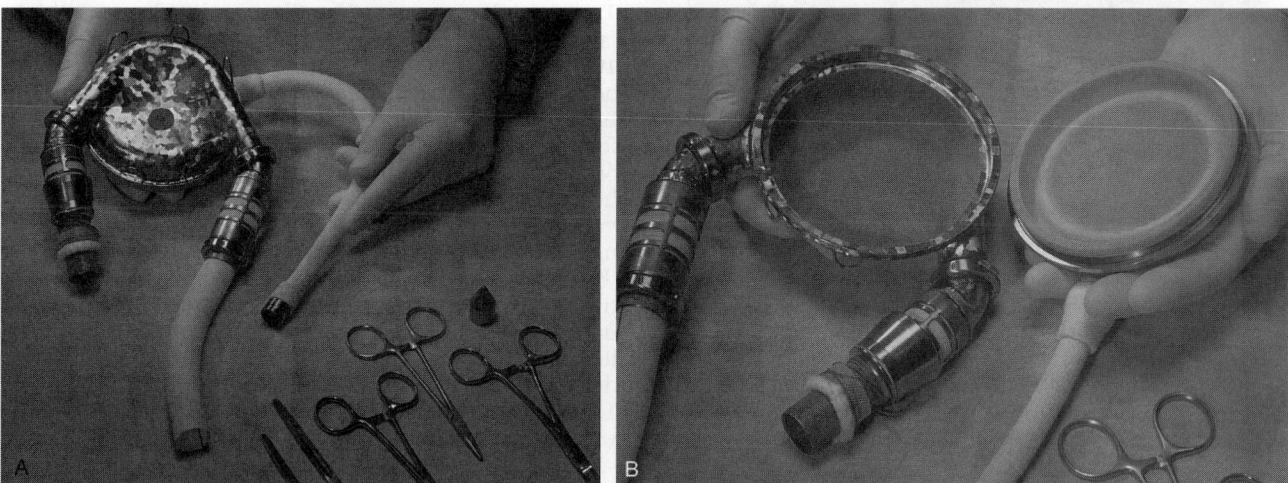

Figure 66-7. TCI HeartMate 1000 IP. (*A*) The titanium encased pump is implanted intraperitoneally in the left upper quadrant, and the percutaneous drive line connects with an external drive console. This device is approved by the Food and Drug Administration only for bridging to cardiac transplantation. Left ventricular apex inlet cannula and aortic outlet cannula pass through the patient's diaphragm. (*B*) Textured blood-contacting surfaces promote formation of a pseudoneointima, reducing the need for anticoagulation. (Courtesy of K.A. Dasse, Thermo Cardiosystems, Inc, Woburn, MA)

diac transplantation (K.A. Dasse, personal communication, May 1996). Eighty percent of transplanted patients are ultimately discharged from the hospital.[56] This bridging device was the first to gain approval for commercial use from the United States Food and Drug Administration (FDA).

Novacor N100. The Novacor N100 left ventricular assist system (Novacor Division, Baxter Healthcare Corp, Oakland, CA) is also designed for bridging to transplantation. This device, implanted in the preperitoneal space or within the abdomen, consists of a polyurethane blood sac compressed by two opposing pusher-plates. Unlike the systems described earlier, the N100 does not use air pulses to compress the blood chamber. Instead, the pump is actuated by a pulsed solenoid energy converter. Bovine pericardial valves direct the flow of blood. An external controller and power console connects with the pump by means of a percutaneous wire, and a percutaneous vent allows the implanted pusher-plates to oscillate freely.[57] Since 1984, more than 200 patients have received the device as part of a multicenter clinical trial (L. Strauss, personal communication, July 1994), and about 60% of the patients went on to cardiac transplantation. Overall, about half of the recipients left the hospital after transplantation.[58] A wearable, electrical control console that allows for improved patient mobility during long-term use (Fig. 66-8) is under clinical investigation. Modifications that make the system appropriate for permanent implantation are also being investigated (see later).

TOTAL ARTIFICIAL HEARTS

A total artificial heart (TAH) consists of orthotopically positioned blood pumps that physically and functionally replace the native left and right ventricles. The primary indication for placement of a TAH is the transplantation candidate with biventricular failure that cannot be corrected through the use of a left VAD and pharmacologic support of the right ventricle. This situation might also be appropriately treated by the implantation of bilateral VADs. When the heart is extremely dilated and lacking much contractility, however, there may be an advantage to excising the theoretically thrombogenic native ventricles. The TAH is also the device of choice for a small number of patients with left-sided failure whose myocardia are so compromised that LVAD placement would be unsafe or ineffective. This subset includes transplantation candidates with ischemic cardiomyopathy who suffer ventricular rupture or who develop an irreparable ventricular septal defect with a large shunt. The decision to use a TAH as opposed to VAD support is not trivial; the implantation of the more complicated TAH puts the patient at increased risk of perioperative morbidity. The procedure, involving cardiectomy, carries a higher risk of bleeding. If the device were to fail, there would be no residual native heart function that might minimally sustain the circulation while corrective measures are taken. Control of a TAH is intrinsically more difficult than that of a VAD. Typically, a VAD maximizes its output in direct proportion to the pump's preload, a function of the intravascular volume status. The equilibrium blood volumes pumped out of the native left and right ventricles are not equal, however. The discrepancy is due in part to a left-to-left shunt of bronchial blood and to differing characteristics of the great vessels. Also, passive pulmonic perfusion, or right-to-left pass-through flow, can occur in the TAH.[59] The TAH control algorithm must therefore be able to respond to differing left and right volume requirements if adequate perfusion is to be maintained. Two TAHs, both pneumatically driven, are under clinical investigation in the United States.

CardioWest C-70 Total Artificial Heart

The CardioWest C-70 (CardioWest Technologies, Inc, Tucson, AZ) represents a smaller, modified version of the Jarvik heart made famous by DeVries and associates in the 1980s.[60] The Jarvik heart, manufactured by Symbion, had been withdrawn from the US market owing to manufacturing difficulties, but it continued to have fairly wide use in foreign countries. In the early 1990s, CardioWest Technologies assumed responsibility for the TAH, and the result has been renewed clinical evaluation of the 70-mL stroke volume device. The C-70 (Fig. 66-9) consists of two pneumatically compressed, polyurethane ventricles placed in the orthotopic position. Percutaneous drive lines connect the pumps to an external drive unit; two mechanical valves in each ventricle ensure the correct direction of blood flow.[61] Since January 1993, 74 patients have received the device as part of an international clinical trial; by May 1996, 48 patients had undergone transplantation, 44 of whom were discharged from the hospital (R.G. Smith, personal communication, May 1996).

Penn State Total Artificial Heart

The Penn State Heart (Fig. 66-10), designed and built by our group at The Pennsylvania State University, consists of two valved, pneumatic ventricles; it shares many features with the Pierce-Donachy VAD also developed at Penn State. Our experience with clinical use of this system is limited; only five patients have presented to our institution thus far with the need for a temporary TAH. One of these patients was supported for 223 days with the device. The device is approved by the FDA for clinical application at Penn State.

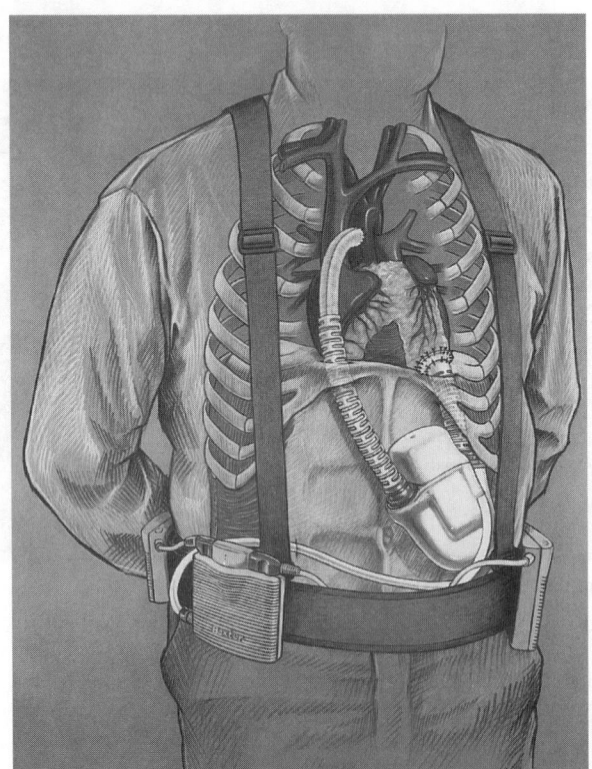

Figure 66-8. Novacor N100. Schematic representation of the electrically actuated left ventricular assist device configured with a wearable, external control package and battery pack. (Courtesy of L. Strauss, Novacor Division, Baxter Healthcare Corp, Oakland)

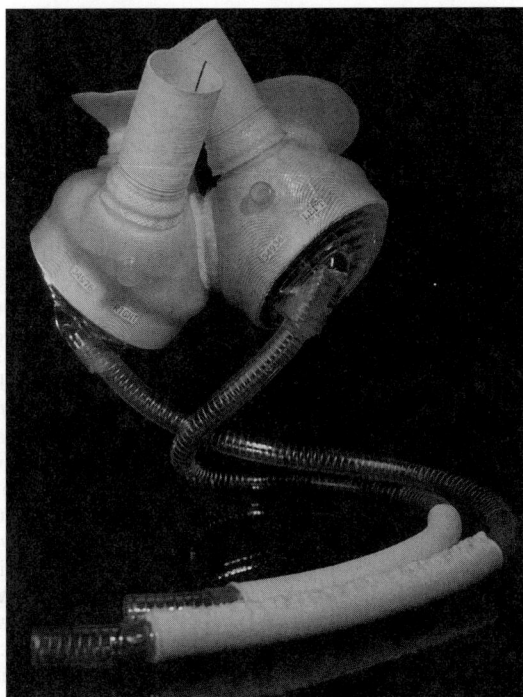

Figure 66-9. CardioWest C-70 total artificial heart. The prosthetic ventricles are implanted orthotopically, and two percutaneous drive lines connect to the pneumatic drive unit. (Courtesy of R. G. Smith, CardioWest Technologies, Inc, Tucson, AZ)

PERMANENT CIRCULATORY SUPPORT SYSTEMS

In the United States alone, between 16,000 and 40,000 patients could benefit each year from cardiac transplantation.[62] Limited donor heart availability, however, means that between 10% and 40% of patients die awaiting transplantation, and donor supply will probably remain the major impediment to broader use of this operation. As experience with bridging techniques has increased, results have improved. The voluntary device registry shows that, from 1983 to 1993, 69% of patients transplanted after mechanical circulatory support were discharged from the hospital. Results in patients with bridging devices suggest outcomes identical to transplantation alone.[57,63,64] Although support strategies are valuable to individual patients, their impact from a public health standpoint is at best minimal. Staged transplantation may raise overall costs, and the relative donor organ shortage will only increase as device use increases. In contrast, a permanently implanted device—one that provides its recipient with a good quality of life at an acceptable cost—could serve as an alternative treatment for heart failure while at the same time do much to ameliorate transplantation's supply/demand disparity. The National Heart Institute (forerunner to the National Heart, Lung, and Blood Institute [NHLBI]) established the Artificial Heart Program in 1964, with the ultimate objective of developing a tether-free, totally implantable device. Since then, NHLBI funding has fostered advances in all types of circulatory assistance, including permanent VADs and TAHs. In 1989, the NHLBI requested the Institute of Medicine to comment on further federal commitment to the TAH and VADs. The Institute of Medicine report recommended cautious but continued government support,[65] and development of both types of device remains an area of active basic and clinical research.

Permanent Left Ventricular Assist Devices

Permanent ventricular assistance offers several advantages over a permanent TAH. Extrapolation from available data suggests that many—perhaps most—candidates for a support device may not need replacement of both right and left ventricles. Residual heart function can provide a "safety net" if a mechanical device fails. Furthermore, if univentricular support could suffice, implantation of a TAH would be inappropriate given the inevitably higher cost and operative risk, more complex control requirements, and greater psychologic burden of biventricular replacement. Although nonpulsatile blood pumps for longer-term use are being developed, the systems specifically targeted as permanent substitutes for transplantation deliver pulsatile blood flow.

HeartMate VE

The HeartMate VE left ventricular assist device (LVAD; Thermo Cardiosystems, Inc) is an electromechanical version of the pneumatically driven unit described earlier.[66] Compression of the diaphragm by means of an implanted electric motor (rather than by air pulses) causes ejection of blood, and filling of the pump occurs passively. The LVAD is externally controlled, with permanent percutaneous wires connecting the pump to a wearable controller/battery pack. A percutaneous vent permits the obligatory displacement of air from within the implanted pump as its diaphragm moves back and forth. This system is being clinically tested under an FDA Investigational Device Exemption for bridging to transplantation; by May 1996, 52 of 70 recipients had undergone transplantation or were awaiting a donor organ (K.A. Dasse, personal communication). Work continues toward a configuration for permanent use that would be well tolerated by patients.

Novacor N100

The implantable Novacor N100 left ventricular assist system described earlier is also being modified to permit its permanent use in patients with end-stage heart failure. The Novacor developers' goal is to create a device without any percutaneous wires or vents. To do so, the system combines their current design with additional components. A transcutaneous energy transmission system

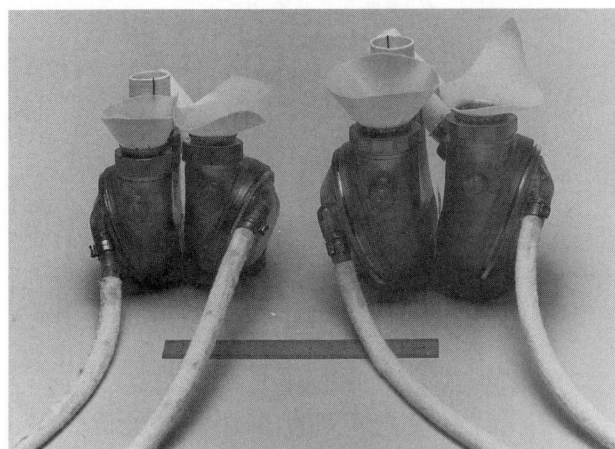

Figure 66-10. Penn State total artificial heart. Two versions of this pneumatic total artificial heart are shown. On the left is a 70-mL stroke volume device that is used clinically for bridging to transplantation. The larger, 100-mL stroke volume device on the right was designed for investigational studies in the calf model.

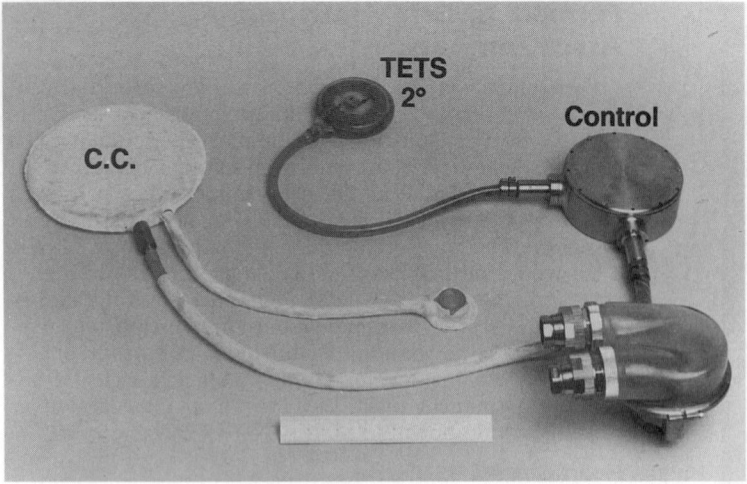

Figure 66-11. Penn State electric left ventricular assist device. The implanted components of the permanent left ventricular assist device are shown. The assist pump is positioned subcutaneously in the abdomen, with inlet and outlet cannulas (not shown) entering the chest through diaphragmatic tunnels. This system is undergoing studies in large animals. C.C., intrathoracic compliance chamber with attached access port; control, implanted electronic controller and backup battery canister; TETS 2°, implanted secondary coil for transcutaneous energy transmission system.

(TETS) powers the system. The TETS consists of two similar wire coils, one implanted underneath the skin and one outside the body.[67] Passing a high-frequency current through the extracorporeal wire coil generates a magnetic field. Placing this coil over the subcutaneously positioned secondary coil induces a current in the implanted system. Rectifying the induced current can then power the LVAD motor. Because this system is not vented, a highly compliant receptacle for gas displaced by the moving pusher-plates is positioned within the pleural space; a conduit connects the compliance chamber with the LVAD pump. Animal studies of this complete system are underway.

Penn State Left Ventricular Assist Device

The Penn State LVAD is a completely implantable device that has been under development at The Pennsylvania State University for more than 15 years (Fig. 66-11). Research efforts are being conducted with an industrial part-

ner, Arrow International (Reading, PA). The LVAD was designed from the outset to operate without percutaneous wires or vents, requiring the patient only to carry a rechargeable, extracorporeal battery pack. A roller-screw mechanism moves the pump's titanium pusher-plate back and forth, permitting ejection and passive filling of a 70-mL blood sac. The seamless blood sacs are solution-cast from segmented polyurethane, and tilting Delrin disk valves direct blood flow. An intrathoracic compliance chamber and implanted controller/back-up battery are included. The TETS is used to power the pump's brushless DC motor as well as to modify the internal controller's algorithm if desired. System telemetry occurs by means of an implanted radio frequency transmitter. Figure 66-12 shows a representation of the implanted LVAD. The pump is placed subcutaneously, and cannulas pass into the mediastinum through the diaphragm. This complete system has been evaluated in Holstein calves, with uninterrupted

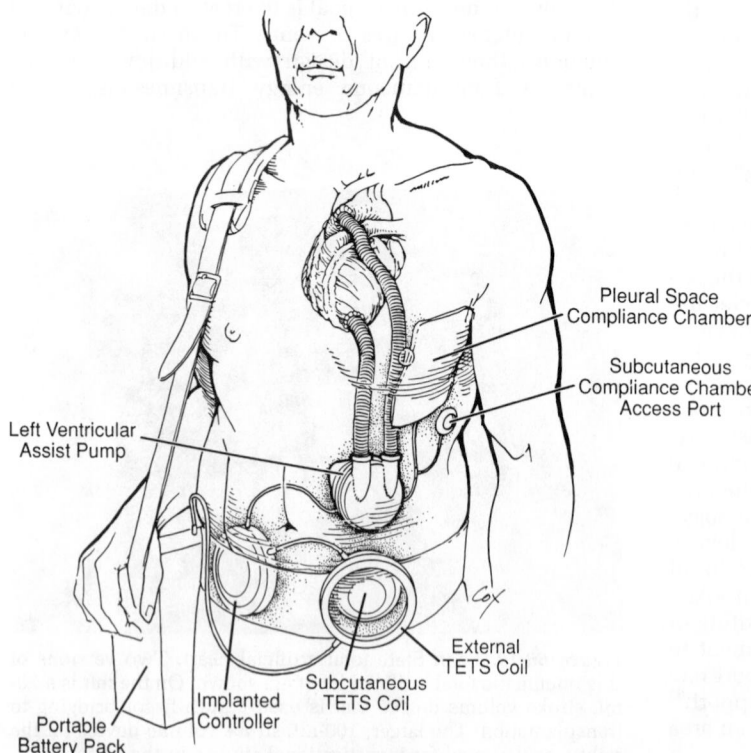

Figure 66-12. Penn State electric left ventricular assist device. This diagram shows the anticipated placement in a human recipient. All implanted components except the cannulas and compliance chamber are positioned subcutaneously. There are no percutaneous wires or external vents for this system. Battery packs are designed to power the system using the transcutaneous energy transmission system (TETS) for 8 hours before recharging.

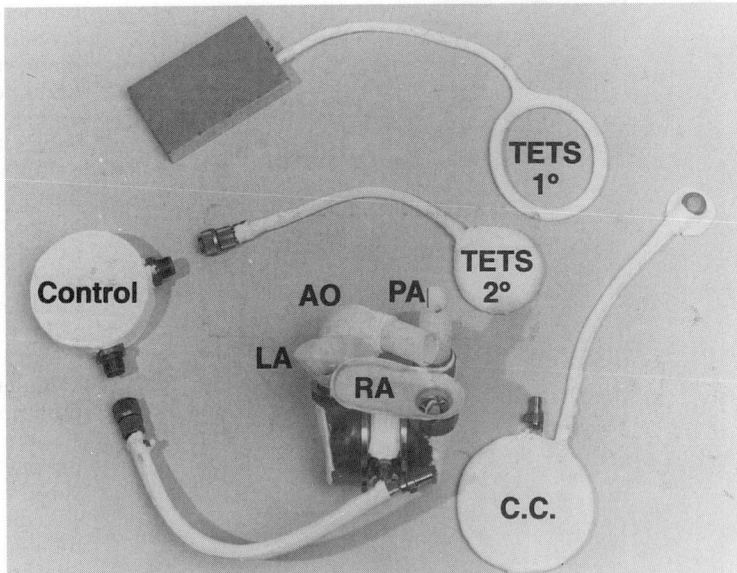

Figure 66-13. PSU/Sarns electric total artificial heart. All implanted components are velour-covered before placement in the body. The orthotopic, 70-mL stroke volume blood pumps and motor are shown in the center. This system's controller/battery canister (Control) incorporates hermetic connectors to eliminate moisture from the electronics. RA, right atrial connector cuff; LA, left atrial connector cuff; PA, right pump outlet and pulmonary artery graft; AO, left pump outlet and aorta graft; C.C., intrathoracic compliance chamber and access port; TETS 1° and 2°, external and implanted coils for transcutaneous energy transmission system.

pumping lasting up to 8 months. Initial clinical study using this system should begin within the next 5 years.

Permanent Total Artificial Hearts

Major governmental contracts targeted at a long-term, implantable TAH were awarded in 1988 to four research teams: Abiomed, Inc, and the Texas Heart Institute (Abiomed/THI); Cleveland Clinic Foundation and Nimbus, Inc (CCF/Nimbus); the University of Utah (Utah); and our group at The Pennsylvania State University along with Sarns/3M Health Care (PSU/Sarns). Stated goals were the initial development and testing of a tether-free device that would offer its recipient a reasonably normal life-style. There were to be no percutaneous lines, and the system was to respond to the varying circulatory demands of everyday activities. The TAH was to be capable of supplying an output of 8 L/min from each ventricle given physiologic preloads and afterloads. Because the system was to work for at least 5 years, biocompatibility was essential. Under this contract, initial systems were designed, and modifications have been implemented on the basis of extensive in vitro and in vivo testing.

Each TAH system has orthotopically positioned blood pumps that alternately eject blood into the pulmonary and systemic vasculature. All four systems use brushless DC motors that are powered by TETS. Implanted nickel–cadmium batteries can also drive the systems in case the external coils detach. These TAHs convert the movements of a motor into the pulsatile pumping of blood by different mechanisms. Using a design similar to the Penn State LVAD, a reversing electric motor in the PSU/Sarns TAH (Fig. 66-13) rotates a roller-screw fixed at either end to circular pusher-plates. In this fashion, the pusher-plates compress the blood sacs, alternately creating left- or right-sided systole and diastole. The Utah TAH has a small, reversing axial flow pump that directs hydraulic oil against flexible diaphragms of the left- and right-sided pumps.[68] The system is volumetrically coupled, meaning that each volume unit of blood outflow is produced by an equivalent displacement of hydraulic fluid. Similarly, the Abiomed/THI TAH (Fig. 66-14) shifts hydraulic fluid to pump blood in a one-to-one fashion.[69] Its unidirectional centrifugal pump, combined with a rotating valve, delivers hydraulic

fluid against one pump's diaphragm while simultaneously withdrawing fluid from the contralateral side. In this fashion, alternating filling and emptying of the pumps with blood occur. The CCF/Nimbus system (Fig. 66-15) contains a unidirectional gear pump to drive a low-volume (16-mL) hydraulic circuit. A spool valve alternately directs the flow of fluid to opposite ends of a piston within the hydraulic chamber. Because the piston is magnetically coupled to a dual pusher-plate assembly outside the hydraulic circuit, compression of left and right pump diaphragms is effected by movement of the piston.[70]

Abiomed/THI pumps are first cast from a solution of proprietary polyetherurethane and then externally reinforced to provide rigidity. The system incorporates 24-mL

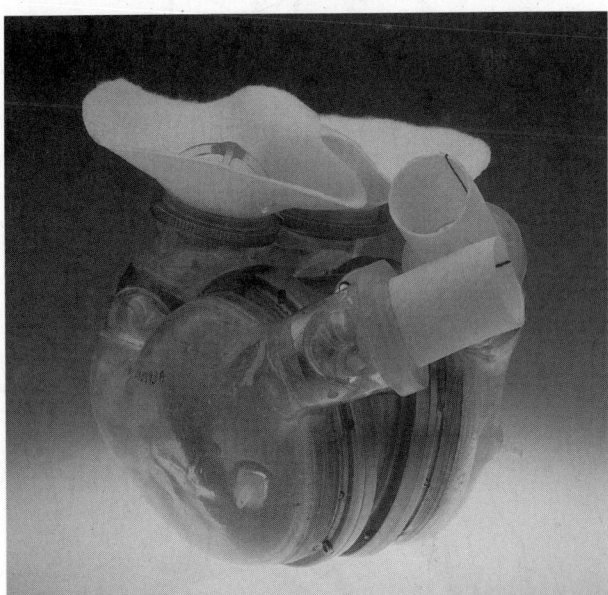

Figure 66-14. Abiomed/THI electric total artificial heart. Orthotopic blood pumps and motor are shown. This system also uses a transcutaneous energy transmission system similar to the type shown in Figure 66. (Courtesy of R. T. V. Kung, Abiomed, Inc, Danvers, MA)

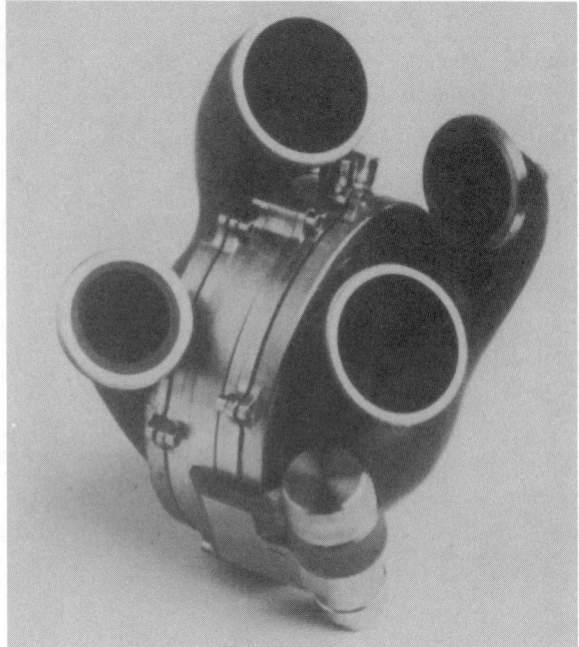

Figure 66-15. CCF/Nimbus electric total artificial heart. This system includes a compliance chamber and transcutaneous energy transmission system similar to those shown in Figure 66-13. (Courtesy of K.C. Butler, Nimbus, Inc, Rancho Cordova, CA)

polyetherurethane trileaflet valves in both the inlet and outlet positions. The Utah group internally coats its rigid pumps with a segmented polyurethane, and tilting disk valves (Medtronic-Hall, 27-mL inlet and 25-mL outlet) ensure the correct direction of blood flow. CCF/Nimbus pumps are fabricated from a reinforced epoxy, and blood-

contacting surfaces are coated with a glutaraldehyde-fixed protein to provide biocompatibility. The use of bioprosthetic valves also decreases the risk of thrombus formation. Rigid polysulfone pumps in the PSU/Sarns TAH surround segmented polyurethane blood sacs. Tilting Delrin disk valves (Bjork-Shiley Monostrut, 27-mL inlet and 25-mL outlet) are placed at the junctions of blood sacs and pump ports.[71]

The control schemes of these systems demonstrate so-called Starling behavior to the extent that increased venous return elicits a commensurate increase in left pump output until a maximum output is reached. The PSU/Sarns system relies on an implanted control algorithm to adjust the left pump's diastolic time period and speed of systole so that complete left pump filling is just barely maintained while pumping rate remains maximized. Hall-effect (magnetic) sensors allow the controller to derive preload and afterload parameters, the time ratio of systole and diastole, and the speed of pump emptying during each ejection cycle. Passive diastolic filling of one pump independent of the contralateral pump's ejection speed can occur because of the attached compliance chamber. Figure 66-16 illustrates the anticipated placement of the PSU/Sarns TAH system within an average-sized patient.

The CCF/Nimbus TAH also requires an intrathoracic compliance chamber. Additionally, the control scheme adjusts motor speed and pumping rate so that the left pump fills to only 90% of maximum. This maneuver provides a buffer to accommodate occasionally increased filling volumes without significant rises in left atrial pressure. This group has also been investigating the use of a mechanical right pump stroke volume limiter to aid with the balance of left and right pump outputs.

The Abiomed/THI TAH modulates motor speed as the principal way to control cardiac output. Optimal pumping rate is made a function of right atrial pressure, inferred

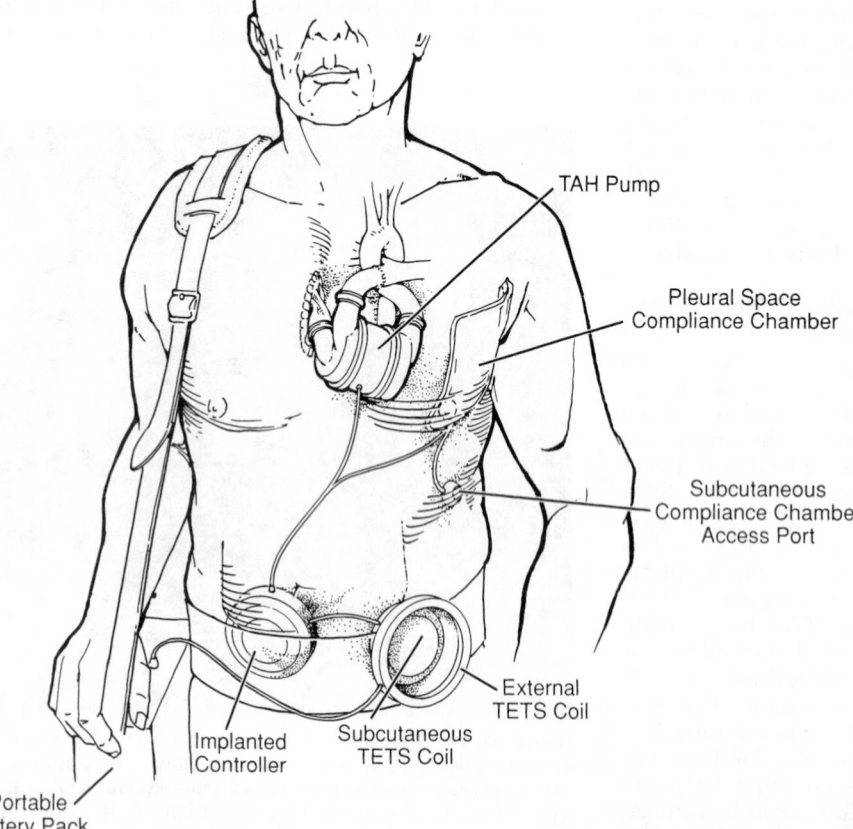

Figure 66-16. PSU/Sarns electric total artificial heart (TAH). This diagram shows the anticipated placement in a human recipient. As with the permanent electric left ventricular assist device, this completely implantable system contains no percutaneous lines or vents. Similar designs are employed for the Abiomed/THI and CCF/Nimbus hearts. TETS, transcutaneous energy transmission system.

from transducer-measured pressure readings within the right hydraulic chamber.[69] Compensation for right and left flow imbalances depends on a flexible, 20-mL hydraulic chamber positioned against the left atrium.[69] This compliance chamber, in continuity with the right pump's hydraulic chamber, exerts negative feedback on right pump filling. As left atrial pressure rises, hydraulic fluid shifts into the right hydraulic chamber, limiting the passive diastolic filling of the right pump's blood chamber. Less blood is then delivered to the left side until left atrial pressure decreases.

To keep its pump output optimal, the Utah system varies both motor speed and the point at which the hydraulic pump reverses. Hydraulic fluid pressure is the primary input parameter for the algorithm.[68] The Utah group's conceptually simple way to correct right and left flow differences depends on an interatrial shunt, analogous to an atrial septal defect. Initial in vivo experiments in calves have been successful; a 4.3-mL diameter shunt provided acceptable flow balance and remained patent for more than 1 month.

Evaluation of the TAH systems includes detailed in vitro analyses on mock circulatory loops and carefully monitored in vivo experiments. Our studies at Penn State have included a 100-mL stroke volume pump specifically designed to support a large animal model, and this system maintained a healthy, growing calf for more than 1 year. An animal that received Penn State's completely implanted, 70-mL stroke volume TAH survived for 160 days; the brisk growth of this calf eventually overwhelmed the perfusion capabilities of this human-sized pump. Development of TAH devices remains costly and complex, in part because the FDA demands extremely stringent testing of devices whose failure could be lethal. Each research group is putting together its concept of the most suitable TAH design, aware that minor or major changes in specifications could have expensive, time-consuming consequences that would jeopardize a device's timely introduction to clinical use. In 1993, the NHLBI awarded new 3-year contracts to three research groups: Abiomed/THI, CCF/Nimbus, and PSU/Sarns. These contracts represent the first phase of a concerted effort by the NHLBI to bring about final development of an effective, reliable TAH.[72] The contracts explicitly outline performance criteria, and the recipient's quality of life is again paramount. Characterization of the three systems is standardized using mock circulatory loops and animal experiments. The NHLBI is maintaining careful oversight throughout the term of the project. The second phase of this project will fund an anticipated two groups for 4 years of device readiness testing and chronic in vivo analysis. During this time, the final system configurations must demonstrate flawless in vitro performance for at least 2 years, as well as failure-free performance in animals for 3 to 5 months. Application to the FDA for an Investigational Device Exemption should follow completion of the second phase, leading to initial human use several years after the turn of the century.

Future of Permanent Circulatory Support Systems

Heart failure patients would benefit greatly from the development of cost-effective, reliable, permanent circulatory support systems that offer reasonably normal lifestyles. Although estimates predict more demand for the LVAD than for the TAH, this a priori allocation may prove to be inappropriate. The native heart's response to mechanical support for a duration on the order of years is unknown, and it is possible that more patients than we suspect may benefit from biventricular support. Moreover, a

TAH has the advantage of orthotopic positioning, thereby eliminating a bulky component from the abdomen. Materials science advances, components miniaturization, and further elucidation of biologic responses to artificial devices will do much to improve a prospective recipient's quality of life. The drive toward cost-containment in the delivery of medical care, however, will temper public enthusiasm for high-technology interventions like mechanical circulatory support. At some point, it will probably be necessary to assign a discrete value to the extended life of a patient with end-stage heart failure. In the meantime, development of completely implantable systems moves ahead, but the issue of cost may prove to be the overriding determinant of how quickly the devices become part of the clinician's armamentarium.

REFERENCES

1. Sarnoff SJ, Braunwald GH, Welch GH, et al. Hemodynamic determinants of oxygen consumption of the heart with special reference to the tension-time index. Am J Physiol 1958; 192:148.
2. Claus RH, Birtwell WC, Albertal G, et al. Assisted circulation, the arterial counterpulsator. J Thorac Cardiovasc Surg 1961;41:447.
3. Moulopoulos SD, Topaz S, Kolff WJ. Diastolic balloon pumping (with carbon dioxide) in the aorta: a mechanical assistance to the failing circulation. Am Heart J 1962;63:669.
4. Kantrowitz A, Tjonneland S, Freed PS, et al. Initial clinical experience with intraaortic balloon pumping in cardiogenic shock. JAMA 1968;203:135.
5. Suga H. Ventricular energetics. Physiol Rev 1990;70:247.
6. Goldberg RJ, Gore JM, Alpert JS, et al. Cardiogenic shock after acute myocardial infarction: incidence and mortality from a community-wide perspective, 1975 to 1988. N Engl J Med 1991;325:1117.
7. Maroko PR, Bernstein EF, Libby P, et al. Effects of intraaortic balloon counterpulsation on the severity of myocardial ischemic injury following acute coronary occlusion. Circulation 1972;45:1150.
8. Roberts AJ, Alonso DR, Combes JR, et al. Role of delayed intraaortic balloon pumping in treatment of experimental myocardial infarction. Am J Cardiol 1978;41:1202.
9. Flaherty JT, Becker LC, Weiss JL, et al. Results of a randomized prospective trial of intraaortic balloon counterpulsation and intravenous nitroglycerin in patients with acute myocardial infarction. J Am Coll Cardiol 1985;6:434.
10. Mueller HS. Role of intraaortic counterpulsation in cardiogenic shock and acute myocardial infarction. Cardiology 1994;84:168.
11. Bardet J, Masquet C, Kahn JC, et al. Clinical and hemodynamic results of intra-aortic balloon counterpulsation and surgery for cardiogenic shock. Am Heart J 1977;93:280.
12. DeWood MA, Notske RN, Hensley GR, et al. Intraaortic balloon counterpulsation with and without reperfusion for myocardial infarction shock. Circulation 1980;61:1105.
13. Ohman EM, Califf RM, George BS, et al. The use of intraaortic balloon pumping as an adjunct to reperfusion therapy in acute myocardial infarction. Am Heart J 1991;121:895.
14. Ishihara M, Sato H, Tateishi H, et al. Intraaortic balloon pumping as the postangioplasty strategy in acute myocardial infarction. Am Heart J 1991;122:385.
15. Gurbel PA, Anderson RD, MacCord CS, et al. Arterial diastolic pressure augmentation by intraaortic balloon counterpulsation enhances the onset of coronary artery reperfusion by thrombolytic therapy. Circulation 1994;89:361.
16. Kahn JK, Rutherford BD, McConahay DR, et al. Supported "high risk" coronary angioplasty using intraaortic balloon pump counterpulsation. J Am Coll Cardiol 1990;15:1151.
17. Olsen PS, Arendrup H, Thiis JJ, et al. Intraaortic balloon counterpulsation in Denmark 1988–1991: early results and complications. Eur J Cardiothorac Surg 1993;7:634.
18. Naunheim KS, Swartz MT, Pennington DG, et al. Intraaortic balloon pumping in patients requiring cardiac operations: risk analysis and long-term follow-up. J Thorac Cardiovasc Surg 1992;104:1654.

19. Creswell LL, Rosenbloom M, Cox JL, et al. Intraaortic balloon counterpulsation: patterns of usage and outcome in cardiac surgery patients. Ann Thorac Surg 1992;54:11.

20. Hedenmark J, Ahn H, Henze A, et al. Intraaortic balloon counterpulsation with special reference to determinants of survival. Scand J Thorac Cardiovasc Surg 1989;23:57.

21. Macoviak J, Stephenson LW, Edmunds LH Jr, et al. The intraaortic balloon pump: an analysis of five years' experience. Ann Thorac Surg 1980;29:451.

22. Dembitsky WP, Moore CH, Holman WL, et al. Successful mechanical circulatory support for noncoronary shock. J Heart Lung Transplant 1992;11:129.

23. Pifarre R, Sullivan H, Montoya A, et al. Comparison of results after heart transplantation: mechanically supported versus nonsupported patients. J Heart Lung Transplant 1992;11:235.

24. Siu SC, Kowalchuk GJ, Welty FK, et al. Intraaortic balloon counterpulsation support in the high-risk cardiac patient undergoing urgent noncardiac surgery. Chest 1991;99:1342.

25. Georgeson S, Coombs AT, Eckman MH. Prophylactic use of the intraaortic balloon pump in high-risk cardiac patients undergoing noncardiac surgery: a decision analytic view. Am J Med 1992;92:1665.

26. Roberts AJ, Hoover EL, Alonso DR, et al. Prolonged intraaortic balloon pumping in *Klebsiella*-induced hypodynamic shock: cardiopulmonary, hematological, metabolic, and pathological observations. Ann Thorac Surg 1979;28:73.

27. Pribble CG, Shaddy RE. Intraaortic balloon counterpulsation in newborn lambs infected with group B *Streptococcus*. Trans Am Soc Artif Intern Organs 1991;37:33.

28. Mercer D, Doris P, Salerno TA. Intraaortic balloon counterpulsation in septic shock. Can J Surg 1981;24:643.

29. Barnett MG, Swartz MT, Peterson GJ, et al. Vascular complications from intraaortic balloons: risk analysis. J Vasc Surg 1994;19:81.

30. Eltchaninoff H, Dimas AP, Whitlow PL. Complications associated with percutaneous placement and use of intraaortic balloon counterpulsation. Am J Cardiol 1993;71:328.

31. Mackenzie DJ, Wagner WH, Kulber DA, et al. Vascular complications of the intraaortic balloon pump. Am J Surg 1992;164:517.

32. Miller JS, Dodson TF, Salam AA, Smith RB III. Vascular complications following intraaortic balloon pump insertion. Am Surg 1992;58:232.

33. Anderson HL, Delius RE, Sinard JM, et al. Early experience with adult extracorporeal membrane oxygenation in the modern era. Ann Thorac Surg 1992;53:553.

34. Karl TR. Extracorporeal circulatory support in infants and children. Semin Thorac Cardiovasc Surg 1994;6:154.

35. Pennington DG. Commentary on circulatory support in infants and children. Semin Thorac Cardiovasc Surg 1994;6:161.

36. Magovern GJ Jr, Magovern JA, Benckart DH, et al. Extracorporeal membrane oxygenation: preliminary results in patients with postcardiotomy cardiogenic shock. Ann Thorac Surg 1994;57:1462.

37. Phillips ST. Resuscitation for cardiogenic shock with extracorporeal membrane oxygenation systems. Semin Thorac Cardiovasc Surg 1994;6:131.

38. Lazar HL, Treanor P, Yang XM, et al. Enhanced recovery of ischemic myocardium by combining percutaneous bypass with intraaortic balloon pump support. Ann Thorac Surg 1994;57:663.

39. Craddock PR, Fehr J, Dalmasso AP, et al. Hemodialysis leukopenia: pulmonary vascular leukostasis resulting from complement activation by dialyzer membrane. J Clin Invest 1977;59:879.

40. Hammerschmidt DE, Stroncek DF, Bowers TK, et al. Complement activation and neutropenia occurring during cardiopulmonary bypass. J Thorac Cardiovasc Surg 1981;81:370.

41. Aufiero TX. Combined registry for the clinical use of mechanical ventricular assist pumps and the total artificial heart. Presented at American Society for Artificial Internal Organs, 40th Anniversary Meeting, San Francisco, April 14, 1994.

42. Chow E, Farrar DJ. Right heart function during prosthetic left ventricular assistance in a porcine model of congestive heart failure. J Thorac Cardiovasc Surg 1992;104:569.

43. Jakob H, Kutschera Y, Palzer B, et al. In-vitro assessment of centrifugal pumps for ventricular assist. Artif Organs 1990;14:278.

44. Purvis NB, Giorgio TD. Flow cytometric analysis of shear-induced platelet activation. Ann Biomed Eng 1993;21(Suppl):44.

45. Kapadvanjwala M, Jy W, Dewanjee MK. Effect of fluid shear on thrombus formation and platelet fragmentation in hemodialyzer. Ann Biomed Eng 1993;21(Suppl):44.

46. Rose DM, Laschinger J, Grossi E, et al. Experimental and clinical results with a simplified left heart assist device for treatment of profound left ventricular dysfunction. World J Surg 1985;9:11.

47. Curtis JJ, Walls JT, Demmy TL, et al. Clinical experience with the Sarns centrifugal pump. Artif Organs 1993;17:630.

48. Ohara Y, Sakuma I, Makinouchi K, et al. Baylor gyro pump: a completely seal-less centrifugal pump aiming for long-term circulatory support. Artif Organs 1993;17:599.

49. Antaki JF, Butler KC, Kormos RL, et al. In vivo evaluation of the Nimbus axial flow ventricular assist system: criteria and methods. ASAIO J 1993;39:M231.

50. Damm G, Mizuguchi K, Bozeman R, et al. In vitro performance of the Baylor/NASA axial flow pump. Artif Organs 1993;17:609.

51. Yamazaki K, Umezu M, Koyanagi H, et al. A miniature intraventricular axial flow blood pump that is introduced through the left ventricular apex. ASAIO J 1992;38:M679.

52. Yozu R, Golding L, Yada I, et al. Do we really need pulse? Chronic nonpulsatile and pulsatile blood flow: from the exercise response viewpoints. Artif Organs 1994;18:638.

53. Pennington DG, McBride LR, Miller LW, Swartz MT. Eleven years experience with the Pierce-Donachy ventricular assist device. Presented at the International Society for Heart and Lung Transplantation, Venice, Italy, March 24, 1994.

54. Guyton RA, Schonberger JPAM, Everts PAM, et al. Postcardiotomy shock: clinical evaluation of the BVS 5000 biventricular support system. Ann Thorac Surg 1993;56:346.

55. Dasse KA, Chipman SD, Sherman CN, et al. Clinical experience with textured blood contacting surfaces in ventricular assist devices. Trans Am Soc Artif Intern Organs 1987;33:418.

56. Frazier OH, Rose EA, Macmanus Q, et al. Multicenter clinical evaluation of the HeartMate 1000 IP left ventricular assist device. Ann Thorac Surg 1992;53:1080.

57. McCarthy PM, Portner PM, Tobler HG, et al. Clinical experience with the Novacor ventricular assist system. J Thorac Cardiovasc Surg 1991;102:578.

58. Portner P. A totally implantable heart assist system: the Novacor program. In: Akutsu T, Koyanagi H, eds. Artificial heart 4: Heart replacement. Tokyo, Springer-Verlag, 1993:71.

59. Jacobs G, Yozu R, Shimomitsu T, et al. "Pass-through" and "inertia" contribution to left-right flow difference (LRFD) in TAH recipients. Trans Am Soc Artif Intern Organs 1985;31:186.

60. DeVries WL, Anderson JL, Joyce LD, et al. Initial human application of the Utah total artificial heart. N Engl J Med 1984;310:273.

61. Arabia FA, Copeland JG, Smith RG. Progress on the total artificial heart. In: Braverman MH, Tawes RL, eds. Surgical technology international II. San Francisco, Surgical Technology International, 1993:251.

62. O'Connell JB, Gunnar RM, Evans RW, et al. 24th Bethesda Conference: organization of heart transplantation in the U.S. J Am Coll Cardiol 1993;22:8.

63. Hill JD, Farrar DJ, Topic N. The Thoratec experience in bridge to cardiac transplantation. In: Ott RA, Gutfinger DE, Gazzaniga AB, eds. Cardiac surgery: state of the art reviews, vol 7. Philadelphia, Hanley & Belfus, 1993;317.

64. Frazier OH. Long-term ventricular support with the HeartMate in patients undergoing bridge-to-transplant operations. In: Ott RA, Gutfinger DE, Gazzaniga AB, eds. Cardiac surgery: state of the art reviews, vol 7. Philadelphia, Hanley & Belfus, 1993:353.

65. Institute of Medicine. The artificial heart: prototypes, policies, and patients. Washington, DC, National Academy Press, 1991.

66. Poirier VL, Sherman CW, Clay WC, et al. An ambulatory, intermediate term left ventricular assist device. Trans Am Soc Artif Intern Organs 1989;35:452.

67. Sherman C, Daly BDT, Dasse K. Research and development of

systems for transmitting energy through intact skin. (Abstract) 1983 Devices and Technology Branch Contractors Meeting, Bethesda, 1984.

68. Rowles JR, Khanwilkar PS, Diegel PD, et al. Development of a totally implantable artificial heart. ASAIO J 1992;38:M713.

69. Yu LS, Finnegan M, Vaughan S, et al. A compact and noise free electrohydraulic total artificial heart. ASAIO J 1993;39:M386.

70. Smith WA, Hete BF, Kiraly RJ, et al. The E4T electric powered total artificial heart (TAH). Artif Organs 1988;12:402.

71. Snyder AJ, Pae WE, Rosenberg G, et al. The Penn State implantable artificial heart: current status. In: Akutsu T, Koyanagi H, eds. Artificial heart 3: heart replacement. Tokyo, Springer-Verlag, 1991;205.

72. National Heart, Lung, and Blood Institute. Request for proposal NHLBI-HV: phased readiness testing of implantable total artificial hearts. Bethesda, National Institutes of Health, Public Health Service, 1992.

SURGERY: SCIENTIFIC PRINCIPLES AND PRACTICE, Second Edition, edited by Lazar J. Greenfield, Michael W. Mulholland, Keith T. Oldham, Gerald B. Zelenock, and Keith D. Lillemoe. Lippincott–Raven Publishers, Philadelphia, © 1997.

CHAPTER 67

CARDIAC ARRHYTHMIAS AND PERICARDIUM

STEVEN F. BOLLING AND JAMES R. STEWART

CARDIAC ARRHYTHMIAS

The surgical management of cardiac arrhythmias is based on knowledge of the underlying anatomy and physiology, which is the basis for treatment of specific patients and arrhythmias, including need for electrophysiologic testing and possible surgical ablation.

Anatomy of the Conduction System

The sinoatrial (SA) node (10 × 12 mm) is superficial beneath the anterolateral junction of the superior vena cava (SVC) and the right atrial appendage. Its blood supply is the sinus node artery, arising from the right (60%) or circumflex coronary artery, which may pass anterior or posterior to the SVC. Although Purkinje cells are seen in atrial muscle, no special conduction path from the SA node to the atrioventricular (AV) node has been identified.[1]

The bean-shaped AV node (1 × 3 × 6 mm) is on the right atrial side of the central fibrous tendon in the muscular AV septum, superior to or rarely in the coronary sinus. From the right atrium, the AV node is within the triangle of Koch, formed by the tricuspid annulus, the tendon of Todaro, and the coronary sinus ostium. The far or left side of the AV node is near the mitral annulus and may be damaged during mitral operations. The AV node blood supply is from the posterior descending coronary artery. The common AV bundle of His is continuous from the AV node and lies on the left side of the ventricular septum in about 80% of humans. It is the only normal muscular connection between the atria and ventricles. The His bundle (1 mm) passes between the septal and anterior leaflets of the tricuspid valve and gives off fibers that form the left and then the right bundle branches. This branching occurs beneath the commissure between the right and noncoronary cusps of the aortic valve. The left bundle branch spreads over the ventricular septum, forming radiations to

the anteroseptal and the posteromedial papillary muscles. The right bundle branch starts at the inferior edge of the membranous septum and passes below the medial papillary muscle, along the septal and moderator bands to the right ventricular wall.[1]

Other areas of anatomy pertinent to surgical management of cardiac arrhythmias include the aortomitral continuity (Fig. 67-1), from the left to the right fibrous trigones, which is part of the central fibrous body and the only place in the AV groove where atrial muscle is not in proximity to the ventricle. Therefore, it is the only area where supraventricular accessory pathways cannot occur. The pyramidal space is bounded by the fibrous trigone, the epicardium, and the posterior superior process of the left ventricle, and contains fat pad, coronary sinus, AV node artery, and possible posterior septal pathways.[1]

Physiology of Arrhythmias

Cardiac electromechanical activity is determined by ion concentration as semipermeable myocyte membranes permit passage of positive cations, such as sodium, potassium, and calcium, but not anionic proteins. Therefore, negatively charged intracellular proteins create a transmembrane electrical potential as the interior of the cell is negatively charged relative to the exterior. Stimulation of cardiac cells produces an action potential, which may last for 300 milliseconds. The standard cardiac muscle action potential has five phases (Fig. 67-2). In phase 4, the resting or diastolic membrane potential is stabilized by active maintenance of the transmembrane potassium and sodium gradients. During phase 0, a physical or electrical stimulus causes the sodium fast channels and the calcium slow channels to open. As positive ions move in, depolarization occurs as the membrane potential rises to threshold and an action potential is generated. Phase 1 is characterized by repolarization to the phase 2 plateau. During phase 2, known as the *effective refractory period,* the slow calcium channels and the fast sodium channels are closed, and the myocardium cannot be excited. During phase 3, potassium

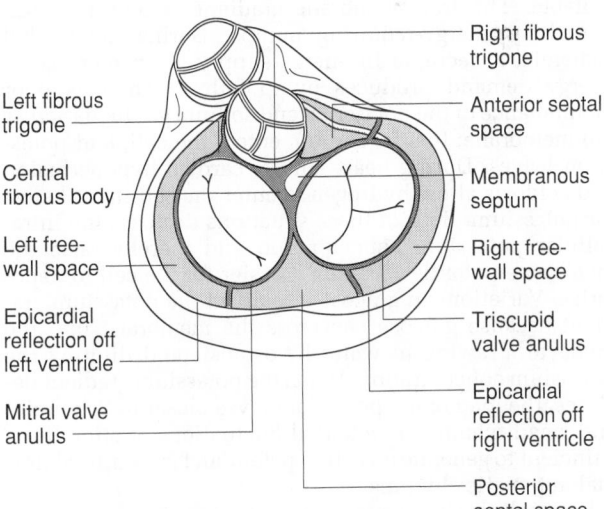

Figure 67-1. View of the heart demonstrating each of the four anatomic areas where accessory pathways can occur. The left free-wall space, the posterior septal space, and the right free-wall space are defined by the adjacent valvular and ventricular structures. (After Cox JL, Ferguson. Surgery for the Wolff-Parkinson-White syndrome: the endocardial approach. Semin Thorac Cardiovasc Surg 1989;1:34)

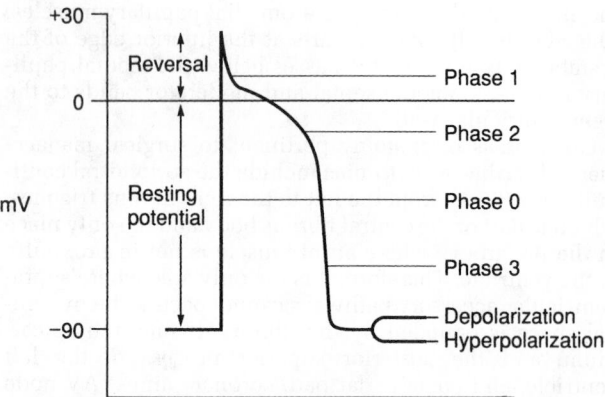

Figure 67-2. A cardiac action potential with a resting potential of −90 mV with respect to the outside. At the peak of the action potential, the inside of the cell becomes about 30 mV positive with respect to the outside. The upstroke of the action potential is called phase 0. The initial rapid repolarization is phase 1, the plateau or period of persisting depolarization is phase 2, and the period of more rapid repolarization is phase 3. A change in membrane potential away from the resting potential toward zero represents depolarization; a change in the membrane potential that makes the inside of the cell more negative is hyperpolarization. (After Cranefield, Erinson. Cardiac arrhythmias: the role of triggered activity in other mechanisms. Mt Kisko, NY, Futura, 1988)

channels reopen, allowing potassium out. Rapid repolarization ensues, reestablishing the myocyte resting membrane potential.[2]

All arrhythmias are caused by automaticity, reentry, or a combination of these mechanisms.[3] Myocardial tissue that depolarizes, reaches threshold, and fires an action potential is termed *automatic;* and stimulation of the surrounding myocytes generates an automatic rhythm. Automatic rhythms are normal and physiologic in the SA and AV nodes. Abnormal automaticity can occur as many pathologic conditions move the resting membrane potential toward threshold, allowing lesser stimuli to achieve threshold and making cardiac muscle hyperexcitable or irritable. The transmembrane gradient of ions is maintained by energy-requiring pumps. During myocardial ischemia, a decrease in energy supply or an increase in energy demand produces pump failure. There is poor maintenance of the potassium and sodium gradients across the membrane; that is, sodium enters the cell, and potassium leaves. During heart failure, cardiac hypoperfusion and acidosis allow hydrogen to enter the cell in exchange for potassium. Both of these situations decrease the intracellular potassium concentration and thereby raise the membrane potential, making it easier for the cell to depolarize. Variations in glucose also affect the potassium gradient because glucose can cross the membrane into the myocyte, drawing in water by osmosis and diluting the potassium concentration. When the potassium gradient declines, the membrane potential moves closer to threshold, and small membrane potential fluctuations or stimuli are sufficient to generate an action potential, facilitating abnormal automatic rhythms.

Extracellular hypokalemia increases the transmembrane potassium gradient. Hypokalemia also increases sodium channel size, promoting sodium influx during phase 0; the result is increased automaticity. Calcium mediates actin and myosin coupling, which produces muscle contraction. High extracellular calcium levels may cause myocardial work to exceed the energy supply and thus impair the membrane pump, enhancing automaticity. Increased cate-

cholamine levels also predispose to automaticity and increase both heart rate and contractility. As with hypercalcemia, elevated catecholamine levels can increase cardiac work beyond the energy supply and cause the membrane potential to move closer to threshold. Also, administration of catecholamines to cardiac myocytes decreases the outward potassium flow, enhancing automaticity. Catecholamines can also produce large spontaneous oscillations in membrane voltage. Digitalis can produce myocardial hyperexcitability, manifested by premature ventricular contractions, which are the most common example of automaticity. Under normal conditions, the SA and AV nodes exhibit faster depolarization and reach threshold sooner than Purkinje fibers. Therefore, the faster SA node is the pacemaker of the heart. Premature ventricular contractions develop when a hyperexcitable automatic cell in the ventricular myocardium undergoes rapid diastolic depolarization and reaches threshold before the next SA node beat.

Reentrant arrhythmias are the second type of arrhythmia.[3] Cardiac tissue has a long refractory period; therefore, few myocytes remain excitable at the end of a beat. Myocardial ischemia, fibrosis, and necrosis slow electrical conduction and produce nonconductive areas that interrupt conduction waves. These areas of differential myocardial conduction (Fig. 67-3) can form a reentrant circuit if the conduction time through this abnormal area exceeds the normal impulse. When a slowed electrical impulse finally leaves the area of abnormal conduction, the surrounding tissue may be able to be stimulated again, thereby setting up an abnormal circuit. Slow conduction of the SA and AV nodes, a shortened refractory period, and anatomic heterogeneity after infarction all favor reentry arrhythmias.

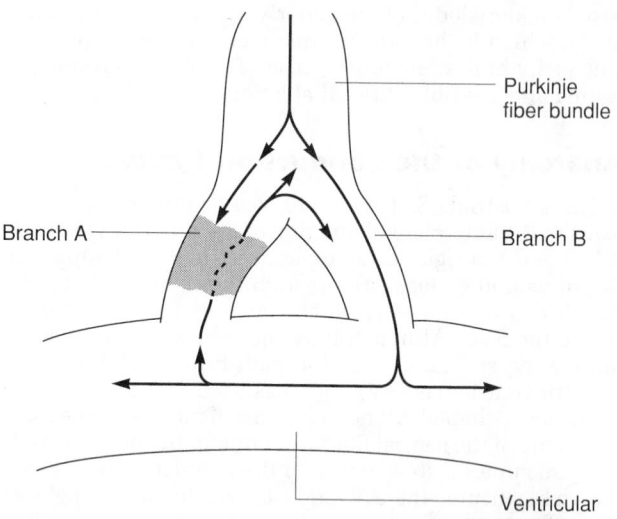

Figure 67-3. Diagram of reentry and circus movement consisting of a fiber bundle that divides into two branches (A and B). Branch A is an area of ischemic injury through which an impulse will not conduct in an antegrade direction but will conduct slowly in a retrograde direction. When an antegrade impulse arrives, it will block in A but will conduct normally through B to activate the ventricular muscle and will enter A in a retrograde fashion. Because retrograde conduction through the area of injury is slowed, the previously depolarized tissue has time to repolarize and become reexcitable. Therefore, when the impulse finally gets through the area of injury, it produces another beat, a ventricular extrasystole (premature ventricular beat). If the impulse continues to go around this reentrant circuit, it will produce a ventricular tachycardia reentrant rhythm. (After Schmitt, Erlanger. J Physiol 1929;87:326)

Electrophysiologic Testing

Electrophysiologic studies are used to document that an arrhythmia is automatic or reentrant, or of ventricular or supraventricular origin. Electrophysiologic testing is performed in a specialized cardiac catheterization laboratory with multiple invasive catheters, both on the venous and arterial sides. Electrophysiologic tests are performed in the fasting state, and all antiarrhythmic medications are discontinued at least 24 hours before the procedure.

For supraventricular arrhythmias, electrophysiologic studies can establish the presence of a Kent bundle causing Wolff-Parkinson-White (WPW) syndrome. Other arrhythmias of atrial origin, including atrial fibrillation and AV nodal reentrant tachycardia, can be diagnosed (Fig. 67-4). For suspected supraventricular arrhythmias, catheters are positioned in the high right atrium, His bundle position, and right ventricle. A catheter is also positioned in the coronary sinus through the right internal jugular vein. Leads V_1, I, and III and the intracardiac electrograms are recorded. Pacing is performed with a programmable stimulator using stimuli that are twice the diastolic threshold and 2 milliseconds in duration. During the electrophysiologic study, the effective refractory periods of the AV node and any accessory AV connections are determined, as are the anterograde and retrograde block cycle lengths of any accessory AV connection. Regional localization of accessory AV connections is made by examination of the α-wave pattern on the electrocardiogram (ECG). Localization also is based on the results of mapping of the coronary sinus and tricuspid annulus. This mapping is undertaken to identify the site of earliest ventricular activation during sinus rhythm or atrial pacing and the site of earliest atrial activation during orthodromic tachycardia or ventricular pacing. Electrophysiologic studies can define the location of the Kent bundle as left free wall if the coronary sinus catheter records earliest atrial activity during reciprocating tachycardia or ventricular pacing and when induced left bundle-branch block prolongs the ventriculoatrial (VA) interval. This location is defined as right free wall if the atrial catheter records the earliest atrial activity during tachycardia or ventricular pacing and induced right bundle-branch block prolongs the VA interval. Also possible is a septal pathway where neither left nor right bundle-branch block prolongs the VA interval.[4]

For arrhythmias of ventricular origin, the electrophysiologic study protocol consists of the introduction of one to three ventricular extrastimuli. The goal is the induction of either a sustained ventricular arrhythmia or multiple episodes of nonsustained ventricular tachycardia. Induced ventricular tachycardia persisting for 100 complexes or requiring pacing or external cardioversion for termination is termed *sustained;* tachycardia persisting for five complexes but terminating spontaneously within 100 complexes is *nonsustained.* Patients with less than five repetitive complexes in response to stimulation are considered to be noninducible. Electrophysiologic testing can also reveal whether areas of reentry are present. Rapid pacing may decrease action potential duration and shorten refractoriness in myocardium with already slowed conduction velocity. Premature or early stimuli may therefore lead to reentrant arrhythmias. Because ventricular reentry does not occur in normal myocardium, all reentrant arrhythmias, whether induced or spontaneous, are pathologic. Reentrant arrhythmias may exist as macroreentry circuits, with unidirectional block in large areas of myocardium, where an appropriate cycle length and refractory period allow the abnormal circuit to depolarize ahead of the normal cardiac impulse. This is typical of arrhythmias after myocardial infarction. More commonly, microreentry exists because of local heterogeneity, which demonstrates unidirectional block and slowed conduction at all cycle lengths. This is typical of arrhythmias due to myocardial ischemia.[5]

Drug Therapy

Antiarrhythmic drug therapy is the fundamental treatment for arrhythmias and generally should precede any surgical therapy. Antiarrhythmic drugs are classified based on their actions. The class 1 drugs are membrane-stabilizing local anesthetics, whose action is sodium channel blockade, inhibiting the rapid influx of sodium ions. Class 1 drugs reduce velocity in phase 0 of the action potential or the rate of membrane depolarization, slowing impulse conduction throughout the myocardium. The slowing of depolarization velocity is seen as an increased QRS interval. Class 1 drugs also prolong the refractory period, reduce membrane excitability, and decrease phase 4 spontaneous depolarization, thereby reducing automaticity. Class 1A drugs (quinidine, disopyramide, procainamide) cause moderate slowing and mildly prolong the QRS interval, but they also prolong the action potential and therefore the QT interval. Class 1B drugs (lidocaine, mexiletine, phenytoin, moricizine (Ethmozine), and tocainide) do not affect membrane depolarization, and the QRS interval is unaltered, but repolarization is prolonged. Class 1C drugs (flecainide, encainide, lorcainide, and propafenone) markedly reduce velocity and impulse conduction, prolonging the QRS.

Class 2 drugs (β-blocking drugs) have an antiarrhythmic action by adrenergic blockade inhibiting β-receptor stimulation through the sympathetic nervous system and circu-

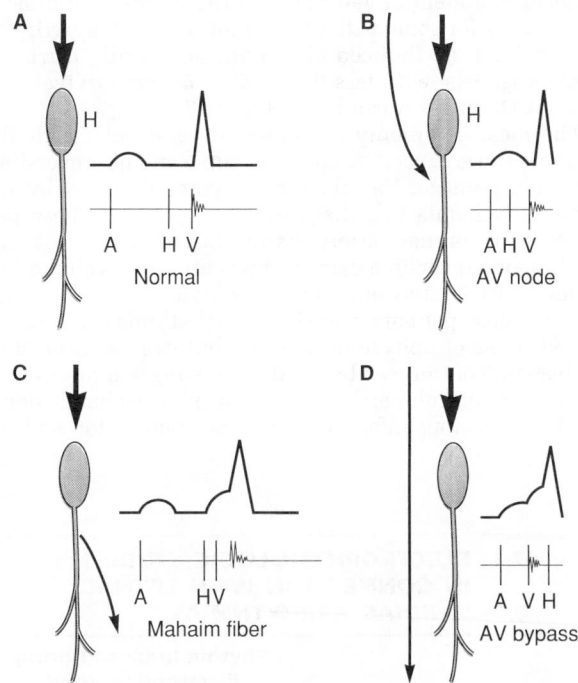

Figure 67-4. Demonstration of the anatomic atrioventricular (AV) connections as well as the surface electrogram and His electrogram for normal AV conduction (*A*), an atrial His bypass tract (*B*), a nodal ventricular bypass or Mahaim fiber (*C*), and a total AV bypass tract as found in Wolff-Parkinson-White syndrome (*D*). (After Lowe JE. Surgical treatment of the Wolff-Parkinson-White syndrome and other supraventricular tachyarrhythmias. J Cardiac Surg 1986;1:119)

lating catecholamines. All β-adrenergic blockers slow the heart rate but may have different side effects as a result of selective receptor stimulation. Class 3 drugs (bretylium, amiodarone, N-acetylprocainamide) affect membrane properties, inhibiting potassium influx into cells. There is prolongation of the action potential duration (phase 2 and 3) and of membrane repolarization. Class 4 drugs (calcium-channel blockers; verapamil, nifedipine, and diltiazem) affect slow, channel-dependent pacemaker tissue (SA and AV nodes) and generate a slowed action potential mediated by calcium ion influxes into the myocardium. Digitalis, although not a slow calcium-calcium blocking drug, also exerts its effects in pacemaker tissue.[6]

Serial drug testing during electrophysiologic testing can be performed to assess the effects of pharmacologic interventions in patients with inducible arrhythmias. Patients are administered intravenous antiarrhythmic agents to a known blood concentration. Suppression of a sustained arrhythmia is defined as the induction of less than 10 complexes in response to the stimulation protocol. Effective suppression of nonsustained ventricular tachycardia is defined as the induction of fewer than five repetitive complexes.

Arrhythmia recurrence rate is lower when drugs are selected by invasive testing.[7] When noninvasive methods are used to evaluate antiarrhythmic drug efficacy, about 40% to 70% of patients appear to respond initially with the elimination of arrhythmias. When electrophysiologically guided testing is used, the response to any antiarrhythmic agent is only 10% to 30%, demonstrating that noninvasive selection of drugs can be misleading.

Postoperative supraventricular arrhythmias (atrial flutter, paroxysmal atrial tachycardia, or atrial fibrillation) are the most common arrhythmias encountered in surgical practice. A long rhythm strip or an atrial lead tracing differentiates these arrhythmias from sinus tachycardia, which rarely exceeds 120 beats/min. Usually, the ventricular response in atrial flutter is 2:1, with a ventricular rate of 150 and an atrial rate of 300, whereas paroxysmal atrial tachycardia has a 1:1 atrium-to-ventricle response. In contrast, atrial fibrillation is an irregularly irregular rhythm. The atrial electrogram varies up to 500 beats/min. Although vagal maneuvers may break paroxysmal atrial tachycardia, the ventricular response in atrial fibrillation and flutter only slows slightly, owing to vagal effects on the AV node. Each of these arrhythmias is capable of producing hypotension and myocardial ischemia; therefore, patients with compromised vital signs, hypotension, heart rate greater than 150 beats/min, or ECG or clinical evidence of myocardial ischemia demand urgent therapy. Patients with stable vital signs can be treated in a less emergent fashion. In either group, the initial goal is ventricular rate control and then conversion to normal sinus rhythm. Once rhythm identification is obtained, an attempt at atrial overdrive pacing should be performed for paroxysmal atrial tachycardia or atrial flutter. In postoperative cardiac surgical patients, this can be accomplished with temporary wires in place. This may result in conversion to normal sinus rhythm. Verapamil, in a test dose of 0.5 mg intravenously, followed by 2.5 mg every 10 minutes, is the most effective method of rate control and often causes cardioversion. Digoxin, 0.5 mg intravenously, is given to adult patients once the potassium level is normal. Digitalization to a dose of 1 to 1.5 mg is completed on a schedule of every 4 hours. Intravenous diltiazem has been shown to be effective for ventricular rate control. Rarely are patients severely compromised by rapid supraventricular tachyarrhythmia to the extent that emergency cardioversion (50 to 400 J) is required. This may occasionally occur and requires mild sedation. Cardioversion of patients on di-

goxin should be undertaken carefully because these patients are prone to ventricular fibrillation. Rate control of supraventricular arrhythmias is achieved when the ventricular response is between 80 and 110. At this point, most patients convert to normal sinus rhythm without the addition of other agents. If the supraventricular arrhythmia continues after 48 hours, addition of a class 1A drug for cardioversion is advised. When treating patients with supraventricular arrhythmias, a ventricular-demand pacemaker should be available in case of bradycardia.

Ventricular Arrhythmias

Some 450,000 people experience sudden cardiac death (SCD) each year in the United States, and although 30% survive this sudden death episode, it is the largest single cause of death in the United States. Although 25% of cases of SCD are due to an acute myocardial infarction, 75% of patients die from ventricular arrhythmias, with a history of previous myocardial infarction. Ventricular arrhythmias during an acute myocardial infarction are common, easily treated, and do not alter the prognosis; however, late ventricular arrhythmias (after 48 hours) are less common, harder to treat (only one third of the patients respond to drugs), and worsen prognosis. The mortality rate of refractory ventricular tachycardia after myocardial infarction is at least 70%; it is the most common rhythm found at electrophysiologic testing, regardless of the rhythm causing SCD[8] (Table 67-1).

Patients with SCD, recurrent ventricular tachycardia, or recurrent syncope from a cardiac arrhythmia have a 30% to 40% recurrence rate of SCD at 1-year follow-up. Survival on empiric antiarrhythmic drug therapy is not improved, and although electrophysiologically guided drug therapy is effective, a large percentage of patients are either noninducible or not controlled by drug therapy alone. Therefore, surgical treatment of ventricular arrhythmias is of utmost importance for some patients. A ventricular tachyarrhythmia that can be induced electrophysiologically carries a poor prognosis, with less than a 50% 5-year survival rate from SCD, unless it can be abolished.[9]

The most commonly encountered ventricular arrhythmias are those caused by both reversible and nonreversible ischemic damage. Ventricular arrhythmia caused by reversible ischemia is a diagnosis of exclusion. These patients have coronary artery disease but no myocardial infarction or irreversible damage, no ventricular wall motion abnormality, and essentially normal left ventricular function. In these patients, ventricular arrhythmias are not induced by electrophysiologic study but can be associated with angina or induced by treadmill testing. Far more common are ventricular arrhythmias caused by ischemic damage from previous infarctions. The mechanism for ventric-

Table 67-1. ELECTROPHYSIOLOGIC STUDIES IN CONNECTION WITH LETHAL CARDIAC ARRHYTHMIAS

Sudden Cardiac Death or Arrest Rhythm	Rhythm Induced During Electrophysiologic Studies (%)	
	Ventricular Tachycardia	Ventricular Fibrillation
Ventricular tachycardia (25%)	83	5
Ventricular fibrillation (65%)	77	10
Unknown (10%)	66	—

ular tachycardia in these patients is usually microreentry found in the nonhomogeneous ischemic border zones of previous infarctions, where normal myocardial fibers are interspersed with scarring. Two thirds to three quarters of these patients have associated ventricular aneurysms, and conversely, 15% of all left ventricular aneurysms have significant ventricular arrhythmias. This morphologic substrate for arrhythmias may be worsened by stresses caused by the aneurysm and the subendocardial scarring, which usually extends beyond the aneurysm. Ventricular fibrillation in these patients with ischemic damage from previous infarctions originates from anterolateral wall in three quarters and inferoposterior wall in one quarter, whereas the septum is the most common site of origin of ventricular tachycardia. Therefore, aneurysmectomy alone is not adequate therapy for arrhythmias associated with aneurysms.[10]

Other underlying causes of ventricular arrhythmias are varied and include idiopathic ventricular tachycardia with no other evidence of cardiac disease. Although results from surgery for idiopathic ventricular tachycardia have generally been poor, occasional cases are amenable to ventriculotomy, excision, or cryoablation, and these patients should undergo electrophysiologic testing. Other causes include nonischemic cardiomyopathy caused by coxsackievirus and sarcoid. These arrhythmias usually originate in the right ventricle, with results of treatment similar to idiopathic tachycardia. A specific cause of ventricular arrhythmia is arrhythmogenic right ventricular dysplasia, which is a congenital transmural infiltration of the right ventricular wall with adipose tissue, causing the right ventricle to bulge, weaken, and form aneurysms. The right ventricular apex, infundibulum, and posterobasal regions are the most commonly affected areas. Uhl syndrome is a variant of arrhythmogenic right ventricular dysplasia and demonstrates complete absence of muscle in the right ventricular free wall, leading to arrhythmias and heart failure. Surgical treatment involves a transmural ventriculotomy to isolate the arrhythmogenic area and may require disconnecting the entire right ventricular free wall.[11] Another unusual cause of ventricular arrhythmias is the long QT-interval syndrome, involving abnormalities of repolarization and associated with torsades de pointes, a polymorphic ventricular tachycardia with a long QT interval on baseline ECG and polymorphic ventricular tachycardia characterized by rhythmic changes in QRS amplitude. The initial beat is usually not premature nor automatic. The long QT-interval syndrome can result from congenital long QT with syncope and deafness as well as viral, ischemic, drug-induced (quinidine, procainamide, disopyramide, thiodiphenylamine (Phenothiazine), and tricyclic antidepressants) and metabolic (starvation and hypokalemia) causes. The treatment of long QT-interval syndrome includes β-blockers, phenytoin (Dilantin), phenobarbital, Mg^{2+}, and automatic internal cardioverter-defibrillator (AICD) placement. There is no specific surgical therapy.

Early surgical approaches to ventricular arrhythmias included indirect approaches such as coronary artery bypass grafting (CABG), sympathectomy, and nonguided aneurysm resection. These resulted in a 20% to 40% mortality rate with up to a 40% recurrence rate. CABG decreases SCD in patients with significant multivessel coronary artery disease and a history of heart failure. These patients had not had prior arrhythmias. The effect of bypass surgery in patients who experienced ventricular tachycardia or ventricular fibrillation before revascularization is unknown. SCD patients with significant multivessel coronary artery disease, who are noninducible for ventricular arrhythmias at electrophysiologic study, have fair survival with revascularization alone. The effect of coronary revascularization in patients who have inducible ventricular arrhythmias is less predictable. Polymorphic ventricular tachycardia or ventricular fibrillation may not be controlled with revascularization, whereas monomorphic ventricular tachycardias usually are not improved and may be an indication for implantation of an AICD.[12]

Management

Reentry as a mechanism for ischemic ventricular tachycardia was proposed in 1927, but it was not until 1962 that studies demonstrated the marked inhomogeneity of injured tissue after infarction, resulting in an ischemic border zone and reentry. This area is responsible for fragmentation of the action potential with microreentry. Macroreentry through large areas is also a mechanism for ventricular arrhythmias after myocardial infarction. Based on this concept, the modern era of ventricular tachycardia surgery has shown improvement in results from intraoperative mapping techniques resulting in aggressive resection aimed at the ischemic border zone, encircling endocardial ventriculotomy, and extended endocardial resection.

Catheter Technique. Catheter ablation for ventricular tachycardia remains disappointing. In two studies of direct-current endocardial ablation in patients with ventricular tachycardia, only about 25% of patients remained free of recurrent arrhythmia when all antiarrhythmic drug therapy was stopped. Complex activation sequence mapping is required because the area of ablation produced by the catheter is much less than that at operation and therefore requires a hemodynamically well-tolerated tachycardia.[13] Other approaches, such as transcoronary chemical and alcohol ablation, have been described, but their success is poor and usefulness limited.

Operative Techniques. Direct surgical approaches are indicated when a patient is refractory to medical treatment, inducible at electrophysiologic testing, an acceptable risk, and has apparent scar or aneurysm. Contraindications to surgery include noninducible at electrophysiologic testing, ventricular failure, poor risk, and recent myocardial infarction. With these guidelines, electrophysiologically guided surgical ablation is efficacious and safe. First reported in 1959, the surgical approach uses preoperative and intraoperative electrophysiologic mapping to identify a specific arrhythmia site of origin. Before surgery, patients undergo catheterization and electrophysiologic study. Both coronary angiography and ventriculography are required to determine whether the patient is suitable and to determine whether other procedures are required (eg, CABG, valve surgery). Monomorphic ventricular tachycardia is the arrhythmia that is most amenable to surgical resection, but some patients who also have inducible ventricular fibrillation are eligible, if the arrhythmia is converted to a monomorphic tachycardia during antiarrhythmic drug therapy.

During surgery, ventricular tachycardia is induced by programmed stimulation after initiation of normothermic cardiopulmonary bypass. Endocardial and epicardial activation sequence maps are obtained by using transmitral balloons with electrodes on the surface or multiple epicardial plunge electrodes. Tachycardia sites are defined as the earliest presystolic electrical diastole. Because patients may have more than one inducible tachycardia, multiple mappings can be obtained between resections and cryoablations.

Modern surgical methods include encircling endocardial ventriculotomy.[14] The myocardium is incised outside the area of scar (1 cm deep on septum, nearly to epicardium on the free wall). Encircling endocardial ventriculotomy is thought to interrupt reentry, isolate abnormal substrate, or make the region totally ischemic and electrically silent because the ischemic border zone between fibrous scarred tissue and normal myocardium is the initiator for most ventricular arrhythmias. By incising circumferentially around an area of infarction, a fibrous barrier might be created, isolating the arrhythmogenic region from the rest of the myocardium. These isolation procedures are simple and do not require detailed mapping and localization of arrhythmias, but they often result in compromised ventricular function. They are not applicable to large areas of scar. Furthermore, one cannot cut closer than 5 mm to the aortic and mitral annuli, so encircling endocardial ventriculotomy is best for focal scars on the left ventricular free wall. Encircling endocardial ventriculotomy is seldom performed because of a higher mortality rate and impairment of left ventricular function.

The surgical procedure of choice is extended endocardial resection, which uses mapping to identify the area of scar to be excised.[15] The aneurysm is opened and endocardial mapping performed. A dissection plane is developed between normal myocardium and the ischemic border zone to resect all endocardial fibroses. Septal involvement may require a septal patch; if aneurysm resection results in a small, distorted left ventricle, an enlarging patch is placed. The papillary muscles and posteroinferior sites of early activation are most likely to lead to recurrence and are probably best treated by endocardial cryoablation.[16] Endocardial cryoablation uses a 1- to 2-cm probe with the tissue cooled to −60C for 2 minutes. This results in loss of cellular viability and electrical activation, whereas collagen matrix and structural integrity are preserved. Endocardial cryoablation is best in areas that cannot be resected (papillary muscles and valve annuli) and in localized ventricular tachycardia of nonischemic origin, but there is a high rate of recurrence if endocardial cryoablation is used alone for septal scars. Laser ablations also have been used with success. Finally, in patients in whom mapping data are poor, a visually guided extended endocardial resection can be performed. Some centers also implant AICD patches in these patients, in case the arrhythmia has not been successfully ablated.

Operative mortality is about 10% for extended endocardial resection for ventricular arrhythmia, whereas the rate for encircling endocardial ventriculotomy remains above 20%. Arrhythmias recur in 20% to 30% of cases, and only 50% can be medically controlled postoperatively. Postoperative inducibility (a positive postoperative electrophysiologic study) is a strong predictor of poor outcome, with early or late death increased by 19-fold if the postoperative electrophysiologic study is positive. With a negative postoperative electrophysiologic study, there is still a late postoperative sudden death rate of 4% over 5 years, and the 5-year survival rate is 60% to 70%.

Favorable intraoperative factors that affect postoperative inducibility include generalized resections, which are more effective than localized ones, map-guided resections, and mapping of the warm, beating heart. In appropriate patients, operative mortality is acceptably low, control of arrhythmia is high, and surgical therapy may be the first-choice therapy.[17]

Implantable Devices. Implantable devices allow treatment of patients with ventricular tachycardia or fibrillation who have unfavorable anatomy or unsuitable arrhythmias for direct surgery. Initially, these devices recognized only ventricular fibrillation, but ventricular tachycardia often precedes ventricular fibrillation, and therefore recognition of ventricular tachycardia with cardioversion capability was included. Since 1980, the AICD has been shown to be effective treatment for patients with both sustained ventricular tachycardia and fibrillation.[18] An AICD includes an arrhythmia detection circuit, a power source, and capacitors capable of storing and releasing electric current. Electrodes are used for cardioversion and defibrillating, rate sensing, and ventricular pacing. The leads are implanted by sternotomy, thoracotomy, or subxiphoid approach tunneled to the generator in a subcutaneous abdominal pouch. Arrhythmia detection by an AICD is based either on rate criterion or ECG morphology analysis. When rate cutoff is used, it is set high enough to distinguish between the highest sinus rate and the patient's ventricular tachycardia rate. QRS morphology analysis recognizes the time that the ECG remains off the isoelectric baseline zone. Once an arrhythmia requiring termination is sensed, the AICD may begin antitachycardia pacing, low-energy cardioversion, high-energy defibrillation, or some combination. Complications of AICDs have included programming errors, component failures, and technical problems, including infections (1% to 5%), generator migration, and skin erosion. Inappropriate shocks due to supraventricular arrhythmias exceeding the rate cutoff and oversensing of nonsustained arrhythmias may also occur. Because arrhythmias still occur with an implanted AICD, patient symptoms occur before arrhythmia termination. This may restrict the patient's life-style and preclude driving or employment. Therefore, the patient may become a candidate for direct ventricular arrhythmia surgery.[19]

Although there have been no randomized controlled trials, survival after AICD is excellent. There is about a 50% improvement in mortality rate when AICD-treated patients are compared with patients treated with drugs. This includes 95% freedom from SCD, as opposed to only 50% in patients without AICD 5 years after implantation.[18] Candidates for AICD implantation include patients with drug-refractory ventricular tachycardia and globally depressed left ventricular function without aneurysm, patients whose arrhythmia is noninducible at electrophysiologic study, and patients who have frequent ventricular tachycardias but who are not candidates for direct resection. Because the AICD is effective in preventing death from malignant ventricular arrhythmias refractory to medical therapy, it has been implanted in patients awaiting cardiac transplantation. The mortality rate of cardiac transplant recipients approaches 65% at 2 years, and four fifths of these deaths are due to dysrhythmia.[20] In one study,[21] despite poor ventricular function (mean ejection fraction, 13%), all patients survived AICD implantation and have either had cardiac transplantation or await transplantation. These patients received a mean of 14 AICD shocks. One patient received 19 shocks in the 24-hour period before transplantation.

Surgical Treatment of Supraventricular Arrhythmias

Supraventricular arrhythmias are caused by automatic or reentrant sources in normally present, although diseased, myocardial tissues or from abnormal anatomy. The diagnosis of abnormal accessory pathways depends on electrophysiologic investigation. Electrophysiologic studies for supraventricular tachycardia (SVT) require placement of catheters in the high right atrium, in the low right atrium, near the bundle of His, in the coronary sinus, and in the right ventricle apex. These catheters can be used to generate a His bundle electrogram, which permits identification of the presence and type of accessory pathway. These abnormal accessory pathways (Fig. 67-5) may include atrial to AV node bypass fibers, Mahaim fibers (His–ventricular or nodoventricular connection), or Kent bundles (complete AV bypass), causing WPW syndrome.

WPW syndrome may account for up to 20% of all cases

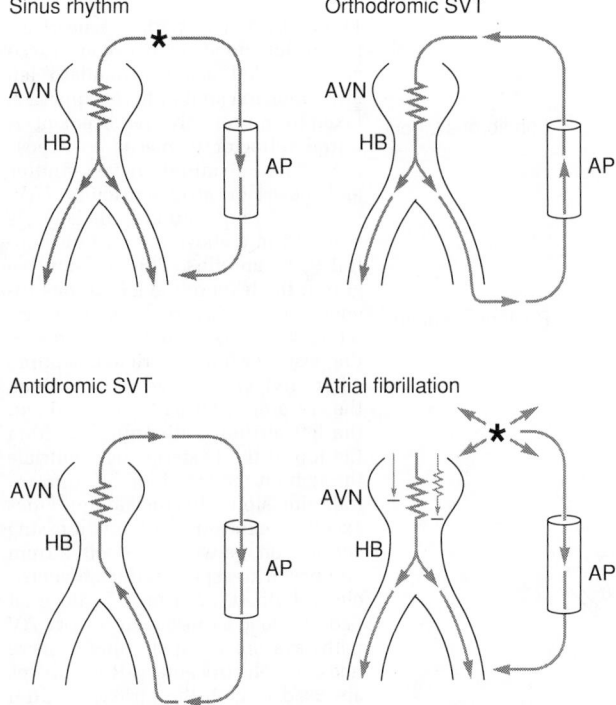

Sinus rhythm   Orthodromic SVT

Antidromic SVT   Atrial fibrillation

Figure 67-5. Schematic representations of the conduction patterns through an accessory pathway (AP) and the normal conduction system (AVN and HB) during sinus rhythm, orthodromic supraventricular tachycardia (SVT), antidromic SVT, and atrial fibrillation. (After Lowe JE. Surgical treatment of the Wolff-Parkinson-White syndrome and other supraventricular tachyarrhythmias. J Cardiac Surg 1986;1:119)

through the AV node and retrograde up the Kent bundle. Kent bundles have short refractory periods that permit rapid and dangerous ventricular responses (by antegrade conduction) to atrial fibrillation or flutter. Although the normal AV node refractory period does not allow a ventricular rate greater than 180, Kent bundles have been observed to conduct up to 400 beats/min and can degenerate to ventricular tachycardia or ventricular fibrillation with lethal consequences (Fig. 67-6).

The clinical features of WPW syndrome include an α wave with short PR interval (<0.12 seconds) on ECG; an α wave can be seen in 0.25% of the population without history of SVT. These patients have normal life expectancies if there is no clinical history of SVT; 75% to 85% present with SVT, including paroxysmal atrial tachycardia, atrial fibrillation, and atrial flutter; and some present with ventricular tachycardia or ventricular fibrillation. The medical therapy of WPW syndrome includes procaine, quinidine, propanolol (Inderal), verapamil, and amiodarone, but it is not particularly successful. The mainstay of treatment is catheter-delivered radiofrequency ablation or the preferred surgical interruption of the Kent bundle. The indication for ablation is primarily recurrent SVT in acceptable-risk patients. Mapping is performed with reference electrodes on the right atrium and ventricle, and with a hand-held or fixed exploring electrode to measure activation times at the AV groove. Normally, the earliest ventricular epicardial breakthrough is on the low anterior right ventricle because this is the point of earliest exit from a normally conducting His bundle. Conventional activation studies localize the accessory pathway along the AV groove but cannot define whether the pathway is epicardial, intramural, or endocardial in depth (Fig. 67-7). Results of histologic studies demonstrate that accessory pathways can originate or insert at any level extending from the endocardium to the epicardium and may cross tangentially. Therefore, intraoperative mapping is performed to reconfirm the location of the bypass tract. In a 1989 report, the atrial and ventricular activation times along the AV groove were measured in 23 patients, and an overlap of

of paroxysmal SVT and may have a prevalence as high as 1 in 500 patients in the general population.[22] Although patients with WPW syndrome may be asymptomatic, some can suffer serious or fatal consequences. Surgical division of an accessory AV pathway for the treatment of WPW syndrome was begun in 1968, and the results in the first 200 patients demonstrated an overall success rate of 86%, including a reoperation rate of about 15%.[23] In most of these patients, the disease became totally asymptomatic. The pathophysiology of the WPW syndrome is the Kent bundle (0.5 to 1 mm wide), of which 10% to 20% are multiple (Table 67-2). Under normal conditions, the accessory pathway conducts antegrade (as does the normal AV node–His bundle) and causes early ventricular excitation, hence the α wave and the short PR interval. Some 15% of patients conduct only retrograde (concealed) and therefore technically do not have WPW syndrome. Reciprocating (reentry) tachycardia impulses usually pass antegrade

Table 67-2. ELECTROCARDIOGRAPHIC INDICATORS OF KENT BUNDLE ACTIVITY

Location of Kent Bundles	Occurrence (%)	Surface ECG
Left free wall	50	Q wave in leads V_4–V_6
Postero septum	25	Q wave in leads II, III, F
Right free wall	15	LBBB
Antero septum	10	LBBB, inferior axis

LBBB, left bundle-branch block.

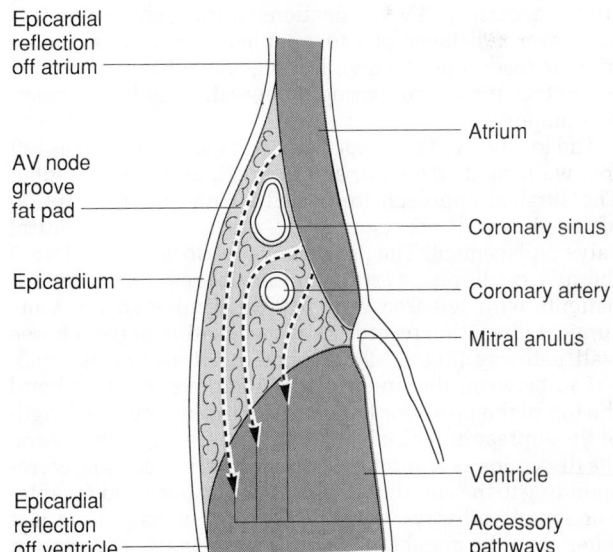

Figure 67-6. Cross-section of the posterior left heart shows the different locations that left free-wall pathways can be located in relation to the mitral annulus and the overlying epicardium at the AV groove. (After Cox JL, Ferguson. Surgery for the Wolff-Parkinson-White syndrome: the endocardial approach. Semin Thorac Cardiovasc Surg 1989;1:34)

Epicardial reflection off atrium

AV node groove fat pad

Epicardium

Epicardial reflection off ventricle

Atrium

Coronary sinus

Coronary artery

Mitral anulus

Ventricle

Accessory pathways

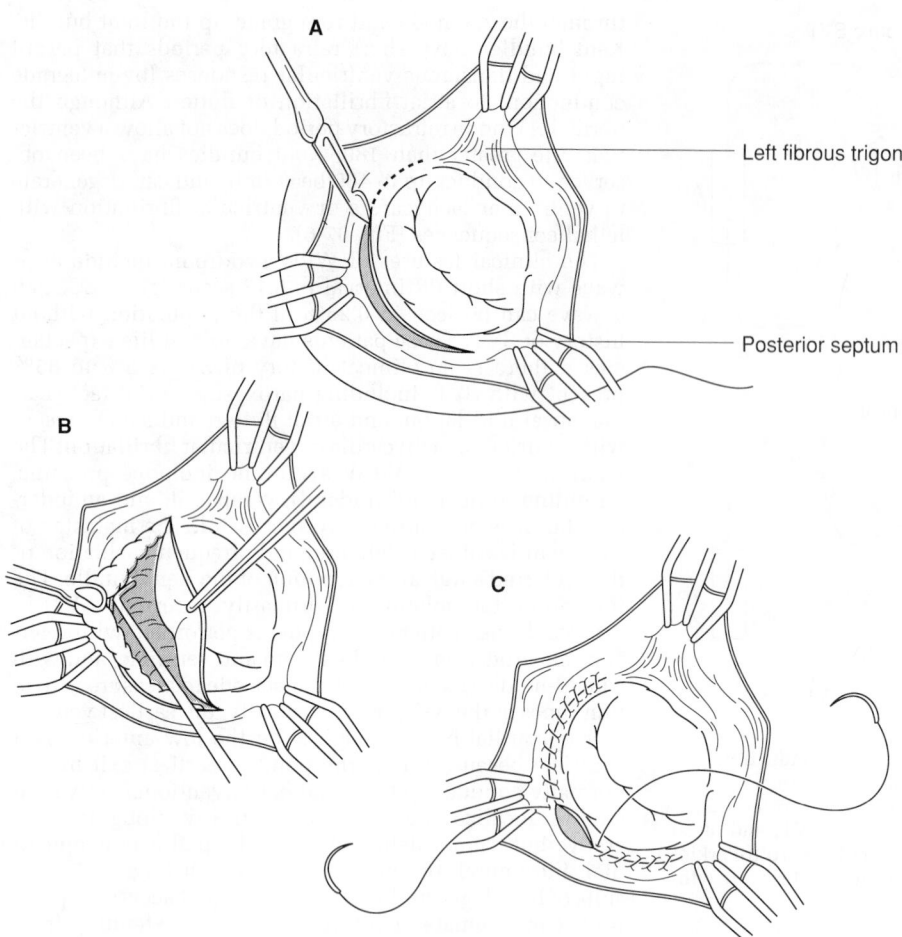

Left fibrous trigone

Posterior septum

Figure 67-7. (*A*) With the heart arrested, left-sided pathways are surgically divided using a standard left atrial incision similar to the approach taken for mitral valve replacement. A mitral retractor is placed to expose the posterior mitral valve annulus and posterior atrioventricular (AV) groove. A supraannular incision is placed 2 mm above the posterior mitral valve annulus. This incision begins at the level of the left fibrous trigone and is carried in a counterclockwise fashion to the area of the posterior interventricular septum. After division of the endocardium, the AV groove fat pad is entered and the left atrium is disconnected from the top of the posterior left ventricle throughout the length of the supraannular incision. This incision provides excellent exposure, and any crossing connection between the left atrium and posterior aspect of the left ventricle is divided. (*B*) The AV groove fat pad has been exposed. Accessory AV pathways are divided using a nerve hook and electrocautery. Ring forceps are used to grab the posterior mitral valve annulus and posterior aspect of the left ventricle. (*C*) After completion of the left-sided dissection, the supraannular incision is closed using a continuous suture. (After Bolling SF, Morady F, Calkins H, et al. Current treatment for Wolff-Parkinson-White syndrome. Ann Thorac Surg 1991; 15:461)

the atrial and ventricular insertions was reported.[24] These observations suggested that wide surgical dissection along the AV groove was more likely to divide the aberrant conduction pathways, even if epicardial mapping disclosed only a discrete area of preexcitation. In a second anatomic study, accessory AV connections were demonstrated to slant over a distance of 1 to 2 cm between atrial and ventricular insertions.[25] These findings have been confirmed in another report comparing preoperative and intraoperative mapping.

The locations of accessory pathways are classified as left free wall, right free wall, anteroseptal, and posteroseptal. The surgical approach to the left atrium for interruption of left free wall accessory pathways is similar to mitral valve replacement. The dissection is performed with hypothermia, cardioplegic arrest, and aortic cross-clamping. All patients with left free wall pathways undergo the same surgical dissection regardless of the location of the left free wall pathway (Fig. 67-8). A plane of dissection is established between the underlying AV groove of fat pad and the top of the posterior left ventricle throughout the length of the supraannular incision. For right free wall pathways, the dissection is around the tricuspid valve annulus, corresponding to the anterior and posterior leaflets; and for anterior septal pathways, an atrial incision is made from just anterior to the membranous portion of ventricular septum clockwise around to the right ventricle free wall.[23] The epicardial approach involves the same concept of completely removing any abnormal AV connections, but the dissection is begun on the epicardial surface. This method has had the same success as the endocardial method but has drawbacks, including injury to the coronary sinus and

missed subendocardial pathways. In a study on the surgical treatment of WPW syndrome in which patients were divided equally into the classic endocardial technique versus the epicardial technique, each group had aberrant pathways successfully ablated in 22 of the 25 patients (88%).[26] Fewer than 20% had even minor postoperative complications. The epicardial approach is now routinely supplemented by cryotherapy. Cryolesions do not appear to cause arrhythmias and also are applicable to AV node bypass and Mahaim fibers.[27]

After the surgical procedure, repeat atrial and ventricular pacing is performed. If the accessory pathway has been divided successfully, the QRS complex is normal, and the AV interval increases progressively during atrial pacing as a Wenckebach phenomenon develops. There should be no evidence of ventricular preexcitation. Retrograde conduction can be assessed by measuring VA intervals during incremental ventricular pacing. About half of patients who have successful division of accessory pathways demonstrate VA block postoperatively. Patients with intact VA conduction should demonstrate a retrograde Wenckebach phenomenon, typical of retrograde conduction through the normal AV conduction system. Failure to demonstrate VA block or decremental retrograde conduction suggests that an accessory pathway is still present, and mapping should be repeated. Rarely, the accessory pathway was traumatized at operation but not divided completely. Abnormal conduction usually recurs within 72 hours postoperatively. Accordingly, incremental atrial and ventricular pacing should be repeated before hospital discharge, and evidence of preexcitation, fixed VA conduction intervals, or initiation of SVT requires that electrophysiologic testing be repeated.

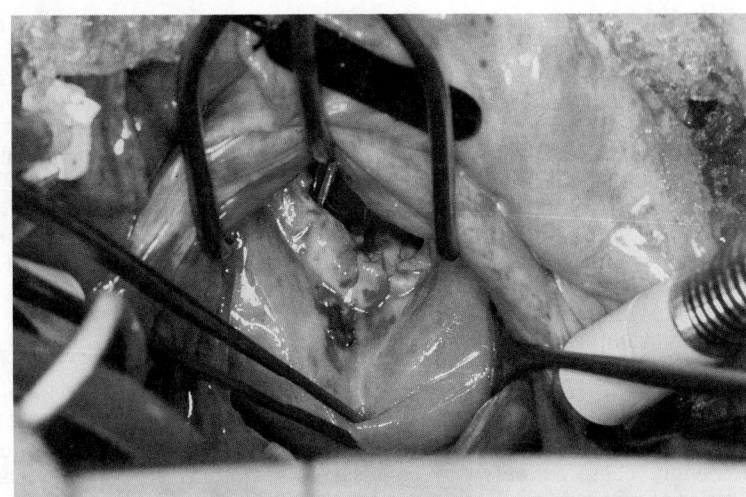

Figure 67-8. Shown is the atrial side of the mitral annulus in a patient who underwent four separate unsuccessful sessions of radiofrequency energy application. There is central hemorrhage and necrosis, with surrounding edema typically seen with radiofrequency lesions. Intraoperative mapping demonstrated that this was the area of accessory conduction. This patient was successfully treated with surgery.

In the first 200 patients undergoing surgery for WPW syndrome, surgical division of the accessory pathway was successful in 98% of right free wall pathways, 92% of left free wall pathways, and 77% of posteroseptal pathways.[23] After 1981, widening the operative field of dissection resulted in an increase in the overall success rate from 86% to 99%, a decrease in reoperation from 19.5% to zero, and a decrease in the incidence of heart block from 10.5% to 0.9%. The mortality rate was 5.5% in one series, but only one death occurred after elective surgery in the absence of associated cardiac anomalies. In a combined series, 20% of patients had multiple accessory pathways, 12% had Ebstein anomaly, 34% had other arrhythmias, 6% had cardiomyopathy, and 6% had coronary artery disease.[23] Since the initial surgical series for WPW syndrome was reported, this procedure has been applied to increasing numbers of patients with the disease, with hundreds of operations being performed each year. Reports have suggested that catheter ablation of accessory AV connections using radiofrequency current can also be accomplished with a high success rate in patients with WPW syndrome.[4,28] Catheter ablation of identified abnormal pathways can be performed using radiofrequency energy at 350 kHz. Twenty-five to 36 watts is delivered for 10 to 20 seconds, or until a sudden rise in impedance indicates coagulum formation (see Fig. 67-8).

One study[22] examined the results of surgical treatment for WPW syndrome and compared and contrasted results with those of patients undergoing radiofrequency catheter ablation. From 1986 to 1991, 123 patients underwent operation for ablation of aberrant conduction pathways (Table 67-3). There were 85 male subjects and 38 female subjects, ranging in age from 11 months to 68 years. Associated abnormalities included Ebstein anomaly, sudden death syndrome, coronary artery disease, cardiomyopathy, abdominal aortic aneurysm, neurofibromatosis, other arrhythmias, and other complex congenital heart disease. Forty-one patients had multiple accessory pathways. Operative results showed a 7% initial failure rate, which dropped to 3% after reoperation. Procedures performed concomitantly included mitral or tricuspid valve repair or replacement, right ventricular conduit replacement, subaortic resection, Fontan repair, corrected transposition repair, CABG, and placement of an AICD. There was no operative mortality, late follow-up was 27 ± 16 months, and complications included mitral regurgitation and myocardial infarction.

By comparison, in 12 months, 124 patients with WPW syndrome underwent catheter ablation using radiofrequency current. There were 9 patients with multiple pathways. One hundred and twelve patients (90%) had all accessory AV connections ablated and have remained free of symptomatic tachycardia. There have been 12 failures (10%), of which 5 have had surgery, and 7 are being treated medically. Mean follow-up was 7 ± 5 months, and complications included circumflex coronary artery occlusion, excessive bleeding, valve perforation, and cerebral vascular accident. This comparison study demonstrated that both surgical ablation (97%) and radiofrequency ablation (90%) offer excellent success with low morbidity for the treatment of WPW syndrome.

Other factors must be considered when comparing and contrasting the two modes of ablation therapy. The first factor is that of cost. In a study of 22 patients with WPW syndrome, the cost of radiofrequency catheter ablation was compared with that of surgical ablation. Catheter ablation was successful in 8 of 11 patients (73%), whereas in the surgical group, the accessory pathway was successfully ablated in all patients. The mean duration of hospitalization was 6 ± 2 days in the catheter group versus 8 ± 4 days in the surgical group. The mean cost per patient expressed in 1988 values was about $14,000 ± $4500 in the radiofrequency catheter group, as compared with $34,000

Table 67-3. SURGERY VERSUS RADIOFREQUENCY CATHETER ABLATION (RFCA) IN THE TREATMENT OF PATIENTS WITH WOLFF-PARKINSON-WHITE SYNDROME

	Surgery	RFCA
Patients	123	124
Age	26 ± 13 y	36 ± 14 y
Male	69%	59%
Duration of symptoms	11 ± 10 y	14 ± 13 y
Failed drugs	2.7 ± 1.8	2.1 ± 1.6
Follow-up	26 ± 7 mo	7 ± 4 mo
Other abnormality	13 (11%)	5 (4%)
Accessory pathways (total)	166	133
Multiple accessory pathways	41	9
Antero septum	10	3
Left free wall	87	85
Right free wall	21	17
Postero septum	43	22
Intermediate septum	5	6

± \$5400 in the surgical ablation group ($P < .001$). The mean time lost from work or school was 10 days in the radiofrequency catheter ablation group and 60 days in the surgical group. Even assuming eventual switch to surgical ablation in the failed radiofrequency catheter ablation patients, the mean cost of therapy in the catheter ablation group was \$24,000 ± \$4700, still significantly less than surgical cost.[29] With the great success of catheter ablation for WPW syndrome and the widespread availability of electrophysiologic diagnostic laboratories, the standard practice for the treatment of WPW syndrome is catheter ablation, with surgery only infrequently used.

Other examples of catheter ablation replacing surgical treatment are for AV nodal reentrant tachycardias and for the creation of complete AV block. Discrete cryosurgery has been performed in patients with AV nodal reentrant tachycardia, which is believed to be a microreentry phenomenon. These patients may have severe symptoms. In a series of cryosurgical cases, postoperative electrophysiologic studies in all patients documented the persistence of only a single AV conduction pathway. Moreover, AV nodal reentry could not be induced postoperatively, nor has it recurred.[30] However, like the treatment for WPW syndrome, most cases of AV nodal reentry are now easily treated by catheter ablation. Furthermore, for the creation of permanent AV block (indicated for some patients with fast rate response to refractory atrial fibrillation), complete surgical division of the bundle of His is frequently unsuccessful, because microscopic His bundle fibers result in continued AV conduction. Early efforts at inducing permanent complete AV block included attempted sharp division of the bundle of His; electrocautery of the bundle of His, the AV node, or both; and suture ligation of the AV node. Electrocautery of the His bundle results more commonly in complete AV block, but this injury can produce atrial septal defects, aneurysms, and VA fistulas. Surgical resection of the AV node is effective in creating permanent AV block but is a difficult and time-consuming procedure. Catheter ablation of the His bundle avoids many of these problems and has evolved as the most rapid and reliable method for producing permanent AV block.

AV nodal reentry and the WPW syndrome are not the only supraventricular arrhythmias that can be approached surgically. Atrial fibrillation affects more than 1 million people in the United States alone, and despite medical treatment for rate control, patients still suffer from irregular rates, impaired hemodynamics from the loss of AV synchrony, and possible thromboembolic phenomena. In the past, surgery for atrial fibrillation was directed toward alleviating the rate-related hemodynamic effects rather than toward ablation of the arrhythmia. Surgical interruption of AV conduction was effective in controlling the ventricular rate response during atrial fibrillation or flutter in patients resistant to medical control. Different investigators have shown, both in animal studies and in human series, that it is possible to perform a series of atrial incisions, known as the *maze procedure,* to prevent atrial reentry and allow sinus node impulses to activate the entire atrial myocardium.[31] A review of the 5-year experience with the maze procedure for atrial fibrillation reported that on 75 patients who underwent the operation. The operative mortality rate was only 1.3%, and at 3-months follow-up, 98% of the patients were shown to be cured of atrial fibrillation and to have restored atrial ventricular synchrony and preserved atrial transport function. The maze procedure was curative without the need for medication in 58 of 65 patients, and 6 other patients remain in normal sinus rhythm on medication.[30] Other series[32] confirm the efficacy of the results of the maze procedure for atrial fibrillation and have documented by two-dimensional echocardiography

the reestablishment of AV synchrony and contraction of both atria. Furthermore, a series of nearly 100 patients from Japan who underwent the maze procedure at the time of mitral valve reconstruction for mitral regurgitation, who were in atrial fibrillation at the time of surgery, showed remarkable long-term recovery of atrial ventricular synchrony.[33] These early results support the conclusion that the maze procedure may be the treatment of choice in patients with medically refractory symptomatic atrial fibrillation. This type of maze surgery for atrial fibrillation appears to be a promising new area of arrhythmia surgery.

PERICARDIUM

The pericardium was described in the Dead Sea Scrolls and by Homer and Galen; however, its function is still not well understood. Schuh in 1840 reported the first successful surgery for pericardial disease, a trocar pericardiocentesis for a pericardial effusion, while Hallopeau in 1898 undertook the first pericardiectomy.

Anatomy and Embryology

The pericardium is a coelomic compartment derived from the embryonic mesenchyme. During the 5th week of gestation, a series of lacunae appear within the mesenchyme and coalesce to form the pericardial coelom. After development, the pericardium is cone-shaped, with the apex ending in continuity with the adventitia of the great vessels and the base attached to the central tendon of the diaphragm. The pericardium is attached to the posterior surface of the sternum by the superior and inferior sternopericardial ligaments securing the heart within the thorax, but separated from the sternum by the lungs and thymus, except for a small area corresponding to the fourth and fifth interspaces anteriorly. The serous pericardium lines the outer fibrous pericardium and consists of a single layer of mesothelial cells. The visceral pericardium, or epicardium, covers the heart and great vessels. The pericardium folds on itself to form the oblique sinus, a cul-de-sac of serous pericardium located behind the left atrium, while the space between the aorta and main pulmonary artery anteriorly and the right and left atria posteriorly forms the transverse sinus. The arterial blood supply to the pericardium is from the internal thoracic arteries and the descending thoracic aorta, while the venous drainage is to the azygos system. Finally, the pericardium is innervated by the vagus and phrenic nerves and both sympathetic trunks.

Physiology

The true function of the pericardium remains speculative because people do well without it. In 1898, Bernard found that hearts without pericardium ruptured at lower distention pressures than those with intact pericardium. The pericardium may serve to protect the heart, prevent acute distention, distribute force, and enforce diastolic coupling of the ventricles. Diastolic coupling theoretically occurs only with an intact pericardium, by linking a pressure rise in the right ventricle to the left ventricle, which then also moves up the Starling curve. The pericardium also serves as an absorptive surface, normally handling 50 mL/d of ultrafiltrate. The absorption of fluid from the pericardial space occurs predominantly through the thoracic duct, but about 20% passes to the pleural space and is absorbed by the right lymphatic duct. The permeability properties of the pericardium have been evaluated[34] and demonstrate fluid transfer from the pericardium to the pleural space with increasing pericardial pressure. The pericardium offers little restriction to the passage of plasma proteins, and the permeability of the pericardium to water is higher than most other tissues. These findings are important in neoplastic and effusive pericardial disease.

Pericardial Diagnostic Studies

Echocardiography is presently the most sensitive means of diagnosing pericardial disease.[35] Two-dimensional echocardiography, surface or transesophageal, provides important information regarding the location, size, distribution, and physiologic effects of effusions. Furthermore, cardiac tamponade can be suspected by echocardiography from a lack of inspiratory collapse of the inferior vena cava, early diastolic collapse of the right ventricle, and late diastolic collapse of the right atrium. The heart can be visualized swinging within the excess pericardial fluid. Also, Doppler estimation of SVC, hepatic venous, and transvalvular flow may show characteristic abnormalities of tamponade. Echo Doppler flow patterns may also be useful in screening for constrictive or restrictive physiology. There is prominent diastolic flow velocity (Y) and smaller systolic velocity (X) with constriction. Echocardiography may also discriminate between pericardial constriction and restrictive cardiomyopathy because with restrictive cardiomyopathy, there is a large inspiratory SVC flow reversal, which generally occurs during expiration with constriction.

Computed tomography (CT), including spiral, ultrafast, and gated studies, provides information regarding pericardial thickness and is also useful to quantitate and localize pericardial effusions. Because tissue attenuation coefficients vary, CT may elucidate the cause of effusions (eg, chyle, blood, exudate). CT may also identify other thoracic lesions that involve the pericardium. Magnetic resonance imaging (MRI) has also been employed in pericardial disease. Although effusions are detected with a high degree of sensitivity, MRI may not be as helpful in determining pericardial thickness because the plane between the epicardial fat and pericardium is often indistinct on MRI. Finally, radionuclide ventriculography is helpful in evaluating constriction and tamponade. The time to peak filling and the filling rate, as indices of diastolic function, are altered with pericardial disease. In addition, pericardial effusions may be diagnosed when a large effusion separates the cardiac and lung images, creating a halo effect around the heart.

Congenital Abnormalities

Congenital absence or defects of the pericardium occur and may be associated with anomalies of the pleura, heart, lung, peritoneum, or kidney.[36] They are more common in males and may involve total absence, but are more frequently partial, particularly on the left side. Partial absence of the pericardium is usually asymptomatic. With right-sided pericardial defects, however, herniation of the right atrium, right ventricle, and lung has been reported and may be associated with ECG changes and a murmur. Congenital total absence of the pericardium is also usually asymptomatic and only an incidental finding at autopsy or operation for other conditions. If there are symptoms or hemodynamic compromise from herniation of one or more cardiac chambers, operation may be indicated. Treatment consists of completion pericardiectomy or replacement of the absent portion with a substitute.

When the embryonic pericardial lacunae fails to fuse, a pericardial cyst occurs, ranging from 1 to 15 cm in diameter. Most cysts occur at the right cardiophrenic angle and are detected on routine chest radiographs. If a communica-tion persists to the pericardium, this becomes a diverticulum. Although pericardial cysts are usually asymptomatic, they rarely cause life-threatening respiratory or hemodynamic compromise in neonates. The diagnosis can usually be made by CT, denoting their usual location at the right cardiophrenic angle. Other conditions in the differential diagnosis include foramen of Morgagni hernia, bronchogenic cyst, lipoma, and other homogeneous benign or malignant lesions of the mediastinum. Operative exploration and removal should be undertaken if the diagnosis is in doubt, if the lesion appears to be enlarging in size, or if it becomes symptomatic.

Neoplasms

Primary malignant neoplasms of the pericardium are rare and include sarcomas, teratomas, pheochromocytomas and mesotheliomas, which usually present with constriction. Benign tumors, including lipomas, hemangiomas, lymphangiomas, leiomyomas, neurofibromas, and thymomas, have also been described. Additionally, the pericardium may be involved by direct extension of lung, esophageal, or primary mediastinal malignancies and clinically present either as constriction or tamponade. This diagnosis is made by CT or MRI. Finally, metastatic involvement of the pericardium is the most common form of neoplasm[37] and is seen in 5% to 10% of patients who die of cancer. It is seen most frequently with lymphoma and lung, breast, and ovarian carcinoma. Although metastatic involvement of the pericardium is commonly treated by radiotherapy, antineoplastic agents have also been instilled into the pericardium, and systemic side effects can occur.[38,39] Tetracycline has been used for chemical pericardiodesis, with control rates of 80% to 90% for malignant effusions.[40] The treatment strategy is to relieve effusion and tamponade and to confirm the diagnosis of malignant pericardial disease. Malignant pericardial disease that presents as cardiac tamponade is an indication for intervention but carries less than a 25% 1-year survival rate. Conversely, in patients in whom prolonged survival is anticipated, operative approach may be preferred to minimize the chance of recurrence or cardiac encasement by metastatic tumor.

Pericarditis

Pericarditis is seen in 2% to 6% of all autopsies and may be present in up to 1% of all admissions.[41] Patients with acute pericarditis may present with chest pain and tamponade-like symptoms of dyspnea, venous hypertension, falling blood pressure, and syncope mimicking the signs of acute myocardial infarction. The predominant sign of pericarditis is chest pain, and although the diagnosis of pericarditis can be difficult, it is of utmost importance that pericarditis be differentiated from myocardial ischemia. The chest pain of acute pericarditis, like that of ischemic chest pain, is precordial or retrosternal and may radiate to the left shoulder and left arm. It differs from ischemic pain in that it can last for days, is pleuritic, and is aggravated by breathing, lying flat, or turning. It is relieved by sitting up or leaning forward. A diphasic (systolic and diastolic) pericardial friction rub is often heard over the entire precordium and sounds like a creaking leather saddle or walking on snow. This rub may be accentuated by leaning forward or inspiration. It may be transient or last for days.

The diagnosis of pericarditis is often made by echocardiogram, which can demonstrate minimal fluid, recognize cardiac tamponade, guide needle pericardiocentesis, and reveal loculations of infectious pericarditis or neoplasms in patients with metastatic cancer. The ECG changes of acute pericarditis are often diagnostic[42] and are thought to be from generalized superficial myocarditis. On ECG, sinus rhythm is present in more than 90% of cases. Patients with atrial fibrillation or flutter may have other underlying heart disease. Typical ECG changes occur in 50% to 70% of cases and evolve in the following four stages: (1) ST-segment elevation without reciprocal depression, (2) return of ST segment to baseline with T-wave change, (3) T-wave negativity, and (4) a return to normal.

Low ECG voltage and electrical alternans may also be observed. The absence of typical ECG changes does not exclude acute pericarditis. Conversely, ST-segment elevation may be from other causes, including normal early repolarization (seldom more than 2 mm). Finally, myocardial ischemia may result in ST-segment elevation that may resemble that of acute pericarditis. Unlike acute pericarditis, however, the changes are less generalized, there is reciprocal ST depression, T waves become negative while ST segments are elevated, and pathologic Q waves develop. Chest radiography is not helpful in the diagnosis of acute pericarditis because there is often little pericardial fluid and a normal configuration. The heart silhouette increases only with larger effusions and may be shaped like a water bottle.

Causes

Metastatic neoplasm is the most common cause of pericardial effusion. Metastatic lung cancer accounts for 33% of cases, breast cancer for 25%, and lymphoma for 15%. The diagnosis may be made by echocardiogram, CT, or MRI, and tumor cells may be identified in aspirated pericardial fluid. Up to half of pericardial effusions in patients with neoplasm are not from metastasis, but from radiotherapy, chemotherapy, or infection.

Idiopathic or nonspecific pericarditis is the second most common cause of pericarditis. Although most patients have prior presumed viral respiratory illness, a viral source can be identified in only 15% to 20% of cases. Chest pain, fever, and general malaise are common. Many cases have evidence of pleural effusions. Cardiac tamponade may occur but is rare. The erythrocyte sedimentation rate is almost universally elevated. Studies for viral antibodies (coxsackievirus A and B, echovirus, and influenza virus), mycoplasma, and histoplasmosis should be sent initially and 4 weeks later. Idiopathic or nonspecific pericarditis usually abates in 1 to 3 weeks, but relapses occur in up to 30% of patients.

Uremic pericarditis is among the most common causes of acute pericarditis in hospitalized patients. Uremic pericarditis is found in about 20% of patients with end-stage renal disease on peritoneal or hemodialysis. Precordial pain is less common in these patients, reported in only 37% of one series. Therefore, uremic patients tend to have undiagnosed pericarditis and have more complications. In a series of 25 uremic patients, 4 developed tamponade, 3 required pericardiectomy, 2 died of heart failure, and 3 developed late constriction. Uremic pericarditis is treated best by more frequent dialysis.[43] Additionally, instillation of steroids into the pericardial sac may be useful.[44] Pericardial resection may be required when there is continued reaccumulation of pericardial fluid.

Acute infectious pericarditis, while not as common as before antibiotics, still occurs frequently and may be a consequence of penetrating injury, hematogenous or lymphatic spread from sepsis, pneumonia, osteomyelitis, or rupture of subphrenic or hepatic abscesses. Clinical manifestations consist of elevated white blood cell count, chest pain, and fever. The most common causes of acute purulent pericarditis are *Staphylococcus* sp, *Pneumococcus* sp, and gram-negative bacteria (especially *Haemophilus influenzae*). Pericarditis from other bacterial organisms, such as meningococcus, salmonella, brucella, legionella, campylobacter, and anaerobic clostridium and streptococcus, have been reported. Pericarditis also can be secondary to viral infection from coxsackievirus A and B, echovirus, influenza, adenovirus, Epstein-Barr virus, chicken pox, psittacosis, mumps, and mononucleosis. Similarly, histoplasmosis, aspergillus, coccidioides, blastomycosis, candida, and nocardial infections may involve the pericardium either by lymphatic spread or direct extension.

Parasitic pericarditis occurs rarely. Amebic pericarditis may result from direct extension of an abscess from the liver and can cause acute tamponade. Echinococcal pericarditis may occur as a result of rupture of a cyst into the pericardial space. This may result in a spectrum of conditions from local pericardial reaction to rapid multiplication of cysts and cardiac compromise. Other opportunistic agents have been reported to cause pericarditis, including toxoplasmosis, *Enterolytica histolytica*, *Tropanzii cruzi*, rickettsia, trichinosis, and microfilaria.

Tuberculous pericarditis is usually secondary to systemic tuberculous infection and results from hematogenous and lymphatic spread or from direct extension from the pleura or lung. Tuberculosis is an uncommon cause of acute pericarditis, due to a declining prevalence of pulmonary tuberculosis. With the increased number of immunocompromised patients, however, there has been an increase in atypical mycobacterial infections from *Mycobacterium avium* or *Mycobacterium intracellulare*, associated with pericarditis. Conversely, in nonindustrialized countries, tuberculosis is the most common cause of pericarditis. Evidence of pulmonary tuberculosis is absent in about 30% of these patients, and pericardial biopsy is used to establish the diagnosis.

Acquired immunodeficiency syndrome may be specifically associated with pericardial disease. One echocardiographic study indicated that 20% of these patients have pericardial effusions related to lymphoma, Kaposi sarcoma, or opportunistic infections.

Pericarditis occurs in about 3% of myocardial infarctions (Dressler syndrome). In a series of 330 patients after acute myocardial infarction, 83 had pericardial effusions, and 38 had a pericardial rub. A similar postpericardiotomy pericarditis syndrome may also occur after cardiac surgery, blunt or penetrating cardiac trauma, pacemaker insertion, or rarely, pulmonary embolism. Signs consist of fever, pain, malaise, and laboratory findings of lymphocytosis and elevated sedimentation rate. This syndrome usually appears 10 days to 2 months after cardiac operation and occurs in up to 30% of patients. Typical ECG changes are present in less than half of cases. A pericardial friction rub is often heard, and pericardial effusion is frequently present. Cardiac tamponade may develop, especially if anticoagulants are used and late constriction is a risk. The cause of postinfarction or postsurgical pericarditis is unknown but may involve an inflammatory reaction to pericardial blood, low-grade infection, or autoantibodies to the myocardium. Treatment is based on severity and usually is limited to aspirin or indomethacin, although steroids may be necessary.

Iatrogenic pericarditis related to drugs or procedures is becoming more common, and the use of warfarin or thrombolytic agents in patients with unrecognized acute pericarditis may lead to fatal tamponade. Other agents have been reported to cause pericarditis, including procainamide, diphenylhydantoin, hydralazine, isonicotinic acid, methysergide, and minoxidil. Pericarditis has also been reported after endoscopic sclerotherapy of esophageal varices, central venous catheter placement, cardiac pacemakers, and internal defibrillator placement.

Acute pericarditis is seen with connective tissue disease, and large effusions are common in patients with acute rheumatic fever or rheumatoid arthritis. About 30% of patients with systemic lupus erythematosus have pericarditis, and it may be the first sign. Cardiac tamponade or constrictive pericarditis may follow. Pericardial effusion is found by echocardiogram in 40% of patients with scleroderma and in 50% of patients with rheumatoid arthritis. Systemic vasculitis and connective tissue diseases that may be associated with pericarditis include scleroderma, systemic lupus erythematosus, Wegener granulomatosis, polyarteritis nodosa, dermatomyositis, ankylosing spondylitis, Reiter syndrome, Behçet disease, and familial Mediterranean fever. Pericarditis associated with connective tissue disease is managed by treating the underlying cause and symptoms.

Treatment

Acute tamponade is uncommon with pericarditis, but large pericardial effusions may develop. Early diagnosis and treatment are important to avoid later fibrous constriction. Acute infectious pericarditis is treated best with a combination of drainage and specific antimicrobial therapy. Drainage may be accomplished using pericardiocentesis, but more complete drainage is ensured with operative placement of a subxiphoid tube. In some infections (pneumococcal pneumonia), pericardial involvement is incidental and resolves as the patient responds to treatment for the primary infection. In others, there may be cardiac tamponade or persistent infection in the pericardium. Alternatively, pericarditis may come to light after the original infection is treated or resolved and no organisms can be found (meningococcemia or histoplasmosis).

Patients with acute pericarditis may be hospitalized for relief of symptoms, diagnostic evaluation, and observation for complications.[45] Specific types of pericarditis are treated for the underlying cause. Chest pain may be relieved with aspirin, 650 mg every 4 to 6 hours; indomethacin, 25 to 50 mg three times daily; or ibuprofen, 400 to 600 mg every 6 hours. For severe pain, narcotics may be required. When the pain does not respond to these agents, prednisone, 20 mg three times daily, nearly always relieves symptoms. The dose is then tapered over 2 to 3 weeks. For relapsing pericarditis or refractory cases, pericardiectomy may be considered and is recommended for an inability to discontinue steroids after 6 months. Finally, colchicine, 1 mg/d, may be useful in the treatment of relapsing pericarditis.[46]

Cardiac Tamponade

Cardiac tamponade occurs when adequate filling of the heart is prevented by compression from fluid or blood in the pericardial space, restricting ventricular filling during diastole, reducing stroke volume and cardiac output, and increasing systemic and pulmonary venous pressure. In acute tamponade, relatively little fluid (100 mL) may produce circulatory collapse, while with chronic pericardial effusions, the pericardium may become stretched and contain liters of fluid before tamponade occurs.[47] The increase in pericardial volume that produces cardiac tamponade results when intrapericardial pressure increases to 20 to 30 mmHg. Compensatory reflex vasoconstriction and catecholamine release lead to an increase in systemic and pulmonary venous pressure that maintains some ventricular filling but with a significantly reduced cardiac output. Right and left atrial, pulmonary artery diastolic and wedge, and biventricular end-diastolic pressures are equal to intrapericardial pressure. Death results when cardiac output declines despite neurohumoral compensatory mechanisms.

Causes and Diagnosis

Cardiac tamponade has the same causes as acute pericarditis: metastatic malignancies, idiopathic pericarditis, renal failure, infections, connective tissue disease, anticoagulants, and complications of procedures. The diagnosis of cardiac tamponade is made clinically and is suspected when a patient with a pericardial effusion has elevated systemic venous pressure, dyspnea, and tachycardia. Three classic clinical signs occur in the setting of acute tamponade: (1) the heart is small and quiet, (2) venous pressure is elevated, and (3) the systemic blood pressure is depressed (the Beck triad). With acute tamponade, shock is evident with a rapid and paradoxical pulse. Cyanosis, especially in the face, may be present as a manifestation of venous stasis. The systemic blood pressure may be normal, low, or even elevated in previously hypertensive patients. The blood pressure is most likely to be normal when the pericardial fluid has accumulated slowly and low when the fluid has accumulated rapidly, as with intrapericardial bleeding. The neck veins are visibly distended and Kussmaul sign is absent. The heart sounds are sometimes faint but may be normal. The cardiac apical impulse is usually not palpable, and cardiac murmurs and gallop rhythm are usually absent. The diagnosis of cardiac tamponade is proved when removal of pericardial fluid relieves symptoms. Aspiration of a few milliliters of pericardial fluid can restore cardiac output and reduce venous pressure. Because reaccumulation of a small amount of fluid may result in sudden hemodynamic decompensation, definitive diagnosis and treatment are mandatory.

Pulsus paradoxus that occurs in tamponade is defined by an inspiratory decrease in systemic blood pressure that exceeds 10 mmHg. During inspiration, right heart volume increases, elevating intrapericardial pressure to an even greater degree. The interventricular septum is deviated to the left, compromising left ventricular filling and stroke volume. It is present in cardiac tamponade, except when there is left ventricular dysfunction or atrial septal defect, or in a postcardiac surgical patient who is receiving positive-pressure respirations. Pulsus paradoxus may also be caused by acute or chronic obstructive airway disease, right ventricular infarction, pulmonary embolism, constrictive pericarditis, tense ascites, and circulatory shock.

The right atrial pressure in cardiac tamponade is usually 15 to 35 mmHg. With hypovolemia, such as seen with postoperative bleeding, central pressures may be low. Intrapericardial pressure, right and left ventricular diastolic pressures, and pulmonary wedge pressure are equally elevated. The systemic venous pulse contour is sensitive to changes in pericardial fluid volume and pressure. Normally, it is composed of three positive deflections and two negative ones (Fig. 67-9). The a wave is generated by atrial systole. The c wave occurs during isovolumic ventricular systole, with displacement of the tricuspid valve apparatus toward the right atrium. The x descent follows and corresponds to a fall in intrapericardial pressure with diminishing ventricular volume and descent of the tricuspid valve apparatus. The v wave occurs with passive venous filling of the atrium from the vena cavae. The y descent occurs during passive right ventricular filling. In tamponade, the right atrial pressure tracing reveals preservation of the x descent and loss of the y descent.

Although the diagnosis of tamponade is made clinically, echocardiographic findings can be helpful. Moderate to large effusions may be present both anterior and posterior to the heart. Furthermore, the two-dimensional echocardiogram is a valuable aid in needle pericardiocentesis. A number of charac-

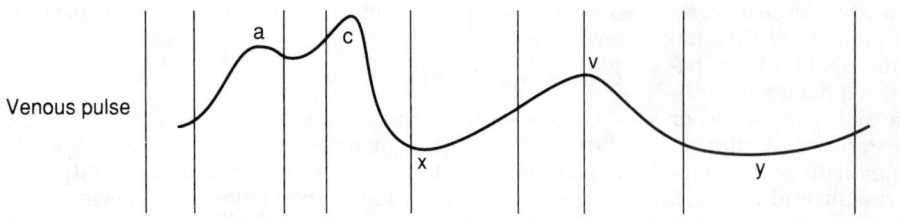

Figure 67-9. The systemic venous pulse contour. (After Berne RM, Levy MN. Cardiovascular physiology, ed 5. St Louis, CV Mosby, 1986:66)

teristic echocardiographic findings are associated with cardiac tamponade, including inspiratory increase of right ventricular dimensions with abnormal inspiratory decrease of left ventricular dimensions, inspiratory decrease of mitral valve excursion, right and left atrial collapse, inspiratory increase of tricuspid valve flow, and abnormal inspiratory decrease of mitral valve flow and inferior vena caval plethora. Localized atrial compression may also cause hemodynamic compromise without characteristic echocardiographic features.

Tamponade Related to Surgery

Although rising filling pressures and falling systemic pressure, urine, and cardiac output may be a manifestation of postoperative myocardial dysfunction, cardiac tamponade can occur early or late after open heart operations and should always be included in the differential diagnosis of low cardiac output. Diagnostic signs favoring tamponade include higher elevation of the central venous pressure in comparison to the pulmonary capillary wedge pressure, poor response to vasopressors and diuretics, enlarging cardiac silhouette, and abrupt increase or cessation of mediastinal drainage. Late postsurgical tamponade is more common in patients on anticoagulants and may present insidiously.[48]

Treatment of cardiac tamponade depends on the cause and the clinical manifestations. When blood pressure is declining, emergency pericardiocentesis must be performed. Needle pericardiocentesis under hemodynamic and echocardiographic monitoring may be done when the etiologic diagnosis is known. When the diagnosis is un-

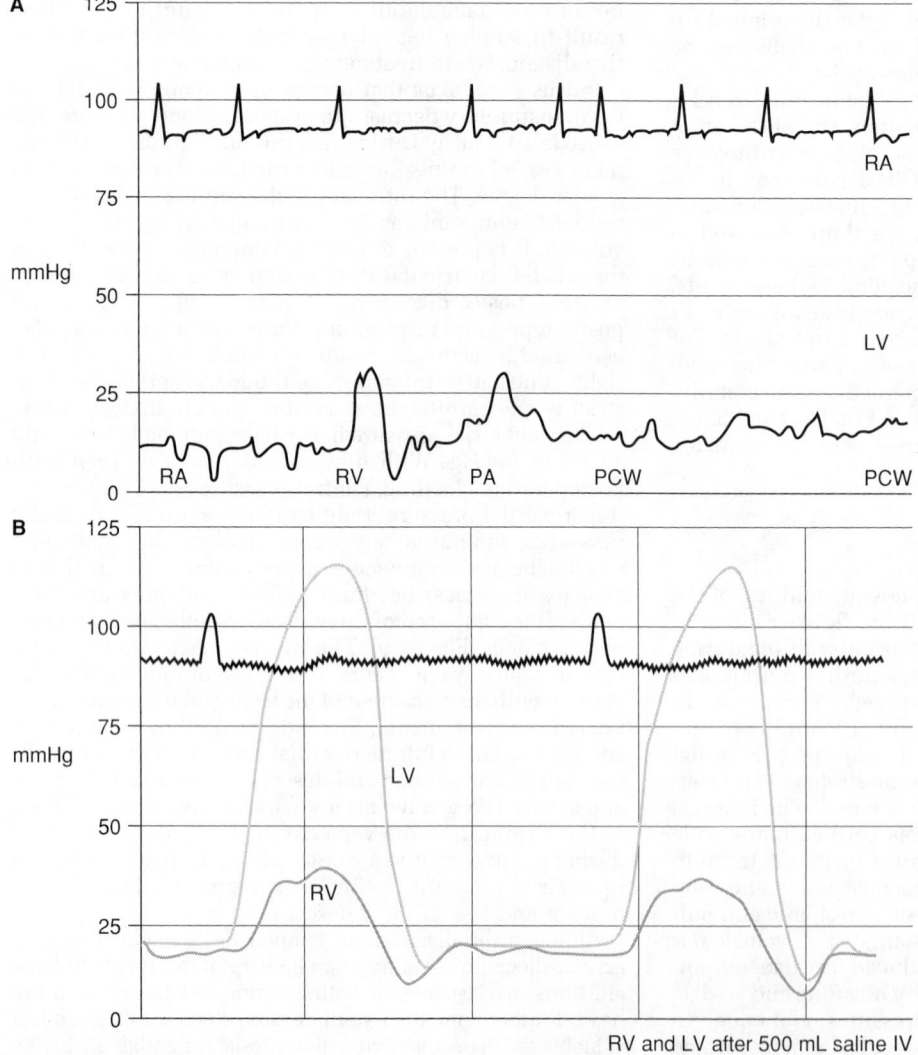

RV and LV after 500 mL saline IV

Figure 67-10. Pressure recordings from a patient with constrictive pericarditis. (*A*) The right atrial (RA) tracing shows elevated pressure and prominent *y* descent. The right ventricular (RV) tracing exhibits the typical dip and plateau pattern, or "square root sign." There is equalization of the RA, RV diastolic, pulmonary artery (PA) diastolic, pulmonary capillary wedge (PCW), and left ventricular (LV) diastolic pressures. (*B*) RV and LV diastolic pressures increase and equalize after administration of 500 mL of saline. (After Brockington GM, Zebede J, Pandian NG. Constrictive pericarditis. Cardiol Clin 1990;8:649)

clear, surgical drainage is a better choice. Patients should be observed carefully for a recurrence of cardiac tamponade, preferably in a cardiac monitoring unit. Recurrent tamponade despite specific treatment is usually an indication for a pericardial window or pericardial resection.

Constriction

Constrictive pericarditis occurs when the heart is compressed by a fibrosis of the pericardium, obliterating the pericardial space. The pericardium may also contain fluid between the fibrotic, thickened visceral and parietal pericardium. The condition usually progresses slowly, producing elevated venous pressure over months to years. Patients present with effort dyspnea, fatigue, abdominal swelling or discomfort, orthopnea, cough, elevated venous pressure, edema, hepatomegaly, ascites, pleural effusion, Kussmaul sign (lack of variation of venous filling with respiration), pericardial knock, pulsus paradoxus, and refractory congestive heart failure despite diuretics. The diagnosis of constriction is made only when coronary disease, hypertension, or valvular disease is ruled out. Constriction is likely if the heart size is normal and the lung fields are clear on chest radiograph. The diagnosis is almost certain if there is pericardial calcification, but calcification is present in only 40% of patients with constriction. Although any type of acute pericarditis can cause constriction, a common cause is radiation. Mediastinal irradiation, however, may also lead to restrictive changes from fibrotic myocarditis. Further causes of constriction include amyloidosis, scleroderma, hemochromatosis, infiltrative neoplasms, sarcoidosis, myocarditis, endomyocardial fibrosis, and pseudoxanthoma elasticum. Conversely, pericardial constriction with effusion is common in suppurative, malignant, and uremic pericardial disease.

Pathophysiology

Constriction limits left ventricular distensibility resulting in inadequate filling despite high end-diastolic pressures. Early diastolic ventricular filling is rapid, quickly reaching the limit of ventricular distensibility, and stroke volume is reduced because of the fusion of myocardium with the pericardium. The right ventricular pressure trace has an early diastolic dip, followed by a rapid increase and plateau (square root sign; Fig. 67-10). The central venous pressure tracing is also abnormal. The ventricle has small end-diastolic volumes with normal left ventricular ejection fractions. The hemodynamic findings are characterized by equal elevation of right and left ventricular filling pressures. As a rule, right atrial and pulmonary wedge pressures, as well as right and left ventricular diastolic pressures, are 15 to 30 mmHg and are roughly equal to each other, with a maximum difference of 4 to 5 mmHg. The right atrial pressure waveform shows prominent x and y descents. Pulmonary arterial systolic pressure usually does not exceed 40 mmHg.

Diagnosis

Ventriculography shows accelerated left ventricular filling in early diastole. During the first one third of diastole, left ventricular filling averages 80% in patients with constrictive pericarditis but only 60% in normal subjects. ECG tends to show low-voltage and nonspecific T-wave changes. About 25% of patients have atrial fibrillation or flutter. Occasionally, there is a pattern of right ventricular hypertrophy owing to fibrotic obstruction of the right ventricular outflow tract or narrowing of the mitral orifice. The echocardiographic changes are not specific. The ventricles are small, with preserved systolic function. There is abrupt halting of ventricular expansion during early diastole, with

diastolic flattening of the left ventricular posterior wall. The inferior vena cava is dilated. More specific findings on Doppler echocardiogram are abnormal inspiratory increase in tricuspid flow and abnormal inspiratory decrease in mitral valve flow.

In patients with effusive–constrictive pericarditis, pericardial fluid collects between the fibrotic visceral and parietal pericardium. The heart tends to be larger on chest radiograph than with constrictive pericarditis. In effusive–constrictive pericarditis, the hemodynamic pattern is characteristic. The atrial and ventricular pressure curves resemble those of cardiac tamponade, with a large x and a small y wave in the right atrium and no prominent early diastolic dip in the ventricular pressure records. If the pericardial fluid is removed by needle, however, the pressure traces then resemble those of constrictive pericarditis, with prominent x and y descents in the right atrium and a prominent early diastolic dip in the ventricular pressure records.

The diagnosis of constrictive pericarditis is made from the characteristic hemodynamic findings in the presence of pericardial thickening (4 mm or more), confirmed by CT or MRI. Restrictive cardiomyopathy may have similar features but does not show increased pericardial thickening. Right atrial and pulmonary wedge pressures may

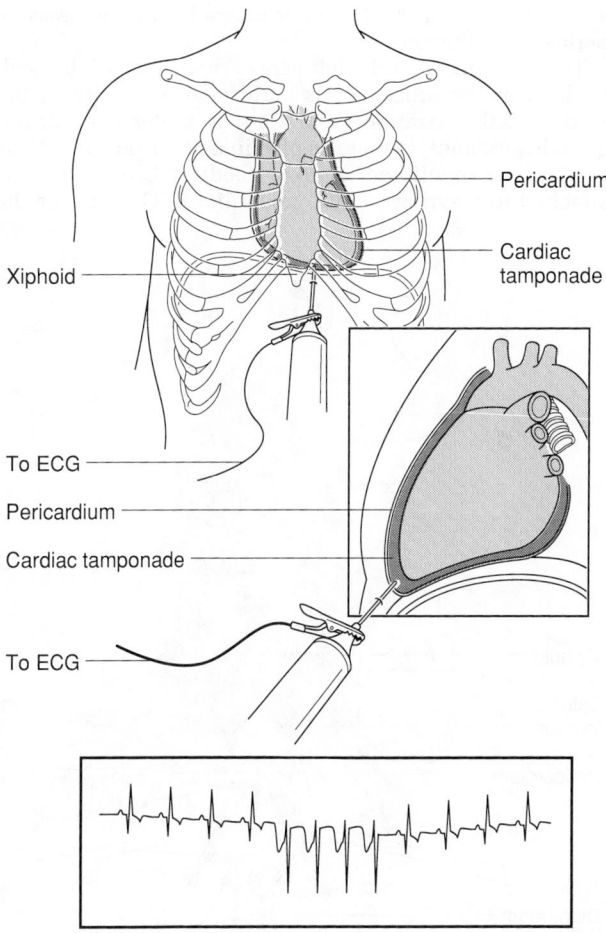

Figure 67-11. Pericardiocentesis. The needle is inserted to the left of the xiphoid and directed toward the left shoulder or midscapular area, posteriorly at a 45-degree angle. The ECG lead is attached to the needle, and the negative deflection of the QRS complex represents contact with the epicardium. (After Ebert PA, Najafi H. In: Sabiston DC Jr, Spencer FC, eds. Gibbon's surgery of the chest, ed 5. Philadelphia, WB Saunders, 1990:1234)

be equal, and there may be an early diastolic dip in the pressure tracings of both left and right ventricles. In some cases, pericardial biopsy may be necessary to confirm the diagnosis because patients who have long-standing constriction with ascites and peripheral edema may be confused with patients who have primary liver disease (eg, Budd-Chiari disease, cirrhosis, or other causes of right-sided heart failure).

Treatment

Although diuretics may offer some improvement in patients with constrictive pericarditis, pericardiectomy is the definitive treatment. The overall mortality rate is 5% to 10%. Operation may be deferred in patients in New York Heart Association (NYHA) functional class I who have a satisfactory quality of life. Operation should not be deferred until the patient is class III, however, because the surgical mortality rate is much higher. Finally, patients with constrictive pericarditis caused by radiation or connective tissue disease may respond poorly because of associated restrictive cardiomyopathy.

Pericardiocentesis

Pericardiocentesis is indicated for patients with acute cardiac tamponade and rapidly falling blood pressure, when purulent pericarditis is suspected because of fever or high white cell count, or for diagnostic purposes when a patient has continued fever or unresolved or progressive pericardial effusion.

The subxiphoid or the left parasternal approach is used. If elective, the procedure is performed optimally in the cardiac catheterization laboratory or under echocardiographic guidance so that the physiologic response to therapy can be monitored. A long needle (12 to 18 cm) is attached to a syringe and a precordial ECG lead. For the

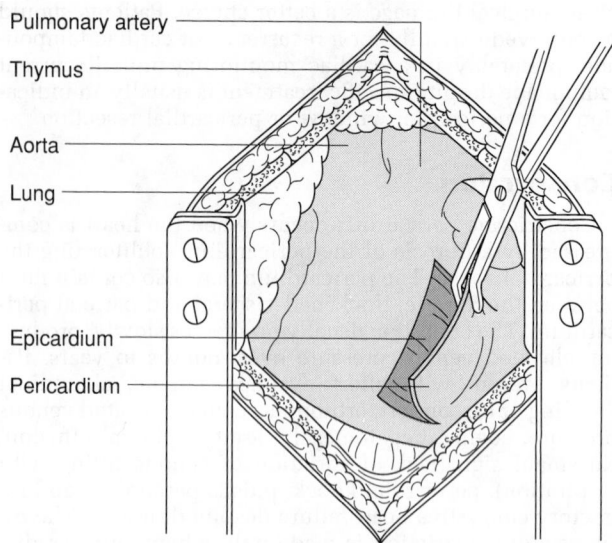

Figure 67-13. The pericardium is exposed through a median sternotomy. The pericardium is incised, and the dissection plane established between the pericardium and epicardium. (After Ebert EA, Najafi H. In: Sabiston DC Jr, Spencer FC, eds. Gibbon's surgery of the chest, ed 5. Philadelphia, WB Saunders, 1990:1242)

subxiphoid approach, the needle is inserted immediately to the left of the xiphoid process and directed posteriorly at a 45-degree angle (Fig. 67-11). The tip may be directed toward the left shoulder or between the scapulas. From the parasternal approach, the aspirating needle is directed posteriorly at 90 degrees to the body, usually in the fourth or fifth intercostal space, 1 to 2 cm to the left of the sternum. The needle is slowly advanced until fluid is encountered or the ECG shows contact with the heart (injury current). Also, air bubble (echocardiography) or radiopaque (fluoroscopy) contrast can be injected to see if the tip of the needle is in the right ventricle or the pericardial space.

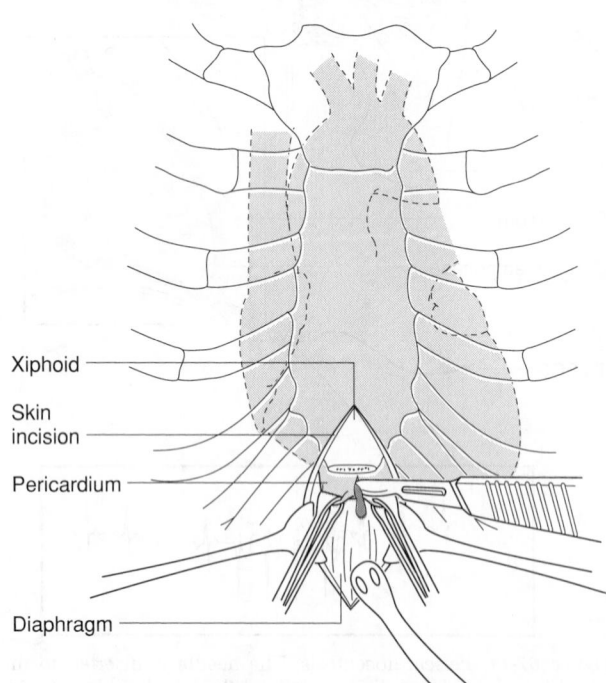

Figure 67-12. The xiphoid is exposed through a midline incision and either retracted or removed. Limited exposure to the pericardium is achieved, and biopsy or drainage is performed. (After Hood RM. Techniques in general thoracic surgery. Philadelphia, WB Saunders, 1985:58)

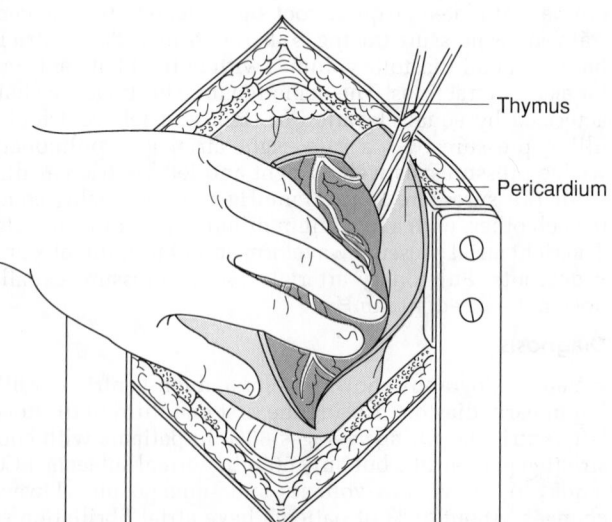

Figure 67-14. The heart is retracted to the right so that complete myocardial decortication can be accomplished. The anterior pericardium from one phrenic nerve to the other will be excised. (After Ebert EA, Najafi H. In: Sabiston DC Jr, Spencer FC, eds. Gibbon's surgery of the chest, ed 5. Philadelphia, WB Saunders, 1990:1242)

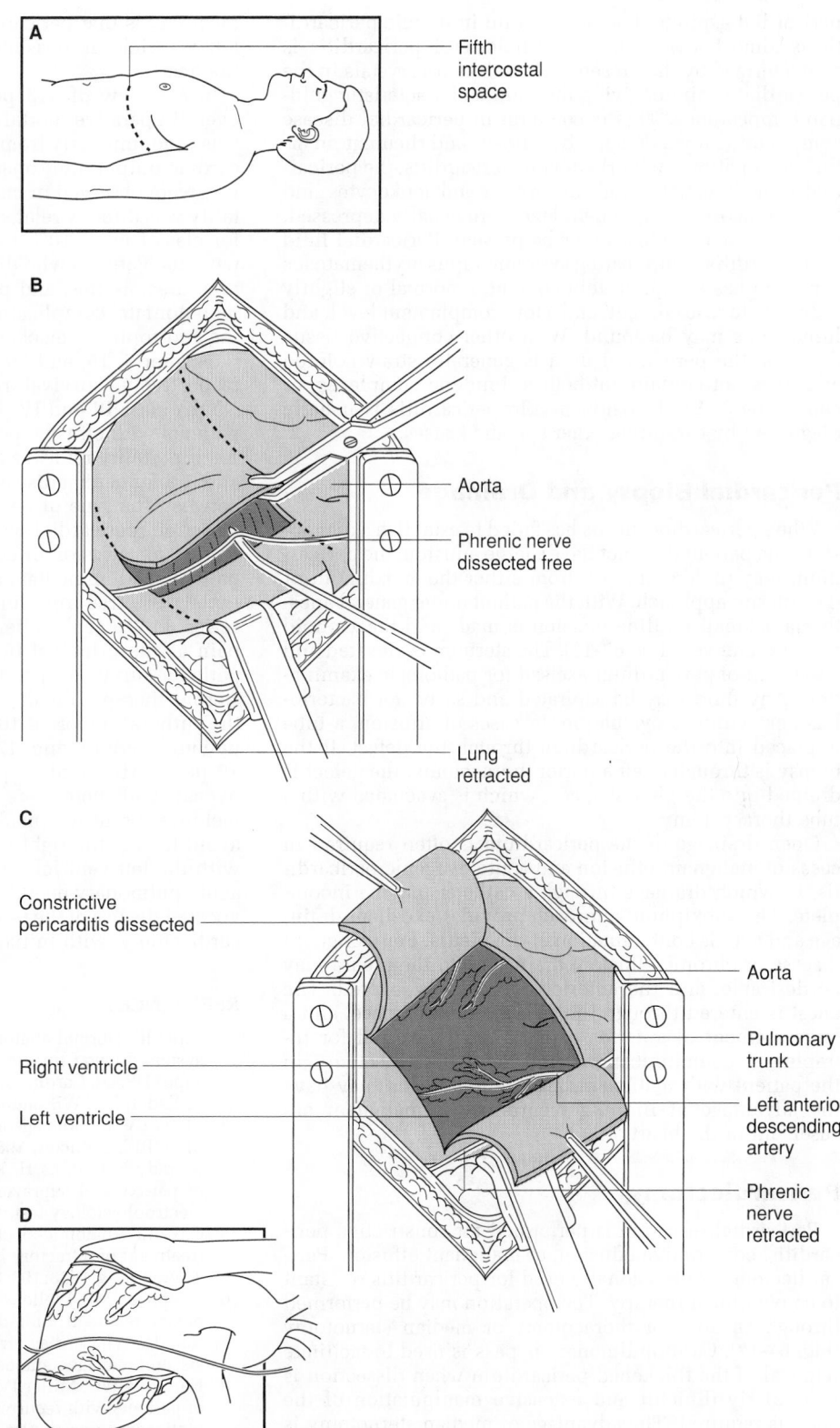

Figure 67-15. Pericardiectomy through an anterolateral left thoracotomy. The heart is exposed through the fifth interspace. The appropriate dissection plane is established and the phrenic nerve mobilized to allow removal of the posterolateral pericardium. (After Kirklin JW, Barratt-Boyes BG. Cardiac surgery. New York, John Wiley & Sons, 1986:1438)

The aspirated fluid should be saved for bacteriologic, cytologic, and chemical analyses. A drainage catheter may be passed through the aspirating needle or over a guide wire to provide for continued drainage, if deemed necessary.

Potential complications of pericardiocentesis include myocardial or coronary arterial laceration or induction of ventricular arrhythmias. Perforation of the lung with resul-

tant pneumothorax and penetration of abdominal viscera may also occur. The use of two-dimensional echocardiography to localize the pericardial effusion before attempted aspiration has reduced the risk of the procedure.

Pericardiocentesis is usually both therapeutic and diagnostic. Infections may be cultured. Tuberculous pericarditis is confirmed by the presence of acid-fast bacilli in the pericardial aspirate. Pericardial fluid in uremic pericarditis is almost always bloody. Cholesterol pericarditis is characterized by the presence of cholesterol crystals in the pericardial aspirate, giving the fluid a characteristic gold-paint appearance. This is common in pericardial disease complicating myxedema, tuberculosis, and rheumatoid arthritis. In patients with rheumatic pericarditis, the pericardial fluid is usually high in protein and leukocytes and low in glucose. Complement levels are usually depressed, and immune complexes may be present. Pericardial fluid in pericarditis complicating systemic lupus erythematosus generally has a high protein content, a normal or slightly reduced glucose content, and a low complement level, and lupus cells may be found. With other connective tissue diseases, the pericardial fluid is generally straw colored and does not contain antibodies, immune complexes, or complement. Viral or nonspecific pericarditis is usually diagnosed by excluding other specific causes.

Pericardial Biopsy and Drainage

When pericardiocentesis has failed to establish a diagnosis or the patient does not have a large effusion, the pericardium may undergo biopsy from either the subxiphoid or the anterior approach. With the patient under general anesthesia, a small midline incision is made and the xiphoid process removed (Fig. 67-12). The sternum is elevated and a segment of pericardium excised for pathologic examination. Any fluid may be aspirated and saved for bacteriologic or cytologic evaluation. In cases of effusion, a tube is placed into the pericardium through the defect. If the biopsy is through a left anterior thoracotomy, the defect is drained into the pleural space, which is evacuated with a tube thoracostomy.

Open drainage of the pericardium is often required in cases of malignant effusion and acute pyogenic pericarditis, in which drainage through a catheter may be incomplete. The subxiphoid approach provides excellent drainage and avoids contamination of the pleura. For malignant disease or chronic effusion, drainage into the pleura may be desirable, and the anterior approach is favored. The chest is entered through the fifth intercostal space, and a large segment of anterior pericardium is excised for intrapleural communication. Anterior pericardiectomy in the patient with malignant or chronic effusion may have the advantage of limiting recurrence or malignant encasement of the heart.

Pericardiectomy

Pericardial resection is performed for constrictive pericarditis, constrictive effusion, or malignant effusion. Pericardiectomy is occasionally used for pericarditis resistant to conventional therapy. The operation may be performed through an anterior thoracotomy or median sternotomy (Fig. 67-13). Cardiopulmonary bypass is used to facilitate removal of the thickened pericardium when dissection is particularly difficult and extensive manipulation of the heart is required. The advantage of median sternotomy is the relative ease of cardiopulmonary bypass. The sternal approach requires extensive manipulation of the heart to reach areas of the pericardium that covers the posterolateral and diaphragmatic aspects of the left ventricle (Fig. 67-14). Cardiopulmonary bypass with heparin is associated with increased bleeding and should be employed with caution. A left anterolateral thoracotomy through the fifth intercostal space, with or without transection of the sternum, is an alternative approach (Fig. 67-15). If required, partial cardiopulmonary bypass may be accomplished using the femoral vessels. The advantage of anterolateral thoracotomy is that pericardial resection, especially over the left ventricle, is possible with minimal manipulation of the heart.

In a review of 313 pericardiectomy procedures,[49] the overall operative mortality rate was 14%. Early mortality was predominantly from myocardial dysfunction and low cardiac output after operation. Cardiac dilation and atrophy were observed in many of these patients. Risk of mortality was directly related to preoperative NYHA class: 1% for class I or II, 10% for class III, and 46% for class IV patients. Patients who died had higher right-sided cardiac pressures, ascites, and peripheral edema. The most common nonfatal complication was low cardiac output requiring inotropic or mechanical support. Actuarial survival rates after 5, 15, and 30 years were 84%, 71%, and 52%, respectively; survival rates were statistically lower in NYHA class III and IV patients. In a further series of 145 patients with effusive pericardial disease, the 30-day hospital mortality rate was 12% (19% for malignant effusion and 5% for benign disease). There was a strong correlation between the type of pericardiectomy (limited pericardial resection, pericardial window) and the incidence of reoperation for effusion or constriction. Eighty-five percent of patients had immediate relief of symptoms, with an additional 10% free from further attacks at 1 year. In another series, 11.7% of all patients requiring pericardiectomy had pain as the principal indication for operation. All seven patients survived operation and were pain free without steroid therapy. Finally, in a series of pericardiectomies, the authors[50] reported 102 patients with 26 neoplasms; 21 patients were uremic, 17 idiopathic, 3 postinfection, and 19 post-CABG. Only 2 patients needed cardiopulmonary bypass, and there were no deaths. In all these series, a technical point was made to free the left ventricle first to avoid having the right ventricle begin pumping normally with the left ventricle still hindered, which can result in acute pulmonary edema. Finally, some authors[51] have advocated the use of the thoracoscope for video-assisted pericardiectomy, with initial good results.

REFERENCES

1. Titus JL. Normal anatomy of the human cardiac conduction system. Mayo Clin Proc 1973;48:24.
2. Zipes DP, ed. Cardiac electrophysiology: from cell to bedside. Philadelphia, WB Saunders, 1990.
3. Platia EV, ed. Management of cardiac arrhythmias. Philadelphia, JB Lippincott, 1987.
4. Morady F, Calkins H, Kadish AH, et al. Diagnosis and cure of paroxysmal supraventricular tachycardia during a single electrophysiology test. N Engl J Med 1991;324:1612.
5. Cox JL. Anatomic-electrophysiologic basis for the surgical treatment of refractory ischemic ventricular tachycardia. Ann Thorac Surg 1983;198:119.
6. Josephson ME, Wellens HJJ. Tachycardias: mechanisms, diagnosis, treatment. Philadelphia, Lea & Febiger, 1984.
7. Mandel WJ. Cardiac arrhythmias: their mechanisms, diagnosis, and management, ed 2. Philadelphia, JB Lippincott, 1980.
8. Hargrove WC, Miller JM. Risk stratification and management of patients with recurrent ventricular tachycardia and on the malignant ventricular arrhythmias. Circulation 1989;79 (Suppl I):178.
9. Elefteriades JA, Biblo LA, Batsford WP, et al. Evolving patterns in the surgical treatment of malignant ventricular arrhythmias. Ann Thorac Surg 1990;49:94.
10. Cox JL. Patient selection criteria and results of surgery for refractory ischemic ventricular tachycardia. Circulation 1989; 79(Suppl I):163.
11. Cox JL, Gust HB, Damiano RJ, et al. Right ventricular isolation procedures for nonischemic ventricular tachycardia. J Thorac Cardiovasc Surg 1985;90:212.
12. Moran JM. Surgery for ventricular arrhythmias. Ann Thorac Surg 1990;49:837.

13. Page P, Cardinal R, Nadeau R. Surgical treatment of ventricular tachycardia: regional cryoablation guided by computerized epicardial and endocardial mapping. Circulation 1989;Suppl I)80:124.

14. Guiraudon G, Fontaine G, Frank R, et al. Encircling endocardial ventriculotomy: a new surgical treatment for life-threatening ventricular tachycardias resistant to medical treatment following myocardial infarction. Ann Thorac Surg 1978;26:438.

15. Moran JM, Kehoe RF, Loeb JM, et al. Extended endocardial resection for the treatment of ventricular tachycardia and ventricular fibrillation. Ann Thorac Surg 1982;34:538.

16. Ott DA, Cooley DA, Moak J, et al. Cryoablative techniques in the treatment of cardiac tachyarrhythmias. Ann Thorac Surg 1987;43:138.

17. Cox JI. The status of surgery for cardiac arrhythmias. Circulation 1985;71:413.

18. Winkle RA, Mead RH, Ruder MA, et al. Long-term outcome with the automatic implantable cardioverter-defibrillator. J Am Coll Cardiol 1989;13:1353.

19. Winkle RA, Cannon DC. Practical aspects of automatic cardioverter/defibrillator implantation. Am Heart J 1984;108:1335.

20. Stevenson LW, Fowler MB, Schroder JS, Stevenson WG, Drucup KA, Fond V. Poor survival of patients with idiopathic cardiomyopathy considered too well for transplantation. Am J Med 1987;83:871.

21. Bolling SF, Deeb GM, Morady F, et al. AICD: new bridge to transplantation. J Heart Lung Transplant 1991;10:562.

22. Bolling SF, Morady F, Calkins H, et al. Current treatment for Wolff-Parkinson-White syndrome: results and surgical implications. Ann Thorac Surg 1991;52:461.

23. Lowe JE. Surgical treatment of the Wolff-Parkinson-White syndrome and other supraventricular tachyarrhythmias. J Cardiac Surg 1986;1:117.

24. Blomstrom P, Jonsson R. The relationship between intraoperatively assessed atrial and ventricular insertions of accessory pathways. Clin Cardiol 1989;12:701.

25. Menasche P, Leclercq JF, Cauchemez B, et al. Surgery for the Wolff-Parkinson-White syndrome in 73 consecutive patients: what have we learnt from intraoperative mapping? Eur J Cardiothorac Surg 1989;3:387.

26. Page PL, Pelletier LC, Kaltenbrunner W, Vitali E, Roy D, Nadeau R. Surgical treatment of the Wolff-Parkinson-White syndrome: endocardial versus epicardial approach. J Thorac Cardiovasc Surg 1990;100:83.

27. Guiraudon GM, Klein GJ, Sharma AD, Jones DL, McLellan DG. Surgery for WPW syndrome: further experience with an epicardial approach. Circulation 1986;74:525.

28. Kuck KH, Kunze KP, Schluter M, Geiger M, Jackman WM. Ablation of a left-sided free-wall accessory pathway by percutaneous catheter application of radiofrequency current in a patient with the Wolff-Parkinson-White syndrome. PACE 1989;12:1681.

29. de Buitleir M, Bove EL, Schmaltz S, Kadish AH, Morady F. Cost of catheter versus surgical ablation in the Wolff-Parkinson-White syndrome. Am J Cardiol 1990;66:189.

30. Sealy WC, Gallagher JJ, Kasell J, et al. His bundle interruption for control of inappropriate ventricular responses to atrial arrhythmias. Ann Thorac Surg 1981;32:429.

31. Cox JL, Boineau JP, Schuesler RB, et al. Operations for atrial fibrillation. Clin Cardiol 1991;14:827.

32. McCarthy PM, Castle LW, Maloney JD, et al. Initial experience with the maze procedure for atrial fibrillation. J Thorac Cardiovasc Surg 1993;105:1077.

33. Cox JL, Boineau JP, Schuesler RB, Kater KM, Lappas DG. Five-year experience with the maze procedure for atrial fibrillation. Ann Thorac Surg 1993;56:814.

34. Pegram BL, Bishop VS. An evaluation of the pericardial sac as a safety factor during tamponade. Cardiovasc Res 1975;9:715.

35. Shabetai R. The pericardium. New York: Grune & Stratton, 1981.

36. Darsee JR, Braunwald E. Diseases of the pericardium. In: Braunwald E, ed. Heart disease: a textbook of cardiovascular medicine. Philadelphia, WB Saunders, 1980:1517.

37. Hancock EW. Neoplastic pericardial disease. Cardiac Clin 1990;8:673.

38. Fiorentino MV, Daneile O, Morandi P, et al. Intrapericardial instillation of platin in malignant pericardial effusion. Cancer 1988;62:1904.

39. Maher E, Buckman R. Intrapericardial instillation of bleomycin in malignant pericardial effusion. Am Heart J 1986;111:613.

40. Shepherd FA, Morgan CD, Evans WK, et al. Medical management of malignant pericardial effusion by tetracycline sclerosis. Am J Cardiol 1987;60:1161.

41. Spodick DH. Pericarditis in systemic diseases. Cardiac Clin 1990;8:709.

42. Spodick DH. Electrocardiogram in acute pericarditis: distributions of morphologic and axial changes by stages. Am J Cardiol 1974;33:470.

43. De Pace NL, Nestico PF, Schwartz AB, et al. Predicting success of intensive dialysis in the treatment of uremic pericarditis. Am J Med 1984;76:38.

44. Buselmeier TJ, Davin TD, Simmons RL, et al. Treatment of intractable uremic pericardial effusion: avoidance of pericardiectomy with local steroid injection. JAMA 1978;240:1358.

45. Carmichael DB, Sprague HB, Wyman SM, Bland EF. Acute nonspecific pericarditis: clinical, laboratory, and follow-up considerations. Circulation 1951;3:321.

46. Fowler NO. Recurrent pericarditis. Cardiac Clin 1990;8:621.

47. Fowler NO. The Pericardium in health and disease. Mt Kisco, NY, Futura Publishing Co, 1985:266.

48. Borkon AM, Schaff HV, Gardner TJ, et al. Diagnosis and management of postoperative pericardial effusions and late cardiac tamponade following open-heart surgery. Ann Thorac Surg 1981;31:512.

49. Tuna IC, Danielson GK. Surgical management of pericardial diseases. Cardiol Clin 1990;8:683.

50. Kutcher MA, King SB, Alimurung BN, Craver JM, Logue RB. Constrictive pericarditis as a complication of cardiac surgery: recognition of an entity. Am J Cardiol 1982;50:742.

51. Hazelrigg SR, Mack MJ, Landreneau RJ, Acuff TE, Seifert PE, Auer JE. Thoracoscopic pericardiectomy for effusive pericardial disease. Ann Thorac Surg 1993;56:792.

ARTERIAL SYSTEM

Basic Considerations in Vascular Disease

SURGERY: SCIENTIFIC PRINCIPLES AND PRACTICE, Second Edition, edited by
Lazar J. Greenfield, Michael W. Mulholland, Keith T. Oldham, Gerald B. Zelenock,
and Keith D. Lillemoe. Lippincott–Raven Publishers, Philadelphia, © 1997.

CHAPTER 68

ATHEROSCLEROSIS AND THE PATHOGENESIS OF OCCLUSIVE DISEASE

ALEXANDER W. CLOWES

Atherosclerosis is a disease of the intima of large arteries that causes luminal narrowing, thrombosis, and occlusion associated with ischemia of the end organ. Throughout much of its course, the disease is not readily detectable. Thrombosis, including vascular occlusion and embolization, produces the clinical events of importance, such as myocardial infarction, stroke, and ischemic gangrene of the extremities. The widespread prevalence of lesions in arteries of asymptomatic people, the chronicity of the process, the suddenness of the terminal vascular events, and the lack of a single etiologic factor make it impossible to give a simple explanation for atherogenesis and atherosclerosis progression. In fact, atherosclerosis might be a form of nonspecific adaptation on the part of large blood vessels to a variety of harmful stimuli, and the clinical consequences (the so-called true disease process) appear when the compensatory mechanisms are overwhelmed.

This chapter described factors that influence the structure of normal arteries and that might also play a role in the development of the atherosclerotic plaque.

NORMAL STRUCTURE OF BLOOD VESSELS

Normal arteries and veins, both large and small, are formed from endothelium, smooth muscle, and extracellular matrix synthesized by vascular wall cells. The vascular

wall is invariably organized into layers (Fig. 68-1). The *intima,* defined as the part of the wall between the blood and the internal elastic lamina, is composed of a monolayer of endothelium at the luminal surface and can overlie one or more layers of smooth muscle. The *media,* lying beneath the intima, constitutes the bulk of the vessel and contains smooth muscle cells arranged in layers and dispersed in a matrix made of elastin, collagen, and proteoglycan. The *adventitia* lies outside the external elastic lamina and forms the outer coat. It is composed of loose connective tissue, fibroblasts, capillaries, neural fibers, and occasional leukocytes. In large arteries with greater than 28 elastic layers, a microvasculature (vasa vasorum) penetrates the media from the adventitial side and provides an alternative nutrient supply to the flux from the luminal surface.[1] In thickened, atherosclerotic vessels, the vasa vasorum are extensive and penetrate into the diseased intima.[2,3]

In the fetus, the vessel wall is derived from mesoderm. A brief review of this process is of interest because many aspects of wound healing and atherogenesis in adult vessels represent a recapitulation of the fetal program of vasculogenesis and angiogenesis. The earliest vascular primordia in the embryo are isolated *hemangioblasts* that display endothelial and hematopoietic immunologic markers.[4,5] The hemangioblasts cluster and form cords and later tubes that become the major vascular conduits. Some of the clusters become blood islands, the precursors for hematopoietic tissues. These structures sprout, grow, and remodel to form the primitive vascular system.[6]

Endothelial cells probably play a central role in the organization and building of vascular structures. They are derived from the hemangioblasts, organize at sites of later vessel development, and are followed by local mesenchymal cells that form the outer layers of the emerging blood vessels. These mesenchymal cells are the precursors of smooth muscle cells and fibroblasts. Once associated with the vessel wall, many of these cells begin to express smooth muscle–specific α-actin. This pattern of endothelial invasion, followed by smooth muscle recruitment, is reactivated in later life during angiogenesis in the presence of tumors and in wounds undergoing repair.

The adult form of blood vessels appears to be established by birth. In large vessels, the number of elastic and smooth muscle layers remains constant, although wall mass increases due to smooth muscle proliferation and matrix synthesis.[7,8] The vascular architecture is probably genetically determined because alterations in animal size by hormonal manipulations (eg, excess growth hormone) are associated with increased wall mass but no change in the number of cell layers.[9] It is likely that the primitive endothelial cell regulates wall architecture because it is involved in the recruitment of the corresponding primitive smooth muscle

This chapter is based in part on Clowes AW. Theories of atherosclerosis. In: White RA, ed. Atherosclerosis and arteriosclerosis: human pathology and experimental animal methods and models. Boca Raton, FL, CRC Press, 1989:3.

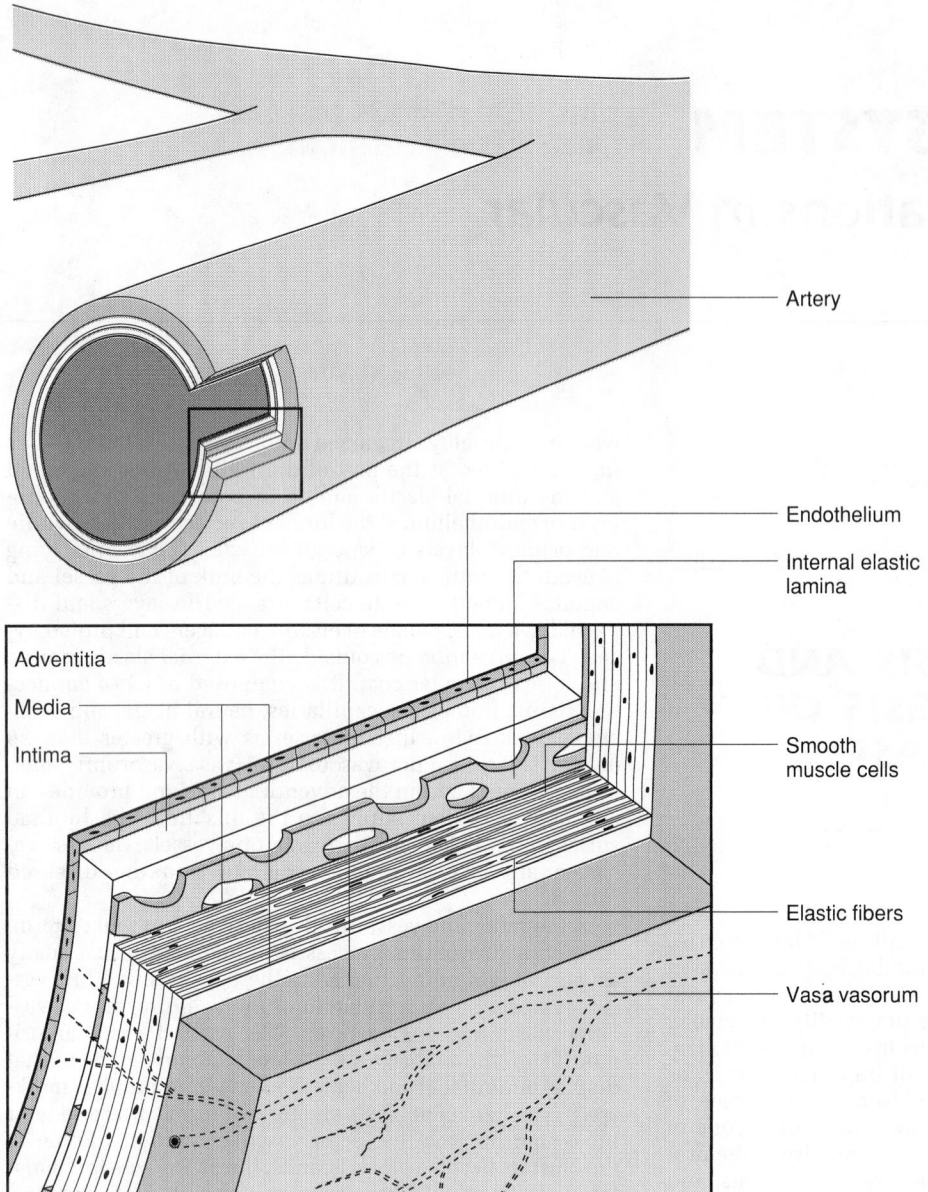

- Artery
- Endothelium
- Internal elastic lamina
- Adventitia
- Media
- Intima
- Smooth muscle cells
- Elastic fibers
- Vasa vasorum

Figure 68-1. The artery wall is made of multiple layers (intima, media, and adventitia) that vary in composition depending on the artery.

cell. As discussed later, these activities of the endothelial cell in the embryo presage its role in determining vascular diameter and mass in normal and diseased adult arteries.

These observations on the embryologic origin of vascular wall cells and the development of blood vessels provide many insights into vascular wall organization and function in the adult and provoke numerous questions that have few answers. What determines the initial organization of the hemangioblasts (the primitive endothelium)? Are they tracking some kind of predetermined scaffolding? What are the signals that regulate proliferation of these cells? How do they go about recruiting the primitive smooth muscle cells? How do the endothelial cells then regulate smooth muscle number and function? Does the molecular language of endothelial–smooth muscle cell discourse extend to other types of cell interactions (eg, between leukocytes or platelets and vascular wall cells)? In the past decade, researches have begun to realize how complex the answers are to these questions and to develop a rudimentary understanding of how vascular cells interact in normal

and disease states. The next section reviews some of the evidence that vascular wall function and structure depend absolutely on cell–cell interactions.

REGULATION OF LUMINAL AREA

This description of the usual arterial wall anatomy gives no clue to how a vessel adjusts its mass and dimensions in response to external stimuli (hypertension, increased blood flow, vascular injury) nor to how it maintains a nonthrombogenic state at the luminal surface. For this, the array of possible physiologic functions of the wall and its cellular components must be considered under normal and abnormal conditions.

Blood vessels, both large and small, become larger during growth and development and as a compensatory mechanism to increased blood flow (or, more appropriately, increased blood velocity; Fig. 68-2). A particularly striking example of this is found in an artery proximal to an arteriovenous fistula; if the fistula is not treated, the artery can

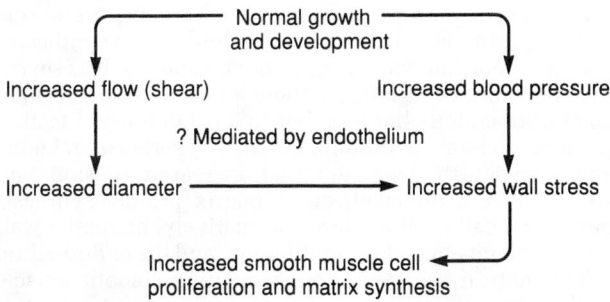

Figure 68-2. Changes in blood flow and pressure can have profound effects on arterial wall structure. In part, the response to hemodynamic changes may be mediated by the endothelium. (After Clowes AW. Theories of atherosclerosis. In: White RA, ed. Atherosclerosis and arteriosclerosis: human pathology and experimental animal methods and models. Boca Raton FL, CRC Press, 1989:3)

become frankly aneurysmal.[10] Similarly, a vessel undergoing stenosis experiences an increase in blood velocity at the point of luminal narrowing. When the stenosis is attributable to intimal thickening or to an atherosclerotic plaque, the vessel dilates at the site of the lesion. For example, a diseased coronary vessel dilates and can maintain the correct luminal dimensions despite changes in wall structure so long as the intimal lesion does not occupy over 40% of the area inside the internal elastic lamina[11] (Fig. 68-3). At this point, pathologic narrowing begins to take place. Why vessels should dilate in each of these instances when the velocity of flow increases has not been determined. One possibility is that the cells in the wall, particularly the endothelium, are somehow capable of sensing changes in blood velocity and shear and can translate this biomechanical information into biochemical signals that then regulate the contractile state of the artery.[12-15] Endothelial cell secretory products play a critical role in smooth muscle cell function.[16] They secrete vasodilating substances (prostaglandin I_2 and E_2, adenosine, endothelium-dependent relaxing factor [EDRF]) and vasoconstricting substances (endothelin). When endothelium is damaged or absent, adherent platelets release the vasoconstrictor thromboxane A_2.

Evidence suggests that EDRF in particular is an important regulator in normal and diseased vessels.[17] It is a short-acting substance or substances. In most circumstances, the predominant EDRF is nitric oxide, which is derived from the metabolic breakdown of arginine.[18-20] A number of factors stimulate endothelial cells to secrete EDRF, including thrombin, acetylcholine, bradykinin, serotonin, and products of platelet release. Hence, when endothelium is present and functional, neighboring thrombotic events are likely to cause vasodilation; whereas when the endothelium is absent or dysfunctional, these same factors cause vasoconstriction. Moreover, when the endothelium is missing, the vessel does not respond normally to changes in blood flow, in either the short or long term.[21] Changes in blood flow affect wall mass.[22-24] In this regard, it is interesting that various factors that affect smooth muscle contraction or relaxation also modulate growth (nitric oxide, endothelin, thrombin, prostaglandins).[25-29] These observations may be the first preliminary evidence that transient signals affecting the diameter of vessels may have, in the long term, more permanent effects on wall structure. Certain pathologic conditions in which endothelium either is missing or is abnormal are associated with acute and chronic vasospasm; it is possible that the acute problems of atypical angina (coronary vasospasm) and

cerebrovasospasm after cerebral hemorrhage are manifestations of abnormal endothelial function and decreased EDRF.[30]

REGULATION OF MEDIAL AND INTIMAL THICKENING

As discussed earlier, for embryonic vessels to form, primitive endothelial cells must migrate and become aligned and then recruit smooth muscle precursors from the surrounding mesenchyme. Because endothelial cells grow as a monolayer, they can proliferate only when the vascular structure is enlarging in circumference (vasodilation), during vascular elongation (angiogenesis), or when injured endothelium is being replaced. Massive denudation and endothelial loss are not normal events and probably occur only during pathologic degeneration of the intima or during surgical instrumentation of the vessel. In any event, endothelial proliferation does not contribute significantly to an increase in wall mass. Smooth muscle cell proliferation does.

Under several circumstances, vessels of adult animals respond by becoming thicker. In hypertensive animals and humans, arteries exhibit medial thickening, while after endothelial denudation or in the presence of hypercholesterolemia, they develop a thick intima.[31,32] Exactly how these responses are regulated is not clear, although it is certain that in each instance proliferation of smooth muscle cells and accumulation of extracellular matrix are important components. In addition, in hypercholesterolemic subjects, the accumulation of lipid and lipid-filled macrophages contributes to the intimal lesion.[33]

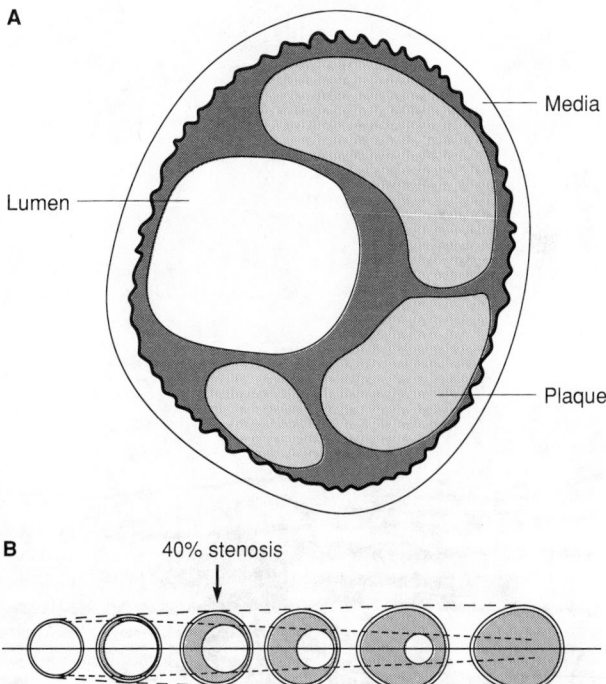

Figure 68-3. (*A*) Coronary arteries dilate as atherosclerotic plaques form and maintain normal luminal dimensions. Luminal narrowing begins only after the plaque occupies more than 40% of the cross-sectional area within the internal elastic lamina and bulges outward at sites of medial atrophy. (*B*) The course of lesion formation and luminal narrowing. (After Glagov S, Weisenberg E, Zarins CK, Stankunavicius R, Kolettis GJ. Compensatory enlargement of human atherosclerotic coronary arteries. N Engl J Med 1987;316:1371)

Vessel wall mass is largely determined by the accumulation of smooth muscle cells and matrix synthesized by smooth muscle cells. Hence, it is important to consider how smooth muscle number is regulated.[34] Under normal circumstances, smooth muscle cells proliferate in the vessels of young animals and enter a quiescent state at maturity. For example, smooth muscle cells in adult rat carotid arteries do not increase in number and turn over at a rate of 0.06% a day.[35] In animal models of disease, these cells can readily be stimulated to enter the growth cycle by induction of hypertension or direct vascular injury. As discussed later, the observations made in these models provide us with insights into possible mechanisms for initiation and progression of vascular disease in humans.

Although hypertension has its greatest impact on the small *resistance vessels*, in fact large arteries are equally affected. In response to increased pressure, the wall thickens.[31,36] Morphometric studies have shown that this increase is largely a medial process and involves all components of the vessel wall, including the mass of smooth muscle cells and matrix. In some forms of hypertension, there is an increase in smooth muscle number, while in others, there is an increase in the DNA content per cell. Tetraploid and octaploid cells have been detected. In venous grafts transposed from a relatively hypotensive venous environment into the normotensive arterial circulation, there is an increase in wall thickness and a corresponding increase in smooth muscle number.[37] In each instance, the change in pressure affects the mass of cells and associated matrix.

How a change in pressure might induce smooth muscle cells to proliferate, to change their ploidy, or to synthesize matrix is not known. In some circumstances (eg, severe hypertension, vein grafting), there is a detectable but small amount of endothelial loss, but this is not a usual feature in more moderate or chronic forms of hypertension. Leung and associates[38] suggested that increased tension and stretch have a direct effect on matrix protein synthesis but not on cell proliferation. Alternatively, increased wall tension might affect the endothelium, and the endothelium might in turn secrete factors regulating smooth muscle mass.

Of the models of smooth muscle growth in vivo, perhaps the best studied is the balloon injury model first developed by Baumgartner.[35,39] In this model, smooth muscle proliferation is stimulated by the passage of an inflated balloon catheter along an artery. The artery is at once stretched and denuded of its endothelium. Immediately thereafter, platelets begin to adhere to the wall wherever endothelium is missing; they then spread and degranulate. In most situations, endothelial denudation and platelet adherence are followed 1 to 2 days later by the onset of medial smooth muscle proliferation. In the ballooned rat carotid (Fig. 68-4), this can be a most dramatic response, with a three-log increase in the thymidine labeling index (a measure of proliferation). This early proliferation in the media does not lead to an increase in wall thickness; the wall thickens only after smooth muscle cells migrate from the media and proliferate in the intima. In normal animals, this process continues for a period and subsides spontane-

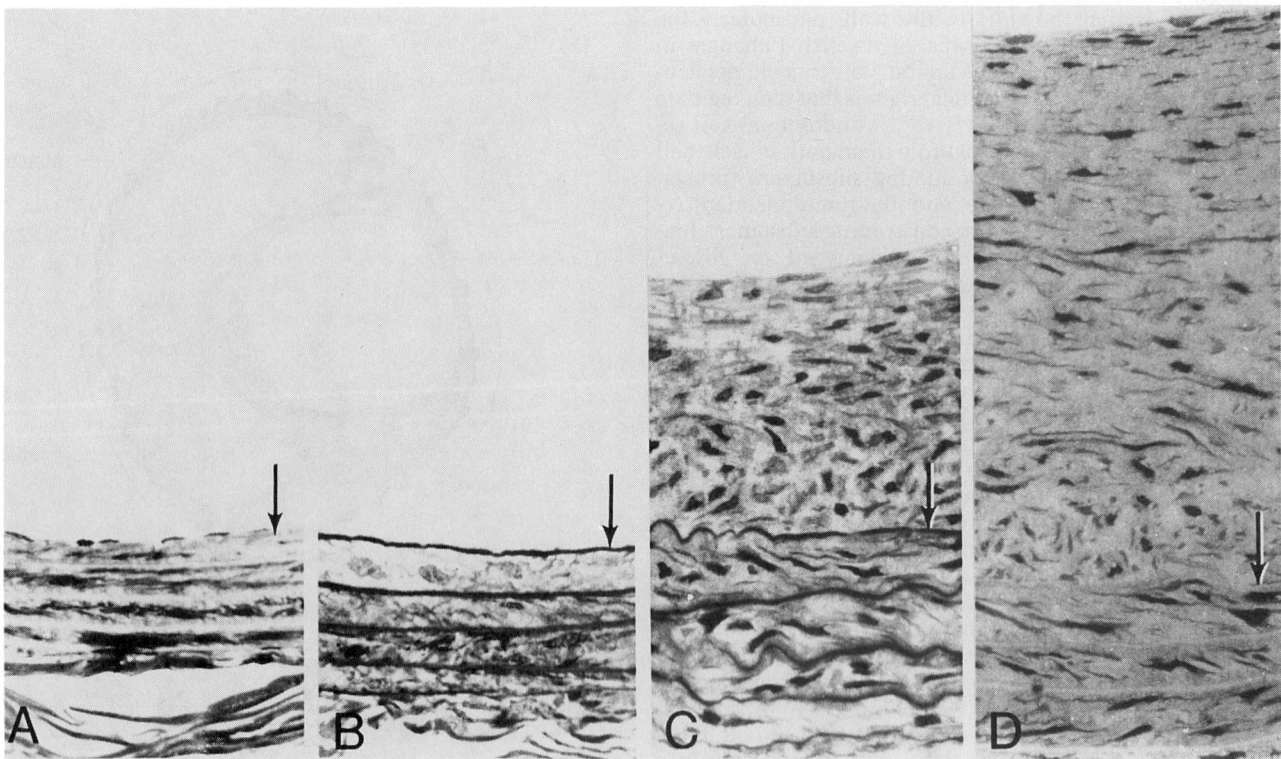

Figure 68-4. Elastic arteries that were injured by the passage of a balloon embolectomy catheter develop substantial intimal thickenings. In this series of histologic cross sections of rat carotid artery before (*A*) and after (*B* through *D*) ballooning, the endothelium is stripped away and the inner layer of medial smooth muscle cells is damaged (*B*). By 2 weeks (*C*), the intima is thickened by the migration and proliferation of smooth muscle cells derived from the media. The mass of cells does not change significantly after this time; nevertheless, the intima is thicker at 3 months (*D*) because of matrix synthesis and accumulation. (Clowes AW, Reidy MA, Clowes MM. Kinetics of cellular proliferation after arterial injury. I. Smooth muscle growth in the absence of endothelium. Lab Invest 1983;49:327)

ously, whether or not endothelium reappears at the luminal surface. The intimal mass is further increased by the accumulation of extracellular matrix synthesized by the smooth muscle cells.[40]

A link between smooth muscle proliferation and earlier platelet granule release has been proposed. Among the proteins released are several growth factors, including platelet-derived growth factor (PDGF), transforming growth factor-beta (TGF-β), and an epidermal growth factor–like (EGF-like) protein.[41] Where these granule proteins go after being released from the platelets is not known. One hypothesis suggests that these factors accumulate in the artery wall and stimulate subsequent smooth muscle growth.[32] This hypothesis (the *reaction-to-injury hypothesis*) was first proposed many decades ago as a general mechanism for atherogenesis and has been refined in view of recent information. Although attractive in theory, it is based on slim evidence mainly derived from experiments in thrombocytopenic animals.[42] Injured arteries in these animals show little intimal thickening.

My colleagues and I reexamined the hypothesis that the decrease in intimal thickening in injured arteries of thrombocytopenic animals is attributable to decreased proliferation of smooth muscle cells.[43] Using the ballooned rat carotid model, these investigators found that even though intimal thickening was diminished in thrombocytopenic animals, smooth muscle proliferation and early cell cycle gene expression were the same as in controls. Our interpretation of these findings is that platelet products play a role in the movement of smooth muscle cells from one vascular compartment to the next (media to intima) but do not affect the initiation of proliferation. Whether platelet factors can influence the growth of intimal smooth muscle has yet to be determined.

Although little is known about what starts or stops the intimal thickening process, several observations are interesting and are perhaps important when considering the theories of atherosclerosis. The first is that the surface of the injured artery accumulates a single layer of platelets. Fibrin and microthrombi are seen only at the luminal surface when the artery is reinjured after an intimal thickening has formed or in small craters in association with adherent macrophages in hypercholesterolemic animals.[44–47] Active, fulminant thrombosis is not a usual feature of injured vessels; when it occurs, it must represent a major aberration of vessel function. Also, in models demonstrating early reendothelialization or partial deendothelialization without medial injury, intimal thickening does not develop, although one or two rounds of medial smooth muscle proliferation can occur.[48] This result suggests that endothelium might play a role in suppressing smooth muscle growth and migration from the media to the intima. It is known that smooth muscle growth inhibitors can be extracted from the vessel wall, endothelium can synthesize a heparin-like molecule that inhibits smooth muscle cell growth in vitro, and heparin can suppress both proliferation and migration of smooth muscle cells in vitro and in vivo.[49] Taken together, these findings suggest that endothelium can inhibit smooth muscle proliferation and that the quiescent state of smooth muscle cells in the normal arteries of adult animals might be actively maintained rather than attributable to the lack of growth factors (Fig. 68-5).

REGULATION OF SMOOTH MUSCLE GROWTH

Platelets have long been considered the major source of mitogen for proliferating smooth muscle. Smooth muscle cells, however, can proliferate in injured and hypertensive

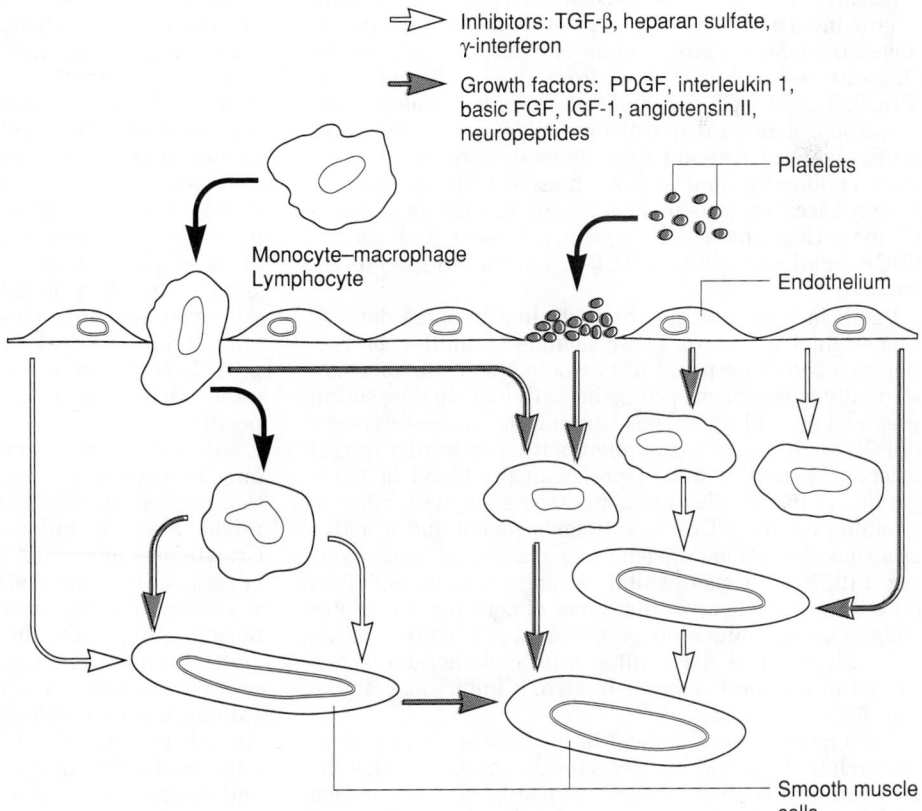

Figure 68-5. Diagram depicting the complexity of the interactions among vascular wall cells (endothelium and smooth muscle), platelets, and blood-borne leukocytes (monocyte–macrophages and lymphocytes). Each cell is capable of synthesizing and releasing several smooth muscle growth factors and inhibitors.

arteries when platelets are absent. If platelet factors are not important, what, then, is the stimulus for smooth muscle growth? Three alternatives are possible: (1) growth factors from vascular wall cells or resident leukocytes; (2) exogenous, neuroendocrine factors; or (3) loss of local inhibitors of smooth muscle proliferation. All three mechanisms may be important. The first alternative is of interest in that when a rat carotid is denuded of endothelium with a balloon catheter, a substantial fraction of the medial smooth muscle cells proliferate (about 20% to 30%), but when denudation is accomplished with a fine nylon wire, there is little proliferation (about 2% to 4%).[50] These procedures differ only in regard to the degree to which the media is damaged. Ballooning destroys 20% of the medial smooth muscle as well as the endothelium, while passage of the nylon wire destroys only the endothelium. Of further interest is that cultured cells, when damaged, release growth-promoting activity.[51,52] The predominant growth-promoting activity is due to fibroblast growth factors (FGFs).[53,54] These factors have been found in a wide variety of tissues and cell types and are synthesized by endothelium and smooth muscle cells. They are distinguished from other polypeptide mitogens by their ability to bind strongly to heparin. Furthermore, both acidic and basic FGFs are potent smooth muscle mitogens in vitro. Finally, FGF can bind to heparin-like molecules so that released FGF might readily be stored in the heparan sulfate proteoglycan-containing matrix at sites of cell death.[55] The experiments of Lindner and colleagues[56,57] provide strong evidence to support the conclusion that basic FGF is the important growth factor for the first wave of proliferation in balloon-injured rat carotid artery. This mechanism of tissue repair is probably relevant for the development of the fibrous cap in advanced atherosclerotic lesions. At these sites, toxic oxidized lipids accumulate, and there is clear evidence of injury and necrosis.[33] The release of cellular FGF could provide the stimulus for smooth muscle proliferation in the overlying fibrous cap.

Because cell death is not necessarily a prominent feature of growing tissues, there must be other means for controlling smooth muscle proliferation. Not only do smooth muscle cells respond to factors from dead cells, platelets (PDGF, TGF-β, EGF-like molecules), and plasma (thrombin, lipoproteins, insulin-like growth factor-1), they also synthesize and respond to their own secreted factors.[34] Both endothelial and smooth muscle cells, as well as macrophages, are potential sources of mitogen. In addition to the FGFs, these cell types synthesize and secrete PDGF, interleukin-1 (IL-1), TGF-β, and insulin-like growth factor-1.

PDGF in particular has been studied in some detail.[58] The original studies on PDGF stemmed from the observation that serum prepared from whole blood contains substantially more growth-promoting activity than does serum prepared from plasma. These findings led to the discovery of PDGF, a basic dimeric protein with a molecular weight of about 30,000. It is transported in the blood in the α granule of the platelet and is released along with other α-granule proteins. PDGF is extremely potent and is active as a smooth muscle mitogen in trace amounts (nanograms per milliliter). It also exhibits a range of other activities on smooth muscle and other types of cells (eg, stimulates smooth muscle migration, contraction, and matrix synthesis), although it is not a mitogen for endothelium. When placed in a wound chamber in vivo, it induces a granulation tissue response.[59]

An important development in the field of growth factor research in the past decade was the demonstration that the structure of the gene for PDGF is nearly identical to that of the oncogene v-*sis*, a gene associated with cellular trans-

formation by the simian sarcoma virus.[60,61] This discovery, coupled with the finding that a variety of cells, including normal cells, synthesize and secrete active PDGF, raises the possibility that normal wound healing and malignant, unscheduled growth of tumor cells might have striking similarities with subtle differences in gene regulation. It also led to a search for growth factors in vascular wall cells. Solid evidence now exists that endothelium, smooth muscle cells, and leukocytes, including macrophages, can express the PDGF gene (c-*sis* or PDGF B chain) in vitro and in vivo.[58] PDGF research is complicated by the observation that PDGF is not a single molecule but is either a heterodimer or homodimer of two isoforms, PDGF A and PDGF B. The cellular receptors are also dimers of two isoforms, α and β, such that PDGF B binds to both α and β, but PDGF A binds only to the α form of the receptor. The implications of this complexity of growth factor and receptor expression have yet to be understood. It is known that human platelets transport mainly PDGF AB, while cultured smooth muscle cells from human plaques, baboon graft intima, and injury-induced rat intimal thickening express mainly PDGF A chain mRNA. This observation is probably not an artifact of cell culture because the primary lesions from which the cells are derived contain relatively large amounts of A chain mRNA. Macrophages in atherosclerotic lesions express PDGF B protein. What role PDGF plays in wall function remains to be determined. It is not clear how the expression of the protein is regulated, nor is it clear whether regulation also occurs at the level of receptor expression. These findings suggest the intriguing possibility that the vascular wall cells, as well as the platelets, are a source of growth factors in the artery wall and, through the endogenous production of growth factors, thus might be able to regulate their own growth (autocrine control) or their neighbor's growth (paracrine control). Alternatively, PDGF might control some other function than proliferation. Experiments from the laboratories of Ross and Clowes provide evidence that, at least after injury, PDGF might act as a chemoattractant and regulate the movement of smooth muscle cells from the media into the intima or from the wall into the overlying thrombus.[62,63]

Another alternative for regulation, in addition to factors from the blood and the cells themselves, is neuroendocrine control of smooth muscle growth.[64,65] Several neurotransmitters affect smooth muscle hypertrophy and proliferation (serotonin, neurokinin A, substance K, substance P). Furthermore, sympathectomy or inhibitors of sympathetic nerve function inhibit the increase in DNA in the media of developing arteries and arteries subjected to hypertension.[66,67] In injury models, prazosin (an α_1-antagonist) and cilazapril (an angiotensin-converting enzyme inhibitor) both inhibit intimal thickening.[68,69] These observations provide some support for the possibility that neuroendocrine factors also influence intimal smooth muscle proliferation.

Although smooth muscle mass may be determined in large measure by the presence or absence of growth factors, that is, positive effectors of growth, smooth muscle mass might also be influenced by endogenous inhibitors. Growth may be viewed as release from quiescence. As discussed earlier, endothelial regeneration in injured arteries is associated with cessation of underlying intimal smooth muscle growth. On the other hand, in healing vascular grafts, intimal smooth muscle cells proliferate *only* underneath the newly formed endothelial surface.[70] These observations are in parallel with studies of endothelial and smooth muscle cells in culture demonstrating that vascular wall cells can synthesize and secrete both inhibitors and promoters of smooth muscle growth.[13] The growth-promoting factors have already been described. Both cell types synthesize heparan sulfate, which, when released from the larger proteoglycan, can inhibit the growth of cultured smooth muscle cells.[71,72] Both cell types synthesize and secrete a TGF-β precursor,[73] and TGF-β can be found in the arterial wall after injury.[74] The precursor molecule can then be activated. In general, TGF-β acts as an inhibitor, although at times it can promote smooth muscle growth. Antibody to TGF-β administered to rats suppresses injury-induced intimal thickening.[75] Other in vivo growth inhibitors might be released by leukocytes present in the vascular wall. Although this mechanism is not important for the regulation of mass in normal artery, it is probably important in diseased vessels. In atherosclerotic plaques, there are large numbers of macrophages and lymphocytes. Hansson and colleagues[76] showed that resident T cells secrete γ-interferon and induce the expression of class II major histocompatibility antigens. γ-Interferon also inhibits smooth muscle growth in culture, and in the injured rat carotid, there is a significant population of I_a-positive, growth-inhibited intimal smooth muscle cells.[77] Although smooth muscle cells make up the bulk of the intimal thickening, 1% or less of the intimal cells are T cells. Because I_a expression is absolutely dependent on the presence of γ-interferon, these observations strongly support the view that γ-interferon is an endogenous regulator of intimal smooth muscle growth. Finally, growth of vascular wall cells might be regulated not only by secreted soluble factors but also by direct cell–cell contact. This inhibitory mechanism is important for endothelium and perhaps less so for smooth muscle cells.

Direct cell–cell communication and the presence of gap junctions have been demonstrated in monolayers of endothelium[78] and in mixed cell populations between endothelium and smooth muscle cells.[79] The significance of these direct links has not been defined, although one study demonstrated that cultured pericytes or smooth muscle cells can inhibit endothelial growth when the cells are in contact with one another. In vivo capillary endothelial cells appear to grow when pericytes are absent and to stop growing when the pericytes reappear. Endothelial cells can also regulate the growth of one another. Plasma membrane preparations from confluent large vessel endothelium actively inhibit growing endothelial cells.[80] The intercellular links might help to regulate endothelial proliferation and endothelial-mediated vascular relaxation in collateral vessels by propagating signals from one cell to the next upstream from a large vessel occlusion. Direct cell–cell communication would also provide a mechanism for a local response in a vessel without the need for the release and wide dissemination of potent vasoactive or growth-regulatory substances.

In summary, the size of a vessel wall depends on the mass of cells and matrix. Because smooth muscle cells and associated matrix proteins make up the bulk of the tissue, an understanding of the regulation of smooth muscle growth during development and in diseased states is extremely important. Smooth muscle cell number and distribution are affected by growth factors from the blood (particularly from platelets and leukocytes), growth factors and inhibitors from the vascular wall cells, and neuroendocrine factors, particularly from sympathetic innervation of the vessel wall. Smooth muscle quiescence in normal adult artery might be maintained by heparin-like inhibitors synthesized by vascular wall cells or by the absence of growth factor. Growth initiation might be due to a shift in the balance of these negative and positive stimuli (see Fig. 68-5). For example, any condition causing injury of vascular wall cells or inducing the influx of macrophages would be expected to set up a favorable environment for smooth muscle growth. Hypercholesterolemia, a significant risk factor for atherosclerosis, is associated with macrophage migration and the accumulation of toxic oxidized low-density lipoprotein (LDL) in susceptible large arteries. Release of endogenous FGF from dying foam cells, as well as release of other growth factors (possibly PDGF) from stimulated endothelium, smooth muscle, and macrophages, would increase the local concentration of growth-promoting activity. Smooth muscle cells would be expected to respond by proliferating and migrating into the intima; if collections of these cells were already present in the intima as a consequence of fetal development, they might be even more responsive. These factors might also regulate the traffic of other leukocytes (macrophages, T cells) in and out of the wall, and these activated cells would in turn amplify or retard the initial smooth muscle response by the production of growth factors or inhibitors. The extent and complexity of these interactions between the cells of the wall and the blood have yet to be unraveled.

REGULATION OF THE ANTICOAGULATED STATE

Blood does not clot in normal arteries even when flow is stopped for prolonged periods. On the other hand, endothelial injury or loss provokes a dramatic thrombotic response. These observations define the importance of the endothelial layer in the maintenance of the anticoagulated state.[81,82] Studies performed primarily on cultured cells have demonstrated that endothelial cells possess an array of anticoagulant and antithrombotic functions, and many of these are of importance in vivo. Endothelial cells also have several procoagulant functions, and the balance between procoagulant and anticoagulant functions is regulated by signals from the blood and from neighboring cells.

On the anticoagulant side of the balance, the endothelium synthesizes a membrane-associated heparan sulfate that, like heparin, increases the affinity of antithrombin III for thrombin.[83] Because this interaction requires the binding of heparan sulfate to antithrombin III, the complex must be active at the level of the endothelial surface. Heparan–antithrombin III then rapidly inactivates circulating thrombin and other activated serine proteases in the clotting cascade, including factors VII, IX, and X. Thus, endothelial-derived heparan sulfate can act to impede two aspects of the injury response: the activation of the clotting cascade and the stimulation of smooth muscle proliferation, referred to earlier. In addition, endothelial cells can inhibit clotting by the protein C pathway.[84] Endothelium synthesizes and secretes a protein called *thrombomodulin,* which in turn is bound to a surface receptor. The receptor–thrombomodulin complex binds thrombin and in so doing inactivates the proteolytic activity for fibrinogen. The thrombomodulin–thrombin complex activates protein C, and the activated protein C binds to protein S on the endothelial surface. The protein C–protein S complex then can inactivate factor Va, thereby inhibiting the clotting cascade. That this pathway is important is amply demonstrated in homozygous protein C–deficient patients who develop spontaneous thrombosis. Finally, endothelial cells can inhibit platelet adhesion and aggregation through the synthesis of prostaglandin I_2 and can degrade formed fibrin by activating plasminogen to plasmin.

On the procoagulant side, endothelial cells synthesize and secrete tissue factor, platelet-activating factor, a plasminogen-activator inhibitor, and von Willebrand factor, and they express a number of receptors for factors of the clotting cascade.[81] When the cells are exposed to a variety of inflammatory mediators derived from the blood or from resident macrophages (eg, endotoxin, IL-1, tumor necrosis factor), endothelial cells respond by changing the balance of anticoagulant–procoagulant activities to favor coagulation. Also, the cells synthesize and express IL-1, which could affect the underlying smooth muscle cells.[85] These conclusions are largely based on in vitro experiments; although they have relevance mainly for the microvasculature, they also might prove to be important for large vessels in view of the evidence that not only macrophages but also different populations of lymphocytes are present in the atherosclerotic plaque. Furthermore, the ability of the vascular wall cells to maintain the anticoagulant state at the luminal surface must have a direct bearing on the thrombotic complications associated with end-stage atherosclerosis.

THEORIES OF ATHEROSCLEROSIS

This chapter has summarized some of the information on vascular wall structure and function that might be relevant to general theories of atherosclerosis. From the foregoing, it should be evident that an artery is not just an inert nonthrombogenic conduit for blood; rather, it is an organ whose structure and function are carefully modulated by interactions among vascular wall cells themselves and between vascular wall cells and the blood. The prevailing theories of atherosclerosis are discussed next.

Atherosclerosis is a disease of the intima characterized by the accumulation of smooth muscle cells and lipid.[85,86] The earliest lesion appears to be a local accumulation of lipid in the vessel wall located either in the extracellular matrix or inside *foam cells* (lipid-filled smooth muscle cells or macrophages). The relation between the *fatty streak*, made up of foam cells, and the pathologic process of atherosclerosis, the fibrous plaque, and the complicated lesion has been the subject of some debate[87] (Fig. 68-6). Fatty streaks are found even in young children. Although atherosclerosis has a predilection for certain countries, the extent of fatty streaks of the aorta and coronary arteries in young people is about the same in countries that have low mortality rates from heart attack as in countries with high rates. The lipid streaks have been found to be just as common in females as in males, although atherosclerosis is more prevalent in males. Finally, even though the lipid

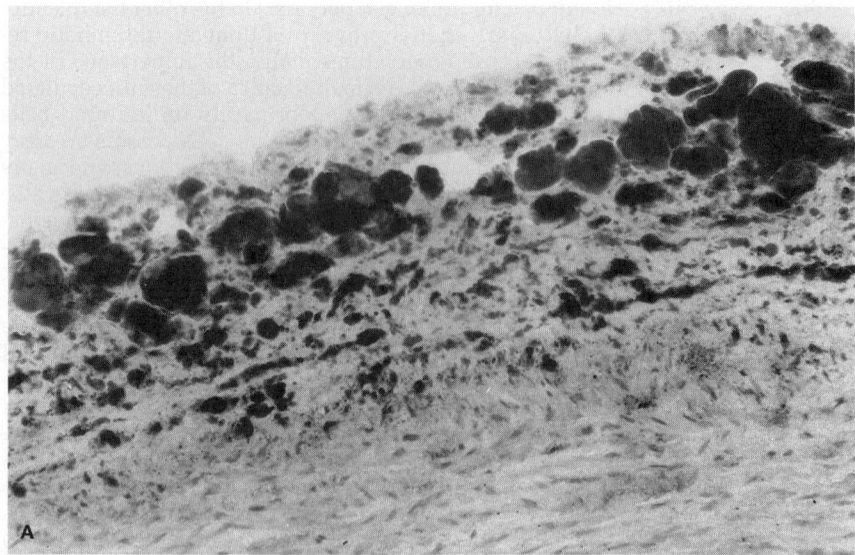

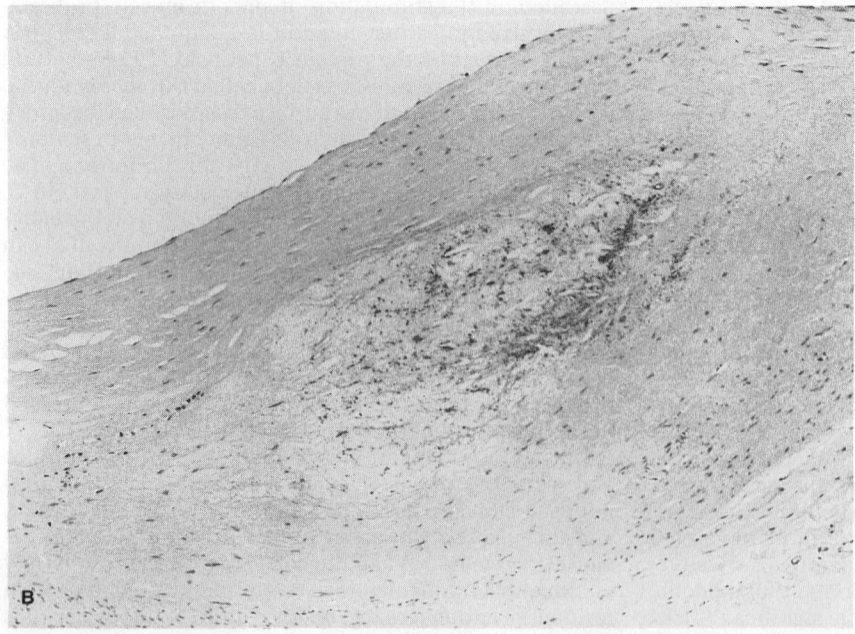

Figure 68-6. Histologic cross sections of a fatty streak containing foam cells stained dark with oil red O (*A*) and atherosclerotic plaque with fibrous cap (*B*). (Courtesy of David Gordon, MD, Department of Pathology, University of Michigan School of Medicine, Ann Arbor).

streaks are distributed throughout the aorta, end-stage disease is mostly confined to the abdominal segment.[88] Hence, if the fatty streak is the precursor of the more advanced lesion, then there must either be a selection process, or the whole concept must be wrong. The issue remains unresolved.

An alternative precursor for the atherosclerotic plaque is the intimal cell mass.[89,90] These focal accumulations of smooth muscle cells are frequently found in the vessels of children in locations where fibrous plaques later develop. In fat-fed swine, the intimal cell masses enlarge and become atherosclerotic.[91] Although the concept of the intimal cell masses as the initial lesion is attractive, there are several problems with it. First, this initial lesion is present in people throughout the world regardless of eventual risk for atherosclerosis. Second, generally there is a gradual thickening of the intima throughout the arterial tree as part of the aging process; this has little to do with atherosclerosis. Finally, it has been difficult to find animal models of atherosclerotic change in intimal masses, while the formation of fibrofatty lesions from fatty streaks has been easily modeled by cholesterol feeding in a number of species. For these reasons, support for the intimal cell mass as the initial lesion has not achieved wide acceptance.

Whatever the initial lesion is in atherosclerosis, it is widely agreed that the lesions characteristic of late atherosclerosis are the fibrous and the complicated plaques. The fibrous plaque is characterized by a thick fibrous luminal cap containing smooth muscle cells and leukocytes overlying a central core of necrotic debris and lipid (the *atheroma*). Animal studies have suggested that there might be either denudation or nondenuding injury of the endothelium at the surface.[46] The functional state of the endothelial and smooth muscle cells and leukocytes in these lesions is not known. Macrophages, by becoming "foamy," clearly play a role in the metabolism of lipid, and activated macrophages also secrete a range of factors that modulate the metabolic and growth states of the vascular wall cells. Macrophages also proliferate locally in the lesions.[92,93] Other leukocytes, particularly T lymphocytes, are also present; because some adjacent smooth muscle cells express the class II antigen HLA-DR, they must be exposed to γ-interferon presumably derived from the neighboring T cells.[94] In addition to inducing the expression of HLA-DR, γ-interferon inhibits smooth muscle proliferation. Hence, in the advanced atherosclerotic lesion, these leukocytes might play a critical role in regulating smooth muscle proliferation and accumulation.[95,96]

The complicated lesion of atherosclerosis is a fibrous plaque with the additional features of ulceration, luminal thrombosis, calcification, and wall hemorrhage (see Fig. 68-6). It is the source of the thromboembolic activities associated with symptomatic disease. Why a fibrous lesion evolves into a complicated plaque is not understood. This process might be accelerated by such risk factors as hypertension, whereas atherogenesis might be affected more by hypercholesterolemia and cigarette smoking. More important, the advent of the inflammatory cells and the release of potent mediators of inflammation must play a role in the development of the complicated lesion. As discussed earlier, growth factors for smooth muscle not only are liberated from platelets but also are synthesized and secreted by macrophages and the vascular wall cells. In addition, potent cytokines, such as IL-1, tumor necrosis factor, and γ-interferon alter the growth state and metabolism of the vascular wall cells. In particular, the anticoagulation–coagulation balance at the surface of the endothelium might be shifted away from anticoagulation and toward coagulation. In the plaque, large amounts of tissue factor and plasminogen activator-1 are present.[97–99] These changes, in addition to frank endothelial desquamation (in response to injurious agents, including oxidized LDL, homocystinemia, and tobacco products), could promote thrombosis in the vessel, an event that is decidedly unusual. Small accretions of thrombus with subsequent fibrotic remodeling and hemorrhage from new blood vessels in the ischemic central region of the plaque could account for the relatively rapid increase in plaque size and luminal narrowing that has been observed in some arterial beds.

During the past century, a number of theories have been advanced to explain how atherosclerosis evolves. In reality, these theories attempt to account for one or more aspects of the disease and are therefore not mutually exclusive. Much of the controversy over these theories has to do with individual opinion concerning which of the aspects of atherosclerosis is most important.

Perhaps the oldest hypothesis, the *lipid insudation hypothesis* states that the lipid in the atherosclerotic lesion is derived from lipoproteins in the blood[33,100]; it thereby links the risk factor hypercholesterolemia directly to the development of the plaque foam cell, the atheroma, and eventually the complicated lesion. There is good evidence now that the lipid in the plaques comes from the blood; there is also substantial evidence correlating severity of hypercholesterolemia (particularly elevated LDL cholesterol) with severity of atherosclerosis both in humans and in animal models. These conclusions are further supported by evidence obtained in mice made hypercholesterolemic by genetic manipulation.[101] Although this hypothesis provides a general concept for how lipid accumulates, it does not explain other features of the lesion, including smooth muscle proliferation and thrombosis.

The *encrustation hypothesis*, like the lipid insudation hypothesis, focuses on one aspect of the disease.[102] This hypothesis proposes that plaque initiation and progression is the consequence of repeated cycles of thrombosis and remodeling. Autopsy studies of vessels of children and experiments with cholesterol-fed animals, however, have shown that thrombosis is not the initial event in atherogenesis; in fact, thrombosis appears to be a feature of advanced disease. Hence, this hypothesis is applicable only to the problem of plaque progression. Furthermore, it does not explain how lipid and smooth muscle cells accumulate in the lesion.

The *reaction-to-injury hypothesis* attempts to explain how smooth muscle growth is regulated in atherogenesis.[32] As originally proposed, it stated that the initial event is some form of injury to the endothelium. In regions denuded of endothelium, platelets adhere and release growth factors; these growth factors accumulate in the wall and stimulate medial smooth muscle proliferation and migration into the intima. As discussed earlier, this theory is based on the observation that platelets carry potent smooth muscle mitogens in their granules and that the injury-induced arterial lesion closely resembles the fibrous cap found in the atherosclerotic plaque. A modified version of this theory suggests that injuries to the endothelium that do not produce denudation might also cause smooth muscle growth by stimulating damaged endothelium to synthesize and release growth factors. Alternatively, monocytes might be attracted to the zone of injury; the monocyte or macrophage might then be activated and start to elaborate growth-promoting activity. The reaction-to-injury hypothesis suggests a possible mechanism for the accumulation of connective tissue cells and matrix; it fails to provide an explanation for the lipid accumulation or the monoclonal nature of the advanced atherosclerotic plaque.

The *monoclonal hypothesis* also focuses on smooth muscle accumulation in the lesion.[103] It states that the cells of any particular plaque are likely to arise as a clone from a single progenitor smooth muscle cell. This hypothesis is based on the observation that individual plaques of human females heterozygote for the X-linked marker glucose-6-phosphate dehydrogenase frequently exhibit one but not both of the glucose-6-phosphate dehydrogenase isotypes. At a certain moment in time, single cells might be stimulated to enter the growth cycle and undergo several rounds of division, leading to the formation of a monoclonal lesion. The mechanism of cell activation leading to such lesions is not evident as yet; the only other known monoclonal cell masses in humans are neoplasias (eg, leiomyomas). This suggests carcinogens or viruses as possible etiologic agents and might explain the link between cigarette smoking and atherosclerosis. An alternative to carcinogenesis as an explanation for monoclonality is the possibility of activation of a susceptible population of stem cells.[104] Smooth muscle cells might have limited replicative capacity, and there might be only a small population of stem cells in the wall capable of responding to growth factors. Whatever the mechanism of activation, any theory attempting to provide a mechanism for the accumulation of smooth muscle cells in atherosclerotic plaques must take into account this observation of monoclonality.

The *intimal cell mass hypothesis* was mentioned earlier and states that the accumulations of intimal smooth muscle cells are one of the two possible initial lesions in atherosclerosis.[89,90] These small accumulations of smooth muscle cells are found in children at sites where atherosclerosis later develops. How they happen to get there is unclear, nor is it evident what makes them susceptible to atherogenic stimuli. It could be that these cells are primordial rests and really are a form of stem cell capable of responding to external mitogenic stimuli. Because the intimal cell masses are found in the vessels of children throughout the world regardless of the prevalence of atherosclerosis, it is likely that atherosclerotic change is largely determined by extrinsic risk factors such as hypercholesterolemia.

Each of these hypotheses attempts to explain one or more aspects of atherogenesis. Each might be applicable at a different time during the development of the lesion (Fig. 68-7). Susceptibility to atherosclerosis might be determined by both intrinsic factors (eg, numbers of intimal masses) and extrinsic factors (eg, hypercholesterolemia, hypertension, diabetes, cigarette smoking). The initial event might be the accumulation of lipid by insudation in regions of increased susceptibility. This would lead to the production of macrophage chemotactic factors and the influx of monocytes from the blood, which, together with the smooth muscle cells, would sequester lipid and become foam cells. LDL oxidized in the wall, as well as other extrinsic injurious agents, could produce some degree of endothelial injury and perhaps at late times even limited denudation. Growth factors might then be released from the endothelium, activated macrophages and other leukocytes, and the smooth muscle cells as well as from adherent platelets; these growth factors could then stimulate proliferation and migration of susceptible smooth muscle cells to form isolated smooth muscle clones and fibrous lesions. Further production of matrix by the smooth muscle would permit continued accumulation of lipid. Like a growing tumor, these lesions would enlarge, develop ischemic cores, and induce an angiogenic response. The thickened plaque with its necrotic lipid core (the atheroma) might not withstand the rigors of continued arterial pulsation and might develop hemorrhage within the lesion on account of the shearing forces on the new capillaries. Breakdown of the surface and a change in the coagulation function of the endothelium would render the plaque more thrombogenic. Such changes would lead to the terminal thrombotic event, the hallmark of all ischemic complications in atherosclerotic patients.

REFERENCES

1. Wolinsky H, Glagov S. Nature of species differences in the medial distribution of aortic vasa vasorum in mammals. Circ Res 1967;20:409.
2. Heistad DD, Armstrong ML. Blood flow through vasa vasorum of coronary arteries in atherosclerotic monkeys. Arteriosclerosis 1986;6:326.
3. Barger AC, Beeuwkes R III, Lainey LL, Silverman KJ. Hypothesis: vasa vasorum and neovascularization of human coronary arteries. N Engl J Med 1984;310:175.
4. Coffin JD, Poole TJ. Embryonic vascular development: immunohistochemical identification of the origin and subsequent morphogenesis of the major vessel primordia in quail embryos. Development 1988;102:735.
5. Pardanaud L, Altmann C, Kitos P, Dieterlen-Lievre F, Buck CA. Vasculogenesis in the early quail blastodisc as studied with a monoclonal antibody recognizing endothelial cells. Development 1987;100:339.
6. Le Douarin NM. Cell migrations in embryos. Cell 1984; 38:353.
7. Wolinsky H, Glagov S. A lamellar unit of aortic medial structure and function in mammals. Circ Res 1967;20:99.
8. Wolinsky H, Glagov S. Structural basis for the static mechanical properties of the aortic media. Circ Res 1964;14:400.
9. Dilley RJ, Schwartz SM. Vascular remodeling in the growth hormone transgenic mouse. Circ Res 1989;65:1233.
10. Zarins CK, Zatina MA, Giddens DP, Ku DN, Glagov S. Shear stress regulation of artery lumen diameter in experimental atherogenesis. J Vasc Surg 1987;5:413.
11. Glagov S, Weisenberg E, Zarins CK, Stankunavicius R, Kollettis GJ. Compensatory enlargement of human atherosclerotic coronary arteries. N Engl J Med 1987;316:1371.
12. Frangos JA, Eskin SG, McIntire LV, Ives CL. Flow effect on prostacyclin production by cultured human endothelial cells. Science 1985;227:1477.

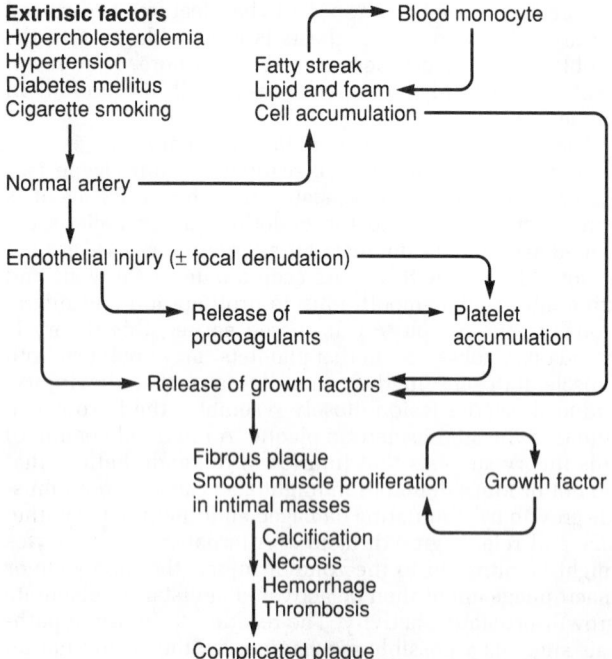

Extrinsic factors
Hypercholesterolemia
Hypertension
Diabetes mellitus
Cigarette smoking

Blood monocyte

Fatty streak
Lipid and foam
Cell accumulation

Normal artery

Endothelial injury (± focal denudation)

Release of procoagulants → Platelet accumulation

Release of growth factors

Fibrous plaque
Smooth muscle proliferation in intimal masses — Growth factor

Calcification
Necrosis
Hemorrhage
Thrombosis

Complicated plaque

Figure 68-7. Atherogenesis and progression of atherosclerosis are probably the consequences of multiple factors acting on the arterial wall. (After Clowes AW. Theories of atherosclerosis. In: White RA, ed. Atherosclerosis and arteriosclerosis: human pathology and experimental animal methods and models. Boca Raton, FL, CRC Press, 1989:3)

13. Gibbons GH, Dzau VJ. The emerging concept of vascular remodeling. N Engl J Med 1994;330:1431.
14. Davies PF, Tripathi SC. Mechanical stress mechanisms and the cell: an endothelial paradigm. Circ Res 1993;72:239.
15. Resnick N, Collins T, Atkinson W, Bonthron DT, Dewey CF Jr, Gimbrone MA Jr. Platelet-derived growth factor B chain promoter contains a cis-acting fluid shear-stress-responsive element. Proc Natl Acad Sci USA 1993;90:4591.
16. Vanhoutte PM. The endothelium: modulator of vascular smooth-muscle tone. N Engl J Med 1988;319:512.
17. Furchgott RF. Role of endothelium in responses of vascular smooth muscle. Circ Res 1983;53:557.
18. Ignarro LJ, Buga GM, Wood KS, Byrns RE, Chaudhuri G. Endothelium-derived relaxing factor produced and released from artery and vein is nitric oxide. Proc Natl Acad Sci USA 1987;84:9265.
19. Palmer RMJ, Ferrige AG, Moncada S. Nitric oxide release accounts for the biological activity of endothelium-derived relaxing factor. Nature 1987;327:524.
20. Ignarro LJ. Biological actions and properties of endothelium-derived nitric oxide formed and released from artery and vein. Circ Res 1989;65:1.
21. Langille BL, O'Donnell F. Reductions in arterial diameter produced by chronic decreases in blood flow are endothelium-dependent. Science 1986;231:405.
22. Kohler TR, Jawien A. Flow affects development of intimal hyperplasia after arterial injury in rats. Arterioscler Thromb 1992;12:963.
23. Kohler TR, Kirkman TR, Kraiss LW, Zierler BK, Clowes AW. Increased blood flow inhibits neointimal hyperplasia in endothelialized vascular grafts. Circ Res 1991;69:1557.
24. Geary RL, Kohler TR, Vergel S, Kirkman TR, Clowes AW. Time course of flow-induced smooth muscle cell proliferation and intimal thickening in endothelialized baboon vascular grafts. Circ Res 1994;74:14.
25. Shultz PJ, Knauss TC, Mené P, Abboud HE. Mitogenic signals for thrombin in mesangial cells: regulation of phospholipase C and PDGF genes. Am J Physiol 1989;257:F366.
26. Bobik A, Grooms A, Millar JA, Mitchell A, Grinpukel S. Growth factor activity of endothelin on vascular smooth muscle. Am J Physiol Cell Physiol 1990;258:C408.
27. Libby P, Warner SJC, Friedman GB. Interleukin 1: a mitogen for human vascular smooth muscle cells that induces the release of growth-inhibitory prostanoids. J Clin Invest 1988;81:487.
28. Nakaki T, Nakayama M, Yamamoto S, Kato R. Endothelin-mediated stimulation of DNA synthesis in vascular smooth muscle cells. Biochem Biophys Res Commun 1989;158:880.
29. Garg UC, Hassid A. Nitric oxide-generating vasodilators and 8-bromo-cyclic guanosine monophosphate inhibit mitogenesis and proliferation of cultured rat vascular smooth muscle cells. J Clin Invest 1989;83:1774.
30. Freiman PC, Mitchell GG, Heistad DD, Armstrong ML, Harrison DG. Atherosclerosis impairs endothelium-dependent vascular relaxation to acetylcholine and thrombin in primates. Circ Res 1986;58:783.
31. Wolinsky H. Long-term effects of hypertension on the rat aortic wall and their relation to concurrent aging changes: morphological and chemical studies. Circ Res 1972;30:301.
32. Ross R. Pathogenesis of atherosclerosis: an update. N Engl J Med 1986;314:488.
33. Steinberg D, Parthasarathy S, Carew TE, Khoo JC, Witztum JL. Modifications of low-density lipoprotein that increase its atherogenicity. N Engl J Med 1989;320:915.
34. Schwartz SM, Campbell GR, Campbell JH. Replication of smooth muscle cells in vascular disease. Circ Res 1986;58:427.
35. Clowes AW, Reidy MA, Clowes MM. Kinetics of cellular proliferation after arterial injury. I. Smooth muscle growth in the absence of endothelium. Lab Invest 1983;49:327.
36. Owens GK. Control of hypertrophic versus hyperplastic growth of vascular smooth muscle cells. Am J Physiol 1989;257:H1755.
37. Zwolak RM, Adams MC, Clowes AW. Kinetics of vein graft hyperplasia: association with tangential stress. J Vasc Surg 1987;5:126.
38. Leung DY, Glagov S, Mathews MB. Cyclic stretching stimu-lates synthesis of matrix components by arterial smooth muscle cells in vitro. Science 1976;191:475.
39. Baumgartner HR, Studer A. Consequences of vessel catheterization in normal and hypercholesterolemic rabbits. Pathol Microbiol 1966;29:393.
40. Kumagai H, Suzuki H, Matsukawa S, Ryuzaki M, Saruta T. Captopril therapy following percutaneous transluminal angioplasty for bilateral renal artery stenosis. Arch Intern Med 1989;149:1973.
41. Bowen-Pope DF, Ross R, Seifert RA. Locally acting growth factors for vascular smooth muscle cells: endogenous synthesis and release from platelets. Circulation 1985;72:735.
42. Friedman RJ, Stemerman MB, Wenz B, et al. The effect of thrombocytopenia on experimental atherosclerotic lesion formation in rabbits: smooth muscle cell proliferation and re-endothelialization. J Clin Invest 1977;60:1191.
43. Fingerle J, Johnson R, Clowes AW, Majesky MW, Reidy MA. Role of platelets in smooth muscle cell proliferation and migration after vascular injury in rat carotid artery. Proc Natl Acad Sci USA 1989;86:8412.
44. Groves HM, Kinlough-Rathbone RL, Richardson M, Jorgensen L, Moore S, Mustard JF. Thrombin generation and fibrin formation following injury to rabbit neointima: studies of vessel wall reactivity and platelet survival. Lab Invest 1982;46:605.
45. Hatton MWC, Moar SL, Richardson M. Deendothelialization in vivo initiates a thrombogenic reaction at the rabbit aorta surface: correlation of uptake of fibrinogen and antithrombin III with thrombin generation by the exposed subendothelium. Am J Pathol 1989;135:499.
46. Faggiotto A, Ross R. Studies of hypercholesterolemia in the nonhuman primate. II. Fatty streak conversion to fibrous plaque. Arteriosclerosis 1984;4:341.
47. Faggiotto A, Ross R, Harker L. Studies of hypercholesterolemia in nonhuman primate. I. Changes that lead to fatty streak formation. Arteriosclerosis 1984;4:323.
48. Reidy MA. A reassessment of endothelial injury and arterial lesion formation. Lab Invest 1985;53:513.
49. Clowes AW, Clowes MM. Regulation of smooth muscle proliferation by heparin in vitro and in vivo. Int Angiol 1987;6:45.
50. Clowes AW, Clowes MM, Fingerle J, Reidy MA. Regulation of smooth muscle cell growth in injured artery. J Cardiovasc Pharmacol 1989;14(Suppl)6:S12.
51. Gajdusek CM, Schwartz SM. Comparison of intracellular and extracellular mitogen activity. J Cell Physiol 1984;121:316.
52. Gajdusek CM, Carbon S. Injury-induced release of basic fibroblast growth factor from bovine aortic endothelium. J Cell Physiol 1989;139:570.
53. Burgess WH, Maciag T. The heparin binding (fibroblast) growth factor family of proteins. Annu Rev Biochem 1989;58:575.
54. Gospodarowicz D, Neufeld G, Schwiegerer L. Fibroblast growth factor: structural and biological properties. J Cell Physiol 1987;(Suppl 5):15.
55. Vlodavsky I, Folkman J, Sullivan R, et al. Endothelial cell-derived basic fibroblast growth factor: synthesis and deposition into subendothelial extracellular matrix. Proc Natl Acad Sci USA 1987;84:2292.
56. Lindner V, Lappi DA, Baird A, Majack RA, Reidy MA. Role of basic fibroblast growth factor in vascular lesion formation. Circ Res 1991;68:106.
57. Lindner V, Reidy MA. Proliferation of smooth muscle cells after vascular injury is inhibited by an antibody against basic fibroblast growth factor. Proc Natl Acad Sci USA 1991;88:3739.
58. Raines EW, Bowen-Pope DF, Ross R. Platelet-derived growth factor. In: Sporn MB, Roberts AB, eds. Handbook of experimental pharmacology: peptide growth factors and their receptors. Heidelberg, Springer-Verlag, 1989.
59. Sprugel KH, McPherson JM, Clowes AW, Ross R. Effects of growth factors in vivo. I. Cell ingrowth into porous subcutaneous chambers. Am J Pathol 1987;129:601.
60. Doolittle RF, Hunkapillar MW, Hood LE, Aaronson SA, Antoniades HN. Simian sarcoma virus oncogene, v-sis, is derived from the gene (or genes) encoding a platelet-derived growth factor. Science 1983;221:275.

61. Waterfield MD, Scrace GT, Whittle N, et al. Platelet-derived growth factor is structurally related to the putative transforming protein p28-sis of simian sarcoma virus. Nature 1983;304:35.

62. Ferns GAA, Raines EW, Sprugel KH, Motani AS, Reidy MA, Ross R. Inhibition of neointimal smooth muscle accumulation after angioplasty by an antibody to PDGF. Science 1991;253:1129.

63. Jawien A, Bowen-Pope DF, Lindner V, Schwartz SM, Clowes AW. Platelet-derived growth factor promotes smooth muscle migration and intimal thickening in a rat model of balloon angioplasty. J Clin Invest 1992;89:507.

64. Blaes N, Boissel JP. Growth-stimulating effect of catecholamines on rat aortic smooth muscle cells in culture. J Cell Physiol 1983;116:167.

65. Dalsgaard CJ, Hultgardh-Nilsson A, Haegerstrand A, Nilsson J. Neuropeptides as growth factors: possible roles in human disease. Regul Pept 1989;25:1.

66. Bevan RD. Trophic effects of peripheral adrenergic nerves on vascular structure. Hypertension 1984;6:III.

67. Bevan RD, Tsuru H. Functional and structural changes in the rabbit ear artery after sympathetic denervation. Circ Res 1981;49:478.

68. Powell JS, Clozel JP, Muller RKM, et al. Inhibitors of angiotensin-converting enzyme prevent myointimal proliferation after vascular injury. Science 1989;245:186.

69. Jackson CL, Bush RC, Bowyer DE. Inhibitory effect of calcium antagonists on balloon catheter-induced arterial smooth muscle cell proliferation and lesion size. Atherosclerosis 1988;69:115.

70. Clowes AW, Reidy MA. Mechanisms of graft failure: the role of cellular proliferation. Ann NY Acad Sci 1987;516:673.

71. Fritze LMS, Reilly CF, Rosenberg RD. An antiproliferative heparan sulfate species produced by postconfluent smooth muscle cells. J Cell Biol 1985;100:1041.

72. Castellot JJ Jr, Addonizio ML, Rosenberg R, Karnovsky MJ. Cultured endothelial cells produce a heparin-like inhibitor of smooth muscle cell growth. J Cell Biol 1981;90:372.

73. Antonelli-Orlidge A, Saunders KB, Smith SR, D'Amore PA. An activated form of transforming growth factor b is produced by cocultures of endothelial cells and pericytes. Proc Natl Acad Sci USA 1989;86:4544.

74. Majesky MW, Lindner V, Twardzik DR, Schwartz SM, Reidy MA. Production of transforming growth factor β_1 during repair of arterial injury. J Clin Invest 1991;88:904.

75. Wolf YG, Rasmussen LM, Ruoslahti E. Antibodies against transforming growth factor-β1 suppress intimal hyperplasia in a rat model. J Clin Invest 1994;93:1172.

76. Hansson GK, Jonasson L, Seifert PS, Stemme S. Immune mechanisms in atherosclerosis. Arteriosclerosis 1989;9:567.

77. Hansson GK, Jonasson L, Holm J, Clowes MM, Clowes AW. Gamma interferon regulates vascular smooth muscle proliferation and Ia expression in vitro and in vivo. Circ Res 1988;63:712.

78. Larson DM, Haudenschild CC, Beyer EC. Gap junction messenger RNA expression by vascular wall cells. Circ Res 1990;66:1074.

79. Orlidge A, D'Amore PA. Inhibition of capillary endothelial cell growth by pericytes and smooth muscle cells. J Cell Biol 1987;105:1455.

80. Heimark RL, Schwartz SM. The role of membrane–membrane interactions in the regulation of endothelial cell growth. J Cell Biol 1985;100:1934.

81. Hawiger JJ. Hemostasis, bleeding, and thromboembolic complications of trauma and infection. In: Clowes GHA Jr, ed. Trauma, sepsis and shock: the physiological basis of therapy. New York, Marcel Dekker, 1988:123.

82. Rodgers GM. Hemostatic properties of normal and perturbed vascular cells. FASEB J 1990;2:116.

83. Marcum J, McKenney J, Rosenberg R. The acceleration of thrombin–antithrombin III complex formation in rat hind quarters via heparin-like molecules bound to endothelium. J Clin Invest 1984;74:341.

84. Esmon CT. The roles of protein c and thrombomodulin in the regulation of blood coagulation. J Biol Chem 1989;264:4743.

85. Cotran RS, Kumar V, Robbins SL. Robbins pathologic basis of disease, ed 4. Philadelphia, WB Saunders, 1989:553.

86. Benditt EP, Gown AM. Atheroma: the artery wall and the environment. Int Rev Exp Pathol 1980;21:55.

87. McGill HC Jr. Persistent problems in the pathogenesis of atherosclerosis. Arteriosclerosis 1984;4:443.

88. PDAY Research Group. Natural history of aortic and coronary atherosclerotic lesions in youth: findings from the PDAY study. Arterioscler Thromb 1993;13:1291.

89. Velican C, Velican D. Intimal thickening in developing coronary arteries and its relevance to atherosclerotic involvement. Atherosclerosis 1976;23:345.

90. Velican C, Velican D. The precursors of coronary atherosclerotic plaques in subjects up to 40 years old. Atherosclerosis 1980;37:33.

91. Thomas WA, Kim DN. Atherosclerosis as a hyperplastic and/or neoplastic process. Lab Invest 1983;48:245.

92. Gordon D, Reidy MA, Benditt EP, Schwartz SM. Cell proliferation in human coronary arteries. Proc Natl Acad Sci USA 1990;87:4600.

93. O'Brien ER, Alpers CE, Stewart DK, et al. Proliferation in primary and restenotic coronary atherectomy tissue: implications for antiproliferative therapy. Circ Res 1993;73:223.

94. Jonasson L, Holm J, Skalli O, Gabbiani G, Hansson GK. Expression of class II transplantation antigens on vascular smooth muscle cells in human atherosclerosis. J Clin Invest 1985;76:125.

95. Stemme S, Rymo L, Hansson GK. Polyclonal origin of T lymphocytes in human atherosclerotic plaques. Lab Invest 1991;65:654.

96. Stemme S, Hansson GK. Immune mechanisms in atherogenesis. Ann Med 1994;26:141.

97. Wilcox JN, Smith KM, Schwartz SM, Gordon D. Localization of tissue factor in the normal vessel wall and in the atherosclerotic plaque. Proc Natl Acad Sci USA 1989;86:2839.

98. Schneiderman J, Sawdey MS, Keeton MR, et al. Increased type 1 plasminogen activator inhibitor gene expression in atherosclerotic human arteries. Proc Natl Acad Sci USA 1992;89:6998.

99. Lupu F, Bergonzelli GE, Heim DA, et al. Localization and production of plasminogen activator inhibitor in human healthy and atherosclerotic arteries. Arterioscler Thromb 1993;13:1090.

100. Page JH. Atherosclerosis: an introduction. Circulation 1954; 10:1.

101. Breslow JL. Insights into lipoprotein metabolism from studies in transgenic mice. Annu Rev Physiol 1994;56:797.

102. Duguid JB. Thrombosis as a factor in the pathogenesis of aortic atherosclerosis. J Pathol Bacteriol 1948;60:57.

103. Benditt EP, Benditt JM. Evidence for a monoclonal origin of human atherosclerotic plaques. Proc Natl Acad Sci USA 1973;70:1753.

104. Schwartz SM, Reidy MA, Clowes AW. Kinetics of atherosclerosis, a stem cell model. Ann NY Acad Sci 1985;454:292.

SURGERY: SCIENTIFIC PRINCIPLES AND PRACTICE, Second Edition, edited by Lazar J. Greenfield, Michael W. Mulholland, Keith T. Oldham, Gerald B. Zelenock, and Keith D. Lillemoe. Lippincott–Raven Publishers, Philadelphia, © 1997.

CHAPTER 69

NONATHEROSCLEROTIC VASCULAR DISEASE

LLOYD M. TAYLOR, JR., RAYMOND W. LEE, E. JOHN HARRIS, JR., AND JOHN M. PORTER

Arteriosclerosis is responsible for most arterial abnormalities encountered by practicing vascular surgeons. This disease process is sufficiently common that the clinical importance of the various nonatherosclerotic causes of arterial pathology might not be immediately apparent. Despite their relative rarity, nonatherosclerotic diseases constitute an extremely important component of vascular surgery. Detailed knowledge of these conditions is essential both to provide requisite surgical treatment and to permit the vascular surgeon to act as a consultation resource because many internal medicine specialists routinely turn to vascular surgeons for information concerning optimal treatment of nonatherosclerotic vascular diseases.

This chapter discusses the major nonatherosclerotic causes of arterial pathology. Other nonatherosclerotic vascular conditions, such as compression and entrapment syndromes, vascular infections, and congenital vascular malformations, are discussed in later chapters.

FIBROMUSCULAR DYSPLASIA

Fibromuscular dysplasia (FMD) is the descriptive term applied to an abnormality characterized by multiple areas of eccentric arterial stenosis alternating with segments of arterial dilation. The angiographic appearance of involved arteries, frequently described as a string of beads, is unmistakable (Fig. 69-1). FMD is thought to be an arterial developmental abnormality, although the cause remains obscure. Multiple stenoses in sequence, as seen in Figure 69-1, are usually present; rarely, FMD causes a single focal stenosis. FMD most frequently involves the renal artery. The carotid and iliac arteries are the next most frequently affected. Mesenteric, subclavian, vertebral, axillary, forearm, and coronary arteries have been reported as rarely occurring sites of FMD involvement. Over 90% of cases occur in female patients, and 80% of the renal artery involvement is on the right side.

The clinical findings of FMD are obviously related to the vascular bed involved. As is true of atherosclerotic obstructive disease, many patients with documented FMD who have no symptoms have been identified. Hypertension caused by renal artery stenosis and transient cerebral ischemic attacks caused by internal carotid artery stenosis are the two most frequently encountered clinical syndromes associated with FMD.

Four distinct variants of FMD are recognized based on differences in histologic appearance—intimal fibroplasia, medial fibroplasia, medial hyperplasia, and perimedial dysplasia.[1] Medial fibroplasia is the most common renal arterial pathologic type of FMD, accounting for 85% of cases, with perimedial dysplasia accounting for 10%. Differentiation of the pathologic groups is determined by the layer of the vessel wall involved as well as by the predominant tissue involved in the dysplastic segment. With medial fibroplasia, infiltration of the media with increased amounts of fibrous connective tissue, collagen, and glycosaminoglycans is seen. Medial hyperplasia is characterized by increased numbers of medial smooth muscle cells; these medial smooth muscle cells define the proliferative changes seen in FMD. As stated earlier, the cause of FMD is unknown, although a number of theories have received varied support including hormonal imbalance, primarily estrogenic; embryologic maldevelopment; immunologic phenomenon; injury from arterial stretching; and abnormal distribution of the vasa vasorum with secondary mural ischemia.

Surgical treatment of FMD is indicated primarily for symptomatic arterial stenoses. Most authorities have not recommended treatment of asymptomatic stenoses; this is particularly true of internal carotid artery FMD, for which the natural history of untreated asymptomatic stenosis is unknown, in contrast to the situation with atherosclerosis. Surgical treatment may also be indicated for true, false, or dissecting aneurysms that can occur in areas of FMD. An example of a rare case involving radial and ulnar artery aneurysms resulting from FMD is seen in Figure 69-2. Surgical treatment methods include arterial dilation, arterial patch angioplasty, and interposition arterial bypass grafting using autogenous or prosthetic materials. Percutaneous transluminal balloon angioplasty has given satisfactory short-term results in treatment of FMD lesions of the main renal artery.[2] Balloon angioplasty has been applied infrequently to the treatment of carotid artery FMD because of appropriate concern about the risk of embolization associated with the procedure.

BUERGER'S DISEASE

Buerger's disease, also known as *thromboangiitis obliterans,* is a clinical syndrome characterized by the occurrence of extensive segmental thrombotic occlusions of small and medium arteries in the lower and, frequently, upper extremities, accompanied by a prominent arterial wall inflammatory cell infiltration.[3] The arterial involvement is often sufficiently severe to produce gangrene and tissue loss. Buerger's disease is clinically and pathologically distinct from immune arteritis and from atherosclerosis. Despite the severe nature of the arterial involvement, life expectancy of patients with Buerger's disease does not differ significantly from that of age-matched controls, indicating an absence of primary coronary arterial involvement. Buerger's disease occurs frequently in the Far East, Middle East, and Asia, but is infrequently encountered in North America. The reason for this striking geographic variance is unknown.

Affected patients are predominantly young male smokers who present with distal limb ischemia, often accompanied by digital (toe or finger) gangrene. Although men are more commonly affected, women represented up to 20% of the patients reported in several North American series. Between 40% and 50% of patients with Buerger's disease have a clear history of superficial migratory thrombophle-

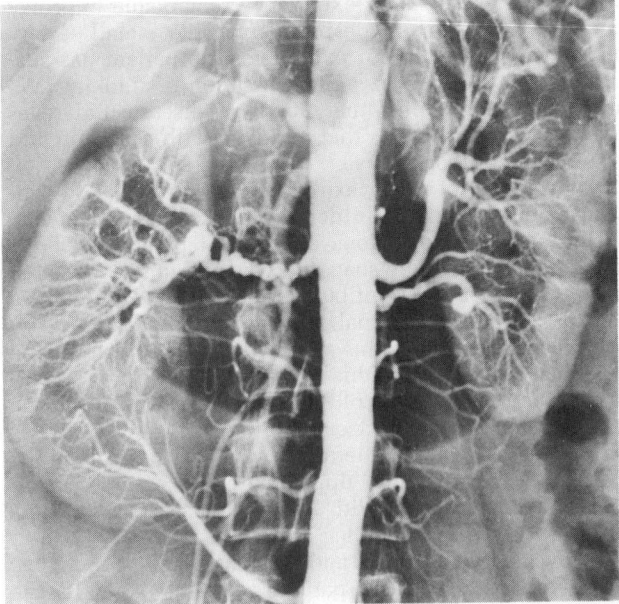

Figure 69-1. Fibromuscular dysplasia involving the right renal artery in a young woman with hypertension. Some changes of fibromuscular dysplasia are also seen in the left segmental renal artery. (Porter JM, Taylor LM Jr, Harris EJ Jr. Nonatherosclerotic vascular disease. In: Moore WS, ed. Vascular surgery: a comprehensive review. Philadelphia, WB Saunders, 1994:111)

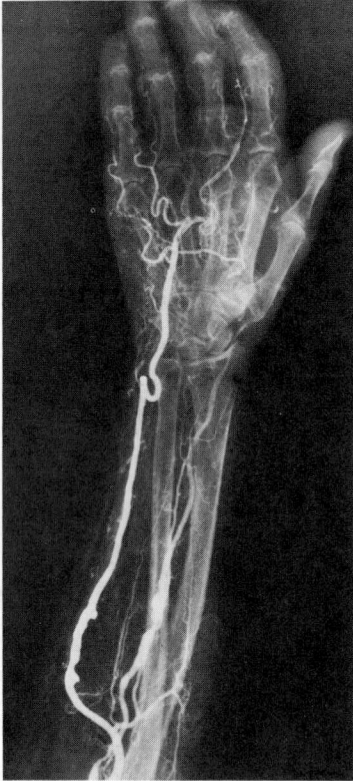

Figure 69-2. Arteriogram showing multiple localized stenotic and aneurysmal formations in a patient with advanced fibromuscular dysplasia of radial and ulnar arteries. (Edwards JM, Antonius JI, Porter JM. Critical hand ischemia caused by forearm fibromuscular dysplasia. J Vasc Surg 1985;2:459)

bitis, or Raynaud syndrome. Although cerebral, coronary, and visceral arterial involvement with Buerger's disease have been reported, in most patients, the disease is limited to extremity vessels distal to the elbow and knee. There have been occasional reports, both arteriographically and pathologically, of iliac artery involvement. In North America, 50% of patients with Buerger's disease have symptoms confined to the lower extremities, 30% to 40% have symptomatic involvement of both the upper and lower extremities, while only 10% of patients have symptomatic involvement confined to the upper extremities.[4]

The acute pathologic lesion of Buerger's disease is a nonnecrotizing panarteritis associated with intraluminal thrombus. In contrast to both atherosclerosis and immune arteritis, the internal elastic lamina remains intact in Buerger's disease. The chronic phase of Buerger's disease includes a decline in hypercellularity with the production of perivascular fibrosis, and frequent recanalization of the luminal thrombus. Adjacent veins and nerves are frequently involved in the perivascular inflammatory process. Although the cause of Buerger's disease remains unknown, the association with heavy tobacco use has been universal.

Diagnostic criteria for Buerger's disease based on clinical, pathologic, and arteriographic criteria have been established as follows[4]:

- Onset of distal extremity ischemic symptoms before 45 years of age
- Absence of an underlying proximal embolic source
- Absence of trauma
- Absence of autoimmune disease (all serologic tests normal)
- Absence of diabetes
- Absence of hyperlipidemia
- Absence of hypercoagulable state
- Normal arteries proximal to the popliteal and brachial arteries
- Objective arteriographic, plethysmographic, or pathologic evidence of distal arterial occlusions

Diagnosis of Buerger's disease requires objective confirmation of occlusive disease of distal arteries as well as absence of disease in more proximal arteries. This can be accomplished through use of noninvasive vascular testing or by arteriography. Exclusion by appropriate testing for hyperlipidemia, diabetes, and autoimmune disease is required for the diagnosis of Buerger's disease.

Vascular laboratory testing for Buerger's disease consists of digit (finger and toe) plethysmography, combined with segmental proximal limb pressures and Doppler analogue waveform recording. Plethysmographic evidence of digital arterial obstruction in all four extremities, combined with normal proximal vessels, is sufficient evidence of intrinsic small artery obstructive disease, and arteriography is not required. Patients with unilateral digital plethysmographic abnormalities should undergo arteriography to rule out proximal arterial lesions as an embolic source of this distal digital ischemia. Arteriography is also advised for patients with vascular laboratory findings that localize the disease to the distal feet and toes, in the presence of normal hand and finger plethysmography, to rule out a proximal arterial embolic source for the ischemia.

Although not pathognomonic, characteristic arteriographic findings have been shown to occur repeatedly in Buerger's disease. The arterial tree appears normal proximal to the popliteal and distal brachial levels. Distally, there is an abrupt transition to occlusion, which is most often segmental rather than diffuse. Extensive digital, palmar, and plantar arterial occlusions are common. The collaterals have a characteristic arteriographic appearance, termed *corkscrew collaterals* (Fig. 69-3).

Treatment of Buerger's disease is most importantly centered on achieving abstinence from tobacco usage. If successful, patients usually experience remarkable improvement in symptoms, despite extensive small artery occlusive disease. In our experience, no patient has sustained further tissue loss after cessation of smoking. We and others have noted that Buerger's disease undergoes remissions and relapses that correlate with cessation and resumption of tobacco use.[5]

Management of upper extremity Buerger's disease consists of minor local débridement of ischemic segments, including partial excisions of exposed phalangeal bone combined with simple soap and water scrubs of ischemic ulcers, together with antibiotics as indicated by culture results. Although regional surgical sympathectomy has been recommended in this setting, we find no convincing evidence in support of this operation and do not recommend it in the treatment of Buerger's disease. Major tissue loss is rare in upper extremity Buerger's disease and is virtually unknown if patients successfully stop smoking.

In marked contrast to upper extremity disease, lower extremity involvement with Buerger's disease often leads to limb loss, with major leg amputation rates of 12% to 31% over 5 to 10 years reported in several large series. Thirty-one percent of our patients with Buerger's disease required leg amputations.[5] Occasionally, patients with Buerger's disease have arteriographically patent distal arterial segments in the calf and foot, suggesting the possibility of arterial bypass grafting. In our experience, such grafts have been universally unsuccessful in achieving prolonged patency or limb salvage and are not recommended.

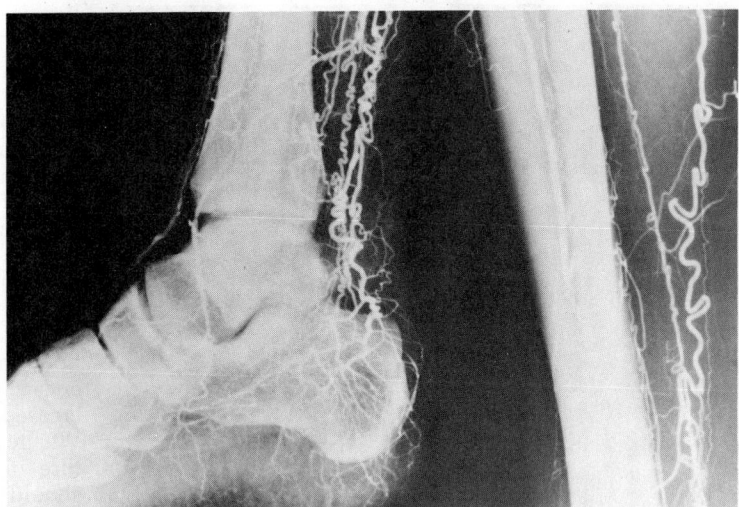

Figure 69-3. Typical arteriogram of patient with Buerger's disease showing abrupt occlusion of proximal normal tibial vessel and characteristic corkscrew collaterals. (Mills JL, Taylor LM Jr, Porter JM. Buerger disease in the modern era. Am J Surg 1987;154:123)

Although several medications have been advocated in the medical treatment of Buerger's disease, including steroids, prostaglandin E_1, vasodilators, hemorrheologic agents, anticoagulants, and antiplatelet agents, no agent has been proved efficacious. Based on mechanism of action, we use nifedipine, pentoxifylline, and aspirin for patients with Buerger's disease. None of these agents has been subjected to a randomized, controlled clinical trial in patients with Buerger's disease.

DISEASES AFFECTING THE ARTERIAL MEDIA

Collagen, elastin, and smooth muscle are found in the arterial media and are responsible for both the strength and resilience of normal arteries. A variety of conditions that affect the amount, strength, or stability of collagen and elastin are surgically important. These conditions all have the presence of medial defects in common.

Cystic Medial Necrosis

In the 1930s, Erdheim[6] described a pathologic condition characterized by uniform hyaline degeneration of the arterial media with replacement by a mucoid-appearing basophilic substance that was clinically associated with aortic dissection. Subsequently, multiple reports of aortic dissection, spontaneous arterial rupture, and disseminated aneurysm formation have been associated with this condition, which Erdheim termed *cystic medial necrosis*. Investigations have identified metabolic aberrations with specific biochemical abnormalities as the cause of the pathologic changes present in many patients with cystic medial necrosis. Syndromes affecting the composition and structure of collagen and elastin and the mucopolysaccharides of the ground substance have been identified. Marfan syndrome, Ehlers-Danlos syndrome, neurofibromatosis, and the mucopolysaccharidoses—Hunter disease, Hurler disease, Sanfillipo disease, and Morquio disease—can all present with the typical arterial lesions of cystic medial necrosis, with its associated pathologic findings.

Most patients identified with cystic medial necrosis have a clinical syndrome characterized by a heritable disorder of collagen metabolism, the most frequent of which have been Marfan syndrome and Ehlers-Danlos syndrome. The most common clinical manifestation of cystic medial necrosis is aortic dissection, with spontaneous arterial rup-

ture and diffuse aneurysm formation occurring less frequently.

Marfan Syndrome

Marfan syndrome is a heterogeneous disorder characterized clinically and biochemically by ocular abnormalities (myopia and lens dislocation), skeletal disproportion (tall stature, chest wall deformities, arachnodactyly, scoliosis), and cardiovascular abnormalities (mitral valve prolapse, aortic dissection with aortic aneurysm formation). A precise biochemical defect has not been identified in Marfan syndrome; rather, a general concept of mutation in the genes controlling the production and use of type I collagen has been proposed as underlying this condition (see Chaps. 89 and 91). Marfan first noted the orthopedic abnormalities of the syndrome in the late 19th century. The ocular abnormalities were identified in the 1940s, and the cardiovascular abnormalities were described by McKusik in the 1950s.[7]

Inheritance of Marfan syndrome is by an autosomal dominant pattern. A number of conditions have been recognized that share some features of Marfan syndrome but have different natural histories. These include homocystinuria (discussed later); contractural arachnodactyly, which is a disorder distinguished by joint stiffness rather than laxity; and the mitral valve prolapse syndrome, a syndrome sharing many of the skeletal abnormalities of Marfan syndrome without ocular manifestations or the propensity for aortic dissection.

Almost all patients with Marfan syndrome develop predictable dilation of the aortic root leading to the development of an ascending aortic aneurysm (Fig. 69-4), which can progress to the development of aortic valvular incompetence. A smaller percentage of patients develop mitral valve prolapse and mitral insufficiency. Untreated, the life expectancy of a patient with Marfan syndrome is about 40 years, with 95% of deaths related to cardiovascular complications. The most common causes of death are aortic insufficiency and ascending aortic dissection and rupture.

Both medical and surgical interventions have been proposed for prophylaxis against aortic dissection and aortic insufficiency. The medical regimens, unproved by clinical trials, are centered around the use of β-adrenergic blockers in a regimen designed to decrease the force of cardiac contraction and reduce blood pressure, potentially protecting the weakened ascending aorta.[8]

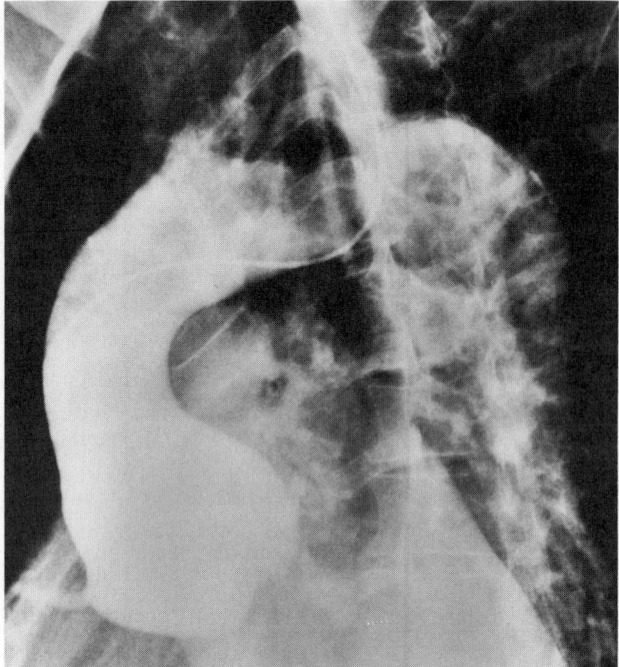

Figure 69-4. Aortogram of a patient with Marfan syndrome showing marked dilation of aortic root and aortic valvular insufficiency. (Porter JM, Taylor LM Jr, Harris EJ Jr. Nonatherosclerotic vascular disease. In: Moore WS, ed. Vascular surgery: a comprehensive review. Philadelphia, WB Saunders, 1994:136)

The surgical treatment has generally consisted of replacement of the ascending aorta and aortic valve with a composite graft. It is recommended that elective repair be performed before either severe aortic insufficiency compromises left ventricular function or the ascending aortic diameter has reached 55 to 60 mm,[9,10] at which point the risk of dissection and rupture increases. With modern surgical techniques in uncomplicated aneurysm replacement, the life expectancy of these patients can be improved considerably, with low morbidity and operative mortality.

Ehlers-Danlos Syndrome

Ehlers-Danlos syndrome is a heterogeneous group of generalized connective tissue disorders, first clearly described by von Meekeren in 1682, characterized by hyperextensible skin, hypermobile joints, fragile tissues, and a bleeding diathesis primarily related to fragile vessels. Detailed genetic and biochemical studies have defined more than 10 types of Ehlers-Danlos syndrome, each with variable signs, symptoms, and patterns of inheritance. For certain types of Ehlers-Danlos syndrome, definable molecular defects have been characterized. It is important to identify correctly the various types because the natural histories differ among them.

Three types of Ehlers-Danlos syndrome—types I, III, and IV—frequently have arterial complications, with type IV, the vascular or ecchymotic type, being most important to the vascular surgeon. Although first recognized as a distinct entity in 1967, the biochemical lesion of Ehlers-Danlos syndrome type IV, which results in abnormalities in the structure, synthesis, and secretion of type III procollagen, was not identified until 1975.[11] These patients produce little or no type III collagen, which is of major structural importance in vessels, viscera, and skin. Clinical features, although not uniformly expressed, consist of a thin translucent skin, easy bruisability, and venous varicosities.

The major vascular complication of Ehlers-Danlos syndrome is arterial rupture, although aneurysm formation (Fig. 69-5) and acute aortic dissection also occur. Spontaneous arterial rupture can lead to stroke, intraabdominal or intrathoracic bleeding, or compartment syndromes in the extremities. The most common site of spontaneous arterial rupture is the abdominal cavity, with smaller visceral arteries more commonly involved than the aorta. Repair of the ruptured vessels is difficult because of their extreme friability, although successful repairs have been reported,[12] emphasizing atraumatic vascular control, gentle dissection, and vessel ligation with plication pledgets. Experienced surgeons advise against arteriography because of increased risk of vessel laceration and hemorrhage.[12] Whenever possible, treatment of spontaneous arterial rupture in patients with Ehlers-Danlos syndrome type IV should be nonoperative, consisting of compression and transfusion. If unsuccessful, the operative objective should be ligation to control hemorrhage. If tissue loss would result, arterial reconstruction can be attempted. Successful arterial reconstructions in patients with Ehlers-Danlos syndrome type IV have been reported.

Most patients with Ehlers-Danlos syndrome type IV have shortened life-spans compared with their unaffected siblings. Death typically occurs in the third or fourth decade, and survival beyond 50 years of age is unusual.

Pseudoxanthoma Elasticum

Pseudoxanthoma elasticum is a group of genetically heterogeneous disorders involving elastic fibers whose basic pathogenetic abnormality remains unknown. Clinical manifestations of the disorder most frequently involve the skin, eyes, and arteries. Pseudoxanthoma elasticum derives its name from the characteristic yellow xanthoma-like cutaneous papules and the loose, baggy skin identified in intertriginous areas such as the axillae, antecubital fos-

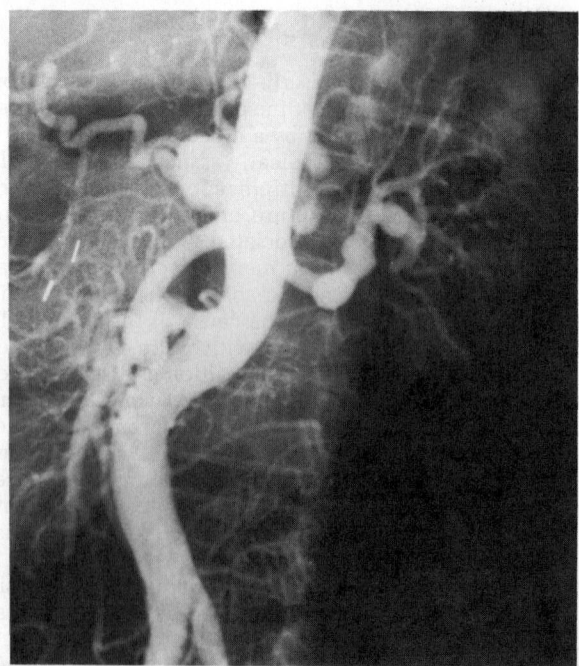

Figure 69-5. Celiac and renal artery aneurysms in a patient with Ehler-Danlos syndrome type III.

sae, and groins. Most patients with pseudoxanthoma elasticum have stenoses or occlusions of the peripheral, cerebral, or coronary arteries, separately or in combination. The basic pathologic change in the arterial wall is the replacement of normal medial elastic fibers by calcium deposits. Clinically, the diminished arterial elasticity and resultant resistance to distention is expressed as weak or absent pulses, which have characteristic plethysmographic tracings.[13] Plain radiographs often identify vascular calcifications in young patients at low risk for the development of atherosclerosis.

Arterial occlusive disease occurs at an early age, usually before the end of the fourth decade. Hypertension is another common manifestation of pseudoxanthoma elasticum. Diffuse arterial elastin degeneration can also involve the visceral arteries, and gastrointestinal hemorrhage is a common complication.[14] Standard techniques of vascular surgery, including autogenous vein bypass and endarterectomy, have been successfully performed in patients with pseudoxanthoma elasticum. Coronary artery bypass surgery has also been successfully performed in affected patients.

Arteria Magna Syndrome

Arteria magna syndrome is a peculiar condition of the aorta and iliofemoral arteries that presents as diffuse arterial elongation, dilation, and tortuosity. Leriche[15] was the first to describe the clinical, angiographic, and operative findings of this arteriopathy in 1943; he termed the condition *dolicho et mega-artere*. Subsequently, numerous reports have described this syndrome with terms such as *arteriomegaly* and *arteria dolicho et magna*. These descriptive terms have been applied to a broad spectrum of findings, ranging from generalized ectasia to contiguous aneurysms from the thoracic aorta to the popliteal trifurcation.[16]

Although the condition was initially thought to be a variant of atherosclerosis, more recent pathologic analysis has suggested the arterial media of these patients are devoid of the usual elastic tissues.[17] Characteristic arteriographic findings include arterial widening and tortuosity, markedly diminished arterial flow velocities with delayed distal arterial filling, and the presence of multiple aneurysms (Fig. 69-6).

Clinical management of patients with arteria magna is centered on detection of aneurysms and replacement using standard vascular surgical techniques. Aneurysms are detected using a combination of physical examination and ultrasound screening of abdominal, femoral, and popliteal sites. Localized aneurysms reaching 2 to 2.5 times the size of the parent artery should be replaced. Embolisms of intraaneurysmal thrombus and thrombotic arterial occlusions are common complications of this diffuse aneurysmal disease and are also an indication for arterial replacement. Coronary artery disease is common in patients with arteria magna, despite the absence of typical arterial occlusive disease elsewhere.[18]

The relation of arteria magna to typical atherosclerosis is uncertain. Pathologically, aneurysms associated with arteria magna have an appearance similar to the typical degenerative aneurysm. The histologic appearance is one of fragmentation of the internal elastic membrane and a profound decrease in the elastic tissue content of the media. There is no inflammatory component in the arterial wall. Although intimal atheromatous changes are often present, they are minimal in comparison to the extensive nature of the medial changes.

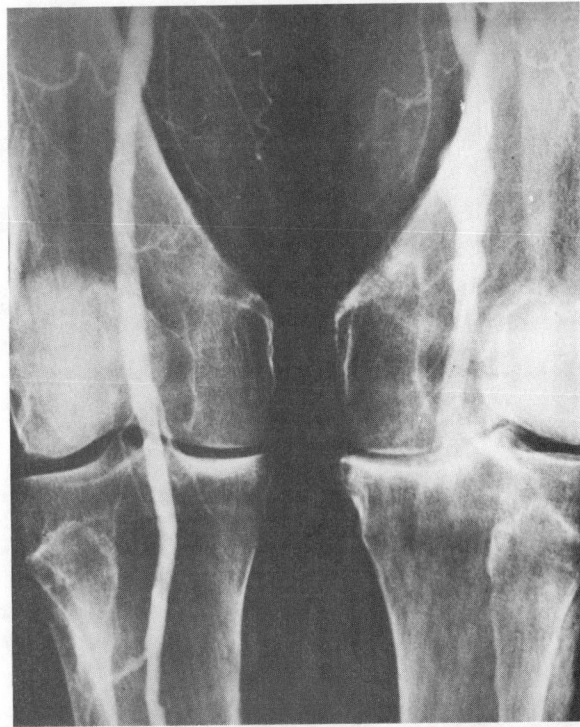

Figure 69-6. Popliteal artery aneurysm in a patient with the arterial magna syndrome. (Porter JM, Taylor LM Jr, Harris EJ Jr. Nonatherosclerotic vascular disease. In: Moore WAS, ed. Vascular surgery: a comprehensive review. Philadelphia, WB Saunders, 1994:137)

ADVENTITIAL CYSTIC DISEASE

Adventitial cystic disease is a rare condition characterized by the presence of single or multiple synovial-like cysts in the subadventitial layer of the arterial wall, with resultant arterial stenosis. These mucin-filled cysts are similar to ganglion cysts. The disease is most often bilateral, usually affects men, and has a median age of presentation of 40 years.[19]

Adventitial cystic disease was initially described by Atkins and Key in 1947, with the first report of successful operative management 7 years later. Although the popliteal artery is by far the most frequently affected artery,[19] adventitial cystic disease has been described in the femoral, radial, ulnar, and branches of the popliteal arteries.

Three etiologic theories have been proposed: (1) repeated arterial microtrauma; (2) the presence within the arterial wall of mucin-secreting cell rests derived embryologically from the synovial anlage of the adjacent joint; and the most popular, (3) the development of true ganglia in the adventitia, arising from an adjacent joint capsule or tendon sheath.[20] The frequent presence of a direct communication from the arterial cyst to the adjacent bony joint supports the latter hypothesis.

Adventitial cystic disease, along with Buerger's disease and popliteal entrapment syndrome, should be considered in any young patient complaining of intermittent claudication. Further examination rarely detects a palpable cyst, and the stigmata of generalized arterial insufficiency are not present. Palpable pulse alterations depending on knee flexion or extension have been described, presumably resulting from variable luminal compression, depending on position. Diagnosis is possible using computed tomographic scanning, magnetic resonance imaging, and ultrasonography. Classically, arteriograms demonstrate a scimi-

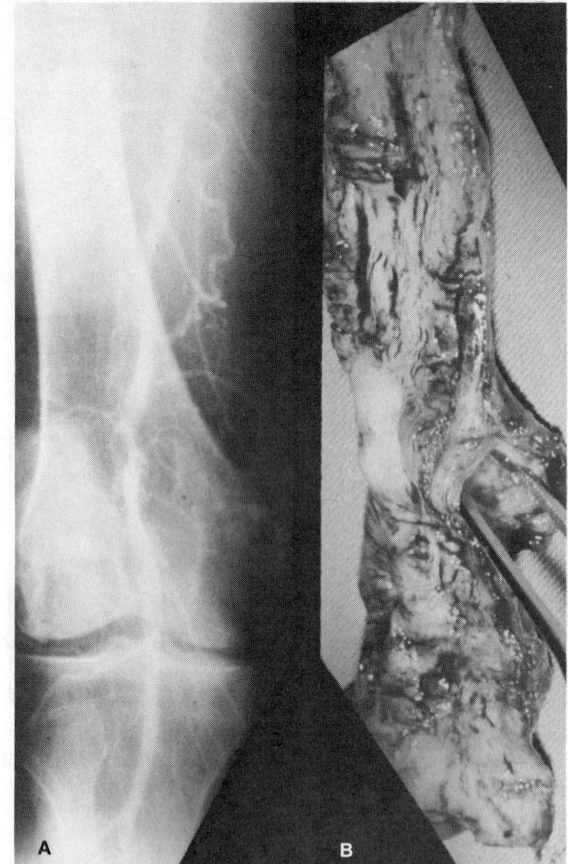

Figure 69-7. Arteriogram (*A*) and operative photograph (*B*) of adventitial cyst of popliteal artery.

tar sign of luminal encroachment by the cyst (Fig. 69-7) in a normally placed vessel with no other signs of occlusive disease.[21]

Several methods of treatment of adventitial cystic disease have been described. When the vessel is not occluded, simple cyst excision, enucleation, or aspiration are acceptable therapies, although there is a 10% recurrence rate. In 30% of patients, there is occlusion of the involved vessel. Resection of the occluded segment with the cystic mass and primary end-to-end anastomosis have been reported, but interposition grafting is usually required and is best accomplished using autogenous saphenous vein. Several reported attempts at percutaneous transluminal angioplasty have been unsuccessful. Computed tomography–guided aspirations of popliteal artery cysts have been reported. The first aspiration was thought to be unsuccessful because no material was aspirated, yet subsequent surgical exploration identified no cyst. Presumably, the aspiration attempt lysed the cyst, relieving the obstructive process. In another report, the cyst was successfully aspirated with restoration of distal arterial flow.[22] There is no long term follow-up for these interesting early reports.

RADIATION-INDUCED ARTERIAL INJURY

Arterial injury resulting from tumoricidal external-beam irradiation in the treatment of regional malignancy is well recognized. Radiation-induced arterial injury has been classified into three pathologic forms. The first type, occurring early in the posttreatment period, is characterized by an intense arterial inflammatory reaction with endothelial sloughing and luminal thrombosis. The second type, developing from 1 to 10 years after radiotherapy, apparently represents the healing phase of the arterial inflammatory response to radiation injury, and consists of intense fibrosis and scar formation within the arterial wall, resulting in areas of arterial stenosis (Fig. 69-8). The third type, developing from 2 to 30 years after radiotherapy, represents accelerated atherosclerosis. The arterial plaque is typically indistinguishable from nonirradiated atherosclerotic plaques.

Most experience with radiation-induced arterial injury has involved the carotid artery.[23] Vascular surgery on these irradiated arteries can be performed with standard techniques. Prosthetic and autogenous bypass grafts, as well as endarterectomy, have been performed satisfactorily.

IMMUNE ARTERITIS

The terms *arteritis* and *vasculitis* properly apply only to necrotizing transmural inflammation of the arterial wall and not to perivascular round cell infiltrates that can be seen in such conditions as livedo reticularis, eczema, cutaneous drug reactions, and Buerger's disease. Substantial evidence indicates that most, if not all, immune vasculitis is associated with the deposition of antigen–antibody immune complexes on the endothelium followed by the production of arterial wall damage. Complement components bind these exposed antigen–antibody complexes, activating the complement cascade. This in turn results in chemotaxis of polymorphonuclear leukocytes, and these leukocytes infiltrate the arterial wall. Leukocyte lysosomal enzymes, including elastase and collagenase, are released within the arterial wall and appear to be the primary cause of the arterial wall necrosis. Thrombosis, aneurysm formation, hemorrhage, and arterial occlusion can all follow or accompany the transmural arterial enzymatic injury.[24] Cell-mediated immune injury can also contribute to the arterial wall damage, yet considerably less information ex-

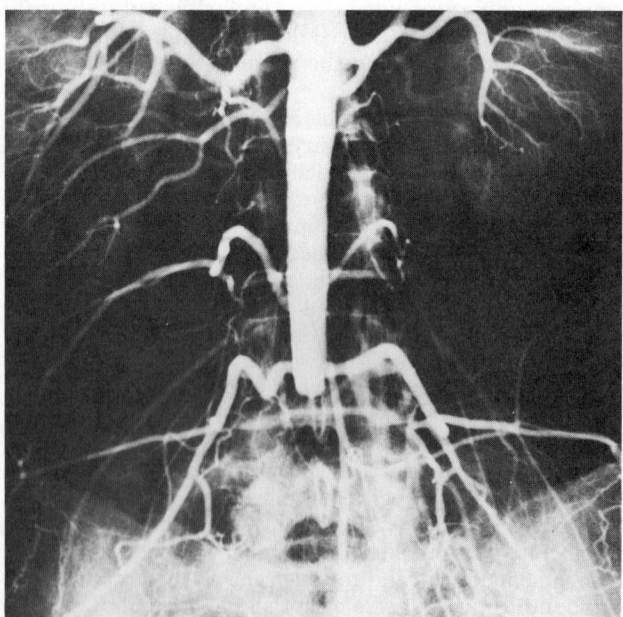

Figure 69-8. Radiation arteritis: abrupt occlusion of normal distal aorta. (Porter JM, Taylor LM Jr, Harris EJ Jr. Nonatherosclerotic vascular disease. In: Moore WAS, ed. Vascular surgery: a comprehensive review. Philadelphia, WB Saunders, 1994:122)

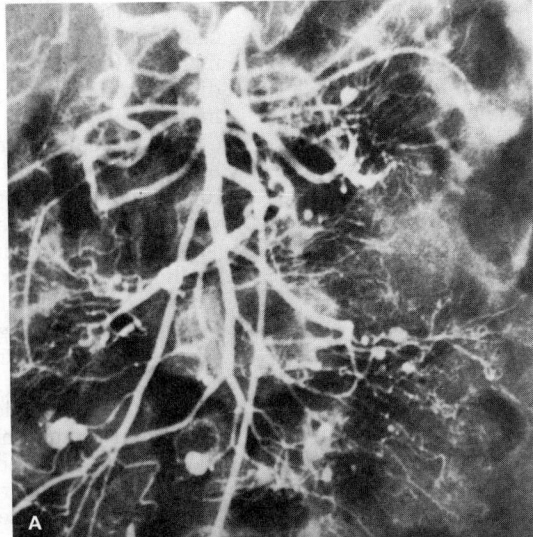
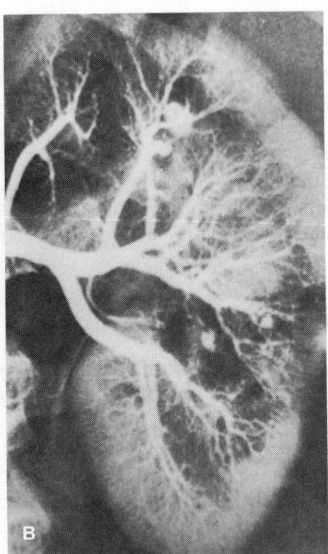

Figure 69-9. Arteriogram showing typical aneurysm formation in medium-sized visceral (*A*) and renal (*B*) arteries in a patient with polyarteritis nodosa. (Porter JM, Taylor LM Jr, Harris EJ Jr. Nonatherosclerotic vascular disease. In: Moore WS, ed. Vascular surgery: a comprehensive review. Philadelphia, WB Saunders, 1994:111)

ists about this mechanism. A suggested classification of the immune arteritides of surgical interest follows:

Polyarteritis Nodosa (PAN) Group (Medium Muscular Arteries)

Classic PAN
Kawasaki disease
Cogan syndrome
Behçet syndrome

Hypersensitivity Angiitis Group (Small Arteries)

Hypersensitivity angiitis
Arteritis of collagen diseases
Mixed cryoglobulinemia
Arteritis of malignancy

Giant Cell Arteritis (Large Arteries)

Temporal arteritis
Takayasu arteritis

Polyarteritis Nodosa

Polyarteritis nodosa is a systemic disease characterized by focal necrotizing arterial inflammatory lesions involving primarily small and medium-sized muscular arteries. There is a 2:1 male/female incidence for this disease process, with the peak incidence in the fifth decade. Aneurysm formation associated with inflammatory destruction of the media was a key finding in the original description of PAN and is still considered a characteristic feature of this disease. Although renal arterial involvement is most frequently reported in PAN, involvement of the heart, lung, liver, gastrointestinal tract, and skin is also recognized (Fig. 69-9). Major lower extremity arterial involvement has been reported. Amazingly, aneurysms associated with PAN have been shown to regress with steroid therapy as assessed by serial arteriograms.[25]

Arteriographic evaluation of patients with PAN has suggested that the presence of an abnormal arteriogram identifies a subset of patients who exhibit more serious disease manifestations.[26] Specific vascular complications of PAN include aneurysm rupture and arterial stenosis or thrombosis with resulting ischemia. Spontaneous rupture of a PAN visceral arterial aneurysm has been well described and usually presents as a surgical emergency because of associated intraperitoneal or retroperitoneal hemorrhage. Interventional radiologic techniques have been success-

fully used to occlude bleeding vessels in this situation. Serious gastrointestinal surgical complications in ischemic segments are frequent, including hemorrhage, perforation, and segmental gangrene.[27]

Kawasaki Disease

Kawasaki disease, also known as *mucocutaneous lymph node syndrome,* is a form of arteritis that occurs in infants and children and is similar to PAN. Although arterial involvement is widespread, the most striking feature of Kawasaki disease is diffuse fusiform and saccular aneurysm formation of the coronary and occasionally brachiocephalic arteries (Fig. 69-10). The coronary artery pathology consists of areas of active arteritis, thrombosis,

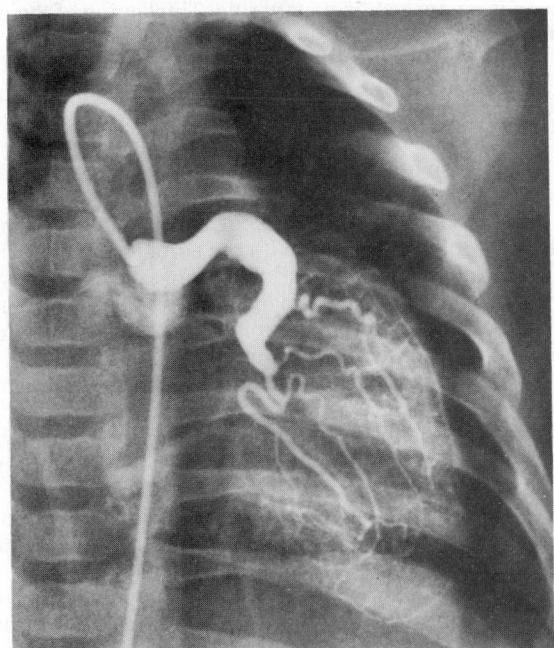

Figure 69-10. Selective coronary arteriogram showing typical aneurysm in a child with Kawasaki disease.

calcification, and stenosis.[28] Although coronary artery rupture can occur, these children usually succumb to acute cardiac arrhythmias or myocardial infarctions. Peripheral arterial involvement is also seen.

As with adult PAN, the role of the vascular surgeon in Kawasaki disease remains unclear. Coronary artery bypass surgery and coronary aneurysmectomy have been successfully performed in several patients. Neither the utility nor the durability of surgery in this setting has been determined.

Cogan Syndrome

Cogan syndrome is a rare condition consisting of nonsyphilitic interstitial keratitis associated with vestibuloauditory symptoms.[29] Cogan syndrome is a disease predominantly of young adults with the mean age of onset in the third decade. The vasculitic component of the disease, present in a minority of patients, is predominantly an aortitis. Aortitis with subsequent development of clinically significant aortic insufficiency occurs in 10% of patients with Cogan syndrome.

Daily administration of high-dose corticosteroids has been successful in reversing both the visual and auditory stigmata of Cogan syndrome and is indicated when aortitis is present. Aortic valve replacement, in the presence of compromised hemodynamic function, has been performed successfully. Long-term prognosis is excellent for Cogan syndrome in the absence of aortic valve involvement.[30]

Behçet Disease

In 1937, Behçet described three patients with iritis and associated oral and genital mucocutaneous ulcerations, and this association has subsequently become known as *Behçet disease.* The underlying pathologic lesion is a vasculitis, with venous thrombotic lesions more frequent than arterial lesions. Lower extremity superficial or deep venous thrombosis occurs in 12% to 27% of patients.[31] The arterial component can consist of occlusive and aneurysmal lesions. When present, the aneurysmal lesions portend mortality rates of up to 20%.

As noted, the predominant pathologic lesion in Behçet disease is a nonspecific panarteritis. Thickening of the endothelium is sometimes seen, whereas disorganization of the elastic fibers within the media and perivascular infiltration by monocytes or lymphocytes are frequently observed. The perivascular infiltration is often associated with luminal thrombosis. The lesions can lead to aneurysmal or occlusive disease, although occlusions are rarely encountered. Aneurysms have been described in numerous locations, including the carotid, subclavian, iliac, femoral, and popliteal arteries, with the aorta as the most frequent site of aneurysm formation. Because of vascular wall disruption and associated fragility of these vessels, aneurysms frequently recur at anastomotic sites after resection with interposition grafts.[32] Arterial puncture can lead to the development of pseudoaneurysms in Behçet disease, rendering diagnostic arteriography hazardous. The arterial aneurysms have a high probability of recurrence elsewhere after repair, necessitating numerous surgical interventions. Unfortunately, interposition bypass grafts have a high incidence of thrombosis in addition to their propensity to develop anastomotic pseudoaneurysms, with long-term graft patency the exception rather than the norm.[33]

This systemic disease largely affects the populations of the Mediterranean area and Japan, suggesting an environmental or genetic factor. Both bacterial and viral infectious causes have been proposed, although definitive evidence is lacking for the implication of infections in the cause of Behçet disease.[34] Autoimmune dysfunction is the likely cause of this condition. Several investigators have identified circulating immune complexes in patients with Behçet disease and have suggested some component of autoimmunity as causative in the vascular changes identified in this diffuse vasculitis. Immune complexes and complement have been demonstrated in the arterial wall and surrounding tissues. The activation of complement within the vascular wall can lead to destruction of the media and subsequent aneurysm formation. An alternate hypothesis implicates vasculitis of the vasa vasorum as the cause of large artery destruction.[32]

Behçet disease might also have a genetic component because there is an increased incidence of the human leukocyte antigen (HLA) B5 in patients with Behçet disease. Specific HLA genetic markers have been identified with the various common clinical subtypes of Behçet disease: HLA-B5 is associated with ocular symptoms, HLA-B27 is associated with arthritic symptoms, and HLA-B12 is associated with the presence of mucocutaneous lesions.

Immunosuppressive agents, including azathioprine, have been used with some success for nonarterial symptoms, as have corticosteroids. Although corticosteroids can suppress symptoms, especially arthritic and ophthalmic symptoms, they do not alter the progression or course of the underlying disease.[35] Reports of corticosteroid prevention of pseudoaneurysm recurrence must therefore be viewed cautiously. Although no uniformly satisfactory therapy exists for Behçet disease, early diagnosis and aggressive reconstructive management of identified arterial aneurysms has provided long-term limb salvage despite arterial graft complications.[34]

Hypersensitivity Angiitis Group

The term *hypersensitivity angiitis group* incorporates a large and heterogeneous group of clinical syndromes characterized by involvement of small arteries in the vasculitic process. The arteritides of this group include classic hypersensitivity angiitis, arteritis of collagen vascular disease, mixed cryoglobulinemia arteritis, and arteritis associated with malignancy. Involved arteries exhibit a thickened basement membrane, swelling of the collagenous and elastic connective tissues, and fragmentation of the elastic fibers. The end result of these conditions is vascular occlusion, which can lead to regional ischemia. This process appears to result from the deposition of immune complexes within the small arteries. In certain of these conditions, the inciting antigen can be identified, such as a drug or chemical, a virus, or a tumor antigen.

The clinical syndromes typically associated with this group of diseases include skin rash, fever, and evidence of organ dysfunction, none of which specifically concerns the vascular surgeon. Vascular surgeons might be called on to evaluate certain patients presenting with arterial involvement substantially limited to the hands and fingers. Plethysmography and arteriography typically identify widespread palmar and digital arterial occlusions, which are frequently associated with digital ischemia.

Our own interest in patients with upper extremity digital ischemia is ongoing, and we have collected detailed clinical and serologic data from more than 150 patients with digital ischemic ulceration. Although certain of these patients have clinically manifested autoimmune disorders, a significant number have no serologic evidence of autoimmune disease, have no clinical evidence of any systemic disease process, and have presented only with the acute onset of hand arterial occlusion and finger ischemia.[36] Each of these patients showed extensive occlusion of the palmar and digital arteries on arteriography. We have had success with a conservative program of local wound care and limited débridement in healing the ischemic lesions (Fig. 69-11). Anecdotally, we have observed clinical improvement in the vasospastic symptomatology in a number of these patients after initiation of vasodilator therapy, principally calcium-channel blockers. Also, healing of digital ischemic ulcers appears to be improved by pentoxifylline.

Giant Cell Arteritis Group

Two easily distinguishable clinical disease patterns occur within the giant cell arteritis group: (1) temporal arteritis, or systemic giant cell arteritis, and (2) Takayasu arteritis. Numerous similarities exist between these two conditions, suggesting to some that these two diseases might represent different expressions of the same disease process. Both conditions consist of localized periarteritis with inflammatory mononuclear infiltrates and giant cells, along with disruption and fragmentation of the elastic fibers of the arterial wall.

Temporal Arteritis

Temporal arteritis, or systemic giant cell arteritis, is predominantly a disease of white women, usually occurring after 55 years of age. This condition is a systemic disease process characterized by chronic inflammation of the aorta and its major branches. The most frequent presenting complaint is headache. Polymyalgia rheumatica, a condition associated with severe pain in the pelvic and shoulder girdles, is often identified in these patients.

Although systemic giant cell arteritis can affect any large artery of the body, the branches of the carotid artery are most frequently involved. The onset of the disease is heralded by a febrile myalgic process, usually involving the back, shoulder, and pelvic regions. The most characteristic complaint is severe pain along the course of the temporal artery, frequently bilateral, accompanied by tenderness and nodularity of the artery with overlying skin erythema.

Visual alterations are severe and occur in over 50% of patients. The disturbances can be secondary to either ischemic optic or retrobulbar neuritis, or occlusion of the central retinal artery. Up to 40% of patients with symptomatic giant cell arteritis experience a permanent partial or complete loss of vision,[37] which can be prevented by early steroid administration. Systemic giant cell arteritis can cause aneurysms or stenoses of the aorta and its main branches. Thoracic aortic aneurysms and aortic dissections are reported, and surgical replacement of these lesions has been successful.

Some have speculated that early high-dose corticoste-

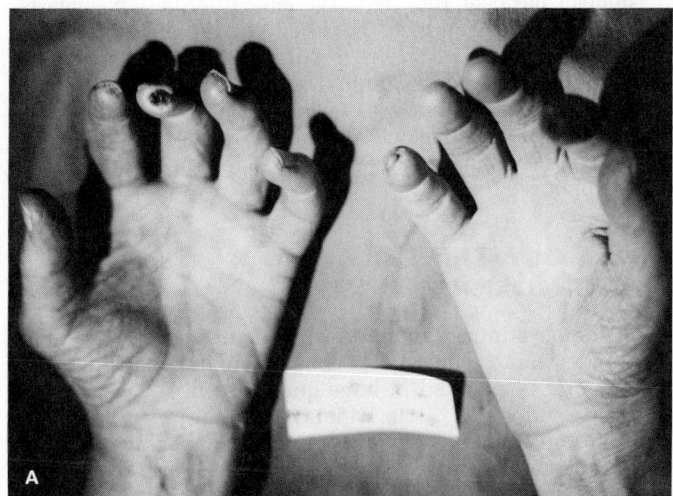

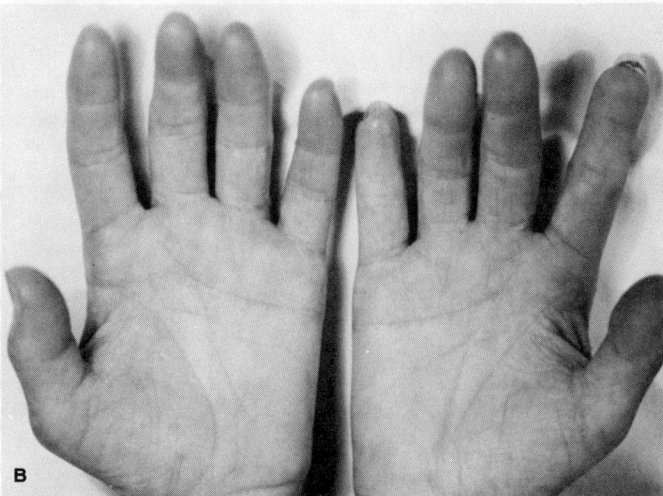

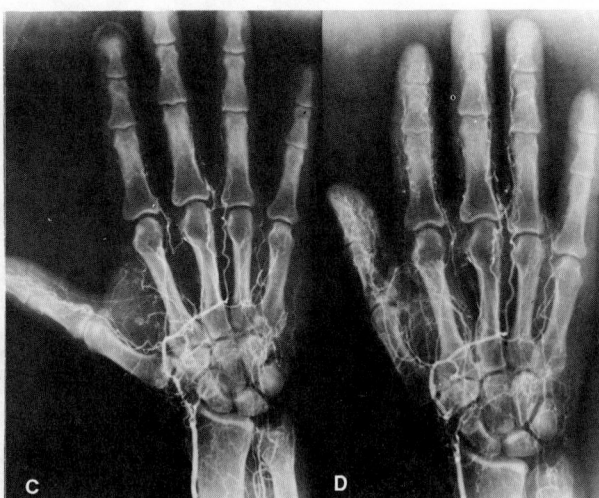

Figure 69-11. (*A*) Hands of a patient with systemic lupus and multiple ischemic finger ulcers. (*B*) Same patient with healed ulcers after 2 months of conservative therapy. (*C*) Arteriogram of same patient, demonstrating extensive palmar and digital arterial occlusions. (*D*) Arteriogram showing formation of collaterals.

roid therapy minimizes the likelihood of aortic lesions, although convincing evidence of this hypothesis is unavailable. The clinical effectiveness of corticosteroid therapy is uniform in that laboratory findings often improve and the patient's constitutional symptoms resolve or improve. Microscopic evaluation of surgical specimens pretreated with steroids fails to identify any effect of steroid therapy on the arterial pathologic features of this disease. Some authors suggest that corticosteroid therapy might increase the chance of aneurysmal rupture.[38] We and others believe that surgical procedures in this disease fail in a high percentage of patients unless accompanied by high-dose steroid administration.[39]

The angiographic features most suggestive of giant cell arteritis include long segments of smooth stenosis interspersed with normal segments, smoothly tapered occlusions, absence of irregular plaques and ulcerations, and distribution of these abnormalities among the subclavian, axillary, and brachial arteries (Fig. 69-12).

Takayasu Arteritis

Takayasu arteritis is a rare primary arteritis of unknown cause that commonly affects the aorta, its major branches, and the pulmonary artery. It occurs predominantly in female patients, with the age of onset between 3 and 35 years. Takayasu arteritis can produce stenosis, occlusion, dilation, or aneurysm formation of the involved artery. Elastic fibers in the arterial wall are involved in an intense periarteritis, characterized by a granulomatous inflammatory process with mononuclear cell infiltration and the formation of multinucleated giant cells.

Although more common in Asia, the disease has a worldwide distribution. Patients present with symptoms of cerebral, visceral, or extremity ischemia. The clinical course of Takayasu arteritis has been described as having two stages. The initial stage is characterized by nonspecific symptoms of fever, myalgia, and anorexia. The second stage can follow closely and consists of a pulseless phase with multiple arterial occlusions and cardiovascular symptoms depending on disease location.[40] Hypertension is common and might be due to aortic coarctation or renal artery stenosis. Neurologic symptoms can result from hypertension or from central nervous system ischemia associated with large artery stenosis or occlusion. Coronary artery involvement is rare in Takayasu disease. The cardiac pathology most frequently found is nonspecific and appears to result from heart failure associated with systemic and pulmonary hypertension.

Takayasu disease has been divided into four types, characterized by their pattern of cardiovascular involvement. Type I is limited to involvement of the aortic arch and arch vessels and occurs in 8.4% of patients. Type II involves the descending thoracic and abdominal aorta and accounts for 11.2% of cases. Type III is the most common and has involvement of the arch vessels and the abdominal aorta and its branches and accounts for 65.4% of cases. Type IV has primarily pulmonary artery involvement with or without the other types and accounts for 15% of patients.[41] Stenosis is the most common angiographic finding in the aorta and its branches, whereas occlusion is the most common pulmonary angiographic finding.

The role of surgery in Takayasu arteritis remains uncertain because no studies have compared operative with nonoperative therapy in a controlled fashion. Surgery has been widely performed, and some conclusions are possible. Endarterectomy has resulted in early failure and generally is not recommended. Successful management requires bypass graft implantation into disease-free arterial segments and continuation of corticosteroid therapy[42] (Fig. 69-13). Percutaneous transluminal angioplasty has provided variable results with no proven long-term efficacy, often requiring several attempts to significantly reduce the stenosis. Successful surgical correction of pulmonary arterial stenosis has been reported. Available information suggests a conservative surgical approach to these patients, although the risk of stroke is sufficiently great that some have recommended prophylactic repair of high-grade brachiocephalic stenoses. Corticosteroid therapy is the key to successful management. Surgical reconstruction has a selective role and produces acceptable long-term relief of symptoms.

HOMOCYSTEINEMIA AND HOMOCYSTINURIA

Homocystinuria, an inborn error of metabolism in which homocysteine accumulates abnormally in plasma and tissues and is excreted in large quantities in the urine, was first described in 1962. Patients with the disorder suffer from multiple abnormalities, including ectopia lentis, mental retardation, rapidly progressive arteriosclerotic vascular disease, and thromboembolic disorders. Evidence

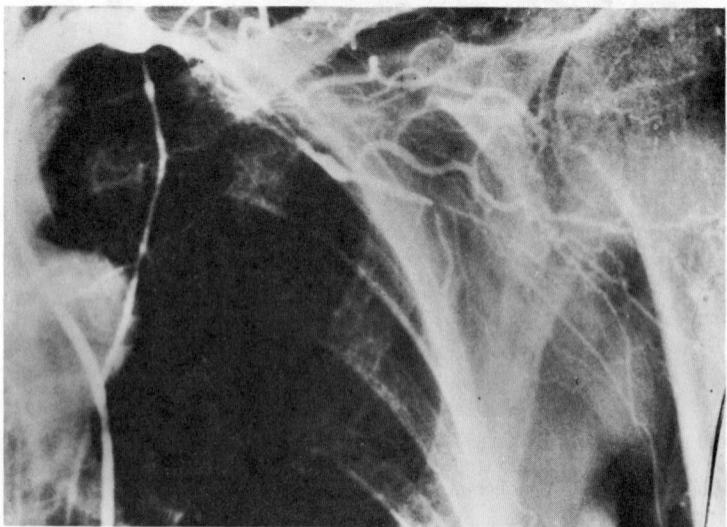

Figure 69-12. Typical tapered stenosis of left axillary artery in giant cell arteritis.

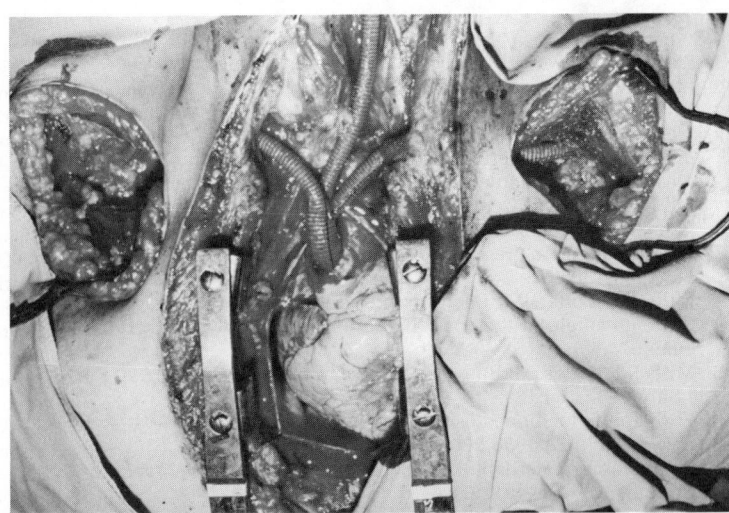

Figure 69-13. Extensive bypass from ascending aorta to left carotid and both axillary arteries in a patient with Takayasu arteritis.

suggests that up to one third of all patients with symptomatic peripheral atherosclerosis have heterozygous homocystinuria. Three specific enzyme deficiencies responsible for homocystinuria have been identified: (1) cystathionine synthetase, (2) homocysteine methyl transferase, and (3) methylene tetrahydrofolate reductase. Additionally, these enzymes require the cofactors pyridoxine, folate, and cobalamin. Deficiencies of any of these cofactors can also cause homocystinuria, initially indistinguishable from an enzyme deficiency. Regardless of the primary cause, all forms of homocysteine accumulation in humans have been associated with premature atherosclerosis, frequently complicated by thrombosis.[43] The arteriosclerotic plaques identified in homocystinura are typical fibrous plaques. Microscopic evaluations reveal medial hypertrophy, elaboration of extracellular matrix and collagen, and degeneration and destruction of the elastic laminae. Lipid deposition in the plaques is characteristically absent.[44]

Although multiple clinical studies have demonstrated the association between homocystinuria and premature atherosclerosis and thrombosis, the exact mechanism of homocysteine-induced atherogenesis and thrombosis is not known. Accumulation of homocysteine leads to the production of homocysteine thiolactone by the liver, and this reduced thiol has been implicated as the toxic substance in homocysteinemic atherogenesis. In vitro, homocysteine induces endothelial cell desquamation, promotes oxidation of low-density lipoproteins, increases monocyte adhesions to vessel wall, and stimulates platelet aggregation. Elevated levels of homocysteine have been shown to enhance factor V activity, decrease protein C activation, diminish fibrinolysis, and increase tissue factor activity, thereby reducing the antithrombotic properties of endothelial cells. The precise in vivo mechanism by which homocysteine might induce acceleration of atherosclerosis and thrombosis remains to be defined.

Homocysteine exists in human plasma in at least three forms: as the mixed disulfide homocysteine-cysteine, as free homocysteine, and as protein-bound homocysteine. Men have higher levels of plasma homocysteine than women, and premenopausal women have lower levels than postmenopausal women.

Evidence has accumulated that mildly elevated levels of plasma homocysteine are associated with symptomatic atherosclerotic disease. Boers and colleagues[45] detected a heterozygous trait they termed *homocysteinemia* in 14 of 70 patients with premature atherosclerotic vascular disease. These investigators performed an oral methionine loading test to aid in the detection of elevated plasma homocysteine in high-risk groups. Kang and associates[46] simplified the investigations when they demonstrated elevated levels of protein-bound homocysteine in patients with coronary artery disease without any requirements for oral methionine loading.

Our own ongoing evaluation of patients with peripheral vascular disease has confirmed elevated total plasma homocysteine levels when compared with age- and sex-matched controls.[47] Investigators have attempted to lower these supranormal plasma homocysteine levels through alteration of the homocysteine-methionine pathways with pharmacologic doses of the cofactors for these enzymatic pathways,[48] namely, folic acid, pyridoxine, vitamin B_{12}, and cobalamin. Although reduction in the plasma homocysteine levels was observed with this therapy, no investigation has established any clinical benefit from this therapy. Intuitively, one would expect clinical improvement or at least cessation of disease progression once the toxic homocysteine levels declined. Serial evaluation of the progression of peripheral vascular disease in groups randomized to treatment and nontreatment is necessary to answer this question; until then, the anecdotal reports appear encouraging.

HYPERVISCOSITY SYNDROMES

Multiple conditions characterized by an increase in the blood viscosity can cause arterial or venous thromboembolism. These are classified as *hyperviscosity syndromes,* and can be divided into two categories.[49] The first group includes pathophysiologic conditions in which a primary blood abnormality causes an increase in the formed elements of the blood, such as the myeloproliferative disorders. The second group includes pathologic conditions that elevate serum proteins, such as myeloma, benign monoclonal gammopathy, macroglobulinemia, cryoglobulinemia, and neoplasia. In our clinical experience, hyperviscosity syndromes result in thrombosis most frequently in the venous system, next most often in the small peripheral arteries (ie, hands and fingers), and least often in the major arteries.

Treatment of these hyperviscosity syndromes is directed at correction of the underlying disorders, with appropriate anticoagulation therapy as needed. Vascular surgery procedures are rarely required in these patients.

REFERENCES

1. Stanley JC, Gewertz BL, Bove EL, et al. Arterial fibrodysplasia, histopathologic character and current etiologic concepts. Arch Surg 1978;110:561.
2. Mahler F, Probst PN, Haertel M, et al. Lasting improvement of renovascular hypertension by transluminal dilation of atherosclerotic and non-atherosclerotic renal artery stenosis: a follow-up study. Circulation 1982;65:611.
3. Buerger L. Thromboangiitis obliterans: a study of the vascular lesions leading to presenile spontaneous gangrene. Am J Med Sci 1908;136:567.
4. Mills JM, Porter JM. Buerger's disease. In: Cameron JL, ed. Current surgical therapy III. Philadelphia, BC Decker, 1989;575.
5. Mills JM, Porter JM. Buerger's disease in the modern era. Am J Surg 1987;154:123.
6. Erdheim J. Medionecrosis aortae idiopathica cystica. Virchows Arch [A] 1930;276:187.
7. McKusick VA. Heritable disorders of connective tissue, ed 4. St Louis, CV Mosby, 1972:61.
8. Pyeritz RE. Propranolol retards aortic root dilatation in the Marfan syndrome. Circulation 1983;68(Suppl III):365.
9. Pyeritz RE, McKusick VA. The Marfan syndrome: diagnosis and management. N Engl J Med 1979;300:772.
10. Gott VL. Pyeritz RF, Magovern GJ, et al. Surgical treatment of aneurysms of the ascending aorta in the Marfan syndrome: results of composite graft repair in 50 patients. N Engl J Med 1986;314:1070.
11. Pope FM, Martin GR, Lichenstein JR, et al. Patients with Ehlers-Danlos syndrome type IV lack type III collagen. Proc Natl Acad Sci USA 1975;72:1314.
12. Hunter GC, Malone JM, Moore WS. Vascular manifestations in patients with Ehlers-Danlos syndrome. Arch Surg 1982;117:495.
13. Carlborg U. Studies of circulatory disturbances, pulse wave velocity, and pressure pulses in large arteries in cases of pseudoxanthoma elasticum and angioid streaks. Acta Med Scand 1944;151(Suppl):1.
14. Carter DJ, Vince FP, Woodward DAK. Arterial surgery in pseudoxanthoma elasticum. Postgrad Med J 1976;52:291.
15. Leriche R. Dilation pathologique des arteres es en dehors des aneurysmes vie tissulaire des arteres. Presse Med 1942;50:641.
16. Rabinov K, Simon M, Sears J. Diffuse arteriectasis of the aorta, iliac, femoral, and popliteal arteries. Vasc Dis 1966;3:122.
17. Thomas ML. Arteriomegaly. Br J Surg 1971;58:690.
18. Hollier LH, Stanson AW, Gloviczki P, et al. Arteriomegaly: classification and morbid implications of diffuse aneurysmal disease. Surgery 1983;93:700.
19. Flannigan DP, Burnham SJ, Goodreau JJ, et al. Summary of cases of adventitial cystic disease of the popliteal artery. Ann Surg 1979;189:165.
20. Savage PEA. Arterial cystic degeneration. Postgrad Med J 1972;48:603.
21. MacFarlane R, Livesey SA, Pollard S, Dunn DC. Cystic adventitial arterial disease. Br J Surg 1987;74:89.
22. Deutsch AL, Hyde J, Miller SM, et al. Cystic adventitial degeneration of the popliteal artery: CT demonstration and directed percutaneous therapy. AJR 1985;145:117.
23. Francfort JW, Gallagher JF, Penman E, et al. Surgery for radiation-induced symptomatic atherosclerosis. Ann Vasc Surg 1989;3:14.
24. Lie JT. The classification and diagnosis of vasculitis in large and medium-sized blood vessels. Pathol Annu 1987;22:125.
25. Robins JM, Bookstein JJ. Regressing aneurysms in periarteritis nodosa. Radiology 1972;104:39.
26. Ewald EA, Griffin D, McCune WJ. Correlation of angiographic abnormalities with disease manifestations and disease severity in polyarteritis nodosa. J Rheumatol 1987;14:952.
27. Cabal E, Holtz S. Polyarteritis as a cause of intestinal hemorrhage. Gastroenterology 1971;61:99.
28. Onouchi A, Shimazu S, Kiyosawa N, et al. Aneurysms of the coronary arteries in Kawasaki disease. Circulation 1982;66:6.
29. Cogan DG. Syndrome of non-syphilitic interstitial keratitis and vestibuloauditory symptoms. Arch Ophthalmol 1945;33:144.
30. Haynes BF, Kaiser-Kupfer MI, Mason P, Fauci AS. Cogan syndrome: studies in thirteen patients, long-term follow-up, and a review of the literature. Medicine 1980;59:426.
31. Chajek T, Fainaru M. Behçet's disease: report of 41 cases and a review of the literature. Medicine 1975;54:179.
32. Bartlett ST, McCarthy WJ, Palmer AS, et al. Multiple aneurysms in Behçet's disease. Arch Surg 1988;123:1004.
33. Jenkins AAL, MacPherson AIS, Nolan B, et al. Peripheral aneurysms in Behçet's disease. Br J Surg 1976;63:199.
34. Sezer FN. Further investigations of the virus of Behçet's disease. Am J Ophthalmol 1956;41:41.
35. O'Duffy JD, Lehner T, Barnes CG. Summary of the Third International Conference on Behçet's Disease. J Rheumatol 1983;10:154.
36. Porter JM, Taylor LM. Small artery disease of the upper extremity. World J Surg 1983;7:326.
37. Hollenhorst RW, Brown JR, Wagener HP, et al. Neurologic aspects of temporal arteritis. Neurology 1960;10:490.
38. Takagi A, Kajiura N, Tada Y, Ueno A. Surgical treatment of non-specific inflammatory arterial aneurysms. J Cardiovasc Surg 1986;27:117.
39. Rivers SP, Baur GM, Inahara T, et al. Arm ischemia secondary to giant cell arteritis. Am J Surg 1982;143:554.
40. Hall S, Barr W, Lie TE, et al. Takayasu arteritis: a study of 32 North American patients. Medicine 1985;64:89.
41. Lupi-Herrera E, Sanchez-Torres G, Marcustiamer J, et al. Takayasu's arteritis: clinical study of 107 cases. Am Heart J 1977;93:94.
42. Joyce JW. The giant cell arteritides: diagnosis and the role of surgery. J Vasc Surg 1986;3:827.
43. McCully KS. Homocysteine theory of atherosclerosis: development and current status. Atherosclerosis Rev 1983;11:157.
44. McCully KS. Vascular pathology of homocysteinemia: implications for the pathogenesis of atherosclerosis. Am J Pathol 1969;56:111.
45. Boers GHJ, Smals AGH, Trijbels FJM, et al. Heterozygosity for homocysteinuria in premature peripheral and cerebral occlusive arterial disease. N Engl J Med 1985;313:709.
46. Kang SS, Wong PWK, Cook HY, et al. Protein-bound homocysteine: a possible risk factor for coronary artery disease. J Clin Invest 1986;77:1482.
47. Harris EJ Jr, Taylor LM Jr, Malinow MR, et al. The association between elevated plasma homocysteine and symptomatic peripheral arterial disease. Surgical Forum 1989;40:307.
48. Olszewski AJ, Szostak WB, Bialkowska M, et al. Reduction of plasma lipid and homocysteine levels by pyridoxine, folate, cobalamin, choline, riboflavin, and troxerutin in atherosclerosis. Atherosclerosis 1989;75:1.
49. Forconi S, Pieragalli M, Guerrini C, et al. Primary and secondary blood hyperviscosity syndromes, and syndromes associated with blood hyperviscosity. Drugs 1987;33(Suppl):19.

SURGERY: SCIENTIFIC PRINCIPLES AND PRACTICE, Second Edition, edited by Lazar J. Greenfield, Michael W. Mulholland, Keith T. Oldham, Gerald B. Zelenock, and Keith D. Lillemoe. Lippincott–Raven Publishers, Philadelphia, © 1997.

CHAPTER 70

OCCLUSIVE DISEASE: THROMBOSIS

G. PATRICK CLAGETT, JR.

Hemostatic mechanisms prevent hemorrhage from occurring at breaks in the vascular system. By localizing the clotting of blood precisely at the site of injury, hemostatic mechanisms also maintain blood fluidity and continued circulation through the vessel. In broad terms, the principal factors that localize hemostatic reactions are (1) antithrombotic properties of vascular endothelium, (2) inhibitory substances in blood that counteract coagulation reactions or lyse clot, and (3) the maintenance of normal laminar and nondisturbed blood flow, which serves to wash away activated coagulation enzymes and platelets and prevents excessive buildup of clot. Imbalances between hemostatic reactions and these protective mechanisms lead to the formation of thrombi that may obstruct the circulation.

LOCATION AND HISTOLOGIC COMPOSITION OF THROMBI

Thrombi may form in the arteries, veins, heart, and the microcirculation. Arterial thrombi may cause tissue ischemia with organ dysfunction or infarction from local obstruction of the vessel or distal embolism. Irregularity in the vessel wall from arterial pathology, most commonly atherosclerosis, is typically found beneath arterial thrombi. One of the most common clinical manifestations of this process is ischemic heart disease. Overwhelming evidence from clinical, angiographic, histologic, and experimental studies suggests that rupture of coronary atherosclerotic plaque with superimposed thrombosis occurs in most patients with unstable angina, myocardial infarction, and sudden death from ischemic heart disease. Similar mechanisms are operative in many patients suffering cerebrovascular and peripheral vascular ischemic syndromes.

Most venous thrombi occur in the lower extremities, where they usually stem from tiny clots found in venous valve sinuses, the cul-de-sac areas located behind venous valves. This is an area of stasis, where blood tends to pool excessively during periods of immobility as may occur postoperatively. Many venous thrombi are clinically silent but may produce symptoms from local inflammation of the vessel wall or obstruction, causing pain and swelling, or they may embolize to the pulmonary circulation.

Intracardiac thrombi usually form on damaged heart valves, infarcted endocardium, or prosthetic valves. Common to all of these conditions is the absence of dysfunction of endocardial endothelium. Flow disturbances frequently contribute to intracardiac thrombus growth in areas of relative stasis and blood pooling found behind obstructed valve orifices, in areas of ventricular dysfunction or aneurysm formation, or during dysrhythmias. Cardiac thrombi are usually asymptomatic until they embolize systemically and produce symptoms according to the site of lodgement and the sensitivity of the vascular bed. Over 80% of patients who present with clinically evident cardiac embolism suffer stroke, blindness, or transient ischemic attacks. Because the cerebral circulation receives only 15% of the cardiac output, most cardiac emboli are probably clinically silent.

In the microcirculation, widespread thrombosis is usually a manifestation of disseminated intravascular coagulation. This may lead to ischemic necrosis and generalized organ failure or consumption of hemostatic elements and secondary diffuse microvascular bleeding.

The histologic composition of thrombi varies according to hemodynamic factors and therefore differs in arterial and venous thrombosis.[1] Thrombi are composed of fibrin and blood cells, including red blood cells (RBCs), leukocytes, and platelets. Arterial thrombi form under conditions of high flow and are frequently composed of platelet aggregates bound loosely by fibrin strands. Venous thrombi form in areas of sluggish blood flow and are composed predominantly of RBCs with large amounts of fibrin and relatively fewer platelets. Because of flow conditions and the relatively small amounts of fibrin that bind the throm-

bus, arterial thrombi break off easily and tend to repetitively embolize small fragments, a pattern that produces clinical manifestations such as unstable angina or cerebral transient ischemic attacks. In contrast, venous thrombi grow to comparatively greater size and tend to embolize large fragments that may produce a single, dramatic clinical event, such as massive pulmonary embolism.

Thrombi undergo constant structural change as they age. Leukocytes are attracted by chemotactic factors released from platelets and incorporate into the thrombus. Aggregated platelets fuse and undergo autolysis and are replaced by fibrin that is lysed by plasma-borne fibrinolytic enzymes as well as leukocyte proteases. Infiltration of the thrombus by fibroblasts and smooth muscle cells leads to remodeling and incorporation into the architecture of the vessel wall. This may contribute to growth of atherosclerotic plaque in the arterial circulation. Detailed study of central portions of atherosclerotic plaques reveals cross-linked fibrin as well as platelet antigens suggesting that arterial thrombus is present early in the growth of the plaque.[2] On the venous side, organization of thrombus may lead to recanalization of the lumen and scarring of the vein wall and valves, rendering them incompetent and leading to chronic venous insufficiency.

MECHANISMS THAT PROTECT AGAINST THROMBOSIS

To better understand the pathogenesis of thrombosis, it is necessary to consider in detail each of the protective mechanisms that limit hemostatic reactions and prevent thrombus formation. These include antithrombotic properties of vascular endothelium, mechanisms that counteract or neutralize coagulation reactions, and laminar nondisturbed blood flow. It is also important to understand the effects of impairment of these protective mechanisms on blood coagulation and platelet reactions. This leads to a rational approach to therapy designed to prevent thrombosis or restore vascular patency after thrombus has formed. In the following sections, each of these mechanisms is considered in detail as well as the consequences of their loss or dysfunction that result in thrombogenesis. Although each of the protective mechanisms are discussed singly, rarely does the loss of a single protective factor lead to clinical thrombosis. For example, a major factor causing postoperative deep venous thrombosis is sluggish venous blood flow with pooling of blood in the lower extremities, but perioperative decreases in antithrombin III, defective fibrinolysis, and venous endothelial damage, especially with orthopedic operations or trauma in areas contiguous with major veins, can be equally important factors. Derangements in combinations of protective mechanisms also stimulate arterial thrombosis. A hemodynamically significant atherosclerotic plaque causing disturbed, nonlaminar blood flow is not particularly thrombogenic as long as its surface is paved with healthy endothelium. However, when endothelial defenses are impaired or endothelium is lost, as occurs with plaque rupture, thrombogenesis ensues. The combination of major rheologic disturbance, loss of endothelium, and exposure of blood to thrombogenic plaque components can result in thrombotic occlusion, distal embolization, or both.

PROTECTIVE MECHANISM: ENDOTHELIUM AND VESSEL WALL REACTIONS
Endothelial Physiology

Endothelial cells play important roles in the regulation of coagulation, fibrinolysis, vascular tone, cellular growth and differentiation, and immune and inflammatory responses.

The normal, intact endothelium is nonthrombogenic and reacts with neither platelets nor blood coagulation factors.[3] The importance of endothelium is apparent when considering that thromboembolic complications are the principal limitations of blood-contacting artificial devices, such as vascular prostheses, arterial and venous catheters, prosthetic heart valves, cardiopulmonary bypass machines, ventricular assist devices, and hemodialysis machines.[4] Antithrombotic properties of endothelium are illustrated in Figure 70-1. Endothelial cells synthesize prostaglandin I$_2$ (prostacyclin), which inhibits platelet aggregation and causes smooth muscle relaxation and vasodilation. Prostacyclin inhibits platelets by increasing platelet adenylate cyclase activity and thereby raising platelet cyclic adenosine monophosphate (cAMP) levels; high cAMP prevents platelet activation. Vasodilation caused by prostacyclin may lead to local increases in blood flow that help to wash away forming platelet aggregates. Another product of endothelial prostaglandin metabolism includes lipoxygenase products that inhibit platelet adhesion. Platelet function is also affected by endothelial ectonucleotidase enzymatic activity that degrades plasma adenosine diphosphate (ADP), a compound that activates platelets and stimulates their aggregation.

Endothelial cells also produce endothelium-derived relaxing factor (EDRF) identified as nitric oxide (NO). Like prostacyclin, EDRF-NO is a potent inhibitor of smooth muscle cell contractions and causes vasodilation. In addition, EDRF-NO inhibits platelet aggregation, stimulates disaggregation, inhibits platelet and monocyte adhesion to endothelial surfaces, and inhibits smooth muscle cell proliferation.[5]

In addition to inhibiting platelet adhesion and aggregation, endothelium also counteracts coagulation enzymatic reactions. Endothelial cells synthesize heparin-like glycosoaminoglycans that possess anticoagulant activity. Endothelial heparan sulfate is capable of activating circulating antithrombin III, which efficiently neutralizes activated factors XII, XI, X, IX, and II (thrombin) in the microenvironment at the cell surface. The principal action of this system is to limit thrombin production. The action of thrombin is also curtailed by binding to an endothelial surface receptor, termed thrombomodulin. Thrombin bound to thrombomodulin loses its substrate specificity and its ability to activate coagulation factors.[6] Thrombin complexed with thrombomodulin is able, however, to activate protein C, which in turn destroys factors Va and VIIIa and stimulates release of plasminogen activator. Thus, the binding of thrombin to thrombomodulin results in loss of its coagulant effects and enhancement of its ability to activate protein C and therefore to inhibit thrombogenesis. Thrombin also stimulates endothelial production of prostacyclin and expression of fibrinolytic activity.

Endothelium synthesizes and secretes plasminogen activator and is the principal in vivo source of tissue plasminogen activator (tPA). tPA in turn converts plasminogen to plasmin, which lyses fibrin. In addition to releasing tPA, endothelial cells possess surface receptors that bind plasminogen and thereby enhance the efficiency of local fibrinolytic mechanisms. Endothelial cells also are the source of plasminogen activator inhibitor (PAI-1), a protein that neutralizes tPA. Thus, endothelium can stimulate or down-regulate local fibrinolytic activity depending on the stimulus.

Vessel Wall Damage

Damage to the vessel wall can lead to endothelium loss and thrombus formation. Endothelial trauma can be direct or indirect. Direct injury includes blunt and penetrating vascular trauma, surgery (injury from application of vascular clamps, endarterectomy, vascular suturing, and manipulation of blood vessels), interventional endovascular therapies (balloon angioplasty, atherectomy), and extreme

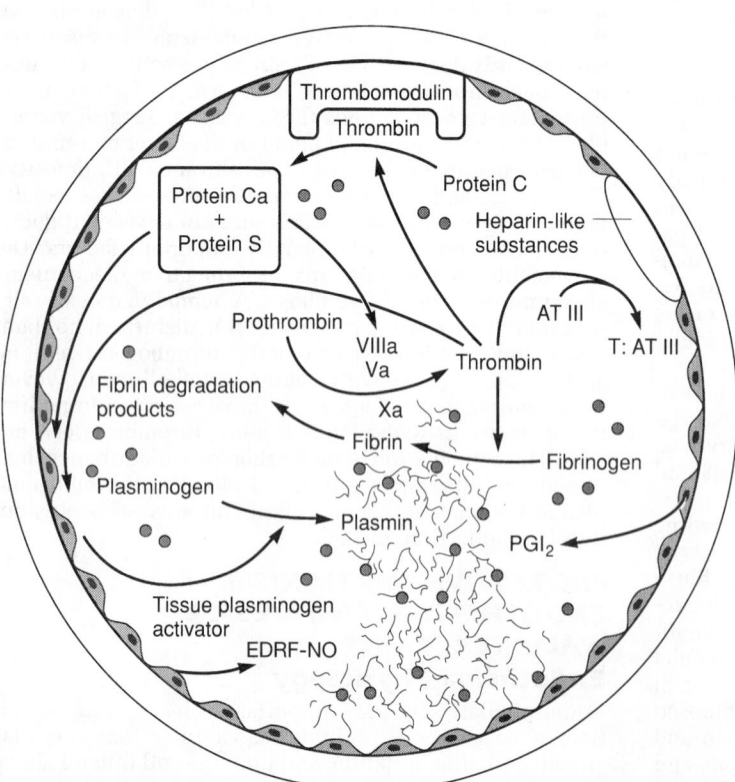

Figure 70-1. Major antithrombotic properties of vascular endothelium.

thermal conditions (burn injury, frostbite). Indirect endothelial injury may occur from immune complexes, viruses or bacteria, hemodynamic stress from localized jetlike flows, tobacco products, high blood cholesterol, elevated blood homocystine, and enzymes released from platelets and leukocytes in inflammatory states.

Loss of endothelium exposes underlying thrombogenic tissues to both platelet and coagulation factors. In addition to frank loss of endothelial cells, many of these conditions induce endothelial *dysfunction,* with thrombus formation occurring on top of intact endothelium. Endothelial dysfunction results in loss of antithrombotic properties, as well as the activation of endothelial mechanisms that promote and enhance thrombosis under certain conditions (Fig. 70-2). Endothelial procoagulant activity is induced by bacterial endotoxin, thrombin, interleukin-1, and tumor necrosis factor.[7] Perturbed endothelial cells not only express tissue factor, but also induce exposure of receptors that bind activated and nonactivated coagulation factors, which enhance local cell-surface clotting. Endothelium is a principal site for production of tissue factor that can act as a cofactor with factor VII to activate the extrinsic coagulation cascade. Factors VII, IX, VIII, and X are bound to the cell surface, resulting in assembled complex that can generate thrombin under certain conditions. These include localized and generalized inflammatory states with tumor necrosis factor and other cytokines providing signaling mechanisms that induce endothelial procoagulant activity.

Reperfusion following ischemia results in the formation of reactive oxygen metabolites, superoxide, and hydrogen peroxide that induce multiple biochemical and functional changes in endothelium.[5] One of the earliest events is a marked reduction in EDRF-NO production. The reduction in EDRF-NO increases neutrophil adhesion and promotes vasoconstriction. This environment also causes endothelial cells to produce platelet-activating factor (PAF), which promotes neutrophil adhesion as well as increases vessel permeability and causes edema. Another biochemical event triggered by reactive oxygen metabolites is the decrease in endothelial cell production of prostacyclin with resulting vasoconstriction and thrombosis. Neutrophils adhere during ischemia reperfusion via expression of endothelial cell adhesion molecules.[8] ICAM-1 belongs to the immunoglobulin G (IgG) super family of proteins and, when expressed, causes neutrophils, lymphocytes, and monocytes to stick to the endothelial surface. P-selectins and E-selectins are also expressed, and this results in neutrophils and monocytes adhering to the endothelial surface. Because platelets can also express P-selectin, as well as stick to neutrophils under these conditions, platelets are also brought to the endothelial surface, and this may be important in promoting local thrombogenesis. The expression of P-selectin on the endothelial surface appears to be important for transient or rolling attachments, which has been likened to a scanning function of polymorphonuclear leukocytes. On the other hand, the expression of ICAM-1 is important for firm attachment of leukocytes.

These ligand–receptor interactions result in profound activation of neutrophils, which is important for transendothelial migration and subsequent damage to organs during ischemia and reperfusion. Neutrophils appear to be the principal cause of tissue injury during reperfusion. Injury occurs through a variety of mechanisms including neutrophil-induced proteolysis from release of elastase, collagenase, and other lytic substances. In addition, leukocytes generate reactive oxygen metabolites that further the vicious cycle of injury. Furthermore, large numbers of white cells accumulating in the microcirculation exacerbate ischemia by plugging the microvasculature and inducing local thrombosis. Microvascular permeability is also increased in the presence of activated white cells and, ultimately, all of these mechanisms result in tissue damage.

Numerous studies have demonstrated that dysfunction in the release of EDRF-NO occurs with hypercholesterolemia and at an early stage in the atherosclerotic process in animals and humans.[9] The impairment in EDRF-NO release may be associated with an increased release of endothelial-derived contracting factors that are functional antagonists of EDRF-NO. The shift in balance of endothelial mediators might contribute in part to the diminution in the protective role of the endothelium and could predispose the blood vessel to vasospasm or to further progression of the atherosclerotic disease process and thrombosis. These mechanisms may in part have a role in certain acute coronary ischemic syndromes as well as other peripheral ischemic problems.[10] Serotonin released from platelets has a vasodilating effect on normal coronary arteries. However, when the endothelium is damaged as in coronary artery disease, serotonin has a direct, unopposed vasoconstricting effect. Serotonin and other vasoactive substances derived from platelets may play an important part in the pathophysiology of a vasoconstriction that accompanies acute thrombosis. The role of endothelium in modulating these effects is an important determinant in the severity of ischemia.

When injured by mechanical or biochemical stimuli, endothelial cells exhibit a spectrum of responses.[11] Acute endothelial responses to injury or to inflammatory stimuli occur within the first 15 minutes of stimulation and are independent of de novo mRNA or protein synthesis. These acute responses include release of prostaglandins, PGI_2 and PGE_2, EDRF-NO, endothelin, and other endothelial-derived contracting factors, endothelial-derived PAF, P-selectin, and peptide leukotrienes that have vasoactive and leukocyte chemotactic properties.

In contrast to these acute responses, endothelial cells also manifest long-term complex responses that require de novo mRNA and protein synthesis. Altered gene regulation in response to injury triggers the acquisition of a new endothelial phenotype. The change in functional properties of endothelium include increased expression of proteins that are adhesive or chemotactic for various immune and inflammatory cells, enhanced capacity to elaborate vasoactive mediators, and the amplified production of various

Figure 70-2. Procoagulant properties of vascular endothelium. Endothelial procoagulant activity is induced by bacterial endotoxin, thrombin, and interleukin-1. Perturbed endothelial cells not only express tissue factor (TF), but also possess specific binding sites for factors VII, IX, VIII, and X. In addition, endothelial cells can synthesize factor V. Binding and activation of these factors results in local thrombin generation.

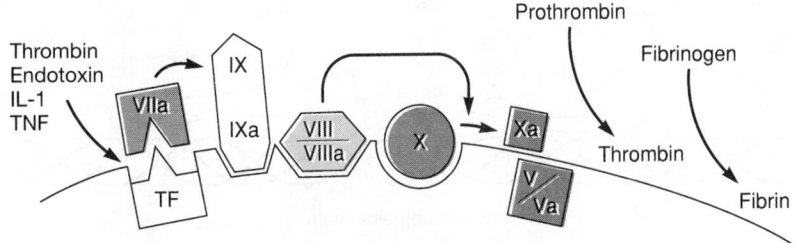

growth factors. The signals that trigger these gene-regulated activities are, for the most part, unknown but are of intense interest because of their role in the pathophysiology of atherosclerosis, thrombosis, immune diseases, and cancer.

Platelet Reactions

Platelet reactions or properties critical to thrombogenesis include the following (Fig. 70-3):

Platelet adhesion, during which platelets adhere to non-endothelialized surfaces
Platelet secretion, when platelets undergo shape change and release their granular contents
Platelet aggregation, during which platelets aggregate to form clumps
Platelet coagulant activity, a property of activated platelets that accelerates coagulation reactions

Platelet adhesion is the initial step in thrombus formation when subendothelial structures are exposed to the circulation following vessel wall injury.[12] Platelets possess several glycoprotein (GP) receptor molecules on their surface that bind with collagen and adhesive proteins located in the vessel. The principal adhesive proteins include von Willebrand factor (vWF), fibronectin, laminin, thrombospondin, and vitronectin. Interaction with these substances depends on shear rate, with platelet adhesion increasing with shear rate. The distribution of blood cells in flowing blood is not uniform; RBCs are concentrated in the middle of the stream and platelets are pushed toward the vessel wall by the much larger, rotating RBCs. This nonhomogeneous distribution is enhanced at increasing shear rates, and this results in more platelet GP receptor-adhesion protein or collagen interaction. Because shear rates are much higher in the arterial circulation, this shear-dependent platelet property partially explains the dominance of platelets in arterial thrombogenesis. The specific platelet GPs involved in these interactions include GPIb:IX, which binds to vWF and GPIa:IIa, which appears to be the principal collagen receptor. Other membrane GPs may also act to facilitate adhesion. vWF and other adhesive proteins are synthesized and secreted by endothelial cells and are bound to subendothelial connective tissue. Adhesion of platelets to polymerizing fibrin, as well as the fibrin network in an established thrombus, is critical to thrombus formation and growth. The GPIIb:IIIa complex is the primary receptor responsible for platelet adhesion to a fibrin network. This receptor ordinarily binds fibrinogen that serves as a molecular bridge between platelets during platelet aggregation. This receptor is not present on the surface of quiescent, circulating platelets and is exposed upon platelet activation.

Platelet secretion, also termed the *platelet release reaction,* is induced by a number of agonists that cause platelet aggregation.[13] The processes of platelet secretion and aggregation are studied separately in vitro systems; however, they most likely occur together in vivo during thrombogenesis and are collectively referred to as "platelet activation." The release reaction is important during thrombogenesis, because many of the substances secreted by platelets cause activation and aggregation of other platelets. Recruitment of other platelets by the products of platelet secretion contributes to the growth of the thrombotic mass. Biochemically, the initial event in platelet activation is binding of an agonist such as thrombin to the extracellular domain of a specific platelet membrane receptor.[14] As in other cells, platelet receptors for agonists and inhibitors are transmem-

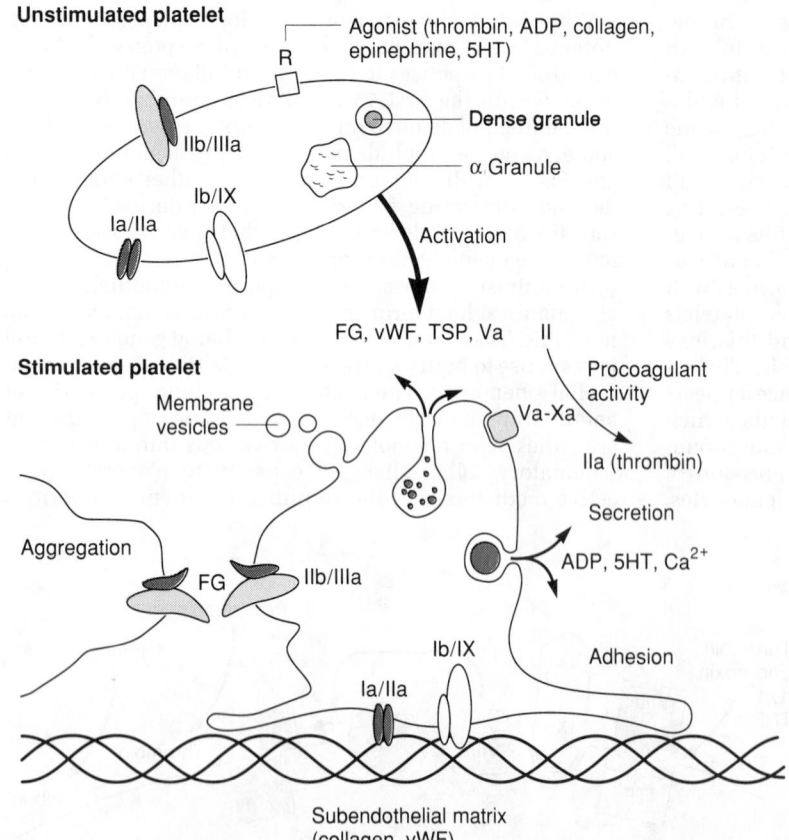

Figure 70-3. The receptor-mediated events of platelet activation, adhesion, secretion, and aggregation. R, receptor; ADP, adenosine diphosphate; 5HT, serotonin; FG, fibrinogen; vWF, von Willebrand factor; TSP, thrombospondin.

brane proteins with cell surface and cytoplasmic components. The signal, initiated by receptor occupancy, is then transmitted by the cytoplasmic domain of the receptor, frequently through guanosine triphosphate-binding regulatory proteins (G proteins), to membrane-bound, signal-generating enzymes such as phospholipase C. Activation of these enzymes generates second messenger molecules. Phospholipase C initiates the phosphoinositide pathway of activation via hydrolysis of the membrane phospholipid phosphatidylinositol 4, 5-bisphosphate (PIP_2). This gives rise to two platelet second messengers—inositol 1, 4, 5-triphosphate (IP_3) and diacylglycerol (DAG). IP_3 induces calcium release from the platelet dense tubular system. A rise in free calcium in the cytosol is a critically important aspect of platelet activation. Diacylglycerol activates protein kinase C, which in turn promotes protein phosphorylation and causes platelet secretion and expression of the fibrinogen receptor (GPIIb:IIIa) on the platelet surface, which leads to platelet aggregation.

Along with thrombin, other agonists that stimulate platelet secretion include collagen, epinephrine, thromboxane A_2, ADP, and PAF. These substances cause platelets to empty their granular contents. Platelet dense granules contain serotonin and ADP, both of which can aggregate platelets. Other platelet granules, termed α-granules, contain multiple proteins that include platelet factor 4 (platelet antiheparin factor), platelet-derived growth factor (PDGF), transforming growth factor β (TGF-β), endothelial cell growth factor (ECGF), β-thromboglobulin, fibrinogen, plasminogen, factor V, vWF, high molecular weight kininogen, fibronectin, thrombospondin, α_2-antiplasmin, α_1-antitrypsin, and α_2-macroglobulin.

Agonists that induce platelet release also activate the platelet prostaglandin synthetic pathway that begins with enzymatic hydrolysis of a membrane phospholipid. Arachidonate, an essential fatty acid, is cleaved from phospholipid largely by catalysis by phospholipase A_2. In the cytosol, arachidonate is enzymatically oxygenated by cyclooxygenase resulting in transient, intermediate, endoperoxides, prostaglandins G_2 and H_2 (PGG_2, PGH_2) which can themselves stimulate platelet secretion and aggregation. PGH_2 is then converted to thromboxane A_2 by thromboxane synthase. Thromboxane A_2 is a potent platelet aggregator and vasoconstrictor.

Platelet aggregation follows or occurs simultaneously with secretion and is induced by virtually the same agonists that cause the release reaction.[15] ADP acts by stimulating the exposure and expression of GPIIb:IIIa, the principal membrane receptor for fibrinogen. The binding of fibrinogen to platelet GPIIb:IIIa is a prerequisite for platelet aggregation, regardless of stimulus, with fibrinogen serving as a molecular bridge between aggregated platelets. The GPIIb:IIIa receptor belongs to the integrin superfamily of adhesive receptors, characterized by their affinity for peptides containing the sequence arginine–glycine–aspartic acid (RGD). The GPIIb:IIIa receptor can recognize and bind the RGD sequence located on the Aα chain, as well as a region in the carboxy terminus of the gamma chain of fibrinogen. The bridging reaction is calcium dependent and may involve the platelet α-granule proteins that contain the RGD sequence including fibronectin, thrombospondin, vitronectin, and vWF.

Thromboxane A_2 stimulates platelet aggregation by triggering release of dense granule ADP that, in turn, causes exposure of the GPIIa:IIIb receptor. Collagen brings about platelet aggregation by activating the prostaglandin metabolic pathway, resulting in thromboxane A_2 production, and by inducing ADP secretion by a mechanism independent of platelet prostaglandin synthesis. In addition to activating phospholipase C, thrombin causes platelet aggregation by directly inducing secretion of ADP and by stimulating thromboxane A_2 production. PAF, synthesized and released from leukocytes and macrophages, causes platelet aggregation by stimulating platelet ADP and serotonin secretion. Thrombogenesis accompanying inflammatory processes may be stimulated by PAF.

The above pathways of platelet activation (secretion and aggregation) are mutually reinforcing and synergistic. They probably all act through a final common pathway, involving intracellular mobilization of calcium from the platelet-dense tubular system in the cytosol and binding of calcium to calmodulin, resulting in activation of protein kinases that trigger other reactions leading to aggregation. Reuptake of calcium into the dense tubular system is cAMP dependent; an increase in cAMP reduces calcium mobilization from all agonists. Drugs that increase levels of cAMP in platelets inhibit platelet release, platelet secretion, and aggregation.

The enzymatic reactions of the coagulation cascade proceed much more efficiently in the presence of platelets. The ability of platelets to enhance coagulation reactions is termed *platelet coagulant activity* and is an important contributing factor during thrombogenesis.[16] Platelet coagulant activity is greatest after activation of platelets by secretion and aggregation stimuli and is thought to be manifest by rearrangement of the platelet lipoprotein surface that accompanies platelet shape change during activation. The interaction of activated factor IX and factor VIII and the interaction of activated factor X and factor V and prothrombin occur on the platelet surface; the rates of these coagulation reactions greatly increase in the presence of platelets. The vitamin K-dependent coagulation factors II, VII, IX, and X bind to the platelet membrane through calcium bridging. The binding of activated factor X (Xa) to Va on the platelet membrane is an important mechanism in promoting coagulation reactions. Va most likely comes from the platelet α granules during secretion. Xa is a pivotal enzyme in the coagulation cascade and, when bound to platelet Va, its efficiency in thrombin generation is dramatically increased. In addition, Xa bound to activated platelets is protected from inactivation by the heparin-antithrombin III complex. All of these properties promote thrombin generation and fibrin formation at sites of platelet thrombogenesis.

Coagulation Reactions

The mechanisms of blood coagulation during hemostasis were reviewed in Chapter 4. Blood coagulation from activation of the intrinsic and extrinsic pathways also occurs during thrombogenesis. Activation of the intrinsic pathway is initiated by the conversion of factor XII to the enzymatic factor XIIa when blood comes into contact with a nonendothelialized vascular surface after vessel wall damage. Factor XII is also activated when blood contacts a prosthetic device, which may be made from a variety of polymers, metals, and other artificial materials, known as biomaterials. The extrinsic pathway is initiated when factor VII, activated by tissue thromboplastin, is expressed by damaged endothelial cells or is released into the bloodstream during extensive tissue damage, as may occur during major surgery or generalized trauma.

PROTECTIVE MECHANISMS: CIRCULATING INHIBITORY PROTEINS AND THE FIBRINOLYTIC SYSTEM
Serine Protease Inhibitors

Activated coagulation factors are serine protease enzymes that are neutralized by circulating protease inhibitors, the most important of which is antithrombin III. This inhibitor scavenges activated blood-clotting enzymes that are free in the microenvironment of a growing clot, thereby limiting its size. Antithrombin III neutralizes thrombin, factor Xa, and factor IXa and is a relatively weak inhibitor of factors XIIa and XIa.[17] The protease inhibitor neutralizes these enzymes by forming a 1:1 stoichiometric complex between the two proteins. Reduction of antithrombin III to less than 50% of normal values predisposes to venous thrombosis. Complex formation occurs at a relatively slow rate in the absence of heparin. The rate of inhibition of these activated coagulation factors by antithrombin III is dramatically accelerated by heparin and, to a lesser extent, by heparan sulfate on the surface of endothelial cells. The latter is a natural catalyst of the inhibitory effects of antithrombin III and thus contributes to the nonthrombogenic properties of endothelium. Heparin compounds bind to lysyl residues on antithrombin III, change the conformation of the protease inhibitor, and make the binding site for serine proteases more readily available.

Protein C is a vitamin K–dependent protein that is activated by thrombin.[6] Along with other vitamin K–dependent coagulation factors, protein C contains γ-carboxyglutamic acid residues, which are required for its normal function. Protein C is activated by thrombin, and this process is greatly facilitated when thrombin is bound to the endothelial cell surface receptor, thrombomodulin. Activated protein C acts as an anticoagulant by destroying coagulation factors Va and VIIIa, especially when these factors are bound to platelet and endothelial membranes. Activated protein C also limits clot formation by facilitating fibrinolysis. The enhancement of fibrinolysis by activated protein C may be due, in part, to its ability to bind to plasminogen activator inhibitor (PAI-1). Protein S is another vitamin K-dependent plasma protein that is a necessary cofactor for the expression of the anticoagulant activity of activated protein C.

Fibrinolytic System

Fibrinolytic activity occurs in circulating blood when the β-globulin plasminogen is converted to the active proteolytic enzyme plasmin by a number of plasminogen activators synthesized by endothelial cells and other tissues or during systemic thrombolytic therapy.[18] Plasmin, in turn, degrades fibrin by hydrolyzing it into soluble polypeptides, termed *fibrin degradation products*. Free plasmin (as may occur with thrombolytic treatment) also hydrolyses and destroys circulating coagulation factors, including fibrinogen. Plasma-borne fibrinolysis is complemented by cellular fibrinolytic activity derived from proteolytic enzymes released from leukocytes that are attracted to thrombus by chemotactic factors released from platelets.

The interactions between components of the fibrinolytic system take place primarily within the environment of a blood clot. During fibrin formation, both plasminogen and tPA, derived from adjacent endothelium, bind specifically to fibrin. tPA converts the clot-bound plasminogen to plasmin. Circulating, native Glu-plasminogen is cleaved to Lys-plasminogen by plasmin, and Lys-plasminogen has greater affinity for fibrin. Fibrin-bound plasmin is partially protected from inhibition by α_2-antiplasmin, the main circulating inhibitor of plasmin. When fibrinolysis occurs, plasmin is released into the blood, where it is rapidly neutralized by α_2-antiplasmin. Excess plasmin is inactivated by α_2-macroglobulin. If both of these inhibitors are overwhelmed, as may occur during the course of thrombolytic therapy, degradation of plasma coagulation factors and fibrinogen occurs.

Endothelium plays an important role in modulating physiologic fibrinolysis. In addition to producing tPA, endothelial cells specifically bind this protein along with Glu-plasminogen, and Lys-plasminogen. Glu-plasminogen is converted to Lys-plasminogen on endothelial cell surfaces and this enhances fibrinolysis because Lys-plasminogen more readily binds to fibrin and is more easily activated to plasmin by both tPA and urokinase. Endothelial cells also oppose fibrinolysis by synthesizing PAI-1. Endothelial cells exposed to thrombin are stimulated to synthesize both PAI-1 and tissue plasminogen activator. Of these two effects, the increase in PAI-1 predominates leading to down-regulation of fibrinolytic activity.

Hypercoagulable Syndromes

Prothrombotic or hypercoagulable states occur when deficiencies of serine proteases or natural anticoagulants exist, when imbalances occur in the fibrinolytic system, when substances are present that accelerate coagulation or platelet reactions, and when diffuse endothelial dysfunction exists.[19] Hypercoagulable states can be classified into two broad categories—hereditary and acquired. The hereditary or congenital coagulation abnormalities, of which antithrombin III and protein C and S deficiencies are examples, are often referred to as inherited thrombophilic disorders. The biochemical abnormalities are generally fixed and persistent, and yet the clinical thrombotic events are episodic. Acquired hypercoagulable states, such as the antiphospholipid syndrome and heparin-associated thrombocytopenia, often accompany another illness. In addition, there are a group of less well-defined acquired hypercoagulable states where multiple complex hemostatic aberrations accompany diverse clinical conditions; examples include malignancy, pregnancy, and the postoperative state. Acquired hypercoagulable states are far more common than congenital thrombophilias.

Inherited thrombophilic disorders are frequently characterized by venous thrombosis, especially in unusual sites, whereas acquired hypercoagulable states may present with venous or arterial thrombosis. Suspicion of an underlying congenital hypercoagulable disorder should be aroused by any of the following characteristics: unexplained venous thrombosis in a person younger than 45 years; recurrent venous thromboembolism; thrombosis of mesenteric, hepatic, portal, renal, or cerebral veins or the inferior vena cava; diffuse cutaneous microvascular thrombosis; and a positive family history of thrombosis.

Arterial thrombosis is a much less common manifestation of hypercoagulable syndromes, and when it does occur, it usually is in patients older than 50 years who have risk factors. In contrast to venous thrombi, which are caused primarily by sluggish blood flow in the presence of hypercoagulable disorders, arterial thrombi result from elevated shear stress at sites of vessel wall injury and are composed predominantly of platelets. Platelet function abnormalities and vessel wall disorders characterized by endothelial dysfunction are the hallmarks of disorders associated with a propensity to arterial thrombosis. Abnormalities of platelets are associated with myeloproliferative disorders and vessel wall abnormalities include homocystinuria and inflammatory vasculopathies. Heparin-induced thrombocytopenia and the antiphospholipid antibody syndrome are examples of hypercoagulable states that are associated with both platelet and vessel wall abnormalities. Thrombin is the most potent physiologic stimulus for platelet aggregation and secretion, and classic hereditary hypercoagulable syndromes that generate thrombin are being increasingly recognized as causing arterial thrombosis as well as venous thrombosis. In addition, arterial thromboembolism is sometimes associated with venous thrombosis and may develop from paradoxical embolism across a patent foramen ovale. In one study, 40% of patients under the age of 55 presenting with ischemic stroke had a patent foramen ovale by microbubble echocardiography compared with 10% of age-matched controls without stroke.[20] This is an increasingly recognized entity and should be considered in patients presenting with "cryptogenic" arterial emboli because clinically occult deep venous thrombosis is common, and paradoxical embolism across a patent foramen ovale can occur in the absence of pulmonary embolism and high pulmonary arterial pressures when there is reversal of the normal interatrial pressure gradient that can occur spontaneously during ventricular systole or from coughing or valsalva maneuver.

Congenital Hypercoagulable States

Antithrombin III Deficiency

Congenital antithrombin III deficiency is inherited as an autosomal dominant trait with equal expression in males and females.[21] The estimated prevalence in the general population is 1 in 2000 to 5000 individuals. Antithrombin III deficiency is found in about 3% of patients presenting with deep venous thrombosis. Heterozygous patients have antithrombin III levels between 30% and 70% of normal; homozygous antithrombin III deficiency is lethal in utero. The major clinical features of antithrombin III deficiency include young age at onset of clinical thrombosis, idiopathic venous thrombosis with no identifiable clinical predisposing conditions such as prolonged immobility, family history of venous thromboembolism, recurrent venous thromboembolism, thrombosis at an unusual site, thrombosis during pregnancy, and thrombosis resistant to heparin therapy. Thrombosis of superficial or deep veins of the leg occurs in over 90% of patients with thromboembolic episodes, and pulmonary emboli are reported in about half of these. Clinical manifestations are somewhat age dependent, with the risk of thrombosis increasing dramatically after age 15 years. The overall prevalence of venous thromboembolism proved by objective tests is about 20% among adult heterozygotes. It has been estimated that by the age of 55 years, venous thrombosis develops in up to 85% of carriers. Although about 50% of episodes of deep venous thrombosis occur without clinically obvious provocation, the remainder are precipitated by factors that may cause thrombosis in nondeficient patients, particularly trauma, surgery, pregnancy, use of oral contraceptives, and infection. Treatment usually entails long-term warfarin therapy.

Two major types of antithrombin III deficiency have been described, one caused by decreased synthesis and the other by synthesis of a defective molecule.[22] The most common abnormality is due to the former problem that stems from various gene mutations. Antigenic and functional antithrombin III levels are reduced in these individuals. Less frequently, functional deficiencies associated with specific molecular abnormalities occur and are diagnosed by reduced antithrombin III biologic activity in functional assays.

Protein C Deficiency

Like antithrombin III deficiency, protein C deficiency is inherited as an autosomal dominant trait with heterozygotes suffering recurrent venous thromboembolism.[23] Protein C deficiency, however, is different in two key ways— the variable expression of thrombosis in carriers and the existence of a homozygous state. Homozygous protein C deficiency causes neonatal purpura fulminans that is extremely difficult to treat and almost always fatal. As with antithrombin III, a moderate reduction to about half of

normal levels can cause devastating thrombotic complications among heterozygotes. The clinical manifestations (young age at onset, venous thrombosis at unusual sites) are similar to those of antithrombin III deficiency. The incidence of venous thromboembolism is 60% to 80% among protein C deficiency kindreds.[24] Although the prevalence of this disorder is unknown, protein C levels below 50% have been found in 0.3% of blood donors. In patients presenting with deep venous thrombosis, protein C deficiency may be more common than antithrombin III deficiency.

Warfarin-induced skin necrosis has occurred in some patients with protein C or protein S deficiency.[25] In this disorder, necrosis and skin infarction appear on the trunk, breasts, extremities, or tip of the penis within a few days of initiating warfarin therapy. The mechanism is probably due to marked reductions in protein C levels from warfarin. Treatment includes immediate heparin, plasma or protein C infusions, and discontinuance of warfarin. Because of the possibility of warfarin-induced skin necrosis in individuals with unrecognized protein C deficiency, heparin should always be administered with warfarin until the prothrombin time is in therapeutic range.

Resistance to Activated Protein C

The most common inherited hypercoagulable condition is activated protein C (APC) resistance.[26] This abnormality is found in 20% to 50% of patients presenting with deep venous thrombosis. In contrast, deficiencies in antithrombin III, protein C, and protein S together account for only 5% to 10% of cases of deep venous thrombosis. APC resistance does not appear to be a major risk factor for arterial thrombosis. The most common cause of APC resistance is a point mutation at nucleotide position 1,691 in the factor V gene that results in replacement of arginine in residue 506 with glutamine (an Arg→Glu mutation).[27] This change in a single amino acid makes the mutant factor V in its activated form resistant to proteolysis by APC. In addition, factor V coagulant activity is not affected by this mutation and thrombosis is favored. APC resistance is an autosomal dominant trait and may be associated with other inherited hypercoagulable conditions, such as protein C and protein S deficiencies. The risk of thrombotic events is higher in such individuals than in patients with single defects. Likewise, homozygous persons are more prone to thrombosis than heterozygotes. The factor V gene mutation is surprisingly common and has been found in 3% to 7% of large populations. In addition to accounting for a large number of cases of so-called spontaneous venous thrombosis, it probably contributes to postoperative venous thrombosis in large numbers of patients. An example of the additive effects of circumstantial and genetic risk factors in stimulating thrombosis are found in pregnancy. It has been estimated that 60% of women who have deep venous thrombosis during pregnancy have APC resistance. Treatment of patients with APC resistance involves anticoagulant therapy. Unlike protein C and antithrombin III deficiencies that usually necessitate indefinite oral anticoagulant treatment, however, APC resistance may only require treatment for as long as an individual is exposed to high-risk situations, such as prolonged immobility or the perioperative state.

Protein S Deficiency

Protein S, the vitamin K-dependent cofactor of activated protein C, is also associated with thromboembolic disease when deficiency states exist.[6] The clinical manifestations of protein S deficiency are similar to those of deficiency of antithrombin III and protein C. In addition to deep venous thrombosis and pulmonary embolism, cerebral venous thrombosis, mesenteric venous thrombosis, portal vein thrombosis, purpura fulminans, subclavian vein thrombosis and arterial thrombosis have been reported in congenital deficiency of protein S.

About 60% of protein S circulates in an inactive form bound to C4b-binding protein. The remaining 40% is free and is the active form. Increased plasma levels of C4b-binding protein decrease the levels of free protein S and can influence thrombotic events. Since C4b-binding protein is an acute phase reactant that increases during inflammatory states and the postoperative period, relative decreases in free protein S may result, predisposing to thrombotic complications. Levels of total protein S in deficient heterozygotes range from 30%–65% and levels of free protein S range from 15%–50% of normal. Those with free protein S levels of less than 5% of normal are considered homozygous. Patients with protein C and S deficiencies who have thromboembolic episodes are best treated with life-long warfarin therapy.

Congenital Fibrinolytic Disorders

Impaired fibrin digestion due to abnormalities in the fibrinolytic system can lead to thrombotic complications. Familial deficiencies and functional abnormalities in plasminogen, defective release of plasminogen activator from vessel walls stemming from defective endothelial synthesis of plasminogen activator, and the presence of excess circulating inhibitors to plasminogen activators have been described. These disorders are rare and the prevalence is unknown. As with the other congenital disorders, fibrinolytic abnormalities usually manifest clinically as venous thromboembolism, and treatment for recurrent thrombosis involves life-long anticoagulant therapy.

Dysfibrinogenemia

Impaired fibrinolysis may be due to the formation of fibrin that is pathologically resistant to plasmin. Congenital functional abnormalities of fibrinogen exist, causing a hypercoagulable state complicated by thrombosis, and the process is transmitted in an autosomal dominant fashion. Patients with dysfibrinogenemia and thrombosis respond to anticoagulant therapy.

Homocystinuria (Cystathionine Synthase Deficiency)

The development of premature atherosclerosis, as well as arterial and venous thromboembolism, are prominent clinical features of homocystinuria. Homocysteine causes endothelial damage and dysfunction. It down-regulates endothelial thrombomodulin function and may also impair endothelial plasmin generation by inhibiting tissue plasminogen activator from binding to its endothelial cell surface receptor.[28] In patients with homozygous cystathionine synthase deficiency, severe vascular disease may appear in childhood, and most patients have thromboembolic events before the age of 40 years. Patients with heterozygous homocystinuria (estimated to be 1 in 70 of the normal population) may develop premature atherosclerosis. It has been estimated that 20% to 40% of patients presenting with premature peripheral vascular disease or stroke have heterozygous homocystinuria.[29] Pyridoxine treatment reduces the incidence of thromboembolic events in homozygous patients. It is not known whether treatment with pyridoxine or other vitamins that influence homocysteine metabolism influence the course of premature atherosclerosis in heterozygotes.

Lipoprotein(a)

Lipoprotein(a) consists of a low-density lipoprotein (LDL) particle enveloped by a unique apolipoprotein, apolipoprotein(a) [apo(a)], disulfide linked to the apolipoprotein B-100 (apo B-100) moiety of LDL.[30] Apo(a) shows remarkable homology with plasminogen, especially in the tandemly repeated sequences that resemble kringle forms of plasminogen. Because of its homology with plasminogen, it has been reported that lipoprotein(a) may compete for binding with fibrin and endothelial cell surface plasminogen thereby blocking fibrinolysis and creating a thrombogenic microenvironment. Lipoprotein(a) is demonstrable in atherosclerotic plaques where it colocalizes with fibrin. Homocysteine enhances the binding of lipoprotein(a) to fibrin, thus providing a biochemical link between thrombosis, atherogenesis, and homocystinemia.[31] Epidemiologic studies have shown increased levels of lipoprotein(a) in approximately 20% of the population and indicated that these elevations, genetically determined, represent a major risk factor for coronary heart disease, occlusion of saphenous vein bypass grafts, and stroke. It appears to be a special risk factor for premature atherosclerosis.

Acquired Hypercoagulable States

Lupus Anticoagulant and Related Antiphospholipid Antibodies

The lupus anticoagulant is an antibody that prolongs phospholipid-dependent coagulation tests, such as the aPTT, by binding to phospholipid. Although initially described in patients with systemic lupus erythematosus—hence its name—the antibody is more frequently encountered in patients without lupus. The paradoxical nature of the term is further compounded by the fact that patients with lupus anticoagulant appear to have a thrombotic, not hemorrhagic, diathesis. Interest has been directed toward a related antiphospholipid antibody known as anticardiolipin antibody. Evidence indicates that lupus anticoagulant and anticardiolipin antibody define two distinct but related patient populations, each associated with an increased risk of arterial and venous thrombosis.[32] It is clear that the lupus anticoagulant and anticardiolipin antibodies are two separate entities. Many individuals with anticardiolipin antibodies do not have a lupus anticoagulant, and many with the lupus anticoagulant do not have anticardiolipin antibodies. About 1% to 2% of individuals in the general population and higher percentages of patients with autoimmune disorders produce a family of circulating antibodies directed against anionic phospholipids. The true incidence and risk of thrombosis is unknown because there are few prospective, longitudinal studies on patients with these antibodies to determine how many will develop thrombosis. The clinical manifestations are diverse and include venous thromboembolism, stroke, myocardial infarction, postoperative thrombosis of arterial reconstructions, and obstetrical complications due to thrombosis of placental vessels. Antiphospholipid antibody syndrome is one of the most common causes of transient cerebral ischemia and stroke in young individuals.

Various potential mechanisms have been proposed to explain the increased risk of thrombosis, including decreased plasma levels of free protein S, a plasma inhibitor of endothelial activation of protein C, a plasma inhibitor of protein C, a plasma inhibitor of factor Va degradation, increased levels of PAI-1, and inhibition of endothelial cell release or production of prostacyclin. All of these biologic activities of the antibodies have been demonstrated in vitro, but it is not clear which mechanisms are responsible for promoting thrombosis in vivo. Diagnostic tests include various coagulation tests (aPTT, the kaolin clotting time, and the dilute phospholipid test), test for antibodies against cardiolipin, and other assays for antibodies against phospholipids. No single test has been demonstrated to be the best predictor of thrombosis, and because the tests may be transiently positive, a positive test result should be repeated after a period of weeks. In patients with systemic lupus erythematosus, persistently positive assays are predictive of thrombosis. In patients who have experienced arterial or venous thrombosis, long-term oral anticoagulant therapy is usually indicated; however, evidence suggests that warfarin therapy does not protect against recurrent thrombosis. Antiplatelet therapy with aspirin or ticlopidine may also be useful.

Heparin-Induced Thrombocytopenia and Thrombosis

Heparin-induced thrombocytopenia is uncommon and occurs in about 6% of patients receiving heparin.[33] Unlike thrombocytopenia due to other drugs, bleeding seldomly occurs; instead, these patients suffer arterial and venous thromboses. Thrombotic complications occur in less than 1% of patients having a drop in platelet count while on heparin therapy. Neither the dosage nor the source (porcine versus bovine) of heparin is related to the severity of the thrombocytopenia or the severity of thrombotic complications. Thrombocytopenia has been reported with all routes of heparin administration, including intravenous, subcutaneous, and even heparin bonded to indwelling venous catheters. The thrombotic complications are diverse and include venous thromboembolism, stroke, myocardial infarction, and peripheral arterial thromboembolism. The mortality rate from thrombotic complications ranges from 20% to 40%, and the morbidity rate in the form of limb loss is 60% to 75%.[34] Peripheral thrombosis frequently manifests in an artery or vein previously damaged by catheterization or instrumentation. The pathogenesis of the disorder appears related to the development of a heparin-dependent IgG antibody that attaches to platelets via the Fc receptor and triggers platelet secretion and aggregation.[35] In addition, heparin-induced antibody binds to endothelial cells and is associated with the expression of tissue factor on the endothelial cell surface. The combination of a potent stimulus for platelet aggregation and secretion, which also alters the thrombogenicity of endothelium, may be the underlying mechanism for thrombosis in some patients with this disorder.

All patients receiving heparin should be monitored with frequent platelet counts. If severe thrombocytopenia or thrombosis develops, heparin should be discontinued. Alternative methods of anticoagulation are necessary in most patients. Substituting a heparin-like compound can be useful. For example, lomoparan is a combination of heparan sulfate and dermatan sulfate that crossreacts very little with most antiheparin antibodies. Iloprost, a prostacyclin analog, has been used to inhibit platelet activation during short periods of heparin administration such as during cardiopulmonary bypass or during vascular reconstructions. Success has also been reported with the use of ancrod, a rapidly acting defibrinogenating agent. In patients presenting with venous thromboembolism as a complication of heparin therapy, placement of a Greenfield filter, systemic thrombolytic therapy, and warfarin therapy are useful.

Myeloproliferative Disorders

The myeloproliferative disorders are a group of related diseases of marrow stem cells and include polycythemia vera, chronic myelogenous leukemia, myeloid metaplasia, and essential thrombocythemia. Arterial and venous thrombosis occur with these diseases and, paradoxically, bleeding complications are prominent.[36] Along with common sites of arterial and venous thrombosis, patients with myeloproliferative disorders may develop thrombosis at unusual sites, such as the splenic, portal, hepatic, and mesenteric veins. Cerebrovascular ischemia may present as stroke or transient cerebral ischemic attacks, and peripheral gangrene from microvascular thrombosis may occur without loss of pulses. These arterial complications are particularly encountered in polycythemia vera and essential thrombocythemia. In polycythemia vera, elevated whole blood viscosity due to increased red cell mass contributes to the risk of thrombosis. The contribution of thrombocytosis, especially in essential thrombocythemia, is unclear. There is no apparent correlation between the platelet count and the risk of thrombosis, but reduction in the circulating number of platelets can dramatically improve symptoms of cerebrovascular or digital ischemia. A variety of morphologic, functional, and metabolic defects of platelets have been described in the myeloproliferative disorders, and these arise from clonal abnormalities of megakaryocytes. These heterogeneous platelet abnormalities are thought to be important in the pathogenesis of arterial and venous thrombosis in these patients as well as the pronounced tendency to bleed. Treatment of thrombosis in patients with myeloproliferative disorders usually involves phlebotomy and cytoreductive therapy to reduce the red cell mass and number of platelets as well as aspirin therapy.

Malignancy

The overall incidence of thrombosis in patients with malignancy is about 5% to 15% but may be as high as 50% with some tumors, notably pancreatic carcinoma.[37] Thrombosis is not equally common in all types of malignancy. The highest incidence of thrombotic manifestations is found in patients with acute promyelocytic leukemia, myeloproliferative disorders, primary tumors of the brain, mucin-secreting adenocarcinomas of the pancreas (especially the body and tail of the pancreas), gastrointestinal tract, lung, and ovary. The overall incidence of thromboembolic manifestations in malignancy bears some relation to the frequency of tumors of particular types. Thus, although an especially high proportion of patients with cancer of the pancreas develop clinically evident thromboembolic disease, cancer of the pancreas is relatively uncommon in comparison with carcinoma of the lung, which, because of its relatively greater frequency, is the tumor most commonly associated with clinically evident thromboembolic disease. Episodes of thrombosis, particularly migratory superficial thrombophlebitis, may antedate by months the clinical diagnosis of cancer in some patients and may be the first clinical indication of the underlying cancer. In addition to venous thromboembolism, arterial embolism from nonbacterial thrombotic endocarditis may develop.

Multiple coagulation abnormalities predisposing to thrombosis have been described in patients with malignancy. These include thrombocytosis, shortening of the prothrombin time and aPTT, elevation of plasma coagulation factors (increases in fibrinogen and factors V, VIII, IX, and XI) and fibrinogen-fibrin degradation products, shortened platelet and fibrinogen survival, decreased antithrombin III levels, and increased PAI-1 activity. Many of these changes reflect generalized activation of the clotting system, resulting in chronic, partially compensated disseminated intravascular coagulation. The clinical expression of these abnormalities may include bleeding and large-vessel thrombosis in complex cases. In addition to these hemostatic abnormalities, there is evidence for platelet activation by tumor cells, the expression of tissue factor by monocytes and macrophages stimulated by tumor antigens, endothelial cell expression of tissue factor by cytokines produced by tumors, and the production of proco-agulants by tumor cells that activate factor X. Other procoagulants may be released, such as thromboplastic substances contained in the granules of leukemic progran-ulocytes. Cytotoxic chemotherapy can also cause release of thromboplastic substances from tumor cells and precipi-tate thrombotic events. An increased risk of thrombosis has been reported with chemotherapy for leukemias, breast cancer, and prostate cancer. In some cases, it appears that cytotoxic agents themselves may contribute to thrombosis.

Postoperative and Inflammatory States

After major surgery or trauma of any nature, several he-mostatic changes occur that predispose to thrombosis. These include elevations in coagulation factors (fibrinogen and factor VIII), moderate (20% to 30%) depression of anti-thrombin III levels, decreases in free protein S levels (due to increases in C4b-binding protein levels), thrombo-cytosis, increased platelet reactivity or stickiness, and re-lease of tissue thromboplastin into the bloodstream.[38] In addition, defective fibrinolysis may occur 48 to 72 hours postoperatively because of elevations in α_2-macroglobulin and other inhibitory proteins. Evidence suggests that post-operative fibrinolytic shutdown is mediated by plasma fac-tors that stimulate endothelial cell PAI-1 biosynthesis.[39] Increases in blood viscosity are also common and are re-lated to fluid shifts and dehydration. When these changes are combined with immobilization and venous pooling in the lower extremities from anesthetics and narcotics, post-operative venous thromboembolism may result.

Inflammatory disorders such as inflammatory bowel dis-ease, rheumatoid arthritis, and chronic infections are asso-ciated with an increased incidence of thrombosis. High levels of inflammatory mediators such as tumor necrosis factor and interleukin-1 that increase the expression of procoagulant properties of the endothelial surface may be involved. In addition, C4b-binding protein is elevated de-creasing levels of free protein S.

Pregnancy

Although pregnancy is associated with an increased risk of venous thromboembolism, the risk increases several-fold immediately after delivery. Multiple anatomic, physi-ologic, and biochemical changes during pregnancy and the postpartum period predispose the patient to venous throm-boembolism. Venous compression by the gravid uterus and increased intraabdominal pressure along with venous smooth muscle relaxation induced by estrogen and other hormonal effects bring about venous pooling of blood in the lower extremities. Fibrinogen levels increase along with concentrations of factors VII, VIII, IX, X, and XII, while antithrombin III levels and protein S levels are mildly decreased. Depression of fibrinolytic activity fur-ther enhances hypercoagulability.

Oral Contraceptives

An increased risk of mortality from cardiovascular dis-ease and particularly venous thromboembolism is seen in persons who use oral contraceptives. Use of newer, low-dose estrogen combination pills reduces but does not elim-inate this risk. The systemic effects induced by oral contra-ceptives are similar to those seen in pregnancy and include increased levels of clotting factors and decreases in anti-thrombin III levels.

Increased Levels of Fibrinogen and Factor VII

Multiple epidemiologic studies have shown an associa-tion between elevated levels of plasma fibrinogen and in-creased levels of factor VII coagulant activity and the risk of ischemic heart disease, stroke, and peripheral vascular disease.[40] A recent metaanalysis suggests that fibrinogen is an independent cardiovascular risk factor. Epidemiologic studies show that smoking is a major determinant of the fibrinogen level, and that dietary fat intake is related to factor VII coagulant activity. Thus two major cardiovascu-lar risks influence coagulation activity and the risk of thrombosis. Fibrinogen is a major determinant of blood viscosity, influences platelet aggregation ability, and inter-acts with the endothelial cell surface to generate fibrin in inflammatory states. The factor VII–tissue factor pathway is a crucial physiologic variable controlling the basal acti-vation state of coagulation.

Nephrotic Syndrome

Patients with the nephrotic syndrome have lowered lev-els of antithrombin III caused by loss in the urine and decreased levels of free protein S due to high circulating levels of C4b-binding protein. In addition, many of these patients have systemic lupus erythematosus and antiphos-pholipid antibodies.

PROTECTIVE MECHANISM: BLOOD FLOW AND THROMBOSIS

Normal, nondisturbed and laminar blood flow discour-ages thrombogenesis. Laminar flow is the type of motion in which the fluid moves as a series of individual layers, with each stratum moving at a different velocity from its neighboring layers (Fig. 70-4A). Laminar blood flow is due to the physical properties of blood. Because blood is vis-cous, its flow near solid boundaries is shear flow. The term *shear* refers to the sliding motion between two contiguous planes. Because of frictional resistance at the blood–vessel wall interface, flow velocity is greater in midstream than at the lumen surface.

Movement of cells and molecules in blood occur by two principal transport processes—convection and diffusion. Convection is transport that occurs because cells and mole-cules move with the fluid surrounding them. Diffusion, in contrast, is transport that occurs when molecules or particles move relative to the motion of the surrounding medium. When convection and diffusion operate simulta-neously, transport is said to occur by convective diffusion. In blood, all cells, particles, and molecules are transported by convective diffusion. Convective diffusion in vessels relies on a combination of convection to effect transport over relatively long distances and diffusion to effect trans-port over relatively short, radial distances.

When blood flow does not follow unidirectional, pre-dictable, and stable linear paths, it becomes nonlaminar and is said to be disturbed. In arteries, disturbed blood flow occurs at vessel orifices, branches, bifurcations, stenoses, irregularities in the vessel wall, and sudden expansions in the lumen radius, as would occur with an aneurysm (see Fig. 70-4B and C). Thrombus formation occurs at these sites in part because of the complex flow patterns that are present. These patterns include areas of flow separation (a portion of the fluid volume moves separately from the main flow), vortices, and zones of recirculation. Thrombo-genesis is favored under these conditions of flow, because activated platelets and coagulation factors have prolonged residence times at one site, platelets collide with each other and other cells and undergo secretion and aggrega-tion, and there is a lack of dilution and clearing of these elements by normal blood-containing inhibitors. In addi-tion, platelets and platelet aggregates are transported to-ward the wall by convective diffusion, especially under conditions of high shear. Diffusion of platelets toward the wall is enhanced at high shear rates by the paddling effect

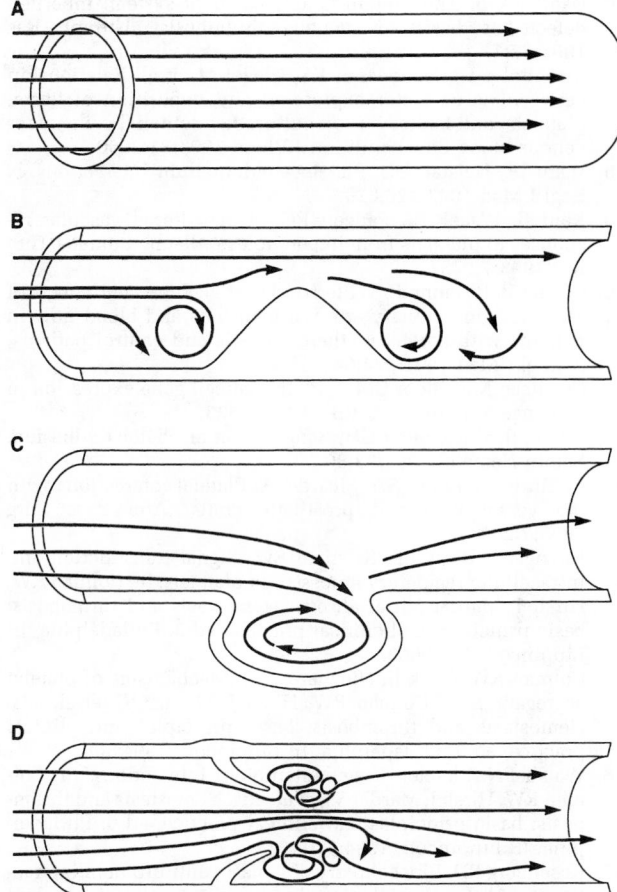

Figure 70-4. (*A*) Nondisturbed laminar blood flow. (*B*) Blood flow at a site of irregularity or stenosis. There are vortices (zones of recirculation) on both sides of the stenosis. In addition, the shear rate is highest at the maximum point of stenosis. (*C*) Vortices occurring in an area of lumen expansion. Arterial pathology causing such areas would include an aneurysm and the crater of an ulcerated atherosclerotic plaque. (*D*) Zone of recirculation formed within a venous valve sinus.

of RBCs that transport platelets radially. In the presence of localized endothelial dysfunction, absence of endothelium, or presence of a reactive surface, such as a polymer, metal, or layer of thrombus, disturbed flow in areas of high shear favor platelet thrombogenesis.

Extreme levels of shear stress exist in close proximity at the most prominent portion of an atherosclerotic plaque that produces a hemodynamically significant narrowing of the lumen. In vessels with intimal injury, platelet deposition increases significantly with increasing stenosis indicating a shear rate-induced cell activation.[41] Further studies have shown that platelet deposition is greatest at the apex of the stenosis and not the flow recirculation zone distal to the apex.

In veins, blood flow is much slower and shear rates are lower. At lower shear rates (below 200 s[1]), blood becomes more viscous because of attractive forces between RBCs in the presence of fibrinogen. Because of these rheologic properties, blood in essence thickens as flow rates are reduced. Sluggish blood flow in veins favors thrombosis primarily because of the prolonged residence time of activated coagulation factors, which allow reactions to proceed to fibrin formation. These reactions are accelerated if there are deficiencies in serine protease

inhibitors, defective fibrinolytic activity, or excess activation of coagulation factors. Disturbed, nonlaminar flow may promote these effects at specific sites. Studies of flow through venous valves have shown that the fluid in the center stream is accelerated, whereas vortices and areas of flow separation form in the pockets (see Fig. 70-4*D*). This area becomes isolated from the already sluggish venous circulation and has been identified as the site of nascent venous thrombi. Because of the lower shear rates in the venous circulation, convective diffusion forces on platelets are not prominent, and platelet thrombogenesis at the vessel wall is not a characteristic feature of venous thrombi.

THERAPEUTIC IMPLICATIONS

Because of its dependency on coagulation reactions resulting in fibrin formation, venous thrombosis is best treated with the anticoagulants heparin and warfarin sodium. The actions of standard heparin have been detailed previously. Low molecular weight heparin is composed of smaller molecular fragments than standard heparin. Because it is more efficient in inactivating Xa than IIa (thrombin), it may effectively impede thrombosis with less hemostatic impairment than standard heparin. Warfarin sodium produces anticoagulation by depressing functional levels of clotting factors II, VII, IV, and X. Heparin and warfarin sodium, given in small doses, prevent the onset of venous thrombosis and can therefore be used successfully as prophylaxis for postoperative deep venous thrombosis in high-risk surgical patients.[42] Agents that are pure inhibitors of platelet function, such as aspirin, are much less successful in prophylaxis for postoperative venous thrombosis. Methods that prevent venous pooling and stasis of blood in the lower extremities are also beneficial in preventing deep venous thrombosis; augmentation of venous emptying by application of intermittent pneumatic compression boots is as effective as anticoagulants. Dextran, another effective agent in reducing venous thromboembolism, acts by increasing blood volume (thereby increasing venous flow), by interfering with fibrin polymerization such that clots are more susceptible to lysis, and by weakly inhibiting platelet function.

In addition to preventing the onset of venous thrombosis, anticoagulants inhibit the growth, propagation, and embolization of established thrombi.[43] In doing so, these agents are the mainstay of therapy in patients with active venous thrombosis who are at risk of pulmonary embolism. Aspirin and other antiplatelet agents are not effective in treating active venous thrombosis.

Intracardiac thromboemboli are also responsive to anticoagulant treatment. These thrombi are fibrin rich and form under the relatively static flow conditions of dilated chambers, obstructed valve orifices, areas of low shear associated with prosthetic valves, ventricular aneurysm formation, and poor pumping action with impaired chamber emptying secondary to cardiac failure or dysrhythmia. Acute treatment with heparin and long-term therapy with warfarin sodium reduces the incidence of symptomatic emboli stemming from intracardiac thrombi.

Antiplatelet agents are effective in preventing thrombogenesis in areas of high shear and disturbed flow in the arterial circulation. This most commonly involves the surface irregularity or stenoses caused by an atherosclerotic plaque. Aspirin is the most widely used antiplatelet agent and has been found to be effective in preventing myocardial infarction in patients with unstable angina and stable coronary disease, stroke and transient ischemic attacks in patients with cerebrovascular arteriosclerosis or after carotid endarterectomy, vein graft thrombosis after coronary artery bypass, and prosthetic bypass thrombosis in patients with femoral popliteal reconstruction.[44] Dipyridamole, often combined with aspirin, has generally been found to be ineffective in rigorous clinical trials. There is no strong indication to use this drug, alone or in combination with aspirin, to prevent arterial thrombosis. Although aspirin retards platelet thrombogenesis on the surface of atherosclerotic plaque, there is no evidence that it prevents plaque formation.

Aspirin acts by acetylating and inhibiting platelet cyclooxygenase, an enzyme that converts arachidonic acid to the endoperoxide intermediates PGG_2 and PGH_2. This inhibits formation of thromboxane A_2. Because platelets do not have the nuclear machinery to replenish cyclooxygenase, platelets exposed to aspirin are permanently affected. Because of differential effects on platelet and endothelial cells (platelets being more sensitive), a great deal of effort has been devoted to finding the lowest possible dose of aspirin that inhibits platelet thromboxane production and allows endothelial prostacyclin production to continue (the production of prostacyclin is dependent on endothelial cyclooxygenase activity, which can also be inhibited by aspirin). These theoretical considerations have not been borne out in data from clinical trials, and it appears that there is no difference in antithrombotic effectiveness between high- and low-dose aspirin. The main advantage to using lower doses of aspirin is that side effects of gastrotoxicity, including gastrointestinal bleeding, are lower.

Ticlopidine is another antiplatelet agent that is effective in preventing platelet-dependent arterial thromboembolism. In patients with cerebrovascular disease, ticlopidine is more effective than aspirin. The principal action of this drug is to prevent fibrinogen binding to the platelet GPIIb:IIIa receptor complex, thereby inhibiting platelet aggregation in response to all agonists.

Fibrinolytic agents include streptokinase, recombinant tPA, and urokinase; all act by accelerating the conversion of plasminogen to plasmin. These substances can be given systemically or regionally by selective infusion through an intraarterial catheter and have been found to be most effective in treating patients with acute myocardial infarction. Clinical trials have demonstrated a reduction in infarct size, preservation of ventricular function, and a reduction in mortality. Clinical benefit has been less consistent in venous thromboembolism, arterial bypass graft thrombosis, and peripheral arterial thrombosis. Because fibrinolytic agents dissolve hemostatic clots along with pathologic clots (thrombi), they are associated with a much higher incidence of bleeding complications than anticoagulants.

REFERENCES

1. Freiman DG. The structure of thrombi. In: Colman RW, Hirsh J, Marder VJ, et al, et al. Hemostasis and thrombosis: basic principles and clinical practice, ed 2. Philadelphia, JB Lippincott, 1987:1123.
2. Woolf N, Davies MJ. Interrelationship between atherosclerosis and thrombosis. In: Fuster V, Verstraete M, eds. Thrombosis in cardiovascular disorders. Philadelphia, WB Saunders, 1992:41.
3. Davies MG, Hagen P. The vascular endothelium: a new horizon. Ann Surg 1993;218:593.
4. Clagett GP, Eberhart RC. Artificial devices in clinical practice. In: Colman RW, Hirsh J, Marder VJ, et al, eds. Hemostasis and thrombosis: basic principles and clinical practice, ed 3. Philadelphia, JB Lippincott, 1994:1486.
5. Lefer AM, Tsao PS, Lefer DJ, et al. Role of endothelial dysfunction in the pathogenesis of reperfusion injury after myocardial ischemia. FASEB J 1991;5:2029.
6. Dahlback B. The protein C anticoagulant system: inherited defects as basis for venous thrombosis. Thromb Res 1995;77:1.
7. Kirchhofer D, Sakariassen KS, Clozel M, et al. Relationship between tissue factor expression and deposition of fibrin, platelets, and leukocytes on cultured endothelial cells under venous blood flow conditions. Blood 1993;81:2050.
8. Ware JA, Heistad DD. Platelet–endothelium interactions. N Engl J Med 1993;328:628.
9. Kaul S, Waack BJ, Padgett RC, et al. Altered vascular responses to platelets from hypercholesterolemic humans. Circ Res 1993;72:737.
10. Golino P, Piscione F, Willerson JT, et al. Divergent effects of serotonin on coronary artery dimensions and blood flow in patients with coronary atherosclerosis and control patients. N Engl J Med 1991;324:641.
11. Gerritsen ME, Bloor CM. Endothelial cell gene expression in response to injury. FASEB J 1993;7:523.
12. Sixma JJ, van Zanten GH, Banga JD, et al. Platelet adhesion. Semin Hematol 1995;32:89.
13. Rubin BG, Santoro SA, Sicard GA. Platelet interactions with the vessel wall and prosthetic grafts. Ann Vasc Surg 1993;7:200.
14. Hawiger J, Brass LF, Salzman EW. Signal transduction and intracellular regulatory processes in platelets. In: Colman RW, Hirsh J, Marder VJ, et al, eds. Hemostasis and thrombosis: basic principles and clinical practice, ed 3. Philadelphia, JB Lippincott, 1994:603.
15. Colman RW, Cook JJ, Niewiarowski. Mechanisms of platelet aggregation. In: Colman RW, Hirsh J, Marder VJ, et al, eds. Hemostasis and thrombosis: basic principles and clinical practice, ed 3. Philadelphia, JB Lippincott, 1994:508.
16. Walsh PN. Platelet–coagulant protein interactions. In: Colman RW, Hirsh J, Marder VJ, et al, eds. Hemostasis and thrombosis: basic principles and clinical practice, ed 3. Philadelphia, JB Lippincott, 1994:629.
17. Rosenberg RD. Biochemistry of heparin antithrombin interactions, and the physiologic role of this natural anticoagulant mechanism. Am J Med 1989;87:25.
18. Bachmann F. The plasminogen–plasmin enzyme system. In: Colman RW, Hirsh J, Marder VJ, et al, eds. Hemostasis and thrombosis: basic principles and clinical practice, ed 3. Philadelphia, JB Lippincott, 1994:1592.
19. Clagett GP. Hematologic factors in arterial thrombotic disease. In: Yao JST, Pearce WH, eds. The ischemic extremity: advances in treatment. Norwalk, CT, Appleton & Lange, 1995:25.
20. Lechat P, Mas JL, Lascault G, et al. Prevalence of patent foramen ovale in patients with stroke. N Engl J Med 1988;318:1148.
21. Hirsh J, Piovella F, Pini M. Congenital antithrombin III deficiency. Am J Med 1989;87:34S.
22. Blajchman MA, Austin RC, Fernandez-Rachubinski F, et al. Molecular basis of inherited human antithrombin deficiency. Blood 1992;80:2159.
23. Esmon CT. The protein C anticoagulant pathway. Arterioscler Thromb 1992;12:135.
24. Allaart CF, Poort SR, Rosendaal FR, et al. Increased risk of venous thrombosis in carriers of hereditary protein C deficiency defect. Lancet 1993;341:134.
25. Comp PC, Elrod JP, Karzenski S. Warfarin-induced skin necrosis. Semin Thromb Hemost 1990;16:293.
26. Svensson PJ, Dahlback B. Resistance to activated protein C as a basis for venous thrombosis. N Engl J Med 1994;330:517.
27. Bertina RM, Koeleman RPC, Koster T, et al. Mutation in blood coagulation factor V associated with resistance to activated protein C. Nature 1994;369:64.
28. Nishinaga M, Ozawa T, Shimada K. Homocysteine, a thrombogenic agent, suppresses anticoagulant heparan sulfate expression in cultured porcine aortic endothelial cells. J Clin Invest 1993;92:1381.
29. Taylor LM Jr., Porter JM. Elevated plasma homocysteine as a risk factor for atherosclerosis. Semin Vasc Surg 1993;6:36.
30. Howard GC, Pizzo SV. Biology of disease. Lipoprotein(a) and its role in atherothrombotic disease. Lab Invest 1993;69:373.
31. Harpel PC, Chang VT, Borth W. Homocysteine and other sulfhydryl compounds enhance the binding of lipoprotein(a) to fibrin: a potential biochemical link between thrombosis, ath-

erogenesis, and sulfhydryl compound metabolism. Proc Natl Acad Sci USA 1992;89:10193.

32. Bick RL, Baker WF. Anticardiolipin antibodies and thrombosis. Hematol/Oncol Clin North Am 1992;6:1287.
33. Schmitt BP, Adelman B. Heparin-associated thrombocytopenia: a critical review and pooled analysis. Am J Med Sci 1993;305:208.
34. Laster J, Cikrit D, Walker N, et al. The heparin-induced thrombocytopenia syndrome: an update. Surgery 1987;102:763.
35. Warkentin TE, Kelton JG. Heparin and platelets. Hematol/Oncol Clin North Am 1990;4:243.
36. Schafer AI. Bleeding and thrombosis in the myeloproliferative disorders. Blood 1984;64:1.
37. Dvorak HF. Abnormalities of hemostasis in malignant disease. In: Colman RW, Hirsh J, Marder VJ, et al, eds. Hemostasis and thrombosis: basic principles and clinical practice, ed 3. Philadelphia, JB Lippincott, 1994:1238.
38. DeLoughery TG, Goodnight SH. The hypercoagulable states: diagnosis and management. Semin Vasc Surg 1993;6:66.
39. Kassis J, Hirsh J, Podor TJ. Evidence that postoperative fibrinolytic shutdown is mediated by plasma factors that stimulate endothelial cell type I plasminogen activator inhibitor biosynthesis. Blood 1992;80:1758.
40. Ernst E. Fibrinogen: an important risk factor for atherothrombotic diseases. Ann Med 1994;26:15.
41. Badimon L, Badimon JJ. Mechanism of arterial thrombosis in non-parallel streamlines: platelet grow at the apex of stenotic severely injured vessel wall. Experimental study in the pig model. J Clin Invest 1989;84:1134.
42. Clagett GP, Anderson FA Jr, Heit J, et al. Prevention of venous thromboembolism. Chest 1995;108:312S.
43. Hyers TM, Hull RD, Weg JG. Antithrombotic therapy for venous thromboembolic disease. Chest 1995;108:335S.
44. Clagett GP, Krupski WC. Antithrombotic therapy in peripheral arterial occlusive disease. Chest 1995;108:431S.

SURGERY: SCIENTIFIC PRINCIPLES AND PRACTICE, Second Edition, edited by Lazar J. Greenfield, Michael W. Mulholland, Keith T. Oldham, Gerald B. Zelenock, and Keith D. Lillemoe. Lippincott–Raven Publishers, Philadelphia, © 1997.

CHAPTER 71

PERIPHERAL ARTERIAL EMBOLISM

LOUIS M. MESSINA

ACUTE ARTERIAL EMBOLISM
Source and Etiology

Between 80% and 90% of acute arterial emboli originate within the heart.[1-4] Of the remaining emboli, the site of origin of half is never identified, and the remainder arise from a variety of uncommon sites (Fig. 71-1). These uncommon sites include arterial aneurysms, most commonly infrarenal aortic and popliteal aneurysms, as well as subclavian aneurysms secondary to thoracic outlet obstruction. Peripheral arterial atherosclerotic plaques can also be the source of macroemboli. Other uncommon sources of arterial emboli include sites of vascular trauma (both iatrogenic and civilian), malignant tumors, and areas of venous thrombosis that cause the so-called paradoxical embolus (ie, venous emboli passing through a patent foramen ovale into the arterial circulation).

Although thrombus can develop on the endothelial surfaces of the heart as a result of a variety of underlying diseases, two thirds arise secondary to atrial fibrillation. In this circumstance, thrombus forms on the endocardial

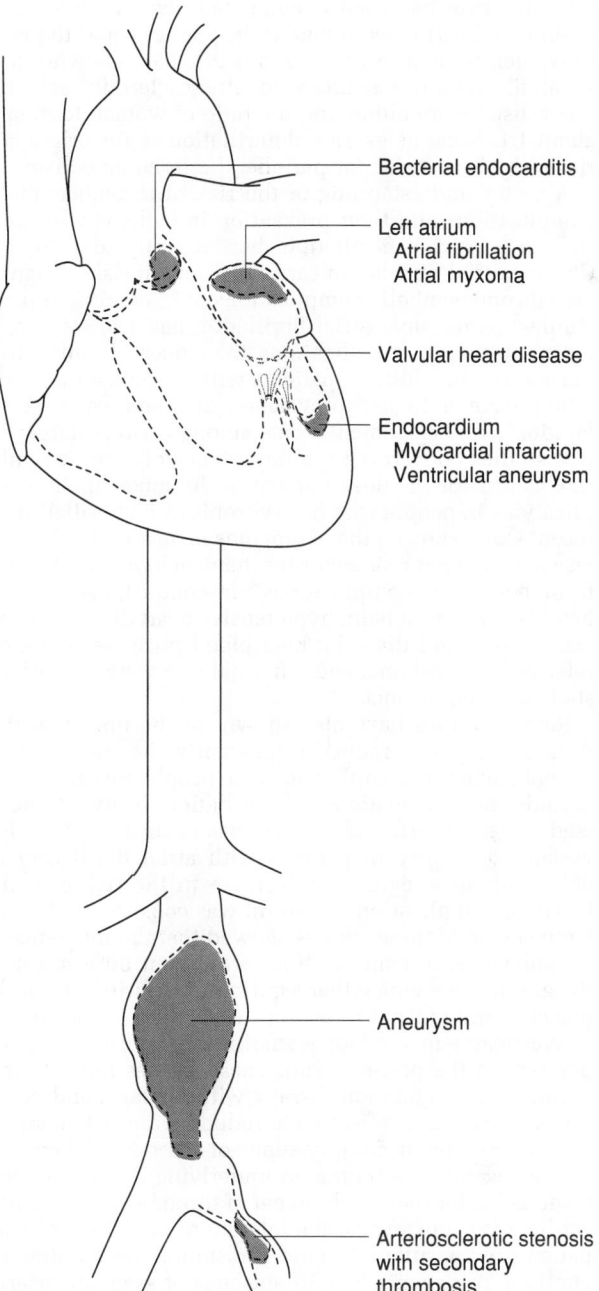

Figure 71-1. Common sources of arterial emboli.

surface of the fibrillating atrium, especially in the large atrial appendage. Historically, rheumatic heart disease was the most common underlying heart disease responsible for atrial fibrillation; more recently, ischemic heart disease has become the most common cause of atrial fibrillation.[1] Other heart diseases that have been implicated in the development of endocardial thrombus formation are acute myocardial infarction, cardiomyopathy, congestive heart failure, and prosthetic heart valves. Rare sources of intracardiac emboli include subacute bacterial endocarditis and cardiac tumors, principally atrial myxomas.

As the relative frequency of rheumatic heart disease has diminished and that of ischemic heart disease has increased as the most common underlying heart disease causing intracardiac thrombus formation, a change in the clinical profile of the patients presenting with acute arterial embolism has been documented. Patients who have rheumatic heart disease tend to be younger, and the ratio of women to men in this group is 2:1. Patients who have atrial fibrillation secondary to atherosclerotic ischemic heart disease are older, and the ratio of women to men is about 1:1. Nonetheless, atrial fibrillation of any origin carries a significant risk for peripheral arterial embolism.

A better understanding of the risk of thromboembolic complications and their prevention in patients with non-rheumatic atrial fibrillation has recently developed.[5] Chronic atrial fibrillation carries an annual risk of significant thromboembolic complications of 3% to 6%. In these studies, paroxysmal atrial fibrillation has a lower risk of thromboembolic complications than does chronic atrial fibrillation. In addition, patients with chronic atrial fibrillation have a higher prevalence of silent cerebral infarction. A disagreement exists among various retrospective studies concerning the importance of cardiovascular risk factors for the development of thromboembolic complications in people who have chronic atrial fibrillation. A recent study showed that a previous myocardial infarction was a significant risk factor for the development of future thromboembolic complications.[6] In contrast, age, gender, heart failure, chest pain, hypertensive heart disease, diabetes, systolic and diastolic high blood pressure, smoking, relative heart volume, and left atrial size were all without statistical significance.

Recent studies have also shown for the first time that drug therapy can reduce significantly the incidence of thromboembolic complications in people suffering from chronic, nonrheumatic atrial fibrillation. In five randomized trials, warfarin reduced the risk of stroke and cardiovascular mortality in patients with atrial fibrillation by 68% without a significant increase in the risk of major bleeding complications.[7] Aspirin was consistently less effective. One of these studies showed that the incidence of thromboembolic complications was about 80% lower in the groups receiving either aspirin or warfarin than in the placebo group (event rates were 1.6% per year in the two active treatment arms of warfarin and aspirin and 8.3% per year in the placebo arm). These studies indicate that chronic anticoagulation therapy with warfarin and possibly with aspirin is effective in reducing the risk of stroke and other systemic complications of acute arterial emboli.

The second most common underlying disease process responsible for the development of thrombus on the endocardium is acute myocardial infarction.[8] In a study of 1277 patients who suffered acute transmural myocardial infarction, 22 patients had 30 episodes of systemic arterial embolism.[9] Postmortem autopsy studies show an even higher, often clinically silent incidence of peripheral arterial embolism after acute myocardial infarction. In most patients, the myocardial infarction is anterolateral in location and accompanied by congestive heart failure. The mortality rate is 55% after the embolism. The risk of emboli after acute myocardial infarction is not indefinite because most emboli occur within 6 weeks of the infarction. Heparin anticoagulation has been shown by some to reduce the clinical incidence of systemic arterial embolism after acute myocardial infarction.

Ventricular aneurysm formation, a complication of acute myocardial infarction, can also be a source of arterial emboli. About half of left ventricular aneurysms are found at the time of surgery to have mural thrombus.[10] Clinically apparent arterial embolism occurs in 5% of patients who develop ventricular aneurysms after acute myocardial infarction. Cardiomyopathies and congestive heart failure are other, less common causes of mural thrombus formation as a source of peripheral arterial emboli.

Various cardiac arrhythmias have been associated with the occurrence of peripheral arterial embolism, particularly the bradycardia–tachycardia arrhythmia, the so-called sick sinus syndrome. A 16% incidence of embolism was found in patients suffering from chronic sinoatrial disorders, whereas only 1.3% of age-matched controls with complete heart block developed peripheral arterial embolism.[11] Patients with idiopathic or alcoholic cardiomyopathy also have a relatively high incidence of arterial embolism.

Arterial aneurysms are an important noncardiac source of peripheral arterial embolism. Thrombus forms along the dilated portion of the artery, and increasing layers of thrombus formation occur as the aneurysm enlarges. Fragments of this laminated thrombus can break loose and obstruct the downstream arterial circulation. The most common arterial aneurysms associated with peripheral arterial embolism are infrarenal abdominal aortic, femoral artery, and popliteal artery aneurysms. Arterial embolism is a common complication of popliteal aneurysms, occurring in about 25% of symptomatic patients.[12] These embolic events are often clinically silent and are detected only after complete obstruction of the outflow arteries of the popliteal artery occurs. Embolism from true femoral artery aneurysms is less frequent, occurring in 5% to 10% of patients. Finally, subclavian artery aneurysms that develop as a consequence of thoracic outlet obstruction or atherosclerosis can give rise to peripheral embolism in up to 33% of patients.

Uncommon cardiac sources of peripheral arterial embolism include bacterial endocarditis, prosthetic heart valves, and cardiac atrial myxomas. In patients suffering from bacterial endocarditis, valvular vegetations fragment and embolize into the arterial circulation, usually obstructing small arteries such as the palmar or plantar arches or the digit arteries. Arterial embolism remains the most common potentially serious complication of bacterial endocarditis. Emboli occur in some 15% to 35% of patients. The vessels of the cerebral circulation are affected most often by acute embolism secondary to bacterial endocarditis.

Prosthetic heart valves can become an important source of arterial emboli. The mitral valve is a more common source of emboli than aortic valves. About 25% of patients who suffer emboli due to prosthetic valves have more than one embolic event. In addition, over 80% of these emboli lodge in the cerebral circulation, and about 10% of these are fatal. Finally, cardiac tumor fragments from an atrial myxoma or an angiosarcoma can also embolize. Because the initial clinical presentation of bacterial endocarditis or atrial myxomas is often an acute arterial embolism, this reinforces the necessity of sending specimens of acute emboli for microscopic analysis and culture after they are removed during surgical embolectomy.

Emboli can also arise from the surface of atherosclerotic plaques (Fig. 71-2). Atherosclerotic plaques give rise to both macroscopic and microscopic emboli. Collectively, they are often referred to as *atheroemboli*. Because the natural history, clinical manifestations, and management of microscopic atheroembolism differ substantially from those of macroemboli composed entirely of thrombus and plaque, they are discussed as a separate entity at the end of this chapter.

Trauma, both civilian and iatrogenic, is an increasingly important cause of peripheral arterial embolism. Gunshot injuries, particularly those to the thorax, can result in the entry of a bullet into the heart or great vessels and then subsequent embolism downstream from the point of arterial entry. This injury is usually identified on the basis of the clinical manifestations of a distal vessel obstruction. After a bullet embolus is identified, it is most important

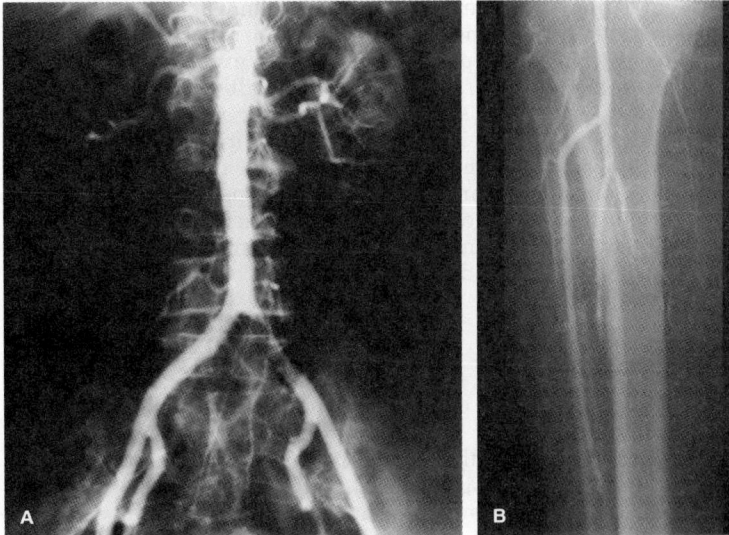

Figure 71-2. (*A*) A thrombus can be seen on the surface of the atherosclerotic plaque in the left common iliac artery. (*B*) Left lower extremity angiogram in the same patient shows occlusion of the anterior tibial, peroneal, and posterior tibial arteries by macroatheroembolus.

to locate the vascular site at which the bullet entered the vascular tree. The site of entry of the bullet is usually a more life-threatening injury than is the ischemia that develops downstream from the level of the bullet obstruction.

Iatrogenic trauma in the form of operative manipulation or as a consequence of diagnostic and therapeutic vascular catheterization is a more important cause of trauma-related arterial embolism. These emboli usually arise from thrombus that forms on the surface of catheters, particularly those that have been indwelling for long periods. These thrombi often obstruct the digital arteries of the hand or foot. In addition to thrombus formation on the catheters, the catheters themselves can fracture and embolize.

Portions of malignant tumors can fragment and embolize into the arterial circulation. Most commonly, these involve primary or metastatic tumors within the lung[13] (Fig. 71-3).

Embolism of lung tumor fragments occurs during surgical manipulation of the tumor or in the immediate postoperative period. These emboli are usually identified in the early postoperative period. Patients suffering from malignant tumor embolism have a good short-term outlook if the emboli are diagnosed and treated promptly.

Finally, arterial embolism can arise from a site of venous thrombosis, the so-called paradoxical embolus. Most commonly, an embolus arises from a site of venous thrombosis and passes through a patent foramen ovale, an atrial septal defect, a patent ductus arteriosus, or a pulmonary arteriovenous fistula. The most common intracardiac defect through which a venous embolus passes to the arterial circulation is a "probe-patent" foramen ovalis. This defect is common but usually results in a left-to-right shunt because left atrial pressure exceeds right atrial pressure. After

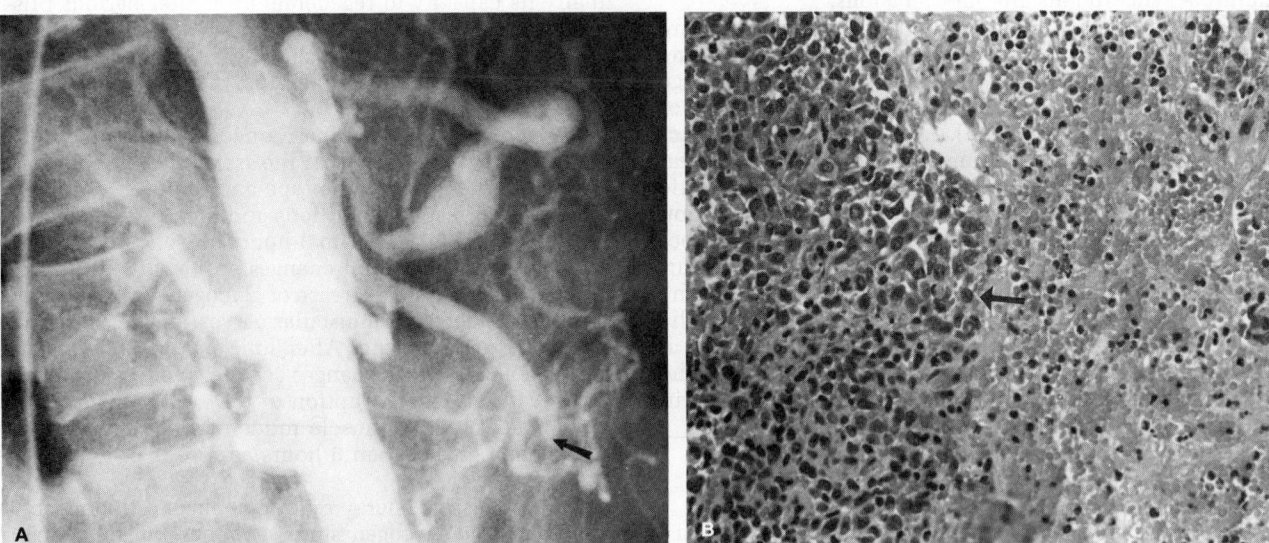

Figure 71-3. (*A*) Arteriogram of a patient who had abdominal pain and acidosis 48 hours after resection of a primary lung tumor. A tumor embolus caused acute occlusion of the superior mesenteric artery at the origins of the middle colic and inferior pancreaticoduodenal arteries. (*B*) Photomicrograph of a tumor embolus, showing poorly differentiated carcinoma (*arrow*) surrounded by organizing thrombus (hematoxylin–eosin, × 40). (*B* courtesy of B. Markey, MD, Department of Pathology, University of Michigan Medical School, Ann Arbor)

a patient suffers pulmonary embolism, pulmonary and right ventricular hypertension can occur. Under these circumstances, right atrial pressure can greatly exceed left atrial pressure. This interarterial pressure gradient facilitates the passage of venous emboli into the arterial circulation. Thus, paradoxical emboli usually occur in patients who have already had clinical manifestations of acute pulmonary embolism or chronic pulmonary hypertension. Paradoxical embolism should be suspected when patients develop acute arterial embolism in the absence of any of the well-defined conditions predisposing to arterial embolism.

Distribution

Arterial emboli do not distribute in the arterial circulation proportionate to the flow rate of a particular artery. Other factors influence their distribution in the arterial tree, including the size and density of the embolus, the arterial diameter, the arterial branch angle, and the shape of arterial bifurcations. A number of factors make it difficult to estimate precisely the distribution of arterial emboli within the arterial circulation, largely because of difficulties in identifying the mechanisms of cerebral infarction. For example, some authors suggest that up to half of arterial emboli go to the cerebral circulation.[14] The frequency of cerebral embolism differs with the type of underlying heart disease. Patients who have rheumatic heart disease complicated by mitral valve disease and atrial fibrillation are at higher risk of developing cerebral embolism and clinical strokes than are patients suffering from the other types of underlying heart disease.

Significant differences exist between autopsy reports of the distribution of arterial emboli and reports based on emboli that are detected clinically. This discrepancy between the incidence and distribution of arterial emboli found at autopsy and those identified on the basis of their clinical manifestations is particularly true for renal emboli. One large study found an autopsy incidence of 1.4% of renal infarction secondary to renal embolism.[15] The diagnosis of acute renal embolism was made in less than 1% of these cases before the patient died. Finally, up to 11% of patients who develop arterial embolism present with multiple synchronous arterial occlusions.[4]

Most arterial emboli lodge at arterial bifurcations, where there is a sudden change in arterial diameter. Excluding carotid embolism, 80% to 90% of all arterial emboli lodge at the bifurcations of large arteries within the upper or lower extremity[4,14] (Fig. 71-4). About 15% of arterial emboli lodge in the upper extremity, 10% within the visceral vessels of the abdomen, and the remainder at the aortic bifurcation or in its more distal branches. The common femoral artery is the most typical site for an arterial embolus to lodge. The next most common site is the aortic bifurcation and the iliac arteries. Arterial emboli lodge in the popliteal arteries in about 10% to 20% of patients. In the upper extremity, three fourths of arterial emboli lodge at the level of the brachial artery. The axillary artery is the site of obstruction in about 20%; the remainder lodge in either the subclavian, radial, or ulnar arteries.

Pathophysiology

The pathophysiology of acute limb ischemia secondary to arterial embolism primarily reflects changes that occur in the skeletal muscle secondary to ischemia and subsequently, after embolectomy, during reperfusion. Although skeletal muscle constitutes 40% of the total body mass, and clinical syndromes involving skeletal muscle ischemia are common, little work has been done until recently to

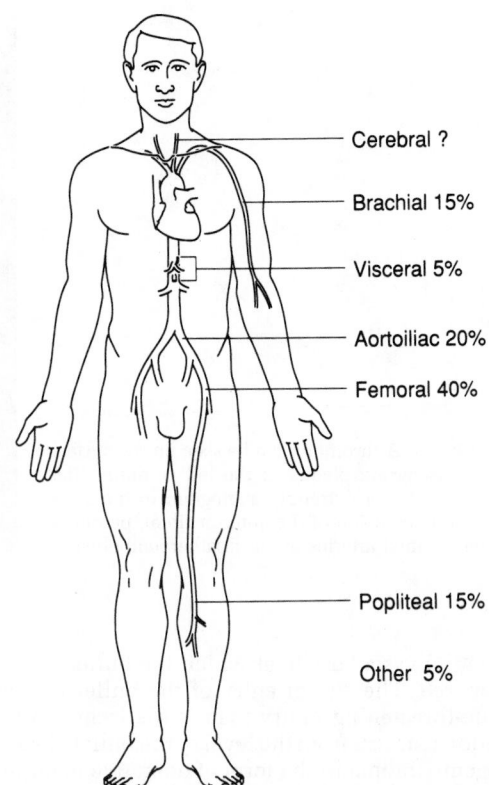

Figure 71-4. Approximate distribution of arterial emboli based on pooled data.

clarify the pathophysiology of skeletal muscle ischemia. Experimental work in both humans and animals shows that skeletal muscle is more tolerant of ischemia than other organs. Skeletal muscle's tolerance to ischemia is due to its low resting metabolic rate, high levels of alternative energy sources such as phosphocreatinine and glycogen, its capacity for anaerobic glycolysis, the tolerance of certain subpopulations of its mitochondria to ischemia, and finally its capacity to regenerate even after periods of severe ischemia.[16] Another important facet of the pathophysiology of skeletal muscle ischemia is the development of the no-reflow phenomenon: that is, the inability to restore perfusion after ischemia.

The extent of skeletal muscle necrosis is a function of the duration and severity of the ischemia, the metabolic rate of the muscle, and the type and duration of reperfusion.[16] Under resting conditions and normothermia, skeletal muscle can tolerate 1 to 3 hours of ischemia. The first detectable ultrastructural changes are those of mitochondrial swelling, and a decrease of glycogen granules within the muscle fibers, intramuscular nerves, and nerve endings of the motor end plate. After long periods of ischemia, irreversible histologic changes occur, including disappearance of the Z-line, disruption of the cell membrane, and vacuolization of the muscle mitochondria. After periods of ischemia greater than 6 hours, autolysis of the muscle fibers occurs.

The low resting energy requirements and the phosphocreatinine and glycogen stores enhance the tolerance of skeletal muscle to ischemia. Adenosine triphosphate (ATP) levels are maintained at a fairly constant level for up to 3 hours of ischemia. During the ischemic period, ATP levels are constantly replenished by the phosphocreatinine-mediated rephosphorylation of adenosine diphosphate. Phosphocreatinine stores then become exhausted at about 3 hours of ischemia. In addition, skeletal muscles that have a high glycogen content can maintain anaerobic glycolysis in the absence of blood flow for up to 6 hours. The linear decline in glycogen levels is paralleled by an increase in lactate levels and thus a decrease in pH. These high lactate levels and the low pH level have a deleterious effect on skeletal muscle membrane integrity. High lactate and low pH levels are associated with a loss of potential across the cellular membranes, resulting in an inability of the cell to maintain proper ionic concentration gradients.[17]

During reperfusion of skeletal muscle that has been ischemic for 4 hours or less, there is a rapid restoration of ATP levels within the first 15 minutes, which are normalized by 3 hours.[18] Phosphocreatinine levels return to normal 30 minutes after reperfusion. Glycogen returns to preischemic levels after 3 hours of reperfusion. In contrast, when ischemia lasts longer than 7 hours, upon reperfusion there is no resynthesis of ATP or phosphocreatinine, and there is no metabolic recovery of the muscle. During this reperfusion period, because there is a loss of cell membrane integrity, extensive edema formation occurs intracellularly and interstitially. In addition, a release of intracellular electrolytes and enzymes into the circulation occurs, particularly potassium, lactic acid, and myoglobin.

The inability to restore microvascular perfusion during reperfusion of ischemic tissue is known as the no-reflow phenomenon.[19] The no-reflow phenomenon has been identified experimentally in the brain, heart, kidney, and adrenal gland. Four mechanisms have been advanced to explain the inability to restore microvascular perfusion during reperfusion: thrombosis of the microcirculation; endothelial cell swelling, resulting in capillary obstruction; extravascular compression of the microcirculation by interstitial edema or hemorrhage; and leukocyte obstruction of capillaries.[16] The precise pathophysiology of the no-reflow phenomenon has not been elucidated; however, obstruction of capillaries by leukocytes is probably a more important mechanism than is capillary thrombosis.

The clinical manifestations of skeletal muscle reperfusion injury are a direct reflection of the cellular and metabolic changes described above. This reperfusion syndrome is characterized clinically by metabolic acidosis, hyperkalemia, myoglobinuria, acute renal tubular necrosis, and muscle edema. The metabolic acidosis, hyperkalemia, and myoglobinuria result from the release of intracellular ions and proteins of skeletal myocytes into the systemic circulation. Both the release of these intracellular constituents and the muscle edema are the consequence of the ischemic injury to the cell membrane. The other clinical manifestations of this reperfusion syndrome are acute tubular necrosis and compartment syndrome. Acute tubular necrosis results from the precipitation of myoglobulin in the renal tubules. Compartment syndromes are caused by compression of nerves, arteries, and veins within the fascial compartments of the lower extremity. Because these compartments have a finite volume, as muscle edema increases, eventual neurovascular compression occurs.

Clinical Manifestations

Sudden occlusion of a peripheral artery by an acute embolus results in unmistakable signs and symptoms of acute limb ischemia, often referred to as the five Ps of acute limb ischemia:

- Pain
- Pallor
- Pulselessness
- Paresthesia
- Paralysis

These signs and symptoms occur in a characteristic distribution, which usually permits accurate localization of the arterial embolus on the basis of physical examination alone.

The pain that occurs as a result of acute arterial occlusion is usually of such sudden onset and severity that the patient can remember precisely its time of onset. The pain is most often described as a severe deep pain, well localized and unremitting. The pain does not dissipate until there is restoration of arterial circulation or irreversible ischemic injury to the sensory nerves. Paresthesias usually appear early after the arterial occlusion and reflect the increased sensitivity of sensory nerves to ischemia. Because small nerve fibers have a relatively increased sensitivity to ischemia, the first loss of sensation is that of light touch.[20] Sensation to deep pain, pressure, and temperature is usually well preserved until late after the acute arterial occlusion. The paresthesia and diminished sensation are not in the cutaneous nerves but rather in a so-called stocking or glovelike distribution. Pallor of the limb appears immediately after the onset of ischemia and is a result of diminished skin blood flow because of the arterial obstruction, as well as reflex vasoconstriction as a secondary response to the tissue ischemia. Although some weakness of the involved extremity can be present early after the onset of ischemia, paralysis of any muscle group is a late feature. In addition to these physical signs, the limb is invariably cool, with the temperature changes becoming greater in the areas more distal to the arterial occlusion. All of these signs and symptoms of acute ischemia progress as the duration of ischemia increases. Eventually, signs of irreversible limb ischemia occur. These signs include loss of sensation or near complete anesthesia of the involved extremity, and rigor mortis when pallor progresses to diffuse mottling of the skin, and the muscles become firm and develop involuntary contraction. The latter findings usually suggest that attempts at restoration of flow in the arterial circulation cannot save the leg and may result in life-threatening complications secondary to reperfusion injury. Complete examination of the patient usually reveals the presence of an acute atrial arrhythmia, most commonly atrial fibrillation. There is no antecedent history of peripheral vascular occlusive disease (ie, no claudication or rest pain). Physical examination of the contralateral limb usually shows normal pulses and no signs of acute or chronic ischemia.

The clinical manifestations of acute arterial embolism are influenced by a number of factors, including the level and duration of arterial occlusion, the adequacy of collateral circulation, the extent of preexisting arterial occlusive disease, the general condition of the patient, the presence or absence of synchronous arterial emboli, and finally the metabolic consequences of the tissue ischemia. Seven percent to 27%[21,22] of patients suffering from acute arterial embolism have no signs or symptoms of arterial occlusion, whereas in others there is an onset of signs and symptoms so gradual that some patients present days and weeks after the embolic occlusion.

When signs and symptoms of acute limb ischemia are present, clinical manifestations usually permit precise localization of the embolus (Fig. 71-5). This is based on the level of absent pulses as well as the level of changes in skin temperature and color. The change in skin temperature is the most sensitive sign of ischemia and is found one skeletal segment below the level of arterial obstruction. Changes in skin color, which initially are usually either a pale yellow or lemon-yellow color, occur one to two skeletal segments below the level of arterial obstruction. Thus, acute occlusion of the distal infrarenal aorta, a so-called saddle embolus, is manifested by the absence of femoral pulses bilaterally, a decrease in skin temperature starting at the

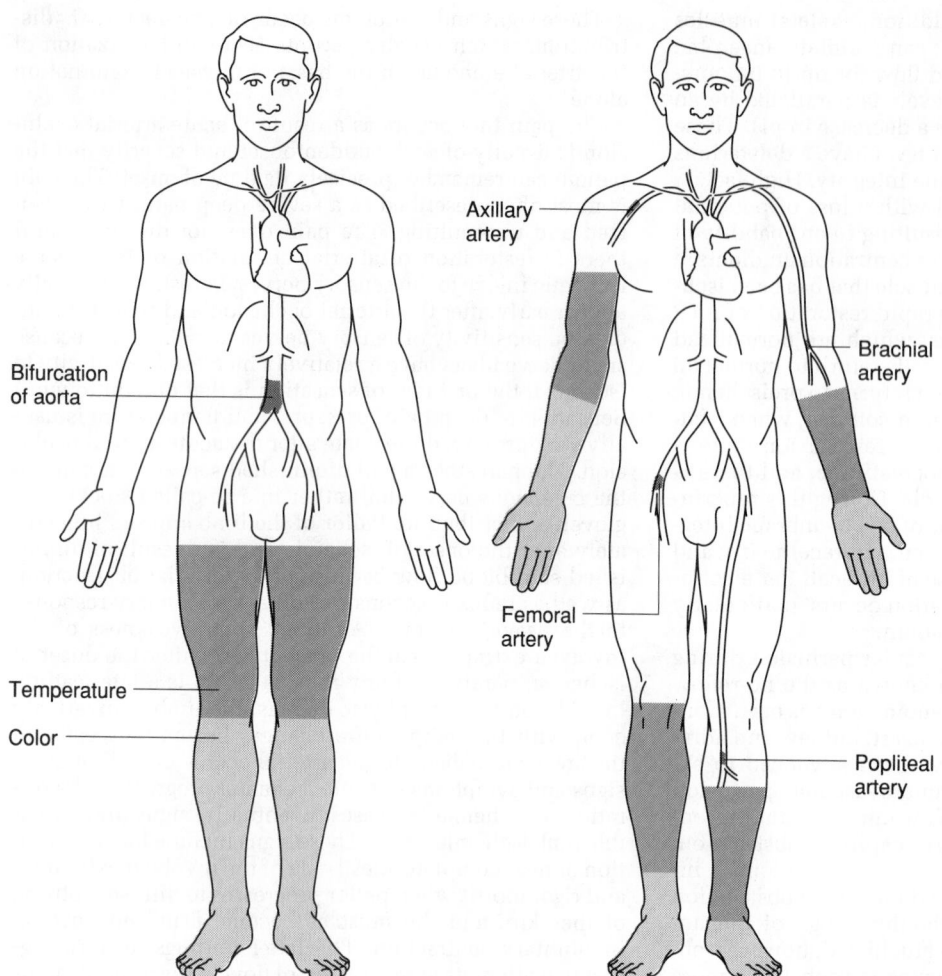

Figure 71-5. The location of an acute arterial embolus can usually be determined precisely based on physical examination of the patient.

level of the upper thigh, and changes in skin color beginning at the level of the knee. Occlusion of the common femoral artery is manifested by a decrease in skin temperature at the level of the lower thigh and a change in skin color starting at the level of the midcalf. Finally, a popliteal occlusion is manifested by a change in skin temperature beginning in the upper calf and a change in skin color beginning at the level of the ankle. The changes in skin temperature and color become more pronounced in areas that are progressively distal to the level of arterial occlusion. A similar relation between the location of the arterial embolus and the changes in skin temperature and color is observed in the upper extremity.

Other factors that influence the clinical manifestations and accurate diagnosis of acute arterial embolism are the general condition of the patient, the presence of synchronous arterial embolism, and the metabolic consequences of the tissue ischemia. Many patients who develop acute arterial embolism have other severe underlying medical illnesses. Common concurrent illnesses are acute congestive heart failure complicated by peripheral edema, acute myocardial infarction, chronic obstructive pulmonary disease, and pneumonia. The general debility of the patient and the presence of concurrent systemic illness can obscure the signs and symptoms of acute limb ischemia, thus preventing rapid diagnosis and treatment. Because up to 20% of patients who develop acute arterial embolism have multiple synchronous emboli, the clinical manifestations of one of the arterial occlusions can obscure the clinical

manifestations of another synchronous lesion. This is particularly true of acute cerebral embolism or acute visceral embolism occurring in patients with acute limb ischemia. There also can be multiple systemic complications because of the metabolic consequences of tissue ischemia. These include the development of systemic acidosis, renal failure, and altered mental status.

There is a subgroup of patients who present for evaluation weeks or months after the embolic event. Most of these patients have evidence of subacute limb ischemia that is not consistent with acute embolic occlusion or chronic occlusive disease. Most of these patients present with a history of a sudden onset of calf claudication or ischemic

Table 71-1. CLINICAL DISTINCTIONS BETWEEN ACUTE ARTERIAL EMBOLISM AND ACUTE ARTERIAL THROMBOSIS

Embolism	Thrombosis
Arrhythmia	No arrhythmia
Sudden onset	Sudden onset
No prior claudication or rest pain	History of claudication or rest pain
Normal contralateral pulses	Contralateral pulses absent
No physical findings of chronic limb ischemia	Physical findings of chronic limb ischemia

limb pain. Less commonly, they are referred for evaluation for presumptive diagnosis of acute deep venous thrombosis. The diagnosis of acute arterial embolism is usually made after arteriography discloses findings consistent with embolic occlusion. Although a significant period of time has elapsed since the onset of their symptoms, these patients can still undergo successful embolectomy in most cases. Thus, recognition of this subacute clinical picture is important in the consideration of any patient who presents with atypical features of either acute or chronic limb ischemia.

Differential Diagnosis

The differential diagnosis of acute limb ischemia includes acute arterial embolism, acute arterial thrombosis, acute aortic dissection, acute venous thrombosis, and arterial spasm. This differential diagnosis is particularly appropriate for consideration in the elderly patient who has generalized atherosclerosis, has no cardiac arrhythmia or acute myocardial infarction, and presents with acute limb ischemia, or in the younger patient who presents with acute limb ischemia and has no cardiac abnormalities.

The most important distinction to make in this differential diagnosis of acute limb ischemia is between acute arterial embolism and acute arterial thrombosis (Table 71-1). The diagnosis of acute arterial embolism is favored when the patient presents with the sudden onset of severe pain, has physical findings consistent with acute ischemia, has no prior history of claudication or rest pain, and when the contralateral extremity has a normal arterial pulse examination. Clinical features that favor the diagnosis of acute arterial thrombosis are a prior history of claudication or rest pain or prior vascular reconstruction, evidence of generalized atherosclerotic occlusive disease, and physical signs of chronic limb ischemia. These signs of chronic ischemia include absence of leg pulses, diminished hair growth, thinning of the skin, thickening of the nails, and the presence of chronic ulceration. In addition, for the same level of arterial occlusion, the signs and symptoms of limb ischemia are usually less than those anticipated in patients with preexisting occlusive disease who suffer an acute thrombosis. Despite these distinguishing features between acute embolic and acute thrombotic occlusion, a correct diagnosis often requires angiography (Figs. 71-6 and 71-7), and occasionally the correct diagnosis can be made only at the time of surgical exploration of the vessel. Although it is frequently assumed that the clinical distinction between these entities is clear-cut, recent studies suggest that the presence of atrial fibrillation is the only reliable clinical sign to distinguish between acute thrombosis and acute embolism.[23]

Management

The diagnosis of acute arterial embolism can be established confidently on the basis of a careful history and physical examination in most patients. Patients who present with the classic signs of acute limb ischemia and have a readily identifiable cardiac abnormality such as atrial fibrillation or acute myocardial infarction need no further evaluation. When the diagnosis is in doubt, particularly if there is a serious question between acute arterial embolism and acute arterial thrombosis, angiography should be used. The first step in the management of patients with acute limb ischemia is immediate heparinization. Heparin prevents proximal and distal propagation of thrombus, maintains patency of collateral vessels, and in addition can have a beneficial effect by reducing the extent of ischemic injury.[24] Although variability is seen among patients, most patients cannot tolerate more than 4 to 6 hours of acute limb ischemia before serious nerve and muscle injury occurs. Thus, prompt diagnosis and expeditious evaluation and treatment are necessary to preserve limb function.

The cornerstone of treatment of acute arterial embolism is thromboembolectomy using arterial embolectomy catheters. Because the perioperative morbidity and mortality for this operation remain high, poor-risk patients such as those who have suffered acute myocardial infarction and who are unstable for transport or who have intractable, severe congestive heart failure should be considered for nonoperative treatment with the use of heparin.[25]

Although the ease of catheter embolectomy makes such an option appear of little value, treatment of arterial embo-

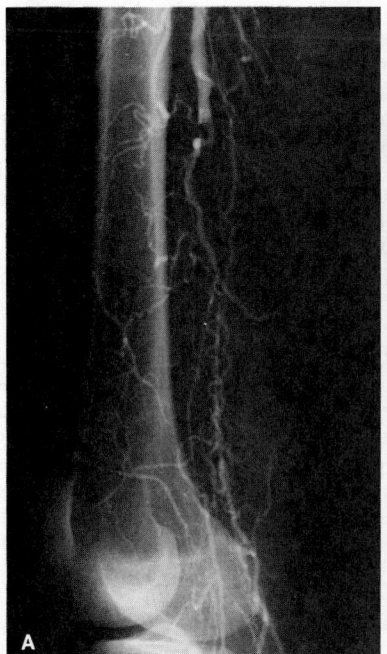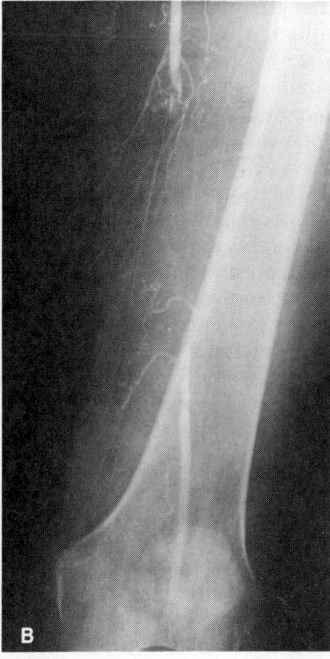

Figure 71-6. (*A*) Angiogram showing a chronic superficial femoral artery thrombosis. Large, preexisting collateral vessels are visible, some of which have a corkscrew appearance. (*B*) Angiogram showing an acute superficial femoral artery embolus. Collaterals are absent, there is a sharp cutoff above the occlusion, and luminal defects show the tail of the obstructing embolus.

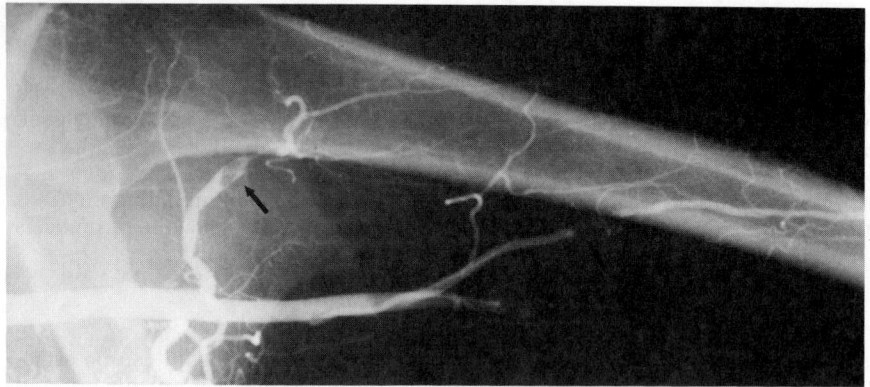

Figure 71-7. Left upper extremity angiogram showing acute embolic occlusion of the brachial artery. The thrombus is obstructing branches of the brachial artery, further reducing arterial inflow to the distal extremity.

lism by catheter embolectomy has the highest morbidity and mortality rate of any vascular operation except for the treatment of ruptured aortic aneurysms. This reflects the seriousness of the underlying illnesses that are found in patients experiencing acute arterial embolism. Some have advocated percutaneous catheter suction embolectomy for high-risk patients. This form of therapy has met with some initial limited success.

The technique of catheter embolectomy is a simple one, but this operation still requires careful planning and execution. After prompt heparinization, all patients should be prepared adequately for the operating room by placing a Foley catheter and arterial and central venous pressure catheters as indicated by the patient's condition. In high-risk patients, cardiac status should be optimized, particularly control of arrhythmias or congestive heart failure. One should always bear in mind the possibility of synchronous embolism, particularly embolism to the viscera, which may not initially be associated with clear signs and symptoms of visceral ischemia.

Catheter embolectomy is undertaken through an artery that provides easy access to the embolus and has a low likelihood of postoperative thrombosis. Most commonly, catheter embolectomy is done through the common femoral artery. Most aortic, iliac artery, superficial femoral artery, and popliteal artery occlusions can be managed successfully through this vessel. After the common femoral artery is exposed and proximal and distal control is obtained, a longitudinal or transverse arteriotomy is made. The transverse arteriotomy is preferred in patients with small arteries so that closure of the arteriotomy does not narrow the vessel. Because acute and chronic complications can occur as a result of injudicious use of embolectomy catheters, catheters should always be passed gently. Catheters are first passed distally until the arterial tree is free of all clot, and then the profunda and proximal aortoiliac vessels are cleared of emboli. When an infrarenal aortic bifurcation occlusion occurs, bilateral femoral artery incisions are used. When severe ischemia of prolonged duration is present, it may be helpful to vent the first 300 to 500 mL of venous outflow into a cell saver.[26] This technique conserves red blood cells but avoids the metabolic consequences of reperfusing a severely ischemic limb. At times, the serum potassium levels are so elevated that they cause cardiac arrest. In addition, the vein parallel to the site of arterial embolectomy should be inspected for venous thrombosis, and venous thrombectomy should be undertaken when clot is found.

When the duration of ischemia has exceeded 4 hours, serious consideration should be given to the use of four-compartment fasciotomy. The consequences of reperfusion of ischemic skeletal muscle are not manifested fully until 12 to 24 hours after operation. Except in patients with congestive heart failure, edema is rarely present at the time of initial operation. Long fasciotomy incisions through relatively small skin incisions can prevent the development of compartment syndrome.

Before leaving the operating room, the patient must have adequate arterial circulation to maintain limb viability and function. This usually can be ascertained adequately by a hand-held continuous-wave Doppler probe evaluation of the pedal pulses. When the viability of the extremity is threatened or when there are no Doppler signals in the distal extremity, intraoperative arteriography or angioscopy should be performed. Retrieving thrombus from the tibial vessels can be difficult from the common femoral artery. Under these circumstances, passing multiple catheters simultaneously permits separate catheterization of the different tibial vessels. Normally, catheters passed from the common femoral artery toward the foot tend to enter the tibial–peroneal trunk. Leaving the catheter that has passed through the peroneal artery to the level of the ankle in place and then passing a second catheter usually allows entry into the posterior tibial artery, and occasionally the anterior tibial artery.

When residual thrombus exists below the popliteal artery, the options are to make a second incision over the popliteal artery or to use intraoperative thrombolytic therapy. Thrombolytic therapy has been shown to be of value in patients with irretrievable clot in small vessels. Angiography is necessary to define the position of the clots so that the catheter can be placed as close to the clot as possible. Thrombolytic therapy is then undertaken for 30 minutes. Concerns remain about the use of fibrinolytic therapy in patients with arterial embolism, because lytic therapy can precipitate the release of more emboli, which can have life-threatening consequences.

Upper extremity emboli are treated in a fashion similar to that for emboli of the lower extremity. An incision can often be made directly over the level of arterial occlusion. This usually involves the axillary or proximal brachial artery. It is frequently necessary to expose the brachial artery bifurcation to selectively catheterize the radial and ulnar arteries. Special care should be taken when thrombectomizing the subclavian or axillary artery so that no clot is dislodged into the common carotid artery or vertebral arteries.

Postoperatively, these patients require careful and close monitoring. They typically have multiple severe underlying medical illnesses and are at risk for complications associated with reperfusion of an ischemic limb (Table 71-2). Thus, the ischemic skeletal muscle can undergo rhabdomyolysis, which results in release of myoglobin into the circulation. Myoglobin can precipitate in the renal tubules,

Table 71-2. MANAGEMENT OF SKELETAL MUSCLE REPERFUSION SYNDROME

Clinical Manifestation	Treatment
Lactic acidosis	Sodium bicarbonate
Hyperkalemia	Insulin and glucose
Myoglobinuria or acute tubular necrosis	Alkalinization of urine to prevent precipitation of myoglobin in renal tubules
Muscle edema or compartment syndrome	Fasciotomy

leading to renal tubular obstruction and acute renal failure. In addition, there is loss of capillary membrane integrity resulting in extensive transudation of fluids and electrolytes. This can lead to a compartment syndrome whereby the increased compartment pressures cause neurovascular compression. In addition, there can be severe hyperkalemia and lactic acidosis. These complications can be minimized by the use of fasciotomy, adequate hydration, the administration of mannitol to maintain a renal diuresis, and intravenous sodium bicarbonate sufficient to alkalinize the urine. Alkalinization of the urine reduces the extent of myoglobin precipitation within the renal tubules. Insulin and glucose given intravenously may be necessary for extreme or sudden elevations in serum potassium levels. Heparin is reinstituted 6 to 12 hours after operation because of a significant incidence of recurrent embolism.

Results

The results of treatment of patients who have suffered acute arterial embolism depend on the location of the embolus, the duration and severity of ischemia, and the seriousness of underlying cardiac and pulmonary disease. In spite of the development of the arterial embolectomy catheter by Fogarty, which has greatly simplified the removal of arterial emboli, and despite significant improvements in the perioperative management of acutely ill patients, there has been only modest improvement in morbidity and mortality rates after arterial embolectomy during the past 40 years.[1] This may reflect the overwhelming impact of the severity of underlying cardiac and pulmonary disease that exists in these patients at the time of the acute arterial embolism. Recent reports of the results of treatment of patients with acute arterial embolism consistently show a high postoperative mortality rate, ranging between 7.5% and 34%.[1,25–30] Amputations are required in about 15% of patients after embolectomy.

The major causes of morbidity after arterial embolectomy are myocardial complications, pulmonary complications including pneumonia and pulmonary embolism, renal failure, and synchronous or recurrent arterial emboli. More than half of the deaths after arterial embolectomy are due to myocardial complications.[27,30] This is particularly true in patients who present with acute myocardial infarction, ventricular aneurysms, or arrhythmias secondary to atherosclerotic heart disease. The second most common cause of death is pulmonary failure due to either pneumonia or pulmonary embolism. In some series, pulmonary embolism is the second most common cause of death.[21] In fact, many instances of pneumonia are thought to be due to underlying pulmonary infarction. This is supported by the study by Darling and associates,[14] which showed that 9 of 76 patients who underwent autopsy study after treatment for arterial embolism had pulmonary embolism; in half of these patients, it was the main cause of death. This significant incidence of pulmonary embolism reflects the

propensity of these patients to develop deep venous thrombosis, which is estimated to occur in 7% to 27% of patients after arterial embolectomy.[21,31]

Other important causes of mortality after arterial embolectomy are renal failure and the cumulative effects of multiple emboli. Acute renal failure is estimated to occur in about 11% of patients after arterial embolectomy.[28] The mortality rate of acute renal failure after arterial embolectomy is about 50%. Finally, an important cause of mortality after arterial embolectomy is the occurrence of synchronous or recurrent arterial embolism. Patients who present with multiple arterial emboli have a substantially increased mortality rate of approximately three times the rate for patients who present with a single embolus to a limb vessel[4,14,32] (Fig. 71-8). This increased mortality rate is often due to the failure to diagnose a visceral embolus in patients presenting with acute limb ischemia.

Complications and limb loss after arterial embolectomy of the upper extremity are lower than those after embolectomy of the lower extremity.[33–36] Mortality rates remain between 10% and 12%, and amputation rates remain at about 7%. In addition, although many of the patients do not undergo amputation, as many as one third have a residual, severe disability.[36] Because of a general impression of reduced mortality and amputation rates in patients with upper extremity arterial embolism, some have advocated nonoperative therapy for many of these patients; nevertheless, Ricotta and associates[35] report a nearly threefold increase in mortality rates in patients treated nonoperatively.

Although the limb salvage rate after arterial embolectomy is usually 85% to 90%, when patients require amputation it most often is at the above-knee level.[27,37] In view of the high level of amputation and the frequent presence of severe underlying cardiac disease, most of these patients never ambulate independently again. Amputation rates after arterial embolectomy and mortality rates are both fre-

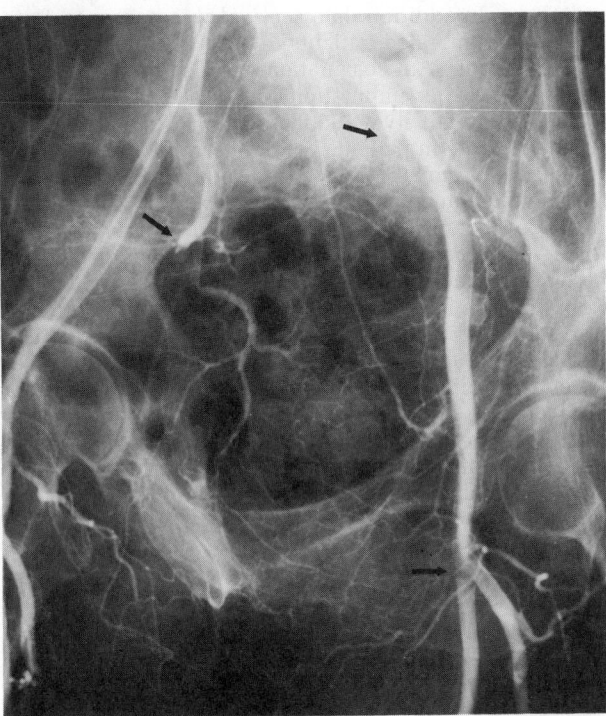

Figure 71-8. Oblique iliac angiogram showing embolic occlusion of the distal right internal iliac artery, the origin of the left internal iliac artery, and the common femoral artery. The patient was also found to have an acute superior mesenteric artery occlusion.

quently related to the level and duration of arterial occlusion, but many studies do not show a constant relation between these variables. Initially, mortality and amputation rates increase with increasing durations of ischemia up to 24 hours after the onset of occlusion. After that, patients presenting more than 24 hours after their initial event often have lower mortality and amputation rates. This so-called harvesting effect is due to the fact that patients presenting days or weeks after the arterial embolism represent a group who survived the early critical period because they have better native collateral circulation as well as less severe underlying cardiac disease. Thus, timeliness of revascularization remains an important goal in the treatment of patients who have acute arterial embolism, but the most important variables in terms of outcome are the duration and severity of the underlying ischemia.

Recurrence of arterial embolism has an important influence on mortality and limb salvage during the immediate postoperative period, as well as on the long-term prognosis of these patients.[1,4,14,38,39] Recurrence rates in patients not receiving anticoagulation vary from 28% to 45.5%.[4,14] The incidence of recurrent embolism appears to be more frequent in patients presenting with acute atrial fibrillation than in patients who present with other cardiac abnormalities, such as acute myocardial infarction.[14] In addition, 31% to 82% of recurrences happen during the initial hospitalization.[38,39] Recurrent embolism has a clear and direct impact on mortality. Mortality rates generally double after each recurrence and are as high as 50% after the third embolic event.

Anticoagulation with heparin or warfarin has been shown convincingly to reduce the rate of recurrent embolism, as well as associated limb loss and mortality. Although heparin reduces the recurrence rate by at least 50% in most studies, significant recurrent embolism occurs even in patients receiving anticoagulation.

Patients receiving anticoagulation after arterial embolectomy had a reduction in early mortality in one series, from 51% in untreated patients to 5% in those receiving anticoagulation.[27] In addition, late survival was improved from 12% in the untreated patients to 43% in those receiving anticoagulation. Anticoagulation has also been shown to reduce the need for amputation from 38% to 0% in patients treated conservatively without operation.[29] In addition, the amputation rate in patients who underwent embolectomy was reduced from 39% to 7% by the addition of anticoagulation in the immediate postoperative period. Most reports show a low complication rate associated with anticoagulation in the immediate postoperative period. On the basis of these results, most patients who develop arterial embolism should receive lifelong anticoagulation. Some recommend short-term therapy in those who develop arterial embolism after an acute myocardial infarction. Patients who suffer acute myocardial infarction usually are at significant risk of developing arterial embolism for only a short period after the acute infarction. In addition, anticoagulation is probably not necessary for people who develop embolism from extracardiac sources, particularly those in whom this source is removed.

Specific complications can occur as a result of the use of balloon catheters in the treatment of arterial embolism. Intimal injury is common after the use of balloon embolectomy catheters. In most patients, this injury is minor and heals spontaneously. Other acute injuries include arterial perforation, vessel wall disruption, the development of arteriovenous fistulas, pseudoaneurysm formation, and the development of arterial stenoses.[40] Diffuse arterial narrowing secondary to intimal hyperplasia has been identified increasingly as a delayed complication of balloon catheter embolectomy[40,41] and occurs with increased frequency

in women. Excessive shear forces are important in the development of a number of these complications. It is recommended that the physician use the smallest catheter that is effective. Important technical points include never passing the catheter against resistance and never withdrawing it under excessive tension. Although complete embolectomy is important, repetitive passing of the catheter increases the incidence of complications.[42]

ATHEROEMBOLISM

Atheroembolism results from the release of cholesterol-rich atheromatous debris from ulcerated atherosclerotic plaques. Most atheroemboli are composed of cholesterol crystals that typically obstruct 200- to 900-μm arterioles. A minority of these emboli are macroemboli that cause large vessel occlusion. Perhaps the most familiar clinical syndrome of atheroembolism is the blue toe syndrome, in which there is obstruction of the digital arteries of the toes. Atheroembolism can have protean clinical manifestations (Fig. 71-9 and Table 71-3), and the diagnosis of atheroembolism is made most frequently at autopsy. Atheroembolism can produce a clinical picture of multisystem organ failure resembling acute polyarteritis nodosa or other acute systemic vasculitides characterized by acute or subacute renal failure, cerebral infarction, retinal embolism, gastrointestinal hemorrhage, pancreatitis, myocardial infarction, and livedo reticularis.

Atheroembolism can occur by at least three mechanisms. It can occur spontaneously, sometimes as a consequence of coughing, tenesmus, or lifting. It can be precipitated by surgical manipulation of the aorta or its major branches.

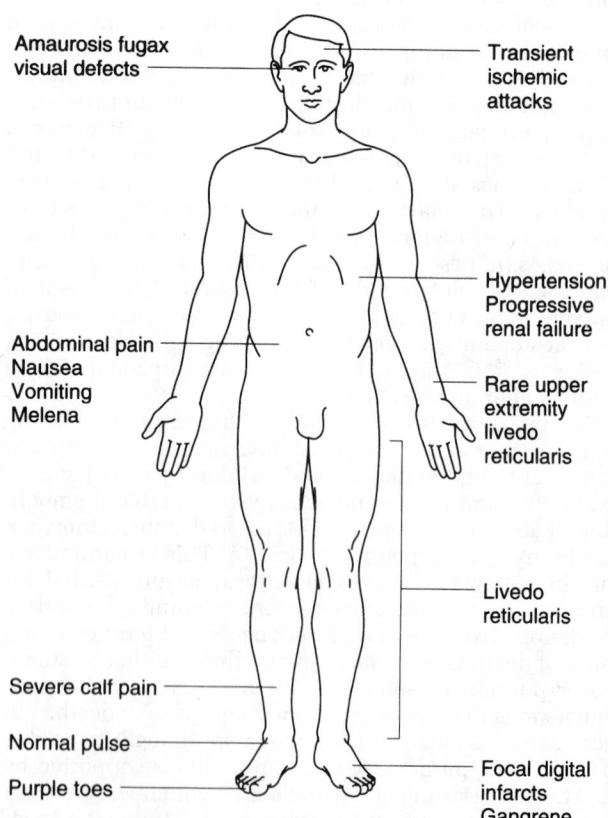

Figure 71-9. Clinical manifestations of multiple cholesterol emboli. (After Kalter X, et al. Livedo reticularis due to multiple cholesterol emboli. J Am Acad Dermatol 1985;13:235)

Table 71-3. LABORATORY ABNORMALITIES ASSOCIATED WITH MULTIPLE CHOLESTEROL EMBOLI

Elevated erythrocyte sedimentation rate
Eosinophilia
Leukocytosis
Abnormal urinalysis—proteinuria, hematuria, albuminuria, granular or hyaline casts
Elevated amylase
Elevated creatinine phosphokinase, aldolase
Azotemia
Findings of disseminated intravascular coagulopathy (rare)
Biopsy of skin, muscle, or kidney—cholesterol clefts in small arteries

(Kalter X, et al. Livedo reticularis due to multiple cholesterol emboli. J Am Acad Dermatol 1985;13:235)

Finally, atheroembolism can be induced by catheter manipulation during angiography.

The true incidence and clinical consequences of atheroembolism remain a matter of conjecture. Florey[43] is responsible for stimulating modern interest in atheroembolism. During an autopsy of a man with extensive aortic atherosclerosis, he first documented atheroembolism to the kidneys, spleen, pancreas, and thyroid. Florey then reviewed the autopsy findings in 267 patients who had significant aortic atherosclerosis and found a 3.4% incidence of atheroembolism. In patients with advanced degenerative atherosclerosis, the incidence was as high as 12.3%. In a later study by Handler[44] of 77 consecutive autopsies of patients who died with severe atherosclerosis, an incidence of 8.6% was found. This study was also the first to call attention to the relation between renal atheroembolism and the onset of severe episodic hypertension and subacute renal failure. Thurlbeck and Castleman[45] found a 77% incidence of atheroembolism to the kidneys in an autopsy study of 22 patients who died after aortic reconstruction during the 1950s at Massachusetts General Hospital. A similar high incidence of atheroembolism was found at autopsy in patients dying with unruptured aortic aneurysms. There was no evidence of atheroembolism in age-matched controls who had minimal atherosclerosis. Studies of necropsies on all patients older than 60 years of age showed that the overall incidence of atheroembolism was 0.8%.[46] Most patients were men whose average age was 76.7 years; 100% had hypertension. In each case of documented atheroembolism, the aorta showed advanced atherosclerosis, sometimes associated with aneurysmal degeneration.

Pathophysiology

Atheroembolism results from the sudden rupture of an atherosclerotic plaque, resulting in showers of cholesterol-rich atheromatous debris into the distal arterial circulation. Depending on the size and concentration of particles, these emboli can either pass through the microcirculation or obstruct a vessel. Most episodes of atheroembolism probably do not result in any detectable clinical sequelae. When the mass of embolus is large, tissue infarction occurs. Cholesterol microemboli can be identified histologically as biconvex, needle-shaped clefts present within the arterial lumen (Fig. 71-10). The birefringent crystals themselves are dissolved during the fixation process, unless special techniques are used to preserve them. Thus, in routine fixation procedures, one sees the shape of the space they occupied, rather than the crystals themselves. These microemboli are found jammed at the arterial bifurcations

with red cells and fibrin adherent to their surface. Typically, the obstructed arteriole is 100 to 900 μm in diameter, the average being 200 μm. At this early stage, the emboli project irregularly into the lumen of the microvessels and have a jagged shape with sharp outlines. Evidence of an acute inflammatory response is found. Intermediate stages are characterized by endothelial and fibroplastic proliferation, an occasional giant cell reaction, and a perivascular lymphocytic infiltration. The surface of the embolus appears smooth and is partially covered with a neoendothelium. The emboli gradually become incorporated into the vessel wall, and eventually an obliterative endarteritis, including intimal and medial thickening and fibrosis, occurs. Cholesterol crystals that have penetrated through the microvessel walls incite a perivascular granulomatous inflammation. Occasionally, a necrotizing angiitis similar to polyarteritis nodosa is present. Both in vitro and in vivo studies have shown that atherosclerotic plaques, particularly ulcerated plaques in which crystalline cholesterol is exposed to circulating plasma, provoke a complement-mediated neutrophil aggregation and inflammatory vasculitis.[47] Patients who have suffered cholesterol embolism syndrome have been shown to have high levels of activated complement cofactors. In addition, it causes aggregation of normal neutrophils, possibly sharing a common mechanism with other causes of vasculitis.

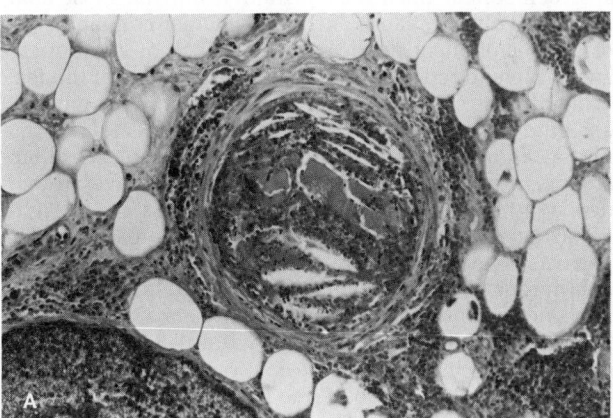
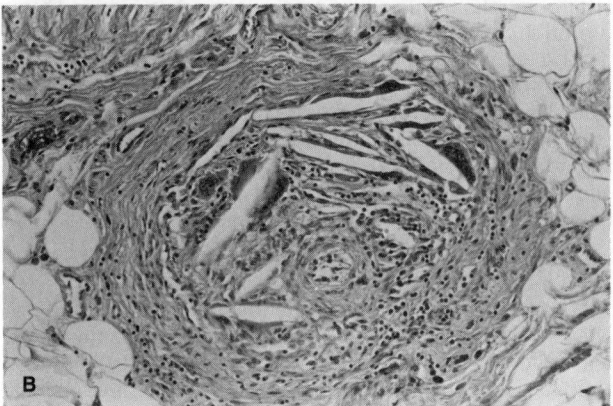

Figure 71-10. (*A*) Fresh atheroembolism. Cholesterol crystals (clear spaces) and amorphous debris from a distant atherosclerotic plaque largely occlude this small arterial branch in the colon (hematoxylin–eosin, ×235). (*B*) Old atheroembolism. Much of the embolus has been organized, but cholesterol crystals remain, with an associated giant cell reaction (hematoxylin–eosin, ×235). (Courtesy of J. Abrams, MD, Department of Pathology, University of Michigan Medical School, Ann Arbor)

Specific Clinical Syndromes

Arterial Catheter–Related Atheroembolism

Atheroembolism can be a serious complication of angiography that is undertaken for diagnostic or therapeutic indications. The frequency of atheroembolism during angiography is unknown. Undoubtedly, many episodes of atheroembolism are asymptomatic. When clinically significant episodes of atheroembolism do occur, they are often not identified correctly because of failure to recognize the clinical syndrome. Thus, the larger and more ridged catheters used for balloon angioplasty have greater potential for dislodging cholesterol emboli. In addition, transfemoral catheterization is associated with a higher incidence of complications than transbrachial catheterization because of the necessity for the transfemoral catheters to traverse the diseased abdominal aorta.

In a retrospective study of autopsy findings of patients who died soon after coronary angiography, it was found that approximately 30% were found to have evidence of atheroembolism.[48] In a series of 70 aged-matched controls who had diffuse atherosclerosis but had not undergone angiography, the incidence of atheroembolism was only 4.3%. Thus, this study confirms the suspicion that cholesterol embolism is not rare during angiography. Because of a delay in the appearance of complications after angiography, a true appreciation of the clinical significance of these complications has not occurred.

A variety of clinical manifestations can be seen after atheroembolism during angiography, but the most commonly involved organ is the kidney. Other common signs of atheroembolism in these patients include the appearance of livedo reticularis and digital infarction in the feet. When diffuse atheroembolism occurs, a clinical picture of episodic or sustained hypertension, fever, and eosinophilia can be seen. The diagnosis of renal cholesterol embolism after angiography can be difficult. The overall incidence of nephrotoxicity after angiography is about 2% in nonazotemic patients and 33% in azotemic patients. The patterns of nephrotoxicity in contrast-induced renal failure and in renal atheroembolism are distinctly different. Contrast-induced nephrotoxicity is usually apparent by elevation of the serum creatinine level within 48 hours of angiography, which reaches its peak 1 week after angiography and usually returns to baseline levels after several weeks in most patients. In contrast, acute renal failure after renal atheroembolism often occurs over a more prolonged time period. In most cases, it is usually not clinically detectable until 1 to 4 weeks after angiography, and then it often pursues a downhill course over the next several weeks.[49] There is no effective therapy for any form of atheroembolism; however, it is important to distinguish between the two forms of renal failure after angiography to provide an accurate prognosis for the patient, and to limit any future angiographic procedures in these patients.

Lower Extremity Atheroembolism

Lower extremity atheroembolism is manifested by sharply demarcated areas of focal ischemia of the lower leg or foot, typically in the toes (see Fig. 71-9). Livedo reticularis can be seen to a variable extent, sometimes extending from the umbilicus to the feet. Thigh and calf myalgias are common and are secondary to atheroembolism of the muscle. The areas of focal ischemia are usually characterized by purplish discoloration of the skin and surrounding petechial hemorrhages (Fig. 71-11). These lesions together represent the so-called blue toe syndrome. Characteristically, these lesions are intensely painful. The areas of bluish discoloration sometimes resemble localized

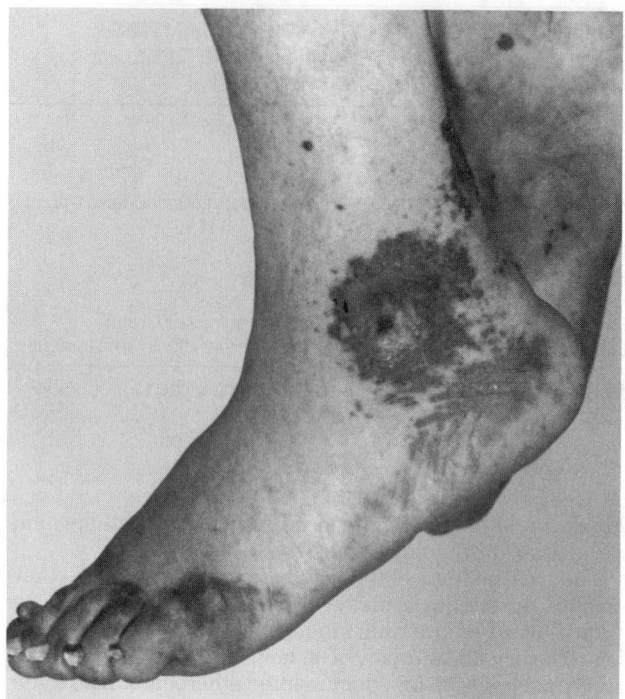

Figure 71-11. Feet of a patient who suffered spontaneous atheroembolism. Well-circumscribed areas of skin discoloration and petechial hemorrhages are visible.

bruising and often are misdiagnosed by both patients and physicians unfamiliar with the syndrome. Pedal pulses may or may not be present.

Atheroembolism of the lower extremities can also result in large vessel obstruction, producing a clinical picture that is indistinguishable from emboli of cardiac origin (see Fig. 71-3). Usually the diagnosis is not made until the time of inspection of the embolus. Although the immediate clinical course after atheromatous macroembolism is the same as that for patients after embolism of cardiac thrombus, these patients must undergo angiography to identify the responsible plaque.

The natural history of microembolism of the extremities is one of repetitive events if left untreated.[50] More than half of the patients have additional complications. Nearly 40% of patients suffering from atheroembolism of an extremity experience some degree of tissue loss. Major amputations are necessary in about 25% of patients. Long-term follow-up shows that up to 20% of these patients die within 1 year of their event. This high mortality rate underlies the severity of the diffuse atherosclerosis in these patients. Because of this poor outlook for patients experiencing extremity atheroembolism, patients should undergo prompt arteriography to delineate possible sources of these emboli. It is important to obtain lateral and oblique films of the aorta and its branches, because many of these lesions are subtle, located on the lateral or posterior walls of the arteries. Although early reports identified aortic lesions, specifically aortic aneurysms, as the most common source of atheroembolism, more recent reports show that the most common source of embolism has been stenotic or ulcerated lesions, or both, of the distal superficial femoral artery.[51,52] In addition, many of these patients have vascular occlusive disease on angiography, which is consistent with reports that show that about half have abnormal pulses. Thus, the emboli can readily pass through collaterals around chronic occlusions of large vessels.

Treatment of arterial lesions identified by arteriography as responsible for the emboli is removal of the lesion by endarterectomy or excision of the diseased portion of the vessel. When these techniques cannot be used, bypass and exclusion of the lesion is an alternative approach. Occasionally there are proximal and distal lesions identified by angiography that could be potentially embologenic. Usually, the lesion that appears more ulcerated and thus more likely to be an embolic source is removed, or, if there are no distinguishing features between multiple lesions, the more distal lesions are removed. Lumbar sympathectomy can be valuable as an adjunctive measure to relieve the cutaneous ischemia, particularly in those patients in whom the arterial source cannot be identified or removed.

There is no effective drug therapy for atheroembolism. Dextran, intraarterial vasodilators, and sympathetic blockers have been used without clear benefit. Some have advocated anticoagulation in these patients. The evidence is contradictory in that there are many reports in which patients have developed these lesions soon after the institution of warfarin therapy for some other purpose. Thus, warfarin itself has been implicated as an etiologic or precipitating factor in the development of embolism by causing sudden hemorrhage into a plaque. Some investigators believe that fibrin platelet emboli are an important component of atheroembolism and on this basis have recommended antiplatelet therapy. There is no evidence that any of these drugs reduce the incidence of recurrent atheroembolism.

Gastrointestinal Microembolism

In view of the predominance of abdominal organ involvement in most autopsy studies of atheroembolism, it is surprising that the gastrointestinal tract has been mentioned relatively infrequently as a separate clinical syndrome. The stomach, small bowel, pancreas, and gallbladder have been affected most frequently by atheroembolism to the gastrointestinal tract. Pathologic studies have shown that atheroembolism usually causes occlusion of multiple submucosal arterioles, which leads to variable degrees of mucosal ischemia. Transmural necrosis of the gut wall can develop, or there can be a pattern of diffuse ulceration. These ulcers undergo cycles of healing and breakdown. Eventually, some ulcers become contracted and fibrotic.

The most common clinical manifestations of atheroembolism to the gastrointestinal tract are diffuse abdominal pain, paralytic ileus, bleeding, and, rarely, small bowel obstruction. Atheroembolism has been implicated as a cause of pancreatitis in patients who have normal biliary and pancreatic ducts. Autopsy studies have shown a correlation between the intensity of the parenchymal evidence of pancreatitis and the degree of associated atherosclerosis in the aorta. Atheroembolism has also been implicated as a cause of perforation of the intestine and gallbladder. Finally, some have drawn an association between cholesterol embolism and the development of angiodysplasia. Cholesterol crystals have been found in areas of angiodysplasia, suggesting that there may be a causal relation. According to this hypothesis, the angiodysplasia is thought to occur as a response of the microvessels to ischemia. In addition, atheroembolism has been implicated as the linking mechanism in patients who are known to have aortic stenosis and gastrointestinal bleeding secondary to angiodysplasia of the right colon.[53] Biopsy in one of these patients showed, in addition to cholesterol emboli and granuloma formation, subepithelial ectasia of vessels and epithelial atrophy. No effective treatment for atheroembolism to the gastrointestinal tract, other than resection of the involved portion, has been developed. Most reports of patients with gastrointestinal involvement secondary to atheroembolism have been autopsy studies.

Coronary Atheroembolism

Atheroembolism of the coronary arteries can cause acute myocardial infarction. It has been reported to occur during cardiopulmonary resuscitation, after strenuous exercise, and, more recently, as a cause of perioperative myocardial infarction during coronary artery bypass grafting. As in other parts of the arterial circulation, atheroembolism results from plaque rupture and the release of cholesterol crystals and other atheromatous debris into the circulation. Histologically, there are areas of arteriolar obstruction. There is an inflammatory response within the vessel walls that is characterized in its later stages by eosinophilic infiltration. The vasculitis is attributed to a hypersensitivity reaction to noncholesterol constituents of atheroma. In patients dying of acute myocardial infarction secondary to coronary atheroembolism, different-aged microinfarcts are found in the myocardium, thus confirming the episodic nature of these emboli prior to the terminal infarction. In addition, atheroembolism has been shown to be an important cause of perioperative myocardial infarction after coronary artery bypass grafting. Recently, 13 fatal cases of perioperative myocardial infarction after coronary artery bypassing were reported and were thought to be secondary to intraoperative atheromatous embolism during manipulation of vein grafts.[54] In somewhat less than half the cases, the emboli originated from ulcerations of the aortic root, rather than the proximal coronary artery. The overall incidence of perioperative myocardial infarction secondary to atheroembolism is approximately 0.22% during redo coronary artery bypass grafting. This increased risk of coronary atheroembolism during cardiac surgery was identified in patients who had severe graft atherosclerosis, rather than in patients who had intimal hyperplasia as a cause of recurrent graft stenosis. To minimize this complication, it has been recommended that the distal vein graft be ligated as early as possible during redo operations.

Renal Atheroembolism

The most frequent organ affected by atheroembolism is the kidney. It is estimated by autopsy studies that renal atheroembolism is found in up to 4% of patients who have minimal aortic atherosclerosis and in 15% of those who have severe aortic atherosclerosis. Histologically, there is extensive occlusion of the arcuate and interlobar arteries, and there can be hyalinization of glomeruli. Variable degrees of inflammatory response within vessel walls, as well as around cholesterol that is outside of vessel walls, can be seen. Renal atheroembolism can be a complication of angiography, it can be a result of manipulation of the aorta or its branches during surgery, or it can occur as a spontaneous event. The clinical picture can be one of acute, subacute, or chronic renal failure. Typically, a patient presents with a recent onset of episodic hypertension or an exacerbation of preexisting hypertension. In a minority of patients, renal atheroemboli do not cause hypertension. An elevated erythrocyte sedimentation rate, peripheral eosinophilia, and urine containing increased protein, white blood cells, and red blood cells can be seen. Generally, the prognosis for patients who develop renal failure secondary to atheroembolism has been poor; only a few cases of reversal of renal failure and survival have been reported. The diagnosis is suspected by identifying predisposing factors of the patients who present with subacute renal failure. Renal biopsy can be performed to confirm the diagnosis. Some have recommended punch biopsy of any skin lesion suspicious for atheroembolism. In the event that the patient recovers from the renal failure, under appropriate clinical circumstances angiography should be done to see if the offending lesion can be removed. For others, management involves appropriate use of dialysis and the treatment of hypertension.

Diffuse Atheroembolism

Diffuse atheroembolism results from showers of cholesterol emboli sufficient to obstruct the microcirculation of multiple organs. Diffuse atheroembolism can mimic many other illnesses, especially polyarteritis nodosa. Many cases of diffuse atheroembolism are misdiagnosed as systemic necrotizing vasculitis, and its true incidence remains unknown. Diffuse atheroembolism is not a rare finding in autopsy studies of patients with severe atherosclerotic disease of the aorta. This syndrome is typically found in patients in the sixth and seventh decades of life who have other manifestations of atherosclerosis. Common signs and symptoms are abdominal pain, lower extremity pain, livedo reticularis, blue toes, neurologic dysfunction, melena, and azotemia. Acute or chronic renal failure can be present. Laboratory studies show elevated erythrocyte sedimentation rate, hematuria, thrombocytopenia, and depletion of complement. The differential diagnosis includes infectious etiologies, especially bacterial endocarditis, disseminated neoplasm, and vasculitis. Diagnosis is made on clinical suspicion of the syndrome as well as on biopsy of the skin, muscle, or kidney. Angiography should be considered with great caution, because this can induce further complications. Again, there is no specific treatment for this disorder. The aortic atherosclerosis is usually diffuse, extending over the thoracic and abdominal aorta. Thoracoabdominal aortic resection is often required. The prognosis of patients with atheroembolism is dismal. The mean interval of survival to death was an average of 2.2 months among 53 patients reported in the literature. In one series, all patients were dead within 6 months of diagnosis.[55]

REFERENCES

1. Abbott WM, Maloney RD, McCabe CC, et al. Arterial embolism: a 44 year perspective. Am J Surg 1982;143:460.
2. Stallone RJ, Blaisdell FW, Caferata HT, Levin SM. Analysis of morbidity and mortality from arterial embolectomy. Surgery 1969;65:207.
3. MacGowan WAL, Mooneeram R. A review of 174 patients with arterial embolism. Br J Surg 1973;60:694.
4. Elliott JP Jr, Hageman JH, Szilagyi E, et al. Arterial embolization: problems of source, multiplicity, recurrence, and delayed treatment. Surgery 1980;88:833.
5. Petersen P. Thromboembolic complications in atrial fibrillation. Stroke 1990;21:4.
6. Petersen P, Boysen G, Godtfredsen J, et al. Placebo-controlled, randomised trial of warfarin and aspirin for prevention of thromboembolic complications in chronic atrial fibrillation: the Copenhagen AFASK study. Lancet 1989;1:175.
7. Risk factors for stroke and efficacy of antithrombotic therapy in atrial fibrillation: pooled data from five randomized controlled trials. Arch Intern Med 1994;154:1449.
8. Arvan S. Mural thrombi in coronary artery disease: recent advances in pathogenesis, diagnosis, and approaches to treatment. Arch Intern Med 1984;144:113.
9. Puletti M, Cusmano E, Testa MG, Borgia C, Fanari F, Curione M. Incidence of systemic thromboembolic lesions in acute myocardial infarction. Clin Cardiol 1986;9:331.
10. Reeder GS, Lengyel M, Tajik AJ, et al. Mural thrombus in left ventricular aneurysm: incidence, role of angiography, and relation between anticoagulation and embolization. Mayo Clin Proc 1981;56:77.
11. Fairfax AJ, Lambert CD, Leatham A. Systemic embolism in chronic sinoatrial disorder. N Engl J Med 1976;295:190.
12. Vermillion BD, Kimins SA, Pace WG, Evans WK. A review of 147 popliteal aneurysms with long term follow-up. Surgery 1981;90:1009.
13. Prioleau PG, Katzenstein AA. Major peripheral arterial occlusion due to malignant tumor embolism: histologic recognition and surgical management. Cancer 1978;42:2009.
14. Darling RC, Austen WG, Linton RR. Arterial embolism. Surg Gynecol Obstet 1967;124:106.
15. Hoxie HJ, Coggin CB. Renal infarction: statistical study of 205 cases and detailed report of unusual case. Arch Intern Med 1949;65:587.
16. Messina LM, Faulkner JA. The skeletal muscle. In: Zelenock GB, D'Alecy LG, Fantone JC, et al, eds. Clinical ischemic syndromes. St Louis, CV Mosby, 1990:457.
17. Haberg H. Intracellular pH during ischemia in skeletal muscle: relationship to membrane potential, extracellular pH, tissue lactic acid, and TNP. Pflugers Arch 1985;404:342.
18. Harris K, Walker PM, Mickle AG, et al. Metabolic response of skeletal muscle to ischemia. Am J Physiol 1986;250:H213.
19. Messina LM. In vivo assessment of microvascular injury after reperfusion of ischemic anterior tibialis of the hamster. Surg Res 1990;48:615.
20. Chin AK, Fogarty TJ. Management of arterial emboli: gleanings from 20 years of experience. Postgrad Med 1987;81:271.
21. Haimovici H. Arterial embolism. In: Haimovici H, ed. The surgical management of vascular diseases. Philadelphia, JB Lippincott, 1970:71.
22. Eastcott HHG. Embolism. In: Eastcott HGG, ed. Arterial surgery, ed 2. Philadelphia, JB Lippincott, 1973:258.
23. Cambria RP, Abbott WM. Acute arterial thrombosis of the lower extremity: its natural history contrasted with arterial embolism. Arch Surg 1984;119:784.
24. Wright JG, Kerr JC, Valeri R, et al. Heparin decreases ischemia-reperfusion injury in isolated canine gracilis muscle. Arch Surg 1988;123:470.
25. Blaisdell FW, Steele M, Allen RE. Management of acute lower extremity arterial ischemia due to embolism and thrombosis. Surgery 1978;84:822.
26. Tawes RL, Harris EJ, Brown WH, et al. Arterial thromboembolism: a 20-year perspective. Arch Surg 1985;120:595.
27. Takolander R, Lannerstad O, Bergqvist D. Peripheral arterial embolectomy, risks and results. Acta Chir Scand 1988;154:567.
28. Bugge M, Jelnes R, Arendrup H, et al. Arterial embolism of the legs and follow-up study of 252 patients. Ann Chir Gynaecol 1985;74:137.
29. Baxter-Smith D, Ashton F, Slaney G. Peripheral arterial embolism: a 20 year review. J Cardiovasc Surg 1988;29:453.
30. Murie JA, Mathieson M. Arterial embolectomy in the leg: results in a referral hospital. J Cardiovasc Surg 1987;28:184.
31. Fogarty TJ. Arterial embolism. In: Dale A, ed. Management of arterial occlusive disease. Chicago, Yearbook Medical Publishers, 1971:329.
32. Jivegard L, Holm J, Schersten T. Acute limb ischemia due to arterial embolism or thrombosis: influence of limb ischemia versus pre-existing cardiac disease on postoperative mortality rate. J Cardiovasc Surg 1988;29:32.
33. Banis JC Jr, Rich N, Col MC, et al. Ischemia of the upper extremity due to noncardiac emboli. Am J Surg 1977;134:131.
34. Kretz JG, Weiss E, Limuris A, et al. Arterial emboli of the upper extremity: a persisting problem. J Cardiovasc Surg 1984;25:233.
35. Ricotta JJ, Scudder PA, McAndrew JA, et al. Management of acute ischemia of the upper extremity. Am J Surg 1983;145:661.
36. Baird RJ, Lajos TZ. Emboli of the arm. Ann Surg 1964;160:905.
37. Hight DW, Tilney NL, Couch NP. Changing clinical trends in patients with peripheral arterial emboli. Surgery 1976;79:172.
38. Green RM, DeWeese JA, Rob CG. Arterial embolectomy before and after the Fogarty catheter. Surgery 1975;77:24.
39. Silvers LW, Royster TS, Mulcare RJ. Peripheral arterial emboli and factors in their recurrence rate. Ann Surg 1980;192:232.
40. Schwarcz TH, Dobrin PB, Mrkvicka R, et al. Balloon embolectomy catheter-induced arterial injury: a comparison of four catheters. J Vasc Surg 1990;11:382.
41. Bowles CR, Olcott CW, Pakter RL, et al. Diffuse arterial narrowing as a result of intimal proliferation: a delayed complication with the Fogarty catheter. J Vasc Surg 1988;7:487.
42. Dobrin PB. Mechanisms and prevention of arterial injuries caused by balloon embolectomy. Surgery 1989;106:457.

43. Florey CM. Arterial occlusions produced by emboli from eroded aortic atheromatous plaques. Am J Pathol 1945; 21:549.

44. Handler FP. Clinical and pathologic significance of atheromatous embolization, with emphasis on an etiology of renal hypertension. Am J Med 1956;20:366.

45. Thurlbeck WM, Castleman B. Atheromatous emboli to the kidneys after aortic surgery. N Engl J Med 1957;257:442.

46. Kealy WF. Atheroembolism. J Clin Pathol 1978;31:984.

47. Hammerschmidt DE, Greenberg CS, Yamada O, et al. Cholesterol and atheroma lipids activate complement and stimulate granulocytes: a possible mechanism for amplification of ischemic injury in atherosclerotic states. J Lab Clin Med 1981;98:68.

48. Ramirez G, O'Neill WM, Lambert R, et al. Cholesterol embolization: a complication of angiography. Arch Intern Med 1978;138:1430.

49. Smith MC, Ghose MK, Henry AR. The clinical spectrum of renal cholesterol embolization. Am J Med 1981;71:174.

50. Wingo JP, Nix ML, Greenfield LJ, et al. The blue toe syndrome: hemodynamics and therapeutic correlates outcome. J Vasc Surg 1986;3:475.

51. Mehigan JT, Stoney RJ. Lower extremity atheromatous embolization. Am J Surg 1976;132:163.

52. Karmody AM, Popwers SR, Monaco VJ, et al. "Blue toe" syndrome. Arch Surg 1976;111:1263.

53. Bank S, Aftalion B, Anfang C, et al. Acquired angiodysplasia as a cause of gastric hemorrhage: a possible consequence of cholesterol embolization. Am J Gastroenterol 1983;78:206.

54. Keon WJ, Heggtveit HA, Leduc J. Perioperative myocardial infarction caused by atheroembolism. J Thorac Cardiovasc Surg 1982;84:849.

55. Kaufman JL, Stark K, Brolin RB. Disseminated atheroembolism from extensive degenerative atherosclerosis of the aorta. Surgery 1987;102:63.

CHAPTER 72

ARTERIAL COMPRESSION SYNDROMES

LLOYD A. JACOBS

Extrinsic compression of vascular structures can produce ischemic injury and cellular death, leading to organ loss or extremity dysfunction. Vascular compression syndromes comprise a heterogeneous group of clinical entities, including some that are poorly described or whose very existence is controversial. Others are well described and well understood but are uncommon or rare. Still others, such as closed compartment syndromes, are common and important to recognize because they profoundly affect clinical outcomes.

Anomalous muscle, tendinous slips, deviant vascular pathways, and congenital osseous abnormalities all can produce extrinsic compression of vascular structures, as can acquired conditions such as osteophytes, benign and malignant tumors, and a host of other conditions. No catalog of vascular compression syndromes can be exhaustive because the compressing structures can occur in unpredictable patterns. Representative vascular compression syndromes include the thoracic outlet syndrome (TOS), vertebral artery compression syndrome, popliteal artery entrapment syndromes, and vascular compression syndromes caused by increased soft tissue pressure within a closed compartment.

THORACIC OUTLET SYNDROMES

Thoracic outlet syndrome occurs when upper extremity neurovascular structures are impinged on by bones or ligaments in the anatomically complex and congested thoracic outlet or within the costal clavicular space (Fig. 72-1). Such compression is usually due to distinct congenital or acquired abnormalities, but occasionally typical symptoms of TOS occur without any demonstrable abnormality.[1-4] Skeletal abnormalities such as a cervical rib, an elongated C-7 transverse process, congenital anomalies of the scalene muscles, or abnormal fibromuscular bands can contribute. Acquired lesions such as excessive callus formation or deformity from a clavicular fracture can also produce TOS. Finally, cervical trauma such as the whiplash deceleration injury can be associated with symptoms of TOS. At times, a demonstrable anatomic abnormality may not be apparent or is extremely subtle. An atypically located scalene tubercle, a hypertrophied or overly broad insertion of the anterior scalene muscle, and a fibrotic, foreshortened scalene muscle can all contribute to TOS (Fig. 72-2). A hypoplastic or anomalous first thoracic rib can also set the stage for TOS. Many TOS patients have multiple anomalies. There was a recent description of a small group of patients who developed compression of the axillary artery by the humeral head during the subluxation that occurs during some athletic activities.

The symptoms of TOS are related to brachial plexus, venous, or arterial compression. Irritation of the brachial plexus is by far the most common presentation of TOS and produces symptoms that are classified in accordance with the nerves and nerve roots involved. Compression of the lower portion of the brachial plexus produces symptoms in the ulnar nerve distribution, whereas compression of the upper portion of the brachial plexus is more likely to produce symptoms in the distribution of the radial nerve. Occasionally, both distributions are involved and there may be associated neck, back, anterior chest, and posterior paraspinous symptoms as well.

Venous compression can produce a chronic picture characterized by intermittent venous obstruction with an increase in upper extremity volume and cyanosis associated with particular movements. More acutely, it can contribute to axillary or subclavian vein thrombosis. This acute complication has been related to periods of strenuous physical activity and is sometimes termed *effort thrombosis*. As this term implies, thrombosis is often preceded by unusually strenuous activity. Acute thrombosis causes pain, cyanosis, and edema and can lead to chronic upper extremity venous insufficiency or, uncommonly, can cause pulmonary embolism. The acute symptoms lessen as compensatory circulation is established.

Arterial complications of thoracic outlet obstruction are the least common of the types outlined earlier but have the most serious prognostic implications (Fig. 72-3). About 5% of the patients operated on for TOS have symptoms related to arterial compression. Long-standing and repeated compressive trauma to the subclavian artery can lead to arterial injury with intimal abnormalities, which can produce stenosis or thrombosis. Alternatively, poststenotic dilation or even aneurysm can occur and can be complicated by embolism or thrombosis. Distal microembolism can produce Raynaud-like phenomena, petechiae, or necrosis of the fingertips. On occasion, the poststenotic dilation can become significantly aneurysmal, and a pulsatile supraclavicular mass can be the presenting complaint. Arterial complications are almost always secondary to

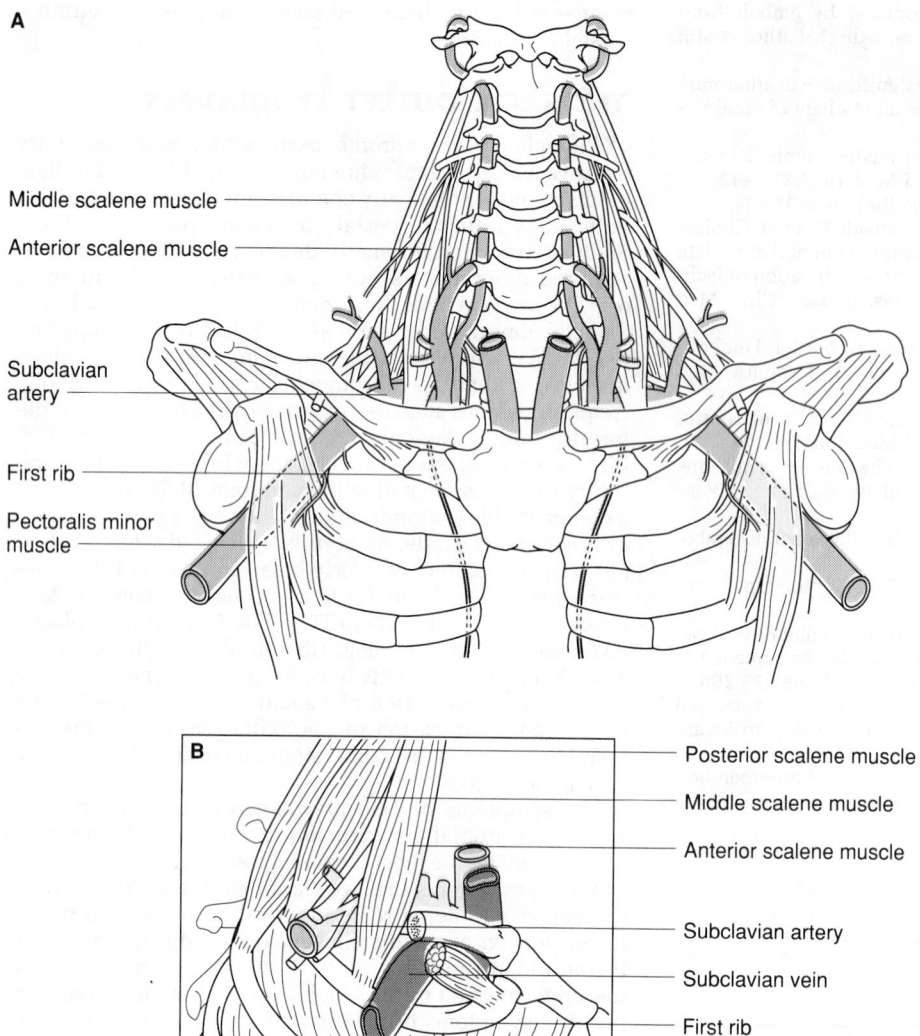

A

Middle scalene muscle

Anterior scalene muscle

Subclavian artery

First rib

Pectoralis minor muscle

B

Posterior scalene muscle

Middle scalene muscle

Anterior scalene muscle

Subclavian artery

Subclavian vein

First rib

Figure 72-1. The normal anatomy of the thoracic outlet in anteroposterior (*A*) and oblique (*B*) views. The brachial plexus and subclavian artery traverse the narrow triangle formed by the anterior and middle scalene muscles and the first rib. The subclavian vein lies anteriorly. (After Zelenock GB. Nonpenetrating subclavian artery injuries. Arch Surg 1985;120:685)

long-standing compression, usually by a bony abnormality, most commonly in the costoscalene passage and somewhat less frequently in the costoclavicular passage of the artery.[1]

In the group of patients with TOS who manifest arterial compression, cervical ribs are common. A complete cervical rib articulates anteriorly to the superior aspect of the first thoracic rib, usually just behind the insertion of the anterior scalene muscle. Incomplete short cervical ribs can be free-floating but invariably are associated with a dense fibrous band that follows the same anatomic course as a complete cervical rib. They have been demonstrated to cause arterial compression. Congenital anomalies of the first thoracic rib are also frequently associated with arterial complications. The most common abnormality is an incomplete first thoracic rib with articulation of its anterior end to the superior aspect of the second thoracic rib. In this situation, the first thoracic rib may be mobile and readily moved by the anterior scalene muscle. Uncommon abnormalities in this area include a bifid first rib or an abnormal tubercle of the first thoracic rib, which can cause compression of the subclavian artery. Congenital bands can also cause arterial compression in this area.

Physical examination findings in patients with acute arterial or venous thrombosis should be obvious. For the former, diminished pulses and a pale or mottled, cool ex-

tremity that fatigues rapidly with exercise should strongly suggest the diagnosis. At times, the upper extremity arterial insufficiency can be even more advanced. In acute venous obstruction, a swollen, tender, congested, and plethoric arm is pathognomonic. A pattern of collateral veins may be apparent across the anterior chest. Unfortunately, TOS most commonly presents with a long prodromic history characterized by intermittent and vague but progressive neurologic symptoms, making diagnosis difficult. These symptoms include pain, paresthesias, and weakness in the neck, shoulder, or hand that may have been exacerbated by certain activities, postures, or unusual exercise. Neurologic examination can be entirely normal or can reveal weakness or atrophy of the triceps or the intrinsic hand muscles. Direct palpation in the supraclavicular fossa or axilla can reproduce the symptoms, as can provocative positioning such as the Adson maneuver, although the latter may not be particularly sensitive or specific.

Many tests have been used to aid in the early diagnosis of TOS. Standard chest roentgenograms and cervical and upper thoracic spine, clavicle, and shoulder films are often obtained. Such plain radiographic studies, in anteroposterior and lateral projections, can display a cervical rib or an abnormal first thoracic rib. Nonunion or hypertrophic callus formation from a clavicular fracture can also be present. Myelograms, electromyograms, nerve conduction

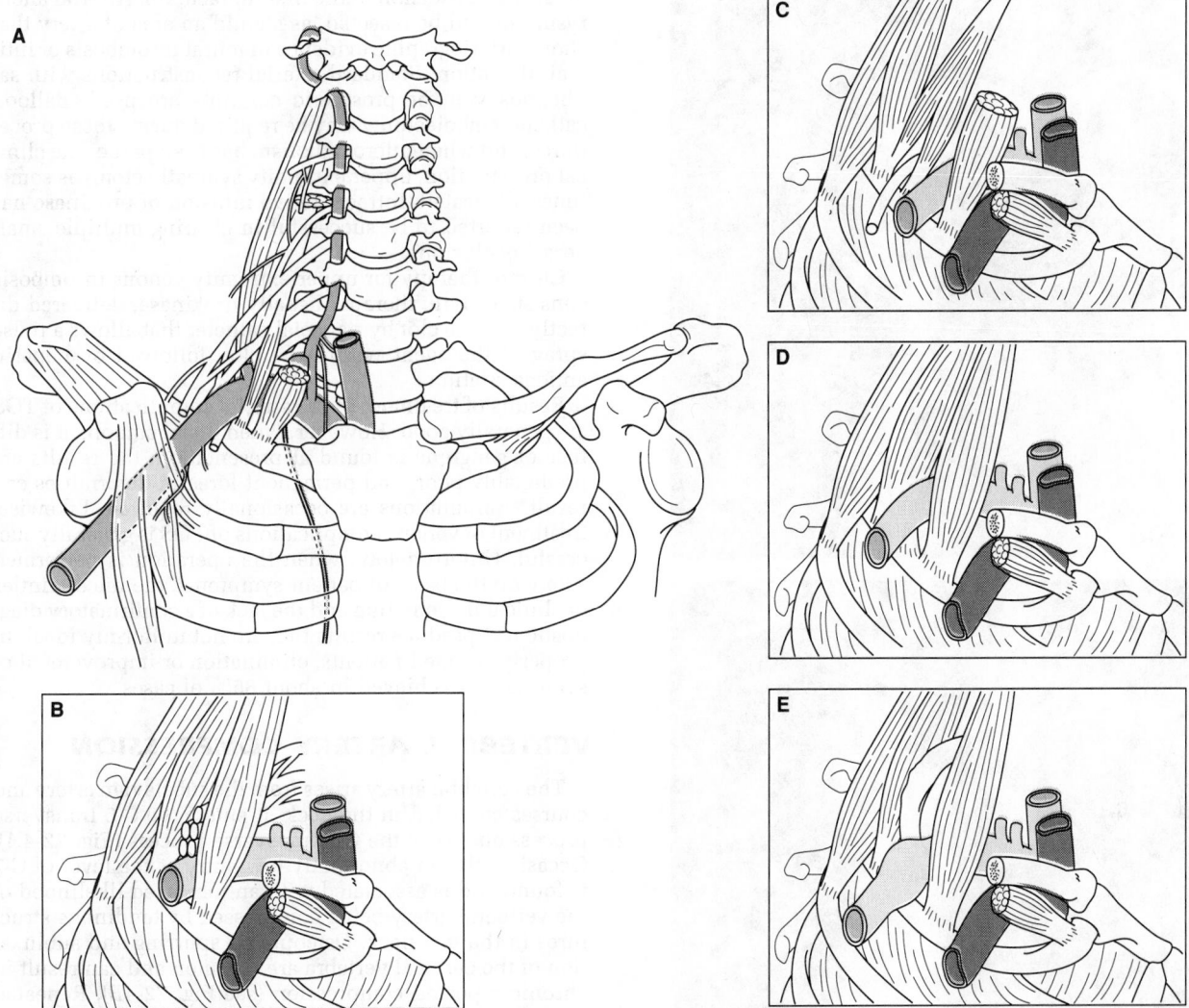

Figure 72-2. (*A*) The anomalous scalene minimus muscle can irritate lower brachial plexus trunks. (*B*) Hypertrophied, fibrosed, and foreshortened scalene muscles elevate the first rib and compress the brachial plexus. (*C*) Unnamed anomalous muscle slips from either the anterior or middle scalene muscle can cause a variable pattern of nerve root compression. (*D*) A broad insertion of the tendon of the middle scalene muscle along the superior aspect of the first rib. (*E*) An anomalous cervical rib or fibrous band is the most common cause of arterial compression. Note the poststenotic subclavian artery aneurysm (see Fig. 72-3). (After Wylie EJ. Manual of vascular surgery, vol 2. New York, Springer-Verlag, 1986)

studies, computed tomography (CT), magnetic resonance imaging, and somatosensory-evoked potentials have all been used in the diagnosis of TOS.[2] These diagnostic tests are seldom definitive, and none has achieved widespread acceptance. They are often most helpful in excluding other causes of the patient's symptoms.

Arterial lesions resulting from TOS are most definitively diagnosed with arteriography. Selective injection of the appropriate subclavian artery is performed, but adequate visualization may require multiple views and subtraction techniques as well as positional maneuvers. Even minor intimal lesions can produce microembolism, and any lesion in this area should be considered significant. Diagnosis is easy when sizable impingements are associated with an abnormal first thoracic rib or cervical rib. In such cases, poststenotic dilation may be obvious and may have progressed to aneurysmal proportions. The presence of mural thrombus within an aneurysm or associated with an intimal lesion is of considerable significance and dictates early

surgical intervention. Occasionally, complete thrombosis of the vessel is seen, and arteriography can be helpful in demonstrating distal embolic occlusions.

Treatment of arterial complications of TOS is always surgical. Emergent operation occasionally is required because of the presence of upper extremity ischemia, continued embolism, or free-floating thrombus in the area. Operation must deal with the underlying arterial compression as well as the complications of aneurysm formation or thromboembolism. Intraarterial thrombolytic therapy followed by definitive operative repair has been used in an attempt to deal with the troublesome distal small vessel thromboses and emboli that have proved difficult for standard surgical approaches.

Several surgical approaches have been advocated for decompressing the thoracic outlet. The transaxillary and anterolateral thoracic approaches provide effective neurologic and venous decompression through a cosmetically acceptable and relatively hidden incision. Arterial compli-

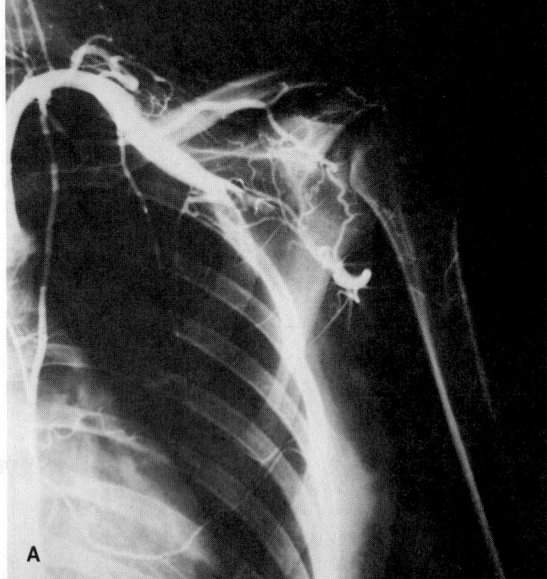

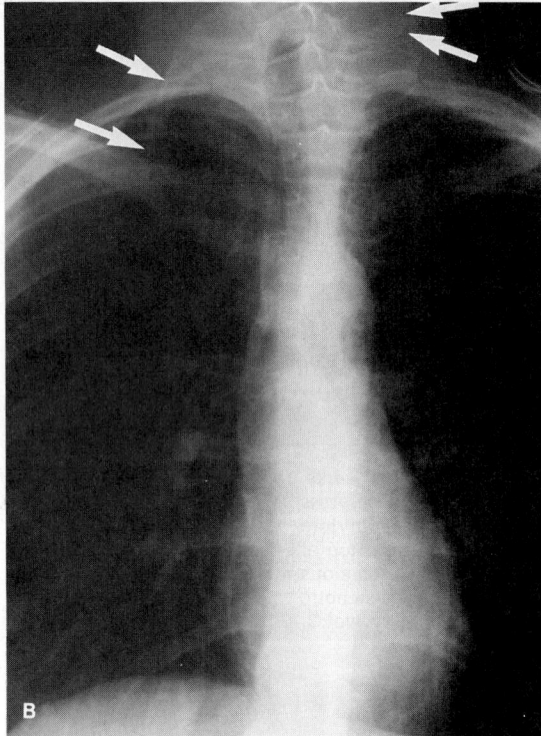

Figure 72-3. (*A*) Upper extremity arteriography demonstrating thromboembolic occlusion of the left axillary artery, the brachial artery, and all forearm arteries (radial, ulnar, and interosseous) as a result of an anomalous cervical rib and a resultant poststenotic subclavian artery aneurysm. (*B*) Immediate postoperative view demonstrating the resected left cervical rib. Also readily seen is a prominent right cervical rib. The resected left subclavian artery aneurysm, which was reconstructed with autogenous saphenous vein, is not seen.

cations of TOS are always best dealt with through the supraclavicular approach, and many surgeons prefer this approach for all TOS procedures. Occasionally, a transclavicular approach can be used when excision of the clavicle is in order because of malunion or excessive callus formation. The goal of thoracic outlet decompression is attained by transection or resection of the anterior scalene muscle and excision of the first thoracic rib. Arterial aneurysms should be resected, as should an area of artery that shows arteriographic evidence of mural thrombosis or intimal ulceration. Standard arterial reconstructions with saphenous vein or prosthetic conduits are used. Balloon catheter embolectomy may be required during these procedures, and when microembolism has been part of the clinical presentation, upper extremity sympathectomy is sometimes advocated. Intraoperative infusion of urokinase has been reported to be successful in clearing multiple small vessel occlusions.

Current therapy for upper extremity venous thrombosis consists of lytic therapy, usually urokinase, delivered directly into the clot by a special catheter that allows a pulse spray of the agent within the clot, followed by heparin anticoagulation.

Results of treatment of the arterial complications of TOS are generally good. However, when distal embolism is diffuse or gangrene is found at presentation, the results are predictably poor, and permanent forearm deformities can result. Amputations are occasionally required. Likewise, treatment of venous complications of TOS is generally successful. Unfortunately, when the operation is performed solely on the basis of patient symptoms, the uncertainties of clinical presentation and the lack of a confirmatory diagnostic test produce results that are not uniformly ideal. In properly selected patients, elimination or improvement of symptoms is achieved in about 85% of cases.

VERTEBRAL ARTERY COMPRESSION

The vertebral artery arises from the subclavian artery and courses cephalad in the neck. It enters the C-6 transverse process and exits the C-2 transverse process (Fig. 72-4*A*). Occasionally, an abnormally low entry at the level of C-7 is found and is associated with an increased likelihood of the vertebral artery being compressed by tendinous structures in the low neck. Osteophytic spurring and subluxation of the cervical vertebra are common and can result in chronic repeated compression (see Fig. 72-4*B*). Repeated trauma to the vessel can cause intimal lesions or a permanent and nonexpandable cicatricial narrowing. In extreme cases, complete occlusion of the vertebral artery can be seen.

Vertebral artery compression can cause vertebrobasilar insufficiency,[5,6] although isolated symptomatic vertebral artery compression is rare. Often, a combination of arteriosclerotic lesions and compression is seen in patients whose symptoms are produced by positional changes of the head and neck. In such cases, one vertebral artery can be occluded by atherosclerotic disease and the other subject to compression on rotation of the head. The symptoms of vertebral basilar insufficiency, whatever the cause, can be vague. Dizziness, vertigo, and paresthesias are fairly commonly reported but are easily confused with other syndromes. Classic drop attacks, in which muscle tone is lost but consciousness is maintained, are uncommon. Alternating or unilateral paresis has also been reported but is likewise uncommon. Because the nonspecific symptoms of vertebral basilar insufficiency are easily confused with symptoms of other origins, the investigation of patients with symptoms of vertebral basilar insufficiency should be systematic and methodical. Efforts to rule out orthostatic and drug-induced hypotension, middle ear labyrinthine disease, and cardiac causes of the patient's symptoms should be undertaken.

Arteriographic study of vertebrobasilar insufficiency requires an evaluation of the entire cerebral vasculature but is indicated only after careful exclusion of other causes of the patient's symptoms. Both the carotids and the intra-

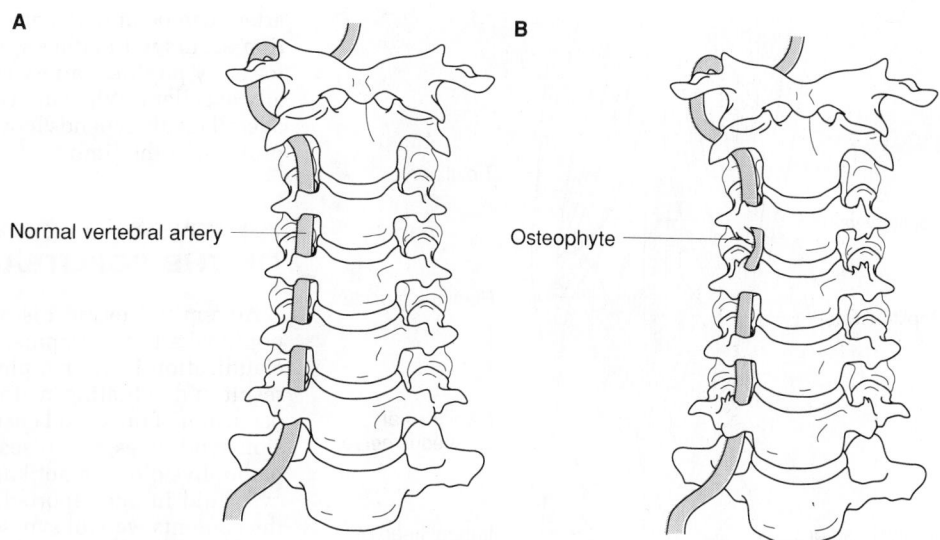

Figure 72-4. (*A*) A normal vertebral artery lying within the vertebral canal. (*B*) A large osteophyte compresses the vertebral artery at the level of C-3. Rotation or flexion–extension can exacerbate the compression.

cranial vasculature, as well as the vertebral system, must be completely visualized. Atherosclerotic lesions of the vertebral artery origins or at other sites within the vertebral system are the most common findings at arteriography, and diffuse extracranial cerebrovascular disease is also common. Evidence of an extrinsic compression of the vertebral artery may require special views and orientations, subtraction techniques, and maneuvers to reproduce the patient's symptoms.

Treatment of symptomatic extrinsic compression of the vertebral artery is operative when symptoms are compelling or when there is any objective evidence of posterior circulation emboli. Relief of the extrinsic compression may require resection of osteophytes, unroofing of the transverse process foramina, or transection of musculotendinous bands associated with the cervical muscles. In the event of an abnormal change in the vertebral artery serving as an embolic source, standard vascular reconstruction should be undertaken.

Osteophytes and other bony abnormalities of the cervical vertebra are exceedingly common, yet symptoms of vertebrobasilar insufficiency are vague, and operations on the vertebral artery have the potential to be overused. In carefully selected patients, judicious operative therapy produces excellent results.

POPLITEAL ARTERY ENTRAPMENT SYNDROME

The popliteal artery entrapment syndrome is an uncommon problem and usually presents as unilateral calf claudication in a young individual.[7–9] Popliteal artery entrapment is most commonly seen in males, with a male-to-female ratio of about 15:1, and tends to occur more frequently in heavily muscled individuals.

Calf claudication is by nature episodic, but patients can frequently relate the onset of symptoms to a specific and intense exercise such as running. During this phase, the artery presumably is compressed intermittently, producing claudication. A more acute phase is entered when repeated trauma damages the intima or when scar tissue envelops the artery and arterial thrombosis occurs. In these cases, acute ischemia of the lower limb develops and the patient can present with a pulseless, cold, painful, and paralyzed extremity.

Patients with popliteal artery entrapment syndrome generally lack the risk factors and secondary signs of atherosclerotic occlusive disease. Those with entrapment but without an occluded popliteal artery frequently have normal foot pulses. These pulses may disappear on passive dorsiflexion of the foot or active plantar flexion against resistance. The sensitivity of this portion of the physical examination can be enhanced by the detection of a decreased Doppler signal or by decreased ankle pressures under similar circumstances in the noninvasive vascular laboratory. An occasional associated popliteal aneurysm is found, presumably a result of the progression of long-standing poststenotic dilation.

The popliteal artery entrapment syndrome usually is associated with a distinct congenital anomaly that was first described more than a century ago. Normally, the popliteal artery passes through the adductor canal and traverses the popliteal space between the medial and lateral heads of the gastrocnemius muscle (Fig. 72-5). Congenital variations of the popliteal artery have been classified into four types (Fig. 72-6). In type I, the popliteal artery deviates medially around the normally located medial head of the gastrocnemius muscle. In type II, the medial head of the gastrocnemius arises from an abnormally lateral position on the femoral condyles so that the popliteal artery descends in a nearly normal course but is still impinged on by the abnormal origin of that muscular head. In type III, the popliteal artery passes through the medial head of the gastrocnemius or between the normal medial head and an accessory muscle slip that originates more laterally. In type IV, the popliteal artery is entrapped by the popliteus muscle, or occasionally the artery is impinged on by a fibromuscular band arising more laterally and joining the gastrocnemius fascia. Other anomalies have been described, and classifications including as many as 10 variants have been given. Schemes recognizing displacement and impingement of the popliteal vein and nerve have also been reported. Popliteal entrapment by the soleus and plantaris tendons has been described. A single case suggestive of popliteal artery compression by hypertrophied calf musculature has been reported. Whatever the precise anatomy, popliteal artery entrapment syndrome should be recognized as an uncommon but important cause of lower extremity arterial occlusive symptoms in healthy young men.

CT scans of the popliteal fossa have been reported to be

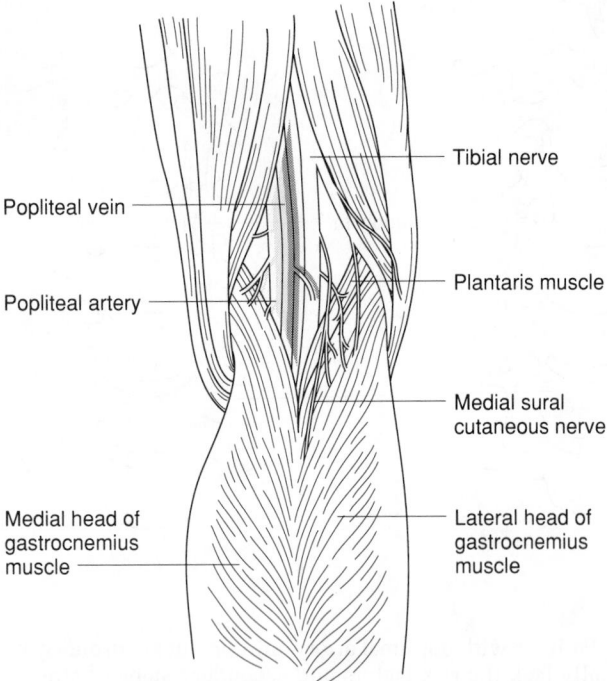

Figure 72-5. The normal anatomy of the popliteal fossa. The popliteal artery and vein and the tibial nerve lie between the medial and lateral heads of the gastrocnemius. The peroneal nerve courses lateral to the head of the gastrocnemius and the head of the fibula.

of value in the diagnosis of popliteal artery abnormalities and, in the hands of a skilled radiographer, may give detailed information about the origin of the head of the gastrocnemius muscle. More experience with the CT scan is necessary before this approach can be considered routine, and the definitive diagnostic procedure in this syndrome is arteriography. Arteriography should be performed bilaterally, because the anomaly is frequently found in the asymptomatic leg as well. In the appropriate setting, medial deviation of the popliteal artery, occlusion of the popliteal artery, and stenosis with poststenotic dilation may confirm the popliteal artery entrapment syndrome.

Treatment of popliteal artery entrapment is surgical, whether the symptoms are minimal or extreme. The grave prognosis and high incidence of limb loss for acute popliteal artery occlusion warrant operative relief of the entrapped artery even with minimal or absent symptoms.

Either a posterior or medial approach to the popliteal artery is acceptable. The posterior approach allows clear visualization of the precise relation between the medial head of the gastrocnemius muscle and the popliteal artery and helps in the recognition of type II, III, and IV anomalies. Most vascular surgeons are more familiar with the medial approach; however, in the case of an occluded vessel, particularly when the occlusion extends distally to the popliteal trifurcation, the medial approach is technically superior. Transection of the compressing portion of the medial head of the gastrocnemius or fascial band relieves the entrapment and is all that is required in most cases. When an intimal lesion has been demonstrated or when stenosis or occlusion has occurred, reconstructive arterial surgery must be performed, usually with autogenous saphenous vein. Most surgeons make no attempt to reconstruct the medial head of the gastrocnemius muscle, although reattachment in a normal relation to the popliteal

artery can be undertaken. Little or no loss of muscle function occurs with either approach. The results of operation for early popliteal artery entrapment syndrome are generally excellent. When arterial thrombosis has occurred, the overall result depends most on the degree of ischemic compromise of the limb.

ADVENTITIAL CYSTIC DISEASE OF THE POPLITEAL ARTERY

Adventitial cystic disease of the popliteal artery, like popliteal artery entrapment syndrome, causes intermittent claudication in young, physically active patients and can result in debilitating symptoms and irreversible damage if occlusion of the vessel ensues. Like other arterial compression syndromes, this disease entity is rare, and its precise pathophysiology is not known (Fig. 72-7). Analysis of the cyst fluid in one reported case led to the suggestion that the contents were of synovial origin,[10] but this view is not widely held. Pulses may be normal in the foot, particularly at rest. The diagnosis of adventitial cystic disease of the popliteal artery has been improved by the use of CT scans of the popliteal space. In addition, CT scanning can help distinguish between popliteal artery entrapment syndrome and a Baker or synovial cyst in the popliteal space. Arteriography is still indicated, particularly if there is a question of distal embolism or thrombosis of the artery. Uncomplicated adventitial cysts of the popliteal artery may be difficult to visualize angiographically, particularly when presented en face. Lateral projection typically demonstrates a smooth indentation into the column of dye and is noteworthy for the lack of atherosclerotic lesions.

Treatment of adventitial cystic disease of the popliteal artery that has become symptomatic is operative. Percutaneous transluminal angioplasty has been attempted, but the results generally have not been satisfactory. Cyst aspiration has not been particularly successful. At operation, the artery and the cystic area should be exposed. The cyst itself can be unilocular or multilocular, and occasionally adventitial cysts appear to contain old blood. The cyst should be incised and its contents removed. This generally completes the operation. Cicatricial stenosis of the artery, poststenotic dilation, or thrombosis may necessitate further procedures. Treatment results in early nonoccluded cases have been uniformly good. When thrombosis has occurred and has progressed distally, the results depend on the degree of ischemia on presentation.

COMPARTMENT SYNDROMES

Compartment syndromes are encountered when increased tissue pressure within a limited anatomic space compromises circulation.[11-14] These syndromes generally occur because of the increasing volume of the compartment's contents but occasionally because the capacity of the compartment is reduced by application of a tight plaster cast or by a tight fascial closure during operation. Compartment syndromes can also be produced by hemorrhage into a closed compartment in association with bleeding disorders, anticoagulant therapy, or trauma. The most common and most important compartment syndromes occur in relation to interruption and subsequent restoration of blood flow to an extremity made ischemic by an embolism, thrombus, trauma, or unusual prolonged positioning.[11] The hyperperfusion and edema that follow ischemic injury doubtless contribute to the development of intracompartmental swelling.[12,13] Swelling of tissue in ischemic and reperfused limbs can be documented by weight gain

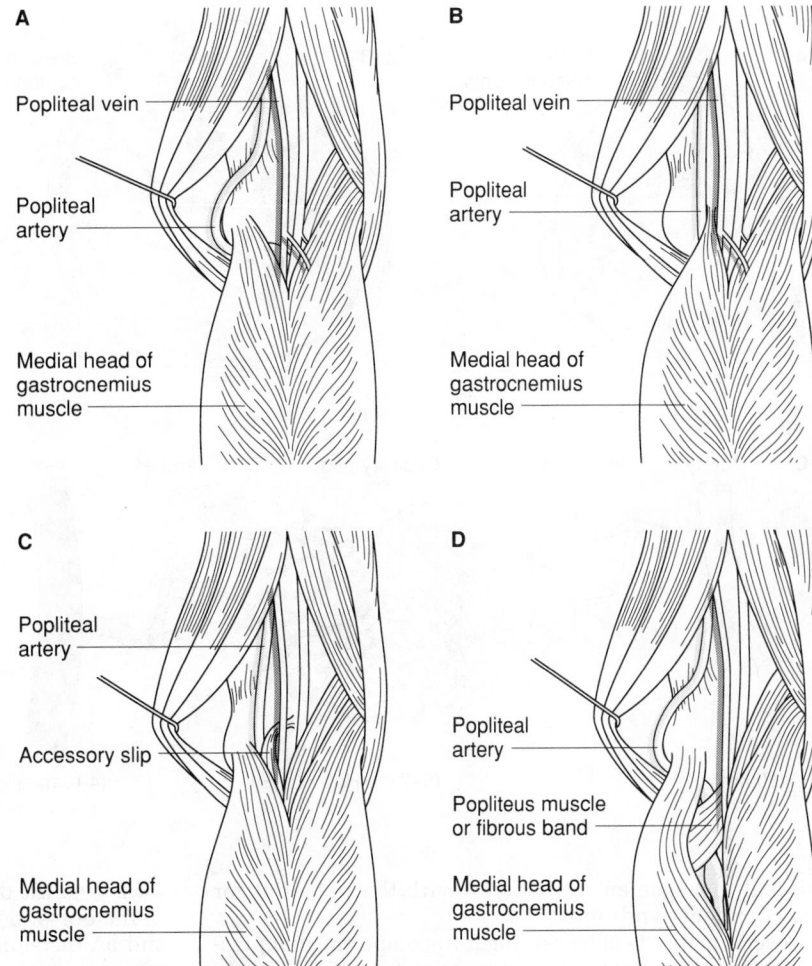

Figure 72-6. (*A*) Posterior view of right popliteal fossa. Normally located medial head of gastrocnemius with deviant medial pathway of popliteal artery (type I). (*B*) In the type II anomaly, an abnormally lateral origin of the medial head of the gastrocnemius muscle places traction on an otherwise normally placed popliteal artery. (*C*) An accessory slip of the gastrocnemius muscle compressing the popliteal artery. (*D*) Medial deviation of the popliteal artery and compression by the popliteus muscle. (After Whelan TJ. Popliteal artery entrapment. In: Rutherford RB, ed. Vascular surgery, ed 3. Philadelphia, WB Saunders, 1989)

of the limb and is due to increased interstitial fluid and intracellular swelling.

The clinical manifestations of compartment syndromes include throbbing and unrelenting pain and the loss of neuromuscular function. The forearm and the leg are the most frequent sites of compression, and each compartment

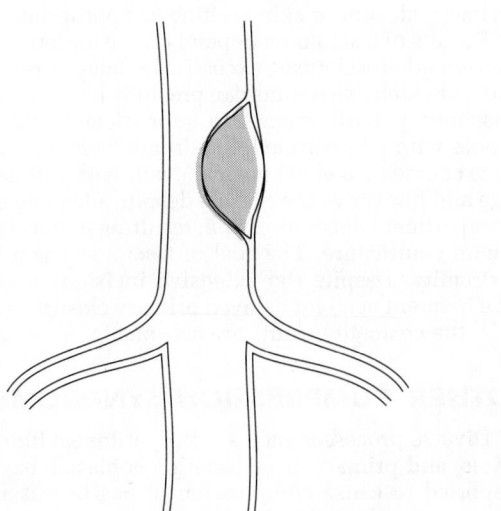

Figure 72-7. Adventitial cystic disease of the popliteal artery causes luminal compromise.

of the forearm and leg contains at least one major peripheral nerve. Careful examination of the hand or foot may disclose neurologic deficits. Subtle sensory changes or paresthesias may be observed before the development of clearcut signs of ischemia. Movement or stretching of the involved muscle by passive motion of the wrist or ankle can produce pain. The only objective signs are a tense, tender, or swollen compartment on direct palpation, and subcutaneous edema or hematoma (Fig. 72-8*A* and *B*). Distal pulses should be assessed, but capillary or venous compression generally precedes the cessation of arterial inflow, and significant tissue damage can occur before intracompartmental pressure exceeds arterial perfusion pressure (see Fig. 72-8*C*). Paralysis of the involved musculature suggests that the compression is advanced.

The most important aspect of the diagnosis of this syndrome is careful repeated clinical evaluations of the involved limb. All patients with major trauma or crush injury should have repetitive neurovascular examination of the involved limb for 48 to 72 hours after injury. During the postoperative period after embolectomy or prolonged reconstructive vascular surgery, similar repetitive examinations are in order. In most cases, such clinical examination is adequate to make the diagnosis of compression in an appropriate time frame. In an unconscious patient, many surgeons prefer intermittent or continuous measurement of intracompartmental pressures.[13] Such compartmental pressure monitoring is the subject of some controversy, and other surgical groups believe that it makes no important contribution to the

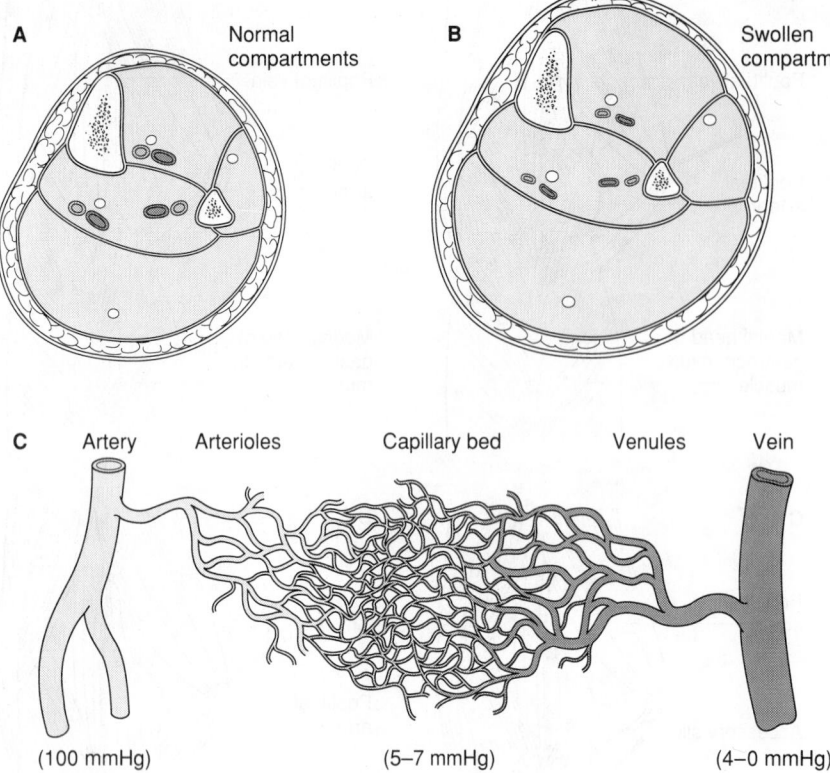

Figure 72-8. (*A*) Compartments of the leg at midcalf. The anterior, lateral, and both the deep and superficial posterior compartments contain major nerves. (*B*) When cellular swelling and interstitial edema develop within the fixed confines of the various compartments, pressure necrosis of the compartment's contents may result. The tissue most sensitive to ischemia is the peripheral nerve. (*C*) As compartment pressures rise to 20 to 40 mmHg, obstruction to flow occurs first at the capillary–venule level. Profound ischemia may then result despite normal distal arterial pulses. (After Mubarak SJ, Hargens AR. Compartment syndromes and Volkmann's contracture. Philadelphia, WB Saunders, 1981)

clinical management of patients with the potential for compartment syndromes.[14]

Several methods of measuring intracompartmental pressure have been described. These range from simple measurements with a central venous manometer to the use of recently developed solid-state pressure transducers small enough to be inserted into the appropriate compartment on a catheter tip. Two other catheter methods are commonly used. The Wick technique uses a catheter kept open with strands of polyglycolic acid suture and a continuous electronic pressure sensor. Others have described a small catheter using a continuous slow infusion and electronic monitoring of the pressure developed by that infusion. Compartmental pressures are normally in the range of 10 mmHg. Pressures exceeding 20 mmHg are considered abnormal, and those exceeding 40 mmHg are dangerous and require decompression.

Fasciotomy is generally performed in the forearm or leg. The leg is composed of four compartments, each nonexpandable and delineated by thick fascia (see Fig. 72-8). The four compartments of the lower extremity include both a deep and a superficial posterior compartment, a lateral compartment, and an anterior compartment. Decompression of all four compartments is the goal. Fibulectomy accomplishes this end, although this operation has been largely supplanted by less extensive procedures. The anterior and lateral compartments should be decompressed through an anterior lateral incision, and the posterior compartments decompressed through a posteromedial incision. These longitudinal incisions are generally left open for delayed primary closure or skin grafting when the edema subsides. An appropriate rehabilitative program is of utmost importance.

Ankle and foot fasciotomy, as an adjunct to leg fasciotomies, is undertaken when continued foot swelling and tenseness over the medial aspect of the proximal foot are encountered.[15] The foot can be decompressed through incisions over the dorsum of the foot and ankle, with incisions in the dorsal deep aponeurosis over the metatarsal spaces and an incision through the distal portion of the inferior extensor retinaculum. A longitudinal incision along the medial and inferior border of the foot allows decompression of the plantar compartment. Ankle and foot fasciotomies appear to be valuable in prolonged reconstructive vascular procedures for arteriosclerotic disease.

Most compartmental syndromes in the forearm are adequately decompressed by a single long volar incision from the antecubital fossa to the proximal palm. Carpal tunnel release is usually included in this procedure, and occasionally a second incision directly over the dorsal compartment of the forearm is necessary. These incisions, like those in the lower extremity, are left open for delayed primary closure or skin grafting as appropriate.

Results of fasciotomy depend on the underlying disease. Severe atherosclerosis, excessively delayed revascularization, or extensive trauma can preclude limb salvage despite fasciotomy. Furthermore, an unpredictable number of patients with compartment syndrome have a slow progressive course of skeletal muscle death with ultimate shrinkage and fibrosis of the muscle despite adequate and timely compartment decompression, resulting in the classic Volkmann contracture. The goal of fasciotomy is a functional extremity. Despite the extensive incisions involved and the frequent need for delayed primary closure or skin grafting, the cosmetic results are acceptable.

OTHER COMPRESSION SYNDROMES

Diverse processes such as retroperitoneal fibrosis, Baker cysts, and primary or metastatic neoplasms have all been reported to cause compression of nearby vascular structures. An exhaustive catalog of these syndromes is not possible. One example is involvement of the carotid bifurcation by metastatic head and neck cancer. In the treatment of selected patients with extensive laryngeal or oropharyngeal cancer, resection and reconstruction of the carotid artery can be used in concert with radical excision of the malignancy. In a recent report, 15 patients were treated with reconstruction or simple ligation for advanced neck cancer. Two of these patients suffered immediate postoperative strokes, and there was one postoperative death. Seven patients were believed to be free of cancer more than 1 year after operation. These data suggest that in selected cases, malignancies compressing adjacent arteries can reasonably be treated by radical excision and concomitant reconstructive vascular surgical techniques.

REFERENCES

1. Cormier JM, Amrane M, Ward A, Laurian C, Gigou F. Arterial complications of the thoracic outlet syndrome: fifty-five operative cases. J Vasc Surg 1989;9:778.
2. Machleder HI, Moll F, Nuwer M, Jordan S. Somatosensory evoked potentials in the assessment of thoracic outlet compression syndrome. J Vasc Surg 1987;6:177.
3. Roos DB. Thoracic outlet nerve compression. In: Rutherford RB, ed. Vascular surgery, ed 3. Philadelphia, WB Saunders, 1989.
4. Wylie EJ, Stoney RJ, Ehrenfeld WK, Effeney DJ, eds. Manual of vascular surgery, vol 2. New York, Springer-Verlag, 1986.
5. Bauer RB. Mechanical compression of the vertebral arteries. In: Berguer R, Bauer RB, eds. Vertebrobasilar arterial occlusive disease: medical and surgical management. New York, Raven Press, 1984:45.
6. Berguer R, Caplan LR. Vertebrobasilar arterial disease. St Louis, Quality Medical, 1992.
7. Collins PS, McDonald PT, Lim RC. Popliteal artery entrapment: an evolving syndrome. J Vasc Surg 1989;10:484.
8. Williams LR, Flinn WR, McCarthy WJ, Yao JST, Bergan JJ. Popliteal artery entrapment: diagnosis by computed tomography. J Vasc Surg 1986;3:360.
9. Whelan TJ. Popliteal artery entrapment. In: Rutherford RB, ed. Vascular surgery, ed 3. Philadelphia, WB Saunders, 1989.
10. Jay GD, Ross FL, Mason RA, Giron F. Clinical and chemical characterization of an adventitial popliteal cyst. J Vasc Surg 1989;9:448.
11. Khalil IM. Bilateral compartmental syndrome after prolonged surgery in the lithotomy position. J Vasc Surg 1987;5:879.
12. Forrest I, Lindsay T, Romaschin A, Walker P. The rate and distribution of muscle blood flow after prolonged ischemia. J Vasc Surg 1989;10:83.
13. Mubarak SJ, Hargens AR. Compartment syndromes and Volkmann's contracture. Philadelphia, WB Saunders, 1981.
14. Skillman JJ, Dohlman LE, Gerhart TN, Ransil BJ. Compartmental pressure monitoring after arterial reconstruction lacks clinical relevance. J Vasc Surg 1986;3:871.
15. Ascer E, Strauch B, Calligaro KD, Gupta SK, Veith FJ. Ankle and foot fasciotomy: an adjunctive technique to optimize limb salvage after revascularization for acute ischemia. J Vasc Surg 1989;9:594.

SURGERY: SCIENTIFIC PRINCIPLES AND PRACTICE, Second Edition, edited by Lazar J. Greenfield, Michael W. Mulholland, Keith T. Oldham, Gerald B. Zelenock, and Keith D. Lillemoe. Lippincott-Raven Publishers, Philadelphia, © 1997.

CHAPTER 73

TISSUE ISCHEMIA

GERALD B. ZELENOCK AND LOUIS G. D'ALECY

Ischemic tissue injury is a basic biologic process of fundamental importance to all surgeons. It is the common pathophysiologic occurrence in many clinical syndromes and is at the root of several vexing technical problems. In the United States and most Western countries, ischemic heart and brain disease (myocardial infarction and stroke) are the first and third leading causes of death, respectively. These disorders result from ischemic injury, cause major morbidity and disability, and exact an enormous personal and societal cost. Operative correction of ischemia is of obvious importance to the vascular and cardiac surgeon and forms the bulk of their efforts. More than 570,000 vascular operations, 1.2 million cardiac procedures, and hundreds of thousands of other interventions are performed annually to alleviate ischemia. The procedures designed to relieve ischemia are themselves associated with an intraoperative risk of ischemic injury during vessel clamping for repair, reconstruction, or bypass. Issues of ischemic injury are crucial in transplantation and donor preservation, resuscitation from shock and trauma, the use of tourniquets and other techniques to obtain a bloodless field, reconstructive surgical procedures with translocation of flaps, and the integrity of anastomoses in gastrointestinal and genitourinary surgery. Ischemia is also the penultimate process of injury in strangulation infarction secondary to hernia, volvulus, adhesions, and other forms of bowel obstruction.

The precise cause of ischemic cell death is not known.

It is almost certainly multifactorial, and the key process may be different in various tissues. Nevertheless, several discrete mechanisms are common and can be used to characterize ischemic injury (Fig. 73-1):

- Energy failure
- Direct parenchymal cell injury
- Vascular (endothelial) injury
- Activation of soluble and cellular inflammatory systems

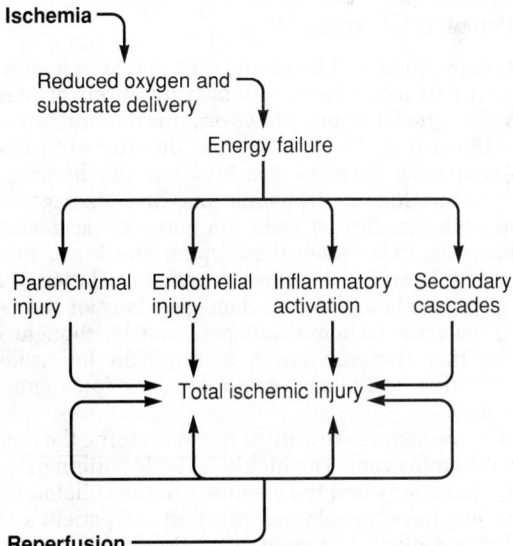

Figure 73-1. Ischemia produces multiple adverse effects. Lack of oxygen and substrate cause failure of energy production for essential cellular processes, resulting in parenchymal and vascular injury, as well as activation of the inflammatory system and secondary cascades. The injury process continues throughout the reperfusion phase.

- Ischemic activation of secondary cascades, such as complement, prostaglandins, and coagulation
- Reperfusion effects

These concepts are complex, and many nuances and subtle interrelations are not fully defined. There are also important organ-specific differences.[1] For the purpose of discussion, each mechanism is considered here as a discrete process, an admittedly artificial intellectual construct. Each mechanism interacts with the others, however, with some factors amplifying and others moderating the overall process. Additional considerations are the mechanisms by which organs tolerate ischemic stress and the process by which localized ischemia causes systemic or remote effects.

TOLERANCE

Ischemia leads to cellular and tissue injury and, ultimately, to organ failure, tissue necrosis, and death. Both the duration and severity of ischemia influence the ultimate clinical outcome. The specific tolerance of various tissues and organs to ischemic injury is highly variable, ranging from minutes in the case of brain to several hours for skeletal muscle, and is influenced by the following factors:

- Duration and severity of ischemic insult
- Resting metabolic rate
- Temperature
- Ability of an organ or tissue to decrease metabolic demand
- The substrate being metabolized during the ischemic episode
- Ability to use alternative substrate (phosphocreatinine, glycogen, ketone)
- Anaerobic glycolysis
- Availability of subtypes of key metabolic enzymes
- Rapidity of development of ischemia
- Efficiency of existing collateral
- Potential for collateral development
- Availability of antioxidants, scavengers, and other defense mechanisms
- The manner in which reperfusion occurs
- Potential for regeneration

The consequence of increased duration of ischemia is for the most part intuitive, with longer durations of ischemia producing greater injury. However, this relation is not simple or linear (Fig. 73-2). With short durations of ischemia, little detectable decrement in function may be produced. At long durations of ischemia, maximal damage is produced such that further ischemia may only accelerate tissue necrosis. In between these upper and lower limits of ischemic tolerance is the *dose-dependent* relation of duration of ischemia and tissue damage. Many of the factors that impact on ischemic outcome can be thought of as shifting this response curve to the right for protective or mitigating influences or to the left for aggravating influences.

Anatomic factors are critical in determining the outcome of an ischemic event. The highly variable pattern of normal vascular anatomy and the adequacy of the collateral circulation may have a profound effect on the patient's ability to tolerate a given ischemic event (Fig. 73-3). Additional anatomic concepts relevant to an occlusion of a particular arterial bed have been recognized: tissues supplied by end arteries may experience watershed effects (Fig. 73-4), and the concept of an *ischemic penumbra* (Fig. 73-5) has been described.

Inherent metabolic factors may also influence ischemic

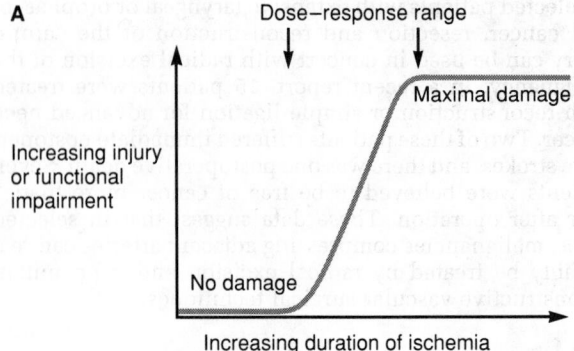

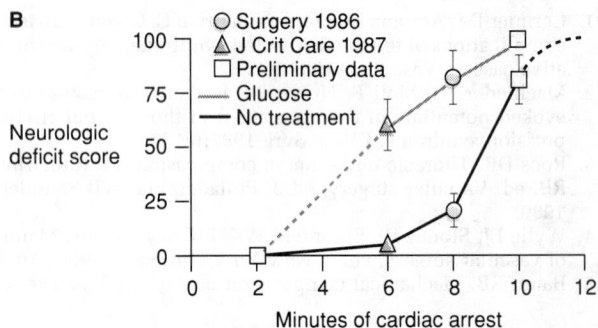

Figure 73-2. (*A*) Theoretical dose–response curve for an ischemic injury. At short durations of ischemia, little or no functional impairment is likely. Above a certain threshold, increasing duration of ischemia results in progressively more severe ischemic injury and functional impairment. Maximal injury to cells, tissues, and organs is not exacerbated by increasing duration of the ischemic event. It does, however, result in permanent impairment or death of cells, tissues, organs, and individuals. (*B*) Actual dose–response curve obtained in a series of experiments in a canine model of timed cardiac arrest (ventricular fibrillation) versus neurologic deficit score. Protective interventions shift the curve to the right, whereas adverse effects, such as glucose administration, shift the curve to the left.

tolerance. Cells and organs with direct and continuous activities, constant energy demand, and a high basal oxygen extraction such as myocardium are less well prepared to meet the demands of an ischemic insult than skeletal muscle, which can markedly diminish its activity, use glycogen stores, increase oxygen extraction, and thus lessen destruction. The substrate metabolized during ischemia is important. Enhanced or exclusive use of glucose during central nervous system (CNS) ischemia worsens neurologic outcomes.[2-5] Conversely, brain ischemia is much better tolerated when ketone is used as the metabolic fuel.[6] In experimental models, lowering ambient blood glucose by administering insulin enhances CNS but not renal tolerance to an ischemic stress.[7-9] The tolerance of an organ may also be influenced by the presence of specific isoenzymes that continue to function under ischemic conditions and allow continued energy production despite a decline in pH. The differential tolerance to ischemia noted between liver and kidney is at least in part attributable to variable concentrations of lactate dehydrogenase isoenzymes. Other anatomic and physiologic factors such as the presence or absence of scavengers, antioxidants, and other protective mechanisms contribute to the variable response of organs and tissues to a given ischemic stress.

The functional severity of ischemic events can be assessed by patient symptoms such as pain (eg, angina pectoris, claudication) or neurologic status (eg, paralysis, amau-

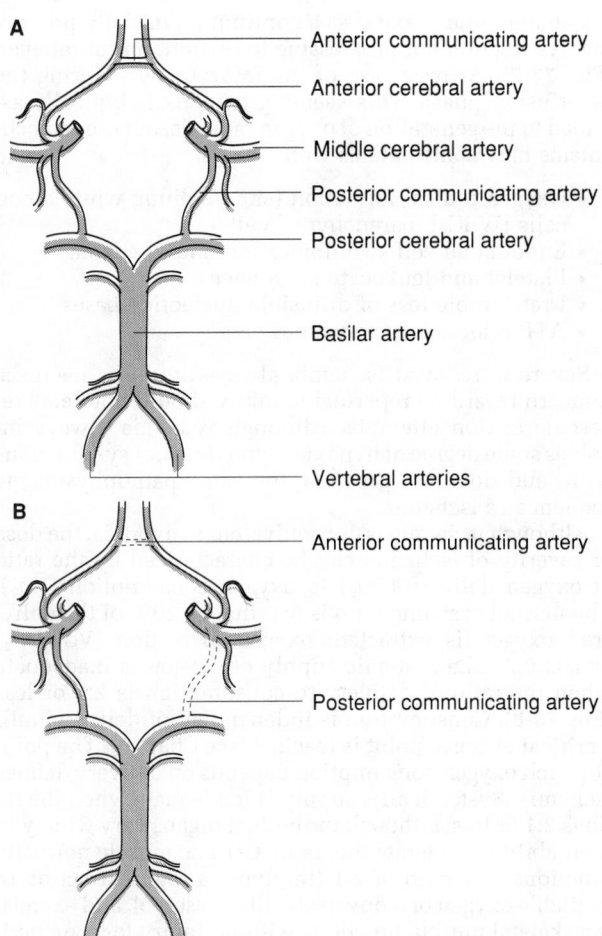

Figure 73-3. (*A*) The normal circle of Willis provides an efficient collateral circulation in the event of internal carotid artery occlusion or clamping. (*B*) An isolated hemisphere with inadequate anterior and posterior communicating arteries places the brain at risk when internal carotid artery occlusion or clamping occurs.

rosis fugax), by physiologic parameters such as pulse–pressure ratios (eg, ankle–brachial index), waveform analysis, or velocity profiles, or by anatomic measures such as angiography or duplex ultrasound scans. The ability to preoperatively assess large-vessel occlusive disease is good, whereas assessment of the relative contribution of small vessel disease is limited. The severity of ischemia (or blood flow restriction) may be a result not only of an increase in large vessel resistance or obstruction, as in atherosclerotic occlusive disease or coarctation, but also a function of the extent of small vessel involvement, as in diffuse arteritis. Unfortunately, operative intervention is generally restricted to the alleviation of large vessel involvement. The degree of success of such interventions depends on the relative contribution of the large and small vessels to the overall ischemic event.

Clinical recognition of an ischemic event occurs at a point when normal physiologic reserves are near exhaustion, even though the ischemic severity in terms of function loss is just becoming clinically apparent (Fig. 73-6). In lower extremity arterial occlusive disease, the occurrence of pain at rest versus exercise-induced claudication indicates an exhaustion of vasodilator reserve and the increased severity of the disease. The range over which tissues tolerate blood flow changes varies substantially. The skin and kidney are tolerant, whereas heart and brain function are more closely linked to blood flow.

There are many paradoxes in the study of ischemic injury (Table 73-1). None of these concepts is so difficult to accept as the concept that a substantial portion of the injury from an ischemic event occurs during reperfusion; this seemingly runs counter to the urgency of revascularization attempts in the clinical setting. That a substantial portion of injury occurs during reflow is indisputable. Similarly, the duration and severity of ischemia have easy to conceptualize relations to the ultimate outcome of an ischemic event when considered separately. The interaction between these two factors is not simple and is only beginning to be explored clinically and experimentally. For example, one might intuit that some minimal blood flow to a tissue might be less damaging than no blood flow over the same

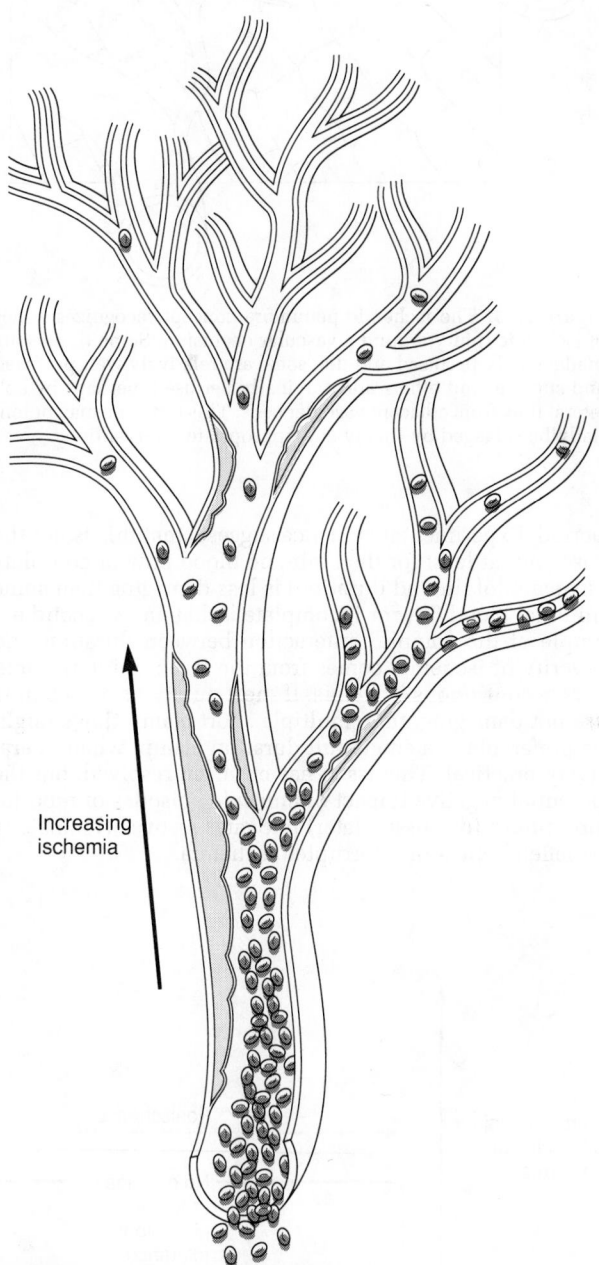

Figure 73-4. Tissues supplied by end arteries may experience watershed infarcts as the most distal tissues become ischemic. The normal decrease in perfusion pressure as one proceeds to the periphery becomes critical as a result of more proximal lesions or periods of systemic hypotension.

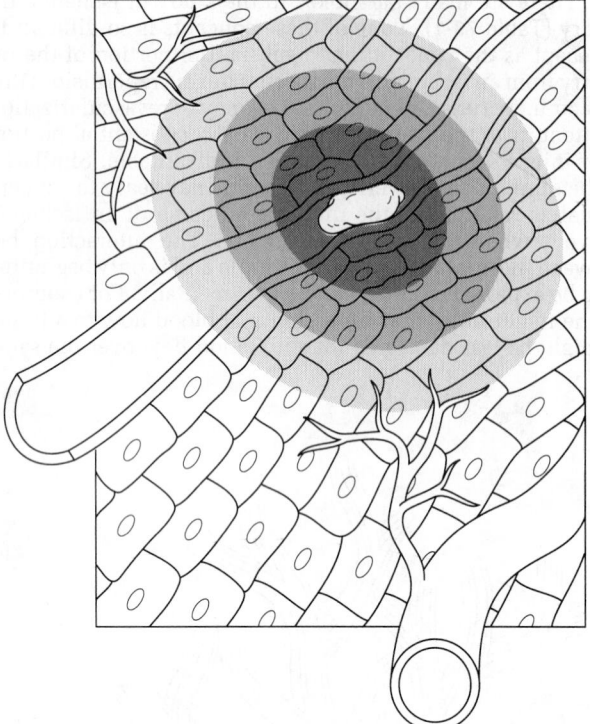

Figure 73-5. The ischemic penumbra concept recognizes zones of ischemic injury around a vascular occlusion. Some tissues are inadequately perfused and die, some are relatively well perfused and survive, and others are marginally perfused, perhaps by collateral flow from adjacent vascular beds. This last zone may potentially be salvaged by timely and appropriate interventions.

period. Experimental evidence suggests that this is not the case and, at least for the brain, no blood flow or complete ischemia (of limited duration) is less damaging than some minimal blood flow or incomplete ischemia. A second example of the complex interaction between duration and severity of ischemia comes from the issue of intermittent versus continuous ischemia. If short durations of ischemia are not damaging, then multiple short clamp times might be preferable to a single full duration clamp, when operatively practical. This issue has not been resolved, but the potential negative impact of multiple episodes of reperfusion injury (discussed later) mitigates or overwhelms any beneficial effect of interrupted ischemia.

Ischemic injury exists as a continuum, initially producing dysfunction but progressing to infarction if unrelieved (Fig. 73-7). At least part of the injury occurs during the reperfusion phase. This seeming paradox is typically ascribed to the generation of oxygen radicals, but other mechanisms may contribute as well:

- Oxygen radical formation (endothelium, white blood cells [WBCs], parenchymal cells)
- Endothelial cell swelling or intramural edema
- Platelet and leukocyte adherence
- Irretrievable loss of diffusible nucleotide bases
- ATP reformation consumes energy

Severe unrelieved ischemia always produces necrosis. Concern regarding reperfusion injury should not delay revascularization attempts. Although ischemia always involves some degree of hypoxia, hypoxia is not synonymous with, and does not produce, the same pathophysiologic sequence as ischemia.

Although ischemia is not equivalent to hypoxia, the dose or severity of ischemia can be characterized by the ratio of oxygen delivery (D_{O_2}) to oxygen consumption (V_{O_2}). The normal systemic ratio is 5:1, that is, 20% of the delivered oxygen is extracted; oxygen extraction (V_{O_2}/D_{O_2}) equals 0.2. The systemic supply of oxygen is inadequate when the ratio of delivery to consumption is 2:1 or less (Fig. 73-8). Consumption is independent of delivery until a critical or break point is reached (see Chap. 8). The point at which oxygen consumption depends on delivery defines ischemia. Systemically, supply is inadequate when the ratio is 2:1 or less, although individual organs vary widely in their ability to tolerate this ratio. Cardiac muscle normally functions at a ratio of 2:1 (implying a high extraction of available oxygen or, conversely, little reserve), and exercising skeletal muscle functions without injury for long periods of time at ratios of less than 2:1.

ENERGY FAILURE

Life depends on the ready availability of free energy. This truism underscores the importance of maintaining essential cellular processes such as membrane stability, ion gradients, electrical activity, biosynthesis, and mechanical work. All such energy-dependent processes obey the thermodynamic laws, balancing production and utilization, and are for the most part brokered through the ATP cycle. Precise regulation occurs by means of hormonal mechanisms, genetic regulation of enzyme synthesis, feedback loops of key enzymes, and factors within the cellular

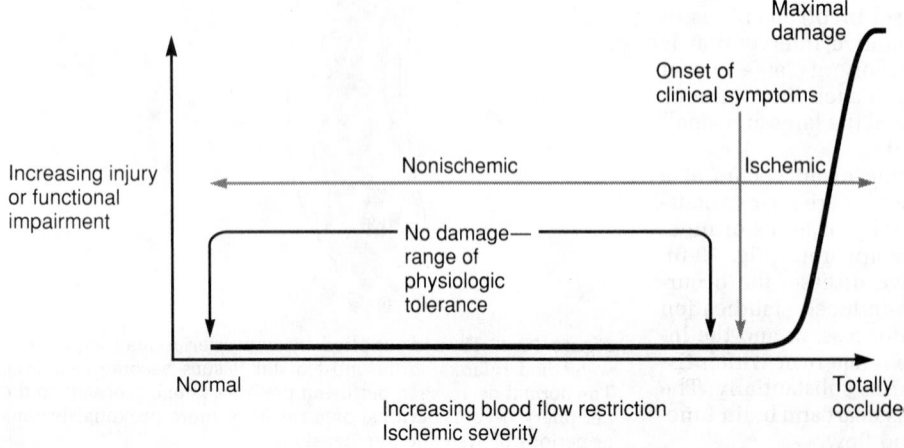

Figure 73-6. Increasing blood flow restriction is usually well tolerated until blood flow restriction becomes severe. Symptoms develop as physiologic reserves are depleted.

**Table 73-1. CLINICAL CAVEATS
AND MECHANISTIC PARADOXES
IN ISCHEMIA AND REPERFUSION**

Hypoxia ≠ ischemia.

Injury continues during reperfusion.

Concern regarding reperfusion injury should not delay prompt relief of ongoing ischemia.

Low flow may be more harmful than no flow.

Oxygen excess is harmful.

Significant reduction in cardiovascular events occurs with control of metabolic factors (ie, cholesterol and homocysteine) despite little change in anatomic severity of stenosis.

Attenuating ischemia and reperfusion injury will probably not be a "silver bullet," but rather a multifaceted approach targeted at basic mechanisms.

milieu. Although ATP is the key high-energy compound, guanine triphosphate, uracil triphosphate, cytosine triphosphate, and creatine phosphates have important roles as well.

Normoxic metabolism is a modestly efficient process. About 44% of the available energy in one molecule of glucose is captured by the coupled reactions of the glyco-

lytic pathway, Kreb cycle, and oxidative phosphorylation (Fig. 73-9, *left*). Each molecule of glucose thus metabolized produces 38 mol of ATP. Anaerobic metabolism is substantially less efficient (see Fig. 73-9, *right*). Rather than 38 mol of ATP, only a net of 2 mol is produced, a 94% reduction in the efficiency of energy production for essential cellular processes. Failure of ion pumping with rapid loss of electrochemical gradients results in translocation of ions, notably Ca^{2+}. The 10,000:1 extracellular-to-intracellular gradient is lost. Free Ca^{2+} rapidly accumulates and triggers many adverse effects including phospholipase activation. Another consequence of failed ion pumping is that intracellular Na^+ accumulates and K^+ is lost to the extracellular fluid. Cell swelling and interstitial fluid accumulation produce edema and increase diffusion distances, further compromising oxygen and substrate delivery.

As ATP degrades under hypoxic conditions, diffusible nucleotides leave the cell. An irreplaceable loss of the pool of nucleotide bases, which are the essential substrate for reforming ATP, may occur. An additional hidden energy cost is incurred when flow is restored. The process of reforming ATP from substrate costs energy, which is diverted from essential cellular processes and adds to the cells metabolic demand while attempting to recover from ischemia.

Other adverse effects of hypoxic energy metabolism are well known.[10,11] The conversion of xanthine dehydroge-

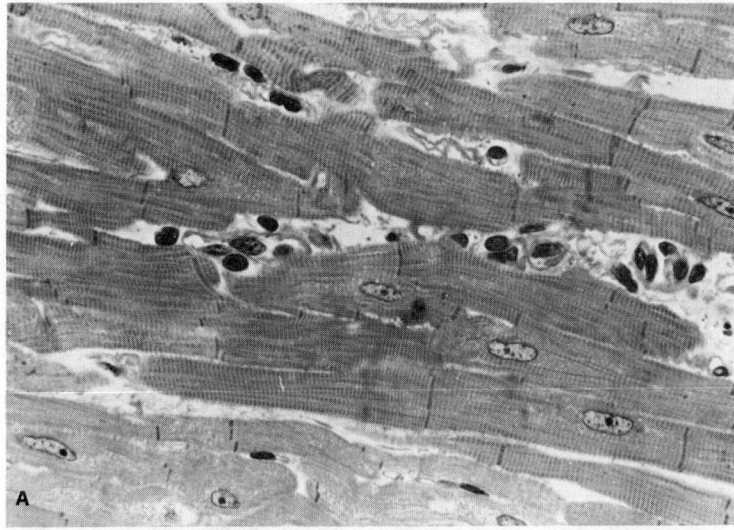

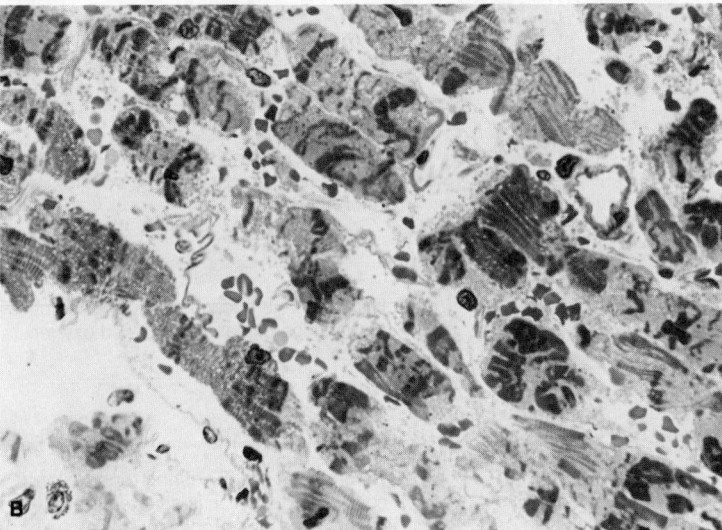

Figure 73-7. (*A*) Photomicrograph of normal myocardial tissue showing intact myocytes with intercollated disks, prominent myocyte cross-striations, and intact myocyte nuclei with nucleoli (×880). (*B*) Photomicrograph of myocardial tissue after ischemia (40 minutes) and reperfusion (4 hours). There is marked disruption of myocardial sarcolemma, prominent contraction bands within myocytes, loss of myocyte nuclei, and hemorrhage (×880). (Courtesy of Joseph C. Fantone, MD, Department of Pathology, University of Michigan, Ann Arbor)

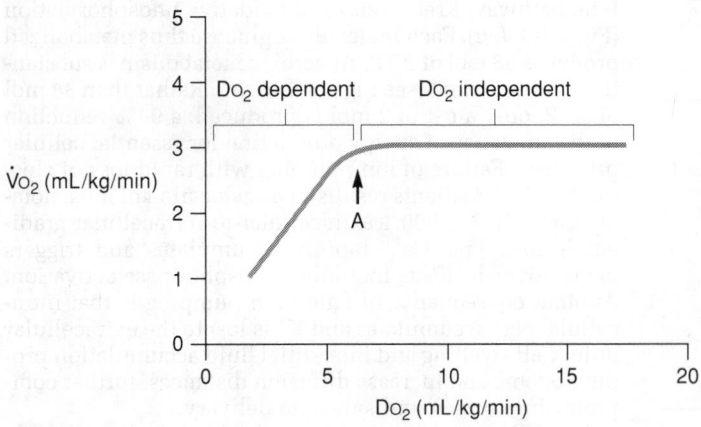

Figure 73-8. The point at which oxygen consumption depends on delivery characterizes ischemia.

nase (XD) to xanthine oxygenase (XO) catalyzes the degradation of hypoxanthine to xanthine and xanthine to uric acid. These are classic reactions for the generation of superoxide anion (O_2^{+-}) and other toxic oxygen species. Further, the accumulation of NADH and NADPH in conjunction with the ready availability of iron facilitates the initiation reactions for producing toxic oxygen species. The clinical and experimental parallel, whereby low-flow ischemia (trickle flow) is more damaging than no-flow ischemia (absolute ischemia), and the seemingly paradoxical finding that a significant portion of an ischemic injury is incurred during reperfusion can be at least partially ex-

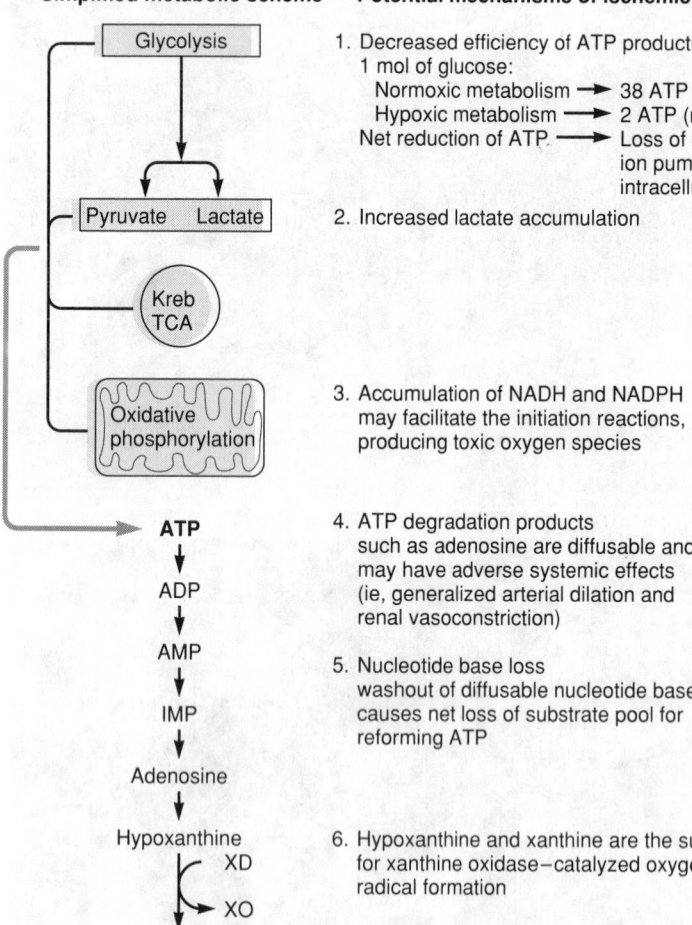

Figure 73-9. (*Left*) Metabolism under normoxic conditions is reasonably efficient. Almost half of the available energy in a molecule of glucose is captured by glycolysis, Krebs cycle, and oxidative phosphorylation, producing 38 mol of ATP. (*Right*) Ischemic metabolism has multiple potential mechanisms to produce cellular, tissue, and organ injury.

plained on the basis of enhanced energy needs to replete a dissipated adenine nucleotide pool. In this regard, it is the total pool of adenine nucleotides, rather than simple measure of ATP or ADP, that is important.

Glucose has a dominant role in normal cellular energy metabolism and is the most thoroughly studied metabolic fuel. Protein and ketone metabolism as substrates for energy production under physiologic and pathologic conditions are less well studied. As the ability to assess systemic energy balance and regional variations increases and experimental evidence identifies a potential role for ketones in hypoxic metabolism, attention is drawn to the potential for a multifuel cellular economy. One substrate may be advantageous (or disadvantageous) under specific circumstances. When considering aerobic versus anaerobic metabolism, we tend inappropriately to restrict our thinking to glucose metabolism and the absolutes of normoxia and anoxia. Absolute anoxia (the total absence of oxygen) is a chemical laboratory phenomenon and is rarely encountered clinically. Likewise, the singular dependence on glucose as a carbon source is an experimental expedient and virtually never occurs clinically. Ketones and to a lesser extent proteins are metabolized for energy whenever they are available to the cell. Thus, when one is considering energy failure as a component of ischemia, the carbon source as well as the oxygen availability needs to be considered. Various substrates markedly influence an organ's ability to tolerate an ischemic insult. Continued or enhanced glucose use adversely affects the outcome in multiple models of CNS, spinal cord, and kidney ischemia.[1–5,12] Provision of alternate substrate (ketone) is beneficial in the experimental setting.[6] The omission of dextrose from resuscitation protocols seems beneficial in experimental models of pure hypoxia, hypoxia and relative ischemia, localized forebrain ischemia, and the global ischemia that accompanies circulatory arrest. Additional experimental work indicates a protective effect for 2-deoxyglucose, a competitive inhibitor of glucose uptake and metabolism (hexokinase) and insulin-induced mild hypoglycemia in neural tissues.[7,8,13,14] The insulin-induced hypoglycemic protective effect is not apparent with renal ischemia models.[9]

PARENCHYMAL CELL INJURY

Hypoxic metabolism is not just inefficient. If allowed to continue it is, in and of itself, injurious. Direct parenchymal cell injury occurs as a result of the ischemic insult. The accumulation of lactic acid has many potentially adverse effects; at levels of 16 to 20 μmol, it may produce a direct injury to organelles. Lesser degrees of lactic acid accumulation with resultant pH changes significantly alter crucial enzyme activity and the shape and configuration of macromolecules. Lactic acid enhances cytokine production by activated macrophages.[15] Increased tumor necrosis factor secretion occurs at lactic acid levels of 5 to 15 μmol, and this effect seems to result from enhanced gene transcription. Whether such increased secretion is a local paracrine effect contributing to angiogenesis and other reparative steps or an endocrine (systemic) effect potentially causing adverse systemic effects has not been determined.

The failure of essential energy-requiring cellular functions produces an inability to maintain ionic gradients and results in cell swelling, increased diffusion distances, and, ultimately, disruption of cell membranes. Leakage of enzymes and other vital components and the continued drop in pH cause important structural and functional changes. Release of proteases, lipases, and other autolytic enzymes cause further irreparable damage. Unmaintained ionic gradients also result in the local accumulation of calcium. The

precise compartmentalization of intracellular Ca^{2+} and the 10^4 extracellular to intracellular gradient is lost, allowing large increases in free intracellular Ca^{2+} (Fig. 73-10). Calcium is an important trigger for phospholipase-catalyzed phospholipid degradation. The essential structure of cellular membranes is thus under direct attack. In addition to loss of essential cell structure and release of autolytic enzymes, membrane disruption releases arachidonic acid and activates secondary cascades such as prostaglandin, thromboxane, and the eicosanoids (Fig. 73-11).

Parenchymal cell injury in ischemia is known to depend on tissue temperature. From cold water drowning to hypothermic cardiac arrest, reports of the salutary effects of profound hypothermia (0 to 15C) in ischemia abound. Such profound cooling has relevance to organ preservation for transplantation or to total circulatory arrest during the repair of complex cardiovascular defects, but it has little applicability to naturally occurring ischemic events or most operations. More sophisticated assessments of cellular energy balance and its role in cell damage have prompted a more precise look at the issue of temperature effects in the setting of ischemia. Even slight reductions in tissue temperature (1 to 2C) can have profound protective effects on the extent of damage to an ischemic tissue. Moderate local cooling can be accomplished without incurring myocardial irritability or compromising hemostasis, thus offering a nonspecific and safe approach to attenuating intraoperative ischemic injury.

The precise cellular origin of the damaging agents in

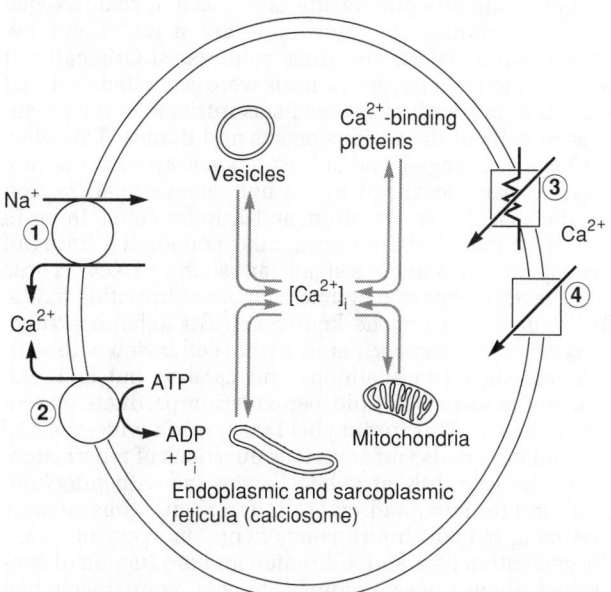

Figure 73-10. The extracellular-to-intracellular Ca^{2+} gradient is approximately 10^4 and is highly regulated (extracellular $[Ca^{2+}]$ is approximately 10^{-3} mol, whereas the intracellular free $[Ca^{2+}]$ is approximately 10^{-7} mol). Calcium can leave cells against this large gradient by Na^+-Ca^{2+} exchange energized by the Na^+ gradient established by the Na^+-K^+-ATPase pump (1). Ca^{2+} can also leave by means of Ca^{2+} ATPases located at the plasma membrane (2). Ca^{2+} can enter cells through voltage-dependent (3) or voltage-independent pathways (4). Within the cell, free Ca^{2+} can exchange with Ca^{2+} in vesicles, endoplasmic and sarcoplasmic reticula, or mitochondria. In addition, dynamic equilibrium exists between free Ca^{2+} and Ca^{2+} associated with Ca^{2+}-binding proteins in the cytosol and intracellular membrane compartments. (After Bonventre JV. Calcium. In: Zelenock GB, ed. Clinical ischemic syndromes mechanisms and consequences of tissue injury. St Louis, CV Mosby, 1990)

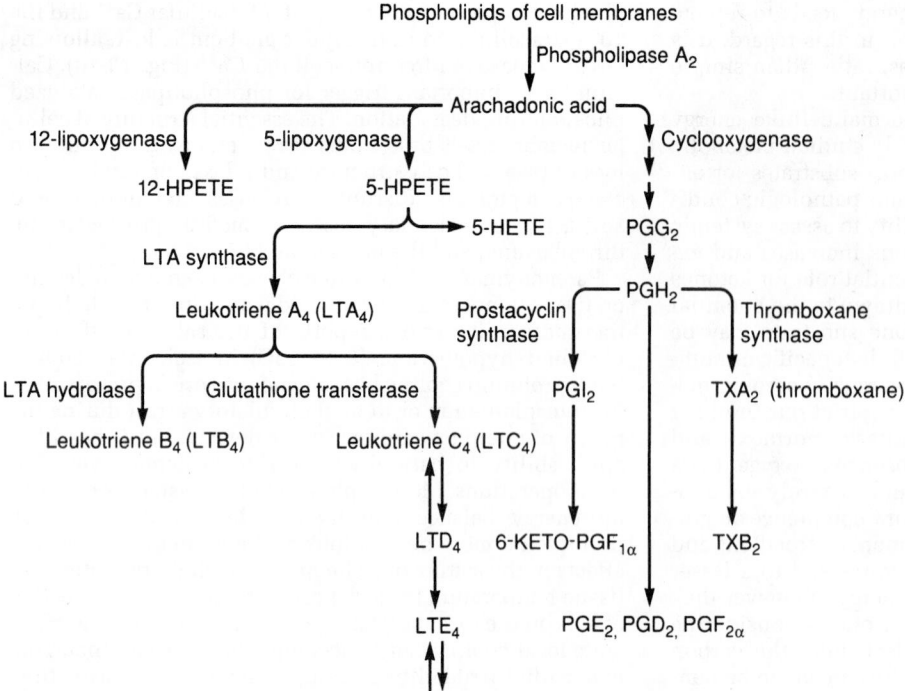

Figure 73-11. Phospholipase activation causes phospholipid degradation and triggers arachidonic acid metabolite cascades.

ischemia and reperfusion is not clearly defined. Lipid peroxidation and other direct effects induced by toxic oxygen species, including the superoxide anion ($O_2^{\bullet-}$) and hydroxyl radical ($\bullet OH$) are prime candidates. Originally, it was assumed that oxygen radicals were generated by direct activation of injurious mechanisms intrinsic to the parenchymal cells of the various organs and tissues. This view has been challenged, and at least in some systems the process has been localized to the nonparenchymal fraction (ie, the vascular endothelium and Kupffer cells). In an in vivo liver model, the microvascular endothelial lining of the hepatic sinusoids is a significant source of XO.[16] These cells have the enzyme system capable of initiating oxidative damage but not the known cellular defense system. By contrast, the hepatic parenchymal cell is rich with antioxidants such as glutathione and catalase but does not generate evidence of lipid peroxidation products (conjugated dienes). This finding held true over a wide range of ischemic intervals and at various durations of reperfusion. It was also true with intact hepatocytes and with mitochondrial, microsomal, and cytosolic fragments, thus reliably localizing oxidant injury components. In every instance, the generation of superoxide anion and production of conjugated dienes was confined to the nonparenchymal fraction.

ENDOTHELIAL INJURY

In many organs, the tissue most susceptible to an ischemic insult is the organ's vasculature, specifically the endothelial tissue.[16] An ischemic stress that causes only a limited injury to the parenchymal cell may greatly injure the endothelium and smooth muscle of the associated vasculature. In this regard, the endothelium and its interaction with formed elements in the blood are major factors contributing to ischemic injury (Fig. 73-12). Activated platelets and WBCs may adhere to vascular endothelium, causing release of cytokines, procoagulants, proteases, oxygen radicals, lysosomal enzymes, and arachidonic acid deriva-

tives. The exposure of highly thrombogenic subendothelial material such as collagen results in enhanced accumulation of platelets and, subsequently, other formed elements in the blood. WBCs are particularly noteworthy with regard to localized destruction and amplification of injury. Aside from direct injurious effects, adherence of granulocytes in the microcirculation in association with swelling of the endothelial and smooth muscle cells of the vessel wall cause obstruction and luminal narrowing, which may significantly impede postischemic blood flow after an ischemic injury. After ischemia, an initial hyperemia typically is replaced by a prolonged period of limited blood flow, often to 20% of baseline values. This no-reflow phenomenon is associated with a markedly increased number of WBCs adherent to the luminal surface of the microcirculation. The luminal compromise due to swelling and granulocyte adherence in turn increases the ischemic stress to the parenchymal cell.

An additional means by which endothelial vascular injury produces parenchymal cell injury is altered production of products produced by normal endothelial cells. Increased parenchymal cell injury would be expected to result from decreased PGI_2 production or enhanced production of thromboxane, procoagulants, or intercellular adherence molecules. The recognition of vascular endothelium as an important and active physiologic tissue rather than a simple thromboresistant lining for distributing conduits is important.[17] Many complex interactions between endothelial cells and blood elements occur. Release of biologically active compounds including tissue plasminogen activator, heparin sulfate, fibronectin, interleukin-1, prostacyclin, endothelial-derived relaxing factor—nitric acid, endothelin-1, and other small molecules occurs in response to physiologic or pathologic stimuli. Several of these molecules may be important in conditions as diverse as hypertension, diabetes, atherosclerosis, endotoxin shock, and subarachnoid hemorrhage, as well as in ischemia and reperfusion.

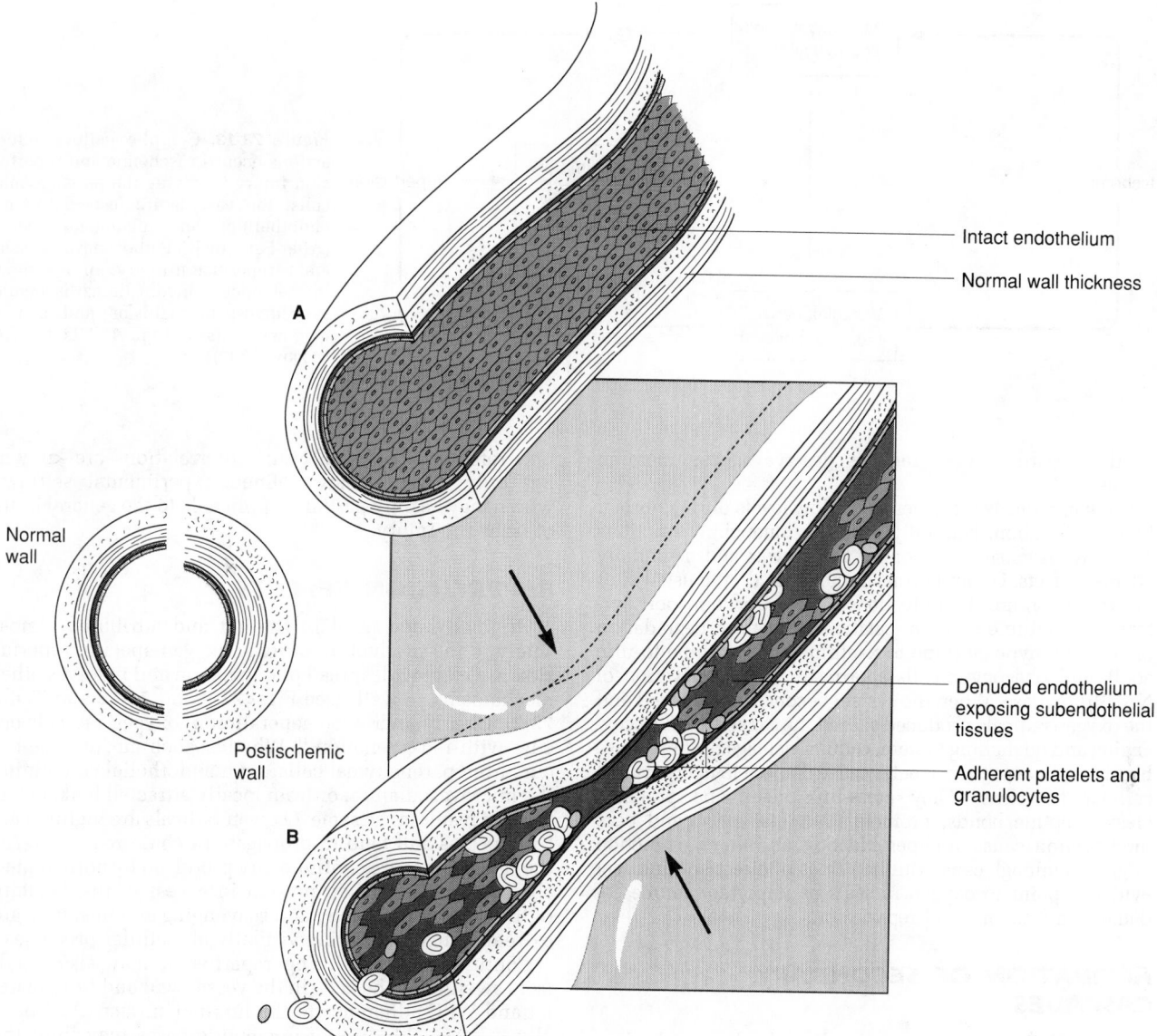

Figure 73-12. (*A*) Normal blood vessel showing normal diameter and wall thickness. The endothelium is intact, produces normal quantities and types of mediators, and resists adherence by granulocytes and platelets. (*B*) Postischemic blood vessel exhibits reduced luminal diameter and increased wall thickness as a result of intramural cell swelling and edema. Sloughing of endothelial cells exposes highly thrombogenic subendothelial tissues, especially collagen. Denuded or injured endothelium results in altered production of mediators with potential adverse effects (ie, loss of PGI_2 and HO and enhanced production of thromboxane A_2 and procoagulants). Granulocyte and platelet adherence result in luminal plugging, reduced flow, and continued injury. Injury to the parenchymal tissues enveloping the blood vessels produces extrinsic compression and reduced flow, exacerbating the original injury.

INFLAMMATORY SYSTEMS

After the initial ischemic insult and resultant metabolic failure with the injury to the parenchymal cell and vascular endothelium, the soluble and cellular inflammatory systems are activated. A number of empirical studies in diverse experimental models have demonstrated attenuation of ischemic damage with antiinflammatory drugs.[18-20] The roles of adherence molecules, chemoattractants, and other mediators that amplify or attenuate this complex process have not been fully defined[21] (Fig. 73-13; see Chaps. 5 and 6). The cellular inflammatory system activated by the ischemic process re-

sults in WBC accumulation and adherence to vascular endothelium. Migration of the cells through the vasculature into the parenchymal matrix and release of proteases, reactive oxygen metabolites, interleukin-1, tumor necrosis factor, and other active mediators results in continued destruction. Originally viewed solely as protection from infecting microorganisms or as a focused mechanism for the removal of injured cells, WBCs are involved in many abnormal processes and are a significant source of toxic oxygen species and cytokines. Removing injured cells, the physiologic function, can be escalated to a more widespread, less controlled effect and thus also contribute to the overall parenchymal injury.

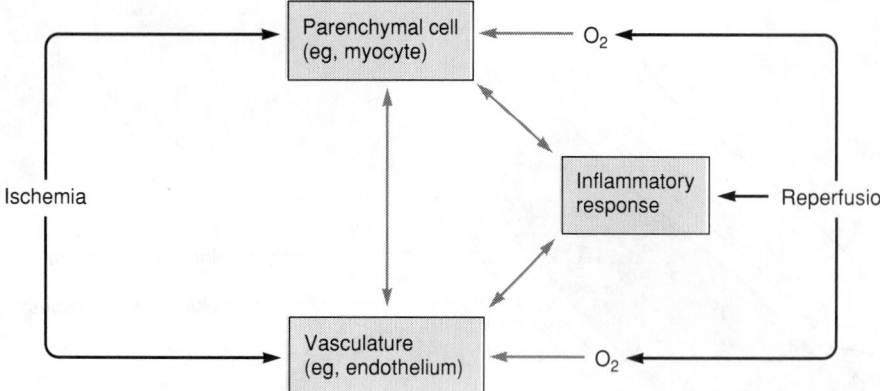

Figure 73-13. Complex cellular interactions occur in ischemia and reperfusion injury involving the parenchymal cells, the vasculature (especially the endothelium), and inflammatory cells. (After Fantone JC. Pathogenesis of ischemia–reperfusion injury: an overview. In: Zelenock GB, ed. Clinical ischemic syndromes: mechanisms and consequences of tissue injury. St Louis, CV Mosby, 1990)

In this regard, oxygen radicals deserve special mention (Table 73-2).

Oxygen radicals are generated at low levels during normal biologic function. Naturally occurring quenching reactions and scavengers serve to control their levels and potentially adverse effects. Under normal circumstances, the usual sites of production are the mitochondrial electron transport system, the xanthine oxidase–catalyzed advanced degradation of ATP (ie, hypoxanthine to xanthine and xanthine to uric acid), and phagocytic cells as a result of the activation of NADPH oxidase. When the system becomes unbalanced and the oxygen radicals produced exceed the capacity of the scavenging and quenching system, cellular damage occurs. These highly reactive oxygen species cause damage to many crucial cellular functions. They cross-link membrane proteins, cleave peptide bonds, promote DNA disruption and base modification, cause lipid peroxidation, and alter the function of glycosaminoglycans. Multiple lines of direct and indirect evidence point to oxygen radicals as important sources of damage in ischemia and reperfusion.

ACTIVATION OF SECONDARY CASCADES

Interactions between the parenchymal cell, vascular (endothelial) cells, and inflammatory cells are increasingly appreciated (see Fig. 73-13). Membrane disruption secondary to phospholipase A_2 activation causes release of arachidonic acid. Subsequent metabolism can produce prostacyclin, thromboxanes, and eicosanoids (see Fig. 73-11). Each of these products has a host of biologically important actions.

In the ischemic environment, the normally fine balance between prostacyclin and thromboxane effects is disrupted. Enhanced production of thromboxane produces vasoconstriction and platelet adherence, favoring continued ischemic injury. Thromboxane A_2 (TXA_2) is also strongly implicated in the systemic and remote effects of lower torso ischemia, particularly the noncardiogenic pulmonary edema that attends aortic reconstruction.[22] This effect of TXA_2 may be initiated by leukotriene B_4 or other mechanisms. It requires WBCs but not complement.[23–25] The coagulation cascade (see Chaps. 4 and 70) is locally activated by exposure of collagen after desquamation of endothelial cells, causing platelet adherence and activation and, by release of tissue factor from injured cells, activating the extrinsic pathway. The inflammatory system's activation (see Chap. 6) and dual involvement as a physiologic and pathologic component of injury is a subject of intense investigation. Precise triggers for activation of complement and WBCs and for immunoglobulin forma-

tion remain ill defined. Many interrelations are known, but only in rigorously defined experimental settings, which may be only partially applicable to the general issue of ischemic injury.

REPERFUSION EFFECTS

Originally described in the gut and attributed almost solely to the production of toxic oxygen species, reperfusion is a more widespread phenomenon and involves other mechanisms as well[1] (see Figs. 73-9 and 73-12 and Table 73-2). Clearly, increased generation of oxygen radicals occurs with reoxygenation.[10] Whether such an increase occurs from parenchymal cells, from endothelial cells lining the microvasculature, or from locally attracted leukocytes, the end result is the same. Oxygen radicals are highly reactive species and tend to propagate in chain reactions. Although radicals are continuously produced by normal metabolic processes, when present in excess of the capacity of the normal quenching and scavenging systems, they are extremely toxic, affecting virtually all cellular processes.

Continued injury during reperfusion may also result from swelling of the cells in the vessel wall and from platelet and WBC adherence to the luminal surface. Additionally, irretrievable loss of nucleotide bases may limit the supply of substrate for ATP reformation. Finally, ATP reformation is an energy-consuming process. At a time when energy stores are critically low, reformation of ATP store competes for available energy with vital cellular processes.

REMOTE OR SYSTEMIC EFFECTS OF ISCHEMIA

For years, the toxic effects of a profound ischemic event involving an extremity or the gut were known to have adverse systemic effects. The experienced clinician recognized and anticipated these effects and adapted management strategies to cope with them when they occurred. This clinical knowledge was at best qualitative and lacked precise mechanistic understanding. At times, the damage appeared organ specific. An elusive myocardial depressant factor was believed to result from gut ischemia. Aortic surgery with lower torso ischemia is associated with renal failure and pulmonary dysfunction, and profound skeletal muscle ischemia with rhabdomyolysis such as occurs in the crush syndrome or with delayed treatment of a thrombosis or embolus regularly produces oliguria and uremia. Understanding the effect of ischemia on remote organ function involves specific mediators. A series of experimental and clinical studies have linked TXA_2 and WBC-mediated pulmonary injury to hind limb and lower torso isch-

Table 73-2. ISCHEMIA AND REPERFUSION, FREE RADICALS, AND TOXIC OXYGEN SPECIES

1. Free radical is any species capable of independent existence that contains one or more unpaired electrons (electrons normally associate in pairs and move in precise relations around the nucleus).
2. Free radical reactions tend to proceed as chain reactions; when reacting with nonradicals (giving up the unpaired electron, removing an electron from the nonradical species, or combining with a nonradical), this still results in an unpaired electron (ie, a radical).
3. Radicals may be involved in biologic processes in addition to ischemia and reperfusion: autoimmune or inflammatory reactions, cancer, heavy metal overload, brain and CNS disorders, vitamin E deficiency, AIDS, eye disorders (retrolental fibroplasia, cataracts, posthemorrhage visual deteriorations), and exposure to various toxins (ozone, asbestos, cigarette smoke).
4. Radicals may have physiologic or beneficial effects.
   NO$^{\bullet}$ relaxes vascular smooth muscle, resulting in vasodilation
   $O_2^{\bullet-}$ participates in the killing and disposal of unwanted material by phagocytes; may serve as a growth regulator; may react with NO$^{\bullet}$ to produce nonradical products and oppose vasodilation
5. Radicals may be formed under physiologic or pathologic circumstances and have a variety of sources.
   Reactive oxygen metabolites

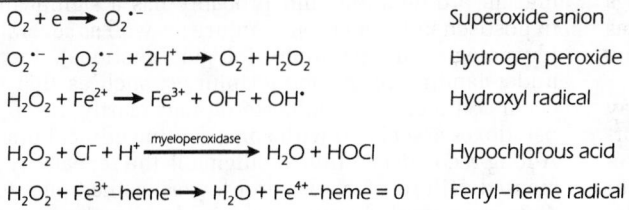

$O_2 + e \rightarrow O_2^{\bullet-}$	Superoxide anion
$O_2^{\bullet-} + O_2^{\bullet-} + 2H^+ \rightarrow O_2 + H_2O_2$	Hydrogen peroxide
$H_2O_2 + Fe^{2+} \rightarrow Fe^{3+} + OH^- + OH^{\bullet}$	Hydroxyl radical
$H_2O_2 + Cl^- + H^+ \xrightarrow{\text{myeloperoxidase}} H_2O + HOCl$	Hypochlorous acid
$H_2O_2 + Fe^{3+}\text{-heme} \rightarrow H_2O + Fe^{4+}\text{-heme} = 0$	Ferryl–heme radical

Sources of reactive oxygen species during reperfusion

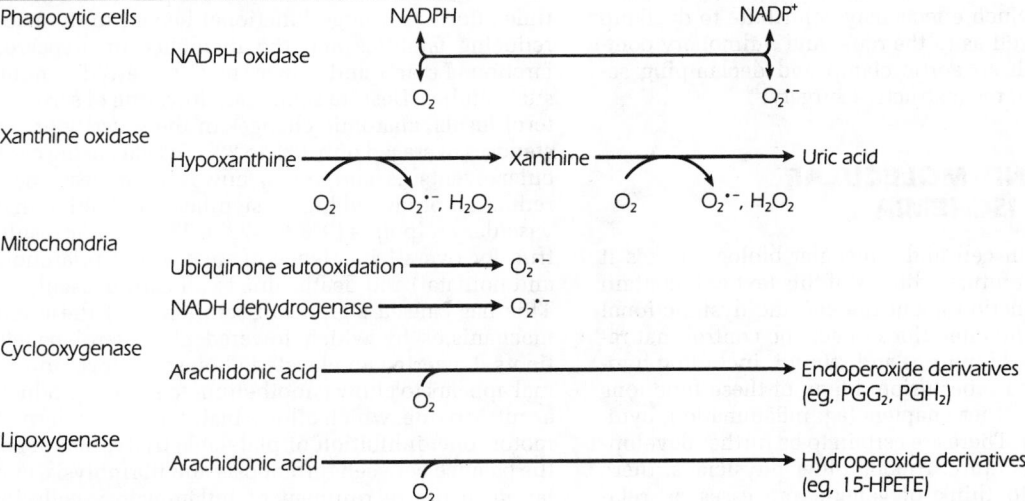

Phagocytic cells

Xanthine oxidase

Mitochondria

Cyclooxygenase

Lipoxygenase

6. Antioxidant defenses:
   Antioxidant enzymes

   $O_2^{\bullet-} + O_2^{\bullet-} + 2H^+ \xrightarrow{\text{superoxide dismutase}} O_2 + H_2O_2$

   $2H_2O_2 \xrightarrow{\text{catalase}} 2H_2O + O_2$

   $H_2O_2 + 2GSH \xrightarrow{\text{glutathione peroxidase}} 2H_2O + GSSG$

   $ROOH + 2GSH \longrightarrow ROH + GSSG + H_2O$

   Minimization of amount of free metal ions (ie, iron and copper)
   Transferrin
   Ferritin
   Ceruloplasmin
   Desferrioxamine
   Antioxidant and quenching reactions
   α-Tocopherol (lipid soluble)
   β-Carotene
   Phytofluene
   Lycopene
   Ascorbic acid
7. Adverse effects of radicals and toxic oxygen species:
   Alter the function of certain enzymes and structural proteins, depolymerization, cleavage of peptide bonds, intramolecular and intermolecular cross-linking of membrane proteins
   Glycosaminoglycan oxidation
   Promote DNA scission and base modifications
   Promote lipid peroxidation

(Modified from Fantone JC. Pathogenesis of ischemia-reperfusion injury: an overview. In: Zelenock GB, ed. Clinical ischemic syndrome: mechanisms and consequences of tissue injury. St. Louis, CV Mosby, 1990; and Halliwell B. Lipid peroxidation, free radical reactions, and human disease. In: Current concepts. Kalamazoo, Upjohn, 1991)

emia.[22-25] One study identified noncardiogenic interstitial pulmonary edema on chest radiograph, an increase in physiologic shunting (9%±2% to 16%±2%), and an increase in peak inspiratory pressure (23±2 cm H_2O to 33±2 cm H_2O) in patients undergoing abdominal aortic aneurysm repair.[22] The operations required infrarenal and suprarenal aortic clamping ranging from 76±27 minutes to 118±25 minutes. These findings were correlated with an increase in TXA_2 generation (measured as TXB_2, its stable metabolite). The increased generation of TXA_2 began with the application of the aortic clamp; however, there was not a significant clamp-associated increase in prostacyclin (measured as 6-keto-PGF_{1a}). Experimental studies in dogs and sheep indicated the change in pulmonary status was WBC dependent and mediated by TXA_2 and leukotriene B_4.[23-25] Complement appeared not to be involved.

Other mechanisms known to occur with ischemia may have adverse systemic effects or compromise the performance of distant organs. As ATP degrades, adenosine release may contribute to systemic hypotension, since in most vascular beds it is a potent vasodilator. Conversely, adenosine is known to cause renal and pulmonary vascular vasoconstriction. Such effects may contribute to declamp hypotension, as well as to the renal and pulmonary compromise seen with an aortic clamp and declamping sequence as in aortic reconstructive surgery.[26]

CELLULAR AND MOLECULAR ASPECTS OF ISCHEMIA

The explosion in cell and molecular biology makes it almost certain that future editions of this text will contain a wealth of information about the specific dysfunctional molecular states and alterations in genetic control that result from a variety of injuries and stimuli, including hypoxia, ischemia, and reperfusion. Many of these functions are touched on in other chapters (eg, inflammation, cytokines, hemostasis). There are certain to be further developments in the near future. Among older physicians, there is a temptation to think of genetic processes as relatively stable and static long-term processes. Evolutionary changes occurring over eons, growth and development occurring over a lifetime, and adaptations to chronic changes in the environment occurring over days to years are clear examples. The recognition that genetic control has both an extremely stable, well-preserved component and an active adaptive role in minute to minute homeostasis makes its vulnerability to hypoxia and ischemia a subject of intense study.

The complex interactions of the nervous system and the endocrine, metabolic, and molecular response to stress have recently been reviewed and summarized by Udelsman and Holbrook.[27] Hypoxia, ischemia-reperfusion sequences and surgical stress activate the hypothalamic-pituitary-adrenal axis, the sympathetic nervous system, and acute-phase reactants. Following activation, the latter three modulate gene expression by formation of transcription factors that interact with certain DNA sequences, affecting the rate of transcription and production of the complementary mRNA. Altered transcription ultimately results in variable production of protein effectors. Transcription factors are themselves proteins and therefore are encoded by genes and also are subject to regulatory processes. Some transcription factors are constitutively expressed, some are inducible, and some accelerate and some inhibit transcription. Multiple transcription factors exist, including heat-shock transcription factor, which is produced by vascular smooth muscle cells in response to several stresses, including shock and ischemia-reperfusion sequences. By altering production of protein effectors, the most basic of cell functions are affected. Several other examples that illustrate the increasingly sophisticated understanding of the basic pathophysiologic mechanisms of ischemic injury and are of importance to clinicians follow.

In most instances, atherosclerosis is the entity that causes ischemic events, and its effects on endothelial function have been aggressively studied. Nitric oxide produced by intact endothelial cells has an integral role in the maintenance of vessel wall smooth muscle vasodilator tone.[28] Nitrous oxide also plays a part in hypertension, is suspected to be important in intimal hyperplasia and smooth muscle proliferation, and probably has a significant role in postischemic reperfusion injury (as well as several other physiologic and pathophysiologic functions). Increased understanding of metabolic injuries, such as that which occurs with elevated cholesterol, may clarify the apparent paradoxes associated with some routine clinical practices. A long-recognized clinical enigma is the repeatedly documented failure of cholesterol-lowering therapies to produce measurable improvement in the severity of stenoses that result from atherosclerotic plaques while at the same time affording a large functional benefit to the patient by reducing fatalities and the incidence of myocardial infarction. Levine and coworkers[29] reviewed a number of such studies. Despite significant lowering of serum cholesterol levels, anatomic changes in the severity of coronary stenoses averaged only 0% to 2%. In trials using cardiovascular events as endpoints, however, modest cholesterol reduction produced highly significant reduction in cardiovascular endpoints (9% to 47%). These latter results hold true for overall incidence of myocardial infarction (fatal and nonfatal) and deaths due to all cardiovascular causes. This has caused significant rethinking of the underlying mechanisms by which lowered cholesterol benefits patients. Lowering an elevated cholesterol level toward normal appears to allow endothelium to secrete products such as nitric oxide, which allows maintenance of normal vasomotor tone, inhibition of platelet activity, maintenance of the balance between thrombosis and fibrinolysis, and regulation of the recruitment of inflammatory cells into the vascular wall. The paradoxical vasoconstriction which occurs with the infusion of acetyl choline in "diseased coronary arteries" is eliminated and returned towards the normal vasodilator response after treatment of hypercholesterolemia. Lowering cholesterol may result in a lesser degree of plaque activation as a process by which a stable atherosclerotic plaque undergoes degeneration and precipitates thrombosis.

Elevated plasma homocysteine has been correlated with arteriosclerotic vascular disease for a number of years. Such elevated homocysteine levels are believed to account for a substantial portion of the vascular disease in the United States. The relation seems consistent for cerebrovascular disease, peripheral vascular occlusive disease, and coronary artery disease. Elevated homocysteine impairs the production of endothelial-derived relaxing factor, stimulates the proliferation of smooth muscle cells and has a prothrombotic effect by changing the expression of thrombomodulin and the activation of protein C. More intriguing, the elevated homocysteine levels can be reduced toward or to normal, simply by provision of folate, vitamins B_{12} and B_6. Somewhat complicating the matter is an inability to agree on the precise definition of an elevated homocysteine concentration, but in all studies, the patients with homocysteine levels in the upper percentiles had increased risks of cardiovascular events. Given the common occurrence of elevated homocysteine levels, a strong correlation with functional outcomes and a plausible pathophysiologic mechanism and relatively benign therapy (ie, the provision of vitamins, a compelling case for prospective clinical trials has been made).[30]

A greatly enhanced understanding of the mechanisms of ischemic injury and the interrelations between the various elements of the many physiologic systems has occurred. Therapeutic strategies for ischemia targeted at the underlying pathophysiology are being devised. Pretreatment to lessen ischemic damage is relevant to surgeons who must clamp blood vessels or interrupt the blood flow to a tissue or organ during their reconstructive procedures. Likewise, pretreatment protocols have significant potential in transplantation and organ preservation. Treatment during or after an ischemic event is more difficult, but potentially of even greater benefit, since most spontaneously occurring ischemic events present as emergencies with little or no warning. The ability to attenuate an ischemic injury or retard its progression is of benefit, because even if the initial therapy only slows the progression of injury or temporarily stabilizes a precarious episode of critical ischemia, it may allow time for diagnostic studies and preparation for more conventional interventions. A note of caution is in order. It is highly unlikely that a single pharmacologic intervention will prove effective or be applicable in all clinical settings. Rather, interventions targeted at several points in the ischemic cascade and focused on the various mechanisms of ischemic injury will be more likely to succeed. Although the clinical problem of brain or heart ischemia may seem to have little to do with acute tubular necrosis or a lower extremity embolus, there are many common pathophysiologic mechanisms.

REFERENCES

1. Zelenock GB, D'Alecy LG, Fantone JC III, Shlafer M, Stanley JC, eds. Clinical ischemic syndromes: mechanism and consequences of tissue injury. St Louis, CV Mosby, 1990.
2. D'Alecy LG, Lundy EF, Barton KJ, Zelenock GB. Dextrose-containing intravenous fluid impairs outcome and increases mortality after eight minutes of cardiac arrest/resuscitation in dogs. Surgery 1986;100:505.
3. Lundy EF, Kuhn JE, Kwon JM, Zelenock GB, D'Alecy LG. Infusion of five percent dextrose increases mortality and morbidity following six minutes of cardiac arrest in resuscitated dog. J Crit Care 1987;2:4.
4. Lundy EF, Ball TD, Mandell MA, Zelenock GB, D'Alecy LG. Dextrose administration increases sensory/motor impairment and paraplegia after infrarenal aortic occlusion in the rabbit. Surgery 1987;102:737.
5. LeMay DR, Neal S, Zelenock GB, D'Alecy LG. Paraplegia in the rat induced by aortic cross clamping: model characterization and glucose exacerbation of neurological deficit. J Vasc Surg 1987;6:383.
6. Lundy EF, Dykstra J, Luyckx B, Zelenock GB, D'Alecy LG. Reduction of neurologic deficit by 1,3-butanediol–induced ketosis in levine rats. Stroke 1985;16:855.
7. LeMay DR, Lu A, Zelenock GB, D'Alecy LG. Insulin protects from paraplegia in the rat aortic occlusion model. J Surg Res 1988;44:352.
8. LeMay DR, Gehua L, Zelenock GB, D'Alecy LG. Insulin administration protects neurologic function in cerebral ischemia in rats. Stroke 1988;19:1411.
9. Podrazik RM, Natale JE, Zelenock GB, D'Alecy LG. Hyperglycemia exacerbates and insulin fails to protect in acute renal ischemia in the rat. J Surg Res 1989;46:572.
10. McCord JM. Oxygen derived free radicals in postischemic tissue injury. N Engl J Med 1985;312:159.
11. Fantone JC, Ward PA. Oxygen-derived radicals and their metabolites: relationship to tissue injury. Kalamazoo, UpJohn, 1985.
12. Moursi MM, Rising CL, Zelenock GB, D'Alecy LG. Dextrose exacerbates acute renal ischemic damage in anesthetized dogs. Arch Surg 1987;122:790.
13. Combs DJ, Reuland DS, Martin DB, Zelenock GB, D'Alecy LG. Glycolytic inhibition by 2-deoxyglucose reduces hyperglycemia-associated mortality and morbidity in the ischemic rat. Stroke 1986;17:989.
14. LeMay DR, Zelenock GB, D'Alecy LG. The role of glucose uptake and metabolism in hyperglycemic exacerbation of the neurologic deficit in the paraplegic rat. J Neurosurg 1989;71:594-.
15. Jensen JC, Buresh C, Norton JA. Lactic acidosis increases tumor necrosis factor secretion and transcription in vitro. J Surg Res 1990;49:350.
16. Walsh TR, Rao PN, Makowka L, Starzl TE. Lipid peroxidation is a nonparenchymal cell event with reperfusion after prolonged liver ischemia. J Surg Res 1990;49:18.
17. Vane JR, Anggard EE, Botting RM. Regulatory functions of the vascular endothelium. N Engl J Med 1990;323:27.
18. Ball TD, Lundy EF, Zelenock GB, D'Alecy LG. Effects of Iodoxamide tromethamine on paraplegia that occurs after infrarenal aortic occlusion in the rabbit. J Vasc Surg 1987;6:572.
19. Kuhn JE, Steimle CN, Zelenock GB, D'Alecy LG. Ibuprofen improves survival and neurologic outcome after resuscitation from cardiac arrest. Resuscitation 1986;14:199.
20. Podrazik RM, Obedian RS, Remick DG, Zelenock GB, D'Alecy LG. Attenuation of structural and functional damage from acute renal ischemia by the 21-amino steroid U74006F in rats. Curr Surg 1989;6:287.
21. Fong Y, Moldawer LL, Shires GT, Lowry SF. The biologic characteristics of cytokines and their implication in surgical injury. Surg Gynecol Obstet 1990;170:363.
22. Paterson IS. Klausner JM, Pugatch R, Allen P, Mannick JA, Shepro D, Hechtman HB. Noncardiac pulmonary edema after abdominal aortic aneurysm surgery. Ann Surg 1989;209:236.
23. Klausner JM, Paterson IS, Kobzik L, Valeri CR, Shepro D, Hechtman HB. Leukotrienes but not complement mediate limb ischemia-induced lung injury. Ann Surg 1989;209:462.
24. Klausner JM, Paterson IS, Valeri R, Shepro D, Hechtman HB. Limb ischemia-induced increase in permeability is mediated by leukocytes and leukotrienes. Ann Surg 1988;208:755.
25. Klausner JM, Anner H, Paterson IS, Kobzik L, Valeri CR, Shepro D, Hechtman HB. Lower torso ischemia-induced lung injury is leukocyte dependent. Ann Surg 1988;208:761.
26. Frank RS, Moursi MM, Podrazik RM, Zelenock GB, D'Alecy LG. Renal vasoconstriction and transient declamp hypotension after infrarenal aortic occlusion: role of plasma purine degradation products. J Vasc Surg 1988;7:515.
27. Udelsman R, Holbrook NJ. Endocrine and molecular responses to surgical stress. Curr Probl Surg 1994;31:657.
28. Moncada S. Higgs A. Mechanisms of disease: the L-arginine–nitric oxide pathway. N Engl J Med 1993;329:2002.
29. Levine GN, Keaney JF, Vita JA. Cholesterol reduction in cardiovascular disease: clinical benefits and possible mechanisms. N Engl J Med 1995;332:512.
30. Selhub J, Jacques PF, Bostom AG, et al. Association between plasma homocysteine concentrations and extracranial carotid-artery stenosis. N Engl J Med 1995;332:286.

SURGERY: SCIENTIFIC PRINCIPLES AND PRACTICE, Second Edition, edited by Lazar J. Greenfield, Michael W. Mulholland, Keith T. Oldham, Gerald B. Zelenock, and Keith D. Lillemoe. Lippincott–Raven Publishers, Philadelphia, © 1997.

CHAPTER 74

ARTERIAL HEMODYNAMICS

JACK L. CRONENWETT AND MARK F. FILLINGER

Hemodynamic principles are the foundation of an understanding of contemporary vascular surgery. The functional success of arterial reconstructive surgery depends on physiologic effects that rely on these principles. Sophisticated noninvasive techniques allow measurement of blood flow velocity and have elevated hemodynamic principles from textbook status to daily application in disease diagnosis. This chapter summarizes the aspects of arterial hemodynamics most commonly applied in vascular surgery. A more detailed discussion can be found in many comprehensive monographs, especially the superb text by Strandness and Sumner.[1-6]

ARTERIAL STRUCTURE AND FUNCTION

The arterial wall is composed primarily of endothelial cells, smooth muscle cells, collagen, and elastin. These basic elements are organized into three recognizable layers of the vessel wall: the intima, media, and adventitia. The intima is composed mostly of endothelial cells and the internal elastic lamina, with few of the other elements intervening. The media carries most of the tensile load and is thus primarily composed of collagen, elastin, and smooth muscle cells arranged in bundles oriented along the lines of greatest tension (circumferentially). The adventitia is primarily fibrous connective tissue, vasa vasorum for nutrient supply to the outer layers of larger arteries, and nerve fibers that regulate medial smooth muscle cell tone. The adventitia generally carries little of the tensile load. When the adventitia does perform a significant support function (eg, in the proximal visceral arteries), it has a larger number of collagen and elastin fibers.

Although the media is responsible for much of the structural integrity of the arterial wall, the elements making up the media are strongly influenced by endothelial cells contained in the intima. The endothelium is much more than an antithrombotic barrier interacting with platelets to promote hemostasis at the site of physical injury. Endothelial cells also produce cell adhesion molecules that are important to local inflammatory responses of the arterial wall. The most important hemodynamic function of endothelial cells, however, is their interaction with smooth muscle cells to regulate acute and chronic lumen diameter.[7-9] Endothelial cells respond to luminal shear stress (the tangential drag force that blood flow causes on the endothelial surface due to friction), and they secrete a number of biologic mediators that maintain shear stress within a narrow range. Mediators of acute vasodilation include endothelial-derived relaxing factor and prostaglandins; endothelin and angiotensin II are among the mediators of acute contraction. When changes in shear stress are chronic, these biologic mediators can produce structural changes in the arterial wall. For example, platelet-derived growth factor can be produced by endothelial cells subjected to low shear, resulting in smooth muscle cell migration and proliferation. Functionally, endothelial

cell–smooth muscle cell interactions allow arteries (and vein grafts placed in the arterial environment[10]) to accommodate acute and chronic changes in blood flow, and they optimize hemostatic and inflammatory mechanisms affected by shear rates.

Adaptive responses to hemodynamic forces are not limited to shear stress. The artery wall is subject to a number of hemodynamic stresses, and its structure must accommodate all of them (Fig. 74-1). These stresses (described in detail later) are primarily controlled by intraluminal blood pressure, blood flow velocity, arterial diameter, and wall thickness. Just as arterial diameter responds to changes in shear stress, the thickness of the arterial wall and the elements within it are regulated to normalize wall tension. Interestingly, the circumferential and longitudinal stresses within the arterial wall are not identical for any given blood pressure (see Fig. 74-1). The structure of the wall, however, makes it *anisotropic;* that is, the wall is stronger circumferentially than it is longitudinally.[11] Tethering of the arteries in situ affects longitudinal stiffness and prevents excessive motion. Acute changes in circumferential wall stiffness are primarily controlled by smooth muscle contraction or relaxation.[6]

Acute and chronic adaptation to hemodynamic stress allows arteries to accommodate changes in blood flow and pressure to a remarkable degree. For example, the arterial system must accommodate five-fold changes in cardiac output between rest and exercise and must alter distribution according to different metabolic demands. Not surprisingly, wall composition varies from central to more peripheral arteries to accomplish specific functions[2,3] (Fig. 74-2). Although the three layers of the arterial wall have different functions, most of the variation occurs in the media. Collagen is primarily responsible for wall strength and increases in proportion to artery diameter. Elastin, which is 5 to 10 times more deformable than rubber, provides stretch to artery walls and also increases with arterial size. The elastin/collagen ratio determines the relative distensibility (compliance) of arteries. Compliance is higher in large central arteries, in which it buffers changes in systemic pressure that occur during the cardiac cycle by allowing expansion during systolic ejection and recoil during diastolic relaxation. As elastin content and distensibility decrease in more peripheral arteries, the content of smooth muscle, the active component of the arterial wall, increases. In medium to large muscular arteries (5 to 10 mm diameter), resting smooth muscle tone does not contribute significantly to peripheral resistance but does decrease arterial compliance. By stiffening these arteries,

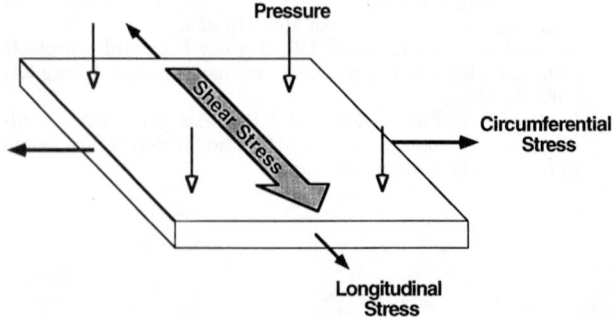

Figure 74-1. Stresses imposed on the arterial wall. Circumferential stress = τ_{circ} = Pr/δ; longitudinal stress = τ_{long} = Pr/2δ; and shear stress = τ_w = 4η Q/(πr^3), where P = pressure (intraluminal blood pressure), r = internal radius of the artery, δ = wall thickness, η = viscosity, and Q = volumetric blood flow rate. Details are presented later in this chapter.

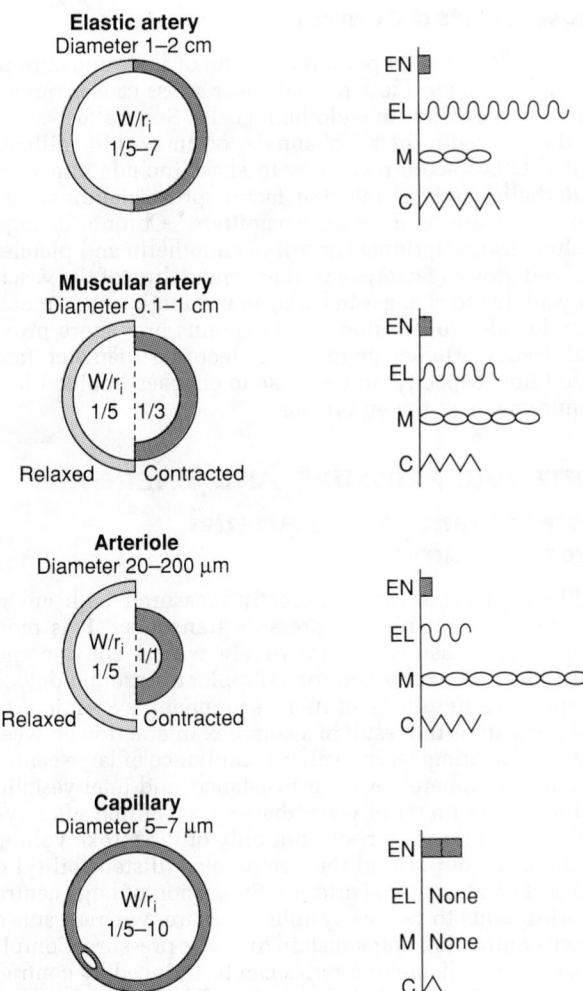

Figure 74-2. Approximate wall composition and relation between wall thickness (W) and internal radius (r_i) in large elastic arteries, medium muscular arteries, arterioles, and capillaries. EN, endothelium; EL, elastin; M, smooth muscle; C, collagen. (After Folkow B, Neil E. Circulation. New York, Oxford University Press, 1971)

resting smooth muscle tone augments systolic pressure and increases pulse-wave propagation rate. In small muscular arteries, arterioles, and precapillary sphincters, smooth muscle tone is the primary determinant of total peripheral resistance, regional blood flow, and the regulation of flow within the microcirculation. Arterioles and precapillary sphincters are well suited to regulate peripheral resistance and capillary perfusion because of their high wall thickness/lumen ratio, which causes maximal lumen constriction with minimal muscle shortening.

Although luminal diameter rapidly decreases from central to peripheral arteries (ie, the aorta, at 2.5 cm, is 1000 times larger than arterioles, at 25 μm diameter), the total cross-sectional area increases in the arteriolar and capillary bed as a result of an even more rapid increase in the number of these vascular channels. In fact, the cross-sectional area of arterioles is estimated to be 50 times that of the aorta, and the cross-sectional area of capillaries is 800 times that of the aorta.[2] This geometry permits rapid blood flow in large central arteries with a high mean velocity (20 to 30 cm/s in the aorta), but extremely low blood flow in capillaries with low mean velocity (0.5 to 1 mm/s). The inverse relation observed between cross-sectional area and

blood velocity is well suited to the distribution function of central arteries and the exchange function of capillaries. The need for a large capillary bed is illustrated by the volume flow through a single capillary of 8 μm in diameter, in which 1 mL of blood flowing at a velocity of 0.5 mm/s would require 15 months to traverse.

BLOOD FLOW CONTROL

Local Control

Vascular smooth muscle has intrinsic tone that is responsible for maintaining partial vascular constriction in the absence of external stimuli. Blood flow remains relatively constant in most organs despite wide changes in perfusion pressure. Two theories of local control mechanisms have been proposed to explain this autoregulation.[2,3,12] The myogenic theory states that vascular smooth muscle contracts in response to stretch caused by increases in intravascular pressure and relaxes in response to decreased stretch when perfusion pressure falls. This direct feedback loop stabilizes organ blood flow by adjusting arteriolar smooth muscle tone to changes in perfusion pressure. The metabolic theory states that tissue blood flow parallels metabolic activity. If the demands of tissue metabolism exceed the blood supply, certain metabolic byproducts accumulate and cause vasodilation of precapillary resistance vessels. Increased flow resulting from this decreased resistance then removes the vasodilating metabolites and restores baseline vascular smooth muscle tone. Factors that have been implicated in metabolic autoregulation include Po_2, Pco_2, pH, adenosine, lactate, K^+, and inorganic phosphate.[12] It is likely that these substances act in concert to produce metabolic vasodilation in response to reduced blood flow, poor systemic oxygen delivery, or increased metabolite production.

The myogenic and metabolic mechanisms of vascular control probably have complementary roles, not only in autoregulation but also during active (exercise) and reactive (postocclusive) hyperemia. In the extreme case of transient arterial occlusion, loss of myogenic tone (due to decreased stretch pressure) and accumulation of vasodilating metabolites results in reactive hyperemia, the near maximal but transient blood flow increase that occurs when blood flow is reestablished. Increased blood flow subsides as metabolites are cleared and myogenic tone restored by perfusion pressure, making the duration and degree of reactive hyperemia proportional to the duration and severity of ischemia.

Nervous System Control

The sympathetic nervous system has primary neural control of vascular smooth muscle tone.[12] Sympathetic adrenergic nerves function primarily by the release of norepinephrine, which stimulates α-adrenergic receptors to produce smooth muscle contraction and vasoconstriction. Basal sympathetic tone is responsible for only 15% to 20% of total vascular resistance, most of which is due to intrinsic myogenic activity (or intrinsic smooth muscle tone). Basal intrinsic arterial tone varies considerably among different organs. It is high in skeletal muscle and other tissues that have a wide range of metabolic rates but low in organs such as kidney or brain that have more stable metabolic rates and flow demands. The density of sympathetic innervation of vascular smooth muscle also varies in different organs, ranging from few fibers in cerebral or coronary arteries to dense innervation of cutaneous arterioles. Density of innervation influences the sensitivity of an organ to sympathetic vasoconstriction. This sensitivity is maximal in the skin, where sympathetic discharge can nearly stop cutaneous blood flow during the fight-or-flight reflex.

Organs also differ in the sensitivity of their vascular smooth muscle to the vasoconstrictor effects of sympathetic innervation and the vasodilator effects of local metabolites. An important example is the difference in sensitivity of precapillary and postcapillary sphincter muscles. Postcapillary sphincter mechanisms are more sensitive to sympathetic innervation than to local metabolic effects, whereas precapillary sphincters respond primarily to accumulating local metabolites and function independent of sympathetic discharge. Although changes in postcapillary sphincter resistance do not contribute significantly to the total resistance of the peripheral circulation, small changes in postcapillary contraction cause large changes in the precapillary-to-postcapillary pressure gradient. This gradient is important for regulating the capillary filtration coefficient and thus the tendency to accumulate peripheral edema or absorb tissue fluids, which is under subtle sympathetic control.

Central nervous system control of sympathetic nerve discharge lies in its cortical–hypothalamic–medullary axis. An important influence on the sympathetic activity that arises from the medullary cardiovascular center is the stretch receptors in the carotid sinus, aortic arch, thyrocarotid junction, and cardiopulmonary vascular bed. These stretch receptors are influenced by the arterial blood pressure and the degree of vascular filling (blood volume). For example, deformation and stretch of carotid sinus receptors stimulates the carotid sinus nerve, a branch of the glossopharyngeal nerve, which excites inhibitor neurons in the medial depressor area of the medulla. This provides negative feedback, or inhibition, of sympathetic activity arising from the medullary cardiovascular center. In addition, bradycardia results from vagal nerve stimulation. Stretch receptors are sensitive to stretch or vascular dilation, as their name suggests, but not to arterial pressure changes. Thus, in a normal artery, increasing arterial pressure increases the stretch of the arterial wall, so that the stretch receptor is stimulated. In an artery prevented from expanding (eg, by arterial calcification in the atherosclerotic patient), increasing arterial pressure does not stimulate this receptor. Removal of the arterial calcification, as occurs during carotid endarterectomy, may expose the adventitial stretch receptor to intense stimulation. This can result in significant inhibition of sympathetic discharge and increased vagal stimulation, causing hypotension and bradycardia.

Local Humoral Control

Many humoral substances also affect vascular smooth muscle tone. Epinephrine, norepinephrine, vasopressin, angiotensin, serotonin, prostaglandins, histamine, and plasma kinins participate in the control of vascular smooth muscle tone under certain circumstances and in specific organ beds.[12] Epinephrine has differential, organ-specific effects based on the predominance of α- or β-adrenergic receptors. Its α effect causes vasoconstriction in kidney, skin, and intestine, whereas its β effect causes vasodilation in the myocardium, skeletal muscle, and liver. These effects are generally minimal when compared with the effect of sympathetic stimulation on blood flow regulation.

Humoral substances, such as endothelial-derived relaxing factor, endothelin, and prostaglandins, play an important role in the regulation of vascular tone in response to hemodynamic stress. In particular, inhibition of endothelial-derived relaxing factor greatly enhances the myogenic response of vasoconstriction to increased blood flow.

Flow-Related Control

Blood flow is an important regulator of acute and chronic arterial diameter. Flow-related shear stress causes numerous biologic effects in endothelial cells. Some effects, such as the activation of K^+ channels, occur within milliseconds.[7] Other acute responses to shear include effects on endothelial-derived relaxing factor, prostaglandins, adenylate cyclase, and neurotransmitters.[7] Chronic changes include transcriptional control of endothelin and platelet-derived growth factor, as well as remodeling of the vascular wall due to changes in collagen production and smooth muscle cell proliferation. This explains how more proximal feeder arteries increase or decrease diameter (and blood flow capacity) in response to changes in blood flow requirements at the end organ.

ARTERIAL PRESSURE AND ENERGY

Determinants of the Arterial Pressure Curve

Blood pressure can be directly measured with an intraarterial catheter and a pressure transducer. It is more frequently measured noninvasively with a sphygmomanometer and a stethoscope or a Doppler ultrasound device. Despite the simplicity of its measurement, systemic arterial pressure is the result of a complex interaction between the cardiac pump, aortic valve, compliance of large central arteries, peripheral vascular resistance, and total vascular volume. The pressure wave that is transmitted after systolic contraction is a result not only of the stroke volume of the heart but also of the compliance (distensibility) of the aorta and proximal arteries. Expansion of large central arteries tends to reduce systolic pressure, whereas subsequent contraction helps sustain diastolic pressure. Compliance of large-diameter arteries can be reduced by contraction of smooth muscle in the walls of these vessels. Thus, sympathetic-mediated vasoconstriction during exercise causes increased pulse pressure (the difference between systolic and diastolic pressure) due to less aortic expansion, resulting in the propagation of a larger systolic pressure wave. Systolic hypertension is produced by a similar mechanism in geriatric patients with calcified and poorly compliant arterial walls.

As arterial pressure waves generated by cardiac contraction proceed peripherally, there is a gradual increase in the pulse pressure amplitude as well as a qualitative change in the shape of these waves (both pressure and flow). This is due primarily to the reflection of pulse waves as they strike the high-resistance segments of the peripheral circulation—the distal arterioles and points of arterial branching. Pulse-wave reflection results in a retrograde flow of each wave, which then interacts with the next prograde-moving pressure wave. The sum of these pressure waves results in an amplification of systolic pressure as each pressure wave proceeds peripherally. The influence of arteriolar resistance is most significant but is also variable, depending on the state of peripheral vasoconstriction. Major arterial branch points contribute the other significant (and constant) resistance for pulse-wave reflection because the sum of the cross-sectional area of the branches (A2) is less than the area of the proximal artery (A1). Minimal wave reflections occur at a bifurcation when the A2/A1 ratio is 1.15 (ie, when the total branch area is slightly greater than the parent artery). In the human aortoiliac bifurcation, this ratio is approached only during infancy (1.11). In the adult aorta, even without atheromatous disease, this ratio becomes progressively smaller, reaching 0.75 in patients between 40 and 50 years of age.[1] This ratio results in a significant reflection of the amplitude of each pulse wave (26%). Although the effect of this reflection is attenuated by the viscoelastic arterial system as it proceeds retrograde, it effectively increases the pressure in the distal abdominal aorta, a factor that may contribute to the predilection for aneurysm formation at this site. Pulse-wave reflection is also responsible for the periods of retrograde flow in peripheral arteries seen immediately after the primary pulse wave has passed, a phenomenon augmented by peripheral vasoconstriction (with increased wave reflection) and decreased by vasodilation (with diminished resistance and decreased wave reflection).

Pressure and Energy

Blood pressure is commonly considered to be the driving force that controls the movement of blood from the heart to various body regions. A more precise and useful concept is that blood flow is controlled by energy gradients, to which arterial pressure makes the largest contribution. Total energy within the circulation results from the sum of potential energy (PE) and kinetic energy (KE), with PE representing the greater portion of total energy during normal blood flow (pressure measured in mmHg (torr) = 1330 dynes/cm^2). PE is the sum of intraarterial pressure and gravitational energy. Intraarterial pressure results primarily from the pressure caused by cardiac contraction (P_c), with a hydrostatic contribution resulting from the weight of the column of blood between the heart and the position of pressure measurement. Hydrostatic pressure is defined as follows:

$$\text{hydrostatic pressure} = P_H = -\rho gh$$

where:
ρ = density of blood (1.056 g/cm^3)
g = acceleration of gravity (980 cm/s^2)
h = height (cm) above a fixed reference point
(atrium) to the point of pressure
measurement

If the point of measurement is below the atrium, then hydrostatic pressure is additive to the pressure due to cardiac contraction. In the legs of an erect human, this position represents a pressure increase (in the neck, it is a pressure decrease). Gravitational PE results from the ability of blood to do work based on its position relative to another location, and is calculated using the term $+\rho gh$. In the human body, the two most relevant points for determining the height, h, in this equation are the atrium and the feet. Using the above units, PE is then expressed as follows:

$$PE \text{ (erg/cm}^3) = P_c + P_H + \rho gh = P + \rho gh \quad (1)$$

As blood moves from the heart to the feet in the erect position, it gains hydrostatic pressure but loses gravitational energy. Thus, arterial pressure measured at the ankle in an upright person is significantly increased by hydrostatic pressure because of the added weight of the upright column of blood. Total PE is unchanged because it is reduced by an equivalent amount as a result of the loss of gravitational PE. Thus, there is no net change in the total driving force (energy) in the erect versus the supine position, despite changes in measured arterial pressure. This explains the apparent paradox of blood flowing against a major pressure gradient, as it does between the heart and the feet in the erect position (Fig. 74-3A).

KE derives from the ability of flowing blood to perform work based on its velocity. In a nonpulsatile flow system with rigid tubing and a Newtonian fluid (see Viscosity and Laminar Blood Flow), KE is defined as follows:

$$KE \text{ (erg/cm}^3) = \tfrac{1}{2}\rho v^2 \quad (2)$$

where:
ρ = density of fluid
v = mean velocity (cm/s)

This definition of KE is valid in an ideal system, but in the human arterial system, it significantly underestimates energy losses due to the pulsatile nature of blood flow, the non-Newtonian characteristics of blood, and many alterations in geometry (eg, those due to atherosclerotic disease). For the purpose of discussion, this formula is useful because it indicates that the total energy of flowing blood is derived in large part from the characteristics of its velocity and hence, flow rate.

Energy in the Ideal System

Bernoulli first characterized the flow of a Newtonian fluid in a frictionless system in which total energy remains constant.[3] Because total energy is equal to PE + KE, Bernoulli stated that total energy at point A is equal to total energy at point B, or

$$PE_A + KE_A = PE_B + KE_B \quad (3)$$

In a horizontal tube, which eliminates gravitational effects (ie, $\rho gh_A = \rho gh_B$), this formula can be expanded using equations 1 and 2 and rewritten as the one-dimensional Bernoulli formula, which relates pressure and velocity:

$$P_A + \tfrac{1}{2}\rho v_A{}^2 = P_B + \tfrac{1}{2}\rho v_B{}^2 \quad (4)$$

This equation explains another apparent paradox, the flow of fluid from a low-pressure to high-pressure region, which results from the conversion of KE to PE in an enlarging tube (see Fig. 74-3B). A clinical example is aortic aneurysm, in which vessel diameter increases from 2 to 6 cm, resulting in the predicted nine-fold decrease in fluid velocity required to maintain constant flow:

$$Q = v \cdot A = v \cdot \pi r^2 \quad (5)$$

where:
Q = flow
v = velocity
A = tube area
r = tube radius

KE thus decreases 81-fold (proportional to v^2), and PE must increase by an equivalent amount to maintain constant energy in this system. This translates into a small increase in pressure (about 1 mmHg) and emphasizes the predominant contribution of PE rather than KE to blood flow in most cases. In a real aneurysm, even this small pressure increase is probably eliminated because of energy lost by flow turbulence at the aneurysm orifice.

ARTERIAL FLOW AND ENERGY LOSS
Measurement

Although arterial blood flow rather than pressure is of ultimate importance for tissue perfusion, flow is more difficult to measure.[1] Most blood flow transducers actually measure instantaneous velocity and calculate the volumetric flow based on vessel diameter. Electromagnetic flow probes detect the voltage generated by charged particles as blood flows through the electromagnetic field created by the probe. Because this technique requires direct access to an artery, it is sometimes useful during surgery but is more often used in experimental laboratories. Clinically, blood flow in an individual artery is usually measured with an ultrasonic flowmeter using the Doppler effect. This technique relies on the shift in frequency of sound waves

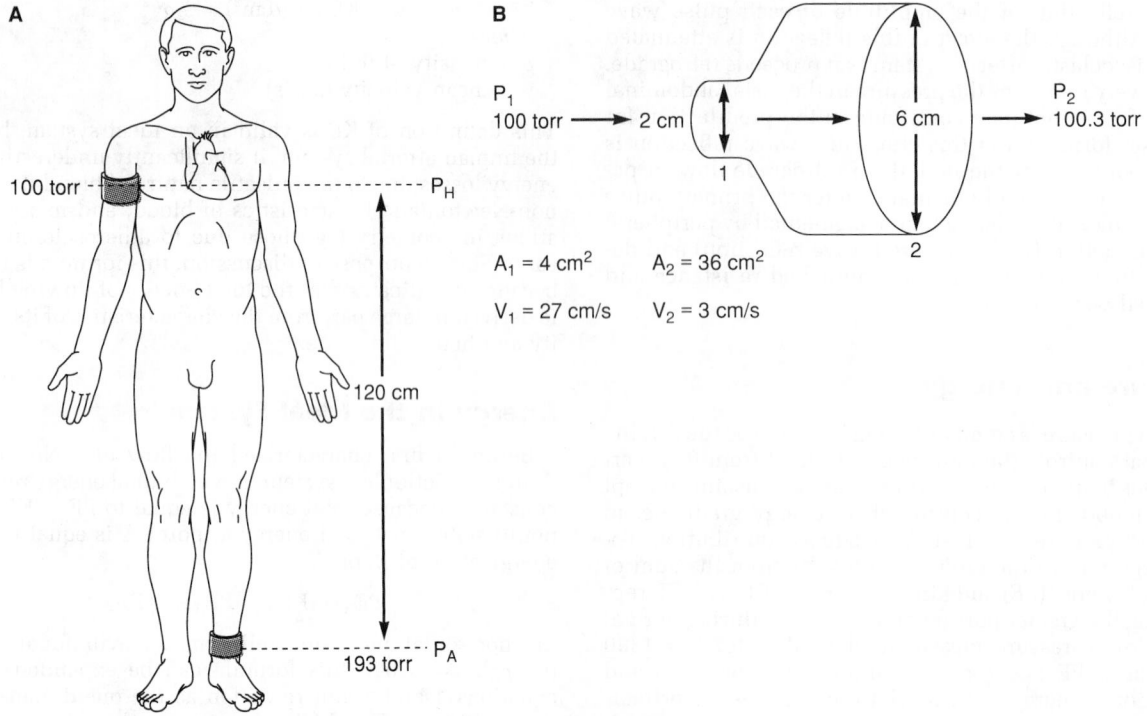

Figure 74-3. (*A*) Effect of gravity on intravascular pressure measured in an erect subject. Pressure at the ankle (P_A) increases substantially compared with pressure at the heart level (P_H) as a result of the weight of the erect column of blood ($P_A = P_H + \rho gh = P_H + [\rho g] [120$ cm]). (*B*) Effect of luminal expansion on intravascular pressure due to conversion of kinetic energy to potential energy as velocity decreases to maintain constant flow. Effect is minimal in a tube with dimensions comparable to a 6-cm diameter aortic aneurysm. (After Sumner DS. Essential hemodynamic principles. In: Rutherford RB, ed. Vascular surgery, ed 3. Philadelphia, WB Saunders, 1989)

when the distance between the sound wave generator and reflector is changing. A Doppler probe detects the shift in frequency of returning versus emitted sound waves, which is proportional to the velocity of blood from which the sound waves reflect.

More complex duplex ultrasound machines calculate volume flow in addition to the velocity of blood flow because they measure artery diameter with B-mode ultrasound. Arterial flow to an entire limb can also be determined by plethysmography (volume measurement). Plethysmographs detect limb volume changes after venous occlusion by measuring electrical impedance, stretch of external wires around the limb (strain gauges), or even fluid displacement. After briefly inflating a proximal pneumatic cuff above venous pressure, the immediate increase in distal extremity volume is proportional to total arterial inflow, expressed as flow per volume of tissue measured by the plethysmograph. Cardiac output is frequently measured by thermodilution techniques according to the Fick principle. Originally based on oxygen consumption, this method calculates flow according to the rate of dilution of a rapidly injected indicator (eg, indocyanine green or cold saline). Other techniques for arterial flow measurement include the rate of tissue uptake of radionuclide-labeled microspheres or the clearance of locally injected, diffusible radiolabeled materials. These latter techniques are generally used only in research applications.

Viscosity and Laminar Blood Flow

Sir Isaac Newton recognized that friction developed between the layers of a flowing fluid and defined viscosity as the lack of slipperiness between adjacent lamina.[4] An ideal fluid with no viscosity (ie, no internal friction between layers) and flowing in a frictionless conduit could have all fluid particles traveling at the same velocity, resulting in a flat velocity profile (Fig. 74-4A). In a real system, cohesive attraction forces develop between the conduit wall and the fluid in contact with the wall, preventing the outermost, infinitesimally thin layer of fluid from moving. Although there is some molecular exchange between the outermost fluid layer and the inner fluid layers, there is no actual movement or slippage of the outermost fluid layer along the conduit wall. Because there is a net fluid movement within the conduit, it follows that there must be a velocity gradient across the conduit, resulting in the maximal velocity being attained at the furthest distance from the conduit wall, the axial center of the tube. Proceeding from this center toward the conduit wall, there is a progressive decrease of the velocity of each lamina of fluid. Zero velocity is reached at the conduit wall, resulting in a parabolic profile for laminar flow of real liquids (see Fig. 74-4B).

Real arteries are not smooth, straight tubes, however. Atherosclerotic plaques, branches, and vessel curvature, together with pulsatile flow, cause significant departures from the parabolic velocity profile of laminar flow. Blood flow disturbances result in disruption of the parallel streamlines characteristic of laminar flow and may produce turbulence. In truly turbulent flow, fluid particles move randomly, and an instantaneous "snapshot" of the fluid velocity vectors would appear chaotic (see Fig. 74-4C). When averaged over time, this turbulent flow produces a mean velocity profile similar to that of laminar flow, only much more blunted (see Fig. 74-4D). The conditions of physiologic blood flow are generally too stable for

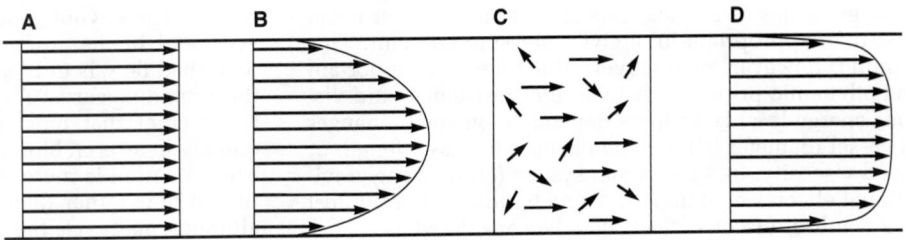

Figure 74-4. (A) Flat velocity profile of an ideal fluid (zero viscosity) in a straight, rigid tube. (B) Parabolic laminar flow profile of a real, Newtonian fluid. (C) Turbulent flow of a real fluid at high Reynolds number. Velocity vectors at any moment in time are random. (D) Time-averaged velocity profile for turbulent flow has a blunted profile when compared with laminar flow.

true turbulence. Flow disturbances do occur, but they tend to dampen out over short distances and are more accurately termed *disturbed flow* rather than *turbulence*. In common use, however, these terms are often applied interchangeably.

When analyzing blood flow, it is best to start with the more straightforward equations related to laminar flow. The stress or force (F) per unit area (A) required to overcome the friction between adjacent fluid layers is defined as shear stress (τ)),[3,4] *where*

$$\tau(dyne/cm^2) = F/A \qquad (6)$$

Shear rate (D) is defined as the velocity gradient (dv) that develops between fluid layers divided by the distance (radius or dr) between adjacent layers:

$$D(s^{-1}) = dv/dr \qquad (7)$$

Thus, shear rate is proportional to velocity. Viscosity (η) is measured in poise, after Poiseuille, or dynes/s^{-1}/cm^2. Viscosity is precisely defined as the ratio of shear stress to shear rate, expressed as follows:

$$\eta = \tau/D = (F \cdot dr)/(A \cdot dv) \qquad (8)$$

Expressed more simply, viscosity is the tangential force required to maintain a constant velocity between two adjacent laminas with area (A) and distance (dr) constant. Commonly, viscosity is conceptualized as the thickness of a liquid (eg, oil has a greater viscosity than water). In reality, viscosity is difficult to measure, depends on the temperature of the fluid, and is probably different in the actual circulation than can be measured in vitro. Approximate viscosities in centipoise (cP) at 37°C are: water, 0.69 cP; plasma, 1.1 to 1.8 cP; and blood, 3 to 5 cP (at high shear rate).[3]

A Newtonian fluid (eg, water) is one in which viscosity is constant despite changes in velocity (shear rate).[2,3] Although plasma may be considered newtonian in behavior, blood may not, primarily because of red blood cells. At low shear rates, red blood cells aggregate and increase viscosity, particularly in the presence of large plasma proteins such as fibrinogen. At high shear rates, red blood cells are drawn into the central high-velocity portion of the flow pattern, which reduces viscosity. Thus, blood viscosity depends primarily on its shear rate (eg, velocity), hematocrit, and plasma protein concentration. Hematocrit, or packed cell volume (PCV), is proportional to the logarithm of viscosity (η), so that at 40% PCV, $\eta = 4$ cP, whereas at 20% PCV, $\eta = 2.2$ cP, and at 60% PCV, $\eta = 8$ cp.[3] Thus, hematocrit elevations above 45% cause disproportionately large increases in viscosity.

Despite these non-Newtonian characteristics, physiologic blood flow often follows Newtonian behavior. The red blood cell aggregation effect at low shear rates has been found to have little or no effect in vessels in which shear can be measured in vivo.[6] The effect at high shear rates due to the size of red blood cells is only important when

the particle size is large in relation to the vessel. Thus, the effect of red blood cells is not measurable until the lumen diameter drops below 1 mm, but it becomes marked when the lumen decreases to 100 to 200 μm.[6] In these very small arteries, the reduction in viscosity is crucial to decreasing the resistance to blood flow. The shear stress that typically defines tube flow is that of wall shear. For laminar flow in a Newtonian fluid:

$$\tau = 4\eta Q/(\pi r^3)$$

where:
τ = shear stress
η = viscosity
Q = volumetric blood flow rate
r = internal radius of the artery

Viscous Energy Loss

As a real fluid flows through a rigid, straight tube, energy is lost in proportion to fluid viscosity as heat generated by friction between layers of the fluid.[4] The details of this relation were empirically determined by Poiseuille in 1846. Using a series of glass microcapillary tubes, Poiseuille derived the relation between pressure and flow in this steady flow system as

$$\Delta P = Q \cdot 8L\eta/\pi r^4 \qquad (9)$$

where:
ΔP = pressure gradient between two points
Q = flow
L = tube length between the points
η = coefficient of viscosity
r = tube radius

The latter term in this formula ($8L\eta/r^4$) represents the resistance to flow in this system according to the generalized hemodynamic formula, pressure = flow × resistance:

$$P = QR \qquad (10)$$

This equation is analogous to Ohm's law of electrical circuits, which states that electromotive force (voltage) = current × resistance (E = IR). Because vascular resistance cannot be directly measured, it is calculated from direct measurements of pressure (P) and flow (Q) according to the relation R = P/Q. Accordingly, resistance is expressed in units of mmHg/cm^3/min, and is defined as a *peripheral resistance unit* for simplicity. The units mmHg/cm^3/s are expressed in standard resistance units of dynes/s^{-1}/cm^5.

Poiseuille's equation reveals that resistance to a steady flow of Newtonian fluid in a straight, rigid tube is proportional to tube length and fluid viscosity but inversely proportional to the fourth power of the tube radius. Poiseuille's law cannot be used to analyze precisely these variables in the human circulatory system because of the non-Newtonian characteristics of blood, the pulsatile nature of arterial flow, and the tapering and elliptic cross-section of nonrigid blood vessels. In general, Poiseuille's equation underestimates resistance, thus calculating a higher mean flow than appropriate for a given pressure gradient. This formula, however, qualitatively illustrates the important hemodynamic principle that vascular resistance (and viscous energy loss) is far more dependent on small changes in vessel diameter (r^4) than on changes in vessel length or blood viscosity. In a horizontal system (eliminating gravitational effects), equations 1, 5, and 9 indicate that PE lost as a result of viscous effects may be considered as

$$PE = Q \cdot 8L\eta/\pi r^4 = v \cdot 8L\eta/r^2 \qquad (11)$$

Inertial Energy Loss

Although Poiseuille stated that changes of pressure in straight tubes were proportional to changes of flow ($\Delta P \propto \Delta Q$), he realized that at high flow rates, larger pressure gradients resulted than could be predicted by his formula. It remained for Osborn Reynolds in 1883 to characterize these additional energy losses and attribute them to flow turbulence.[2] Reynolds injected dye into the axial stream of a long, rigid, cylindric tube and showed that turbulence disrupted the laminar flow pattern of parallel streamlines when the flow rate reached a certain critical value. From these experiments, he derived the formula:

$$Re = \rho Dv/\eta \qquad (12)$$
where:
Re = a dimensionless number (Reynolds number)
ρ = fluid density (g/cm^3)
D = diameter (cm)
v = fluid velocity (cm/s)
η = viscosity (cP)

In steady (nonpulsatile) flow, v is taken to be the mean cross-sectional fluid velocity, whereas in pulsatile systems, the peak Reynolds number (calculated using the cross-sectional velocity at peak flow) is often used. Reynolds demonstrated that in long, straight, rigid tubes, turbulence occurred when Re exceeded 2000 during steady flow (referred to as the *critical Reynolds number*). Turbulence within an artery may result in an audible noise, or bruit, as a result of vibration of the arterial wall. Severe wall vibration in superficial arteries may be palpated as a thrill. Reynolds' observation indicates that turbulence is more likely with increased velocity and decreased viscosity. The former explains the frequent association of bruits with arterial stenoses because of markedly increased blood velocity as the flow stream narrows to accommodate the stenosis. Viscosity may be decreased sufficiently in patients with severe anemia to produce turbulence and a bruit in an otherwise normal artery. Furthermore, the Reynolds number predicts the lack of turbulence observed in arterioles and capillaries that have low velocities and minimal vessel diameters.

As with Poiseuille's formula, the critical value of the Reynolds number cannot be exactly applied to the arterial circulation because of the assumptions inherent in its derivation. In the human arterial system, the Reynolds number does not exceed 2000 except in the ascending aorta. The classic value of the critical Reynolds number, however, was derived for steady flow in straight, smooth, rigid, cylindric tubes. The critical Reynolds number depends on a number of factors, including the roughness of the conduit walls, the shape of the conduit, and the presence of discontinuities such as branches or step-offs. It can vary from 100 to 50,000 (depending on inlet, conduit, and flow characteristics).[13] In the arterial circulation, pulsatile flow, compliant vessels, arterial branching, wall irregularities, stenoses, and the non-Newtonian characteristics of blood

all affect the critical Reynolds number at which turbulence occurs. The Reynolds number is a useful parameter, however, and in the absence of pathologic lesions, severely disturbed flow is only associated with cardiac valves and the ascending aorta.[6] Physiologic values of Reynolds number predict that most disturbances would dampen out quickly in arterial blood flow, and this is usually the case. This situation is more appropriately characterized as disturbed flow rather than true, fully developed turbulence, although many use the terms interchangeably.

In addition to viscous energy losses (equation 11), real fluids lose inertial (kinetic) energy as a result of changes in velocity that cause turbulence or flow disturbance (equation 2). Because velocity is a vector quantity, pulsatile blood flow and altered arterial geometry result in complex velocity directional changes. These are virtually impossible to measure in vivo, so energy losses cannot be accurately calculated. Inertial energy losses are directly proportional to the second power of velocity (equation 2), whereas viscous energy losses are proportional to the first power of velocity (equation 11). Thus, at low flow velocities, viscous forces predominate, and pressure gradients are more linearly proportional to flow (ie, Poiseuille's law). At high flow velocities, inertial energy losses predominate because of the rapidly increasing magnitude of v^2. As predicted by Reynolds, turbulence occurs beyond a certain critical velocity and imparts significantly more energy loss than predicted by Poiseuille's formula for viscous energy losses alone.

Local Effects of Turbulent Flow

Changes in geometry at an arterial bifurcation result in altered velocity vectors that create subtle but important local turbulence or disturbed flow.[1,4] These effects have been studied in clear glass tubes and specially prepared arteries in which flow-streaming and turbulence can be observed by injecting colored dyes. During normal laminar flow, a boundary layer of fluid with essentially zero velocity exists at the fluid–vessel interface because of the viscous properties discussed earlier. At a bifurcation, where there is a sudden change in the direction of flow, local pressure gradients develop, and the laminar velocity profile changes, being skewed with higher velocities toward the central flow divider. This results in a new region of zero velocity separated from the arterial wall, termed *boundary layer separation* (Fig. 74-5). Flow between this boundary layer and the arterial wall is low or stagnant, until more typical laminar flow is reestablished downstream from the bifurcation (boundary layer separation is not synonymous with turbulence). This region of low flow (and low shear stress) at the site of boundary layer separation has been shown to correspond to the region of the carotid artery bifurcation, where atherosclerosis develops and is predominant.[14] Conversely, the flow divider, the site of high shear stress, is not usually the site of atherosclerosis. This has led to speculation that increased particle residence time, which occurs at sites of boundary layer separation, may accelerate atherosclerosis because of more prolonged contact of the arterial wall with blood-borne stimulants derived from platelets and other blood elements. As discussed previously, low shear is also a stimulus for endothelial cells to increase production of biologic mediators that induce narrowing of the vessel lumen through vasoconstriction, smooth muscle cell proliferation, and extracellular matrix production.[7]

ARTERIAL STENOSES
Energy Loss

Atherosclerotic occlusive disease primarily affects the circulation through energy loss at arterial stenoses or occlusions. As blood flow encounters a fixed stenosis within

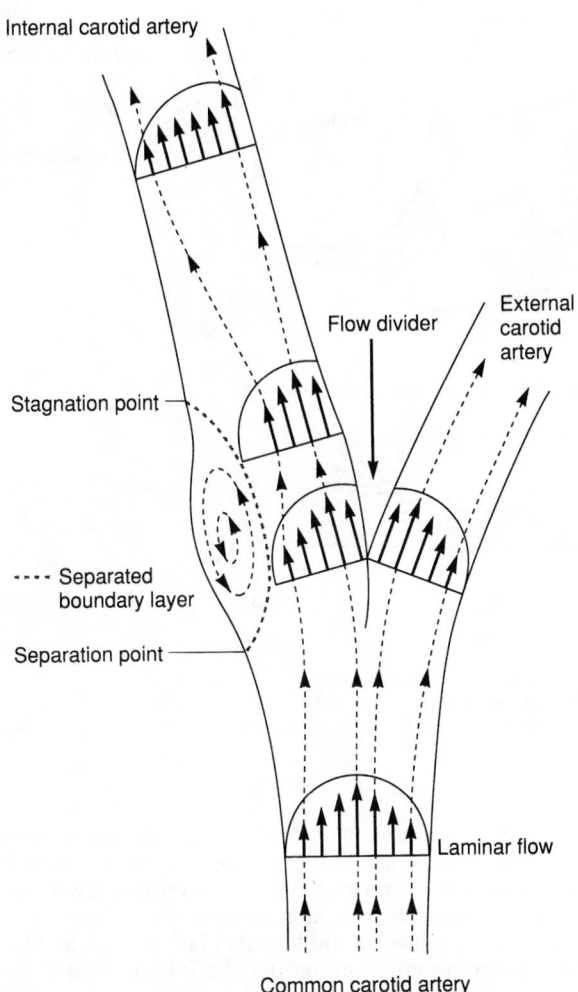

Internal carotid artery

External carotid artery

Flow divider

Stagnation point

---- Separated boundary layer

Separation point

Laminar flow

Common carotid artery

Figure 74-5. Alteration in flow at the human carotid artery bifurcation resulting in boundary layer separation and stagnant flow along the outer wall of the internal carotid artery. This corresponds to the region of development of atherosclerotic plaque. (After Zarins CK, Giddens DP, Bharaduaj BK, Sottiurai VS, Mabon RF, Glagov S. Carotid bifurcation atheroscleroses: quantitative correlation of platelet localization with flow velocity profiles and wall shear stress. Circ Res 1983;53:502)

an artery, its velocity must increase across the stenosis to maintain constant flow (equation 5). This is a consequence of conservation of mass and the fact that blood is an essentially incompressible fluid. Inertial energy is lost when the velocity changes at the entrance and exit from the stenosis.[4,5] Considerably less flow disturbance results at the convergence of a stenosis than at its divergence, although precise calculations of energy loss depend on factors such as abruptness of tapering, roughness, and tortuosity, which are practically impossible to measure in vivo. For practical considerations, the inertial energy losses at a stenosis are proportional to the second power of the change in velocity (Δv^2), as predicted by equation 2. Because the change in velocity is inversely proportional to the second power of the change in radius ($1/\Delta r^2$; equation 5), it follows that inertial energy lost at an arterial stenosis is inversely proportional to the fourth power of the change in radius ($1/\Delta r^4$). Although Poiseuille's law was derived for long, straight tubes rather than short arterial stenoses, it provides a useful approximation of the viscous energy lost at an arterial stenosis, which is also proportional to $1/\Delta r^4$ (equation 9). These estimates of inertial and viscous energy lost

at an arterial stenosis would predict that a 50% reduction in luminal diameter would cause at least a 16-fold energy loss. Inertial effects (turbulence), which depend on v^2, contribute significantly more to this energy loss than do viscous effects, which depend on v (Fig. 74-6). At the exit of a stenosis, the loss of KE due to turbulence has been estimated as follows:

$$\Delta P = k\rho(v_s - v_e)^2/2 \qquad (13)$$

where:
k depends on the exact geometric configuration
v_s = velocity in the stenosis
v_e = velocity after the exit of the stenosis
ρ = fluid density

This formula can be rewritten as

$$\Delta P = kv^2[(r/r_s)^2 - 1]^2 \qquad (14)$$

where:
v = velocity after stenosis
r = radius of the uninvolved artery
r_s = radius of the stenosis

This formula emphasizes that the energy lost at an arterial stenosis is proportional to the fourth power of the change in radius and the second power of the velocity within the normal artery. This illustrates that the energy lost at any fixed stenosis increases exponentially with increasing blood flow or velocity (Fig. 74-7).

Critical Stenosis

Experimental studies have investigated the above relation between blood flow and pressure lost at an arterial stenosis to determine the clinical significance of varying degrees of stenosis. A pressure gradient or flow reduction does not occur until a rather significant arterial stenosis is reached, usually a 75% to 90% reduction of the artery cross-sectional area, which corresponds to a 50% to 70% reduction in diameter, assuming that the stenosis is symmetric.[1,15] An arterial stenosis is termed *critical* at the point at which it reduces distal pressure or flow. This point depends on the blood flow (velocity) within the artery. A stenosis that is not critical at lower flow might become critical at high flow (hence the term *subcritical stenosis*). It is impossible to predict that a certain percentage arterial stenosis will result in a significant pressure gradient unless the flow rate is specified (see Fig. 74-7). Under normal circumstances, a generous margin is incorporated into the size of large and medium transport arteries, resulting in such a large value of r^4 (and therefore low resistance) that the pressure gradient approaches zero regardless of flow. Based on the normal relation between artery size and flow demand of the particular organ supplied, a flow-limiting stenosis generally occurs in the clinical setting at about a 50% diameter reduction and becomes exponentially worse beyond that point.

Subcritical Stenosis

The fact that arterial stenoses become increasingly significant at higher flow velocities is central to an understanding of the hemodynamic changes responsible for the symptoms of peripheral arterial occlusive disease. A stenosis that is subcritical during resting conditions (low blood flow) may become critical during the increased blood flow associated with exercise. This is easily conceptualized using the general formula P = QR (equation 10). If flow (Q) increases across a fixed stenosis (resistance, R), the pressure gradient across the stenosis (P) must increase accordingly. This results in reduced distal blood pressure, which

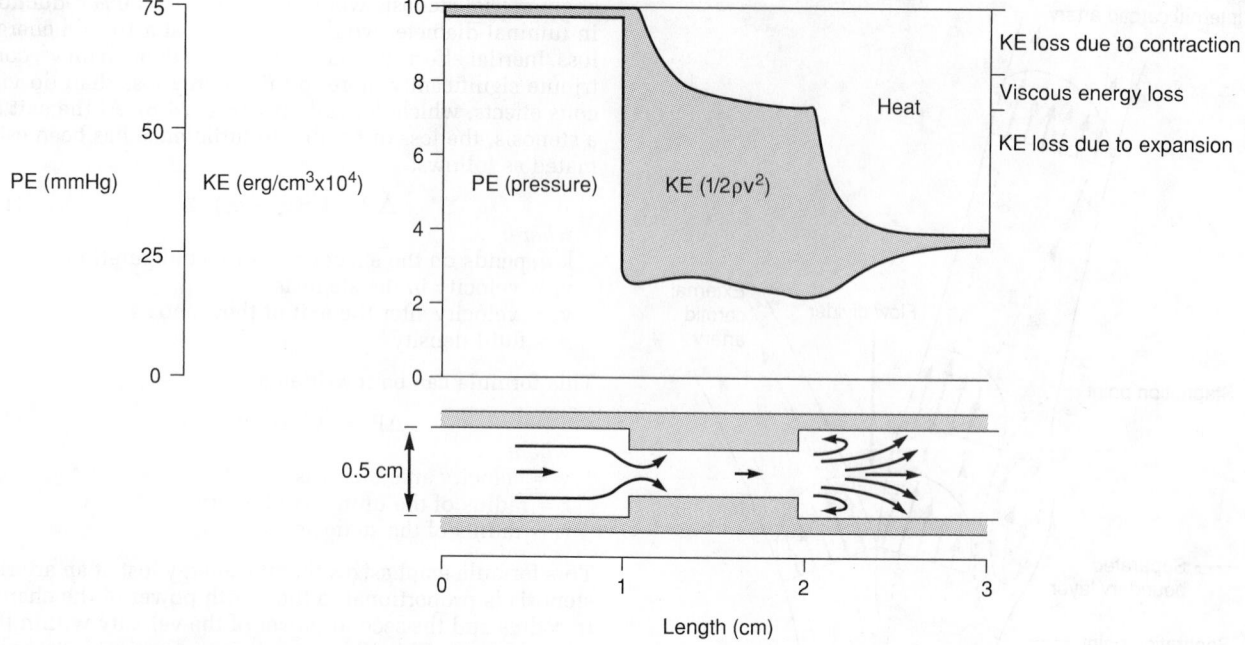

Figure 74-6. Kinetic energy (KE) and potential energy (PE) losses resulting from blood passing through a fixed stenosis under steady flow conditions. Most energy is lost at the stenosis exit, with little loss of viscous energy. (After Sumner DS. Essential hemodynamic principles. In: Rutherford RB, ed. Vascular surgery, ed 3. Philadelphia, WB Saunders, 1989)

limits the blood flow increase that would otherwise occur to meet the increased metabolic demands of exercise. Inadequate blood flow then leads to metabolite accumulation and pain (claudication). Only when exercise stops is resting blood flow sufficient to remove accumulated metabolites and relieve pain.

If a lower extremity arterial stenosis is subcritical during resting conditions, systolic cuff pressure measured at the ankle demonstrates no gradient when compared with central arterial pressure (commonly estimated by brachial artery pressure, hence the ankle–brachial index). The distal blood pressure reduction that results from increased flow across a subcritical stenosis can be used to detect such a stenosis. Immediately after or during exercise, the ankle–brachial index decreases in proportion to the reduction in blood flow, returning gradually toward normal after cessation of exercise (Fig. 74-8). This principle is used clinically

Figure 74-7. The effect of increasing blood flow rate (Q) on inertial energy loss (expressed as change in pressure) at the exit of a stenosis in a tube with a radius of 0.5 cm. At low flow, a greater percentage area of stenosis is required to reduce pressure. The curves demonstrate the exponential effect of stenosis radius ($1/r^4$) on pressure loss at any given flow. Calculations based on equation 14. (After Sumner DS. Essential hemodynamic principles. In: Rutherford RB, ed. Vascular surgery, ed 3. Philadelphia, WB Saunders, 1989)

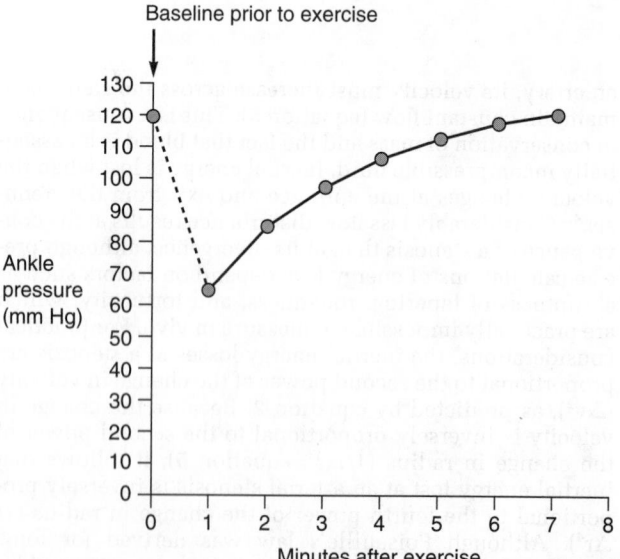

Figure 74-8. Decrease in blood pressure at the ankle during exercise, revealing the presence of a stenosis that is subcritical at rest. This type of plot is obtained with a treadmill exercise test.

to detect subcritical stenoses and to verify the presence of early arterial occlusive disease in patients who manifest claudication but who do not have reduced resting blood pressure. Exercise hyperemia is induced by having the patient walk at a fixed rate and grade on a treadmill until claudication symptoms occur. Then distal (ankle) pressures are measured and compared with arm and resting ankle pressure measurements. Increased blood flow across a suspected subcritical stenosis can also be induced with reactive hyperemia. Transient arterial occlusion in the extremity is created by cuff inflation for 3 to 5 minutes at the thigh or upper calf, resulting in dilation of arterioles distal to the cuff. The resulting decrease in peripheral resistance causes a sudden flow increase after cuff release, during which ankle pressure measurements are made. Patients with subcritical stenoses often have normal or only slightly reduced ankle or femoral pulses palpable at rest. These pulses may actually disappear during and immediately after exercise because of the pressure reduction that occurs as flow increases across the proximal stenoses.

Multiple Stenoses

Because atherosclerotic occlusive disease is a diffuse process, it is unlikely that an isolated arterial stenosis will occur but rather that multiple sequential stenoses will eventually develop. Theoretically, resistances in series are additive:

$$R_T = R_1 + R_2 + R_3 \tag{15}$$

Resistances in parallel (eg, in collateral vascular beds) are additive as an inverse function:

$$1/R_T = 1/R_1 + 1/R_2 + 1/R_3 \tag{16}$$

Multiple factors, such as the distance between stenoses, the Reynolds number, the stenosis contour, stenosis severity, and other intervening geometric variables prevent exact calculation of the contribution of sequential stenoses in a real arterial system. Experimental results indicate that multiple sequential stenoses generally have an additive effect, although each subsequent stenosis contributes less resistance.[15] In practice, the single most critical stenosis largely determines any limitation of blood flow. Multiple subcritical stenoses can produce the effect of a single critical stenosis.

It is clinically expedient to divide the lower extremity into three major subsegments—the aortoiliac, femoropopliteal, and distal (below-the-knee) circulations. Frequently, significant stenoses occur in more than one of these segments, resulting in complex influences on distal arterial pressure. It is important to determine the hemodynamic significance of stenoses in each of these areas to reconstruct optimally arterial occlusive disease and achieve maximal clinical effects with minimal intervention. Although arteriography provides an anatomic representation of atherosclerotic disease, it is frequently impossible to measure the severity of stenoses accurately because of irregularities of their geometry and three-dimensional asymmetry that confound single-plane or even biplane arteriography. For these reasons, measurement of segmental pressure gradients in the lower extremity, by placing blood pressure cuffs at different levels, is an important part of the clinical evaluation.

It is possible to illustrate the effect of sequential stenoses on segmental pressures in the lower extremity by assuming fixed arterial resistances (stenoses) without changes in collateral blood flow (Fig. 74-9). Aortoiliac and superficial femoral artery stenoses result in progressive pressure decrements because resting flow is maintained in the extremity by compensatory increases in peripheral vasodilation.

During exercise, peripheral resistance is further decreased by dilation of arterioles in skeletal muscle to augment flow required by local metabolism. The resulting flow increase causes a larger pressure gradient across the first (proximal) fixed stenosis in the aortoiliac segment, so that the pressure "head" seen by the superficial femoral system is even further reduced. This ultimately results in inadequate flow to calf muscles despite maximal vasodilation, so that calf claudication occurs. This distal watershed depletion explains the calf claudication that can occur with aortoiliac occlusive disease before buttock and thigh claudication.

Collateral Circulation

Assessment of an arterial stenosis by measuring the resultant pressure gradient is further complicated by collateral arteries that may improve blood flow around a major stenosis or occlusion. Blood flow through collateral arteries results when an energy gradient occurs across the stenosis in a major artery, inducing flow through collaterals from the proximal, higher energy level to the distal, lower energy level.[16] Chronically, this leads to dilation and perhaps proliferation of collateral arteries. Because collateral arteries develop as a result of flow limitation through the major artery, they are generally maximally dilated and represent a relatively fixed resistance. The presence of an effective collateral circulation, however, limits the impact of a major arterial stenosis. In reality, clinical pressure and flow measurements cannot separate the contribution of flow across the stenosis and the collateral flow. Instead, they determine the overall flow reduction and pressure gradient in affected extremities.

Because collateral arteries are considerably smaller than the primary diseased vessel, a much larger number of collateral vessels is required to compensate for the resistance change caused by stenosis of a large artery. Resistance is an inverse function of the radius to the fourth power; therefore, a 50% stenosis in a 0.5-cm artery would require 625 collateral arteries of 1 mm in diameter to compensate completely for this stenosis. The inability to achieve this compensation results in the necessity for surgical bypass or endovascular intervention to restore the original conduit diameter and relieve symptoms.

ARTERIAL ANEURYSMS

Although the factors responsible for aneurysm development are complex, there is a well-defined hemodynamic contribution to aneurysm expansion and rupture. Expansion occurs as a result of tangential stress (τ) within the wall of an aneurysm, and rupture occurs when τ exceeds the wall tensile strength. In a cylindric tube, circumferential wall tensile stress (τ_c) is defined by

$$\tau_c = P \cdot r/\delta \tag{17}$$

where:
P = pressure
r = internal radius
δ = wall thickness

This is a modification of LaPlace's law for cylinders with negligible thickness, expressed as

$$T = P \cdot r \tag{18}$$

In a sphere, circumferential wall tensile stress is defined by the formula:

$$\tau_c = P \cdot r/2\delta \tag{19}$$

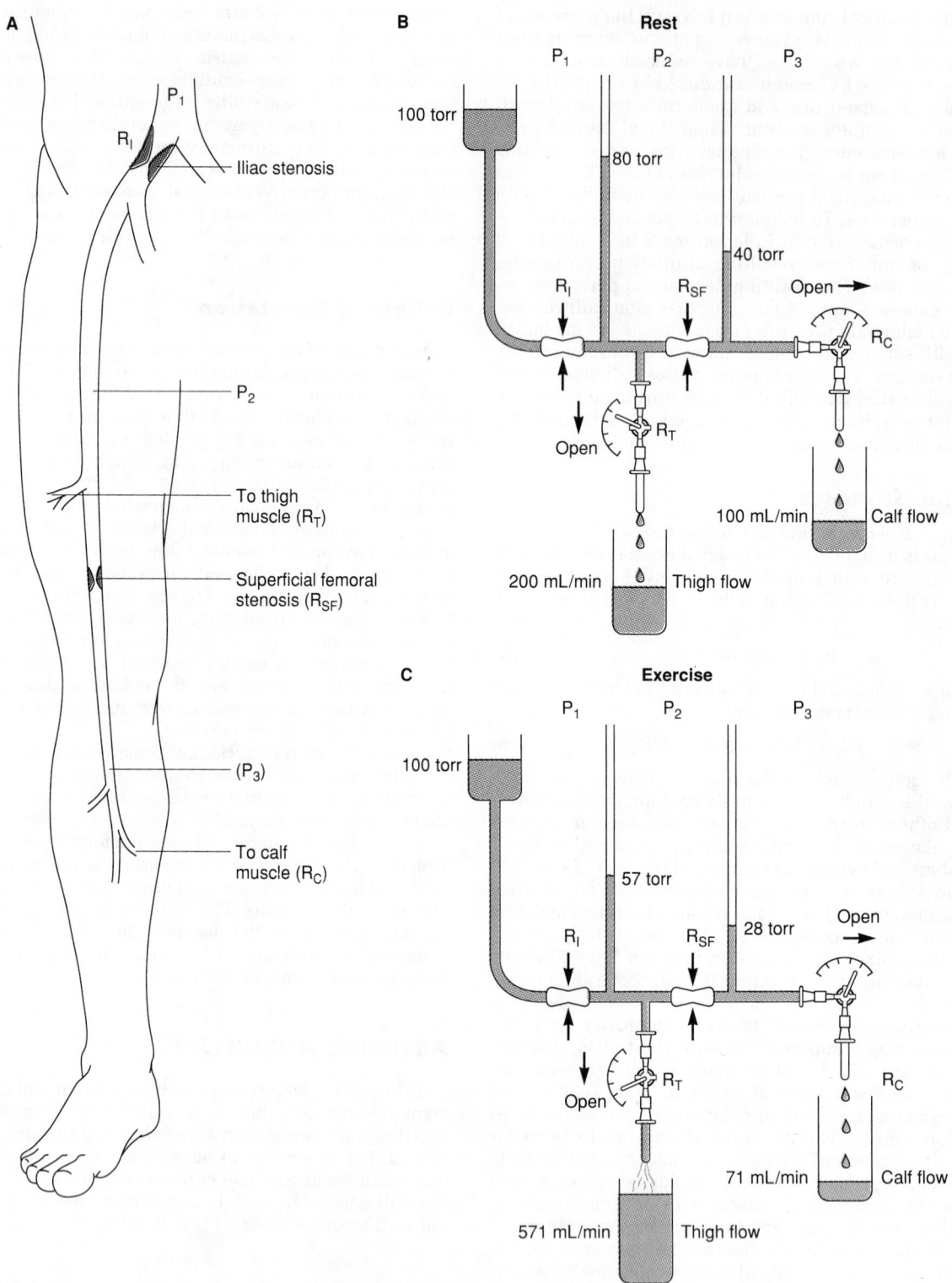

Figure 74-9. (*A*) Atherosclerosis producing common iliac and superficial femoral artery stenoses with fixed resistances (R_I and R_{SF}). Arterioles in the thigh and calf muscle control muscle flow with variable resistances (R_T and R_C). Intravascular pressure is measured at points shown (P_1, P_2, P_3). (*B*) Hydraulic model illustrating the effect of iliac and superficial femoral artery stenoses on resting thigh and calf muscle flow. Pressure reduction across R_I results in diminished P_2, which forces decreased R_C to provide sufficient calf muscle flow. (*C*) Exercise causes decreased R_T, which increases thigh muscle flow across fixed R_I and results in even lower P_2. This causes reduction in calf muscle flow because R_C is already maximally dilated and pressure at P_2 cannot overcome fixed R_{SF}. The calculation is based on equation 10. (After Sumner DS. Essential hemodynamic principles. In: Rutherford RB, ed. Vascular surgery, ed 3. Philadelphia, WB Saunders, 1989)

According to these formulas, increased arterial blood pressure and aneurysm size (radius) are linearly proportional to the wall tensile stress and, therefore, to the risk of aneurysm expansion and rupture. Conversely, aneurysm wall thickness is inversely proportional to wall stress, making thinner aneurysms more prone to rupture (Fig. 74-10). These mathematically derived risk factors for aneurysm rupture, hypertension, and aneurysm size have been confirmed by clinical observation.[17] Unfortunately, the wall thickness (and strength) of real aneurysms is not homogeneous and cannot be accurately measured. Of interest is the predicted difference between wall stress in a fusiform versus a saccular aneurysm. Fusiform aneurysms are best approximated by cylinders, whereas saccular aneurysms are more analogous to spheres. Comparison of equations

17 and 19 predicts that saccular aneurysms would experience about half the circumferential wall stress of a fusiform aneurysm. These analogies are oversimplifications, however, because real aneurysms have complex shapes and variable wall thickness.

A more accurate method to estimate aneurysm wall stress uses finite element analysis.[18] Results using this technique also predict greater circumferential stress in cylindric compared with spheric aneurysms, although longitudinal stress is equivalent. Furthermore, the tensile stress in an aneurysm wall is inversely related to the size of the native (proximal) aorta if wall thinning occurs during aneurysm expansion. Thus, a 6-cm aneurysm arising from a 1-cm aorta would experience three to four times greater wall stress than a 6-cm aneurysm arising from a 3-cm aorta. Unfortunately, none of these techniques allows precise calculation of aneurysm rupture risk in individual patients. They do, however, emphasize the contribution of aneurysm size and blood pressure to this outcome.

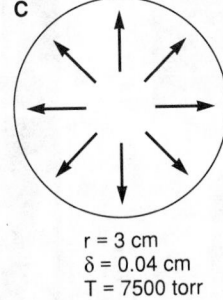

Cylinder $T = P \cdot r/\delta$

A

P = 100 torr

r = 1 cm
δ = 0.2 cm
T = 500 torr

B

P = 100 torr

r = 3 cm
δ = 0.2 cm
T = 1500 torr

C

P = 100 torr

r = 3 cm
δ = 0.04 cm
T = 7500 torr

Figure 74-10. Cross-sectional views of cylinders representing normal diameter infrarenal aorta (*A*) and 6-cm diameter aortic aneurysms (*B* and *C*) to demonstrate the effect of radius (r) and wall thickness (δ) on circumferential wall stress (T; τ_c elsewhere in chapter) at constant pressure (r = 100 torr). Expansion of a 2-cm diameter cylinder (*A*) to 6-cm diameter with no change in wall thickness (*B*) increases wall tensile stress by six-fold. If expansion occurs without increasing wall mass, wall thinning occurs (*C*), which results in even greater tensile stress within the wall.

REFERENCES

1. Strandness DE, Sumner DS. Hemodynamics for surgeons. New York, Grune & Stratton, 1975.
2. Folkow B, Neil E. Circulation. New York, Oxford University Press, 1971.
3. Burton AC. Physiology and biophysics of the circulation, ed 2. Chicago, Year Book Medical Pub, 1972.
4. Daugherty RL, Franzini JB. Fluid mechanics with engineering application, ed 7. New York, McGraw-Hill, 1977.
5. Sumner DS. Essential hemodynamic principles. In: Rutherford RB, ed. Vascular surgery, ed 3. Philadelphia, WB Saunders, 1989.
6. Nichols WW, O'Rourke MF. McDonald's blood flow in arteries, ed 3. Philadelphia, Lea & Febiger, 1990.
7. Davies PF, Robotewskyj A, Griem ML, Dull RO, Polacek DC. Hemodynamic forces and vascular cell communication in arteries. Arch Pathol Lab Med 1992;116:1301.
8. Giddens DP, Zarins CK, Glagov S. Response of arteries to near-wall fluid dynamic behavior. Appl Mech Rev 1990;43:S96.
9. Langille BL, O'Donnell F. Reductions in arterial diameter produced by chronic decreases in blood flow are endothelium-dependent. Science 1986;231:405.
10. Fillinger MF, Cronenwett JL, Besso S, Walsh DB, Zwolak RM. Vein adaptation to the hemodynamic environment of infrainguinal grafts. J Vasc Surg 1994;19:970.
11. Dobrin PB. Biaxial anisotropy of dog carotid artery. J Biomechanics 1986;19:351.
12. McGrath MA, Verhaeghe RH, Shepard JT. The physiology of limb blood flow. In: Jaergens JL, Spittel JA Jr, Fairbairn JF II, eds. Peripheral vascular diseases. Philadelphia, WB Saunders, 1980.
13. Whitmore RL. The flow of fluids. In: Whitmore RL, ed. Rheology of the circulation. New York: Pergamon Press, 1968:37.
14. Zarins CK, Giddens DP, Bharaduaj BK, Sottiurai VS, Mabon RF, Glagov S. Carotid bifurcation atheroscleroses: quantitative correlation of platelet localization with flow velocity profiles and wall shear stress. Circ Res 1983;53:502.
15. Karayannacos PE, Talukder N, Nerem RM, Roshon S, Vasko JS. The role of multiple noncritical arterial stenoses in the pathogeneses of ischemia. J Thorac Cardiovasc Surg 1977; 73:458.
16. Strandness DE Jr. Collateral circulation in clinical surgery. Philadelphia, WB Saunders, 1969.
17. Cronenwett JL, Sargent SK, Wall MH, Hawkes ML, Freeman DH, Dain BJ, et al. Variables that affect the expansion rate and outcome of small abdominal aortic aneurysms. J Vasc Surg 1990;11:260.
18. Stringfellow MM, Lawrence PF, Stringfellow RG. The influence of aorta-aneurysm geometry upon stress in the aneurysm wall. J Surg Res 1987;42:425.

SURGERY: SCIENTIFIC PRINCIPLES AND PRACTICE, Second Edition, edited by Lazar J. Greenfield, Michael W. Mulholland, Keith T. Oldham, Gerald B. Zelenock, and Keith D. Lillemoe. Lippincott–Raven Publishers, Philadelphia, © 1997.

CHAPTER 75

VASCULAR DIAGNOSTICS

DAVID S. SUMNER

The physician faced with a patient suspected of having arterial disease must answer the following questions: Is the disease present, and if so, what is its location and extent? What are the physiologic effects? What is the likely prognosis? Clinical assessment provides valuable clues to the diagnosis, but the history is often unreliable, and symptoms may be mimicked by other nonarterial conditions; the physical examination is subjective and heavily dependent on the skill and experience of the examiner; and arteriography—formerly the next step—is expensive, time-consuming, and carries some risk. During the past three decades, the gap between clinical assessment and arteriography has been increasingly filled by noninvasive testing procedures. Originally, these tests used simple instruments that contributed little more than basic physiologic information, but now that technology has become more sophisticated, they provide anatomic information as well. These noninvasive methods have become widely accepted and are considered an integral part of the diagnostic process.[1–4]

PHYSIOLOGIC AND ANATOMIC BASIS

Obstructive lesions introduce an impediment to blood flow that is manifested as a decrease in arterial pressure, as a distortion of the normal pressure and flow waveforms, and as a change in the velocity of blood flow. When the obstruction becomes sufficiently severe, flow may be compromised to the extent that tissues are deprived of nutrition, and metabolic effects appear. These perturbations can be detected and their severity evaluated with noninvasive testing methods. Other lesions may serve as the source of emboli, which in turn obstruct the more distal vascular tree. Still other lesions, such as aneurysms and arterial dissections, carry the potential of rupture and exsanguination as well as the possibility of secondarily causing obstruction. The newer imaging techniques are useful for diagnosing and evaluating these problems.

DIAGNOSTIC METHODS AND INSTRUMENTS

A vast array of diagnostic methods and instruments have been introduced.[1] Some have withstood the test of time; others have been discarded because of inaccuracy or because they were superseded by better methods. This chapter concentrates only on those of proven value or those with promising features.

Ultrasound

Of all diagnostic methods, those that employ ultrasound are the most widely applicable. Doppler flow detectors emit an ultrasonic beam at a frequency of 2 to 10 MHz. When the beam encounters a moving red blood cell, its frequency is changed in proportion to the velocity of the moving particle and the cosine of the angle (θ) that the beam makes with the velocity vector. Because the frequency shift is in the audible range, listening to the Doppler signal provides a quick and simple method of assessing blood flow transcutaneously. More information can be obtained by subjecting the Doppler signal to spectrum analysis. The resulting spectra are depicted graphically with frequency on the vertical axis, time on the horizontal axis, and amplitude as increasing intensity of a gray scale. The display not only shows the direction and contour of the flow pulse but also demonstrates flow disturbances, which produce a broadening of the normally narrow band of frequencies that parallel the flow envelope. If the angle θ is known, it is possible to estimate the velocity of blood flow at any part of the cardiac cycle (Fig. 75-1).

Real-time B-mode devices measure the time required for a pulse of ultrasound to reach an acoustic interface and return to the transducer. Intensity of the echoes is shown on a gray scale, and time is shown on an axis perpendicular to the probe. As the sound beam is swept over the area of interest (either mechanically or electronically) a two-dimensional image appears on the video screen, corresponding to a "slice" of the underlying tissue (Fig. 75-2). With these devices, the interface of the vessel wall and blood is easily imaged.

Duplex scanning, which combines real-time B-mode imaging and Doppler flow detection, has significant advantages over either of the techniques used alone. The image permits accurate placement of the Doppler sample volume, and the Doppler signal facilitates identification of the vessel being imaged. Color-flow imaging superimposes in real time a flow map on the B-mode image. Color (red or blue) identifies the direction of flow, and color saturation corresponds to velocity. Slow flow gives a deep color, whereas high velocities give a pale color approaching white. Color-flow scanning aids in the differentiation of arteries and veins and immediately identifies areas of increased velocity and flow disturbances.

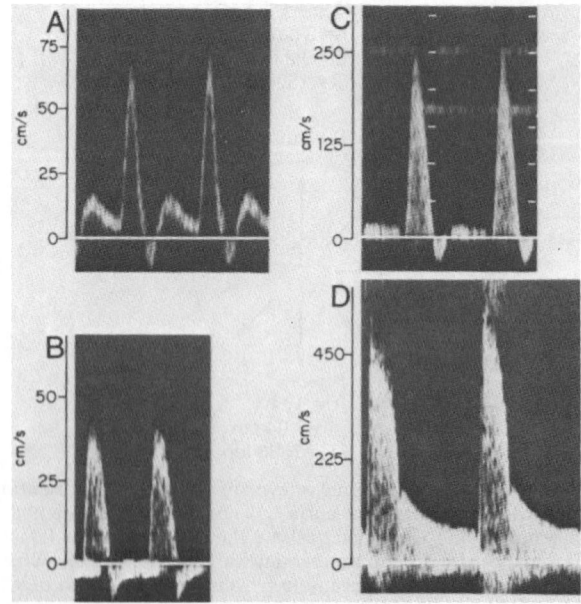

Figure 75-1. Spectral analysis of Doppler flow signals: (*A*) normal, (*B*) 1% to 19% stenosis, (*C*) 20% to 49% stenosis, and (*D*) 50% to 99% stenosis. (Kohler TR, Nance DR, Cramer MM, Vandenburghe N, Strandness DE. Duplex scanning for diagnosis of aortoiliac and femoropopliteal disease: a prospective study. Circulation 1987;76:1075)

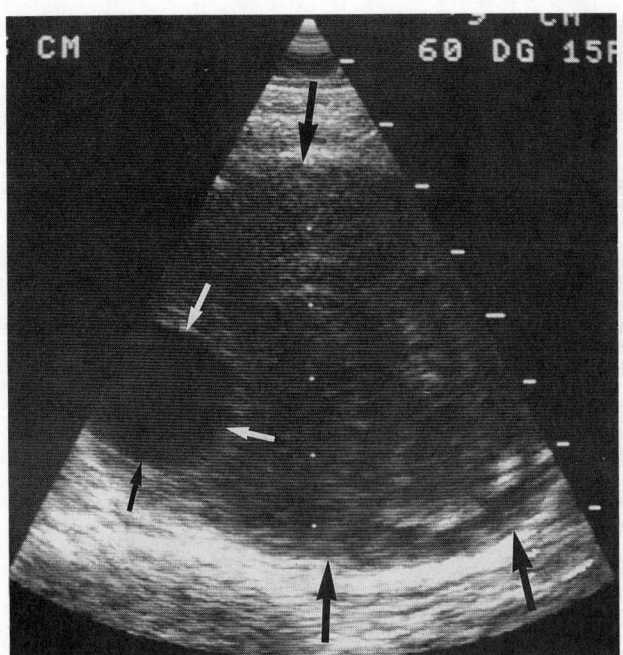

Figure 75-2. Real-time B-mode scan of cross section of a 5.6-cm abdominal aortic aneurysm. Lumen is largely filled with clot; hypoechogenic residual lumen is clearly defined. (Sumner DS. Ultrasonic screening for the detection of abdominal aortic aneurysms. Surg Clin North Am 1989;69:715)

technologic innovation that permits construction of three-dimensional displays of vascular structures. By manipulating the image on a computer screen, one can obtain views in multiple projections (Fig. 75-3). Early reports indicate that spiral CT scanning may be helpful in evaluating anatomic relations between abdominal aortic aneurysms and associated visceral arteries, thus obviating the need for arteriography.[5] Other potential applications include assessing disease in renal and visceral arteries.

Magnetic resonance (MR) imaging, which uses no ionizing radiation and is completely noninvasive, is now widely available. The images are comparable to those obtained with CT and, in many cases, are superior.[6] In addition to cross-sectional views, sagittal and coronal displays can also be obtained. Unlike CT, MR imaging can be used to assess blood flow. Although specialized instruments have been developed that produce recordings of pulsatile blood flow similar to those obtained invasively with an electromagnetic flowmeter, they provide less information than can be obtained with Doppler techniques and must be considered investigational. On the other hand, MR angiography, which generates an image of the flow stream that closely resembles a conventional arteriogram, promises to assume a prominent role in vascular diagnosis[7,8] (Fig. 75-4). Both cross-sectional and longitudinal images can be obtained in any desired plane. MR angiography has been reported to be more sensitive than conventional arteriography for visualizing distal runoff vessels in limbs with extensive obstructive disease, but this is debated. One drawback of MR angiography is that it tends to overestimate stenoses, owing to signal drop-out in vessels with slow or disturbed flow.

Plethysmography

Plethysmographs are instruments designed to measure volume change. Because volume changes in all organs (except the lungs) is a function of blood content, plethysmography can be used to measure fluctuations in venous blood volume and arterial pressure pulsations. Among the devices still in use for assessing arterial disease are the mercury strain gauge, the air plethysmograph (pulse volume recorder), and the photoelectric plethysmograph.

Other Vascular Laboratory Methods

Polarographic electrodes and the laser Doppler flowmeter are two instruments that are gaining acceptance in the vascular laboratory. When applied to the skin, polarographic electrodes can be used to measure oxygen tension ($TcPO_2$) or carbon dioxide tension ($TcCO_2$) in the underlying cutaneous vascular bed. The laser Doppler flowmeter, a device that amplifies shifts in the frequency of monochromatic light caused by motion of red blood cells, provides a qualitative assessment of cutaneous blood flow. Because of the complex geometry of capillaries in the skin and the multiple angles involved, quantitative measurements are not possible with this instrument.

Computed Tomography and Magnetic Resonance Imaging

Computed tomography (CT) plays a valuable but limited role in vascular diagnosis as a method for accurately displaying the dimensions and anatomic relations of larger vascular structures, particularly in the abdomen and thorax. It also provides the most convenient method for assessing the anatomic extent of ischemic lesions in the brain and for demonstrating intracranial hemorrhage, vascular malformations, or tumors. Spiral (helical) CT scanning is a

PHYSIOLOGIC MEASUREMENTS

The symptoms and signs of arterial disease are largely the result of impaired blood flow. The mere presence of arterial disease, however widespread, is of little immediate relevance. Consequently, physiologic measurements are of paramount importance in vascular diagnosis.[3]

Indirect Measurement of Blood Pressure

Of all the diagnostic methods available, none is more informative than measurement of peripheral arterial blood pressure. Fortunately, this is also one of the easiest and most accurate noninvasive tests. A pneumatic cuff is wrapped around the limb, and a Doppler probe is positioned over a peripheral artery (usually the radial artery at the wrist or the dorsalis pedis or posterior tibial artery at the foot; Fig. 75-5). The cuff is inflated to supersystolic pressure, and then slowly deflated. The pressure in the cuff when flow resumes is equal to the systolic pressure in the arteries underlying the cuff.

Ankle Pressure

In normal subjects and in those with lesions that do not reduce the diameter of the arterial lumen by over 50%, the resting ankle pressure usually exceeds the brachial blood pressure. Because the ankle systolic blood pressure varies with central aortic pressure, values may be normalized by dividing the ankle pressure by the brachial blood pressure. This ratio, commonly referred to as the *ankle–brachial index* (ABI), normally averages about 1.1 (Fig. 75-6). An ABI of less than 0.92 almost invariably signifies the presence of hemodynamically significant arterial disease. Claudicants have a wide range of ABIs, with average values of 0.60±0.15. In limbs with rest pain, the mean ABI is typi-

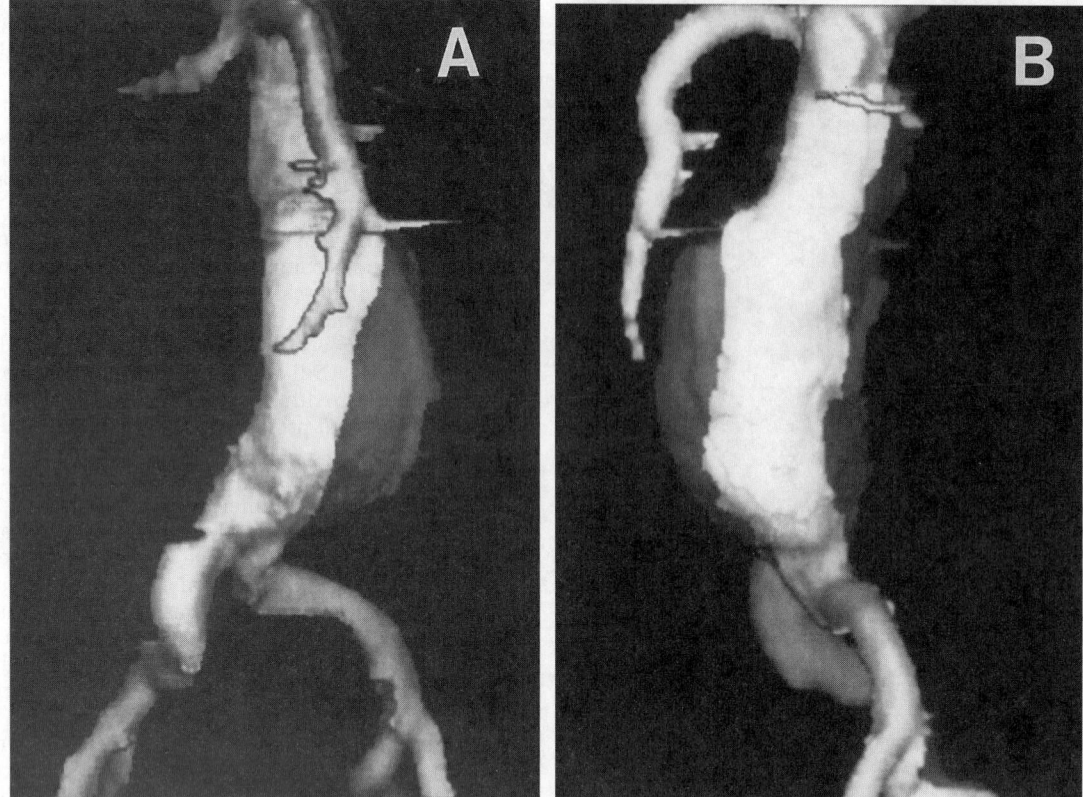

Figure 75-3. Spiral CT scan showing right anterior oblique (*A*) and left lateral (*B*) projection of an abdominal aortic aneurysm. Superior mesenteric artery, residual lumen, intraluminal thrombus, and both iliac arteries are seen. Highly stenotic left renal artery is poorly visualized.

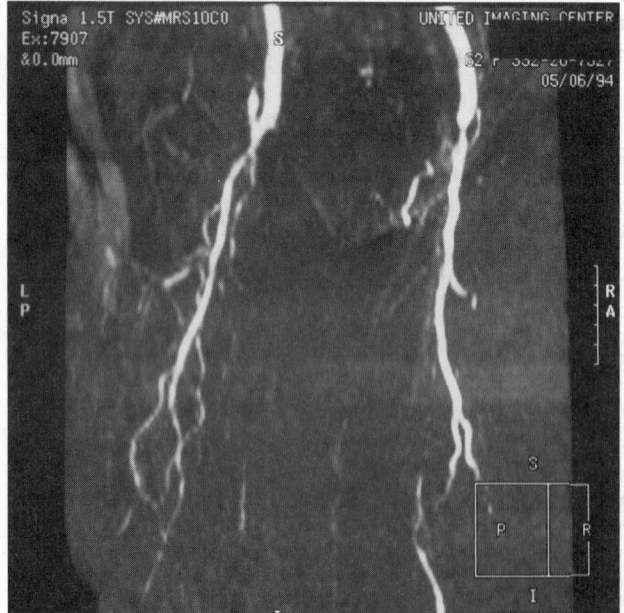

Figure 75-4. MR arteriogram (posterolateral projection) showing groin and thigh segments of a patient with an aortofemoral bifurcation graft, occlusions of both superficial femoral arteries, and short stenoses of both profunda femoris arteries near their origin. The right popliteal artery is patent above the knee.

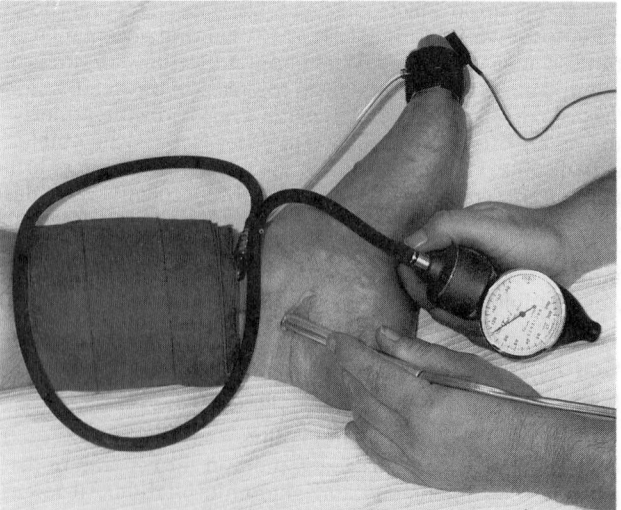

Figure 75-5. Measurement of ankle and toe blood pressure by the pneumatic cuff method. Flow in the posterior tibial artery is sensed with a Doppler probe, and toe pulses are detected with a photoplethysmograph.

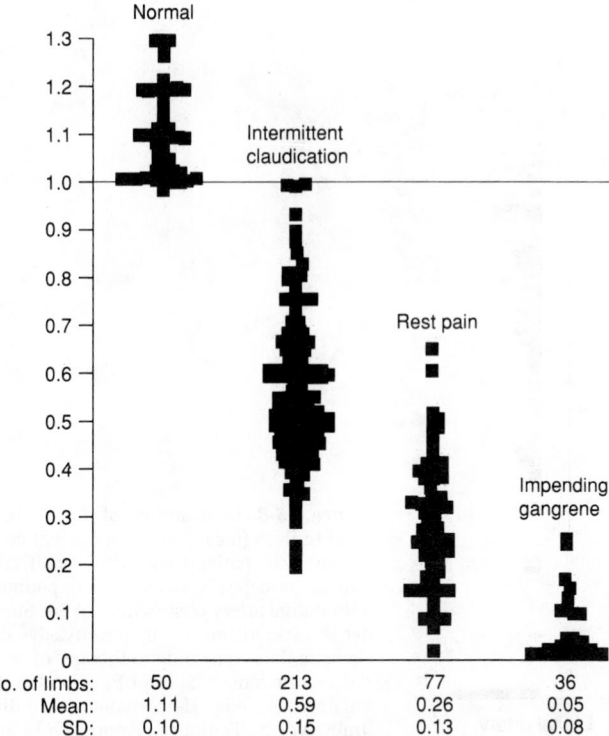

Figure 75-6. Relation of ankle–brachial index to the severity of functional impairment produced by arterial obstruction. (After Yao ST. Haemodynamic studies in peripheral arterial disease. Br J Surg 1970;57:763)

cally 0.25±0.13; and in limbs with impending gangrene, ABIs seldom exceed 0.2 and average about 0.05±0.08.

Absolute ankle pressures of less than 40 mmHg indicate severe arterial compromise, regardless of the ABI. When the arteries at the ankle are incompressible due to calcification (a condition often seen in diabetic patients), spuriously high ankle pressures may be obtained.

Toe Pressure

Systolic blood pressure in toe arteries can be measured by a method analogous to that used at the ankle (see Fig. 75-5). A small pneumatic cuff is wrapped around the proximal toe, and a photoplethysmograph, applied to the terminal phalanx, is used to sense the return of blood flow. Toe pressures are normally lower than ipsilateral ankle pressures. They are particularly valuable for identifying lesions confined to the pedal or digital arteries and are more reliable than ankle pressures in diabetic extremities. A toe pressure less than 30 mmHg indicates severe ischemia (Fig. 75-7).

Segmental Leg Pressures

Arterial pressure can be estimated in the upper thigh, above the knee, and in the upper calf by placing pneumatic cuffs at the appropriate levels. Comparison of pressures measured at the same level in the two legs or between levels in the same leg may help identify the location of the obstructive process. A difference of 20 to 30 mmHg is considered significant. Unfortunately, cuff pressures measured at these levels, especially those at the upper thigh, are frequently unreliable. The use of segmental pressures for locating arterial obstructions has largely been superseded by more accurate methods.

Upper Extremity Pressure Measurements

A pressure difference exceeding 15 to 20 mmHg between arms at the brachial, forearm, or wrist levels signifies the presence of proximal arterial obstruction. Gradients between levels should be less than 15 mmHg. Finger pressures are measured in the same fashion as toe pressures, using cuffs placed around the proximal phalanx and a photoplethysmograph attached to the fingertip. The finger–brachial index is calculated by dividing the finger pressure by the ipsilateral brachial pressure. In the absence of

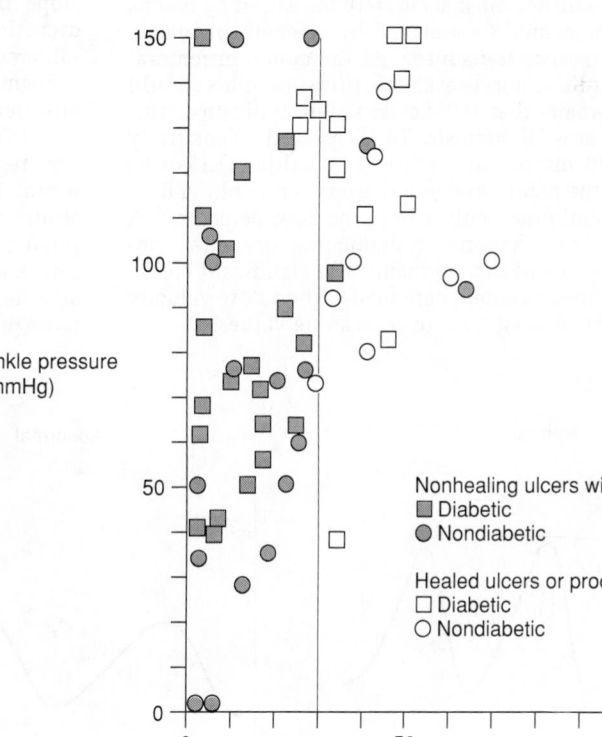

Figure 75-7. Ankle and toe pressures in limbs in which ulcers healed with local therapy compared with those in which healing did not occur. Few lesions heal when the toe pressure is below 30 mmHg. (After Ramsey DE, Manke DA, Sumner DS. Toe blood pressure: a valuable adjunct to ankle pressure measurement for assessing peripheral arterial disease. J Cardiovasc Surg 1983;24:47)

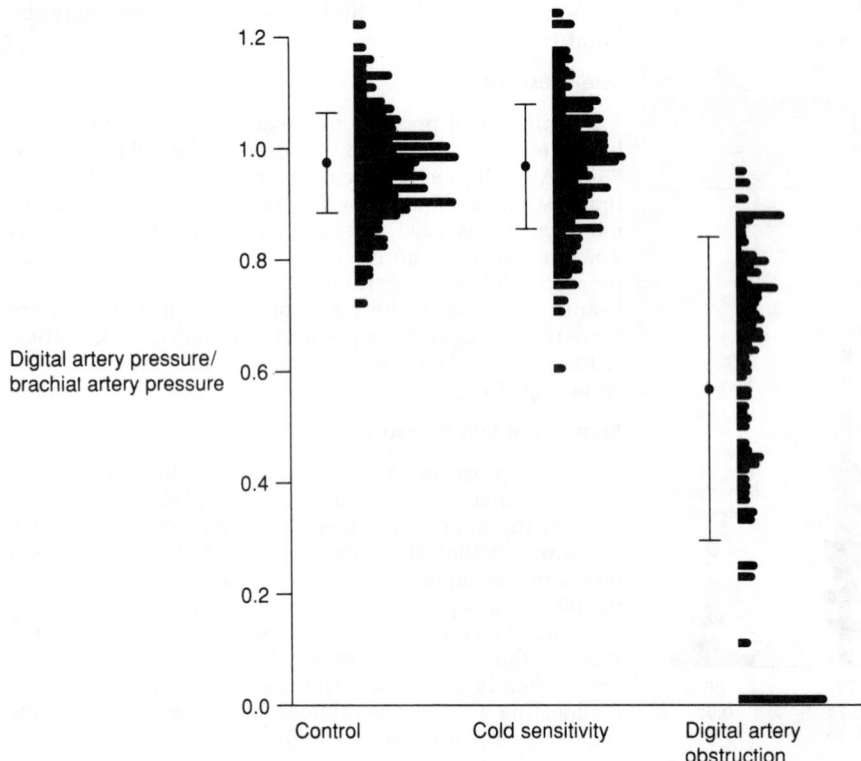

Figure 75-8. Distribution of finger–brachial indices (mean ± SD) in normal control subjects, patients with cold sensitivity due to vasospastic disease, and patients with digital artery obstruction. (After Sumner DS. Algorithms using non-invasive diagnostic data as a guide to therapy of arterial insufficiency. In: Puel P, Boccalon H, Enjalbert A, eds. Hemodynamics of the limbs, vol 1. Toulouse, France, GEPESC, 1979:544)

arterial obstruction, the finger–brachial index averages 0.97±0.09 (Fig. 75-8). Values less than 0.8 indicate obstruction of the digital, palmar, or more proximal arteries.[9]

Direct Measurement of Blood Pressure

Arterial pressure is most accurately measured by means of a needle or cannula connected by a length of plastic tubing to a pressure transducer. At the common femoral level, the systolic femoral–systemic pressure index should normally be greater than 0.9. Lesser values indicate a critical proximal arterial stenosis. To increase the sensitivity of the test, 30 mg of papaverine (a vasodilator) may be injected into the common femoral artery while blood flow velocity is monitored with a Doppler flow detector.[10] A 15% decrease in the femoral–systemic pressure index confirms the presence of hemodynamically significant stenosis, provided measurements are made when flow velocity is increased by at least 50% over baseline values.

Plethysmographic Studies

Plethysmographic pulses normally have a rapid upslope, a sharp peak, and a downslope that bows toward the baseline (Fig. 75-9). A dicrotic notch or wave is usually present on the downslope. Distal to an obstruction, the pulse becomes more rounded, has a slow upslope, and has a downslope that bows away from the baseline and loses the dicrotic wave. In severe ischemia, pulses may be imperceptible.

Segmental plethysmography is performed by applying air-filled cuffs to the thigh, calf, and ankle. These studies, known as *pulse volume recordings*, provide some information regarding the location of disease (Fig. 75-10). More useful is digital plethysmography, which uses mercury strain gauges or photoplethysmographic transducers applied to the tips of the fingers or toes to act as volume sensors. An abnormal or absent plethysmographic tracing signifies the presence of disease in the digital arteries or more proximal vessels. Digital plethysmography is particu-

Normal

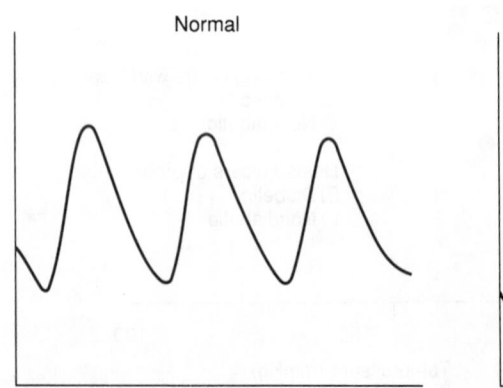

Abnormal

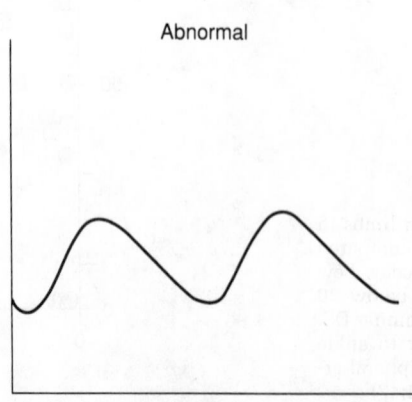

Figure 75-9. Toe plethysmographic pulses, normal and abnormal (distal to an arterial obstruction). Tracings on the right were recorded at a sensitivity twice that of those on the left.

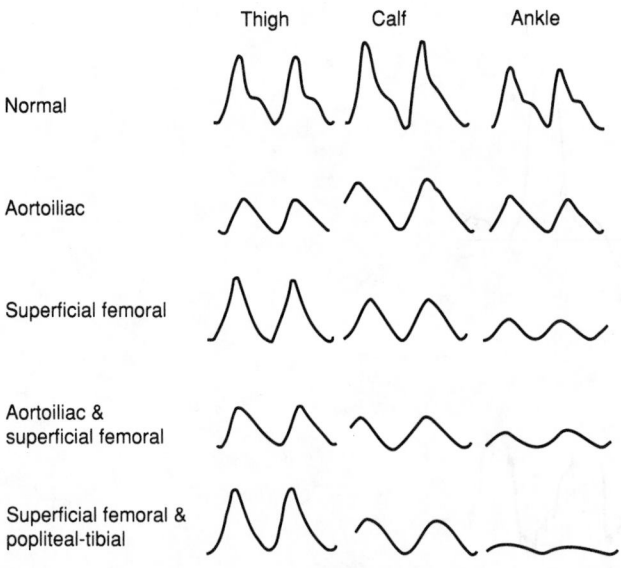

Figure 75-10. Segmental plethysmographic pulses from normal limbs, limbs with obstruction confined to the aortoiliac and superficial femoral segments, and limbs with multilevel obstruction involving the aortoiliac and superficial femoral arteries and superficial femoral and popliteal–tibial arteries. (After Rutherford RB, Lowenstein DH, Klein MF. Combining segmental systolic pressures and plethysmography to diagnose arterial occlusive disease of the legs. Am J Surg 1979;138:216)

larly valuable in conjunction with digital pressures for assessing disease distal to the wrist or ankle. The amplitude of the digital pulse, which is roughly proportional to blood flow, provides an index of local tissue perfusion.

Flow Studies

The normal peripheral arterial flow pulse is characterized by a rapid acceleration in early systole that culminates in a typically sharp peak velocity, followed by a rapid deceleration phase during which velocities fall to zero, a short period of flow reversal in early diastole, and a low-level forward flow phase extending throughout the remainder of diastole (Fig. 75-11). These fluctuations in velocity produce a characteristic triphasic audible Doppler signal that is easily recognized by the experienced observer. Beyond an obstruction, the flow pulse becomes more rounded, the acceleration phase is less rapid, the peak is less clearly defined, the reversed flow component disappears, and velocities remain well above baseline levels throughout diastole (see Fig. 75-11). Audible signals have a lower peak frequency, sound more noisy, and become monophasic. As the Doppler probe is passed over a stenotic area, the frequency of the signal increases commensurate with the increase in velocity. Absence of a signal indicates a totally occluded artery.

Spectral analysis of the Doppler flow signal, usually performed in conjunction with duplex scanning, provides a more accurate and more comprehensive method of assessing blood flow patterns (see Fig. 75-1). In peripheral arteries and bypass grafts, an increase in velocity of 100% or more and the loss of the reversed flow component identifies the presence of a stenosis with a diameter reduction exceeding 50%.[11,12] The presence of spectral broadening in the absence of a velocity increase distinguishes normal from minimally diseased arteries (1% to 19% stenosis), and a velocity increase of 30% to 100% suggests lesions

in the moderate stenosis category (20% to 50% diameter reduction).[11]

Different criteria are applied to studies of the carotid circulation. Flow in the internal carotid artery, which feeds a low-resistance bed, is positive throughout the cardiac cycle; there is no reversal of flow. External carotid flow patterns resemble those obtained from peripheral arteries. In the internal carotid artery, a peak velocity exceeding 130 cm/s suggests a stenosis greater than 50%, and an end-diastolic velocity greater than 120 cm/s suggests a stenosis exceeding 80%.[13] An internal carotid/common carotid peak systolic velocity ratio of 4 or more and an end-diastolic velocity of 100 cm/s have been proposed as criteria for identifying diameter stenoses of the internal carotid artery that exceed 70%, the cutoff point for severe disease employed by the North American Symptomatic Carotid Endarterectomy Trial.[14,15] Again, the presence of spectral broadening differentiates vessels with low-grade stenoses (15% to 49% stenoses) from normal or minimally diseased vessels. These studies are highly accurate, having sensitivities and specificities that exceed 90% for all categories of disease severity.

Color-coded flow mapping is a third way of assessing velocity patterns.[13] Color mapping is helpful primarily for rapidly identifying areas of flow disturbance or increased velocity (see Color Fig. 75-1). Spectral analysis must still be performed to assess accurately the degree of arterial stenosis.

Laser Doppler tracings obtained from normal skin exhibit three major characteristics: pulse waves that coincide with the cardiac cycle; vasomotor waves that occur four to six times per minute; and a mean flow velocity represented by an elevation of the tracing above the baseline. Arterial obstruction attenuates pulse waves, decreases mean velocity, and reduces vasomotor waves.

Oxygen Tension

Because the quantity of oxygen available for diffusion to the skin depends on the quantity delivered by the influx of blood and that extracted to meet metabolic demands, $TcPO_2$ levels provide an index of the adequacy of tissue perfusion. Measurements may be made from any region of interest, usually the dorsum of the foot or upper calf. Because oxygen supply is a function of arterial PO_2, cardiac output, and age, peripheral measurements should be compared with $TcPO_2$ levels from a well-perfused central area, such as the infraclavicular skin. In normal limbs, $TcPO_2$ averages about 60 mmHg (about 90% of the infraclavicular value) and is relatively independent of the site of measurement. Whereas many claudicants have resting values in the normal range, measurements made from the feet of patients with limb-threatening ischemia are usually less than 20 mmHg and frequently approach zero.

Exercise Testing and Reactive Hyperemia

Walking on a treadmill at 2 mph at a 10% grade provides an estimation of the severity of claudication. Subjects with normal limbs ordinarily walk for 5 minutes without experiencing leg pain, whereas those with arterial obstruction usually are forced to stop after about 2 to 3 minutes. In normal limbs, ankle pressures remain unchanged after exercise. A decrease in the ankle pressure measured immediately after exercise indicates the presence of arterial obstruction, the severity of which is roughly proportional to the pressure drop and to the time required for pressure to return to preexercise levels (which may exceed 20 minutes

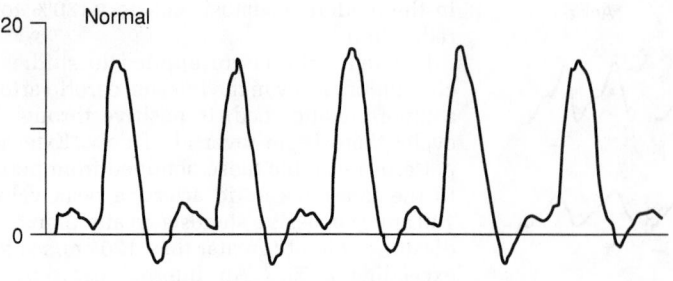

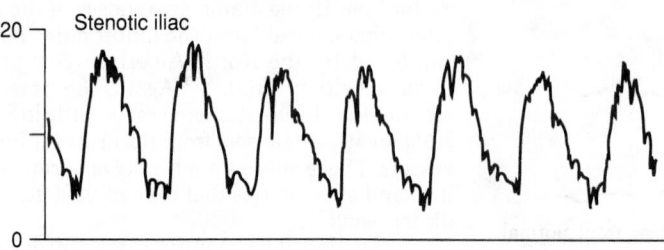

Velocity (cm/s)

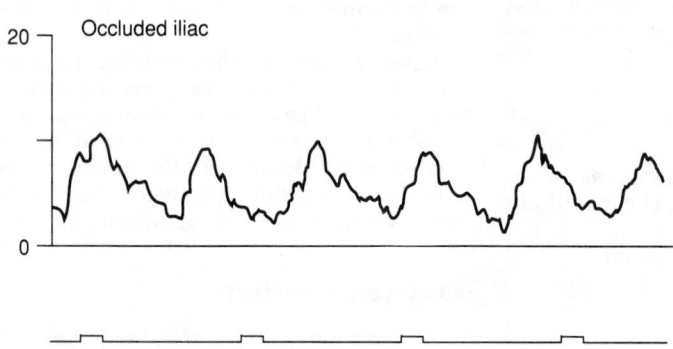

Figure 75-11. Analogue recordings of Doppler signals obtained from the common femoral artery of a normal subject, a patient with an iliac artery stenosis, and a patient with occlusion of the iliac artery. (After Strandness DE Jr, Sumner DS. Hemodynamics for surgeons. New York, Grune & Stratton, 1975:257)

in severely diseased extremities). The test is sensitive and capable of detecting arterial disease in patients in whom the resting ankle pressure appears normal. Reactive hyperemia may be used as a substitute for treadmill exercise.

Reactive hyperemia is produced when a pneumatic cuff placed around the limb has been inflated to supersystolic pressures for 3 to 5 minutes and is then quickly deflated. The increase in blood flow is commensurate with the ability of the terminal arterioles to dilate in response to ischemia. Normally, the digital plethysmographic pulse reaches peak amplitude in a few seconds, and the maximum excursion is more than double that measured during the control period. In limbs with arterial obstruction, pulse reappearance time is delayed, and there is little increase in pulse amplitude.

CLINICAL APPLICATIONS

All of the tests described need not be used in every patient; indeed, to do so would waste time, energy, and valuable resources. The selection of tests should be dictated by the history and physical findings and should be designed to answer specific questions pertinent to the diagnosis, prognosis, or treatment of the individual patient.

Lower Extremity Peripheral Arterial Obstruction

When the presenting complaints are compatible with intermittent claudication, an abnormal ABI usually is sufficient to establish the diagnosis, and no other tests are required (Fig. 75-12). If the symptoms are atypical or the ABI is normal (or nearly so), treadmill exercise is helpful. Failure of the ABI to drop rules out arterial obstruction, and another explanation for the patient's symptoms must be sought. Pseudoclaudication, caused by spinal stenosis, can be identified in this way. When the decrease in ABI seems inconsistent with the severity of the symptoms or when the patient stops because of angina, dyspnea, or pain localized to the knee or hip, the limiting defect should be addressed before considering treatment of the arterial disease. If calcification of the ankle arteries renders the ABI falsely high, arterial disease may be detected and evaluated by digital or segmental plethysmography, by Doppler flow studies, or by duplex scanning.

Severe Ischemia

The diagnostic approach is different in patients presenting with rest pain, nonhealing ulcers, or gangrene (Fig. 75-13). It is important not only to identify the presence of arterial disease and determine its severity but also to assess the potential for healing. Again, the first step is to measure the ankle pressure; there is no need for exercise testing. If the ankle pressure is in the ischemic range (below 30 to 40 mmHg), the diagnosis is established, and spontaneous healing is unlikely. When the ankle pressure is normal or above the ischemic range (due to arterial calcification or pedal artery disease), digital plethysmography, toe pressures, laser Doppler studies, or $TcPO_2$ measurements should be obtained. If these tests are normal or have values above the ischemic

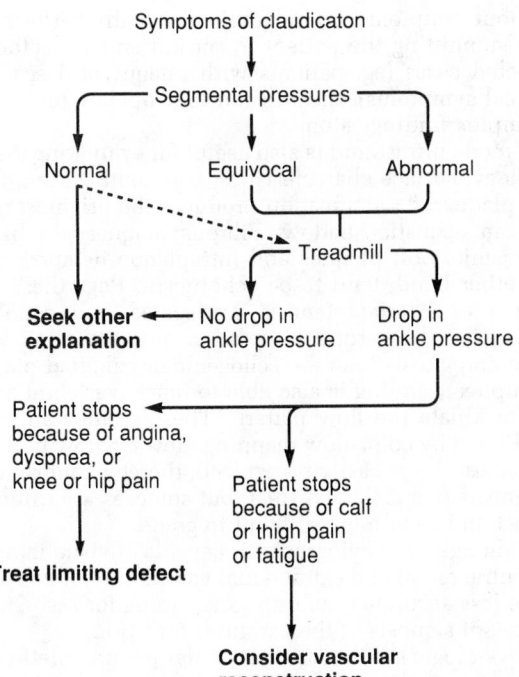

Figure 75-12. Diagnostic approach to patients with intermittent claudication. (After Sumner DS, Lambeth A, Russell JB. Diagnosis of upper extremity obstructive and vasospastic syndromes by Doppler ultrasound, plethysmography, and temperature profiles. In: Puel P, Boccalon H, Enjalbert A, eds. Hemodynamics of the limbs, vol 1. Toulouse, France, GEPESC, 1979:369)

range, it is unlikely that the pain or ulcers are caused by ischemia. Although atheroemboli constitute an exception to this rule, even in these cases, measurements obtained from the affected toe should be abnormal.

Ankle pressures above the ischemic range do not reliably predict healing. Toe pressures, in my experience, are reli-

able: healing is unlikely when toe pressures are less than 30 mmHg and likely when pressures exceed this level (see Fig. 75-7). $TcPO_2$ levels of less than 10 mmHg and laser Doppler velocities below 40 mV also portend poor healing, but these values vary from one laboratory to the next. Despite extensive research, no firm criteria have been developed for predicting the failure of below-the-knee amputations. However, a calf pressure greater than 40 mmHg, an ankle pressure greater than 30 mmHg, and a $TcPO_2$ greater than 35 mmHg provide reasonable assurance of healing.

Locating Sites of Obstruction

Before the development of imaging techniques, noninvasive vascular methods were limited in their ability to locate major arterial stenoses or obstructions. Although segmental pressure measurements, Doppler surveys, and plethysmographic studies might suggest that disease is confined to the aortoiliac, femoropopliteal, or below-knee segments (or to some combination of these areas), the results are too imprecise to be used as a guide to interventional therapy. Duplex scanning and color-flow imaging, on the other hand, have proved to be reliable methods for identifying arterial stenoses and for evaluating their severity.[11,16,17] These studies have proved useful for distinguishing between extensive occlusions that require surgery and short stenoses that are suitable for transluminal angioplasty. Even so, once the decision to intervene has been made, arteriography is almost always necessary. Arteriography provides no physiologic information and, when limited to one view, may seriously underestimate or overestimate disease severity. The hemodynamic significance of lesions in the aortoiliac segment is especially hard to assess arteriographically. Use of invasive pressure measurements at the common femoral level is recognized as a reliable method for determining whether a lesion in the iliac artery requires reconstructive therapy.[10] In skilled hands, duplex scanning coupled with Doppler spectral analysis may also suffice.

MR angiography, which has the advantages of being noninvasive and of providing multiple views, may prove suf-

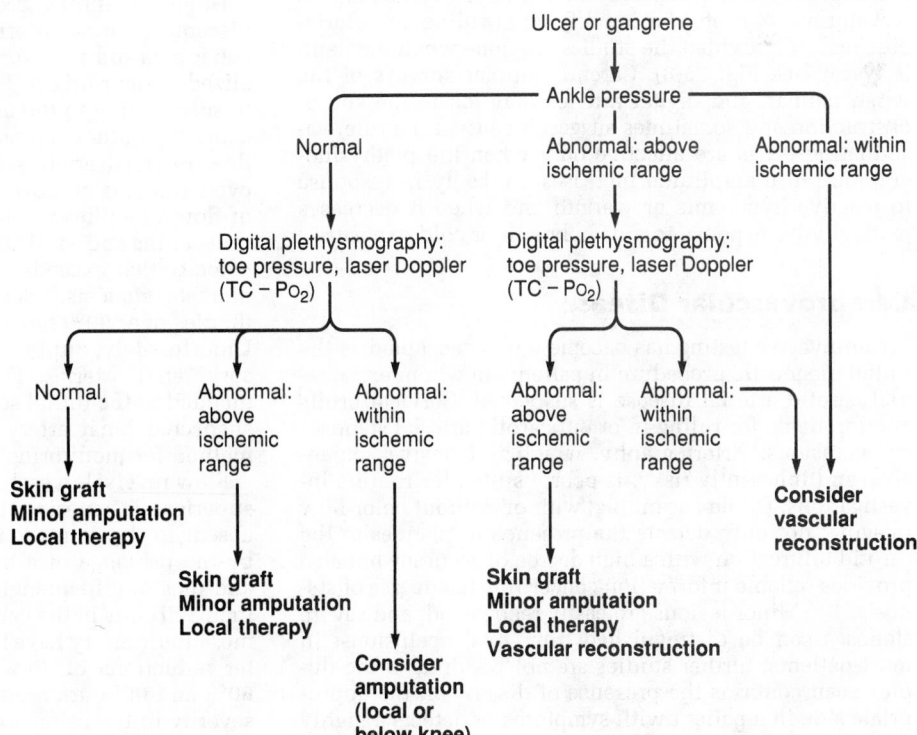

Figure 75-13. Diagnostic approach to patients with foot ulcers or gangrene.

ficiently accurate to supplant conventional arteriography in selected patients[7] (see Fig. 75-4).

Acute Arterial Obstruction and Trauma

Although acute ischemia is easily recognized clinically, it may be difficult to distinguish between embolic and thrombotic occlusion. Abnormal noninvasive test results in the opposite extremity indicate the presence of preexisting chronic arterial disease and suggest that the acute occlusion may be thrombotic. When the occlusion is embolic, a quick Doppler survey usually identifies the site of obstruction with sufficient accuracy to obviate the need for preoperative arteriography. If Doppler signals are present in the terminal arteries of the involved extremity and if distal pressures (ankle or wrist) exceed 30 mmHg, it is safe to delay surgical intervention, provided the symptoms are not severe. The time gained may be used to administer thrombolytic therapy, which is frequently useful in cases of graft thrombosis.

Decreased pressure and reduced or absent Doppler signals in arteries distal to the site of penetrating or blunt trauma indicate arterial trauma or spasm. In such cases, arteriography or surgical exploration must be undertaken. Negative noninvasive studies do not exclude arterial trauma when there is major hemorrhage, hematoma formation, fractures, or penetrating wounds in the vicinity of a major artery.

Vasospastic Disease

Vasospasm of the digital arteries in response to cold or to emotional stimuli (Raynaud phenomenon) is a common complaint of patients referred to the vascular laboratory. The presence of fixed obstruction (due to autoimmune disease, trauma, or many other conditions) in the digital or more proximal arteries of the upper extremity distinguishes secondary Raynaud phenomenon from Raynaud disease, in which arterial obstruction is purely vasospastic.[9] Digital arterial pressures and digital plethysmographic waveforms are useful for identifying or ruling out arterial obstruction, provided the studies are done when the hand is warm (see Fig. 75-8). Careful Doppler surveys of the wrist, palmar, and digital arteries may locate the site of obstruction and sometimes suggest a cause. As a rule, vasodilating drugs are effective only when the plethysmographic pulse amplitude increases markedly in response to reactive hyperemia or warmth and when it decreases markedly in response to a deep breath or cold exposure.

Cerebrovascular Disease

Noninvasive testing has become widely accepted as the initial diagnostic procedure in patients in whom extracranial carotid arterial disease is suspected. Cervical bruits are unreliable for ruling in or out carotid arterial stenoses or occlusions. Arteriography, which is invasive, expensive, and inherently risky, is poorly suited for routine investigations. Duplex scanning, with or without color-flow imaging, not only detects the presence of plaques at the carotid bifurcation with a high degree of accuracy but also provides reliable information concerning the degree of stenosis.[13-15] Minor lesions are easily recognized, and severe stenoses can be distinguished from total occlusions. In most patients, further studies are not required. If the duplex scan confirms the presence of disease on the appropriate side in a patient with symptoms or detects a highly stenotic plaque (over 80% diameter reduction) in a patient

without symptoms, arteriography is usually performed before submitting the patient to carotid endarterectomy. In selected cases (eg, patients with unequivocal scans and typical symptoms), the surgeon may operate on the basis of duplex findings alone.[18]

B-mode ultrasound is also useful for evaluating the morphology, surface characteristics, and composition of arterial plaques.[19] Calcification produces the brightest echoes and an acoustic shadow. Fibrous plaques are likewise echogenic. Soft plaques and intraplaque hemorrhage, on the other hand, tend to be echolucent. Regardless of the degree of arterial stenosis, variegated and echolucent plaques at the carotid bifurcation are associated with a worse prognosis than are echogenic or calcified plaques.

Duplex scanning is also able to image vertebral arteries and evaluate the flow pattern. These studies are greatly facilitated by color-flow mapping. Reverse flow in the vertebral arteries is easily recognized, thereby confirming the diagnosis of subclavian steal; but stenoses are difficult to detect and even more difficult to grade.

Although MR angiography is capable of visualizing both the intracranial and extracranial vasculature, it has proved to be less accurate than duplex scanning for assessing the degree of stenosis at the carotid bifurcation.[8]

Physiologic studies, such as ocular pneumoplethysmography, are sensitive only to stenoses that exceed 50% diameter reduction, cannot distinguish between severe stenosis and total occlusion, and furnish no morphologic information. These methods are seldom used today.[20] Transcranial Doppler, which is capable of recording flow velocities in the anterior, middle, and posterior cerebral and basilar arteries, provides more information than ocular pneumoplethysmography and is becoming the preferred method for assessing the intracranial circulation.[21] Although neurosurgeons have found many applications for the transcranial Doppler, its role in the evaluation of patients for carotid endarterectomy remains to be defined.[22]

Visceral Arterial Obstruction

Duplex scanning provides a method for studying the visceral and renal arteries noninvasively.[23,24] Although the celiac axis and superior mesenteric arteries are easily visualized at their origins, the renal arteries are more difficult to scan, owing to the angle they make with the aorta. Because the kidney represents a low-resistance vascular bed, flow in renal arteries is positive throughout the cardiac cycle (there is no flow reversal in early diastole). Absence of flow identifies a total occlusion, and marked spectral broadening and a ratio of renal artery to aortic peak systolic velocity that exceeds 3.5 indicate the presence of a 60% diameter stenosis.[24] Sensitivities exceeding 80% and specificities over 90% have been reported using these criteria. Unfortunately, duplex scanning often fails to detect accessory renal arteries. Duplex scanning has been recommended as the initial screening technique in patients with suspected renal artery hypertension and as an accurate method for monitoring renal artery reconstructions.

Flow reversal in early diastole typically is present in the superior mesenteric artery during the fasting state but is absent in the celiac axis.[23] Severe stenoses are identified by the presence of a high-velocity jet with high systolic and diastolic frequencies. Peak systolic velocities greater than 200 cm/s in the celiac axis or 275 cm/s in the superior mesenteric artery have been found to correlate with diameter reductions of 70% or more.[25] Accuracies exceeding 80% and 90% are reported for identifying disease of this severity in the celiac axis and superior mesenteric artery, respectively.

Aneurysms

Magnetic resonance imaging and CT are unexcelled for diagnosing and evaluating the dimensions of aneurysms or dissections of the thoracic and abdominal aorta[5,6] (see Fig. 75-3). Although the images obtained with B-mode ultrasound are less well defined, this method is useful for detecting and sizing abdominal and peripheral aneurysms and has the advantages of being more readily available and less expensive (see Fig. 75-2). Coupled with color-flow imaging, B-mode ultrasound readily differentiates femoral, popliteal, and upper extremity true and false aneurysms from hematomas, cysts, enlarged lymph nodes, and other masses in the same location. If the decision is made not to operate, the aneurysm should be monitored noninvasively to detect growth. In addition, the arteries peripheral to the aneurysm should be investigated noninvasively to detect and locate any concomitant atherosclerotic stenoses or emboli. These findings may affect the decision to operate and the design of the surgical procedure.

When the relation between an abdominal aortic aneurysm and the renal or visceral arteries requires better definition, or when obstructive disease of these arteries or the iliofemoral vessels is suspected, arteriography is necessary. MR angiography may provide sufficient detail in patients who are poor candidates for arteriography.[26]

Follow-Up Studies

Duplex scanning provides the best method for monitoring bypass grafts. A graft-threatening defect can be detected before the patient develops symptoms and before the ankle pressure begins to drop. The lesion can be localized to the inflow or outflow arteries, to the anastomoses, or to the graft. The addition of color-flow mapping facilitates these studies by immediately identifying areas in which the velocity of flow is increased or the flow patterns are disturbed[27] (see Color Fig. 75-1). A localized increase in systolic velocity greater than 100% of that in the graft above or below the lesion identifies a diameter reduction of over 50%.[12] Peak systolic velocities of less than 40 cm/s found throughout the graft are also an ominous sign.[28] To preserve graft function when either of these findings are observed, arteriography should be performed and the lesion, if found, corrected. Arteriovenous fistulas associated with in situ bypass grafts create flow disturbances that are easily recognized with duplex scanning or color-flow imaging. Blood flow velocities are increased at and above the side of the fistula and are decreased below.

Noninvasive follow-up studies also furnish objective information regarding the hemodynamic efficacy and longevity of arterial reconstruction. Even a properly functioning graft may not correct the primary defect, and there may be disease progression remote from the graft. Recurrent carotid arterial stenosis occurs with surprising frequency, a fact that was unappreciated until the advent of duplex scanning.[29,30] Most patients with vascular disease do not require operation, but they should be followed up noninvasively to detect or confirm progression and to provide information concerning the natural history of the disease.

1. Bernstein EF, ed. Vascular diagnosis, ed 4. St Louis, CV Mosby, 1993.
2. Kempczinski RE, Yao JST, eds. Practical noninvasive vascular diagnosis, ed 2. Chicago, Year Book Medical Pub, 1987.
3. Zierler RE, Sumner DS. Physiologic assessment of peripheral arterial occlusive disease. In: Rutherford RB, ed. Vascular surgery, ed 4. Philadelphia, WB Saunders, 1995:65.
4. Fronek A. Noninvasive diagnostics in vascular disease. New York, McGraw-Hill, 1989.
5. Gomes MN, Davros WJ, Zeman RK. Preoperative assessment of abdominal aortic aneurysm: the value of helical and three-dimensional computed tomography. J Vasc Surg 1994;20:367.
6. Tennant WG, Hartnell GG, Baird RN, Horrocks M. Radiologic investigation of abdominal aortic aneurysm disease: comparison of three modalities in staging and the detection of inflammatory change. J Vasc Surg 1993;17:703.
7. Carpenter JP, Baum RA, Holland GA, Barker CF. Peripheral vascular surgery with magnetic resonance angiography as the sole preoperative imaging modality. J Vasc Surg 1994;20:861.
8. Wesbey GE, Bergan JJ, Moreland SI, et al. Cerebrovascular magnetic resonance angiography: a critical verification. J Vasc Surg 1992;16:619.
9. Sumner DS. Evaluation of acute and chronic ischemia of the upper extremity. In: Rutherford RB, ed. Vascular surgery, ed 4. Philadelphia, WB Saunders, 1995:918.
10. Flanigan DP, Ryan TJ, Williams LR, et al. Aortofemoral or femoropopliteal revascularization? A prospective evaluation of the papaverine test. J Vasc Surg 1984;1:215.
11. Kohler TR, Nance DR, Cramer MM, et al. Duplex scanning for diagnosis of aortoiliac and femoropopliteal disease: a prospective study. Circulation 1987;76:1074.
12. Grigg MJ, Nicolaides An, Wolfe JHN. Detection and grading of femorodistal vein graft stenoses: duplex velocity measurements compared with angiography. J Vasc Surg 1988;8:661.
13. Londrey GL, Spadone DP, Hodgson KJ, et al. Does color-flow imaging improve the accuracy of duplex carotid evaluation? J Vasc Surg 1991;13:659.
14. Moneta GL, Edwards JM, Chitwood RW, et al. Correlation of North American Symptomatic Carotid Endarterectomy Trial (NASCET) angiographic definition of 70% to 99% internal carotid artery stenosis with duplex imaging. J Vasc Surg 1993;17:152.
15. Faught WE, Mattos MA, van Bemmelen, et al. Color-flow duplex scanning of carotid arteries: new velocity criteria based on receiver operator characteristic analysis for threshold stenoses used in the symptomatic and asymptomatic carotid trials. J Vasc Surg 1994;19:818.
16. Moneta GL, Yeager RA, Antonovic R, et al. Accuracy of lower extremity arterial duplex mapping. J Vasc Surg 1992;15:275.
17. Hatsukami TS, Primozich JF, Zierler RE, et al. Color Doppler imaging of infrainguinal arterial occlusive disease. J Vasc Surg 1993;16:527.
18. Dawson DL, Zierler RE, Strandness DE Jr, et al. The role of duplex scanning and arteriography before carotid endarterectomy: a prospective study. J Vasc Surg 1993;18:673.
19. Langsfeld M, Gray-Weale AC, Lusby RJ. The role of plaque morphology and diameter reduction in the development of new symptoms in asymptomatic carotid arteries. J Vasc Surg 1989;9:548.
20. Martin KD, Patterson RB, Fowl RJ, et al. Is the continued use of ocular pneumoplethysmography necessary for the diagnosis of cerebrovascular disease? J Vasc Surg 1990;11:235.
21. Schneider PA, Rossman ME, Torem S, et al. Transcranial Doppler in the management of extracranial cerebrovascular disease: implications in diagnosis and monitoring. J Vasc Surg 1988;7:223.
22. Comerota AJ, Katz ML, Hosking JD, et al. Is transcranial Doppler a worthwhile addition to screening tests for cerebrovascular disease? J Vasc Surg 1995;21:90.
23. Nicholls SC, Kohler TR, Martin RL, Strandness DE Jr. Use of hemodynamic parameters in the diagnosis of mesenteric insufficiency. J Vasc Surg 1986;3:507.
24. Taylor DC, Kettler MD, Moneta GL, et al. Duplex ultrasound scanning in the diagnosis of renal artery stenosis: a prospective evaluation. J Vasc Surg 1988;7:363.
25. Moneta GL, Lee RW, Yeager RA, et al. Mesenteric duplex scanning: a blinded prospective study. J Vasc Surg 1993;17:79.
26. Prince MR, Narasimham DL, Stanley JC, et al. Gadolinium-enhanced magnetic resonance angiography of abdominal aortic aneurysms. J Vasc Surg 1995;21:656.
27. Mattos MA, van Bemmelen PS, Hodgson KJ, et al. Does correction of stenoses identified with color duplex scanning improve infrainguinal graft patency. J Vasc Surg 1993;17:54.
28. Bandyk DF, Kaebnick HW, Bergamini TM, et al. Hemodynam-

ics of in situ saphenous vein arterial bypass. Arch Surg 1988;123:477.

29. Healy DA, Zierler RE, Nicholls SC, et al. Long-term follow-up and clinical outcome of carotid restenosis. J Vasc Surg 1989;10:662.

30. Mattos MA, van Bemmelen PS, Barkmeier LD, et al. Routine surveillance after carotid endarterectomy: does it affect clinical management? J Vasc Surg 1993;17:819.

SURGERY: SCIENTIFIC PRINCIPLES AND PRACTICE, Second Edition, edited by Lazar J. Greenfield, Michael W. Mulholland, Keith T. Oldham, Gerald B. Zelenock, and Keith D. Lillemoe. Lippincott–Raven Publishers, Philadelphia, © 1997.

CHAPTER 76

DIAGNOSTIC ANGIOGRAPHY

DAVID M. WILLIAMS AND KYUNG J. CHO

Angiography is the study of blood vessels. In conventional percutaneous angiography, radiographs are made as blood is displaced by contrast medium injected through a catheter that has been selectively placed in an artery or vein. When the lumina of vessels become visible as branching columns of contrast medium, subtle inferences can be made about the vessels themselves, their surroundings, and the organs or tumors they supply. Transcatheter angiography (hereafter called angiography, unqualified by a technical modifier) is unrivaled in its global, high-resolution demonstration of vascular anatomy and remains the gold standard by which newer vascular imaging modalities are judged. Angiography is used to demonstrate vascular anatomy, to identify abnormalities of the vascular wall and lumen, and to guide interventional vascular radiologic procedures.

ANGIOGRAPHIC TECHNIQUE

The percutaneous catheterization technique pioneered by Seldinger in 1953 provides vascular access for most diagnostic and therapeutic angiographic procedures.[1] The percutaneous transfemoral route is the preferred approach for most diagnostic and therapeutic procedures.[2] The transaxillary or transbrachial route is used when it offers a mechanical advantage for selective catheterization of aortic branches or when severe aortoiliac disease precludes the transfemoral approach. When severe occlusive disease, a recent surgical procedure, or local infection precludes catheterization of the femoral or brachial arteries, the translumbar route may be used for evaluation of the aorta and arteries of the lower extremities. This route limits the options for selective aortic branch injections.

After the route of catheterization is chosen, the puncture site is determined by palpation. In the absence of a palpable pulse, fluoroscopically visualized bone landmarks or Doppler ultrasound may assist in puncturing the nonpalpable artery. The artery is punctured with a quick thrust of an 18- or 19-gauge needle (20- or 21-gauge for children). The needle is slowly withdrawn, and, after pulsatile arterial blood return is observed, a guide wire is advanced through the needle into the aorta. The needle is replaced over the wire by a catheter with a preformed tip, and the wire is removed. In general, central (eg, aortic) injections of contrast medium are made before selective injections,

especially when ostial lesions are a concern or when a global view of arterial anatomy is desired. Aortic injections are made with a pigtail catheter, which has an end hole that allows the catheter to track over a guide wire. A preformed terminal pigtail-shaped curve prevents intimal laceration during catheter recoil, and multiple side holes are distributed symmetrically around the shaft just proximal to the pigtail to achieve radially uniform contrast injection. Aortic branch artery injections are made after the pigtail catheter is exchanged for one with an end hole and tip conforming to the proximal course of the artery of interest.

Contrast medium is introduced into the artery by a power injector at a rate sufficient to replace blood for several cardiac cycles. The blood flow rate in the artery is estimated by fluoroscopic observation of a hand injection of contrast medium. Underinjection of contrast medium results in dilution of the contrast by blood and poor filling of the arterial bed of interest. Overinjection results in reflux of contrast medium into the aorta or adjacent branch arteries and visualization of irrelevant or potentially confusing vessels. In the adult, typical iodinated contrast injection rates are 25 to 35 mL/s for 2 seconds in the thoracic aorta and 6 to 8 mL/s for 1.5 seconds in the renal artery. In general, filming or image recording proceeds rapidly during the arterial phase at the onset of contrast injection and more slowly during the capillary and venous phases. In the thoracic aorta, typical filming sequences are three exposures per second for 3 or 4 seconds (no capillary or venous phase); in the renal artery, typical sequences are two per second for 3 seconds, one per second for 3 seconds, and one every other second for 6 seconds.

Tissue detail on angiograms can often be enhanced by photographic subtraction. The negative of a film exposed just before the contrast medium is injected is photographically added to films exposed subsequently. This technique is useful in subtracting bone to enhance visualization of arteries, veins, or tumor stain (Fig. 76-1). It can also be used to salvage overexposed films caused by poor radiographic technique or nonuniform tissue density. Subtraction films must be interpreted with care, because photographic misregistration artifacts resulting from peristaltic and diaphragmatic motion during the exposure sequence can mimic vessels or tumor blush.

DIGITAL ANGIOGRAPHY

Conventional (film, screen-based) angiography combines high-spatial-resolution vascular imaging with sturdy and simple equipment. Certain clinical questions can be resolved without the high-resolution imaging of film, such as graft patency, presence of an arteriovenous fistula, and pattern of arterial branching as a reference for guide wire or catheter placement. In digital angiography, image recording is on an image intensifier rather than on film, at the sacrifice of high spatial resolution. The intensifier image is electronically read and stored on a computer disk. An image recorded before the injection of contrast medium can be used as a mask and subtracted, in real time, from images recorded as the contrast bolus passes through the circulatory bed of interest. Simple translations of the mask can be performed after the study to reduce small misregistration artifacts from cardiac, respiratory, and peristaltic motion. The accumulation of multiple masks allows one to choose the best mask (in place of the initial default mask) to subtract from a given postcontrast image. The images demonstrating the pertinent arterial and venous anatomy are recorded on film.

When used in the subtraction mode, digital angiography provides high visual contrast resolution, which may reduce the amount of iodinated contrast medium required

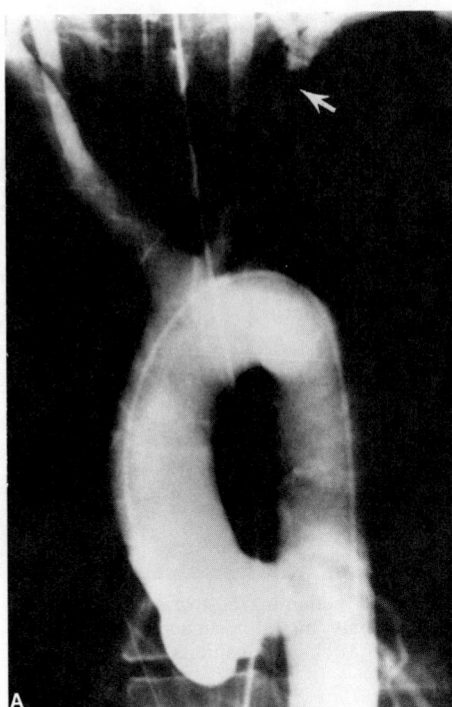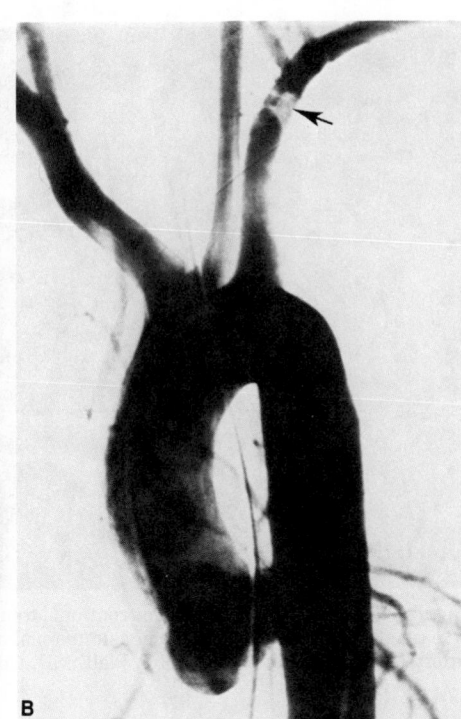

Figure 76-1. Value of photographic subtraction technique in thoracic aortography in a patient with chest trauma. An intimal injury in the left subclavian artery is barely appreciable on the conventional angiogram (*A*), but it is evident after photographic subtraction (*B*).

for an angiogram and even allows the use of carbon dioxide gas as a contrast medium (see later). Digital angiography provides images promptly, streamlining the conduct of vascular interventional procedures, and reduces film costs because only images showing the pertinent anatomy are transferred to film (usually multiple images on a single sheet of film). Digital subtraction angiography (DSA) with an intravenous injection of contrast medium is technically simple. When used to demonstrate arteries, however, it requires the injection of a large volume of contrast medium (40 to 50 mL) into the cava or right atrium and sacrifices the selectivity of the intraarterial exam. DSA with a peripheral venous injection is useful for studying venous abnormalities such as subclavian vein thrombosis or the venous side of dialysis fistulas. DSA with an intraarterial injection of contrast medium uses smaller volumes of contrast medium to produce angiograms and is superior in quality to intravenous DSA. Intraarterial DSA can be performed with small-bore catheters (3F to 4F); in conventional angiography, larger-bore catheters must be used. The significant disadvantages of digital angiography compared with film or screen angiography are its inferior spatial resolution and its motion-induced misregistration artifact.

HELICAL COMPUTED TOMOGRAPHY ANGIOGRAPHY

In conventional computed tomography (CT), contiguous axial images are obtained by alternating table movement and rotation of the x-ray tube or detector gantry. In helical CT, table movement and rotation of the x-ray tube or detector are continuous, so that the path traced by the x-ray beam on a cylindrical patient is a helix rather than a series of circles. Eliminating the delays required for table movement allows the acquisition of many slices in a single breath hold. With proper timing of the contrast injection, initiation of data acquisition, and choice of slice thickness and table speed, images can be obtained during peak arterial opacification. After image reconstruction, the vas-

cular system is displayed by computer interaction using contrast thresholds, regions of interest, and other picture-processing tools. There is a trade-off between the resolution of the image (how small a vessel can be reliably detected) and the volume imaged (how long a segment of the aorta is included). Helical CT angiography (CTA) seems reliable for visualizing the aorta and the first- and second-order vessels. Selection of the proper imaging protocol requires clear communication of the clinical question to be answered. Indications for helical CTA include preoperative evaluation of thoracic and abdominal aortic disease; in some institutions, this study has already replaced conventional aortography. Helical CTA evaluation of prospective renal donors and the screening of patients with normal renal function for renovascular hypertension are promising and under investigation at many institutions[3] (Fig. 76-2).

MAGNETIC RESONANCE ANGIOGRAPHY

Magnetic resonance (MR) imaging has revolutionized musculoskeletal radiology and neuroradiology. Using the same basic technology and exploiting motion-sensitive pulse sequences, MR angiography provides an unparalleled noninvasive demonstration of vascular anatomy. Cardiac and respiratory artifacts have been reduced by gating data acquisition and adding compensatory pulses to the imaging train. Patient compliance with the requirements of immobility and breath holding can be enhanced with intravenous sedation, hyperventilation with oxygen-rich air, and verbal encouragement. Imaging of the arterial system is significantly improved by carefully coordinating the intravenous injection of a magnetic resonance contrast agent with data acquisition. With careful attention to detail, impressive demonstration of the aorta and first-order branches is feasible, even in patients unable to hold their breath (Fig. 76-3). As in helical CT, there is a trade-off between resolution (the smallest vessel imaged) and the

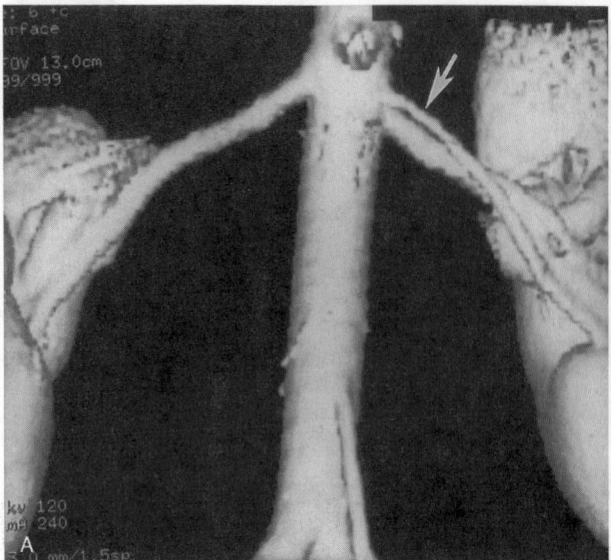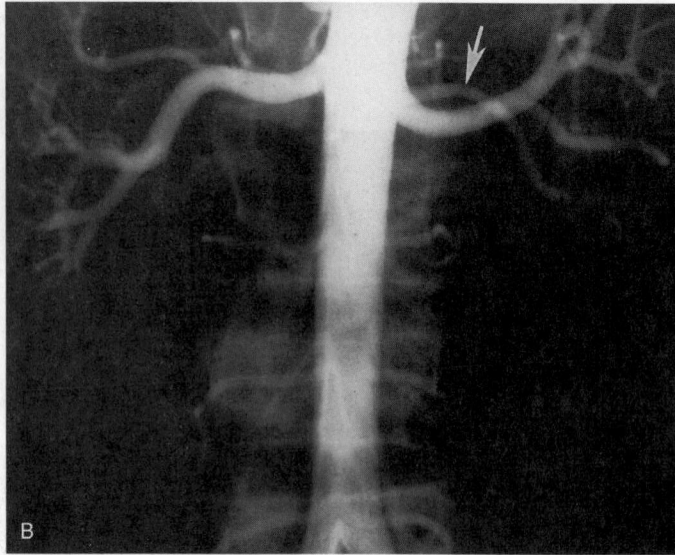

Figure 76-2. Helical CT (*A*) and conventional transcatheter (*B*) abdominal aortograms in a prospective renal donor. Both images demonstrate renal artery anatomy, including an accessory left renal artery (*arrows*). (Courtesy of Joel F. Platt, MD, University of Michigan Hospitals, Ann Arbor)

patient volume surveyed. The indications for MR angiography include the diagnosis and preoperative evaluation of thoracic aortic disease, abdominal aortic aneurysms, adult renovascular hypertension, and carotid artery disease. On the venous side, MR angiography is useful to evaluate deep venous thrombosis involving the portal, iliocaval, and lower extremity venous systems.[4-6] Contraindications to MR angiography include pacemakers and certain metallic devices adjacent to easily traumatized critical structures such as the eye and brain.

CONTRAST MEDIA

The contrast medium used for conventional angiography is a viscous, water-soluble, radiopaque liquid that is injected at the time of the angiogram. There are two general classes of contrast agents—the conventional high-osmolality ionic agents, which dissociate into a radiopaque anion and a cation, and the newer low-osmolality nonionic agents. Examples of the ionic agents are sodium methylglucamine diatrizoate and methylglucamine iothalamate; examples of the nonionic agents are iohexol and iopamidol. Sodium methylglucamine ioxaglate is an example of an ionic, low-osmolality agent. The high-osmolality agents are associated with direct cardiac and renal toxicity, idiosyncratic anaphylactoid reactions, and an uncomfortable tissue response (eg, coughing during pulmonary artery injection and pain during injection of arteries supplying the body wall or extremities). The nonionic agents appear safer in every respect, although they have shown no conclusive advantage in patients with renal failure.[7-9] If the question of safety were compelling, nonionic agents would be used exclusively. Universal adoption of the nonionic agents, which are about 10 times more expensive than the ionic agents, would increase the cost of medical care and, in an institution with a fixed budget, would exert financial pressure on other medical programs.[10] In practice, nonionic agents are reserved for patients with a history of contrast reactions or cardiac or renal failure, for children, and for potentially painful injections.

Carbon dioxide gas is also a suitable contrast agent for many peripheral applications.[11] Because of its inherent bi-

ocompatibility, it is especially useful in patients with a history of a severe contrast reaction and in those with renal failure. Its low viscosity permits the use of small-bore catheters, but its high compressibility makes it difficult to achieve uniform injection rates without the use of a special injector, which is not yet commercially available in the United States. It has been used safely as a contrast agent for abdominal aortography and lower extremity arteriography, for inferior vena cavography to guide placement of vena cava filters, and for venous opacification to guide placement of venous access devices such as Hickman catheters. It has not been used for thoracic aortography because of the potential risk of neurologic complications. Carbon dioxide angiography must be performed with the use of DSA (Fig. 76-4).

Contrast materials for magnetic resonance angiography are typically gadolinium-based compounds. These are expensive, but patent expiration may reduce their cost in the near future. They have no documented renal toxicity. For angiographic applications, the volumes of contrast material (20 to 60 mL) required for an adequate magnetic resonance signal from blood are relatively small; therefore, the risk of fluid overload is reduced compared with conventional angiography, which requires 100 to 200 mL of hyperosmolar liquid.

COMPLICATIONS

The overall rate of serious complications with diagnostic angiography is less than 5%.[2] The complications of angiography occur at the puncture site, in conjunction with catheterizing and injecting the selected vessel, or in association with the contrast medium. Puncture site complications include hematomas, dissections, pseudoaneurysms, arteriovenous fistulas, thrombosis, and, when applicable, graft infection. The frequency and severity of these complications depend on the experience of the angiographer, the attention to postprocedure hemostasis, the size of the catheter or sheath, the choice of puncture site, the number of catheter exchanges, and the duration of the procedure. Patients with uncontrolled hypertension, obesity, severe atherosclerosis, precariously compensated renal or cardiac

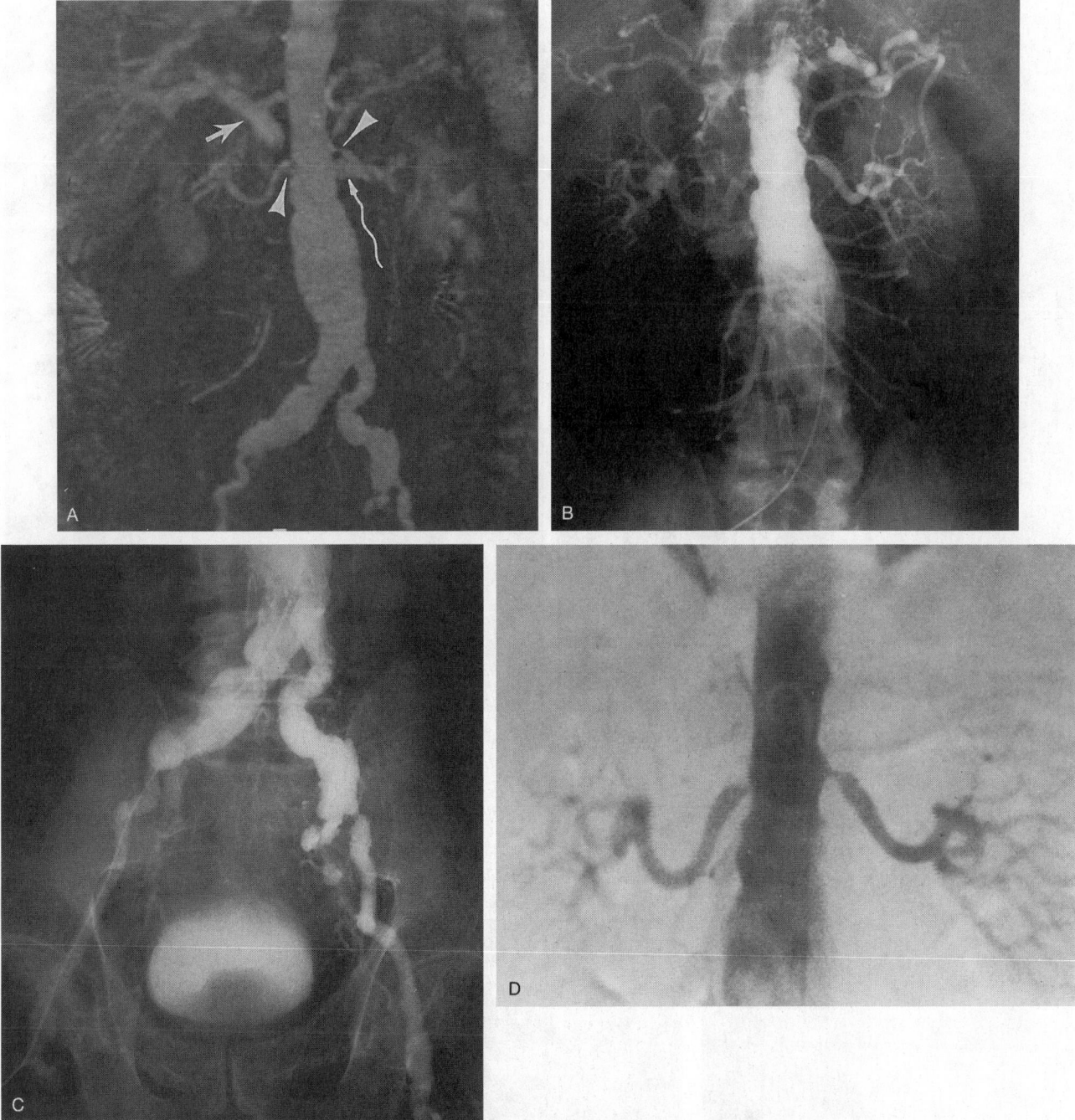

Figure 76-3. (*A*) Gadolinium-enhanced MR abdominal aortogram shows, in a coronal reconstruction, an infrarenal aortic aneurysm with proximal stenoses involving bilateral single renal arteries (*arrowheads*). Iliac artery aneurysms are also present. The celiac and superior mesenteric artery origins were demonstrated on a sagittal reconstruction of the dataset (not shown). Gadolinium has reached the portal (*straight arrow*) and left renal (*wavy arrow*) veins, but in this instance the study is not compromised. (*B* and *C*) Transcatheter aortography (using three injections) confirms the extent of the aneurysm. (*D*) Digital subtraction angiography with rapid image acquisition rate confirms the renal artery anatomy. (*E*) In another patient, gadolinium-enhanced MR abdominal aortogram shows the celiac and superior mesenteric origins (*arrowheads*) in profile. At the level of the left renal vein (*straight arrow*), an infrarenal aortic aneurysm buckles anteriorly; other reconstructions showed that the aneurysm extended to the bifurcation (not shown). Mural thrombus is apparent anteriorly and posteriorly (*open arrows*). (*F*) Conventional aortogram confirms visceral artery anatomy, but the caudal extent of the aneurysm is poorly opacified, even on later films in this sequence, because of contrast medium layering in the dependent posterior aspect of the aorta. (*A* to *D* from Prince M, Narasimham D, Stanley J, et al. Gadolinium-enhanced magnetic resonance angiography of abdominal aortic aneurysms. J Vasc Surg 1995;21:656; *E* and *F* from Prince M. Gadolinium-enhanced MR aortography. Radiology 1994;191:155. Courtesy of Martin R. Prince, MD, University of Michigan Hospitals, Ann Arbor) (*continues*)

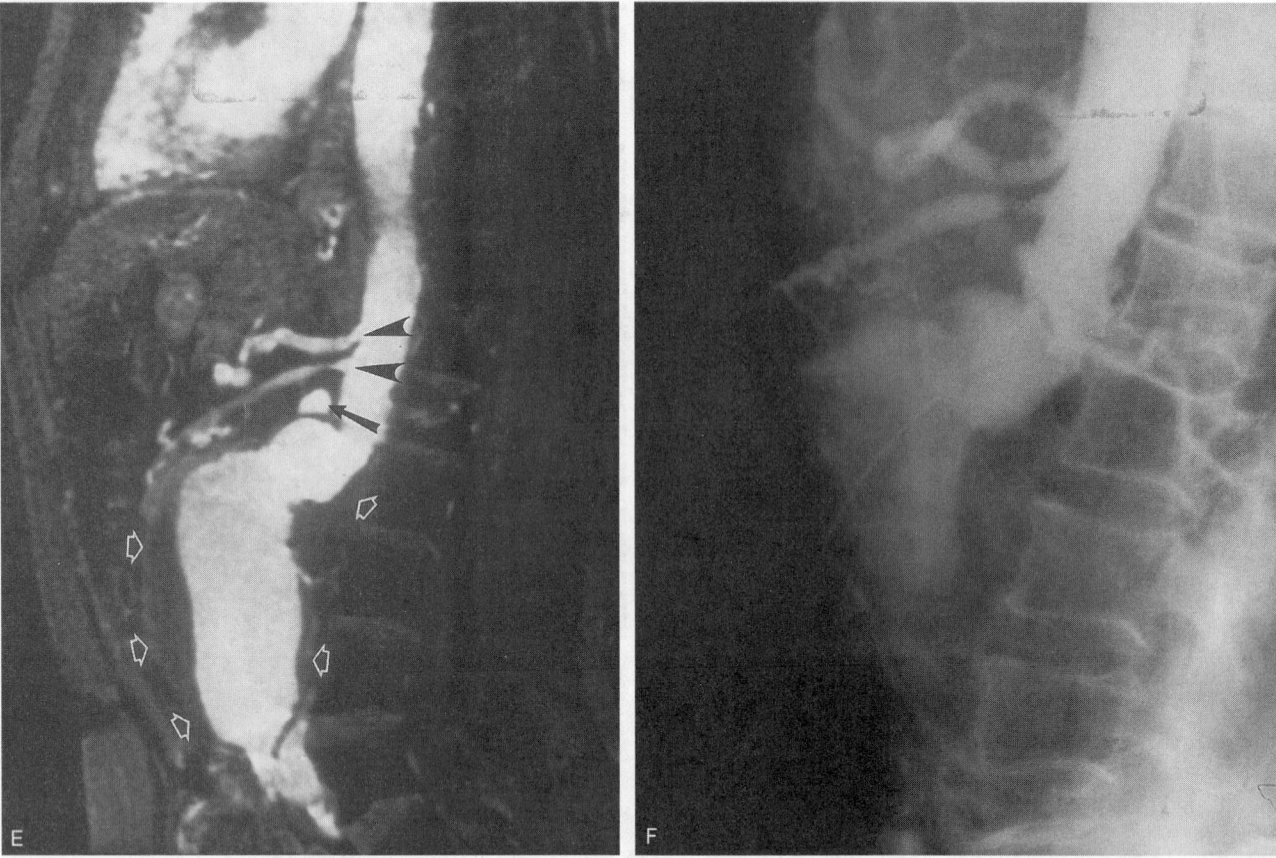

Figure 76-3. (Continued.)

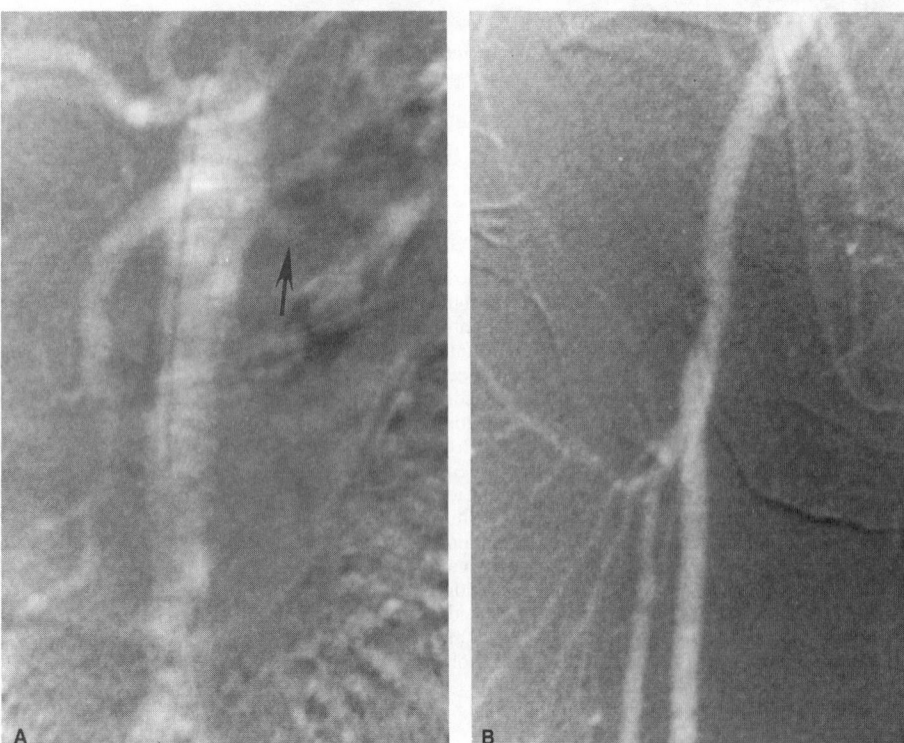

Figure 76-4. Carbon dioxide gas used as a contrast medium. A lumbar aortogram (*A*) and right common femoral arteriogram (*B*) were made during hand injection of carbon dioxide gas using digital subtraction angiography. The renal and lumbar arteries, which course posteriorly, are generally not filled by the buoyant gas with the patient in the supine position. The left renal artery is incompletely opacified (*arrow*).

disease, spasm-prone vessels, or poor coagulation status are at increased risk of complications.

Catheterization and injection complications include arterial dissection, perforation, and embolism (including stroke). The risks depend on the experience of the angiographer, anatomic variations affecting the ease of selective catheterization, the vessel catheterized, and intrinsic arterial disease. Thus, embolic stroke is associated with catheter manipulation or contrast injection in the aortic arch or brachiocephalic arteries. The gravity of a given complication such as arterial dissection or thrombosis depends on the vessel involved and the integrity of collaterals. For example, celiac artery dissection is usually well tolerated, but superior mesenteric artery (SMA) dissection may require urgent surgical repair.

The complications related to the administration of contrast medium include renal failure, fluid overload and congestive heart failure, transverse myelitis, and anaphylactoid reactions. These complications can be minimized by adequate hydration of the patient, careful catheter placement, and the appropriate use of a steroid preparation (eg, 32 mg of oral methylprednisolone 12 and 2 hours before the procedure) or nonionic contrast medium, or both.[12,13]

As a result of recent improvements in catheter and guide wire technology, the complication rate of diagnostic angiography has been reduced. Small-diameter (3F and 4F) catheters have fewer puncture-site complications and have made outpatient arteriograms a routine procedure in low-risk patients. Coaxial catheter systems and guide wires with excellent torque control and atraumatic radiopaque tips facilitate superselective catheterization for both diagnostic and therapeutic angiography.

CONTRAINDICATIONS

There are no absolute contraindications to angiography. Relative contraindications include severe hypertension, poor coagulation status, severe renal or cardiac failure, and a history of severe contrast reaction. Reversible medical conditions affecting the risks of the procedure should be corrected before the angiographic procedure.

OUTPATIENT ANGIOGRAPHY

Outpatient angiography is a safe procedure and a realistic option for elective procedures in many patients.[14] The use of small-bore catheters, postprocedure patient monitoring for 4 to 6 hours by radiology nursing staff, and discharge of the patient to attendant care by a family member or friend minimize the risk of puncture-site hematomas. Intraarterial DSA and hydration with intravenous or oral fluids reduce the nephrotoxicity of the contrast medium. In selected patients, uncomplicated procedures such as angioplasty may be appropriate on an outpatient basis.[15] Communication between the surgery and angiography departments well in advance of the procedure is desirable to ensure that the patient is properly prepared for the examination. Such preparation includes review of the clinical history and screening laboratory tests, the appropriate use of prophylactic antibiotics, preprocedure hydration, and arrangements for observed care after discharge from the outpatient facility. Patients at increased risk for puncture-site complications or renal failure (see Complications, earlier) should probably undergo angiography as inpatients.

FUTURE DEVELOPMENTS

Helical CT and MR angiography are in their technical adolescence, and it is difficult to predict their final impact on conventional diagnostic angiography. With further technological advances, helical CT and MR angiography will likely be capable of visualizing the aorta and vena cava and their first- to third-order branches. The role of angiography would then be limited to the hemodynamic evaluation of vascular lesions and the guidance of endovascular therapy, and to the diagnosis of medium- and small-vessel disease. Moreover, it would share the interventional monitoring functions with intravascular ultrasound and angioscopy. In interventional angiography, stent grafts appear poised to revolutionize the treatment of aortic disease, although the ideal combination of stent, cover, fixation device, and delivery system has yet to be found. All stents and possibly stent grafts are plagued by restenosis at the transition zone between the stented and unstented vessel wall. Effective therapy for neointimal hyperplasia is required before these devices can be used for routine treatment rather than just for salvage-type procedures.

VASCULAR ANATOMY AND IMPLICATIONS

Although a detailed description of the vascular anatomy of individual organs is beyond the scope of this chapter, a brief discussion of vascular anatomy is important for both the performance and interpretation of angiograms.

Thoracic Aorta

Thoracic aortography is indicated for the study of congenital anomalies and acquired diseases of the thoracic aorta and its major branches (eg, aneurysm, dissection, traumatic laceration, aortic valvular disease, and aortic arch syndrome). It is performed with use of the right posterior oblique, anteroposterior, and lateral projections, with injection of contrast medium into the aortic root. Thoracic aortography should demonstrate the thoracic aorta from the aortic root to the level of the diaphragm, the innominate artery, and the subclavian, common carotid, and vertebral arteries. Other branches of the thoracic aorta, which usually require selective catheterization for visualization, are the bronchial and intercostal arteries and the anterior radiculomedullary artery. The bronchial arteries arise from the ventral surface of the upper part of the thoracic aorta or from the upper intercostal arteries between the fifth and seventh thoracic vertebrae. They become dilated in a variety of conditions, including pulmonary thromboembolism, chronic inflammatory disease of the lung, and congenital heart diseases associated with a decrease in pulmonary artery blood flow. Because the anterior radiculomedullary artery (artery of Adamkiewicz) may arise anywhere from the descending thoracic and proximal lumbar aorta, extreme care should be exercised to avoid spinal cord injury during bronchial and intercostal angiography. Precautions include the use of nonionic contrast medium, scrupulous care not to wedge the catheter in the bronchial or intercostal artery during contrast injection, prompt removal of the catheter from the artery after injection, and meticulous inspection of diagnostic arteriograms for the characteristic appearance of the spinal artery.

Abdominal Aorta

Abdominal aortography is performed to demonstrate the abdominal aorta and its branches, including the celiac, mesenteric, renal, lumbar, and iliac arteries. The celiac and superior mesenteric arteries arise from the ventral surface of the aorta proximal to the renal arteries between the 12th thoracic body and the first lumbar vertebral body.

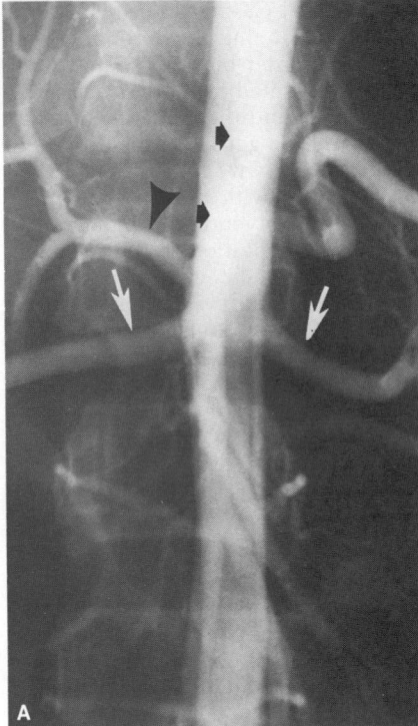 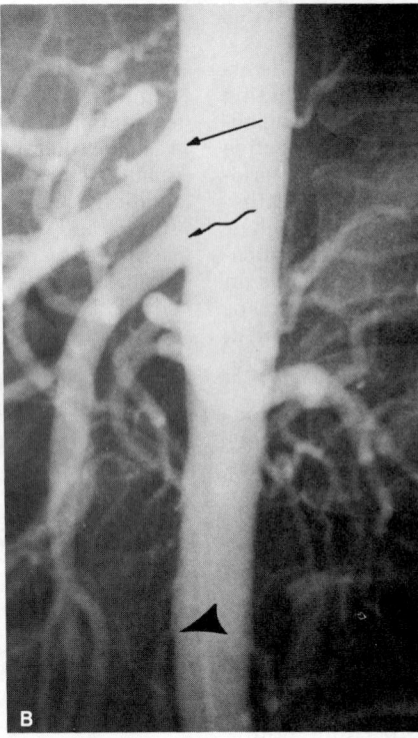

Figure 76-5. Biplanar aortography reveals visceral artery origins in optimal projection. (*A*) Anteroposterior aortogram shows the renal artery origins (*white arrows*) in profile. The celiac and superior mesenteric artery origins (*solid arrows*) project over the aorta. The common hepatic artery (*arrowhead*) originates from the superior mesenteric artery. (*B*) Lateral aortogram (different patient) shows the celiac (*straight arrow*) and superior (*wavy arrow*) and inferior mesenteric artery origins in profile. Mild stenosis is visible at the inferior mesenteric artery origin (*arrowhead*).

Thus, lateral aortography is necessary to see their origins (Fig. 76-5).

The renal arteries arise from the lateral margins of the aorta below the origin of the SMA, and their orifices are seen by aortograms obtained in the anteroposterior and slight left anterior oblique projections. Each kidney usually has a single renal artery. In about 20% to 30% of cases, more than one renal artery supplies a kidney (Fig. 76-6). The supplementary renal arteries are usually smaller than the main renal artery and may arise from anywhere between the 11th thoracic vertebral body and the iliac arteries. It is important to identify the origins of supplementary arteries before surgery for aortic aneurysm, aortoiliac occlusive disease, and renal artery stenosis. The arterial supply of ectopic and fused kidneys is variable in the origin, number, and course of renal arteries, and multiple injections of contrast may be necessary for complete evaluation. The lumbar arteries are ordinarily small and supply the body wall, retroperitoneum, paravertebral muscles, and spine. They provide collateral flow to the pelvis and lower extremities in the presence of aortoiliac occlusive disease. Supplemental collateral flow to the lower trunk can also develop from the subclavian artery by way of the internal mammary artery and from the axillary artery by way of the lateral thoracic artery.

Pelvic Arteries

Pelvic arteriography is indicated for suspected abnormalities of the common, external, internal iliac, and femoral arteries, and as part of the arteriographic study of the lower extremities. Contrast material is injected into the distal abdominal aorta. Optimal evaluation of the bifurcations of the common iliac and femoral arteries requires oblique pelvic arteriograms. Selective catheterization of the branches of the internal iliac artery is done for visualization of the penile arteries in the workup of impotence and for embolization in pelvic neoplasms and hemorrhage. Proximal embolization of the branches of the internal iliac artery with particulate materials can be performed safely because of the availability of abundant collateral circulation. Liquid materials, such as alcohol, sclerosing agents, and tissue adhesives, are generally not used because of the potential for tissue necrosis and sciatic nerve paralysis. Anastomoses of the external and internal iliac arteries with their contralateral mates and with branches of the lumbar and deep femoral arteries allow collateral reconstitution

Figure 76-6. Multiple renal arteries. Lumbar aortogram shows normal right and left main renal arteries (*arrowheads*). In addition, two accessory right lower pole arteries arise from the aortic bifurcation and mid-portion of the right common iliac artery (*white arrows*). Multiple jejunal arteries arising from the superior mesenteric artery are seen below the level of the left renal artery.

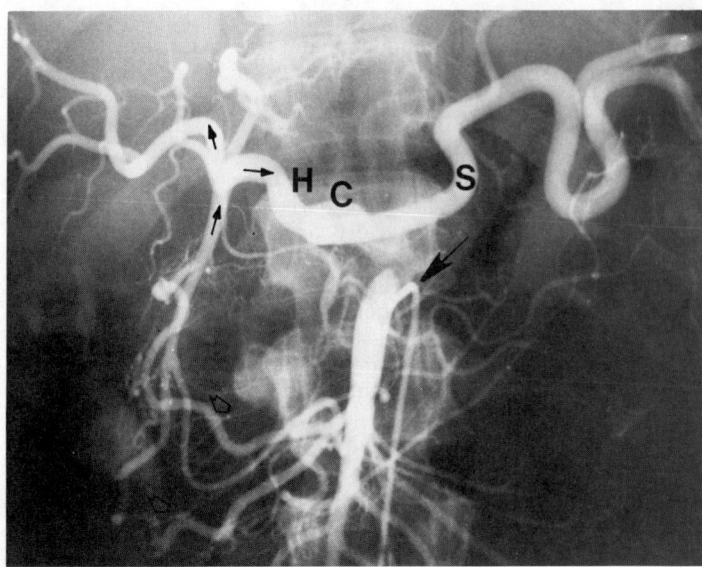

Figure 76-7. Celiac occlusion (C). Superior mesenteric artery injection (catheter, *large arrow*) fills the hepatic (H) and splenic (S) arteries from the superior mesenteric artery through the enlarged gastroduodenal and pancreatic arcade arteries (*open arrows*). Blood flows in the gastroduodenal artery toward the liver and in the common hepatic artery toward the spleen (*small arrows*). (Courtesy of James Andrews, MD, University of Michigan Hospitals, Ann Arbor)

of major pelvic vessels in the event of proximal occlusive disease.

Visceral Arteries

The three major arteries supplying the abdominal visceral organs are the celiac artery, SMA, and inferior mesenteric artery (IMA). Celiac artery and SMA angiography are routinely performed for any suspected abnormalities of the gastrointestinal tract, liver, pancreas, and mesentery, including tumors, aneurysms, cysts, occlusive disease, and bleeding. Knowledge of the many normal variants in arterial anatomy of abdominal organs is crucial to planning surgical procedures.

In standard anatomy, the celiac artery divides into the splenic and common hepatic arteries after giving rise to the left gastric artery (Fig. 76-7). The inferior phrenic and dorsal pancreatic arteries may also arise from the celiac axis. The common hepatic artery divides into the right, middle, and left hepatic arteries distal to the origin of the gastroduodenal artery. The right hepatic artery divides into the anterior and posterior segmental arteries, which further subdivide into superior and inferior subsegmental branches. The middle hepatic artery arises from the right, proper, or left hepatic arteries and supplies blood to the medial segment of the left lobe of the liver. The left hepatic artery divides into two subsegmental branches.

In about half of the population, the liver receives blood from aberrant hepatic arteries. The aberrant hepatic artery may be a lobar (or replaced) hepatic artery or a segmental (accessory) hepatic artery. At least 10 basic types of hepatic artery variations have been demonstrated angiographically or in dissection studies of human cadavers. Both replaced (10% incidence) and accessory (5% incidence) right hepatic arteries usually originate from the SMA, but in rare cases they arise from other branches of the celiac artery and SMA (Fig. 76-8). Most replaced (12% incidence) and accessory (12% incidence) left hepatic arteries originate from the left gastric artery. Thus, the left gastric artery should be visualized to determine the presence of an aberrant left hepatic artery. The left gastric artery generally originates from the ventral surface of the celiac axis distal to the origin of the inferior phrenic artery and gives rise to mural branches to the stomach while coursing along the lesser curvature of the stomach. In 3% of cases, the left

gastric artery has an aberrant origin from the aorta. Because the left gastric artery freely anastomoses with the right gastric, short gastric, and gastroepiploic arteries, embolization of its branches can be performed safely to control arterial bleeding from the stomach. The gastroduodenal artery usually arises from the hepatic artery but may have an aberrant origin from other branches of the celiac artery or SMA. It supplies blood to the duodenum and pancreas through the anterior and posterior pancreatic arcade arteries and to the stomach through the gastroepiploic artery. The anterior and posterior arcade arteries anastomose with the inferior pancreaticoduodenal artery, arising either sep-

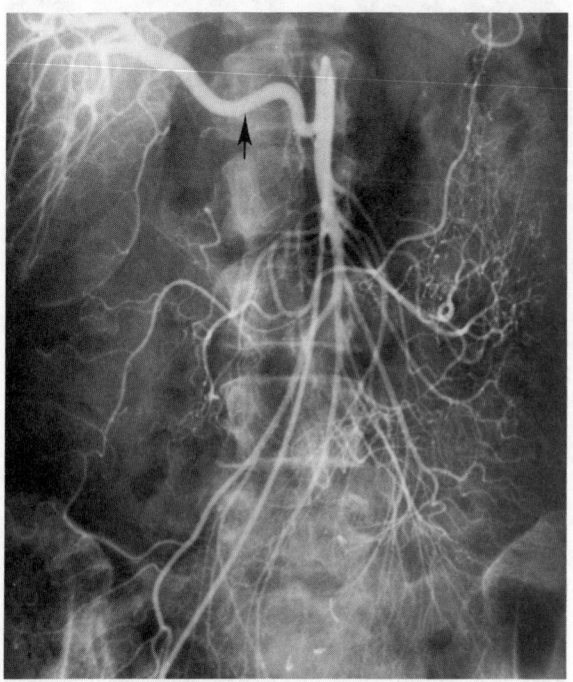

Figure 76-8. Replaced right hepatic artery. The right hepatic artery (*arrow*) originates from the superior mesenteric artery. (Courtesy of James Andrews, MD, University of Michigan Hospitals, Ann Arbor)

arately or as a common trunk with the first jejunal artery from the SMA. The gastroduodenal and pancreatic arcade arteries are the main collateral pathways in celiac artery and SMA occlusion (see Fig. 76-7). When angiography is performed for the diagnosis and embolization of duodenal bleeding, injections into both the celiac artery and SMA are necessary to complete the examination.

The dorsal pancreatic artery may arise from the splenic artery, celiac artery, hepatic artery, or SMA. It usually divides into the transverse and anastomotic branches immediately after its origin. These branches in turn anastomose with the branches of the pancreatic arcade and splenic arteries. While coursing along the pancreas, the splenic artery gives rise to numerous branches to the pancreas, the most important of which are the pancreatica magna and caudal pancreatic arteries.

The SMA runs posterior to the pancreas after its origin from the ventral surface of the aorta between the celiac and renal arteries. It then gives rise to jejunal, ileal, and colic branches (Fig. 76-9). Occasionally, the dorsal pancreatic and retroportal arteries arise from the main trunk of the SMA proximal to the origin of the middle colic artery. The middle colic artery arises from the ventral surface of the SMA at or distal to the origin of the first jejunal artery and divides into the right and left branches, which anastomose with the right colic, ileocolic, and left colic arteries by way of the arc of Riolan and the marginal artery of Drummond. The IMA originates from the anterolateral surface of the aorta between the left renal artery and the aortic bifurcation. It divides into the sigmoidal and superior hemorrhoidal arteries after giving rise to its first branch, the left colic artery (Fig. 76-10). The superior hemorrhoidal artery anastomoses with the middle and inferior hemorrhoidal arteries of the internal iliac artery and provides collateral blood flow to the lower extremities when there is aortic and iliac occlusion.

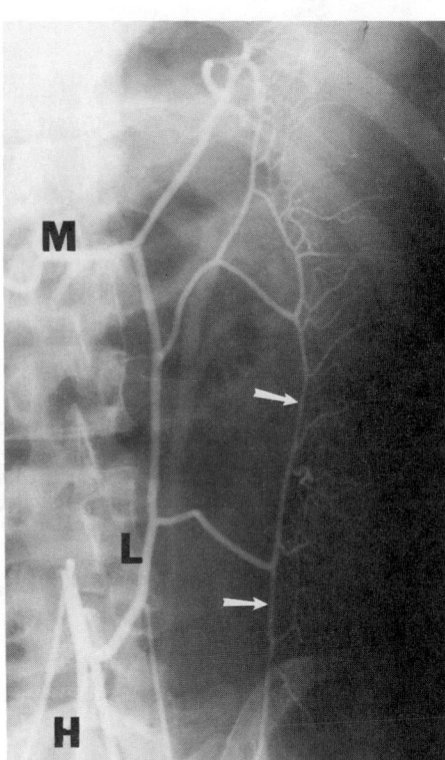

Figure 76-10. Inferior mesenteric arteriogram demonstrates the left colic (L), middle colic (M), and superior hemorrhoidal (H) arteries and the marginal artery of Drummond (*arrows*).

Visceral Veins

The portal venous system can be demonstrated by injection of contrast medium into the celiac artery, splenic artery, and SMA. Earlier techniques such as splenoportography and umbilical vein cannulation are rarely used for opacification of the portal venous system. Percutaneous transhepatic portal vein catheterization is an alternative approach in the evaluation of the portal vein and its hemodynamics; it provides access to the coronary vein for embolization of bleeding esophageal varices (Fig. 76-11).

The portal vein commences at the junction of the splenic and superior mesenteric veins. It runs anterior to the inferior vena cava toward the porta hepatis, where it divides into the right and left portal branches. In normal conditions, the blood in the portal vein and its tributaries (ie, the coronary and inferior mesenteric veins) flows toward the liver. Reversal of blood flow in any of the portal venous tributaries indicates the presence of portosystemic collaterals induced by portal hypertension. Angiography continues to play a major role in the evaluation of patients with portal hypertension before and after a portosystemic shunt procedure.

The hepatic veins lie between hepatic segments or lobes and join the inferior vena cava either separately or as a single trunk, just before the right atrium. The hepatic veins can be catheterized through the femoral, jugular, or peripheral arm veins. In the presence of a postsinusoidal block such as alcoholic cirrhosis, manometry through a catheter wedged in the hepatic vein reflects portal vein pressure. Hepatic venography is indicated for evaluation of the hepatic venous drainage pattern before hepatic resection for liver tumor or hepatic venoocclusive disease. Wedged hepatic venography is useful for visualizing the portal vein when indirect portography (after intraarterial injection of contrast medium) has failed to do so.

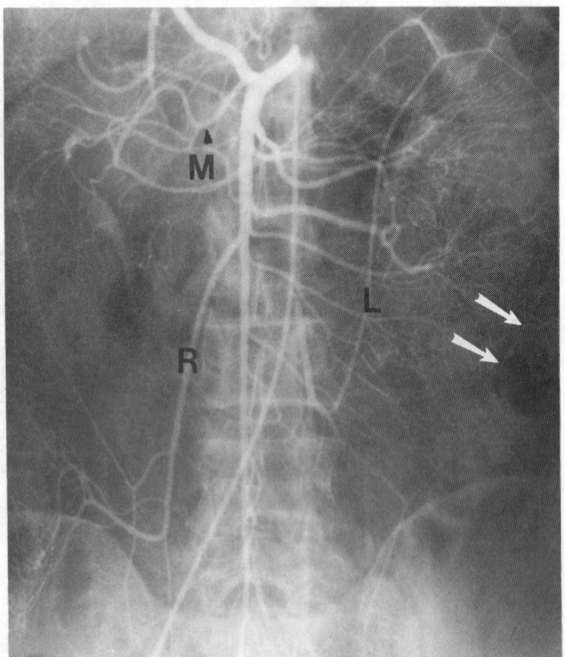

Figure 76-9. Superior mesenteric arteriogram demonstrates right (R), middle (M), and left (L) colic arteries. The marginal artery of Drummond (*arrows*) can be seen adjacent to the gas-filled descending colon. The common hepatic artery originates from the superior mesenteric artery.

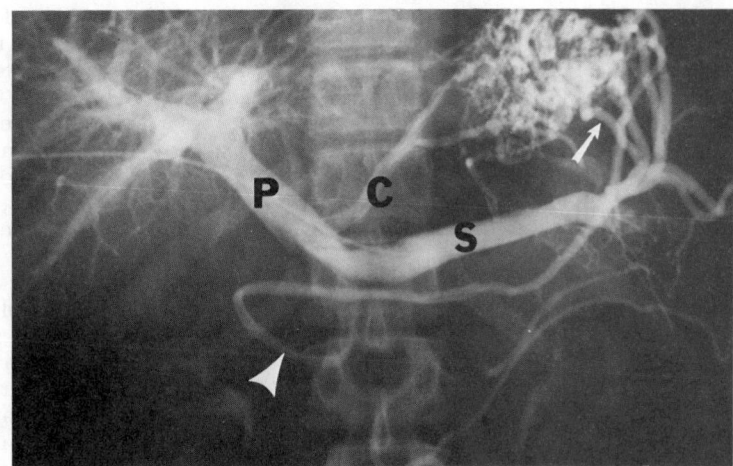

Figure 76-11. Transhepatic splenic venography demonstrates splenic (S), portal (P), and coronary (C), or left gastric, veins. The gastrocolic trunk (*arrowhead*) and short gastric veins (*arrow*) are also demonstrated. All these veins are normally demonstrated during the venous phase of celiac angiography.

The renal veins, usually one from each kidney, join the inferior vena cava. Knowledge of both normal and variant anatomy is important for renal vein renin sampling, preoperative evaluation of a renal transplant donor, and splenorenal shunt placement for portal hypertension. The right renal vein joins the inferior vena cava directly and may be multiple. The left renal vein is usually joined by the adrenal and gonadal veins before running anterior to the aorta and joining the inferior vena cava. Rarely, the renal vein may run behind the aorta (retroaortic renal vein), or both preaortic and retroaortic renal veins may exist together (circumaortic renal vein).

Arteries of the Upper Extremities

Upper extremity arteriography is indicated for the study of suspected arterial abnormalities of the shoulder, arm, forearm, and hand. The study usually begins with arch aortography using standard cut-film technique or DSA to demonstrate the innominate and subclavian arteries, followed by selective injections into the axillary artery to see the brachial, ulnar, radial, and digital arteries.

The brachial artery gives off the deep brachial artery and divides into the ulnar, radial, and interosseous arteries below the level of the neck of the radius. In about 10% of cases, the bifurcation arises in the upper arm or even from the axillary artery; this variation can be confused with an arterial occlusion if the injection of contrast material is distal to the aberrant origin. The deep brachial artery provides the main collateral flow to the arm in the presence of brachial artery occlusion.

In the forearm, the ulnar artery gives rise to the common interosseous artery (which divides into the anterior and posterior interosseous arteries) and the anterior and posterior ulnar recurrent arteries. The radial artery supplies a recurrent artery near the elbow as well as muscular branches distally. The median artery is an embryologic remnant that can originate from the proximal ulnar, radial, or interosseous arteries and normally runs with the median nerve.

Terminology of palmar arch arterial anatomy varies among authors and will not be discussed here.[16,17] Digital angiography is usually performed with the injection of a vasodilator such as tolazoline (usual dose, 25 to 50 mg) before contrast injection. Direct magnification filming (airgap technique) is useful for identifying the distal ulnar and radial artery contributions to the wrist and hand circulation through the superficial and deep palmar arches. Arteries are usually opacified as far distally as the fingertip plexus. The radial, ulnar, and digital arteries anastomose with each other through the palmar arches.

Arteries of the Lower Extremities

Lower extremity arteriography is indicated for suspected arterial abnormalities in the thigh, calf, and foot. In patients at risk for arteriosclerotic occlusive disease, arteriography is usually preceded by abdominal aortography and pelvic arteriography. Both extremities can be studied simultaneously by injecting contrast material into the distal abdominal aorta and recording the image with conventional film or DSA. In some circumstances, such as evaluation of distal anatomy for placement of a free flap, a single-leg outflow study is performed with an injection into the external iliac artery from either the ipsilateral or contralateral femoral artery approach. In patients with poor cardiac output, significant aneurysmal disease, or multilevel occlusive disease, visualization of distal calf vessels and the plantar arch is often poor with aortic injections of contrast medium. Visualization of these vessels is crucial when surgical bypass for limb salvage is contemplated, and it can be enhanced by augmenting distal flow (by intraarterial vasodilators, postischemic hyperemia, or contrast injection distal to an occlusion balloon) or by using DSA.

The common femoral artery bifurcates into the deep and superficial femoral arteries several centimeters distal to the inguinal ligament. In most patients, the bifurcation is best seen on the ipsilateral anterior oblique projection. Angiographically, the superficial femoral artery courses in a medial and anterior direction, and the deep femoral artery courses in a lateral and posterior direction. Numerous communications between branches of the deep femoral and internal iliac arteries above and the genicular branches below emphasize the importance of the deep femoral artery in reconstituting lower extremity outflow in the presence of aortoiliac or femoropopliteal occlusive disease. The superficial femoral artery continues at the adductor hiatus as the popliteal artery. Major branches of the popliteal artery include the "trifurcation" branches (peroneal and anterior and posterior tibial arteries) and the genicular complex with its important anastomoses with the deep femoral artery above and the recurrent tibial branches below. The posterior tibial artery terminates in the foot as the lateral and medial plantar arteries. The anterior tibial artery continues at the foot as the dorsalis pedis, whose terminal deep plantar branch connects with the lateral plantar artery to form the plantar arch. Two distal branches of the peroneal artery, the anterior and posterior perforating branches, anastomose with the anterior and posterior tibial arteries and are important sources of collateral blood flow when occlusive disease affects these vessels. The arteries of the distal calf and foot are best seen in the lateral projection.

NORMAL VARIATIONS SIMULATING DISEASE

Anatomic variations and artifacts of the angiographic procedure can simulate arterial occlusions, arterial encasement, and parenchymal perfusion defects. Such confusion can be minimized by knowledge of the normal variations in arterial anatomy and common artifacts encountered during angiography. Failure to fill the expected arterial pattern of an organ or limb may be due to arterial occlusion or to an avascular mass, but it may also result from a contrast injection that fails to fill aberrant or accessory arteries. Catheter- and guide wire–induced spasm can mimic neoplastic encasement; thus, selective catheterization should be preceded by proximal arterial injections to demonstrate true arterial narrowing (Fig. 76-12). For example, aortography should precede renal arteriography, and celiac arteriography should precede gastroduodenal arteriography. Contrast injection occasionally demonstrates an

ill-understood phenomenon called *standing waves*, in which the arterial lumen is distinguished by smooth, regular, alternating bands of mild narrowing and expansion (Fig. 76-13). This condition can be distinguished from drug-induced (Fig. 76-14) or hypovolemic vasoconstriction and from arterial fibrodysplasia (see Fig. 76-28A) by the monotonous regularity of the alternating bands. The high specific gravity of contrast material compared with blood contributes to incomplete mixing of the contrast during injection, especially at the head and tail of the contrast bolus. When mixing is incomplete, contrast material tends to pool along the dependent surface of large vessels such as the aorta or along the mural surface of small arteries. This layering of contrast is responsible for visualization of lumbar arteries on abdominal aortograms after visceral and renal arteries have cleared (Fig. 76-15). In small arteries, the mural layering of contrast material with nonopacified blood flowing in the center of the lumen can simulate an embolus (Fig. 76-16).

DIAGNOSTIC ANGIOGRAPHY: INDICATIONS AND FINDINGS

Hemorrhage and ischemia, real or threatened, are the indications for most diagnostic angiography. Other indications include the demonstration of vascular anat-

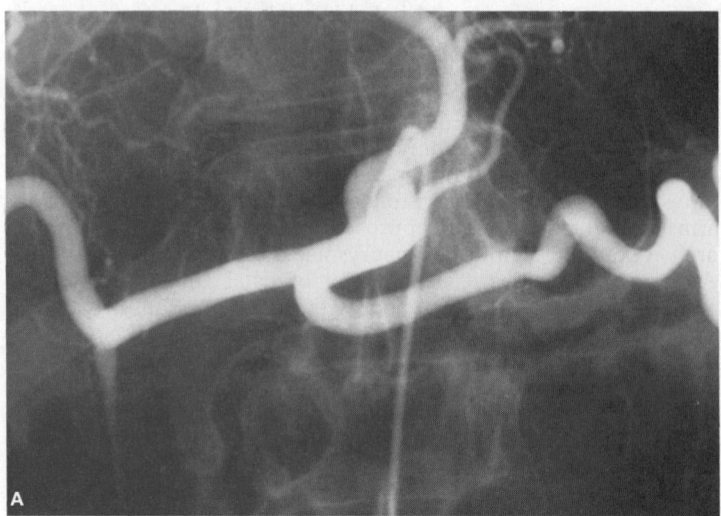

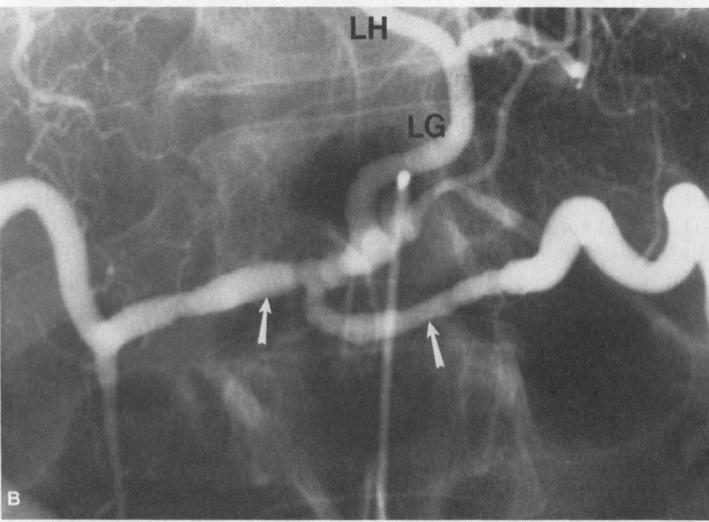

Figure 76-12. Guide wire–induced arterial spasm in a patient with pancreatitis. Celiac arteriograms made before (*A*) and after (*B*) catheterization of the splenic artery. Irregular narrowing of the splenic and common hepatic arteries (*arrows in B*) can be seen, mimicking tumor encasement. The left hepatic artery (LH) originates from the left gastric artery (LG).

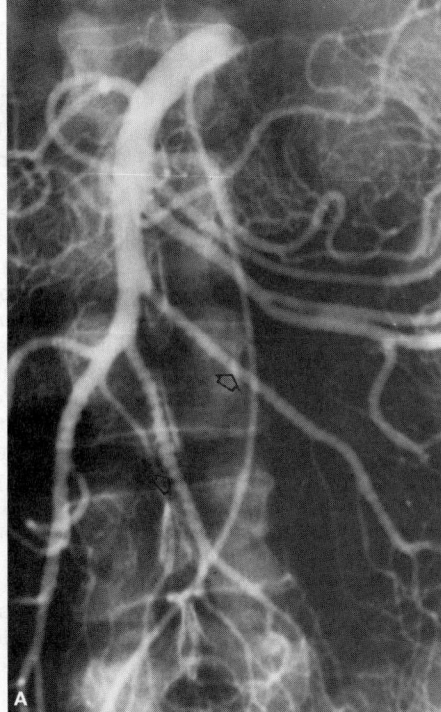
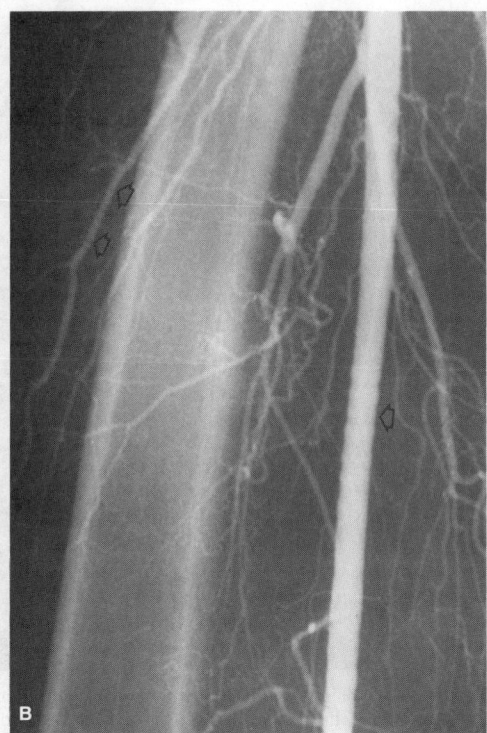

Figure 76-13. Arterial standing waves. Smooth repetitive bands of mild narrowing (*open arrows*) are demonstrated in branches of the superior mesenteric (*A*) and superficial femoral (*B*) arteries during contrast injection.

omy before surgical or transcatheter intervention and venous thromboembolism. Hemorrhage, except in association with catastrophes such as a ruptured aneurysm, is an indication for both diagnostic and therapeutic angiography and is discussed in the next section. The clinical presentation of ischemia depends on the organ involved and includes stroke, angina, renovascular hypertension, mesenteric ischemia, and limb claudica-

tion. Neurologic and cardiac disease are not discussed in this chapter. The prototypical ischemic diseases are macroemboli and nonaneurysmal atherosclerosis. Although aneurysms, arterial fibrodysplasia, dissection, arteritis, and trauma may present as ischemic disease (or as hemorrhage), the angiographic findings and workup of the primary disease are distinct enough to merit separate discussion.

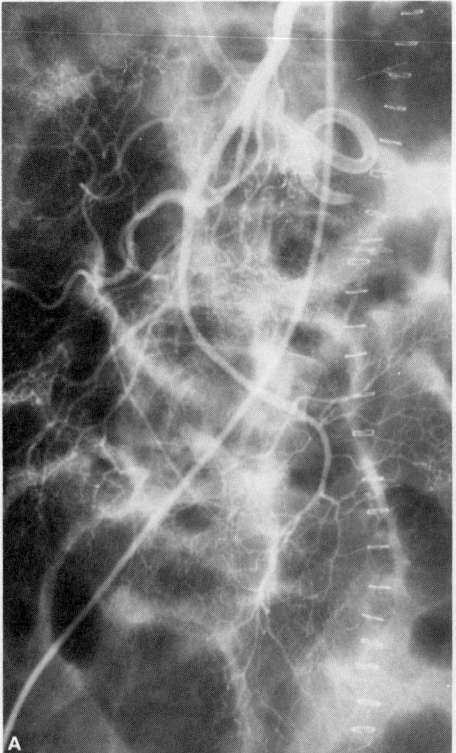
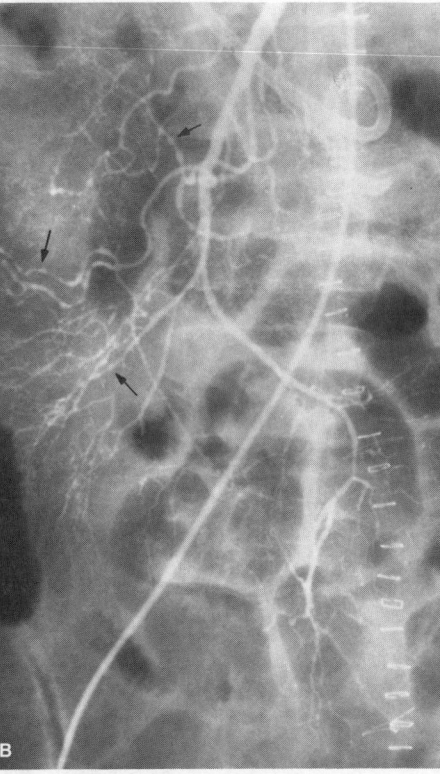

Figure 76-14. Vasopressin-induced arterial spasm in a woman with gastrointestinal bleeding and multiple vascular ectasias in the small bowel. (*A*) Celiac and superior mesenteric arteriograms show no vascular abnormalities. (*B*) A second mesenteric arteriogram after 12 hours of vasopressin infusion into the superior mesenteric artery (0.2 IU/min) shows diffuse arterial vasoconstriction. Multiple focal vasodilated segments (*small arrows*) reflect uneven response to vasopressin.

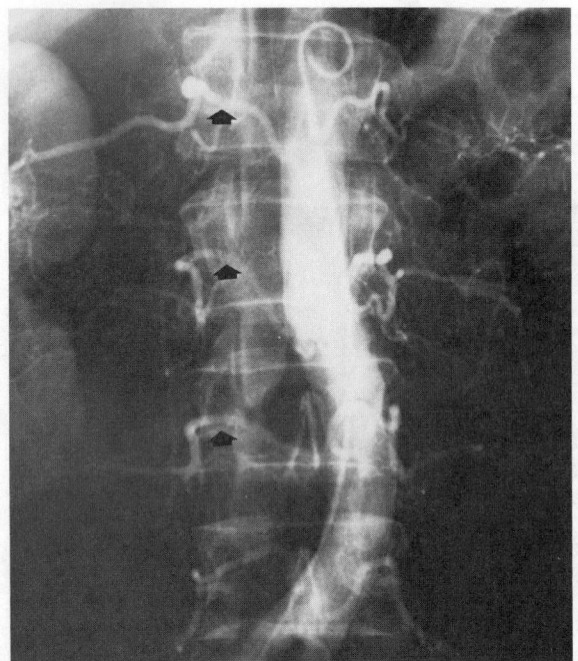

Figure 76-15. Dependent layering of contrast material. Late arterial phase of a lumbar aortogram demonstrates contrast material pooling along the posterior surface of the aorta in a patient in the supine position. Contrast material continues to fill lumbar arteries (*arrows*) after it has cleared from renal and mesenteric branches.

Macroembolism

Most macroemboli involving the abdominal viscera or the extremities are cardiac in origin and present as one of the acute ischemic syndromes. The indications for angiography in acute ischemia are to document the cause of acute occlusion (such as arterial emboli), to show arterial anatomy proxi-

mal and distal to significant occlusions, and to demonstrate associated or incidental pathology. If emboli are documented, angiography should search for an aortic or arterial source such as an aneurysm or atherosclerotic plaque or ulcer (Fig. 76-17). The search for a cardiac source of emboli requires echocardiography. The appropriateness of intraarterial lytic therapy should be considered at the time of diagnostic angiography. If no emboli are found, other causes of acute ischemia should be considered, including mesenteric arterial spasm or in situ thrombosis secondary to a low flow state. Dissection and trauma may also cause acute ischemia but are usually suggested by the clinical history.

Contrast medium surrounding the leading or trailing edge of an arterial clot indicates acute occlusion, either embolic or thrombotic (Figs. 76-18 and 76-19). It may be impossible to distinguish between acute embolism and in situ thrombosis unless multiple sites of acute occlusion due to random embolism are demonstrated. The distinction between acute and chronic occlusion is usually based on the size of the collaterals bridging the occlusion; they are small when the occlusion is acute and large when long-standing.

If the patient history and presentation suggest embolic disease, the angiographic workup includes thoracic and biplane abdominal aortography to search for a source of emboli, and selective arteriography tailored to the clinical problem (eg, mesenteric, renal, lower extremity, and so forth).

Nonaneurysmal Atherosclerosis: Renal, Mesenteric, and Peripheral

Atherosclerosis is a progressive, systemic disease primarily affecting large and medium-sized arteries. The ischemic syndrome varies with the organ involved and disease severity. Renal arteriosclerosis may present as hypertension or renal failure; mesenteric ischemia as postprandial epigastric pain, weight loss, and bowel infarction; and peripheral occlusive disease as claudication, rest pain, and gangrene.

The purposes of angiography are to document hemody-

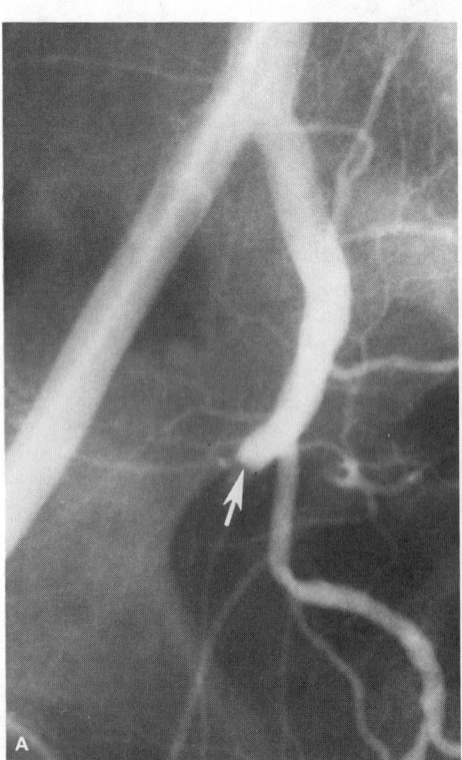

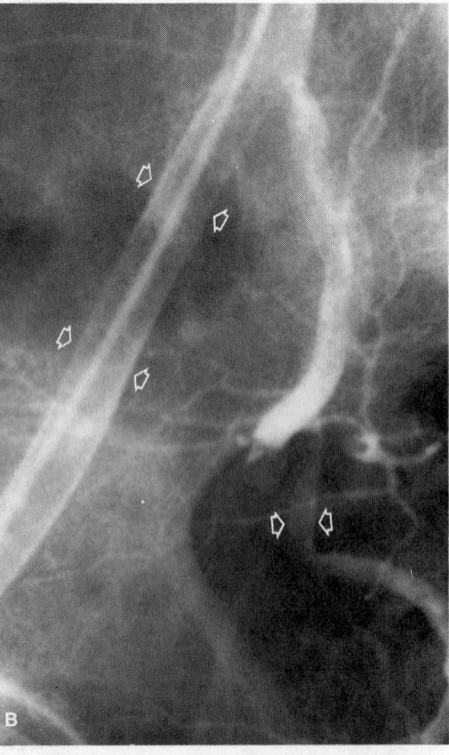

Figure 76-16. Residual contrast material simulating thrombosis in an artery. (*A*) Right common iliac arteriogram demonstrates embolic occlusion of the superior gluteal artery (*arrow*). (*B*) Later in the filming sequence, after unopacified blood has replaced the center of the contrast column, residual contrast outlines the walls of the external iliac artery and anterior division of the internal iliac artery, simulating thrombus (*open arrows*). This artifact can be confusing when the artery in question has been underinjected or receives collateral blood supply from unopacified arteries.

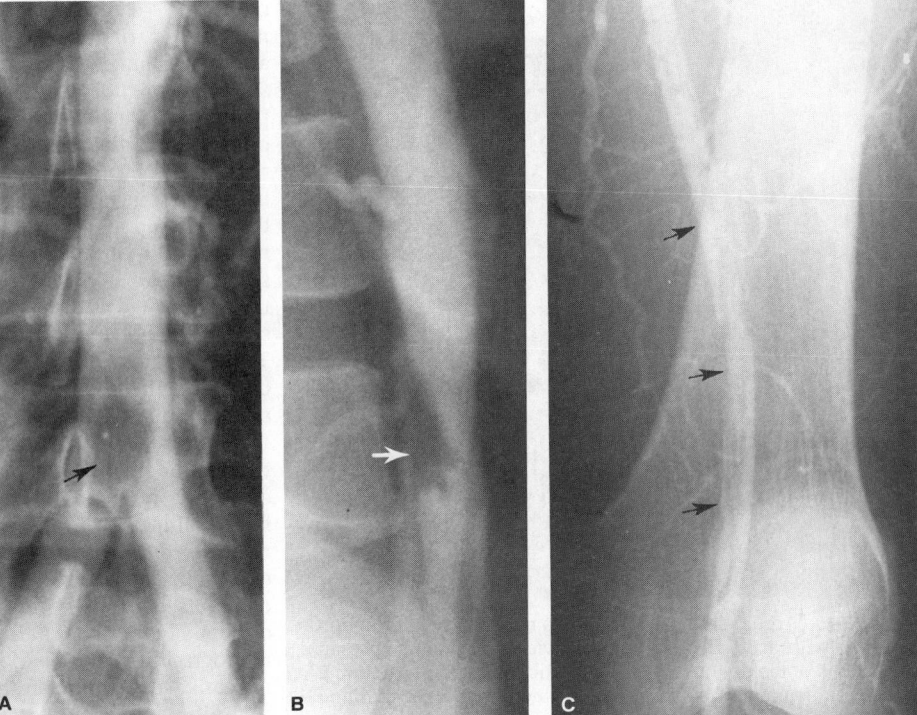

Figure 76-17. Recurrent lower extremity macroemboli from an atherosclerotic plaque in a man with recurrent lower extremity emboli, in whom surgical embolectomy failed to restore peripheral pulses. Biplanar aortogram shows a large irregular posterior plaque (*arrow*) at the aortic bifurcation, subtle on the frontal film (*A*) but evident on the lateral film (*B*). (*C*) A detail from the lower extremity outflow study shows extensive thromboemboli (*arrows*) in the left popliteal artery.

namically significant occlusive disease, to show the arterial anatomy of the donor and receptor sites of a prospective revascularization graft, and to demonstrate associated or incidental pathology. The appropriateness of transcatheter interventional procedures such as percutaneous angioplasty should be considered at the time of diagnostic angiography.

Atherosclerosis is characterized angiographically by ulcers (pocket-like collections of contrast communicating with the arterial lumen), irregular or smooth narrowing and occlusions of large and medium-sized arteries, and the presence of collaterals. Atherosclerotic stenoses may be confused with neoplastic encasement or arterial fibrodysplasia (see later). Angiographic features of stenoses fa-

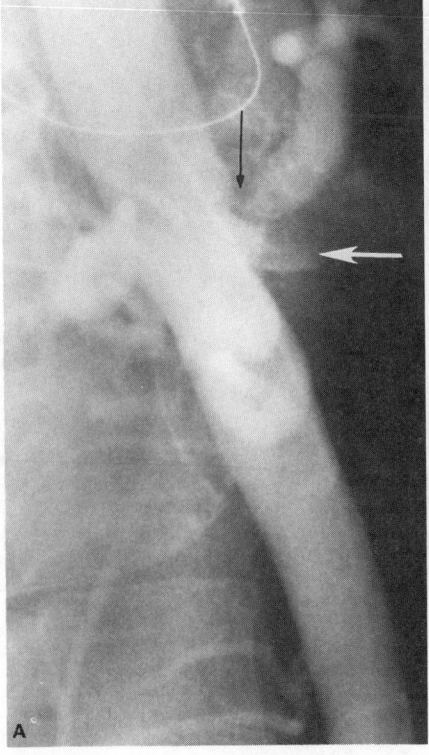
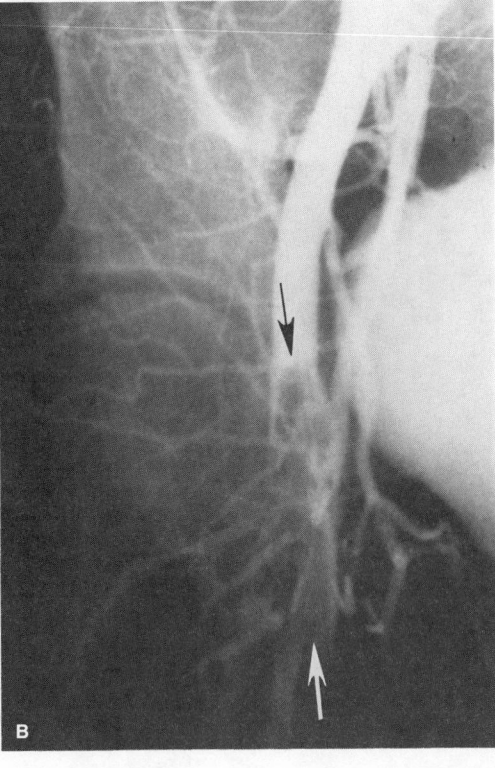

Figure 76-18. Arterial emboli in a woman with right lower extremity ischemia. (*A*) Lateral aortogram shows median arcuate ligament compression on the celiac axis (*black arrow*) and an embolus in the superior mesenteric artery (*white arrow*). (*B*) An embolus is also visible at the bifurcation of the common femoral artery (*arrows*).

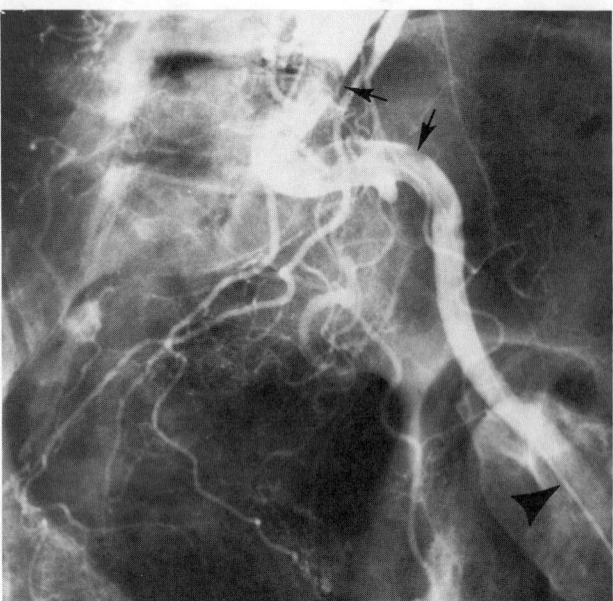

Figure 76-19. Aortic saddle embolism in a man in atrial fibrillation presenting with acute right leg pain. Pelvic arteriogram shows an acute saddle embolus (*arrows*) at the aortic bifurcation, extending into the left common iliac artery and occluding the right common iliac artery. Despite the large amount of thrombus in the left common iliac artery, the left femoral pulse was palpable, allowing the transfemoral approach for catheter access (*arrowhead*).

voring atherosclerosis are eccentricity, calcification, a tendency to involve the ostium or branch points, evidence of atherosclerosis in other vessels, and normal associated veins. An arterial stenosis is considered significant when associated with bridging collaterals, poststenotic dilation, a pressure gradient exceeding 10 mmHg, or, in the appropriate clinical setting, ipsilateral renal vein renin hyperse-

cretion.[18–20] Stenoses of questionable hemodynamic significance during baseline blood flow should be reassessed after augmenting flow by pharmacologic or physiologic stimulation such as vasoactive drugs or postischemic hyperemia.[21] Vasospasm (diffuse narrowing of an arterial bed) may be distinguished from severe diffuse arteriosclerotic narrowing by its involvement of collaterals and branch arteries in the affected distribution, which are relatively spared in arteriosclerosis. Vasospasm is not a prominent finding on angiograms of atherosclerosis and should suggest drug toxicity (eg, ergot, digitalis), Raynaud phenomenon, cellulitis or compartment syndrome, heavy smoking, or other conditions with increased vascular tone. The angiographic findings and workup of arteriosclerotic occlusive disease vary with the duration of the occlusion and the organ system involved.

Renovascular occlusive disease resulting in hypertension or renal failure is most commonly due to atherosclerosis (Fig. 76-20). Other causes include arterial fibrodysplasia, abdominal or thoracic aortic coarctation, neurofibromatosis, aortic dissection, and trauma. The indication for angiography is to document a hemodynamically adequate conduit from the aortic root to the renal parenchyma. If aortic coarctation or arterial stenoses are present, angiography should document their hemodynamic significance and demonstrate vascular anatomy necessary for planning a revascularization or angioplasty procedure. In an older adult, an abdominal aortogram that demonstrates all renal artery origins in profile along the aorta or iliac artery is usually sufficient to rule out a surgically correctable stenosis. In children and young adults, hypertension may be due to renal artery branch stenoses that could require selective renal artery injections with magnification filming for convincing documentation. Alternatively, hypertension may be due to aortic coarctation. Revascularization in the presence of densely calcified or severely ulcerated aortic and iliac vessels may require use of the splenic or hepatic–gastroduodenal artery. Consequently, a lateral

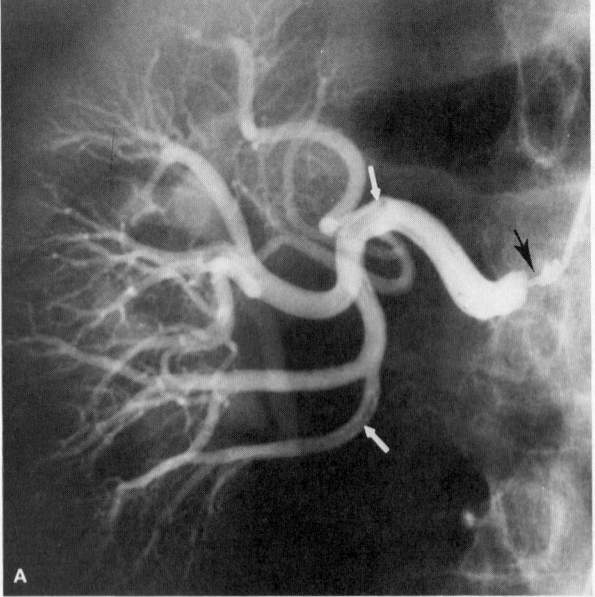
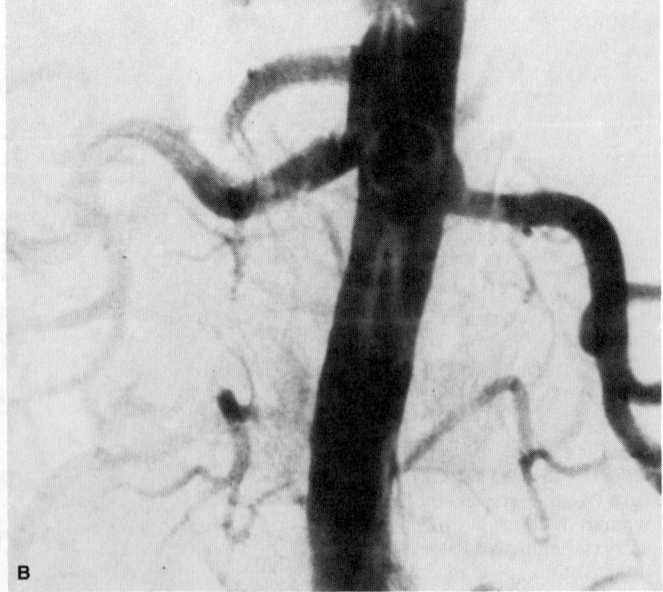

Figure 76-20. Atherosclerotic renal artery stenosis. (*A*) Right renal arteriogram shows a tight concentric proximal stenosis of the renal artery (*black arrow*). The linear filling defects in the main renal artery and its segmental branches (*white arrows*) represent flow defects caused by unopacified blood flowing retrograde from nonparenchymal renal artery branches. The presence of collateral flow to the kidney indicates that the stenosis is hemodynamically significant. (*B*) Lumbar aortogram after percutaneous angioplasty shows significant improvement in the caliber of the arterial lumen.

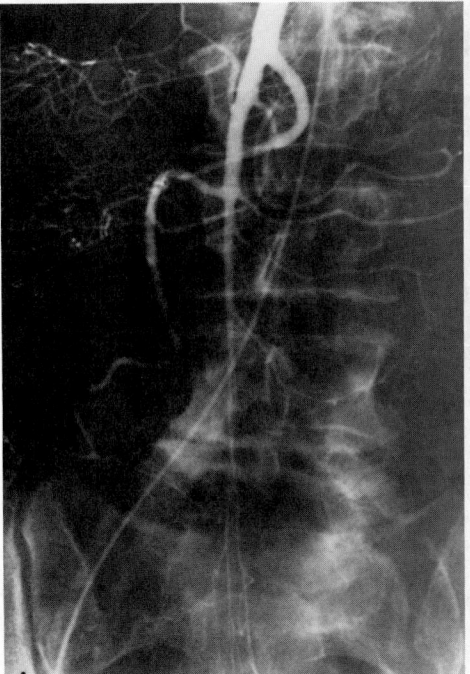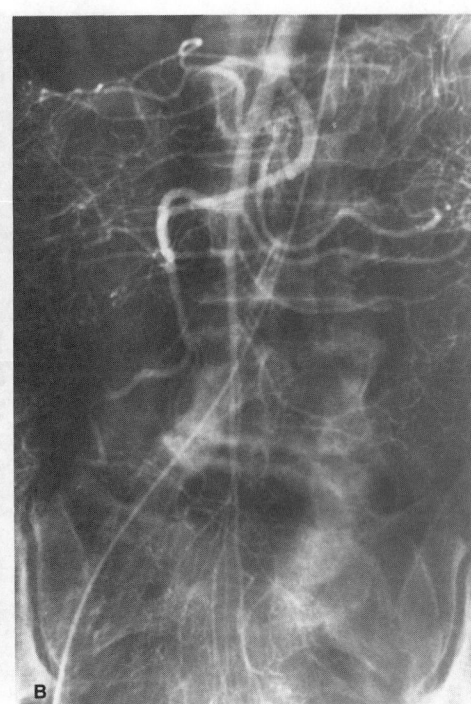

Figure 76-21. Nonocclusive mesenteric ischemia. (*A*) Superior mesenteric angiogram shows diffuse arterial vasoconstriction without occlusion. (*B*) A second arteriogram after injection of 50 mg of tolazoline into the superior mesenteric artery shows decreased vasoconstriction.

aortogram must be obtained to rule out celiac artery stenosis.

Mesenteric ischemia may be acute or chronic, occlusive or nonocclusive.[22] Biplane aortography demonstrates the celiac artery and SMA origins. It is useful in documenting proximal stenosis or embolic occlusion and in demonstrating mesenteric collateral flow. Selective injections into the celiac artery, SMA, and IMA may be necessary to demonstrate distal emboli, branch occlusions, or unsuspected neoplasm mimicking ischemic bowel disease. The mesenteric injection rates should be large enough to document patency of the mesenteric and portal veins. Acute embolic occlusion appears as a filling defect in the contrast column, usually at branch points. The angiogram in nonocclusive mesenteric ischemia may show diffuse vasoconstriction of the SMA and its branches (often drug related) with slowing of blood flow and decreased contrast accumulation in the bowel wall, or it may be distressingly normal (Fig. 76-21). Isolated celiac artery or SMA occlusion is common and usually asymptomatic because of abundant, short (and therefore low-resistance) peripancreatic collaterals (see Fig. 76-7). Proximal SMA stenosis may also be relieved by collateral supply from the IMA through the left colic to middle colic anastomosis. In general, at least two of the three visceral arteries must be occluded or significantly narrowed before mesenteric ischemia develops. The angiogram should document collateral supply reconstituting the bowel at risk; such collaterals are usually sparse and long compared with those in simple celiac stenosis.

Lower extremity ischemia can be documented noninvasively by blood pressure measurements and pulse waveforms. Angiography is reserved for planning surgical or percutaneous revascularization procedures and demonstrates the distribution of disease, the distribution of relatively healthy arteries (necessary for planning surgical bypass procedures), and the status of collaterals. A complete study consists of an aortogram to demonstrate renal artery anatomy and distal aortic disease, one or both oblique pelvic arteriograms to display the iliac and femoral artery bifurcations, and a lower extremity outflow study to demonstrate thigh and calf vessels. Visualization of distal calf vessels may be technically difficult, especially in the presence of severe proximal disease. If a femoral to distal tibial or peroneal bypass is contemplated, additional studies, including

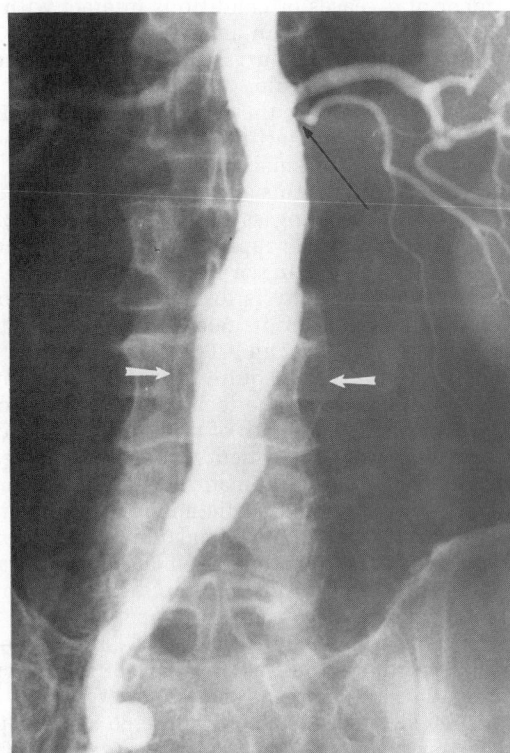

Figure 76-22. Abdominal aortic aneurysm in a 67-year-old man. Lumbar aortogram demonstrates an infrarenal aortic aneurysm. The opacified lumen underestimates the true diameter of the aneurysm, here outlined by a shell of intimal calcification (*white arrows*). The orifice of the accessory lower pole left renal artery is narrowed (*black arrow*).

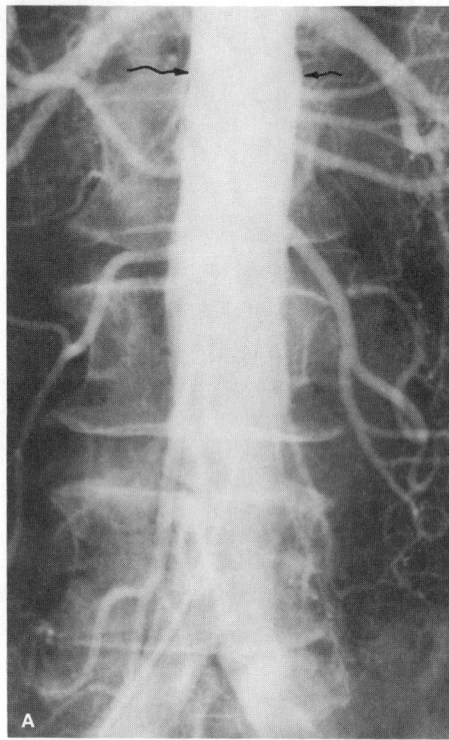 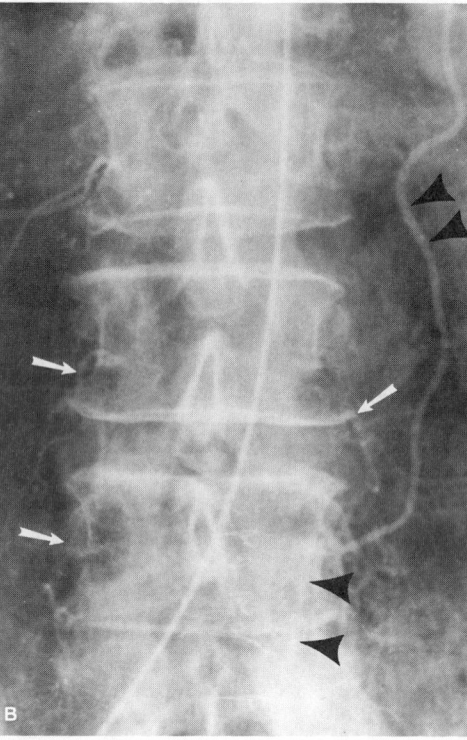

Figure 76-23. Abdominal aortic aneurysm in a 74-year-old man. (*A*) Lumbar aortogram shows subtle widening of the infrarenal aortic lumen (*wavy arrows*). Renal and superior mesenteric artery branches are normal, but infrarenal aortic branches are apparently missing. (*B*) A later film shows filling of lumbar (*arrows*) and inferior mesenteric (*arrowheads*) arteries through collaterals, as a result of occlusion of these vessels by mural thrombus in the aneurysm.

occlusive angiography or DSA, may be used to demonstrate the optimal site for the distal graft anastomosis.

Aneurysmal Disease

A number of diseases or conditions interact with the arterial system and result in aneurysm formation. The size and distribution of aneurysms vary with the underlying disease. For example, atherosclerosis typically causes aneurysms along the aorta and its proximal branches, whereas polyarteritis nodosa may result in microaneurysms along the small branches of the renal and visceral arteries. Aneurysms and pseudoaneurysms may present as slowly growing asymptomatic masses or as masses of indeterminate or rapid growth with symptoms due to intermittent bleeding or impending rupture. The indication for angiography is to demonstrate the exact origin of the aneurysm and its relation to nearby critical normal vessels (Figs. 76-22 and 76-23). Safe and effective deployment of stent grafts requires an accurate depiction of aneurysm dimensions, the location of critical aortic branch origins, and the length of the aneurysm "necks" between the margins of the aneurysm and branch vessel origins. Other relevant information includes the presence of inflammatory or mycotic aneurysms and aneurysmal rupture. Three-dimensional rendering of aneurysms and periaortic inflammatory changes are best seen with CT. Mycotic aneurysms have no distinctive angiographic appearance other than an unusual location and configuration (Fig. 76-24; see Fig. 76-32C). Rupture of an atherosclerotic thoracic or abdominal aortic aneurysm is an indication for emergent surgical intervention. The patient is usually too unstable to undergo angiography, which in any case is less sensitive than CT in demonstrating the periaortic hematoma. In intermittent hemorrhage, by definition, the mural defect has resealed and the lumen is intact; the angiogram can only suggest the site of rupture when asymmetric nipple-like projections of contrast extend radially from the principal axis of the vessel.

Angiographically, aneurysms appear as dilations in the arterial lumen. With extensive mural thrombus, the caliber of the lumen may be normal, and the presence of the aneurysm may only be inferred from mural calcification or stereotypical thrombosis of arterial branches such as lumbar arteries.

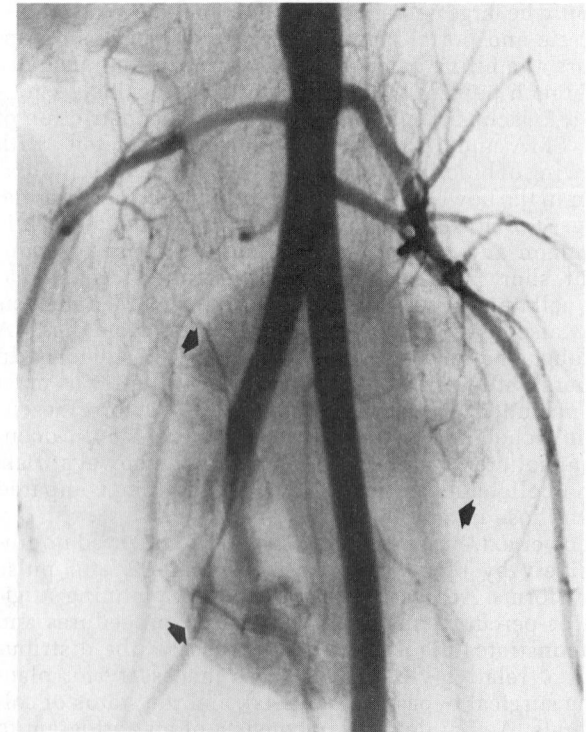

Figure 76-24. Mycotic pseudoaneurysm. Left common femoral arteriogram shows a saccular pseudoaneurysm (*arrows*) originating from the deep femoral artery.

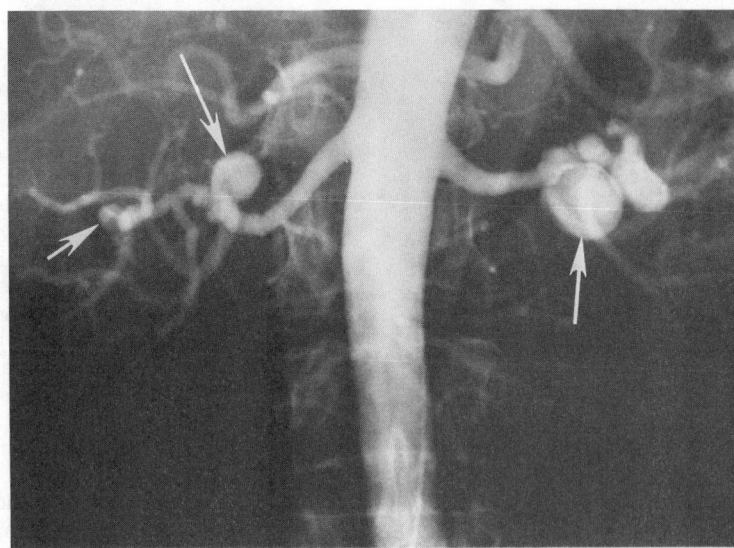

Figure 76-25. Renal artery aneurysms. Lumbar aortogram in a normotensive woman demonstrates multiple bilateral renal artery aneurysms (*arrows*) associated with renal arterial fibrodysplastic disease.

Large atherosclerotic aneurysms of the thoracic and abdominal aorta may distort the axis of the aorta and quickly dilute the injected bolus of contrast medium. Additional contrast injections or filming projection may be required to demonstrate branch artery anatomy. The angiogram, then, is a compromise between a thorough anatomic study and the contrast medium load. The thoracic aortogram should demonstrate the coronary and brachiocephalic artery origins. The abdominal aortogram should demonstrate the visceral and renal artery origins, with specific attention focused on multiple renal arteries. Thoracic aortic aneurysms are studied from the aortic root to the diaphragm; abdominal aneurysms are studied from the diaphragm to the inguinal ligaments. If infrainguinal arterial disease is suspected clinically, an arterial runoff study is obtained.

Renal or visceral artery aneurysms are studied with selective injections of the parent artery, often in multiple projections. Angiography should demonstrate the relation of the aneurysms to nearby branch arteries. When relevant, the adequacy of collateral arteries should be demonstrated in sufficient detail to plan surgical reconstruction or resection or percutaneous embolization (Fig. 76-25).

Arterial Dissections

Dissections can occur as spontaneous intramural hematomas (in the presence of arterial medial disease) or as the result of intimal trauma (usually iatrogenic). Spontaneous dissections are most common in the thoracic aorta and represent a surgical or medical emergency (Fig. 76-26). In

Figure 76-26. Type I aortic dissection in an 86-year-old hypertensive woman with acute onset of back pain. (*A*) Arch aortogram, performed from a right brachial artery approach, shows early opacification of the true lumen. The jet of contrast material is opacifying the intimal tear that initiated the dissection (*black arrow*). The false lumen extends retrograde, compressing the ascending aorta along its right lateral margin, narrowing the origin of the right coronary artery (*white arrow*), and undermining the aortic valve leaflets with secondary aortic insufficiency (*open arrows*). (*B*) A few seconds later, the entire false lumen is opacified, and the dissection septum appears as a radiolucent line (*open arrows*) between the false and true lumens. The dissection extends into the descending aorta with involvement of the innominate artery.

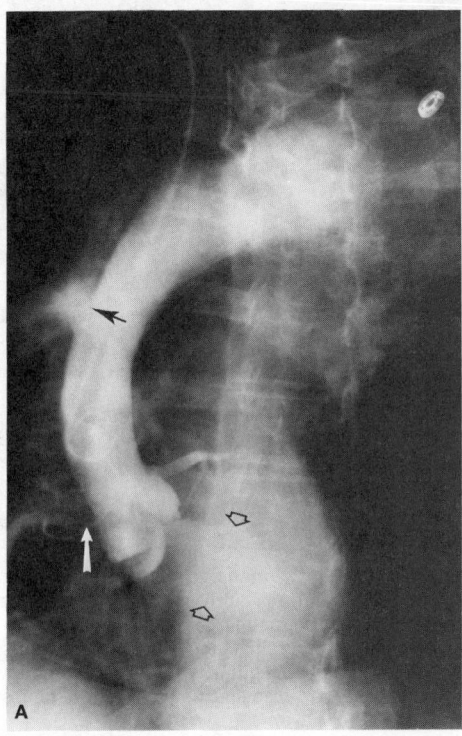

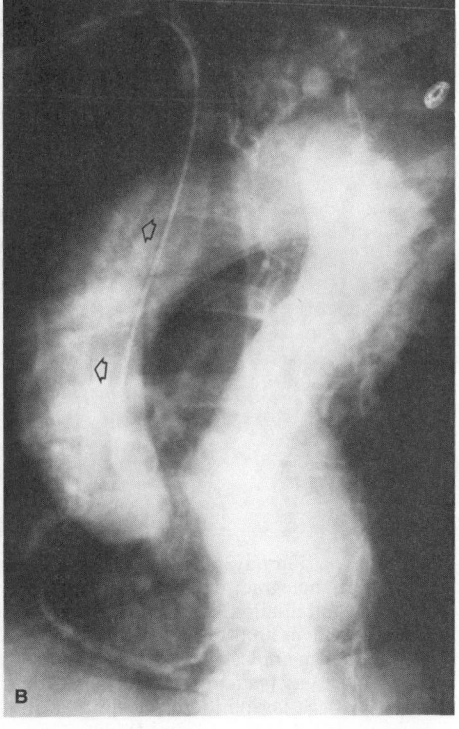

A

B

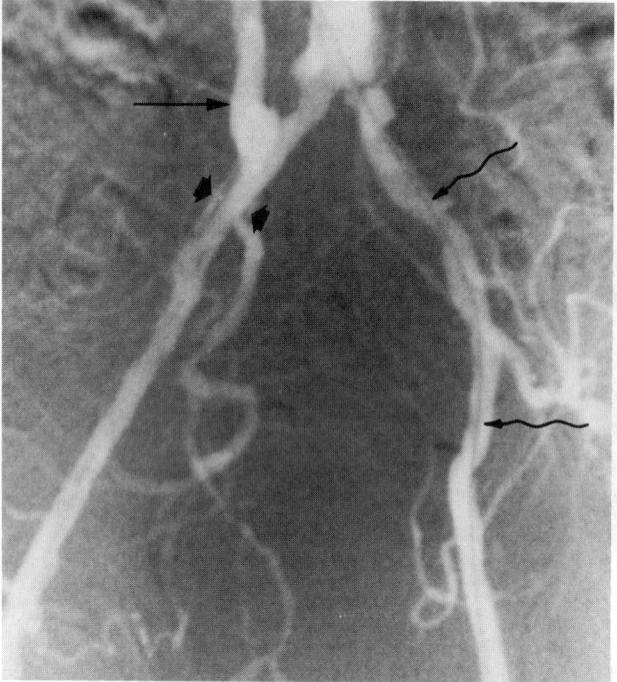

Figure 76-27. Iatrogenic dissection in a 70-year-old woman with cholesterol emboli following cardiac catheterization. Pelvic arteriogram performed with digital subtraction angiography demonstrates a linear collection of contrast medium outside the arterial lumen, representing a dissection. The dissection extends into the common iliac artery (*solid arrows*), stopping short of the origin of the iliorenal bypass graft (*straight arrow*). The linear filling defect in the left iliac artery (*wavy arrows*) is produced by the angiographic catheter.

the typical aortic dissection, the normal (or true) lumen communicates by way of the intimal tear with an intramedial (or false) lumen. The tear is usually several centimeters above the aortic valve or just distal to the subclavian artery. As the false lumen spirals longitudinally both antegrade and retrograde in the aorta, normal aortic branches may be spared, occluded, or sheared from their true lumen origins. The false lumen may expand because of its thin and fragile outer wall and compress the true lumen. The diagnosis of aortic dissection and its classification with respect to involvement of the ascending aorta are usually established by transesophageal echocardiography, CT, or MR angiography. The indications for transcatheter aortography are to resolve equivocal or discordant findings by cross-sectional imaging tests, to evaluate the hemodynamic significance of branch vessel compromise by the dissection, and to plan and perform endovascular treatment of ischemic and aneurysmal complications of dissection. The angiographic appearance of aortic dissection depends on the site of contrast injection and the vagaries of the dissection in a given patient. If the injection is upstream from the intimal tear or a reentry point, it fills the true and false lumina, usually at different rates, and outlines the intervening septum as a linear filling defect in the contrast column. If the injection is remote from a transseptal communication and fills a single lumen, the margins of the lumen are variable, smoothly scalloped as the septum is seen in profile, and normal or possibly aneurysmal elsewhere. Involvement of aortic branches may be difficult to demonstrate unless the lumen perfusing the branches in question can be catheterized directly. Manometry, interpreted in the context of peripheral limb pressures, may help determine the hemodynamic significance of a given branch artery stenosis.

The angiographic workup of dissections in the renal or

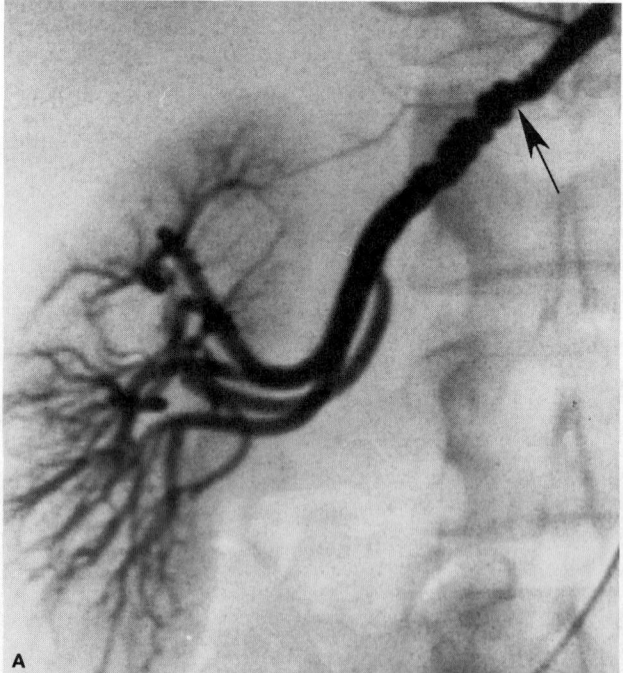
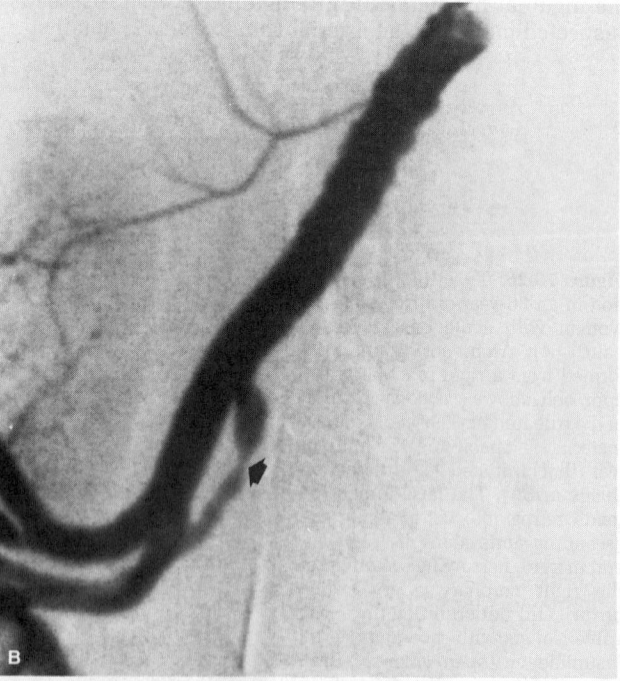

Figure 76-28. Fibrodysplasia of the renal artery in a 51-year-old hypertensive woman. (*A*) Digital subtraction angiogram of the right renal artery shows a ptotic kidney with alternating bands of narrowing and dilation in the middle third of the main renal artery (*arrow*), in the so-called string-of-beads configuration of medial fibroplasia. (*B*) A second arteriogram made after percutaneous transluminal angioplasty shows improvement in the arterial lumen. Irregularity in the small branch of the renal artery (*solid arrow*) represents transient guide wire–induced spasm. (Courtesy of James Shields, MD, St Joseph Mercy Hospital, Ann Arbor)

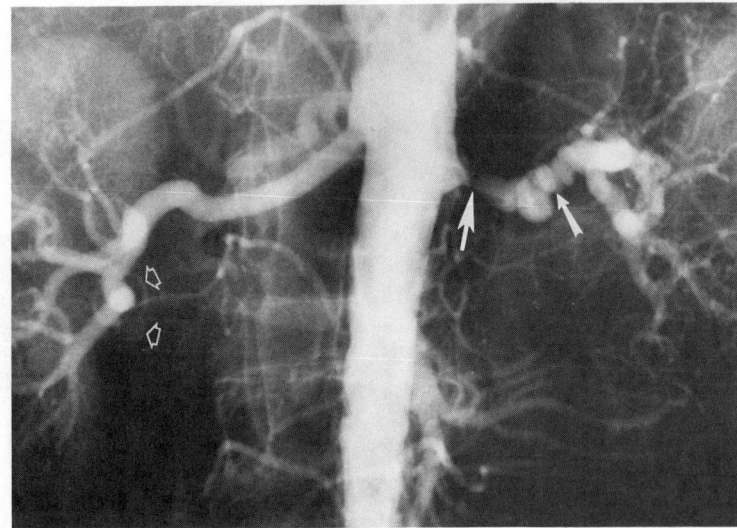

Figure 76-29. Concurrent atherosclerotic and dysplastic renal artery stenoses in a 60-year-old hypertensive woman. Lumbar aortogram shows smooth concentric narrowing of the proximal left renal artery (*large arrow*) and alternating constrictions and aneurysmal dilations in the distal main renal artery (*small arrow*). A calcified bilobed aneurysm involves the right renal artery (*open arrows*).

visceral arteries is analogous to the workup of occlusive and aneurysmal disease. Angiography should document the hemodynamic significance of arterial narrowing, the extent of the dissection, the relation of the dissection to nearby normal branches, and the integrity of the collateral circulation. Dissections in these medium-sized arteries appear as long, smooth narrowings of the artery, with smooth sigmoid contour changes or socklike dead ends reflecting the spiral course of the dissection, which usually terminates at a branch point of the parent artery. A double lumen is not always seen.

Occasionally, an atherosclerotic ulcer penetrates the media and results in intramedial dissection.[23] This penetrating ulcer may be associated with a pseudoaneurysm or a false lumen and may simulate a classic dissection clinically. The dissecting hematoma or pseudoaneurysm of the penetrating aortic ulcer tends to originate in the distal thoracic aorta.

Iatrogenic dissections result from the intraarterial manipulation of guide wires or catheters, percutaneous angioplasties, and cannulation of the aorta during bypass (Fig. 76-27). The significance of these dissections depends on the vessel involved, the status of the collateral circulation, and the direction of dissection with respect to blood flow. Celiac artery dissection is usually well tolerated because of the immediate recruitment of collateral blood supply (through the pancreatic arcades) and because of the dual blood supply to the liver. SMA dissection extending beyond the origins of the first jejunal and middle colic arteries requires surgical intervention. Retrograde iliac artery dissection (such as that caused by subintimal passage of a guide wire) usually heals spontaneously and remains asymptomatic unless blood flow is significantly altered. Flow-limiting dissections in the iliac, renal, or mesenteric arteries can sometimes be treated by the use of intravascular prostheses such as the Palmaz stent or Wallstent (see Fig. 76-43).

Arterial Fibrodysplasia

Arterial fibrodysplasia is a disease of medium-sized muscular arteries that is of uncertain etiology, although retrospective reviews have documented significant associations with cigarette smoking, a history of hypertension, HLA type, and female gender. Arterial fibrodysplasia most commonly affects

the renal, carotid, and external iliac arteries but may be found in the coronary, vertebral, mesenteric, and brachial arteries as well. Histologic classification of the disease is based on the type and distribution of dysplastic material in the arterial wall.[24] The accumulation and proliferation of this material can result in narrowing of the arterial lumen or weakening of the arterial wall and loss of elastic material, which may result in secondary dissection or widening of the lumen and even aneurysm formation. The patients present with organ-related symptoms associated with arterial stenoses, dissections, or aneurysms. These symptoms include hypertension,

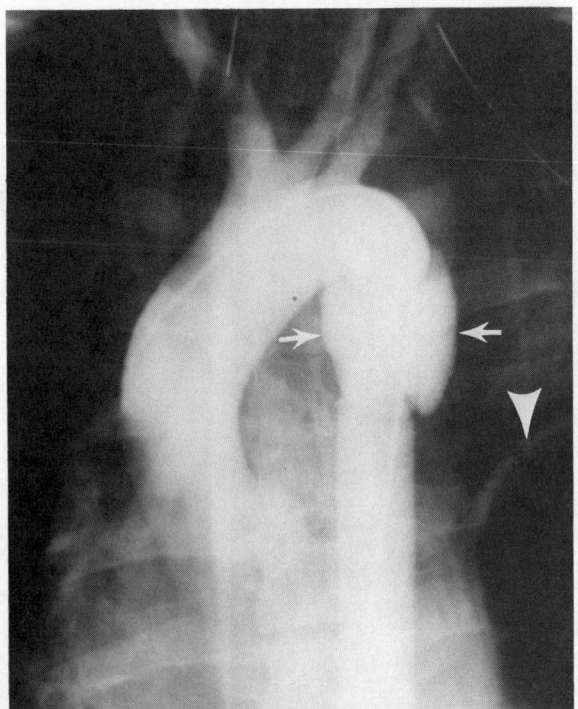

Figure 76-30. Traumatic thoracic aortic rupture in a 30-year-old man involved in a motor vehicle accident. Arch aortogram shows a contained rupture of the proximal descending aorta (*arrows*), just distal to the origin of the left subclavian artery. A ruptured left hemidiaphragm with herniation of the stomach (*arrowhead*) is visible.

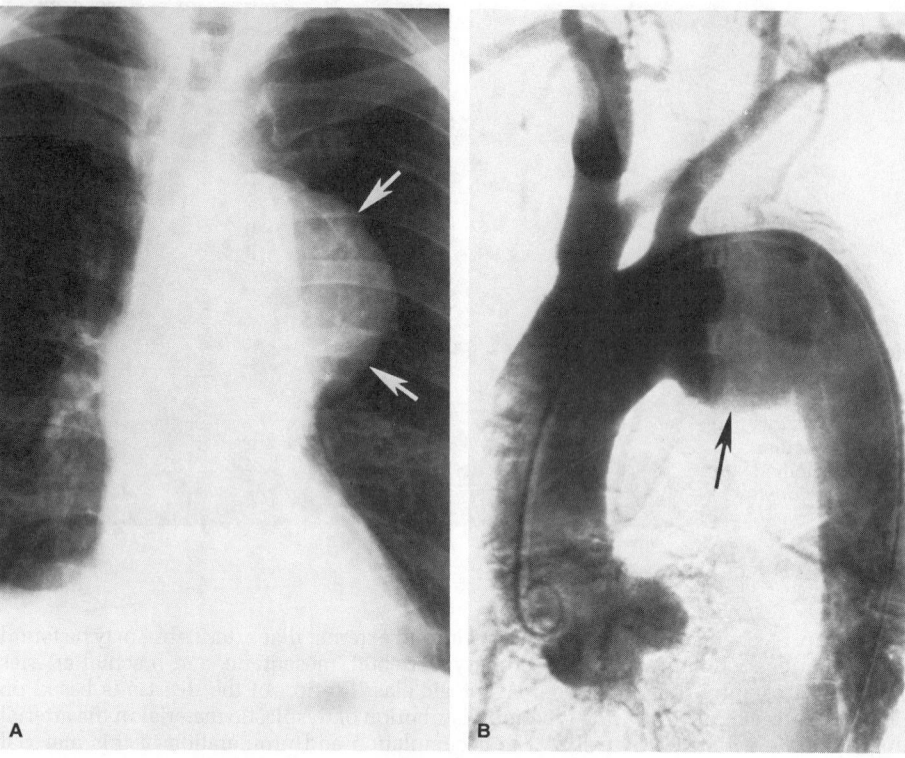

Figure 76-31. Posttraumatic chronic aortic pseudoaneurysm in a 71-year-old man with a 6-week history of increasing hoarseness. (*A*) Chest film shows localized enlargement of the aortic knob (*arrows*). (*B*) Arch aortogram in the right posterior oblique position shows focal dilation of the thoracic aorta just distal to the left subclavian artery (*arrow*). The rupture was successfully repaired surgically.

stroke, and claudication. Angiography is directed at the presenting symptoms, and the indications for angiography parallel those for atherosclerosis, aneurysms, and dissections. The histologic changes lead to an angiographic appearance of arterial fibrodysplasia that is easily distinguished from atherosclerosis, except when the disease is focal or in an unusual location. The classic angiographic appearance of arterial fibrodysplasia is the "string of beads" appearance of medial

fibroplasia, the most common histologic type of the disease (Figs. 76-28 and 76-29). Angiographic findings in renal arteries that favor fibrodysplasia include the following:

- Long, smooth narrowing
- Long, irregular, beaded narrowing often with associated poststenotic dilation or large aneurysms
- Discrete, weblike stenoses

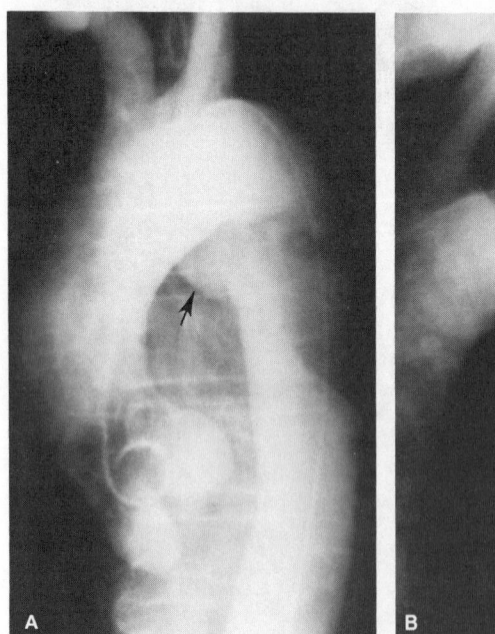
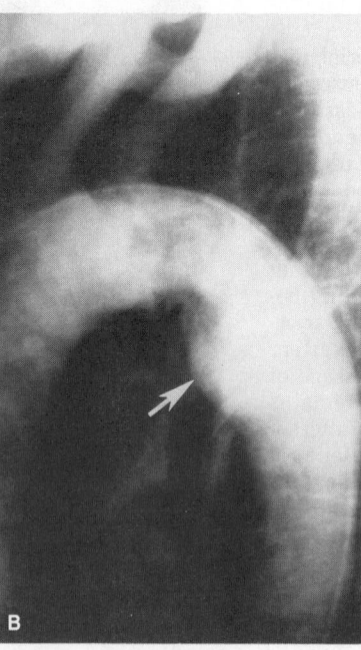
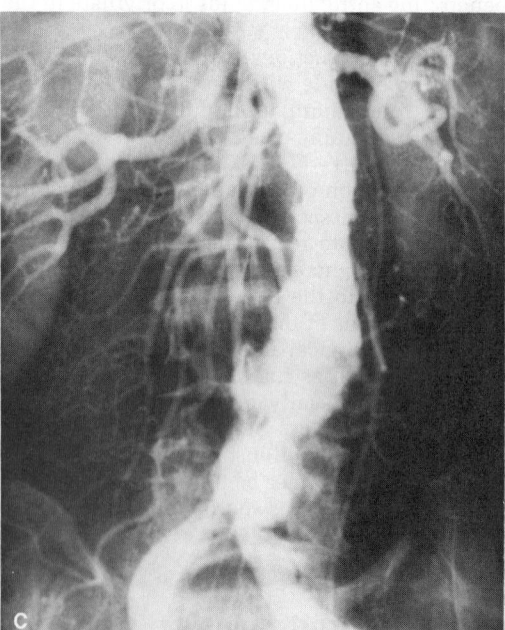

Figure 76-32. Prominent ductus bump simulating a posttraumatic aortic pseudoaneurysm in a man with septic peripheral emboli. (*A* and *B*) Biplanar arch aortograms show focal bulging from the anteromedial surface of the descending aorta at the ligamentum arteriosum (*arrow*). (*C*) Abdominal aortogram shows an irregular infrarenal aneurysm with mural debris. At exploration, the thoracic aorta was normal, and a mycotic abdominal aortic aneurysm was resected. Angiographically, this mycotic aneurysm cannot be distinguished from a bland atherosclerotic aneurysm.

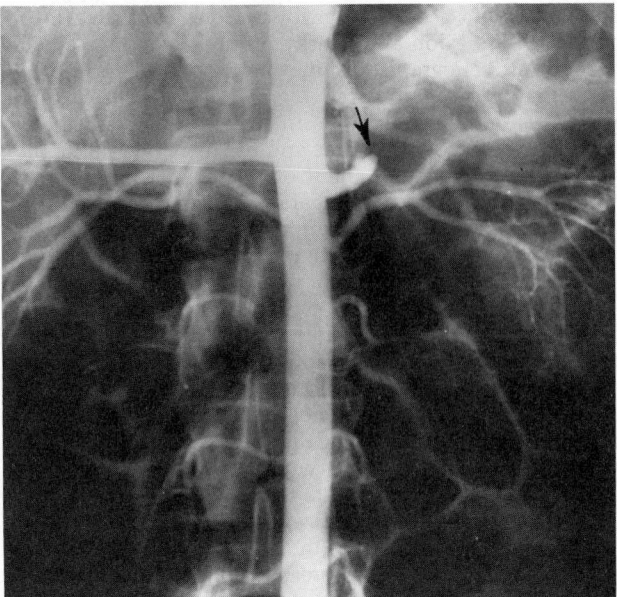

Figure 76-33. Traumatic renal artery occlusion in a 20-year-old male victim of a motor vehicle accident. Abnormal nephrogram was demonstrated on an abdominal film obtained after arch aortography. A subsequent lumbar aortogram confirmed left renal artery occlusion (*arrow*). The lower pole artery, fortuitously originating separately from the aorta, is irregular and deformed secondary to a retroperitoneal hematoma.

- Spontaneous dissections
- Involvement of the middle and distal thirds of the main trunk that often extends into segmental arteries[25]

These findings are typical of the disease in other arteries as well.

Arteritis

Inflammatory arteritis becomes a surgical problem in the presence of arterial insufficiency syndromes, hemorrhage, or threatened tissue loss. The indication for angiography in inflammatory arteritis is to determine the extent of disease and to demonstrate the status of the proximal and distal circulation for a prospective vascular reconstruction procedure. At times, angiography is helpful in the primary diagnosis of an inflammatory arteritis. The angiogram may demonstrate diffuse spasm or microaneurysms in active disease. Arterial stenoses, occlusions, and prominent collaterals may be present in active or quiescent disease. The vessels involved range in size from the aorta and pulmonary arteries in Takayasu arteritis to the renal interlobar arteries of necrotizing arteritis. Small-caliber vessels found on muscle or skin biopsy are too small to be seen by standard angiographic techniques.

Trauma

Blunt and penetrating trauma can result in acute ischemia or hemorrhage, either immediate or delayed. Deceleration injuries (eg, motor vehicle accidents, falls) are associated with injuries to the thoracic aorta or brachiocephalic vessels. Penetrating wounds are associated with vascular injuries along the track of the foreign body (eg, knife, low-speed bullets). Shock waves radiated through tissue by high-speed missiles may injure vessels remote from the missile track. The role of angiography is to demonstrate the extent of the arterial injury and the status of the proximal and distal normal circulation. Angiographic findings include pseudoaneurysm, arterial or venous occlusions, arteriovenous fistulas, and contrast extravasation indicating active hemorrhage. The workup for traumatic occlusive disease parallels that of the preceding discussions. Certain traumatic vascular injuries warrant specific comments.

Aortic rupture is best demonstrated by thoracic aortogra-

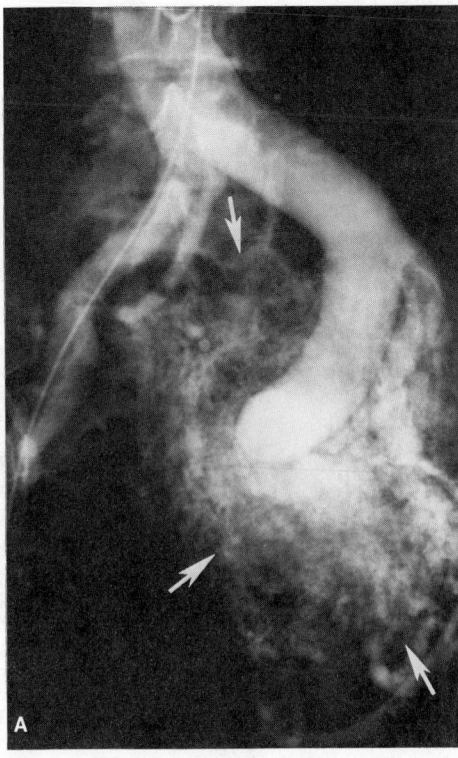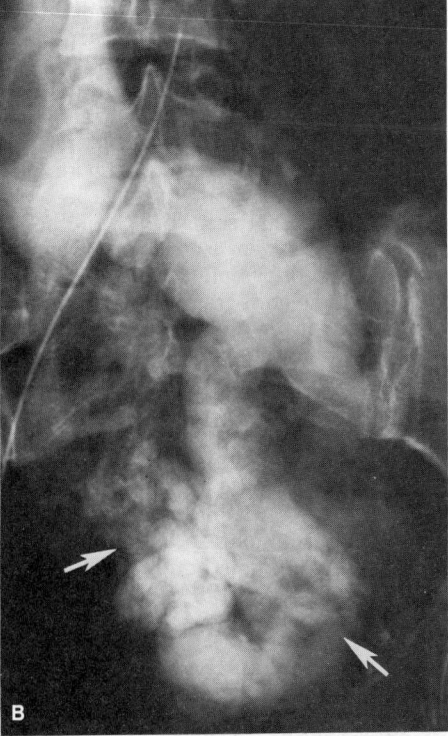

Figure 76-34. Arteriovenous malformation in a 50-year-old schizophrenic woman. Cardiac output measured 16 L/min. (*A*) The arterial phase of the pelvic angiogram shows gross asymmetry of the common iliac arteries, with a massively dilated left internal iliac artery supplying a large nidus of innumerable small arteries (*arrows*). Other arterial injections documented contributions from the left external, deep femoral, and right internal iliac arteries. (*B*) A large tangle of tortuous veins (*arrows*) empties into dilated left iliac veins.

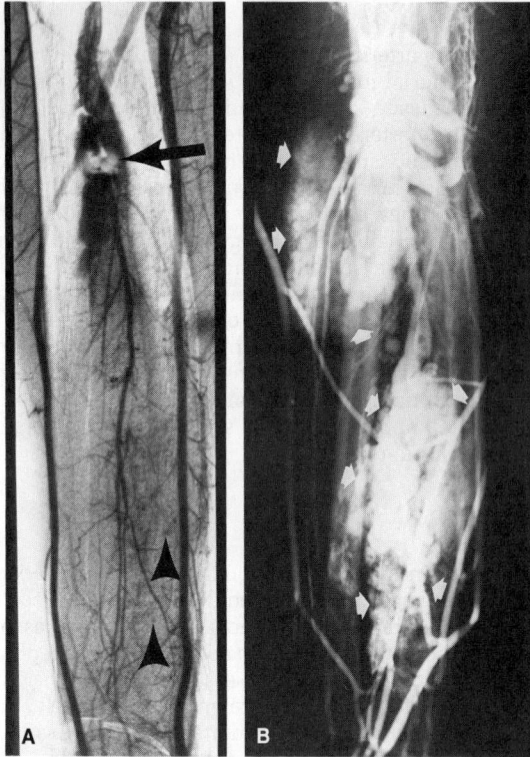

Figure 76-35. Venous angioma in a 19-year-old woman with symptoms of recurrent right forearm venous thrombosis and a mass noticed at age 6 years. (*A*) Photographic subtraction of the capillary phase of the forearm arteriogram shows normal radial, ulnar, interosseous, and muscular arteries; faint scattered punctate areas of contrast pooling (*arrowheads*); and draining vein containing thrombus (*arrow*). (*B*) A closed-system venogram provides much better documentation of the component of the angioma (*solid arrows*).

phy in the right posterior oblique projection. The most common site of rupture is at the level of the ligamentum arteriosum, at the transition between the relatively immobile descending aorta and the relatively mobile arch (Figs. 76-30 and 76-31). The diagnosis of a subtle injury is occasionally difficult in the presence of an unusual ductus diverticulum or atherosclerotic plaque (Fig. 76-32). Multiple views of the aorta may be helpful in clarifying the unusual normal variant. Other sites of cardiovascular decelerating injury are the aortic root, the aorta at the level of the diaphragm, and the proximal innominate artery. Preliminary reports of the diagnosis of aortic rupture by CT scanning have been published. No prospective study of CT scans or DSA in the diagnosis of aortic rupture has sufficient statistical power to justify replacing conventional aortography at this time.

The thoracic aortogram is followed routinely by supine radiographs of the abdomen to evaluate the kidneys and bladder. If renal injury is suspected, an abdominal aortogram is obtained (Fig. 76-33).

In the angiographic workup of traumatic hemorrhage, therapeutic considerations may require extension of the diagnostic examination. For example, if occlusive therapy is contemplated (either surgical ligation or transcatheter embolism), the status of the collateral circulation and the arterial bed distal to the arterial injury should be carefully evaluated before intervention.

Hemangiomas and Vascular Malformations

Hemangiomas and vascular malformations constitute a spectrum of neoplasms and congenital vascular dysplasias, including capillary, venous, and arteriovenous lesions.[26,27]

Angiography is used to identify and describe the arterial supply to the lesion and nearby normal structures. In the extremities, venography is often performed in addition to arteriography to demonstrate the deep veins. This is done because some malformations in the limbs are associated with deep-vein abnormalities and because the relation between the venous component of the lesion and the deep veins is important if sclerotherapy is to be used. CT and MR imaging are useful in demonstrating the three-dimensional relation between the malformation or hemangioma and the normal structures.

Angiographic findings in an arteriovenous malformation consist of tortuous and enlarged feeding arteries, a nidus of innumerable small arteries, and large draining veins (Fig. 76-34). When rapid flow throughout the malformation is demonstrated, venography is not indicated. In a venous malformation, the arterial phase of the angiogram may be normal. Veins are large and tortuous with slow flow; occasionally, large venous lakes are present. The venous malformation is best studied by closed-system venography or by direct injection of contrast material into the malformation (Fig. 76-35). No persistent tissue stain is present after contrast injections in arteries supplying pure venous or arteriovenous malformations. The arteries supplying and the veins draining a capillary hemangioma may be normal or mildly enlarged. Selective injection of contrast into feeding arteries results in a dense and persistent tumor stain.

Neoplasm

In the past, angiography was performed to identify and stage neoplasms and inflammatory masses. Over the past 15 years, tests that are more sensitive than angiography in these diagnostic applications have been developed, including CT, ultrasound, and MR imaging. Angiography is usually performed after CT or MR imaging has defined the location of the primary tumor, the presence of metastases, or both. Angiography no longer has a prominent role in

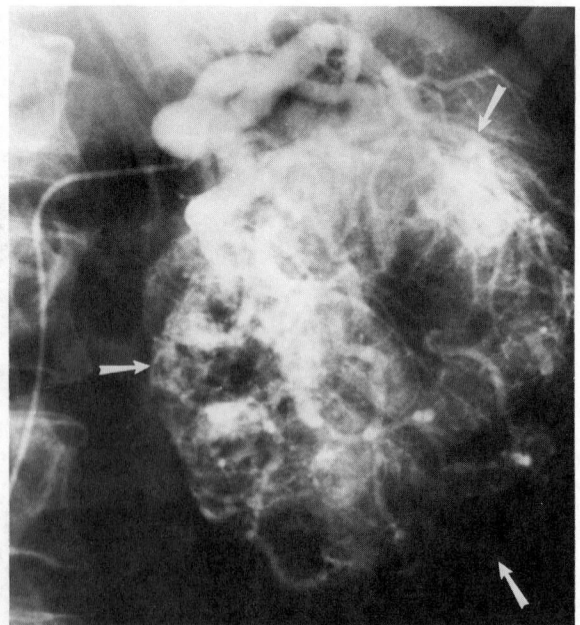

Figure 76-36. Tumor neovascularity in a 52-year-old man with a hypernephroma. Left renal arteriogram demonstrates a large hypervascular tumor in the lower pole of the left kidney (*arrows*) with abundant neovascularity and intense contrast accumulation (tumor stain).

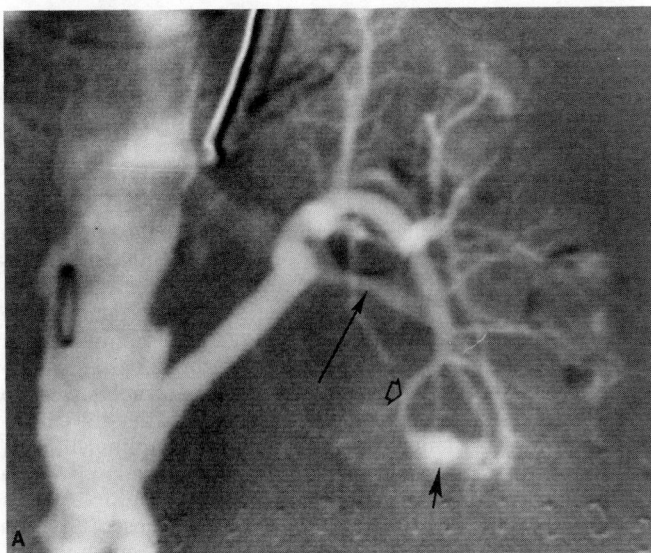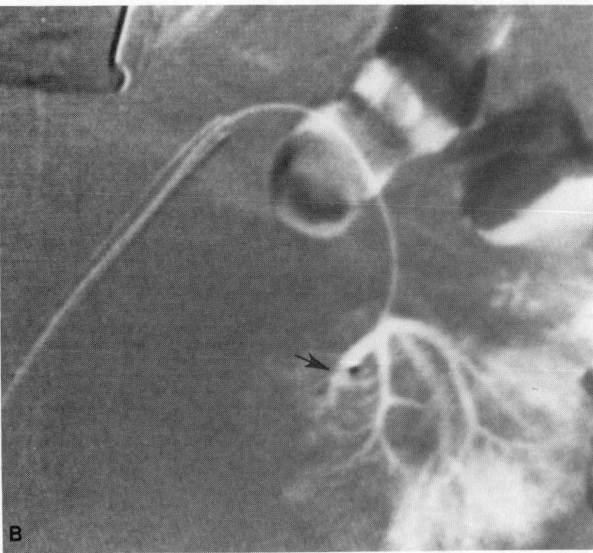

Figure 76-37. Postoperative renal artery pseudoaneurysm with an arteriovenous fistula in a woman with hematuria 1 day after a left aortorenal revascularization procedure. (*A*) Lumbar aortogram with digital subtraction angiography demonstrates a lower-pole pseudoaneurysm (*short arrow*) supplied by a normal-sized segmental artery (*open arrow*). Early venous filling is present (*long arrow*). The segmental artery supplying the pseudoaneurysm was subselectively catheterized with a 3F coaxial catheter system and embolized with polyvinyl alcohol (Ivalon) particles. (*B*) A segmental arteriogram after embolization shows successful occlusion of the pseudoaneurysm (*arrow*), with sparing of the adjacent arteries.

the diagnosis of tumors, although it is more sensitive than cross-sectional studies in the demonstration of small (5-mm) hypervascular tumors and is useful in the study of large tumors growing at the interface of two abdominal structures (eg, the mesentery and omentum, or liver and adrenal gland). Angiography is commonly used to provide

a vascular road map before resection of abdominal neoplasms, especially in the pancreas and liver; to document vascular invasion by nonresectable tumors; to answer specific clinical questions such as resectability of pancreatic or hepatic masses; and in conjunction with transcatheter chemotherapy.

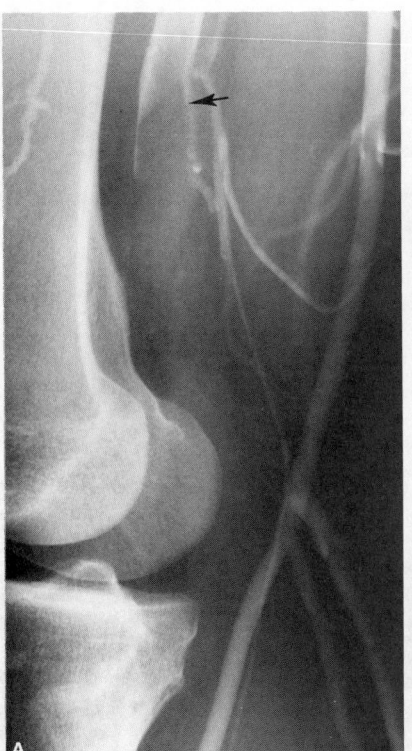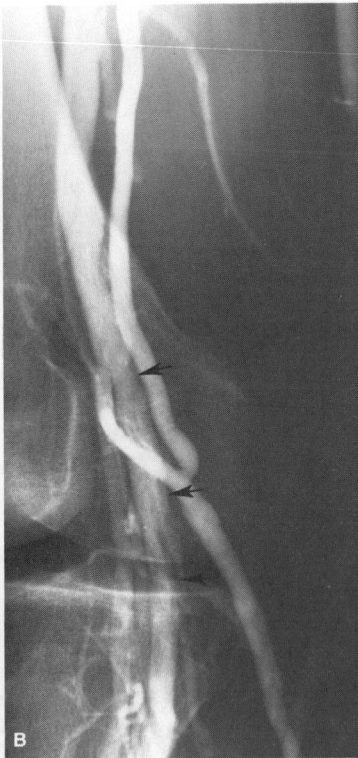

Figure 76-38. Acute and chronic deep venous thrombosis in a 19-year-old man who presented with acute right calf swelling. (*A*) An ascending leg venogram shows acute thrombus in the popliteal vein. The patient was examined 25 months later for right calf pain. (*B*) A second venogram shows recanalization of the popliteal vein with residual linear filling defects (*arrows*), representing organized clot. No valves are seen in this segment of popliteal vein.

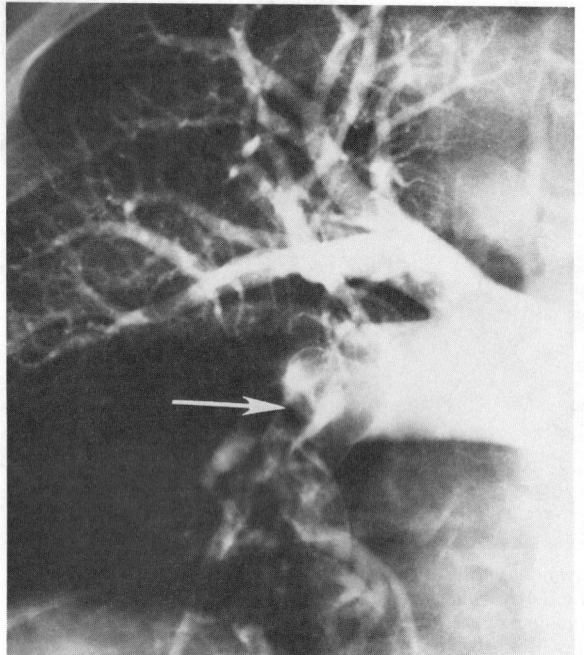

Figure 76-39. Acute pulmonary embolism in a 39-year-old man with a renal transplant. A selective right pulmonary arteriogram shows a large saddle embolus in the right main pulmonary artery with occlusion of the middle lobe arteries and a cast of thrombus (*arrow*) in the lower lobe arteries.

Neoplasms are characterized angiographically as avascular, hypovascular, or hypervascular, depending on the number and size of tumor vessels and on the intensity of contrast-medium stain in the tumor (tumor blush) relative to surrounding normal tissue. Tumor vessels are somewhat disorderly and meandering compared with normal parenchymal branches, which branch systematically. The con-

tour of tumor vessels may be smooth, somewhat beaded in appearance, or highly irregular and serrated. Early or intense venous opacification is common with hypervascular tumors such as hepatomas, hypernephromas, and leiomyomas (Fig. 76-36).

Postsurgical Follow-Up

Angiography is often performed after a surgical procedure to establish a vascular baseline (after a revascularization procedure), to rule out a surgical complication (after transplantation, revascularization, or shunt surgery), or to demonstrate progression of disease (Fig. 76-37). Vascular complications consist of stenoses, occlusions, dissections, pseudoaneurysms, and arteriovenous fistulas. The angiographic workup proceeds as in the earlier discussions, except that the examination may be tailored on the basis of the clinical signs, the surgeon's impression of a specific complication, and the known preoperative anatomy. In addition, multiple views may be necessary to observe vascular anastomoses in profile to exclude arterial strictures (especially after renal revascularization or transplant surgery).

Peripheral Venous Disease

Venography is the most accurate means of diagnosing deep-vein thrombosis and incompetent lower extremity venous valves. It is also the best way to demonstrate venous anatomy in certain vascular malformations or hemangiomas, or before dialysis shunt construction or venous reconstructive procedures. When injections are in a peripheral vein, venography can demonstrate deep and superficial veins of the extremity. Inferior vena cavography is usually performed by the percutaneous transfemoral venous approach. For the diagnosis of deep-vein thrombosis (when the display of global venous anatomy is of secondary interest), conventional contrast venography has been largely replaced by duplex (Doppler and B-mode imaging) or color-flow ultrasonography for the extremities and mag-

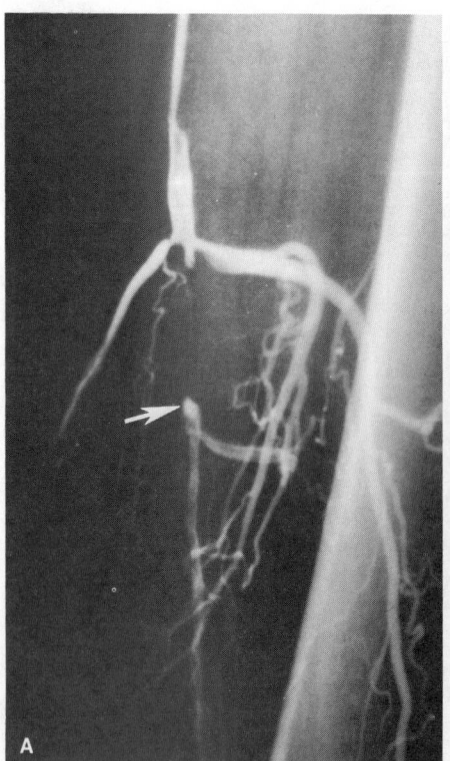
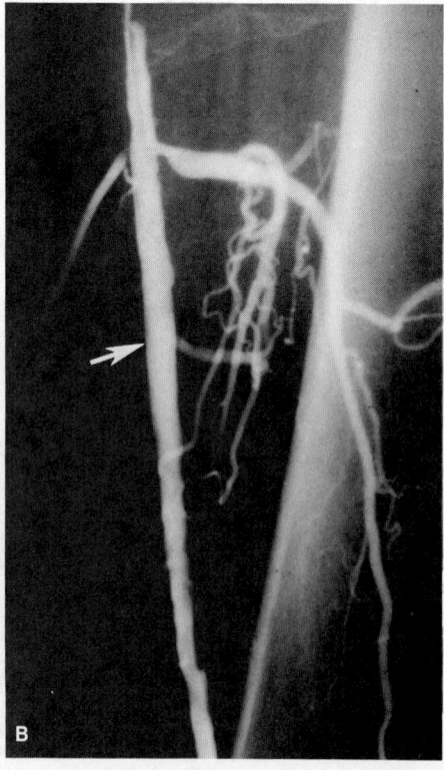

Figure 76-40. Percutaneous transluminal angioplasty of a superficial femoral artery occlusion in a 60-year-old man with claudication. Superficial femoral arteriograms before (*A*) and after (*B*) recanalization and angioplasty of a distal superficial femoral artery occlusion. The caliber of the popliteal artery (*arrow*) is increased after inflow has been improved.

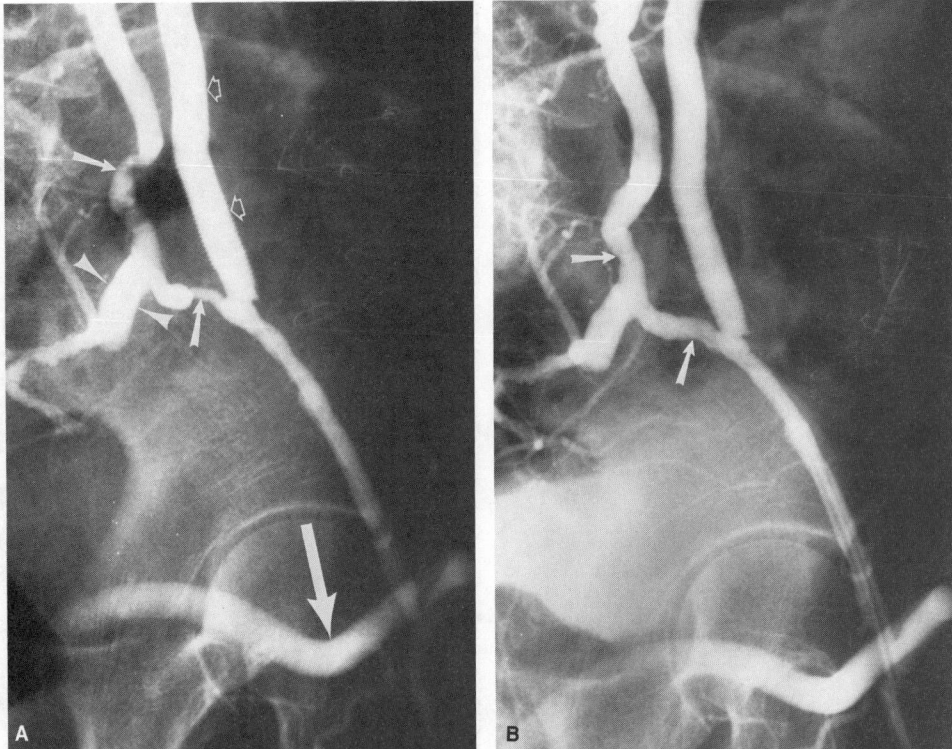

Figure 76-41. Percutaneous transluminal angioplasty of the iliac arteries in a man with right buttock claudication after aorto–left external iliac bypass and left-to-right femorofemoral bypass. (*A*) Lumbar aortogram shows a patent aortoiliac graft (*open arrows*) in continuity with the mid-external iliac artery and the femorofemoral graft (*large arrow*). The graft did not fill the right pelvis, which was perfused by transpelvic collaterals from the left internal iliac artery (*arrowheads*). Tight stenoses in the common iliac and proximal external iliac arteries (*small arrows*) limit internal iliac perfusion. (*B*) Both stenoses responded to percutaneous angioplasty (*arrows*), and buttock claudication resolved.

Figure 76-42. Percutaneous transluminal angioplasty (PTA) of brachiocephalic vein strictures in a 70-year-old woman with superior vena cava syndrome after radiation for breast cancer. CT scans (not shown) showed no tumor in the mediastinum. (*A*) Bilateral upper extremity venogram demonstrates strictures of the right and left brachiocephalic veins at their confluence (*arrows*). The strictures were dilated by simultaneous inflation of two 10-mm angioplasty balloons, one across each stricture. (*B*) Venogram after PTA shows improved appearance of the brachiocephalic vein confluence (*arrows*). Pressure gradients from the brachiocephalic vein to the superior vena cava were improved from 27 cm of saline to 2 cm on the right and from 21 to 4 cm on the left.

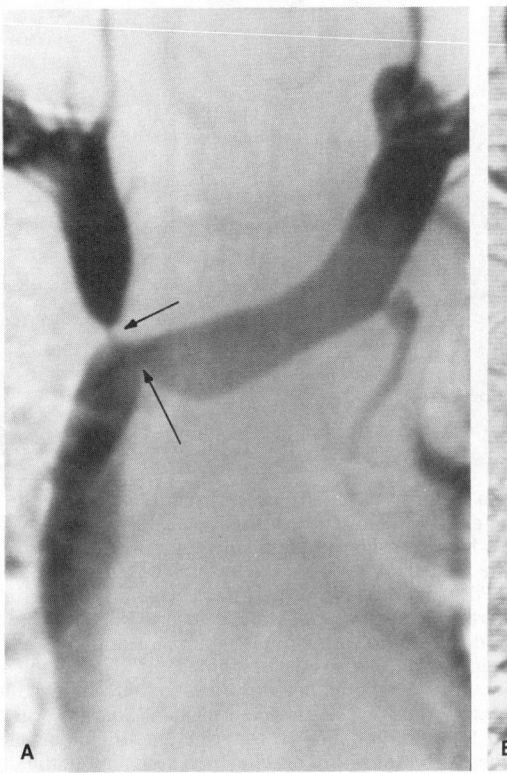

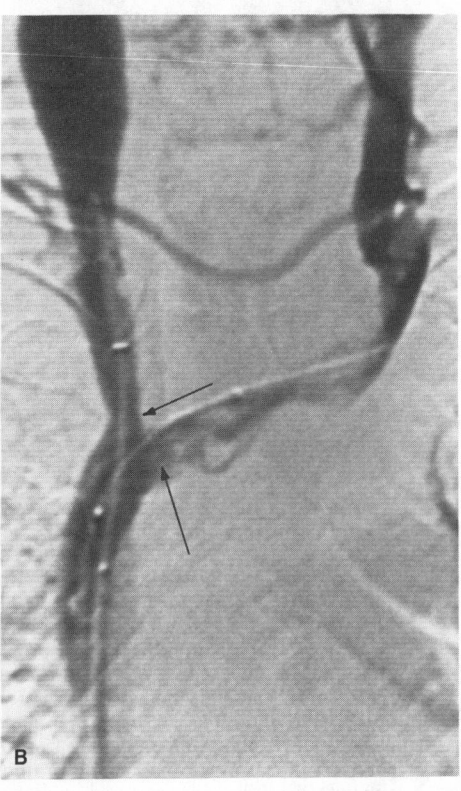

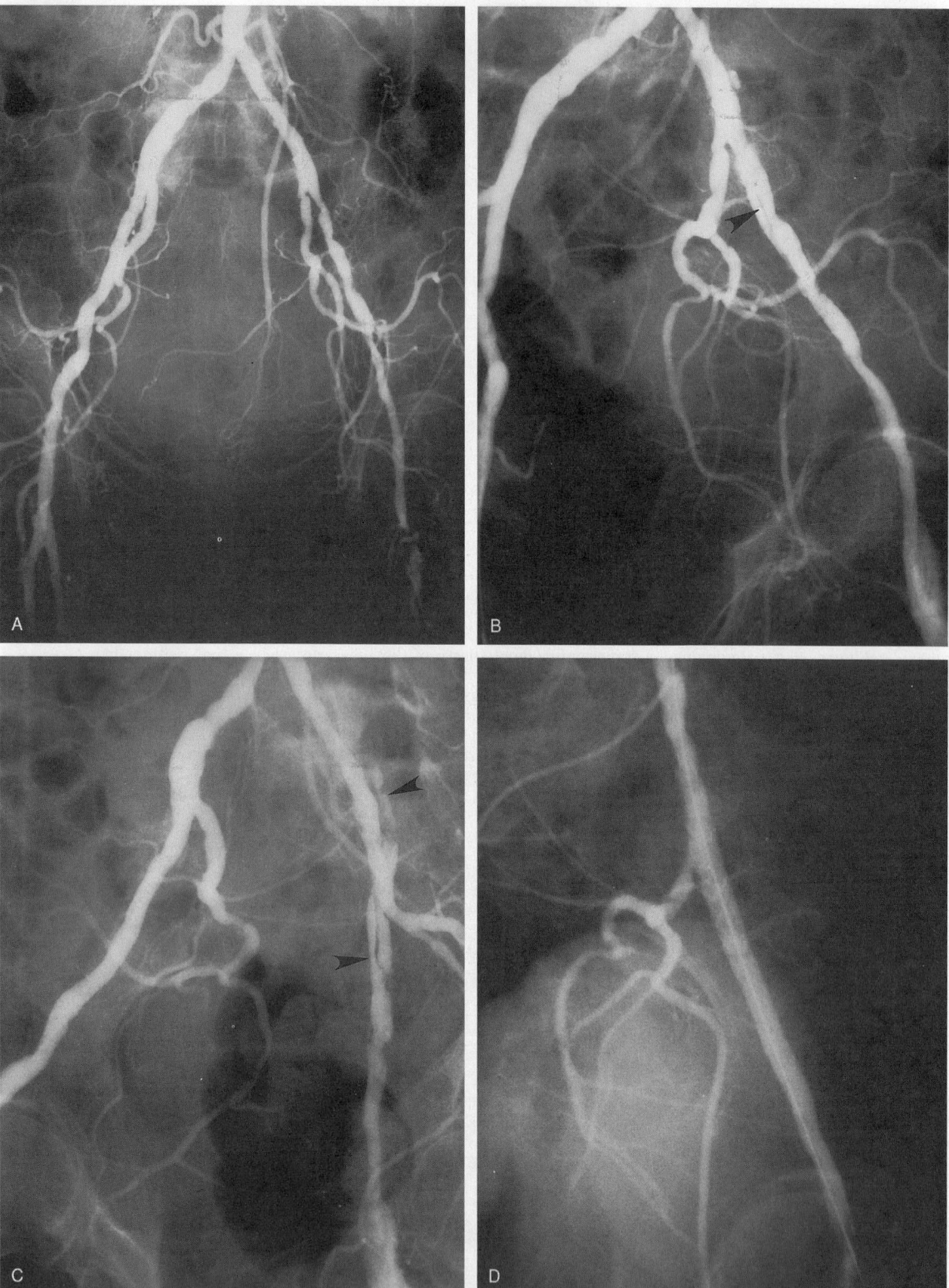

Figure 76-43. Serial pelvic arteriograms in a patient with left lower extremity occlusive disease. (*A*) Initial outflow study shows moderate external iliac artery occlusive disease. The superficial femoral artery was occluded. Inflow was judged to be adequate, and the patient underwent a femoropopliteal bypass graft. Several days after the operation, the left ankle–brachial index reverted to the preoperative level. (*B* and *C*) Postoperative oblique pelvic arteriograms show a dissection involving the external iliac artery (*arrowheads*) and reflecting a Fogarty catheter–induced injury sustained during the surgical procedure. The femoropopliteal graft is occluded as a result of compromised inflow. With fluoroscopic guidance and injections of contrast from the right transfemoral catheter, the left femoral artery was punctured between the endarterectomized hood of the femoropopliteal graft and the inguinal ligament. The dissected segment of artery was then paved with Palmaz stents tapering from 7 to 6 mm in diameter. (*D*) After stent deployment, left common iliac artery injection shows unobstructed flow; the aortofemoral pressure gradient was ablated. Distal flow was restored by operative thrombectomy of the graft.

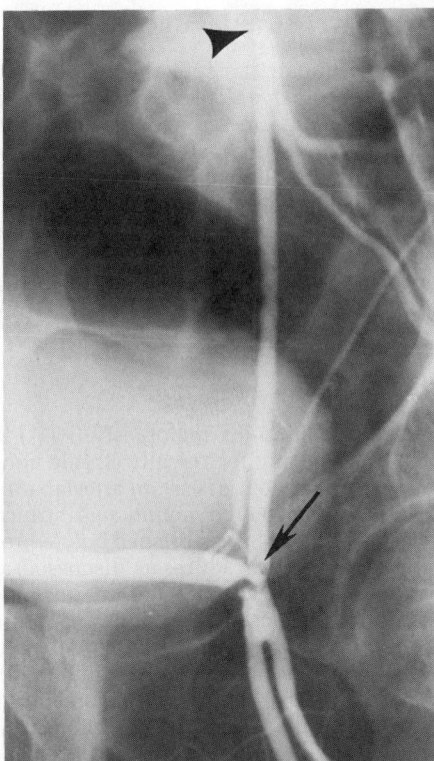

Figure 76-44. Lytic therapy with urokinase. A 50-year-old man presented with occluded right axillofemoral and right-to-left femorofemoral bypass grafts. With use of a right brachial artery approach, flow in the axillofemoral graft was reestablished after 12 hours of urokinase infusion at 2000 IU/min. With use of a right femoral artery approach, flow in the femorofemoral graft was reestablished after 6 hours of urokinase infusion at 2000 IU/min through a catheter with the tip just distal to the graft origin. Angiogram made at the termination of the procedure shows narrowing of the distal graft lumen and a filling defect in the left common femoral artery (*arrow*). Because of the angle of the graft insertion site (nearly 90 degrees) and the filling defect above and below the anastomosis, this lesion is not suitable for angioplasty or atherectomy from the right femoral approach. A mound of intimal hyperplasia was removed during surgical revision of the anastomosis. The left internal iliac artery fills through retrograde flow in the external iliac artery (*arrowhead*).

netic resonance venography for the iliocaval, portal, and renal systems.

Lower extremity ascending venography requires injection of contrast medium in a dorsal foot vein with the leg relaxed and dependent.[28] In an adult patient, 100 mL of 43% contrast medium fills deep and superficial veins from the foot to the inguinal ligament. Visualization of the external and common iliac veins and the caudal inferior vena cava can be enhanced by maneuvers that evacuate the contrast medium from the calf, such as weight bearing. Acute deep-vein thrombosis appears as a castlike filling defect in the contrast column within the deep veins (Fig. 76-38*A*). Acute thrombosis may be so extensive that contrast does not enter the deep system. Absence of deep-vein filling in acute deep-vein thrombosis is distinguished from that in chronic deep-vein thrombosis by the size of the superficial veins and venous collaterals; they are small when accompanying acute disease and large when accompanying chronic disease. In the patient with chronic deep-vein thrombosis, venography demonstrates linear or weblike intraluminal filling defects representing organized thrombus, occluded deep veins with large collaterals, or, rarely, no abnormality (see Fig. 76-38*B*).

Lower extremity descending venography is performed to evaluate the competence of the valves in the saphenous, femoral, and popliteal veins. The study can be performed by retrograde catheterization of the opposite femoral vein and manipulation of the catheter tip across the iliac confluence into the external iliac vein on the side of interest. If the femoral vein cannot be punctured, venous access may be obtained by use of an antecubital vein puncture. Contrast medium is then injected at the level of the inguinal ligament under fluoroscopic observation as the patient breathes quietly or performs the Valsalva maneuver. Reflux in the greater saphenous, deep femoral, and superficial femoral veins is assessed and graded from 0 (no reflux) to 4 (reflux below the knee).[29] A global view of venous anatomy (necessary if a venous bypass or valvuloplasty procedure is planned) requires ascending venography.

Closed-system extremity venography may be required for demonstration of the full extent of a venous malformation or hemangioma.[30,31] A vein distal to the lesion is cannulated with a soft angiocatheter. A tight elastic wrap is then applied to the limb beginning at the angiocatheter. It is wrapped proximally, compressing the lesion and evacuating venous blood centrally. A blood pressure cuff is then inflated above

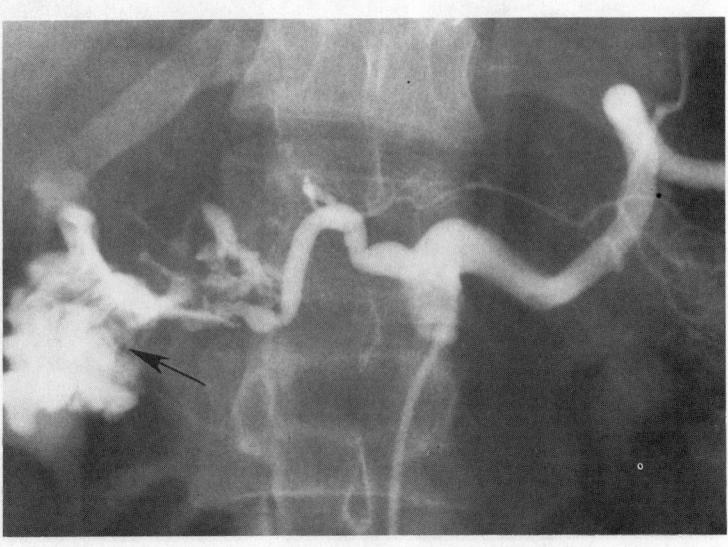

Figure 76-45. A 31-year-old man with a peptic ulcer and a previous vagotomy, antrectomy, and Billroth II procedure presented with massive upper gastrointestinal bleeding. Selective celiac arteriogram shows contrast extravasation into the second portion of the duodenum (*arrow*). Celiac stenosis was present, and retrograde flow in the common hepatic artery (temporarily reversed by the power injection of contrast) precluded safe transcatheter embolization of the bleeding artery. (Courtesy of James Andrews, MD, University of Michigan Hospitals, Ann Arbor)

systolic pressure (250 to 300 mmHg) proximal to the lesion, preventing arterial refilling of the lesion, and the elastic wrap is removed. Contrast medium is then injected during fluoroscopic observation of the limb. The closed-system venogram demonstrates contrast filling in the capillary and venous components of a malformation or hemangioma as well as deep and superficial venous anatomy of the limb distal to the blood pressure cuff (see Fig. 76-35*B*).

Pulmonary Embolism

The diagnosis of pulmonary embolism often requires confirmation by pulmonary angiography because of the low specificity of ventilation and perfusion scans in certain clinical settings. In addition to documenting the presence of pulmonary emboli, angiography can demonstrate alternative pathology that explains abnormalities on chest radiographs or ventilation and perfusion scans. Pulmonary artery injections are preceded by the measurement of pulmonary artery pressures, because the risk of sudden cardiac decompensation is increased in the presence of right ventricular or pulmonary artery hypertension.[32] When mean pulmonary artery pressure exceeds 40 mmHg, the injection rate (ordinarily 25 mL/s for 2 seconds in a main pulmonary artery) is reduced to match decreased pulmonary flow as estimated at fluoroscopy (eg, 16 mL/s for 3 seconds). The angiographic findings of acute pulmonary embolism consist of intraarterial filling defects, arterial cutoffs, and perfusion defects (Fig. 76-39). The angiographic findings of chronic pulmonary embolism are intraluminal webs, arterial stenoses and cutoffs, collateral reconstitution of occluded vessels, and perfusion defects. Arterial cutoffs, perfusion defects, and slow arterial flow are nonspecific for pulmonary embolism (acute or chronic).

INTERVENTIONAL ANGIOGRAPHY

A large number of percutaneous therapeutic options for acute or chronic occlusive disease, active or intermittent hemorrhage, and neoplasm are available, and others are under investigation. Transcatheter therapy should be considered in appropriate clinical circumstances at the time that diagnostic angiography is undertaken because the mechanical constraints of the therapeutic catheter system affect the choice of puncture site and because thorough pretherapy evaluation may require additional diagnostic injections.

Angioplasty

Percutaneous transluminal angioplasty (PTA) is generally accepted as a safe and technically simple nonsurgical alternative for the treatment of certain arterial and venous occlusive lesions. The hemodynamic significance of the lesion in question should be established before proceeding with an interventional procedure, as discussed above in the section on nonaneurysmal atherosclerosis. PTA requires crossing the stenosis or occlusion with a guide wire. After the intraluminal position of the guide wire is confirmed, the balloon (chosen so that the inflated diameter is about 20% greater than the normal diameter of the vessel) is advanced over the wire across the stenosis or occlusion and inflated. Balloon inflation is observed at fluoroscopy. Adequate dilation is assessed by intraarterial manometry, ankle–brachial pressure indices, or improvement in the luminal diameter of the vessel as judged by post-PTA angiography. PTA is often performed for femoropopliteal (Fig. 76-40), iliac (Fig. 76-41), and renal occlusive lesions. It is less commonly performed for infrapopliteal, mesenteric, and aortic lesions, and only occasionally for subclavian and carotid lesions.[33,34] PTA has also been performed for renal transplant anastomotic strictures, renal

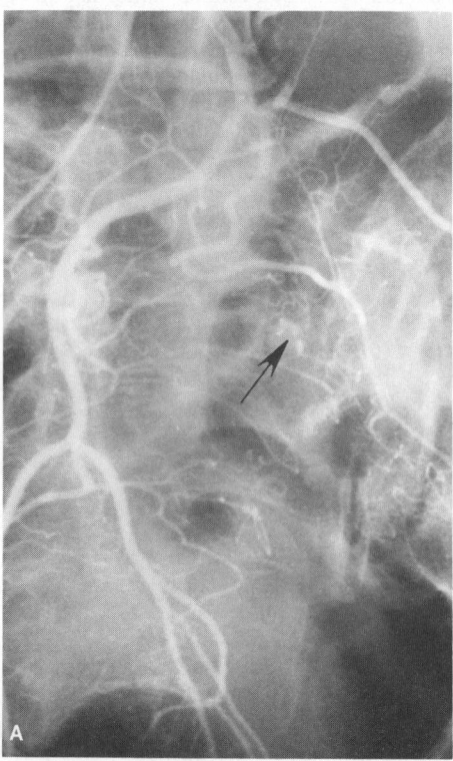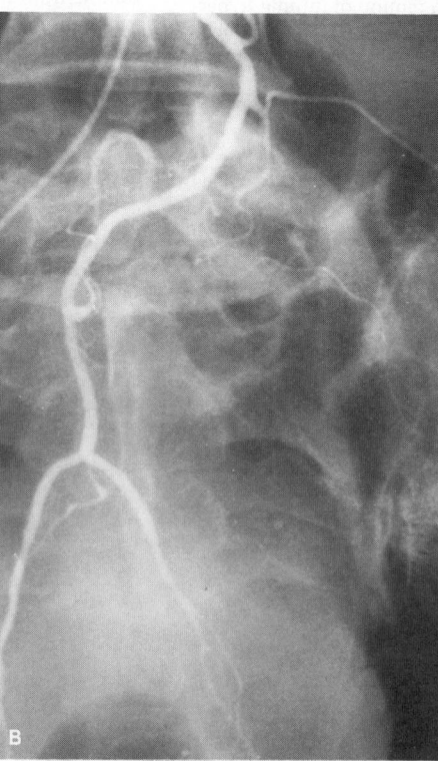

Figure 76-46. Lower gastrointestinal bleeding. A 72-year-old man presented with hematochezia after endoscopic polypectomy. (*A*) Inferior mesenteric arteriogram shows extravasation of contrast from a sigmoidal branch. (*B*) A second arteriogram after a 30-minute infusion of vasopressin at 0.2 IU/min shows arrest of the bleeding and marked constriction of all sigmoidal and rectal branches. Superselective embolotherapy would have been indicated if the hemorrhage had failed to respond to vasopressin.

or limb revascularization anastomotic strictures, dialysis graft stenoses, and venous stenoses (Fig. 76-42). The ideal PTA lesion is the renal fibromuscular dysplastic lesion without associated aneurysms (see Fig. 76-28), or concentric, nonostial, noncalcified atherosclerotic lesions. Complications of PTA include thrombosis, perforation, dissection, and distal embolism.

Late failures of PTA are due to restenosis at the PTA site or progression of disease. Percutaneous approaches to reducing the restenosis rate have not shown proven benefits. These approaches include debulking the lesion (laser-assisted PTA or various atherectomy devices) or physically stenting the lesion with meshlike prostheses.[35] Intravascular stents are approved for use in the iliac arteries, but there are numerous reports of their use in the aorta and visceral and brachiocephalic arteries. The indications for their use include restenosis at a site of angioplasty, elastic recoil of a lesion that just underwent angioplasty, and flow-limiting dissection at a site of angioplasty or other arterial injury[36,37] (Fig. 76-43). There is preliminary evidence that primary stenting of iliac lesions has a higher long-term patency rate than unassisted percutaneous angioplasty.

Thrombolytic Therapy

Embolic or thrombotic occlusion of vascular conduits can often be managed by thrombolytic therapy.[38] The success of such therapy (measured by clot lysis and minimal complications) depends on the composition of the occlusive material (thrombus versus atheroembolus), the duration of occlusion, the vascular structure involved, the thrombolytic agent, and the route and duration of infusion. Complications of thrombolytic therapy include hemorrhage (remote or at the puncture site), distal embolism, and reperfusion injury. Clot lysis depends on surface interaction between the thrombus and the lytic agent. Lysis may be enhanced (shortening infusion time and perhaps decreasing hemorrhagic complications) by increasing the plasma concentration of the lytic agent at the plasma–clot interface and maximizing the molecular interface at which it may act. Numerous strategies have been described to enhance clot lysis, including transcatheter delivery of the lytic agent at the leading (upstream) edge of the clot or within the clot, the use of coaxial catheters with simultaneous proximal and distal infusion of the lytic agent within the clot, and breaking up the clot with a guide wire or with high-pressure radial sprays of a lytic agent. Because of potentially catastrophic hemorrhagic complications, transcatheter lytic therapy requires close observation of the patient in the intensive care unit and scrupulous angiographic monitoring with respect to the remaining clot burden.

Diagnostic angiography should precede lytic therapy in order to define vascular anatomy, and it should follow lytic therapy to identify the cause of arterial occlusion or graft failure (Fig. 76-44). Judicious choice of the initial puncture site (based on the patient's symptoms and, if known, the arterial and bypass anatomy) may greatly simplify placement of the infusion catheter in the occluded conduit and the subsequent percutaneous management of the underlying cause of occlusion. Acute embolic occlusion of a vessel presents additional considerations. Emboli are often multiple, precluding efficient lysis even when they are accessible by catheter. Emboli may be composed of organized material less susceptible to lytic agents. The symptomatic embolus in the leg may mask a more serious embolus in the bowel or kidney, and a cardiac source of emboli may shower additional emboli during the lytic state.

Agents in common use include urokinase, streptokinase, and tissue plasminogen activator, which are reviewed in detail elsewhere.[39,40] Urokinase is the lytic agent of choice for peripheral arterial and graft occlusions. A widely accepted protocol is initial high-dose infusion of urokinase at 4000 IU/min for 2 to 4 hours, and then reduced infusion at 1000 to 2000 IU/min for 6 to 8 hours.[41,42] The concomitant use of heparin (5000-IU bolus and 500 IU/h) may be necessary when a long segment of catheter is exposed upstream from the urokinase infusion in a low flow conduit. Close clinical monitoring of the patient, laboratory determination of coagulation status, and frequent angiographic inspection of progress are important to avoid complications and maintain the necessary surface contact between the catheter tip and the remaining thrombus. The infusion is terminated when complete recanalization of the vessel is achieved, as long as no complication supervenes. If an underlying lesion is discovered, appropriate endovascular or open surgical treatment is undertaken.

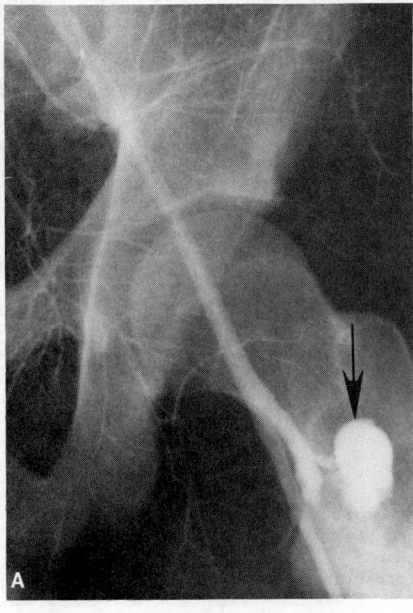 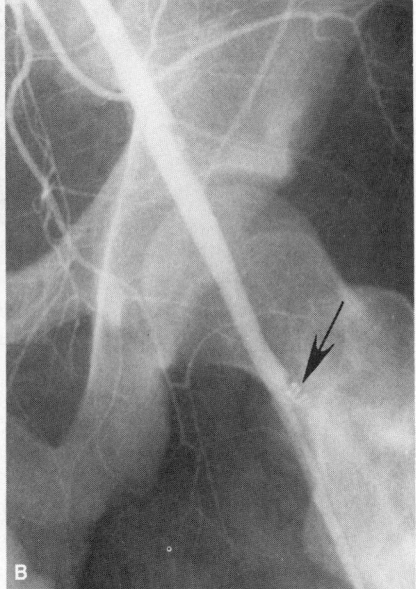

Figure 76-47. Posttraumatic hemorrhage. A 17-year-old male presented with an enlarging left groin hematoma after a gunshot wound. (*A*) Left pelvic arteriogram shows extravasation of contrast medium (*arrow*) from the deep femoral artery. The deep femoral artery was selectively catheterized from the right femoral artery approach and occluded with Gelfoam pledgets and two 3-mm Gianturco steel coils. (*B*) Pelvic arteriogram after embolization shows the coil in the proximal deep femoral artery with arrest of the bleeding. The superficial femoral artery remains patent.

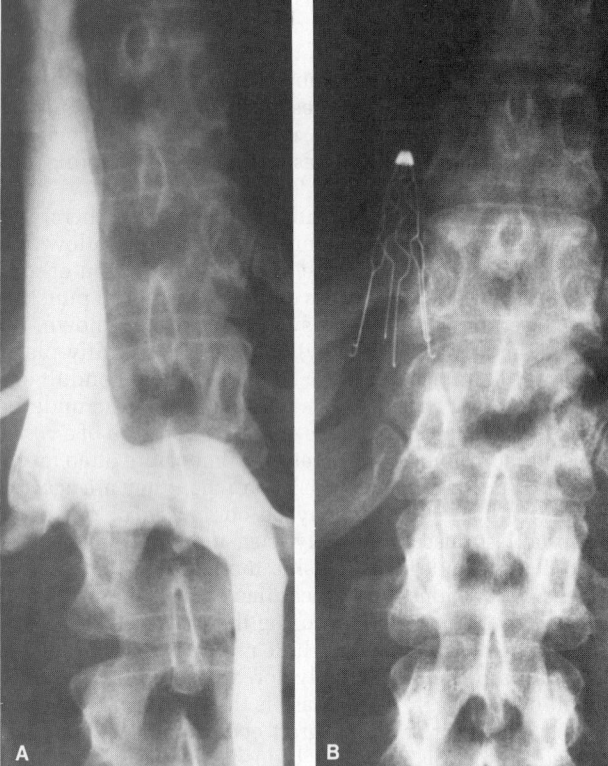

Figure 76-48. Suprarenal Greenfield filter placement through the left inferior vena cava. (*A*) Vena cavogram demonstrates a left-sided inferior vena cava joining the left renal vein and suprarenal cava. A 24F carrier was advanced into the suprarenal cava with use of the percutaneous left transfemoral approach. (*B*) Abdominal film after filter placement shows the filter in satisfactory position.

Embolotherapy

Transcatheter delivery of embolic agents has proved useful in managing life-threatening hemorrhage and in certain devascularization procedures. With the use of steerable guide wires and coaxial catheter systems, superselective catheterization of vessels as small as 1 mm in diameter is possible. Two clinical considerations guide the choice of embolic materials—the level of occlusion required, either proximal (corresponding to surgical ligation) or distal, and the duration of occlusion desired (either permanent or temporary). A variety of embolic agents is available for the combination best suited to the clinical problem and to the proximity of accessible vessels in the area of interest.[43,44] As with other interventional procedures, embolotherapy should be preceded by thorough diagnostic angiography to document the pertinent vascular anatomy and to predict the hemodynamic effect of embolization with respect to target organ infarction, recanalization of vessels, and recruitment of collaterals (Fig. 76-45). Indications for embolotherapy include treatment of gastrointestinal (Fig. 76-46) or traumatic (Fig. 76-47) hemorrhage,[45,46] management of vascular malformations and arteriovenous fistulas,[47–49] and tumor therapy (devascularization or vascular redistribution to optimize perfusion therapy).[50,51] The principal complications of embolotherapy (in addition to those of selective angiography) include abscess formation and infarction of normal tissue due to inadvertent reflux of embolic material. A postinfarction syndrome of fever, pain, and leukocytosis may follow extensive embolic procedures in solid organs.[50] Antibiotic coverage depends on the immune status of the patient, the level of occlusion, and the amount and type of tissue infarcted.

Caval Interruption

The indications for caval interruption procedures are discussed in Chapter 96. Placement of an inferior vena cava filter should be preceded by cavography to identify

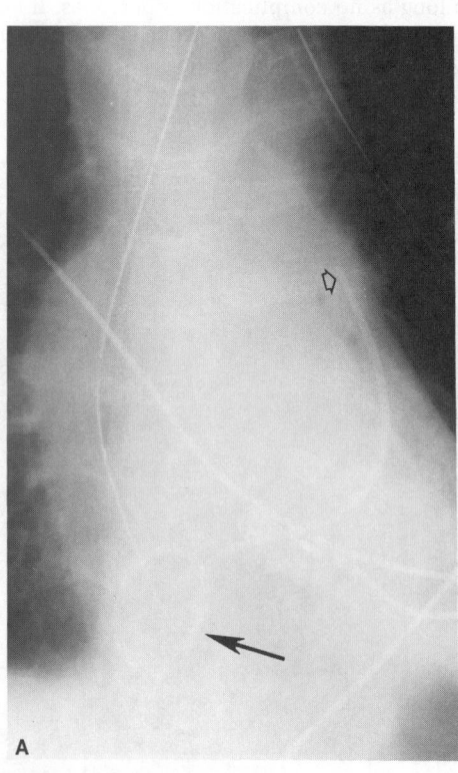

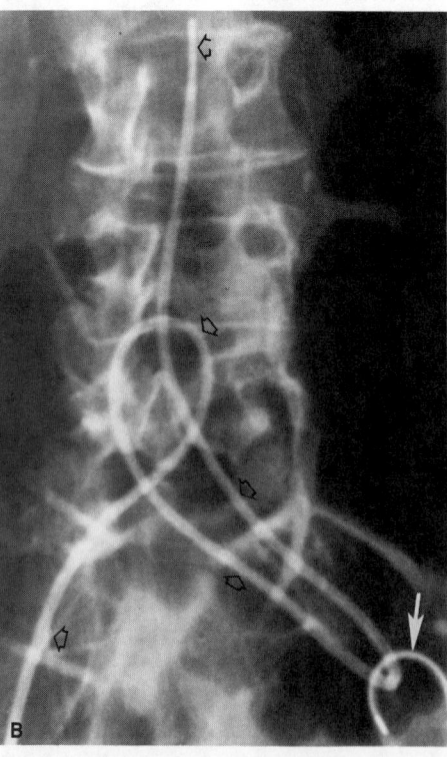

Figure 76-49. Knotted Swan-Ganz catheter. (*A*) Chest film shows an overhand loop (*arrow*) in the shaft of a right transfemoral Swan-Ganz catheter. The catheter tip is in the main pulmonary artery (*open arrow*); the knot is in the right atrium. (*B*) From the right groin, the catheter knot was retracted into the iliac vein confluence, where the knot (*open arrows*) was engaged and teased loose by a left transfemoral catheter (*arrow*).

inferior vena cava anomalies and anatomic variations in the renal veins (Fig. 76-48). Percutaneous placement of caval filters is best accomplished through the right femoral or internal jugular approach.

Transjugular Intrahepatic Portosystemic Shunt

In the transjugular intrahepatic portosystemic shunt (TIPS) procedure, an 8- to 12-mm conduit between intrahepatic portal and hepatic venous branches (usually the right hepatic and right portal veins) is created through a percutaneous transjugular approach and buttressed open with intravascular stents.[52,53] Indications for TIPS construction include variceal bleeding unresponsive to medical and endoscopic therapy (sclerotherapy or banding), recurrent variceal bleeding that has failed endoscopic therapy, and intractable ascites. Technical success rates are about 80% to 90%. Restenosis of the TIPS, usually at the hepatic venous end, occurs in about 60% of patients by 6 months. This usually responds to repeat angioplasty and stenting. Because the TIPS requires relatively vigilant follow-up and angiographic maintenance, its role in terms of surgical portosystemic shunting in the management of the stable patient with good liver function requires further study.

Miscellaneous Interventional Procedures

Percutaneous retrieval of catheter fragments in the arterial or venous system is usually straightforward (Fig. 76-49). The use of a Check-Flo sheath at the puncture site facilitates atraumatic removal of the snared fragment.

Indwelling central venous access devices (peripherally inserted central catheters, Hickman catheters, or subcutaneous ports) may be placed with the help of fluoroscopic guidance for localization of the venous entry (eg, brachial vein or the infrarenal inferior vena cava), for optimal catheter placement in the right atrium or superior vena cava—atrium junction, and for guidance across chronic thromboses or venous strictures.[54] Venous access procedures are preceded by diagnostic venography to ensure venous patency.

Percutaneous treatment of the ischemic complications of aortic dissection has been described. These procedures include fenestration of the aortic septum, balloon dilatation of a compressed true lumen, and internal stenting of the aortic true lumen or affected branch arteries.[55,56]

REFERENCES

1. Seldinger S. Catheter replacement of needle in percutaneous arteriography: new technique. Acta Radiol 1953;39:368.
2. Hessel S, Adams D, Abrams H. Complications of angiography. Radiology 1981;138:273.
3. Rubin G, Dake M, Semba C. Current status of three-dimensional spiral CT scanning for imaging the vasculature. Radiol Clin North Am 1995;33:51.
4. Edelman R. MR angiography: present and future. AJR 1993;161:1.
5. Prince M. Gadolinium-enhanced MR aortography. Radiology 1994;191:155.
6. Prince M, Narasimham D, Stanley J, et al. Gadolinium-enhanced magnetic resonance angiography of abdominal aortic aneurysms. J Vasc Surg 1995;21:656.
7. Dawson P. Chemotoxicity of contrast media and clinical adverse effects: a review. Invest Radiol 1985;20:S84.
8. Palmer F. The RACR survey of intravenous contrast media reactions: final report. Aust Radiol 1988;32:426.
9. Katayama H, Yamaguchi K, Kozuka T, Takashima T, Seez P, Matsuura K. Adverse reactions to ionic and nonionic contrast media. Radiology 1990;175:621.
10. Fischer H, Spataro R, Rosenberg P. Medical and economic considerations in using a new contrast medium. Arch Intern Med 1986;146:1717.
11. Hawkins I. Carbon dioxide digital subtraction arteriography. AJR Am J Roentgenol 1982;139:19.
12. Eisenberg R, Bank W, Hedgcock M. Renal failure after major angiography can be avoided with hydration. AJR 1981;136:859.
13. Lasser E, Berry C, Talner L, et al. Pretreatment with corticosteroids to alleviate reactions to intravenous contrast material. N Engl J Med 1987;317:845.
14. Block P, Ockene I, Goldberg R, et al. A prospective randomized trial of outpatient versus inpatient cardiac catheterization. N Engl J Med 1988;319:1251.
15. Rogers W, Kraft M. Outpatient angioplasty. Radiology 1990;174:753.
16. Coleman S, Anson B. Arterial patterns in the hand based upon a study of 650 specimens. Surg Gynecol Obstet 1961;113:409.
17. Lippert H, Pabst R. Arterial variations in man. New York, Springer-Verlag, 1985:121.
18. Stanley J, Whitehouse W. Occlusive and aneurysmal disease of the renal arterial circulation. Dis Mon 1984;30:7.
19. Neiman H, Bergan J, Yao J, Brandt T, Greenberg M, O'Mara C. Hemodynamic assessment of transluminal angioplasty for lower extremity ischemia. Radiology 1982;143:639.
20. Mannick J. Evaluation of chronic lower-extremity ischemia. N Engl J Med 1983;309:841.
21. Bookstein J, Ernst C. Vasodilatory and vasoconstrictive pharmacoangiographic manipulation of renal collateral flow. Radiology 1973;108:55.
22. Boley S, Brandt L, Veith F. Ischemic disorders of the intestines. Curr Probl Surg 1978;15:1:
23. Stanson A, Kazmier F, Hollier L, et al. Penetrating atherosclerotic ulcers of the thoracic aorta: natural history and clinicopathologic correlations. Ann Vasc Surg 1986;1:15.
24. Stanley J, Gewertz B, Bove E, Sottiurai V, Fry W. Arterial fibrodysplasia: histopathologic character and current etiologic concepts. Arch Surg 1975;110:561.
25. Bookstein J, Abrams H, Buenger R, et al. Radiologic aspects of renovascular hypertension. I. Aims and methods of the radiology study group. JAMA 1972;220:1218.
26. Mulliken J, Glowacki J. Hemangiomas and vascular malformations in infants and children: a classification based on endothelial characteristics. Plast Reconstr Surg 1982;69:412.
27. Burrows P, Mulliken J, Fellows K, Strand R. Childhood hemangiomas and vascular malformations: angiographic differentiation. AJR 1983;141:483.
28. Rabinov K, Paulin S. Roentgen diagnosis of venous thrombosis in the leg. Arch Surg 1972;104:134.
29. Ackroyd J, Thomas M, Browse N. Deep vein reflux: an assessment by descending phlebography. Br J Surg 1986;73:31.
30. Geiser J, Eversmann W. Closed system venography in the evaluation of upper extremity hemangiomas. J Hand Surg 1978A;3:173.
31. Braun S, Moore A, Mills S, et al. Closed-system venography in the evaluation of angiodysplastic lesions of the extremities. AJR Am J Roentgenol 1983;141:1307.
32. Mills S, Jackson D, Older R, et al. The incidence, etiologies and avoidance of complications of pulmonary angiography in a large series. Radiology 1980;136:295.
33. Becker G, Katzen B, Dake M. Noncoronary angioplasty. Radiology 1989;170:921.
34. Casarella W. Noncoronary angioplasty. Curr Probl Cardiol 1986;11:138.
35. Waller B. "Crackers, breakers, stretchers, drillers, scrapers, shavers, burners, welders and melters:" the future treatment of atherosclerotic coronary artery disease? A clinical-morphologic assessment. J Am Coll Cardiol 1989;13:969.
36. Becker G. Intravascular stent. General principles and status of lower-extremity arterial applications. Circulation 1991;83(Suppl I):122.
37. Martin E. Percutaneous therapy in the management of aortoiliac disease. Semin Vasc Surg 1994;7:17.
38. Motarjeme A. Thrombolytic therapy in arterial occlusion and graft thrombosis. Semin Vasc Surg 1989;2:155.

39. Marder V, Sherry S. Thrombolytic therapy: current status, part 1. N Engl J Med 1988;318:1512.
40. Marder V, Sherry S. Thrombolytic therapy: current status, part 2. N Engl J Med 1988;318:1585.
41. McNamara T, Fischer J. Thrombolysis of peripheral arterial and graft occlusions: improved results using high-dose urokinase. AJR Am J Roentgenol 1985;144:769.
42. McNamara T. Technique and results of "higher-dose" infusion. Cardiovasc Intervent Radiol 1988;11:S48.
43. Kunstlinger F, Brunelle F, Chaumont P, Doyon D. Vascular occlusive agents. AJR 1981;136:151.
44. Amplatz K, Coleman C. Therapeutic embolization of thorax and abdomen. Semin Intervent Radiol 1984;1:95.
45. Ben-Menachem Y. Logic and logistics of radiography, angiography, and angiographic intervention in massive blunt trauma. Radiol Clin North Am 1981;19:9.
46. Keller F. Nonoperative management of gastrointestinal hemorrhage. Semin Intervent Radiol 1988;5:1.
47. Gomes A, Mali W, Oppenheim W. Embolization therapy in the management of congenital arteriovenous malformations. Radiology 1982;144:41.
48. Yakes W, Haas D, Parker S, et al. Symptomatic vascular malformations: ethanol embolotherapy. Radiology 1989;170:1059.
49. White R, Lynch-Nyhan A, Terry P, et al. Pulmonary arteriovenous malformations: techniques and long-term outcome of embolotherapy. Radiology 1988;169:663.
50. Wallace S, Chuang V, Swanson D. Embolization of renal carcinoma: experience with 100 patients. Radiology 1981;138:563.
51. Chuang V, Wallace S. Hepatic arterial redistribution for intra-arterial infusion of hepatic neoplasms. Radiology 1980;135:295.
52. Kerlan R, LaBerge J, Gordon R, Ring E. Transjugular intrahepatic portosystemic shunts: current status. AJR 1995;164:1059.
53. Coldwell D, Ring E, Rees C, et al. Multicenter investigation of the role of transjugular intrahepatic portosystemic shunt in management of portal hypertension. Radiology 1995;196:335.
54. Andrews J, Walker-Andrews S, Ensminger W. Long-term central venous access with a peripherally placed subcutaneous infusion port: initial results. Radiology 1990;176:45.
55. Akaba N, Ujiie H, Umzawa K, et al. Management of acute aortic dissections with a cylinder-type balloon catheter to close the entry. J Vasc Surg 1986;3:890.
56. Williams D, Brothers T, Messina L. Relief of mesenteric ischemia in type III aortic dissection by percutaneous fenestration of the aortic septum. Radiology 1990;174:450.

SURGERY: SCIENTIFIC PRINCIPLES AND PRACTICE, Second Edition, edited by Lazar J. Greenfield, Michael W. Mulholland, Keith T. Oldham, Gerald B. Zelenock, and Keith D. Lillemoe. Lippincott–Raven Publishers, Philadelphia, © 1997.

CHAPTER 77

NONOPERATIVE TREATMENT OF ATHEROSCLEROSIS

JOSEPH H. RAPP, LINDA M. REILLY, AND WILLIAM C. KRUPSKI

The epidemic of atherosclerotic cardiovascular disease in North America and Europe is essentially a 20th-century phenomenon. In 1977, the reported incidence of cardiovascular disease among men aged 35 to 74 years in Canada, the United States, and England was more than 600 per 100,000 people, whereas in Japan, it was less than 100 per 100,000 people.[1] It is well recognized that certain risk factors are major contributors to the development of ath-

erosclerosis and that eliminating these risks can slow or even reverse progression of the disease. It is not always possible to translate epidemiologic trends or clinical trials of a complex multifactorial disease into decisions for an individual patient. However, general principles of conservative treatment of atherosclerosis are emerging. It has become clear that the natural history of this disease can be significantly altered by successfully altering a primary causative factor.

RISK FACTORS FOR ATHEROSCLEROSIS

Certain behaviors and metabolic traits have long been associated with an increased risk for cardiovascular disease, although the term *risk factor* was first introduced in reports from the Framingham Study in 1961.[2] Risk factors are categorized as behavioral or metabolic. The two primary behaviors that increase the risk for atherosclerosis are consuming a diet high in animal fat and smoking cigarettes. The data linking a sedentary life-style, aggressive, high-stress (type A) behavior, and alcohol use are much less clear. The metabolic traits that increase risk are primarily hyperlipidemia, hypertension, and diabetes. Homocysteinemia may also be an independent variable.

Neither the metabolic nor the behavioral factors appear to have a threshold effect. For example, both the Framingham and the larger Multiple Risk Factor Intervention Trial demonstrate a progressive increase in the incidence of coronary heart disease, with levels of plasma cholesterol and hypertension above the 20th percentile of the population.[3] The rate of rise becomes logarithmic at about the 85th percentile, representing a serum cholesterol of 253 mg/dL and a diastolic pressure of 94 mmHg. Similar observations have been made about cigarette smoking and cardiac disease.[4]

With the exception of cigarette smoking, which may contain components that directly alter the artery wall, the personal behaviors that increase cardiovascular risk probably do so by modifying metabolic parameters. Increased physical activity may decrease risk by improving resting blood pressure and lipid profiles, thus raising levels of high-density lipoprotein (HDL). A reduction in type A behavior also may reduce blood pressure levels. Finally, a diet high in cholesterol and saturated fats may increase plasma total, levels of low-density lipoprotein (LDL) cholesterol, and the production of β-VLDL (very low-density lipoprotein), an atherogenic remnant of triglyceride-rich lipoprotein metabolism.

Hyperlipidemia

Lipoproteins and Atherosclerosis

The thrust of research on atherosclerosis has begun to move from describing plasma lipid levels to examining the metabolism of the artery wall, resulting in a clearer picture of the role hyperlipidemia plays in the atherogenic process. When animals are made hyperlipidemic, the initial change is a migration of macrophages through the endothelium and into the media. Later, these cells engorge the lipids carried into the wall by lipoproteins and presumably elaborate chemoattractants, growth factors, and cytokines, which initiate the complex events that culminate in the formation of an atherosclerotic plaque.[3]

Although the process is not solely regulated by lipids, the movement of lipids, primarily cholesterol esters and free cholesterol, has a central role in this process. Much of the confusion regarding the role of lipids in atherosclerosis results from a lack of appreciation of what constitutes a physiologically normal cholesterol level. In countries where the total plasma cholesterol level averages 150 mg/dL—for example, Japan in 1960—atherosclerosis is not a public health problem.[5] In the Japanese population that has moved across the Pacific, however, both plasma cholesterol level and rate of cardiovascular disease have increased to meet that of US citizens of European descent, who have a mean cholesterol level of more than 210 mg/dL at age 50 years.[6]

Although a high level of LDL cholesterol is an important risk factor for atherosclerosis, epidemiologic studies have shown that levels of apolipoprotein B (Apo B), the primary protein constituent of LDL, VLDL, and chylomicrons, correlate more accurately with atherosclerotic risk. There may be several reasons for this. Smaller LDLs (ie, lipoproteins with less lipid and proportionately more Apo B) are associated with an increased risk. Lipoproteins other than LDL that contain Apo B, such as VLDL and b-VLDL, also are involved in the atherosclerotic process. In support of this theory, particles resembling VLDL and intermediate-density lipoprotein (IDL) have been identified within the atherosclerotic plaque.[7]

Another lipoprotein, Lp(a), an LDL-like particle that contains a nonfunctional protein analogue of plasminogen bound to the Apo B, has also been found in the arterial wall, suggesting a mechanistic basis for its known association with atherosclerosis. Whether the lipoproteins residing in the artery wall are actively involved in the atherosclerotic process may depend on their degree of oxidation. In vitro, this is clearly correlated with increased uptake by the macrophage scavenger receptor and the creation of foam cells,[4] although in vivo validation of lipoprotein oxidation as a unifying concept of atherogenesis is lacking.

HDLs appear to oppose the depositing of cholesterol by participating in a centripetal transport of cholesterol to the liver. Thus, low levels of HDL correlate with reduced centripetal transport of cholesterol and an increased risk of atherosclerosis. Subfractions of HDL, HDL-2 and HDL-3, can be separated by ultracentrifugation, and a reduction in the amount of cholesterol in the HDL-2 fraction correlates closely with higher atherosclerotic risk. As with Apo B, the best correlations with risk occur when the primary apolipoprotein associated with HDL, Apo A-I, is measured.

Lipoproteins

There are many lipid disorders, each characterized by an excess of specific lipoproteins. Treatment strategies vary depending on which lipoprotein fraction is found in excess.

Chylomicrons are the largest of the lipoproteins. Formed in the gut primarily from dietary fat, they range from 1000 to 5000 Å, depending on the amount of fat in the meal. Taken to the blood by way of the thoracic duct, chylomicrons release their triglyceride load by interacting with lipoprotein lipase, an enzyme located on the endothelium. After removal of the triglyceride, the cholesterol ester–enriched chylomicron remnants are formed. An accumulation of chylomicrons in plasma constitutes type I hyperlipidemia. This is a rare genetic disorder and does not appear to increase the risk of developing atherosclerosis.

VLDL is a triglyceride-rich lipoprotein secreted by the liver and possibly the intestine. It ranges in size from 350 to 1000 Å. Accumulation of VLDL characterizes type IV hyperlipidemia, which results from an overproduction of VLDL rather than a clearance defect. Type IV is a common condition often found in diabetic persons and may be the most common lipid abnormality found in peripheral vascular disease.

Endothelial-bound lipoprotein lipase is also involved in the clearance of VLDL triglyceride and the production of

the VLDL remnant. Remnants of both chylomicrons and large VLDL are cleared by the liver, whereas small VLDL remnants are further metabolized to the smaller, denser LDL. Accumulations of chylomicron and VLDL remnants characterize type III hyperlipidemia, an unusual condition that includes both premature peripheral vascular disease and coronary heart disease. A combination of metabolic influences and an abnormal Apo E reduces the lipoprotein's affinity for the Apo B–E receptor.

The cholesterol ester–rich LDLs are removed from the circulation primarily in the liver by means of the Apo B–E receptor. Receptor-mediated clearance reduces the de novo production of cholesterol by inhibiting the activity of hydroxymethylglutaryl coenzyme A (HMG CoA), which reduces the rate-limiting step in cholesterol synthesis. Elevations of LDL alone constitute type IIa (familial) hypercholesterolemia, whereas type IIb (familial combined) hyperlipidemia is characterized by elevations of both LDL and VLDL. Both IIa and IIb are typically associated with coronary artery disease, although these patients may also have peripheral vascular lesions. The incidence of heterozygous familial hypercholesterolemia in the population is about 1 in 500. These individuals have defective cellular Apo B receptors and therefore a reduced clearance of LDL. In this rare genetic abnormality, individuals have plasma cholesterol levels of 350 mg/dL or higher. Familial combined hyperlipidemia, or type IIb, is more frequent, occurring in as many as 1 in 50 people, and is probably caused by an overproduction of VLDL.

Lp(a) is an LDL-like particle with a unique apolipoprotein, Apo(a). Apo(a) has virtual sequence homology with plasminogen but lacks lytic activity. It can reduce the lysis stimulated by TPA and may be a link between lipids, thrombosis, and atherosclerosis. Lp(a) appears to be synthesized by the liver, and the particle probably is secreted intact with the Apo(a) attached to Apo B. The frequency of elevated Lp(a) levels in the population is not known, but higher levels are associated with both coronary and peripheral atherosclerosis. Little is known about Lp(a) metabolism.

Lipid-Lowering Therapy

For many individuals, aggressive dietary change alone is adequate. Substantial dietary change is difficult without high patient motivation and support, however, and many clinics provide both dietetic and behavioral counseling. Restrictions of saturated fat and cholesterol intake can lower cholesterol levels by 20% or more. Caloric restrictions can cause normalization of triglyceride levels.

Drug therapy for hypercholesterolemia includes the bile acid–binding resins cholestyramine and colestipol. These drugs interrupt the enterohepatic recycling of bile acids, increase the synthesis of bile acids from cholesterol in the liver, and increase the receptor clearance of LDL. These agents may also stimulate an increased production of VLDL, the precursor of LDL. Therefore, combination therapy with niacin, which reduces VLDL production, is particularly effective. The usual dose of bile salt–binding resin is 15 to 20 g/d. Larger doses of up to 30 g/d may be required in heterozygous familial hypercholesterolemia but are associated with more side effects, most commonly gastric distress and constipation.

Niacin can be used both as a single agent and in combination therapy. The decreased VLDL seen with niacin therapy is associated with a rise in HDL levels. Niacin also may affect thrombogenicity, with flushing as the most common side effect. Although serious hepatic toxicity is rare, elevated transaminases are common. Abdominal discomfort may require that niacin be taken with meals or with antacids. Patients with gout or diabetes mellitus may need to avoid this drug since it can raise uric acid and glucose levels. Treatment begins with low doses that are slowly increased to 3 to 6 g/d.

The fibric acid derivatives effectively reduce plasma VLDL levels, probably by increasing lipoprotein lipase activity. They are useful in treating hypertriglyceridemia and are usually the drugs of choice for type III hyperlipidemia. In some instances, LDL levels may rise and HDL minimally increases. Nausea and abdominal discomfort may occur, and these drugs potentiate sodium warfarin (Coumadin) activity. Clofibrate and gemfibrozil are the fibric acid derivatives available in the United States. Dosages are 1 g/d for clofibrate and 600 mg/d for gemfibrozil.

Lovastatin is the first of a new class of compounds that are structural analogues of HMG CoA reductase and inhibit the synthesis of cholesterol. It is clearly the most effective of the lipid-lowering agents and allows a single drug therapy for moderate hypercholesterolemia. In combination with bile salt—binding resins or niacin, complete normalization of lipid values in heterozygous familial hypercholesterolemia is possible. Initially thought to be safe, side effects of lovastatin are now recognized. Mild elevations in liver enzymes are common, and a serious hepatitis can occur in up to 2% of patients, making the drug contraindicated in anyone with hepatic dysfunction. Mild elevations of creatine kinase are also common, and about 1% of patients develop painful, tender muscles. The risk of developing this myopathic syndrome is increased by concomitant use of cyclosporin, fibric acid derivatives, erythromycin, or niacin. Although rare, these complications are not trivial and require that anyone on lovastatin receive close follow-up. The dosage is 20 to 80 mg/d in divided doses.

Several clinical trials have shown a relation between the reduction in lipoprotein risk profile and a reduction in cardiac events. The Coronary Primary Prevention Trial demonstrated a decrease in fatal and nonfatal myocardial infarctions with cholestyramine treatment.[8] A 20% reduction in LDL cholesterol yielded more than a 30% reduction in coronary events. In the Helsinki Heart Study, treatment with gemfibrozil reduced LDL cholesterol by 8% and triglycerides by more than 35%, while causing a nearly 15% increase in HDL cholesterol.[9] Statistically, nearly half of the protective effect of gemfibrozil treatment was due to the increase in HDL.

Several studies have shown a benefit of lipid lowering on the angiographic morphology of lesions in the coronary circulation. Lipid effects on the artery wall appear to be a key element in atherosclerosis, but lipids also affect platelet aggregation, fibrinogen levels, and vascular reactivity. All of these may be important in the clinical manifestations of atherosclerosis, making the potential benefits of an aggressive treatment of hyperlipidemia all the more attractive. In addition, hypercholesterolemia appears to be an important factor in restenosis after carotid endarterectomy.

Smoking

Despite the national attention given to the hazards of cigarette smoking by the American Lung Association, the American Heart Association, and other public and private groups, many Americans do not associate tobacco use with the complications of atherosclerosis. Cigarettes cause one in six deaths in the United States.[10] Most of the excess mortality related to tobacco use is due to cardiovascular disease. As a group, smokers have 70% more coronary artery disease than nonsmokers, and the risk of developing cardiovascular disease exhibits a dose-response relation. Risk increases with increased duration of smoking, increased quantity of cigarettes smoked, and the increased

depth of inhalation of smoke[11] (Fig. 77-1). Cardiovascular risks of smoking are multiplicative, not simply additive, to other coronary risk factors, such as hypertension, hypercholesterolemia, diabetes, and use of oral contraceptives. For example, a 40-year-old smoker with a serum cholesterol level greater than 260 mg/dL and a diastolic blood pressure greater than 95 mmHg has more than 2.5 times the risk for myocardial infarction compared with a similar smoker without those additional risk factors.[12]

Smoking is an especially important risk factor for peripheral vascular occlusive disease. Symptoms of intermittent claudication are 15 times more likely to develop in men smokers than nonsmokers, and 7 times more likely in women smokers than nonsmokers. In the Framingham cohort, smokers had a 0.65% prevalence of peripheral vascular disease compared with 0.22% for nonsmokers.[13] Moreover, patients with established peripheral vascular disease who smoke cigarettes are more likely to suffer disease progression and graft failure than those who do not. There is an 11-fold increase in amputation rate among smokers in patients observed for claudication.

In addition to causing occlusive peripheral vascular disease, tobacco smoking induces abdominal aortic aneurysm formation. Smokers have a two- to three-fold increase in incidence of death from aneurysms compared with nonsmokers.[11] An autopsy study of aortas from elderly men revealed an eight-fold increase in the incidence of aortic aneurysms in those who had smoked cigarettes compared with those who did not.[14]

Smokers, notably women smokers, have a higher risk of stroke than nonsmokers. In the Framingham cohort, heavy smokers (ie, more than 40 cigarettes per day) were almost twice as likely to suffer strokes than nonsmokers, independent of presence of hypertension.[15] In a study of almost 120,000 women nurses, those who smoked 25 or more cigarettes per day had a relative risk for stroke of 3.7 compared with those who did not.[16] Use of tobacco and oral contraceptives is a particularly dangerous combination. The risk of stroke for a woman smoker who uses oral contraceptives has been found to be 21.9 times the risk of a nonsmoking woman.[16]

The mechanisms by which smoking exerts its deleterious effect on blood vessels are complex. Because tobacco smoke contains more than 2000 recognized substances, identification of a single toxic agent is not likely. Morbidity and mortality from arterial disease is a consequence of a complex interplay between the fixed lesions of atherosclerosis and dynamic factors such as vasomotor tone and platelet aggregation. Smoking is thought to increase the risk of atherosclerosis by its direct effects on the vascular wall and on circulating lipoproteins.[17] Vasoconstriction, increased heart rate, increased blood pressure, decreased regional myocardial blood flow, and a negative inotropic effect result from cigarette smoking and influence both acute and chronic symptoms of vascular disease.[18] Tobacco smoke also affects platelets, red blood cells, leukocytes, and fibrinogen. The net result is a tendency toward thrombosis through increases in these elements (and thereby in blood viscosity) and through increased platelet aggregation accompanied by decreased platelet sensitivity to prostacyclin.[19]

Twenty-five years have elapsed since the first Surgeon General's Advisory Committee Report on Smoking and Health. The prevalence of smoking among adults decreased from 40% in 1965 to less than 29% in 1987; nearly half of all living adults who ever smoked have quit. It has been estimated that over 90% of cigarette smokers would like to stop smoking and that most cigarette smokers have tried unsuccessfully to quit several times. Failure to quit smoking is attributable in large part to the addictive prop-

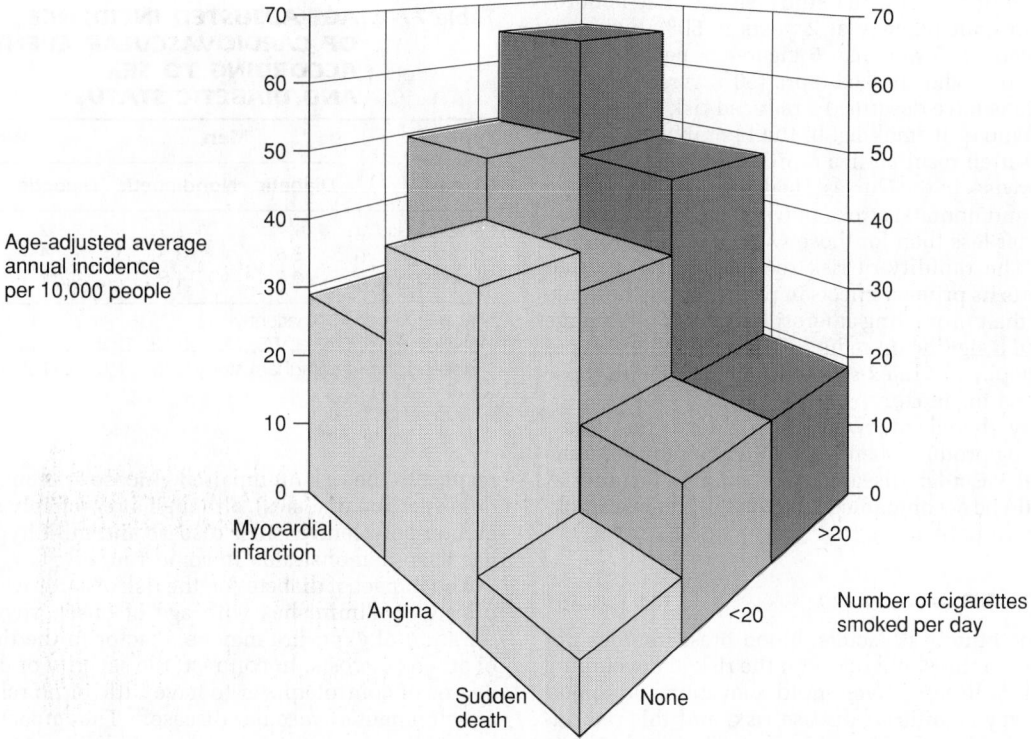

Figure 77-1. Cardiovascular manifestations of cigarette smoking. (After Kuller L, Meilahn E, Ockene J. Smoking and coronary disease. In: Connor WE, Bristow JD, eds. Coronary disease: prevention, complications, and treatment. Philadelphia, JB Lippincott, 1985:67)

erties of nicotine. Thus, interventions to decrease the physiologic nicotine withdrawal syndrome are important adjuncts to traditional behavioral approaches for smoking cessation.

Many comprehensive reviews of smoking cessation strategies have been published. It is impossible to recommend a specific approach because of design limitations in reported studies with few randomized controlled trials of any method. There are six major smoking cessation methods—behavior modification, education and commercial programs, hypnosis, acupuncture, multiple risk factor reduction programs, and drug therapy. Unfortunately, although initial quit-rates average almost 45%, relapse rates are 40% to 50%. Regardless of the cessation method chosen, physicians are in a unique position to identify their patients who smoke and to motivate them to quit. Brief counseling achieves smoking cessation only in a small percentage of well patients but is more effective in patients with smoking-related illnesses. Thus, using the patient's clinical condition (eg, newly diagnosed claudication) as a springboard for counseling increases effectiveness.

Pharmacologic treatment of tobacco dependence is based on the symptoms observed after smoking cessation, including cravings for cigarettes, irritability, anxiety, difficulty concentrating, coughing, and constipation. By blocking withdrawal symptoms, nicotine gum, introduced in the United States in 1964, can assist smokers in long-term abstinence. When combined with behavioral counseling in smoking cessation clinics, nicotine gum doubles quit-rates, with long-term abstinence ranging from 12% to 70%.[20] In the medical practice setting, nicotine gum has been less effective in actuating smoking cessation. Moreover, some patients have difficulty weaning from nicotine gum after the recommended 2- to 6-month therapy period.

Clonidine, an α-noradrenergic agonist first used as an antihypertensive, is another drug that may help smokers quit. A transdermal patch form of the medication decreases its side effects. Clonidine reduces the intensity of tobacco craving and the severity of tobacco-withdrawal symptoms, presumably by its effect on the adrenergic receptors of the central nervous system. In one controlled trial, clonidine treatment for 6 weeks was more effective than placebo as an aid to smoking cessation.[21]

Cessation of smoking may significantly influence the effects of medical and surgical therapy on peripheral vascular disease. Several large observational epidemiologic studies, including the Framingham Study, the Kaiser-Permanente Health Plan, and the British Physicians' Study have demonstrated a substantial reduction in risk of heart attack within 1 or 2 years after smoking cessation. The Surgeon General's report in 1983 concluded that in 1 year, the risk for a first myocardial infarction decreases by 50% if a smoker quits; after 10 years of not smoking the risk for myocardial infarction of an ex-smoker approaches that of a nonsmoker.[11] One large case-control study of women aged 25 to 64 years confirmed that in women as in men, the risk of myocardial infarction attributable to cigarette smoking is largely reversible within a few years.[22] Unfortunately, American women have been less successful than men in quitting smoking. The proportion of men smokers has decreased by almost half in the past two decades (from 51% to 29%), whereas the proportion of women smokers has decreased by less than 30% (from 33% to 24%).

The beneficial effects of smoking cessation on peripheral vascular occlusive disease are well known. Several studies have shown improvement in claudication symptoms and avoidance of rest pain in smokers who quit. Smoking cessation also has a favorable effect after arterial reconstruction is performed. Aortofemoral bypass grafts are three times more likely to occlude if patients continue to smoke than if they quit.[23] The same study shows that femoro-popliteal vein graft patency at 2 years is 50% higher in those who smoked fewer than 5 cigarettes per day compared with those who smoked more (90% versus 60%).

Investigations have described a reduced risk of stroke in individuals who quit smoking. In the Framingham Study, smoking cessation resulted in a rapid reduction in risk for stroke.[15] Likewise, in the Nurses' Health Study, the relative risk for fatal and nonfatal stroke in women who quit smoking was 1.6, far less than for those women who continued to smoke.[16] The rapidity of risk reduction suggests that smoking exerts its primary effects in precipitating the acute event rather than promoting atherosclerosis. Another large study showed a significant reduction in mean thickness of carotid artery plaques in ex-smokers compared with those who continued to smoke.[24]

In summary, there is overwhelming evidence that cessation of smoking produces beneficial effects on the outcome of peripheral vascular disease. All therapies for arterial disease should be accompanied by efforts to achieve smoking cessation in patients.

Hypertension

As with the other risk factors, blood pressure does not appear to exert a threshold effect on the risk of developing cardiovascular disease. Even mild elevations in blood pressure convey significant disease risk, and this risk increases with the degree of hypertension. This morbidity is due to the strong relation of hypertension to stroke, but hypertension also promotes the development of both peripheral and coronary atherosclerosis. Although blood pressure reduction is of clear benefit in reducing the incidence of stroke, renal failure, and congestive heart failure, the incidence of myocardial infarction is not affected if other risk factors, particularly hyperlipidemia, remain untreated. Unfortunately, both β-adrenergic receptor–blocking agents and thiazide diuretics, the most commonly used antihypertensive agents, can have negative effects on a patient's lipid profiles. This, coupled with the fact that aggressive blood pressure reduction in patients with ischemic heart disease may actually increase mortality and morbidity, explains why earlier multiple risk factor reduction trials failed to show a decrease in cardiovascular events with blood pressure reduction. Blood pressure reduction has been shown to be a significant factor both in decreasing cardiovascular events in long-term follow-up[25] and in promoting lesion regression by angiography.

Diabetes Mellitus

Epidemiologic and morphologic studies have confirmed that atherosclerotic occlusive disease is more prevalent in patients with insulin-dependent or non–insulin-dependent diabetes than in the general population[26] (Table 77-1). In fact, atherosclerosis is the most common complication of diabetes, developing in 84% of patients surviving more than 20 years after diagnosis.[27] Furthermore, atherosclerosis is the cause of death in 75% of diabetic persons, in striking contrast to about one third of all deaths in the general population.[28] After myocardial infarction, diabetic persons have a higher rate of in-hospital mortality than nondiabetic persons (31% versus 19%) as well as a higher 5-year mortality rate (62% to 75% versus 25% to 50%). Additionally, the long-term survival rate among diabetic persons with claudication is less than among nondiabetic persons (50% versus 75%). Finally, late survival of diabetic persons after virtually any type of revascularization procedure is worse than for nondiabetic persons[29-31] (Table 77-2). The picture is less clear with

Table 77-1. AGE-ADJUSTED INCIDENCE OF CARDIOVASCULAR EVENTS ACCORDING TO SEX AND DIABETIC STATUS*

Type of Arterial Disease	Men		Women	
	Diabetic	Nondiabetic	Diabetic	Nondiabetic
Cerebrovascular	4.7	1.9	6.2	1.7
Coronary	12.6	3.3	8.4	1.3
Claudication	24.8	14.9	17.8	6.9

* Incidence per 100 patient-years
(Adapted from Kannel WB, McGee DL. Diabetes and cardiovascular disease: the Framingham study. JAMA 1979;241:2035)

respect to the risk of impaired glucose tolerance (chemical or borderline diabetes), although a reasonably strong association between vascular disease and mild hyperglycemia has been demonstrated in some studies.

The impact of diabetes on the risk of cardiovascular complications diminishes with age of onset, suggesting that duration of exposure may be a factor in the development of atherosclerosis. In contrast, the severity of diabetes and degree of control appear to have little or no relation to the development of vascular disease.[27] The impact of diabetes on cardiovascular risk is substantially greater for women than for men[26,28] (see Table 77-1). For men, diabetes has the smallest impact of all the major risk factors; for women, the impact exceeds that of cigarette smoking.[32] As a consequence, among diabetic persons the usual protective effect of gender is lost.

Although diabetes increases the risk of atherosclerosis at almost any anatomic site, the most dramatic effect is seen in the arteries of the lower extremities.[26,32] Although only 1% to 2% of the population is diabetic, diabetes is present in 65% to 75% of patients undergoing operations for infrageniculate occlusive disease. Multiple tibioperoneal vessel involvement by occlusive lesions is present in 69% of diabetic persons but in only 35% of nondiabetic persons. Arteriographic studies before revascularization demonstrate a complete major pedal arch in only 25% of diabetic persons, and diabetic persons are three times more likely to have involvement of metatarsal arteries.[33] Furthermore, profunda femoris artery involvement by atherosclerosis is three times as common among diabetic persons as nondiabetic persons,[27] whereas aortic involvement is only half as common.[34]

In addition to influencing the pattern of atherosclerotic disease, diabetes also influences the severity of the disease. Diabetic persons develop occlusive arterial lesions about 10 years earlier than nondiabetic persons. Inoperable coronary artery disease is more frequent among diabetic persons (12% versus 4.5%). The prevalence of lower extremity ulceration or gangrene at presentation is almost twice as great among diabetic persons as among nondiabetic persons. Diabetic persons with claudication are more likely to require amputation ultimately[35,36] (see Table 77-2). Finally, after distal arterial reconstruction, diabetic persons are less likely to experience long-term graft patency or limb salvage.

Results of Treatment

Control of hyperglycemia corrects many of the metabolic abnormalities that occur in diabetes. Improved glycemic control of type I diabetes results in a reduction of abnormally elevated plasma triglycerides and cholesterol and a restoration of normal LDL internalization and degradation

Table 77-2. SURVIVAL AND AMPUTATION RATES ACCORDING TO TREATMENT AND DIABETIC STATUS

Patient Category	Follow-Up (y)	Survival Rate (%)		Amputation Rate (%)	
		Diabetic	Nondiabetic	Diabetic	Nondiabetic
Claudication	9	54.4	75.7	27.1	3.8
	6	50.0	74.0	12.8	0.5
	6	—	—	46.0	1.0
Revascularization					
Aortic	9	36.0	73.0	—	—
Femoropopliteal	10	8.0	35.0	—	—
Femorotibial	6	66.0	79.0	—	—

by fibroblasts.[37] Additionally, some investigators have shown that HDL cholesterol rises with improved control in type II diabetes.[38] Abnormally elevated plasma fibrinogen levels and fibrinogen turnover rates have been found to decrease toward normal with treatment. Abnormalities of platelet function in diabetic persons may sometimes be corrected by improved diabetic control. Morphologic changes in the endothelium of diabetic animal models, decreased endothelial prostacyclin production, and increased histamine production can all be prevented by insulin administration. Finally, the diminished activity of acid cholesterol ester hydrolase seen in the aorta of diabetic rats can be restored to normal by treatment with insulin.

Despite these observations, there is little evidence that oral hypoglycemic agents or insulin treatment reduces the incidence of cardiovascular sequelae in diabetic persons.[27,28,32] Tight glycemic control is feasible for many diabetic persons because of the availability of home blood-glucose monitoring, the increased use of infusion pumps, and the use of multiple-dose insulin regimens, but it remains to be seen whether it diminishes the risk of atherosclerosis. Since macrovascular disease occurs in diabetic persons with minimal degrees of hyperglycemia, more appears to be gained by multifactorial risk factor intervention than by attention to early detection and control of hyperglycemia alone.[39]

This treatment approach is supported by International Atherosclerosis Project's demonstration that the effect of diabetes is most marked in societies and groups in which the prevalence of atherosclerosis is high even in the absence of diabetes.[32] In general, these are societies with high prevalences of other atherogenic factors. Thus, the impact of diabetes on cardiovascular risk is not uniform in all populations; rather, it seems to parallel the population in which the diabetic person finds himself, augmenting or facilitating the other risk factors.[40] In fact, diabetic persons tend to have higher levels of other cardiovascular risk factors than do nondiabetic persons.[32] Additionally, within populations of diabetic persons, those at greatest risk of atherosclerosis (type II diabetic persons and type I diabetic persons with renal impairment) also demonstrate a greater prevalence of other atherogenic factors than those diabetic persons who are at lesser risk of vascular disease. Although the cardiovascular risk of diabetes cannot be completely ascribed to its facilitating effect on other risk factors, diabetic persons with optimal levels of other risk factors appear to have little excess risk of atherosclerosis.[32] Clearly, further definition of the mechanisms responsible for atherosclerosis in diabetes is required. Future studies need to standardize the inclusion criteria for patients (definition of diabetes), distinguish between subpopulations of diabetic persons, control for secondary atherogenic factors, and investigate cerebral and peripheral vascular disease to a greater extent.

Homocysteine

Although the causal relation between hyperlipidemia and atherosclerosis is well established, only about half of symptomatic patients younger than 60 years, and even fewer older than 60, have hyperlipidemia. It has been argued that an atherogenic diet is a major contributor in these patients with normal fasting lipid levels. Other factors such as hypertension, smoking, and diabetes may promote atherosclerosis without hyperlipidemia. Elevated levels of homocysteine, a thiol-containing amino acid formed from the metabolism of methionine, also may play a role in atherosclerosis. Homocysteinuria is an inborn error in metabolism in which homocysteine and related compounds accumulate and are excreted in the urine. These individuals have severe and usually fatal atherosclerosis in childhood. A simplified technique for screening homocysteine is available and has shown that elevated homocysteine levels are associated with an increased incidence of coronary artery disease. Elevated homocysteine levels were more common in symptomatic patients with peripheral vascular disease than asymptomatic controls.[41]

Moderate increases in plasma homocysteine levels can be treated simply. In general, simple folate normalizes levels regardless of whether the patient is folate deficient. More research is needed to clarify the role of homocysteine, but it may be an important contributor to atherosclerotic risk in certain patients.

NONOPERATIVE TREATMENT FOR CLAUDICATION
Exercise Training

The effectiveness of exercise training in the treatment of intermittent claudication has been acknowledged for years, although the mechanism of symptomatic improvement is not known. The earliest proposed explanation was simply increased calf blood flow, secondary to increased collateral development. Subsequently, numerous studies have failed to document any increased calf blood flow after exercise training. The largest of these studies (148 patients) measured significantly improved calf blood flow after training in patients with inflow disease (aortoiliac lesions), but not in patients with outflow disease (femoropopliteal lesions) or combined level disease.[42] Most studies suggest that there is improved metabolic efficiency of the calf muscles after exercise training. Trained muscle extracts more oxygen as reflected by decreased popliteal and femoral venous oxygen saturation. Additionally, other investigators have shown an increase in aerobic metabolism as manifested by decreased venous lactate levels, increased incorporation of glucose into glycogen and lipids with decreased incorporation into lactate, and increased muscle succinic oxidase activity. Finally, a study by Ernst and Matrai[43] documented that exercise training in claudicators is associated with a significant reduction in blood viscosity and red cell aggregation. This is an intriguing effect since it is the proposed mechanism for the improvement seen in patients treated with pentoxifylline (discussed later).

Among the many studies investigating exercise training and claudication in the past 25 years, only five are controlled clinical trials (Table 77-3). These studies generally focus on middle-aged men with stable claudication of at least 2 years' duration that limited the patient to less than a 500-meter walking distance. The exercise regimen was similar in these five studies and consisted of supervised, regularly scheduled dynamic leg exercises. Only two studies randomized patients, and blinding was not feasible. All of these studies reported a significant improvement in both pain-free and maximal walking distances in the groups subjected to exercise training.[44-48] Data from both controlled and uncontrolled studies suggest that age, gender, presence of diabetes, and level of obstructive lesion do not prevent improvement in walking distance. Patients with angina or chronic obstructive pulmonary disease are likely to show a lesser degree of improvement. There are no absolute contraindications to the use of exercise training in treating claudication, except for the presence of advanced limb ischemia (rest pain or gangrene) and significant comorbid conditions. It does require a high degree of patient commitment over a prolonged period. Exercise training is time-intensive and is particularly difficult for younger patients with an active life-style. Finally, a treatment that only improves the symptoms of claudication rather than eradicating them is rarely viewed as successful by the patient.

Pharmacologic Treatment of Claudication

Pentoxifylline

Pentoxifylline is the only hemorrheologic agent approved for treating intermittent claudication in the United States. It is a methylxanthine derivative and has been reported to increase the flow of erythrocytes through capillaries by increasing red blood cell ATP content,[49] thus improving erythrocyte deformability.[50] Further, it reduces platelet aggregation and hyperactivity,[51] probably indirectly by stimulating prostacyclin formation in the vessel wall.[52] Plasma hypercoagulability is reduced by restoring levels of antithrombin III and plasmin and antiplasmin activities to near-normal,[53] as well as by reducing fibrinogen levels.[51,53,54] It is presumably because of these changes that pentoxifylline reduces blood viscosity.[52,55] Perhaps as

a result of improved viscosity, limb blood flow increases[56] and direct micropipette measurements show increased tissue PO_2 in ischemic muscle after treatment with pentoxifylline.[49] The clinical significance of such changes is not completely understood.

Of the many clinical trials of pentoxifylline, 12 were prospective, randomized, double-blind, and controlled studies.[56,57-66] In almost all published series, improvement in pain-free and maximal walking distances was observed in pentoxifylline-treated patients[48,55] (Table 77-4). In a number of studies, this improvement was not significantly different from that observed in the control (usually placebo) group. Furthermore, some trials only demonstrated increased walking distances in certain subpopulations of the study groups.[60,66] For instance, a significant difference between groups for percentage change from baseline at the end of the treatment period was not shown, but a significant difference was achieved when analyzing the mean percentage changes from baseline at each 2-week interval during the study.[58] Analysis of the improved walking distances achieved by some investigators shows that the magnitude of the effect is usually small, leading several investigators to emphasize that statistical significance does not establish clinical significance.[48,55] The available data do not allow a definitive conclusion about the significance of any clinical effect of pentoxifylline in the average patient with claudication. This agent may be appropriate for patients with severely impaired walking who are not candidates for revascularization or exercise treatment because of anatomic constraints or serious comorbid conditions.

Levocarnitine

Levocarnitine (L-carnitine) is a metabolic agent that is thought to enhance pyruvate oxidation, and hence energy production, by stimulating the activity of pyruvate dehydrogenase. As a consequence, production of lactate decreases and generation of ATP increases. This ability of levocarnitine to improve the efficiency of metabolism in terms of energy production might allow for improved muscle function in ischemic limbs. A double-blind, crossover study of 18 patients documented a significant increase in walking distance in treated patients compared with placebo (306±122 m versus 174±63 m).[67] A significant reduction in popliteal venous lactate concentration after exercise in levocarnitine-treated patients was also seen (54%±32% increase in treated patients versus 107%±16% increase in the control group). Subsequently, a multicenter, randomized, double-blind, placebo-controlled study of levocarnitine in about 50 patients with intermittent claudication failed to confirm these results (unpublished data). The clinical usefulness of levocarnitine in intermittent claudication has yet to be proved.

Table 77-3. RESULTS OF PROSPECTIVE, CONTROLLED CLINICAL TRIALS OF THE EFFECTIVENESS OF EXERCISE TRAINING

Study	Patients	Treatment Duration (mo)	Improvement	Pain-Free Walking Distance (% Improvement)		Maximal Walking Distance (% Improvement)	
				Treated	Control	Treated	Control
Dahllof et al[43]	18	6	Yes	190	—	117	—
Larsen and Lassen[44]	14	6	Yes	155	−14	178	−6
Ericsson et al[45]	13	11	Yes	104	−22	95	17
Ernst and Matrai[46]	42	2	Yes	103	19	121	16
Mannarino et al[47]	16	6	Yes	88	18	67	14

(Adapted from Radack K, Wyderski RJ. Conservative management of intermittent claudication. Ann Intern Med 1990;113:135)

Table 77-4. RESULTS OF PROSPECTIVE, RANDOMIZED, DOUBLE-BLIND CONTROLLED CLINICAL TRIALS OF THE EFFECTIVENESS OF PENTOXIFYLLINE

Study	Patients		Treatment Duration (wk)	Improvement	Pain-Free Walking Distance (% Improvement)		Maximal Walking Distance (% Improvement)	
	Initially	At Completion			Treated	Control	Treated	Control
Accetto[56]	60	47	8	Yes	—	—	46	3
Bollinger and Frei[57]	26	19	8	Yes	—	—	208	53
Detorri et al[58]	74	59	52	NI	189	142	—	—
Di Perri and Guerrini[59]	24	24	8	Yes	—	—	61	3
Gallus et al[60]	50	38	8	No	76	68	33	14
Perhoniemi et al[61]	35	31	12	No	19	19	17	43
Porter et al[62]	128	82	24	NI	59	36	38	25
Reilly et al[63]	30	25	12	No	—	—	27	89
Roekaerts and Deleers[64]*	20	20	24	Yes	124	28	101	9
Roekaerts and Deleers[64]*	16	16	24	Yes	137	−25	121	−15
Strano et al[65]	18	18	12	Yes	45	4	—	—
Tonak et al[66]	60	55	4	NI	126	38	—	—

NI, no significant improvement was noted unless analysis was restricted to the proportion of patients whose walking distance improved by at least 25%[58] or 50%[66] over baseline, or unless analysis of multiple points during treatment course was used.[62]
* Two groups treated in crossover study.
(Adapted from Radack K, Wyderski RJ. Conservative management of intermittent claudication. Ann Intern Med 1990;113:135)

Aspirin

Because platelets are thought to contribute to a variety of abnormal processes, ranging from acute coronary artery occlusion to failure of vascular reconstructive operations, the use of platelet inhibitors to prevent the complications of vascular disease has gained wide acceptance. Aspirin, the most frequently used antiplatelet agent, inhibits platelet aggregation by blocking cyclooxygenase.[68] Generation of the potent platelet-aggregating agent thromboxane A_2 from arachidonic acid is prevented by acetylation of a serine residue in the active site of the enzyme. Aspirin also prevents the vasoconstriction caused by thromboxane A_2. Platelets have no nuclei and are incapable of synthesizing new cyclooxygenase, so aspirin affects platelets throughout their life-spans. In contrast, endothelial cell cyclooxygenase, which is also inhibited by aspirin, can be regenerated, restoring the cell's ability to produce prostacyclin (PGI_2). PGI_2 and thromboxane A_2 exert opposite effects on platelets, and therapeutic strategies have been directed toward using these different actions to achieve a net balance that favors production of PGI_2 and inhibition of thromboxane A_2 synthesis. Although there is a general consensus that low doses of aspirin (80 to 325 mg/d) achieve this favorable balance, more than 30 randomized trials of antiplatelet treatment for patients with transient ischemic attacks, strokes, unstable angina, or myocardial infarctions have failed to document increased efficacy of one regimen over another.[69]

Aspirin and other antiplatelet agents that inhibit cyclooxygenase (eg, indomethacin, phenylbutazone, ibuprofen, fenoprofen, naproxen, and sulfinpyrazone) do not interfere with ADP-induced aggregation, adherence of platelets to collagen, release of granule contents from platelets adherent to collagen, or thrombin-induced aggregation and release.[70] Thus, thrombus formation in which any or all of these mechanisms are dominant is unaffected by these drugs. Moreover, because release of α-storage granules is unaffected by aspirin, mitogenic factors present therein are released from adherent platelets. It is not surprising that aspirin does not predictably prevent smooth muscle cell proliferation in response to vessel damage.

Potential indications for aspirin treatment can be grouped into three broad categories: (1) prevention of complications of atherosclerosis; (2) therapy for established disease; and (3) improvement in results of invasive treatments for atherosclerosis. Two large prospective randomized studies have addressed the first of these categories. In a US study, 22,000 male physicians of 40 to 84 years were randomly assigned to receive buffered aspirin, 325 mg, or placebo and were observed for an average of 4.8 years.[71] Although aspirin had no effect on the total number of vascular deaths or deaths from all causes, when the numbers of important vascular events were combined (nonfatal myocardial infarctions plus nonfatal strokes plus deaths from all causes), those receiving aspirin had a significant 23% reduction in risk. In contrast, aspirin treatment resulted in no significant reduction in disabling stroke or vascular death in a randomized study of 5139 healthy British male physicians.[72]

For treating established atherosclerosis, evidence of a beneficial effect for aspirin treatment is more convincing. The effect of 990 mg/d of aspirin on the progression of peripheral arterial occlusive disease was evaluated by serial arteriography.[73] Although aspirin alone had no effect, aspirin plus dipyridamole resulted in significantly decreased progression of disease. The clinical relevance of these findings is unclear because no true outcome data (eg, progression of symptoms or need for operation) were reported. A meta-analysis of 31 randomized trials of antiplatelet treatment for patients with a history of transient ischemic attack (TIA), occlusive stroke, unstable angina, or myocardial infarction involved more than 29,000 patients with established vascular disease and showed that antiplatelet treatment reduced vascular mortality rate (death due to myocardial infarction and stroke) by 15% and nonfatal stroke and myocardial infarction rates by 30%.[69] There have been four major prospective randomized and blinded clinical trials of aspirin in the treatment of patients with transient ischemic attacks. In an American study, aspirin reduced the incidence of TIAs but not strokes or deaths.[74] In a Canadian study, aspirin reduced TIAs and the combination of strokes and deaths.[75] In a French study, aspirin decreased the incidence of completed strokes.[76] In a Danish study, aspirin had no significant effect on the incidence of TIAs, strokes, or deaths.[77]

Aspirin may be beneficial after operative or endovascular treatment of atherosclerosis. Many clinical trials of aspirin with or without dipyridamole in patients undergoing aortocoronary or femoropopliteal bypass grafting or percutaneous transluminal angioplasty have been published. Although results vary, the following generalizations can be drawn from the data:

1. There is no clear advantage of aspirin plus dipyridamole over aspirin alone.
2. The optimal dosage of aspirin has not been determined.
3. Antiplatelet therapy is most effective when drugs are administered either preoperatively or immediately after surgery.
4. Aspirin is more effective in preventing early graft failure (1 month postoperatively) than late failure (1 year postoperatively).
5. Aspirin is of particular benefit when grafts are placed to arteries already well supplied by competing collaterals.
6. Antiplatelet therapy is not as effective for femorodistal bypass grafts as for aortocoronary grafts, but aspirin therapy started before operation may improve patency of lower extremity bypasses, particularly when a vascular prosthesis is implanted.
7. Aspirin should probably be used both preoperatively and postoperatively in patients undergoing carotid endarterectomy.
8. Pretreatment with antiplatelet agents before transluminal angioplasty reduces thrombotic complications.

In addition to aspirin and the other cyclooxygenase inhibitors already mentioned, some alternative antiplatelet agents are available. Dipyridamole indirectly increases platelet cyclic adenosine monophosphate (cAMP) levels by blocking the enzyme phosphodiesterase, which converts cAMP to AMP. Resultant increased levels of cAMP inhibit platelet aggregation caused by adenosine diphosphate (ADP). Calcium channel blockers may interfere with the effect of calcium flux on the release of phospholipase from the platelet membrane. Imidazole blocks thromboxane synthetase, thus reducing the production of thromboxane A_2. Ticlopidine is a novel platelet antiaggregant that functions primarily as an inhibitor of the adenosine diphosphate pathway of platelet aggregation. It was shown to be somewhat more effective than aspirin in preventing strokes in one randomized trial,[78] although the risks of side effects were greater.

REGRESSION

The first clear demonstration of regression of atherosclerotic lesions was reported in primates in 1970.[79] Substantial reductions in experimental atherosclerosis were found in rhesus monkeys when their atherogenic egg yolk and cholesterol diet was changed to a diet low in cholesterol and fat. In the ensuing decade, this model of atherosclerotic regression was repeated many times with a variety of diet and drug regimens. Studies with cynomolgus monkeys do not demonstrate the same ease of regression, a finding attributed to the extent of lesion invasion of the media in this species. Because advanced human atherosclerosis also has extensive involvement of media, the degree to which these primate data can be extrapolated to humans has been uncertain.

Clinical trials in humans can be separated into studies examining femoral arteries and those examining the coronary circulation. Two studies have compared groups treated with aggressive lipid lowering to controls using a computerized wall contour analysis technique. Measurable regression of femoral atherosclerosis with drug treatment was noted in 9 of 25 patients, and regression or nonprogression was significantly correlated with reduced serum lipid levels.[80] In the only double-blind study examining the effects of lipid lowering on peripheral vascular disease, a significant reduction in disease progression was found with aggressive lipid lowering.[81]

Four trials have used angiography to examine the changes in atherosclerotic lesions as a consequence of aggressive lipid-lowering therapy (Table 77-5). Three trials used medications[82-84] and one study (POSCH) used partial ileal bypass to reduce plasma lipid values.[85] Although the POSCH report did not achieve as dramatic a normalization of lipid levels, particularly of HDL cholesterol, it is notable for having nearly 10 years of follow-up. These studies show less disease progression, more lesion regression, and a greater reduction in morbidity and mortality than in the control groups. Aggressive lipid lowering alone can not only slow disease progression but can also create atherosclerotic lesion regression in both men and women. The time course for this appears to be rapid, with measurable changes occurring within 2 years. More importantly, these angiographic changes with lipid lowering have been correlated with a significant reduction in clinical events.

Table 77-5. RESULTS OF AGGRESSIVE LIPID LOWERING ON ATHEROSCLEROSIS*

Study	Subjects	Controls	Males/Females	Sx CAD	Progression (%) Rx	Progression (%) No Rx	Regression (%) Rx	Regression (%) No Rx	LDL Cholesterol (% Change)§ Rx	LDL Cholesterol (% Change)§ No Rx	HDL Cholesterol (% Change) Rx	HDL Cholesterol (% Change) No Rx
Kane et al[82]*	40	32	31/41	1/72	28	53	53	38	−39	−12	+26	—
Brown et al[83]†	74	46	All male	All	23	46	36	11	−39	−7	+29	+5
Blankenhorn et al[84]‡	80	82	All male	All	39	61	16	2	−43	−5	+37	+2

Sx CAD, symptomatic coronary artery disease

* The percentage regression and progression represent the number of individuals whose global scores coincided with an increase or reduction in luminal diameter.
† Two treatment groups are combined.
‡ These patients underwent postcoronary artery bypass. Both the native arteries and bypass grafts were examined in determining disease progression and regression.
§ There were also substantial reductions in triglycerides in these groups, which may help to explain the substantial increases in HDL.

REFERENCES

1. Report of the Intersociety Commission for Heart Disease Resources. Optimal resources for primary prevention of atherosclerotic diseases. Circulation 1984;70(Suppl):1.
2. Kannel WB, Dawber TR, Kagan A, et al. Factors of risk in the development of coronary heart disease: six-year follow-up experience—the Framingham study. Ann Intern Med 1961;55:33.
3. Matsuda J, Ross R. Atherogenesis during low level hypercholesterolemia in the nonhuman primate. I. Fatty streak formation. Arteriosclerosis 1990;10:164.
4. Steinberg D, Parthasarathy S, Carew TW, et al. Beyond cholesterol: modifications of low density lipoprotein that increase its atherogenicity. N Engl J Med 1989;320:915.
5. Leaf A. Management of hypercholesterolemia: are preventive interventions advisable? N Engl J Med 1989;321:680.
6. Marmot MG, Syme SL, Kagan A, et al. Epidemiologic studies of CHD and stroke in Japanese men living in Japan, Hawaii, and California: prevalence of coronary and hypertensive heart disease and associated risk factors. Am J Epidemiol 1975; 102:514.
7. Rapp JH, Harris HW, Hamilton RL, et al. Particle size distribution of lipoproteins from human atherosclerotic plaque. J Vasc Surg 1989;9:81.
8. Lipid Research Clinics Program. The lipid research clinics' coronary primary prevention trial results. II. The relationship of reduction in incidence of coronary heart disease to cholesterol lowering. JAMA 1984;251:365.
9. Frick MH, Elo O, Haapa K, et al. Helsinki heart study: primary prevention trial with gemfibrozil in middle-aged men with dyslipidemia. N Engl J Med 1987;317:1237.
10. A Report of the Surgeon General. Reducing the health consequences of smoking: 25 years of progress. Washington, DC, Department of Health and Human Services, 1989.
11. A Report of the Surgeon General. The health consequences of smoking: cardiovascular disease. Rockville, MD, Department of Health and Human Services, 1983.
12. Kuller L, Meilahn E, Ockene J. Smoking and coronary heart disease. In: Connor WE, Bristow JD, eds. Coronary heart disease: prevention, complications, and treatment. Philadelphia, JB Lippincott, 1985.
13. Kanel WB. Update on the role of cigarette smoking in coronary artery disease. Am Heart J 1981;101:319.
14. Auerbach O, Garfinkel L. Atherosclerosis and aneurysm of aorta in relation to smoking habits and age. Chest 1980; 78:805.
15. Wolf PA, D'Agostino RB, Kannel WB, et al. Cigarette smoking as a risk factor for stroke: the Framingham study. JAMA 1988;259:1025.
16. Golditz GA, Bonita R, Stampfer MJ. Cigarette smoking and risk of stroke in middle-aged women. N Engl J Med 1988;318:937.
17. Krupski WC, Olive GC, Weber CA, et al. Comparative effects of hypertension and nicotine on injury-induced myointimal thickening. Surgery 1987;102:409.
18. McGill HC. The cardiovascular pathology of smoking. Am Heart J 1988;115:250.
19. Krupski WC, Rapp JH. Smoking and atherosclerosis. Perspect Vasc Surg 1988;1:103.
20. Lam W, Sze PC, Sacks HS, et al. Meta-analysis of randomized controlled trials of nicotine chewing gum. Lancet 1987;2:27.
21. Glassman AH, Stetner F, Walsh BT, et al. Heavy smokers, smoking cessation, and clonidine: results of a double-blind, randomized trial. JAMA 1988;259:2863.
22. Rosenberg L, Palmer JR, Shapiro S. Decline in the risk of myocardial infarction among women who stop smoking. N Engl J Med 1990;322:213.
23. Myers KA, King RB, Scott DF, et al. The effect of smoking on the late patency of arterial reconstructions in the legs. Br J Surg 1978;65:267.
24. Tell GS, Howard G, McKinney WM, et al. Cigarette smoking cessation and extracranial carotid atherosclerosis. JAMA 1989;261:1178.
25. Samuelsson O, Wilhelmsen L, Andersson OK, et al. Cardiovascular morbidity in relation to change in blood pressure and serum cholesterol levels in treated hypertension: results from the primary prevention trial in Goteborg, Sweden. JAMA 1987;258:1768.
26. Kannel WB, McGee DL. Diabetes and cardiovascular disease: the Framingham study. JAMA 1979;241:2035.
27. Stemmer EA. Influence of diabetes on patterns of peripheral vascular disease. Surg Rounds 1990;13:43.
28. Steiner G. Diabetes and atherosclerosis: an overview. Diabetes 1981;30(Suppl 2):1.
29. Bartlett FF, Gibbons GW, Wheelcock FC Jr. Aortic reconstruction for occlusive disease. Arch Surg 1986;121:1150.
30. Imparato AM, Kim GE, Madayag M, et al. Angiographic criteria for successful tibial arterial reconstructions. Surgery 1973;74:830.
31. DeWeese JA, Rob CG. Autogenous venous grafts ten years later. Surgery 1977;82:775.
32. Kannel WB, Schatzkin A. Risk factor analysis. Prog Cardiovasc Dis 1983;26:309.
33. Ferrier TM. Comparative study of arterial disease in amputated lower limbs from diabetics and nondiabetics. Med J Aust 1967;1:5.
34. Strandness DE, Priest RE, Gibbons GW. Combined clinical and pathologic study of diabetic and nondiabetic peripheral arterial disease. Diabetes 1964;13:366.
35. Schadt DC, Hines EA Jr, Juergens JL, Barker NW. Chronic atherosclerotic occlusion of the femoral artery. JAMA 1961; 175:937.
36. Jonason T, Ringqvist I. Diabetes mellitus and intermittent claudication. Acta Med Scand 1985;218:271.
37. Lopes-Virella MF, Sherer GK, Lees AM, et al. Surface binding internalization and degradation by cultured human fibroblasts of low density lipoproteins isolated from type I (insulin dependent) diabetic patients: changes with metabolic control. Diabetologia 1982;22:430.
38. Calvert GD, Mannik T, Graham JJ, et al. Effects of therapy on plasma high density lipoprotein cholesterol concentration in diabetes mellitus. Lancet 1981;1:66.
39. Kannel WB, Doyle JT, Ostfeld AM, et al. Optimal resources for primary prevention of atherosclerotic diseases. Circulation 1984;70:153A.
40. Keen H, Ashton CE. Mechanisms of excess cardiovascular mortality in diabetes. Postgrad Med J 1989;65(Suppl 1):S26.
41. Malinow MR, Kang SS, Taylor LM Jr, et al. Prevalence of hyperhomocysteinemia in patients with peripheral arterial occlusive disease. Circulation 1989;79:1180.
42. Ekroth R, Dahllof AG, Gendevall B, et al. Physical training of patients with intermittent claudication: indications, methods and results. Surgery 1978;84:640.
43. Dahllof AG, Bjorntorp P, Holm J, et al. Metabolic activity of skeletal muscle in patients with peripheral arterial insufficiency. Eur J Clin Invest 1974;4:9.
44. Larsen OA, Lassen NA. Effect of daily muscular exercise in patients with intermittent claudication. Lancet 1966;2:1093.
45. Ericsson B, Haeger K, Lindell SE. Effect of training on intermittent claudication. Angiology 1970;21:188.
46. Ernst EE, Matrai A. Intermittent claudication, exercise, and blood rheology. Circulation 1987;76:1110.
47. Mannarino E, Pasqualini L, Menna M, et al. Effect of physical training on peripheral vascular disease: a controlled study. Angiology 1989;40:5.
48. Radack K, Wyderski RJ. Conservative management of intermittent claudication. Ann Intern Med 1990;113:135.
49. Ehrly AM. Improvement of the flow properties of blood: a new therapeutical approach in occlusive arterial disease. Angiology 1976;27:188.
50. Angelkort B, Maurin N, Boateng K. Influence of pentoxifylline on erythrocyte deformability in peripheral occlusive arterial disease. Curr Med Res Opin 1979;6:255.
51. Muller R, Lehrach F. Haemorrheological role of platelet aggregation and hypercoagulability in microcirculation: therapeutic approach with pentoxifylline. Pharmatherapeutica 1980; 2:372.
52. Spittell JA Jr. Pentoxifylline and intermittent claudication. Ann Intern Med 1985;102:126.
53. Angelkort B, Kiesewetter H. Influence of risk factors and coagulation phenomena on the fluidity of blood in chronic arterial occlusive disease. Scand J Clin Lab Invest 1981; 156(Suppl):185.
54. Solerte SB, Ferrari E. Diabetic retinal vascular complications

and erythrocyte filterability: results of a 2-year follow-up study with pentoxifylline. Pharmatherapeutica 1985;4:341.

55. Taylor LM Jr, Porter JM. Drug treatment of claudication: vasodilators, hemorrheologic agents and antiserotonin drugs. J Vasc Surg 1986;3:374.

56. Accetto B. Beneficial hemorrheologic therapy of chronic peripheral arterial disorders with pentoxifylline: results of double blind study versus vasodilator-nylidrin. Am Heart J 1982;103:864.

57. Bollinger A, Frei C. Double blind study of pentoxifylline against placebo in patients with intermittent claudication. Pharmatherapeutica 1977;1:557.

58. Dettori AG, Pini M, Moratti A, et al. Acenocoumarol and pentoxifylline in intermittent claudication: a controlled clinical study—the APIC study group. Angiology 1989;40:237.

59. Di Perri T, Guerrini M. Placebo controlled double blind study with pentoxifylline of walking performance in patients with intermittent claudication. Angiology 1983;34:40.

60. Gallus AS, Morley AA, Gleadow F, et al. Intermittent claudication: a double-blind crossover trial of pentoxifylline. Aust N Z J Med 1985;15:402.

61. Perhoniemi V, Salmenkivi K, Sundberg S, et al. Effects of flunarizine and pentoxifylline on walking distance and blood rheology in claudication. Angiology 1984;35:366.

62. Porter JM, Cutler BS, Lee BY, et al. Pentoxifylline efficacy in the treatment of intermittent claudication: Multicenter controlled double-blind trial with objective assessment of chronic occlusive arterial disease patients. Am Heart J 1982;104:66.

63. Reilly DT, Quinton DN, Barrie WW. A controlled trial of pentoxifylline (Trental 400) in intermittent claudication: clinical, hemostatic and rheological effects. NZ Med J 1987;100:445.

64. Roekaerts F, Deleers L. Trental 400 in the treatment of intermittent claudication: results of long-term, placebo-controlled administration. Angiology 1984;35:396.

65. Strano A, Davi G, Avellone G, et al. Double-blind, crossover study of the clinical efficacy and the hemorrheological effects of pentoxifylline in patients with occlusive arterial disease of the lower limbs. Angiology 1984;35:459.

66. Tonak J, Knecht H, Groitl H. Treatment of circulatory disturbances with pentoxifylline: a double-blind study with Trental. Pharmatherapeutica 1983;3(Suppl 1):126.

67. Brevetti G, Chiariello M, Ferulano G, et al. Increases in walking distance in patients with peripheral vascular disease treated with L-carnitine: a double-blind, cross-over study. Circulation 1988;77:767.

68. Salzman EW. Aspirin to prevent arterial thrombosis. N Engl J Med 1982;307:113.

69. Antiplatelet Trialists Collaboration. Secondary prevention of vascular disease by prolonged antiplatelet treatment. BMJ 1988;296:320.

70. Packham MA, Mustard JF. Pharmacology of platelet-affecting drugs. Circulation 1980;62(Suppl V):5.

71. Steering Committee of the Physician's Health Study Research Group. Preliminary report: findings from the aspirin component of the ongoing physicians' health study. N Engl J Med 1988;29:318.

72. Peto R, Gray R, Collins R, et al. Randomized trial of prophylactic daily aspirin in British male doctors. BMJ 1988;296:313.

73. Hess H, Mietaschik A, Deichsel G. Drug-induced inhibition of platelet function delays progression of peripheral occlusive arterial disease: a prospective double-blind arteriographically controlled trial. Lancet 1985;1:416.

74. Fields WS, Lemak NA, Frankowski RF, et al. Controlled trial of aspirin in cerebral ischemia. Stroke 1977;8:301.

75. Canadian Cooperative Study Group. Randomized trial of aspirin and sulfinpyrazone in threatened stroke. N Engl J Med 1978;299:53.

76. Bousser MG, Eschwege JE, Haguenau M, et al. AICLA controlled trial of aspirin and dipyridamole in the secondary prevention of atherothrombotic cerebral ischemia. Stroke 1983;14:5.

77. Sorensen RS, Pedersen H, Marquardsen J, et al. Acetylsalicylic acid in the prevention of stroke in patients with reversible cerebral ischemic attacks: a Danish cooperative study. Stroke 1983;14:15.

78. Hass WK, Easton JD, Adams HP, et al. A randomized trial comparing ticlopidine hydrochloride with aspirin for the prevention of stroke in high-risk patients. N Engl J Med 1989;321:501.

79. Armstrong ML, Warner ED, Connor WE. Regression of coronary atheromatosis in rhesus monkeys. Circ Res 1970;27:59.

80. Barndt R, Blankenhorn DH, Crawford DW, et al. Regression and progression of early femoral atherosclerosis in treated hyperlipoproteinemic patients. Ann Intern Med 1977;86:139.

81. Duffield RG, Lewis B, Miller ME, et al. Treatment of hyperlipidemia retards progression of symptomatic femoral atherosclerosis: a randomized controlled trial. Lancet 1983;1:639.

82. Kane JP, Malloy MJ, Ports TA, et al. Regression of coronary atherosclerosis during treatment of familial hypercholesterolemia with combined drug regimens. JAMA 1990;264:3007.

83. Brown G, Albers JJ, Fisher LD, et al. Regression of coronary artery disease as a result of intensive lipid-lowering therapy in men with high levels of apoprotein B. N Engl J Med 1990;323:1289.

84. Blankenhorn DH, Nessim SA, Johnson RL, et al. Beneficial effects of combined colestipol-niacin therapy on coronary atherosclerosis and coronary venous bypass grafts. JAMA 1987;257:3233.

85. Buchwald H, Varco RL, Mattis JP, et al. Effect of partial ileal bypass surgery on mortality and morbidity from coronary heart disease in patients with hypercholesterolemia: report of the program on the surgical control of the hyperlipidemias (POSCH). N Engl J Med 1990;323:946.

SURGERY: SCIENTIFIC PRINCIPLES AND PRACTICE, Second Edition, edited by Lazar J. Greenfield, Michael W. Mulholland, Keith T. Oldham, Gerald B. Zelenock, and Keith D. Lillemoe. Lippincott–Raven Publishers, Philadelphia, © 1997.

CHAPTER 78

VASCULAR INFECTIONS

DENNIS F. BANDYK

Infection has been the nemesis of vascular surgery throughout its history. Early surgeons relied on ligature and, when feasible, excision to deal with spontaneously occurring mycotic aneurysms and contaminated vascular battlefield injuries. At the turn of the century, Carrel[1] developed arterial reconstruction techniques, including vein bypass grafting, but adoption of these procedures in the preantibiotic era was delayed because of disastrous experiences with infection.

Vascular infection is an uncommon and dreaded clinical condition. Infected arterial aneurysms are identified in 0.4% of postmortem examinations and is a presenting manifestation in 3% of patients with abdominal aortic aneurysm.[2,3] Diagnosis and eradication of the infectious process are among the most challenging therapeutic problems a physician can encounter. Delays in recognition and treatment significantly increase morbidity due to sepsis, artery wall erosion into adjacent organs, or hemorrhage after aneurysmal rupture. In his Gulstonian lectures of 1885, Osler vividly described the clinical manifestations and sequelae of mycotic aneurysms that resulted from bacterial endocarditis.[4] Abscesses involving artery walls had been described earlier in the 19th century, but Osler was the first to recognize the propensity of bacterial vegetations on the aortic valves to embolize and infect remote arteries. Infection can also occur after arterial reconstructive surgery, or cannulation of arteries and veins for drug administration, pressure monitoring, diagnostic studies, or therapeutic endovascular procedures (transluminal angioplasty, atherectomy, stent or vena cava filter placement).

The invasive nature of modern medicine and, unfortunately, increasing drug abuse have resulted in a resurgence of vascular infections from penetrating wounds that introduce contamination at the vessel wall puncture or into an adjacent hematoma. The incidence of infection after endovascular procedures is rare (less than 1%), and after arterial surgery ranges from 0.7% to 3.5%. Risk of infection increases with implantation of a prosthetic graft and when arterial surgery is performed under emergency conditions. The true incidence of postoperative vascular infections may be as high as 5% if both early (within 4 months) and late infections are included. Approximately one half of vascular graft infections develop months to years after implantation and are typically caused by less virulent microorganisms. If the early infection rate after autologous or prosthetic arterial reconstruction by an individual surgeon or institution exceeds 1.5% (the expected incidence of wound infection for clean surgical cases), review of operative technique, operating room environment and personnel, and antibiotic prophylaxis is indicated.[5]

Classification

Vascular infections can be classified based on the mechanisms by which infecting organisms invade the vessel wall, preexisting status of the arterial segment, and anatomic site[6]:

Mycotic Aneurysm

Intravascular
Extravascular
Embolomycotic
Cryptogenic

Vascular Graft Infection

Perigraft (early versus late appearing)
Graft-enteric erosion or fistula
Aortic stump sepsis

Suppurative (Septic) Thrombophlebitis

Osler used the term *mycotic aneurysm* to denote any vascular infection caused by microorganisms, including fungal infections. In contemporary vascular surgery, the term mycotic aneurysm encompasses both false or pseudoaneurysms caused by arterial infection and true aneurysms that have become secondarily infected. These lesions are fulminant infections and are distinct from positive cultures of aneurysm sac contents without local or systemic signs of infection. Mycotic aneurysms can occur by three mechanisms: direct extension of an adjacent suppurative focus (extravascular); bacterial colonization of diseased arterial segments (intravascular); and septic emboli as a result of endocarditis (embolomycotic) or septicemia with organisms entering the vessel wall at sites of damaged endothelium or the vasa vasorum (cryptogenic). Infections involving vascular grafts are classified based on anatomic signs (perigraft, graft-enteric erosion or fistula), mode of onset (early versus late), and pathogen involved. Aortic stump sepsis is a unique vascular lesion, produced by residual artery wall infection after excision of an infected aortic graft or aneurysm and ligation of the aorta. Finally, suppurative thrombophlebitis is an important infection involving the venous system. Infection usually develops at an intravenous cannulation site, but can also occur in the deep veins in the pelvis, lower limb, and neck.

Anatomic Distribution

No artery is immune to infection. Improved diagnosis and treatment of bacterial endocarditis and syphilis have altered the anatomic distribution of mycotic aneurysms.

The classic luetic aortic aneurysm is now rarely seen in the Western world, whereas it used to be responsible for half of all aneurysms. In the preantibiotic era, the proportion of aortic to peripheral mycotic aneurysms was relatively high. Infection frequently occurred at the site of preexisting arterial disease (congenital lesion, atherosclerotic aneurysm) and was a complication of untreated endocarditis. Although embolomycotic aneurysms still occur, most mycotic aneurysms are now extravascular or intravascular in origin, the most frequent being the result of direct trauma (drug abuse, endovascular procedures) and concomitant bacterial contamination. Collected series of mycotic aneurysms indicate the femoral artery is the prevalent location, followed by the abdominal aorta and visceral vessels[7-10] (Fig. 78-1). Mycotic aortic aneurysms tend to be saccular and develop in the transverse aortic arch or in the thoracoabdominal aorta especially in the region posterior to the origin of the visceral vessels.

Infection can follow any vascular reconstruction procedure, but is more common when prosthetic material is used and when the grafting procedure extends into the groin[11-15] (Table 78-1). The propensity of graft infection in groin wounds is not unexpected, considering the microflora in this region of the body, the frequency of poor hygiene in obese patients, and the colonization of lymphatics-draining infected lesions of the foot. Most vascular graft infections originate from a wound infection. Infection after placement of an aortic graft confined to the abdomen is rare (incidence is below 1%). Those that occur follow repair of a ruptured abdominal aortic aneurysm or a postoperative intraabdominal complication (colon or intestinal ischemia, bowel perforation, cholecystitis, appendicitis).

Clinical Manifestations

Presenting symptoms and signs of vascular infection are varied and often subtle. The triad of back or groin pain, a pulsatile mass, and fever suggests the presence of an infected arterial aneurysm. A history of bacterial endocarditis, other source of septicemia, or recent penetrating trauma is important, although no source of infection can be identified in approximately one quarter of patients. When located in the extremities, the mycotic aneurysm can be palpated in most patients (over 80%). Petechial skin lesions and septic arthritis can occur because of peripheral embolism, and a systolic bruit may be present over the lesion. If the infection is deeply situated, the aneurysm is not palpable and clinical presentation is a fever of unknown origin. Abdominal pain is present in only 35% of patients with infected abdominal aortic aneurysms, with the aneurysm palpable in half of cases. Myalgias, arthalgias, episodes of fever and chills, or progressive weakness can persist for weeks before the diagnosis of mycotic aneurysm is made. Intracerebral aneurysms present with lateralizing hemispheric deficits secondary to rupture or with lethargy and confusion due to abscess formation.

The presentation of vascular graft infections depends on graft site, time interval after operation, infecting pathogen, and extent of graft involvement. Most patients present with anastomotic false aneurysm, anastomotic or gastrointestinal hemorrhage (aortoenteric fistula), graft thrombosis, or signs (local or systemic) of infection.[16-18] Early (within 4 months of operation) graft infections are apparent on clinical grounds with sepsis (fever, leukocytosis, bacteremia), a draining or pulsatile mass in the operative incision, or graft–artery anastomotic dehiscence. If graft material is visible in the wound after drainage of an abscess, diffuse involvement of a vascular prosthesis should be assumed. Infection of grafts confined to the abdomen (aortic interpo-

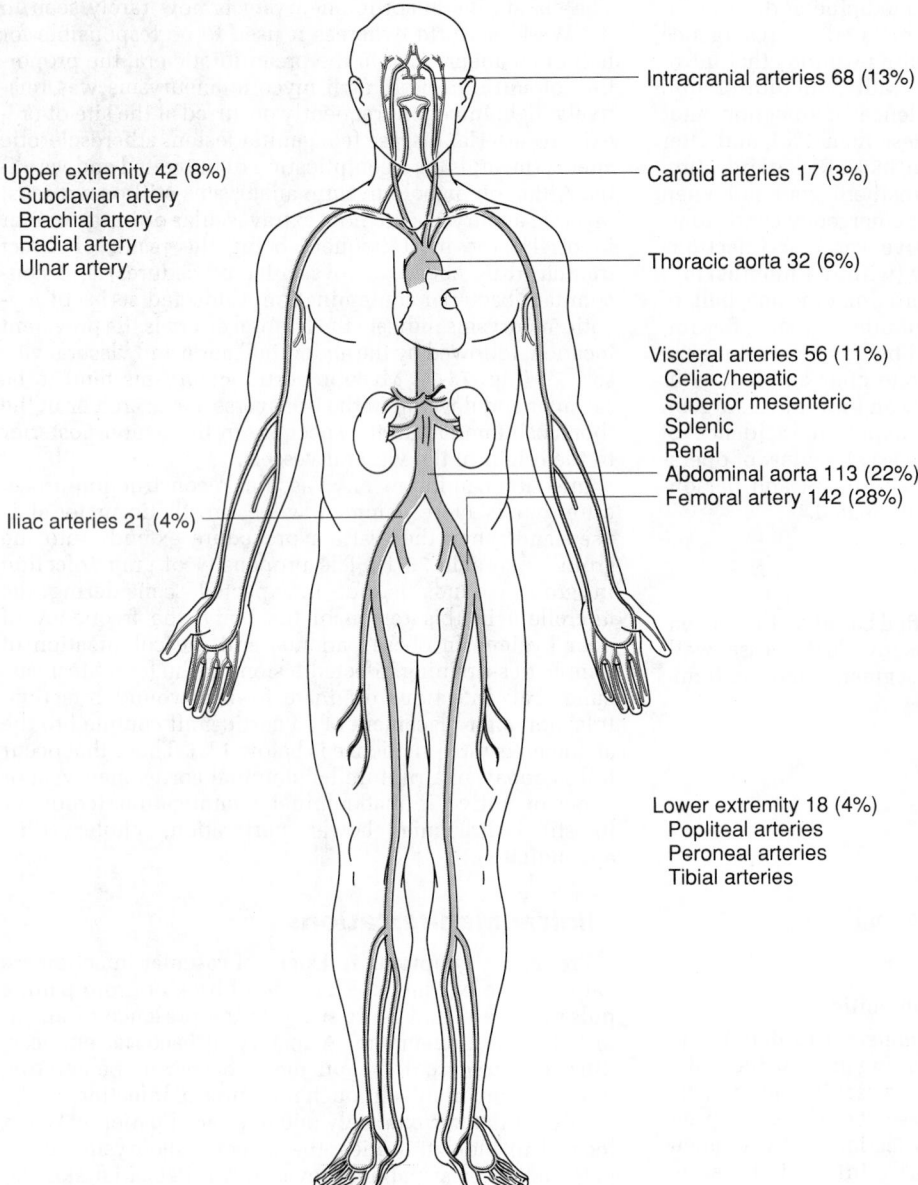

Intracranial arteries 68 (13%)

Upper extremity 42 (8%)
  Subclavian artery
  Brachial artery
  Radial artery
  Ulnar artery

Carotid arteries 17 (3%)

Thoracic aorta 32 (6%)

Visceral arteries 56 (11%)
  Celiac/hepatic
  Superior mesenteric
  Splenic
  Renal
Abdominal aorta 113 (22%)
Femoral artery 142 (28%)

Iliac arteries 21 (4%)

Lower extremity 18 (4%)
  Popliteal arteries
  Peroneal arteries
  Tibial arteries

Figure 78-1. Anatomic distribution of 510 mycotic aneurysms from collected series.

sition, aortoiliac) can present as unexplained sepsis, prolonged postoperative ileus, or abdominal distention and tenderness as the only clinical signs.

Most aortic graft infections are recognized beyond 1 year of graft implantation.[17-20] About two thirds of patients have perigraft infections. Common clinical manifestations include an inflammatory process (sinus tract, perigraft exudate) involving the groin incision of an aortofemoral graft or an anastomotic false aneurysm. In the remaining one third of patients, the graft infection is manifest as an erosion into the upper or lower gastrointestinal tract. Pathologic interaction between the prosthesis and bowel may involve direct communication of an infected graft–artery anastomosis (graft-enteric fistula [GEF]) or exposure of the prosthesis within the bowel lumen (graft-enteric erosion [GEE]). Half the patients with GEF or GEE have acute bleeding episodes manifested as either hematemesis or melena, accompanied by hypotension. These bleeding episodes occur over a period of hours to days.

The signs and symptoms of suppurative thrombophlebitis can mimic aseptic venous thrombosis.[21,22] Swelling, erythema, and induration extend along the involved vein or

at sites of cutdown and cannulation. Purulence may be present at the site of cannulation. Persistent fever and chills in a patient with no apparent cause should suggest the diagnosis of septic thrombophlebitis. Systemic sepsis with positive blood culture occurs when suppuration involves the thrombosed segment of vein. At this stage, the entire vein is inflamed, extremely painful, and fluctuant.

Pathophysiology of Vascular Infections

Although infection can occur in any artery, there is a predilection for atherosclerotic lesions, in particular aneurysms, vascular reconstructions in which a prostheses is implanted, and sites of iatrogenic, accidental, or self-induced penetrating arterial trauma. There is considerable evidence to indicate bacteremia alone rarely causes infection in a normal artery, although important exceptions include particulate embolism from a proximal septic focus and arteritis produced by syphilis and tuberculosis. Direct arterial trauma is the prevalent etiologic factor for mycotic

Table 78-1. INCIDENCE OF VASCULAR GRAFT INFECTIONS

Study	Graft Type	Location	Incidence (%)
Hoffert et al, 1965[11]	Prosthetic	Aortoiliac/ femoral	2.2
		Femoropopliteal	12.0
Szilagyi et al, 1972[12]	Prosthetic	Aortoiliac	0.7
		Aortofemoral	1.6
		Femoropopliteal	3.0
	Vein	Femoropopliteal	0.4
Goldstone & Moore, 1974[13]	Prosthetic	Aortofemoral	1.5
		Axillofemoral	3.1
Lorentzen et al, 1985[14]	Prosthetic	Aortoiliac	0.0
		Aortofemoral	3.0
		Femoropopliteal	3.5
O'Hara et al, 1986[18]	Prosthetic	Aortoiliac	0.4
		Aortofemoral	1.3
Durham et al, 1986[15]	Prosthetic	Femoropopliteal	2.8

aneurysms diagnosed and treated in clinical practice. A common form involves infection of a surgically created arteriovenous fistula for chronic hemodialysis. Inoculation of the vessel wall can occur at the time of an injury or operative manipulation, from a contiguous septic process via periarterial lymphatics or vasa vasorum, or by embolism of septic microemboli to arterial branch points or arterial vasa vasorum. Intercurrent bacteremia from any source can establish infection in any intimal defect, especially vessels with atherosclerotic plaque and mural thrombus. In the case of salmonellal bacteremia, normal arterial intima may be invaded by the infectious process. Whether an infection becomes established depends on the quantity and virulence of the pathogens and host resistance. Traumatized tissue and collections of blood can provide nourishment, whereas foreign bodies (vascular prostheses) adversely affect local host-defense mechanisms.

The presence of a foreign body potentiates the infectivity of bacteria by adhering to biomaterial surfaces and forming a bacteria-laden biofilm that protects enclosed organisms against antibiotics, antibiodies, and phagocytes. Experimental models have demonstrated that the risk of foreign body infections can be predicted by using the following formula:

$$\text{risk of infection} = \frac{\text{dose of bacterial contamination} \times \text{virulence}}{\text{host resistance}}$$

Gram-positive organisms, such as staphylococcal species, produce an extracellular glycocalyx or "mucin" that promotes adherence and biofilm formation. The addition of suture lines and mural thrombus also increases bacterial adherence. Once a prosthetic graft is incorporated with surrounding tissue and a luminal psuedointima is established, it is less susceptible to colonization via bacteremia or adjacent infection.

The ultimate manifestation of arterial or vascular graft infection, regardless of location, is wall or anastomotic disruption and hemorrhage. Vascular infections are complex processes involving activation of host defenses by the microorganisms, their products of metabolism, and foreign bodies, if present. Tissue invasion by the microorganism into vessel walls with an accompanying inflammation weakens tensile strength. Aneurysm formation or local, contained rupture can result in deposition of mural throm-

bus, forming a septic nidus for continuous bacteremia. Less virulent pathogens, such as *Staphylococcus epidermidis* and other coagulase-negative staphylococci have a limited capacity to produce an invasive vascular infection and, in general, require the presence of a foreign body (intravascular catheter, prosthetic graft). Unlike *Staphylococcus aureus* and gram-negative bacteria, coagulase-negative staphylococci sequester and grow primarily within biofilms adherent to prosthetic surfaces, do not produce toxins capable of producing tissue autolysis, and in the presence of intact host defenses, do not invade surrounding tissue. Bacteria colonization may be confined only to biomaterial surfaces as bacterial biofilm. These indolent infections typically produce no systemic signs of infection when host defenses are normal.

Predisposing Factors

More than 90% of patients have one or multiple risk factors for the development of mycotic aneurysms, graft infection, or suppurative thrombophlebitis. The most common entities are arterial trauma, depressed immunocompetence, and concurrent sepsis or bacterial endocarditis:

Arterial Trauma

Accidents
Surgical manipulation
Parenteral drug abuse
Invasive diagnostic procedures
Endovascular procedures

Depressed Immunocompetence

Malignant neoplasms
Lymphoproliferative disorders
Chronic alcoholism
Corticosteroid administration
Chemotherapy
Chronic renal failure
Autoimmune disease
Diabetes mellitus

Bacterial Endocarditis
Concurrent Sepsis

Salmonellal bacteremia
Tuberculous lymphadenitis
Syphilitic gumma

Wound Healing Complications

Hematoma
Lymphocele
Dermal necrosis

Vascular Prosthesis
Congenital Cardiovascular Defects

Patent ductus arteriosus
Coarctation of the thoracic aorta

Emergency Arterial Revascularization

One quarter of patients with mycotic aneurysms have documented cellular or humeral immunodeficiency.[8,10] The rarity of mycotic aneurysms in the absence of obvious risk factors attests to the immunity of the normal artery wall to invasive bacterial infection. Salmonellal septicemia usually occurs in elderly patients with predisposing factors such as autoimmune diseases, diabetes, and steroid or immunosuppressive medication.

Early vascular graft infections are usually the result of wound sepsis, with important risk factors being a break in aseptic surgical technique, reoperation for hematoma, concomitant remote infection (eg, foot sepsis, pneumonia, urinary tract infection), and impaired immunocompetence. A characteristic of patients with late-appearing graft infections is a history of multiple operations for complications of postoperative hematoma, graft thrombosis, or false aneurysm.[17]

Bacteriology

Although virtually any organism can infect the vascular system, *S aureus* is the prevalent pathogen (Table 78-2). Approximately 80% of early postoperative vascular infections are caused by staphyococcal or streptococcal sp.[23] Over the past two decades, the microbiology of mycotic aneurysms and graft infections has changed. The frequency of infections due to gram-negative organisms, such as *Escherichia coli, Pseudomonas* sp, *Klebsiella* sp, *Enterobacter* sp, *Proteus* sp, and fungi (*Candida, Aspergillus*), have increased and account for one third of infections involving arteries, veins, or vascular grafts. Aneurysms infected with gram-negative organisms have an increased rupture rate (80%) compared with infections due to gram-positive organisms (10%). Infections due to *Pseudomonas* sp are particularly virulent because of the organisms' ability to produce destructive endotoxins (elastase, alkaline protease) that act against elastin and collagen in artery and vein graft walls to compromise structural integrity. Coagulase-positive staphylococci and streptococci sp. Also produce lysins that are hemolytic and result in cell necrosis and necrosis of mobilized leukocytes. Infections produced by *S aureus* and gram-negative bacteria involve invasion of tissue and are associated with a high concentration of bacteria (10^5 to 10^7 colony-forming units [CFU]). Most patients with fungal vascular infections are either immunosuppressed or have established fungal infections elsewhere. The importance of coagulase-negative staphylococci, especially *S epidermidis,* has also been recently emphasized in the pathogenesis of late-appearing vascular prostheses infection and infections of intravascular catheters. The microbiologic confirmation of vascular infections due to coagulase-negative staphylococci require a sensitive culture techniques (broth media, disruption of surface biofilms). Swabs of tissue, fluid, and perigraft exudate imprinted on agar media can be associated with significant sampling error if low (less than 10^4 CFUs) numbers of bacteria are present. Microbiologic sampling error results in negative cultures in up to one quarter of patients with mycotic aneurysms or vascular graft infections.[7,10,13,17]

Salmonella sp are the infecting pathogen in most intravascular mycotic aneurysms involving the thoracic or abdominal aorta, with staphylococci and other gram-positive cocci second in incidence. Contaminated water, poultry, and meat products are the most important sources of these gram-negative, flagellated bacteria, which have a predilection for diseased arterial walls. The portal of entry is the gastrointestinal tract and the biliary tree, with the subsequent clinical course determined by extent of mucosal invasion, serotype involved, and host resistance. Children and adults with lymphoproliferative disorders or sickle cell anemia are particularly vulnerable to develop salmonellal bacteremia and extravascular metastatic sites of infection (osteomyelitis of lumbar vertebrae, paravertebral abscesses, meningitis). There are more than 2200 serotypes, but *Salmonella choleraesuis, typhimurium,* and *enteritidis* account for two thirds of arterial infections.

Diagnostic Modalities

Prompt diagnosis and treatment of vascular infections are essential to avoid complications (septic emboli, rupture) and fatal outcomes. Blood cultures are positive in 50% to 75% of patients with mycotic infections, but the incidence is lower in patients with vascular graft infections. Leukocytosis and increased erythrocyte sedimentation rate are common but nonspecific findings in patients with vascular infections and fever. By contrast, all laboratory testing may be normal in patients with late-appearing perigraft infections due to *S epidermidis.*

Vascular imaging is vital in evaluating patients with suspected or proven vascular infection. Both anatomic and functional diagnostic imaging techniques may be necessary to confirm the presence of infection, plan management, and assess operative sites for residual or recurrent infection:

Anatomic Imaging Techniques

Ultrasonography
Computed tomography (CT)
Magnetic resonance imaging/angiography (MRI/MRA)
Digital subtraction/conventional contrast arteriography

Functional Imaging Techniques

Techneium^{99m} (^{99m}Tc)-hexametazime–labeled leukocytes
Indium-111 (^{111}In)–labeled leukocyte scan
^{111}In-labeled immunoglobulin G (IgG) scan

Anatomic and functional radioisotope imaging techniques are equally valuable in assessing patients with suspected mycotic aneurysms or arterial graft infections. Anatomic definition of the infectious process demonstrates the extent of infection, allows anticipation of technical difficulties, identifies safe locations for vascular clamp placement, and minimizes the likelihood of vascular injury or organ ischemia secondary to unsuspected anatomic anomalies or concomitant arterial occlusive disease. A caveat in patients with gastrointestinal hemorrhage after aortic graft placement is that a negative diagnostic imaging study does not exclude infection and presence of a graft-enteric erosion or fistula.

Ultrasonography

Ultrasound scans can accurately locate aneurysms and identify presence of perigraft fluid. Color Doppler flow imaging is particularly useful in evaluating pulsatile masses to differentiate between fluid collection or hematoma and

Table 78-2. BACTERIOLOGY OF VASCULAR INFECTIONS

Microorganism	Incidence from Collected Series (%)		
	Mycotic Aneurysm	Graft Infection	Suppurative Thrombophlebitis
Streptococcus sp	10	10	5
Staphylococcus aureus	28	36	50
Staphylococcus epidermidis	<5	25	10
Salmonella sp	20	<1	—
Pseudomonas sp	10	2	1
Escherichia coli	10	12	20
Proteus sp	4	4	2
Klebsiella sp	3	6	5–30
Enterobacter sp	3	4	5
Enterococcus group	2	1	2
Serratia sp	3	3	2
Candida sp	2	1	5
Mycobacterium tuberculosis	1	—	—
Other species	5–10	2–5	<5
Cutlure-negative	15–20	15–25	

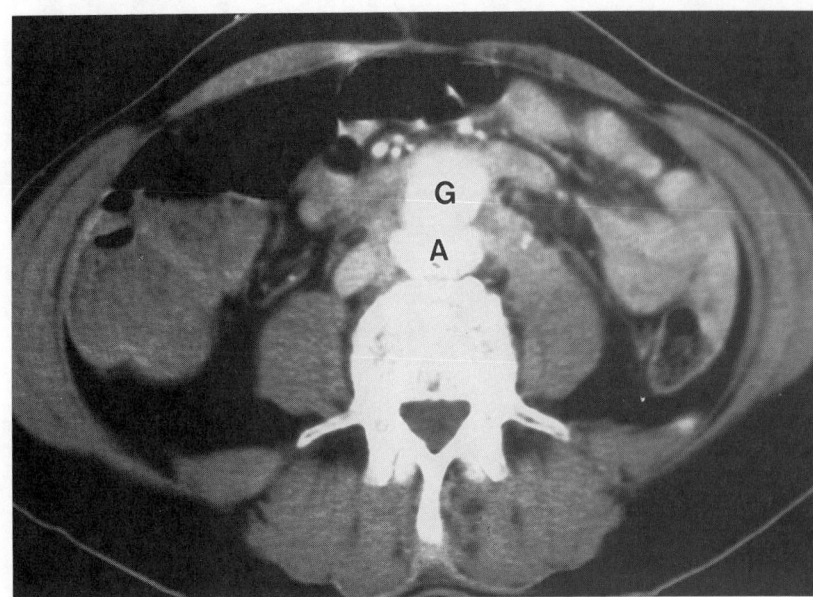

Figure 78-2. CT scan of infected aortic aneurysm with gas (*arrow*) present within the aorta and adjacent soft tissue. Infected, confined aneurysmal rupture was found at operation.

false aneurysm formation. Diagnostic accuracy relies on the examiner's skill, but the widespread availability of duplex scanners, coupled with the ability to perform bedside examinations of critically ill patients, makes ultrasonography a useful initial diagnostic technique to verify vessel patency and size and to assess pulsatile masses adjacent to peripheral vessels and grafts, especially in the groin and limbs. Imaging of the venous system is used to identify suitable-sized saphenous and femoral veins for use as autologous grafts.

Computed Tomography

Contrast-enhanced CT scanning is the preferred imaging technique in patients with suspected infection involving the aorta, visceral arteries, or abdominal vascular grafts. Diagnostic criteria of infection include well-localized vessel dilatation with paucity of calcification, abnormal collections of fluid or air around vessels or grafts, or an encasing mass that contains air, adjacent vertebral osteomyelitis, or juxtaaortic retroperitoneal abscess.[24] CT-guided needle aspiration of perigraft fluid collections is useful in identifying the infecting pathogen. CT scans are superior to ultrasound in assessing aneurysm wall integrity and in detecting inflammation or infection involving the aneurysm sac (Fig. 78-2). Scanning can be performed with sufficient speed to be useful in evaluating symptomatic but hemodynamically stable patients with suspected rupture or with graft-enteric fistula or erosion. Many hemorrhagic, embolic, and ischemic complications associated with operative management can be avoided by preliminary CT imaging. Arterial segments not involved in the inflammatory process can be accurately located and should be used as initial sites for dissection, vascular control, and placement of occluding clamps.

Magnetic Resonance Imaging

MRI is another vascular imaging technique that affords anatomic delineation in multiple planes and provides information about tissue characterization (eg, presence of fluid, inflammation). These features result in improved resolution between tissue and fluid interfaces compared to CT imaging. Patients with suspected infection of the aorta can be scanned in transverse, sagittal, and coronal planes (Fig. 78-3). Multiplanar reconstruction of vascular anatomy permits evaluation of complex aortic aneurysms and infectious complications after aortic surgery. Anatomic information available includes lumen dimensions, rate of blood flow, quality of the aortic wall, cephalad and caudal extension, and involvement of branch vessels and neighboring structures. MRI has been demonstrated to be superior to CT imaging in identifying the presence and extent of infection involving aortic grafts.[25] The ability to perform

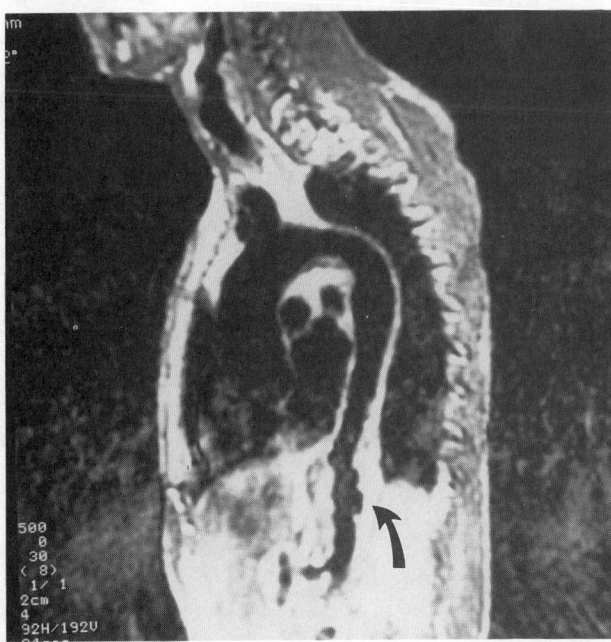

Figure 78-3. MR scan of thoracic and suprarenal aorta in a patient with tuberculous aortitis. Saccular dilatation of aorta was demonstrated in the sagittal view (*arrow*).

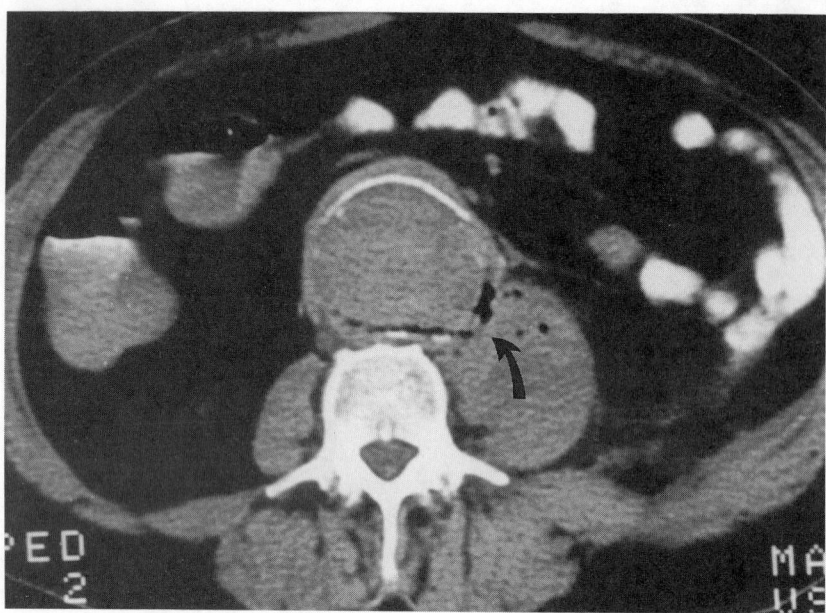

Figure 78-4. Contrast-enhanced CT image of an aortic interposition graft in a patient with gastrointestinal bleeding. False aneurysm at graft (G) to aorta (A) anastomosis and perigraft inflammation were consistent with diagnosis of graft-enteric erosion. The corresponding aortograms are shown in Figure 78-5.

MRA with the scan data supports more widespread use of this modality for initial patient evaluation.

Angiography

Biplanar angiography should be performed on all patients with confirmed or suspected arterial infections. Angiograms can identify pseudoaneurysms, assess patency of involved vessels or grafts, and evaluate the status of proximal and distal vessels (Figs. 78-4 and 78-5). A saccular or lobulated aneurysm of the aorta with otherwise normal vasculature is pathognomonic of a mycotic aneurysm (Figs. 78-6 and 78-7). The diagnosis of intracranial or visceral mycotic aneurysms can only be made reliably by angiography. In most patients with arterial or vascular graft

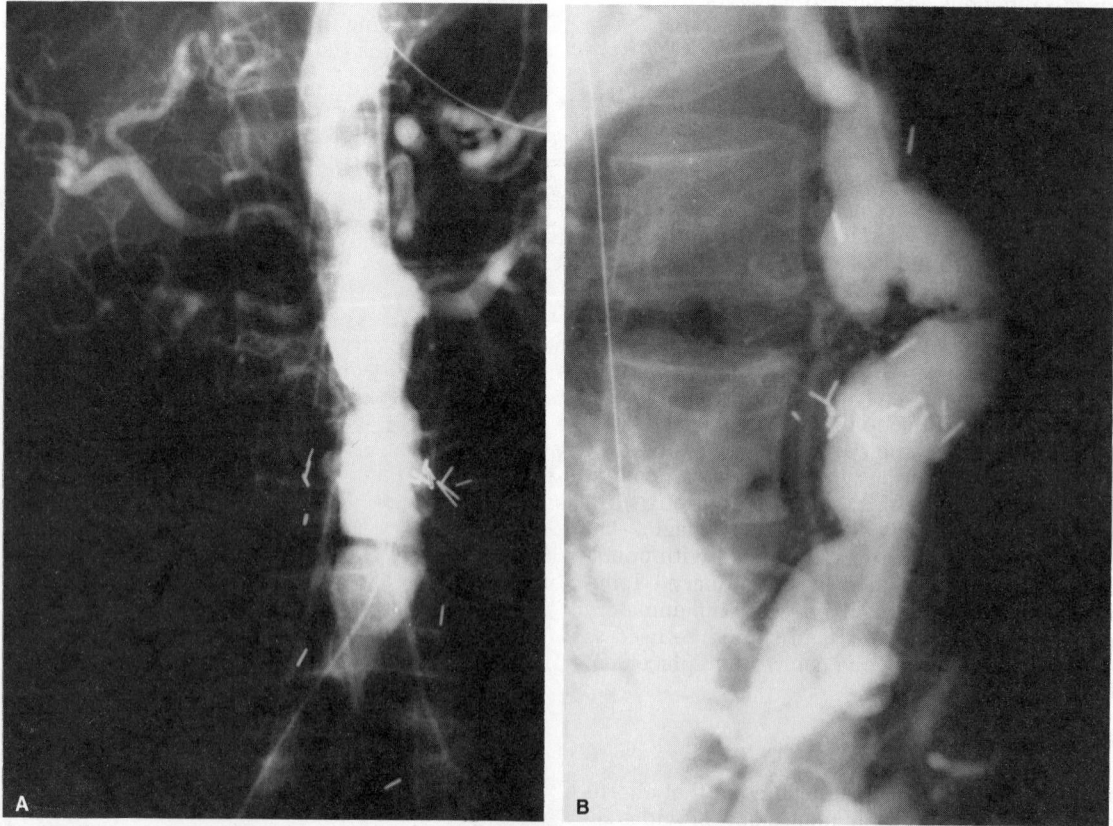

Figure 78-5. Anteroposterior (*A*) and lateral (*B*) aortograms of an interposition graft 11 months after aortic endoaneurysmorrhaphy. False aneurysm is present at the distal anastomosis with kinking of the graft. Graft-enteric erosion was found at operation.

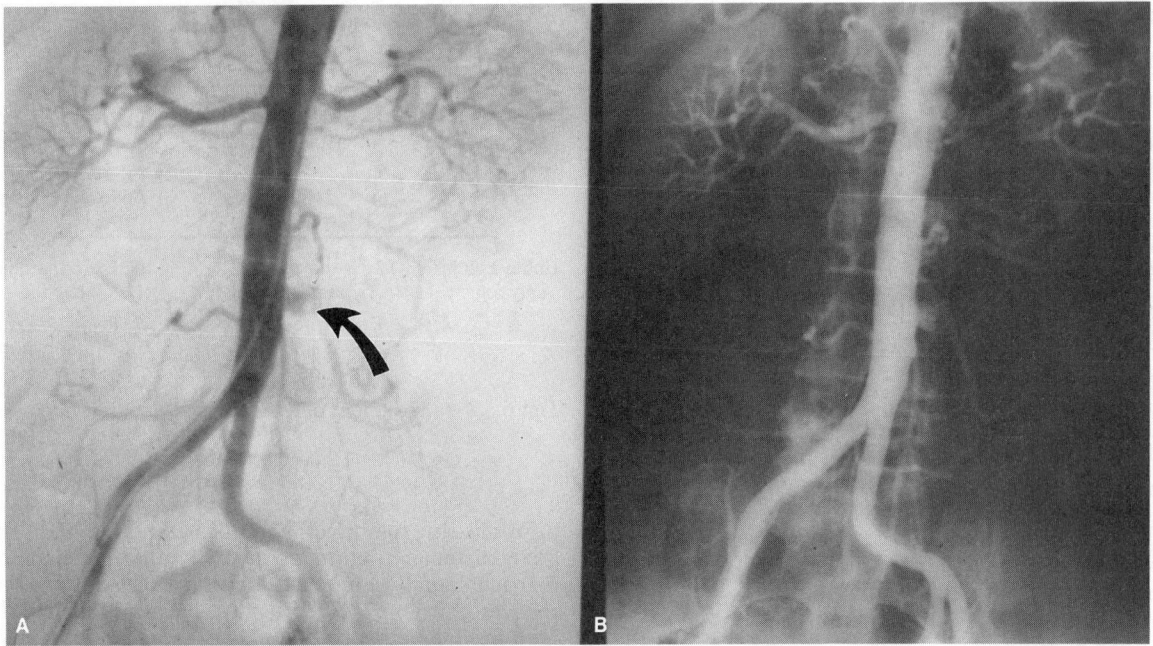

Figure 78-6. Positive (*A*) and negative (*B*) aortograms demonstrating two mycotic aneurysms (*arrows*) in a patient with streptococcal septicemia.

infections, angiography is used to aid in planning surgical therapy and to answer specific questions posed by results of clinical examination or CT and MRI. If the facilities are available, intraarterial digital subtraction arteriography is the preferred initial angiographic technique.

Functional Imaging Techniques

Radionuclide scans using ^{99m}Tc-labeled leukocytes, ^{111}In-labeled leukocytes, or polyclonal human IgG show accumulation at sites of infection. Although used extensively to diagnose prosthetic graft infections, functional imaging studies do not reliably predict infection because of the low specificity of the test, particularly in the early postoperative period.[26] False-positive accumulation of ac-

tivity can occur in hematomas, pseudoaneurysms, tumors, and other sites of inflammation. False-negative studies are unusual, so exclusion of early perigraft infection is possible, but normal studies have been reported in late-appearing aortic graft infections complicated by GEF or GEE. IgG scans are preferred over leukocyte scans because of ease of preparation, lack of staff exposure to patient blood, absence of concomitant erythrocyte and platelet imaging, and long shelf life. Functional imaging studies can be used with MRI and CT imaging to accurately delineate the extent of infection. In asymptomatic patients after aortic graft placement, the finding of a positive radioisotope scan but normal CT imaging indicates a low-grade infection, and parenteral antibiotic administration followed by

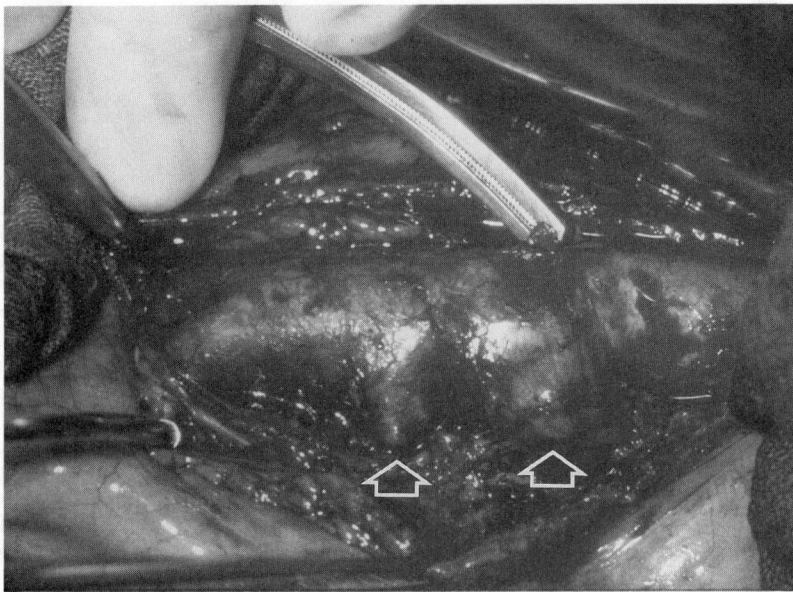

Figure 78-7. Operative appearance of mycotic aneurysms (*arrows*) visualized by the aortograms in Figure 78-6.

careful, serial patient examination is recommended. Accuracy of radioisotope scans has not been evaluated in confirming the diagnosis of infected aneurysm.

Microbiologic Testing

Recovery of microorganisms from sites of suspected vascular infection is necessary to confirm the diagnosis and to select antibiotic therapy. Appropriate microbiologic culture technique is important for the reliable recovery of anaerobic bacteria, fungi, and coagulase-negative staphylococci from vascular prostheses. Gram stain of tissue or perigraft fluid showing no organisms is not sufficient to exclude the presence of infection. Low numbers and virulence of infecting microorganisms, concomitant antibiotic administration, absence of tissue invasion, surface biofilm formation on prosthetic surfaces, and activation of host defenses contribute to the sampling error of routine culture techniques. Use of tryptic soy broth media and mechanical (tissue grinding) or ultrasonic disruption of explanted tissue or graft material reliably increases the recovery of microorganisms.[17,27] Culture tubes containing graft/tissue specimens should be maintained for 5 to 7 days to exclude growth of coagulase-negative staphylococci.

Principles of Management

Mycotic aneurysms and most vascular graft infections are uniformly fatal if not treated by aggressive surgical and antibiotic therapy. The spectrum of vascular infection requires surgeons to individualize therapy based on the clinical presentation of the patient and the anatomic and microbiologic characteristics of the infectious process (Figs 78-8 and 78-9). The quantity and virulence of pathogens, adequacy of local and systemic host defense mechanisms, and extent of the infectious process are critical factors that influence outcome. Residual arterial infection is the major cause of morbidity and mortality and the reason local treatment methods and in situ grafting procedures often fail. Local control of infection is more successful when gross purulence is absent, cultures are negative, or *S epidermidis* is recovered. Infections caused by gram-negative organisms, especially *Salmonella* sp and *Pseudomonas aeruginosa,* are associated with a high incidence (more than 50%) of rupture, morbidity, and operative mortality (Table 78-3).

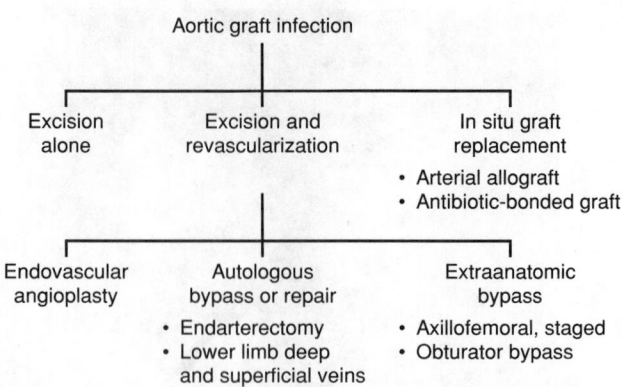

Figure 78-9. Treatment options for vascular graft infections.

Eradicating the infectious process and maintaining adequate distal circulation are the two important principles of management. Systemic antibiotics bacteriocidal to bacteria recovered from blood or wound cultures, aspirated perigraft fluid, or expected pathogens should be administered. Patients must be physiologically and psychologically prepared for operation. Surgical control of infection is a priority when sepsis is present because antibiotic administration alone is insufficient. In cases of ruptured aneurysms or graft-enteric fistula, operation should be undertaken immediately. The infected artery, aneurysm, or vascular graft must be totally excised and arterial reconstruction, if necessary, meticulously performed as either a staged or simultaneous procedure. Wide débridement of infected tissues, including the artery adjacent to the infection, antibiotic irrigation and placement of drains, reconstruction of vital arteries through uninfected tissue planes, and prolonged postoperative antibiotic administration are established surgical tenets. Total excision of infected prosthetic grafts is associated with the lowest incidence of persistent or recurrent infection. If a vascular infection can be excised without limb or organ loss, this treatment option is always preferred. In situ graft replacement (autologous vein, arterial homograft, antibiotic-impregnated prosthesis) is best suited for treating lower-grade, late-appearing infections without extensive perivascular infection.

Aorta

For infrarenal aortic infections, preliminary axillobifemoral bypass is the preferred initial procedure in hemodynamically stable patients if the diagnosis can be established.[33,36,37] This approach avoids lower limb ischemia and the necessity to keep the patient heparinized during excision of the aortic aneurysm or graft and closure of the aortic stump. The aorta should be débrided to normal-appearing tissue and closed using monofilament sutures. A pedicle of omentum is carefully positioned around the aortic stump and bed of excised aorta and graft (Fig. 78-10). Closed suction drains are left in the retroperitoneum and brought out of the flank opposite the axillofemoral graft. Collected series over the past two decades strongly support the strategy of resection and remote bypass, but reoperation for extraanatomic graft complications (thrombosis, infection) and residual aortic infection manifest as aortic stump blowout remain major problems in treating infected aortic aneurysm and grafts (Table 78-4).

In situ prosthetic reconstruction has been used successfully in carefully selected patients with both primary and secondary aortic infections, but relapsing infection is common with gram-negative infections, especially *Salmonella.*

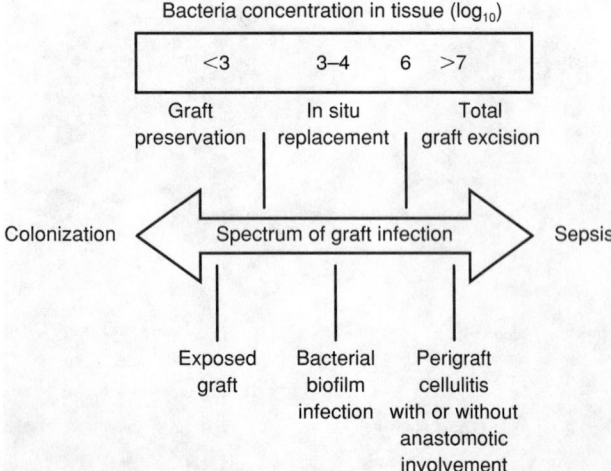

Figure 78-8. The spectrum of vascular graft infection. Clinical manifestation and treatment options depend on the bacteria virulence and concentration in tissue.

Table 78-3. OUTCOME OF TREATED MYCOTIC ANEURYSMS

Study	Etiology	Location (No.) Aorta	Location (No.) Peripheral	Prevalent Pathogen	Survivors
Jarrett et al, 1975[28]	Infected AAA	12	—	Staphylococcus Salmonella	7 [59%]
Wilson et al, 1978[7]	Endocarditis	8	18	Streptococcus Staphylococcus	18 (75%)
Mendelowitz, 1979	Bacteremia	25	—	Salmonella	5 (25%)
Brown et al, 1984[10]	Bacteremia	4	6	S aureus	6 (60%)
Taylor et al, 1988[30]	Infected AAA	5	—	Staphylococcus Salmonella	5 (100%)
Chan et al, 1989[29]	Infected AAA	22	—	S aureus Salmonella	19 (86%)
Atnip, 1989	Bacteremia	21	—	Salmonella	16 (72%)
Oz et al, 1989[35]	Bacteremia	21	—	Salmonella Staphylococcus	13 (62%)
Feldman & Berguer, 1983[31]	Drug abuse	—	53	S aureus	52 (2%)
Johnson et al, 1983[32]	Drug abuse	—	52	S aureus	52 (100%)
Reddy et al, 1986[33]	Drug abuse	—	54	S aureus	54 (100%)

AAA, abdominal aortic aneurysm.

In the absence of gross purulence and sepsis, or when a low-grade infection is encountered (ie, Gram stain is negative for bacteria; coagulase-negative staphylococci are suspected as the infecting pathogen; adjacent artery wall is normal), in situ reconstruction using autologous reconstruction may be preferable to remote bypass using a prosthetic graft.[38,39] This treatment option, which uses either arterial allograft or splices segments of lower extremity veins together, is not feasible in all patients. The procedures are technically demanding and associated with perioperative morbidity similar to total graft excision and ex situ bypass. Benefits of this approach include a reduced amputation rate, no aortic stump rupture, and avoidance of late complications (thrombosis, infection) of ex situ bypasses; however, reoperation for vein graft/allograft stricture or thrombosis has been required in one third of patients. In situ graft replacement has been used successfully to treat both primary and secondary aortoenteric fistula. Patients with GEE and minimal retroperitoneal infection fared best, particularly when treatment included débridement of the proximal aorta to histologically normal wall before graft replacement and interposition of the greater omentum between the graft and bowel. Long-term survival can be expected in 75% of patients, and the incidence of

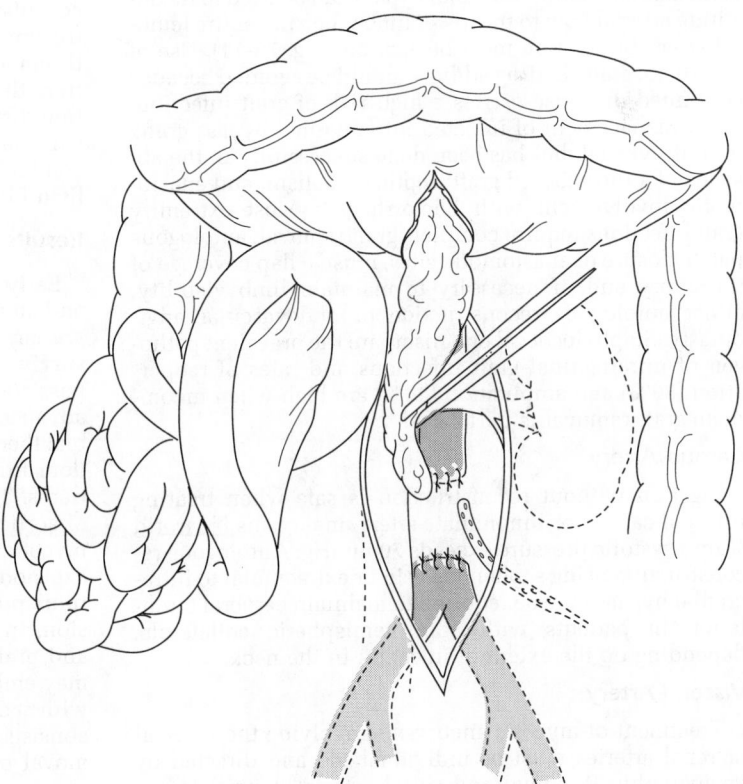

Figure 78-10. Schematic representation of the retroperitoneum after excision of an aortic mycotic aneurysm or infected aortic graft and closure of the aorta. Pedicle of omentum is brought through transverse mesocolon and interposed between the aortic stump and bowel. Closed suction drain is placed in the graft bed and brought out the left flank.

Table 78-4. OUTCOME OF TREATED AORTIC GRAFT INFECTIONS

Investigators	Cases	Operative Mortality Rate (%)	Results		1-Year Survival Rate (%)
			Amputation (%)	Stump Blowout	
GRAFT EXCISION AND EXTRAANATOMIC BYPASS OR AUTOLOGOUS RECONSTRUCTION					
Bandyk et al, 1984[17]	18	11	11	0/14	66
O'Hara et al, 1986[18]	84	18	27	13/58	58
Reilly et al, 1987[19]	92	14	14	9/70	73
Schmitt et al, 1990[36]	20	15	5	1/16	75
Yeager et al, 1993[34]	38	26	10	1/28	77
Bunt, 1990[42]	22	9	14	—	—
IN SITU GRAFT REPLACEMENT (GRAFT, VEIN, ALLOGRAFT)				**Reinfection**	
Walker et al, 1987[20]	23	22	0	3/15	75
Clagett et al, 1993[38]	17	10	10	0/20	80
Kieffer et al, 1993[39]	43	12	0	2/36	78
Towne et al, 1994[43]*	20	0	0	2/20	90

* Late-appearing *Staphylococcus epidermidis* biofilm graft infections.

late graft infection and thrombosis is low. When infection involves thoracic or suprarenal aorta and its branches, in situ graft replacement is the only practical approach. Use of a rifampin-impregnated Dacron graft is recommended when staphylococcal organisms are involved.[40] Successful outcome has been reported in patients with gram-negative infection, including *Salmonella* after in situ prosthetic reconstruction, accompanied by thorough drainage and débridement, prolonged parenteral antibiotic therapy, and permanent suppressive oral antibiotics.

Femoropopliteal Arterial Segment

Collateral circulation is usually sufficient to maintain limb viability after excision and ligation of infected femoral artery aneurysms, particularly if limited to a single arterial segment that is common, superficial, or deep. Autologous reconstruction using saphenous vein or the extraanatomic obturator canal bypass can be used to reconstitute arterial flow to the lower limb when the entire femoral artery bifurcation must be excised (Fig. 78-11). Use of prosthetic grafts in drug addicts should be avoided because continued drug use carries a high risk of graft infection. Local management of infected infrainguinal bypass grafts is controversial, but has been done successfully in the absence of a thrombosed graft, septic embolism, and anastomotic involvement with hemorrhage.[42] Most extremity graft infections require complete graft removal, autologous patch closure of anastomotic sites, muscle flap coverage of the artery and, if necessary to maintain limb viability, either autologous reconstruction or endovascular angioplasty. Staphylococcal organisms are the prevalent pathogen of infrainguinal graft infections and rates of reoperation (80%) and amputation (40%) are high when incomplete graft removal is performed.[44]

Carotid Artery

Ligation without reconstruction is safe when treating infected carotid or innominate artery aneurysms if carotid stump systolic pressure exceeds 70 mmHg. Autologous reconstruction using saphenous vein or extracranial to intracranial bypass may be required to maintain cerebral circulation in patients with poor hemispheric collaterals, depending on the extent of infection in the neck.

Visceral Artery

Treatment of mycotic aneurysms involving the visceral or renal arteries must be individualized and directed by angiography. Proximal and distal arterial control is obtained and the aneurysm excised if possible. Endoaneurysmorrhaphy with oversewing of the orifices of afferent and efferent vessels should be used when excision is not possible and for treatment of saccular aneurysms without purulence. This technique produces less damage to the collateral blood supply. Aneurysm excision and ligation of superior mesenteric, hepatic, celiac, and splenic arteries is the preferred procedure. Renal artery reconstruction is required to maintain organ function without exception.

Suppurative Thrombophlebitis

Wide excision of the infected vein to normal-appearing, patent vein and débridement of all devitalized tissue are required for local control of the infection. Surgical wounds should be left open and packed with sterile, saline-soaked gauze. Secondary closure is performed when the infection is resolved and granulation tissue develops. Systemic anticoagulation with heparin is a necessary component of treatment, with antibiotic administration for suppurative thrombophlebitis involving deep veins of the pelvis or extremities. If pulmonary septic emboli develop, venous ligation distal to the infected deep venous segment should be considered. Favorable results have also been obtained by combining surgical drainage or thrombotomy and Greenfield filter insertion (see Chap. 97).

Results and Late Outcome

Early diagnosis coupled with careful evaluation before and after surgery to assess etiology and extent of infection are key elements for successful treatment and long-term survival. Results after both excision and extraanatomic bypass and in situ reconstruction have improved because of advances in surgical technique and prolonged antimicrobial therapy (see Table 78-4). Long-term survival with freedom from infection can be expected in over 75% of patients. The amputation rate is 5% to 10% after treatment of aortic infections, 11% to 17% after excision of femoral mycotic aneurysm in drug addicts, and 30% to 50% after excision of infected infrainguinal bypass grafts. If the infectious process can be eradicated with artery or graft excision, in situ replacement using implantation techniques and graft material that minimizes bacterial colonization may emerge as the preferred treatment option. In patients with secondary aortoenteric fistula, the optimal treatment consists of extraanatomic revascularization followed by removal of the infected graft. Vascular infections will decrease as surgeons develop a clearer understanding of etio-

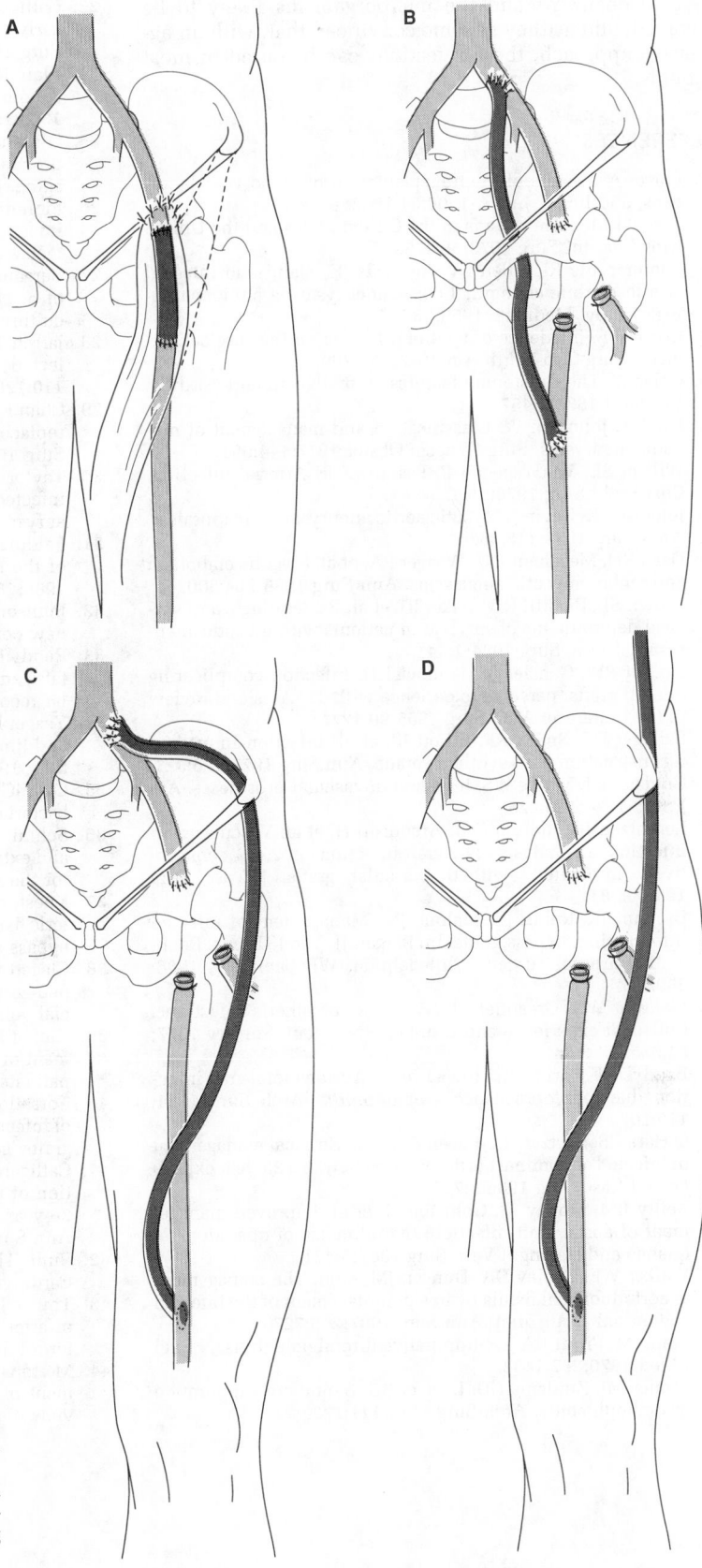

Figure 78-11. Methods of femoral artery reconstruction after excision and ligation of femoral mycotic aneurysm. (*A*) Interposition vein autograft with sartorius muscle flap coverage. (*B*) Obturator bypass. (*C*) Lateral femoral bypass. (*D*) Unilateral axillofemoral bypass. (After Reddy DJ, Smith RF, Elliott JP Jr, et al. Infected femoral artery false aneurysms in drug addicts: evolution of selective vascular reconstruction. J Vasc Surg 1986;3:718)

logic mechanisms and the microorganisms likely to be involved, and as they become convinced that, with an aggressive approach, these infections can be cured in most patients.

REFERENCES

1. Carrel A. Results of the transplantation of blood vessels, organs, and limbs. JAMA 1908;51:1662.
2. Farooki MA. Aneurysms in the United States and the United Kingdom. Int Surg 1973;58:475.
3. Sommerville RI, Allen EV, Edwards JE. Bland and infected arteriosclerotic abdominal aortic aneurysms: a clinicopathologic study. Medicine 1959;38:207.
4. Cruse PJE. Incidence of wound infection on the surgical services. Surg Clin North Am 1973;55:1269.
5. Osler W. The Gulstonian lectures on malignant endocarditis. Br Med J 1885;1:467.
6. Patel S, Johnston W. Classification and management of mycotic aneurysms. Surg Gynecol Obstet 1977;144:691.
7. Wilson SE, VanWagenen P, Passaro E Jr. Arterial infection. Curr Probl Surg 1978;15:1.
8. Johansen K, Devin J. Mycotic aortic aneurysms: a reappraisal. Arch Surg 1983;118:583.
9. Dean RH, Meacham PW, Weaver FA, et al. Mycotic embolism and embolomycotic aneurysms. Ann Surg 1986;204:300.
10. Brown SL, Busittil RW, Baker JD, et al. Bacteriologic and surgical determinants of survival in patients with mycotic aneurysms. J Vasc Surg 1984;1:541.
11. Hoffert PW, Gensler S, Haimovici H. Infection complicating arterial grafts: personal experience with 12 cases and review of the literature. Arch Surg 1965;90:427.
12. Szilagyi DE, Smith RF, Elliott JP, et al. Infection in arterial reconstruction with synthetic grafts. Ann Surg 1972;176:321.
13. Goldstone J, Moore WS. Infection in vascular prostheses. Am J Surg 1974;128:225.
14. Lorentzen JE, Nielsen OM, Arendrup H, et al. Vascular graft infection: an analysis of 62 graft infections in 2,411 consecutively implanted synthetic vascular grafts. J Vasc Surg 1985;98:81.
15. Durham JR, Rubin JR, Malone JM. Management of infected infrainguinal bypass grafts. In: Bergan JJ, Yao JST, eds. Reoperative arterial surgery. Philadelphia, WB Saunders, 1986:359.
16. Liekweg WG, Greenfield LJ. Vascular prosthetic infections. Collected experience and results of treatment. Surgery 1977;81:335.
17. Bandyk DF, Berni GA, Thiele L, et al. Aortofemoral graft infection due to Staphylococcus epidermidis. Arch Surg 1984;119:102.
18. O'Hara CS, Hertzer NR, Beven EG, et al. Surgical management of infected abdominal aortic grafts: review of a 25-year experience. J Vasc Surg 1986;3:725.
19. Reilly LM, Stoney RJ, Goldstone J, et al. Improved management of aortic graft infection: the influence of operation sequence and staging. J Vasc Surg 1987;5:421.
20. Walker WE, Cooley DA, Duncan JM, et al. The management of aortoduodenal fistula by in situ replacement of the infected abdominal aortic graft. Ann Surg 1987;205:727.
21. Stein JM, Pruitt BA Jr. Suppurative thrombophlebitis. N Engl J Med 1970;282:1452.
22. Zinner MJ, Zuidema GD, Lowery BD. Septic nonsuppurative thrombophlebitis. Arch Surg 1976;111:122.
23. Calligaro KD, Veith FJ, Schwartz ML, et al. Differences in early versus late extracavitary arterial graft infections. J Vasc Surg 1995;22:680.
24. Blair RH, Resnik MD, Polga JP. CT appearance of mycotic abdominal aortic aneurysms. J Comput Assist Tomogr 1989;13:101.
25. Olofsson PA, Auffermann W, Higgins CB, et al. Diagnosis of prosthetic aortic graft infection by magnetic resonance imaging. J Vasc Surg 1988;8:99.
26. Fiorani P, Speziale F, Rizzo L, et al. Detection of aortic graft infection with leukocytes labelled with technetium 99m hexametazime. J Vasc Surg 1993;17:87.
27. Bergamini TM, Bandyk DF, Govostis D, et al. Identification of S. epidermidis vascular graft infections: a comparison of culture techniques. J Vasc Surg 1989;9:665.
28. Jarrett F, Darling RC, Mundth ED, et al. Experience with infected aneurysm of the abdominal aorta. Arch Surg 1975;110:1281.
29. Chan FY, Crawford ES, Coselli JS, et al. In situ prosthetic graft replacement for mycotic aneurysm of the aorta. Ann Thorac Surg 1989;47:193.
30. Taylor LM Jr, Deitz DM, McConnell DB, et al. Treatment of infected abdominal aneurysms by extraanatomic bypass, aneurysm excision, and drainage. Am J Surg 1988;155:655.
31. Feldman AJ, Berguer R. Management of an infected aneurysm of the groin secondary to drug abuse. Surg Gynecol Obstet 1983;157:519.
32. Johnson JR, Ledgerwood AM, Lucas CE. Mycotic aneurysm: new concepts in therapy. Arch Surg 1983;118:577.
33. Reddy DJ, Smith RF, Elliott JP Jr, et al. Infected femoral artery false aneurysms in drug addicts: evolution of selective vascular reconstruction. J Vasc Surg 1986;3:718.
34. Yeager RA, Moneta GL, Taylor LM Jr, et al. Improving survival and limb salvage in patients with aortic graft infection. Am J Surg 1990;159:466.
35. Oz, MC, Brener BJ, Buda JA, et al. A ten-year experience with bacterial aortitis. J Vasc Surg 1989;10:439.
36. Schmitt DD, Seabrook GR, Bandyk DF, et al. Graft excision and extra-anatomic revascularization: the treatment of choice for the septic aortic prosthesis. J Cardiovasc Surg 1990;327.
37. Kuestner LM, Reilly LM, Jicha DL, et al. Secondary aortoenteric fistula: contemporary outcome with use of extraanatomic bypass and infected graft excision. J Vasc Surg 195;21:184.
38. Clagett GP, Bowers L, Lopez-Viego MA, et al. Creation of a neo-aortoiliac system from lower extremity deep and superficial veins. Ann Surg 1993;218:239.
39. Kieffer E, Bahnini A, Koskas F, et al. In situ allograft replacement of infected aortic prosthetic grafts: results in forty-three patients. J Vasc Surg 1993;17:349.
40. Torsello G, Sandmann W, Gehrt A, et al. In situ replacement of infected vascular prostheses with rifampin-soaked vascular grafts: early results. J Vasc Surg 1993;17:768.
41. Calligaro KD, Veith FJ, Schwartz ML, et al. Selective preservation of infected prosthetic grafts arterial grafts: analysis of a 20-year experience with 120 extracavitary-infected grafts. Ann Surg 1994;220:461.
42. Bunt TJ. Vascular graft infection: a personal experience. Cardiovasc Surg 1993;1:489.
43. Towne JB, Seabrook GR, Bandyk DF, et al. In situ replacement of arterial prostheses infected with bacterial biofilms: long-term followup. J Vasc Surg 1994;19:226.
44. Mertens RA, O'Hara PJ, Hertzer NR, et al. Surgical management of infrainguinal arterial prosthetic graft infections: review of a 35-year experience. J Vasc Surg 1995;21:782.

SURGERY: SCIENTIFIC PRINCIPLES AND PRACTICE, Second Edition, edited by Lazar J. Greenfield, Michael W. Mulholland, Keith T. Oldham, Gerald B. Zelenock, and Keith D. Lillemoe. Lippincott–Raven Publishers, Philadelphia, © 1997.

CHAPTER 79

ENDOVASCULAR SURGICAL TECHNIQUES

RODNEY A. WHITE

Endovascular surgical therapy is a minimally invasive procedure that has the potential to revascularize ischemic tissues, avoiding the morbidity and cost of major operations. This development is particularly beneficial for patients who have significant cardiovascular disease since they have a higher morbidity and mortality associated with surgery.[1] A theoretical and controversial advantage of endovascular therapy is its use to treat lesions that produce minor symptoms such as claudication that are not normally considered indications for conventional operations. Endovascular therapy has a limited but potentially expanding role in the treatment of vascular disease.

Removing arterial occlusions by an endoluminal approach was one of the first methods devised by surgeons to treat atherosclerotic disease. Plaque removal was accomplished by techniques that enabled endovascular endarterectomy, such as metal strippers, or by intramural or intraplaque introduction of gas to separate the lesion from the vessel wall. Radiologists and cardiologists have focused primarily on enlarging the vessel lumen by dilating the vessel, compacting the lesions, or lysing constituents. In comparison with dilatation, endarterectomy yields a more durable repair. For endarterectomy, 30% to 60% recurrences of longer lesions are reported at 5 years for occluded superficial femoral arteries, whereas 20% to 30% of balloon dilatations of similar lesions restenose at 1 year.

Many surgeons are skeptical of the value of endovascular angioplasty devices, believing that the patency rates reported for endarterectomy represent the best estimate of the potential for the new technologies and that these results are inadequate when compared with patencies obtained from reconstructive operations. Certain lesions respond favorably to endarterectomy, and many surgeons prefer this approach in these sites. Patency rates for endarterectomy of isolated lesions in large-diameter vessels such as the iliac artery are comparable to bypasses. In some settings (eg, carotid bifurcation), endarterectomy is preferred.

An analysis of the potential patency of endovascular procedures compared with survival of high-risk cardiovascular patients suggests that potential benefit might be derived by appropriate use of this technology. Comparing the incidence of reocclusion (about 10% per year for endarterectomized arteries) to the 10% death rate per year in this group of symptomatic patients, most patients could be maintained by minimal, low-risk endovascular procedures, with recurrent symptomatic lesions managed by an alternative method. Endoluminal devices also have the potential to treat arterial disease in locations such as small-diameter vessels (2 to 4 mm) where methods such as prostheses, thrombolytics, and rheologic agents have particularly poor results. Autogenous vein bypasses also remain an option in this setting.

Endovascular surgical procedures can be used to treat selected lesions, and successful recanalizations are limited by early recurrence. Improved guidance techniques, including angioscopy and intraluminal ultrasound, reduce failures in two ways—by eliminating initial failures caused either by perforations or by an inability to cross the lesions and also by improving removal of lesions so that hemodynamics are restored while preserving sufficient vessel wall to prevent aneurysm formation. Achieving long-term patency of endarterectomy-like recanalizations comparable to conventional reconstructions using autogenous vein awaits the ability to control the fundamental cellular mechanisms causing recurrences.

DISTRIBUTION OF ATHEROSCLEROTIC LESIONS TO THE APPLICATION AND DEVELOPMENT OF ENDOVASCULAR INTERVENTIONAL METHODS

Atherosclerosis occurs initially in areas of low shear stress, in transition sites, and at the orifices and bifurcations of branch arteries. Some 70% of both coronary and peripheral lesions develop in an eccentric position within the vessel so that the residual lumen is usually off center in relation to the walls of the artery[2] (Fig. 79-1).

Conventional vascular reconstructions bypass heavily diseased or occluded arterial segments by connecting relatively normal areas proximal and distal to the lesions. Endarterectomy relies on the eccentric, usually posterior, localization of lesions so that complete removal can be accomplished through an incision in the anterior surface of the artery, removing the plaque with a smooth transition to the adjacent luminal surface. Eccentric positioning of the atherosclerotic lesions within the artery wall predisposes to controlled fracture of the thinner portion of the plaque by balloon dilatation, displacing most of the mass to create a neolumen[3] (Fig. 79-2).

An additional factor that enhances the success of transluminal recanalizations beyond what might be estimated from preintervention angiography is the localized nature of atherosclerotic lesions in the artery. Clot and softer organized material fills the lumen proximal and distal to the lesion up to the site of patent branch arteries (Fig. 79-3). Thus, most long occlusions on angiography have significant portions of the vessel obstructed by acute and chronic thrombosis. For this reason, the length of many vascular lesions can be markedly reduced by thrombolytic therapy. The significant component of soft material in an arterial occlusion also enables guide wires to pass across long obstructions. The success rates of devices are enhanced by this factor, whereas failures are related to imprecise passage and guidance of devices and inadequate debulking of

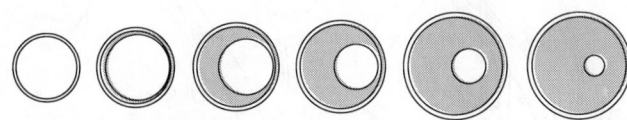

Figure 79-1. Diagrammatic representation of a possible sequence of changes in atherosclerotic arteries leading eventually to lumen narrowing. The artery enlarges initially (left to right in diagram) in association with plaque accumulation to maintain an adequate, if not normal, lumen area. Early stages of lesion development may be associated with overcompensation. At more than 40% stenosis, however, the plaque area continues to increase to involve the entire circumference of the vessel, and the artery no longer enlarges at a rate sufficient to prevent narrowing of the lumen. (After Glagov S, Weisenberg E, Zarins C, et al. Compensatory enlargement of human atherosclerotic coronary arteries. N Engl J Med 1987;316:1374)

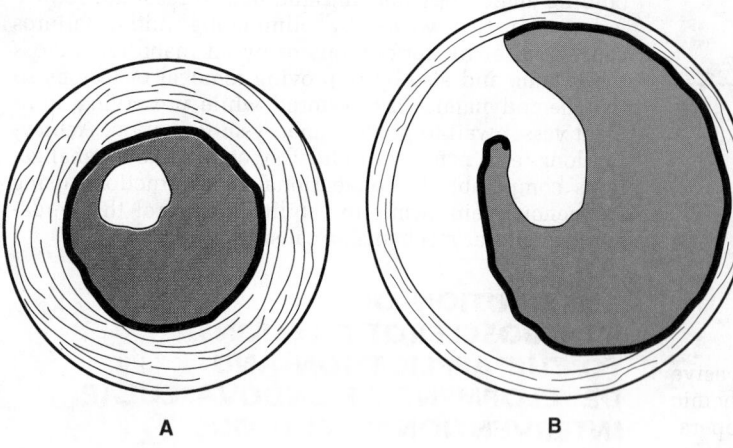

Figure 79-2. Mechanism of balloon dilatation of an arterial stenosis. (*A*) Eccentric atherosclerotic arterial lesion. (*B*) The weakest point of the eccentric lesion is fractured and displaced by expansion of the balloon.

lesions in segments occluded by fibrotic or calcified material (Fig. 79-4). The following discussions highlight this principle as a limiting factor that requires special attention in the development of new devices.

INTRALUMINAL ACCESS TECHNIQUES

Access to the artery being treated by an endovascular device may be gained by percutaneous catheter techniques or by intraoperative exposure and opening of the vessel. Percutaneous vascular access is usually obtained by the Seldinger technique. A beveled needle is introduced through the arterial wall through a small skin incision to facilitate subsequent insertion of vessel dilators and instruments. The needle is slowly withdrawn until the return of arterial blood is achieved. A guide wire is then introduced

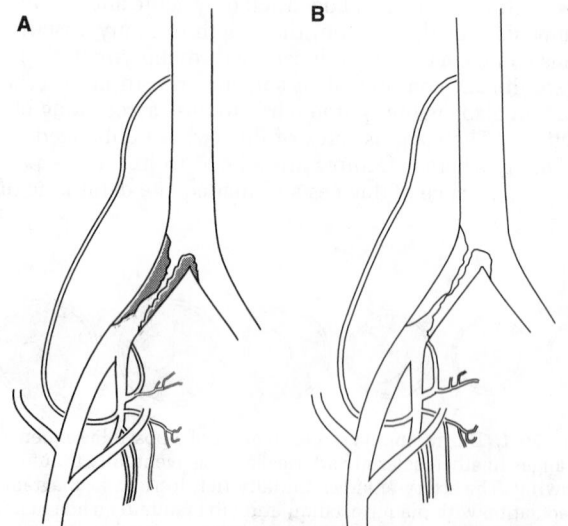

Figure 79-3. (*A*) Schematic drawing of a localized fibrocalcific atherosclerotic lesion in the right common iliac artery. (*B*) Occlusion of the artery proximal and distal to the lesion with clot and softer organized thrombus (*blue area*) to the site of patent branch arteries. (After White RA, White GH. The atherosclerotic lesion and balloon angioplasty. In: Color atlas of endovascular surgery. London, Chapman & Hall, 1990:13)

through the lumen of the needle and positioned under fluoroscopic control. For many procedures, an introducer sheath is threaded over the guide wire after passage of a vascular dilator. The diameter of the sheath is determined by the size of the device to be passed through the sheath lumen into the artery.

Access for many percutaneous procedures is obtained by cannulation of the common femoral artery. Lesions of the infrarenal aorta, iliac bifurcation, and iliac arteries are most effectively approached by ipsilateral retrograde puncture of the femoral artery. Lesions of the infrainguinal vessels are frequently approached antegrade by way of the ipsilateral femoral artery. Lesions close to the femoral puncture site require careful consideration to determine the best access. A contralateral approach may often be preferred for treating lesions of the distal external iliac artery, common femoral artery, or proximal segments of the superficial femoral and profunda arteries. Alternative entry approaches include the axillary, brachial, superficial femoral, and popliteal arteries or direct puncture of bypass grafts. Puncture of the external iliac artery above the inguinal ligament may facilitate antegrade access to the femoral vessels, but is associated with a risk of retroperitoneal hemorrhage.

Guide wires establish a channel through lesions and facilitate introduction and atraumatic passage and exchange of endovascular devices. The ideal guide wire is atraumatic and steerable and passes with minimal resistance. The guide wire must transmit torque readily, while having strength to cross the lesion and then to provide a sturdy track for the treatment device to follow. Wire strength and stiffness are closely related to diameter.

There are several types of guide wires. A standard guide wire consists of a solid wire core inside and an outer spiral wire. A Teflon coating is usually applied to reduce friction. These wires are nonsteerable, of varying stiffness, and frequently have a distal taper, which gives flexibility to the tip. J-shaped guide wires may have a movable inner core that can be retracted or extended to allow the tip to bend, soften, or extend. Floppy-tip guide wires have no core wire in the distal 10 to 15 cm, conveying maximum flexibility. Steerable guide wires combine an angulated distal tip with a stiff proximal shaft to transmit torque. An exchange wire is longer (145 to 260 cm) to allow withdrawal and insertion of devices without moving the distal portion of the wire from a secure position through a lesion. Hydrophilic guide wires or so-called slippery or eel wires are coated with a polymer that make them slick when wet. This characteristic results in low friction between the guide wire and ath-

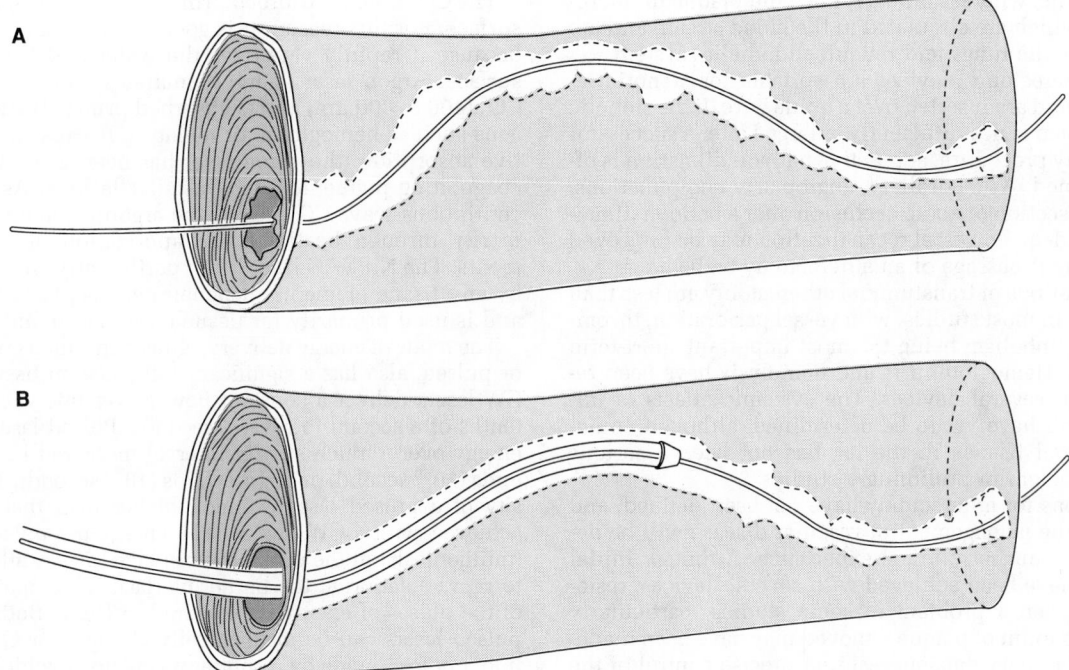

Figure 79-4. Placement of a guide wire through the meandering, eccentric lumen of an atherosclerotic vessel (*A*) limits the ability of a device passed over the guide wire (*B*) to adequately remove the lesion without causing vessel wall perforation as a result of being maintained in the eccentric position by the guide wire.

erosclerotic lesions and facilitates passage of another catheter or device over the wire. Angiographic delivery or guiding catheters are small-diameter tubes used to introduce or exchange guide wires and inject contrast material. To traverse difficult lesions, a fine guide wire is frequently passed through the lesion, followed by an angiography catheter over this wire. The thin guide wire is then easily exchanged by way of the catheter for a more substantial wire that supports and directs a device more effectively.

ENDOVASCULAR SURGICAL DEVICES AND TECHNIQUES

Transluminal Dilation

Transluminal dilation of stenotic atherosclerotic arterial lesions was initially advocated by Dotter in 1964. Dilatation was performed using successively larger coaxial polyethylene catheters (ie, a 12F catheter over an 8F catheter). Staple and van Andel later used tapered catheters to reduce trauma to the arterial wall caused by the blunt-tipped devices Dotter used.

Dotter subsequently postulated that balloon dilatation of an atherosclerotic lesion might effectively enlarge the lumen. In 1965, he successfully dilated a stenosed iliac artery using a Fogarty balloon embolectomy catheter. The concept of balloon dilatation was advanced by Gruntzig in 1974 using a double-lumen polyvinyl balloon catheter. Subsequent design modifications include the development of stronger noncompliant, nonelastomeric balloons that can withstand inflation pressures of 12 to 15 atm without distorting shape or overstretching diameter. Increased catheter flexibility and decreased catheter diameters have improved the maneuverability of the devices and the ability to cross tight stenotic regions, including those in small tortuous arteries of the lower leg and coronary circulation.

After placement of the balloon at the site of an athero-sclerotic narrowing, the weakest point in the plaque is fractured by expansion of the balloon, enlarging the arterial lumen.[3] Measurements of pressure gradients across a lesion before and after dilatations are helpful in determining the success of an angioplasty procedure. Residual gradients greater than 20 mmHg suggest that inadequate flow has been achieved. Pressure gradients across a lesion may be measured simultaneously with dual catheters or separately by measuring the pressure as a catheter is passed through the lesion.

Balloon angioplasty is especially effective for localized, short stenotic lesions or short-length occlusions of the iliac arteries, with about 90% initial recanalization and long-term patency of 60% to 70% at 4 years.[4] Percutaneous balloon angioplasty of infrainguinal arterial disease is not as effective as for aortoiliac disease; about 10% of patients becoming clinically worse if the procedure fails. Factors that predict success are short, localized lesions with patent arteries in the distal vascular bed. In general, satisfactory results can be obtained if patients are selected carefully.

Balloon angioplasty is also used to treat disease in the branches of the abdominal aorta, particularly the renal and mesenteric arteries. Renovascular disease is amenable to dilatation if there is a short, focal stenosis of the renal artery that does not involve the ostium. Lesions of the orifice of the renal artery formed by an extension of aortic plaque are less favorable and more difficult to treat successfully, as are totally occlusive lesions of the renal artery.

Atherectomy

Atherectomy devices are designed to remove atherosclerotic plaque from the vessel by cutting, drilling, or pulverizing atheroma. This produces a luminal surface different from balloon dilatation or open surgical endarterectomy. Some atherectomy devices have mechanisms for extracting the fragments, whereas others reduce the plaque to micro-particles, which are circulated in the blood stream and are removed by the lungs and reticuloendothelial system.

Most atherectomy devices are suitable for stenotic lesions only and are inserted over a guide wire. If the stenotic arterial lumen is not sufficiently enlarged after a successful atherectomy procedure, adjunctive balloon dilatation is often performed. As a corollary, angioplasty complications, such as dissection or acute occlusion after a balloon dilatation, or inadequate vessel recanalization may be improved by subsequent passage of an atherectomy catheter.

Complications of transluminal atherectomy are less than 5% to 10% in most studies, with vessel perforation, thrombosis, and embolism being the most important short-term limitations. Hemoglobinuria and hemolysis have been reported with several devices. The systemic effects of microembolism have yet to be determined, although embolism to distal tissues in the leg has not been a serious clinical problem in preliminary studies.

Indications for atherectomy have not been defined, and its role in the management of vascular disease will be determined by further clinical experience. Although initial successes have been achieved with several devices, restenosis has been a problem in some studies, particularly when the amount of plaque removed may have been inadequate. Preliminary data suggest that precise control of the removal of the lesion within the arterial wall dramatically improves the follow-up patency and hemodynamic results. If this finding is substantiated, development of this principle could improve the results of endovascular recanalizations.

Laser Therapy

The concept of using lasers to remodel stenotic lesions and recanalize arterial occlusions is based on the unique qualities of laser light. Many of the early industrial prototypes (eg, CO_2, argon, and Nd:YAG lasers) have developed into commercially available units that are used clinically. For this reason, these were the first lasers to be evaluated for cardiovascular ablation. Other prototypes are becoming available as special requirements are identified.

There are several characteristics of laser delivery systems that have an important effect on the energy delivered to the tissue interface. To enable precise delivery of laser energy at some distance from the source, such as at the operating table, flexible delivery systems are desirable. For certain types of lasers (Nd:YAG, argon, dye) this is easily accomplished using quartz fiberoptics. For wavelengths that are absorbed by the quartz or those that destroy fibers by high-peak energies, such as the CO_2 laser, the energy is delivered by articulating arms or hollow wave guides.

When laser energy interacts with tissue, the effects depend on how the laser energy is dissipated and on the absorption characteristics of the tissue for the particular wavelength of energy. Laser energy can be described according to a wave theory, that is, as having a wavelength and frequency, or it can be described as particles or photons with each having a quantum of energy corresponding to the particular wavelength. If the photons of laser light do not have enough energy to break chemical bonds, they cause vibration and collision of nearby atoms, producing heat, or a photothermal effect. This causes tissue burning and vaporization if enough energy is delivered. If the emitted photons have enough energy to break chemical bonds, tissue ablation occurs by ionization of atoms and molecules, or by a photochemical effect. The energy absorbed may also be reemitted as photons with the same or less energy than those that were absorbed, and is called *laser-induced fluorescence*.

The CO_2 laser is absorbed primarily by water at the tissue surface. For this reason, it is good for cutting applications because it rapidly vaporizes the water and tissue at the surface. Argon laser energy penetrates more deeply than CO_2 (400 to 800 μm) and is absorbed primarily by chromogens such as hemoglobin or melanin. Because of its selective absorption, the argon laser has been used widely for coagulating pigmented and vascular lesions. As with the continuous-wave CO_2 lasers, the argon mechanism is primarily through heating and vaporization of tissue elements. The Nd:YAG laser is not particularly well absorbed by any tissue elements. It penetrates deeply (1 to 4 mm) and is used primarily for tissue coagulation and necrosis.

The mode of energy delivery, either continuous wave (CW) or pulsed, also has a significant influence on tissue effects. CW lasers deliver a constant power over intervals of a few tenths of a second to several seconds. Pulsed lasers deliver energy over a much shorter interval measured in microseconds (10^{-6} second) or nanoseconds (10^{-9} second). The intensity of a pulsed laser is much higher than that typically achieved with a CW device. The energy per pulse is small (millijoules), but the peak power is high (megawatts) leading to rapid ablation at the tissue interface. The repetition rate of the pulses of energy is measured in Hertz. Both CW and pulsed lasers can be mechanically chopped or Q-switched into a pulsed mode by a shutter mechanism, which releases the pulse of energy over a short interval. In the Q-switch mode, the energy builds up rapidly and can be released in a short interval with an intensity increased by several orders of magnitude. It has been well documented that pulsed energy from certain types of lasers at a low repetition rate can simulate a photochemical effect. Thus, thermal injury can be avoided, even in certain types of lasers that ablate by a thermal mechanism, if the time of thermal diffusion of the tissue is less than the pulse interval.

To provide reproducible laser–tissue interactions with fiberoptic delivery, the depth of tissue penetration for each particular wavelength is an additional key parameter. The ultraviolet wavelengths (up to 380 nm) provide precise tissue ablation due to the photochemical tissue ablation and have a shallow depth of penetration (2 to 4 μm). At 380 to 2000 nm, the depth of tissue penetration is much deeper (ie, up to 2 to 4 mm for the Nd:YAG laser at 1060 nm). Above 2000 nm, the penetration is again shallow, permitting precise ultraviolet-like ablation.

Laser spectroscopic analysis of atherosclerotic tissues can enhance guidance and target specificity. Preliminary evidence suggests that the pattern of reemitted energy from irradiated tissues may be tissue specific. Normal arteries have spectroscopic patterns that are different from atherosclerotic lesions. An additional method to enhance local tissue absorption of laser energy and thus produce more specific tissue ablation is with chromophores. A chromophore is a substance that specifically absorbs a particular laser wavelength. Carotenoids (endogenous fats) are chromophores that are present in early atherosclerotic lesions and selectively absorb the 460- to 480-nm wavelength. Hematophorin derivative (HPD) or its concentrated form, photofrin II, selectively absorbs argon laser energy. HPD has several characteristics that demonstrate the potential application of chromophores. This compound has an affinity for vascular structures and binds to mitochondria and the plasma membrane of the cell. On absorbing the argon light, HPD fluoresces pink and causes cell death by singlet oxygen toxicity.

Role of Laser Angioplasty in Endovascular Therapy

Laser angioplasty is a controversial technology because it was rapidly applied to clinical practice shortly after the first clinical trials in 1984. The technique then quickly fell into disfavor because of many problems that developed during the early development and application of the method. The rapid acceptance, application, and subsequent disfavor of the laser devices highlight the considerations and controversies involved in the evolution of endovascular angioplasty devices and are reviewed briefly to outline the mechanisms of failure of devices and to highlight the possible attributes that may need further use of lasers if clinical need arises.

The initial trials of laser angioplasty using argon or Nd:YAG continuous-wave energy demonstrated the ability to ablate atherosclerotic lesions, but the method was limited by a significant rate of vessel perforation from excessive thermal damage. As a solution to this problem, an ovoid metal cap was attached to the end of the fiberoptic catheter to limit the diffusion of heat and eliminate some of the perforations caused by the fiber. Initial clinical evaluations of the hot-tip or laser-thermal angioplasty systems were performed using 1.5- and 2-mm diameter solid metal caps and were designed to compare the efficiency and safety of the technique to the conventional balloon angioplasty methods. For this reason, about 60% of the procedures were performed on stenotic femoropopliteal lesions without making comparisons with standard surgical procedures. Since the laser probes create a channel that is smaller than the size of the metal cap (channel size is estimated to be 60% to 70% of the tip diameter), the initial recanalizations were followed by balloon dilation to further enlarge the lumen. Thus, the technique is correctly called laser-thermal–assisted balloon angioplasty.

Impressive preliminary reports of successful recanalizations using the laser-thermal devices lead to optimism regarding the usefulness of this method. The complication rates, including vessel perforations, groin hematomas, and so forth, were about 6% to 10%, but the incidence decreased after the initial learning experience, which occurs in almost all institutions. From these initial studies, it appeared that combined laser thermal balloon angioplasty was applicable in a higher percentage of cases and could recanalize a higher percentage of long segment occlusions compared with balloon angioplasty alone. As a result of the initial enthusiasm for the method, rapid development followed, including larger diameter laser devices, combined thermal and free-energy or hybrid probes, and high-energy pulsed systems such as the excimer or holmium:YAG lasers.

The preliminary reports of the successful use of laser thermal and controlled free-energy devices were performed primarily by cardiologists and radiologists for stenotic lesions or short occlusions. When surgeons began to use these devices for longer occlusions in patients with conventional indications for surgery, the incidence of arterial wall perforations, reocclusions, and early restenosis increased dramatically.[5]

Laser angioplasty remains an investigational method with limited applications that is undergoing rapid evolution. Its success rate is inferior to that of conventional surgical methods. An analysis of the cases in which laser angioplasty has been performed suggests that the indications include arterial stenoses and short occlusions, iliac lesions, chronically occluded polytetrafluoroethylene (PTFE) grafts, patients at high risk for conventional surgery, or patients in whom interval patency may improve operability at a later date. Criteria for choosing patients as candidates for laser angioplasty, as for any investigational endovascular technique, should include conventional surgical indications with the therapy being administered by an experienced operator. One reason to be conservative when treating minimal disease with state-of-the-art devices is that short stenoses or occlusions can be converted to long occlusions if imprecise technique is used or if complications occur.

Additional Endovascular Recanalization Devices

Subsequent to the preliminary reports of success using laser thermal devices, several other more cost-effective nonlaser thermal angioplasty systems were developed. These include radiofrequency and electric and catalytic thermal systems, which may be alternatives to the laser thermal devices if thermal ablation remains acceptable.

Ultrasonic ablation of atherosclerotic plaques has been evaluated as a method to remove abnormal tissue while preserving normal arterial wall. Pulsed and continuous forms of energy have been delivered to plaques by wire probes, with histologic evidence of tissue ablation that conforms to the shape of the probe tip. Other intriguing methods of plaque dissolution have been identified, for example, a pulsatile, high-velocity water jet. It is likely that other modalities will also develop as angioplasty continues to evolve.

THROMBOLYTIC THERAPY

Thrombolytic therapy involves the use of drugs to lyse thrombus in the arterial or venous systems.[6] The fibrinolytic system, which is responsible for clot lysis, is activated when plasminogen is converted to plasmin by mediators such as tissue-type plasminogen activator. Fibrinolysis can also be initiated by exogenous activators such as urokinase (UK) and streptokinase (SK). Plasmin degrades fibrin and fibrinogen into fragments, some of which have antithrombotic activity. The fibrinolytic system is most effective on fresh thrombus, but has also been shown to be effective in more organized thromboses.

Plasminogen and plasmin exist in free-circulating and thrombus-bound forms. To protect against the development of a generalized fibrinolytic state, the plasma contains antiplasmins: α_2-antiplasmin, which instantly neutralizes free plasmin; α_2-microglobulin, a slower, more stable inhibitor of plasmin; α_1-antitrypsin; antithrombin III; and C1 inactivator. The plasmin bound within thrombus is protected from neutralization by the antiplasmins and is free to degrade fibrin. Thus, the interaction between plasmin and antiplasmin provides a system of selective fibrinolysis.

SK is a lytic agent purified from a preparation of bacterial proteins elaborated by group C, β-hemolytic streptococci. It is supplied as a water-soluble, white lyophilized powder. It has two peaks of activity—one at 16 minutes and the other at 83 minutes. SK combines with plasminogen to form SK-plasminogen. This complex then unites with another plasminogen molecule to form plasmin. Since each molecule of SK uses two molecules of plasminogen to generate one molecule of plasmin, it is less efficient and also causes greater plasminogen depletion than UK. Because SK plasminogen is a more potent activator than UK, fibrinogen degradation is also greater than during UK administration. Streptococcal antibodies produced during an earlier bacterial infection directly inactivate the agent by forming an irreversible complex. Therefore, all the antibody sites must be saturated by an initial loading dose of SK before a subsequent dose can be active systemically. A standardized loading dose of 250,000 IU of SK has been found to neutralize antibodies in 90% of the US population. As a foreign protein, SK causes a pyretic reaction in 5% to 10% of patients. Anaphylaxis and serum sickness have been reported, but serious reactions are rare.

UK is an enzyme with thrombolytic activity produced by the kidney and found in the urine. There are two forms of UK that differ in molecular weight but have similar clinical effects. Abbokinase (injectable UK) is a thrombolytic agent obtained from human kidney cells by tissue culture techniques and is primarily the low molecular weight form. UK differs significantly from SK in several aspects. First, there are no antibodies to cause inactivation, so no loading dose is necessary. In addition, UK is a direct plasminogen activator. All plasminogen activated by UK is converted to plasmin. UK is nonantigenic and does not induce an allergic response. Its half-life is short, averaging 14 minutes.

Thrombolytic therapy was first used systemically in the mid-1950s for thromboembolic peripheral arterial occlusions. Although complete or partial thrombolysis was achieved in 20% to 50% of the patients, the high incidence of hemorrhagic complications led investigators to explore methods to perform selective local treatment. Local intraarterial infusion was described and subsequently the angiographic technique for intraarterial infusion of thrombolytic agent (SK) was used to treat arterial thromboembolic disease.

In most reports, UK is considered safer and more effective than SK and is the preferred thrombolytic agent. The most popular method of administration consists of initial continuous intrathrombus infusion of 4000 IU/min with serial advance of the catheter into any remaining occluded segment at 1- to 2-hour intervals until antegrade flow is achieved. After restoration of flow, the catheter tip is repositioned proximal to any residual clot, and the dosage is decreased to 1000 IU/min and continued for an additional 8 to 12 hours before reexamination. The infusion is continued until complete clot lysis has been accomplished, unless complications or the patient's degree of ischemia requires cessation and operative intervention. Heparinization (about 1000 IU/h) is maintained during UK infusion to prevent thrombus development along the delivery catheter.

Recombinant human tissue-type plasminogen activator is being evaluated for local thrombolysis in peripheral arterial or bypass graft occlusions. This tissue plasminogen activator, produced by recombinant DNA technology, is an enzyme that has the property of fibrin-enhanced conversion of plasminogen to plasmin. It produces limited conversion of plasminogen in the absence of fibrin. When introduced into the systemic circulation at pharmacologic concentrations, it binds to fibrin in a thrombus and converts the entrapped plasminogen in plasmin. This initiates local fibrinolysis, but also produces limited systemic proteolysis.

Pro-urokinase (pro-UK), or kidney plasminogen activator, is a single-chain zymogen form of UK that is naturally present in the body in the same concentration as native tissue-type plasminogen activator. Pro-UK has a longer half-life and higher enzyme activity then tissue-type plasminogen activator, so smaller doses are required. The effectiveness of pro-UK in humans is under investigation.

Thrombolytic agents, particularly UK, have been used extensively as adjuncts to endovascular procedures. They are useful for lysing acute and chronic thrombus in occluded vessels to localize atherosclerotic lesions that may be amendable to endovascular treatment by balloon dilation, other recanalization devices, or intravascular stents. The utility of this approach in occluded aortoiliac segments, in which lytic therapy is used to clear the vessel lumen followed by dilation and stent reinforcement of recanalized lesions, has been particularly impressive in preliminary clinical evaluation.[7] Demonstration of the long-term efficacy of this approach awaits the results of additional investigations.

An additional possible application of thrombolysis under wide investigation is the use of lytic agents as an alternative to conventional surgical management of acute arterial occlusions. Preliminary studies have suggested that the survival rate is higher and the morbidity rate lower in patients undergoing lytic therapy followed by surgical thrombectomy than in patients who receive conventional surgical treatment alone.[8] This concept is being investigated by controlled, randomized studies to determine the utility of this approach in routine care. The use of thrombolytic agents has increased as an adjunct to both endoluminal and conventional surgical management of vascular lesions.

The complications of thrombolytic therapy include allergic reactions to SK, localized bleeding and bruising, systemic fibrinolysis causing diffuse hemorrhage, gastrointestinal hemorrhage or cerebral bleeding, and embolism of dislodged clot to distal arteries.

ENDOVASCULAR IMPLANTS
Intravascular Stents

Vascular stents or intraluminal splints were first investigated by Dotter in 1969 when he used nonexpanding stainless steel coils placed in canine femoral arteries. His work prompted studies by other investigators using a variety of stent designs. Early prototypes suffered from many limitations including bulky configurations, unpredictable expansion of the stent, migration, abrupt thrombosis, and gradual restenosis from intimal hyperplasia.

There are three basic designs—stainless steel spring-loaded stents, thermally expanded memory metal stents, and balloon expandable stents. The last is the most popular because it can be inserted at the time of concomitant balloon angioplasty. In animal studies, intraarterial stents can prevent elastic recoil of the vessel wall and maintain luminal diameter by plaque compression after angioplasty. Although stents become incorporated in the vessel wall and are covered by endothelium, preliminary histologic studies performed 12 months after placement reveal that the stented segments show thinning of the media and neointimal proliferation over the stent.

Stents are most beneficial clinically in large-diameter, high-flow vessels. Stenting of lesions in iliac arteries and veins and superior vena caval stenoses has been particularly useful. Intravascular stents have been shown to improve the patency of iliac artery stenoses and occlusions beyond balloon angioplasty alone,[9] with the major limitation of routine use beyond the cost of the stent. Their suitability in medium-caliber vessels of lower velocity, such as the femoral and popliteal arteries, is unknown. The value of stents may be to manage acute reclosure of angioplasties from residual thrombotic material, flaps, dissections, or recoil of the vessel wall. Preliminary clinical evaluation of these devices has demonstrated a benefit in saving patients who have abrupt closure of coronary balloon angioplasties by restoring patency and preventing myocardial infarctions. Prevention of restenosis by stent therapy remains to be demonstrated; therefore, using stents for this indication remains controversial, particularly with the risks of chronic thrombosis, dislodgement and migration, or embolism.

Endoluminal Grafts

Repairing vascular lesions using devices that are deployed intraluminally by catheter delivery systems has been investigated for many years. Although this an appealing concept, a method of fixation of the prosthesis within the arterial lumen has been a limitation to further advances. In recent years, the development of intravascular stents offers a solution to this technical problem (Fig. 79-5).

Several investigators have demonstrated the potential to place vascular prostheses intraluminally in normal vessels and in aneurysm models using catheter-based deployment systems and stent fixation to adjacent vessels.[10] Both tubular and bifurcated devices have been developed, with rapid healing in animal models by tissue incorporation in 3 to 4 weeks and with patency of 6 to 12 months being shown in selected evaluations.

After the successful use of endoluminal grafts in animal studies, the first human application was report by Parodi[10] in 5 high-risk patients. He reported no deaths in these patents and successful deployment in 4. Encouraged by these promising results, Parodi treated 8 more patients (for a total of 13), for a total of 12 with abdominal aortic aneurysms and 1 with a subclavian posttraumatic arteriovenous fistula. In a follow-up period of 3 to 23 months (mean, 10 months) there were no deaths and no postprocedure problems on the basis of clinical findings, CT scanning, and duplex scanning. A recent unpublished follow-up of Parodi's series included more than 40 patients being treated with intravascular prostheses. The results of this series continue to be promising, with the unresolved issues that need further investigations being related to imaging techniques, graft deployment, fixation of the device, and wound healing.

Recent updates on other investigators clinical experience substantiates the probable clinical utility of endoluminal grafts. Transluminal placement of prosthetic graft-stent devices has been used in more than 60 patients with a variety of vascular lesions in an Australian experience reported by May and White.[10] Chuter[10] reported on 26 cases of aortic aneurysm treated with bifurcated prostheses, and Marini and Veith[10] described more that 50 graft-stent procedures for treatment of a variety of vascular lesions. Investigators at Stanford University have also reported the use of intravascular grafting to treat 14 patients with thoracic aortic aneurysms or dissections.[10] The outcome of these initial studies awaits further follow-up and

formal reporting, although the preliminary data are promising.

Knowledge about endoluminal prostheses is expanding rapidly because of the experimental laboratory and clinical testing of several prototype devices. Significant in vitro and in vivo experimental animal data are available. Most of the clinical experience is based on devices constructed by combining available stents and prostheses, which are subsequently used in off-label applications of the devices. In addition, several prototype prostheses are being evaluated in clinical series conducted outside the United States. There is only one FDA-approved human protocol in the United States (endovascular Technologies, Menlo Park, CA), so there is tremendous variability in the data that are available from the studies that are being conducted. In addition, many of the investigations are being conducted with prototype devices undergoing significant evolution in variable patient groups, with many different indications for the procedures. These studies are also affected by varying levels of investigator skill and variability in the available imaging methods and the quality of imaging equipment.

In general, studies of endoluminal grafts show a remarkably good outcome, with patency of up to 1 year indicating significant potential for further development.

INTRALUMINAL IMAGING TECHNIQUES

Precise guidance of intraluminal angioplasty devices, particularly through high-resistance, completely occlusive lesions, is a limiting factor that must be addressed by future development if instruments and clinical results are to be improved. Recanalization of distal, small-diameter peripheral arteries and coronary lesions requires control with a sensitivity equivalent to the thickness of vessel wall. This degree of precision is required to enable passage of devices through the vessel without causing perforations or false aneurysm formation. Thus, methods that permit reproducible concentric recanalization of the vessel yet preserve a uniform thickness of the media and adventitia are needed. In addition to spectroscopy and angioscopy, advances in fluoroscopic equipment and ultrasound (both transcutaneous external and intraluminal systems) promise to improve precise intraluminal guidance.

Cinefluoroscopy

Cinefluoroscopy is readily available and is the standard method to measure the luminal anatomy of the arterial disease. It provides a detailed outline of the location and severity of stenoses and occlusions and is uniformly used to guide devices and to determine the success of interventional procedures. With the development of endovascular treatment methods, cinefluoroscopy is being used widely in both interventional radiology and cardiology suites and in the operating room to perform these procedures. Other chapters in this text are devoted to the diagnostic and therapeutic applications of angiography, and the inclusion of this discussion in this chapter is only to emphasize the role that the method and the evolution of cine imaging systems has had on endovascular approaches, particularly in the operating room.

Standard angiographic techniques, which often lack good spatial and contrast resolution, may require multiple reinjections to follow the progress of the dye. Digital subtraction techniques have increased contrast sensitivity and allow detection of low levels of iodinated contrast. Many digital units have freeze-frame and road-mapping features

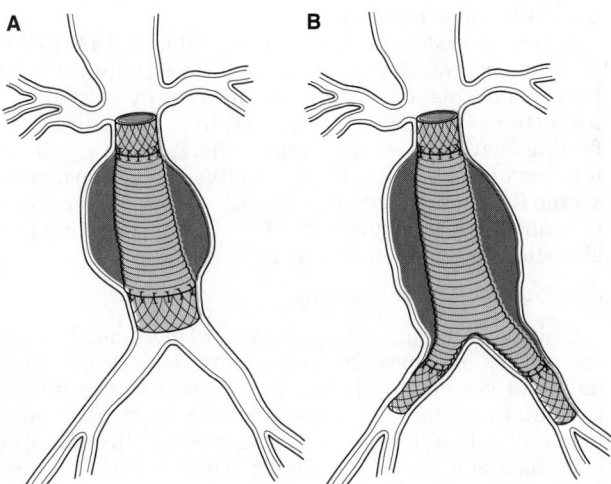

Figure 79-5. Schematic of an intraluminal prosthesis for treatment of abdominal aortic aneurysms in tubular (*A*) and bifurcated (*B*) configurations. Fixation at the ends of the prostheses is by intravascular metal stents.

that permit a subtracted contrast image of a vessel to be superimposed on a live fluoroscopic image.

The quality of equipment available for radiologic imaging of procedures varies from conventional C-arm fluoroscopes to sophisticated image-intensifying tubes, high-resolution intensifiers, and video monitoring systems in interventional radiology suites, cardiac catheterization laboratories, and operating rooms. Immediate image replay systems can improve the accuracy of information conveyed and the safety of interventional procedures. Unfortunately, this type of equipment is expensive and is not available in many facilities, particularly operating rooms. Advances in computerized image-processing systems have extended the advantages of digital imaging technology to C-arm fluoroscopy by enabling modular addition of contrast enhancement, image-holding, and road-mapping during angiographic procedures. The use of cinefluoroscopy in the operating room as an integral component of endovascular procedures requires that the quality of equipment and images be enhanced. This limitation is being addressed at many institutions.

Cinefluoroscopy is limited as a diagnostic and therapeutic guidance method during endovascular procedures by the fact that atherosclerotic occlusions of arteries develop with eccentric positioning within the vessel lumen in about 70% of coronary and peripheral lesions. Because of the asymmetric location of the residual lumen, contrast radiography has significant variability in the estimation of the percentage of luminal stenosis, since it only visualizes the vessel in one dimension. An additional consequence of the eccentric positioning of atherosclerotic lesions is that angiography is unable to determine the transmural component of a lesion. This limitation is being addressed by other endovascular imaging methods that detail the luminal and transmural anatomy of vessels, including angioscopy and intraluminal ultrasound.

Angioscopy

Angioscopy, the endoscopic examination of the luminal anatomy of blood vessels, is used to establish the diagnosis and etiology of vascular diseases, to evaluate the technical accuracy of vascular reconstructions, and to visualize intraluminal instrumentation. Attempts to perform cardiac endoscopy were reported in the early 1900s using rigid tubes passed into the cardiac chambers. Vascular endoscopy was initially attempted in the 1960s after development of modern flexible arthroscopes and choledochoscopes. Newly developed 0.8- to 3.3-mm diameter angioscopes feature improved fiberoptic imaging systems and light sources, enabling intraluminal inspection of smaller diameter vessels.

Equipment

For angioscopy of peripheral vessels more than 3 mm in diameter, multichannel endoscopic catheters are optimal because they incorporate a fluid channel for irrigating the vessel lumen to keep the field of view and the lens free of blood. Angioscopes that include a fluid channel are about 2.5 mm in diameter. This channel or additional channels in larger devices can be used to pass guide wires, snares, laser fibers, or other instruments. The larger angioscopes (2.5 to 3.3 mm) are suited for most peripheral vascular procedures, whereas 0.5- to 1.8-mm instruments are required for smaller vessels, such as the tibial or coronary arteries. The smaller designs sacrifice the fluid lumen to provide a narrower catheter diameter.

Angioscopic visualization is enhanced by coupling the scopes to a video camera. The field of view can be projected on a video monitor and magnified 40 to 200 times. Using the improved angioscopes and video display, intravascular detail with greater than 0.2-mm spatial resolution at 5 mm is achieved, and the minimum focal distance ranges from 2 to 6.5 mm. A light source of at least 300 watts is required to provide sufficient illumination to obtain adequate images through the fine fiberoptics. The power of light sources available in hospitals for gastrointestinal and surgical endoscopy is usually about 100 to 150 watts. Newer angioscopes are being developed that function well with less illumination to enable use of available light sources.

The angioscopes, video camera, and cables are gas sterilizable and are set up on a sterile field on a side table before the procedure. At all times, these instruments must be handled with care because of the fragility of the optical fibers. Immediately after use, blood is cleared from the tubing and internal channels of the devices to avoid deterioration of the optics. Ethylene oxide gas sterilization and airing procedures take 12 to 18 hours, so each nondisposable angioscope can usually be used in only one procedure each day.

Technique

For percutaneous angioscopic examination, access to the lumen is obtained by passing the scope through an introducer catheter. Percutaneous angioscopy is used to define the mechanisms and accuracy of angioplasties and to evaluate vessel trauma when angiograms provide equivocal information. Achieving good images with percutaneous angioscopes is limited by stiff systems that make control and centering of the devices difficult. To aid manipulation of the tip of the scope, a steering mechanism in at least one plane is desirable. Control of proximal blood flow in the area being examined can be achieved by inflation of a balloon on the tip of the catheter. A rapid flow of irrigating solution through the delivery catheter is then required to control blood from collateral vessels. Back-bleeding from the distal circulation can be limited by having an assistant apply external pressure over the vessels in a distal extremity.

Angioscopy can be performed intraoperatively in 10 minutes or less through an opening in the vessel. To perform the intraluminal inspection, vascular occlusion is obtained by conventional operative means or by a balloon on the end of the angioscope. Infusion of saline under pressure of about 300 mmHg (30 to 75 mL/min), through an irrigation channel in the angioscope or by a coaxial catheter, clears the intraluminal blood and enables visualization in 80% to 90% of cases.

Several investigators have reported that in 15% to 30% of vascular procedures, angioscopy reveals clinically important information that is not apparent by extraluminal inspection, probing, or angiography. The angioscopic findings have altered the surgical therapy in a significant number of these cases. In prospective evaluations, angioscopic findings differed significantly from preoperative or intraoperative angiograms in 24% of cases, resulting in an alteration in the operation in 17% of cases.

Angioscopic Thrombectomy

Embolectomy and thrombectomy of peripheral vessels are greatly enhanced by angioscopy. Unless the whole length of vessel is occluded, the angioscope can initially be introduced through the arteriotomy to inspect the lumen and define the exact site and extent of thrombosis or embolism and also to determine whether there is preexisting atherosclerotic disease. Fogarty catheters can then be passed beside the angioscope if the arterial lumen is large enough to accommodate both devices. Balloon inflation and the detachment and removal of thrombus and debris can then be visually monitored.

Direct visual observation of the degree of balloon inflation is important because it determines the amount of balloon distention necessary to adequately remove the lesion without causing injury to the vessel wall. Balloon catheters frequently slide over thrombi that adhere to the wall, leaving large fragments that may or may not be removed with repeated passes and that are frequently not demonstrated adequately by completion arteriograms. When adherent thrombus is observed, further attempts at retrieval can be made by positioning the balloon just distal to the clot and by oscillating it back and forth over the site. If this is not successful, a decision should be made whether further attempts at extraction are warranted using other instruments such as flexible grasping forceps, rotary atherectomy devices, or vascular brushes. Another alternative is the intraoperative use of fibrinolytic agents.

When thromboembolectomy is considered complete, a final angioscopic inspection of the entire artery is made. Angiographic examination of the smaller runoff vessels can be obtained by injecting contrast medium through the fluid channel of the angioscope before the scope is withdrawn. One of the advantages offered by angioscopy is that complications and technical errors, such as retained thrombus or intimal flaps, can be corrected while the arterial lumen is still open and before blood flow is restored. The angiogram usually fails to demonstrate the smaller irregularities of the wall caused by intimal flaps or adherent thrombus and may underestimate larger lesions as well.

Transfemoral thromboembolectomy of the iliac artery is performed by initially clearing about 80% of the length of occlusion with the Fogarty catheter and then introducing the angioscope to inspect the lumen for retained thrombus, mural defects, and atherosclerotic plaque. After the remainder of the iliac segment has been reopened, a Fogarty catheter is inflated at the level of the aortic bifurcation to impede blood flow and enable inspection of the thrombectomized vessel. If there is good collateral flow through branches of the iliac artery, it may be difficult to overcome the blood in the field to obtain an adequate view. Similar techniques are used for thromboembolectomy in an occluded limb of an aortobifemoral graft. In this case, the absence of blood flow from branch vessels ensures a blood-free field.

Femoropopliteotibial thromboembolectomy is performed through a groin incision and by obtaining exposure and control of the common femoral, profunda, and superficial femoral arteries. An arteriotomy is performed, and the angioscope is inserted into the profunda femoris artery, where it usually passes easily to a distance of 20 to 25 cm. Because of the narrow diameter of this artery, the Fogarty catheter cannot be inserted at the same time, so the angioscopic monitoring of thromboembolectomy of the profunda is limited to inspection before and after passage of the balloon.

In the superficial femoral artery, and within prosthetic bypass grafts in this position, the Fogarty catheter passes comfortably alongside the angioscope. At the distal popliteal level, the orifices of each of the tibial arteries can be identified, and selective cannulation with the Fogarty catheter is often possible. This is achieved by slightly bending the catheter tip to enhance cannulation. It is more difficult to access the anterior tibial artery because of the severe angle. On occasion, selective cannulation of the tibial artery can avert exposure of the vessels below the knee to retrieve embolic or thrombotic material.

In prosthetic grafts, extensive buildup of neointimal hyperplasia may be difficult to differentiate from chronic thrombus. Alternative instruments such as forceps, curettes, and brushes to extract intraluminal lesions are prob-

ably safer here than in the native vessels. Inspecting the distal anastomosis is important because this is often the site of hyperplastic stenosis. Twists or kinks of the graft can also be identified by angioscopic inspection.

Thrombectomy of the iliac and femoral veins using angioscopic visualization has been reported to be superior to venograms for demonstrating residual thrombus, poor operative result, and the presence of venous spurs in the left common iliac vein. When incomplete thrombectomy is demonstrated endoscopically, a temporary peripheral arteriovenous fistula may be indicated to improve patency rates.

Residual thrombus has been identified angioscopically within arteries and grafts after standard thromboembolectomy procedures in about 80% of cases. The direct, three-dimensional view provides significantly more information regarding luminal compromise than does contrast radiologic imaging. In many cases, the missed clot is small and probably of no significance. This is most likely with soft mural thrombus, which is closely attached to the wall and is not stenotic. In some instances, thrombectomy catheters have also been observed to pass between the vessel wall and the clot without dislodging it. With lesser amounts of thrombus, especially nonobstructing mural thrombus, it is difficult to judge whether further attempts at removal are indicated. Mural thrombus often simulates spasm on angiograms, and thus good backflow does not necessarily correlate with a satisfactory removal of thrombus. It is likely that many of these minor defects would normally be resolved by the natural fibrinolytic and healing processes. During angioscopic thrombectomy, the infusion of the irrigating fluid simulates blood flow, thus giving a dynamic representation of potential flaps and loose debris. In some cases, severe dissections or atherosclerotic stenosis or occlusion identified by endoscopy can not be treated endoluminally, indicating that the best therapy is to proceed immediately to vascular bypass rather than persist with unproductive attempts at thrombectomy.

Angioscopy-Assisted in Situ Vein Bypasses

Observing the completeness of valvulotomy in in situ vein bypasses has improved the technical accuracy of the procedure and reduced the operative time by ensuring complete incompetence of valve cusps. The valvulotome is inserted through a side branch of the upper segment of the saphenous vein or through the vein lumen at the distal end. The valvulotome is passed proximally from the distal vein through the most proximal valve, and the angioscope is inserted proximally and passed distally until the valvulotome can be seen at the valve site. Low profile valvulotomes such as a Mills valvulotome can be easily seen and controlled by angioscopic inspection (Fig. 79-6). Incompetence of valve cusps is easily tested under direct vision by distending the vein with saline infusion and compressing the vein lumen by external pressure. As valve cusps are serially disrupted the valvulotome and angioscope are advanced distally to the next valve.

Intraluminal identification of tributary veins during the procedure can help limit dissection and isolation of the vein and prevent tears in the vein caused by hooking a side branch with the valvulotome. Several manufacturers are developing microinstruments that can be passed through a lumen in an angioscope or coaxial to the scope to enhance accurate and expedient valvulotomy under direct vision. During the procedure, extreme care must be taken to prevent damaging the vein by the intraluminal instruments. Angioscopes too large to pass easily through the lumen can produce severe trauma to the vein wall.

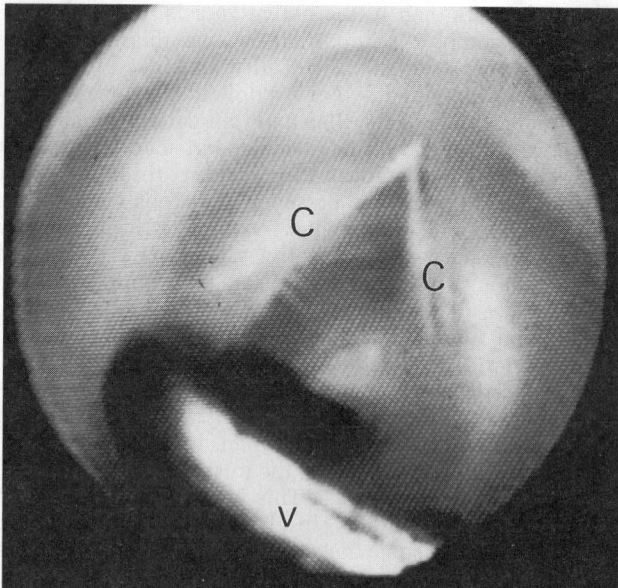

Figure 79-6. Angioscopic visualization of in situ vein valvulotomy. C, valve cusp; v, vein valve.

Angioscopic Monitoring of Angioplasty Procedures

Angioscopy monitoring of angioplasty procedures has advantages compared with arteriography because it removes the hazards of radiation exposure and contrast reactions and allows immediate detection and correction of technical complications. Arteriography tends to underestimate wall irregularities and stenosis. Angioscopic inspection under magnification and video control enables placement of angioplasty devices without deviation into collateral vessels. Proximal stenotic lesions or tapering of the vessel near the site of an occlusion limits angioscopic inspection and prevents clear visualization of an occlusion. Angioscopy after angioplasty has been extremely helpful in determining the adequacy of recanalizations, inspecting the surface for fragments, and determining the mechanism of action of recanalization devices. Inspection of the treated arteries frequently demonstrates intimal flaps, mural thrombus, balloon dilatation cracks, and other intraluminal features not apparent by angiographic studies (Fig. 79-7).

An additional benefit of angioscopy during angioplasty procedures is that the examination is conducted before restoration of blood flow and may help to prevent embolism of arterial wall or thrombus fragments. Angioscopy examinations are limited in that assessment of smaller distal vessels is usually not possible because of the angioscope diameters. Examining normal vessels beyond the treated segment may cause intimal lesions or induce spasm. Angiography of the distal vasculature can be performed by injecting contrast through a channel in the scope. This allows direct correlation of the angiogram and angioscopic image.

Angioscopy has limited benefits during an angioplasty procedure or in preventing perforations because visualization of the device is obviated once it has entered an occlusion. Another limitation of angioscopy is that there is no way to evaluate the vessel thickness or concentricity of lesions. In the future, a combination of angioscopy with intraluminal ultrasound may provide a three-dimensional perspective of the vessel lumen and transmural vessel wall anatomy.

Intravascular Ultrasound

Intracardiac ultrasound catheters were first built in 1956. During the following two decades, delineation of intracardiac dimensions and cardiac images improved with the devices. Recent advances in catheter-based technology have led to intravascular ultrasound devices that generate images of the transmural anatomy of blood vessels using 20- to 50-MHz transducers incorporated into the tip of the catheter.[11] Although higher frequency has limited tissue penetration, it is adequate to produce images when used in an intraluminal position. At 20 MHz, the usable depth of penetration in blood is about 2 to 4 cm^3. At 50 MHz, the resolution of the images is finer but has less penetration.

Ultrasound images are generated from piezoelectric transducers by mechanically rotating either an echotransducer or a mirror on the tip of a catheter or by scanning an array of stationary elements (Fig. 79-8). The rotating intraluminal devices are more simple to manufacture, but the rotating transducer prototypes are more difficult to use in tortuous vessels because of the necessity for rotating connecting wires. This disadvantage is eliminated by the rotating mirror design or the multielement phase array configurations, although the increased electronic connection required in phase array devices is difficult to miniaturize. Integrated circuits at the catheter tip may permit sequenced transmission while improving flexibility and simplifying manufacturing by reducing the number of wires in the catheter. Ultrasound images produced by side-viewing devices display the transmural anatomy of the arterial wall. Potential forward-viewing catheters are being developed, although the interpretation of the wall thickness and lesion location are complicated by images obtained in a plane that is not perpendicular to the vessel wall.

Clinical application of intraluminal ultrasound devices is easily accomplished in any procedure where introduction of a 5F to 9F catheter is possible. Catheters as small as 3F are also being evaluated. Several prototype catheters

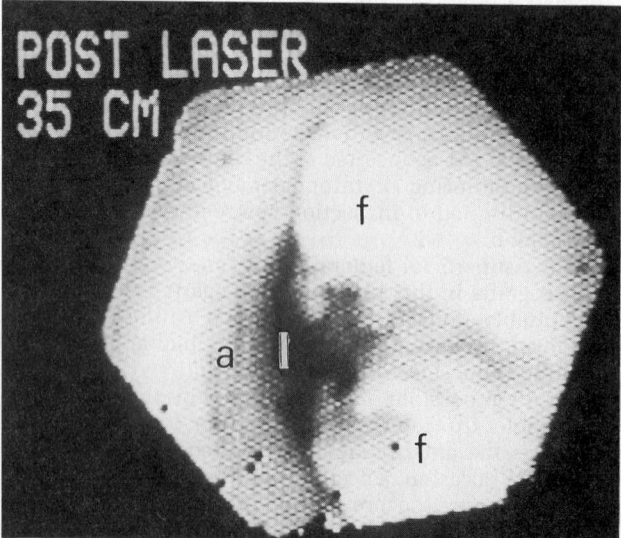

Figure 79-7. Angioscopic view of laser-thermal–assisted balloon angioplasty of the superficial femoral artery demonstrating residual cracks, intimal flaps and fissures in an atherosclerotic plaque. l, artery lumen; f, intimal flap; a, artery wall.

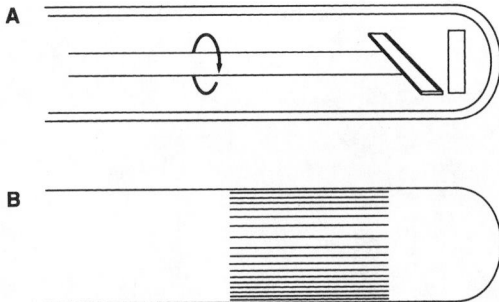

Figure 79-8. (*A*) Schematic depiction of a prototype mechanical ultrasound device with both rotating and fixed elements. Either the tranducer or the mirror may be fixed with the other element in the rotating position. (*B*) Schematic diagram of a phased array device with elements arranged circumferentially around the tip of the catheter. (After White RA. Indications for fiberoptic angioscopy and intraluminal ultrasound. Comprehens Ther 1990; 16:23)

can be passed over a guide wire, which enhances central positioning and imaging with the device. The images produced by intravascular devices outline the luminal and adventitial surfaces of normal or minimally diseased arterial segments within 0.1-mm accuracy. Determination of outside diameter of the vessels is less accurate, with a margin of error up to 0.5 mm. Preliminary experimental and clinical studies using intravascular ultrasound catheters have demonstrated the devices' ability to identify intraluminal thrombus, intimal flaps, and artery wall dissections (Figs. 79-9 and 79-10). In muscular arteries, distinct layers of the vessel wall may be visible, with the lumen and adventitia more echogenic than the media. Small intimal lesions are well defined in muscular arteries because of

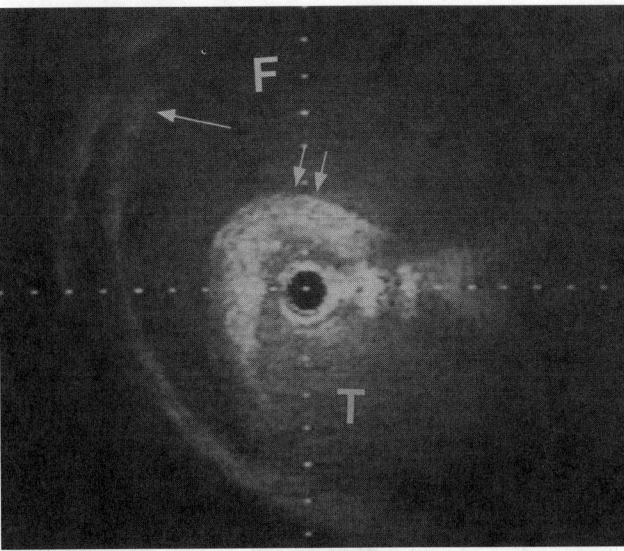

Figure 79-10. Intravascular ultrasound image of a human thoracic aortic dissection (*arrow*) surrounded by aortic wall (*double arrows*). T, true lumen; F, false lumen; u, ultrasound probe. (Cavaye DM, French WJ, White RA, et al. Intravascular imaging of acute dissecting aortic aneurysm: a case report. J Vasc Surg 1991;13:510)

the fibrous tissue content. Four basic types of plaque contours can be distinguished by in vitro intravascular ultrasound imaging of human atherosclerotic arteries. Hypoechoic images denote a significant deposit of lipid. Soft echoes reflect fibromuscular tissue (intimal proliferation) as well as lesions that consist of fibromuscular tissue and diffusely dispersed lipid. Bright echoes denote collagenrich fibrous tissue, and bright echoes with shadowing behind the lesion represent calcium.

Most intravascular ultrasound devices produce clear images of the vessel anatomy under optimal conditions. Careful positioning of catheter tips and appropriate size ratios of probe to vessel are required to optimize visualization in clinical situations. Image quality is best when the catheter is perpendicular to the wall, and minor angulations may affect image quality. Eccentric positioning makes the near wall appear more echogenic and thicker. Methods to precisely identify the location and orientation of the probes are also required. With further development of these instruments, the limitations related to image resolution and position sensitivity will be resolved.

Intravascular ultrasound evaluations are adding a new perspective to available vascular diagnostic modalities. This benefit is apparent in two respects: for defining the distribution of disease within the arterial lumen by visualizing transmural anatomy of the vessel and by providing control cross-section information about vessel luminal and wall morphology before and after intervention. This is of particular importance in addressing the phenomenon involved in restenosis after angioplasty.

Several investigators have compared the sensitivities of intravascular ultrasound and of coronary angiography for the diagnosis of coronary atherosclerosis.[10] In segments of arteries determined to be normal angiographically, calculations of luminal cross-sectional area by both methods were essentially the same. In contrast, intravascular ultrasound revealed a substantial amount of atheroma within the wall in either a concentric or smooth eccentric distribution involving some 40% of the available area bounded by the vessel wall media, demonstrating that, compared with in-

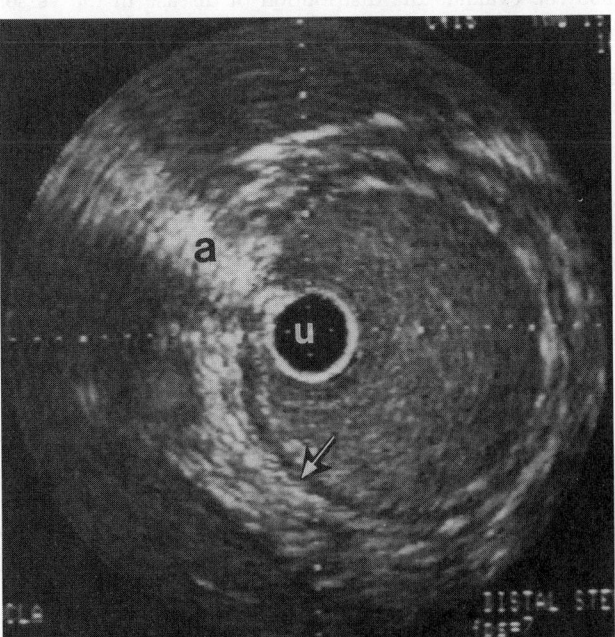

Figure 79-9. Intravascular ultrasound image of a normal human iliac artery demonstrating three-layered appearance of the wall. The medium is indicated by the arrow. u, ultrasound probe; a, imaging artifact used for positioning the catheter in the vessel.

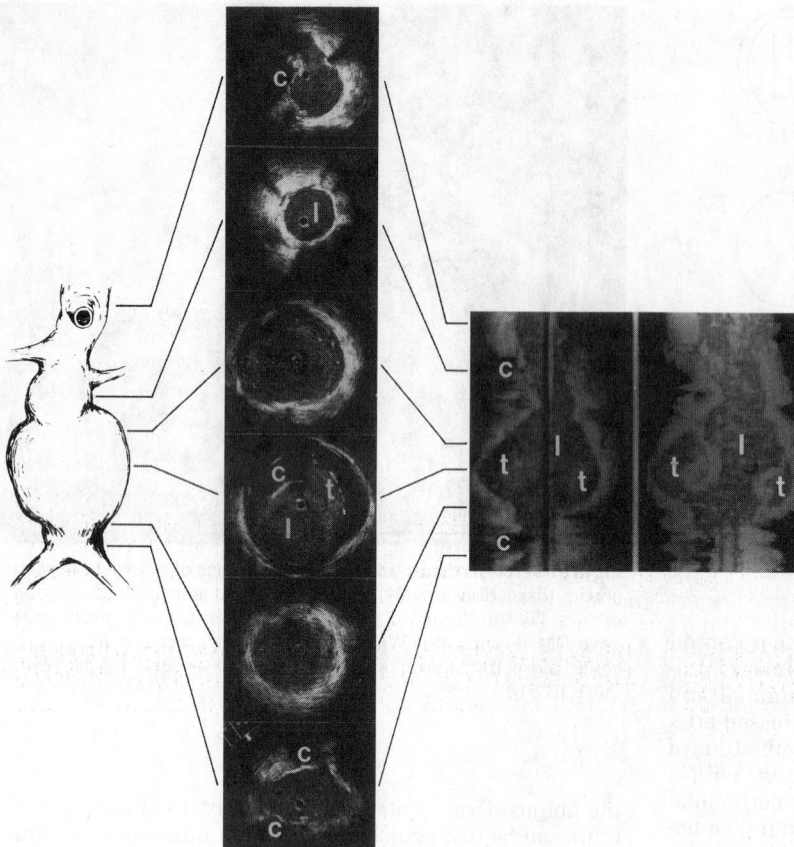

Figure 79-11. Selected cross-sectional images of the aorta and aneurysm at various levels (*center*) compared with a schematic diagram of the lesion (*left*) and the longitudinal gray-scale and three-dimensional IVUS images (*right*) of the aneurysm. There is evidence of thrombus (t) and calcification (c) at several levels throughout the length of the vessel. l, lumen. (White RA, et al. Innovations in vascular imaging: angiography, 3D CT, and 2D and 3D intravascular ultrasound of an abdominal aortic aneurysm. Ann Vasc Surg 1994;8:285)

travascular ultrasound, angiography underestimates the extent of disease in coronary arteries.

Comparison of intravascular ultrasound and angiographic images of coronary balloon angioplasties demonstrates that intravascular ultrasound is more sensitive in defining the extent of atherosclerosis and calcification. Tears and dissections occurred in 80% of vessels, and the mean cross-sectional lumen area after dilation measured by ultrasound correlated poorly with the value calculated by angiography. The inaccuracy of determination of luminal area using cineangiography questions the reliability of this method as the standard for evaluating lesion recurrence. The investigators also reported that intravascular ultrasound documented that the mean residual atheroma area at the site of previous dilation was 73% of the available arterial cross-sectional area of the artery; they postulated that this finding may explain the high incidence of restenosis after percutaneous coronary angioplasty. These data highlight the inaccuracies of conventional cineangiographic systems in providing adequately sensitive data about the distribution and consistency of lesions and the outcome of current methods. In this regard, it is questionable whether this method should still be used as the gold standard for quantitating restenosis, particularly since intravascular ultrasound offers a more precise alternative and also can evaluate the distribution of disease in the vessel wall.

Preliminary investigators have confirmed the utility of angioscopy and intravascular ultrasound in identifying the distribution and cross-sectional analysis of plaque morphology before and after atherectomy. These data will be useful in quantitating the amount of plaque removed and in redefining the recurrence of lesions based on these observations.

Intravascular ultrasound has also been used to help define the morphology of lesions in the arterial wall during catheter-based interventions, such as stent repairs of aortic dissections. The use of intravascular ultrasound real-time imaging during endovascular procedures is appealing from several perspectives. It provides improved precision for

Table 79-1. ENDOVASCULAR SURGERY MODALITIES

Method	Mechanism	Applications	Advantages
Thrombolysis	Clot lysis	Thromboses of variable lengths	Thrombis removal without a surgical procedure
Balloons	Lesion displacement	Stenoses and short occlusions	Cost-effective
			Percutaneous angioplasty
Lasers	Tissue ablation	Stenoses and occlusions	Tissue removal
			Miniature delivery systems
Atherectomy	Tissue removal	Stenoses and some occlusions	Tissue removal
Stents	Maintain lumen patency by fixed lesion displacement	Stenoses, occlusions, dissections, lesion recoil, etc	Maintains luminal patency and treats some complications of other devices

quantitating disease, choosing appropriate interventional methods, and assessing the outcome of an intervention. Its role in enhancing the interpretation of preoperative angiographic and CT imaging studies is exemplified in Figure 79-11.

FUTURE PERSPECTIVES

Table 79-1 summarizes the mechanisms and potential applicability of various endovascular surgical modalities to intravascular therapy. Combined approaches using thrombolysis, luminal dilatation, and tissue ablation or removal have unique potentials if improved guidance and delivery systems become available. Future angioplasty instrument delivery catheters may combine angioscopy for visually inspecting the lumen, spectroscopy for characterizing the tissue elements, and ultrasound for determining the vessel wall and lesion dimensions. Improved intraluminal ultrasound devices will provide not only improved visualization of cross-sectional vessel wall anatomy but also three-dimensional longitudinal reconstruction of the vasculature by storing a sequence of ultrasound images. Improved guidance of angioplasty catheters will help to eliminate the primary causes of failure of recanalizations and recurrence of lesions, vessel wall perforation, and inadequate debulking of lesions. This advance is required as the first step toward solving the limitations of technology, such as inaccurate guidance of devices and limited tissue removal. Further improvement will occur as the fundamental processes responsible for restenosis of lesions are elucidated and methods of control become available.

REFERENCES

1. Hertzer NR. Natural history of peripheral vascular disease: implications for management. Circulation. 1991;83 (Suppl I):12.
2. Glagov S, Weisenberg E, Zarins C, et al. Compensatory enlargement of human atherosclerotic coronary arteries. N Engl J Med 1987;316:1371.
3. Zimmerman JH, Fogarty TJ. Adjunctive intraoperative dilatation (angioplasty). In: Wilson SE, Veith F, Hobson R, et al, eds. Vascular surgery: principles and practice. New York, McGraw-Hill, 1986:297.
4. Johnson KW. Balloon angioplasty: predictive factors for long-term success. Semin Vasc Surg 1989;2:113.
5. White RA, Grundfest WS, eds. Lasers in cardiovascular disease: clinical applications, alternative angioplasty devices and guidance systems, ed 2. Chicago, Year Book Medical Publishers, 1989.
6. Clagett GP, Genton E, Salzmon E. Antithrombotic therapy in peripheral vascular disease. Chest 1989;95:1285.
7. Diethrich EB. Endovascular techniques for abdominal aortic occlusions. Int Angiol 1993;12:270.
8. Ouriel K, Shortell CK, DeWeese JA, et al. A comparison of thrombolytic therapy with operative revascularization in the initial treatment of acute peripheral arterial ischemia. J Vasc Surg 1994;19:1021.
9. Palmaz J, Rivera F, Encarnacion C. Intravascular stents. In: Whittemore A, Bandyk D, Cronenwett J, et al, eds. Advances in vascular surgery. St Louis, Mosby–Year Book, 1993:107.
10. Chuter T, Donayre C, White R, eds. Endoluminal vascular prostheses. Boston, Little, Brown, 1995.
11. Cavaye DM, White RA. Intravascular ultrasound imaging. New York, Raven Press, 1993.

Occlusive Disease Involving Specific Vascular Territories

SURGERY: SCIENTIFIC PRINCIPLES AND PRACTICE, Second Edition, edited by Lazar J. Greenfield, Michael W. Mulholland, Keith T. Oldham, Gerald B. Zelenock, and Keith D. Lillemoe. Lippincott–Raven Publishers, Philadelphia, © 1997.

CHAPTER 80

CEREBROVASCULAR OCCLUSIVE DISEASE

LOUIS M. MESSINA AND GERALD B. ZELENOCK

Cerebrovascular disease encompasses a variety of clinical disorders of the extracranial cerebral arteries that cause transient ischemia or stroke. In the past, most causes of strokes were considered untreatable. Nowhere has the progress been greater in reducing mortality from stroke than that achieved by surgical treatment of extracranial cerebrovascular disease.

The first carotid endarterectomy was performed in 1954. By 1984, it had become the most common vascular surgical procedure performed and the third most common of any operation performed in the United States. Nonetheless, much controversy surrounded the operation owing to the publication of a number of clinical reports that showed wide variability in mortality and morbidity rates after carotid endarterectomy, leading many to question its efficacy. Recently, publication of prospective randomized studies comparing the efficacy of carotid endarterectomy plus optimal medical treatment to optimal medical treatment alone has established unambiguously the efficacy of carotid endarterectomy in the management for cerebrovascular disease.

This chapter reviews the epidemiology, anatomy, pathophysiology, diagnosis, and treatment of cerebrovascular disease of the extracranial arteries.

EPIDEMIOLOGY

Stroke remains the third most common cause of death in the United States, and atherosclerotic occlusive disease of the extracranial portion of the carotid artery is the most common cause of stroke. Stroke is a devastating illness in every respect. Five hundred thousand people suffer strokes each year, and of these 200,000, die as a consequence of stroke (Fig. 80-1). Of the remaining patients who survive stroke, two thirds are disabled and one third require prolonged hospitalization due to residual disability (Table 80-1). The disability caused by stroke is greater than that encountered with other ischemic disorders, such as myocardial infarction. Neurologic deficits causing paralysis, blindness, and aphasia compromise the stroke victim's ability to perform many normal daily functions and to live a satisfying existence. The cumulative public health cost for disabilities caused by strokes are enormous, exceeding $16 trillion a year.[1]

Although the incidence of stroke in the general population is declining, the prevalence is increasing. The decrease in the incidence of stroke is thought to reflect improved management of risk factors for stroke, particularly hypertension. Because the US population is aging, however, the prevalence remains high and is increasing. The effect of an aging population on the incidence of stroke is seen in the fact that in the general population the incidence of stroke is 195 per 100,000 but increases dramatically to 1440 per 100,000 in the 75- to 84-year-old age range. Thus, stroke, owing to its frequency in the population and its personal and financial costs, will remain an exceedingly important public health issue in the years to come.

ANATOMY

The embryonic derivation of the brain's rich blood supply is complex (Fig. 80-2). This rich blood supply to the brain reflects the high oxygen requirement of neural tissue. Although the brain constitutes only 2% of total body

Table 80-1. RESIDUAL DISABILITY IN 119 STROKE SURVIVORS: FRAMINGHAM STUDY

Disability Level	Occurrence (%)
Institutionalized	16
Dependent in self-care activities	31
Dependent for mobility	20
Dependent for vocational activity	71
Decreased socialization	62

(Adapted from Gresham GE, et al. Residual disability in stroke survivors: the Framingham study. N Engl J Med 1975;293:954)

weight, it uses 17% of cardiac output and 20% of the available oxygen supply.[2] A clinical implication of these high oxygen requirements by neural tissue is that necrosis of this tissue can occur within minutes of loss of arterial circulation.

In adults, the ascending aorta rises from the left ventricle, coursing anteriorly in the mediastinum. The branches of aortic arch are the brachiocephalic or innominate artery, the left common carotid artery, and the left subclavian artery. These arteries supply arterial blood to the head and neck, both upper extremities, and the proximal trunk. The aortic arch crosses the upper mediastinum in an oblique fashion from a right anterior to a left posterior position. The brachiocephalic artery is the first and most anterior branch of the aortic arch. Beneath the head of the right clavicle, the brachiocephalic bifurcates to form the right subclavian artery and the right common carotid artery. It is this anterior position of the brachiocephalic artery that makes it accessible for reconstruction through a median sternotomy. The left common carotid artery arises within 1 cm of the brachiocephalic and courses posteriorly into the left of the base of the neck. In 10% of the normal population, the left common carotid artery arises directly from the brachiocephalic artery. Finally, the left subclavian artery arises from its posterior location at the distal end of the aortic arch. Because of this distal and posterior location, it is not easily reached through median sternotomy and is best approached through a high left anterior or anterolateral thoracotomy.

The brain is supplied by the paired internal carotid arteries anteriorly and the vertebral arteries posteriorly (Fig. 80-3). Under normal conditions, the paired carotid arteries supply about 80% to 90% of total cerebral blood flow, whereas the paired vertebral arteries supply 10% to 20% of total cerebral flow. The common carotid artery bifurcates at the angle of the mandibles into the internal and external carotid arteries. The branches of external carotid artery include the ascending pharyngeal, which supplies the hypopharynx and oropharynx; the superior thyroid; the lingual; the occipital; and the posterior auricular. Its final terminal branches are the internal maxillary and the superior temporal arteries.

The internal carotid artery can be divided into four segments: cervical, intrapetrosal, intracavernous, and supraclinoid. The cervical, extracranial portion of the internal carotid artery has no branches. The intracavernous and supraclinoid portions are referred to clinically as the carotid siphon. The first major branch of internal carotid artery is the ophthalmic artery. The supraclinoid portion of the internal carotid artery gives rise to the major branches of internal carotid artery, including the ophthalmic, posterior communicating, and anterior choroidal arteries. Eventually, the internal carotid artery bifurcates into its terminal branches, the anterior cerebral and the

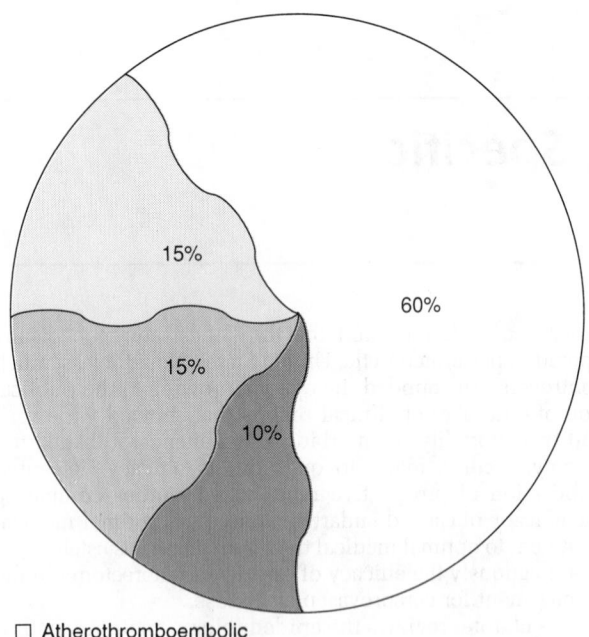

15%
60%
15%
10%

☐ Atherothromboembolic
☐ Cardiocerebral embolic
▨ Hemorrhagic—subarachnoid, intracerebral
▨ Other

Figure 80-1. The precise distribution of causes of stroke varies among reports, but the most common causes are atherothromboembolic events that originate from the extracranial arteries, from cardiac sources, and from intraparenchymal or subarachnoid hemorrhage. (After Zelenock GB, D'Alecy LG. The brain. In: Zelenock GB, D'Alecy LG, Fantone JC III, et al. Clinical ischemic syndrome mechanisms and consequences of tissue injury. St Louis, CV Mosby, 1990)

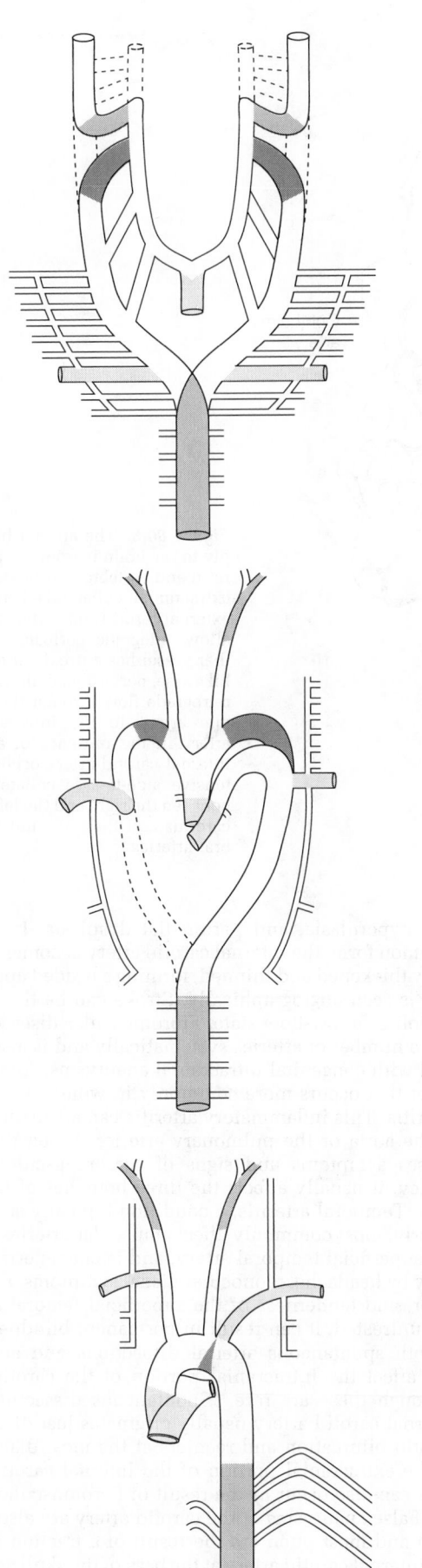

Figure 80-2. Development of the great arteries: (*A*) 5th week; (*B*) 7th week; (*C*) 9th week. (After Barry A. The aortic arch derivatives in the human adult. Anat Rec 1951;111:221)

middle cerebral arteries. The anterior communicating artery joins the comparable vessel from the contralateral hemisphere; similarly, the posterior communicating arteries are continuous with the posterior cerebral branches of the basilar artery. These branches form the circle of Willis, which is composed of an anterior communicating artery that connects the right and left anterior cerebral arteries of the internal carotid artery system with the posterior cerebral arteries of the vertebrobasilar system by way of the posterior communicating artery (Fig. 80-4). Variations in the anatomy of the circle of Willis occur in 50% to 80% of the normal population. About 15% of the population have no anastomoses between the anterior and the posterior cerebral circulations, and as many as 35% are missing the anastomotic channels between either the anterior and posterior circulations or the right and left hemispheric circulations. Deficiency of this collateral pathway has important clinical consequences when one of the four major cerebral arteries become occluded.

The vertebral arteries arise from the first portion of the subclavian artery and enter the transverse cervical process at the level of the sixth cervical vertebra and ascend in the transverse foramen, eventually piercing the posterior allantoid–occipital membrane and coursing into the posterior fascia through the foramen magnum. The vertebral arteries course along the lateral border of the medulla and unite to form the basilar artery. The extracranial portion of the vertebral artery has segmental spinal and muscular branches. The basilar artery terminates as the right and left posterior cerebral arteries, from which arise the posterior communicating arteries of the circle of Willis.

A number of clinically important collateral pathways exist between cerebral arteries. These collaterals become significant sources of arterial flow to the brain when arterial occlusive disease develops in one of the four major arteries supplying arterial blood to the brain. Branches of the external carotid artery, particularly the facial, internal maxillary, and superficial temporal arteries, may anastomose with the intraorbital and supraorbital arteries. These anastomotic networks become important sources of blood flow into the intracranial portions of the internal carotid artery when a hemodynamic stenosis occurs at the carotid bifurcation in the cervical portion of the internal carotid artery. Communication between these external carotid artery branches and the ophthalmic artery branch of internal carotid artery is the most important of these collateral networks. This collateral pathway may be identified angiographically or by using a directional Doppler probe. Similarly, the vertebral artery gives off numerous muscular branches in the neck. If the proximal vertebral artery is occluded, collateral arteries from the external carotid artery may anastomose to the distal vertebral artery by way of these branches. In addition, a patient who experiences a common carotid artery occlusion may receive blood flow from the vertebral artery through the external carotid artery branches into the internal carotid artery, thereby maintaining antegrade internal carotid artery blood flow. Finally, branches of the left and right external carotid arteries may anastomose freely across the face.

PATHOPHYSIOLOGY

Although there are many causes of stroke (Tables 80-2 and 80-3), most strokes are the result of a few distinct pathologic processes. Atherosclerosis remains the most common cause of stroke in adults. Less common pathologic processes include aneurysms of the internal carotid artery; anatomic abnormalities, including coils, which are loops or gentle curves in the internal carotid artery; kinks, which are acute bends in the internal carotid artery that

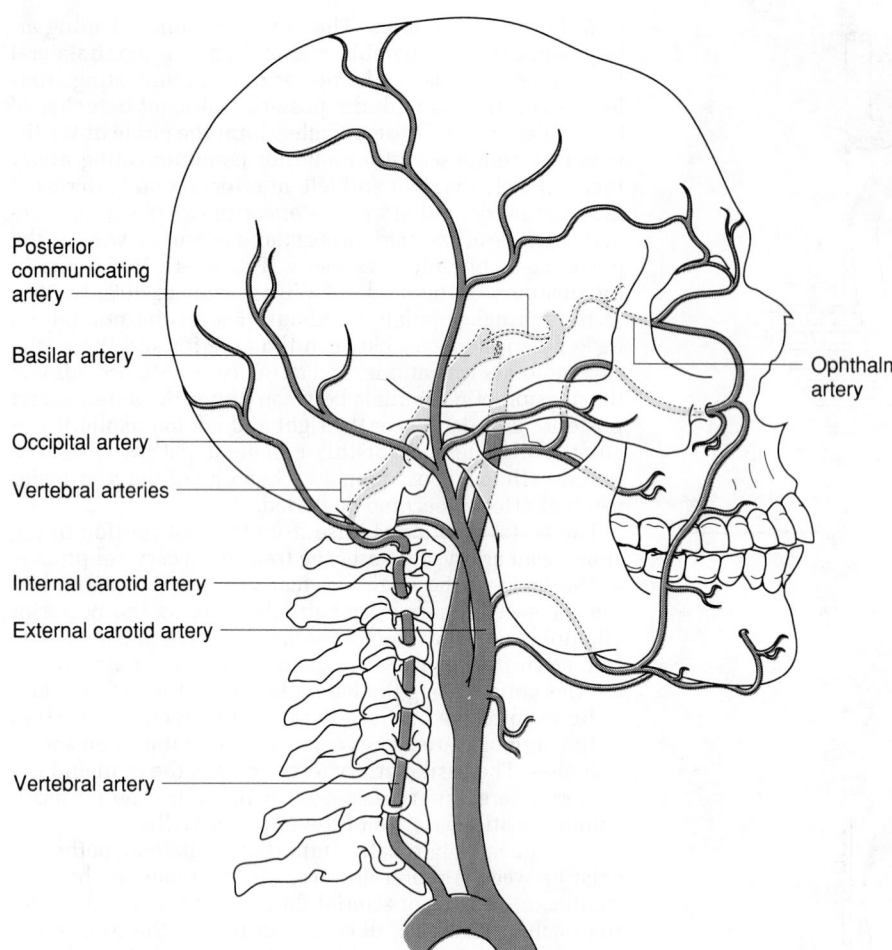

Figure 80-3. The arterial blood supply to the brain is from the paired carotid and vertebral arteries. Extensive extracranial collaterals between the external carotid and vertebral systems allow antegrade perfusion when either vessel has a proximal occlusion. Likewise, periorbital collateral allows retrograde flow through the ophthalmic artery to the internal carotid artery in the presence of a cervical internal carotid artery occlusion. Extensive side-to-side collateral exists between the right and the left external carotids and the right and left vertebral arteries.

result in the carotid artery folding up in itself. Fibromuscular dysplasia is a vessel wall abnormality that occurs typically in women 30 to 50 years of age and involves the cervical internal carotid artery distal to the carotid bifurcation.[3,4] Fibromuscular dysplasia is usually subdivided into four categories: intimal fibroplasia, medial fibroplasia, me-

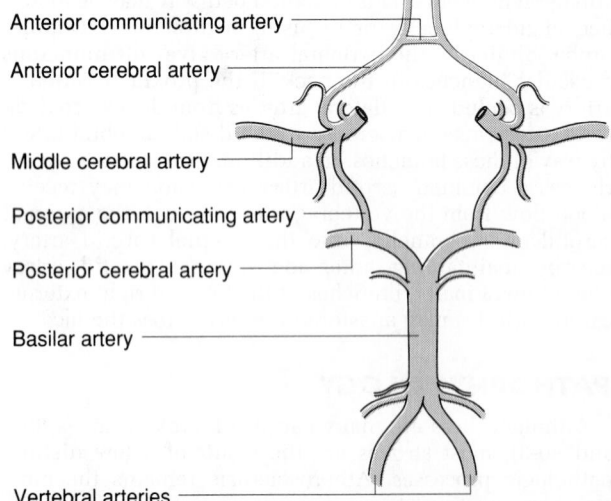

Figure 80-4. The circle of Willis is a highly efficient intracranial collateral network; however, multiple important variations occur, and an incomplete circle producing an isolated hemisphere is not uncommon.

dial hyperplasia, and perimedial dysplasia. In its most common form, the internal carotid artery becomes alternatingly thickened and thinned, forming a beaded appearance that is seen angiographically. Stroke can be the result of emboli or a low-flow state. Fibromuscular disease can affect a number of arteries systematically and is also associated with congenital intracranial aneurysms. Another disorder that occurs more commonly in women is Takayasu arteritis. This inflammatory arteritis can affect any branch of the aorta or the pulmonary arteries. When this entity causes symptoms and signs of cerebrovascular insufficiency, it usually affects the three branches of the aortic arch. Temporal arteritis, a condition typically seen in the elderly, most commonly affects muscular arteries, such as the superficial temporal artery, and is characterized clinically by headache, monocular visual symptoms, low-grade fever, and tenderness of the superficial femoral artery. If left untreated, it can result in permanent blindness.

Both spontaneous arterial dissections and aneurysms can affect the intracranial portion of the carotid artery, although these are rare.[5] Spontaneous dissection of the internal carotid artery usually originates just distal to the carotid bifurcation and reenters at the most distal aspect of the extracranial portion of the internal carotid artery. This can also occur as the result of fibromuscular dysplasia. False aneurysms of the carotid artery are also uncommon and most often are the result of a traction injury to the internal carotid artery at the base of the skull associated with forceful flexion and extension of the neck. Spontaneous dissections and aneurysm of the internal carotid artery

Table 80-2. CAUSES OF CEREBRAL ISCHEMIA AND INFARCTION

ISCHEMIC

Atherothromboembolic

High-grade stenoses and occlusions
Emboli
Plaque
Platelet-fibrin debris
Intraplaque hemorrhage

Cardioembolic

Arrhythmias (atrial fibrillation; other arrhythmias)
Myocardial infarction with mural thrombus
Mitral valve prolapse; calcified annulus
Rheumatic heart disease (valvular, nonvalvular)
Prosthetic heart valves
Other (myopathy, atrial myxoma, subacute bacterial endocarditis, paradoxical emboli)

Systemic

Cardiac arrest and resuscitation
Profound shock
Cardiopulmonary bypass

Venous Thromboses

Dural venous sinuses
Bilateral jugular vein occlusions

Miscellaneous Causes

Lacunar infarcts
Lipohyalinosis
Fibrinoid necrosis
Charcot-Bouchard aneurysms
Migraine and vasospasm
Diabetes
Moyamoya
Kawasaki syndrome
Amyloid degeneration
Fibromuscular disease
Giant cell arteritis
Spontaneous dissections
Trauma (extracranial cerebral vessels)
  Blunt
  Penetrating
Hypercoaguable states
Binswanger encephalopathy
Substance abuse

HEMORRHAGIC

Intraparenchymal Hemorrhage

Hypertensive encephalopathy
Amyloid angiography
Arteriovenous malformation
Trauma

Subarachnoid Hemorrhage

Berry aneurysms
Arteriovenous malformation
Trauma

EXTRACRANIAL

Atherosclerosis
  Great vessels
  Carotid artery
Fibromuscular dysplasia
Trauma
Aortic aneurysms
  Dissecting
  Atherosclerotic
  Traumatic
Takayasu panarteritis
Temporal arteritis
Carotid dissections
  Spontaneous
  Trauma associated
Carotid aneurysms

(Modified from Zelenock GB. The brain. In: Clinical ischemic syndromes: mechanisms and consequences of tissue injury. St Louis, CV Mosby, 1990)

are most often complicated by thromboembolic events causing transient ischemia or stroke.

Atherosclerosis is the pathologic process most responsible for symptoms of cerebrovascular insufficiency. The cause of atherosclerosis in the cerebral arterial circulation or in any portion of the systemic arterial circulation remains incompletely understood.[6] Clinically, atherosclerosis tends to be a segmental disease, usually developing at areas of local turbulence, such as vessel bifurcations, thereby causing focal vessel wall injury. Thus, the origin of the great vessels from the aortic arch or the proximal cervical bifurcation of these vessels is involved frequently. Typically, the common carotid artery is spared. The ca-

rotid bifurcation is the most common location of atherosclerosis in the cerebral circulation. The predilection of atherosclerosis for the carotid bulb is thought to be secondary to the turbulent blood flow generated by the carotid bifurcation, resulting in areas of *low* shear stress and increased particle residence time. Grossly, the atherosclerotic plaque is thickest at the carotid bifurcation and extends 2 cm into the distal internal carotid artery. The plaque occupies the media and intima, sparing the outer media and adventitia. Usually, the plaque tapers from the media into the normal intima. This tapering often permits a smooth surface after endarterectomy. Finally, atherosclerotic stenosis can occur at the origins of the anterior and middle cerebral arteries, but these lesions are significantly less common than those found in the cervical portion of the internal carotid artery.

The atherosclerotic plaque at the carotid bifurcation, as at other locations in the systemic arterial circulation, initially appears as a *fatty streak*, which is largely an intimal lesion characterized by fat deposition but some mononuclear and foam cell infiltration. Fatty streaks do not cause hemodynamically significant stenoses of the vessel, and not all fatty streaks develop into complex plaques. As plaques increase in size, they may intermittently ulcerate or suffer intraplaque hemorrhage; both processes can result in emboli or thrombosis of the artery. Mature atherosclerotic plaques are characterized by endothelial cell damage and denudation, intimal hyperplasia secondary to smooth muscle cell proliferation, and then a gradual increased deposition of collagen matrix and extensive intracellular and extracellular lipid accumulation. These mature atherosclerotic plaques are usually covered by a *fibrous cap*. Disruption of the fibrous cap is often a precipitating event that causes a plaque to become symptomatic. Disruption of fibrous caps can occur secondary to a number of processes, including progressive growth of the atherosclerotic lesion, increased blood flow velocity and shear stress, hemorrhage into the plaque, or rupture of vasa vasorum. Loss of the fibrous cap secondary to intraplaque hemorrhage or surface disruption due to mechanical forces results in a loss of endothelial cell coverage, exposing the underlying necrotic core of the plaque to the circulating blood. These changes promote platelet deposition and thrombus formation on the ulcerated surface. Disrupted mature, complex plaques may then result

Table 80-3. CLASSIFICATION OF SYMPTOMS

HEMISPHERIC

Contralateral hemiparesis
Contralateral paresthesias or hemisensory changes
Ipsilateral monocular visual changes
Aphasia

NONHEMISPHERIC

Vertigo
Ataxia
Diplopia
Bilateral visual symptoms
Shifting pareses or paresthesias
Drop attacks
Dysarthria
Syncope
Dizziness
Light-headedness
Decreased mentation
Headache
Personality change
Tinnitus
Seizures

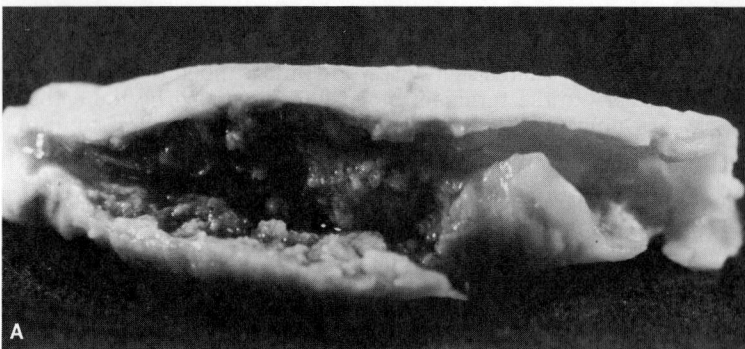

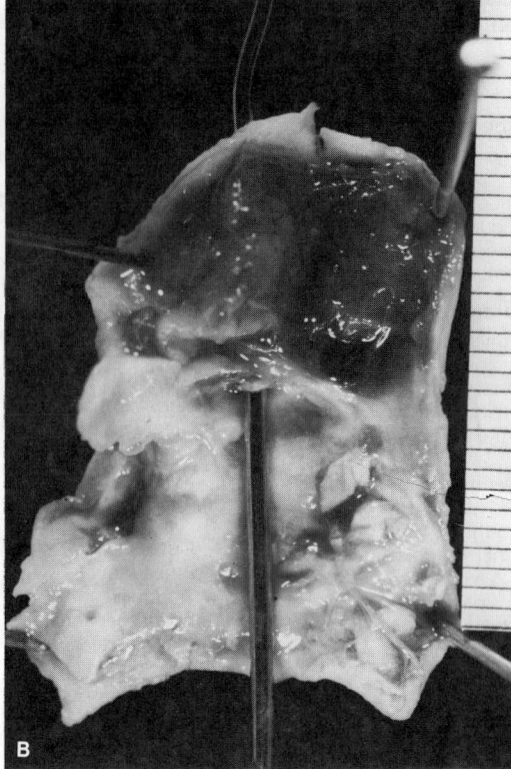

Figure 80-5. Endarterectomy specimens. (*A*) The thickened atherosclerotic plaque is almost totally occluded with intraluminal thrombus. This patient had symptoms of repeated embolization. (*B*) Hemorrhage is seen within the plaque, not in the lumen. If this hemorrhagic plaque excavates into the lumen, an ulceration will form.

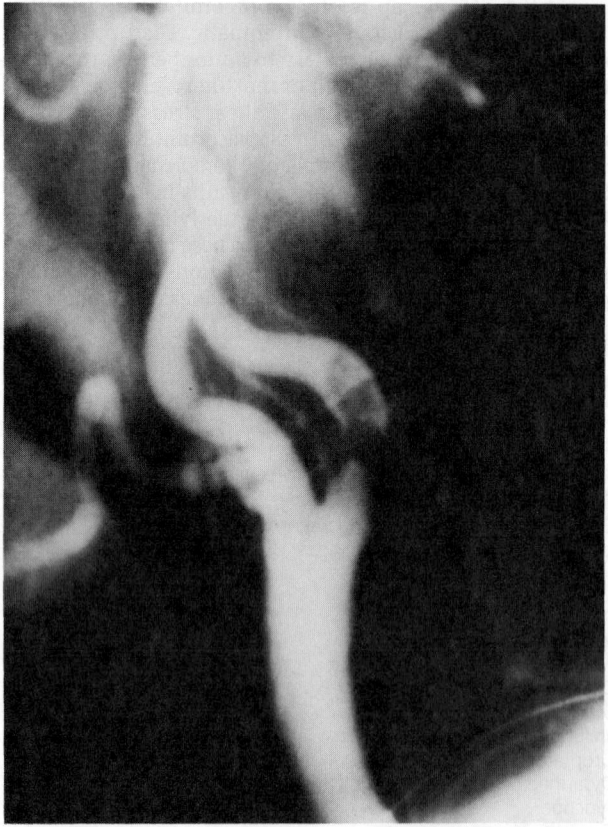

Figure 80-6. An isolated atherosclerotic lesion at the origin of the internal carotid artery. Free-floating intraluminal thrombus can be seen distal to the atherosclerotic plaque in this patient with crescendo transient ischemic attacks.

in stroke through embolization of atheromatous debris or platelet-fibrin aggregates (Figs. 80-5 and 80-6). Alternatively, thrombosis of the artery can result in ischemic necrosis when there is insufficient collateral blood flow.

Some of these pathologic changes can be seen by the carotid duplex scan. When a mature plaque is hard and calcified, the plaque is highly echogenic, whereas a mature plaque complicated by intraplaque hemorrhage or loss of the fibrosis cap is normally anechoic and is called *soft plaque*. Some prospective studies have shown a correlation between the presence of soft plaque and transient ischemia and stroke and between the presence of hard, calcified plaque and lack of associated symptoms.

The predilection of atherosclerosis to occur at the carotid bifurcation is most likely due to a variety of hemodynamic changes.[7] Atherosclerotic plaques tend to occur along the outer wall, not the inner wall, of the carotid bifurcation, often sparing or only involving the most proximal portion of the external carotid artery. At the outer wall of the carotid bifurcation, there is disruption of normal laminar blood flow, resulting in flow separation, flow stasis, increased particle residence time, and increased shear stress oscillations, that is, areas of high and low shear stress. The clinical risk factors for the development of carotid artery atherosclerotic lesions are the same as those for coronary artery disease and include age, hypertension, diabetes mellitus, hyperlipidemia, hypercoaguable states, positive family history, and tobacco abuse. A strong correlation between carotid plaque and elevated plasma homocysteine levels has been identified.[8]

Stroke secondary to cerebrovascular disease can occur by two distinct mechanisms—ischemia due to low-flow states and embolism. Cerebral ischemia due to low-flow states occurs secondary to the development of hemodynamically significant stenosis, often involving multiple cerebral arteries or secondary to a stenosis in an artery supplying a vascular territory for which is there is a poor collateral network. Although the earliest reports linking stroke and extracranial carotid occlusive disease occurred in the 19th century, it was not until the 1950s that Fisher and colleagues[9] and Milliken[10] established the correlation between extracranial coronary artery occlusive disease and stroke. These investigators established that most strokes caused by carotid artery occlusive disease were due to cholesterol or platelet–fibrin emboli that dislodged from atherosclerotic plaques within the extracranial carotid artery and subsequently occluded distal branches of the internal carotid artery. Their hypothesis differed substantially from the conventional dogma that most strokes occurred as a result of cerebral ischemia due to reduced cerebral perfusion. One way in which this hypothesis was established was by the identification of *Hollenhorst plaques*, which are platelet–fibrin aggregates or cholesterol crystals obstructing branches of the retinal artery.[11]

CLINICAL PRESENTATION

The most common clinical presentations of cerebrovascular occlusive disease are transient ischemic attack (TIA) and hemispheric stroke. Cerebrovascular disease resulting in atheroemboli or thrombosis accounts for up to 60% of patients suffering cerebral infarctions (see Fig. 80-1). A TIA is the sudden onset of a focal neurologic deficit that resolves completely within 24 hours of its onset. TIAs can occur as transient hemispheric ischemic attacks or transient mononuclear blindness. Transient hemispheric attacks present clinically as contralateral motor and sensory deficits or as a pure motor or pure sensory deficit. The specific clinical presentation depends on the anatomic location of the area of cerebral ischemia. Transient mononuclear blindness also known as *amaurosis fugax*, which is a transient loss of vision secondary to mechanical obstruction of a branch of the retinal artery by either a cholesterol crystal or a Hollenhorst plaque.[10] When most patients are examined immediately after an episode of amaurosis fugax, however, most are found to have a normal retinal circulation. Transient ischemia can occur in the distal distribution of the posterior circulation of the brain, causing transient *vertebrobasilar insufficiency*. This can present as binocular visual loss; *drop attacks*, in which the patient does not lose consciousness but collapses to the floor; dysarthria; vertigo; dysphasia; incoordination; and other signs of cerebellar insufficiency. The differential diagnosis of patients suffering TIAs includes cerebral tumor, hypoglycemia, hyponatremia, hypercalcemia, and hepatic or renal failure. In addition, vasospasm, particularly that associated with migraine headache, can present as transient ischemia. A significant clinical finding in patients suffering TIAs secondary to atheroemboli is that the TIA is usually short, less than 15 minutes. Although the distinction between a TIA and a completed stroke is sharply defined, serial computed tomographic (CT) scans of patients suffering TIAs have shown that as many as 25% have had strokes in the distribution of their symptoms.[12]

A stroke is an acute neurologic deficit that lasts more than 24 hours. As is true of TIAs, most strokes are due to embolic occlusion of a branch of the middle cerebral artery by atheromatous debris or a platelet–fibrin aggregate. Alternatively, a minority of strokes occur after internal carotid artery occlusion and subsequent cerebral infarction in a "watershed" distribution due to low flow. The watershed areas are located at the border areas between the anterior and posterior cerebral circulation, typically between the superior parietal and the posterior temporooccipital lobes of the ipsilateral hemisphere. When strokes occur in this area, they are characterized clinically by a contralateral sensorimotor deficit more pronounced in the proximal than in the distal limb, a prominent visual field defect, aphasia, and features of partial inattention.[13]

Stroke in the distribution of the anterior cerebral artery is characterized by weakness or paralysis at the contralateral limbs, numbness and tingling in the contralateral limbs, sparing of the face, dyspraxia, and abnormalities of higher cerebral function due to frontal lobe involvement. The latter is manifested by the presence of a grasp reflex, behavior disorder, poor concentration, and slowness of response. Strokes in the distribution of the middle cerebral artery are characterized by sensorimotor deficits in the contralateral limbs and homonymous hemianopsia. Strokes in the distribution of the anterior choroidal artery are characterized by contralateral hemiplegia, hypesthesia, and homonymous hemianopsia. Anterior circulation strokes should be distinguished clinically from lacunar strokes and vertebrobasilar strokes. Lacunar strokes are usually characterized by pure motor or sensory dysfunction in the contralateral limb in patients with hypertension. The term *lacunar* is derived from the Latin word for "hole" or "cavity" and refers to the appearance of infarcted tissue within the substance of the brain on gross examination. The pathophysiology of lacunar strokes is usually a reflection of disease of small, 200-μm arterioles. Pathologically, lamellae of lipohyalinosis are often found. Finally, patients with vertebrobasilar strokes present with ipsilateral cranial nerve deficits; contralateral sensorimotor deficits; signs of cerebellar insufficiency, including ataxia, vertigo, nystagmus, diplopia, and drop attacks. Symptoms of global cerebral ischemia can be difficult to distinguish from those of vertebrobasilar dysfunction.

DIAGNOSIS

Despite the development of multiple sophisticated diagnostic technologies, the clinical diagnosis of patients with symptomatic cerebrovascular occlusive disease remains centered on a carefully performed neurologic examination before obtaining any of these diagnostic studies. Of paramount importance is to establish the distinction between a focal and a nonfocal neurologic deficit, such as dizziness. The history and physical examination should localize the area of cerebral ischemia responsible for the neurologic deficit. The neurologic examination of the patient should be complemented by a more complete physical examination to determine the presence of vascular occlusive disease in either the coronary or peripheral arteries as well as to define the other risk factors for stroke, such as acute arrhythmia.

A wide variety of noninvasive and invasive diagnostic studies can be performed to determine the cause and effect of stroke. Color-flow duplex scanning uses real-time B-mode ultrasound and color-enhanced pulsed Doppler flow measurements to determine the extent of the carotid stenosis with reliable sensitivity and specificity[14,15] (Color Figs. 80-1 and 80-2). Real-time B-mode imaging permits localization of the disease and determination of the presence or absence of calcification within the plaque. Determination of the extent of stenosis is based largely on velocity criteria. The Doppler technique uses an ultrasonic frequency that is transmitted at predetermined frequencies. The emitted sound frequency is then reflected by the moving red blood cells within a vessel back to a receiver crystal within the probe. The *Doppler effect,* which is the delay between the emission and reception of the ultrasonic frequency, is proportional to a velocity of the red cells. As the stenosis increasingly obliterates the lumen of the vessel, the velocity of blood must increase in the area of the stenosis so that the total volume of flow remains constant within the vessel. Thus, the velocity is correlated with the extent of carotid artery stenosis (see Color Fig. 80-1). Typically, the internal carotid artery velocity profile is one of a low-resistance artery characterized by a significant period of carotid blood flow during diastole. Low-resistance velocity profiles also occur in the hepatic and renal arteries. In contrast, the external carotid artery reflects a signal typically found in a high-resistance muscular artery, such as the common femoral artery, in which little blood flow occurs during diastole.

A carotid duplex scan requires considerable skill and experience in both its performance and interpretation. Duplex scanning is most accurate in the estimation of carotid artery stenosis of greater than 50% diameter reduction. Color-flow duplex scanning has been refined sufficiently such that some clinicians now proceed to carotid endarterectomy without preoperative angiography. As mentioned earlier, the hypoechoic presence of calcium within the carotid wall may have prognostic significance.

Transcranial Doppler

Transcranial Doppler uses a low-frequency probe and the thinness of the temporal bone to focus a directional Doppler probe on the anterior, middle, and posterior cerebral arteries. Transcranial Doppler is of particular clinical value in patients suffering vasospasm after subarachnoid hemorrhage. In patients with cerebrovascular disease, transcranial Doppler complements duplex scanning by assessing the presence of significant intraarterial stenoses as well as patterns of collateral flow. Transcranial color-flow duplex imaging is also available.

Angiography

Angiography remains the gold standard for the diagnosis of cerebrovascular disease. Angiography permits visualization of the arterial system by injection of a radiopaque dye from an intraarterial catheter. Angiography remains the only method that allows complete and detailed visualization of both the intracranial and extracranial arterial circulations. Nonetheless, angiography remains a painful study for the patient and has serious inherent risks, such as dye allergy; renal toxicity, particularly in patients with diabetes mellitus; chronic renal insufficiency; and neurologic complications, such as stroke (2% to 4% of patients). Digital subtraction angiography has reduced the need for selective carotid artery catheterization and thus reduced the risk of these neurologic complications.

Computed Tomographic Scanning and Magnetic Resonance Imaging

Computed tomographic scanning of the brain is a valuable test for patients suffering TIAs or stroke. Contrast-enhanced scans that assess density changes, the presence of edema, and the presence of mass effect can determine the location and the extent of a stroke and can rule out other causes. A CT scan of the brain distinguishes accurately between cerebral hemorrhage and infarction. Hemorrhage is associated with areas of increased density on a CT scan, whereas infarction is associated with areas of decreased density that do not appear until at least 8 hours after the occurrence of the stroke.

Magnetic resonance (MR) imaging and MR angiography are highly sensitive techniques for the evaluation of patients with symptomatic cerebrovascular disease. MR imaging is more sensitive than CT scanning for the detection of an acute stroke. MR imaging can detect a stroke immediately after the infarction occurs, whereas CT scanning can-

not. Cerebral hemorrhage, however, is less well identified by MR imaging than by CT scan. MR angiography, which is evolving rapidly, permits evaluation of both the extracranial and intracranial cerebral circulations. The precision of MR angiography in determining the extent of stenosis, although improving rapidly, remains inferior to that achieved by conventional angiography. Nonetheless, MR angiography probably will play an increasingly important role in the diagnostic evaluation of patients with cerebrovascular disease.

NATURAL HISTORY OF CAROTID ARTERY OCCLUSIVE DISEASE

Symptomatic Disease

Although many studies have been undertaken to define the natural history and clinical consequences of TIAs and strokes, a variety of methodologic problems have limited the conclusions that can be drawn from these studies. Despite limitations, it is clear that there is a substantial risk of stroke after a carotid territory TIA or stroke. In community-based studies, the risk of stroke in the first 3 years after TIA varies from 12% to 17%.[16,17] In hospital-based studies, the risk of stroke after TIA varies from 10% to 30% after the first year, and then patients have a 6% risk of stroke each year for the subsequent 5 years. The cumulative risk of stroke after TIA at 5 years was 30% to 50%. More important is the very high mortality rate secondary to coronary artery disease: one third of the patients died within 5 years after TIA, usually of coronary occlusive disease. The natural history of patients after ischemic stroke is ominous. The initial stroke carries a 20% to 30% hospital mortality rate and the risk of recurrent stroke is high, ranging from 5% to 40%, of which 30% are fatal.[18,19]

Asymptomatic Disease

Because only 10% of patients who experience stroke of any cause have an antecedent TIA, defining clearly the natural history of asymptomatic carotid artery disease attains significant clinical importance. Much of the early literature that addressed this issue studied asymptomatic carotid *bruits*, which are relatively common and have been reported to occur in about 5% of the population older than 50 years.[20] Unfortunately, carotid bruits do not always arise from significant carotid artery stenosis; they can be due to radiation of cardiac murmurs or denote the presence of mild carotid artery disease associated with calcification of the arterial wall. In fact, the poor correlation between the presence of a bruit and stenosis is illustrated by the fact that only 23% of patients identified to have bruits on physical examination have a significant (over 50%) carotid stenosis.[21] With the wide availability of relatively inexpensive but accurate noninvasive studies to determine the presence and degree of carotid artery stenosis, the presence of a carotid bruit has little significance relative to the neurologic prognosis of the patient. The presence of a carotid bruit, however, remains a significant predictor of symptomatic life-threatening coronary artery disease.

The development of carotid duplex ultrasonography has permitted a more accurate assessment of the prevalence of asymptomatic carotid stenosis in older and high-risk populations. The prevalence of internal carotid artery stenosis is 30% in patients older than 50 years; however, the prevalence of carotid stenosis greater than 50% diameter reduction was only 3.7%, and only 0.9% of patients had a diameter reduction of over 80%.

Studies that have examined the natural history of patients with asymptomatic carotid artery stenosis do not

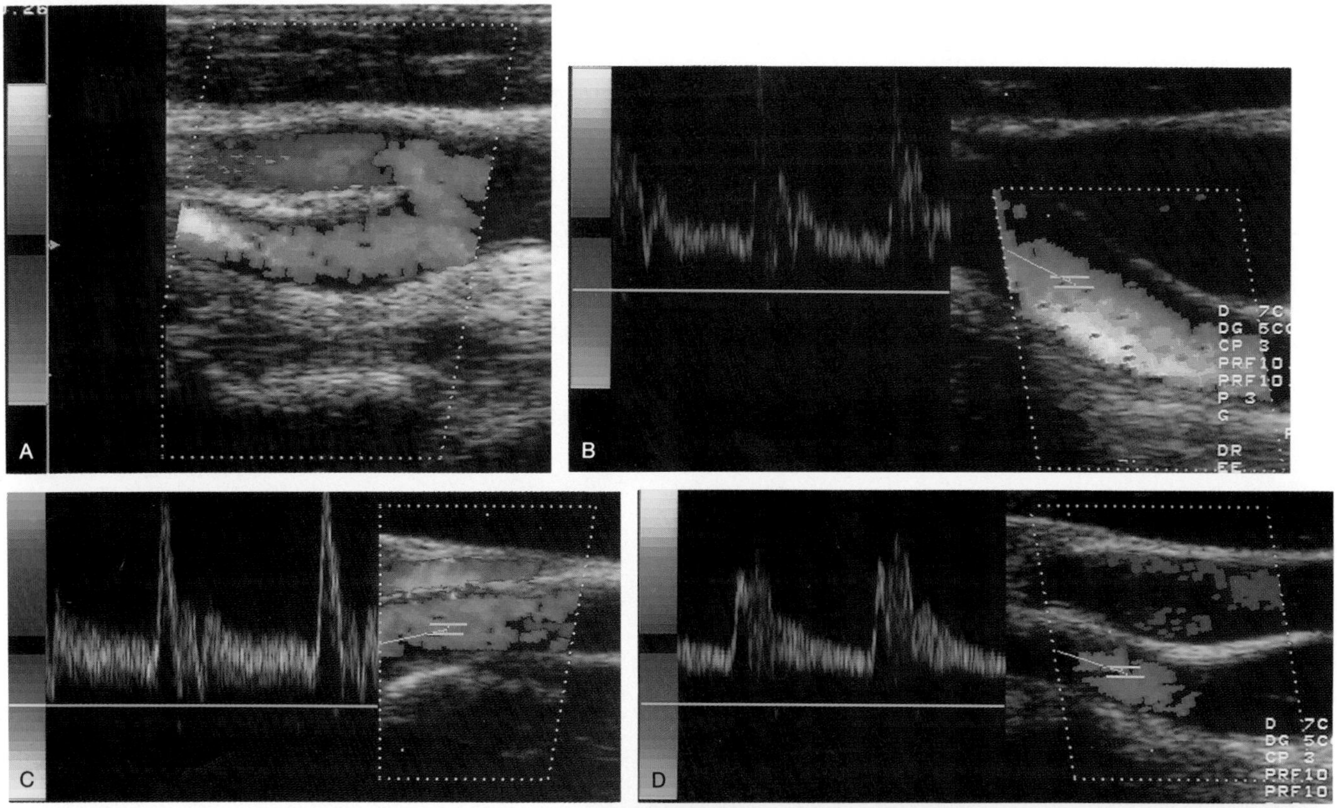

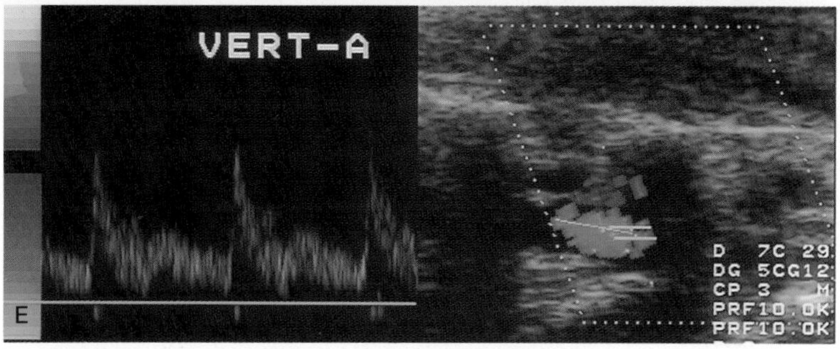

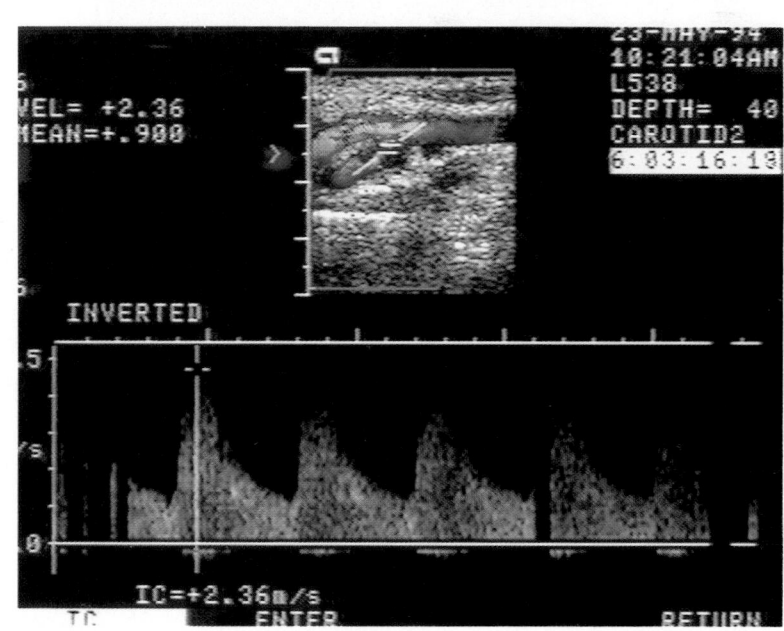

Color Figure 80-1. (*A*) Color-flow duplex scan showing a normal carotid artery bifurcation, the external carotid artery, and the internal carotid artery. (*B* to *D*) Duplex B-mode and analogue waveform of the common carotid artery (*B*), external carotid artery (*C*), and internal carotid artery (*D*). There is a typical high-resistance waveform of the external carotid artery, which has reversal of flow in early diastole and minimal diastolic flow. In contrast, the internal carotid artery has a classic low-resistance waveform characterized by continuous flow throughout diastole. (*E*) Color flow duplex image and analogue waveform of the vertebral artery.

Color Figure 80-2. Color-flow duplex scan and analogue waveform of a high-grade internal carotid artery stenosis. Note acoustic shadowing in the region of the stenosis caused by calcification of the artery wall. Doppler taken at midstream of the jet of flow through the stenosis shows marked elevation of the peak systolic velocity (236 cm/s).

provide a clear and definitive estimate of the risk of stroke in these patients. Studies do show, however, that the risk of stroke appears to be proportionate to the degree of stenosis in that the highest risk patients are those with stenosis of greater than 80% diameter reduction. In addition, in studies that employed serial carotid duplex scans, 85% of patients experienced progression in the extent of the stenosis during follow-up. For patients who are found to have a 75% to 80% stenosis, the risk of stroke varies from 18% and 46%.[21,22]

An important clinical question is whether the presence of a severe but asymptomatic carotid artery stenosis increases the risk of stroke in patients who undergo a major surgical procedure, such as coronary artery bypass grafting or peripheral vascular surgery. For noncardiac surgery, most studies found that the perioperative risk of stroke is not increased; but when the patients were followed up carefully, a high neurologic complication rate was identified.[23] Most studies that specifically addressed the issue of preoperative stroke after coronary artery bypass grafting found that unilateral asymptomatic high-grade stenoses do not increase the risk of stroke.[24-27] Consideration for prophylactic repair is recommended, however, when bilateral high-grade asymptomatic stenosis are present.

MANAGEMENT

Medical Treatment

Both asymptomatic and symptomatic carotid artery occlusive disease are virtually always caused by atherosclerosis, a systemic disease. As with symptomatic atherosclerosis in other parts of the systemic arterial circulation, it is important to make every effort to modify risk factors to prevent progression of disease. The most important risk factor for stroke that should be controlled is hypertension. In addition, cessation of smoking, management of lipid disorders, attainment of ideal body weight, and regular exercise should be undertaken. No drug therapy has been shown to reduce the risk of stroke in patients with asymptomatic carotid artery occlusive disease. A number of studies have examined the role of antiplatelet drugs as well as anticoagulation to reduce the risk of stroke in patients after TIA or stroke.[1] No study has shown definitive evidence that systemic anticoagulation reduces the risk of stroke in patients with significant carotid artery occlusive disease who experienced a TIA and stroke. The role of aspirin is less controversial. Aspirin, by reducing platelet adhesion and aggregation, has been shown to reduce morbidity and mortality from symptomatic coronary artery occlusive disease. A number of studies have shown a reduction in the risk of stroke and death in patients treated with aspirin. A number of serious methodologic criticisms of these studies have been made, however, and a metaanalysis of the prospective placebo-controlled trials of antiplatelet and anticoagulant therapies concluded that therapeutic benefit for either treatment could not be established and that anticoagulants probably had an adverse effect.[28]

Surgical Treatment

The major indications for reconstruction of the cerebrovascular arteries hemispheric TIA, stroke that leaves minimal residual neurologic deficits, and high-grade asymptomatic carotid artery stenosis. Less common indications include global cerebral ischemia, which usually occurs when three of the four major cerebral arteries have hemodynamically significant stenosis. These patients should undergo extensive evaluation for other possible explanations for their global symptoms, such as cardiac arrhythmia and middle ear abnormalities.

Technique of Carotid Endarterectomy

Although carotid endarterectomy has been performed for more than 40 years and is the most commonly performed vascular operation, variability still exists in certain aspects of this procedure, particularly in the type of anesthetic and the methods used for determining the adequacy of cerebral perfusion during transient internal carotid artery occlusion. Anesthesia for carotid endarterectomy can be either general endotracheal anesthesia, regional cervical block, or local anesthesia. Proponents of general anesthesia argue that the anesthetized, motionless patient makes the operation safer and allows more direct control of hemodynamic variables. In addition, general anesthesia reduces the cerebral metabolic rate and therefore may increase the threshold for ischemia. Proponents of regional or local anesthesia believe that these techniques minimize the risk of perioperative myocardial infarction caused by general anesthesia and provide a more accurate assessment of the adequacy of cerebral perfusion during the period of transient internal carotid occlusion.

Surgical exposure of the carotid artery can be achieved through an incision along the medial border of the sternocleidomastoid muscle or by an oblique transverse incision through a skin crease. During dissection and mobilization of the common carotid artery and its branches, it is important to proceed with gentle dissection and minimal manipulation of the carotid bulb to prevent embolization from the atherosclerotic plaque. After systemic heparinization of the patient, the carotid artery is occluded, and a lateral arteriotomy is made from just proximal to the plaque in the common carotid artery to just beyond the distal extent of the plaque in the internal carotid artery (Fig. 80-7). The success of carotid endarterectomy is based on the unique location of arterial atherosclerotic plaques, which occupy the intima and the media, usually sparing the adventitia of the involved arterial wall. In addition, atherosclerotic plaques are segmental in nature and taper from within the deep media into the intima of the diseased artery distally. The cleavage plane for the endarterectomy is chosen at the thickest portion of the plaque, usually in the carotid bulb. This plane is then extended proximally and circumferentially, and the proximal plaque is transected. As the endarterectomy is extended toward the internal carotid artery, it is important to identify the transition zone of the plaque from within the deep media to the intima. This usually allows a plaque to be feathered distally, leaving a naturally molded arterial wall in the internal carotid artery distally. The operation is completed by performing an eversion endarterectomy of the portion of the plaque that extends into the proximal external carotid artery. The plaque in the external carotid artery usually ends at the first bifurcation of this artery. At the completion of the endarterectomy, any loose fragments of artery wall are removed, and if there is any residual shelf or loose intima distally, tacking sutures are placed to avoid a flap being raised during restoration of blood flow. The carotid arteriotomy is closed using a running suture, and if the internal carotid artery is small, a patch angioplasty can be performed (see Fig. 80-7).

Some surgeons believe that patch angioplasty should be performed routinely after carotid endarterectomy to reduce the incidence of recurrent carotid stenosis. An objective technique to assess the patency of the endarterectomy should be undertaken at the completion of this procedure using continuous-wave Doppler assessment, B-mode ultrasound, or intraoperative arteriography. The patient should be monitored carefully for the first 12 to 24 hours after endarterectomy to evaluate for hemodynamic stability as

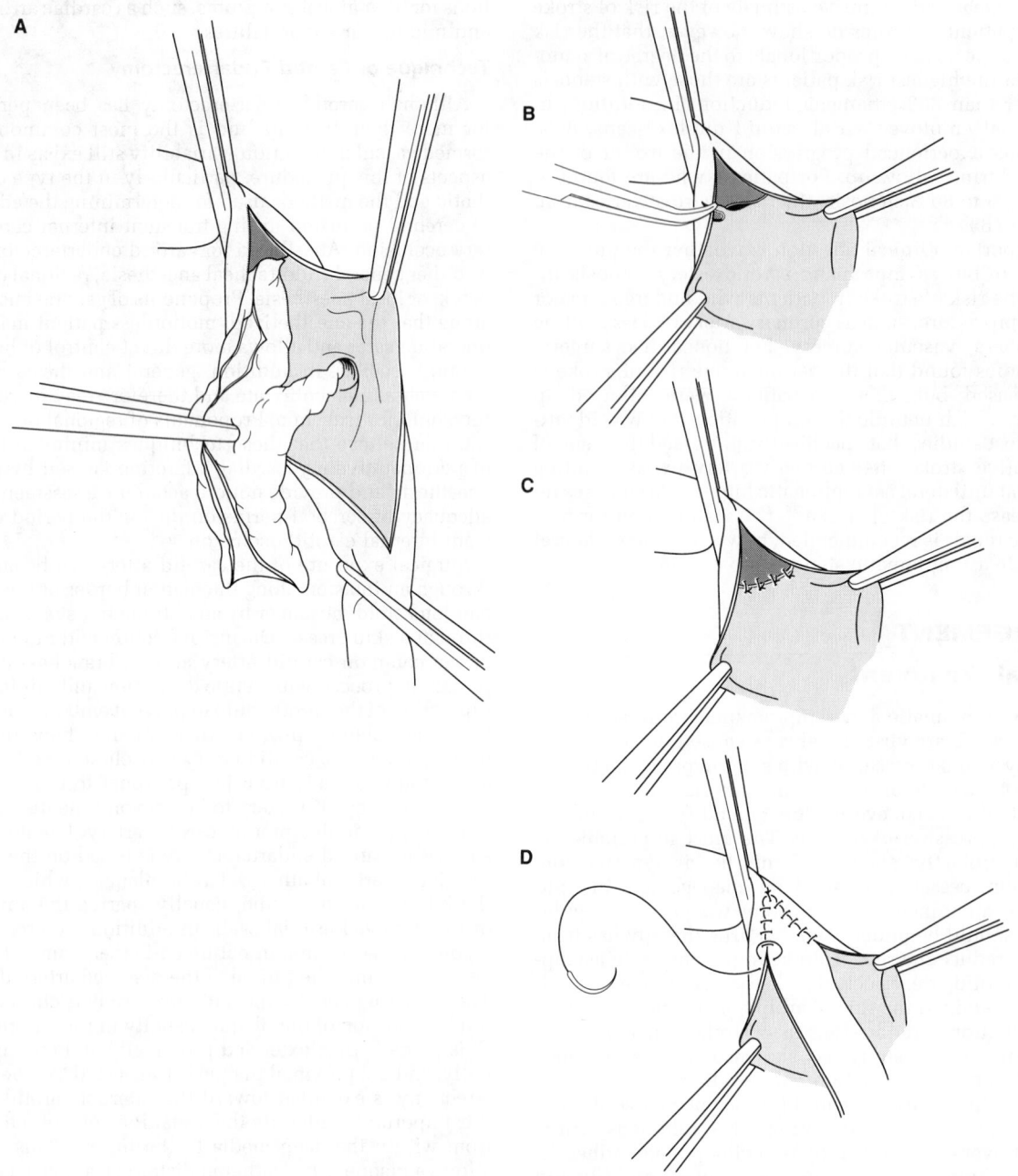

Figure 80-7. Carotid endarterectomy. (*A*) The atheroma is transected proximally and teased out of the external and internal carotid arteries. The distal internal carotid endpoint must be directly visualized to ensure that it feathers into normal intima. (*B*) Any loose pieces of atheroma or strands of media are removed. (*C*) If necessary, the distal normal intima is tacked in place with vertically oriented stitches. (*D*) Although direct closure is often possible, patch angioplasty may be required when the carotid is small or in cases of reoperation.

well as to monitor neurologic status. Most patients tolerate this procedure well and can be discharged 48 to 72 hours after the operation.

Depending on the surgeon's preference, a variety of methods can be used to monitor the adequacy of cerebral perfusion during the period of temporary internal carotid artery occlusion. The commonly employed options include using temporary shunts or undertaking some method to determine the adequacy of cerebral perfusion during carotid cross-clamping. These methods include neurologic assessment of the awake patient being operated on under regional cervical or local block, assessment of the internal carotid artery back

pressure in the anesthetized patient, or using continuous bilateral electron encephalographic monitoring.

Complications of Carotid Endarterectomy

Neurologic Complications. Stroke can occur during or after carotid endarterectomy secondary to a variety of mechanisms, including inadequate collateral blood flow to the brain during temporary internal carotid artery occlusion, embolization during dissection of the carotid artery, or embolism or thrombosis of the reconstruction during the early postoperative period. Thrombosis after carotid endarterectomy usually is a result of sudden intimal dissection due to a loose flap or inadequate distal endarterectomy endpoint. Embolization after carotid endarterectomy is usually secondary to platelet aggregates forming on the surface of the endarterectomized vessel. Finally, stroke can be caused by intracerebral hemorrhage, which appears to occur more commonly in patients who have multivessel involvement preoperatively and tends to occur on the second or third postoperative day.

Postoperative cranial nerve dysfunction can occur in up to 39% of patients undergoing carotid endarterectomy.[29] Only 60% of these injuries produce clinical symptoms, such as hoarseness, difficulty in swallowing, or change in speech patterns. Common cranial nerve injuries include dysfunction of the recurrent laryngeal nerve causing hoarseness, dysfunction of the hypoglossal nerve causing deviation of the tongue toward the side of the injury, and superior laryngeal nerve dysfunction causing easy fatigability of the voice. Less common is injury of the marginal mandibular nerve, which results in drooping of the nasolabial fold ipsilateral to the injury. Also vulnerable to injury are the greater auricular nerve, the spinal accessory nerve, and the glossopharyngeal nerve.

Most cranial nerve injuries resolve completely within 6 months of operation. Particularly important are bilateral injuries, which may occur after bilateral endarterectomy. All patients who undergo carotid endarterectomy should be subjected to careful cranial nerve examination before and after operation. For second-stage contralateral carotid endarterectomies, it is mandatory to obtain preoperative indirect laryngoscopy to assess the vocal cord ipsilateral to the previous operation. If a bilateral recurrent laryngeal nerve injury occurs, the patient may require emergency tracheostomy.

Nonneurologic Complications. Carotid endarterectomy may also result in a number of nonneurologic complications. Significant hemorrhage occurs after carotid endarterectomy in about 1% to 5% of patients. A somewhat higher postoperative hemorrhage rate is noted in patients receiving aspirin perioperatively. Patients may also experience episodes of hypertension and hypotension.[30] Hypotension and bradycardia occur secondary to increased baroreceptor reflex activity during dissection of the carotid artery or stimulation of the sinus nerve after removal of a rigid atheromatous plaque. Hypertension may be caused by the interruption of the carotid sinus nerve, owing to either its transection or changes in arterial wall compliance. Episodes of severe hypertension or hypotension are associated with an increased risk of neurologic deficits.[30] Finally, myocardial infarction remains the most common source of non-stroke-related morbidity and mortality after carotid endarterectomy. Death secondary to myocardial infarction accounted for 20% to 100% of all deaths after carotid endarterectomy.[31] Myocardial infarction is also the most common cause of late death in patients who have undergone prior carotid endarterectomy. The 10-year cumulative survival rate after carotid endarterectomy in patients with coronary artery disease who underwent coronary artery bypass grafting before carotid endarterectomy was 55%, but only 32% in patients in whom the disease remained uncorrected.[32]

Recurrent carotid stenosis is a relatively common but only infrequently serious complication after carotid endarterectomy (Fig. 80-8). Residual or recurrent carotid artery stenosis can be detected in up to 30% of patients undergoing careful postoperative surveillance with carotid duplex

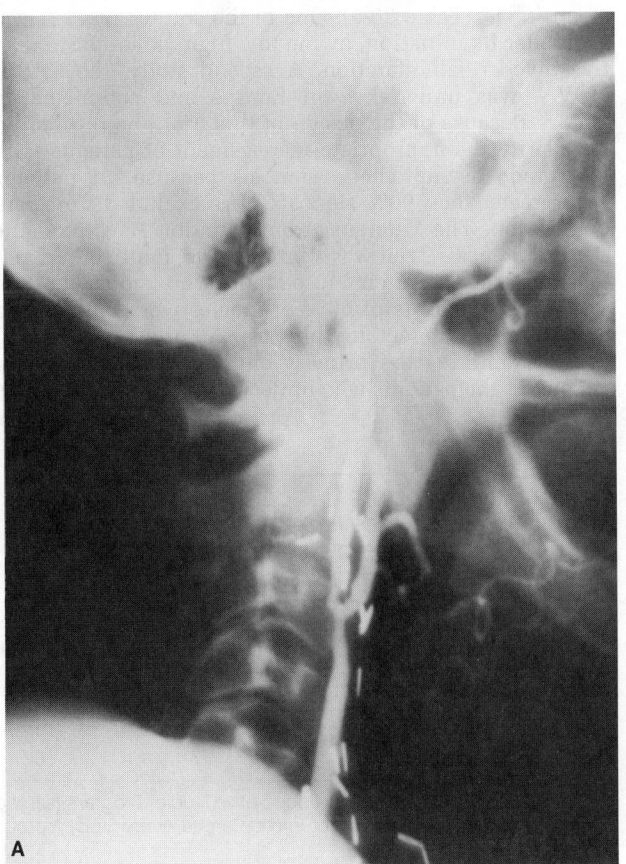
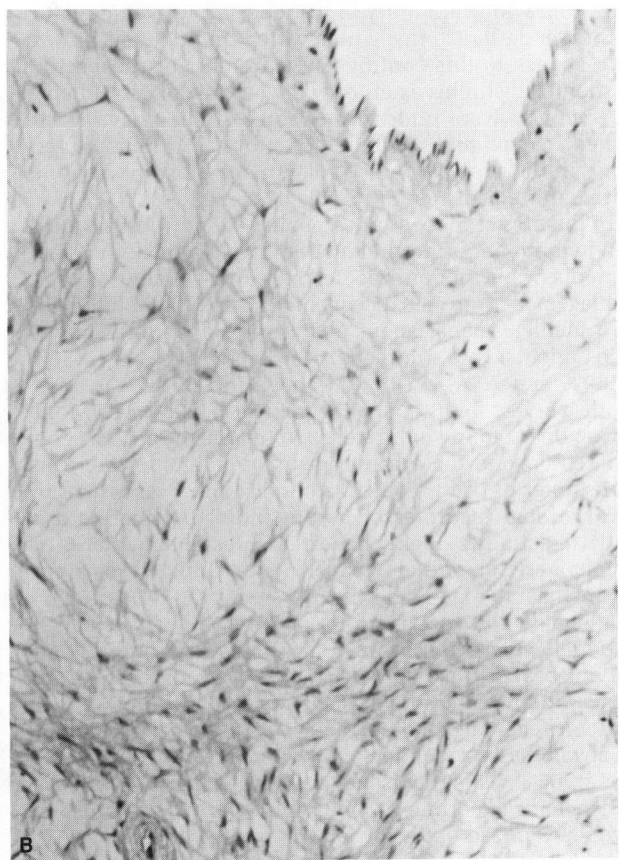

Figure 80-8. (*A*) Angiogram showing recurrent carotid stenosis. (*B*) This fibrous hyperplastic lesion was excised at operation.

Table 80-4. OUTCOME OF CLINICAL TRIALS OF CAROTID ENDARTERECTOMY IN PATIENTS WITH SYMPTOMATIC HIGH-GRADE CAROTID ARTERY STENOSIS

Study	Mean Follow-Up	Ipsilateral Stroke Rate (%)		Risk Reduction (%)	
		Surgical	Nonsurgical	Absolute	Relative
NASCET	2 y	9*	26	17	65
ECST	3 y	12.3*	21.9	9.6	56
VA CSP #309		7*	19.4†	11.7	63

NASCET, North American Symptomatic Carotid Endarterectomy Trial; ECST, European Carotid Surgery Trial; VA CSP, VA Cooperative Study.
* Significantly different from nonsurgery, $P < .05$
† Included episodes of crescendo transient ischemic attack in addition to stroke as major endpoint of study

scanning; however, less than 3% of patients experience symptomatic recurrence. Two forms of recurrent disease have been identified.[33] Recurrent carotid stenosis that occurs within 6 months of the initial endarterectomy usually is secondary to intimal hyperplasia characterized by both proliferation of vascular smooth muscle and increased matrix deposition. When the recurrent stenosis develops 2 years or longer after endarterectomy, recurrent atherosclerosis is usually found at the time of reoperation. The risk of recurrent carotid stenosis has been documented to be higher in women and in patients with hypercholesterolemia.

Efficacy of Carotid Endarterectomy in the Prevention of Stroke

In the past, much controversy surrounded the efficacy of carotid endarterectomy in the prevention of strokes in patients with carotid stenosis. This controversy arose in part from wide variability in the reported stroke rates after carotid endarterectomy, which varied from 1% to 24.4%.[34] In response to this controversy, a number of prospective randomized studies examining the efficacy of carotid endarterectomy were undertaken. Three studies have established unambiguously the efficacy of carotid endarterectomy in the prevention of stroke in symptomatic patients with carotid stenosis[35-37] (Table 80-4).

In the first of these studies published, the North American Symptomatic Carotid Endarterectomy Trial (NASCET), patients were randomized to the best available medical management or to an experimental group that included the best medical management plus carotid endarterectomy.[35] The patients were stratified by the degree of stenosis, 30% to 69% and 70% to 99%. Although the study was to include a 5-year follow-up, in February 1991, the Data Monitoring Board found a difference in treatment that was considered beyond the preapproved stop points for the trial. Thus, after only 18 months, a clinical alert was issued by the National Institutes of Health indicating that carotid endarterectomy is highly beneficial in patients with recent hemispheric or retinal TIAs or nondisabling strokes and an ipsilateral high-grade carotid stenosis (70% to 99%). The conclusion was based on an interim analysis of 328 patients undergoing carotid endarterectomy and 331 receiving best medical therapy alone. At 18 months, the incidence of stroke in surgical patients was 9%, but 26% in patients receiving medical therapy alone. This represented an absolute risk reduction of 17% and a relative risk reduction of 65%. This represents one of the largest differences between the experimental and control groups in a prospective randomized clinical trial. An even greater risk reduction was seen in the group of patients who experienced major or fatal ipsilateral stroke, in which there was an 81% relative risk reduction in patients undergoing carotid

endarterectomy. The benefit accrued to the patients undergoing carotid endarterectomy held up under all subgroup analyses. Of clinical importance, the benefit of surgery was seen within 3 months of operation. The implication of this finding is that many of the strokes occurred soon after randomization. Thus, when a patient is identified to have a symptomatic high-grade carotid artery stenosis, evaluation for surgery should begin immediately. The results of the NASCET trial were supported by a second trial, the European Carotid Surgery Trial, as well as by a trial undertaken at 16 university-affiliated Veterans Administration medical centers, the Veterans Administration Cooperative Study 309. Nearly identical results were found in these studies, further substantiating the significant efficacy of carotid endarterectomy in symptomatic patients.[36,37]

A number of studies have also been undertaken to evaluate the efficacy of carotid endarterectomy in the prevention of stroke in patients who have asymptomatic carotid artery stenosis[38-40] (Table 80-5). One of the studies was aborted soon after its initiation, owing to a high rate of postoperative myocardial infarction. A second study, the CASANOVA, was undertaken in Europe and completed in 1988.[38] Because of the design of this trial, the results did not clarify the appropriate management of patients with high-grade asymptomatic stenosis because all patients with greater than 90% stenosis were excluded from randomization. The Veterans Administration Asymptomatic Carotid Stenosis Trial was a prospective, multicenter, randomized trial in which 440 patients who had asymptomatic carotid stenosis of 50% or greater were randomized to carotid endarterectomy plus aspirin or aspirin alone.[39] When examining the primary endpoint of this study, a benefit for the patients who underwent carotid endarterec-

Table 80-5. OUTCOME OF CLINICAL TRIALS OF CAROTID ENDARTERECTOMY IN PATIENTS WITH ASYMPTOMATIC CAROTID STENOSIS

Study	Rate of Ipsilateral Neurologic Event (%)		Risk Reduction (%)	
	Surgical	Nonsurgical	Absolute	Relative
VA CSP*	8*	20.6	12.6	38
ACAS†	4.8*	10.6	5.8	55

VA CSP, Veterans Administration Cooperative Studies Program (carotid stenosis ≥ 50%); ACAS, Asymptomatic Carotid Artery Study (carotid stenosis ≥ 60%).
* Transient ischemic attacks and stroke were endpoints.
† Stroke was only endpoint.
†† $P ≤ .05$ compared with nonsurgical group.

tomy was identified. At the time of analysis, 8% of the patients undergoing carotid endarterectomy experienced a TIA or stroke, whereas 20.6% of patients who received aspirin alone experienced a neurologic complication, a statistically significant difference. When excluding the patients who experienced TIA and only examining the patients who experienced ipsilateral stroke, no significant difference between the two groups was identified. The latter finding is not surprising because once patients in the nonsurgical group experienced TIAs, they usually underwent carotid endarterectomy. Thus, this was the first well-designed prospective randomized study that showed that carotid endarterectomy plus aspirin was more effective than aspirin alone in reducing the frequency of TIA or stroke in patients with asymptomatic carotid stenosis.

The Asymptomatic Carotid Artery Stenosis Trial is a prospective study sponsored by the National Institutes of Health similar to the NASCET study for symptomatic carotid stenosis.[40] This study was also interrupted because of a significant benefit identified in patients undergoing carotid endarterectomy. Patients were randomized with asymptomatic stenosis of 60% or greater to either carotid endarterectomy and aspirin or aspirin alone. At the time of interruption of the study, a relative reduction in stroke rate by 50% was observed by patients undergoing carotid endarterectomy. The benefit was much greater in men than women. This study used stroke as its primary endpoint. This group has since substantiated unequivocally the effectiveness of carotid endarterectomy in good-risk patients identified to have high-grade stenosis.

These prospective randomized studies established the role of carotid endarterectomy in the prevention of strokes in patients with both symptomatic and asymptomatic high-grade carotid artery stenosis. All the patients in these studies were carefully selected, good-risk patients, and the complication rates of surgeons performing these operations were extremely low. For patients to receive benefit from this operation, it must be performed at this very low complication rate by experienced surgeons.

External Carotid Endarterectomy

External carotid endarterectomy is recommended in patients with ipsilateral internal carotid artery occlusion and clinical evidence of retinal or hemispheric TIAs or stroke. Many of these patients have a large cul-de-sac in the proximal internal carotid artery that may serve as a source of emboli (Fig. 80-9). These are relatively uncommon clinical occurrences, but external carotid endarterectomy has been shown to be safe and effective in these patients.

Direct Aortic Arch Reconstruction

Atherosclerotic lesions at the origin of the great vessels can result in TIA or stroke. Most commonly involved are the brachiocephalic or left common carotid arteries. When such lesions are identified, they can be repaired by direct reconstruction through a median sternotomy. For brachiocephalic artery lesions, the option of endarterectomy or aortobrachiocephalic bypass grafting using a synthetic graft are available. Often, it is necessary to undertake revascularization of both the brachiocephalic and left common carotid arteries. Despite the complexity of these operations, they are, in general, attended by low complication rates and a neurologic morbidity rate of 2% or less.

Vertebral Artery Reconstruction

Atherosclerosis at the origin of the vertebral arteries can become symptomatic, causing TIA or stroke in the posterior cerebral circulation. When appropriate indications exist, a variety of techniques are available for reconstruction of the vertebral arteries. Vertebral artery endarterectomy

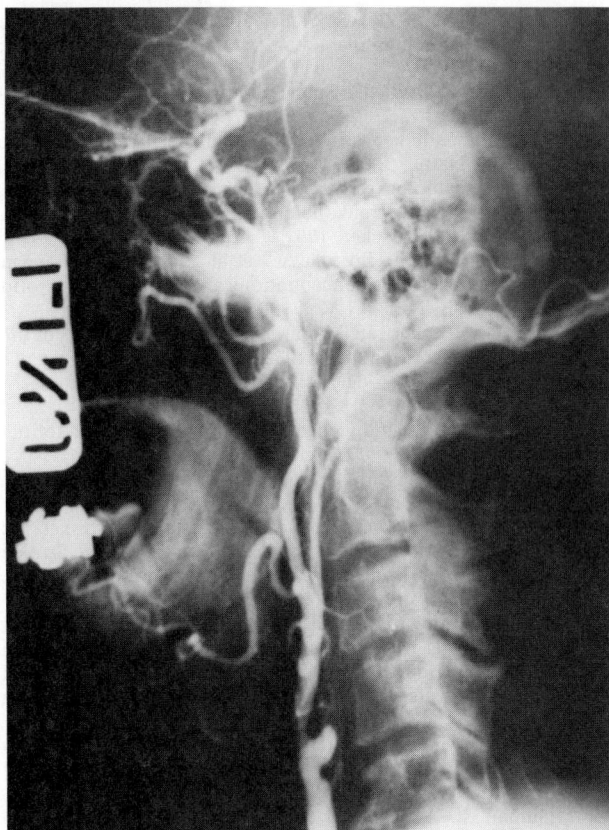

Figure 80-9. A totally occluded internal carotid artery with a residual stump may be a source of emboli. Note the periorbital collateral circulation.

can be undertaken through an arteriotomy in the subclavian artery. Alternatively, the vertebral artery can be ligated at its origin and replanted into a normal ipsilateral common carotid artery. Less commonly, distal vertebral artery reconstructions are accomplished with a carotid–vertebral bypass using saphenous vein.

Nonanatomic Bypass

Patients with atherosclerotic stenosis at the origin of the aortic arch vessels may present with not only neurologic implications but also symptoms related to ischemia of the upper extremities. For patients who are not candidates for direct aortic arch reconstruction, a variety of alternative, nonanatomic bypasses can be undertaken, such as a subclavian–carotid, carotid–subclavian, axillary–axillary, carotid–carotid, and even femoral–axillary bypass operations. Some have suggested that synthetic Dacron grafts have a superior patency to saphenous vein grafts. Saphenous vein grafts are preferred by some surgeons, however, owing to a theoretically lower rate of platelet embolization. Most of these nonanatomic reconstructions have good long-term patency rates.

REFERENCES

1. Marshall RS, Mohr JP. Current management of ischaemic stroke. J Neurol Neurosurg Psych 1993;56:6.
2. Carpenter MB. Blood supply of the central nervous system. In: Core text of neuroanatomy. Baltimore, Williams & Wilkins 1974:231.
3. Stanley JC, Gerwertz BL, Bove EL, Sottiurai VS, Fry WJ. Arterial fibrodysplasia, histopathological character, and current etiologic concepts. Arch Surg 1975;11:561.

4. Effeney DJ, Ehrenfeld WK, Stoney RJ, Wylie EJ. Why operate on carotid fibromuscular dysplasia? Arch Surg 1980;115:1261.

5. Ehrenfeld WK, Wylie EJ. Spontaneous dissection of the internal carotid artery. Arch Surgery 1976;111:1294.

6. Ross R. The pathogenesis of atherosclerosis: a perspective for the 1990's. Nature 1993;362:801.

7. Zarins CK. Pathology of carotid atherosclerosis. In: Ernst CB, Stanley JC, eds. Current therapy in vascular surgery, ed 2. Philadelphia, BC Decker, 1991:1.

8. Selhub J, Jaques PF, Bostom AG, et al. Association between plasma homocysteine concentrations and extracranial carotid artery stenosis. N Engl J Med 1995;332:286.

9. Fisher CM, Pritchard JE, Mathews WH. Arteriosclerosis of the carotid arteries. Circulation 1952;6:457.

10. Milliken CH. The pathogenesis of transient focal cerebral ischemia. Circulation 1965;32:438.

11. Hollenhorst RW. Significance of bright plaques in the retinal arteries. JAMA 1961;178:23.

12. Norris JW, Zhu CA. Silent stroke and carotid stenosis. Stroke 1992;23:483.

13. Mohr JP, Barnett HJM. Classification of ischemia strokes. In: Barnett HJM, Mohr JP, Stein BM, Yatsu FM, eds. Stroke: pathophysiology, diagnosis, and management. New York, Churchill Livingstone, 1986:281.

14. Moneta GL, Edwards JM, Chitwood RW, et al. Correlation of North American Symptomatic Carotid endarterectomy trial (NASCET) angiographic definition of 70% to 99% internal carotid artery stenosis with duplex scanning. J Vasc Surg 1993;17:152.

15. Londrey GL, Spadone DP, Hodgson, et al. Does colorflow imaging improve the accuracy of duplex carotid evaluation. J Vasc Surg 1991;13:659.

16. Friedman GD, Wilson WS, Mosier JM, et al. Transient ischemic attacks in a community. JAMA 1969;210:1428.

17. Whisnant JP, Matsumoto N, Elveback LR. Transient cerebral ischemic attacks in a community. Mayo Clin Proc 1973;48:194.

18. Matsumoto N, Whisnant JP, Kurland LT, et al. Natural history of stroke in Rochester, Minnesota, 1955 through 1969: an extension of a previous study, 1945 through 1954. Stroke 1973;4:20.

19. Bardin JA, Bernstein EF, Humbert PB, et al. Is carotid endarterectomy beneficial in prevention of recurrent stroke? Arch Surgery 1982;117:1401.

20. Mohr JP. Asymptomatic carotid artery disease. Stroke 1982;13:431.

21. Chambers BR, Norris JW. Outcome in patients with asymptomatic neck bruits. N Engl J Med 1986;315:860.

22. Roederer GO, Langlois YE, Jager KA, et al. The natural history of carotid arterial disease in asymptomatic patients with cervical bruits. Stroke 1984;15:605.

23. Barnes RW, Marzalek PB. Asymptomatic carotid disease in the cardiovascular surgical patient: is prophylactic endarterectomy necessary? Stroke 1981;12:497.

24. Brener BJ, Brief DK, Alpert J, et al. The risk of stroke in patients with asymptomatic carotid stenosis undergoing cardiac surgery: a follow-up study. J Vasc Surg 1987;5:269.

25. Breslau PJ, Fell G, Ivey TD, et al. Carotid arterial disease in patients undergoing coronary artery bypass operations. J Thorac Cardiovasc Surg 1981;82:765.

26. Ivey TD, Strandness DJ Jr, Williams DB, et al. Management of patients with carotid bruit undergoing cardiopulmonary bypass. J Thorac Cardiovasc Surg 1984;87:183.

27. McCann RL. Surgical management of carotid artery atherosclerotic disease. South Med J 1993;86:2S23.

28. Ramirez-Lassepas M, Cipolle RJ. Medical treatment of transient ischemic attacks: does it influence mortality? Stroke 1988;19:397.

29. Hertzer NR. Postoperative management and complications of extracranial carotid reconstruction. In: Rutherford RM, ed. Vascular surgery. Philadelphia, WB Saunders, 1984:1300.

30. Bove EL, Fry WJ, Gross WS, et al. Hypotension and hypertension as consequences of baroreceptor dysfunction following carotid endarterectomy. Surgery 1979;85:633.

31. O'Donnell TF, Callow AD, Willett C, et al. The impact of coronary artery disease on carotid endarterectomy. Ann Surg 1983;198:705.

32. Hertzer NR, Arison R. Cumulative stroke and survival ten years after carotid endarterectomy. J Vasc Surg 1985;2:661.

33. Stoney RJ, String ST. Recurrent carotid stenosis. Surgery 1976;80:705.

34. Easton JP, Sherman DG. Stroke and mortality rate in carotid endarterectomy: 228 consecutive operations. Stroke 1977; 8:565.

35. North American Symptomatic Carotid Endarterectomy Trial Collaborators. Beneficial effect of carotid endarterectomy in symptomatic patients with high-graft carotid stenosis. N Engl J Med 1991;325:445.

36. European Carotid Surgery Trialists' Collaborative Group. MRC European Carotid Surgery Trial: interim results for symptomatic patients with severe (70–99%) or with mild (0–29%) carotid stenosis. Lancet 1991;337:1235.

37. Mayberg MR, Wilson SE, Yatsu F, et al, for the Veterans Affairs Cooperative Studies Program 309 Trialist Group. Carotid endarterectomy and prevention of cerebral ischemia in symptomatic carotid stenosis. JAMA 1991;266:3289.

38. The CASANOVA Study Group. Carotid surgery vs medical therapy in asymptomatic carotid stenosis. N Engl J Med 1993;328:221.

39. Hobson RW II, Weiss DG, Fields WS, et al. Efficacy of carotid endarterectomy for asymptomatic carotid stenosis. N Engl J Med 1993;328:221.

40. Executive Committee for the Asymptomatic Carotid Atherosclerosis Study. Endarterectomy for asymptomatic carotid artery stenosis. JAMA 1995;273:1421.

SURGERY: SCIENTIFIC PRINCIPLES AND PRACTICE, Second Edition, edited by Lazar J. Greenfield, Michael W. Mulholland, Keith T. Oldham, Gerald B. Zelenock, and Keith D. Lillemoe. Lippincott–Raven Publishers, Philadelphia, © 1997.

CHAPTER 81

UPPER EXTREMITY OCCLUSIVE DISEASE

JAMES S.T. YAO

Upper extremity arterial occlusive disease encompasses a wide spectrum of diseases that can cause ischemic symptoms. Accurate diagnosis requires a thorough history, a careful physical examination, and the liberal use of ancillary diagnostic tests. Appropriate surgical treatment depends on the location of the occlusive lesion and the nature of the underlying occlusive process. In general, proximal arterial lesions involving the subclavian, axillary, and brachial arteries are more amenable to reconstructive surgery.

HISTORY TAKING

Taking an appropriate history is the most important initial step in the workup of a patient with upper extremity ischemia. In addition to a careful delineation of the patient's symptoms, appropriate inquiry should include occupational, pharmacologic, and athletic risks, and pertinent medical history. Table 81-1 lists conditions and risks related to the development of upper extremity ischemic symptoms.

Symptoms

The presenting symptoms of upper extremity occlusive disease include evidence of arterial emboli, Raynaud phenomenon, pain, and exercise-related forearm fatigue. Embolic symptoms include gangrene of the tips of the fingers, petechiae of the skin, splinter hemorrhages of the nail bed, and livedo reticularis. The term *Raynaud phenomenon* refers to episodic

Table 81-1. CONDITIONS AND RISKS FOR UPPER EXTREMITY ISCHEMIA

OCCUPATIONAL INJURY	MEDICAL CONDITIONS
Vibration syndrome	Atherosclerosis
Pneumatic tools	Arteritis
Chain saws	Collagen disease
Grinders	Scleroderma
Electrical burns	Rheumatoid arteritis
Hypothenar hammer syndrome	Systemic lupus
Mechanical work or auto	erythematosus
repair	Dermatomyositis
Lathe operation	Allergic necrotizing arteritis
Carpentry	Takayasu disease
Electrical work	Giant cell arteritis
Occupational acroosteolysis-	Blood dyscrasias
polyvinylchloride	Cold agglutinins
exposure	Cryoglobulins
	Polycythemia vera
ATHLETIC ACTIVITIES	Behçet syndrome
Thoracic outlet compression	Antiphospholipid syndrome
Baseball pitching	Thoracic outlet syndrome
Kayaking	Congenital arterial wall defects
Weight lifting	Pseudoxanthoma elasticum
Rowing	Ehlers-Danlos syndrome
Butterfly swimming	Fibromuscular dysplasia
Golfing	Iatrogenic injury
Hand ischemia	Arterial blood gas and
Baseball catching	pressure monitoring
Frisbee	Cardiac catheterization
Karate	Arteriography
Handball	Frostbite
	Renal transplantation and related
PHARMACOLOGIC HISTORY	problems
Ergot poisoning	Azotemic arteriopathy
β-Blockers	Hemodialysis shunts
Drug abuse, cocaine use	Radiation
Cytotoxic drugs	Breast carcinoma
Dopamine overdose	Hodgkin disease
	Aneurysms of the upper
	extremity

digital color changes provoked by stimuli such as cold or emotion. The digits first exhibit pallor, followed by cyanosis and then by a reactive hyperemia. The pathophysiology of the color changes from white to blue to red is thought to be digital ischemia (due to vasospasm), followed by desaturation of hemoglobin (which produces cyanosis), and then by a reactive hyperemia. Raynaud phenomenon should not be confused with Raynaud disease. The former is a secondary process, whereas the latter is a primary disease without known cause. The diagnosis of primary Raynaud disease is made only after exclusion of all the etiologic factors listed in Table 81-1 and after symptoms persist for at least 2 years in the absence of other conditions that might be causal. Raynaud phenomenon secondary to an underlying cause can be unilateral or bilateral. In patients with unilateral Raynaud phenomenon, organic arterial occlusive disease should be suspected. In contrast, bilateral symptoms are often due to systemic disease causing vasospasm. The precise classification of primary and secondary Raynaud phenomenon is often difficult, and the terminology is imprecise. Many physicians prefer to use the term *Raynaud syndrome* to characterize all patients with episodic vasospastic disease of the hands. Raynaud phenomenon should also be distinguished from acrocyanosis, a disorder characterized by painless, persistent, diffuse cyanosis of the fingers and hands.

Clinical Examination

Physical examination of the patient should include examination of the thoracic outlet and the entire upper extremity. Palpation of the supraclavicular region may help to detect the presence of a subclavian aneurysm or a cervical rib. Auscultation of the subclavian artery with the stethoscope placed just below the midclavicular region, and listening for the presence of a bruit with the arm placed in neutral (or abduction) and external rotation (or hyperabduction) help to establish the diagnosis of thoracic outlet compression to the artery. Pulse palpation begins with the subclavian artery in the supraclavicular fossa and continues with the axillary artery under the armpit, the brachial artery at the upper arm and elbow, and the radial and ulnar arteries at the wrist level. A decreased or absent pulse in any site other than the supraclavicular fossa indicates major artery occlusion. Conversely, a readily palpable pulse in the supraclavicular fossa can represent a subclavian artery aneurysm.

Examination of the hand is not complete unless an Allen test is performed. The examiner stands beside or facing the subject. The radial and ulnar arteries of one wrist are compressed by the examiner's fingers. The subject is asked to open and close the hand rapidly for 1 minute to empty blood out of the hand and then to extend the fingers quickly. The radial or the ulnar artery is released, and the hand is observed for capillary refilling and return of color. The test is judged normal if refilling of the hand is complete within a short period (less than 6 seconds). Any portion of the hand that does not blush is an indication of incomplete continuity of the arch. Hyperextension of the fingers must be avoided because it produces a false-positive result. In addition to the Allen test, examination of the hand must include palpation of the palm for a pulsatile mass or excess scar tissue. Assessment of the patency of digital arteries by palpation is often difficult and unreliable. Upper extremity digital capillary refill is nearly instantaneous in normal subjects.

Noninvasive Examination

Several noninvasive tests, including plethysmography, transcutaneous Doppler, and duplex scan, are available for objective evaluation of patients with upper extremity ischemia.[1] Of these, the Doppler examination is the most straightforward and consists of audible signal interpretation, waveform recording with spectral analysis, and systolic pressure measurements. Bilateral examinations should be done for comparative purposes. Because many of the diseases affecting the hand are symmetric, the asymptomatic hand often will have significant disease also.[2] This is especially true in patients with systemic disease causing hand ischemia.

Because both the axillary and the brachial arteries are superficial vessels, they lend themselves to Doppler examination. Any change from normal signals (triphasic) to abnormal signals (monophasic) indicates the presence of an occlusive lesion. Distal to the elbow, arterial signals are more difficult to obtain. At the wrist, both the radial and ulnar arteries become superficially situated once again. Palpation of the ulnar artery can be difficult, and Doppler examination is helpful in determining the patency of this artery. In the hand, Doppler examination of the palmar arches is performed best at the mid-thenar and hypothenar regions. The common digital vessels should be examined at the base of the fingers at their division into the proper digital arteries, which lie along the shaft of the proximal phalanx of each finger. Waveform recording is useful in both analysis and record keeping.

For segmental upper extremity pressures, a pneumatic cuff is placed at the upper arm, as in routine blood pressure recording. Brachial artery blood pressure reflects all proximal arteries and should be within 10 to 20 mmHg of that in the opposite extremity. A greater difference signifies innominate, subclavian, axillary, or brachial stenosis. If brachial artery occlusion is suspected, a pressure cuff is applied to the forearm and the pressure recorded in a similar manner with the radial artery used for signal detection. A pressure drop of 20 to 30 mmHg signifies an obstruction distal to the brachial artery. For finger pressure measurement, a 2.5-cm cuff is placed at the base of the finger, and the return of Doppler signals after cuff deflation is monitored at the fingertip. An arterial occlusion distal to the palmar arch is defined by a pressure gradient between the fingers of greater than 15 mmHg or a wrist-to-digit difference of 30 mmHg.

The Doppler technique is of particular value in determining palmar arch patency in a patient who is unconscious or is uncooperative in performing an Allen test. Before arterial line placement, this simple test may help to avoid hand ischemia. In the modified Allen test, the Doppler probe is placed over the radial artery while the ulnar artery is compressed. If the signal disappears, the arch depends on the ulnar artery for supply. If the signal remains strong, the arch is complete. A similar maneuver is repeated over the ulnar artery while compressing the radial artery.

The plethysmograph is used to record finger pulse contours for analysis and to differentiate normal, obstructive, and vasospastic disease.[1] For aneurysms, the duplex scan is helpful in establishing the diagnosis.

Laboratory Examination

In severe bilateral hand ischemia, a systemic cause of the arterial lesions should be sought. Laboratory tests include serologic, immunologic, and hematologic studies to help establish the diagnosis:

- Erythrocyte sedimentation rate
- Rheumatoid factor
- Antinuclear antibody
- Immunoglobulin electrophoresis
- Cryoglobulins
- Cold agglutinins
- VDRL test
- Complement (C3, C4)
- Anticardiolipin antibody
- Blood counts

The erythrocyte sedimentation rate remains a useful screening test to aid in the diagnosis of various forms of arteritis. The presence of a positive antinuclear antibody test is helpful in detecting connective tissue disease and other arteritides. When the antinuclear antibody titer is abnormal, immunofluorescent pattern analysis of antibodies can help to establish the diagnosis of various connective tissue disorders. The speckled pattern antibody is more specific for systemic lupus erythematosus. A nucleolar pattern suggests the presence of scleroderma. A positive anticardiolipin antibody is diagnostic for antiphospholipid syndrome, which is characterized by thromboembolic events in young adults.[3]

Radiologic Examination

A combination of laboratory and radiologic testing may be needed to establish the proper diagnosis of systemic disease. Radiologic examination includes soft tissue radiograph of the hand, chest film, esophageal barium swallow and motility test, and arteriography. The soft tissue radiograph of the hand may reveal calcinosis, which is diagnostic for the CREST syndrome, or diffuse calcified arteries in diabetic or azotemic arteriopathy (Fig. 81-1). The chest

film is essential to detect bony anomalies of the thoracic outlet such as cervical ribs (Fig. 81-2), anomalous first ribs, and healed fractures of the first rib or clavicle. Pulmonary fibrosis seen on the chest film is another indication of systemic sclerosis.

Arteriography is useful in defining the vascular anatomy of the hand and in calculating the degree of peripheral ischemia. In the investigation of upper extremity ischemia, arteriography must include all arteries from the aortic arch to the hand.[4] Liberal use of subtraction techniques, multiple views, and magnification films should provide proper detail. In addition to the state of the inflow arteries, the anatomic characteristics of the palmar arches may aid in determining the degree of hand ischemia. Anatomic variation of upper extremity arteries, especially the palmar arches (superficial and deep), is well known,[5] and incomplete palmar arches play a significant role in ischemic disease and contribute to digital ischemia. In general, the deep palmar arch is formed primarily by the terminal part of the radial artery, and the superficial arch by the ulnar artery. The variations of the arches, based on the manner in which the contributing arteries join, are divided into complete arches and incomplete arches. There are many subtypes and variations of the superficial and deep palmar arches[6] (Fig. 81-3). In a study of 500 hand arteriograms,

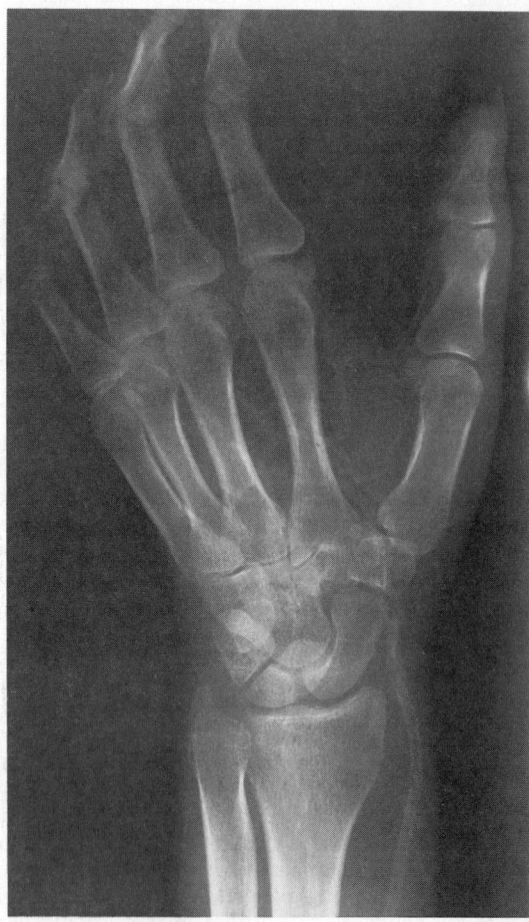

Figure 81-1. Typical appearance of azotemic arteriopathy (calciphylaxis) in a diabetic patient with a renal transplant. All digital arteries are distinctly seen on plain film. The radial artery has a pipestem appearance. An arteriogram shows multiple digital artery occlusions. (Yao JST. Arterial surgery of the upper extremity. In: Haimovici H, Callow AD, DePalma RG, et al, eds. Vascular surgery: principles and techniques, ed 3. Norwalk, CT, Appleton & Lange, 1989:863)

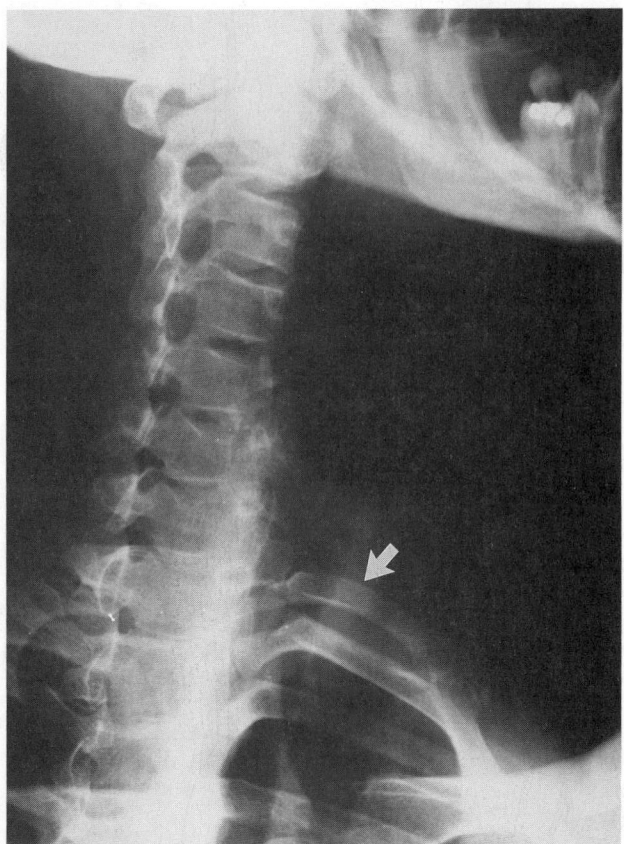

Figure 81-2. Cervical rib (*arrow*) in a patient with subclavian aneurysm caused by thoracic outlet compression.

the deep palmar arch appeared complete in 95.2% of the cases.[6] The finding is similar to that reported in earlier studies using classic techniques of anatomic dissection.[5] Because the ulnar artery is the dominant artery in the blood supply of the hand, the completeness of the superficial palmar arch is the determining factor in hand ischemia. In contrast to the deep arch, there are many variations of the superficial palmar arch. Six types of complete arch are known; however, the complete superficial palmar arch occurred in only 42.4% of cases in the angiographic study.[6] In contrast, the anatomic dissection study found a complete superficial arch in 78.5% of cases.[5] Such discrepancies are important and undoubtedly are due to the methods used. Arteriographic studies allow substantially better visualization of arteries of small caliber and increased recognition of luminal obstruction contributing to the incomplete arch. The angiographic studies, however, were performed in patients with symptoms. Thus, a higher frequency of incomplete arches might be expected.

DIAGNOSIS

The diagnosis of large artery occlusion is usually not difficult, and careful pulse examination often helps to establish the diagnosis. In distal arterial lesions causing hand or finger ischemia, the use of noninvasive testing to detect digital artery occlusion helps to distinguish Raynaud phenomenon from Raynaud disease. The diagnosis of primary Raynaud disease should not be made until secondary causes of Raynaud phenomenon have been eliminated. Furthermore, because the onset of Raynaud phenomenon may precede other manifestations of underlying systemic disease by many years, the

diagnosis of Raynaud disease is usually not made until 2 years have elapsed with no appearance of systemic disease. If this strict criterion is followed, most patients will be found to have Raynaud phenomenon (secondary) rather than Raynaud disease (primary).

Diagnosis is facilitated by classification of arterial lesions into proximal and distal sites of involvement. Proximal lesions are those involving arteries above the elbow, and distal lesions are those involving arteries below the elbow, predominantly in the wrist and hand.

Proximal Arterial Lesions

Atherosclerosis is the most common cause of upper extremity occlusive lesions. The most common site of involvement is the first part of the subclavian artery, and the innominate artery is also a common site of disease. Lesions include total occlusion with or without associated steal phenomena, high-grade stenoses, and ulcerating plaques causing distal embolism.

Arteritis producing upper extremity ischemic symptoms includes such diverse processes as Takayasu arteritis, giant cell arteritis, temporal arteritis, and polymyalgia rheumatica. Takayasu arteritis is a nonspecific inflammatory process of unknown cause affecting segmentally the aorta and its main branches. The disease process can affect carotid, subclavian, axillary, and pulmonary arteries and is noted most often in young women from 10 to 30 years of age.

The most frequently recognized clinical features of giant cell arteritis (cranial, temporal, and granulomatous arteritis) result from involvement of cranial arteries. For temporal arteritis and polymyalgia rheumatica, the subclavian or axillary arteries are common sites of involvement. In addition to upper extremity ischemic symptoms, patients with arteritis often present with fever, malaise, headache, and joint pains. The erythrocyte sedimentation rate is often elevated. Some serologic tests can also become positive, but none are sufficiently sensitive or specific to be considered diagnostic.

Arteriographic examination in patients with upper extremity occlusive symptoms is often diagnostic. Multiple artery involvement and a well-developed network of collaterals are characteristic of Takayasu disease; the pulmonary artery is affected in more than 45% of patients. Characteristic arteriographic findings in giant cell arteritis include long segments of smooth arterial stenosis alternating with areas of normal or increased caliber, smoothly tapered occlusions, and the absence of irregular plaques and ulcerations (Fig. 81-4).

Thoracic outlet syndrome is by far the most common condition producing upper extremity vascular complications in young adults. Possible compression sites include the costoclavicular space formed by the first thoracic rib and clavicle; the interscalene triangle; the angle between the insertion of the pectoralis minor tendon and the coracoid process in the axilla; and the humerus head in extreme external rotation. Thoracic outlet compression may be due to bony anomalies such as a cervical rib or an abnormal first thoracic rib, or it may be secondary to hypertrophy of the anterior scalene muscle. Although a cervical rib is found in 0.5% to 1% of the population, less than 10% of such persons have symptoms of neurovascular compression (Fig. 81-5). Arterial complications include aneurysm formation, poststenotic dilation, thrombosis, and distal embolism. The latter can cause digital gangrene or severe hand ischemia. Aneurysm formation is not confined to the subclavian or axillary arteries; repetitive trauma to branch arteries, such as the posterior circumflex humeral artery, has been reported to lead to aneurysm formation in baseball pitchers and volleyball players.[7] In such

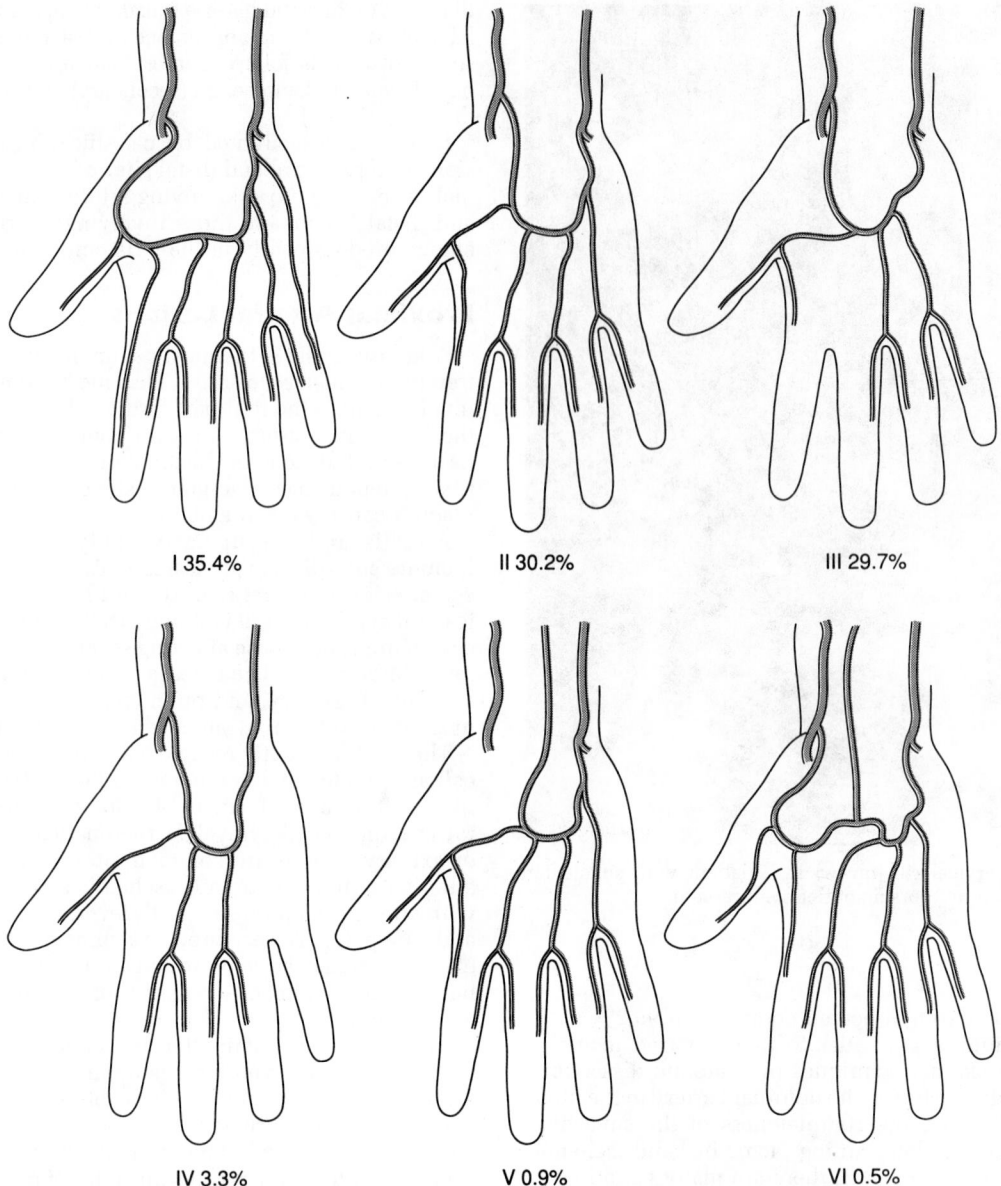

I 35.4%   II 30.2%   III 29.7%

IV 3.3%   V 0.9%   VI 0.5%

Figure 81-3. Different types of complete superficial palmar arch found on 500 hand arteriograms. (After Janevski BK. Angiography of the upper extremity. The Hague, Amsterdam, Martinus Nijhoff, 1982)

individuals, Raynaud phenomenon is often an initial complaint and is often unilateral. Neurologic symptoms and upper extremity venous thrombotic complications are more common presentations of thoracic outlet syndrome than are arterial complications, but the latter symptoms are more threatening to limb and function and are always an urgent indication for arteriography.

Distal Arterial Lesions

Several collagen vascular disorders produce distal upper extremity ischemia, including scleroderma, rheumatoid arthritis, systemic lupus erythematosus, polyarteritis nodosa, and dermatomyositis. All have systemic symptoms and present upper extremity symptoms ranging from Raynaud phenomenon to gangrene of the digits. Extensive involvement of the palmar arches or digital arteries is common (Fig. 81-6).

Buerger's disease (thromboangiitis obliterans) was first described in 1879, but its existence as a distinct entity is still questionable. It was initially described in male patients of Mediterranean origin who presented with digital gangrene without occlusion of larger arteries, but contemporary practice recognizes that men and women of many ethnic backgrounds can be affected. A persistent characteristic of the disease is a strong association with heavy smoking of a particularly addictive nature. Diagnosis of Buerger's disease depends on histologic examination with involvement of arteries as well as veins. The latter can be manifested clinically as migrating phlebitis. Characteristic arteriographic findings are occlusion of the small arteries of the digits and abundant collaterals. The typical corkscrew appearance of the collaterals and the lack of large vessel plaques characteristic of atherosclerosis are strongly suggestive of Buerger's disease. Not only does the symptomatic hand demonstrate digital artery occlusions, but the asymptomatic hand may show them as well.

Blood dyscrasias, such as cold agglutinins, cryoglobulin,

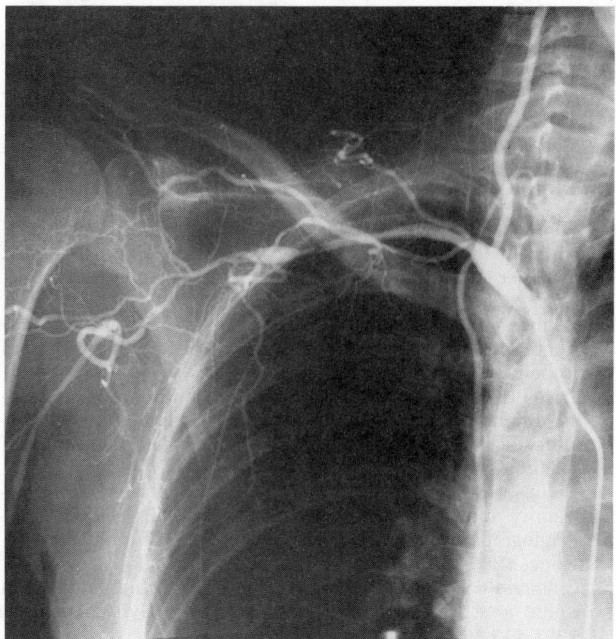

Figure 81-4. Characteristic long segmental narrowing of the sub-clavian artery in a patient with giant cell arteritis. (Yao JST. Arterial surgery of the upper extremity. In: Haimovici H, Callow AD, DePalma RG, et al, eds. Vascular surgery: principles and techniques, ed 3. Norwalk, CT, Appleton & Lange, 1989:858)

and polycythemia vera, are the most common forms of blood dyscrasias associated with occlusion of the arteries of the hand. The cause of small artery occlusion is generally thought to be local thrombosis or embolism. Specific immunologic and blood tests help to establish the diagnosis.

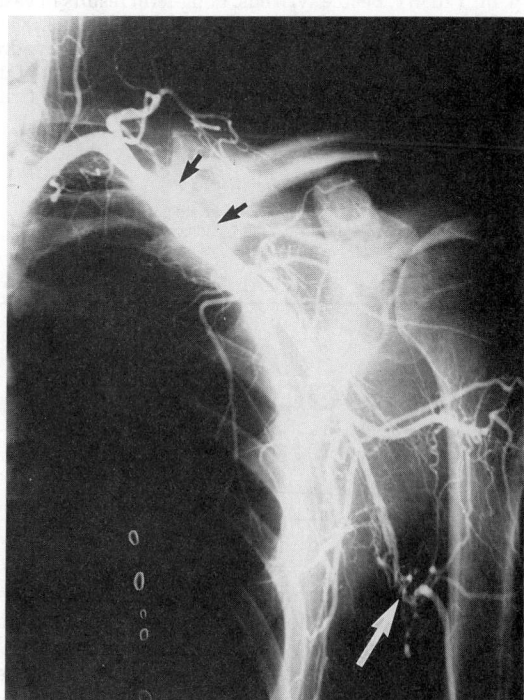

Figure 81-5. Arteriogram in a patient with subclavian aneurysm (*black arrows*) caused by a cervical rib. Multiple distal arterial occlusion has occurred as the result of embolization (*white arrow*).

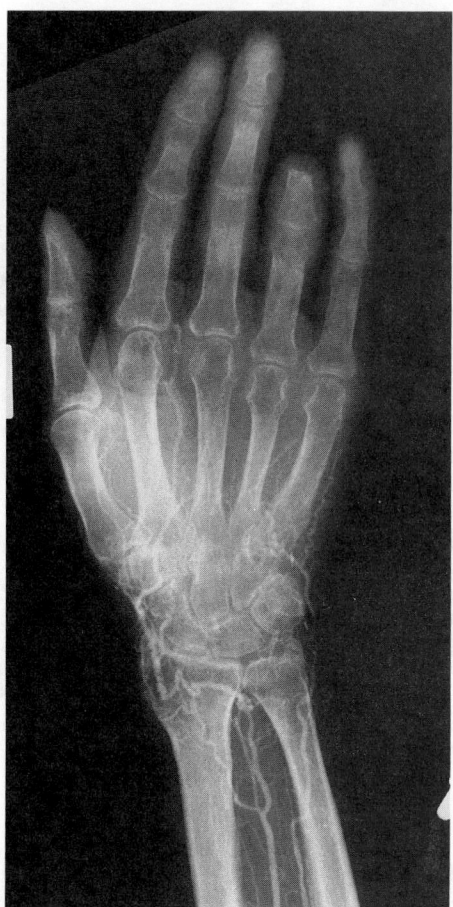

Figure 81-6. Arteriogram of a patient with scleroderma and digital gangrene. The extensive small artery occlusion involves the palmar arch and digital arteries.

Catheter injuries with damage to the radial and brachial arteries have become more common because of increasing use of diagnostic and therapeutic procedures involving catheterization. These are especially troublesome when an incomplete palmar arch is not recognized before placement of a catheter in the radial artery. Gangrene or severe ischemia can occur as a result of the injury.

Vibration syndrome causing blanching and numbness of the hands after the use of pneumatic drills is a well-recognized clinical entity causing hand ischemia. The so-called vibratory white finger is a form of occupational trauma. Repetitive trauma to the digital arteries that initially causes spasm but ultimately causes thrombosis and permanent occlusion is believed to be the primary factor responsible for ischemic symptoms.

Hypothenar hammer syndrome is another form of occupational trauma commonly seen in mechanics and carpenters. The mechanism of injury is the repetitive use of the palm of the hand in activities that involve pounding, pushing, or twisting. The anatomic location of the ulnar artery at the area of hypothenar eminence places it in a vulnerable position. When this area is repeatedly traumatized, ulnar artery occlusion or aneurysm formation can result (Fig. 81-7). Digital artery occlusion is a result of embolism from the injured artery.

Calciphylactic arteriopathy in diabetic patients or patients with chronic renal failure can produce heavily calcified arteries, leading to gangrene or severe ischemia of the hand. The so-called azotemic exteriography (calciphylaxis) is characterized by calcification of the media of the digital arteries resulting in a pipestem pattern on plain film.

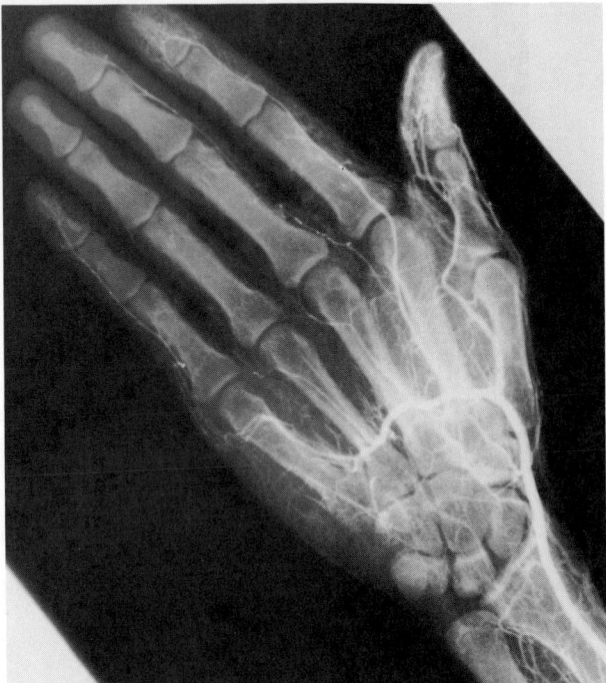

Figure 81-7. Occlusion of the ulnar artery over the hamate bone in a patient with hypothenar hammer syndrome.

TREATMENT

The treatment of upper extremity ischemic vascular disorders is directed toward the underlying cause. Proximal large vessel stenosis or embologenic lesions usually require surgical therapy. The type of reconstructive procedure depends on the nature and location of the lesion. Arterial complications due to thoracic outlet obstruction often require a bypass procedure after resection of the subclavian aneurysm and removal of the cervical rib.[8] A bypass graft with autogenous vein (saphenous or cephalic) often relieves occlusion of the brachial artery and its major branches.[9-11] A short segmental occlusion of either the radial or ulnar artery is best treated by thrombectomy or endarterectomy with a vein patch. An aneurysm in the hand can be resected and continuity restored by end-to-end anastomosis or an interposed vein graft.

The result of bypass grafts for the upper extremity is rather similar to that for lower extremity revascularization; that is, proximal grafts fare better than distal grafts. In a recent report, overall 5-year patency was 52.2% in 43 patients.[12] The patency for anastomosis proximal to the brachial artery bifurcation was better than that for more distal placement (61.9% versus 34.8%). Unlike lower extremity surgery, major amputation is not often required, even after graft occlusion.

Steroid therapy may be needed if there is arteritis with systemic symptoms. Iatrogenic drug-induced ischemia must be treated by cessation of the drug. Dramatic improvement can occur in patients with ergot poisoning.

Distal lesions with occlusion at or distal to the palmar arch are unlikely to be amenable to direct surgical treatment. In these patients, conservative treatment with the use of a calcium blocker (eg, nifedipine) may reduce the severity and frequency of attacks. A host of medications have been recommended.[13] Unfortunately, none have proved consistently effective.

In all patients with upper extremity ischemia from any cause, cessation of smoking is an important step. Tobacco smoke has many constituents with adverse vascular ef-

fects. It clearly causes vasoconstriction, and this effect seems prominent in the upper extremity. Likewise, general protective measures such as avoiding exposure to cold temperatures and avoiding mechanical trauma have beneficial effects when scrupulously applied.

REFERENCES

1. Sumner DS. Noninvasive assessment of upper extremity ischemia. In Bergan JJ, Yao JST, eds. Evaluation and treatment of upper and lower extremity circulatory disorders. Orlando, Grune & Stratton, 1984:75.
2. Erlandson EE, Forrest ME, Shields JJ, et al. Discriminant arteriographic criteria in the management of forearm and hand ischemia. Surgery 1981;90:1025.
3. Love PE, Santoro SA. Antiphospholipid antibodies: anticardiolipin and the lupus anticoagulant in systemic lupus erythematosus (SLE) and in non-SLE disorders. Ann Intern Med 1990;112:682.
4. Yao JST, Bergan JJ, Neiman HL. Arteriography for upper extremity and digital ischemia. In: Neiman HL, Yao JST, eds. Angiography of vascular disease. New York, Churchill Livingstone, 1985:353.
5. Coleman SS, Ansun BJ. Arterial patterns in the hand based upon a study of 650 specimens. Surg Gynecol Obstet 1961;113:409.
6. Janevski BK. Angiography of the upper extremity. The Hague, Amsterdam, Martinus Nijhoff, 1982.
7. Durham JR, Yao JST, Pearce WH, Nuber GM, McCarthy WJ. Arterial injuries in the thoracic outlet syndrome. J Vasc Surg 1995;21:57.
8. Yao JST, Flinn WR, McCarthy WJ, et al. Upper extremity revascularization. In: Bergan JJ, Yao JST, eds. Techniques in arterial surgery. Philadelphia, WB Saunders, 1990:328.
9. Garrett HE, Morris GC, Howell FJ, et al. Revascularization of upper extremity with autogenous vein bypass graft. Arch Surg 1965;91:751.
10. Whitehouse WM Jr, Zelenock GB, Wakefield TN, et al. Arterial bypass grafts for upper extremity ischemia. J Vasc Surg 1986;3:569.
11. McCarthy WJ, Flinn WR, Yao JST, et al. Result of bypass grafting for upper limb ischemia. J Vasc Surg 1986;3:741.
12. Mesh CL, Yao JST. Upper extremity bypass: five-year follow-up. In: Yao JST, Pearce WH, eds. Long-term results in vascular surgery. Norwalk, CT, Appleton & Lange, 1993:353.
13. Porter JM, Rivers SP. Management of Raynaud's syndrome. In: Bergan JJ, Yao JST, eds. Evaluation and treatment of upper and lower extremity circulatory disorders. Orlando, Grune & Stratton, 1984:181.

SURGERY: SCIENTIFIC PRINCIPLES AND PRACTICE, Second Edition, edited by Lazar J. Greenfield, Michael W. Mulholland, Keith T. Oldham, Gerald B. Zelenock, and Keith D. Lillemoe. Lippincott–Raven Publishers, Philadelphia, © 1997.

CHAPTER 82

VISCERAL OCCLUSIVE DISEASE

GERALD B. ZELENOCK

The relatively complex functions of the abdominal viscera are subserved by a circulation uniquely adapted for absorbing and distributing nutrients. As organogenesis proceeds in fetal development, the primitive dual arterial supply to the abdominal viscera changes such that the ventral anastomosis disappears and the paired segmental vitelline arteries fuse. The 10th arterial pair form the celiac trunk; the 13th, the superior mesenteric artery (SMA); and the 21st or 22nd, the inferior mesenteric artery (IMA; Fig. 82-1). Variations in the persistence or regression of parts of the primitive ventral anastomosis result in anatomic variations and recognized patterns of collateral circulation. A common celiomesenteric trunk, the replaced hepatic branches from the celiac artery to the SMA, or a persistent ventral anastomosis producing an arch of Bühler are commonly occurring anatomic variations that are important to surgeons.

VASCULAR ANATOMY OF THE ABDOMINAL VISCERA

The vascular anatomy of the abdominal viscera follows well-described patterns. The celiac artery typically gives rise to three branches—the splenic, the common hepatic,

and the left gastric arteries (Fig. 82-2). In addition, it gives rise to the inferior phrenic arteries in about 55% of the population. The splenic artery originates from the celiac artery, distal to the origin of the left gastric artery. The splenic artery is closely associated with the pancreas and provides arterial input to the spleen, the pancreas (dorsal pancreatic artery, transverse pancreatic artery, pancreatic magna artery, caudal pancreatic artery, and other small unnamed pancreatic branches), and the stomach by way of the short gastric and left gastroepiploic arteries. The common hepatic artery divides into the gastroduodenal and proper hepatic arteries. Through its proper hepatic branch, it typically gives rise to both the right and left hepatic arteries. In about 25% of the population, the left hepatic artery is derived from the left gastric artery. In

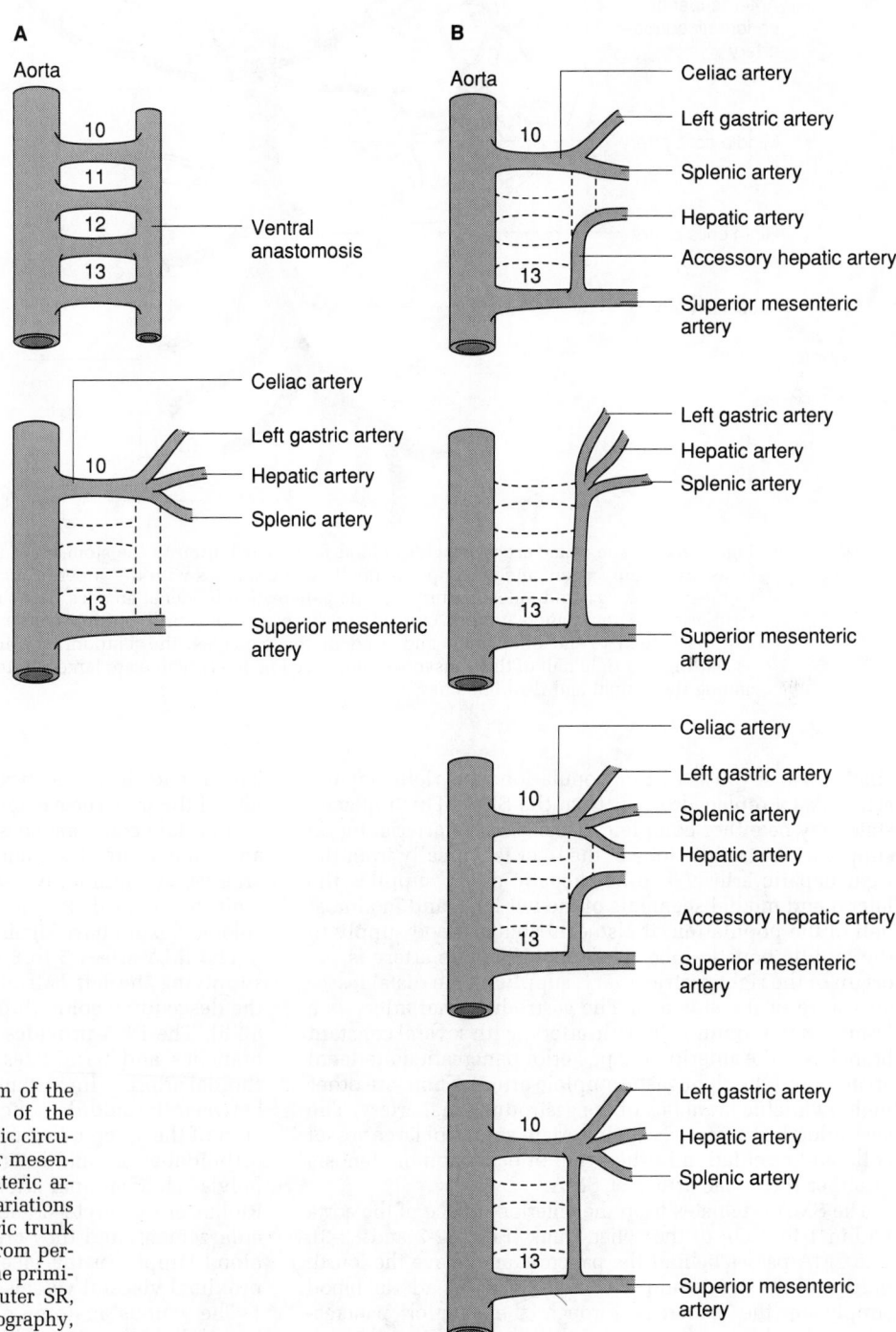

Figure 82-1. (*A*) Schematic diagram of the normal embryologic development of the three main branches of the splanchnic circulation—the celiac axis, the superior mesenteric artery, and the inferior mesenteric artery. (*B*) Recognized anatomic variations such as a common celiacomesenteric trunk or a replaced hepatic artery result from persistence or abnormal regression of the primitive ventral anastomosis. (After Reuter SR, Redman HC. Gastrointestinal angiography, ed 2. Philadelphia, WB Saunders, 1977)

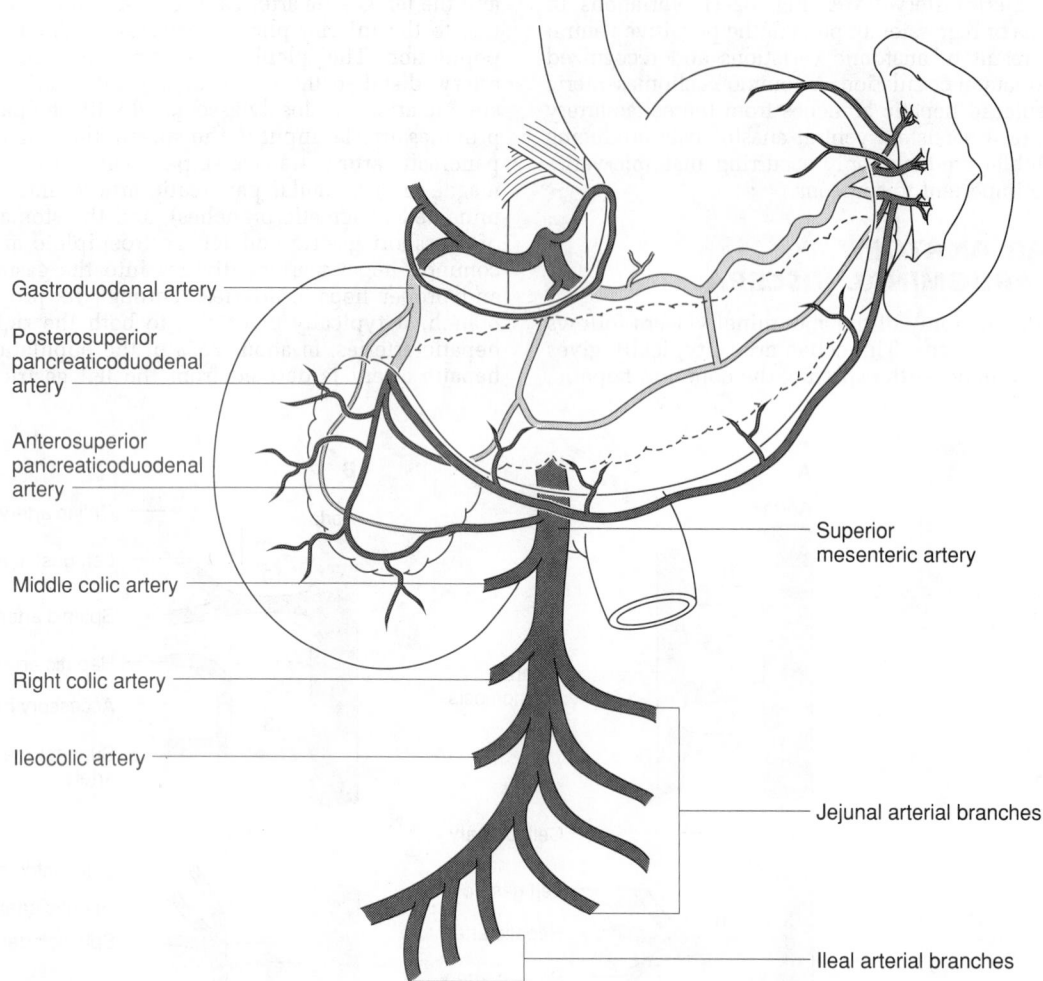

Gastroduodenal artery

Posterosuperior pancreaticoduodenal artery

Anterosuperior pancreaticoduodenal artery

Middle colic artery

Right colic artery

Ileocolic artery

Superior mesenteric artery

Jejunal arterial branches

Ileal arterial branches

Figure 82-2. The celiac artery provides blood flow distribution to the stomach, duodenum, pancreas, liver, and spleen, and has important collateral branches with the superior mesenteric artery by means of the gastroduodenal artery and the pancreaticoduodenal arcades. The superior mesenteric artery is retropancreatic but crosses anteriorly to the fourth portion of the duodenum. It supplies blood to the duodenum and head of the pancreas, the jejunum, the ileum, and the ascending and right half of the transverse colon (see Fig. 82-3). There are large anastomotic arcades among the jejunal and ileal branches.

about 15% to 20% of the population, the right hepatic artery has a replaced origin from the SMA. This replaced state may be either complete or partial. The arterial blood supply to the middle lobe of the liver is typically from the right hepatic artery. The left hepatic artery supplies the lateral and medial segments of the left lobe, and in almost half of the population, it also contributes blood supply to the middle hepatic lobe. The proper hepatic artery is the origin of the right gastric artery, supplying the distal lesser curvature of the stomach. The gastroduodenal artery is a branch of the common hepatic artery, with several constant branches—the anterior and posterior pancreaticoduodenal arcades and the right gastroepiploic artery. There are other highly variable branches of the gastroduodenal artery. The gastroduodenal artery is an important source of large vessel collateral circulation in the event of occlusion or stenosis of either the celiac artery or SMA.

The SMA originates from the anterior surface of the aorta within 1 to 2 cm of the celiac trunk (Figs. 82-2 and 82-3). The SMA passes behind the pancreas and above the fourth portion of the duodenum. The vessel provides arterial blood supply to the pancreas through the inferior pancreaticoduodenal artery, to most of the small intestine through

jejunal and ileal branches, and to the ascending and right half of the transverse colon through its ileocolic, right colic, and middle colic branches. There are extensive large vessel anastomotic arcades among the 10 to 20 jejunal and ileal arteries. In addition, well-defined anastomoses between the main branches of the SMA and IMA in the region of the splenic flexure have significant implications for surgeons.

The IMA arises 5 to 6 cm distal to the SMA, typically supplying the left half of the transverse colon and all of the descending colon through the left colic artery (see Fig. 82-3). The IMA provides a variable number of sigmoidal branches and terminates as the paired superior hemorrhoidal arteries. Important SMA to IMA anastomoses occur between the middle colic and left colic arteries in the region of the splenic flexure and between the superior hemorrhoidal artery and internal iliac branches supplying the pelvis. The marginal artery of Drummond and the arch of Riolan are discrete branch vessels capable of significant enlargement, and they are important sources of collateral blood supply in the face of occlusion or stenosis of the proximal visceral vessels (Fig. 82-4).

The venous anatomy of the gastrointestinal tract tends to parallel the arterial blood supply and drains into the

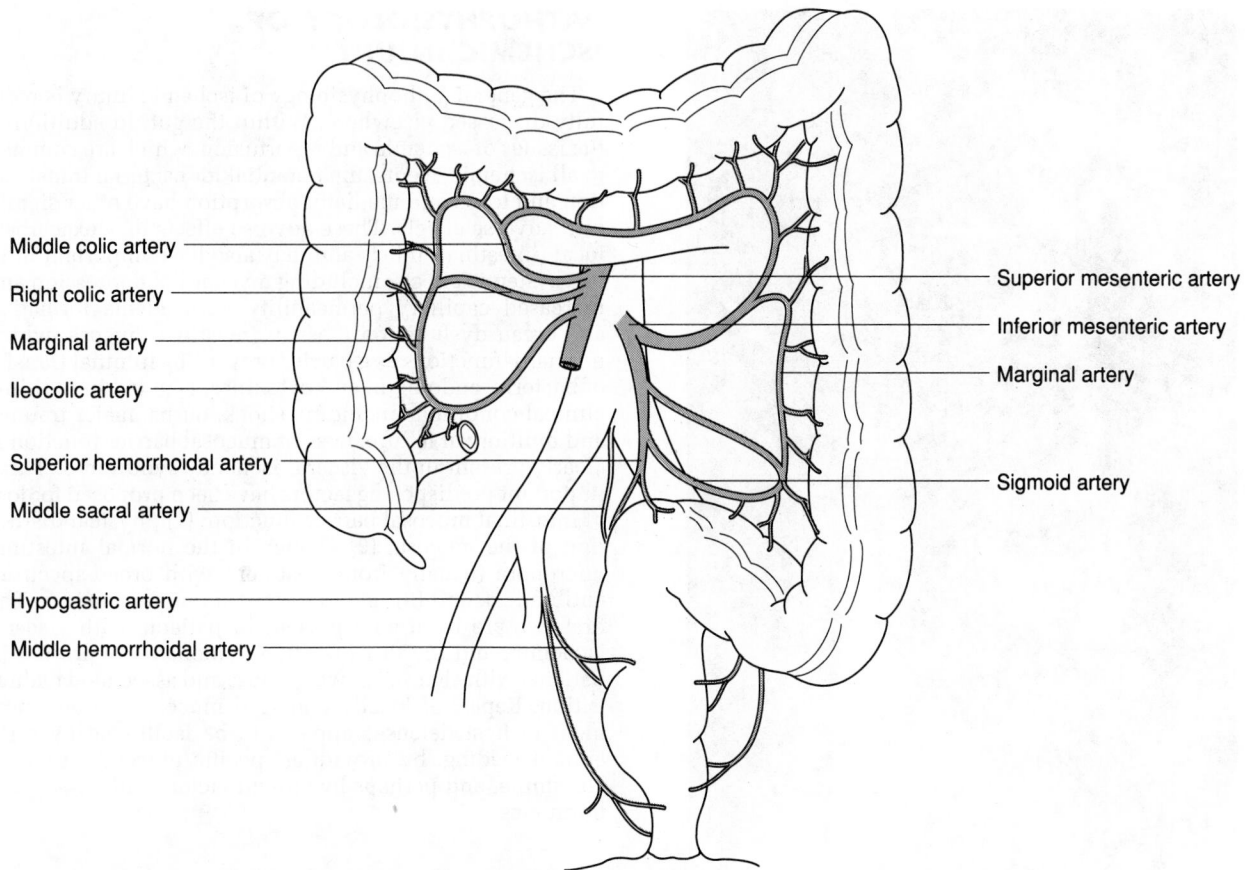

Middle colic artery

Right colic artery

Marginal artery

Ileocolic artery

Superior hemorrhoidal artery

Middle sacral artery

Hypogastric artery

Middle hemorrhoidal artery

Superior mesenteric artery

Inferior mesenteric artery

Marginal artery

Sigmoid artery

Figure 82-3. The inferior mesenteric artery (IMA) provides blood supply to the left half of the transverse colon and all of the descending colon, including the sigmoidal and superior hemorrhoidal branches. The left branch of the middle colic artery from the superior mesenteric artery and the ascending portion of the left colic artery from the IMA form a collateral network in the region of the splenic flexure. The IMA serves as an important source of collateral blood supply when the proximal two visceral vessels are occluded.

portal venous system perfusing the liver. The inferior mesenteric vein drains into the splenic vein. The splenic vein anastomosis with the superior mesenteric vein forms the origin of the portal vein. The portal vein subdivides into right and left portal veins and by repetitive subdivision supplies the liver parenchyma. Hepatic venous blood is drained by right, middle, and left hepatic veins, which enter the vena cava. Portal–systemic anastomoses are common and are of considerable importance in the presence of portal hypertension.

Extensive visceral–visceral and visceral–systemic collaterals, as well as the "redundancy" built into the system by normal anatomic patterns, afford a measure of protection from vascular occlusion (Fig. 82-5). Virtually every visceral organ has multiple sources of blood supply and venous drainage. Further, the extensive collateral circulation is enhanced by the arcade arrangement as well as frequently encountered collateral patterns. The left and right gastric and right and left gastroepiploic blood vessels, the anterior and posterior, superior and inferior pancreaticoduodenal arcades, and the anastomosis between the middle and left colic arteries are almost invariably observed. Furthermore, visceral–systemic collaterals, such as occur between the IMA and the hypogastric artery or between the celiac axis and the systemic vessels by way of phrenic, esophageal, and intercostal arteries, are well described. An extensive intramural plexus and the specialized circulation within the mucosa and villus tip allow

the intestinal circulation to perform its physiologic function but also account for the unique vulnerability of the mucosal tip.

A variety of techniques in humans and experimental studies have been used to quantify intestinal blood flow. Electromagnetic flow meters, indicator dilution techniques, microspheres, aminopyrine, inert gases, pulsed Doppler ultrasound flow meters, and angiographic techniques, such as spill-over or videodilution, all have had some applicability to measuring intestinal blood flow. Using such techniques, typical large-vessel intestinal blood flow in humans has been estimated to be between 500 and 1200 mL/min, or about 10% to 20% of the cardiac output. Recent advances in noninvasive vascular diagnostic technology allow visualization and volume flow determinations within the celiac artery and SMA. Duplex scanning, combining Doppler blood flow velocity determinations with B-mode ultrasonography, allows precise measurement of cross-sectional areas and enables calculation of volumetric flows (Fig. 82-6). Such technology is useful in diagnosing intestinal vascular disorders but also allows repetitive physiologic investigations in humans without resort to operative implantation of flow transducers or the intraarterial injection of dyes and tracers. Baseline flow in fasted human subjects and the response to standard meals are shown in Table 82-1. Minimal but nonsignificant changes in celiac artery blood flow occur with all meal types, whereas significant

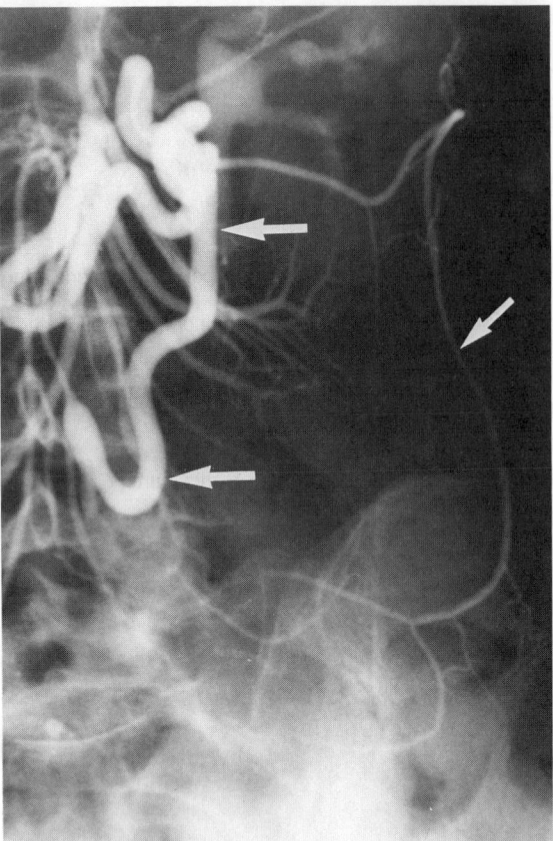

Figure 82-4. Selective inferior mesenteric artery angiography demonstrates the marginal artery of Drummond and the larger, more functionally important arc of Riolan or central anastomotic artery. (Zelenock GB. Splanchnic arteriosclerotic disease and intestinal angina. Arch Surg 1980;115:497)

increases in SMA blood flow are seen 20 to 30 minutes after eating and persist for up to 90 minutes after ingestion. The earliest maximal blood flow response occurs with a carbohydrate meal, whereas the largest overall increase in blood flow occurs after ingesting a mixed meal containing carbohydrate, protein, and fat. Better definition of the factors involved in regulation of intestinal blood flow under physiologic and pathologic conditions should be possible as investigations proceed.

Within the wall of the intestine, most blood flow is to the mucosa. This tissue, representing 50% of the mass of the intestine, receives about 75% of the resting blood flow. The muscular and serosal layers of the intestine receive the remaining 25%. Control of blood flow in the splanchnic circulation is affected by the sympathetic nervous system as well as by metabolic, myogenic, and extrinsic factors. Stimulation of sympathetic nerves increases vascular tone and decreases splanchnic blood flow. Parasympathetic nerve fibers appear to have little direct effect on blood flow. Numerous intrinsic hormonal regulators (eg, secretin, gastrin, cholecystokinin, glucagon, and vasoactive intestinal peptide), as well as substances such as histamine, serotonin, and bradykinin and the prostaglandins, may play important physiologic roles in the regulation of blood flow. Circulating hormones and regulatory substances (eg, epinephrine, norepinephrine, and angiotensin), as well as many commonly used pharmaceuticals, may also have important effects on the splanchnic circulation (Table 82-2).

PATHOPHYSIOLOGY OF ISCHEMIC INJURY

The general pathophysiology of ischemic injury is more fully discussed elsewhere. Within the gut, in addition to the issues of ischemia and reperfusion, which are common to all ischemic events, the potential for bacterial translocation and toxin and mediator absorption have other significant adverse effects. These adverse effects may exacerbate local (intestinal) injury and may also have important indirect systemic effects, including myocardial depression and increased capillary permeability with edema formation and organ dysfunction. Loss of intestinal mucosa, which normally functions as a barrier preventing luminal transfer of bacteria, endotoxin, and cytokines, is noted in multiple clinical conditions including shock, burns, major trauma, and multiorgan failure. Loss of mucosal barrier function is clearly present in the visceral ischemic syndromes. Three important predisposing factors have been proposed for loss of intestinal mucosal barrier function: (1) physical disruption of the mucosa, (2) change in the normal intestinal microflora (usually from treatment with broad-spectrum antibiotics), and (3) impaired host immune defenses. The first two are invariably present in patients with visceral ischemia, and the third is often demonstrably present in patients with significant weight loss and associated malnutrition. Repair of locally damaged mucosa and enhancement of host defenses appears to be facilitated by early enteral feeding, by providing specific nutrients, such as glutamine, and perhaps by growth factors and gut trophic hormones.

CLINICAL SYNDROMES

The visceral ischemic syndromes are most conveniently considered as acute or chronic (subacute) with respect to their clinical presentation. Acute visceral ischemic syndromes include mesenteric embolism, mesenteric thrombosis, low-flow nonocclusive mesenteric ischemia, and iatrogenic ischemia. These are always serious and potentially life-threatening events; the mortality attending such processes is typically in excess of 70%. Chronic, or subacute, visceral ischemic syndromes include visceral angina, mesenteric venous thrombosis, and perhaps the median arcuate ligament syndrome. The designation of "chronic" visceral ischemia is questioned by some and is perhaps a misnomer since even when the clinical presentation is chronic, the underlying pathophysiology is characterized by repetitive near-critical ischemic events. The traditional designations are used in this chapter, but the severity of the ischemic process and the precarious and profoundly threatening nature of chronic visceral ischemia are recognized.

Acute Visceral Ischemic Syndromes

Mesenteric Embolism

Mesenteric embolism accounts for about half of cases of acute mesenteric ischemia. Typically, the embolus arises from a cardiac source. Classically, atrial fibrillation or a myocardial infarction with mural thrombus formation is the source of the embolus, but virtually any arrhythmia or anatomic cardiac defect may result in a mesenteric embolus. Embolism of intracardiac tumor, such as an atrial myxoma or a paradoxical embolus, is another possible cause but is extraordinarily uncommon.

Acute mesenteric embolism tends to cause the sudden onset of severe epigastric or mid-abdominal pain, which is followed promptly by evacuation of the gut, either

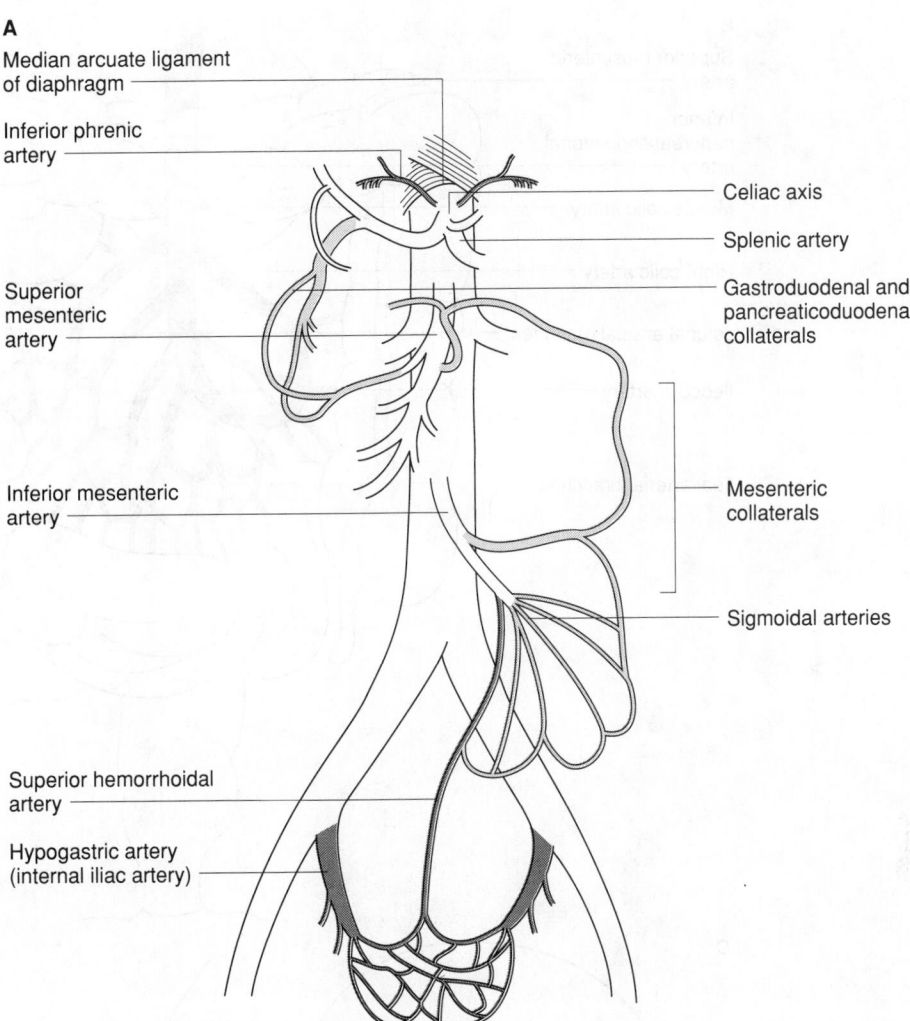

A

Median arcuate ligament of diaphragm

Inferior phrenic artery

Superior mesenteric artery

Inferior mesenteric artery

Superior hemorrhoidal artery

Hypogastric artery (internal iliac artery)

Celiac axis

Splenic artery

Gastroduodenal and pancreaticoduodenal collaterals

Mesenteric collaterals

Sigmoidal arteries

Figure 82-5. (*A*) The collateral circulation to the intestine occurs at several levels. Well-recognized visceral–visceral and visceral–parietal collateral branches and anastomoses are important. The unnamed intestinal arcades (*B*) and the intramural anastomoses (*C*) are effective short-segment collaterals. *(continues)*

through emesis or explosive diarrhea. Typically, the patient felt well before the onset of pain and can often precisely pinpoint the onset of the pain. Fully 25% of patients have had previous embolic events. The general physical examination may indicate the underlying cardiac disorder. An unusual irregular rhythm indicating atrial fibrillation, the classic murmur of mitral stenosis, or an enlarged heart all support the diagnosis. The abdominal examination may reveal signs of an acute abdomen or may be normal. Slight to moderate abdominal distention is common. Bowel sounds are highly variable, as are findings on palpation. A well-recognized presentation of acute mesenteric insufficiency is severe abdominal complaints out of proportion to the physical findings. Peritoneal signs or blood in the stool are late and ominous signs, implying severe ischemia with infarction.

There are no pathognomonic laboratory tests. An electrocardiogram may confirm cardiac abnormalities suspected from the history and physical examination, or a cardiac echo or ultrasound scan may demonstrate mural thrombus. Such tests are helpful but not diagnostic. Standard hematology and biochemical evaluation are unrewarding early in the clinical course. Late evaluation may demonstrate hemoconcentration, acidosis, leukocytosis, and serum phosphorus or transaminase elevations. None of these abnormalities need be present even with a major mesenteric embolus. None is sufficiently sensi-

tive or specific to confirm the diagnosis. Diagnosis depends on clinical suspicion followed by diagnostic angiography. Emboli tend to lodge at branch points of the SMA. In this regard, the origin of the SMA is typically spared, and the lodging point is in proximity to the origin of the inferior pancreaticoduodenal artery or the middle colic artery (Fig. 82-7).

After diagnosis, the patient is heparinized, volume-resuscitated, and taken emergently to the operating room. Prophylactic antibiotics and full hemodynamic monitoring are required. The SMA is approached beneath the transverse mesocolon. Proximal and distal control are obtained, and Fogarty catheter embolectomy through either a transverse or longitudinal arteriotomy is performed. Patch closure of the SMA is not usually required with a transverse arteriotomy, but it is used if the SMA is small or if a longitudinal incision was used. In most instances, this approach should result in prompt return of visceral blood flow. An assessment of intestinal viability is made. After restoration of blood flow, an important consideration is the possibility of multiple emboli lodging in distal branches of the SMA.

Mesenteric Thrombosis

Mesenteric thrombosis is a common cause of acute visceral ischemia. The presentation is that of an acute intestinal catastrophe with the progressive develop-

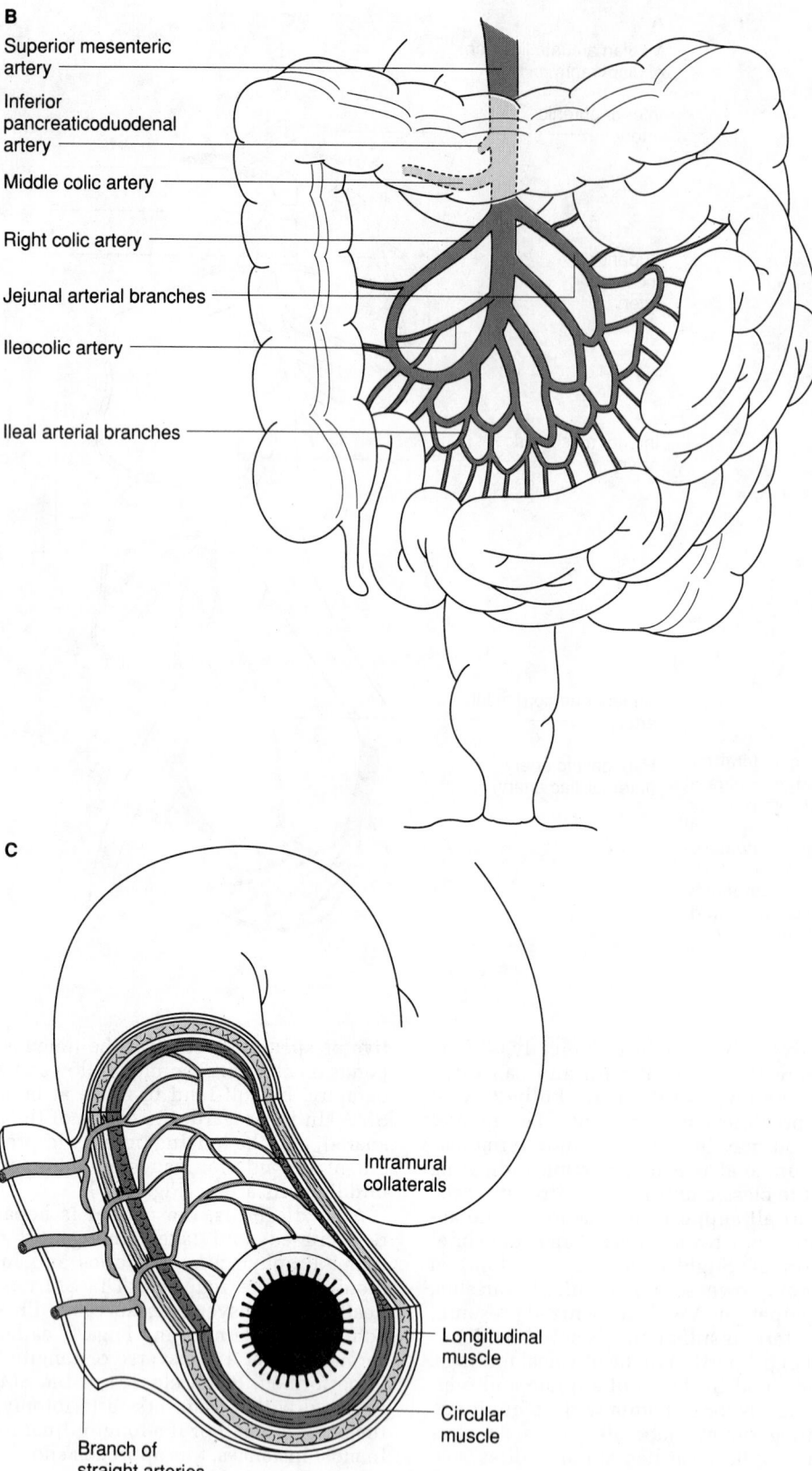

B

Superior mesenteric artery

Inferior pancreaticoduodenal artery

Middle colic artery

Right colic artery

Jejunal arterial branches

Ileocolic artery

Ileal arterial branches

C

Intramural collaterals

Longitudinal muscle

Circular muscle

Branch of straight arteries

Figure 82-5. (Continued)

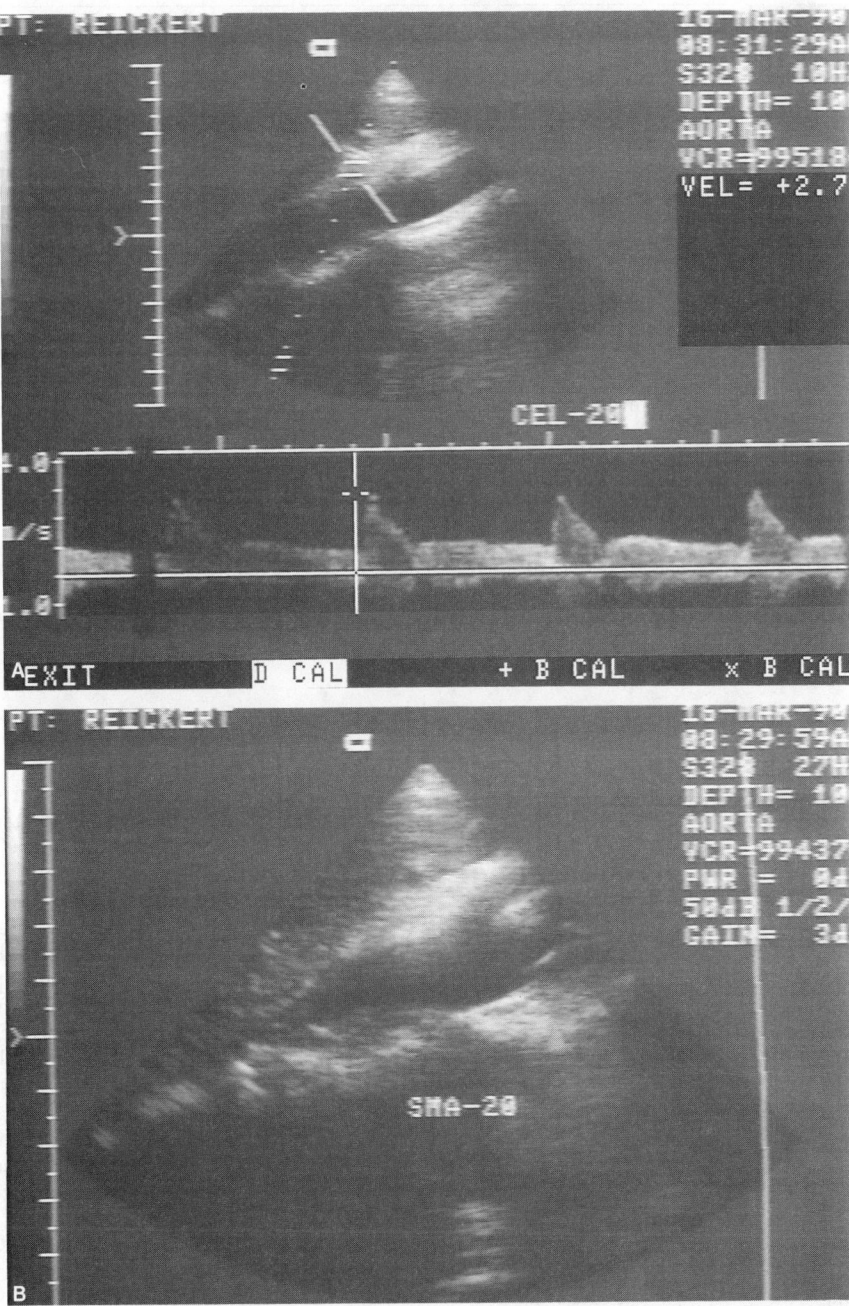

Figure 82-6. Duplex scan of celiac (*A*) and superior mesenteric (*B*) arteries. Vessel diameter, flow velocity, calculated volumetric blood flow, spectral analysis, and the response to physiologic stimuli allow a precise assessment of the visceral circulation.

ment of severe mid-abdominal pain. Acute symptoms may be superimposed on a background of chronic intestinal angina or may occur without antecedent symptoms. Usually, the onset is less abrupt than with SMA embolus. If the patient has a history of postprandial abdominal pain associated with meals, substantial weight loss is common. The weight loss is typically due to fear of eating, which precipitates the pain. A history compatible with motility disturbances causing symptoms such as nausea, diarrhea, or constipation is much more common than malabsorption syndromes. Often, the patient has undergone an extensive diagnostic evaluation to rule out the possibility of an underlying gastrointestinal malignancy.

Urgent visceral angiography is required for diagnosis and involves lateral aortography in addition to standard anteroposterior views (Fig. 82-8). The occlusive process is always more widespread than may be apparent on angiography. Multiple-branch stenoses and occlusions within the intestinal arcades are not well demonstrated on standard arteriography.

Reperfusion of the visceral circulation is a major priority. Until recently, mesenteric thrombosis has been an urgent indication for operation. However, in these acutely ill patients, recent massive weight loss with attendant nutritional, wound-healing, and immunologic compromise make a major operative procedure extraordinarily hazardous. Reperfusion to temporarily maintain intestinal viability may sometimes be accomplished by infusion of thrombolytic agents or other angioplastic techniques, and if successful restoration of blood flow is obtained, vigorous hyperalimentation allows optimization of the patient's condition and an elective surgical procedure. The latter approach is not

Table 82-1. DUPLEX MEASUREMENT OF INTESTINAL BLOOD FLOW

Vessel	Average Diameter (Range)	Characteristics on Duplex Scan	Calculated Fasting Volume Flow (mL/min)	Calculated Volume Flow Change From Fasting by Type of Meal* (%)					
				Mixed	Cholesterol	Fat	Protein	Mannitol	Water
Celiac artery	0.66 cm (0.4– 0.8 cm)	Continuous forward flow; no reverse flow; end-diastolic velocity about $1/3$ peak systolic velocity No significant changes with meals	1083 ± 75	18 ± 4	1 ± 4	10 ± 8	21 ± 6	37 ± 19	14 ± 5
Superior mesenteric artery	0.59 cm (0.44– 0.68 cm)	Early diastolic flow reversal; forward diastolic flow; end-diastolic velocity about 0 After eating, loss of reverse flow and increased peak systolic and end-diastolic velocities are noted	538 ± 37	164 ± 30	118 ± 23	117 ± 25	78 ± 15	48 ± 11	24 ± 8

* Calculated volume flow changes that occurred after meals were not significantly increased in the celiac artery but were significantly increased with all meals except water in the superior mesenteric artery.
(Moneta GL, Taylor DC, Heiton WS, et al. Duplex ultrasound measurement of postprandial intestinal blood flow: effect of meal composition. Gastroenterology 1988;95:1294)

Table 82-2. EFFECTS OF VARIOUS SUBSTANCES ON MESENTERIC CIRCULATION AND MOTOR ACTIVITY

Substance	Intestinal Blood Flow	Intestinal O_2 Uptake	Intestinal Motility
Acetylcholine	Increase	Increase	Increase
Adenosine	Increase	Variable	—
Angiotensin II	Decrease	—	Increase
Bradykinin	Variable	—	Increase
Ca^{2+}, high levels	Decrease	—	Increase
Ca^{2+} antagonists	Increase	—	Decrease
Dopamine	Variable	Decrease	—
Epinephrine	Variable	Variable	—
Gastrin	Increase	Increase	Increase
Glucagon	Increase	Increase	Decrease
Histamine	Increase	Increase	Increase
Isoproterenol	Increase	Variable	—
K^+ high levels	Decrease	—	Increase
Mg^{2+}	Increase	—	—
Nitroprusside	Increase	—	—
Norepinephrine	Decrease	Decrease	—
Papaverine	Increase	No change	—
PGE_1	Increase	Increase	—
$PGF_{2\alpha}$	Decrease	Variable	Increase
PGI_2	Increase	—	—
Secretin	Variable	No change	—
Serotonin	Variable	Variable	Variable
Somatostatin	Decrease	—	Decrease
Vasopressin	Decrease	Decrease	Variable
Vasoactive intestinal polypeptide	Increase	Increase	—

(Wakefield TW, Stanley JC. The intestine. In: Zelenock GB, D'Alecy LG, Schlafer M, et al, eds. Clinical ischemic syndromes: mechanisms and consequences of tissue injury. St Louis. CV Mosby, 1990)

often used in clinical practice and is never appropriate when frankly necrotic bowel requiring resection is a consideration. Used selectively, however, this combined approach has potential benefit.

Operations for acute mesenteric thrombosis must be individualized. Emergent revascularization procedures ideally should parallel those used to treat chronic visceral ischemia. Contemporary opinion favors multiple-vessel revascularization and short antegrade conduits (prosthetic or vein) whenever possible. Nevertheless, in the acute setting, a variety of alternative surgical techniques, including single-vessel revascularization and the use of vein and retrograde conduits, have resulted in survival and are appropriate in certain circumstances. In the presence of frankly necrotic bowel requiring resection, autogenous conduits are always preferred.

Low-Flow Nonocclusive Mesenteric Ischemia

Low-flow nonocclusive mesenteric ischemia seems to have diminished in frequency and severity in recent years. Vasoconstriction in mesenteric blood vessels is the underlying mechanism most commonly cited as the cause of low-flow nonocclusive ischemia. This vasoconstriction occurs in response to diminished cardiac output, shock, hypovolemia, dehydration, and the use of medications known to diminish splanchnic blood flow. Virtually all vasoconstrictors and many inotropic agents have been implicated. Other drugs may also have significant effects on intestinal blood flow (see Table 82-2). Diagnosis is typically suspected in critically ill, intensive care unit patients, often with unstable hemodynamics secondary to shock, congestive heart failure, cardiac arrhythmia, recent myocardial infarction, or valvular insufficiency. These problems often coexist with renal or hepatic disease. There may be a suggestion of gastrointestinal bleeding or guaiac-positive secretions noted in nasogastric aspirates. Diagnosis in these instances may require angiography (Fig. 82-9). Because there is no definitive surgical therapy other than resection of necrotic intestine, the focus of intervention is

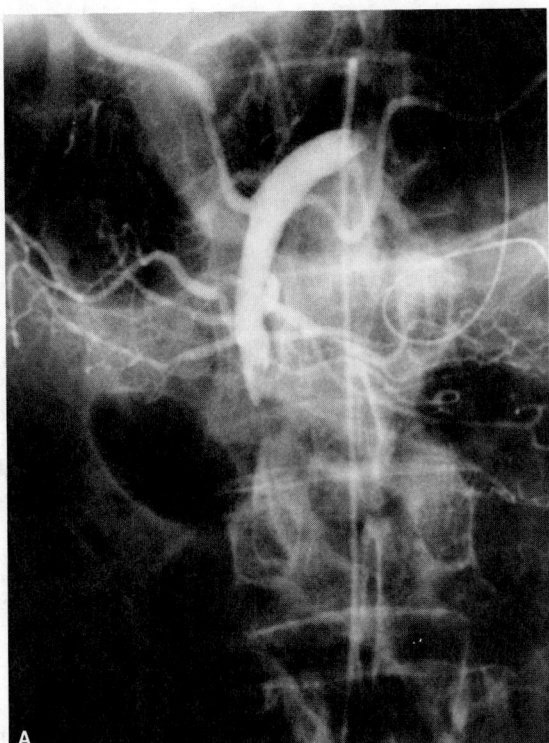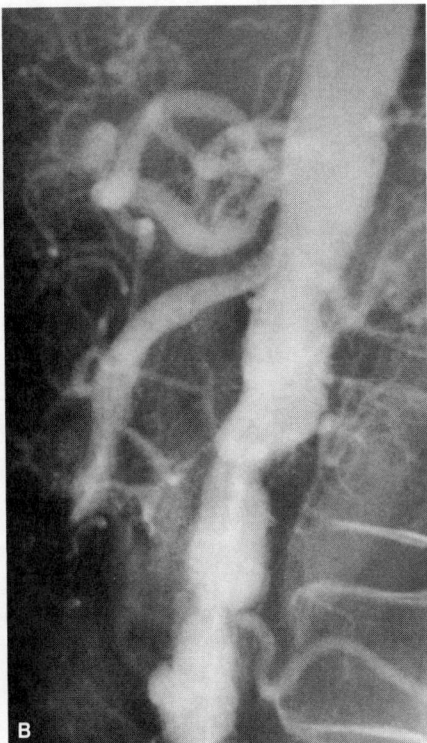

Figure 82-7. (*A*) Anteroposterior view of the typical superior mesenteric artery (SMA) embolus lodging distal to the origin of the middle colic and first jejunal branches of the SMA. The pattern of injury typically spares the first few inches of the jejunum and the colon distal to the midtransverse colon. (*B*) Lateral aortogram demonstrates embolus with sparing of proximal SMA. This pattern is distinct from SMA thrombosis.

on pharmacologic support of the circulation with relief of splanchnic vasoconstriction. Treatments include optimizing hemodynamic and volume status, correcting contributing medical conditions, and eliminating (when possible) adverse pharmacologic agents. Under some circumstances, infusion of vasodilators is appropriate. Papaverine (30 to 60 mg/h) is used by some groups but requires selective intraarterial infusion to avoid systemic hypotension. Glucagon (2 to 4 mg/h), which selectively increases splanchnic blood flow, may be given by peripheral venous infusion and has positive inotropic effects; it may therefore be more suitable in some settings.

Iatrogenic Visceral Ischemia

Iatrogenic visceral ischemia can occur after operations, diagnostic procedures, or with the use of certain pharmacologic agents. Digitalis preparations clearly decrease intestinal blood flow, as do ergotamines and virtually all pressor agents. Diagnostic or therapeutic angiography may cause iatrogenic visceral ischemia by means of embolization, and selective mesenteric angiography has the potential for intimal flap formation or dissection.

Aortic aneurysm resection is the prototypical surgical procedure associated with iatrogenic intestinal ischemia. Its potential for compromise of the colonic and occasionally the intestinal circulation is underappreciated and may occur with or without ligation of the IMA. Intestinal ischemia is more common with ruptured aneurysms, when occlusive and aneurysmal disease coex-

ist, and when important collateral vessels are compromised by the aortic procedure (Fig. 82-10). After aneurysm repair, colonic ischemia is clinically apparent in 1% to 2% of cases and has been detected endoscopically in upward of 6% to 8% of cases. Patients present with diarrhea, often bloody or guaiacpositive. When hemorrhagic diarrhea occurs, immediate colonoscopy is indicated. When ischemia is confined to the mucosa and submucosa and subsequently heals, the patient typically survives, but stricture formation results (Fig. 82-11). When the ischemia is more profound and transmural infarction occurs, resection is required, and the mortality rate approaches 60%. The incidence of colonic ischemia after aortic surgery can be decreased by aggressive colonic and pelvic revascularization. Other operative procedures, such as extensive resections for gastrointestinal and genitourinary cancer, also can provide iatrogenic compromise of intestinal blood flow.

Miscellaneous Causes of Acute Visceral Ischemia

Acute visceral ischemia can occur with an aortic dissection, traumatic injuries, inflammatory arteriopathy, or vasculitis (Table 82-3). The clinical presentation in each instance usually depends on the underlying cause, with superimposed symptoms of abdominal distention, an acute abdomen, or gastrointestinal bleeding. Diagnosis depends on recognizing the potential for intestinal ischemia and often is confirmed by angiography. The treatment in these instances must be highly individualized. Branch revascularization in the setting of acute

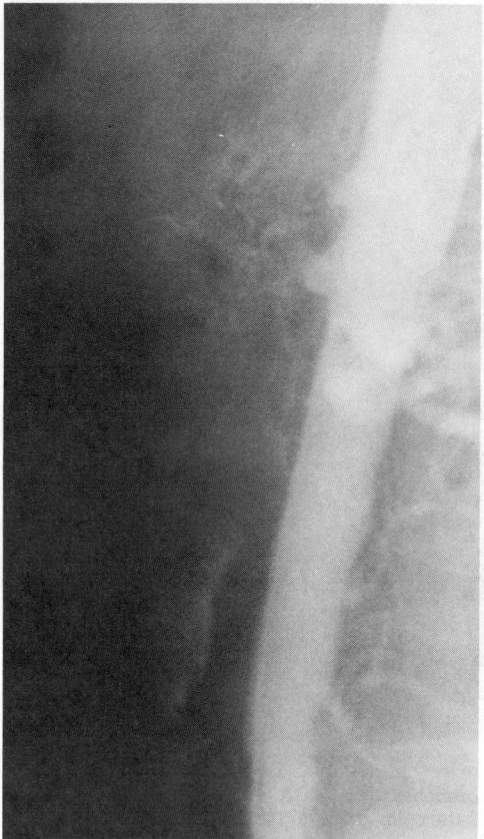

Figure 82-8. Lateral aortogram demonstrating acute celiac and superior mesenteric artery thrombosis, which results in widespread necrosis of the abdominal viscera.

aortic dissection is essential when ischemia is profound. Likewise, traumatic injuries require acute surgical intervention. Inflammatory arteriopathy and vasculitis, however, require treatment of the underlying medical condition with operation reserved for resection of clearly nonviable segments of bowel.

Recognition of Intestinal Viability

Any acute intervention for visceral occlusive disease raises the issues of intraoperative recognition of viability, the appropriate limits to resection, and consideration of a second-look procedure. Recognition of viable versus nonviable intestine might seem straightforward; it is not. When critical lengths of intestine are compromised, decisions regarding how much to resect are of paramount importance. Clinical parameters of color, spontaneous peristalsis, and the presence or absence of palpable pulses are not sensitive nor specific enough to allow precise and confident clinical decisions. A variety of techniques to assess intestinal viability have been described. These techniques range from straightforward but relatively insensitive to more sensitive but cumbersome or complex, requiring technologies not regularly available at the time of an acute problem (Table 82-4). Commonly used techniques are not necessarily sensitive or specific, nor do they directly assess viability or reversibility of injury. They do have the advantage of ready availability and ease of application. The infrequently used techniques often are cumbersome, rela-

tively unavailable, and not yet widely accepted in clinical practice.

By far, the most common adjunctive technique to aid in clinical decisions regarding the margin of resection is Doppler ultrasonic assessment. Although Doppler detects blood flow signals and not necessarily viability, ease and availability make its use commonplace. Fluorescein dye or Wood lamp analysis is also frequently used.

Second-Look Procedures

If resection of large segments of ischemic small intestine is performed, the potential exists for creation of the short-gut syndrome, a condition in which insufficient intestinal mucosal surface remains for adequate nutrient absorption. A dilemma then exists in dealing with damaged but potentially viable intestine. In this specialized circumstance, a second-look procedure may be beneficial. Contemporary clinical practice is to leave all definitely viable and marginally viable intestine, resecting only unequivocally necrotic tissue. At the original operation, the decision for a planned second-look surgical procedure is made, and the patient is prepared for a return to the operating room in 24 to 48 hours to further evaluate the status of the intestine. Innovative technical advances, such as laparoscopy and peritoneoscopy, may prove valuable in this setting but have not been fully evaluated.

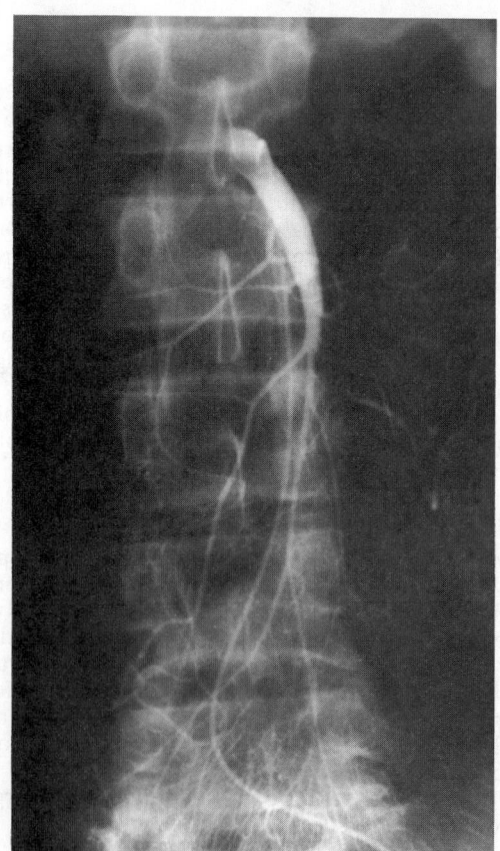

Figure 82-9. Low-flow nonocclusive ischemia causes profound vasoconstriction within the mesenteric arcades. This may be sufficient to cause mucosal necrosis or transmural infarction if unrelieved.

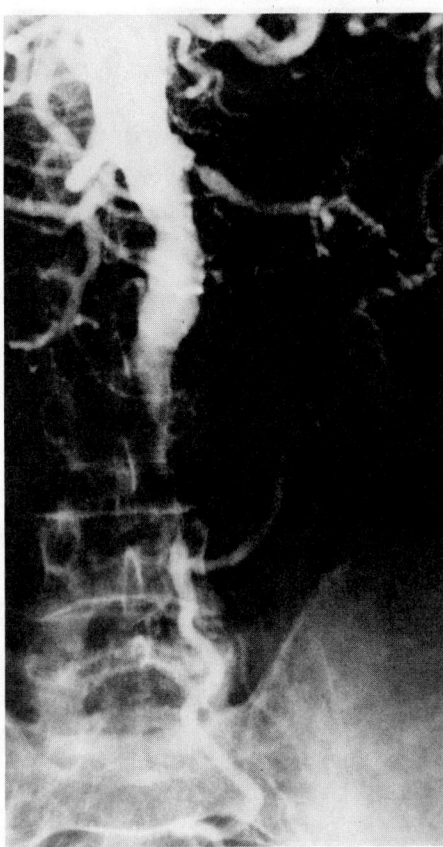

Figure 82-10. There are multiple causes of iatrogenic visceral ischemia, including medications, diagnostic and therapeutic angiographic procedures, and surgical procedures. A common surgical cause is aortic aneurysm resection. Coexistent aneurysmal and occlusive disease as seen in this aortogram identify a patient at high risk.

Chronic Visceral Ischemic Syndromes

The chronic, or subacute, presentation of visceral occlusive disease includes visceral angina, mesenteric venous thrombosis, and possibly the median arcuate ligament syndrome. Although some authorities question the latter, the first two are well established.

Visceral Angina

Visceral angina secondary to arteriosclerotic occlusive disease of the splanchnic trunks causes midepigastric pain 30 to 45 minutes after eating. The responsible anatomic lesions usually involve the origins of at least two of the three visceral vessels (Fig. 82-12), but the occlusive process also is relatively widespread throughout the mesenteric arcades. The patient is typically either atherosclerotic or relatively young (usually a woman) with an extensive cigarette smoking habit. The latter produces a proliferative overflow of adjacent aortic intima into the origins of the visceral vessels. Affected patients have "food fear" and have often modified their pattern of eating so they avoid solid food altogether or consume small quantities of food at any one time. This small-meal syndrome may be erroneously reported by the patient as "eating all the time." Patients with chronic visceral ischemia almost always have a profound weight loss (11 kg on average), raising the

specter of an intraabdominal malignancy. Weight loss represents avoidance of food secondary to pain rather than a malabsorption problem. Many times, an extensive series of gastrointestinal contrast studies, endoscopies, and scans have been undertaken and are normal. Occasionally, nonproductive exploratory laparotomies are noted in the history.

The progression from symptoms to infarction is unpredictable. Many patients with intestinal infarction are discovered, in retrospect, to have had preexisting symptoms of visceral angina. Although delayed recognition is the rule, diagnostic and therapeutic interventions must proceed expeditiously because progress from symptomatic visceral angina to visceral thrombosis with transmural infraction is attended by an 80% mortality rate.

Aortography, including both anteroposterior and lateral views, confirms the clinical suspicion (Fig. 82-13). Multiple proximal vascular trunks have either total occlusion or a high-grade, hemodynamically significant stenosis. In some clinical series, 85% of the potential sites within the celiac, superior mesentery, and inferior mesentery arteries were totally occluded or severely stenosed. Although diseased, the IMA frequently serves as the major source of intestinal blood supply.

Confidence is developing in the ability of the noninvasive vascular diagnostic laboratory to image the celiac and mesenteric blood vessels. Expeditious screening of patients with postprandial pain and weight loss may enable more timely diagnosis.

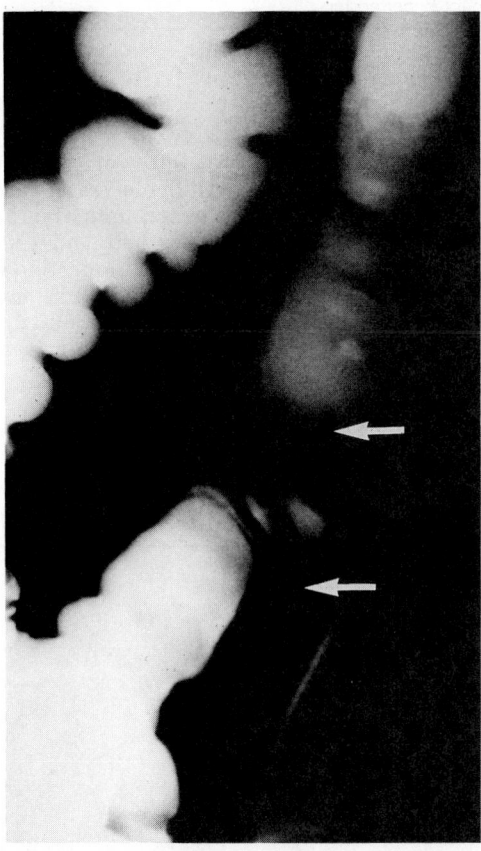

Figure 82-11. Stricture formation resulting from sigmoid colon ischemia after repair of a ruptured aortic aneurysm. There is loss of haustrations through the descending colon and the fixed narrowing in mid–sigmoid colon (*arrows*).

Table 82-3. MISCELLANEOUS CAUSES OF VISCERAL ARTERY OCCLUSION

MECHANICAL CAUSES

Aortic dissection
Blunt and penetrating trauma

COLLAGEN VASCULAR AND INFLAMMATORY VASCULOPATHY

Polyarteritis
Dermatomyositis
Rheumatoid arthritis
Sjögren syndrome
Henoch-Schönlein purpura
Essential mixed cryoglobulinemia
Wegener granulomatosis
Giant cell arteritis
Hepatitis B–associated antigens
Typhoid
Inflammatory bowel disease

LOCALIZED INJURY

Cholesterol embolization
Radiation
Enteric-coated potassium salts

SYSTEMIC VASCULOPATHY

Diabetes mellitus
Polycythemia vera
Köhlmeier-Degos syndrome

REACTIVE VASCULOPATHY

Estrogen–progesterone compounds
Pheochromocytoma
Carcinoid syndrome
Ergotism
Buerger disease
Associated with renal vascular hypertension or accelerated phase of
  malignant hypertension

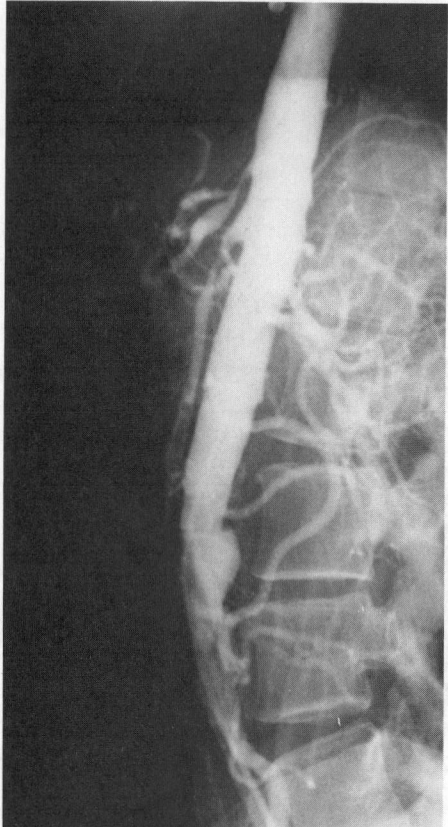

Figure 82-12. High-grade stenoses of the celiac and superior mesenteric arteries are apparent in this lateral aortogram. (Zelenock GB. Splanchnic arteriosclerotic disease and intestinal angina. Arch Surg 1980;115:497)

Elective but relatively urgent intestinal revascularization is standard therapy. Multiple-vessel revascularizations with short, antegrade conduits of either autogenous saphenous vein or prosthetic material are favored (Fig. 82-14). A variety of techniques, however, have resulted in long-term relief of symptoms and may be appropriate in some circumstances (Fig. 82-15). End-arterectomy through a trap-door aortotomy is appropriate after thoracoabdominal exposure (Figs. 82-16 and

Table 82-4. TECHNIQUES FOR ASSESSING INTESTINAL VIABILITY

COMMONLY USED

Clinical assessment
Intraoperative Doppler
Fluorescein dye or Wood lamp

INFREQUENTLY USED

Surface oximetry
Laser Doppler
Radiolabeled microspheres
Ultrasonography of intestinal wall
Intraluminal tonometry
Electronic contractility monitor (ECM)

SECOND-LOOK PROCEDURES

Surgery
Laparoscopy or peritoneoscopy

82-17) and is particularly effective when multiple proximal intestinal arterial stenoses or occlusions and concomitant renal artery lesions are present. In selective settings, a percutaneous angioplastic procedure may suffice, but long-term follow-up and collected series of patients treated in this fashion are lacking.

Mesenteric Venous Thrombosis

Mesenteric venous thrombosis is most often subacute in its presentation. A vague prodrome of crampy abdominal pain, abdominal distention, nausea, and malaise may occur over a few days to several weeks. Alternatively, in the presence of widespread and major vessel venous occlusions, the presentation may be more acute. Mesenteric venous thrombosis may be secondary to an underlying condition or may present without recognized cause. Associated conditions include intraabdominal inflammatory processes, peritonitis, portal hypertension, hypercoagulable states, and the use of oral contraceptives. Plain films reveal edema of the bowel wall. Computed tomographic scanning may demonstrate thrombus within the portal vein or the superior mesenteric vein. The venous phase of a selective mesenteric arteriogram may also reveal the thrombus. In most instances, however, the diagnosis is made intraoperatively. At exploration, a bloody ascites may be present. The intestine appears dusky and feels thick and rubbery. Arterial pulses are palpable in the mesentery. The small mesenteric veins feel cordlike and exude clot

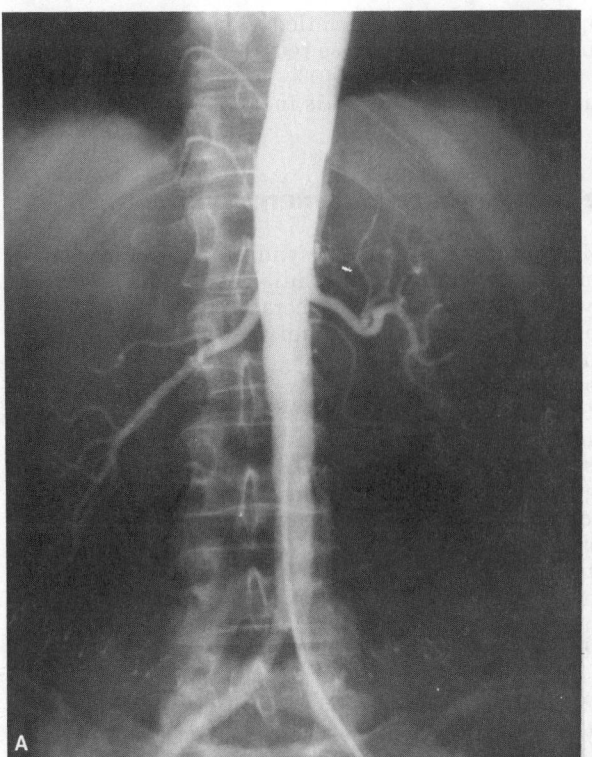
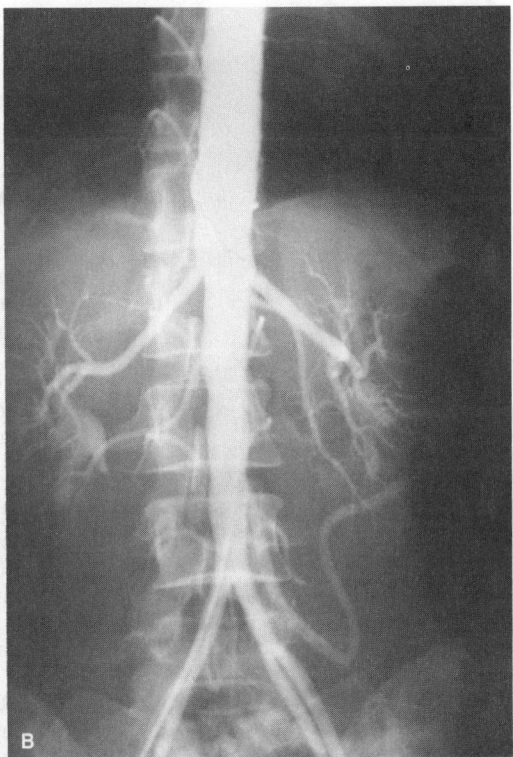
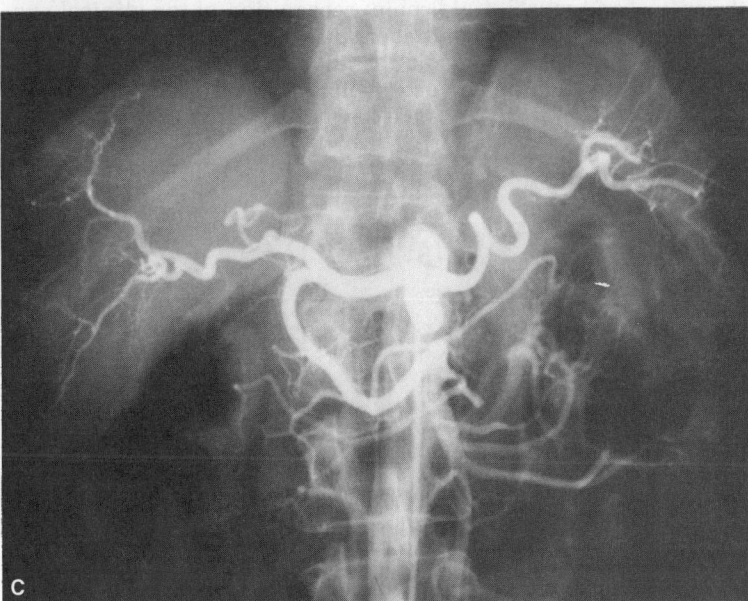

Figure 82-13. Chronic visceral ischemia producing visceral angina occurs in the presence of multiple occlusions of major splanchnic blood vessels. Lack of apparent intestinal blood flow (*A*) and an unusually prominent inferior mesenteric artery (*B*) are angiographic signs of chronic visceral ischemia. This selective celiac injection (*C*) also fills the superior mesenteric artery distribution secondary to proximal superior and inferior mesenteric artery occlusions.

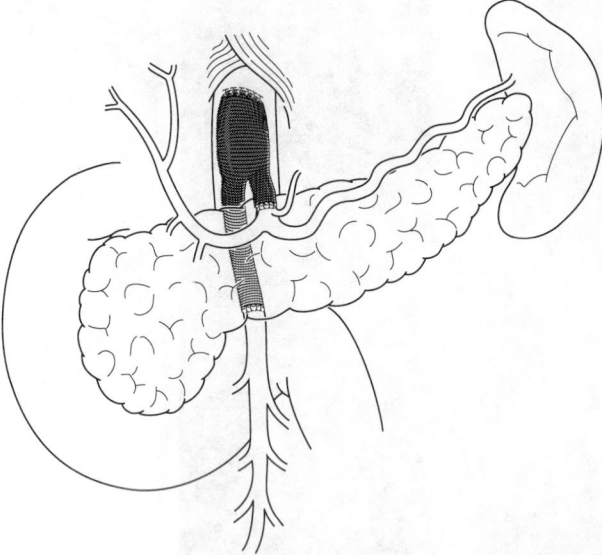

Figure 82-14. Bypass grafts to the visceral vessels may be originated from the supraceliac aorta. Short antegrade conduits and multiple-vessel revascularization are favored.

when cut. Surgical therapy consists of resection of nonviable intestine, occasional large-vessel venous thrombectomy, and the use of anticoagulants. Correcting any predisposing cause and investigating hypercoagulable states, such as antithrombin III and protein C and S deficiencies and the lupus anticoagulant, are always ap-

propriate. Postoperative anticoagulant therapy is continued indefinitely because recurrent venous thrombosis occurs in 30% to 40% of untreated patients; anticoagulation reduces this incidence to 3% to 5%.

Median Arcuate Ligament Syndrome

Median arcuate ligament syndrome is controversial. Symptoms include postprandial abdominal pain but may or may not represent visceral ischemia. An alternative pathophysiologic mechanism may represent irritation of neural tissue overlying the origin of the celiac artery. Patients typically present with abdominal pain, and in the course of their evaluation, arteriography demonstrates a significant compression of the celiac axis by the median arcuate ligament of the diaphragm (Fig. 82-18). Other visceral vessels seldom show involvement with an occlusive process. Lysis of the overlying median arcuate ligament and surrounding neural tissue affords relief of symptoms in many instances, provided alternative causes for the patients' symptoms have been thoroughly and exhaustively evaluated.

The acute and chronic visceral ischemic syndromes may be dramatic or pedestrian in presentation. Unattended, they are associated with substantial mortality and morbidity. Prompt recognition of the clinical syndromes, early and liberal use of diagnostic angiography, urgent or emergent operative intervention, vigorous resuscitation, and use of ancillary pharmacologic support offer the best chance for patient survival.

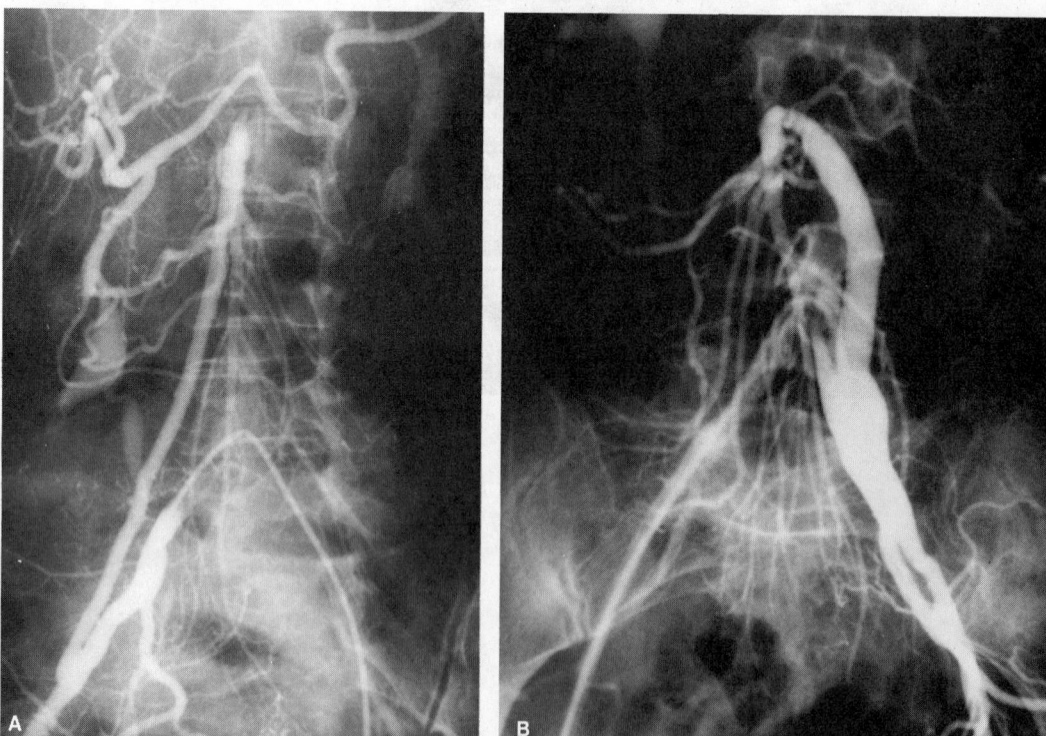

Figure 82-15. Retrograde conduits are an alternative bypass, and even single-vessel revascularization may provide effective long-term relief of symptoms in selected circumstances. (*A*) Retrograde right external *iliac* artery to superior mesenteric artery (SMA) vein graft. There is excellent filling throughout the distribution of the SMA and to the branches of the celiac artery by collateral flow through the gastroduodenal artery. (*B*) A left common iliac artery–SMA bypass.

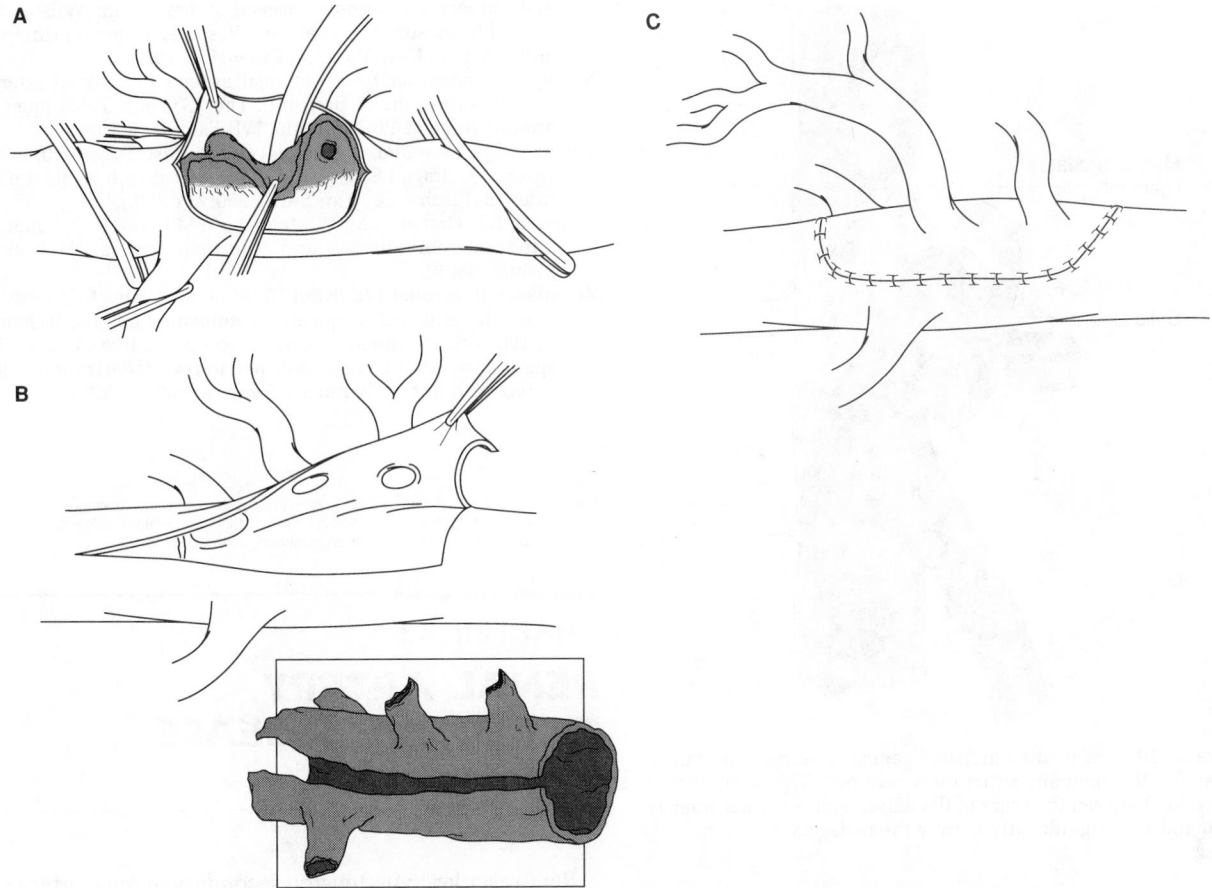

Figure 82-16. Endarterectomy of the celiac and superior mesenteric arteries is performed through a longitudinal trapdoor aortotomy. (After Wylie EJ. Manual of vascular surgery, vol 1. New York, Springer-Verlag, 1980)

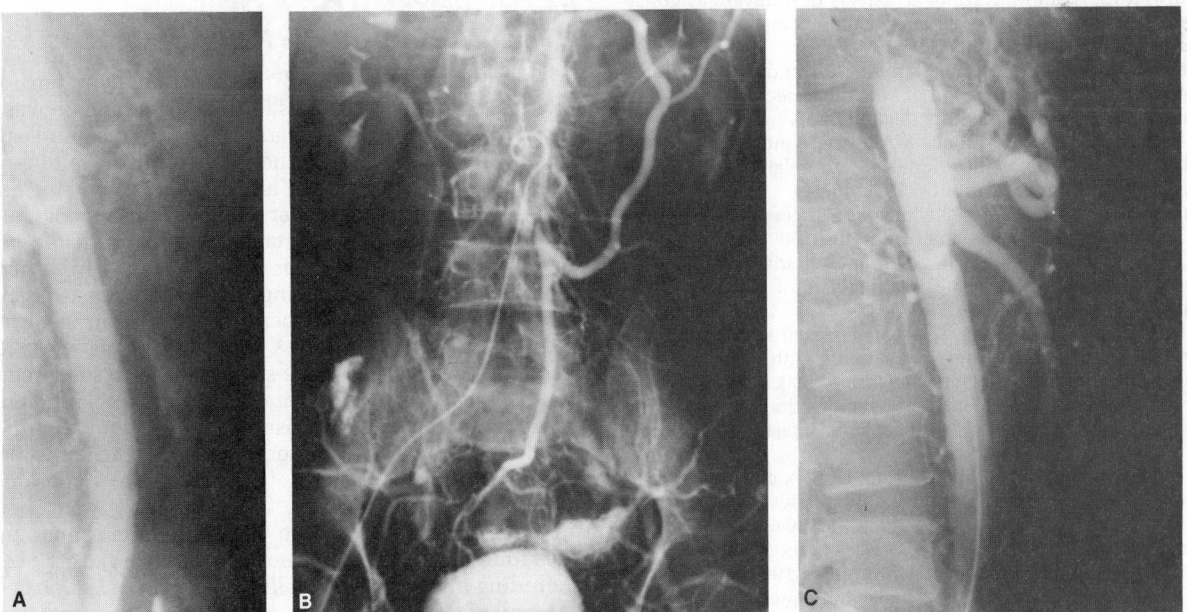

Figure 82-17. (A) Preoperative lateral aortogram demonstrating total occlusion of the celiac and superior mesenteric arteries. (B) Anteroposterior view with selective injection, demonstrating large inferior to superior mesenteric artery collateral flow. (C) Postoperative angiography demonstrates widely patent celiac and superior mesenteric arteries after transaortic endarterectomy.

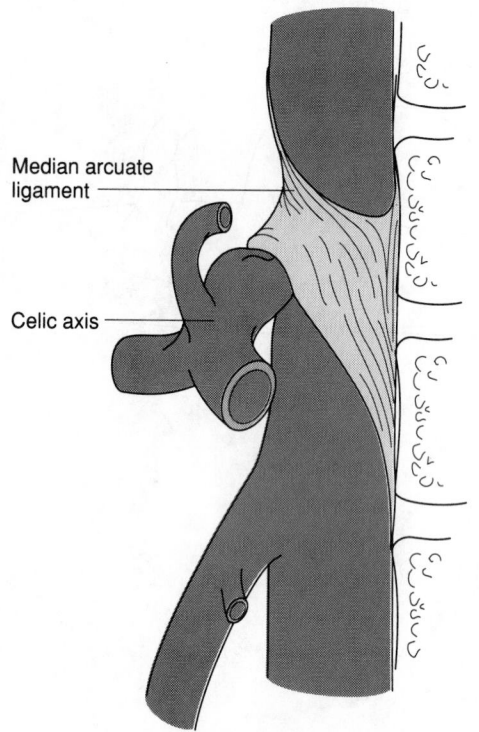

Median arcuate
ligament

Celic axis

Figure 82-18. The median arcuate ligament syndrome is controversial, but the anatomic structure is very real. This firm, fibrous connection between the crura of the diaphragm is extraordinarily strong and may significantly narrow the celiac axis.

BIBLIOGRAPHY

Boley SJ, Borden EB. Acute mesenteric vascular disease. In: Wilson SE, Veith FJ, Hobson RW, et al, eds. Vascular surgery: principles and practice. New York, McGraw-Hill, 1987.

Brolin RE, Semmlow JL, Sehonanda A, et al. Comparison of five methods of assessment of intestinal viability. Surg Gynecol Obstet 1989;168:6.

Cronenwett JL, Ayad M, Kazmer A. Effects of intravenous glucagon on the survival of rats after acute occlusive mesenteric ischemia. J Surg Res 1985;38:445.

Deitch EA. The role of intestinal barrier failure and bacterial translocation in the development of systemic infection and multiple organ failure. Arch Surg 1990;125:403.

Garcia JG, Rollan CM, Enrinquez MAR, et al. Improved survival in intestinal ischemia by allopurinol not related to xanthine-oxidase inhibition. J Surg Res 1990;48:144.

Landreneau RJ, Fry WJ. The right colon as a target organ of nonocclusive mesenteric ischemia. Arch Surg 1990;125:591.

Levy PJ, Krausz MM, Manny J. Acute mesenteric ischemia: improved results—a retrospective analysis of ninety-two patients. Surgery 1990;107:372.

Levy PJ, Krausz MM, Manny J. The role of second-look procedures in improving survival time for patients with mesenteric venous thrombosis. Surg Gynecol Obstet 1990;170:287.

Mesh CL, Gewertz BL. The effect of hemodilution on blood flow regulation in normal and postischemic intestine. J Surg Res 1990;48:183.

Moneta GL, Taylor DC, Helton WS, et al. Duplex ultrasound measurement of postprandial intestinal blood flow: effect of meal composition. Gastroenterology 1988;95:1294.

Oshima A, Kitajama M, Sakai N, et al. Does glucagon improve the viability of ischemic intestine? J Surg Res 1990;49:524.

Park PO, Haglund U, Bulkley GB, et al. The sequence of development of intestinal tissue injury after strangulation ischemia and reperfusion. Surgery 1990;107:574.

Reuter SR, Redman HC. Gastrointestinal angiography, ed 2. Philadelphia, WB Saunders, 1971.

Stoney RJ, Reilly LM, Ehrenfeld WK. Chronic mesenteric ischemia

and surgery for chronic visceral ischemia. In: Wilson SE, Veith FJ, Hobson RW, et al, eds. Vascular surgery: principles and practice. New York, McGraw-Hill, 1987.

Stoney RJ, Schneider PA. Technical aspects of visceral arterial revascularization. In: Bergan JJ, Yao, JST, eds. Techniques in arterial surgery. Philadelphia, WB Saunders, 1990.

Taylor LM Jr. Mesenteric ischemia. Semin Vasc Surg 1990;3:141.

Thompson JS, Bragg LE, West WW. Serum enzyme levels during intestinal ischemia. Ann Surg 1990;211:369.

Zelenock GB, Graham LM, Whitehouse WM Jr., et al. Splanchnic arteriosclerotic disease and intestinal angina. Arch Surg 1980;115:497.

Zelenock GB, Strodel WE, Knol JA, et al. A prospective study of clinically and endoscopically documented colonic ischemia in 100 patients undergoing aortic reconstructive surgery with aggressive colonic and direct pelvic revascularization, compared with historic controls. Surgery 1989;106:771.

SURGERY: SCIENTIFIC PRINCIPLES AND PRACTICE, Second Edition, edited by Lazar J. Greenfield, Michael W. Mulholland, Keith T. Oldham, Gerald B. Zelenock, and Keith D. Lillemoe. Lippincott–Raven Publishers, Philadelphia, © 1997.

CHAPTER 83

RENAL ARTERY OCCLUSIVE DISEASE

JAMES C. STANLEY

Renovascular hypertension secondary to renal artery occlusive disease is the most common form of surgically correctable hypertension. Systemic blood pressure elevations in these patients follow reductions in renal perfusion with activation of the renin–angiotensin system. Although this physiologic response tends to restore the renal circulation toward normal, it does so in a pathologic manner by producing hypertension in the systemic circulation.

PATHOPHYSIOLOGY OF RENOVASCULAR HYPERTENSION

The physiologic basis of renovascular hypertension is relatively well defined. This form of hypertension was first recognized more than 60 years ago by Goldblatt and associates,[1] who produced sustained hypertension in dogs after gradual reductions in renal artery blood flow using an externally controlled vascular clamp. Subsequent studies have discounted the importance of renal ischemia per se as the cause of renovascular hypertension, with other hemodynamic signals appearing essential in increasing renin release, the most obvious being a decrease in mean renal artery perfusion pressure. A stenosis causing an 80% reduction in renal artery cross-sectional area, a so-called critical stenosis, induces a pressure gradient sufficient to cause increased renin release from the kidney. Renin and its effects on angiotensin and aldosterone account for the elevated blood pressure of renovascular hypertension (Fig. 83-1).

Renin is produced by the juxtaglomerular apparatus of the kidney. This anatomic area consists of a variety of cells, including *myoepitheloid cells* or *granular cells,* located on the wall of the afferent arterioles; the *macula densa,* which is composed of specialized tubular epithelial cells in the glomerular hilus at the transition of the loop of Henle to the distal convoluted tubule; and *lacis cells,* located in the region of the efferent glomerular arteriole and the macula

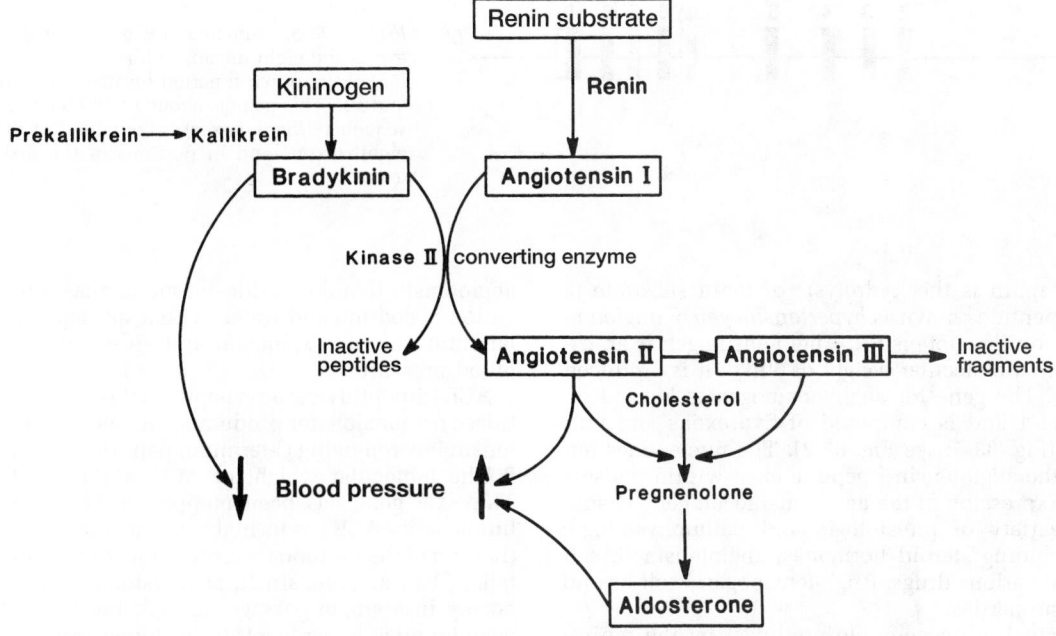

Figure 83-1. Renin–angiotenin system interrelation with aldosterone and bradykinin in regulation of blood pressure. (After Stanley JC, Graham LM, Whitehouse WM Jr. Renovascular hypertension. In: Miller TA, Rowland BJ, eds. Physiologic basis of modern surgical care. St Louis, CV Mosby, 1988:734)

densa. Lacis cells are intimately associated with the glomerulus and are anatomically similar to mesangial cells. The interrelations between the macula densa, glomerular arteriole vasomotion, and renal tubular function are important in understanding renin kinetics.

Regulation of renin production and its release from the kidney at the cellular and molecular level is complex.[2-4] Renal baroreceptors, acting as stretch receptors, affect the release of renin from juxtaglomerular cells. Activation of these receptors appears to involve the calcium ion, with increasing evidence that renin release and intracellular levels of calcium are inversely related. Alternatively, renin release can occur with changes in pressure at the afferent renal arteriole level as well as with changes in renal interstitial volume and pressure.

Renin is a proteolytic enzyme, active at a neutral pH on its only known substrate, angiotensinogen. The renin gene is located on chromosome 1[5] (Figs. 83-2 and 83-3). This gene is composed of nine exons and an additional miniexon, interrupted by eight introns.[6] Transcription of the renin gene to renin mRNA is followed by its translation into a preprorenin molecule with a molecular weight of 45 kd.[7] Subsequent cleavage and glycosylation of this molecule in the rough endoplasmic reticulum produces prorenin with a molecular weight of 47 kd. Prorenin is transferred into the Golgi complex, where it is secreted and processed to active renin. Renin is a single-chain polypeptide with a molecular weight of about 38 kd.[8] It is stored as granules within the juxtaglomerular cells and, in some instances, as granules within the arteriolar wall.

Renin has a half-life of 20 to 30 minutes. Under usual circumstances of normal sodium balance, the sum of renin activity measured in both renal veins is about 48% greater than that in the infrarenal vena cava or peripheral arterial and venous circulations.[9] The renin levels in the peripheral circulation appear to be in a steady state because of this relatively constant 48% contribution of renin from the kidneys. The liver is the primary site for removal and clearance of renin.[10] Extrarenal renin or renin-like en-

zymes (isorenins) exist in the submaxillary salivary gland, uterus, placenta, and brain, but there is no evidence that these substances are functionally important in elevating blood pressure.

The biochemistry of the renin–angiotensin system has been well defined (Fig. 83-4). The primary, if not sole,

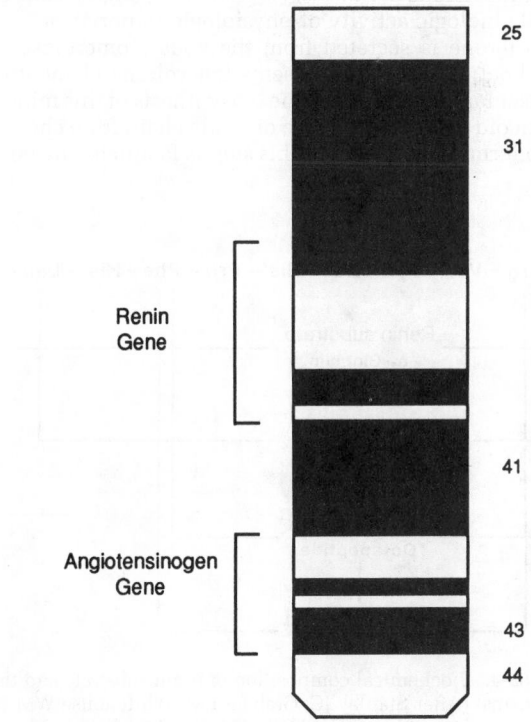

Figure 83-2 Chromosome 1 contains both the human renin and angiotensinogen genes.

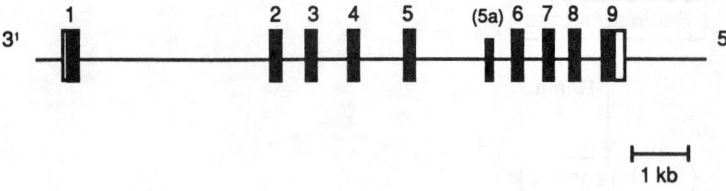

Figure 83-3. Human renin gene, consisting of nine exons and eight introns, with a 9–base pair miniexon (5a) of unknown function located between exons five and six. This gene is about 12.18 kb long. The coding sequence (*black boxes*) is contained in the second to eighth exons and in portions of the first and ninth exons.

function of renin is the hydrolysis of renin substrate (a circulating peptide known as *hypertensinogen* or *angiotensinogen*) to form angiotensin I. Angiotensinogen is an α_2-globulin with a molecular weight of 60 kd. It is produced in the liver. The gene for angiotensinogen is located on chromosome 1 and is composed of five exons and four introns[11,12] (Fig. 83-5; see Fig. 83-2). The nucleotides encoding for the angiotensin I peptide exist within the second exon. Expression of the angiotensinogen gene is subject to a variety of physiologic and pathophysiologic stimuli, including steroid hormones, angiotensin II, salt loading, and various drugs. Angiotensinogen itself has no vasoactive properties.

Angiotensin I, a decapeptide produced by the renin–renin substrate reaction, has little vasoactivity. It does exert an effect on the adrenal medulla, the sympathetic and central nervous systems, and the renal arterioles. Angiotensin II is formed when two C-terminal peptides are cleaved from angiotensin I by the carboxypeptidase, angiotensin-converting enzyme (ACE). Angiotensin II, an octapeptide, represents the vasoconstrictive element of renovascular hypertension. Although angiotensin II stimulates liver production of renin substrate, in normal subjects, it provides a continuous negative feedback on renal release of renin.[13] Angiotensin II has a half-life of about 4 minutes.[14] Angiotensin III, a heptapeptide, is produced with the aminopeptidase cleavage of angiotensin II to I-desaspartyl-angiotensin II. Angiotensin III is known to inhibit angiotensin II, but its most relevant effect is to increase aldosterone synthesis. Nevertheless, angiotensin III has little biologic activity of physiologic importance.

Aldosterone is secreted from the zona glomerulosa of the adrenal cortex and represents the volume element of renovascular hypertension. The biosynthesis of this mineralocorticoid includes cleavage of a side chain from cholesterol to form pregnenolone. This step is facilitated by both

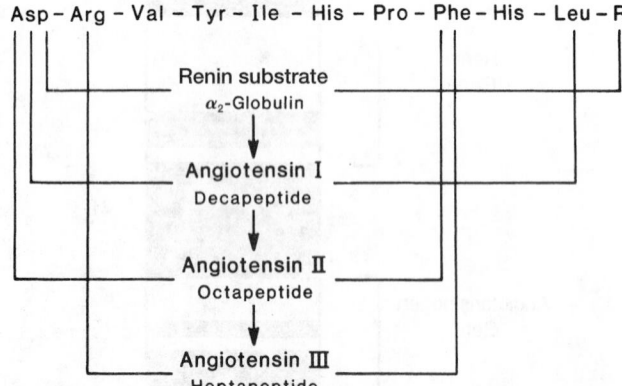

Figure 83-4. Biochemical composition of renin substrate and the angiotensins. (After Stanley JC, Graham LM, Whitehouse WM Jr. Renovascular hypertension. In: Miller TA, Rowland BJ, eds. Physiologic basis of modern surgical care. St Louis, CV Mosby, 1988:734)

angiotensin II and III. Aldosterone increases renal conservation of sodium and water, with a subsequent extracellular fluid volume expansion and an eventual increase in blood pressure.

ACE (dipeptidylcarboxypeptidase) is a zinc metallopeptidase responsible for producing angiotensin II from angiotensin I by removing C-terminal peptides from angiotensin I. The molecular weight of ACE is 150,000 to 180,000. The ACE gene has been mapped to chromosome 17 in humans.[15,16] ACE has its highest concentration in the endothelium of the pulmonary circulation. Conversion of angiotensin I to angiotensin II, at physiologic concentrations, occurs in a single passage through the lungs.[17] ACE has been found at lower levels in the blood and kidney as well as in other vascular beds. ACE is also important in the metabolism of the vasodepressor bradykinin. At least two enzymes appear to inactivate bradykinin. The first is kinase I, which acts by cleaving the carboxy-terminal arginine of bradykinin. The second, kinase II, acts by cleaving the carboxy-terminal dipeptide group, Phe-Arg. Kinase II and ACE appear to be the same in that they have nearly identical substrate specificities, cofactor requirements, and antigenic specificities.[18]

The most common means of determining plasma renin activity is the measurement of angiotensin I generation using a modified radioimmunoassay. Renin activity is expressed as the hourly amount of angiotensin I generated per volume of plasma assayed. The assay involves two phases: (1) an incubation of plasma to generate angiotensin I and (2) the actual radioimmunoassay of generated angiotensin I. Assay techniques vary among laboratories, often making interlaboratory comparisons difficult. Renin secretion is calculated as the renal arteriovenous difference in renin activity multiplied by renal plasma flow and is expressed as nanograms per milliliter per hour.

The actions of angiotensin on cardiac activity, vascular smooth muscle reactivity, and sodium and water metabolism contribute to increased arterial pressure (Fig. 83-6). The most important consequence of renal artery occlusive disease is the production of angiotensin II, which is one of the most potent pressor substances known. Angiotensin II acts directly on arteriolar smooth muscle of nearly all vascular beds; the splanchnic, renal, and cutaneous circulations are most sensitive to its effects. Despite an acceptance of the central importance of angiotensin in the generation of renovascular hypertension, the exact role of cellular or locally secreted renin and generated angiotensin in this clinical setting remains undetermined.

Hemodynamic responses to an activated renin–angiotensin system depend on the rate of alterations in renal blood flow as well as on whether one or both kidneys are affected. Acute reductions in renal blood flow result in rapid increases in plasma renin and blood pressure. In the case of unilateral renovascular disease with a normal opposite kidney, the hypertension is characterized by renin hypersecretion from the affected kidney and suppression of renin production in the contralateral kidney.[19,20] Sodium retention within the affected kidney is counterbalanced by continuous sodium excretion from the normal

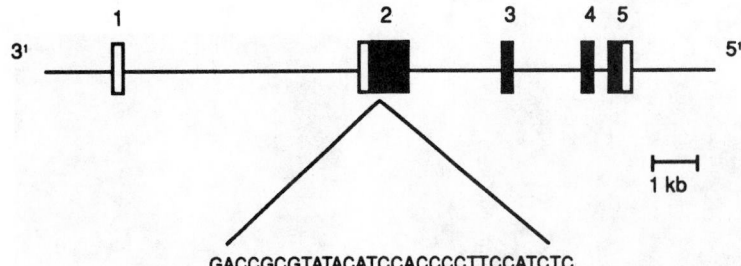

Figure 83-5. Human angiotensinogen gene, which consists of five exons and four introns. This gene is about 14.55 kb long. The coding sequence (*black boxes*) for angiotensinogen is contained in the second to fifth exon. The second exon contains the coding sequence for angiotensin I.

contralateral kidney, resulting in relative intravascular volume depletion. This vasoconstrictive form of hypertension is angiotensin II dependent and responds to ACE inhibitors.

Pathophysiologic alterations in the case of bilateral renovascular disease, or unilateral disease of a solitary kidney, relate to changes other than vasoconstriction. Angiotensin II causes sodium retention, diminutions in glomerular filtration, stimulation of aldosterone production, and stimulation of norepinephrine release from the adrenergic nervous system. In chronic bilateral or unilateral renovascular hypertension in patients with only one kidney, sodium retention accounts for late reductions in renin secretion, although it is possible that absolute renin activity is abnormally high with regard to the existing sodium balance. Blood pressure elevations do not appear as dependent on the renin–angiotensin system in sodium-replete chronic renovascular hypertension. In this setting, ACE inhibitors are more effective in reducing elevated blood pressures with sodium depletion.[21]

PATHOLOGY OF RENAL ARTERY OCCLUSIVE DISEASE

Different macrovascular occlusive diseases affect the renal arterial circulation, the most common being arteriosclerosis and arterial fibrodysplasia.[22] Developmental renal artery narrowings are a rare cause of renovascular hypertension. Although uncommon, renal artery emboli, spontaneous dissections, and traumatic occlusions are occasionally associated with acute renin-mediated hypertension.

Arteriosclerosis

Arteriosclerotic renal artery occlusive disease accounts for about 95% of reported cases of renovascular hypertension (Fig. 83-7). This type of renovascular hypertension may be even more common because most reported experiences are surgical series that exclude many older patients who are not operative candidates. Arteriosclerotic renovascular disease most commonly presents during the sixth decade of life. Men are affected twice as often as women. Although some degree of arteriosclerotic renal artery stenotic disease affects nearly half of the elderly population, it is not always associated with elevated blood pressures. Many of these patients exhibit occlusive disease of the coronary, cerebral, mesenteric, or extremity circulation.[23–26] This is particularly the case in black patients, who exhibit more severe extrarenal arteriosclerotic vascular disease.[27]

Arteriosclerotic renal artery occlusive disease characteristically affects the proximal third of the vessel in the form of eccentric or concentric stenoses. In nearly 80% of cases, these lesions occur as spillover of diffuse aortic atherosclerosis. Arteriosclerotic renal artery lesions are bilateral in

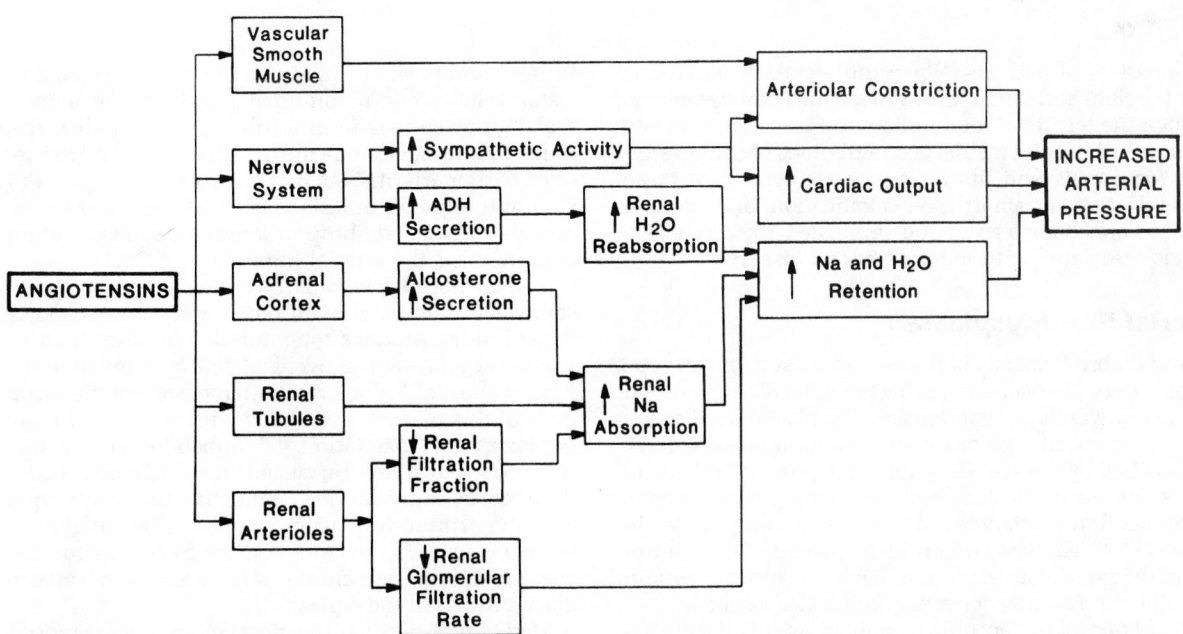

Figure 83-6. Effects of angiotensins contributing to increased arterial pressure. (After Stanley JC, Graham LM, Whitehouse WM Jr. Renovascular hypertension. In: Miller TA, Rowland BJ, eds. Physiologic basis of modern surgical care. St Louis, CV Mosby, 1988:734)

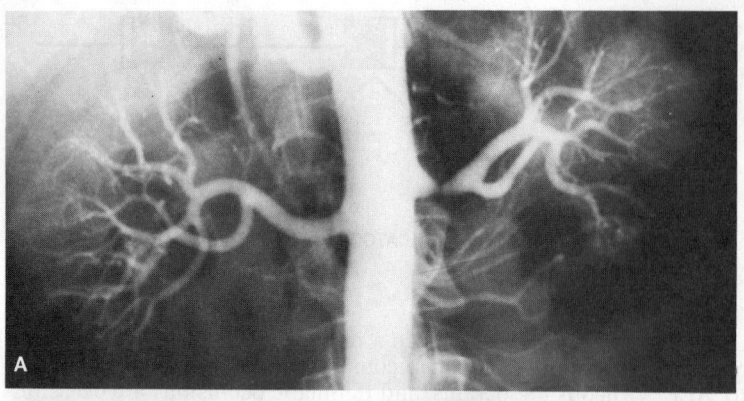
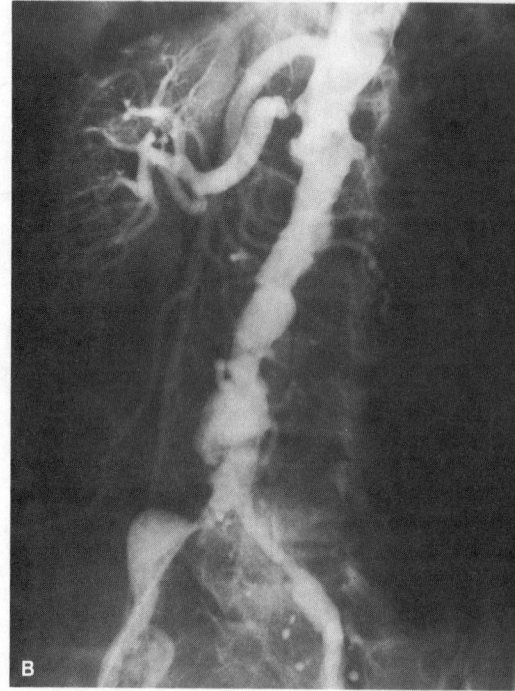
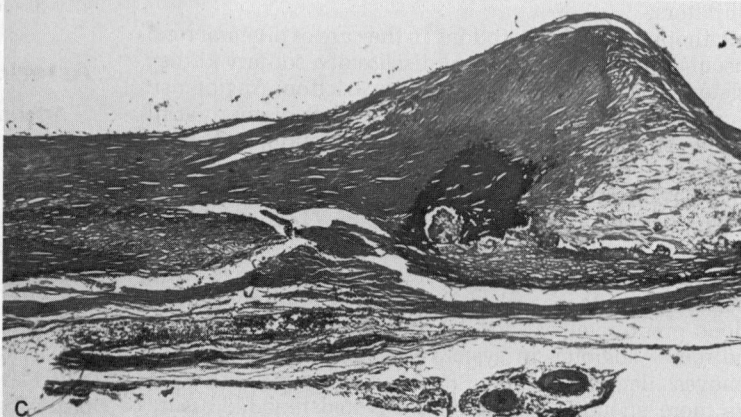

Figure 83-7. Renal artery arteriosclerosis. (*A*) Intrinsic focal lesion of proximal renal artery. (*B*) Severe aortic spill-over disease affecting renal artery orifice and entire abdominal aorta. (*C*) Complicated renal artery plaque exhibiting collections of cholesterol, extensive fibrosis, and calcification (hematoxin–eosin, ×60). (*A* and *C* from Stanley JC. Morphologic, histopathologic and clinical characteristics of renovascular fibrodysplasia and arteriosclerosis. In: Bergan JJ, Yao JST, eds. Surgery of the aorta and its body branches. New York, Grune & Stratton, 1979:355; *B* from Stanley JC, Graham LM, Whitehouse WM Jr. Renovascular hypertension. In: Miller TA, Rowland BJ, eds. Physiologic basis of modern surgical care. St Louis, CV Mosby, 1988:734)

three-quarters of patients. When unilateral, these lesions affect the right and left renal arteries with equal frequency, although the left renal artery often appears more severely diseased. Intimal and medial accumulations of cholesterol-laden foam cells and fibrous tissue are typical of these lesions. Necrosis, hemorrhage, calcification, and luminal thrombus are characteristic of complicated atherosclerotic plaques associated with more advanced disease.

Arterial Fibrodysplasia

Arterial fibrodysplasia is the second most common type of renal artery disease, accounting for about 5% of reported cases of renovascular hypertension. Dysplastic renal artery stenoses represent a heterogenous group of lesions. They are classified by the specific pathologic process and vessel wall region most affected. Included among these lesions are intimal fibroplasia, medial fibroplasia, and perimedial dysplasia.[28,29] The last two entities appear to be a continuum of the same disease process. Each category has certain characteristic features deserving individual comment.

Intimal fibroplasia accounts for about 5% of all dysplastic renal artery stenoses[29] (Fig. 83-8). These lesions occur in children and young adults more often than the elderly, and they affect both genders equally. The cause of primary

intimal fibroplasia is unknown but may be related to persistent embryonic myointimal cushions. Secondary intimal fibroplasia has been attributed to flow disturbances, blunt abdominal trauma during childhood, and the sequela of an earlier arteritis, such as occurs with rubella. Progression of intimal fibroplasia may cause turbulent blood flow and an accelerated fibroproliferative response that rapidly compromises the arterial lumen.

Intimal fibroplasia usually presents as a smooth, focal stenosis of the distal main renal artery. In some patients, these lesions produce long, tubular stenoses, and in rare cases, they present as webs affecting segmental arteries. Proximal ostial lesions most often represent the secondary form of this disease, associated with abdominal aortic hypoplasia and coarctation.[30,31] Subendothelial accumulations of irregularly arranged mesenchymal cells surrounded by loose fibrous connective tissue are typical of all intimal fibrodysplastic lesions.[28] The internal elastic lamina is usually intact, but partial fragmentation may occur. Medial and adventitial structures are normal in primary intimal fibrodysplasia.

Medial fibroplasia is the most commonly diagnosed dysplastic renal artery disease, accounting for 85% of these lesions[29] (Fig. 83-9). Medial fibroplasia is invariably found in women, with encounters in men being anecdotal. The

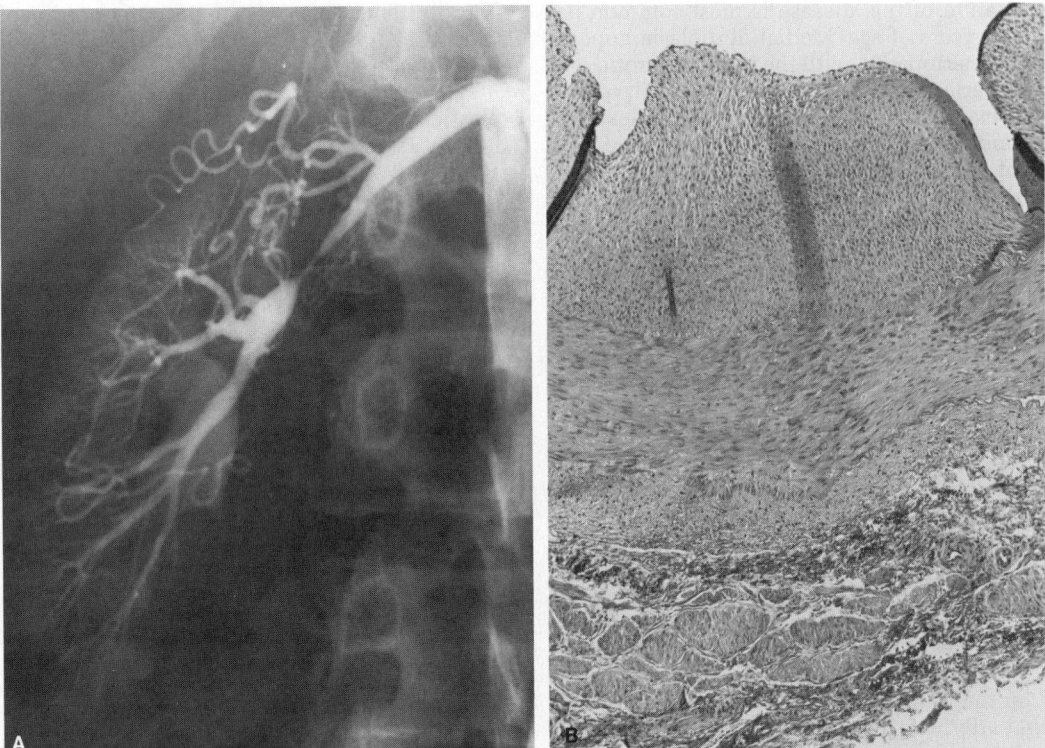

Figure 83-8. Intimal fibroplasia. (*A*) Focal stenosis of main renal artery mid-portion. (*B*) Subendo-thelial mesenchymal cells within a loose fibrous connective tissue matrix are noted above an intact internal elastic lamina, normal media, and normal adventitial tissues (hematoxin–eosin, ×120). (*A* from Stanley JC, Fry WJ. Renovascular hypertension secondary to arterial fibrodysplasia in adults: criteria for operation and results of surgical therapy. Arch Surg 1975;110:922; *B* from Stanley JC. Morphologic, histopathologic and clinical characteristics of renovascular fibrodysplasia and arteriosclerosis. In: Bergan JJ, Yao JST, eds. Surgery of the aorta and its body branches. New York, Grune & Stratton, 1979:355)

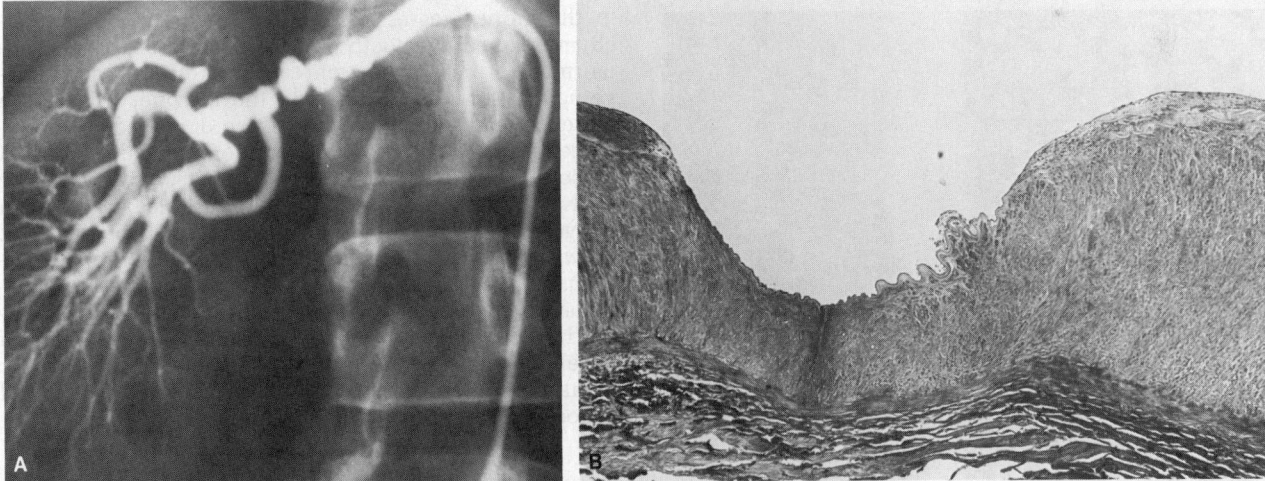

Figure 83-9. Medial fibroplasia. (*A*) Serial stenoses alternating with mural aneurysms, producing a string-of-beads appearance in the mid-portion and distal main renal artery. (*B*) Diffuse form of medial fibroplasia exhibiting regions of excess fibroproliferation with intervening area of medial thinning (Masson stain, ×60, longitudinal section). (Stanley JC. Morphologic, histopathologic and clinical characteristics of renovascular fibrodysplasia and arteriosclerosis. In: Bergan JJ, Yao JST, eds. Surgery of the aorta and its body branches. New York, Grune & Stratton, 1979:355)

clinical presentation of this disease is most common between 25 and 45 years of age. Medial fibroplasia appears to be a systemic arteriopathy, with the internal carotid and external iliac arteries representing the extrarenal vessels most often affected. The cause of medial fibroplasia remains poorly understood but appears to be associated with modification of smooth muscle to myofibroblasts due to estrogenic stimuli during the reproductive years, unusual traction forces on affected vessels, and mural ischemia from impairment of vasa vasorum blood flow.[28] The physical forces contributing to medial fibroplasia may be attributed to ptotic kidneys with stretching of the renal arteries (Fig. 83-10). The fact that renal ptosis occurs more often in women than in men may explain the almost unique involvement of the renal artery with medial fibroplasia in women.

Morphologic appearances of medial dysplasia range from solitary stenoses to multiple constrictions with intervening mural dilations affecting the middle and distal main renal artery. The latter are responsible for this lesion's classic string-of-beads appearance. Actual macrovascular aneurysms occurring at branchings affect nearly 13% of patients with arterial fibrodysplasia,[32] but these are an unusual cause of a hypertensive state.[33] Stenotic disease of segmental branches occurs in about 25% of cases. Bilateral disease affects nearly 60% of patients and is usually most severe on the right. Unilateral lesions affect the left and right renal arteries in 10% and 30% of cases, respectively. Progression of disease occurs in about 20% of patients and is most evident among premenopausal women.

Gradations in medial fibroplasia exist, including diffuse and peripheral forms of the disease in the same vessel.[28] Diffuse medial fibroplasia is typified by severe disorganization of medial smooth muscle cells, which appear to be transformed to myofibroblasts.[34] These latter secretory cells generate accumulations of ground substances that encroach on the vessel lumen. These stenoses often alternate with areas of medial thinning and mural dilations. Peripheral medial fibroplasia is typified by a limitation of the fibroproliferative process to the outer portion of the media, causing stenoses less severe than those occurring with diffuse disease.

Perimedial dysplasia accounts for nearly 10% of dysplastic renal artery stenotic disease[29] (Fig. 83-11). These lesions invariably occur in women, usually between the ages of 30 and 50 years. Perimedial dysplasia is bilateral in 20% of patients and appears to be more progressive than medial fibrodysplasia. Perimedial dysplasia is characterized by solitary or multiple constrictions, without intervening dilations. Most stenoses involve the distal main renal artery, without segmental branch involvement. Certain histologic features are common to both perimedial dysplasia and medial fibroplasia, and they may represent different manifestations of the same pathologic entity. Although unusual accumulations of elastic tissue in inner adventitial regions is the most prominent abnormality in perimedial dysplasia, increases in medial ground substances may also accompany this type of dysplastic disease.[28]

Developmental Renal Artery Disease

Developmental renal artery stenoses are a rare cause of renovascular hypertension[29–31] (Fig. 83-12). These lesions are encountered most often in children and young adults. About 40% of children with renovascular hypertension are thought to have developmental renal artery stenoses.[35,36] Similarly, nearly 20% of adults with intimal fibroplastic renal artery disease have stenoses that can be attributed to developmental defects. Both genders are affected equally. These stenotic lesions represent true hypoplasia of the renal artery, exhibiting an external hourglass appearance. Developmental lesions usually occur at the aortic origin of the artery. Sparse medial tissue, intimal fibroplasia, fragmentation and duplication of the internal elastic lamina, and disproportionate excesses in adventitial elastic tissue are the most common histologic abnormalities in these diminutive vessels.[29,31]

Developmental renal artery narrowings may be attributed to certain embryonic events occurring as the two fetal dorsal aortas fuse and all but one of their lateral branches to the kidney regress.[30] Abnormal transition of mesenchyme to medial smooth muscle at that time, or later impairment of its growth, can cause both aortic and renovascular anomalies. Vessels to the mesonephros within mesenchymal tissue around the two dorsal aortas are replaced during fetal growth by a more cephalic group of vessels to the metanephros. A solitary artery to each kidney evolves from these arteries in 75% of people because of an obligate hemodynamic advantage over adjacent channels. Flow changes in the region where single central renal arteries usually arise may afford coexisting polar arteries hemodynamic advantages that ensure their persistence. Supporting such a hypothesis concerning the cause of developmental lesions is the fact that multiple stenotic renal arteries exist in up to 70% of patients with central abdominal aortic coarctation or hypoplasia.[30,31]

CLINICAL FEATURES OF RENOVASCULAR HYPERTENSION

The frequency of renovascular hypertension among patients who have diastolic blood pressures higher than 100 mmHg is about 2%. It is much more common in patients with more severe diastolic blood pressure elevations; as many as 5% of such patients are found to have a renovascular cause of their hypertension.

Findings suggestive of renovascular hypertension in-

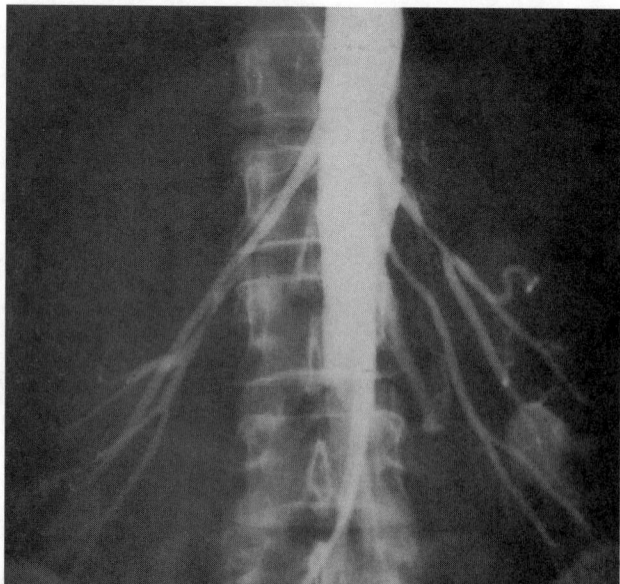

Figure 83-10. Medial fibrodysplasia manifest as irregular narrowings to ptotic kidneys affecting the mid-portion of the main renal artries, which appear stretched during upright aortography. (Stanley JC, Wakefield TW. Arterial fibrodysplasia. In: Rutherford RB, ed. Vascular surgery, Philadelphia, WB Saunders, 1995:264)

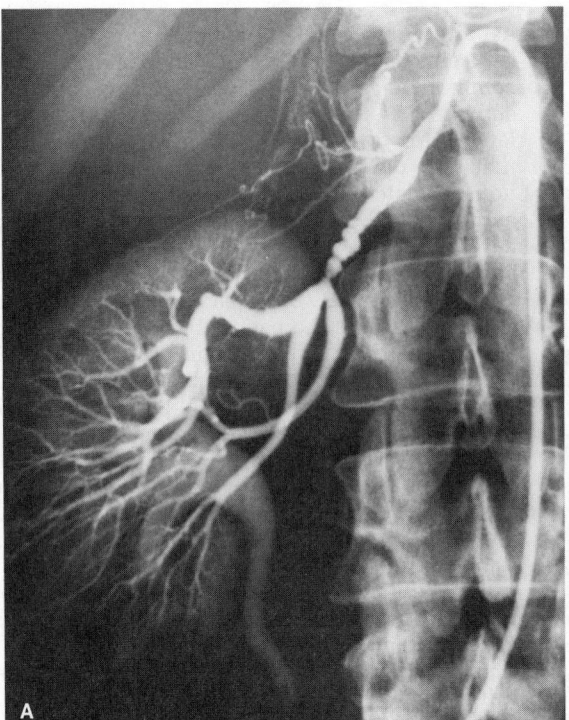
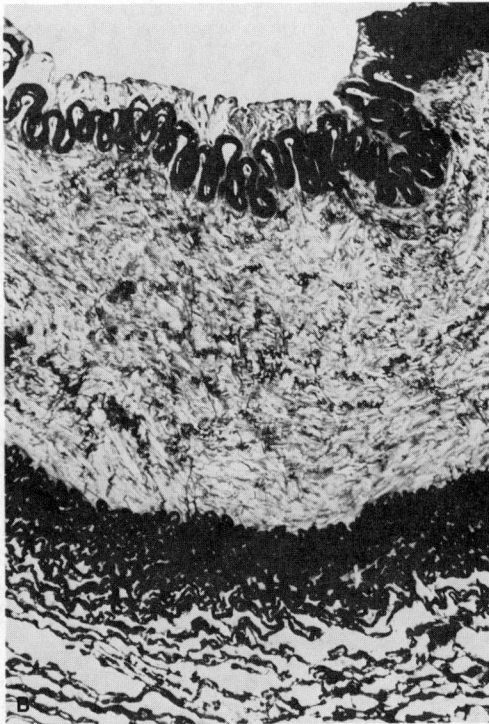

Figure 83-11. Perimedial dysplasia. (*A*) Multiple stenoses without mural aneurysms in the midportion of the renal artery are characteristic of these lesions. (*B*) These lesions are due to excessive accumulations of elastic tissue at medial–adventitial junction (Verhoeff stain, ×120). (Stanley JC. Morphologic, histopathologic and clinical characteristics of renovascular fibrodysplasia and arteriosclerosis. In: Bergan JJ, Yao JST, eds. Surgery of the aorta and its body branches. New York, Grune & Stratton, 1979:355)

clude systolic and diastolic upper abdominal bruits; initial diastolic blood pressures greater than 115 mmHg; a sudden worsening of mild to moderate essential hypertension; development of hypertension during childhood; or rapid onset of high blood pressure after the age of 50 years. Hypertension resistant to drug therapy and malignant hypertension are also more likely to be associated with this form of secondary hypertension. Similarly, patients who exhibit deterioration in renal function while receiving multiple antihypertensive drugs, especially ACE inhibitors, may have underlying renal artery stenotic disease. The costs and errors incumbent to indiscriminate evaluations for this form of hypertension are prohibitive.[37] A decision algorithm based on the presenting degree of hypertension and presence or absence of clinical and laboratory evidence of renovascular hypertension is necessary for contemporary practice (Fig. 83-13).

DIAGNOSIS OF RENAL ARTERY STENOSIS AND SECONDARY HYPERTENSION

Most diagnostic and prognostic tests for renovascular hypertension assess either the anatomic stenosis or derangements of renal function attributed to the stenosis. The usefulness and limitations of these tests become relevant in the proper selection of patients for surgical intervention.[37]

Conventional arteriography is central to the evaluation of patients in whom renovascular hypertension is suspected. Oblique aortography and multiple-plane selective renal arteriography have improved the recognition of the morphologic character and extent of renal artery stenoses in this disease entity. Collateral vessels circumventing a

renal artery stenosis are evidence of the lesion's hemodynamic importance. A pressure gradient of about 10 mmHg is necessary for collateral vessel development, and the same degree of pressure change is associated with activation of the renin system. Thus, the functional importance of an otherwise benign-appearing stenosis is established when collateral vessels are evident (Fig. 83-14). Intraarterial digital substraction angiography is a useful modification of conventional studies in assessing the presence of renal artery stenotic disease. The latter allows use of smaller quantities of contrast agents compared with conventional arteriography or intravenous digital substraction arteriography, and it lessens the potential of contrast-induced nephrotoxicity. This is of particular relevance in patients with compromised renal function.

Magnetic resonance angiography, especially with gadolinium enhancement, has the potential to provide high-resolution images of diseased renal arteries.[38-40] Further refinements in magnetic resonance angiography will undoubtedly evolve before it becomes widely used in assessing patients suspected of renovascular hypertension. Its noninvasiveness and lack of nephrotoxicity make it an attractive diagnostic test.

Deep abdominal renal artery ultrasonography may identify hemodynamically significant renal artery narrowings by directly imaging the renal arteries and characterizing flow velocity patterns through these vessels.[41,42] Existence of a stenosis appears established when peak systolic velocities are in the range of 180 to 200 cm/s and the ratio of these velocities to those in the aorta approaches 3.5. Unfortunately, ultrasonography does not discriminate among renal artery stenoses exceeding 60% cross-sectional narrowing. Failure to identify a main renal artery in the

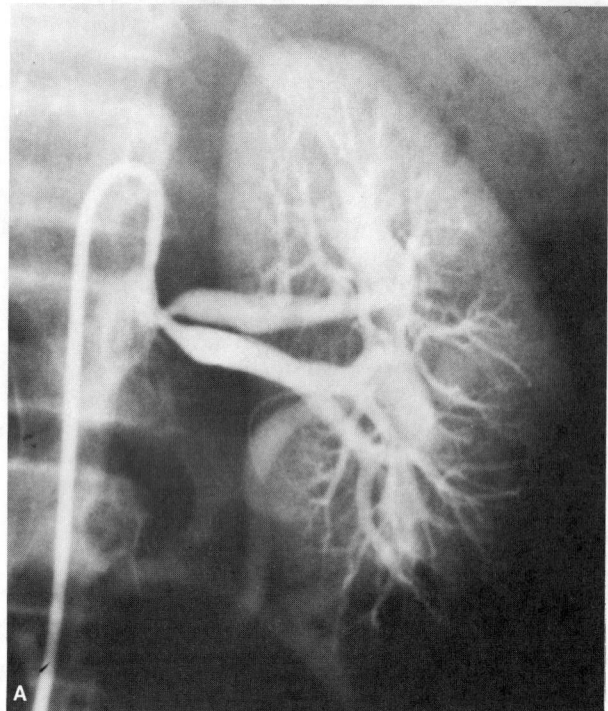

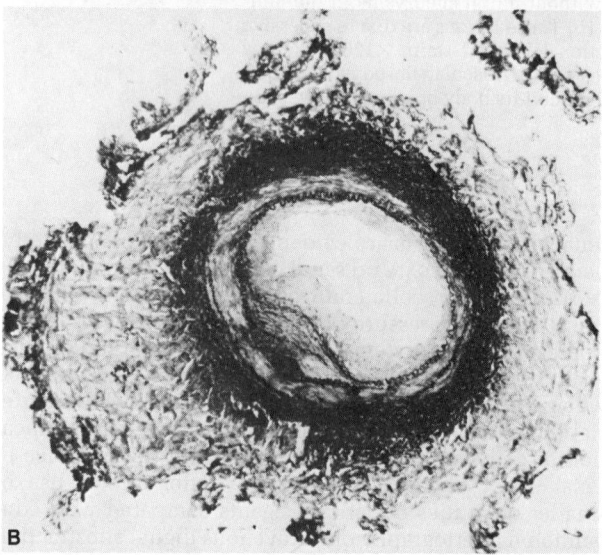

Figure 83-12. Developmental renal artery stenoses. (*A*) Proximal vessel stenosis in a patient with neurofibromatosis and infrarenal aortic hypoplasia. (*B*) Fragmentation and duplication of the internal elastic lamina and deficient medial tissues characterize these lesions. Intimal fibroplasia encroaches on the vessel lumen, which is less than 1 mm in diameter. Adventitial elastic tissues appear excessive (Movat stain, ×100). (*A* from Stanley JC, Fry WJ. Pediatric renal artery occlusive disease and renovascular hypertension: etiology, diagnosis, and operative treatment. Developmental occlusive disease of the abdominal aorta and the splanchnic and renal arteries. Arch Surg 1981;116:669; *B* from Stanley JC, Graham LM, Whitehouse WM Jr, et al. Developmental occlusive disease of the abdominal aorta and the splanchnic and renal arteries. Am J Surg 1981;142:190)

absence of any parenchymal flow signal suggests main renal artery occlusion. An occluded accessory or segmental renal artery, however, may not be recognized and, thus, contributes to this technology's false-negative assessments.

Renin activity of peripheral and renal venous blood is a recognized means of detecting functionally important re-

nal artery disease. Peripheral blood renin assays may not be useful unless they are related to sodium balance. More common practice involves assessments of renal vein renin activity. The renin–angiotensin system should be stimulated before sampling to reduce interpretive errors of data that may otherwise result from minimal fluctuations in nonstimulated basal renin activity. In most adults, this is accomplished by limiting sodium intake to 20 mEq/d and administering a diuretic for 3 days before testing. Renin-suppressing drugs, such as β-blockers, are discontinued whenever possible. Blood samples for renin assays should be obtained with the patient tilted to an upright position. The role of ACE inhibitors in stimulating renin release and improving test results remains to be further defined in patients with renovascular hypertension. Renin activity is usually reported as either a ratio or index.

The *renal vein renin ratio* (RVRR) is calculated by dividing the renin activity in venous blood from the affected kidney by that from the contralateral kidney. A RVRR of greater than 1.48 is indicative of functionally important renovascular stenotic disease.[19,20] Because this test compares one kidney to another, it may not be useful in patients with bilateral disease if both kidneys exhibit elevated but equal degrees of abnormally high renin secretion. This is believed to be the case in the 15% of patients benefiting from operation in whom the RVRR is less than 1.48 (Fig. 83-15).

The *renal:systemic renin index* (RSRI) is calculated by subtracting systemic renin activity from individual renal vein renin activity and dividing the remainder by systemic renin activity.[19] It is an expression of individual kidney renin release. In nonrenovascular essential hypertensive patients, renal vein renin activity from each kidney is usually 24% higher than systemic activity.[9] Thus, the total of both kidneys' activity is usually 48% higher than systemic activity. This figure of 48% represents a steady state of renal renin release.

In renovascular hypertension, the RSRI of the affected kidney is greater than 0.24. In mild degrees of renal artery disease, an increase in ipsilateral renin release is normally balanced by suppression of the contralateral kidney renin production, with a drop in its RSRI to less than 0.24. Bilateral renal artery disease may cause this servomechanism to be lost, and the autonomous release of renin from both kidneys may cause the sum of the individual RSRIs to be considerably greater than 0.48. Renin production then exceeds the capacity of normal hepatic degradation, and a hyperreninemic form of hypertension evolves.

The usefulness of ischemic kidney renin hypersecretion (RSRI more than 0.48) and contralateral kidney renin suppression (RSRI less than 0.24, approaching 0.0) as a means of discriminating between expected cured and improved operative outcomes has been well established[19,20,43] (Fig. 83-16). The prognostic accuracy of RSRI appears limited in that nearly 8% of patients who are cured do not exhibit contralateral renin suppression.[43] Renin secretion from the nonoperated kidney must be suppressed if a cure is to be expected. Although the RSRI represents an important refinement in the use of renin data in managing renovascular hypertensive patients, these data must be applied cautiously to clinical decision making.

Hypertensive urography is not a good diagnostic test for renovascular hypertension because of its limited sensitivity.[44] Bilateral or segmental disease often interferes with the recognition of gross differences in contrast excretion between the two kidneys. Nevertheless, rapid-sequence urography may contribute to a diagnosis of renovascular hypertension in the following circumstances: (1) there is at least a 1-minute delay in contrast appearance within the

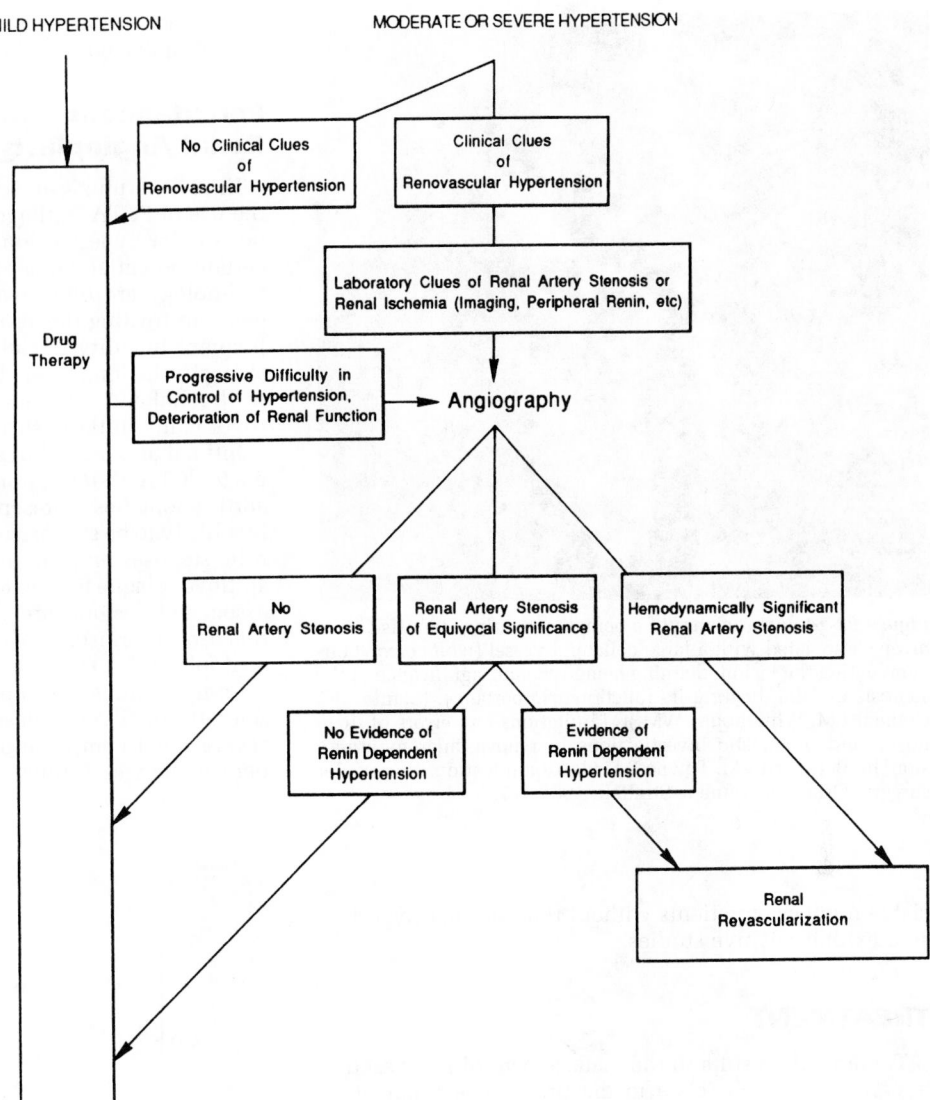

Figure 83-13. Management algorithm for renovascular hypertension. (After Stanley JC. Renal artery stenosis and hypertension. In: Brewster DC, ed. Common problems in vascular surgery. Chicago, Year Book, 1989:187)

collecting system of the affected kidney compared with that of the contralateral kidney; (2) a discrepancy in renal length exists, with the right kidney being 2 cm shorter than the left or the left being 1.5 cm shorter than the right; and (3) there is hyperconcentration of contrast in the collecting system of the affected kidney evident on late radiographs. Ureteral or pelvic irregularities owing to the presence of large collateral vessels may accompany the aforementioned urographic findings. In a large series of patients with proven renovascular hypertension, urograms were abnormal in 27% of children, 48% of adults with arterial fibrodysplastic disease, and about 72% of adults with atherosclerotic lesions.[45] Thus, continued use of hypertensive urography as a diagnostic or prognostic test for renovascular hypertension appears unjustified.

Isotopic renography allows both renal imaging and analysis of the washout curve of a number of radioactive tracers. The most common compounds used for these studies include ^{99m}Tc-DTPA, ^{123}I- or ^{131}I-orthoidohippurate, ^{99m}Tc-MAG$_3$, ^{99m}Tc-DMSA, and ^{99m}glucoheptonate. These studies provide an assessment of renal blood flow as well as excretory function. Unfortunately, different states of hydration and intrarenal vascular resistance often contribute to flow abnormalities and false-positive studies in nonrenovascular hypertensives. The specificity and sensitivity of these studies are both about 75%. Administration of ACE inhibitors improves the sensitivity and specificity by blocking the compensatory change in glomerular filtration, causing it to fall in the affected kidney. The widespread use of this modified technology has not occurred, although some view ACE inhibitor-modified studies to be of greater value.[46] Renal perfusion/excretion ratios and more sophisticated computer analyses offer a potential means of increasing the predictive value of radionuclide screening for renovascular hypertension.

Split renal function studies were among the earliest tests used in evaluating patients with suspected renovascular hypertension.[47] These studies necessitate ureteral catheter placement for sampling of urine from each kidney. The two studies used most widely are: (1) the Howard test, which documents reduced urine volume as well as increased sodium and creatinine concentration from the affected kidney; and (2) the Stamey test, which reveals a smaller volume of urine and a greater concentration of paraaminohippurate from the affected kidney. A liberalization of diagnostic criteria for split renal function studies has been proposed, with a constant lateralization to the affected kidney, evident by 25% less urine volume and a 15% increase in creatinine concentration. The diagnostic sensitivity using these criteria is improved, but an appre-

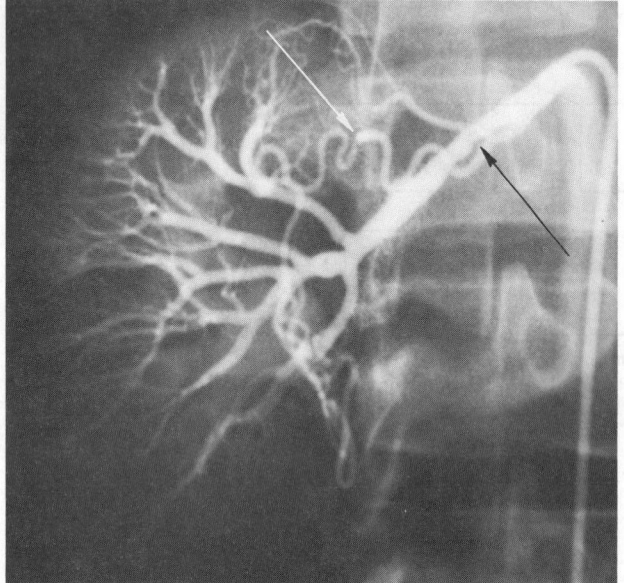

Figure 83-14. Arteriogram of a benign-appearing stenosis (*black arrow*) associated with a large collateral vessel (*white arrow*) circumventing the lesion, defining hemodynamic significance of the stenosis and implicating its functional importance. (Stanley JC, Graham LM, Whitehouse WM Jr. Limitations and errors of diagnostic and prognostic investigations in renovascular hypertension. In: Bernhard VM, Towne JM, eds. Complications in vascular surgery. Orlando, Grune & Stratton, 1984:213)

ciable number of patients without renovascular hypertension exhibit positive studies.

TREATMENT

Therapeutic results in the management of renovascular hypertension often relate to the proper execution of an appropriate intervention. Treatment options include drug therapy, percutaneous transluminal angioplasty (PCTA), transcatheter renal infarction, a vascular reconstructive procedure, and nephrectomy.

Drug Therapy

Antihypertensive drugs are often successful in the initial management of patients with renovascular hypertension. β-Blocking agents, such as propranolol and atenolol, are commonly used as first-line therapy. Refractory hypertension, especially due to bilateral disease or unilateral lesions with contralateral parenchymal disease, may respond to the addition of a thiazide diuretic, although with impaired renal function, the use of a loop diuretic such as furosemide is more effective. ACE inhibitors, such as captopril and enalapril, have proved to be the most effective drugs in treating renovascular hypertension. Unfortunately, ACE inhibitors may have a deleterious effect on renal function by critically decreasing intrarenal blood pressure and altering intrarenal autoregulation. Certainly, ACE inhibitors should be used cautiously when the entire renal parenchymal mass is at risk, as occurs in renovascular hypertensive patients who have bilateral disease or a solitary kidney. Because stenotic disease of the renal artery often progresses with concomitant loss of renal mass and function, a definitive means of restoring normal renal blood flow may be more logical therapy than drug treat-

ment, once a diagnosis of renovascular hypertension has been established.

Percutaneous Transluminal Renal Angioplasty

In 1978, Gruntzig and colleagues[48] were the first to report the use of PCTA in the management of arteriosclerotic renovascular hypertension. This method of treatment offers certain potential patient benefits, but certain facets of this technology are often overlooked, including clear differences in treating the various types of renal artery disease, frequent inability to catheterize or dilate a given type of stenosis, the long-term effects of angioplasty on the vessel wall, renal and extrarenal complications, and the durability of many initially successful dilations.

Intimal and medial dysplastic stenoses are most amenable to PCTA. Ostial lesions associated with developmental aortic anomalies represent true hypoplastic vessels that are less likely to be successfully dilated.[49] PCTA of atherosclerotic stenoses may be limited by an inability to dilate the spillover plaque from extensive aortic disease. These aorta-associated lesions are responsible for the high recurrence of arteriosclerotic occlusive stenoses after balloon angioplasty.[50]

Complications accompanying dilation of either arteriosclerotic or fibrodysplastic lesions are uncommon, with severe renal complications occurring in less than a few percent of cases. Intimal disruption occurs more often with

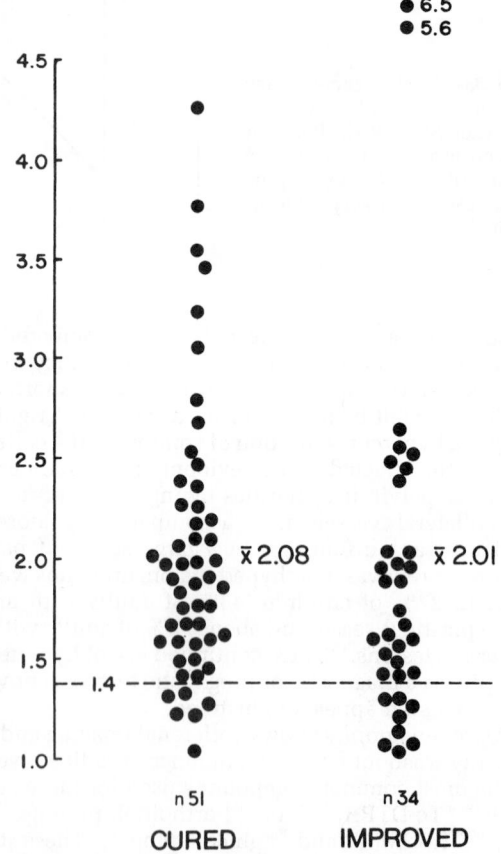

Figure 83-15. Renal vein renin ratios, reflecting their limited diagnostic and prognostic value. (After Stanley JC, Gewertz BL, Fry WJ. Renal:systemic renin indices and renal vein renin ratios as prognostic indicators in remedial renovascular hypertension. J Surg Res 1976;20:149)

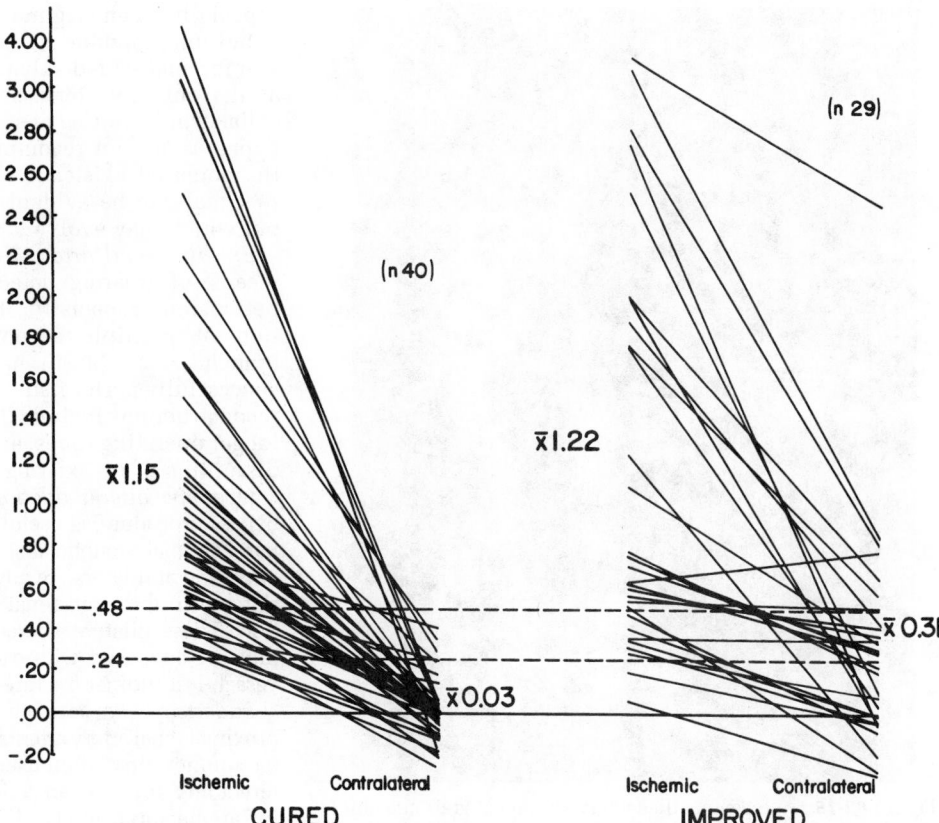

Figure 83-16. Renal–systemic renin indices, depicting their prognostic usefulness. (Stanley JC, Fry WJ. Surgical treatment of renovascular hypertension. Arch Surg 1977;112:1291)

proximal renal artery dilation, in which elasticity of the vessel is greater and medial disruption is less likely. Medial tears are more common with distal renal artery dilation because vascular elasticity is less. Extrarenal complications usually relate to hemorrhage at the site of arterial catheterization. This is rarely limb- or life-threatening. Early benefits after successful PCTA in certain categories of patients approach 90%.[51,52] Renal PCTA in properly selected patients must be considered an alternative therapy for managing renovascular hypertension.[53–55]

Renal Revascularization

Operative treatment of patients with renovascular occlusive disease has become relatively well defined.[56–62] It is important that the primary revascularization procedure be successful. This is underscored by the fact that nephrectomy accompanies nearly half of the reoperations for failed initial reconstructions.[63] Careful preoperative assessment of extrarenal occlusive disease in patients with arteriosclerotic renovascular disease is mandatory to ensure the patient's ability to undergo complex renal artery surgery.[23–27] Operative details vary when treating the different subgroups of renal artery disease.[63]

Aortorenal bypass in adults with arteriosclerotic and fibrodysplastic occlusive disease is most often performed using autologous reversed saphenous vein (Fig. 83-17). Dacron or expanded polytetrafluoroethylene conduits may also be used in reconstructing these vessels. Because vein grafts in children often become aneurysmal,[35,36,64] autologous hypogastric artery grafts and direct aortic reimplanta-

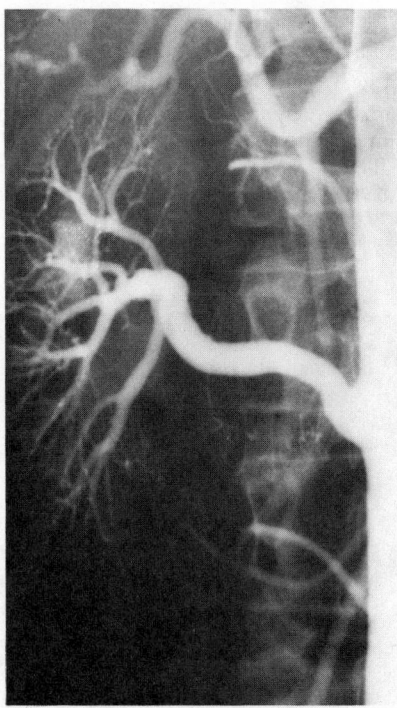

Figure 83-17. Autogenous saphenous vein aortorenal graft. (Stanley JC, Graham LM. Renovascular hypertension. In: Miller DC, Roon AJ, eds. Diagnosis and management of peripheral vascular disease. Menlo Park; CA, Addison-Wesley, 1981)

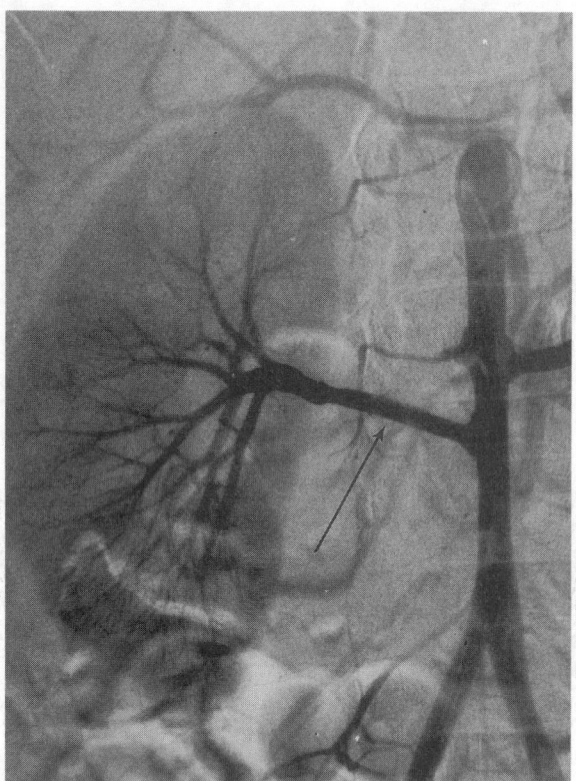

Figure 83-18. Autogenous iliac artery aortorenal graft in a child. (Stanley JC, Zelenock GB, Messina LM, Wakefield TW. Pediatric renovascular hypertension: a thirty-year experience of operative treatment. J Vasc Surg 1995;21:212)

tions of the renal artery are favored in children (Figs. 83-18 and 83-19).

Nonanatomic bypass procedures are important in treating many patients with renovascular hypertension.[65-68] The hepatic artery or iliac arteries may be used as sites of origin for bypass grafts to the renal artery,

especially when originating a graft from the aorta would entail unacceptable risks.[66] Use of the splenic artery in situ for a left-sided splenorenal bypass is appropriate in adults, but only after ascertaining that this vessel and the celiac trunk are free of stenotic disease.[67,69] Splenorenal bypasses are not recommended in children because of the potential existence of a celiac artery growth arrest that may not be evident at the time of reconstruction, but which may evolve later.

Ex vivo renal artery reconstruction is an alternative means of treating select cases of renovascular hypertension, especially those involving revascularization of multiple second- or third-order segmental branches.[59,70,71] Most renal artery reconstructions can be successfully performed in situ. Disadvantages of ex vivo reconstructions include the necessity to cool the kidney, longer operating times, and perhaps most important, the disruption of preexisting collateral channels.

Operative arterial dilation, alone or in conjunction with a bypass procedure, is useful in the treatment of fibrous intraparenchymal stenotic disease. In this setting, sequentially larger metal dilators are advanced through a transverse arteriotomy in the main renal artery after heparin anticoagulation. These dilators, increasing in size by 0.5 increments, must be advanced with care in order not to overdilate the vessel, lest intimal fracture occur.

Endarterectomy is often the preferred means of treating proximal renal artery arteriosclerotic disease.[58,62,72-74] The two techniques most often used are (1) transaortic renal endarterectomy through an axial aortotomy or the transected infrarenal aorta, and (2) direct renal artery endarterectomy. The extent of aortic and renal artery disease, as well as the need to perform coexistent aortic reconstructive surgery, dictates which of these procedures is most appropriate. In most cases, a linear aortotomy is begun just to the left of the superior mesenteric artery and extended in the midline to below the renal arteries. The diseased aortic intimal and medial tissues are elevated, and with gentle traction, the renal artery atheroma is extracted. This type of endarterectomy is particularly useful in treating bilateral disease (Fig. 83-20) or when the disease affects multiple renal arteries. Extensive plaque of the more distal renal artery, especially when involving bifurcations, may be better treated by a

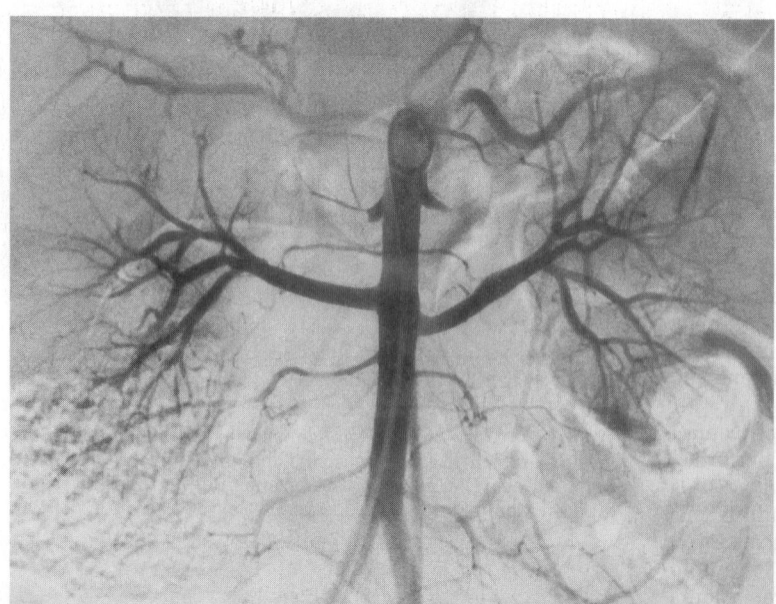

Figure 83-19. Aortic reimplantation of main renal arteries, beyond orificial stenoses in a child. (Stanley JC, Zelenock GB, Messina LM, Wakefield TW. Pediatric renovascular hypertension: a thirty-year experience of operative treatment. J Vasc Surg 1995;21:212)

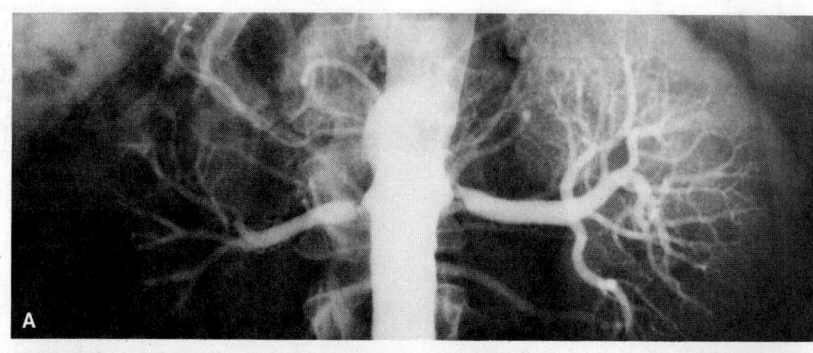

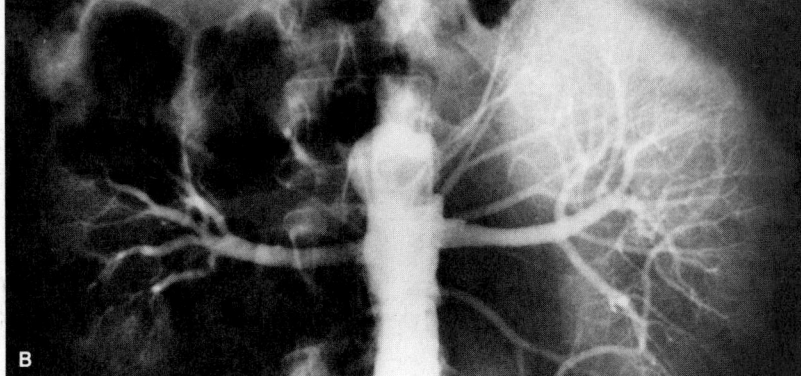

Figure 83-20. Transaortic bilateral renal artery endarterectomy. Preoperative (*A*) and postoperative (*B*) autography. (Stanley JC, Messina LM, Wakefield TW, et al. Renal artery reconstruction. In: Bergan JJ, Yao JST, eds. Techniques in arterial surgery. Philadelphia, WB Saunders, 1990:247)

direct renal artery arteriotomy and endarterectomy with a patch-graft closure.

Results of Operative Therapy

Renal preservation and maintenance of renal function are important in assessing clinical experiences.[75-80] Nephrectomy may provide good early results but obviously leaves the patient at considerable risk if contralateral disease occurs later. Cumulative primary and secondary nephrectomy rates in any given practice should not exceed 10%. Improved renal function after revascularization is well recognized and is most likely to occur among patients exhibiting arteriosclerotic disease with marked preoperative impairment in renal function.

Surgical treatment of renovascular hypertension affords excellent outcomes.[60,61] Differences among most individual experiences reflect variations in the prevalence of different renovascular disease categories (Table 83-1). Renovascular hypertension in childhood is most likely to exhibit a salutary outcome after restoration of normal renal blood flow (Table 83-2). Arterial fibrodysplastic renovascular hypertension (Table 83-3) is more likely to benefit from operation than is arteriosclerotic renovascular hypertension (Table 83-4). This is probably a reflection of coexistent essential hypertension in older patients with arteriosclerotic disease. Arteriosclerotic renovascular hypertension occurs in two subgroups of patients: (1) those with focal renal artery disease whose only clinical manifestation of arteriosclerosis is secondary hypertension, and (2) those with clinically overt extrarenal arteriosclerosis affecting the coronary, carotid, aorta, or extremity vessels. The se-

Table 83-1. RESULTS OF SURGICAL TREATMENT OF RENOVASCULAR HYPERTENSION IN SPECIFIC PATIENT SUBGROUPS, UNIVERSITY OF MICHIGAN EXPERIENCE

Subgroup	Patients	Postoperative Status*			Operative Mortality Rate (%)
		Cure Rate (%)	Improvement Rate (%)	Failure Rate (%)	
Pediatric disease	34	85	12	3	0
Arterial fibrodysplasia	144	55	39	6	0
Arteriosclerosis					
Focal renal artery disease	64	33	58	9	0
Overt extrarenal disease	71	25	47	28	8.5

* Represents outcome of 415 operations (346 primary, 59 secondary), including initial nephrectomy in 17 patients. *Cure:* Blood pressures were 150/90 mmHg or less for a minimum of 6 months postoperatively, during which no antihypertensive medications were administered. *Improvement:* Normotensive while on drug therapy, or if diastolic blood pressures ranged between 90 and 100 mmHg but were at least 15% lower than preoperative levels. *Failure:* Diastolic blood pressures greater than 90 mmHg but less than 15% lower than preoperative levels or greater than 110 mmHg. Lower pressure standards were used in evaluating children. (Stanley JC, Whitehouse WM Jr, Graham LM, Cronenwett JL, Zelenock GB, Lindenauer SM. Operative therapy of renovascular hypertension. Br J Surg 1982;63[Suppl]:S63)

Table 83-2. RENOVASCULAR HYPERTENSION IN CHILDREN

Institution	Patients	Operative Outcome (%)			Surgical Mortality Rate (%)
		Cured	Improved	Failed	
University of Michigan	57	79	19	2	0
Cleveland Clinic	27	59	18.5	18.5	4
University of California, Los Angeles	26	84.5	7.5	4	4
Vanderbilt University	21	68	24	8	0
University of Pennsylvania	17	76.5	23.5	0	0
Argentinian Institute, Buenos Aires	15	53	13	27	7
University of California, San Francisco	14	86	7	0	7

(Modified from Stanley JC. The evolution of surgery for renovascular occlusive disease. Cardiovasc Surg 1994;2:195)

Table 83-3. FIBRODYSPLASTIC RENOVASCULAR HYPERTENSION IN ADULTS

Institution	Patients	Operative Outcome (%)			Surgical Mortality Rate (%)
		Cured	Improved	Failed	
University of Michigan	144	55	39	6	0
Baylor College of Medicine	113	43	24	33	0
Cleveland Clinic	92	58	31	11	Unstated
University of California, San Francisco	77	66	32	1.3	0
Mayo Clinic	63	66	24	10	Unstated
University Hospital Leiden, The Netherlands	53	53	34	13	2
Vanderbilt University	44	72	24	4	2.3
Columbia University	42	76	14	10	Unstated
Bowman Gray	40	33	57	10	0
University of Lund, Malmo, Sweden	40	66	24	10	0

(Modified from Stanley JC. The evolution of surgery for renovascular occlusive disease. Cardiovasc Surg 1994;2:195)

Table 83-4. ARTERIOSCLEROTIC RENOVASCULAR HYPERTENSION IN ADULTS

Institution	Patients	Operative Outcome (%)			Surgical Mortality Rate (%)
		Cured	Improved	Failed	
Baylor College of Medicine	360	34	31	35	2.5
Bowman Gray	152	15	75	10	1.3
University of Michigan	135	29	52	19	4.4
University of California, San Francisco	84	39	23	38	2.4
Cleveland Clinic	78	40	51	9	2
Columbia University	67	58	21	21	Unstated
University of Lund, Malmo, Sweden	66	49	24	27	0.9
Hospital Aiguelongue, Montpellier, France	65	45	40	15	1.1
Vanderbilt University	63	50	45	5	9

(Modified from Stanley JC. The evolution of surgery for renovascular occlusive disease. Cardiovasc Surg 1994;2:195)

verity and duration of hypertension, age, and gender in these two subgroups are similar, yet the surgical outcome regarding amelioration of hypertension is worse in patients with overt extrarenal arteriosclerotic disease. Salutary outcomes justify surgical intervention in properly selected patients with renovascular hypertension.

REFERENCES

1. Goldblatt H, Lynch J, Hanzal RF, et al. Studies on experimental hypertension. I. The production of persistent elevation of systolic blood pressure by means of renal ischemia. J Exp Med 1934;59:347.
2. Hackentahl E, Paul M, Ganten D, et al. Morphology, physiol-

ogy, and molecular biology of renin secretion. Physiol Rev 1990;70:1067.

3. Lynch KR, Peach MJ. Molecular biology of angiotensinogen. Hypertension 1991;17:263.

4. Morris BJ. Molecular biology of renin. I. Gene and protein structure, synthesis and processing. J Hypertens 1992;10:209.

5. Griffiths LR, Board PG, Zwi MB, et al. The B subunit of coagulation factor VIII is linked to renin and the Duffy blood group to α-spectrin on human chromosome 1. Hum Hered 1989;39:107.

6. Hobart PM, Fogliano M, O'Connor BA, et al. Human renin gene: structure and sequence analysis. Proc Natl Acad Sci USA 1984;81:5026.

7. Pratt RE, Ouellette AJ, Dzau VJ. Biosynthesis of renin: multiplicity of active and intermediate forms. Proc Natl Acad Sci USA 1983;80:6809.

8. Pratt RE, Carleton JE, Richie JP, et al. Human renin biosynthesis and secretion in normal and ischemic kidneys. Proc Natl Acad Sci USA 1987;84:7837.

9. Sealey JE, Buhler FR, Laragh JH, et al. The physiology of renin secretion in essential hypertension: estimation of renin secretion rate and renal plasma flow from peripheral and renal vein renin levels. Am J Med 1973;55:391.

10. Schneider EG, Davis JO, Baumber JS, et al. The hepatic metabolism of renin and aldosterone: a review with new observations on the hepatic clearance of renin. Circ Res 1970;26/27(Suppl 1):175.

11. Gaillard-Sanchez I, Mattei MG, Clauser E, et al. Assignment by in situ hybridization of the angiotensinogen gene to chromosome band 1qr, the same region as the human renin gene. Hum Genet 1990;84:341.

12. Fukamizu A, Takahashi S, Seo MS, et al. Structure and expression of the human angiotensinogen gene. J Biol Chem 1990;265:7576.

13. Samuels AI, Miller ED Jr, Fray JCS, et al. Renin-angiotensin antagonists and the regulation of blood pressure. Fed Proc 1976;35:2512.

14. Semple PF, Boyd AS, Dawes PM, Morton JJ. Angiotensin II and its heptapeptide (2), hexapeptide (3), and pentapeptide (4) metabolites in arterial and venous blood of man. Circ Res 1976;39:671.

15. Hubert C, Houot AM, Corvol P, et al. Structure of the angiotensin I–converting enzyme gene. J Biol Chem 1991;15:377.

16. Mattei MG, Hubert C, Alhene-Gelas F, et al. Angiotensin-I converting enzyme is on chromosome 17. Cytogenet Cell Genet 1989;51:1041.

17. Oparil S, Tregear GW, Koerner TJ, et al. Mechanism of pulmonary conversion of angiotensin I to II in the dog. Circ Res 1971;29:682.

18. Oshima G, Gecse A, Erdos EG. Angiotensin I–converting enzyme of the kidney cortex. Biochim Biophys Acta 1974;350:26.

19. Stanley JC, Gewertz BL, Fry WJ. Renal:systemic renin indices and renal vein renin ratios as prognostic indicators in remedial renovascular hypertension. J Surg Res 1976;20:149.

20. Vaughan ED Jr, Buhler FR, Laragh JH, et al. Renovascular hypertension: renin measurements to indicate hypersecretion and contralateral suppression, estimate renal plasma flow, and score for surgical curability. Am J Med 1973;55:402.

21. Gavras H, Brunner HR, Vaughan ED Jr, et al. Angiotensin-sodium interaction in blood pressure maintenance of renal hypertensive and normotensive rats. Science 1973;180:1369.

22. Stanley JC. Pathologic basis of macrovascular renal artery disease. In: Stanley JC, Ernst CB, Fry WJ, eds. Renovascular hypertension. Philadelphia, WB Saunders, 1984:46.

23. Louie J, Isaacson JA, Zierler RE, et al. Prevalence of carotid and lower extremity arterial disease in patients with renal artery stenosis. Am J Hypertens 1994;7:436.

24. Missouris CG, Buckenham T, Cappuccio FP, et al. Renal artery stenosis: a common and important problem in patients with peripheral vascular disease. Am J Med 1994;96:10.

25. Valentine RJ, Clagett GP, Miller GL, et al. The coronary risk of unsuspected renal artery stenosis. J Vasc Surg 18:433.

26. Valentine RJ, Martin JD, Myers SI, et al. Asymptomatic celiac and superior mesenteric artery stenoses are more prevalent among patients with unsuspected renal artery stenoses. J Vasc Surg 1991;14:195.

27. Novick AC, Zaki S, Goldfarb D, Hodge EE. Epidemiologic and clinical comparison of renal artery stenosis in black patients and white patients. J Vasc Surg 1994;20:1.

28. Stanley JC, Gewertz BL, Bove EL, et al. Arterial fibrodysplasia: histopathologic character and current etiologic concepts. Arch Surg 1975;110:551.

29. Stanley JC, Wakefield TW. Arterial fibrodysplasia. In: Rutherford RB, ed. Vascular surgery. Philadelphia, WB Saunders, 1995;264.

30. Graham LM, Zelenock GB, Erlandson EE, et al. Abdominal aortic coarctation and segmental hypoplasia. Surgery 1979;86:519.

31. Stanley JC, Graham LM, Whitehouse WM Jr, et al. Developmental occlusive disease of the abdominal aorta and the splanchnic and renal arteries. Am J Surg 1981;142:190.

32. Stanley JC, Fry WJ. Renovascular hypertension secondary to arterial fibrodysplasia in adults. Arch Surg 1975;110:922.

33. Stanley JC, Rhodes EL, Gewertz BL, et al. Renal artery aneurysms: significance of macroaneurysms exclusive of dissections and fibrodysplastic mural dilations. Arch Surg 1975;110:1327.

34. Sottiurai V, Fry WJ, Stanley JC. Ultrastructure of smooth muscle, myofibroblasts and fibroblasts in human arterial dysplasia. Arch Surg 1978;113:1280.

35. Stanley JC, Fry WJ. Pediatric renal artery occlusive disease and renovascular hypertension: etiology, diagnosis, and operative treatment. Arch Surg 1981;116:669.

36. Stanley JC, Zelenock GB, Messina LM, et al. Pediatric renovascular hypertension: a thirty-year experience of operative treatment. J Vasc Surg 1995;21:212.

37. Stanley JC, Graham LM, Whitehouse WM Jr. Limitations and errors of diagnostic and prognostic investigations in renovascular hypertension. In: Bernhard VM, Towne JM, eds. Complications in vascular surgery. Orlando, Grune & Stratton, 1984:213.

38. Hertz SM, Holland GA, Baum RA, et al. Evaluation of renal artery stenosis by magnetic resonance angiography. Am J Surg 1994;168:140.

39. Kent KC, Edelman RR, Kim D, et al. Magnetic resonance imaging: a reliable test for the evaluation of proximal atherosclerotic renal arterial stenosis. J Vasc Surg 1991;13:311.

40. Prince MR, Narasimham DL, Stanley JC, et al. Breath-hold 3D gadolinium MRA: new developments for imaging the abdominal aorta and its major branches. Radiology 1995;197:785.

41. Hansen KM, Tribble RW, Reavis SW, et al. Renal duplex sonography: evaluation of clinical utility. J Vasc Surg 1990;12:227.

42. Kohler TR, Zierler RE, Martin RL, et al. Noninvasive diagnosis of renal artery stenosis by ultrasonic duplex scanning. J Vasc Surg 1986;4:450.

43. Stanley JC, Fry WJ. Surgical treatment of renovascular hypertension. Arch Surg 1977;112:1291.

44. Thornbury JR, Stanley JC, Fryback DG. Hypertensive urogram: a nondiscriminatory test for renovascular hypertension. AJR 1982;138:43.

45. Stanley JC, Whitehouse WM Jr, Graham LM, et al. Operative therapy of renovascular hypertension. Br J Surg 1982;63(Suppl):S63.

46. Meier GH, Sumpio B, Setaro FJ, et al. Captopril renal scintigraphy: a new standard for predicting outcome after renal revascularization. J Vasc Surg 1993;17:280.

47. Dean RH, Rhamy RK. Split renal function studies in renovascular hypertension. In: Stanley JC, Ernst CB, Fry WJ, eds. Renovascular hypertension. Philadelphia, WB Saunders, 1984:135.

48. Gruntzig A, Vetter W, Meier B, et al. Treatment of renovascular hypertension with percutaneous transluminal dilatation of a renal-artery stenosis. Lancet 1978;1:801.

49. Martin EC, Diamond NG, Casarella WJ. Percutaneous transluminal angioplasty in nonatherosclerotic disease. Radiology 1980;135:27.

50. Grim CE, Luft FC, Yune HY, et al. Percutaneous transluminal dilatation in the treatment of renovascular hypertension. Ann Intern Med 1981;95:43.

51. Sos TA, Pickering TG, Sniderman K, et al. Percutaneous transluminal renal angioplasty in renovascular hypertension due

to atheroma or fibromuscular dysplasia. N Engl J Med 1983;309:274.

52. Tegtmeyer CJ, Kellum CD, Ayers C. Percutaneous transluminal angioplasty of the renal artery: results and long-term follow-up. Radiology 1984;153:77.

53. Canzanello VJ, Millan VG, Spiegel JE, Ponce PS, Kopelman RI, Madias NE. Percutaneous transluminal renal angioplasty in the management of atherosclerotic renovascular hypertension: results in 100 patients. Hypertension 1989;13:163.

54. Klinge J, Mali WP, Puijlaert CB, et al. Percutaneous transluminal renal angioplasty: initial and long-term results. Radiology 1989;171:501.

55. Weibull H. Percutaneous transluminal renal angioplasty versus surgical reconstruction of atherosclerotic renal artery stenosis: a prospective randomized study. J Vasc Surg 1993; 18:841.

56. Anderson CA, Hansen KJ, Benjamin ME, et al. Renal artery fibromuscular dysplasia: results of current surgical therapy. J Vasc Surg 1995;22:207.

57. Cambria RP, Brewster DC, L'Italien G, et al. Simultaneous aortic and renal artery reconstruction: evolution of an eighteen-year experience. J Vasc Surg 1994;21:916.

58. Hansen KJ, Starr SM, Sands RE, et al. Contemporary surgical management of renovascular disease. J Vasc Surg 1992; 16:319.

59. Murray SP, Kent KC, Salvatierra O, Stoney RJ. Complex branch renovascular disease: management options and late results. J Vasc Surg 1994;20:338.

60. Stanley JC. The evolution of surgery for renovascular occlusive disease. Cardiovasc Surg 1994;2:195.

61. Stanley JC, Ernst CB, Fry WJ. Surgical treatment of renovascular hypertension: results in specific patient subgroups. In: Renovascular hypertension. Philadelphia, WB Saunders, 1984: 363.

62. Stanley JC, Messina LM, Wakefield TW, Zelenock GB. Renal artery reconstruction. In: Bergan JJ, Yao JST, eds. Techniques in arterial surgery. Philadelphia, WB Saunders, 1990;247.

63. Stanley JC, Whitehouse WM Jr, Zelenock GB, et al. Reoperation for complications of renal artery reconstructive surgery undertaken for treatment of renovascular hypertension. J Vasc Surg 1985;2:133.

64. Stanley JC, Ernst CB, Fry WJ. Fate of 100 aortorenal vein grafts: characteristics of late graft expansion, aneurysmal dilatation, and stenosis. Surgery 1973;74:931.

65. Cambria RP, Brewster DC, L'Italien GJ, et al. The durability of different reconstructive techniques for atherosclerotic renal artery disease. J Vasc Surg 1994;20:76.

66. Chibaro EA, Libertino JA, Novick AC. Use of the hepatic circulation for renal revascularization. Ann Surg 1984;199:406.

67. Khauli RB, Novick AC, Ziegelbaum M. Splenorenal bypass in the treatment of renal artery stenosis: experience with 69 cases. J Vasc Surg 1985;2:547.

68. Novick AC, Stewart R, Hodge EE, Goldfarb D. Use of the thoracic aorta for renal arterial reconstruction. J Vasc Surg 1994;19:605.

69. Moncure AC, Brewster DC, Darling RC, Atnip RG, Newton WD, Abbott WM. Use of the splenic and hepatic arteries for renal revascularization. J Vasc Surg 1986;3:196.

70. Brekke IB, Sodal G, Jakobsen A, et al. Fibro-muscular renal artery disease treated by extracorporeal vascular reconstruction and renal autotransplantation: short- and long-term results. Eur J Vasc Surg 1992;6:471.

71. van Bockel JH, van den Akker PJ, Chang PC, Aarts JCNM, Hermans J, Terpstra JL. Extracorporeal renal artery reconstruction for renovascular hypertension. J Vasc Surg 1991; 13:101.

72. Dougherty MJ, Hallett JW Jr, Naessens J, et al. Renal endarterectomy vs. bypass for combined aortic and renal reconstruction: is there a difference in clinical outcome? Ann Vasc Surg 1995;9:87.

73. McNeil JW, String ST, Pfeiffer RB Jr. Concomitant renal endarterectomy and aortic reconstruction. J Vasc Surg 1994;20:331.

74. Stoney RJ, Messina LM, Goldstone J, Reilly LM. Renal endarterectomy through the transected aorta: a new technique for combined aortorenal arteriosclerosis—a preliminary report. J Vasc Surg 1989;9:224.

75. Dean RH, Lawson JD, Hollifield JW. Revascularization of the poorly functioning kidney. Surgery 1979;85:44.

76. Dean RH, Shack RB, Rhamy RK, Wilson JP, Foster JH. The effect of renal revascularization on kidney function. J Surg Res 1977;22:443.

77. Hallett JW Jr, Textor SC, Kos PB, et al. Advanced renovascular hypertension and renal insufficiency: trends in medical comorbidity and surgical approach from 1970 to 1993. J Vasc Surg 1995;21:750.

78. Hansen KJ, Thomason RB, Craven TE, et al. Surgical management of dialysis-dependent ischemic nephropathy. J Vasc Surg 1995;21:197.

79. Jamieson GG, Clarkson AR, Woodroffe AJ, Faris I. Reconstructive renal vascular surgery for chronic renal failure. Br J Surg 1984;71:338.

80. Whitehouse WM Jr, Kazmers A, Zelenock GB, et al. Chronic total renal artery occlusions: effects of treatment on secondary hypertension and renal function. Surgery 1981;89:753.

SURGERY: SCIENTIFIC PRINCIPLES AND PRACTICE, Second Edition, edited by Lazar J. Greenfield, Michael W. Mulholland, Keith T. Oldham, Gerald B. Zelenock, and Keith D. Lillemoe. Lippincott-Raven Publishers, Philadelphia, © 1997.

CHAPTER 84

AORTOILIAC DISEASE

DAVID C. BREWSTER

Arteriosclerotic occlusive disease involving the infrarenal abdominal aorta and iliac arteries is a common cause of symptomatic arterial insufficiency of the lower extremities. Because arteriosclerosis is usually a generalized process, obliterative disease in the aortoiliac segment frequently coexists with disease in the infrainguinal vessels. Nonetheless, correction of hemodynamic problems in the inflow system alone frequently provides clinical relief of leg ischemic symptoms. In addition, careful evaluation of the adequacy of arterial inflow is important even in patients whose primary difficulty lies in the femoropopliteal outflow segment. Despite its generalized nature, chronic arteriosclerotic disease is usually segmental in distribution and is usually amenable to effective surgical treatment.

During the four decades since the introduction of surgical methods of arterial reconstruction for aortoiliac disease, great progress has been achieved. More accurate physiologic assessment of the extent and severity of the disease process is possible, whereas advances in preoperative evaluation of patient risk in terms of coronary artery disease and other associated medical conditions has led to improved patient selection. Improvements in prosthetic materials, simplification of surgical techniques, and refinements in perioperative care all have contributed to a steady reduction of operative morbidity and mortality and to excellent long-term results. A variety of methods of revascularization are available for use, depending on the extent of disease, patient risk, and other clinical variables. With selection of the most appropriate treatment in each individual patient, safe and effective symptom relief can be achieved in almost all patients.

ANATOMY

The major arteries supplying blood flow to the lower extremities are the abdominal aorta, iliac arteries, and the femoral, popliteal, anterior and posterior tibial, and peroneal artery of each limb (Fig. 84-1). Although patients with clinical

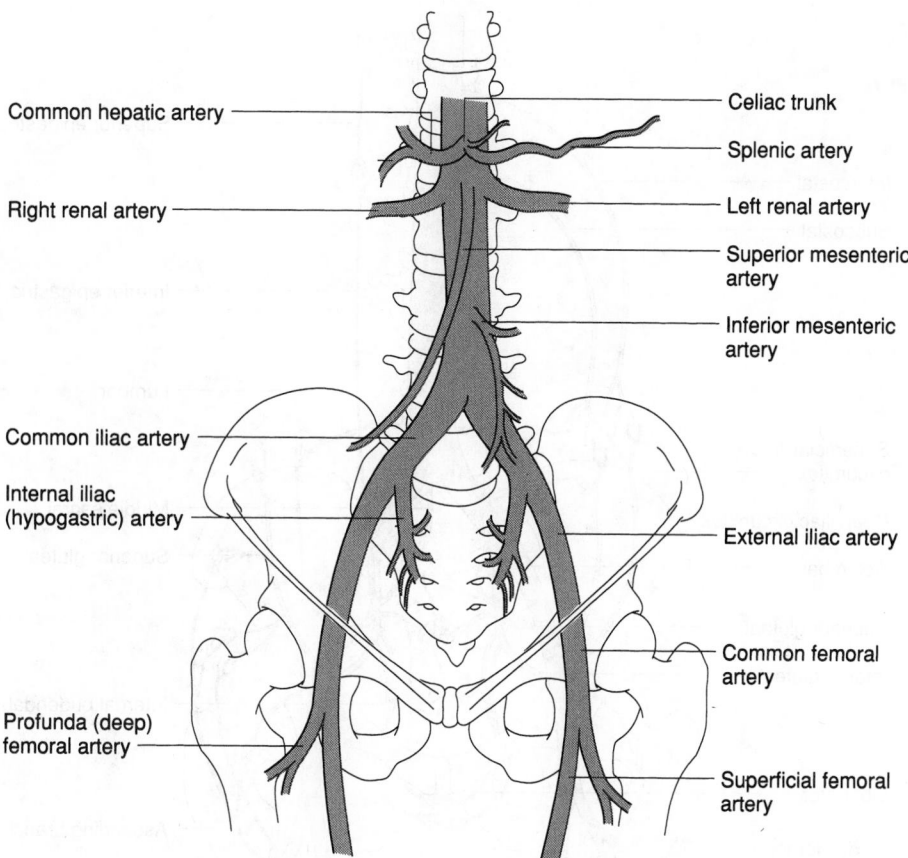

Figure 84-1. Anatomy of the abdominal aorta and iliac arteries.

Labels (clockwise):
Common hepatic artery — Celiac trunk — Splenic artery — Left renal artery — Superior mesenteric artery — Inferior mesenteric artery — External iliac artery — Common femoral artery — Superficial femoral artery — Profunda (deep) femoral artery — Internal iliac (hypogastric) artery — Common iliac artery — Right renal artery

symptoms of arterial insufficiency often have disease in more than one area, it is useful to consider evaluation and management of obliterative disease in different segments of the arterial tree separately. Therefore, this chapter focuses on chronic occlusive disease in the inflow vessels (aorta and iliac arteries); the following sections deal with lesions in the infrainguinal femoropopliteotibial outflow tract.

The abdominal aorta begins at the aortic hiatus of the diaphragm, in front of the lower border of the last thoracic vertebra, and descends in front of the vertebral column slightly to the left of midline. As it courses distally, it diminishes in size as a consequence of the many large visceral and parietal branches that arise from this conduit vessel. The most important of these branches are the celiac trunk, superior mesenteric artery (SMA), right and left renal arteries, inferior mesenteric artery, and about four sets of paired lumbar arteries. The abdominal aorta generally terminates at the level of the fourth lumbar vertebra by bifurcating into the common iliac arteries. Topographically, this usually corresponds to the approximate level of the umbilicus on the abdominal wall.

Because of its deep posterior retroperitoneal location, surgical exposure of the abdominal aorta is often difficult. This is particularly true of its upper aspect, the suprarenal aortic segment from the diaphragm to the renal artery level. Here, the aorta is enveloped by the muscular crura of the diaphragm as they insert onto the lumbar vertebrae, and is covered anteriorly by the lesser omentum, stomach, pancreas, and left renal vein. The latter generally crosses the aorta anteriorly but is retroaortic in about 5% of cases. Mobilization of the suprarenal aorta is further complicated by the origin of the celiac axis and SMA from the anterior wall of the aorta. Exposure of the infrarenal aorta requires opening of the overlying retroperitoneal tissue and displacement of

the inferior aspect of the duodenum and overlying small bowel mesentery. The inferior vena cava is often closely approximated to the right side of the infrarenal aorta.

The common iliac arteries diverge from the aortic bifurcation and pass downward and lateral. They are usually about 5 cm in length before dividing into the internal (hypogastric) and external iliac arteries. The former supplies the viscera and parietes of the pelvis; the latter supplies the lower extremity. The femoral artery is the direct continuation of the external iliac artery, beginning at the level of the inguinal ligament. About 4 to 5 cm below the inguinal ligament, the common femoral artery divides into its superficial and deep (profunda) branches. Because of the high incidence of concomitant occlusive disease in the superficial femoral artery in patients with aortoiliac disease, the profunda femoris branch is important to the surgeon for revascularization procedures.

Potential pathways of collateral circulation to compensate for aortoiliac disease include both visceral and parietal routes, such as internal mammary to inferior epigastric; intercostal and lumbar arteries to circumflex iliac and hypogastric networks; hypogastric and gluteal branches to common femoral and profunda femoral arteries; and superior mesenteric to inferior mesenteric and superior hemorrhoidal pathways by means of the marginal artery of Drummond (meandering mesenteric artery) and arch of Riolan (Figs. 84-2 and 84-3).

PATHOPHYSIOLOGY

Arteriosclerosis can produce partial or complete occlusion of the aorta and iliac arteries. As progressive narrowing of these vessels reduces blood flow to the

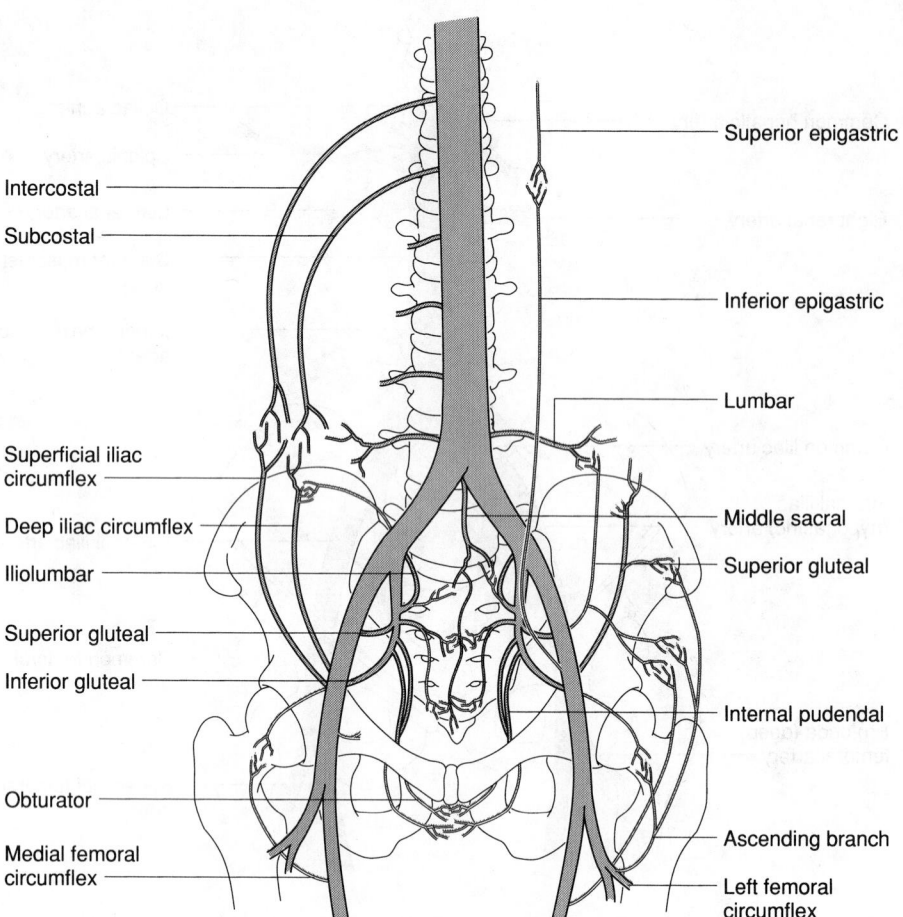

Intercostal

Subcostal

Superficial iliac circumflex

Deep iliac circumflex

Iliolumbar

Superior gluteal

Inferior gluteal

Obturator

Medial femoral circumflex

Superior epigastric

Inferior epigastric

Lumbar

Middle sacral

Superior gluteal

Internal pudendal

Ascending branch

Left femoral circumflex

Figure 84-2. Major pathways of parietal collateral circulation in aortoiliac occlusive disease.

pelvic viscera and lower extremities, characteristic symptom complexes develop. The disease process is commonly centered around the aortic bifurcation, and hence disease is usually maximal in the lower infrarenal aorta, aortic bifurcation, and common iliac arteries (Fig. 84-4). As is typical of arteriosclerotic disease in general, the occlusive process is often most pronounced at arterial bifurcations. Plaque is also generally more extensive on the posterior arterial wall, causing the distal lumbar arteries and median sacral vessel to be occluded at an earlier stage of disease.

It is distinctly unusual for clinically significant occlusive disease to involve the suprarenal aorta. Similarly, the aorta immediately distal to the renal arteries is usually relatively spared from advanced occlusive disease, an important feature that is exploited in aortic reconstructive surgery.

Because of the abundant potential for collateral circulation, distal blood flow to the lower extremities is rarely critically reduced as long as the occlusive process is restricted to the intraabdominal aortoiliac segment. Claudication or sexual impotence is commonly present, but blood flow at rest remains adequate, and the viability of the extremity is rarely threatened. More advanced ischemic symptoms nearly always indicate additional distal disease.

Symptoms result when progressive narrowing of the vessel lumen and consequent reduction of distal tissue perfusion outpace the ability of collateral circulation to compensate adequately. Claudication or crampy, aching discomfort with exercise is almost always the

earliest manifestation, a logical consequence of collateral blood flow being sufficient for tissue nutrition at rest but unable to accommodate for the 5- to 10-fold increase in blood flow associated with maximal exercise in the normal leg. More advanced ischemic symptoms, such as ischemic pain at rest or ischemic tissue necrosis (ulceration or digital gangrene; Fig. 84-5), occur when resting blood flow is insufficient to satisfy basic metabolic requirements for nonexercising tissue.

With progressive stenosis of a diseased vessel, blood flow may be reduced to a point that total thrombosis of the diseased segment occurs, often accounting for a sudden worsening in symptomatology in a patient with previously mild ischemic manifestations. Similarly, degeneration or ulceration of plaques can lead to distal embolism of thrombin or platelet aggregations that have accumulated on its irregular surface, or to dislodgement of actual atherosclerotic debris from the plaque itself, a process referred to as *atheromatous embolism* (Fig. 84-6).

PATTERNS OF DISEASE AND CLINICAL MANIFESTATIONS

The symptoms, natural history, and choice of optimal method of surgical reconstruction are strongly influenced by the extent and distribution of occlusive disease (Fig. 84-7). Disease truly confined to the distal aorta and proximal iliac vessels (type I) is relatively

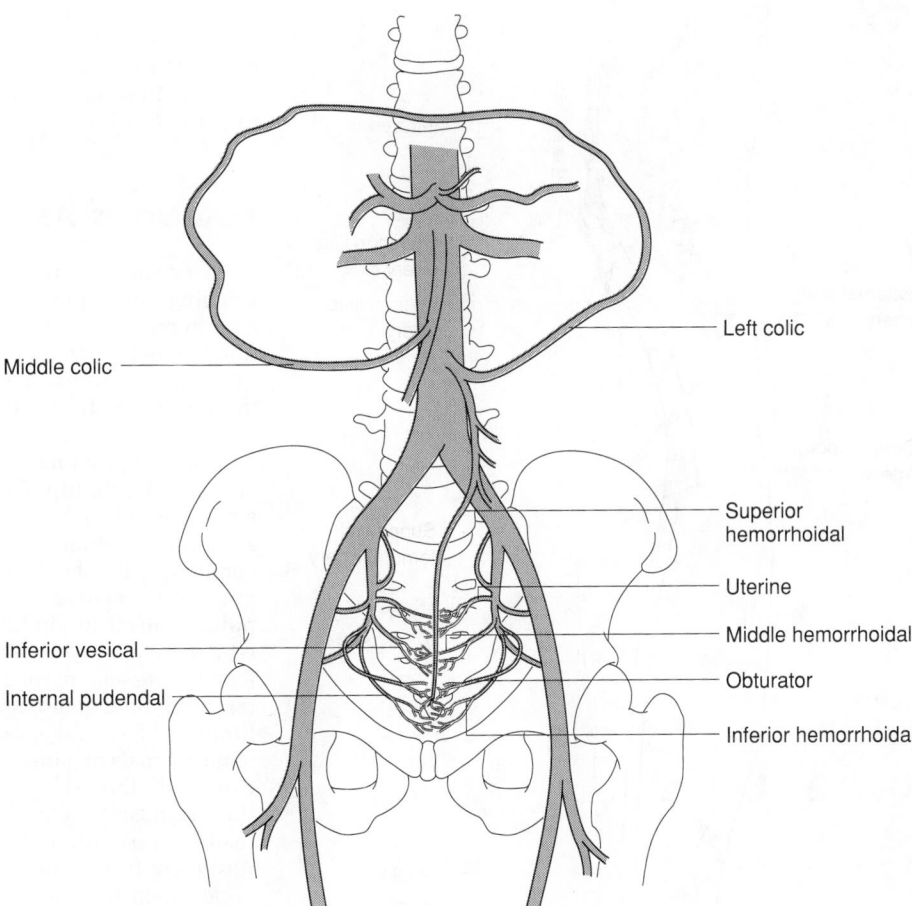

Figure 84-3. Major visceral collateral networks available for compensation of aortoiliac disease.

Labels: Middle colic, Left colic, Superior hemorrhoidal, Uterine, Middle hemorrhoidal, Inferior vesical, Obturator, Internal pudendal, Inferior hemorrhoidal

infrequent, seen in about 10% of surgical candidates. These data are derived from arteriographic findings in patients with sufficiently severe symptoms to warrant surgical intervention. It is likely that such localized disease is more commonly present earlier in the disease process, when symptoms are few; therefore, invasive investigation often is not undertaken.

In localized aortoiliac disease, patients typically present with claudication alone, often involving primarily the proximal musculature of the thigh, hip, or buttock area. More advanced ischemic complaints are absent unless distal atherosclerotic disease is also present or atheroembolic complications have occurred. Impotence is often an associated complaint, present in varying degrees of severity in at least 30% to 50% of men with aortoiliac disease.

Patients with a type I disease pattern are characteristically younger, with a relatively low incidence of hypertension or diabetes, but commonly are noted to have abnormal blood lipids. In contrast to the usual male predominance in chronic peripheral vascular disease, almost half of those patients with localized aortoiliac disease are women, often with small aortic, iliac, and femoral vessels; such a characteristic clinical picture is often termed the *hypoplastic aorta syndrome.*

Disease initially isolated to the bifurcation region commonly progresses to cause occlusion of one iliac artery or extends to involve the external iliac or femoral vessels, usually by a posterior tongue of atheroma. Although circulation to both lower extremities may be maintained by hypogastric collateral networks of the stenotic limb, this pattern of disease is relatively unstable. Occlusion of the

remaining common iliac artery can result in thrombus propagating to the groin, which causes severe ischemia of both lower extremities and precipitates the need for emergency intervention, otherwise rarely necessary in chronic aortoiliac disease.

Bilateral occlusion of the common iliac arteries leads to propagation of thrombus and total occlusion of the infrarenal aorta. Complete aortic occlusion extends to the level of the inferior mesenteric artery (Fig. 84-8A); or if this vessel has undergone prior obliteration, superimposed thrombus extends proximally to a juxtarenal level (see Fig. 84-8B), with the renal vessels acting as an outflow tract for the proximal aorta. Rarely, further proximal extension of clot compromises the renal arteries or SMA, but this is unusual unless these vessels are stenotic secondary to associated occlusive disease. About 5% to 10% of patients undergoing aortoiliac surgery for occlusive disease have a totally occluded aorta.

Most patients who are candidates for aortoiliac operations have diffuse disease. About 20% to 25% have a type II pattern, with occlusive disease still confined largely to the abdominal vessels but also involving the external iliac and perhaps common femoral arteries. Diffuse occlusive disease involving both inflow and infrainguinal outflow arterial segments (type III) affected 66% of patients in one review[1] and constitutes half to two thirds of most major surgical series.[2-5] Patients with such multilevel disease (also frequently referred to as *combined segment* or *tandem* disease) are typically older, more commonly male (about a 6:1 ratio), and much more likely to have diabetes, hypertension, and associated atherosclerotic disease involving the coronary, cerebral, or visceral arteries. Most

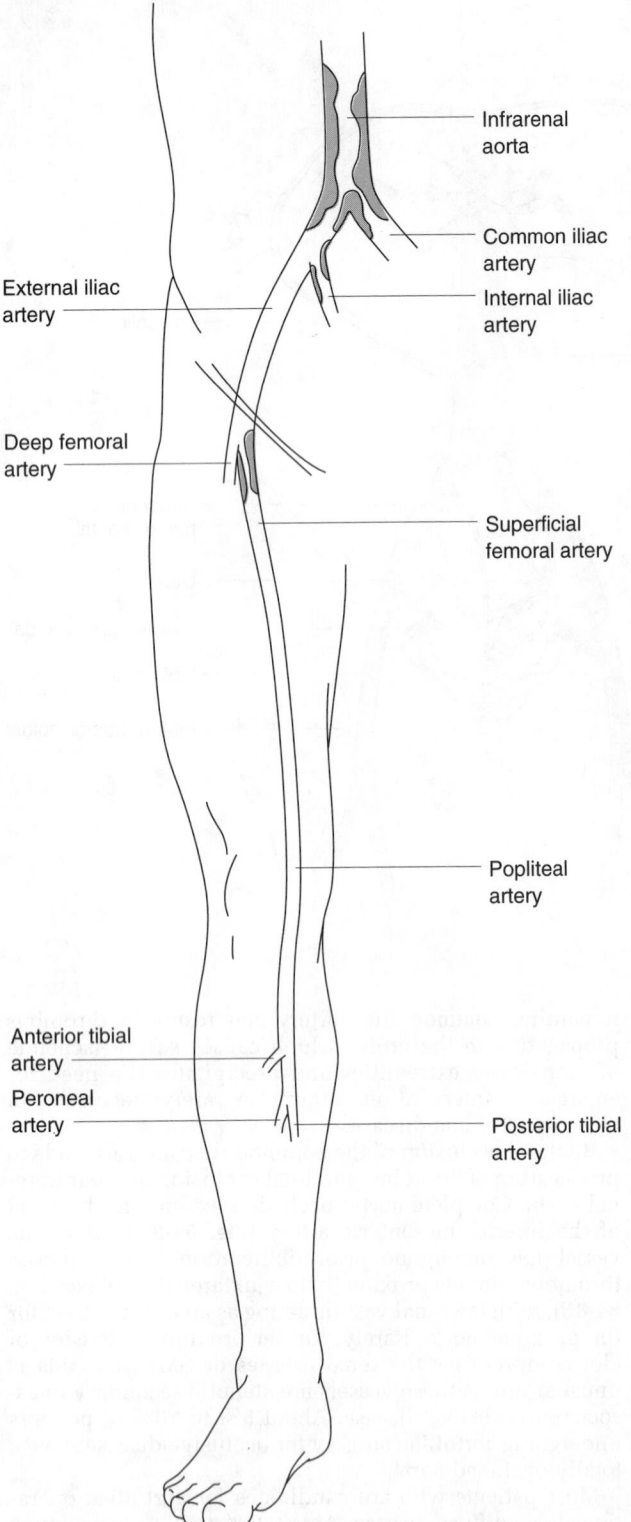

External iliac artery

Deep femoral artery

Infrarenal aorta

Common iliac artery

Internal iliac artery

Superficial femoral artery

Popliteal artery

Anterior tibial artery

Peroneal artery

Posterior tibial artery

Figure 84-4. Common sites of arteriosclerotic lesions in aortoilio-femoral occlusive disease. Although often a generalized process, partially segmental distribution of major disease, most prominent at arterial bifurcations, usually allows surgical revascularization.

patients with multilevel disease manifest symptoms of more advanced ischemia, such as ischemic pain at rest or varying degrees of actual tissue necrosis, and operation is more often undertaken for limb salvage than simply for relief of claudication. The higher incidence of associated atherosclerotic disease and other comorbid conditions in patients with multilevel disease increases the morbidity and mortality risks of revascularization procedures. In addition, these characteristics lead to a decrease in life expectancy of 10 or more years, whereas it may be near normal in patients with more localized aortoiliac disease.[6]

DIAGNOSIS AND EVALUATION

An accurate history and carefully performed physical examination can establish the diagnosis of aortoiliac disease in most instances. A reliable description of claudication in one or both legs, possible decreased sexual potency in men, and diminished or absent femoral pulses define the characteristic triad often referred to as the *Leriche syndrome.*

Although proximal claudication symptoms in the distribution of thigh, hip, and buttock musculature are usually a reliable indicator of clinically important inflow disease, a significant number of patients with aortoiliac disease complain only of calf claudication, particularly those with multilevel disease. In addition to diminished femoral pulses, physical findings often include audible bruits, which frequently are heard over the lower abdomen or femoral vessels, particularly after exercise. Elevation pallor, rubor on dependency, shiny atrophic skin in the distal limbs and feet, and occasionally areas of ulceration or ischemic necrosis or gangrene may be noted, depending on the extent of atherosclerotic impairment. In some instances, the diagnosis of aortoiliac occlusive disease may not be readily apparent, and certain complaints can cause diagnostic confusion. In some patients, pulse evaluation and appearance of the feet may be judged to be entirely normal at rest, despite the presence of proximal stenoses that are physiologically significant with exercise. This is often the case in patients presenting with distal microemboli secondary to atheroembolism. In other instances, complaints of exercise-related pain in the leg, hip, buttock, or even low back may be mistaken for symptoms of degenerative hip or spine disease, nerve root irritation caused by lumbar disk herniation or spinal stenosis, diabetic neuropathy, or other neuromuscular problems. Many of these patients may be distinguished from patients with true claudication by the fact that their discomfort is often relieved only by sitting or lying down, as opposed to simply stopping walking. In addition, the typical sciatic distribution of the pain and the fact that often the complaints are brought on by simply standing, as opposed to walking a certain distance, suggest nonvascular causes. In many such circumstances, use of noninvasive vascular laboratory testing modalities, including treadmill exercise, may be helpful.

Use of various noninvasive physiologic tests such as segmental limb Doppler pressure measurements and plethysmography (see Chap. 75) may be of considerable help in diagnosis and provide quantification of the severity of the disease process. For instance, these tests have clinical importance in differentiating diabetic neuropathic foot pain from true ischemic rest pain or in predicting the likelihood that a foot lesion may heal without revascularization. Noninvasive studies may also serve as a reliable and objective baseline by which a patient's course can be followed.

Duplex scanning has also been used to evaluate aortoiliac occlusive disease. Although such studies may provide additional information regarding the presence of occlusive disease and its severity, the anatomic imaging is generally too imprecise to serve as a definitive guide to interventional therapy, and arteriography is almost always necessary if revascularization is planned.

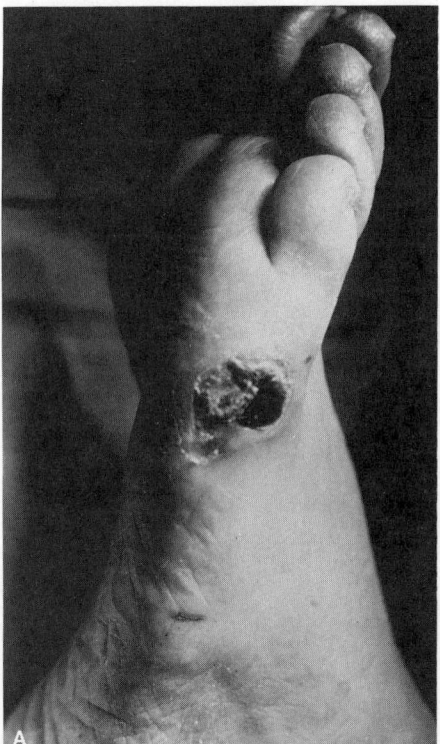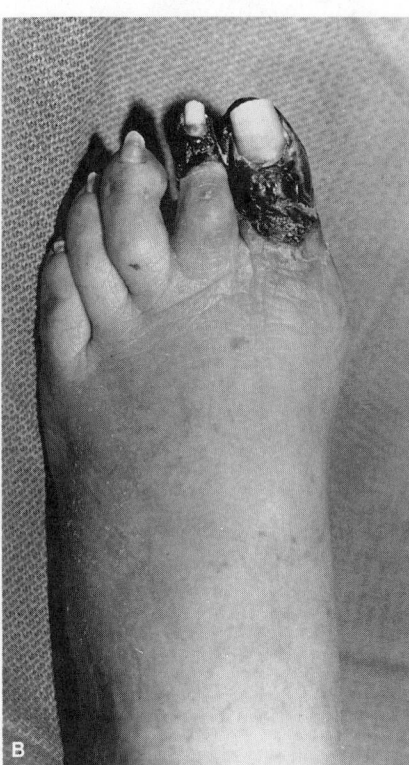

Figure 84-5. Examples of ischemic tissue necrosis. (*A*) Ischemic ulceration. (*B*) Digital gangrene.

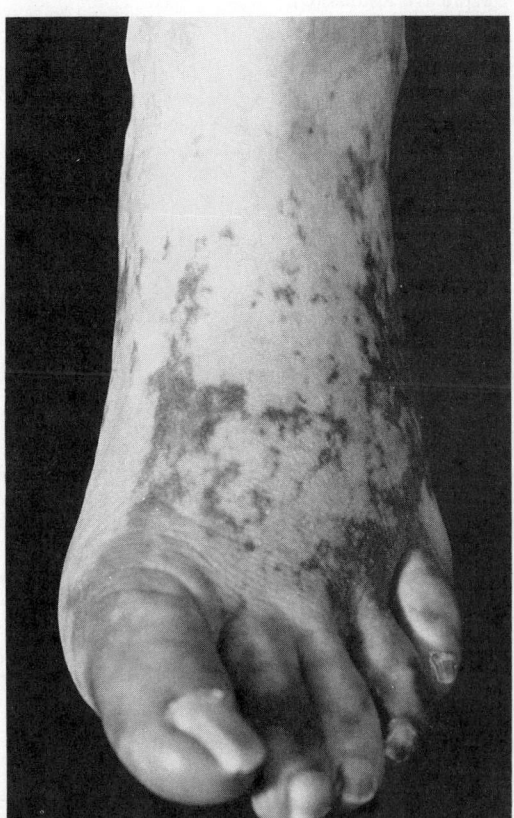

Figure 84-6. Typical appearance of foot in a patient with distal atheroembolism (blue-toe syndrome).

Arteriography

If clinical evaluation suggests that the patient is a likely candidate for arterial reconstructive surgery, arteriography is performed to obtain the anatomic information necessary for the surgeon to select the best method of revascularization and properly plan an operative procedure. In addition to noting the anatomic distribution of occlusive disease in the aortoiliac segment and distal vessels, the surgeon should examine the films for critical anatomic variations or associated occlusive lesions in the renal, visceral, or runoff vessels. For example, an enlarged meandering left colic artery often is an indicator of associated occlusive disease in the SMA; this can usually be appreciated only on a lateral view. Failure to recognize this can lead to catastrophic bowel infarction if the inferior mesenteric artery is ligated at the time of aortic reconstruction.

For most patients, a full and complete arteriographic survey of the entire intraabdominal aortoiliac segment and infrainguinal runoff vessels is advisable. In general, runoff views are obtained to at least the level of the middle calf. In selected patients with advanced distal disease and threatened limbs, more distal views, including the distal leg, ankle, and even foot, may be advisable if the possibility of very distal infrapopliteal bypass grafting is considered likely.

The major risk of conventional contrast angiography is contrast-induced renal dysfunction. Although the incidence of this difficulty may be minimized by adequate hydration and limitation of contrast volume, certain high-risk patients, such as diabetic patients with preexistent chronic renal insufficiency, may represent a significant hazard. In such instances, alternative imaging modalities may be considered. Development of magnetic resonance angiography has substantial promise as a satisfactory substitute for conventional arteriography, both for diagnosis and planning of therapy.[7]

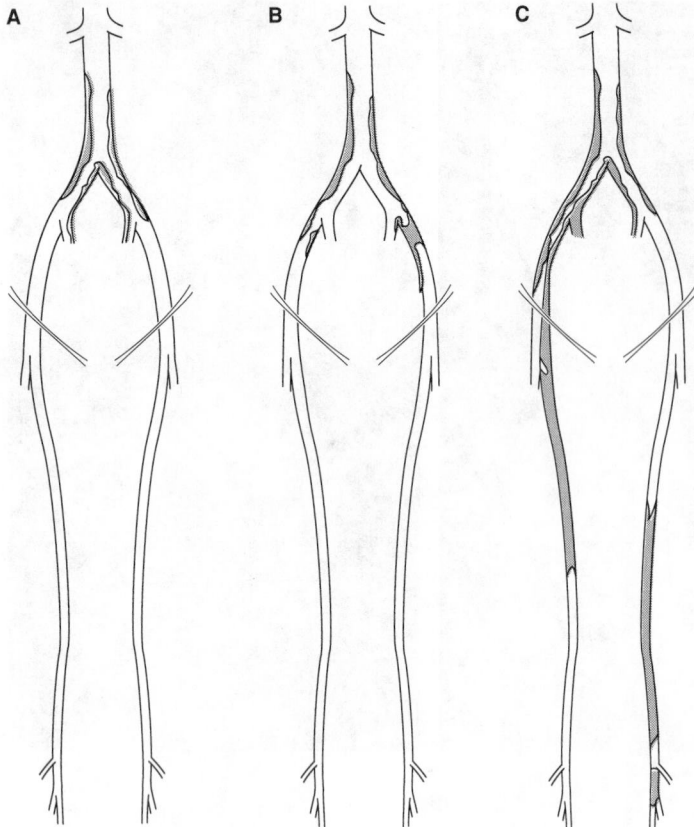

Figure 84-7. Patterns of aortoiliac disease. (*A*) In type I, localized disease is confined to the distal aorta and common iliac arteries. More widespread intraabdominal disease is present in type II (*B*), whereas a type III pattern signifies multilevel disease with associated infrainguinal occlusive lesions (*C*).

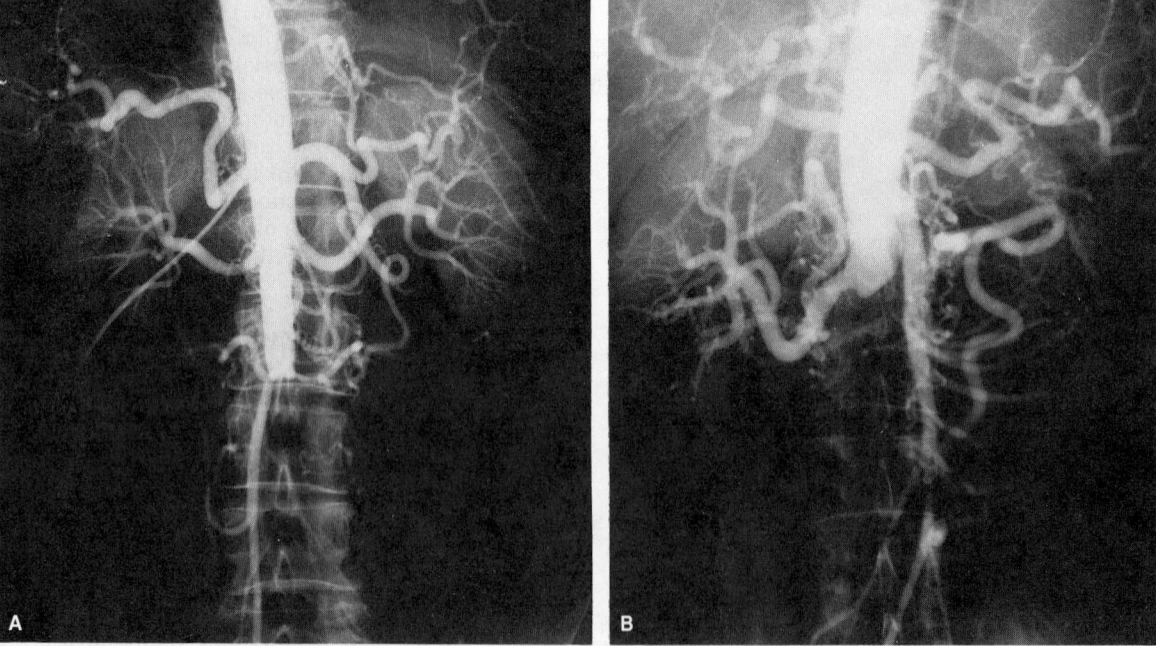

Figure 84-8. Arteriographic examples of complete aortic occlusion. (*A*) Occlusion to mid-infrarenal aorta, with patency of upper infrarenal aortic segment maintained by inferior mesenteric and lumbar artery runoff. (*B*) Complete juxtarenal aortic occlusion with retrograde thrombosis to the level of renal artery runoff.

Pressure Measurements

Although an accurate assessment of occlusive disease is possible by traditional clinical evaluation and good quality arteriography in most patients, difficulty can exist in patients with multilevel occlusive disease. Assessment of the hemodynamic significance of occlusive disease at each segmental level is obviously of critical importance in selection of an appropriate reconstructive procedure.

For this purpose, actual measurement of femoral artery pressure often is of considerable value.[5,8] Peak systolic pressure in the femoral artery is compared with distal aortic or brachial systolic pressure. A resting systolic pressure difference greater than 5 mmHg or a fall in femoral artery pressure greater than 15% with reactive hyperemia induced pharmacologically or by inflation of an occluding thigh cuff for 3 to 5 minutes implies hemodynamically significant inflow disease (Fig. 84-9). If revascularization is indicated in such patients, attention should first be directed at correction of the inflow lesions. With a negative study, the surgeon more confidently can proceed directly with distal revascularization without fear of premature compromise or closure of the distal graft and without subjecting the patient to an unnecessary inflow operation.

TREATMENT

Indications for Operation

Ischemic pain at rest or actual tissue necrosis, including ischemic ulcerations or frank digital gangrene, are well accepted as indicative of advanced ischemia and threatened limb loss. Although true ischemic rest pain or ulceration occasionally resolves because of collateral development, this is infrequent. An exception is ischemia that occurs after an acute thrombotic event, such as terminal thrombosis of a previously stenotic artery. Improvement of collateral circulation over a period of days to a few weeks may result in lessened ischemia and only claudication symptoms.

Untreated, most patients with limb-threatening ischemic symptoms eventually require a major amputation. These symptoms are therefore clearcut indications for arterial reconstruction, if anatomically feasible. Age alone is rarely an important consideration. Even elderly or frail patients or patients at high risk from multiple associated medical problems generally can be revascularized by alternative surgical methods if direct aortoiliac reconstruction is deemed inadvisable.

Some controversy remains concerning operation for claudication symptoms alone. In each patient, these decisions must be individualized, with consideration of age, associated medical disease, employment requirements, and life-style preferences. Claudication that jeopardizes the livelihood of a patient or significantly impairs the desired life-style of an otherwise low-risk patient may be considered to be a reasonable indication for surgical correction, assuming that a favorable anatomic situation for operation exists. If this more liberal approach is undertaken, it is desirable that symptoms can be attributed to isolated proximal inflow disease, as opposed to more distal disease in the femoropopliteal arterial segment. This seems logical and appropriate because of the generally excellent and long-lasting results achieved by aortoiliac reconstruction, at a low risk to the patient. A less frequent but recognized indication for surgical intervention is distal atheromatous embolization from proximal aortoiliac disease. If the clinical presentation is consistent with this diagnosis and arteriography demonstrates shaggy or ulcerated atherosclerotic plaques in the aortoiliac system, which are the likely source of such embolic debris, treatment by means

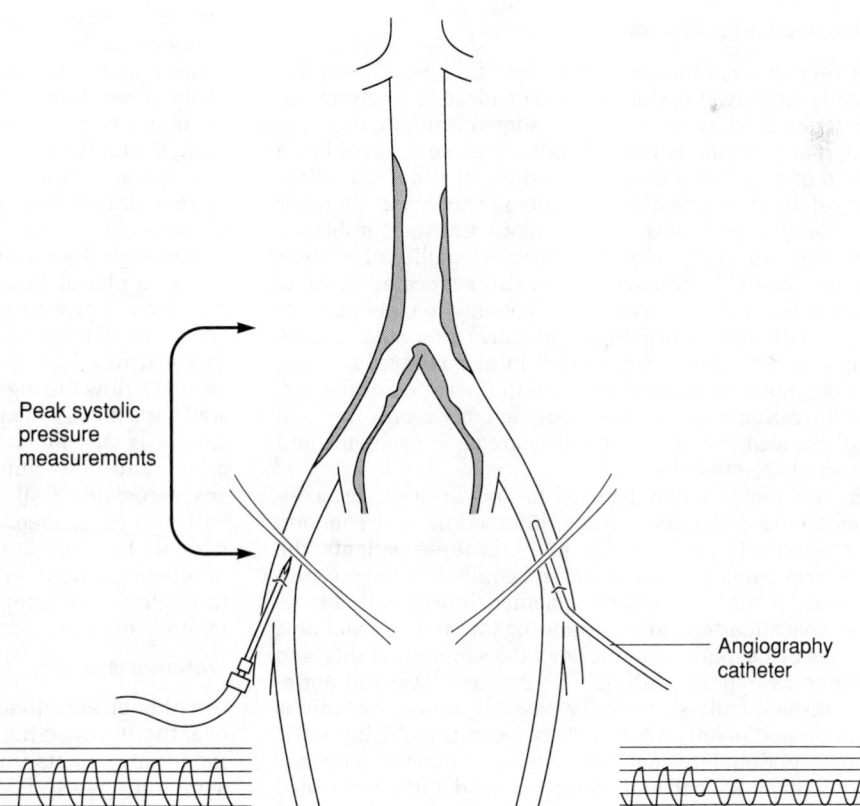

Figure 84-9. Femoral artery pressure measurement to assess hemodynamic significance of aortoiliac disease. A significant decrease in peak systolic pressure is recorded on the left as the catheter is withdrawn across the diseased segment in the left iliac arterial system.

Peak systolic pressure measurements

Angiography catheter

of endarterectomy or grafting with exclusion of the segment may be advisable.

Procedure Selection

A variety of operative approaches and methods are available for the management of aortoiliac disease. In each instance, the decision of what procedure is best in a particular patient is based on the general condition of the patient, the extent and distribution of occlusive disease, and the experience and training of the surgeon. Methods of direct bilateral aortoiliac reconstruction, usually employing prosthetic bypass grafts, offer the most successful and durable results. Remote (extraanatomic) procedures are generally reserved for the relatively small group of patients with concomitant serious medical problems, most often advanced coronary disease, which places them at high risk for conventional anatomic reconstruction. Remote procedures may also be employed in circumstances of infection or other problems creating a "hostile abdomen" that may hamper standard, direct operation. Finally, more limited procedures may be employed for truly unilateral iliac disease if clinical considerations or patient condition suggest that such an approach may be most prudent.

In addition to the anatomic distribution and extent of occlusive disease, careful assessment of patient risk is generally the most important consideration in selecting the most appropriate operative procedure. Preoperative evaluation of pulmonary and renal function is routine. Evaluation of cardiac status, particularly ischemic heart disease secondary to associated atherosclerotic coronary artery disease, is most important because coronary artery disease is the major cause of both early and late death after aortic operations. In patients with aortoiliac disease, the incidence of coronary artery disease exceeds 50% and may be asymptomatic in 10% to 20% of patients.[9]

Direct Aortic Reconstruction

Aortoiliac Endarterectomy

Although aortoiliac endarterectomy (Fig. 84-10) was frequently employed in the early era of aortic reconstruction, it is rarely used by most vascular surgeons in practice. The principal potential benefit of endarterectomy is avoidance of use of prosthetic grafts, with their possible complications of dilation, infection, anastomotic aneurysm, or other degenerative problems. These are all unusual problems, however, especially with the improved quality of modern vascular grafts. Endarterectomy is also advocated by some as more likely to improve sexual potency in male patients by more directly improving hypogastric artery blood flow. This has not been demonstrated in any study, however, and the more extensive dissection in the region of the aortic bifurcation required in endarterectomy seems likely to result in a higher incidence of neurogenic problems and retrograde ejaculation.

Endarterectomy may be used for localized disease confined to the distal aorta, aortic bifurcation, and common iliac arteries (type I, see Fig. 83-7). In these patients, the long-term patency is excellent and equivalent to graft procedures.[1] It has been well documented, however, that more extensive endarterectomy extending into the external iliac arteries or beyond does not have the same durability and patency as bypass grafting.[1,10,11] Because localized aortoiliac disease truly suitable for possible endarterectomy is encountered in only 5% to 10% of patients requiring aortic reconstruction, most patients with more extensive disease are not amendable to endarterectomy and are better treated by graft insertion.

In addition, in the past decade, use of percutaneous transluminal angioplasty, atherectomy, stent insertion, and other "less invasive" endovascular procedures has increasingly replaced surgical correction of such localized disease. Finally, endarterectomy is acknowledged to be a technically demanding procedure. Most vascular surgeons trained within the past 15 to 20 years have little or no training and experience with this technique.

Endarterectomy is also contraindicated in several other circumstances. Any evidence of aneurysmal change in the aorta makes endarterectomy ill advised because of possible continued aneurysmal degeneration of the endarterectomized segment. Second, if extensive occlusive disease extends superiorly close to the level of the renal arteries, transsection of the aorta close to the renal vessels with thromboendarterectomy of the aortic cuff below the clamp followed by graft insertion is easier, faster, and more definitive.

Endarterectomy remains useful for a small number of patients with localized disease, particularly young patients with a projected life-span of 20 to 30 years in whom a higher incidence of possible graft-related problems might be anticipated, or in patients who might have an increased risk of infection with a nonautogenous reconstruction.

Aortobifemoral Bypass Grafts

Prosthetic bypass grafting from the infrarenal aorta to femoral arteries (Fig. 84-11) is the most frequently used reconstructive procedure for aortoiliac occlusive disease and offers the most effective and durable method of revascularization available.

The proximal aortic anastomosis may be either end-to-end or end-to-side. End-to-end anastomosis is clearly indicated in patients with coexisting aneurysmal disease or complete aortic occlusion up to the renal arteries. It is also preferred by many surgeons for routine use in most cases because of perceived better long-term patency, although there have been no randomized or controlled series. End-to-side proximal anastomosis appears advantageous if the surgeon wishes to preserve a patent inferior mesenteric artery or sizable accessory renal artery, or if the anatomic pattern of disease suggests that end-to-end bypass will likely devascularize both hypogastric arteries and hence the pelvic region (Fig. 84-12). Irrespective of the technique used, the important principle is to place the proximal anastomosis as high as possible in the infrarenal aorta, where there is almost always a lesser amount of occlusive disease, to minimize the incidence of recurrent difficulties.

Although the distal anastomosis of the graft may sometimes be placed in the external iliac artery in the pelvis, it is almost always preferable in patients with aortoiliac occlusive disease to carry the graft to the femoral level. The fear of a higher incidence of infection if grafts were carried below the inguinal ligament has not been substantiated by extensive experience. At the femoral level, exposure is usually much better, the anastomosis is technically easier, and most important, assessment and correction of any associated profunda origin disease are most expediently accomplished. Because such a high percentage of patients have associated occlusive disease of the femoropopliteal segment, establishment of adequate graft outflow through the profunda femoris artery (Fig. 84-13) is of paramount importance in both early and late results.[1,4,5,11]

Iliofemoral Grafts

Although aortoiliac disease is generally a diffuse process eventually involving both iliac arteries, it is not uncommon that patients initially present with largely unilateral symptoms, with a fairly normal femoral pulse and minimal to no clinical symptoms in the contralateral leg. If arteriog-

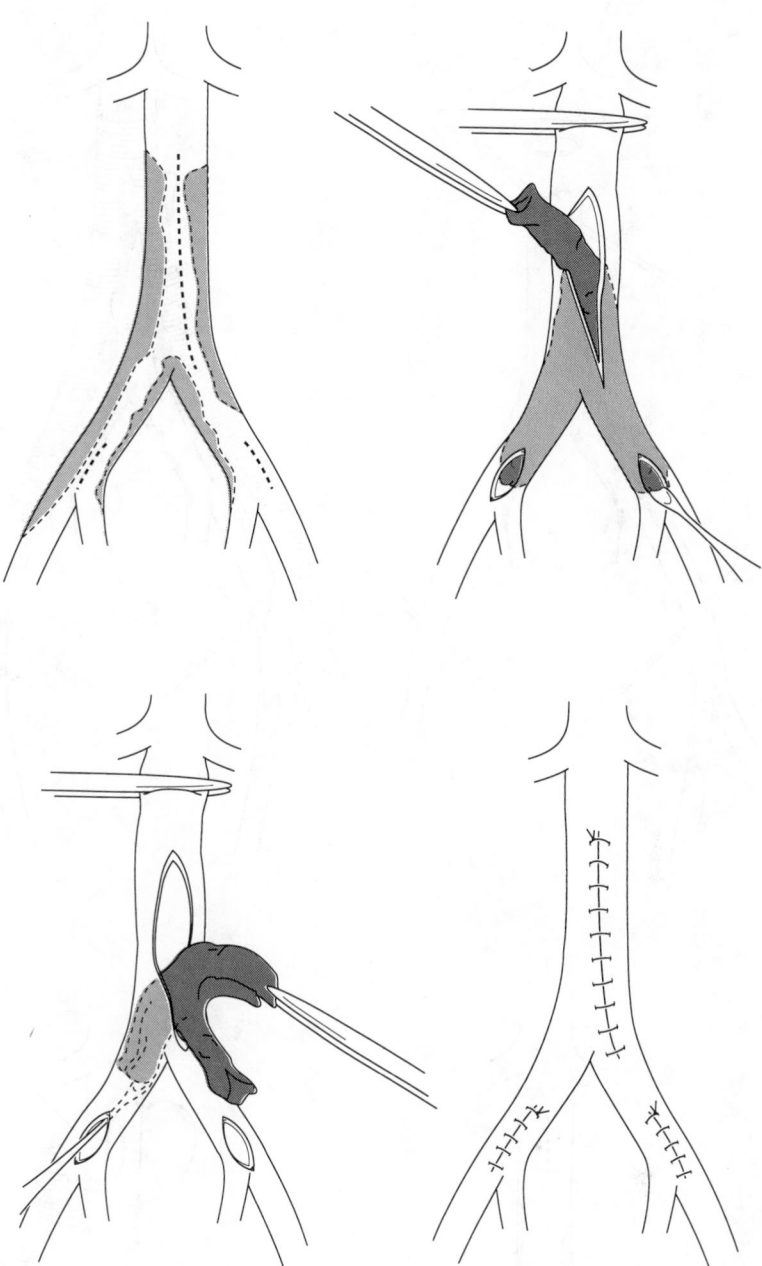

Figure 84-10. Aortoiliac endarterectomy.

raphy confirms largely unilateral iliac disease, more limited arterial reconstruction by means of an iliofemoral bypass may be considered.

Ipsilateral iliofemoral grafts are useful principally for patients with disease confined to the external iliac artery of the symptomatic extremity, with a fairly good common iliac artery that can be used for proximal graft anastomosis. A retroperitoneal approach through an oblique lower abdominal incision (Fig. 84-14) provides good exposure and can be carried out with low morbidity. The advantages of iliofemoral grafts are that they provide a direct in-line reconstruction with potentially better late patency rates than indirect extraanatomic (femorofemoral) grafts, do not involve procedures on the asymptomatic iliofemoral system, and carry less morbidity and mortality risk than conventional aortobifemoral grafts. As such, iliofemoral grafts are a useful and effective alternative in appropriate patients.[12]

Concern regarding the possible progression of disease in the contralateral untreated iliac system requiring later reoperation has led many authorities to regard aortobifemoral grafts as the definitive reconstruction option, even in patients with mostly unilateral iliac disease, particularly in younger, good-risk patients.[13] The frequency with which such progression has required reoperation has been cited to be as high as 30% to 40% of patients, but several reports suggest that this occurs in only about 10% of patients.[14]

Indirect Revascularization Methods

Bypass grafting that uses significantly different anatomic pathways than the native vessels the grafts are meant to replace was originally devised as a compromise procedure for unusual or frequently desperate clinical problems such as infection or serious complications of aortoiliac reconstruction. Within a short time, their potential application for revascularization in patients at potentially prohibitive

(text continues on page 1808)

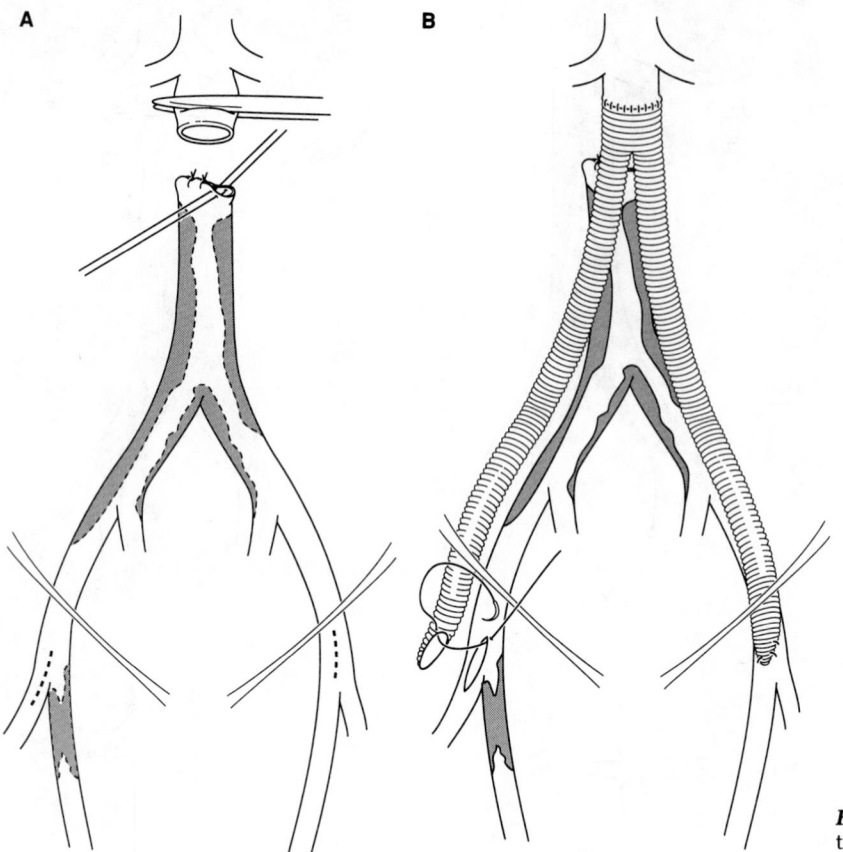

Figure 84-11. Aortobifemoral graft reconstruction. (*A*) Oversewing distal aorta. (*B*) Proximal end-to-end anastomosis.

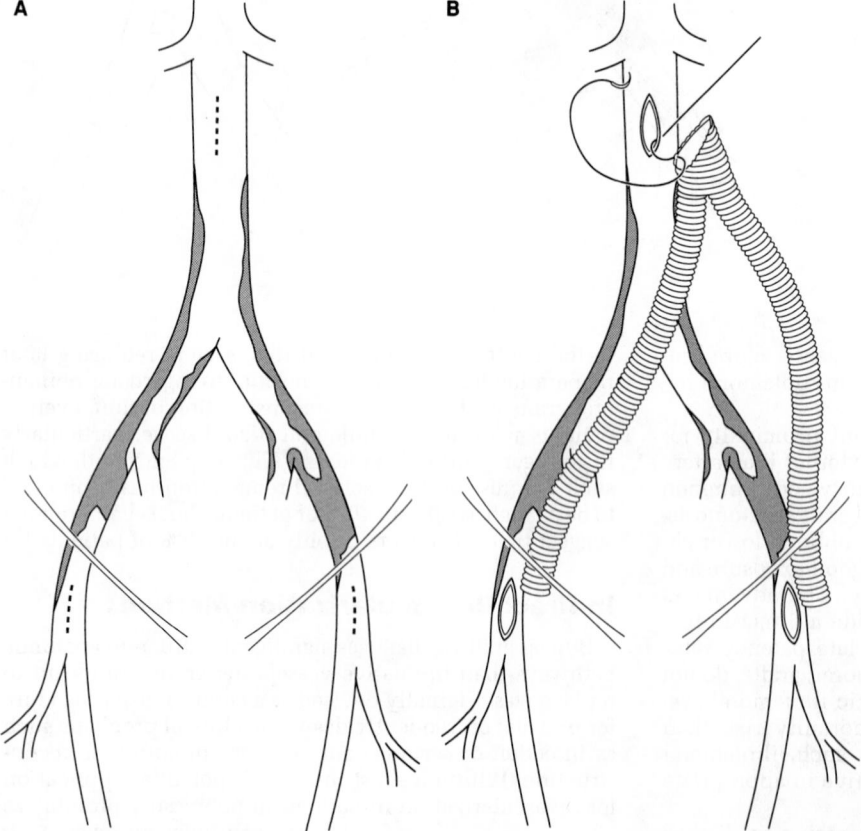

Figure 84-12. (*A*) Anatomic circumstances favoring end-to-side aortic anastomosis include large accessory renal arteries arising from the lower aorta, an enlarged patent inferior mesenteric artery, or occlusive disease confined largely to external iliac arteries that precludes retrograde pelvic perfusion. (*B*) Both proximal and distal anastomoses are end to side.

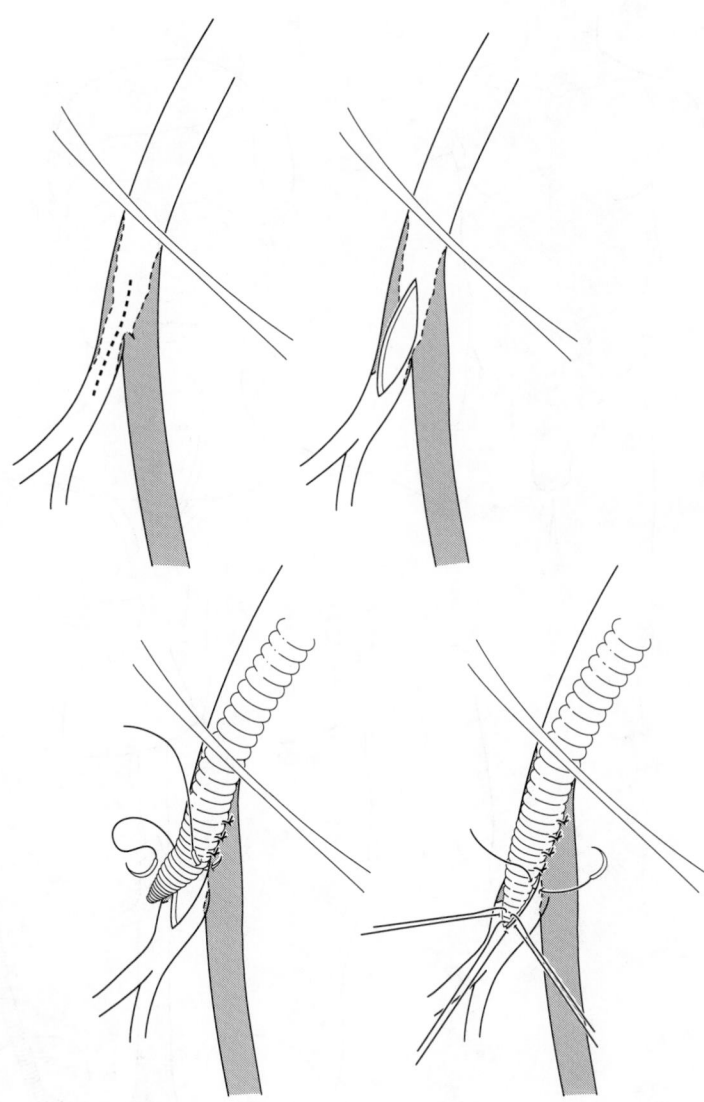

Figure 84-13. In patients with multilevel disease, runoff through the profunda femoris artery is essential. Any disease of profunda origin should be corrected by endarterectomy or by extending the tongue of the beveled graft tip into the profunda beyond the stenosis.

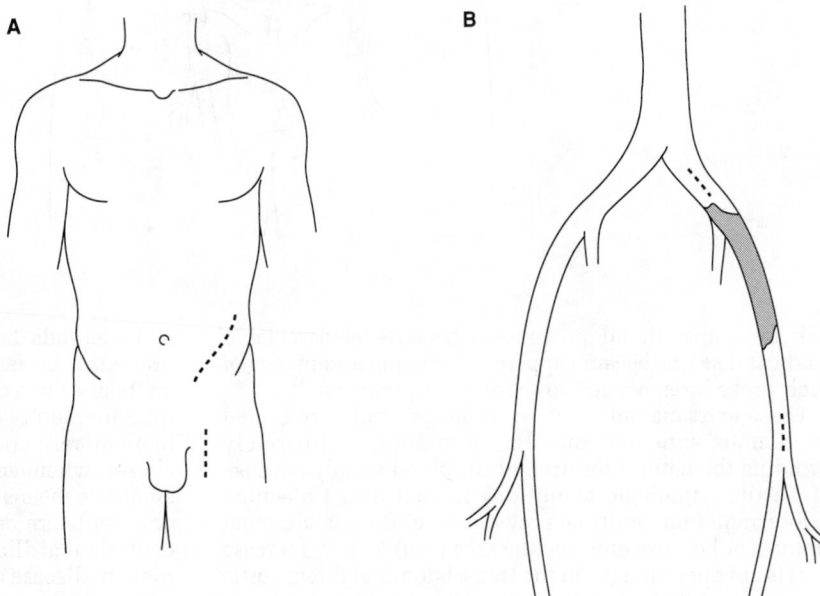

Figure 84-14. Iliofemoral bypass is applicable for unilateral iliac disease confined largely to the ipsilateral external iliac artery. (*A*) Skin incision for retroperitoneal approach. (*B*) Typical lesion producing ischemic symptoms.

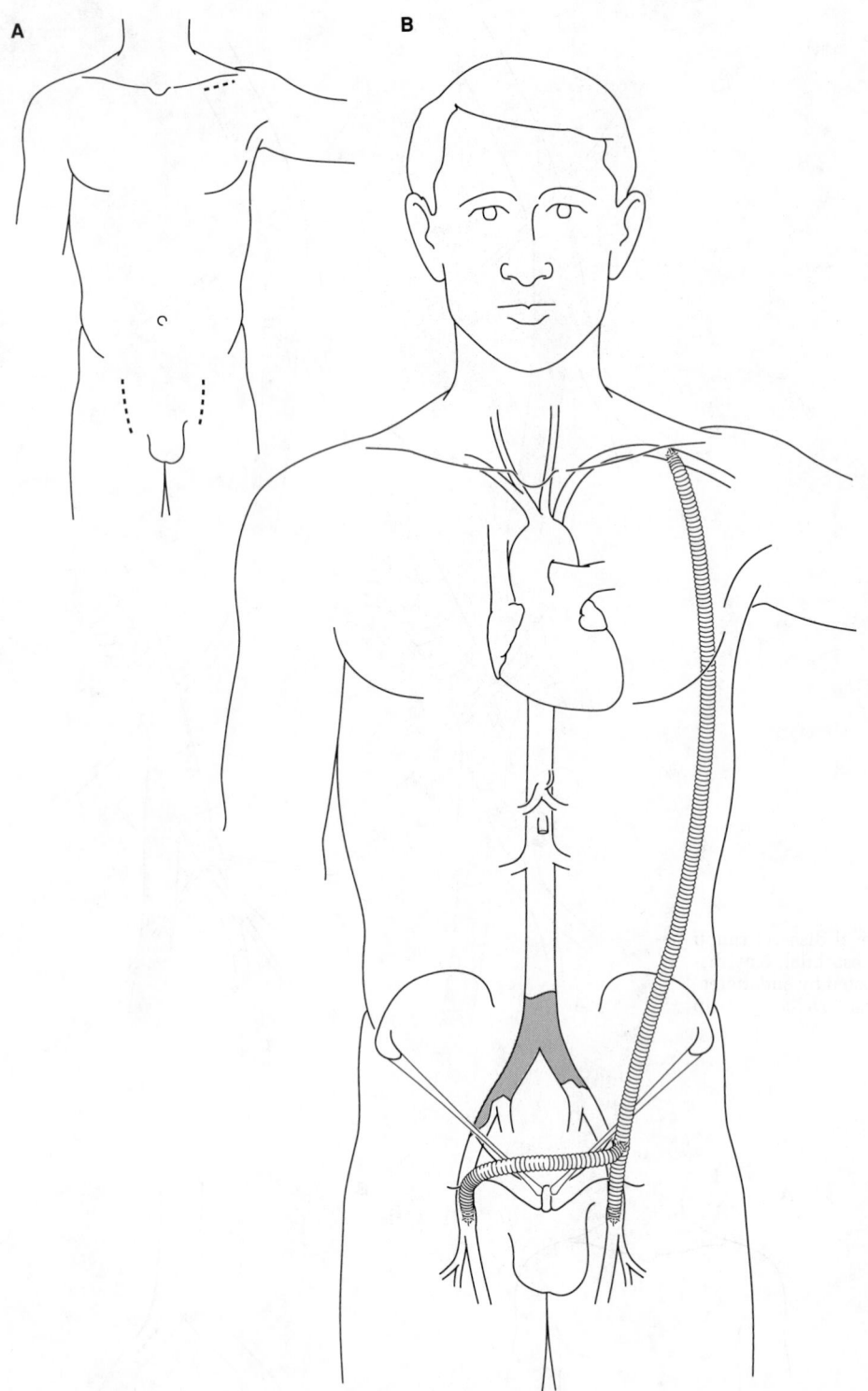

Figure 84-15. Extraanatomic methods of revascularization in aortoiliac disease. (*A*) Skin incisions for axillobifemoral bypass. (*B*) Completed bypass. (*C*) Skin incisions for femorofemoral bypass. (*D*) Completed bypass.

(continues)

risk for conventional procedures because of associated medical diseases became apparent. Growing acceptance of such procedures has led to more widespread use.[15]

These extraanatomic bypass grafts generally are routed in remote subcutaneous tissue planes, deliberately avoiding the natural location of the blood supply because of hostile pathologic conditions in that area (infection, prior irradiation, multiple previous operations, abdominal stomas) or because entering the area would likely increase the risk of operation (as in the transabdominal direct aortic approach). Although a large number of ingenious routes

and methods have been described for different clinical problems, by far the most frequently used extraanatomic grafts are the axillofemoral and femorofemoral bypass, or their frequently employed combination, the so-called axillobifemoral bypass (Fig. 84-15). Axillobifemoral grafts are chosen whenever bilateral iliac disease requires an extraanatomic means of inflow restoration, whereas femorofemoral grafts are employed for unilateral iliac disease if the contralateral iliac artery is free of hemodynamically significant disease and can adequately serve as a donor inflow source. If disease in the contralateral iliac artery is focal,

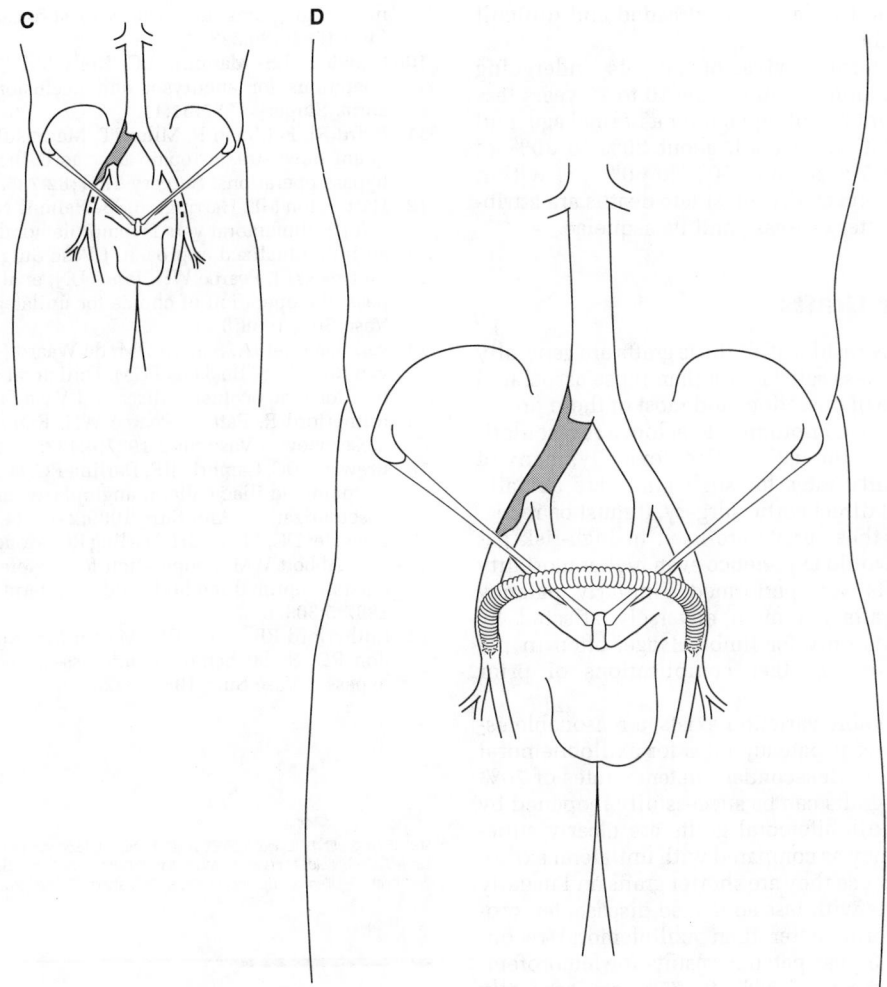

Figure 84-15. *(Continued)*

percutaneous transluminal balloon angioplasty on this side may be carried out to establish adequate inflow for a femorofemoral graft.[16] Femorofemoral grafts are also believed by many vascular surgeons to be a most expedient and successful method of managing occlusion of one limb of an aortobifemoral graft that cannot be successfully reopened by thrombectomy.[17]

RESULTS OF AORTOILIAC SURGICAL REVASCULARIZATION

Direct Reconstruction

Excellent early and late results of anatomic aortoiliofemoral operations can be anticipated, at acceptable patient morbidity and mortality rates. Most large series in the modern era clearly document that it is reasonable to expect about 85% to 90% 5-year graft patency rates and 70% to 75% 10-year patency rates.[1-4] Perioperative mortality rates well below 5% are now uniformly achieved, with many experienced centers reporting operative mortality of only 1% to 2%. Mortality risks for direct reconstruction in patients with relatively localized aortoiliac disease can be expected to be extremely low, whereas those patients with more widespread, multilevel disease have somewhat higher mortality risks, as would be expected from their greater age and more frequent associated atherosclerotic disease in coronary, carotid, and visceral vessels.

In patients with relatively localized disease, successful direct reconstructive procedures afford relief of symptoms in nearly all patients. Because most operative candidates have more diffuse multilevel disease, symptom relief may be incomplete in 25% to 30% of patients.[4,5,18]

Major early complications of direct aortic operation occur in 5% to 10% of patients. Many are largely technical in nature and therefore infrequent with an experienced surgeon and operating team. Bleeding that requires reoperation or acute limb ischemia secondary to graft thrombosis or distal thromboembolism are each encountered in 1% to 2% of patients. Acute renal failure is infrequent with recognition of the importance of provision of adequate fluid volume during surgery, optimization of cardiac function intraoperatively, and avoidance of declamping hypotension. Spinal cord and bowel ischemia are much more difficult to predict but fortunately are rare occurrences. Nonfatal myocardial infarction is noted in about 3% to 5% of patients, often with little hemodynamic compromise. Significant pulmonary insufficiency is unusual in the absence of severe preoperative chronic lung disease.

The frequency of late complications depends largely on the length of follow-up. During a 10-year period, 10% to 20% of patients may experience occlusion of a graft limb.[17] Anastomotic aneurysm is the second most common late complication of aortic graft insertion, seen in 3% to 5% of patients, almost always at the femoral anastomosis. Graft infection and enteric fistula remain dreaded and difficult late problems, but they are infrequent.

Cumulative long-term survival of patients undergoing aortoiliac reconstruction remains some 10 to 15 years less than that which might be anticipated for a normal age- and sex-matched population. Overall, about 20% to 30% of patients die within 5 years, and 50% to 60% die within 10 years.[2,3,6] Not unexpectedly, most late deaths are attributable to coronary artery disease and its sequelae.

Extraanatomic Grafts

Long-term patency results of all these grafts are generally acknowledged to be less satisfactory than those associated with direct methods of operation, and most of these procedures are selected as a compromise to achieve revascularization at lower risk to the patient. Paradoxically, many of the reported mortality rates for such grafts are actually higher than those of direct aortic surgery. It must be recognized that most of these grafts are used in high-risk patients, who clearly would experience even higher mortality if aortofemoral grafts were performed. Similarly, patency results of these grafts are often adversely affected by use of such methods only for limb salvage, often in patients with infection or other complications of prior reconstruction.

Although considerable variation exists, a reasonable estimate of primary 5-year patency rates for axillobifemoral grafts is about 50%, with secondary patency rates of 70% to 75% if occluded grafts can be successfully reopened by thrombectomy.[15] Axillobifemoral grafts are clearly superior in terms of patency as compared with unilateral axillofemoral bypass. Because they are shorter grafts and usually employed in patients with less advanced disease, femorofemoral grafts perform better than axillofemoral reconstructions. Primary 5-year patency results for femorofemoral grafts in the range of 65% to 75% are generally reported.[15] For all results of extraanatomic grafts, detailed breakdown of results according to indication and runoff explains the wide variance of reported results and provides a better perspective of their application in different clinical settings.[15]

REFERENCES

1. Brewster DC, Darling RC. Optimal methods of aortoiliac reconstruction. Surgery 1978;84:739.
2. Crawford ES, Bomberger RA, Glaeser DH, Saleh SA, Russell LL. Aortoiliac occlusive disease: factors influencing survival and function following reconstructive operation over a 25-year period. Surgery 1981;90:1055.
3. Szilagyi DE, Elliott JP Jr, Smith RF, Reddy DJ, McPharlin M. A 30-year survey of the reconstructive surgical treatment of aortoiliac occlusive disease. J Vasc Surg 1984;3:421.
4. Malone JM, Moore WS, Goldstone J. The natural history of bilateral aortofemoral bypass grafts for ischemia of the lower extremities. Arch Surg 1975;110:1300.
5. Brewster DC, Perler BA, Robison JG, Darling RC. Aortofemoral graft for multilevel occlusive disease: predictors of success and need for distal bypass. Arch Surg 1982;117:1593.
6. Malone JM, Moore WS, Goldstone J. Life expectancy following aortofemoral arterial grafting. Surgery 1977;81:551.
7. Cambria RP, Yucel EK, Brewster DC, et al. The potential for lower extremity revascularization without contrast arteriography: experience with magnetic resonance angiography. J Vasc Surg 1993;17:1050.
8. Flanigan DP, Williams LR, Schwartz JA, Schauler JJ, Gray B. Hemodynamic evaluation of the aortoiliac system based on pharmacologic vasodilatation. Surgery 1983;93:709.
9. Hertzer NR, Beven EG, Young JR, et al. Coronary artery disease in peripheral vascular patients: a classification of 1000 coronary angiograms and results of surgical management. Ann Surg 1984;199:223.
10. Crawford ES, Manning LG, Kelly TF. "Redo" surgery after operations for aneurysm and occlusion of the abdominal aorta. Surgery 1977;81:41.
11. Baird RJ, Feldman P, Miles JT, Madras PM, Gurry JF. Subsequent downstream repair after aorta-iliac and aorta-femoral bypass operations. Surgery 1977;82:785.
12. Harrington ME, Harrington EB, Haimov N, Schanger H, Jacobson JH. Iliofemoral versus femorofemoral bypass: the case for an individualized approach. J Vasc Surg 1992;16:841.
13. Piotrowski J, Pearce WH, Jones DN, et al. Aortobifemoral bypass: the operation of choice for unilateral iliac occlusion? J Vasc Surg 1988;8:211.
14. van der Vliet JA, Scharn DM, de Waard J-WD, Roumen RMH, van Roye SFS, Buskens FGM. Unilateral vascular reconstruction for iliac occlusive disease. J Vasc Surg 1994;19:610.
15. Rutherford R, Patt A, Pearce WH. Extra-anatomic bypass: a closer view. J Vasc Surg 1987;6:437.
16. Brewster DC, Cambria RP, Darling RC, et al. Long-term results of combined iliac balloon angioplasty and distal surgical revascularization. Ann Surg 1989;210:324.
17. Brewster DC, Meier GH, Darling RC, Moncure AC, LaMuraglia GM, Abbott WM. Reoperation for aortofemoral graft limb occlusion: optimal methods and long-term results. J Vasc Surg 1987;5:303.
18. Rutherford RB, Jones DN, Martin MS, Kempczinski RF, Gordon RD. Serial hemodynamic assessment of aortobifemoral bypass. J Vasc Surg 1984;4:428.

SURGERY: SCIENTIFIC PRINCIPLES AND PRACTICE, Second Edition, edited by Lazar J. Greenfield, Michael W. Mulholland, Keith T. Oldham, Gerald B. Zelenock, and Keith D. Lillemoe. Lippincott–Raven Publishers, Philadelphia, © 1997.

CHAPTER 85

FEMOROPOPLITEAL AND INFRAPOPLITEAL OCCLUSIVE DISEASE

LLOYD M. TAYLOR, JR., JOHN M. PORTER, AND PHILIPPE A. MASSER

Symptomatic lower extremity ischemia is frequently encountered in the aging population, and patients with generalized cardiovascular disease, diabetes, and renal failure are particularly likely to have lower extremity arterial occlusive disease. Each year, 100,000 operations for lower extremity revascularization and an estimated 50,000 major lower extremity amputations are performed in the United States. Clearly lower extremity ischemia represents a major health problem. This chapter discusses lower extremity ischemia caused by atherosclerotic disease below the inguinal ligament and addresses the relevant anatomy, pathophysiology, and natural history as well as diagnostic evaluation and nonoperative and operative treatment.

ANATOMY

The common femoral artery begins at the inguinal ligament as the direct extension of the external iliac artery. It lies midway between the anterosuperior iliac spine and the symphysis pubis (Fig. 85-1). In the proximal thigh, the common femoral artery is superficial, covered by skin and subcutaneous tissue; the femoral nerve is lateral to the artery and the femoral vein is medial. Between 2 and 5 cm below the inguinal ligament, the common femoral artery divides into the more lateral and posterior deep femoral artery and the more medial superficial femoral artery. The medial and lateral circumflex femoral arteries, as well as four to six perforating muscular arteries to the upper thigh, normally originate from the deep femoral artery, which terminates in the middle thigh.

The superficial femoral artery continues anteromedially beneath the sartorius muscle. In the middle third of the thigh, it enters the adductor (Hunter) canal, which is an aponeurotic tunnel formed by fascial contributions from the vastus medialis, adductor longus, and adductor mag-

nus muscles. The popliteal artery emerges from the adductor canal and proceeds posteriorly behind the knee between the lateral and medial heads of the gastrocnemius muscle. The popliteal artery divides into two major branches just distal to the knee. The first is the anterior tibial artery, which passes laterally, pierces the interosseous membrane between the tibia and fibula, and lies anterior to this membrane in the anterior compartment of the calf, eventually terminating in the foot as the dorsalis pedis artery. The tibial-peroneal trunk is the direct continuation of the popliteal artery and quickly divides into the posterior tibial and peroneal arteries. The posterior tibial artery continues distally in the calf behind the tibia, entering the foot between the medial malleolus and the Achilles tendon, where it divides into the medial and lateral plantar arteries. The peroneal artery courses deep in the substance of the calf, descending along the medial aspect of the fibula, and ends in terminal branches above the ankle. All three vessels supply the calf, with the anterior tibial and posterior tibial arteries continuing onto the foot as its primary blood supply.

COLLATERAL CIRCULATION

The superficial femoral artery is the artery in the leg most likely to be obstructed by atherosclerosis with the popliteal, deep femoral, common femoral, and calf arteries involved less frequently. Atherosclerotic disease in diabetics is distributed slightly more distally, frequently with primary involvement of the popliteal and calf arteries. Arterial collaterals become important and occur by enlargement of preexisting arterial connections, rather than by growth of new vessels when obstruction of the major arteries prevents normal lower extremity blood flow.

When the common femoral artery is obstructed, collateral circulation to the upper thigh occurs through the internal pudendal and obturator branches of the internal iliac artery as well as through the deep circumflex and inferior epigastric branches of the external iliac artery (Fig. 85-2).

When the superficial femoral artery is obstructed, the popliteal artery is supplied from the branches of the profunda femoris artery, the lateral femoral circumflex, and a number of muscular perforating branches. Occlusion of the popliteal artery leads to filling of the tibial vessels by the medial and lateral geniculate arteries. The peroneal artery fills an important collateral bed with reconstitution of the plantar arch when the dorsal pedal and posterior tibial arteries are obstructed at the ankle.

PATHOPHYSIOLOGY

The redundant collateral arterial circulation of the lower extremity described earlier means that atherosclerotic obstruction of leg arteries is well tolerated, at least initially. Resting blood flow in the lower extremity must increase 2- to 10-fold in response to exercise. Specific muscle blood flow may increase as much as 100-fold. The profound increase in muscle blood flow induced by exercise results from a profound decrease in arterial resistance in exercising muscle which occurs in response to complex neurohumoral stimuli. Moderate arterial obstruction produces no change in resting flow but restricts the ability of arterial flow to increase normally in response to exercise. The clinical result of this restriction is called *intermittent claudication*, which is defined as lower extremity muscular pain occurring with exercise and relieved by short periods of rest (minutes). The site of the symptoms is always one level

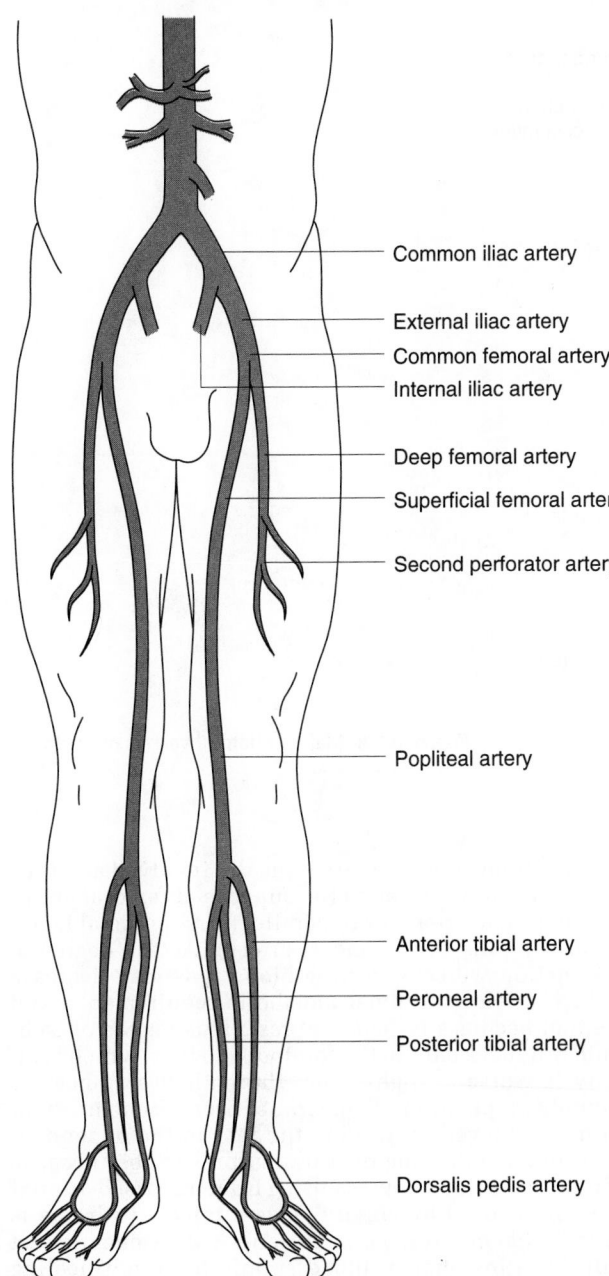

Common iliac artery

External iliac artery
Common femoral artery
Internal iliac artery

Deep femoral artery

Superficial femoral artery

Second perforator artery

Popliteal artery

Anterior tibial artery

Peroneal artery

Posterior tibial artery

Dorsalis pedis artery

Figure 85-1. Anatomy of the arterial circulation to the lower extremity.

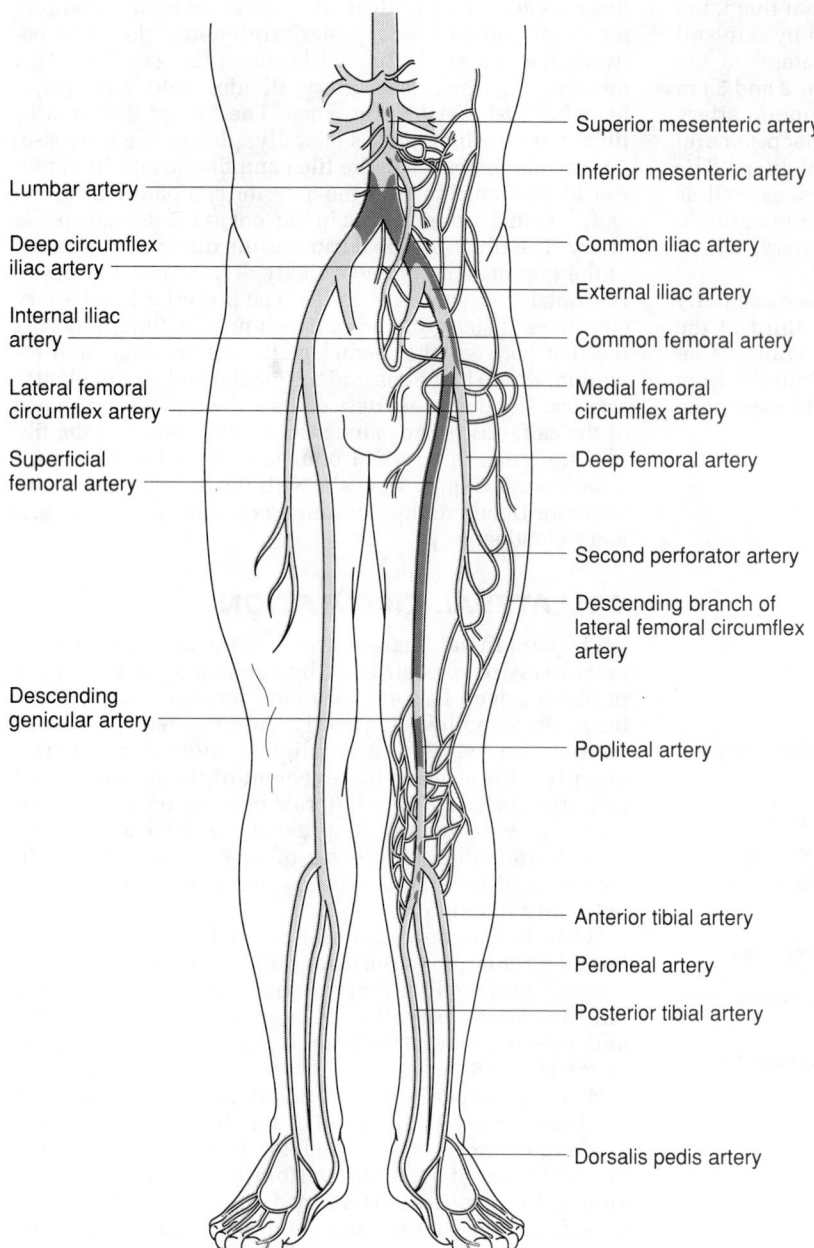

Figure 85-2. Major collateral vessels of the lower extremity.

Labels (clockwise):
Superior mesenteric artery
Inferior mesenteric artery
Common iliac artery
External iliac artery
Common femoral artery
Medial femoral circumflex artery
Deep femoral artery
Second perforator artery
Descending branch of lateral femoral circumflex artery
Popliteal artery
Anterior tibial artery
Peroneal artery
Posterior tibial artery
Dorsalis pedis artery

Lumbar artery
Deep circumflex iliac artery
Internal iliac artery
Lateral femoral circumflex artery
Superficial femoral artery
Descending genicular artery

distal to the site of arterial obstruction, that is, superficial femoral artery obstruction in the thigh produces calf claudication. Most patients with intermittent claudication have lower extremity arterial obstruction at a single site (Table 85-1).

As atherosclerotic disease becomes more severe, the lower extremity arteries are typically involved at multiple levels either in series (ie, superficial femoral artery plus popliteal artery) or in parallel (ie, superficial femoral artery plus deep femoral artery). As the degree of obstruction worsens, resting blood flow may decrease to levels below minimal metabolic requirements, and the foot becomes ischemic at rest. This degree of ischemia produces pain in the forefoot and toes, which typically is worse at night when the patient assumes the recumbent position. Some relief from ischemic foot pain is achieved by placing the foot in the dependent position, as in sitting or walking, presumably because of increased blood flow resulting from increased arterial pressure caused by gravity. This clinical syndrome is called *ischemic rest pain.* Patients with ischemic rest pain have insufficient blood supply to permit healing of minor traumatic lesions, such as cuts, scrapes, and bruises. These lesions are then referred to as *ischemic ulcers.* As resting blood flow levels decrease even fur-

Table 85-1. SYMPTOMS PRODUCED BY ARTERIAL OBSTRUCTION IN THE LOWER EXTREMITY

Symptom	Site of Arterial Obstruction	Ankle/Brachial Pressure Ratio
Claudication	Single level	>0.5
Ischemic ulcer	Multiple level	0.3–0.5
Gangrene	Multiple level	<0.3

Table 85-2. SURVIVAL RATES FOR PATIENTS WITH CHRONIC LOWER EXTREMITY ISCHEMIA

Investigator	Patients	Mean Follow-Up (y)	Survival Rate (%) 5 y	10 y	15 y
Bloor, 1961	1476	7	79	54	—
		72	35	—	—
		60	20	—	—
Silbert, 1958	1198	12	94.7	71	52
Kallero, 1981	193	9.7	—	52	—
Schadt, 1961	362	9	76	59	—
Leferve, 1959	500	5	57	—	—
Hansteen, 1975	307	8–16	70	50	37
Crawford, 1981	949	0–25	74	50	30
Szilagyi, 1986	1648	0–30	70	64	25
Hertzer, 1981	256	6–11	80	60	—
Malone, 1977	180	0–15	80	43	26
Veith, 1981	551	5	48	—	—
Edwards, 1990	82	2	12	—	0

ther, spontaneous necrosis of the distal toes and forefoot occurs, giving rise to *gangrene*.

NATURAL HISTORY OF INFRAINGUINAL ATHEROSCLEROSIS

Considerable published experience and traditional teaching assign a relatively benign prognosis to intermittent claudication with fewer than one fourth of claudicant persons experiencing significant worsening leading to the need for vascular surgical repair. Less than 10% ever require ischemic limb amputation. Patients with ischemic rest pain, ischemic ulcers, and gangrene, however, have traditionally been considered to have a uniformly poor prognosis, with amputation the inevitable result unless the ischemia is relieved by surgical revascularization. Recent experience suggests that arbitrarily assigning patients to one of two prognostic categories based on symptoms alone is inappropriate. The presence and severity of lower extremity ischemia are more readily and accurately assessed by quantitative means noninvasively, and the prognosis for chronic lower extremity ischemia is more closely related to the results of objective testing than to subjective description of symptoms. Thus, patients with

claudication and an ankle/brachial arterial pressure index (ABI) of less than 0.5 are about 3.5 times more likely to require revascularization than those with a higher ABI. Multiple studies have demonstrated that the outcomes for patients with chronic lower extremity ischemia can be predicted most accurately by the severity of disease, as assessed by simple ankle blood pressure measurement. Revascularization is rarely necessary and amputation is virtually unheard of in patients with ABIs greater than or equal to 0.55, whereas one of these outcomes is close to inevitable for patients with ABIs less than 0.3.

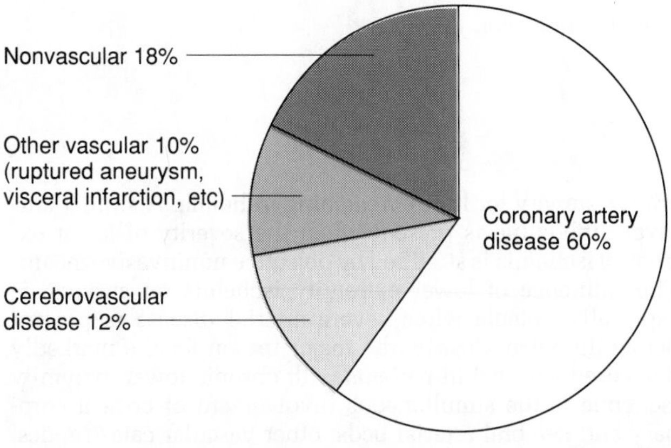

Nonvascular 18%

Other vascular 10% (ruptured aneurysm, visceral infarction, etc)

Cerebrovascular disease 12%

Coronary artery disease 60%

Figure 85-3. Causes of death in patients with chronic lower extremity ischemia. (After Taylor LM Jr. Porter JM. Natural history and nonoperative treatment of chronic lower extremity ischemia. In: Rutherford RB, ed. Vascular surgery, ed 3. Philadelphia, WB Saunders, 1989:653)

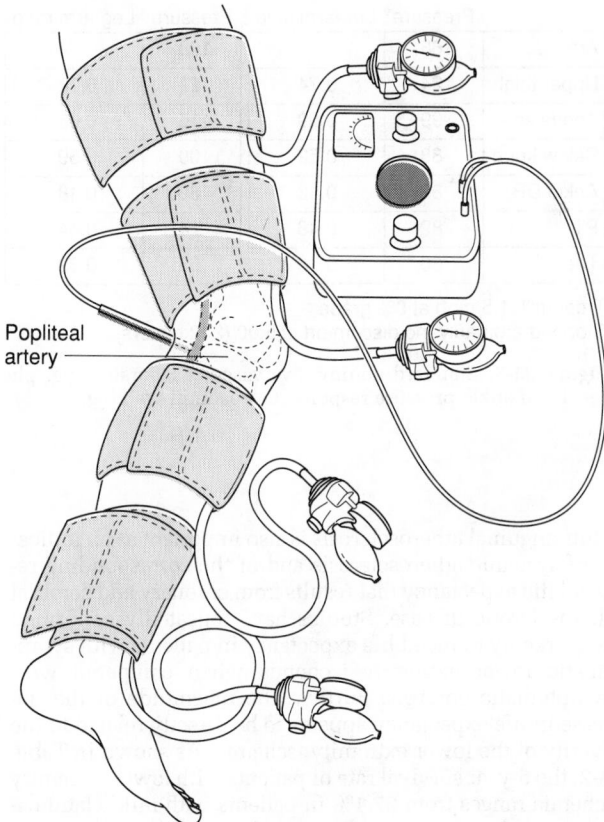

Popliteal artery

Figure 85-4. Technique of segmental pressure measurements using a Doppler ultrasonic flow detector.

Peripheral arterial examination

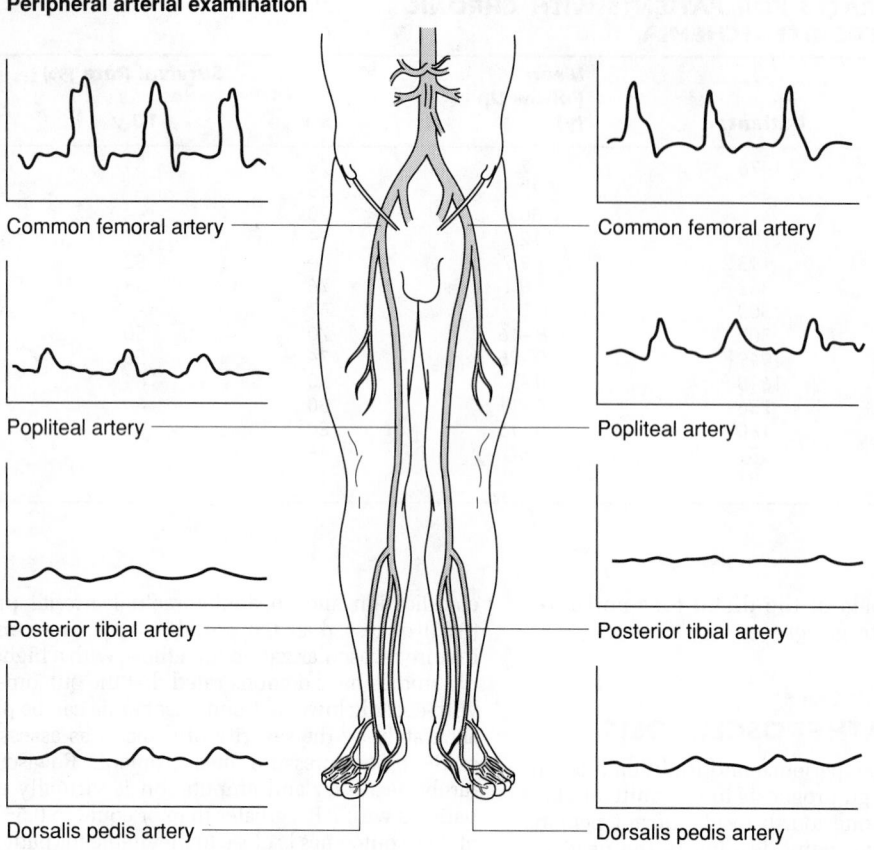

Resting segmental blood pressures

	Right		Left	
	Pressure	Leg/arm ratio	Pressure	Leg/arm ratio
Arm	168		168	
Upper thigh	124	0.74	127	0.76
Above knee	99	0.59	115	0.68
Below knee	88	0.52	100	0.59
Ankle DP	82	0.48	80	0.48
PT	82	0.48	74	0.44
Toe	60	0.36	66	0.39

Treadmill: 1.5 mph at 0% grade
Stopped arbitrarily; no discomfort at 5:00 (202 meters)

Right

Arm	165	150	156	150
Ankle	50	65	70	72

Left

Arm				
Ankle	98	90	60	90

Figure 85-5. Standard noninvasive vascular laboratory peripheral arterial examination includes results of ankle pressure response to treadmill walking.

Infrainguinal atherosclerosis is also important as an indicator of systemic atherosclerosis and of the corresponding reduced life expectancy that results from coronary and cerebral atherosclerotic disease. Studies have repeatedly confirmed the markedly reduced life expectancy in patients with symptomatic lower extremity ischemia when compared with asymptomatic controls. Further, the magnitude of the decrease in life expectancy appears to be directly related to the severity of the lower extremity ischemia. As shown in Table 85-2, the 5-year survival rate of patients with lower extremity ischemia ranges from 97.4% in patients with mild claudication treated nonoperatively, to 80% in patients requiring operation for claudication, to 48% in patients with limb-threatening ischemia, to only 12% in patients requiring reop-

erative surgery for limb-threatening ischemia. A similar survival differential is present when the severity of lower extremity ischemia is stratified by objective noninvasive means. The influence of lower extremity ischemia on survival is especially notable when severe arterial disease is present below the knee. Clearly, the major reason for the markedly decreased survival in patients with chronic lower extremity ischemia is the simultaneous involvement of critical coronary and cerebral arterial beds; other vascular catastrophes, including ruptured aneurysm and visceral infarction (Fig. 85-3), are also important. Awareness of the significantly diminished anticipated life-span in patients with symptomatic lower extremity atherosclerosis is important to selecting optimal therapy.

Table 85-3. IMPROVEMENT IN WALKING DISTANCE RESULTING FROM EXERCISE PROGRAMS IN CLAUDICANT PATIENTS

Author	Patients	Duration of Exercise Program (wk)	Improvement (%)
Clifford, 1980	21	4	75
Dahllof, 1976	23	140	20
Sorlie, 1978	10	15	78
Ernst, 1987	42	82	80
Carter, 1989	56	16	70

PATIENT EVALUATION

Complete evaluation of patients with symptomatic infrainguinal atherosclerosis requires complete history and physical examination as well as objective testing for both the presence and severity of arterial obstructive disease.

The historic features of intermittent claudication include the uniform onset of symptoms when walking, the reproducibility of symptoms when repeating the same distance walk, and the reliable relief of symptoms with a few minutes rest. Symptoms confined to the calf suggest occlusive disease limited to below the inguinal ligament. Ischemic rest pain is usually confined to the forefoot and toes, is provoked by elevating the foot, and is relieved by dependency. In addition to these specific symptoms, the history obtained from patients suspected of having infrainguinal atherosclerosis must include careful questioning regarding arterial disease at other sites, especially coronary and cerebral arterial ischemic symptoms. A history of angina pectoris, myocardial infarction, coronary bypass, cerebral transient ischemic attacks, stroke, or carotid surgery must be specifically addressed.

Physical examination of patients with infrainguinal atherosclerosis must include careful palpation of all peripheral pulses. Classic signs of lower extremity ischemia include pallor, hair loss, dependent rubor, abnormal nail growth, and slow capillary filling. These signs are subjective and may be influenced by environmental conditions. Measurement of blood pressure using a Doppler ultrasound flow detector in both arms and at both ankles is a routine part of the examination of all patients with suspected lower extremity ischemia.

Noninvasive testing in the vascular laboratory should be regarded as a critical extension of the physical examination and is obtained in all patients with suspected infrainguinal occlusive disease. The basic examination consists of segmental pressure measurements and Doppler arterial waveform tracings recorded from the upper-thigh, above-knee, below-knee, and ankle levels (Fig. 85-4). Pressures and waveforms recorded by plethysmography from the toes are useful in patients with distal arterial disease as well as in those with extensive calcification of proximal arteries, which makes pressure measurements invalid, a condition

frequently present in diabetics. In some cases, ankle pressure measurements are repeated immediately after treadmill walking. The presence of a decrease in ankle pressure after treadmill walking is distinctly abnormal and provides objective confirmation of the diagnosis of claudication. Vascular claudication is always associated with at least a 20% decrease in the ABI at the time of occurrence of symptoms (Fig. 85-5). Absence of this finding raises serious questions about the diagnosis and should lead to a search for other causes of leg pain. Duplex scanning, a combination of B-mode ultrasound imaging and Doppler spectral analysis, allows examination of specific lesions in the lower extremities, with determination of their precise location, length, and degree of stenosis. Because of the frequency of associated coronary and cerebrovascular disease, evaluations of patients with infrainguinal atherosclerosis should include assessment of the coronary circulation and noninvasive examination of the carotid bifurcations, which may seriously affect prognosis. For a more detailed description of noninvasive testing of the arterial system, refer to Chapter 75.

NONOPERATIVE TREATMENT OF LOWER EXTREMITY ISCHEMIA

At least 2% to 3% of the population over age 50 years and as many as 10% over age 70 years have symptomatic lower extremity ischemia, but only 100,000 vascular surgical procedures are performed to treat lower extremity ischemia in the United States each year. It is clear from these figures that most symptomatic patients are treated nonoperatively. Nonoperative treatment consists of exercise, risk factor modification, and pharmacologic therapy.

Exercise

Patients with intermittent claudication typically curtail walking markedly because of the inevitable discomfort. In addition, many assume that the pain of claudication indicates damage and that additional walking might produce harm. In fact, the opposite is true. Walking produces a predictable and significant improvement in symptoms of claudication. The improvement in walking distance resulting from a program of regular exercise averages about 75% after 8 weeks of training (Table 85-3). It was formerly assumed that this improvement resulted from increased collateral development induced by exercise, but sophisticated studies have conclusively shown that this is not the case. Patients with improved walking distance after exercise do not have increased blood flow to the limb, nor do they have improvement in ABIs after exercise training. What does appear to change is the amount of oxygen extracted from the blood (femoral arterial and venous oxygen difference is increased), which is associated with increased efficiency of muscle function (popliteal venous lactate levels are reduced). These changes induced by exercise probably can best be thought of as analogous to athletic training and can be reliably predicted in nearly all patients who

Table 85-4. RESULTS OF PENTOXIFYLLINE TREATMENT IN CONTROLLED TRIALS

	Patients Treated	Patients With <50% Improvement (%)	Patients With 50%–100% Improvement (%)	Patients With >100% Improvement (%)
Pentoxifylline	375	45	24	31
Placebo	354	76	15	9

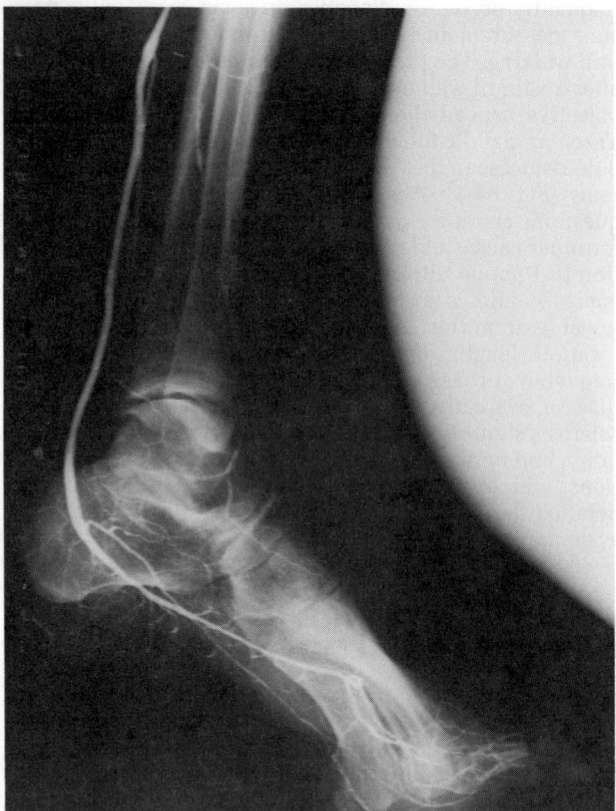

Figure 85-6. Successful reversed saphenous vein graft to lateral plantar artery performed to treat gangrene in the foot of a diabetic patient. This graft has been patent for 18 months.

exercise consistently. Given the age group in which claudication occurs, a realistic prescription for exercise is necessary. Patients are advised to walk at a comfortable pace to the point of claudication, then to stop and rest until symptoms are relieved, then to walk again, and to repeat this cycle for 1 hour each day. Patients who follow this advice experience noticeable improvement in comfortable walking distance within 2 to 3 months.

Cessation of Smoking

Although nonsmokers occasionally experience symptomatic lower extremity ischemia, this occurrence is uncommon and always indicates the presence of other major risk factors for atherosclerosis such as diabetes, congenital hyperlipidemia, or a hypercoagulable state. With these exceptions, the association between tobacco use and lower extremity ischemia is monotonously consistent. Thus, 90% of claudicant persons are smokers, and 95% of patients requiring lower extremity amputation for ischemia are smokers. Tobacco use is such a sufficiently powerful risk factor for lower extremity ischemia that, for practical purposes, it can be considered the most important or even the only important risk factor most patients need to modify. Despite this overwhelming association, most patients are curiously unaware of the relation between smoking and lower extremity ischemia. Most recognize only lung cancer or perhaps bronchitis and emphysema as risks of smoking. In view of this, the obvious first duty of physicians is to inform patients of the causative relation between smoking and limb ischemia. This information should be given to patients in a specific, unqualified, and conclusive

manner that leaves no doubt or room for rationalization. Patients should simply be told: "The cause of your problem is cigarette smoking." This should be repeated at every patient encounter. Physicians' unwavering and repetitive advice to stop smoking has been shown to have a powerful effect on patient behavior, with as many as one third of smokers achieving abstinence based on this approach alone.

Physicians must be aware that cigarette smoking represents a powerful addiction and that achieving abstinence usually involves multiple cycles of smoking cessation and resumption. Physician–patient interactions regarding smoking should be positively oriented. Patients should be told of the many positive effects that result from successful smoking cessation. Besides the obvious reduction in mortality from cancer and myocardial infarction, there are multiple direct beneficial effects on symptoms of lower extremity ischemia. Smokers with claudication who successfully stop smoking experience and immediate improvement in walking distance that averages 100% to 150% as well as an eight-fold reduction in the risk of eventual need for lower extremity amputation. Former smokers are less likely to suffer occlusion of vascular interventions, whether balloon angioplasty or bypass surgery.

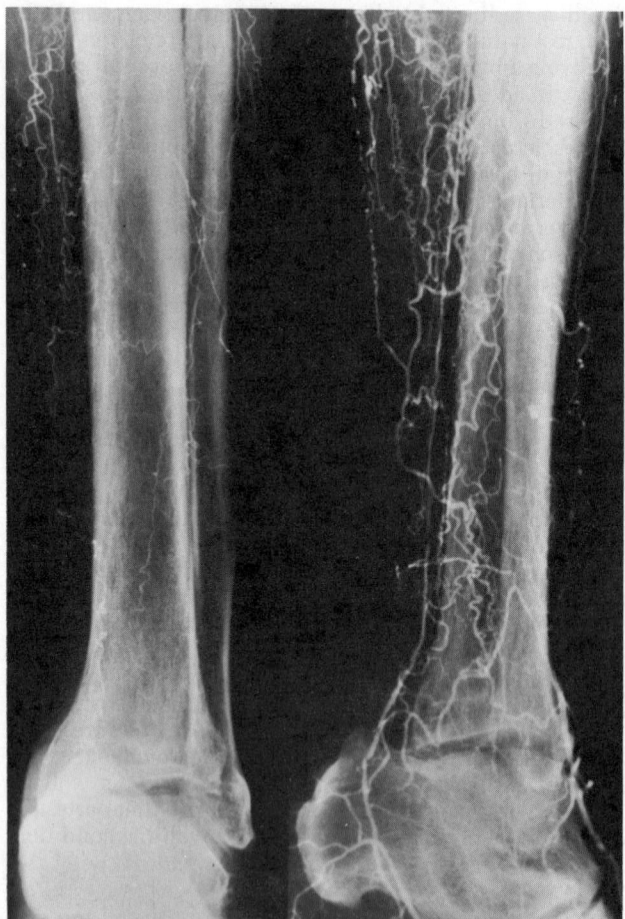

Figure 85-7. (*Left*) Initial arteriogram fails to show graftable distal vessels. The patient was considered to be inoperable. (*Right*) A second arteriogram using selective injection, external warming, and intraarterial vasodilator demonstrates graftable distal posterior tibial artery. The patient's foot was salvaged by a successful bypass graft. (Taylor LM Jr, Edwards JM, Phinney ES, Porter JM. Reversed vein bypass to infrapopliteal arteries. Ann Surg 1987;205:90)

The combined beneficial effects of regular walking and cessation of smoking are sufficient enough that patients with claudication who successfully comply with these recommendations rarely, if ever, require any other treatment for lower extremity ischemia. Nevertheless, these changes are difficult to achieve, and many patients require more extensive treatment, including pharmacologic and interventional therapy.

PHARMACOLOGIC TREATMENT OF INFRAINGUINAL ISCHEMIA

Hemorrheologic Drugs

In the past, knowledge of the critical relation between vessel diameter and flow led to a search for vasodilating agents to treat symptoms of lower extremity ischemia. A multitude of agents has been tried, none with objective proof of success. No vasodilators are approved for use in the United States to treat lower extremity ischemia. Interest in pharmacologic treatment is centered on *hemorrheology*, a term describing the study of the flow characteristics of blood. In large vessels, the important flow characteristic is viscosity. Reducing blood viscosity through hemodilution results in a reproducible improvement in claudicant

patients' walking distance. In the microcirculation, cellular deformability is a critical determinant of blood flow. Because erythrocytes are 6 to 8 μm in diameter and leukocytes are 6 to 15 μm, they must deform considerably to pass through typical 4- to 5-μm capillaries. Another important determinant of microcirculatory flow is the degree of aggregation of erythrocytes, leukocytes, and platelets.

Pentoxifylline appears to affect blood viscosity, cellular deformability, and cellular aggregation, and it appears to act through hemorrheologic mechanisms to improve the symptoms of chronic lower extremity ischemia, specifically claudication. A large number of prospective double-blind trials in the United States and Europe have convincingly shown that pentoxifylline significantly improves treadmill walking distance in one third to one half of claudicant patients. Pentoxifylline has few side effects (primarily nausea) and is well tolerated by most patients. The results of two double-blind trials evaluating pentoxifylline in the treatment of claudication are summarized in Table 85-4.

Metabolism-Enhancing Drugs

A second approach to improving symptoms of chronic lower extremity ischemia involves the use of drugs that beneficially affect the metabolism of ischemic tissues. Car-

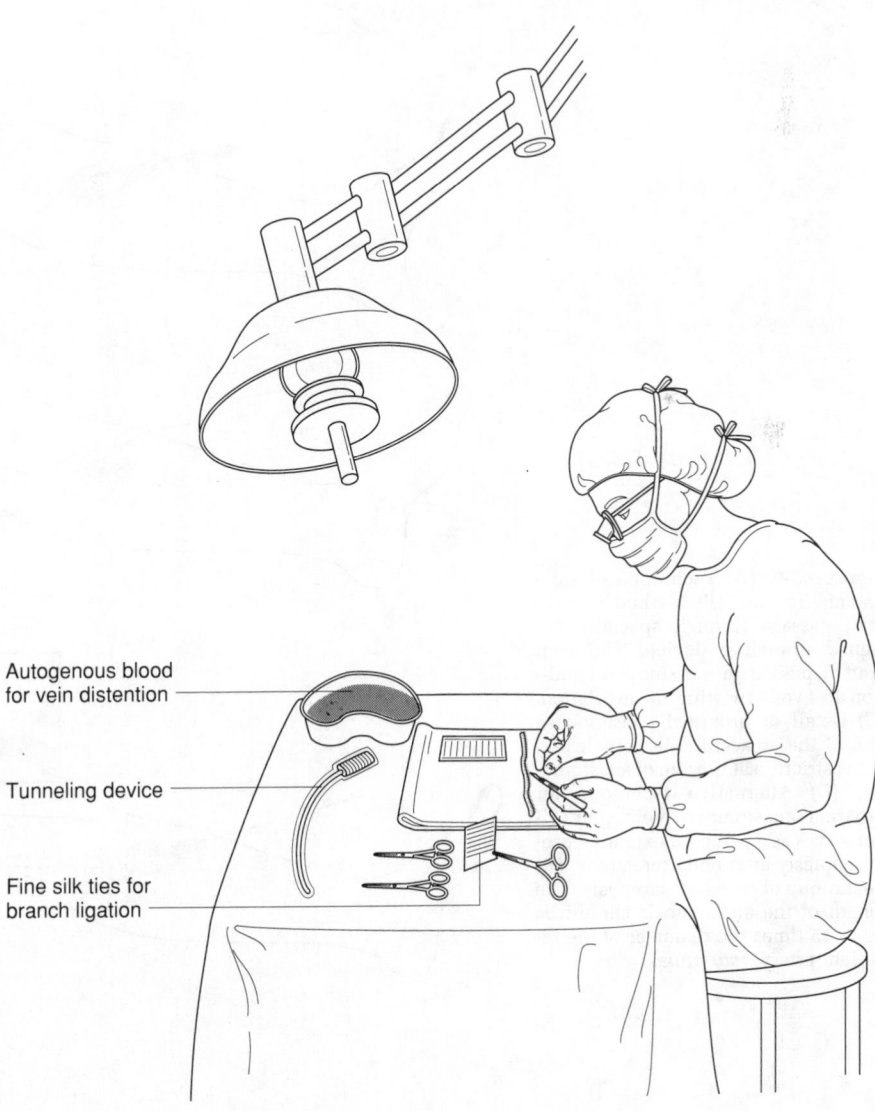

Autogenous blood for vein distention

Tunneling device

Fine silk ties for branch ligation

Figure 85-8. Vein graft preparation is performed on a separate operating bench equipped with adequate lighting, magnification, and microinstruments.

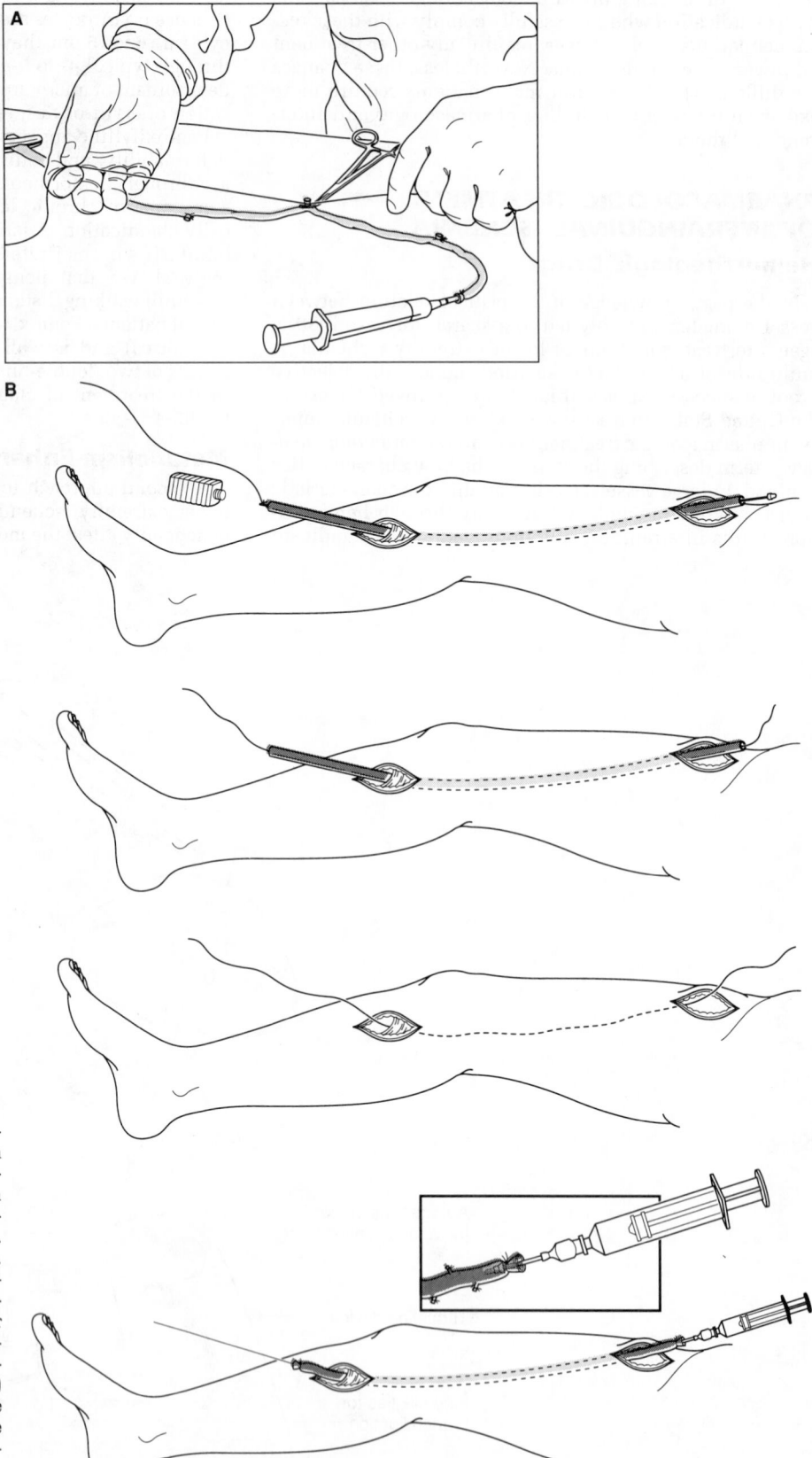

Figure 85-9. (A) Technique of side-branch ligation. (B) Method of vein graft passage through specially designed tunneling device. The vein graft is passed in a distended condition to avoid twisting or angulation. (C) Detail of proximal anastomosis. Use of the adjacent side branch prevents stricture at the site of anastomosis. (D) Alternative technique for proximal anastomosis. Vein graft origin serves as a patch for extended profundaplasty after endarterectomy. (E) Technique of distal anastomosis. The length of the anastomosis should be 10 to 15 times the diameter of the recipient artery. *(continues)*

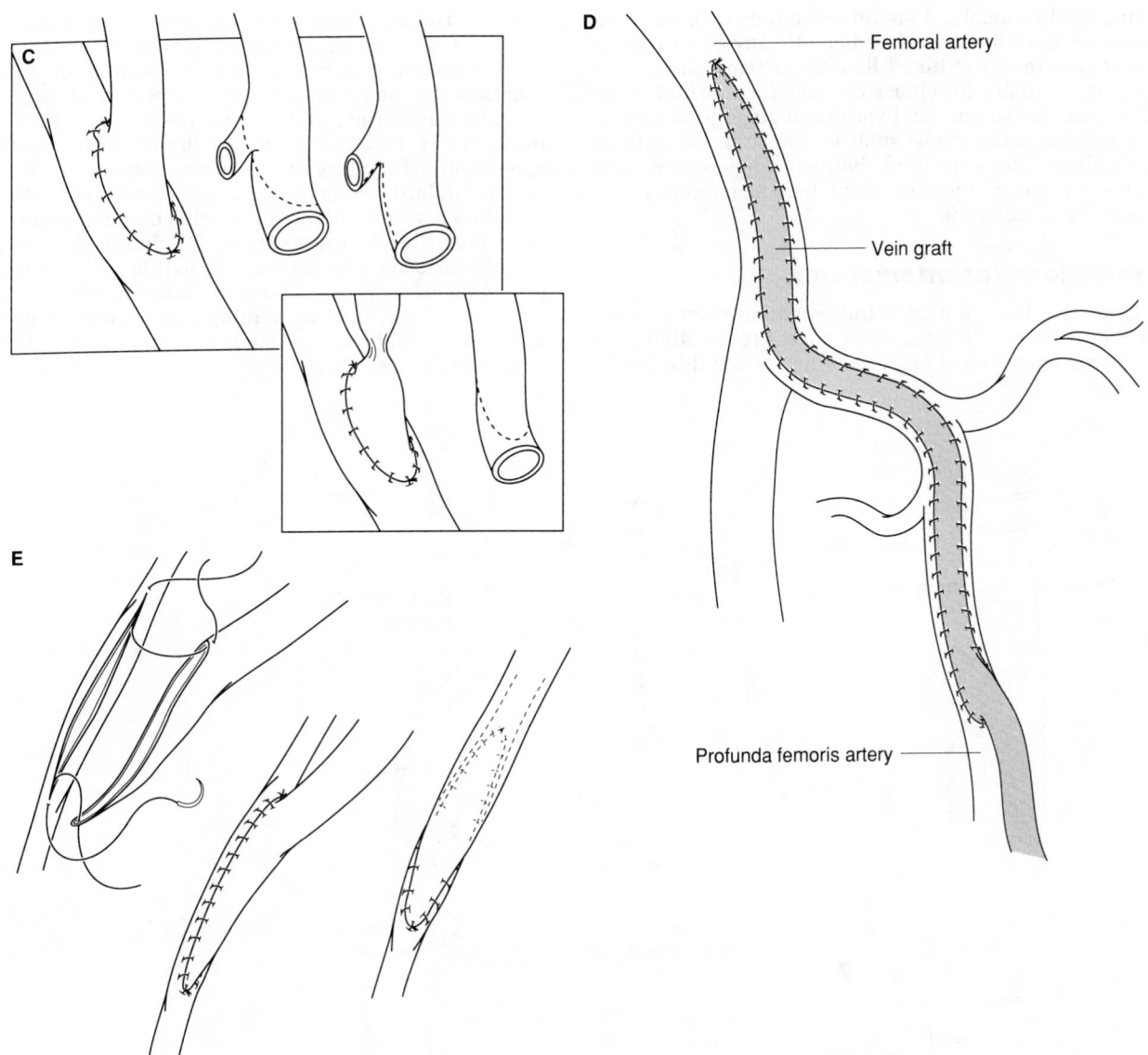

Figure 85-9. (Continued)

nitine is a naturally occurring substance that facilitates aerobic metabolism by promoting entry of pyruvate into the citric acid cycle and by enhancing the transport of fatty acids. These effects result in the production of greater amounts of adenosine triphosphate and, therefore, in greater amounts of available energy from the same amount of oxygen. Carnitine also has been shown to significantly increase claudicant persons' treadmill walking distance, accompanied by a significant decrease in popliteal venous lactate levels.

Antiplatelet Agents

Aspirin affects platelet function by irreversibly acetylating the enzyme cyclooxygenase, thus blocking the formation of thromboxane A_2 and eliminating an important stimulus of platelet aggregation and release. The use of aspirin in patients with chronic lower extremity ischemia is strongly supported by a multitude of studies involving more than 29,000 patients in total, which clearly demonstrated improved survival in patients with symptomatic vascular disease. This treatment results in an overall reduction of 15% in the vascular mortality rate, with reduc-

tions in nonfatal stroke and myocardial infarction of 15% and 30%, respectively. In addition to its effect on survival, aspirin apparently benefits the patency of vascular repairs, especially if the drug is begun preoperatively. Based on this evidence, many clinicians feel that all patients with symptomatic lower extremity ischemia should receive aspirin, 325 mg/d, unless contraindicated by allergy or intolerable side effects.

Ticlopidine is a newer antiplatelet agent that apparently acts by both inhibiting platelet adenosine diphosphate receptors and stimulating the enzyme adenyl cyclase. A recent double-blind trial of this drug in patients with claudication demonstrated significant improvement in both treadmill walking distance and in ABIs in treated patients. If these findings are confirmed, ticlopidine may become an important agent for treating claudication.

OPERATIVE TREATMENT OF INFRAINGUINAL OCCLUSIVE DISEASE

The nonoperative measures described in the preceding sections of this chapter are sufficient to adequately relieve symptoms in most patients with symptomatic infrainguinal ischemia. A significant minority of patients, however, have symptoms sufficiently severe to require direct restoration of blood flow to ischemic areas. The methods available to achieve this goal include both operative vascular surgery and various angiographic and interventional techniques, such as transluminal balloon angioplasty, laser-assisted balloon angioplasty, and catheter atherectomy. The role of these techniques is discussed in Chapter 79.

Indications for Intervention

Operative intervention is indicated for lower extremity ischemia that is sufficiently severe to threaten limb survival. The clinical symptoms indicating this condi-

tion are ischemic rest pain, ischemic ulceration, and gangrene. Objective findings confirming the presence of limb-threatening ischemia usually include an ABI of less than 0.4, nonpulsatile distal extremity plethysmographic waveforms, and a great toe/brachial pressure index of less than 0.25. Although there is near universal agreement with these indications, there is no recognized standard for the timing of intervention in patients with less severe ischemia producing claudication only. Most practitioners limit surgery for claudication to patients whose symptoms interfere significantly with employment or to those whose walking distance is less than one block, thus producing severe impairment of daily tasks. Objectively, such patients nearly always have ABIs of less than 0.55.

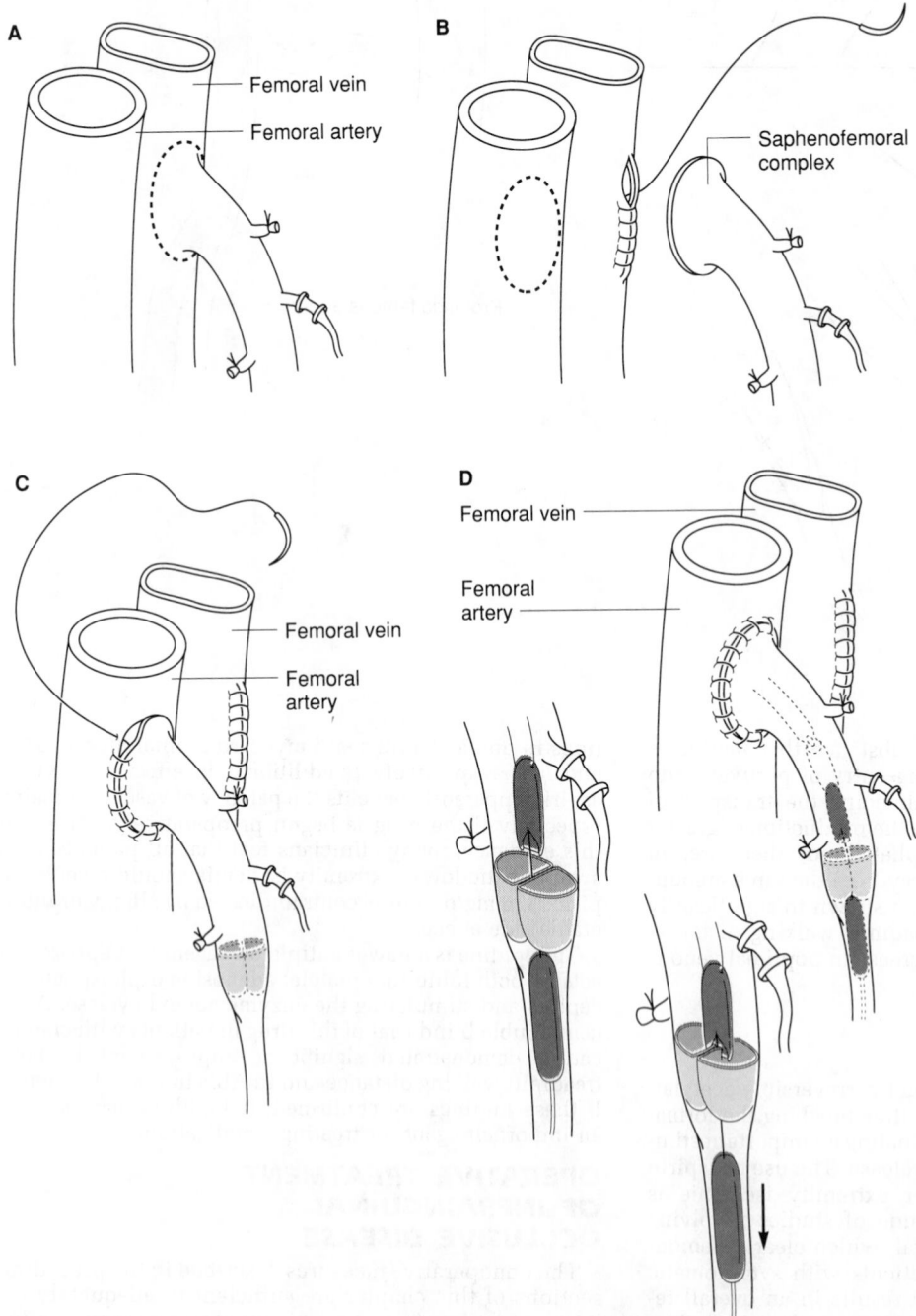

Figure 85-10. (A) The saphenofemoral complex is detached from the femoral vein. (B) The femoral vein harvest site is oversewn. (C) The proximal end-to-side anastomosis is completed. The valve is intact. (D) The valve cutter is passed retrograde through the valves and pulled distally, engaging and cutting the valves. (After LeMaitre G. In situ grafting made easy. Arch Surg 1988;123:102)

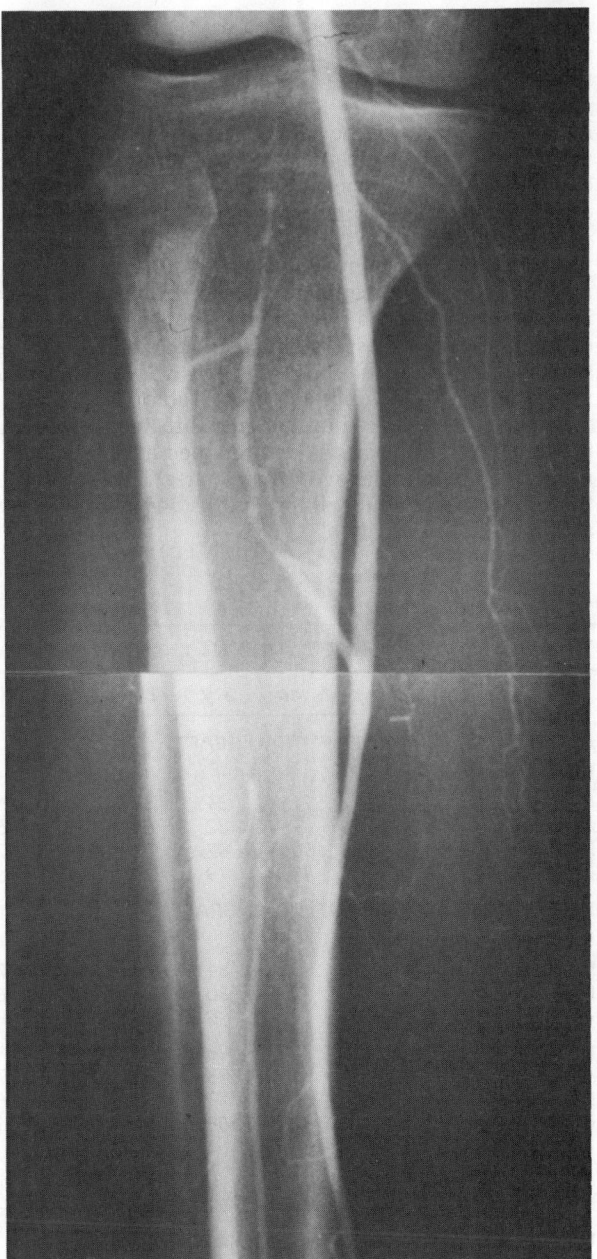

Figure 85-11. Operative completion arteriogram demonstrating a satisfactory reversed saphenous vein graft to the distal posterior tibial artery.

vasodilator injections, digital subtraction techniques, and femoral occlusion balloon angiography have all been used to improve distal arteriographic visualization. Rarely, visualization of distal vessels is possible using only operative angiography, but the advantages of foreknowledge of the anatomy and intended procedure are sufficiently great that surgeons should insist on adequate preoperative studies. It may be necessary to obtain repeat arteriograms to answer specific questions critical to operative planning in patients with severe ischemia once the initial arteriogram has been examined.

Primary Amputation

Occasionally, patients have limb ischemia from arterial obstructive disease that is so advanced that no revascularization is possible. In the past, large numbers of these patients were considered to have inoperable disease, and busy vascular surgeons might have performed primary amputation in as many as 30% to 50% of all patients presenting with gangrene of the lower extremities. This situation is rare today. Distal bypass grafts to the ankle and foot arteries are now routine (Fig. 85-6). Patients must not be assigned to primary amputation until adequate arteriography using the described techniques fail to reveal distal vessels suitable for bypass. Simple lack of visualization of distal vessels cannot be used as a criterion of inoperability. An arteriogram can only rule out the possibility of distal bypass if unnamed collateral vessels in the region of the main arteries are visualized by contrast, confirming that contrast would have outlined the named arteries had they been patent (Fig. 85-7). Of 600 ischemic limbs in 500 patients with limb-threatening ischemia encountered over 10 years, only 14 limbs (2%) were found to have no possibility for revascularization and underwent primary amputation.

Vein Bypass Grafting

Saphenous vein bypass for treating infrainguinal atherosclerosis has been expanded to include almost any conceivable site. As arteriography, sutures, lighting, instruments, and surgical training have improved, the potential sites for bypass grafting have been extended from the popliteal artery below the knee to the tibial and peroneal arteries of the calf and the arteries of the ankle and foot.

Vein bypass is possible if there is arterial inflow to the level of the femoral artery and a patent distal vessel suitable for anastomosis. Two techniques are used to construct lower extremity vein bypasses—the reversed technique

Arteriography

In contrast to nonoperative treatment, selecting appropriate operative therapy for lower extremity arterial disease requires detailed visualization of the obstructive lesions as well as the proximal and distal vessels. This requires arteriography, although in the future, duplex scanning or magnetic resonance imaging may replace arteriography.

Technically adequate studies to permit proper procedural planning are essential. Consistent visualization of all leg arteries requires great skill and expertise by the arteriographer. In particular, visualization of patent vessels in the distal calf and foot in the presence of extensive proximal occlusive disease is technically demanding. Selective catheterization of distal vessels, external warming,

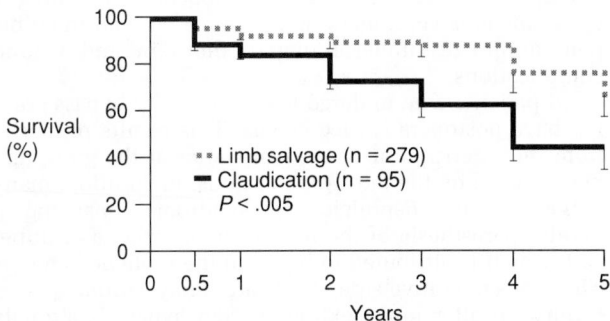

Figure 85-12. Survival of patients undergoing reversed venous bypass for limb salvage versus for claudication. (After Taylor LM Jr, Porter JM. Current status of the reversed saphenous vein graft. In: Bergan JJ, Yao JST, eds. Arterial surgery. Orlando, Grune & Stratton, 1988:494)

and the in situ technique. In reversed vein grafting, the saphenous vein is removed by gentle dissection, reversed in direction to permit blood flow in the direction allowed by the venous valves, distended with physiologic solution, and passed through the leg in an appropriate tunnel, after which anastomoses to proximal and distal vessels are performed (Figs. 85-8 and 85-9). With the in situ technique, the upper greater saphenous vein is detached from the common femoral vein and anastomosed to the common femoral artery, after which the vein is allowed to fill with blood under arterial pressure, and the valve sites are successively identified and incised until unobstructed arterial flow arrives at the chosen level of distal anastomosis. The saphenous vein branches that become arteriovenous fistulas must be individually occluded (Fig. 85-10).

Whichever technique is used to construct lower extremity vein grafts, the immediate success of the procedure is confirmed by using one or more techniques, including electromagnetic flow measurements, continuous wave or pulsed Doppler confirmation of normal flow, or operative completion arteriography (Fig. 85-11).

For patients with absent or unusable greater saphenous veins, grafting using the in situ technique is impossible. These patients can still undergo reversed vein grafting using alternate vein sources, such as arm veins, lesser saphenous veins, and superficial femoral veins.

Complications of Lower Extremity Vein Grafting

For most elective extremity operations, operative mortality is negligible, but this is not true for lower extremity arterial bypass grafting. The patient population undergoing these procedures is elderly, frequently diabetic, and has a significant incidence of associated coronary and cerebrovascular arteriosclerotic disease. It is therefore not surprising that myocardial infarction is the most frequently encountered morbid complication of lower extremity bypass grafting and is responsible for most operative deaths. In our patients operated on since 1980, the operative mortality rate was 1.3% (86% from myocardial infarction, 14% from stroke).

Complications related to the extensive incisions required for vein harvest and preparation, as well as exposure of proximal and distal arterial sites, occur frequently after lower extremity vein bypass. These complications include delayed wound healing and skin edge necrosis, and they occur to some extent in 25% to 30% of patients. Although these complications are rarely serious in patients undergoing reversed vein grafts in which the bypass grafts are tunneled deep within the leg, they may lead to severe complications after in situ grafts, in which the bypass grafts are located superficially and may be exposed by wound complications with subsequent graft infection, necrosis, hemorrhage, or occlusion. Preoperative mapping of the saphenous vein, marking its course with an indelible pen, minimizes undermining of the skin and wound complications.

All patients who undergo lower extremity bypass grafting have postoperative leg edema. This results primarily from the interruption of leg lymphatics at the groin and knee caused by the multiple incisions. In addition, many patients have a neuralgic pain syndrome consisting of painful paresthesia of the medial thigh, knee, and upper calf, which is attributed to injury to the saphenous nerve. These postoperative side effects are rarely serious.

Survival after lower extremity vein bypass is strongly influenced by the indication for operation. Patients operated on for claudication have significantly better long-term survival than those treated for limb-threatening ischemia because the severity of the systemic atherosclerotic process is accurately mirrored by the severity of the leg atherosclerosis (Fig. 85-12). Most patient deaths after vascular surgery are caused by vascular disease, especially myocardial infarction.

Long-term patency of lower extremity vein grafts is related to the quality of the vein conduit, the site of the distal anastomosis, the indication for operation, as well as the experience and skill of the operating team. Primary patency (defined as uninterrupted patency of the conduit without the need for further treatment or revision) at 5 years ranges from about 80% for femoropopliteal grafts performed for claudication to 60% for grafts to tibial arteries performed for limb salvage in patients who already had one failed bypass. Despite considerable controversy, there seems to be little difference in patency whether the reversed or in situ technique is used (Table 85-5).

For patients operated on for limb-threatening ischemia, the long-term limb salvage rate (defined as absence of the need for amputation above the metatarsal level, preserving the ability to ambulate without a prosthesis) is about 80% at 5 years after operation.

Table 85-5. VEIN GRAFT PATENCY RATES (%)

	1 mo	6 mo	1 y	2 y	3 y	4 y
ABOVE-KNEE FEMOROPOPLITEAL GRAFTS						
Primary Patency						
RSV	99	91	84	82	73	69
Arm vein	99	—	82	65	60	60
HUV	95	90	82	82	70	70
PTFE	—	89	79	74	66	60
BELOW-KNEE FEMOROPOPLITEAL GRAFTS						
Primary Patency						
RSV	98	90	84	79	78	77
ISVB	95	87	80	76	73	68
Secondary Patency						
ISVB	97	96	96	89	86	81
Arm vein	97	—	83	83	73	70
HUV	88	82	77	70	61	60
PTFE	96	80	68	61	44	40
Limb Salvage						
RSV	100	92	90	88	86	75
ISV	97	96	94	84	83	—
INFRAPOPLITEAL GRAFTS						
Primary Patency						
RSV	92	81	77	70	66	62
ISVB	94	84	82	76	74	68
Secondary Patency						
RSV	93	89	84	80	78	76
ISVB	95	90	89	87	84	81
Arm vein	94	—	73	62	58	—
HUV	80	65	52	46	40	37
PTFE	89	58	46	32	—	21
Limb Salvage						
RSV	95	88	85	83	82	82
ISVB	96	—	91	88	83	83
RTFE		76	68	60	56	48
AT-KNEE OR BELOW-KNEE GRAFTS						
Primary Patency						
RSV	95	85	81	—	—	—
Secondary Patency						
RSV	96	90	85	81	76	—
ISVB	93	93	92	82	72	—
Foot Salvage	99	94	93	87	84	—

RSV, reverse saphenous vein; HUV, human umbilical vein; PTFE, polytetrafluoroethylene; ISVB, in situ vein bypass.

It is clear from the data described here, and in view of the survival information discussed previously, that for most patients, a lower extremity bypass graft results in limb salvage and graft patency for life. For some patients, however, venous conduit adequate to perform the indicated bypass may not be present for a variety of reasons. These include previous vein removal for treatment of venous disease or for use as coronary or peripheral vein grafts, and primary venous disease, such as varicosities or episodes of superficial venous thrombosis. For these patients, bypass grafting is still possible using prosthetic conduits.

Prosthetic Lower Extremity Bypass

Prosthetic arterial substitutes have been in use for more than 30 years. Dacron and polytetrafluoroethylene (PTFE) grafts are the conduits of choice for replacing diseased abdominal and thoracic vessels. In the extremities, however, this is not the case. Patency rates achieved using prosthetic conduits at all locations in the lower extremities are significantly lower than those achieved with autogenous veins. Several other materials have been evaluated, including Dacron, Teflon, nylon, PTFE, and a variety of biologic materials such as bovine carotid arteries, umbilical veins, and cryopreserved human saphenous veins, each of which must undergo treatments to increase strength and destroy antigenicity. None of these materials has demonstrated results superior to PTFE, which is the prosthetic conduit preferred by most surgeons for lower extremity grafting. Because of the lower patency rates achieved with prosthetic grafting, most surgeons reserve these materials for patients in whom no autogenous veins are available. Considerable evidence indicates that long-term warfarin anticoagulation improves the patency of prosthetic lower extremity grafts, especially with distal anastomoses below the knee. The improvement, although significant, is not equivalent to the results of autogenous vein grafting and is accompanied by the considerable complications of anticoagulation.

BIBLIOGRAPHY

Dalman RD, Taylor LM Jr. Basic data related to infrainguinal revascularization procedures. Ann Vasc Surg 1990;4:309.

Dormandy J, Mahir M, Ascady G, et al. Fate of the patient with chronic leg ischemia. J Cardiovasc Surg 1989;30:50.

Flinn WR, Rohrer MJ, Yao JST, et al. Improved long-term patency of infragenicular polytetrafluoroethylene grafts. J Vasc Surg 1988;7:685.

Hertzer NR, Beven EG, Young JR, et al. Coronary artery disease in peripheral vascular patients: a classification of 1000 coronary angiograms and results of surgical management. Ann Surg 1984;199:223.

Kim YW, Taylor LM Jr, Porter JM. Circulation-enhancing drugs. In: Rutherford RB, ed. Vascular surgery, ed 3. Philadelphia, WB Saunders, 1995:324.

Leather RP, Shah DM, Chang BB, Kaufman JL. Resurrection of the in situ saphenous vein bypass: 1000 cases later. Ann Surg 1988;208:435.

Taylor LM Jr, Edwards JM, Porter JM. Present status of reversed vein bypass: five-year results of a modern series. J Vasc Surg 1990;11:193.

Taylor LM Jr, Porter JM. Natural history and nonoperative treatment of chronic lower extremity ischemia. In: Rutherford RB, ed. Vascular surgery, ed 4. Philadelphia, WB Saunders, 1995:751.

Veith FJ, Gupta SK, Ascer E, et al. Six-year prospective multicenter randomized comparison of autologous saphenous vein and expanded polytetrafluoroethylene grafts in infrainguinal arterial reconstructions. J Vasc Surg 1986;3:104.

CHAPTER 86

LOWER EXTREMITY AMPUTATION

THOMAS S. HUBER

Amputations of the lower extremity are among the most important operations performed by the general and vascular surgeon. The significance is reflected both by the number of procedures and the magnitude of the impact on the patient (Table 86-1). Amputations are often considered a treatment failure and relegated to the junior members of the surgical team, but this is not appropriate on either account. Amputations should be viewed as another treatment option for the underlying disease process. Furthermore, they are a reconstructive procedure that should be regarded as the first step toward rehabilitation. The responsibility for both the operative procedure and the postoperative rehabilitation lies with the primary surgeon. Indeed, the success of the operation has been correlated to the experience of the surgeon.[1] An amputation may be considered a success when the patient returns to his or her previous ambulatory and functional capacity. This outcome can only be ensured by a long-term commitment from both the primary surgeon and the health care team.

INDICATIONS

Most lower extremity amputations are performed for the complications of either diabetes or arterial insufficiency (Table 86-2). Chronic infection and trauma account for a small percentage of the procedures; miscellaneous indications, including neuroma, frostbite, malignancy, chronic pain, congenital deformity, arterial embolization, and venous insufficiency, account for the balance.

Amputation is indicated in dysvascular and diabetic patients for gangrene (dry gangrene), gangrene with infection (wet gangrene), unremitting and unreconstructable rest pain, and nonhealing ulcers. The specific objectives for

Table 86-1. TOTAL AMPUTATIONS EACH YEAR IN THE UNITED STATES

Type of Amputation	Number	Percentage
Phalangeal	36,800	32
Foot	11,500	10
Below-knee	33,350	29
Above-knee	33,350	29
Total	115,000	100

(Frang RD, Tayor LM, Porter JM. Amputations. In: Porter JM, Taylor LM, eds. Basic data underlying clinical decision making in vascular surgery. St Louis, Quality Medical Publishing, 1994:153)

Table 86-2. **INDICATIONS FOR LOWER EXTREMITY AMPUTATION**

	Percentage
Complications of diabetes mellitus	60–80
Nondiabetic infection with ischemia	15–25
Ischemia without infection	5–10
Chronic osteomyelitis	3–5
Trauma	2–5
Miscellaneous (neuroma, frostbite, tumor, pain, nonhealing)	5–10

(Malone JM. Lower extremity amputation. In: Moore WS, ed. Vascular surgery: a comprehensive review. Philadelphia, WB Saunders, 1993:810)

Table 86-3. **AMPUTATION MORTALITY**

Category	Percentage	Number
Below-knee	2	25/1200
Above-knee	9	54/609
Diabetic vs nondiabetic	No difference	
After amputation revision	5.5	12/218

(Frang RD, Taylor LM, Porter JM. Amputations. In: Porter JM, Taylor LM, eds. Basic data underlying clinical decision making in vascular surgery. St Louis, Quality Medical Publishing, 1994:154)

these indications are to remove all nonviable tissue, relieve the source of ischemic rest pain, ensure primary wound healing, and facilitate rehabilitation. The role of amputation in this population has evolved because of the aggressive emphasis on revascularization. Revascularization is often performed concomitant with amputation for gangrene or gangrene with infection, while amputation is reserved for rest pain and nonhealing ulceration if revascularization is either precluded or unsuccessful. Veith and colleagues[2] reported that 96% of all patients who undergo arteriography for limb-threatening infrainguinal arteriosclerosis are candidates for arterial revascularization. Patients with organic brain syndrome and extensive local gangrene were excluded from this study.

Amputation is occasionally indicated as the primary treatment for lower extremity trauma. This decision requires experienced clinical judgment and is based on the severity of the injury, the overall status of the patient, and the ultimate rehabilitation potential. Although the goal is to save both the patient's life and the extremity, heroic efforts to salvage a severely injured extremity with a poor prognosis are not appropriate. Furthermore, both penetrating and blunt extremity injuries are frequently complicated by associated nerve, vascular, bone, and soft tissue injuries. Several treatment guidelines for the injured extremity have been reported. Lange and coworkers[3] recommended primary amputation for open tibial fractures with associated vascular injuries if the posterior tibial nerve was disrupted in adults or if the injury resulted from a crush mechanism and the duration of warm ischemia was greater than 6 hours. Additionally, they reported that primary amputation was relatively indicated with associated polytrauma, severe ipsilateral foot trauma, and an anticipated protracted postoperative course. Similarly, Johansen and colleagues[4] devised a Mangled Extremity Severity Score to predict the need for amputation based on the extent of skeletal or soft tissue damage, limb ischemia, shock, and patient age.

PREOPERATIVE MANAGEMENT

Medical Evaluation

The preoperative evaluation of all patients before lower extremity amputation is similar to that for any major surgical procedure. Evaluation should include a complete history and physical examination, routine laboratory studies, a chest radiograph, an electrocardiogram, and additional diagnostic studies and consultations as indicated. Special attention should be directed at the cardiac, respiratory, and renal systems in light of the inherent comorbid medical problems of the patient population. The importance of the preoperative evaluation cannot be overemphasized. The mortality rates for lower extremity amputations equal or exceed those for most other general and vascular surgical procedures (Table 86-3), while the long term survival for dysvascular patients undergoing amputation is significantly less than that for age-matched controls (Table 86-4).

Management of Infectious Problems

Foot and lower extremity infections in dysvascular and diabetic patients are common. They present as a clinical spectrum ranging from insignificant to life-threatening, but they all merit serious attention in light of their potential. All patients with evidence of cellulitis or wet gangrene of either the digits, forefoot, or foot should be admitted emergently. All wounds should be cultured, and empiric broad-spectrum antibiotics effective against gram negative, gram-positive, and anaerobic organisms should be initiated against a presumed polymicrobial infection.[5] The specific antibiotic choices should be dictated by the severity of the infection; regimens including a third-generation cephalosporin, an aminoglycoside, or both should be reserved for the more extensive infections. The empiric, broad-spectrum antibiotic coverage may ultimately be narrowed according to the results of the culture if the patient's clinical course improves. Additionally, plain radiographs of the extremity should be obtained at the time of presentation to rule out gas in the soft tissue, osteomyelitis, fractures, and foreign bodies.

Definitive management of the affected extremity depends on the extent of the infectious involvement, the presence of systemic signs, and the severity of the vascular occlusive disease. Cellulitis often can be treated successfully with a course of systemic antibiotics in a well-vascularized extremity. In the presence of peripheral vascular occlusive disease, the blood supply may be inadequate to eradicate the infection, and revascularization should be considered. Cellulitis associated with systemic signs is more worrisome and mandates further interven-

Table 86-4. **SURVIVAL AFTER AMPUTATION FOR ISCHEMIA**

Time (y)	Survival Rate (%)
1	75
2	60
3	50
4	45
5	37

(Frang RD, Taylor LM, Porter JM. Amputations. In: Porter JM, Taylor LM, eds. Basic data underlying clinical decision making in vascular surgery. St Louis, Quality Medical Publishing, 1994:155)

tion to rule out a plantar space soft tissue abscess as the septic source. All infected, gangrenous tissue of the digits, forefoot, or foot should be débrided and cultured. This often can be performed at the bedside for limited wounds, particularly in diabetic patients with peripheral neuropathy and a minimally sensate foot. More extensive involvement requires emergent operative débridement and open drainage. In the presence of extensive wet gangrene of the foot, a guillotine amputation through the distal tibia fibula may be indicated. Lower extremity revascularization to salvage ischemic but viable tissue is frequently necessary for patients who present with wet gangrene. The presence of gas in the soft tissues of the foot or lower extremity is a life-threatening emergency that requires high-dose broad-spectrum antibiotics and aggressive operative débridement or amputation of all the involved tissue.

Diabetic patients are particularly prone to foot and lower extremity infections as a result of a compromised immune system, associated vascular occlusive disease, and peripheral neuropathy. These infections are difficult to treat and emphasize the need for an aggressive therapeutic approach and the importance of patient education and prevention. The treatment algorithms were outlined earlier. The sensory deficit associated with the peripheral neuropathy frequently leads to ulceration of the foot over the metatarsal heads and bony prominences. Although these ulcerations are not necessarily infectious in origin, they may become secondarily infected and involve the underlying bone. Treatment of these ulcerations requires stopping the inciting trauma and any weight bearing on the affected surfaces until resolution. Furthermore, patients should be evaluated by the orthotist and fit with proper shoes before resuming ambulation. The presence of a peripheral neuropathy complicates the selection of the ultimate amputation level because forefoot amputations in patients with decreased foot sensation are potentially ulcerogenic.[6-8] Fortunately, the incidence of primary wound healing after below-knee amputations in diabetic patients equals or exceeds that in nondiabetic patients.[9,10]

Potential for Revascularization

All patients with peripheral vascular occlusive disease who present for possible amputation should be evaluated for lower extremity arterial revascularization. Revascularization and limb salvage are associated with numerous physiologic and psychologic advantages. Successful revascularization frequently allows the patients to maintain their functional status, but the choice between revascularization and amputation must be individualized. The patient's functional status, associated medical problems, and rehabilitation potential all must be factored into this decision. The operative mortality rates for lower extremity arterial revascularizations range from 2.8% to 3.8%.[2,11,12] These rates are comparable to those for a below-knee amputation and are less than those for an above-knee amputation. Comparison of the operative mortality rates is not appropriate, however, owing to the inherent selection bias because amputations have traditionally been performed in patients with multiple comorbid medical conditions.

The recent emphasis on revascularization and limb salvage has illustrated several important points. Initial studies reported that a failed distal bypass procedure compromised the ultimate amputation level and necessitated a more proximal one.[13-15] More recent studies, however, have contradicted this contention,[16-18] and this argument should not be used as justification for amputation over revascularization. Failure to visualize the distal vasculature on preoperative imaging studies does not preclude a lower extremity bypass. Patients presenting for possible amputation usually have multilevel occlusive disease. Nonvisualization of the distal vasculature with standard contrast angiography may result from proximal stenoses or occlusions and dilution of the contrast agent.[19,20] Intraoperative angiography or preoperative magnetic resonance angiography may be useful in this setting.[21,22] Additionally, failed vascular reconstructive procedures do not necessarily equate with amputation because reported limb salvage rates exceed those for graft patency.[2,23,24] A bypass procedure may provide a bridge to facilitate wound healing despite limited long-term patency. Furthermore, reoperative procedures are often successful, although their associated long-term patency rates are usually less than for the primary procedure. The possibility of lower extremity amputation should be considered at the time of revascularization, and the skin incisions should be planned accordingly. Fortunately, the incisions to expose the infragenicular vessels correspond to the posterior flap used for most below-knee amputations. Finally, multiple studies have reported that the financial cost of revascularization is comparable to that of amputation.[25-27]

Selection of Amputation Level

The amputation level is contingent on the indication for the procedure, the underlying medical condition of the patient, the rehabilitation potential of both the patient and the proposed amputation level, and the potential for wound healing. The ultimate goal is to provide the most functional extremity that satisfies the indications for the procedure and does not require additional operations. The common amputation levels for the lower extremity are shown in Figure 86-1. Although not inclusive, these levels are preferred owing to their wound healing potential and ability to fit a prosthesis. Advances in prosthetic construction have made amputations at the level of the ankle (Syme amputation) and the knee (knee disarticulation) more feasible.

The amputation level selected must satisfy the indication for the procedure. As noted earlier, most lower extremity amputations are performed for complications of either diabetes or arterial insufficiency. The specific objectives for these indications are to remove all nonviable, painful tissue while ensuring primary wound healing and maximal rehabilitation. Similarly, amputations for extremity trauma must be performed at a level proximal to the necrotic, nonviable tissue. Fortunately, most trauma patients do not have underlying vascular disease, and therefore, wound healing is likely in the absence of infection. Selection of the amputation level for extremity malignancies is dependent on the biologic characteristics of the tumor type and the extent of the disease.

The general medical condition and rehabilitation potential of the patient must factor into the decision-making process of selecting the amputation level. The severity and significance of the comorbid medical conditions, however, must be individualized because there are no set guidelines for recommending either an amputation or an amputation at a specific level. The level with the greatest likelihood of maintaining ambulation and independence should be selected. If the patient is not ambulatory, has limited rehabilitation potential, or has overwhelming comorbid medical conditions, the level should be dictated by the primary wound healing rate. An above-knee amputation is favored in this setting. Aggressive attempts to salvage a more distal amputation level are not appropriate for patients who are unlikely to ambulate on a prosthesis. This includes both patients with joint contractures greater than 15 degrees that preclude a functional prosthesis and patients with paraplegia. Indeed, below-knee amputations are relatively

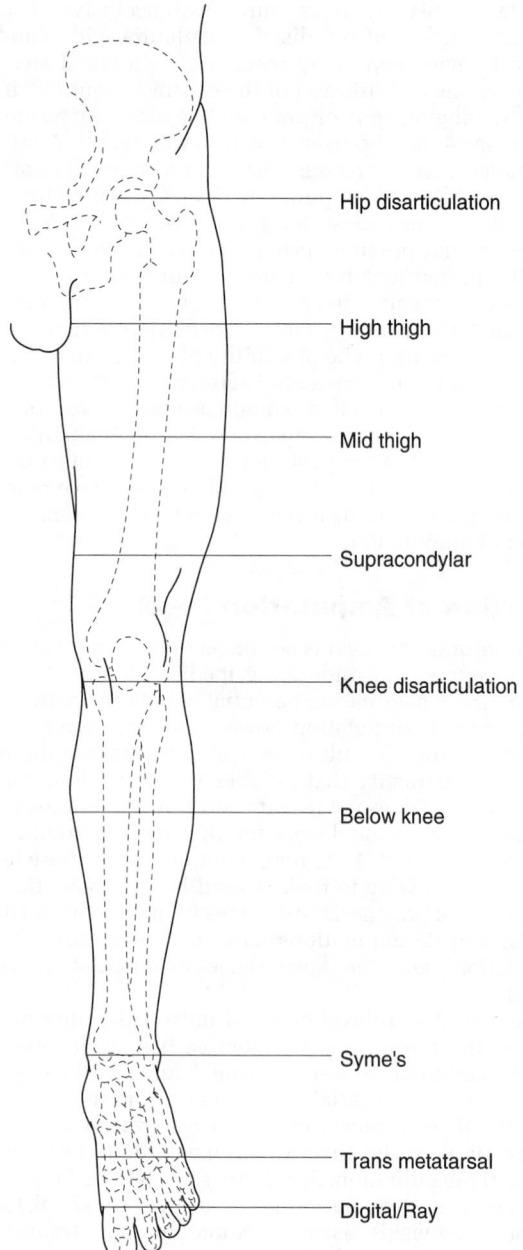

- Hip disarticulation
- High thigh
- Mid thigh
- Supracondylar
- Knee disarticulation
- Below knee
- Syme's
- Trans metatarsal
- Digital/Ray

Figure 86-1. Common amputation levels for the lower extremity.

contraindicated in patients with paraplegia because of the propensity to develop flexion contractures at the knee and subsequent stump ulcerations.

The likelihood of a patient ambulating on a prosthesis after a lower extremity amputation varies inversely with the proximity of the level. This inverse relation results from the increased energy required to ambulate on a more proximal residual extremity. Most important, there is a marked increase in the energy requirements between the below-knee and the above-knee levels (Table 86-5). The energy requirement for ambulating on bilateral below-knee prostheses is less than for a unilateral above-knee prosthesis. Ambulation on an above-knee prosthesis requires the use of muscle groups poorly suited for that purpose. These energy concerns are not as relevant for young, otherwise healthy patients who require amputation for either traumatic or malignant indications. These increased energy requirements however, represent a considerable obstacle

for dysvascular and diabetic patients and frequently are prohibitive. Arterial revascularizations to ensure that a below-knee amputation will heal are occasionally indicated. Additionally, even a relatively short below-knee amputation is superior to an above-knee amputation from an energy requirement standpoint. Although suboptimal, it is possible to fit a below-knee amputation at the level of the tibial tuberosity.

Clinical judgment and a variety of adjunctive studies have been used in dysvascular and diabetic patients to predict wound healing at a specific amputation level. The primary preoperative consideration for wound healing is the adequacy of skin and muscle blood flow. Healing is contingent on multiple other factors, however, including the operative technique, the patient's nutritional status, and the presence of infection. The most frequent concern is whether a below-knee amputation will heal or whether a more proximal amputation will be required. Similar considerations are appropriate for every amputation level because failure of the wound to heal requires an additional procedure and a more proximal amputation. The clinical judgment of an experienced surgeon accurately predicts healing of a below-knee amputation in about 80% of cases.[9,28] A palpable pulse at the level immediately above the selected amputation site almost always ensures wound healing,[29] but the converse is not true because the absence does not equate with nonhealing. A variety of adjunctive preoperative tests have been used to predict the appropriate amputation level and thus improve the primary wound healing rates. Indeed, a combination of clinical judgment and adjunctive tests predict healing at the below-knee level with an accuracy of 94%.[30] Systolic blood pressure measurements have been used most commonly,[31] but they are frequently inaccurate in the presence of diabetes and medial sclerosis owing to the noncompressibility of the vessels. Digital pressures may be helpful in this setting because the digital vessels are frequently spared from the sclerotic changes. A variety of nuclear medicine techniques have been applied to assess skin perfusion as an adjunct to selecting the amputation level,[32-34] but these have been limited by the lack of reproducibility among centers and the availability of the isotopes. Similarly, skin blood flow has been quantified with fluorescein, although the technique did not correlate with amputation healing in a blinded study.[35] Transcutaneous oxygen and carbon dioxide tension measured at the surface of the skin using a miniature Clark electrode compare favorably with the other adjunctive tests and hold significant promise as a predictor of wound healing.[36] Furthermore, a variety of other adjunctive tests, including laser Doppler velocimetry,[37] photoplethysmography,[38] skin temperature measurements,[39] and pulse volume recordings,[40] have all been applied with mixed results.

The perfect adjunctive study has not been described.

Table 86-5. REHABILITATION ENERGY COST OF AMPUTATION AT VARIOUS LEVELS

Amputation Level	Energy Cost
Digital or ray	Minimal (except first ray)
Transmetatarsal	Minimal during normal walking
Below-knee amputation	30%–60% increase in energy required for ambulation
Above-knee amputation	60%–100% increase in energy required for ambulation
Hip disarticulation	100%–110% increase in energy required for ambulation

Most tests have been verified by selecting the amputation level based on clinical criteria and then analyzing the predictive value. The limitation of both this approach and the adjunctive tests is that they fail to predict the most distal level that may heal. Despite their limitations, the various adjunctive tests are helpful and should be used in the preoperative assessment of the patient. The specific criteria for each amputation level are further discussed in subsequent sections.

Timing of Operative Intervention

The timing of the operative procedure is contingent on the indication. The timing for amputations performed for either trauma or malignancy is usually evident. There are specific concerns in the timing for amputations performed for acute ischemia, chronic ischemia, and chronic ischemia with infection.

All patients presenting with evidence of acute ischemia should be considered candidates for immediate revascularization, and the appropriate workup and treatment should be initiated. Arterial embolism and thrombosis account for most of these acute episodes. The heart is by far the most common source of peripheral arterial emboli, and aortoiliac and peripheral aneurysms account for the remainder.[41] In situ arterial thrombosis results most often from severe peripheral vascular occlusive disease and less frequently from peripheral aneurysms. The cause of the acute ischemia (embolus versus thrombus) can be determined in most cases by the history and physical examination. The extremity is revascularized with either embolectomy, distal bypass, or lytic therapy, as appropriate. Unfortunately, not all patients presenting with acute ischemia are candidates for revascularization. Revascularization may be precluded by the severity of the patient's comorbid medical conditions, the extent of the ischemia or necrosis, or the presence of systemic signs.

Amputations for acute extremity ischemia should ideally be postponed until completion of the preoperative evaluation. The morbidity and mortality rates for amputations performed emergently for acute ischemia generally exceed those performed electively.[30] These increased rates are a result of multiple factors. The urgency of the procedure frequently precludes adequate medical management of the associated comorbid conditions. Additionally, critically ill patients may develop an acutely ischemic extremity as a complication of their underlying medical conditions. Furthermore, ischemic breakdown products may be released from the extremity and cause systemic complications as manifested by cardiovascular compromise, respiratory insufficiency from adult respiratory distress syndrome, and renal insufficiency or failure from myoglobinuria. Finally, the ischemic extremity may become secondarily infected and cause a similar spectrum of septic complications. Delaying the operative procedure also allows the ischemic or necrotic tissue to demarcate completely and potentially salvages additional viable tissue and a more distal amputation. The feasibility of postponing the operative procedure is contingent on the absence of systemic symptoms attributable to the extremity. Manifestation of these symptoms requires initiation of the appropriate medial therapy for the involved organ and urgent amputation. A "medical amputation" may be performed if the patient's condition is so tenuous that operative intervention is precluded; a tourniquet is applied proximally to the involved tissue and the extremity packed in ice.

The operative timing for amputations indicated for chronic ischemia is not nearly as crucial. Dry gangrene by definition is noninfectious and should not result in any systemic symptoms, so these patients can undergo complete preoperative evaluation. As described earlier, all patients with dry gangrene should be evaluated for possible revascularization to salvage additional tissue or a more distal amputation. Gangrene localized to the digits alone may be treated operatively or nonoperatively by simply allowing the digits to mummify and autoamputate. This nonoperative approach relieves the concern about primary wound healing and frequently permits salvage of additional tissue, but it can take 6 to 12 months for completion. Gangrene proximal to the digits should be treated operatively.

The infectious process dictates the operative timing for amputations indicated for chronic ischemia with infection (wet gangrene). The goal in this setting is to treat the infection and salvage the greatest amount of viable tissue. All infected wounds should be initially débrided to remove the necrotic tissue. The viable, infected tissue should be preserved in the hope that the parenteral antibiotics are effective. Simultaneously, the patient should be evaluated for a distal arterial revascularization. If the infection resolves with the débridement and antibiotics, the resultant dry gangrene can be treated as outlined for chronic ischemia, and the definitive amputation can be delayed until after the appropriate preoperative evaluation. The presence of systemic symptoms, extensive infection, or failure of the débridement and antibiotic treatment necessitate emergent amputation. The magnitude of this problem cannot be overemphasized. An infected extremity in dysvascular and diabetic patients is both a limb- and life-threatening problem. A wider débridement or guillotine amputation should be performed as part of a staged procedure in this setting to remove additional necrotic or grossly infected tissue. It is not necessary, however, to remove all the cellulitic tissue because removal of the necrotic and grossly infected tissue with appropriate antibiotic treatment is often sufficient to treat the cellulitis, potentially salvaging a more distal amputation. A second-stage definitive amputation can then be performed after the infectious process has resolved. Staged guillotine amputation before definitive below-knee amputation has resulted in a decrease of the wound infection rate from about 22% to 3% or less.[42,43]

Multidisciplinary Evaluation

Amputation of the lower extremity has a profound impact on the patient from a physiologic, psychologic, and social standpoint. The magnitude is dependent on the level of amputation and the preoperative functional status. All patients should be evaluated and treated within the context of a multidisciplinary team composed of surgeon, internist, physiatrist, prosthetist, physical therapist, and social worker. This multidisciplinary approach facilitates assessment of the patient's functional status, provides a mechanism for patient and family education, and ensures adequate psychologic preparation. The net result is a smoother transition to the rehabilitation process.

OPERATIVE MANAGEMENT
General Considerations

Amputations of the lower extremity are major operative procedures with significant associated morbidity and mortality rates. Attention to detail is pivotal and favorably impacts primary wound healing and the likelihood of salvaging a more distal amputation. The techniques of the specific operations are discussed after an introduction to the principles.

The techniques of amputation surgery are based on the

surgical principles and apply to all levels. Strict aseptic technique should be used as with any operative procedure. Postoperative wound infections after amputations are particularly detrimental and may necessitate a more proximal amputation. All gangrenous tissue should be draped outside of the operative field using either an adhesive drape or a bowel bag. Proximal tourniquets should not be used for dysvascular and diabetic patients because they may compromise an already tenuous blood supply and cause tissue damage. They are both acceptable and helpful for amputations performed for other indications, including trauma and malignancy. Incisions should be made perpendicular to the plane of the skin to avoid undermining and potentially creating poorly vascularized flaps. The subcutaneous tissues and muscle layers may be incised either sharply or with the electrocautery, although the former is preferred distally owing to the potential to damage adjacent tissues with the electrocautery. All major blood vessels should be identified, dissected free, and suture ligated. The major nerves should be placed under tension, transected, suture ligated, and then allowed to retract. The ligation prevents bleeding from the vaso nervorum, while the retraction ensures that the nerve end and the resultant neuroma are neither incorporated into the incisional scar nor in contact with a potential weight-bearing surface. Excessive tension should be avoided, however, because it can lead to postoperative neuralgias. Similarly, all tendons should be transected sharply under tension and allowed to retract. Amputations through joint articular surfaces should be avoided due to their poor vascular supply. The periosteum adjacent to the proposed level of bone transection should be elevated proximally no more than necessary in an attempt to prevent excessive bone overgrowth. Although both manual and reciprocating air-driven power saws may be used, the latter is preferred owing to the precision of the cut. All bone edges should be filed smooth to prevent damage to the soft tissue. Bone wax should be avoided because it is a foreign body and a potential nidus for infection. Similarly, all prosthetic material from previous bypass procedures should be removed because it has been shown to result in a significantly lower postoperative wound infection rate.[44,45] All wounds should be aggressively irrigated with saline solution containing antibiotics, and hemostasis should be confirmed. Postoperative hematomas can compromise the amputation level and predispose to wound infections. The fascial and skin layers should be reapproximated atraumatically without tension, and the use of forceps on the skin should be avoided. Either nonreactive, permanent monofilament sutures or staples can be used for the skin closure. The wound should be left open and packed with saline-soaked gauze if there is any concern that the tissues are infected. These open wounds can be allowed to heal by secondary intention or closed as a delayed primary. The skin staples or sutures should be left intact for 4 to 6 weeks.

Digital and Ray Amputations

Digital and ray (metatarsal) amputations are commonly performed for gangrene resulting from the complications of diabetes and arterial insufficiency. The noninvasive criteria to predict primary wound healing are shown in Table 86-6. The choice between the two is determined by the extent of bone and soft tissue involvement. A digital amputation is indicated for gangrene involving the distal or midphalanx, while a ray amputation is indicated for gangrene extending to the digital crease. A ray amputation is contraindicated if multiple digits are involved; a transmetatarsal amputation is indicated in this setting. Additionally, a ray

Table 86-6. PREOPERATIVE LEVEL SELECTION: TOE AMPUTATION

Selection Criteria	Successful Healing, Primary and Secondary/Total
Empiric	86/115 (75%)
Presence of pedal pulses	357/365 (98%)
Doppler toe pressure >30 mm*	47/60 (78%)
Doppler ankle pressure >35 mm*	44/46 (96%)
Photoplethysmographic digit or TMA pressure >20 min*	20/20 (100%)
^{133}Xe skin blood flow >2.6 mL/100 g tissue/min	5/6 (83%)

* Systolic pressure (mmHg).
TMA, transmetatarsal.
(Durham JR. Lower extremity amputation levels: indications, methods of determining appropriate level, technique, prognosis. In: Rutherford RB, ed. Vascular surgery, ed 3. Philadelphia, WB Saunders, 1989:1693)

amputation is relatively contraindicated for neurotropic ulcers owing to the high likelihood of recurrence.

The technique used for digital amputation through the proximal phalanx is illustrated in Figure 86-2*A*. A circumferential skin incision is made proximal to the gangrenous tissue over the distal aspect of the proximal phalanx, and the incision is extended to the bone. The tendons and nerves are transected under tension and allowed to retract. The proximal phalanx is transected with either the handheld bone cutter or the reciprocating air-driven power saw. The wound is closed horizontally without tension after irrigation and hemostasis. The proximal phalanx should be transected more proximally, or a ray amputation should be performed if either the skin or soft tissue cannot be closed without tension. A variety of skin and soft tissue flap designs are suitable, and the choice may be dictated by the extent of the underlying process.

The technique for ray amputations is similar and is illustrated in Figure 86-2*B*. A racquet-shaped skin incision is created with the circular component extending circumferentially around the digit at the margins of the viable tissue and the longitudinal component extending proximal to the head of the metatarsal. This longitudinal component should be made over the dorsum of the foot for resection of the second, third, and fourth metatarsal heads and over the medial and lateral aspects of the foot for resection of the first and fifth metatarsal heads, respectively. The skin incision is extended to the bone, and the tendons and nerves are transected under tension. The soft tissue is dissected from the metatarsal bone, the periosteum is minimally elevated, and the metatarsal bone is transected proximal to the head. Care should be used during the dissection and transection to prevent damaging the skin flap and to prevent entering both the deep tendon compartments and the joint spaces of the adjacent digits. The longitudinal component of the incision is closed along its axis while the circumferential incision is closed perpendicularly.

The immediate postoperative course after both digital and ray amputations is usually uneventful and the necessary care minimal. A soft incisional dressing is adequate, and ambulation may be resumed 2 to 3 weeks after operation.

Transmetatarsal Amputation

Transmetatarsal amputations are indicated when the underlying gangrenous or infectious process involves multiple digits or the forefoot. The noninvasive criteria used to

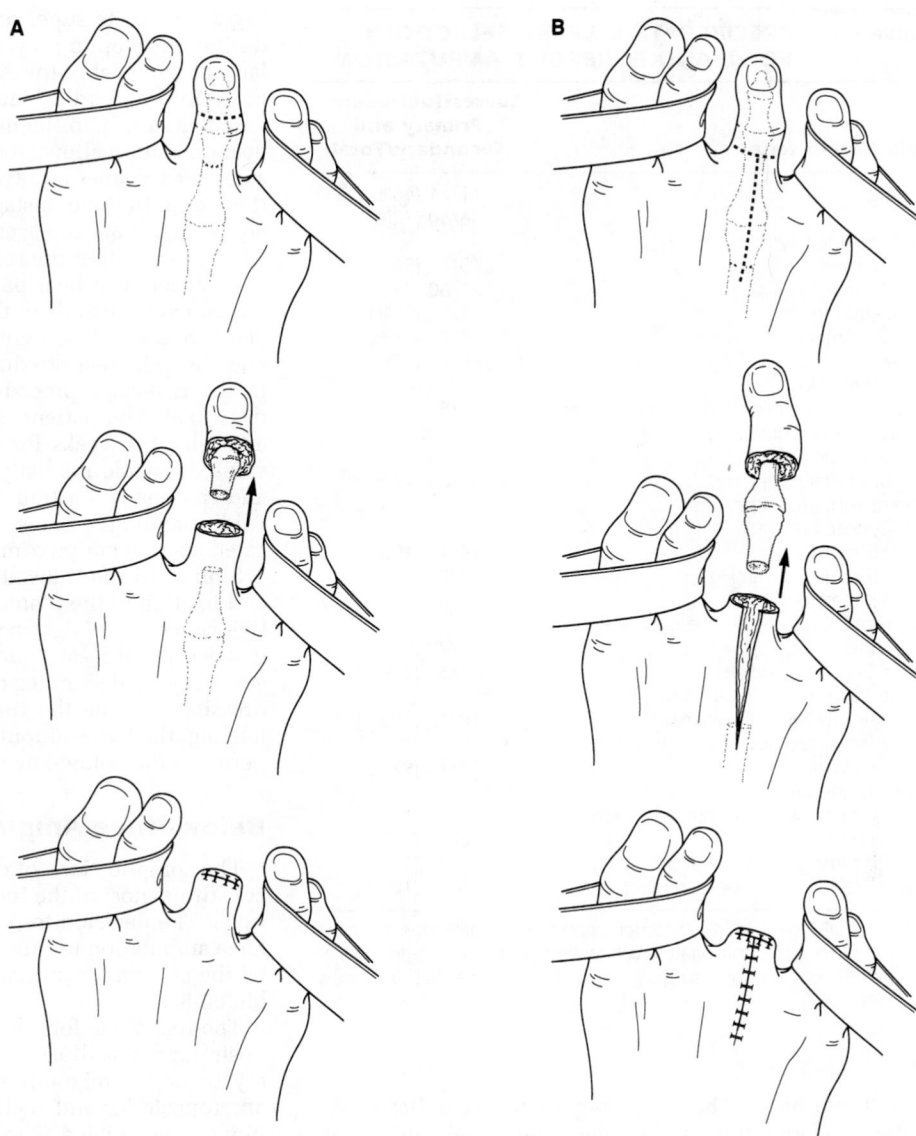

A

B

Figure 86-2. (*A*) Digital amputation. A circumferential skin incision is made proximal to the gangrenous process. The proximal phalanyx is transected and the soft tissue approximated. (*B*) Metatarsal head resection (ray amputation). A racquet-shaped skin incision is made with the circular component extending circumferential around the digit and the longitudinal component extending proximal to the metatarsal head. The metatarsal is transected proximal to the head and the soft tissue approximated.

select the level and predict primary wound healing are shown in Table 86-7. A transmetatarsal amputation is contraindicated when the underlying process extends to the proposed skin incisions or when it involves the plantar surface of the forefoot. In the latter situation, a guillotine amputation through the metatarsal bones can be performed and either allowed to heal by secondary intention or subsequently covered with a split-thickness skin graft. Split-thickness grafts, however, are not durable in this location and are prone to break down with ambulation; consideration should be given to a more proximal amputation. Additionally, a transmetatarsal amputation is relatively contraindicated in patients with neurotrophic sensory losses owing to the propensity for further ulceration.

The technique used for a transmetatarsal amputation is shown in Figure 86-3. The skin incision is made on the dorsum of the foot immediately proximal to the metatarsal heads and extended onto the medial and lateral aspects of the foot to a point midway between the plantar and dorsal surfaces. The plantar incision is made along the digital crease and extended diagonally over the medial and lateral aspects of the foot to connect the dorsal incision. The dorsal skin incision is then extended to the metatarsal bones and the periosteum elevated. The metatarsal bones are

transected about 5 mm proximal to the skin incision, creating a small dorsal flap. The metatarsal heads are then separated from the plantar flap sharply along a horizontal plane immediately deep to the bone, and the forefoot is removed. Caution should be exercised during this step to stay in the proper plane and to keep the plantar flap as thick as possible. The nerves and tendons are then transected under tension and allowed to retract. The plantar flap is rotated anteriorly and all redundant tissue excised. The flap is apposed with absorbable sutures and the skin reapproximated atraumatically.

The primary immediate postoperative concerns after a transmetatarsal amputation are the adherence and healing of the plantar flap. Ambulation should be delayed for 1 month. Either a soft dressing or a short leg cast is a suitable postoperative dressing.

Syme Amputation

The Syme amputation is one of the more technically demanding amputations. It is a foot amputation in which the ends of the tibia and fibula are covered by the preserved heal pad. The selection criteria used to ensure wound healing are the same as those used for the transmetatarsal level

Table 86-7. PREOPERATIVE LEVEL SELECTION: FOOT AND FOREFOOT AMPUTATION

Selection Criteria	Successful Healing, Primary and Secondary/Total
Empiric	11/24 (46%)
	36/50 (72%)
Doppler ankle systolic pressure	
<40 mmHg	5/9 (56%)
>40 mmHg	20/60 (33%)
40–60 mmHg	4/5 (80%)
>50 mmHg	14/21 (66%)
>60 mmHg	68/91 (75%)
>70 mmHg	70/93 (75%)
Doppler toe systolic pressure >30 mmHg	4/5 (80%)
Doppler ankle–brachial pressure index	
>0.45 (nondiabetic)	
>0.50 (diabetic)	58/60 (97%)
Photoplethysmographic toe systolic pressure	
>55 mmHg	14/14 (100%)
>45 and <55 mmHg	2/8 (25%)
<45 mmHg	0/8 (0%)
Fiberoptic fluorometry (dye fluorescence index >44)	18/20 (90%)
Laser Doppler velocimetry	2/6 (33%)
[125]I iodopyrine skin blood flow >8 mL/100 g tissue/min	18/18 (100%)
[133]Xe skin blood flow >2.6 mL/100 g tissue/min	23/25 (92%)
Transcutaneous P_{O_2}	
>10 mm (or a >10 mm increase on F_{IO_2} = 1.0)	6/8 (75%)
>28 mmHg	3/3 (100%)
Transcutaneous P_{CO_2} <40 mmHg	3/3 (100%)

(Durham JR. Lower extremity amputation levels: indications, methods of determining appropriate level, technique, prognosis. In: Rutherford RB, ed. Vascular surgery, ed 3. Philadelphia, WB Saunders, 1989:1695)

(see Table 86-7). The Syme amputation is indicated for extensive foot trauma and for the usual diabetic or dysvascular indications when the gangrenous or infectious processes preclude a transmetatarsal amputation. Predictably, a Syme amputation is rarely an option for diabetic or dysvascular patients because the processes that preclude a transmetatarsal amputation usually require a below-knee amputation. The Syme amputation is useful in children because it preserves the epiphyseal growth plates. As noted earlier, amputation at this level is relatively contraindicated in patients with neurotrophic sensory changes.

The Syme amputation can be performed as either a one- or a two-stage procedure; both are illustrated in Figure 86-4. The advantage of the two-stage procedure is that it results in a square stump that is both cosmetically more appealing and easier to fit with a prosthesis. The initial steps for both techniques are identical with the exception of the skin incision. The incision for the one-stage procedure connects the medial and lateral malleoli in both the horizontal and vertical planes. The incision for the two-stage procedure is similar but is located 1.5 cm further distally. The dorsal incision is extended to the bone, the tendons are transected under tension, and the anterior tibial artery is identified and suture ligated. The incision is extended into the tibiotalar joint space, and the foot is placed in forced plantar flexion. The ligamentous structures are incised and the talus dislocated. The plantar incision is then extended to the calcaneus, and the calcaneus is sharply dissected from the densely adherent plantar fascia beginning at its superior aspect. Care must be exercised during this step to prevent injuring the heel pad, particularly at the level of the Achilles tendon. Additionally, the posterior tibial artery must be preserved because it is the vascular supply to the heel pad. Completion of the calcaneal dissection allows removal of the foot. The subsequent steps for the one- and two-stage procedures diverge from this point. In the one-stage procedure, the medial and lateral malleoli are transected flush with the tibiotalar joint space using either the reciprocating air-driven power saw or a chisel. The heel pad is rotated anteriorly and positioned over the ends of the tibia and fibula. The deep fascial layers are closed with interrupted absorbable sutures and the skin reapproximated. After the foot is removed in the two-stage procedure, the heel pad is apposed as described. The patient is returned to the operating room after about 6 weeks for the second stage. Elliptical incisions are made medially and laterally over the malleoli, and the bones are transected flush with the ankle joint. Additionally, the flares over the distal tibia and fibula located about 6 cm proximal to the ankle joint are removed.

Similar to the transmetatarsal amputation, the healing and fixation of the plantar flap are the primary postoperative concerns. Weight bearing on the heel pad should be delayed for at least 1 month to allow fixation, and either a soft or a rigid short leg cast is adequate as a postoperative dressing. Despite the limitations associated with wound healing, the Syme amputation has been reported to be superior to the below-knee amputation.[46]

Below-Knee Amputation

The complications of diabetes and arterial insufficiency constitute most of the indications for below-knee amputations. The decision to perform a below-knee or an above-knee amputation in this setting is crucial and is facilitated by the criteria for primary wound healing outlined in Table 86-8.

The technique for a below-knee amputation based on a posterior flap is illustrated in Figure 86-5. Although a variety of flap configurations are possible, including equal anteroposterior and sagittal flaps, the posterior flap technique is associated with the highest incidence of wound healing and is therefore preferred.[47,48] This increased incidence of wound healing presumably reflects the fact that the posterior flap is better vascularized. The gastrocnemius and soleus muscles that compose the posterior flap are supplied from the sural arteries that originate proximal to the knee. Despite this advantage, the flap construction is occasionally dictated by the underlying ischemic process and the previous incisions. The proposed skin incisions are drawn on the extremity with a marker. The optimal level for tibial transection is 10 cm distal to the tuberosity. The anterior skin incision is made 1 cm distal to the point selected for the tibial transection and extended circumferentially around the calf both medially and laterally to the midpoint of the calf in the anteroposterior axis. The skin incision is extended distal from this midpoint along the longitudinal axis of the calf both medially and laterally for a distance 2 cm greater than the diameter of the calf at the point of the anterior, proximal incision. The distal medial and lateral incisions are connected posteriorly by extending the incision circumferentially around the calf. Redundant tissue at the medial and lateral aspects of the completed amputation ("dog ears") may be avoided by rounding the distal corners of the posterior flap. The muscles in the anterior compartment are incised flush with the anterior skin incision either sharply or with the electrocautery. The anterior tibial neurovascular bundle is identified during this step and suture ligated. The tibia is dissected

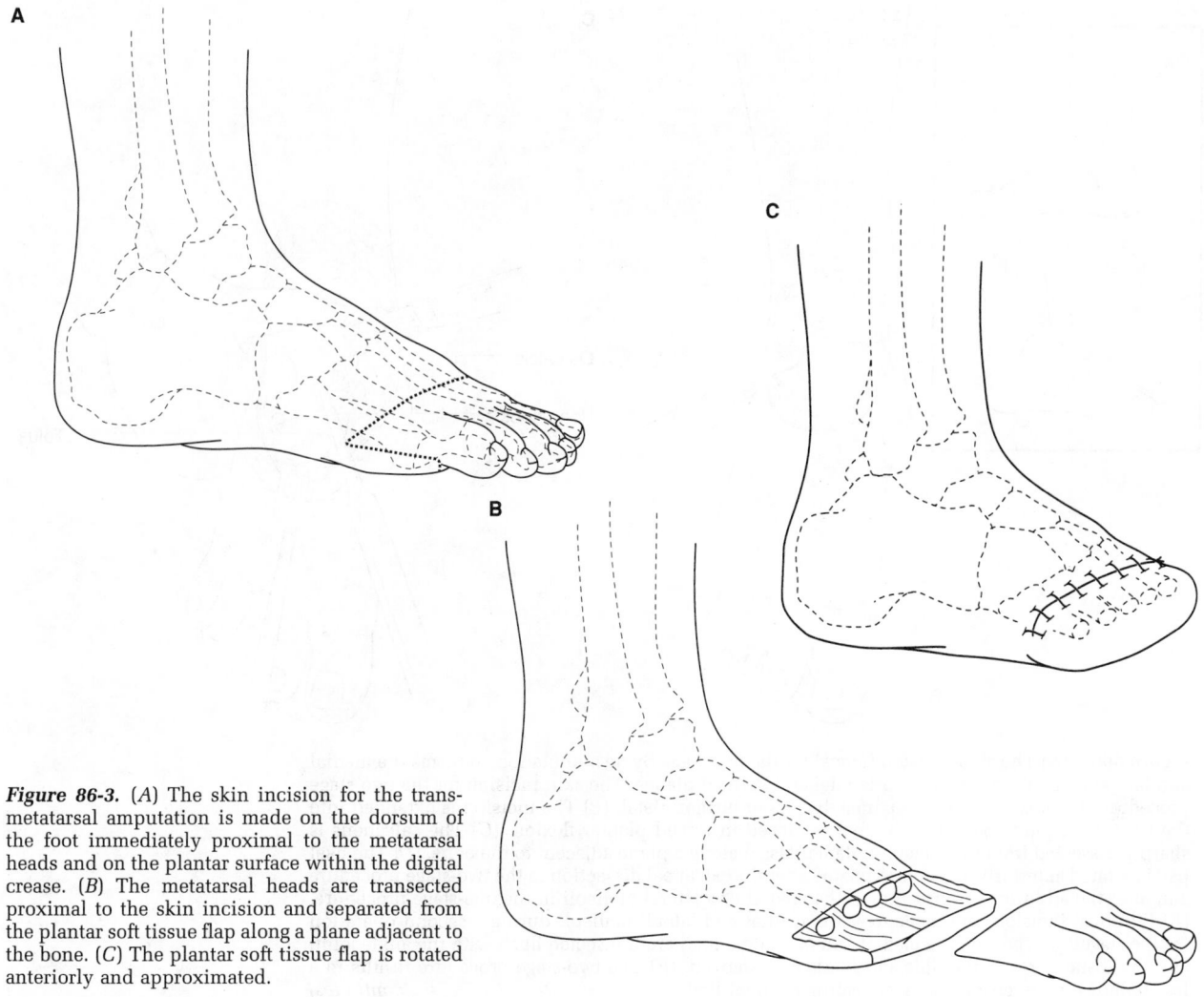

Figure 86-3. (*A*) The skin incision for the trans-metatarsal amputation is made on the dorsum of the foot immediately proximal to the metatarsal heads and on the plantar surface within the digital crease. (*B*) The metatarsal heads are transected proximal to the skin incision and separated from the plantar soft tissue flap along a plane adjacent to the bone. (*C*) The plantar soft tissue flap is rotated anteriorly and approximated.

circumferentially and the adherent periosteum elevated proximally. The tibia is then transected 1 cm proximal to the skin incision with either the manual or reciprocating air-driven power saw, while the skin and soft tissues are retracted for protection. Similarly, the fibula is transected 1 cm proximal to the level of the tibia. Transecting the fibula at this level results in a cylindric stump. The posterior tibial and common peroneal neurovascular structures are then identified and suture ligated. The tibia and the fibula are retracted anteriorly, and the posterior musculature is incised along the plane of the skin incision with the amputation knife. Caution should be exercised during this step to prevent inadvertently injuring the posterior flap. The specimen is removed from the operative field, and all remaining neurovascular structures are suture ligated. The posterior flap is then rotated anteriorly to confirm that both the length and size are suitable. Frequently, the posterior flap skin and musculature need to be debulked to allow a tension-free closure. Conversely, if the posterior flap length is inadequate, the tibia and fibula can be transected more proximally. After the flap is deemed appropriate, the anterior aspect of the tibia is beveled about 45 degrees through the mid-portion of the transected bone, and the edges of the tibia and fibula are filed smooth. The posterior flap is rotated anteriorly, the fascia is approximated with absorbable suture, and the skin is closed atraumatically. Large dog ears should be excised at this step,

although smaller ones can be left because they resolve as the stump shrinks and the muscles atrophy.

Several technical points merit additional comment. If the infectious or gangrenous process involves the skin incisions outlined for the posterior flap, a shorter below-knee stump can be created using the same flap design but a more proximal anterior incision. Although suboptimal, a short below-knee amputation is superior to an above-knee amputation. In the most extreme condition, a below-knee prosthesis can be fit for a stump in which the tibia is transected at the tuberosity. If the tibia is transected at this level, the fibula should be removed to prevent angulation. Additionally, the biceps tendon and collateral ligament should be sutured to the tibia, and the common peroneal nerve should be transected above the knee. A guillotine below-knee amputation should be performed as part of a staged procedure in the presence of an extensive foot infection. A guillotine amputation is essentially a large débridement. A circumferential incision is made in the distal calf and then extended through the underlying fascia. The tibia and fibula are dissected free, the periosteum is elevated, and the bones are transected flush with the skin incision. All major neurovascular structures are suture ligated and the remaining soft tissue incised to complete the amputation. The wound is left open, and the second-stage, definitive below-knee amputation is delayed until the infectious process resolves. Alternatively, a for-

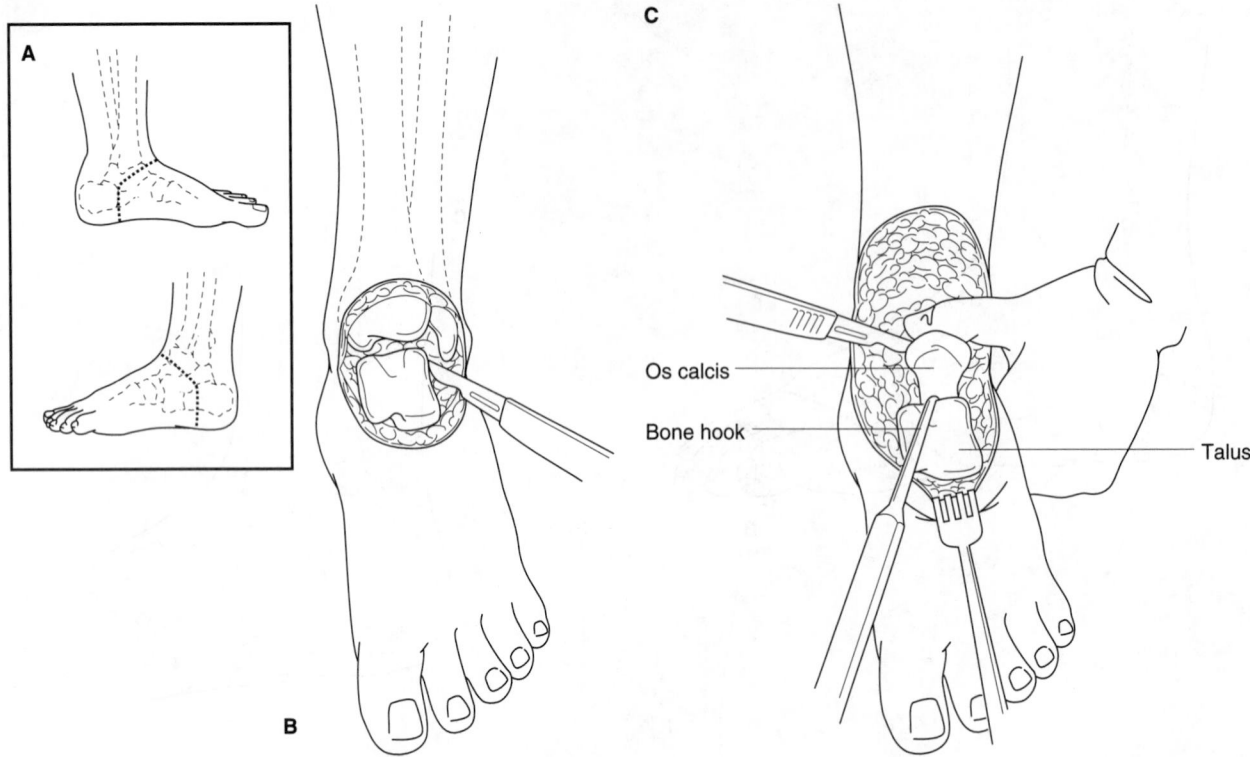

Figure 86-4. (*A*) The skin incision (*black*) for the one-stage Syme amputation connects the medial and lateral malleoli in both the horizontal and vertical planes. The skin incision for the two-stage procedure (*blue*) is located approximately 1.5 cm further distal. (*B*) The incision is extended into the tibial-talar joint space and the foot is placed in forced plantar flexion. (*C*) The calcaneus is sharply dissected from the adherent plantar fascia along a plane adjacent to the bone. (*D*) The heel pad is rotated anteriorly and approximated after the calcaneal dissection in the two-stage procedure and after the additional transection of the medial and lateral malleoli in the one-stage procedure. (*E*) Elliptical incisions are made over the medial and lateral malleoli during a second operation for the staged procedure. The medial and lateral malleoli are transected flush with the ankle joint, and the distal flares of the tibia and fibula are removed. (*F*) The two-stage procedure results in a less bulbous, more cosmetically appealing residual limb.   (*continues*)

mal below-knee amputation can be performed in the presence of an extensive foot infection, with the skin and soft tissue flap left open. The flap can be closed subsequently with a delayed primary technique after resolution of the infectious process. The skin and soft tissue flap should be left slightly longer than usual in this setting to allow for contraction. Occasionally, patients require an emergent amputation yet have overwhelming medical problems that preclude any operative intervention. A temporizing medical amputation is indicated in this setting. Simply, a tourniquet is applied proximal to the infectious or gangrenous process and the extremity packed in dry ice. This effectively prevents the release of all systemically active ischemic breakdown products and allows the definitive amputation to be delayed for a few days until stabilization of the medical condition occurs.

A rigid postoperative dressing is preferred after a below-knee amputation, although soft dressings with elastic support have been used traditionally. The rigid dressings have several reported advantages, including stump protection, stump molding, prevention of edema, acceleration of wound healing, improved patient comfort, and prevention of contractures.[30,49] Additionally, they afford the potential to attach an immediate-fit prosthesis. The technique for applying the rigid dressing is straightforward. After the sterile dressing is applied to the incision, the distal stump is covered with fluffed gauze. A knitted, sterile sock is then placed over the stump, and the potential pressure points over the bony prominences, including the patella, the head of the fibula, and the tibial condyles, are padded with felt. The knee is then positioned in about 10 degrees of flexion, and a cast is constructed to the high thigh with graded compression. The inner layers of the cast are constructed from elastic plaster, while the outer layers are constructed with fiberglass. The cast is suspended with a strap and waist belt. A rigid removable dressing is an excellent alternative to the thigh-high rigid dressing.[50] The technique is essentially the same, but the trim line for the cast is below the patella anteriorly and slightly further distally posteriorly, thus allowing knee flexion. An additional knitted sock is placed over the cast, and the dressing is suspended from the thigh by a Velcro strap. The rigid removable dressing allows early examination of the wound in addition to the other advantages reported for the high-thigh dressing. The wound is first examined with the high-thigh dressing after 10 days during the first cast change unless the patient is febrile or there are specific wound concerns.

Above-Knee Amputation

The indications for an above-knee amputation are similar to those for the below-knee level. The noninvasive criteria used to select the above-knee level are shown in Table 86-9. As can be seen, the primary wound healing rates are excellent.

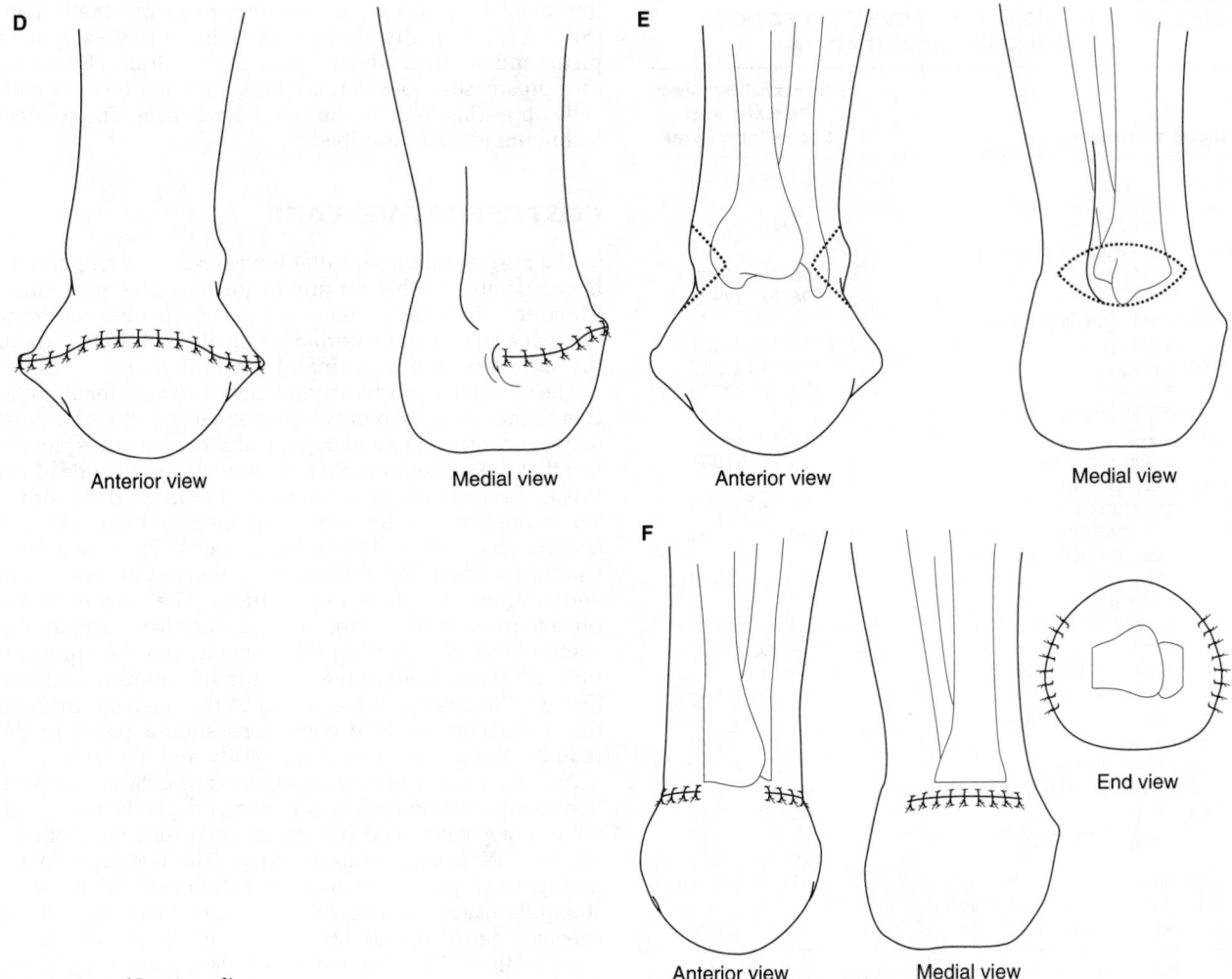

D   Anterior view   Medial view

E   Anterior view   Medial view

F   Anterior view   Medial view   End view

Figure 86-4. (Continued)

Amputation at the above-knee level has historically been favored over the below-knee level in dysvascular patients because of the primary wound healing rate. Although this approach essentially ensures primary wound healing, it denies the patient the advantages of the below-knee amputation. A more aggressive approach to knee salvage has resulted in an above-knee/below-knee amputation ratio of less than 1.[51] An above-knee amputation is contraindicated if the infectious or gangrenous process extends above the proposed amputation level, but this situation is infrequent owing to the length of the femur. An above-knee amputation can be performed at the distal, middle, or proximal femur, depending on the extent of the underlying process. Although the failure of an above-knee amputation to heal is infrequent, it can be associated with fatal complications. Bunt[52] identified three scenarios in which an above-knee amputation is relatively contraindicated: (1) acute thrombosis of both an inflow and an outflow procedure, (2) occlusion of the superficial femoral artery in the presence of a diseased profunda, and (3) the absence of palpable femoral pulses, with no detectable high-thigh pulse volume recording. An arterial inflow procedure, a profundaplasty, or both should be performed before or concomitant to the above-knee amputation in these settings.[52,53]

The technique for an above-knee amputation is illustrated in Figure 86-6. Equal-length anterior and posterior skin and soft tissue flaps are preferred, although both circular and sagittal flaps are acceptable. The distal extent of the anterior and posterior flaps and thus the length of the stump is dictated by the underlying process. Long above-knee stumps are favored owing to the increased potential for ambulation despite the associated marginally decreased wound healing rate. If the ischemic or infectious processes are limited to below the knee, a point immediately proximal to the patella is chosen as the distal extent of the flaps. The midpoint of the thigh in the anteroposterior axis is identified both medially and laterally, and equal-length 3-cm flaps are created. The skin incision is extended into the soft tissue and fascia, and the anterior musculature is incised either sharply or with electrocautery along the line of the skin incision. The femur is dissected free circumferentially, and the periosteum is elevated proximal to the level of the proposed transection at the intersection of the anterior and posterior flaps. The femur is transected with the reciprocating air-driven power saw, and the remaining major neurovasculature structures are identified and suture ligated. The posterior musculature is incised along the line of the skin incision, and the specimen is removed from the operative field. The edges of the transected femur are filed smooth. The fascial edges of the anterior and posterior flaps are approximated with absorbable, interrupted sutures, and the skin edges are reapproximated.

The immediate postoperative care of patients after above-knee amputation is similar to that for below-knee amputation. Soft dressings with elastic support are applied intraoperatively. A rigid dressing may be applied, although it does not confer the same advantages at the above-knee level and is significantly more difficult to apply.

Table 86-8. PREOPERATIVE LEVEL SELECTION: BELOW-KNEE AMPUTATION

Selection Criteria	Successful Healing, Primary and Secondary/Total	
Empiric	794/974	(82%)
Doppler ankle systolic pressure		
>30 mmHg	66/70	(94%)
Doppler calf systolic pressure		
>50 mmHg	36/36	(100%)
>68 mmHg	96/97	(99%)
Doppler thigh systolic pressure		
>100 mmHg	31/31	(100%)
>80 mmHg	104/113	(92%)
Fluorescein dye	24/30	(80%)
Fiberoptic fluorometry (dye fluorescence index >44)	12/12	(100%)
Laser Doppler velocimetry	8/8	(100%)
Skin perfusion pressure		
^{99m}Tc pertechnate	24/26	(92%)
^{131}I or ^{125}I antipyrine >30 mm	60/62	(97%)
Photoelectric skin perfusion pressure		
>20 mm	60/71	(85%)
^{133}Xe skin blood flow		
Epicutaneous >0.9 mL/100 g tissue/min	14/15	(93%)
Intradermal >2.4 mL/100 g tissue/min	83/89	(93%)
Intradermal >1 mL/100 g tissue/min	11/12	(92%)
Transcutaneous Po_2 = 0	0/3	(0%)
>10 mmHg (or >10 mm increase on Fio_2 = 1.0)	76/80	(95%)
>10 and <40 mmHg	5/7	(71%)
>20	25/26	(96%)
>35 mmHg	51/51	(100%)
Transcutaneous Po_2 index >0.59	17/17	(100%)
Transcutaneous Pco_2 <40 mmHg	7/8	(88%)

(Durham JR. Lower extremity amputation levels: indications, methods of determining appropriate level, technique, prognosis. In: Rutherford RB, ed. Vascular surgery, ed 3. Philadelphia, WB Saunders, 1989:1700)

Hip Disarticulation

Amputation of the lower extremity at the level of the hip (hip disarticulation) is performed infrequently. The indications include malignancy, trauma, the complications of arterial insufficiency, and infected hip prostheses. Hip disarticulations are rarely performed for complications of arterial insufficiency because a high above-knee amputation heals in most cases. Furthermore, hip disarticulation performed for an ischemic above-knee amputation stump is associated with a high incidence of complications in the absence of revascularization.[53] There are no noninvasive criteria to predict primary wound healing at this level because of the infrequency of the procedure and the limited alternatives. The surgical technique is well described.[54-57]

Other Amputation Levels

The operative procedures described are not all-inclusive. Additional foot and forefoot amputations have been described, although they are inferior to the transmetatarsal, Syme, and below-knee amputations. An amputation at the level of the knee (knee disarticulation) is occasionally indicated for patients in whom below-knee amputation is not possible. Knee disarticulations are superior to above-knee amputations and allow end weight bearing,

improved proprioception, and improved prosthetic control.[30,58] Additionally, they preserve the epiphyseal growth plates and are thus advantageous for children. The necessary prostheses, however, are bulky and are less cosmetically appealing than for the below-knee level. The surgical technique is well described.[59]

POSTOPERATIVE CARE

The postoperative care after lower extremity amputation is comparable to that for any major operative procedure. Three specific areas of concern that merit further emphasis are management of comorbid medical conditions, care of the extremity, and initiation of rehabilitation.

The associated morbidity and mortality rates for amputation of the lower extremity equal or exceed those for most major general and vascular surgical procedures despite the fact that the procedures are not associated with large blood losses, hemodynamic instability, nor large fluid shifts. These rates reflect the underlying medical condition and general physiologic state of the patients. These problems should be identified during the preoperative evaluation and optimized before intervention. The operative approach from both a surgical and anesthetic standpoint should be devised within this context, and the optimization of these underlying conditions should continue through the postoperative period. A thorough approach to the underlying medical conditions should result in the reduction of the associated morbidity and mortality.

Ambulation on a prosthesis requires a well-healed amputation stump. Wound healing is primarily dependent on a variety of preoperative and intraoperative factors, but there are several postoperative considerations. The objectives in the postoperative period are to prevent stump edema, allow for stump shrinkage, maintain full range of joint motion, maintain adequate nutrition, and aggressively anticipate and treat all complications.[50] The wound should be inspected daily and all hematomas or evidence of cellulitis treated appropriately. Edema of the stump should be prevented because it limits tissue perfusion and inhibits wound healing. It may be prevented with either elastic compression wraps or a rigid dressing. As noted earlier, rigid dressings are preferred after below-knee amputation. Stump shrinkage results from both resolution of soft tissue edema and atrophy of the musculature and is expedited by the appropriate dressing. Contractures across the joint spaces can develop quickly and can preclude ambulation on a prosthesis. Early initiation of joint range of motion exercises is the key to preventing contractures.

The rehabilitation process should be initiated immediately after operation within the context of a multidisciplinary approach. This ensures the greatest likelihood of patients returning to their previous ambulatory and functional status.

COMPLICATIONS
Mortality

The operative mortality rate after amputation of the lower extremity is dependent on both the indication for the procedure and the level of the amputation. The reported operative mortality rates for major lower extremity amputations in dysvascular and diabetic patients have ranged from 0% to 35%.[30] The mortality rates for these patients are shown in Table 86-3 and were determined from multiple series with appropriate weighting for the patient numbers.[51] As can be seen, the mortality rate increases significantly for above-knee amputations. Cardiovascular causes are responsible for two thirds of these postoperative deaths, with one third of the deaths resulting from myocar-

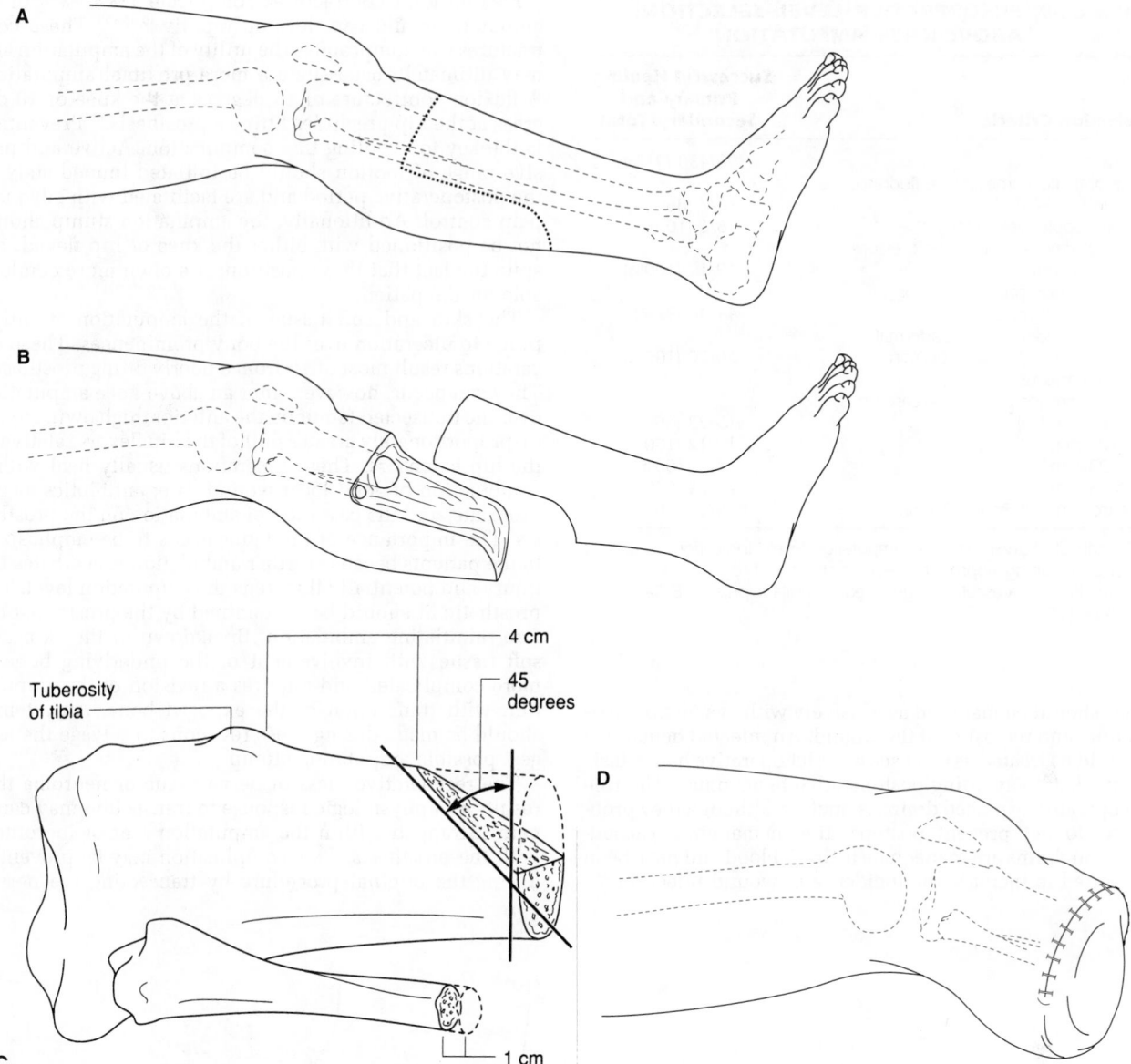

Figure 86-5. (*A*) The skin incision for a below-knee amputation based on a posterior flap is made 11 cm distal to the tibial tuberosity and extended medially and laterally to the mid-point of the calf. The length of the posterior flap is about 2 cm longer than the diameter of the calf at the point of the proximal incision. (*B*) The tibia is transected 1 cm proximal to the skin incision. The fibula is transected an additional 1 cm proximal to the level of the tibial transection, and the posterior calf muscles are incised along the plane of the skin incision. (*C*) The anterior aspect of the tibia is beveled at an angle of about 45 degrees, and the bone edges are filed. (*D*) The posterior flap is rotated anteriorly and approximated.

dial infarction.[30] The operative mortality rate for amputations performed for the other indications should be less.

The long-term survival after lower extremity amputation in the dysvascular population is shown in Table 86-4. The 5-year survival rate of 37% is markedly less than the 85% expected 5-year survival rate for the age-adjusted normal population.[10] Sixty percent of the deaths are secondary to complications of cardiovascular disease, with myocardial infarction accounting for about 50% of these.[30] This poor long-term survival emphasizes the necessity of long-term medical follow-up.

Stump Complications

A small percentage of amputations do not heal, despite the prediction based on preoperative noninvasive testing. Amputation at the next most proximal level is usually suc-

cessful in this setting, but the preoperative noninvasive tests should be repeated.

Postoperative wound infections complicate 12% to 28% of all amputations and vary with the indication for the procedure.[60,61] The rates are highest among the subset of patients who undergo amputations with active infectious processes. The incidence of wound infection may be reduced in this setting by staged local débridement or guillotine amputation before the definitive procedure.[42,43] Postoperative wound infections should be handled in the standard fashion with a combination of intravenous antibiotics, wound exploration and drainage, and dressing changes. Unfortunately, they are often ominous and portend amputation at a more proximal level. Similarly, wound hematomas can become secondarily infected and compromise the amputation level. All significant hemato-

Table 86-9. PREOPERATIVE LEVEL SELECTION: ABOVE-KNEE AMPUTATION

Selection Criteria	Successful Healing, Primary and Secondary/Total
Empiric	390/430 (91%)
Fiberoptic fluorometry (dye fluorescence index >44)	6/7 (86%)
Laser Doppler velocimetry	6/6 (100%)
Photoelectric skin perfusion pressure >21 mm	19/19 (100%)
Skin perfusion pressure (^{131}I or ^{125}I antipyrine)	44/48 (92%)
^{133}Xe skin blood flow intradermal >2.6 mL/100 g tissue/min	20/20 (100%)
Transcutaneous P_{O_2}	
>10 mm (or 10 mm increase on F_{IO_2} = 1.0)	15/23 (65%)
>20 mm	12/12 (100%)
>23 mm	2/2 (100%)
>35 mm	21/24 (88%)
Transcutaneous P_{CO_2} <38 mm	5/5 (100%)

(Durham JR. Lower extremity amputation levels: indications, methods of determining appropriate level, technique, prognosis. In: Rutherford RB, ed. Vascular surgery, ed 3. Philadelphia, WB Saunders, 1989:1707)

mas should be managed aggressively with evacuation, irrigation, and reclosure of the wound. An infected hematoma should be treated as an abscess. Strict operative hemostasis is the key to avoiding postoperative hematomas. The role of operatively placed drains is unclear, although they probably do not prevent postoperative hematomas. Closed-suction drains are inadequate to drain blood and have been reported to increase the incidence of wound infection.[62]

Flexion joint contractures complicate 1% to 3% of all amputations and can develop rapidly.[10,63–65] These contractures can compromise the utility of the amputation and may ultimately necessitate a more proximal amputation. A flexion contracture of 15 degrees at the knee or 10 degrees at the hip precludes fitting a prosthesis.[66] Prevention is the key to avoiding this complication. Active and passive range of motion should be initiated immediately in the postoperative period and are facilitated with adequate pain control. Additionally, the amputation stump should not be positioned with either the knee or hip flexed, despite the fact that these positions are often more comfortable for the patient.

The skin and soft tissue of the amputation stump is prone to ulceration over the bony prominences. These ulcerations result most often from a poorly fitting prostheses. They can occur, however, after an above-knee amputation over the transected femur on the anterior thigh owing to the disproportionately greater pull of the hip flexors relative to the hip extensors. These ulcerations usually heal with a combination of good local wound care, antibiotics as appropriate, and the cessation of ambulation on the prosthesis. The importance of the latter needs to be emphasized to the patients because further ambulation exacerbates the injury and potentially threatens the amputation level. The prosthetic fit should be reexamined by the prosthetist before reinitiating ambulation. Breakdown of the skin and soft tissue with involvement of the underlying bone is more complicated and requires a revision of the amputation with transection of the exposed bone. An attempt should be made during these revisions to salvage the longest possible amputation stump.

The regenerative mass of nerve tissue or neuroma that results as a physiologic response to transection may cause pain if trapped within the amputation scar or in contact with the prosthesis. This complication may be prevented during the original procedure by transecting the nerves

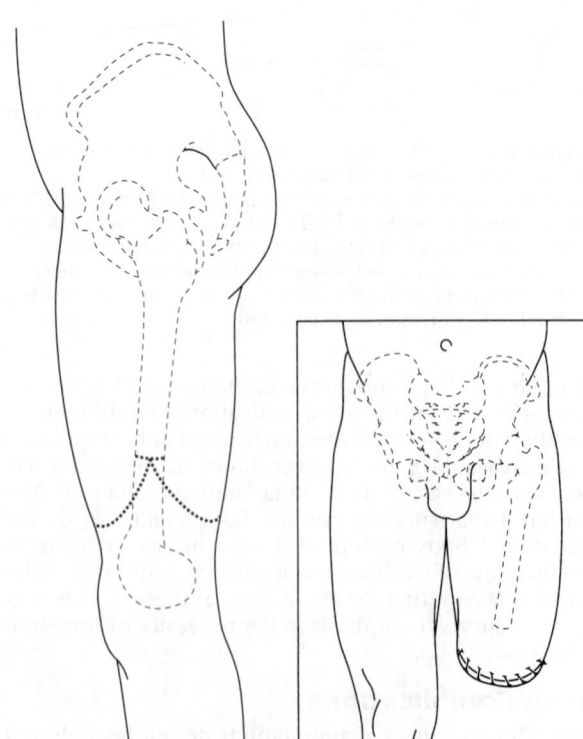

Figure 86-6. (*A*) Equal length anterior and posterior flaps are made for the above-knee amputation, and the femur is transected at the level of the angle formed by the flaps. (*B*) The anterior and posterior thigh soft tissues are incised along the plane of the skin incision, and the flaps are approximated.

under tension and allowing them to retract into the wound. Symptomatic neuromas should be treated by proximal resection of the nerve because excision of the neuroma is rarely adequate.

Phantom extremity pain occurs after essentially all lower extremity amputations. Sherman and colleagues[67,68] reported that 85% of all amputees surveyed reported significant phantom pain, although the complaints were not always related to the responsible physician. Furthermore, severe, disabling phantom pain was reported by 5% to 30% of patients surveyed.[67-71] This pain is believed to be part of a central pain syndrome and unrelated to either a neuroma or the perception of an intact extremity. Several treatment modalities have been tried, including medication, transcutaneous nerve stimulation, and ablative neurologic procedures, although they have been uniformly unsuccessful.[67,68] There is no effective treatment for chronic phantom pain. Malone[30] reported that disabling phantom pain may be reduced to less than 5% by an aggressive postamputation rehabilitation program with immediate prosthetic fitting.

Deep Venous Thrombosis and Pulmonary Embolus

The incidence of deep venous thrombosis after lower extremity amputation ranges from 4% to 38%[10,63] while that for pulmonary embolus ranges from 1% to 3%.[10,72] Both immobility and prior attempts at arterial revascularization with injury to the deep venous system increase the risk of these complications. Prophylactic measures, including subcutaneous heparin, early mobility, and pneumatic compression devices, should be used routinely.

Additional Limb Loss

The incidence of additional limb loss in dysvascular and diabetic patients is significant. Little and colleagues[73] reported that a more proximal amputation was required in 75% of all dysvascular patients within 3.5 years after toe amputation. The incidence of contralateral limb loss in dysvascular and diabetic patients ranges from 15% to 33% 5 years after a major lower extremity amputation.[74-76] These additional procedures reflect the systemic nature of the underlying disease process and emphasize the importance of appropriate foot care, patient education, and close medical surveillance.

REHABILITATION AND PROSTHETIC MANAGEMENT

General Considerations

Rehabilitation

The goal of the rehabilitation process is to restore patients to their optimal functional capacity. Ideally, this means ambulation on a prosthesis and an independent lifestyle. This is not realistic for all patients, however, and the rehabilitation program must be individualized to help each patient reach his or her optimal level, whether ambulation or transfer to a wheel chair.

Successful ambulation on a prosthesis is dependent on the physiologic status of the patient. As noted earlier, the energy requirements for ambulation on a prosthesis increase with the proximity of the amputation level (see Table 86-5). Successful ambulation requires sufficient physiologic reserve to overcome these increased requirements. Interestingly, crutch walking requires more energy than ambulating on a unilateral below-knee prosthesis.[77] Pre-

dictably, the likelihood of a diabetic or dysvascular patient ambulating on a prosthesis varies inversely with the proximity of the level (Table 86-10). The likelihood is good for patients who undergo below-knee amputations but decreases significantly for above-knee amputations. Furthermore, the likelihood decreases with increasing patient age and longer duration of the rehabilitation process.[75,77,78] The progression from below-knee amputation to ambulation averages 133 days for dysvascular and diabetic patients and is longer after above-knee amputation.[63]

Prostheses

The prosthesis should provide an acceptable extremity substitute from both a functional and cosmetic standpoint. The prosthetic requirements vary considerably with the level of the amputation. A prosthesis for the more proximal amputation levels requires several components. It must include a socket that comfortably interfaces with the residual extremity and effectively transmits the forces necessary for ambulation. It requires a suspension mechanism that allows it to maintain the contact and alignment with the residual extremity. Furthermore, it requires an endoskeletal system that is lightweight yet sufficiently strong to withstand daily use. Finally, the prosthesis must include the necessary joints.

Specific Levels

Digit and Ray Amputation

No specific rehabilitation nor prosthesis is required after a digital or ray amputation. All patients should be able to resume their preoperative functional levels. The first digit and the metatarsal head are important for weight bearing and for the push-off component of ambulation. These functions may be effectively reproduced with an orthosis that inserts into the shoe.

Transmetatarsal Amputation

Rehabilitation after a transmetatarsal amputation is excellent because there is no increased energy expenditure required for ambulation. All patients should be able to resume their preoperative activity levels once the wound has healed. The loss of the digits and metatarsal heads results in the loss of the push-off motion during ambulation. This may be reproduced with either a steel shank or a rigid, roller-soled shoe, and the void in the shoe created by the loss of the digits can be filled with an insert.

Table 86-10. AMBULATION AFTER LOWER EXTREMITY AMPUTATION FOR DIABETES OR OCCLUSIVE DISEASE

Amputation Level	Postoperative Ambulation (%)
Digit or ray	100
Transmetatarsal	100
Syme amputation	90–100
Below-knee	75
Above-knee	39
Hip disarticulation	<10

(Data from Malone JM. Lower extremity amputation. In: Moore WS, ed. Vascular surgery: a comprehensive review. Philadelphia, WB Saunders, 1993:809; Frang RD, Taylor LM, Porter JM. Amputations. In: Porter JM, Taylor LM, eds. Basic data underlying clinical decision making in vascular surgery. St Louis, Quality Medical Publishing, 1994:153)

Syme Amputation

All patients undergoing a Syme amputation should be able to return to their preoperative functional levels because ambulation requires only a 10% increase of energy expenditure.[30] The usual prosthesis is composed of a non-motion foot attached to a leg shaft. The shaft is constructed with a medial window that allows the end of the residual extremity to fit easily through the more narrow section. The net result is a bulbous ankle that is less cosmetically appealing than the below-knee prosthesis. Unlike the more proximal amputations, the end of the residual extremity serves as the weight-bearing surface. Limited ambulation is permitted within the home on the stump using a cup slipper.

Below-Knee Amputation

The rehabilitation potential after a below-knee amputation is good. About 75% of all patients requiring a below-knee amputation for complications of arterial occlusive disease are able to ambulate on a prosthesis.[51] Furthermore, patients ambulatory at the time of admission and operated on within 30 days should remain ambulatory.[30] A variety of prosthetic design options are available to satisfy the patient's preferences and functional requirements. The patellar tendon and the medial and lateral tibial flares are the primary weight-bearing surfaces for most of these prostheses. The prosthesis may be suspended using either a patellar tendon strap, elastic-strap waist belt, suction, a thigh lacer with external hinges, or a supracondylar clip. The exoskeleton is commonly made of wood, plastic, or both. Similarly, a variety of foot designs are available and potentially permit extension, flexion, rotation, and energy storage. The solid ankle cushion heel foot is commonly used and is composed of a sponge rubber heel and flexible keel that bends when weight is applied and recoils as it is removed, facilitating push-off.

Above-Knee Amputation

Successful ambulation on an above-knee prosthesis is achieved in less than 40% of all patients who require amputation for the complications of arterial insufficiency.[51] Furthermore, the likelihood of these patients ambulating on bilateral above-knee amputations is less than 10%.[79] The ischial tuberosity is the primary weight-bearing surface for the common above-knee prostheses, and they are suspended using either a belt or a suction socket. The latter mechanism is useful for the young amputee although frequently more difficult for the dysvascular patient owing to previous groin incisions. The prosthetic knee design is dependent on the physiologic state of the patient and the patient's relative thigh strength. A prosthetic knee that engages during the stance phase of gait is commonly used in the geriatric population owing to its added stability. The remaining components of above-knee prostheses are similar to those for below-knee prostheses.

REFERENCES

1. Falstie-Jensen N, Christensen KB. A model for prediction of failure in amputation of the lower limb. Dan Med Bull 1990;37:283.
2. Veith FJ, Gupta SK, Samson RH, et al. Progress in limb salvage by reconstructive arterial surgery combined with new or improved adjunctive procedures. Ann Surg 1981;194:386.
3. Lange RH, Bach AW, Hansen ST, et al. Open tibial fractures with associated vascular injuries: prognosis for limb salvage. J Trauma 1985;25:203.
4. Johansen K, Daines M, Howey T, et al. Objective criteria accurately predict amputation following lower extremity trauma. J Trauma 1990;30:568.
5. Fierer J, Daniel D, Davis C. The fetid foot: lower-extremity infections in patients with diabetes mellitus. Rev Infect Dis 1979;1:210.
6. Effeney DJ, Lim RC, Schecter WP. Transmetatarsal amputation. Arch Surg 1977;112:1366.
7. McKittrick LS, McKittrick JB, Risley TS. Transmetatarsal amputation for infection or gangrene in patients with diabetes mellitus. Ann Surg 1949;130:826.
8. Wagner FW Jr. The Syme amputation. In: American Academy of Orthopaedic Surgeons, eds. Atlas of limb prosthetics: surgical and prosthetic principles. St Louis, CV Mosby, 1981:326.
9. Keagy BA, Schwartz JA, Kotb M, et al. Lower extremity amputation: the control series. J Vasc Surg 1986;7:321.
10. Roon AJ, Moore WS, Goldstone J. Below-knee amputations: a modern approach. Am J Surg 1977;134:153.
11. Hobson RW, Lynch TG, Jamil Z, et al. Results of revascularization and amputation in severe lower extremity ischemia: a five year clinical experience. J Vasc Surg 1985;2:174.
12. Reichle FA, Rankin KP, Tyson RR, et al. Long term results of 474 arterial reconstructions for severely ischemic limbs: a fourteen year followup. Surgery 1979;85:93.
13. Kazmers M, Satiani B, Evans WE. Amputation level following unsuccessful distal limb salvage operations. Surgery 1980;87:683.
14. Ramsburgh SR, Lindenauer SM, Weber IR, et al. Femoropopliteal bypass for limb salvage surgery. Surgery 1977;81:453.
15. Szilagyi DE, Hageman JH, Smith RF, et al. Autogenous vein grafting in femoropopliteal atherosclerosis. Surgery 1979;86:836.
16. Bartlett ST, Olinde AJ, Flinn WR, et al. The re-operative potential of infrainguinal bypass: long-term limb and patient survival. J Vasc Surg 1987;5:170.
17. Bloom RJ, Stevick A. Amputation and distal bypass salvage of the limb. Surg Gynecol Obstet 1988;166:1.
18. Light JT, Rice JC, Kerstein MD. Sequelae of limited amputation. Surgery 1988;103:294.
19. Patel PR, Semel L, Clauss RH. Extended reconstruction rate for limb salvage with intraoperative prereconstruction angiography. J Vasc Surg 1988;7:531.
20. Ricco JB, Pearce WH, Yao JST, et al. The use of operative prebypass arteriography and Doppler ultrasound recordings to select patients for extended femoro-distal bypass. Ann Surg 1983;198:646.
21. Cambria RP, Yucel EK, Brewster DC, et al. The potential for lower extremity revascularization without contrast arteriography: experience with magnetic resonance angiography. Radiology 1993;187:637.
22. Owens RS, Carpenter JP, Baum RA, et al. Magnetic resonance imaging of angiographically occult runoff vessels in peripheral arterial occlusive disease. N Engl J Med 1992;326:1577.
23. Brewster DC, LaSalle AJ, Robison JG, et al. Femoropopliteal graft failure: clinical consequences and success of secondary reconstructions. Arch Surg 1983;118:1043.
24. DeWeese JA, Rob CG. Autogenous venous grafts ten years later. Surgery 1977;82:775.
25. Callow AD, Mackey WC. Costs and benefits of prosthetic vascular surgery. Int Surg 1988;73:237.
26. Gregg RO. Bypass or amputation? Am J Surg 1985;149:397.
27. Rabiola CA, Nichter LS, Baker JD, et al. Cost of treating advanced leg ischemia. Arch Surg 1988;123:495.
28. Cederburg PA, Pritchard DJ, Joyce JW. Doppler-determined segmental pressures and wound healing in amputations for vascular disease. J Bone Joint Surg 1983;65A:363.
29. Dwars BJ, Van Den Broek TA, Ravwerda JA, et al. Criteria for reliable selection of the lowest level of amputation in peripheral vascular disease. J Vasc Surg 1992;15:536.
30. Malone JM. Lower extremity amputation. In: Moore WS, ed. Vascular surgery: a comprehensive review. Philadelphia, WB Saunders, 1993:809.
31. Yao JST, Bergen JJ. Application of ultrasound to arterial and venous diagnosis. Surg Clin North Am 1974;54:23.
32. Holloway GA, Burgess EM. Cutaneous blood flow and its relation to healing of below knee amputation. Surg Gynecol Obstet 1978;146:750.
33. Kostuik JP, Wood D, Hornby R, et al. Measurement of skin blood flow in peripheral vascular disease by the epicutaneous application of xenon-133. J Bone Joint Surg 1964;58:833.

34. Moore WS. Determination of amputation level: measurement of skin blood flow with xenon-133 clearance. Arch Surg 1973;107:798.
35. Burnham ST, Wagner WH, Keagy BH, et al. Objective measurement of limb perfusion by dermal fluorometry: a criterion for healing of below knee amputation. Arch Surg 1990; 125:513.
36. Malone JM, Anderson GG, Halka SC, et al. Prospective comparison of noninvasive techniques for amputation level selection. Am J Surg 1987;154:179.
37. Holloway GA, Watkins BW. Laser Doppler measurement of cutaneous blood flow. J Invest Dermatol 1977;69:300.
38. Schwartz JA, Schuler JJ, O'Connor RJA, et al. Predictive value of distal perfusion pressure in the healing of amputation of the digits and the forefoot. Surg Gynecol Obstet 1982;154:865.
39. Golbranson FL, Yu EC, Gleberman RH. The use of skin temperature determinations in lower extremity amputation level selection. Foot Ankle 1982;3:170.
40. Gibbons GW, Wheelock FC, Hoar CS, et al. Predicting success of forefoot amputations in diabetics by noninvasive testing. Arch Surg 1979;114:1034.
41. Mills JL, Porter JM. Acute limb ischemia. In: Porter JM, Taylor LM, eds. Basic data underlying clinical decision making in vascular surgery. St Louis, Quality Medical Publishing, 1994:134.
42. McIntyre KE, Bailey SA, Malone JM, et al. The nonsalvageable infected lower extremity: a new look at guillotine amputation. Am J Surg 1985;117:58.
43. Fischer DF, Clagett GP, Fry RE, et al. One stage versus two-stage amputation for wet gangrene of the lower extremity: a randomized study. J Vasc Surg 1988;8:428.
44. Rubin JR, Yao JST, Thompson RG, et al. Management of infection of major amputation stumps after failed femorodistal grafts. Surgery 1985;98:810.
45. Rubin JR, Marmen C, Rhodes RS. Management of failed prosthetic grafts at the time of major lower extremity amputation. J Vasc Surg 1988;7:673.
46. Warren R, Kihn RB. A survey of lower extremity amputations for ischemia. Surgery 1968;63:107.
47. Burgess EM, Roman RL, Zettl JH, et al. Amputation of the leg for peripheral vascular insufficiency. J Bone Joint Surg 1971;53A:875.
48. Burgess EM, Mason FA. Current concepts to review: determining amputation level in peripheral vascular disease. J Bone Joint Surg 1981;63A:1493.
49. Shea JD. Surgical techniques of lower extremity amputation. Orthop Clin North Am 1972;3:287.
50. Leonard JA, Andrews KL. Rigid removable dressings, immediate postoperative prostheses, and rehabilitation of the amputee. In: Ernst CB, Stanley JC, eds. Current therapy in vascular surgery, ed 2. Philadelphia, BC Decker, 1991:708.
51. Frang RD, Taylor LM, Porter JM. Amputations. In: Porter JM, Taylor LM, eds. Basic data underlying clinical decision making in vascular surgery. St Louis, Quality Medical Publishing, 1994:153.
52. Bunt TJ. Gangrene of the immediate postoperative above-knee amputation stump: role of emergency revascularization in preventing death. J Vasc Surg 1985;2:874.
53. Kwaan JHM, Connolly JE. Fatal sequelae of the ischemic amputation stump: a surgical challenge. Am J Surg 1979;138:49.
54. Endean ED, Schwarz TH, Barker DE, et al. Hip disarticulation: factors affecting outcome. J Vasc Surg 1991;14:398.
55. Boyd HB. Anatomic disarticulation of the hip. Surg Gynecol Obstet 1947;84:346.
56. Hogshead HP. Experience with hip disarticulation and hemipelvectomy procedure. J Bone Joint Surg 1971;53A:1031.
57. Wu KK, Guise ER, Forst, HM, Mitchell CL. The surgical technique for hindquarter amputation: report of 19 cases. Acta Orthop Scand 1977;48:479.
58. Houghton A, Allen A, Luff R, McColl I. Rehabilitation after lower extremity amputation: a comparative study of above-knee, through knee and Gritti-Stokes amputations. Br J Surg 1989;76:622.
59. Burgess EM. Disarticulation of the knee: a modified technique. Arch Surg 1977;112:1250.
60. Berardi RS, Keonin Y. Amputations in peripheral vascular occlusive disease. Am J Surg 1978;135:231.
61. Wray CH, Still JM, Moretz WH. Present management of amputations for peripheral vascular disease. Am Surg 1972;38:87.
62. Malone JM. Complications of lower extremity amputation. In: Bernhard VM, Towne J, eds. Complications in vascular surgery. Orlando, Grune & Stratton, 1985:445.
63. Malone JM, Moore WS, Goldstone J, et al. Therapeutic and economic impact of a modern amputation program. Ann Surg 1979;189:798.
64. Malone JM, Moore WS, Leal JM, et al. Rehabilitation for lower extremity amputation. Arch Surg 1981;116:93.
65. Malone JM, Leal JM, Moore WS, et al. The "gold standard" for amputation level selection: xenon-133 clearance. J Surg Res 1981;30:449.
66. Gottschalk FA, Fisher DF. Complications of amputations. In: Rutherford RB, ed. Vascular surgery, ed 3. Philadelphia, WB Saunders, 1989:1713.
67. Sherman RA, Sherman CJ, Gall NG. A survey of current phantom limb pain treatment in the United States. Pain 1980; 18:83.
68. Sherman RA, Sherman CJ, Parker L. Chronic phantom and stump pain among American veterans: results of a survey. Pain 1984;18:83.
69. Abramson AS, Feibel A. The phantom phenomenon: its use and disuse. Bull NY Acad Med 1981;57:99.
70. Parkes CM. Factors determining persistence of phantom pain in the amputee. J Psychosomat Res 1973;17:97.
71. Sherman RA. Published treatment of phantom pain. Am J Phys Med 1980;59:232.
72. Huston CC, Bivins BA, Ernst CB, Griffen WO. Morbid implications of above-knee amputations: report of a series and review of the literature. Arch Surg 1980;115:165.
73. Little JM, Stephen MS, Zylstra PL. Amputation of the toes for vascular disease: fate of the affected leg. Lancet 1976;2:1318.
74. Malone JM, Snyder M, Anderson GG, Bernhard VM, Holloway GA, Bunt TJ. Prevention of amputation by diabetic education. Am J Surg 1989;158:520.
75. Mazet R, Schiller FJ, Dunn OJ, Alonzo NJ. The influence of prosthesis wearing on the health of the geriatric patient. Project 431. Washington, DC, Office of Vocational Rehabilitation, Department of Health, Education and Welfare, March 1963.
76. Whitehouse FW, Jurgensen C, Block MA. The later life of the diabetic amputee: another look at fate of the second leg. Diabetes 1968;17:520.
77. Waters RL, Perry J, Antonelli D, et al. Energy cost of walking amputees: the influence of level of amputation. J Bone Joint Surg 1976;58A:42.
78. Harris PL, Read F, Eardley A, et al. The fate of elderly amputees. Br J Surg 1974;61:665.
79. Malone JM. Above the knee amputation and hip disarticulation. In: Ernst CB, Stanley JC, eds. Current therapy in vascular surgery, ed 2. Philadelphia, BC Decker, 1991:699.

Aneurysmal Disease

SURGERY: SCIENTIFIC PRINCIPLES AND PRACTICE, Second Edition, edited by
Lazar J. Greenfield, Michael W. Mulholland, Keith T. Oldham, Gerald B. Zelenock,
and Keith D. Lillemoe. Lippincott–Raven Publishers, Philadelphia, © 1997.

CHAPTER 87

PATHOGENESIS OF ANEURYSMS

M. DAVID TILSON, ANIL P. HINGORANI,
AND ANITA K. GREGORY

An aneurysm is a permanent, localized dilation of a blood vessel. Lending precision to this definition, the Committee for Reporting Standards of the major North American vascular societies recommended a definition of a 50% increase in the diameter of a vessel compared with its expected normal diameter.[1] Normal arterial diameters within the aortoiliac and femoral popliteal segments are shown in Figure 87-1. Aneurysms can occur throughout the arterial tree, in central vessels (thoracic and abdominal aorta), peripheral vessels (femoral and popliteal arteries), cerebral vessels, and mesenteric and renal vessels. The most common location for an aneurysm is in the infrarenal aorta. This chapter focuses on the abdominal aortic aneurysm (AAA), but many of the concepts apply to aneurysms of the thoracic aorta as well as the femoral and popliteal arteries.

AAAs are the 15th leading cause of death in the United States,[2] and their incidence has been steadily increasing.[3–6] Accordingly, the cause, pathogenesis, and methods for possible prevention of AAAs have been subjects of increasing concern and investigation. The view that aneurysms may develop from the pulsation of blood on a weakened arterial wall, based on the late development of aneurysms after trauma, goes back to the time of Galen. In 1804, the cause of AAA was attributed to atherosclerotic degeneration by Scarpa,[7] based on the gross finding of atherosclerotic plaque on the intimal surface. Since then, most authors have attributed the formation of AAAs to atherosclerosis, and the term *atherosclerotic aneurysm* has been frequently used. Unfortunately, this expression is not scientifically informative in the sense of defining the necessary cause, as in the usage *syphilitic aneurysm*.[8] Studies have led to consideration of genetic, biochemical, and immune factors that are unique to AAA development.

INCIDENCE

About 15,000 deaths are due to AAA disease every year in the United States.[2] Autopsy studies show that the prevalence ranges from 1.8% to 6.6%.[9–12] Studies using ultrasound as a screening test suggest that the prevalence of clinically significant AAAs is about 2% to 3%.[13,14] In a study of 45,000 patients, the incidence was found to have increased seven-fold during a 30-year period to a high of 36.5 per 100,000 person-years.[6] This increase may be due in part to better diagnostic ability and an aging population, but the study also found that the incidence of symptomatic aneurysms had doubled.

This increase in incidence took place despite an overall decrease in the rate of coronary artery disease and strokes.[15,16] Thus, the increasing incidence of AAA, combined with the decrease in the rate of atherosclerotic disease, suggests that aneurysmal disease of the aorta may have a different cause than stenosing disease.

Certain groups are more likely to develop AAAs than others. The male/female ratio of AAA ranges from 2:1 to 8:1.[17–19] Some data suggest that the peak prevalence is delayed in females.[20] White males have a three times higher incidence than black males and females.[21–24] A person with a family history of AAA in a first-order relative is also more likely to develop an AAA.[25–30] Patients with AAA tend to be taller and older than typical atherosclerotic patients.[18,31]

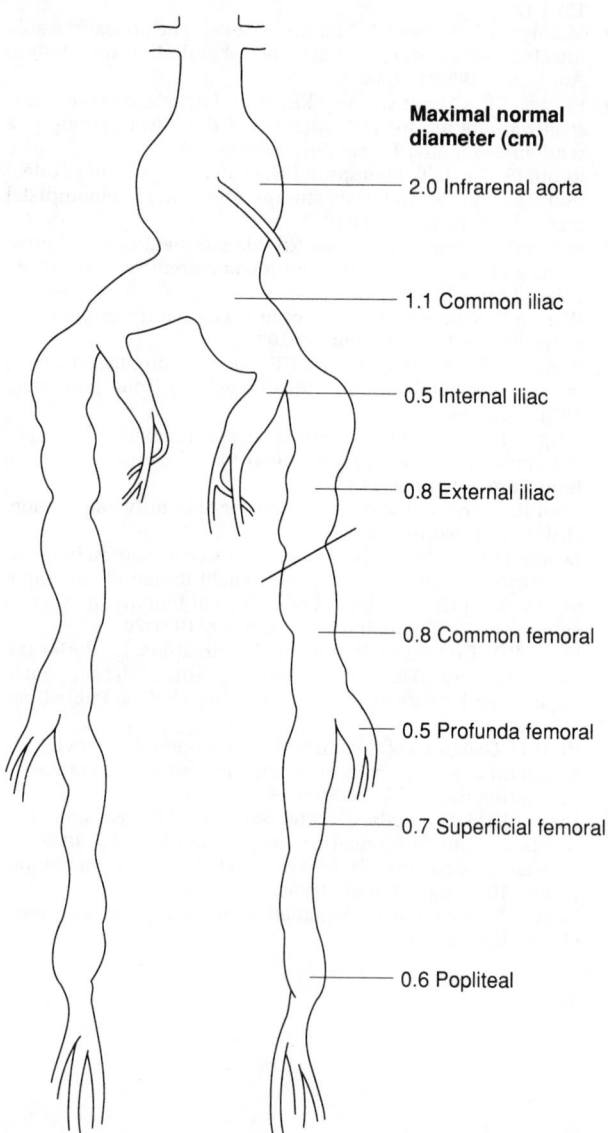

Maximal normal diameter (cm)

- 2.0 Infrarenal aorta
- 1.1 Common iliac
- 0.5 Internal iliac
- 0.8 External iliac
- 0.8 Common femoral
- 0.5 Profunda femoral
- 0.7 Superficial femoral
- 0.6 Popliteal

Figure 87-1. Normal arteriographic sizes of arteries. An aneurysm is defined as a 50% increase in the diameter of the vessel (After Hollier LH, Stanson AW, Gloviczki P, et al. Arteriomegaly: classification and morbid implications of diffuse aneurysmal disease. Surgery 1983;93:700)

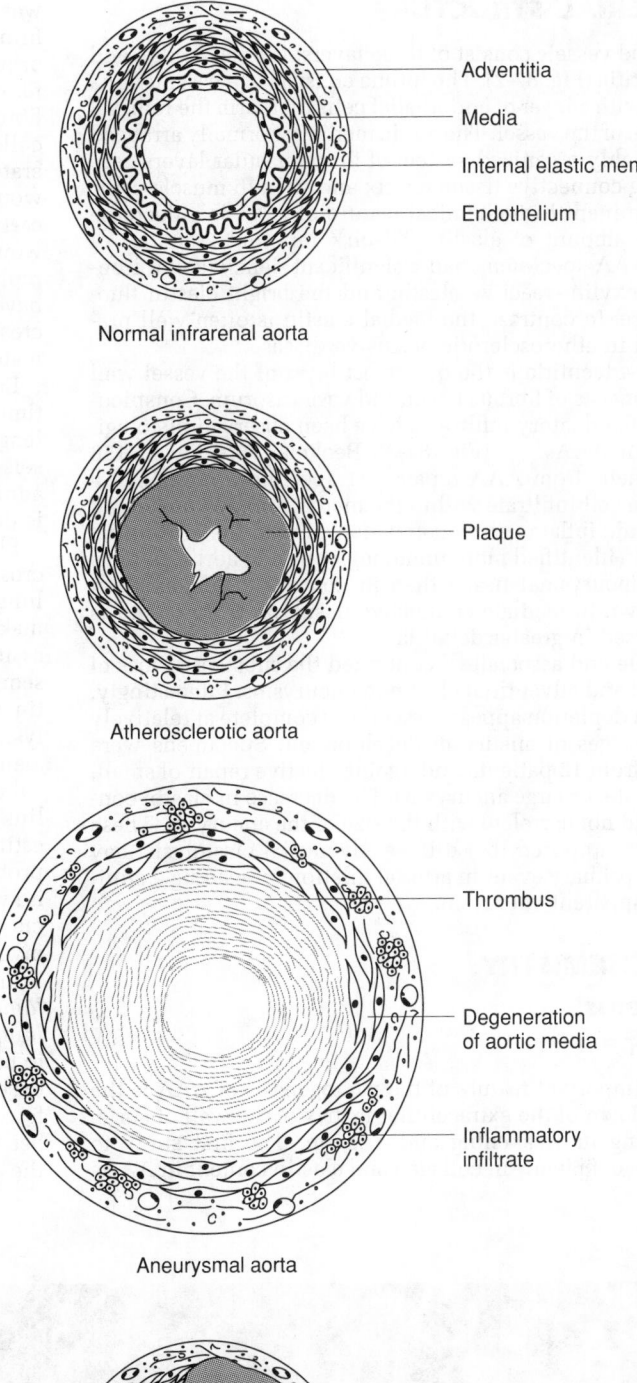

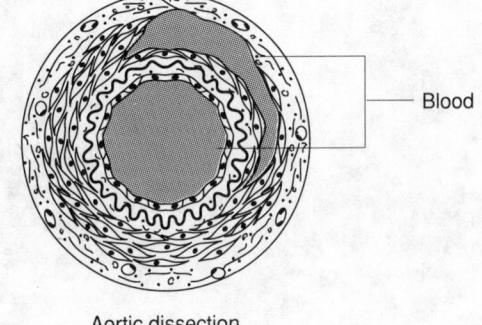

Figure 87-2. Schematic representation of the normal aorta with three distinct layers—intima, media, and adventitia. Atherosclerosis results in intimal thickening secondary to the formation of plaque. An aneurysm is dilation of an artery with degeneration of the media. The inner lining is a layer of thrombus. Aortic dissection results from an intimal tear and a consequent plane of blood cleaving the media.

ARTERIAL STRUCTURE

Blood vessels consist of three layers: intima, media, and adventitia (Fig. 87-2). The intima consists of a basal lamina lined with a layer of endothelial cells that form the luminal surface of the vessel. The aortic media is normally arranged in a highly organized system of fibromuscular layers containing connective tissue matrix and smooth muscle cells. A prominent histochemical feature of AAA is a decrease in the amount of elastin. Tilson[32] reported that four of nine AAA specimens had a significant deficiency of iron-hematoxylin–reactive elastin and the bright elastin fluorophore. In contrast, the medial elastin is often well preserved in atherosclerotic occlusive disease.

The adventitia is the outermost layer of the vessel wall and consists of fibrous tissue and vasa vasorum. Conspicuous inflammatory infiltrates have been observed histologically in AAAs[33–35] (Fig. 87-3). Beckman[36] reviewed 156 specimens from AAA repairs; 31 specimens contained a plasma cell infiltrate within the media, and 106 contained a chronic inflammatory component within the adventitia. We also identified more immunoglobulin in aortic extracts from aneurysmal tissue than in controls.[33] Inflammation is known to mediate connective tissue proteolysis and is discussed in greater detail later.

White and associates[37] confirmed the substantial loss of medial and adventitial elastin in aneurysms. Interestingly, elastin depletion appears essentially complete at relatively early stages of aneurysm development. Specimens were taken from 12 patients undergoing elective repair of small, moderate, or large aneurysms. The decrease in elastin content did not correlate with the size of the aneurysm. These authors proposed that diffuse adventitial elastolysis may be the primary event in arterial dilation, preceding a clinically apparent aneurysm.

BIOCHEMISTRY

Proteins

Elastin

An important feature of the pathogenesis of AAA is the breakdown of the extracellular matrix of the wall of aorta, resulting in weakening and dilation. The first study to show a deficiency in collagen and elastin content in AAAs was published 25 years ago.[38] Further studies have confirmed deficiency of elastin as a percentage of total mass or protein.[39–42] The amount of collagen, however, has been found to be normal or increased,[43–45] most likely because fibroblasts have a substantial capacity to synthesize new collagen to repair deficiencies. Human tissues do not generate much new elastin after the first decade of life.[46] This would imply that if elastin were not synthesized properly early in development or if it were broken down, the body would have limited capacity to synthesize new elastin to replace it. Studies of the cross-links of aneurysm elastin have not substantiated the hypothesis that there is a decrease in the number of cross-links in the residual material.[41,42]

Elastin has a remarkable ability to extend to two to three times its resting length and quickly return to its original length. In an ex vivo model of human iliac arteries,[47] vessels treated with elastase dilated and became stiffer. An additional study confirmed that the recoil of AAA tissue is decreased compared with normal tissue.[48]

Elastin is a 74-kd molecule characterized by its lysine cross-links formed by lysyl oxidase.[49] Skin, ligaments, lung, and the walls of arteries are rich in elastin. Glycine makes up about one third of the amino acids of elastin, as it does in collagen, but without the regular repeating sequence of collagen. Proline makes up about 11% of elastin, but elastin has little hydroxyproline and no hydroxylysine. Elastin is rich in nonpolar amino acids, such as alanine, valine, leucine, and isoleucine, which may contribute to its insolubility along with its extensive cross-linking through lysine residues.[50] Elastin's half life is estimated to be 70 years.[51] This remarkable stability is probably due to the abundance of its cross-links. Elastin is synthesized by mesenchymal cells, such as smooth muscle cells, chondroblasts, mesothelial cells, fibroblasts, and myofibroblasts.

In the aortic media, elastin is arrayed in layers called *lamellae,* which are separated by smooth muscle cells. The number of lamellae in mammalian aortas has been found to be directly proportional to the load that the aorta bears, except in the human abdominal aortas, where there are fewer lamellae than expected.[52] This decrease in the number of lamellae may explain why the abdominal aorta is the most frequent site of aneurysms in humans. Zatina

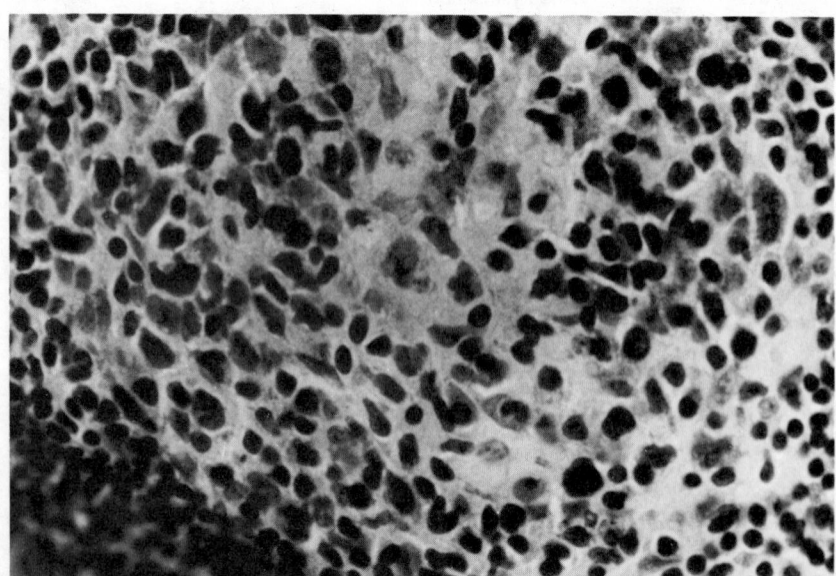

Figure 87-3. Microscopic section from a patient with a nonspecific abdominal aortic aneurysm. Marked mononuclear inflammatory infiltrate is visible (hematoxylin–eosin, ×40).

and colleagues[53] reduced the number of lamellae in pig thoracic aorta by a crush injury to induce aneurysm formation. Study results suggested that if the number of lamellae were reduced by 50%, aneurysms would develop. Because collagen and the other matrix components were also crushed, however, it is not clear that the reduction in the elastic lamellae was the most important factor resulting in the aneurysms.

Collagen

The fibrillar collagens are a family of structural proteins of extracellular matrix with repetitive sequences of amino acids in the format Gly-X-Y, where the amino acid in the X position is frequently proline and the amino acid in the Y position is frequently hydroxyproline.[54] About 1000 amino acids long, the backbone forms a left-handed helix called an α chain. Three of these chains are coiled around each other after a right-handed twist to form a procollagen molecule.[55] Numerous other nonfibrillar collagens contain noncollagenous domains in addition to the characteristic Gly-X-Y repeats. The glycine placed at every third residue plays an important role in the stability of collagen. Glycine, a small flexible amino acid, is the only one that can fit in turns of the coil. A mutation that changes this amino acid to another results in a conformational change, reducing the thermal stability of the molecule. Substitution of an arginine residue for the glycine at position 691 in the procollagen III gene has been found to cosegregate with aneurysm disease in one family.[56]

The tensile strength of collagen is four orders of magnitude (10^4) that of elastin.[57] Collagen contributes to the tensile strength of the aorta, and its failure is probably important to the development of AAAs.[58] In isolated human iliac arteries, treatment with collagenase results in aneurysm formation and rupture.[47] Tilson and associates[8,58] have suggested that failure of the collagen is a sentinel event in the chain of causal factors that result in aneurysmal dilation. Based on known arterial mechanics and experimental observations, it is postulated that elastin bears the load at small diameters, but as the arterial diameter increases, it is the collagen that actually prevents further progression to aneurysmal proportions. Biomechanical studies have shown that the adventitia, after removal of the media, can maintain normal maximal aortic diameter throughout a range of expected pressures. Clinically, vessels that undergo endarterectomy do not typically undergo aneurysmal degeneration, probably owing to the much greater tensile strength of collagen than elastin.

Fibrillin

Fibrillin is a 350-kd glycoprotein that makes up the microfibrillar structure of the extracellular matrix.[59] The microfibrillar structure appears to act as the scaffolding for the deposition of elastin during elastogenesis.[60] The two general strategies of modern molecular genetics simultaneously led to identification of fibrillin mutations as the cause of Marfan syndrome. In the candidate gene approach, fibrillin was found to be deficient, and the candidate gene was identified.[61] A mutation was then found in the gene for fibrillin in two patients with Marfan disease.[62] The reverse genetic approach correlated different portions of genetic material that were segregating with Marfan disease in a series of Finnish families.[63] These techniques led to the identification of the gene on the long arm of chromosome 15. Considering the potential significance of a change in the scaffolding for elastin throughout the aorta and the occasional association of Marfan syndrome with AAAs, fibrillin should be considered a candidate gene in AAA disease.

Other Extracellular Matrix Proteins

The extracellular matrix was long thought to be an inert framework in which cells carry on their functions. More recent evidence suggests that the matrix does not play simply a passive role but may be an active player in a wide range of functions, including the response to injury, filtration of solutions, inflammatory states, clotting cascade, and host defenses against spread of tumor and infection. Other matrix components, such as laminin, glycosaminoglycans, proteoglycans, and fibronectin may also play as yet unidentified roles in the cause of AAAs.

Proteases

Elastase

Studies that showed decreased amounts of elastin in AAA tissue led investigators to determine whether elastase activity was increased. In 1982, Busuttil and colleagues[64] found that elastase activity was increased in AAA tissue. Cannon and Read[65] found elevated blood elastolytic activity and decreased serum antiproteolytic activity in AAA patients who smoked. They suggested that the elastase was leukocyte elastase. In 1988, Dubick and colleagues[66] suggested that pancreatic elastase was the source of the increased elastolytic activity of AAA tissue. Cohen and colleagues[67] suggested that the elastolytic activity might be attributed to a serine protease from smooth muscle cells.

Other studies suggested that a nonserine elastase was present. Brown and colleagues[68] suggested that a thiol, carboxyl, or metalloenzyme was present. Campa and associates[40] found that the elastase did not react with an antibody to leukocyte elastase. Finally, Herron and colleagues[69] found several serine proteinases and gelatinolytic metalloproteinases in AAA tissue.

Our group confirmed inhibition of the principal elastase with ethylenediamine tetracetic acid, suggesting metalloproteolytic activity.[70] The enzyme was partially purified by its affinity to recombinant tissue inhibitor of metalloproteinase-1 (TIMP-1).[71] Antibody to matrix metalloproteinase 9 (MMP9) reacts with the purified enzyme on Western blot and immunoprecipitates the enzymatic activity.[72] Others have found that MMP9 has elastolytic activity,[73,74] so we believe that MMP9 is an excellent candidate for assignment as the "killer elastase" of AAA, but the possibility of additional elastases has not been ruled out.

Collagenase

Given the importance of collagen in the structural integrity of arterial wall, some investigators have studied the presence of collagenases in AAA that would weaken the aorta and cause it to become aneurysmal. In 1980, Busuttil and associates[75] found increased collagenase activity in AAA tissue. Another group confirmed the activity but was not able to extract it under nondenaturing conditions.[76] Menashi and associates[77] found collagenolytic activity to be elevated in ruptured AAA or explant cultures but did not detect it in nonruptured AAA. Finally, Herron and colleagues[69] did not detect collagenase (MMP1). On the other hand, Vine and Powell[78] reported the presence of collagenase by carbon-14 collagen assay and by specific antibody in extracts of AAA tissue. Some confusion has resulted because collagenase binds to its natural inhibitor TIMP and because there have been variations in the specificities of the antibodies that have been used for detection. By performing polyacrylamide gel electrophoresis and immunoblots on AAA extracts, we have detected MMP1 (interstitial collagenase) in several complexes and isoforms and strongly immunoreactive bands at the expected molecular weights of MMP1.[79]

Other Matrix Metalloproteinases

The MMPs are a family of extracellular proteinases that digest components of the matrix. They can break down collagens, elastin, fibronectin, laminin, and proteoglycans. They are zinc dependent and have major areas of homology. These proteinases have been found to be important in inflammatory states, organogenesis, and tumor invasion. They can be synthesized by macrophages, mesenchymal cells, and vascular smooth muscle cells. MMP3 (stomelysin) is known to activate the precursor forms of MMP1 and MMP9. MMP3 has been found by specific antibody to be present in AAA tissue in our laboratory.[72] MMP3 might have a special role in the cascade of the pathogenesis of AAA.

Plasmin

Plasmin has also been implicated in the development of AAA. Aortic infusion of plasmin and thioglycolate (a macrophage stimulator) produced aneurysms in an in vivo rat model, in which neither alone produced aneurysms.[80] Macrophages can be induced to secrete plasminogen activator.[81] Plasmin is known to degrade extracellular matrix and activate MMP9, MMP3, and MMP1.[82] We have detected plasmin by immunoblots in AAA tissue.[83] Furthermore, tissue plasminogen activator has been found to be elevated in AAA[84] and also induces secretion of MMP9 by macrophages.[85] Thus, plasmin has the potential to play an important role in the pathogenesis of AAA, and research continues to explore this issue.

Protease Inhibitors

As some studies have looked at the increase of proteolytic activity in AAA disease, others have examined whether a deficiency in antiproteolytic activity might play a role. AAAs have been associated with smoking. In the development of emphysema, smoking is known to cause methylation and inactivation of the active site of α_1-antitrypsin, a major serum antiprotease.[86] A similar role for smoking in AAA pathogenesis has been suggested, resulting in overactivity of proteases and in weakening of the extracellular matrix.[87] Indeed, an important risk factor for rupture of an AAA appears to be the degree of concomitant chronic obstructive pulmonary disease.[88]

Two inhibitors have been found to be specific for members of the MMP family: TIMP-1 and TIMP-2. Both are small glycosylated proteins produced by cells of the extracellular matrix, with 30% of the molecular weight being attributed to carbohydrate.[89] MMPs have been found to be secreted in complexes with TIMP in the extracellular matrix, which suggests an in vivo regulatory mechanism of TIMP and lends support to the idea that the controversy over the presence of MMP1 in AAA may have stemmed from MMP1 complexing to TIMP.[90] We have found immunoreactive TIMP to be reduced in AAA tissue,[91] but its gene expression appears to be normal in dermal fibroblasts from AAA patients.[92]

EXPERIMENTAL ANEURYSMS

Dobrin and associates[93] found that ex vivo infusion of elastase into an arterial wall resulted in vessel wall dilation, which did not progress to aneurysmal dimensions unless collagenase was also infused. An in vivo variation of this theme in a rat model was later developed, in which aneurysms were induced by perfusing an isolated segment of rat abdominal aorta with pancreatic elastase.[94] All elastase-perfused aortas developed local aneurysmal dilation, while saline-perfused controls did not. Perfusion with other proteases, such as papain, trypsin, or chymotrypsin, also produced elastic tissue disruption and smaller microaneurysms. Passive transfer of thioglycolate-activated macrophages or activation of native macrophages within the aortic media by thioglycolate infusion produced similar histologic results. Plasmin appeared to facilitate the interaction between elastase and its substrate, but it has no independent elastolytic activity.

These experimental aneurysms reveal a marked inflammatory cell infiltrate composed primarily of macrophages and T lymphocytes. Several days after elastase infusion in the rat, the aorta dilated nearly 300%, with large numbers of activated macrophages and T cells seen in the media. At 6 days after infusion, the vessel enlarged 421%, with persistent immunohistologic demonstration of macrophages, polymorphic neutrophils, and T lymphocytes. Regression of the inflammatory cell infiltrate to control levels occurred by day 12. These results imply that inflammatory cells may play a crucial role in the destruction of the vessel wall, leading to aneurysm formation.

Work in our laboratory using the Anidjar/Dobrin rat model has confirmed this significant inflammatory cell infiltrate during the evolution of abdominal aortic aneurysms along with the induction of endogenous proteases.[95] Quantitative analysis of the inflammatory cell response was performed using immunohistochemical methods. Antibodies to T cells (CD4, CD5, CD8), macrophages or monocytes (ED2), B cells (LCA), immunoglobulin M, and immunoglobulin G revealed a progressive stepwise infiltration of the aortic wall with various inflammatory cell subsets. Localized deposition of immunoglobulin M along the elastic lamina may represent a specific cell-mediated immune response to a given extracellular matrix component.

ROLE OF INFLAMMATION

The presence of inflammatory cells in experimentally induced aneurysms parallels the histologic findings in human AAA disease. Beckman,[36] in a review of 156 aortic aneurysm specimens, documented a significant inflammatory cell infiltrate in more than two thirds of the specimens examined. Using immunophenotypic analysis, Koch and associates[34] observed T lymphocytes, B lymphocytes, and macrophages in human aneurysmal adventitia. Macrophages are present in aortas with aneurysms and atherosclerotic occlusive disease, but T lymphocytes are less frequently seen in the normal or occlusive vessels. Our laboratory has confirmatory evidence for these changes using the technique of fluorescence-activated cell counting.[96] The lymphocytes present in aneurysmal tissue are known to secrete various cytokines, including γ-interferon, tumor necrosis factor-α (TNF-α), and interleukins (ILs). These factors can increase macrophage proteolytic activity and thereby potentiate aneurysmal dilation and rupture.

We have coined the names *aneurysm-infiltrating macrophages* (AIM cells) and *aneurysm-infiltrating lymphocytes* (AIL cells) to focus attention on these interesting cells.[96] Not only can AIM cells initiate proteolysis through MMP release, they also might be important in signal activation of mesenchymal and other inflammatory cells in the extracellular matrix. The production of tissue proteinases has been shown to be significantly affected by a number of soluble cytokines, in particular IL-1β and TNF-α.[97] IL-1β is produced by macrophages, B cells, endothelial cells, and fibroblasts, causing induction of MMP and prostaglandin synthesis. TNF-α is produced by activated macrophages or monocytes, lymphocytes, and vascular smooth muscle cells, causing induction of IL-1β and MMP expression. These effects on proteinase expression and vascular smooth muscle suggest that soluble cytokines are likely to have a role in AAA pathogenesis. An increase in IL-1β secretion from aortic aneurysmal cells in culture has been demonstrated by Pearce and coworkers.[98] Work in our laboratory has confirmed elevation of IL-1β and demonstrated statistically significant elevation of TNF-α in AAA extracts when compared with controls.[99] Assays for these two cytokines were performed on seven AAA and five control aortic tissue extracts using enzyme-linked immunosorbent assay methods. Immunoblotting also demonstrated known forms of TNF-α and IL-1β in the AAA extracts.

Western blot analysis of aortic extracts incubated with protein A revealed a significant amount of immunoglobulin in aneurysmal tissue when compared with controls.[33] Aggregates of extruded immunoglobulin are seen in histologic section as Russell bodies.[33] Work in our laboratory suggests that IgG is an immune response specifically directed against an aortic antigen with a molecular weight of about 70 kd. In others words, there is evidence for autoimmunity in the nonspecific AAA (unpublished observations).

A COMPREHENSIVE THEORY

Human Genetics

Many hypotheses of AAA etiology have emerged from the biochemical and cellular research of aortic aneurysm tissue, but a comprehensive theory must also encompass genetic, mechanical, and environmental contributions. Observations have documented that many aortic aneurysms are familial, so genetic factors might be important in their pathogenesis. A genetic basis for aneurysmal disease was postulated in 1981 by Tilson and Dang,[31] who cited the familial predisposition and preponderance of male over female patients as evidence of an inherited disorder. Johansen and Koepsell,[100] in a study comparing the family histories of 250 patients with AAA and 250 patients with atherosclerotic occlusive disease, confirmed that a genetic component exists in AAA disease. The risk/odds ratio for AAA among first-degree relatives in aneurysm patients was six times that of the controls. Retrospective reviews have shown a positive history of an affected first-degree relative in 11% to 20% of cases.[101,102] Darling and colleagues[103] found that identifying a female family member with an aneurysm appears to mark those families at significantly higher risk (63% versus 37%) for developing a potentially fatal ruptured aneurysm, leading to the term *black widow syndrome*.

Screening studies have established that the overall prevalence of significant AAAs (larger than 4 cm) is 2% to 3%.[13,14] Autopsy results corroborate this finding. The incidence of a previously undiagnosed AAA in first-degree relatives of AAA patients, however, is much higher. Collin and Walton[28] reported that 29% of brothers of AAA probands had abdominal aneurysms by ultrasound screening. Webster and colleagues[30] found a similar incidence, with 25% of male siblings and 6.9% of female siblings having a previously undiagnosed AAA. These observations all support a genetic predisposition to AAA disease.

Pedigree analyses have not led to a unified interpretation of the mode of inheritance. Tilson and Seashore[27] concluded that if a single aneurysm gene exists, it is likely autosomal, but X-linked inheritance is possible if there is molecular heterogeneity. A statistical evaluation by Majmunder and colleagues[104] supports recessive inheritance. Powell and Greenhalgh[105] proposed that inheritance of AAA is multifactorial, with an estimated heritability factor of 70%.

Candidate Genes

Because of the extensive connective tissue matrix remodeling documented in AAA vessels, the genes involved in synthesis and degradation of connective tissue proteins have been the primary targets of investigation for a genetic cause of AAA disease. The genetic loci coding for haptoglobin, cholesterol–ester transfer protein, α_1-antitrypsin, type III collagen, TIMP, elastin, and fibrillin have all been suggested as candidates for further study.

The frequency of the haptoglobin α_1-gene and variations at the cholesterol–ester transfer protein locus were reported by Powell and associates[106] to be significantly higher in AAA patients when compared with controls. Neither of these genes directly encode connective tissue proteins, but they are in close proximity to gelatinase B (type IV collagenase), which is known to degrade several proteins, including elastin.

Several studies have documented altered antiprotease activity in AAA patients, following the suggestion of Cannon and Read[65] that failure of the protease inhibitor mechanism may be involved in AAA pathogenesis. Cohen and colleagues[107] found that patients with ruptured AAA had the highest elastase activity and lowest α_1-antitrypsin activity when compared with patients undergoing elective AAA repair or aortic bypass procedures for atherosclerotic occlusive disease. The frequency of an α_1-antitrypsin deficiency phenotype in AAA patients, reported from merged data from our group and Cohen and colleagues,[108] was not confirmed in subsequent screening study by St. Jean and coworkers.[109]

The first evidence for a causative collagen mutation in AAA disease was reported in 1990.[56] A single-base mutation, which converted the codon for glycine at position 619 to the codon for arginine in type III procollagen, was found in a family who had aortic aneurysms but no definitive stigmata of Ehlers-Danlos or Marfan syndrome. The enthusiasm generated by this report was down-modulated by a later study, in which sequencing of the cDNA from 50 additional patients revealed only one nucleotide substitution that changed the type III procollagen structure.[110] Thus, mutations in the triple-helical domain of type III procollagen account for no more than a small subset of the entire AAA population.

Our research group was keen on TIMP-1 as a candidate gene; however, it was not found to have global abnormalities on Southern blotting techniques in AAA, and it appeared to be normally expressed by skin fibroblasts. Sequence analysis of the TIMP cDNA revealed an identical point mutation in two of the six AAA patients. This nucleotide substitution did not change the amino acid encoded, however, so the discovery turned out to be trivial.[92]

Mutations in the elastin gene have not been reported, although a transgenic mouse with a mutated elastin gene was found to have an aortic perforation consistent with rupture of an aneurysm.[111] Mutations in the fibrillin gene, which affect the functional integrity of the protein, have been discovered in patients with Marfan syndrome. This microfibrillar protein is an important component of the aorta and other connective tissues. Whether fibrillin mutations contribute to AAA pathogenesis remains to be seen.

Formulation of a hypothesis of AAA pathogenesis that encompasses all of the knowledge from known cellular, molecular, biochemical, and genetic studies of AAA disease must be tentative, but much progress has been made during the past decade. A schematic representation of some proven and potential interactions contributing to disruption of the extracellular matrix and eventual aneurysm development is offered in Figure 87-4. Our present models oversimplify the complex interactions that are likely oc-

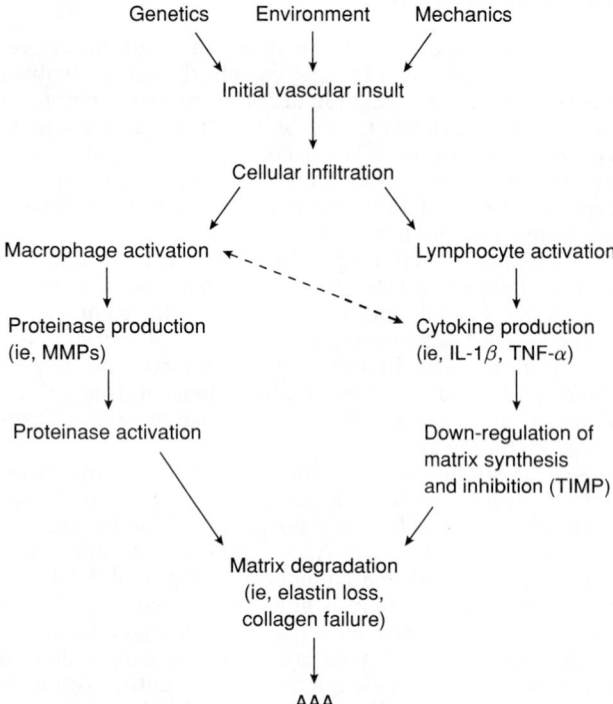

Figure 87-4. This schematic represents an overview of numerous influences on the expression of aneurysm disease as discussed in this chapter. We believe that a genetic susceptibility will eventually be discovered to be the necessary cause of abdominal aortic aneurysms, with environmental factors such as smoking and mechanical factors such as hypertension being potential contributing causes. An initial injury occurs, triggering an inflammatory response that results in a chain of causative events, eventually resulting in matrix degradation and failure of the tensile properties of collagen that prevent aneurysms from occurring under normal conditions.

curring among genetic, environmental, proteolytic, and inflammatory mechanisms to produce the cascade of events that culminates in the clinical expression of an abdominal aortic aneurysm.

POTENTIAL APPROACHES FOR INTERVENTION

Several potential areas for therapeutic or preventative measures can be considered. Early detection is the first step toward preventing the morbidity and mortality of AAA disease. If the putative AAA gene were identified, a screening test, such as the polymerase chain reaction on salivary DNA, could identify patients with a genetic susceptibility before expression of the disease. Once the population at risk is identified, patients can be followed by serial ultrasound examinations.

Propranolol has been shown to delay the formation of aortic aneurysms in the male Blotchy mouse, possibly by a direct effect on collagen cross-linking.[112] Retrospective study of the effect of β-adrenergic blockade on the growth rate of aneurysms in humans suggests that future randomized prospective studies should be considered to evaluate the effects of specific pharmacologic interventions.[113,114]

The presence of inflammatory cells, with their known induction of proteases and production of cytokines, may be another target for intervention. Soluble cytokines downregulate proteolytic inhibitory mechanisms and matrix

synthesis. Perhaps some intervention as simple as aspirin, or some other antiinflammatory agent, could block some of the inflammatory responses that potentiate matrix destruction.

Finally, when the antigen responsible for the antibody response in the aneurysmal wall is identified, it may be possible to induce tolerance in patients. This approach has been taken in patients with rheumatoid arthritis in whom type II collagen has been found to be autoantigenic. In a randomized, double-blind study of 60 patients with severe, active rheumatoid arthritis, subjects fed type II collagen for 3 months reported significant decreases in the number of tender and swollen joints when compared with the group who received a placebo.[115] Four of the collagen-fed subjects reported complete remission of their symptoms. Thus, an approach to induce immune tolerance might also be clinically efficacious in patients at high risk for AAA disease.

REFERENCES

1. Johnston KW, Rutherford RB, Tilson MD, Shah DM, Hollier L, Stanley JC. Suggested standards for reporting on arterial aneurysms. J Vasc Surg 1991;12:444.
2. Silverberg E, Boring CC, Squires TS. Cancer statistics, 1990. Cancer J Clin 1990;40:9.
3. Melton L, Bickerstaff L, Hollier L, et al. Changing incidence of abdominal aortic aneurysms: a population based study. Am J Epidemiol 1984;120:379.
4. Maniglia R, Gregory JE. Increasing incidence of arteriosclerotic aortic aneurysms: analysis of six thousand autopsies. Arch Pathol 1952;54:298.
5. Fowkes FGR, MacIntyre CCA, Ruckley CV. Increasing incidence of aortic aneurysms in England and Wales. Br Med J 1989;298:33.
6. Lillienfeld DE, Gunderson PD, Sprafka JM, et al. The epidemiology of abdominal aortic aneurysms: mortality trends in the United States 1951. Arteriosclerosis 1987;7:637.
7. Scarpa A. Treatise on the anatomy, pathology, and surgical treatment of aneurism, with engravings. Translated from the Italian by John Henry Wishart, FRCS. Edinburgh, 1808.
8. Tilson MD. Causality and the problem of aneurysms. Chron Dis Can 1994;15(Suppl):S18.
9. Auerbach O, Garfinkel L. Atherosclerosis and aneurysm of the aorta in relation to smoking habits and age. Chest 1980;78:805.
10. Matsushita S, Kuroo M, Takagi T, et al. Cardiovascular disease in the aged: overview of an autopsy series. Jap Circ J 1988;52:442.
11. McFarlane MJ. The epidemiologic necropsy for abdominal aortic aneurysm. JAMA 1991;265:2085.
12. Turk K. Post-mortem incidence of abdominal aortic aneurysms. Proc R Soc Med 1965;58:869.
13. Collin J, Araujo L, Lindsell D. Screening for abdominal aortic aneurysms. Lancet 1987;2:736.
14. Collin J, Araujo L, Walton J, Lindsell D. Oxford screening programme for abdominal aortic aneurysm in men aged 65 years. Lancet 1988;2:613.
15. Elveback LR, Connolly DC, Kurkland LT. Coronary heart disease in residents of Rochester, Minnesota. II. Mortality, incidence, and survivorship, 1950. Mayo Clin Proc 1981;56:665.
16. Garaway WM, Whisnat JP, Furlan AJ. The declining incidence of stroke. N Engl J Med 1979;300:449.
17. Morris T, Bouhoutos J. ABO blood groups in occlusive and ectatic arterial disease. Br J Surg 1973;60:892.
18. Tilson MD, Stansel HC. Differences in results for aneurysms vs. occlusive disease after bifurcation grafts: results of 100 elective grafts. Arch Surgery 1980;115:1173.
19. Bickerstaff LK, Hollier LH, Ban Peenan HJ, et al. Abdominal aortic aneurysms: the changing natural history. J Vasc Surg 1984;1:6.
20. Bengtsson H, Bergqvist D, Sternby NH. Increasing prevalence of abdominal aortic aneurysms, a necropsy study. Eur J Surg 1992;158:19.

21. Johnson G, Avery A, McDougal G, et al. Aneurysms of the abdominal aorta: incidence in blacks and whites in North Carolina. Arch Surg 1985;120:1138.

22. Gore I, Hirst AE Jr. Arteriosclerotic aneurysms of the abdominal aorta: a review. Prog Cardiovasc Dis 1973;16:113.

23. Halpert B, Willms RK. Aneurysms of the aorta: an analysis of 249 necropsies. Arch Pathol Lab Med 1962;74:163.

24. Kitchen ND. Racial distribution of aneurysms in Zimbabwe. J R Soc Med 1989;82:136.

25. Tilson MD, Seashore MR. Human genetics of abdominal aortic aneurysm. Surg Gynecol Obstet 1984;15:129.

26. Tilson MD, Seashore MR. Ninety-four families with clustering of abdominal aortic aneurysms (AAA). Circulation 1984;70:141.

27. Tilson MD, Seashore MR. Fifty families with abdominal aortic aneurysms in two or more first-order relatives. Am J Surg 1984;147:551.

28. Collin J, Walton J. Is abdominal aortic aneurysm a familial disease? Br Med J 1989;299:493.

29. Bengtsson H, Norrgard O, Angquist KA, Eckberg O, Obereg L, Bergqvist D. Ultrasonographic screening of the abdominal aorta among siblings of patients with abdominal aortic aneurysms. Br J Surg 1989;76:589.

30. Webster MW, Ferrell RE, St. Jean PL, et al. Ultrasound screening of first-degree relatives of patients with an abdominal aortic aneurysm. J Vasc Surg 1991;13:9.

31. Tilson MD, Dang C. Generalized arteriomegaly: a possible predisposition to the formation of abdominal aortic aneurysms. Arch Surg 1981;16:1030.

32. Tilson MD. Histochemistry of aortic elastin in patients with non-specific aortic aneurysmal disease. Arch Surg 1988;123:503.

33. Brophy CM, Reilly JM, Smith GJW, Tilson MD. The role of inflammation in nonspecific abdominal aortic aneurysm disease. Ann Vasc Surg 1991;5:229.

34. Koch AE, Haines GK, Rizzo RJ, et al. Human abdominal aortic aneurysms: immunophenotypic analysis suggesting an immune-mediated response. Am J Pathol 1990;137:1199.

35. Brophy CM, Smith GJW, Tilson MD. Pathology of nonspecific abdominal aortic aneurysm disease. In: Ernst CB, Stanley JC, eds. Current therapy in vascular surgery, ed 2. Philadelphia, BC Decker, 1991;238.

36. Beckman EN. Plasma cell infiltrates in abdominal aortic aneurysm. Am J Clin Pathol 1986;85:21.

37. White JV, Haas K, Phillips S, Comerota AJ. Adventitial elastolysis is a primary event in aneurysm formation. J Vasc Surg 1993;17:371.

38. Sumner DS, Hokanson DE, Standness DE. Stress-strain characteristics and collagen-elastin content of abdominal aortic aneurysms. Surg Gynecol Obstet 1970;130:459.

39. Dubick MA, Hunter GC, Perez-Lizano I, Mar G, Geokas MC. Assessment of the role of pancreatic proteases in human abdominal aortic aneurysms and occlusive disease. Clin Chim Acta 1988;177:1.

40. Campa JS, Greenhalgh RM, Powell JT. Elastin degradation in abdominal aortic aneurysms. Atherosclerosis 1987;65:13.

41. Baxter BT, Mcgee GS, Shively VP, et al. Elastin content, cross-links, and mRNA in normal and aneurysmal human aorta. J Vasc Surg 1992;16:192.

42. Gandhi R, Keller S, Cantor J, et al. Analysis of elastin cross-links in the insoluble matrix of aneurysmal abdominal aorta. Surgery 1994;115:617.

43. Menashi S, Campa JS, Greenhalgh RM, et al. Collagen in abdominal aortic aneurysm: typing, content, and degradation. J Vasc Surg 1987;6;578.

44. Rizzo RJ, McCarthy WJ, Dixit SN, Lilly MP, Shively VP, Flinn WR. Collagen types and matrix protein content in human abdominal aortic aneurysms. J Vasc Surg 1989;10:365.

45. Hunter GC, Dubick MA, Keen CL, Eskelson CD. Effects of hypertension on aortic antioxidant status in human abdominal aneurysmal and occlusive disease. Proc Soc Exp Biol Med 1991;196:273.

46. Mecham RP. Elastin synthesis and fiber assembly. Annals NY Acad Sci 1991;624:137.

47. Dobrin PB. Pathophysiology and pathogenesis of aortic aneurysms: current concepts. Surg Clin North Am 1989;69:687.

48. MacSweeney STR, Young G, Greenhalgh RM, Powell JT. Mechanical properties of the aneurysmal aorta. Br J Surg 1992;79:1281.

49. White, A. In: Principles of biochemistry, ed 6. New York, McGraw-Hill, 1978:110.

50. Lefevre M, Rucker RB. Aorta elastin turnover in normal and hypercholesterolemic Japanese quail. Biochim Biophys Acta 1980;630:519.

51. Rucker RB, Tinker D. Structure and metabolism of arterial elastin. Int Rev Exp Pathol 1977;17:1.

52. Wolinsky H, Glagov S. Comparison of abdominal and thoracic aortic medial structure in mammals: deviation of man from the usual pattern. Circ Res 1969;29:677.

53. Zatina MA, Zarins CZ, Gerertz BL, Glagov S. Role of medial lamellar architecture in the pathogenesis of aortic aneurysms. J Vasc Surg 1984;1:442.

54. Prockop DJ, Kivirikko KI. Heritable disease of collagen. N Engl J Med 1984;311:376.

55. Kivirikko KI. Collagens and their abnormalities in a wide spectrum of disease. Ann Med 1993;25:113.

56. Kontusaari S, Tromp G, Kuivaniemi H, et al. A mutation in the gene for type III procollagen (COL3A1) in a family with aortic aneurysms. J Clin Invest 1990;86:1465.

57. Dobrin PB. Mechanical properties of arteries. Physiol Rev 1978;58:397.

58. Tilson MD, Elefteriades J, Brophy CM. Tensile strength and collagen in abdominal aortic aneurysm disease. In: Greenhalgh RM, Mannick JA, Powell JT, eds. The cause and management of aneurysms. London, WB Saunders, 1990;97.

59. Hollister DW, Godfrey M, Sakai LY, Pyeritz RE. Immunohistologic abnormalities of the microfibrillar-fiber system in the Marfan syndrome. N Engl J Med 1990;323:152.

60. Cleary EG. The microfibrillar component of the elastic fibers: morphology and biochemistry. In: Uitto J, Perejda AJ, eds. Connective tissue disease: molecular pathology of the extracellular matrix. New York: Marcell Dekker, 1987;55.

61. Lee B, Godfrey M, Vitale E, et al. Linkage of Marfan syndrome and a phenotypically related disorder to two different fibrillin genes. Nature 1991;352:330.

62. Dietz HC, Cutting GR, Pyeritz RE, et al. Marfan syndrome caused by a recurrent de novo missense mutation in the fibrillin gene. Nature 1991;352:337.

63. Kainulainen K, Pulkkinen L, Savolainen A, Kaitila I, Peltonen L. Location on chromosome 15 of the gene defect causing Marfan syndrome. N Engl J Med 1990;323:35.

64. Busuttil RW, Rinderbriecht H, Flesher A, Carmack C. Elastase activity: the role of elastase in aortic aneurysm formation. J Surg Res 1982;32:214.

65. Cannon DJ, Read RC. Blood elastolytic activity in patients with aortic aneurysm. Ann Thorac Surgery 1982;34:10.

66. Dubick MA, Hunter GC, Perez-Lizano E, Mar G, Geokas MC. Assessment of the role of pancreatic proteases in human abdominal aortic aneurysms and occlusive disease. Clin Chim Acta 1988;177:1.

67. Cohen JR, Sarfati I, Dana D, Wise L. Elastase secretion by smooth muscle cells grown in culture from human aortic aneurysm explants. Surg Forum 1990;41:328.

68. Brown SL, Backstrom B, Busuttil FW. A new serum proteolytic enzyme in aneurysm pathogenesis. J Vasc Surg 1982;2:393.

69. Herron GS, Unemori E, Wong M, et al. Connective tissue proteinases and inhibitors in abdominal aortic aneurysms. Arterioscl Thromb 1991;11:1667.

70. Reilly JM, Brophy CM, Tilson MD. Characterization of an elastase from aneurysmal aorta which degrades intact aortic elastin. Ann Vasc Surg 1992;6:499.

71. Newman KM, Malon AM, Shin RD, Scholes JV, Ramey WG, Tilson MD. Matrix metalloproteinases in abdominal aortic aneurysm: characterization, purification, and their possible sources. Connect Tissue Res 1994;30:265.

72. Newman KM, Ogata Y, Malon AM, et al. Identification of matrix metalloproteinases 3 (stromelysin) and 9 (gelatinase B) in abdominal aortic aneurysm. Arterioscl Thromb 1994;14:1315.

73. Senior RM, Griffin GL, Fliszar CJ, Shapiro SD, Goldberg GL, Welgus HG. Human 92- and 72-kilodalton type IV collagenases are elastases. J Biol Chem 1991;266:7870.

74. Murphy G, Cockett MI, Ward RV, Docherty AJP. Matrix me-

talloproteinase degradation of elastin, type IV collagen, and proteoglycan. Biochem J 1991;277:277.

75. Busuttil RW, Abou-Zamzam AM, Machleder HI. Collagenase activity of the human aorta: a comparison of patients with and without abdominal aortic aneurysms. Arch Surg 1980;115:1373.

76. Webster MW, McAuley CE, Steed DL, Miller DD, Evans CH. Collagen stability and collagenolytic activity in the normal and aneurysmal human abdominal aorta. Am J Surg 1991;161:635.

77. Menashi S, Campa JS, Greenhalgh RM, et al. Collagen in abdominal aortic aneurysm: typing, content, and degradation. J Vasc Surg 1987;6;578.

78. Vine N, Powell JT. Metalloproteinases in degenerative aortic disease. Clin Sci 1991;81:233.

79. Irizarry E, Newman KM, Gandhi RH, et al. Demonstration of interstitial collagenase in abdominal aortic aneurysm disease. J Surg Res 1993;54:437.

80. Anidjar S, Salzmann JL, Gentric D, Lagneau P, Camilleri JP, Michel JB. Elastase induced experimental aneurysms in rats. Circulation 1990;82:973.

81. Gordon S, Unkeless JC, Cohn Z. Induction of macrophage plasminogen activator by endotoxin stimulation and phagocytosis. J Exp Med 1974;140:995.

82. He C, Wilhelm SM, Pentland AP, et al. Tissue cooperation in a proteolytic cascade activating human interstitial collagenase. Proc Natl Acad Sci USA 1989;86:2632.

83. Jean-Claude J, Newman K, Li H, Gregory AK, Tilson MD. Possible key role for plasmin in the pathogenesis of abdominal aortic aneurysms. Surgery 1994;116:472.

84. Reilly JM, Sicard GA, Lucore CL. Differential expression of plasminogen activators in abdominal aortic aneurysm and occlusive disease. Circulation 1992;16(Suppl I):139.

85. Tryggvason K, Huhtala P, Tuuttila A, et al. Structure and expression of type IV collagenase genes. Cell Differ Develop 1990;32:307.

86. Cohen AB, James HL. Reduction of the elastase inhibitory capacity of α antitrypsin by peroxides in cigarette smoke. Lung Res 1980;1:225.

87. Tilson MD. Aortic aneurysms and atherosclerosis. Circulation (Editorial) 1992;85:378.

88. Cronenwett JL, Sargent SK, Wall MH, et al. Variables that affect the expansion rate and outcome of small abdominal aortic aneurysms. J Vasc Surg 1990;11:260.

89. Cawston TE. Protein inhibitors of metallo-proteinases. In: Barret AJ, Salvesen G, eds. Proteinase inhibitors. Amsterdam, Elsevier, 1986:589.

90. Goldberg GI, Strongin A, Collier IE, Genrich LT, Mahmer BL. Interaction of 92-kDa type IV collagenase with the tissue inhibitor of metalloproteinases prevents dimerization, complex formation with interstitial collagenase, and activation of the proenzyme with stromelysin. J Biol Chem 1992;267:4583.

91. Brophy CM, Marks WH, Reilly JM, Tilson MD. Decrease tissue inhibitor of metalloproteinases (TIMP) in abdominal aortic tissue: a preliminary report. J Surg Res 1991;50:653.

92. Tilson MD, Reilly JM, Brophy CM, Webster EL, Barnett TR. Expression and sequence of the gene for tissue inhibitor of metalloproteinases in patients with abdominal aortic aneurysms. J Vasc Surg 1993;18:266.

93. Dobrin PB, Baker WH, Gley WC. Elastolytic and collagenolytic studies of arteries: implications for the mechanical properties of arteries. Arch Surg 1984;119:405.

94. Anidjar S, Dobrin PB, Eichorst M, Graham GP, Chejfec G. Correlation of inflammatory infiltrate with the enlargement of experimental aortic aneurysms. J Vasc Surg 1992;16:139.

95. Nackman GB, Halpern V, Gandhi R, Irizarry E, Ramey WG, Tilson MD. Induction of endogenous proteinases and alterations of extracellular matrix in a rat model of aortic aneurysm formation. Surg Forum 1992;43:348.

96. Tilson MD, Newman KM. Proteolytic mechanisms in the pathogenesis of aortic aneurysms. In: Yao JST, Pearce WH, eds. Aneurysms: new findings and treatments. Norwalk CT, Appleton & Lange, 1994:3.

97. Lefebvre V, Peeters-Jorris C, Vaes G. Production of gelatin-degrading matrix metalloproteinases (type IV collagenases) and inhibitors by articular chondrocytes during their dedifferentiation by serial subcultures and under stimulation by interleukin and tumor necrosis factor-α. Biochim Biophys Acta 1991;1094:8.

98. Pearce WH, Sweis I, Yao JST, McCarthy WJ, Koch AE. Interleukin-1β and tumor necrosis factor-α release in normal and diseased human infrarenal aortas. J Vasc Surg 1992;16:784.

99. Newman KM, Johnson CJ, Jean-Claude JM, Li H, Ramey WG, Tilson MD. Cytokines which activate proteolysis are increased in abdominal aortic aneurysms. Circulation 1994;90:224.

100. Johansen K, Koepsell T. Familial tendency for abdominal aortic aneurysms. JAMA 1986;256:1934.

101. Cole CW, Barber GC, Bouchard AG, et al. Abdominal aortic aneurysms: Consequences of a positive family history. Can J Surg 1989;32:117.

102. Norrgard O, Rais O, Angquist A. Familial occurrence of abdominal aortic aneurysms. Surgery 1984;95:650.

103. Darling RC III, Brewster DC, Darling RC. Are familial aortic aneurysms different? J Vasc Surg 1989;10:39.

104. Majmunder PP, St. Jean PL, Ferrell RE. On the inheritance of abdominal aortic aneurysm. Am J Hum Genet 1991;48:164.

105. Powell JT, Greenhalgh RM. Multifactorial inheritance of abdominal aortic aneurysm. Eur J Surg 1987;1:29.

106. Powell JT, Bashir A, Dawson S. Genetic variation on chromosome 16 is associated with abdominal aortic aneurysm. Clin Sci 1990;78:138.

107. Cohen JR, Mandell C, Margolis I, Chang J, Wise L. Altered aortic protease and antiprotease activity in patients with ruptured abdominal aortic aneurysms. Surg Gynecol Obstet 1987;164:355.

108. Cohen JR, Sarfati I, Ratner L, Tilson MD. Alpha antitrypsin phenotypes in patients with abdominal aortic aneurysms. J Surg Res 1990;49:319.

109. St. Jean PL, Ferrell RE, Majmunder PP, Steed DL, Webster MW. Abdominal aortic aneurysm (AAA): association with α-antitrypsin, haptoglobin, and type III collagen. J Cardiovasc Surg 1991;32:38.

110. Tromp G, Wu Y, Prockop DJ, et al. Sequencing of cDNA from 50 unrelated patients reveals that mutations in the triple-helical domain of type III procollagen are an infrequent cause of aortic aneurysm. J Clin Invest 1993;91:2539.

111. Tilson MD. Abdominal aortic aneurysm surgery: something old and something new. J Cardiovasc Surg 1994;2:159.

112. Brophy CM, Tilson JE, Tilson MD. Propranolol delays the formation of aortic aneurysms in the male blotchy mouse. J Surg Res 1988;44:687.

113. Leach SD, Toole AL, Stern H, et al. Effect of β-adrenergic blockade of the growth rate of abdominal aortic aneurysms. Arch Surg 1988;123:606.

114. Gadowsky GR, Pilcher DB, Ricci MA. Abdominal aortic aneurysm expansion rate: effect of size and beta-adrenergic blockade. J Vasc Surg 1994;19:727.

115. Trentham DE, Dynesius-Trentham RA, Orav EJ, et al. Effects of oral administration of type III collagen on rheumatoid arthritis. Science 1993;261:1727.

SURGERY: SCIENTIFIC PRINCIPLES AND PRACTICE, Second Edition, edited by
Lazar J. Greenfield, Michael W. Mulholland, Keith T. Oldham, Gerald B. Zelenock,
and Keith D. Lillemoe. Lippincott–Raven Publishers, Philadelphia. © 1997.

CHAPTER 88

EXTRACRANIAL CAROTID, INNOMINATE, SUBCLAVIAN, AND AXILLARY ANEURYSMS

PATRICK J. O'HARA

GENERAL CONSIDERATIONS

Incidence

Aneurysmal degeneration of the innominate, extracranial carotid, subclavian, and axillary arteries is rare.[1-3] The explanation for this is unknown, and reliable data regarding the natural history of these lesions are unavailable because no large series of untreated cases have been published. Most information has been derived from small series of treated patients or individual case reports.

Anatomy

The normal anatomy and embryologic development of the aortic arch and the brachiocephalic arterial system are depicted in Figure 88-1. During development, the dorsal aortas are paired, lie on either side of the trachea proximally, and are fused distally. Although never present simultaneously, six pairs of aortic arches form, some of which regress. Normally, the right dorsal aorta also regresses and the fourth aortic arches form the subclavian arteries.[4] Variations in the origins of the arteries arising from the arch are not unusual. One of the most common aberrations, found in 1 of every 200 autopsies, is an anomalous origin of the right subclavian artery arising as the fourth or last branch of the aortic arch.[5-7] As it courses to the right, it is retroesophageal in 80% of patients, between the trachea and the esophagus in 15%, and anterior to the trachea in 5%.[8]

Definition and Etiology

Classically, an aneurysm is defined as dilatation of an artery to more than twice its normal diameter, whereas ectasia is similar dilatation to less than twice normal diameter. The etiologies usually proposed for brachiocephalic aneurysms are atherosclerosis, trauma, and infection.[1-3] Among carotid aneurysms, about half are associated with atherosclerosis, which may produce fusiform or saccular aneurysms.[9] The remainder are caused by penetrating or nonpenetrating trauma, infection, dissection, connective tissue disease, or fibromuscular disease.[1,10] Among axillo-subclavian aneurysms, about half are thought to result from atherosclerosis; chronic trauma and extrinsic compression are also frequent causes.[2,9,11,12] Chronic injury of the arterial wall from a cervical rib or fibrous band at the thoracic outlet or from improper crutch use may lead to poststenotic dilatation or frank aneurysm formation.[2,13-16] Aneurysms involving an aberrant right subclavian artery are now recognized with increasing frequency.[17-21] In the preantibiotic era, mycotic aneurysms secondary to syphilitic arteritis were the most common type observed. Luetic

aneurysms are extremely rare, and mycotic aneurysms are more likely to be related to infected arterial puncture sites associated with parenteral drug abuse.[22] Other less common etiologies include various forms of medial degeneration,[23] fibromuscular disease, arteritis, and congenital anomalies.[23]

Pathophysiology

The pathophysiology of these lesions has certain common features. In general, rupture is rare, although it has been reported in each location, usually associated with catastrophic consequences.[1-3,9,24] Depending on the location, size, and rate of expansion of the aneurysm, symptoms of nerve, tracheal, esophageal, or venous compression from its mass effect may prevail. The most threatening aspect of these aneurysms is the propensity for embolism and thrombosis, which can lead to end-organ ischemia or infarction.[1-3] Extracranial carotid aneurysms may produce focal cerebrovascular symptoms, whereas subclavian and axillary aneurysms are associated with upper extremity ischemic symptoms. Emboli from innominate aneurysms may cause right hemispheric or right upper extremity ischemic symptoms.

Therapeutic Objectives

The therapeutic objectives with all brachiocephalic aneurysms are similar. Foremost is the preservation of life and neurologic function, followed closely by preservation or restoration of end-organ function. Optimally, the embolic source is eliminated or excluded, and perfusion is maintained by resection and arterial reconstruction or ligation and bypass.

CAROTID ANEURYSMS

Incidence

Although aneurysmal degeneration of the intracranial carotid arteries and their branches is frequently encountered, extracranial carotid aneurysms are uncommon lesions. Most involve the common and internal carotid arteries. Only seven cases of isolated atraumatic extracranial vertebral artery aneurysm and only 2 cases of isolated atraumatic external carotid aneurysm have been reported.[25-28] The true prevalence of extracranial carotid aneurysms is unknown because most early reports are anecdotal, and more recent series from single institutions contain relatively few patients. Furthermore, many reports combine patient experience with atherosclerotic as well as traumatic, postsurgical, and mycotic aneurysms[10,27,29-37] (Table 88-1). In some instances it may be difficult to distinguish the cause of the reported aneurysms. There is general agreement that the incidence of nontraumatic carotid aneurysms is probably low. Only 6 patients were found to have undergone surgical correction of extracranial aneurysms at a busy clinic from 1977 to 1984, during which time more than 1500 carotid endarterectomies for occlusive disease were performed. This yielded a relative incidence of surgically correctable carotid occlusive disease of less than 0.4%.[38] In another report, 19 carotid aneurysms were encountered; only 5 were atherosclerotic and only 13 were surgically corrected. During this period, more than 500 carotid reconstructions for occlusive disease were performed, for a relative incidence of surgically correctable carotid occlusive disease of less than 3.8%.[31] Relative to other peripheral aneurysms, fusiform and saccular carotid aneurysms are uncommon. Only 21 carotid aneurysms were diagnosed from a pool of 1118 peripheral arterial

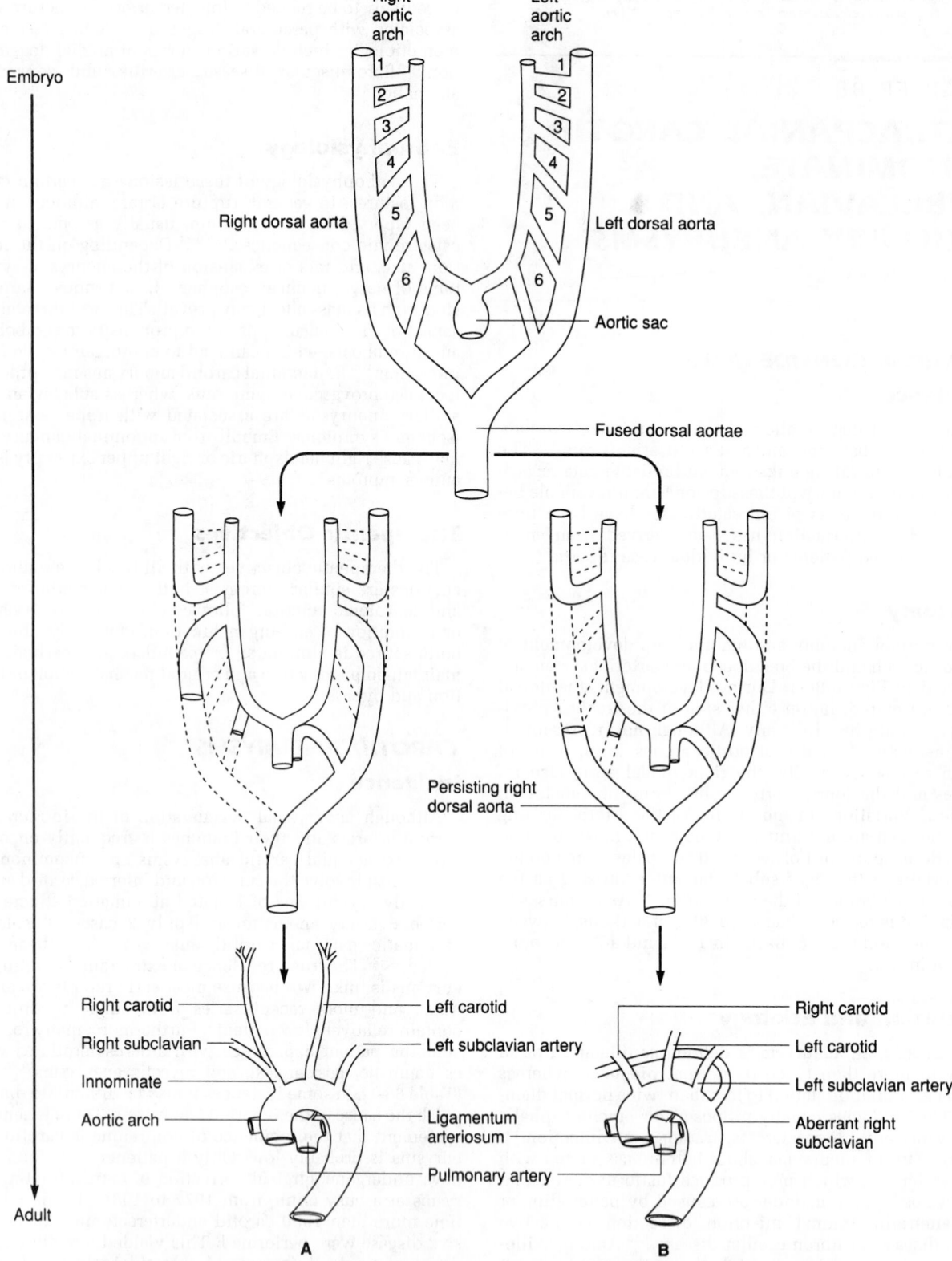

Figure 88-1. Diagrammatic representation of the embryologic development and anatomy of the aortic arch and brachiocephalic arterial systems. (*A*) Normal pattern. (*B*) Anomalous origin of the right subclavian artery. (After Langman J. Arterial system. In: Medical embryology. Baltimore, Williams & Wilkins, 1963:171)

aneurysms, for a relative incidence of 1.9% of all peripheral aneurysms.[34] In another report, only 37 carotid aneurysms, 16 of which were atherosclerotic, were diagnosed during a time when some 8500 aneurysms of the arterial tree were treated surgically. Thus, the incidence of surgically treated peripheral aneurysms was about 0.4%.[30]

Etiology

The most common causes of extracranial carotid aneurysms are atherosclerosis and trauma. Atherosclerosis accounted for 26% to 84% of the carotid aneurysms in several large, selected series. Pseudoaneurysms, traumatic and postsurgical, constituted 12% to 58% of the aneurysms in these series[10,27,29-37] (see Table 88-1). Other less common causes include infection, cystic medial necrosis, fibromuscular dysplasia, and congenital anomalies.[39]

Clinical Manifestations

Symptomatic extracranial carotid aneurysms most commonly present with stroke, focal transient ischemic attacks (TIAs), amaurosis fugax, or evidence of retinal infarction. All of these are manifestations of the propensity for embolization from these lesions. In seven selected series, the incidence of associated focal neurologic symptoms ranged from 15% to 67%[10,27,29-31,33-38,40] (Table 88-2). A pulsatile neck mass, with or without associated discomfort, was present in 13% to 100% of the patients in the selected series in which such information was available. In these series, rupture was distinctly uncommon, occurring in only three patients, although it has been reported anecdotally in the past. Associated abdominal aortic and peripheral arterial aneurysms were reported in up to 26% of the patients.[29-31,36,40] Other less commonly reported symptoms include dysphagia, respiratory stridor, Horner syndrome, and symptoms of cranial nerve compression, presumably from the mass effect of large aneurysms.[1,3]

Diagnosis

A careful history alone is important but is seldom sufficient to confirm the diagnosis of extracranial carotid aneurysm. The presence of a pulsatile mass in the neck on physical examination should raise the suspicion of aneu-

rysmal disease; the most frequent explanation for this finding is a prominent, tortuous carotid artery, commonly observed in elderly, hypertensive women.[1,3] The differential diagnosis also includes carotid body tumors, lymphadenopathy, cystic hygromas, salivary gland tumors, metastatic tumors, cervical lymphoma, lipomas, peritonsillar abscesses, and brachial cleft cysts.[1,3] Careful examination often is sufficient to distinguish these entities from aneurysm, and duplex scanning usually provides the definitive diagnosis. If carotid duplex scanning confirms the presence of an aneurysm, or if the diagnosis is still in doubt, intraarterial digital subtraction angiography of the arch and both carotid arteries with intracranial filming is required. Until the diagnosis of carotid aneurysm has been ruled out, incision and drainage or biopsy of a neck mass is unwise because of the risk of hemorrhage, which may be substantial and difficult to control.

Indications for Intervention

Because of the rarity of these lesions, definitive data about the natural history of untreated extracranial carotid aneurysms are unavailable and will remain so for the foreseeable future. A 1925 review of 106 reported cases of extracranial aneurysm of the internal carotid artery provides some insights. The aneurysms were classified as 42 spontaneous, 18 erosive, 26 traumatic, 19 arteriovenous, and 1 unclassified. Of the 105 patients available for follow-up, 35 were treated conservatively and 25 died. Seventy patients underwent surgical therapy consisting of carotid artery ligation, which resulted in 21 deaths (30%). Forty-eight patients (68%) were either cured or improved, and 1 operative survivor was not improved.[41] Because many of the reported patients probably harbored mycotic aneurysms, the applicability of these data to atherosclerotic aneurysms remains problematic. In the modern era, over a mean follow-up period of 6.3 years, atherosclerotic extracranial carotid artery aneurysms were associated with a 50% (3 of 6 patients) ipsilateral stroke rate if treated nonoperatively.[36] Two of these strokes occurred in patients with focal TIAs, although 1 patient had an asymptomatic carotid aneurysm on initial presentation. Because of the significant

Table 88-1. ETIOLOGY OF EXTRACRANIAL CAROTID ANEURYSM IN 11 SELECTED REPORTS

Investigators	Year	Duration	Aneurysms	Patients	Atherosclerotic Aneurysms	Pseudoaneurysms	Other Aneurysms*
Rhodes et al[29]	1976	1959–1975	23	19	70	30	0
McCollum et al[30]	1979	1956–1977	37	34	44	56	0
Busuttil et al[31]	1980	1954–1978	19	19	26	58	16
Pratschke et al[27]	1980	1960–1979	28†	27	46	36	18
Mokril et al[32]	1982	1979–1981	7	6	4	2	1
Krupski et al[33]	1983	1960–1982	22	21	8	10	4
Welling et al[34]	1983	1952–1982	25‡	20	84§	12	4
Dehn & Taylor[35]	1984	1968–1982	9	9	5	2	2
Zwolak et al[36]	1984	1957–1983	52	NA	46	NA	NA
Sahlman et al[37]	1991	1963–1989	18	18	6	2	10
Bour et al[10]	1992	1977–1990	8‖	8	0	0	8‖

NA, not available.

* Includes mycotic, congenital, and unknown.
† Includes 5 external carotid aneurysms.
‡ Excludes 16 spontaneous dissections.
§ Includes 15 fusiform and 16 saccular aneurysms presumed atherosclerotic.
‖ All fibromuscular dysplasia.

Table 88-2. CLINICAL MANIFESTATIONS OF EXTRACRANIAL CAROTID ANEURYSM IN 12 SELECTED REPORTS

Investigators	Year	Patients	Neck Mass	Rupture or Bleeding	Focal Neurologic Symptoms	Associated Aneurysms	Bilateral
Kaupp et al[40]	1972	8	1 (13%)	0 (0%)	2 (25%)	0 (0%)	5 (63%)
Rhodes et al[29]	1976	19	13 (68%)	0 (0%)	9 (47%)	4 (21%)	4 (21%)
McCollum et al[30]	1979	34	34 (100%)	0 (0%)	5 (15%)	8 (24%)	3 (9%)
Busuttil et al[31]	1980	19	5 (26%)	0 (0%)	12 (63%)	5 (26%)	0 (0%)
Pratschke et al[27]	1980	27	26 (96%)	2 (7%)	12 (44%)	NA	1 (4%)
Krupski et al[33]	1983	21	18 (22%)	4 (18%)	7 (32%)	NA	1 (5%)
Welling et al[34]*	1983	20	NA	1 (5%)	4 (20%)	NA	5 (25%)
Dehn & Taylor[35]	1984	9	5 (56%)	0 (0%)	3 (33%)	2 (22%)	0 (0%)
Zwolak et al[36]	1984	21	7 (33%)	0 (0%)	12 (57%)	3 (14%)	3 (14%)
Painter et al[38]	1985	6	1 (17%)	0 (0%)	4 (67%)	NA	1 (17%)
Sahlman et al[37]	1991	18	6 (33%)	0 (0%)	6 (33%)	3 (17%)	0 (0%)
Bour et al[10]	1992	8	2 (25%)	0 (0%)	5 (63%)	NA	0 (0%)

NA, not available.
* Excludes 16 spontaneous dissections.

potential for neurologic morbidity, extracranial carotid aneurysms should be treated when the diagnosis is made.

Treatment Options

The procedure of choice for the treatment of extracranial carotid aneurysms is direct reconstruction.[31,36,38] The reconstructive methods may vary, depending on the local anatomy. Often, the internal carotid artery is sufficiently redundant to allow resection of the aneurysm and primary anastomosis. Figure 88-2 illustrates this approach, which is used in the treatment of a saccular internal carotid aneurysm. Fusiform aneurysms involving the carotid bifurcation can be managed by resection, end-to-end anastomosis of the internal and common carotid arteries, and reimplantation of the external carotid artery, as shown in Figure 88-3. When insufficient redundant internal carotid artery remains to allow primary anastomosis, a saphenous vein interposition graft may be used in a variety of configurations, as demonstrated in Figure 88-4. Although synthetic grafts can be used for this purpose, autogenous reconstruction is usually preferable. Intraluminal shunting may be required and has been used routinely by some groups during carotid artery reconstruction. The graft can be threaded over the shunt, allowing better alignment and avoiding the problem of kinking due to excessive graft length.[38]

Operative exposure of the distal internal carotid artery can be facilitated by the use of nasotracheal intubation, which, without an oral airway, allows the mouth to close and the mandible to swing anteriorly, providing valuable additional distal exposure of the internal carotid artery above the angle of the mandible. Further exposure can be obtained by anterior subluxation of the mandible with the use of arch bars and intramaxillary fixation. Mastoidectomy can provide even more distal exposure but may require the sacrifice of some auditory acuity; this procedure is usually not required.

Some authors have proposed aneurysmorrhaphy or resection with patch angioplasty as a feasible alternative, especially in the treatment of saccular aneurysms.[29-31] If interposition grafting or patch angioplasty is required, the graft material of choice is autogenous saphenous vein, although redundant internal carotid artery may occasionally be used as autogenous patch material. Others have described the transposition of the distal internal carotid artery to the external carotid artery, although this option sacrifices the distal outflow of the external carotid artery, which may be a useful collateral source.[29,36] In the absence of adequate autogenous graft material, synthetic prostheses may be required.

Before the development of safe techniques for carotid artery reconstruction, ligation was the procedure of choice for the management of extracranial carotid aneurysms.[41] Rarely, occlusion of the internal carotid artery by suture ligation or balloon catheter placement may be required for the management of nonreconstructible aneurysms extending to the base of the skull or beyond. Although this approach may have an occasional role, it has been associated with substantial mortality and morbidity.[1,29,31,38] If carotid artery ligation or occlusion is required, postoperative anticoagulation is recommended to minimize the risk of embolism from retrograde thrombosis.[1] In this unusual setting, extracranial to intracranial bypass may be beneficial.[31,38]

Results

Because of the lack of large series of patients with extracranial carotid aneurysms treated at a single center, early and late data regarding the effectiveness of treatment are sparse. The collected early results of 66 procedures performed from 1972 to 1985 for the correction of atherosclerotic extracranial carotid aneurysms reported that ligation appears to be associated with a 40% incidence of both mortality and morbidity, although only 5 patients were treated in this manner.[38] Of the 61 patients who underwent direct carotid artery reconstruction, 13 (8%) sustained transient neurologic deficits and 8 (5%) had permanent strokes. The single death in this subset yielded a mortality rate of 1.6%. One patient in the collected series was reported to exhibit late postoperative ipsilateral hemispheric TIAs.[36,38]

These results suggest that the repair of extracranial atherosclerotic carotid aneurysms probably has a higher morbidity risk than does standard carotid endarterectomy performed for the correction of occlusive disease. This observation may be explained by the more extensive dissection required for the treatment of aneurysmal disease compared with that for occlusive lesions, and by the propensity for embolism of atheromatous debris from within many of these aneurysms. Thus, careful surgical technique and avoidance of unnecessary manipulation of the aneurysm are essential during dissection and repair.[29,36,38]

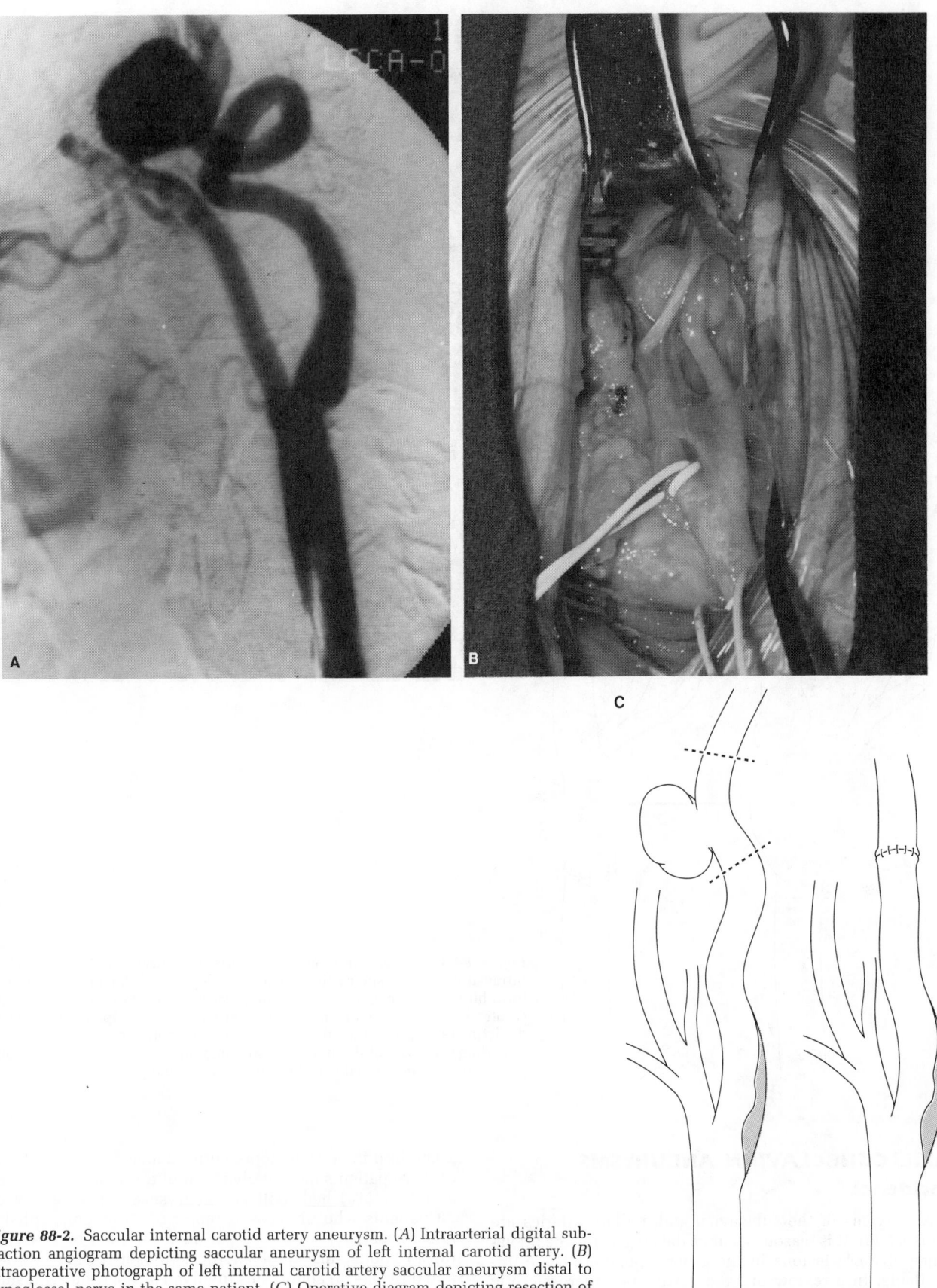

Figure 88-2. Saccular internal carotid artery aneurysm. (*A*) Intraarterial digital subtraction angiogram depicting saccular aneurysm of left internal carotid artery. (*B*) Intraoperative photograph of left internal carotid artery saccular aneurysm distal to hypoglossal nerve in the same patient. (*C*) Operative diagram depicting resection of left internal carotid artery saccular aneurysm with end-to-end arterial carotid anastomosis in the same patient.

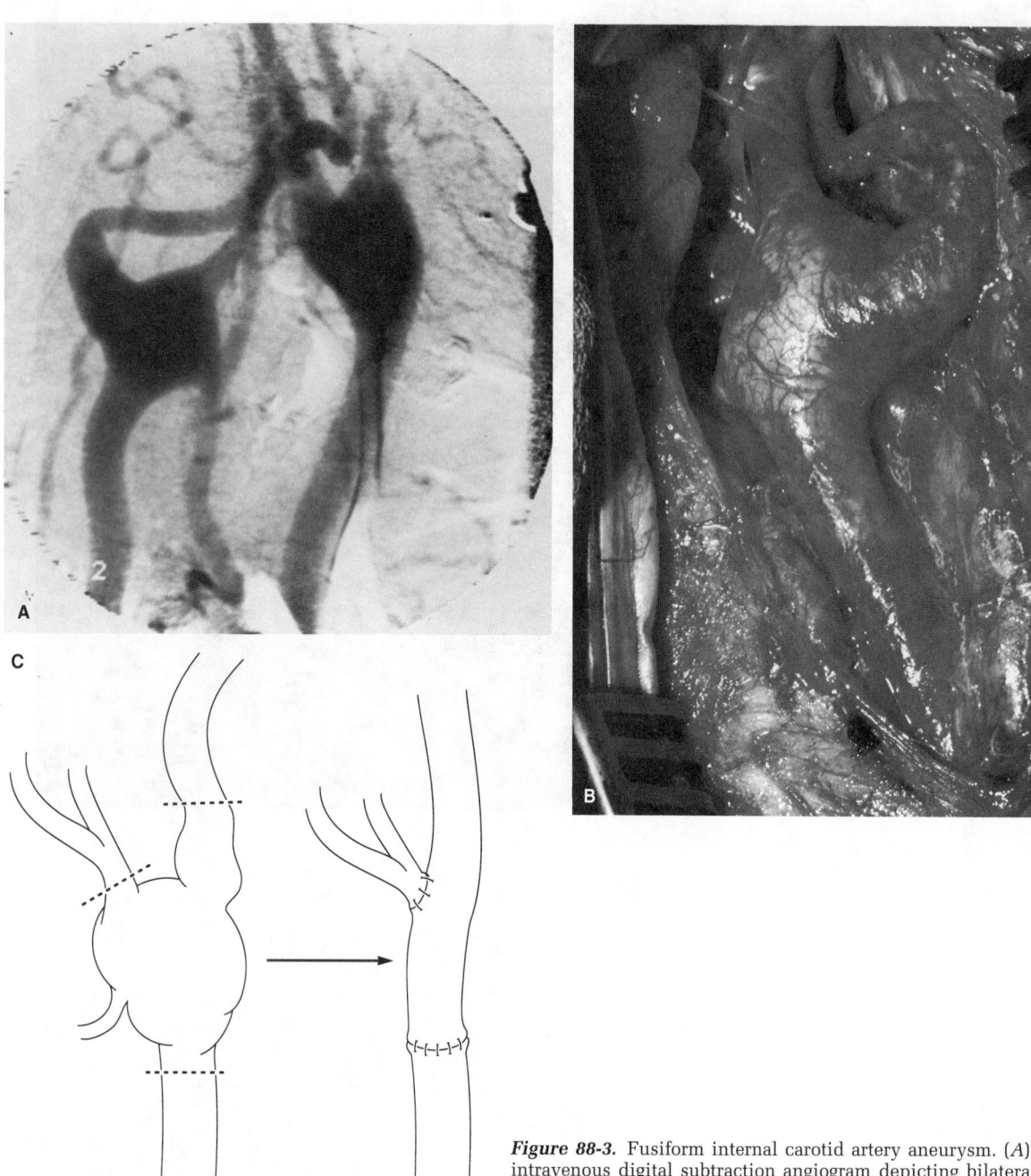

Figure 88-3. Fusiform internal carotid artery aneurysm. (*A*) Good-quality intravenous digital subtraction angiogram depicting bilateral fusiform carotid bifurcation aneurysms. (*B*) Intraoperative photograph of fusiform left carotid bifurcation aneurysm in the same patient. (*C*) Operative diagram depicting resection of the fusiform left internal carotid aneurysm with end-to-end anastomosis of the internal and common carotid arteries and reimplantation of the external carotid artery in the same patient.

AXILLOSUBCLAVIAN ANEURYSMS

Incidence

Aneurysms of the subclavian and axillary arteries are unusual. For this reason, accurate data regarding the prevalence of these lesions in the general population are unavailable. In a review of 1488 peripheral atherosclerotic aneurysms treated from 1960 to 1971, 52 were multiple aneurysms (3.5% of the patients); only 2 subclavian aneurysms were reported.[42] Another extensive review identified 195 axillosubclavian aneurysms, 171 (88%) of which involved the subclavian artery and 24 (12%) of which involved the axillary artery.[2] A 20-year review from 1960 to 1980 described 31 patients with 32 aneurysms; 14 (45%) of these patients had involvement of the subclavian artery and 17 (55%) had axillary aneurysms.[24] In a review of 73 patients who underwent repair of 73 brachiocephalic aneurysms over a 40-year period from 1950 to 1990, 38 (52%) aneurysms involved the axillosubclavian arteries and only 3 (4%) aneurysms involved an aberrant right subclavian artery.[28]

Etiology

Axillosubclavian aneurysms are most commonly caused by trauma or atherosclerosis, although other less common etiologies, such as infection (especially syphilis in the

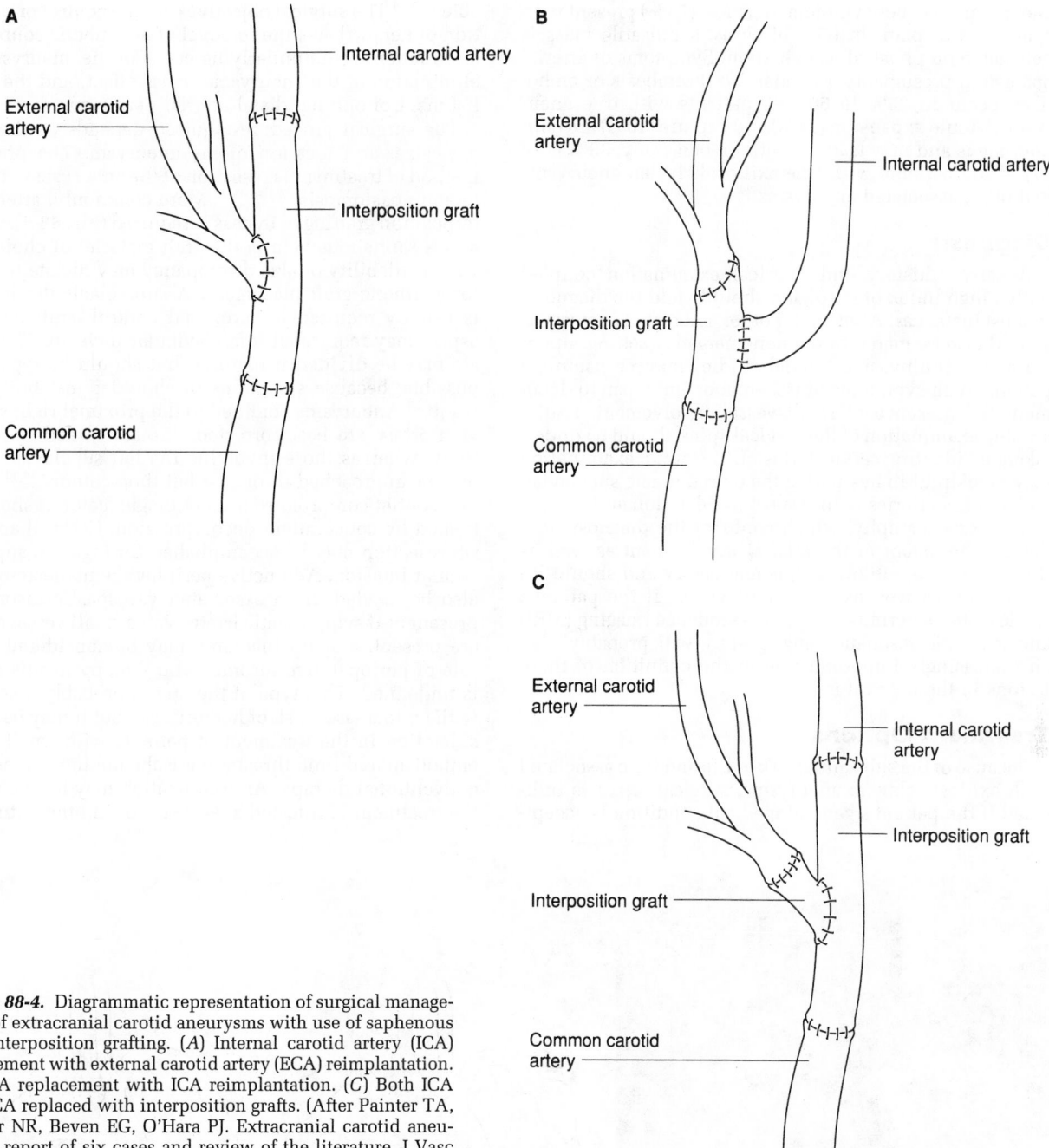

Figure 88-4. Diagrammatic representation of surgical management of extracranial carotid aneurysms with use of saphenous vein interposition grafting. (*A*) Internal carotid artery (ICA) replacement with external carotid artery (ECA) reimplantation. (*B*) ECA replacement with ICA reimplantation. (*C*) Both ICA and ECA replaced with interposition grafts. (After Painter TA, Hertzer NR, Beven EG, O'Hara PJ. Extracranial carotid aneurysms: report of six cases and review of the literature. J Vasc Surg 1985;2:312)

past), arteritis, medial degeneration, fibromuscular disease, and congenital anomalies, account for occasional aneurysms.[2,24,43] Of the traumatic aneurysms, most are caused by chronic pressure producing intimal damage and poststenotic dilatation. In the subclavian region, the usual etiology is thoracic outlet obstruction related to cervical ribs or other causes of thoracic outlet syndrome.[2,13,15,24,43] In the axillary region, improper long-term crutch usage has been associated with the development of axillary artery aneurysms.[2,14] Eighty percent of subclavian and 67% of axillary arterial aneurysms were related to these causes, whereas only 15% were thought to be secondary to atherosclerosis.[2] In another report, 10 patients (32%) had pseudoaneurysms secondary to penetrating or crush injuries, whereas the remaining patients had aneurysms secondary to athero-

sclerosis (39%), thoracic outlet obstruction (19%), infection (6%), and Ehlers-Danlos syndrome (3%).[24]

Clinical Manifestations

Axillosubclavian aneurysms may be asymptomatic but are usually associated with symptoms of peripheral embolism or pressure from the presence of a pulsatile mass against surrounding neurovascular structures.[2,24,44] Rupture is relatively uncommon.[2,24,43] Rarely, dysphagia or respiratory distress can occur from esophageal or tracheal compression secondary to atherosclerotic aneurysmal degeneration of an aberrant right subclavian artery originating from the distal aortic arch (see Fig. 88-1).[4-8]

Although up to 25% of patients with axillosubclavian

aneurysms may be asymptomatic, most (74%) present with symptoms of pain. In 65% of cases, a pulsatile mass is detectable on physical examination. Symptoms of arterial occlusion, presumably secondary to thrombosis or embolism, occur in 25% to 68% of patients with true aneurysms.[2] Acute expansion (14%) and rupture (10%) are ominous signs and may lead to death. In one study, 33% (7 of 21) of the patients with true axillosubclavian aneurysms had other associated aneurysms.[24]

Diagnosis

A careful history and physical examination coupled with a high index of suspicion should yield the diagnosis in most instances. A search for other associated aneurysms should also be made. In the nonemergency setting, upper extremity noninvasive arterial studies may be useful in patients with symptoms of ischemia or embolism to document the presence of small vessel involvement. Radiographic examination of the cervical spine should be undertaken to identify cervical ribs. Ultrasound examination may be helpful in evaluating the extrathoracic subclavian and axillary arteries with respect to dilatation and intimal injury. Arteriography, which confirms the diagnosis and defines the extent of the arterial involvement as well as the state of the outflow bed, is mandatory and should include arch as well as full runoff views, if the patient's clinical status permits. Magnetic resonance imaging (MRI) and magnetic resonance angiography will probably play an increasingly important role in the definition of these lesions in the near future.

Treatment Options

Because of the substantial risk to life and limb associated with axillosubclavian aneurysms, surgical repair is indicated if the patient's general medical condition is accept-able.[2,24,43] The surgical objectives are the control or prevention of hemorrhage, the removal of an embolic source, the elimination of the underlying cause of the aneurysm, the elimination of the aneurysmal mass effect, and the establishment of optimal distal arterial perfusion.

The surgical procedure required depends on the etiology, size, and location of the aneurysm. The preferred method of treatment is resection of the aneurysm with end-to-end anastomosis.[2,24,43,45,46] More commonly, arterial interposition grafting or bypass is required (Fig. 88-5). Autogenous saphenous vein is the graft material of choice, but vein availability or size discrepancy may dictate the need for synthetic graft placement. A supraclavicular incision is usually required for proximal control, and the distal aspect may require an infraclavicular incision. The clavicle may be divided if required but should be repaired if possible, because symptoms of shoulder instability may result.[24] Aneurysms confined to the proximal right subclavian artery are best corrected through a median sternotomy, whereas those involving the left subclavian artery may be approached through a left thoracotomy.[44,46] If thoracic outlet compromise is an etiologic factor, it should be treated by concomitant decompression. Cervical and first rib resection may be accomplished through the supraclavicular incision. Adjunctive peripheral embolectomy may also be needed. If an associated vasospastic disorder is present or if symptomatic irretrievable small vessel emboli are present, a sympathectomy may be considered.[24] The role of perioperative thrombolytic therapy in this setting is undefined. This type of therapy is probably associated with an increased risk of hemorrhage, but it may be a consideration in the treatment of patients with small vessel embolism and limb-threatening ischemia unresponsive to conventional therapy. Arterial ligation may have a role in the treatment of infected aneurysms or in other situations

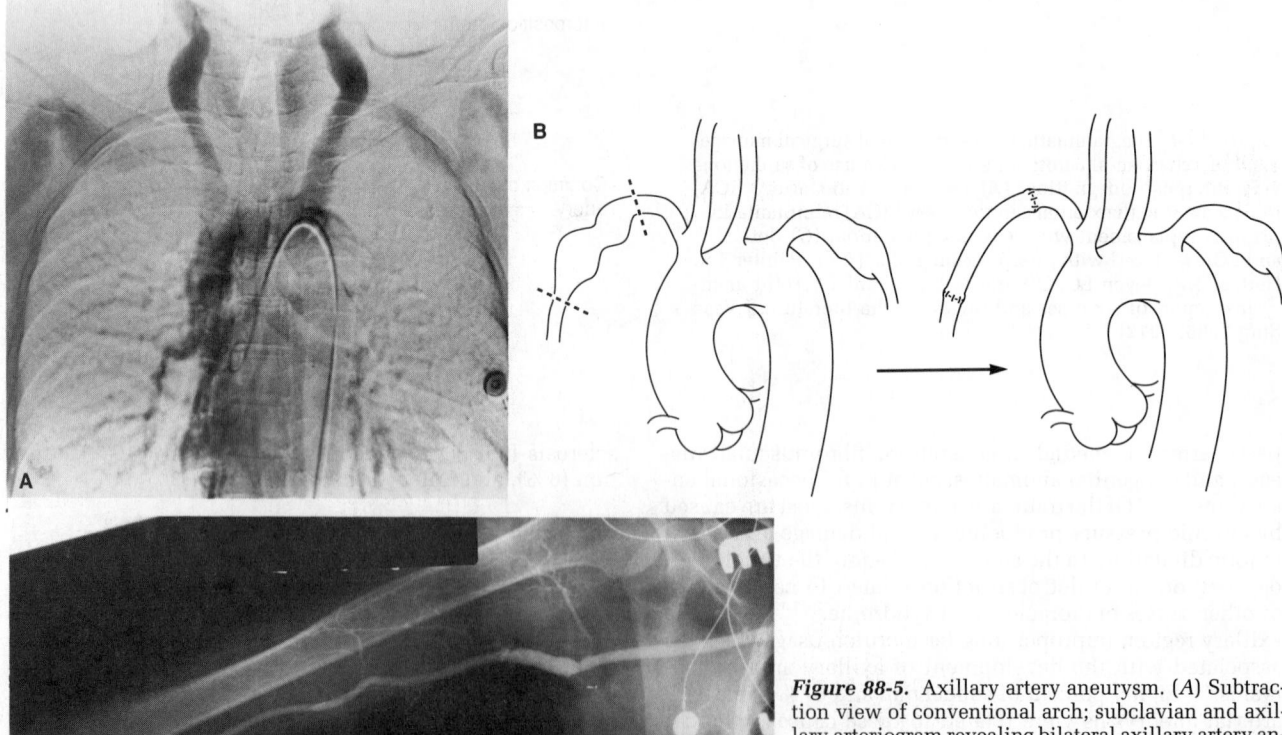

Figure 88-5. Axillary artery aneurysm. (*A*) Subtraction view of conventional arch; subclavian and axillary arteriogram revealing bilateral axillary artery aneurysms. (*B*) Operative diagram depicting repair with reversed saphenous vein axillobrachial interposition graft. (*C*) Intraoperative right axillobrachial arteriogram revealing functioning interposition graft.

in which reconstruction is not feasible, but it is accompanied by a 25% incidence of effort-related upper extremity ischemic symptoms.[24] Axilloaxillary bypass may be a useful adjunct in this unusual situation.[47] The rare patient with an aberrant right subclavian artery aneurysm is probably best treated by preliminary extraanatomic bypass to the right subclavian artery followed by a left thoracotomy for ligation of the aneurysm, since it is difficult or impossible to control the origin of the aberrant right subclavian artery from a right thoracotomy or median sternotomy[7] (see Fig. 88-1).

Finally, it should be emphasized that patients who have required repair of axillary aneurysms for chronic crutch trauma should be retrained to use the Canadian-style elbow-supporting crutches to avoid further trauma to the arterial reconstruction.[14]

Results

Late follow-up (mean, 9.2 years) of 31 patients in one series included 3 patients who were not operated on and 28 who underwent operative repair. Of the 27 operative survivors, 1 required a forearm amputation 6 days after aneurysm repair because of distal arterial thrombosis. Eighteen other operative survivors who underwent aneurysm repair and arm revascularization had no recurrence of aneurysm or signs of ischemia at late follow-up. The 4 remaining patients who underwent thoracic outlet decompression alone had no late evidence of embolism or aneurysm rupture.[24] Cumulative 5- and 10-year survival rates for patients who underwent axillosubclavian aneurysm repair have been reported to be 87% and 62%, respectively.[28]

INNOMINATE ANEURYSMS

Incidence and Etiology

Innominate artery aneurysms are unusual lesions; for this reason, the actual incidence is unknown. A 1940 report described 10 innominate aneurysms in a review of 1147 cases of aneurysm, for an incidence of 0.9%.[48] Many of these aneurysms were probably luetic, because syphilitic arteritis was relatively common at that time. Only a few cases of atherosclerotic innominate aneurysm have been reported. In a review of 71 surgical reconstructions of the innominate artery performed from 1964 to 1984, three patients who underwent operation for the repair of innominate aneurysm were identified.[49] In a review of 73 patients who underwent repair of 73 brachiocephalic aneurysms over a 40-year period from 1950 to 1990, only 6 aneurysms (8%) involved the innominate artery. Five of the 6 patients in that series had other, associated aneurysms.[28]

Clinical Manifestations

Patients with innominate artery aneurysms either have chest discomfort, have hoarseness caused by recurrent laryngeal nerve dysfunction, or are asymptomatic. Two thirds of innominate artery aneurysms recently reported were detected during preoperative evaluation for abdominal aortic aneurysm repair.[49] Occasionally, multiple symptoms are present. A case of innominate artery aneurysm in a woman presenting with hoarseness, dysphagia, mediastinal mass, and a right hemispheric stroke has been reported.[50]

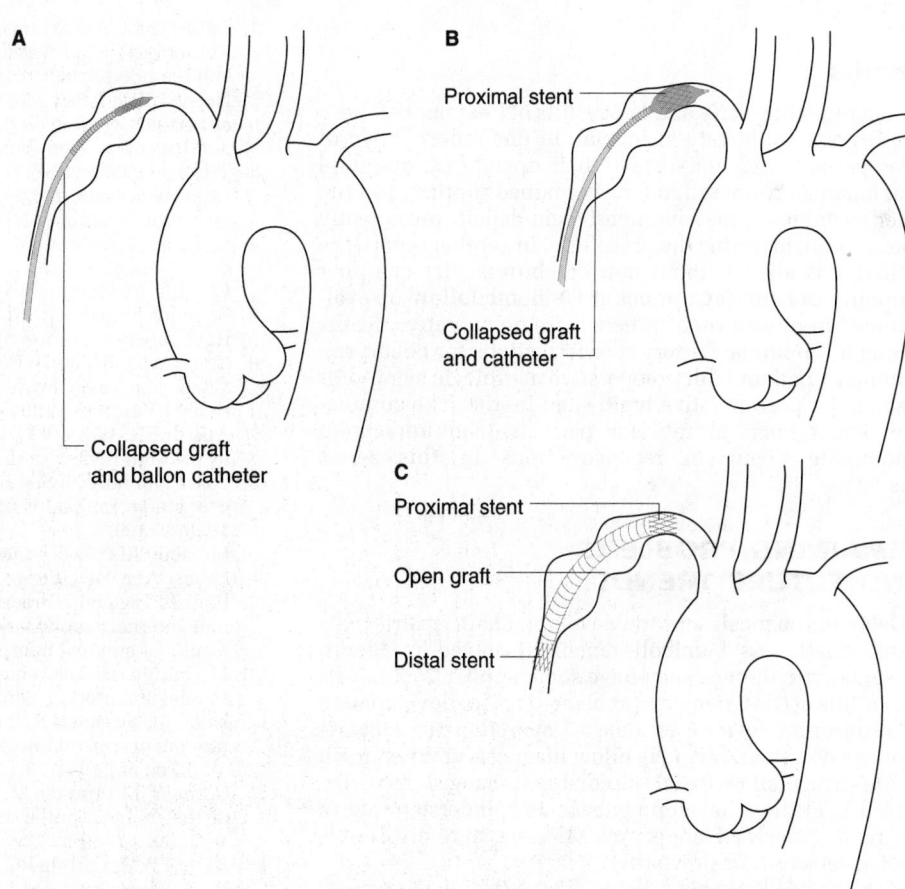

A

Collapsed graft and ballon catheter

B

Proximal stent

Collapsed graft and catheter

C

Proximal stent

Open graft

Distal stent

Figure 88-6. Intraluminal stent–graft placement for treatment of an axillosubclavian aneurysm. (*A*) Catheter delivery of the stent–graft. (*B*) Balloon deployment of the proximal stent to anchor the graft proximally. (*C*) Graft in place after deployment of the distal anchoring stent.

Diagnosis

The diagnosis can be suspected when chest radiography reveals a mediastinal mass. MRI or contrast-enhanced computed tomographic scanning of the chest differentiates aneurysm from tumor mass. Arch aortography confirms the pathologic arterial anatomy and allows planning of therapy.

Treatment

Because of the risks of embolism and rupture, surgical repair is indicated, especially if the aneurysm is symptomatic, the aneurysm is large or enlarging, and the patient is an acceptable surgical risk.

Optimal therapy involves excision of the aneurysm and restoration of both upper extremity and cerebral perfusion. On occasion, it may be acceptable to restore flow only to the right carotid artery. The aneurysm can be approached through a median sternotomy, which can be extended along the anterior border of the right sternocleidomastoid muscle for additional exposure. Resection of a small aneurysm with end-to-end anastomosis has been reported.[50] More often, replacement of the aneurysmal innominate artery with a synthetic interposition graft or a bifurcated graft to the right common carotid and subclavian arteries is performed. Alternatively, autogenous saphenous vein grafts from the aorta to the right subclavian artery and from the aorta to the right common carotid artery can be used if the vein size is adequate. Cardiopulmonary bypass is not required for elective innominate aneurysm repair but may be a necessary adjunct in the event of a rupture.[50] Ligation of the innominate artery is well tolerated by the upper extremity; however, cerebral injury has occurred after occlusion of the common carotid artery. Ligation is rarely performed and is certainly less preferable than direct reconstruction.

Results

Data regarding early and late results of treatment of these rare lesions are largely anecdotal. In one report,[49] two of three patients did not survive their operations; one died after emergency operation for a contained rupture, and the other sustained a massive neurologic deficit, presumably from embolism during the procedure. In another report, the patient was alive without new cerebrovascular or upper extremity ischemic symptoms at a 9-month follow-up evaluation.[50] In a third report, there were no operative deaths among 6 innominate artery reconstructions for aneurysm, although 1 patient with preoperative neurologic symptoms sustained a postoperative brain-stem infarct. The cumulative 5-year survival rate for patients who underwent innominate aneurysm reconstructions in this series was 63%.[28]

REMAINING PROBLEMS AND FUTURE TRENDS

Delay in diagnosis and the development of irretrievable distal small vessel emboli remain unsolved problems. Thrombolytic therapy may have some application, but its use in this setting remains problematic. The development of ultrasonic devices to detect asymptomatic embolic showers noninvasively may allow diagnosis and treatment before irreversible distal circulatory changes have occurred.[51] Further developments in the understanding of the pathogenesis of aneurysmal disease may also allow earlier detection or prevention.

It seems unlikely that reliable data regarding the natural history of untreated lesions will be available in the foreseeable future. Until then, reliance on collective reviews of individual and small group experiences is required. Definitive guidelines for the optimal treatment of these rare aneurysms await the accumulation of data on sufficiently large numbers of patients with brachiocephalic aneurysms to allow statistical analysis. Because these lesions are rare, the development of large patient registries will probably be required to provide such data.

Recent progress in the development of endovascular catheter techniques for the placement of intraluminal prosthetic grafts may simplify considerably the treatment of brachiocephalic aneurysms.[52-54] The graft–stent device is introduced through a peripheral artery, and the synthetic graft is fixed to the arterial lumen proximally and distally by means of a balloon-expandable stent (Fig. 88-6). Originally envisioned for use in the aorta, a transluminal prosthetic graft–stent device for treatment of a subclavian artery aneurysm has been reported.[55] The applicability of this approach to the treatment of many aneurysms may be limited by the requirement of an artery neck of normal caliber proximal and distal to the aneurysm that is adequate to allow fixation by the intraluminal stent. Furthermore, the widespread application of this technique is limited by the size and restricted flexibility of the graft–stent device and its introducer. Atheromatous embolization has also been reported with the use of this device in the abdominal aorta. Questions remain regarding the durability of intraluminally fixed grafts because further dilatation of the aneurysm neck may allow dislodgment and migration of the graft. Nevertheless, further refinements of this technique seem likely to permit its more widespread application.

REFERENCES

1. Goldstone J. Aneurysms of the extracranial carotid artery. In: Rutherford RB, ed. Vascular surgery, ed 3, vol 2. Philadelphia, WB Saunders, 1989:1418.
2. Hobson RW, Israel MR, Lynch TG. Axillosubclavian arterial aneurysms. In: Bergan JJ, Yao JST, eds. Aneurysms: diagnosis and treatment. New York, Grune & Stratton, 1982:435.
3. Trippel OH, Haid SP, Kornmesser TW, et al. Extracranial carotid aneurysms. In: Bergan JJ, Yao JST, eds. Aneurysms: diagnosis and treatment. New York, Grune & Stratton, 1982:493.
4. Langman J. Arterial system. In: Medical embryology: human development—normal and abnormal. Baltimore, Williams & Wilkins, 1963:171.
5. Schmidt FE, Hewitt RL, Flores AA. Aneurysm of anomalous right subclavian artery. South Med J 1980;73:255.
6. Stone WM, Brewster DC, Moncure AC, et al. Aberrant right subclavian artery: varied presentations and management options. J Vasc Surg 1990;11:812.
7. Austin EH, Wolfe WG. Aneurysm of aberrant subclavian artery with a review of the literature. J Vasc Surg 1985;2:571.
8. Poker N, Finby N, Steinberg I. The subclavian arteries: roentgen study in health and disease. AJR Am J Roentgenol 1958;80:193.
9. McCann RL. Basic data related to peripheral artery aneurysms. Ann Vasc Surg 1990;4:411.
10. Bour P, Taghavi I, Bracard S, et al. Aneurysm of the extracranial internal carotid artery due to fibromuscular dysplasia: results of surgical management. Ann Vasc Surg 1992;6:205.
11. McCollum CH, DaGama AD, Noon GP, et al. Aneurysm of the subclavian artery. J Cardiovasc Surg 1979;20:159.
12. Israel M, Sussman B, Ibrahim IM, et al. Subclavian and axillary aneurysms: etiology, manifestations and management. J Med Soc N J 1981;78:173.
13. Cormier JM, Amrane M, Ward A, et al. Arterial complications of the thoracic outlet syndrome: fifty-five operative cases. J Vasc Surg 1989;9:778.
14. Abbott WM, Darling RC. Axillary artery aneurysms secondary to crutch trauma. Am J Surg 1973;125:515.

15. Mathes SJ, Salam AA. Subclavian artery aneurysm: sequela of thoracic outlet syndrome. Surgery 1974;76:506.

16. Sanders RJ, Haug C. Review of arterial thoracic outlet syndrome with a report of five new instances. Surg Gynecol Obstet 1991;173:415.

17. Harrison LH, Batson RC, Hunter DR. Aberrant right subclavian artery aneurysm: an analysis of surgical options. Ann Thoracic Surg 1994;57:1012.

18. Kieffer E, Bahnini A, Koskas F. Aberrant subclavian artery: surgical treatment in thirty-three adult patients. J Vasc Surg 1994;19:100.

19. Kiernan PD, Dearani J, Byrne WD, et al. Aneurysm of an aberrant right subclavian artery: case report and review of the literature. Mayo Clin Proc 1993;68:468.

20. Verkroost MW, Hamerlijnck RP, Vermeulen FE. Surgical management of aneurysms at the origin of an aberrant right subclavian artery. J Thorac Cardiovasc Surg 1994;107:1469.

21. Esposito RA, Khalil I, Spencer FC. Surgical treatment for aneurysm of aberrant subclavian artery based on a case report and review of the literature. J Thorac Cardiovasc Surg 1988;95:888.

22. Miller CM, Sanguiolo P, Schanzer H, et al. Infected false aneurysms of the subclavian artery: a complication in drug addicts. J Vasc Surg 1984;1:684.

23. Fee HJ, Gewirtz HS, O'Connell TX, et al. Bilateral subclavian artery aneurysm associated with idiopathic cystic medial necrosis. J Thorac Cardiovasc Surg 1978;26:387.

24. Pairolero PC, Walls JT, Payne WS, et al. Subclavian–axillary artery aneurysms. Surgery 1981;90:757.

25. Rifkinson-Mann S, Laub J, Haimov M. Atraumatic extracranial vertebral artery aneurysm: case report and review of the literature. J Vasc Surg 1986;4:288.

26. Johnson JN, Helsby CR, Stell PM. Aneurysm of the external carotid artery. J Cardiovasc Surg 1980;21:105.

27. Pratschke E, Schafer K, Reimer J, et al. Extracranial aneurysms of the carotid artery. Thorac Cardiovasc Surg 1980;28:354.

28. Bower TC, Pairolero PC, Hallett JW, et al. Brachiocephalic aneurysm: the case for early recognition and repair. Ann Vasc Surg 1991;5:125.

29. Rhodes EL, Stanley JC, Hoffman GL, et al. Aneurysms of extracranial carotid arteries. Arch Surg 1976;111:339.

30. McCollum CH, Wheeler WG, Noon GP, et al. Aneurysms of the extracranial carotid artery: twenty-one years' experience. Am J Surg 1979;137:196.

31. Busuttil RW, Davidson RK, Foley KT, et al. Selective management of extracranial carotid arterial aneurysms. Am J Surg 1980;140:85.

32. Morki B, Piepgras DG, Sundt TM Jr, et al. Subject review: extracranial internal carotid artery aneurysms. Mayo Clin Proc 1982;57:310.

33. Krupski WC, Effeney DJ, Ehrenfeld WK, et al. Aneurysms of the carotid arteries. Aust N Z J Surg 1983;53:521.

34. Welling RE, Taha A, Goel T, et al. Extracranial carotid artery aneurysms. Surgery 1983;93:319.

35. Dehn TCB, Taylor GW. Extracranial carotid artery aneurysms. Ann R Coll Surg 1984;66:247.

36. Zwolak RM, Whitehouse WM, Knake JE, et al. Atherosclerotic extracranial carotid artery aneurysms. J Vasc Surg 1984;1:415.

37. Sahlman A, Salo J, Kostiainen S, et al. Extracranial carotid artery aneurysms. Vasa 1991;20:369.

38. Painter TA, Hertzer NR, Beven EG, et al. Extracranial carotid aneurysms: report of six cases and review of the literature. J Vasc Surg 1985;2:312.

39. Hammon JW, Silver D, Young WG Jr. Congenital aneurysm of the extracranial carotid arteries. Ann Surg 1971;176:777.

40. Kaupp HA, Haid SP, Jurayj MN, et al. Aneurysms of the extracranial carotid artery. Surgery 1972;72:946.

41. Winslow N. Extracranial aneurysm of the internal carotid artery: history and analysis of the cases registered up to Aug. 1, 1925. Arch Surg 1926;13:689.

42. Dent TL, Lindenauer SM, Ernst CB, et al. Multiple atherosclerotic arterial aneurysms. Arch Surg 1972;105:388.

43. Hobson RW, Sarkaria J, O'Donnell JA, et al. Atherosclerotic aneurysms of the subclavian artery. Surgery 1979;85:368.

44. Salo JA, Ala-Kulju K, Keikkinen L, et al. Diagnosis and treatment of subclavian artery aneurysms. Eur J Vasc Surg 1990;4:271.

45. Neumayer LA, Bull DA, Hunter GC, et al. Atherosclerotic aneurysms of the axillary artery. J Cardiovasc Surg 1992;33:172.

46. Coselli JS, Crawford ES. Surgical management of aneurysms of the intrathoracic segment of the subclavian artery. Chest 1987;91:704.

47. Anderson CA, Collins GJ Jr, Rich NM. Axillo-axillary bypass for complications of an axillary arterial aneurysm: a case report. Am Surg 1977;43:464.

48. Matas R. Personal experience in vascular surgery: statistical synopsis. Ann Surg 1940;112:802.

49. Brewster DC, Moncure AC, Darling RC, et al. Innominate artery lesions: problems encountered and lessons learned. J Vasc Surg 1985;2:99.

50. Schumacher PD, Wright CB. Management of arteriosclerotic aneurysm of the innominate artery. Surgery 1979;85:489.

51. Spencer MP, Thomas GI, Nicholls SC, et al. Detection of middle cerebral artery emboli during carotid endarterectomy using transcranial Doppler ultrasonography. Stroke 1990;21:415.

52. Sayers RD, Thompson MM, Bell PRF. Endovascular stenting of abdominal aortic aneurysms. Eur J Vasc Surg 1993;7:225.

53. Parodi JC, Palmaz JC, Barone HD. Transfemoral intraluminal graft implantation for abdominal aortic aneurysms. Ann Vasc Surg 1991;5:491.

54. Marin ML, Veith FJ, Panetta TF, et al. Transluminally placed endovascular stented graft repair for arterial trauma. J Vasc Surg 1994;20:446.

55. May J, White G, Waugh R, Yu W, Harris J. Transluminal placement of a prosthetic graft-stent device for treatment of subclavian artery aneurysm. J Vasc Surg 1993;18:1056.

SURGERY: SCIENTIFIC PRINCIPLES AND PRACTICE, Second Edition, edited by Lazar J. Greenfield, Michael W. Mulholland, Keith T. Oldham, Gerald B. Zelenock, and Keith D. Lillemoe. Lippincott-Raven Publishers, Philadelphia, © 1997.

CHAPTER 89

THORACIC AORTIC ANEURYSMS

R. SCOTT MITCHELL

The incidence of aneurysmal disease of the thoracic aorta appears to be increasing. Whether this reflects an actual increase in incidence, an increase in diagnosis through improved diagnostic modalities, or an increasing population at risk remains unknown. True aneurysmal dilatation of the aorta involves all three layers of the arterial wall (intima, media, and adventitia) and can be fusiform or saccular. False aneurysms, conversely, exhibit an intimal disruption contained only by adventitial layers and surrounding reactive fibrosis. Arteriosclerotic aneurysms typically demonstrate degenerative changes within the aortic media, whereas intrinsic abnormalities of connective tissue account for the degenerative aneurysms found in Marfan syndrome and Ehlers-Danlos syndrome, wherein all parts of the aorta, including the sinuses of Valsalva, are involved. These entities are to be differentiated from aortic dissections, wherein an intimal tear allows a high-pressure entry point into the subadventitial layer, which can then propagate proximally and distally, possibly leading to rupture or branch vessel compromise. In a patient with Marfan syndrome, the risk of aortic dissection appears directly related to the extent of aneurysmal dilatation of the aortic root.

The development of cardiopulmonary bypass and synthetic graft materials has allowed tremendous progress in the management of these life-threatening disorders. DeBakey and Cooley[1] pioneered many of the techniques that have been accepted and refined by surgeons throughout the world. The use of new graft materials (including aortic homografts), composite valve–graft conduits, new suture materials, modern techniques of cardiopulmonary bypass, and more effective myocardial and cerebral protection has allowed acceptable survival after surgical treatment of even the most severe disease of the thoracic aorta.

ARTERIOSCLEROTIC ANEURYSMS

Only slightly less common than abdominal aortic aneurysms, aneurysmal disease of the thoracic aorta is increasingly detected in aging populations with associated hypertension and chronic obstructive lung disease. Most commonly, these aneurysms are asymptomatic and are discovered on routine chest radiographs or during evaluation for another medical problem. Males are affected more commonly than females (3:1), and involvement of the descending aorta is more common than that of the ascending aorta. A positive family history for many patients with thoracic aortic aneurysms raises the question of whether these aneurysms, like their abdominal aortic counterparts, may have a genetic basis.

Once aneurysmal dilatation of the aorta has begun, it tends to progress. Whether this represents a gradual but constant increase in size or episodic incremental increases is unknown, but both appear likely. Concomitant hypertension contributes to continued expansion in two ways: increased radial pressure results in increased wall tension, and there is ongoing damage to the structural integrity of the aortic wall through accelerated arteriosclerotic change. Unlike the classic natural history studies of abdominal aortic aneurysms,[2] no such studies exist for aneurysms of the thoracic aorta. However, in a series of over 600 patients with thoracic aneurysms described before operative repair was possible, 66% of patients died as a result of their aneurysms. A 1980 study reinforced the dismal outcome of patients managed nonoperatively after discovery of a large thoracic aneurysm.[3] The high rupture rates for aneurysms greater than 10 cm in diameter and for symptomatic aneurysms were alarming. The mean survival after diagnosis was only 2.6 years, and only 20% of patients survived 5 years. Aneurysm rupture accounted for 40% of deaths, with an additional 30% resulting from other cardiovascular causes. Signs and symptoms of rapid expansion, including hemoptysis, hematemesis, hoarseness, stridor, and an increase in chest pain, warrant surgical intervention. We also favor repair for thoracic aortic aneurysms greater than 7 cm in diameter, for aneurysms greater than twice the diameter of the normal adjacent aorta, and for aneurysms with a rapid increase in size.

Several new diagnostic modalities allow much closer monitoring and detection of thoracic aneurysms than was previously possible. Although the routine biplane diagnostic chest radiograph can alert the clinician to the presence of an aneurysm (Fig. 89-1), the cross-sectional images available through computed tomography (CT) scanning and magnetic resonance imaging (MRI) allow much more accurate sizing of the aneurysm and can differentiate between aneurysmal chronic dissections and true arteriosclerotic or degenerative aneurysms. This differentiation is important because chronic dissections tend to be more extensive, and their operative repair more complex. Once an aneurysm is suspected, imaging of the entire thoracic and abdominal aorta must be performed, because multiple aneurysms can exist in as many as 40% of patients. Because angiography delineates only the aortic lumen within the laminated thrombus, it can seriously underestimate aneurysm size and extent; thus, it is only of minimal usefulness for ongoing clinical assessment.

Operative Management

Once the necessity for operation has been determined, and cardiac evaluation completed, aneurysm replacement with an interposition graft or cardiopulmonary bypass is the treatment of choice. Proper anesthetic management of these patients is critical and requires arterial, central venous, and pulmonary arterial pressure monitoring, urinary catheters, and double-lumen endotracheal intubation. Additionally, large-volume intravenous infusion lines and central infusion ports for vasoactive drugs are essential. Transesophageal echocardiography has also been extremely helpful in assessing regional wall motion and in-

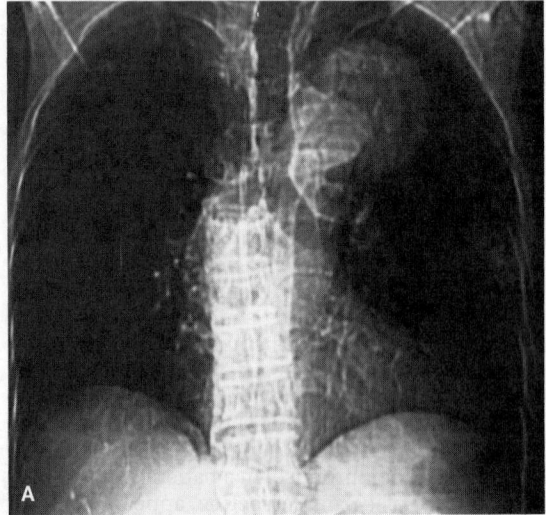 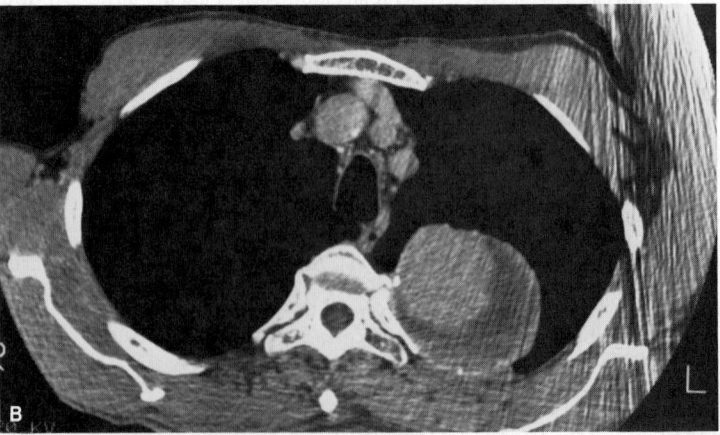

Figure 89-1. (*A*) Large asymptomatic descending thoracic aortic aneurysm discovered incidentally on routine chest radiograph. A peripheral left upper zone pulmonary mass is also apparent. (*B*) CT scan of the thorax allows precise determination of aneurysm size and location, frequently obviating the necessity for angiography.

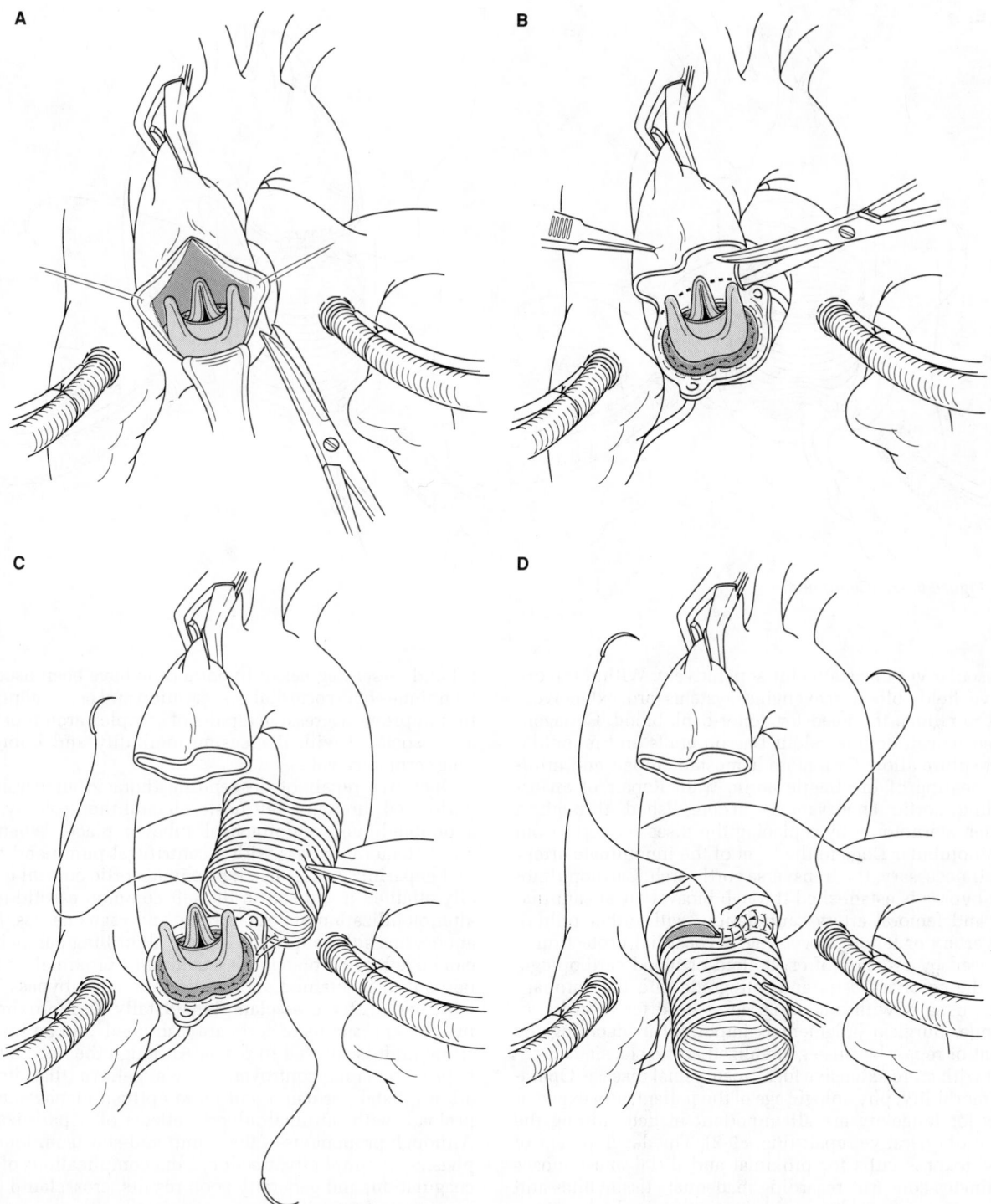

Figure 89-2. (*A*) Operative repair of ascending aortic aneurysm without degenerative aortic disease. Valve replacement, if indicated, is performed after cardiac arrest with cardioplegia and during continuous topical hypothermia. (*B*) A full-thickness cuff of proximal aorta is developed by meticulous dissection of the aorta off the pulmonary artery, and the aorta is transected just distal to the coronary ostia. (*C*) The posterior suture line begins to the left of the left main coronary ostium, and proceeds rightward, over the ostium. Meticulous hemostasis is mandatory, because repair sutures in this area can narrow the left main coronary artery. (*D*) Completion of the posterior suture line demonstrates the exposure attained by extensive mobilization of the aorta and pulmonary artery. (*E*) The anterior suture line may compromise the right coronary artery in the atrioventricular groove. (*F*) Careful measurement of graft length ensures a tension-free distal anastomosis. (After Frist WH, Miller DC. Repair of ascending aortic aneurysms and dissections. J Cardiac Surg 1986;1:33) *(continues)*

E F

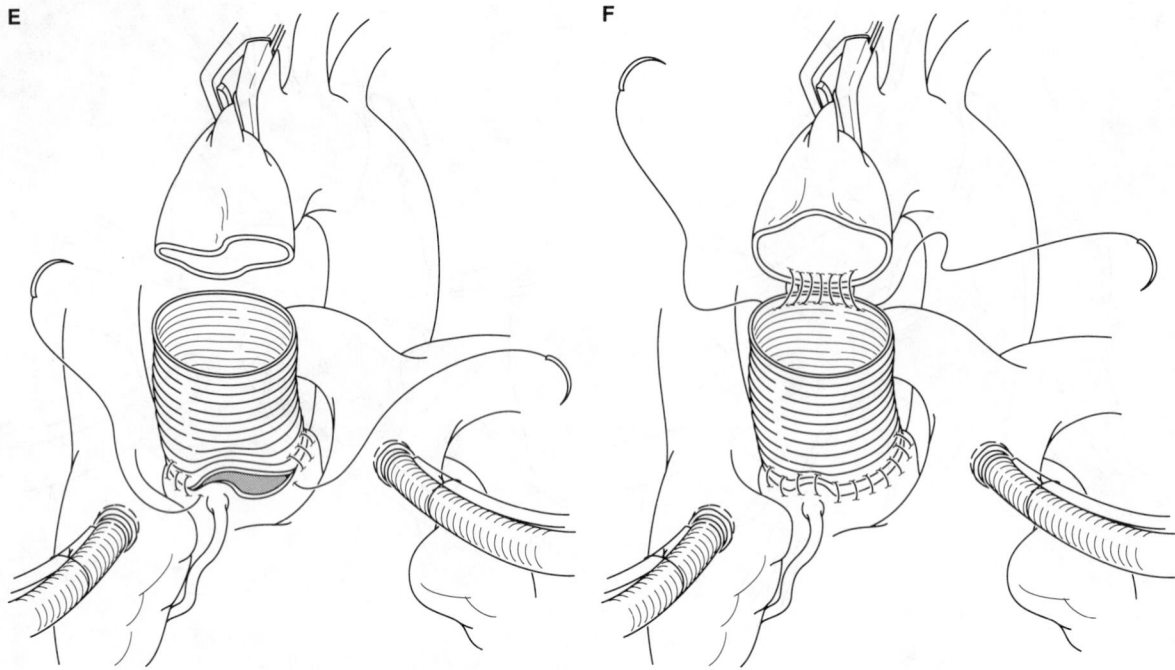

Figure 89-2. *(Continued)*

travascular volume status intraoperatively. Within the operative field, blood scavenging systems are extensively used to reduce the need for donor-bank blood. Collagen-coated woven double-velour Dacron grafts and monofilament suture allow for a more hemostatic repair and minimize tearing of the fragile aortic wall. Repair of an ascending aortic aneurysm is accomplished through a median sternotomy by replacing the diseased aorta from the sinotubular ridge to the level of the innominate artery and, if necessary, the transverse aortic arch. Cardiopulmonary bypass is established through bicaval atrial cannulation and femoral artery cannulation, with either pulmonary artery or left atrial venting. Myocardial protection is achieved by infusion of crystalloid or blood cardioplegia into the coronary ostia and retrograde into the coronary sinus, usually with a cooling jacket used for local hypothermia. Surgical judgment is important in deciding the extent of repair because generalized aortic ectasia can coexist with more extensive focal aneurysmal disease. Operative morbidity, physiologic age of the patient, and expectations for longevity are all important in determining the extent of operative repair (Fig. 89-2). The development of full-thickness cuffs for proximal and distal anastomoses eliminates concerns regarding inadequate tissue bites and the subsequent problems with hemostasis and false aneurysm formation that can result from use of the inclusion technique. Management of the degenerative aneurysms of Marfan disease and of aortic dissections requires additional technical considerations and is covered separately. After rewarming is accomplished, all air is removed from the left side of the heart and graft, and the aortic crossclamp is removed. After a sufficient period of resuscitation, with continuous venting of the ascending aorta for entrapped air, the patient is weaned from cardiopulmonary bypass. Avoidance of postoperative hypertension is critical to avoid excessive bleeding or anastomotic disruption.

Operations on the transverse aortic arch are usually performed with profound hypothermic circulatory arrest with retrograde cerebral venous perfusion. Alternatively, separate arterial cannulation of a single nondiseased arch ves-

sel and lesser degrees of hypothermia have been used. As techniques of myocardial preservation and cerebral protection improve, aggressive repairs of complex arch problems are associated with decreasing morbidity and improved long-term survival.

Operative repair of descending thoracic aneurysms is performed through a left posterolateral thoracotomy with a double-lumen endotracheal tube in place. When left atrial–femoral bypass with a centrifugal pump and minimal heparinization is used, proximal aortic control is usually attained just distal to the left common carotid artery after mobilization of both phrenic and vagus nerves. Large aneurysms adherent to the chest wall or lung parenchyma can be left incompletely dissected until proximal and distal control is attained and cardiopulmonary bypass is established. After crossclamping distally and proximally, full-thickness cuffs of aorta are fashioned, and an interposition graft is sutured in place. Although the necessity for bypass remains controversial, we believe that its use allows distal perfusion and more optimal management of preload, with minimal adverse effects of heparinization. Although proponents of the clamp-and-sew technique emphasize its simplicity, freedom from complications of anticoagulation, and generally good results, crossclamp times in excess of 30 minutes are associated with an increased risk of paraplegia, a dreaded complication of operations on the distal thoracic aorta.[4]

Bypass techniques using heparin-bonded shunts, while avoiding the bleeding complications of full-dose heparin, may deliver variable and inadequate flows for distal perfusion. Left atrial to femoral artery partial bypass with a centrifugal pump and minimal heparinization is an attractive alternative to the full heparinization required for partial (venoarterial) cardiopulmonary bypass. No single technique, however, obviates the possibility of postoperative paraplegia. Multiple adjunctive techniques have been explored, both clinically and in the laboratory, in an effort to protect the spinal cord, including monitoring of evoked potentials, perfusion of cord with cooled blood, drainage of spinal fluid to lower intrathecal pressure, the use of

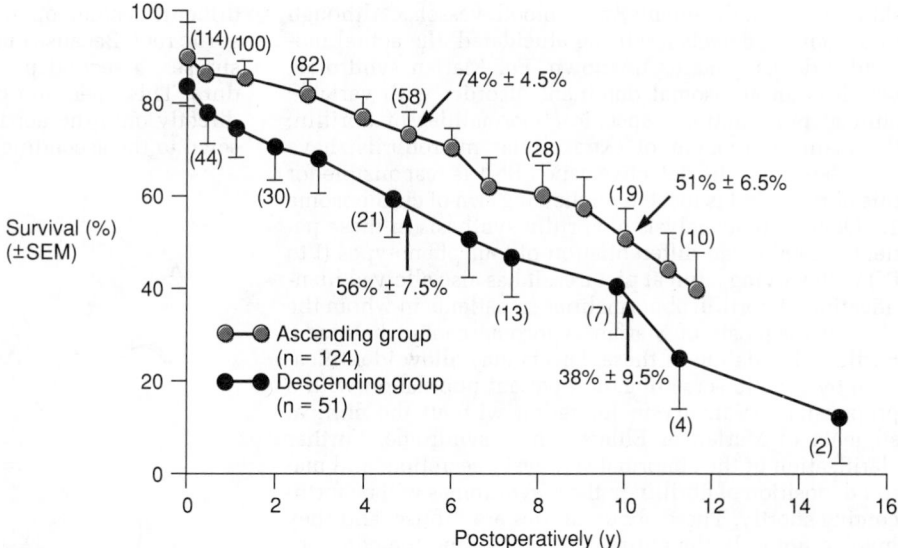

Figure 89-3. Actuarial survival curves for patients with thoracic aortic aneurysms treated operatively. (After Moreno-Cabral CE, Miller DC, Mitchell RS, et al. Degenerative and atherosclerotic aneurysms of the thoracic aorta. J Thorac Cardiovasc Surg 1984;88:1025)

neuroprotective agents, local and systemic hypothermia, reimplantation of critical intercostal vessels, and corticosteroid administration. Although all of these adjuncts can lessen the incidence of paraplegia, none confers absolute protection. Research continues in an effort to prevent this complication.

Multivariate analysis of preoperative variables has been attempted in an effort to identify significant clinical predictors of early and late mortality for all aneurysms of the ascending and descending aorta.[5] The operative mortality rate for ascending aneurysm repair was 7%, with a range of 5% to 15% reported in large series in the literature. Only emergency operation and age over 62 years were independent predictors of increased mortality. For aneurysms of the descending aorta, the operative mortality rate

was 17%, and it correlated significantly with emergency operation and preoperative congestive heart failure. The survival rate after 10 years for this group was about 50% (Fig. 89-3), which reflects diffuse involvement with arteriosclerotic cardiovascular disease. Thirty percent of patients suffered late deaths due to myocardial failure, cerebrovascular accidents, or aneurysm rupture. For all patients, the possibility of late survival was significantly diminished by increased age at the time of operation and by the preoperative presence of congestive heart failure and renal dysfunction.

DEGENERATIVE ANEURYSMS

Aneurysms classified as degenerative are those thought to be secondary to defective formation of collagen, the fibrous ground substance that is the main constituent of

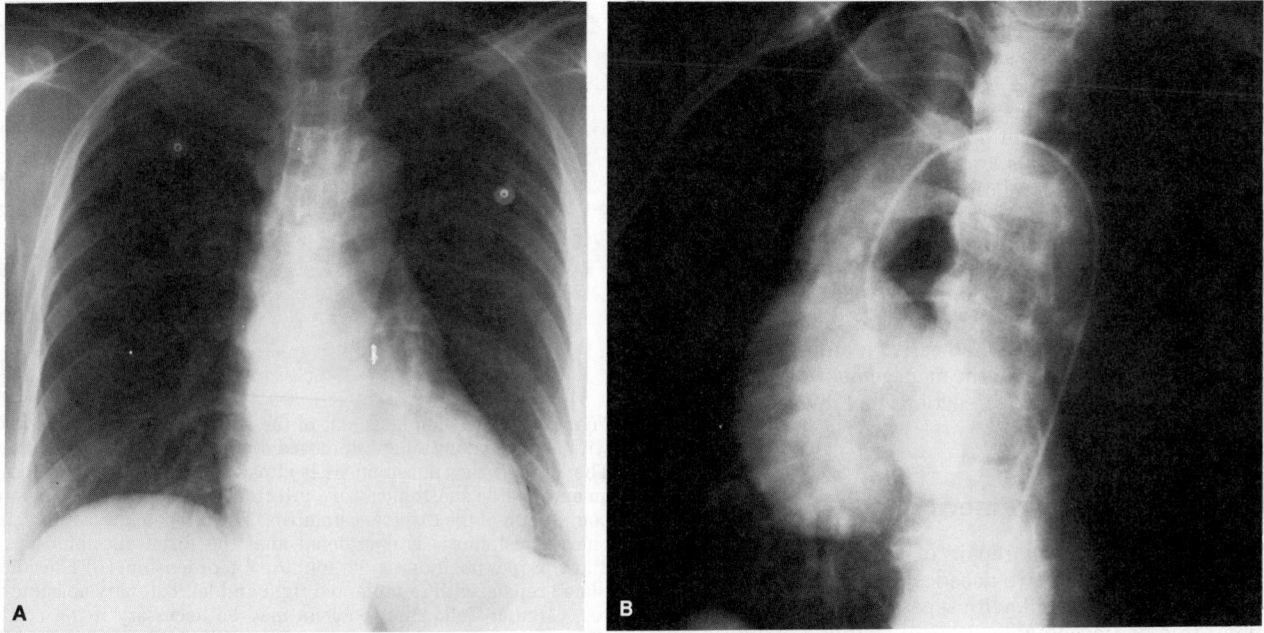

Figure 89-4. (*A*) Dilation of the proximal aorta may be hidden by mediastinal structures on routine posteroanterior chest radiograph. (*B*) Aortography reveals dilation of the entire ascending aorta, including the coronary sinuses, as well as aortic regurgitation.

skin, tendons, ligaments, and blood vessels. Although these genetic defects are being elucidated, the actual molecular defect remains unknown. For Marfan syndrome, which is an autosomal dominant disorder with variable clinical presentations, specific abnormalities of fibrillin, the main component of extracellular microfibrils, have been detected. The defective gene FBN1 is responsible for this fibrillin and is located on the long arm of chromosome 15. Quantitative analysis of fibrillin synthesis in these patients has allowed differentiation of four phenotypes (I to IV) with varying clinical pictures. It has also allowed identification of fibrillin abnormalities in patients in whom the clinical diagnosis of Marfan syndrome cannot be made. Further elucidation of these defects may allow identification, by genetic screening, of a patient population with a propensity for aneurysm formation without the clinical stigmata of Marfan or Ehlers-Danlos syndrome. Further clarification of the abnormal synthesis, secretion, and matrix deposition of fibrillin in these syndromes will be forthcoming shortly. These abnormalities are diffuse, and they involve not only the entire aorta, including the coronary sinuses, but also the cardiac valvular tissues. In contrast to arteriosclerotic aneurysmal disease, the aortic aneurysms found in Marfan patients begin at the level of the aortic annulus, involve the coronary sinuses as well as the supracoronary aorta, and necessitate replacement of the entire aortic root. Because these changes may not be obvious on serial diagnostic chest radiographs (Fig. 89-4), echocardiography, CT scanning, or MRI may be required for serial evaluation.

In patients with the obvious stigmata of Marfan syndrome (ie, long extremities, hyperextensible joints, ectopic lenses, and pectus deformity of the sternum), the diagnosis of Marfan syndrome may be straightforward. In a significant number of patients, however, the diagnosis may not be obvious. The criteria from the Johns Hopkins registry have been used to identify patients with Marfan syndrome.[6] Patients were considered to have the syndrome if they had an affected family member or had evidence of lens dislocation, aortic insufficiency, or musculoskeletal involvement. Historically, the severely diminished longevity of both males and females with Marfan syndrome has been graphically illustrated, with fewer than half of patients surviving past the age of 45 years. Cardiac deaths account for over 90% of early deaths of known cause, and 75% of these deaths are secondary to aortic root dilatation or aortic dissections and their complications.

These dismal statistics prompted recommendations for prophylactic replacement of the aortic root before rupture or dissection, despite its known attendant morbidity and mortality. The direct relation between increasing aortic root size and the propensity for both rupture and dissection supports prophylactic aortic root replacement for aneurysmal dilation greater than 6 cm. As surgical results improve, and the durability of these repairs is documented, these criteria may be revised downward so that prophylactic repair can be accomplished early, avoiding the morbidity associated with long-term management of aneurysmal dilation of chronic aortic dissections that involve the entire aorta.

Operative Management

Methods of surgical repair of the Marfan aorta have evolved over the past two decades. Initially, the supracoronary aorta was replaced, with separate aortic valve replacement; this had acceptable surgical results. Long-term follow-up, however, demonstrated progressive aneurysmal dilatation of the aortic sinuses, frequently necessitating a difficult second operation for replacement of the entire aortic root. Because of the known involvement of the aortic sinuses, a second procedure evolved, the Bentall procedure. This operation consisted of a valved conduit sewn directly onto the aortic annulus, with the coronary ostia sewn to the ascending graft in a side-to-side fashion. Late

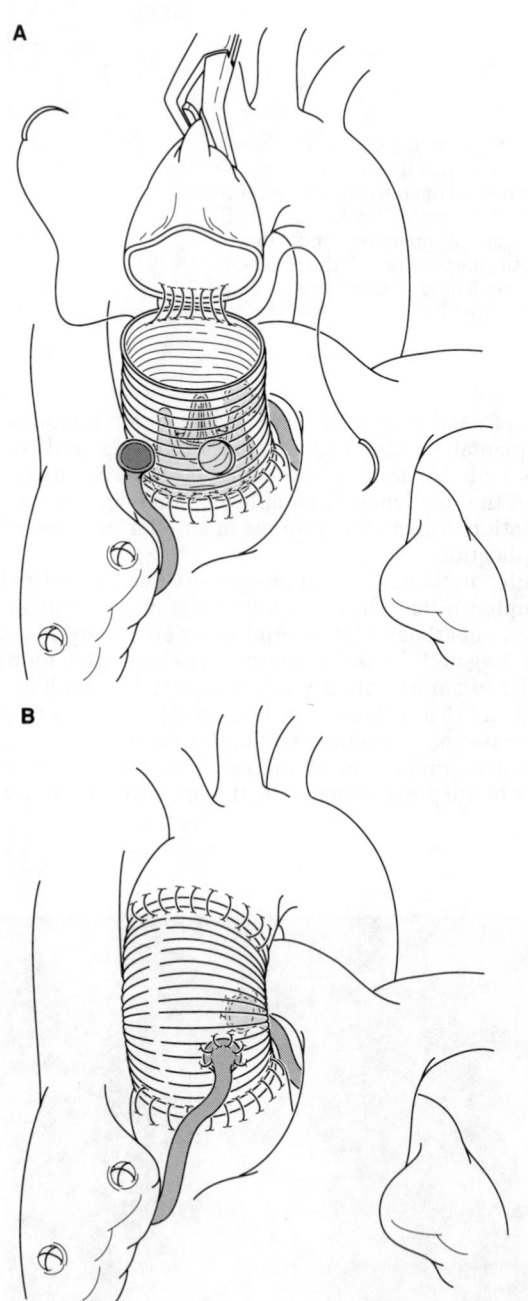

Figure 89-5. (*A*) Replacement of the aortic root is accomplished with a valved conduit anastomosed directly to the aortic annulus. The left coronary anastomosis is already complete, performed as an end-to-side anastomosis of a full-thickness aortic button before completion of the distal anastomosis. The full-thickness right coronary anastomosis is completed after the distal anastomosis to allow proper positioning without torsion or tension. (*B*) The completed repair, with reimplanted right and left coronary anastomoses. Circular Teflon felt bolsters may be necessary if the aortic tissues are unduly friable. (After Frist WH, Miller DC. Repair of ascending aortic aneurysms and dissections. J Cardiac Surg 1986;1:33)

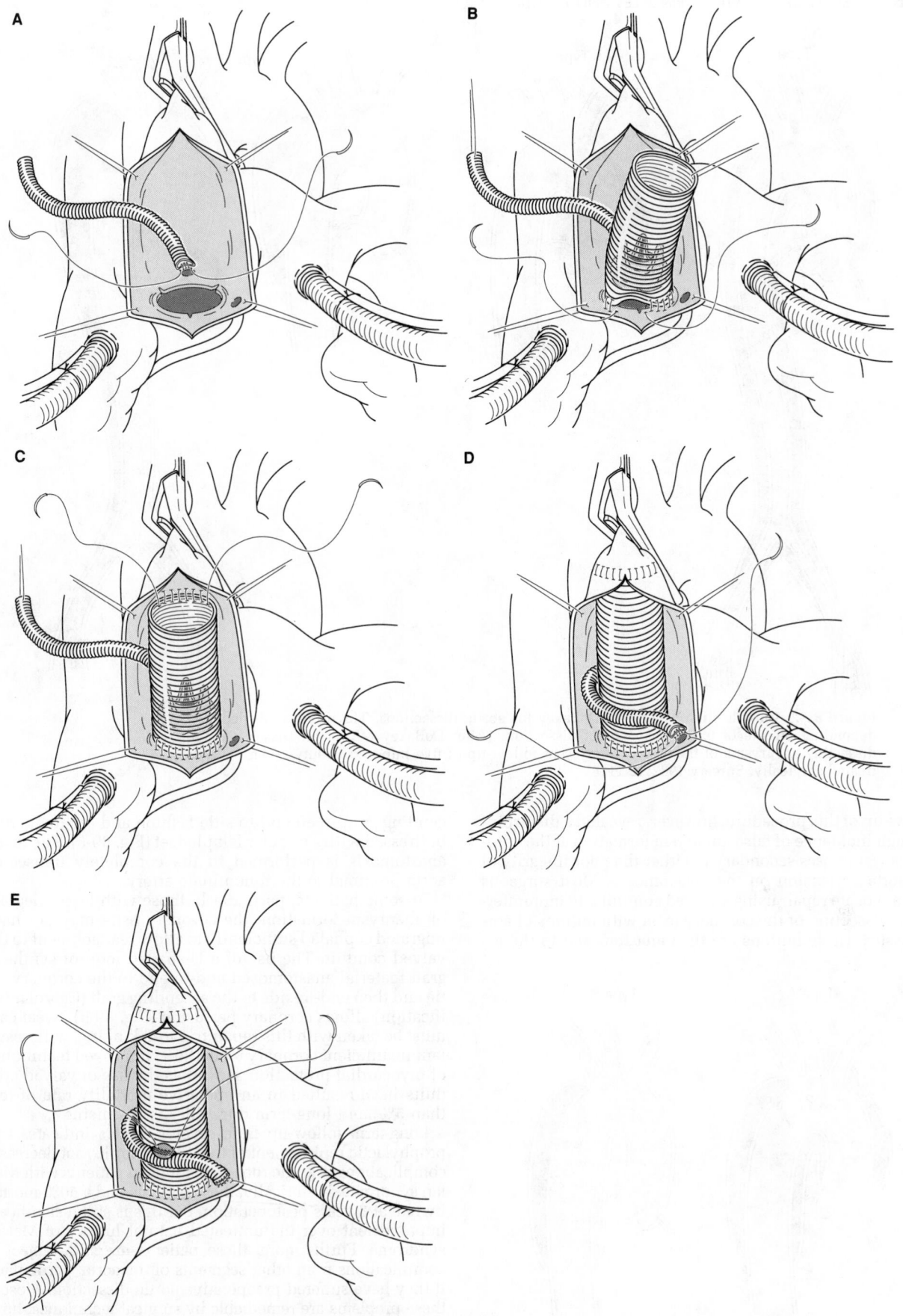

Figure 89-6. (*A*) The low-lying left main coronary ostia can be anastomosed end to side to a Dacron graft. (*B*) The valved conduit is sewn directly to the aortic annulus. (*C*) The distal anastomosis is then constructed, preferably to the transected distal aorta with full-thickness bites. (*D*) The right coronary anastomosis to the Dacron graft is completed without tension. (*E*) A side-to-side anastomosis between the ascending graft and the coronary graft is fashioned without distortion. (After Cabrol C, Gandjbakhc I, Pavie A. Surgical treatment of ascending aortic pathology. J Cardiac Surg 1988;3:167)

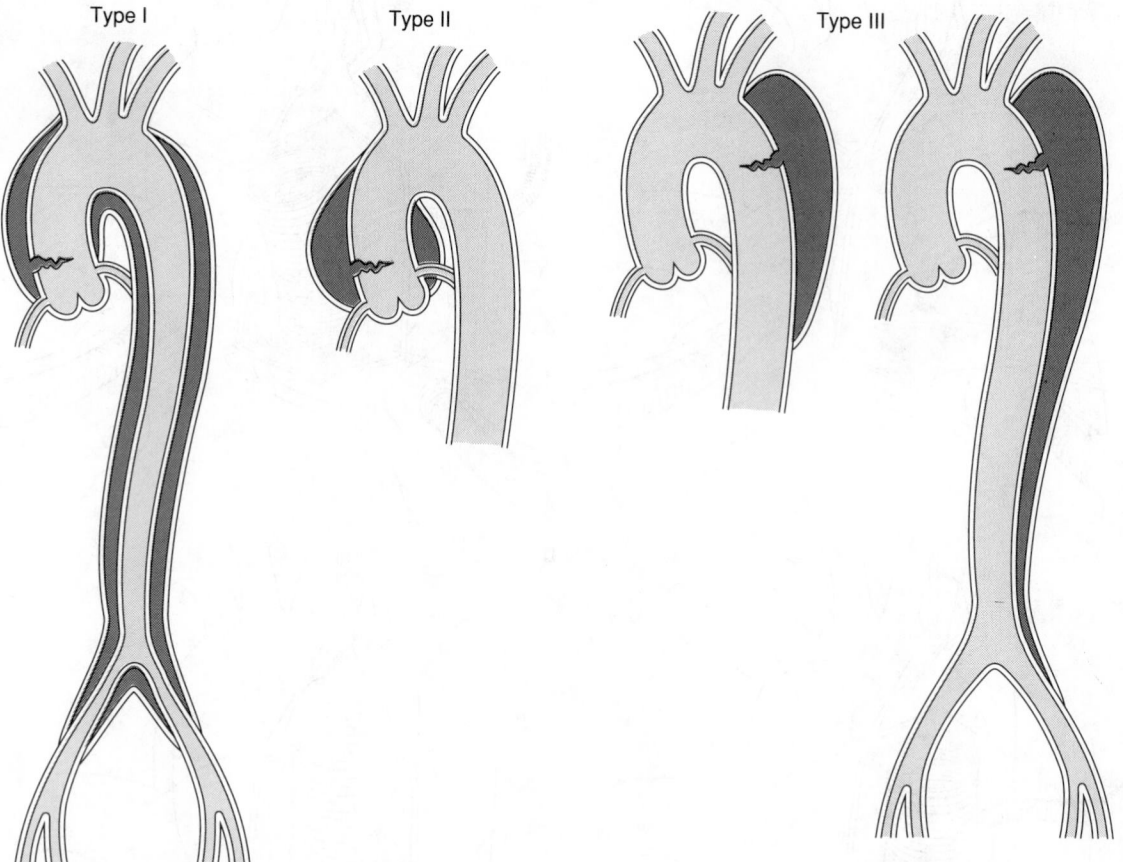

Figure 89-7. Classification scheme of DeBakey for aortic dissections. Three types are depicted depending on site of tear and extent of dissection. (After DeBakey ME, et al. Dissection and dissecting aneurysms of the aorta: twenty-year follow-up of five hundred twenty-seven patients treated surgically. Surgery 1982;92:1118)

follow-up of this procedure, however, revealed a disturbingly high incidence of false aneurysm formation at the coronary anastomoses secondary to either the poor integrity of the aorta or tension on the anastomoses. Most surgeons now advocate repair using a valved conduit and circumferential dissection of the coronary ostia with buttons of aortic tissue. These buttons are then anastomosed to the as-

cending graft in an end-to-side fashion and are frequently buttressed with a circular felt pledget (Fig. 89-5). The distal anastomosis is performed to the completely transected aorta proximal to the innominate artery.

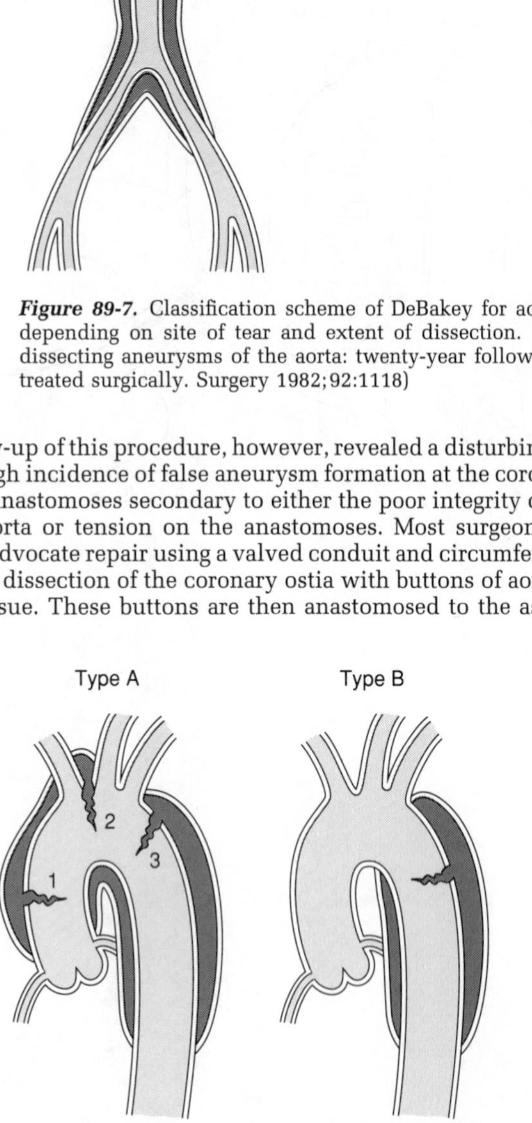

In some patients, particularly those with lesser degrees of aneurysm formation, the coronary ostia may not have migrated cephalad sufficiently to allow reattachment to the valved conduit. The use of a U-shaped loop of synthetic graft material anastomosed end-to-end to the coronary ostia and then end-to-side to the ascending graft (Cabrol modification) allows coronary perfusion (Fig. 89-6). Great care must be taken with this repair to avoid kinking, with resultant insufficient coronary blood flow. Improved techniques of myocardial protection as well as the use of valved conduits have resulted in an operative mortality rate of less than 5%, and long-term durability is promising.

Long-term follow-up from several centers indicates that prophylactic replacement of the dilated aortic root decreases complications of aortic root dissections in patients with Marfan syndrome. Historically, these patients had a 50% mortality rate at 8 years postoperation, but this is still a significant improvement over the untreated natural history of Marfan syndrome. Furthermore, these patients are still subject to complications from other segments of the aorta, particularly if they have suffered preoperative aortic dissection. Most of these problems are remediable by surgical techniques, however, and aggressive follow-up is advocated so that problem areas can be repaired or replaced before a new catastrophic event occurs. Dramatic progress in the understanding of the syndrome and the development of surgical approaches to the marfanoid aorta have allowed significant improvement in a morbid natural history.

Figure 89-8. Stanford classification of aortic dissections based on the presence or absence of involvement of the ascending aorta. Numbers indicate possible locations of the site of primary intimal tear. (After Miller DC, et al. Operative treatment of aortic dissections. J Thorac Cardiovasc Surg 1979;78:365)

AORTIC DISSECTIONS

Acute dissection of the thoracic aorta remains the most frequent catastrophe involving the aorta, with an incidence almost double that of ruptured abdominal aortic aneurysm. Failure to diagnose this entity probably accounts, at least in part, for the lack of appreciation of its prevalence. Most commonly affected are middle-aged and elderly men with coexistent hypertension, although younger women, particularly during the third trimester of pregnancy, can also be affected, as can patients with Marfan disease.

Classification

Multiple classification systems from various institutions have been promulgated, based primarily on anatomic features. Involvement of the ascending aorta remains the most important single feature of acute dissections because this alone predicts the unfavorable clinical behavior of this entity. Neither the exact location of the primary tear nor the distal extent of the dissection exerts as significant an effect on subsequent clinical behavior. Therefore, classification schemes should be based on anatomic features as they relate to clinical behavior or management. Thus, Stanford type A, Massachusetts General proximal, University of Alabama ascending, and DeBakey type 1 all connote involvement of the ascending aorta, whereas Stanford type B, Massachusetts General distal, University of Alabama descending, and DeBakey type 3 connote dissections not involving the ascending aorta (Figs. 89-7 and 89-8).

Acute aortic dissection can present with protean signs and symptoms, mimicking other more common illnesses. Typically, affected patients experience the sudden onset of severe, sharp retrosternal or intrascapular pain, which may then migrate. Occasionally, it is entirely silent, the diagnosis becoming apparent only after the onset of a secondary effect, such as congestive heart failure subsequent to aortic regurgitation or limb ischemia caused by arterial occlusion. A high index of suspicion for seemingly unrelated signs and symptoms remains the key to timely diagnosis, which is critical to avoid the 1% to 2% *per hour* mortality rate during the first 24 to 48 hours after acute dissection of the ascending aorta. When ascending dissection is undiagnosed, the mortality rate approaches 90% at 3 months; the prognosis for type B or descending dissections is somewhat less ominous. Unfortunately, even in the modern era, as many as one third of cases may go undiagnosed.

Diagnosis

A careful history and physical examination can produce subtle clues to suggest the diagnosis; a new murmur of aortic regurgitation or an absent pulse can provoke the critical further evaluation.

The single best definitive diagnostic technique remains unclear. Given the critical importance of early diagnosis and treatment, however, the best diagnostic test may be the one most rapidly available. Contrast-enhanced dynamic CT scanning, MRI, biplane aortography and cineangiography, and multiplanar transesophageal echocardiography all have sufficient diagnostic accuracy, especially regarding involvement of the ascending aorta, to allow accurate therapeutic decisions. The precise choice of diagnostic modality is based on availability and individual expertise. Although aortography and CT scanning have been the traditional gold standards, they have 5% to 10% false-negative rates. Transesophageal echo with color-flow mapping, especially with multiplanar capability, may become the preferred diagnostic modality (Fig. 89-9). The

ascending aorta is easily and clearly imaged, and a flap is readily detected. Advantages include high diagnostic accuracy and the fact that the machine can be brought to the patient, allowing continuous monitoring and treatment and avoiding transport of a critically ill patient to a distant radiology suite. If ascending repair is required, the transducer can be left in place and used to ascertain retrograde flow in the transverse arch during bypass and to monitor cardiac segmental wall motion and aortic valve function after repair. Because of the constraints on medical instrumentation within a strong magnetic field, MRI is more appropriate for the evaluation and long-term management of patients with chronic dissection. Intravascular ultrasound offers dramatic diagnostic capabilities, but it also requires patient transport to a radiology suite.

Hemodynamic stabilization, with particular attention paid to control of hypertension to levels just adequate for maintenance of cerebral, myocardial, and renal perfusion, is the immediate goal of medical therapy. Blunting the rate of pressure increase ($\Delta P/\Delta T$) is also advocated. Although the intravenous titration of sodium nitroprusside has been the traditional pharmacologic therapy of choice, intravenous esmolol more effectively reduces the aortic and left ventricular hyperdynamic state and may allow a stable interval during which definitive diagnosis can be attained and appropriate therapy instituted.

After stabilization and diagnosis, appropriate treatment should be directed toward correcting the life-threatening aspects of the dissection. For dissections involving the ascending aorta (type A), this involves replacement of the supracoronary aorta to prevent rupture of the proximal root into the pericardium with subsequent tamponade, which is the cause of death in over 90% of patients with ascending dissections. Correction of aortic regurgitation and replacement of the dissected aorta also limit morbidity. Ascending dissections in patients with Marfan disease

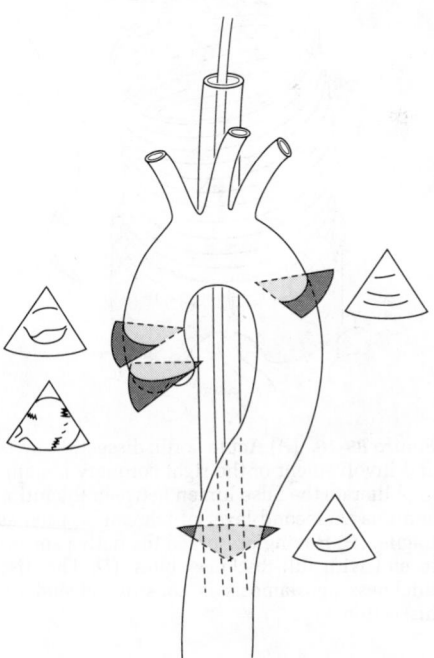

Figure 89-9. Transesophageal two-dimensional echocardiography with color-flow mapping accurately detects an intimal flap in the ascending, transverse, and descending aorta. (After Erbel RB, et al. Detection of aortic dissection by transesophageal echocardiography. Br Heart J 1987;58:45)

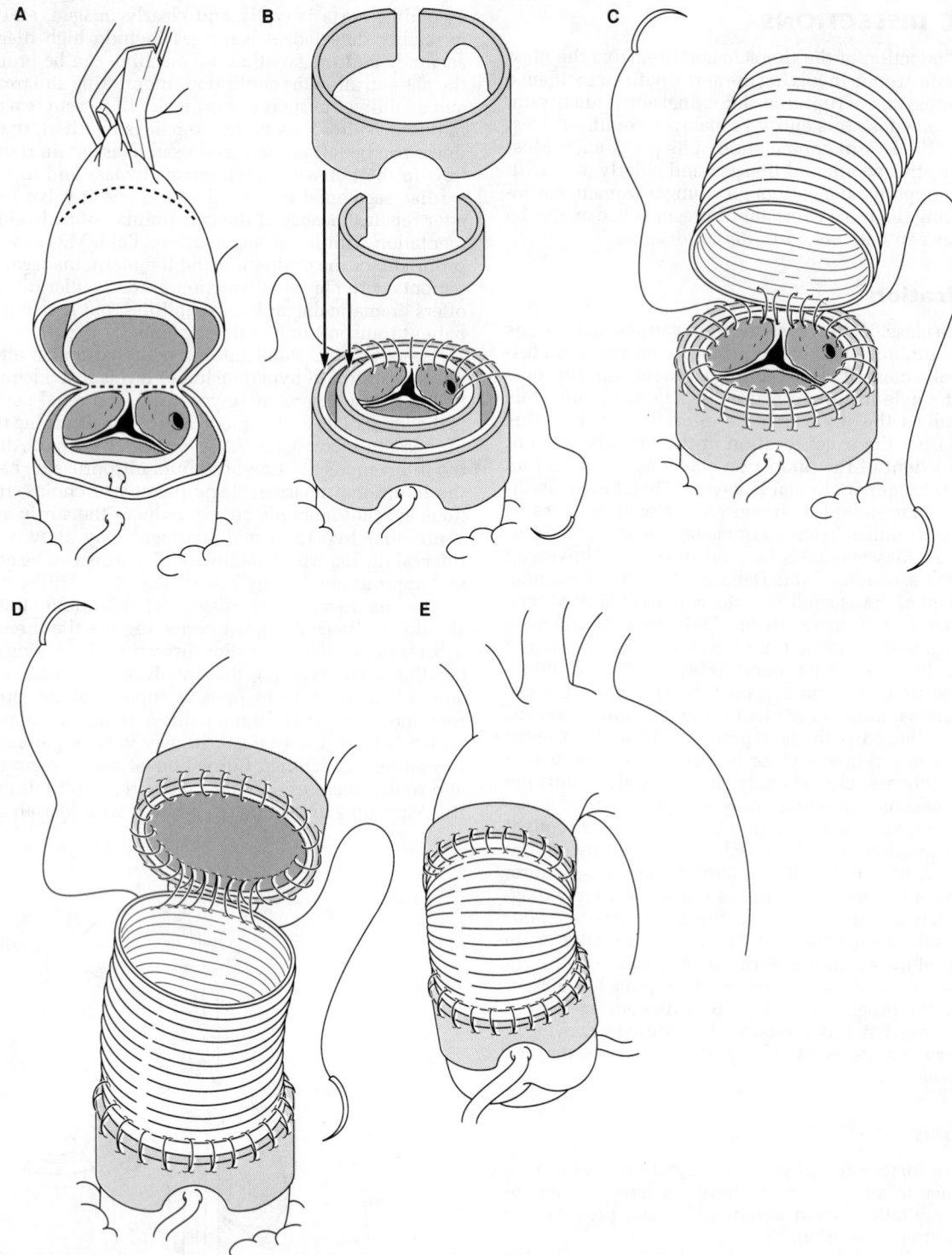

Figure 89-10. (*A*) Acute aortic dissection involving the ascending aorta. The false lumen, septum, and involvement of the right coronary are apparent. (*B*) A strip of Teflon felt is carefully tailored to obliterate the false lumen between the intima and adventitia, extending proximally to the aortic annulus. A second layer of felt can be used as an adventitial support if the vessel is particularly fragile. (*C*) Having preserved the native aortic valve, the proximal anastomosis is constructed end to end with full-thickness bites. (*D*) The distal false lumen is similarly obliterated, and a full-thickness anastamosis is constructed end to end. (*E*) Completed repair after ascending aortic dissection.

or annuloaortic ectasia are treated by aortic root replacement with a valved conduit, as previously described.

For patients with acute type B dissections, the optimal management is more controversial. An aggressive surgical approach for younger, good-risk patients is advocated in an effort to prevent proximal extension of the dissection, to resect the intimal tear, and to direct flow into the distal true lumen. Surgical therapy instituted only after failure of medical management, usually because of limb, renal, or mesenteric ischemia, is associated with excessive morbidity and mortality. An analysis of the combined Duke and Stanford data base revealed that about 22% of patients with acute descending dissections presented with a compelling indication for surgical repair. The presence of another major concomitant disease excluded an additional 37% from surgical consideration. Of the remaining 40% of patients for whom either surgical or medical therapy was a viable option, multivariate analysis failed to detect any treatment-related benefit for either early or late survival. Only advanced age was an independent predictor of poor outcome after a surgical repair, supporting a bias toward surgical repair in young, healthy patients.

Operative Management

The ascending aorta is approached through a median sternotomy, and cardiopulmonary bypass is achieved by bicaval atrial cannulation and femoral arterial cannulation into the true arterial lumen. Cardiopulmonary bypass with full heparinization is established, and the left ventricle is vented. The latter is especially important in cases with significant aortic regurgitation. Rapid cooling to 15°C is commenced, with atraumatic clamping of the mid–ascending aorta used if left ventricular distention occurs after the onset of fibrillation (Fig. 89-10). Myocardial protection is achieved with retrograde coronary sinus perfusion and a hypothermia blanket. After a core and tympanic membrane temperature of 15°C is attained, circulatory arrest is instituted, the crossclamp removed, and the distal aorta assessed regarding the extent of dissection and presence of arch tear to determine the site of distal anastomosis. This distal aorta is then fashioned so as to allow a full-thickness end-to-end anastomosis buttressed by Teflon felt strips. Usually, this requires only 20 to 25 minutes of circulatory arrest time, after which circulatory support and rewarming can commence. Retrograde cerebral perfusion is used to flush air and particulate debris from the brachiocephalic vessels and to provide some additional cerebral protection. The distal graft is then clamped just proximal to the anastomosis, and the arterial perfusion is repositioned into the distal graft to allow antegrade perfusion. The proximal anastomosis and any aortic valve repairs are then accomplished during this subsequent period of systemic rewarming. Absolute surgical hemostasis is mandatory to avoid a cascading coagulopathy or the late development of false aneurysms.

Surgical repair of descending dissections is accomplished through a left posterolateral thoracotomy with an interposition graft of woven Dacron. Access for cardiopulmonary bypass is established through cannulation of the femoral artery and the left atrial appendage, and proximal control of the aorta is obtained just distal to the left carotid artery. Only a short segment of aorta, the most severely affected, is resected, unless a known single intimal tear exists more distally. After reestablishing intimal and adventitial continuity with an interposed medial layer of Teflon felt, the interposition graft is sewn carefully to full-thickness cuffs, and the patient is immediately weaned from cardiopulmonary bypass.

Patients with tears of the transverse arch represent a small (5%) but perplexing proportion of acute dissections. Medical management alone is associated with substantial mortality. Concomitant surgical repair with either an ascending or descending dissection can double the operative mortality. Nevertheless, given the adverse impact of the unresected arch tear on both short- and long-term survival, arch replacement under profound hypothermic circulatory rest may be justified in young, otherwise healthy patients who would sustain the greatest long-term benefit (Fig. 89-11).

RESULTS OF SURGICAL THERAPY

In spite of continued improvements in surgical technique, operative mortality remains high for this complex problem.[7] In the most recent Stanford analysis (Fig. 89-12), operative risk was 7%±5% for type A dissections, with preoperative renal failure, tamponade, and renal or visceral ischemia heralding a poor outcome. For patients with acute type B dissection, older age, aortic rupture, and renal or visceral ischemia were independent predictors of perioperative death.

The 5-year actuarial survival rate for discharged patients was relatively good—78%±6% for type A dissections. For type B dissections, the actuarial 5-year survival rate for discharged patients was 80%±12%, and, significantly, the survival rate at 10 years was no different from that of an age- and sex-matched population.

Given the frequent complications from aneurysmal disease elsewhere in the thoracic and abdominal aorta, long-term follow-up and aggressive medical therapy are critical for patients after acute dissections. Operative procedures remain palliative at best, designed only to curtail lethal complications. Serial CT or MRI scans should be performed on a regular basis indefinitely to detect progressive aneurysmal dilatation and to allow timely elective repair. In a 20-year follow-up, aortic rupture accounted for nearly one third of late deaths, a situation that clearly can be improved. Progressive dilation of the false lumen of chronic aortic dissections (Fig. 89-13) should be managed like other aneurysmal diseases of the thoracic aorta.

Penetrating atherosclerotic ulcers of the thoracic aorta have a clinical presentation that can closely mimic acute aortic dissection or rupturing aneurysm of the thoracic aorta.[8] Evaluation of these patients may demonstrate only a localized area of subintimal hemorrhage along the thoracic aorta, with an enhancing subadventitial layer on MRI. Although the long-term sequelae of this entity remain unknown, we have been impressed with the rapid progression to aneurysmal dilatation in the short term, prompting the recommendation of careful aggressive follow-up and surgical repair for any patient with continued pain or evidence of enlargement.

MISCELLANEOUS CONDITIONS

Trauma is perhaps the most common cause of nondegenerative disease affecting the thoracic aorta. Whether the apparent increase in incidence of thoracic aortic injuries represents a real increase in injuries secondary to high-speed vehicular trauma or an increase in diagnoses incidental to the increased use of CT scanning in blunt trauma is unknown. Regardless, during sudden deceleration, the untethered aortic arch and descending aorta can flex anteriorly, stretching the aorta against the ligamentum, with a resultant partial or complete circumferential intimal disruption. For the 10% to 20% of patients who survive this acute event, the rupture is partially contained by the aortic adventitia and pleura, but the risk of subsequent hemorrhage is ongoing; thus, early diagnosis is essential.

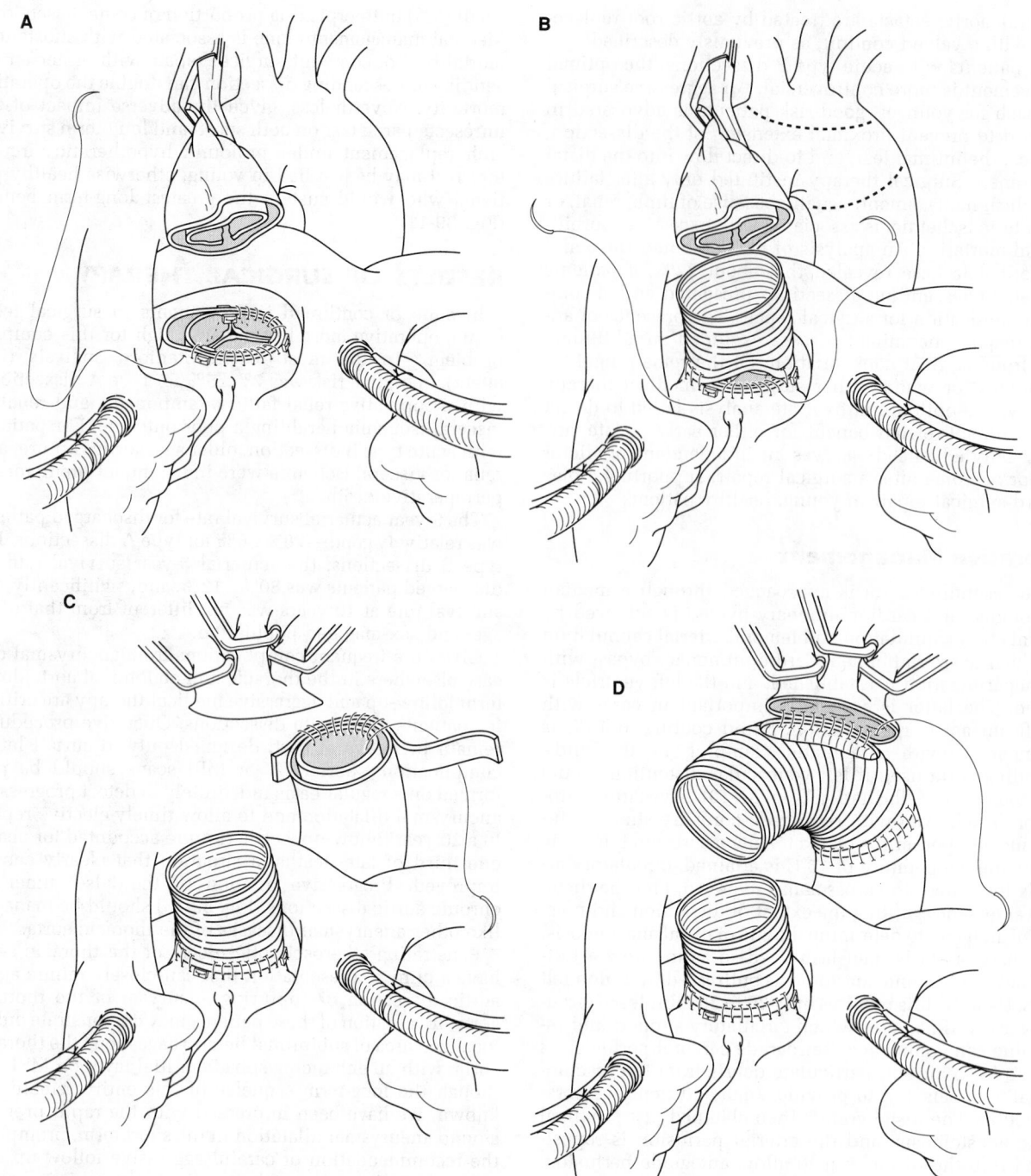

Figure 89-11. (*A*) Repair of dissection of the ascending and transverse arch of the aorta. Administration of cardioplegia and repair of ascending dissection, with aortic resuspension, is completed with the crossclamp in place. (*B*) Ascending graft is sutured in place while core cooling continues. (*C*) During a period of profound hypothermic circulatory arrest (18°C), distal aortic repair is accomplished, and a button of aorta containing the origin of the cerebral vessels is fashioned. (*D*) Distal graft anastomosis and aortic button are completed. (*E*) Crossclamp is placed proximally, rewarming is instituted, and proximal and distal grafts are joined. (*F*) Completed repair before decannulation. (After Griepp RB, et al. Prosthetic replacement of the aortic arch. J Thorac Cardiovasc Surg 1975;70:1051)

(*continues*)

The diagnosis should be suspected in any patient with a history of sudden deceleration, with a severe chest injury, or with other evidence of thoracic trauma, such as multiple posterior rib fractures, thoracic spine fractures, or fracture of the scapula. Remarkably, aortic transection can exist in patients with known sudden deceleration who have no other signs of chest trauma. Given the rapidly lethal nature of the undiagnosed injury, suggestive clinical or radiographic findings should prompt further investigation. The subsequent diagnostic test remains problematic. Many imaging techniques, including biplane aortography or cineangiography, dynamic contrast-enhanced CT scan-

E   F

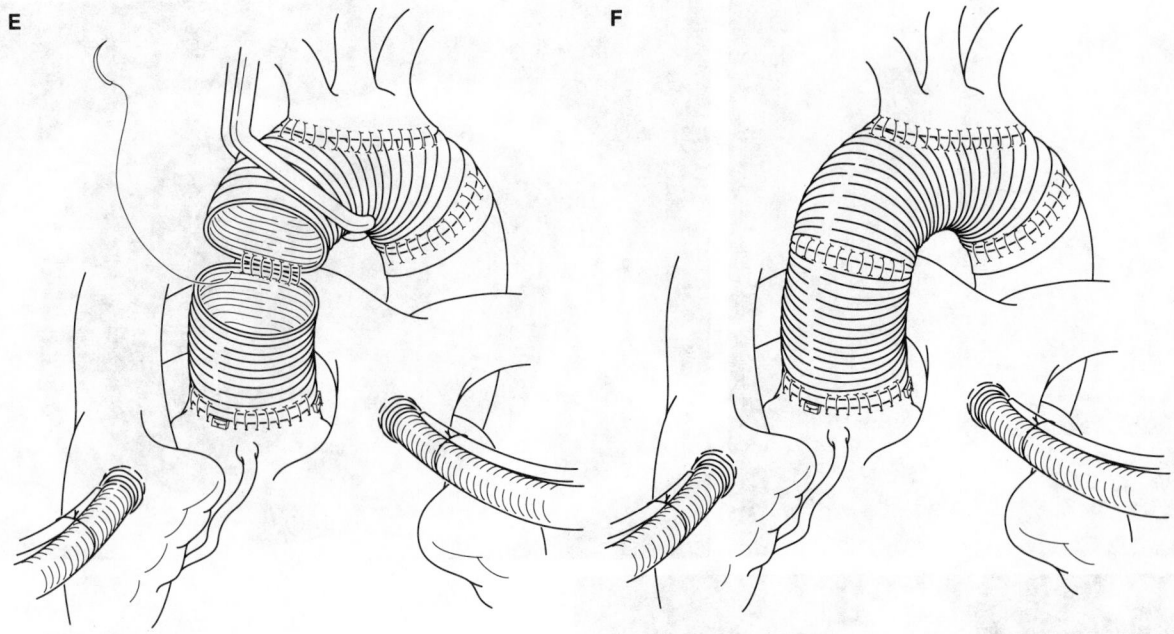

Figure 89-11. *(Continued)*

ning, MRI, and intravascular ultrasound, have demonstrated adequate sensitivity in experienced hands. These techniques, however, all require transfer from the emergency department, with loss of monitoring capabilities and the ongoing potential for hemodynamic instability or catastrophic hemorrhage. Omniplane transesophageal echocardiography may allow adequate visualization of the distal transverse arch. This technique is advantageous because the equipment is transportable to the emergency department and because rapid data acquisition is possible.

After initial evaluation and stabilization, the first prior-

ity is recognition and management of all life-threatening injuries, including intracranial or intraabdominal trauma. In the patient with multiple trauma, mature judgment regarding priorities for diagnostic studies and the sequence of therapeutic interventions is required. If the patient is stable and if the initial evaluation indicates the necessity for abdominal or cranial CT scan, the patient should be expediently transported to the radiography suite, where a rapid-sequence, contrast-enhanced CT scan of the thorax, abdomen, or brain can be performed. If no other injuries are suspected, efforts focus on the aortic injury, and the

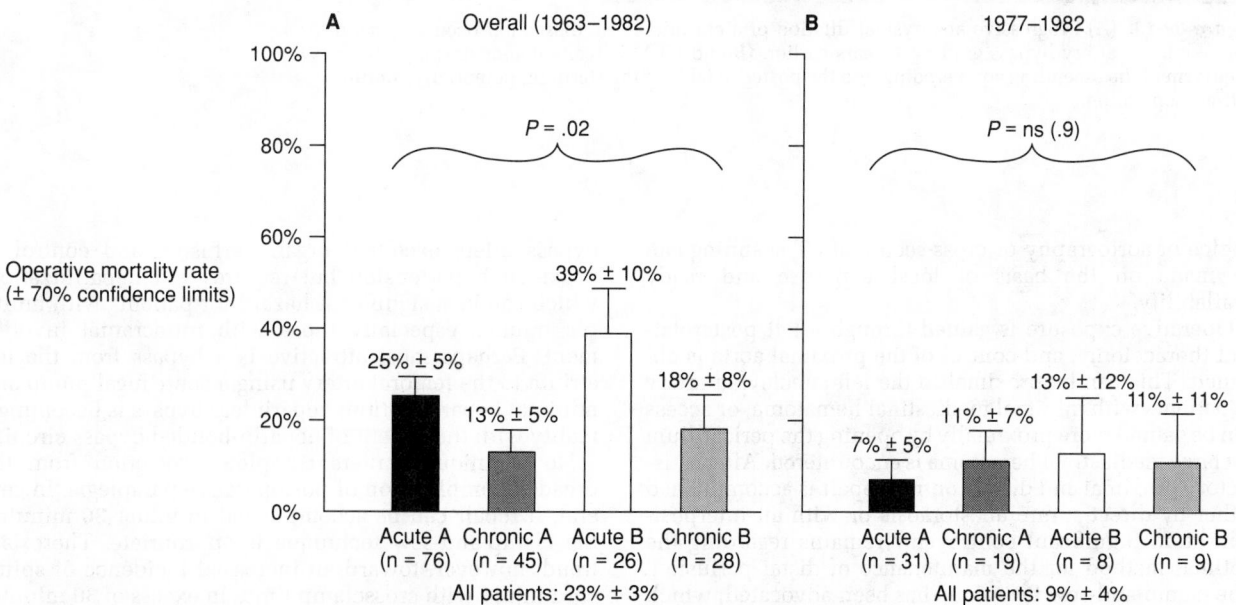

Figure 89-12. *(A)* Operative mortality rates for aortic dissections from the time frame 1963 to 1982. *(B)* The operative mortality rate was reduced by almost 50% in the more recent interval 1977 to 1982. (After Frist WH, Miller DC. Ascending aortic aneurysms and dissections. J Cardiac Surg 1986;1:50)

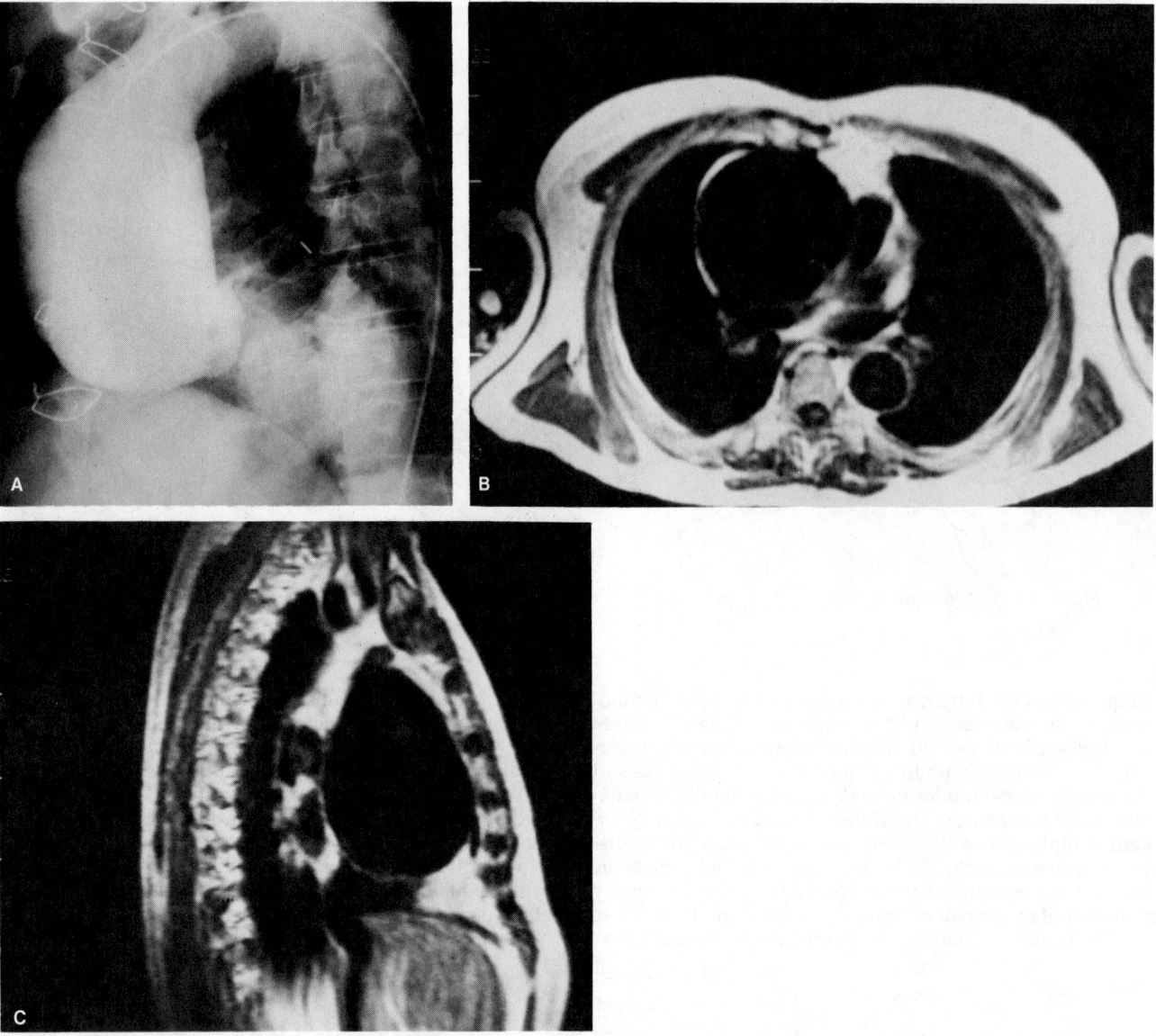

Figure 89-13. (*A*) Progressive aneurysmal dilation of a chronic aortic dissection occurring soon after coronary artery bypass grafting 7 years earlier. (*B* and *C*) MRI scans demonstrating a huge aneurysm of the ascending aorta eroding into the posterior table of the sternum, potentially complicating reoperation.

choice of aortography or cross-sectional CT scanning can be made on the basis of local expertise and ready availability.

Operative exposure is gained through a left posterolateral thoracotomy, and control of the proximal aorta is obtained. This can be proximal to the left subclavian artery in patients with minimal mediastinal hematoma, or access can be gained more proximally by opening the pericardium if a large mediastinal hematoma is encountered. After satisfactory proximal and distal control, repair is accomplished either by direct-suture anastomosis or with an interposition graft. Significant controversy remains regarding the optimal method for the maintenance of distal perfusion. The clamp-and-sew technique has been advocated, which avoids the complications of heparin and complex bypass procedures. Others have recommended a heparin-bonded shunt, which avoids systemic heparinization but results in inconstant shunt flows. Femorofemoral cardiopulmonary

bypass offers excellent organ perfusion and control of proximal hypertension but requires full heparinization, which can be a significant hazard for patients with multiple trauma, especially those with intracranial involvement. Perhaps most attractive is a bypass from the left atrium to the femoral artery using a centrifugal pump and minimal heparinization; heparinless bypass is becoming a reality with the advent of heparin-bonded bypass circuits.

No technique confers complete protection from the dreaded complication of postoperative paraplegia. In general, if repair can be accomplished in under 30 minutes, the clamp-and-sew technique is appropriate. There is a trend, however, toward an increased incidence of spinal cord injury with crossclamp times in excess of 30 minutes (Fig. 89-14). A 1988 review of a 15-year experience emphasized the priority of repair and observed that increasing age was the only significant adverse factor for postoperative survival. Typically, if the patient reaches the operating

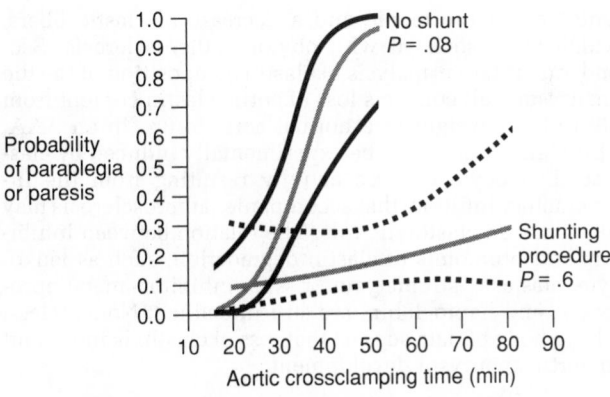

Figure 89-14. The probability of spinal cord dysfunction appeared directly related to aortic crossclamp time. (After Katz NM, Blackstone EH, Kirklin JW, et al. Incremental risk factors for spinal cord injury following operation for acute traumatic aortic transection. J Thorac Cardiovasc Surg 1981;81:669)

room in stable condition, a successful procedure can be performed in most cases. Thirty to 50% of patients who reach the hospital alive, however, die before definitive therapy, which emphasizes the need for a rapid and complete evaluation.

Mycotic aneurysms, although unusual, can result from endocarditis, bacteremic seeding of existing aneurysms, contiguous pleural and mediastinal infections, or contaminated intravenous injections. In general, the essential nature of the brachiocephalic and visceral vessels precludes resection and extraanatomic bypass. Intensive preoperative antibiotic therapy, combined with extensive surgical débridement, in situ grafting, and long-term antibiotics, especially for distal thoracic aneurysms and thoracoabdominal aneurysms infected with *Salmonella* organisms, may allow long-term survival. For infections arising in the ascending aorta, or for ascending grafts contaminated by mediastinitis, débridement, graft replacement, and a vascularized omental wrap may confer more protection than transposed muscle flaps alone.[9] Early diagnosis, isolation of the infective organism, institution of appropriate antibiotic therapy, and débridement and repair of the infection before aneurysm rupture are essential for any realistic hope for success.

Aneurysms of the ductus diverticulum have been reported in a small number of patients, usually presenting as an asymptomatic mass in the aortopulmonary window on an incidental chest radiograph. Hoarseness has been a presenting complaint in a significant number of patients, secondary to stretching of the recurrent laryngeal nerve. Erosion into the esophagus or bronchus can provoke life-threatening hemorrhage.

Contrast-enhanced CT scanning or MRI confirms the diagnosis in most patients and allows planning of the operative approach. Aortography adds little additional information, especially if the aneurysm lumen is thrombosed. Because of the relatively narrow aneurysm neck, repair frequently can be accomplished by Dacron patch closure on cardiopulmonary bypass. Although repair can be accomplished through a median sternotomy, superior exposure can be attained through a left lateral thoracotomy if there is no necessity for a concomitant cardiac procedure. Generalized atherosclerosis and obstructive pulmonary disease may limit long-term survival in these patients.

REFERENCES

1. DeBakey ME, Cooley DA. Successful resection of aneurysm of thoracic aorta and replacement by graft. JAMA 1953;152:673.
2. Szilagyi DE, Smith RF, DeRusso FJ, et al. Contribution of ab-dominal aortic aneurysmectomy to prolongation of life. Ann Surg 1966;164:678.
3. Pressler V, McNamara JJ. Thoracic aortic aneurysm. J Thorac Cardiovasc Surg 1980;79:489.
4. Cartier R, Orszulak TA, Pairolero PC, et al. Circulatory support during crossclamping of the descending thoracic aorta. J Thorac Cardiovasc Surg 1990;99:1038.
5. Moreno-Cabral CE, Miller DC, Mitchell RS, et al. Degenerative and atherosclerotic aneurysms of the thoracic aorta. J Thorac Cardiovasc Surg 1984;88:1020.
6. Murdoch JL, Walker BA, Halpern BL, et al. Life expectancy and causes of death in the Marfan syndrome. N Engl J Med 1972;286:804.
7. Miller DC, Mitchell RS, Oyer PE, et al. Independent determinants of operative mortality for patients with aortic dissection. Circulation 1984;70(Suppl I):153.
8. Cooke JP, Kazmier FJ, Orszulak TA. The penetrating aortic ulcer: pathologic manifestations, diagnosis, and management. Mayo Clin Proc 1988;63:718.
9. Coselli JS, Crawford ES, Williams TW, et al. Treatment of postoperative infection of ascending aorta and transverse arch, including use of viable omentum and muscle flaps. Ann Thorac Surg 1990;50:868.

SURGERY: SCIENTIFIC PRINCIPLES AND PRACTICE, Second Edition, edited by Lazar J. Greenfield, Michael W. Mulholland, Keith T. Oldham, Gerald B. Zelenock, and Keith D. Lillemoe. Lippincott–Raven Publishers, Philadelphia, © 1997.

CHAPTER 90

THORACOABDOMINAL AORTIC ANEURYSMS

DANIEL J. REDDY, CALVIN B. ERNST, AND ALEXANDER D. SHEPARD

Thoracoabdominal aortic aneurysms (TAAAs) are unusual but not rare. In frequency, they rank behind infrarenal aortic aneurysms, popliteal aneurysms, and femoral artery aneurysms. Like all aneurysms, TAAAs are a threat to life and limb since they may rupture, erode into adjacent structures, and initiate peripheral embolism. Because of the extent of aortic involvement, successful TAAA repair is complex and requires substantial technical expertise and a coordinated team effort. Consequently, this procedure is usually performed in major medical centers that can provide the necessary support. Advances in anesthetic management and perioperative care coupled with recent operative technical innovations allow TAAA repairs to be accomplished with an acceptable morbidity and mortality. This chapter addresses the natural history, pathophysiology, clinical manifestations, and management of nonspecific (atherosclerotic) TAAAs. Aneurysms of the ascending aorta and transverse arch, dissecting thoracic aneurysms, aneurysms limited to the descending thoracic aorta or abdominal aorta, and aneurysms associated with Marfan syndrome, infection, or trauma are discussed elsewhere.

MAGNITUDE OF THE PROBLEM

Reliable epidemiologic data on TAAAs are not available, largely because of the low prevalence of these lesions. Incidence is also difficult to determine because estimates are based on autopsy studies from urban areas and reflect a biased referral pattern. It is known that purely thoracic aortic aneurysms are uncommon. In a relatively stable patient population, 5.3 persons with new thoracic aneurysms per 100,000 person-years were identified.[1] A companion study of abdominal aortic aneurysms (AAAs) found an incidence of 21.8 aneurysms per 100,000 person-years and noted that the incidence of abdominal aortic aneurysms has been increasing because of increased longevity, improved diagnostic methods, or both.[2] Based on data from these two studies, it is logical to infer that the magnitude of the problem of TAAA is low.

NATURAL HISTORY

Just as the prevalence of TAAA can only be inferred from data regarding thoracic and abdominal aortic aneurysms, so too the natural history of TAAA is not precisely known. No prospective or randomized clinical trials of treated and untreated patients with TAAAs have been reported. Consequently, one must rely on retrospective reviews from large referral centers to determine their natural history. Retrospective analyses of abdominal, thoracic, and thoracoabdominal aneurysms combined may place the problem of TAAA in a proper perspective for the surgeon, the patient, and the patient's family.

In a study published in the mid-1960s evaluating the contribution of abdominal aortic aneurysmectomy to the prolongation of life, there was only a 19.2% 5-year actuarial survival for unselected patients with AAAs.[3] The comparable 5-year survival rate for patients undergoing aneurysm repair was 52.9%. The poor outcome in untreated patients resulted mainly from aneurysm rupture. Among 72 untreated patients with thoracic aortic aneurysms collected over a 30-year period, aneurysm rupture occurred in 18 of 27 (67%) of those with descending thoracic aneurysms.[1] The overall rupture rate for all nondissecting thoracic aneurysms was 51%.

In the only large series of patients with TAAAs, the natural history of untreated TAAAs appeared to parallel that of thoracic and abdominal aortic aneurysms.[4] The investigators observed 94 untreated patients with TAAAs and compared their fates with those of 579 patients who underwent aneurysm repair. Of untreated patients, 64 (68%) died; of these, 41 (57%) died of aneurysm rupture. Only 18 (19%) untreated patients survived 5 years, whereas 341 (59%) of those undergoing TAAA repair survived 5 years.

These retrospective data suggest that untreated TAAAs eventually rupture and cause death. Therefore, if elective TAAA repair can be accomplished with reasonable operative mortality and morbidity, surgical therapy is warranted to prevent death from aneurysm rupture. Contemporary operative mortality rates for elective TAAA repair range from 8.5% to 15%.[5–7] This is a striking contrast to the high mortality rates for untreated TAAAs.

ETIOLOGY

Aside from the unusual dissecting thoracic aneurysm that evolves into the thoracoabdominal variety and the rare patient with Marfan syndrome, most TAAAs probably result from atherosclerotic degenerative disease. Because the role of atherosclerosis in aneurysm development has been questioned, such aneurysms are best designated nonspecific rather than atherosclerotic. Elastic degeneration also weakens the aorta, and since elastin is not resynthesized, such degeneration may prove to be the main factor in aneurysm genesis.

There are three commonly cited sources of evidence that aortic aneurysmal dilatation is associated with loss of elastin, a scleroprotein with a biologic half-life of 70 years.[8] First, histologic examinations of aneurysm walls find attenuation of the media and a decrease of elastic fibers, which are associated with obvious atherosclerosis. Second, quantitative analysis of elastin composition of the the aneurysm wall confirms loss of aortic elastin content from 36% of dry weight in a normal aorta to 8% in an AAA. Third, aneurysms may be experimentally induced by elastase. Leukocyte elastase activity resulting from the inflammatory infiltrate that accompanies atherosclerosis may play such an elastolytic role. The relation between inhibitors and promoters of elastin degradation, such as leukocyte elastase, stromelysin, tissue inhibitor metalloproteases, and haptoglobin, are still undefined. Nonetheless, a large body of data suggest that loss of elastin is important in aortic aneurysm development.

PATHOPHYSIOLOGY

Mural degeneration with fragmentation of elastin and subsequent dilation leads to fusiform TAAA development. For unknown reasons, saccular aneurysms may develop, especially in the thoracic aorta. This saccular configuration may provide a therapeutic advantage near the origins of the celiac, superior mesenteric, and renal arteries. If the spatial orientation of the origins of these vessels remains reasonably normal and close together, repair is facilitated because these vessel origins may be reconstructed as a continuous inclusion patch into the aortic prosthesis.

As the aneurysm inexorably expands, flow velocity at the wall is reduced and thrombus is deposited and eventually becomes organized and partially fills the aneurysmal sac. Occasionally, bits of thrombus may dislodge to become peripheral emboli. Emboli from TAAAs are particularly troublesome because, unlike emboli from AAAs, they may lodge in vital visceral vessels such as the superior mesenteric or renal arteries.

CLASSIFICATION

Because the extent of aortic involvement has a significant impact on methods of repair and results, a practical classification has been proposed that stratifies TAAAs into four different types[5] (Fig. 90-1). Each type occurs with a frequency of about 25%. Type I involves most of the descending thoracic aorta and upper abdominal aorta down to the celiac axis. In type II, which is the most extensive, most or all of the descending and abdominal aorta is aneurysmal from the left subclavian artery to the abdominal aortic bifurcation. Type III involves the distal half of the descending aorta and most of the abdominal aorta, including the celiac, superior mesenteric, and renal arteries. In type IV, only the abdominal aorta is aneurysmal, including the origins of all visceral vessels. Other investigators have proposed a classification of three types of TAAA that is less precise but reflects the extent of aortic involvement.[6] The importance of a uniform classification is to provide valid comparisons between diagnostic and treatment methods.

CLINICAL MANIFESTATIONS
Symptoms

Small TAAAs of less than 5 cm in diameter are usually asymptomatic. As they increase in size, most TAAAs become symptomatic before rupture occurs. Clinical manifestations include expansion, rupture, embolism, and thrombosis. Consequently, a wide variety of symptoms may develop, the most common of which is pain in the chest, back, abdomen, or flank.

Ideally, TAAAs should be identified before catastrophic complications develop. Unfortunately, diagnosing an

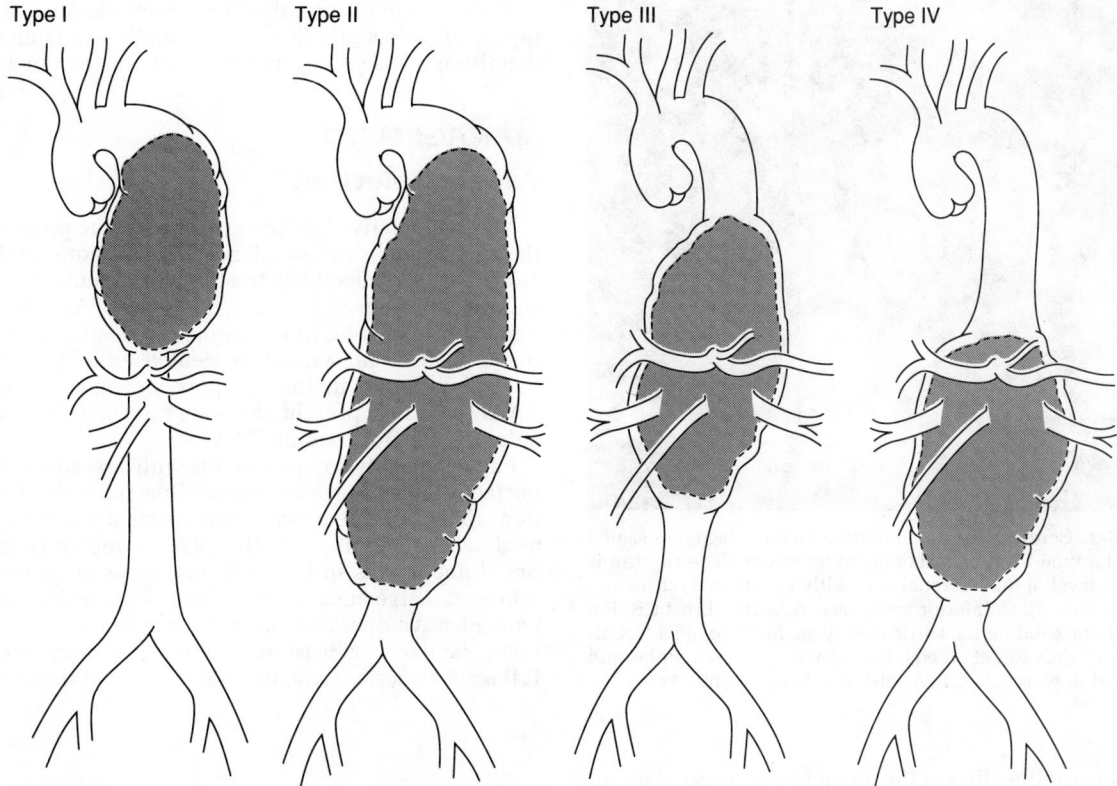

Figure 90-1. Four types of thoracoabdominal aortic aneurysms. (After Ernst CB, Reddy DJ. Thoracoabdominal aortic aneurysm. In: Haimovici H, Callow AD, DePalma RE, et al, eds. Vascular surgery: principles and practice, ed. 3. Norwalk, CT, Appleton & Lange, 1989:613)

asymptomatic TAAA is not as easy as diagnosing an asymptomatic AAA, which is frequently identified during palpation of the abdomen. Although a large abdominal component of the TAAA may be palpable, the cephalad extent of the aneurysm may be indistinct in the upper abdomen, particularly in obese patients or those with narrow costal margins. Occasionally, an asymptomatic TAAA is identified by chest radiograph, ultrasonography, or computed tomographic (CT) scans of the chest or abdomen during evaluation for other problems.

About three quarters of patients have symptoms when first encountered. Almost half present with frank rupture or severe back and chest pain secondary to a contained rupture. A similarly high symptomatic rate but a lesser rate of rupture (less than 5%) has been noted in other reports.[5] Patients with symptomatic TAAAs usually complain of back, chest, abdominal, or flank pain. The differential diagnosis includes several diseases that present as an acute abdomen, including a perforated viscus, acute cholecystitis, and colonic diverticulitis. Extraabdominal differential diagnoses include angina pectoris, acute myocardial infarction, esophagitis with cardiospasm, esophageal perforation, vertebral osteoarthritis, pulmonary embolus, pneumonia, aortic dissection, and urinary tract disease.

Additional symptoms result from compression of adjacent structures by the aneurysm or branch artery occlusion as a result of thrombosis or embolism. Renal insufficiency or accelerated hypertension may result from renal artery involvement. Spinal cord ischemia resulting in paraparesis or paraplegia is more commonly associated with thoracic aortic dissection, but it may result from nonspecific TAAAs as well. Distal embolism of aneurysmal contents may result in acute leg ischemia. Less common symptoms associated with TAAAs include airway or esophageal com-

pression and hoarseness from left recurrent laryngeal nerve compression. Erosion of TAAAs into the digestive or pulmonary tracts may produce dramatic hematemesis or hemoptysis with profound hypovolemic shock. Diffuse intravascular coagulation and a consumptive coagulopathy with thrombocytopenia may develop in association with large TAAAs.

Associated Diseases

Most patients with TAAAs are elderly (median age, 65 years), and they frequently have associated degenerative diseases such as hypertension, renal insufficiency, arteriosclerotic heart disease, heart failure, chronic obstructive pulmonary disease (COPD), cerebrovascular disease, or peripheral arterial occlusive disease. Risk factors that may be improved by intensive preoperative therapy include arteriosclerotic heart disease, COPD, and renal insufficiency, and such physiologic corrections favorably influence surgical results. The extent of associated vascular occlusive or aneurysmal disease influences the extent and type of TAAA repair and must also be delineated preoperatively.

DIAGNOSIS

Precise determination of the extent of thoracoabdominal aortic involvement, including type of aneurysm and extent of branch vessel involvement, is essential to successful management. It allows estimation of operative risk and precise planning of the optimal operative approach. Such information is readily obtained by noninvasive means such as contrast-enhanced CT scanning and magnetic resonance (MR) imaging. Ultrasonography is of limited or no value in managing TAAA disease because it fails to pro-

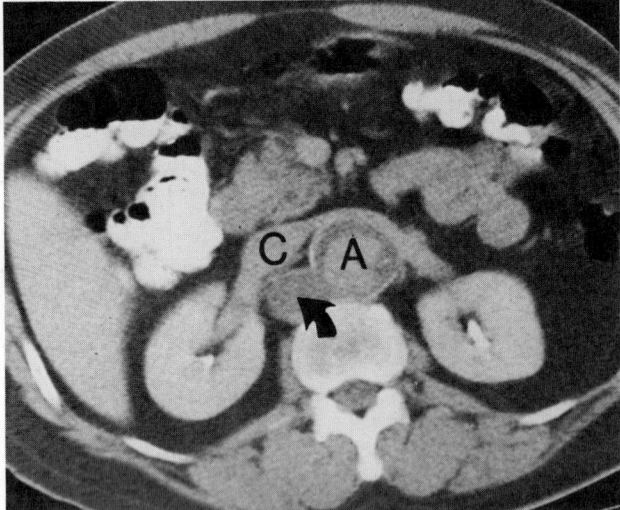

Figure 90-2. Contrast-enhanced transverse CT image of a sealed rupture of a type III thoracoabdominal aneurysm. The rupture is seen at the level of the left renal vein with a contained retroaortic hematoma (*arrow*). C, inferior vena cava: A, aorta. (Ernst CB, Reddy DJ. Thoracoabdominal aortic aneurysm. In: Haimovici H, Callow AD, DePalma RE, et al, eds. Vascular surgery: principles and practice, ed 3. Norwalk, CT, Appleton & Lange, 1989:614)

The future holds promise for magnetic resonance angiography but this study is still not widely available and the definition of its precise utility awaits further analysis.

MANAGEMENT

Patient Selection

No nonoperative therapy can prevent the progression of the aneurysmal process. Management options are limited, and other than effectively treating the patients' other medical problems, operative correction of the TAAA is the only treatment available. In the future, endovascular interventions, such as placement of stented endoluminal grafts, may play a role in the complex strategies required for TAAA repair. At present, there are no established endovascular options for treating TAAAs.

Physiologically sound patients with a reasonable life expectancy (at least 2 years) are candidates for elective operation. Extent of aneurysmal involvement must be considered when deciding whether TAAA repair is required. Small aneurysms in high-risk patients can be cautiously followed. Large aneurysms in low-risk patients require repair. Elective operation is recommended when the aneurysm diameter is at least twice that of the uninvolved aorta. If the entire aorta is aneurysmal (mega aorta), operation is

vide precise delineation of the thoracic and upper abdominal aorta.

CT imaging provides an excellent assessment of the proximal and distal extent of aneurysmal involvement, but it fails to yield detailed information regarding location, number, and patency of visceral and renal arteries. CT imaging may also be misleading and overestimate the aortic diameter, particularly when images include an obliquely positioned segment of aorta, an anatomic variant that is not uncommonly observed at the diaphragmatic hiatus. Contrast-enhanced CT imaging is especially helpful in diagnosing a contained rupture of a TAAA (Fig. 90-2).

Because of shortcomings of ultrasound and CT, aortography is routinely obtained before TAAA repair unless the aneurysm has clearly ruptured. Either conventional or digital subtraction techniques are appropriate. Because aortography may underestimate the size of the aneurysm because of laminated clot lining its walls, optimal diagnosis requires both CT imaging and aortography. These studies are complementary and provide the information necessary to plan aneurysm repair and aortic, intercostal, and visceral vessel reconstruction (Fig. 90-3).

Highly selective arteriography may help to identify crucial spinal cord circulation, which may require reconstruction to minimize the incidence of cord ischemia and subsequent paraplegia or paraparesis after TAAA repair. For practical reasons, not the least of which is contrast medium–induced transverse myelitis, preoperative arteriographic delineation of spinal cord circulation has not gained wide acceptance.

MR imaging holds promise for noninvasive diagnosis and classification of TAAAs. From transaxial images, the aneurysm diameter and length, the extent of luminal thrombus, and the amount of associated atherosclerotic occlusive disease can often be determined. Parasagittal MR images can document the proximal and distal limits of the aneurysm (Fig. 90-4). Unfortunately, MR imaging is not yet precise enough to reliably determine the size, number, location, and patency of arteries arising from the TAAA. CT scanning and aortography remain the mainstays for diagnosing and planning TAAA repair.

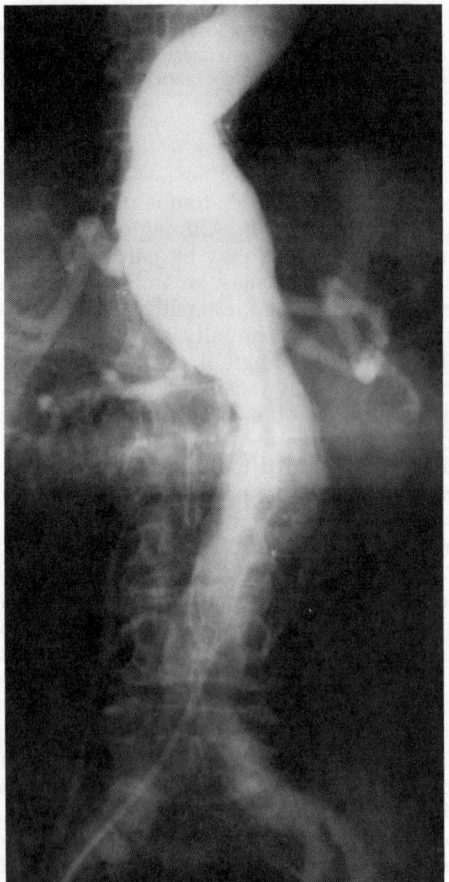

Figure 90-3. Aortogram documenting visceral branches from a type III thoracoabdominal aortic aneurysm. The aneurysm extends from the distal descending thoracic aorta into the abdominal aortic bifurcation. (Ernst CB, Reddy DJ. Thoracoabdominal aortic aneurysm. In: Haimovici H, Callow AD, DePalma RE, et al, eds. Vascular surgery: principles and practice, ed 3. Norwalk, CT, Appleton & Lange, 1989:616)

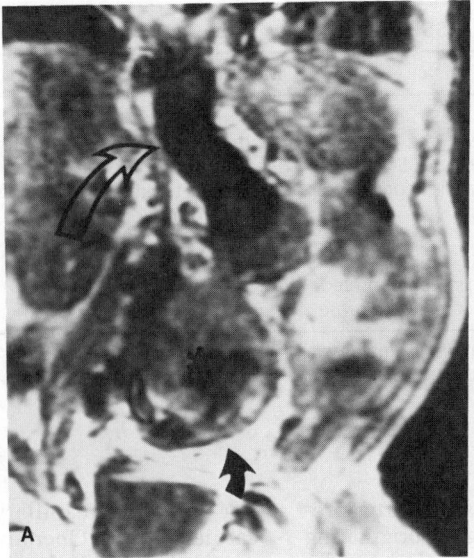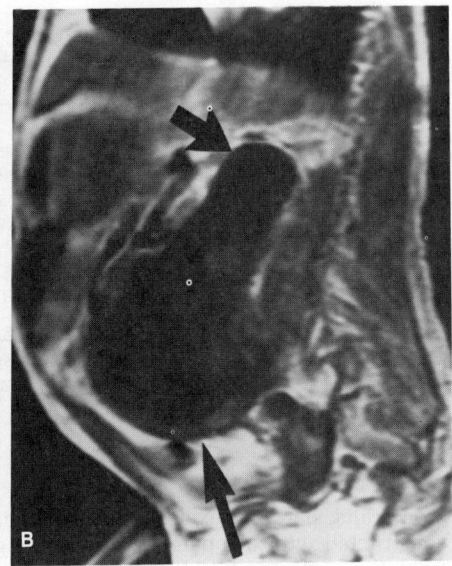

Figure 90-4. (*A*) Anteroposterior MR scan of a type IV thoracoabdominal aortic aneurysm documenting the proximal (*open arrow*) and distal (*closed arrow*) extents of the aneurysm with a large saccular infrarenal component (*asterisk*). (*B*) Parasagittal image documenting the proximal (*short arrow*) and distal (*long arrow*) extents of the aneurysm. (Ernst CB, Reddy DJ. Thoracoabdominal aortic aneurysm. In: Haimovici H, Callow AD, DePalma RE, et al, eds. Vascular surgery: principles and practice, ed 3. Norwalk, CT, Appleton & Lange, 1989:617)

advised when the aneurysm exceeds twice the expected size of the aorta.

Operative mortality and morbidity rates are related to the extent of aortic involvement and associated medical problems. Type II aneurysms are the most extensive and technically the most demanding to repair. This is reflected by increased mortality and morbidity, especially paraplegia or renal failure requiring chronic dialysis.

If life expectancy appears limited by associated diseases, operation is deferred until major aneurysmal complications mandate repair. Increased age (more than 80 years), severe COPD, chronic renal insufficiency, and extensive arteriosclerotic heart disease preclude TAAA repair. If hypertension, the most common associated disease, or pulmonary, hepatic, cardiac, renal, and cerebrovascular diseases can be successfully treated, they do not contraindicate operation.

Risk Factor Assessment

Operative outcome is directly influenced by associated risk factors. Objective assessment of the patient's cardiopulmonary reserve is important in deciding for or against operation. In an experience with 605 patients undergoing TAAA repairs, the most important risk factors influencing results were patient age, aortic clamp time, and presence of COPD.[5] The leading cause of death among the 54 patients who died within 30 days of operation was cardiac complications (44% of the deaths). Therefore, accurate assessment of cardiopulmonary reserve and appropriate selection of patients is the key to successful treatment.

A negative cardiac history and normal electrocardiogram (ECG) suggest minimal cardiac risk.[9] Most patients with TAAAs have a positive cardiac history or an abnormal ECG and therefore require further evaluation. Several objective tests are available to determine cardiac risk and reserve[10] (Table 90-1). Stress ECG testing is reliable and is the least expensive and easiest to perform. Unfortunately, many patients with TAAAs also have significant peripheral vascular occlusive disease that precludes effective exercise (ability to achieve 85% predicted heart rate). Consequently, other studies such as radionuclide ventriculography, radionuclide myocardial imaging, and coronary arteriography may be required to determine the extent of cardiac disease and functional reserve. Patients who demonstrate

redistribution with thallium-201 imaging or ejection fractions of less than 35% should be considered at high risk and may be candidates for coronary arteriography and possible coronary artery reconstruction before TAAA repair (see Table 90-1).

Preoperative pulmonary function studies have been advocated, but no reports have documented their role in assessing pulmonary risk in patients with TAAAs. An estimate of pulmonary risk can be determined by such studies (Table 90-2). In patients with CO_2 retention or a 1-second forced expiratory volume of less than 1 L, operation is not advised.[5] High-risk patients with COPD, asthma, or bronchitis benefit from preoperative pulmonary therapy consisting of cessation of smoking 1 month before operation, chest physiotherapy, and bronchodilator therapy.

Renal dysfunction and cerebral vascular occlusive disease also must be evaluated to estimate operative risk. Because the extent of renal arterial occlusive disease impacts significantly on outcome,[5] thorough assessment of renal circulation by detailed arteriography is mandatory. Such assessment alerts the surgeon to the need for concomitant renal arterial reconstruction during TAAA repair.

For patients in whom operation is not indicated or is refused, regular follow-up with periodic CT scans is appropriate. If symptoms develop or increasing size is documented, the need for TAAA repair should be reconsidered.

Surgery

During the past two decades, refinements in operative techniques have simplified TAAA repair. Operations require much attention to detail and coordination of a large and diverse group of professionals. Operations should not be attempted without necessary support, such as expert anesthesia, a responsive blood bank, and experienced nursing.

Several surgical techniques have been described for repairing TAAAs. Essential to successful outcome is removal of the aneurysm from the circulation and rapid, precise reconstruction of vital visceral vessels including the celiac, superior mesenteric, and renal arteries. In addition, special attention must be directed to restoring blood flow to large proximal lumbar or intercostal arteries that are essential to spinal cord viability.

Before the mid-1970s, TAAAs were bypassed with Da-

Table 90-1. PREOPERATIVE CARDIAC ASSESSMENT

	Low Risk	Minimal Risk	High Risk
Stress ECG	Normal ECG, >85% predicted maximal heart rate	Abnormal ECG, 75%–85% predicted maximal heart rate	Abnormal ECG, <75% predicted maximal heart rate
Radionuclide angiocardiography	Ejection fraction > 55%	Ejection fraction 36%–55%	Ejection fraction < 35%
Dipyridamole–thallium scan	No defect or redistribution	Fixed defect without redistribution (scar from prior infarction)	Thallium redistribution, especially with congestive heart failure, angina, prior infarction, or diabetes mellitus
Coronary angiography	No disease, mild compensated disease, or corrected disease	Advanced but compensated disease	Severe uncorrected or inoperable disease

(Stanley JC, Wakefield TW. Cardiopulmonary assessment for major vascular reconstructive procedures. In: Haimovici H, Callow AD, DePalma RE, et al, eds. Vascular surgery: principles and practice, ed 3. Norwalk, CT, Appleton & Lange, 1989:196)

cron grafts, partially excised, and each visceral artery reconstructed with a separate Dacron side graft originating from the aortic graft. The graft inclusion technique described in 1974 revolutionized TAAA repair.[11] With this method, blood flow to visceral and selected intercostal vessels is reestablished from inside the opened aneurysm by anastomosing the arterial ostia of these vessels to elliptical incisions in the Dacron aortic graft. Because of its simplicity and safety, this technique has been adopted by most major surgical centers.

Preoperative Preparation

The patient is admitted to the hospital the day before operation or earlier if pulmonary, renal, and cardiac problems require special attention. The evening before the operation, the patient should take a shower with antibacterial soap and the bowel should be purged. Optimal circulatory volume loading and testing of cardiodynamics can be performed in the intensive care unit. An appropriate prophylactic antibiotic is given the morning of operation along with the preanesthetic medications.

Operative Technique

The patient is placed supine on the operating table and arterial cannulas are placed in both radial arteries to monitor systemic blood pressure continuously and to provide access for blood sampling and measurement of arterial blood gases, hemograms, and coagulation parameters during the operation and early postoperative period. A pulmonary artery flow-directed balloon catheter is placed to monitor pulmonary capillary wedge pressures and to measure cardiac output. Operative imaging of left ventricular wall motion by two-dimensional transesophageal echocardiography provides information about ventricular function. This is particularly important when the descending aorta is clamped and unclamped. Large intravenous cannulas are also inserted into the patient's upper extremities for infusion of fluids, drugs, and blood products. A spinal drainage catheter is inserted at the L-1 to L-2 level for cerebrospinal fluid (CSF) drainage during aortic cross-clamping. Also mandatory is a responsive blood bank well stocked with blood and blood components, such as platelets and fresh frozen plasma, and a device for salvaging shed blood that permits processing and reinfusion of large volumes of blood or washed, packed red blood cells during operation.

After placing intraarterial and intravenous cannulas, a urinary catheter, and a nasogastric tube, the patient is anesthetized using a double-lumen endotracheal tube, which allows controlled collapse of the left lung during intrathoracic portions of the operation. Reinflation of the left lung without hyperinflation of the right lung is possible when intrathoracic exposure is no longer required. After intubation and anesthesia, the patient is positioned in a right lateral decubitus position with the left chest elevated about 75 degrees. This position may be modified slightly by rotating the hips posteriorly when the need for iliac or femoral arterial exposure is anticipated for distal anastomoses.

A posterolateral thoracoabdominal incision is used (Fig. 90-5). For low aneurysms, the ninth interspace is entered. For more proximal lesions, an incision is made through the sixth interspace. A posterolateral approach to the aorta with the left kidney, spleen, pancreas, and colon reflected to the right provides excellent exposure of the thoracoabdominal aorta. The left hemidiaphragm is divided radially or circumferentially down to the aortic hiatus, and the crus of the diaphragm is further divided with electrocautery and dissected from the aneurysm. Because extraperitoneal exposure limits ability to inspect the intraabdominal viscera, a retroperitoneal–transperitoneal approach is occasionally used so that the abdominal viscera may be inspected on completion of the operation. This approach also facilitates assessment of the celiac, superior mesenteric, and right renal arterial pulses after reconstruction. The retroperitoneal–transperitoneal approach is appropriate for all types of thoracoabdominal aneurysms, but a retroperitoneal approach is preferred for type III and IV aneurysms, since extension into the peritoneal cavity may also be required. Occasionally, heparin sodium, shunts, bypasses, circulatory arrest, hypothermia, renal cooling, or vessel perfusion techniques are employed. Precise rapid

Table 90-2. PREOPERATIVE PULMONARY ASSESSMENT

	Normal	High Risk
Vital capacity	30–50 mL/kg; >80% predicted	<30%–50%
Forced expiratory volume in 1 second	>80% predicted	<40%–50%
Maximal midexpiratory flow	150–200 L/min; >80% predicted	<35%–50%
Maximal voluntary ventilation	150–500 L/min; >80% predicted	<35%–50%
PaO_2, room air	85 ± 5 mmHg	<50–55 mmHg
$PaCO_2$, room air	40 ± 4 mmHg	>45–55 mmHg

(Stanley JC, Wakefield TW. Cardiopulmonary assessment for major vascular reconstructive procedures. In: Haimovici H, Callow AD, DePalma RE, et al, eds. Vascular surgery: principles and practice, ed 3. Norwalk, CT, Appleton & Lange, 1989:200)

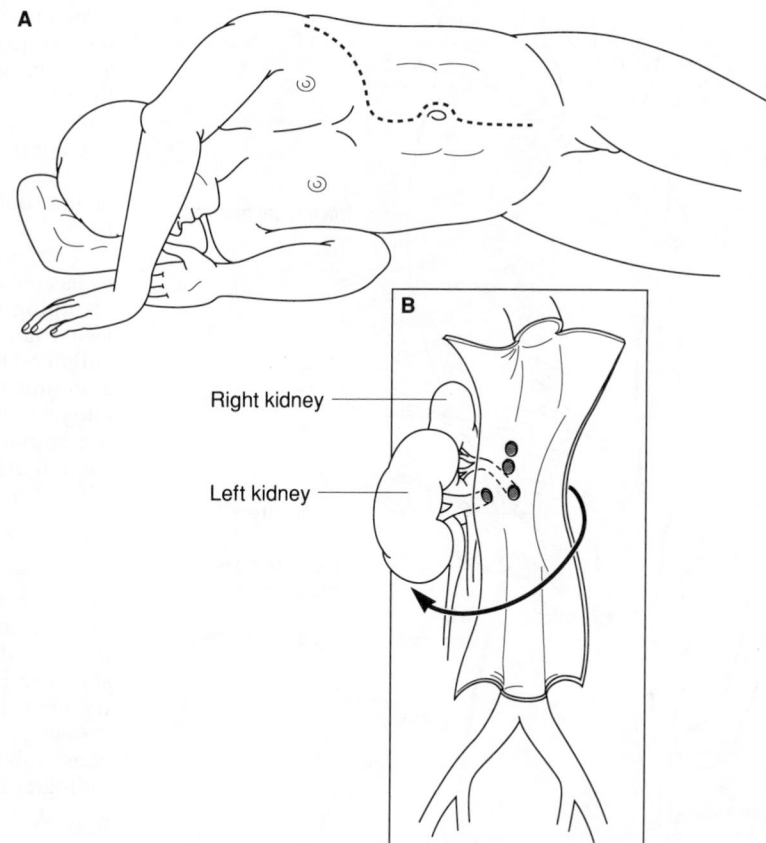

Figure 90-5. Incision and operative approach for a thoracoabdominal aortic aneurysm. (*A*) The patient lies in the right lateral semidecubitus position. The chest incision is made anywhere from the sixth the the ninth interspace, depending the on the type of aneurysm. The retroperitoneal structures and left kidney are mobilized to the right. (*B*) Open aneurysm with ostia of the visceral vessels seen. (After Ernst CB, Reddy DJ. Thoracoabdominal aortic aneurysm. In: Haimovici H, Callow AD, DePalma RE, et al, eds. Vascular surgery: principles and practice, ed 3. Norwalk, CT, Appleton & Lange, 1989:618)

suturing while clearing the field with the autotransfusion suction device has worked well and simplifies the operative procedure, reducing blood loss and transfusion requirements and minimizing postoperative bleeding.

To minimize proximal hypertension and left ventricular strain during aortic cross-clamping, nitroglycerin is infused intravenously just before application of the proximal aortic clamp. Careful coordination between the surgeon and anesthesiologist is required to titrate cardiac preload reduction and avoid left ventricular strain and iatrogenic hypotension once the occluding clamps are removed. About 30 minutes before proximal aortic clamping, the anesthesiologist measures the CSF pressure and drains it to maintain a CSF pressure of less than 10 mmHg. The pressure is monitored throughout the procedure and immediate postoperative period. Additional CSF is drained as necessary.

After the proximal aortic clamp is placed, the aorta is opened posterolaterally throughout the length of the aneurysm (Fig. 90-6). Laminated clot and intraaneurysmal debris are removed. After precisely identifying the ostia of the visceral vessels, balloon occlusion catheters are placed into these branches and gently inflated to control backbleeding from the celiac, superior mesenteric, and renal arteries. Occasionally, vigorous back-bleeding occurs from a few intercostal arteries and these are similarly occluded. Back-bleeding from the distal aorta is usually minimal but can be easily controlled by gentle external pressure by an assistant or by placing intraluminal balloons in the distal aorta or iliac arteries.

Ordinarily, the proximal aortic anastomosis is completed in an end-to-end fashion. Identifiable intercostal vessels are reimplanted by the inclusion technique to elliptic holes cut in the graft (see Fig. 90-6). The graft is then clamped distal to the reimplanted intercostal vessels and the aortic clamp slowly removed, restoring intercostal arterial blood flow in the hope of minimizing spinal cord ischemia. Additional elliptic holes are then cut in the prosthesis to accommodate the visceral vessels. Usually the celiac, superior mesenteric, and right renal arteries can be reimplanted as a single button containing all three ostia. Occasionally the left renal artery may also be included with the other three ostia in a single inclusion anastomosis. If the right and left renal arterial ostia are widely separated and diseased aortic wall would remain by including the two in the same patch, the left renal artery is reimplanted separately. Carefully select the site to avoid kinking this vessel when the viscera are returned to their normal anatomic positions. It may be necessary to reconstruct the left renal artery with a short 6-mm prosthetic side limb between the aortic graft and the end of the renal artery, which is readily accessible throughout its length.

After visceral vessel reconstruction, the proximal clamp is temporarily released to flush out debris. A second clamp is placed beneath the reconstructed visceral vessels, and the proximal occluding clamp is slowly released to test the integrity of the various anastomoses. The occlusion balloon catheters that have been inflated and left in place during the anastomosis and brought out through separate small openings in the suture line are then deflated and removed one by one, restoring blood flow to the visceral vessels. With restoration of blood flow to the gut as well as the kidneys, there is a transient decrease in the blood pressure. Flow to visceral vessels is confirmed visually by return of color and peristalsis, by palpating pulses, by using the Doppler ultrasound to check large vessel flow, and by listening over the parenchyma of the kidney and liver and at the antimesenteric border of the gut. Renal blood

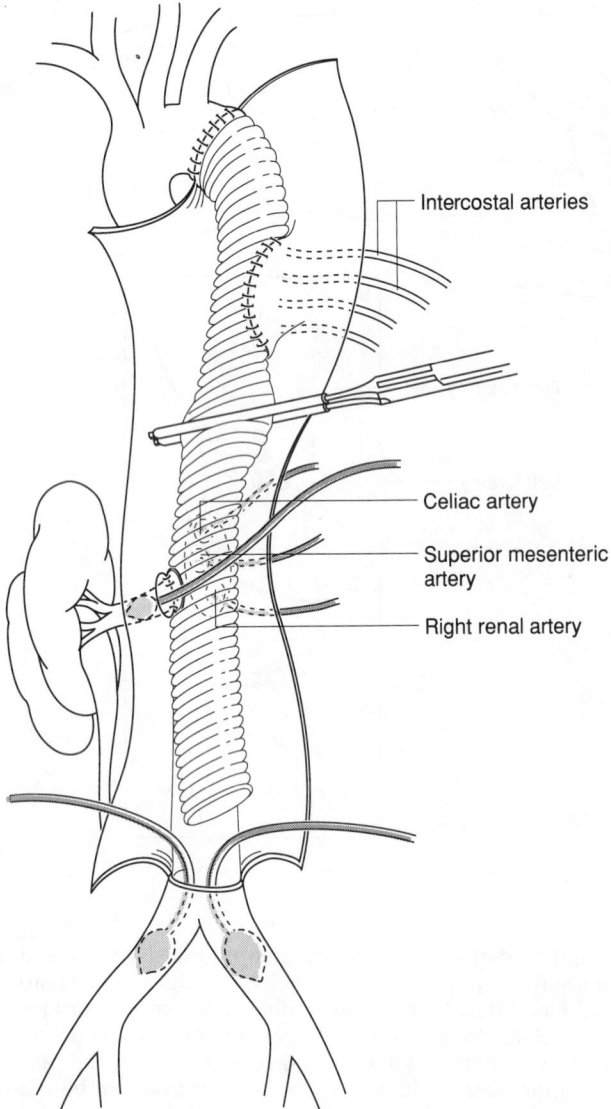

— Intercostal arteries

— Celiac artery

— Superior mesenteric artery

— Right renal artery

Figure 90-6. Various operative maneuvers used in the repair of thoracoabdominal aortic aneurysms. Intercostal arteries are implanted into the Dacron graft and reperfused before completion of the renal and gut anastomoses. The graft is clamped distal to the intercostal repairs, and the celiac, superior mesenteric, and right renal arteries are implanted as a single unit into the graft. The left renal artery reconstruction follows separately. The kidneys and gut are reperfused before the distal aortic anastomosis is begun. Balloon occlusion catheters minimize back bleeding during the anastomosis. (After Ernst CB, Reddy DJ. Thoracoabdominal aortic aneurysm. In: Haimovici H, Callow AD, DePalma RE, et al, eds. Vascular surgery: principles and practice, ed 3. Norwalk, CT, Appleton & Lange, 1989:619)

flow is more precisely evaluated by intravenously injecting 5 mg of indigotindisulfonate sodium (indigo carmine) and noting its appearance in the urine about 30 minutes later, during which time the distal anastomosis is constructed.

Depending on the extent of aneurysmal involvement, the distal anastomosis is constructed end-to-end to the aorta immediately proximal to the bifurcation (see Fig. 90-6). If disease extends into the iliac vessels, a separate bifurcated graft is anastomosed to the aortic Dacron graft and the distal anastomoses are made either to the common iliac or to the common femoral arteries.

Before restoring visceral blood flow, several units of

platelets and fresh frozen plasma are infused to counteract the coagulopathy that develops. After inspection of the anastomoses to ensure that all are intact and hemostatic, the diaphragm is closed with nonabsorbable sutures. The abdominal viscera are returned to their normal position, two chest tubes are placed in the left side of the chest, and the lung is slowly reinflated. The incisions are closed in layers. Before leaving the operating room, the lower extremities are examined carefully to be sure that the peripheral circulation is satisfactory. In recent years, some have suggested distal aortic perfusion during the period of aortic clamping in an effort to decrease the risk of paraplegia. Distal aortic perfusion is designed to provide protective collateral blood flow to the spinal cord during clamp occlusion and reconstruction of the aorta, its major branches, and available segmental intercostal arteries, which supply the spinal cord. Such distal aortic perfusion techniques use left atrial femoral bypass using an extracorporeal centrifugal pump.[12]

Postoperative Management

Postoperative management for these cases is more demanding and complicated than with many other operations because of the extent of TAAA repair. Careful attention is directed to maintaining optimal hemodynamic status and to monitoring renal function and lower extremity neurologic status. Reexpansion of the left lung and proper positioning of the pulmonary artery catheter and chest tubes are documented regularly by portable chest radiographs.

Results

Refinements in operative technique and anesthetic management have led to progressively improved results for TAAA repair. An experience with more than 1000 TAAA repairs over 25 years revealed a 9% operative mortality rate and survival rates of 60% and 32% at 5 and 10 years, respectively.[13] No other reports of comparable breadth or length of follow-up are available for comparison, but impressive results have also been reported by several other groups. The first included 101 patients and reported an overall 15% operative mortality rate with only a 10% operative mortality rate for patients undergoing elective TAAA repair.[6] The other large series included 50 patients undergoing TAAA repair. For 27 elective TAAA repairs, the operative mortality rate was 15%, but for the 23 emergency procedures, the operative mortality rate was 48%.

Major complications after TAAA repair include postoperative bleeding, respiratory insufficiency, renal failure, and spinal cord ischemia with paraparesis or paraplegia. Postoperative bleeding may result from the incision and dissected tissues, from the anastomoses, or from disordered coagulation. Although mechanical causes of bleeding may require reoperation in about 5% to 8% of patients, dilutional coagulopathy associated with massive blood replacement or platelet dysfunction is the most common cause of postoperative bleeding.[5,6] Liberal and prompt administration of clotting factors and platelets are necessary both during and after operation to avoid this complication and its 26% mortality rate.[5] Because coagulopathy is almost universal with TAAA repair, most authorities advise against heparin anticoagulation during aortic reconstruction.

Respiratory complications occur from left lung collapse or atelectasis and from right lung congestion due to its dependent position during operation. Pulmonary parenchymal injury may occur during dissection of adherent lung from large aneurysms. Preexisting COPD is a predictor of postoperative death in up to 14% of patients.[5] In one series, the most common postoperative complication was respiratory insufficiency, which developed among 33 of 101 patients, 10 of whom required tracheostomy. Such pulmonary complications emphasize that pulmonary function should be optimized before operation.

Mesenteric ischemia and lower extremity ischemia seldom occur after TAAA repair. Renal failure requiring dialysis develops in about 5% of patients.[5,6] Paraparesis or paraplegia resulting from spinal cord ischemia is a major and as yet unsolved postoperative problem. This devastating complication is unpredictable, unpreventable, and untreatable once established.[14] It is directly related to the extent and causes of aneurysmal disease. Frequencies of postoperative paraplegia for type I, II, III, and IV nondissecting TAAAs are 6%, 15%, 3%, and 2%, respectively.[14] Paraparesis frequencies were 6%, 12%, 2%, and 1%, respectively. Combined, paraparesis and paraplegia rates for the four types were 12%, 27%, 4.6%, and 3%. In addition to spinal cord ischemia, other factors influencing development of neurologic complications postoperatively include the patient's age (more than 65 years), duration of aortic clamp time (longer than 60 minutes), and postoperative hypotension.[5]

Several measures have been suggested to prevent or modify these neurologic complications, but none has proved effective. The combination of cerebral spinal fluid drainage and distal aortic perfusion holds promise, but both techniques need further study.[12] Despite the mortality and morbidity related to TAAA repair, elective aortic reconstruction is advised in good-risk patients with a reasonable life expectancy. Preventing premature death from aneurysmal rupture by operative repair can significantly lengthen life.

REFERENCES

1. Bickerstaff LK, Pairolero PC, Hollier LH, et al. Thoracic aortic aneurysms: a population-based study. Surgery 1982;92:1103.
2. Bickerstaff LK, Hollier LH, Van Peenen HJ, et al. Abdominal aortic aneurysms: the changing natural history. J Vasc Surg 1984;1:6.
3. Szilagyi DE, Smith RF, DeRusso FJ, et al. Contribution of abdominal aortic aneurysmectomy to prolongation of life. Ann Surg 1966;164:678.
4. Crawford ES, DeNatale RW. Thoracoabdominal aortic aneurysm: observations regarding the natural course of the disease. J Vasc Surg 1986;3:578.
5. Crawford ES, Crawford JL, Safi HJ, et al. Thoracoabdominal aortic aneurysms: preoperative and intraoperative factors determining immediate and long-term results of operations in 605 patients. J Vasc Surg 1986;3:389.
6. Hollier LH, Symmonds JB, Pairolero PC, et al. Thoracoabdominal aortic aneurysm repair. Arch Surg 1988;123:871.
7. Ernst CB, Reddy DJ. Thoracoabdominal aortic aneurysm. In: Haimovici H, Callow AD, DePalma RE, et al, eds. Vascular surgery: principles and practice, ed 3. Norwalk, CT, Appleton & Lange, 1989:612.
8. Powell JT. Dilatation through loss of elastin. In: Greenhalgh RM, Mannick JA, Powell JT, eds. The cause and management of aneurysms. Philadelphia, WB Saunders, 1990:89.
9. Golden MA, Whittemore AD, Donaldson MC, et al. Selective evaluation and management of coronary artery disease in patients undergoing repair of abdominal aortic aneurysms: a sixteen-year experience. Ann Surg 1990;212:415.
10. Stanley JC, Wakefield TW. Cardiopulmonary assessment for major vascular reconstructive procedures. In: Haimovici H, Callow AD, DePalma RE, et al, eds. Vascular surgery: principles and practice, ed 3. Norwalk, CT, Appleton & Lange, 1989:195.
11. Crawford ES. Thoracoabdominal and abdominal aortic aneurysms involving renal, superior mesenteric, and celiac arteries. Ann Surg 1974;179:763.
12. Safi HJ, Bartoli S, Hess KR, et al. Neurologic deficit in patients at high risk with thoracoabdominal aortic aneurysms: the role
of cerebral spinal fluid drainage and distal aortic perfusion. J Vasc Surg 1994;20:434.
13. Crawford ES. Thoraco-abdominal and proximal aortic replacement for extensive aortic aneurysmal disease. In: Greenhalgh RM, Mannick JA, Powell JT, eds. The cause and management of aneurysms. Philadelphia, WB Saunders, 1990:351.
14. Crawford ES, Svensson LG, Hess KR, et al. A prospective randomized study of cerebrospinal fluid drainage to prevent paraplegia after high risk surgery on the thoracoabdominal aorta. J Vasc Surg 1991;13:36.

SURGERY: SCIENTIFIC PRINCIPLES AND PRACTICE, Second Edition, edited by Lazar J. Greenfield, Michael W. Mulholland, Keith T. Oldham, Gerald B. Zelenock, and Keith D. Lillemoe. Lippincott–Raven Publishers, Philadelphia, © 1997.

CHAPTER 91
ABDOMINAL AORTIC ANEURYSMS
JERRY GOLDSTONE

Aneurysms of the abdominal aorta are common. Their incidence has been estimated at between 30 and 66 per 1000 persons and is increasing. This trend has been noted in the United States and other western countries and probably reflects the increasing age of the population and improved diagnostic methods.[1,2] The incidence varies with the population studied and is lowest in unselected groups and highest in patients with other atherosclerotic lesions. For example, aortic aneurysms are found in about 1.5% of routine autopsies and in 5% of patients over 50 years of age who are seen in a cardiology follow-up clinic.[3,4] In a community study, 2.8% of men aged 65 to 79 years who were screened by ultrasound had aortic aneurysms. In a similar study that included women, the incidence was 2.7%. In contrast, 5% of patients with coronary artery disease had aortic aneurysms, and in patients with atherosclerotic femoral or popliteal aneurysms, the incidence was as high as 53%.

Abdominal aortic aneurysms (AAAs) have a propensity for sudden rupture, leading to 15,000 deaths per year and making these aneurysms the 13th leading cause of death in the United States. Data from Great Britain indicate that 1 in 70 men between the ages of 60 and 84 years dies of ruptured AAAs. The only way to prevent these deaths is surgery, so it is important to establish the presence of aortic aneurysms before they rupture.

CLASSIFICATION

An aneurysm is a permanent localized dilation of an artery to 1.5 times or more its normal diameter. Some limit the term *aneurysm* to any dilation that equals or exceeds twice the normal diameter of the affected vessel. Either definition is acceptable. Ectasia implies dilation of an arterial segment to a diameter greater than 50% of normal, whereas arteriomegaly represents diffuse enlargement of an artery without specific aneurysm formation.[5] Arteriomegaly is rare and must be distinguished from diffuse aneurysmal disease, which is rarer still. Arteriomegaly often affects the external iliac, profunda femoris, and superficial femoral arteries, all of which are rarely the site of true aneurysms. In some patients with AAAs, the entire aortoiliofemoral arterial tree is arteriomegalic or ectatic. Thus, an aorta of any given diameter might be dilated, ectatic, or an aneurysm, depending on the size of the normal aorta above the dilated segment.

A classification of AAAs is shown in Figure 91-1. Degenerative aortic aneurysms are almost always fusiform in shape, and 95% arise below the origin of the renal arteries and are termed *infrarenal AAAs*. Aneurysms in which there is no normal segment of infrarenal aorta and the renal arteries are not involved are termed *juxtarenal* or *juxtarenal, infrarenal.* When aneurysmal involvement extends cephalad to involve the renal artery origin (but not the superior mesenteric artery), the aneurysms are known as *pararenal* and are a type of *suprarenal* aortic aneurysm. Thoracoabdominal aneurysms, which account for 2% to 2.5% of aortic aneurysms, involve a variable extent of the descending thoracic and abdominal aorta and usually involve at least some of the visceral vessels. The importance of this classification is the implications for surgical management. For example, infrarenal aneurysms require infrarenal aortic cross-clamping and infrarenal repair, whereas pararenal aneurysms require suprarenal (or supra–superior mesenteric artery) clamping for renal artery and infrarenal repair.

Aneurysms of the infrarenal aorta are by far the most common arterial aneurysms encountered in clinical practice. Men are affected more often than women by a ratio of 4:1. Other aneurysms frequently coexist, including common or internal iliac aneurysms (41% of patients) and fem-

oropopliteal aneurysms (about 15% of patients).[4] Conversely, popliteal aneurysms are markers of AAAs. Aortic aneurysms can be found in about 8% of patients who present with a unilateral popliteal aneurysm and in more than 33% of patients who have bilateral popliteal aneurysms.[6] In at least one group of patients with carotid atherosclerosis, there was a 10% incidence of AAA. In another group of patients with tortuous internal carotid arteries, a 40% incidence of aortic aneurysms was found.

PATHOGENESIS

True aneurysms of the abdominal aorta can be caused by cystic medial necrosis, dissection, Ehlers-Danlos syndrome, and syphilis. Most are associated with significant aortic atherosclerosis, which has traditionally been considered the cause. One observation casting doubt on atherosclerosis as the cause of aortic aneurysms is that patients with aneurysmal disease do not usually have aortoiliac occlusive disease. Only about 25% of aortic aneurysms are associated with significant occlusive disease. Biochemical studies have shown decreased quantities of both elastin and collagen in the wall of aneurysms. This has been correlated with the histopathologic features of a thin, dilated wall with replacement of the elastin in the media by a much thinner layer of collagen. This thinned-out aortic wall contains calcium as well as typical atherosclerotic lesions, rendering the wall weak and brittle. Laminated thrombus lines the lumen concentrically, resulting in a nearly normal flow channel but providing no structural strength. Elongation of aneurysms occurs as they enlarge, causing them to become bowed and tortuous. Mature elastin is a major structural constituent of the aortic wall in humans, and alterations of its metabolism within the aortic wall have been implicated in the pathogenesis of AAAs.[7] Weakening and fragmentation of the elastic lamellae (elastin) permits this lengthening. Thus, failure of elastin to provide sufficient retractive force in the circumferential and longitudinal directions allows for both the increased diameter and length, respectively, of aneurysms. Collagen is the other principal structural fiber responsible for the integrity of the aortic wall. It makes up about 25% of the wall of an atherosclerotic aorta, but only 6% to 18% of an aneurysmal aortic wall. Thinning of collagen and the fragmentation of other components (elastin) of the aortic wall contribute to weakening and a propensity to rupture.

Several investigators have discovered genetically linked enzyme deficiencies that are associated with aneurysms in experimental animals. Deficiency of a copper-containing enzyme, lysyl-oxidase, which is important in collagen cross-linking, has caused aortic aneurysms in a strain of mice.[8] This enzyme defect is sex chromosome–linked, and in human studies several large families have been found in which virtually every male member had an aortic aneurysm, supporting the concept of genetic susceptibility.[9] According to one report, there is a 19.2% chance that patients with AAA have a first-degree family member who also has one.

Other nonatherogenic mechanisms that disrupt collagen or elastin in the aortic wall have been proposed by other investigators. These mechanisms involve excessive protease activity (collagenase or elastase) or reductions in their naturally occurring inhibitors (antiprotease) in the aortic wall. Hemodynamic (mechanical) factors may also play a role in aneurysm development. The abdominal aorta is subjected to large pulsatile stresses because of its tapering geometry, increased stiffness, and the reflected pressure waves from the peripheral vessels. Reductions in the number of elastic lamellae and the virtual lack of vasa vasorum in the media of the distal abdominal aorta (compared with

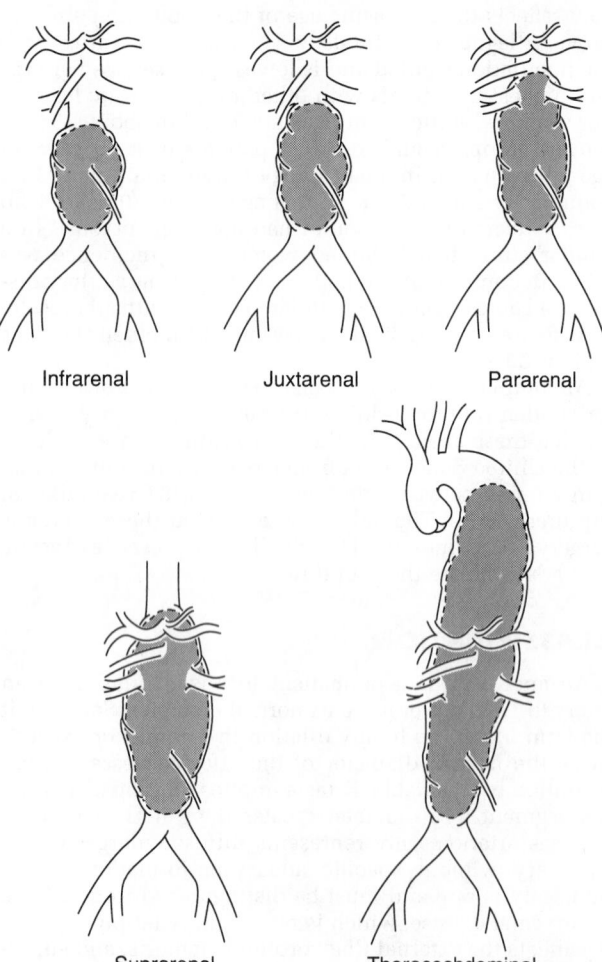

Infrarenal   Juxtarenal   Pararenal

Suprarenal   Thoracoabdominal

Figure 91-1. Classification of abdominal aortic aneurysms.

the thoracic aorta) may also favor aneurysmal formation in this segment of the arterial tree by making the aorta structurally less well adapted to handle the increased hemodynamic stresses that occur there.

Cigarette smoking correlates with the presence of aortic aneurysms, with an 8:1 preponderance of aneurysms in smokers compared with nonsmokers. Hypertension is found in up to 40% of patients with aortic aneurysms. The importance of these factors in the pathogenesis of aneurysms is not known. It is probably more accurate to consider the etiology of aortic aneurysms to be multifactorial and to refer to them as degenerative rather than atherosclerotic. They account for over of AAAs.

Once an aneurysm develops, its enlargement is governed by physical principles. For a given transmural pressure, the wall tension is proportional to the radius. Once dilation of the aorta has started, the law of LaPlace explains why aortic enlargement is enhanced, why large aneurysms are more prone to rupture than small ones, and why hypertension (increased transmural pressure) is an important risk factor for rupture. Tripling the aortic radius from 2 to 6 cm results in a 12-fold increase in wall tension. When this tension exceeds the tensile strength of the collagen in the aortic wall, disruption occurs.

CLINICAL MANIFESTATIONS

Seventy to 75% of all infrarenal AAAs are not symptomatic when diagnosed. They are most often discovered during a routine physical examination or during an imaging study performed for some other reason (eg, upper gastrointestinal series, barium enema, intravenous pyelogram, lumbosacral spine radiographs, or abdominal computed tomography [CT] or ultrasound examination). Occasionally, an aneurysm is detected during an unrelated abdominal operation, or by the patient, who notices a prominent abdominal pulsation.

When symptoms are associated with AAAs, they may be due to rupture or expansion, pressure on adjacent structures, distal embolism, thrombosis, or dissection. Abdominal or back pain is the most common symptom and can be elicited in up to one third of patients. Any type of abdominal, flank, or back pain can be caused by an aneurysm, a fact that often delays diagnosis. Large aneurysms can actually erode the spine and cause severe back pain in the absence of rupture. Compression of adjacent bowel can cause early satiety and even nausea and vomiting.

The abrupt onset of severe pain in the back, flank, or abdomen is characteristic of aneurysmal *rupture* or acute *expansion*. It is not clear why pain is produced by an expanding but unruptured aneurysm. The best explanation is sudden stretching of the layers of the aortic wall with pressure on adjacent somatic sensory nerves. In most surgical series, symptomatic but unruptured aneurysms account for 6% to nearly 40% of cases (the average of five series totaling 311 patients was 13.7%). Ruptured aneurysms constitute between 20% and 25% of most series.[10,11] The nature and duration of symptoms varies with the type of rupture. Small tears of the aneurysm wall may result in a small leak that seals temporarily with minimal blood loss. This is usually followed within a few hours by frank rupture, which usually produces a catastrophic medical emergency although chronic, contained ruptures have been reported. Rupture most frequently occurs in the posterolateral aortic wall into the retroperitoneal space and less commonly into the free peritoneal cavity. The incidence of this latter type of rupture is probably higher than indicated in most surgical series because most of these patients die before reaching the hospital. Rarely, the aneurysm ruptures into the inferior vena cava or one of the iliac veins, producing an aortocaval (or aortoiliac) fistula, or into the gastrointestinal tract producing a primary aortoenteric fistula.

The classic clinical manifestations of ruptured aortic aneurysm are severe, mild, or diffuse abdominal pain, shock, and a pulsatile abdominal mass. The pain may be more prominent in the back or flank or may radiate to the groin or thigh. The severity of the shock varies from mild to profound, depending on the amount and rapidity of blood loss, and may last for a few minutes or more than 24 hours. The pain of expanding but intact aneurysms may closely mimic that of ruptured ones. The pain tends to be severe, constant, and unaffected by position. Hypotension and shock do not usually occur in the absence of rupture.

The diverse and nonspecific nature of the pain caused by expanding and leaking aneurysms all too often leads to errors and delays in diagnosis. Catastrophic rupture in the midst of a diagnostic procedure is a well-known occurrence. Occasionally, a patient with a contained rupture arrives in the emergency room complaining of angina pectoris, a result of blood loss and reflex tachycardia, and is rapidly transferred to a coronary care unit without the abdominal examination that would identify the true cause of the chest pain. Most diagnostic errors are due to failure to palpate the expanding and pulsatile epigastric mass.

DIAGNOSTIC METHODS

Except in thin patients, an AAA must be about 5 cm in diameter to be detected on a routine physical examination. Physical examination alone establishes the correct diagnosis in 30% to 90% of patients, but even when the aneurysm is detected, determination of its size by palpation is imprecise. Obesity, ascites, and lack of patient cooperation impair aneurysmal detection by physical examination. On the other hand, tumors or cystic lesions adjacent to the aorta, unusual aortic tortuosity, and excessive lumbar lordosis can lead to an erroneous diagnosis of an aneurysm. The expansile nature of a pulsatile mass is the key element in deciding whether a palpable abdominal mass is an aneurysm.

Objective methods are necessary to measure size accurately and identify smaller aneurysms. Determination of size is especially important since size is the primary determinant of management decisions. The oldest objective method for accomplishing this purpose is the plain abdominal and lateral spine radiograph. Enough calcium is visible in the aortic wall to diagnose an aneurysm in 67% to 75% of cases, but accurate determination of maximal aortic size is possible in only about two thirds of these cases. Therefore, a negative or inadequate plain film cannot be relied on to exclude this diagnosis.

Imaging Modalities

Several imaging modalities are widely available for establishing the presence and accurately determining the size of an aortic aneurysm—ultrasound, CT, and magnetic resonance (MR) imaging.[12]

Real-time, B-mode ultrasound is available in most hospitals. It employs no ionizing radiation, provides structural detail of vessel walls and atherosclerotic plaques, and can accurately measure aneurysm size in both longitudinal and cross-sectional directions[13] (Figs. 91-2 and 91-3). When compared with intraoperative measurements, ultrasound is accurate to within 3 mm. Many studies have documented the ability of B-mode ultrasound to establish the diagnosis and to determine accurately the size of abdominal and peripheral aneurysms.[14] Ultrasonography has not been as useful for imaging the thoracic or suprarenal aorta

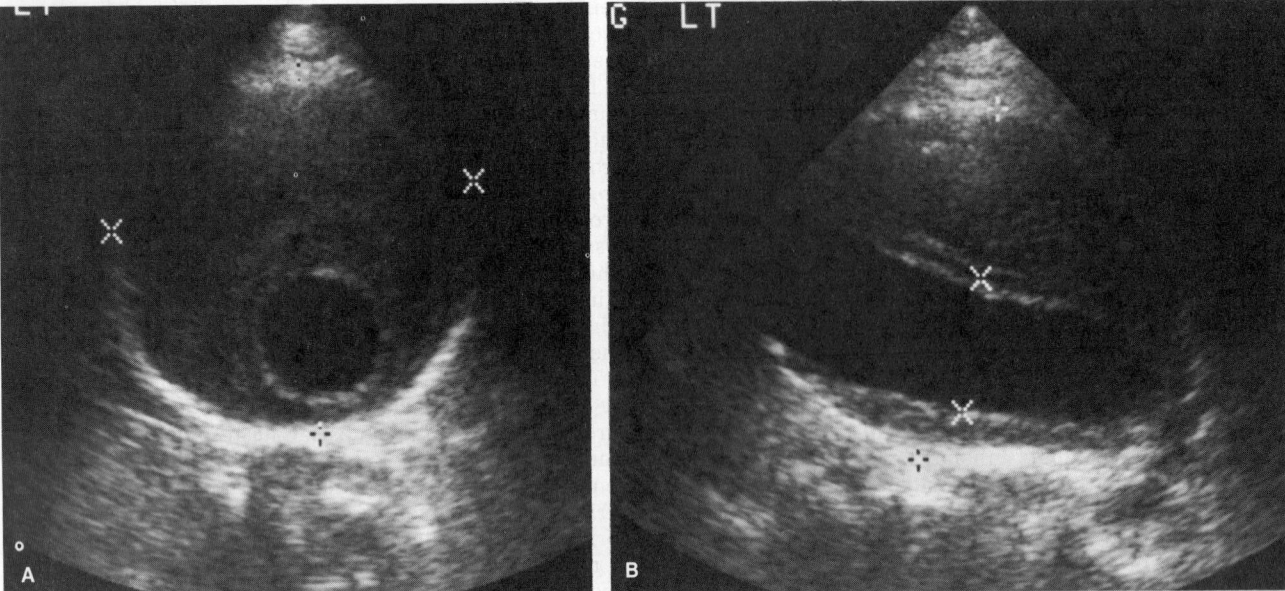

Figure 91-2. B-mode ultrasound scan showing large aortic aneurysm. (*A*) Transverse view, maximum diameter 83.3 mm (X to X). Note the dark, smaller lumen surrounded by mural thrombosis. (*B*) Longitudinal view showing flow channel (X to X).

because of the overlying air-containing structures. A transesophageal ultrasound transducer can largely avoid this problem but is not practical for routine evaluation of abdominal aortic disease. Because ultrasound can obtain images in longitudinal, transverse, and oblique projections, it is especially useful in differentiating a tortuous aorta from an aneurysm, but it is not reliable in defining the relation between AAAs and the renal arteries.

Ultrasound images are impaired by obesity, intestinal gas, or barium in the bowel. Overlying bowel gas also interferes with evaluation of the iliac arteries. Ultrasound studies can be performed quickly, and the portability of the machines is advantageous for the emergency room evaluation of suspected ruptured aneurysms. These factors make ultrasound the modality of choice for the initial evaluation of pulsatile abdominal or peripheral masses and for follow-up of aneurysms to determine increase in size.

CT scans use ionizing radiation to obtain cross-sectional images of the aorta and other body structures. Although computer programs can reconstruct sagittal, coronal, and oblique images from cross-sectional CT data, these are complex and generally not available. CT images provide reliable information about the size of the entire aorta, including the thoracic aorta, so the size and extent of an aneurysm can be accurately measured.[15] Modern CT scanners possess sufficient spatial resolution to allow identification of celiac, superior mesenteric, renal, and iliac arteries and their relation to the aneurysm and to adjacent organs. Major venous structures, including surgically important anomalies, can also be identified by CT. The administration of intravenous contrast allows CT to evaluate the size of the aortic lumen, the amount and location of mural thrombus, and, in the presence of dissection, differentiation of the true from the false lumen (Fig. 91-4). Contrast-enhanced CT scans are also useful for assessing the retroperitoneum and can identify retroperitoneal hematoma (aneurysmal rupture) and the periaortic fibrosis associated with inflammatory aneurysms. CT images are degraded by patient motion and the presence of metallic objects such as surgical clips. CT scanning requires more time and is more expensive than ultrasound and only provides images in one (transverse) plane, but it provides more information about other abdominal and retroperitoneal structures than ultrasound. One of the most helpful uses of CT scanning is to define the relation of an aneurysm to the renal artery origins. This definition is not always accurate, however, especially when there is forward buckling of the aorta so that the superior border of the aneurysm ascends anterior to the aorta. Overall, CT scans are the most useful imaging method for evaluating the abdominal aorta. Many physicians believe CT should be performed as part of the preoperative evaluation of all patients with aortic aneurysms.

MR imaging is the newest imaging modality available for evaluating aortic aneurysms.[14,16] It uses radiofrequency energy and a strong magnetic field to produce images in longitudinal, transverse, and coronal planes. Because the instruments are new and expensive, they are not as widely

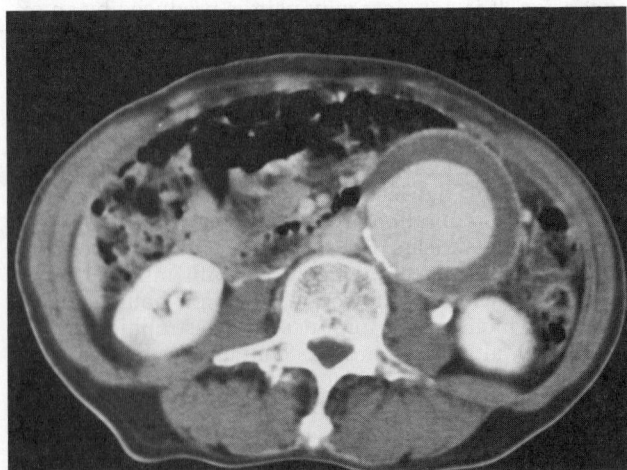

Figure 91-3. Abdominal CT scan showing large abdominal aortic aneurysm. 70 mm in diameter, with contrast-filled lumen surrounded by mural thrombus.

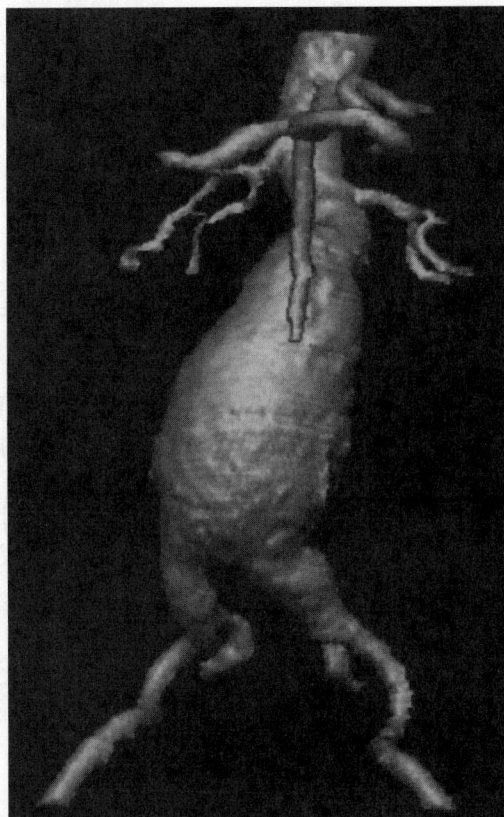

Figure 91-4. Ultrafast (spiral) CT scan of large infrarenal aortic aneurysm, with three-dimensional showing relation of renal and visceral vessels to aneurysm neck.

available as ultrasound or CT, and their interpretation requires considerable experience and skill. The spatial resolution is limited (about 0.8 mm), and the presence of metallic surgical clips, cardiac pacemakers, or monitoring equipment makes MR imaging impossible. Also, MR imaging is more expensive than either CT or ultrasound. Nevertheless, MR imaging clearly distinguishes arteries and veins from viscera and other surrounding tissue. MR images of aortic aneurysms have excellent agreement with ultrasonograms and CT images in determining aortic diameter, and MR images better show involvement of branch vessels. This is especially true for the renal arteries; some authors have reported visualization of the renal arteries in more than 90% of cases. Other advantages of MR imaging over CT are the absence of ionizing radiation, its ability to obtain multiplane images, and the large field of image. It is not necessary to use potentially toxic contrast agents for MR imaging to achieve intravascular enhancement, but paramagnetic contrast agents, such as gadolinium, are available and may prove useful. Advances in signal acquisition and computer programs allow MR imaging instruments to measure blood flow and construct images that look like conventional angiograms (MR angiography). When these techniques become routinely available, MR imaging may become the only imaging method necessary for most patients with aortic disease of any type.

Objective documentation of the size should be accomplished with one of these imaging modalities in all patients with suspected AAA before performing an elective aneurysm operation. Each method can establish an accurate diameter measurement. An initial scan can be used for comparison with subsequent scans to determine aneurysmal enlargement. For routine situations, ultrasound is probably the method of choice because of its widespread availability, lower cost, and lack of ionizing radiation. When there is suspicion of suprarenal or thoracoabdominal aortic involvement or dissection, MR imaging and CT are preferable.

For symptomatic aneurysms, MR imaging and CT also have advantages over ultrasound because they are better able to identify contained rupture. CT and MR imaging probably have equally superior capability to demonstrate unexpected features such as venous anomalies, perianeurysmal fibrosis, and horseshoe kidney, although the ureters are not easily identified by MR imaging.

Aortography

The limitations of aortography for diagnosing and evaluating aortic aneurysms, like plain film roentgenograms, are well known. Because of the mural thrombus, which is nearly always present and tends to reduce the aneurysmal lumen size towards normal, aortography cannot be relied on to determine the diameter of an aneurysm or even to establish its presence. Thus, aortography should not be used as a diagnostic method for AAAs. It is used to define the extent of aneurysm formation, especially suprarenal and iliac involvement, and of the associated arterial lesions involving renal and visceral vessels, including distal stenotic lesions[17] (Table 91-1 and Fig. 91-5). Although many of these associated lesions are detectable and manageable intraoperatively, preoperative identification of such lesions is useful in planning operative strategy, and routine preoperative aortography has been advocated by some surgeons. Aortography is essential in patients with AAA and the following indications:

- Clinical suspicion of visceral ischemia
- Occlusive iliofemoral vascular lesions
- Severe hypertension or impaired renal function in a patient in whom a concomitant renal artery stenosis would be repaired if discovered
- Suspicion of a horseshoe kidney
- Suspicion of suprarenal or thoracoabdominal aneurysm
- Presence of femoral or popliteal aneurysms

Aortography is not used simply to determine presence or size of an abdominal aneurysm.

Risks associated with aortography include potential renal toxicity from the large contrast volumes that are sometimes required to adequately fill a large aneurysm and the branch vessels. In addition, manipulation of a retrograde catheter past the laminated mural thrombus risks distal embolization, and there is always the possibility of local complications at the arterial puncture site where the angiographic catheter is introduced. The use of digital subtraction angiographic techniques has decreased but not eliminated these risks.

RISK OF ANEURYSM RUPTURE

Most AAAs are discovered in asymptomatic patients or during evaluation of an unrelated problem. They are being discovered at a smaller size than when the original studies on their natural history were first published by Estes,[18] Wright and colleagues,[19] Szilagyi and coworkers,[20] and others.[21] Although aneurysms can cause symptoms and serious consequences from thrombosis or distal embolism, rupture is the most important risk. Aneurysm size directly correlates with risk; the larger the aneurysm, the greater the risk of rupture. For example, the yearly risk of rupture for aneurysms of 5 cm or less in diameter is about 4.1%. For aneurysms between 5 and 7 cm, risk increases to 6.6%

and increases even further to 19% for aneurysms larger than 7 cm in diameter. Calculated as 5-year rupture rates, these numbers become 20.5%, 33%, and 95%, respectively. The steepness of a curve plotting these data increases sharply at a diameter of about 6 cm, but this value should not be used as an absolute size for recommending an elective aneurysm operation. Autopsy studies have shown that 23.4% of aneurysms between 4.1 and 5 cm rupture, and the same may be true for up to 10% of aneurysms less than 4 cm in diameter. Data such as these have led surgeons to recommend operation for almost all aortic aneurysms in good-risk patients.

There is little debate about the appropriateness of elective aneurysm surgery for patients with large aneurysms (those greater than 6 to 7 cm in diameter) because of the high risk of rupture and its associated mortality. Two recent reports have questioned the need to operate on small asymptomatic aneurysms.[22,23] In a population-based study from Rochester, Minn., the mean enlargement rate for aneurysms less than 5 cm in diameter was only 0.32 cm/y, and after 5 years of observation, no aneurysm less than 5 cm ruptured. Rupture occurred in 25% of patients whose aneurysm measured 5 cm or more, and elective repair of aneurysms 5 cm or more in diameter was recommended. In a study of small nonoperated aneurysms, chronic obstructive pulmonary disease and systolic hypertension were predictors of increased risk of rupture.[24] In that study, the rate of enlargement of small aneurysms was unpredictable, but increased systolic pressure or decreased diastolic pressure (ie, increased pulse pressure) were both associated with an increased rate of aneurysm expansion. The average rate of expansion was 0.4 cm/y in anteroposterior dimensions and 0.5 cm/y in lateral dimensions. Other studies have shown that aneurysms are frequently elliptic rather than round and that aneurysmal expansion is initially more rapid in the lateral direction. Aneurysm rupture most frequently occurs in the lateral wall.

A collected review of four series described the outcome of 378 patients with small aortic aneurysms initially treated nonoperatively.[24] After an average follow-up study of 31 months, 27% of the patients were alive with an intact aneurysm, 29% had died of other causes, 39% had had elective aneurysm operations because their aneurysm diameter reached 5 or 6 cm, and 4% suffered aneurysm rupture or acute expansion leading to emergency operation. Overall, there was a mean 5-year survival of 54% in these patients. It appears that most patients can be carefully observed using serial ultrasound measurements until an aneurysm size of 5 cm is reached. The 4% to 6% annual rupture rate of aneurysms smaller than this is similar to the 5% operative mortality rate reported in this collective

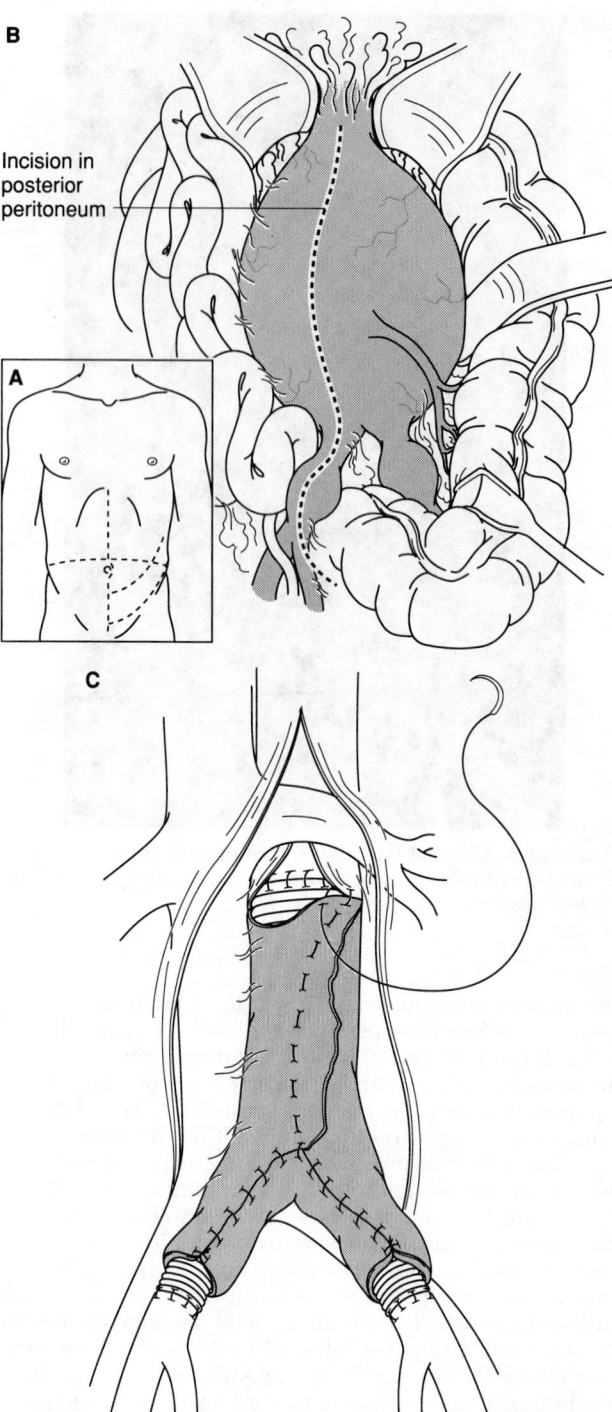

Figure 91-5. Operative repair of abdominal aortic aneurysm. (*A*) Suitable incisions. (*B*) Dissected aneurysm showing line of incision into aneurysm sac. (*C*) Closure of aneurysm wall over prosthetic graft.

Table 91-1. **ANGIOGRAPHICALLY DETECTED LESIONS ASSOCIATED WITH ABDOMINAL AORTIC ANEURYSMS**

Findings	Total Patients	Patients With Lesions
Suprarenal extension	680	46 (6.7%)
Renal stenosis and occlusion	763	138 (18.0%)
Accessory and multiple renal arteries	680	92 (13.5%)
Celiac and superior mesenteric artery stenosis	628	87 (13.8%)
Iliofemoropopliteal stenosis and occlusion	680	298 (43.8%)
Iliofemoropopliteal aneurysm	680	243 (34.2%)

experience and appears to support this approach, although several authors have reported essentially no mortality for small aneurysms.

Although the risk of aneurysm rupture correlates with aneurysm size and the average rate of aneurysmal enlargement is known (0.4 to 0.5 cm/y), it is impossible to predict when a small aneurysm will rupture in any given patient. Therefore, even small, asymptomatic AAA are not harmless.

SURGICAL TREATMENT RISKS

Long-term survival after surgical treatment of AAAs has been documented, including steady improvement in operative results for elective operations.[25] Several large, contemporary series have reported operative mortality rates between 0.9% and 5% for university medical centers and only slightly higher rates for community hospitals.[26,27] Operative mortality in this range (5% or less) justifies elective repair, even for small aneurysms. Most of the deaths, even in elective operations, occur in high-risk patients. Chronologic age is not as important as physiologic age in assessing operative risk, so patients should not be denied elective operation based solely on age.[28] Most vascular surgeons have successfully treated ruptured aneurysms in patients previously rejected for elective operation because they were too old. The major risks for elective AAA resection are similar to those for other major intraabdominal operations and include cardiopulmonary and renal dysfunction. High-risk patients are those with unstable, or rest, angina, cardiac ejection fraction less than 25% or 30%, congestive heart failure, serum creatinine greater than 3 mg/dL, and pulmonary disease manifested by room air PO_2 of less than 50 mmHg or elevated PCO_2. Even in these high-risk patients, aneurysm resection has been carried out with an operative mortality rate of less than 6%, using intensive perioperative monitoring and support.[29] Thus, large abdominal aneurysms should be considered for elective treatment, even in high-risk patients if the appropriate support facilities are available, since a substantial percentage of these high-risk patients die of ruptured aneurysm and not from the diseases that led to their categorization as high risk.

The operative results for ruptured aneurysms are not nearly as favorable and have not improved over the years as have the results of elective aneurysm operations. Although there are a few series with better results, nearly 50% of patients die after being operated on for rupture. The nature of the rupture influences the results. Less than 10% of patients presenting in shock with free intraperitoneal rupture survive, but stable patients with small contained leaks have a better than 80% survival rate. Although the incidence of aneurysm rupture has decreased as a result of aggressive elective resection programs, a substantial percentage (about half) of patients with ruptured aneurysms die before reaching a medical facility. Another 24% arrive at a hospital alive but die before a definitive operation can be performed. Thus, operative mortality figures underestimate the true significance of aneurysmal rupture.

Several factors are responsible for failure in the treatment of ruptured AAA.[30] The most important are failure to perform elective aneurysmectomy in patients with known aneurysms, delay in performing operation due to errors in diagnosing rupture, technical errors committed during the operation (eg, venous injuries), and undue delays in inducing anesthesia. These factors are all preventable. Discrepancies in operative mortality between various reports are due in part to failure to categorize patients and types of rupture properly. Many of these series also fail to distinguish patients with unruptured but symptomatic aneurysms who undergo emergency operations. The operative morbidity and mortality rate for this group falls between that of elective, asymptomatic patients and those with frank rupture, averaging 16% to 19%. The reason for this increased mortality may be the omission of thorough preoperative evaluation and preparation necessitated by the emergency operation.

LATE SURVIVAL

The most common cause of death among patients with AAA is rupture. Elective surgical repair prevents rupture and is associated with markedly improved survival rates.

Several long-term studies using actuarial methods have reported 5-year survival rates ranging from 49% to 84%, with an average of 61%. These data are far better than the survival of patients not undergoing operation, but they are still somewhat below the survival expected for the normal age-matched population. For example, the Canadian experience reported a 50% survival of 7.4 years for patients surviving operative treatment, whereas the survival in the US general population was 15.7 years and that for North Carolina was 14.5 years.[31] Most of the excess mortality can be attributed to coronary artery disease. This has led some centers to pursue an aggressive coronary evaluation and treatment protocol before elective aortic aneurysm operations. Several large surveys have shown that the safety of vascular surgical procedures for patients who have had previous coronary revascularization is comparable to that for patients with no evidence of ischemic cardiac disease, but this has not been evaluated by randomized clinical trials.[32-34]

ASSESSMENT OF CARDIAC RISK

Severe coronary artery disease is angiographically documented in about 50% of patients with AAAs in whom coronary disease is suspected clinically. The prevalence is 20% in patients who have no traditional clinical indicators of coronary disease.[35] Coronary artery disease is responsible for at least 50% to 60% of all perioperative and late deaths after operations on the abdominal aorta. The incidence of fatal myocardial infarction (MI) after elective AAA surgery has been reported to be as high as 4.7%, and nonfatal MI occurs in up to 16% of patients. The high-risk cardiac patient can be identified using clinical assessment, exercise stress testing, radionuclide angiography (MUGA scan), echocardiography, thallium scanning, continuous portable electrocardiographic (ECG) monitoring, and coronary angiography.[36,37]

Clinical factors predictive of increased risk for postoperative cardiac complications include a history of previous MI, congestive heart failure, angina pectoris, abnormal preoperative ECG, diabetes mellitus, and advanced age. Dipyridamole–thallium myocardial scanning has replaced exercise stress testing for these elderly patients in many hospitals. It identifies areas of myocardium that are reversibly ischemic and is sensitive for identifying patients most likely to have perioperative cardiac complications; unfortunately, its specificity is low. Determining left ventricular ejection fraction by radionuclide angiography identifies patients with poor ventricular function. Although ejection fractions less than 30% have been associated with increased cardiac complications, they do not predict postoperative MI or death. Continuous portable ECG monitoring of vascular surgical patients for silent ischemia associated with ST-T wave changes has been shown to correlate with postoperative MI in some series, but additional studies are needed to verify the value of this technique.

Routine preoperative screening of all aortic aneurysm patients with coronary angiography is not feasible or prudent, although Hertzer[32] reported a nearly five-fold increase in the operative mortality rate (5.1%) of aneurysm patients with suspected coronary disease compared with those without coronary disease (1.1% mortality) or corrected coronary artery disease (0.44% mortality). Late survival was also better in the groups with no or corrected coronary artery disease. Despite these data, no single means accurately predicts perioperative cardiac risk after aortic aneurysmorrhaphy. Each modality has its own usefulness as well as limitations. Older patients with congestive heart failure, active angina pectoris, previous MI, or markedly abnormal noninvasive cardiac studies must receive a thorough cardiac evaluation before elective aortic aneurysm surgery. Younger patients with normal ECG and without overt cardiac disease probably do not need this type of evaluation. The difficult decisions are in patients who fall between these two extremes and in whom unexpected coronary events occur. Because the ultimate objective of a cardiac evaluation is to identify and to correct dangerous coronary artery lesions, the results of the subsequent interventions (ie, coronary artery bypass grafting, percutaneous transluminal angioplasty) must be considered and balanced against the low MI rates that can be achieved in patients who do not undergo coronary revascularization. Preliminary myocardial revascularization before aortic aneurysm repair should be necessary in only about 10% of patients.

ABDOMINAL AORTIC ANEURYSM REPAIR

Indications

The natural history of unoperated AAAs and the excellent results achieved by conventional surgical treatment justify a vigorous diagnostic and therapeutic approach. The objectives of surgical treatment are to relieve symptoms, if present, to prevent rupture, and to prolong life. These goals are best accomplished when operations are performed electively under optimal conditions.

Emergent operation should be performed on almost all patients with known or suspected rupture, regardless of the size of the aneurysm or the patient's age. The coexistence of another fatal illness, such as metastatic cancer, may be sufficient reason to choose a nonoperative approach. Emergent operation is also indicated for symptomatic aneurysms without signs of rupture, since it is frequently impossible to determine whether an aneurysm has in fact ruptured or is just expanding. Although CT scanning and MR imaging can detect the presence of periaortic blood in most cases, the absence of this finding should not lead to unnecessary delays in operating since actual rupture can occur at any time.

Elective aneurysm repair should be considered for asymptomatic patients with aneurysms greater than 5 cm in diameter who are acceptable operative risks and who have an estimated life expectancy of 2 years or more. Elective operation may also be prudent for aneurysms less than 5 cm diameter in good-risk patients, especially if they are hypertensive or live in a remote area where proper medical care would not be readily available should signs and symptoms of rupture develop. Aneurysms between 4 and 5 cm in diameter that have shown documented enlargement by serial imaging studies should also be treated surgically.

High-risk patients (eg, the elderly and those with nonreconstructible coronary disease or poor left ventricular function) with small aneurysms should be observed until the aneurysm becomes symptomatic or large. High-risk patients with large aneurysms require thorough evaluation for the condition that puts them in the high-risk category. Frequently, such evaluations fail to substantiate the original degree of presumed risk, and less than 50% of these patients die of the disease for which they were denied aneurysm repair.

Because of excessively high operative mortality in some high-risk patients with large abdominal aneurysms, nonresectional therapy (extraanatomic bypass with induced thrombosis of the aneurysm) has been proposed by several surgeons.[38] Thrombosis of the aneurysm was thought to eliminate the risk of rupture, and the extraanatomic bypass would lower operative mortality by avoiding the risks of a major intraabdominal operation. Nonresective therapy has not proved as successful as hoped. Rupture still occurs in about 20% of patients, and operative mortality has been more than 10%, far in excess of the mortality reported in a similar but highly selected groups of patients subjected to conventional aneurysm operations. Fortunately, nonresective therapy for abdominal aneurysms is being abandoned, even by some of its earlier proponents.[39]

Operative Technique

There are three incision options for AAA operations: a full-length midline incision, a wide transverse incision, or an oblique incision from the left 11th intercostal space to the edge of the rectus abdominus muscle[40,41] (see Fig. 91-5A).

The choice of incision remains largely a matter of personal preference. Factors to consider in making this choice include the extent of the aneurysm, the status of the iliac arteries, the degree of obesity and pulmonary disease, previous abdominal operations and the necessity to inspect intraperitoneal structures (especially in patients with atypical symptoms), and the speed with which aortic control must be attained. Surgeons should be familiar with all three approaches to take advantage of each when appropriate.

Extensive perioperative monitoring is used for patients undergoing AAA repair and includes continuous recording of ECG, intraarterial pressure, body temperature, urine output, and central venous or pulmonary artery pressures.[42] In high-risk patients, especially if the aorta must be occluded above the renal arteries, transesophageal two-dimensional echocardiographic monitoring of left ventricular function may be superior to measurements of pulmonary artery pressure for evaluating intravascular volume status. Blood components should be monitored, including arterial oxygen and carbon dioxide, as well as pH, glucose, electrolytes, and coagulation parameters. Monitoring the clotting system is especially important in ruptured aneurysms and in cases when large volumes of blood and blood products have been replaced. Autotransfusion should be routine to minimize the amount of homologous blood administered. For elective operations, patients should be encouraged to donate their own blood for autologous transfusion in the perioperative period.

When midline or transverse incisions are used, the aorta is exposed by a retroperitoneal incision slightly to the left of the midline (see Fig. 91-5B). The duodenum must be carefully reflected laterally along with the rest of the small bowel.

Regardless of the infrarenal extent of the aortic aneurysm, graft replacement should begin just below the renal arteries to prevent recurrent aortic abnormalities. The degree of disease in the iliac arteries determines the distal extent of the graft. In some recent series, up to 80% of patients were successfully treated with a straight tube (aortoaortic) graft, although in our experience only about one third of patients have suitable anatomy for this approach. There does not appear to be a significant incidence of subsequent iliac aneurysm formation when tube grafts are used. The choice of graft material, Dacron or polytetrafluoroethylene, and its construction, knitted or woven, is a controversial but unimportant issue. There is no proven superiority of one graft type for aortic replacement.

Systemic heparin is almost always administered during the occlusive phase of aneurysm operations. Most surgeons believe it provides an added margin of safety from distal thrombosis. The distal clamps should be applied before the proximal aortic clamp to prevent distal embolism. The aorta is opened longitudinally and either partially or completely transected at the site of the proximal anastomosis (see Fig. 91-5*B*). In a short neck, temporary proximal aortic clamping above the renal arteries is required. The proximal anastomosis can be done with a continuous or interrupted suture technique. The former is quicker. If the aorta is especially weak or friable, the sutures can be supported with prosthetic felt pledgets.

The distal anastomoses can be end-to-end or end-to-side, depending on their location and the status of the common and internal iliac arteries. All mural thrombus and atheroma should be débrided from the aneurysm wall. Several studies have shown a surprisingly high incidence of positive bacterial cultures of this material, occurring in 10% to 40% of patients.[43] The significance of these positive cultures is unknown, but most have been coagulase-negative *Staphylococcus* sp, an organism commonly found in aortic graft infections. Backbleeding lumbar vessels can cause significant blood loss and should be suture ligated from within the aortic sac. If the inferior mesenteric artery is patent and actively backbleeding, it can also be ligated within the aneurysm. If backbleeding is meager, the vessel should be preserved and reassessed after distal flow is reestablished, especially if internal iliac flow is compromised. Reimplantation of the inferior mesenteric artery is easy to perform using the Carrel patch technique.

All anastomoses should be constructed with permanent, synthetic sutures. Braided Dacron and monofilament polypropylene are the most commonly used. Fears about late fracture of polypropylene sutures have not been substantiated. If suprarenal clamping is necessary, the clamp can be moved onto the graft below the renal arteries to minimize renal ischemia after ensuring that the proximal anastomosis is secure. The distal anastomoses are then constructed as indicated by the distal disease. It is sometimes easier to control iliac artery backbleeding by using intraluminal balloon catheters and to oversew the common iliac arteries from within the opened aortic or iliac aneurysm. In unusual circumstances, external iliac disease necessitates making the anastomosis to the common femoral artery.

Declamping hypotension is an unusual event in elective aortic aneurysm surgery. Communication with the anesthesiology team must be maintained so that depth of anesthesia and blood and fluid replacement can be adjusted in anticipation of lower extremity reperfusion. Even though the graft and native vessels are flushed and backbled before reestablishing distal flow, it is preferable to reestablish flow first into one hypogastric artery to minimize the chances of distal embolism to the leg. Before abdominal closure, the adequacy of lower extremity and left colon perfusion should be ensured by direct inspection or noninvasive assessment. The graft should be insulated from the overlying bowel by careful closure of the aneurysm sac over the graft (see Fig. 91-5*C*). This is sometimes impossible when the aneurysm is small. In this situation, a flap of the aneurysm wall or a vascularized omental pedicle can be used to separate the graft from the duodenum. If additional vascular procedures are required, such as renal or visceral artery reconstruction, appropriate modifications in technique are required.[44]

For ruptured aneurysms, the first priority is to gain proximal control of the aorta. Usually, it is better to have the patient prepared and draped, with the surgical team ready to make a rapid entry into the abdomen, before anesthesia is induced. The induction of anesthesia in these circumstances is often associated with sudden and severe hypotension when the tamponade effects are relieved by relaxation of the abdominal wall. If the rupture is contained, proximal aortic control is best achieved at the level of the supraceliac aorta through the lesser omentum. The hematoma can then be entered and the clamp repositioned distally after the aortic neck is identified. The hematoma usu-

ally makes this portion of the dissection easy, but caution must be exercised to avoid injury to major venous structures, since this is one of the most common causes of excessive hemorrhage and subsequent death. In a free intraperitoneal rupture, the aorta can be quickly compressed at the diaphragm with an assistant's hand or a compression device without formally dissecting this area. An infrarenal clamp or an intraluminal balloon occluding catheter can be substituted as soon as possible. After bleeding is controlled, adequate blood and volume replenishment should be achieved before attempting to restore flow to the lower extremities. Heparin is best avoided for ruptured aneurysms, since bleeding and coagulopathy are frequently associated with the massive blood loss and replacement that occur. The proper use of blood and blood products, including platelets and fresh frozen plasma, is essential for survival of these patients.

Complications of Aortic Aneurysm Repair

Survival after aortic aneurysm surgery was discussed earlier. Mortality rates range from up to 3% for patients with uncomplicated aneurysms operated on electively to more than 80% for patients with rupture, hypotension, or oliguria. The most frequent cause of death is myocardial dysfunction, which is usually ischemic in origin. Nonfatal MI is also fairly common, even after elective aortic aneurysm repair, occurring in 3% to 16% (average, 7%) of patients in reported series.

Several other major complications can occur during or after aortic aneurysm operations. Hemorrhage is a constant threat, most often from injury to iliac or lumbar veins. It can be severe and extremely difficult to control, especially if it involves the left common iliac vein where it passes beneath the right common iliac artery. Injury to the left renal vein or one of its tributaries can also be associated with brisk bleeding, particularly when there are venous anomalies such as a retroaortic left renal vein or a circumaortic venous collar. Postoperative hemorrhage can occur in any patient, and hemodynamic instability and evidence of continued blood loss should lead to early reexploration of the abdomen.

Declamping hypotension is not as frequent or severe a problem as it once was. Better understanding of its pathophysiology, more aggressive management of intravascular volume, and better monitoring and anesthetic techniques have all reduced the incidence and seriousness of this problem. Gradual declamping, coordinated with the anesthesiologist, minimizes this complication. Nonetheless, declamping hypotension can still be a serious problem, especially in the setting of a ruptured aneurysm in a cold, hypovolemic patient with poor cardiac performance.

Renal failure is another complication that occurs much less frequently than it once did. At one time, 3% to 12% of operative deaths after elective AAA operations and an even higher percentage after emergency operations for rupture were attributable to acute renal failure. Renal failure or less severe renal dysfunction can occur even when there is no hypotension and the proximal aortic clamp was infrarenal in location. The causes of renal dysfunction in these situations is poorly understood but is thought to involve reflex renal vasoconstriction and intrarenal redistribution of blood flow. Atheromatous embolism from clamping or manipulation of the pararenal aorta is a potential contributing factor as is temporary suprarenal clamping. The large contrast load of an aortogram performed a day or two preoperatively can cause renal dysfunction that only becomes apparent postoperatively. Mannitol is commonly administered before aortic cross-clamping to increase urine output and prevent renal failure. Although this seems reasonable, studies have shown that intraoperative urine volume does not predict postoperative renal function. Renal failure caused by acute tubular necrosis is much more common after ruptured aortic aneurysms, occurring in 21% of survivors of operation in one series. Unfortunately, the mortality rate associated with this complication remains high, varying from 50% to 70% despite acute hemodialysis and adequate nutritional support.

Injury to the bowel or ureters can cause catastrophic infectious complications involving the newly implanted prosthetic graft. This is most likely to occur when there are adhesions from previous operations or when the structures are in an unusual position (eg, the ureters are displaced anteriorly and laterally by the aneurysm). Such injuries should be meticulously repaired and the area irrigated with antibiotic solution. Ureteral injuries should be stented, but in some situations, nephrectomy is the safest course to avoid possible graft contamination.

Gastrointestinal complications of a functional nature regularly occur after aortic aneurysm surgery. Ileus is the rule for at least 3 or 4 days after transperitoneal surgery. Typically, gastric and colonic ileus persists longer than small bowel ileus. Occasionally, duodenal obstruction persists for longer periods. Hematoma and edema in the vicinity of the proximal anastomosis may contribute to this problem. Postoperative pancreatitis is common, as determined by elevated serum amylase levels, although clinically apparent pancreatitis is unusual. The most serious gastrointestinal complication is ischemia of the left colon and rectum.[45] The incidence of ischemic colitis after aortic reconstruction is about 2% (range, 0.2% to 10%). It is three or four times more common after operations for aortic aneurysm than after operations for occlusive disease, and the incidence is several times higher in patients studied prospectively with colonoscopy after sustaining a ruptured aneurysm.

Ligation of the inferior mesenteric artery is thought to be an important pathophysiologic mechanism, but the inferior mesenteric artery is already occluded in most patients with abdominal aneurysms. Ligating the inferior mesenteric artery too far away from the wall of the aneurysm can contribute to this complication by interfering with collateral blood supply to the rectosigmoid. When possible, it is important to maintain antegrade perfusion in at least one internal iliac artery after arterial reconstruction for aortic aneurysm. Most patients with occlusion of both internal iliac arteries and the inferior mesenteric artery have adequate colonic perfusion, but postoperative hypotension, bowel distention, and mesenteric vessel compression by hematoma can all contribute to postoperative colonic ischemia. The ischemia can involve the mucosa only, which usually causes a transient, mild form of ischemic colitis, or it can involve mucosa and muscularis, which may result in fibrous healing and stricture formation. The most severe and dreaded form is transmural ischemia, which occurs in more than 60% of the reported cases of postaneurysmectomy colonic ischemia.

The clinical manifestations of bowel ischemia depend on the severity of ischemia. Diarrhea, especially if it is bloody, is one of the earliest manifestations and usually begins within 48 hours of operation. It is an indication for colonoscopy to assess the status of the colonic mucosa. Findings indicative of bowel gangrene and peritonitis demand prompt reoperation, resection of all compromised bowel, and creation of appropriate stomas. During bowel resection, efforts should be made to isolate the underlying aortic prosthesis from the surgical field, although this is usually impossible, setting the stage for subsequent prosthetic infection. If the graft becomes grossly contaminated, it should be removed and lower extremity perfusion restored by axillofemoral bypass. Less severe degrees of colonic ischemia can be managed nonoperatively, although subsequent correction of a colonic stricture may be required.

The mortality rate for postoperative colon ischemia after aortic aneurysm surgery is about 50% but increases to 90% when full-thickness colonic gangrene and peritonitis occur. Preoperative evaluation of the blood supply to the colon and intraoperative assessment of colonic perfusion by Doppler device or inferior mesenteric artery back pressure measurements might help to identify patients at highest risk for this disastrous complication.

Paraplegia due to spinal cord ischemia, a well-recognized complication of thoracoabdominal aneurysm repair, is a rare event after operations confined to the infrarenal aorta, with only slightly more than 50 cases reported, an incidence of 0.2% in more than 3000 aortic operations.[46] It occurs 10 times more frequently in patients with ruptured aneurysms, suggesting that hypotension is a contributing factor in most cases even though injury to an unusually located arteria magna radicularis (artery of Adamkiewicz) to the spinal cord may be the primary event. Unfortunately, this complication is not preventable, predictable, or treatable. Although the severity of the clinical manifestations varies and about 50% of affected survivors recover some neurologic function, the associated mortality is 50%.

Ischemia of the lower extremities can occur after aortic aneurysm surgery. It can be caused by embolism of dislodged mural thrombus from the aneurysm itself, from thrombosis of a vessel due to distal stasis, or by creation of an intimal flap or crushed atherosclerotic plaque. The use of heparin during the occlusive phase of aneurysm repair does not prevent embolic events from occurring but may limit the propagation of thrombus and should prevent formation of stasis thrombi in the distal vascular beds.

Microembolism can also occur, resulting in small patchy areas of ischemia, usually on the plantar aspect of the feet. Pedal pulses are usually still palpable in this situation. This condition is known as *trash foot*, and if recognized intraoperatively, the passage of small balloon catheters can sometimes retrieve at least some of the atheromatous debris. Lumbar sympathectomy may also help to limit or to prevent full-thickness tissue loss.

Infection of the prosthetic graft used to restore aortic continuity occurs in less than 6% of patients and is more common after treating ruptured aneurysms. It may be associated with a graft—enteric fistula, which is more common after surgery for aortic aneurysm than aortic occlusive disease. These infections usually become manifest months to years after graft implantation and are among the most challenging vascular surgical problems to treat.

MYCOTIC AORTIC ANEURYSMS

Mycotic aneurysm refers to an aneurysm of infectious etiology. It does not imply fungal etiology but relates to the mushroom-shaped false aneurysm of the arterial wall that is typically found. Mycotic aneurysms usually occur as a consequence of bacterial or septic emboli lodging at a point on the intimal surface of an artery in sufficient number to produce a locally invasive infection that then spreads to become a transmural arteritis. This can occur in normal arteries but more commonly affects atherosclerotic vessels, which tend to be large major vessels, and their branches. A septic embolus may also lodge in a vasa vasorum and initiate a necrotic process in the arterial wall. A third mechanism is arterial invasion from a septic focus adjacent to a major artery. In recent years, traumatic contamination of an artery has replaced endocarditis as the most common cause, often as a result of drug abuse.

In the largest collective review of mycotic aneurysms, the abdominal aorta was the second most frequent site (31%), exceeded only by the femoral artery (38%).[47] One series of 22 mycotic aortic aneurysms in 2585 patients suggests an incidence of 0.85%.[48] Coincident with the change in cause, there has been a change in the bacteriology of mycotic aneurysms, with *Salmonella* sp declining and *Staphylococcus* sp increasing, but together, these are still the most frequently cultured organisms from aortic mycotic aneurysms. The predilection for the infrarenal abdominal aorta probably relates to the frequent occurrence of atherosclerotic plaques in that location.

The triad of abdominal pain, fever, and a pulsatile abdominal mass should suggest the diagnosis of mycotic aneurysm, but most patients present with a nonspecific febrile illness of variable duration. Many do not have a palpable aneurysm, and only about one third have abdominal pain. Leukocytosis is a common finding. Many mycotic aneurysms are detected by CT scans performed for evaluation of undiagnosed fever. They appear as a mass located on one side of the aorta rather than a circumferential enlargement. They are enhanced with intravenously administered contrast, but their significance can be difficult to appreciate. Angiography demonstrates the characteristic lobulated saccular aneurysm, which may be multiple and contiguous. These are false aneurysms, contained by compressed periaortic tissue. The aneurysm wall tends to be thin and friable and associated with contiguous lymphadenopathy and obvious inflammation. Blood clot of varying age is present both within and outside the aneurysmal sac because there is a high incidence of rupture, although it is usually contained. Periaortic abscess may also be present. The opening between the aorta and the aneurysm tends to be irregular or ragged.

Mycotic aneurysms are a fulminant infectious process and must be treated vigorously and promptly. Control of clinical sepsis does not appear to be necessary for successful surgical treatment, and delays in operative intervention are associated with aneurysmal rupture. Proper antibiotic therapy must be combined with resection of the infected arterial segments, débridement of all adjacent necrotic tissue, and arterial reconstruction. Control of infection by antibiotics does not prevent rupture of the aneurysm, so excision is mandatory and should be carried out promptly. Many of these aneurysms involve the upper abdominal aorta, where it is not always possible to avoid use of prosthetic arterial grafts. In situ prosthetic replacement is necessary when renal or visceral perfusion would be compromised by aortic excision. For the infrarenal aorta, if the intraoperative Gram stains are negative and there is no periaortic purulence, in situ prosthetic grafting is also the procedure of choice. It should be followed with 6 to 8 weeks of specific antibiotic therapy, and, in the case of salmonellal infections, probably lifelong antibiotics. Frank periaortic pus or gram-positive infrarenal mycotic aneurysm can be managed successfully by aortic débridement and ligation, extraanatomic bypass, and a shorter course of antibiotics. Alternatively, the in situ grafting technique described above can be used, and recent data tend to favor this in situ method. Using these principles, an operative survival rate of 86% with only one recurrent infection has been reported.[48]

ILIAC ARTERY ANEURYSMS

Common iliac artery aneurysms often appear in continuity or in association with AAAs. As isolated lesions they are rare, accounting for less than 1% of all aneurysms involving the aortoiliac segment. Most are atherosclerotic and occur in the atherosclerosis age group, but some develop during pregnancy in the absence of atherosclerosis. Iliac aneurysms usually involve the common or internal iliac arteries and are multiple in more than 33% of patients.[49,50] Isolated external iliac aneurysms are rare. Because they are in the pelvis, iliac aneurysms are difficult to detect by abdominal examination and tend to be large or symptomatic when they are eventually discovered. This accounts for the unusually high incidence of rupture, which averages 33% in collected series, but was 51% in the largest review. Symptoms are most often due to rupture (77%) or pressure on adjacent pelvic structures (eg, urinary tract, lower GI tract, lumbosacral nerves, pelvic veins). Lower abdominal, flank, and groin pain are common.[51] Most symptoms are not those usually attributed to the arterial system, which contributes to delay in diagnosis.

Some large iliac aneurysms can be palpated on abdominal, rectal, or pelvic examination. CT, ultrasound, and MR imaging can be expected to establish the correct diagnosis in most patients. Arteriography documents the presence of most iliac aneurysms but, as with aneurysms elsewhere, often underestimates the size because of laminated thrombus. Other useful tests are proctoscopy, barium enema, cystoscopy, and plain abdominal radiograph.

Iliac aneurysms tend to be large when diagnosed. In a collected review, the average size at operation or autopsy was 8.5 cm, and the incidence of rupture of the entire series of 83 iliac aneurysms was 51%.[49] The natural history of iliac aneurysms is unfavorable. The operative mortality rate in patients with rupture is high, 59% compared with only 11% for elective operations. Thus, isolated iliac aneurysms should be treated surgically when they are discovered to avoid the high mortality associated with rupture.

The treatment of choice for internal iliac aneurysms is proximal ligation and endoaneurysmorrhaphy. For aneurysmal involvement of the common iliac artery, graft replacement is recommended. Because the external iliac artery is rarely aneurysmal, these grafts can be confined to the abdomen. If both common iliac arteries are aneurysmal or if the aneurysm extends to the aortic bifurcation, an aortoiliac bifurcation graft should be inserted.

The concept of endoluminal treatment of abdominal aortic aneurysms, first reported by Parodi and colleagues in 1991, has become a clinical reality.[52] Several hundred patients have now been treated worldwide using a variety of stent–graft combinations that are undergoing clinical evaluation.[53–56] Most insertions require femoral arteriotomy. The goals of endoluminal repair are to achieve successful treatment (prevention of rupture) of aortic aneurysms with reduced morbidity and mortality, and lower cost. To be successful, this method of repair has to permanently exclude arterial flow and pressure from the aneurysm sac and prevent further aneurysmal growth and rupture. Early results are encouraging, but no long-term follow-up data (ie, 5 years) are available, and several problems remain unresolved. The two most important are the fate of the aneurysm sac itself (whether it continues to be at risk for enlargement and rupture) and the fate of the aortic wall where the devices are attached. Not all patients with aortic aneurysms are suitable for endoluminal repair, usually because of anatomic reasons such as vessel size or tortuosity or an inadequate aneurysm neck in which to secure the device. Nevertheless, it is estimated that about 40% to 50% of abdominal aortic aneurysms ultimately are treatable in this manner.

REFERENCES

1. Bickerstaff LK, Hollier LH, Van Peenen HJ, et al. Abdominal aortic aneurysm: the changing natural history. J Vasc Surg 1984;1:6.

2. Castleden W, Mercer J. Abdominal aortic aneurysms in Western Australia: descriptive epidemiology and patterns of rupture. Br J Surg 1985;72:109.

3. Darling RC, Messina CR, Brewster DC, et al. Autopsy study of unoperated aortic aneurysms. Circulation 1977;6(Suppl 2):161.

4. Taylor LM, Porter JM. Basic data related to clinical decision-making in abdominal aortic aneurysms. Ann Vasc Surg 1986;1:502.

5. Hollier LH, Stanson AW, Glovicski P, et al. Arteriomegaly: classification and morbid implications of diffuse aneurysmal disease. Surgery 1983;93:700.

6. Vermilion BD, Kimmins SA, Pace WG, et al. A review of 147 popliteal aneurysms with long-term follow-up. Surgery 1981;90:1009.

7. Dobrin PB. Pathophysiology and pathogenesis of aortic aneurysms: current concepts. Surg Clin North Am 1989;69:687.

8. Tilson MD, Seashore MR. Human genetics of the abdominal aortic aneurysm. Surg Gynecol Obstet 1984;158:129.

9. Collin J, Walton J. Is abdominal aortic aneurysm familial? Br Med J 1989;299:493.

10. Lawrie GM, Crawford ES, Morris GC Jr, et al. Progress in the treatment of ruptured abdominal aortic aneurysm. World J Surg 1980;4:653.

11. Rutherford RB, McCroskey BL. Ruptured abdominal aortic aneurysms: special considerations. Surg Clin North Am 1989;69:4:859.

12. Goldstone J. Vascular imaging techniques. In: Rutherford RB, ed. Vascular surgery, ed 3. Philadelphia, WB Saunders, 1989:119.

13. Gomes MN, Choyke PL. Pre-operative evaluation of abdominal aortic aneurysms: ultrasound or computed tomography? J Cardiovasc Surg 1987;28:159.

14. Amparo EG, Hoddick WK, Hricak H, et al. Comparison of magnetic resonance imaging and ultrasonography in the evaluation of abdominal aortic aneurysms. Radiology 1985;154:451.

15. Weinbaum FI, Dubner S, Turner JW, et al. The accuracy of computed tomography in the diagnosis of retroperitoneal blood in the presence of abdominal aortic aneurysm. J Vasc Surg 1987;6:11.

16. Lee JKT, Ling D, Heiken JP, et al. Magnetic resonance imaging of abdominal aneurysms. AJR 1984;143:1197.

17. Rich NM, Clagett GP, Salander JM, et al. Role of arteriography in the evaluation of aortic aneurysms. In: Bergan JJ, Yao JST, eds. Aneurysms: diagnosis and treatment. New York, Grune & Stratton, 1982:233.

18. Estes JE Jr. Abdominal aortic aneurysm: a study of 102 cases. Circulation 1950;2:258.

19. Wright IS, Urdenata E, Wright B. Re-opening the case of the abdominal aortic aneurysm. Circulation 1956;13:754.

20. Szilagyi DE, Elliott JP, Smith RF. Clinical fate of the patient with asymptomatic abdominal aortic aneurysm and unfit surgical treatment. Arch Surg 1972;104:600.

21. Bernstein EF, Chan EL. Abdominal aortic aneurysm in high risk patients: outcome of selective management based on size and expansion rate. Ann Surg 1984;200:255.

22. Cronenwett JL, Murphy TF, Zelenock GB, et al. Actuarial analysis of variables associated with rupture of small aortic aneurysms. Surgery 1985;98:472.

23. Nevitt MP, Ballard DJ, Hallett JW Jr. Prognosis of abdominal aortic aneurysms. N Engl J Med 1989;321:1009.

24. Cronenwett JL, Sargent SK, Wall, et al. Variables that effect the expansion rate and outcome of small abdominal aortic aneurysms. J Vasc Surg 1990;11:260.

25. Crawford ES, Saleh SA, Babb III JW, et al. Infrarenal abdominal aortic aneurysm: factors influencing survival after operation performed over a 25 year period. Ann Surg 1981;193:699.

26. Hertzer NR, Avellone JC, Farrel CJ, et al. The risk of vascular surgery in a metropolitan community. J Vasc Surg 1984;1:13.

27. DeBakey ME, Crawford ES, Cooley DA, et al. Aneurysm of abdominal aorta: analysis of results of graft replacement therapy one to eleven years after operation. Ann Surg 1964;160:622.

28. O'Donnell TF, Darling RC, Linton RR. Is 80 years too old for aneurysmectomy? Arch Surg 1976;111:1250.

29. Hollier LH, Reigel MM, Kozmier FJ, et al. Conventional repair of abdominal aortic aneurysm in the high-risk patient: a plea for abandonment of nonresective treatment. J Vasc Surg 1986;3:712.

30. Hiatt JCG, Barker WF, Machleder HI, et al. Determinants of failure in the treatment of ruptured abdominal aortic aneurysm. Arch Surg 1984;119:1264.

31. Johnson G Jr, Gurri JA, Burnham SJ. Life expectancy after abdominal aortic aneurysm repair. In: Bergan JJ, Yao JST, eds. Arterial aneurysms: diagnosis and treatment. New York, Grune & Stratton, 1982:279.

32. Hertzer NR. Fatal myocardial infarction following abdominal aortic aneurysm resection: 343 patients followed 6–11 years postoperatively. Ann Surg 1980;190:667.

33. Crawford ES, Morris GC Jr, Howell JF, et al. Operative risk in patients with previous coronary artery bypass. Ann Thorac Surg 1978;26:215.

34. Reul GJ Jr, Cooley DA, Duncan MJ, et al. The effect of coronary bypass on the outcome of peripheral vascular operation in 1093 patients. J Vasc Surg 1986;3:788.

35. Bevan EG. Routine coronary angiography in patients undergoing surgery for abdominal aortic aneurysm and lower extremity occlusive disease. J Vasc Surg 1986;3:682.

36. Yeager RA, Moneta GL. Assessing cardiac risk in vascular surgical patients: current status. Perspect Vasc Surg 1989;2:18.

37. Cheitlin MD. Finding the high-risk patient with coronary artery disease. JAMA 1988;259:2271.

38. Karmody AM, Leather RP, Goldman M, et al. The current position of non-resective treatment for abdominal aortic aneurysm. Surgery 1983;94:591.

39. Inahara T, Beary GL, Mukherjee D, et al. The contrary position to the nonresective treatment for abdominal aortic aneurysm. J Vasc Surg 1985;2:42.

40. Cambria RP, Brewster DC, Abbott WM, et al. Transperitoneal versus retroperitoneal approach for aortic reconstruction: a randomized, prospective study. J Vasc Surg 1990;11:314.

41. Chang BB, Shan DJ, Paty PS, et al. Can the retroperitoneal approach be used for ruptured abdominal aortic aneurysm? J Vasc Surg 1990;11:326.

42. Goldstone J. Intraoperative monitoring in aortic surgery. In: Bergan JJ, Yao JST, eds. Arterial surgery: new diagnostic and operative techniques. Orlando, Grune & Stratton, 1988:257.

43. Macbeth GA, Rubin JR, McIntyre KE, et al. The relevance of arterial wall microbiology to the treatment of prosthetic graft infections: graft infection versus arterial infection. J Vasc Surg 1984;1:754.

44. Tarazi RY, Hertzer NR, Bevan EG, et al. Simultaneous aortic reconstruction and renal revascularization: risk factors and late results in 89 patients. J Vasc Surg 1987;5:707.

45. Ernst CB, Hagihara PF, Daughorty ME, et al. Ischemic colitis incidence following abdominal aortic reconstruction: a prospective study. Surgery 1976;80:417.

46. Szilagyi DE, Hagemen JH, Smith RF, et al. Spinal cord damage in surgery of the abdominal aorta. Surgery 1978;83:38.

47. Brown SL, Busuttil RW, Baker JD, et al. Bacteriologic and surgical determinants of survival in patients with mycotic aneurysms. J Vasc Surg 1984;1:541.

48. Chan FY, Crawford ES, Coselli JS, et al. In situ prosthetic graft replacement for mycotic aneurysms of the aorta. Ann Thorac Surg 1989;47:193.

49. Schuler JJ, Flanigan DP. Iliac artery aneurysms. In: Bergan JJ, Yao JST, eds. Arterial aneurysms: diagnosis and treatment. New York, Grune & Stratton, 1982:469.

50. Lowry SF, Kraft RO. Isolated aneurysms of the iliac artery. Arch Surg 1978;113:1289.

51. Richardson JW, Greenfield LJ. Natural history and management of iliac aneurysms. J Vasc Surg 1988;8:165.

52. Parodi JC, Criado FJ, Barone HD, et al. Endoluminal aortic aneurysm repair using a ballon-expandable stent–graft device: a progress report. Ann Vasc Surg 1994;8:523.

53. Goldstone J. Initial human results with a Spikes, stented endoluminal graft to treat abdominal aortic aneurysms. In: Veith, FJ, ed. Current critical problems in vascular surgery, vol 6. St Louis, Quality Medical Publishing, 1994:127.

54. May J, White GH, Waugh RC, et al. Endoluminal repair of abdominal aortic aneurysms. Med J Aust 1994;161:541.

55. Moore, WS, Rutherford, RB. Transfemoral endovascular re-

pair of abdominal aortic aneurysm: results of the North American EVT phase I trial. J Vasc Surg 1996;23:543.

56. Yousef SW, Baker DM, Chuter TA, et al. Transfemoral endoluminal repair of abdominal aortic aneurysm with bifurcated graft. Lancet 1994;334:650.

SURGERY: SCIENTIFIC PRINCIPLES AND PRACTICE, Second Edition, edited by Lazar J. Greenfield, Michael W. Mulholland, Keith T. Oldham, Gerald B. Zelenock, and Keith D. Lillemoe. Lippincott–Raven Publishers, Philadelphia, © 1997.

CHAPTER 92

SPLANCHNIC ARTERY ANEURYSMS

JAMES C. STANLEY

Splanchnic artery aneurysms are uncommon, but the more frequent use of arteriography, computed tomography (CT), and ultrasonography has resulted in increasing clinical recognition of these lesions. These aneurysms are clearly important considering that nearly 22% present as surgical emergencies, including 8.5% that result in the patient's death. The splanchnic vessels involved with these macroaneurysms, in decreasing order of frequency, are the splenic, hepatic, superior mesenteric, celiac, gastric–gastroepiploic, jejunal–ileal–colic, pancreaticoduodenal–pancreatic, and gastroduodenal arteries (Table 92-1). The clinical manifestations and management of these aneurysms have been better defined in recent years.[1,2]

SPLENIC ARTERY ANEURYSM

Splenic artery aneurysms account for 60% of all splanchnic artery aneurysms.[3] The higher frequency of these aneurysms in the splenic artery cannot be accounted for by the greater length of this vessel compared with other splanchnic arteries; the frequency instead reflects a peculiar predisposition for this vessel to undergo aneurysmal change. The occurrence of these lesions in the general population is probably similar to the 0.78% incidence in nearly 3600 consecutive patients undergoing abdominal arteriographic studies for reasons other than suspected aneurysmal disease.[3] Women are four times more likely than men to develop these aneurysms.

Three distinct factors may contribute to the development of splenic artery aneurysms, including two that account for their unusual female predilection. The first factor is medial fibrodysplasia, which usually occurs in women and is most often manifested by renal artery stenosis and secondary hypertension. As many as 4% of patients with dysplastic renal artery disease have splenic artery aneurysms, and all of these patients have been women.[3] The second factor relates to the deleterious consequences of pregnancy, with its known increase in splenic blood flow and reproductive hormone-related changes in elastic vascular tissue. This becomes a particular problem with repeated pregnancies. Some 45% to 55% of women harboring these lesions have completed six or more pregnancies.[3,4] The third factor is evident in the nearly 10% of patients with portal hypertension and splenomegaly who develop splenic artery aneurysms.[3] In these cases, the vessel wall integrity may be compromised by increased splenic blood flow[5] and excessive estrogen activity occurring as a conse-

Table 92-1. SPLANCHNIC ARTERY MACROANEURYSMS

Aneurysm Location	Frequency Within Splanchnic Circulation	Male/Female Ratio	Frequency of Reported Rupture	Mortality Rate With Rupture	Treatment
Splenic artery	60%	1:4	2% (bland aneurysms)	25% (bland aneurysms); during pregnancy— 70% maternal and 75% fetal	Splenectomy; aneurysm exclusion or excision without splenectomy
Hepatic artery	20%	2:1	20%	35%	Aneurysmectomy with and without hepatic artery reconstruction; hepatic territory resection; transcatheter aneurysm obliteration
Superior mesenteric artery	5.5%	1:1	Uncommon (thrombosis more common)	50%	Aneurysmectomy with superior mesenteric artery reconstruction; ligation if collateral circulation is adequate
Celiac artery	4%	1:1	13%	50%	Aneurysmectomy with celiac artery reconstruction; ligation if circulation is adequate
Gastric and gastroepiploic arteries	4%	3:1	90%	70%	Aneurysm excision with involved gastric tissue; ligation if extramural
Pancreaticoduodenal, pancreatic, and gastroduodenal arteries	3.5%	4:1	75% Inflammatory 50% Noninflammatory	50%	Aneurysm excision with false aneurysms (pseudocyst-related); pancreatic resection; ligation if extrapancreatic
Jujunal, ileal, and colic arteries	3%	1:1	30%	20%	Aneurysm excision with involved intestine; ligation if extramural

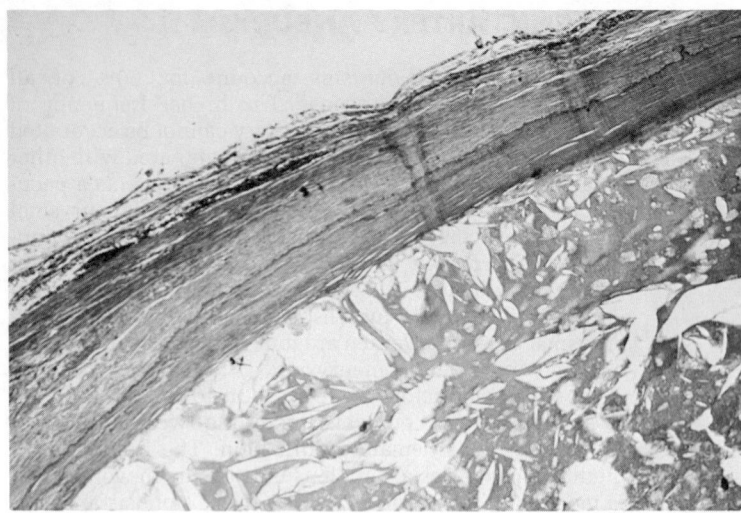

Figure 92-1. Splenic artery aneurysm exhibiting marked fibrosis with cholesterol clefts and calcific arteriosclerosis (hematoxylin-eosin, decalcified, ×32). (Stanley JC, Fry WJ. Pathogenesis and clinical significance of splenic artery aneurysms. Surgery 1974; 76:898)

quence of the underlying cirrhosis. No sex predilection exists in this latter subgroup of patients. Although splenic artery aneurysms have been described with regularity among patients after orthotopic liver transplantation, it is speculative as to whether these represent preexisting aneurysms associated with portal hypertension or have arisen as a consequence of the transplant itself and attendant drug therapy, such as steroids.[6]

Certain splenic artery aneurysms exhibit extensive arteriosclerosis (Fig. 92-1). The fact that calcific arteriosclerotic changes appear limited to the aneurysm and not the intervening artery suggests that this is more likely a secondary event, rather than a primary etiologic process (Fig. 92-2). Arterial disruptions due to periarterial inflammatory disease, such as chronic pancreatitis, or penetrating trauma are less common causes of these aneurysms. Microaneurysms of smaller intraparenchymal splenic arteries are usually due to a systemic vasculitis, such as polyarteritis nodosa, and appear to be of less clinical importance as a vascular disease than extraparenchymal aneurysms attributed to other causes.

Nearly all splenic artery aneurysms associated with arterial fibrodysplasia, multiple pregnancies, or portal hypertension are saccular and occur at branchings. At such sites, discontinuities exist in the internal elastic lamina of normal vessels, and any subsequent degenerative events involving elastic tissue, as might occur with arterial fibrodysplasia or pregnancy, are likely to produce aneurysmal changes (Fig. 92-3). Splenic artery branch aneurysms are multiple in 20% of cases. Proximal aneurysms of the main splenic artery are usually solitary and are frequently associated with pancreatitis-related pseudocysts (Fig. 92-4).

Vascular calcifications on plain abdominal radiographs are often the first clinical evidence of a splenic artery aneurysm.[7] The most characteristic of these findings are signet-ring calcifications (Fig. 92-5). Contemporary diagnosis of splenic artery aneurysms usually follows their arteriographic demonstration during studies for nonvascular diseases. Ultrasonography, CT, and magnetic resonance imaging (MRI) occasionally establish the presence of these lesions and are often useful in identifying bleeding aneurysms. These noninvasive studies are most valuable for determining size changes in asymptomatic (bland) aneurysms.

Left upper quadrant or epigastric pain occurs in an occasional patient with an intact splenic artery aneurysm. In cases of rupture, bleeding is usually initially contained within the lesser sac, but free hemorrhage eventually occurs into the peritoneal cavity and causes vascular collapse. This represents the so-called double-rupture phenomenon attributed to splenic artery aneurysms. Pancreatitis-related aneurysms are not usually associated with intraperitoneal bleeding; more often, they are a source of intestinal hemorrhage after rupture into the stomach or pancreatic ductal system.[8-11] Arteriovenous fistula formation after rupture of a splenic artery aneurysm into an adjacent splenic vein is rare. Gastrointestinal hemorrhage from esophageal varices associated with left-sided portal hypertension may accompany these fistulas.

The risk of splenic artery aneurysm rupture depends on a number of confounding and poorly defined factors. In general, rupture of bland aneurysms occurs in less than 2% of cases.[3] Rupture appears just as likely when the aneu-

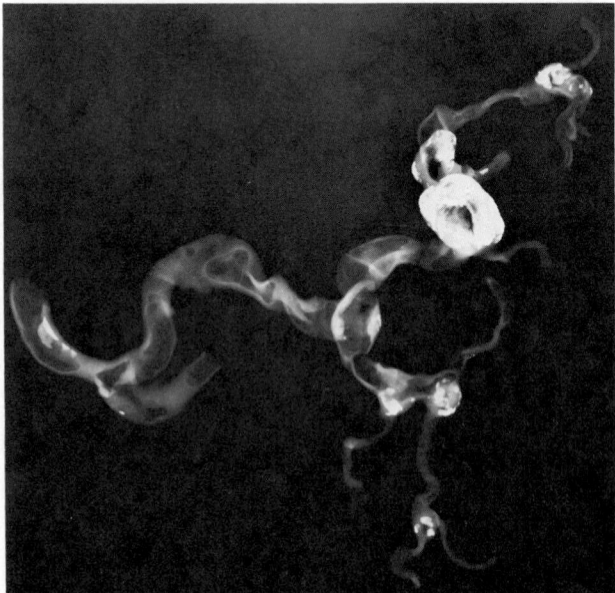

Figure 92-2. Splenic artery aneurysm. Marked calcific arteriosclerosis limited to splenic artery aneurysms occurring at vessel bifurcations (specimen roentgenogram) is seen. Intervening arterial segments are unaffected by advanced arteriosclerotic changes. (Stanley JC, Thompson NW, Fry WJ. Splanchnic artery aneurysms. Arch Surg 1970;101:689)

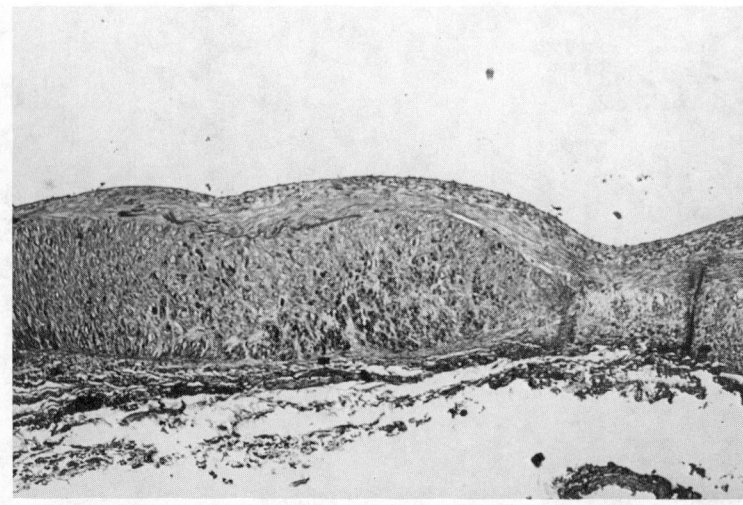

Figure 92-3. Splenic artery aneurysm exhibiting fragmentation of internal elastic lamina and medial dysplasia in patient having renal arterial fibrodysplasia (Masson stain, ×32). (Stanley JC, Fry WJ. Pathogenesis and clinical significance of splenic artery aneurysms. Surgery 1974;76:898)

rysm is calcified, occurs in a normotensive patient, or occurs in the very elderly patient. Pregnancy is a major risk factor; nearly 95% of aneurysms recognized during pregnancy have ruptured.[3,12,13] The maternal mortality rate approaches 75%, and the fetal mortality rate exceeds 95% in these cases.[14] Pregnancy-related rupture occurs most often during the third trimester (69%) and is less common during the first two trimesters (12%), during labor (13%), or postpartum (6%).[13] Given the fact that most women develop these aneurysms with repeated pregnancies, it is reasonable to assume that most aneurysms in pregnant women go unrecognized and do not rupture. Nevertheless, splenic artery aneurysms in pregnant patients must be considered a threat to the life of the mother and fetus.

The reported mortality rate accompanying operation for rupture of a splenic artery aneurysm is 25%.[4] Thus, it would seem ill advised to undertake elective operative intervention for an asymptomatic splenic artery aneurysm if the surgical mortality rate exceeds 0.5%. This latter figure represents the product of the known 25% risk of operative death and 2% rupture rate of bland aneurysms. If intervention becomes necessary in higher risk patients, then percutaneous transcatheter embolization of the aneurysm may represent an acceptable alternative.[15-17]

Splenectomy has been the most common form of surgical therapy for splenic artery aneurysms. Because of the immunologic importance of the spleen even in the aged, simple ligature obliteration or excision of these aneurysms appears preferable to splenectomy. As technologic advances continue, laporoscopic ligation of these aneurysms may prove quite feasible.[18] Treatment of splenic artery aneurysms embedded in pancreatic tissue may require distal pancreatectomy. In some of these cases, especially false aneurysms due to pseudocyst erosion into the artery, treatment may entail incising the aneurysmal sac and ligating entering and exiting vessels from within. Pancreatic resection or cyst drainage in these latter cases must be individualized and depends on the extent and chronicity of the associated pancreatic inflammatory disease.

HEPATIC ARTERY ANEURYSM

Hepatic artery aneurysms account for 20% of all previously reported splanchnic artery aneurysms[2,19] (Fig. 92-6). These aneurysms are being encountered more fre-

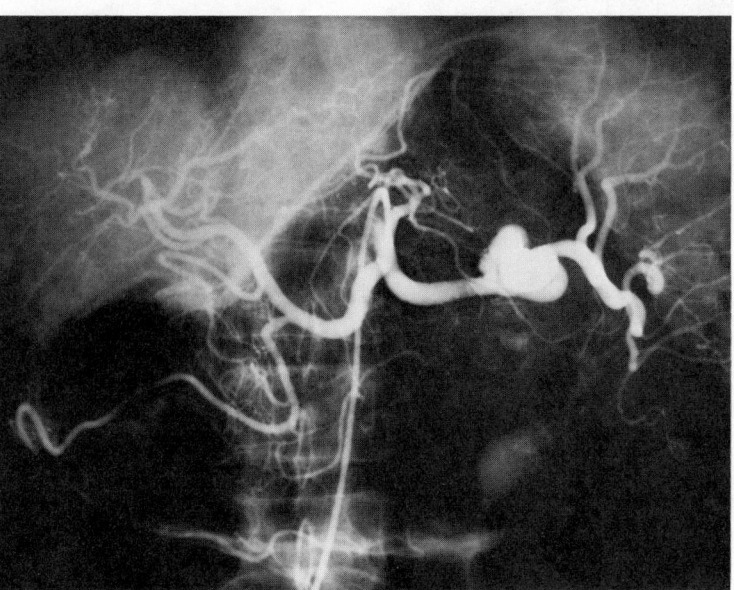

Figure 92-4. Splenic artery aneurysm. Arteriogram documents a pancreatitis-related aneurysm affecting the mid-splenic artery. (Stanley JC, Frey CF, Miller TA, et al. Major arterial hemorrhage: a complication of pancreatic pseudocysts and chronic pancreatitis. Arch Surg 1976;111:435)

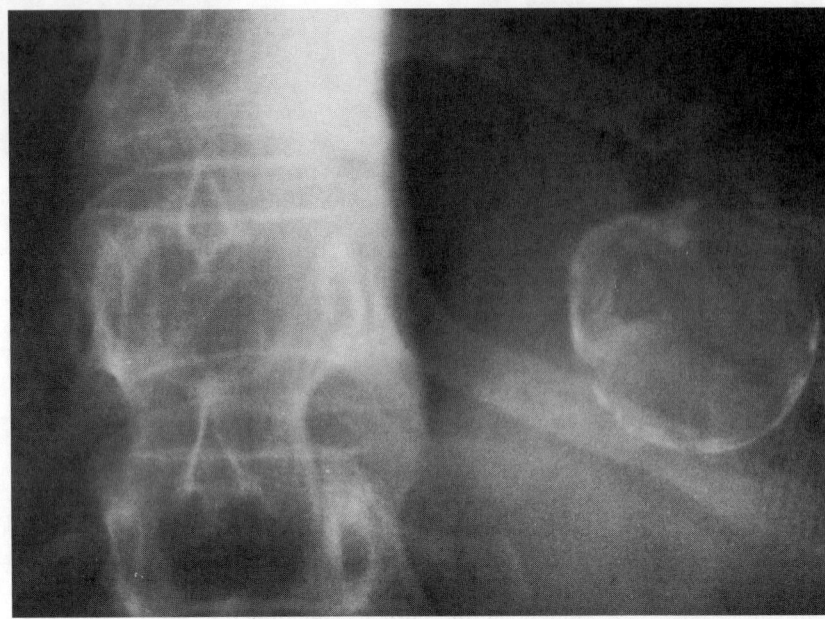

Figure 92-5. Splenic artery aneurysm. Curvilinear signet ring–like calcification in the left upper quadrant characteristic of a splenic artery aneurysms. (Stanley JC, Thompson NW, Fry WJ. Splanchnic artery aneurysms. Arch Surg 1970;101:689)

quently in contemporary times, and in some experiences, they outnumber splenic artery aneurysms. Men are twice as likely to be affected as women. Most noninfectious and nontraumatic aneurysms are usually first recognized during the sixth decade of life. The cause of many hepatic artery aneurysms is poorly defined. Two facts regarding the etiology of these aneurysms are noteworthy. First, arteriosclerosis most likely represents a secondary event rather than a primary cause of these aneurysms. Most of these lesions probably occur as a result of medial degeneration. Second, with increasing societal violence and intravenous substance abuse, the number of reported traumatic and infection-related aneurysms has markedly increased (Fig. 92-7). One of the most common causes of intrahepatic pseudoaneurysms is arterial injury accompanying invasive percutaneous diagnostic and therapeutic procedures involving penetration of the liver.[20,21] Systemic arteriopathies, such as periarteritis nodosa, have been incriminated as a cause of occasional macroaneurysms, but are more often associated with intraparenchymal microaneurysms.

Hepatic artery macroaneurysms are usually solitary. Large aneurysms tend to be saccular, and aneurysms less than 2 cm are usually fusiform. These aneurysms are extrahepatic in nearly 80% of cases and intrahepatic in 20%.

Hepatic artery aneurysms may be suspected because of displacement of or indentations on intestinal structures noted on barium contrast studies. Most contemporary diagnoses of these aneurysms result from their incidental recognition during arteriography, CT, or ultrasonography for nonvascular disease. Few hepatic artery aneurysms are symptomatic. When they become symptomatic, most present with right upper quadrant or epigastric pain. Rapid expansion of these aneurysms may cause severe discomfort similar to that of acute pancreatitis. Large aneurysms have been reported to cause obstructive jaundice, although most hepatic artery aneurysms are too small to compress the major bile ducts.[22] These lesions rarely present as pulsatile abdominal masses.

The reported incidence of hepatic artery aneurysm rupture approaches 20%, but the actual incidence may be less.

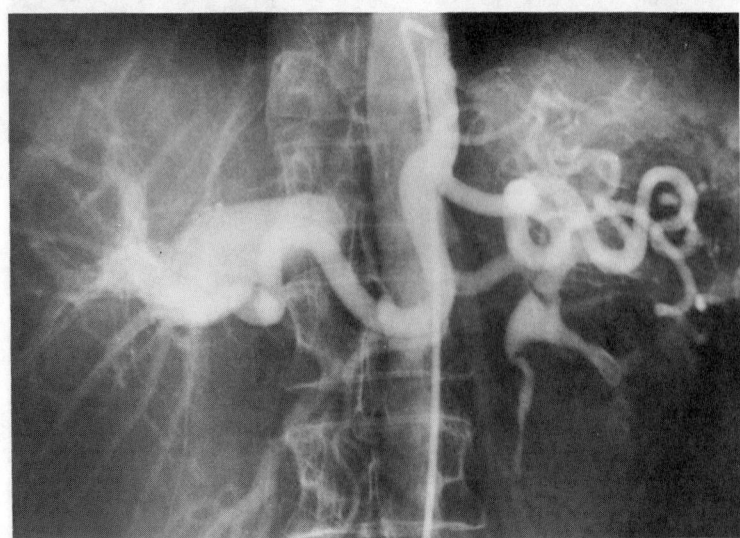

Figure 92-6. Hepatic artery aneurysm. Selective celiac arteriogram demonstrates a large saccular aneurysm at the bifurcation of the proper hepatic artery. (Stanley JC, Zelenock GB. Splanchnic artery aneurysms. In: Rutherford RB, ed. Vascular surgery. Philadelphia, WB Saunders, 1995:1124)

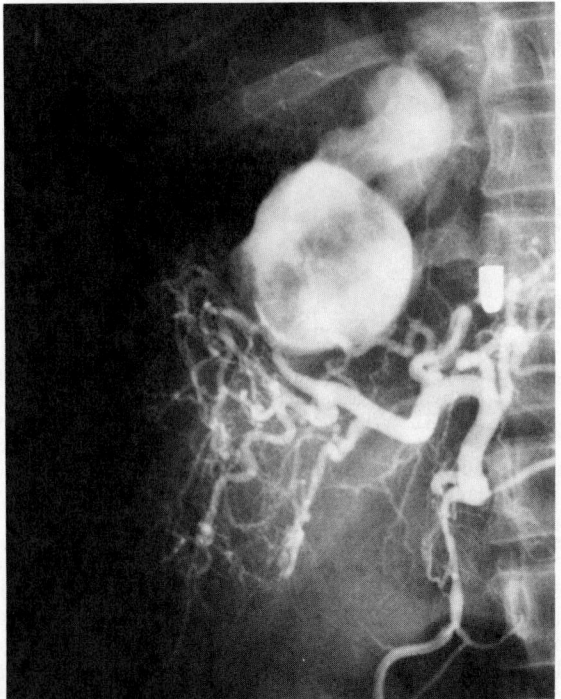

Figure 92-7. Traumatic hepatic artery aneurysm. Blunt abdominal injury and gunshot wounds cause most traumatic lesions. (Whitehouse WM Jr, Graham LM, Stanley JC. Aneurysms of the celiac, hepatic, and splenic arteries. In: Bergan JJ, Yao JST, eds. Aneurysms: diagnosis and treatment. New York, Grune & Stratton, 1981:405)

It is certainly less than the often-quoted rupture rate of 44% in cases reported a few decades ago.[4] Aneurysm rupture is associated with a 35% mortality rate. Bleeding from ruptured hepatic artery aneurysms occurs with equal frequency into the biliary tract and peritoneal cavity. Hemobilia accompanies the former, being manifest by biliary colic, hematemesis, and jaundice.[23] Chronic, relatively asymptomatic hemorrhage is an uncommon sequela of aneurysm rupture into the biliary tract. Intraperitoneal bleeding is usually due to rupture of inflammatory-related false aneurysms.

Common hepatic artery aneurysms may often be treated by aneurysmectomy or aneurysm exclusion, without arterial reconstruction. The extensive hepatic arterial collateral circulation and the parallel portal venous circulation often ensure adequate blood flow to the liver with interruption of the proximal common hepatic artery. Liver necrosis is more likely to follow ligation of arteries in the more distal hepatic circulation. Nevertheless, even in the latter vessels, complex arterial reconstructions should be avoided and simple ligation undertaken if temporary intraoperative occlusion of the involved artery does not result in obvious hepatic ischemia. If liver blood flow appears inadequate with such a maneuver, then hepatic artery reconstruction should be undertaken using either prosthetic or autologous vein grafts. In the case of intraparenchymal aneurysms, hepatic territory resection may be necessary therapy. However, percutaneous transcatheter obliteration of the aneurysm with balloons, coils, or nonreabsorbable thrombogenic matter, may be preferable to surgical intervention in many patients.[16,21]

SUPERIOR MESENTERIC ARTERY ANEURYSM

Aneurysms of the proximal superior mesenteric artery (SMA) account for 5.5% of all splanchnic artery aneurysms.[2] These lesions occur in men and women equally.

Infection from a cardiac source is the most common cause of these aneurysms.[24] Nonhemolytic streptococci, as well as many common pathogens accompanying parenteral substance abuse, cause bacterial endocarditis and are the underlying source of infection in these cases. Many of these aneurysms are associated with intramural dissections (Fig. 92-8). SMA aneurysms may also be caused by medial degeneration, periarterial inflammation, and trauma. Arteriosclerosis, as in the case of other splanchnic aneurysms, is usually a secondary process. SMA aneurysms have been recognized in contemporary times most often during arteriographic studies for nonvascular disease.

Although many patients with SMA aneurysms are asymptomatic, an equal number have abdominal discomfort, often suggestive of intestinal angina. SMA aneurysm rupture is rare.[25] The mortality rate with rupture approaches 50%. Gastrointestinal hemorrhage associated with these aneurysms often accompanies their acute occlusion with bleeding into areas of intestinal infarction. Location of most aneurysms near the origins of the inferior pancreaticoduodenal and middle colic arteries isolates the distal mesenteric circulation when dissections or occlusions occur. In these circumstances, intestinal ischemia develops because the usual collateral network from the adjacent celiac and inferior mesenteric arterial circulations is lost.

Operative management of SMA aneurysms is best accomplished by aneurysmectomy or aneurysm exclusion, followed by intestinal revascularization with an aortomesenteric graft. Because of potential infection when bowel ischemia is present, autologous vein or artery is favored over prosthetic conduits for these reconstructions. Aneurysmorrhaphy may be performed in certain cases.[26]

SMA aneurysm ligation without arterial reconstruction may be successful in patients who have developed an ade-

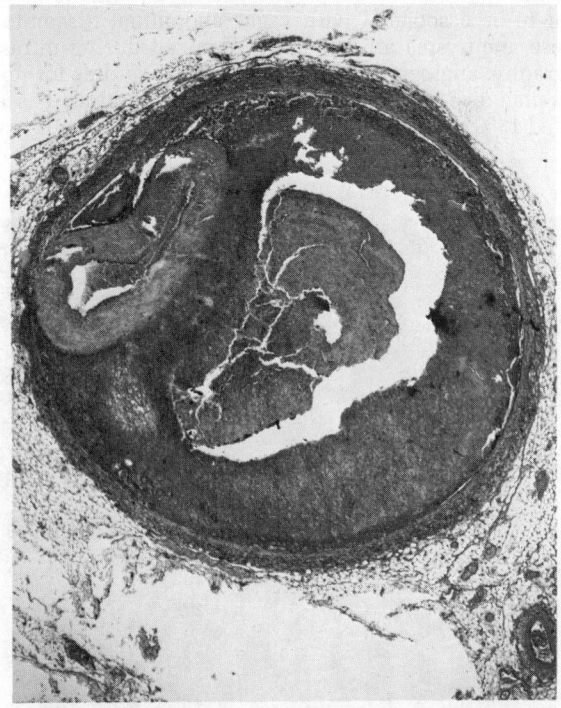

Figure 92-8. Superior mesenteric artery aneurysm. Microscopic cross-section of a dissecting aneurysm affecting the proximal superior mesenteric artery (hematoxylin-eosin, ×20). (Stanley JC, Zelenock GB. Splanchnic artery aneurysms. In: Rutherford RB, ed. Vascular surgery. Philadelphia, WB Saunders, 1995:1124)

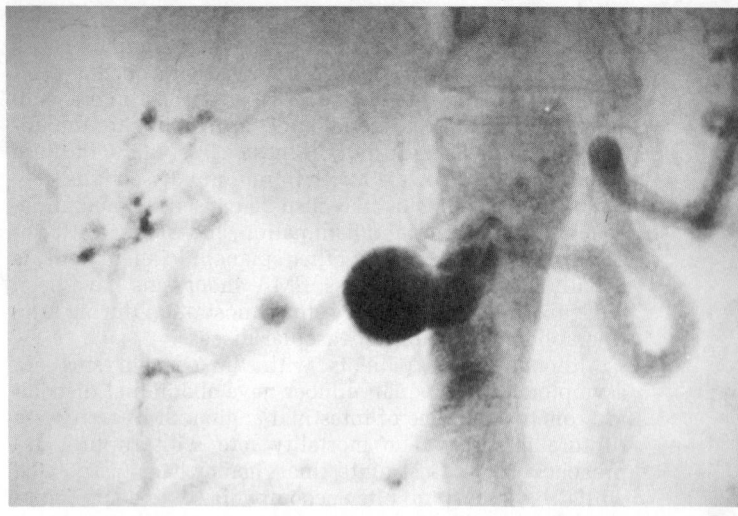

Figure 92-9. Celiac artery aneurysm. Aortogram reveals saccular aneurysm that exhibited medial degenerative changes and secondary arteriosclerosis. (Stanley JC, Whitehouse WM Jr. Aneurysms of the splanchnic and renal arteries. In: Bergan JJ, Yao JST, eds. Surgery of the aorta and its body branches. Orlando, Grune & Stratton, 1979:497)

quate collateral circulation to their midguts. In fact, ligation and aneurysmorrhaphy have been the most commonly reported means of managing these aneurysms.[27] Temporary intraoperative occlusion of the SMA with Doppler documentation of adequate intestinal blood flow should be undertaken before proceeding to ligation of the SMA.

CELIAC ARTERY ANEURYSM

Celiac artery aneurysms account for 4% of all splanchnic artery aneurysms.[2,28] Men and women appear equally affected. Most aneurysms encountered in contemporary times have been associated with medial degeneration. Arteriosclerosis is a common histologic finding that is considered a secondary event rather than an etiologic process. Celiac artery aneurysms are usually saccular, and most are located in the distal vessel (Fig. 92-9).

Most celiac artery aneurysms are asymptomatic or appear to be associated with vague abdominal discomfort. These aneurysms are usually recognized during ultrasonography, angiography, or other imaging studies for nonvascular diseases. In more recent times, rupture has affected 13% of these aneurysms and carried a mortality rate of 50%.[28] In contrast, rupture rates published before 1950 were often higher than 80%. Rupture usually causes exsanguinating intraperitoneal hemorrhage. Although rare, gastrointestinal bleeding may follow rupture of the aneurysm into the stomach or pancreatic ductal system.

Aneurysmectomy with celiac artery reconstruction is the preferred treatment for these lesions, although aneurysm exclusion with ligation of its branches has been performed successfully in select patients.[28,29] When simple ligature is undertaken, the adequacy of the liver's collateral circulation must be documented. If liver ischemia is apparent after temporary intraoperative celiac artery occlusion, then hepatic revascularization becomes mandatory. An aortoceliac artery bypass in these circumstances is best performed with either an autologous vein or prosthetic graft. Surgical therapy of celiac artery aneurysmal disease has been successful in more than 90% of cases.

GASTRIC AND GASTROEPIPLOIC ARTERY ANEURYSMS

Gastric and gastroepiploic artery aneurysms account for 4% of all splanchnic artery aneurysms[2] (Fig. 92-10). Gastric artery aneurysms occur 10 times more often than gas-

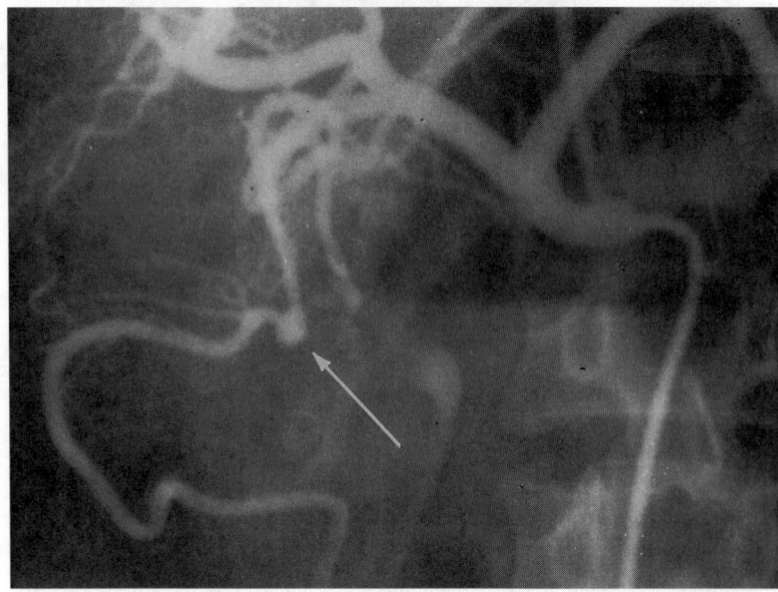

Figure 92-10. Gastroepiploic artery aneurysm. Selective celiac arteriogram revealing small aneurysm responsible for massive gastrointestinal hemorrhage. (Stanley JC, Thompson NW, Fry WJ. Splanchnic artery aneurysms. Arch Surg 1970; 101:689)

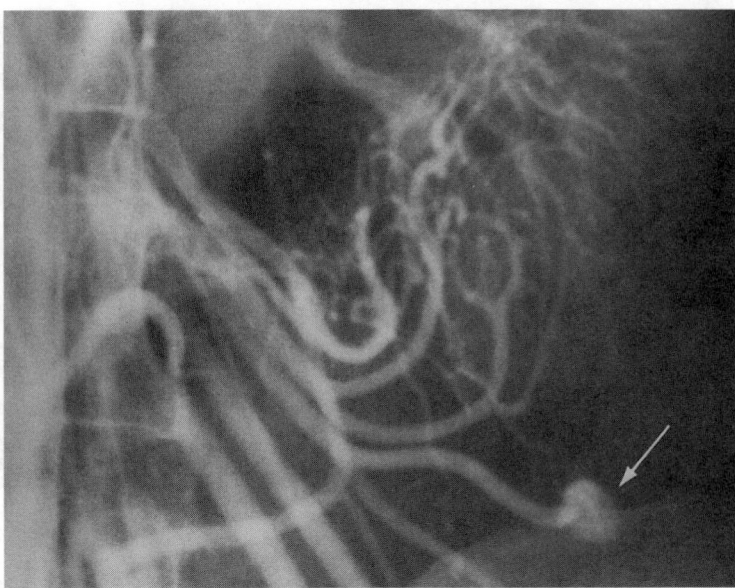

Figure 92-11. Ileal artery aneurysm. Mesenteric arteriogram documenting saccular aneurysm of distal ileal artery (Stanley JC, Zelenock GB. Splanchnic artery aneurysms. In: Rutherford RB, ed. Vascular surgery. Philadelphia, WB Saunders, 1995:1124)

troepiploic artery aneurysms. Men are three times more likely than women to develop these aneurysms. Most of these perigastric lesions have been encountered in patients more than 50 years of age. These aneurysms usually are solitary, occurring as a result of periarterial inflammation or medial degeneration. In many cases, there is an antecedent history of peptic ulcer disease. Arteriosclerosis, when present, is considered a secondary event, not a cause of these lesions.

Most reported gastric or gastroepiploic artery aneurysms have been symptomatic when initially recognized, frequently presenting as emergencies.[30] Rupture has accompanied more than 90% of reported cases, with gastrointestinal bleeding occurring slightly more than twice as often as intraperitoneal hemorrhage. Rupture carries a 70% mortality rate.[4]

Surgical treatment is recommended for all gastric and gastroepiploic artery aneurysms. Vascular reconstructive surgery is not required in these cases. Intramural gastric aneurysms may be excised with a small segment of involved stomach, whereas extramural aneurysms can be treated by arterial ligation alone, with or without aneurysm excision. Certain lesions may be treated by a laporoscopic approach.[31] Intraoperative identification of these small aneurysms is often tedious if preoperative localization has not been established by arteriographic studies.

JEJUNAL, ILEAL, AND COLIC ARTERY ANEURYSMS

Aneurysms of the jejunal, ileal, and colic arteries account for 3% of all splanchnic artery aneurysms[2] (Fig. 92-11). They usually occur in patients more than 60 years of age, with men and women affected equally. Multiple aneurysms have been encountered in 10% of cases. Acquired medial defects cause most of these lesions. Although arteriosclerosis is present with 20% of these aneurysms, it is considered to represent a secondary event, not an etiologic process. An increasing number of mycotic aneurysms affect these vessels, developing as the sequela of infected emboli originating from subacute bacterial endocarditis.[32] Periarteritis nodosa is a common underlying cause of multiple aneurysms affecting these intestinal branch arteries.[33] Inferior mesenteric artery aneurysms are

so rare and the etiology so varied that their clinical importance has not been clearly established.[34]

Many aneurysms of these vessels are first recognized as incidental findings during arteriography for gastrointestinal bleeding. Jejunal, ileal, and colic artery aneurysms are reported to have ruptured in 30% of cases, but actual rupture rates are probably a third of those previously published. Rupture continues to be associated with a mortality

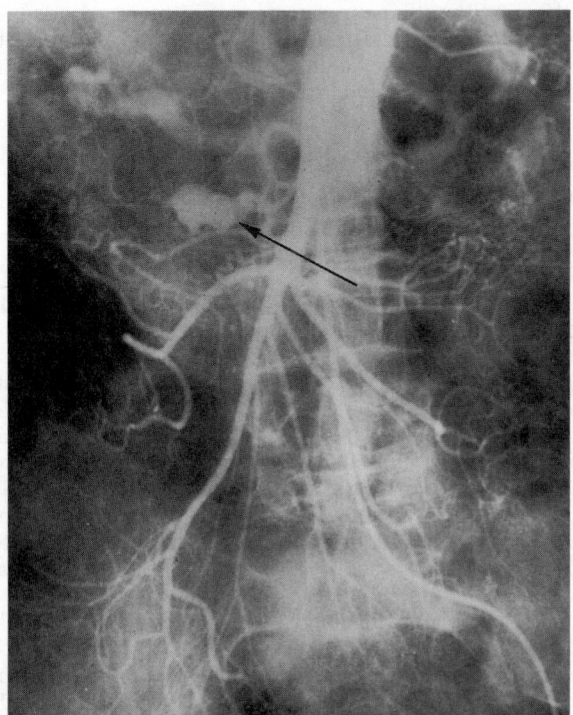

Figure 92-12. Inferior pancreaticoduodenal artery aneurysm. Selective superior mesenteric arteriogram revealing false aneurysm secondary to pseudocyst erosion of artery. (Stanley JC, Frey CF, Miller TA, et al. Major arterial hemorrhage: a complication of pancreatic pseudocysts and chronic pancreatitis. Arch Surg 1976;111:435)

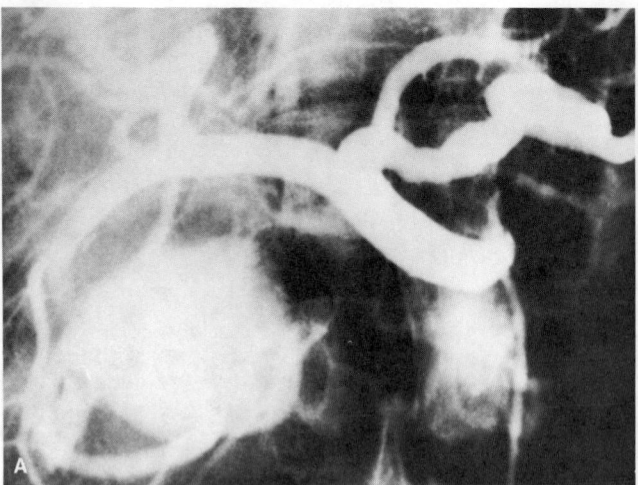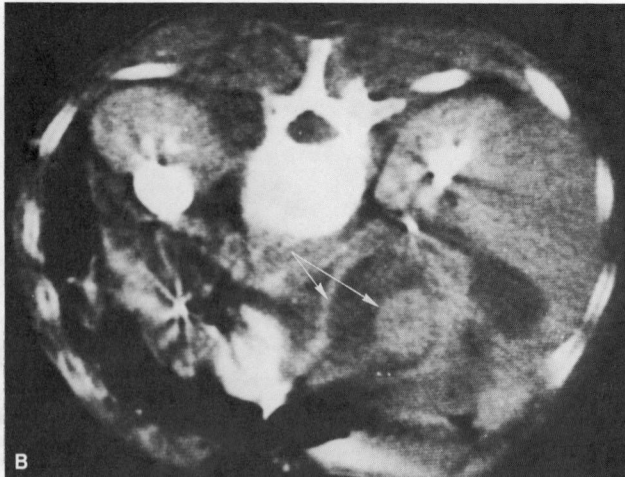

Figure 92-13. Gastroduodenal artery aneurysm. (*A*) Selective celiac arteriogram. (*B*) CT scan of a pancreatic pseudocyst (*short arrow*) containing the aneurysm (*long arrow*). (Eckhauser FE, Stanley JC, Zelenock GB, et al. Gastroduodenal and pancreaticoduodenal artery aneurysms: a complication of pancreatitis causing spontaneous gastrointestinal hemorrhage. Surgery 1980;88:335)

rate of 20%.[4] Aneurysmal rupture usually occurs into the gastrointestinal tract. Rupture into the mesentery or peritoneal cavity is uncommon. Regardless of this fact, these small mesenteric branch aneurysms are more apt to cause abdominal apoplexy than any other splanchnic artery aneurysm.

Operation for intestinal branch aneurysms is recommended in all instances, except for treating bland aneurysms associated with connective-tissue diseases. Expeditious surgical therapy requires careful preoperative localization with arteriographic studies. Arterial ligation, with or without aneurysmectomy, is recommended in treating extraintestinal lesions, whereas intramural aneurysms and those associated with bowel infarction require resection of the involved intestine.

PANCREATICODUODENAL, PANCREATIC, AND GASTRODUODENAL ARTERY ANEURYSMS

Pancreatic and pancreaticoduodenal artery aneurysms (Fig. 92-12) account for 2% of all splanchnic artery aneurysms, and gastroduodenal artery aneurysms (Fig. 92-13) represent an additional 1.5% of these aneurysms.[2] Men are four times more likely than women to develop these lesions. Most patients with these aneurysms are older than 50 years. Most of these lesions are associated with pancreatitis-related vascular necrosis or vessel erosion by an adjacent pancreatic pseudocyst. Medial degeneration and trauma are less common causes of these aneurysms. Arteriosclerosis is invariably a secondary, not a causative, process.

These peripancreatic aneurysms are often difficult to diagnose and treat. Most are associated with epigastric pain and discomfort, which may be due to the underlying pancreatic inflammatory disease that accompanies about 60% of gastroduodenal and 30% of pancreaticoduodenal artery aneurysms.

Gastroduodenal and pancreaticoduodenal aneurysm rupture has affected more than half of the reported cases, occurring in 75% of inflammatory and 50% of noninflammatory lesions. Hemorrhage usually occurs into the

stomach, the biliary tract, or pancreatic ductal system; bleeding into the peritoneal cavity is less likely. Arteriography usually establishes the presence of these aneurysms, but CT scanning and MRI are of increasing importance in their recognition. These latter noninvasive studies are especially important in detecting rupture or associated pancreatic pathology. The mortality rate with rupture approaches 50% despite operative intervention.

Surgical treatment is recommended for all but the poorest risk patients with gastroduodenal, pancreaticoduodenal, or pancreatic arterial aneurysms.[35–38] Pancreatitis-related false aneurysms are usually treated by arterial ligation from within the aneurysmal sac, rather than extraaneurysmal arterial ligation. Extensive dissection of the pancreas affected by dense inflammatory adhesions in such circumstances is hazardous. In situations in which a pancreatic pseudocyst or abscess has eroded the artery, a drainage procedure should be undertaken. Distal pancreatectomy, or even pancreaticoduodenectomy, may be the safest mode of treatment in select cases. Transcatheter embolization and electrocoagulation have been recommended for treating very high-risk patients with these aneurysms.[39] Unfortunately, rebleeding after such therapy decreases the usefulness of this type of intervention.[40]

REFERENCES

1. Jorgensen BA. Visceral artery aneurysms: a review. Dan Med Bull 1985;32:237.
2. Stanley JC, Zelenock GB. Splanchnic artery aneurysms. In: Rutherford RB, ed. Vascular surgery, ed 3. Philadelphia, WB Saunders, 1995:1124.
3. Stanley JC, Fry WJ. Pathogenesis and clinical significance of splenic artery aneurysms. Surgery 1974;76:898.
4. Stanley JC, Thompson NW, Fry WJ. Splanchnic artery aneurysms. Arch Surg 1970;101:689.
5. Nishida O, Moriyasu F, Nakamura T, et al. Hemodynamics of splenic artery aneurysm. Gastroenterology 1986;90:1042.
6. Ayalon A, Wiesner RH, Perkins JD, et al. Splenic artery aneurysms in liver transplant patients. Transplantation 1988; 45:386.
7. Trastek VF, Pairolero PC, Joyce JW, et al. Splenic artery aneurysms. Surgery 1982;91:694.
8. deVries JE, Schattenkerk ME, Malt RA. Complications of splenic artery aneurysm other than intraperitoneal rupture. Surgery 1982;91:200.

9. Stabile BE, Wilson SE, Debas HT. Reduced mortality from bleeding pseudocysts and pseudoaneurysms caused by pancreatitis. Arch Surg 1983;118:45.

10. Stanley JC, Frey CF, Miller TA, et al. Major arterial hemorrhage: a complication of pancreatic pseudocysts and chronic pancreatitis. Arch Surg 1976;111:435.

11. Wagner WH, Cossman DV, Treiman RL, et al. Hemosuccus pancreaticus from intraductal rupture of a primary splenic artery aneurysm. J Vasc Surg 1 994;19:158.

12. Lowry SM, O'Dea TP, Gallagher DI, et al. Splenic artery aneurysm rupture: the seventh instance of maternal and fetal survival. Obstet Gynecol 1986;67:291.

13. MacFarlane JR, Thorbjarnason B. Rupture of splenic artery aneurysm during pregnancy. Am J Obstet Gynecol 1966; 95:1025.

14. Cailloutte JC, Merchant EB. Ruptured splenic artery aneurysm in pregnancy. Twelfth reported case with maternal and fetal survival. Am J Obstet Gynecol 1993;168:1810.

15. Baker KS, Tisnado J, Cho SR, et al. Splanchnic artery aneurysms and pseudoaneurysms: transcatheter embolization. Radiology 1987;163:135.

16. Salam TA, Lumsden AB, Martin LG, et al. Nonoperative management of visceral aneurysms and pseudoaneurysms. Am J Surg 1992;164:215.

17. Waltman AC, Luers PR, Athanasoulis CA, et al. Massive arterial hemorrhage in patients with pancreatitis: complementary roles of surgery and transcatheter occlusive techniques. Arch Surg 1986;121:439.

18. Hashizume M, Ohta M, Veno K, et al. Laparoscopic ligation of splenic artery aneurysm. Surgery 1993;113:352.

19. Guida PM, Moore SW. Aneurysm of the hepatic artery: report of five cases with a brief review of the previously reported cases. Surgery 1966;60:299.

20. Czerniak A, Thompson JN, Hemingway AP, et al. Hemobilia: a disease in evolution. Arch Surg 1988;23:718.

21. Okazaki M, Higashihara H, Ono H, et al. Percutaneous embolization of ruptured splanchnic artery pseudoaneurysms. Acta Radiologica 1991;32:349.

22. Lal RB, Strohl JA, Piazza S, et al. Hepatic artery aneurysm. J Cardiovasc Surg 1989;30:509.

23. Stauffer JT, Weinman MD, Bynum TE. Hemobilia in a patient with multiple hepatic artery aneurysms: a case report and review of the literature. Am J Gastroenterol 1989;84:59.

24. Friedman SG, Pogo GJ, Moccio CG. Mycotic aneurysm of the superior mesenteric artery. J Vasc Surg 1987;6:87.

25. Blumenberg RM, David D, Skovak J. Abdominal apoplexy due to rupture of a superior mesenteric artery aneurysm: clip aneurysmorrhaphy with survival. Arch Surg 1974;108:223.

26. Olcott C, Ehrenfeld WK. Endoaneurysmorrhaphy for visceral artery aneurysms. Am J Surg 1977;133:636.

27. DeBakey ME, Cooley DA. Successful resection of mycotic aneurysm of superior mesenteric artery: case report and review of the literature. Am J Surg 1953;19:202.

28. Graham LM, Stanley JC, Whitehouse WM Jr., et al. Celiac artery aneurysms: historical (1745–1949) versus contemporary (1950-1984) differences in etiology and clinical importance. J Vasc Surg 1985;2:757.

29. Hertzer NR, Mullally PH. Celiac artery aneurysmectomy with hepatic artery ligation. Arch Surg 1972;104:337.

30. Witte JT, Hasson JE, Harms BA, et al. Fatal gastric dissection and rupture occurring as a paraesophageal mass: a case report and literature review. Surgery 1990;107:590.

31. Uchikoshi F, Sakamoto T, Imabunn S, et al. Aneurysm of the right gastroepiploic artery: a case report of laporoscopic resection. Cardiovasc Surg 1993;1:550.

32. Trevisani MF, Ricci MA, Michaels RM, et al. Multiple mesenteric aneurysms complicating subacute bacterial endocarditis. Arch Surg 1987;122:823.

33. Selke FW, Williams GB, Donovan DL, et al. Management of intra-abdominal aneurysms associated with periarteritis nodosa. J Vasc Surg 1986;4:294.

34. Graham LM, Hay MR, Cho KJ, et al. Inferior mesenteric artery aneurysms. Surgery 1985;97:158.

35. Eckhauser FE, Stanley JC, Zelenock GB, et al. Gastroduodenal and pancreaticoduodenal artery aneurysms: a complication of pancreatitis causing spontaneous gastrointestinal hemorrhage. Surgery 1980;88:335.

36. Chiou AC, Josephs LG, Menzoian JO. Inferior pancreaticoduodenal artery aneurysm: report of a case and review of the literature. J Vasc Surg 1993;17:784.

37. Gadacz TR, Trunkey D, Kieffer RF. Visceral vessel erosion associated with pancreatitis: case reports and a review of the literature. Arch Surg 1978;113:1438.

38. Iyomasa S, Matsuzaki Y, Hiei K, et al. Pancreaticoduodenal artery aneurysm: a case report and review of the literature. J Vasc Surg 1995;22:161.

39. Mandel SR, Jaques PF, Mauro MA, et al. Nonoperative management of peripancreatic arterial aneurysms: a 10-year experience. Ann Surg 1987;205:126.

40. Lina JR, Jaques P, Mandell V. Aneurysm rupture secondary to transcatheter embolization. AJR 1979;132:553.

SURGERY: SCIENTIFIC PRINCIPLES AND PRACTICE, Second Edition, edited by Lazar J. Greenfield, Michael W. Mulholland, Keith T. Oldham, Gerald B. Zelenock, and Keith D. Lillemoe. Lippincott–Raven Publishers, Philadelphia, © 1997.

CHAPTER 93

RENAL ARTERY ANEURYSMS

JAMES C. STANLEY

Aneurysms of the renal artery are unusual vascular lesions that have been encountered with increasing frequency.[1-7] Although our understanding of these aneurysms has improved, their clinical importance is still controversial.[7-10] In part, this relates to the fact that complications of these aneurysms have been overestimated in reports that usually describe operative experiences rather than population-based experiences. Other misperceptions regarding the importance of these aneurysms reflect unrecognized differences among their four principal categories: (1) true renal artery aneurysms,[7] (2) dissecting renal artery aneurysms,[11,12] (3) aneurysmal dilations occurring with medial fibrodysplastic disease,[13] and (4) arteritis-related microaneurysms.[14] The two renal artery macroaneurysms most relevant to clinical practice, true aneurysms and those associated with dissections, deserve individual discussion (Table 93-1).

TRUE RENAL ARTERY ANEURYSMS

The precise incidence of true renal artery aneurysms in the general population approaches 0.09%. This figure was derived in the mid-1970s from incidental demonstration of these aneurysms in some 8500 patients subjected to arteriographic studies for nonrenal disease at the University of Michigan.[7] The group being studied bears greatly on the reported frequency of these lesions. For example, macroaneurysms were identified in 0.7% of patients undergoing arteriographic studies directed at renal disease,[15] and in 2.5% of those being evaluated for hypertension.[7] The occurrence of these lesions in 9.2% of hypertensive adults with renal artery fibrodysplasia emphasizes the importance of patient selection in determining their incidence.[13]

Women are affected with renal artery aneurysms 1.2 times more often than men. However, when aneurysms in patients with arterial fibrodysplasia are excluded there appears to be no gender predilection. Furthermore, the predisposition of these aneurysms to affect the right renal

Table 93-1. **TRUE AND DISSECTING RENAL ARTERY ANEURYSMS**

Lesion	Males/Females	Contributing Factors	Rate of Rupture	Mortality With Rupture	Treatment
True aneurysm	1/1.2	Congenital defects Arterial fibrodysplasia Hypertension	3%	10% (during pregnancy— 55% maternal, 85% fetal)	Aneurysmectomy with renal artery reconstruction Aneurysmorrhaphy Nephrectomy for ruptured aneurysms
Dissecting aneurysm	10/1	Blunt trauma Arterial catheterization Arterial fibrodysplasia Arteriosclerosis	Uncommon	Undefined	Renal artery reconstruction

artery may be a reflection of the greater incidence of right-sided medial fibrodysplastic disease in women.[13]

True renal artery aneurysms are usually located at renal artery bifurcations (Fig. 93-1). Most of these aneurysms are saccular. The average diameter of true aneurysms in one large series was 1.3 cm.[13] Extraparenchymal aneurysms are very common, accounting for more than 90% of cases, with more than 75% occurring at first- or second-order branchings of the main renal artery.

Two distinct histologic categories of true renal artery aneurysms exist. The first type appears to be associated with a congenital elastic tissue defect or medial degenerative process (Fig. 93-2). Internal elastic lamina fragmentation, excessive accumulations of collagen and other ground substances, a paucity of elastic tissue, and a loss

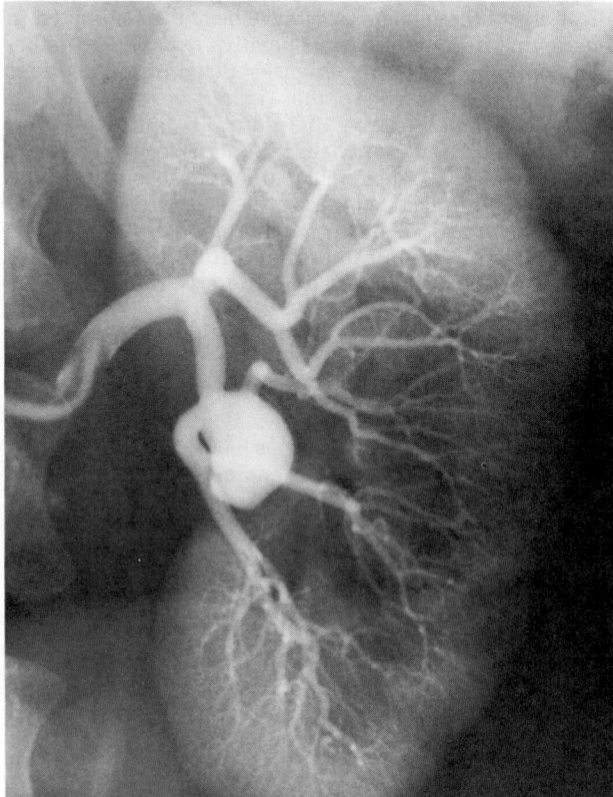

Figure 93-1. Renal artery aneurysm at a second-order branch. (Stanley JC, Whitehouse WM Jr. Renal artery macroaneurysms. In: Bergan JJ, Yao JST, eds. Aneurysms. New York, Grune & Stratton 1982:417)

of recognizable medial smooth muscle characterize these lesions.

The second type of aneurysm exhibits arteriosclerosis (Fig. 93-3). Hemorrhage, calcium deposition, collections of cholesterol, necrotic debris, and a matrix of fibrous tissue typify these lesions. Such atheromatous changes often occur at irregular intervals in these aneurysms, with intervening areas composed of thin, collagenous acellular fibrous tissue. Severe arteriosclerosis of the adjacent renal artery is uncommon. When present in an aneurysm, arteriosclerosis is considered a secondary event rather than a primary etiologic event. The fact that arteriosclerotic changes affect some but not all aneurysms in patients who have multiple lesions suggests a nonarteriosclerotic cause of most renal artery aneurysms.[7,15]

Both congenital and acquired factors appear to contribute to the formation of true renal artery aneurysms. Discontinuity of the internal elastic lamina is a common finding at branchings of normal muscular arteries. The fenestrations resulting from these discontinuities may contribute to the development of aneurysms considered congenital in origin. The reported increase in the frequency of aneurysms with age is a likely sequela of further loss of the integrity of the elastic tissue at these already weakened branchings.[15]

The high incidence of renal artery aneurysms associated with medial fibrodysplasia is well recognized (Fig. 93-4). In the latter disease state, further fragmentation and disruption of elastic tissue with loss of smooth muscle at bifurcations leaves little more than a thin layer of fibrous connective tissue to contain blood flow. The greater incidence of aneurysms among patients with hypertension secondary to dysplastic renal artery stenoses, in comparison with those with arteriosclerotic stenoses, supports the tenet that arterial fibrodysplasia is a direct contributor to aneurysmal changes.[7]

Blood pressure elevations occur in 80% of patients with renal artery macroaneurysms and may also play a role in aneurysm development. Increased mural tension in these cases, especially in the presence of preexisting internal elastic deficiencies at bifurcations, may further compromise the structural integrity of the renal artery.

In the case of pediatric patients, most aneurysms occur in poststenotic locations.[16,17] Most of these latter aneurysms have an amorphous globular configuration with thinning of all vessel wall elements. The more typical saccular aneurysms seen at bifurcations in older patients account for approximately a third of renal artery aneurysms seen in childhood.

Clinical manifestations of intact renal artery aneurysms are poorly defined. Most renal artery aneurysms appear to be asymptomatic.[8-10] Aneurysmal expansion, compression of nearby structures, and renal infarction from dislodged thrombus may cause flank or abdominal pain. Hematuria

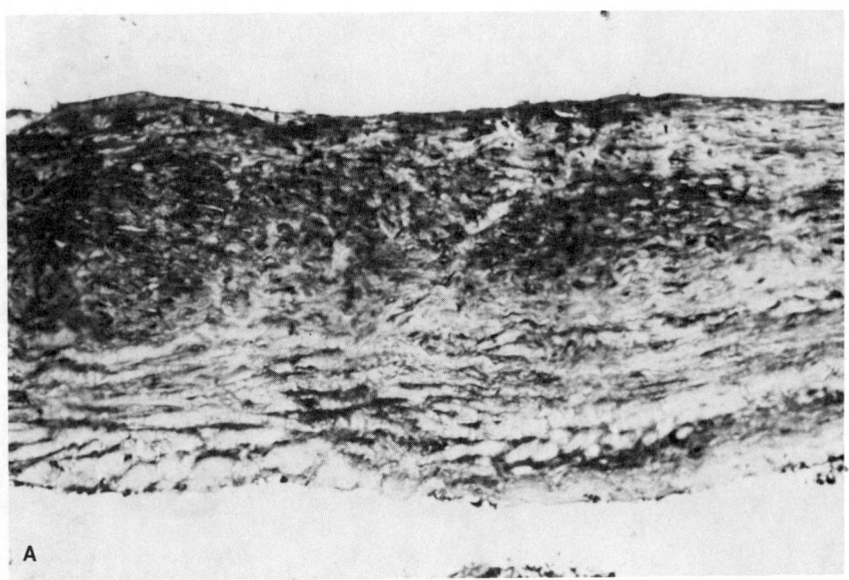

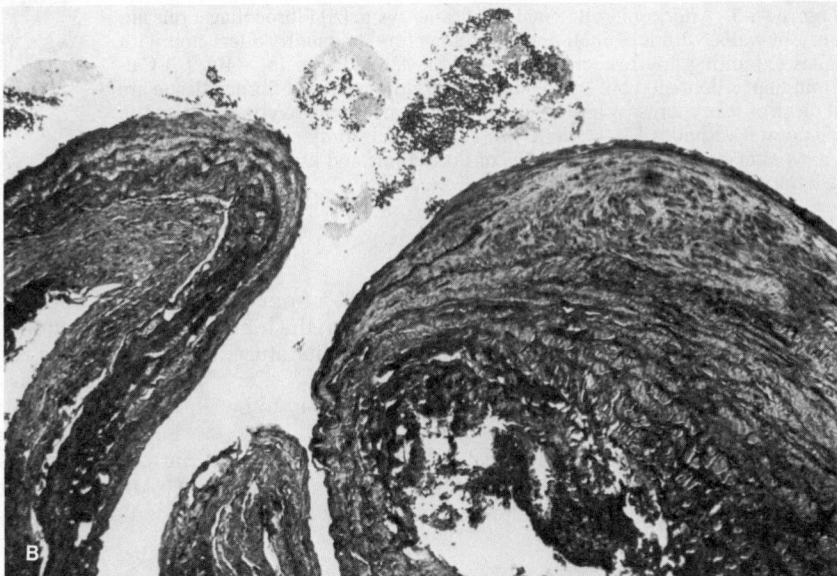

Figure 93-2. Renal artery aneurysm of undetermined etiology. (*A*) Excessive collagen and accumulation of ground substance with loss of smooth muscle characterize most such aneurysmal walls (Movat stain, ×40). (*B*) Interruption of internal elastic lamina (*arrow*) demonstrated at orifice of saccular renal artery aneurysm. Defects in elastic lamella have been related to the development of renal artery aneurysms (Movat stain, ×60). (Stanley JC, Rhodes EL, Gewertz BL, et al. Renal artery aneurysms: significance of macroaneurysms exclusive of dissections and fibrodysplastic mural dilations. Arch Surg 1975;110:1327)

and abdominal bruits have been attributed to certain of these lesions, but in most instances, these findings result from nonaneurysmal disease. Although quite rare, covert rupture of renal artery aneurysms into an adjacent vein may be associated with hematuria and hypertension.

The potential for renal artery aneurysms to cause hypertension has been a subject of continual controversy.[5,6,18–20] Embolization of aneurysmal thrombus or thrombotic occlusion of an adjacent artery may result in renal ischemia and renovascular hypertension (Fig. 93-5). This is uncommon. Atheromatous plaque ulceration within large aneurysmal sacs may predispose to embolic complications. This was a clear cause of secondary hypertension in only 3 of 118 patients with renal artery aneurysms in one series.[7] If the kidney segment affected by embolization is totally infarcted, the patient may not become hypertensive. However, if the tissue simply becomes hypoperfused, then it may be the source of considerable renin and the cause of severe secondary hypertension. Small aneurysms without calcific arteriosclerosis are less likely sources of such renal arterial occlusions. Compression or kinking of a neighboring artery causing flow reductions have been proposed

as causes of renovascular hypertension but have rarely been documented in the literature.[21]

Renal artery occlusive disease in the vicinity of aneurysms may account for certain cases of secondary hypertension in these patients. Because of this possibility, one should search for existence of occult stenoses in hypertensive patients with aneurysms. Assessments of renin activity with determination of renal:systemic renin indices among patients with hypertension and isolated renal artery aneurysms may establish the presence of renovascular hypertension.

Rupture is the most serious complication attending renal artery aneurysms. Exsanguinating hemorrhage from a ruptured renal artery aneurysm occurs less often than suggested in earlier reports.[3,4,22] The mortality rate with rupture is approximately 10%. Loss of a kidney is a near universal outcome of rupture.[7,20] Rupture among renal artery aneurysms approaches 3%, according to the literature. This relatively high rupture rate likely reflects the surgical nature of most published experiences. In fact, overt extraparenchymal rupture occurred in 2.8% of patients harboring these lesions, and covert rupture causing renal arterio-

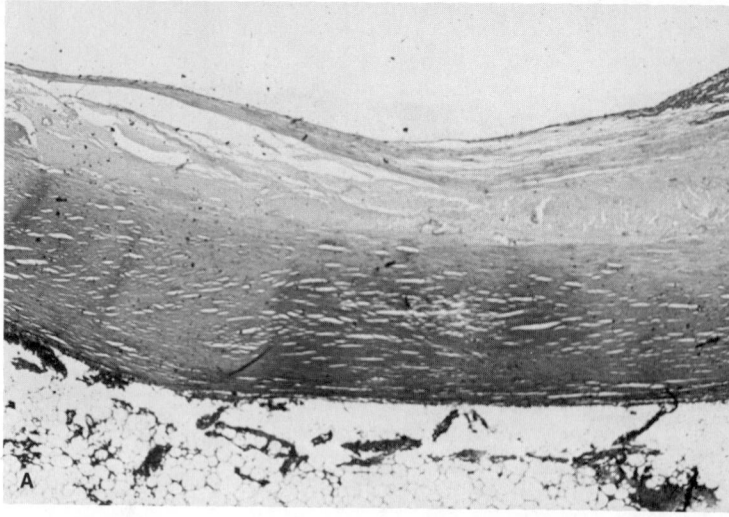

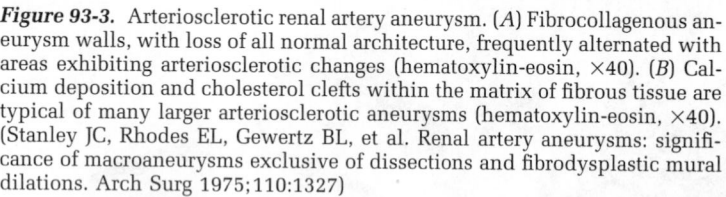

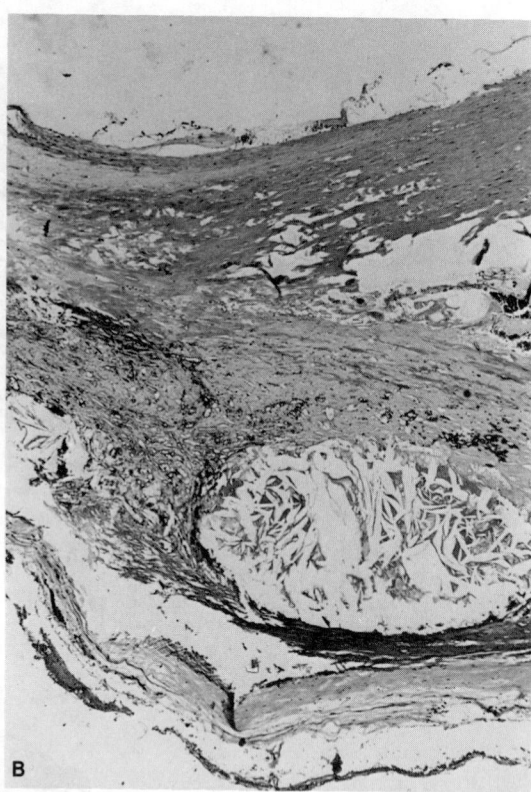

Figure 93-3. Arteriosclerotic renal artery aneurysm. (*A*) Fibrocollagenous aneurysm walls, with loss of all normal architecture, frequently alternated with areas exhibiting arteriosclerotic changes (hematoxylin-eosin, ×40). (*B*) Calcium deposition and cholesterol clefts within the matrix of fibrous tissue are typical of many larger arteriosclerotic aneurysms (hematoxylin-eosin, ×40). (Stanley JC, Rhodes EL, Gewertz BL, et al. Renal artery aneurysms: significance of macroaneurysms exclusive of dissections and fibrodysplastic mural dilations. Arch Surg 1975;110:1327)

venous fistulas occurred in an additional 2.8% of one of the largest series from a surgical group.[7] However, the high frequencies of rupture, as noted in the earlier literature, have not been confirmed in more recent reports.[3,4,7] Certainly, bland renal artery aneurysm rupture is likely to be considerably less than 3%.

Rupture of renal artery aneurysms during pregnancy is an exception to the generally accepted benign nature of most bland aneurysms.[23–26] These ruptures during pregnancy do not appear related to age, increased blood pressure, or number of pregnancies.[24] Rupture of renal artery aneurysms is responsible for fetal death in nearly 85% of cases and is associated with a 55% maternal mortality rate.[24] Parenthetically, there is not any obvious relation between repeated pregnancies and the evolution of renal artery aneurysms as is seen with splenic artery aneurysms.

An increased risk of renal artery aneurysm rupture has been attributed to large size, absence of calcification, and

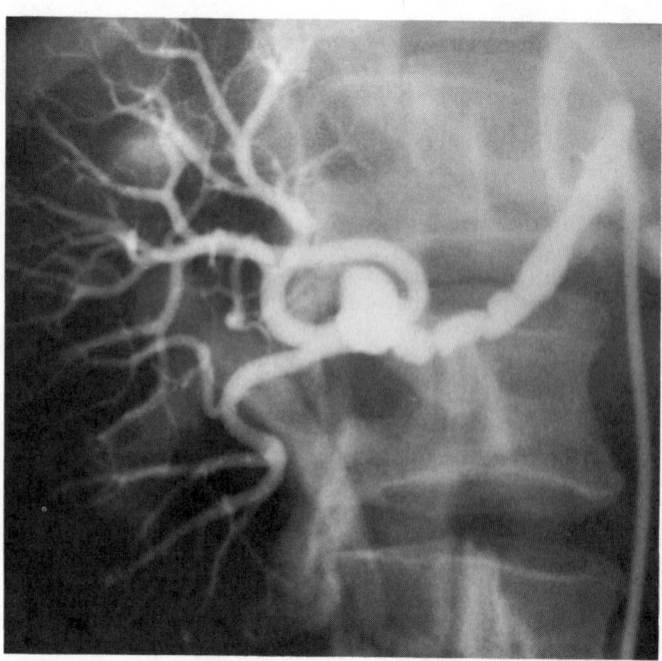

Figure 93-4. Saccular renal artery aneurysm occurring at the primary bifurcation of a main renal artery exhibiting medial fibroplasia. (Stanley JC, Whitehouse WM Jr. Renal artery macroaneurysms. In: Bergan JJ, Yao JST, eds. Aneurysms. New York, Grune & Stratton 1982;417)

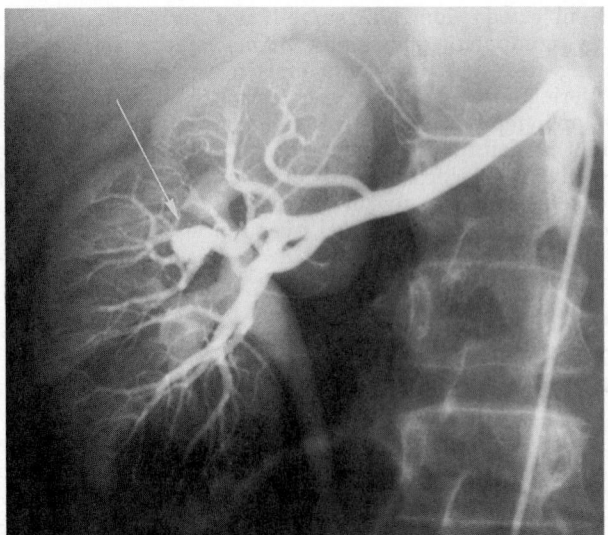

Figure 93-5. Small nonatherosclerotic intraparenchymal aneurysm associated with segmental thromboembolic renal ischemia and cortical infarct (*arrow*). (Stanley JC, Whitehouse WM Jr. Renal artery macroaneurysms. In: Bergan JJ, Yao JST, eds. Aneurysms. New York, Grune & Stratton 1982:417)

elevated blood pressure. These factors are not always relevant. In fact, overt rupture often has occurred in normotensive patients as well as with calcific atherosclerotic aneurysms.[7] Similarly, size is of limited prognostic value as an indicator of rupture potential; the statistical validity of rupture occurring in larger aneurysms has not been clearly proved in the literature. Nevertheless, a larger size remains a logical reason to assign a greater risk of rupture.

Indications for surgical intervention for true renal artery aneurysms are reasonably well defined. Patients suspected of symptomatic aneurysmal expansion are operative candidates. Similarly, patients with aneurysms and coexisting functionally important renal artery stenoses causing secondary hypertension are best treated operatively. Surgical intervention is also justified for aneurysms harboring thrombus, particularly if distal embolization is evident. Because of catastrophes accompanying aneurysm rupture during pregnancy, surgical therapy is recommended for all women who might conceive at a later time. Although large size is a controversial indication for operative intervention, many would recommend such therapy for aneurysms greater than 1.5 cm in diameter in otherwise healthy patients. Size is a soft indication for surgical therapy and should probably be espoused only by those experienced in renovascular reconstructive surgery. Cautious surgical intervention in properly selected patients with renal artery aneurysms appears justified because of the small but unpredictable incidence of rupture with its attendant loss of kidney and life.

The objective of surgical therapy is to eliminate the aneurysm without losing the kidney or compromising its function.[7,27-30] Renal artery reconstruction after aneurysmectomy is often complex and should be individualized depending on the size and location of the aneurysm.[30] Most of these aneurysms are best approached with a transabdominal, extraperitoneal exposure of the renal vasculature following medial displacement of the overlying colon and foregut viscera.

Large aneurysms of the main renal artery can usually be excised with simple primary closure of the artery, but excision of smaller aneurysms often requires arterial closure with a vein patch (Fig. 93-6). More extensive renal artery reconstructions using autogenous saphenous vein or internal iliac artery as aortorenal grafts for bifurcation

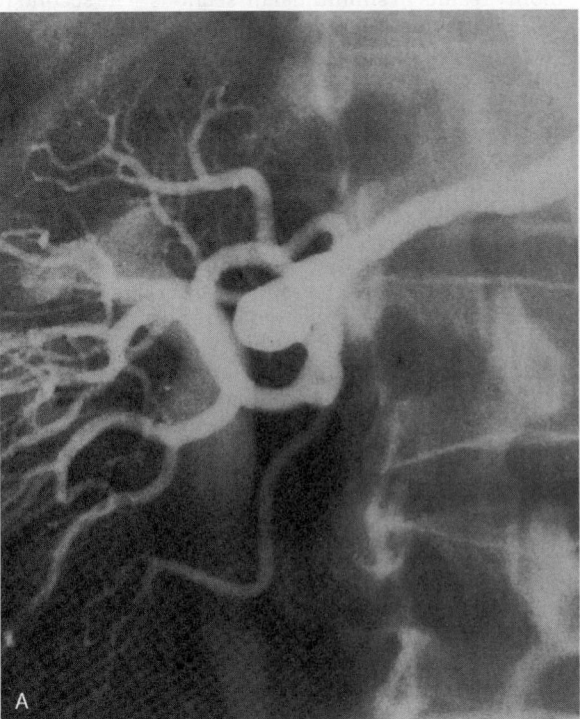
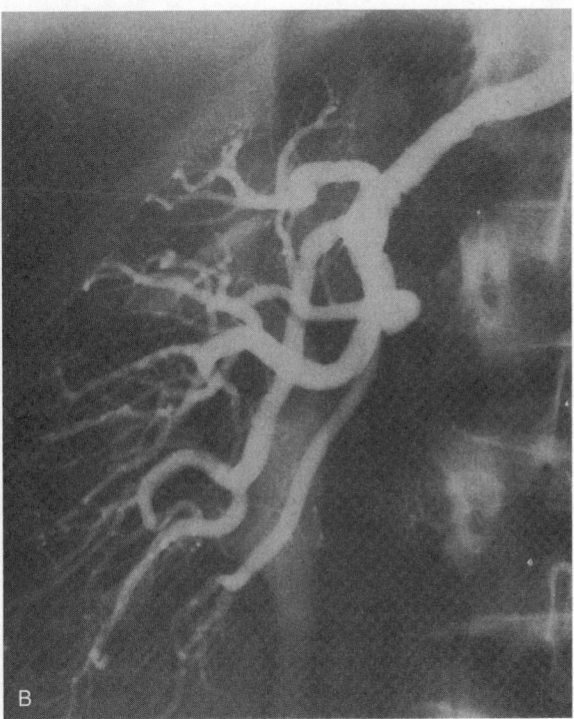

Figure 93-6. Renal artery aneurysm located at bifurcation of main renal artery (*A*). Surgical treatment included aneurysmectomy and vein patch graft closure of the artery (*B*). (Stanley JC. Renal artery aneurysms and dissections. In: Veith FJ, ed. Current critical problems in vascular surgery, vol 3. St Louis, Quality Medical Publishing, 1991;311)

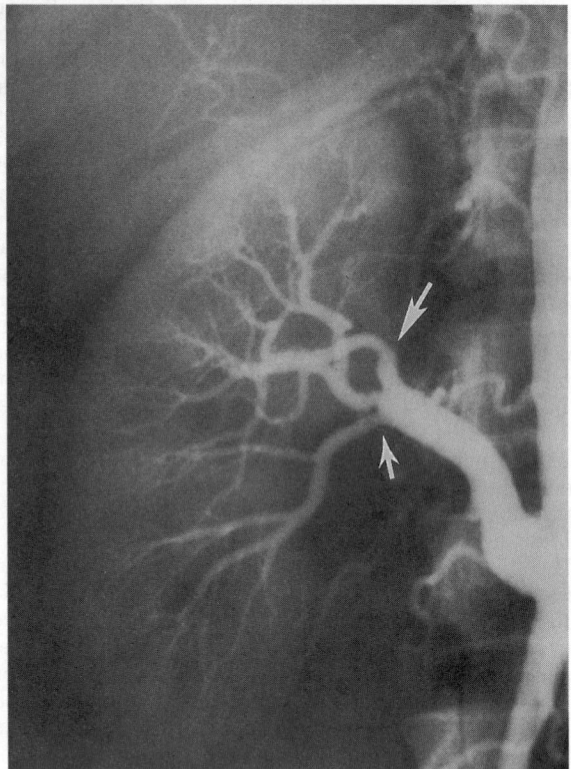

Figure 93-7. Aortorenal bypass with reversed autogenous saphenous vein, following excision of an aneurysm in a fibrodysplastic vessel (same patient as in Figure 93-4), with end-to-end anastomosis to one first-order segmental branch (*large arrow*) and end-to-side implantation of the other first-order segmental branch (*small arrow*). (Ernst CB, Stanley JC, Fry WJ. Multiple primary and segmental renal artery revascularization utilizing autogenous saphenous vein. Surg Gynecol Obstet 1973;137:1023)

aneurysms, especially those associated with functionally important stenoses (Fig. 93-7), are favored over other complex reconstructions.[7,30,31]

Aneurysmectomy with reimplantation of the involved vessel or vessels into a normal adjacent or proximal renal artery is appropriate for treating many first- and second-order branch aneurysms (Fig. 93-8). These procedures are usually undertaken in situ, although ex vivo reconstructions may be preferred in certain cases. Lastly, renal artery aneurysms 2 to 3 mm in diameter may be plicated by way of a closed aneurysmorrhaphy using a fine running cardiovascular suture. These very small aneurysms are often encountered as incidental lesions when treating larger aneurysms. Ex vivo repairs are appropriate in selected cases, especially when repair of coexistent segmental renal artery stenotic disease is necessary.[31-33]

Nephrectomy is the usual therapy for managing ruptured aneurysms. However, arterial reconstruction should be considered in those rare instances when the kidney has not been irreparably injured from ischemia due to the rupture. Partial nephrectomy may be required when aneurysmal erosion has occurred into adjacent veins causing a chronic arteriovenous fistula. Acute arteriovenous fistulas can occasionally be treated by conventional means with local excision and arterial reconstruction. Interventional arteriography with transcatheter embolization may be an effective alternative to subtotal nephrectomy in treating those aneurysms not amenable to conventional aneurysmectomy and vascular reconstruction.

Renal artery aneurysms not treated by operation must be subjected to long-term surveillance. Serial ultrasonography, computed tomography, or magnetic resonance imaging are useful in establishing an aneurysm's stability. Arteriography should be considered in patients who develop symptoms suggestive of aneurysmal expansion, exhibit hematuria, or become hypertensive. Because of the relatively low incidence of complications attending most renal artery aneurysms, noninvasive studies performed on a regular basis are favored over repeated arteriographic studies, which may carry risks exceeding those of the aneurysmal disease.

DISSECTING RENAL ARTERY ANEURYSMS

Isolated renal artery dissections causing aneurysms are rare.[11,12,34,35] Dissections are usually classified into two categories—those due to blunt abdominal trauma or intraluminal catheter-induced injury and those occurring spontaneously (Fig. 93-9). Nearly one third of renal artery dissections are bilateral.[11]

Dissections of the renal artery affect men nearly 10 times as often as women.[36] In part, this reflects the greater frequency of trauma-induced dissections that occur in men. Although an overall predilection for right renal artery involvement exists, trauma-related dissections more commonly affect the left renal artery. Blood viscosity, shear forces, and flow turbulence are common contributors to the propagation of all dissections, but inadequate structural integrity due to injury or disease initiates the dissection. Other factors contributing to dissecting aneurysms vary among the different categories of dissection.

Blunt abdominal trauma contributes to renal artery dissections by two specific mechanisms. The first is violent displacement of the kidney with deceleration causing marked stretching of the artery with fracture of the intima, which is the least elastic vessel wall component. This commonly results in subintimal dissections. The second relates to the unyielding posteriorly located vertebral bodies and direct vessel trauma. Compression of the renal arteries against the vertebra may cause deeper medial hemorrhage and false aneurysm formation in this setting because of vasa vasorum rupture or actual vessel wall disruption.

Iatrogenic catheter-related renal artery injury occurring during diagnostic arteriography is another recognized cause of these lesions. This is a very uncommon complication. In one series, only four renal artery catheter dissections were encountered among more than 11,000 abdominal diagnostic arteriographic examinations, including more than 2200 selective renal arteriograms.[12] These iatrogenic dissections are more likely to affect arteriosclerotic arteries than dysplastic renal arteries and usually occur within the inner media or subintimal tissues. Needless to say, dissections accompanying therapeutic catheterizations during balloon angioplasty are common, although few cause critical narrowings or occlusion of the renal artery.[37]

Primary or spontaneous dissections causing pseudoaneurysms, affect the renal arteries more than any other peripheral artery. Most are related to coexistent arteriosclerotic or dysplastic renovascular disease.[7,38] A 9% incidence of dissections in patients with fibrodysplastic renal arteries has been reported in some studies,[39] whereas others have reported only a 0.5% incidence in similar cases.[12] Differences in interpreting arteriographic or histologic studies may account for such divergent observations. Spontaneous dissections usually occur within the outer media adjacent to the external elastic lamina (Fig. 93-10). They occur less commonly within the central media. In

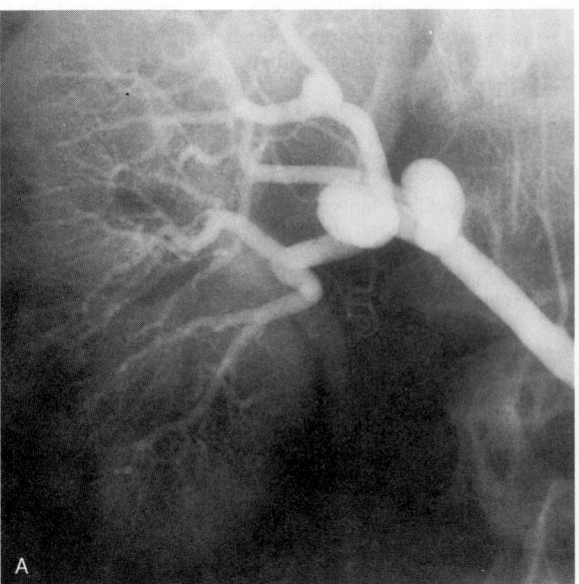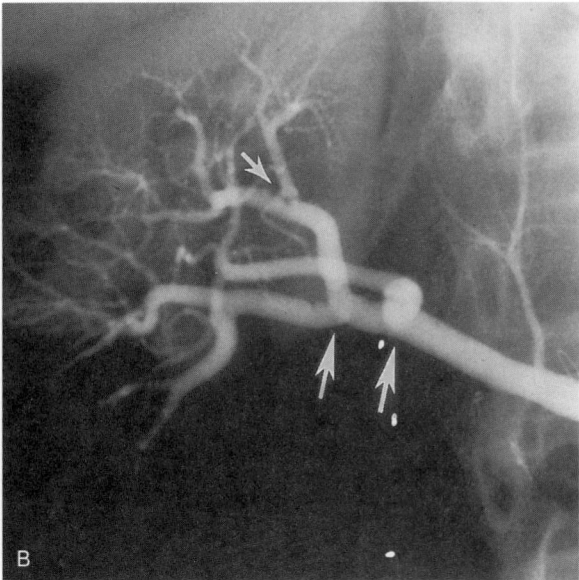

Figure 93-8. Renal artery aneurysms involving multiple segmental artery branchings (*A*). Surgical treatment included aneurysmectomy and end-to-side reimplantation (*large arrows*) of segmental vessels into the adjacent artery and closed aneurysmorrhaphy (*small arrow*) (*B*). (Stanley JC. Renal artery aneurysms and dissections. In: Veith FJ, ed. Current critical problems in vascular surgery, vol 3. St Louis, Quality Medical Publishing, 1991;311)

many instances, these dissections have been attributed to rupture of abnormal vasa vasorum. It is possible that the dissecting intramural hematoma in these circumstances increases medial ischemia and contributes to further aneurysm formation. Spontaneous renal artery dissections usually affect proximal vessels and terminate at branchings.

Clinical manifestations of renal artery dissections are rather protean. Pain, hematuria, and elevated blood pressure frequently accompany acute dissections regardless of

the cause.[12,36,40] Chronic renal artery dissections, when clinically relevant, are usually associated with renovascular hypertension or impaired renal function. Certain dissections may be self-limited, asymptomatic, and of no functional importance.

An incorrect initial clinical diagnosis is common, occurring in over half of patients having renal artery dissections.[40] Intravenous pyelography has been advocated for evaluating patients suspected of serious renal hilar injuries including dissecting aneurysms. However, some have noted a false-negative excretory urogram in approximately 12% of patients who have documented major renal artery injury.[41] Furthermore, minor perirenal hematomas and cortical contusions frequently impair contrast excretion and may cause one third to one half these studies to be false-positive. Because of this fact and the need for prompt diagnosis to improve results of surgical therapy, intravenous urograms should be deferred in favor of earlier arteriographic examinations.

Arteriography is necessary to diagnose and define the extent of renal artery dissections. Dissection is radiographically diagnosed when the following are recognized[38]:

- Luminal irregularities with aneurysmal dilatation or saccular dissections associated with segmental stenoses
- Extension of the dissections to the first renal artery branching
- Cuffing at branchings
- Variable degrees of reversibility documented on serial arteriographic studies

Trauma-related dissections warrant emergent primary arterial reconstructions once a hemodynamic narrowing or occlusion of the main renal artery or a major segmental branch is recognized.[12,34] Delayed repair is necessary for less obvious trauma-related injuries if hypertension persists or renal function deteriorates. Spontaneous dissecting aneurysms, when acute, are technically easier to treat than traumatic lesions and should be subjected to surgical therapy soon after hemodynamically significant stenoses or

Figure 93-9. Saccular dissecting main renal artery aneurysm. (Gewertz BL, Stanley JC, Fry WJ. Renal artery dissections. Arch Surg 1977;112:409)

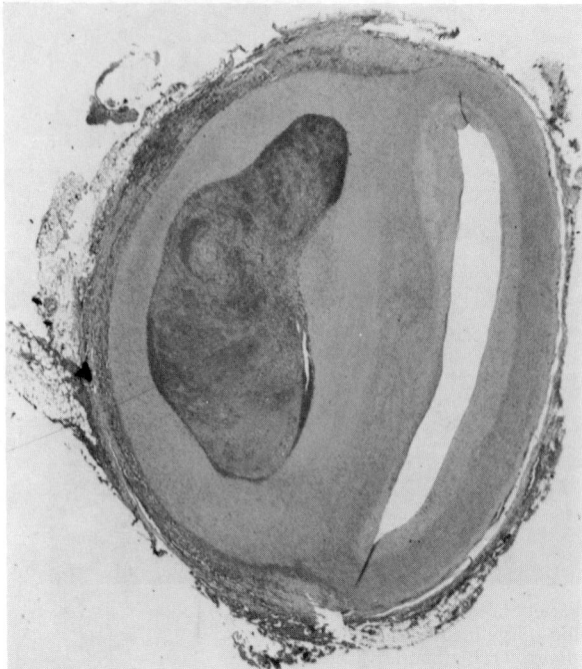

Figure 93-10. Dissection exhibiting deep mural hematoma and compression of adjacent lumen (hematoxylin-eosin, ×60). (Stanley JC. Pathologic basis of macrovascular renal artery disease. In: Stanley JC, Ernst CB, Fry WJ, eds. Renovascular hypertension. WB Saunders, Philadelphia, 1984:46)

occlusions are recognized. Operative intervention is also pursued for chronic spontaneous dissections associated with severe renovascular hypertension or deteriorating renal function.

Kidney preservation is very important in patients with renal artery dissections, especially because renal artery disease of the contralateral kidney may be present in half the cases related to blunt abdominal trauma.[12] Nephrectomy under such circumstances should be avoided. Although many dissections are not amenable to operative repair, arterial reconstructions in the form of aortorenal bypass using autogenous saphenous vein or hypogastric artery, with ex vivo repairs in selected cases, provide reasonable kidney salvage rates.

REFERENCES

1. Debakey ME, Lefrak EA, Garcia-Rinaldi R, et al. Aneurysm of the renal artery: a vascular reconstructive approach. Arch Surg 1973;106:438.
2. Dzsinich C, Gloviczki P, McKusick MA, et al. Surgical management of renal artery aneurysm. Cardiovasc Surg 3:243, 1993.
3. Hageman JH, Smith RF, Szilagyi DE, et al. Aneurysms of the renal artery: problems of prognosis and surgical management. Surgery 1978;84:563.
4. Hubert JP Jr, Pairolero PC, Kazmier FJ. Solitary renal artery aneurysm. Surgery 1980;88:557.
5. Martin RS III, Meacham PW, Ditesheim JA, et al. Renal artery aneurysm: selective treatment for hypertension and prevention of rupture. J Vasc Surg 1989;9:26.
6. Soussou ID, Starr DS, Lawrie GM, et al. Renal artery aneurysm: long-term relief of renovascular hypertension by in situ operative correction. Arch Surg 1979;114:1410.
7. Stanley JC, Rhodes EL, Gewertz BL, et al. Renal artery aneurysms: significance of macroaneurysms exclusive of dissections and fibrodysplastic mural dilations. Arch Surg 1975; 110:1327.
8. Henriksson C, Bjorkerud S, Nilson AE, et al. Natural history of renal artery aneurysm elucidated by repeated angiography and pathoanatomical studies. Eur Urol 1985;11:244.
9. Henriksson C, Lukes P, Nilson AE, et al. Angiographically discovered, non-operated renal artery aneurysms. Scand J Urol Nephrol 1984;18:59.
10. Tham G, Ekelund L, Herrlin K, et al. Renal artery aneurysms: natural history and prognosis. Ann Surg 1983;197:348.
11. Edwards BS, Stanson AW, Holley KE, et al. Isolated renal artery dissection: presentation, evaluation, management and pathology. Mayo Clin Proc 1982;57:564.
12. Gewertz BL, Stanley JC, Fry WJ. Renal artery dissections. Arch Surg 1977;112:409.
13. Stanley JC, Gewertz BL, Bove EL, et al. Arterial fibrodysplasia: histopathologic character and current etiologic concepts. Arch Surg 1975;110:561.
14. Smith DL. Spontaneous rupture of a renal artery aneurysm in polyarteritis nodosa: critical review of the literature and report of a case. Am J Med 1989;87:464.
15. Edsman G. Angiography and suprarenal angiography. Acta Radiol 1965;(Suppl 155):104.
16. Sarkar R, Coran A, Lindenauer SM, et al. Arterial aneurysms in children: a clinicopathologic classification. J Vasc Surg 1991;13:47.
17. Stanley JC, Zelenock GB, Messina LM, et al. Pediatric renovascular hypertension: a thirty-year experience of operative treatment. J Vasc Surg 1995;21:212.
18. Cummings KB, Lecky JW, Kaufman JJ. Renal artery aneurysms and hypertension. J Urol 1973;109:144.
19. Ruberti U, Miani S, Scorza R, et al. Aneurysm of the renal artery. Int Angiol 1987;6:407.
20. Vaughan TJ, Barry WF, Jeffords DL, et al. Renal artery aneurysms and hypertension. Radiology 1971;99:287.
21. Youkey JR, Collins GJ, Orecchia PM, et al. Saccular renal artery aneurysm as a cause of hypertension. Surgery 1985; 97:498.
22. Garritano AP. Aneurysm of the renal artery. Am J Surg 1957;94:638.
23. Burt RL, Johnson FR, Silverthorne RG, et al. Ruptured renal artery aneurysm in pregnancy: report of a case with survival. Obstet Gynecol 1956;7:229.
24. Cohen JR, Shamash FS. Ruptured renal artery aneurysms during pregnancy. J Vasc Surg 1987;6:51.
25. Cohen SG, Cashdan A, Burger R. Spontaneous rupture of a renal artery aneurysm during pregnancy. Obstet Gynecol 1972;39:897.
26. Rijbroek A, Dijk AV, Roex AJM. Rupture of renal artery aneurysm during pregnancy. Eur J Vasc Surg 1994;8:375.
27. Dayton B, Helgerson RB, Sollinger HW, et al. Ruptured renal artery aneurysm in a pregnant uninephric patient: successful ex vivo repair and autotransplantation. Surgery 1990;107:708.
28. Huppt, T, Allenberg JR, Post K, et al. Renal artery aneurysms: surgical indications and results. Eur J Vasc Surg 1992;6:477.
29. Mercier C, Piquet P, Piligian F, et al. Aneurysms of the renal artery and its branches. Ann Vasc Surg 1986;1:321.
30. Stanley JC, Messina LM, Wakefield TW, et al. Renal artery reconstruction. In: Bergan JJ, Yao JST, eds. Techniques in arterial surgery. Philadelphia, WB Saunders, 1990:247.
31. Ortenberg J, Novick AC, Straffon RA, et al. Surgical treatment of renal artery aneurysms. Br J Urol 1983;55:341.
32. Bugge-Asperheim B, Sdal G, Flatmark A. Renal artery aneurysm: ex vivo repair and autotransplantation. Scand J Urol Nephrol 1984;18:63.
33. Dubernard JM, Martin X, Gelet A, et al. Aneurysms of the renal artery: surgical management with special reference to extracorporeal surgery and autotransplantation. Eur Urol 1985;11:26.
34. Reilly LM, Cuningham CG, Maggisano R, et al. The role of arterial reconstruction in spontaneous renal artery dissection. J Vasc Surg 1991;14:468.
35. Smith BM, Holcomb GW, Richie RE, et al. Renal artery dissection. Ann Surg 1984;200:134.
36. Bakir AA, Patel K, Schwartz MM, et al. Isolated dissecting aneurysm of the renal artery. Am Heart J 1978;96:92.
37. Stanley JC. Surgery of failed percutaneous transluminal renal artery angioplasty. In: Bergan JJ, Yao JST, eds. Reoperative arterial surgery. Orlando, Grune & Stratton, 1986:441.

38. Hare WSC, Kincaid-Smith P. Dissecting aneurysm of the renal artery. Radiology 1970;97:255.
39. Harrison EG Jr, Hunt JC, Bernatz PE. Morphology of fibromuscular dysplasia of the renal artery in renovascular hypertension. Am J Med 1967;43:97.
40. Rao CN, Blaivas JG. Primary renal artery dissecting aneurysm: a review. J Urol 1977;118:716.
41. Scott R Jr, Carlton CE Jr, Goldman M. Penetrating injuries of the kidney: an analysis of 181 patients. J Urol 1969;101:247.

SURGERY: SCIENTIFIC PRINCIPLES AND PRACTICE, Second Edition, edited by Lazar J. Greenfield, Michael W. Mulholland, Keith T. Oldham, Gerald B. Zelenock, and Keith D. Lillemoe. Lippincott–Raven Publishers, Philadelphia, © 1997.

CHAPTER 94

FEMORAL AND POPLITEAL ANEURYSMS

CHARLES L. MESH AND LINDA M. GRAHAM

PERIPHERAL ANEURYSMS

Incidence

Femoral and popliteal artery aneurysms, although far less common than abdominal aortic aneurysms, are the most frequently encountered peripheral aneurysms. The exact incidence of femoral and popliteal aneurysms is difficult to define, but in a large series from a single medical center, arteriosclerotic aortic aneurysms were identified in 0.5% of hospitalized patients, femoral artery aneurysms in 0.01%, and popliteal aneurysms in 0.01%.[1] Of the 1488 total patients with arteriosclerotic aneurysms, 1470 (99%) had abdominal aortic aneurysms, 37 (2.5%) had femoral aneurysms, and 36 (2.4%) had popliteal aneurysms. Of patients with aortoiliac aneurysms, 3% also had peripheral aneurysms, whereas more than 70% of patients with peripheral aneurysms had concomitant abdominal aortic aneurysms. Men are afflicted with arteriosclerotic femoral and popliteal artery aneurysms far more frequently than women; the male/female ratio in these patients is about 20:1. This predilection for men is markedly different from the usual incidence of aortic aneurysmal and peripheral arteriosclerotic occlusive disease, for which the male/female ratios are about 5:1 and 3:1, respectively.

Pathogenesis

The cause of femoral and popliteal aneurysms has changed distinctly since they were first recognized centuries ago. Once primarily mycotic, syphilitic, or traumatic in origin, most true aneurysms are now of arteriosclerotic cause, whereas false aneurysms are related to surgery or trauma. The frequency of peripheral aneurysms appears to be increasing as the average age of the population increases and as iatrogenic and violent arterial trauma become more common.

The cause of arteriosclerotic aneurysms of the femoral and popliteal vessels is not clear. One factor believed to contribute to aneurysm formation is turbulent flow past a relative stenosis. At the femoral level, this results in poststenotic dilation beyond the inguinal ligament. At the popliteal position, such dilation occurs distal to tendinous hiatus of the adductor magnus.[2] Arterial wall fatigue due to vibration and turbulence proximal to a major branching or due to stress and kinking during hip and knee flexion can also contribute to aneurysm formation.[3] These factors do not explain the multiplicity of aneurysms in these patients nor the male predilection for the disease. The latter observation has prompted suggestions that aneurysm formation may be due, in part, to a sex-linked, genetic abnormality similar to that seen in the aneurysm-prone blotchy mouse.[4] Other investigators have noted enhanced collagen synthesis, relative elastin dilution, and disturbed architecture in aneurysms and explained the multiplicity of peripheral aneurysms as a reflection of a systemic abnormality in the arterial wall.[5]

Clinical Manifestations

Femoral and popliteal aneurysms are frequently asymptomatic and thus only discovered as an incidental finding on routine physical examination. When symptomatic, they commonly present with lower extremity ischemia due to thrombosis or distal embolization. Local pain may be due to enlargement, whereas leg pain and edema can result from compression of the adjacent nerve and vein, respectively. Because the natural histories and complication rates of femoral and popliteal aneurysms differ, they are considered separately.

FEMORAL ARTERY ANEURYSMS

Femoral artery aneurysms are the most common peripheral aneurysm if one includes both true and false aneurysms. Their clinical importance rests in the fact that they are limb-threatening lesions and can jeopardize the viability of the leg if thrombosis, embolization, or rupture occur. They gain additional importance for their frequent association with limb-threatening popliteal aneurysms and life-threatening abdominal aortic aneurysms. Most true aneurysms are arteriosclerotic lesions, whereas false aneurysms are anastomotic, traumatic, or mycotic in origin. Rarely, femoral aneurysms develop secondary to connective tissue disorders. The femoral region is the most common site for both anastomotic, traumatic, and mycotic pseudoaneurysms. The presentation and surgical repair of these lesions are considered separately in this chapter.

Arteriosclerotic Aneurysms

Incidence

The exact incidence of arteriosclerotic femoral artery aneurysms remains undefined in the general population; however, 3% of all patients with abdominal aortic aneurysms have femoral aneurysms, and 85% of patients with femoral artery aneurysms have abdominal aortic aneurysms.[6] Multiple aneurysms are common in patients with femoral artery aneurysms. In a series of 100 patients with femoral artery aneurysms, 72% of patients had bilateral femoral artery aneurysms.[6] In addition, aortoiliac aneurysms were detected in 85% of patients, thoracic aortic aneurysms in 6%, and popliteal aneurysms in 44%.

Femoral aneurysms frequently involve the common femoral artery. They can be classified as type I, those limited to the common femoral artery, or type II, those involving the orifice of the profunda femoris artery.[7] Type I and II aneurysms occur with nearly equal frequency, but type II aneurysms generally require more complex reconstruction. Isolated lesions of the profunda femoris artery are rare (2% of femoral artery aneurysms), difficult to diagnose at the asymptomatic stage, and thus prone to rupture.

Clinical Manifestations

The typical patient with an arteriosclerotic femoral artery aneurysm is a man in his seventh decade of life. These patients have the usual risk factors for atherosclerosis; 86% are cigarette smokers, 36% have hypertension, and 14% have diabetes mellitus.[6] Associated cardiovascular disease is common, with clinical manifestations of coronary artery and cerebrovascular disease present in 34% and 7% of patients, respectively.

The clinical manifestations of femoral artery aneurysms cover the spectrum from asymptomatic to severe ischemia of the lower extremity. Although 40% of patients are asymptomatic at the time of diagnosis, most present with either local symptoms or complaints of lower extremity ischemia.[6] Local pain or appreciation of a groin mass is the only symptom in 18% of patients. Lower extremity venous disease is present in 8%, and is attributable to venous obstruction by the femoral artery aneurysm in half of these. Symptoms of claudication, rest pain, or gangrene are present in 42% of patients.

As with aneurysms in other locations, femoral artery aneurysms can be complicated by embolism, thrombosis, or rupture. The rates of complication are variable among reported series and tend to be higher in those consisting primarily of surgical experience. Peripheral microembolization can produce signs as mild as spotty discoloration of the toes and as severe as peripheral gangrene, or it may be diagnosed unexpectedly at angiography. Although embolism is reported in about 10% of femoral aneurysms, the femoral artery may not be the source of these emboli because many of these patients have a concomitant popliteal aneurysm.[6] In larger clinical series, 1% to 16% of patients with arteriosclerotic femoral artery aneurysms presented with acute thrombosis, whereas 1% to 16% had a chronically thrombosed lesion.[6,7] Rupture is reported in 1% to 14% of lesions.[6,7]

Diagnosis

In most cases, the diagnosis of femoral aneurysm is suspected by the finding of a pulsatile groin mass on physical examination. Although a radiograph of the region may occasionally demonstrate the calcified rim of the aneurysm, only ultrasonography, computed tomography (CT), or magnetic resonance imaging (MRI) can reliably diagnose femoral artery aneurysms. These modalities define the size of the femoral artery while simultaneously excluding the presence of associated aneurysmal disease in the distal aorta and popliteal arteries. The diagnostic accuracy of arteriography is limited because it only outlines the residual lumen and may miss large aneurysms filled with mural thrombus. The importance of arteriography is its capacity to define the anatomy of the femoral region and distal vasculature for planning operative therapy (Fig. 94-1).

Natural History

The natural history of arteriosclerotic femoral artery aneurysms is poorly defined because most series review aneurysms in patients from a surgical service, many of which were subjected to operation. A small asymptomatic femoral artery aneurysm does not appear to pose the same threat to the limb as does a popliteal artery aneurysm. In a series of 100 patients with femoral artery aneurysms, serious limb-threatening complications were documented in only 2.9% of the 172 aneurysms followed nonoperatively.[6] This was, however, a preselected group in which many symptomatic aneurysms were excluded from follow-up because operative intervention was undertaken after initial diagnosis.

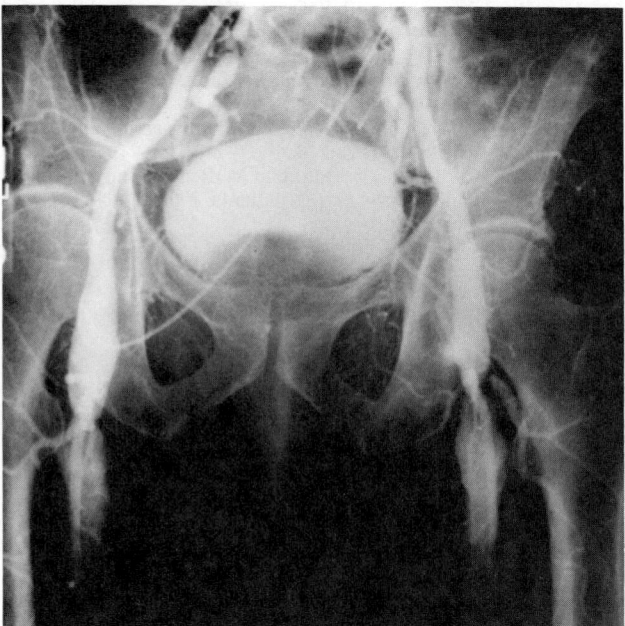

Figure 94-1. Arteriogram demonstrating bilateral femoral artery aneurysms that extend into the superficial femoral arteries. Unlike many patients with femoral artery aneurysms, this patient did not have associated aortic or popliteal aneurysms.

Treatment

Indications. Operative treatment is indicated for all symptomatic femoral aneurysms. Asymptomatic aneurysms greater than 2.5 cm in diameter should also be repaired unless the patient is a prohibitive risk for operative intervention. If nonoperative management is selected, the size of the aneurysm should be documented and the patient should be followed with careful serial examination and duplex scans.

Surgical Strategy. Femoral artery aneurysms are usually approached through a vertical groin incision. Occasionally, an unusually large aneurysm or ruptured aneurysm requires proximal control of the external iliac artery through a retroperitoneal approach. After proximal and distal arterial control is obtained, the aneurysmal sac is opened and the atheromatous debris removed. Small aneurysms can be excised, but routine excision of large aneurysms is not recommended because these lesions can adhere to adjacent vein and nerve. Type I aneurysms are reconstructed with an interposition graft of Dacron or expanded polytetrafluoroethylene extending from the external iliac artery to the femoral bifurcation. For type II aneurysms with patent superficial and profunda femoris arteries, an interposition graft from the external iliac artery to the superficial femoral artery with reimplantation of the profunda femoris artery is a standard configuration. If the superficial femoral artery is chronically occluded and the patient has minimal symptoms, an interposition graft to the profunda femoris is performed. If recent emboli or in situ thrombosis have occluded the outflow tract, catheter thromboembolectomy, thrombolytic therapy, or both are useful adjuvants.

Femoral artery aneurysms can be associated with either concomitant occlusive disease or other aneurysms. In patients with multiple asymptomatic aneurysms, treatment is staged. Life-threatening aortoiliac aneurysms are addressed before limb-threatening femoral and popliteal aneurysms. A femoral aneurysm can be treated at the time of an aortofemoral bypass by performing the distal anastomosis either beyond the aneurysm or into a femoral interposition graft. In the patient with severe lower extremity ischemia, the femoral aneurysm is treated with an interposition graft, from which the proximal anastomosis of required femoropopliteal or femorotibial reconstruction is based.

Results. Results of surgical therapy depend on the patency of the distal vasculature. In asymptomatic patients, excellent long-term results can be expected in over 80%, whereas 68% of those presenting with lower extremity ischemia achieve satisfactory long-term outcomes.[6] Operative mortality rates for repair of isolated femoral artery aneurysms approach 0%. Reported mortality rates of up to 4% are a reflection of concomitant aortic reconstruction.[6]

Anastomotic Pseudoaneurysms

Incidence

Anastomotic aneurysms result from a disrupted suture line between a graft and the host artery. The incidence varies with the location of the anastomosis and the type of graft used. Anastomotic aneurysms at the femoral artery account for nearly 80% of these lesions, and 3% of all femoral anastomoses ultimately develop false aneurysms. After aortofemoral bypass, 6% of femoral anastomoses are complicated by pseudoaneurysm, as compared with only 0.2% of aortic anastomoses.[8,9] After infrainguinal bypass, 6% of femoral Dacron anastomoses develop aneurysms, as compared with 1% of autogenous venous anastomoses.[8] Anastomotic aneurysms are a late complication of bypass procedures, and the mean interval from primary procedure to recognition is more than 6 years.[10,11]

Pathogenesis

The factors contributing to anastomotic aneurysm formation include weakness of the arterial wall, type of graft material, type of suture, presence of infection, method of anastomotic construction, and stress on the suture line from hypertension, leg motion, or excess tension on the graft limb.[8,10,11] Progressive atherosclerotic degeneration of the recipient artery can cause anastomotic aneurysms, but their incidence is increased after local endarterectomy. False aneurysms occur more commonly with synthetic vascular grafts than with saphenous vein grafts and may reflect the more complete healing with autogenous tissue. When silk suture was used for vascular anastomoses, suture breakdown was a common cause of anastomotic aneurysm formation. With the advent of synthetic suture, anastomotic aneurysms due to loss of suture integrity are rare unless the suture is mishandled during the procedure. Although most anastomotic aneurysms are not accompanied by overt graft infection, occult infections with coagulase-negative *Staphylococcus* sp may be an important factor in development of anastomotic aneurysms.[11] A higher incidence of anastomotic aneurysms is noted in patients with wound healing complications. Some studies suggest that anastomotic aneurysms are more common with an end-to-side anastomosis than with an end-to-end anastomosis, although other reports do not verify this. Finally, hypertension, joint motion, or excessive tension on the graft limb can place stress on the suture line and cause anastomotic disruption.

Clinical Manifestations

Femoral anastomotic aneurysms usually present as a pulsatile groin mass that can be accompanied by pain, redness, or symptoms of venous obstruction. Acute complications of anastomotic aneurysms include hemorrhage, embolism, and occlusion. When false aneurysms accompany graft sepsis, the manifestations occur earlier in the postoperative period.

Diagnosis

The diagnosis of a false aneurysm is usually made on physical examination when a pulsatile groin mass is detected in a patient who has undergone a femoral arterial reconstructive procedure. The differential diagnosis must include other nonpulsatile groin masses (hernia, lymphocele, and abscess) through which pulsation from the normal underlying femoral artery is being transmitted. The presence of an anastomotic femoral aneurysm necessitates the search for other anastomotic aneurysms. Multiple lesions are found in at least 30% of patients,[10] and their presence implies infection. Complete evaluation of an anastomotic aneurysm should include ultrasound, CT, or MRI, with examination of all anastomoses of the involved graft. Angiography is obtained before repair of the anastomotic aneurysm to define the proximal and distal arterial anatomy (Fig. 94-2).

Treatment

Surgical Strategy. Because of the progressive nature of anastomotic aneurysms, surgical treatment is undertaken for all lesions except small (less than 2 cm in diameter), asymptomatic aneurysms in high-risk patients. The principles of surgical treatment include proximal and distal control and replacement of the aneurysmal segment. Securing proximal control may require division of the inguinal ligament to isolate the graft limb. Distal control is easily obtained with intraluminal balloon occlusion catheters, or control of the superficial and deep femoral arteries can be facilitated by dissection distal to the previous exposure. After débridement of the degenerated artery, an interposition graft is placed between the limb of the prosthetic graft and the healthy native artery. Cultures of the graft and

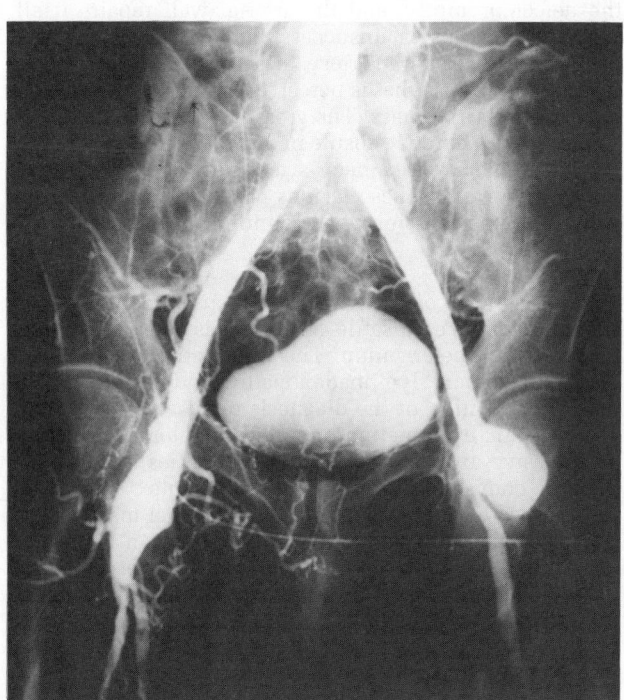

Figure 94-2. Arteriogram demonstrating bilateral femoral anastomotic aneurysms after an aortofemoral bypass and a left femoropopliteal bypass.

vessel wall are essential to exclude infection as an etiologic factor in the aneurysmal degeneration. In the presence of obvious infection, graft sepsis is managed by the removal of all infected prosthetic material. The reestablishment of blood flow, if necessary, is accomplished with a bypass through uninfected tissue planes.

Results. Results of elective operations on uncomplicated anastomotic aneurysms are excellent, with 2% operative mortality, 97.5% graft patency at 2 years, and 2% amputation within 2 years of surgery.[10] Recurrence occurs in less than 16% of cases.[8,9] Patients presenting with aneurysms complicated by hemorrhage, occlusion, or embolism have significantly increased operative morbidity and mortality.

Catheter-Induced Pseudoaneurysms

Incidence

The femoral artery is the preferred site of arterial access for both diagnostic angiography and interventional endovascular therapy. In recent years, diagnostic studies for coronary and peripheral artery occlusive disease have increased, as have the subsequent endovascular interventions.[12] Because these techniques often require prolonged arterial cannulation, large-bore sheaths, and anticoagulation, a relatively fixed rate of arterial complications is to be expected. Review of recent experiences shows that pseudoaneurysm formation can be expected in about 0.05% of diagnostic catheterizations and in up to 0.4% of more complex procedures.[13]

Pathogenesis

Pseudoaneurysms from iatrogenic catheter trauma meet the classic definition for pseudoaneurysm in that they are collections of blood in continuity with the arterial system, unenclosed by all three layers of the arterial wall. These lesions form because of failed hemostasis at the arterial wall defect created by catheter insertion. Normally, hemostasis, aided by direct focal application of pressure, seals the defect promptly, and the arterial wall repairs itself. When hemostasis is unsuccessful, blood under arterial pressure leaks from the artery, dissects surrounding tissue planes, and forms what is perceived on physical examination as a pulsatile mass. The gross findings at surgery are a blood-filled, fibrous capsule in direct continuity with the arterial lumen by a catheter-sized mural defect. Like all pseudoaneurysms, these lesions can cause symptoms by rupture or compression of surrounding structures.

Diagnosis

The diagnosis of catheter-induced pseudoaneurysm is suspected when a pulsatile groin mass is noted after femoral arterial catheterization. The differential diagnosis includes hematoma, lymphadenopathy, and abscess. In the past, confirmation of the diagnosis required either repeat angiographic examination or surgical exploration. Today, noninvasive axial scanning with modalities such as CT, MRI, or conventional and color-flow duplex technology can delineate the extent of these periarterial mass lesion. Of these tests, MRI and color-flow duplex can define the communication between the mass and the arterial lumen. Color-flow duplex is relatively inexpensive and is thus the investigative test of choice.

Natural History

Color-flow duplex scanning provides accurate diagnosis, localization, and sizing of catheter-induced false aneurysms. Using color-flow duplex scanning, Kresowik and colleagues[14] monitored 144 groins suspected of complications after percutaneous transluminal angioplasty. They found seven pseudoaneurysms, all of which went on to spontaneous thrombosis. Kent and colleagues[15] prospectively evaluated 16 duplex-confirmed, catheter-induced femoral pseudoaneurysms. Nine of these lesions closed spontaneously, but 30% required surgical repair. In the latter series, thrombosis was less likely in anticoagulated patients and in those with pseudoaneurysms more than 1.8 cm in diameter. These natural history studies have documented that groin pseudoaneurysms do spontaneously develop thrombi, and suggest that asymptotic aneurysms may be more common than previously suspected.

Treatment

Traditional therapy of catheter-induced pseudoaneurysms has been early surgical repair.[16] This is performed under local anesthesia, necessitates proximal and distal arterial control, and rarely requires more than one to two sutures in the arterial defect. Several investigators have used the duplex scanner as an instrument to treat catheter-induced pseudoaneurysms. In these studies, pseudoaneurysms were identified with color-flow scanners and then compressed with the scan head. Real-time observation of flow in the underlying artery prevented arterial occlusion. Pseudoaneurysm thrombosis was documented by absence of flow signals on release of scan-head pressure. In a series of 17 pseudoaneurysms, Feld and colleagues[17] reported successful obliteration in 88% of cases, but noted only a 29% success rate in anticoagulated patients. The average time of compression was less than 1 hour, and thrombosis was not dependent on the size of the pseudoaneurysm. Cox and colleagues[18] have reported the largest series of pseudoaneurysms treated with ultrasound-guided compression. In 100 consecutive pseudoaneurysms, they achieved thrombosis in 86% of anticoagulated patients and in 98% of those not anticoagulated. These authors reported a 20% immediate (less than 24 hours) recurrence rate in anticoagulated patients, and cautioned that their outstanding results were due, in part, to meticulous post-compression follow-up and early immobilization. Size had no influence on outcome, but long-standing pseudoaneurysms were less likely to respond to compression therapy. Surgical therapy is still mandatory for all catheter-induced pseudoaneurysms that are acutely expanding, compressing adjacent nerves, or compromising overlying skin. For all other such lesions, if an ultrasonographer skilled in compression is available, initial obliteration with ultrasound-guided compression should be attempted.

Mycotic Aneurysms

The term *mycotic aneurysm* is used to refer to any infected aneurysm. Today, mycotic femoral aneurysms are most commonly complications of trauma due to either parenteral drug abuse or invasive medical procedures. In the past, septic emboli from bacterial endocarditis were a major cause of mycotic femoral aneurysm. In the era of antibiotics, nontraumatic mycotic aneurysms of infectious cause (bacterial, syphilitic, or tuberculous) are exceedingly rare. As the cause of mycotic aneurysms has changed, their location has shifted from central to peripheral arteries, with the femoral artery now the most common site.[19,20]

Pathogenesis

The causes of mycotic aneurysms fall into four major categories.[19] First, septic emboli from bacterial endocarditis may lodge in normal arteries, causing infection that weakens the arterial wall and results in aneurysm formation. Second, during an episode of bacteremia, microorganisms may lodge in a preexisting atherosclerotic plaque or aneurysm, multiply, and cause aneurysmal degeneration. A third cause of mycotic aneurysms is the contiguous spread of bacteria from a local abscess, with the inflammatory process causing destruction of the arterial wall and pseudoaneurysm formation. Finally, trauma to the artery with concomitant contamination may result in formation of an infected pseudoaneurysm.

The bacteriology of arterial infections depends on the cause of the lesion. In the preantibiotic era, aneurysms secondary to bacterial endocarditis grew *Pneumococcus, Streptococcus,* and *Enterococcus* sp. Today, staphylococci, *Salmonella, Escherichia coli,* and *Proteus* organisms are the most frequent isolates.[20] *Staphylococcus aureus* is found in up to 65% of patients with mycotic femoral artery aneurysms secondary to trauma and drug abuse.[21] In this population, about 50% of *S aureus* organisms are resistant to methicillin, and polymicrobial groin infections are common.

Clinical Manifestations

The typical patient with a mycotic femoral aneurysm presents with the triad of chills, fever, and a tender, enlarging, pulsatile groin mass. Lower extremity edema may occur secondary to venous obstruction. The patient often has a history of intravenous drug use, recent penetrating trauma, or bacterial endocarditis. Local signs of infection, such as erythema, warmth, and tenderness, are present on physical examination. Evidence of septic embolization may include petechial skin lesions, splinter hemorrhages, cutaneous abscesses, or even signs of septic arthritis. A small sentinel bleed may herald impending free-rupture and uncontrollable, life-threatening hemorrhage.

Diagnosis

The diagnosis of mycotic femoral aneurysm is usually straightforward, but distinguishing an abscess adjacent to the femoral artery from a femoral mycotic aneurysm is occasionally difficult. In the patient with a pulsatile groin mass, laboratory findings, including leukocytosis, elevated erythrocyte sedimentation rate, and positive blood cultures, are suggestive but not specific for a mycotic aneurysm. Ultrasonography, CT, and MRI are helpful in diagnosis of aneurysms but cannot distinguish infected from bland lesions. Arteriography may confirm the presence of an aneurysm, but more important, it serves to delineate the proximal and distal arterial anatomy in planning the operative intervention (Fig. 94-3). Ultimately, the diagnosis of mycotic aneurysm can only be confirmed at operation by either the demonstration of organisms on Gram stain or by positive cultures of the aneurysm wall.

Treatment

A mycotic femoral aneurysm represents a life- and limb-threatening entity because of its natural history of expansion and rupture. All mycotic femoral aneurysms therefore are treated surgically. The goals of treatment include eradication of infection and restoration of distal circulation.

The complexity of the operative procedure varies with the location and extent of the aneurysm. Although a direct approach to the femoral artery can be taken, a retroperitoneal exposure of the distal external iliac artery is preferred for large or proximal femoral lesions. An infected femoral artery aneurysm that is confined to only the common, superficial, or deep femoral artery can be excised with proximal and distal arterial ligation. Amputation is unusual when an isolated arterial segment is ligated without reconstruction. When the infectious process involves the femoral artery bifurcation and necessitates multiple arterial resections, most patients experience significant lower extremity ischemia followed by gradual improvement as

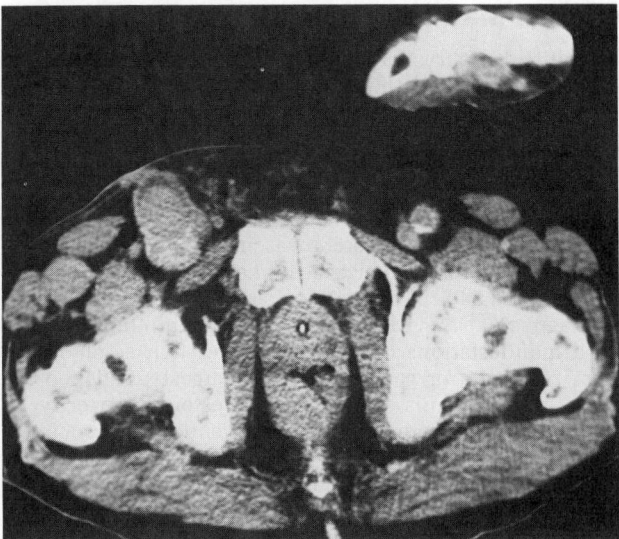

Figure 94-3. CT scan of an infected right femoral anastomotic aneurysm diagnosed 5 years after aortofemoral graft placement.

collateral circulation increases. Unfortunately, about one third of such patients require amputation if the limb is not urgently revascularized.[21] In patients whose sepsis can be adequately controlled at the initial procedure by excision of the aneurysm and aggressive débridement of adjacent tissue, Reddy and colleagues[21] have recommended immediate revascularization with an autogenous saphenous vein graft. Such a bypass, from healthy common femoral to healthy superficial femoral artery distal, is covered with a sartorius muscle flap. Using this approach, 54 infected false aneurysms in drug abusers were treated with an 11% amputation rate and no mortality.

In patients whose sepsis cannot be locally controlled at the time of initial arterial resection, in situ reconstruction is not an alternative. If limb-threatening ischemia persists for 24 hours after arterial ligation, revascularization through uninfected tissue planes using the lateral femoral or obturator route must be undertaken to avoid amputation. Use of prosthetic material is avoided because of the high incidence of early and late septic complications. Antibiotics are begun preoperatively, modified according to sensitivities from intraoperative cultures, and continued for at least 6 weeks.

POPLITEAL ARTERY ANEURYSMS

Incidence

Popliteal artery aneurysms are the most common arteriosclerotic peripheral aneurysm. They occur slightly more frequently than femoral artery lesions, but are diagnosed with one fortieth the frequency of abdominal aortic aneurysms.[1] As in patients with femoral lesions, multiple aneurysms commonly accompany popliteal aneurysms. Extrapopliteal degeneration occurs in up to 55% of patients,[22-26] with abdominal aortic and femoral lesions found in 40% to 50% and 40%, respectively.[27-29] Fifty to 70% of patients have bilateral popliteal aneurysms, and abdominal aortic aneurysms are found in 70% of these patients.[22,23,25 27-29] Popliteal artery aneurysms are clinically more important than femoral aneurysms because the former are more prone to limb-threatening complications.

Clinical Manifestations

Popliteal aneurysmal degeneration occurs almost exclusively in men, and the typical patient is in his seventh decade of life. Risk factors for atherosclerosis are common in these patients, and consequently there is a high incidence of other cardiovascular diseases. Of patients with popliteal aneurysms, 50% are smokers, 40% to 60% have hypertension, about 15% have diabetes mellitus,[27–29] 10% have manifestations of cerebrovascular disease[27], and over 40% have evidence of significant cardiac disease.[27]

Twenty to 54% of patients are asymptomatic at the time of diagnosis.[22–27,29] Most patients with symptoms present with manifestations of limb ischemia, such as claudication, rest pain, or gangrene. In the largest published reports, this ischemia was of limb-threatening severity in 44% to 95% of patients,[23,24] and frequently was associated with an acute event such as popliteal aneurysm thrombosis. Blue-toe syndrome is relatively common and is an reliable sign of microembolization. Nonischemic symptoms include the presence of a popliteal mass and local pain, leg swelling, or phlebitis secondary to compression of adjacent neural or venous structures.

Natural History

Popliteal artery aneurysms may be complicated by thrombosis, embolism, or rupture. Thrombosis and embolization both cause obliteration of the distal tibial vasculature and occur in 40% and 25% of patients, respectively.[28,30] Of patients developing these complications, up to 25% come to early amputation.[22,24,26,28] Rupture occurs in less than 5% of popliteal aneurysms.[27,28] In such cases, hemorrhage is usually confined to the popliteal space and does not preclude successful arterial reconstruction.

The natural history of asymptomatic popliteal aneurysms has been defined by observation of medically compromised patients with popliteal aneurysms. In most large surgical series of popliteal aneurysms, about 21% to 30% of patients are not operated on because of poor medical status.[23,26,29–31] Of these patients, about 30% die shortly after aneurysm discovery,[23,30] a finding consistent with their compromised medical condition. Of the remaining patients, 31% to 57% become symptomatic within 3 years.[23,26–30] Although some authors have correlated the risk of asymptomatic patients developing complications with the size of the aneurysm[22,29,31,32] and with the presence of mural thrombus,[23,27] it is critical to realize that small popliteal aneurysms are not free from such complications.[33]

Diagnosis

The diagnosis of popliteal aneurysm is usually first suspected after physical examination. In two thirds of patients with popliteal aneurysms, palpation of the popliteal space with the knee flexed reveals a pulsatile mass. Small aneurysms may not be palpable, and if thrombosis has occurred, only a nonpulsatile mass may be felt. Radiographs of the knee, demonstrating mural calcium, may suggest but not confirm the diagnosis. Only ultrasonography, CT, or MRI can exclude the other entities in the differential diagnosis of a popliteal fossa mass (tumor and Baker cyst), while confirming the presence of popliteal artery aneurysm. Once the diagnosis of popliteal artery aneurysm is made, a search for associated, life-threatening aortic and other limb-threatening peripheral aneurysms must be undertaken. Because abdominal aortic aneurysms can be missed during physical examination, investigation with CT and MRI is most efficient. Angiography can be misleading in the diagnosis of aneurysms because of the presence of intraluminal thrombus. Once repair is planned, however, angiography is essential to define the patency of distal vasculature (Fig. 94-4).

Treatment

Surgical Strategy

Early surgical treatment is recommended when a popliteal aneurysm is diagnosed because of the high incidence of complications. Operation is deferred in favor of observation only in patients with either inordinately high operative risk or severely limited life expectancy due to malignancy.

The goals of surgical treatment are to eliminate the potential for complications and to restore adequate lower extremity blood flow. In patients with multiple aneurysms, life-threatening aortic aneurysms are treated first, followed by repair of limb-threatening popliteal aneurysms. Conversely, if a limb-threatening complication has occurred, treatment of the popliteal aneurysm takes precedent, followed by expeditious aortic aneurysm repair.

Most popliteal artery aneurysms are easily exposed through standard medial thigh and calf incisions. Occasionally, for those lesions confined to the popliteal fossa, the posterior approach is effective. Most aneurysms are left in situ, bypassed, and then ligated. The conduit of choice is reversed saphenous vein, harvested from the thigh for good size match and tunneled along the course of popliteal artery. The proximal and distal anastomoses may be either end to end or end to side. When an end-

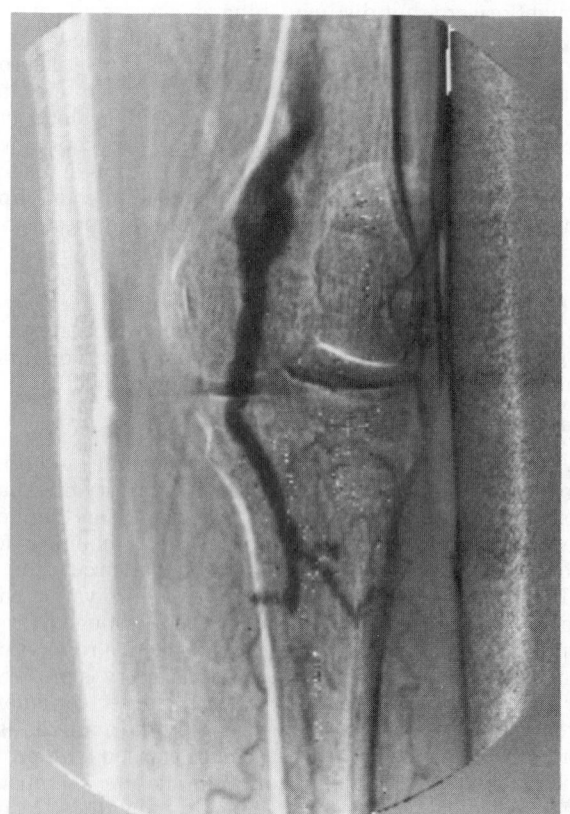

Figure 94-4. Arteriogram demonstrating a popliteal aneurysm associated with occlusion of the outflow tract, presumably from repeated episodes of embolism. A bypass to the distal posterior tibial artery was successful.

to-side configuration is chosen, the aneurysm must be excluded from the circulation by both proximal and distal ligation. When the distal popliteal and proximal tibial vessels are occluded with recent emboli, they may be cleared with a balloon catheter, intraoperative thrombolytic therapy, or both. In many of these cases, standard bypass grafts to the distal tibial vessels may be necessary.

If the aneurysm is large and causes local symptoms, the sac is opened, the thrombus evacuated, and the redundant portion of the wall removed. Alternatively, an obliterative endoaneurysmorrhaphy may be performed, thus avoiding trauma to the popliteal veins. For extensive femoral and popliteal aneurysmosis, in situ saphenous vein bypass, combined with proximal and distal aneurysmal ligation, preserves arterial continuity and avoids the potential of venous and neurologic injury associated with graft tunneling adjacent to large popliteal aneurysms.

The approach to the patient with an acutely ischemic extremity and a thrombosed popliteal aneurysm is controversial.[22,34-39] Preoperative thrombolysis of an occluded popliteal artery aneurysm was first described by Schwartz and colleagues in 1984.[40] Recommendations range from the use of lytic therapy in all ischemic extremities with a popliteal artery aneurysm[35] to its use in only those extremities with thrombosed popliteal artery aneurysms and absent runoff.[22] Because thrombolysis may unmask a runoff vessel suitable for distal bypass and thus allow a directed surgical approach, it is useful as a diagnostic adjuvant to angiography. In the setting of a critically ischemic limb, rapid access to angiographic personnel facile with the techniques of high-dose, pulse-spray thrombolysis is mandatory for the successful application of preoperative lytic therapy. In the absence of such support staff, or in the case of an extremity with severe neurologic compromise, standard on-table angiography, surgical cutdowns, and intraoperative instillation of lytic agents are necessary to define inflow and outflow sites.

Results

Excellent results can be expected in patients with asymptomatic aneurysms with intact distal vasculature.[22-29] Patients with thrombosed aneurysms or those in whom emboli have occluded the tibial arteries have less optimal results.[22,24,27,29] Operative mortality rates range from 0% to 6%,[22-25,27,32] with contemporary series nearly free from operative deaths. Most series report greater than 90% early patency and limb salvage for revascularization performed before ischemic complications. In contrast, in patients with ischemic symptoms, early patency rates range from 59% to 85%, with limb salvage rates of about 70% to 80%.[22-27] Series of popliteal artery aneurysms indicate that in the setting of acute ischemia, most limb loss occurs early after failed reconstruction[22,24,32] and bears little relation to whether one, two, or three named runoff vessels are present. The utility of lytic therapy, therefore, may lie in the identification of more limbs that can be salvaged with bypass to single vessel tibial outflow, and not in restoring multivessel outflow in limbs with single vessel runoff already suitable for bypass. After successful vascular reconstruction, overall long-term patency of vein grafts approaches 75%, with improved patency rates noted in extremities with preserved runoff.[22-27] Overall limb salvage rates exceed 90%.[22-27]

REFERENCES

1. Dent TL, Lindenauer SM, Ernst CB, Fry WJ. Multiple arteriosclerotic aneurysms. Arch Surg 1972;105:338.
2. Gedge SW, Spittel JA, Ivins JC. Aneurysm of the distal popliteal artery and its relationship to the arcuate popliteal ligament. Circulation 1961;24:270.
3. Newman DL, Gosling RG, Bowden NLR. Pressure amplitude increase on unmatching the aortoiliac junction of the leg. Cardiovasc Res 1972;6:1.
4. Brophy CM, Tilson JE, Braverman IM, Tilson MD. Age of onset, pattern of distribution, and histology of aneurysm development in a genetically predisposed mouse model. J Vasc Surg 1988;8:45.
5. Baxter BT, Halloran BG. Matrix protein metabolism in abdominal aortic aneurysms. In: Yao JST, Pearce WH, eds. Aneurysms: new findings and treatments. Norwalk CT, Appleton & Lange, 1994:25.
6. Graham LM, Zelenock GB, Whitehouse WM. Clinical significance of arteriosclerotic femoral artery aneurysms. Arch Surg 1980;115:502.
7. Cutler BS, Darling RC. Surgical management of arteriosclerotic femoral aneurysms. Surgery 1973;74:764.
8. Szilagyi DE, Smith RF, Elliott JP, Hageman JH, Dall'Olmo CA. Anastomotic aneurysms after vascular reconstruction: problems of incidence, etiology, and treatment. Surgery 1975;78:800.
9. Szilagyi DE, Elliott JP, Smith RF, Reddy DJ, McPharlin M. A 30-year survey of the reconstructive surgical treatment of aortoiliac occlusive disease. J Vasc Surg 1986;3:421.
10. Dennis JW, Littooy FN, Greisler HP, Baker WH. Anastomotic pseudoaneurysms: a continuing late complication of vascular reconstructive procedures. Arch Surg 1986;121:314.
11. Seabrook GR, Schmidtt DD, Bandyk DF, Edmiston CE, Krepel CJ, Towne JB. Anastomotic femoral pseudoaneurysm: an investigation of occult infection as an etiologic factor. J Vasc Surg 1990;11:629.
12. Babu SC, Piccorelli GO, Shah PM, Stein JH, Clauss RH. Incidence and results of arterial complications among 16,350 patients undergoing cardiac catheterization. J Vasc Surg 1989;10:113.
13. Messina LM, Brothers TE, Wakefield TW. Clinical characteristics and surgical management of vascular complications in patients undergoing cardiac catheterization: interventional versus diagnostic procedures. J Vasc Surg 1991;13:593.
14. Kresowik TF, Khoury MD, Miller BV, et al. A prospective study of the incidence and natural history of femoral vascular complications after percutaneous transluminal coronary angioplasty. J Vasc Surg 1991;13:328.
15. Kent KC, McArdle CR, Kennedy B, Baim DS, Anninos E, Skillman JJ. A prospective study of the clinical outcome of femoral pseudoaneurysms and arteriovenous fistulas induced by arterial puncture. J Vasc Surg 1993;17:125.
16. Mills JL, Wiedeman JE, Robison JG, Hallet JW. Minimizing mortality and morbidity from iatrogenic arterial injuries: the need for early recognition and prompt repair. J Vasc Surg 1986;4:22.
17. Feld RE, Patton GM, Carabasi A, Alexander A, Merton D, Needleman L. Treatment of iatrogenic femoral artery injuries with ultrasound-guided compression. J Vasc Surg 1992;16:832.
18. Cox GS, Young JR, Gray BR, Grubb MW, Hertzer NR. Ultrasound-guided compression repair of postcatheterization pseudoaneurysms: results of treatment in one hundred cases. J Vasc Surg 1994;19:683.
19. Anderson CB, Butcher HR, Ballinger WF. Mycotic aneurysms. Arch Surg 1974;109:712.
20. Brown SL, Busuttil RW, Baker JD, Machleder HI, Moore WS, Barker WF. Bacteriologic and surgical determinants of survival in patients with mycotic aneurysms. J Vasc Surg 1984;1:541.
21. Reddy DJ, Smith RF, Elliott JP, Haddad GK, Wanek EA. Infected femoral artery false aneurysms in drug addicts: evolution of selective vascular reconstruction. J Vasc Surg 1986;3:718.
22. Carpenter JP, Barker CF, Roberts B, Berkowitz HD, Lusk EJ, Perloff LJ. Popliteal artery aneurysms: current management and outcome. J Vasc Surg 1994;19:65.
23. Varga ZA, Locke-Edmunds JC, Baird RN. A multicenter study of popliteal aneurysms. J Vasc Surg 1994;20:171.
24. Shortell CK, DeWeese JA, Ouriel K, Green RM. Popliteal artery

aneurysms: a 25-year surgical experience. J Vasc Surg 1991;14:771.

25. Lilly MP, Flinn WR, McCarthy WJ, Courtney DF, Yao JST, Bergan JJ. The effect of distal arterial anatomy on the success of popliteal aneurysm repair. J Vasc Surg 1988;7:653.

26. Dawson I, van Bockel JH, Brand R, Terpstra JL. Popliteal artery aneurysms: long-term follow-up of aneurysmal disease and results of surgical treatment. J Vasc Surg 1991;13:398.

27. Anton GE, Hertzer NE, Beven EG, O'Hara PJ, Krajewski LP. Surgical management of popliteal aneurysms: trends in presentation, treatment, and results from 1952 to 1984. J Vasc Surg 1986;3:125.

28. Vermilion BD, Kimmins SA, Pace WG, Evans WE. A review of one hundred forty-seven popliteal aneurysms with long-term follow-up. Surgery 1981;90:1009.

29. Whitehouse WM Jr, Wakefield TW, Graham LM. Limb-threatening potential of arteriosclerotic popliteal artery aneurysms. Surgery 1983;93:694.

30. Wychulis AR, Spittell JA, Wallace RB. Popliteal aneurysms. Surgery 1970;68:942.

31. Schellack J, Smith RB III, Perdue GD. Non-operative management of selective popliteal aneurysms. Arch Surg 1987; 122:372.

32. Bouhoutsos J, Martin P. Popliteal aneurysm: a review of 116 cases. Br J Surg 1974;61:469.

33. Inahara T, Toledo AC. Complications and treatment of popliteal aneurysms. Surgery 1978;84:775.

34. Ferguson LJ, Faris I, Robertson A, Lloyd JV, Miller JH. Intra-arterial streptokinase therapy to relieve acute limb ischemia. J Vasc Surg 1986;4:205.

35. Bowyer RC, Cawthorn SJ, Walker WJ, Giddings AEB. Conservative management of asymptomatic popliteal aneurysm. Br J Surg 1990;77:1132.

36. Taylor LM, Porter JM, Baur GM, Hallin RW, Peck JL, Eidemiller LR. Intraarterial streptokinase infusion for acute popliteal and tibial artery occlusion. Am J Surg 1984;147:583.

37. Kissin MW, Pullan R, Scott DJA, Horrocks M, Baird RN. Popliteal aneurysms presenting as acute limb ischemia. Br J Surg 1989;76:416.

38. Lancashire MJR, Torrie EPH, Gallard RB. Popliteal aneurysms identified by intra-arterial streptokinase: a changing pattern of presentation. Br J Surg 1990;77:1388.

39. Walker WJ, Giddings AEB. A protocol for the safe treatment of acute lower limb ischemia with intra-arterial streptokinase and surgery. Br J Surg 1988;75:1189.

40. Schwarz W, Berkowitz H, Taormina V, Gatti J. The preoperative use in intraarterial thrombolysis for a thrombosed popliteal artery aneurysm. J Cardiovasc Surg 1984;25:465.

SURGERY: SCIENTIFIC PRINCIPLES AND PRACTICE, Second Edition, edited by Lazar J. Greenfield, Michael W. Mulholland, Keith T. Oldham, Gerald B. Zelenock, and Keith D. Lillemoe. Lippincott–Raven Publishers, Philadelphia, © 1997.

CHAPTER 95

VASCULAR MALFORMATION AND ARTERIOVENOUS FISTULA

S. MARTIN LINDENAUER

An arteriovenous fistula (AVF) is an abnormal connection between an artery and vein that bypasses a capillary bed. AVFs are classified as either acquired or congenital. An acquired fistula is almost always caused by penetrating trauma such as a stab or bullet wound or the physician's or surgeon's needle or trocar. On rare occasions, an acquired AVF may be nontraumatic in origin, resulting from the erosion of an aneurysmal artery into an adjacent vein or by infection or a neoplasm. The acquired arteriovenous connection is usually single, and only occasionally is a second or third communication encountered. Congenital AVF is usually present at birth, although it may not be immediately apparent. It is to be distinguished from an acquired fistula by the multiple connections that are sometimes too numerous to count (Fig. 95-1).

An acquired fistula usually results in early dilation of both the artery and vein leading to and from the fistula site (Fig. 95-2). The extent of the dilation is related to the size of the fistula, its location (central versus peripheral), and its duration. A fistula of long duration is associated with degenerative changes in the proximal arterial wall (Fig. 95-3) and with premature arteriosclerosis and calcification. Despite elimination of the fistula, aneurysmal dilation and even late rupture of the dilated artery proximal to the fistula have occurred.[1,2]

Although almost all congenital fistulas have a multitude of arteriovenous connections, there are some specific exceptions, such as cardiac atrial and ventricular septal defects, patent ductus arteriosus, and the rare peripheral arteriovenous malformation (AVM) with a solitary connection.

Purposeful construction of AVFs are sometimes used for therapeutic purposes, such as vascular access for hemodialysis, chemotherapy, and long-term parenteral nutrition. The dialysis fistula, first introduced by Brescia and associates in 1966,[3] can be easily accomplished by the creation of a side-to-side radial artery to cephalic vein anastomosis and should be attempted initially if suitable vessels are present. Prosthetic material can also be used to join the radial or brachial artery to the cephalic vein in either a linear fashion or in a circular configuration in the antecubital fossa. Care must be exercised in the construction of

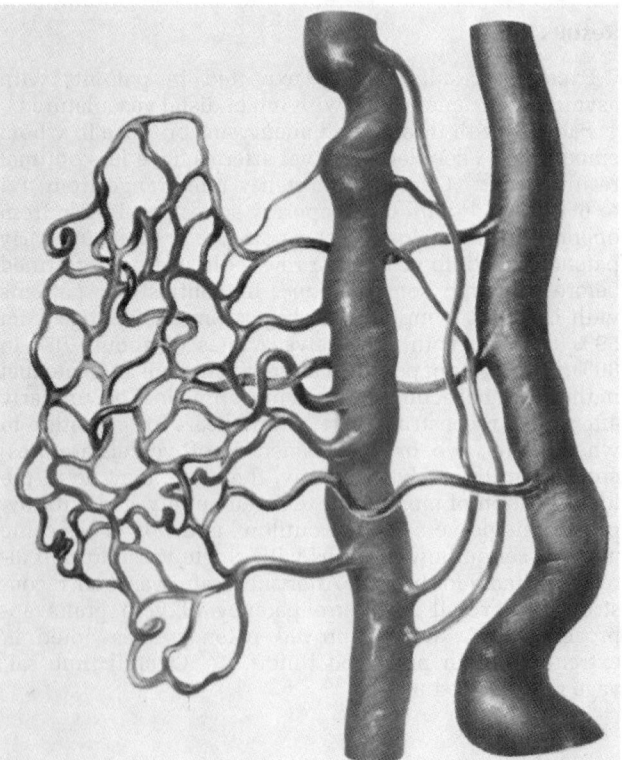

Figure 95-1. Artist's rendition of multiple connections between an artery and vein in a congenital arteriovenous fistula (Malan E, ed. Vascular malformations. Milan, Carlo Erba Foundation, 1974:34)

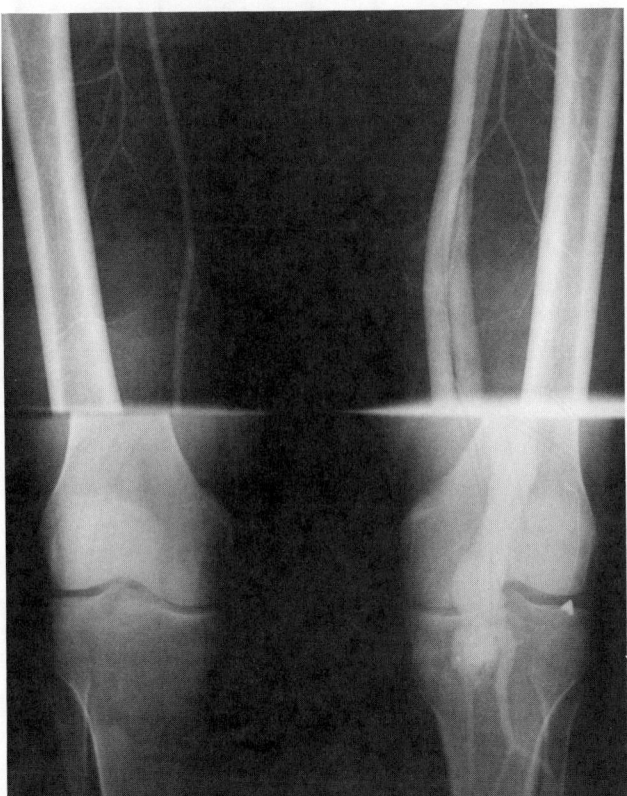

Figure 95-2. Radiograph of popliteal arteriovenous fistula, showing dilation of proximal artery and vein. (Lindenauer SM, Thompson NW, Kraft RO, Fry WJ. Late complications of traumatic arteriovenous fistulas. Surg Gynecol Obstet 1969;129:530)

such a fistula to avoid distal ischemia and venous hypertension, which causes discomfort and swelling, both of which can be troublesome. Such fistulas may stay open for prolonged periods, despite the chronic trauma caused by puncturing them frequently with large-caliber needles needed for hemodialysis. If the fistula is initially too small, early failure results; if it is too large, undesirable hemodynamic effects are created.

AVFs have been used in children to increase limb length; but this practice has been largely abandoned, particularly subsequent to the introduction of orthopedic bone-lengthening techniques, first reported in the Soviet Union. AVFs have also been created as an adjunct to enhance the patency of a low-flow distal bypass and in venous reconstruction.

Normal limbs contain arteriovenous shunts that bypass capillary beds and are present in the skin and subcutaneous tissue of the extremities. They are largely under adrenergic control, are nonnutritive, and play an important role in temperature regulation of the extremities.[4] The evidence that they are present in significant numbers in the viscera is controversial. They may play a role in hyperdynamic sepsis.[5] They normally account for less than 5% of total limb flow but can cause the early venous fill sometimes observed in severely ischemic extremities. They are thought by some authors to be related to the origin of venous varicosities.[6,7]

A growing number of acquired AVFs are associated with percutaneous procedures performed in the groin for a variety of diagnostic and therapeutic cardiac and radiographic procedures as well as for solid-organ percutaneous needle biopsy for the diagnosis of solid-organ disease and of transplant rejection.

The abnormal hemodynamics of an AVF result in local, peripheral, and systemic effects, all of which are influenced by the size of the fistulous connection and its location and duration. In general, centrally located AVFs are more likely to produce heart failure; whereas in distal AVFs, ischemia may be more troublesome. Congenital AVFs tend to produce less dramatic peripheral and systemic manifestations, whereas the local changes may be more striking.

HEMODYNAMIC ALTERATIONS

The predominant feature of an AVF is the significant decrease in peripheral resistance created by bypassing the capillary bed distal to the fistulous connection. The length and diameter of the fistula influence the degree of the reduction in peripheral resistance. Peripheral resistance is decreased less by the greater length of the abnormal connection between the artery and vein, such as in an H-type fistula, than by a side-to-side fistula of equal diameter. Peripheral resistance is inversely proportional to the diam-

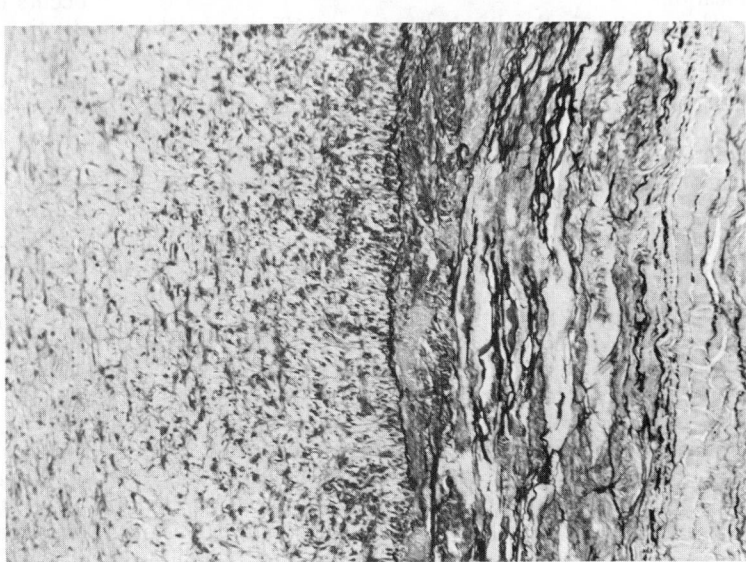

Figure 95-3. Photomicrograph of segment of subclavian artery proximal to traumatic brachial arteriovenous fistula of 21 years' duration. Thickened intima is seen on the left, and the fragmented elastic fiber is stained black (elastic tissue stain, ×127). (Lindenauer SM, Thompson NW, Kraft RO, Fry WJ. Late complications of traumatic arteriovenous fistulas. Surg Gynecol Obstet 1969;192:527)

eter of the connection in an AVF. There is no further decrease in peripheral resistance, however, when the diameter of the connection is greater than the diameter of the proximal artery. The multiple small connections of a typical congenital AVF usually do not significantly lower peripheral resistance.

Local Hemodynamic Effects

The most significant local hemodynamic change in an AVF is the increase in volume flow through the proximal artery, which is consistently present. Not only is the overall flow increased, but the reversed flow normally seen in diastole is absent. Although both systolic and diastolic flow are greatly increased, the relatively greater increase in diastolic flow results in markedly reduced pulsatility. The flow in the proximal vein increases significantly and becomes pulsatile, coinciding with arterial systole and diastole. This is usually most evident close to the fistulous connection and becomes less prominent at increasing distance from the fistulous site.

The direction of flow in the proximal artery is toward the fistula, whereas the flow in the proximal vein is directed proximally. After several weeks, arterial and venous collateral circulation develop around the fistula. The arterial and venous collateral flow initially bypass the fistula.

Flow in the distal artery and vein may be either proximal or distal, depending on the specific anatomic arrangement, and it can change over time. The direction of the venous flow distal to the fistula changes as the venous valves become incompetent, allowing reversed venous flow.

In a small AVF with minimal arterial collaterals, the flow in the distal artery usually continues in an antegrade fashion. In a large chronic AVF, the well-developed arterial collaterals bypassing the fistula result in reversal of the flow in the distal artery. Sometimes, the flow in the artery distal to the AVF is relatively stagnant, depending on the balance between the peripheral resistance and the degree of arterial collateral development. Distal arterial flow seldom becomes stagnant enough to cause thrombosis. Retrograde distal arterial flow contributes to the peripheral ischemia that occurs in an AVF.

Arterial pressure may be normal in the proximal artery; when the fistulous connection is large and associated with increased volume flow and decreased peripheral resistance, the arterial pressure may be lower than normal. As the proximal artery dilates, the pressure increases and can become greater than in a normal artery at a comparable location.

The pressure in the distal artery of an AVF is invariably reduced and is associated with retrograde arterial flow. The decreased distal pressure is offset by the increase in the collateral vessels that develop. Collateral formation around a chronic AVF can be striking. The increased collateral flow further decreases arterial outflow resistance and increases the flow reversal in the distal artery (Fig. 95-4).

Because of the nature of the venous capacitance, the pressure in the vein proximal to an AVF tends to rise minimally despite the large increase in volume flow. The pressure in the distal vein tends to rise acutely when the venous valves are still competent; over time, distal venous resistance falls because of dilation and subsequent venous valve incompetence associated with the formation of venous collateral around the fistula. The distal venous collateral may be equally extensive and the striking varicosities that are sometimes encountered may be the feature that brings the patient to clinical attention.

A unique characteristic of an AVF is the thrill and bruit created by the turbulent flow and resultant wall vibration

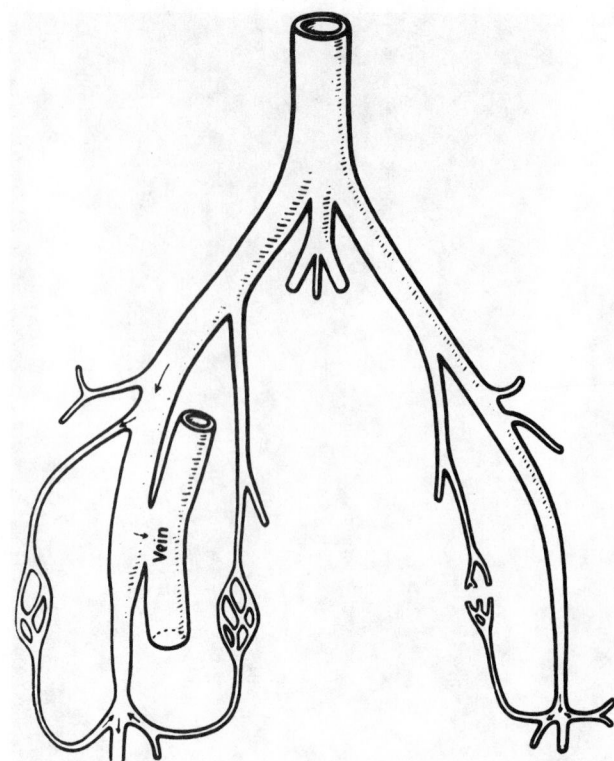

Figure 95-4. Illustration of collateral formation around a femoral arteriovenous fistula that is contributing to flow reversal in the arterial segment distal to the fistula. (Holman E. Abnormal arteriovenous connections. Springfield, IL, Charles C Thomas, 1968:62)

created in this unusual hemodynamic environment. It is similar but usually more marked than the turbulence in the area of bifurcations, aneurysms, and abrupt changes in lumen diameter.

Generally, AVFs that are small may not come to clinical attention and may close spontaneously. This occurs in small AVFs associated with in situ vein bypass grafts. The reason for this is unclear but may relate to the volume flow through such small AVFs and the capacity of the venous outflow bed. Many small acquired AVFs in the groin secondary to femoral catheterization resolve spontaneously.[8] In clinically apparent AVFs, the characteristic change that occurs in the proximal artery and in the draining vein is dilation. Over time, this leads to structural changes in the arterial wall.[9] On occasion, the structural damage can result in aneurysm formation, which can occur even after the fistula has been disconnected (Fig. 95-5). Because of the structural damage, the loss of strength in the arterial wall can make repair of a chronic AVF technically difficult, and suture disruption of the anastomosis has been reported both with closure of the AVF and with repair of an arteriovenous aneurysm, if present. The cause of the degenerative changes is unclear but is probably related to the altered hemodynamics created by the AVF.

The dilated proximal vein becomes elongated, tortuous, and thickened (Fig. 95-6), and degenerative changes of the vein wall are sometimes pronounced. It is in this setting that the rarely encountered venous aneurysm occurs[10,11] (Fig. 95-7).

The venous wall that is exposed to the forceful jet of arterial blood at the fistula site is invariably damaged and can be the locus of bacterial endarteritis. Dilation of the distal vein can be progressive, and the valves in the deep system, as well as the perforating and superficial vein

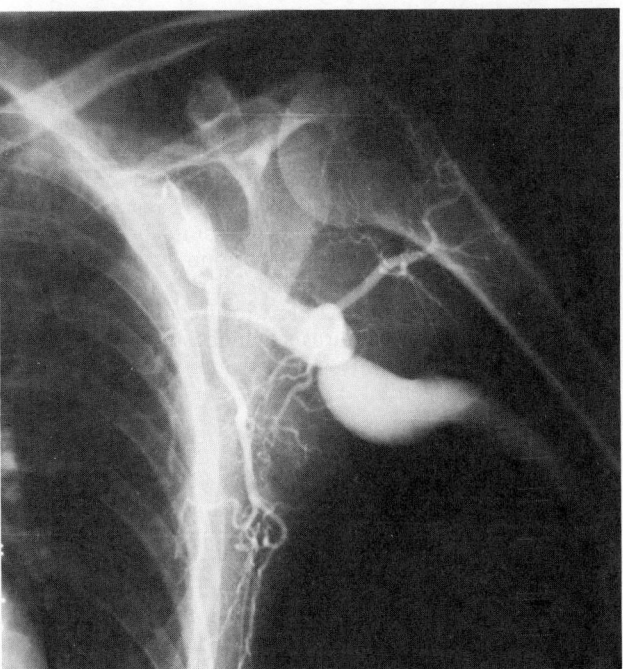

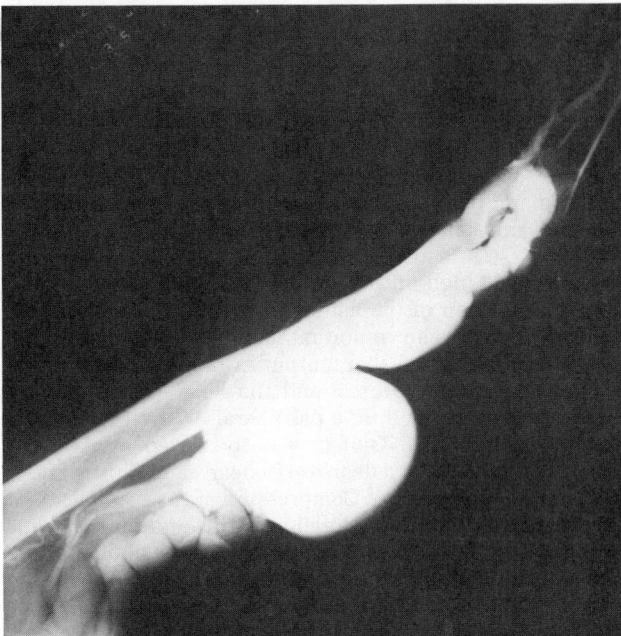

Figure 95-5. Radiograph of an axillary artery aneurysm proximal to a brachial arteriovenous fistula of 21 years' duration. (Lindenauer SM, Thompson NW, Kraft RO, Fry WJ. Late complications of traumatic arteriovenous fistulas. Surg Gynecol Obstet 1969;192:526)

Figure 95-7. Radiograph of a brachial venous aneurysm proximal to a chronic antecubital arteriovenous fistula. (Thompson NW, Lindenauer SM. Central venous aneurysm and arteriovenous fistula. Ann Surg 1969;170:853)

valves, ultimately become incompetent. A serious consequence of this is the development of venous varicosities, chronic venous valvular insufficiency, and chronic venous ulceration. When there is distal arterial insufficiency associated with an uncorrected AVF, the ulcer can have both an arterial and venous component. Correction of the fistula

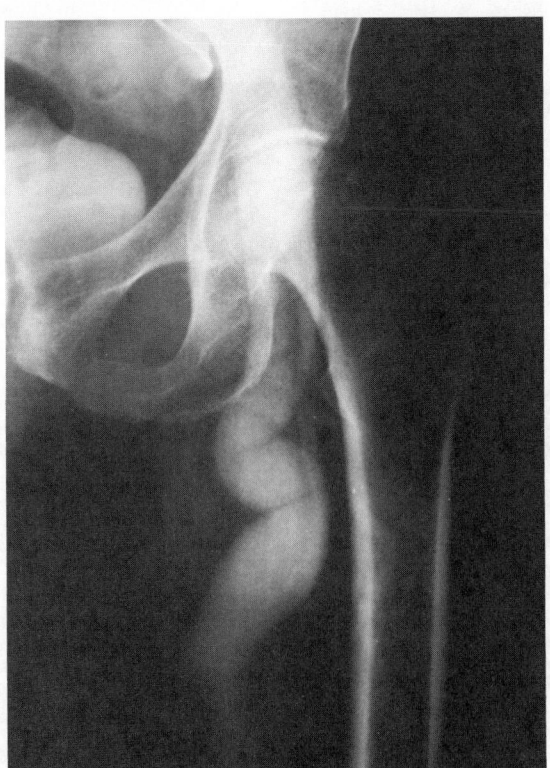

Figure 95-6. Radiograph of dilated and tortuous ileofemoral vein proximal to a chronic arteriovenous fistula.

can eliminate the arterial component, but the chronic venous changes are not usually reversible, and a venous ulcer can persist and result in considerable morbidity.

Depending on the particular anatomic arrangement, the abnormal arteriovenous connection can enlarge and form a frank aneurysm (an arteriovenous aneurysm), which may even undergo calcification.

Systemic Hemodynamic Effects

The most important systemic abnormality of an AVF is a drop in total peripheral resistance. The systemic response to this change is an increase in cardiac output achieved by an increase in both heart rate and stroke volume. The enhanced stroke volume is related to greater venous return and a larger total blood volume. In hemodynamically significant AVFs, the blood volume, cardiac output, heart rate, and stroke volume are always increased. In most AVFs after a relatively short period, there is a decrease in systemic diastolic pressure with a larger pulse pressure, which may sometimes be appreciated by the astute clinician as a "water-hammer pulse."

Because of the ability of the venous circulation to accommodate to a greater blood volume without a rise in venous pressure, the increased blood volume that occurs in an AVF is not associated with an increase in central venous pressure.

The increase in cardiac output in the presence of an AVF appears almost immediately and rapidly reaches maximal levels. Abrupt compression or occlusion of an AVF rapidly decreases cardiac output. In a large fistula, the increase in cardiac output may not equal the increased flow through the fistula. In such a circumstance, there is a decrease in systemic arterial flow as a result of peripheral vasoconstriction. If this compensatory mechanism is insufficient, systemic arterial pressure can fall and high-output cardiac failure can rapidly and dramatically ensue. This is typically seen in an acute aortocaval fistula, as can occur with erosion of an aortic aneurysm into the inferior vena cava. Rupture into an iliac vein or renal vein has been reported but is a less frequent occurrence. Aortocaval fistula occurs most often from aneurysmal rupture into the inferior vena cava, whereas trauma and iatrogenic causes occur only rarely. Dramatic unresponsive cardiac failure and death usually occur unless the aortocaval fistula is promptly diagnosed and treated. Fortunately, most AVFs are more peripheral and smaller, and these changes are less severe. The increase in cardiac output and blood volume and the occurrence of high-output cardiac failure are related to the size and location of the fistula; the amount of preexisting cardiac disease is an important factor as well.

The increase in cardiac output is due primarily to an increase in stroke volume, and the heart rate may only be minimally elevated. In a peripheral AVF, the proximal artery or the fistula itself may be occluded by external pressure, resulting in a decrease in heart rate. This is know as the Branham sign.[12,13] Compression of the fistula causes a slight rise in systemic arterial pressure, and the resultant bradycardia (which may be minimal) can be abolished by the administration of atropine, which suggests that this phenomenon is a vagus-mediated response of the baroreceptors in the carotid sinus and aortic arch. Other baroreceptors, such as those present in the heart and lung, can also be involved.

The increased stroke volume contributing to the elevated cardiac output in an AVF is associated with the increased venous return that is present. It may also reflect enhanced cardiac contractility due to elevated catecholamine levels and adrenergic stimulation.

Cardiomegaly is almost always seen in patients with a hemodynamically significant AVF (Fig. 95-8). The degree of cardiomegaly is directly related to the size of the fistula and its duration and is far more common in patients with acquired fistulas than in those with congenital fistulas. The cardiomegaly is usually reversed when the fistula is eliminated. The increase in cardiac size represents both dilation and hypertrophy.

The increase in total blood volume in a large AVF may be striking. It correlates with the size of the AVF and the increase in cardiac output. The increase in total blood volume is due to a disproportionate increase in plasma volume. This occurs through the normal sodium- and water-retaining mechanisms that are activated in response to the fistula, in which systemic arterial pressure changes stimulate the renin–angiotensin–aldosterone system. The occurrence of high-output congestive heart failure is a liability of all large, chronic AVFs. Closure of the fistula is associated with urinary diuresis, which is sometimes striking. High-output congestive heart failure seldom occurs in patients with congenital AVFs.

SIGNS AND SYMPTOMS

The signs and symptoms of an AVF are often striking, yet patients may fail to come to clinical attention for prolonged periods. There is almost always a history of penetrating injury; this may on occasion be overlooked despite the usually dramatic circumstances surrounding a gunshot wound or stabbing. There may be evidence of a prior injury in the form of a cutaneous scar at the site of the fistula. The development of an AVF due to blunt trauma is highly unlikely but presumably could occur, for example, by the occult penetration of an adjacent artery and vein by a bone fragment associated with a fracture. Usually a pulsating mass, a vibration, or a buzzing sound can be felt and sensed by the patient. There is increased warmth at the site of the fistula, and the extremity distal to the AVF is cool.

The arterial circulation distal to an AVF is invariably diminished, and there is impaired venous return. This can be observed clinically by the appearance of edema, diminished pulses, pallor, and varicosities. There may be pain, symptoms of intermittent claudication, paresthesia, cuta-

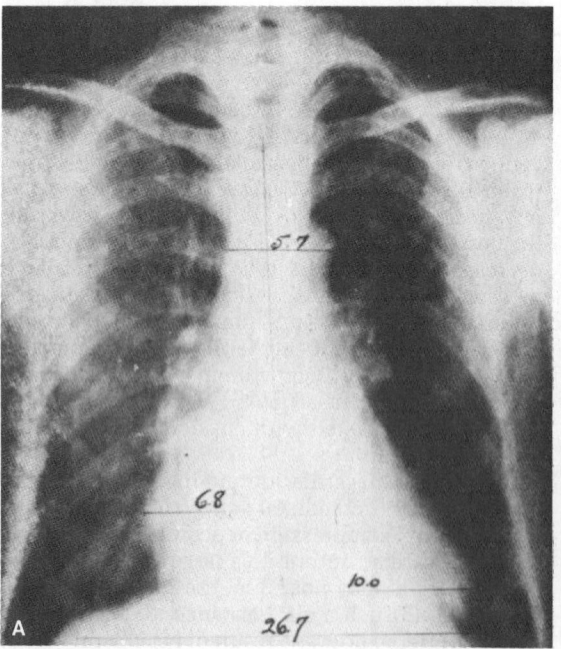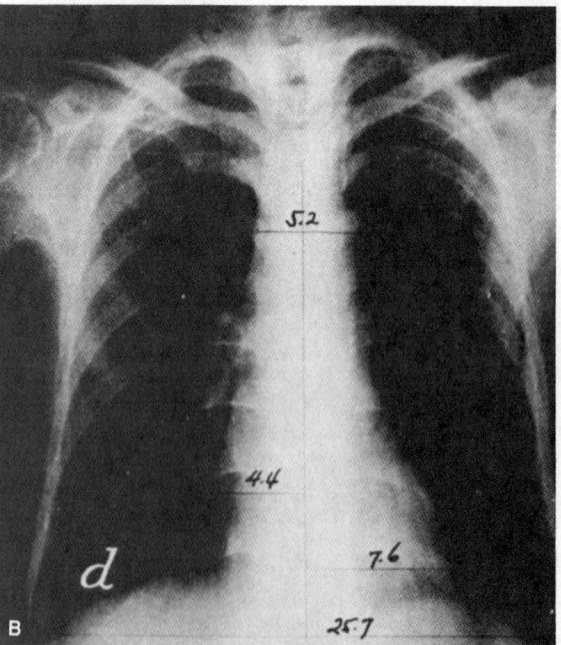

Figure 95-8. (*A*) Chest radiograph demonstrating cardiomegaly with a femoral arteriovenous fistula. (*B*) Chest radiograph demonstrating normal heart size after closure of a femoral arteriovenous fistula. (Holman E. Abnormal arteriovenous connections. Springfield, IL, Charles C Thomas, 1968:62)

neous ulceration, or frank gangrene of the digits. In large fistulas with well-developed collateral circulation, temporary occlusion of the proximal artery further decreases distal arterial pressure. This phenomenon explains the poor results previously obtained in treatment of AVFs by proximal artery ligation. Edema due to impaired arterial perfusion or inefficient venous return may be present. The reduction in arterial flow and pressure distal to the fistula site is related to the size of the fistula, and the hemodynamic significance can be easily assessed by measurement of the distal artery pressure using the Doppler velocity meter. The signs and symptoms of high-output cardiac failure usually occur only in larger, more centrally located AVFs and are a late phenomenon.

A loud murmur is usually heard directly over the fistula, and a thrill is frequently present. The loudness and duration of the murmur are equal during systole and diastole; the murmur is sometimes referred to as a *machinery murmur.* There may also be some systolic accentuation. The veins distal to the fistula, particularly in the leg, are dilated and varicose and demonstrate incompetent valves. There may be an increase in limb girth. In young children, extremity AVF can lead to limb length inequality if the AVF is present before epiphyseal fusion. The veins in the region of the fistula may pulsate and exhibit a thrill and murmur. Compression of the artery proximal to the fistula or compression of the fistulous connection produces the Branham sign.

Carotid cavernous sinus fistula is an uncommon AVF in which tearing of the cavernous portion of the carotid artery occurs.[14] It can be due to basilar skull fracture, penetrating injuries, carotid aneurysm rupture, collagen vascular disease, surgical trauma, and fibromuscular dysplasia. Most carotid cavernous fistulas present with orbital bruit, retro-orbital pain, chemosis, proptosis, visual loss, cerebral ischemia, and subarachnoid hemorrhage.

Vertebral AVFs are also uncommon.[15] They may result from penetrating wounds of the neck or iatrogenic trauma. Symptoms of vertebral artery steal can occur, with a thrill and bruit over the fistula site.

Hepatic artery–portal venous fistula[16] can result from erosion of a portal vein by a hepatocellular carcinoma, from a hepatic artery aneurysm, or from blunt or penetrating hepatic trauma. This type of fistula can cause portal hypertension and result in esophageal varices, upper gastrointestinal bleeding, ascites, splenomegaly, hemobilia, and right upper quadrant pain. A thrill or bruit in the region of the liver is uncommon, and liver function is usually normal.

DIAGNOSIS

Noninvasive techniques offer several important opportunities to document the presence of an AVF. The decrease in artery pressure distal to an AVF in an extremity can easily be measured by a Doppler velocity meter. Further evidence of an AVF is an increase in distal arterial pressure with manual compression of the fistula and an immediate increase in pulse volume. If there is a reversal of flow in the distal artery, compression just distal to the suspected AVF results in an increase in arterial pressure in the distal extremity. Distal arterial pressure also increases with compression at the proximal or distal vein and is strong clinical evidence of the presence of an AVF. The finding of normal distal arterial pressure does not rule out an AVF; but if an AVF is present, the normal pressure suggests that the AVF is not large and that compensating mechanisms are sufficient to prevent significant hemodynamic abnormalities. Plethysmographic techniques (pulse volume recorder, photoplethysmograph, mercury strain gauge) that measure

limb or digital volume distal to a suspected AVF are usually decreased. Not only is Doppler flow velocity increased in the artery proximal to an AVF, the quality of the signal is also different—the normal triphasic flow is replaced by a higher pitched, more continuous signal that is prolonged in diastole without reversal of flow. Phasic pulsatile flow may also be heard in the larger proximal and distal veins adjacent to the fistula. The continuous quality of the abnormal bruit heard directly over the fistulous connection with the stethoscope is even more striking with Doppler auscultation.

Direct measurement of skin temperature with a thermistor documents the decreased temperature distal to the fistula and the increased temperature in the area of the fistula. Oxygen saturation measured in the venous blood draining an AVF is usually elevated when compared with the venous oxygen saturation of the contralateral limb.

The increased cardiac output can be measured by thermal dilution techniques. Compression of the fistulous connection causes a decrease in cardiac output, and the amount of the difference provides a good estimate of the volume flow through the fistula.

Technetium-labeled albumin microspheres larger than a dilated capillary (10 μm) when injected into the proximal artery pass through an AVF and are then trapped in the lung, where they can be monitored with an external gamma detector. The normally occurring arteriovenous shunts in the skin and subcutaneous tissues of the extremities usually represent less than 5% of total extremity flow. With careful mixing during injection, the fraction of microspheres that are detected over the lung provide a qualitative assessment of the volume flow through the fistula. Care must be taken to account for the effect of sympatholytic drugs and sympathetic denervation, which increase the normal arteriovenous shunting in an extremity to as much as 40% of total limb flow.[17]

This technique may be most useful in distinguishing congenital AVFs from those congenital anomalies in which an arteriovenous component is minimal or absent. Although this can usually be accomplished by arteriography, smaller hypodynamic congenital AVFs are sometimes not visible on an arteriogram and can easily be missed if exposure timing of the arteriogram is incorrect.

The most important modality for both the diagnosis and treatment of AVF is arteriography, which not only provides information about the precise site, number, and size of fistulous connections but also indicates the functional status of the abnormality and the extent of collateral circulation (Fig. 95-9). Multiple radiographs taken at a rapid rate are necessary to capture the rapid clearance of the contrast through the fistula. The status of the proximal arterial vessels can be assessed, and their degree of dilation, their tortuosity, and the presence of aneurysmal disease can be defined. Similar information regarding the draining veins can be obtained as well. In profoundly ischemic extremities, there may be exaggeration of the flow through the normally occurring arteriovenous anastomoses, and in the same radiograph, simultaneous visualization of large arteries and veins may be possible. The absence of the other signs and findings of an AVF and the presence of profound ischemia should allow the clinician to avoid such confusion.

The angiographic diagnosis of congenital AVFs can be more difficult than that of traumatic AVFs because small hypodynamic AVFs may not be visible. A number of indirect signs of abnormal arteriovenous connections may be helpful, such as increased flow in the proximal artery, decreased peripheral arterial flow, and early venous filling. The larger, more hyperdynamic connections in a congenital AVF create a confusing maze of vessels, and it is usually

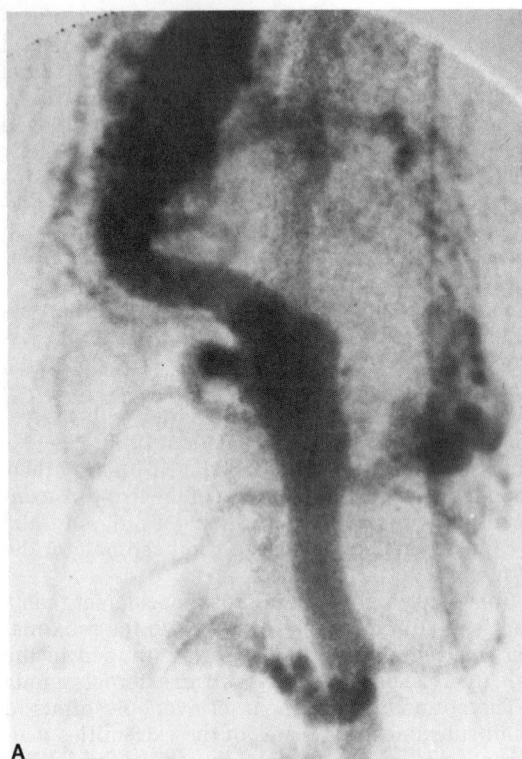

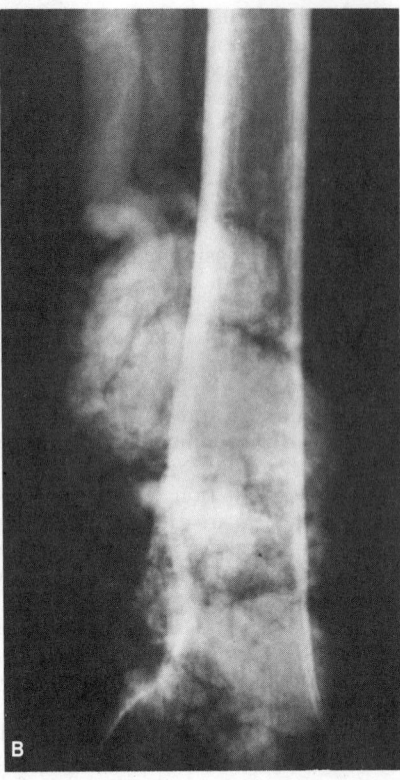

Figure 95-9. (*A*) Radiograph taken during the early phase of arteriography of congenital arteriovenous fistula of distal thigh, showing multiple abnormal dilated and tortuous arteries. (*B*) Radiograph from the later phase of arteriography in the same patient. There is a mass of abnormal vascular channels, and simultaneous visualization of the dilated proximal artery and vein is possible.

impossible to distinguish arteries from veins from fistulous connections. It is not possible, except in a general qualitative fashion, to ascertain the magnitude of the arteriovenous connections in a congenital AVF.

Duplex scanning can identify the enlarged artery and vein leading to a peripheral fistula as well as the increased flow velocity. If there is a single, large connection, it can be easily identified, and so can the arteriovenous aneurysm joining the vessels, if present. Congenital fistulas present a more complex picture, but duplex scanning may be useful in identifying an enlarged proximal artery and draining vein. Patients with an acquired AVF or with the more common femoral pseudoaneurysm secondary to femoral catheterization can be followed with duplex scanning, and many such lesions resolve spontaneously.[8]

Computed tomography (CT) with contrast may be particularly useful in demonstrating the sometimes troublesome multiple connections present in muscle and bone in a congenital fistula.

Congenital fistulas can also be visualized by magnetic resonance imaging (MRI), which provides views in both transverse and longitudinal section. MRI allows precise anatomic localization and provides details concerning the size and extent of a congenital AVF. The relation to specific muscle groups, bones, and vascular structures can be accurately determined.[18] The MRI appearance of a congenital AVF consists of dilated tortuous vessels infiltrating or replacing involved tissues. MRI allows differentiation among fat, muscle, tendon, bone, and blood vessels based on signal characteristics. In this manner, the true extent of a congenital AVF can be visualized. Although enlarged vessels are seen, the exact arteries and veins supplying and draining the lesion frequently cannot be ascertained.

In contrast, arteriography is usually unable to show the relation of a congenital AVF to muscle groups, fascial planes, and nerves. Angiography frequently underestimates the extent of a congenital AVF and the amount of abnormal tissue present.

MRI and angiography are complementary in the evaluation of congenital AVF and in treatment planning.

TREATMENT

The principles underlying the treatment of traumatic and congenital AVFs are distinctly different. Traumatic AVFs exhibit unpredictable increases in size; congenital AVFs may progress to involve areas previously clinically uninvolved, confounding treatment.

Historically, the treatment of traumatic AVF was delayed to allow the formation of sufficient collateral so that ligation of the fistula would not cause distal ischemia. This is no longer necessary because four-vessel ligation is reserved for small fistulas involving unimportant vessels in areas where the blood supply is redundant, and ligation does not interfere with overall perfusion. Using standard vascular surgery techniques, preservation of arterial flow is a goal that is easily attained. Small veins may be ligated with impunity; larger veins should be reconstructed to preserve venous flow, not to worsen an already damaged venous circulation.

Delay in treatment exposes the patient to a number of significant complications, such as progressive cardiomegaly, high-output congestive heart failure, bacterial endarteritis at the site of the fistula, weakening of the arterial wall with aneurysm formation, possible venous aneurysm formation, venous valve insufficiency, venous hypertension and swelling with impairment of function, chronic venous insufficiency, chronic venous ulcer, distal arterial ischemia, and ischemic neuritis. These unpleasant sequelae make correction of a traumatic AVF mandatory, and treatment should be undertaken promptly after the diagnosis is made. This can be accomplished by either percutaneous embolization, surgical excision, or a combination of both, which requires the close collaboration of the angiographer and the vascular surgeon. An additional reason for the prompt repair of a traumatic fistula is the occasional difficulty encountered in the repair of the proximal artery, whose wall is invariably weakened and structurally damaged if the fistula has been present for many years.

Standard vascular surgical techniques must be scrupulously followed. The arterial defect almost always can be closed primarily. If this is not possible, a vein patch can be used if primary closure compromises the arterial lumen. An end-to-end repair can occasionally be performed, particularly if there is redundancy in a tortuous vessel that allows sufficient mobilization to bridge a fistula that is resected. Adjacent soft tissue is usually interposed over the suture line to provide an additional buttress to avoid recurrence of the fistula. Most often, what is believed to be recurrence is an overlooked additional connection. During surgical excision of AVFs, a sterile intraoperative Doppler probe can be extremely useful in ascertaining whether residual fistulous connections are present that had been overlooked.

Duplex scanning allows femoral AVFs and pseudoaneurysms to be followed and evaluated serially in a noninvasive fashion. Thus, the natural history of these catheter-related lesions may be observed. Surgical repair of a femoral AVF is recommended for cases of an enlarging lesion, acute arterial thrombosis, evidence of femoral nerve compression, and the inability to provide continuing follow-up for the patient. Femoral artery AVF that persist beyond 3 months should be repaired electively to avoid further complications. Stable, painless hematomas related to femoral percutaneous puncture usually can be managed nonoperatively.

An aortogram is extremely useful in the treatment of aortocaval fistula, but the clinical status of the patient may preclude the time necessary to obtain it. In the stable patient, arteriography is indicated. It can delineate rupture into the renal or iliac veins and demonstrate the presence of an intraluminal clot, which is particularly important. The mortality rate of patients operated on with an aortocaval fistula (40% to 50%) is similar to that for patients with ruptured aortic aneurysms. Attempts to improve the patient's congestive heart failure or renal failure are seldom successful until the aortocaval fistula is corrected. The potential for pulmonary embolism requires that special care be taken during mobilization of the aneurysm. Occlusion of the inferior vena cava is important to prevent thromboembolism or air embolus and to control vena caval bleeding. After vena caval control, the aneurysm is opened, and the fistula can be identified by the venous blood coming from an obvious orifice in the side of the cava, which can usually be repaired from within the aneurysm. Once the vena cava is repaired, the aneurysm resection can proceed in a routine fashion. After successful fistula repair, the cardiac and other physiologic manifestations of the AVF clear rapidly. There is marked diuresis, weight loss, prompt improvement in dyspnea and tachycardia, reduction of limb edema, normalization of blood pressure, and distal arterial perfusion.

Certain fistulas present technical difficulty in surgical closure and can be more safely eliminated by arterial embolization. The emboli are injected so that they lodge at the site of the fistulous connection. Embolization can be useful in wounds caused by shotgun blasts with multiple injuries to the femoral arterial system. Embolic occlusion of the profunda femoris artery in these circumstances is tolerated when the superficial femoral artery is intact. Fistulas between the hypogastric artery and vein may also be difficult to control and can more easily be dealt with by embolization.

Embolization is not without complications; distal ischemia, infarction, embolization to an undesired artery, and transvenous migration with pulmonary embolism have been reported. Embolization should be reserved for selected instances in which surgical exposure would be hazardous.

Hepatic artery–portal vein fistulas may result from erosion or trauma. Although resection of the affected liver segment is possible, embolization of the involved artery is safer and more easily accomplished.

Similar to AVF in other areas, a carotid cavernous sinus AVF can not be cured by simple proximal arterial ligation. Direct arterial access for detachable balloon occlusion therapy is the procedure of choice in this difficult location, allowing selective elimination of the AVF with the preservation of normal arterial flow. A balloon attached to a catheter and introduced through the carotid artery can be placed precisely at the site of the fistula. The balloon is then filled with a silicone monomer that solidifies at body temperature and keeps the balloon in place. The catheter is then detached and removed. In the presence of a proximally occluded carotid artery, transvenous embolization is an alternative.

Detachable balloons, although widely used as embolization devices in neurovascular AVFs, are seldom used outside the head.[19] Detachable balloons offer a safe and precise method of embolization because they can be sited accurately, deflated, and repositioned if appropriate occlusion is not initially obtained. The two most common problems with the use of detachable balloons are the possibility of early deflation and premature detachment.

Local complications of femoral artery catheterization occur in institutions where angiography and cardiac catheterization is performed frequently. Complications result from an increase in the complexity of interventional techniques, the use of larger catheters, and the use of anticoagulation and thrombolytic agents. Femoral artery complications include hematoma, pseudoaneurysm, AVF, arterial obstruction, lymphocele, and abscess. High-resolution B-mode gray-scale ultrasonography with color-flow Doppler imaging can easily diagnose an AVF of the femoral vessels in the groin. The groin fistula can be treated by manual external compression of the AVF track with the ultrasound transducer. Real-time imaging allows precise localization and occlusion of the fistula. The amount of compression needed can be determined by noting the disappearance of flow on the Doppler image. After 30 minutes of compression, Doppler imaging usually reveals occlusion of the fistula.[20] Factors that increase the chances of successful compression therapy are the age of the fistulous track (endothelialized tracks are more difficult to thrombose) and the anatomic characteristics of the track (long, thin tracks are easier to compress than short, broad tracks). Inadvertent femoral artery occlusion can be avoided by color-flow Doppler imaging during compression or by monitoring distal pulses. Because as many as one third of femoral AVFs due to catheterization spontaneously close, operation should be reserved for lesions that increase in size or that exhibit continued patency after 2 months.[8,21]

Repair of a femoral AVF by endovascular placement of an intraluminal graft-covered stent has been described.[22] The balloon expandable stented graft was used to obliterate an AVF caused by a bullet injury to the superficial femoral artery and vein.

Occasionally, the construction of an AVF for hemodialysis may create undesirable complications. Depending on the size and the location of the fistula, there may be troublesome distal ischemia or even frank rest pain. This can be managed by decreasing the size of the fistula flow by constricting arterial inflow with a band of prosthetic material. An easy way to determine the degree of constriction necessary to relieve the ischemia is to monitor the distal artery while constricting the proximal artery until distal retrograde flow is eliminated. An occasional patient with heart disease experiences congestive heart failure as a result of an AVF created for hemodialysis, and the increased cardiac output may be decreased by reducing the fistula flow volume.

Some patients also experience excessive swelling of the hand or of one or more digits after creation of a side-to-side radial artery–cephalic vein fistula constructed at the wrist. The fistula may have been too large at the time it was created or may have subsequently undergone excessive enlargement. The increased venous pressure causing the swelling and discomfort often subsides. If it does not, it is best treated by removal of the fistula and restoration of normal arterial and venous continuity.

Congenital AVFs are much more difficult to treat because of the many connections (Fig. 95-10) and the propensity of some congenital fistulas to infiltrate muscle groups and bone (Fig. 95-11). Furthermore, inactive microscopic connections that cannot be seen grossly are often left behind and account for the invariable recurrence, unless the fistula is unusually well localized. Ligation of major feeding vessels may result in significant peripheral ischemia and also limits the opportunity subsequently to embolize such fistulas percutaneously. Most congenital AVFs are best treated conservatively unless they are small, well localized, and easily accessible.[23–25]

Treatment of congenital AVFs should be reserved for pressing, specific indications. Treatment may be required because of ulceration, bleeding, cardiac failure, and occasionally excessive limb growth in a prepubertal child. Treatment often can be accomplished by percutaneous em-

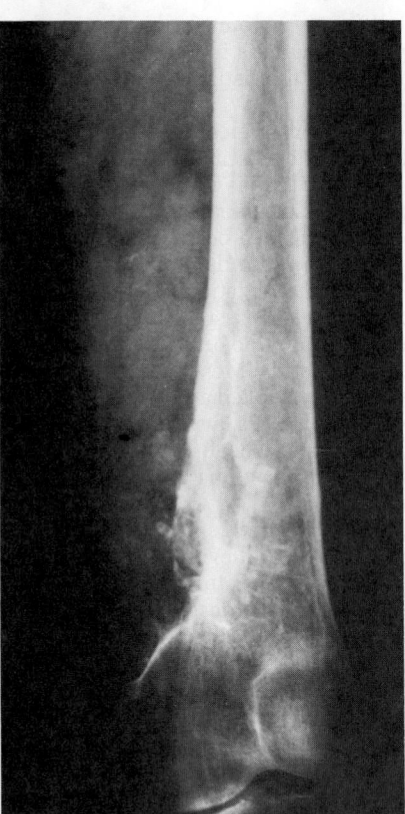

Figure 95-11. Radiograph of femur involved with congenital arteriovenous fistula, showing bony erosion.

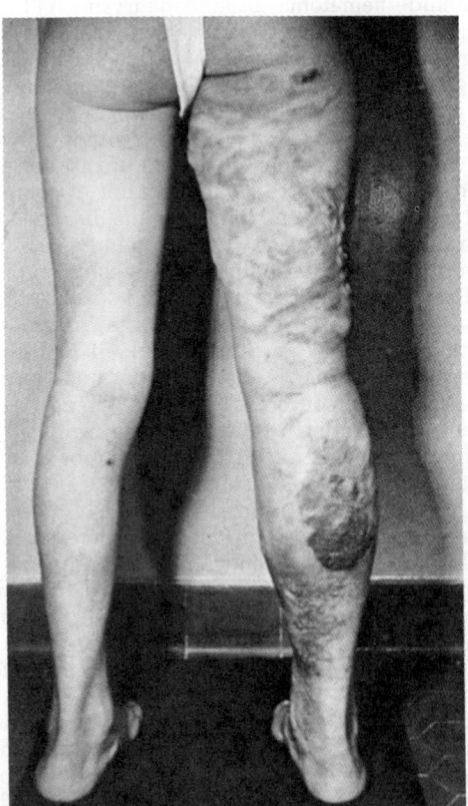

Figure 95-10. Massive congenital arteriovenous fistula that involves the entire right lower extremity in a 23-year-old man. Both the length and girth of the leg are increased. (Malan E, ed. Vascular malformations. Milan, Carlo Erba Foundation, 1974:61)

bolic occlusion and limited resection. Compulsive attempts to remove all of the fistula frequently result in an ischemic or nonfunctional extremity and excessive hemorrhage, and sometimes in unnecessary amputation. Recurrence of a congenital fistula should not be viewed as a failure of therapy but as inevitable, particularly in a large, hyperdynamic fistula.

A variety of permanent occlusive devices may be introduced percutaneously to occlude either traumatic or congenital AVFs, and these have proved to be extremely effective both as primary treatment and as an adjunct to subsequent surgical therapy. Metal coils, detachable balloons, thrombin-soaked Gelfoam, autologous muscle, alcohol, and liquid acrylic adhesive can be employed. These devices are most useful in the management of congenital AVFs with a multiplicity of arteriovenous connections.

Successful repair of a traumatic fistula reverses the abnormal hemodynamics of both the arterial and venous components of the circulation. Cardiac output usually falls dramatically, and there can be a significant decrease in heart size, relief of congestive heart failure, and decrease in blood volume with urinary diuresis.

The surgical correction of AVF can be deceptively difficult for numerous reasons: the abundant collateral circulation is usually underestimated; scarring associated with the original injury may be encountered; and the vessels are sometimes unduly fragile and difficult to suture. AVFs are sufficiently uncommon to provide limited experience for the average surgeon, who may be unfamiliar with the difficulty of and indications for surgical intervention.

VASCULAR MALFORMATIONS

The classification of congenital vascular malformations (CVMs) remains difficult and somewhat controversial. These lesions can most simply be divided into those that are primarily venous and those in which an AVF is present. Both may include a lymphatic component, which may vary in extent. The older literature is confusing because of the inclusion of colorful, descriptive terms that are of little value (eg, cirsoid aneurysm, arteriovenous angioma, cavernous angioma, racemose angioma, phlebectasia, phlebarteriectasia, port wine stain, nevus flammeus). Contemporary diagnostic modalities can almost always categorize these malformations as either primarily venous or containing abnormal arteriovenous connections. It may be useful to subdivide the AVMs into those that contain overt large hyperdynamic arteriovenous connections and those that are small (perhaps even microscopic) and are functionally hypodynamic. Hyperdynamic AVMs are frequently diffuse and appear to cross natural tissue boundaries and invade muscle and bone, whereas hypodynamic AVMs more often are small and well circumscribed.

Etiology

Congenital vascular malformations result from an abnormality in which there is an arrest of the normal embryologic development of the vascular system. The primary capillary network present in the early developing embryo normally grows simultaneously with the development and differentiation of all mesodermal, endodermal, and ectodermal structures. The normal vascular system results from a complex development sequence in which there is an orderly regression of vascular elements and the disappearance of portions of the original diffuse capillary network. Although specific capillaries remain, others enlarge and fuse to form the major vascular trunks. This complex differentiation process occurs early in embryonic development and is essentially complete by the 10th week of fetal growth.

The factors that cause abnormal development of peripheral arteries and veins are not known. Potential exogenous causes include viral infection, poorly defined medication effects, and other external factors. With few exceptions, the cause of the abnormal persistence of arteriovenous connections, capillary angiomas, or venous agenesis is unknown. Furthermore, the cause of associated phenomena such as increased bone length, and increased extremity girth with CVMs remains speculative. The increased blood flow, hyperemia, increased local oxygen concentration, and venous hypertension that are frequently associated with these lesions have not clearly been shown to be the cause of hypertrophy. Furthermore, hypertrophy is seen in the absence of hyperemia and increased oxygen tension, such as in patients with Klippel-Trenaunay syndrome with impaired venous return.

CVMs are seldom encountered by most surgeons and hence are poorly understood and frequently not well managed. The CVMs that are primarily arteriovenous generally exhibit a different biologic life history and pathophysiology, and their prognosis and therapy are different from traumatic or acquired AVFs, from which they need to be clearly distinguished. Congenital AVMs are present from birth and represent abnormal vascular development or an arrest in normal development. The arteriovenous connections are multiple, yet they seldom produce significant systemic effects. It is unclear whether certain lesions, such as capillary hemangiomas, are actually hypodynamic or nonfunctional AVMs. Examination of such lesions histologically does not shed additional light on this question. Congenital AVMs may be either diffuse or circumscribed. The fistulous connections in the latter are usually small and without hemodynamic significance, whereas diffuse fistulas usually have large connections and are more likely to produce hemodynamic changes. Mulliken and Glo-

wacki[26] observed that certain cutaneous hemangiomas in children can be distinguished from other vascular malformations. These hemangiomatous lesions appear shortly after birth, proliferate for the first year of life, and involute by age 5 or 6 years. These lesions are associated with endothelial hyperplasia and an increase in the number of mast cells present during their proliferative phase and by fibrosis, diminished cellularity, and a normal mast cell count during involution. Arteriographically, these lesions demonstrate rapid blood flow and occasional arteriovenous shunting, and they appear similar to a vascular neoplasm with a parenchymal appearance. In rare instances, in a rapidly enlarging hemangioma, there may be an associated thrombocytopenic purpura, a microangiopathic hemolytic anemia, and a consumptive coagulopathy. The primary pathologic event is trapping of platelets within the vascular lesion (Kasabach-Merritt syndrome[27]).

Aside from isolated case reports, the first comprehensive review of CVMs was reported in 1920.[28] Features that distinguish congenital AVMs from acquired AVFs[29] and an initial embryologic basis for congenital AVMs were similarly reported.[30] The developing vasculature that first appears in the fetus is an undifferentiated network of blood spaces in the mesenchyme of the embryo. If an arrest in development occurred at this stage, a lack of differentiation might result in a hemangioma. This type of undifferentiated capillary network is sometimes seen in hemangiomas. Normal embryonic development proceeds with differentiation due to absorption and coalescence of vascular spaces, resulting in separate arterial and venous conduits, which have been defined as the *retiform stage* of vascular development. This stage is marked by the presence of large plexiform structures that form from the original capillary network. Developmental arrest at this stage might result in an arteriovenous aneurysm with arteriovenous connections that may vary in size. These vessels often appear developmentally mature and may be present in large numbers. Further embryonic development produces vascular stems that are interconnected; if further development does not occur, these vessels persist as arteriovenous connections. The bony and soft tissue hypertrophy frequently seen in congenital AVMs may be secondary to the altered hemodynamics that accompany such lesions or may represent an additional primary component of such anomalies. These lesions are equally distributed between males and females but are several times more common in the lower extremity than in the upper. Congenital AVMs are present at birth but are not always clinically evident. Unlike the hemangioma of infancy, they seldom undergo spontaneous involution.

Signs and Symptoms

Cutaneous AVMs can present with a mass, discoloration of the skin, enlarged veins, unequal limb length and girth, and occasionally hemorrhage or ulceration. It is unclear what stimuli may activate lesions that have been dormant, but the hormonal changes incident to the onset of puberty or pregnancy have sometimes coincided with the clinical recognition of these lesions and their exacerbation. The increased size and deformity caused by these lesions in an extremity give the appearance of invasion of adjacent tissues, but there is no histologic evidence of cellular proliferation or other evidence of neoplasia.

In addition to the lower extremities, congenital AVMs are frequently encountered in the pelvis and head. They may affect the viscera but are usually clinically silent. The most common presenting feature of visceral AVMs are hemoptysis, hematuria, hematemesis, and melena. Only rarely do large, hyperdynamic AVMs cause changes in car-

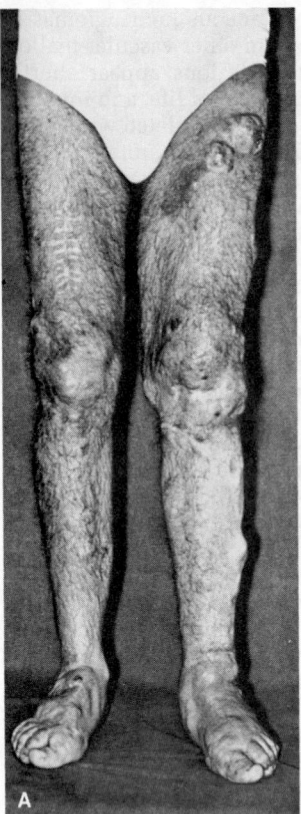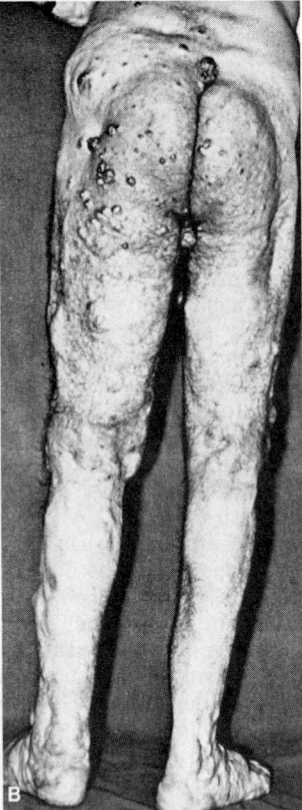

Figure 95-12. Photograph of a 25-year-old man with congenital venous malformation. Striking cutaneous manifestations are seen. (Malan E, ed. Vascular malformations. Milan, Carlo Erba Foundation, 1974:92)

diac output or other significant local or systemic hemodynamic abnormalities. There may be increased warmth of the lesion, and if there is a significant arteriovenous component, the mass does not decrease with elevation and is more firm than a venous anomaly. Occasionally, one may encounter pulsating veins and a thrill and bruit, but they are not consistently present. If there is significant hemodynamic alteration, the area distal to the lesion may be cool with diminished pulses. Occasionally, arterial ischemia and ulceration, chronic venous stasis changes, and venous ulceration are present.

Patients may be aware of heaviness, throbbing, pulsation, and vibration in a hyperdynamic AVM and may feel increased local warmth. The extremity may exhibit a strik-

ing increase in length and girth resulting from hypertrophy of both bony and soft tissue. Significant increases in cortical bone thickness may occur, and bony defects may be seen in plain films when there has been involvement and erosion of bony tissue by active AVMs.

An increase in limb length and girth can occur in the absence of an active AVF. Limb enlargement is always due to an AVF if a thrill or bruit can be detected. Pain is an uncommon symptom but can occur with involvement or direct compression of peripheral nerves by the lesion.

The cutaneous manifestations are often striking, with a mass of dilated vessels and extremely large venous varicosities (Figs. 95-12 and 95-13). Venous pulsations may occasionally be visible. A cutaneous hemangioma may be present and varies in extent and appearance. The hemangioma can be cavernous or capillary and can vary from a subtle pink blush to a deep red or reddish blue color. Its surface may be smooth or irregular, depending on the size of the vascular channels (Fig. 95-14). There may be gross distortion of the contour of the limb, which may appear grotesquely deformed (Fig. 95-15). The mass, when present, does not always represent an arteriovenous connection (or a vascular lesion), and if a palpable thrill and continuous bruit are not evident, the nature of the mass may require further investigation. Varicosities may not become apparent until a child begins to stand and walk. The varicosities are not in the normal distribution of the greater and lesser saphenous veins and are atypical in location and appearance. Limb hypertrophy, varicosities, and a hemangioma of the skin may be present with or without a demonstrable AVF.[31] When there is an absence of deep veins and no arteriovenous communication, this combination of findings corresponds to what has been described as the Klippel-Trenaunay syndrome[24] (Figs. 95-16 through 95-18). The thrill and continuous machinery-like murmur with systolic accentuation invariably present with a traumatic AVF are not always evident in congenital lesions. When present, the bruit is loudest directly over areas of arteriovenous shunting but may also be heard some distance away.

The Branham sign (slowing of the pulse with compression of the arteriovenous communication of the major proximal artery) may be elicited. Because of the multiple connections, it may be difficult to sufficiently compress the appropriate vessels. When there is involvement of muscle and bone, such compression is not feasible.

Localized hypoactive microfistulous AVMs usually are not associated with limb enlargement, thrill, bruit, or Branham sign. These lesions may present as an asymptomatic localized mass, and their vascular nature may not be apparent until they are excised. Dilated veins are sometimes present as well as a cutaneous hemangioma.

Doppler examination can provide clearcut evidence of

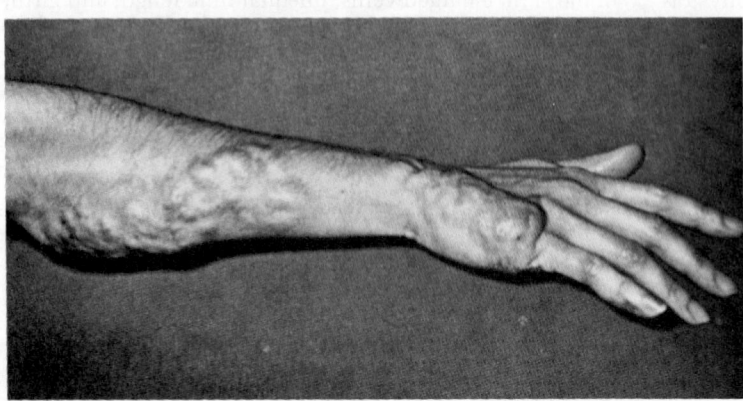

Figure 95-13. Photograph of a 21-year-old woman with congenital venous malformation of arm. Large atypical varicosities are visible. (Malan E, ed. Vascular malformations. Milan, Carlo Erba Foundation, 1974)

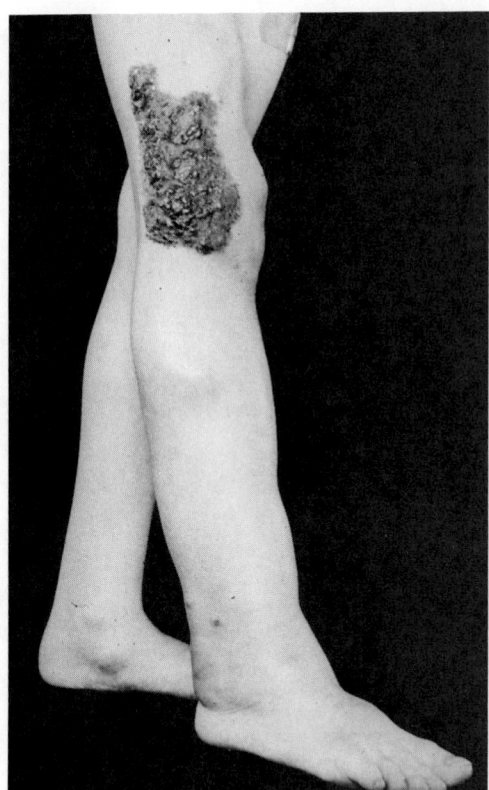

Figure 95-14. Photograph of a 6-year-old girl with congenital vascular malformation. Cutaneous cavernous hemangioma and distortion of limb contour are seen.

a congenital AVM. The extent of the lesion can sometimes be defined, and a continuous Doppler signal may be present over cutaneous veins. The Doppler signal may disappear with compression of an afferent artery. There may be little alteration in the audible signal because of the many arteriovenous connections.

Only rarely do congenital AVMs produce cardiac manifestations. This may be true even in large, hyperdynamic, congenital AVMs and is difficult to understand. The many connections might be expected to produce a significant bypass of the capillary bed and to result in the pathophysiologic alterations that occur in a traumatic AVF. This usually does not occur, possibly because of greater resistance to flow in the many long and sometimes tortuous connections in a congenital AVM. Less than 10% of congenital AVMs are associated with high-output cardiac failure.[32]

The diagnosis of a congenital AVM can be made on the basis of clinical signs and symptoms, but arteriography is essential to delineate the number, location, and extent of the abnormalities (Fig. 95-19). Additional imaging modalities, such as CT and MRI, have proved to be extremely useful in assessing congenital vascular lesions. MRI provides information and understanding in diagnosing CVMs of the extremities. MRI can determine the character of blood flow and also can define the anatomy of a lesion. The flow through the anomaly can be characterized, and important feeding arteries and draining veins can be identified. The involvement of muscle and bone can be defined by MRI, which usually shows more extensive disease than is shown by physical examination or arteriography. MRI is the most informative diagnostic maneuver in managing AVMs (Fig. 95-20). Slow-flow venous malformations can be distinguished from high-flow AVFs on the basis of MRI signal characteristics. Hemangiomas show postcapillary

dilated venous spaces associated with stagnant flow, lack of normal venous valves, and the absence of arteriovenous shunting. A tendency for orientation of the lesion along the long axis of affected extremities and a tendency to follow the neurovascular distribution associated with enlargement of the adjacent subcutaneous fat suggest that a more diffuse congenital tissue dysplasia exists rather than a dysplasia isolated to vascular tissue.

The complete extent of the vascular malformation must be assessed before any treatment is contemplated. This can be easily demonstrated by MRI, which can show the malformation more accurately than can be achieved using a combination of arteriography and venography. The abnormal vascular spaces of a venous malformation are best visualized by closed-system venography. The area most suitable for direct-puncture venography can be delineated by MRI. Closed-system venography is a useful technique in which percutaneous puncture of a venous lesion is accomplished in the distal portion of the extremity after the use of a blood pressure cuff and an Esmarch bandage to exsanguinate the limb. The lesion under study is then visualized with contrast injected under fluoroscopic control. This technique is simple to perform and well tolerated by the patient. MRI is helpful in assessing the presence of residual fistulous connections and in following such patients. Because of the complexity of a congenital AVM, duplex scanning may be less useful than in traumatic or acquired AVF. Venous oxygen saturation draining an AVM is usually elevated compared with the uninvolved extremity.

Arteriography should always be performed if therapeutic intervention is considered. It usually shows one or more dilated proximal arteries and draining veins as well as the multiple fistulous connections. It may be difficult or impossible to distinguish arteries, veins, or connecting channels. In a hypodynamic fistula, the only abnormality may be early venous opacification. Other indirect arteriographic findings suggestive of a hypodynamic microfistulous AVM include increased flow through afferent arterial trunks and accumulation of the injected contrast in the area of the suspected fistula.

Histologic examination of removed tissue sometimes sheds little light on the true nature of the lesion, and what can be seen are simply blood-filled spaces lined by endothelial cells. They are clearly vascular structures but are difficult to identify further because of secondary changes that alter the appearance of the normal vascular wall. It may be difficult to distinguish thick-walled veins from atrophic arteries, deficient in smooth muscle and elastic tissue.

The Klippel-Trenaunay syndrome is a fairly specific congenital venous anomaly that was described in 1900.[33] It is usually confined to a single lower extremity, with varying degrees of venous varicosities that are atypical in location and extent. A cutaneous hemangioma or port wine stain is usually present and may vary from a faint pink to the dark color of port wine. The hemangioma has a variegated irregular margin and often involves the buttock and lower back but seldom crosses the midline of the lower trunk. Increased length and girth of the affected extremity are common. The lesion is usually present at birth but may become manifest only when the child begins to stand or walk. It is found equally in boys and girls, is seen as an isolated anomaly, and does not occur in siblings or other family members. There may be a varying amount of lymphatic involvement and, inexplicably, the affected extremity may, on occasion, be smaller in length and girth. The deep venous system is frequently absent or abnormal[31] (Figs. 95-21 and 95-22). Careful arteriographic studies do not show the presence of an AVF.[24] The presence of a

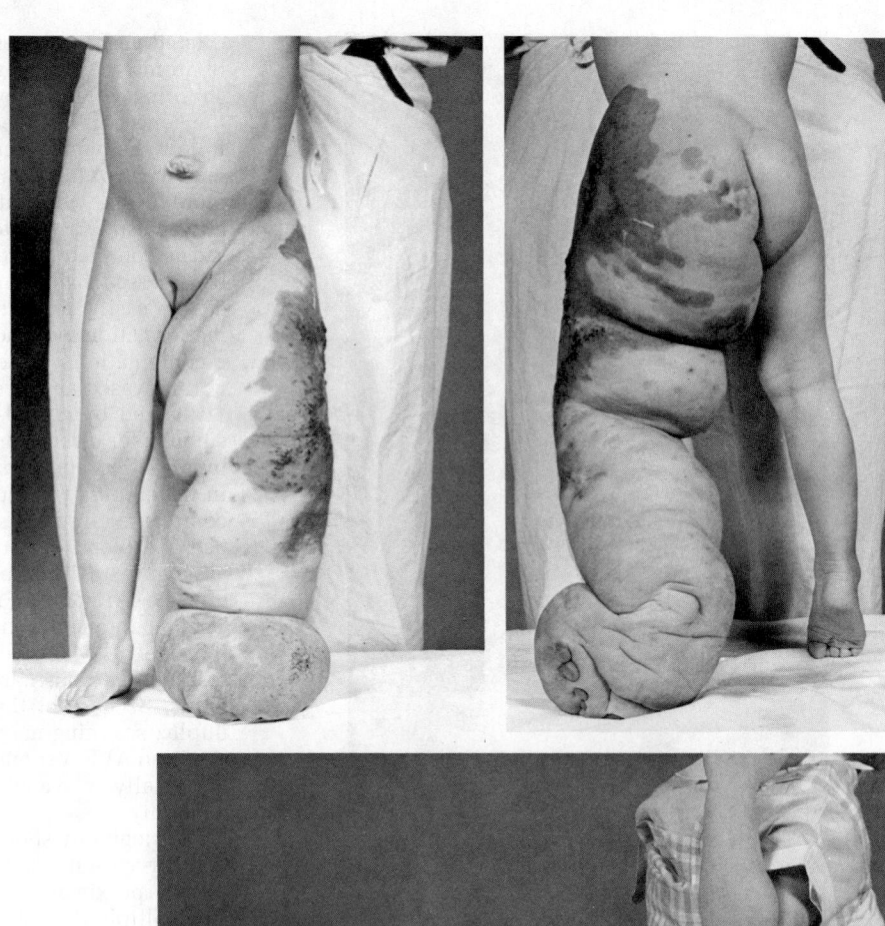

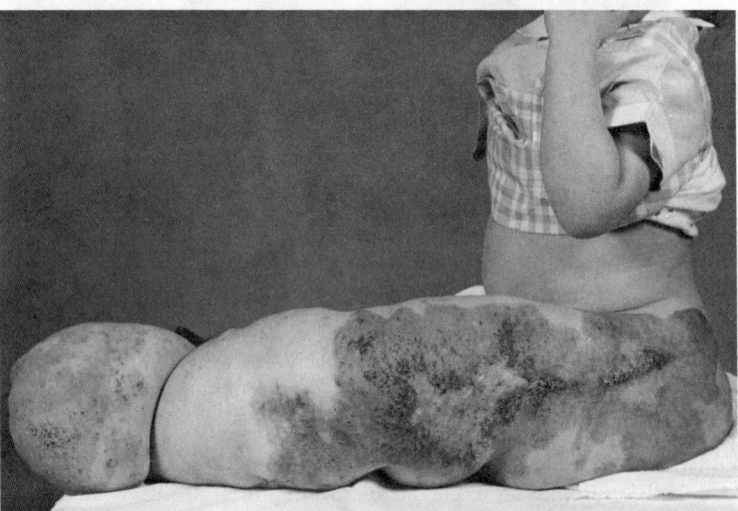

Figure 95-15. Photograph of a 3-year-old girl with congenital vascular malformation, showing a grotesquely deformed left leg.

congenital AVF associated with the Klippel-Trenaunay triad (varicosities, cutaneous hemangioma, and hypertrophy) is more properly designated Parkes-Weber syndrome.[34,35]

Plain radiographs of the extremities usually demonstrate phleboliths (round calcified nodules within dilated veins). The lesion may be extensive when imaged by CT scan or MRI. The cavernous hemangioma or the varicosities of the Klippel-Trenaunay syndrome can also be visualized by direct percutaneous puncture.

Treatment

The major emphasis of management of all CVMs is conservative.[32] Certainly, asymptomatic lesions, once identified as CVMs, require no therapy and usually exhibit no progression. Treatment should not be rendered simply because of the presence of the abnormality. The major form of conservative therapy is the use of well-fitted elastic support hose, which can reduce flow through arteriovenous malformations to a significant degree. Specific indications for surgical therapy include hemorrhage, ischemia, congestive heart failure, nonhealing ulcers, functional impairment, and limb-length inequality.

Hemorrhage from cutaneous lesions subject to minor trauma can be troublesome and a source of difficulty for schoolage children, who are invariably sent home with the appearance of the smallest blood staining of their clothing. Bleeding in the gastrointestinal and urinary tracks may be the source of chronic anemia, which can be occult and require diligent search and appropriate extirpation. If the abnormal vessels can be localized angiographically, embolization should be considered. Initial embolization can make subsequent surgical excision easier, less extensive, or not necessary. Overzealous use of either modality may result in ischemia and an undesirable amputation or visceral resection or a nonfunctional extremity. Therefore, incomplete excision avoiding ischemia should be viewed as a desirable goal rather than as a treatment failure. In either circumstance, such therapeutic interventions must

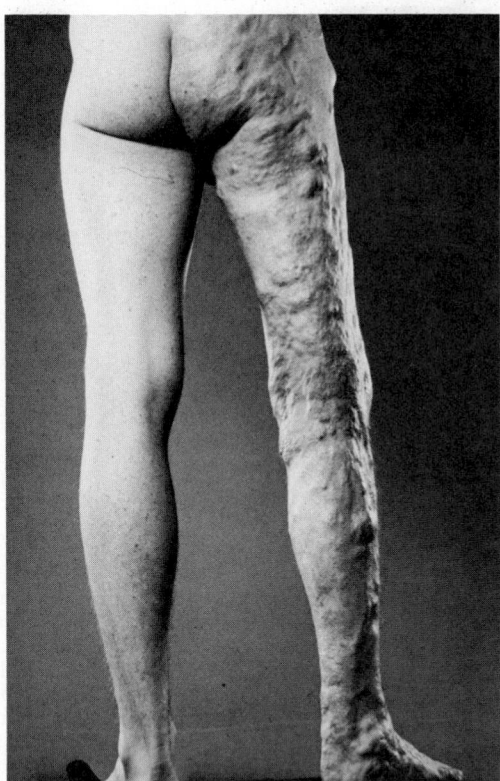

Figure 95-16. Photograph of an 18-year-old man with Klippel-Trenaunay syndrome. Prominent varicosities are seen in atypical locations.

be viewed as temporary because AVMs invariably recur. Even if all overt diseased tissue is excised, the residual microfistulous connections subsequently are activated by unknown stimuli to enlarge and create the false impression of the surgeon having overlooked a component of the lesion when complete excision is attempted (Fig. 95-23).

Complex AVMs located in the pelvis are usually impossible to remove and are associated with major blood loss and potential injury to vital structures, such as the ureter, bladder, rectum, and pelvic nerves. Although significantly safer and easier, percutaneous embolization, if too extensive, can result in ischemic necrosis of vital organs. Permanent embolic materials, such as stainless steel coils, tissue adhesive, polyvinyl alcohol particles (Ivalon), and detachable balloons, can be used. Care must be taken that occlusion of large-caliber feeding vessels does not preclude subsequent embolization, should that be necessary. Most complex lesions should be embolized in stages because of the time-consuming nature of the undertaking and the large volumes of contrast material that are required for localization. Embolization complications include passage through an arteriovenous communication, resulting in pulmonary embolism, inadvertent embolization of normal tissue, and ischemic neuritis.

Hypoactive AVMs that are small, localized, and not hemodynamically significant can be difficult to diagnose before removal. They usually present as an asymptomatic subcutaneous mass, and excision is necessary for histologic examination and diagnosis. Once the nature of the mass is identified, further excision is not required because recurrence is common, and the mere presence of the lesion is not associated with any long-term undesirable effects.

Cutaneous hemangiomas that are present at birth as an isolated lesion frequently regress by the age of 5 or 6 years and simply require observation because over 90% of such lesions spontaneously disappear. Occasionally, a cutaneous hemangioma may exhibit rapid or atypical growth or be associated with thrombocytopenia and require surgical excision or embolization, if possible. Some authors have advocated the use of heparin, corticosteriods, or antifibrinolytic agents in addition to general supportive measures. The rare CVM that involves a joint can be troublesome in a young, active person with recurrent episodes of hemarthrosis. Excision may significantly limit joint function, and such lesions are best treated by limited emboliza-

Figure 95-17. Photograph of a 10-year-old boy with Klippel-Trenaunay syndrome, showing varicosities, cutaneous hemangioma, and increased length. (Lindenauer SM. The Klippel-Trenaunay syndrome. Ann Surg 1965; 162:309)

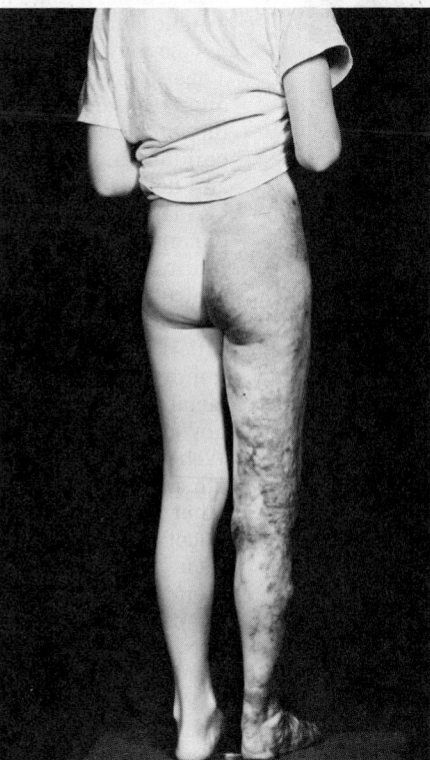
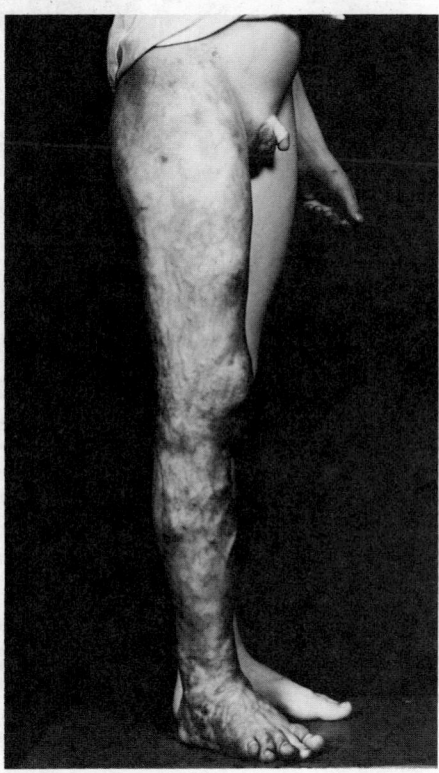

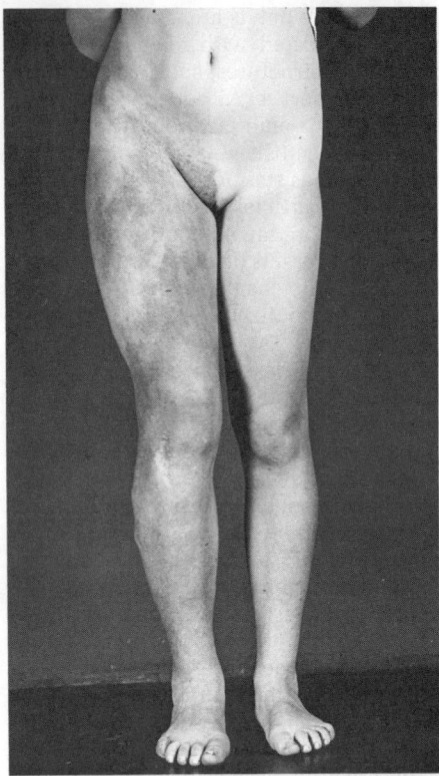
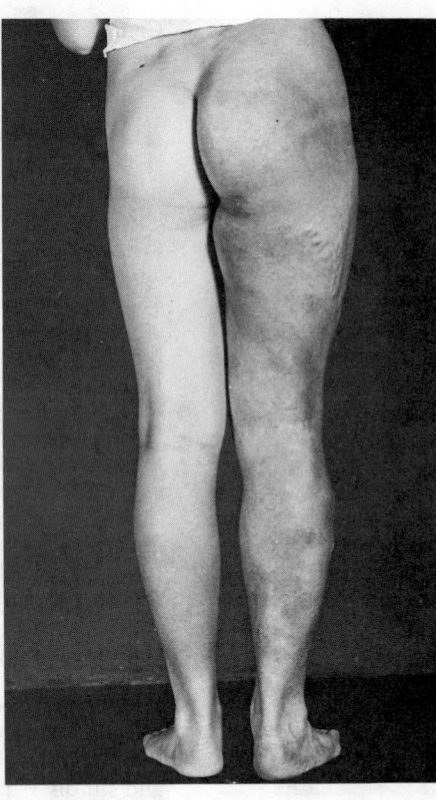

Figure 95-18. Photograph of an 11-year-old girl with Klippel-Trenaunay syndrome, showing marked cutaneous hemangioma, increased length and girth, and minimal varicosities. (Lindenauer SM. The Klippel-Trenaunay syndrome. Ann Surg 1965;162: 309)

tion and avoidance of contact sports. CVMs cause limb lengthening that may require treatment. Generally, the limb lengthening seldom exceeds 5 cm. Shoes of different sizes may be required if there is significant hypertrophy of the foot. A lift may be inserted in the shoe on the normal side. Sometimes, the toes are grotesquely distorted. Finding a properly fitting shoe may be impossible, requiring a custom-fitted orthotic shoe. Marked leg-length inequality can cause a pelvic tilt and low back pain, which, if it cannot be corrected with a simple insert in the shoe, may require epiphysiodesis of the affected leg to slow the rate of growth. Conceivably, the newer orthopedic techniques of limb lengthening may be used to lengthen the uninvolved extremity.

The lesions of the Klippel-Trenaunay syndrome seldom cause symptoms. They are best treated conservatively with elastic hose; if there is a large lymphatic component that is troublesome, intermittent use of a pneumatic compression device may provide symptomatic relief. In the absence of a deep venous system, the removal of superficial veins has often resulted in worsening of the patient's symptoms and therefore should be scrupulously avoided.[24] Women of childbearing age can expect to carry a pregnancy to term and deliver vaginally without any unusual complications.

A large experience has been reported in which a variety of constricting-type bands that interfere with deep venous return have been found and released.[36] Removal of these obstructing lesions is said to provide relief of symptoms. This assertion has not been substantiated by others.

Port wine stains are always present on the affected extremity in the Klippel-Trenaunay syndrome and are rarely facial in location. Facial port wine stains may be found, however, as isolated lesions or associated with Sturge-Weber syndrome (encephalotrigeminal angiomatosis) and other rare syndromes with central nervous system and other organ involvement. Facial port wine stains can produce a significant psychologic burden for a young patient.[37] Attempts to obliterate port wine stains with laser therapy have had mixed results, including replacement of the port wine stain with undesirable scarring. The pulsed-dye laser has shown some promising results. It was developed and approved specifically for the treatment of port wine stains. By careful tuning of the wavelength of the laser, it emits a burst of yellow light that is selectively absorbed by oxyhemoglobin in blood vessels within 2 mm

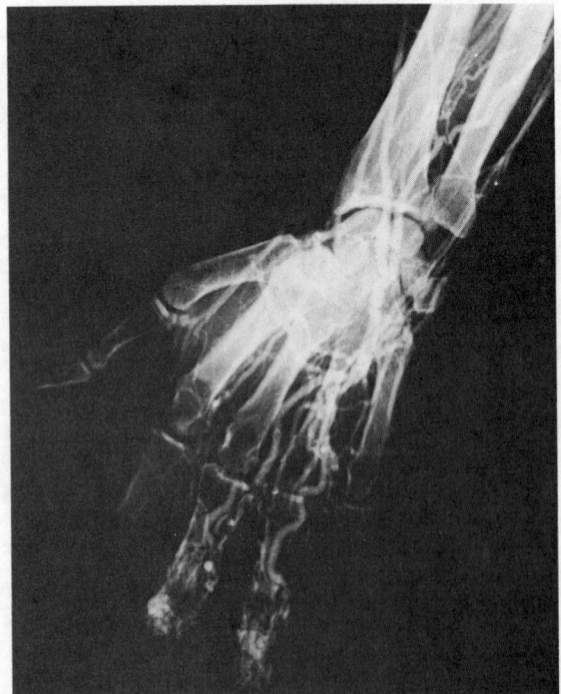

Figure 95-19. Radiograph of congenital arteriovenous fistulas confined to the distal portions of the third and fourth fingers of a young man.

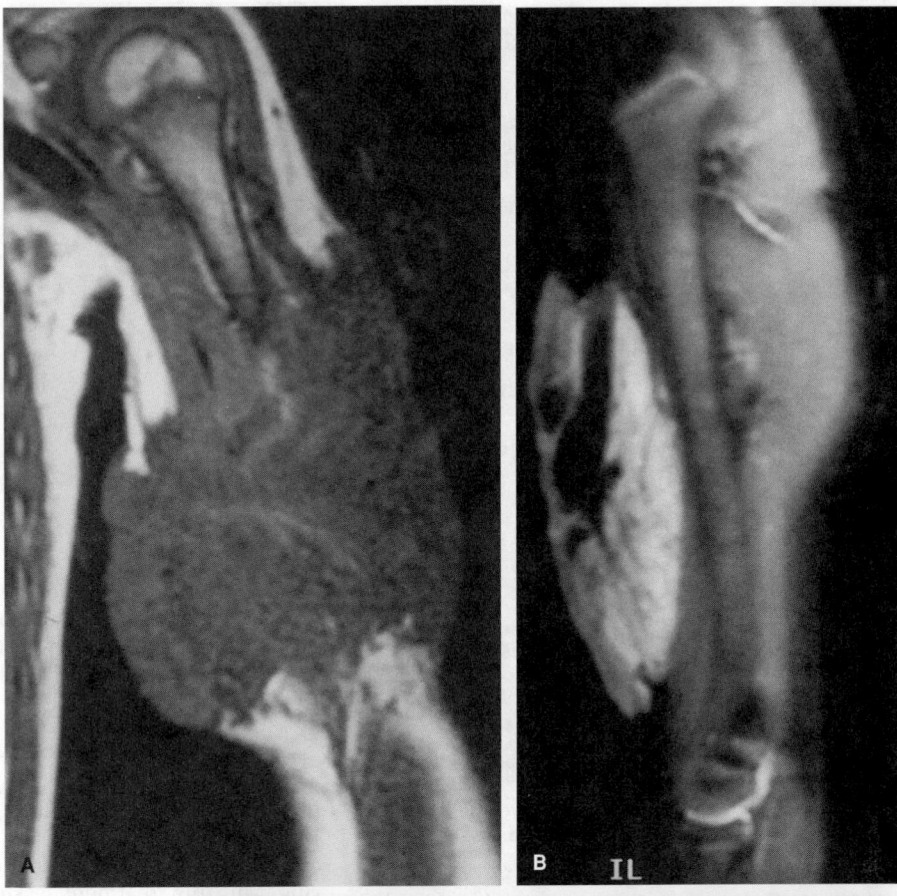

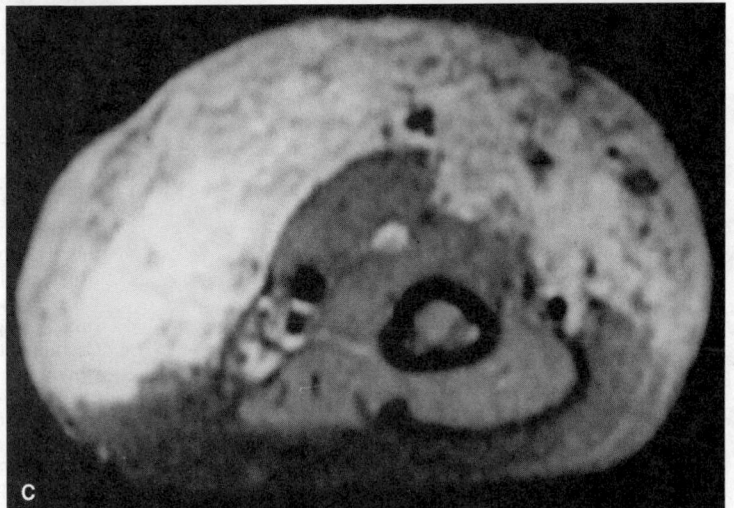

Figure 95-20. (A) MRI, T₁ technique, demonstrating soft tissue mass of congenital arteriovenous fistula seen in sagittal plane of mid-upper arm in 2-year-old girl. No contrast was used. (B) MRI, short T₁ inversion recovery, sagittal view. In same patient, white image in medial upper arm is congenital AVF vessel mass. Large black medial vertical channel is single abnormal vein. No contrast was used. (C) MRI, proton density technique, coronal view. In same patient, white image is mass of congenital arteriovenous vessels. Intensity of white color is proportional to blood velocity. Involvement of muscle tissue is visible laterally. No contrast was used.

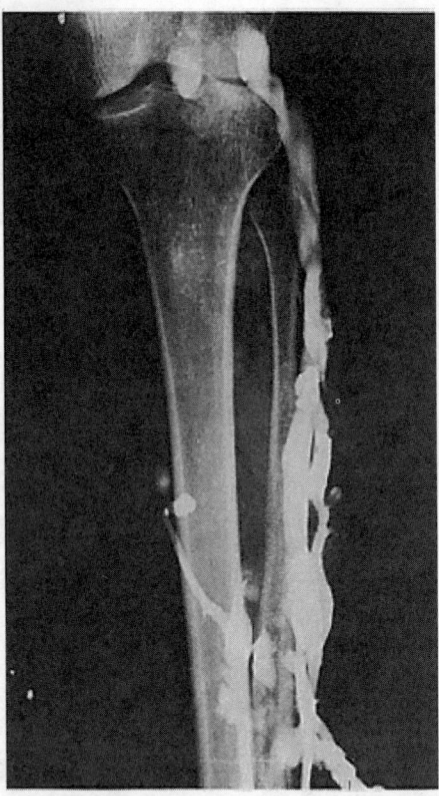

Figure 95-21. Radiograph of a venogram of a 30-year-old woman with Klippel-Trenaunay syndrome. The deep veins of the leg are absent up to the level of the popliteal vein.

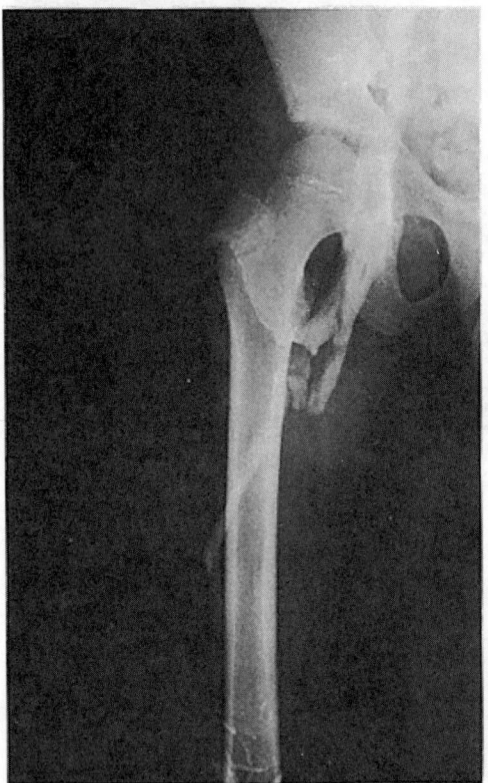

Figure 95-22. Radiograph of a venogram of a 9-year-old boy with Klippel-Trenaunay syndrome. The deep thigh veins are absent to the level of the common femoral vein.

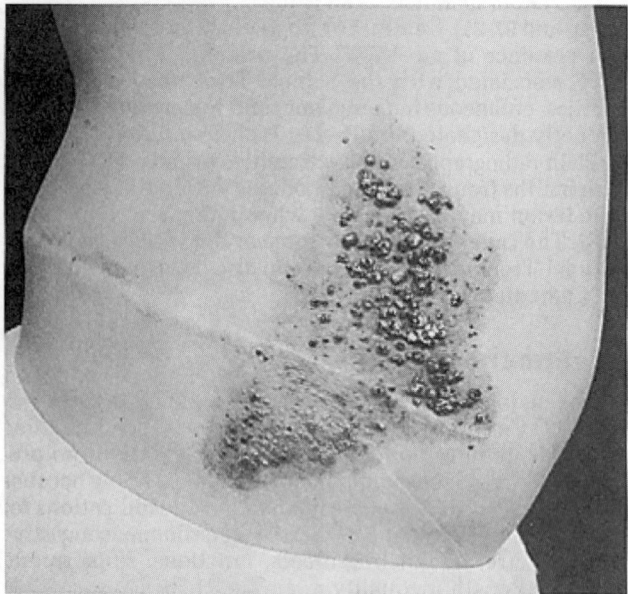

Figure 95-23. Recurrent cutaneous congenital vascular malformation in a 4-year-old girl. It was previously removed because of bleeding (scar is from earlier "complete" excision).

of the skin surface, which is where 90% of the vessels in the port wine stain are located. Extremely brief light pulses limit the spread of destructive heat energy, permitting precise treatment with minimal destruction and residual scarring. Multiple treatment sessions are required because the pulse spot is only 5 mm in diameter. Recurrence of the port wine stain has not been reported, but the possibility of long-term soft tissue damage has yet to be assessed.

REFERENCES

1. Gerbode F, Holman E, Dickenson EH, Spencer FC. Arteriovenous fistulas and arterial aneurysms. Surgery 1952;2:259.
2. Hunter W. The history of an aneurysm of the aorta with some remarks on aneurysms in general. Med Observ Inq 1757;1:323.
3. Brescia MJ, Cimino JE, Appel K, et al. Chronic hemodialysis using venipuncture and surgically created arteriovenous fistula. N Engl J Med 1966;275:1089.
4. Cronenwett JL, Lindenauer SM. Direct measurement of arteriovenous anastomotic blood flow after lumbar sympathectomy. Surgery 1977;82:82.
5. Cronenwett JL, Lindenauer SM. Direct measurement of arteriovenous anastomotic blood flow in septic canine hind limbs. Surgery 1979;85:275.
6. DeLaney JP. Control of arteriovenous anastomoses in the limb. In: Rutherford RB, ed. Vascular surgery. Philadelphia, WB Saunders, 1977;785.
7. Haimovici H, Steinman C, Caplan LH. Role of arteriovenous anastomoses in vascular disease of the lower extremity. Ann Surg 1966;164:990.
8. Kent KC, McArdel CR, Kennedy B, Baim DS, Anninos E, Skillman JJ. A prospective study of the clinical outcome of femoral pseudoaneurysms and arteriovenous fistulas induced by arterial puncture. J Vasc Surg 1993;17:125.
9. Lindenauer SM, Thompson NW, Kraft RO, Fry WJ. Late complications of traumatic arteriovenous fistulas. Surg Gynecol Obstet 1969;129:525.
10. Thompson NW, Lindenauer SM. Central venous aneurysms and arteriovenous fistula. Ann Surg 1969;170:852.
11. Lindenauer SM. Treatment of venous aneurysms. In: Ernst CB, Stanley JC, eds. Current therapy in vascular surgery, ed 2. Toronto, BC Decker, 1991:1019.
12. Nicoladoni C. Phlebarteriestasie der rechten oberen extremitat. Arch Klin Chir 1875;18:252.

13. Branham HH. Aneurysmal varix of the femoral artery and vein following a gunshot wound. Int J Surg 1890;3:250.

14. Kwan E, Hieshima GB, Higashida RT, Halbach VV, Wolpert SM. Interventional neuroradiology in neuro-ophthalmology. J Clin Neuroophthalmol 1989;9:83.

15. Peeters FL, Kromhout JG, Reekers JA, Koster PA. Treatment of solitary arteriovenous fistulas. Surgery 1991;109:220.

16. Redmond PL, Kumpe DA. Embolization of an intrahepatic arterioportal fistula: case report and review of the literature. Cardiovasc Intervent Radiol 1988;11:274.

17. Cronenwett JL, Lindenauer SM. Direct measurement of arteriovenous anastomotic blood flow after lumbar sympathectomy. Surgery 1977;82:82.

18. Cohen JM, Weinreb JC, Redman HC. Arteriovenous malformations of the extremities: MR imaging. Radiology 1986;158:475.

19. DeSouza NM, Reidy JF. Embolization with detachable balloons: applications outside the head. Clin Radiol 1992;46:170.

20. Fellmeth BD, Roberts AC, Bookstein JJ, et al. Postangiographic femoral artery injuries: nonsurgical repair with US-guided compression. Radiology 1991;178:671.

21. Allen BT, Munn JS, Stervern SL, et al. Selective non-operative management of pseudoaneurysms and arteriovenous fistulae complicating femoral artery catheterization. J Cardiovasc Surg 1992;33:440.

22. Marin ML, Veith FJ, Panetta TF, et al. Percutaneous transfemoral insertion of a stented graft to repair a traumatic femoral arteriovenous fistula. J Vasc Surg 1993;18:299.

23. Szilagyi DE, Smith RF, Elliott JP, et al. Congenital arteriovenous anomalies of the limbs. Arch Surg 1976;111:423.

24. Lindenauer SM. The Klippel-Trenaunay syndrome: varicosity, hypertrophy, and hemangioma with no arteriovenous fistula. Ann Surg 1965;162:303.

25. Lindenauer SM. Congenital arteriovenous fistula. In: Rutherford RB, ed. Peripheral vascular surgery. Philadelphia, WB Saunders, 1977:793.

26. Mulliken JB, Glowacki J. Hemangiomas and vascular malformations in infants and children: a classification based on endothelial cell characteristics. Plast Reconstr Surg 1984;12:41.

27. Kasbach HH, Merritt KK. Capillary hemangioma with extensive purpura. Am J Dis Child 1940;59:1063.

28. Callander CL. Study of arteriovenous fistula with an analysis of 447 cases. Ann Surg 1920;71:428.

29. DeTakats G. Vascular anomalies of the extremities. Surg Gynecol Obstet 1932;55:227.

30. Wollard HH. The development of the principal arterial stems in the forelimb of the pig. Contrib Embryol 1922;14:139.

31. Lindenauer SM. Congenital arteriovenous fistula and the Klippel-Trenaunay syndrome. Ann Surg 1971;174:248.

32. Szilagyi DE, Elliott JP, DeRusso FJ, Smith RF. Peripheral congenital arteriovenous fistulas. Surgery 1965;57:61.

33. Klippel M, Trenaunay P. Du noevus variqueux osteohypertrophique. Arch Gen Med Paris 1900;185:641.

34. Parkes-Weber F. Hemangiectatic hypertrophy of limbs: congenital phlebarteriectasia and so-called congenital varicose veins. Br J Child Dis 1918;15:13.

35. Parkes-Weber F. Further rare diseases and debatable subjects. London, Staples Press, 1949.

36. Servelle M. Klippel and Trenaunay's syndrome: 768 operated cases. Ann Surg 1985;201:365.

37. Silverman RA. Hemangiomas and vascular malformations. Pediatr Clin North Am 1991;38:811.

VENOUS AND LYMPHATIC SYSTEMS

SURGERY: SCIENTIFIC PRINCIPLES AND PRACTICE, Second Edition, edited by
Lazar J. Greenfield, Michael W. Mulholland, Keith T. Oldham, Gerald B. Zelenock,
and Keith D. Lillemoe. Lippincott–Raven Publishers, Philadelphia, © 1997.

CHAPTER 96

VENOUS PHYSIOLOGY AND DISORDERS OF THE SUPERFICIAL AND DEEP VEINS

THOMAS W. WAKEFIELD AND LAZAR J. GREENFIELD

The superficial veins of the lower extremity consist of the greater and the lesser saphenous veins. They contain multiple valves and exhibit significant variability in branching and location. The greater saphenous vein begins anterior to the medial malleolus with the joining of superficial draining veins from the medial aspect of the dorsum of the foot with veins from the medial aspect of the sole. It travels subcutaneously, usually in a straight line on the anteromedial aspect of the lower leg 1 or 2 cm posterior to the tibia, and passes along the medial aspect of the knee. The greater saphenous vein continues in a straight line to the thigh, where it joins the femoral vein 2 to 4 cm lateral to the pubic tubercle and inferior to the inguinal ligament at the fossa ovalis (Fig. 96-1). In the leg, the greater saphenous vein lies adjacent to and sometimes is crossed by the saphenous branch of the femoral nerve, providing cutaneous sensation to the medial aspect of the lower leg.

The location of the saphenous nerve places it at risk during procedures involving the use or removal of the greater saphenous vein. The junction of the greater saphenous vein with the femoral vein is sometimes missed, since the greater saphenous vein may appear to continue proximally if the superficial inferior epigastric vein or the superficial circumflex iliac vein joins the saphenous vein vertically and is large in size. The superficial external pudendal vein joins the saphenous vein medially, although the arrangement of this branch and other superficial saphenous venous tributaries is not constant. Usually, there are four to five branches off of the saphenous vein at this location. The saphenous vein receives a variable number of tributaries draining the posteromedial and anterolateral aspects of the leg. The medial and lateral greater saphenous branches may be large and can be confused with the main greater saphenous trunk. The greater saphenous vein may be duplicated and exist as two separate trunks that join to form a single vein at its origin and termination. This occurs in as many as 5% to 10% of patients. The lesser saphenous vein arises behind the lateral malleolus, from the conflu-

ence of veins draining the lateral aspect of the foot. It curves toward the midline of the posterior calf and then ascends in a straight line vertically to join the popliteal vein behind the knee near the head of the gastrocnemius muscle, although it has been demonstrated to terminate above the level of the knee crease in 7% to 8% of cases.[1] The lesser saphenous vein lies in the subcutaneous tissues just below the skin. It may continue upward in the posterior region of the thigh and connect with tributaries of the greater saphenous vein.

The greater and lesser saphenous veins are joined in the foot by a superficial dorsal venous arch. The deep veins of the sole of the foot consist of lateral and medial plantar veins. They are joined through communicating veins to a cutaneous arch and come together to form the posterior tibial vein (Fig. 96-2). Multiple communicating veins connect the superficial to the deep veins in the foot. The deep veins of the lower leg consist of vena comitantes that accompany the anterior tibial, posterior tibial, and peroneal arteries. Each of the deep veins consist of two or three vena comitantes adjacent to the artery with multiple connections that cross and surround the artery. These connecting veins make surgical exposure of the tibial arteries difficult. The anterior tibial venous drainage arises from the dorsum of the foot and lies in the anterior compartment of the calf next to the interosseous membrane. The posterior tibial veins, which drain the superficial and deep plantar veins, are inferior to the medial malleolus and follow the course of the posterior tibial artery. The peroneal veins lie directly behind and medial to the fibula and ascend along the peroneal artery (Fig. 96-3). These deep veins of the calf have frequent interconnections. The soleal muscle sinusoids are without valves and are referred to as *venous lakes*. The venous lakes in the calf are a common site of early thrombus formation. They coalesce to join the posterior tibial and peroneal veins. These sinusoids are less apparent in the gastrocnemius muscle, where the veins tend to be linear and exhibit valves. The paired vena comitantes merge to form single trunks that unite at the knee to form the popliteal vein. Sometimes the junction occurs above the knee, resulting in a dual popliteal vein system.

The popliteal vein continues proximally as the superficial femoral vein in proximity to the superficial femoral artery in the adductor canal. It is joined below the inguinal ligament by the deep femoral (profunda) vein and then continues as the common femoral vein. The deep femoral vein frequently connects directly or through tributary veins to the popliteal vein. The anatomy of the popliteal and femoral veins is variable, and duplication is common. The common femoral vein runs medial to the common femoral artery beneath the inguinal ligament and continues as the external iliac vein. The greater saphenous vein usually joins the common femoral vein 2 to 4 cm proximal to the junction of the deep and superficial femoral vein at the fossa ovalis. The external iliac vein is the continuation in the pelvis of the common femoral vein and is joined at

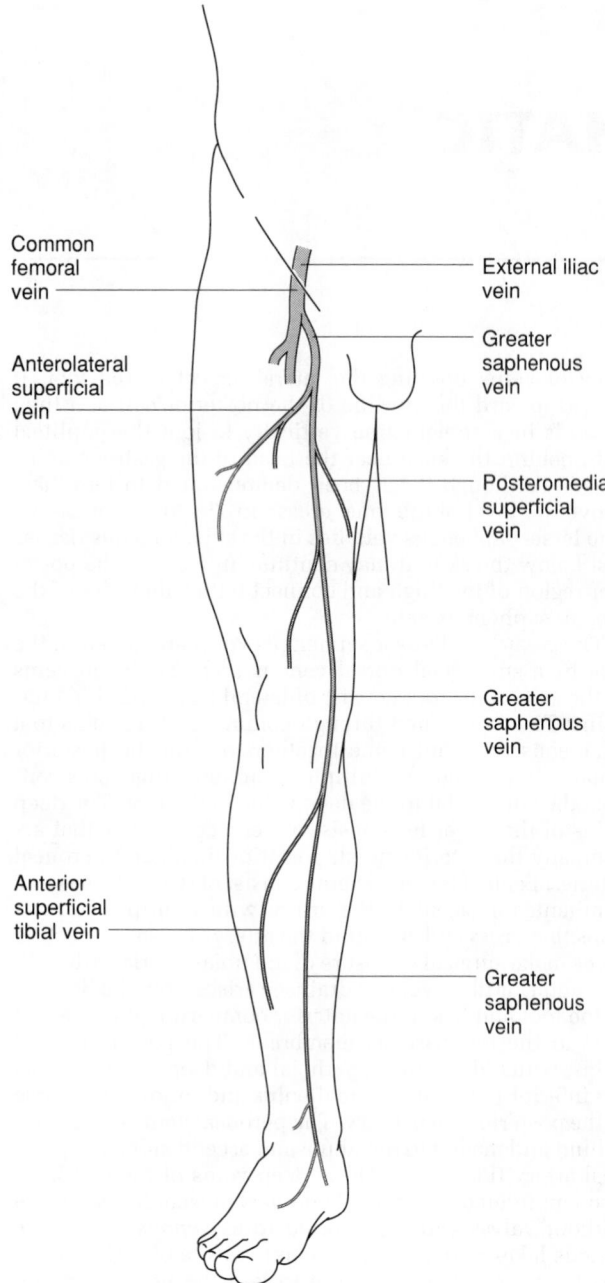

Common femoral vein

External iliac vein

Anterolateral superficial vein

Greater saphenous vein

Posteromedial superficial vein

Greater saphenous vein

Anterior superficial tibial vein

Greater saphenous vein

Figure 96-1. Greater saphenous vein and its branches.

the level of the sacroiliac joint medially by the internal iliac vein (hypogastric) draining the pelvis. Both internal iliac veins form a generous collateral network within the pelvis and include connections with the gluteal, obturator, and internal pudendal veins, a large number of unnamed vessels, as well as multiple extrapelvic collateral pathways. The common iliac veins arise from the joining of the external and internal iliac veins. They ascend in a medial direction and join on the right side of the fifth lumbar vertebra and the aorta forming the inferior vena cava. The right common iliac vein ascends in an almost straight line to the inferior vena cava, whereas the left common iliac vein is more transversely oriented and joins the right iliac vein at an angle of approximately 90 degrees. The left common iliac vein may be compressed between the convexity of the lumbosacral spine posteriorly and the anterior crossing of the right common iliac artery. This variable degree

of compression may be seen on venography (Fig. 96-4) and probably accounts for the higher incidence of left-sided deep venous thrombosis, varicose veins, and varicocele in men.

The inferior vena cava ascends from the level of the fifth lumbar vertebra and ends at the right atrium. It lies to the right of the midline and lateral to the aorta and receives a variable number of paired lumbar veins that connect with the vertebral and paravertebral venous plexus. At the level of the L-1 to L-2 interspace, the renal veins join the inferior vena cava. More proximally, the hepatic veins join the inferior vena cava. The inferior vena cava may be duplicated below the level of the renal veins, with a left-sided cava draining into the left renal vein, which then joins to form a single proximal inferior vena cava. If unsuspected, this anomaly can cause confusion at operation and inadvertent injury may result. The incidence of inferior vena caval and renal vein anomalies is significant. Duplication of the inferior vena cava occurs in 0.2% to 3% of cases, transposition or left-sided inferior vena cava occurs in 0.2% to 0.5%, a retroaortic left renal vein in 1.2% to 2.4%, and a circumaortic left renal vein in 1.5% to 8.7%.[2] The left renal vein normally crosses the aorta on its anterior surface, but it occasionally crosses posteriorly and may result in confusion and unexpected injury. Collateral circulation around an obstructed inferior vena cava occurs through many alternate pathways, including the vertebral plexus, gonadal veins, ureteral veins, the azygos system, and the extensive superficial collaterals, which include the superficial epigastric, circumflex iliac veins, and the lateral thoracic and intercostal veins.

Important communicating veins exist at the termination of the greater and lesser saphenous veins where they join the deep venous system in the popliteal fossa and in the fossa ovalis. The perforating veins of the lower leg are important to the pathophysiology of venous disease and chronic venous insufficiency, especially the three or four perforating veins at the level of the medial and lateral malleolus in the so-called gaiter area of the lower leg. Other perforating veins are located in the upper medial calf and along the posterolateral aspect of the lower leg, connecting the lesser saphenous vein with the deep veins of the calf. A small but variable number of communications exist in the mid-thigh between the greater saphenous vein and the superficial femoral vein. The locations of perforating veins can only be accurately determined by venous duplex imaging or venography.

Venous valves direct the flow of blood to the heart and prevent valvular reflux. These valves consist of two thin and delicate leaflets composed of an intimal fold with a small amount of connective tissue in between. Venous valves in the lower extremity are more numerous in the distal extremity, decrease in number proximally, and are absent in the superior and inferior vena cava. The valves in the upper extremity appear less important for venous function, and the influence of the venous muscle pump is less significant. The loss of valvular function in the upper extremity after thrombosis less frequently produces problems, in marked contrast to the lower extremity, where the valves play an important role. There are no valves present in the soleal and gastrocnemius sinusoids, but all other deep veins of the calf contain multiple valves. The popliteal vein contains one or two valves whose function is essential to the normal venous return from the calf. Valves in the deep veins of the thigh vary in number and position. There is a constant valve in the femoral vein just distal to its junction with the deep femoral vein and in the proximal portion of the popliteal vein just distal to the adductor hiatus. The greater and lesser saphenous systems contain 8 to 10 valves with a constant valve present at the proximal

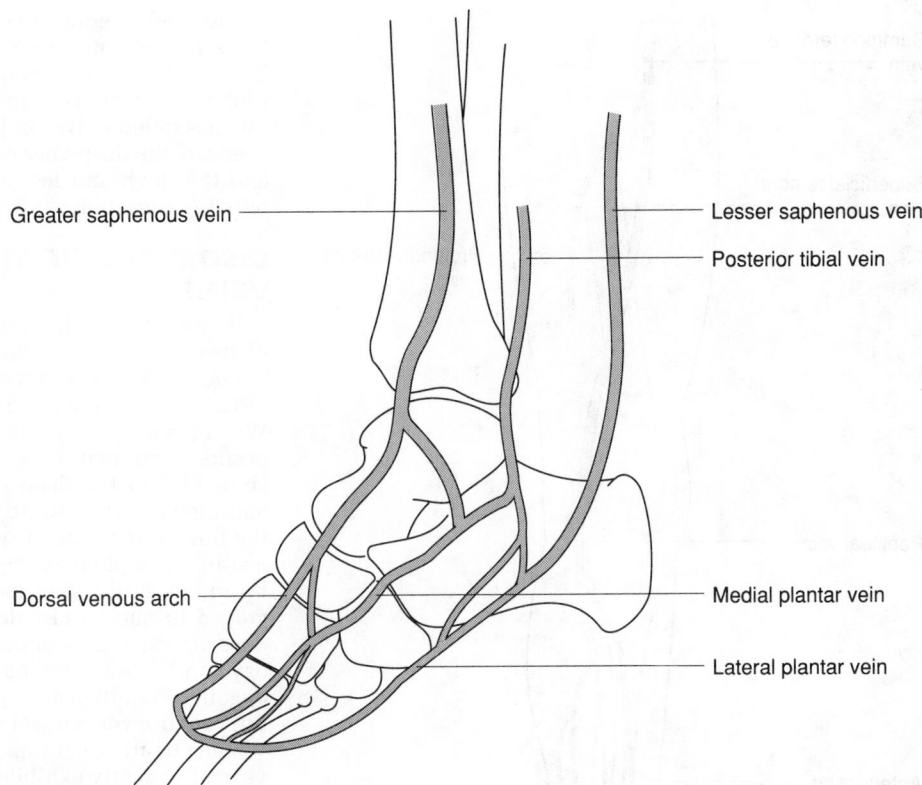

Figure 96-2. Veins of the foot.

end of the greater saphenous vein just at or slightly distal to its junction with the common femoral vein. A third set of valves is present in the perforating veins, which communicate between the superficial and deep veins. Valves are oriented so that they direct venous flow from the superficial to the deep system and, in the deep system, from the foot to the heart. They prevent reflux of the higher pressure deep venous circulation into the superficial saphenous system. The valves in these perforating veins lie both deep and superficial to the muscle fascia.

VENOUS PHYSIOLOGY

Foot vein pressure is influenced by the patient's position in either the supine or erect posture. When measured supine, venous pressure is the residual kinetic energy of the heart reduced by capillary and arteriolar resistance. This residual pressure is approximately 15 mmHg and results in a pressure gradient of 13 to 15 mmHg returning blood to the heart, since the right atrial pressure usually ranges between 0 to 2 mmHg. When foot vein pressure is measured in the erect position, the hydrostatic pressure caused by the weight of the column of blood that extends from the heart to the foot must be included. Therefore, foot vein pressure in the erect posture is the sum of the hydrostatic pressure and the kinetic pressure of 15 mmHg. In a person 6 feet tall, the hydrostatic pressure equals about 100 mmHg. Therefore, in the upright posture, the pressure measured in a foot vein is approximately 115 mmHg. Hydrostatic pressure is also exerted on the arterial circulation so that the net pressure is still the difference in pressure across the capillary bed.

Assuming the erect posture increases venous volume, and the volume of the calf increases about 2% to 3%. In the leg veins, the upright position increases capacitance by about 500 mL of blood, which arises from the central circulation and fills the veins. Orthostatic hypotension

may result in patients with a low blood volume. This increment is returned to the central circulation with exercise in the presence of a normal calf muscle pump. For patients at bed rest, wearing graded compression stockings increases the velocity of venous return and reduces the venous volume pooling in the legs, reducing stasis and also decreasing the potential for venous thrombosis.

The vein wall is composed of collagen, elastic tissue, and smooth muscle fibers. The smooth muscle fibers are responsible for active venous tone. Venous capacity is influenced by variations in transmural pressure and, to a lesser extent, by the contractility of the smooth muscle in the venous wall. This is particularly true when the veins are collapsed and the transmural pressure is low. When there is further filling, the veins assume a circular configuration, and the smooth muscle venous tone assumes greater importance in regulating venous volume. The venous system can accommodate significant variations in volume with little change in pressure. This ability allows alterations in blood volume to occur with minimal change in central venous pressure. When the venous capacitance is exceeded, however, the central venous pressure rises significantly.

Empty veins are flat. As they fill, they evolve from an elliptical to a circular form in cross section. Initially, there is little resistance to flow as veins distend and their shape changes. During early filling, as veins assume a circular configuration, more blood can be accommodated with little increase in venous pressure. Once veins assume a circular configuration, the pressure per unit of volume increase rapidly increases and reaches a plateau (Fig. 96-5). The transmural pressure, which causes distention, is the difference between the intraluminal pressure and the external tissue pressure. With outflow obstruction, a small volume increment results in a disproportionate increase in pressure in the veins.

Venous flow is affected by a number of factors, including

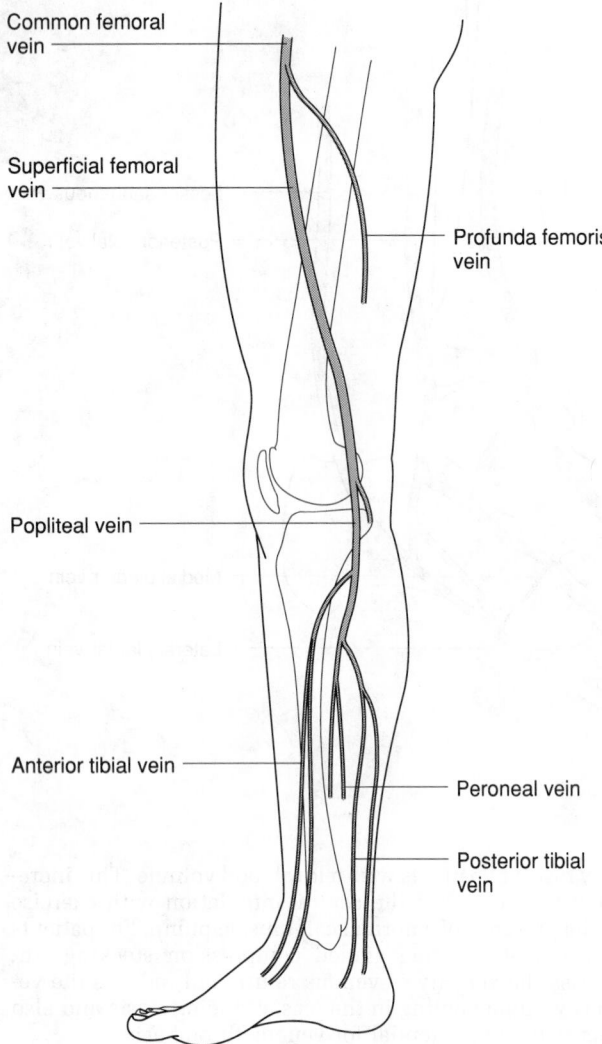

Figure 96-3. Deep veins of the lower leg.

respiration, body position, calf muscle pump function, and the arterial circulation. For example, flow is at its minimum during peak inspiration. A unique feature of the venous circulation is the presence of bicuspid valves that direct the flow of venous blood toward the heart and prevent reflux (Fig. 96-6). The valve cusps of the superficial veins are oriented so that they lie parallel to the skin surface. The normal valve sinus is wider than the diameter of the vein, and it is believed that the valve cusps do not lie flat against the vein wall when open. The open valve cusps are easily engaged by retrograde blood flow, and the slightly greater valve diameter ensures a tight seal that prevents valvular reflux. A crucial set of valves is found in the perforating veins. The balloon-like appearance of the vein wall around the confluence of a vein valve may reflect differences in the tensile strength of the vein wall. The distention at the site of the valve spreads and places tension on the commissures, causing the valve cusp edges to tighten, further enhancing valvular competency.

Normally, veins can accommodate large volume changes with only small pressure changes. This does not occur in many patients, however, so that with calf muscle pump dysfunction, venous pressures do not normalize but remain chronically elevated. Additionally, any dissipation of pressure is quickly overcome by a return to preexercise pressure levels when walking stops. It is this chronic state of elevated venous pressure (venous hypertension) that leads to the state of chronic venous insufficiency (CVI). The syndrome of venous claudication occurs when the iliofemoral venous segment is obstructed by thrombosis that has failed to lyse or by an anatopic abnormality. With exercise, the deep venous system fills but does not empty, and the thigh and leg become heavy and painful with a bursting sensation.

DISORDERS OF THE SUPERFICIAL VEINS

Varicose veins that arise spontaneously in the absence of deep venous involvement are referred to as *primary varicose veins*, whereas veins arising as the outward manifestation of CVI are referred to as *secondary varicose veins*. When the deep veins are competent, a circular flow circuit occurs such that flow down the saphenous system is shunted into the deep system by competent perforators and then returns toward the heart. However, a portion of the flow at the femoral vein level reverses down the leg, leading to saphenous vein insufficiency during exercise; up to one fifth of the total femoral vein flow may be involved in such a circular motion.[3] This circular motion does not exist in secondary varicose veins. The epidemiology of varicose veins has been determined as part of the ongoing Framingham study.[4] During 16 years of follow-up, varicose veins developed in 629 women and 396 men. Women of all age groups, except those between 80 and 89 years, frequently exhibited varicose veins, and the highest incidence was in women aged 40 to 49 years. Women with varicose veins were more often obese, physically inactive, hypertensive, and older at menopause. In men, varicosities were associated with smoking and physical inactivity. Although there was no independent direct relation to atherosclerosis, patients with the risk factors mentioned are clearly at greater risk for atherosclerosis than patients without these characteristics.

Treatment

Treatment for both primary and secondary varicose veins involves a program of CVI management including elastic stocking support, periodic leg elevation, and exer-

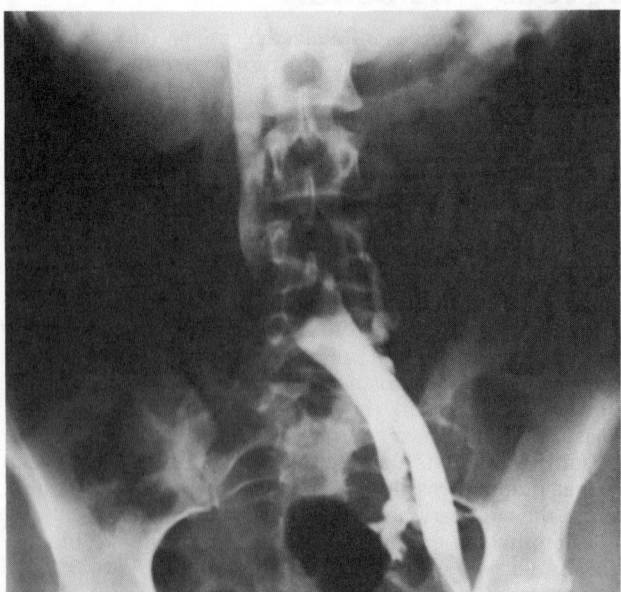

Figure 96-4. Phlebogram showing compression of the left common iliac vein by the right common iliac artery.

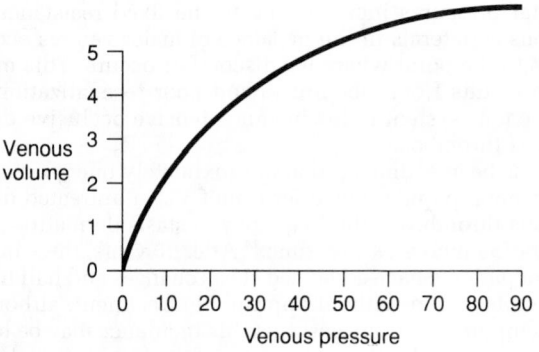

Figure 96-5. Relation between venous volume and venous pressure.

cise wearing stocking support. The elastic hose coapts the vein walls, preventing further distention of the already dilated superficial veins. Indications for surgical treatment of varicose veins include pain over the varicosities themselves (to be distinguished from the discomfort of underlying deep venous insufficiency), superficial thrombophlebitis in the varicosities, erosion of the overlying skin with bleeding, disabling edema with or without subcutaneous cellulitis, induration or lipodermatosclerosis associated with the varicosities, and manifestations of CVI (especially ulceration) related to incompetency of the superficial saphenous system and the varicosities. Contraindications to varicose vein ligation and stripping include a cosmetic improvement only, varicose veins secondary to CVI from deep venous insufficiency in which the CVI is causing the patient's symptoms, and varicose veins associated with other chronic disease states which are the cause of the patient's symptoms, such as degenerative arthritis, arterial occlusive disease, neurogenic syndromes, lymphedema, congestive heart failure, and obesity. Ligation and stripping should also be avoided for varicose veins associated with an underlying arteriovenous fistula or underlying congenital venous abnormalities, such as the Klippel-Trenaunay syndrome. Injection sclerotherapy may be indicated for small varicosities but more frequently for "spider" telangiectactic veins. Indications for injection sclerotherapy include direct pain over the varicose or spider telangiectactic veins, symptoms of venous insufficiency related to the varicose or spider telangiectactic veins (especially symptoms before or during menstruation), previous thrombophlebitis in small varicose veins, bleeding from the varicose or spider telangiectactic veins, and trophic changes related to the spider telangiectactic veins. These are essentially the same indications as for larger varicose veins. Contraindications to injection sclerotherapy include active thrombophlebitis, pregnancy during the first and second trimester, the postpartum period for approximately 3 months after termination of lactation, significant leg edema, inability to participate in physical activity after injection therapy, a concomitant bed-ridden condition, severe arterial occlusive disease, the inability to wear properly applied bandages after injection sclerotherapy, and cosmetic effect only without underlying symptoms.

Preoperative testing should include documenting an intact deep venous system by venous ultrasound duplex imaging. Reflux testing, such as photoplethysmographic (PPG) examination, may be indicated to help predict the overall success of the varicose vein removal and the need for postoperative elastic support. If CVI is present, the patient is best instructed to follow a program of CVI management. The classic procedure of high ligation and stripping

of the entire saphenous system has been replaced by more selective vein removal, and the stab evulsion technique has gained popularity. High ligation alone with careful perforator interruption has been recommended with excellent long-term results[5] as has ambulatory stab evulsion phlebectomy for truncal varicosities.[6] In this technique, after high ligation of the greater saphenous vein, small stab wounds 1.5 to 3 mm long are made along the premarked varicosities. Specially designed hooks are used to remove trunk and tributary varicosities. Although this technique may work well for primary varicose veins, in the presence of significant secondary varicosities, larger incisions and perforating vein interruption and ligation are important technical considerations. In the presence of secondary varicosities in which varicose clusters are related primarily to deep venous insufficiency and perforator incompetence, high ligation is usually not necessary. With careful patient selection and properly tailored operative techniques, the recurrence rate should be 10% or lower.[7] Major complications include hematoma, infection, sural nerve irritation (from lesser saphenous stripping), and saphenous nerve irritation (minimized by removing a stripper if used from proximal to distal). A combination of surgical and sclerotherapy techniques yields optimal functional and cosmetic results.[8]

DISORDERS OF THE DEEP VEINS

CVI has traditionally been considered a consequence of previous deep venous thrombosis in most cases and of congenital or hereditary venous valvular incompetence in a few cases, although more recent reports have suggested a more equal incidence of these two causes of CVI. Other causes include cavernous hemangioma, congenital arteriovenous fistula, and pelvic tumors.

With valvular incompetence, the standing column of blood produces elevated venous pressures leading to CVI. Furthermore, patients with CVI have little if any venous pressure reduction during exercise in contrast to the normal response, and with venous obstruction, the venous pressure may actually rise with exercise. After exercise, the venous pressure returns much faster than it should so

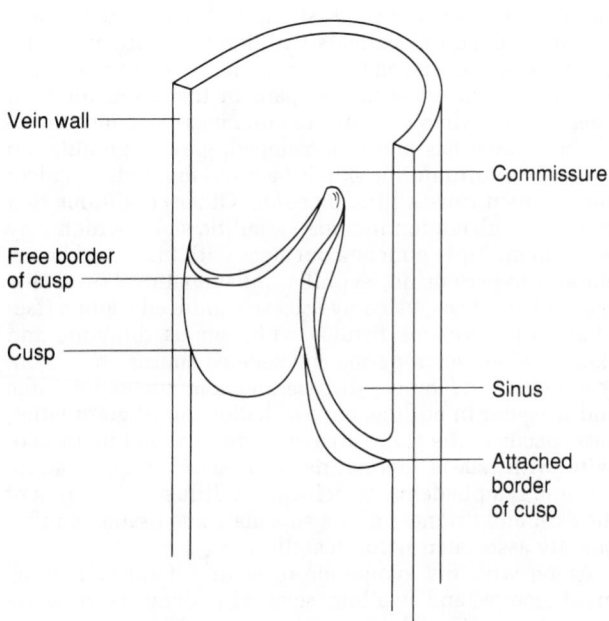

Figure 96-6. Structure of a venous valve.

that the lower leg and ankle region is exposed chronically to elevated venous pressures.[9] There are two important reasons why the changes of CVI (including stasis pigmentation, stasis dermatitis, and ulceration) occur in the gaiter area. First, incompetent perforating veins produce extreme venous hypertension in the ankle region. Second, the ankle has little soft tissue support. Elevated venous pressures lead to brawny edema from plasma fluid constituents in the interstitial space along with plasma proteins and red blood cells. These constituents produce low-grade inflammation, the red cells break down to produce a dark pigment called hemosiderin, and eventually, the subcutaneous tissues become scarred and fibrotic. Due to the fibrosis in the subcutaneous tissue, skin perfusion decreases, leading to skin ischemia facilitating ulceration. Leukocytes also play an important role as they become sequestered in the microcirculation of the leg with elevated venous pressures, possibly leading to capillary occlusion.[10] In the capillaries, these leukocytes become activated and destroy tissue by releasing superoxide radicals and proteolytic enzymes.[11] Macrophages and T lymphocytes are the cell types most often involved.[12] The inflammatory response initiated by these cells is more important in the pathogenesis of the skin changes than microvascular occlusion as leukocytes "trapped" in the capillaries during venous hypertension are released within 10 to 20 minutes of resumption of a supine position.[10]

Although severe changes of CVI have traditionally been considered to be associated only with deep venous insufficiency and not saphenous vein insufficiency, more and more studies are suggesting that even isolated saphenous vein incompetence can lead to the CVI syndrome. According to the pathophysiology discussed earlier, the symptoms of CVI begin with edema. The edema usually occurs at and above the ankle without involvement of the forefoot or toes. It usually responds well to leg elevation. Characteristically, the patient has worse edema at night than in the morning, and eventually, dermatitis, stasis pigmentation, brawny induration and ulceration may occur. Other causes of ulceration must be distinguished from venous ulceration, including neurotrophic and ischemic ulceration. *Neurotrophic* ulcers are painless and bleed with manipulation. They are deep, indolent, and surrounded by chronic inflammatory tissue reaction appearing as callous. They are usually located over pressure points, commonly the plantar surface of the first and fifth metatarsal heads, and are common in patients with long-standing neuropathy. *Ischemic* ulcers, on the other hand, are extremely painful and associated with rest pain in the distal forefoot. These ulcers when chronic are circumscribed, and the ulcer base often has poorly developed, grayish granulation tissue. The surrounding skin is pale and mottled, and ulcer débridement causes little bleeding. Other conditions that may cause ulceration include vasculitic states which may result in multiple punched out areas with indurated bases, chronic hypertension, syphilis, inflammatory bowel disease, tuberculosis, osteomyelitis self-induced trauma (factitial), arteriovenous fistulas with venous dilations and skin erosion, scleroderma, myxedema, burns, radiation, lymphoma, and fungal diseases. *Venous* ulcers are large and irregular in outline, have a shallow moist granulation base, occur in the gaiter area, and are involved in areas of skin with stasis dermatitis and stasis pigmentation. Chronic lymphedema, which causes diffuse thickening of the skin and firmness of the subcutaneous tissue, is infrequently associated with ulceration.

Along with the symptoms of aching, fatigue, itching, night cramps, and swelling, selected patients describe venous claudication.[13] As venous volume increases to near maximum with exercise, leg distention and intracompartmental pressures increase due to the fixed resistance of venous collaterals in the presence of major venous occlusions to the point where leg discomfort occurs. This most often results from incomplete and poor recanalization of the venous system following an extensive occlusive deep venous thrombosis.

It has been estimated that approximately one quarter of the general population suffer from CVI. In untreated deep venous thrombosis, the frequency of stasis dermatitis and ulceration increases over time.[14] After 10 years, three quarters of patients have advanced stasis changes and half have stasis ulceration without appropriate treatment, although contemporary data suggest that this incidence may be less. The mean time for the appearance of the first stasis-related venous ulcer is two to three years. Interestingly, it has been found that valvular reflux after deep venous thrombosis progresses over time. Of extremities 1 week after thrombosis, 17% reveal reflux while greater than two thirds of extremities show reflux at 12 months, not limited to the area of initial thrombosis.[15] This suggests that mechanisms other than valve entrapment in scar must exist for the development of CVI.

Treatment

Once venous insufficiency has developed, it is an incurable but manageable problem. Most of the changes of CVI in the leg are due to chronic swelling. Elastic compression stockings improve but do not prevent swelling. Elevating the legs above the heart level, which CVI patients should do two to three times per day, is important to decrease venous hypertension. Additionally, elastic support should be applied before the patient gets out of bed in the morning and taken off before the patient goes to sleep at night. The manner in which elastic compression improves the symptoms of CVI has not been absolutely established. However, recent studies suggest that external compression may restore competency of the dilated valve cusps[16] or may affect the venoarterial reflex.[17] Exercise such as walking and bicycling with proper support applied and swimming is excellent for patients with CVI. If stasis ulceration eventually develops, it usually improves with leg elevation and local wound care, especially with occlusive dressings. In some cases, these ulcers may become superinfected and require antibacterial treatment although the routine use of topical antibiotics is not indicated.[18] The unna boot has been the traditional treatment and includes a gauze dressing impregnated with gelatin, zinc oxide, and caladryl. Application of the unna boot is followed by dry gauze and an elastic wrap and is usually repeated on a weekly basis. We have found a combination of occlusive dressings under the unna boot to be extremely effective for most venous ulcers.[19,20] The hypothesis about the effectiveness of occlusive dressings is that collagen synthesis and reepithelialization of tissue are increased in wounds beneath these dressings because they prevent the removal of new epidermis with each change. Granulation tissue forms quickly under these occlusive dressings because they are oxygen impermeable, and wound angiogenesis is inversely proportional to the ambient oxygen tension.

Most patients with CVI can be treated nonsurgically. However, 1% to 2% of patients benefit from operative correction. The two basic categories of operation are venous bypass for obstruction and valve restoration procedures for reflux. Before operative therapy is considered, the diagnosis of CVI must be confirmed objectively. Noninvasive laboratory studies include complete venous Doppler exams, PPG, and air plethysmography (APG). The PPG exam is qualitative and not quantitative whereas the APG is quantitative. The APG test measures many aspects of lower leg

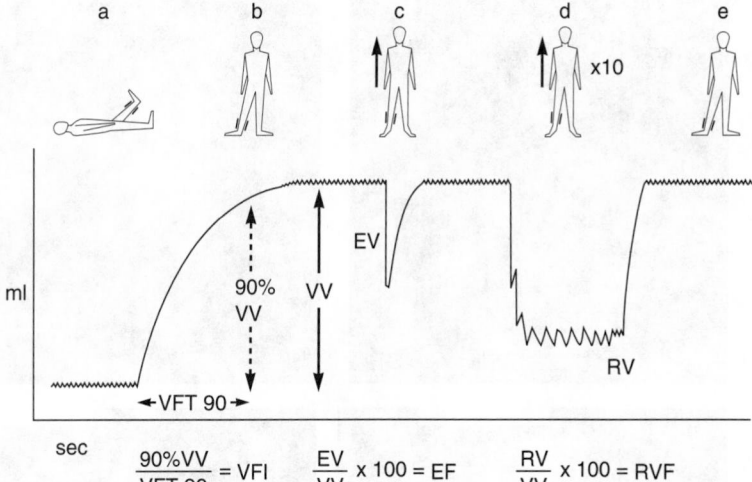

Figure 96-7. Diagram of typical recording of changes in the APG with patient supine with leg elevated (*a*), standing with weight on contralateral leg (*b*), after a single tiptoe (*c*), after 10 tiptoes (*d*), and returning to standing with weight on the contralateral leg (*e*). RVF, residual volume fraction; EF, ejection fraction; RV, residual volume; EV, ejection volume; VFI, volume filling index; VFT, venous filling time. (After Christopoulous DG, Nicolaides AN, Szendro G, et al. Air-plethysmography and the effects of elastic compression on venous hemodynamics of the leg. J Vasc Surg 1987;5:150)

$$\frac{90\%VV}{VFT\ 90} = VFI \qquad \frac{EV}{VV} \times 100 = EF \qquad \frac{RV}{VV} \times 100 = RVF$$

physiology at one time including venous obstruction, venous reflux, and calf muscle pump function and thus gives an overall assessment of the leg as a whole.[21] It can be used during exercise, is easily and readily repeated, and can also be used to differentiate superficial from deep venous insufficiency (Fig. 96-7). The residual volume fraction generated by this test correlates closely with ambulatory venous pressure.[21] Additionally, duplex imaging of closing times of individual venous valves indicates venous reflux.[22] Although outflow obstruction can be assessed by APG, it is best determined by the arm/foot pressure gradient measured directly. In normal limbs, the arm/foot pressure differential is less than 4 mmHg at rest and less than 6 mmHg with reactive hyperemia.[23] The invasive measurement of ambulatory venous pressure for reflux, however, is rarely needed because of the availability of the above noninvasive tests.

After the vascular laboratory tests, ascending phlebography is used to assess the patency of the tibial, popliteal, superficial femoral, common femoral, iliac, inferior vena cava, and perforating veins. A thin tourniquet placed at the ankle at 120 to 140 mmHg pressure is used to test for perforator incompetence.[24] Combined with ascending phlebography, descending phlebography requires placement of a catheter into the common femoral vein with the weight borne by the contralateral leg on a 60-degree footdown tilt table. A steady stream of contrast medium is injected into the femoral vein, and the valves are tested during normal breathing and with a forced Valsalva. Descending phlebography provides visual information about the function of the valves. Using this technique, pathologic reflux in patients with postthrombotic damage is found in about 31% of cases.[25] Thus, a combination of venous noninvasive testing and phlebography define the distribution of venous valvular incompetence in patients with CVI. Isolated proximal valvular incompetence is present in only 5% of limbs with severe disease in patients undergoing Doppler evaluation for CVI. Distal incompetence is found in 67% of those with proximal venous incompetence and in 57% of patients with competent proximal valves.[26] Thus, most patients with severe CVI have venous valvular incompetence that is more closely associated with distal deep venous valvular incompetence either alone or in combination with proximal valvular involvement.

Perforating vein ligation is indicated in patients who have recurrent or recalcitrant venous ulcers when there are large incompetent perforating veins under the area of ulceration (Fig. 96-8). Perforator ligation does not change the venous hemodynamics of the limb and is indicated to allow for ulcer healing so the patients may then follow a standard conservative program including stocking support, exercise, and leg elevation. Patients must understand that after perforator ligation, a standard aggressive conservative program needs to be followed. Other indications for

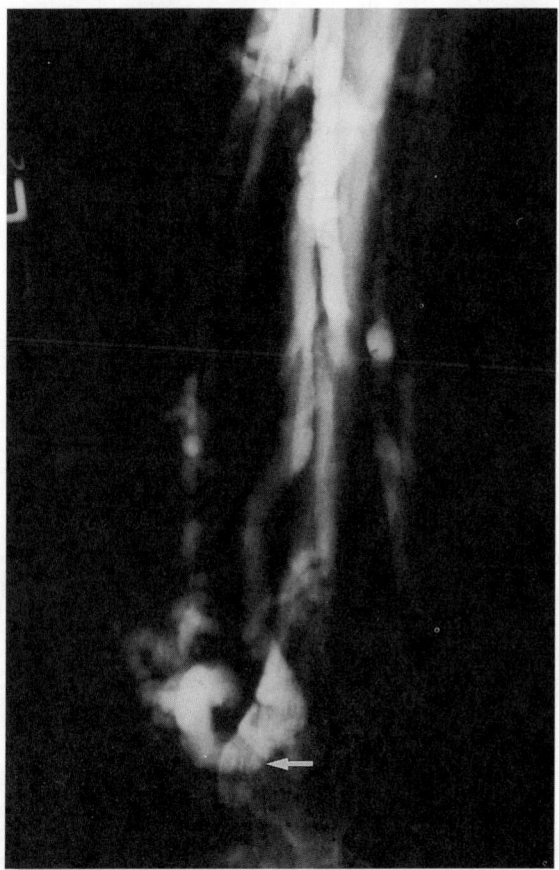

Figure 96-8. Large incompetent perforator (*arrow*) underneath an area of recurrent venous ulceration on the medial aspect of ankle. Ligation of the perforator resulted in ulcer healing. (Wakefield TW. Venous disorders. Probl General Surg 1994)

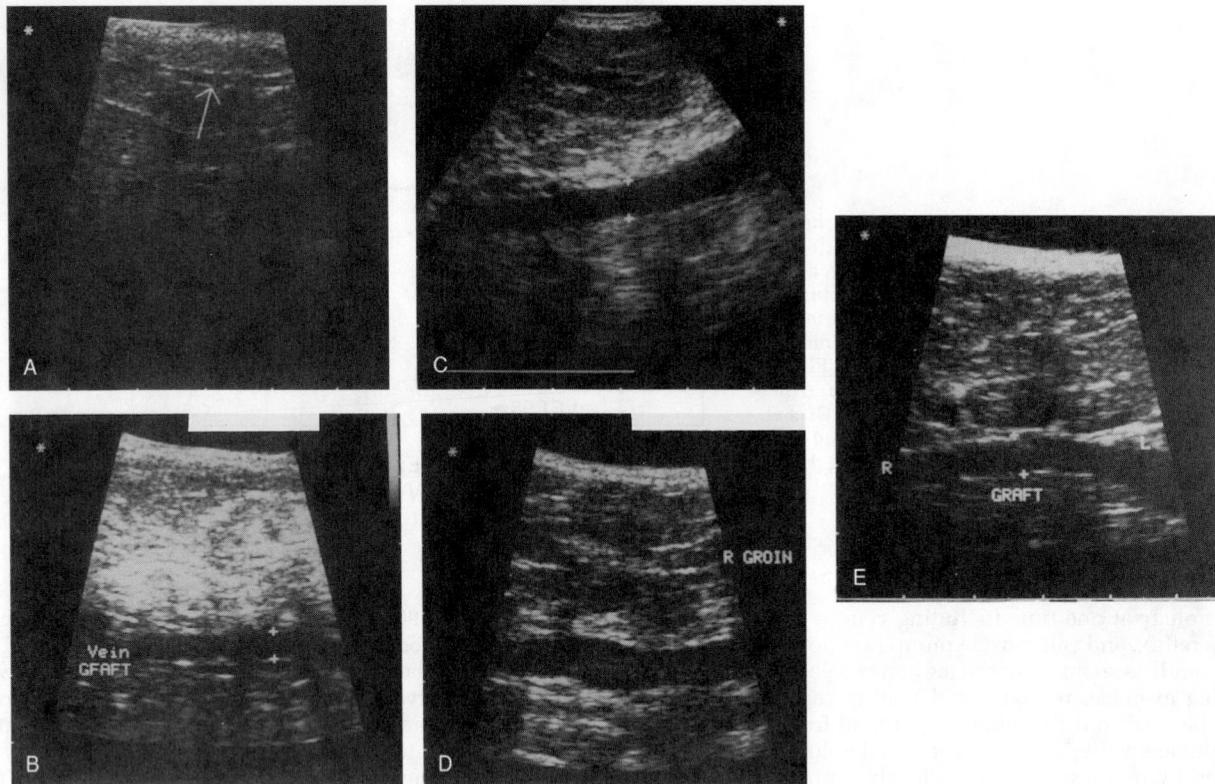

Figure 96-9. Increasing size of femorofemoral crossover bypass (*arrow in A*) from time of insertion (*A*), through 1 month (*B*), 4 months (*C*), and 13 months (*D* and *E*) postoperatively. (Wakefield TW. Venous disorders. Probl General surg 1994)

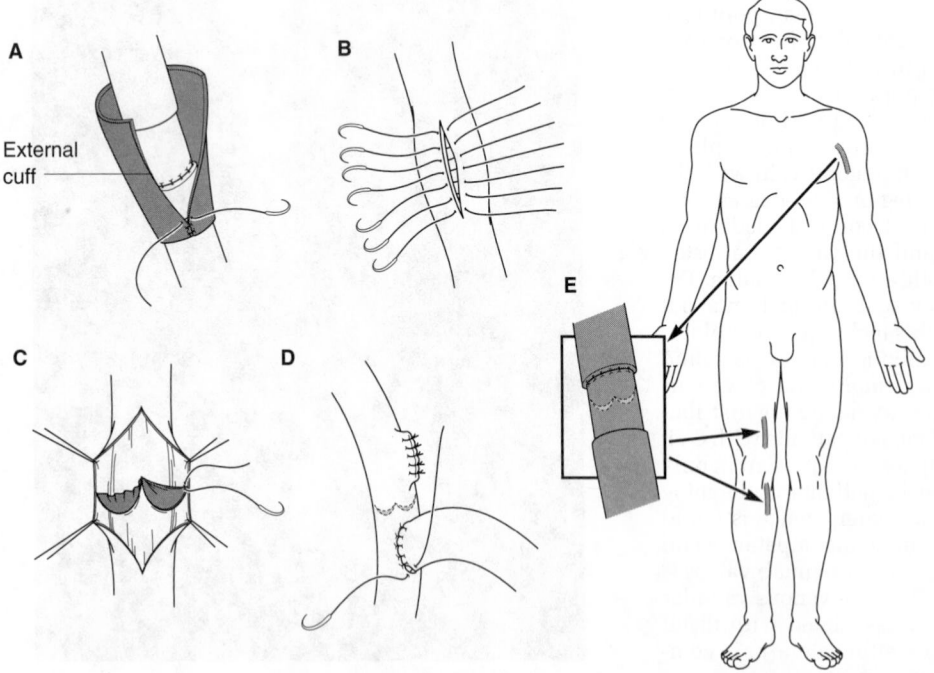

Figure 96-10. Methods of reflux correction. (*A*) External cuff banding. (*B*) Vein wall plication. (*C*) Valvuloplasty. (*D*) Transposition of an incompetent superficial femoral vein into a competent profunda femoris veins, and (*E*) Valve transplantation. (After Eriksson I. Reconstructive surgery for deep vein incompetence in the lower limb. Eur J Vasc Surg 1990;4:214)

perforator ligation include persistent pain in the region of a previous venous ulcer with an underlying incompetent perforating vein and repeated failure of skin graft healing in an area of venous ulceration. Patients with proximal deep venous occlusion should have this proximal occlusion resolved before or at the same time as perforator ligation. Contraindications to perforator ligation include the failure to demonstrate an appropriate perforator under the ulcer and such severe stasis disease of the skin and subcutaneous tissue that the incision for the procedure would not be expected to heal. Among 650 patients with 1799 limbs reported, the ulcer recurrence rate was 15% with a 17% postoperative wound complication rate with perforator ligation.[27]

Indications for direct venous reconstructive surgery include significant venous claudication associated with venous outflow obstruction; significant symptoms of venous reflux including severe aching, fatigue, and swelling; recurrent venous ulceration not responsive to conservative therapy or perforator ligation, resulting from either venous obstruction or reflux; such significant combined superficial and deep venous insufficiency that the patient's symptoms cannot be relieved with superficial venous surgery alone; and failure of maximal conservative therapy to relieve severe symptoms of deep venous insufficiency. Contraindications to direct venous surgery include venous obstruction as seen on phlebography that is not associated with symptoms; CVI that has not been treated with an aggressive conservative management program; symptoms associated with chronic diseases, such as degenerative arthritis and peripheral vascular occlusive disease from nonvenous origins; and symptoms of CVI that cannot be documented with any of the anatomic or physiologic tests described earlier.

For venous obstruction, two bypasses have been described—the femorofemoral and saphenopopliteal. The crossover femorofemoral venous bypass (Palma procedure) was first described in 1958. After dividing the ipsilateral saphenous vein distally, this vein is tunneled suprapubically to the opposite femoral vein. Prosthetic material for this bypass has also been advocated. This procedure is indicated for relief of persistent unilateral iliac vein obstruction. In 303 patients reported on (277 from postthrombotic problems and 26 from extrinsic compression), results were excellent in 187 (62%), good in 39(13%), and poor in 77 (25%)[28]. The ipsilateral saphenopopliteal bypass (May-Husni procedure) may benefit patients with superficial femoral vein occlusion. In 65 patients reported, 75% were improved while 15% were not.[28] For both of these bypasses, concomitant procedures such as perforator ligation, saphenous vein stripping, and creation of distal arteriovenous fistulas have been advocated (the latter if prosthetic conduits are used). In both of these procedures, the saphenous vein when used as a conduit tends to dilate over time (Fig. 96-9).

Venous valvular operations for reflux include valvuloplasty,[29,30] venous segment transposition,[31,32] venous valvular autotransplantation,[33] external banding, and vein wall plication[34] (Fig. 96-10). In the experience of Kistner, the best results with valvuloplasty have occurred when combined with perforator ligation. Reported results of valvuloplasty in 155 limbs with 1 to 13 year follow-up have revealed good clinical results in 77% of cases.[34] Valvuloplasty may use external cuffs or bands, suture techniques not requiring incision into the vein, vein wall plication, and repair using the angioscope. Venous segment transposition procedures have reported good early results but deteriorating later results.[35] Of 46 limbs reported with follow-up for 1 to 6 years, 63% revealed good clinical results. Finally, valvular autotransplantation has been shown to be successful in nearly 80% of the cases in one series[33] but curative in only about 50% in another series.[30] The transplanted vein valve may thus

develop the same problems over time as the original failed valve. Interestingly, the valve transfer now believed to be most important is the popliteal valve rather than the femoral valve. Of the 176 limbs reported with follow-up to 6 years, good clinical results have been reported in 66%. Importantly, O'Donnell documented improvement in venous hemodynamics as assessed by APG after popliteal vein transplantation.[36] A final procedure to mention is the substitute valve operation (Psathakis procedure) using a Silastic tendon spacer behind the knee.[37]

In all of these procedures for CVI, there is often discrepancy between hemodynamic and clinical results, making it difficult to evaluate results objectively. In addition, the relative infrequency of isolated proximal venous valve incompetence in patients with CVI and the importance of distal vein valvular reflux suggest that most patients who have proximal valve reconstruction will need additional surgical correction for distal valves or incompetent perforating veins.

Acknowledgments

We wish to acknowledge S. Martin Lindenauer, MD, for his contributions to this chapter in the first edition of this book.

REFERENCES

1. Chang BB, Paty PS, Shah DM, et al. The lesser saphenous vein: an unappreciated source of autogenous vein. J Vasc Surg 1992;15:152.
2. Goidano JM, Trout HH. Anomalies of the inferior vena cava. J Vasc Surg 1986;3:924.
3. Sumner DS. Hemodynamics and pathophysiology of venous disease. In: Rutherford RB, ed. Vascular surgery, ed 4. Philadelphia, WB Saunders, 1995:1673.
4. Brand FN, Dannenberg AL, Abbott RD, et al. The epidemiology of varicose veins: the Framingham study. Am J Prev Med 1988;4:96.
5. Hammarsten J, Pedersen P, Cederlund C-G, et al. Long saphenous vein saving surgery for varicose veins: a long-term follow-up. Eur J Vasc Surg 1990;4:361.
6. Goren G, Yellin AE. Ambulatory stab evulsion phlebectomy for truncal varicose veins. Am J Surg 1991;162:166.
7. Burnham SJ. Varicose veins: patient selection and treatment, In: Rutherford RB, ed. Vascular surgery, ed 3. Philadelphia, WB Saunders, 1989:1512.
8. Lary BG. Varicose veins and intracutaneous telangiectasia: combined treatment in 1,500 cases. South Med J 1987; 80:1105.
9. Zierler RE, Strandness DE Jr. Hemodynamics for the vascular surgeon. In: Moore WS, ed. Vascular surgery: a comprehensive review, ed 4. Philadelphia, WB Saunders, 1993:179.
10. Thomas PR, Nash GB, Dormandy JA. White cell accumulation in the dependent legs of patients with venous hypertension: a possible mechanism for trophic changes in the skin. Br Med J 1988;296:1693.
11. Coleridge Smith PD, Thomas P, Scurr JH, et al. Causes of venous ulceration: a new hypothesis. Br Med J 1988;296:1726.
12. Wilkinson LS, Bunker C, Edwards JC, et al. Leukocytes: their role in the etiopathogenesis of skin damage in venous disease. J Vasc Surg 1993;17:669.
13. Killewich LA, Martin R, Cramer M, et al. Pathophysiology of venous claudication. J Vasc Surg 1984;1:507.
14. Bauer G. A roentgenological and clinical study of the sequelae of thrombosis. Acta Chir Scand 1942;86(Suppl 74):1.
15. Markel A, Manzo RA, Bergelin RO, et al. Valvular reflux after deep venous thrombosis: incidence and time of occurrence. J Vasc Surg 1992;15:377.
16. Sarin S, Scurr JH, Coleridge Smith JD. Mechanism of action of external compression on venous function. Br J Surg 1992;79:499.
17. Belcaro G, Grigg M, Vasdekis S, et al. Evaluation of the effects of elastic compression in patients with postphlebitic limbs by laser-Doppler flowmetry. Phlebologie 1988;41:797.

18. The Alexander House Group. Consensus paper on venous leg ulcer. J Dermatol Surg Oncol 1992;18:592.

19. Kikta MJ, Schuler JJ, Meyer JP, et al. A prospective, randomized trial of unna's boot versus hydroactive dressing in the treatment of venous stasis ulcers. J Vasc Surg 1988;7:478.

20. Cordts PR, Hanrahan LM, Rodriguez AA, et al. A prospective, randomized trial of unna's boot versus duoderm CGF hydroactive dressing plus compression in management of venous leg ulcers. J Vasc Surg 1992;15:480.

21. Christopoulos DG, Nicolaides AN, Szendro G, et al. Air-plethysmography and the effect of elastic compression on venous hemodynamics of the leg. J Vasc Surg 1987;5:148.

22. Strandness DE, van Bemmelen P. Quantitation of venous reflux using duplex scanning. In: Bergan JJ, Yao JST, eds. Venous disorders. Philadelphia, WB Saunders, 1991:137.

23. Raju S. New approaches to the diagnosis and treatment of venous obstruction. J Vasc Surg 1986;4:42.

24. Kistner RL. Diagnosis of chronic venous insufficiency. J Vasc Surg 1986;3:185.

25. Ackroyd JS, Lea Thomas M, Brouse NL. Deep vein reflux: an assessment by descending phlebography. Br J Surg 1986; 73:31.

26. Moore DJ, Himmel PD, Sumner DS. Distribution of venous valvular incompetence in patients with the postphlebitic syndrome. J Vasc Surg 1986;3:49.

27. Silver D, Cikrit DF. Operative management of perforator vein incompetence. In: Rutherford RB, ed. Vascular surgery, ed 3. Philadelphia, WB Saunders, 1989:1608.

28. Lalka SG. Management of chronic obstructive venous disease of the lower extremity. In: Rutherford RB, ed. Vascular surgery, ed 4, Philadelphia, WB Saunders, 1995:1862.

29. Kistner RL. Surgical repair of the incompetent femoral vein valve. Arch Surg 1975;110:1336.

30. Raju S. Venous insufficiency of the lower limb and stasis ulceration. Changing concepts and management. Ann Surg 1983;197:688.

31. Kistner RL, Sparkuhl MD. Surgery in acute and chronic venous disease. Surgery 1979;85:31.

32. Ferris EB, Kistner RL. Femoral vein reconstruction in the management of chronic venous insufficiency: a 14-year experience. Arch Surg 1982;117:1571.

33. Taheri SA, Lazar L, Elias SM, et al. Vein valve transplant. Surgery 1982;91:28.

34. Eriksson I. Reconstructive surgery for deep vein valve incompetence in the lower limb. Eur J Vasc Surg 1990;4:211.

35. Bergan JJ, Yao JS, Flinn WR, et al. Surgical treatment of venous obstruction and insufficiency. J Vasc Surg 1986;3:174.

36. O'Donnell TF. Popliteal vein valve transplantation for deep venous valvular reflux: rationale, method, and long-term clinical, hemodynamic, and anatomic results. In: Bergan JJ, Yao JST, eds. Venous disorders. Philadelphia, WB Saunders, 1991:273.

37. Psathakis N, Psathakis D. Rationale of the substitute "valve" operation by technique II in the treatment of chronic venous insufficiency. Int Angiol 1985;4:397.

SURGERY: SCIENTIFIC PRINCIPLES AND PRACTICE, Second Edition, edited by Lazar J. Greenfield, Michael W. Mulholland, Keith T. Oldham, Gerald B. Zelenock, and Keith D. Lillemoe. Lippincott–Raven Publishers, Philadelphia, © 1997.

CHAPTER 97

VENOUS THROMBOSIS AND PULMONARY THROMBOEMBOLISM

LAZAR J. GREENFIELD

Venous thrombosis involving the deep veins is a major medical problem in the United States, affecting more than 2.5 million people each year. The most serious complication of the disorder is pulmonary thromboembolism, which is estimated to cause or to be associated with 50,000 to 200,000 deaths per year. The true mortality rate is impossible to determine because of the difficulty in diagnosing pulmonary embolism with certainty in the absence of an autopsy, and because of the difficulty in determining the contribution of an embolic event in a patient with another serious disease. A recent decline in the death rate may be due to improved management of the disorder. Most patients with deep venous thrombosis (DVT) respond to treatment, but in half of these patients thrombus resolution is associated with chronic valvular dysfunction. Less commonly, residual thrombus obstructs the vein. Either event can result in the postthrombotic syndrome. This syndrome of edema, pain, occasional ulceration, and increased susceptibility to infections is a debilitating and costly disorder (see Chap. 98). Our understanding of DVT began with the description by Virchow in 1856 of the relation between venous thrombosis and pulmonary thromboembolism. He also developed the most widely accepted concept of the genesis of intravascular thrombosis.

ETIOLOGY AND PATHOGENESIS

The basic factors leading to the development of venous thrombosis as defined in the Virchow triad include changes in the vessel wall, stasis, and thrombogenic changes in the blood. Some controversy about the role of stasis remains, but in surgical patients, stasis is perhaps the most treatable of the causative factors. Other risk factors associated with DVT include the following:

- Age over 40 years
- Male sex
- Obesity
- Malignancy
- Previous history of DVT or pulmonary embolism
- Procedure
    Orthopedic
    Neurosurgical
    Urologic
    Any operation over 2 hours long
- Pregnancy
- Oral contraceptive use
- Nephrotic syndrome
- Lupus anticoagulant
- Dysfibrinogenemia
- Inherited deficiency or disorder
    Protein C deficiency or resistance
    Protein S
    Antithrombin III
    Plasminogen
- Drug abuse

When contrast medium is injected into the foot veins of supine, immobilized patients, it may remain in the soleal vein valve sinuses for as long as an hour. This is also the typical location for the formation of a nidus of thrombus. The thrombus begins with a small platelet accumulation on the vessel wall, but it is not known whether previous damage to the endothelium is necessary for thrombus formation. Stagnant hypoxemia is capable of causing endothelial injury, and stasis retains all the procoagulant factors locally leading to successive regional activation of the co-agulation cascade and further platelet and fibrin deposi-tion. As the thrombus propagates, it can become attached to the opposite wall, obstructing venous flow and produc-ing retrograde thrombosis and signs of venous stasis in the extremity (Fig. 97-1). As venous pressure increases dis-tally, edema develops subcutaneously and in the confines of the deep fascia, producing pain. More commonly, the thrombus propagates without obstructing flow and devel-ops a long floating tail that is susceptible to breaking loose from its tenuous anchor within the valvular sinus. This sequence of events is the most dangerous aspect of the disorder, because pulmonary embolism can and does oc-cur without premonitory signs or symptoms at its point of origin.

In addition to stasis, hypercoagulability (more appropri-ately called the *prothrombotic state*) must be included as a causative factor. Although preoperative coagulation tests cannot identify patients who will develop DVT, there are inherited disorders that clearly predispose patients to de-velop DVT. The most important inhibitor of activated fac-tor X is antithrombin III, a serine protease usually de-creased in plasma after surgery or trauma. Congenital deficiency of antithrombin III predisposes patients to ve-nous thrombosis and pulmonary thromboembolism. Simi-lar susceptibility occurs with deficiencies of protein C, protein S, or heparin cofactor II (see Chap. 4). Resistance to activated protein C can also occur and has recently been found to relate to an abnormal coagulation factor V that occurs as a result of a single point mutation at Arg^{506}.[1] This is believed to account for up to one third of hitherto idiopathic recurrent venous thrombosis cases. The associa-tion of thrombosis with cocaine use has also been corre-lated with an increase in plasminogen activator inhibitor-1 (PAI-1) activity.[2] Other unexplained prothrombotic states are associated with trauma, major surgical proce-dures in proportion to the length of operation, obesity, advanced age, and sepsis. The association of DVT and ma-lignancy (Trousseau syndrome) has been clarified recently with the demonstration that some tumors release tissue factor into the circulation. Tissue factor appears to be de-rived not only from neoplastic cells but also from regional infiltration of activated macrophages around the tumors. This thrombogenic effect of malignant cells is of more con-cern in patients receiving chemotherapy, another factor associated with an increased incidence of thromboembolic disease.

In addition to an increase in coagulability of the blood after trauma or operation, systemic plasma fibrinolytic ac-tivity is reduced for as long as 10 days. This is known to be a significant factor in the development of DVT, and preoperative evidence of reduced fibrinolytic activity also has been correlated with postoperative evidence of DVT. The conversion of plasminogen to plasmin is required for fibrinolysis to occur and results from the action of throm-bin and another activator in the venous endothelium. A measurable inhibitor of this process, PAI is associated with the prothrombotic state. In addition, the presence of an abnormally structured plasminogen has been associated with both arterial and venous thrombotic disorders. There is less fibrinolytic activity in the veins of the lower extremi-ties than in those of the upper extremities, increasing the predisposition of thrombi to originate in the lower extremities.

The third and final causative factor in the Virchow triad is vessel wall damage, which usually is not demonstrable in areas of thrombosis. One theory suggests that the veno-dilation that occurs under general anesthesia can disrupt the endothelial lining, exposing the thrombogenic suben-dothelial surface. Direct damage to the endothelium by

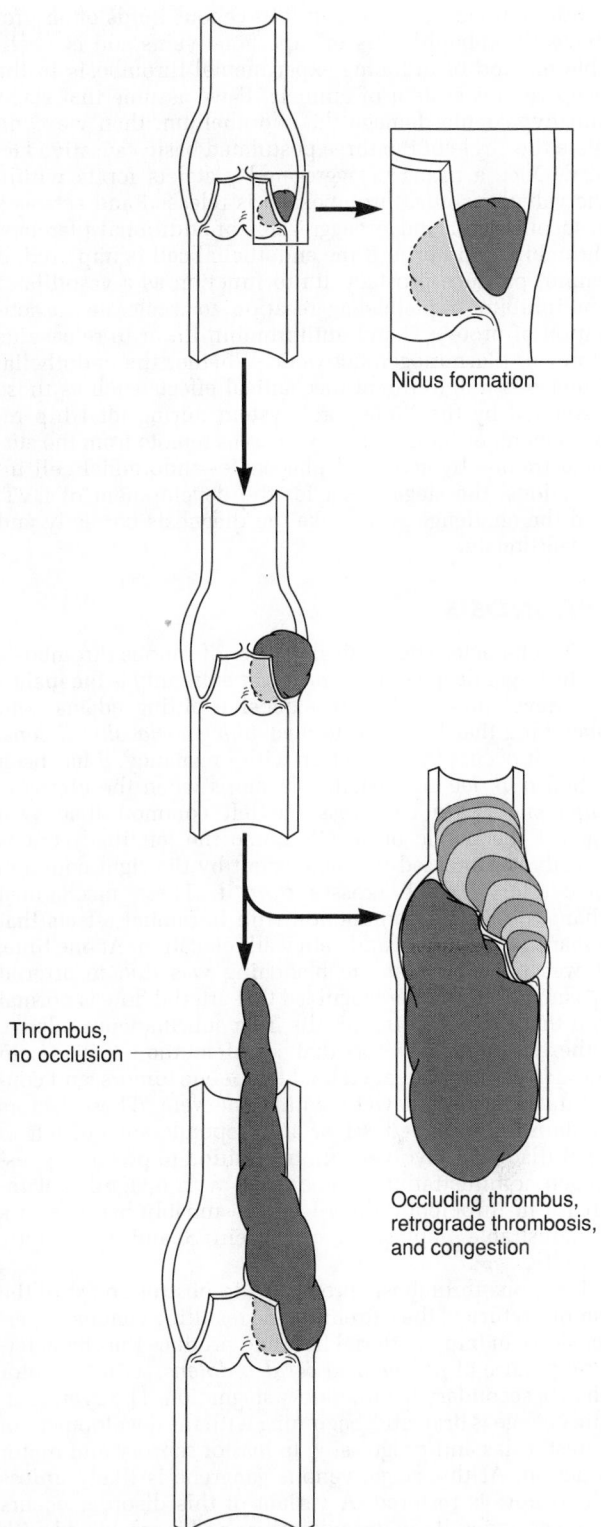

Nidus formation

Thrombus, no occlusion

Occluding thrombus, retrograde thrombosis, and congestion

Figure 97-1. The nidus of thrombus that forms in a valvular sinus can lyse or continue to propagate. If it propagates without ob-structing the lumen, it remains clinically silent and is susceptible to detachment, producing pulmonary thromboembolism. If it propagates to obstruct the lumen, it is likely to produce venous hypertension, retrograde thrombosis, and symptoms of deep ve-nous thrombosis.

acidic or toxic substances in intravenous fluids often produces thrombophlebitis in superficial veins and is a reliable method of inducing experimental thrombosis in the deep venous system of animals. If we assume that stasis and hypoxemia damage the endothelium, then we complete the circle of the three postulated basic causative factors. Once a nidus of aggregated platelets forms within the valvular sinus, thromboxane is released and acts as a vasoconstrictor and proaggregator of additional platelets, thrombin, and fibrin. If the endothelial cell is impaired, it cannot produce prostacyclin to function as a vasodilator and inhibitor of platelet aggregation, to accelerate the activation of protein C and antithrombin III, or to release its stores of plasminogen activator. Whether the endothelial damage is due to direct mechanical effects such as those sustained by the iliofemoral system during total hip replacement, or indirect injury in areas remote from the surgical trauma by activated phagocyte–endothelial cell interactions, the stage is set for the development of DVT, and the challenge is to make the diagnosis correctly and expeditiously.

DIAGNOSIS

The characteristic clinical picture of venous thrombosis of the larger deep veins of the lower extremity is the insidious development of pain, extensive pitting edema, and blanching that has been termed *phlegmasia alba dolens*. When it occurs in association with pregnancy, it has been called *milk leg* and usually develops when the uterus is large enough to compress the left common iliac vein against the pelvic brim. Of course the left iliac vein is already compressed to some extent by the right common iliac artery, which crosses over it. These mechanical changes occur in conjunction with hormonal effects that enhance coagulation and vein wall relaxation. At one time, it was believed that the blanching was due to arterial spasm, but it is now recognized that arterial flow is normal and that the blanching results from subcutaneous edema. Other mechanical factors that can affect the left iliac vein include an overdistended bladder, pelvic tumors, and congenital or acquired webs within the vein. These factors explain the observed 3:1 or 4:1 preponderance of left to right iliac vein involvement. In addition to pregnancy, estrogen administration is associated with a significant increase in thrombotic disorders, presumably because of a demonstrable depression of protein S and fibrinolytic activity.

If venous thrombosis progresses to obstruct most of the venous return of the extremity, the resulting venous hypertension can impair arterial flow and produce the characteristic picture of *phlegmasia cerulea dolens*, with the color change secondary to circulatory stagnation. The symptomatic change is dramatic, beginning with the development of paresthesias and progressing to loss of sensory and motor function. At this stage, venous gangrene is likely unless blood flow is restored. A variant of this disorder occurs more peripherally in the extremities and is associated with concurrent malignant disease and a high mortality rate.

The physical findings in DVT are determined by the level of venous obstruction, with overt signs of edema and discoloration occurring below the level of occlusion. Thus, superficial femoral vein DVT produces pain and swelling below the knee, whereas uniform swelling of the extremity reflects iliofemoral occlusion. Unfortunately, the clinical findings are nonspecific and are readily mimicked by cellulitis, trauma, and other inflammatory and mechanical disorders. One of the most overrated and unreliable signs is that of Homans, who described a limitation in passive dorsiflexion of the foot in association with calf vein DVT.

Reliance on these findings alone for the diagnosis results in an error rate that exceeds 55%. Furthermore, once a patient is diagnosed as having DVT, all subsequent complaints are likely to be treated by a course of anticoagulation, with its inherent risks. Therefore, the diagnosis must be established objectively to confirm the clinical impression.

Venography

Historically, venography was considered the gold standard for providing an accurate, anatomic diagnosis of DVT. The test consists of the injection of contrast medium into a vein in the foot. A tourniquet on the lower leg promotes filling of the deep venous system. Failure to fill the deep system with passage of contrast medium into the superficial system or demonstration of discrete filling defects represents a positive study (Fig. 97-2). A supplementary injection into the femoral veins may be required to visualize the iliofemoral system. Failure to fill the deep venous system does not provide information concerning the proximal extent of the thrombus. Disadvantages of the test are the need for transport to the radiology suite, patient discomfort, expense, and time commitment. In addition, the contrast material itself can be thrombogenic unless it is flushed out of the extremity with heparinized saline. Inadequate filling of the venous system and interobserver variations in interpretation reduce the accuracy of the study. The study is currently used to determine if there is new thrombus formation when the duplex evaluation is not diagnostic or when there is old disease.

The procedure can also be performed with the use of iso-

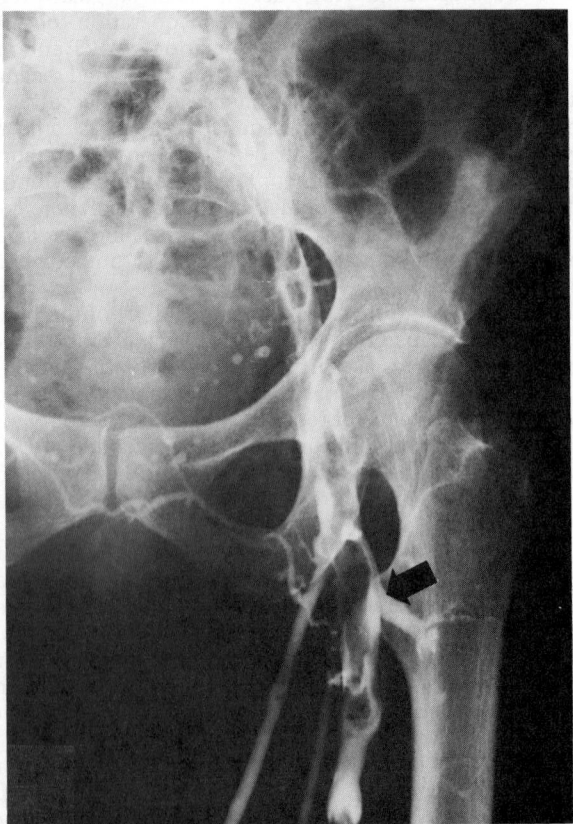

Figure 97-2. Contrast venogram showing a filling defect produced by thrombus within the femoral vein (*arrow*) and extension into the iliac veins.

tope rather than contrast injection and with use of a γ-scintillation counter to record the flow pattern of the isotope. Delayed imaging of persistent hot spots may indicate isotope incorporation at the sites of thrombus. This latter option allows a perfusion lung scan to be obtained concurrently for baseline comparison and to detect silent embolism. The reluctance to use isotopes and the observer variability in scan readings have created interest in alternative noninvasive tests, the most effective of which is the duplex examination.[3]

Duplex Study

The determination of venous flow by a combination of Doppler analysis and B-mode ultrasound has been termed a *duplex study.* Color-enhanced Doppler imaging has added to the speed and accuracy of the measurements. The advantages of duplex scanning include its bedside use, its noninvasive and nonthrombogenic nature, and its sensitivity and specificity, which are comparable to those of venography. The ease with which the test can be repeated adds a new dimension to monitoring the course of the thrombotic process.

The Doppler probe alone can be used at the bedside to detect DVT with a high degree of accuracy if the examiner is skilled and experienced (Fig. 97-3). The principle is based on the impairment of an accelerated flow signal by the presence of an intraluminal thrombus. The examination begins at the ankle with identification of the posterior tibial vein signal, which should be enhanced by compression distally and interrupted by proximal compression. The same maneuvers are repeated over the superficial femoral and popliteal veins. Failure to augment flow on compression distally or release of compression proximal to the probe suggests venous thrombi. The sensitivity of the Doppler examination exceeds 90%, but the specificity is 10% lower because of interference with venous flow by other mechanical problems, such as hematoma or a Baker cyst. A negative Doppler study is reassuring, but a positive or equivocal test should be confirmed by B-mode ultrasound or contrast venography. A negative test is not reassuring when pulmonary thromboembolism is suspected because the thrombus may have been evacuated from the extremity. The test is also less sensitive to calf vein thrombi but can be used in patients who are wearing a plaster cast.

B-mode ultrasonography allows direct visualization of venous valvular movement, accelerated blood flow in the presence of a thrombus, and even imaging of the thrombus itself, depending on its age. Fresh thrombi are not echogenic but can be identified when pressure of the probe fails to compress the walls of the vein, as would be expected normally. The affected vein is also larger than expected and can be compared with the vein in the opposite extremity. Chronic thrombi show brighter echogenicity, heterogeneity, and an irregular surface (Fig. 97-4). The duplex examination is the most appropriate initial screening test for clinically suspected DVT, and if it is negative, it will safely exclude the diagnosis of DVT in the area studied.

Impedance Plethysmography

Impedance plethysmography measures the volume response of the extremity to temporary occlusion of the venous system. The diagnosis of venous thrombosis depends on the changes in venous capacitance and on the rate of

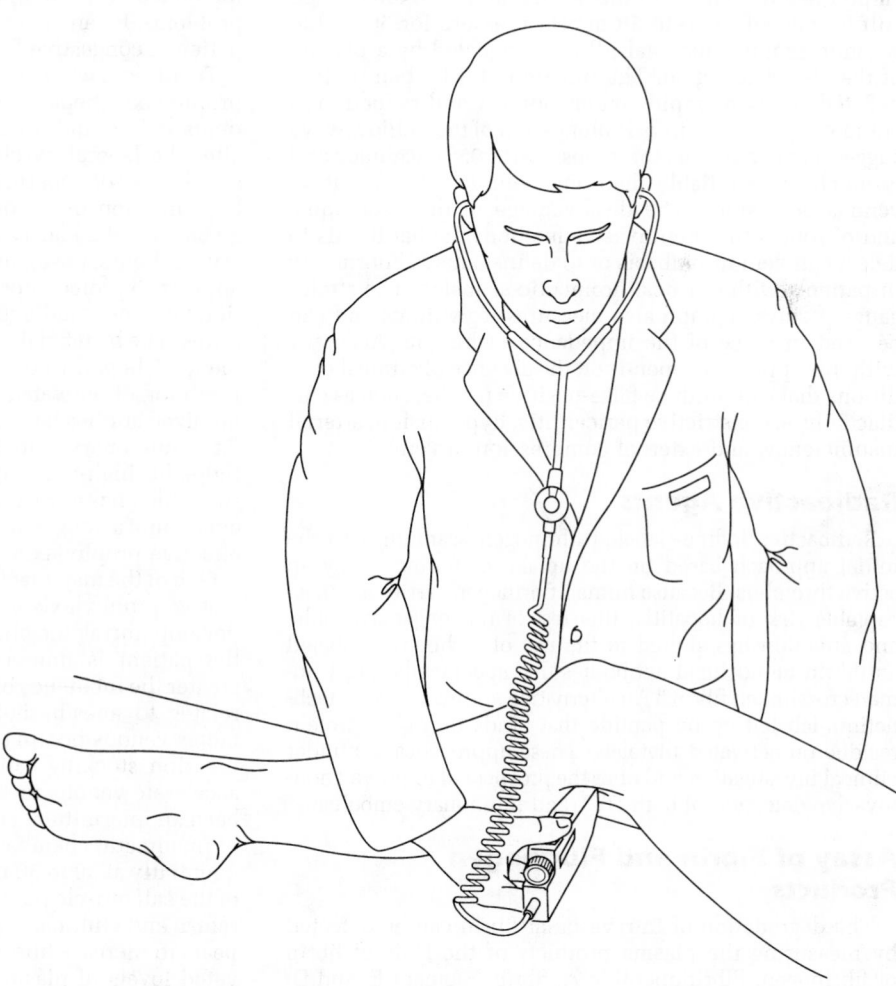

Figure 97-3. Bedside Doppler examination with the ultrasound stethoscope applied to detect flow in the popliteal vein. In the duplex study, the Doppler examination is paired with B-mode ultrasound imaging of the veins.

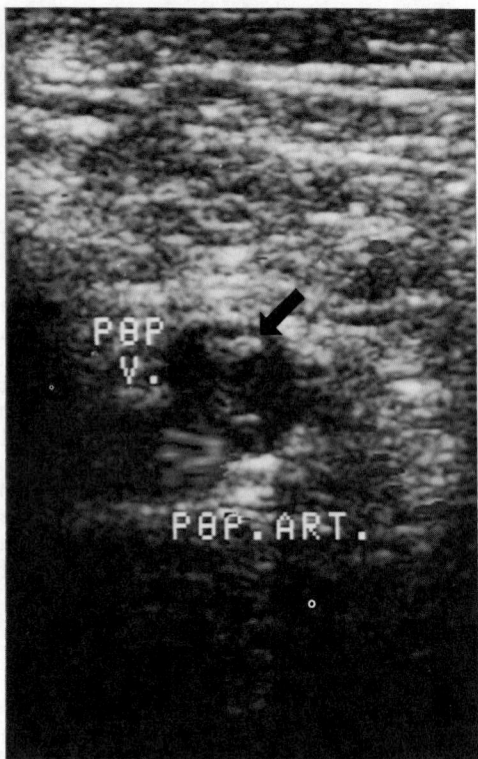

Figure 97-4. B-mode ultrasound image of the popliteal vein, showing an echogenic mature thrombus within the lumen (*arrow*).

emptying after release of the occlusion. A proximal thigh cuff is inflated to 40 to 50 mmHg pressure for 50 to 120 seconds or until maximal filling is signaled by a plateau of the electrical signal. The inflation cuff is then rapidly deflated, allowing rapid venous outflow and reduction of volume in a normal limb. Prolongation of the outflow wave suggests major venous thrombosis with 95% accuracy and is much more reliable than any voluntary technique of venous occlusion.[4] The disadvantage of this technique, and of some other noninvasive methods, is that it fails to detect calf vein thrombosis or to define a new abnormality in patients with old postthrombotic sequelae. The strain-gauge plethysmograph also measures leg volume and can be used in place of the impedance technique. Accuracy with this approach depends on the absence of clinical conditions that can produce false-positive results, such as cardiac failure, constrictive pericarditis, hypotension, arterial insufficiency, and external compression of veins.[5]

Radioactive Agents

Radioactive iodine–labeled fibrinogen scanning was the initial approach based on the uptake of fibrinogen by an active thrombus. Because human fibrinogen carries an unacceptable risk of hepatitis, this test is no longer available, and attention has shifted to the use of technetium-labeled antifibrin monoclonal antibodies that specifically target human crosslinked fibrin.[6] An alternative approach uses a technetium-labeled cyclic peptide that binds to a glycoprotein residue on activated platelets. These approaches are under clinical investigation and offer the prospect of improved noninvasive detection of both DVT and pulmonary embolism.

Assay of Fibrin and Fibrinogen Products

The degradation of intravascular fibrin can be detected by measuring the plasma products of the lysis of fibrin or fibrinogen. Fibrinopeptide A, fibrin fragment E, and D-dimer can be detected by radioimmunoassay but are not specific for acute venous thrombosis. A negative test result could have some value in ruling out the diagnosis, but the tests are difficult and require more investigation and simplification. A recent study in patients with proved pulmonary embolism showed that D-dimer values were 100% sensitive but only 16% specific, having only negative predictive value.[7] This does suggest a potential role for the simpler latex assays as a screening test.

PROPHYLAXIS

In theory, the formation of venous thrombi can be prevented either by eliminating or reducing venous stasis or by altering blood coagulability. The belief that early ambulation prevents stasis and reduces the formation of thrombi is controversial and was not supported by studies using radiolabeled fibrinogen. One explanation is that early ambulation may actually consist of having the patient walk to a chair and sit, reducing venous return from the legs.

There has been considerably more interest in the prophylactic use of anticoagulants, antiplatelet agents, and drugs such as aspirin and dipyridamole, although reports of the effectiveness of antiplatelet agents are contradictory.[8,9] Convincing data support the use of preoperative oral anticoagulation therapy with coumarin derivatives in high-risk patients. Unfortunately, this also increases the risk of surgical hemorrhage, and with the added difficulty of laboratory control of prothrombin time, the approach has not been widely accepted. The administration of dextran 40, which has many inhibitory effects on platelets and clotting factors, has been demonstrated to reduce the incidence of thrombi, but it too can produce hemorrhagic problems. It can also cause allergic reactions and, in older patients, congestive heart failure.

To minimize the problems associated with anticoagulant prophylaxis, heparin is recommended for appropriate patients before and after surgery in low doses that do not alter the laboratory clotting profile. The rationale is that small doses of heparin block the activation of the thrombin by inhibition of factor Xa. Generally, a 5000-IU dose is given subcutaneously 2 hours preoperatively and then every 12 hours postoperatively for 5 days. This treatment appears to protect most high-risk patients, with the exception of those undergoing orthopedic or urologic procedures. The beneficial effect is probably due to the enhancement of heparin cofactor (antithrombin III) as a natural inhibitor of activated factor X. Many prospectively randomized studies have shown significant protection against fatal pulmonary embolism, as well as against DVT. In orthopedic high-risk patients, low-molecular-weight heparin, which has a greater anti-Xa effect, less platelet interference, and a longer half-life, has been shown to provide effective prophylaxis.

One of the major factors limiting the efficiency of postoperative prophylaxis is that nearly half of thrombi actually develop during the operative procedure. In fact, the longer the patient is immobilized on the operating table, the greater the incidence of thrombus formation. This probably relates to anesthesia-induced venodilation, which promotes venous pooling and stasis. Although a graded compression stocking can help counteract venodilation and accelerate venous return, the most effective approach has been an intermittent compression device. Through a series of pneumatic chambers encircling the leg and inflated sequentially at 30 to 50 mmHg, the device mimics the effects of the calf muscle pump. In addition to accelerating venous return and eliminating venostasis, the massaging effect appears to increase fibrinolysis. This is demonstrated by elevated levels of plasma fibrin split products and reduced circulating plasminogen, whether pneumatic compression is applied to the upper or lower extremity. Patients who develop DVT despite this treatment have an 85% prevalence of an intrinsic defect in the fibrinolytic system that is not observed in patients who remain thrombus-free.

For the general population of surgical patients younger than age 40, the risk of DVT is low, and prophylaxis can be limited to leg elevation and early ambulation with or without graduated compression stockings. For patients older than age 40 who undergo major surgical procedures, the risk is moderate, and prophylaxis such as intermittent pneumatic compression or low-dose heparin administered subcutaneously twice daily should be considered. The patients at highest risk (age over 40 and obese, with malignant disease, history of DVT, or major trauma) need more protection. This protection might include low-dose heparin, intermittent pneumatic compression, oral anticoagulants, or dextran, with the recognition that pharmacologic therapies result in a 3% increase in hemorrhagic complications. Low-dose heparin should not be used in neurosurgical patients because of the consequences of intracranial bleeding. For these patients, external pneumatic compression is the prophylaxis of choice. In high-risk orthopedic patients the risk extends beyond the period of hospitalization; thus, prophylaxis should be extended for 1 to 2 months.

TREATMENT

Management of the patient with DVT has three objectives—to minimize the risk of pulmonary embolism, to limit further thrombosis, and to facilitate resolution of existing thrombi and avoid the postthrombotic syndrome. The patient is initially placed at bed rest, with the foot of the bed elevated 8 to 10 inches, ideally by using the Trendelenburg position to maintain a pressure gradient between the legs and the heart. Pain, swelling, and tenderness generally resolve over 4 or 5 days with anticoagulation, when ambulation with continued elastic stocking support can be permitted. Standing still and sitting should be prohibited to avoid increased venous pressure and stasis. Some clinical studies suggest that ambulatory patients with DVT can be treated on an outpatient basis.

Anticoagulation

Therapy for DVT is based on adequate systemic anticoagulation, initially with heparin and then with warfarin for prolonged protection against recurrent thrombosis. Unless there are specific contraindications, heparin should be administered in an initial dose of 100 to 150 IU/kg intravenously. Heparin is an acid mucopolysaccharide that neutralizes thrombin, inhibits thromboplastin, and reduces the platelet release reaction. It can be administered in continuous or intermittent intravenous doses and monitored by whole blood or partial thromboplastin clotting time. Bleeding complications can be minimized with no loss of effectiveness by using doses of heparin that prolong the laboratory clotting determinations by about twice as long as normal. Continuous intravenous infusion regulated by an infusion pump seems to minimize the total dose required for control and is associated with a lower incidence of complications.

The potential problems associated with heparin treatment include bleeding, thrombocytopenia, hypersensitivity, arterial thromboembolism, and osteoporosis. Bleeding is more likely to occur in elderly females, in patients treated with aspirin, or after recent surgery or trauma. It has been well demonstrated that bleeding due to the effect of heparin on platelets can occur when the results of laboratory monitoring tests are within the therapeutic range.

Arterial thromboembolism can complicate heparin administration by any route and is more common in the elderly. It tends to occur after 7 to 10 days of therapy and is associated with thrombocytopenia. This complication carries high morbidity and mortality rates and requires immediate cessation of heparin treatment. Thrombocytopenia is due to an immune reaction and is rapidly reversed when heparin is stopped, usually within 2 days. Hypersensitivity to heparin can take the form of a skin rash or, rarely, can produce anaphylaxis. Subcutaneous injections that show urticaria can become necrotic in an unusual form of sensitivity. Osteoporosis has been observed in patients on long-term heparin therapy in excess of 6 months. It is probably due to a direct effect on bone resorption and can be avoided by shorter periods of treatment and a dosage of less than 15,000 IU/d.

Oral administration of anticoagulants is begun shortly after initiation of heparin therapy because several days are usually required to bring the prothrombin time within the therapeutic range of 2.0 to 3.0 international normalized ratio, or 1.3 to 1.5 times the control value, and to provide the optimal antithrombotic effect. A maintenance dose is preferable to a larger loading dose when initiating therapy. This avoids suppression of the natural anticoagulant, protein C. The coumarin derivatives block the synthesis of several vitamin K–dependent clotting factors, and prolongation of the prothrombin time beyond the range suggested is associated with a high incidence of bleeding complications. Nonhemorrhagic side effects are uncommon but include skin necrosis, dermatitis, and a syndrome of painful erythema in areas of large amounts of subcutaneous fat. Most changes are reversible if the drug is stopped. Also, the administration of fresh frozen plasma rather than vitamin K usually restores the prothrombin time. After an episode of acute DVT, anticoagulation should be maintained for a minimum of 3 months, although some investigators favor 6 months for thrombi in the larger veins. Many drugs interact with the coumarin derivatives (eg, barbiturates); thus, a routine for regular monitoring of prothrombin time is essential after the patient leaves the hospital. Oral anticoagulants are teratogenic and should not be used during established or planned pregnancy. In the pregnant patient, heparin is the drug of choice; for long-term management, subcutaneous self-administration should be taught. This regimen allows a normal delivery and can be continued postpartum.

Fibrinolysis

There has been great interest in the use of fibrinolytic agents to activate the intrinsic plasmin system (see Chap. 4). Tissue plasminogen activator, streptokinase, and urokinase have been used clinically and have been found effective, although they are associated with a high incidence of hemorrhagic complications. Ten percent of patients treated with streptokinase suffer allergic reactions, which vary from urticaria to anaphylaxis. In addition, streptokinase offers no advantage over heparin in the treatment of recurrent venous thrombosis or when thrombosis has existed for more than 72 hours. Lytic agents are contraindicated in the postoperative or posttraumatic patient. Rarely, the fibrinolytic agent has appeared to lyse the attachment of the thrombus, allowing it to embolize. Silent pulmonary embolism also occurs and has been documented prospectively in patients treated for DVT with tissue plasminogen activator.[10] Even when thrombolysis is complete, preservation of valvular function is not ensured. Randomized trials have demonstrated no benefit of fibrinolytic treatment over conventional anticoagulation in terms of preventing the development of the postthrombotic syndrome.[11] Catheter-

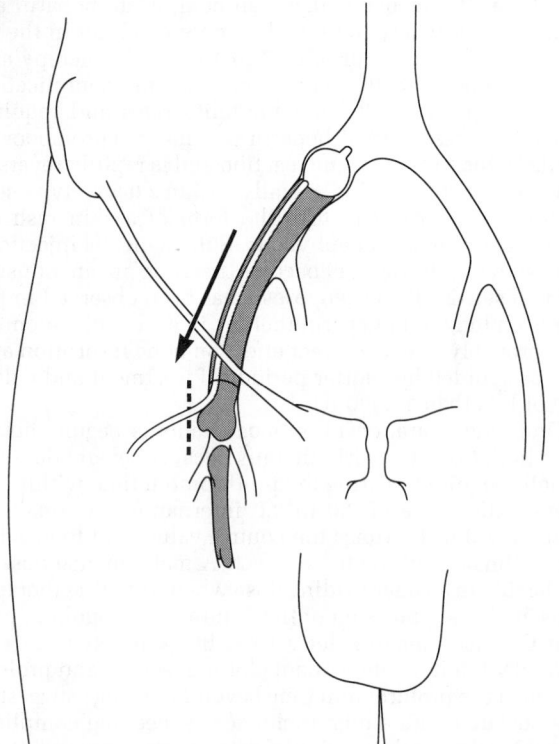

Figure 97-5. The Fogarty balloon catheter technique for venous thrombectomy allows evacuation of thrombus in the iliofemoral system proximal to the incision. Distal thrombus is evacuated by an elastic wrap that squeezes the thrombus proximally.

directed thrombolysis with direct infusion of urokinase into the thrombus may offer more effective lysis with less complications.[12]

SURGICAL APPROACHES

Operative Thrombectomy

A direct surgical approach to remove thrombi from the deep veins of the leg by way of the common femoral vein has been facilitated by the use of Fogarty venous balloon catheters for extraction of the proximal thrombus and by an elastic wrap for milking the extremity to extrude the distal thrombus (Fig. 97-5). Although the operative results are impressive, venograms obtained before discharge from the hospital show rethrombosis in many patients. Only a few reports show a lessened incidence of postthrombotic syndrome. Consequently, the procedure is customarily reserved for limb salvage in the presence of phlegmasia cerulea dolens and impending venous gangrene.

Vena Cava Interruption

Adequate anticoagulation usually is effective in managing DVT, but if recurrent pulmonary embolism occurs during anticoagulant therapy or if there is a contraindication to anticoagulation, a means of mechanical protection is necessary. Mechanical protection is also indicated as prophylaxis against recurrence of embolism for patients who have required pulmonary embolectomy and for some high-risk patients who cannot tolerate recurrence.

INDICATIONS FOR INSERTION OF A VENA CAVA FILTER

- Recurrent thromboembolism despite adequate anticoagulation

- DVT or documented thromboembolism in a patient who has a contraindication to anticoagulation
- Complication of anticoagulation that forces therapy to be discontinued
- Recurrent pulmonary embolism with associated pulmonary hypertension and cor pulmonale
- Immediately after pulmonary embolectomy for massive pulmonary embolism
- Previous device or ligation failure with recurrent embolism
- Relative indications
  Patient who has occlusion of more than half of the pulmonary vascular bed and who cannot tolerate additional embolism
  Patient with a propagating iliofemoral thrombus despite anticoagulation
  High-risk patient with a large free-floating iliofemoral thrombus on venogram

Early surgical efforts to prevent recurrence of pulmonary embolism were directed at the common femoral vein, which was ligated bilaterally. This approach had an unacceptable rate of recurrent embolism. The next approach was ligation of the inferior vena cava below the renal veins, which had the adverse effect of a sudden reduction in cardiac output. This effect, coupled with stasis sequelae and recurrent embolism through dilated collateral veins, led to efforts to compartmentalize the vena cava by means of sutures, staples, and external clips to provide filtration without occlusion.

The cone-shaped Greenfield filter was developed to maintain patency after trapping emboli and to permit continued flow to avoid stasis and facilitate lysis of the embolus (Fig. 97-6). It can be inserted percutaneously through either the jugular or femoral vein. The recurrent embolism rate with this device is 3% to 4%.[13,14] Its long-term patency rate of 95% to 98% allows it to be placed above the renal veins when necessary for embolism control (eg, when thrombus is within the renal veins or vena cava itself) or in the superior vena cava.

The complications of any filter device range from minor wound hematoma due to early resumption of anticoagulation to potentially lethal migration of some devices into the pulmonary artery. The most common complication with the stainless steel Greenfield filter was misplacement, which occurred in 7% of cases prior to the use of a guidewire. When the filter is misplaced below the diaphragm, the patient has inadequate protection, but the location (re-

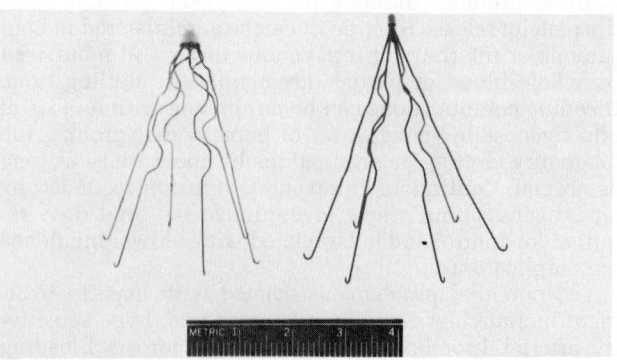

Figure 97-6. The standard stainless-steel Greenfield filter (*left*) is a cone-shaped device designed for operative insertion through the jugular or femoral vein into the inferior vena cava. A titanium modification of the design (*right*) allows percutaneous insertion using a smaller carrier system.

nal or iliac vein) poses no circulatory problem because the filter can be expected to remain patent.

Recurrent embolism after filter placement occurs in 2% to 4% of cases and may be due to a source of thrombus outside of the filtered flow, such as the pelvic veins, by way of the ovarian vein, the upper extremities, or the right atrium. Recurrent embolism is an indication for inferior venacavography to evaluate the filter for possible entrapped and propagating proximal thrombus. The latter is a rare finding and can be managed either by thrombolytic therapy if the amount of thrombus is small or by placement of a second filter in the suprarenal vena cava.

Sepsis is not a contraindication to filter insertion. Secondary infection of captured thrombus within a Greenfield filter has been produced experimentally, but it was possible to sterilize the stainless steel filter and thrombus with a 2-week course of antibiotic therapy. The capture of a large embolus within a filter can suddenly occlude the vena cava and cause a precipitous fall in blood pressure. In a patient with known prior pulmonary embolism, this event can be mistaken for recurrent pulmonary embolism, with disastrous results if vasopressor therapy is initiated rather than fluid volume replacement. The basic distinction between functional hypovolemia of caval occlusion and right ventricular overload from recurrent pulmonary embolism can be made at the bedside by the measurement of central venous pressure and arterial oxygen tension. The response to volume resuscitation for the patient with sudden vena caval occlusion should be dramatic.

Percutaneous Filter Insertion

The advantages of the percutaneous approach with dilators over use of a guidewire and a sheath have prompted the development of modified stainless steel and titanium Greenfield filters that can be inserted either through a 14F sheath or operatively (see Fig. 97-6). Clinical studies have confirmed that these devices remain effective and safe for long-term protection against pulmonary thromboembolism.

PULMONARY THROMBOEMBOLISM

The most serious complication of DVT is pulmonary thromboembolism, which is estimated to cause more than 50,000 deaths per year in the United States. It is difficult to know the exact incidence of the disorder, because the clinical diagnosis is inherently inaccurate and often confused with myocardial infarction, pneumothorax, sepsis, or pneumonia. It is estimated that 5 of every 1000 adults undergoing major surgery die from massive pulmonary embolism. This is of particular concern to surgeons whose patients are prone to develop DVT in the immediate postoperative period.

Just as with DVT, our understanding of the pathophysiology of pulmonary embolism dates back to Virchow, who first recognized the association between the two events. It also became obvious in early reports by pathologists that pulmonary embolism could be well tolerated by some patients who then died of other causes. In fact, the full spectrum of the disorder ranges from asymptomatic minor embolism to sudden death from massive embolism.

Diagnosis

Clinical Presentation

The signs and symptoms of an embolic episode depend primarily on the quantity of embolus involved and, to a lesser extent, on the cardiopulmonary status of the patient. In the classic presentation, the patient suddenly develops chest pain, cough, dyspnea, tachypnea, and marked anxiety. Although hemoptysis has traditionally been associated with pulmonary embolism, it is an uncommon sign. When present, it usually occurs late in the course of the disease and represents pulmonary infarction. Objectively, the patient with major embolism usually shows tachycardia, an increased pulmonary second sound, cyanosis, prominent jugular veins, and varying degrees of collapse. Less commonly, there can be wheezing, a pleural friction rub, splinting of the chest wall, rales, low-grade fever, ventricular gallop, and wide splitting of the pulmonic second sound. The prevalence of these findings is shown in Table 97-1.

Because the differential diagnosis includes esophageal perforation, pneumonia, septic shock, and myocardial infarction, all of which are life-threatening, it is imperative that an orderly approach be formulated to establish the correct diagnosis. Laboratory studies in general are not helpful in the differential diagnosis, although a white blood cell count of less than $15,000/\mu L$ can help rule out pneumonitis when a pulmonary infiltrate is present. The following examinations are particularly useful in the evaluation of suspected major pulmonary embolism.

Electrocardiography

The most common electrocardiographic findings associated with pulmonary embolism are nonspecific ST-segment and T-wave changes (66% of patients). More specific signs of right ventricular overload such as the often quoted S_1-Q_3-T_3 pattern are seldom seen. In patients with proved pulmonary embolism, the observed electrocardiographic changes do not correlate with increased right ventricular systolic pressure or end diastolic diameter.[15] Consequently, the primary value of the electrocardiogram is to exclude the presence of a myocardial infarction. Unfortunately, the finding of a myocardial infarction does not exclude the diagnosis of pulmonary embolism, and in some cases a lung scan or pulmonary angiogram may be required to clarify the problem.

Chest Radiography

Although the chest radiograph can suggest the diagnosis of pulmonary embolism because of central vascular enlargement, asymmetry of the vascular markings with segmental or lobar ischemia (Westermark sign), or pleural effusion, these signs are nonspecific. The chest radiograph

Table 97-1. CLINICAL MANIFESTATIONS OF MAJOR PULMONARY EMBOLISM

Clinical Manifestations	Prevalence (%)
SYMPTOMS	
Dyspnea	80
Apprehension	60
Pleural pain	60
Cough	50
Hemoptysis	27
Syncope	22
SIGNS	
Tachypnea	88
Tachycardia	63
Accentuated P_2	60
Rales	51
S_3 or S_4	47
Pleural rub	17

(Data from Urokinase Pulmonary Embolism Trial. A national cooperative study. Circulation 1973;14[Suppl II]:86)

then serves to exclude other diagnostic possibilities, such as pneumonia, pneumothorax, esophageal perforation, or congestive heart failure. It is crucial in the interpretation of a lung scan because radiographic density or evidence of chronic lung or cardiac disease makes a perfusion defect less likely to represent pulmonary embolism.

Arterial Blood Gases

Frequent measurement of blood gases and pH in all critically ill patients can provide important support for the diagnosis of pulmonary embolism. Hypoxemia with PaO_2 of less than 60 mmHg is found in most patients. Contributing factors are shunting by overperfusion of a nonembolized lung, a diffusion impairment, and a widened alveolar–arterial oxygen gradient due to reduced cardiac output. Careful clinical studies have shown the latter to be the most important contributing factor. The reduction in $PaCO_2$ that follows major embolism is the most discriminating finding, because hypoxemia is present in several disorders likely to be misdiagnosed as massive embolism (eg, septic shock). If concurrent hypoxemia and hypocarbia are not present, the diagnosis of major embolism in the severely ill patient is unlikely, and an alternative diagnosis should be sought.

Central Venous Pressure

In the patient with systemic hypotension, central venous pressure measurement can supply valuable information. In addition, the venous catheter provides access for administration of drugs and fluids. A low central venous pressure virtually excludes pulmonary embolism as the primary cause of the hypotension, because massive embolism almost always is accompanied by right ventricular overload and elevated right atrial pressures. Elevated right ventricular filling pressures can be transient, however, as hemodynamic accommodation occurs. In subacute or chronic embolism, the central venous pressure can be normal.

Lung Scan

The availability and widespread use of lung photoscanning have led to an overemphasis on this test and a tendency to overdiagnose pulmonary embolism. In a nonhypotensive patient with a normal chest radiograph, the lung scan is a valuable screening test that has increasing validity as the size of the perfusion defect approaches lobar distribution. Smaller peripheral perfusion defects are much more difficult to interpret, because pneumonitis, atelectasis, or other ventilation abnormalities alter pulmonary perfusion. A normal lung scan, on the other hand, usually excludes the diagnosis of pulmonary embolism. Adding a ventilation scan for combined ventilation–perfusion imaging increases the accuracy of the diagnosis of thromboembolism, provided that there are at least two moderate size areas or one large area of ventilation–perfusion mismatch and no history of embolism. This high-probability reading is found in few cases and overlooks 59% of patients who show thromboembolism on angiogram.[16] The assumption that the underperfused regions of the lung after embolism remain normally ventilated, producing the mismatch in the scans, is clouded by the known physiologic effect of bronchoconstriction produced by embolism. When the additional variable of wide variance in scan interpretation among observers is considered, the diagnosis is much more reliable when based on arteriography.

Pulmonary Vascular Imaging

Selective pulmonary arteriography is the most accurate method of confirming the presence, size, and distribution of pulmonary emboli. The procedure is invasive, requiring passage of a catheter into the pulmonary artery for injection of a bolus of contrast medium. A rapid film changer produces a series of radiographs that outline areas of decreased perfusion and usually show filling defects or the rounded trailing edge of impacted emboli (Fig. 97-7). Straight cutoffs of the smaller pulmonary arteries are more difficult to interpret, particularly if there is associated chronic lung disease that tends to obliterate pulmonary vessels. The procedure can be performed with low risk, although pulmonary hypertensive and cardiac patients are at highest risk for this type of study, which usually carries a 0.3% to 0.5% mortality rate. Avoiding the injection of contrast medium into the main pulmonary artery minimizes the complications and mortality rates. Additional useful information is obtained before contrast injection by measurement of pulmonary arterial pressures. A normal pulmonary angiogram excludes the diagnosis of pulmonary embolism. Dynamic contrast-enhanced magnetic resonance angiography has been introduced and does not require breath-holding or cardiac gating. It provides multiplanar, rapid, dynamic visualization of the pulmonary arteries and is an accurate method for detecting pulmonary embolism in the proximal portions of the pulmonary arteries. Unfortunately, it does not detect peripheral thromboembolism. Similarly, transesophageal echocardiographic visualization of massive pulmonary embolism has been reported. Because this can be performed at the bedside under emergency circumstances, it offers a new approach to making or excluding the diagnosis, although more experience will be required to determine its appropriate role.

Pathophysiology

Although DVT precedes pulmonary embolism, less than 33% of patients with documented pulmonary embolism show clinical signs of venous thrombosis. Despite this, it is estimated that 85% to 90% of all pulmonary emboli originate from the veins of the lower extremity, and the remainder arise from the right side of the heart or other veins. In addition, the emboli from a recent thrombus tend to be multiple, fragmenting either in the right side of the heart or during impaction into the pulmonary vascular bed. Older thrombi contain laminated fibrin layers that make them more solid and more difficult to lyse.

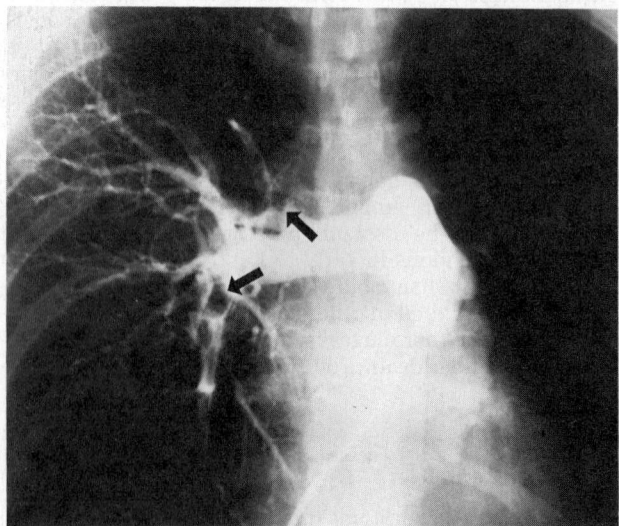

Figure 97-7. Pulmonary arteriogram demonstrating no flow to the left lung and filling defects in the right lower and upper lobar pulmonary arteries (*arrows*).

Once the embolus has lodged and interrupted pulmonary blood flow, the ratio of regional ventilation to perfusion increases. The lung responds by bronchoconstriction to reduce mismatched ventilation. This response is mediated by a local reduction in CO_2 output, because it can be prevented by ventilation with an increased concentration of CO_2. Some experimental studies also suggest a generalized neural reflex vasoconstriction, but even if this occurs in humans, it is not likely to be as significant a factor in survival as the mechanical effect of major vascular occlusion. Similarly, the effects of vasoactive humoral agents can be demonstrated in animals. There is evidence that serotonin, which is elaborated from platelets adherent to the embolus, also contributes to the bronchoconstriction. The ability of heparin to inhibit the release of serotonin further justifies the early use of this drug. Other vasoactive agents such as bradykinin, histamine, and prostaglandins can play a role in humans, but the net effect is a reduction in size of peripheral airways, reduced lung volume, and reduced static pulmonary compliance.

The hypoxemia that characterizes major embolism is thought to be due to the increased alveolar–arterial oxygen gradient reducing the mixed venous Po_2, although the findings in some patients resemble true arteriovenous shunting. Such shunting is anatomically possible if there is a patent foramen ovale that opens in the presence of elevated right atrial pressures. Such an opening can also allow passage of a venous embolus into the systemic circulation; it then is termed *paradoxical embolism*. Although there may be some improvement in Pao_2 after supplemental oxygen is administered, the effects usually are minimal. The return of pulmonary blood flow effected by embolectomy restores respiratory gas exchange, but the ischemia can result in loss of capillary integrity, causing interstitial pulmonary edema or overt pulmonary hemorrhage.

Pulmonary infarction as a consequence of embolism is rare and is associated clinically with problems of poor systemic perfusion, such as shock and congestive heart failure. In these patients, the symptoms include pleuritic chest pain, dyspnea, cough, and hemoptysis. The signs include fever, tachycardia, splinting, and occasionally a friction rub. There is usually prominent leukocytosis, an elevated lactic dehydrogenase level, and hyperbilirubinemia. A wedge-shaped density usually is seen on chest radiography.

The pulmonary vascular and cardiac effects of embolism are a more direct consequence of the degree of filling of the pulmonary vascular bed. Occlusion of over 30% of the vascular tree is required to elevate mean pulmonary artery pressure, and usually over 50% occlusion is required to reduce systemic arterial pressure. The degree of pulmonary hypertension produced is proportional to the extent of angiographic vascular occlusion, but in a previously normal patient the limit of pressure elevation has a mean of about 40 mmHg.

The fate of pulmonary embolism in patients is not easy to predict, although a great deal of experimental work in animals has been reported. Injection of autologous thrombi into the pulmonary circulation of dogs is followed by rapid recovery of pulmonary function and objective evidence of lysis over a period of weeks. Activation of plasminogen to plasmin, which is found in high concentration in the pulmonary circulation, promotes this fibrinolytic effect. Unfortunately, the resolution of aged thrombi proceeds more slowly and is hampered further by impaction of the embolus and isolation from pulmonary blood flow. Consequently, resolution after massive embolism in patients is unpredictable and often incomplete. It is not unusual to find residual fibrin strands or webs in the pulmonary arteries at autopsy as remnants of prior embolism.

Management of acute, massive pulmonary thromboembolism depends on an accurate diagnosis that documents the presence and location of intravascular thrombus. This usually requires angiography, which has the added advantage of allowing blood pressure measurement in the pulmonary circulation. Because of the inherent nonspecificity of the perfusion lung scan, scans are most useful as a screening test to exclude the diagnosis in patients with minor degrees of embolism. In suspected massive embolism, the patient should receive intravenous heparin sodium (150 to 200 IU/kg) and be taken directly to the angiographic suite for selective pulmonary angiography. In addition to insertion of the angiographic catheter, usually through the femoral vein, a radial artery cannula is inserted for monitoring arterial blood gases. Anesthesia standby is requested if the patient requires intubation and ventilatory control. If the patient's condition is too unstable for angiography and there are other objective signs of venous thrombosis or embolism, such as a previous scan showing large or multiple defects, it is reasonable to proceed to the operating room where the diagnosis can be confirmed under fluoroscopy by injection of contrast material through an embolectomy catheter.

Classification and Management

Anticoagulation

With use of the hemodynamic variables mentioned above, embolism can be classified into four grades of severity, providing a useful guide to therapy and prognosis (Table 97-2). Minor embolism can usually be managed by anticoagulants alone with a satisfactory outcome. Heparin is selected for initial treatment in a dose designed to prolong the partial thromboplastin time to at least twice that of normal. A dose of about 150 IU/kg provides adequate protection against further attachment of thrombus and platelets to the embolus. Heparin should be administered intravenously by pump-regulated continuous infusion. Some authors have advocated higher doses of heparin to prolong the activated clotting time to 150 to 190 seconds with no increase in bleeding complications but improved control of recurrent embolism. Heparin control of recurrent embolism is imperfect, and recurrence is reported in 10% to 16% of patients with a bleeding complication rate of 20% to 27%. Nonetheless, heparin remains the initial treatment of choice. Most clinicians also begin oral anticoagulation therapy at the same time to allow the drugs several days to overlap as prothrombin time is extended into the therapeutic range.

Thrombolytic Therapy

Thrombolytic therapy has been advocated for the treatment of both DVT and pulmonary embolism. Several plasminogen activators, including streptokinase, urokinase, and tissue plasminogen activator, are available and can be effective, as documented in several large clinical trials. The drugs are administered by intravenous infusion after a loading dose, and beneficial effects in thromboembolism usually can be seen in 12 to 24 hours. Laboratory tests that confirm the presence of a lytic state following streptokinase or urokinase administration have not proved useful in predicting the therapeutic response to these drugs or in preventing hemorrhagic complications. Unfortunately, there are hemorrhagic side effects judged to be significant in 30% of the patients treated with both drugs, half of whom require transfusion. The use of streptokinase for pulmonary embolism has been associated with bleeding complications as well as with allergic reactions, fever, and adult respiratory distress syndrome. Also, after the first

Table 97-2. STRATIFICATION OF PULMONARY THROMBOEMBOLISM

Category	Signs and Symptoms	Gases	PA Occlusion (%)	Hemodynamics
Minor	Anxiety Hyperventilation	$Pao_2 < 80$ mmHg $Paco_2 < 35$ mHg	20–30	Tachycardia
Major	Dyspnea Collapse	$Pao_2 < 65$ mmHg $Paco_2 < 30$ mmHg	30–50	CVP elevated; PA pressure > 20 mmHg; responds to resuscitation
Massive	Dyspnea Shock	$Pao_2 < 50$ mmHg $Paco_2 < 30$ mmHg	>50	CVP elevated; PA pressure > 25 mmHg; requires pressors, inotropes
Chronic	Dyspnea Syncope	$Pao_2 < 70$ mmHg $Paco_2$ 30–40 mmHg	>50	CVP elevated; PA pressure > 40 mmHg; fixed low cardiac output

CVP, central venous pressure; PA, pulmonary artery.

2 weeks of a multicenter trial, there was no significant difference between urokinase and heparin treatment in the recurrence rate of embolism or in the mortality rate.

More recently, recombinant human tissue-type plasminogen activator (rtPA) has become available as a fibrin-specific thrombolytic agent. In a series of 36 patients with documented pulmonary embolism by angiography, peripheral infusion of 50 mg over 2 hours improved the angiographic score by 21%. An additional 40 mg over 6 hours improved the average score by 49%. Because patients with hypotension were excluded, the initial pulmonary arterial pressure was only moderately elevated to 22 mmHg and declined to 17 mmHg after infusion. Significant groin hematomas were seen in 5 patients, hematuria in 2 patients, and periodontal oozing in 3 patients. Two patients had major hemorrhage requiring operative treatment, and 1 patient required relief of pericardial tamponade 8 days after coronary artery bypass. One patient had recurrent embolism and died, for an overall mortality rate of 3% and a morbidity rate of 33% in patients with submassive embolism. There was hope that this agent would be specific for thrombus fibrin, but plasma fibrinogen declined 55% in patients who received two-chain rtPA and 34% in those who received one-chain rtPA.

The advantage of thrombolytic therapy may well be to improve the ultimate resolution of major thromboembolism. Follow-up studies in patients treated with urokinase or streptokinase have shown a restoration of pulmonary–capillary blood volume and diffusing capacity after 2 weeks that is better than that in patients treated with heparin and anticoagulants alone. The reason for the continued improvement that was seen at 1 year is not clear, but it was believed to be related either to more complete early resolution of the embolic condition, allowing more effective natural lytic processes, or to more complete clearance of peripheral venous thrombi, preventing silent recurrent embolism. Therefore, the patient who is not in shock and who has no clear contraindication to the use of thrombolytic therapy would probably benefit from its use.

Pulmonary Hypertension

Pulmonary emboli can accumulate gradually over a prolonged period if they do not undergo lysis and obliteration of the pulmonary vascular bed. The clinical picture in this case is one of chronic cor pulmonale, because significant pulmonary hypertension results from changes in the pulmonary vascular bed (see Table 97-2). The presentation can be subtle with only dyspnea or syncope on exertion, but there is a loud P_2 and right-sided strain on the electrocardiogram. The sequence can also occur unaccompanied by significant respiratory symptoms, and this may explain the etiology in some of the patients considered to have primary pulmonary hypertension. When the diagnosis is made, life expectancy is usually limited to 2 years, but the patient may benefit from a vena caval filter to prevent further embolism even if the disorder is primary pulmonary hypertension. The rationale is that right ventricular failure ultimately develops, predisposing the patient to pulmonary embolism that is lethal even if small. When acute cardiopulmonary decompensation occurs in these patients after embolism, they are not good candidates for embolectomy because of fixation of the older thrombi to the pulmonary arterial wall. They should be classified separately as chronic and managed by long-term anticoagulation therapy. Some cases can be considered for delayed thrombectomy or heart–lung transplantation.

Pulmonary Embolectomy

For those patients who sustain massive embolism producing systemic hypotension, management must be a rapidly coordinated effort, because survival may be only a matter of minutes. The initial approach to thromboembolism in patients who have either transient collapse or persistent systemic hypotension should include full heparinization and administration of inotropic drugs, if necessary, to support the circulation while the diagnosis is confirmed angiographically. Either dopamine or isoproterenol can be used for circulatory support initially, the latter because of its bronchodilator, vasodilator, and positive inotropic cardiac effects, although it can provoke arrhythmias. For the patient with thromboembolism who responds to heparin sodium and does not require vasopressors to maintain systemic blood pressure or urine output (major pulmonary embolism), careful monitoring is essential to determine whether anticoagulation alone can control the disorder. Often the additional protection of a vena caval filter is indicated in the high-risk patient who cannot tolerate another pulmonary embolic event.

The high mortality associated with the Trendelenburg procedure of thoracotomy for pulmonary embolectomy prompted the use of extracorporeal circulation to bypass the impacted pulmonary circulation. Experience in persistently hypotensive patients (massive pulmonary embolism) shows that partial bypass support under local anesthesia using the femoral artery and vein can provide initial support to allow general anesthesia (Fig. 97-8). Once the sternotomy is accomplished, the partial bypass can be converted to total bypass by insertion of a superior vena caval catheter. The pulmonary emboli can then be removed through a pulmonary arteriotomy (Fig. 97-9).

Although open pulmonary embolectomy is effective, it still has a mortality rate in excess of 40%. The most serious complication is uncontrollable pulmonary parenchymal hemorrhage, which can follow restoration of pulmonary perfusion. Consequently, open pulmonary embolectomy is most appropriate for patients who require closed cardiac

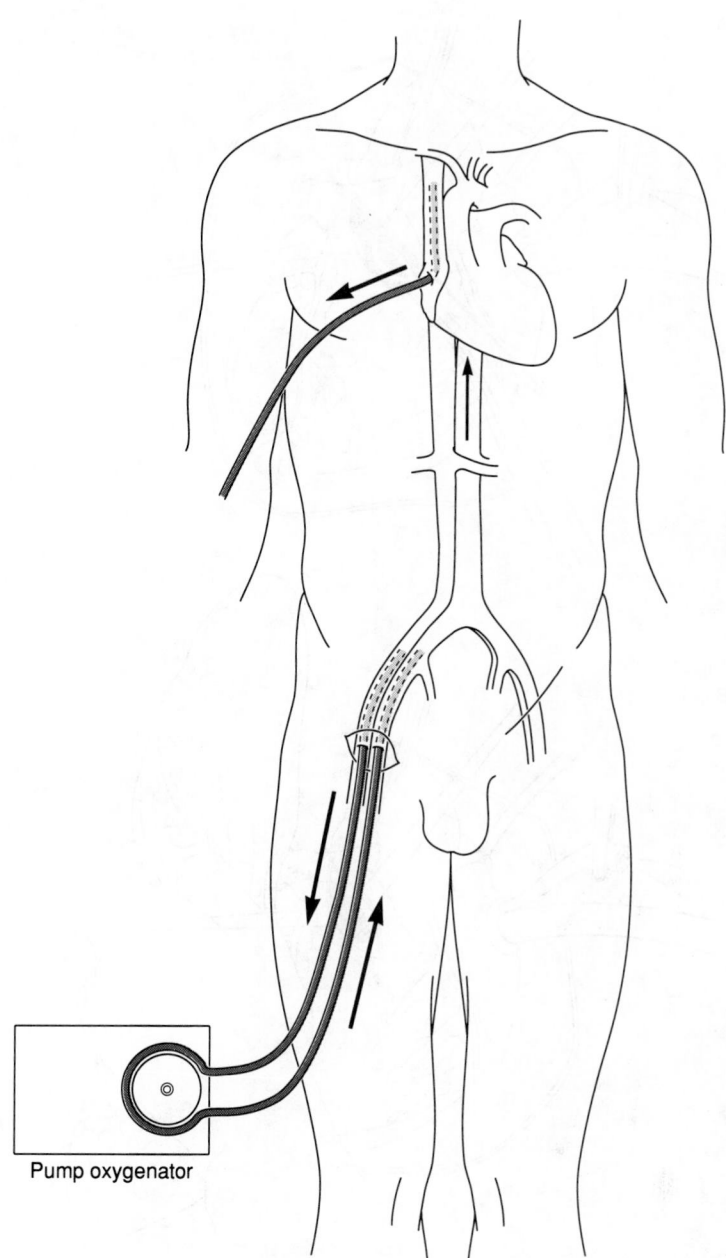

Figure 97-8. For a deteriorating patient with massive pulmonary embolism and systemic hypotension, circulatory support can be achieved by cannulation of the femoral artery and vein under local anesthesia for partial cardiopulmonary bypass. The patient can then tolerate general anesthesia and sternotomy, which allows insertion of a superior vena caval cannula for total bypass and pulmonary embolectomy (see Fig. 97-9).

Pump oxygenator

massage to maintain blood pressure or for patients in whom the catheter embolectomy procedure fails to remove thrombi.

Transvenous Catheter Embolectomy

An alternative approach to open embolectomy on cardiopulmonary bypass has been developed for transvenous removal of pulmonary emboli under local anesthesia. A cup device attached to a steerable catheter is inserted in either the jugular or the femoral vein, and the cup is positioned under fluoroscopy adjacent to the embolus seen on arteriography (Fig. 97-10). The position is verified by injection of contrast medium through the catheter. Syringe suction is then applied to aspirate the embolus into the cup, where it is held by suction vacuum as the catheter and captured embolus are withdrawn (Fig. 97-11). Clinical experience in a series of 46 patients demonstrated that the best results were obtained for patients with major or massive embolism (31

of 37 or 84% successful), and the worst results were found in patients with chronic pulmonary embolism (5 of 9 or 56% successful).[17] Emboli could not be removed when they had been impacted for more than 72 hours or if the patient suffered cardiac arrest at the time of angiography, in which case open embolectomy was required. Placement of a Greenfield vena caval filter after removal of sufficient emboli to produce near normal hemodynamics protected the patients from recurrent embolism.

Chronic Pulmonary Embolism and Pulmonary Hypertension

Recurrent thromboembolism can lead to progressive obliteration of the pulmonary vascular bed if the thrombi fail to undergo lysis. The resultant pulmonary hypertension produces exertional dyspnea and signs of right heart strain with cor pulmonale. With further progression of right heart overload, tricuspid insufficiency can develop.

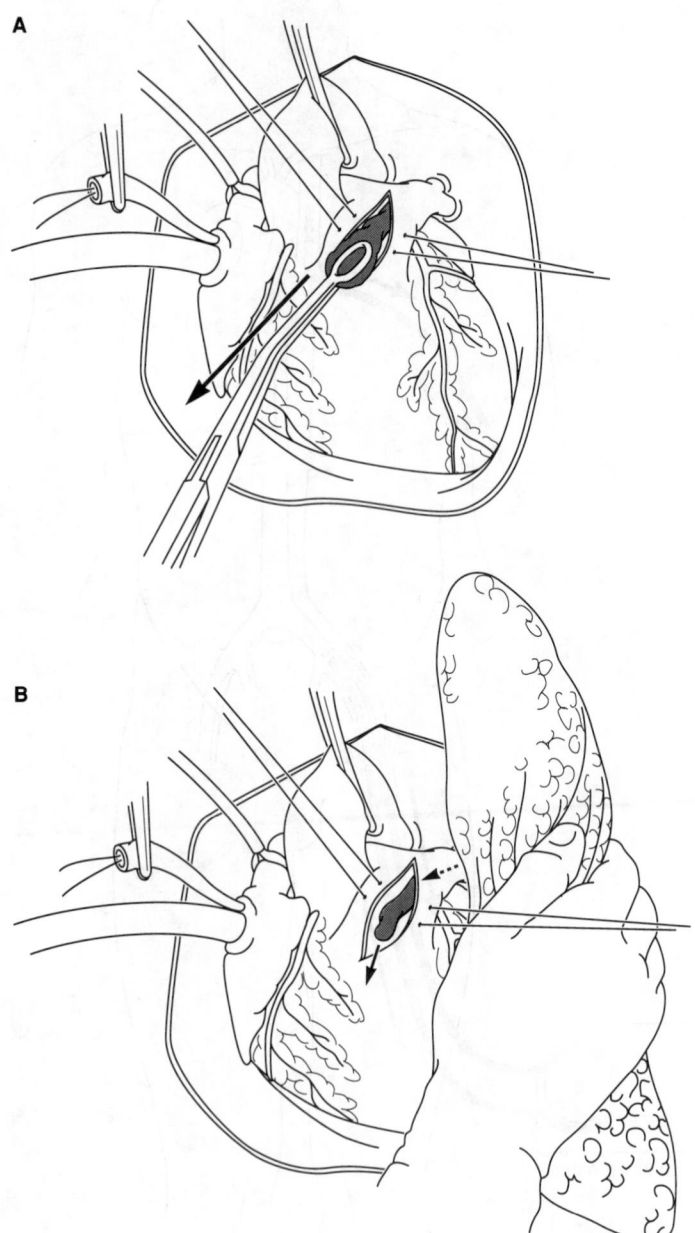

Figure 97-9. (*A*) A patient with massive pulmonary embolism on total cardiopulmonary bypass (see Fig. 97-8) can undergo pulmonary embolectomy through the opened main pulmonary artery. (*B*) More peripheral emboli can be retrieved by balloon embolectomy and compression of the lung.

This disorder can be difficult to distinguish from primary pulmonary hypertension, although the latter is more likely to be found in women younger than 20 years without a history of DVT.

Open thrombectomy for chronic pulmonary artery occlusion was first performed in 1958 and remains a means of improving pulmonary blood flow. Unfortunately, for the procedure to be feasible, the occlusion must involve the proximal portion of the pulmonary arterial tree, and the distal bed must be patent. The physiologic basis for continued distal patency after proximal occlusion is bronchial arterial collateral flow. The historically high mortality rate with this has been reduced by the use of deep hypothermia with circulatory arrest, but it remains around 9%.[18] For most patients with severe pulmonary hypertension, the outlook is poor unless they receive maximal protection from recurrent embolism, which in our experience requires both anticoagulation therapy and vena caval filter placement.

OTHER TYPES OF VENOUS THROMBOSIS

Thrombophlebitis

The term *thrombophlebitis* is typically applied to a disorder of the superficial veins that is characterized by a usually aseptic local inflammatory process. The cause in the upper limb is usually intravenous acidic fluid infusion or prolonged cannulation. In the lower extremities, it is frequently associated with varicose veins and can coexist with DVT. The association of additional venous thrombosis with the injection of contrast material can be minimized by washout of the contrast material with heparinized saline.

Thrombophlebitis Migrans

Thrombophlebitis migrans, a condition of recurrent episodes of superficial thrombophlebitis, has been associated with visceral malignancy, systemic collagen vascular dis-

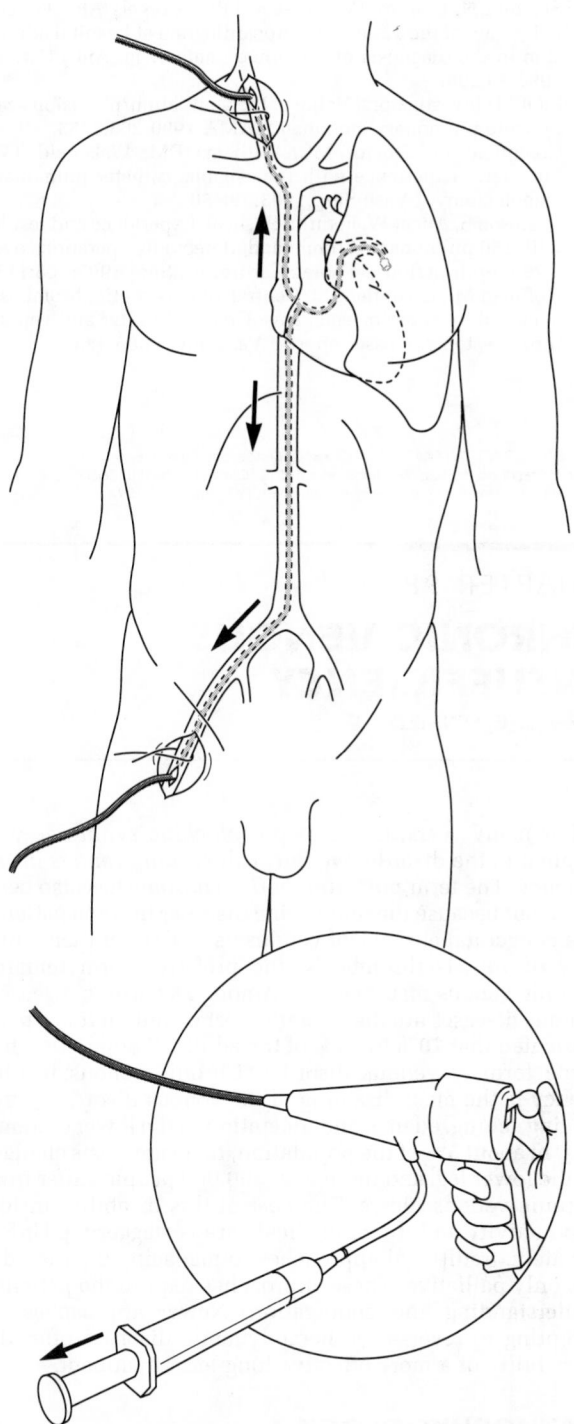

son (effort thrombosis), presumably as a result of injury at the thoracic outlet. If the patient is seen late, there is usually a satisfactory response to elevation and anticoagulation, although some venous insufficiency and discomfort with exercise can persist. Pulmonary thromboembolism can occur from these thrombi, with a prevalence of 12% reported in two series. We have inserted a Greenfield filter in the superior vena cava in an inverted position, although this is rarely necessary.[19]

Increased use of the axillary and subclavian veins for diagnostic and therapeutic procedures has resulted in a higher incidence of traumatic and foreign body thrombosis. Often these thrombi are asymptomatic because of gradual onset, short-segment involvement, or only partial occlusion. Thrombolytic therapy can be of value and should be considered with any acute subclavian vein thrombosis occurring within 3 or 4 days of onset of symptoms. If the thrombus lyses, a contrast venogram should be obtained to outline any anatomic site of compression that could be treated surgically. Direct operative thrombectomy with first rib or medial clavicular excision can be used and should be considered for younger patients and manual laborers. Thrombectomy should always be performed in conjunction with the creation of an ipsilateral arteriovenous fistula for angioaccess if there is proximal venous thrombosis. If the fistula is made without recognizing the proximal occlusion, the extremity can be endangered by massive edema. Operative correction is still possible without loss of the fistula, even if a jugular venous bypass is necessary, because the fistula assists in maintaining patency of the repair or bypass.

Abdominal Vein Thrombosis

Thrombosis of the inferior vena cava can result from tumor invasion or propagating thrombus from the iliac veins. Most often, it results from ligation, plication, or insertion of occluding caval devices. Thrombosis of the renal vein is most likely to be associated with the nephrotic syndrome. It can be a source of thromboembolism and has been treated successfully by suprarenal placement of the Greenfield filter.

Figure 97-10. Access for catheter pulmonary embolectomy can be obtained under local anesthesia from either the right jugular vein or the femoral vein. The steerable cup-catheter is then positioned under fluoroscopy in proximity to the embolus. Syringe suction is applied to capture the embolus within the cup, which is then withdrawn.

ease, and blood dyscrasias. Involvement of the deep veins and the visceral veins has also been described.

Subclavian Vein Thrombosis

Subclavian vein thrombosis is most likely to be secondary to an indwelling catheter and can occur in children. It can also occur as a primary event in a young, athletic per-

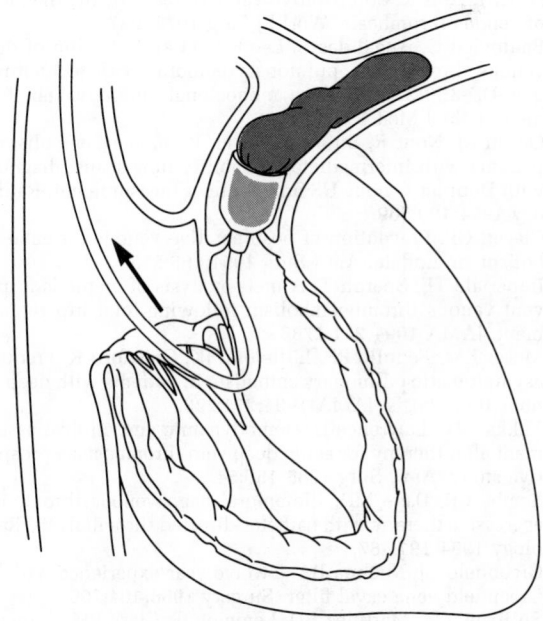

Figure 97-11. Once the embolus is captured within the embolectomy catheter cup (see Fig. 97-10), the catheter is withdrawn while syringe suction is maintained to hold on to the embolus.

Portal vein thrombosis can occur in the neonate, usually secondary to propagating septic thrombophlebitis of the umbilical vein. Collateral development leads to the creation of esophageal varices. Thrombosis of the portal, hepatic, splenic, or superior mesenteric vein in an adult can occur spontaneously, but usually it is associated with hepatic cirrhosis. Thrombosis of mesenteric or omental veins can simulate an acute abdomen but usually results in prolonged ileus rather than intestinal infarction.

Hepatic vein thrombosis (Budd-Chiari syndrome) usually produces massive hepatomegaly, ascites, and liver failure. It can be associated with a congenital web, endophlebitis, or polycythemia vera. Although some success has been reported with use of a direct approach to the congenital webs, the usual treatment is a side-to-side portacaval shunt to allow decompression of the liver or liver transplantation. The development of pelvic sepsis after abortion, tubal infection, or puerperal sepsis can lead to septic thrombophlebitis of the pelvic veins and septic thromboembolism. Ovarian vein and caval ligation have been the traditional treatment, but the emphasis should be on drainage or excision of the abscesses and appropriate antibiotic therapy. The Greenfield filter can also been used for septic thrombosis because the filter is inert stainless steel or titanium and does not lead to the development of an intraluminal abscess, which could occur after the traditional approach of ligation of the vena cava.

REFERENCES

1. Voorberg J, Roelse J, Koopman R, et al. Association of idiopathic venous thromboembolism with single point-mutation at Arg[506] of factor V. Lancet 1994;343:1535.
2. Moliterno DJ, Lange RA, Gerard RD, Willard JE, Lackner C, Hillis LD. Influence of intranasal cocaine on plasma constituents associated with endogenous thrombosis and thrombolysis. Am J Med 1994;96:492.
3. Flanagan LD, Sullivan ED, Cranley JJ. Venous imaging of the extremities using real-time B-mode ultrasound. In: Bergan J, Yao JST, eds. Surgery of the veins. New York, Grune & Stratton, 1985:89.
4. Wheeler HB, Mullick SC. Detection of venous obstruction in the leg by measurement of electrical impedance. Ann NY Acad Sci 1970;170:804.
5. Hirsh J, Hull R. Comparative value of tests for the diagnosis of venous thrombosis. World J Surg 1978;2:27.
6. Bautovich G, Angelides S, Lee F-T, et al. Detection of deep venous thrombi and pulmonary embolus with technetium-99m-DD-3B6/22 anti-fibrin monoclonal antibody Fab' fragment. J Nucl Med 1994;35:195.
7. Quinn RJ, Nour R, Butler SP, et al. Pulmonary embolism in patients with intermediate probability lung scans: diagnosis with Doppler venous US and D-dimer measurement. Radiology 1994;190:509.
8. Clagett GP. Prevention of postoperative venous thromboembolism: an update. Am J Surg 1994;168:515.
9. Imperiale TF, Speroff T. A meta-analysis of methods to prevent venous thromboembolism following total hip replacement. JAMA 1994;271:1780.
10. Moser KM, Fedullo PF, LittleJohn JK, Crawford R. Frequent asymptomatic pulmonary embolism in patients with deep venous thrombosis. JAMA 1994;271:223.
11. Kakkar VV, Lawrence D. Hemodynamic and clinical assessment after therapy for acute deep vein thrombosis: a prospective study. Am J Surg 1985;150:54.
12. Semba CP, Dake MD. Iliofemoral deep venous thrombosis: aggressive therapy with catheter-directed thrombolysis. Radiology 1994;191:487.
13. Greenfield LJ, Michna BA. Twelve year experience with the Greenfield vena caval filter. Surgery 1988;104:706.
14. Sullivan TM, Martinez BD, Lemmon G, Clark PM, Schwartz RA, Bondy B. Clinical experience with the Greenfield filter in 193 patients and description of a new technique for operative insertion. J Am Coll Surg 1994;178:117.
15. Sreeram N, Cheriex EC, Smeets JLRM, Gorgels AP, Wellens HJJ. Value of the 12-lead electrocardiogram at hospital admission in the diagnosis of pulmonary embolism. Am J Cardiol 1994;73:298.
16. PIOPED Investigators. Value of the ventilation/perfusion scan in acute pulmonary embolism. JAMA 1990;263:2753.
17. Greenfield LJ, Proctor MC, Williams DM, Wakefield TW. Long-term experience with transvenous catheter pulmonary embolectomy. J Vasc Surg 1993;18:450.
18. Jamieson S, Auger W, Fedullo PF, et al. Experience and results with 150 pulmonary thromboendarterectomy operations over a 29-month period. J Thorac Cardiovasc Surg 1993;106:116.
19. Hoffman MJ, Greenfield LJ. Central venous septic thrombosis managed by superior vena cava Greenfield filter and venous thrombectomy: a case report. J Vasc Surg 1986;4:606.

SURGERY: SCIENTIFIC PRINCIPLES AND PRACTICE, Second Edition, edited by Lazar J. Greenfield, Michael W. Mulholland, Keith T. Oldham, Gerald B. Zelenock, and Keith D. Lillemoe. Lippincott–Raven Publishers, Philadelphia, © 1997.

CHAPTER 98

CHRONIC VENOUS INSUFFICIENCY

LAZAR J. GREENFIELD

For many years, the term *postphlebitic syndrome* was applied to the disorder we now call *chronic venous insufficiency*. The term *postthrombotic syndrome* has also been used, but because the underlying disorder in some patients is a congenital absence of venous valves rather than a history of venous thrombosis, the preferred term remains chronic venous insufficiency. Among 28 chronic diseases, venous diseases are the seventh most common. It has been estimated that 10% to 35% of the adult US population has some form of venous disorder. Chronic venous insufficiency is the most disabling of the venous disorders, producing aching, edema, and ulceration in the lower extremities. In about 5% of the population, there are stasis changes in the lower leg, and more than 500,000 people suffer from chronic venous ulcers. The cost of this disability in lost productivity and direct medical care is staggering. Unfortunately, traditional approaches to managing the disorder are only palliative. These approaches require the patient's understanding and cooperation. Newer approaches attempting to reverse the hemodynamic disorder offer the possibility of a more effective long-term treatment.

PATHOPHYSIOLOGY

In the upright human, large hydrostatic pressure loads oppose the return of venous blood from the lower extremities. The delicate-appearing venous valves are actually strong and support the hydrostatic pressure, facilitating unidirectional venous return in response to the calf muscle pump. The bicuspid valves also direct flow from the superficial veins into the deep venous system by way of the perforating veins. Valvular incompetence in the superficial veins produces varicose veins, and venous malformations can cause skin changes and venous insufficiency (see Chap. 96).

In the absence of normal venous valvular function, chronic venous insufficiency is produced by reflux of blood into the superficial system through incompetent perforating veins. This reflux is compounded by muscle contraction, which pushes blood distally within the incompetent deep system. As a result, ambulation fails to produce the normal physiologic decrease in venous pressure, instead causing ambulatory venous hypertension. Recorded distal venous pressures typically show a drop of less than 20%, whereas the normal decrease is about 70%. After termination of exercise in the normal patient, more than 20 to 30 seconds are required for venous pressure to return to the resting level by distal refill. In chronic venous insufficiency, proximal reflux produces a rapid elevation of pressure after cessation of exercise. Absence of valvular function is usually due to destruction from venous thrombosis with or without proximal venous obstruction, but it may also be due to congenital absence of the valves.

Chronic venous hypertension results in increased hydrostatic pressure at the capillary level, causing transudation of fluid and protein and diapedesis of erythrocytes. Hemosiderin from these erythrocytes is responsible for the typical brownish skin pigmentation. Excessive melanocyte activity secondary to chronic inflammation may also contribute to the discoloration. The chronic dermatitis that develops is termed *venous eczema* and produces the pruritis that is often seen initially by dermatologists. The histologic picture shows increased capillary proliferation, fat necrosis, and fibrosis in skin and subcutaneous tissue, together known as *lipodermatosclerosis*.[1] The condition may even progress to calcification, which can be seen on radiographs. The capillaries also show perivascular layering with fibrin and fibrinogen, a result of increased extravasation in the presence of venous hypertension. Fibrinolysis in the area is impaired because of decreased levels of fi-

brinolytic activator and the presence of a fibrinolytic inhibitor. The latter is a primary systemic defect found commonly in patients with a history of deep-vein thrombosis. The pericapillary fibrin layer may act as a barrier to oxygen transport to the cells, resulting in slow tissue death and replacement by scar tissue (Fig. 98-1). At the least, it impairs wound healing. Since there is some evidence that the pericapillary rings do not interfere with oxygen transport, a more recent and popular concept is that leukocyte trapping with stasis, obstruction to flow, extravasation of toxic products, and anoxia produce inflammation and tissue necrosis.[2] Evidence for this has been seen by fluorescence video microscopy and intravital microscopy.

Although the lymphatic vessels in the area of lipodermatosclerosis may be abnormally permeable, the total lymphatic return from an extremity with venous hypertension is two or three times normal. The lymphatic contribution to the disorder is secondary to the changes in skin and subcutaneous tissues. The typical venous ulcer occurs on the medial leg above the ankle, where venous pressure is highest in proximity to a perforating vein. The skin around the ulcer is indurated, and there may be adjacent cellulitis (Fig. 98-2).

If venous obstruction persists after an episode of deep-vein thrombosis or for any other mechanical reason, persistent lower extremity edema may be complicated further by disabling pain with exercise. This venous claudication is produced by elevated interstitial pressures in the muscle and fascial compartments of the extremity from the hyperemia of exercise. Extensive subcutaneous venous collaterals can be seen over the leg and trunk and demonstrated by

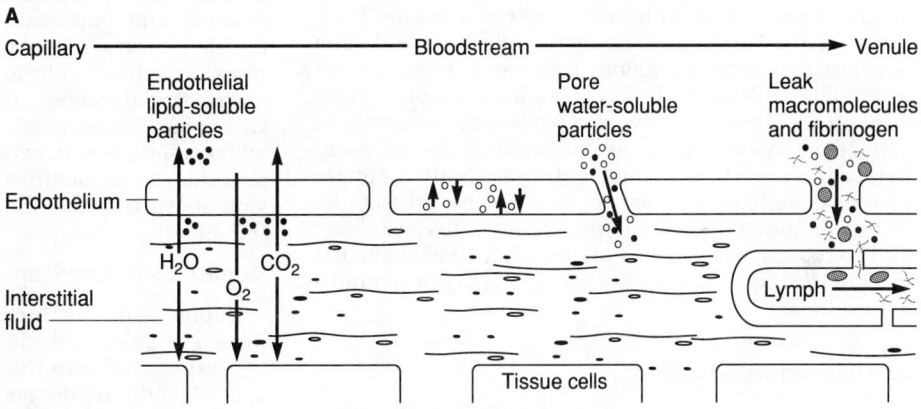

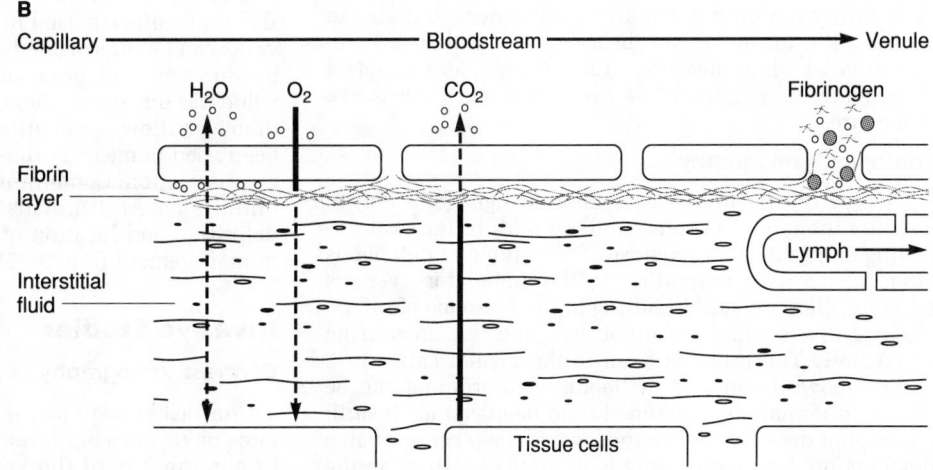

Figure 98-1. Schematic representation of normal lymphatic function (*A*) and the changes that occur after lymph stasis and the accumulation of a fibrin layer (*B*). The passage of oxygen and nutrients to the cells is impaired by the fibrin, leading to cellular anoxia and further replacement of skin and subcutaneous tissue by scar tissue (lipodermatosclerosis). (After Browse NL, Burnard KG, Thomas ML, eds. Diseases of the veins. London, Edward Arnold, 1988)

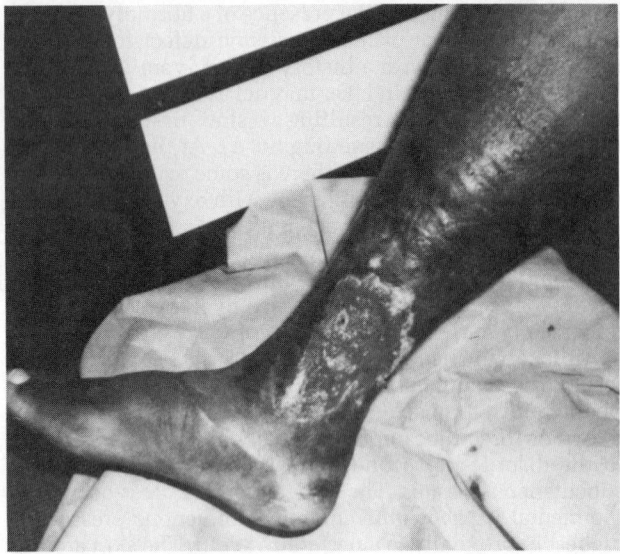

Figure 98-2. Chronic venous stasis ulcer seen in the typical location on the distal medial leg. The skin around the ulcer is usually indurated and pigmented.

venography. In evaluating this disorder, segmental arterial pressure must be measured to ensure there is no arterial insufficiency.

DIAGNOSIS

The patient with suspected chronic venous insufficiency must be examined in both the upright and supine positions, and the location of edema should be noted. The discrimination between venous stasis and lymph edema can often be made on the basis of whether the foot and toes are involved, since such involvement is a characteristic of lymphedema. Venous stasis edema begins at the ankle and extends to involve the lower leg and occasionally the thigh. Superficial varicosities may or may not be present depending on the competence of perforating veins (see Chap. 96). The typical venous ulcer occurs on the posteromedial aspect of the lower leg but may occur laterally or in multiple locations.

Noninvasive Studies

In many cases of chronic venous insufficiency, the diagnosis can be made on the basis of patient history and examination. The value of noninvasive venous studies lies in their ability not only to confirm the diagnosis but also to measure the extent of the disorder, to establish a baseline from which to measure future changes, and to detect those patients who might be candidates for a corrective procedure.

Photoplethysmography

Photoplethysmography uses infrared light (805 nm) to measure the rate of venous capillary refill in the skin following emptying after exercise. The volume of cutaneous blood changes in proportion to the ambulatory venous pressure, showing rapid refilling in the presence of reflux. Photoplethysmography cannot be used for measuring blood flow. The probe is fixed to the medial calf 4 to 5 inches above the medial malleolus. A tourniquet can be used to differentiate superficial from deep venous insufficiency, but does not isolate the level of deep venous valve dysfunction. The patient sits with the feet resting on the floor and then performs heel raises without weight bearing. The refilling time is measured in seconds or to 50% maximum (Fig. 98-3).

Outflow Plethysmography

Venous volume of the lower extremity can be measured by impedance, strain-gauge, or air plethysmography. Application of a proximal tourniquet with compression above resting venous pressure produces an increase in leg volume as the leg becomes congested. With release of the tourniquet, there should be a rapid return to the baseline value achieving 50% reduction within 2 seconds. Any obstruction to venous return, whether intraluminal or extraluminal, retards outflow and prolongs emptying time. Therefore, a fracture hematoma or a pelvic tumor can produce a false-positive test, although the reported accuracy is about 90% for femoral vein thrombosis.

Air plethysmography is the most valuable test for venous function since it measures calf venous volume changes in response to active and passive maneuvers in the supine and erect positions. The venous filling index measures the volume of blood refluxing into the calf as the best index of overall valvular incompetence. The calf ejection fraction and the residual volume fraction measure calf muscle pump effectiveness and residual volume in the calf respectively after 10 tiptoe exercises. Both APG and duplex examinations are evolving as quantitative documentation of the extent of chronic venous insufficiency.

Doppler Study

The bidirectional Doppler probe is useful for detecting directional flow in accessible veins, such as the saphenous, femoral, and popliteal.[3] Accelerated flow produced by transient obstruction above the level insonated or by compression below confirms patency and the absence of an obstructing thrombus. Reversal of flow occurs when the valves are incompetent. False-positive results can occur when collateral veins are insonated. Incompetent perforator veins can be identified using a tourniquet and compression above it to test the competency of the deep system (Fig. 98-4).

Duplex Colorflow Scan

Duplex scans combine B-mode ultrasound imaging and pulsed Doppler analysis of flow. It has become the screening test of choice in the diagnosis of DVT (see Chaps. 96 and 97) and provides accurate assessment of both superficial and deep venous systems in chronic venous insufficiency. The addition of color flow provides imaging of forward or reverse flow in real time. When rapid inflation–deflation cuffs are used in the standing position, the major veins can be interrogated and extent of reflux documented by duration and peak and by mean reverse blood flow velocities that occur after cuff deflation. Knowledge of vein diameter allows a quantitative estimation of reflux that has been used to measure the effectiveness of venous valvular reconstruction. Combining the duplex evaluation with the findings on APG provides a physiologic approach to the definition and location of the venous disorder as a guide to management (Fig. 98-5).

Invasive Studies

Contrast Venography

Contrast venography is useful in determining the presence or absence of normal or abnormal valves, the extent of abnormality of the veins, and the estimated amount

Venous Reflux

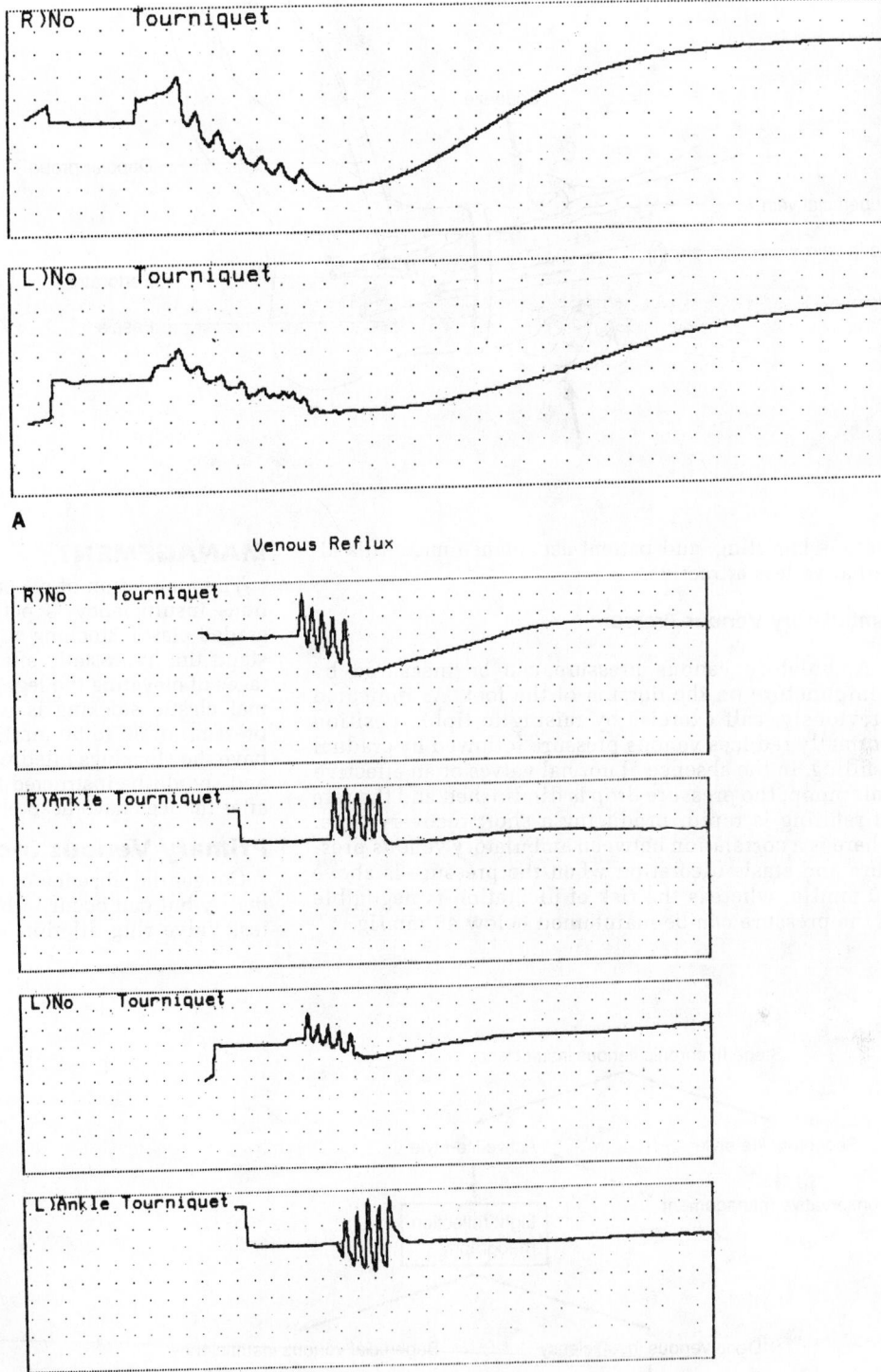

Figure 98-3. (*A*) Photoplethysmographic (PPG) tracing showing decreases in cutaneous blood volume with calf muscle exercise followed by gradual recovery over 18 seconds as a normal response in both lower extremities in the absence of a tourniquet. (*B*) PPG tracing showing deep venous insufficiency in both lower extremities as reflected by minimal decreases in cutaneous blood volume with exercise and rapid refilling time (10 seconds) unimproved by the addition of a tourniquet.

of venous reflux. Reflux is induced by table tilting or by injecting contrast medium in an iliac vein while the patient does the Valsalva maneuver. Reflux can then be graded according to how far distally the contrast is seen, with the most severe grade recorded when contrast is seen below the level of the knee (Fig. 98-6). In addition to descending venography, an ascending study should be performed by injecting contrast medium in the foot to demonstrate the status of veins below the knee for evidence of thrombus, recanalized veins, and incompetent perforating veins. Contrast medium can be thrombogenic unless it is washed out of the extremity by a flush of heparinized saline. Newer nonionic contrast materials of lower osmolality are less thrombogenic. Radioisotopes also can be used for imaging the venous system and for plethysmography, but problems with expense,

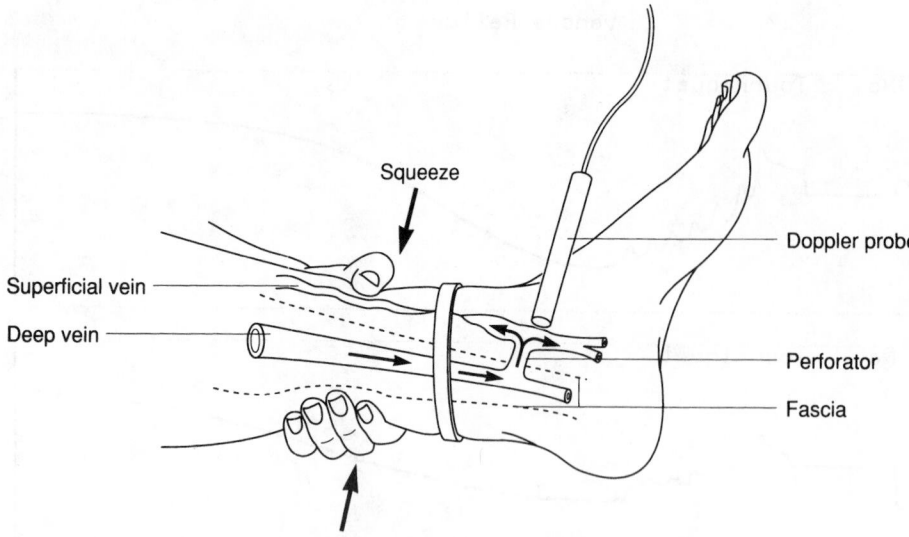

Figure 98-4. The bidirectional Doppler probe detects incompetent perforating veins when superficial venous flow is arrested by the tourniquet and deep venous pressure is increased by squeezing the leg above the tourniquet. Reflux also depends on incompetence of the deep vein valves.

isotope handling, and patient acceptance make this alternative less attractive.

Ambulatory Venous Pressure

Ambulatory venous pressure can be measured by venipuncture on the dorsum of the foot. As indicated previously, calf exercise by raising to tiptoe position normally reduces venous pressure followed by gradual refilling. In the absence of normal valves or an effective calf pump, the pressure drop is diminished and the rate of refilling is rapid, producing a short recovery time. There is a correlation between ambulatory venous pressure and stasis ulceration when the pressure is above 60 mmHg, whereas the risk of ulceration is negligible if the pressure can be maintained below 45 mmHg.

MANAGEMENT

The foundation of effective management of chronic venous insufficiency is patient education combined with graded elastic stocking support. The patient must understand the hydrostatic effects of standing and the advantages of elevating the legs above the heart level. The optimal elastic stocking is calf length with a compression pressure of 30 to 50 mmHg at the ankle. Patients should have the stockings fitted when the legs are not edematous and should be instructed to put them on daily on arising after the legs have been elevated overnight.

Primary Venous Incompetence

Congenital absence of venous valves is a rare abnormality but can occur in both upper and lower extremities. Valve ring dilation with valvular incompetence is

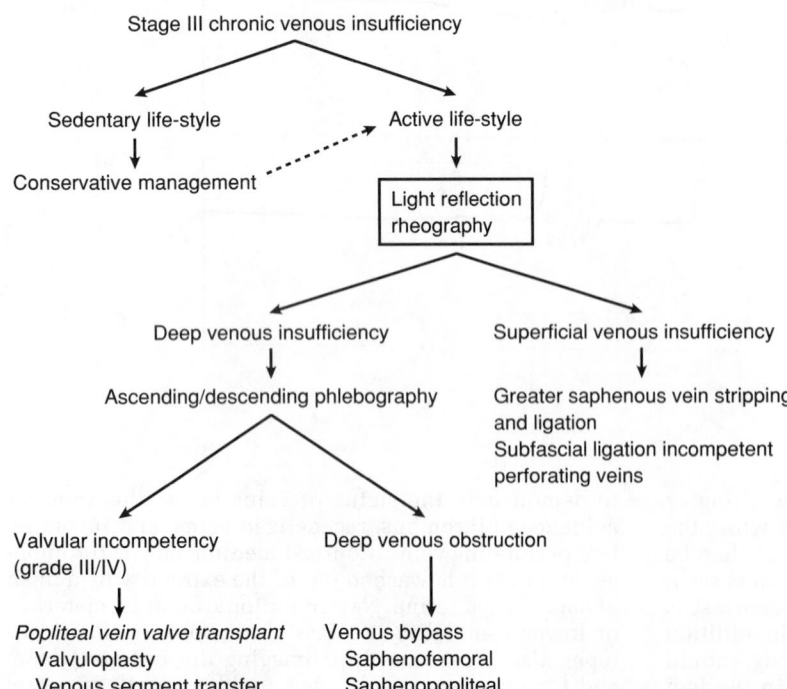

Figure 98-5. Algorithm for the management of chronic venous insufficiency using air plethysmography and duplex scanning. (After Ernst CB, Stanley JC. Current therapy in vascular surgery, ed 3. St Louis, CV Mosby, 1995:918)

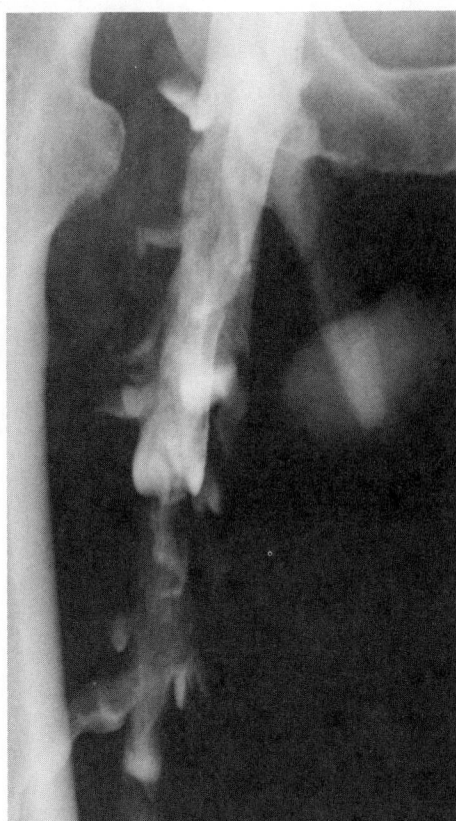

Figure 98-6. Contrast venography can be used to measure venous reflux by proximal injection while the patient is tilted upright or is increasing venous pressure by the Valsalva maneuver. Contrast medium was injected above the inguinal ligament in this case, which shows reflux into both superficial and profunda veins, indicating valvular incompetence. The most severe grade of reflux occurs when contrast is seen below the knee.

more common in superficial than deep veins. It can occur during overdistention of the vein (eg, distal to an arteriovenous fistula or during pregnancy). Changes in the valves to produce thickening or fixation usually are post-thrombotic, but these changes have been described in the absence of a history of venous thrombosis and may be due to other unknown abnormal events. Primary vein valve prolapse due to the floppy valve described by Kistner appears to result from a congenital abnormality that leads to lengthening of the free edge of the valve cusp.[4] This allows the valve to evert, rendering it incompetent. In this situation, it may be possible to repair the valve by a plication technique that restores normal length and support for the valve leaflet (Fig. 98-7). The benefit of this procedure has been difficult to evaluate because it has usually been combined with ligation of perforating veins and excision of varicosities, but good to excellent results have been reported in 80% of cases.

In the absence of suitable valves, there are two other approaches that have been used for patients with chronic venous insufficiency whose disability is refractory to conservative management. These are vein segment transfer or transposition and autologous vein valve transplantation. In the transposition procedure, a vein segment in the extremity with normal valvular function is identified and becomes the recipient of flow from the incompetent vein by implanting it distal to the competent valve. For example, an incompetent superficial femoral vein could be divided and reattached to a competent

greater saphenous vein to take advantage of the valvular support in the saphenous system (Fig. 98-8). Combinations of vein transpositions can be used with or without associated valvular repairs (Fig. 98-9). The lack of an available adjacent competent vein becomes the indication for considering vein valve transplantation.[5] In this approach, a short segment of brachial vein with a competent valve is removed from the arm and interposed into the femoral system distally or at the upper end of the popliteal vein. This procedure is still considered investigational and longer follow-up is needed to determine its appropriate role. Cryopreserved and living vein allografts have been studied experimentally but usually

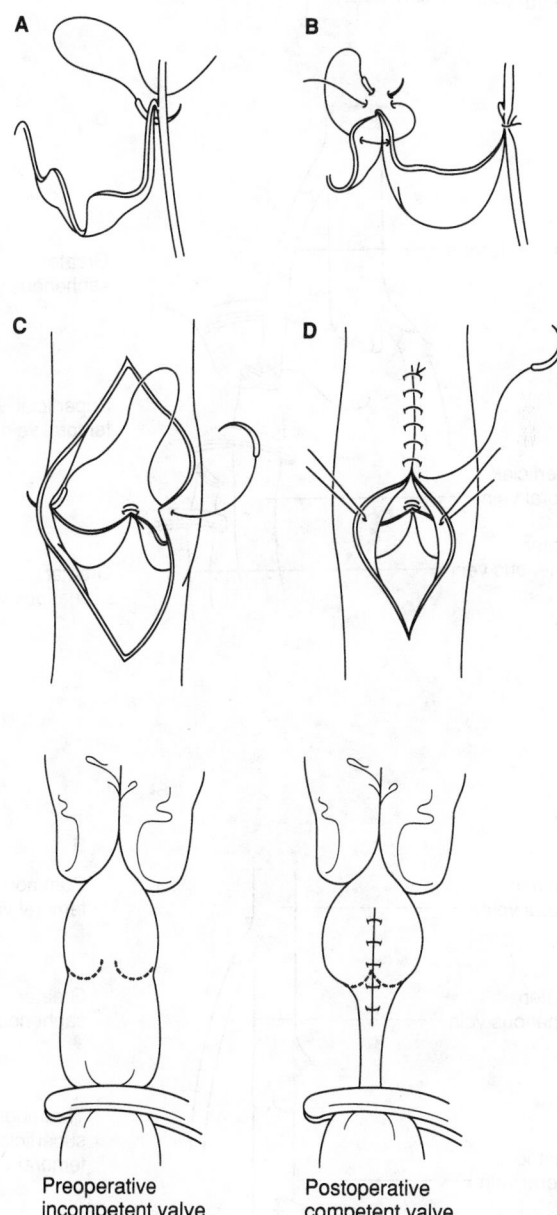

Figure 98-7. (*A* and *B*) Direct repair of an incompetent floppy valve can be accomplished by shortening the face edges of the valve cusp at the commissures. (*C*) To achieve this access, it is necessary to open the vein precisely at one commissure. (*D*) After closure, the competency of the valve can be tested by proximal compression of the distally occluded vein. (After Bergan J, Yao J, eds. Operative techniques in vascular surgery. Orlando, Grune & Stratton, 1980)

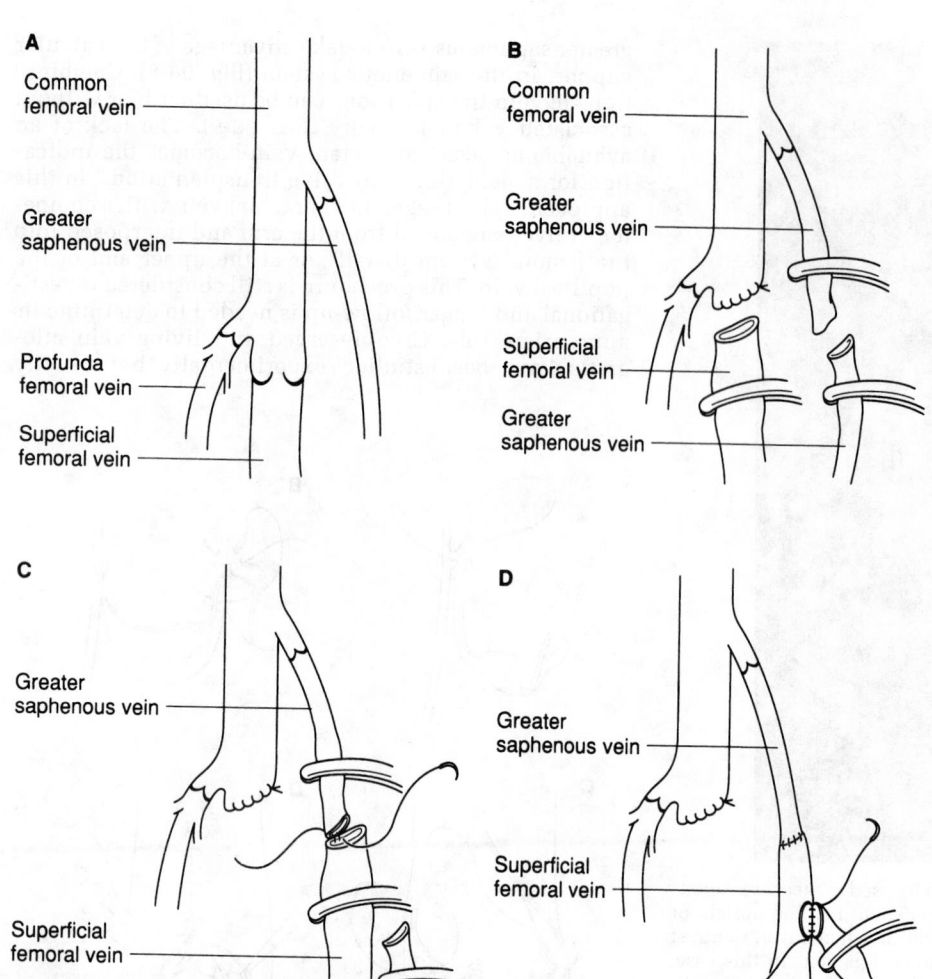

Figure 98-8. Functional venous competency can be restored by transposing an incompetent superficial femoral vein (SFV; *A*) to the divided greater saphenous vein (GSV; *B* and *C*), which has a competent proximal valve. The distal GSV is then reattached to the SFV (*D*). (After Bergan J, Yao J, eds. Operative techniques in vascular surgery. Orlando, FL, Grune & Stratton, 1980)

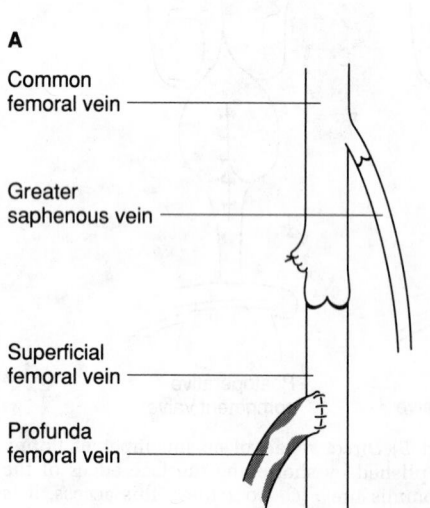
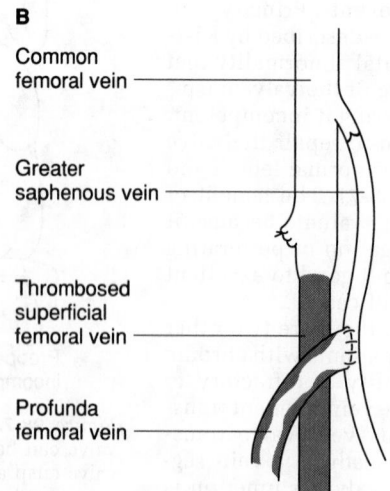

Figure 98-9. The transposition procedure can also be used with a stenotic and incompetent profunda femoral vein (*A*) attached to a competent superficial femoral vein (*B*) or, if that vein is thrombosed, to the competent greater saphenous vein (*B*).

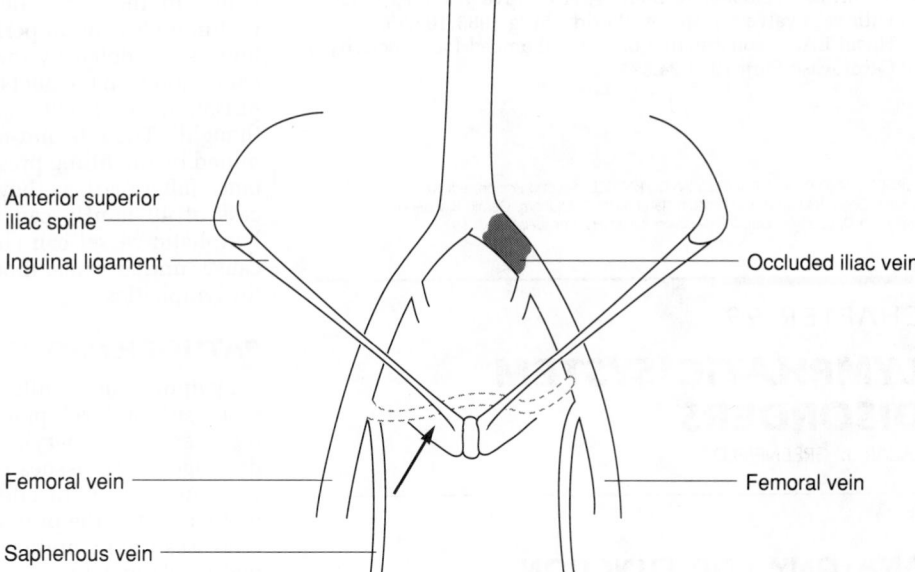

Figure 98-10. Chronic iliofemoral venous obstruction can be relieved by using the saphenous vein from the contralateral normal leg as a bypass graft. The vein is mobilized and divided distally, then tunneled behind the pubis (*arrow*) for attachment to the obstructed femoral vein.

show signs of rejection despite immunosuppression and have a high rate of thrombosis.

Venous Ulceration

The natural history of chronic venous stasis ulcers is that they tend to remain unhealed for many years. With standard therapy of paste bandages and elastic compression, about 80% heal and the remainder can be healed by split-thickness skin grafts with or without ligation of adjacent perforating veins. Unfortunately, the ulcers have a high rate of recurrence, depending to a large extent on how well the patient maintains effective elastic stocking support. Little evidence justifies the use of antibacterial agents, antiseptics, or enzymes in the management of stasis ulcers. In fact, recent evidence suggests that the best results are obtained with a totally occlusive dressing combined with graded elastic support. When skin grafts are used, it is advisable to fenestrate the graft or to use mesh or pinch grafts to allow evacuation of serous wound drainage. The patient should remain at bed rest until the ulcer is completely healed. The most useful measures to prevent ulcer recurrence include saphenous vein ligation when this system is incompetent, ligation of perforating veins, permanent elastic stocking support, and, in some reports, stanozolol to enhance fibrinolytic activity.

Venous Obstruction

Most venous obstruction is postthrombotic, although the same clinical picture can be produced by tumors in the pelvis and by structural changes such as iliac artery compression of the left common iliac vein. Because collateral circulation usually improves over time, few patients are candidates for bypass procedures. The most common procedure used is the saphenous vein crossover graft described by Palma in 1959 to bypass iliofemoral obstruction[6] (Fig. 98-10). The saphenous vein is mobilized from the normal contralateral extremity and divided distally. Then, it is tunneled suprapubically and anastomosed to the femoral vein. The failure rate with this procedure exceeds 20% and has prompted some surgeons to use prosthetic graft material for the bypass. Because prosthetic grafts are thrombogenic in the venous system, a temporary arteriovenous fistula often is used to promote flow and patency until a compatible graft lining is developed. The saphenous vein has also been used for popliteal-to-femoral venous bypass when the superficial femoral vein is obstructed. Described by Warren and Thayer in 1954,[7] the procedure is often referred to as the *Husni bypass* on the basis of his reported experience. The success rate for this approach is only about 60%, which explains its infrequent use.

Venous bypass of the inferior vena cava has also been reported using externally supported PTFE grafts. The external ring support of the graft is necessary to prevent its compression by abdominal pressure. It also requires use of an arteriovenous fistula to remain patent. Only a limited experience has been reported with a high late thrombosis rate after closure of the fistula. In considering patients for venous bypass where a fistula may be necessary, the ankle–arm pressure index should be greater than 0.75 to avoid arterial insufficiency, and the fistula should not exceed 4 mm to avoid distal venous hypertension, valvular damage, and overload of cardiac output. Arteriovenous fistulas can preserve patency of a prosthetic bypass graft. They also dilate collateral veins, which remain effective when the fistula is closed after 2 or 3 months. Closure of the fistula is facilitated by leaving a ligature around the fistula in the subcutaneous tissue where it can be retrieved under local anesthesia. Direct operative approaches to webs and scarring of the left common iliac vein have not had acceptable long-term results and have been abandoned.

REFERENCES

1. Browse NL, Burnand KG, Thomas ML, eds. Diseases of the veins: pathology, diagnosis and treatment. London, Edward Arnold, 1988.
2. Moyses C, Cedarholm-Williams SA, Michel CC. Hemoconcentration and accumulation of white cells in the feet in venous stasis. Int J Microcirc Clin Exp 1987;5:331.
3. Bernstein EF. Future prospects in the treatment of venous disease. World J Surg 1986;10:959.
4. Kistner RL, Sparkuhl RD. Surgery in acute and chronic venous disease. Surgery 1979;85:31.
5. Dale WA. Venous bypass surgery. Surg Clin North Am 1982;62:391.

6. Taheri SA, Heffener R, Budd T, et al. Five years' experience with vein valve transplant. World J Surg 1986;10:935.

7. Husni EA. Reconstruction of veins: the need for objectivity. J Cardiovasc Surg 1983;24:525.

SURGERY: SCIENTIFIC PRINCIPLES AND PRACTICE, Second Edition, edited by Lazar J. Greenfield, Michael W. Mulholland, Keith T. Oldham, Gerald B. Zelenock, and Keith D. Lillemoe. Lippincott–Raven Publishers, Philadelphia, © 1997.

CHAPTER 99

LYMPHATIC SYSTEM DISORDERS

LAZAR J. GREENFIELD

ANATOMY AND FUNCTION

Embryologists disagree on the origin of the lymphatic vessels. One group traces the vessels to the venous system, whereas another group favors an origin by fusion of mesenchymal spaces or clefts. Regardless of origin, there are paired lymph sacs in the neck and lumbar region by the sixth week of gestation and a developing cisterna chyli by the eighth week. Communicating channels connect these systems to form the thoracic duct by merger of the right lymphatic duct with the left across the fourth to sixth thoracic vertebrae to connect with and drain into the left subclavian vein. Smaller lymphatic ducts persist, draining into the right subclavian vein. Developmental arrest or abnormalities can result in primary hypoplasia or absence of ducts and lymph nodes. Abnormal growth of jugular lymph sacs can produce unilocular or multilocular lymph cysts termed *cystic hygromas*. Most often found in the neck, these cysts can also be found in the axilla, mediastinum, retroperitoneum, or intestinal mesentery. Hyperplastic changes can also occur and produce lymphangiomas with or without other vascular malformations.

The function of the lymphatic system begins with lymphatic capillaries, which collect fluid and protein from the extravascular spaces. This is a significant responsibility because more than 50% of the circulating albumin is lost into the interstitial space every 24 hours. During this period, as much as 4 pounds of lymph is returned to the venous system.[1] In addition to the proteins that cannot be reabsorbed by the venules, red cells and bacteria as well as other large particles can only be evacuated through the lymphatics. This unique permeability is facilitated by the absence of a basement membrane beneath the lymphatic endothelial cells. The lymphatic capillaries are found beneath the epidermis in the superficial dermis. These vessels drain into valved channels in the deep dermis and subdermal tissues, forming larger channels that follow the vascular pathways superficial to the deep fascia. Although lymphatics can be found in the intermuscular fascia, they are absent in muscles, tendon, cartilage, brain, and cornea.

Lymph is transported by afferent vessels to regional lymph nodes, which vary in size according to their function and activity (Fig. 99-1). Within the medullary sinuses of the node, circulating lymphocytes are replaced and initial contact between foreign material and the immune system is made. Efferent lymph leaves the node by way of hilar channels. These channels are less numerous than the afferent channels that enter the convex side of the node. In addition to direct thoracic duct drainage into the subcla-

vian vein, there are other lymphovenous communications within nodes and in peripheral vessels. Central lymphatic flow is promoted by the lymphatic valves and muscular contractions in the ducts rather than by respiration, arterial pulsation, and external massage, as was previously thought.[2] The rate and force of the contractions are determined by the filling pressures (preload) and outflow resistance (afterload), as they are in the heart. Pressures in excess of 40 mmHg can be generated, and an obstructed lymphatic vessel can show pressures over 60 mmHg because, unlike veins, there is not a good collateral system for lymphatics.[3]

PATHOPHYSIOLOGY

Lymphedema results from obstruction of lymph ducts as a result of developmental defects (primary) or acquired disorders (secondary). The effect of inadequate lymph drainage in the tissues is an increase in protein and fluid accumulation, with additional fluid retained by the osmotic effect of the protein. Protein content in edema fluid increases from a normal range of 0.1 to 0.5 g/dL to abnormal levels of 1 to 5 g/dL, which stimulate tissue fibrosis in the subcutaneous tissue, skin thickening, and hyperkeratosis. The microlymphatics of human skin show network enlargement in primary lymphedema of late onset, whereas they are aplastic or ectatic in congenital lymphedema.[4] Although the edema is initially soft and pitting, it becomes more indurated and rubbery with time and progresses to involve the entire extremity in a picture resembling elephantiasis. The differentiation of lymphedema from venous stasis edema is possible because there is usually no hyperpigmentation or ulceration in lymphedema, and the edema does not decrease significantly with overnight elevation. Also, it is more common for lymphedema to involve the dorsum of the foot and toes and to be associated with recurrent episodes of cellulitis and lymphangitis after trivial trauma. The latter complication presents with erythema, pain, and red streaks on the extremity. Lymphangitis may be accompanied by systemic signs of infection, typically by a β-hemolytic *Streptococcus* organism.

The most common serious complication of lymphedema is lymphangiosarcoma, which is usually seen in the upper extremity in a patient with chronic lymphedema after mastectomy for carcinoma (Fig. 99-2). Multiple raised bluish red or purple lesions are seen in the skin or subcutaneous tissue, and they can progress to an ulcerating mass lesion if untreated. Lymphangiosarcoma is thought to arise from lymphatic endothelium and has a poor prognosis, with most patients dying from the disease in less than 2 years. The tumor can occur on the lower extremity as a nonhealing ulcer with hemorrhagic nodules, pointing out the necessity of biopsy of any suspicious nonhealing lesion.

Because lymphedema occurs as the result of an abnormality of the lymphatic system, use of the term should be restricted to situations in which other causes of edema have been excluded or a specific lymphatic abnormality has been demonstrated. The presence of bilateral dependent pitting edema usually indicates a renal or cardiac etiology. Other generalized hypoproteinemias can be idiopathic or can be seen in malnutrition, cirrhosis, and protein-losing enteropathy. Allergies or hereditary causes are unusual. In unilateral edema, venous disease is the most likely cause (see Chap. 98).

DIAGNOSIS

The patient with lymphedema complains of swelling and fatigue. Limb size increases during the day and decreases at night but is never normal. It is important to

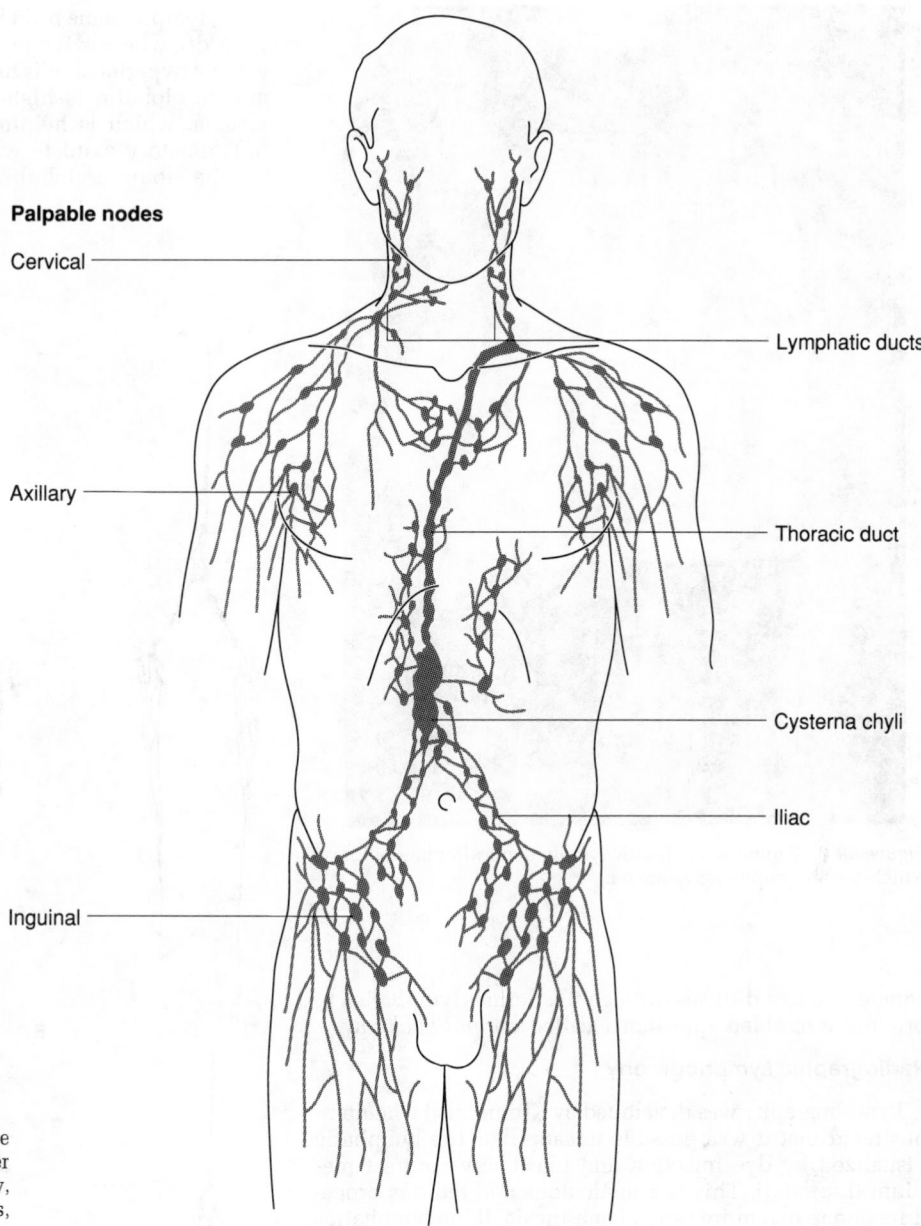

Palpable nodes

Cervical

Lymphatic ducts

Axillary

Thoracic duct

Cysterna chyli

Iliac

Inguinal

Figure 99-1. Major lymph node groups and collecting ducts. (After Basmajian JV. Primary anatomy, ed 7. Baltimore, Williams & Wilkins, 1976:293)

determine whether there is a family history of primary lymphedema and whether the patient has visited any countries where filariasis is endemic. Weight loss and diarrhea suggest small bowel lymphangiectasia. On examination, lymphedema is characteristically firm and rubbery but nonpitting. Lymph vesicles may be present, containing fluid with a high protein concentration. Complications of lymphedema, such as infection, cellulitis, erythema, and hyperkeratosis, may be present. It is important to document limb size to identify isolated limb gigantism and the Klippel-Trenaunay syndrome, which may have hypoplastic lymphatics in addition to venous abnormality, capillary nevus, and limb elongation. The patient should be examined for upper extremity and genital lymphedema, hydroceles, and amelogenesis imperfecta.

The differential diagnosis of lower extremity edema includes systemic disorders such as congestive heart failure and acute and chronic venous abnormality. In congestive heart failure, there is a generalized increase in venous pressure with distended neck veins and an enlarged liver. The question of venous disease can be most easily resolved by noninvasive duplex examination using Doppler and B-mode ultrasound imaging (see Chap. 97). In the absence of these disorders, the patient usually can be managed on the basis of the clinical diagnosis of lymphedema. Only rarely is it necessary to confirm the diagnosis by lymphatic visualization.

Lymphatic Visualization

Lymphatics can be visualized by dye injection in the extremities and mesentery. Ingestion of cream or milk enables visualization of intestinal lacteals and major ducts.

Dye Injection

A highly diffusible dye such as patent-blue or sky-blue dye can be injected in 0.2-mL amounts subcutaneously into each interdigital web. Massaging the skin and moving the joints usually defines a network of fine intradermal lymphatics. If the collecting vessels are obstructed or inad-

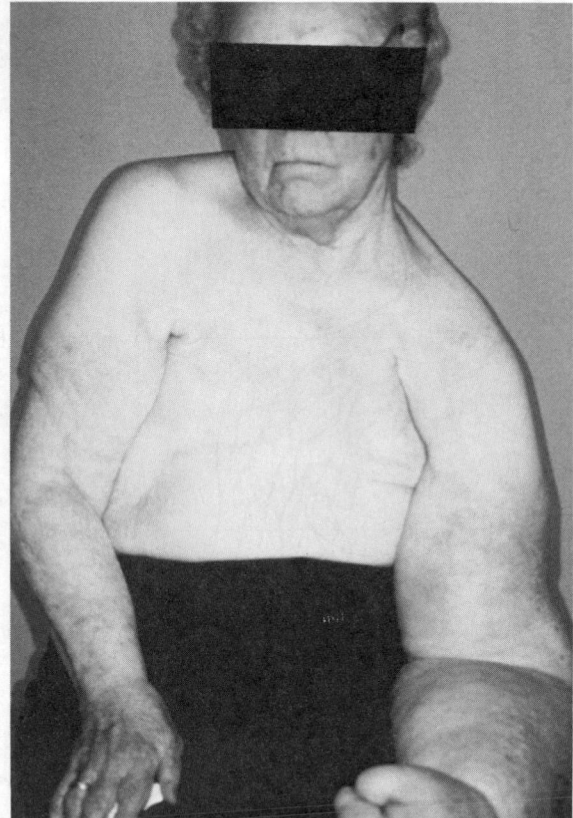

Figure 99-2. Patient with chronic lymphedema after mastectomy, which led to lymphangiosarcoma.

cally, lymphedema fluid has a protein content of more than 1.5 g/dL, whereas the protein content of edema fluid from venous hypertension is usually less. Also, the ratio of albumin to globulin is higher in lymphedema fluid than in plasma, which is helpful in the differentiation from an inflammatory exudate where the protein content is high but the albumin/globulin ratio is normal.

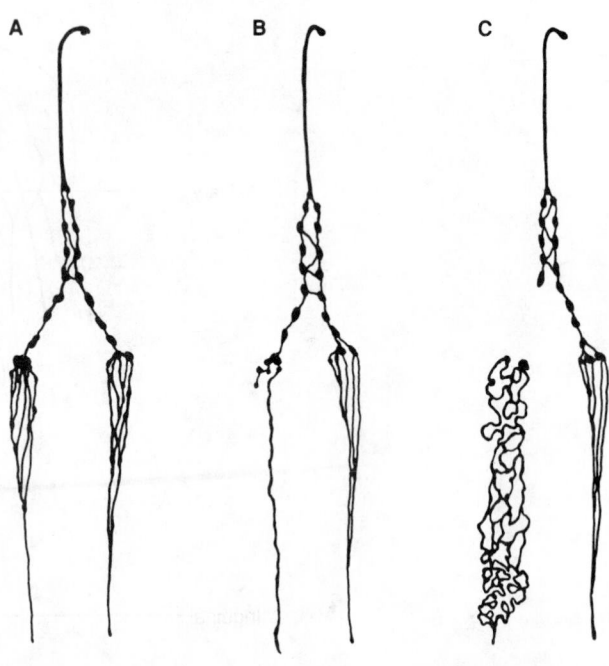

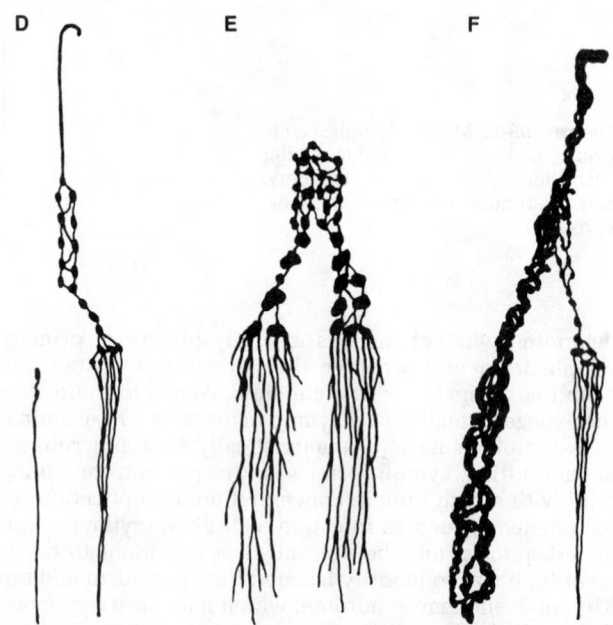

Figure 99-3. Diagrammatic representation of lymphographic patterns from feet to thoracic duct as seen in a normal person (*A*), in distal hypoplasia (*B*, right lower extremity), in proximal hypoplasia with distal distention (*C*, right limb), in combined proximal and distal hypoplasia (*D*), in bilateral hyperplasia (*E*), and in megalymphatics (*F*) often seen with a large, incompetent thoracic duct. (After Kinmonth JP. The lymphatics: surgery, lymphography and diseases of the chyle and lymph systems, ed 2. London, Edward Arnold, 1982:134)

equate, the dye diffuses through the dermal lymphatics to produce a marbled appearance called *dermal backflow*.

Radiographic Lymphography

Lymphography was developed by Kinmonth,[1] who demonstrated that it was possible to cannulate the lymphatic visualized by dye injection and inject oily contrast medium (Lipiodol). This is a meticulous and tedious procedure and may require general anesthesia. If the lymphatics in the foot are not usable, it is possible either to cannulate lymphatics adjacent to groin nodes or to inject the node directly. With adequate visualization, the lymphatics in the extremity can be identified. They often appear as parallel tracks of uniform size that bifurcate as they proceed proximally, in contrast to the venous system (Fig. 99-3). Normally, there is some dilation at the level of the valves.

Radionuclide Lymphatic Clearance

Radionuclide scanning using human serum albumin labeled with radioactive iodine or technetium-99m colloid has been used to monitor lymphatic clearance by serial scanning. Although the technique is simpler than standard lymphography, its disadvantages are haziness of the scan, radiation dosage, and distribution of the radionuclide into the extracellular fluid, making calculations of clearance dependent on leg volume.

Analysis of Tissue Fluid

Tissue fluid or lymph can be aspirated or collected from a tube in the subcutaneous tissues, but its analysis contributes little to the diagnosis of lymphedema. Characteristi-

TRAUMA

The lymphatics are delicate vessels vulnerable to operative and penetrating trauma. Disruption of larger lymphatic ducts can result in pseudocysts, fistulas, or lymph collection in body cavities such as pleura, pericardium, or peritoneum.

Lymphocysts

Pseudocysts that form after operation or trauma are termed *lymphocysts* and can progressively enlarge, producing pressure symptoms. Lymphocysts typically occur after radical node dissections and in association with kidney transplantation. Although some can involute or respond to aspiration, it is usually necessary to explore the cyst and suture ligate the draining ducts. Identification of the ducts can be facilitated by distal subcutaneous injection of blue dye. Wound drainage and a pressure dressing enhance the healing of the area.

Thoracic Duct Trauma

Injury to the thoracic duct is usually the result of operative or penetrating trauma and produces chylothorax. In rare cases, spontaneous rupture of the thoracic duct can occur in patients with mediastinal lymphoma or congenital malformations of the duct. Treatment initially consists of thoracostomy tube drainage for injured ducts as opposed to thoracotomy to suture ligate the involved vessels, which is usually necessary for spontaneous rupture of a malformation. The volume of chylous drainage can be reduced significantly by an elemental diet and by medium-chain triglyceride administration. If the lung fails to expand or if drainage persists for longer than a week, thoracotomy should be performed to ligate the thoracic duct. The thoracic duct can be identified by the preoperative administration of milk and cream or the intraoperative injection of blue dye into the distal wall of the esophagus. Chylopericardium can be managed similarly, although it usually responds to external drainage and dietary control.

Chylous Ascites and Chyluria

Chylous ascites occurs most often as a result of congenital abnormalities or malignant tumors involving the retroperitoneum. It does not often result from trauma. Proximal obstruction of the thoracic duct can be responsible for persistent leakage and can make spontaneous closure less likely. Lymphography may be necessary to clarify the situation anatomically if a congenital abnormality is suspected. Management is similar to that described for chylothorax. Chyluria can result from filariasis or congenital abnormalities and is diagnosed by the finding of milky urine. Lymphangiography is usually necessary to define the anatomy for operative correction.

CLASSIFICATION OF LYMPHEDEMA

The original Allen classification distinguished two types of lymphedema—primary lymphedema, in which there was no known cause, and lymphedema secondary to a known disease or disorder.[1] The primary lymphedemas were called *congenital* when present at birth and *praecox* when the onset was in childhood. When the onset was delayed into later life, Kinmonth added the term *tarda*. With the advent of lymphography, it became possible to classify the primary lymphedemas structurally into *hyperplasias* and *hypoplasias* (see Fig. 99-3). The classification proposed by Kinmonth is as follows:

Primary Lymphedema
- Primary hypoplastic
  Distal hypoplasia or aplasia
  Proximal hypoplasia
  Proximal and distal hypoplasia
- Primary hyperplastic
  Bilateral hyperplasia
  Megalymphatic

Secondary Lymphedema
- Malignancy
- Radiation
- Trauma or surgical excision
- Inflammation or parasitic invasion
- Paralysis

The primary lymphedemas are hypoplastic in 92% of cases. Their subgroups are defined by lymphography and behave differently. Patients with distal hypoplasia have a mild, nonprogressive form of the disorder, provided that their proximal pathways are normal. Most of these patients are female, in a ratio of 3:1. The onset at puberty (lymphedema praecox) represents 80% of cases. Only 10% of cases are present at birth (congenital lymphedema). The remaining 10% present after age 35 (lymphedema tarda). In proximal hypoplasia, the lymphedema is more extensive and involves the entire extremity. It occurs with equal frequency among males and females. The combination of proximal and distal hypoplasia shows features of both groups and tends to be progressive.

The primary hyperplastic lymphedemas are uncommon (8%), and those with bilateral hyperplasia can usually be recognized by diffuse capillary angiomata on the lateral sides of the feet. Lymphography shows dilated lymphatics with normal valves, in contrast to the findings in the megalymphatic group where no valves can be seen. In this latter group, chylous reflux can produce chylometrorrhea, skin vesicles, or chyluria.

The most common cause of secondary lymphedema in the United States is malignant disease metastatic to lymph nodes. Another common cause is surgical removal of nodes, especially when combined with radiation therapy, which produces lymphatic fibrosis. In tropical and subtropical countries, filariasis is the most common cause of secondary lymphedema, producing the typical appearance of elephantiasis. Other infective or chemical agents (eg, silica) can enter the lymphatic system by means of barefoot walking and cause fibrosis of lymphatics and lymph nodes.

MANAGEMENT OF LYMPHEDEMA
Conservative Treatment

There are significant anatomic and physiologic limitations to the treatment of lymphedema. Physiologically, diuretic removal of fluid is not as effective in lymphedema as in edema due to other causes because of the residual protein in lymphedema. From an anatomic standpoint, the development of fibrosis produces irreversible changes in the subcutaneous tissues. Therefore, the options are limited, and the primary objectives are to control the edema, to maintain healthy skin, and to avoid the complications of cellulitis and lymphangitis.

To control edema, the leg can be elevated and sequential pneumatic compression boots can be used to massage the leg. These treatments can be done at home with equipment rented for this purpose. Once the leg has reached optimal size, the patient should be fitted with firm elastic stockings. For lymphedema, a full-length leotard should be used, in contrast to the calf-length hose recommended for venous insufficiency. The stockings should be removed at night and the foot of the bed elevated 6 to 8 inches to maintain the pressure gradient from leg to right atrium. For more severe forms of the disorder, a 2- to 3-day period of hospitalization has been recommended by Pappas and O'Donnell[5] with use of a high-pressure pneumatic compression pump to reduce the size of the extremity. Subsequent control of the edema by elastic compression stockings was successful initially in 90% and then declined to 53% at a mean follow-up of 25 months.

A red streaking up the leg and the onset of pain and swelling usually signify early cellulitis or lymphangitis. The causative organism is most often *Staphylococcus* or β-hemolytic *Streptococcus* and must be treated vigorously, usually with intravenous antibiotics. The extremity should be immobilized, and warm, moist compresses should be applied to provide symptomatic relief. In the absence of treatment, the infection can obliterate more lymphatics and can produce constitutional signs of fever, malaise, nausea, and vomiting. Another frequent complication is eczema, which usually responds to hydrocortisone cream. Antifungal agents may be necessary, both topically and systemically for chronic infections, particularly between the toes. Ulceration is unusual, in contrast to the stasis edema of venous insufficiency, although fissures and lymph fistulas may develop and require surgical excision.

Secondary lymphedemas may lend themselves to treatment of the underlying disorder. Diethylcarbamazine can be used for filariasis, and appropriate antibiotics can be used for tuberculosis or lymphogranuloma venereum. In rare cases of long-standing secondary lymphedema, a lymphangiosarcoma can develop and can appear as a raised blue or reddish nodule. Satellite tumors and early metastases can develop if the malignancy is not recognized and widely excised. Improvement in tissue softening and volume reduction has been reported in a randomized, double-blind study using a benzopyrone (5,6-benzo-(alpha)-pyrone), which is thought to stimulate tissue macrophages to reduce intercellular protein concentration.[6] Treatment for 6 months produced a 20% reduction in upper limb volume and an 8% reduction in lower limb volume, with reduced skin temperature and fewer episodes of infection. This drug has not been approved for use in the United States.

Operative Treatment

Only 10% to 15% of patients with primary lymphedema are candidates for operative treatment, which usually is directed to reducing leg size. The indications for operation are related to functional rather than cosmetic improvement, because the appearance of the extremity even after a successful debulking procedure will still be abnormal. The best results are obtained when the bulk of the extremity has severely impaired movement or when there have been recurrent attacks of cellulitis. Although some efforts have been made to improve techniques for lymphatic drainage, most of the established procedures consist of excisional operations.

Three of these excisional procedures were based on the incorrect assumption that the deep fascia acted as a barrier to lymphatic drainage. The efforts of Kondoleon, Sistrunk, and Thompson to excise fascia and to insert a dermal flap into muscle proved ineffective in improving lymphatic drainage.[1] The original procedure devised by Charles consists of wide excision of lymphedematous tissue followed by skin grafting and is useful when the overlying skin is in poor condition, as in elephantiasis. The procedure used most often is Kinmonth's modification of Homans' procedure, in which skin flaps are raised to allow excision of the underlying subcutaneous tissues.[1]

The most logical, albeit technically demanding, approach has been to establish lymphaticovenous anastomoses. Initial efforts in this area were made in 1968 by Nielubowicz, who divided a lymph node, removed the pulp under magnification, and then sutured the node capsule with its afferent lymphatics into a vein. This procedure is more suitable for secondary lymphedema than for primary lymphedema, in which the disorder lies in the lymphatic channels themselves. Another promising technique of direct lymphovenous connection was developed by Cardeiro and modified in 1974 by Degni,[7] who used a special needle to insert lymphatic vessels directly into veins and fix them there by a single suture.

Microlymphatic bypass for secondary lymphedema continues to be investigated. Encouraging results have been found in several series, such as the report by Huang and coworkers[8] of improvement in 79% of 91 patients. Gloviczki and colleagues[9] reported improvement in 4 of 7 patients with secondary lymphedema but only one of eight patients with primary lymphedema. Another large series was reported from Australia, where O'Brien and associates[10] performed lymphovenous anastomoses for chronic lymphedema in 90 patients. Although a significant number of patients also underwent excisional operations, 74% of the group could discontinue use of elastic stockings. The procedure has also been used to treat chyluria and scrotal lymphangial fistula.[11] Confidence in the durability of the procedure awaits better long-term results with demonstration of patency of the lymphovenous anastomoses. A more practical approach consisting of liposuction curettage was reported by Louton and Terranova in 1989.[12] This procedure is performed through multiple small incisions at the knee, ankle, and calf to debulk the leg, and redundant tissue is excised 4 days later. Again, the long-term results of such an approach are unknown, but it seems likely that repeated liposuction will be necessary to maintain the reduction in limb size.

It is difficult to evaluate the results of such procedures when combined with resectional operations,[13] and in the absence of postoperative lymphography it is difficult to demonstrate patency of the lymphovenous anastomoses. The deleterious effects of lymphangiographic contrast on lymphatics were well demonstrated in 1981 by O'Brien, who measured limb volume after lymphangiography in 100 patients and found that 32% had a significant increase in leg volume and 19% developed lymphangitis. Therefore, it seems advisable to use lymphangiography only for diagnostic studies and not for preoperative or postoperative evaluation until safer contrast material becomes available.

REFERENCES

1. Kinmonth JB. The lymphatics: surgery, lymphography and diseases of the chyle and lymph systems, ed 2. London, Edward Arnold, 1982.
2. Reddy NP. Lymph circulation: physiology, pharmacology and biomechanics. CRC Crit Rev Biomed Eng 1986;14:45.
3. Roddie IC. Lymph transport mechanisms in peripheral lymphatics. News Physiol Sci 1990;5:85.
4. Bollinger A. Microlymphatics of human skin. Int J Microcirc Clin Exp 1993;12:1.
5. Pappas CJ, O'Donnell TF Jr. Long term results of compression treatment for lymphedema. J Vasc Surg 1992;16:555.
6. Casley-Smith JR, Morgan RG, Piller NB. Treatment of lymphedema of the arms and legs with 5,6-benzo-(alpha)-pyrone. N Engl J Med 1993;329:1158.
7. Degni M. New techniques of lymphatic-venous anastomosis for the treatment of lymphedema. Vasa 1974;3:479.
8. Huang G-K, Ru-Qi H, Zong-Zhao L, Yao-Liang S, Tie-De L, Gong-Ping P. Microlymphaticovenous anastomosis in the

treatment of lower limb obstructive lymphedema: analysis of 91 cases. Plast Reconstr Surg 1985;76:671.

9. Gloviczki P, Fisher J, Hollier LH, et al. Microsurgical lympho-venous anastomosis for treatment of lymphedema: a critical review. J Vasc Surg 1988;7:647.

10. O'Brien BM, Mellow CG, Khazanchi RK, et al. Long term results after microlymphatico-venous anastomoses for treatment of obstructive lymphedema. Plast Reconstr Surg 1990; 85:562.

11. Ji YZ, Zheng JH, Chen JN, Wu ZD. Microsurgery in the treatment of chyluria and scrotal lymphangial fistula. Br J Urol 1993;72:952.

12. Louton RB, Terranova WA. The use of suction curettage as adjunct to the management of lymphedema. Ann Plast Surg 1989;22:354.

13. Servelle M. Surgical treatment of lymphedema: a report on 652 cases. Surgery 1987;101:485.

SURGERY: SCIENTIFIC PRINCIPLES AND PRACTICE, Second Edition, edited by Lazar J. Greenfield, Michael W. Mulholland, Keith T. Oldham, Gerald B. Zelenock, and Keith D. Lillemoe. Lippincott–Raven Publishers, Philadelphia, © 1997.

CHAPTER 100

NEONATAL AND PEDIATRIC PHYSIOLOGY

SAMUEL M. MAHAFFEY

The physiologic responses of children to injury or operation vary dramatically, depending on maturation (the functional state of development of various organ systems), anatomic abnormalities, and underlying metabolic disorders. In many instances, the physiology of neonates more closely resembles that of fetuses than that of adults.

This chapter summarizes those aspects of physiology relevant to the perioperative management of premature and term neonates, infants, and children, and offers strategies for clinical management.

GROWTH AND MATURATION

High-Risk Pregnancy, Premature Birth, and Intrauterine Growth

Intrauterine growth is one of the most important clinical signs of fetal well-being. At delivery, categorization of the infant by birthweight is a useful assessment of fetal growth.[1] Low-birthweight infants are defined as those infants with a birthweight of less than 2500 g, and very-low-birthweight infants are those with a birthweight of less than 1500 g. Perhaps a more useful assessment is the expression of birthweight relative to gestational age (an age assessment based on the physical and neurologic characteristics of the infant in addition to obstetric dates): the weight of small-for-gestational-age infants is less than the 10th percentile for the population, large-for-gestational-age infants weigh more than the 90th percentile, and appropriate-for-gestational-age infants make up the remainder.

The term *intrauterine growth retardation* (IUGR) is used to describe a pathophysiologic process that results in restriction of fetal growth. IUGR can result from any combination of fetal, placental, and maternal abnormalities. Congenital anomalies are common. Placental size and functional capacity may be limiting factors in nutrient transport to the fetus, or maternal nutrient delivery to the placenta may be inadequate owing to decreased uteroplacental blood flow or reduced oxygen or nutrient concentrations. IUGR infants are a heterogeneous population. They tend to have neonatal problems related more to their gestational ages than to their birthweights, including perinatal asphyxia, hypoglycemia, hypothermia, pulmonary hemorrhage, necrotizing enterocolitis, and complications related to specific syndromes or congenital anomalies.

Prematurity is defined by the World Health Organization as a gestational age at birth of less than 37 weeks. Premature birth of infants whose weight is appropriate for their preterm gestational age is often due to medical conditions in which there is inability of the uterus to retain the fetus, interference with the course of the pregnancy, premature separation of the placenta, or stimulus to effective uterine contractions before term.

Complications of prematurity account for about 85% of fetal deaths. These deaths are commonly due to perinatal asphyxia, respiratory failure, and infection. Morbidity is also much higher in premature neonates compared with term neonates; they are more susceptible to oxygen-induced lung (bronchopulmonary dysplasia) and eye (retinopathy of prematurity) injury, intracranial hemorrhage, hypothermia, sepsis, necrotizing enterocolitis, hyperbilirubinemia, and renal tubular acidosis.

Postnatal Growth and Development

After the complex physiologic and metabolic adaptation to extrauterine life, the fetus undergoes a phase of rapid postnatal growth and development that is unparalleled at any stage of later postnatal development. This dramatic change in physical size occurs simultaneously with complex maturational events. A significant deviation in somatic growth may, in fact, be the first indication of an underlying functional abnormality.

During the first year of life, a typical infant increases in weight by about 200% and in length by 50%. Genetic and environmental factors, such as parental size, nutritional status, overall health status, and socioeconomic factors, have been shown to have roles in determining the rate of postnatal growth.

Growth in stature is largely controlled by hormones and growth factors. Growth hormone, or somatotropin, is essential for the balanced growth of the body to normal adult size. Like other peptide hormones and growth factors, growth hormone exerts its effects by binding to specific receptors on the cell membrane of target cells.[2] The mechanism of signal transduction, however, is unclear. Growth hormone has short-term metabolic effects much like those of insulin, including stimulation of amino acid transport and protein synthesis.[3] Long-term administration and conditions of excessive growth hormone production produce insulin-antagonistic effects and glucose intolerance.[4] Growth hormone appears to exert its growth-promoting effects through intermediates, including insulin-like growth factor I (formerly known as somatomedin C) and insulin-like growth factor II.

Insulin exerts a prominent influence on fetal and neonatal growth, best illustrated by disorders at the extremes of abnormal insulin secretion. Hyperinsulinemia in the fetus, such as can occur in infants born of poorly controlled diabetic mothers, results in visceromegaly and increased body fat, whereas hypoinsulinemic infants born with insulin resistance or pancreatic agenesis are severely growth stunted and depleted of body fat. In postnatal life, poorly controlled diabetes is associated with remarkable growth failure (Mauriac syndrome).[5] Insulin effects on growth are likely mediated through direct, metabolic effects mediated by the insulin receptor and indirect, mitogenic effects mediated primarily through the structurally homologous insulin-like growth factor I receptor.[6]

Thyroid hormones also have direct metabolic effects and other effects due to induction of genes that more directly affect cell growth and function. Thyroid hormone receptors are more akin to steroid hormone receptors than the receptors of other peptide hormones; they exist in the cytoplasm and regulate the transcription of other genes by binding to regulatory regions of DNA.[7] Many of the developmental effects of thyroid hormone result from induction of the genes for other hormones and growth factors. Congenital hypothyroidism occurs about once in every 5000 newborns. Affected infants may have prolonged icterus, feeding difficulties, and sluggishness. Growth is stunted, the extremities are short, and mental and physical development is retarded. The potentially catastrophic consequences of delayed diagnosis until clinical symptoms are recognized underscores the necessity for routine neonatal screening programs. Congenital hyperthyroidism is generally confined to the offspring of mothers with Graves disease. Hyperthyroidism in utero results in somatic overgrowth, depletion of fat stores, tachycardia, and hyperalertness.

Nutrient Requirements

An adequate supply of nutrients is essential to fulfill resting energy requirements, provide for growth, and provide necessary metabolic intermediates. The traditional approach to perioperative nutritional support attempts to prevent stress-induced catabolism due to injury or operation and to allow for normal growth. A contemporary approach to nutritional support includes the recognition that certain nutrients function as pharmacologic agents, with essential roles in the regulation of growth, immunologic activity, and antioxidant activity, which helps protect cells from the adverse effects of oxidative metabolism and the pathologic effects of free radicals. The clinician must recognize the variability in nutrient stores and requirements resulting from immaturity to provide appropriate nutritional support in a given clinical situation.

Water

Optimal water intake is a function of obligatory water loss and the amount retained for somatic growth. Obligatory water losses are closely correlated with the functional maturity of the major organs of water loss, the kidney and the integument, and thus vary considerably during gestation and postnatal development.

Fetal body water content is a function of the fetal growth rate and the relative proportion of fat to fat-free body mass. The percentage of water content and the ratio of intracellular to extracellular water progressively decrease during fetal development.[8]

Postnatal water requirements include insensible water loss, urine loss, and accretion of lean body mass. Insensible water loss is primarily due to evaporation from the lung and the skin and averages 1.5 to 3 g/kg/h. Evaporation is the primary means for the dissipation of heat produced by oxidative metabolism. The rate of transepithelial water loss is a function of skin thickness, body surface area/mass ratio, ambient temperature, subcutaneous tissue water-vapor pressure, and ambient humidity. Thus, the premature infant's thin skin barrier and large body surface area/mass ratio tend to enhance evaporative water loss. The other major water requirement is for the excretion of dissolved solute in the urine. Neonatal renal function is discussed in more detail later.

Taking all factors into account, total daily water requirements are estimated to be 100 mL/100 kcal ingested, assuming an insensible loss of 50 mL/kg/d and a growth requirement of 15 mL/kg/d.[9]

Energy

Energy expenditure is usually expressed in kilocalories per kilogram of body weight. Expressed in this manner, the energy expenditure of normal neonates is about twice that of normal adults (50 kcal/kg/d versus 25 kcal/kg/d). This method of expression ignores body composition, which can largely explain the lower resting metabolic rate per kilogram of body weight in adults compared with neonates.[10]

Energy requirements are determined by measurement of energy balance[11]:

$$\text{Energy balance} = \text{energy intake} - \text{energy expenditure}$$

This equation, although deceptively simple, has many components, making accurate measurement of energy balance extremely difficult. Determination of *metabolizable energy* depends on accurate measurement of energy intake and loss, including losses in the urine and stool. Energy expenditure is the summation of multiple components, which can be difficult to separate. The major component of energy expenditure (65% to 70%) is the resting metabolic rate, which is measured during the period of quiet inactivity in the postabsorptive state. Resting metabolic rate is more useful, practical, and predictive than the basal metabolic rate,[12] which occurs transiently during the early morning hours of deep sleep, has little influence on total energy requirements, and is nearly impossible to measure in neonates.

Other substantial determinants of energy expenditure include dietary intake, ambient temperature, activity, and the energy cost of growth. Dietary intake has an immediate effect on energy expenditure, referred to as *diet-induced thermogenesis;* this is thought to represent the energy necessary for absorption and assimilation of nutrients.[13] There is also a longer-term effect of dietary intake on energy expenditure, with higher intake leading to increased levels of expenditure.[14,15] The mechanisms underlying this increase have not been well defined. Energy expenditure for thermogenesis is associated with lower environmental temperatures.[16] Because infants sleep 80% to 90% of the time, energy requirements for physical activity are proportionally lower in infants compared with adults. Activity is estimated to contribute about 10% to energy expenditure in the neonatal period.

The total energy cost of growth consists of a storage component (the energy value of the substrates retained) and an energy expenditure component (the energy required for absorption, metabolism, and assimilation). Neither the total energy cost of growth nor the energy expenditure component can be measured directly. The estimated energy cost of growth in neonates ranges from 1.2 to 6 kcal/g.[17]

Significant variability can be found in estimates of energy requirements, a reflection of the multiple factors affecting energy intake and expenditure. In premature infants, recommended energy intake ranges from 90 to 160 kcal/kg/d. Estimated energy requirements during infancy are likewise variable.[18]

Energy is provided from either dietary carbohydrates or lipids. At birth, the constant maternal supply of glucose is interrupted, and newborns must then meet the metabolic demand for glucose by mobilization of stored carbohydrate (glycogen) or by synthesis of glucose. Glycogen stores are relatively limited and are quickly depleted; thus, an exogenous glucose source is required to prevent injury to organs that require glucose for fuel (eg, the brain).[19]

One method for estimating carbohydrate requirements is to examine the intake of normal, breastfed infants, assuming that breastfeeding provides optimal nutrient intake. All carbohydrate is provided in breast milk in the form of lactose. Although lactose concentrations vary somewhat in breast milk, overall lactose intake ranges from 7.5 to 10 g/kg/d, or about 40% of the total energy intake during the first 4 months of life.[20] Carbohydrate requirements can also be estimated by measurement of endogenous carbohydrate production during periods when an exogenous source is not available. Endogenous, steady-state (fasting) glucose release can be measured by constant tracer infusion methods; glucose production rates in term newborns are about 4 to 6 mg/kg/min (5.8 to 8.6 g/kg/d), and are similar in premature infants.[21,22] This methodology yields a minimal glucose requirement and does not take into account the requirements for growth.

Another consideration is the relative contribution of carbohydrate to overall energy intake. These types of studies have been performed on infants receiving parenteral nutrition for various reasons, in which the relative proportions of carbohydrate and fat are altered, while the provision of protein remains constant. In most circumstances, high carbohydrate/low fat ratios result in high rates of energy expenditure and decreased nitrogen retention, while low carbohydrate/high fat ratios result in excessive fat deposition. A balanced ratio (about 40% carbohydrate) provides the highest rate of nitrogen retention and is consistent with the proportion of carbohydrate found in breast milk and with the estimates of minimal carbohydrate needs determined by isotope infusion studies.[23]

Dietary lipid serves multiple metabolic needs; it is a source of energy, a source of essential fatty acids (which are metabolized to prostaglandins and leukotrienes, and serve structural functions), a component of structural membranes, and a carrier for fat-soluble vitamins. Dietary lipid is an efficient package of metabolizable energy. Lipids are carried in the bloodstream by lipoproteins and are cleared by the activity of the enzyme lipoprotein lipase. Reduced activity of this enzyme may account for the inability of neonates (especially premature and small-for-gestational-age neonates) to clear large fat loads.[24] Long-chain fatty acids are metabolized within the mitochondria by β-oxidation. Transport into the mitochondria is accomplished by the enzyme carnitine palmitoyl transferase, which requires carnitine as a cofactor. Carnitine must be supplied from the diet or synthesized from lysine and methionine; it is lacking in soy-based formulas and most parenteral nutrition solutions. Term infants not supplemented with carnitine have decreased entry of long-chain fatty acids into mitochondria. The requirement for exogenous carnitine has not been defined.[25,26]

An absolute requirement has been defined for certain polyunsaturated ("essential") fatty acids. A deficiency state has been described due to linoleic acid (18:2 ω6).[27] Linolenic acid (18:3 ω3) is also described as essential, although the deficiency state has been described on only one occasion. Recommendations include a total intake of 3.3 g of dietary lipid per 100 kcal, of which 1% should be ω6 fatty acids.[28] Requirements in premature infants may be considerably higher.

Based on plasma and tissue fatty acid profiles, it has been speculated that the metabolic pathways for elongation and desaturation of fatty chains may not be fully functional for weeks to months after birth.[29] This is of consider-

able importance in determining dietary requirements because the developing central nervous system incorporates a substantial quantity of polyunsaturated fatty acids with more than 20 carbons, primarily during the third trimester of pregnancy. Human milk, although variable in fat content and fatty acid profile due to maternal dietary intake, contains appropriate amounts of linoleic acid (8% of total fat) and long chain (more than 20 carbons) fatty acids. The fat content of premature infant formulas is based on vegetable oils, which contain a large amount of linoleic acid and a significant amount of linolenic acid. Likewise, intravenous lipid emulsions prepared from soybean or safflower oil contain large amounts of linoleic acid. Although the infant receiving these preparations is at little risk of fatty acid deficiency, the metabolic pathway for elongation and desaturation necessary for accretion into the central nervous system may be lacking. There is also cause for concern when linoleic and linolenic acid intake is excessive owing to inhibition of the metabolism of the ω6 and the ω9 series, which could result in abnormal lipid profiles and altered cell membrane composition.

Protein

Assessment of protein metabolism and requirements is difficult, and evaluation of different endpoints often leads to different dietary recommendations. Various measurements of "growth" may reflect nutritional adequacy, although in an indirect and nonspecific fashion. It is difficult to achieve growth studies in separate populations that differ only in protein intake; however, assessment of growth may still be a useful method to determine broad protein requirements in specific populations. In premature infants, this generally means achieving the rate of intrauterine growth, which may or may not be appropriate in a given physiologic circumstance.

Protein requirements may also be based on the premise that breastfeeding from well-nourished mothers provides adequate (although not necessarily optimal) protein intake. Protein intake, however, is difficult to quantify in terms of volume and composition. The protein composition of human milk is variable, and some components (lactoferrin, lysozyme and secretory immunoglobulin A [IgA]) may not be available for absorption.

The factorial approach to estimation of protein requirements is based on the concept that protein requirement should equal the quantity of protein needed for growth plus the quantity needed to replace inevitable losses (a concept analogous to energy balance).[30,31] Data examining inevitable losses in urine, feces, skin, and secretions are limited, but estimates range from 0.4 to 0.9 g/kg/d. The estimated protein increment for growth is based on limited infant body composition data and does not include high intraindividual variability in use and accretion. A final component of the factorial model is the efficiency of dietary protein use, which is estimated to be about 70%. Based on this methodology, a joint committee of the Food and Agriculture Organization, World Health Organization, and United Nations University estimated protein requirements for infants ranging from 2.5 g/kg/d in newborns to 1.25 g/kg/d at 1 year of age.[32] A similar approach can be used for premature infants, in whom estimated protein requirements range from 2.5 to 3.9 g/kg/d in infants weighing less than 2.5 kg.[33]

A final approach to estimation of protein requirements is normalization of plasma amino acid profiles, again based on the assumption that breastfed infants exhibit ideal plasma amino acid concentrations (the standard for premature infants remains controversial).[34] Normalization of

Table 100-1. **VITAMIN REQUIREMENTS AND FUNCTIONS**

Vitamin	Recommended Intake*	Function	Deficiency State
Ascorbic acid	8 mg	Hydroxylation reactions, including carnitine and collagen	Scurvy
Thiamine	40 μg	Coenzyme in oxidative decarboxylation	Beriberi
Riboflavin	60 μg	Electron transport	Stomatitis, glossitis, cheilosis, seborrheic dermatitis
Vitamin B$_6$	35 μg	Interconversions of amino acids, synthesis of heme, metabolic reactions (brain)	Anemia, CNS abnormalities, vomiting, diarrhea
Niacin	0.8 mg NE	Metabolic intermediate (NAD, NADP)	Pellagra
Biotin	1.5 μg	Coenzyme	Dermatitis, conjunctivitis, seizures, ataxia, hearing loss, developmental delay
Pantothenic acid	0.3 mg	Integral part of coenzyme A	Cardiovascular instability, lethargy, depression
Vitamin B$_{12}$	0.5 μg†	Synthesis of nucleotides, methyl transfers	Megaloblastic anemia, neurologic changes
Folate	50 μg†	Acceptor and donor of one-carbon units in amino acid and nucleotide metabolism	Hypersegmentation of neutrophils, megaloblastic changes, poor growth
Vitamin D	400 IU†	Stimulates absorption of Ca and P	Rickets
Vitamin A	420 μg†	Growth and differentiation of epithelial tissues; vision	Night blindness, keratoconjunctivitis, dermatitis and growth failure
Vitamin E	0.5 mg α-TE	Antioxidant	

NE, niacin equivalent; α-TE, α-tocopherol equivalent.
* Minimum units per 100 kcal/d.
† Units/d.
(Committee on Nutrition, American Academy of Pediatrics. Nutritional needs of low-birth-weight infants. Pediatrics 1985;75:976)

Table 100-2. **COMPOSITION AND USE OF INFANT FORMULAS**

Formula	Distribution of Calories	Carbohydrate Source	Protein Source	Fat Source	Osmolality	Use
HUMAN MILK AND STANDARD INFANT FORMULAS						
Human milk	Carbohydrate 38% Protein 7% Fat 55%	Lactose	Whey 80% Casein 20%	Human milk fat	300	Normal infants, premature infants
Enfamil, SMA	Carbohydrate 41%–43% Protein 9% Fat 48%–50%	Lactose	Nonfat cow's milk, whey Whey 60% Casein 40%	Coconut, soy, oleo, or safflower	278–305	Normal infants
Similac	Carbohydrate 43% Protein 9% Fat 48%	Lactose	Nonfat cow's milk Casein 82% Whey 18%	Coconut, soy	290	Normal infants
SOY-BASED INFANT FORMULAS						
Isomil Nursoy Prosobee	Carbohydrate 40% Protein 12%–13% Fat 47%–48%	Corn syrup solids, sucrose, or both	Soy isolate	Soy, coconut, corn, or safflower	150–296	Intolerance of lactose or cow's milk proteins
SPECIFIC-USE INFANT FORMULAS						
Nutramigen	Carbohydrate 54% Protein 11% Fat 35%	Corn syrup solids, corn starch	Casein hydrolysate	Corn oil	320	Lactose or cow's milk protein intolerance; malabsorption syndromes
Pregestimil	Carbohydrate 41% Protein 11% Fat 40%	Corn syrup solids, glucose, tapioca starch	Casein hydrolysate	MCT 60% Corn oil 20% Safflower 20%	300	Malabsorption syndromes; short gut
Portagen	Carbohydrate 46% Protein 14% Fat 40%	Corn syrup solids, sucrose	Sodium caseinate	MCT 88% Corn 12%	220	Malabsorption
Alimentum	Carbohydrate 41% Protein 11% Fat 48%	Surcrose, tapioca starch	Casein hydrolysate	MCT 50% Safflower, soy	370	

MCT, medium-chain triglycerides.

amino acid profiles is an important consideration in the design of parenteral amino acid solutions. Differences in plasma amino acid profiles, however, do not necessarily translate into differences in growth rates, and factors unrelated to nutritional intake (disease, enzyme deficiencies, sampling) may influence the plasma amino acid concentration.

Vitamins

Water-soluble vitamins function as enzyme cofactors, and requirements are dependent on energy intake and energy use. Although water-soluble vitamins generally are not stored, transplacental gradients favor accumulation in the fetus. This helps protect newborns from the development of vitamin deficiencies in the immediate postnatal period, although urinary losses and decreased dietary intake during the first weeks of life predispose the infant (particularly the premature infant) to vitamin deficiencies.

The fat-soluble vitamins A, D, E, and K participate primarily in cell differentiation and growth. Intestinal absorption is mediated through the same mechanisms as the absorption of dietary lipid, and a carrier mechanism (usually lipoproteins) is required for solubility in the blood. Depletion times for the fat-soluble vitamins are usually considerably longer than those of the water-soluble vitamins owing to tissue storage.

Vitamin functions, deficiency states, and requirements are summarized in Table 100-1.

Trace Elements and Minerals

The most abundant of the major elements—calcium, phosphorus, and magnesium—are primary constituents of the skeleton and are important components of extracellular fluid, cell membranes, muscle, and soft tissue. About 99% of all calcium is located in the skeleton, with about one third of this in a readily exchangeable pool with the extracellular fluid. By term, a newborn accumulates between 20 and 30 g of elemental calcium, 80% in the last trimester.[35] Ionized calcium is

the physiologically active form, playing important roles in nerve transmission, neurotransmitter release, coagulation, and muscle contraction. Serum calcium homeostasis is maintained through the interaction of parathyroid hormone, calcitonin, and vitamin D.

Term newborns experience a physiologic fall in serum calcium concentration. In the last trimester of pregnancy, the hormonal milieu (low parathyroid hormone level and high calcitonin) promotes bone deposition, and the serum calcium in fetal blood exceeds maternal levels.[36] At birth, placental transfer of mineral is halted, and the infant must increase bone resorption and decrease mineralization to maintain homeostasis. Concomitant with the fall in serum calcium, serum parathyroid hormone levels increase, and usually after 24 to 48 hours of life, the serum calcium stabilizes. The ability of the parathyroid glands to respond is a function of gestational and postnatal age; the incidence of neonatal hypocalcemia increases with decreasing gestational age.[37] Signs of pathologic hypocalcemia in newborns include irritability, jitteriness, tremors, seizures, and nonspecific symptoms that may suggest sepsis.

Preterm infants are deficient in calcium and phosphorus because they miss the peak period of skeletal mineralization, which is often complicated by inadequate supply postnatally. Evidence of poor bone mineralization or fractures is present in up to 30% of very-low-birthweight infants.

Trace elements (less than 0.01% of body weight) of established physiologic importance include iron, iodine, fluoride, zinc, copper, manganese, chromium, molybdenum, selenium, and cobalt. The function of these elements is often related to enzyme systems, in which they serve as cofactors for metal ion–activated enzymes, as constituents of metalloenzymes, or as constituents of other proteins. Other trace elements, including vanadium, silicon, arsenic, nickel, lithium, lead, tin, bromide, and cadmium, are thought to be essential, but their importance in human nutrition has not been delineated.

Table 100-3. NUTRIENT REQUIREMENTS FOR PARENTERAL NUTRITION

Component	Infant	Child (10–30 kg)	Older Child (7–12 y)	Adolescent
Water	120–150 mL/kg	1800–2000 mL/m^2/d	2000 mL/m^2/d	2000 mL/m^2/d
Energy	60–120 kcal/kg	75–90 kcal/kg	60–75 kcal/kg	30–60 kcal/kg
Dextrose (3.4 kcal/g)	40%–60%	60%–75%	60%–75%	60%–75%
Lipid emulsion (20%, 2.0 kcal/mL)	Up to 60% (max 4 g/kg/d)	25%–40%	25%–40%	25%–40%
Amino acids	2.5–3.5 g/kg	2.0–2.5 g/kg	1.5–2.0 g/kg	1.0–1.5 g/kg
Electrolytes				
Sodium	2–4 mEq/kg	2–5 mEq/kg	60–150 mEq/d	0–150 mEq/L
Potassium	2–4 mEq/kg	2–6 mEq/kg	90–240 mEq/d	0–80 mEq/L
Calcium	0.1–0.5 g/kg/d	1–4 g/d	2–3 g/d	0–10 mEq/L
Phosphorus	1–1.5 mM/kg/d	6–50 mM/d	30–50 mM/d	0–20 mmol/L
Magnesium	0.25 mEq/kg/d	4–24 mEq/d	8–24 mEq/d	0–15 mEq/L
Trace elements				
Zinc	Preterm 400 µg/kg <3 mo 250 µg/g >3 mo 100 µg/kg	50 µg/kg	2.5–5.0 mg/d	
Copper	20 µg/kg	20 µg/kg	0.5–1.5 mg/d	
Manganese	1 µg/kg	1 µg/kg	0.15–0.8 mg/d	
Chromium	0.20 µg/kg	0.2 µg/kg	10–15 µg/d	
Molybdenum	0.25 µg/kg	0.25 µg/kg		
Selenium	2 µg/kg	2 µg/kg		
Iodide	1 µg/kg	1 µg/kg		
Fluoride	—			
Iron	—			
Vitamins	2–3 mL/d MVI Pediatric	5 mL/d MVI Pediatric	10 mL/d MVI Pediatric	

Clinical Considerations

Enteral Feeding

Consumed in adequate quantities, breast milk from a well-nourished mother is thought to be sufficient in all nutrients, with the possible exception of vitamins D and K, fluoride, and iron. Human milk contains lactose as the primary carbohydrate, whey and casein (80:20) as the protein source, and human milk fat. Human milk provides 67 kcal/dL (20 kcal/oz) of metabolizable energy. The composition or caloric density may be modified by the addition of skimmed components from donor human milk or by the addition of commercial human milk fortifiers.

Standard infant formulas are adequate for normal infants who are not breastfed. These formulas are prepared from nonfat cow's milk, with carbohydrate (lactose) and vegetable oil added to simulate the caloric distribution and digestibility of human milk. Specialized formulas are modified for use in certain clinical situations, such as intolerance to one or more components of standard formula. In soy-based formulas, the protein is soy protein isolate; the carbohydrate is corn syrup solids (glucose polymers, hydrolyzed corn starch), sucrose, or a mixture of both; and the fat is from vegetable oils. Protein hydrolysate formulas are designed to minimize the risk of adverse response to cow's milk or soy protein; the protein is hydrolyzed to amino acids or short-chain polypeptides. Other formulas are specifically modified to manage malabsorption of certain components (such as fat malabsorption due to deficiency of pancreatic enzymes or bile salts) or inborn errors of metabolism (phenylketonuria, maple syrup urine disease, tyrosinemia, homocystinuria). The composition and use of infant formulas are summarized in Table 100-2.

Healthy term newborns nipple feed on demand every 3 to 4 hours. Preterm infants often suck a nipple, but rarely have a coordinated suck and swallow until 33 to 34 weeks of gestation. Gavage feedings are appropriate for infants who have immature suck and swallowing reflexes or medical conditions that preclude nipple feeding. Intragastric feedings are usually given intermittently (every 3 to 4 hours in term infants, more frequently in smaller infants) but may be given by continuous infusion. Transpyloric feeding tubes are used for infants who do not tolerate intragastric feedings or who are at high risk of aspiration.

Parenteral Nutrition

Parenteral nutrition is a technique for the intravenous administration of the nutrients required for basal metabolism and growth. Parenteral nutritional support is required when the gastrointestinal tract is not available or not functional to provide adequate digestion and absorption of required nutrients. The objective of total parenteral nutrition (TPN) is to achieve a normal rate of growth and body composition with minimal morbidity. Because of the high concentration of nutrients in these solutions, they must be administered into the central circulation through an indwelling central venous catheter. Peripheral parenteral nutrition is used for nutritional supplementation in patients who are receiving some enteral nutrition or who have a short-term requirement for parenteral nutritional support (less than 2 weeks). These solutions are less concentrated (maximum of 12.5% dextrose) and may be administered through a peripheral vein.

Nutrient requirements for TPN vary substantially, depending on patient age, baseline nutritional status, and energy expenditure. Guidelines for fluid, energy, protein, electrolytes, vitamins, and minerals are given in Tables 100-3 and 100-4. These guidelines should be considered a starting point and must be tailored to the individual patient response.

Table 100-4. SUGGESTED INTAKE OF PARENTERAL VITAMINS IN TERM AND PRETERM INFANTS

Vitamin	Full-Term Infants and Children (dose/d)*	Preterm Infants (dose/kg body weight)	
		Practical Suggestion†	Best Estimate
LIPID-SOLUBLE VITAMINS			
A (µg)	700	280	500
E (µg)	7	2.8	2.8
K (µg)	200	80	80
D (IU)	400	160	160
WATER-SOLUBLE VITAMINS			
Ascorbic acid (mg)	80	32	25
Thiamin (mg)	1.2	0.48	0.35
Riboflavin (mg)	1.4	0.56	0.15
Pyridoxine (mg)	1.0	0.4	0.18
Niacin (mg)	17	6.8	6.8
Pantothenate (mg)	5	2.0	2.0
Biotin (µg)	20	8.0	6.0
Folate (µg)	140	56	56
Vitamin B$_{12}$ (µg)	1.0	0.4	0.3

* Equivalent to one vial (5 mL) MVI Pediatric (Armour).
† Practical recommendations based upon 2 mL MVI Pediatric (Armour). (Green HL, Hambidge KM, Schanler R, et al. Guidelines for the use of vitamins, trace elements, calcium, magnesium and phosphorus in infants and children receiving total parenteral nutrition: report of the Subcommittee on Pediatric Parenteral Nutrient Requirements from the Committee on Clinical Practice Issues of the American Society for Clinical Nutrition. Am J Clin Nutr 1988;48:1324)

The protein source for parenteral nutrition requires an additional comment. Early solutions of the hydrochloride salts of crystalline amino acids (which resulted in acidosis) have been replaced with their acid equivalents. These solutions (FreAmine [McGaw], Aminosyn [Abbott], and Travasol [Baxter]) are suitable for general use, although the content of glycine is high, and cystine and tyrosine contents are low. Special-purpose solutions have been developed based on metabolic studies of specific populations, such as Hepatamine (McGaw) for patients with liver disease and Nephramine (McGaw) for patients with renal disease. Pediatric amino acid solutions (Aminosyn-PF [Abbott], TrophAmine [McGaw], and Neopham [KabiVitrum]) were developed to support normal growth and plasma amino acid concentrations in neonates, while decreasing complications such as cholestasis. These solutions contain higher concentrations of tyrosine and histidine, which are considered essential amino acids for neonates. Cysteine is also thought to be essential for premature infants but is not included in commercial formulations owing to solubility limitations. Weight gain and nitrogen retention are similar in studies comparing these formulations. Only TrophAmine results in normalization of the amino acid profile compared with normal infants receiving breast milk. TrophAmine has also been associated with a lower incidence of cholestasis.[38]

Lipid emulsions are used as an energy source and for prevention of essential fatty deficiency. The high caloric density of lipid emulsions (2 kcal/mL for 20% solutions) allows for provision of substantial energy substrate by the peripheral route or when fluid intake is restricted. Lipid emulsions are composed of triglycerides, egg yolk phospholipids, and glycerol. The emulsified fat particles are cleared from the circulation in the same manner as naturally occurring chylomicrons; the resulting triglycerides and phospholipids are then hydrolyzed by lipoprotein lipase to free fatty acids. Allergy to egg proteins, hyperphosphatemia, thrombocytopenia, and deposition of fat emboli in the pulmonary capillaries are potential complications of the use of intravenous lipid emulsion. In neonates, the fatty acids produced by hydrolysis may displace bilirubin from albumin-binding sites, resulting in kernicterus; lipid emulsions should be used with care in infants with hyperbilirubinemia.

A number of technical and metabolic complications are associated with parenteral nutrition. Technical problems are usually related to the central venous catheter and include infection, air embolism, and catheter malposition resulting in pericardial or pleural effusion. Metabolic complications include fluid overload, hyperglycemia, hypoglycemia, electrolyte imbalance, nutritional deficiencies, hyperlipidemia, rickets, and cholestasis, which may lead to chronic liver dysfunction. Careful nutritional assessment before initiation of support (physical examination, growth curves, anthropometrics, immune function, and visceral proteins such as albumin, transferrin, transthyretin [prealbumin] and retinol-binding protein), along with careful monitoring during therapy (Table 100-5), may help to minimize the adverse effects of parenteral nutrition. In this regard, a dedicated team of physicians, nurses, clinical pharmacists, and dietitians is invaluable. The best way to avoid the complications of parenteral nutrition is to avoid using it.

THERMOREGULATION

The fetus exists within a warm, thermally favorable environment. In fact, the high metabolic activity of the fetus (by adult standards) results in excessive heat production, which must be transferred to the mother for dissipation. This is accomplished through placental heat transfer and conductance through the fetal skin to the amniotic fluid and uterine wall. Fetal heat transfer is closely regulated, and fetal and maternal temperature are tightly linked. This link is referred to as a *heat clamp* and prevents independent temperature regulation before birth.[39]

After birth, heat transfer from the infant to the environ-

Table 100-5. MONITORING NUTRITIONAL SUPPORT

ASSESSMENT AT INITIATION OF NUTRITIONAL SUPPORT AND DAILY

Body weight
Intake and output
Chemstrips or urinalysis for glucose and ketones
Medication changes
Serum electrolytes (until stable)

ASSESSMENT AT INITIATION OF NUTRITIONAL SUPPORT AND WEEKLY*

Serum electrolytes, calcium, magnesium, and potassium
Serum albumin
Total or direct bilirubin
Alkaline phosphatase
Hepatic transaminases
Complete blood count

ASSESSMENT AS INDICATED

Trace elements (zinc, copper, iron)
Ammonia

---

* Every 2 to 4 weeks if long-term and stable.

ment occurs through four mechanisms: conduction, convection, radiation, and evaporation. *Conduction* is the direct transfer of heat between solid bodies in contact (such as the infant and the mattress). The rate of heat transfer is dependent on the thermal gradient between the two bodies and their thermal conductivity. When infants are placed on a thick mattress pad, which is an excellent insulator and can be warmed within an incubator or radiant warmer, conductive heat loss is expected to be low. *Convection* is the transfer of heat from the infant's skin to the surrounding air. The heated air expands and is displaced upward by the heavier surrounding air, resulting in bulk flow of heated gas away from the infant's skin. Convection is related to the air velocity around the infant and the surface temperature. Convection is also related to surface area, resulting in substantially larger convection heat losses in small, premature infants compared than in term infants. *Radiation* heat loss is due to the emission of electromagnetic energy from an object (the infant); the spectrum of emitted radiation is a function of the temperature of the object. *Evaporation* is physically similar to convection, except that water is transported from the skin surface rather than kinetic energy. The skin of term infants provides a substantial barrier to the transport of water and thus to evaporative water loss. Premature infants, however, have thin skin, which provides little resistance to evaporative water loss.[40]

Exposure to environmental cold stress evokes compensatory thermogenic responses. Principal among these responses is nonshivering thermogenesis of brown fat, mediated by the sympathetic nervous system. Sympathetic stimulation results in the release of norepinephrine onto the surface of adipose cells, activation of β-receptors, and activation of intracellular lipoprotein lipase, which in turn releases free fatty acids for hydrolysis. Nonshivering thermogenesis becomes quantitatively less important during maturation. Shivering mechanisms are intact in newborns, although these mechanisms are of lesser importance in infants than adults. During shivering, random muscle contractions result in hydrolysis of adenosine triphosphate and dissipation of energy as heat, without associated mechanical work.

The components of the temperature regulatory mechanism are intact in the human neonate; no substantial differences in neuronal or hormonal control mechanisms have been described between neonatal and adult thermoregulatory systems. The capacity of the metabolic systems to control temperature in term infants is comparable to adults when the metabolic rate is related to body mass, but it is too small to compensate for heat loss in as wide a range of ambient temperatures.[41] In premature infants, thermoregulatory responses can be evoked, but either the capacity of the effector systems or the afferent or processing mechanisms are not sufficiently adjusted to the smaller body size to affect temperature stability.[42] This, combined with substantially increased heat loss due to convection and evaporation, places the premature infant at substantial risk for temperature instability and cold stress.

Reducing metabolic rate by keeping premature infants warm favorably affects morbidity and mortality and favorably influences growth. Although swaddling may be effective for healthy term infants, ill infants must be exposed to provide access to their caregivers. Temperature stabilization is usually provided by either an incubator (a closed plastic system with servo-controlled heated and humidified atmosphere) or a radiant warmer (an open platform with low plastic sides, and a servo-controlled heating coil that warms the infant's skin by convection). An effort is made to provide a thermoneutral environment; that is, no increase in resting metabolic rate is required to maintain temperature stability. The servo-regulation is generally based on probes placed on the skin, however, and the appropriate set-point skin temperature needed to achieve thermoneutrality is unclear.

CARDIOVASCULAR PHYSIOLOGY

The cardiovascular system plays the central role of oxygen and substrate delivery to the tissues and removal of carbon dioxide and waste products. During the course of fetal development and transition to postnatal life, many changes in cardiac function and the central circulation are required to perform this function efficiently. Adequate respiratory function is essential to this process. In fact, in postnatal life, the pulmonary and systemic vascular beds are in series, and the physiology of the systems is interdependent. In this section, the function of the heart and central circulation are considered through the various phases of fetal development and transition to postnatal life.

Fetal Circulation

The placenta is the organ of gas exchange, the source of substrates, and the organ of end-product removal for the fetus. To achieve the most efficient circulatory function, blood returning to the right ventricle should be relatively desaturated and lower in substrate concentration; right ventricular output should be directed to the umbilical–placental circulation. Blood flowing to the left ventricle should be more highly saturated and higher in substrate concentration; left ventricular output should be directed to the fetal body, allowing the left ventricle to fulfill its role as the oxygen delivery ventricle. This is accomplished through various streaming patterns. The nonuniform flow of blood is achieved by the anatomic structure of the atria and the foramen ovale and by the presence of central vascular channels—the ductus arteriosus and the ductus venosus (Fig. 100-1).

Desaturated blood returning to the heart from the brain and upper body (through the superior vena cava) and the heart (through the coronary sinus) flows through the atrium and across the tricuspid valve into the right ventricle. Blood in the inferior vena cava is derived from two sources: (1) desaturated blood from the lower body and splanchnic circulation (which largely flows across the tricuspid valve into the right ventricle), and (2) oxygenated blood from the umbilical–placental circulation, which enters the inferior vena cava primarily from the ductus venosus. The more highly oxygenated blood streams along the medial aspect of the inferior vena cava and is directed across the foramen ovale into the left atrium.

Because pulmonary vascular resistance is high, only a fraction of right ventricular output flows to the lungs (about 13% in fetal lambs). The remaining right ventricular output flows across the ductus arteriosus to the descending aorta. About one third of this blood flows to the fetal body; the remaining blood flows to the placenta for oxygenation and substrate uptake.

Left ventricular output is even more efficiently streamed. Left ventricular blood is directed primarily to the head and upper extremities. About 80% of the relatively highly saturated left ventricular output is delivered to the fetal body for oxygen and substrate use.

Transitional Circulation

Major changes in central blood flow patterns occur at birth. Many of the changes are a direct result of expansion of the lungs, which results in increased pulmonary blood flow and increased arterial oxygen tension. The initial fall

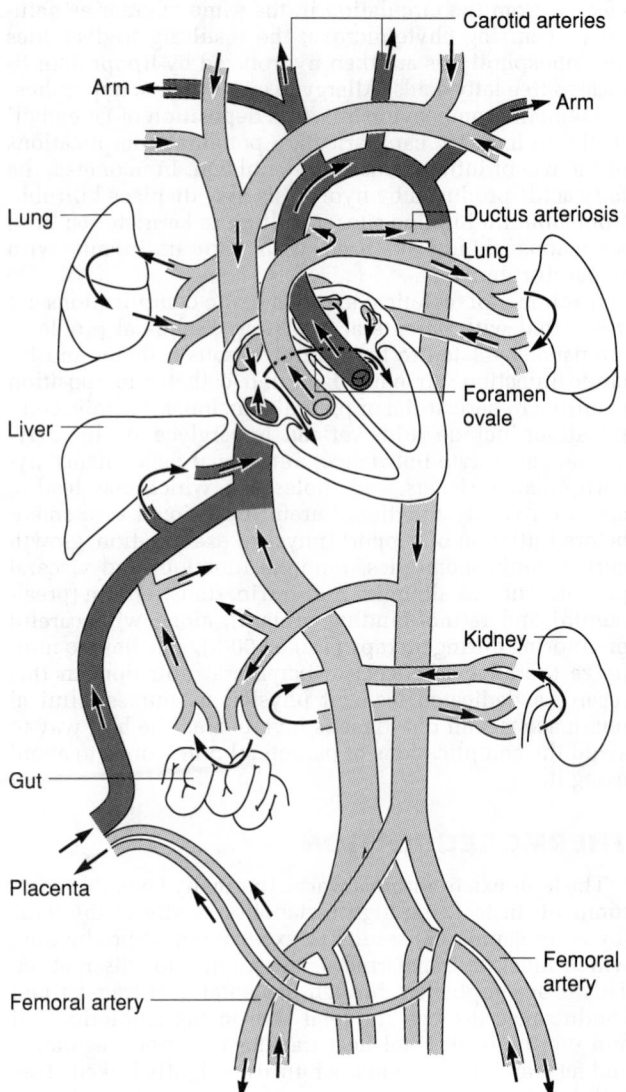

Figure 100-1. Persistent fetal circulation.

in pulmonary vascular resistance is probably due to mechanical factors; continued decreases may be related to prostaglandin release or local changes in PO_2 or PCO_2. Oxygenation causes pulmonary venous return to increase, raising left atrial pressure above right atrial pressure, functionally closing the valvelike flap of the foramen ovale. Closure of the ductus arteriosus begins shortly after birth. The mature ductus arteriosus is responsive to increased oxygen concentration and a variety of other hormonal factors. The final major mechanical event associated with birth is clamping of the umbilical cord. Clamping of the umbilical cord increases systemic vascular resistance, but its effect on central circulatory patterns is limited.

Ventricular output increases dramatically at birth, in part reflecting enhanced left ventricular filling from increased pulmonary venous return. Maturational changes are demonstrable in both right and left ventricular function with increasing gestational age, at birth, and during postnatal development.[43] This maturational process includes architectural changes in the immature myocyte,[44] changes in expression of various isoforms of contractile proteins,[45–49] maturation of membrane systems, and changes in the passive mechanical properties of the heart (specifically, the immature heart is less compliant than the adult heart[50]).

Shape factor analysis of the ventricles demonstrates a transition from an elongated ellipsoid in fetuses to a more rounded shape in newborns. During fetal development, the interventricular septum is buckled into the left ventricle; the echocardiographic appearance is that of right ventricular overload. At birth, right ventricular work decreases, and left ventricular work increases substantially, resulting in "physiologic hypertrophy" of the left ventricle. In both ventricles, there is a shift of ventricular filling from late to early diastole. Right ventricular function has a profound influence on left ventricular mechanics in neonates. Atrial contraction makes an important contribution to ventricular filling in neonates; arrhythmias that result in loss of normal atrioventricular synchrony can significantly impair ventricular filling.

Monitoring and Hemodynamic Assessment

Aerobic metabolism is dependent on a constant and adequate supply of oxygen. The goal of cardiorespiratory support (systems with an integrated and interdependent role in tissue oxygen delivery) is to ensure adequate oxygen delivery (DO_2) to the tissues to meet oxygen demand:

$$DO_2 = CaO_2 \times CI$$

where:
oxygen content (CaO_2) = [Hgb (g/dL) $\times$ 1.36 (mL O_2/g Hgb) $\times$ %O_2 sat] + [PaO_2 (mmHg) $\times$ 0.003 (mL O_2/mmHg)]; CI = cardiac index

Thus, the primary mechanisms for increasing oxygen delivery are increasing hemoglobin concentration, increasing arterial saturation, and increasing cardiac output.

This approach to cardiorespiratory support (ie, adequate oxygen delivery to meet or exceed oxygen demand) applies to certain types of shock states, such as hypovolemia, profound anemia, arterial hypoxia due to failed alveolar gas exchange or transpulmonary shunt, or cardiogenic shock. The adequacy of oxygen delivery must be assessed and interventions tailored to correct the suboptimal components of the oxygen delivery equation. This assessment may be straightforward (such as transfusion to correct profound anemia) or extremely complex, particularly when multiple factors contribute to failure of oxygen delivery.

The adequacy of oxygen delivery to the cells is not easily assessed. This determination is made by a combination of clinical assessment, noninvasive monitoring, laboratory evaluation, and, if indicated by the patient's condition, invasive monitoring. In the course of this assessment, the physician gains insight into which components of the oxygen delivery equation require intervention.

Clinical assessment includes examination of the patient, review of vital signs and trends (Table 100-6), and evaluation of end-organ function. A great deal of information can be garnered by assessment of organ perfusion and function, including mentation, warmth and perfusion of the skin, determination of capillary refill, quality of peripheral pulses, and quality and quantity of urine production. Noninvasive monitoring includes the use of devices that do not require indwelling catheters or probes. Continuous electrocardiographic monitoring is routinely indicated in the pediatric or neonatal intensive care unit for the rapid identification of arrhythmias or bradycardia. Echocardiography may be used to assess ventricular performance as well as to evaluate structural abnormalities of the heart and great vessels; since echocardiography is not available continuously, it is of limited utility in monitoring. Arterial oxygen saturation may be determined by pulse oximetry and "arterialized" tissue gases measured by continuous transcutaneous monitoring of PO_2 and PCO_2.[51]

Laboratory assessment is also helpful in evaluating the adequacy of oxygen delivery, usually by measurement of the products of anaerobic metabolism (direct measurement of lactic acid in serum or determination of base deficit during arterial blood gas analysis). Other major components of the oxygen content component of the oxygen delivery equation are hemoglobin concentration and oxygen saturation, which should be measured by automated blood count and arterial blood gas sampling, respectively. PO_2 is a relatively minor contributor to oxygen content; however, PO_2 is an important indicator of pulmonary gas exchange.

In infants and children with uncertain hemodynamic status or in whom the appropriate interventions remain unclear after clinical and noninvasive assessment, invasive monitoring is indicated. *Arterial catheterization,* using a peripheral artery or one of the umbilical arteries in infants, allows continuous measurement of arterial blood pressure and access for sampling of arterial blood. Umbilical catheters can be introduced into the vessel through the umbilical stump or by cutdown on the umbilicus. The catheter should be positioned with its tip below the renal arteries, near the middle of the L3 vertebra. Infection and vascular complications (arterial insufficiency, thrombosis, and embolization) are the main disadvantages of arterial catheterization. *Central venous catheters* may be placed for hemodynamic monitoring, when peripheral venous access cannot be established, for infusion of TPN, or for administration of drugs that cannot be given peripherally. Measurement of central venous pressure from the superior vena cava or right atrium presupposes a proportional relation between right heart and left heart filling pressures. Pulmonary disease, cardiac lesions, positive-pressure ventilation, pneumothorax, abdominal distention, and pericardial tamponade may disturb this relation and limit the accuracy of central venous pressure in assessing filling pressures. *Pulmonary artery catheters* are used for the mea-

---

Table 100-6. NORMAL RANGE OF VITAL SIGNS

Age	Heart Rate (beats/min)	Systolic Blood Pressure (mmHg)	Diastolic Blood Pressure (mmHg)	Respiratory Rate (breaths/min)
Premature infant				
1 kg	120–140	36–58	18–38	40
3 kg	120–140	50–72	26–46	40
Term infant	120	65–80	30–50	40
0–12 mo*	100–120	105	65	40
1–6 y*	100	105–110	70	30
6–12 y*	80	110–125	70–80	20

* 90th percentile.
(Adapted from Horan MJ. Report of the Second Task Force on Blood Pressure Control in Children—1987. Pediatrics 1987;79:1)

surement of central venous pressure, pulmonary artery occlusion pressure, and cardiac output (by thermodilution technique). Pulmonary artery occlusion pressure reflects left ventricular filling pressure, an indication of preload. Resistance in the pulmonary and systemic vascular beds can be calculated from the pressure and cardiac output data. Pulmonary artery catheters are available in 4F (double lumen) and 5F and 8F (triple lumen) sizes and can be placed in even the smallest infant.

Perhaps the single most sensitive indicator of oxygen delivery is *venous oxygen saturation monitoring* (venous oximetry). Using reflectance spectrophotometry technology, reflected light from red blood cells is transmitted by fiberoptic bundles in a special pulmonary artery catheter. The wavelengths of light are selected to measure oxyhemoglobin and deoxyhemoglobin to determine the percentage saturation of hemoglobin in the mixed venous blood. Measurement of oxygen saturation in the blood (SvO_2) returning to the right side of the heart reflects not only oxygen delivery but also oxygen use in the tissues. Normal mixed venous oxygen saturation (68% to 78%) reflects an appropriate balance between oxygen delivery and oxygen use. Uncompensated changes in oxygen delivery (decreased cardiac index, arterial desaturation, or anemia) result in decreased venous oxygen saturation, while peripheral arteriovenous shunting or decreased oxygen use (as seen in systemic sepsis or cyanide toxicity) result in increased saturation.

Systemic sepsis differs dramatically from other shock states. Rather than the uncompensated decrease in oxygen delivery seen with most shock states, sepsis causes maldistribution of blood flow and inefficient oxygen use within the cells, often leading to a hyperdynamic state. Mediators of the septic response and the unique features of sepsis in the immature patient are discussed later.

A final look at the oxygen delivery equation helps to develop an algorithm for management of shock states due to inadequate oxygen delivery:

$$DO_2 = CaO_2 \times CI$$

Correction of abnormalities of the primary components of the oxygen content part of the equation—hemoglobin concentration and oxygen saturation—is intuitive. The effect of hemoglobin concentration on oxygen content is depicted in Figure 100-2. Oxygen saturation may be enhanced by respiratory support techniques, which are detailed in the next section. After these components of the oxygen delivery equation have been optimized, enhancement of oxygen delivery by improving cardiac index becomes the major objective of hemodynamic monitoring and support.

Cardiac output, the volume of blood ejected from the heart each minute, is the product of the stroke volume (the amount ejected with each beat) and the heart rate (beats per minute). Throughout maturation, ventricular output is the result of complex interactions among heart rate, diastolic filling, the inotropic state of the myocardium, and afterload.

In fetuses and neonates, the maximum rate of rise of ventricular pressure (dP/dt_{max}) is positively affected by an increase in heart rate, in a fashion similar to that observed in adults.[52] This rate-induced increase in dP/dt_{max} occurs over a wide range of heart rates, despite a rate-induced fall in ventricular end-diastolic volume.[53] Endogenous stimulation of heart rate often has a positive effect on ventricular output because the same stimuli often enhance inotropy and venous return. Isolated increases in heart rate (as by atrial pacing), however, may actually decrease ventricular output through a heart rate–induced decrease in diastolic filling time and thus a decrease in end-diastolic volume.

The Frank-Starling relation (correlating contractile force with initial fiber length) can be demonstrated in the immature heart, although its functional importance is controversial. When dP/dt_{max} is used to assess the effects of changes in end-diastolic volume (preload), there is a positive effect of volume loading on ventricular function.[54] When ventricular output is used to assess the effect of volume infusions, little functional reserve in the Frank-Starling relation is demonstrated.[55] This finding may be due to the relatively low compliance of the fetal myocardium; changes in filling pressures may result in trivial changes in end-diastolic volume and therefore initial fiber length. Thus, a combination of maturational changes in ventricular size, compliance, and ventricular interaction may contribute to the quantitative differences in the effect of preload observed between the immature and the adult heart.[50,56]

The immature myocardium responds to inotropic interventions in a manner qualitatively similar to that in adults. The overall effect of a given inotropic agent on ventricular performance is dependent on concurrent alterations in afterload, heart rate, and end-diastolic volume.

Ventricular function of the immature heart is also influenced by afterload in a manner similar to that in adults, although there are quantitative differences. When shortening against the same load, the immature myocardium shortens more slowly and by a smaller amount than the adult myocardium. This difference is probably due to structural differences in the ventricular myocardium.[53]

Persistent Pulmonary Hypertension of the Newborn

A number of in utero and perinatal insults result in the reestablishment of a fetal circulatory pattern in newborns. This is caused by increases in pulmonary vascular resistance, often resulting in increases in pulmonary arterial pressure to suprasystemic levels. This results in shunting of unsaturated blood from the pulmonary circulation to the systemic circulation through the patent ductus arteriosus or the foramen ovale. The pulmonary hypertension results in increased right ventricular strain and ultimately right ventricular failure; buckling of the interventricular septum into the left ventricle impedes filling of the left ventricle, eventually leading to biventricular failure. The combined effects of decreased cardiac output and arterial desaturation result in decreased oxygen delivery to the tissues and, eventually, failure of cellular oxidative metabolism.

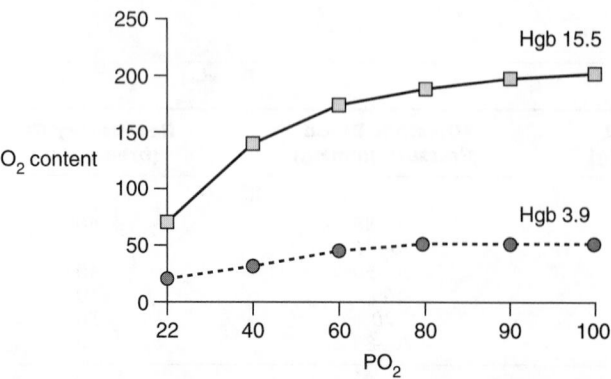

Figure 100-2. Oxygen content as a function of hemoglobin concentration.

In some instances, the increase in pulmonary vascular resistance appears to be primarily due to abnormal reactivity of the pulmonary vasculature (meconium aspiration syndrome, sepsis, idiopathic pulmonary hypertension). Hypoxia has been recognized since the 1960s to elicit an intense vasoconstrictor response in the pulmonary arterioles. The role of other mediators, including prostaglandins and endothelins, has been difficult to study. Developmental abnormalities, including space-occupying lesions in the chest (congenital diaphragmatic hernia, congenital cystic adenomatoid malformation of the lung), often result in pulmonary hypoplasia and abnormal development of the pulmonary vasculature (decreased total cross-sectional area, increased perivascular smooth muscle, and abnormal extension of the smooth muscle in the pulmonary arteries beyond the level of the terminal bronchioles). Mechanical injury resulting from positive-pressure ventilation can result in similar changes and in the development of pulmonary hypertension over an extended period.

Pulmonary hypertension resulting in right-to-left shunting often causes a vicious cycle of progressive hypoxia and worsening pulmonary hypertension, which can rapidly lead to death. Management has focused on factors recognized to lower pulmonary vascular resistance, including alkalosis[57] and hyperventilation.[58] Unfortunately, the effect of alkalinization does not appear to be sustained,[59] and the high ventilatory pressures required to achieve hyperventilation often result in significant barotrauma. Studies have demonstrated that an increase in both alveolar oxygen concentration (PAO_2) and arterial oxygen (PaO_2), by increasing inspired oxygen concentration, can result in reduction of pulmonary vascular resistance.[58] Vasodilators, such as tolazoline and prostaglandin E, have not been consistently useful in treatment because they are not selective for the pulmonary circulation and often result in severe systemic hypotension.[60] Addition of nitric oxide to the respiratory gases is a promising new therapy. Inhaled nitric oxide promptly relaxes pulmonary vascular smooth muscle; nitric oxide is rapidly inactivated by hemoglobin, so there is little, if any, systemic effect.[61,62] When the predicted mortality rate exceeds 80%, extracorporeal life support techniques may be the only rescue available.

RESPIRATORY PHYSIOLOGY

Development of the lung includes the processes of growth and maturation.[63] Lung growth is primarily influenced by physical factors, including intrathoracic space, lung liquid volume and pressure, and amniotic fluid volume. Lung liquid volume is particularly critical for lung growth. Experimentally, fetal tracheal ligation has been shown to increase retention of lung fluid and intratracheal pressure, resulting in lung hyperplasia.[64] This effect can reverse the experimental pulmonary hypoplasia associated with congenital diaphragmatic hernia and oligohydramnios and thus may be relevant to the prenatal management of these entities clinically.

Structural maturation of the lung (multiplication and thinning of the alveolar walls) is also regulated by physical factors. Physical factors that produce hypoplasia also produce structurally immature lungs, while factors that produce hyperplasia result in structurally mature lungs. *Biochemical maturation* of the lungs refers primarily to the maturation of the surfactant system, which appears to be hormonally mediated (adrenocorticotropin, cortisol, thyroid hormones, and others). This effect is exploited clinically by the use of steroids to promote lung maturation in preterm infants.

Respiratory Mechanics and Gas Exchange

Although a complete discussion of pulmonary mechanics is beyond the scope of this chapter, a basic knowledge of lung volumes and respiratory mechanics is necessary to understand the age-related variations in pulmonary function parameters (Fig. 100-3).

There are four primary lung volumes. The *tidal volume* is the volume of gas inspired or expired during each respiratory cycle. *Expiratory reserve volume* is the volume of gas that can be expired from the end of tidal respiration. *Residual volume* is the volume of gas remaining in the lungs at the end of maximal expiration. *Inspiratory reserve volume* is the volume of gas that can be inspired from the end of tidal inspiration.

There are also four lung capacities, which are combinations of two or more of the primary lung volumes. The *total lung capacity* is the volume of gas in the lungs at the end of maximal inspiration. The total lung capacity is equal to the sum of the residual volume, expiratory reserve volume, tidal volume, and inspiratory reserve volume. The *vital capacity* is the maximal volume of gas that can be expelled from the lung by forceful effort after maximal inspiration. The vital capacity is equal to the sum of the inspiratory reserve volume, tidal volume, and expiratory reserve volume. *Inspiratory capacity* is the maximal volume of gas that can be inspired from resting expiration. Inspiratory capacity is equal to the sum of tidal volume and inspiratory reserve volume. *Functional residual capacity* (FRC) is the volume of gas remaining in the lungs at the end of tidal expiration and is equal to the sum of expiratory reserve volume and residual volume. A critical relation exists between between FRC and the volume of gas in the lung at which conducting airways begin to collapse, which is called the *closing capacity*.

Diseases or conditions that decrease FRC below closing capacity or that increase closing capacity above FRC result in collapse of the involved areas of the lung, adversely affecting gas exchange. In normal children and adults, FRC is well above closing capacity. Closing capacity exceeds FRC in infants, which explains in part the frequency with which young children with respiratory disease progress to acute respiratory failure. In disease processes characterized by decreased FRC (pulmonary edema, adult or infantile respiratory distress syndrome, pneumonitis), respiratory interventions are designed to increase lung volumes

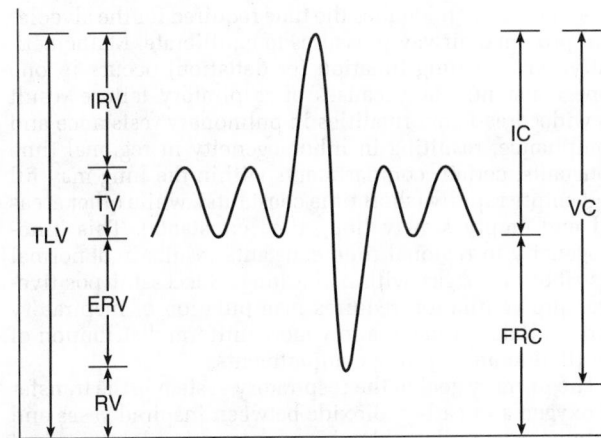

Figure 100-3. Lung volumes and capacities: inspiratory reserve volume (IRV), tidal volume (TV), expiratory reserve volume (ERV), residual volume (RV), total lung volume (TLV), vital capacity (VC), inspiratory capacity (IC), and functional residual capacity (FRC).

toward normal FRC (continuous positive airway pressure [CPAP] or positive end-expiratory pressure [PEEP]). Conditions resulting in increased closing capacity (bronchiolitis, asthma) are managed using bronchodilators and by control of pulmonary secretions.

The rate of entry and exit of gas from the lung is determined by compliance and resistance. Compliance is a measure of the elasticity or distensibility of the lung. The *static compliance* (C_s) is the change in lung volume over the plateau pressure, measured when there is no flow in the airway or the lung. *Dynamic compliance* (C_{dyn}) is the ratio of the change in volume to pressure change at a time when flow in the airway is zero:

$$C_{dyn} = \frac{\Delta V_T}{\Delta P_{TP}}$$

Decreased lung compliance is the most striking abnormality in infants with respiratory distress syndrome and in children with adult respiratory distress syndrome. For gas flow to occur, a pressure gradient must be generated to overcome the nonelastic airway *resistance* of the lungs. Resistance (R) is defined by the pressure gradient (ΔP) required to generate a given flow of gas (V):

$$R = \frac{\Delta P}{V}$$

Physically, resistance results from the friction of movement of gas molecules within the airways (airway resistance) as well as from the friction from motion of the lung and chest wall (tissue viscous resistance). Total airway resistance is determined by a number of factors, including the cross-sectional area of the airway. In adults and older children, the peripheral airways have a large cross-sectional area, and only 20% of the total airway resistance is contributed by airways smaller than 2 mm.[65] In this circumstance, considerable small airway disease may result in little change in total airway resistance. In infants and children, small airways account for about half of total airway resistance, and diseases that alter small airways (eg, bronchiolitis) can lead to dramatic alterations in resistance and significant obstruction to gas flow.

The interaction between compliance and resistance largely determines the distribution of ventilation within the lungs. This interrelation is defined as the *time constant* (TC), the product of the resistance (R) and compliance (C_{dyn}):

$$TC = C_{dyn} \times R$$

The time constant defines the time required for the alveolar and proximal airway pressures to equilibrate. Mathematically, 63% of lung inflation (or deflation) occurs in one time constant. Many causes of respiratory failure result in widespread abnormalities in pulmonary resistance and compliance, resulting in inhomogeneity in regional time constants; certain compartments within the lung may fill and empty rapidly (short time constants), while other areas fill and empty slowly (long time constants). This inhomogeneity in regional time constants results in abnormal distribution of gas within the lung. Successful positive-pressure ventilation requires manipulation of inspiratory and expiratory time to allow more uniform distribution of ventilation among lung compartments.

The primary goal of the respiratory system is the transfer of oxygen and carbon dioxide between inspired gases and pulmonary capillary blood across the alveolus (terminal gas exchange unit). During inspiration, gas is entrained into the respiratory tract, and a portion is distributed to the alveoli; this portion contributes to gas exchange. The remaining gas that does not contribute to alveolar ventila-

tion is referred to as *dead-space ventilation*. Dead-space ventilation can be further defined by the location of the nonparticipating gas; *anatomic dead space* refers to gas contained within the conducting airways, while *alveolar dead space* refers to gas that enters the alveolus but does not contribute to gas exchange. The tidal volume is thus distributed between the total, or physiologic, dead space and those alveoli that participate in gas exchange ($V_{alveolar}$):

$$\text{Tidal volume} = V_{D\ anatomic} + V_{D\ alveolar} + V_{alveolar}$$

An increase in alveolar dead space occurs in a variety of pathophysiologic conditions, such as adult respiratory distress syndrome. Ventilatory strategies may be designed to recruit alveolar dead space for supplemental gas exchange.

Assessment of alveolar ventilation is important in evaluating the adequacy of cardiorespiratory function. The PaO_2 is not a good indicator of alveolar ventilation because it is affected primarily by right-to-left intracardiac or intrapulmonary shunts. Alveolar ventilation is adequately assessed by measurement of the $PaCO_2$. A 50% reduction in pulmonary blood flow results in only a slight increase in the $PaCO_2$, but a 50% reduction in alveolar ventilation results in a doubling of the $PaCO_2$.

Gas exchange across the alveolar–capillary membrane occurs by the process of *diffusion*. Gases move from an area of high partial pressure to an area of low partial pressure. The amount of gas transferred across a semipermeable membrane (Q) is dependent on the partial pressure difference (P1 – P2), the surface area available for diffusion (S), and the diffusion coefficient for the gas (K), and it is inversely related to the distance of diffusion (D):

$$Q = \frac{(P1 - P2) \times K \times S}{D}$$

The diffusion coefficient is directly dependent on the solubility of the gas and inversely proportional to the square of the molecular weight of the gas. The high solubility of carbon dioxide results in a rate of diffusion 20 times that of oxygen, despite the small partial pressure difference between the alveolus and pulmonary capillary.

Efficient gas exchange requires matching of ventilation and perfusion within the lung. Mismatch of ventilation and perfusion is the major cause of arterial hypoxemia associated with respiratory diseases. Blood flow to underventilated alveoli results in increased $PaCO_2$ and decreased PaO_2. carbon dioxide can be eliminated from overventilated alveoli, however, although the PaO_2 is not substantially increased. Thus, ventilation–perfusion mismatch can result in arterial hypoxemia with a normal or even low $PaCO_2$. Respiratory interventions intended to improve ventilation–perfusion inequality include increased concentration of oxygen in inspired gases (FIO_2) or the use of positive airway pressure.

Surfactant

The architecture of the alveolus, and the unique physical–chemical interface created by the interaction of respiratory gases with the surface cells of the respiratory epithelium, creates a region of high surface tension. The pulmonary surfactant complex lowers surface tension, stabilizing the alveolus even at low lung volumes (and thus preventing atelectasis). Surfactant is a complex material, secreted by the type II alveolar cells lining the distal respiratory epithelium. Surfactant is composed primarily of phospholipid (80% to 90%) and unique surfactant-associated proteins (10%). The most abundant phospholipid is phosphatidylcholine, which is uniquely enriched in disaturated forms of palmitoylphosphatidylcholine (DPPC).[66] The molecular structure of the phospholipids, with polar head groups and long, hydrophobic fatty acid chains, is essential to their surface tension—reducing properties; the molecules are inherently insoluble in aqueous environments and tend to form complex bilayers, monolayers, and micelles. Surfactant proteins appear to play a critical role in the organization of the phospholipid molecules and modify the surface active properties of the lipids. Three surfactant proteins have been identified: SP-A, SP-B, and SP-C. In addition to their interactions with the phospholipids, surfactant proteins play a role in the uptake and recycling of surfactant by the type II alveolar cells.

Phospholipid synthesis and secretion and the expression of surfactant proteins increase with advancing gestation. The phosphatidylcholine content of amniotic fluid increases substantially during the later one third of human gestation. The ratio of lecithin (phosphatidylcholine) to sphingomyelin (L/S ratio) has been useful in the clinical assessment of respiratory distress syndrome.[67] Amniotic fluid surfactant, phosphatidylglycerol, and DPPC have been used to predict pulmonary maturity.[68]

Surfactant deficiency is the primary factor in the pathophysiology of the neonatal respiratory distress syndrome,[69] and changes in the phospholipid content and the relative abundance of phospholipid species also accompany respiratory failure in older children and adults.[70] The use of exogenous surfactant replacement therapy is under investigation for the treatment of neonatal respiratory distress syndrome. Several types of replacement surfactants are available, including surfactant obtained by lung lavage (which cannot be sterilized), surfactant from amniotic fluid (difficult to harvest enough for widespread use), and organic extracts of surfactant. Phospholipids, such as DPPC, and combinations of DPPC and other phospholipids have also been used. The best known of these is artificial lung-expanding compound, which consists of 70% DPPC and 30% phosphatidylglycerol.[71] The most commonly used replacements in the United States are: Exosurf, a combination of DPPC and two spreading agents (hexadecanol and tyloxapol); and Survanta, an organic extract of minced cow lungs modified for improved dispersion and storage. Other surfactant replacements are under investigation in Japan (Surfactant-TA) and Europe (Curosurf).

Evaluation of Respiratory Function

Clinical examination is important in the assessment of respiratory function. The clinical signs of impending respiratory failure include increased respiratory rate, altered respiratory pattern (including deep, shallow, or irregular breaths), use of accessory muscles, nasal flaring, and expiratory grunting. Auscultation of the chest may help define the nature and location of pulmonary pathology. During the initiation of positive-pressure ventilation, physical examination is important in the assessment of the adequacy of delivered tidal volume, the appropriate inspiratory and expiratory time, and patient–ventilator synchrony.

The chest radiograph is also helpful in evaluating pulmonary pathophysiology. The lung fields should be evaluated for the adequacy of lung volumes and the presence of local underexpansion or overexpansion. The parenchyma should be evaluated for the presence of edema, atelectasis, or consolidation. Finally, the appropriate location of tubes and catheters should be confirmed.

Pulse oximetry is a noninvasive method of determining oxygen saturation. Pulse oximetry technology uses infrared light absorption to compare saturated and unsaturated hemoglobin; oxygen saturation is derived from this comparison. The determination is accurate between 70% and 100% saturation. Adequate perfusion of the region where the probe is located is essential for accurate measurement. Oximetric monitoring should be provided for all patients requiring assisted ventilation or supplemental oxygen and during sedation or anesthesia.

Capnography is the graphic display of airway CO_2 during the respiratory cycle. The maximum CO_2 during exhalation is defined as the end-tidal CO_2. In normal subjects, the end-tidal CO_2 closely approximates the $Paco_2$. Monitoring end-tidal CO_2 is helpful during weaning and in ventilator-dependent patients, and can reduce the required number of arterial blood gas determinations.

Bedside measurement of respiratory mechanics is an exciting new development in evaluation of respiratory function. Traditional spirometry is impractical and requires an awake, cooperative patient. Contemporary systems permit continuous display of gas flow, airway pressures, delivered tidal volume, and calculated compliance, airway resistance, and time constants of the lung. Monitoring of respiratory mechanics allows assessment of the effectiveness and adverse effects of respiratory interventions. The continuous display rapidly indicates alveolar overdistention, stacking of breaths, excessive or inadvertent PEEP, and patient–ventilator dyssynchrony.

Direct measurement of arterial pH, Pco_2, and Po_2 by blood gas analysis is the most accurate method of evaluating the adequacy of gas exchange. Blood gas analysis requires arterial puncture or an indwelling arterial catheter. Another disadvantage of this method is the intermittent nature of the sampling.

Ventilatory Support

Classification of Positive-Pressure Ventilators

A mechanical ventilator is a life-support system designed to replace or support lung function. A ventilator is designed to alter, transmit, and directly apply energy in a predetermined way to perform the work of the thorax and lungs. This section briefly describes the classification of ventilators relevant to clinical respiratory care in infants and children.

Ventilator control variables address the physical qualities adjusted, measured, or used to manipulate the ventilatory cycle. The four common types of control variables are *flow, pressure, volume,* and *time.* Inspiratory flow pattern determines the characteristics of the gas flow delivery during a positive-pressure breath and the distribution of the breath within the respiratory system (Fig. 100-4). Airway pressures are dependent on the mechanical properties of the lungs and the movement of gas into the lungs. The selection of an appropriate inspiratory flow pattern, based on the patient's pulmonary pathophysiology, improves the effectiveness of ventilation, reduces peak inspiratory pressures, minimizes mean airway pressure, and promotes patient–ventilator synchrony.[72]

Ventilatory Modes

Ventilatory modes describe specific breathing patterns used during positive-pressure ventilation and include spontaneous breaths, mechanical breaths, or combinations of both.

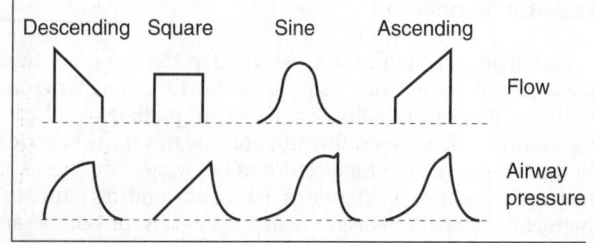

Figure 100-4. Waveform patterns in positive-pressure ventilation

CPAP maintains a constant positive airway pressure above baseline throughout the respiratory cycle to support spontaneous breaths. Raising the expiratory pressure above atmospheric pressure traps a volume of gas in the lungs proportional to the pressure applied and lung compliance. This gas volume augments the expiratory reserve volume and FRC of the lung. CPAP can be used alone or in combination with mechanical breaths.

Pressure support ventilation provides a preset level of inspiratory pressure that is delivered with each spontaneous effort. The tidal volume delivered in this mode varies with changes in lung compliance, airway resistance, and level of pressure support. Pressure support can also be used alone or in combination with other modes.

Positive-pressure breaths can be delivered in a *controlled* or *assist-controlled* manner. During controlled breaths, ventilator cycles are delivered at a preset rate. Inspiratory and expiratory times are fixed and are dependent on the ventilator rate and the preset I:E ratio. The patient cannot trigger additional positive-pressure breaths. Sedation or paralysis may be required to minimize patient–ventilator dyssynchrony. Assisted modes deliver a patient-triggered ventilator breath with each spontaneous effort. The ventilator sensitivity determines the amount of effort required by the patient to trigger the mechanical breath. Control and assisted breaths may be limited by either volume or pressure. The various combinations include *volume control* (a predetermined breath rate is delivered, the breaths are volume limited); *volume assist* (mechanical breaths are volume limited, the patient triggers breaths in excess of the preset rate); *pressure control* (a preset breath rate is delivered with preset pressure limits); and *pressure assist* (a breathing pattern whereby the patient may trigger breaths in excess of the preset rate, and the breaths are pressure limited). A new mode of ventilation that combines these features is *pressure-regulated volume control*; the ventilator monitors the airway resistance and compliance of the lungs and adjusts the inspiratory pressure level to deliver a preset volume limit.

Intermittent mandatory ventilation and *synchronized intermittent mandatory ventilation* modes combine mechanical breaths with spontaneous breathing. In the synchronized mode, the initiation of the mechanical breath is synchronized with the patient's spontaneous effort to prevent stacking of breaths and overdistention of the alveoli.

Neonatal Ventilation

Contemporary neonatal ventilators are flow controlled, time triggered, time cycled, and pressure controlled. Neonatal ventilators provide continuous flow at preset values, and therefore a square wave flow pattern. The square wave flow pattern may increase the risk of barotrauma in patients with immature lungs and abnormal lung parenchyma. Advances in neonatal ventilator design provide the option of volume-controlled synchronized intermittent mandatory ventilation.

Pediatric Ventilation

Pediatric ventilators are essentially the same as those used in adults but are used at lower ranges of flow and volume. The variable flow capability of pediatric and adult ventilators allows pressure and volume to vary in response to the pneumatic characteristics of the lungs. Pressure control and pressure assist modes use a decelerating ramp flow pattern, which decreases peak inspiratory pressures and increases mean airway pressure to recruit collapsed alveoli.[73]

Nonconventional Modes of Ventilation

High-frequency ventilation refers to a group of technologies that use low tidal volumes and high ventilatory rates to minimize the adverse effects of high airway pressures. Adequate alveolar ventilation must be maintained despite delivered tidal volumes that are usually less than the dead-space volume.

High-frequency jet ventilation systems use a high-pressure, air and oxygen gas source to generate gas flow. A solenoid valve interrupts gas flow, regulating the frequency of ventilation between 150 and 600 breaths/min. A specially designed endotracheal tube is required. A second ventilator is also required in tandem to provide PEEP and "sigh" breaths. The mechanism of gas exchange during high-frequency jet ventilation has not been well defined, although convection streaming and molecular diffusion are known to occur.[74] Convection streaming is the bulk flow of gas to the level of the alveoli. Exhalation is passive and is promoted by an extremely short inspiratory time (20 to 40 ms) and relatively long exhalation time. The slower-moving exhaled gas is pushed to the side of the airway lumen by the rapidly moving inspired gas, resulting in a continuous stream of exhaled gas around the inspired gas. Lung volumes remain static around the mean lung volume because the peak pressures are low and the inspiratory times are short. Oxygenation is primarily dependent on mean airway pressures; increasing airway pressure increases lung volumes and improves V/Q mismatching. The primary physiologic advantage is reduction in the peak airway pressures produced compared with conventional positive-pressure ventilation.

High-frequency oscillatory ventilation uses a piston diaphragm oscillator to alternate positive and negative pressures in the airway. Tidal volumes of 1 to 3 mL/kg are generated, with cycles ranging from 900 to 300 breaths/min. Inspiration and expiration are both active, resulting in an increase in overall mean airway pressure. High-frequency oscillatory ventilation has been used successfully in infants with respiratory distress syndrome.[75]

Complications of Ventilatory Support

Oxygen is toxic to the central nervous system, the retina, and the respiratory system. Contributing events include the FIO_2, the duration of exposure, and the underlying respiratory pathophysiology. Oxygen-induced injury in the lung begins with the capillary endothelial cell and eventually leads to destruction of the type I pneumatocyte. Progression of oxygen toxicity results in hyperplasia of type II pneumatocytes, interstitial fibrosis, and eventually end-stage pulmonary fibrosis. Medical management is limited to prevention by limiting inspired oxygen exposure.

Barotrauma is an all-inclusive term that describes pathologic changes resulting from alveolar overdistention. Predisposing factors in the development of barotrauma include preexisting lung pathology, high peak airway pressures, and high levels of PEEP. Barotrauma presents in a variety of forms, including pneumothorax, pneumomediastinum, pneumoperitoneum, pulmonary interstitial emphysema, subpleural air cysts, and hyaline membrane formation.

RENAL PHYSIOLOGY
Renal Function

Unlike the embryogenesis of most organs, which develop as a direct process from a clearly defined anlage, the differentiation of the definitive kidney, or metanephros, requires the successive formation and involution of two embryonic kidneys, the pronephros and mesonephros.[76] In the human, the *pronephros* is a primitive, nonfunctional kidney that appears during the 3rd week of development and regresses by the 5th week. The pronephric duct, which arises from fusion of pronephric tubular buds, persists after pronephric regression to form the mesonephric duct, which in turn evolves into the ureteric bud. The *mesonephros* appears in the 3rd to 4th week of gestation, immediately caudal to the last of the pronephric tubules. The mesonephros develops a filtering apparatus and tubular system. The mesonephros degenerates from the 5th to the 12th week of gestation. Residual mesonephric structures give rise to the ureteric bud and other components of genitourinary development. The *metanephros* develops from the interaction of the ureteric bud with the mesenchymal nephrogenic blastema. The patterned migration and division of the ureteric bud determines the elaborate three-dimensional architecture of the kidney (renal architectonics[77]) and is responsible for the formation of the collecting system. The specific induction of the nephrogenic blastema by the ureteric bud is responsible for individual nephron formation (nephrogenesis). The two processes of architectonics and nephrogenesis occur simultaneously from week 6 through week 36 of gestation. Nephrogenesis is complete at birth in term infants, but nephron formation, along with elongation of the loop of Henle and convolutions of the proximal tubule, continue after birth in preterm infants.[78,79]

Total renal blood flow increases from 2% to 3% of cardiac output in the fetus to 6% to 18% in the 1st month of postnatal life and to 20% to 25% in the adult due to significant decreases in renal vascular resistance.[80] There are also important developmental changes in the intrarenal distribution of blood flow, with increasing blood flow to the outer cortex that parallels the centrifugal morphologic development of the kidney (ie, from medulla to cortex). Glomerular filtration (GFR) is lower in fetuses and preterm infants than in term infants. In absolute terms, GFR in very-low-birthweight infants is only about 40 mL/h, compared with 300 mL/h in term infants. An abrupt increase in GFR is observed coincident with the changes in renal blood flow that occur with the completion of nephrogenesis at 34 to 36 weeks postconceptual age; this increase is observed regardless of whether completion of nephrogenesis is an in utero or a postnatal event.[81] In turn, GFR is substantially decreased in term infants when compared with older children or adults.[82,83]

Tubular function has generally been considered to lag behind glomerular function (glomerulotubular imbalance); however, studies indicate adequate tubular function, even in the preterm neonate. Fractional excretion of sodium (FE_Na) can be useful in the assessment of renal function:

$$FE_{Na} = \frac{\text{urine Na}}{\text{serum Na}} \times \frac{\text{serum Cr}}{\text{urine Cr}} \times 100$$

Studies suggest a steady decline in FE_{Na} during the transition from fetal to postnatal life, from 3.3% in infants less than 34 weeks' gestation, to 1.2% at 34 to 37 weeks' gestation, to 0.4% at term.[84] Urinary sodium losses may be high, however, in preterm infants, particularly those who are critically ill.[85]

Immaturity of tubular function may contribute to alterations in acid–base balance, particularly the development of a metabolic acidosis and difficulty handling an acid load. Newborn infants have a decreased threshold for HCO_3^- reabsorption[86] as well as increased permeability, which may allow backflux of HCO_3^- and thus diminished net resorption.[87] Preterm infants may also have decreased ability to produce NH_3 and may lack urinary buffers to excrete titratable acid.[87]

Neonates generally handle water load appropriately, achieving maximal dilution of urine (30 to 50 mOsm/L). The ability to concentrate the urine, however, is limited to the range of 400 to 600 mOsm/L, probably secondary to diminished tonicity of the medullary interstitium (ie, a poorly established corticomedullary concentrating gradient).

In addition to immaturity of renal function, one must also consider extrarenal factors when attempting to correct fluid and electrolyte abnormalities. For example, positive-pressure ventilation and CPAP have been shown to impair renal perfusion and glomerular filtration.[88,89] In the preterm infant in whom that GFR is already low, these effects can be significant.

Fluid Spaces

The total body water is distributed between the intracellular and extracellular spaces. The extracellular space is further divided into two compartments: the plasma (intravascular) and the interstitial (extravascular) compartments. The intracellular space includes the red blood cell volume as well as the water content of all the noncirculating cells. Together, the plasma and red blood cell volumes add up to the total blood volume.

In the early fetal period, water constitutes about 95% of the fetus. Although the accumulation of water with fetal growth is roughly linear, accretion of solids results in a decrease in the proportion of body water relative to body weight throughout gestation, to 80% at 7 months and 75% at term. Concurrently, there is redistribution of body water among the compartments as the percentage of the body that is extracellular fluid (largely interstitial fluid) sharply declines, while there is a more gradual rise in the percentage of intracellular fluid. This is attributable to changes in cell density, deposition of ground substance in the extracellular matrix, and deposition of body fat in late gestation. This changing distribution continues throughout the neonatal period. Total body water content decreases until about 9 months of age, when it reaches 62%; intracellular water reaches its maximum at 43% of body weight, and the extracellular fluid declines to 30% of body weight. Blood volume is considerably larger in fetuses than in newborns; about one third of the fetal blood volume is contained within the placenta and cord. Blood volume in term newborns is about 80 mL/kg.

Abnormal fetal development can significantly impact the total body water content and the distribution among the compartments. IUGR infants are characterized by increased total body water and extracellular water compared with normal gestational peers. *Hydrops fetalis* is the accumulation of excess fluid in the fetus, producing generalized edema, ascites, and pleural and pericardial effusions. Hydrops varies in severity from mild edema to massive edema and effusions that can result in utero death. Hydrops fetalis develops most commonly as the end stage of severe alloimmune hemolytic anemia (erythroblastosis fetalis), usually due to maternofetal incompatibility for the D antigen in the Rh system. There is a severe hemolytic anemia and enlargement of the liver and spleen from extramedullary hematopoiesis. The pathophysiology underlying the development of hydrops is still not well defined. In some infants, intrauterine transfusion of packed red blood cells into the umbilical vessels may reverse hydrops.[90,91] Nonimmune hydrops occurs in association with a wide variety of conditions, including other anemias, cardiac arrhythmias, structural heart disease, vascular malformations, chest masses (eg, teratomas, adenomatoid malformations, and sequestrations) and storage diseases.[92] The prognosis for nonimmune hydrops is poor; only 20% survive to de-

Table 100-7. ASSESSMENT OF VOLUME STATUS

HISTORY
Underlying illnesses
Nature, magnitude, and duration of fluid loss
Therapeutic interventions

PHYSICAL EXAMINATION
Mild to Moderate Volume Depletion (<10%)

Mild tachycardia
Dry mucous membranes and tears
Concentrated urine and oliguria
Decreased skin turgor
Sunken eyeballs and fontanelle

Severe Volume Depletion (>10%)

Increased severity of above signs
Hypotension
Absent or poor-quality peripheral pulse
Delayed capillary refill
Cool, clammy skin
Anuria
Depressed mentation

---

livery, and only 40% to 50% of those liveborn ultimately survive.

Fluid and Electrolyte Management

The combination of immature glomerular and tubular function, changes in distribution of body fluids, and altered requirements for water and major electrolytes due to growth and enhanced losses make fluid and electrolyte management of preterm and term infants and children particularly challenging. This is especially true when injury due to trauma or operation, infection, or other underlying disease is superimposed on already complex fluid and electrolyte requirements.

Correct assessment of fluid and electrolyte status (and therefore determination of the correct interventions) requires a review of the patient history, physical examination, laboratory studies, and monitoring data (Table 100-7). Evaluation of the *history* should include known underlying illnesses and the nature, magnitude, and duration of fluid and electrolyte losses. The number of wet diapers during the past 24 hours may indicate the hydration status. It is also important to review therapy that was administered at home or by another physician. Often, an easily recognizable pattern of fluid and electrolyte abnormalities is apparent from the history alone. For example, chronic vomiting due to gastric outlet obstruction (such as pyloric stenosis) results in a hypokalemic, hypochloremic metabolic alkalosis due to the loss of hydrochloric acid, while intractable diarrhea often results in substantial loss of HCO_3^-, resulting in metabolic acidosis.

The *physical examination* gives important information on total body water status and the distribution of fluid between compartments. Documented changes in body weight are an important indicator of overall fluid status. Tenting of the skin, dry mucous membranes, and sunken fontanelle (in infants) are all indicators of moderate dehydration. Hemodynamic instability, manifested by tachycardia, hypotension, cool and clammy skin, delayed capillary refill, decreased quality of peripheral pulses, or altered end-organ function (eg, mentation, urine output) is indicative of severe volume losses that require immediate correction. Volume overload is suggested by dependent soft tissue edema or evidence of pulmonary edema.

Useful laboratory studies include the serum electrolyte profile (Na^+, K^+, Cl^-, CO_2), blood urea nitrogen, creatinine, lactic acid, and arterial blood gas analysis (pH, base deficit or excess). These studies, however, are useful only in the context of the history and physical examination; for example, hyponatremia may be the result of excessive sodium loss with inadequate replacement (perhaps due to diuretic therapy) or water intoxication.

Fluid and electrolyte therapy is initiated when the patient assessment is completed and a plan is formulated. (Resuscitation of hemodynamically compromised patients should begin immediately, with modifications to the plan as necessary.) Therapy is conveniently divided into *maintenance* requirements, correction of existing *deficits,* and *replacement* of ongoing losses. When the plan is formulated and therapy initiated, the most important factor in successful fluid and electrolyte management comes into play: frequent evaluation of the success of therapy, with modifications of the plan as necessary. This evaluation should include review of vital signs, urine output, accurate input and output data, weight, and repeat laboratory assessment as necessary.

Maintenance Requirements

Maintenance therapy refers to the administration of water and major electrolytes for growth and replacement of obligatory losses resulting from respiration, evaporation (transepithelial water loss), metabolism, and renal excretion of wastes. Maintenance requirements reflect the total of *insensible* losses (eg, respiration, evaporation) and *sensible* (or measurable) loss of water, such as urine or stool.

Maintenance water requirements can be estimated based on body weight or surface area (Table 100-8). Water requirements in infants less than 10 kg are roughly 100 mL/kg/24 h or 1500 to 1800 mL/m^2/24 h. Maintenance fluids are often decreased in the first 48 hours of life (60 to 80 mL/kg/24 h), reflecting the rapid decrease in the extracellular fluid compartment that occurs after birth and the decreased ability of the immature kidney to excrete a water load. Water requirements may be substantially increased in premature infants (120 to 160 mL/kg/24 h) due to increased transepithelial water loss, particularly when there is increased evaporative loss (radiant warmer). In older infants and children, water requirements can be calculated based on body weight according to the following formula: 100 mL/kg/24 h (first 10 kg) + 50 mL/kg/24 h (second 10 kg) + 20 mL/kg/24 h (more than 20 kg).

Sodium requirements are about 2 to 3 mEq/kg/24 h (30 to 50 mEq/m^2/24 h). Sodium requirements may be slightly increased in premature infants owing to decreased tubular resorption. Potassium requirements are about 2 to 4 mEq/kg/24 h. Calcium is not usually required in maintenance fluids because of to the large skeletal stores. Hypocalcemia,

---

Table 100-8. MAINTANENCE WATER AND ELECTROLYTE REQUIREMENTS

	Holliday-Segar Method*	Body Surface Area Method
Water	<10 kg: 100 mL/kg 10–20 kg: 1000 mL + 50 mL/kg over 10 >20 kg: 1500 mL + 20 mL/kg over 20	1500–1800 mL/m^2/24 h
Sodium	3 mEq/100 mL H$_2$O/24 h	30–50 mEq/m^2/24 h
Potassium	2 mEq/100 mL H$_2$O/24 h	20–40 mEq/m^2/24 h

* Caloric expenditure estimates based on body weight alone; assumes 100 mL H$_2$O is required for each 100 kcal metabolized.

however, is common in newborns (see earlier), and calcium supplementation may be required for several days.

Correction of Existing Deficits or Excesses

The second component of fluid and electrolyte management is correction of existing deficits or excesses. Again, this requires assimilation of the history, physical findings, and laboratory studies to assess the relative magnitude of water and electrolyte loss or excess and therefore to determine the appropriate composition of the replacement fluid.

The principal extracellular cation is Na^+, and it is convenient and relevant to express the magnitude of water gain or loss relative to the loss of Na^+. Significant increase in total body water relative to total body Na^+ results in hyponatremia due to *water intoxication*. Water intoxication may occur due to excessive intake of free water (eg, freshwater drowning, use of tap water for enemas) or inappropriate retention of free water, most commonly due to secretion of antidiuretic hormone, often seen after head injury. The appropriate therapy in this circumstance is water restriction. A significant decrease in total body water relative to Na^+ results in volume *contraction* and hypernatremia; common causes include inadequate free water intake or failure of tubular reabsorption of free water (usually due to inadequate antidiuretic hormone or *diabetes insipidus*). Appropriate therapy depends on the underlying cause; free water intake should be increased, and exogenous ADH should be considered in cases of diabetes insipidus.

Increased total body Na^+ relative to total body water results in volume *expansion* and hypernatremia. The most common cause is excessive Na^+ intake, often administered inadvertently (there is a substantial amount of Na^+ in some antibiotics and in sodium bicarbonate solutions administered for the correction of acidosis). Sodium restriction is the appropriate management. Sodium deficit relative to total body water results in hyponatremia and volume contraction; common causes include inadequate replacement of sodium losses and increased sodium excretion due to diuretic therapy. The sodium deficit can be calculated from the measured serum Na^+ and the volume of distribution of sodium:

$$Na^+_{deficit} = (Na^+_{desired} - Na^+_{measured}) \times weight\ (Kg) \times 0.6$$

Potassium is principally an intracellular cation; serum levels do not reflect total body stores. The serum level is critical to muscle (including myocardial) and nerve function, however, and must be maintained within relatively close limits. Hypokalemia most often results from increased renal potassium loss associated with diuretic therapy. Other causes include inadequate intake, unreplaced gastrointestinal losses, and alkalotic states in which K^+ is transported intracellularly in exchange for H^+. Clinically, hypokalemia can result in hypotonia, tetany, and decreased concentrating ability. Electrocardiographic changes include ST-segment depression, flattened T waves, and the presence of U waves. Treatment includes modification of diuretic therapy (if appropriate) and oral or intravenous K^+ supplementation. It is generally safe to administer 1 mEq/kg as potassium chloride or phosphate; the bolus should be administered slowly, with continuous ECG monitoring.

False hyperkalemia occurs commonly, the result of hemolysis of the sample when blood is withdrawn through small-gauge needles. True hyperkalemia is associated with renal insufficiency, excessive potassium intake, use of potassium-sparing diuretics, and severe acidosis. Hyperkalemia often occurs in the course of critical illness, associated with massive cellular injury. ECG changes include peaked T waves, widening of the QRS complex, and flattened P waves. Untreated hyperkalemia can progress to ventricular fibrillation and cardiac standstill. Treatment includes cessation of exogenous potassium supplementation, use of a cation exchange resin such as polystyrene sulfonate (Kayexalate), administration of supplemental Ca^{2+} (10% calcium gluconate, 0.5 mL/kg), administration of glucose and insulin (glucose, 2 g/kg plus insulin 0.5 U/kg), or alkalinization by the administration of sodium bicarbonate (2 to 3 mEq/kg). Life-threatening hyperkalemia may require exchange transfusion or dialysis.

Acidosis due to inadequate oxygen delivery should be corrected by improving oxygen delivery, using the strategies discussed previously. The administration of sodium bicarbonate should be reserved for refractory acidosis (pH below 7.10) or for correction of unreplaced loss of bicarbonate in the urine (renal tubular acidosis, carbonic anhydrase inhibitors) or from the gastrointestinal tract (diarrhea, excessive ostomy output, fistula). An estimation of the amount of bicarbonate required to correct the pH to 7.40 can be calculated based on the base deficit (from blood gas analysis) and the volume of distribution:

$$mEq\ HCO_3^- = base\ deficit \times weight\ (Kg) \times 0.3$$

Replacement of Ongoing Losses

The final component of fluid and electrolyte management is replacement of ongoing losses. These includes losses from nasogastric tubes, thoracostomy tubes, drains, excessive gastrointestinal losses (diarrhea, ostomies, fistulas), biliary or pancreatic drainage, or leakage of peritoneal fluid (eg, abdominal wall defects). These losses may be substantial and are of relatively greater importance in smaller patients (premature and term newborns, infants). In general, the safest approach is replacement of these losses on a milliliter by milliliter basis with a fluid of comparable composition (Table 100-9). Pleural and peritoneal fluid losses can result in the loss of a substantial amount of protein, which must be replaced to maintain plasma oncotic pressure. This may be accomplished by use of a protein-containing replacement solution or by administration of exogenous albumin (1 g/kg 25% albumin) on an as-needed basis as determined by the serum albumin and total protein. The administration of exogenous albumin is advocated solely for the maintenance of oncotic pressure and should be accompanied by adequate nutritional support. In the face of protein catabolism, the circulating half-life of exogenous albumin is short, and it becomes an expensive method of supplementing protein intake.

The most difficult ongoing loss to replace appropriately is the third-space loss, which results from the movement of intravascular fluid to the extravascular space owing to loss of capillary integrity associated with injury, operation, or sepsis. The resulting loss of cardiac preload adversely effects hemodynamics and oxygen delivery. As discussed earlier, restoration of circulating intravascular volume (and thus preload) is the first goal of hemodynamic support (see Monitoring and Hemodynamic Assessment).

The fluid lost to the third space is essentially plasma, so the replacement solution should be comparable in composition. A balanced salt solution (such as lactated Ringer solution) or colloid solution (such as Plasmanate) is an appropriate replacement solution. The replacement should be administered as a bolus; a volume of 10 to 20 mL/kg is almost always an appropriate starting point.

Again, fluid and electrolyte management is a dynamic process, requiring frequent reassessment of the patient's status and response to management, with appropriate modification of the management strategy.

Table 100-9. COMPOSITION OF BODY FLUIDS

Source	Na$^+$ (mEq/L)	K$^+$ (mEq/L)	Cl$^-$ (mEq/L)	HCO$_3^-$ (mEq/L)	Protein (g/dL)	Suggested Replacement
Gastric	20–80	5–20	100–150	—	—	0.45% NaCl + 10 mEq/L Cl
Pancreatic	120–140	5–15	40–80	115	—	LR or 0.45% NaCl + 50 mEq/L NaHCO$_3$
Bile	120–140	5–15	80–120	100–115	—	LR or 0.45% NaCl + 50 mEq/L NaHCO$_3$
Ileostomy	45–135	3–15	20–115	30–50	—	LR or 0.45% NaCl + 25 mEq/L NaHCO$_3$
Diarrhea	10–90	10–80	10–110	30–50	—	LR or 0.45% NaCl + 25 mEq/L NaHCO$_3$
Pleural or peritoneal	140	5	100	25	6–8	LR + 5% albumin or plasmanate

LR, lactated Ringer solution.

HEPATIC PHYSIOLOGY

The development of the liver begins during week 3 or 4 of gestation and is presented in detail in Chapter 103. Even when substantially immature, hepatocytes begin secretion of hepatic proteins, such as α-fetoprotein, α_1-antitrypsin, and transferrin.[93,94] Maturation of lipid and carbohydrate synthetic function lags behind that of proteins. The bile ducts are derived from the primitive hepatocytes.[95] These cells tend to form small cysts close to the portal vein branches, which fuse to form contiguous bile ducts.[96] Formation of the ducts begins at the hilum and extends peripherally. About 70% to 80% of the total hepatic blood flow in utero is contributed by the highly oxygenated blood of the umbilical vein. The umbilical vein enters the liver through the falciform ligament, makes connections with the portal vein, and continues on as the ductus venosus. The remainder of the blood flow to the fetal liver is unsaturated blood from the portal vein, with a negligible contribution from the hepatic artery.[97]

After formation during the first trimester, the liver grows linearly throughout the remainder of gestation. Bile secretory function is decreased during fetal life, and studies suggest metabolic and secretory functions related to bile acid metabolism remain immature in neonates, leading to a particular susceptibility to cholestasis.[98] In addition, a number of hepatic enzyme systems are functionally immature in term infants and almost nonexistent in extremely preterm infants,[99] leading to alterations in the metabolism and excretion of endogenous and exogenous substrates and xenobiotics.

Enzyme Function and Pharmacokinetics

A number of factors affect the metabolism and elimination of drugs in newborns. The apparent volume of distribution of drugs is altered by the differences in total body water and the low percentage of body fat. These differences in apparent volume of distribution can influence the loading doses of various drugs. Qualitative and quantitative differences in plasma proteins can influence protein binding and thus the availability of free drug to the infant. Immature glomerular and tubular function can influence the renal elimination of drugs. Finally, immature hepatic enzyme systems can influence biotransformation reactions, which then affect the elimination of any drug that cannot be excreted in an unchanged form.

Two main categories of biotransformation reactions are important in drug elimination: nonsynthetic reactions (oxidation, reduction, hydrolysis) and conjugation or synthetic reactions. Although the enzymes mediating these reactions are present at birth, the functional immaturity of the newborn liver limits its ability to perform these functions.[99] Premature infants have even greater impairment of enzymatic functions. Certain drugs, such as phenobarbital, have been used clinically to stimulate hepatic microsomal enzyme function nonspecifically during the neonatal period.

A particularly important set of hepatic microsomal oxidative functions is performed by the cytochrome P-450 monooxygenase system. Enzyme activity in fetuses and newborns is about 20% to 40% of adult values; there is a positive relation between monooxygenase activity and postconceptual age. Immaturity of this system results in the prolonged half-life of phenytoin, phenobarbital, and theophylline in neonates and necessitates careful monitoring of serum drug levels.

Drugs that cannot undergo biotransformation must be excreted unchanged by the kidney. Renal elimination is influenced by the functional immaturity of the kidney, including decreased renal blood flow, decreased GFR, and immature tubular function. The aminoglycosides are not metabolized and are excreted unchanged, primarily by glomerular filtration. This results in prolongation of the serum half-life of this class of antibiotics, which is directly related to gestational age, postnatal age, and creatinine clearance.[100]

Bilirubin Metabolism

Hyperbilirubinemia is common in newborns, perhaps the most common diagnosis in otherwise well newborns. The origin is usually idiopathic and the outcome usually benign. High levels of unconjugated bilirubin, however, result in deposition of unbound bilirubin in the central nervous system and central nervous system toxicity, or *kernicterus*. The toxicity is related to the level of unbound bilirubin, the potential for displacement of unbound bilirubin from albumin-binding sites, and the integrity of the blood–brain barrier (which is likely to be compromised by prematurity or illness).

Bilirubin is the product of heme degradation, primarily from the destruction of senescent or hemolyzed red blood cells. Bilirubin is released from the hepatocytes or the reticuloendothelial cells into the circulation, where it is tightly but reversibly bound to albumin. Circulating bilirubin is rapidly taken up by hepatocytes through a carrier-mediated membrane transport system.[101] The bilirubin is then conjugated to form monoglucuronides and diglucuronides by an enzyme system that transfers a glycosyl group from a uridine diphosphate–sugar nucleotide to bilirubin (uridine diphosphate–glucuronosyltransferase).[102] Most of the hydrophilic bilirubin monoconjugates and diconjugates are then excreted in bile.

In the fetus, unconjugated bilirubin is transferred to the maternal circulation through the placenta; the fetal liver has a relatively minor role in bilirubin excretion. After birth, the newborn liver must assume the role of bilirubin conjugation and excretion. Bilirubin production rates in newborns are more than twice those in adults,[103] and the conjugating enzyme systems are immature. This leads to elevation of serum unconjugated bilirubin level, which usually peaks between the third and fifth days of life and gradually decreases to adult levels (physiologic jaundice). Unconjugated bilirubin concentration may increase to toxic levels as a result of increased bilirubin production (commonly due to hemolytic disease in newborns) or impaired conjugation and excretion, which is more marked in premature infants.

Therapy is required when the level of unconjugated bilirubin is rising rapidly or approaching toxic levels. Phototherapy is usually the initial treatment. Absorption of a photon of light results in photochemical conversion of the bilirubin molecule.[104] The resulting configurational or structural isomerization of the bilirubin molecule increases water solubility, allowing the bilirubin to be excreted by the kidneys. This is not particularly efficient (only 2 of 10 bilirubin molecules undergo photoconversion); if the level of unconjugated bilirubin continues to rise, exchange transfusion may be required.

Breast milk feeding is also associated with neonatal hyperbilirubinemia. As many as 6.8% of healthy, breastfed neonates develop unexplained serum bilirubin levels greater than 15 mg/dL.[105] The pathophysiology of breast milk jaundice is unclear but theoretically could involve increased bilirubin production, decreased excretion, or a combination of the two mechanisms. There is no evidence to suggest increased bilirubin production in breast-fed infants compared with formula-fed infants. Theories have focused on decreased fluid intake, inhibitors of hepatic bilirubin excretion that may be present in breast milk, and enhanced intestinal resorption of bilirubin as possible mechanisms.[106]

DEVELOPMENTAL IMMUNOLOGY AND INFECTION

Ontogeny of the Immune System

The development of the immune system begins early in gestation and is not complete until after birth. The structural (organized tissues of the immune system, including thymus, bone marrow, spleen, mucosa-associated immune tissue, and peripheral lymph nodes) and circulating (lymphocytes, macrophages, neutrophils, eosinophils, and mast cells) components of the mature immune system are all present at birth. However, there are differences between neonatal and adult immunity. In term newborns, these differences are due primarily to immunologic immaturity and lack of previous antigen exposure. Extremely premature infants are not only immunologically immature but also immunologically incompetent because of inadequate development of the structural, cellular, and humoral components of the immune system. This translates to a 60-fold increase in the incidence of sepsis in premature infants compared with term infants.[107] A recent review of the ontogeny of the cellular and structural components of the immune system has much to say on this subject.[108]

A number of factors adversely effect the immune response of the immature patient. Certain cell subpopulations may not be present or may not be fully developed. Newborns have no "immunologic memory"; thus, the initial exposure to antigen results in a primary immune response, which differs in kinetics, magnitude, and quality from secondary responses.[109] Neonatal serum has been found to have decreased opsonic activity for a variety of organisms because of decreased levels of specific IgG and IgM, all the components of the classic complement pathway, C3 proactivator, and properdin.[110,111]

Neonates have a full complement of mature, functional T lymphocytes at birth. Quantitatively, the T-cell response is weak owing to the small number of specific T cells for any antigen. Subsequent responses are more vigorous owing to clonal expansion after antigenic exposure. Transplantation immunity is fully developed in term and premature neonates,[112] although experience suggests that less immunosuppression is required in neonates than in mature recipients.[113,114] Neonates, however, clearly have increased susceptibility to some viral pathogens.[115]

Phagocytic activity and inflammation are limited in term newborns. Although peripheral granulocyte counts in normal newborns usually exceed those of normal adults, the storage pool is relatively small. In addition, neonatal granulocytes have defective chemotaxis in response to inflammatory mediators[116] and microbicidal activity, particularly in stressed newborns.[117,118]

Maternal Transfer of Humoral Immunity

Throughout gestation, humoral immunity is passively transferred to the fetus in the form of IgG. Late in gestation, IgG is actively transferred to achieve serum levels that exceed maternal levels. IgG levels in cord blood of premature neonates are decreased in proportion to the degree of immaturity.[119] IgG levels gradually decrease over 4 to 6 months, resulting in a physiologic hypogammaglobulinemia. Small amounts of IgM are present in the fetus early in gestation, and small amounts are synthesized by the normal fetus. In the absence of congenital infection, IgM levels remain low but increase rapidly after birth.

Neonates also benefit immunologically from breastfeeding. Human colostrum and breast milk contain an array of cellular and humoral elements important in immune competence, including T and B lymphocytes, phagocytic cells, immunoglobulins, complement components, interferon, and other microbial inhibitors.[120]

Neonatal Sepsis

Neonatal sepsis is defined as a generalized bacterial infection accompanied by a positive blood culture during the 1st month of life.[107] Early-onset sepsis occurs during the 1st week of life and is due primarily to maternal organisms, such as group B streptococcus, *Escherichia coli*, or *Listeria monocytogenes*. Maternal infection can be transmitted transplacentally (maternal bacteremia or viremia), by direct contamination of the amniotic fluid after prolonged rupture of membranes, or during passage through the birth canal. The mortality rate of early-onset sepsis is 50%. Late-onset sepsis is due primarily to hospital-acquired organisms, such as *Staphylococcus epidermidis*, *Staphylococcus aureus*, or *Pseudomonas* sp, and is often related to indwelling tubes and catheters. The mortality rate of late-onset sepsis is 20%.

The signs and symptoms of neonatal sepsis are subtle and nonspecific.[121] Early signs include lethargy, irritability, temperature instability, change in the respiratory pattern, or change in the feeding pattern. Hematologic changes are variable and include thrombocytopenia, leukocytosis, or leukopenia; bandemia is often present. Hemodynamic changes are late manifestations of sepsis. The classic findings of fever and leukocytosis seen in mature patients are often not present in neonates. The clinician is advised to have a low index of suspicion, to obtain appropriate cultures (including cerebrospinal fluid), and to initiate presumptive therapy promptly. Presumptive therapy should be based on the suspected organism, but often includes ampicillin or an antistaphylococcal agent plus an aminoglycoside. Granulocyte transfusion[122,123] and immunoglobulin administration[124,125] have met with mixed results in the treatment of neonatal sepsis.

Viral Sepsis

Most neonatal viral infections are acquired transplacentally. Congenital infections from the TORCH complex (*to*xoplasmosis, *r*ubella, *c*ytomegalovirus, and *h*erpesvirus) often present with hepatosplenomegaly, a petechial rash, thrombocytopenia, and central nervous system manifestations such as calcifications and seizures.

Vertical transmission of the human immunodeficiency virus (HIV) is an emerging problem. About 30% of infants born to HIV-infected mothers are positive for the virus. The factors affecting placental transmission of the HIV virus and congenital infection have not been well delineated.

REFERENCES

1. Sparks JW, Cetin I. Intrauterine growth and nutrition. In: Polin RA, Fox WW, eds. Fetal and neonatal physiology. Philadelphia, WB Saunders, 1992:179.
2. Leung DW, Spencer SA, Cachianes G, et al. Growth hormone receptor and serum binding protein: purification, cloning and expression. Nature 1987;330:537.
3. MacGorman LR, Rizza RA, Gerich JE. Physiological concentrations of growth hormone exert insulin-like and insulin antagonistic effects on both hepatic and extrahepatic tissues in man. J Clin Endocrinol Metab 1981;53:556.
4. Rizza RA, Mandarino LJ, Gerich JE. Effects of growth hormone on insulin action in man: mechanisms of insulin resistance, impaired suppression of glucose production, and impaired stimulation of glucose utilization. Diabetes 1982; 31:663.
5. Lee RGL, Bode HH. Stunted growth and hepatomegaly in diabetes mellitus. J Pediatr 1977;91:82.
6. Russell WE. Endocrine and other factors affecting growth. In: Polin RA, Fox WW, eds. Fetal and neonatal physiology. Philadelphia, WB Saunders, 1992:204.
7. Evans RM. The steroid and thyroid hormone receptor superfamily. Science 1988;240:889.
8. Shaffer SG, Bradt SK, Meade VM, Hall RT. Extracellular fluid volume changes in very low birth weight infants during the first 2 postnatal months. J Pediatr 1987;111:124.
9. Winters RW. Principles of pediatric fluid therapy, ed 2. Boston, Little, Brown, 1982:71.
10. Holliday MA. Metabolic rate and organ size during growth from infancy to maturity and during late gestation and early infancy. Pediatrics 1971;47:169.
11. Putet G, Senterre J, Rigo J, Salle B. Energy balance and composition of body weight: energy metabolism, nutrition and growth in premature infants. Biol Neonate 1987;52(Suppl 1):17.
12. Owen OE. Resting metabolic requirements of men and women. Mayo Clin Proc 1988;63:503.
13. Danforth E. Diet and obesity. Am J Clin Nutr 1985;41:1132.
14. Chessix P, Reichman BL, Verellen GJE, et al. Influence of postnatal age, energy intake, and weight gain on energy metabolism in the very low-birth-weight infant. J Pediatr 1981;99:761.
15. Schulze KF, Stefanski M, Masterson J, et al. Energy expenditure, energy balance, and composition of weight gain in low birth weight infants fed diets of different protein and energy content. J Pediatr 1987;110:753.
16. Hey EN, O'Connell B. Oxygen consumption and heat balance in the cot-nursed baby. Arch Dis Child 1970;45:335.
17. Whyte RK, Sinclar JC, Bayley HS, et al. Energy cost of growth of premature infants. Acta Paediatr Acad Sci Hung 1982; 23:85.
18. Denne SC. Energy requirements. In: Polin RA, Fox WW, eds. Fetal and neonatal physiology. Philadelphia, WB Saunders, 1992:215.
19. Jones MD Jr. Energy metabolism in the developing brain. Semin Perinatol 1979;3:121.
20. Denne SC. Carbohydrate requirements. In: Polin RA, Fox WW, eds. Fetal and neonatal physiology. Philadelphia, WB Saunders, 1992:234.
21. Bougneres PF, Castano L, Rocchiccioli F, Pham Gia H, Leluyer B, Ferre P. Medium-chain fatty acids increase glucose production in normal and low birth weight newborns. Am J Physiol 1989;256:E692.
22. Cowett RM, Anderson GE, Maguire CA, Oh W. Ontogeny of glucose homeostasis in low birth weight infants. J Pediatr 1988;112:462.
23. Nose O, Tipton JR, Ament ME, Yabuuchi H. Effect of the energy source on changes in energy expenditure, respiratory quotient, and nitrogen balance during total parenteral nutrition in children. Pediatr Res 1987;21:538.
24. Dhaniready R, Hamash M, Sivasubramanian KN, Chowdhry P, Scanlon JW, Hamash P. Postheparin lipolytic activity and intralipid clearance in very low birth weight infants. J Pediatr 1981;98:617.
25. Schmidt-Sommerfeld E, Penn D, Wolf H. Carnitine blood concentrations and fat utilization in parenterally alimented premature newborn infants. J Pediatr 1982;100:260.
26. Warshaw JB, Curry E. Comparison of serum carnitine and ketone body concentrations in breast and in formula fed newborn infants. J Pediatr 1980;97:122.
27. Burr GO, Burr MM. A new deficiency disease produced by the rigid exclusion of fat from the diet. J Biol Chem 1929;82:345.
28. American Academy of Pediatrics Committee on Nutrition. Nutritional needs of low birth weight infants. Pediatrics 1985;75:976.
29. Clandinin MT, Chappell JE, Leong S, Heim T, Swyer PR, Chance GW. Intrauterine fatty acid accretion rates in human brain: implications for fatty acid requirements. Early Hum Dev 1980;4:121.
30. Beaton GH, Chery A. Protein requirements of infants: a reexamination of concepts and approaches. Am J Clin Nutr 1988;48:1403.
31. Fomon SJ. Protein requirements of term infants. In: Fomon SJ, Hierd WC, eds. Energy and protein needs during infancy. New York, Harcourt Brace Jovanovich, 1986:55.
32. Food and Agriculture Organization, World Health Organization, United Nations University. Energy and protein requirements: report of a joint expert consultation. WHO technical report series no. 724. Geneva, World Health Organization, 1985.
33. Denne SC. Protein requirements. In: Polin RA, Fox WW, eds. Fetal and neonatal physiology. Philadelphia, WB Saunders, 1992:223.
34. Hanning RM, Zlotkin SH. Amino acid and protein needs of the neonate: effects of excess and deficiency. Semin Perinatol 1989;13:131.
35. Halbert KE, Tsang RC. Neonatal calcium, phosphorus, and magnesium homeostasis. In: Polin RA, Fox WW, eds. Fetal and neonatal physiology. Philadelphia, WB Saunders, 1992:1745.
36. Mimouni F, Tsang RC. Pathophysiology of neonatal hypocalcemia. In: Polin RA, Fox WW, eds. Fetal and neonatal physiology. Philadelphia, WB Saunders, 1992:1761.
37. Tsang RC, Light IJ, Sutherland JM, Kleinman LI. Possible pathogenetic factors in neonatal hypocalcemia of prematurity: the role of gestation, hyperphosphatemia, hypomagnesemia, urinary calcium loss, and parathyroid hormone responsiveness. J Pediatr 1973;82:423.
38. Adamkin DH, McLead R, Marchildon M, et al. Comparison of two neonatal intravenous amino acid formulations in preterm infants: multicenter study. (Abstract) Pediatr Res 1989;25:283A.
39. Power GG. Fetal Thermoregulation: animal and human. In: Polin RA, Fox WW, eds. Fetal and neonatal physiology. Philadelphia, WB Saunders, 1992:477.
40. Hammarlund KG, Sedin G, Stromberg B. Transepidermal water loss in newborn infants, VIII. Acta Paediatr Scand 1983;72:721.

41. Bruck K. Neonatal thermal regulation. In: Polin RA, Fox WW, eds. Fetal and neonatal physiology. Philadelphia, WB Saunders, 1992:477.
42. Bruck K. Temperature regulation in the newborn infant. Biol Neonate 1961;3:65.
43. Reed KL. Fetal and neonatal cardiac assessment with Doppler. Semin Perinatol 1987;11:347.
44. Nassar R, Reedy MC, Anderson PAW. Developmental changes in the ultrastructure and sarcomere shortening of the isolated rabbit ventricular myocyte. Circ Res 1987; 61:465.
45. Anderson PAW, Oakeley AE. Immunological identification of five troponin T isoforms reveals an elaborate maturational troponin T profile in rabbit myocardium. Circ Res 1989; 65:1087.
46. Cummins P, Lambert SJ. Myosin transitions in the bovine and human heart: a developmental and anatomical study of heavy and light chain subunits in the atrium and ventricle. Circ Res 1986;58:846.
47. Humphreys JE, Cummins P. Regulatory proteins of the myocardium: atrial and ventricular tropomyosin and troponin-I in the developing and adult bovine and human heart. J Mol Cell Cardiol 1984;16:643.
48. Lompre AM, Mercadier JJ, Wisnewsky C, et al. Species- and age-dependent changes in the relative amounts of cardiac myosin isoenzymes in mammals. Dev Biol 1981;84:286.
49. Sweeney LJ, Nag AC, Eisenberg B, Manasek FJ, Zak R. Developmental aspects of cardiac contractile protein. Basic Res Cardiol 1985;80(Suppl 2):123.
50. Romero T, Covell J, Friedman WF. A comparison of pressure–volume relations of the fetal, newborn and adult heart. Am J Physiol 1972;222:1285.
51. Vidyasagar D. Transcutaneous PO2 and PCO2 monitoring in the neonate. In: Shoemaker WC, Ayres S, Grenvik A, Holbrook PR, Thompson WL, eds. Textbook of critical care, ed 2. Philadelphia, WB Saunders, 1989:280.
52. Anderson PAW, Manring A, Serwier GA, et al. The force-interval relationship of the left ventricle. Circulation 1979; 60:334.
53. Anderson PAW. Physiology of the fetal, neonatal and adult heart. In: Polin RA, Fox WW, eds. Fetal and neonatal physiology. Philadelphia, WB Saunders, 1992:722.
54. Anderson PAW, Manring A, Crenshaw C. Biophysics of the developing heart. II. The interaction of the force-interval relationship with inotropic state and muscle length (preload). Am J Obstet Gynecol 1980;138:44.
55. Thornburg KL, Morton MJ. Filling and arterial pressures as determinants of left ventricular stroke volume in fetal lambs. Am J Physiol 1986;251:H961.
56. Minczak BM, Wolfson MR, Santamore WP, Shaffer TH. Developmental changes in diastolic ventricular interaction. Pediatr Res 1988;23:466.
57. Malik AB, Kidd SL. Independent effects of changes in H+ and CO2 concentrations on hypoxic pulmonary vasoconstriction. J Appl Physiol 1973;34:318.
58. Drummond WH, Gregory GA, Heyman MA, Phibbs RA. The independent effects of hyperventilation, tolazoline, and dopamine in infants with persistent pulmonary hypertension. J Pediatr 1981;98:603.
59. Gordon JB, Martinez FR, Keller PA, Tod ML, Madden JA. Differing effects of acute and prolonged alkalosis on hypoxic pulmonary vasoconstriction. Am Rev Respir Dis 1993; 148:1651.
60. Drummond WH, Lock JE. Neonatal pulmonary vasodilator drugs. Dev Pharmacol Ther 1984;7:1.
61. Roberts JD, Chen TY, Kawai N, et al. Inhaled nitric oxide reverses pulmonary vasoconstriction in the hypoxic and acidotic newborn lamb. Circulation Res 1993;72:246.
62. Roberts JD, Lang P, Bigatello LM, Vlahakes GJ, Zapol WM. Inhaled nitric oxide in congenital heart disease. Circulation 1993;87:447.
63. DiFiore JW, Wilson JM. Lung development. Semin Pediatr Surg 1994;3:221.
64. DiFiore JW, Fauza DO, Wilson JM. Experimental fetal tracheal ligation reverses the structural and physiological effects of pulmonary hypoplasia in congenital diaphragmatic hernia. J Pediatr Surg 1994;29:248.
65. Rutter N, Milner AD, Hiller J. Effects of bronchodilators on respiratory resistance in infants and young children with bronchiolitis and wheezy bronchitis. Arch Dis Child 1975; 50:719.
66. Shelley SA, Balis JU, Paciga JE, Espinoza CG, Richman AV. Biochemical composition of adult human lung surfactant. Lung 1982;160:195.
67. Gluck L, Kulovich MV, Borer RC Jr, Brenner PH, Anderson GG, Spellacy WN. Diagnosis of respiratory distress syndrome by amniocentesis. Am J Obstet Gynecol 1971;109:440.
68. Hallman M. Antenatal diagnosis of lung maturity. In: Robertson B. Van Golde LMG, Batenburg JJ., eds Pulmonary surfactant. Amsterdam, Elsevier, 1984:419.
69. Avery ME, Mead J. Surface properties in relation to atelectasis and hyaline membrane disease. Am J Dis Child 1959;97:517.
70. Hallman M, Spragg R, Harrell JH, Moser KM, Gluck L. Evidence of lung surfactant abnormality in respiratory failure: study of bronchoalveolar lavage phospholipids. Surface activity, phospholipase activity and plasma myoinositol. J Clin Invest 1982;70:673.
71. Morley DJ, Miller N, Bangham AD, Davis JA. Dry artificial surfactant and its effect on very premature babies. Lancet 1981;1:64.
72. Rau JL. Inspiratory flow patterns: the shape of ventilation. Respir Care 1993;38:132.
73. McIntyre NR, Li-Ing Ho. Effects of initial flow rate and breath termination criteria on pressure support ventilation. Chest 1991;99:134.
74. Bunnell JB. High-frequency jet ventilation. Neonatal Intensive Care 1990:28.
75. Boynton BR, Mannino FL, Davis RF, Kopotic RF, Friederichsen G. Combined high-frequency oscillatory ventilation and intermittent mandatory ventilation in critically ill neonates. J Pediatr 1984;105:297.
76. Avner ED. Embryogenesis and anatomic development of the kidney. In: Polin RA, Fox WW, eds. Fetal and neonatal physiology. Philadelphia, WB Saunders, 1992:1181.
77. Oliver J. Nephrons and kidneys: a quantitative study of development and evolutionary mammalian renal architectonics. New York, Harper & Row, 1968.
78. Kleinman LI. Developmental renal physiology. Physiologist 1982:25;103.
79. Spitzer A. The developing kidney and the process of growth. In: Seldin DW, Giebisch G, eds. The kidney: physiology and pathophysiology. New York, Raven Press, 1985:1979.
80. Robillard JE, Nakamura KT, Matherne GP, Jose PA. Renal hemodynamics and functional adjustments to postnatal life. Semin Perinatol 1988;12:143.
81. Engle WD. Development of fetal and neonatal renal function. Semin Perinatol 1986;10:113.
82. Goldsmith DI. Clinical and laboratory evaluation of renal function. In: Edelmann CM Jr, ed. Pediatric kidney disease. Boston, Little, Brown, 1978.
83. Leake RD, Trygstad CW. Glomerular filtration rate during the period of adaptation to extrauterine life. Pediatr Res 1977;11:959.
84. Arant BS Jr. Developmental patterns of renal functional maturation compared in the human neonate. J Pediatr 1978; 92:705.
85. Engleke SC, Shah BL, Vasan U, Raye JR. Sodium balance in very low-birth-weight infants. J Pediatr 1978;93:837.
86. Edelmann CM Jr, Soriano JR, Boichis H, Gruskin AB, Acosta MI. Renal bicarbonate reabsorption and hydrogen ion excretion in infants. J Clin Invest 1967;46:1309.
87. Spitzer A. Renal physiology and functional development. In: Edelmann CM Jr, ed. Pediatric kidney disease. Boston, Little, Brown, 1978:25.
88. Moore ES, Galvez MB, Paton JB, Fisher DE, Behrman RE. Effects of positive pressure ventilation on intrarenal blood flow in infant primates. Pediatr Res 1974;8:792.
89. Tulassay T, Machay T, Kiszel J, Varga J. Effects of continuous positive airway pressure on renal function in prematures. Biol Neonate 1983;43:152.
90. Grannum PA, Copel JA, Plaxe SC, Scioscia AL, Hobbins JC. In utero exchange transfusion by direct intravascular injec-

tion in severe erythroblastosis fetalis. N Engl J Med 1986; 314:1431.

91. Socol ML, MacGregor SN, Pielet BW, Tamura RK, Sabbagha RE. Percutaneous umbilical transfusion in severe rhesus isoimmunization: resolution of fetal hydrops. Am J Obstet Gynecol 1987;157:1369.

92. Phibbs RH. Hydrops fetalis and other causes of neonatal edema and ascites.In: Polin RA, Fox WW, eds. Fetal and neonatal physiology. Philadelphia, WB Saunders, 1992: 1319.

93. Luzzatto AC. Hepatocyte differentiation during early fetal development in the rat. Cell Tissue Res 1981;215:133.

94. Jones CT, Rolph TP. Metabolism during fetal life: a functional assessment of metabolic development. Physiol Rev 1985;65:357.

95. Shiojiri N. Enzymo- and immunocytochemical analyses of the differentiation of liver cells in the prenatal mouse. J Embryol Exp Morph 1981;62:139.

96. Shiojiri N, Katayama H. Secondary joining of the bile ducts during the hepatogenesis of the mouse embryo. Anat Embryol 1987;177:153.

97. Rudolph AM. Hepatic and ductus venosus blood flows during fetal life. Hepatology 1983;3:254.

98. Tavoloni N. Bile secretion and its control in the mature and immature organism.In: Polin RA, Fox WW, eds. Fetal and neonatal physiology. Philadelphia, WB Saunders, 1992: 1123.

99. Aranda JV, Stern L. Clinical aspects of developmental pharmacology and toxicology. Pharmacol Ther 1983;20:1.

100. Nagourney BA, Aranda JV. Physiologic differences of clinical significance.In: Polin RA, Fox WW, eds. Fetal and neonatal physiology. Philadelphia, WB Saunders, 1992:169.

101. Paumgartner G, Reichen J. Kinetics of hepatic uptake of unconjugated bilirubin. Clin Sci Mol Med 1976;51:169.

102. Fevery J, Leroy P, Geirwegh KPM. Enzymic transfer of glucose and xylose from uridine diphosphate glucose and uridine diphosphate xylose to bilirubin by untreated and digitonin-activated preparations from rat liver. Biochem J 1972; 129:619.

103. Maisels MJ, Pathak A, Nelson NM, Nathan DG, Smith CA. Endogenous production of carbon monoxide in normal and erythroblastic newborn infants. J Clin Invest 1971;50:1.

104. Lightner DA, McDonagh AF. Molecular mechanisms of phototherapy for neonatal jaundice. Acc Chem Res 1984;17:417.

105. DeAngelis C, Sargent J, Chun MK, et al. Breast milk jaundice. Wis Med J 1980;79:40.

106. Gourley GR. Pathophysiology of breast-milk jaundice. In: Polin RA, Fox WW, eds. Fetal and neonatal physiology. Philadelphia, WB Saunders, 1992:1173.

107. Speck WT, Aronoff SC, Fanaroff AA. Neonatal infections. In: Klaus MH, Fanaroff AA, eds. Care of the high-risk neonate, ed 3. Philadelphia, WB Saunders, 1986:262.

108. Flake AW. Ontogeny of fetal immunity. In: Fonkalsrud EW, Krummel TM, eds. Infections and immunologic disorders in pediatric surgery. Philadelphia, WB Saunders, 1993:9.

109. Kincade PW, Gimble JM. B Lymphocytes. In: Paul WE, ed. Fundamental immunology. New York, Raven Press, 1989:41.

110. Kohler PF. Maturation of the human complement system. I. Onset of the time and site of fetal C1q, C4, C3 and C5 synthesis. J Clin Invest 1973;52:671.

111. Dossett JH, Williams RC Jr, Quie PG. Studies on interaction of bacteria, serum factors and polymorphonuclear leukocytes in mothers and newborns. Pediatrics 1969;44:49.

112. Soloman J. Fetal and neonatal immunology: frontiers of biology. Amsterdam, Elsevier-North Holland, 1971:234.

113. Najarian JS, Frey DJ, Matas AF, et al. Renal transplantation in infants. Ann Surg 1990;212:353.

114. Mavroudis C, Harrison H, Klein JB, et al. Infant orthotopic cardiac transplantation. J Thorac Cardiovasc Surg 1988; 96:912.

115. Overall JC, Glasgow LA. Virus infections in the fetus and newborn infant. J Pediatr 1970;77:315.

116. Pahwa SG, Pahwa R, Grimes E, Smithwick E. Cellular and humoral components of monocyte and neutrophil chemotaxis in cord blood. Pediatr Res 1977;11:677.

117. Boner A, Zeligs BJ, Bellanti JA. Chemotactic responses in various differentiational stages of neutrophils from human cord and adult blood. Infect Immun 1982;35:921.

118. Hill HR. Biochemical structural and functional abnormalities of polymorphonuclear leukocytes in the neonate. Pediatr Res 1987;22:375.

119. Berg T. Immunoglobulin levels in infants with low birth weights. Acta Paediatr Scand 1968;57:369.

120. Ogra SS, Weintraub D, Ogra PL. Immunologic aspects of human colostrum and milk. III. Fate and absorption of cellular and soluble components in the gastrointestinal tract of newborns. J Immunol 1977;119:245.

121. Siegel JD, McCracken GH Jr. Sepsis neonatorum. N Engl J Med 1981;304:642.

122. Baley JE, Stork EK, Warkentin PI, Shurin SB. Buffy coat transfusions in neutropenic neonates with presumed sepsis: a prospective randomized trial. Pediatrics 1987;80:712.

123. Cairo MS. Granulocyte transfusions in neonates with presumed sepsis. Pediatrics 1987;80:738.

124. Christensen RD, Brown MS, Hall DC. Effect on neutrophil kinetics and serum opsonic capacity of intravenous administration of immune globulin to neonates with clinical signs of early-onset sepsis. J Pediatr 1991;118:606.

125. Berger M. Use of intravenously administered immune globulin in newborn infants: prophylaxis, treatment, both, or neither? J Pediatr 1991;118:557.

SURGERY: SCIENTIFIC PRINCIPLES AND PRACTICE, Second Edition, edited by Lazar J. Greenfield, Michael W. Mulholland, Keith T. Oldham, Gerald B. Zelenock, and Keith D. Lillemoe. Lippincott–Raven Publishers, Philadelphia, © 1997.

CHAPTER 101

PEDIATRIC HEAD AND NECK

JOHN R. WESLEY

Surgical lesions of the head and neck range from trivial to life-threatening and comprise a broad spectrum of anatomic defects. The more common problems include airway obstruction, branchial cleft remnants, thyroglossal duct remnants, hemangiomas, cystic hygroma, lymphangioma, and lymphadenopathy.

AIRWAY OBSTRUCTION

Many lesions, both congenital and acquired, may produce airway obstruction in infants and children. They may be intrinsic or extrinsic to the airway and vary from clinically insignificant to universally fatal.[1]

Congenital Obstruction

The first significant sign of respiratory distress in an infant is restlessness, followed by tachypnea, chest wall retraction, and cardiorespiratory arrest. It is crucial to establish an adequate airway and to administer respiratory support while proceeding with the diagnostic evaluation. This may consist of simple positioning of the infant, endotracheal intubation, or, in extreme cases, tracheostomy. Work-up includes a careful history, physical examination, chest radiograph, evaluation of arterial blood gases, and passage of a nasogastric tube with a radioopaque marker. Newborn infants breathe primarily through their nostrils, especially when sleeping. Oral breathing is a learned response that may take weeks or months to develop. Therefore, obstruction of the nasal passages, nasopharynx, or pharynx may cause respiratory arrest.

Clinical findings in upper airway obstruction are similar for diverse causes such as nasal encephalocele, heterotopic brain, tumor, and choanal atresia. Tachypnea and suprasternal, intercostal, and costal margin retraction are prominent, but there is no apparent difficulty exhaling, and the voice and cry are normal. Emergency management consists of placing an oropharyngeal airway. An orogastric feeding tube facilitates feeding, and a tracheostomy may be necessary until the nasal airway obstruction has been corrected either by dividing the septum that occludes the posterior nares, as in the case of choanal atresia, or by excising the nasopharyngeal mass.

Airway obstruction at the level of the oral cavity may be caused by macroglossia due to muscular hyperplasia and hypertrophy or to diffuse involvement by lymphangioma, neurofibromatosis, or hemangiopericytoma.[2] Micrognathia as a result of Pierre Robin syndrome may cause airway obstruction, particularly during feeding. Most infants respond to being placed in the prone position, allowing the posterior prolapsed tongue to fall forward. Cysts or tumors of the pharynx (eg, a dermoid or a bronchogenic cyst arising in the wall of the pharynx or a mass arising at the base of the tongue such as a lingual thyroid) may produce a lesion large enough to obstruct the glottis.[3]

The trachea and larynx may become obstructed by tumors or cysts originating in the neck. Hemangiomas, lymphangiomas, cystic hygromas, and teratomas are the most common cervical tumors in infants and children. Enteric duplications and unilateral cervical bronchogenic or cervical thymic cysts are less common causes of airway obstruction. Emergency management of these lesions frequently requires placement of an endotracheal tube, which can be difficult if the larynx is displaced. After stabilizing the airway, further diagnostic evaluation includes neck and chest radiographs, computed tomography (CT), ultrasonography, and laryngobronchoscopy. Although tumors and cysts require excision, hemangiomas may involute with time or may be removed endoscopically with laser resection.

Acquired Obstruction

In addition to foreign body aspiration (see Chap. 102), acute epiglottitis is a common cause of acquired airway obstruction in the pediatric age group. *Haemophilus influenzae* type B is nearly always the causative organism, and most children are toxic at presentation with an elevated temperature and an increased pulse and respiratory rate. Prolonged inspiratory stridor that worsens in the supine position is characteristic. The child usually sits erect, anxious, and drooling and becomes increasingly exhausted with air hunger. No attempt should be made to visualize the larynx outside of the operating room because of the risk of sudden airway occlusion with aspiration of secretions and cardiac arrest. If the child's condition permits, lateral neck roentgenograms with soft tissue technique are obtained to confirm the presence of the swollen epiglottis. These are valuable in ruling out other causes of acute airway obstruction, particularly foreign bodies of the hypopharynx, larynx, and trachea. The standard therapy is short-term endotracheal intubation performed in the operating room with general anesthesia and a tracheostomy tray at the ready. The inflammatory process resolves rapidly with intravenous antibiotics, and intubation is seldom required beyond 3 days. In the past, tracheostomy was the standard therapy, but comparative reviews demonstrate that short-term endotracheal intubation is associated with less morbidity and fewer complications.[4]

BRANCHIAL CLEFT REMNANTS

Cysts, sinuses, and fistulas of the neck derived from branchial cleft remnants are common in children. Sinuses and fistulas are encountered more frequently than cysts, and branchogenic cysts occur more often in older children and young adults.[5]

ANATOMY AND EMBRYOLOGY

Remnants of the first and second branchial cleft are the most common, and abnormalities of the second cleft outnumber those of the first cleft by six to one. A simple knowledge of head and neck embryology is helpful in understanding these abnormalities (Fig. 101-1). The region of the developing neck in the embryo presents a series of ridges and furrows known as the branchial arches and the branchial clefts, respectively. The arches coalesce during the growth of the embryo, and part of the first branchial cleft remains open as the eustachian tube and auditory canal. The second branchial cleft normally closes completely; however, either branchial cleft may form a sinus tract or cyst during coalescence. Remnants of the first branchial cleft occur along the base of an imaginary fold extending from the auditory canal behind and below the angle of the mandible to a point just below the midpoint of the cleft. Second branchial cleft remnants are found along any part of a line extending from the tonsillar fossa down to a point on the lower third of the anterior border of the sternocleidomastoid muscle (Fig. 101-2).

Cysts or infections arising from the third or fourth branchial arch and cleft are rare but now well-defined entities that offer diagnostic and therapeutic challenges not encountered with the anomalies of the first and second branchial remnants. The etiology for both presentations is a fistula tract from the pyriform sinus, most commonly on the left side, occurring as a result of a persistent remnant from the third or fourth branchial pouch[5] (Fig. 101-3).

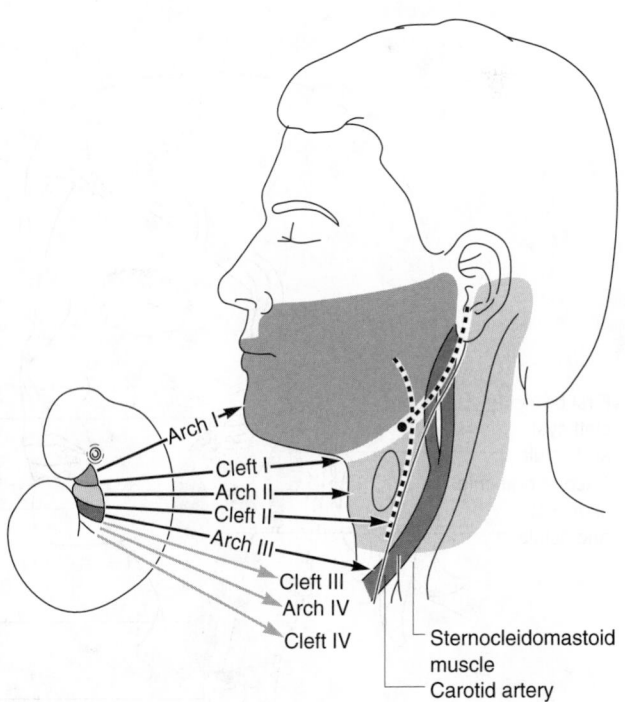

Figure 101-1. Derivation of various areas of the head and neck from the branchial arches and clefts of the embryo.

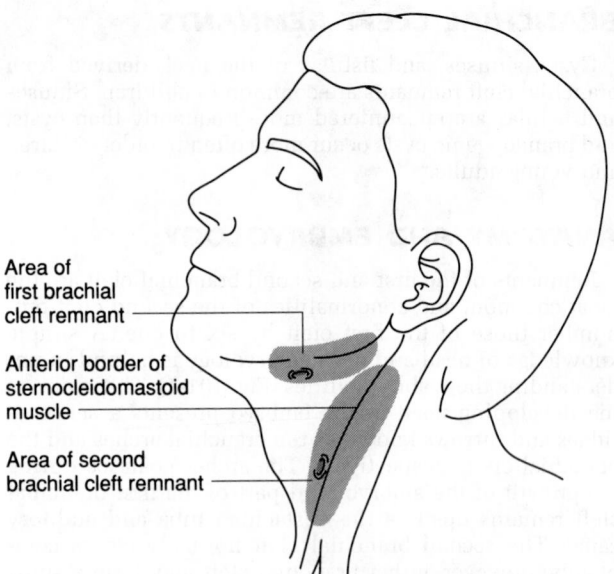

Figure 101-2. Areas of the neck in which cysts and sinuses from the first and second branchial clefts are usually found.

CLINICAL ISSUES

Clinically, first branchial cleft lesions present as a sinus opening near the angle of the mandible. The more common second branchial cleft anomalies present as a pinpoint opening on the anterior border of the sternocleidomastoid muscle, one fourth to one third of its length cephalad from the sternum. Attention is usually drawn to the defects by the appearance of small drops of clear fluid at the opening of the tract or by the occurrence of infection in the tract itself. The anomaly may be either unilateral or bilateral. Less frequently, an oval mass may present, overlying the surface of the parotid gland or anterior to the upper portion of the sternocleidomastoid muscle, representing the first or second branchial clefts, respectively. Tracts that have an exterior opening rarely become infected, although infection is a more common problem in the older age group.

Cysts or sinuses arising from third or fourth branchial arch or cleft present as an air-containing inflammatory lateral neck mass in the neonate or as acute suppurative thyroiditis in the infant or child. Barium studies may demonstrate the presence of a pyriform sinus fistula, particularly after a course of antibiotics and resolution of the surrounding inflammation. CT has also proved useful in diagnosing lesions of the third or fourth branchial cleft origin. If imaging techniques are not successful after resolution of the inflammation, then with recurrent inflammation, compression of the pus-filled cyst during endoscopy may reveal the origin of the fistula as pus exudes from the pyriform sinus.[6]

OPERATIVE CONSIDERATIONS AND OUTCOME

Management of branchial cleft lesions consists of surgical excision. The use of sclerosing solutions is not indicated and may be dangerous. The operation may be performed at any age, usually at the time of diagnosis. If active infection is present, a course of antibiotics is administered first.

The operation for the common second branchial cleft lesions begins with an elliptical transverse incision at the sinus opening, and cephalad dissection of the tract to its furthest extent. The tract is more substantial and more easily dissected in an older patient, usually extending all the way to the tonsillar fossa. The length of the dissection is shorter in the younger child; therefore, the operation is readily accomplished through a single shorter incision. The dissection is kept directly on the tract to avoid injury to contiguous structures such as the internal jugular vein, the internal or external carotid arteries, and the hypoglossal nerve. The operation can almost always be carried out through a single cosmetic elliptic incision if the tract is

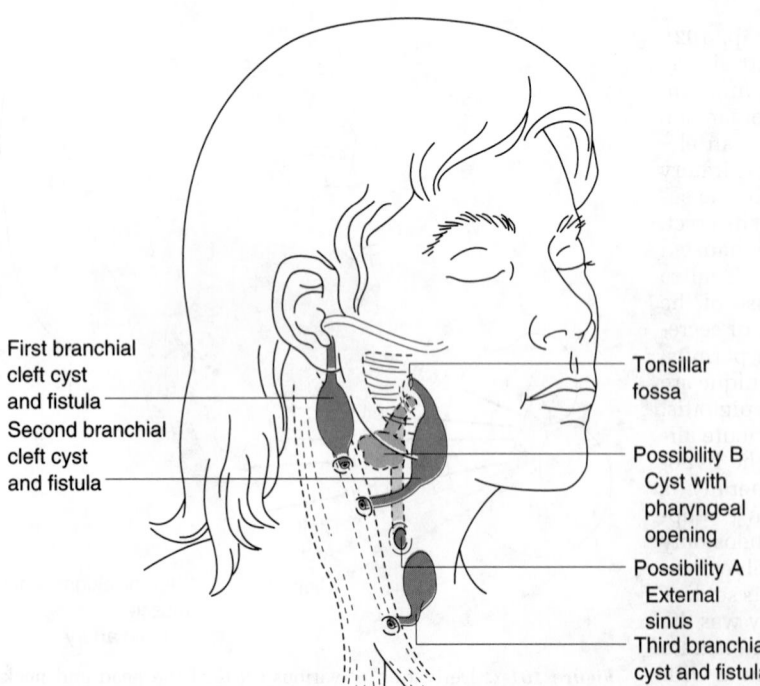

First branchial cleft cyst and fistula

Second branchial cleft cyst and fistula

Tonsillar fossa

Possibility B Cyst with pharyngeal opening

Possibility A External sinus

Third branchial cyst and fistula

Figure 101-3. Types of first, second, and third branchial cleft remnants. Sinuses and fistulas are seen most often in infants and young children, whereas cysts usually appear at a later age.

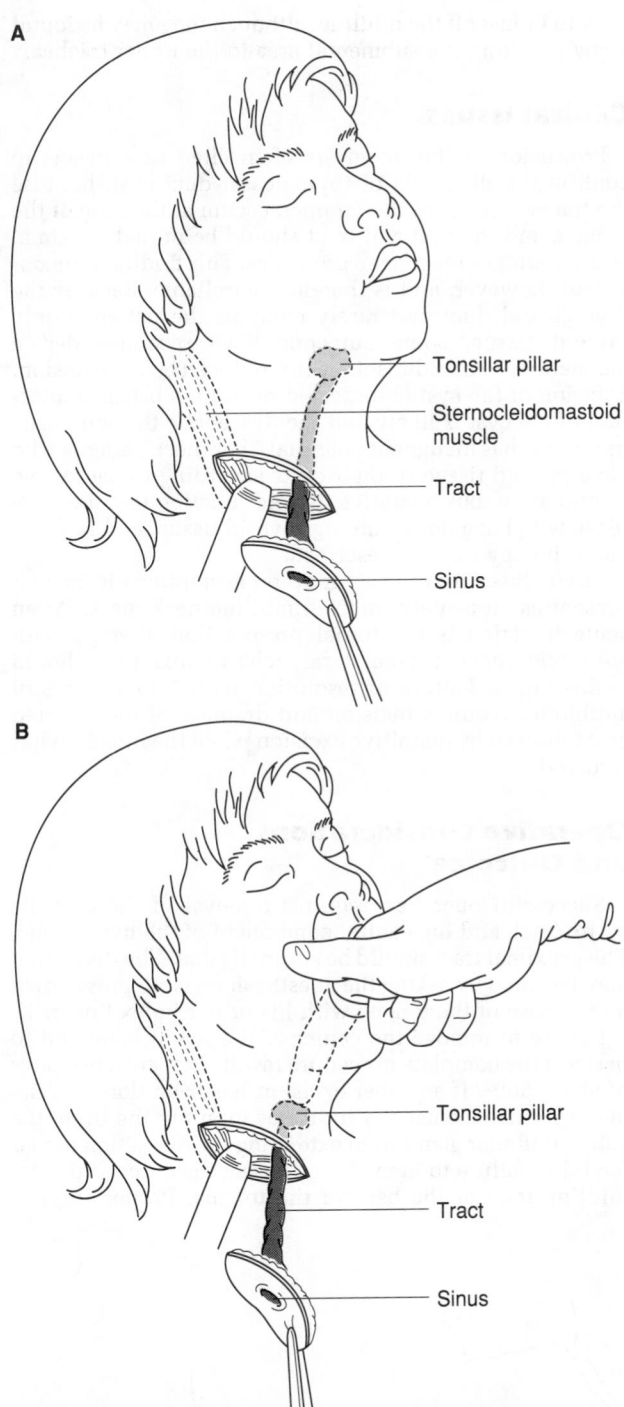

Cysts and sinuses of the first branchial cleft are less common than those of the second and are frequently misdiagnosed, incompletely removed, and subject to repeated infection. The sinus tract opening usually presents just beneath the center of the body of the mandible. The tract consists of stratified squamous epithelium, which may contain hair follicles, and extends upward just behind the angle of the mandible to end blindly at the cartilage of the external auditory canal (Fig. 101-5).

Repeated infection often leads to the diagnosis of a first branchial cleft cyst or sinus, but adequate drainage and antibiotic treatment of the infection must be carried out before excision is attempted. An elliptic incision is made around the opening of the sinus and dissection of the tract carried upward to the lower portion of the auditory canal. Care should be taken during the dissection to avoid injury to the facial nerve, particularly its mandibular branch.

If the dissection has been carefully performed and the lesion is not infected, it is not necessary to leave a drain after excising either a first or second branchial cleft anomaly. Failure to excise the cyst or sinus completely may lead to its recurrence.

In all cases of third or fourth branchial lesions, the acute

Figure 101-4. (*A*) Single incision in the lower part of the neck with the sinus tract developed to usual length. (*B*) The anesthesiologist's finger depresses the tonsillar fossa, facilitating complete dissection of the sinus tract through the single incision.

kept under gentle traction and the anesthesiologist places a finger in the tonsillar fossa and exerts downward pressure toward the field of dissection. In addition, the anesthesiologist's finger helps to localize the tonsillar fossa as the endpoint of dissection where the sinus tract is suture-ligated and divided (Fig. 101-4). Dissection of the sinus tract may be facilitated by passing a fine silver probe or piece of heavy nylon suture through the length of the tract and clamping this in position as the dissection progresses.

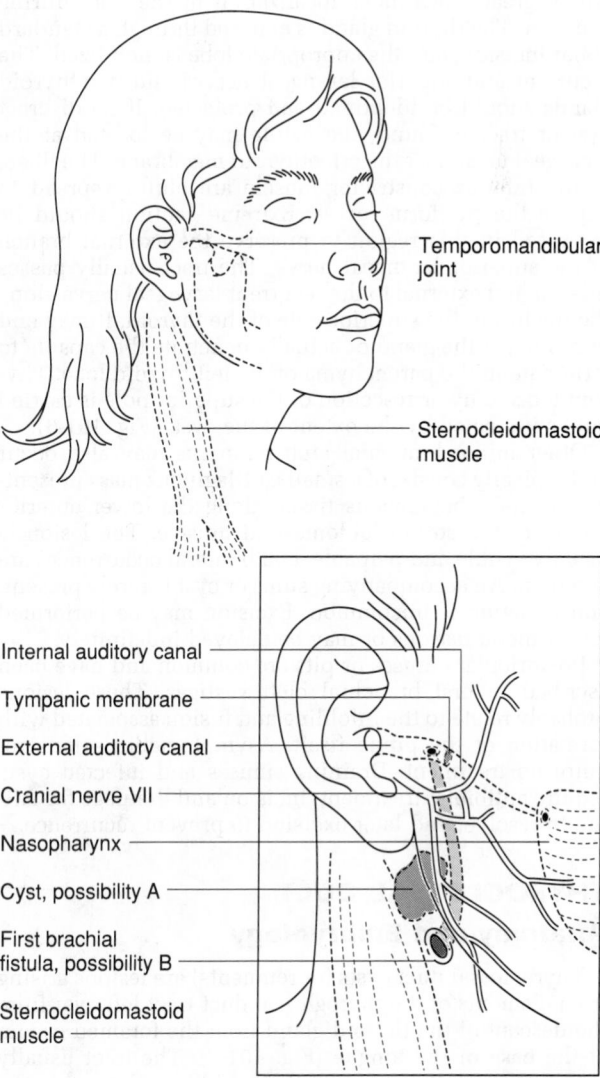

Figure 101-5. Relations of cyst or sinus of the first branchial cleft. Note especially the proximity to the facial nerve and external auditory canal.

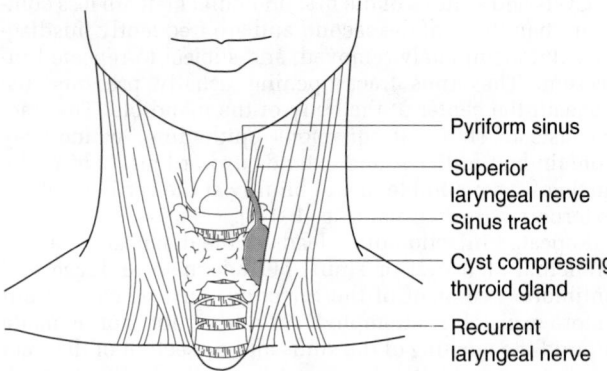

Figure 101-6. Relations of the third or fourth branchial cleft cyst or sinus to the thyroid gland and pyriform sinus.

infection should first be treated, followed by surgical extirpation. Exploration of the neck with excision of the entire tract to the level of the pyriform sinus is necessary to prevent recurrence. Operative endoscopy at the start of the operation may enable cannulation of the tract from above, which greatly facilitates localization of the tract during excision. The thyroid gland is exposed through a standard collar incision, and the appropriate lobe is mobilized. The recurrent and superior laryngeal nerves and parathyroid glands should be identified and protected. If no discreet cyst or tract is found, the fistula may be located at the laryngeal level near the cricothyroid membrane. The fibers of the inferior constrictor muscle are bluntly spread to expose the pyriform recess. Extreme caution should be exercised in this region to preserve the external branch of the superior laryngeal nerve. The tract usually passes inferior and external to the recurrent laryngeal nerve along the trachea to the superior pole of the thyroid. It may end blindly near the gland or actually penetrate the capsule to terminate in the parenchyma of the left thyroid lobe. Thyroid lobectomy or resection of the superior pole is carried out as indicated by the extent of the cyst[7] (Fig. 101-6).

Other minor branchial arch remnants may also occur and typically consist of a small cartilaginous mass presenting in the subcutaneous tissue along the lower anterior border of the sternocleidomastoid muscle. The lesion is usually visible and palpable, and bilateral occurrences are common. An accompanying sinus or cyst is rarely present, and infection is uncommon. Excision may be performed for cosmetic reasons or may be delayed indefinitely.

Preauricular sinuses or pits are common and have been ascribed to first branchial cleft vestiges. These lesions probably relate to the infolding and fusion associated with formation of the pinna itself. Asymptomatic lesions require no treatment. Draining sinuses and infected cysts require antibiotic treatment, incision and drainage for failure to resolve, and later excision to prevent recurrence.

THYROGLOSSAL DUCT
Anatomy and Embryology

Thyroglossal duct cysts (or remnants) are lesions arising from elements of the thyroglossal duct tract left over from the descent of the thyroid gland from the foramen cecum at the base of the tongue (Fig. 101-7). The tract usually passes through the center of the hyoid bone but may pass in front of or behind it. These lesions usually present in late infancy or early childhood and are rarely apparent at birth. They are typically located in the hyoid area of the

neck in or just off the midline, although they may be found anywhere from the submental area to the upper trachea.

Clinical Issues

Protrusion of the tongue is often cited as a means to confirm the diagnosis of thyroglossal duct cyst, because the tract connects to the foramen cecum at the base of the tongue, and the cyst and tract should be pulled proximal and superior as the tongue protrudes. This finding is inconsistent, however, and is therefore unreliable. Because the thyroglossal duct cyst rarely contains the patient's only thyroid tissue, some surgeons have recommended a technetium-99m radioisotope thyroid scan before excision. Excision of the cyst is indicated regardless because infection of the cyst is likely and the dysgenetic thyroid tissue in the cyst has malignant potential.[8] For those patients who have thyroid tissue in their cysts according to pathologic examination, postoperative thyroid function tests identify those who have no remaining thyroid tissue, and replacement therapy can be prescribed.

Thyroglossal duct cysts may be asymptomatic or first present as an acutely infected midline neck mass. When acute infection is the initial presentation, therapy with antibiotics that cover oral flora, such as amoxicillin, should be instituted. Failure of resolution with 7 to 10 days of antibiotics requires incision and drainage of the infected cyst followed by definitive excision when the infection has resolved.

Operative Considerations and Outcome

Successful operation requires removal of the cyst, its entire tract, and the central component of the hyoid bone. The proximal tract should be suture ligated. The dissection may be aided by asking the anesthesiologist to press down on the base of the tongue with his or her index finger.

Failure to remove the center of the hyoid bone and to perform the complete procedure results in recurrence rates of about 50%. If a proper excision has been done, subsequent recurrence usually indicates injury to the tip of the submandibular gland from extending the dissection too far lateral or failure to identify and resect the entire proximal midline tract at the base of the tongue. Proper surgical

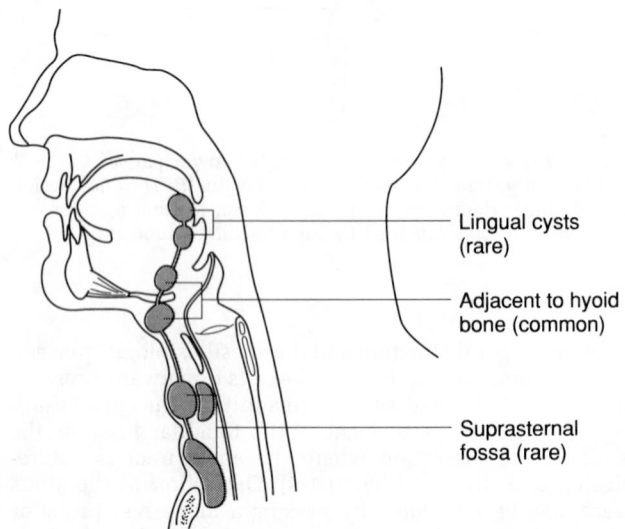

Figure 101-7. Locations of thyroglossal duct cysts.

removal should result in recurrence rates of less than 10%, and any subsequent infection should be treated initially with antibiotics. Often, complete resolution follows, eliminating the need for a second surgical procedure.[9]

A low neck mass near the midline may represent a cervical thymic cyst or bronchogenic cyst. Ultrasound or CT scanning demonstrates the cystic or solid characteristics of the cyst and determines whether it extends into the mediastinum. Complete surgical removal is indicated, and a successful outcome can be anticipated.

LYMPHANGIOMA AND CYSTIC HYGROMA
Anatomy and Embryology

About the sixth week of gestation, a system of clefts develops in the cervical mesenchyme and subsequently forms lymph channels. These channels give rise to jugular lymph sacs that form cervical lymph nodes and lymphatics, ultimately draining into the internal jugular venous system (Fig. 101-8). If portions of these lymphatic channels fail to develop communications with the internal jugular system, masses of disorganized dilated lymph channels form. These are *lymphangiomas.* They are most commonly found in the lateral cervical and submandibular region along the jugular chain of lymphatics. They vary in size from a few centimeters in diameter to massive tumor-like lesions extending into the mediastinum. The larger lesions with dilated cystic lymphatic channels are often referred to as *cystic hygromas.*

Clinical Issues

About 65% of cystic hygromas are apparent at birth. These may be diagnosed prenatally with the increasing use of ultrasonography as a part of obstetric care. These lesions

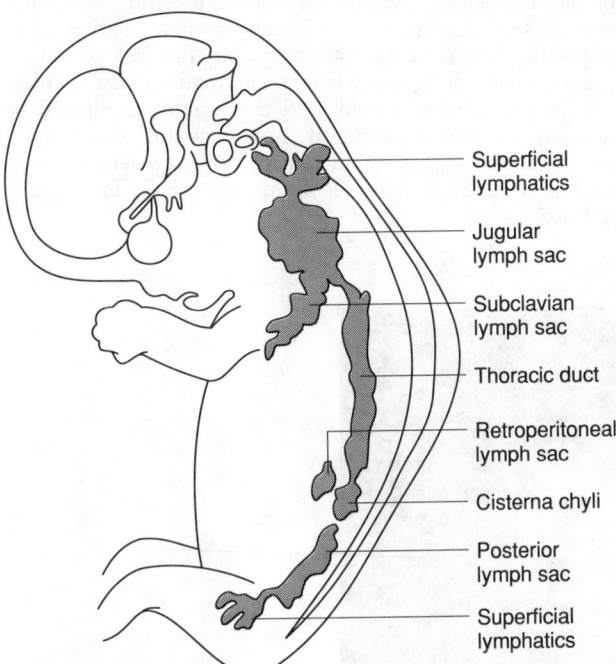

Figure 101-8. Lymphatic system in an 8-week-old human embryo. Development of the major and minor lymphatic sacs is well underway. The jugular lymphatic sac in the neck is prominent. Sequestration of tissue from any of the developing lymphatic structures leads to formation of a lymphangioma or cystic hygroma.

Superficial lymphatics

Jugular lymph sac

Subclavian lymph sac

Thoracic duct

Retroperitoneal lymph sac

Cisterna chyli

Posterior lymph sac

Superficial lymphatics

are generally soft, fluctuant, multiloculated, and in the newborn, may result in significant airway compromise or esophageal and pharyngeal obstruction. In the presence of hypopharyngeal and supraglottic involvement, endotracheal intubation may be difficult, and in extreme cases, early tracheostomy may be required.

Although small lesions may be missed at birth, about 90% are diagnosed by age 2 years. As lymph accumulates, they may gradually increase in size. Dramatic enlargement may occur hours or days after acute occlusion of draining lymphatics or acute hemorrhage into the lesion. Although a smaller lesion may be confused with hemangioma or branchial cleft cyst, ultrasonography demonstrates the cystic multiloculated character of the lesion, and radionuclide scans or angiography can confirm its vascularity. Spontaneous regression of these lesions is unusual but may occur after acute inflammation.

Operative Considerations and Outcome

As a rule, definitive surgical excision is indicated. Ionizing radiation and various sclerosing agents have been used but have their own morbidity and are not recommended. Most lymphangiomas and cystic hygromas are readily excised with little attendant morbidity. Large cystic hygromas may extend across tissue planes, infiltrate muscle, distort nerves and vessels, or otherwise involve vital structures that cannot be resected. When complete resection is not possible, the lesions should be unroofed and well drained with the expectation that recurrence and further surgical excision may be required in the future. Occasionally, lesions treated in this way scar and involute with a good cosmetic result. Radical surgery that risks major disability is not warranted generally.

LYMPHADENOPATHY

Palpable lymph nodes are common during childhood. A recent study of 223 children between the ages of 3 weeks and 6 years, who were attending an outpatient clinic for routine health maintenance (47%) or for acute illness (53%), demonstrated an overall prevalence of 55% with palpable lymph nodes.[10] The nodes most commonly enlarged were cervical in 30% of children, followed by occipital (15%) and submandibular (14%) nodes. Only 8% of the children had palpable postauricular nodes. The location of lymphadenopathy varied greatly with age, with occipital nodes most common in infants and cervical nodes most common in older children.

Acute suppurative lymphadenitis related to bacterial pathogens is generally straightforward to diagnose. Most often, there is accompanying infectious illness, such as an upper respiratory infection, pharyngitis, or facial rash. The node or nodes enlarge rapidly, are tender, and erythema of the overlying skin is present. Fever and an elevated white blood count with a left shift are usually present. Fluctuant nodes can be aspirated with a large bore needle to obtain material for culture, and removing the central necrotic infected material by aspiration often hastens resolution and avoids the need for incision and drainage.

Inflammatory nodes of the subacute variety are more difficult to diagnose and treat. These are often deeper, may appear suddenly, or enlarge slowly over days and weeks. If present, tenderness is minimal, and there may be no systemic signs. Lymph node hyperplasia can occur in response to any viral or bacterial infection and may not respond to antibiotics. The most common causes for subacute inflammatory nodes in the United States are atypical

Mycobacterium and cat-scratch disease.[11] *Mycobacterium tuberculosis* is uncommon in the United States, but when it is the source of lymphadenopathy, it is usually accompanied by positive findings on chest roentgenogram since the lung is the site of first entry of the organism. Atypical *Mycobacterium* enters through the oral pharynx and is not associated with pulmonary findings. The first-strength tuberculosis skin test (purified protein derivative) is often negative with atypical *Mycobacterium,* but because of antigen cross-reactivity, the intermediate-strength test may be positive. In some institutions, atypical antigens are available for skin testing. Cat-scratch antigens are not widely available.

It is common, therefore, for the pediatrician to encounter asymptomatic lymph node enlargement and not have the diagnostic armamentarium to determine the cause. A reasonable first response is to prescribe a 5- to 10-day course of an antibiotic to which *Streptococcus* and most nosocomial *Staphylococcus* organisms are sensitive. If the adenopathy fails to resolve in 2 to 3 weeks, the patient should have an excisional biopsy. An enlarged nonsuppurative lymph node that fails to resolve after a short course of antibiotics should be considered lymphoma until proven otherwise by biopsy. If this rule is strictly followed, lesions of major consequence will not be missed.

Operative Considerations and Outcome

Excisional lymph node biopsy should be done in the operating room and, in most cases, under general anesthesia so that deep dissection to obtain the most involved lymph node is well tolerated. The specimen should be handled by a pathologist familiar with electron microscopy and the protocols and preservation techniques for obtaining tumor markers necessary to characterize lymphomas properly. Samples of the node should be sent for routine bacterial, viral, fungal, tuberculosis, and atypical mycobacterial culture. Lymph nodes suspected of infection with atypical mycobacterial organisms must be completely excised or a draining fistula may result. A child presenting with multiple enlarged nonsuppurative lymph nodes should be evaluated for infectious mononucleosis and other diseases associated with Epstein-Barr virus by appropriate serum assays. If these are negative, Hodgkin disease or non-Hodgkin lymphoma must be strongly suspected.

HEMANGIOMA

Hemangiomas may occur anywhere on the head and neck and fall into one of three classifications: capillary, with a significant dermal component; cavernous, which are primarily subcutaneous; and mixed. Any dermal capillary component helps to confirm by inspection that the underlying mass is a hemangioma. A flow-directional ultrasound may demonstrate the vascular component of a complex mass when the tell-tale dermal component is missing.

Clinical Issues

Hemangiomas often grow rapidly during the first 6 to 12 months of life, after which they stabilize and begin to involute. The natural history is generally one of spontaneous resolution by thrombosis and epithelialization, during which the capillary component changes from bright red to gray as regression takes place. Therefore, most hemangiomas of the head and neck region can be treated by watchful waiting and by reassuring the family that resolution is probable (Fig. 101-9). Periodic clinic visits reassure the parents and child and ensure detection and treatment of the occasional hemangioma that begins to interfere with function by deforming an eyelid or obstructing an ear canal.

Treatment and Outcome

Lesions that grow uncontrollably or impair function should be treated first with a course of steroids (about 30% effective before the age of 10 months).[12] Treatment with daily injections of recombinant α_1-interferon has shown dramatic results with involution in 90% of patients whose lesions are characterized by an extensive spindle-cell component.[13] In the past, occasional massive lesions were helped by low-dose radiotherapy, but the risk of subsequent thyroid malignancy from such treatment is considerable in the head and neck and this treatment should be avoided. If medical treatment is unsuccessful, careful surgical excision may be required. In certain selected cases, tunable laser therapy is effective, particularly for superficial lesions.[14]

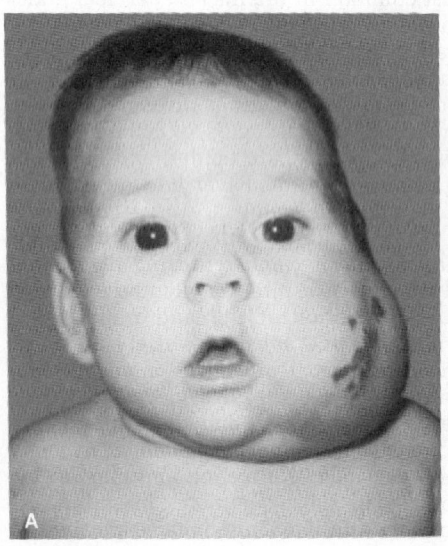
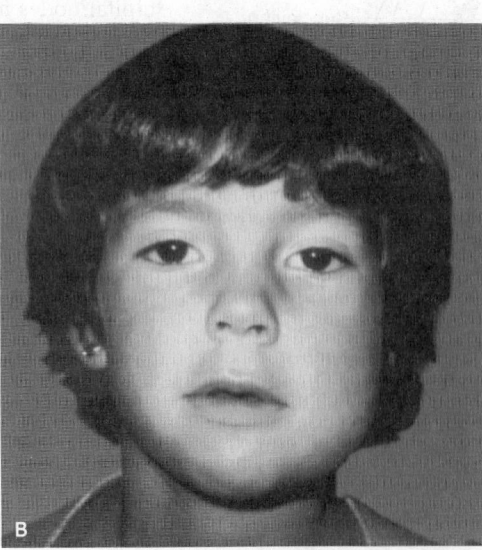

Figure 101-9. Spontaneous resolution of a capillary hemangioma over a 6-year period. (*A*) Appearance at age 1 month. (*B*) Appearance at age 6 years.

REFERENCES

1. DeLorimer AA. Congenital malformations and neonatal problems of the respiratory tract. In: Welch KJ, Randolph JG, Ravitch MM, O'Neill JA, Rowe MI, eds. Pediatric surgery, ed 4. Chicago, Year Book, 1986:631.

2. Alpers CE, Rosenau W, Finkbeiner WE, et al. Congenital (infantile) hemangiopericytoma of the tongue and sublingual region. Am J Clin Pathol 1984;81:377.

3. Wider DJ, Parker W. Lingual thyroid: review, case reports, and therapeutic guidelines. Ann Otol Rhinol Laryngol 1977; 86:841.

4. Kinnefors A, Olofsson J. Acute epiglottitis in children: experiences with tracheostomy and intubation. Clin Otolaryngol 1983;8:25.

5. Soper RT, Pringle KC. Cysts and sinus of the neck. In: Welch KJ, Randolph JG, Ravitch MM, O'Neill JA, Rowe MI, eds. Pediatric surgery, ed 4. Chicago, Year Book, 1986:539.

6. Rosenfeld RM, Biller HF. Fourth branchial pouch sinus: diagnosis and treatment. Otolaryngol Head Neck Surg 1991; 105:44.

7. Miller D, Hill JL, Sun CC, O'Brien DS, Haller JA Jr. The diagnosis and management of pyriform sinus fistulae in infants and young children. J Pediatr Surg 1983;18:377.

8. Page CP, Kemmerer WT, Haff RC, et al. Thyroid carcinoma arising in thyroglossal ducts. Ann Surg 1974;180:799.

9. Filston HC: Common lumps and bumps of the neck in infants and children. Pediatr Ann 1989;18:180.

10. Hartzog LW. Prevalence of lymphadenopathy of the head and neck in infants and children. Clin Pediatr 1983;22:485.

11. Zitelli DJ. Neck masses in children: adenopathy and malignant disease. Pediatr Clin North Am 1981;28:813.

12. Bartoshesky LE, Bull M, Feingold M. Corticosteroid treatment of cutaneous hemangiomas: how affected? Clin Pediatr 1978;17:625.

13. Orchard PJ, Smith CN, Woods WG, Day DL, Dehner LP, Shapiro R. Treatment of hemangioendotheliomas with alpha interferon. Lancet 1989;2:565.

14. Oon TT, Gilchrest BA. Laser therapy for selected cutaneous vascular lesions in the pediatric population: a review. Pediatrics 1988;82:652.

SURGERY: SCIENTIFIC PRINCIPLES AND PRACTICE, Second Edition, edited by Lazar J. Greenfield, Michael W. Mulholland, Keith T. Oldham, Gerald B. Zelenock, and Keith D. Lillemoe. Lippincott–Raven Publishers, Philadelphia, © 1997.

CHAPTER 102

PEDIATRIC THORAX

ARNOLD G. CORAN AND KEITH T. OLDHAM

Chest Wall, Lung, and Mediastinum

ARNOLD G. CORAN

CHEST WALL DEFORMITIES

Congenital deformities of the chest wall vary considerably in appearance. Generally, the clinical presentations focus on cosmetic and psychological issues rather than physiologic disability. Indeed, demonstrable pulmonary function abnormalities often are insignificant. These deformities are not infrequent in incidence. The anomalies discussed in this chapter include sternal clefts, pectus excava-

tum, pectus carinatum, and Poland syndrome. The most common of these deformities, pectus excavatum, represents about 90% of the lesions, and its management serves as the basis for considering the other malformations.

Embryology

The sternum develops during the sixth week of gestation from two parallel mesenchymal primordia lateral to the midline. These paired primordia, called *sternal bands*, converge superiorly and become progressively chondrified as they fuse from cephalad to caudad. The ribs develop independently from the individual somites and gradually approach the sternal bands during the midline fusion process. After this initial fusion, transverse divisions of the cartilaginous sternum differentiate into segments opposite each end of rib pairs. At birth, the sternum is cartilaginous, except for small centers of ossification. The marrow spaces in the sternum appear by the third year of life, and final ossification is usually complete by 14 to 16 years of age. The process is sufficiently predictable that sternal ossification is considered one reliable method of determining bone age.

STERNAL CLEFTS

Congenital sternal clefts result from failure of midline fusion of the paired sternal bands. The most common form of sternal cleft is a defect in the superior portion of the sternum, sometimes extending to, but not including, the xiphoid (Fig. 102-1). These defects are extremely rare, with fewer than 100 operated cases reported. Although the defects are generally asymptomatic, the concept is that repair protects underlying mediastinal structures. This is best done in the immediate neonatal period when approximation of the two halves of the sternal cleft is accomplished more easily. Surgical repair is straightforward, consisting of subcutaneous mobilization and midline approximation of the fibrocartilagenous sternal bars. If a cleft is incomplete, it must be completed by surgically dividing the intact portion so that closure does not lead to buckling of the inferior portion of the sternum. It is necessary to dissect the pericardium from the underside of the sternal bars before approximation, but this is easily done. Although it is extremely uncommon, approximation of the two sternal

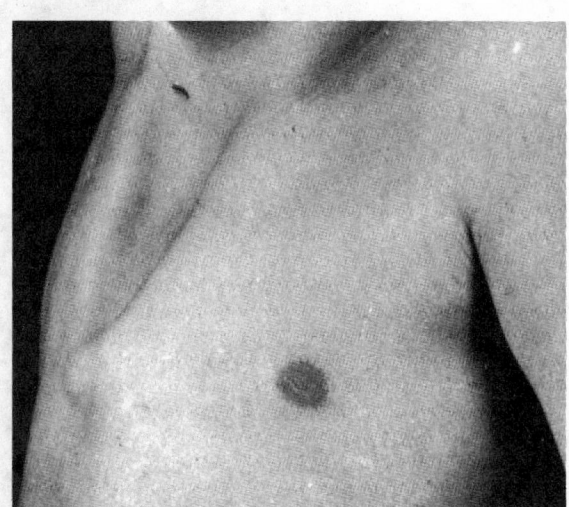

Figure 102-1. Incomplete, large V-shaped sternal cleft. (Sabiston DC. J Thorac Cardiovasc Surg 1958;35:118)

bars may result in significant respiratory compromise. If necessary, synthetic material or autogenous cartilage may be used to close the sternal defect. The cosmetic and functional results with repair are excellent. An unusual form of sternal cleft occurs with the Cantrell pentalogy. This syndrome consists of a distal sternal cleft, an omphalocele, a diaphragmatic defect, a pericardial defect, and an intracardiac abnormality, and usually a ventricular septal defect or a left ventricular diverticulum. Other congenital heart anomalies have also been described with this syndrome. Exstrophy of the heart may occur and has been uniformly lethal until recently.

PECTUS EXCAVATUM

The pectus excavatum deformity is characterized by a posterior curve in the body of the sternum, beginning at the manubrium and extending to the xiphoid (Fig. 102-2). The lower costal cartilages bend dorsally to create the depression. The pathogenesis is thought to be related to primary abnormalities in the regulation of cartilagenous growth in the costal cartilages. Although the deformity is usually symmetric, asymmetric forms are not rare.[1] The most common variation is a significant rotation of the sternum to the right, which may be as much as 90 degrees. The deformity is usually present at birth and can be progressive, with significant worsening during childhood. On the other hand, many patients remain stable throughout childhood and adult life. In the younger child, a potbelly appearance is characteristic, and by adolescence, a stoopshouldered posture is frequent. Concurrent scoliosis is not uncommon and is best corrected after pectus excavatum repair. Marfan syndrome is often associated with pectus excavatum.

Although the exact incidence is not recorded in the literature, pectus excavatum is common, with equal distribution between the genders. Most children with pectus excavatum are asymptomatic. There have been numerous efforts to detect associated cardiac and pulmonary abnormalities, but objective data do not show that pectus excavatum has consistently important physiologic consequences.[2–4] A well-controlled study showed that pulmonary function is not improved by surgical repair of the defect.[5] As a result, the indications for repairing pectus excavatum are essentially cosmetic and psychological. The importance of these, however, should not be minimized in a largely adolescent population.

The operative repair requires general anesthesia, and although the procedure takes several hours, blood transfusion is not usually required. Although timing of repair is controversial, it is best done in older childhood or adolescence because the risk of recurrence may be less after growth is nearly complete. In addition, a form of iatrogenic acquired thoracic dystrophy is reported following repair in preschool children. The original description has undergone innumerable modifications but retains some common features. For cosmetic reasons, the repair is done through a transverse submammary incision, which provides adequate exposure for all age groups. The pectoral muscles are detached from the sternum and elevated laterally to expose the costal cartilages on both sides. The deformed costal cartilages, usually three through seven, are resected subperichondrially bilaterally. The xiphoid is then divided from the sternum, and the rectus muscles are detached inferiorly. The undersurface of the sternum is freed from the anterior surface of the pericardium, with care taken not to enter either pleural cavity. An anterior osteotomy is created just below the manubrium, and the posterior cortex of the sternum is fractured. The sternum is then elevated, and the anterior osteotomy is closed with interrupted sutures to maintain the new sternal position. This is generally followed by the placement of a strut beneath the sternum for additional stability. The choice of material is highly variable, but use of a metallic or plastic strut requires operative removal after 6 to 8 weeks. The wound is closed by reattaching the pectoral muscles and the rectus muscles to the sternum over a sump drain, which is left in place for 3 to 5 days.

The results with this type of repair are excellent. One personal experience with more than 500 patients, ranging in age from 2 months to 40 years at the time of operation, has shown essentially no recurrence of the deformity.[6] Similar results are reported in most institutions.

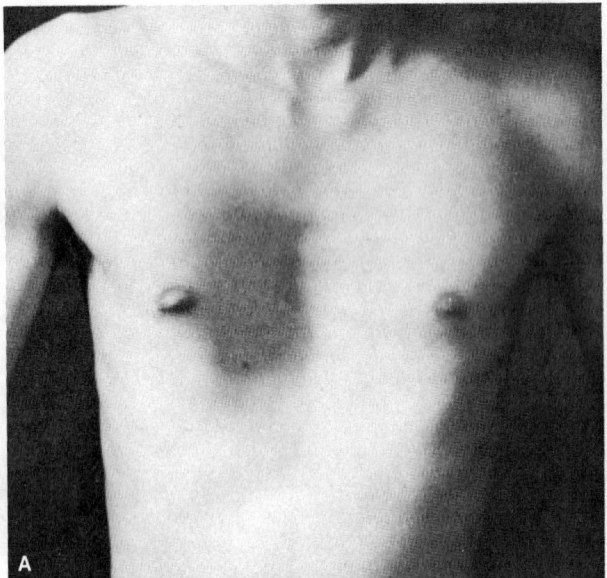
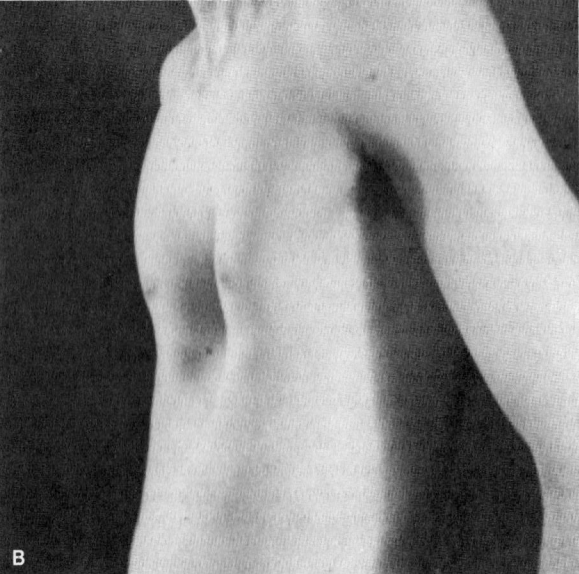

Figure 102-2. Anterior (*A*) and lateral (*B*) views of a typical pectus excavatum deformity.

PECTUS CARINATUM

Pectus carinatum (pigeon breast) occurs much less frequently than pectus excavatum (one tenth the incidence of pectus excavatum). Because the thoracic cavity is larger than expected, there are no physiologic impairments. The clinical presentation is typically for cosmetic concerns. The origin of both pectus excavatum and pectus carinatum appears to be related to excessively rapid growth of the costal cartilages. Buckling of the sternum results in the excavatum deformity, whereas elevation of the sternum leads to the carinatum deformity (Fig. 102-3). The operative repair of pectus carinatum is similar to that described for pectus excavatum; however, the sternum requires depression to achieve the normal position. There is typically no need for a sternal strut with this deformity. Results after surgery are similar to those seen with pectus excavatum, with recurrence being rare.

POLAND SYNDROME

In 1841, Poland noted the classic findings of the syndrome that would bear his name in a cadaver. Features include absence of the sternal portions of the pectoralis major muscle; absence of the pectoralis minor muscle; absence of portions of the serratus anterior and external oblique muscles; hand deformities, usually syndactyly and absence of the phalanges; ipsilateral hypoplasia of the nipple, breast, and subcutaneous tissue; absence or deformity of costal cartilages two through five; and hairlessness of the skin of the axilla on the affected side. In many cases of Poland syndrome, hand deformities are not present. This syndrome is far less common than pectus excavatum or pectus carinatum and is asymptomatic in virtually all patients.

The operative approach to the chest deformity of Poland syndrome is similar to that used for pectus excavatum and pectus carinatum repair. The tendency of the sternum to rotate in an axial plane toward the affected side, however,

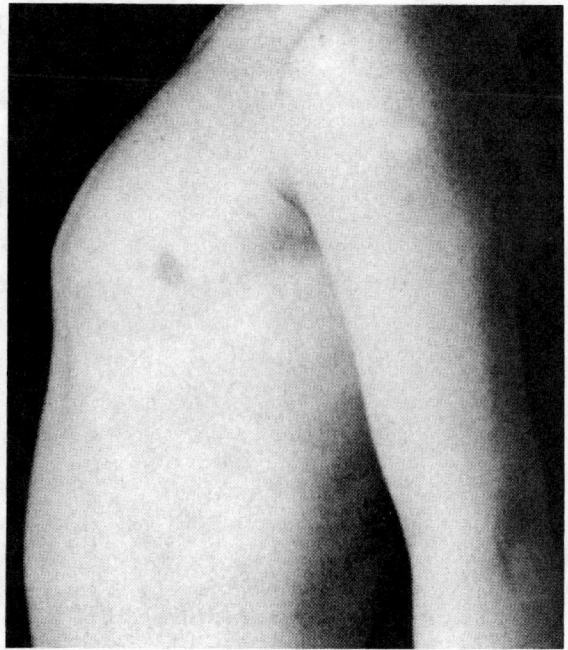

Figure 102-3. Lateral view of a prominent pectus carinatum deformity. (Ravitch MM. In: Welch KJ, ed. Pediatric surgery, ed 4. Chicago, Year Book, 1986:579)

requires placement of a substernal strut in all cases to prevent this rotation. In the female, a mammary implant is usually required after puberty to compensate for the asymmetry or the absence of the breast on the affected side. The cosmetic results after surgery are generally good, although the additional abnormalities make a normal appearance more difficult to achieve.

CYSTS AND TUMORS

Congenital Cystic Disease of the Lung

Pulmonary sequestration, cystic adenomatoid malformation (CAM), congenital lobar overinflation, and bronchogenic cyst are four congenital lesions of the tracheobronchial tree that may present as abnormal cystic areas in the pleural cavity in early life.[7] They share similar clinical and embryologic features, are frequently difficult to diagnosis, and are all best managed surgically.[8]

Embryology

By the end of the third week of gestation, the laryngotracheal groove can be seen at the proximal end of the foregut. While the laryngotracheal groove is forming, there is proliferation of the mesenchyme of the primitive (mediastinal) mesentery. The cartilage, muscle, and connective tissue of the lungs develop from this mesenchymal tissue. By 4 to 5 weeks' gestation, the buds of the secondary bronchi are present, and separation of the trachea and esophagus is well underway. This separation is complete by 6 weeks' gestation, at which time three to five orders of bronchi are present.

Initially, the level of the tracheal bifurcation is high in the cervical region. With first trimester growth, it descends to the level of the first thoracic vertebra, and at birth, it is at the level of the fourth or fifth thoracic vertebra. The lungs, which are at first dorsal to the heart, grow lateral and ventral to surround it. All major bronchial buds are present before closure of the pleuroperitoneal canals. Until the third gestational month, the right lung grows faster than the left, being larger and having more generations of bronchial branching. These differences persist, and the right lung remains slightly larger than the left throughout life.

Cartilage appears in the trachea and primary bronchi at about the 10th week. By the 16th week, the cartilage has progressed distally to the segmental bronchi, completing development of the conducting airways. Respiratory epithelial glands appear during the 11th gestational week and achieve maturity by the 13th week. Alveoli undergo a substantial proportion of their growth and development during the latter portion of gestation and the first few years of life. There is a rapid increase in the number of alveoli up to 6 months of age and a slower increase until maturity at 8 to 10 years. During this maturation, the number of generations of airways increases from 21 to 23, principally in the first few years of life. The mean size of an alveolus in the neonate is 150 μm, whereas it is about 280 μm in the adult. The most distal bronchioles undergo transformation into alveolar ducts by centripetal formation of new alveoli during the first 2 months of postnatal life. Formation of alveoli themselves occurs up to the fourth year. At birth, the infant has about 24×10^6 alveoli; the adult has 296×10^6 alveoli.

Types of Abnormality

Pulmonary Sequestrations. These are collections of abnormal lung tissue with anomalous systemic blood supply that do not communicate with the tracheobronchial tree by normally related bronchi. The embryologic origin of a

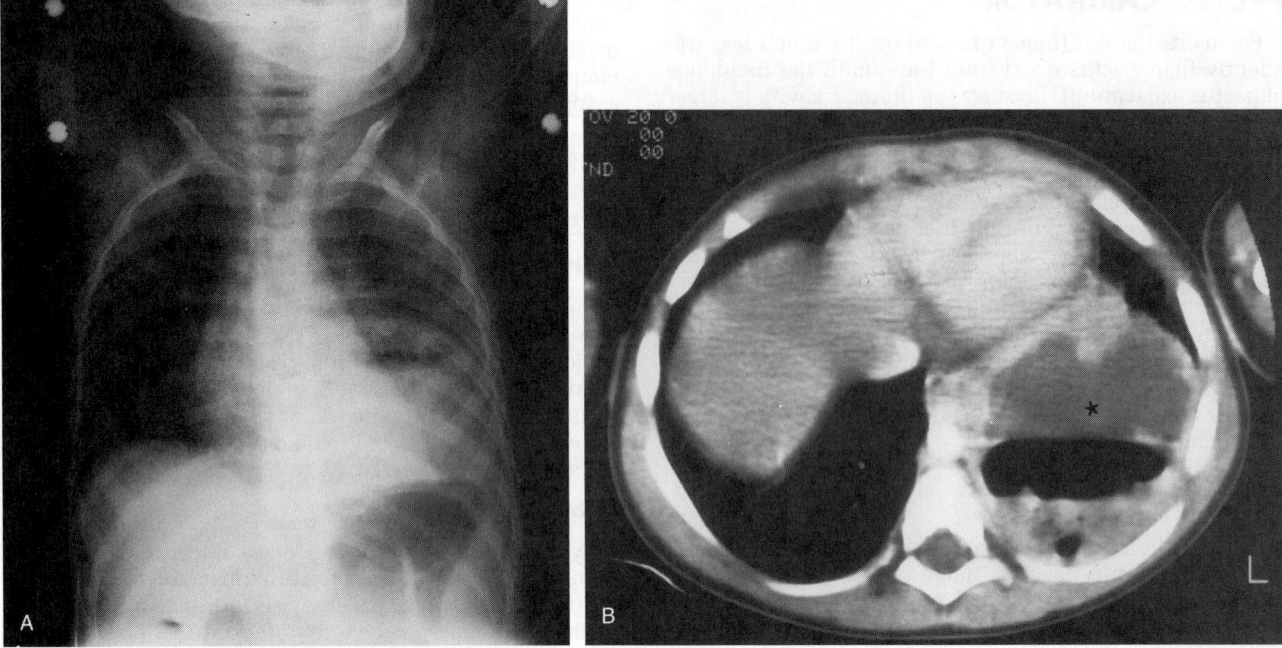

Figure 102-4. (*A*) Plain chest radiograph of a child with fever and cough who had an infected intralobular sequestration of the left lower lobe. (*B*) CT scan of the same lesion (*asterisk*).

pulmonary sequestration is uncertain. One plausible hypothesis is that the pulmonary artery fails to develop appropriate blood supply for the whole of the growing lung, leading to formation (or persistence) of collateral aortic blood supply by means of the anomalous artery. This abnormal parenchyma may be either intralobar or extralobar, depending on the relation with the normal lung.

An intralobar sequestration lies within a lobe of the lung, invested by its visceral pleura (Fig. 102-4). Venous drain-

age from either an intralobar or extralobar type of sequestration can be into either the pulmonary or systemic circulation. The anomalous arterial supply usually comes from the thoracic or abdominal aorta and may penetrate the diaphragm to supply the sequestration. Microscopically, the intralobar sequestration may be normal-appearing lung parenchyma intersected by many large blood vessels in a random fashion. In the usual case, however, there is exten-

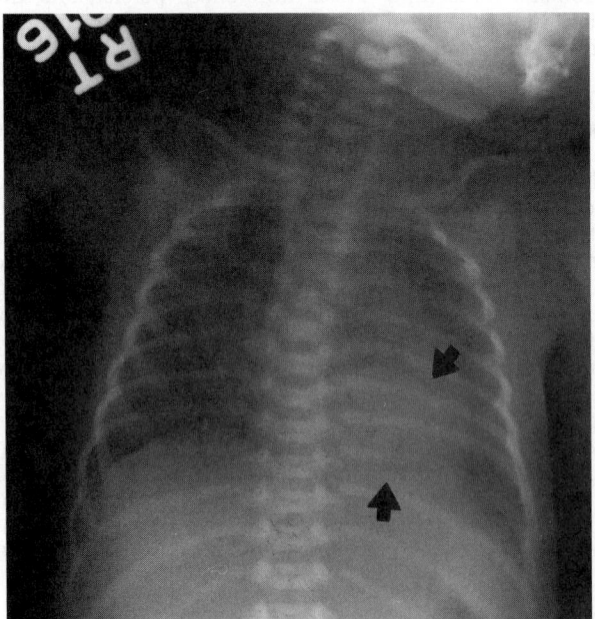

Figure 102-5. Chest radiograph of an extralobular pulmonary sequestration (*arrow*) in the left lower thorax. The contour of the retrocardiac left hemidiaphragm has been obliterated. This was a newborn with no symptoms whose lesion was first noticed on prenatal maternal ultrasound.

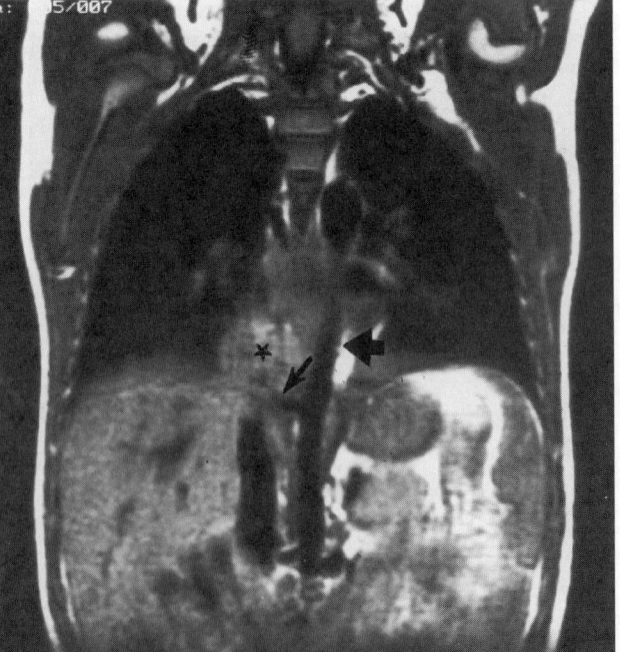

Figure 102-6. MR image of a right lower lobe extralobar pulmonary sequestration (*asterisk*), with the descending aorta shown (*thick arrow*) and clear demonstration of the systemic arterial blood supply to the sequestration (*thin arrow*).

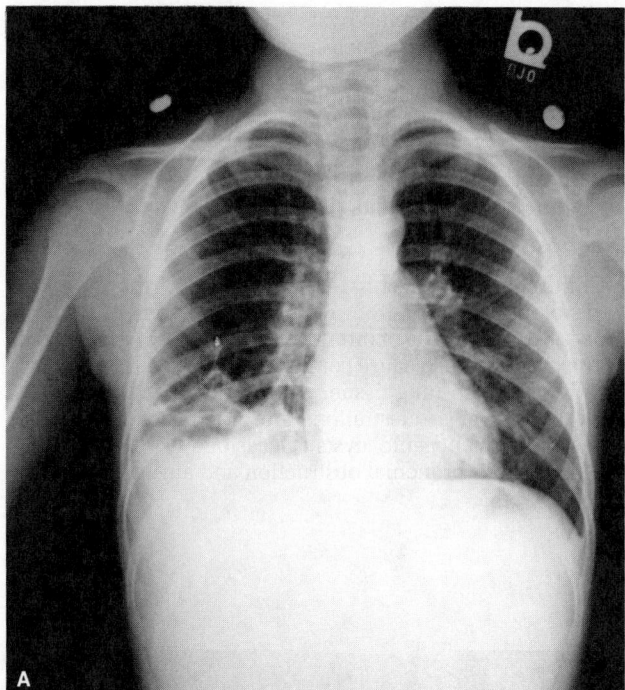

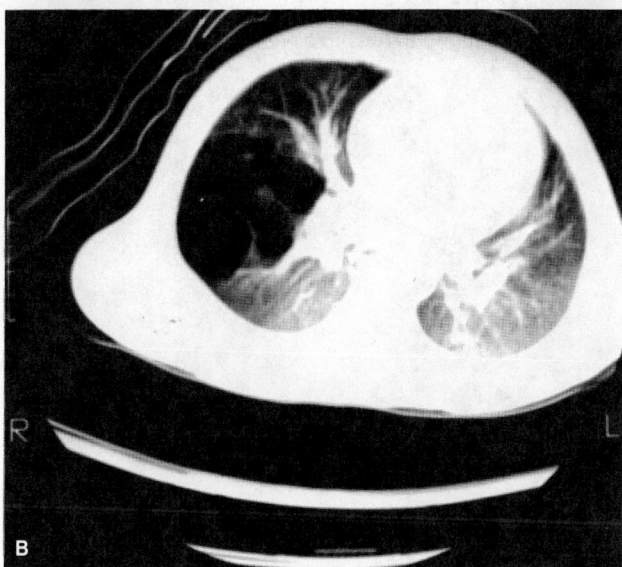

Figure 102-7. (*A*) Chest radiograph showing a cystic adenomatoid malformation of the right lower lobe. (*B*) Axial, intravenous contrast-enhanced CT scan showing the mass involving the right lower lobe.

sive acute and chronic inflammation and fibrosis so that little normal tissue remains. The remainder of the lobe around the sequestration is often sharply demarcated in its normality. Lobectomy is usually definitive.

The extralobar sequestration is a spongy tissue mass within its own investing pleura and outside the normal lung parenchyma (Figs. 102-5 and 102-6). This may be at various positions within the thorax or beneath the diaphragm; adjacent to the left lower lobe is the most common position. The parenchyma may be normal, dysplastic, or immature, with areas of interstitial edema and dilated lymphatics. Infection is rarely prominent. These may be asymptomatic or may be associated with hemorrhage, arteriovenous shunting, mediastinal compression, or occa-

sionally malignancy. Excision is straightforward and recommended.

Cystic Adenomatoid Malformations. CAMs are solid, cystic, or mixed lung parenchymal masses that communicate with the normal tracheobronchial tree. They typically occur in a lung lobe and rarely have an anomalous systemic blood supply (Fig. 102-7). Embryologically, CAMs result from excessive proliferation of bronchial structures without alveoli during gestation. The three types of CAMs are characterized by size, shape, spacing of the cysts, and histologic appearance. Type I CAMs are composed of cysts with large, irregular, and widely dispersed spaces with lining cells of cuboidal or low columnar epithelium and occasional foci of mucous cells. Type II CAMs have smaller cysts that are closer together and more numerous (Fig. 102-8). Histologically, the cysts resemble closely packed, dilated bronchioles. Type III CAMs have cysts that may be so small as to be unrecognizable on gross inspection. These have closely packed, curved channels lined by cuboidal epithelium that resemble late-gestation fetal lung. Types II and III may also be found in extralobar sequestrations. Cartilage is essentially lacking in all three types of CAMs. Prenatal diagnosis is now common, and successful in utero resection of the affected lobe is reported for infants who develop fetal hydrops.[9,10] This remains an area of controversy, however, as the criteria for patient selection and the natural history of these lesions are unclear.[11] In particular, spontaneous in utero resolution occurs in one fourth to one third of these patients. At present, most patients are delivered at term in institutions with a full range of respiratory support options where postpartum lobectomy and appropriate ventilatory support are provided.

Congenital Lobar Overinflation. In congenital lobar overinflation, the lesion is one of air-trapping, with histologic examination showing a normally formed acinus with greatly overexpanded alveoli. There is no tissue destruction, and the vascular supply is normal. There is usually a normally placed, although partially obstructed, bronchus. Embryologically, the cartilage of the involved bronchus fails to develop, leading to focal collapse with expiration and air-trapping (Fig. 102-9). Progression to hemodynamic instability can occur rapidly and dictate emergency thoracotomy, at which time overdistended lung or lobe must be resected to decompress the thorax.

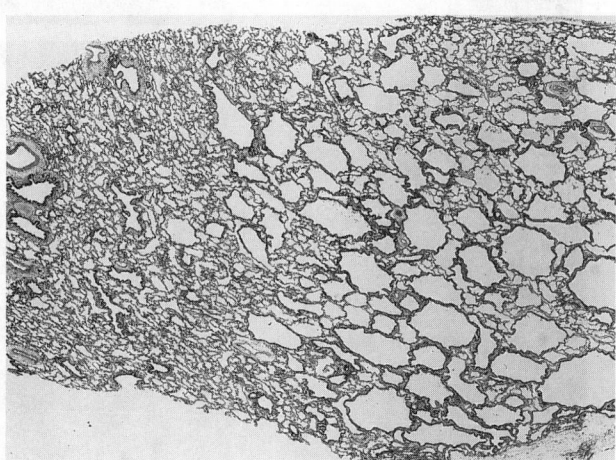

Figure 102-8. Congenital cystic adenomatoid malformation type II. Numerous small cysts are separated by alveolar-like spaces and merge with normal parenchyma (hematoxylin-eosin, ×12). (Courtesy of Kay Washington, MD, Duke University Medical Center, Durham)

Bronchogenic Cysts. Embryologically, bronchogenic cysts originate before bronchial formation and persist after birth. Hilar and carinal bronchogenic cysts represent groups of epithelial cells from the developing trachea and lung buds that have become separated from the tracheobronchial tree. Unlike the isolated bronchial buds around which sequestered lobes of the lung form, these do not originate distal enough to reach the pulmonary mesenchyme, on which further development is dependent. Earlier separation results in the formation of bronchogenic cysts and enterogenous cysts, or esophageal duplications, whereas later separation results in sequestration of the lung or accessory lungs. The earliest separation is usually dorsal, from the presumptive esophageal portion of the foregut, whereas the later separations are from the ventral or tracheal portion of the foregut. The rare paratracheal cysts have been considered to be derived from tracheal diverticula that are subsequently sequestered from the par-

ent organ. Bronchogenic cysts are usually but not exclusively extrapulmonary masses (Figs. 102-10 and 102-11). They do not communicate with a normal tracheobronchial tree, nor do they have a unique blood supply. Also, distal lung structures (alveoli) are absent. On microscopic examination, they are lined by ciliated columnar epithelium and have a fibrous tissue wall that contains nests of cartilage and sometimes bronchial glands.

Diagnosis

Children with congenital cystic disease of the lung tend to develop symptoms from recurrent infections in the cyst. This is especially true of intralobar sequestrations and CAMs. These cysts can also cause compression and collapse of adjacent bronchi and lung tissue, with resultant respiratory distress. Extralobar sequestrations are often asymptomatic, as are most bronchogenic cysts. Occasionally, bronchogenic cysts can cause bronchial obstruction and air-trapping in the

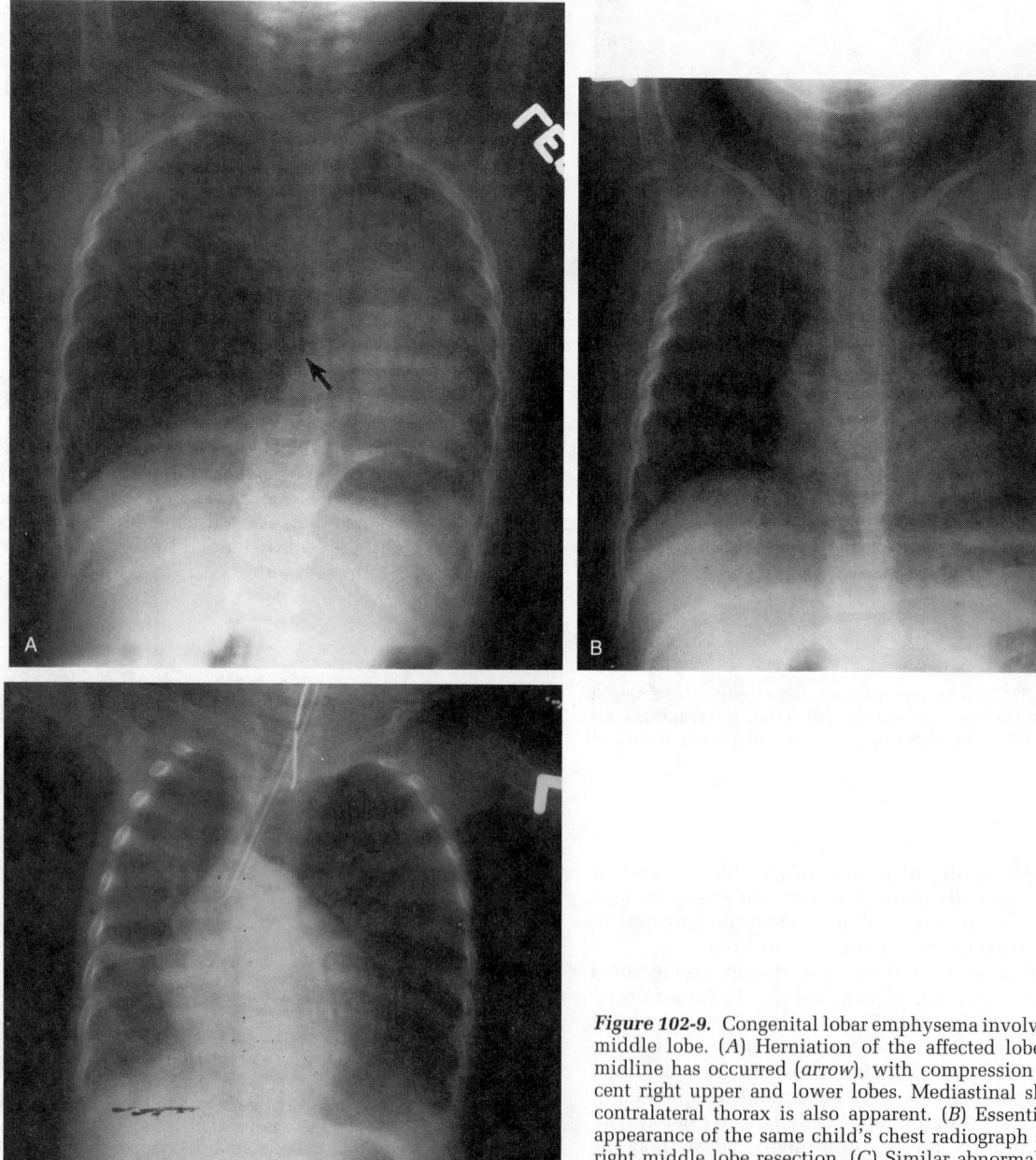

Figure 102-9. Congenital lobar emphysema involving the right middle lobe. (*A*) Herniation of the affected lobe across the midline has occurred (*arrow*), with compression of the adjacent right upper and lower lobes. Mediastinal shift into the contralateral thorax is also apparent. (*B*) Essentially normal appearance of the same child's chest radiograph shortly after right middle lobe resection. (*C*) Similar abnormalities in a 4-month-old girl with involvement of the left upper lobe, the most common site of congenital lobar emphysema.

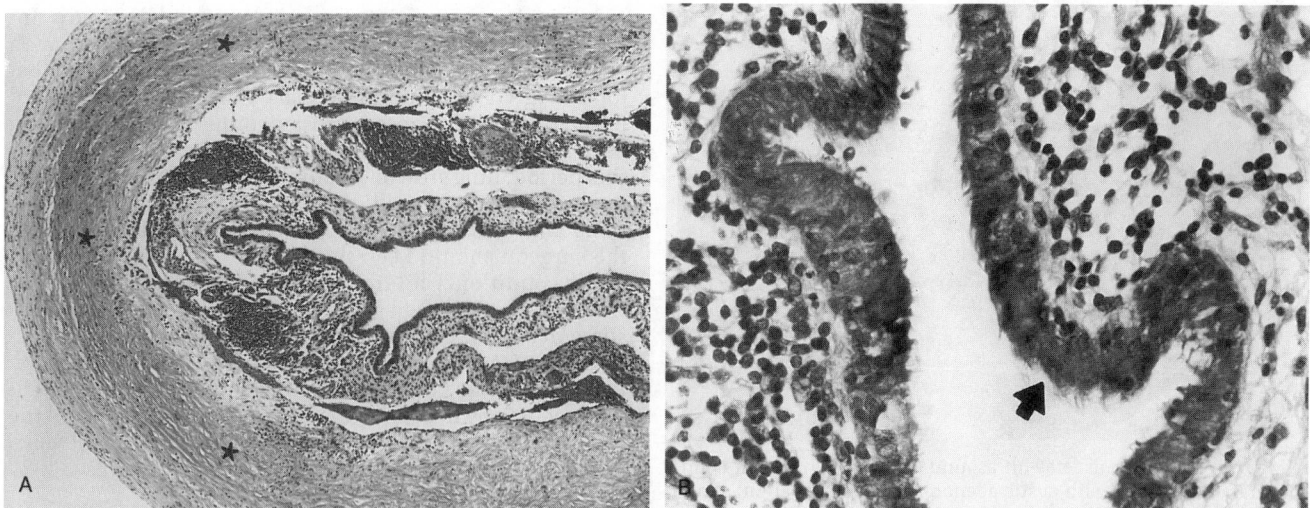

Figure 102-10. Bronchogenic cyst. (*A*) The wall of this cyst consists of dense fibrous tissue (*asterisks*). Cartilage and seromucinous glands were also present (not shown) (Masson trichrome, ×52). (*B*) The cyst is lined by ciliated pseudostratified columnar epithelium (*arrow*) (Masson trichrome, ×400). (Courtesy of Kay Washington, MD, Duke University Medical Center, Durham)

newborn, resulting in severe respiratory distress. Congenital lobar overinflation usually causes marked air-trapping and respiratory distress within the first 48 hours of life. Plain film radiography is the first imaging study performed and remains a cornerstone of diagnosis and follow-up for this family of lesions. The selective use of additional imaging studies may help in arriving at an accurate differential diagnosis and in planning a surgical approach. Computed tomography (CT) can separate cystic from solid components in a radiopaque lung mass. This is the single most useful diagnostic study available, although magnetic resonance imaging yields excellent information as well.[12] Intravenous contrast administration enhances a cyst wall solid parenchyma and thereby differentiates it from fluid. Dynamic scanning during a bolus

contrast injection may show the aberrant systemic artery feeding a pulmonary sequestration. Even without contrast, CT scans may show lung markings or septations within a hyperlucent portion of the lung. In cases in which a soft tissue or water-dense mass is adjacent to the chest wall, ultrasonography can differentiate solid tissue from fluid (Fig. 102-12). Ultrasonography is less costly and more readily performed than CT and, in selected cases, may be as sensitive. Ultrasound images at the level of the diaphragm may show an aberrant systemic artery arising from the aorta with pulmonary sequestration. Although both CT scan and ultrasound are useful, they overlap in diagnostic efficacy. Prenatal ultrasound diagnosis of many of these lesions is now routine.[13]

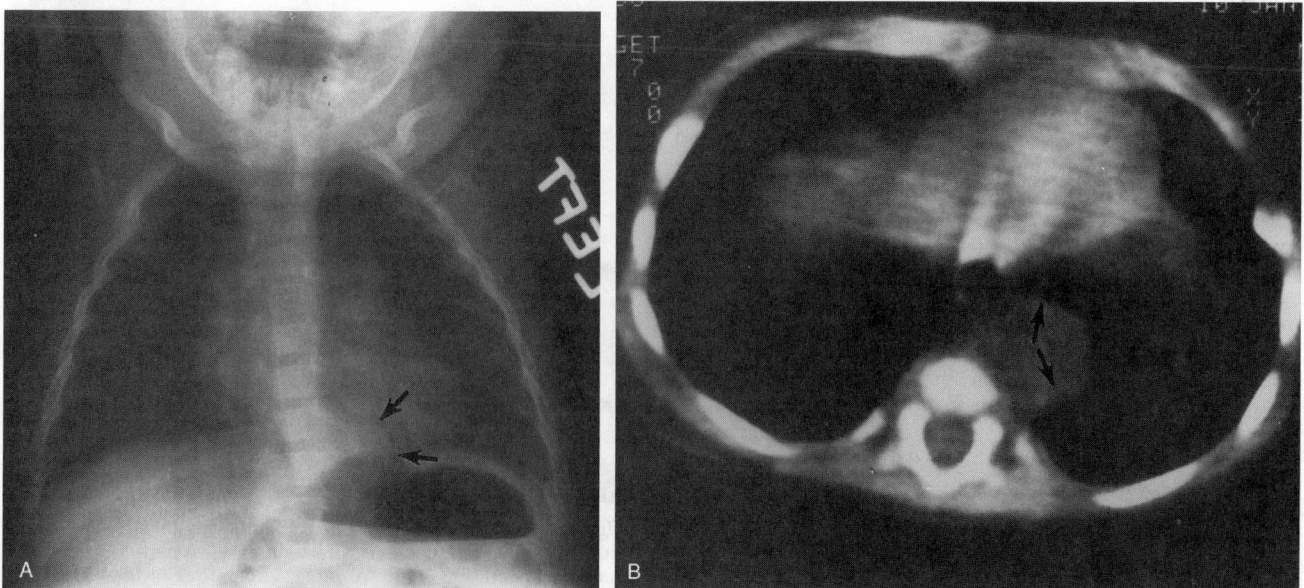

Figure 102-11. (*A*) Plain chest radiograph of a child with a mediastinal bronchogenic cyst (*arrows*). (*B*) CT appearance of the same lesion (*arrows*). (Courtesy of Don Frush, MD, Duke University Medical Center, Durham)

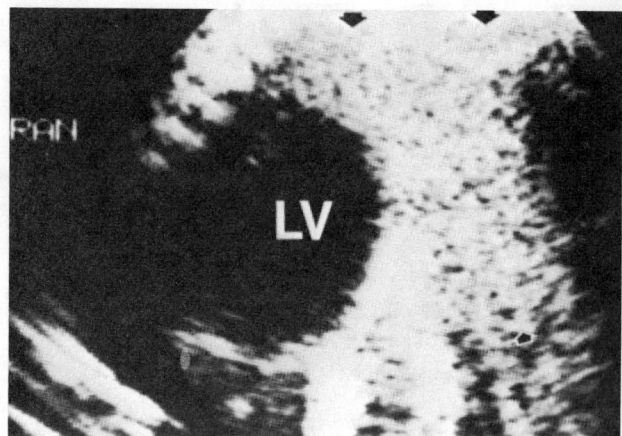

Figure 102-12. Transverse ultrasound scan through the left hemithorax of a patient with cystic adenomatoid malformation, showing a solid echogenic mass (*arrows*) adjacent to the heart. LV, left ventricle. (Wesley JR, Heidelberger KP, DiPietro MA, et al. Diagnosis and management of congenital cystic disease of the lung in children. J Pediatr Surg 1986;21:205)

Barium esophagogram is indicated in patients with dysphagia and may also warn the surgeon of an abnormal communication with the gastrointestinal tract. Segmentation anomalies of the spine in this group of patients suggest a neurenteric cyst. Thoracic and upper abdominal aortography may be useful to demonstrate an anomalous systemic arterial vessel. These vessels usually originate from the descending thoracic aorta or upper abdominal aorta below the diaphragm. Angiography is not used regularly because the aberrant blood supply is readily identifiable at surgery without the aid of a preoperative study. If necessary, computer-enhanced digital subtraction angiography may demonstrate the vascular anatomy. This technique reduces the morbidity associated with an arterial puncture and catheterization, especially in infants (Fig. 102-13).

Treatment

With improved safety of pediatric anesthesia and the development of sophisticated noninvasive diagnostic techniques, there should be no delay in operating on a symptomatic infant with congenital cystic disease of the lung. Asymptomatic pulmonary cysts generally require removal because of their tendency to become infected. Another reason for their removal is the rare association of congenital pulmonary cysts and malignant neoplasms.[14] Embryonal rhabdomyosarcoma and other malignancies are reported. Any cyst that is enlarging on serial chest films should be resected because of the respiratory compromise that may ensue and the propensity for infection either in the cyst or in the adjacent compressed lung tissue. If a congenital cyst is infected at the time of diagnosis, it can be safely removed once tissue levels of broad-spectrum antibiotics have been established. Unless the patient is an exceptional surgical risk, the only reason for following a lesion long-term would be if serial radiographs demonstrated progressive resolution, indicating the possibility of an acquired infectious cyst that has the potential for complete resolution.

Surgical management should include complete lobectomy for patients with intralobar pulmonary sequestration and CAMs. Segmental resection carries a prohibitively high complication rate. Successful thorascopic resection of selected lesions is reported as well.[15] Complications include prolonged air leaks and recurrent infection, which

may require reoperation to complete the lobectomy. Infants and children tolerate lobectomy extremely well, with growth and expansion of the remaining lung tissue, so that total lung volume and pulmonary function return toward normal.[16] This response is most vigorous in the very young because new acini and alveoli form for several years. After this period, lung growth is achieved principally by enlargement of existing alveoli. Extralobar pulmonary sequestrations may be associated with a diaphragmatic hernia, and the surgeon should keep this in mind when operating for either condition. Children with congenital lobar overinflation require complete resection of the affected lobe. The surgeon should be present at the time of anesthetic induction because patients with congenital lobar overinflation may not tolerate positive pressure ventilation. Rapid thoracotomy may be necessary to relieve the compression of the remaining normal lung tissue and the heart and great veins to prevent cardiopulmonary collapse.

Cysts of the Mediastinum

Cysts and tumors of the mediastinum are not rare in infancy and childhood. Although most of these are asymptomatic at presentation, surgical resection is usually required. When present, symptoms may include chest pain, cough, respiratory distress, hemoptysis, and dysphagia. The more common cystic lesions include thymic cysts, enterogenous cysts, dermoid cysts, pericardial cysts, and cystic lymphangiomas (cystic hygromas).

Thymic Cysts

Thymic cysts are usually asymptomatic and generally have both mediastinal and cervical components. These are benign lesions lined by ciliated columnar epithelium that

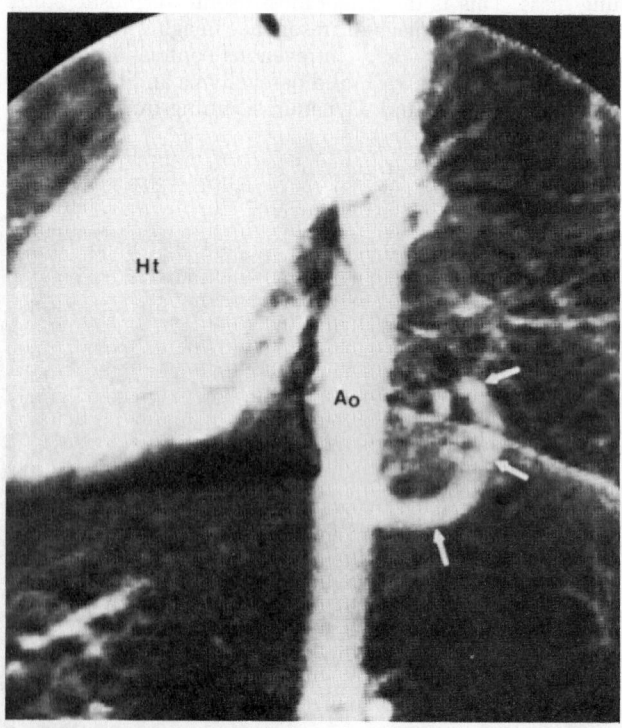

Figure 102-13. Lateral view of intravenous digital subtraction angiogram after intravenous contrast showing an extralobar pulmonary sequestration with a large anomalous systemic artery (*arrows*) arising from the aorta (Ao) at the level of the diaphragm. Ht, heart. (Wesley JR, Heidelberger KP, DiPietro MA, et al. Diagnosis and management of congenital cystic disease of the lung in children. J Pediatr Surg 1986;21:206)

are thought to be congenital in origin. Lymphocytes and cholesterol crystals are prominent characteristics of the cyst wall. Clinical problems are usually the result of rapid expansion from either hemorrhage or infection. Symptoms are generally related to compression of adjacent structures. Most are incidental discoveries. In general, excision is needed either to establish the diagnosis or to relieve symptoms.

Enterogenous Cysts

Enterogenous cysts, or esophageal duplications, occur in the posterior mediastinum and consist of smooth muscle with intestinal epithelium, often gastric mucosa, lining the cyst. Commonly, cervical or upper thoracic vertebral anomalies, particularly hemivertebrae, are associated with these cysts. In rare instances, enterogenous cysts may attach to or communicate with the spinal canal. It is common for a patient with a mediastinal enterogenous cyst to have an intraabdominal intestinal duplication. These cysts may penetrate the diaphragm, ending blindly in the peritoneal cavity or communicating with the jejunum.[17] The presence of gastric epithelium within these cysts may result in an acid–ulcer diathesis and bleeding within the cysts. Perforation of the cyst with erosion into a bronchus or the adjacent esophagus has been reported. Removal is recommended to avoid these possible outcomes as well as to establish the diagnosis.

Cystic Hygromas

Cystic hygromas are benign, multilocular, thin-walled cysts derived from the primitive lymphatic sacs (see Chap. 101). They are commonly found in the neck, axilla, and mediastinum. They contain lymph and are composed of dilated and dysplastic lymphatic channels. Hemorrhage, enlargement, or infection within these cysts warrants elective removal. These mediastinal lesions may present complex technical problems related to involvement of the great vessels or tracheal compression in the neonate. The operative principle is to resect from lesions without sacrificing physiologically important structures. Recurrence because of residual disease is an important potential problem.

Pericardial Cysts

Pericardial cysts are almost always asymptomatic lesions discovered as incidental findings in the cardiophrenic angle on routine chest radiography. These are thin-walled cysts that contain clear serous fluid and are lined by flattened mesothelium. Resection is straightforward and is considered standard therapy.

Cystic Teratomas

Second in frequency only to mediastinal tumors of neurogenic origin, teratomas, including both cystic and solid types, represent some of the largest mediastinal tumors seen in children. The term *dermoid cyst* applies to cystic teratomas composed entirely of ectodermal derivatives. This is the most common lesion. The typical dermoid cyst is a thick-walled fibrous sac lined by squamous epithelium in which the various skin appendages, including hair, teeth and caseous detritus, are found. The tumors are found almost invariably in the anterior mediastinum and occasionally within the pericardium. These lesions may become malignant, with the malignancy being a carcinoma rather than a sarcoma. Removal of these cysts is warranted because of the risks of infection, rupture into the pleura or pericardium, local compression, and malignancy.

Thoracic Tumors

Thoracic tumors in infants and children should be considered as either lung tumors or extrapulmonary (mediastinal) tumors. Both benign and malignant primary lung tumors are rare in childhood, whereas extrapulmonary neoplasms are uncommon.[18]

Lung Tumors

Primary Tumors. Bronchial adenomas are the most common primary lung tumors of childhood. Nevertheless, they are quite rare. Typically, they are low-grade adenocarcinomas that are classified histologically as carcinoids, cylindromas, mucoepidermoid tumors, or bronchomucous gland adenomas. Carcinoid tumors are the most common bronchial adenomas and represent more than 80% of the total. Adenomas usually arise in a primary or secondary bronchus and typically produce persistent cough, hemoptysis, and bronchial obstruction with secondary pulmonary infection and atelectasis. Chest radiographs may show a pneumonic process or atelectasis and occasionally air-trapping. (Figs. 102-14 and 102-15) CT may demonstrate the lesion, but this should be considered fortuitous. The most important diagnostic test remains bronchoscopy. On endobronchial evaluation, the typical carcinoid tumor is friable and prone to bleed. For this reason, biopsy must be done with great care, and the surgeon must be prepared to do an emergency thoracotomy to control hemorrhage if necessary. The carcinoid syndrome has been documented only once with a bronchial carcinoid tumor, even though these tumors may produce serotonin. Carcinoids have been removed bronchoscopically; however, most adenomas require pulmonary resection, usually a lobectomy, for complete removal. Occasionally, a segmental resection of the involved bronchus suffices for a small adenoma. About 5% to 10% of children with bronchial adenomas show evidence of malignancy through local invasion and metastases to regional nodes. These bronchial carcinoids generally respond to radiotherapy.

Although common in adults, bronchogenic carcinoma

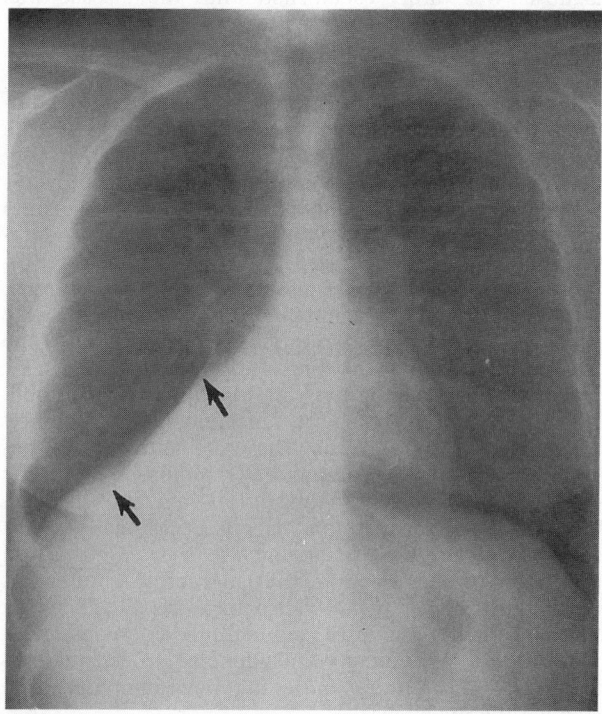

Figure 102-14. Chest radiograph of a 15-year-old girl with a 3-week history of refractory pneumonia. Right middle and lower lobe collapse is obvious (*arrows*). At bronchoscopy, this patient had a nearly completely obstructing carcinoid tumor of the bronchus intermedius.

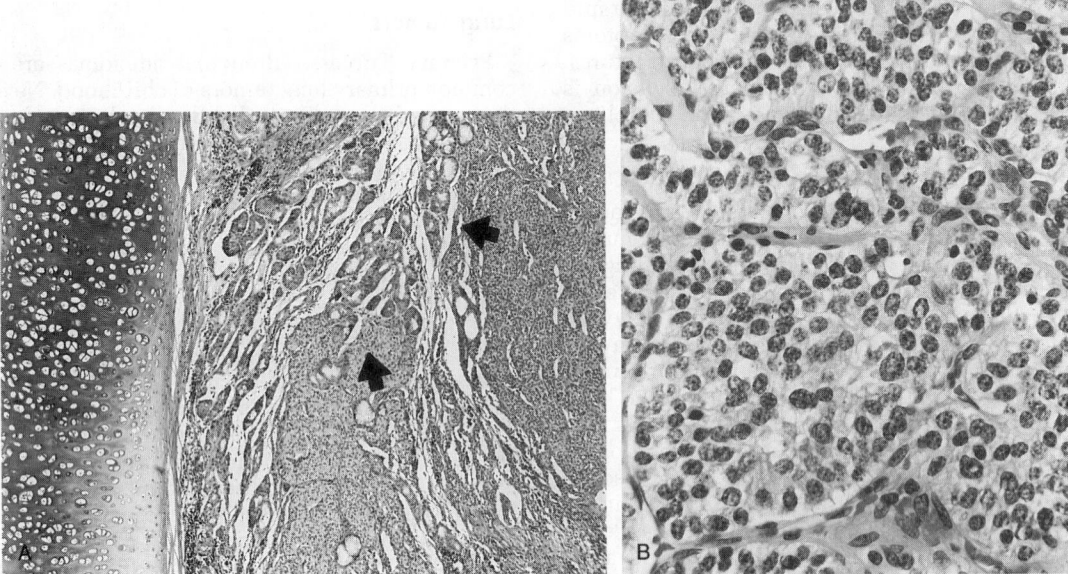

Figure 102-15. The patient in Figure 102-14 underwent resection of the endobronchial lesion with the right middle and lower lobes. The right upper lobe was preserved. The pathology was consistent with an endobronchial carcinoid. (*A*) The carcinoid tumor arising in the submucosa of the bronchus infiltrates among submucosal glands (*arrows*) (hematoxylin–eosin, ×52). (*B*) This carcinoid tumor consisted of uniform cells with round or oval nuclei and abundant pale or eosinophilic cytoplasm. The cells are arranged in nests, and the trabeculae are separated by a fine vascular network. This is a typical carcinoid appearance. (Courtesy of Kay Washington, MD, Duke University Medical Center, Durham)

of the lung is extremely rare in childhood. A review of the world's literature in 1983 summarized 47 such carcinomas in children between 5 months and 16 years of age.[19] The diagnosis was rarely established until the disease was widespread. Cough and dyspnea associated with a pleural effusion were the common presenting symptoms. With early discovery, tumor resection for cure was possible.

Pulmonary blastoma is a malignant lung tumor composed of cells that histologically resemble fetal lung. Its incidence is actually highest in adults, although it may develop at any age. The site of this lesion is almost always in the periphery of the lung. Pulmonary lobectomy results in cure in more than half of these cases. Other rare malignant tumors of the lung seen in children include neurofibrosarcoma, embryoma, mesothelioma, fibrosarcoma, rhabdomyosarcoma, and endothelial sarcoma. Lobectomy or pneumonectomy are appropriate for these lesions if the disease is localized at the time of diagnosis.

Benign tumors of the lung are also rare in childhood. The most common of these benign tumors are pulmonary hamartomas or chondromas. These are found in the periphery of the lung and are normally composed of fibrous tissue, adipose tissue, bronchial epithelium, and cartilage. They are usually asymptomatic but occasionally cause bronchial obstruction. If symptomatic, they can be cured by a limited wedge resection. The usual surgical indication is related to the need to establish a diagnosis. Other benign tumors of the lung in childhood include leiomyoma, leiomyoblastoma, and mucus gland adenoma. In general, surgical resection is required either to relieve symptoms or to establish the diagnosis.

Metastatic Tumors. Lung metastases are most common in children with Wilms tumor and osteogenic sarcoma. About half of children with Wilms tumor develop pulmonary metastases. If metastases are present at the time of

the initial diagnosis of Wilms tumor, nephrectomy with chemotherapy and radiotherapy are initiated. Surgical removal of the metastatic lung tumor is generally undertaken if the pulmonary metastases remain or recur after adequate initial treatment. Using this approach, more than half of children with pulmonary metastases from Wilms tumor can be saved.

Pulmonary metastases commonly occur from osteogenic sarcoma. Adjuvant chemotherapy in the management of osteogenic sarcoma has reduced the incidence of these metastases from 80% to about 20%. Protocols include an aggressive surgical approach to pulmonary metastases after adequate chemotherapy and after appropriate resection of the primary tumor. About 40% of patients with pulmonary metastases from osteogenic sarcoma can be saved with surgical resection, which may require multiple thoracotomies.

Mediastinal Tumors

Mediastinal tumors include lymphomas, neurogenic tumors, teratomas, thymomas, and a variety of rare lesions.

About 25% of children with Hodgkin lymphoma present with an anterior mediastinal mass. Cough, respiratory obstruction, or superior vena cava syndrome may be the presenting symptoms. Usually, cervical adenopathy is also present. In general, the surgical requirement for these patients is to provide tissue for diagnosis, usually through cervical lymph node biopsy. In addition, a staging laparotomy may be appropriate, although the current role for this is limited. Other lymphomas also present in this fashion, but biopsy is necessary to distinguish among the different cell types.

Neurogenic Tumors. Tumors of neurogenic origin represent the most common thoracic tumors of infancy and childhood. The benign tumors, ganglioneuroma and neurofibroma, may grow large without producing any symptoms. Horner syndrome or symptomatic tracheal displacement may provide the first clinical signs of these lesions. Neuroblastoma is the principal malignant tumor of neurogenic origin (see Chap. 105). These mediastinal lesions are often asymptomatic, although they may cause pain from involvement of nerve roots or symptoms from distant metastases. Occasionally, a neuroblastoma may erode through the chest wall, producing a visible thoracic mass. Acute cerebellar ataxia, characterized by opsomyoclonus and chaotic nystagmus, has been observed in some of these cases. This neurologic syndrome is associated with a better prognosis.

Ganglioneuromas Ganglioneuromas are the most common neurogenic mediastinal tumors. Most cases have been reported in infants and children. These tumors can reach a large size before discovery. Histologically, they are usually well encapsulated and are composed of cells that have the appearance of a typical ganglion cell, indicating their sympathetic chain origin. These tumors frequently widen the intercostal spaces and may extend into the spinal canal. Symptoms are related to compression of adjacent structures. Because these lesions are well encapsulated, they usually can be removed readily. All these masses require routine resection for diagnosis.

Neurofibromas Neurofibromas arise from nerves in the posterior mediastinum, such as intercostal nerves, the phrenic nerve, the vagus nerve, or the sympathetic chain. They may occur as isolated tumors or in association with neurofibromatosis or von Recklinghausen disease. Scoliosis is often associated with neurofibromas because of widening and displacement of the vertebral foramina. Isolated tumors are usually well encapsulated and readily removed. Tumors associated with neurofibromatosis, however, tend to extend along nerve sheaths so that total removal is often impossible. Malignant degeneration can occur, which usually takes place in large tumors; therefore, periodic monitoring is mandatory.

Teratomas. Teratomas are second in frequency to neurogenic tumors in the mediastinum. By definition, teratomas contain derivatives of all three embryonic germ layers. They may be cystic, solid, or both. They are almost always found within the anterior mediastinum and occasionally within the pericardium. Surgical resection is generally straightforward. The incidence of malignancy in these tumors is low, but this possibly represents a compelling surgical indication. When present, the malignant lesion is carcinoma (usually adenocarcinoma rather than sarcoma). Symptoms are generally related to direct extension into adjacent structures.

Thymomas. Thymomas are extremely rare in childhood and are managed as they are in the adult population (see Chap. 62).

Other Neoplasms. Several other neoplasms of the mediastinum have been described in childhood, but none is common. These include hemangioma, lipoma, embryonal rhabdomyosarcoma, osteochondroma, pheochromocytoma, and a group of anaplastic carcinomas and sarcomas. Surgical extirpation or biopsy are generally required.

CONGENITAL ABNORMALITIES OF THE TRACHEA AND ESOPHAGUS
Esophageal Atresia and Tracheoesophageal Fistula
Embryology

The trachea first appears as a ventral diverticulum of the foregut at 22 to 23 days of gestation. As the diverticulum elongates, lateral masses of endodermal cells coalesce to form ridges of tissue that ultimately divide the foregut into a separate ventral trachea and dorsal esophagus. This process begins at the carina and progresses in a cephalad direction. By the 26th day of gestation, the esophagus and trachea have completely separated to the level of the larynx. It is probably during the 4th week of gestation that an interruption in this separation process results in the development of a tracheoesophageal fistula. The explanation for the development of esophageal atresia is less clear. One theory suggests that the elongation of the trachea in a caudal direction is occasionally so rapid that, when there is a fistula producing fixation of the esophagus to the trachea, the dorsal wall of the esophagus is drawn forward and downward to be incorporated into the trachea. As a result, atresia of the esophagus may result because of the presence of the fistula.

By the 6th week of gestation, the circular muscular coat of the esophagus appears, and the vagus nerves develop shortly thereafter. Segmental blood vessels from the aorta appear by the 7th week, and the longitudinal muscle of the esophagus is discernible by the 9th week of gestation. The lining of the esophagus is initially ciliated, but by the 20th week of gestation, this is largely replaced by stratified squamous epithelium. These events are considered further in subsequent sections.

Classification

Figure 102-16 depicts the classic anatomic variations of this anomaly. Historically, alphabetical and numeric schemes were presented by Gross and Haight. In general, descriptive terminology is now used. Esophageal atresia with distal tracheoesophageal fistula is by far the most common type of esophageal atresia. This anatomic variant accounts for 85% to 90% of all cases. Esophageal atresia without tracheoesophageal fistula occurs in 5% to 7% of these anomalies and is the second most common variety. Tracheoesophageal fistula without esophageal atresia, the H-type fistula, is third in frequency and accounts for 2% to 6% of all cases. Other, more rare forms of this anomaly include esophageal atresia with proximal tracheoesophageal fistula and esophageal atresia with both proximal and distal tracheoesophageal fistula. The frequency of these latter variants is than 1% in most reports.

Incidence

The incidence of esophageal atresia in Washtenaw County, Michigan, is estimated to be 1 in 4425 live births.[20] A similar incidence is reported in Australia. The incidence reported in Finland is somewhat higher at 1 in 3000 live births.

Pathophysiology

The clinical manifestations of the most common variant of esophageal atresia, that is, esophageal atresia with distal tracheoesophageal fistula, are reviewed later. In general, significant respiratory symptoms develop soon after birth. The esophageal atresia prevents normal swallowing and results in the accumulation of saliva in the proximal esophageal pouch, where eventual aspiration occurs. In addition, because these children are usually asymptomatic at birth, feedings are given, but vomiting with aspiration invariably results if feedings are not stopped. Pneumonia is inevitable without treatment.

The distal tracheoesophageal fistula produces the most serious physiologic disturbances. Because most newborns have free gastroesophageal reflux, gastric secretions reflux unimpeded into the tracheobronchial tree and generate acid-induced pneumonitis. This is exacerbated by gastric distention resulting from the passage of air from the trachea into the fistula and into the stomach with each breath.

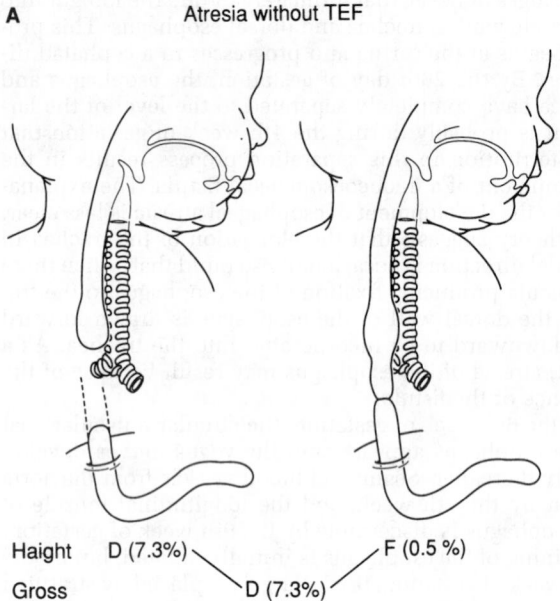

A Atresia without TEF

Haight   D (7.3%)   F (0.5 %)

Gross   D (7.3%)

B Proximal TEF and distal pouch

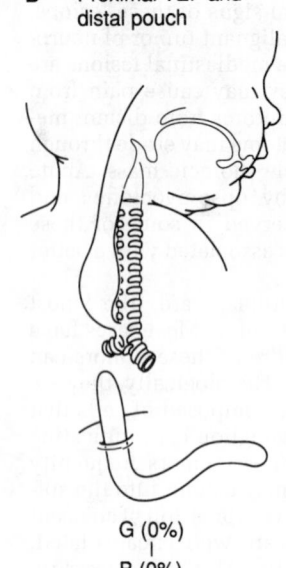

G (0%)

B (0%)

Figure 102-16. The anatomy of the possible variants of esophageal atresia (EA) and tracheoesophageal fistula (TEF). Both the Haight and the Gross classification systems are shown, with approximate incidence of occurrence. (After Manning PB, Morgan RA, Coran AG, et al. Fifty years' experience with esophageal atresia and tracheoesophageal fistula. Ann Surg 1986;204:446) *(continues)*

This distention is occasionally so severe that it limits excursions of the diaphragm and seriously impairs the neonate's ventilation.

Diagnosis

Maternal polyhydramnios is an expected feature of the history with this anomaly, especially when isolated esophageal atresia is present. Given the increasing use of prenatal ultrasound screening, this anomaly is often detected before delivery. Postpartum, infants with esophageal atresia tend to drool and to accumulate excessive secretions in the posterior pharynx. This is typically associated with the early onset of choking, coughing, and episodes of cyanosis, especially with feedings.

The simplest way to establish the diagnosis of esophageal atresia is to attempt to pass a catheter through the mouth or nose into the stomach. If the tube encounters an obstruction, a plain radiograph in the frontal and lateral projections is used to document the atresia (Fig. 102-17). Contrast studies can then be carried out to confirm the diagnosis. Usually 0.5 to 1 mL of thin barium is injected through the tube into the upper pouch. Experience in performing this procedure is necessary to prevent inadvertent tracheobronchial aspiration of barium. This injection typically outlines a blind-ending, smooth upper esophageal pouch. It is important to examine this study for evidence of the rare proximal pouch fistula. In addition, the abdomen should be examined on plain radiograph to determine whether intestinal gas is present. A gasless abdomen confirms the diagnosis of esophageal atresia without tracheoesophageal fistula.

Isolated tracheoesophageal fistula without atresia is much more difficult to diagnose in the newborn; therefore, these children are typically older at diagnosis, often several months of age. The history usually includes recurrent respiratory symptoms, including pneumonia and choking with feedings. A properly done cine esophagogram with barium by an experienced radiologist usually shows the communication between the trachea and esophagus. If the contrast study is normal, yet the clinical suspicion is high, then simultaneous bronchoscopy and esophagoscopy almost always identify the fistula.

Associated Anomalies

Patients with esophageal atresia and tracheoesophageal fistula frequently have associated anomalies. The incidence of recognizable defects associated with this esophageal malformation is about 30% to 50% in most reports (Table 102-1). The anomalies vary from minor skeletal deformities to uncorrectable cardiac defects. The most common associated anomalies are cardiac and gastrointestinal, especially imperforate anus (10%). Most important, every newborn with an imperforate anus should be carefully examined for the presence of esophageal atresia, and vice versa. Of interest are infants with VACTERL syndrome, who have vertebral, anal, cardiac, tracheoesophageal, renal, and limb anomalies (see Chap. 103).

Preoperative Treatment

Pneumonitis is the most critical problem in the immediate preoperative period for these children. The pneumonitis results from aspiration of pharyngeal contents and from the reflux of gastric juice into the tracheobronchial tree. Preoperative treatment involves preventing further aspiration and reflux as well as treating any pneumonitis that may be present. This is best accomplished by placing a sump catheter into the upper pouch, placing the infant upright, and if necessary, performing a gastrostomy under local anesthesia. In addition, the infant is placed on broad-spectrum antibiotic coverage. The infant is kept in an upright position until definitive surgery is carried out, which may be a matter of several weeks in a premature infant with esophageal atresia.

Surgical Treatment

The goal of modern operative therapy is to correct the anomaly completely with one operation. This includes division of the tracheoesophageal fistula and a primary esophagoesophagostomy. This approach was first performed successfully in 1941 by Haight and has remained the standard treatment since that time.[21] Gastrostomy is not routinely performed, either preoperatively or postoperatively. Prematurity, significant pneumonia, and severe associated congenital anomalies all increase the risk of operation and the postoperative morbidity. The concept of staging the

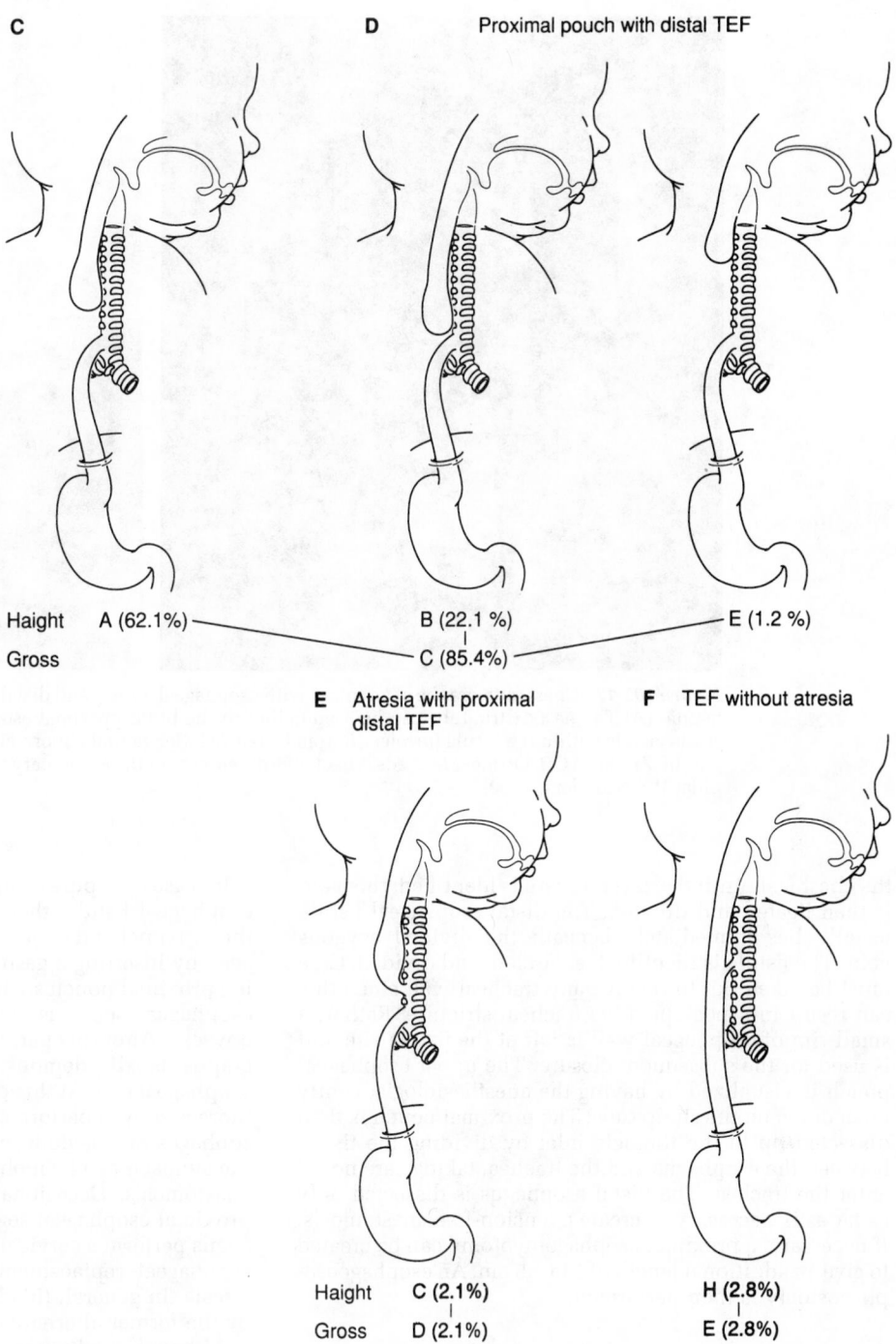

C

D   Proximal pouch with distal TEF

| Haight | A (62.1%) | B (22.1 %) | E (1.2 %) |
| Gross | | C (85.4%) | |

E   Atresia with proximal distal TEF

F   TEF without atresia

| Haight | C (2.1%) | H (2.8%) |
| Gross | D (2.1%) | E (2.8%) |

Figure 102-16. *(Continued)*

operation in high-risk patients has been largely abandoned in recent years. This approach involved the extrapleural division of the distal tracheoesophageal fistula and the placement of a gastrostomy tube. Proximal pouch suction was used to prevent aspiration pneumonia. This allowed treatment of the pneumonia, prematurity, and the other anomalies to proceed before definitive anastomosis of the esophagus (Fig. 102-18). The disadvantages of this staged approach were that it precluded the use of the extrapleural route for the esophageal anastomosis and also required two operations. Most high-risk infants with esophageal atresia and tracheoesophageal fistula are now treated with a gastrostomy for gastric decompression, proximal esophageal suction, and parenteral nutrition. Once stable, an extrapleural thoracotomy is used for division of the tracheo-

esophageal fistula and primary repair of the esophageal atresia. The results with this approach have been better than those with the staged operation.[21]

Operative Technique. A right posterolateral, extrapleural thoracotomy is used unless a right-sided aortic arch is identified preoperatively, which occurs in about 5% of cases and for which a left thoracotomy is preferred. Although most centers use the extrapleural approach to reduce the incidence of postoperative empyema from an esophageal anastomotic leak, a few pediatric surgeons still use the transpleural route.

The chest is entered through the fourth intercostal space, and the intercostal muscles are separated carefully until the pleura is visualized. The pleura is then dissected from

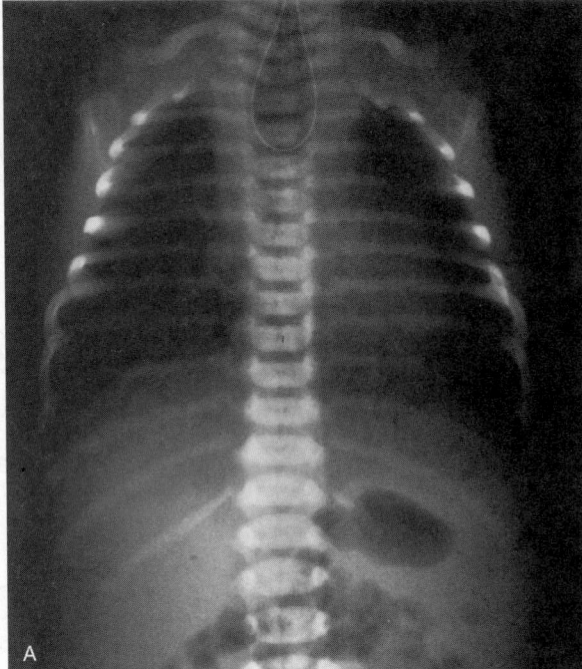
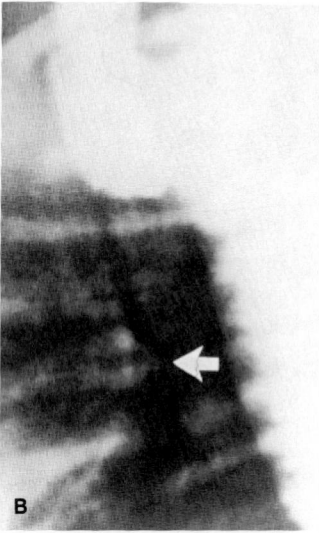

Figure 102-17. Chest radiographs of an infant with esophageal atresia and distal tracheoesophageal fistula. (*A*) The nasogastric tube can be seen coiled in the blind proximal esophageal pouch. (*B*) Air is visible within the fistula (*arrow*). (*B* from Coran AG. Congenital abnormailites of the esophagus. In: Zuidema GD, Orringer MD, eds. Shackelford's surgery of the alimentary tract, ed 2. Philadelphia, WB Saunders, 1990)

the chest wall until the azygous vein is identified; this vein is then ligated and divided. The distal esophageal fistula usually lies immediately beneath the divided azygous vein. The fistula is identified, encircled, and divided. Care must be taken not to remove any tracheal wall since this can result in a postoperative tracheal stricture. Rather, a small rim of esophageal wall is left at the fistula site and is used for the subsequent closure. The upper esophageal pouch is visualized by having the anesthesiologist gently push down on the sump tube. The proximal pouch is then dissected up to the thoracic inlet by dividing the tissue between the esophagus and the trachea, taking care not to enter the trachea. The distal esophagus is dissected only as far as is necessary to create a tension-free anastomosis. If necessary, a proximal esophagomyotomy can be created to give an additional length of 1 to 1.5 cm. An esophagoesophagostomy is then performed.

In cases of pure esophageal atresia without tracheoesophageal fistula, there is typically a long gap between the proximal and distal esophagus. These infants are managed by inserting a gastrostomy for feeding and establishing proximal pouch suction drainage. After this, the upper esophageal pouch is elongated using bougienage for 3 to 6 weeks. After this period of stretching and growth, radiographs usually demonstrate significant shortening of the esophageal gap. At this point, a standard right extrapleural thoracotomy is performed. If possible, primary esophagoesophagostomy is done, even if under tension. If necessary, the stomach can be mobilized into the thorax to allow the anastomosis. Occasionally, an esophagomyotomy of the proximal esophageal segment may be required. Some surgeons perform a cervical esophagostomy and a subsequent esophageal replacement procedure for pure esophageal atresia. In general, this latter approach has been replaced by the former alternatives.

Although tracheoesophageal fistula without esophageal atresia is relatively rare, it is important to be familiar with the technical differences this lesion presents. Endoscopy is considered routine to identify and cannulate the fistula. Cannulation is best done from the trachea, because this orifice is proximal to the esophageal orifice. Division of the fistula with tracheal and esophageal closure is straightforward and usually is accomplished by a cervical incision on the right.

Complications.   Three major complications are related to the esophageal anastomosis—leak, stricture, and recurrent fistula. The incidence of leak varies from 10% to 20%, depending on the type of anastomosis done and the degree of tension. A distinct advantage of an extrapleural anastomosis is the predictable resolution of these leaks if adequately drained. Similarly, the stricture rate varies between 10% and 25%, again depending on the type of anastomosis done. Many infants require one or two dilations, but few have sig-

Table 102-1. CONGENITAL ANOMALIES ASSOCIATED WITH ESOPHAGEAL ATRESIA AND TRACHEOESOPHAGEAL FISTULA

Area	1935–1966	1966–1976	1976–1985
Cardiovascular	44	12	10
Gastrointestinal	31	8	10
Neurologic	9	1	2
Genitourinary	4	1	1
Orthopedic	0	0	0
Other	3	1	1
TOTAL	91 (31.6%)	23 (27.3%)	24 (34%)

(Manning PB, Morgan RA, Coran AG, et al. Fifty years' experience with esophageal atresia and tracheoesophageal fistula. Ann Surg 1986;204:446)

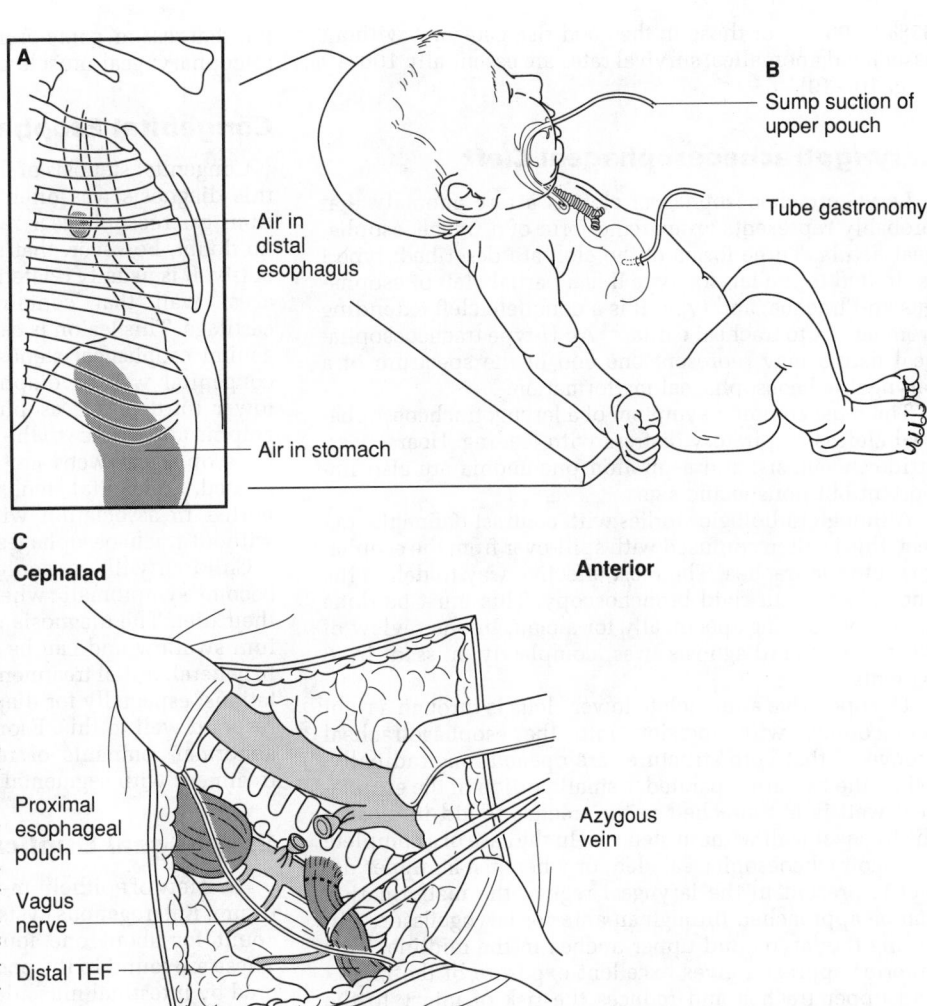

Figure 102-18. (*A*) Schematic illustration of the most common anatomy—esophageal atresia with distal tracheoesophageal fistula. (*B*) The initial management of this anomaly includes upright posture, sump suction of the blind esophageal pouch, and, possibly, placement of a gastrostomy tube. (*C*) The right extrapleural operative approach. After division and closure of the fistula, primary esophagoesophagostomy is performed. (*B* after Coran AG. Congenital abnormalities of the esophagus. In: Zuidema GD, Orringer MD, eds. Shackelford's surgery of the alimentary tract, ed 2. Philadelphia, WB Saunders, 1990)

nificant long-term problems. The incidence of recurrent esophageal fistula is difficult to determine since few authors emphasize this technical problem, but it appears to be about 10% in most reports (Table 102-2).

Two other postoperative conditions that are not technical complications are gastroesophageal reflux and tracheomalacia. The gastroesophageal reflux is probably secondary to dysmotility of the distal esophagus and can sometimes be

treated with simple medical maneuvers. A significant number of these infants (25% to 30% or more), however, are refractory to medical therapy and require surgical fundoplication. Gastroesophageal reflux may also manifest as a recurrent anastomotic stricture. The problem here is related to acid-induced inflammation. In these infants, a surgical antireflux procedure is usually necessary. Tracheomalacia has been reported with increasing frequency as a complication of the malformation, not of the repair. This appears to result from intrinsically inadequate cartilagenous tracheal rings at the level of the fistula. Although the incidence is likely constant, increasing recognition has resulted in an incidence of 25% in some recent series. Most infants with tracheomalacia improve with growth and time, but a small percentage develop severe respiratory difficulty, which can result in respiratory arrest and death. These latter patients may require surgical aortopexy, a procedure in which the aortic arch is sutured to the undersurface of the sternum to suspend and open the adjacent trachea. This is generally successful in patients with focal tracheomalacia. Intraoperative endoscopic assessment of the tracheal configuration is an important technical necessity.

Results of Operations

Most children born with esophageal atresia and tracheoesophageal fistula can look forward to survival with a normal existence. Current overall survival rates range from

Table 102-2. COMPLICATIONS AFTER REPAIR OF ESOPHAGEAL ATRESIA AND TRACHEOESOPHAGEAL FISTULA, 1956–1985

Type of Repair	Leak	Stricture	Recurrence
One-layer (n = 47)	8 (17%)	1 (4.3%)	3 (6.4%)
Two-layer (n = 177)	11 (6.2%)	41 (23.2%)	11 (6.2%)
	P < .03*	P < .002*	

* P values represent statistically significant differences between one- and two-layer repair.
(Manning PB, Morgan RA, Coran AG, et al. Fifty years' experience with esophageal atresia and tracheoesophageal fistula. Ann Surg 1986;204:446)

85% to 90%. For those in the good-risk category, without associated anomalies, survival rates are essentially 100%[21] (Fig. 102-19).

Laryngotracheoesophageal Cleft

Laryngotracheoesophageal cleft is a rare anomaly that probably represents an extreme form of a tracheoesophageal fistula. Three forms of the cleft are described: type I is limited to the larynx; type II is a partial cleft of esophagus and trachea; and type III is a complete cleft extending from larynx to tracheal carina.[22] An H-type tracheoesophageal fistula may represent one end of the spectrum of a laryngotracheoesophageal malformation.

The most common symptom of a laryngotracheoesophageal cleft is respiratory distress with feeding. Hoarseness, stridor, cyanosis, and aspiration pneumonia are also important but nonspecific signs.

Although radiologic studies with contrast define the defect, this is often confused with spill-over from the esophagus into the trachea. The most effective way to define the anomaly is with rigid bronchoscopy. This must be done carefully, looking specifically for a cleft. In one review of 33 cases, the diagnosis was completely missed in 6 patients.

The operative approach to lower clefts is through a right thoracotomy with incision into the esophagotracheal groove so that both structures are opened longitudinally. When the two are separated, a small portion of the esophageal wall is left attached to the trachea to aid in closing the tracheal wall without stenosis. In the case of a complete laryngotracheoesophageal cleft, or when just an upper defect is present in the laryngeal region, the malformation can be approached through an anterior laryngofissure, dividing the larynx and upper trachea in the midline. This anterior approach gives excellent exposure of the larynx and upper trachea and reduces the risk of injury to the recurrent laryngeal nerve. Postoperative laryngeal instability can result, however, requiring prolonged intubation.

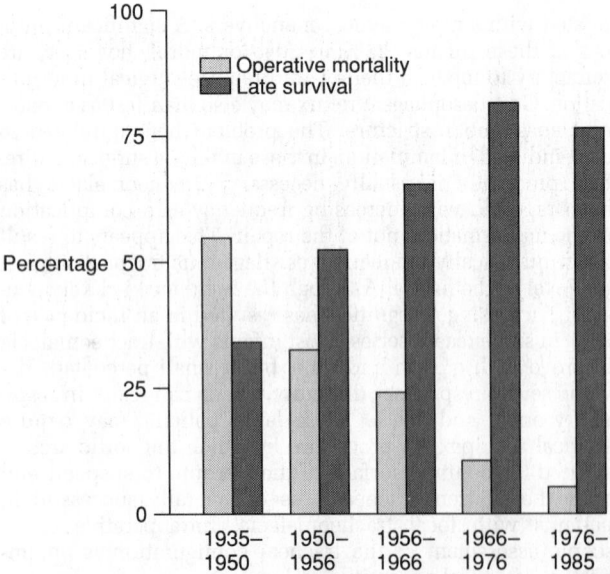

Figure 102-19. Trends in operative mortality and late survival for esophageal atresia and tracheoesophageal fistula during the past 50 years. (After Manning PB, Morgan RA, Coran AG, et al. Fifty years' experience with esophageal aresia and tracheoesophageal fistula. Ann Surg 1986;204:446)

For that reason, some prefer a lateral approach through the cricopharyngeal muscle and lateral pharyngeal wall.

Congenital Esophageal Stenosis

Congenital stenosis of the esophagus is rare. Historically, this diagnosis was often given when in fact esophagitis from gastroesophageal reflux was the problem. There is no doubt, however, that esophageal stenosis is a discrete entity. It is usually related to abnormal tissue in the esophageal wall that contains respiratory epithelium and cartilage. This lesion is certainly of congenital origin. Congenital esophageal stenosis may also take the form of a congenital web or diaphragm located in the middle to lower third of the esophagus. This has a similar radiographic appearance to the Schatzki ring in adults. Congenital esophageal webs are usually thin and can be easily dilated. Congenital stenosis of the esophagus has been reported in association with esophageal atresia with and without tracheoesophageal fistula.

Children with congenital esophageal stenosis typically become symptomatic when solid foods are introduced into their diet. The diagnosis can usually be made with a barium swallow and can be confirmed with esophagoscopy. In general, initial treatment should consist of repeated dilatations, especially for diaphragms or webs, which usually respond well to this. Esophageal stenosis associated with abnormal remnants of respiratory tissue often requires treatment with segmental resection.

Esophageal Duplications

A variety of epithelium-lined cysts appear in the mediastinum. Enterogenous cysts, or esophageal duplications, account for about one fourth of these mediastinal cysts. These are found in the posterior mediastinum and are covered by intestinal muscular wall. They are generally lined by intestinal epithelium, often gastric epithelium, although ciliated respiratory epithelium may also be present (see previous discussion). Occasionally, the cysts may be attached to or communicate with the spinal canal and are termed neurenteric cysts. They usually have no communication with the lumen of the esophagus and are generally filled with mucoid-type material. Gastric epithelium can lead to acid–peptic ulceration of these cysts, with resultant substernal pain, erosion into the bronchus or esophagus, and pulmonary hemorrhage.

Most often, symptoms result from compression of adjacent viscera. In general, these lesions are best excised. This is accomplished readily by dissecting the cyst from the adjacent esophagus.

Vascular Rings

Vascular rings, a relatively rare cause of esophageal obstruction, result from faulty embryologic development of the aortic arch. These rings are either complete or incomplete and result in obstruction of the trachea, the esophagus, or both.[23]

Complete Rings

The double aortic arch represents the most common type of complete vascular ring. It results from persistence of both the right and left embryologic aortic arches. The double aortic arch arises from the ascending aorta and bifurcates, with one branch going to the right and dorsal to the trachea and esophagus with the other going to the left and ventral to the trachea. These two arches join again to form the descending aorta. Each arch gives rise to a common carotid and subclavian artery; the innominate artery is usually absent. The ductus arteriosus may be on the left, on the right, or bilateral. The arch size varies, but the anterior, left arch is usually smaller.

The other form of complete ring is a right arch with a left ligamentum arteriosum or ductus arteriosus. A complete ring is formed by the ascending aorta and pulmonary artery anteriorly, with the aortic arch on the right, and either the ductus arteriosus or the ligamentum arteriosum and the left subclavian artery on the left.

Incomplete Rings

An aberrant right subclavian artery is the most common vascular anomaly of the aorta and occurs in about 0.5% of the normal population. The aberrant artery arises as the last branch of the aortic arch and passes behind the esophagus to reach the right arm. This is rarely symptomatic but may cause dysphagia lusoria.

A pulmonary artery sling is the result of an aberrant left pulmonary artery arising from the right pulmonary artery posteriorly and passing anterior to the right main-stem bronchus, causing compression of the right main-stem bronchus and the distal trachea. This is a rare anomaly that does not cause esophageal compression. Likewise, an anomalous innominate artery, which results from an innominate artery that arises more distal than normal from the aorta, causes only tracheal compression.

The symptoms of vascular rings are due to compression of the trachea, the esophagus, or both. The child with a double aortic arch generally is the most symptomatic, and most patients have symptoms early in infancy. The typical clinical picture is one of inspiratory wheezing, coughing, noisy breathing, shortness of breath, stridor, and frequent bouts of pneumonia. Feeding problems become apparent when solid foods are started. The most important screening test is the barium swallow, although CT or magnetic resonance imaging are definitive. Angiography and endoscopy are usually not needed to make a definitive diagnosis.

Any patient who is symptomatic from a vascular ring should be treated surgically.[24] Most of these anomalies can be approached through a left lateral thoracotomy in the fourth interspace. In the case of a double aortic arch, the ductus arteriosus or ligamentum arteriosum is divided. The smaller arch is then divided distal to the origin of the left subclavian artery when the anterior (left) arch is hypoplastic, and it is divided near its junction with the descending aorta when the posterior (right) arch is hypoplastic. When the arches are equal in size, the right or posterior arch is preferentially divided. After division of the arch, the fibrous tissue around the esophagus and trachea must be completely divided to allow expansion of these two structures. An aortic arch with a left ligamentum arteriosum is managed by division of the ligament and appropriate lysis of the fibrous bands around the esophagus and trachea. A symptomatic aberrant right subclavian artery should be divided at its origin from the aorta through a left posterolateral thoracotomy.

Congenital Tracheal Stenosis

Congenital stenosis of the distal trachea usually has been considered a fatal disease, although nonlethal forms have been described. Failure of tracheal growth can manifest itself over a wide spectrum of severity, ranging from mild, generalized hypoplasia to a specific stenosis, to pulmonary agenesis. Most forms are associated with complete tracheal rings at the level of the stenosis and various degrees of disorganization of cartilage formation. The diagnosis is confirmed by bronchoscopy. Therapy depends on the anatomy of the lesion. Segmental stenoses have been handled by resection and end-to-end anastomosis. Longer stenoses

have been managed with rib, pericardial, or synthetic grafts. Overall experience with these types of reconstructive operations is limited.[25]

FOREIGN BODIES OF THE TRACHEOBRONCHIAL TREE

Foreign bodies of the tracheobronchial tree are frequently encountered in pediatric patients. Reports from the National Safety Council estimate that about 600 children die each year from complications related to the aspiration or ingestion of foreign bodies. Under the age of 4 years, foreign body aspiration or ingestion is one of the four leading causes of accidental death. The incidence of death from this cause approaches 2 per 100,000 children, and it has not changed significantly in the last 20 years. A number of instruments and techniques for foreign body extraction from the airway have been described over the years. The most significant advance in the safe and successful treatment of tracheobronchial foreign bodies was the development in the 1970s of the Hopkins rod lens optical system with fiberoptic illumination. The incorporation of this system into the rigid endoscope has resulted in a reliable method for most foreign body extractions.[26]

Pathophysiology

Physiologically, bronchial foreign bodies create a ball–valve phenomenon in the affected bronchus. This usually allows bidirectional but unequal flow of air. More air flows into the bronchus with inspiration than flows out with expiration. The result is significant air-trapping and hyperinflation in the affected lobe or lung. This, in turn, leads to a mediastinal shift to the opposite side. Total blockage of the bronchus by the foreign body results in loss of volume in the affected lobe or lung, with atelectasis and shift of the mediastinum to the ipsilateral side.

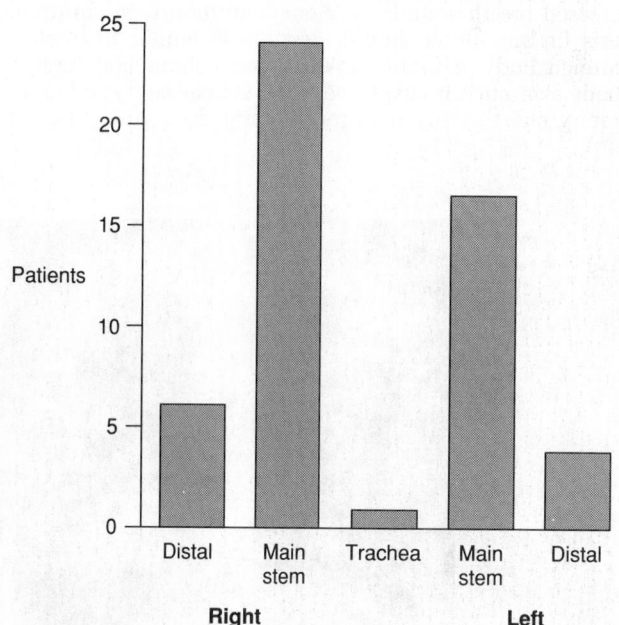

Figure 102-20. Distribution of foreign bodies in the tracheobronchial tree. (After Manning PB, Wesley JR, Polley TZ Jr, et al. Esophageal and tracheobronchial foreign bodies in infants and children. Pediatr Surg Int 1987;2:346)

Table 102-3. CLINICAL FINDINGS OF TRACHEOBRONCHIAL FOREIGN BODIES

Signs and Symptoms	Incidence (%)
SYMPTOMS	
Cough	70
Wheezing	50
Dyspnea	30
Fever	20
Emesis	6
Pain	6
SIGNS	
Unilateral decreased breath sounds	50
Unilateral wheezing	45
Rhonchi	10
Cyanosis	10
Pneumonia	6

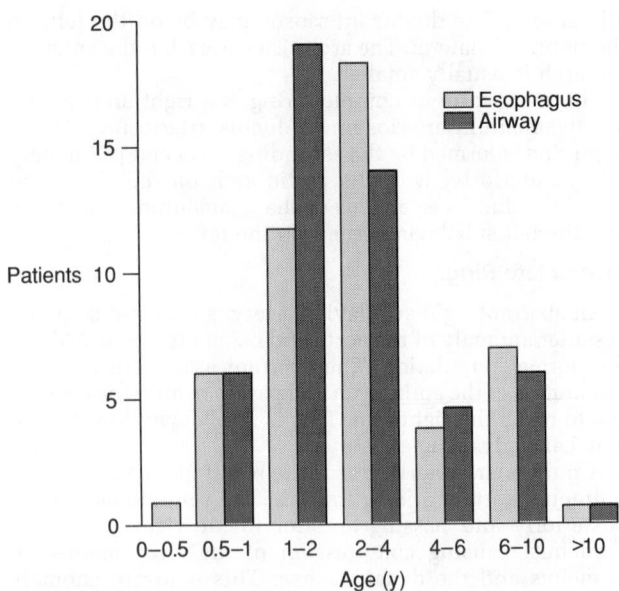

Figure 102-21. Age distribution of patients with tracheobronchial and esophageal foreign bodies. (After Manning PB, Wesley JR, Polley TZ Jr, et al. Esophageal and tracheobronchial foreign bodies in infants and children. Pediatr Surg Int 1987;2:346)

Clinical Picture

The location of offending objects distributed in the tracheobronchial tree is shown in Figure 102-20. Peanuts constitute the single most common foreign body (33%) and are particularly troublesome because of the accompanying inflammatory reaction and their hygroscopic characteristics, which cause them to become soft and thus require piecemeal removal. Other common foreign bodies include food, such as carrots and popcorn, and toy parts, such as pins, wood, paper, and plastic.

The clinical signs and symptoms of tracheobronchial foreign bodies are listed in Table 102-3. The most common problems are coughing, wheezing, dyspnea, and fever. Most affected children are less than 4 years of age (Fig. 102-21). It is unusual for a child with a tracheobronchial foreign body to be asymptomatic with no related physical findings. A suggestive history, however, is an adequate indication to proceed with bronchoscopy. The physical examination typically demonstrates wheezing or decreased breath sounds over one hemithorax. In children, this finding alone should alert the examiner to suspect foreign body aspiration. When tracheobronchial foreign body aspiration is suspected, routine inspiratory and expiratory chest radiographs (or bilateral decubitus views of the chest in patients not old enough to cooperate) should be obtained. These radiographs usually demonstrate hyperinflation on the affected side (Fig. 102-22).

Management

When the diagnosis is confirmed by radiographs showing hyperinflation or a radiopaque foreign body, or when the history is sufficiently worrisome, immediate rigid bronchoscopy is indicated. Although the flexible bronchoscope is used by some, visualization is not nearly as good as with the rigid scope, and the extraction process is considerably more difficult and perhaps impossible.

Most bronchial foreign bodies can be extracted with the optical forceps (Fig. 102-23). If this technique is unsuccessful, then the flexible wire grasper or a Fogarty catheter can be used, especially if the foreign body has migrated into a

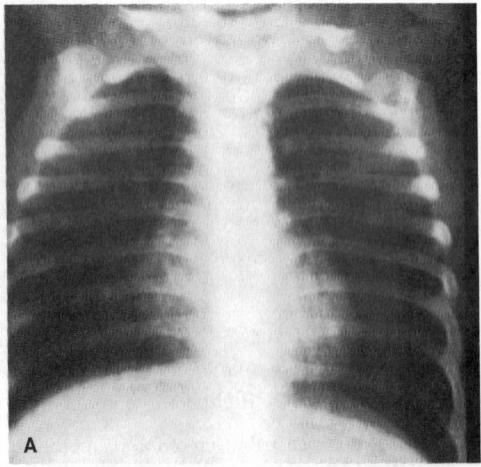
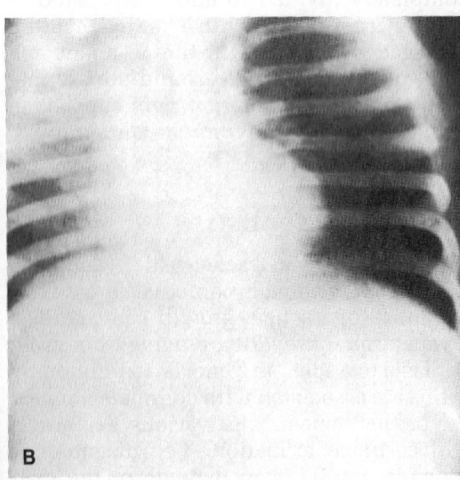

Figure 102-22. Inspiratory (*A*) and expiratory (*B*) chest radiographs in a child with a tracheobronchial foreign body. Air-trapping on the left is demonstrated during expiration.

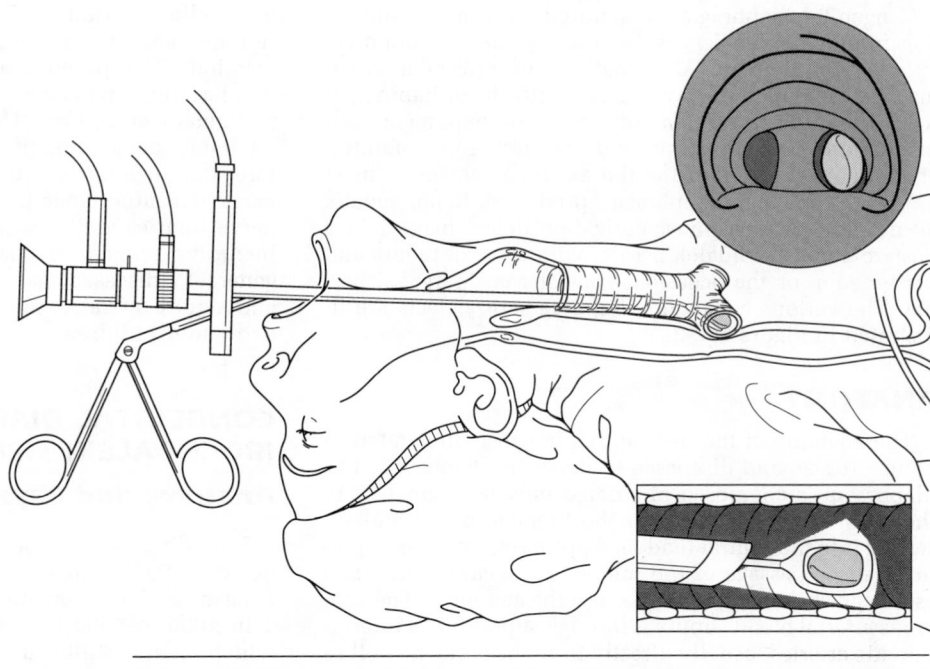

Figure 102-23. Schematic illustration of a peanut foreign body being extracted from the right mainstem bronchus under direct vision.

segmental bronchus. Rarely, when the foreign body cannot be visualized with the bronchoscope, the procedure is done under fluoroscopy to guide the flexible wire grasper to the foreign body.

Despite the advances made in the equipment and techniques for extracting tracheobronchial foreign bodies from children, education leading to prevention remains the most important goal.

Congenital Abnormalities of the Diaphragm

KEITH T. OLDHAM

EMBRYOLOGY

The human diaphragm forms between the fourth and eighth gestational weeks, dividing the primitive coelom into pleural and peritoneal cavities.[27] The initial contribution is from the transverse septum, a mesenchymal condensation at the caudal aspect of the pericardial sac that ultimately gives rise to the central tendon of the adult diaphragm. During the eighth week, posterolateral pleuroperitoneal membranes fuse with the centrally placed transverse septum to complete separation of the pleural and peritoneal cavities by an intact diaphragm (Fig. 102-24). Failure of this fusion may result in a posterolateral diaphragmatic defect, a foramen of Bochdalek hernia. In addition, a Bochdalek hernia may result from premature return of the extracoelomic gut into the abdomen, with intestinal herniation into the pleural cavity before diaphragmatic closure. Closure of the right hemidiaphragm normally precedes that of the left. This asynchronous closure and the presence of the liver on the right account for the finding that 85% to 90% of congenital diaphragmatic hernias involve the left hemidiaphragm.

After initial fusion, the muscular portion of the diaphragm develops circumferentially around the membranous central tendon. The muscular diaphragm is derived in part from the innermost layer of thoracic mesoderm. It also appears to benefit from contributions of migratory myoblasts derived from cervical, infrahyoid mesoderm. This inference is drawn because diaphragmatic innervation is provided by the phrenic nerve to which cervical nerves III, IV, and V contribute. Because muscles retain their embryonic segmental innervation regardless of ultimate location or modification, it follows that a portion of the diaphragmatic muscular mass is derived from these cervical myoblasts.

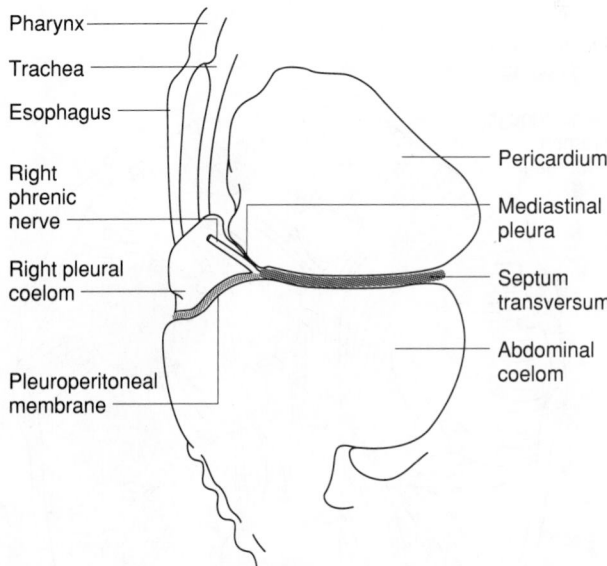

Figure 102-24. Embryogenesis of the diaphragm (6 weeks' gestation). The components of the developing diaphragm are illustrated. In particular, the relation of the transverse septum and the pleuroperitoneal membrane is shown.

Congenital diaphragmatic abnormalities may result either from fusion defects as described earlier or from muscularization defects. Abnormalities of muscularization may be focal or may involve an entire hemidiaphragm. Regardless, the result is a portion of the diaphragm with insufficient strength to prevent the herniation of intraabdominal viscera into the thorax. Involvement of most or all of one hemidiaphragm produces diaphragmatic eventration. A focal muscularization defect may yield a posterolateral Bochdalek hernia, with a sac of pleura and peritoneum, or the occasional parasternal Morgagni hernia. The various congenital diaphragmatic defects are illustrated in Figure 102-25.

ANATOMY

The anatomy of the normal diaphragm is illustrated in Figure 102-26 and discussed in detail in Chapter 62. The diaphragm is composed of striated muscle originating in the chest and body walls at the thoracic outlet and inserting into the central tendon. Appropriately named apertures allow passage of the inferior vena cava, aorta, and esophagus between the thorax and the abdomen. The generous arterial blood supply is through superior and inferior phrenic arteries, usually directly from the aorta, as well as the musculophrenic and pericardiophrenic arteries. Venous drainage generally follows the arterial supply, with drainage primarily into the inferior vena cava or azygous vein on the right and into either the adrenal or renal and hemiazygous veins on the left. Innervation is principally by the phrenic nerve. In addition, there are minor contributions from the lower thoracic nerves bilaterally. The phrenic nerves descend from their cervical origins along the ventral surface of the scalenus anterior muscle between the subclavian vein and the subclavian artery. The right phrenic nerve passes lateral and immediately adjacent to the brachiocephalic vein and superior vena cava, descending across the pericardium anterior to the pulmonary hilum. The left phrenic nerve passes directly posterior to the thoracic duct and subclavian vein, descending across the pericardium in a course similar to that on the right. The phrenic nerves enter the muscular diaphragm in an-

teromedial locations and promptly give off sternal, posterior, and anterolateral branches with a roughly radial orientation. The phrenic nerve is vulnerable to surgical trauma from a wide variety of cervical, thoracic, and diaphragmatic procedures. Unlike adults, infants may depend on diaphragmatic function for adequate ventilation. Therefore, the anatomic relations of the phrenic nerve are of particular importance in the pediatric age group. Phrenic nerve injuries and a variety of neuromuscular disorders, including primary myopathies and anterior horn cell degenerative diseases, may produce diaphragmatic paralysis and require operative plication of the diaphragm in infants and young children.

CONGENITAL DIAPHRAGMATIC (BOCHDALEK) HERNIA

Anatomy and Physiology

Excluding esophageal hiatal hernias, the posterolateral defect at the foramen of Bochdalek is the most common congenital diaphragmatic hernia. The incidence is about 1 in 4000 to 5000 live births. Population-based studies, which include stillbirths and early deaths, suggest an incidence as high as 1 in 2000 conceptions. The defect is variable in size, ranging from a hernia 1 to 2 cm in diameter to complete agenesis of the hemidiaphragm. Prognosis is not necessarily related to defect size but rather to the degree of associated pulmonary hypoplasia. Most commonly, a ventral and medial leaf of diaphragm is found with a smaller, posterior muscular portion enveloped by pleura and peritoneum. A hernia sac is present in 10% to 20% of cases but has no physiologic significance. The usual left-sided hernia contains small bowel, spleen, stomach, and colon, whereas hernias on the right typically contain liver and may include intestine (Fig. 102-27). Recent observations with sequential ultrasound examinations demonstrate that the intrauterine visceral displacement from the peritoneal to the pleural cavity is a dynamic process with considerable variability as to timing and degree. This may account for the spectrum of pulmonary hypoplasia observed in infants with diaphragmatic hernias. It is suggested that hernias associated with polyhydramnios, those occurring early in gestation, and those with more intrathoracic liver or intestine (eg, stomach) have more severe pulmonary hypoplasia and a worse prognosis. Because perinatal management options range from termination of pregnancy to in utero repair, patient selection based on anticipated outcome is a critical consideration. Data are limited, and there is no consensus as to how prognosis is best estimated in utero.

After parturition, respiration is accompanied by air swallowing, which distends the gut so that the anatomic displacement of abdominal viscera into the thorax is exacerbated in the first hours of extrauterine life. The air-filled intestine contributes to the acute respiratory distress because of ipsilateral pulmonary compression as well as mediastinal shift into the contralateral thorax. Physiologically, this scenario is equivalent to a tension pneumothorax, although in this case, the air is contained within the intestinal lumen. Decompression of the gastrointestinal tract is an essential and immediate requirement for these infants.

Malrotation is an expected finding with diaphragmatic hernia because intestinal herniation into the thorax normally precedes the fixation of the gut to the posterior body wall between the 10th and 12th gestational weeks. It is prudent to correct this at the time of initial transabdominal repair of the diaphragmatic hernia. Midgut volvulus asso-

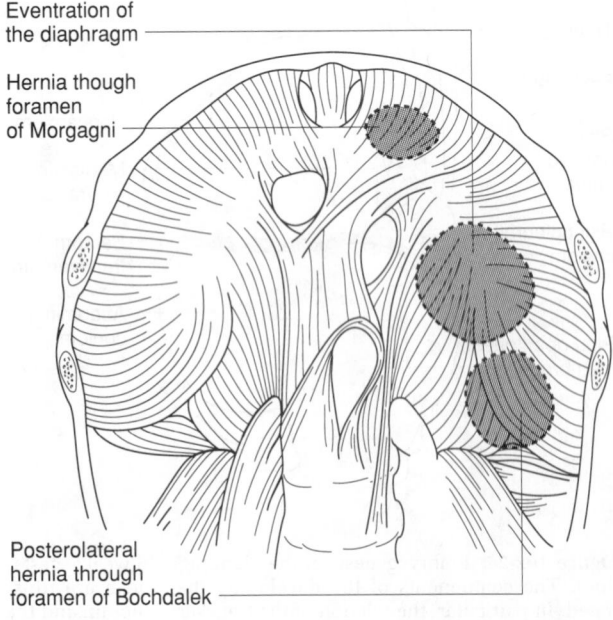

Eventration of the diaphragm

Hernia though foramen of Morgagni

Posterolateral hernia through foramen of Bochdalek

Figure 102-25. Locations of congenital diaphragmatic defects.

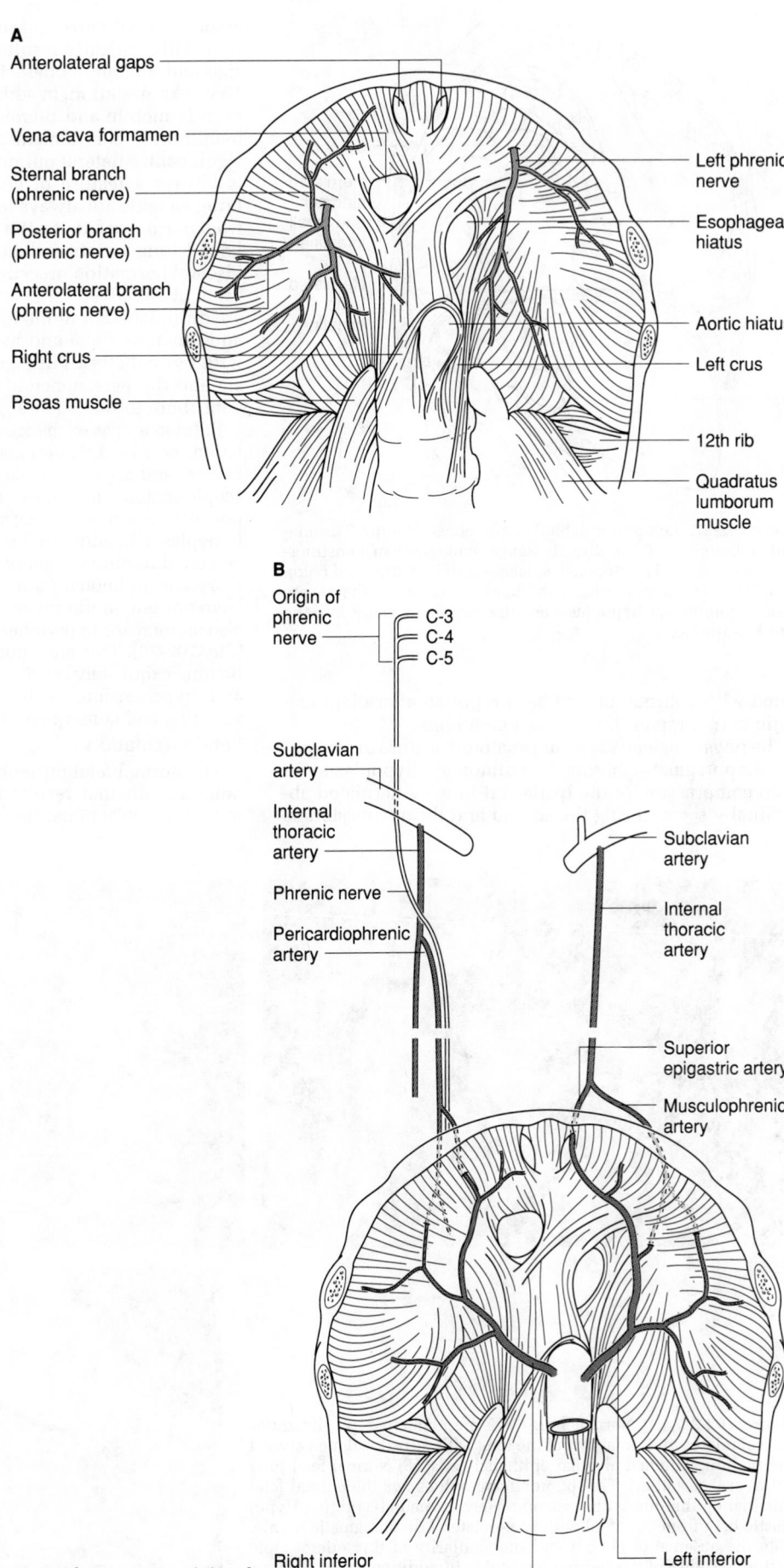

A

Anterolateral gaps

Vena cava formamen

Sternal branch
(phrenic nerve)

Posterior branch
(phrenic nerve)

Anterolateral branch
(phrenic nerve)

Right crus

Psoas muscle

Left phrenic
nerve

Esophageal
hiatus

Aortic hiatus

Left crus

12th rib

Quadratus
lumborum
muscle

B

Origin of
phrenic
nerve

C-3
C-4
C-5

Subclavian
artery

Internal
thoracic
artery

Phrenic nerve

Pericardiophrenic
artery

Subclavian
artery

Internal
thoracic
artery

Superior
epigastric artery

Musculophrenic
artery

Right inferior
phrenic artery

Left inferior
phrenic artery

Figure 102-26. Intact normal diaphragm with innervation (*A*) and
arterial blood supply (*B*).

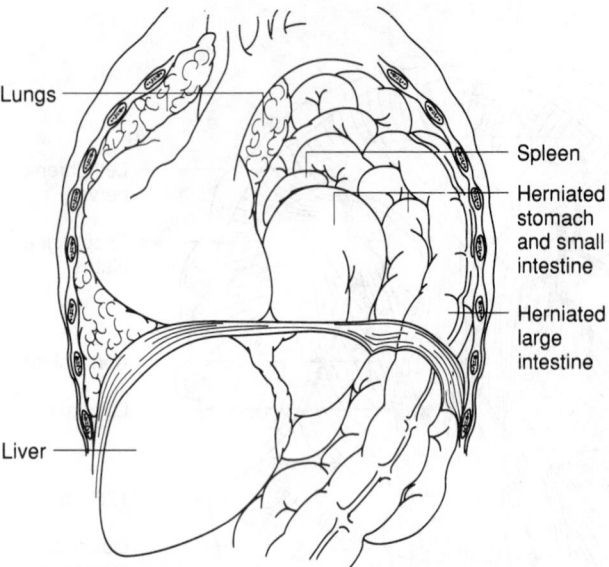

Figure 102-27. Left posterolateral diaphragmatic hernia. The anatomic relations are taken directly from a photograph of a postmortem examination. The stomach, spleen, small intestine, and colon occupy the left hemithorax. Particularly notable are the severe bilateral pulmonary hypoplasia and the mediastinal shift into the right hemithorax.

ciated with malrotation has been reported after diaphragmatic hernia repair, but it is not common.

The physiologically relevant anatomic feature of congenital diaphragmatic hernia is pulmonary hypoplasia. In utero compression of the ipsilateral lung by herniated abdominal viscera during the second and third trimesters is associated with arrest of pulmonary parenchymal maturation. This typically results in an ipsilateral lung with the size and anatomic characteristics of a fetal lung of 14 to 16 weeks' gestation. In addition, because the fetal mediastinum is mobile and therefore displaced into the opposite hemithorax, contralateral pulmonary hypoplasia may be significant. Bilateral pulmonary hypoplasia of some degree is always a feature of congenital diaphragmatic hernia. Lung weights are always low; as much as a 90% reduction from normal occurs on the ipsilateral side, whereas contralateral lung weight reductions are more modest. Because visceral herniation precedes the development of segmental bronchi and alveoli, the alveoli in these hypoplastic lungs are diminished in number as well as abnormal in structure and function. Fetal and hypoplastic alveoli are contrasted with normal alveoli in Figure 102-28. The severe hypoplasia and the persistence of embryonic alveolar epithelium contribute to inadequate gas exchange.

Pulmonary gas exchange relies on adequate alveolar ventilation, normal diffusion across the alveolar–endothelial interface, and appropriate capillary blood flow. As the microscopic anatomy in Figure 102-28 suggests, neither ventilation nor diffusion proceeds normally in infants with pulmonary hypoplasia. In addition, the hypoplastic pulmonary vascular bed is a diminutive, high-resistance circuit with reduced capillary and pulmonary artery blood flow. The affected lungs have not only a diminished arterial cross-sectional area but also an increase in peripheral arteriolar smooth muscle mass (Fig. 102-29). This anatomic variation renders the hypoplastic lung exquisitely sensitive to pulmonary artery vasospasm and hypertension, with the development of right-to-left shunting and consequent respiratory failure.

Fetal Circulation

The normal fetal pulmonary vascular bed is a high resistance circuit that results in the intrauterine shunting of more than 90% of cardiac output from right to left by way

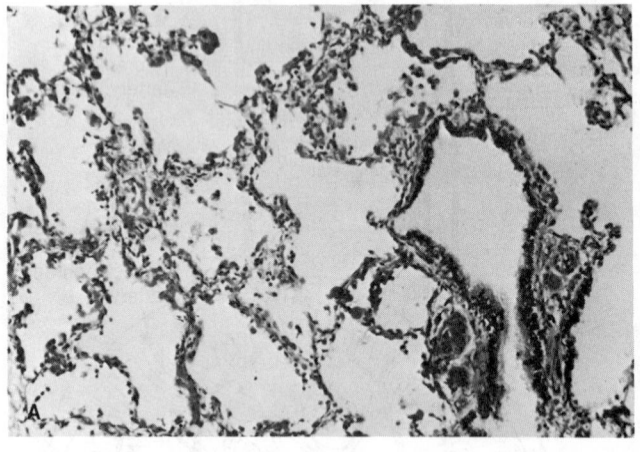

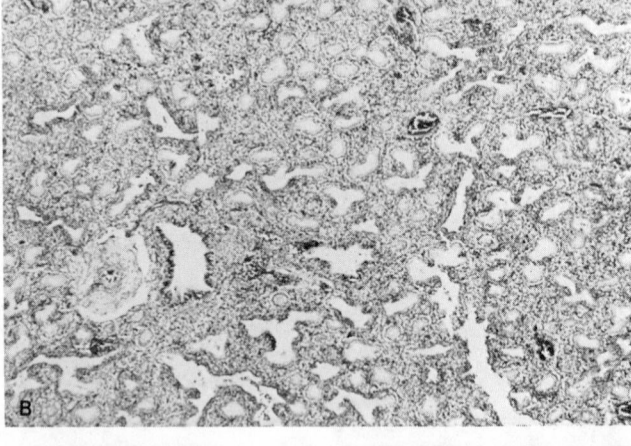

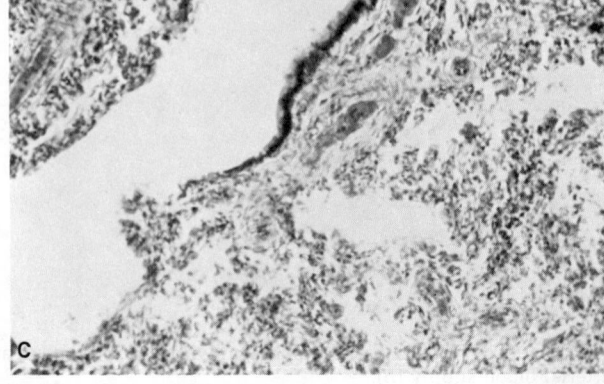

Figure 102-28. (*A*) Normal lung. This photomicrograph illustrates normal microscopic anatomy of the lung with fully developed alveoli and mature, flattened alveolar epithelial cells. (*B*) Normal fetal lung (20 weeks' gestation). This photomicrograph shows the normal fetal cuboidal epithelium within incompletely formed alveoli. (*C*) Hypoplastic lung from an infant with posterolateral diaphragmatic hernia. Note the absence of alveoli and the similarity of this microscopic anatomy to that of the normal fetal lung. In addition to the obvious developmental arrest, the number of alveoli is markedly reduced.

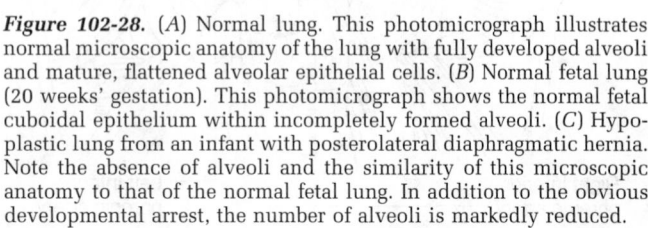

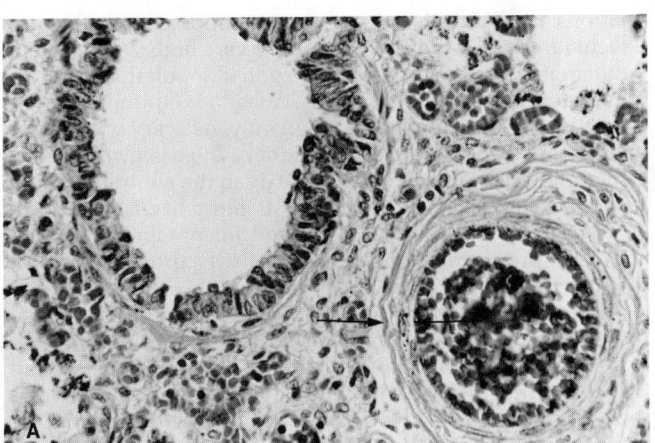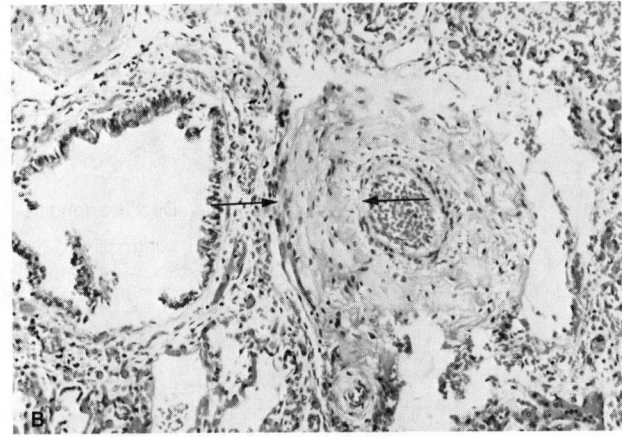

Figure 102-29. Histology of pulmonary artery. Pulmonary artery branches of similar size and location are shown in a normal infant (*A*) and in an infant with Bochdalek diaphragmatic hernia (*B*). In particular, there is increased muscle mass associated with the arterial wall in *B* (*arrows*). This vascular smooth muscle is exquisitely sensitive to chemical, hormonal, and paracrine mediators in the neonatal period. Pulmonary arterial vasospasm is an important cause of persistent fetal circulation and respiratory failure.

of either the foramen ovale (right atrium to left atrium) or the patent ductus arteriosus (pulmonary artery to aorta; Fig. 102-30). With an infant's first breaths at parturition, alveoli inflate, alveolar capillaries open, and pulmonary vascular resistance and right atrial pressure fall. When the low-resistance placenta is removed from the circulation, systemic resistance, left atrial pressure, and aortic blood pressure increase acutely. Normally, the ductus arteriosus closes functionally at birth and is anatomically obliterated within hours or days. The foramen ovale becomes functionally closed, and significant right-to-left shunting ceases shortly after birth. The control mechanisms for these complex events are not entirely known. It is clear, however, that the pulmonary vascular smooth muscle mass is particularly sensitive to a variety of chemical and hormonal signals during this perinatal transitional period. The increase in pulmonary artery oxygen tension from fetal levels of about 20 mmHg to extrauterine levels of 90 to 100 mmHg is normally associated with profound pulmonary artery vasodilation. Conversely, perinatal hypoxia, hypercarbia, and acidosis induce pulmonary artery vasospasm, reducing pulmonary blood flow as much as 90% experimentally. Within days of birth, both this sensitivity and the size of the pulmonary arterial wall muscle mass diminish.

Persistence of pulmonary hypertension with major right-to-left shunting has been termed *persistent fetal circulation* or, more recently, *persistent pulmonary hypertension of the newborn* (PPHN). The terms refer to the physiologic phenomenon, whether it results from a diaphragmatic hernia, meconium aspiration, or any other cause of respiratory failure in the newborn period. Some degree of PPHN is virtually always present in infants with diaphragmatic hernias. It is a potentially self-perpetuating process in which right-to-left shunting exacerbates hypoxemia, leading to further pulmonary vasoconstriction and more shunting. The cycle is not easily interrupted, and the attendant mortality remains high.

Arterial oxygen tension is the single most important determinant of pulmonary vascular tone, but many other chemical, endocrine, and paracrine mediators are involved. Temperature, Pa_{CO_2}, and pH are other important chemical signals. Catecholamines appear to be clinically relevant endocrine vasoconstrictors; and endocrine vasodilators include histamine and glucagon. Among the paracrine signals, arachidonic acid products, particularly the

prostaglandins and nitric oxide, appear to be relevant mediators of the transitional circulation. The data regarding these substances are controversial and not easily interpreted, in part because some of these mediators are derived from pulmonary artery endothelial cells, and their local actions on the adjacent vascular smooth muscle may be independent of the plasma concentrations that are usually measured. In addition, the perinatal transitional circulation is neither simple nor static with regard to these control mechanisms. Prostaglandins E_1, E_2, and prostacyclin induce pulmonary artery vasodilation, with prostacyclin arguably the most potent.[28] E-series prostaglandin infusions are clinically useful to reduce pulmonary artery hypertension or to prevent closure of the ductus arteriosus in infants with congenital heart disease who are shunt dependent. It appears that the thromboxanes (A_2 and B_2), leukotrienes, and F-series prostaglandins are pulmonary vasoconstrictors. Complement products and cytokines may also be involved in regulating pulmonary blood flow. Nitric oxide is a potent vasodilator in the pulmonary and other circulations. The net physiologic effect of these mediators is exerted through a complex series of interactions with the target vascular smooth muscle, but their individual specific roles in infants with diaphragmatic hernias are not known.

Pharmacologic management of persistent pulmonary hypertension in the newborn has remained problematic. In general, the clinical strategy has been to provide exogenous vasodilators to interrupt the cycle of pulmonary vasospasm and hypoxemia. In this effort, acetylcholine, histamine, the E-series prostaglandins, bradykinin, nitroprusside, general anesthetics, fentanyl, tolazoline, inhaled nitric oxide, and other agents have been tried. The largest clinical experience has been with tolazoline, which acts directly by relaxing vascular smooth muscle. Unfortunately, the clinical experience is characterized by inconsistent and unpredictable results. Although most patients respond to intravenous tolazoline infusion with pulmonary vasodilation, about one third do not. In addition, systemic hypotension and tachyphylaxis are limiting clinical problems. Tolazoline and other vasodilator drugs are used as adjuncts to mechanical ventilatory support, but pharmacologic treatment alone is not sufficient for treating the infant with PPHN. Inhaled nitric oxide has been shown to reduce pulmonary hypertension and improve oxygenation in

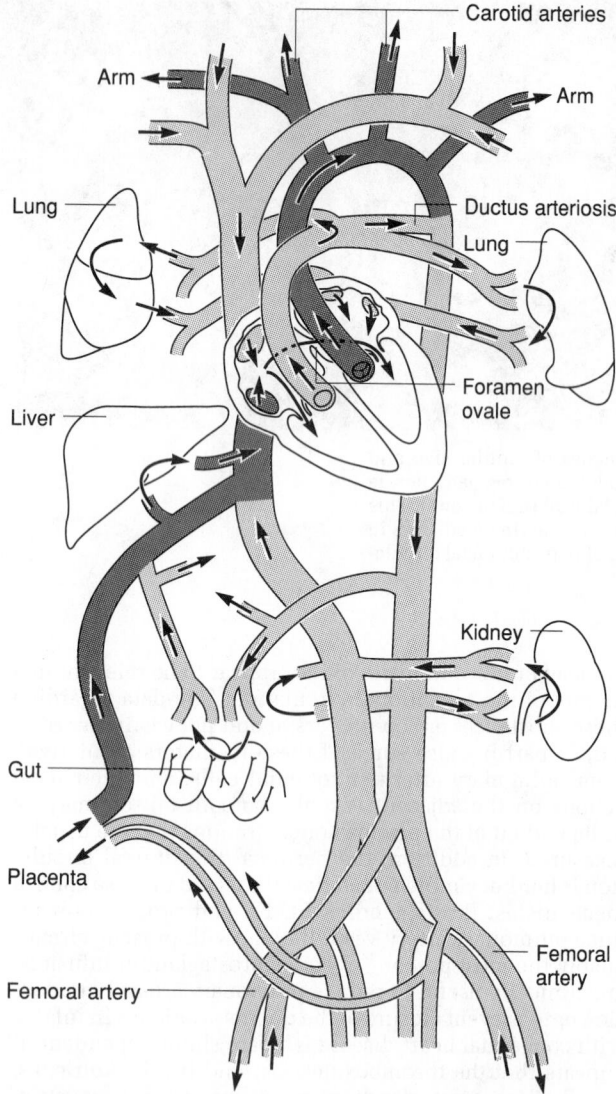

Figure 102-30. Schematic illustration of normal fetal circulation. At parturition, the placenta is removed from the circuit, and the pulmonary vascular resistance drops. Failure of pulmonary resistance to decrease leads to right-to-left shunting through the foramen ovale and ductus arteriosus, and persistent fetal circulation or persistent pulmonary hypertension of the newborn results.

these infants, but to date, survival does not appear to be improved.[29] Inotropic agents may also be useful in these infants to increase systemic blood pressure and minimize right-to-left shunting through the patent ductus arteriosus. Unfortunately, this too is rarely sufficient. The conclusion must be that pharmacologic management is sometimes helpful, but other approaches are necessary to successfully treat infants with persistent pulmonary hypertension.

Clinical Management

Diagnosis

Increasingly, diaphragmatic hernias are discovered before birth during maternal ultrasound examinations. This finding presents a dilemma and is the source of considerable controversy. The probability of fetal survival and successful neonatal correction may be as low as 20% and as high as 75%.[30,31] The variability is related in part to different popu-

lations in different series. Series composed of highly selected referred patients tend to have very high risk and poor outcomes.[32,33] Series based on regional populations are less biased and have higher survival rates.[34-36] Options include elective termination of the pregnancy, delivery with ventilatory support and cardiopulmonary bypass available for the infant, and in utero surgery. Given the complex nature of the problem and the attendant mortality, it is appropriate to have these mothers cared for prospectively in a facility prepared to provide definitive perinatal care for both mother and infant.

Most cases of diaphragmatic hernia in infants are discovered because of severe respiratory distress, either immediately in the delivery suite or within the first few hours of life. For the 10% to 15% who develop symptoms beyond 24 hours of age, or who are asymptomatic when discovered, repair is predictably uneventful and the outcome good. The remainder of this review deals with infants who are physiologically unstable at, or shortly after, birth. Afflicted infants are typically delivered at term with a maternal history remarkable for polyhydramnios in two thirds of cases. The infant abdomen is scaphoid and the ipsilateral chest prominent because of the intrathoracic, air-filled intestine. The cardiac impulse is displaced to the contralateral side, usually the right. Breath sounds are diminished or absent on the ipsilateral side. Bowel sounds may be heard over the chest, but this sign is not usually present. The diagnosis is best confirmed with a plain chest radiograph. Air-filled loops of intrathoracic intestine with a paucity of abdominal intestine, a nasogastric tube within an intrathoracic stomach, a small ipsilateral lung, no diaphragmatic silhouette, and a contralateral mediastinal shift are all characteristic (Fig. 102-31). It may occasionally be difficult to differentiate this picture from primary pulmonary pathology, such as a CAM, lobar emphysema, or parenchymal pneumatoceles. A barium upper gastrointestinal tract series resolves the uncertainty in these instances.

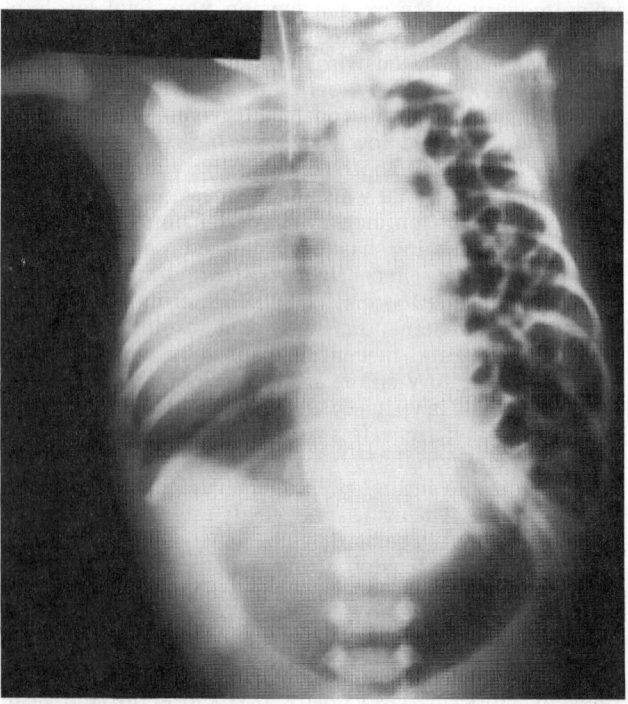

Figure 102-31. Appearance of a classic left posterolateral diaphragmatic hernia on a plain chest radiograph.

Associated Anomalies

Between 15% and 25% of infants with a diaphragmatic hernia have an associated anomaly, the most important being cardiovascular abnormalities. Although ventricular septal defects and aortic coarctations are most common, virtually all cardiac and great vessel anomalies have been reported. Cardiac ultrasound screening examinations are therefore routine. Every infant with a diaphragmatic hernia has a patent ductus arteriosus because of the pulmonary artery hypertension. This may require surgical ligation but usually does not. Indeed, ligation of the ductus arteriosus eliminates a potentially critical right-to-left shunt and has been associated with sudden right ventricular failure and death. Central nervous system malformations, gastroesophageal reflux, pulmonary sequestration, chromosomal abnormalities (trisomy 13 and 18), and other more rare anomalies have also been associated with diaphragmatic hernias.

Medical Management

All posterolateral diaphragmatic hernias in infants require operative repair. Unfortunately, operative repair alone usually does not resolve the respiratory failure. Outcome is determined by the degree of pulmonary hypoplasia and pulmonary artery hypertension rather than by the details of the surgical repair. With this in mind, the clinical emphasis should be on maximizing medical treatment, primarily respiratory support, and on carefully selecting an optimal time for operative repair. Preoperative management requires effective nasogastric tube decompression of the intrathoracic intestine. Prompt endotracheal intubation and appropriate ventilatory support are required since acidosis and hypoxemia exacerbate the tendency to develop persistent pulmonary hypertension. Hyperventilation-induced respiratory alkalosis designed to reduce pulmonary artery vasospasm has been a standard approach until recently. In the last several years, a strategy of permissive hypercapnia has evolved with results that appear encouraging. The concept is that by tolerating moderate hypoxemia and hypercarbia (without acidosis), iatrogenic lung injury related to positive pressure ventilation can be minimized.[37] Induced metabolic alkalosis is less helpful but rational and occasionally beneficial. Paralysis and fentanyl-induced anesthesia have been used to ensure total control of ventilation and may directly reduce pulmonary artery pressure. Vasodilators, particularly tolazoline, may be used therapeutically, or perhaps diagnostically, to provide a period of improved pulmonary artery blood flow. Inotropic agents, most notably dopamine, are useful to increase aortic blood pressure and to further diminish right-to-left shunting. Inhaled nitric oxide is being evaluated in several centers and a multiple-institution trial of liquid ventilation with a perflurocarbon emulsion is beginning as well. Insufficient data are available at present to reach conclusions as to their utility.

Arterial blood gases are best monitored using both a preductal sampling site, usually the right radial artery, and a postductal site, usually the descending aorta by way of an umbilical artery catheter. Comparison of blood gas data from these sites allows assessment of the degree of right-to-left shunting through the ductus arteriosus. Contralateral pneumothorax is always a risk in view of the high airway pressures required for ventilation during the first hours of life. Given the bilateral pulmonary hypoplasia and the extremely poor tolerance of even transient hypoxemia, some advocate prophylactic contralateral chest tube placement.

Infants with diaphragmatic hernias have considerable variation in the degree of respiratory distress. Some appear simply to have inadequate alveolar surface area for gas exchange; these newborns die promptly after birth regardless of treatment. Most, however, have one or more periods of adequate gas exchange, the so-called honeymoon period. A definition of adequate gas exchange has not been uniformly agreed on, but one reasonable definition includes a single blood gas determination with a postductal PaO_2 greater than 80 mmHg or a $PaCO_2$ less than 40 mmHg.[38] It has been suggested that a honeymoon period, regardless of the medical support required, implies the presence of adequate alveolar surface area and is consistent with potentially reversible respiratory failure and possible survival.[39] This concept emphasizes the pathogenic importance of pulmonary artery vasospasm. Conversely, the absence of a honeymoon period may imply an irreversible degree of pulmonary hypoplasia. This observation has been used in clinical practice as the basis for withholding or modifying treatment, but the data are controversial.

Operative Management

The operative repair of a diaphragmatic hernia is usually straightforward (Fig. 102-32). A transabdominal approach through a left subcostal incision is standard, although repair is also possible through the thorax, if required. A transthoracic approach may be preferable for right-sided lesions. Reduction of the herniated viscera is done with gentle traction and is distinctly more simple using the transabdominal approach. Suture repair of the defect is the procedure of choice and is usually uneventful. Large diaphragmatic defects may occasionally require a transversus abdominis muscle flap, purposeful deformation of the chest wall, or insertion of prosthetic material to obtain closure. A diminutive peritoneal cavity resulting from the in utero displacement of abdominal viscera may present an abdominal wall closure problem similar to that seen in a child with an omphalocele or gastroschisis. Stretching the abdominal wall musculature is usually sufficient to effect closure; however, prosthetic material or a staged closure occasionally may be required. An ipsilateral chest tube may be placed before diaphragmatic closure, but some have advocated that thoracic drainage tubes not be used

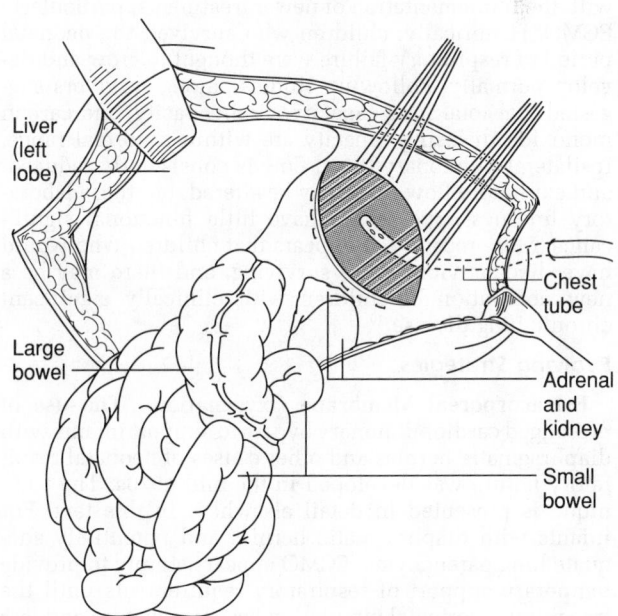

Figure 102-32. Operative repair typically involves simple suture closure of the diaphragm after reduction of abdominal viscera.

routinely. If chest tubes are used, water seal or minimal suction drainage must be used judiciously to avoid acute mediastinal shifts.

The controversial issue with regard to operative treatment of diaphragmatic hernia is that of optimal timing for repair. Traditionally, infants were rushed emergently to the operating room for reduction of the herniated viscera and diaphragmatic closure. Because effective preoperative decompression of the intestine is usually possible, and because it has become clear that the underlying pulmonary hypoplasia is not reversed by emergency operation, the sense of urgency has diminished. Most surgeons now commit themselves to preoperative stabilization, which is used to confirm the diagnosis, optimize ventilation and oxygenation, correct the usual acidosis, institute inotropic support, resuscitate the infant, and insert appropriate intravenous and intraarterial lines. Operative repair is then undertaken when these goals have been achieved and when the patient is physiologically stable. The accumulating data suggest delaying for hours or days so that the risks of general anesthesia, transportation, and the postoperative reduction in chest wall and lung compliance are incurred later when the transitional pulmonary circulation may not be so vulnerable to vasoconstrictive stimuli. Experience with this latter approach suggests at least an equivalent outcome.[40-47] The issue is further complicated by the availability of long-term extracorporeal membrane oxygenation (ECMO) and controversy over its application and timing. In general, ECMO appears best reserved for infants who cannot be stabilized using less invasive respiratory support strategies. The current recommendation is that operative repair be undertaken in a stable patient who is nearing extubatable levels of ventilatory support, regardless of which means of support has been used. Therefore, repair is done at or after the end of cardiopulmonary bypass in some infants.

Results

Overall survival rates for infants with diaphragmatic hernias symptomatic in the first few hours of life remained stable at about 50% during the 1960s and 1970s. Selected series, which excluded early deaths outside of tertiary referral centers, may have incorrectly suggested higher survival rates. Survival may have improved to the 75% range with the implementation of newer treatments, particularly ECMO. Historically, children who survived the neonatal period of respiratory failure were thought to grow and develop normally. Follow-up studies among survivors suggested that total lung capacity, vital capacity, and carbon monoxide diffusing capacity are within a normal range. Ipsilateral pulmonary blood flow is consistently reduced, and expiratory flow rates may be altered, but these laboratory findings appeared to have little functional significance. More recently, it appears that children who would have died previously are surviving, and there may be a new population of children with clinically significant chronic lung disease.[48]

Evolving Strategies

Extracorporeal Membrane Oxygenation. The use of prolonged cardiopulmonary bypass to support infants with diaphragmatic hernias and other causes of neonatal respiratory failure was developed in the mid-1970s. The technique is presented in detail elsewhere in this text. For infants with diaphragmatic hernias and potentially adequate lung parenchyma, ECMO appears simply to provide temporary support of respiratory requirements until the transitional perinatal circulation becomes mature and less sensitive to vasoconstrictive stimuli. The alternative hypothesis, that new alveoli grow and develop adequately to support gas exchange during a 1- or 2-week period of ECMO, appears less tenable. ECMO allows respiratory support without the risks of barotrauma and oxygen toxicity associated with conventional ventilation. Although there have been no prospective randomized trials of ECMO specifically for infants with diaphragmatic hernias, most major children's hospitals in the United States have adopted the technique for infants who fail conventional ventilatory support. This is a controversial and rapidly changing issue, but survival rates as high as 80% to 90% in selected high-risk patients are reported.[49] In general, oxygenation, pH, and airway pressure criteria have been developed to estimate prognosis. Infants with projected mortality rates of over 80% have been considered for treatment with ECMO. Some institutions are reporting overall survival rates for children with congenital diaphragmatic hernias of 70% to 75%, compared with historical figures of about 50%.[31,49-51]

High-Frequency Ventilation. This approach includes the use of either high-frequency oscillation or high-frequency jet ventilation to support infants with diaphragmatic hernias. The techniques are based on the concept that adequate gas exchange can be achieved with diminshed barotrauma by using a pattern of very rapid, low-volume inspirations. High-frequency ventilation, like ECMO, may make it possible to provide adequate gas exchange and defer surgical repair beyond the early neonatal period when the pulmonary vascular bed is so exquisitely sensitive to vasospasm. For infants with diaphragmatic hernias, the techniques have proved effective at reducing the $PaCO_2$ but less so at improving oxygenation.[52] Unfortunately, the experience is limited and does not suggest improvement in overall survival rates.

In Utero Repair of Diaphragmatic Hernia. Appropriately timed in utero correction of a simulated diaphragmatic hernia in fetal lambs results in improved lung growth and better neonatal survival. These experimental data, coupled with the apparently poor prognosis for the human fetus with a diaphragmatic hernia, have led to attempts at surgical repair in the human fetus.[31,53,54] In a report of 14 such fetal repairs performed between 1989 and 1991 from a referral population of 61 patients, 4 infants survived to term.[55] This is an approach of great interest to both the lay and scientific communities, but it is not clear where this line of investigation will lead. Substantial ethical and technical issues remain as well as major concerns related to the problem of appropriate patient selection. This approach should be considered experimental at this time.

More recently, data suggest that in utero tracheal occlusion reverses important aspects of pulmonary hypoplasia in experimental congenital diaphragmatic hernia models. This observation suggests a new and more simple strategy for in utero therapy for the fetus with a diaphragmatic hernia.[56] This too is an area of active investigation that has now been applied to a few human fetuses.

Pulmonary Transplantation. Pulmonary transplantation has recently achieved a level of predictable success such that it can be considered a reasonable clinical option for selected adults with chronic respiratory failure.[57] This evolution has generated experimental work that confirms the technical feasibility of neonatal single-lung or segmental transplantation. Because of the continuing high mortality of infants with diaphragmatic hernias, several surgical groups are pursuing this approach. Successful neonatal lung transplantation for congenital diaphragmatic hernia has been achieved but remains reportable.[58]

Liquid Ventilation. Liquid ventilation using perflubron is an experimental strategy undergoing clinical trials for acute respiratory failure in both adults and children. It has been used in limited preliminary trials for infants with congenital diaphragmatic hernia. Oxygenation and pulmonary compliance respond very favorably; however, no meaningful long-term data or survival statistics are available.[59] A multiple-institution clinical trial is in progress.

MORGAGNI DIAPHRAGMATIC HERNIAS

This diaphragmatic hernia results from a defect in the anterior retrosternal muscle at one, or occasionally both, of the minor apertures where the superior epigastric arteries traverse the diaphragm. The location is parasternal rather than midline (see Fig. 102-25). It is a rare defect, representing 5% or less of all congenital diaphragmatic hernias. Patients are generally asymptomatic, and discovery typically results from diagnostic imaging undertaken for unrelated reasons. Air-filled viscera in the mediastinum on plain chest radiograph is the single most common scenario. Given the lack of symptoms, these patients are generally older than those with Bochdalek hernias. The hernia most often contains liver, but transverse colon, stomach, and small intestine are all possible. Incarcerated hollow viscera usually account for any related symptoms. Operative repair is straightforward and involves a transabdominal approach, reduction of involved viscera, and simple suture closure of the diaphragm to the posterior sheath of the rectus abdominis muscle.

EVENTRATION OF THE DIAPHRAGM

Diaphragmatic eventration is defined as the abnormal elevation of a portion of an intact diaphragm. This most often involves an entire hemidiaphragm but may be more focal. Congenital eventration is associated with an embryonic defect in muscularization, yielding an intact membranous diaphragm with an inadequate or abnormal muscular component. Acquired eventration is associated with neuromuscular dysfunction of the diaphragm. Most commonly, this results from injury to the phrenic nerve and may occur secondary to trauma, inflammation, or local neoplastic invasion. Patients with acquired eventration have a normally formed but paralyzed hemidiaphragm, which undergoes muscular atrophy with time.

The incidence of diaphragmatic eventration is low, but precise estimates are not available since all reported series have some selection bias. Furthermore, many patients with eventration are asymptomatic and never discovered. The defect usually involves the left hemidiaphragm and therefore may be difficult to differentiate from a diaphragmatic hernia. Fluoroscopy or ultrasound differentiates patients with eventrations, who characteristically have an intact hemidiaphragm with paradoxical motion on inspiration. Occasionally, a barium upper gastrointestinal tract series is needed to make the distinction. When symptoms are present in older children and adults, they are usually related to either compression of the ipsilateral lung or displacement of the stomach into the chest with gastroesophageal reflux or gastric outlet obstruction. Infants, however, may develop respiratory failure secondary to impaired function of the diaphragm. In general, symptomatic patients benefit from surgical stabilization of the diaphragm; asymptomatic patients are best observed.

The surgical approach may be through either the abdomen or chest. For unilateral eventration, the excellent transthoracic exposure is usually preferable. The operative management consists of suture plication of the diaphragm, fixing it in an expiratory position. It is sometimes expedient to resect a portion of the redundant diaphragm to accomplish this. The procedure is straightforward and the outcome predictably good.

REFERENCES

1. Ochsner A, DeBakey M. Chone-chondrosternum. J Thorac Surg 1938;8:469.
2. Beiser GD, Epstein SE, Stampfer M, et al. Impairment of cardiac function in patients with pectus excavatum with improvement after operative correction. N Engl J Med 1972; 287:267.
3. Morshuis WJ, Folgering HT, Barentsz JO, et al. Exercise cardiorespiratory function before and one year after operation for pectus excavatum. J Thorac Cardiovasc Surg 1994;107:1403.
4. Kaguraoka H, Ohnuki T, Itaoka R, et al. Degree of severity of pectus excavatum and pulmonary function in preoperative and postoperative periods. J Thorac Cardiovasc Surg 1992; 104:1483.
5. Wynn SR, Driscoll DJ, Ostrom NK, et al. Exercise cardiorespiratory function in adolescents with pectus excavatum. J Thorac Cardiovasc Surg 1990;99:41.
6. Ravitch MM. Congenital deformities of the chest wall and their operative correction. Philadelphia, WB Saunders, 1977.
7. Buntain WL, Isaacs H, Payne VC, et al. Lobar emphysema, cystic adenomatoid malformation, pulmonary sequestration, and bronchogenic cysts in infancy and children: a clinical group. J Pediatr Surg 1974;9:85.
8. Coran AG, Drongowski R. Congenital cystic disease of the tracheobronchial tree in infants and children: experiences with 44 consecutive cases. Arch Surg 1994;129:521.
9. Adzick NS, Harrison MR, Flake AW, et al. Fetal surgery for cystic adenomatoid malformation of the lung. J Pediatr Surg 1993;28:806.
10. Revillion Y, Jan D, Plattner V, et al. Congenital cystic adenomatoid malformation of the lung: prenatal management and prognosis. J Pediatr Surg 1993;28:1009.
11. Budorick NE, Pretorius DH, Leopold GR, et al. Spontaneous improvement of intrathoracic masses diagnosed in utero. J Ultrasound Med 1992;11:653.
12. Stein SM, Cox JL, Hernanz-Schulman M, et al. Pediatric chest disease: evaluation by computerized tomography, magnetic resonance imaging, and ultrasonography. Southern Med J 1992;85:735.
13. Dolkart LA, Reimers FT, Helmuth WV, et al. Antenatal diagnosis of pulmonary sequestration: a review. Obstet Gynecol Surv 1992;47:515.
14. Domozio P, Liesner RJ, Dicks-Mireaux C, et al. Malignant mesenchymoma associated with a congenital lung cyst in a child: case report and review of the literature. Pediatr Pathol 1990;10:785.
15. Rodgers BM. Thoracoscopy. In: Holcomb GW III, ed. Pediatric endoscopic surgery. Norwalk, Appleton & Lange, 1994:103.
16. McBride JT, Wohl MEB, Strieder DL, et al. Lung growth and airway function after lobectomy in infancy for congenital lobar emphysema. J Clin Invest 1980;66:962.
17. Pokorny WJ, Goldstein IR. Enteric thoracoabdominal duplications in children. J Thorac Cardiovasc Surg 1984;87:821.
18. Silverman NA, Sabiston DC Jr. Primary tumors and cysts of the mediastinum. Curr Probl Cancer 1977;2:1.
19. Hartman GE, Shochat SJ. Primary pulmonary neoplasms of childhood: a review. Ann Thorac Surg 1983;36:108.
20. Manning PB, Morgan RA, Coran AG, et al. Fifty years' experience with esophageal atresia and tracheoesophageal fistula. Ann Surg 1986;204:446.
21. Coran AG. Congenital abnormalities of the esophagus. In: Zuidema GD, Orringer MB, eds. Shackelford's surgery of the alimentary tract: the esophagus, ed 4. Philadelphia, WB Saunders, 1990.
22. Donahoe PK, Gee PE. Complete laryngotracheal cleft: management and repair. J Pediatr Surg 1984;19:143.
23. Gross RE. The surgery of infancy and childhood. Philadelphia, WB Saunders, 1953:913.
24. Richardson JV, Doty DB, Rossi NP, et al. Surgical management of vascular ring. Ann Surg 1981;31:426.
25. DeLorimmer AA, Harrison MR, Hardy K, et al. Tracheobron-

chial obstructions in infants and children: experience with 45 cases. Ann Surg 1990;212:277.

26. Manning PB, Wesley JR, Polley TZ Jr, et al. Esophageal and tracheobronchial foreign bodies in infants and children. Pediatr Surg Int 1987;2:346.

27. Gray SW, Skandalakis JE. Embryology for surgeons. Philadelphia, WB Saunders, 1972:359.

28. Anderson KD. Congenital diaphragmatic hernia. In: Welch KJ, Randolph JG, Ravitch MM, et al, eds. Pediatric surgery. Chicago, Year Book, 1986:589.

29. Shah N, Jacob T, Exler R, et al. Inhaled nitric oxide in congenital diaphragmatic hernia. J Pediatr Surg 1994;29:1010.

30. Harrison MR. Fetal diaphragmatic hernia. In: Puri P, ed. Congenital diaphragmatic hernia. New York, Karger, 1989:130.

31. Stolar CJH. Repair in utero of a fetal diaphragmatic hernia. N Engl J Med 1990;323:1279.

32. Sharland GK, Lockhart SM, Heward AJ, et al. Prognosis in fetal diaphragmatic hernia. Am J Obstet Gynecol 1992;166:9.

33. Harrison MR, Adzick NS, Estes JM, et al. A prospective study of the outcome for fetuses with diaphragmatic hernia. JAMA 1994;271:382.

34. Wenstrom KD, Weiner CP, Hanson JW: A five-year statewide experience with congenital diaphragmatic hernia. Am J Obstet Gynecol 1991;165:838.

35. Wilson JM, Fauza DO, Lund DP, et al. Antenatal diagnosis of isolated congenital diaphragmatic hernia is not an indicator of outcome. J Pediatr Surg 1994;29:815.

36. Steinhorn RH, Kriesmer PJ, Green TP, et al. Congenital diaphragmatic hernia in Minnesota. Impact of antenatal diagnosis on survival. Arch Pediatr Adolesc Med 1994;148:626.

37. Wung JT, Sahni R, Moffitt ST, et al. Congenital diaphragmatic hernia: survival treated with very delayed surgery, spontaneous respiration, and no chest tube. J Pediatr Surg 1995;30:406.

38. Schumacher RE, Oldham KT. Congenital diaphragmatic hernia. In: Faix RG, Donn SM, eds. Neonatal emergencies. New York, Futura, 1990:297.

39. Bohn DJ, James I, Filler RM, et al. The relationship between $PaCO_2$ and ventilation parameters in predicting survival in congenital diaphragmatic hernia. J Pediatr Surg 1984;19:666.

40. Coughlin JP, Drucker DE, Cullen ML, et al. Delayed repair of congenital diaphragmatic hernia. Am Surg 1993;59:90.

41. Charlton AJ, Bruce J, Davenport M. Timing of surgery in congenital diaphragmatic hernia. Low mortality after preoperative stabilization. Anaesthesia 1991;46:820.

42. West KW, Bengston K, Rescorla FJ, et al. Delayed surgical repair and ECMO improves survival in congenital diaphragmatic hernia. Ann Surg 1992;216:454.

43. Iwanaka T, Tamura M, Tanaka K, et al. Congenital diaphragmatic hernia treated by perinatal stabilization. Asia Oceania J Obstet Gynaecol 1994;20:115.

44. Goh DW, Drake DP, Brereton RJ, et al. Delayed surgery for congenital diaphragmatic hernia. Br J Surg 1992;79:644.

45. Adolph V, Flageole H, Perreaultt T, et al. Repair of congenital diaphragmatic hernia after weaning from extracorporeal membrane oxygenation. J Pediatr Surg 1995;30:349.

46. Breaux CW Jr., Rouse TM, Cain WS, et al. Improvement in survival of patients with congenital diaphragmatic hernia utilizing a strategy of delayed repair after medical and/or extracorporeal membrane oxygenation stabilization. J Pediatr Surg 1991;26:333.

47. Wilson JM, Lund DP, Lillhei CW, et al. Delayed repair and preoperative ECMO does not improve survival in high-risk congenital diaphragmatic hernia. J Pediatr Surg 1992;27:368.

48. Nakayama DK, Motoyama EK, Mutich RL, et al. Pulmonary function in newborns after repair of congenital diaphragmatic hernia. Pediatr Pulmonol 1991;11:49.

49. Heiss K, Manning P, Oldham KT, et al. Reversal of mortality for congenital diaphragmatic hernia with ECMO. Ann Surg 1989;209:225.

50. Rasheed K, Coughlan G, O'Donnell B. Congenital diaphragmatic hernia in the newborn: outcome in 59 consecutive cases over a ten year period (1980–1989). Ir J Med Sci 1992;161:16.

51. Butt W, Mee R, McDougall P, et al. ECMO in newborn infants: the Melbourne experience. J Paediatr Child Health 1992; 28:426.

52. Bohn D, Tamura M, Perrin D, et al. Ventilatory predictors of pulmonary hypoplasia in congenital diaphragmatic hernia,

confirmed by morphologic assessment. J Pediatr 1987; 111:423.

53. Harrison MR, Adzick NS, Longaker MT, et al. Successful repair in utero of a fetal diaphragmatic hernia after removal of herniated viscera from the left thorax. N Engl J Med 1990;322:1582.

54. Oldham KT. Congenital diaphragmatic hernia. Curr Opin Pediatr 1991;3:489.

55. Harrison MR, Adzick NS, Flake AW, et al. Correction of congenital diaphragmatic hernia in utero. VI. Hard-earned lessons. J Pediatr Surg 1993;28:1411.

56. Bealer JF, Skarsgard ED, Hedrick MH, et al. The "PLUG" odyssey: adventures in experimental fetal tracheal occlusion. J Pediatr Surg 1995;30:361.

57. Grossman RF, Frost A, Zamel N, et al. Results of single-lung transplantation for bilateral pulmonary fibrosis. N Engl J Med 1990;322:727.

58. Van Meurs KP, Rhine WD, Benitz WE, et al. Lobar lung transplantation as a treatment for congenital diaphragmatic hernia. J Pediatr Surg 1994;29:1557.

59. Pranikoff T, Gauger P, Hirschl RB. Partial liquid ventilation in newborn patients with congenital diaphragmatic hernia. J Pediatr Surg 1996;31:613.

SURGERY: SCIENTIFIC PRINCIPLES AND PRACTICE, Second Edition, edited by Lazar J. Greenfield, Michael W. Mulholland, Keith T. Oldham, Gerald B. Zelenock, and Keith D. Lillemoe. Lippincott–Raven Publishers, Philadelphia. © 1997.

CHAPTER 103

PEDIATRIC ABDOMEN

KEITH T. OLDHAM, ARNOLD G. CORAN, AND JOHN R. WESLEY

Abdominal Wall Defects

JOHN R. WESLEY

Defects of the abdominal wall are generally obvious at birth, and therapy is either emergent, urgent, or elective, depending on the type of defect, the condition of the herniated gastrointestinal viscera, and the overall condition of the infant, including any associated anomalies. The present discussion includes gastroschisis, omphalocele, umbilical hernia, inguinal hernia, and hydrocele.

GASTROSCHISIS

Anatomy, Embryology, and Pathophysiology

Gastroschisis is a full-thickness defect of the abdominal wall with herniation of a variable amount of uncovered intestine. Its size is variable, but the defect most often is 2 to 3 cm in diameter. The liver generally is normally positioned within the abdominal cavity, but occasionally the herniated intestines are accompanied by a portion of the liver, spleen, stomach, fallopian tubes, ovaries, or testes. The defect almost always occurs immediately to the right of an otherwise normally formed umbilicus. There is no sac or remnant of peritoneum, and the intestine is edematous, frequently matted together, and covered with a gelatinous exudate. The edema and inflammatory exudate are apparently secondary to chemical irritation caused by substances in the amniotic fluid during the 36th to 40th weeks of gestation (Fig. 103-1). The intestine is frequently foreshortened, malrotated, and temporarily nonfunctional because of the thick serosal exudate.

The incidence of gastroschisis has been estimated at 1 in 3000 to 8000 live births and may be increasing.[1] Associated anomalies are uncommon, with an incidence of 10%, and largely consist of related intestinal defects, such as intestinal stenosis and atresia.

Although the embryology has been debated over the years, the most likely explanation for gastroschisis is based on experimental evidence that the anatomic defect is related to the umbilical vein or the adjacent abdominal wall. Early in development, the umbilical veins are paired structures, consisting of a left and right vein. As the intestine is reduced from the umbilical cord, the right umbilical vein is resorbed, leaving the left vein and a thin membrane on the right. This membrane can stretch to form a hernia of the umbilical cord, with the umbilical vein on the stronger, left side of the defect. Gastroschisis can be the result of a prenatal tear or rupture through the membranes of the early hernia, with evisceration of intestine through the defect. At this early stage of development, the bowel is not fully rotated and fixed, and extensive evisceration can occur. This sequence recently was substantiated by serial antenatal ultrasonography showing the transformation of an in utero ruptured hernia of the umbilical cord into a typical gastroschisis at birth.[2] The fact that the defect is a simple mechanical one, rather than a major defect in embryogenesis, is further supported by the low incidence of associated anomalies in infants born with gastroschisis.

OMPHALOCELE

Anatomy, Embryology, and Pathophysiology

Omphalocele is a 2- to 15-cm defect of the abdominal wall with herniation of varying amounts of abdominal viscera into a translucent sac composed of amnionic membrane and peritoneum. The umbilical cord is attached to the sac, but it can be eccentric and near the abdominal wall (Fig. 103-2). Although the sac can be ruptured and in remnants, it is always present. The size of the defect determines the amount and type of visceral herniation. A

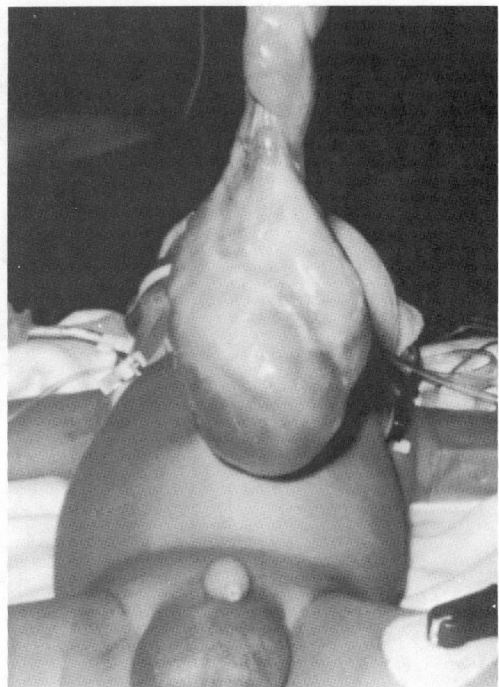

Figure 103-2. Omphalocele. The intact sac, with attached umbilicus, contains liver and intestine.

small defect results in only a small portion of herniated intestine. When the fascial defect and external sac are large, however, there can be massive extrusion of the intestine, stomach, liver, and spleen, leaving a small, underdeveloped peritoneal cavity (Fig. 103-3). The intestine generally is malrotated but appears relatively normal because it has not been exposed to the proinflammatory stimuli of the amniotic fluid. The incidence of omphalocele is estimated at 1 in 6000 to 10,000 births.

Synonyms for omphalocele include *amniocele, exomphalos, celosomia,* and *hernia of the umbilical cord,* reflecting years of confusion over the embryology, terminol-

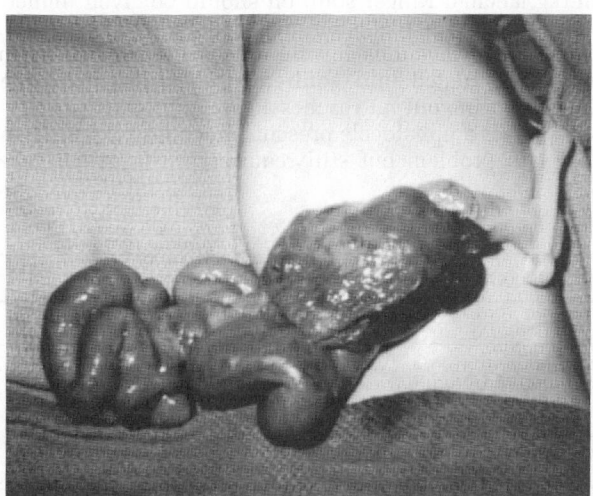

Figure 103-1. Gastroschisis. The normal umbilicus is attached to the abdominal wall to the left of the defect.

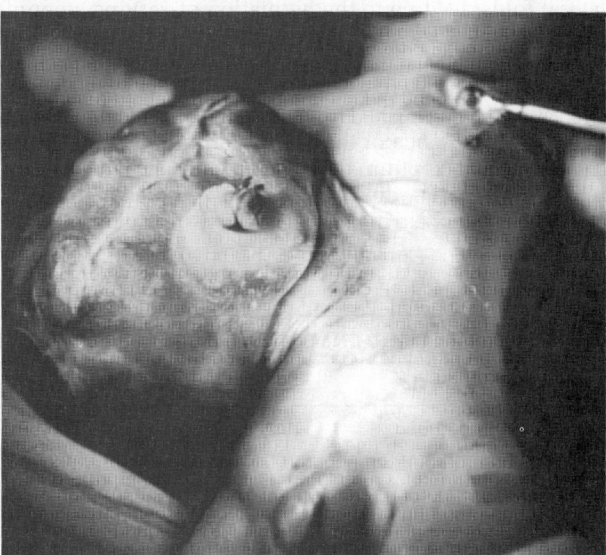

Figure 103-3. Giant omphalocele with small, underdeveloped abdominal cavity.

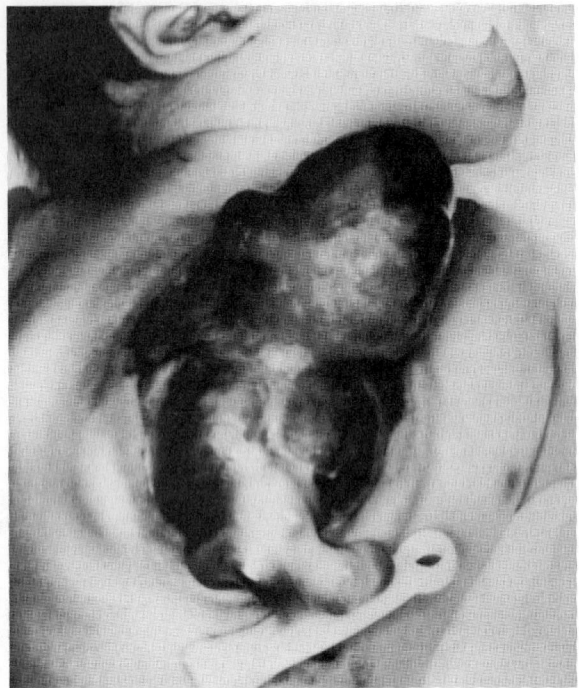

Figure 103-4. Ectopia cordis—supraumbilical omphalocele and sternal defect with herniated, abnormal heart.

ogy, and classification of congenital malformations of the anterior abdominal wall. The common feature, however, is incomplete closure of the anterior abdominal wall of the embryo at the umbilicus. During the 4th week of gestation, the midgut grows and elongates more rapidly than the embryo and is contained in the yolk sac outside the embryonic coelom. During the 10th week, as the embryo continues to grow, the midgut returns to the abdominal cavity and undergoes rotation and posterior fixation to the body wall. Final closure of the abdominal wall depends on normal return of the midgut along with proper growth and fusion of the four body folds (cephalic, caudal, and two lateral) as they meet at the base of the umbilical cord.[3]

The most common form of omphalocele (middle celosomia) is caused by failure of migration and fusion of the lateral folds, leading to the herniation of varying amounts of abdominal viscera. Failure of growth and fusion of the cephalic fold is termed *upper celosomia* and leads to either ectopia cordis (Fig. 103-4) or a constellation of five defects, described by Cantrell.[4] This *pentalogy of Cantrell* consists of a cleft or absence of the lower sternum, absence of the diaphragmatic septum transversum, absence of the diaphragmatic pericardium, congenital cardiac anomalies, and an omphalocele in the epigastric portion of the abdom-

inal wall. These are always severe defects and are frequently incompatible with life.

Given the relation of abnormal embryogenesis to omphalocele development, it is expected that major associated anomalies are much more common with omphalocele than with gastroschisis. Fifty to 60% of infants with omphalocele have at least one associated anomaly.[5] Most of these involve organ systems other than the gastrointestinal tract, and many are related to significantly increased morbidity and mortality. Infants with omphalocele commonly have cardiac, neurologic, genitourinary, skeletal, and chromosomal anomalies. In addition, malrotation, Meckel's diverticulum, and intestinal atresia are more frequent than in the normal population. The important similarities and differences for gastroschisis and omphalocele are summarized in Table 103-1.

CLINICAL ISSUES

The management of infants with gastroschisis and omphalocele from the time of delivery through transport and up until the time of operation is nearly identical. Immediately after birth, the stomach should be aspirated and a nasogastric sump catheter placed to reduce the amount of intestinal distention that will otherwise occur as the infant begins to breathe and swallow air. This helps to prevent vomiting and aspiration during transport. Equally important, gastric decompression reduces bowel distention, thereby easing the operative task of replacing the herniated viscera into the abdominal cavity. The avoidance of additional contamination and prevention of hypothermia are essential. The herniated viscera should be wrapped with warm, saline-soaked gauze and covered with a plastic drape to prevent evaporative heat loss. In the case of gastroschisis, the intestine should be supported in such a way that the blood supply is not compromised as bowel loops and mesentery are draped over the edge of the abdominal defect. The infant initially should be placed under an external warmer and then transported in a warm humidified incubator to maintain normal body temperature. An intravenous cannula should be inserted early and 5% or 10% dextrose given for maintenance. Broad-spectrum intravenous antibiotics should be started immediately.

With gastroschisis, the large, exposed surface area of inflamed intestine risks rapid and extensive fluid and heat loss with the development of hypovolemic shock and hypothermia if intravenous fluids and appropriate covering of the intestines are delayed. An intravenous bolus of 20 mL/kg lactated Ringer solution should be given immediately, along with 10% albumin at 10 mL/kg as needed. A follow-up intravenous infusion at two to four times the infant's calculated fluid requirement should be maintained until the urine output reaches 1 to 2 mL/kg/h.

An intact omphalocele presents much less of a fluid and heat loss problem but still requires sterile saline gauze

Table 103–1. COMPARISON OF GASTROSCHISIS AND OMPHALOCELE

Characteristic	Gastroschisis	Omphalocele
Defect size	2–3 cm	2–15 cm
Sac	Never	Always; may be torn, with remnants
Umbilical cord	Left of defect, on abdominal wall	Attached to sac
Herniated viscera	Small bowel; occasionally stomach, colon	Small bowel, colon, stomach, liver
Malrotation	Yes	Yes
Quality of bowel	Edematous, stiff, with inflammatory exudate	Normal
Alimentation	Delayed	Normal
Associated anomalies	Uncommon (10%)	Common (50%)

wraps and a plastic barrier drape. Because cardiac or renal anomalies can affect the anesthetic management and timing of closure, investigation for associated anomalies, including chest radiograph and cardiac and renal ultrasound, is an important part of the preoperative evaluation. Operative closure may be more elective than with gastroschisis, and protection of the sac should continue until the decision regarding the timing and method of repair has been made. If the membrane is ruptured, immediate closure or coverage is necessary.

OPERATIVE CONSIDERATIONS, SUBSEQUENT MANAGEMENT, AND OUTCOME

Prenatal ultrasound has enabled the diagnosis of gastroschisis and omphalocele before delivery. This also has greatly improved the management of these infants by allowing prospective preparation by the neonatology and surgical services and by allowing for predelivery counseling for the parents. It might be expected that the management of gastroschisis and the incidence of complications, particularly sepsis, would be improved by elective cesarean section in infants diagnosed by prenatal ultrasound. A prospective study alternating vaginal delivery with elective cesarean section, however, has demonstrated no important differences in outcome.[6] Therefore, a careful vaginal delivery generally remains the birthing method of choice.

The timing of delivery may be important. Fitzsimmons and colleagues[7] described little bowel thickening when infants with gastroschisis were delivered at 36 weeks' gestation after lung maturity had been established. In this study, 12 of 14 of these infants had successful primary abdominal wall closure and an earlier return of bowel function. Their average hospital stay was 20 days.

After delivery, stabilization, and assessment of other anomalies, preparations are made for correcting the defect in the operating room. Primary closure after reduction of the herniated viscera is the desired goal, and this is possible in 60% to 70% of infants with either anomaly, provided that the abdominal wall is well stretched and that a feeding gastrostomy is not performed. A feeding gastrostomy takes up considerable space in the left upper abdomen and has given way to decompression of the gastrointestinal tract with a soft orogastric or nasogastric tube. Care must be taken not to generate excessive intraabdominal pressure when performing a primary abdominal wall closure. Potential problems include reducing venous return by compressing the vena cava, creating bowel ischemia by reducing splanchnic blood flow, and compromising respiratory function by limiting diaphragmatic excursion. Both experimentally and clinically, maintenance of the intragastric pressure below 20 cm H_2O, as measured through a nasogastric tube, gastrostomy, or the intraperitoneal bladder, ensures safe reduction that is physiologically tolerable to the infant.[8] If the herniated viscera cannot be reduced primarily, a Silastic pouch is constructed to temporarily contain the extraabdominal bowel, and a series of daily or twice-daily partial reductions is begun. The measurement of intraabdominal pressure can be used as a guide to the amount and frequency of reduction. In most cases, complete reduction can be obtained in 3 to 5 days, and the patient can be returned to the operating room for removal of the Silastic sheeting and final closure of the abdominal wall (Fig. 103-5). Generally, antibiotics are continued until after the abdominal wall is closed.

Adequate nutritional support by means of total parenteral nutrition (TPN) is another important part of the suc-

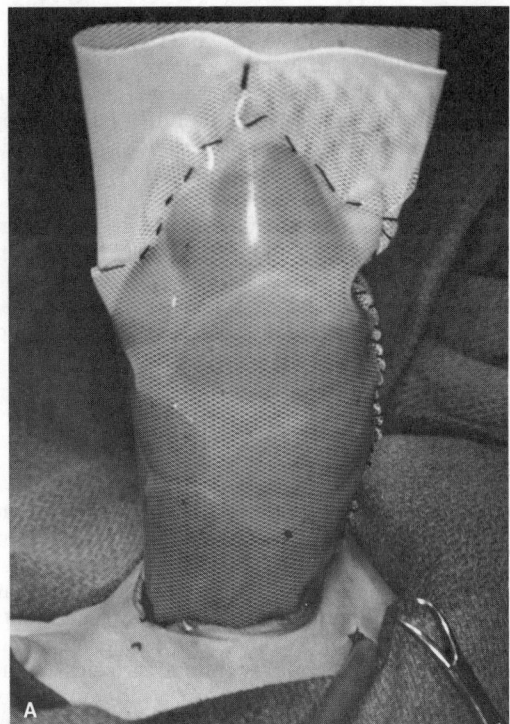

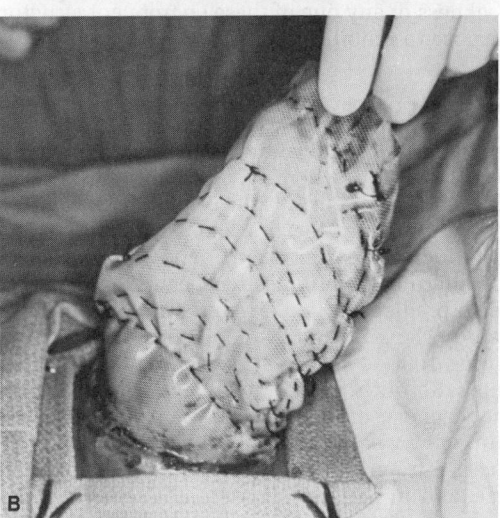

Figure 103-5. (*A*) Infant with gastroschisis with temporary Silastic chimney enclosing herniated bowel. (*B*) Four days after twice-daily serial reduction, the Silastic material is ready for operative removal with closure of remaining defect.

cessful treatment of infants with gastroschisis or giant omphalocele. Together with introduction of the Silastic chimney, this has been responsible for the marked reduction in morbidity and mortality in these infants since the late 1960s. With omphalocele, once reduction has been completed, normal bowel function usually returns promptly, and enteral feedings can be started. For infants with gastroschisis, it is not unusual to require 3 to 5 weeks of TPN after reduction has been completed to provide sufficient time for resolution of the inflammatory process and subsequent resumption of bowel function. This prolonged period of TPN support is not without risks, however, and irreversible cholestasis and liver failure have developed in some patients from the effects of the intravenous nutrition before normal bowel function returned. In most instances, hepatocyte function returns to normal once enteral feeding has resumed, and the degree of liver toxicity can be reduced by matching intravenous caloric support to energy needs by means of indirect calorimetry measurement. In addition, introducing a small amount of enteral feedings with dilute, lactose-free formula as soon as practicable probably exerts an additional protective effect for the liver by stimulating the enterohepatic circulation.[9]

In addition to hepatic toxicity and liver failure, late sequelae of gastroschisis include short bowel syndrome, necrotizing enterocolitis, gastroesophageal reflux, and poor bowel motility.[10] The latter, in its extreme, results in a condition termed *pseudoobstruction* with prolonged and sometimes permanent reliance on TPN.

UMBILICAL HERNIA

Anatomy and Embryology

Congenital umbilical hernias are the most common of the abdominal wall defects in infants and children and seldom present as an emergency except in the rare instance of an associated infected vitelline or urachal remnant, or incarceration. The umbilical ring begins to contract soon after birth and is normally reinforced by the lateral umbilical ligaments (obliterated umbilical arteries), urachus, round ligament (umbilical vein), and a subumbilical extension of the transversalis fascia. Incomplete development or weakness of any one of these component structures can predispose to umbilical herniation.

Clinical Issues

The incidence of congenital umbilical hernia is reported to be 6 to 10 times higher in blacks than in whites. Its incidence ranges from 25% to 50% in blacks and from 4% to 9% in whites in the first months of life.[11] There is a definite increased familial incidence, but no specific genetic pattern of inheritance has been identified. Prematurity also predisposes to congenital umbilical hernia, with one study showing an 84% incidence in newborn infants weighing 1000 to 1500 g at birth, compared with 21% in infants with birthweights over 2500 g.[12]

The diagnosis of umbilical hernia usually is easily made within a few weeks of umbilical cord separation. The defect varies from a few millimeters to several centimeters in size, and in children the hernia is rarely symptomatic. It is almost always easily reducible. No definitive, long-term prospective study has evaluated a stable population with umbilical hernia from birth to adulthood in whom hernia repair was withheld. The following conclusions, however, can be drawn from the many imperfect studies on the subject:

1. Most congenital umbilical hernias close spontaneously within the first 3 years of life.
2. Small-diameter umbilical hernias close earlier than large-diameter umbilical hernias.
3. Some umbilical hernias that are still present at ages 4 to 5 years close by the onset of puberty.
4. Claims that strapping helps cure umbilical hernia are not supported by available data.[13]

Operative Considerations and Outcome

Because of the high incidence of spontaneous closure, surgical repair of congenital umbilical hernia generally is not performed within the first 2 years of life. Subsequent to this, the timing of repair is individualized. Indications for earlier repair include incarceration, symptoms clearly referable to the hernia, and, in selected instances, parental and patient preference when the protrusion is large and the child is self-conscious about it. Surgical repair is safe, the incidence of recurrence is low, and the cosmetic result is gratifying.

INGUINAL HERNIAS AND HYDROCELE

Anatomy, Embryology, and Pathophysiology

Because of their frequency and potential morbidity, inguinal hernias in the pediatric population constitute a major health problem. Three types of hernias occur in the inguinal region—indirect or congenital (99% in infants and children), direct or acquired (0.5%), and femoral (less than 0.5%).[14] An *indirect inguinal hernia* is an abnormal protrusion of the peritoneal lining through the internal inguinal ring along the line of testicular descent, extending caudally with the spermatic cord within the cremasteric fascia for varying distances. The sac can lie completely within the inguinal canal or can protrude through the external inguinal ring to the level of the testicle or below. Its origin is lateral to the deep inferior epigastric artery and veins. A *direct inguinal hernia* disrupts the posterior wall of the inguinal canal, medial to the deep inferior epigastric artery and veins, attenuating the transversalis fascia. It can exit the inguinal canal through the external inguinal ring and extend into the scrotum, always external to the cremasteric fascia or tunica vaginalis. A *femoral inguinal hernia* protrudes medial to the femoral vein into the femoral canal. A femoral hernia always occurs deep and inferior to the inguinal ligament and never enters the scrotum or labia.

The testicle begins its development and descent adjacent to the mesonephros (developing kidney) and enters the scrotum during the third trimester. Descent of the testicle on the right side can be impeded by the retroperitoneal tissue formed by the developing vena cava and external iliac vein, accounting for the higher incidence of right-sided indirect inguinal hernias. The extension of the peritoneum (processus vaginalis) follows the chorda gubernaculum, extending from the testicle in the retroperitoneum to the scrotum during the third month of gestation. During the third trimester, the testicle descends into the scrotum, where the processus vaginalis forms a serous covering around the testicle (tunica vaginalis). Close to the time of birth, the segment of the processus vaginalis between the testicle and the abdominal cavity is normally obliterated. If this process is not complete, as is more frequently the case when an infant is born prematurely, a variety of anatomic conditions can occur (Fig. 103-6).

In a large autopsy study of newborn infants, Snyder and Greanly[15] reported an 80% to 94% incidence of a patent processus vaginalis. The incidence of a patent processus in adults without a history of hernia is 20% to 30%. It is apparent, therefore, that the presence of a patent processus vaginalis by itself does not constitute a hernia. It implies, however, that the size of the sac is of clinical significance. Rowe and colleagues[16] studied 2764 patients with unilateral inguinal hernias and found that the contralateral processus vaginalis remained patent 60% of the time during the first few months of life. Twenty percent of these were obliterated by the age of 2 years, and half of the remaining 40% became clinical hernias.

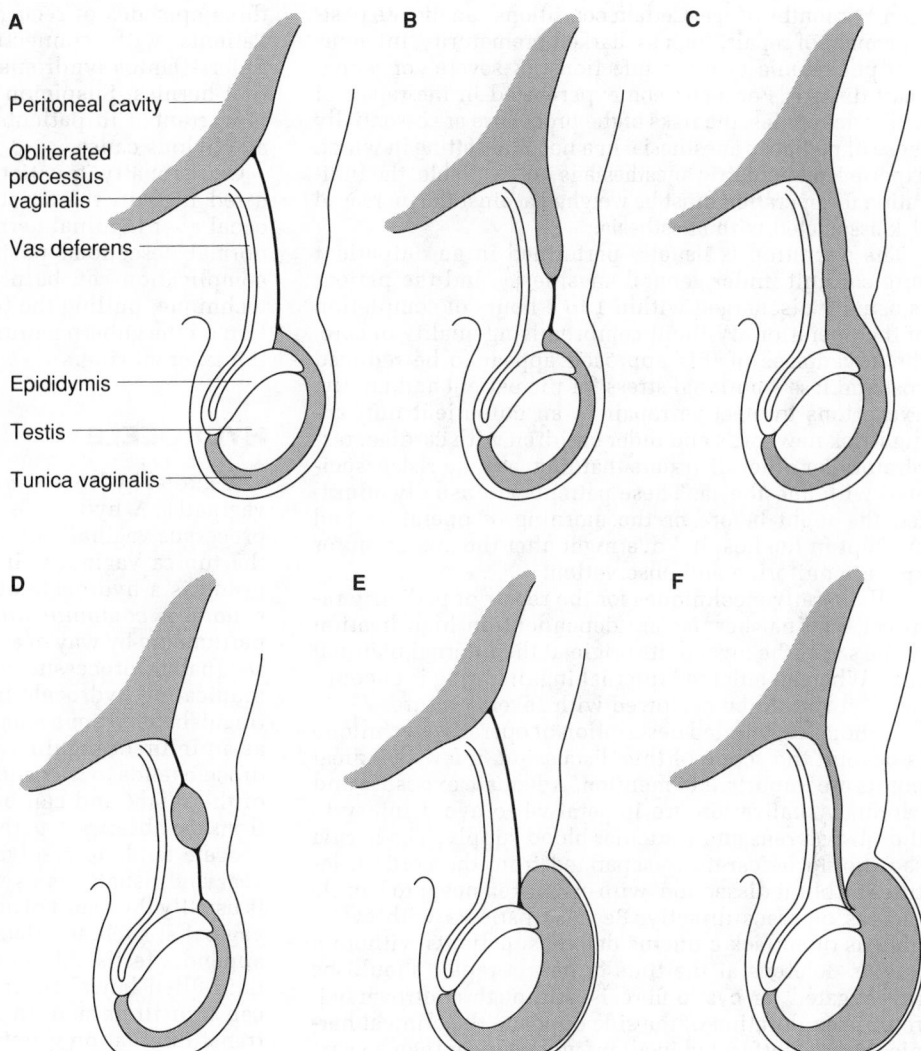

Figure 103-6. Diagrammatic representation of the different forms of inguinal hernia and hydrocele that occur with different degrees of obliteration of the processus vaginalis. (*A*) Normal; obliterated processus vaginalis. (*B*) Proximal sac; distal obliterated processus. (*C*) Hernia sac extending into scrotum; no obliteration. (*D*) Proximal and distal obliteration with hydrocele of the cord. (*E*) Hydrocele of scrotum. (*F*) Patent processus with communicating hydrocele.

Clinical Issues

Inguinal hernias occur in 1% to 3% of all children and in 3% to 5% of infants born prematurely. Of these infants, 11.5% have a family member with a hernia, although there is no known hereditary factor. There is a 6:1 predominance of males over females, and 36% of these infants are younger than 6 months old at the time of operation. For the embryologic reasons outlined earlier, the presentation is right-sided 56.2% of the time, left-sided 27.5%, and bilateral 16.2%. There is an increased incidence of inguinal hernias in patients with connective tissue disorders, such as Ehlers-Danlos syndrome or Marfan syndrome, and in patients with ventriculoperitoneal shunt.[17]

The clinical presentation usually consists of an intermittent bulge in the groin, scrotum, or labia, noted at times of increased intraabdominal pressure. The mass usually reduces spontaneously or with gentle external pressure. In the female infant, the hernia can present as a firm, discrete, nontender mass in the labia, containing a fallopian tube and ovary. A characteristic history is usually sufficient to make a definitive diagnosis of inguinal hernia, even in those patients in whom the hernia cannot actually be demonstrated at the time of examination.

An incarcerated inguinal hernia presents as a mass in the labia or scrotum that does not reduce spontaneously.

If the incarceration has been present for several hours, symptoms of intestinal obstruction (crampy pain, abdominal distention, vomiting, and cessation of stool) are usually present. An incarcerated hernia must be distinguished from an acute hydrocele or inguinal lymphadenitis. As a general rule, if the mass has been present for longer than 24 hours without symptoms or radiographic evidence of intestinal obstruction, it is unlikely to be an incarcerated hernia. Inguinal lymphadenitis is frequently associated with a recent infection in the lower extremity, and fever and redness are common. A palpably normal cord structure above the scrotal mass excludes an incarcerated hernia. When the mass cannot be reduced and an incarcerated hernia cannot be ruled out, an urgent operation is indicated.

Operative Considerations and Outcome

The presence of an inguinal hernia in the pediatric age group constitutes the indication for operative repair. An inguinal hernia does not resolve spontaneously and must be repaired because of the high risk of incarceration. Rowe and Clatworthy[18] found that 71% of incarcerated hernias requiring operative reduction occurred in infants younger than 11 months of age. Certain conditions can dictate postponement of repair, such as marked prematurity, intercurrent pneumonia or other infections, or severe congenital heart disease. For a surgeon experienced in the repair of pediatric hernias, the risks of the procedure are essentially those of pediatric anesthesia. In a hospital setting in which experienced pediatric anesthesia is not available, the indication for operation must be weighed against the increased risk associated with anesthesia.

The operation is usually performed in an outpatient surgical unit under general anesthesia, and the patient is usually discharged within 1 to 2 hours of completion of the operation. Without compromising quality of care, the advantages of this approach appear to be reduced cost and less emotional stress for the patient and family. Exceptions to elective repair in an outpatient unit are high-risk newborns and older children with cardiac, respiratory, or other disorders that increase the risk associated with anesthesia. These patients are usually admitted the night before or the morning of operation and are kept in the hospital overnight after the operation for apnea monitoring and observation.

All operative techniques for the repair of pediatric indirect inguinal hernias are dependent on high ligation of the sac at the level of its origin at the internal inguinal ring. When an enlarged internal inguinal ring is encountered, it should be narrowed with several sutures.

Although a detailed description of operative technique is beyond the scope of this discussion, a few technical points are important to mention. Adequate exposure and careful visualization are imperative to avoid injury to the vas deferens and testicular blood supply. The hernia sac should be carefully separated from the cord structures by blunt dissection, with care taken never to handle the vas deferens directly. Because patients with cystic fibrosis often lack a ductus deferens, patients without a ductus deferens at the time of hernia repair should be investigated for cystic fibrosis. Although controversial, routine exploration of the side opposite the clinical hernia is often performed in all infants younger than 2 years of age because of the high incidence of a patent processus vaginalis (60%) on the contralateral side.[19] With the development of contemporary laparoscopic techniques, it is now feasible to evaluate the contralateral internal inguinal ring endoscopically, and this approach is gaining acceptance in some centers.[20] In females, the fallopian tube is routinely visualized on the clinical side to rule out the testicular feminization syndrome (male pseudohermaphroditism with absent uterus and short vagina). The use of subcuticular absorbable sutures to close the skin incision, along with a collodion or plastic film dressing, minimizes the risk of wound infection, even in the infant without bladder or bowel control, and ensures an excellent cosmetic result.

All incarcerated hernias should be reduced, if possible, and the hernia repaired promptly, electively, after the edema has resolved. Sedation and elevation of the patient's buttocks on a pillow can help to reduce the incarcerated hernia, but ice packs should not be applied to the groin. Although manual reduction of strangulated nonviable bowel is possible in an adult patient, this is a rare occurrence in the pediatric patient. If there is any difficulty with reduction, the patient should be admitted to the hospital for observation. If the hernia cannot be reduced, prompt surgical exploration is indicated. Occasionally, suspected incarcerated hernias prove at operation to be an acute hydrocele of the cord or inguinal lymphadenitis.

Recurrent hernias are much less common in children than in adults. Of 1000 reported patients, there were three episodes of recurrent indirect inguinal hernias.[21] Patients with connective tissue disorders, such as Ehlers-Danlos syndrome, are particularly prone to recurrent hernias. Suspicion of a connective tissue disorder is warranted in patients with recurrent hernia without an obvious cause.

Occasionally, a patient is found to have a testicle located high in the scrotum or trapped in the inguinal canal after inguinal herniorrhaphy, when it had been in normal descended position before the operation. This complication can be prevented by careful attention to technique, pulling the testicle into the scrotum by traction on the gubernaculum rather than pushing it through the external ring.

HYDROCELE

A scrotal hydrocele is a collection of fluid in the tunica vaginalis. A hydrocele of the cord is a remnant of the processus vaginalis filled with fluid and separated from the tunica vaginalis. In the female, the corresponding lesion is a hydrocele of the canal of Nuck in the labia majora. A *communicating hydrocele* connects with the peritoneum by way of a narrow opening into a peritoneal sac (patent processus vaginalis; see Fig. 103-6). A communicating hydrocele is, therefore, anatomically indistinguishable from a small hernia and is treated the same as an indirect inguinal hernia. The communicating hydrocele tends to wax and wane depending on the activity of the infant and can be identified by a careful history from an observant parent. The noncommunicating hydrocele tends to resolve spontaneously by the age of 1 year and usually is asymptomatic. An *acute hydrocele* is usually the result of an acute process within the tunica vaginalis, such as infection or torsion of the testicle or appendix testis. Although a hydrocele transilluminates, fluid-filled bowel in an incarcerated infant hernia sac can transilluminate in an identical fashion. Therefore, transillumination is not a reliable differential diagnostic tool. Aspiration of a hydrocele is mentioned only to be condemned. It is ineffective as a therapeutic measure and can be catastrophic if the suspected hydrocele proves to be an incarcerated loop of bowel. The one exception is the postoperative recurrent hydrocele. Because the possibility of hernia should not exist in this condition, aspiration is safe and frequently effective in controlling a small reaccumulation of fluid. A simple, noncommunicating scrotal hydrocele that has not resolved spontaneously by 1 year of age is excised electively. Operation should always use the inguinal approach so that an accompanying hernia, if present, can be identified and repaired.

Gastrointestinal Disorders

KEITH T. OLDHAM

NEONATAL INTESTINAL OBSTRUCTION

A variety of congenital anatomic defects, inherited metabolic disorders, and acquired physiologic abnormalities present with intestinal obstruction in the 1st

Table 103-2. NEONATAL INTESTINAL OBSTRUCTION

Diagnosis	History	Physical Examination	Relevant Studies
Intestinal atresia or stenosis	Bilious vomiting	Abdominal distention Acholic meconium	Plain radiograph Barium enema
Congenital duodenal obstruction	Bilious vomiting	Gastric distention Trisomy 21	Plain radiograph Upper GI study
Imperforate anus	Failure to pass meconium Bilious vomiting (late)	Abdominal distention Nonpatent anus	Evaluate for VATER syndrome and cardiac anomalies
Necrotizing enterocolitis	High-risk, premature infant Bilious vomiting	Abdominal distention Guaiac-positive stool	Plain radiograph Contrast studies contraindicated
Meconium ileus	Bilious vomiting Cystic fibrosis	Abdominal distention Acholic meconium	Plain radiograph Barium enema
Malrotation	Full-term, healthy infant Bilious vomiting	No abdominal distention	Plain radiograph Upper GI study Barium enema
Hirschsprung disease	Bilious vomiting Delayed passage of meconium Family history	Abdominal distention Trisomy 21	Barium enema Suction rectal biopsy
Uncommon causes of neonatal obstruction (intussusception, Meckel diverticulum duplications)	Variable	Incarcerated hernia Mass	Variable
Medical conditions associated with bilious vomiting and ileus	Variable	Variable	Sepsis Hypothyroidism Meconium plug syndrome Others

month of life. The cardinal clinical manifestation of neonatal bowel obstruction is bilious vomiting, often in conjunction with abdominal distention. These signs in the newborn must be considered to be the result of mechanical obstruction until proved otherwise. Table 103-2 provides an overview of the possible diagnoses with some important generalizations regarding the history, physical examination, and relevant diagnostic studies. These are discussed in detail later.

Considerable variability exists in the clinical presentations of these disorders. Distal obstructions are almost invariably characterized by abdominal distention, whereas proximal obstructions are not. Partial obstructions may produce minimal or no physical findings. The anatomic relation of the obstruction to the ampulla of Vater determines whether bile is present in the stool or in the gastric contents. Generally, clinical clues provide enough information for a preliminary diagnosis and thus direct the diagnostic approach for an individual infant. Because malrotation with midgut volvulus is part of this differential diagnosis, the imaging evaluation must be considered an emergency and must be pursued until malrotation is eliminated as a possibility.

Table 103-3. IMAGING EVALUATION FOR SUSPECTED NEONATAL INTESTINAL OBSTRUCTION

Plain abdominal radiographs

Contrast enema

Upper gastrointestinal series

Fortunately, establishment of a diagnosis is ordinarily straightforward using a combination of readily available imaging studies, including plain abdominal radiographs, barium enema, and upper gastrointestinal (GI) contrast series. More complex diagnostic strategies provide little additional information and generally have a limited role. In the absence of specific clinical clues, the imaging sequence for suspected neonatal intestinal obstruction should begin with plain radiographs, followed by a barium enema and an upper GI study (Table 103-3). The information obtained with each study determines the next requirement. For example, a plain film with pneumatosis intestinalis may be diagnostic of necrotizing enterocolitis (NEC) and therefore sufficient. Both Hirschsprung disease and malrotation have classic abnormalities on barium enema that are essentially diagnostic. With many forms of small bowel obstruction, however, the barium enema simply demonstrates a nonspecific microcolon, which is actually an unused and diminutive but normal colon. Therefore, an upper GI study may provide additional information. An upper GI series is most helpful in evaluating suspected malrotation or possibly proximal and incomplete obstructions.

Although the classic surgical causes of neonatal bilious vomiting are considered in detail later, other medical problems and a variety of less common anatomic obstructions also present with a similar clinical picture. These are briefly considered in Table 103-3. Of the less common obstructive lesions noted, only incarcerated hernia is typical in the neonatal age group. This is considered elsewhere in detail and is excluded here because it does not generally present a diagnostic dilemma. Simple inspection ordinarily yields this diagnosis. Infants with a wide variety of medical illnesses may also develop ileus with bilious vomiting. These diseases may be common, such as sepsis; some are rare, such as congenital hypothyroidism. These topics are not within the scope of this review but do represent important considerations for the clinician once mechanical obstruction is ruled out. The meconium plug syndrome is a benign but important problem relevant to these neonates and is discussed later.

Intestinal Atresia or Stenosis

Atresia or stenosis of the intestine can occur in any location. Lesions affecting the jejunum, ileum, and colon are considered jointly.

Embryology and Anatomy

The embryonic intestine is identifiable by the 3rd gestational week and is divided into three segments_the foregut, midgut, and hindgut. The transverse septum demarcates the caudal extent of the foregut; the hindgut is within the primitive tail fold; and the midgut is between the two. Developmental issues relevant to this discussion are limited to the midgut.[22] This can be considered a simple tubular structure that undergoes elongation, herniation into and reduction from the coelom, rotation, and ultimately, fixation to the posterior body wall (see section on malrotation).

The different forms of intestinal atresia suggest several common patterns of abnormal embryogenesis.[23] Type I atresia is an intraluminal diaphragm that can be either complete or fenestrated. Types II and IIIa atresia can result from one of several in utero vascular accidents, such as intussusception, segmental volvulus, or thromboembolism. These types of atresia can be reproduced experimentally by interrupting the appropriate blood supply in the intestinal mesentery.[24] More rare and complex types of atresia are also described. These include the apple-peel or Christmas tree deformities and multiple segmental atresia (types IIIb and IV; Fig. 103-7). These appear to be related to major or multiple interruptions of proximal mesenteric blood flow during gestation.

Ninety percent or more of infants with congenital jejunoileal obstructions have complete atresia, and the remainder have stenoses or perforated intraluminal diaphragms. The single most common location is in the distal ileum, but any site is possible, and the overall distribution is roughly equal between jejunum and ileum. More than one jejunal or ileal atresia is reported in 6% to 20% of these infants, mandating a complete intraoperative assessment of intestinal patency.[25] Infants with perforated intraluminal diaphragms may have a small, often eccentric, opening, perhaps only millimeters in diameter. Nevertheless, the diagnosis often is not apparent in the neonatal period because symptoms of incomplete obstruction may be minimal or absent for months or even years. The discrepancy between orifice size and symptoms is often remarkable.

In general, examination of the microscopic anatomy adds little to the evaluation or treatment of patients with small intestinal atresia. Proximal muscular hypertrophy is predictable. Enterocyte morphology appears relatively normal, and the simple restoration of intestinal continuity eventually allows normal functional recovery in most infants.

Unlike congenital small bowel atresia, colonic atresia is a rare lesion. Otherwise, it is without fundamental differences in terms of pathogenesis, clinical presentation, and management. It may be associated with skeletal or cardiac anomalies, abdominal wall defects, or other intestinal atresias.

Clinical Presentation

Published incidence estimates for congenital small bowel atresia range from 1 per 300 to 400 births to 1 per 20,000 births.[25,26] Jejunoileal atresia occurs most frequently without a discernible cause, but evidence of in utero bowel injury secondary to intussusception, hernia, malrotation with volvulus, and meconium ileus should be sought.

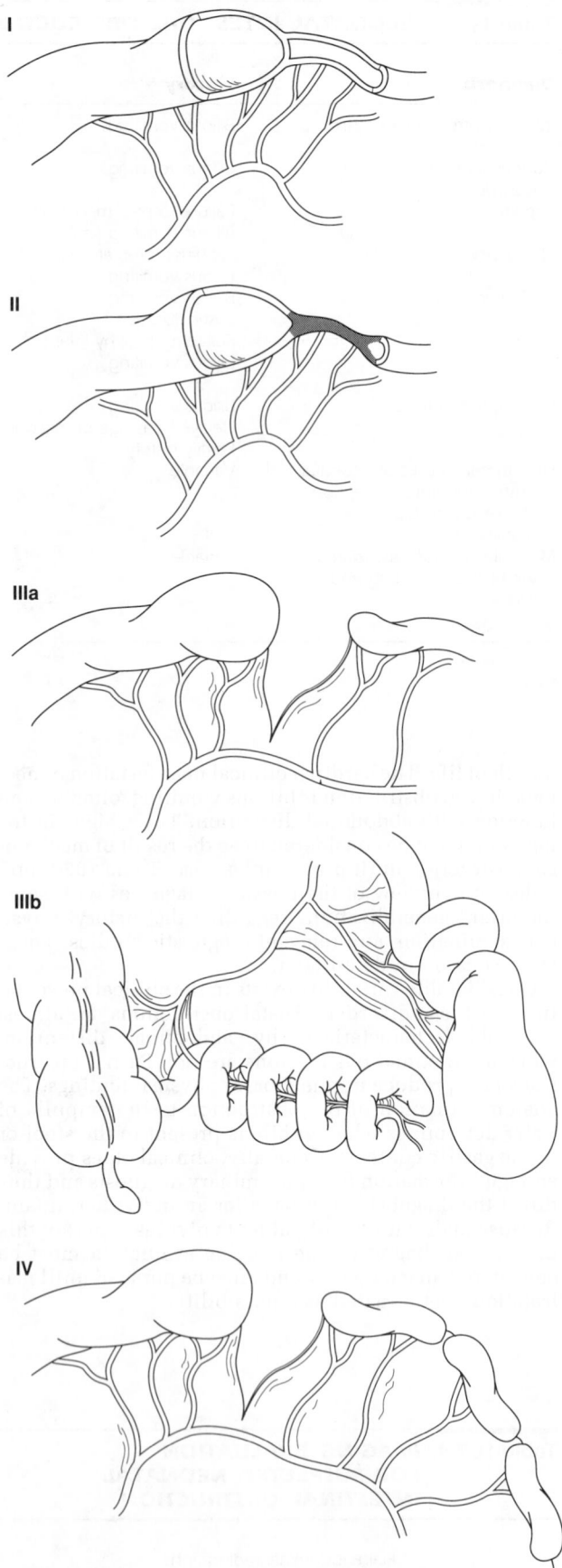

Figure 103-7. Classification of intestinal atresias. Type I, muscular continuity with a complete web. Type II, mesentery intact, fibrous cord. Type IIIa, discontinuous muscle and mesentery. Type IIIb, apple-peel deformity. Type IV, multiple atresias[25].

About 15% to 20% of infants with abdominal wall defects have either congenital or neonatally acquired atresia or stenosis. With this exception, infants with jejunoileal atresia generally have a low incidence (less than 10%) of significant associated anomalies.

Congenital bowel obstructions produce proximal intestinal distention that is predictably detectable with prenatal ultrasound screening techniques. Maternal polyhydramnios related to interruption of normal amniotic fluid absorption in the fetal gut is a sign of proximal intestinal obstruction, and its development is a specific indication for prenatal ultrasound examination. The classic postnatal presentation for small bowel obstruction includes bilious vomiting, abdominal distention, and failure to pass meconium. The degree of distention is dependent on the level of obstruction, postpartum age, and efficacy of proximal decompression. More distal obstructions and longer postpartum times are associated with more distention of the proximal small bowel. Proximal jejunal or duodenal obstructions produce significant vomiting, but distention may be minimal because of effective gastric emptying by this route. On physical examination, it is common to be able to palpate individual loops of proximal intestine through the thin neonatal abdominal wall. In even the smallest premature infant, a rectal examination should be performed when bowel obstruction is suspected. In the case of complete congenital intestinal obstruction distal to the ampulla of Vater, the rectum typically contains white mucus rather than bile-stained meconium. Normal green meconium in the rectum suggests proximal intestinal patency, although obstruction developing late in gestation may be an occasional exception.

Diagnosis

After the history and physical examination, investigation begins with plain abdominal radiographs. The plain film in jejunoileal atresia shows marked distention of proximal intestinal loops with gasless distal small bowel and colon. Because haustral markings are not normally apparent in the neonatal colon, this cannot be differentiated from small bowel without intraluminal contrast. Generally, a contrast enema is obtained to confirm the diagnosis. A diminutive and unused but otherwise normal colon is characteristic of jejunoileal obstructions. Reflux of contrast into the infant small bowel is achieved with relative ease, and a specific point of obstruction in the small intestine may be demonstrable. The diagnosis of colonic atresia is readily made by barium enema as well. Contrast studies of the upper GI tract are generally unnecessary and probably unwise in view of the impending need for operative enterotomy. Incomplete obstruction from a partial web or diaphragm may be difficult to diagnose without a more sophisticated approach such as enteroclysis, but this is typically a problem in infants or children beyond the neonatal period.

Treatment

The treatment for all types of congenital intestinal obstruction is operative. With the exception of malrotation with volvulus, life-threatening physiologic disturbances and bowel loss are not ordinarily associated with these obstructions. Therefore, it is generally appropriate to treat urgent associated problems, to confirm the suspected diagnosis, and to prepare the infant for general anesthesia. Delay in operation beyond this serves no purpose, and proximal perforation can occur.

The operative strategy for congenital bowel obstructions is simply to reestablish intestinal continuity while preserving length and normal anatomy as nearly as possible. A transverse supraumbilical incision provides excellent exposure for all these lesions. Simple end-to-end or end-oblique anastomosis, short segmental bowel resection, and diaphragm excision are employed whenever possible (Fig. 103-8). The size discrepancy between the proximal and distal lumens is usually considerable, and postoperative bowel function may be slow to develop. This has led some to adopt procedures designed to hasten the establishment of normal motility. These include a variety of plication, reduction, and resection techniques that reduce the diameter of the dilated proximal bowel segment. These techniques may be helpful, but the need to preserve intestinal length and absorptive surface area limits their application. Multiple or complex atresias require individualized plans and sometimes multiple anastomoses. The risk for short bowel syndrome may be substantial with these more complex cases; therefore, reestablishment of intestinal continuity is done without resection and regardless of the number of anastomoses required. Preservation of the ileocecal valve is an important objective; the minimal length of bowel necessary to sustain adequate enteral nutrition is reduced by about half if this can be done (ie, from about 40 cm to 15 to 20 cm in the neonate).[27]

The management of colonic atresia is straightforward, and the principles are essentially no different than those summarized for the small bowel. Staged reconstructions

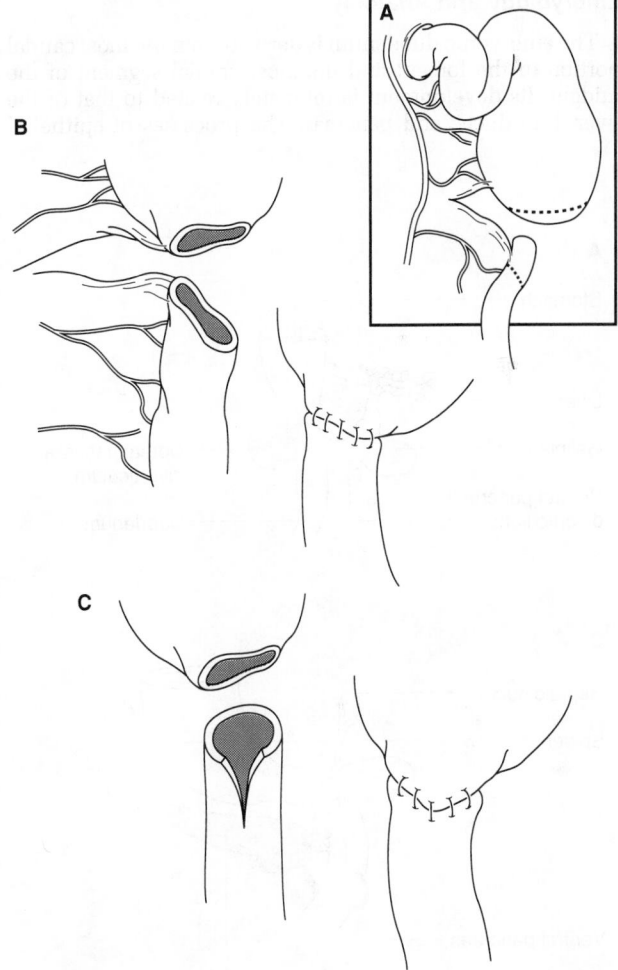

Figure 103-8. (*A* and *B*) The end-oblique anastomosis for small bowel atresia. (*C*) An antimesenteric extension of the distal enterotomy may be used to equalize the proximal and distal lumens.

were advocated in the past, but this is usually unnecessary in contemporary practice.

Results and Complications

The survival rate after surgery for uncomplicated intestinal atresia or stenosis is essentially 100%.[25] The incidence of technical anastomotic problems, such as leak or stricture formation, is as high as 10% to 15% in some published reports, but the current experience is more nearly 5%, which is probably not significantly different than that for adult enteroenterostomy. In modern pediatric surgical practice, morbidity and mortality are generally limited to that imposed by concurrent illness, such as prematurity, congenital heart disease, abdominal wall defects, or other associated problems. Prolonged dysfunction of the proximal gut is relatively common and, as mentioned, may persist for days or weeks. In this regard, total parenteral nutrition (TPN) may be life-saving. Cholestatic jaundice related to parenteral hyperalimentation in the neonate is common but usually reversible with the establishment of enteral feedings.

Congenital Duodenal Obstruction

Congenital duodenal obstruction (duodenal atresia or stenosis and annular pancreas) can result from a pure atresia, an intraluminal diaphragm, or an annular pancreas. Embryonic origins, clinical presentations, and treatment strategies are related; therefore, all three are considered jointly here.

Embryology and Anatomy

The embryonic duodenum is derived from the most caudal portion of the foregut and the most cranial segment of the midgut. Its development is intimately related to that of the liver, bile ducts, and pancreas. The processes of epithelial proliferation and recanalization are similar in the duodenum and the midgut. The pancreas arises from paired dorsal and ventral foregut diverticula during the 6th gestational week. The dorsal anlage gives rise to the body and tail of the gland as well as the main pancreatic duct. The ventral anlage migrates 180 degrees to fuse with the dorsal gland, forming the uncinate process and the distal portion of the duct of Wirsung (Fig. 103-9). An annular pancreas is characterized by circumferential persistence of the gland around the duodenum at the site of the embryonic ventral anlage. It is invariably associated with intrinsic duodenal obstruction and a patent accessory pancreatic duct[28] (Fig. 103-10).

Arrest of normal pancreatic development, failure of duodenal recanalization, vascular accidents, and possibly other events appear to be responsible for the several forms of congenital duodenal obstruction. Unlike congenital jejunoileal obstructions, duodenal anomalies are about evenly divided between intraluminal webs or stenoses and complete atresia. Atresia may occur with or without muscular continuity. Duodenal webs may or may not be fenestrated. Although the site of obstruction may be anywhere within the duodenum, the most frequent location is in the descending duodenum, classically near the ampulla of Vater. Most series report a 5% to 10% incidence of preampullary obstruction. This is an important variant because the vomitus is nonbilious; therefore, this cardinal manifestation of neonatal intestinal obstruction is lacking. Other important variants are periampullary webs or diaphragms that project distally within the duodenal lumen, forming a wind-sock deformity (Fig. 103-11). In this instance, the ampulla is vulnerable to surgical injury because of its proximity or even incorporation into the web.

Clinical Presentation

The incidence of congenital duodenal obstruction is 1 in 10,000 to 40,000 births. Twenty to 40% of these infants also have trisomy 21.[25] Because this syndrome is not al-

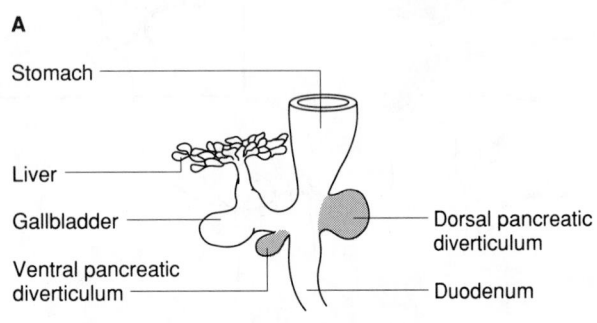

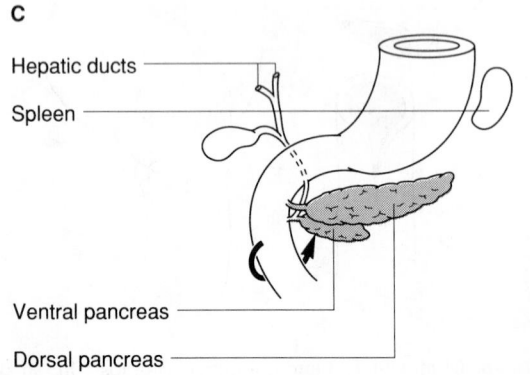

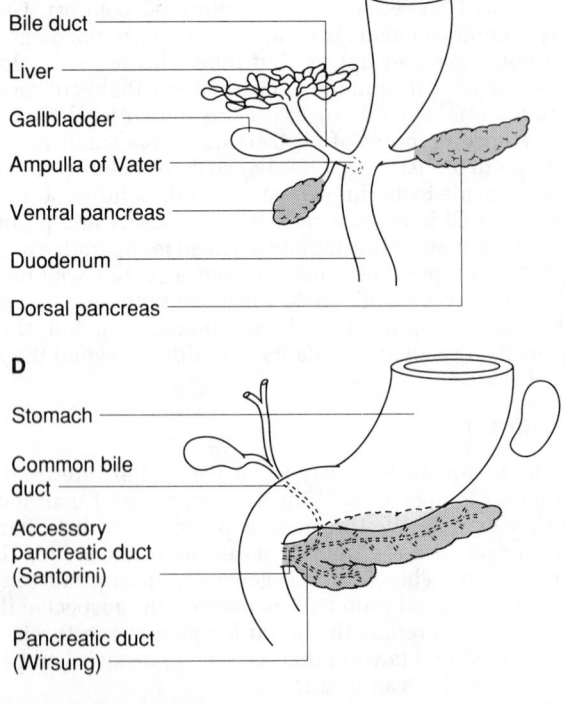

Figure 103-9. The normal embryologic development of the pancreas and bile ducts. (*A*) Fifth gestational week. (*B*) Sixth week. (*C*) Seventh week. (*D*) Eighth week.

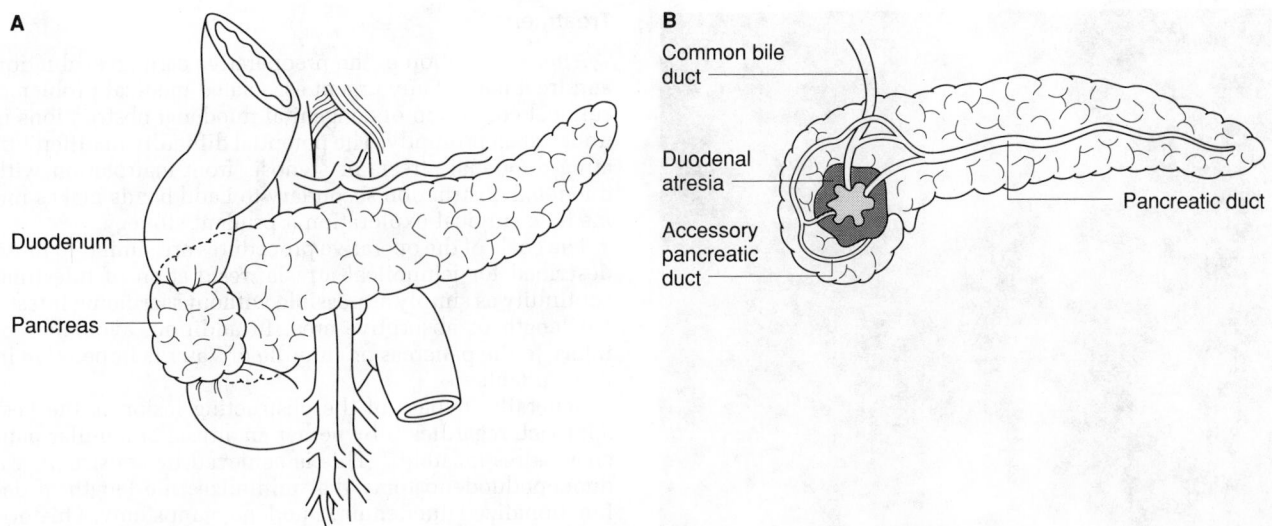

Figure 103-10. Schematic depiction of the annular pancreas. (*A*) The associated duodenal atresia is shown. (*B*) The patent accessory pancreatic duct is shown in cross-section.

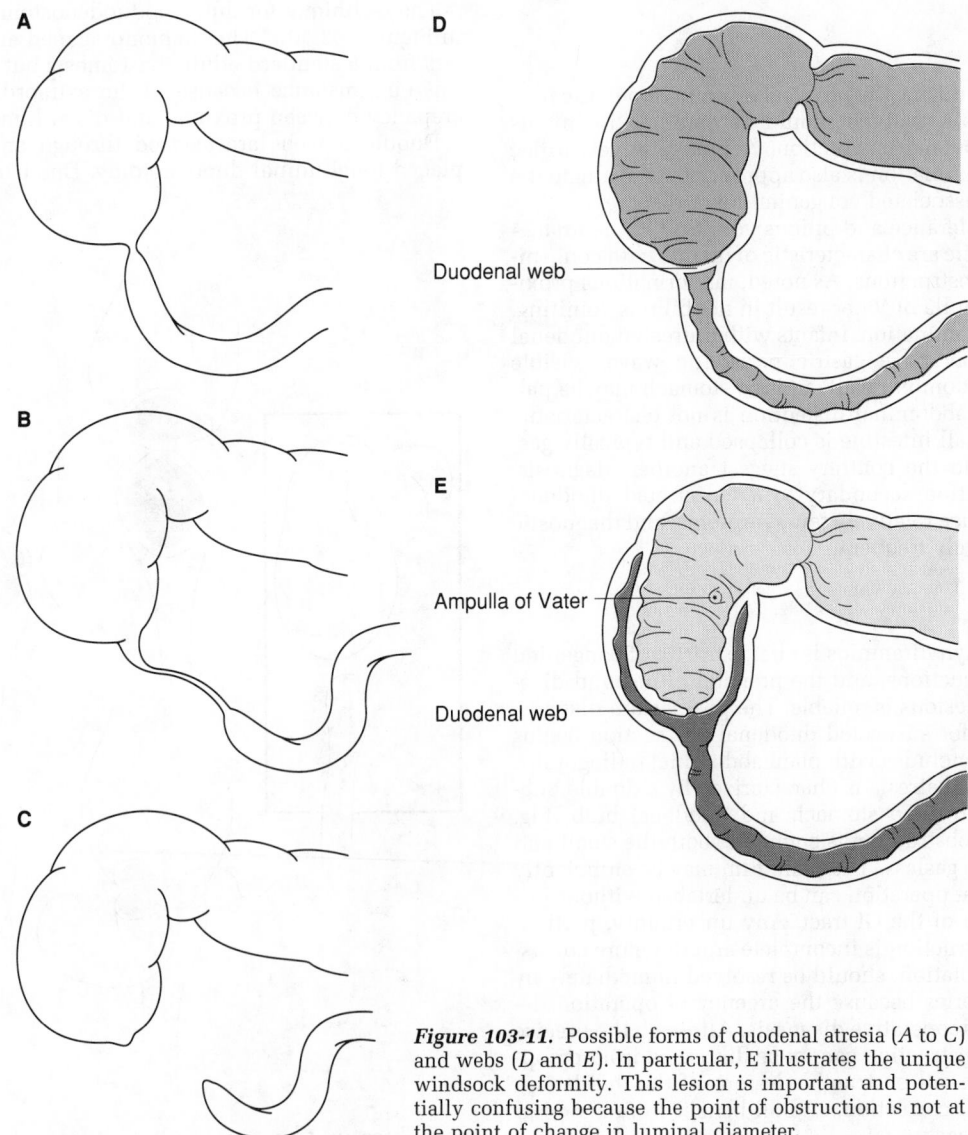

Figure 103-11. Possible forms of duodenal atresia (*A* to *C*) and webs (*D* and *E*). In particular, E illustrates the unique windsock deformity. This lesion is important and potentially confusing because the point of obstruction is not at the point of change in luminal diameter.

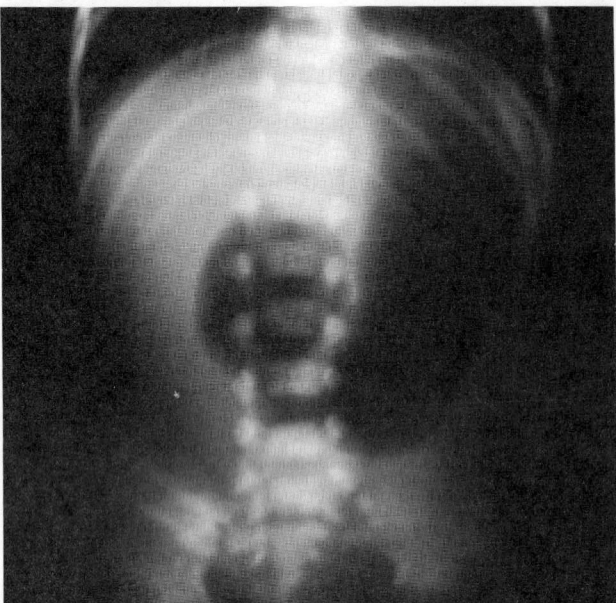

Figure 103-12. Classic radiographic appearance of duodenal atresia. There is a double bubble of the stomach and proximal duodenum with no air in the distal gastrointestinal tract.

ways apparent during the physical examination of the neonate, a routine karyotype should be obtained in infants born with duodenal obstruction. A preoperative cardiac ultrasound examination is also appropriate to evaluate the possibility of associated congenital heart disease.

Feeding intolerance and bilious vomiting in the first 24 to 48 hours of life are characteristic of infants with congenital duodenal obstructions. As noted, malformations proximal to the ampulla of Vater result in nonbilious vomiting. On physical examination, infants with untreated duodenal obstruction may have gastric peristaltic waves visible through the abdominal wall, and the stomach may be palpable. Diffuse abdominal distention is not characteristic. Indeed, the small intestine is collapsed and typically gasless; findings to the contrary suggest another diagnosis. Partial obstruction secondary to a fenestrated duodenal web may produce relatively few symptoms, and diagnostic delay is relatively frequent.

Diagnosis

Maternal polyhydramnios is characteristic of congenital duodenal obstructions, and the prenatal ultrasound diagnosis of these lesions is reliable. The postpartum diagnostic evaluation for suspected duodenal obstruction begins and perhaps concludes with plain abdominal radiographs. Classic duodenal atresia is characterized by a double bubble, with an air-filled stomach and duodenal bulb (Fig. 103-12). If the obstruction is complete, both the small and large bowel are gasless. The plain film may be sufficiently informative that operation can be undertaken without further evaluation of the GI tract. Any uncertainty, particularly if the obstruction is incomplete and therefore consistent with malrotation, should be resolved immediately by an upper GI series because the urgency of operation depends on the preoperative diagnosis. Although the precise nature of the obstruction cannot be discerned from preoperative imaging, all obstructive lesions of the duodenum require surgical correction, and all benefit from a similar operative approach.

Treatment

After completion of the preoperative cardiac evaluation and treatment of any urgent associated medical problems, surgical correction of congenital duodenal obstructions is undertaken promptly. The potential difficulty in differentiating duodenal atresia or stenosis from malrotation with duodenal obstruction secondary to Ladd bands makes immediate surgical exploration a prudent strategy.

The goals of the operative procedures are similar to those described for jejunoileal atresia: restoration of intestinal continuity as simply as possible without sacrificing intestinal length or absorptive area. In addition, avoidance of injury to the pancreas or ampulla of Vater is imperative in these infants.

Generally, bypass of the obstructing lesion is the best approach regardless of whether an atresia or annular pancreas is responsible.[28] This is achieved by constructing a duodenoduodenostomy that minimizes the length of defunctionalized duodenum. Duodenojejunostomy, a historically preferred procedure, is generally reserved for obstructing lesions in the distal duodenum. The treatment strategy for an annular pancreas is also to provide a bypass using a duodenoduodenostomy. The certainty of accessory pancreatic ductal injury and the underlying duodenal atresia preclude any lesser procedure, such as division of the circumferential pancreatic gland.

The technique for duodenoduodenostomy is illustrated in Figure 103-13.[29] The diamond-shaped anastomosis differs from a standard adult anastomosis but is preferred in this circumstance because of the extraordinary size discrepancy between proximal and distal lumens.

Duodenal webs are excised through an appropriately placed longitudinal duodenotomy. Duodenotomy closure

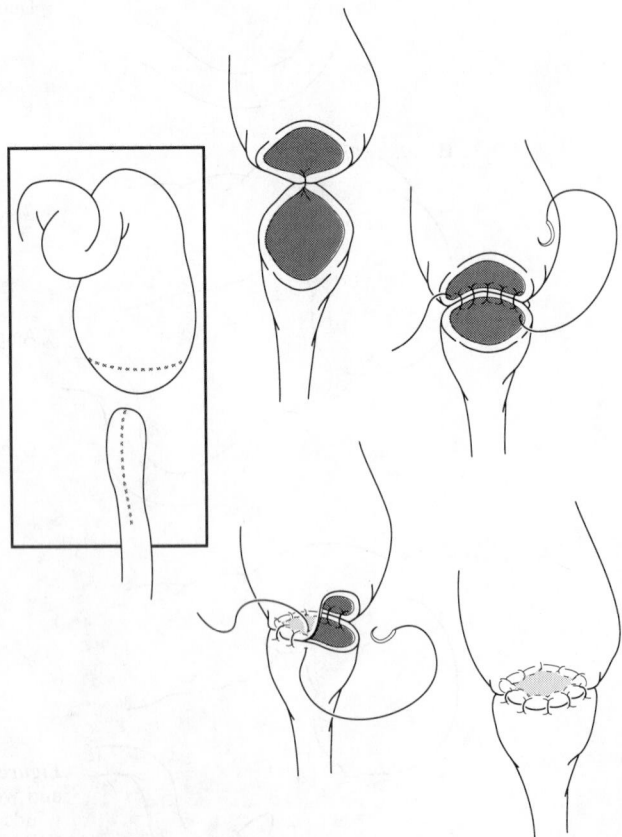

Figure 103-13. Diamond-shaped duodenoduodenostomy.

is obtained transversely and may require a duodenoduodenostomy as well. The wind-sock type of web malformation can be a problem because the visible transition from proximal distended duodenum to diminutive duodenum may be several centimeters distal to the actual base of the web. Traction applied to the apex of the web deforms the duodenum at its point of attachment and allows careful, complete excision. Careful definition of the anatomy of the entire duodenum is required for each of these procedures. In particular, the papilla of Vater must be unequivocally identified intraoperatively to avoid injury because it is often adjacent to or even incorporated into the web.

As with jejunoileal obstructions, the marked distention of the proximal duodenum has prompted some to advocate a variety of procedures designed to plicate or otherwise reduce the diameter of the proximal pouch to expedite postoperative function. Given the hazards of surgical complications in this area, these procedures are viewed with limited enthusiasm, and data about efficacy are not available.

Results and Complications

After operation, it is common for infants with congenital duodenal obstructions to require an adaptive period of several weeks before enteral feeding is tolerated. Parenteral nutrition is routinely necessary during this period. Once GI function is established, the clinical course is predictably uneventful.

The surgical outcomes after operative repair of congenital duodenal obstructions typically are excellent.[30] Mortality is confined to those infants with other serious medical problems, particularly trisomy 21 and congenital heart disease. The relevant issues are no different than those discussed for jejunoileal atresia.

Anorectal Malformations (Imperforate Anus)

Embryology

By the 5th week of gestation, the fetal cloaca is identifiable with the adjacent hindgut, allantois, and vestigial tailgut[22] (Fig. 103-14). Normally, the mesoderm of the proximal urorectal septum grows caudally to fuse with the cloacal closing plate. This occurs in conjunction with fusion of lateral cloacal ridges to form the completed urorectal septum. The caudal aspect of the urorectal septum forms the perineal body. The cloaca is thus divided into a dorsal rectum and a ventral urogenital sinus. With regard to the rectum, the process is normally completed when the anal membrane ruptures during the 8th gestational week. The urogenital sinus participates in the formation of the urethra and bladder. In female development, an additional contribution from the müllerian ducts gives rise to the adjacent uterus and vagina. Developmental arrest at any one of several stages during normal embryogenesis appears to account for the anatomic variations seen with anorectal malformations.

Anatomy and Classification

The normal anatomy of the anus and rectum is reviewed in Chapters 44 and 52. The anatomy relevant to this discussion concerns the funnel of striated muscle within the center of the pelvis, through which the rectum normally descends to the perineum. This striated muscle complex is under voluntary control and is responsible for fecal continence (Fig. 103-15). Traditional labels assigned to specific but anatomically indistinct portions of this funnel-shaped muscular complex include *levator ani* (the cranial portion of the funnel), *external sphincter* (the caudal portion), *puborectalis*, and others. Peña[31] has provided convincing clinical and anatomic data for a unified concept.

Many different classification systems have been developed to describe the various anatomic features of anorectal malformations. Each has specific merits and failings. The 1984 Wingspread International Classification is summarized in Table 103-4.[32,33] This is a simple, current, anatomically descriptive, and well-accepted classification system.

A limited summary provides the fundamentals for the remaining discussion, but a more detailed anatomic description of these anomalies and their classification systems is beyond the scope of this overview. Briefly, the two common variants in the male are low imperforate anus with a perineal fistula (Fig. 103-16) and high anorectal agenesis with a rectoprostatic urethral fistula (Fig. 103-17). It appears that either early or late embryonic arrest of the

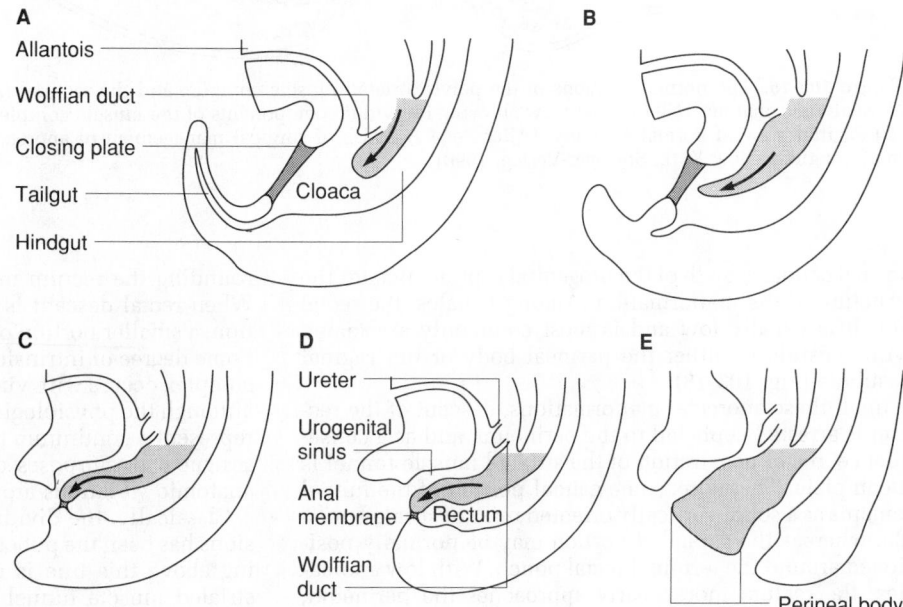

A
Allantois
Wolffian duct
Closing plate
Tailgut
Hindgut
Cloaca

B

C

D
Ureter
Urogenital sinus
Anal membrane
Rectum
Wolffian duct

E
Perineal body

Figure 103-14. Normal embryologic division of the cloaca by the urorectal septum into the ventral urinary tract and the dorsal rectum. This process is normally completed by the 9th or 10th week of gestation.

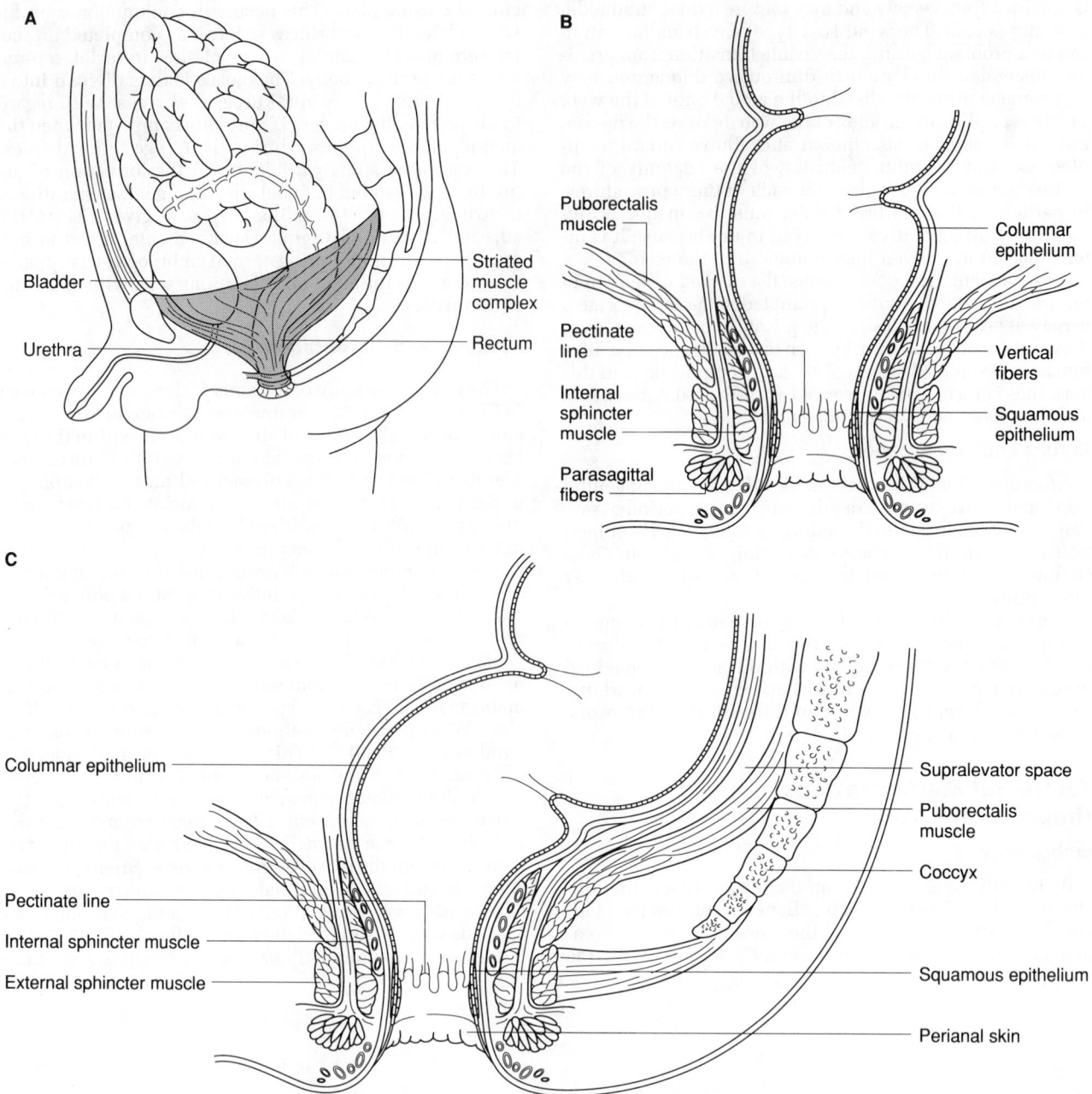

Figure 103-15. The normal relations of the pelvic striated muscle complex and the rectum. (*A*) Normal male anatomy. (*B*) Coronal view showing individual components of the muscle complex. (*C*) Sagittal view of normal anatomy. (After Peña A. Atlas of surgical management of anorectal malformations. New York, Springer-Verlag, 1990)

normal caudal growth of the urogenital septum dictates the structure of the malformation. Among females, the rectal pouch is usually low and is most commonly associated with a fistula to either the perineal body or the vaginal vestibule (Fig. 103-18).

In all these anorectal malformations, descent of the rectum is arrested cephalad to the perineum, and as a consequence, rectal penetration of the striated muscle funnel is incomplete. Therefore, some caudal portion of the funnel remains as a solid, vertically oriented mass of striated muscle, whereas the cephalad portion may be normally positioned around the terminal rectal pouch. With low anomalies, the rectum more nearly approaches the perineum; therefore, the configuration of the muscle complex sur-

rounding the rectum more closely approximates normal. When rectal descent is arrested in a high cephalad position, a smaller portion of the funnel surrounds the rectum. Some degree of intrinsic hypoplasia of the striated muscle complex occurs with virtually all anorectal malformations, although the physiologic effects can vary. These anomalies represent a continuum to which arbitrary terms have been assigned for purposes of communication. Individualized anatomic variations are to be expected.

Classically, the dividing line between high and low lesions has been the pubococcygeal line. A rectal pouch ending above this line is considered to be cephalad to the striated muscle funnel (or levator ani). In reality, some descent into the cranial portion of the funnel is also fre-

Table 103-4. ANATOMIC CLASSIFICATION OF ANORECTAL MALFORMATIONS

Female	Male
High	High
Anorectal agenesis	Anorectal agenesis
With rectovaginal fistula	With rectoprostatic urethral fistula*
Without fistula	Without fistula
Rectal atresia	Rectal atresis
Intermediate	Intermediate
Rectovestibular fistula	Rectobulbar urethral fistula
Rectovaginal fistula	Anal agenesis without fistula
Anal agenesis without fistula	
Low	Low
Anovestibular fistula*	Anocutaneous fistula*
Anocutaneous fistula*†	Anal stenosis*‡
Anal stenosis‡	
Cloacal malformations§	Rare malformations
Rare malformations	

* Relatively common lesion.
† Includes fistulas occurring at the posterior junction of the labia minora, often called *fourchette fistulas* or *vulvar fistulas*.
‡ Previously called *covered anus*.
§ Previously called *rectocloacal fistulas*. Entry of the rectal fistula into the cloaca may be high or intermediate, depending on the length of the cloacal canal.

(Modified from Templeton JM, O'Neill JA. Anorectal malformations. In: Welch KJ, Randolph JG, Ravitch MM, et al. eds. Pediatric surgery, ed 4. Chicago, Year Book, 1986:1022)

quent (see Fig. 103-17). This latter group of lesions is appropriately placed in an intermediate category for descriptive purposes, but clinical management is similar to that of high lesions. Low lesions are those in which the rectal pouch descends below the lower border of the ossified ischium. This correlates with more complete investment within the striated muscle funnel. Because fecal continence is determined by competence of the muscular funnel, this degree of descent has important and salutary functional consequences.

Associated Anomalies

As many as 70% of all infants with anorectal malformations have associated anomalies, the incidence being greatest among those with high malformations.[33] The VATER (or VACTERL) associations are most important. *Vertebral* anomalies are common. These may be inconsequential, but sacral dysplasia and agenesis are associated with sacral autonomic dysfunction and are particularly common in high malformations. These infants have a poorer prognosis for fecal continence and a high incidence of neurogenic urologic dysfunction. *Anorectal* malformations are the subject of this review. *Tracheoesophageal* fistulas occur in about 10% of infants with anorectal malformations, and esophageal patency should be confirmed specifically to rule out esophageal atresia. *Renal* or lower genitourinary tract malformations are the most common associated anomalies with anorectal malformations and may take virtually any form. Screening for both upper and lower tract anomalies is required. A broad range of *cardiac* anomalies are also reported, and screening echocardiography is considered routine. *Limb* or other skeletal anomalies, particularly those involving the radius, are well described.

Finally, a variety of spinal cord malformations have been associated with high anorectal malformations and sacral abnormalities. These include anomalies such as a tethered spinal cord and a variety of myelodysplastic syndromes. In the neonate, these can be identified routinely using either ultrasound or magnetic resonance imaging (MRI).

Clinical Presentation

The incidence of anorectal malformations is about 1 in 5000 births, with a slight male preponderance. High anomalies are at least twice as common in males, an important feature of the initial clinical assessment. These malformations should be apparent at birth when the infant is given a routine physical examination that includes inspection of the perineum and a digital rectal examination. If not recognized, the signs and symptoms are those of bowel obstruction. Abdominal distention and bilious vomiting occur if the obstruction is complete, but these may require 24 hours or more to develop in view of the distal location of the obstruction. In addition, meconium is not passed if obstruction is complete. In infants with low malformations, however, the passage of meconium through a perineal or vestibular fistula at about 24 hours of age is common; indeed, it is diagnostic. These infants may have a large enough fistula that the anomaly is noted only after an obstructive stooling pattern becomes apparent during a period of weeks or months. Meconium or air may be passed in the urine through a urethral or bladder fistula associated with a high malformation.

With experience, the physical examination is the most helpful method of estimating whether a malformation is high or low. In males, 95% of low malformations are associated with either a thin anal membrane or a perineal or scrotal midline fistula. A bucket-handle skin bridge in the area of the anus implies a low lesion. Signs of a high malformation include the absence of normal anal skin features and the absence of external sphincter contraction with cutaneous stimulation. In addition, abnormal gluteal contour produces a characteristic flat-bottom appearance. In girls, 90% to 95% of low malformations have a perineal or vaginal vestibular fistula. Regardless of gender, external fistulas may not become apparent until 12 to 24 hours of age when meconium moves distally into the rectum.

Diagnosis

No single physical sign or diagnostic test consistently defines the anatomy, so it is prudent to make use of the several complementary procedures outlined later. The pri-

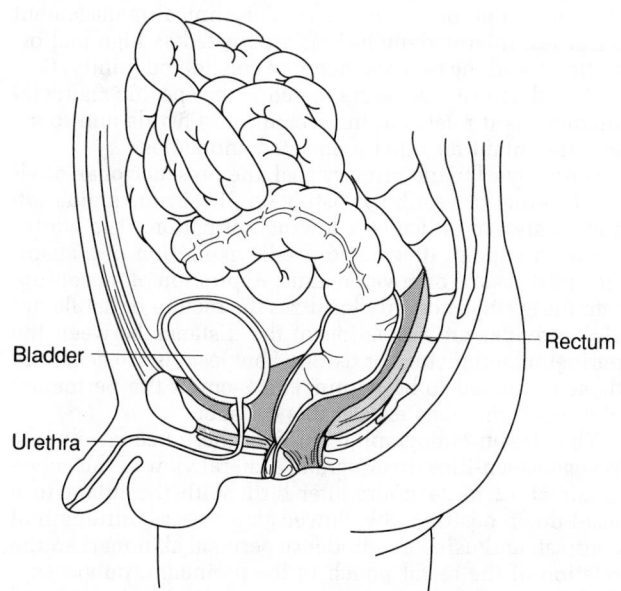

Figure 103-16. Boy with low imperforate anus and perineal fistula.

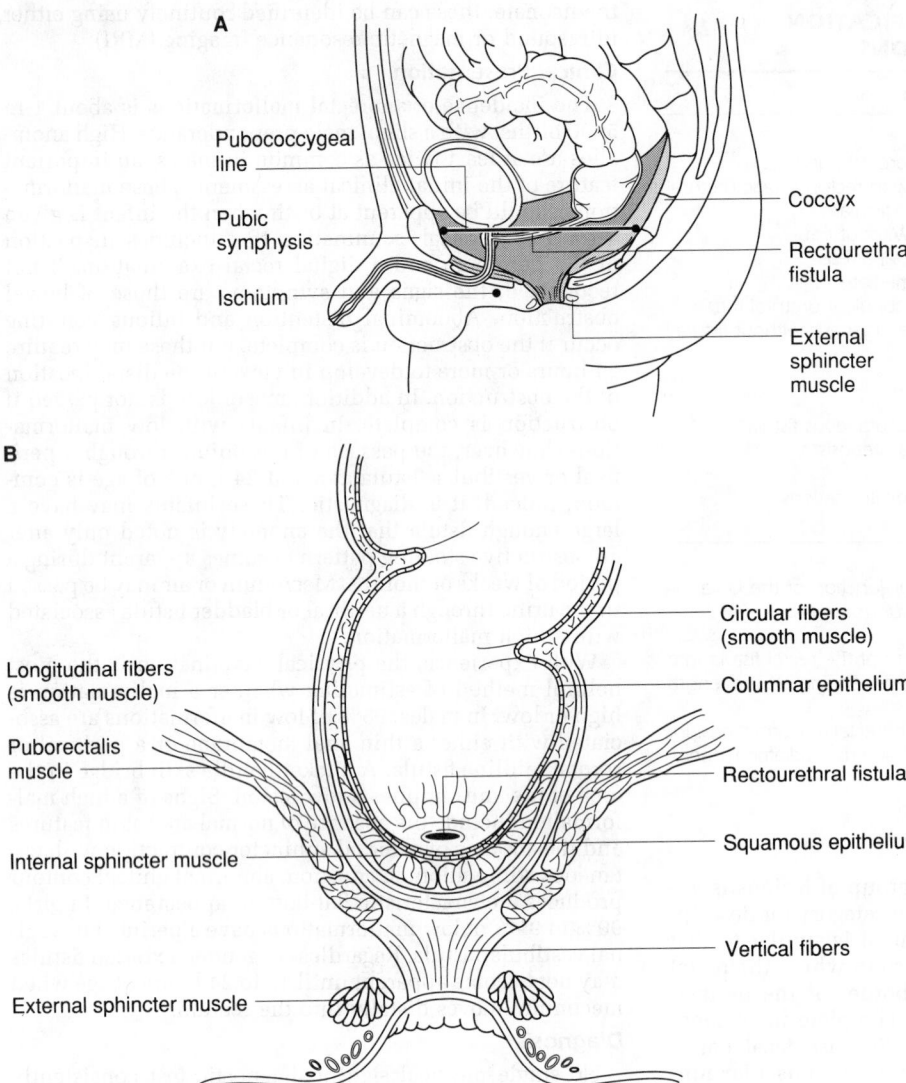

Figure 103-17. Boy with high imperforate anus, showing the pubococcygeal line, ischium, and striated muscle complex. (*A*) The rectal pouch ends cephalad to the pubococcygeal line. This location of the rectourethral fistula is typical. (*B*) Coronal view showing incomplete investment of the rectal pouch in the striated muscle complex. The rectourethral fistula is also clearly shown. This perspective illustrates the major advantage of the posterior sagittal surgical approach—improved visualization of the anatomy. (After Peña A. Atlas of surgical management of anorectal malformations. New York, Springer-Verlag, 1990)

mary goal of the diagnostic evaluation is to place the anomaly into a high or low category. For clinical management purposes, intermediate lesions are treated as high malformations, and the two are therefore considered jointly. Secondary diagnostic goals are to define the specific anorectal anatomy as it relates to the rectourinary fistula and to assess the infant for other associated anomalies.

With regard to the primary goal, the presence of an obvious external or vestibular fistula on physical examination almost always indicates a low malformation. It is worthwhile to attempt diagnostic needle aspiration of a suspicious fistula site or covered anus. Aspiration of meconium into the syringe not only localizes the rectum or fistula but also provides an estimation of the distance between the perineum and rectum or fistula. Low lesions are generally those estimated to be within 1 to 2 cm of the perineum; high malformations exceed this distance.

The classic radiographic study of these neonates is the Wangensteen-Rice invertogram, a lateral view of the pelvis obtained 12 to 24 hours after birth with the infant in a head-down position. Swallowed air serves as intraluminal contrast, and using a radiodense perineal skin marker, the relation of the rectal pouch to the perineum, pubococcygeal line, and ischium is assessed as previously outlined (see Fig. 103-17). The procedure can be accurate if carried out by a technically skilled and experienced examiner.

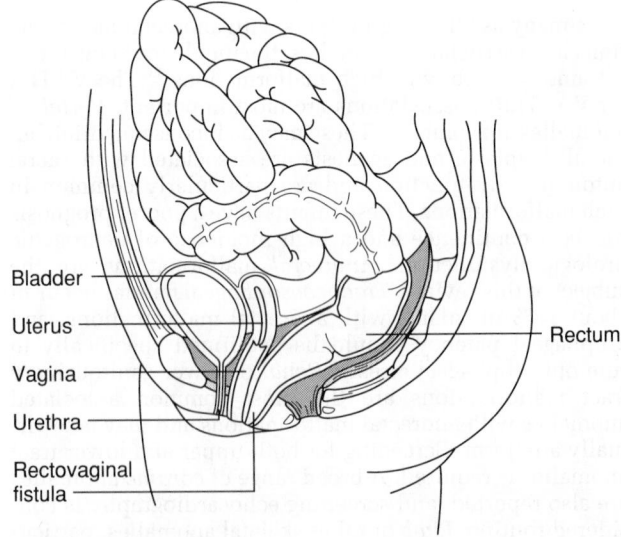

Figure 103-18. Girl with low imperforate anus and fistula to the vaginal vestibule.

Incomplete filling of the rectum with air and caudal prolapse of the rectal pouch with crying or straining are potentially misleading technical problems that diminish the accuracy.

Ultrasound examination of the perineum is preferred to visualize the anatomic relations described earlier. The advantage of real-time dynamic observation is that the precise definition of the distal rectal pouch at a time when the infant is not crying or straining is simplified. Experience with this is substantial, and it is now routinely employed. When data derived from the physical examination, plain film, ultrasound, and needle aspiration are combined, almost all these infants can be placed into a high or low group. As detailed later, any child not clearly found to have a low anomaly should be considered to have a high or intermediate lesion.

Definition of the anatomy of the rectourinary fistula is generally best done with contrast studies. A preoperative voiding cystourethrogram fills most fistulas into the bladder or urethra. A postoperative barium contrast study of the distal colostomy limb serves a similar purpose, although this approach tends to be less successful. Endoscopic visualization of the urinary orifice of the fistula is generally possible as well and may be done at the time of the initial anesthesia. Anatomic definition of the tract is often limited with this approach.

The striated muscle complex in anorectal malformations can be assessed using computed tomography (CT) or MRI to evaluate the degree of intrinsic hypoplasia. Prognostic and therapeutic guidelines are being developed, but this approach appears to have particular merit in potential reoperative situations because the position of a previously pulled-through rectal pouch can be assessed with regard to the muscular complex. MRI has the additional advantage of assessing the spine and spinal cord for abnormalities, which are common in patients with high lesions.

The high incidence of associated anomalies dictates that all these infants undergo comprehensive preoperative evaluation. This includes specific assessment of both upper and lower urinary tracts. Renal ultrasound examination and voiding cystourethrography together quickly accomplish this. Other possible skeletal, esophageal, and cardiac anomalies require screening as previously outlined.

Treatment

Treatment of anorectal malformations is always surgical, but it is not a matter of life-threatening urgency. Delay for 12 to 24 hours may actually simplify the diagnostic effort as the meconium enters the distal rectum or fistula. In addition, cardiac, genitourinary, and other evaluations can be completed and treatment instituted if necessary.

Low Malformations. Low malformations are definitively repaired in the newborn period with relatively simple perineal procedures that do not require a proximal diverting colostomy. Because the objective is to relieve the obstruction, simple dilation of a fistula or unroofing of a covered anus under local anesthesia may be sufficient. For more problematic stenoses or anterior fistulas, a variety of formal but simple perineal anoplasties are done. Most common is the cutback anoplasty, in which the anterior fistula or anal orifice is opened posteriorly, simply dividing the perineum to the external sphincter. More complex alternatives may be preferred in females with low vaginal or anterior perineal anal openings. These generally involve the circumferential mobilization of the anterior fistula with transposition to the site of the external sphincter and reconstruction of the perineal body. This type of transfer anoplasty is designed to position the neoanus at the center of the external sphincter and separate the anal opening from the vaginal introitus.

Intermediate and High Malformations. Neonates with intermediate, high, or indeterminate anorectal malformations require a diverting colostomy when the diagnostic evaluation is complete. The colostomy may be placed in either the sigmoid colon or the transverse colon as long as the selected site provides adequate distal length for an eventual pull-through of the rectal pouch to the perineum. The colostomy is best divided to divert the fecal stream from the urinary fistula.

The pull-through procedure usually is performed between 9 and 18 months of age or when the infant weighs about 10 kg or 20 lb. Many different approaches have been described, and considerable personal and institutional variation is the rule. No single approach has superior results, and all have important drawbacks. All the procedures share four objectives: (1) to place the rectal pouch on the perineum, (2) to eliminate rectal obstruction, (3) to position the pulled-through rectum as normally as possible within the striated muscle complex, and (4) to close the rectourinary fistula.

Perhaps the most widely employed procedure in the United States is the posterior sagittal anorectoplasty as described by Peña.[31] The important technical features of this procedure illustrate the principles outlined earlier. A posterior sagittal incision is used, and a meticulous midline division of the external sphincter and striated muscle complex is accomplished, carrying the incision directly down to the rectal pouch. The use of a nerve stimulator is required to map the striated muscle complex precisely for purposes of symmetric division as well as reconstruction. Once identified, the rectal pouch can generally be mobilized adequately to reach the perineum by means of the sacral approach without need for a laparotomy. A particular advantage of this approach is that the mobilized rectum is opened and the rectourinary fistula identified and closed under direct vision. The distended rectum is then tapered and placed centrally within the striated muscle funnel, which is reconstructed circumferentially around the pulled-through rectum. The neoanus is centered within the external sphincter.

Other repairs with broad acceptance include the Stephens and Smith[32,34] sacroperineal approach and the Rehbein[35] endorectal dissection. Both are characterized by a blind pull-through of the rectum to the perineum without direct visualization of the striated muscle complex. Fistula closure using these procedures is also accomplished with more limited exposure. Mollard and colleagues[36] proposed a combined abdominal and anterior perineal approach, again with a relatively blind pull-through of the rectum between the urethra and puborectalis portion of the striated muscle complex.

Personal preference and experience rather than clear differences in outcome generally dictate the selection of procedure. Regardless of the type of pull-through performed, the proximal colostomy is preserved until healing is complete and any narrowing resolved, after which elective colostomy closure can be performed.

Results and Complications

Mortality is rarely the direct result of anorectal malformations, but it is related to other concurrent medical problems. Regardless, reported mortality rates for these children range from 11% to 35%.[33]

Potential complications are similar to those associated with any GI procedure. For the posterior sagittal anorectoplasty in particular, the long posterior suture line required for the tapering rectoplasty is subject to leak or stricture formation in 5% to 10% of infants. Generally, these are easily managed problems because of the proximal fecal diversion. Most infants with this posterior rectoplasty require rectal dilations, at least transiently.

The major issue for these infants and children is related to long-term functional outcomes. Virtually all infants with low malformations have excellent outlooks with regard to fecal continence, as would be expected with the relatively normal descent of the rectum within the striated muscle funnel. Children with high and intermediate malformations have much less predictable outcomes with poorer functional results. As noted, the outcomes appear to be independent of the particular surgical repair used. This is consistent with the fundamental problems of inadequate rectal descent, hypoplasia of the striated muscle complex, and abnormal sacral innervation. Few or perhaps none of these children have completely normal bowel habits after operation. About half (range, 30% to 80%) have good results, with few episodes of accidental soilage and relatively simple management using enemas and cathartics.[37] The remainder of these children are divided more or less evenly into categories generally labeled fair and poor. Although precise definitions vary, these children may require major adjustments in life-style, with complex and possibly disruptive medical management requirements. Occasionally, a permanent diverting colostomy is required.

Necrotizing Enterocolitis

Pathophysiology

Neonatal NEC is an idiopathic clinical condition characterized by an initial mucosal intestinal injury that may progress to transmural bowel necrosis. Despite its frequency and an extensive descriptive literature, the pathogenesis remains obscure and the treatment empiric.

Many clinical conditions have been reported with NEC, and virtually all are simply descriptive of a population of critically ill, premature infants. Among these associations are respiratory failure, sepsis, hypothermia, hypotension, acidosis, hypoxemia, and structural cardiac defects. Cocaine exposure[38] and indomethacin treatment[39] are particular pharmacologic risk factors. This variety suggests that many stimuli may initiate the process and that the observed clinical and pathologic events may result from nonspecific stress responses among particularly susceptible neonates. Intestinal mucosal injury appears to be fundamental to the initial development of NEC. It is probable in the clinical setting that several factors usually participate, but it is also possible that a single extraordinary stimulus can independently generate the initial mucosal injury. After mucosal injury is established, a variety of additive infectious and inflammatory events may occur. Irreversible bowel injury and progressive systemic illness may result.

Relevant mucosal injury may result from ischemia related either to chronic hypoperfusion or to a discrete ischemic event followed by reperfusion. With regard to the former, the premature neonate may be at particular risk. The normal neonatal transitional circulation is characterized by rapid structural and physiologic changes in pulmonary and systemic vascular smooth muscle (see Chap. 102). The critically ill, premature infant appears to be exceptionally vulnerable to vasoconstriction, and this may include the splanchnic circulation. In addition, stresses such as hypoxemia, acidosis, and hypothermia are associated with acute pulmonary hypertension and right-to-left shunting through a patent ductus arteriosus. This shunting may well exacerbate the physiologic problem of inadequate peripheral and visceral oxygen delivery. Hyperviscosity, low cardiac output, and other events may contribute further to chronic intestinal hypoperfusion in the premature infant.

It appears that discrete ischemic events, such as episodic hypotension and arterial embolism, are linked to NEC. Similar acute intestinal ischemia–reperfusion events are well characterized experimentally and may be clinically relevant. Oxygen radical–mediated mucosal injury occurs by both xanthine oxidase–and NADPH oxidase–dependent pathways after ischemia–reperfusion events.[40] Generation of these oxidant species is also associated with important systemic events, such as complement activation, endotoxin and cytokine release, and bacterial translocation from the intestine. These events appear to be important mediators of the systemic inflammatory response and of multiorgan dysfunction.

The mucosal injury in NEC has been correlated clinically to a variety of infectious and feeding-related events. More than 90% of cases of NEC occur after the initiation of feedings. Although controversial, it appears that hyperosmolar medications and formulas may increase the risk of NEC, whereas breast milk, which contains maternal immunoglobulin A (IgA), lymphocytes, and macrophages, may confer some protection. Indeed, the oral administration of monomeric IgG may diminish the incidence of NEC in high-risk infants.[41]

The concept of an infectious cause of or contribution to NEC is based largely on epidemiologic data that show periodic temporal and geographic clustering of cases. Aggressive bacteriologic investigation during these epidemics has suggested that a variety of organisms from the normal gut microflora have phlogistic potential. Among these organisms are several *Clostridium* sp (including *C difficile*) *Pseudomonas aeruginosa, Enterobacter cloacae, Staphylococcus aureus,* some *Klebsiella* sp, and others. Most cases of NEC cannot be linked to a single specific pathogen. Indeed, for any given patient, it is not possible to differentiate whether systemic sepsis is a cause or an effect of NEC.

The characteristic pathologic findings of NEC are virtually indistinguishable from those of ischemic necrosis. Mucosal involvement alone produces a histologic picture that has been likened to postmortem autolysis, with enterocyte dissolution but a remarkable absence of an inflammatory response.[42] More advanced disease includes submucosal edema, hemorrhage, and microvascular thrombosis. Pneumatosis intestinalis, the presence of gas within the bowel wall, is the classic radiographic sign of NEC and appears to result from dissection of intraluminal air through the disrupted basement membrane of injured mucosa. Initially, the air appears in the submucosa or lymphatic channels but may later dissect into the muscularis, the portal venous circulation, or subserosal locations. The penultimate histologic finding of NEC is transmural necrosis involving the muscularis, which may be followed by frank intestinal perforation.

The distribution of involvement is variable on both macroscopic and microscopic levels (Fig. 103-19). NEC has a general predilection for patchy regional involvement of the terminal ileum and colon, but virtually any distribution is possible. Children without discernibly different clinical risk factors may have a range of involvement, from confluent transmural necrosis of the entire bowel, to isolated, full-thickness necrosis of the terminal ileum, to self-limited and reversible mucosal injury. The histopathology of NEC resembles that of experimental intestinal ischemia, with areas of reversible mucosal injury often found immediately adjacent to areas of transmural necrosis.

We are left with the somewhat vague concept that many clinical factors determine the premature infant's response to a variety of intestinal (mucosal) stresses. The relevance of the individual initiating events, the regulation of the endogenous responses, and the clinical outcomes remain unknown (Fig. 103-20).

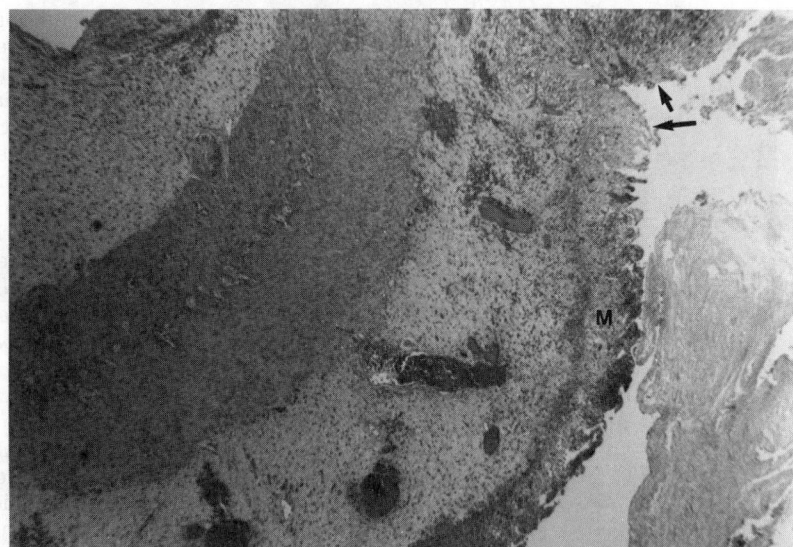

Figure 103-19. Photomicrograph of intestine in an infant with necrotizing enterocolitis. An area of epithelial slough (*arrows*) is adjacent to injured but surviving mucosa (M). Despite the obvious injury, the muscular mucosa is not infarcted.

Clinical Presentation

The classic clinical signs of NEC include abdominal distention, bilious vomiting, and either occult or gross blood in the stool. As expected with a primary mucosal injury, bleeding into the GI tract is common (80% to 90% of cases) but rarely hemodynamically significant. The affected infant is typically premature, has concurrent medical problems, and has had feedings initiated recently. Low birthweight and low gestational age are clear risk factors, though not absolute prerequisites. Half of all infants with NEC have birthweights less than 1500 g, and 80% of these infants weigh less than 2500 g at birth. In one large study, the mean gestational age of infants who developed NEC was 31 weeks, and the mean birthweight was 1460 g.[43] A number of important clinical risk factors for the development of NEC were noted earlier.

The incidence of NEC is difficult to determine because it is a subjective clinical diagnosis and definitions are not uniform. Many infants have only minimal evidence of disease; most have no pathognomonic laboratory findings. Thus, individual patients may be excluded from retrospective institutional reviews. Most major centers estimate an incidence of 1 to 2 in 1000 live births.[44] In addition, data suggest that substantial variation in incidence is probably related to individual clinical practice patterns.[45] NEC is relatively common and represents the single most frequent surgical emergency in neonates in North America. The physical examination is not specific. Abdominal tenderness with distention is common, and individual loops of thickened or fixed bowel may be palpable. A fixed abdominal mass and abdominal wall edema, erythema, or crepitus suggest intestinal necrosis, perforation, or an abscess. Hematochezia or guaiac-positive stools are expected. Systemic signs of sepsis, such as bradycardia, apnea, oliguria, hypoxemia, thrombocytopenia, acidosis, and temperature instability, are common. The primary goal of the initial clinical evaluation is to differentiate reversible mucosal injury from transmural necrosis because this finding dictates treatment. No single physical finding or laboratory test makes this distinction, but a number of relevant observations are discussed later.

Diagnosis

Assignment of the NEC diagnosis is always a clinical judgment based on appropriate findings in the correct setting. Confirmation requires only plain abdominal radiographs. In fact, contrast studies may be hazardous and are contraindicated during the acute illness.

The classic radiographic finding of pneumatosis intestinalis (Fig. 103-21) confirms the diagnosis in appropriate clinical circumstances, but the incidence of unequivocal radiographic findings ranges from 20% to 98%. Pneumatosis intestinalis is often found in the right lower quadrant and reflects terminal ileal or cecal involvement, but it is also common in the sigmoid colon and can occur anywhere. Other important radiographic observations include the presence of portal vein gas, fixed or thickened small bowel loops, and ascites. Of importance is periodic screening for free intraperitoneal air. The critical nature of this finding mandates that sequential screening films, including a left lateral decubitus or upright film, be obtained every 6 to 8 hours during the early course of the disease. If present, pneumoperitoneum confirms intestinal perforation and requires exploratory laparotomy. Up to

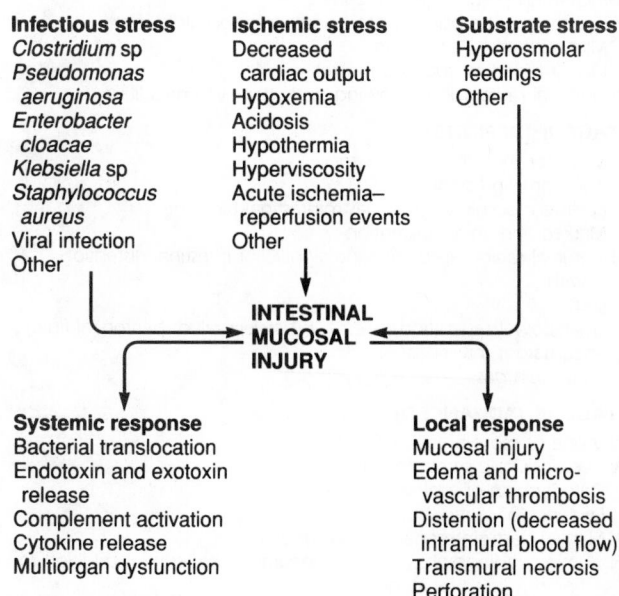

Infectious stress	Ischemic stress	Substrate stress
Clostridium sp	Decreased	Hyperosmolar
Pseudomonas	cardiac output	feedings
aeruginosa	Hypoxemia	Other
Enterobacter	Acidosis	
cloacae	Hypothermia	
Klebsiella sp	Hyperviscosity	
Staphylococcus	Acute ischemia–	
aureus	reperfusion events	
Viral infection	Other	
Other		

INTESTINAL MUCOSAL INJURY

Systemic response	Local response
Bacterial translocation	Mucosal injury
Endotoxin and exotoxin	Edema and micro-
release	vascular thrombosis
Complement activation	Distention (decreased
Cytokine release	intramural blood flow)
Multiorgan dysfunction	Transmural necrosis
	Perforation

Figure 103-20. Schematic summary of the pathogenesis of necrotizing enterocolitis.

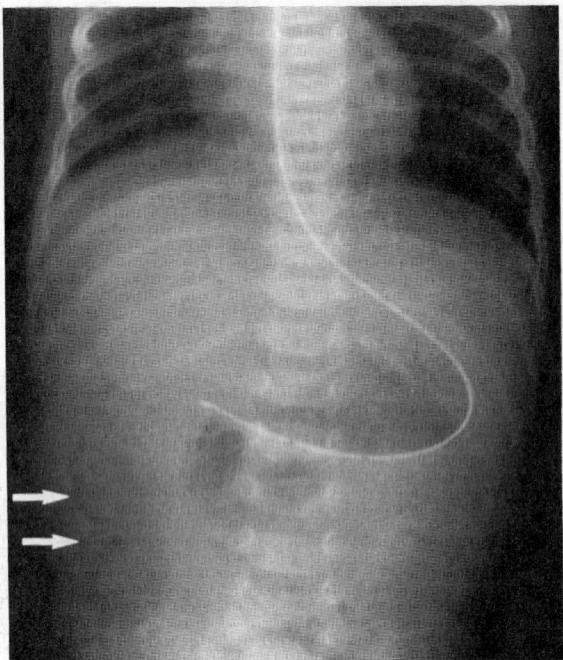

Figure 103-21. Plain radiograph showing pneumatosis intestinalis (*arrows*) in an infant with necrotizing enterocolitis.

half of infants with perforations do not have discernible pneumoperitoneum.

Radionuclide scanning of the intestine with technetium-99m (^{99m}Tc) diphosphate has been used in an effort to provide an objective differentiation between reversible injury and transmural necrosis. In the laboratory setting, the technique appears to be sensitive and moderately specific. In one clinical trial, however, the combined error rate was 12%.[46] Generally, the technique adds little to the clinical assessment and is not widely used. This distinction remains dependent on a difficult series of subjective clinical judgments.

Treatment

Nonoperative. Up to 90% of infants with NEC can be managed successfully nonoperatively, but this is widely variable among institutions because of differing referral patterns and interinstitutional variations in assigning this diagnosis. With regard to the latter issue, several clinical classification systems have been developed. Table 103-5 provides a summary of the staging system most widely used in the United States.[47]

The initial management of infants with NEC consists of nasogastric decompression, broad-spectrum antibiotic administration, and correction of hypoxemia, hypotension, acidosis, fluid and electrolyte disorders, and any other reversible medical problems. In particular, optimizing cardiac performance is necessary, and this may specifically require surgical closure of a patent ductus arteriosus. As noted, monitoring for progression of the disease and perforation includes sequential plain abdominal radiographs (every 6 to 8 hours) to screen for pneumoperitoneum. Serial physical examinations, platelet counts, lactate levels, and arterial blood gases are the most useful indicators of progressive sepsis.

Indications to abandon medical management are controversial but fundamentally include evidence of either intestinal perforation or temporal clinical deterioration consistent with refractory sepsis. Perforation is best documented

by pneumoperitoneum on plain film. Evidence of persistent or progressive sepsis may include thrombocytopenia, acidosis, hypoxemia, temperature instability, bradycardia, hypoglycemia, neutropenia, portal vein gas, and abdominal wall erythema or crepitus. The subtle and subjective nature of the clinical deterioration criteria accounts for the controversy regarding operative indications for NEC. It remains an experience-dependent judgment. Abdominal paracentesis in the presence of ascites, or peritoneal lavage in its absence, may demonstrate bacteria or intestinal contents if an NEC-induced perforation has occurred. These are occasionally helpful diagnostic maneuvers in complex individual patients but are not considered routine. The presence of a fixed mass suggests intestinal perforation with a localized abscess and may be a relative indication for operative therapy.

Most infants improve with the simple medical treatment outlined, and typically, the distention and ileus resolve during a period of days. Signs of systemic sepsis generally resolve promptly. Antibiotics usually can be discontinued after 10 to 14 days. Enteral alimentation is resumed at this time, but it is not unusual for this to require a lengthy period of trial-and-error feeding. This may result in part from additional enterocyte dysfunction imposed by the disease itself. Because of this, it is prudent to initiate TPN routinely by means of a central venous catheter promptly after the diagnosis of NEC is made. Clinical progression of the disease is an exception after medical treatment is initiated, but if it occurs, it typically becomes obvious within 24 to 36 hours. It is unusual to have an appropri-

---

Table 103-5. **NECROTIZING ENTEROCOLITIS**

STAGE I (SUSPECTED)

Any one or more historical factors producing perinatal stress
Systemic manifestations
    Temperature instability
    Lethargy
    Apnea
    Bradycardia
Gastrointestinal manifestations
    Poor feeding
    Increasing pregavage residuals
    Emesis (may be bilious or test positive for occult blood)
    Mild abdominal distention
    Occult blood in stool (no fissure)
Abdominal radiographs showing distention with mild ileus

STAGE II (DEFINITE)

Any one or more historical factors
Above signs and symptoms, *plus*
    Persistent occult or gross gastrointestinal bleeding
    Marked abdominal distention
Abdominal radiographs showing significant intestinal distention
    with:
    Ileus
    Small bowel separation (edema in bowel wall or peritoneal fluid)
    Pneumatosis intestinalis
    Portal vein gas

STAGE III (ADVANCED)

Any one or more historical factors
Above signs and symptoms, *plus*
    Deterioration of vital signs
    Evidence of septic shock
    Marked gastrointestinal hemorrhage
Abdominal radiographs showing pneumoperitoneum in addition to
    findings listed for stage II

(Bell MJ, Kosloske A, Benton C, et al. Neonatal necrotizing enterocolitis in infancy: prevention of perforation. J Pediatr Surg 1973;8:6013)

ately treated patient with NEC develop bowel necrosis after a period of initial stability.

Operative. A principle that governs all operative decisions for these fragile, premature infants is that complications are tolerated poorly. The operative indications are invariably associated with dead bowel, with or without perforation. This generally requires that segmental resection of nonviable bowel be done with proximal and distal exteriorization. This may require multiple resections and multiple enterostomies. Because of the tenuous blood supply and diminutive bowel size in these small infants, formal maturation of the stomas is avoided. If possible, the ileocecal valve is preserved, and every effort is made to conserve bowel length because the risk of the short gut syndrome can be substantial. If a major portion of the intestine is involved, it is rational to preserve marginal areas and plan formal operative reexploration at a later time for reassessment. Measurement of remaining bowel length is appropriate for informational and prognostic purposes, but the length of bowel resected is determined by the extent of necrosis rather than by the surgeon's preference. Several reports have suggested that bowel resection with a primary anastomosis may be safely done in selected low-risk patients with limited bowel involvement. This remains a controversial issue, but the initial generalization that complications are not well tolerated is relevant. Necrosis of the entire small bowel and colon is an unfortunate but not uncommon finding at laparotomy for NEC. Faced with the dilemma of certain death or the short bowel syndrome, some surgeons have reported survival with reconstructible gut after proximal jejunal diversion without enterectomy. The mortality rate in this desperate circumstance remains high. Some have advocated limited peritoneal drainage rather than laparotomy for very-high-risk low-birthweight infants, and this may be advantageous for selected patients.[48]

Results and Complications

Nonoperative treatment for NEC is sufficient in 50% to 90% of infants.[49] For infants in this category, morbidity and mortality are related primarily to prematurity. Neonatal cholestatic jaundice secondary to parenteral nutrition occurs commonly, but it is generally reversible. The major complication relates to progression of disease such that laparotomy becomes necessary. The predictable infectious complications associated with bowel necrosis include bacterial peritonitis, systemic sepsis, and intraabdominal abscess formation. Progression of disease is also possible after surgical therapy, particularly if marginally viable intestine has been conserved and exteriorized. Operative reexploration may be necessary in this circumstance.

Technical surgical problems related to intestinal leaks, fistula formation, and nonviable stomas are all more likely to occur in these extremely small infants with preexisting intestinal injury. Disorders related to extraordinary fluid and electrolyte losses from proximal intestinal stomas may become important or even life-threatening in infants whose circulating plasma volume is less than 50 to 100 mL. This is potentially a compelling reason to close the intestinal stomas promptly after the peritonitis is resolved and the infant made stable. Virtually every infant with NEC has some complication or at least an important associated medical problem. The overall incidence of surgical complications is about 20% to 40%.

An important additional complication unique to this setting is late stricture formation, which must be considered whether the patient has been managed operatively or nonoperatively. Given the segmental nature of the disease, it is not unusual to have areas of deep or transmural necrosis

adjacent to viable bowel. Strictures may develop at these sites. It is difficult to ascertain the frequency of stricture formation related to NEC, largely because of the issue of diagnostic accuracy previously discussed. Stricture formation is clearly related to severity of disease. Radiographic evidence of stricture formation is reported in as many as 11% to 36% of infants in some retrospective series.[42] Most cases occur in infants who have had advanced clinical disease. Seventy percent of these strictures occur in the colon, most commonly the sigmoid colon, with terminal ileum and other small bowel sites involved less frequently. Generally, asymptomatic strictures can be followed and resolve with time and normal growth. Symptomatic strictures usually require segmental resection with anastomosis, although balloon catheter dilation has been reported. Routine screening barium enema examinations for infants who have had NEC have been advocated, and this approach has been adopted in some institutions.

Overall survival rates for neonates with NEC are about 60% to 80% for both operative and nonoperative management groups.[50,51] This represents a substantial improvement from the 20% to 30% survival probability for premature infants when NEC was first recognized 30 to 40 years ago. This is attributable to continuing improvements in neonatal care, TPN, and particularly aggressive early treatment. Most neonatal units initiate treatment for any infant with even a suspicion of NEC, and this approach yields a high nonoperative treatment rate. In general, the long-term outcome for infants who survive NEC is good, or at least no different than for other premature infants. Survivors may well have residual neurologic, pulmonary, or other developmental problems, but morbidity related to the GI tract is generally limited. Those with related problems are usually infants with the short gut syndrome. These children present complex technical and ethical issues that are discussed elsewhere.

Meconium Ileus

Meconium ileus refers to the characteristic obstruction of the small intestine in neonates with cystic fibrosis. Some 10% to 20% of infants with cystic fibrosis present initially with meconium ileus. A brief review of the pathophysiology of cystic fibrosis is provided and is followed by a more detailed clinical discussion of meconium ileus.

Cystic Fibrosis

Cystic fibrosis is the most common fatal hereditary disease in European and North American populations. It is an autosomal recessive disorder with a heterozygote incidence of 1 in 20 to 25 whites. Therefore, the incidence of the homozygous gene is about 1 in 2000 to 2500 in these populations.[52] The cystic fibrosis gene has been cloned and the most common single mutation characterized.[53,54]

DNA analysis identifies the most common point mutation, a three–base-pair deletion that is present in 70% to 75% of the cystic fibrosis carrier population. This appears as a deletion of a phenylalanine residue in the 508 position of the gene product. About 200 additional, more rare mutations that produce clinical cystic fibrosis disease have been identified. This has important practical implications in attempting to apply this information to the problem of developing screening tests for carriers. Because there are many rare cystic fibrosis mutations, only about half the couples at risk can be identified prospectively; therefore, carrier screening in the general population is not recommended by the National Institutes of Health.[52] Rather, carrier testing using DNA samples from families known to be afflicted with cystic fibrosis is recommended. In this setting, carrier discovery approaches 100%, and appropriate genetic counseling can be provided. Similarly, prenatal and immediate postnatal DNA analyses applied selectively to families at risk or to new families with clinically suspected disease should allow prompt confirmation of virtually all cystic fibrosis homozygotes. The role of the traditional diagnostic sweat chloride test is appropriately diminished (see later).

In addition to the issue of cystic fibrosis screening, continuing evolution in the field of cystic fibrosis–related molecular biology raises the real possibility of effective gene therapy.[55] This is a rapidly changing area of active investigation.

Pathophysiology.   Cystic fibrosis is characterized by an electrolyte transport defect of epithelium that is the result of impermeability to the chloride (Cl⁻) ion.[56] It has been believed that the defect occurs in the epithelia of the sweat glands and airways, although the pancreas, gut, and liver are also affected. In the sweat glands, failure of normal Cl⁻ reabsorption in the distal tubule after β-adrenergic stimulation leads to an obligate sodium chloride loss despite a normal ATP-dependent, sodium–potassium membrane pump. This is the basis for both the historical clinical observation that cystic fibrosis infants have a salty taste as well as the traditional diagnostic sweat test.

The electrochemical effects in the airways are more complex, but reduced Cl⁻ permeability leads to both diminished secretion volumes and increased absorption of sodium chloride. The clinical effect is the production of an inadequate volume of viscid airway secretions. These are poorly cleared and lead in turn to chronic and recurrent infections with bronchitis, bronchiectasis, and progressive parenchymal lung destruction. *P aeruginosa* colonization of the airways is a certainty, and other similar infections are routine. Ninety percent of cystic fibrosis deaths are related directly to this chronic pulmonary disease. Although treatable, it is not curable, and the mean life expectancy with cystic fibrosis is about 26 years. The effects of cystic fibrosis on the pancreas are similar to those in the airways. Impaired exocrine function secondary to duct obstruction from viscid and inadequate secretions appears to be followed by secondary autolysis, acinar atrophy, and pancreatic glandular fibrosis. Exocrine pancreatic insufficiency is a predictably early and characteristic clinical feature of cystic fibrosis that may lead to the initial diagnosis. Fortunately, exocrine enzyme replacement is accomplished relatively easily, and endocrine insufficiency is a later, more rare event.

Some data suggest that the Cl⁻ ion transport defect may not be present in the intestinal epithelium of patients with cystic fibrosis as previously believed.[56] Impaired pancreatic exocrine secretion, with or without primary abnormalities of intestinal epithelial secretion and absorption, is the apparent explanation for the GI manifestations of cystic fibrosis. In particular, the lack of pancreatic proteinases leads to the neonatal phenomenon of meconium ileus, which is characterized by abnormally thick and viscid, protein-laden meconium that obstructs the GI tract, classically in the terminal ileum proximal to the ileocecal valve (Fig. 103-22). In this circumstance, the terminal ileum is filled with inspissated concretions composed of pale, non-bilious meconium. The colon is small and unused but intrinsically normal. Immediately proximal to the obstruction, the meconium is of variable consistency with tarry, thick material and air mixed together. The most proximal intestine is often normal in gross and microscopic appearance. Immediately proximal to the obstruction, muscular hypertrophy is present, and mucous glands are distended with prominent goblet cells.

One half to one third of fetuses with meconium ileus

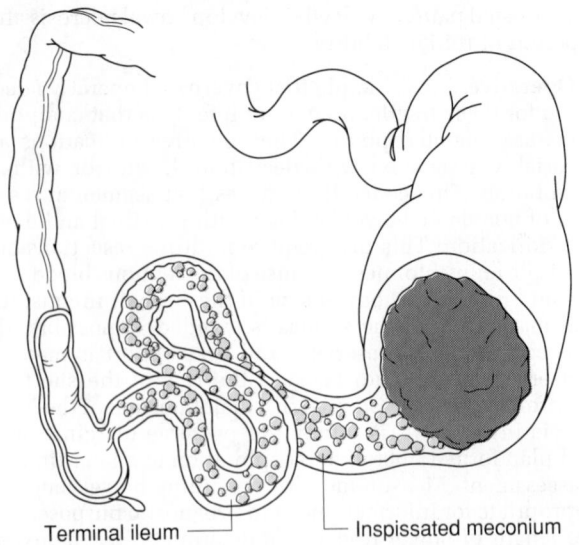

Figure 103-22.   Meconium ileus–induced obstruction of the terminal ileum.

have related in utero complications, such as proximal volvulus, perforation, or atresia. A classic finding is intestinal perforation with sterile meconium peritonitis and the formation of a calcified pseudocyst (Fig. 103-23). GI manifestations of cystic fibrosis presenting outside the neonatal time frame occur in 10% of affected children. These may include acute appendicitis, distal small bowel obstruction (meconium ileus equivalent), and volvulus. All appear to be related to the presence of abnormally viscid, obstructive stool in the distal ileum. Medical management is generally successful for these older infants and children with meconium ileus equivalent and is similar to that outlined later for neonates. Pancreatic enzyme replacement is always a necessity. Rectal prolapse and intussusception may also occur with cystic fibrosis, apparently related to the chronic motility alterations that result from difficulty in clearing the gut lumen. Additionally, patients with cystic fibrosis appear to be vulnerable to a cholestasis syndrome initiated by obstruction of small intrahepatic bile ducts and followed by chronic inflammation. Ultimately, hepatic fibrosis with cirrhosis may result. Clinical presentation with evidence of liver failure and portal hypertension occurs in about 5% of patients with cystic fibrosis.

Diagnostic Evaluation.   Historically useful screening tests for cystic fibrosis are being replaced by specific DNA analyses for the cystic fibrosis gene, as outlined earlier. The analysis of the sodium chloride content of sweat has been the historical standard for cystic fibrosis detection. The most reliable technique involves the pilocarpine iontophoresis method, with positive test results showing sodium and chloride concentrations in excess of 60 mEq/L.[57] The test is often unhelpful before 4 to 6 weeks of age because the normal neonate does not reliably conserve sodium chloride in sweat. Other sweat test techniques have unacceptably high rates of false-negative and false-positive results. Other evaluations have included stool analyses for trypsin or protein content, but these lack specificity and have not achieved broad clinical acceptance.

Meconium Ileus

Clinical Presentation.   Historically, only 10% to 33% of infants with meconium ileus were known prospectively to have a family history of cystic fibrosis.[25] Accurate prena-

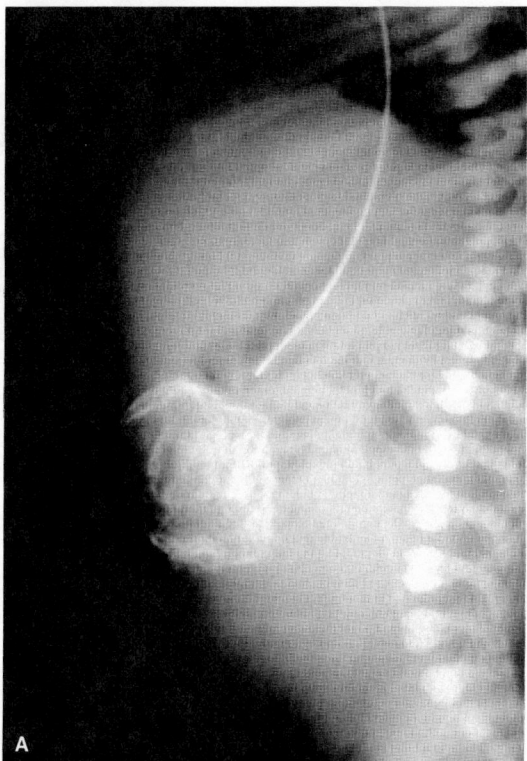

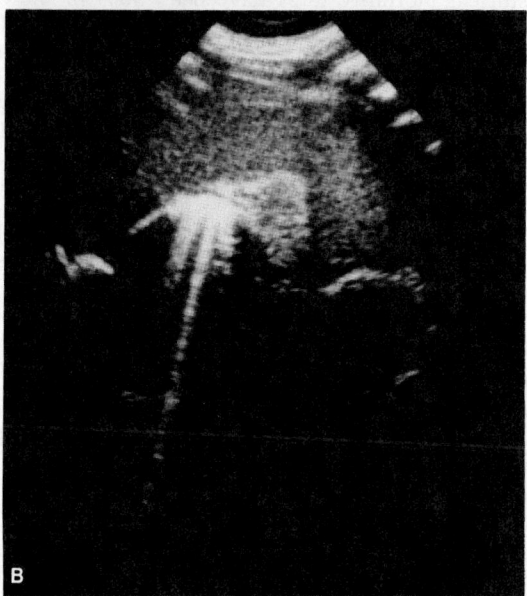

Figure 103-23. (*A*) Radiograph of meconium pseudocyst with calcification. (*B*) In utero ultrasound scan demonstrating a calcified meconium pseudocyst.

tal ultrasound diagnosis of meconium ileus, particularly in its complicated forms, is now feasible; together with fetal DNA screening, this should improve the likelihood for prospective discovery. After birth, affected infants develop signs and symptoms of ileal obstruction with abdominal distention and bilious vomiting, usually beginning in the first day of life. The physical examination is notable for doughy loops of palpable distended intestine filled with meconium. On rectal examination, white mucus or thick gray meconium without bile is typical, but this does not differentiate meconium ileus from other causes of proximal intestinal obstruction. Prenatal intestinal perforation

with meconium cyst formation may cause a palpable abdominal mass. In this instance, speckled calcifications on plain radiograph or ultrasound examination are diagnostic. Postnatal volvulus or perforation related to meconium ileus predictably results in peritonitis and sepsis. In this latter circumstance, systemic signs of infection occur in conjunction with the intestinal obstruction. Intestinal atresia may be associated with complex meconium ileus, but generally, other anatomic malformations are uncommon.

Diagnosis. The diagnosis of meconium ileus may be possible with plain radiographs alone (Fig. 103-24*A*). Typically, multiple distended loops of intestine are seen. These usually vary in size and may be filled with fluid or meconium mixed with air to give a characteristic soap-bubble appearance. Classic air–fluid levels are not an expected finding because the meconium is viscid and adheres tenaciously to the intestinal wall. Prenatal spillage of sterile meconium leads to intraperitoneal calcifications, as seen in Figure 103-23 and discussed earlier.

The imaging evaluation is best continued with a contrast enema, which typically shows a small, unused colon (see Fig. 103-24*B*). Reflux of contrast into the terminal ileum is often possible and confirms the presence of intraluminal meconium concretions adjacent to the ileocecal valve. Taken together with a family history and plain films, this is sufficient evidence to confirm the diagnosis of meconium ileus. Upper GI tract contrast studies are generally unnecessary and may complicate therapeutic efforts.

Treatment
Nonoperative. The nonoperative relief of distal small bowel obstruction is possible in about 60% to 70% of infants with simple meconium ileus.[25] Once the diagnosis is confirmed by contrast enema, the strategy consists of enema instillation of one of several irrigation solutions into the obstructed terminal ileum. Saline, hyperosmolar contrast agents, dilute *N*-acetylcysteine, and a variety of other solutions have been used. The initial experience with this approach emphasized the need for hyperosmolar solutions in the belief that the resultant flux of fluid into the intestinal lumen was necessary to clear the inspissated meconium. It appears, however, that simple mechanical irrigation with saline is equally effective with any of the specific solutions, without irritant or toxic effects. Sequential enemas may be necessary to disimpact effectively the inspissated meconium from the terminal ileum; generally, these are continued as long as clinical progress is made. Nasogastric tube instillation of mucolytic agents, such as *N*-acetylcysteine, may also be useful, but the mucosal inflammation induced makes this unappealing because the GI tract may need to be opened if operation becomes necessary.

The obvious important advantage of the enema and irrigation approach is elimination of the need for general anesthesia and laparotomy, thereby reducing the incidence of postoperative pulmonary problems. Possible complications of this approach include intestinal perforation, toxic injury to intestinal mucosa, and failure to relieve the obstruction.

Long-term management for cystic fibrosis–related GI tract problems associated with meconium ileus includes pancreatic enzyme replacement, aggressive nutritional support, periodic enemas if obstructive symptoms develop, and avoidance of intravascular volume or sodium chloride depletion.

Operative. Failure to relieve the ileal obstruction with enema irrigations and the development of complicated meconium ileus are the usual indications for operative management of this problem. For persistent obstruction with simple meconium ileus, the principal goals at laparotomy are to disimpact the terminal ileum and evacuate the meco-

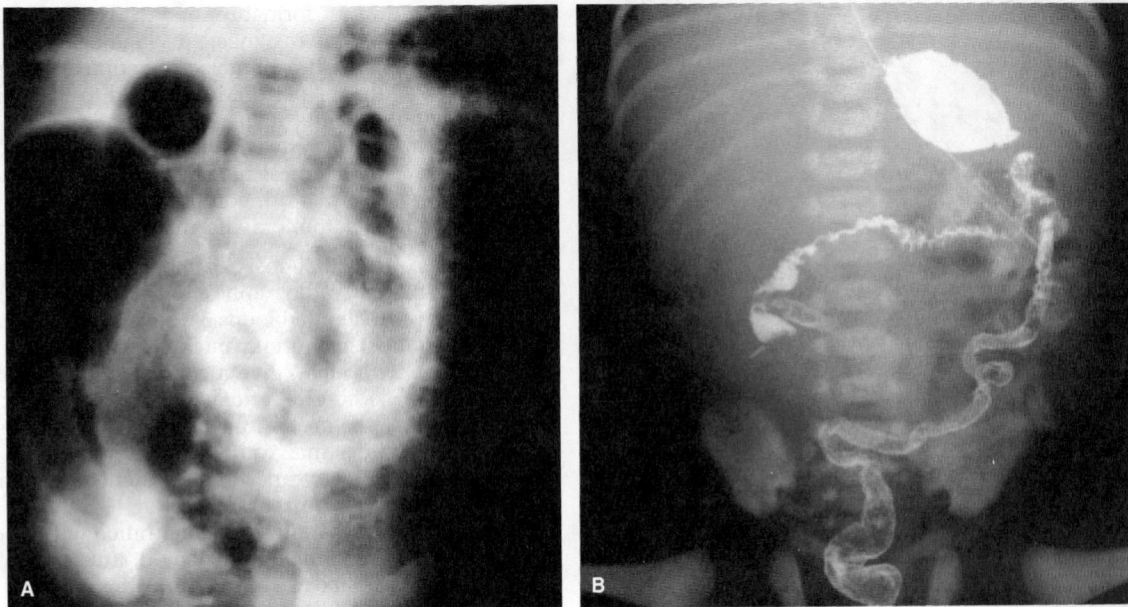

Figure 103-24. (*A*) Plain radiograph from neonate with meconium ileus. (*B*) Barium enema in an infant with meconium ileus typically shows an unused but intrinsically normal microcolon.

nium from the small intestine. These may be accomplished by external massage or transmural needle installation of irrigation solutions, but enterotomy or enterostomy with direct irrigation generally is required. Simple closure of the enterotomy is preferable, but segmental intestinal resection may be necessary if marginal or compromised intestine is found. Simple end-to-end anastomosis is the preferable form of reconstruction after segmental resection for obstruction. A temporary enterostomy may be necessary, and a variety of techniques for exteriorization have been described. These are principally of historical interest with simple meconium ileus.

Complicated forms of meconium ileus occur in about one third of patients. Segmental volvulus, atresia, stenosis, bowel necrosis, perforation, and meconium cyst formation are possible. In these circumstances, nonviable, stenotic, or perforated intestine is resected and intestinal continuity reestablished, if possible. As with other, similar conditions, concurrent medical problems or established peritonitis may preclude a safe primary anastomosis. In this case, exteriorization of the proximal and distal intestine is indicated. Closure of these stomas can be done promptly after resolution of the underlying problems. Generally, appendectomy is performed at the time of laparotomy for meconium ileus because of the relatively high frequency of subsequent appendicitis and possible confusion with the meconium ileus equivalent syndrome. Small bowel atresia is associated with meconium ileus and should be specifically excluded at laparotomy by demonstrating patency of the small bowel throughout its length.

Postoperative Care and Results. If the GI tract has not been opened surgically, dilute *N*-acetylcysteine may be given through the nasogastric tube or by enema during the postoperative period to keep the ileum patent. Recurrent ileal obstruction due to inspissated meconium is a potential problem. Oral pancreatic enzyme replacement and an elemental diet are routine in the postoperative period after the ileus resolves. Perhaps most important in the postoperative period is aggressive pulmonary therapy that includes postural drainage, mucolytic agents, and prophylactic and specific antibiotics as indicated.

Historical mortality rates have been 50% or more for infants requiring operation for meconium ileus, largely as a result of the pulmonary complications. Perioperative care has improved to the extent that a number of institutions have recently reported 70% to 100% survival rates after surgery.[25,58–60] The mean survival age for cystic fibrosis is well into the third decade of life and is primarily determined by the course of the pulmonary disease rather than GI problems. The late sequelae of portal hypertension represent the one important exception to this generalization. Techniques directed at treatment of the pulmonary problems, such as pharmacologic therapy, lung transplantation, and possibly gene therapy, may ultimately improve this outlook.

Meconium Plug Syndrome

Meconium plug syndrome is generally considered independently of meconium ileus, because few of these infants have cystic fibrosis. The potential confusion of the two entities clinically, however, and their occasional association make it appropriate to consider this syndrome briefly here. Meconium plug syndrome affects normal and preterm neonates with immature gut motility patterns, and is characterized by meconium plugs that functionally obstruct the colon or rectum. Unlike meconium ileus, these plugs are composed of normal meconium, and the colon is of normal caliber. The infants are discovered within the first days of life when they develop abdominal distention and bilious vomiting. The meconium is bile stained and normal, but spontaneous passage through the rectum is often absent. Rectal examination may be therapeutic because the offending plug may be delivered digitally. The diagnosis is confirmed by contrast enema, which may also be therapeutic by irrigating the colon and rectum. The importance of the syndrome is related to its relative frequency and the need to differentiate it from other causes of neonatal intestinal obstruction. Although most of these infants are normal, meconium ileus and Hirschsprung disease are important associations. Cystic fibrosis screening and a suction rectal biopsy are therefore appropriate routine diagnostic studies for infants who present with meconium plug syndrome.

Malrotation

Embryology

Disproportional growth and elongation of the midgut beginning in the 5th gestational week results in three important and distinct stages of intestinal positioning that are relevant to this review of congenital rotational abnormalities. Initially, herniation of the primary midgut loop occurs into the base of the umbilical cord, where it remains until the 10th gestational week. The axis of the loop is the superior mesenteric artery (SMA), and the omphalomesenteric duct is at the apex. This loop rotates 180 degrees in a counterclockwise direction so that the proximal prearterial half of the loop passes posterior to the SMA. The cranial portion of the prearterial segment gives rise to the proximal duodenum, which lies to the right of the midline. The more distal prearterial segment passes behind and to the left of the SMA. This transverse segment develops into

the third and fourth portions of the duodenum, normally becoming fixed to the left of the aorta at the ligament of Treitz, having rotated 270 degrees in a counterclockwise arc from its original position. The jejunoileal segment undergoes dramatic elongation, forming about six primary intestinal loops. The embryonic postarterial segment, which gives rise to the cecum and right colon, also rotates 270 degrees in a counterclockwise direction. Thus, the cecum is positioned initially to the left, then anterior, and finally to the right of the SMA before reaching its final adult location.[22] This is illustrated in Figure 103-25.

The second stage of midgut development, reduction of the extracoelomic gut, occurs between 10 and 12 weeks of gestation when the rotation of both prearterial and postarterial segments approximates 180 degrees from their original positions. At this time, the duodenojejunal junction has passed posterior to the SMA, the small bowel is to the right of the midline, and the cecum and ascending colon

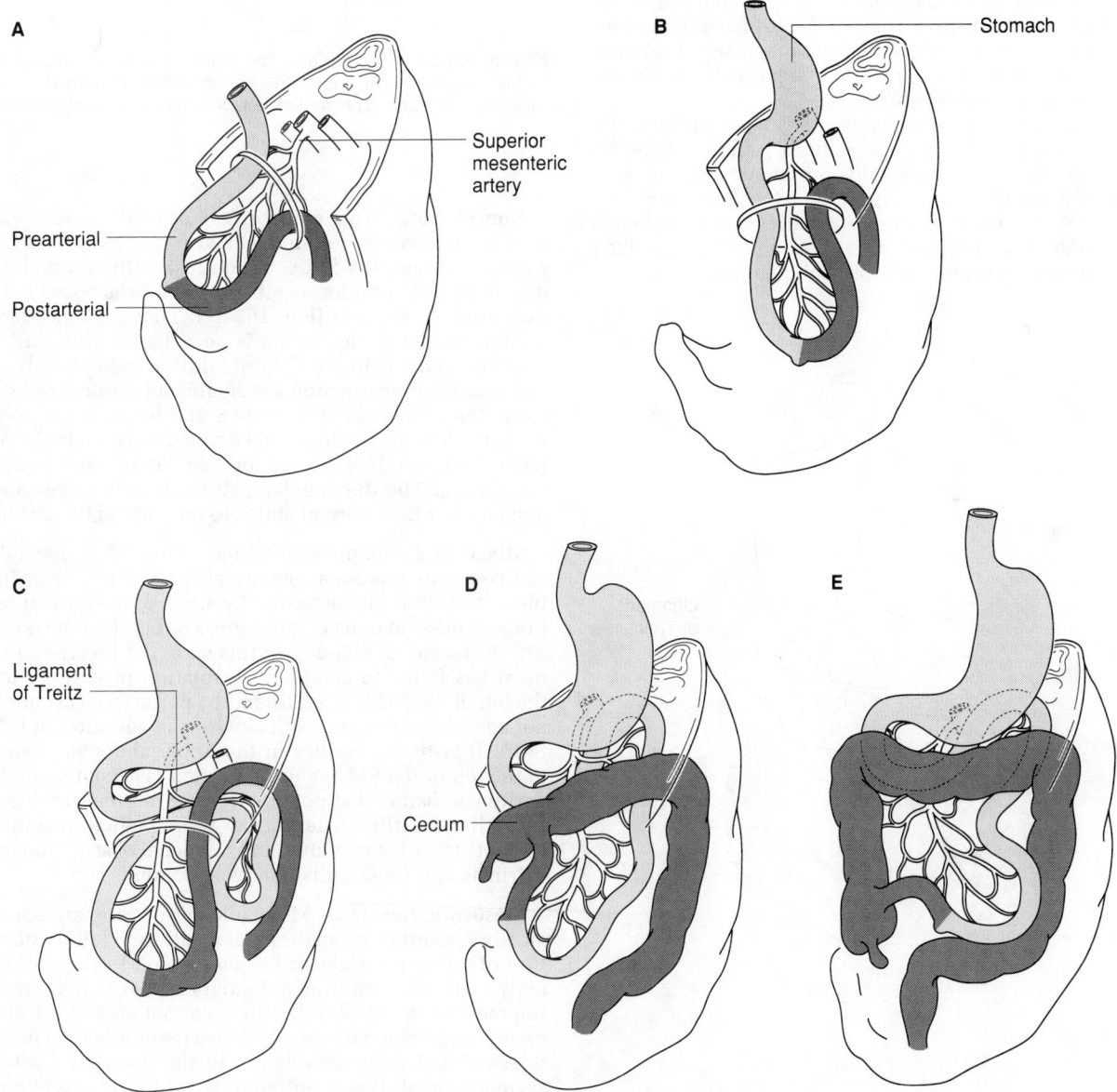

Figure 103-25. Normal midgut rotation is shown with appropriate positioning of the stomach, duodenum, small intestine, and cecum from the fifth gestational week (A) through completion by the 12th week (E).

are anterior to the SMA after reduction into the left abdomen. Many common abnormalities of position occur as a result of arrested development during this 2-week period.

The final step in the positioning process is *fixation* of the intestine to the posterior body wall after the 12th gestational week. Cecal descent occurs at this time. Normal points of fixation include the cecum in the right iliac fossa and the duodenojejunal junction at the ligament of Treitz just to the left of the aorta and anterior to the left renal vein (Fig. 103-26). The resulting intestinal mesentery is fixed with a broad base and is therefore not at risk for volvulus. In contrast, the base of the mesentery, with the positional abnormalities described later, is neither fixed nor broad, and the midgut may therefore be at risk for volvulus.

Anatomy

Interruption of normal intestinal positioning may occur at any stage in development, and the resulting anomalies therefore represent a spectrum of findings with many individual variations. Developmental arrest before reduction of the extracoelomic gut results in an omphalocele. Anomalies such as gastroschisis and congenital diaphragmatic hernia also allow displacement of the gut from the peritoneal cavity before completion of the processes of rotation and fixation. Therefore, positional abnormalities are expected in each of these situations.

The imprecise term *malrotation* has been irretrievably incorporated into clinical usage and is generally taken to encompass the several surgically important malformations reviewed later. For practical purposes, the discussion here is limited to the more common anomalies that an embryologist would more properly classify as nonrotation, mixed or incomplete rotation, and mesocolic hernia.

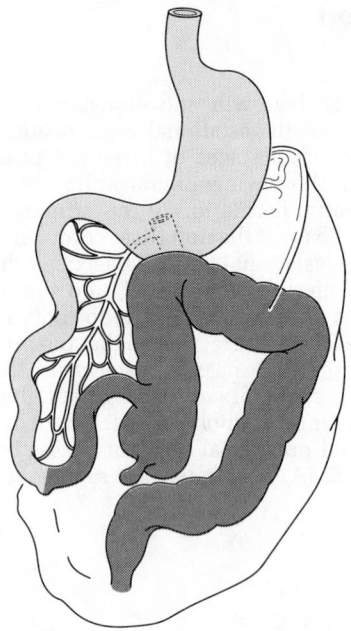

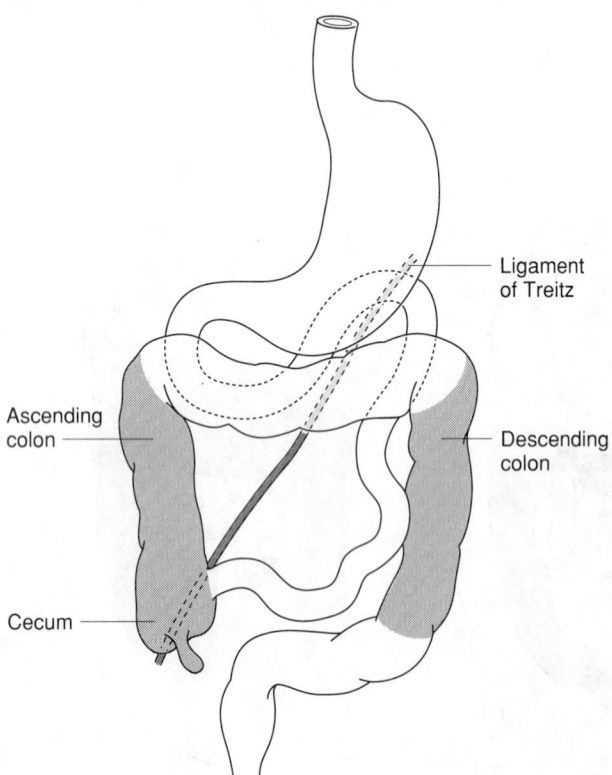

Figure 103-26. Normal oblique fixation of the midgut mesentery at the ligament of Treitz and in the right lower quadrant. The blue portions of the colon are retroperitoneal.

Figure 103-27. Nonrotation. The small bowel (prearterial segment) resides on the right side of the abdomen, and the colon (postarterial segment) is on the left. Neither has rotated normally.

Nonrotation. This common abnormality is characterized by inadequate counterclockwise rotation of the midgut loop around the SMA. In contrast to the normal 270-degree arc, the rotation is either absent or arrested before exceeding 90 degrees (Fig. 103-27). The colon resides in the left abdomen, the cecum is near the midline, and the small intestine is to the right of midline. Midgut volvulus and duodenal obstruction are significant clinical risks because the SMA pedicle is narrow and because the peritoneal attachments (Ladd bands) fixing the cecum to the posterior body wall pass anterior and lateral to the distal duodenum. The duodenojejunal juncture is more caudal and anterior than normal and is to the right of the midline.

Mixed or Incomplete Rotation. This is the second of the common rotational abnormalities. Mixed or incomplete rotation is characterized by arrest of the normal rotational process at or near 180 degrees rather than the normal 270 degrees (Fig. 103-28). In this case, the prearterial segment has failed to complete its rotation posterior and to the left of the SMA. In addition, the postarterial cecum has not completed its counterclockwise passage anterior to the SMA. It typically resides in the upper abdomen, usually to the left of the SMA, and its fixation is accomplished by peritoneal bands that potentially obstruct the duodenum, as outlined earlier. The narrow SMA pedicle places the midgut at risk for volvulus, and duodenal obstruction from extrinsic compression is relatively common.

Mesocolic Hernias. Mesocolic hernias are rare but surgically important anomalies that result from failure of fixation of either the right or left mesocolon to the posterior body wall. The resulting potential cavities may allow entrapment of the small intestine on either side of the abdomen. A right-sided mesocolic defect (paraduodenal hernia) is associated with nonrotation of the prearterial midgut segment. Small bowel entrapment behind the right colon and cecum may occur. Similar entrapment of the small intestine may occur behind an incompletely fixed left mesocolon but is associated with normal positioning of the

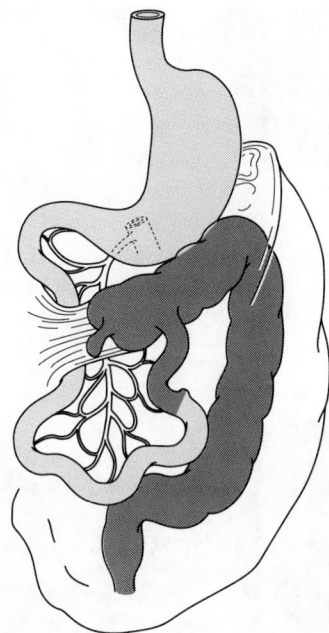

Figure 103-28. Incomplete rotation. The prearterial segment has failed to rotate and is on the right. The postarterial segment has rotated to reside anterior to the duodenum so that cecal bands to the posterior abdominal wall may compress and obstruct the duodenum.

colon and cecum. In this latter case, entrapped small intestine is contained within a hernia sac with a neck composed of the inferior mesenteric vein and peritoneal bands extending to the posterior body wall. As with any hernia, obstruction, incarceration, and strangulation are potential risks.

Clinical Presentation

The autopsy prevalence of rotational abnormalities may be as high as 1% of the total population, but the absence of symptoms in many patients yields a much lower clinical incidence. The discovery of malrotation usually results from clinical evidence of duodenal obstruction or midgut volvulus. Duodenal obstruction is a consequence of Ladd peritoneal bands fixing the abnormally positioned cecum to the posterior body wall at or near the level of the duodenum. These bands cross anterior and lateral to the distal duodenum and may cause extrinsic compression. It follows that the clinical signs and symptoms include gastric and proximal duodenal distention with bilious vomiting. In the neonate, relatively little small bowel gas is present distally because of the partial obstruction, and abdominal distention is not typically found on physical examination.

Midgut volvulus often exacerbates the obstructive symptoms, but its life-threatening consequence is vascular insufficiency of the intestine supplied by the SMA. Guaiac-positive stool from mucosal injury is a common early finding. If transmural necrosis develops, acidosis, thrombocytopenia, and frank sepsis may ensue. The clinical outcome for midgut volvulus is clearly time dependent, and this is the fundamental reason that signs and symptoms of neonatal intestinal obstruction must be pursued aggressively until a diagnosis is obtained.

Fifty to 75% of malrotations are discovered in the 1st month of life, and about 90% occur in children younger than 1 year old.[25,61] Affected neonates and infants are usually without other medical problems. All require emergency surgical exploration and correction. Older children

and adults may present with acute volvulus, episodic obstructive symptoms, or chronic abdominal pain. In addition, patients with minimal or no symptoms may be discovered at the time of coincidental GI imaging or surgery. In general, it is safest to correct these malformations surgically because the complications of volvulus may be lethal and the risk appears to persist, although it is diminished in older children and adults.

Diagnosis

The diagnostic evaluation for neonatal intestinal obstruction begins with a plain abdominal radiograph. The classic findings with malrotation include a distended stomach and proximal duodenal bulb with a paucity or absence of small bowel air, all consequences of the partial duodenal obstruction (Fig. 103-29*A*). The plain film may not distinguish malrotation from duodenal atresia or a duodenal stenosis. In most instances of duodenal obstruction, an upper GI series is the second and conclusive imaging study (see Fig. 103-29*B*) and almost always differentiates these lesions. Typically, malrotation produces an incomplete obstruction with a corkscrew or coiled appearance in the third or fourth portions of the duodenum. Duodenal atresia can occur anywhere within the duodenum but tends to be more proximal, without the contour of extrinsic compression typical of Ladd bands. Complete absence of distal air is typical of duodenal atresia, whereas diminished but discernible distal air is characteristic of malrotation. Duodenal stenosis with incomplete obstruction, particularly if located in a more atypical distal location, may be indistinguishable from malrotation.

Additional important findings with malrotation are suggested by the earlier descriptions of the anatomy and embryology. Malposition of the duodenojejunal junction is diagnostic. In particular, this includes a location to the right of the midline. Additionally, failure to achieve normal posterior and cephalad fixation is typical and often is best evaluated with lateral films. The small bowel resides in the right abdomen, and the colon and cecum are on the left (see Fig. 103-29*C*). Attempts to differentiate malrotations with and without volvulus radiographically may be unreliable and therefore hazardous in clinical practice.

A barium enema is helpful in evaluating children with neonatal and intestinal obstruction, although it may not be the study of first choice if malrotation is suspected. The classic finding of malrotation with contrast enema is malposition of the cecum, usually in the upper abdomen, and most often on the left.

Treatment

There is no role for the nonoperative management of malrotation or an internal hernia in the neonate. Assessment, resuscitation, and preoperative preparation should be conducted concurrently so that a diagnosis of malrotation can be followed immediately by laparotomy. The urgency is derived from the fact that a delay measured in hours may represent the difference between viable or infarcted midgut at laparotomy. The latter finding is ordinarily survivable only with permanent or long-term parenteral hyperalimentation. In older, asymptomatic patients discovered coincidentally, operation may be approached more electively because the risk of volvulus diminishes with age. Although controversial, surgical correction appears to be indicated in these children as well.

Operative repair of malrotation is achieved nearly universally by the Ladd procedure.[62] The goals of the procedure are two-fold. The first is to relieve the midgut volvulus. This is initially accomplished by delivery and detorsion of the affected midgut, usually in a counterclockwise direction. Recurrence of the volvulus is pre-

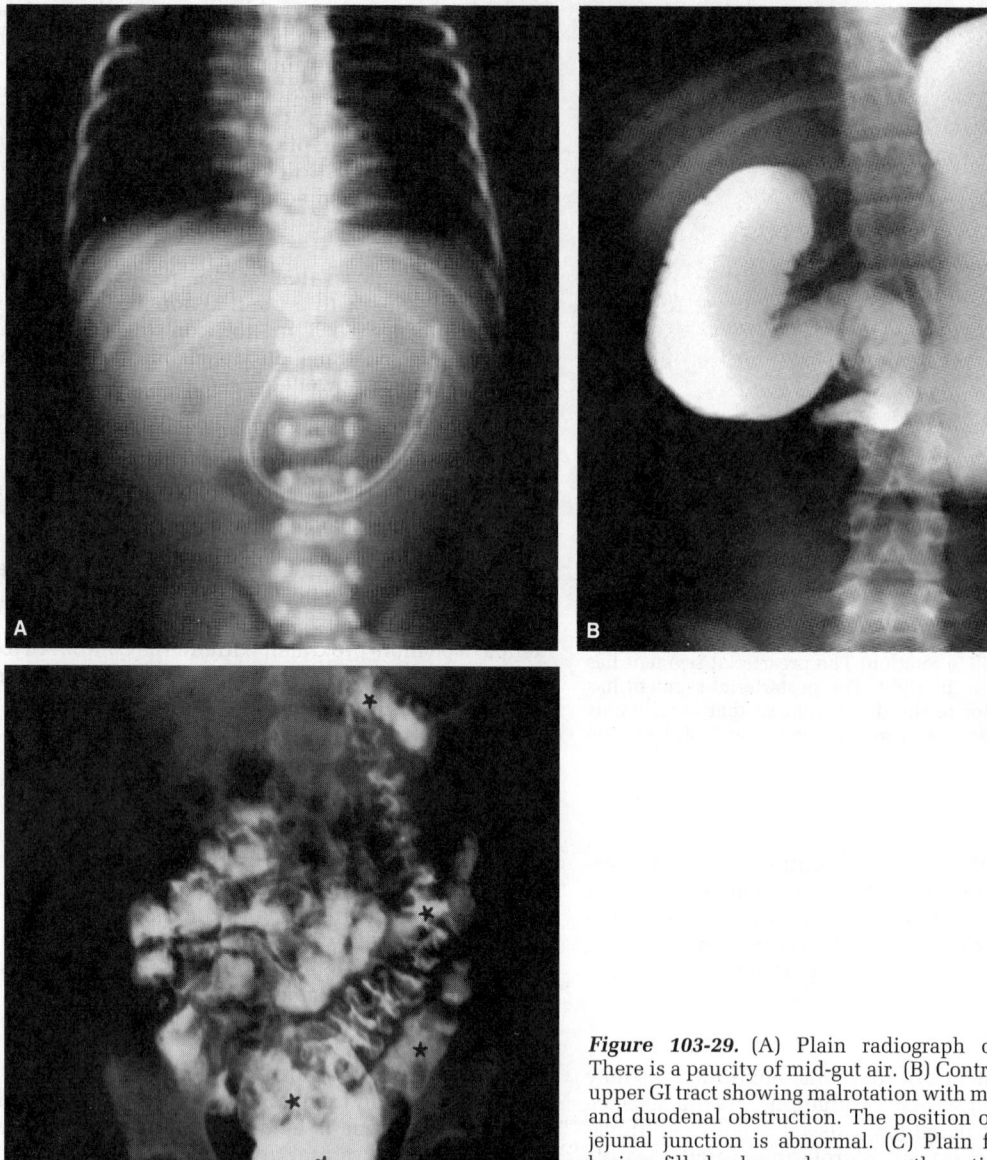

Figure 103-29. (A) Plain radiograph of malrotation. There is a paucity of mid-gut air. (B) Contrast study of the upper GI tract showing malrotation with mid-gut volvulus and duodenal obstruction. The position of the duodeno-jejunal junction is abnormal. (C) Plain film showing a barium-filled colon and cecum on the patient's left (*asterisks*). The entire small intestine is to the right of midline. These are typical findings of malrotation.

vented by broadening the base of the mesenteric vascular pedicle by dividing the peritoneal bands that tether the cecum, small bowel mesentery, mesocolon, and duodenum around the base of the SMA (Fig. 103-30). Properly done, the mesenteric leaves and mesocolon open widely. Efforts to fix the mesentery by cecal or duodenal attachment to the body wall have been largely abandoned for lack of supportive data. Properly opened, the mesenteric pedicle is at low risk for recurrent volvulus. Postoperative small bowel obstructions are reported in about 10% of patients, but virtually all are the result of simple adhesion formation.

The second operative objective is to divide the Ladd peritoneal bands to relieve the extrinsic compression and obstruction of the distal duodenum. This is done by meticulous and complete mobilization of the entire duodenum with division of all anterior, lateral, and posterior attachments, essentially a modified Kocher maneuver. Duodenal and distal small bowel patency should also be demonstrated using intraluminal air or saline because concurrent cases of atresia have been reported.

When nonviable intestine is found at laparotomy, the principle is to preserve whatever length is possible. Decisions regarding resection, exteriorization, or primary anastomosis are necessarily individualized, but principles are not different than for other situations in which nonviable intestine is encountered. In situations in which the entire midgut is lost and long-term survival is doubtful, difficult intraoperative ethical decisions must be made with the parents.

An incidental appendectomy is usually performed in infants with rotational abnormalities to eliminate potential future confusion if acute appendicitis develops in the malpositioned appendix.

Right mesocolic hernias are corrected simply by dividing the lateral peritoneal attachments of the cecum and right colon to eliminate this potential space. In addition, the SMA pedicle should be broadened as much as possible using the techniques outlined earlier. Left mesocolic hernias present a more difficult problem. These patients require mobilization of the inferior mesenteric vein, reduction of small bowel from the hernia sac, and closure

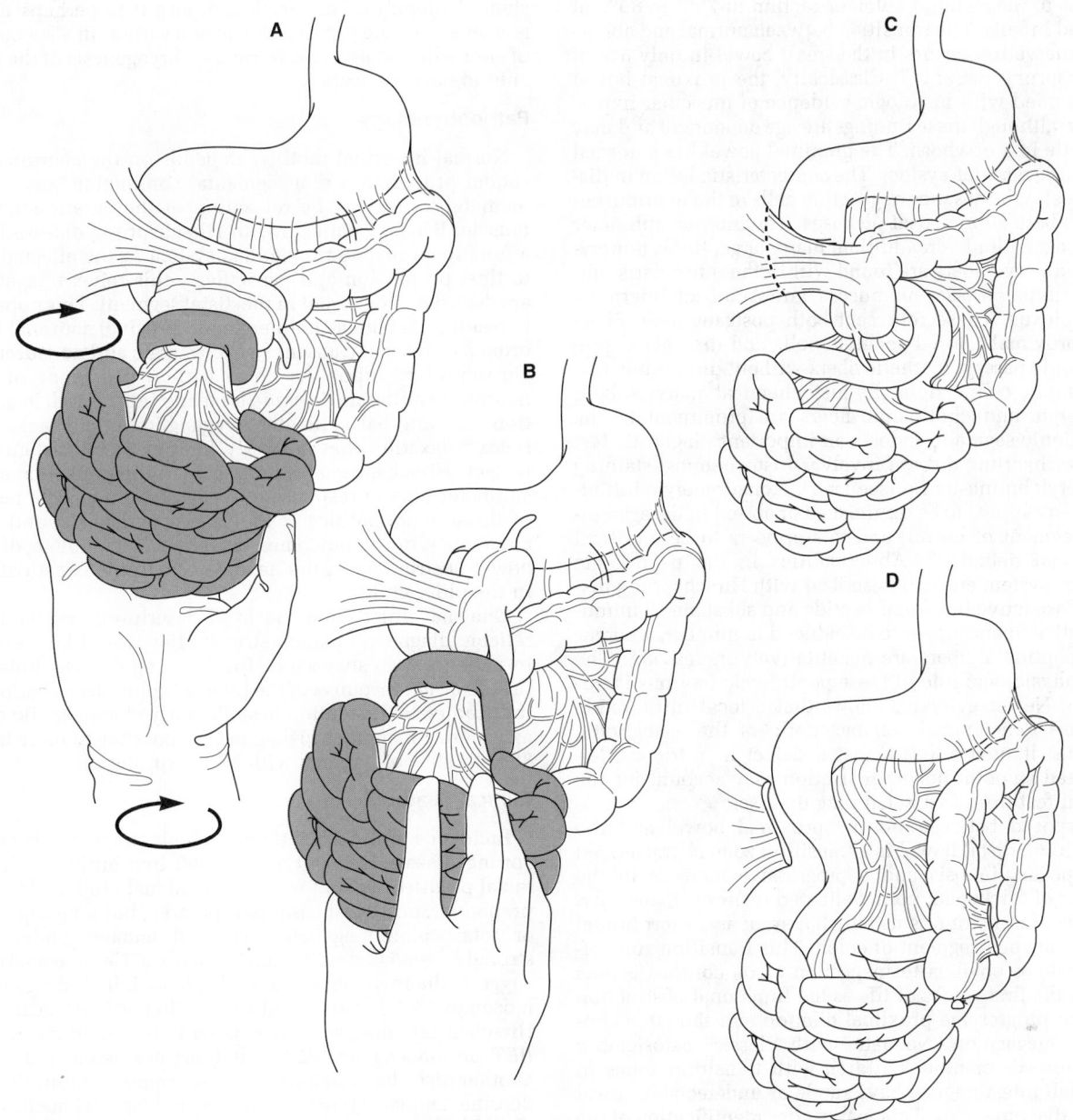

Figure 103-30. Correction of malrotation. (*A* and *B*) Derotation. (*C* and *D*) Division of cecal (Ladd) bands.

of the neck of the mesocolic sac to eliminate the potential space.

Results and Complications

The results after surgical correction for all rotational anomalies should be excellent, with normal life expectancy in the absence of compromised bowel at the time of the initial procedure. The reported incidence of adhesive small bowel obstruction after surgical correction of malrotation is 1% to 10%. Recurrent volvulus and recurrent duodenal obstruction are rare if the initial procedure is technically complete.

Congenital Aganglionosis (Hirschsprung Disease)

Embryology

Congenital aganglionosis of the intestine (Hirschsprung disease) is the result of disordered embryogenesis involving the myenteric nervous system, but the precise patho-genic mechanisms involved are unknown. Normally, neuroblasts derived from neural crest precursors become discernible in the foregut by the 5th gestational week. After maturation and caudal migration with vagal nerve fibers, these neuroblasts form the ganglion cells of the myenteric nervous system. The initial caudal migration of neuroblasts in an intermuscular plane is followed by intramural dispersal into both superficial and deep submucosal nerve plexuses. Functional maturation normally continues well into infancy. Anatomically normal ganglion cells can be identified in the esophagus at 6 weeks' gestation, in the transverse colon at 8 weeks' gestation, and in the rectum by 12 weeks' gestation.[63]

Anatomy

Hirschsprung disease is characterized by migratory arrest of the neuroblasts within the gut. The distal extent of the normal myenteric nervous system is variable but reaches to the sigmoid colon or rectum in 75% to 80% of affected infants. The transition between normal and abnormal innervation occurs in the small bowel in only 5% of Hirschsprung patients.[64] Classically, the proximal bowel is distended with histologic evidence of muscular hypertrophy, although these findings are age dependent and may be subtle in a newborn. The proximal bowel has a normal myenteric nervous system. The characteristic lesion in distal bowel is the absence of ganglion cells in the intermuscular and both submucosal plexuses. The internal sphincter is also aganglionic. In addition, many large, thick, nonmyelinated nerve fibers are found within the muscularis mucosa, lamina propria, submucosa, and Auerbach intermuscular plexus. These represent both postganglionic fibers from proximal normal ganglion cells and disordered preganglionic parasympathetic fibers without discernible distal synaptic connections. By histochemical analysis, both adrenergic and cholinergic fibers are prominent in the aganglionic segment. Indeed, an important diagnostic test for Hirschsprung disease involves histochemical staining for acetylcholinesterase (see later). Nonadrenergic inhibitory fibers appear to be diminished or absent in the aganglionic segment of bowel, and this appears to be a critical functional deficit.[65,66] Abnormalities in the peptidergic nervous system are also described with Hirschsprung disease. Vasoactive intestinal peptide and substance P immunoreactive fibers appear to be reduced in number, whereas neuropeptide Y fibers are quantitatively increased.[67] The pathophysiologic role of these peptidergic neurons is unknown. Newer evidence shows that a local nitric oxide synthase deficiency is characteristic of the aganglionic segment. It now appears that a defect in nitric oxide–mediated smooth muscle relaxation may account for the clinical features of Hirschsprung disease.[68,69]

Interposed between normal proximal bowel and the aganglionic distal bowel is a transition zone characterized by hypoganglionosis and a progressive increase in the number of thickened, nonmyelinated neurons. Externally, the area of transition is usually apparent as a short funnel or cone-shaped segment of colon. This transition zone often becomes obvious to inspection or on contrast enema during the first weeks of life as the functional obstruction leads to progressive proximal dilation and thus to a congenital megacolon. Neonates with classic rectosigmoid aganglionosis or older children with transition zones in the small intestine may have subtle or undetectable bowel lumen discrepancies. This may render identification of the transition zone problematic for either the surgeon or radiologist. In addition, the correlation between gross and microscopic anatomy is not necessarily precise, so histologic confirmation of the level of ganglion cell transition is always necessary for surgical decision making. Although a few reports of discontinuous aganglionosis have appeared, most evidence supports the concept that Hirschsprung disease results from interruption of the normal craniocaudal neuroblast migratory process. Therefore, continuous distal aganglionosis is expected, and the distal rectum is always affected. Even though the rectal segment involved may be short, a correctly done rectal biopsy demonstrating ganglion cells 2.5 to 3 cm cephalad to the pectinate line and normal myenteric axons precludes the existence of Hirschsprung disease.

An entity similar to or perhaps associated with Hirschsprung disease has been described; neuronal intestinal dysplasia.[70–72] As the name suggests, the characteristic histologic findings are those of a dysplastic myenteric nervous system, but ganglion cells can be identified. Clinical presentation and treatment are generally similar to those of classic Hirschsprung disease. There is considerable controversy regarding even the existence of the entity; but a substantial literature has developed, and it is perhaps most reasonable to suggest that this is one variant in a spectrum of anomalies related to abnormal embryogenesis of the myenteric nervous system.

Pathophysiology

Normal intestinal motility depends on the coordinated caudal propagation of a segmental contraction wave, immediately preceded by relaxation of the enteric smooth muscle. Because patients with Hirschsprung disease lack a functional myenteric nervous system in the affected intestine, propulsion and particularly this reflex relaxation are disordered or absent in the distal segment. This appears to result from both a cholinergic (propulsive) neuronal disorder as well as the absence of adrenergic and nonadrenergic inhibitory input. As noted earlier, deficiency of the neurotransmitter nitric oxide is clearly implicated. In addition, the internal sphincter is aganglionic and lacks the reflex relaxation that normally follows rectal distention. In fact, Hirschsprung patients actually exhibit increased sphincter tone in response to rectal distention. The result of these abnormalities is ineffective peristalsis, and the common clinical outcomes are either incomplete distal bowel obstruction in the neonate or chronic constipation in the older child.

One may infer from the brief description earlier that reliable diagnostic manometric studies would be feasible in patients with suspected Hirschsprung disease. Indeed, the abnormal response of the internal sphincter to balloon-induced rectal distention is sufficiently characteristic that an accurate manometric diagnosis is possible in more than 85% to 90% of patients with Hirschsprung disease.

Clinical Features

Incidence and Associations. The incidence of Hirschsprung disease is about 1 per 5000 live births, with no racial predilection, but with a marked male-to-female (4:1) preponderance. Most cases are sporadic, but long-segment or total colonic aganglionosis and female gender are strongly associated with familial disease. Genetic analysis suggests the involvement of multiple loci, including chromosomes 13q22, 21q22, and 10q.[73,74] In particular, familial Hirschsprung disease is associated with mutations of the *RET* protooncogene. *RET* mutations are associated with another disorder of neural crest development, multiple endocrine neoplasia types 2A and 2B, and familial medullary thyroid carcinoma, which are occasionally associated with Hirschsprung disease. Other rare anomalies have been reported with Hirschsprung disease, but the consistent important association is a 5% to 15% incidence of trisomy 21.[75] Cardiac malformations occur in 2% to 5% of infants with Hirschsprung disease. For unknown reasons, prematurity is uncommon (less than 5%) among affected infants, and this is an important clinical observation. The meconium plug syndrome and neonatal appendicitis are not common presentations of Hirschsprung disease, but the possible association should lead to a screening suction rectal biopsy in either case.

Presentation. Most infants with Hirschsprung disease do not have normal passage of meconium in the first 24 to 48 hours of life, although this is frequently noted only in retrospect. In addition, the neonatal presentation is characterized by abdominal distention and bilious vomiting, both nonspecific signs of intestinal obstruction. About half the patients with Hirschsprung disease in the United States are diagnosed in the neonatal period; most of the remainder are discovered before the age of 2 years. In older children or in the occasional adult, Hirschsprung disease may be discovered during evaluation for chronic constipation.

Symptoms range from minimal to disabling, but chronic abdominal distention is characteristic. Malnutrition and failure to thrive may also be seen, but these are relatively uncommon in developed countries.

The physical examination of patients with Hirschsprung disease is nondiagnostic, although the rectal examination may be helpful. Spasm of the rectum on the initial digital examination may be discernible to an experienced clinician. If present, enterocolitis may be associated with characteristic forceful decompression of gray liquid stool at the time of rectal examination.

Ten to 30% of children with Hirschsprung disease develop enterocolitis, and this may be the initial clinical presentation. This event is characterized by an inflammatory process involving the colon. Although the pathogenesis is unknown, stasis and bacterial overgrowth are thought to be important contributors. *C difficile* has been implicated as an important pathogenic organism[76]; diagnostic and treatment plans should therefore take this possibility into consideration. The early clinical presentation of Hirschsprung enterocolitis includes fever, abdominal distention, and diarrhea, which may be explosive, distinctively malodorous, and bloody. Systemic sepsis, transmural intestinal necrosis, and perforation are all possible later findings. The clinical progression can be rapid, with death in as few as 12 to 24 hours if untreated. Infants appear particularly vulnerable to this complication of Hirschsprung disease, and it continues to have a 25% to 30% mortality rate. Enterocolitis accounts for virtually all Hirschsprung disease–induced mortality in modern pediatric surgical practice. Treatment of Hirschsprung enterocolitis consists of intravenous fluid resuscitation, broad-spectrum antibiotic treatment, possibly colonic irrigation, and intestinal decompression with an appropriate enterostomy, usually a colostomy proximal to the transition zone.

Diagnosis

Because mortality for Hirschsprung disease is essentially confined to the undiscovered neonate or infant who develops enterocolitis, every effort should be made to establish this diagnosis in the newborn period. Although predictable radiographic and manometric findings do occur, any infant suspected of having Hirschsprung disease must have a rectal biopsy performed.

Plain Abdominal Radiographs. In the neonate with Hirschsprung disease, air-filled and distended bowel typically occupies the entire abdomen on plain radiograph. This is a nonspecific finding, and because the small intestine and large intestine are not easily differentiated on plain films at this age, it is simply indicative of distal bowel obstruction. The older child may have a feces-filled megacolon on plain film, but this too is nonspecific. Pneumatosis intestinalis may accompany enterocolitis. Because plain films are nonspecific, they are never sufficient when Hirschsprung disease is suspected.

Contrast Enema. A contrast enema generally should follow plain radiographs when a distal bowel obstruction is present in an infant. The neonatal enema is performed without a rectal balloon to minimize the risks of perforating or obscuring the rectal findings. In older children, the enema should be obtained with an unprepared colon because conventional laxative and enema preparations temporarily eliminate or obscure the transition zone. The classic radiographic finding with Hirschsprung disease is that of a transition zone (Fig. 103-31). This may not be apparent in the neonate because proximal dilation requires some time to develop. In addition, short-segment aganglionosis and total colonic involvement may not have obvious transitions. In these cases, a lateral view of the rectum is usu-

ally abnormal, classically showing spasm with a unique spiculated appearance (see Fig. 103-31*B*). Barium retained in the colon more than 24 hours after a contrast study may also indicate Hirschsprung disease. In general, Hirschsprung disease can be detected by barium enema with a high degree of certainty in newborns as well as older children. It is not sufficient, however, to initiate surgical treatment without histologic confirmation of the diagnosis.

Rectal Biopsy. Rectal biopsy is the diagnostic standard for Hirschsprung disease and should always be obtained. A suction biopsy using one of several commercially available instruments can be obtained routinely in a clinic or at the bedside without anesthesia in all newborns and children up to several years of age. The requirement for neonatal diagnosis and the technical simplicity of the procedure dictate liberal use in all suspected or at-risk infants. Indeed, when suction biopsy is used appropriately, 85% to 90% or more of infants who undergo the procedure do not have Hirschsprung disease. The potential complications of bleeding and rectal perforation are rare and should not dissuade one from an aggressive diagnostic approach. Using the suction technique, a biopsy of mucosa and submucosa is obtained. This is sufficient to establish the diagnosis because ganglion cells are absent from all intramural plexuses in patients with Hirschsprung disease. The biopsy must be taken between 2 and 3 cm proximal to the pectinate line because of normal physiologic hypoganglionosis in the most distal rectum. Full-thickness rectal biopsy under general anesthesia is reserved for older children and those in whom suction biopsy has been inadequate.

Involvement of an experienced pediatric pathologist is essential for this procedure to achieve maximal accuracy. The examination requires both a search for ganglion cells and evaluation of the axons of the myenteric neurons (Fig. 103-32). This may be done using either conventional techniques or histochemical staining for acetylcholinesterase, as illustrated. Similar histochemical techniques have been used to test for nitric oxide synthetase deficiency. The histochemical techniques have the advantage of providing an unequivocal positive finding rather than simply demonstrating the absence of ganglion cells in a small specimen. The overall accuracy of diagnosis for Hirschsprung disease can be 100% with a correctly done suction rectal biopsy and an experienced pediatric pathologist.[77]

Anorectal Manometry. As noted, characteristic manometric findings are demonstrable in most patients with Hirschsprung disease. This diagnostic approach has been adopted in many areas of the world, perhaps most successfully in Japan. Because of the general availability and absolute accuracy of the suction rectal biopsy technique, however, alternative approaches such as this have not achieved wide use in the United States.

Treatment

Although an occasional undiagnosed patient survives with tolerable symptoms until adolescence or adulthood, obstructive symptoms generally dictate that surgical decompression be provided immediately on discovery of Hirschsprung disease. The approach for the neonate is to obtain proximal diversion by means of a colostomy (or enterostomy if necessary) placed in normal, ganglionated intestine. The colostomy is usually provided as a loop in an effort to preserve marginal collateral vessels for the subsequent pull-through. For classic rectosigmoid disease, a leveling colostomy is typically placed just proximal to the transition zone after intraoperative mapping with sequential frozen-section biopsies. This approach is generally combined with a two-stage operative strategy, subse-

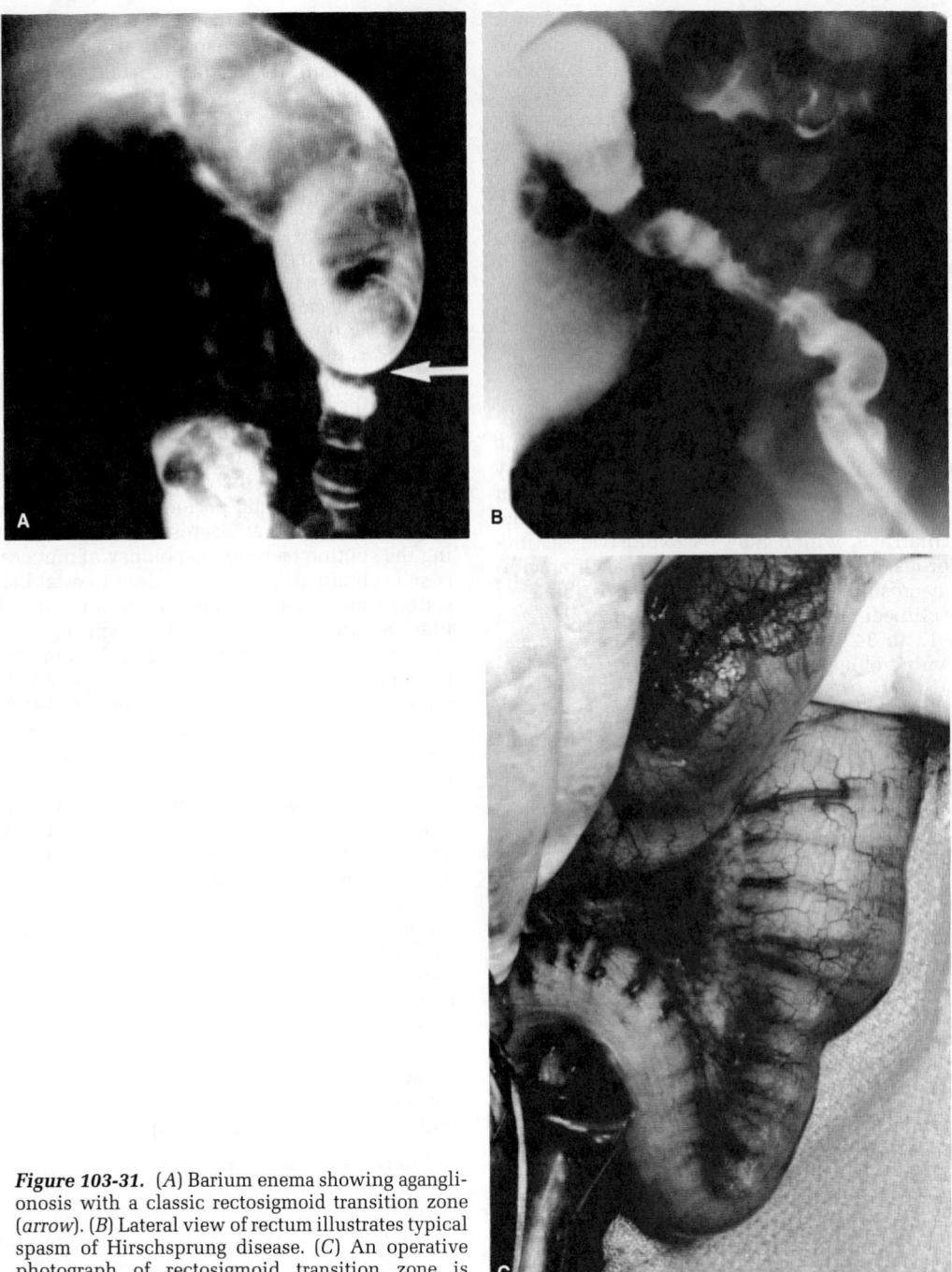

Figure 103-31. (*A*) Barium enema showing aganglionosis with a classic rectosigmoid transition zone (*arrow*). (*B*) Lateral view of rectum illustrates typical spasm of Hirschsprung disease. (*C*) An operative photograph of rectosigmoid transition zone is shown.

quently performing the definitive pull-through operation without proximal diversion. A right transverse colostomy may also be done after confirming the presence of ganglion cells at this site. This approach is usually selected when a three-stage approach is planned, leaving the proximal colostomy for a separate operative closure after the definitive pull-through procedure is completed.

The strategy has generally been to provide diversion in neonates until about 9 to 12 months of age or in older children until the colon is decompressed to about normal caliber. After this, a definitive pull-through procedure is done. More recently, a one-stage approach has been advocated that involves performing a pull-through procedure at the time of discovery without proximal diversion. This has been applied to neonates as well as older infants if the caliber of the colon

is sufficiently small.[78] Results among the three different approaches appear roughly equivalent when patients are carefully selected. A limited experience using laparoscopic technique for definitive endorectal pull-through in neonates has been reported.[79]

For children presenting with enterocolitis, colon irrigation for decompression can be an acceptable temporizing measure while resuscitation and broad-spectrum antibiotics are provided. Proximal diversion is still required promptly but is best done when the patient is not systemically toxic.

Definitive Operations for Hirschsprung Disease

Definitive operations for congenital aganglionosis all depend on resection or bypass of the distal aganglionic rectum in conjunction with a low rectal anastomosis to nor-

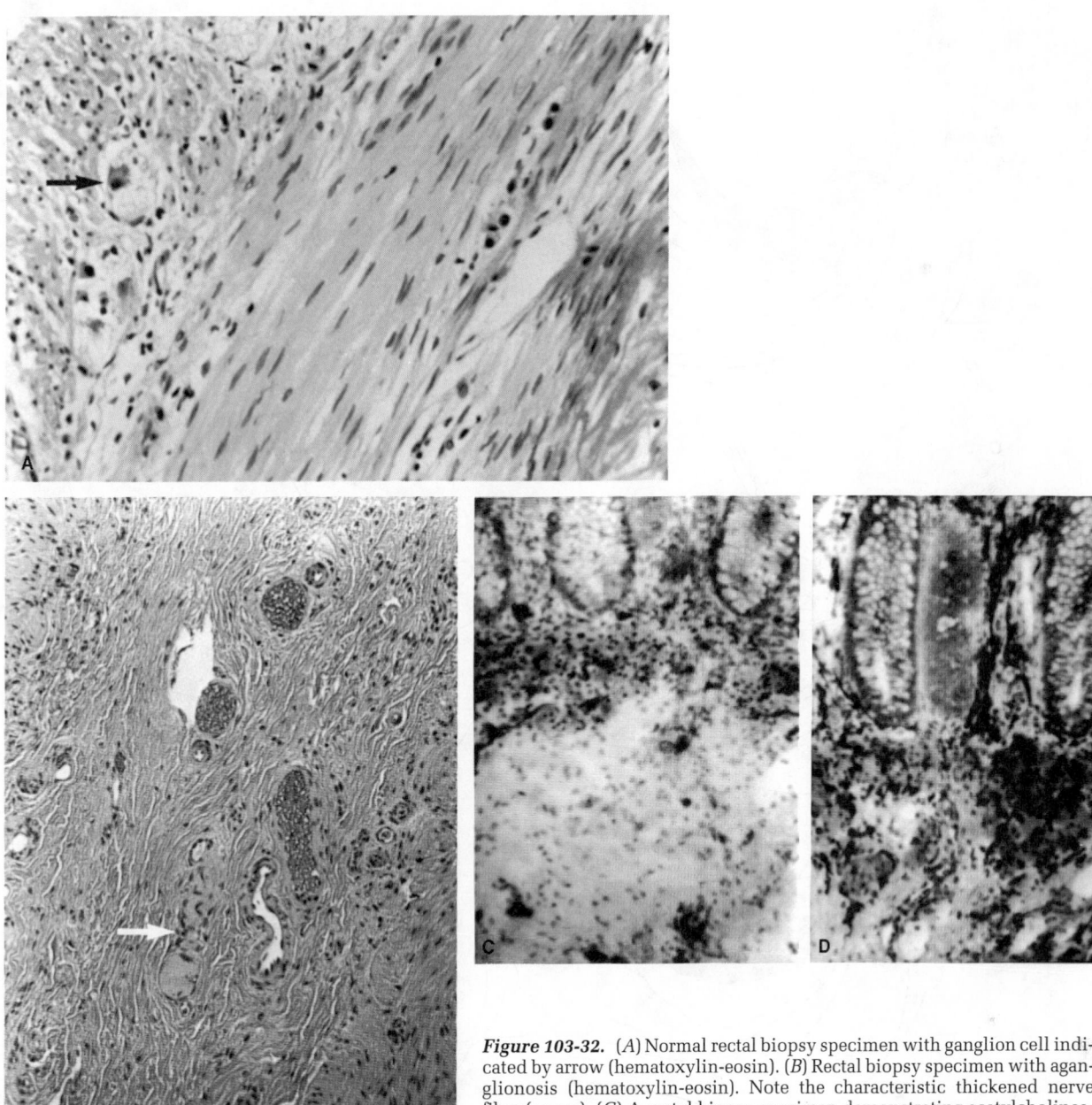

Figure 103-32. (*A*) Normal rectal biopsy specimen with ganglion cell indicated by arrow (hematoxylin-eosin). (*B*) Rectal biopsy specimen with aganglionosis (hematoxylin-eosin). Note the characteristic thickened nerve fiber (*arrow*). (*C*) A rectal biopsy specimen demonstrating acetylcholinesterase histochemical staining in a normal patient. (*D*) Similarly stained specimen from a patient with Hirschsprung disease. Many thickened submucosal nerve fibers stain densely black.

mally innervated pulled-through proximal intestine. Because the eponymous references are indelibly fixed in the literature and in daily use, they are reviewed here briefly. The principal procedures were described by Duhamel, Soave, and Swenson. Generally, selection among these depends on a surgeon's individual training and preference rather than compelling differences in outcome.[80]

Duhamel Procedure (Martin Modification). The Duhamel procedure is illustrated in Figure 103-33. After a minimal pelvic dissection, resection of aganglionic colon is done. A retrorectal pull-through of normally innervated proximal colon is performed, and the aganglionic rectum is left in situ. A colorectal anastomosis is performed. The original operation left the defunctionalized rectal pouch as shown, and this proved problematic. The procedure has since been modified by Martin to include a long side-to-

side colorectal anastomosis, variants of which are now considered standard around the world. Advantages of this procedure include its relative ease and the limited pelvic dissection. Adoption of the stapled anastomosis has simplified this procedure significantly.

Soave Procedure. The Soave procedure is illustrated in Figure 103-34. After resection of aganglionic bowel, an endorectal dissection in the submucosal plane is performed from the proximal rectum to the anus. This endorectal dissection is generally straightforward and technically much more simple than the similar dissection in a patient with ulcerative colitis. Normal proximal bowel is pulled through the residual rectal muscular cuff, and an anastomosis is performed to the most distal rectum, usually after everting the dissected rectal mucosal tube onto the perineum. Although the original report described a

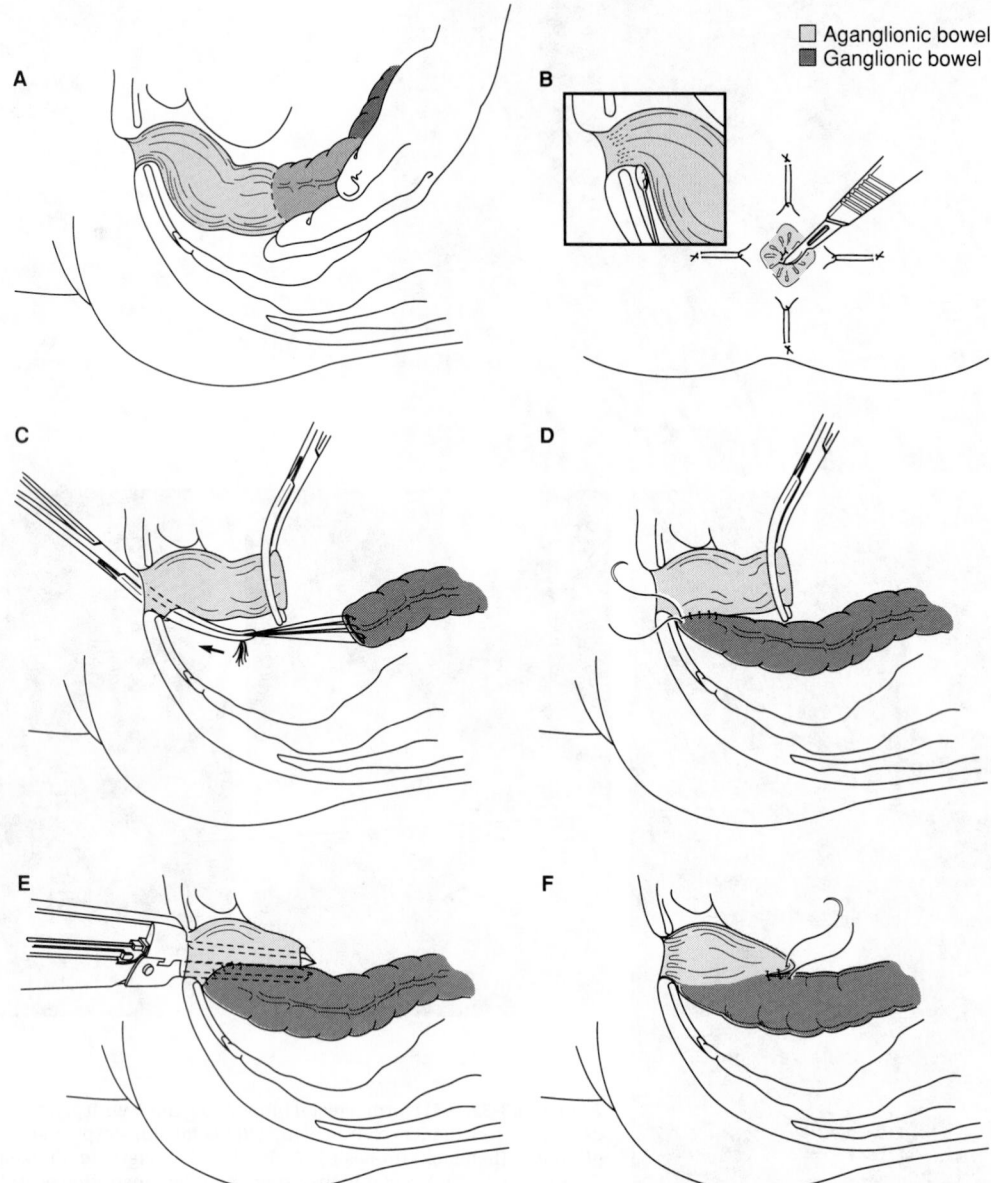

☐ Aganglionic bowel
■ Ganglionic bowel

Figure 103-33. Duhamel procedure (Martin modification). (*A*) Blunt retrorectal dissection. (*B*) Incision in the posterior wall of the aganglionic rectum. (*C*) Retrorectal pull-through after resection of aganglionic segment. (*D*) End-to-side colorectal anastomosis preserving aganglionic rectum (as originally described). (*E* and *F*) Stapled conversion of anastomosis into an extended side-to-side colorectal anastomosis (Martin modification).

pull-through without a formal anastomosis, this is essentially always done now using a conventional sutured anastomosis. This procedure is roughly equivalent to the Duhamel procedure in terms of ease, operative time, and outcome.

Swenson Procedure. Although the Swenson procedure was the original curative pull-through procedure for Hirschsprung disease, it has fallen into relative disfavor because it appears to be technically more problematic and to have a higher incidence of postoperative complications, particularly enterocolitis. It can be predictably curative, however, if precisely done. The fundamentals include resection of aganglionic colon, then careful and nearly complete extramural rectal dissection with a pull-through of

normal proximal bowel, followed by an anastomosis of colon to low rectum. The anastomosis is done on the perineum after full-thickness eversion of the dissected rectum (Fig. 103-35).

Laparoscopically Assisted Endorectal Pull-Through. A limited experience with an endoscopically assisted primary neonatal endorectal pull-through has been reported. The early results suggest an outcome similar to those of the well-established procedures. The procedure is shown in Figure 103-36.

Rectal Myectomy. Rectal myectomy for Hirschsprung disease refers to the resection of a longitudinal strip of the posterior muscular wall of the rectum. This procedure has

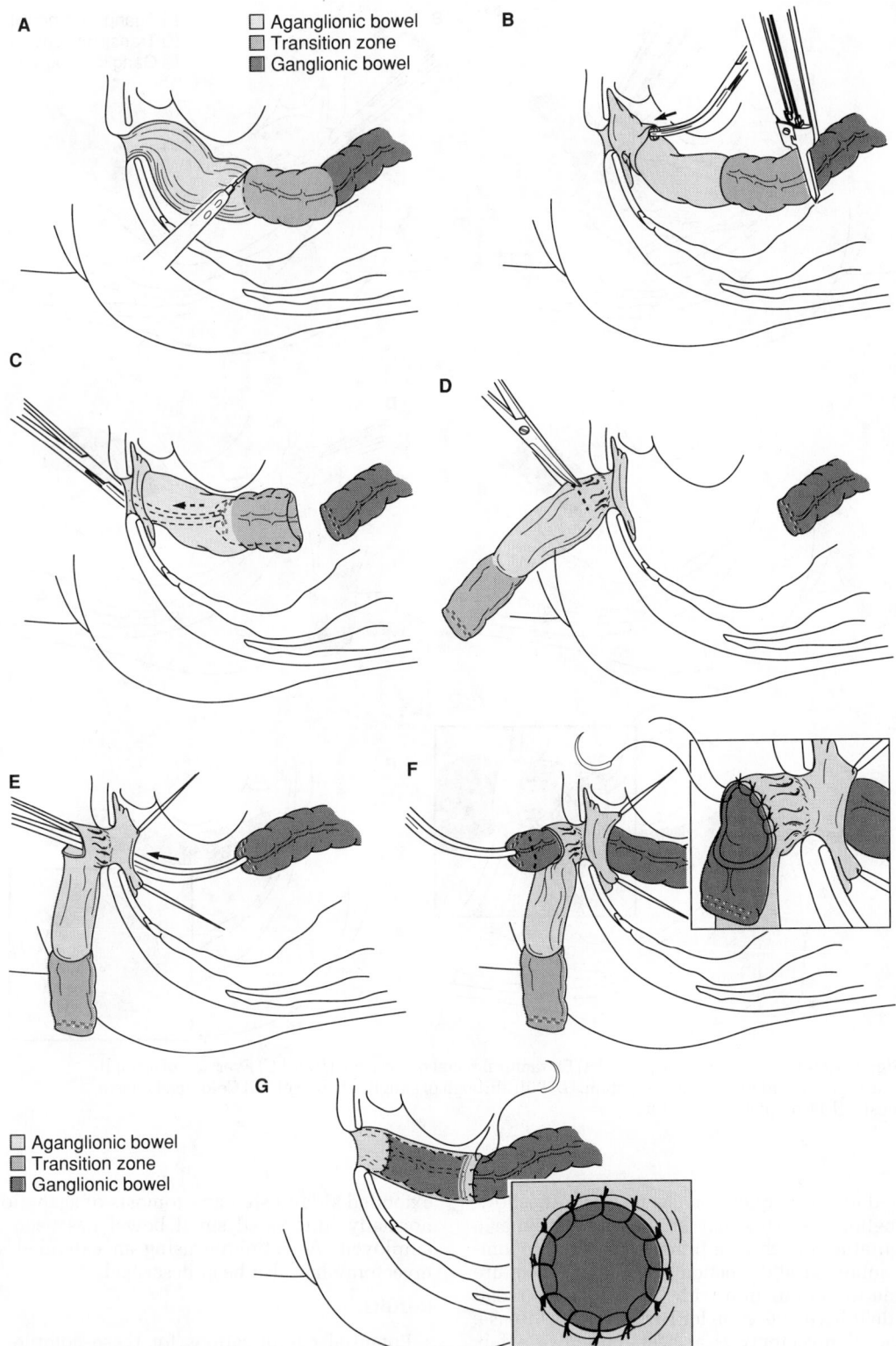

Figure 103-34. Soave (endorectal) procedure. (*A*) Endorectal dissection initiated. (*B*) Endorectal dissection complete. (*C*) Eversion of aganglionic segment and rectal mucosal tube. (*D*) Incision of everted rectal tube. (*E*) Endorectal pull-through. (*F*) Colorectal anastomosis. (*G*) Completed procedure.

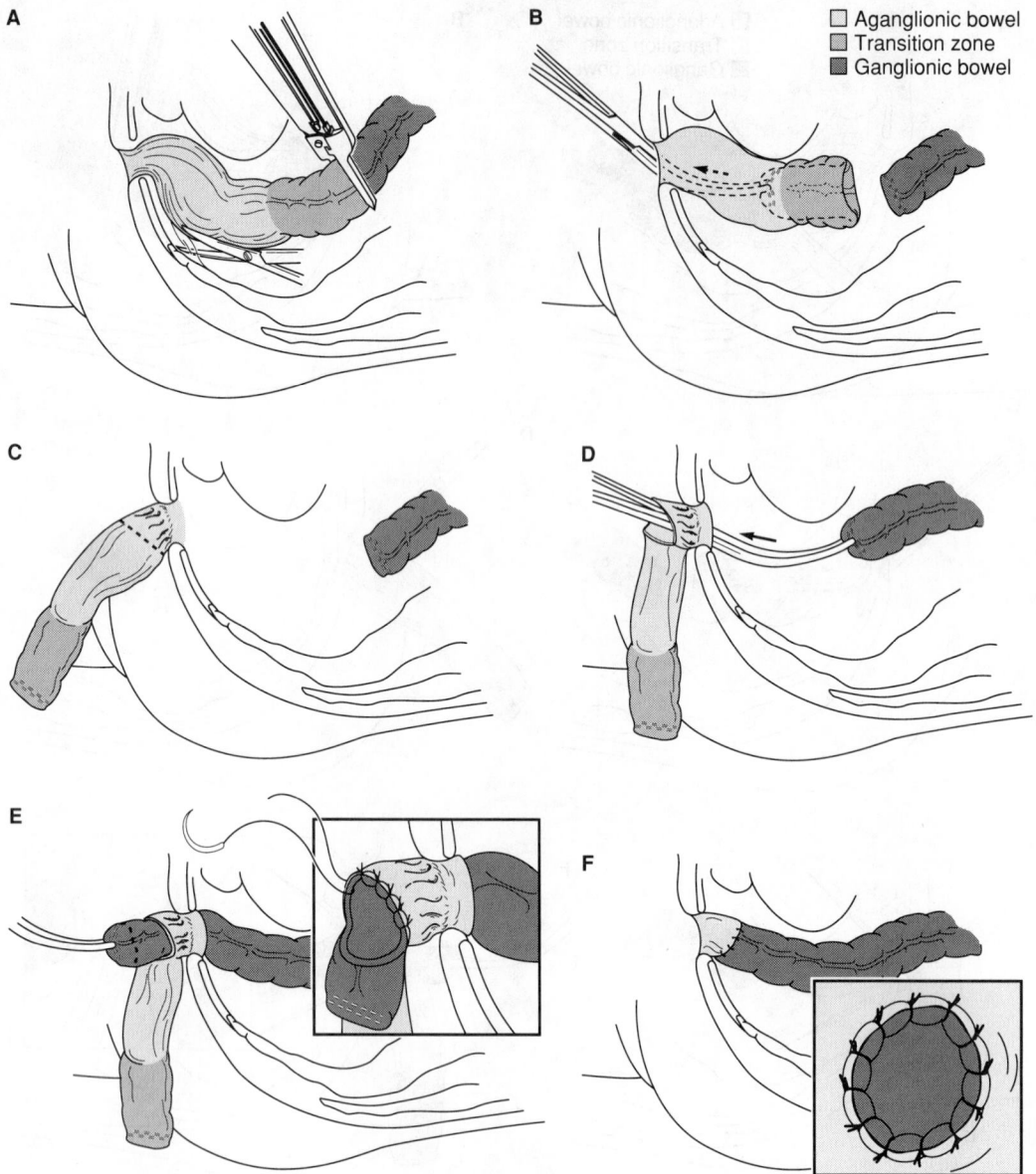

Figure 103-35. Swenson procedure. (*A*) Extramural rectal dissection. (*B* and *C*) Eversion of aganglionic segment and full-thickness rectum. (*D*) Pull-through of ganglionic bowel. (*E*) Colorectal anastomosis. (*F*) Completed procedure.

been advocated for the surgical management of ultrashort-segment aganglionosis. This may be done using either a posterior sagittal approach or a transanal approach combined with a submucosal dissection. This latter procedure has been done in conjunction with the diagnostic rectal biopsy. As a definitive operation for Hirschsprung disease, the role of rectal myectomy is at best limited to a few patients with ultrashort-segment aganglionosis. Many experienced pediatric surgeons believe that it has no role at all. Available data are too limited for an objective evaluation.

Total Colonic Aganglionosis

Total colonic aganglionosis is a complex and rare disorder. Several different operative procedures are described, and each patient is best considered individually. The endorectal pull-through with ileoanal anastomosis has been used with good success when most or all of the small bowel is preserved. For extensive small bowel aganglionosis, an extended side-to-side anastomosis of aganglionic colon to normally innervated small bowel has been successfully employed. A technique using an extended small bowel myectomy has also been described.

Results

Potential complications for these complex procedures include the entire spectrum of problems seen in GI surgery. The following problems occur (with their approximate incidence): anastomotic leak, 5%; anastomotic stricture, 5% to 10%; intestinal obstruction, 5%; pelvic abscess, less than 5%; and other wound problems, 10%. In experienced hands, these generic complications occur with roughly equal frequency for each of the operations. Mortality is rare from Hirschsprung disease in modern practice unless enterocolitis is a presenting clinical feature or there is some associated problem, such as cardiac disease. Some clinical series report no mortality attributable directly to Hirschsprung disease.

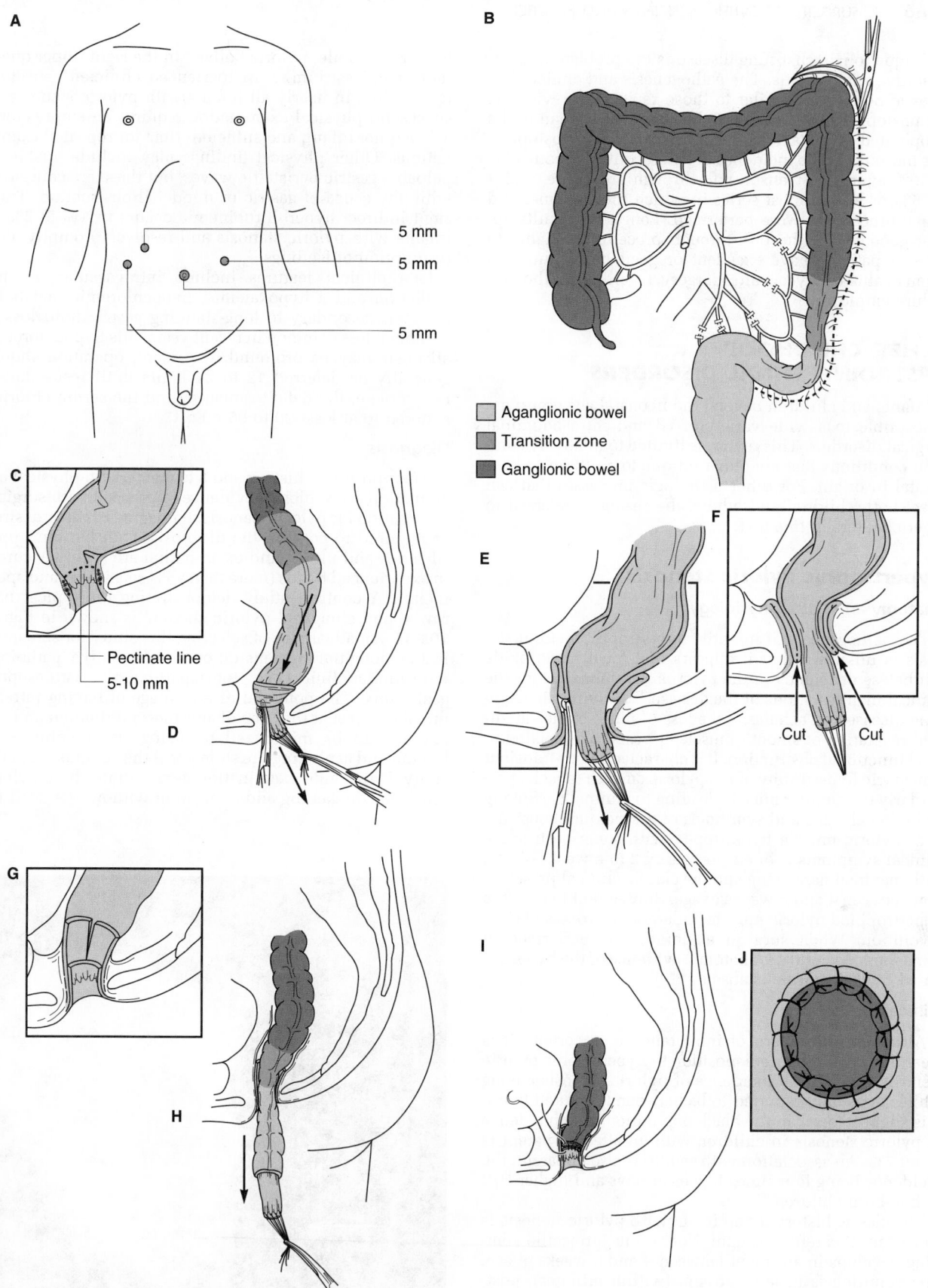

Figure 103-36. The technique for laparoscopically assisted pull-through for Hirschprung disease is shown. (*A*) Insertion sites for trocars. (*B*) Division of colon and rectal mesentary with mobilization of proximal colon. (*C*) A circumferential incision is made in the rectal mucosa 5 to 10 mm cephalad to the pectinate liver. (*D*) Transanal traction sutures are placed in the mucosa to facilitate dissection from the muscular rectal cuff. (*E*) The transanal submucosal dissection is continued cephalad to meet the caudal extent of the transperitoneal rectal mobilization. (*F*) An incision is placed in the rectal muscular cuff posteriorly to meet the dissection from above, and this is extended circumferentially. (*G*) The rectal cuff is split posteriorly down to the planned anastomotic site to accommodate the ganglionated colon pulled down through the cuff. (The pulled-through colon is not shown here to clarify this maneuver.) (*H*) The rectum and sigmoid colon are pulled down through the rectal cuff to the anastomotic site. (*I*) Control of appropriate mesenteric blood supply and full-thickness biopsy specimen for frozen section are obtained transanally. The colon is transected at an appropriate site in normal ganglionated bowel, and a transanal single layer end-to-end anastomosis is done. (*J*) The completed anastomosis.

Unique to Hirschsprung disease is the problem of postoperative enterocolitis. The pathogenesis and clinical features appear to be similar to those reviewed previously, but postoperatively, it tends to be less virulent than in the unoperated patients. It is an important cause of postoperative morbidity. The incidence of enterocolitis is about 15% to 30% after the Swenson pull-through procedure, and it is 15% or less in most series in which the Duhamel and Soave procedures were performed. Long-term results appear good for all the pull-through procedures. Eighty to 90% of patients have excellent or good bowel function when evaluated 5 years after surgery, regardless of the procedure employed.

OTHER CHILDHOOD GASTROINTESTINAL DISORDERS

Infants and children beyond the neonatal age group are susceptible to a wide variety of GI and intraabdominal surgical disorders. This review is limited to relatively common conditions that are either unique to children or congenital in origin. For other pathologic processes that can affect both children and adults, the reader is referred to other chapters in this text.

Hypertrophic Pyloric Stenosis

Anatomy and Pathophysiology

The pathogenesis of infantile hypertrophic pyloric stenosis is unknown, but it appears that focal nitric oxide synthetase deficiency in the pylorus is responsible for the clinical manifestations of the disease.[81] As with Hirschsprung disease and achalasia, the loss of nitric oxide–mediated relaxation of smooth muscle appears to be related to focal functional obstruction. It is characterized by transient concentric hypertrophy of the pyloric smooth muscle, particularly the circular muscle, leading to luminal narrowing and clinical signs and symptoms of gastric outlet obstruction. Pyloric muscle hypertrophy with some obstructive clinical symptoms is often present by 2 to 4 weeks of age, with maximal narrowing and the classic clinical presentation between 4 and 8 weeks of age. Subsequent to this, the hypertrophied pyloric muscle undergoes a process of slow involution. When surgical exploration is performed at some remote later date, anatomic evidence of the hypertrophied pyloric muscle is absent.

Clinical Presentation

Although the pattern of inheritance is uncertain, it is clear that a familial predisposition to hypertrophic pyloric stenosis occurs. The incidence of pyloric stenosis among whites is usually reported to be between 0.1% and 0.4%; it is slightly lower in the black population. The incidence of pyloric stenosis in children with an affected parent is about 7%. An association with gender is also apparent, the incidence being four times higher in boys and higher still in first-born children.[82]

The classic history for an infant with pyloric stenosis is consistent if carefully sought. Nonbilious, projectile vomiting develops in an infant between 4 and 6 weeks of age. The vomiting is usually prompt (within minutes), postprandial, and progressive. Cessation of feedings typically eliminates the vomiting. The infant appears generally well and feeds eagerly until late in the course. Presentation is rarely outside of a period between 2 weeks and 3 months of age. In retrospect, most afflicted infants have progressive feeding intolerance, the onset of which predates diagnosis by a number of days.

The pathognomonic physical finding is that of a palpable, firm, mobile, pyloric "olive" in the right upper quadrant or epigastrium. An experienced clinician can elicit this finding in nearly all infants with pyloric stenosis. A successful physical examination requires an empty stomach, a quiet infant, and sufficient time for repeated examinations. Other physical findings may include visible or palpable gastric peristaltic waves, but these are consistent with any cause of gastric or duodenal obstruction. Transient indirect hyperbilirubinemia occurs in 1% to 2% of infants with pyloric stenosis and resolves promptly after resumption of feedings.

Late clinical features include intravascular volume depletion and a hypokalemic, hypochloremic metabolic alkalosis secondary to long-standing gastric fluid losses. Although less common in recent years, this hypochloremic alkalosis may be profound. If present, operation should generally be deferred 12 to 24 hours until resuscitation is complete, the deficit replaced, and the serum chloride restored to at least 90 to 95 mEq/L.

Diagnosis

An appropriate history and a characteristic physical examination are sufficient evidence to proceed with surgical exploration for pyloric stenosis. If imaging is either desired or required to confirm the diagnosis, both barium upper GI series and ultrasound examination are highly accurate in experienced hands (more than 95% sensitivity and specificity). A contrast study demonstrating the typical narrowed and elongated pyloric channel is shown in Figure 103-37. An advantage of selecting this study for screening is the potential demonstration of alternative pathology with similar clinical symptoms, particularly gastroesophageal reflux. The potential disadvantage of having intraluminal contrast at the time of anesthesia induction and operation can be minimized by using small volumes of barium and aspirating the stomach at the conclusion of the study. Ultrasound examination demonstrates both pyloric muscular thickening and elongation without the need for

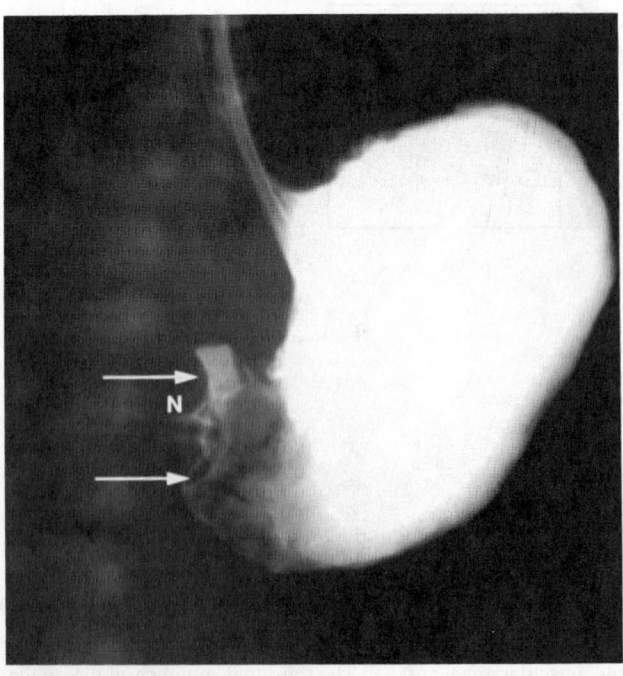

Figure 103-37. Hypertrophic pyloric stenosis is reliably diagnosed with a barium upper gastrointestinal series showing pyloric channel narrowing (N) and elongation with antral shouldering (*arrows*).

irradiation or intragastric barium and is preferred in many institutions.

Treatment

The pyloric muscular hypertrophy is known to be transient, and nonoperative treatment of pyloric stenosis has been successfully achieved using both long-term enteral and parenteral hyperalimentation. From a practical standpoint, however, the potential morbidity and the predictable cost preclude this approach. The Ramstedt pyloromyotomy has achieved essentially universal acceptance because it is curative in virtually all infants with negligible morbidity (Fig. 103-38). The procedure is performed when the patient is adequately resuscitated and hypochloremia and hypokalemia corrected. The operation is straightforward. The hypertrophied pylorus is delivered through a limited right upper quadrant incision. The pyloromyotomy consists of a single longitudinal incision in the hypertrophied pyloric muscle. It is necessary to divide all the hypertrophied circular muscle from the normal stomach to the junction with the proximal duodenum. Adequacy of the pyloromyotomy is demonstrated with herniation of the submucosa into the myotomy site (see Fig. 103-38).

Postoperative care is predictably uneventful, and feedings generally can be resumed within 6 to 8 hours after operation. Nasogastric suction is not required. Most patients are discharged from the hospital within 24 hours of operation. Postoperative complications are rare and generally represent technical failures related either to an inadequate pyloromyotomy or inadvertent entry into the duodenum or stomach. Avoidance of the former requires meticulous division of the entire segment of hypertrophied muscle. Rarely, repeat pyloromyotomy (on the posterior

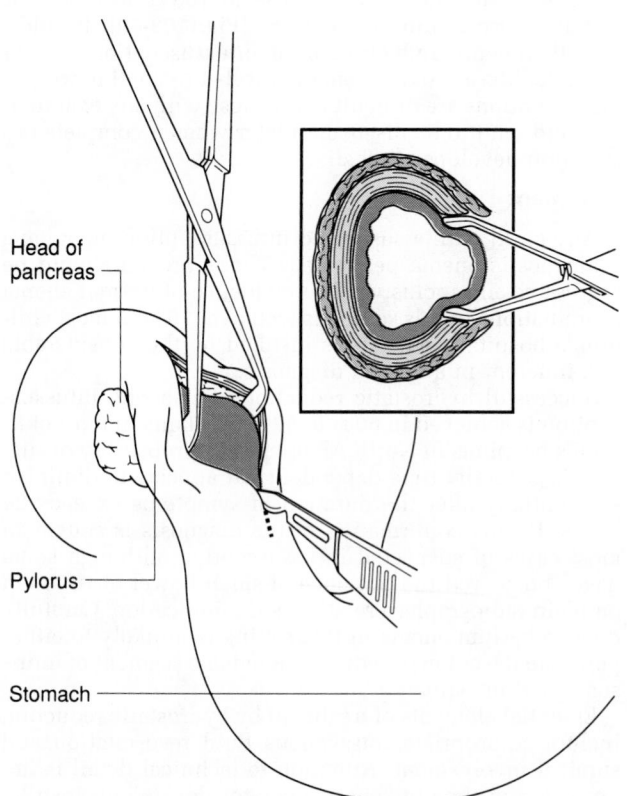

Figure 103-38. A pyloromyotomy. The cross-sectional view shows herniation of the submucosa into the myotomy site, indicative of an adequate myotomy.

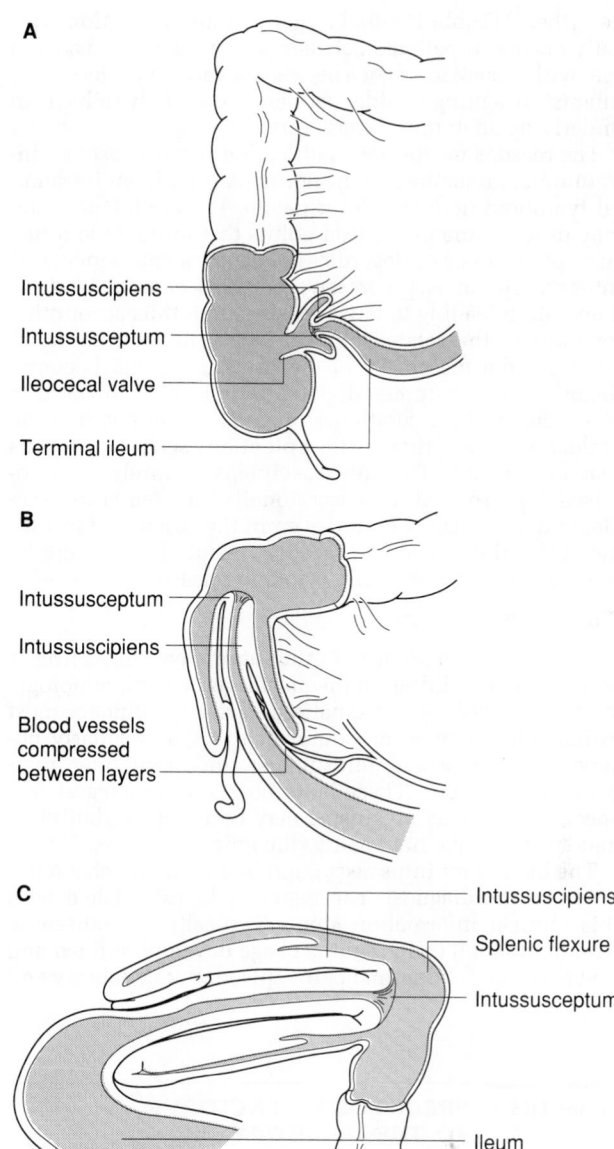

Figure 103-39. Ileocolic intussusception is shown, with intussusceptum and intussuscipiens indicated.

pyloric wall) may be required. Inadvertent duodenotomy or gastrotomy is also rare but easily repaired if recognized. Mortality should be essentially nonexistent in these infants in the absence of concurrent associated illness.

Intussusception

Anatomy and Pathophysiology

Intussusception is defined as the invagination of a proximal segment of intestine into an adjacent distal segment (Fig. 103-39). The invaginated proximal bowel is referred to as the *intussusceptum,* and the recipient distal bowel is the *intussuscipiens.* This process usually originates in the small intestine, typically at or near the ileocecal valve, causing passage of the terminal ileum through the ileocecal valve into the colon (ileocolic intussusception). In 95% of cases, no intrinsic anatomic abnormality is found (idiopathic intussusception), although many associations are described[25] (Table 103-6). Idiopathic intussusception typically occurs in patients between 3 months and 3 years of age, with a peak incidence between 6 and 9 months of age. Infants presenting at older ages are more likely to have an underlying anatomic abnormality.

The reasons for the age predilection remain obscure. Intraluminal projections of the normally prominent intramural lymphoid nodules (Peyer patches) in the infant ileum may provide functional lead points that initiate the intussusception process. Regardless of cause, a consequence of intussusception is progressive edema formation and inflammation leading to bowel obstruction, thus accounting for most of the related clinical signs and symptoms. In addition, the mesentery of the intussusceptum becomes distorted and compressed, potentially leading to vascular insufficiency. Incarceration, strangulation, and perforation of the intussusceptum are the potentially serious problems that may result. The intussuscipiens is rarely compromised. Hyperpyrexia and occasionally bacteremia are associated with intussusception even in the absence of intestinal infarction. These probably result from bacterial translocation and systemic cytokine release.

Clinical Presentation

The clinical incidence of intussusception ranges from 1 to 4 per 1000 children in the most rigorous epidemiologic studies available. Referral patterns strongly influence most estimations. A male predominance (3:2) is regularly observed, and seasonal midsummer and midwinter incidence peaks occur. These latter observations suggest that specific infectious organisms may be involved, but clear data for this have not been forthcoming.

The history for intussusception is sufficiently characteristic that the diagnosis can regularly be established with this clinical information alone. Typically, an otherwise healthy infant 6 to 18 months of age develops sudden and severe colicky abdominal pain. Episodes of irritability and crying are associated with drawing the legs up onto the abdomen for several minutes during a 20- to 30-minute cycle. Between bouts of colic, the infant is often lethargic or sleepy. The unwary examiner may conclude that a sleeping infant who has a benign abdominal examination between bouts of colic is well, when in reality the child is simply exhausted. Vomiting occurs in most of these infants, and particularly in nonverbal younger children, this tends to be the principal presenting complaint. Intractable vomiting and abdominal distention associated with complete bowel obstruction are relatively late occurrences, generally requiring 24 hours or more to develop. Volume depletion may become profound in this circumstance. Guaiac-positive stool is present in most infants with intussusception (up to 90% to 95%) because of ischemic mucosal injury to the intussusceptum. Hematochezia is less common, but classically, blood mixed with mucus (currant-jelly stool) may be passed. Physical findings may include a palpable, sausage-shaped mass in the right upper quadrant in as many as 80% to 90% of patients, but this is often subtle and therefore not appreciated. The intussusceptum is occasionally palpable on rectal examination and may present with prolapse through the anus.

Diagnosis

Plain abdominal radiographs are generally nonspecific for intussusception. Early findings may include an empty right lower quadrant with a mass suggested in the region of the hepatic flexure. Late findings are those of mechanical small bowel obstruction with proximal distention and air-fluid levels. Ultrasound examination reliably demonstrates a mass with two lumens that resembles a bull's eye, corresponding to the intussusceptum within the intussuscipiens. Enthusiasm for this approach is limited because it only confirms the diagnosis without the therapeutic potential of an air or contrast enema. Both air and contrast enemas are diagnostic with close to 100% accuracy for classic ileocolic intussusceptions (Fig. 103-40). In addition, therapeutic reduction of the intussusception is often possible. More proximal small bowel-to-small bowel intussusceptions are difficult to diagnose with any examination and tend to be discovered later when a complete obstruction develops clinically.

Treatment

Any child with a suspected intussusception must have a diagnostic enema performed. The approach should be aggressive and inclusive. The incidence of normal enema examinations in this setting is well over 75% in most children's hospitals, but this is justified by the considerable risk inherent in a missed diagnosis.

Successful hydrostatic reduction of ileocolic intussusception is achieved in 60% to 80% of infants in most children's hospitals in North America. The probability of success is generally time dependent but appears to diminish substantially after the duration of symptoms exceeds 24 hours. Enema confirmation of the diagnosis is sought in most cases of suspected intussusception, although some have considered the presence of small bowel obstruction on plain radiographs a relative contraindication. Carefully done, a barium enema in this setting is unlikely to either perforate the colon or reduce a nonviable segment of intussuscepted intestine.

Essential elements of treatment by hydrostatic reduction include appropriate intravenous fluid resuscitation and surgical involvement. Attention to technical detail is important, and the outcome is operator dependent. Instillation of barium is through a balloon rectal catheter from a reservoir placed no more than 1 m above the patient. This should be continued or repeated as long as progressive

---

Table 103-6. PREDISPOSING FACTORS TO THE DEVELOPMENT OF INTUSSUSCEPTION

ANATOMIC LEAD POINTS
Meckel's diverticulum
Polyp
Hypertrophied Peyer patch
Appendix
Duplication or enteric cyst
Lymphoma
Other neoplasm
Ectopic pancreas

ASSOCIATED INFECTIONS
Adenovirus
Rotovirus
Others

BLEEDING DISORDERS*
Henoch-Schönlein purpura
Hemophilia
Leukemia

TRAUMA*
Blunt abdominal trauma
Major retroperitoneal operative procedures

OTHER
Cystic fibrosis

*These factors are more likely to be associated with small bowel-to-small bowel intussusception than with ileocolic intussusception.

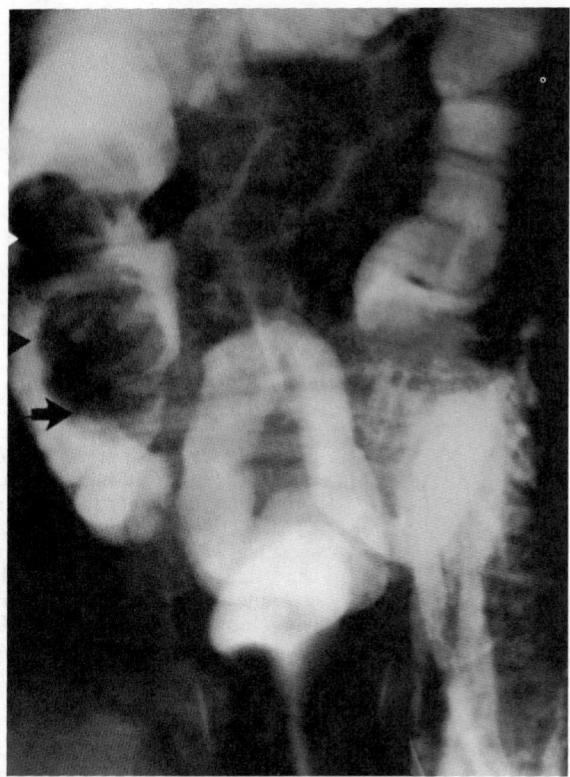

Figure 103-40. A barium enema demonstrates a classic ileocolic intussusception with the intussusceptum in the ascending colon (*arrows*).

reduction is achieved. Successful ileocolic intussusception reduction must be confirmed by demonstrating the free flow of contrast into the terminal small bowel. Inability to show this suggests incomplete reduction and mandates surgical exploration.

Air contrast enemas also may be used to diagnose and successfully treat intussusception. After reports from China of successful air pressure enema reductions of intussusception, many Western children's hospitals have adopted this approach. Done under fluoroscopic control with air pressure monitoring, the results appear comparable to the traditional hydrostatic reduction process.

Operative Management. Laparotomy is required immediately for either failed or uncertain enema reduction of an intussusception. The operative strategy is dictated by the findings. Spontaneous reduction of the intussusception occurs in up to 20% to 30% of children during the process of preparing for the operating room and administering general anesthesia. In this case, exploration confirming the reduction is sufficient. In the event that the intussusception persists and the bowel is viable, manual reduction of the intussusception is undertaken. If this cannot be done, or if the bowel is clearly necrotic, a segmental resection and primary anastomosis are done. When the bowel is clearly nonviable, attempts at reduction should be avoided to minimize the risk of perforation and allow a noncontaminated procedure. Exteriorization of the bowel is seldom required if this is done. Appendectomy is considered routine in all these infants who undergo operation.

Results

Hydrostatic or pneumatic reduction is successful in about 60% to 80% of infants with idiopathic ileocolic intussusception. Because the failure rate increases substantially after 24 hours, institutional success rates may reflect more about referral patterns than technical proficiency. Generally, a child is admitted to the hospital for 24 hours of intravenous fluids and possibly antibiotics after intussusception reduction. Recovery and the resumption of oral feedings is predictably straightforward. When a bowel resection is required, the course is several days but generally no different than for other similar GI procedures. Recurrence after either operative or hydrostatic reduction of an idiopathic intussusception occurs in about 5% of the infants. This problem can often be resolved with a repeat enema. Mortality from intussusception is rare in modern practice and is virtually always the result of systemic sepsis and hypovolemia secondary to neglected strangulated intestine.

Meckel's Diverticulum and Related Disorders

Embryology and Anatomy

The most frequent congenital anomaly of the GI tract is Meckel's diverticulum, one of several malformations that result from persistence of the embryonic yolk stalk. (Synonymous terms include the *vitelline duct* and the *omphalomesenteric duct*.) The embryonic yolk stalk connects the yolk sac and the developing midgut (Fig. 103-41). Involution normally occurs between the 5th and 7th gestational weeks as the yolk sac disappears and the stalk becomes fused with the umbilical cord. Failure or interruption of yolk sac involution creates a spectrum of anomalies dependent on the timing of the event. The possible structural variations are summarized in Figure 103-42. Ninety-five percent or more of the anomalies are Meckel's diverticula. The eponym describes a true diverticulum derived from the intestinal end of the yolk stalk, usually arising from the antimesenteric border of the small bowel in the terminal ileum. The site of origin is generally 40 to 50 cm proximal to the ileocecal valve in adults and proportionately closer in children. The size of the diverticulum is variable with regard to both length and diameter. The blood supply is derived from the persistent vitelline vessels, which are supplied from the SMA. Up to 25% of patients have attach-

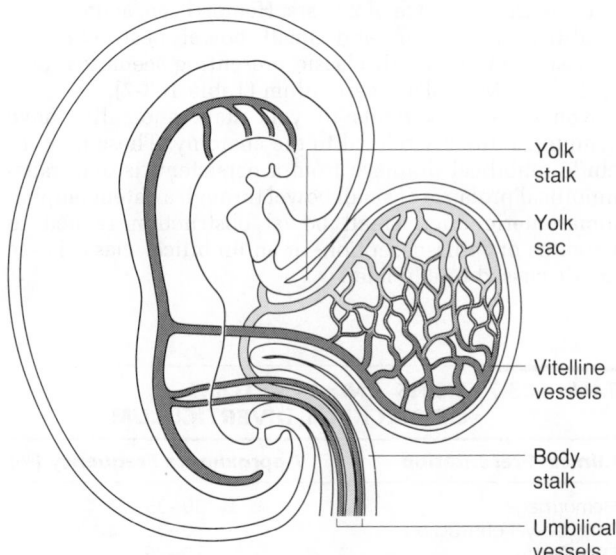

Figure 103-41. Normal embryologic relations of the embryonic yolk sac, yolk stalk, and gut.

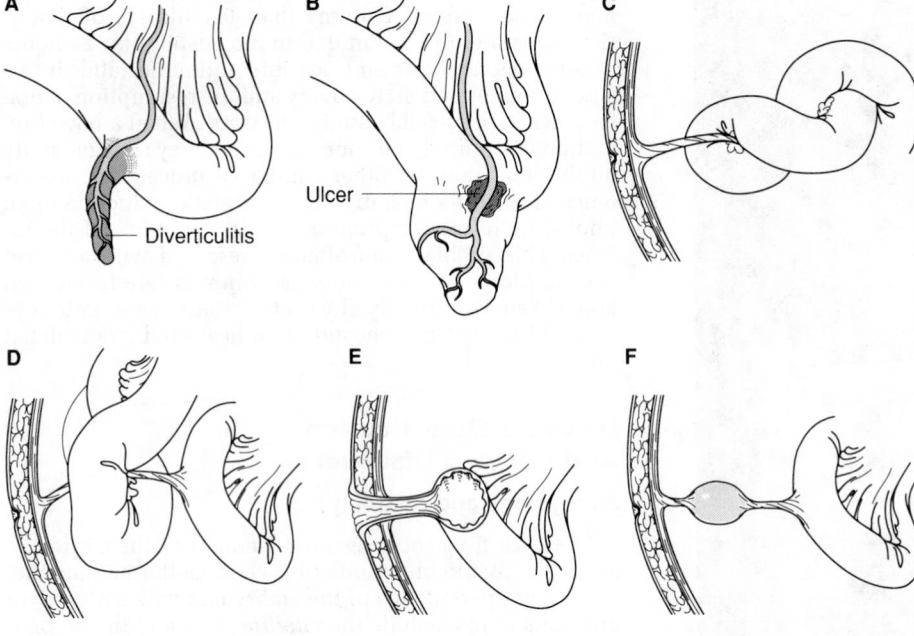

Figure 103-42. Common variants of yolk stalk malformations are illustrated. (*A* and *B*) Meckel diverticulum can result in symptoms from diverticulitis and acid-induced ulcer formation with hemorrhage. (*C* and *D*) Meckel diverticulum may be associated with an abdominal wall band that predisposes to volvulus and intestinal obstruction. (*E*) Patent omphalomesenteric duct. (*F*) Omphalomesenteric sinus and cyst.

ment of the Meckel's diverticulum to the anterior abdominal wall by means of a fibrous or vascular band at the umbilicus; the remainder are unattached.

In addition to the normal ileum, which comprises the diverticulum, heterotopic gastric mucosa or pancreatic tissue is found in about half the Meckel's diverticula examined at autopsy. Gastric mucosa is present in 75% of patients who develop symptoms referable to the diverticulum. Generally, symptoms result from peptic ulceration of adjacent ileal mucosa, leading to bleeding or perforation.

Clinical Presentation

The incidence of Meckel's diverticula is about 2% in the general population, with a 2:1 male/female predominance. Most of these people remain asymptomatic throughout life. Estimations of the frequency with which symptoms develop among people with Meckel's diverticula vary from 4% to 30%, but it is clear that the risk diminishes substantially with age. About half of those who become symptomatic are under the age of 2 years. Hemorrhage, acute diverticulitis, perforation, and small bowel obstruction or intussusception are all classic presenting scenarios for a child with Meckel's diverticulum (Table 103-7).

Non-Meckel's variants of yolk stalk anomalies have symptoms directly related to the anatomy. These may include umbilical drainage from a persistent fistula, transumbilical prolapse of small bowel through a patent omphalomesenteric duct, small bowel obstruction related to volvulus or intussusception, or an umbilical mass. These are discussed briefly later.

Hemorrhage. Hemorrhage related to Meckel's diverticulum results from acid-induced peptic ulcer disease involving the vulnerable adjacent ileal mucosa. The bleeding is typically painless and episodic, with the character of the rectal blood reflecting the rate of blood loss. Bright red or brick red rectal bleeding is characteristic and reflects relatively brisk bleeding, but Meckel's-associated hemorrhage is not often exsanguinating at the initial presentation. Melena is not characteristic. Confirmation of the diagnosis is best pursued with a ^{99m}Tc-pertechnetate radioisotope scan when the presenting symptom is hemorrhage. Because of the affinity of the isotope for gastric mucosa and the high probability that gastric acid–induced ulceration is responsible for the hemorrhage, the diagnostic accuracy is 90% or more in patients with Meckel's-related hemorrhage. Selective angiography may be diagnostic in the event that isotope scanning is unsuccessful and the hemorrhage active. Contrast studies of the small intestine and endoscopy are predictably unhelpful when the problem is hemorrhage related to a Meckel's diverticulum. Arteriovenous malformations, polyps, coagulopathic bleeding, intestinal duplications, and hemangiomas are all causes of GI hemorrhage that may share some clinical features with Meckel's-related hemorrhage.

Obstruction. Small bowel obstruction related to Meckel's diverticulum usually results from either intussusception or a volvulus around an attachment to the abdominal wall. Occasionally, other mechanical causes of obstruction related to peritoneal bands or hernias are encountered. Five to 10% of patients with symptomatic Meckel's diverticula present with intussusception. Of patients with Meckel's diverticula who present with small bowel obstruction, about half have intussusception, and the remainder have volvulus, internal hernias, or some other mechanical cause. Attempted hydrostatic reduction of intussusception associated with a Meckel's diverticulum has a reduced likelihood of success. For infants with Meckel's diverticulum–related small bowel obstruction, the correct diagnosis is usually obtained at laparotomy.

Diverticulitis. A long Meckel's diverticulum with a narrow base is predisposed to intraluminal obstruction. Distal inflammation, necrosis, and perforation may result in a manner analogous to that of acute appendicitis. Alter-

---

Table 103-7. SIGNS AND SYMPTOMS OF MECKEL'S DIVERTICULUM

Clinical Presentation	Approximate Frequency (%)
Hemorrhage	30–35
Small bowel obstruction	30–35
Diverticulitis	20–25
Umbilical fistula	10
Other	Uncommon

natively, free perforation of a Meckel's peptic ulcer may result in both local inflammation and diffuse peritonitis. Clinical signs and symptoms of Meckel's diverticulitis are virtually indistinguishable from those of acute appendicitis, and a correct diagnosis is rarely made preoperatively. In retrospective analyses of symptomatic Meckel's diverticulum patients, acute diverticulitis accounts for about one third of the presentations.

Umbilical Anomalies. Up to 10% of patients with Meckel's diverticula or yolk stalk remnants present with umbilical abnormalities. These may include a mucosal polyp mistaken for an umbilical granuloma, a patent omphalomesenteric duct, or other related cysts and sinuses. Intestinal mucosa or persistent drainage at the umbilicus are the usual clinical presentations of these lesions. The diagnosis is best established by intubation and contrast injection of any umbilical orifice or tract. Ultrasound examination may demonstrate cystic remnants of the yolk stalk. Surgical exploration of the umbilicus may be required to define the anatomy.

Meckel's Diverticulum as an Incidental Finding. The management of Meckel's diverticulum discovered coincidentally at laparotomy is controversial. The presence of heterotopic gastric mucosa is generally considered a clear indication for resection because of the frequency of associated complications related to peptic ulceration. This is detected simply by palpation because gastric mucosa is thicker than ileal mucosa. Attachment to the abdominal wall should be eliminated either by diverticulectomy or division of the appropriate intraperitoneal band. A relative indication for resection is the presence of a long diverticulum with a narrow orifice that is judged to be at risk for luminal obstruction. Patients younger than 2 years of age are at higher risk for developing Meckel's diverticulum–related complications, whereas adults are unlikely to do so. The decision whether to perform excision should include an assessment of the relative risks and the primary operative indications.

Treatment

Patients with umbilical abnormalities generally do not present with acute illness. Elective umbilical exploration and possibly laparotomy are performed. Excision of the yolk stalk remnant and appropriate primary bowel closure are the two principal goals. These are generally limited and straightforward procedures with little morbidity and essentially no mortality.

Many people with Meckel's diverticula remain asymptomatic and undiscovered, but the development of clinical symptoms is an absolute indication for surgical management. Exploration can be done through a variety of incisions, but if the diagnosis is anticipated, a transverse subumbilical incision provides excellent exposure. For the usual diverticulum, treatment consists simply of excision. This may be accomplished using either an antimesenteric wedge resection of the ileum or a segmental small bowel resection. Both procedures are accompanied by primary small bowel closure without enterostomy. Laparoscopic resection of Meckel's diverticulum has been described[83] and is no doubt appropriate in selected patients. As with most other children requiring GI surgery in modern practice, an excellent functional result with virtually no mortality is predictable in the absence of other medical problems.

Foreign Bodies

Foreign body ingestions among infants and children are usually the result of the natural processes of oral exploration and accidents rather than psychological disorders.

Most occur in the toddler age group, generally from 9 months to several years of age. The outcomes are generally benign despite the diverse nature of the objects involved. The location of the foreign body in the GI tract determines symptoms and dictates management.

Esophagus

Foreign bodies, such as coins and small toys, are commonly entrapped in the esophagus. Impaction usually occurs at the anatomically narrow esophageal segments, the cricopharyngeus, the site of the left main-stem bronchus, and the diaphragmatic hiatus (Fig. 103-43). Previous sites of esophageal surgery or injury are also potential points of foreign body lodgement. This is an important consideration in children with previous tracheoesophageal fistula repairs, gastroesophageal reflux, or caustic esophageal injuries.

Clinical symptoms are generally referable to esophageal obstruction. Unlike objects in the more distal GI tract, those entrapped in the esophagus generally produce symptoms such as drooling, dysphagia, and substernal chest pain. Longstanding foreign bodies and sharp or unusually configured objects may penetrate or erode through the esophagus so that mediastinitis may be the presenting clinical picture. The diagnosis is readily apparent on plain radiographs if the object is metallic or otherwise radiodense. Radiolucent foreign bodies usually require a barium swallow to confirm the diagnosis. A lateral view of the chest or neck may be helpful in differentiating esophageal and tracheal foreign bodies because of contrast provided by the intratracheal air column. Because the potential complications of untreated esophageal obstruction include aspiration, erosion, perforation, and late stricture, these foreign bodies must all be removed. Foreign body extraction is usually accomplished using either a balloon catheter under fluoroscopic control or endoscopic retrieval with direct visualization. Balloon catheter extraction has an overall success rate of about 75% if performed within 24 hours of the ingestion. Beyond this time, local inflammation and mucosal edema, coupled with the lack of direct visualization, make the technique problematic and potentially hazardous. Balloon extractions are generally limited to smooth objects such as coins that pose little risk of esophageal laceration during retrieval. The most important risk is the absence of airway control as the foreign body traverses the pharynx. For this reason, the procedure must be carefully performed in the prone position with adequate assistance and preparation to prevent secondary aspiration. Occasionally, it is appropriate to push vegetable, meat, or other irretrievable objects into the stomach and allow them to pass distally.

Endoscopic retrieval of esophageal foreign bodies is generally straightforward, although children usually require general anesthesia. Either flexible or rigid fiberoptic endoscopy systems may be used with predictable success and minimal morbidity. Modern instruments include foreign body forceps designed to grasp a variety of specific objects under direct vision (see Fig. 103-43). Esophageal perforation is the major risk of either of these extraction techniques but fortunately is uncommon, with an incidence of 5% or less in most reports.

Distal Gastrointestinal Tract

Passage of an ingested foreign body beyond the gastroesophageal junction is associated with a 95% probability of uneventful distal transit. The character of the foreign body is largely irrelevant with regard to this, but some specific exceptions are noted here. Generally, a radiodense foreign body in an asymptomatic patient can be followed with periodic abdominal radiographs for a number of weeks. The stool should be routinely screened to confirm passage of the foreign body. Empiric clinical guidelines

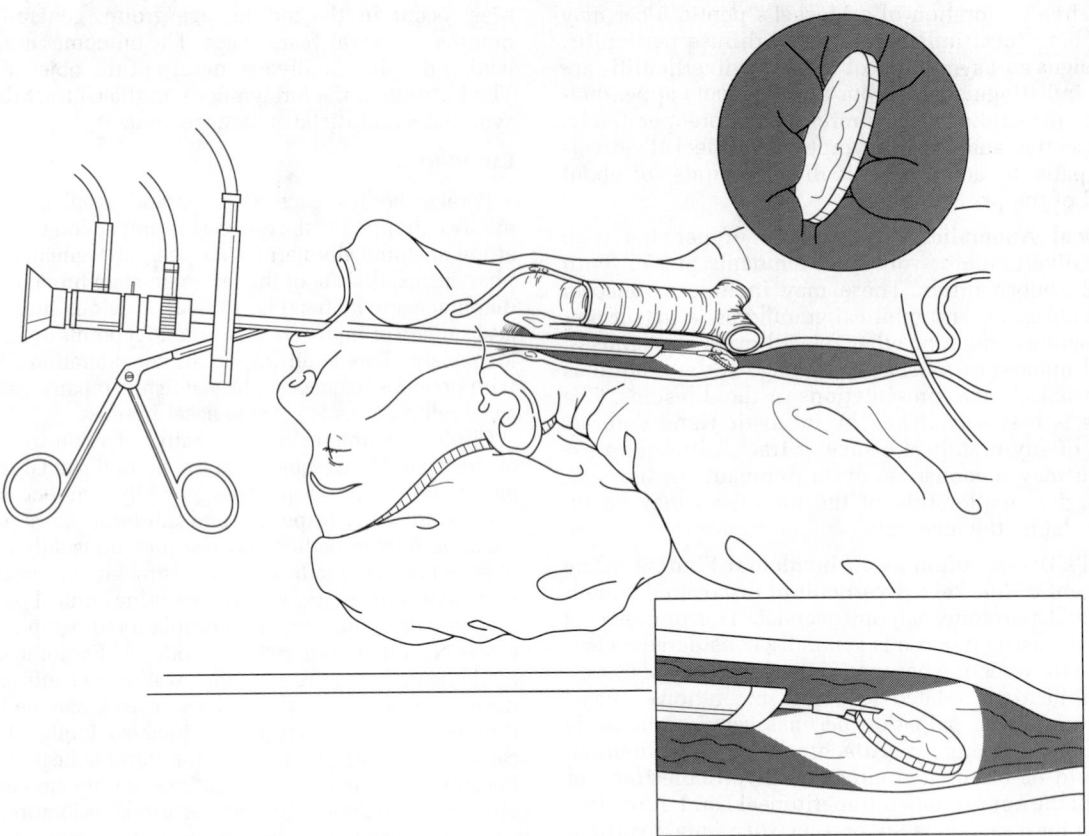

Figure 103-43. Schematic illustration of foreign body extraction from the esophagus. Foreign bodies typically become entrapped at the cricopharyngeus, at the point where the left main-stem bronchus narrows the adjacent esophagus, or at the diaphragmatic hiatus.

for undertaking open or endoscopic removal of distal GI foreign bodies are summarized:

1. The development of symptoms suggesting perforation, obstruction, or intestinal injury (pain, vomiting, fever, peritonitis) requires prompt foreign body removal.

2. Failure of an object to pass from the stomach into the small intestine within 3 to 4 weeks is a relative indication for endoscopic extraction. Objects with configurations that are exceptionally long, sharp, or judged unlikely to transverse the pylorus should be extracted endoscopically more promptly. This judgment is best reserved for the experienced pediatric surgeon because remarkably complex and improbable objects routinely transit the GI tract uneventfully.

3. Failure of a foreign body to continue to progress distally is a relative indication for intervention. One week or more in a fixed position suggests that erosion and perforation are possible.

4. Batteries, particularly alkaline disc batteries, present a potentially serious hazard to children and may require a more aggressive approach.[84] A number of reports have documented the unique risk of intestinal perforation resulting from disruption of the battery casing and associated spillage of the toxic contents. Although some have advocated routine immediate removal, this does not appear necessary. If the battery is endoscopically accessible in the esophagus, it should be removed when recognized. Cathartics and enemas may help expedite passage of batteries discovered when already in the small or large bowel.

Failure of distal progression for more than a few days, casing rupture on plain radiograph, or symptoms of any kind require extraction. Despite the risks, most batteries pass without these sequelae.

Gastrointestinal Hemorrhage

The general subject of GI hemorrhage is discussed in detail in Chapter 50. This brief review is designed to emphasize the principal clinical differences in the diagnostic approach to children and adults.[85] Management principles are discussed elsewhere. The causes of pediatric GI hemorrhage are diverse and age-dependent. Tables 103-8 and 103-9 summarize sites and sources of hemorrhage as they relate to age.

Neonates (0 to 30 Days)

A variety of rare structural lesions can produce upper GI hemorrhage in neonates, but the most common cause is gastritis. Fifty to 75% of neonates evaluated endoscopically for upper GI hemorrhage prove to have gastritis. About 10% of neonates have an underlying coagulopathy, and 10% to 15% have swallowed maternal blood in the process of parturition. Specific anatomic lesions for which surgical control of hemorrhage is required are rare (1% to 5%). The occasional peptic ulcer in this age group is almost invariably secondary to some other process, such as sepsis, congenital heart disease, steroid treatment, or intracranial hypertension.

Lower GI tract hemorrhage commonly takes the form of benign anorectal bleeding and, in the absence of other

Table 103-8. **CAUSES OF UPPER GASTROINTESTINAL HEMORRHAGE***

Patient Age Group	Common Causes	Less Common Causes
Neonate (0–30 d)	1. Gastritis 2. Esophagitis 3. Ingested maternal blood 4. Peptic ulcer	1. Iatrogenic trauma 2. Primary coagulopathy 3. Vascular malformations (hemangioma, telangiectasia, arteriovenous malformations) 4. Nasal or pharyngeal bleeding 5. Miscellaneous structural abnormalities (leiomyoma, gastric polyp, duplications)
Infant (30 d to 1 y)	1. Gastritis 2. Esophagitis 3. Peptic ulcer	Same as for neonate, with addition of: 1. Drugs (salicylates, steroids) 2. Foreign body or caustic ingestion 3. Esophageal varices
Child (1–12 y)	1. Esophageal varices 2. Esophagitis 3. Peptic ulcer	Same as for infant, with addition of: 1. Acquired thrombocytopenia (chemotherapy)
Older child and adolescent (12 y to adulthood)	1. Esophageal varices 2. Esophagitis 3. Peptic ulcer	Same as for child

* Order of appearance approximates clinical frequency
(Modified from Oldham KT, Lobe TE. Gastrointestinal hemorrhage in children. Pediatr Clin North Am 1985;32:1247)

symptoms in this age group, does not require aggressive investigation. NEC, malrotation, and an incarcerated hernia are potentially serious problems associated with lower GI tract bleeding. These situations are almost invariably associated with characteristic histories and physical findings that are discussed in detail elsewhere.

Infants (30 Days to 1 Year)

The likelihood of disease amenable to specific therapy is high enough in infants, unlike neonates, that an aggressive endoscopic investigation should be undertaken for upper GI tract hemorrhage. Specific lesions are considered in Table 103-8.

Intussusception and a bleeding Meckel's diverticulum must be considered when children of this age present with lower GI tract hemorrhage. The magnitude of blood loss associated with intussusception is usually minor, but the associated vomiting and bowel obstruction may lead to significant volume depletion with hemoconcentration. The magnitude of the hemorrhage is usually more significant with Meckel's diverticulum. Infectious diarrheas may also occur in this age group. Typically, signs and symptoms include fever and ileus with bloody diarrhea. The diagnosis is confirmed with stool examination for leukocytes and cultures for specific pathogens.

Children (1 to 12 Years)

Portal hypertension with esophageal variceal bleeding has been an important cause of upper GI hemorrhage that generally first appears in this age group. The frequency varies among institutions, but biliary atresia and extrahepatic portal vein obstruction have been the most important causes. The emergence of liver transplantation has reduced the number of children requiring care for variceal hemorrhage. The strategy for this acute problem in almost all children is to temporize using endoscopic sclerotherapy and then to proceed with hepatic transplantation if appropriate. Portosystemic shunts or esophageal devascularization procedures are not commonly required in pediatric surgical practice.

Sources of lower GI hemorrhage in this age group are summarized in Table 103-9. Of the lesions not considered elsewhere in this review, juvenile polyps are most important. These benign hamartomas are the single most

common source of lower GI bleeding in children. Twenty to 30% are palpable on rectal examination, although a small, soft polyp can be subtle. The characteristic hemorrhage is bright red, episodic with bowel movements, and usually not massive. Hemorrhage results from the involution and sloughing of a pedunculated polyp, so it is relatively common to pass tissue with the stool. With a classic history of painless, episodic, minor rectal bleeding, the initial investigation in this age group is an air contrast barium enema. The alternative, colonoscopy, often requires general anesthesia. Endoscopic snare polypectomy is feasible for lesions up to 2 to 3 cm in diameter and is the standard treatment. In the case of multiple juvenile polyps not amenable to endoscopic polypectomy, management can be expectant based on a benign natural history characterized by involution during adolescence. These lesions must not be confused with adenomatous polyps, which are seen with familial polyposis or Gardner syndrome and are discussed in detail in Chapter 46.

Older Children and Adolescents (Older Than 12 Years)

Common causes of both upper and lower GI hemorrhage in older children are generally familiar to adult practitioners. Perhaps the most important addition to this age group in Tables 103-8 and 103-9 is inflammatory bowel disease. Specific pediatric considerations for these diseases are discussed in the appropriate chapters.

Diagnosis

In keeping with the age divisions presented earlier, several principles govern the diagnostic approach to pediatric patients with GI hemorrhage:

1. A specific source and site of GI hemorrhage can be identified in more than 95% of infants and children. Pediatric fiberoptic endoscopy, arteriography, and radioisotope imaging are widely available, safe, and applicable in any age group, including the newborn.
2. The investigation of choice for upper GI hemorrhage is flexible fiberoptic endoscopy, preferably within the first 24 hours after cessation of active hemorrhage. This may require general anesthesia for compliance as well as for airway protection, but bedside examination with sedation can often be accomplished.

Table 103-9. CAUSE OF LOWER GASTROINTESTINAL HEMORRHAGE*

Patient Age Group	Common Causes	Less Common Causes
Neonate (0–30 days)	1. Benign anorectal lesions (anal fissure) 2. Upper GI hemorrhage 3. Milk allergy 4. Necrotizing enterocolitis 5. Midgut volvulus 6. Incarcerated hernia	1. Iatrogenic trauma 2. Primary coagulopathy 3. Vascular malformations 4. Enterocolitis (Hirschsprung disease, others) 5. Miscellaneous structural abnormalities (lymphoma, duplication, lymphangiectasia)
Infant (30 d to 1 y)	1. Benign anorectal lesions 2. Idiopathic intussusception 3. Meckel diverticulum 4. Infectious diarrhea 5. Upper GI hemorrhage 6. Milk allergy	Same as for neonate, with addition of: 1. Acquired thrombocytopenia (drug-induced, aplastic anemia, disseminated intravascular coagulation, sepsis) 2. Ingestion of red foodstuffs (guaiac test mandatory)
Child (1–12 y)	1. Benign anorectal lesions 2. Juvenile polyp 3. Intussusception 4. Meckel diverticulum 5. Infectious diarrhea 6. Upper GI hemorrhage	Same as for infant, with addition of: 1. Juvenile polyposis coli 2. Familial polyposis coli 3. Hemolytic–uremic syndrome 4. Henoch-Schönlein purpura 5. Systemic vasculitis (dermatomyositis, lupus) 6. Acquired thrombocytopenia (as above plus idiopathic thrombocytopenic purpura)
Older child and adolescent (12 y to adulthood)	1. Juvenile polyps 2. Benign anorectal lesions 3. Inflammatory bowel disease 4. Upper GI hemorrhage	Same as for child, but: 1. Henoch-Schönlein purpura and hemolytic–uremic syndrome less likely 2. Meckel diverticulum

* Order of appearance approximates clinical frequency
(Modified from Oldham KT, Lobe TE. Gastrointestinal hemorrhage in children. Pediatr Clin North Am 1985;32:1247)

3. As in adults, radiographic contrast studies are often unhelpful in the evaluation of active upper GI hemorrhage. With the exception of suspected intussusception or juvenile polyps, contrast studies of the colon for evaluation of bleeding have also been replaced by endoscopy.

4. Significant and sometimes massive upper GI hemorrhage in a newborn infant may occur in the absence of a demonstrable anatomic lesion. This is usually the result of self-limited gastritis, and treatment is with appropriate blood replacement, correction of any coagulopathy, and appropriate supportive care.

5. Newborns, infants, and children with lower GI hemorrhage that is minor and anorectal in character are best evaluated with simple digital rectal examination and anoscopy. Sigmoidoscopy is rarely helpful and may require general anesthesia.

6. Massive lower GI hemorrhage in an infant or child beyond the newborn period is most likely related to a Meckel's diverticulum.

7. Lower GI hemorrhage from juvenile polyps is common in children between the ages of 3 or 4 years and adolescence. It is rarely massive, usually painless, and often episodic. Hypochromic microcytic anemia may occur.

8. Pain is an uncommon symptom with GI hemorrhage. It implies a more complex problem, such as ischemic or obstructed bowel. If these signs and symptoms are present, the need to establish a specific diagnosis becomes urgent.

9. Unlike adults, children rarely have GI bleeding secondary to a GI neoplasm.

These generalizations provide a framework within which to evaluate the child with GI hemorrhage. Specific treatments and outcomes are dependent on the sources of hemorrhage and are discussed in detail elsewhere in the text.

Miscellaneous Disorders

Duplications

The term *duplication* incorporates many older descriptive names, such as *enteric* or *enterogenous cyst, reduplication, giant diverticulum, ileum duplex,* and others. In current use, it is applied to both cystic and tubular GI duplications.

Cystic Malformations. Cystic duplications may be found anywhere in the GI tract, but they are most common in the midgut distribution, stomach, duodenum, and small intestine. The single most common location is in the ileum, particularly near the ileocecal valve. Terminal ileal lesions represent more than 75% to 80% of small intestinal duplications. The embryogenesis is controversial, but most authors believe that a discrete diverticulum or a sequestered portion of the embryonic gut containing primitive pleuripotential endodermal cells develops adjacent to the primary gut. The resulting lesions are found along the mesenteric border of the gut within the leaves of the mesentery, and the blood supply is shared with the functional intestine, an important surgical issue (Fig. 103-44A). All types of gut-derived epithelia are found, but the clinically relevant finding is ectopic gastric mucosa. The muscular wall is typically well developed and intimately attached to the functional gut. Communication between a cystic duplication and the gut lumen is not usual.

Cystic duplications are also found in the esophagus and are not rare. These appear to result from a different embryologic process involving the sequestration of both foregut endoderm and primitive notochord elements. This mechanism appears to explain the periodic association of thoracic spinal cord or vertebral defects with these cysts. Unlike duplications in the small bowel, these lesions are not intimately attached to the functional esophagus and therefore lend themselves to simple excision. Similar simple

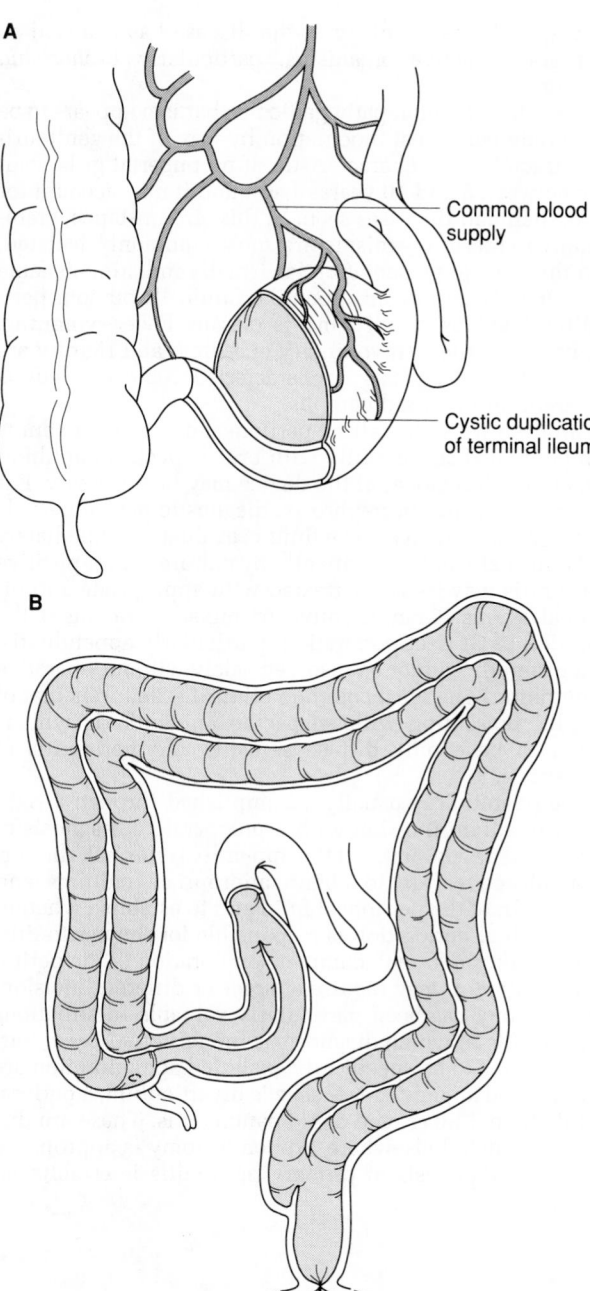

Figure 103-44. (*A*) Cystic duplication of terminal ileum. (*B*) Tubular duplication of terminal ileum and colon.

cystic duplications may be associated with the hindgut, particularly the rectum.

The clinical presentations of cystic duplications are protean, but discovery often results from the coincidental observation of an asymptomatic mass during imaging. Ultrasound, abdominal CT, and GI contrast studies are potential means of discovery. In addition, routine perinatal or prenatal ultrasound screening is the source of an increasing number of cases.

Hemorrhage related to ectopic gastric mucosa and an acid–ulcer diathesis, intussusception, infection, obstruction, perforation, torsion, and occasional malignant degeneration are all important possible presenting clinical scenarios. In general, mediastinal and rectal duplications are more likely to remain asymptomatic than those in the midgut. Treatment for all these lesions is operative. Even in asymptomatic patients, uncertainty regarding the cause of the mass lesion and the potential for subsequent problems dictates that surgical exploration be performed.

Treatment can usually be limited to simple excision of mediastinal or rectal cysts without resection of adjacent gut. This is more difficult or perhaps impossible in the small bowel, and short segmental resections with primary anastomoses are generally required. Cystic lesions not amenable to resection with simple reconstruction, particularly those involving the duodenum and stomach, require individualized plans. One approach involves marsupialization with resection of the redundant duplication wall and preservation of the common wall and its blood supply. When employed, this is combined with a submucosal dissection and stripping of the remaining epithelium from the cyst wall. Internal drainage (cystoduodenostomy) has been used successfully as well; however, this is usually unnecessary, and long-term drainage is potentially a problem.

Tubular Malformations. Tubular duplications may also occur anywhere in the GI tract. These are more rare than cystic duplications and are most likely to occur in the terminal ileum and colon. The embryogenesis is thought to be related to disordered recanalization after epithelial proliferation obliterates the intestinal lumen during the 6th or 7th gestational week. Anatomic features include a shared blood supply and a common wall with the functional gut. Communication between lumens is common. The lesion may be extensive, involving long segments of ileum or colon (see Fig. 103-44*B*). Malformations involving the entire colon and rectum are associated with genitourinary anomalies, particularly doubling of the external genitalia or bladder. These latter anomalies appear to represent an aborted embryologic twinning process.

Clinical presentations are diverse and in this respect are similar to those of cystic duplications. In particular, peptic ulceration and obstruction account for most clinical symptoms. The surgical treatment of these malformations requires an individualized plan directed to the specific anatomy. Simple resection may pose unacceptable risks because of the length of involved gut. The technique of marsupialization with submucosal stripping of the epithelium is potentially helpful when ectopic gastric mucosa is present and acid–ulcer disease is an issue. Obstruction may result from a long, blind-ending, parallel duplication that communicates with the functional gut lumen. In this circumstance, a distal enteroenterostomy (a reentry procedure) affords a straightforward solution without requiring a complex resection.

As with most other childhood surgical conditions of the GI tract, the outcomes are predictably excellent if the problem is confined to the single organ system. Postoperative morbidity and mortality are dependent on the location and anatomy of the lesion.

Mesenteric and Omental Cysts

Mesenteric and omental cysts are rare cystic malformations that appear to result from the sequestration of embryonic lymphatic tissue within the mesentery or omentum. Unlike duplications, mesenteric cysts are typically thin walled without surrounding smooth muscle. The cyst lining is typically composed of endothelial cells but is often incomplete. Both mesenteric and omental cysts may be filled with either chyle or serous fluid. Both may be either multilocular or unilocular. A mesenteric location is twice as frequent as an omental origin.

Most patients with mesenteric and omental cysts are discovered before the age of 10 years. The cysts vary in size but may become extraordinarily large before becoming symptomatic. Abdominal pain is the most important historical finding, and the finding of a soft, mobile abdominal mass is classic on physical examination. Like patients with duplications, these children may remain asymptomatic and are discovered incidentally at routine physical examination or at the time of diagnostic imaging for unrelated reasons. Hemorrhage, obstruction, volvulus, cyst rupture, and infection are all possible alternative presentations (Fig. 103-45). Ultrasound and CT imaging should discover all these lesions, although the specific diagnosis may not be possible. Ascites, pancreatic pseudocysts, duplications, and large ovarian cysts are among the lesions that may have a similar appearance. Peripheral calcifications and recent hemorrhage are two characteristics of these cysts that may be diagnostic during the imaging evaluation.

Treatment consists of simple cyst excision if possible, and if necessary for mesenteric cysts, resection of adjacent intestine. It may be impossible to differentiate a cystic duplication from a mesenteric cyst even under direct vision at laparotomy. Surgically, the distinction is worthwhile because simple mesenteric cysts can often be excised without bowel resection. Occasionally, partial excision of the cysts with marsupialization may be appropriate, but total excision is generally preferable.

The only morbidity or mortality of these lesions is related to concurrent problems associated with the intestine. In particular, mesenteric cysts may be associated with volvulus, and this in turn introduces all the potential related hazards of intestinal infarction.

Primary Peritonitis

Bacterial peritonitis without a specific identifiable cause is correctly referred to as *primary peritonitis.* In this century, this phenomenon in childhood has diminished 10-fold in frequency, now representing fewer than 1% of all cases of peritonitis in childhood. Use of the term has been modified to include patients who develop peritonitis secondary to a clearly identifiable cause, such as a peritoneal dialysis catheter or a ventriculoperitoneal shunt. In addition, children with ascites or nephrosis who develop spontaneous bacterial peritonitis are included with these patients. Bacterial inoculation of protein-laden ascitic fluid through a hematogenous route appears to be the mechanism by which this latter process occurs. The offending organisms are classically gram-positive; a variety of streptococcal, staphylococcal, and other species have been im-

plicated. The bacteriology of the disease has changed so that gram-negative organisms, particularly *Escherichia coli,* predominate.[86]

The other common pathogenic mechanism appears to be retrograde peritoneal inoculation by way of the genitourinary tract. This is characteristic of prepubertal girls, usually between 5 and 10 years of age, and it may account for more than half the cases seen. In this circumstance, gram-negative enteric organisms are most commonly isolated, and the clinical presentation is virtually indistinguishable from that of a perforated appendix. Clinically obvious peritonitis develops rapidly and is classic. Fever, vomiting, diffuse tenderness, involuntary guarding, and rigidity are expected. Leukocytosis is characteristic, and an ileus is apparent on plain radiographs.

Children with indwelling peritoneal catheters or shunts can be treated successfully with broad-spectrum antibiotics, although removal of the device may be necessary. For those with ascites or nephrosis, diagnostic paracentesis is an essential maneuver. The fluid is evaluated immediately by Gram stain and subsequently by culture. Gram-positive peritonitis may be safely treated with appropriate antimicrobial agents. Gram-negative or mixed flora raises the question of GI tract perforation, particularly appendicitis, and generally cannot be resolved safely without operative exploration. The most common clinical scenario is that of a child presenting with suspected appendicitis who is found to have only diffuse serositis and peritonitis at operation.

The operation is usually accomplished through a right lower quadrant incision with a preoperative diagnosis of perforated appendicitis. If the appendix is normal, the surgical objectives are to obtain appropriate cultures and Gram stain of the peritoneal fluid and to establish whether an intestinal perforation is responsible for the peritonitis. This requires a formal, complete exploration of the peritoneal cavity and may require a larger or different incision. Laparoscopy has been particularly valuable in situations such as this in which diagnosis is the principal need. Surgical lesions to be specifically excluded at exploration are a perforated appendix or Meckel's diverticulum, a perforated duodenal ulcer, and acute pancreatitis. These are discussed in detail elsewhere. Appendectomy is appropriate when the diagnosis of primary peritonitis is established operatively.

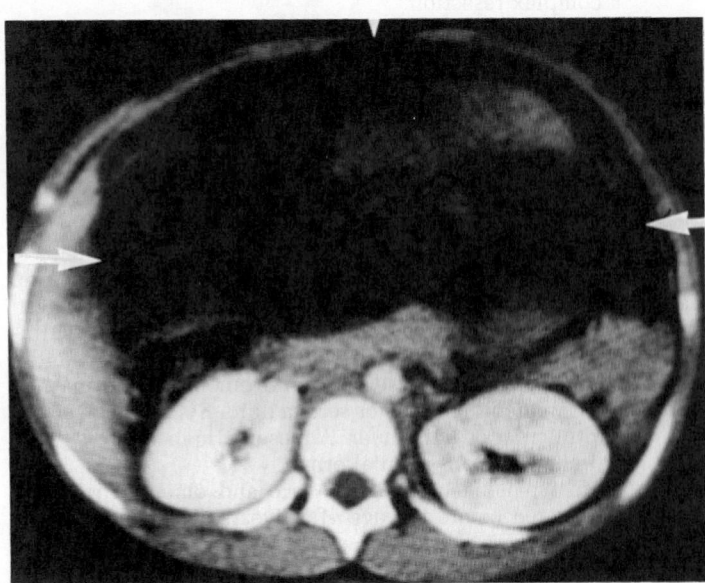

Figure 103-45. CT image from a child after abdominal trauma. Hemorrhage into large omental cyst is apparent (*arrows*).

Peritoneal fluid cultures are positive in about half the children with primary peritonitis and almost invariably reveal a single organism. Treatment consists of specific antibiotics for about 10 days and is predictably uneventful. If operation is required, the morbidity and recovery are essentially no different than after appendectomy. Mortality rates are near zero if treatment is promptly instituted.

Ascites

Infants and children with ascites are easily recognized by their characteristic physical findings, particularly abdominal distention with bulging flanks. The diagnosis is confirmed by ultrasound or CT. In addition, this diagnosis may be established in utero. A partial inventory of the many possible causes of neonatal and childhood ascites is presented in Tables 103-10 and 103-11.

The diagnostic effort begins with paracentesis and examination of the ascitic fluid. The physical, biochemical, and microbiologic characteristics of the ascitic fluid are important determinants of the evaluation and treatment (see Table 103-11). Chylous ascites is characterized by a milky appearance, a high lymphocyte count, and a high triglyceride content. In unfed neonates, the characteristics of the fluid are similar to serous ascites, and a diagnostic trial of feeding may be appropriate. Bile staining is characteristic of biliary ascites, a high amylase content indicates pancreatic ascites, and a low protein count (less than 3 g/dL) is consistent with serous ascites. Elevated urea nitrogen levels or creatinine levels suggest a renal origin, but these findings may be absent. Cytologic examination should be performed routinely to evaluate the possibility of malignancy, and cultures are appropriate to rule out an infectious cause.

In the absence of a diagnosis from the initial fluid examination, a comprehensive imaging evaluation should include examinations of the heart, kidneys and lower urinary tract, liver and biliary tract, and pancreas. Echocardiography, abdominal CT or ultrasound, and a voiding cystourethrogram assess many of the possibilities enumerated in Tables 103-10 and 103-11.

The primary diagnosis dictates specific treatment. Many of the issues related to ascites are discussed elsewhere in detail. Specific and important treatment principles that are unique to infants and children are summarized briefly here.

1. Administration of parenteral hyperalimentation, or possibly enteral alimentation limited to medium-

Table 103-10. COMMON CAUSES OF NEONATAL ASCITES

Maternal–fetal Rh incompatibility (now rare)
Structural malformations
  Urinary obstructions
  Congenital heart disease
  Malrotation, duplications, cysts (associated with intestinal volvulus)
  Biliary perforation
  Ovarian ascites
  Pulmonary abnormalities
Chylous ascites
Hematologic disorders
  α-Thalassemia
Infection
  Toxoplasmosis
  Cytomegalovirus
  Others
α_1-Antitrypsin deficiency
Idiopathic

Table 103-11. CHARACTERISTICS AND CAUSES OF CHILDHOOD ASCITES

SEROUS ASCITES

Cirrhosis
Budd-Chiari syndrome
Nephrosis
Right-sided heart failure
Postoperative ascites (after renal transplantation, peritoneal dialysis, ventriculoperitoneal shunts)
α_1-Antitrypsin deficiency
Other rare metabolic diseases

CHYLOUS ASCITES

Malrotation with volvulus
Small bowel obstruction
Incarcerated hernia
Lymphangioma
Trauma (including surgical trauma)

BILIARY ASCITES

Neonatal bile duct perforation
Cystic fibrosis
Biliary atresia
Hepatitis
Cytomegalovirus infection

URINARY ASCITES (7:1 MALE PREDOMINANCE)

Urinary obstruction
Posterior urethral valves
Bladder perforation
Ureterocele
Neurogenic bladder

PANCREATIC ASCITES

Acute pancreatitis (drugs, trauma, gallstones, infection)
Pancreatic pseudocysts

OVARIAN ASCITES

Cysts (torsion, rupture)
Tumors

MALIGNANT ASCITES

Any intraperitoneal neoplasm

IDIOPATHIC

chain triglycerides, leads to spontaneous resolution of chylous ascites in 50% to 75% of cases if no anatomic lesion is present. Persistence of the ascites beyond 4 to 6 weeks is a relative indication for surgical exploration with an attempt to repair or ligate the cisterna chyli.

2. Neonatal biliary ascites may result from spontaneous bile duct perforation. Cystic fibrosis with transient bile plugging must be considered in this circumstance. The perforation is typically found at the junction of the cystic duct and common bile duct. External drainage is predictably successful, and efforts at complex biliary tract reconstruction are technically hazardous and unnecessary.

3. The presence of urinary ascites in a male infant requires a voiding cystourethrogram to rule out posterior urethral valves, the cause in as many as two thirds of these patients. Relief of any cause of obstructive uropathy provides resolution of urinary ascites.

4. Pancreatic ascites ordinarily resolves in the absence of a correctable anatomic lesion, such as a pancreatic duct injury or obstruction. Treatment is designed to provide symptomatic relief. Formal internal drainage procedures, external drainage, and percutaneous aspiration have been successfully used for persistent pancreatic ascites.

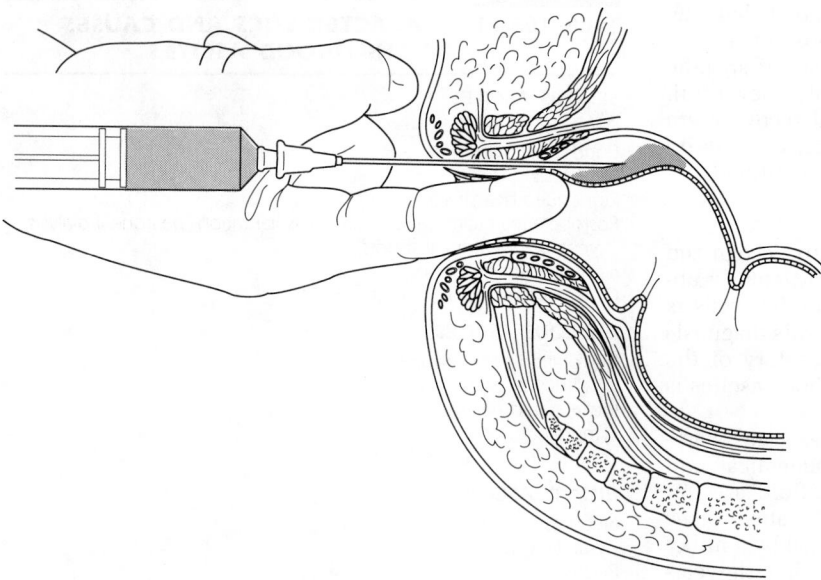

Figure 103-46. Four-quadrant injection of sclerosant into the submucosa is an effective treatment for rectal prolapse in children.

5. Ascites related to liver or cardiac disease in children is not fundamentally different than similar problems in adults. Treatment is directed at providing symptomatic relief and correcting the underlying problem.

In neonates, inadequate ventilation may result from interference with diaphragmatic breathing. Morbidity and mortality related to ascites, however, are generally linked to the prognosis of the underlying disease process rather than to the ascites itself. Intractable ascites can be managed in children as in adults, with peritoneal–venous shunting. The 10% incidence of serious coagulopathy, the need to use smaller (obstruction prone) shunt tubing, and the rarity of the problem have combined to limit the experience with these procedures in children.

Rectal Prolapse

Rectal prolapse in adults is discussed in detail in Chapter 52. Only the relevant and different childhood clinical considerations are reviewed here.

In preschool-aged children, spontaneous prolapse of the rectum is relatively common, with a peak incidence at or near the time of toilet training. Although the cause is controversial, important childhood clinical associations include straining at stool for any reason, cystic fibrosis, colorectal polyps, and Hirschsprung disease.

Appropriate diagnostic evaluations for each of these possibilities are discussed elsewhere. Children with myelodysplasia or other causes of sacral neuropathy also have a higher incidence of rectal prolapse than normal infants. In addition, children with congenital anorectal malformations are at increased risk. Most children with rectal prolapse, however, have no associated abnormalities.

The diagnosis of rectal prolapse is ordinarily straightforward, although it is frequently entirely dependent on the parental history. Protrusion of mucosa or full-thickness rectum through the anus is usually described in graphic terms. In children, the only other lesion with a similar appearance is intussusception with passage of the intussusceptum through the anus. Children with rectal prolapse rarely have other symptoms, whereas signs and symptoms of intussusception are usually obvious in the latter group. In addition, the rectal examination is diagnostic. If the prolapsed intestine is an intussusceptum, a finger can be placed adjacent to it within the rectum. This is not possible with rectal prolapse.

Unlike the situation for adults, nonoperative management should be tried in all infants or children with rectal prolapse. Initially, manual reduction, stool softeners, parental instruction, and taping of the buttocks may all be undertaken. The usual result is spontaneous resolution over a period of weeks, and an operative procedure is not often indicated. For refractory or unsuccessful situations, many operative approaches have been proposed. The principle in children is to avoid complex operations involving laparotomy with bowel resection or suspension. Generally, any strategy that creates a perirectal inflammatory process creates enough fibrosis to fix the rectum in position and eliminate the propensity to prolapse. Therefore, the approach is to proceed as simply as possible. The most useful and common procedure involves submucosal rectal injections using a sclerosant while the patient is under general anesthesia. Five percent phenol, 5% sodium morrhuate, hypertonic glucose or saline, peanut oil, and many other sclerosants have been used with good effect. This is routinely done on an outpatient basis. About 90% of children can be successfully treated with a single four-quadrant submucosal injection procedure, but occasionally, several injection sessions are necessary[25] (Fig. 103-46). Linear submucosal electrocoagulation achieves the same end but may have a higher incidence of associated bleeding or stricture formation and usually requires a short period of hospitalization. A variety of other limited perineal or transanal procedures have been described, with the objective being to create a local extraperitoneal, perirectal inflammatory process. Most have had excellent results and little morbidity. Resectional procedures and complex fixations or suspensions are widely used in adults but have little or no place in the management of rectal prolapse in children.

Pediatric Liver

ARNOLD G. CORAN

TUMORS OF THE LIVER

Primary liver tumors are uncommon in children. Of these tumors, about one third are benign, and two thirds are malignant[87] (Table 103-12). The most common presenting feature of pediatric liver neoplasms is an asymptomatic abdominal mass. Other symptoms, such as pain, hemorrhage, precocious puberty, and hypertension, are more rare. The diagnostic evaluation of a child with a suspected liver mass includes an initial plain radiograph of the abdomen to determine whether calcification is present. Although not pathognomonic, this finding may suggest echinococcal disease or other specific diagnoses. Ultrasound differentiates solid and cystic masses and is easily obtained. Computed tomography (CT) and magnetic resonance (MR) imaging of the abdomen are the most definitive diagnostic tests. An experienced radiologist can usually differentiate benign and malignant tumors preoperatively. CT and MR imaging also demonstrate the anatomic location and relations of the tumor within the liver, providing the surgeon with an assessment of resectability that previously could be obtained only by angiography. Laparotomy is necessary in most patients, both to establish the diagnosis and to allow resection or other therapy.

Benign Tumors of the Liver

About one third of primary pediatric liver tumors are benign. In approximate order of frequency, these neoplasms include vascular tumors such as hemangiomas and hemangioendotheliomas, mesenchymal hamartomas, cysts, focal nodular hyperplasia, and hepatic adenomas. Vascular tumors account for about half of the total.[88]

Vascular Tumors

Hemangiomas consist of disordered, dilated vascular structures with flattened endothelium, whereas hemangioendotheliomas are tumors composed principally of endothelial cells that have formed vascular channels but maintain a diffuse hypercellular pattern. Cavernous hemangiomas are the most frequent benign hepatic tumors. These may occur in either children or adults. In contrast to hemangioendotheliomas, typically discovered in the first months or years of life, hemangiomas are more likely to present in the adolescent and young adult populations. Generally, these neoplasms are asymptomatic and noted as an abdominal mass or an incidental finding. A large proportion of these are found only at autopsy. Some are associated with hemangiomas in other parts of the body. The diagnosis is readily made by ultrasound and CT scan or MR imaging.

Vascular lesions in the liver do not require routine operative management. Complications such as high-output congestive heart failure, thrombocytopenia, or rupture and hemoperitoneum are potential operative indications. Congestive heart failure usually can be managed medically, and thrombocytopenia is potentially improved with the use of corticosteroids. Relevant treatment strategies include irradiation, selective arterial ligation or embolization, sclerosis, treatment with recombinant α-interferon, and surgical resection. Because spontaneous involution is common and the lesions are rare, no clear prospective data are available to compare these therapies. Surgical resection is generally reserved for ruptured lesions with active hemorrhage, for masses with an uncertain diagnosis, and for symptomatic locally approachable lesions. Therapy using systemic α-interferon administration has been used with impressive responses in some diffuse, nonresectable vascular malformations.[89] Treatment remains highly individualized.

Hemangioendotheliomas tend to present before 6 months of age. These neoplasms vary in size, ranging from less than 1 cm to more than 15 cm in diameter, and they may be solitary or multiple (Fig. 103-47). The presentation may be as an asymptomatic abdominal mass, although hepatomegaly and congestive heart failure are more frequent. Symptoms include tachycardia, tachypnea, and cyanosis. A thrombocytopenic coagulopathy due to sequestration of platelets within the tumor (Kasabach-Merritt syndrome) develops in about half of these children. In addition, spontaneous rupture with bleeding into the peritoneal cavity is not uncommon. A significant percentage of these patients have cutaneous hemangiomas as well. CT or MR imaging is the definitive diagnostic test. As with cavernous hemangiomas, treatment is required for the management of specific symptoms, such as congestive heart failure unresponsive to medical therapy, and for coagulopathy unresponsive to corticosteroids. The response to systemic steroids is highly variable. In general, the treatment options are those outlined briefly earlier. The probability of significant symptoms is higher in these lesions, and the lesions are more likely to be extensive; therefore, the approach is more aggressive but still individualized.

Mesenchymal Hamartomas

Mesenchymal hamartomas of the liver are rare, although they represent about one third of the benign neoplasms in children. The presentation usually occurs within the first year of life. These tend to be solitary lesions, possibly with both solid and cystic components, and they are often large. The presentation is usually as an asymptomatic abdominal mass. The definitive diagnosis can often be made with ultrasonography, CT scan, or MR image, although differentiation from a malignant hepatoblastoma usually requires surgical exploration. Surgical resection is the recommended therapy. Resection is often done by simple enucleation of the encapsulated tumor, but occasionally a formal lobectomy is necessary. Recurrence is rare after an adequate resection. Spontaneous involution has been described, and therefore nonresectional therapy may be appropriate, particularly when complete resection would engender a high-risk procedure.

Table 103-12. INCIDENCE OF LIVER TUMORS IN CHILDHOOD

Tumor Type	Incidence (%)
BENIGN	
Vascular tumors	13
Hemangioma	9
Hemangioendothelioma	4
Mesenchymal hamartoma	6
Focal nodular hyperplasia	2
Adenoma	2
Teratoma	2
Other	3
MALIGNANT	
Hepatoblastoma	43
Hepatocellular carcinoma	23
Malignant mesenchymal tumor	4
Sarcoma	2
Embryonal rhabdomyosarcoma	1
Angiosarcoma	1

(Adapted from Dehner LP. Hepatic tumors in the pediatric age group: a distinctive clinicopathologic spectrum. In: Rosenberg HS, Bolande RP. Perspectives in pediatric pathology. Chicago, Year Book, 1978)

Focal Nodular Hyperplasia

Focal nodular hyperplasia is usually a well-defined solitary hepatic mass, generally larger than 5 cm in diameter. Although the cause is unknown, there may be an association with oral contraceptives or focal hepatic injury. The tumor occurs principally in females and in adults, although 15% of patients are children younger than 15 years.[90] Discovery is often the result of finding an asymptomatic abdominal mass. The tumor has a characteristic angiographic vascular pattern, but the diagnosis is usually made from ultrasonography and CT scanning. It is sometimes difficult to differentiate focal nodular hyperplasia from hepatic adenomas. Biopsy may be necessary to establish the diagnosis. Histologically, these tumors are composed of normal hepatocytes surrounded by fibrous tissue with an inflammatory infiltrate. The clinical picture is one of micronodular cirrhosis with hyperplastic regenerative nodules. Surgery is not generally required, although spontaneous rupture and hemoperitoneum have been reported to require emergency laparotomy and resection for hemorrhage control.

Hepatic Adenomas

Hepatic adenomas are also rare, representing less than 5% of the benign childhood hepatic lesions. They may be associated with oral contraceptives, anabolic androgenic steroids, or glycogen storage disease type I (von Gierke disease). Hepatic adenomas tend to be large (10 cm or more) solitary lesions, generally found in the right lobe of the liver. Microscopically, they consist of a uniform field of hepatocytes without abnormal nuclei, vascular structures, or bile ducts. These patients often present with an asymptomatic abdominal mass, and spontaneous rupture and hemoperitoneum are reported in 20% to 25% of cases. In general, operative indications are hemorrhage or diagnostic uncertainty. Biopsy and enucleation or local resection of the adenoma usually are possible, and recurrence is rare.

Liver Cysts

Congenital nonparasitic cysts of the liver may be either solitary or multiple. If multiple, they are often associated with polycystic kidney disease. This hereditary disease is of uncertain cause, and liver and kidney failure are possible outcomes. Transplantation may be necessary for one or both of these problems. Histologically, multiple and solitary cysts are similar and may be lined with cuboidal, columnar, or squamous epithelium.[91] Embryologically, these cysts probably represent the failure of the intralobular or interlobular biliary ducts to fuse. Most children with these lesions are asymptomatic and generally do not require surgical therapy. The diagnosis can be made definitively with ultrasonography. During the diagnostic evaluation, hepatic hydatid disease must be considered. Calcification and compartmentalization of the cyst are typical and highly suggestive findings. The diagnosis can be confirmed with an accuracy of 80% or more using one or more serologic tests, including indirect hemagglutination, complement fixation, dot immunobinding, or enzyme-linked immunosorbent assay. Therapy for echinococcal cysts requires injection of hypertonic saline or other scolicidal agents into the parent cyst before surgical resection or marsupialization. Perioperative mebendazole therapy is recommended as well. Congenital cysts that are asymptomatic require no therapy. Resection, marsupialization, or internal drainage may be necessary. Communication of the cyst with the biliary tract must be investigated, usually with contrast injection of the cyst. If present, this necessitates internal drainage into the gut.

Teratomas

Teratomas of the liver are extremely rare, with fewer than 50 cases reported. Because these can be either benign or malignant, resection is recommended.

Malignant Tumors

Most primary hepatic tumors in children are malignant. Hepatoblastoma represents about half of these malignant childhood neoplasms, followed in frequency by hepatocellular carcinoma and sarcomas.[92]

Hepatoblastoma

Hepatoblastomas are malignant neoplasms composed of immature hepatocytes of variable developmental age. Most are discovered within the first 2 years of life. The tumor is twice as common in boys and usually presents as an abdominal mass or with GI symptoms related to compression of adjacent viscera, such as the stomach or duodenum. In most of these children, the tumor can be palpated on physical examination. Although there may be slight abnormalities in plasma transaminase or alkaline phosphatase levels, jaundice is rare. Plasma α-fetoprotein levels are elevated in more than 90% of children with hepatoblastoma and are therefore a useful tumor marker for postoperative surveillance. Occasionally, precocious puberty or virilization, secondary to excess androgen secretion, is seen in children with hepatoblastoma. In addition, the incidence of hepatoblastoma is increased among patients with hemihypertrophy and with Beckwith-Wiedemann syndrome. Plain films of the abdomen may show calcifications within the liver mass, but the definitive diagnostic test is a contrast-enhanced CT scan or MR imaging. These studies show the extent and location of the tumor, eliminating the need for preoperative angiographic mapping of vascular anatomy (Fig. 103-47).

Complete excision is necessary for cure, and an aggres-

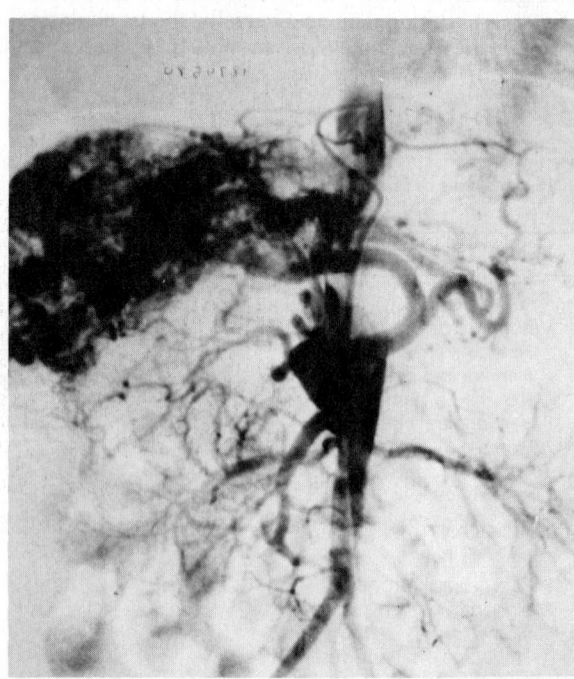

Figure 103-47. Subtraction image angiogram with an aortic injection showing a vascular malformation in a neonate with congestive heart failure. This is consistent with a hemangioendothelioma involving the right and left lobes of the liver.

sive surgical approach is appropriate. Generally, formal lobectomy or extended lobectomy is performed for localized tumors (Fig. 103-49). Extensive, unresectable tumors are treated with aggressive multidrug chemotherapy for cytoreduction, after which a delayed resection is generally attempted. This approach yields a 65% to 75% probability of cure if histologically clear resection margins can be achieved.[93] Cure with chemotherapy and radiation without resectional surgery is not expected. Adjuvant chemotherapy is also given to any child who has undergone excision of a hepatoblastoma.

Hepatocellular Carcinoma

Hepatocellular carcinoma generally occurs among adults but is also a disease of adolescents and children. It is not common in children younger than the age of 3 or 4 years. As with hepatoblastoma, there is a male predominance in childhood of 2 to 1. The clinical presentation is not different from hepatoblastoma except for the older age predilection. Hepatoblastoma and hepatocellular carcinoma are indistinguishable by imaging analysis. Liver function studies are much more likely to be abnormal with hepatocellular carcinoma, and jaundice is also more likely. Concurrent cirrhosis is found in about 5% of children with hepatocellular carcinoma but in about 80% of adult patients. Patients with hepatitis B infection, cirrhosis, type 1 glycogen storage disease, Fanconi syndrome, Beckwith-Wiedemann syndrome, cerebral giantism, and hemihypertrophy all have an increased risk of hepatocellular carcinoma. In addition, pharmacologic agents such as anabolic steroids, oral contraceptives, and methotrexate have been associated with hepatocellular carcinoma.

Hepatocellular carcinoma tends to be multicentric in origin. The prognosis is poor, with a survival rate of less than 10% regardless of radical surgery and intensive chemotherapy. Complete surgical resection is a prerequisite for cure. A rare variant of hepatocellular carcinoma in children is fibrolamellar carcinoma. As in adults, it has a much better prognosis than classic hepatocellular carcinoma.

Malignant Mesenchymal Tumors

Malignant mesenchymomas are rare childhood hepatic tumors. These neoplasms tend to occur in children between 5 and 10 years of age and usually present as symptomatic abdominal masses associated with pain and fever. These tumors are often large with multiple cystic areas throughout on imaging. Treatment requires complete excision with adjuvant chemotherapy and irradiation. The

prognosis for children with this lesion is no better than that of hepatocellular carcinoma.

Sarcoma

Sarcomas are the rarest primary malignant tumors of the liver in children. These tumors can take the form of embryonal rhabdomyosarcoma of the biliary tract, classically presenting with obstructive jaundice, or of angiosarcoma, possibly resulting from exposure to hepatotoxins such as arsenic or thorium dioxide in a young child. In general, the prognosis for both of these tumors is dismal, although long-term survival has been reported with aggressive extirpative surgery.

Liver Resection in Infants and Children

The operative technique for hepatic resection is covered elsewhere in this text. Several technical aspects of the procedures unique to the pediatric population are reviewed here.[94,95] Intraoperative monitoring using arterial and central venous catheters is more critical than in adults because of the small blood volume in infants and children. Almost all pediatric liver resections can be safely accomplished through an abdominal incision alone, so a thoracoabdominal incision is unnecessary. Care must be taken not to angulate and obstruct the inferior vena cava during resection because minimal changes can cause a significant loss in venous return to the right atrium and a child with a small blood volume is sensitive to systemic hypotension. Both the right and left hepatic veins of young children can be very short, and if they are not safely approached after extrahepatic dissection, they should be controlled within the liver parenchyma from an anterior approach (Fig. 103-50). Finally, the extrahepatic bile ducts of young children are very small, and T-tubes are not used for postoperative drainage because they can produce biliary strictures. Hepatic lobectomy in infants and children is carried out under normothermic vascular occlusion (about 1 hour) in which the suprahepatic vena cava, infrahepatic vena cava above the renal veins, and the portal vein and hepatic artery are cross-clamped. This diminishes the blood loss during and after the resection.

HEPATIC INFECTIONS

Hepatic parenchymal infections are rare in children. Management is generally similar to that discussed for adult patients. One important association is chronic granulomatous disease and pyogenic liver abscesses.

Pyogenic Abscess

In the preantibiotic era, pyogenic hepatic abscesses occurred most frequently after perforated appendicitis. This complication is rarely seen today. Chronic granulomatous disease of childhood is the most common condition associated with hepatic abscess.[96] This disease is the result of a genetically transmitted deficiency of oxidant-mediated bacterial killing by circulating granulocytes. Children with chronic granulomatous disease often develop abscesses in sites such as regional cervical and axillary lymph nodes, liver, lungs, and other soft tissues. In the pediatric age group, 40% of pyogenic liver abscesses occur in children with chronic granulomatous disease, and another 30% occur in children with other immunodeficiencies, most commonly leukemia. Other rare causes of liver abscesses in children are umbilical vein catheter-induced infection, omphalitis, and other biliary diseases.

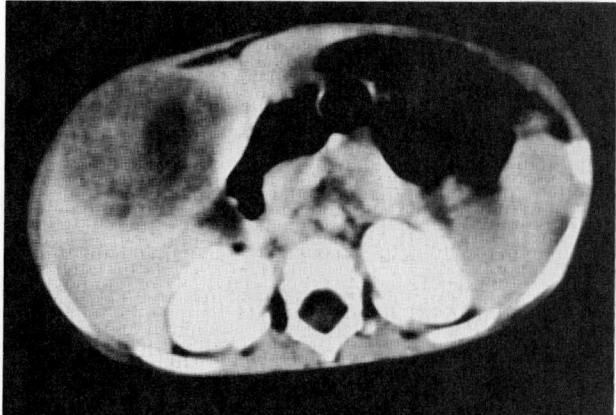

Figure 103-48. Contrast-enhanced CT scan of an infant with a hepatoblastoma in the right lobe of the liver.

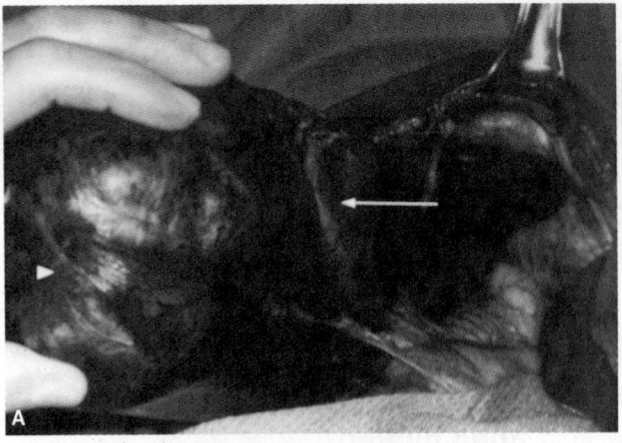

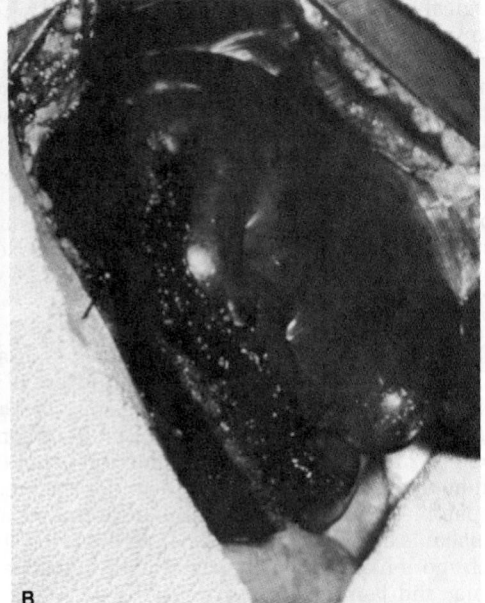

Figure 103-49. (*A*) Hepatoblastoma (*arrowhead*) arising in the right lobe of the liver seen at operation. The gallbladder (*long arrow*) is indicated for orientation. (*B*) The liver after the right hepatic lobectomy in *A*.

The clinical picture usually includes fever, leukocytosis, and jaundice associated with hepatosplenomegaly. The diagnosis is made with ultrasound, contrast-enhanced CT scan, or MR image. The most common pathogenic organisms are *Staphylococcus aureus, Streptococcus* sp, and *Escherichia coli.* Occasionally, anaerobic bacteria are responsible, and gram-negative organisms have become more frequent in the past decade. Multiple small abscesses are best treated with appropriate broad-spectrum intravenous antibiotics, often for as long as 4 to 6 weeks. Single abscesses or large multiple abscesses can be drained percutaneously using ultrasound or CT guidance. Open operative drainage is only rarely necessary. Intraoperative ultrasound may be helpful in this circumstance. The outcome

for pyogenic liver abscesses has improved substantially, but reported mortality rates have ranged from 25% to 40%.

Amebic Abscess

Amebic abscess of the liver is caused by the parasite *Entamoeba histolytica.* This parasite enters the liver through the portal circulation of patients with amebic dysentery. Although this condition is uncommon in the United States, it is endemic in Latin America, Asia, and South Africa. It is not uncommon to see children with an amebic abscess present to an American hospital after travel from their native country. These patients tend to have a chronic illness characterized by low-grade fever, malaise, and right upper quadrant tenderness. The abscess can usu-

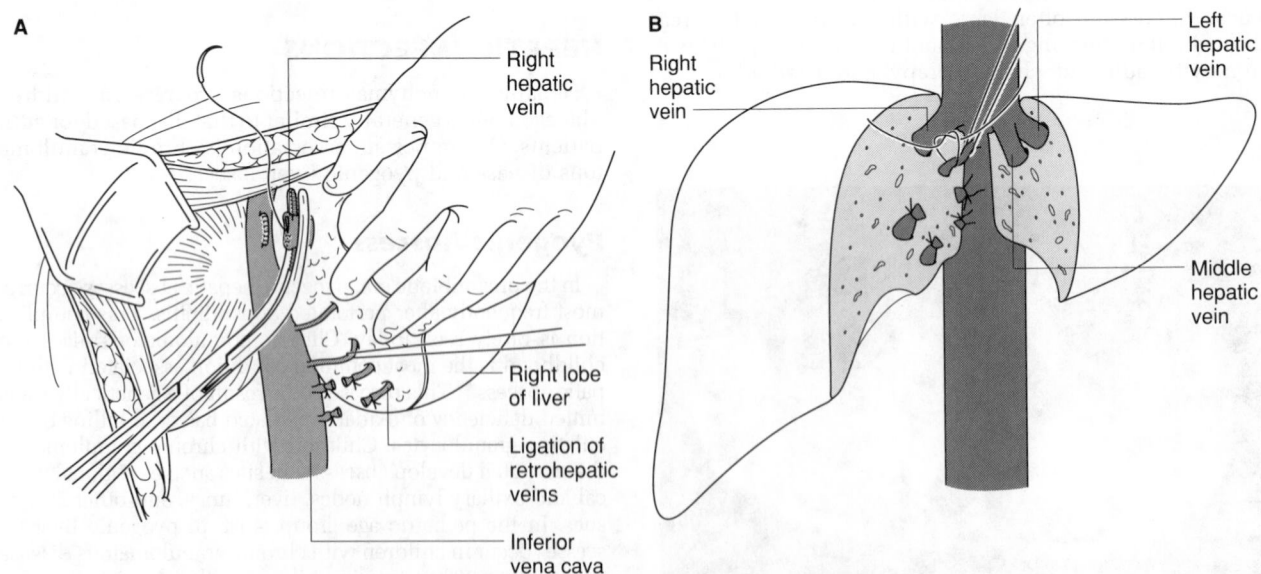

Figure 103-50. (*A*) The hepatic veins in infants and children may be extremely short, precluding extrahepatic control as is conventional in adults. (*B*) Intrahepatic control of the hepatic veins may be a safer approach in infants and children.

ally be diagnosed by CT scan and a serum fluorescence antibody test or by immunoelectrophoresis study. Spontaneous rupture of these abscesses is reported in up to 10% of patients.[97] Almost all patients with amebic abscesses can be effectively treated with metronidazole. Surgical or percutaneous drainage is usually unnecessary.

Pediatric Biliary Tract

KEITH T. OLDHAM

The spectrum of biliary tract pathology in infants and children includes many congenital, neoplastic, inflammatory, infectious, and gallstone-related disorders. The two common problems unique to children are biliary atresia and congenital cystic disease of the biliary tract (choledochal cysts).

EMBRYOLOGY

The fetal liver and biliary tract develop between the 4th and 10th gestational weeks, combining an endodermal contribution from a foregut diverticulum with a mesodermal component from the transverse septum.[98] Hepatocytes differentiate from cords of endodermal cells at the distal extent of the hepatic diverticulum. These cords grow into the surrounding mesenchyme, which ultimately gives rise to the endothelium of the hepatic sinusoids. The bile ducts are derived from the more proximal hepatic diverticulum (Fig. 103-51).

The distal extrahepatic biliary tract, which includes the gallbladder, cystic duct, and common bile duct, forms from the caudal (proximal) portion of the hepatic diverticulum. Intrahepatic and proper hepatic ducts develop from either a cranial portion of the hepatic diverticulum or possibly from primitive hepatocytes. The embryonic intrahepatic and extrahepatic ductal systems unite to form an arborizing system of cords composed of primitive ductular epithelial cells. These epithelial cells assume a concentric orientation with luminal polarity established between 6 and 8 weeks of gestation. Ductal patency is normally apparent between 6 and 12 weeks, and bile flow is demonstrable by the beginning of the second trimester. It appears that this embryologic sequence takes place normally in most infants with biliary atresia. That is, the process is not truly an atresia resulting from failure of ductal recanalization during embryogenesis but rather an acquired defect involving a dynamic obliterative inflammatory process.

The embryogenesis of choledochal cysts is unknown. Abnormalities in the process of bile duct recanalization may initiate cyst formation, although simple bile duct obstruction does not appear to be causative either experimentally or clinically. The association with an anomalous extramural junction of the pancreatic and common bile ducts is common, indeed expected, with type I choledochal cysts. Reflux of activated pancreatic proteases into the common bile duct through this long common channel may be a contributing factor. The association of biliary atresia and choledochal cysts in some patients and in Asian populations suggests that these cysts may share pathogenic features.

BILIARY ATRESIA

Anatomy

Biliary atresia has been termed either *correctable* or *uncorrectable*, with many variations described[99] (Fig. 103-52). The former atresia is characterized by hepatic duct patency suitable for conventional anastomosis to an enteric conduit, whereas the latter is not. Most patients have a form of biliary atresia with complete obstruction of the extrahepatic bile ducts and gallbladder, whereas 10% to 15% have obstruction of the proximal system with gallbladder and distal common bile duct patency. This surgically inspired nomenclature is relatively unhelpful for three reasons. First, the correctable variation is rare. Some early studies suggested that this anatomy occurred in 10% to 15% of patients, but the true incidence is closer to 1% or 2% of all infants with biliary atresia. Given an incidence of biliary atresia of about 1 per 15,000, few infants have this anatomy. Second, bile drainage is actually achieved by portoenterostomy in most infants with so-called uncorrectable biliary atresia. Last, the natural history of the liver disease and patient outcome are not necessarily good even when a biliary conduit is provided surgically in patients with correctable biliary atresia.

The surgical approach, portoenterostomy, is similar for all these variants, and thus the semantic distinction between correctable and uncorrectable has little practical value. An important point, however, is the differentiation of biliary atresia from biliary hypoplasia. The latter term applies to a diminutive but patent biliary system, a finding that may result from many underlying conditions (eg, neonatal hepatitis, Alagille syndrome, and α_1-antitrypsin deficiency). Because this finding invariably includes abnormalities of both the intrahepatic and extrahepatic biliary tracts, surgical procedures such as portoenterostomy that replace only the extrahepatic bile ducts are not helpful, and the outcome depends on the course of the underlying disease.

Microscopic Anatomy

The extrahepatic bile ducts in biliary atresia are replaced with dense fibrous tissue containing evidence of both acute and chronic inflammation.[100] Typically, the entire extrahepatic biliary tract, including the gallbladder, is obliterated. The degree of inflammation and fibrosis varies greatly but generally increases with age, suggesting a dynamic, inflammatory process. The proximal resection margin of the fibrous biliary cord in the porta hepatis is usually examined separately at the time of surgical exploration for portoenterostomy. The presence of patent bile ducts with normal cuboidal epithelium rather than biliary glands or obliterated ducts may confer a better prognosis. This examination is usually done intraoperatively on a frozen-section specimen, so the surgeon can revise the site of transection

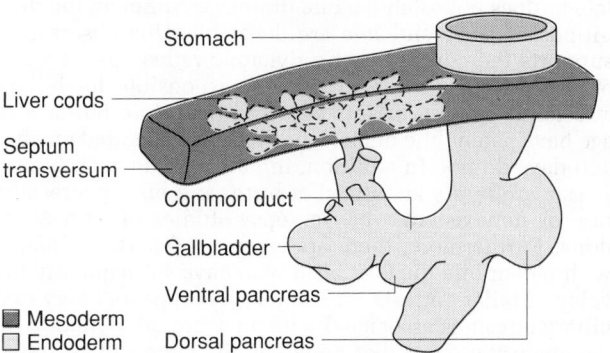

Figure 103-51. The embryonic liver and biliary tract, with contributions from the foregut diverticulum (endoderm) and transverse septum (mesoderm) at about 5 to 6 weeks' gestation.

Labels: Stomach, Liver cords, Septum transversum, Common duct, Gallbladder, Ventral pancreas, Dorsal pancreas, ■ Mesoderm, □ Endoderm

more proximally if only inadequate or obliterated bile ducts are demonstrable (Fig. 103-53). In addition, the luminal diameter of the hilar bile ducts may have prognostic value. Type I bile ducts are defined by a diameter greater than 150 μm and appear to be associated with up to a 90% to 95% probability of postoperative bile flow. Type II bile ducts are patent but have luminal diameters less than 150

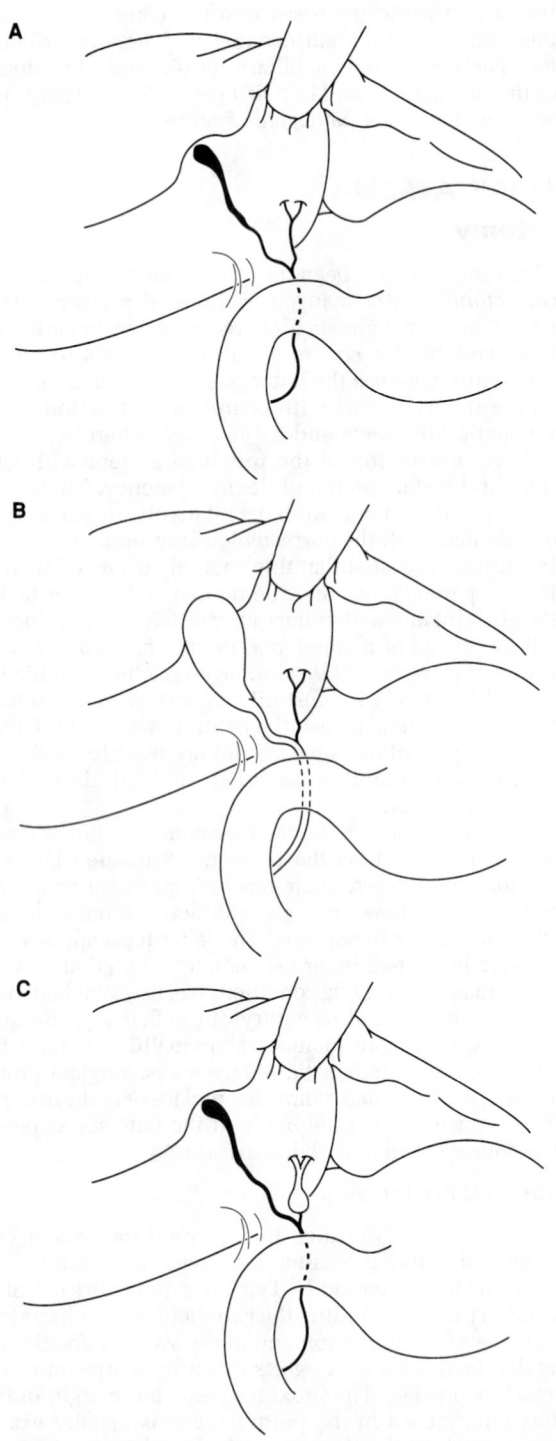

Figure 103-52. Several abnormalities in the anatomy of the biliary tract are seen in biliary atresia. (*A*) The most common variant is considered uncorrectable with a conventional mucosa-to-mucosa biliary enteric anastomosis. (*B*) Proximal atresia with distal bile duct patency occurs in 10% to 15% of patients. (*C*) Correctable anatomy is rare.

μm and have a probability of postoperative bile drainage in the range of 60% to 80%. Type III bile ducts are completely obliterated by the fibrotic process and are associated with a poor prognosis.[101] This classification system is not universally accepted[102] but has intuitive appeal and retains support in the literature.

Biliary atresia is associated with predictable liver parenchymal injury and possibly intrahepatic bile duct obliteration, but there is no single pathognomonic histologic feature. Neocholangiogenesis, the formation of disorganized, nonpatent bile ductules within the liver, is highly suggestive of biliary atresia in the appropriate clinical setting but is not specific (Fig. 103-54). Also typical of biliary atresia is bile pigment deposition, which may occur within bile canaliculi, intralobular bile ducts, or individual hepatocytes. The presence of multinucleated giant cells and periductal inflammation is a frequent finding but is also consistent with neonatal hepatitis. The absence of specific histologic findings is one important reason that diagnostic percutaneous liver biopsy has not been adopted uniformly for the evaluation of neonatal jaundice (see later).

The histologic features within the liver appear to be age-related but vary from patient to patient and from one biopsy to another in a single patient. Early biliary atresia is characterized by acute periportal inflammation with neutrophils and few mononuclear cells (see Fig. 103-54*A*). Older infants typically have evidence of chronic inflammation with dense fibrosis (see Fig. 103-54*C*). Intermediate forms of liver injury with periportal bridging fibrosis are common. Progressive disease ultimately results in biliary cirrhosis with all of its clinical sequelae. Although the rationale for surgical portoenterostomy is to establish bile drainage in the expectation that this will arrest or reverse the process of liver injury, the point at which the injury becomes irreversible is unknown. In clinical practice, most infants beyond 3 or 4 months of age appear to be irreversibly injured, whereas most of the long-term successes have been achieved in patients younger than 2 or 3 months of age at the time of surgery. Almost all patients with biliary atresia have some histologic evidence of residual liver injury.

Pathophysiology

The pathogenesis of biliary atresia is unknown. Experience appears to contradict the concept that biliary atresia results from failure of the extrahepatic bile ducts to recanalize or from primary failure of organogenesis. The accumulated data from the portoenterostomy procedures during the past three decades indicate that early establishment of sustained bile drainage may be associated with reversal of liver injury and long-term survival, whereas cirrhosis and a poor outcome are predictable if surgical intervention is late or does not establish bile drainage. Although the definitions of *early* and *late* are debatable, this observation supports the concept that a dynamic rather than a static or preexisting disease process is responsible for biliary atresia. Typically, infants operated on before 60 days of age have patent bile ducts, whereas those operated on after 120 days do not. In addition, infants who develop biliary atresia are rarely jaundiced at birth, and biliary atresia is rare or nonexistent when autopsy studies of fetuses are done. Furthermore, there are scattered reports of infants with patent bile ducts at birth who have subsequently developed biliary atresia. In summary, it appears likely that biliary atresia is associated with an acquired, dynamic inflammatory process that preferentially targets the extrahepatic biliary ducts of the neonatal infant. In this regard, it shares some clinical and morphologic features of sclerosing cholangitis in adults. The initiating events are unknown, al-

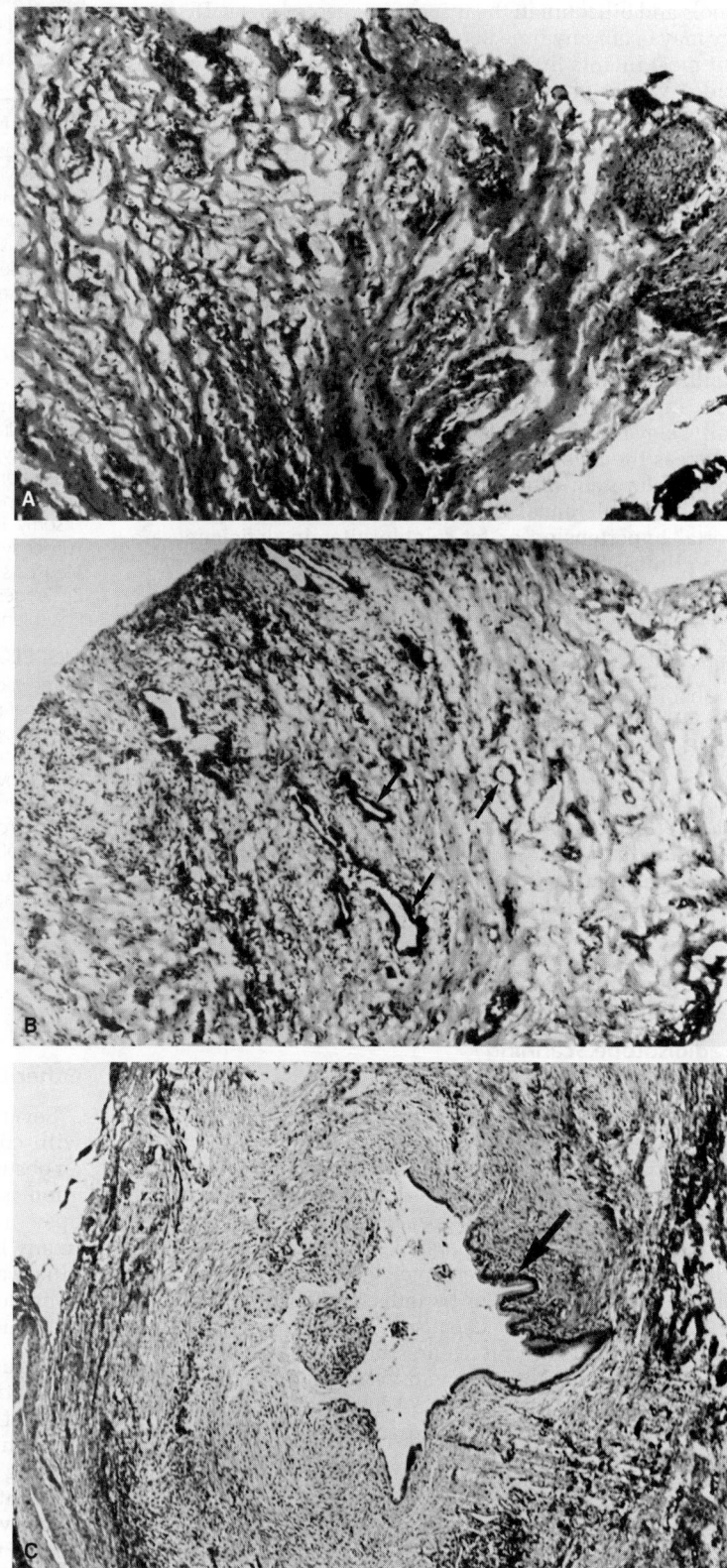

Figure 103-53. Frozen sections of the fibrous biliary tract remnant at the proximal point of transection. (*A*) Complete absence of patent bile ducts with fibrous obliteration of the extrahepatic biliary tract. (*B*) Many patent but small ducts (*arrows*). (*C*) Larger duct with periductal inflammation and fibrosis with loss of normal biliary epithelium (*arrow*). Any of these variations may be found with biliary atresia. (Courtesy of K. Heidelberger, MD, University of Michigan, Ann Arbor)

though there are experimental mouse data and human epidemiologic data to suggest that neonatal reovirus type 3 and other infections may be stimuli.[103-105] Other nonspecific inflammatory stimuli that are not infectious are also implicated.[106] This concept of neonatal biliary tract targeting by an inflammatory process may help explain the frequent progression of intrahepatic biliary injury and liver disease after apparently successful surgical portoenterostomy.

Clinical Presentation and Diagnosis

The incidence of biliary atresia is about 1 per 15,000 infants and may be slightly higher in female and Japanese infants. Patients have typically been anicteric full-term infants without maternal or perinatal difficulties. The cardinal manifestation of the disease is progressive neonatal jaundice with an onset in the first weeks of life. Acholic stools and bilirubin in the urine are expected signs. Discovery may occur any time between birth and 3 months of age, but most infants first become visibly jaundiced between 2 and 4 weeks of age. Infants with biliary atresia usually have a normal physical examination except for the icterus and perhaps mild hepatosplenomegaly. Specific attention is required to exclude the physical findings of Alagille syndrome (eg, biliary hypoplasia associated with peripheral pulmonic stenosis, abnormal facies, growth retardation, and vertebral defects) because the syndrome does not benefit from surgical exploration.

Conjugated hyperbilirubinemia is characteristic of obstructive jaundice. In general, a direct fraction of more than 50%, or greater than 2 mg/dL, requires investigation. Neither serum bilirubin or other biochemical markers of liver injury, however, are specific for biliary atresia. Typically, elevations in levels of serum transaminases are mild, whereas the level of alkaline phosphatase is more significantly elevated, often in the range of 500 to 1000 IU/L. Feeding intolerance, growth failure, and the stigmata of portal hypertension or fat-soluble vitamin deficiency are late clinical findings of biliary atresia.

Neonatal physiologic jaundice is most often a self-limited process related to the normal postpartum delay in the maturation of the glucuronyl transferase system by which hepatocytes conjugate bilirubin. Because of this probability, the rarity of neonatal obstructive jaundice, and the absence of a single definitive diagnostic test for biliary atresia, the diagnosis of biliary atresia has often been delayed. The traditional evaluation of the jaundiced neonate has included longitudinal clinical follow-up and a complex series of diagnostic tests designed to evaluate the differential diagnosis outlined in Table 103-13. The resultant delay in diagnosis and treatment has generally been at least 1 or 2 weeks and frequently longer. The considerations in Table 103-13 are relevant and appropriate in the overall evaluation of the jaundiced neonate, but the time-dependent results after surgery for biliary atresia require a sense of urgency in the diagnostic evaluation.

Radioisotope Scanning

The development of technetium-99m–iminodiacetic acid (^{99m}Tc-IDA) analogues for hepatobiliary imaging has provided a sensitive and specific test for biliary atresia in the appropriate clinical setting. The sensitivity of this examination can be 100% for biliary atresia, with a specificity as high as 94%.[107] To achieve this specificity, a 5- to 7-day course of oral phenobarbital preparation, 5 mg/kg/d, is required. Phenobarbital appears to enhance the study by virtue of its choleretic effect as well as by inducing hepatic microsomal enzymes and increasing hepatocyte processing of ^{99m}Tc-IDA. Interpretation of the scan requires an assessment of excretion (ie, the appearance of isotope in the extrahepatic bile ducts, gallbladder, or intestine up to 24 hours after injection) and an evaluation of hepatocyte extraction of the isotope from plasma. Normally, a patient with a patent extrahepatic biliary tree has isotope promptly excreted into the gut. With biliary atresia, efficient uptake and retention of the tracer within liver parenchyma are expected because the hepatocytes are initially well preserved; however, there is no excretion into the gut. Patients with primary hepatocellular disorders characteristically have impaired isotope extraction, poor hepatocyte definition, and delayed excretion (Fig. 103-55). The reliability of radioisotope scanning in experienced hands has made it possible to conduct this study simultaneously with the traditional neonatal jaundice evaluation and thereby to diminish the diagnostic delay. In addition, the radioisotope biliary scan reliably provides a definitive diagnosis of a choledochal cyst, the other important cause of neonatal obstructive jaundice.

Table 103-13. CAUSES AND ASSOCIATIONS OF NEONATAL CHOLESTATIC SYNDROMES

CONGENITAL INFECTIOUS CAUSES

Cytomegalovirus*
Rubella virus*
Herpes virus
Hepatitis virus B*
Echovirus 14, 19
Coxsackievirus B
Toxoplasmosis
Syphilis

GENETIC ASSOCIATIONS

Galactosemia
Tyrosinemia
Congenital fructose intolerance
α_1-Antitrypsin deficiency
Cystic fibrosis
Niemann-Pick disease
Trisomy 17, 18, 21
Turner syndrome
Menkes syndrome
Zellweger syndrome
Polysplenia syndrome†

MISCELLANEOUS ASSOCIATIONS

Hemolytic disease
Bacterial sepsis
Pyelonephritis
Parenteral hyperalimentation
Congestive heart failure
Hypoplastic left-sided heart syndrome
Postnecrotizing enterocolitis, gastroschisis, omphalocele
Neonatal hypopituitarism
Inspissated bile syndrome (without hemolysis)—neonatal shock, respiratory distress syndrome, acidosis

* Rarely reported with biliary atresia
† Frequently associated with biliary atresia

Other Diagnostic Tests

Several additional studies are appropriate for infants with conjugated hyperbilirubinemia suspected of having an obstructive cause. The principle that governs this evaluation is that prompt laparotomy or laparoscopy, liver biopsy, and operative cholangiogram should be performed in any indeterminate situation or for any patient in whom biliary atresia is suspected. Failure to adopt this aggressive approach may lead to inappropriate delay and a poorer outcome than might otherwise have been achieved.

Ultrasound. An abdominal ultrasound examination evaluating the liver and biliary tract should be performed promptly as a standard part of the evaluation of the jaundiced neonate. For infants with biliary atresia, the typical finding is an absent, diminutive, or obliterated gallbladder without associated intrahepatic bile duct dilation. Additionally, ultrasound reliably demonstrates a cystic mass within the hepatoduodenal ligament if a choledochal cyst is the cause of the biliary obstruction. If other, more rare causes of extrahepatic biliary obstruction are present, proximal bile dilation is likely to be apparent. To be reliable, this evaluation requires an examiner familiar with neonatal ultrasound findings.

Liver Biopsy. The histologic findings of biliary atresia are sufficiently nonspecific that a diagnosis is not possible in 20% to 25% of affected infants subjected to percutaneous liver biopsy. Given this difficulty and the utility of radioisotope scanning, the emphasis on preoperative per-

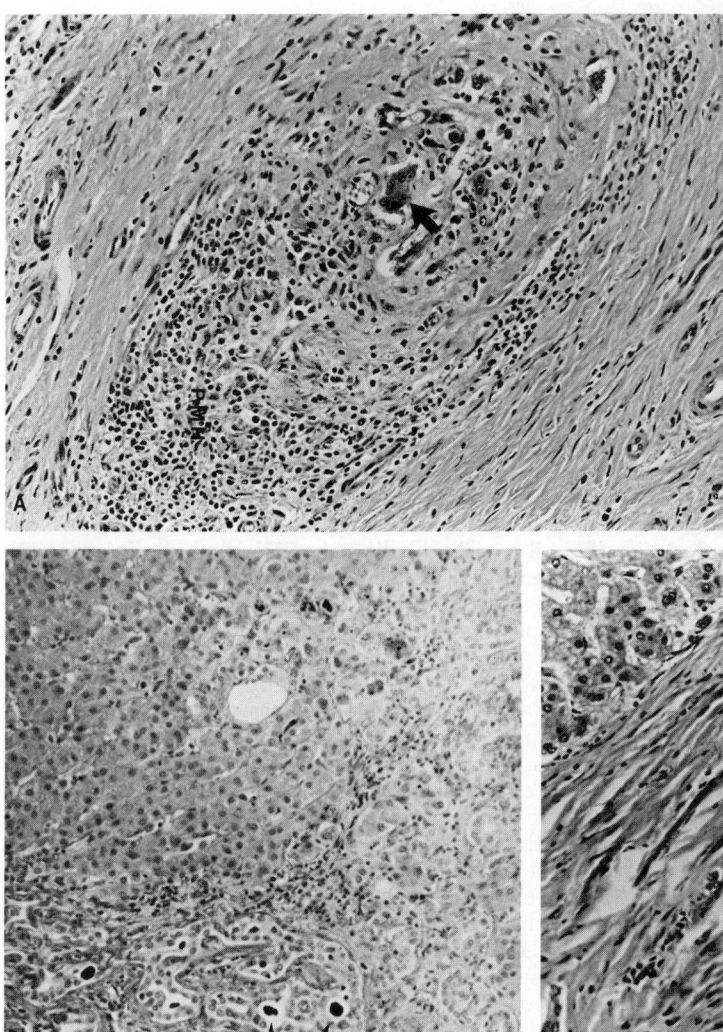

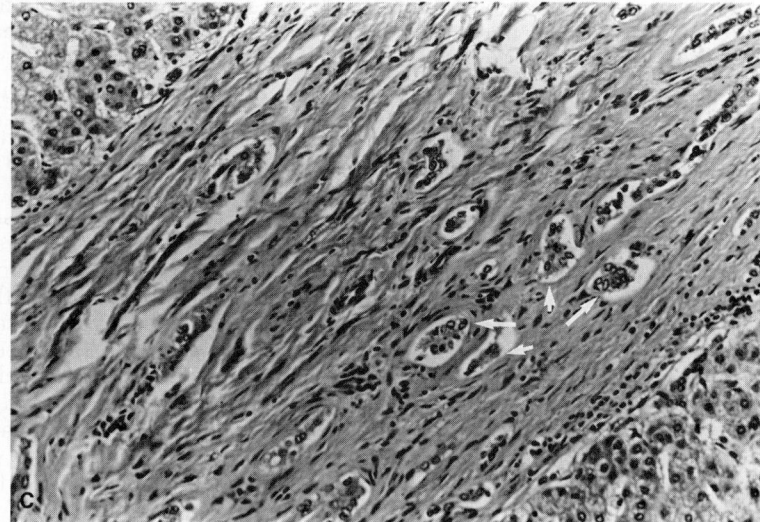

Figure 103-54. Liver morphology from patients with biliary atresia shows evidence of neocholangiogenesis, the disordered proliferation of nonpatent bile ductules, and bile plugs. The degree of inflammation and cirrhosis vary greatly. (*A*) Liver histology at an early stage characterized by acute periportal neutrophil infiltration and giant cell formation (*arrow*). (*B*) Classic bile plug formation (*arrows*). (*C*) Liver histology in an older child with biliary atresia and cirrhosis. There is nearly complete replacement of normal hepatocytes with fibrosis and prominent neocholangiogenesis (*arrows*).

cutaneous liver biopsy has diminished. Its best use is probably in the jaundiced infant likely by history to have a nonsurgical cause of cholestatic jaundice, in whom the percutaneous biopsy can confirm the diagnosis without the need for anesthesia and laparotomy.

α_1-**Antitrypsin Deficiency.** α_1-Antitrypsin deficiency is the single most important medical condition that may be difficult or impossible to differentiate from biliary atresia using the approach outlined earlier. For this reason, all jaundiced infants should have plasma α_1-antitrypsin levels determined before surgical exploration for suspected biliary atresia.

Treatment

Although the choice between operative and nonoperative treatment was a subject of controversy two decades ago, the 100% mortality rate associated with medical man-

agement of biliary atresia has led to a consensus that all infants with biliary atresia should undergo surgical therapy. Medical therapy is directed to the postoperative management of chronic liver disease. Debate is centered on the relative merits and appropriate roles for portoenterostomy and hepatic transplantation.

Portoenterostomy

Before the development of the portoenterostomy procedure in Japan in the late 1950s, all infants with biliary atresia succumbed to chronic liver disease and biliary cirrhosis.[108] The procedure was adopted in Europe and North America 10 to 15 years later and is the recommended surgical procedure for the initial management of infants with biliary atresia. Primary transplantation is advocated by a few surgeons but generally is reserved for infants with delayed diagnosis and with established cirrhosis at initial presentation. Most biliary atresia patients undergoing hepatic transplantation have failed portoenterostomy procedures.[109,110]

The approach for the usual infant in whom biliary atresia is discovered within the first 90 days of life is to confirm the suspected diagnosis by operative cholangiogram at laparotomy, then proceed with portoenterostomy. Previous enthusiasm for sequential operations to construct and close complex exteriorized biliary conduits has diminished because there appears to be little additional benefit and multiple operations are associated with increased technical risks at transplantation.

Failure is predictable with the portoenterostomy procedure if certain technical requirements are not fulfilled; unfortunately, correct surgical technique does not ensure success. The procedure is performed through a right upper quadrant incision. A liver biopsy is routinely performed to document the extent of preexisting hepatic parenchymal injury. A cholangiogram is attempted through the gallbladder but is often not successful because the gallbladder and cystic duct are obliterated. The distal extrahepatic biliary tree is patent in 10% to 15% of infants, but because of proximal obstruction, these infants also require portoenterostomy. In this circumstance, use of the patient's gallbladder and cystic duct for the biliary conduit is feasible, but it appears to have a high incidence of technical failure related to mechanical obstruction of the cystic duct. Inspection of the hepatoduodenal ligament most often reveals a nonpatent fibrous cord rather than a normal common bile duct. This remnant is divided distal to the cystic duct, and dissection into the porta hepatis is taken cephalad to the bifurcation of the portal vein. The fibrous cord is transected sharply at this level without the use of cautery or hemostatic sutures so as to preserve any patent bile ducts. Evaluation of the bile ducts on frozen section allows intraoperative confirmation of the level of the transection and potentially allows a more proximal dissection if necessary. A short (about 15 to 30 cm) retrocolic Roux-en-Y jejunal conduit is constructed. No clear advantage has been shown for longer or otherwise modified conduits with regard to concerns of ascending infection leading to cholangitis. In addition, cyclosporin A absorption is potentially diminished by the use of longer defunctionalized conduits.[111] The biliary enteric portoenterostomy does not yield a gratifying union of biliary and intestinal mucosa (Fig. 103-56).

Whether the conduit should be exteriorized or not has been an issue of considerable debate. No clear consensus has emerged, and many modifications are in use (Fig. 103-57). It appears that exteriorized conduits may have a slightly lower incidence of postoperative cholangitis and that bile flow is more easily monitored. Disadvantages of exteriorization include the need for a second procedure to close the stoma, parastomal variceal bleeding, possibly a higher incidence of bowel obstruction, high bile outputs requiring bile refeeding, and possibly fluid and electrolyte abnormalities.[112] There are no survival differences between patients with exteriorized and closed conduits. Given the emphasis on simplicity and that many of these infants ultimately come to transplantation, there is a trend toward the selection of simple closed conduits.

Results and Complications. Bile flow may require weeks or even months to develop after portoenterostomy, but eventually about 66% to 75% of infants operated on when younger than 60 days of age have clinical evidence of bile flow. The likelihood of bile flow diminishes with increased age at operation, so that the probability approaches zero in infants older than 120 days of age.[113]

Postoperative cholangitis is the most important late complication after portoenterostomy. It is defined as fever and leukocytosis associated with diminished bile flow in the absence of other systemic illness. The incidence is reported to be as low as 40% to 50% after portoenterostomy, but most patients have some evidence of this if carefully monitored. Cholangitis is characterized by evidence of a systemic inflammatory process and is thought to be associated with progressive liver disease. There is no convincing evidence that this cholangitis results from ascending bacterial infection, but the traditional and successful treatment approach includes broad-spectrum antibiotic administration and intravenous fluid resuscitation. Steroids and other antiinflammatory agents may occasionally be useful; reoperation or endoscopic revision of the portoenterostomy usually is not. Postoperatively, patients may be empirically maintained on prophylactic broad-spectrum antibiotics and choleretic agents such as phenobarbital in an attempt to diminish the incidence of cholangitis. Ursodeoxycholate is appropriate for these children as well as for others with cholestatic liver disease. It has been shown to protect the liver from harmful bile acids, to improve symptoms,

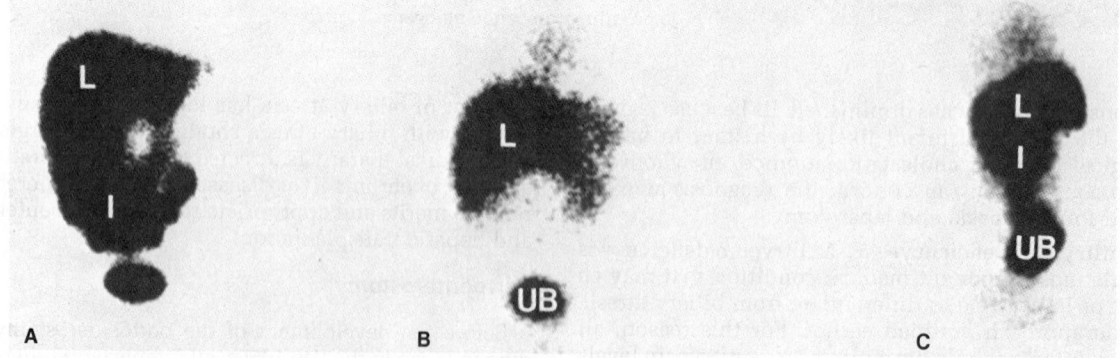

Figure 103-55. (*A*) Normal scan using PIPIDA as the hepatobiliary scanning agent. At 45 minutes, isotope is clearly visible in the liver (L) and intestine (I). (*B*) PIPIDA scan (after phenobarbital administration) from a patient with biliary atresia. Even after 8 hours, isotope is apparent only in the liver and urinary bladder (UB). No evidence is seen of biliary or intestinal excretion. (*C*) PIPIDA (after phenobarbital administration) from a patient with cholestatic jaundice. At 65 minutes, isotope is visible in the liver (L) and intestine (I). Hepatocyte extraction is variable but is usually decreased or normal, whereas gastrointestinal excretion is predictably present with cholestatic jaundice or hepatocellular disease.

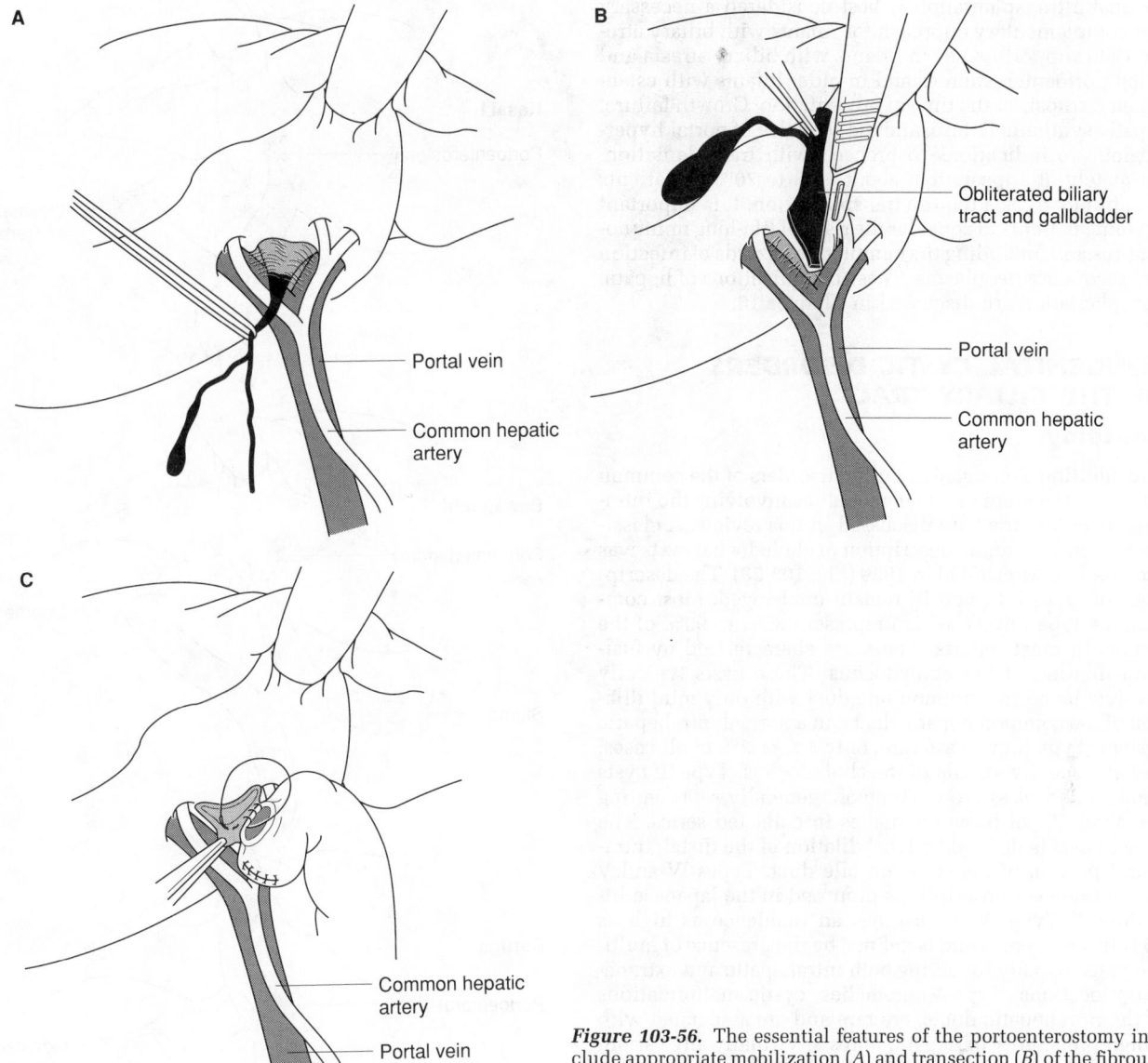

A

Portal vein

Common hepatic artery

B

Obliterated biliary tract and gallbladder

Portal vein

Common hepatic artery

C

Common hepatic artery

Portal vein

Figure 103-56. The essential features of the portoenterostomy include appropriate mobilization (*A*) and transection (*B*) of the fibrous biliary tract remnant. (*C*) Creation of a Roux-en-Y jejunal conduit with biliary enteric anastomosis completes the procedure.

and to delay the onset of liver failure and complications of cirrhosis.[114]

Almost all patients with biliary atresia have some degree of residual liver injury. Portal hypertension with esophageal variceal bleeding, hypersplenism, hepatic synthetic failure, and vitamin D, E, A, and K deficiencies have all been problems. These problems are best treated with hepatic transplantation with the exception of the vitamin deficiencies, which can be treated with oral supplementation. The strategy for acute variceal hemorrhage should be to temporize with esophageal sclerotherapy if necessary but to avoid operative portosystemic shunts to simplify subsequent transplantation.

Most institutions report 5-year survival rates between 40% and 60% for portoenterostomy.[99] In general, survival appears to be inversely related to age at the time of operation. After portoenterostomy, about one third of patients have good long-term results with bile drainage, stable or inconsequential liver disease, and normal growth and development. One third do poorly postoperatively and require prompt hepatic transplantation for survival. The remaining third have serious liver disease, progressive

cirrhosis, or both but maintain growth and development for a period of months or years before requiring transplantation. These data provide the principal argument for the continued use of portoenterostomy procedures rather than transplantation for the initial treatment of biliary atresia.[115–117] Although the portoenterostomy failure rate is high, the possibility of long-term success and the likelihood of a period of normal growth have led most centers around the world to continue with this approach.

Hepatic Transplantation

Hepatic transplantation is discussed in detail in Chapter 16. With regard to biliary atresia, early transplantation in infants after a failed portoenterostomy is technically feasible, with acceptable complication rates and 1-year graft survival rates of 70% to 80%, which are similar to adult results.[109,110,118] In addition, the ability to use reduced-size donor livers, including those from living, related donors, provides hope for reducing the overall donor organ shortage. In part because of these latter approaches, the mortality rate for these infants while on transplantation waiting lists has fallen from about 50% to 10% or less.[119]

Hepatic transplantation is best considered a necessary and complementary approach for infants with biliary atresia. Data support its use in infants with biliary atresia and failed portoenterostomies and in older infants with established cirrhosis at the time of presentation. Growth failure, hepatic synthetic failure, and the sequelae of portal hypertension are indications to proceed with transplantation. Ultimately, it appears that about 60% to 70% of patients with biliary atresia require transplantation. It is important in young patients to consider the risks of life-long immunosuppression, including the cumulative hazards of infection and secondary neoplasms. These complications of hepatic transplantation are discussed in Chapter 16.

CONGENITAL CYSTIC DISORDERS OF THE BILIARY TRACT

Anatomy

In addition to congenital cystic disorders of the common bile duct, the more unusual anomalies involving the intrahepatic biliary tract are discussed in this review. A classification and anatomic description of choledochal cysts was provided by Alonso-Lej in 1959 (Fig. 103-58). The descriptions of types I, II, and III remain unchanged. Most common are type I cysts, which represent 85% to 90% of the lesions in most reports. These are characterized by fusiform dilation of the choledochus. These cysts typically involve the entire common bile duct with only mild dilation of the common hepatic duct and a normal intrahepatic system. Type II cysts are rare, only 1% or 2% of all cases, and are true diverticula of the choledochus. Type III cysts (choledochoceles) are uncommon, generally representing less than 2% of these anomalies in collected series. The type III cyst is defined by local dilation of the distal, intramural portion of the common bile duct. Types IV and V are more recent descriptions proposed in the Japanese literature.[120] Type IV disease has an incidence as high as 15% in some series and is defined by the presence of multiple cysts, usually involving both intrahepatic and extrahepatic locations. Type V anomalies, cystic malformations of the intrahepatic ducts, are rare and are associated with a high probability of hepatic fibrosis. Virtually any variant or combination of these anomalies is possible, including a rare association with biliary atresia.

Type I cysts are typically large, extending from the porta hepatis into the pelvis and displacing adjacent viscera. The proximal extent of the cyst is at the origin of the common bile duct, with only mild or moderate dilation of the hepatic ducts. The most distal common bile duct is a diminutive structure often located considerably cephalad and medial to the inferior pole of the cyst. The associated distortion of the distal duct and its typical 1- or 2-mm caliber explain the propensity for clinical presentation with obstructive jaundice. The junction of the distal common bile duct and the pancreatic duct is not in a normal intramural duodenal position but is located proximal to the duodenal wall and the sphincter of Oddi (Fig. 103-59).

With the exception of the choledochocele (type III), microscopic anatomy is similar for all cysts. Normal biliary epithelium is either absent or replaced by abnormal and sometimes dysplastic columnar epithelium. The wall of the cyst contains normal smooth muscle but with a variable degree of inflammation and fibrosis. Infants and young children often have less evidence of inflammatory change, whereas adolescents and adults typically have established inflammation extending to the adjacent structures in the hepatoduodenal ligament. This feature of the disease and its technical surgical risks led to the historic reliance on internal drainage procedures for treatment. Type III cysts

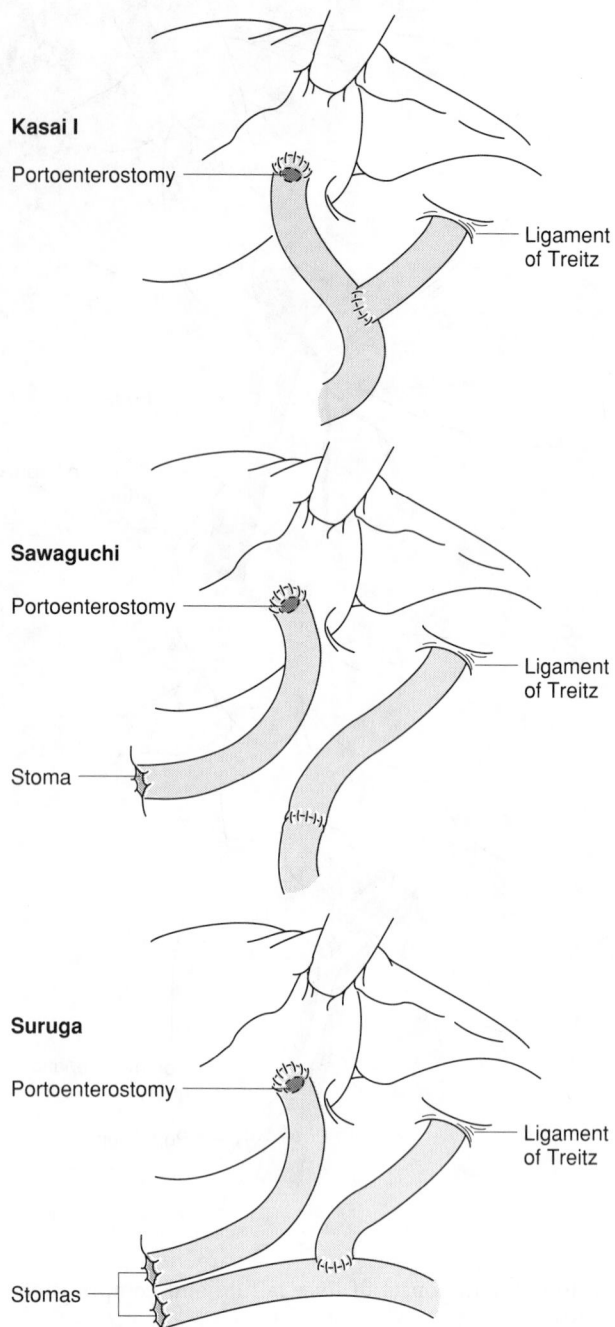

Figure 103-57. Many types of conduits have been used for biliary drainage after portoenterostomy. There are relatively few data to select among these, and current trends emphasize simplicity. The primary importance of this issue is that the reoperative surgeon must be familiar with the anatomic possibilities. These are the three most commonly used conduits.

are usually but not always lined by normal duodenal mucosa and are considered separately.

Pathophysiology

The pathogenesis of cystic lesions of the bile ducts is obscure, but the now routine prenatal discovery of the lesions makes an embryonic origin a certainty. Whether this is related to abnormal recanalization of the primitive bile duct cords, reflux of pancreatic secretions into the

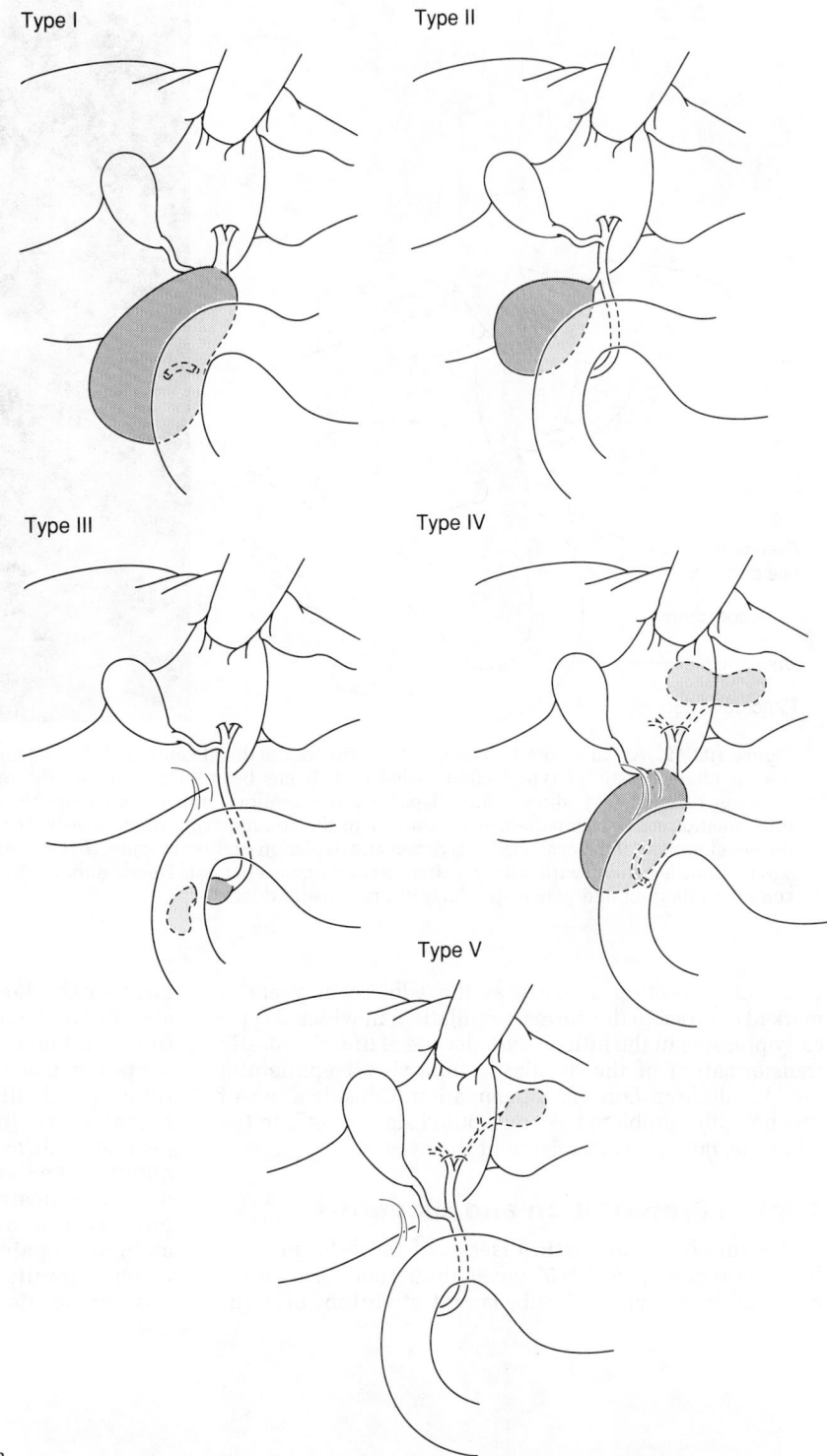

Type I

Type II

Type III

Type IV

Type V

Figure 103-58. Choledochal cyst classification.

common bile duct, a primary inflammatory process, or some other mechanism is not known. The physiologic consequences of choledochal cysts are generally associated with obstruction to bile flow or occasionally with extrinsic compression of adjacent viscera. Obstructive jaundice is an expected presenting finding. Liver injury is usually reversible, and progression to biliary cirrhosis is rare. An exception is type V disease, which for unknown reasons is associated with a high incidence of hepatic fibrosis. Gallstone formation and secondary acute bacterial cholangitis, presumably related to inadequate bile drainage and stasis,

are common presentations for choledochal cysts. Acute pancreatitis, particularly with type III cysts, is well described and is likely secondary to partial obstruction of the distal pancreatic duct. A rare clinical presentation is the development of portal hypertension on the basis of chronic extrinsic portal vein compression.

Adenocarcinoma of the biliary tract develops in 3% to 5% of patients who have choledochal cysts. Although this represents a small number of patients, the total number reported exceeds 50 and the incidence is about 1000 times that of the normal population.[121] In addition, the carci-

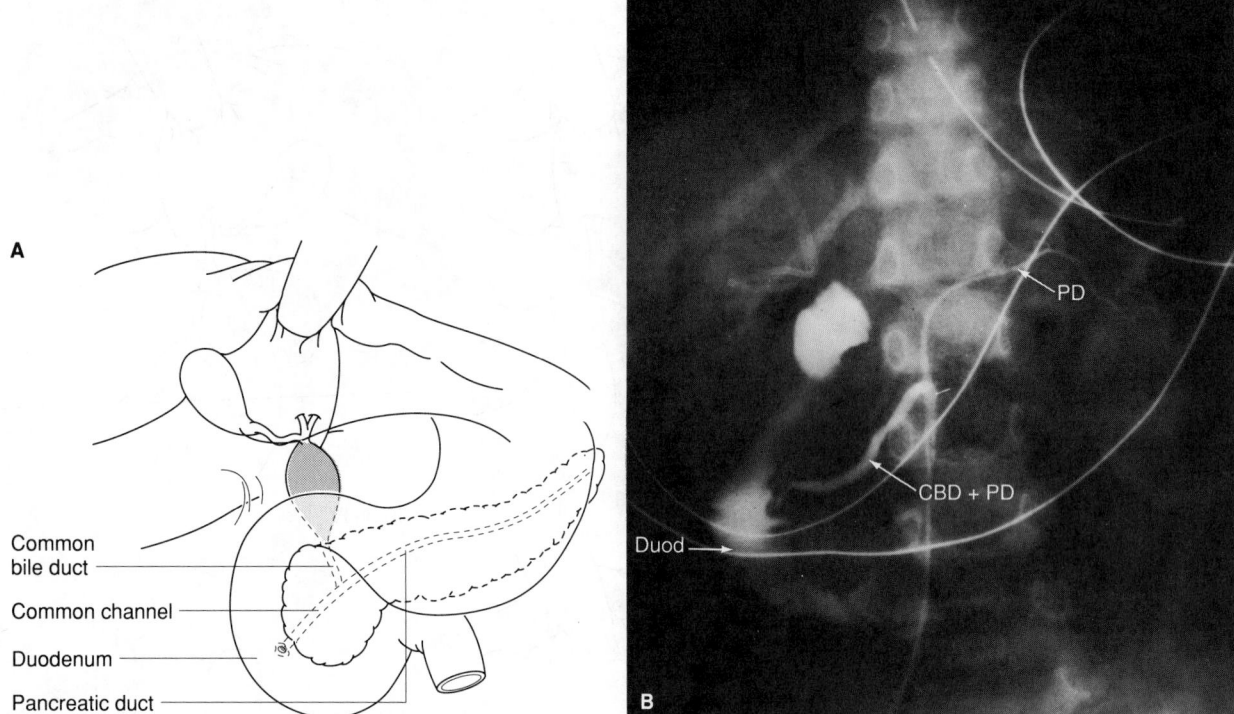

Figure 103-59. An anomalous, extramural junction of the distal common bile duct and pancreatic duct is characteristic of type I choledochal cyst. It has been suggested that the resulting long common channel may allow reflux of pancreatic secretions into the choledochus, resulting in inflammation and proteinase-mediated injury to the common bile duct, possibly contributing to the development of the cyst itself. (*A*) Schematic depiction of this anatomy. (*B*) Operative cholangiogram from a patient with a long extramural common channel. Duod, duodenum; CBD + PD, common bile duct and pancreatic duct; PD, pancreatic duct.

noma may develop as early as the adolescent years, a marked contrast to the normal population, in which it typically presents in the fifth or sixth decade of life. Neoplastic transformation of the dysplastic biliary cyst epithelium may result from chronic inflammation. Consideration of this potential problem has contributed significantly to the emphasis on surgical excision of the cysts.

Clinical Presentation and Diagnosis

The incidence of cystic disease of the bile ducts is low. As recently as 1975, fewer than 1000 cases were reported worldwide.[122] Subsequent attention, particu-

larly in the Japanese literature, has shown that these are not rare lesions in tertiary care and pediatric institutions, and more than 300 cases have been reported. Presentation can occur at any age, but discovery during infancy and childhood is most common, particularly in recent years. Infants may be diagnosed as a result of perinatal ultrasound screening examinations or subsequent to the development of neonatal obstructive jaundice. Classically, older children and adults develop a clinical triad of a right upper quadrant mass, episodic abdominal pain, and jaundice, but these three findings coexist simultaneously in less than one half of patients. Physical examination may also demonstrate hepato-

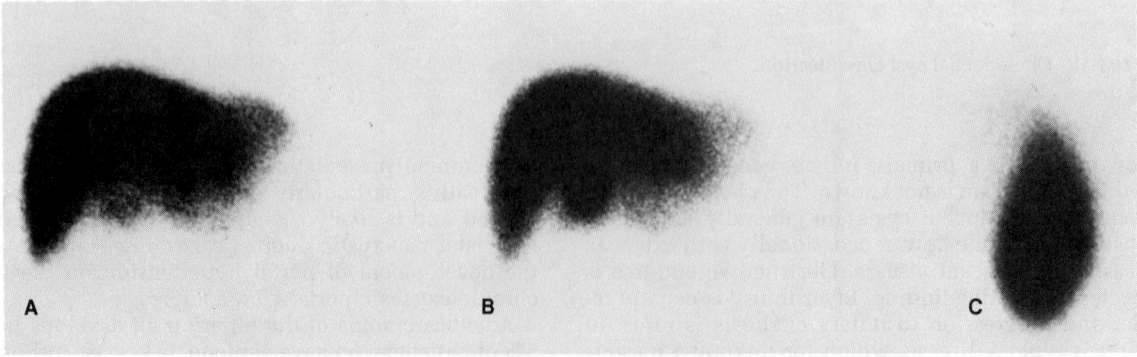

Figure 103-60. Typical HIDA scan from a child with a type I choledochal cyst. Images were made 5 minutes (*A*), 30 minutes (*B*), and 3 hours (*C*) after isotope injection. The isotope is retained within the choledochal cyst more than 24 hours, and the pattern of hepatocyte extraction is normal.

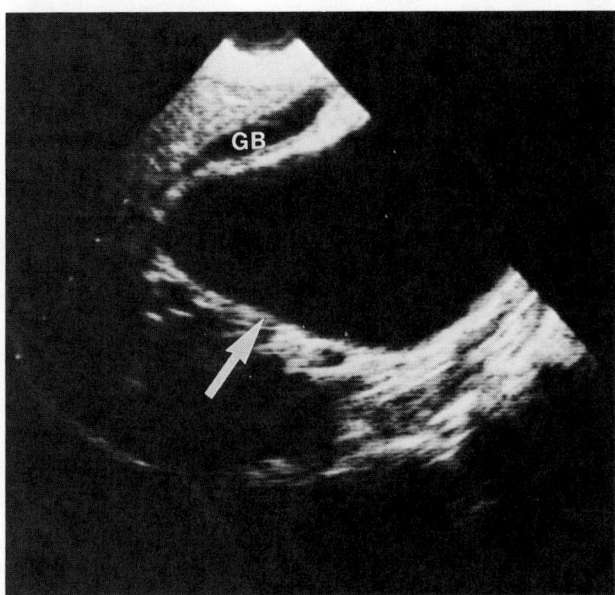

Figure 103-61. Ultrasound demonstration of a type I choledochal cyst (*arrow*; longitudinal image). The gallbladder (GB) is also shown.

megaly or occasionally evidence of portal hypertension. Diagnosis in neonates and infants is definitively obtained using ^{99m}Tc-IDA scans and ultrasound examinations (Figs. 103-60 and 103-61). In older patients, endoscopic retrograde cholangiopancreatography is a highly accurate and readily available technique to confirm the diagnosis but generally is not necessary. Because of the nonspecific clinical features of choledochal cysts, other diagnostic tests are invariably the means by which some patients are discovered. An upper GI series may show medial and anterior displacement of the duodenum by a type I cyst or intraluminal projection of a type III cyst at the ampulla of Vater. Indeed, these latter patients may present with signs and symptoms of partial duodenal obstruction. Percutaneous transhepatic cholangiography defines intrahepatic biliary tract anatomy more precisely than a retrograde approach in some complex patients. Abdominal computed tomography scans and magnetic resonance imaging demonstrate biliary dilation and other intraabdominal anatomy, although generally they are not as helpful as the approaches already considered. Liver biopsy, regardless of the method, has little role other than to document the extent of established liver injury. Diagnostic imaging techniques are sufficiently precise that a correct preoperative diagnosis of a choledochal cyst is usually possible.

Treatment

Type I Cysts

Treatment of cystic disease of the biliary tree is always surgical and depends on the specific anatomic abnormality. Operative procedures should routinely commence with cholangiography, usually by way of the gallbladder, but contrast injection into the common bile duct is sometimes necessary. Cholecystectomy is standard. Internal drainage procedures without cyst resection (eg, cyst duodenostomy, cyst gastrostomy, and cyst jejunostomy of any construction) were routinely performed for type I choledochal cysts until the 1970s. The rate of failure (eg, stricture, recurrent cholangitis, stone formation, pancreatitis) ranged from 30% to 75%, depending on the length of follow-up and the type of procedure. As these late complication rates became apparent, the risk of bile duct adenocarcinoma in the residual cyst also became widely recognized. In addition, the operative and anesthetic risks of primary excision diminished. For these reasons, a consensus has developed in the last two decades that primary excision of a type I cyst with reconstruction using a Roux-en-Y hepaticojejunostomy is the surgical procedure of choice (Fig. 103-62). Cyst excision is preferentially a total transmural excision that is routinely done in infants and almost always possible in older patients as well. Occasionally, adults with severe inflammation and fibrosis may require intramural cyst dissection, leaving the posteromedial outer wall of the cyst in situ to protect the adjacent portal vein and hepatic artery.

Other Types of Cysts

Type II cysts are excised and the common bile duct closed. Type III choledochoceles require a transduodenal approach with marsupialization of the cyst into the duodenum and generally a formal sphincteroplasty to ensure adequate drainage of biliary and pancreatic secretions. The presence of intrahepatic cystic disease requires an individualized strategy. In general, unilobar or focal cystic disease can be either resected or adequately drained using a Roux-en-Y jejunal reconstruction. Bilobar intrahepatic disease, particularly if associated with hepatic fibrosis, may be difficult or impossible to adequately drain. Fortunately, it is rare.

Complications and Results

Recurrent cholangitis, stricture, stone formation, and pancreatitis may complicate any of the surgical procedures for choledochal cysts. The incidence of complications, mortality, and reoperation for the different procedures is summarized in Table 103-14.[122] Most important are the morbidity and reoperation data, which show a clear advantage for cyst excision. The shift away from internal drainage procedures took place partly as a result of this 1975 analysis, which showed no increase in mortality rates with primary cyst excision.[122] Subsequently, operative mortality has continued to diminish, with no mortality in a number of recent reports, thus emphasizing the safety and desirability of total transmural excision of choledochal cysts.[123,124]

Operation	Cases	Morbidity	Reoperation	Mortality
Cyst excision and hepaticojejunostomy	83	7 (8%)	0	6 (7%)
Cyst jejunostomy (Roux)	53	18 (34%)	7 (13%)	9 (17%)
Cyst jejunostomy (loop)	12	6 (50%)	5 (42%)	1 (3%)
Cyst duodenostomy	93	55 (58%)	35 (38%)	6 (5%)

(Data from Flanigan DP. Biliary cysts. Ann Surg 1975;182:635)

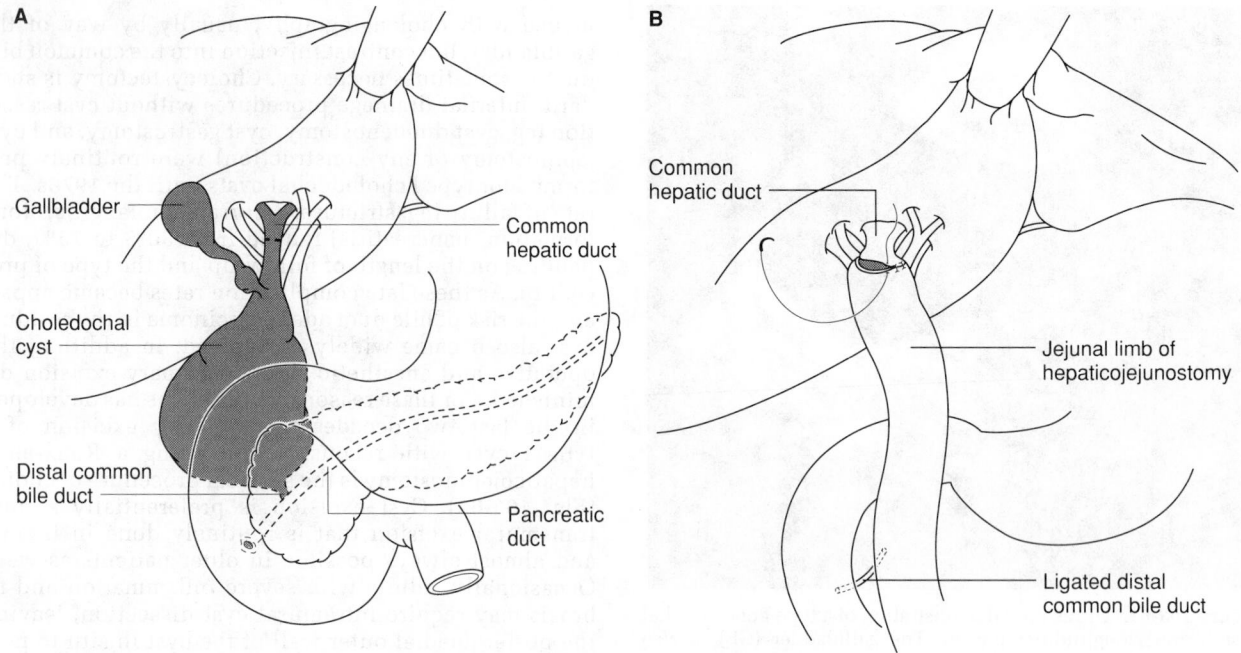

Figure 103-62. The preferred operative treatment of a type I choledochal cyst consists of total transmural cyst excision with Roux-en-Y hepaticojejunostomy.

Pediatric Pancreas
ARNOLD G. CORAN

In comparison with diseases of the liver and biliary system, pancreatic problems in infants and children are rare. Because they are rare, they are often overlooked in the differential diagnosis of acute abdominal pain and abdominal masses. It is important to understand the issues specific to infants and children with regard to pancreatitis (acute and chronic), pancreas divisum, pancreatic cysts, pancreatic neoplasms, and endocrine lesions of the pancreas.[125]

EMBRYOLOGY

Between the fourth and seventh weeks of fetal life, paired primordia arise from the duodenum and become the dorsal and ventral anlage of the pancreas. The ventral pancreas grows around from the right side of the duodenum and fuses with the dorsal pancreas, which forms the body and tail of the pancreas (Fig. 103-62). The independent ductal systems of the pancreatic anlage fuse, and the dorsal (Santorini) duct opens directly into the duodenum (persisting in 10% to 15% of normal patients). The ventral (Wirsung) duct opens into the duodenum by way of the common bile duct. The dorsal duct, draining the body and tail, fuses with ventral duct just to the right of the mesenteric vessels. Occasionally, the ventral duct disappears, and the entire gland is drained by the accessory duct of Santorini.

Both acinar cells and islet cells differentiate from primitive duct cells of the pancreas. The earliest islets are visible at the end of the second gestational month, just before the acini appear. The islet cells regress after the fifth month. Although a few of these primary islets may remain in the pancreas of premature infants, usually all have disap-peared by the time of birth. Secondary islets arise from centroacinar cell proliferation during the third gestational month. These cells appear to migrate out of the acini in which they are formed, developing into islets that remain connected to the duct by a thin cellular stalk (the tubule of Bensley). The primary islets are located in the interlobular connective tissue, whereas the secondary islets are found among the acini within lobules.

Rare anomalies of the exocrine pancreas arise from defective embryogenesis. The most common of these defects is the annular pancreas, which is thought to result from interrupted migration of the ventral pancreas during embryogenesis. Less common defects include anomalies of the ductal system, intrapancreatic enteric duplications, pancreatic–splenic fusion, heterotopic pancreatic tissue, and congenital agenesis of portions of the pancreas such as the body and tail.

ACUTE PANCREATITIS

Although acute pancreatitis is a common cause of acute abdominal pain in the adult population (see Chap. 31), it is seldom considered in the child who presents with abdominal pain. It is the most common disorder of the pancreas in infants and children. Although adult pancreatitis is usually related to cholelithiasis or alcohol ingestion, pediatric causes are considerably more varied. Fifty to 80% of childhood acute pancreatitis is either idiopathic or posttraumatic in origin. These causes occur with about equal frequency, and the problem is most common in adolescents. Other causes of pancreatitis in children include biliary stone disease, hyperlipidemia, cystic fibrosis, choledochal cyst or other anatomic abnormality, juvenile diabetes mellitus, ethanol ingestion, duodenal ulcer, mumps, coxsackievirus infection, and collagen vascular disease such as lupus erythematosus. Immunosuppressive agents, especially high-dose corticosteroids, have been associated with acute pancreatitis in children. Indeed, steroid-induced acute pancreatitis follows only trauma and idiopathic causes for pancreatitis in most children's hospitals. Additional drugs associated with acute pancreatitis include chlorthiazide, tetracyclines, oral contraceptives, azathioprine, and L-asparaginase. The anticonvulsant valproic acid is related to a particularly virulent form of necrotizing pancreatitis that may be fatal. Occasionally, infectious mononucleosis and acute pancreatitis are associated, although the pathogenic basis for this is unknown.

The diagnosis of acute pancreatitis is based on the clinical picture of epigastric abdominal pain, fever, leukocytosis, and elevated plasma levels of amylase and lipase. The serum amylase determination alone is not sufficient because it is not specific and it may not be elevated despite the occurrence of acute pancreatitis. In these situations, the amylase/creatinine clearance ratio may help improve diagnostic accuracy. Ultrasonography, computed tomographic (CT) scanning, and magnetic resonance (MR) imaging have improved diagnostic specificity. With each imaging technique, acute pancreatitis is characterized by edema and enlargement of the gland. Occasionally, ductal dilation is demonstrable with ultrasound. Endoscopic retrograde cholangioscopic pancreatography (ERCP) is not indicated during the acute inflammatory phase of the illness because exacerbation of the pancreatitis can result. Its principal role is to evaluate patients for the cause of acute pancreatitis after recovery.

Management of acute pancreatitis in childhood is similar to that of adults in that nonoperative management is emphasized. This includes pain relief, parenteral fluids, parenteral nutrition, and pancreatic rest by nasogastric decompression and possibly anticholinergic agents, although the latter have never been proved efficacious. Similarly, somatostatin analogues have been used, but their efficacy remains to be demonstrated convincingly. If hypocalcemia occurs, calcium supplementation is needed. Almost all children with pancreatitis have simple edematous pancreatitis. Hemorrhagic or necrotizing pancreatitis is rare in children who are immune competent.

Therapy is usually supportive and nonoperative. Parenteral nutrition and ventilatory support are provided as necessary. Operation is reserved for complications related to acute pancreatitis. Occasionally, surgical exploration is undertaken for diagnostic purposes such as suspected acute appendicitis.

Recurrent acute pancreatitis in childhood is usually associated with a specific physiologic cause or anatomic abnormality. For this reason, a child with recurrent disease should be investigated aggressively, including the use of ERCP, even in infants. This approach yields a specific diagnosis in more than half of children in several small series.

PANCREAS DIVISUM

Pancreas divisum is an anatomic variation that results when the dorsal and ventral ducts do not fuse normally. As previously noted, the dorsal gland is normally drained by the duct of Santorini and the ventral component the duct of Wirsung, which joins the distal common duct and enters the duodenum as a common channel (Fig. 103-64A). The presence of two completely separate pancreatic ducts is not unusual and occurs in about 10% to 15% of normal children. About 5% to 10% of asymptomatic patients undergoing ERCP show two complete ductal systems. The anatomic variant of pancreas divisum is not necessarily abnormal. If the orifice of the accessory papilla is stenotic, however, pancreatitis can result.[126] About 25% of these patients ultimately develop pancreatitis. Stenosis of the lesser papilla is probably developmental because there is

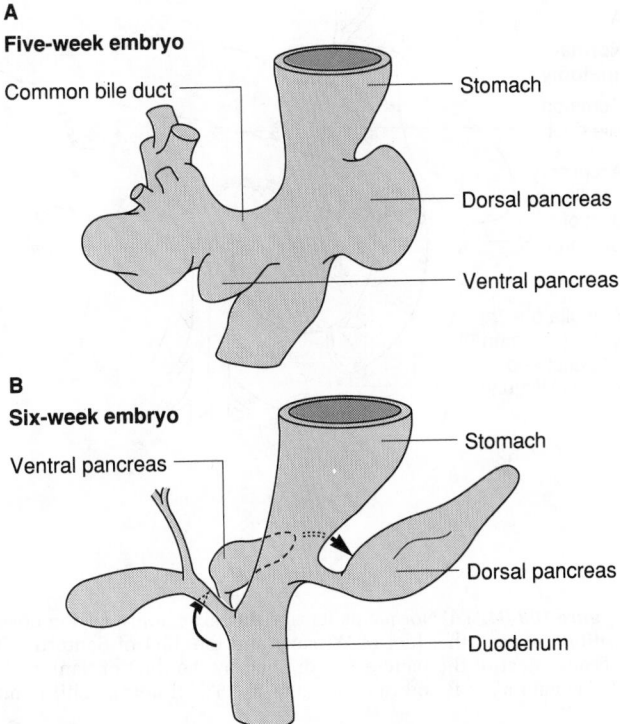

A
Five-week embryo

Common bile duct — — Stomach

— Dorsal pancreas

— Ventral pancreas

B
Six-week embryo

Ventral pancreas — — Stomach

— Dorsal pancreas

— Duodenum

Figure 103-63. Embryology of the pancreas. (*A*) In the 5-week embryo, the ventral pancreatic bud lies caudal to the dorsal pancreatic bud. The common bile duct and the duct of the ventral pancreas drain into the duodenum through the major papilla and the dorsal pancreatic duct drains through the accessory papilla. Persistence of this anatomy results in pancreas divisum. (*B*) At 6 weeks' gestation, the dorsal and ventral pancreas fuse. The duct of Wirsung (to the ampulla of Vater) becomes the main pancreatic drainage duct, although the accessory papilla may persist.

usually a diminutive orifice without evidence of inflammation. Most reported cases have been in adults, but children with recurrent pancreatitis and pancreas divisum have been described.[127,128] With ERCP evaluation of ductal anatomy in children, this diagnosis should be made more frequently in younger patients.

ERCP is necessary to establish the diagnosis of pancreas divisum. Visualization of both major and minor papillae through the endoscope is required. The radiologic appearance of pancreas divisum demonstrates a short duct of Wirsung that does not communicate with the duct of Santorini (see Fig. 103-64B). The duct of Wirsung is entirely absent in about 5% of cases. A definitive diagnosis of pancreas divisum can be made with this demonstration of two separate, parallel ductal systems.

Determining the physiologic relevance of pancreas divisum has also been proposed by using intravenous secretin stimulation of pancreatic secretions, while performing real-time ultrasound imaging of the pancreatic ducts. A functional stenosis of the accessory papilla with secretion-induced proximal ductal dilation is thought to be characteristic of clinically significant pancreas divisum.[129] This remains controversial.

Only 14 patients younger than 18 years with pancreatitis and pancreas divisum requiring operation have been reported. Most of these patients were girls. These children generally presented with mid-epigastric abdominal pain and hyperamylasemia. Improvement with medical management was routine, but recurrent bouts of pancreatitis

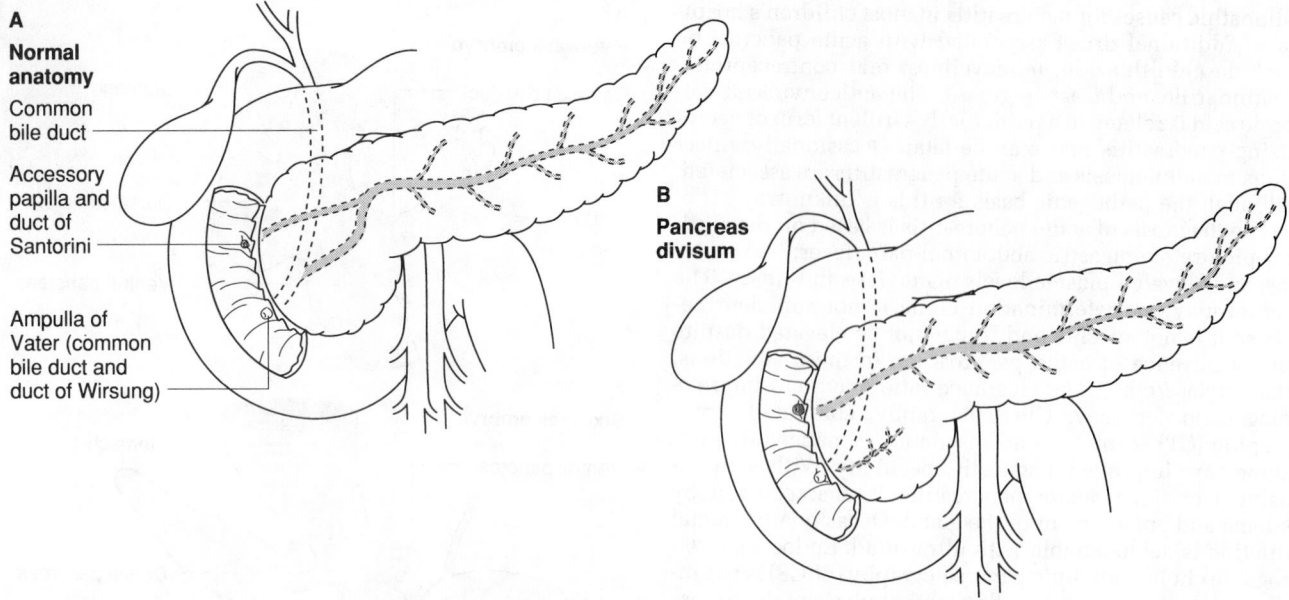

A
Normal anatomy

Common bile duct

Accessory papilla and duct of Santorini

Ampulla of Vater (common bile duct and duct of Wirsung)

B
Pancreas divisum

Figure 103-64. (*A*) Normal pancreatic ductal anatomy. (*B*) Pancreas divisum. There is no communication between the duct of Wirsung and the duct of Santorini. The duct of Wirsung is short or absent. Most of the pancreas is drained by the duct of Santorini through the accessory ampulla. This anatomy is found in about 10% to 15% of normal children.

followed. Operative indications generally have been recurrent pancreatitis with appropriate anatomy and no other explanation of cause. The surgical outcome was good in the handful of children for whom the outcome was reported.

The primary goal of surgery is to obtain adequate drainage of the duct of Santorini by performing a sphincteroplasty of the accessory duct.[130] Endoscopic sphincterotomy is associated with a high incidence of restenosis, so that open sphincteroplasty is favored. Some have also advocated sphincteroplasty of the ostium of the duct of Wirsung, which is accomplished by opening the ampulla of Vater. Because sphincteroplasty of the ampulla of Vater interferes with normal filling and emptying of the gallbladder, cholecystectomy is also performed to avert stasis and stone formation in this circumstance.

PANCREATIC CYSTS

Pseudocysts of the pancreas occur most commonly after trauma in children. Pseudocysts are usually diagnosed after a history of blunt abdominal trauma or an episode of pancreatitis. Symptoms include epigastric pain associated with nausea, vomiting, and weight loss. The cyst is often palpable on abdominal examination. In the past, the diagnosis was made with an upper GI series showing anterior displacement of the stomach. The diagnosis is easily made now with either ultrasound, CT scanning, or MR imaging.

A number of small pancreatic pseudocysts disappear spontaneously without causing symptoms during involution. The larger cysts usually require formal drainage. These cysts may or may not have demonstrable communication with the pancreatic duct. Potential complications

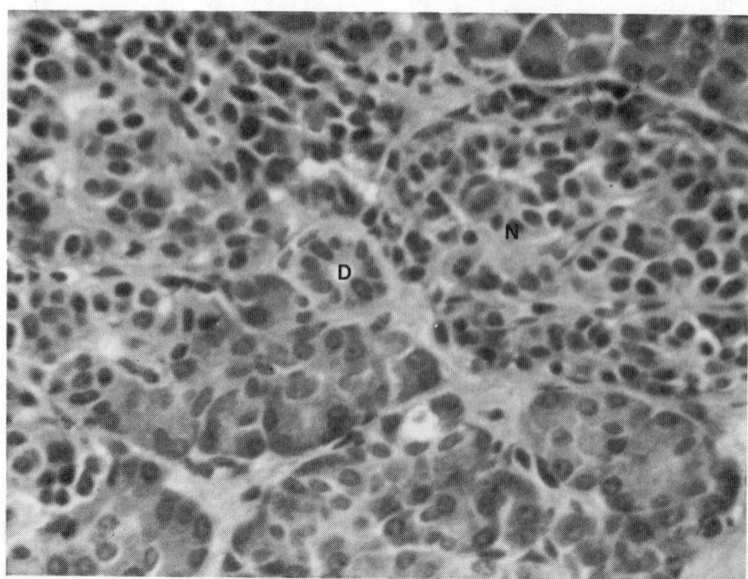

Figure 103-65. Nesidioblastosis showing neoislet (N) formation from primitive pancreatic ductules (D).

include internal hemorrhage, infection, perforation with peritonitis, and gastric, duodenal, or biliary obstruction. External drainage is successful in about 75% of these patients and has had a resurgence in interest because it is easily done with percutaneous drainage techniques employing ultrasound or CT guidance. Internal drainage into the stomach or jejunum and distal pancreatectomy are occasionally needed alternative approaches.[131]

Except for posttraumatic pseudocysts, cysts arising from the pancreas are rare in children. These cysts are classified as congenital, retention, neoplastic, and parasitic. Congenital cysts may be unilocular or multilocular and are frequently associated with cysts in other organs. An example are the cysts seen in von Hippel–Lindau disease, which is characterized by hereditary cerebellar cysts, hemangiomas of the retina, and cysts of the pancreas and other organs. Congenital cysts are lined by epithelium and acinar tissue and are most commonly seen in the body and tail of the pancreas. They are usually asymptomatic unless they cause significant extrinsic pressure on adjacent viscera such as the stomach and the transverse colon. Treatment of congenital cysts consists of either total excision or internal drainage into the stomach or jejunum.

Retention cysts are occasionally found as a result of chronic ductal obstruction. These are lined by epithelium unless it has been destroyed by chronic inflammation. Management consists of excision or internal drainage. Occasionally, a duplication cyst of the stomach or duodenum can mimic a pancreatic cyst and may be intimately attached to the pancreas and the pancreatic duct. These enteric cysts can communicate with the pancreatic duct. Treatment consists of excision or, if necessary, distal pancreatectomy including the enteric cyst.

Cystadenoma, cystadenocarcinoma, and rhabdomyosarcoma in association with a pancreatic cyst have been reported. These are all rare lesions and are treated with excision with or without associated pancreatic resection. Histologic confirmation of these diagnoses is always necessary.

PANCREATIC NEOPLASMS

Malignant pancreatic neoplasms in childhood are rare. Fewer than 100 such neoplasms have been reported.[132] Islet cell carcinoma is the most common of these, followed by adenocarcinoma. Other types of malignancies encountered are differentiated carcinoma, cylindric cell carcinoma, ductal cell carcinoma, simplex carcinoma, medullary carcinoma, and cystadenosarcoma. These tumors almost always present as an asymptomatic abdominal mass, although occasionally obstructive jaundice occurs if the site of origin is in the head of the pancreas. Regardless of histology, resection with partial pancreatectomy or a total pancreatectomy is appropriate for local disease. Even pancreaticoduodenectomy is appropriate if it allows complete resection of the tumor. As in adults, the prognosis for these childhood malignancies is poor. One form of adenocarcinoma, termed *pancreaticoblastoma,* appears to have a much more favorable prognosis than the standard form of adenocarcinoma and appears to have histologic features of embryonic acinar cells.

ENDOCRINE LESIONS OF THE PANCREAS

Zollinger-Ellison Syndrome

Since the Zollinger-Ellison syndrome was described in 1955, fewer than 50 patients have been children. The symptoms in children are similar to those in adults,

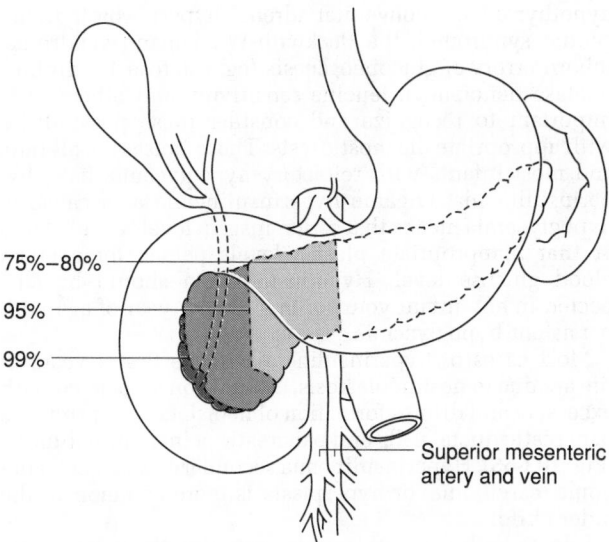

Figure 103-66. Schematic illustration of various degrees of pancreatic resection.

namely, a severe ulcer diathesis secondary to marked gastric hypersecretion. This is associated with diarrhea in about 35% of patients. As in adults, the diagnosis is confirmed by demonstration of elevated levels of gastrin in the serum. Basal acid hypersecretion is also typical. An exaggerated response of the serum gastrin to intravenous calcium stimulation and a paradoxical rise in the serum gastrin after intravenous secretin confirm the diagnosis in doubtful cases. Historically, treatment has emphasized total gastrectomy, as for adults. Resection of the primary tumor has been emphasized along with the use of histamine antagonists such as cimetidine and ranitidine. Omeprazole is a selective inhibitor of the parietal cell proton pump, and it is also an important pharmacologic aid in the treatment of Zollinger-Ellison syndrome.

When the pancreatic tumor cannot be resected because of metastases or other problems, total gastrectomy may be necessary, although this is not often the case. Gastrectomy may also be appropriate if partial resection, histamine antagonists, and omeprazole are unsuccessful.

Gastrinomas and Zollinger-Ellison syndrome may be part of the multiple endocrine neoplasia syndrome, which is caused by an autosomal dominant gene with a high degree of penetrance. Ninety percent of these patients have hyperparathyroidism secondary to hyperplasia of the parathyroid glands. Fifty to 85% have gastrinomas of the pancreas, 30% have pituitary adenomas, and 30% to 50% have adrenocortical hyperplasia. A few patients with insulinoma have also been reported[133] (see Chap. 57).

Childhood tumors of the endocrine pancreas are rare. The most common of these tumors are gastrinoma (see earlier) and insulinoma (see later). Other endocrine tumors of the pancreas are also reported in children, but these are exceedingly rare and do not differ fundamentally from their adult presentation and management. These tumors are characterized by their peptide products and have included glucagonomas, vipomas, apudomas producing excess pancreatic polypeptide, and tumors producing motilin and somatostatin.

Hypoglycemia

Hypoglycemia in infancy and childhood has several extrapancreatic causes. These include panhypopituitarism, isolated growth hormone deficiency, adrenal insufficiency, hypothyroidism, congenital adrenal hyperplasia (adreno-genital syndrome), the Beckwith-Wiedemann syndrome, inborn errors of gluconeogenesis (eg, fructose-1,6-diphosphatase deficiency), leucine sensitivity, and others. It is important to recognize and consider these possibilities with appropriate diagnostic tests. These causes are all rare, and most infants with refractory hypoglycemia have hyperinsulinemia. Organic hyperinsulinemia as a cause of hypoglycemia means that serum insulin levels are elevated or that inappropriate plasma levels persist for a given blood glucose level. Hyperinsulinemia should be suspected in any infant younger than than 1 year of age with persistent hypoglycemia.

Most cases of hyperinsulinemia in the first 2 years of life are due to nesidioblastosis, a condition associated with excessive and diffuse formation of neoislets from primitive pancreatic ductal cells and pancreatic acinar epithelium[134] (Fig. 103-65). Hyperinsulinemia secondary to islet cell adenoma, carcinoma, or hyperplasia is more common in the older child.

Infants with nesidioblastosis present with symptomatic hypoglycemia most commonly. Frank seizures or other neurologic symptoms are typical. These children have fasting blood glucose levels below 40 mg/dL. Nesidioblastosis is associated with multiple endocrine neoplasia syndrome, and this possibility must be investigated.

Organic hyperinsulinemia is suspected clinically if Whipple triad is demonstrated: (1) mental status changes or dizziness are precipitated by fasting or exercise; (2) fasting blood glucose concentrations are below 40 to 50 mg/dL; and (3) symptoms are relieved by oral or intravenous administration of glucose. The diagnosis is confirmed by the simultaneous measurement of plasma insulin and glucose levels with the finding of an insulin level inappropriately high for the level of blood glucose. An insulin/glucose ratio (insulin in IU/mL divided by glucose in mg/dL) that is greater than 0.5 with fasting is highly suggestive of this disease. In infants and children, the absolute ratio of insulin to glucose is not so important as in adults, but an insulin level of greater than 5 IU/mL in the presence of hypoglycemia is diagnostic. Low serum levels of β-hydroxybutyrate have been considered diagnostic of organic hyperinsulinemia in infants and children as well.

Infants with nesidioblastosis initially are managed medically with maintenance of blood glucose levels above 40 mg/dL. This is best carried out by the infusion of hypertonic glucose solutions through a permanent central venous catheter. In addition, diazoxide, 15 mg/kg/d, may be administered to counteract the effects of insulin and raise plasma glucose levels. Cortisone growth hormone and adrenocorticotropic hormone temporarily increase the blood glucose levels but are not definitive therapy. Streptozocin, a potent antibiotic that destroys islet cells, improves the hypoglycemia but is generally reserved for patients with metastatic islet cell carcinoma because of its significant toxicity and permanent effects. Once a patient has been stabilized medically, surgery should be considered early because of the risk of serious permanent neurologic impairment.

Definitive management of nesidioblastosis may require a pancreatic resection.[135] The abdomen is explored through a long upper abdominal transverse incision, and the lesser omentum is opened to expose the entire pancreas. If an islet cell adenoma is found, it should be removed without further resection of the pancreas. Often, an adenoma can be diagnosed preoperatively with a CT scan or with selective venous sampling and measurement of insulin from the pancreas. If no adenoma is found, the patient is assumed to have nesidioblastosis or islet cell hyperplasia. Intraoperative ultrasound examination of the pancreas may be useful in this evaluation. The next step in the surgical algorithm is a 95% pancreatectomy with preservation of the spleen. The entire pancreas from the tail to the head is resected, including the uncinate process, leaving a small rim of pancreatic tissue with the C loop of the duodenum. If a child remains hypoglycemic after a 95% pancreatectomy, a 99% or near-total pancreatectomy with preservation of the duodenum is required (Fig. 103-66). This procedure involves removal of essentially all pancreatic tissue except for the region of the distal common bile duct and the region of the duodenal arterial arcade. The entire common bile duct is exposed so that it remains undamaged during the dissection.

After a 95% or 99% pancreatectomy, a child tends to be hyperglycemic for some time. In the case of the 95% pancreatectomy, the patient normally returns to euglycemia. In contrast, with the 99% pancreatectomy, diabetes mellitus may result, and insulin therapy may be required. An 80% (subtotal pancreatectomy) has no place in the management of nesidioblastosis or islet cell hyperplasia in infancy and childhood. A more aggressive resection of the pancreas is required for adequate therapy. More than 90% of infants with nesidioblastosis are rendered permanently euglycemic with a 95% pancreatectomy.[136] The remainder (10%) may need conversion to a 99% pancreatectomy for a good outcome.

REFERENCES

1. Caniano DA, Starr J, Ginn-Pease ME. Extensive short-bowel syndrome in neonates: outcome in the 1980s. Surgery 1989;105:119.
2. Glick LG, Harrison MR, Adzick NS, et al. The missing link in the pathogenesis of gastroschisis. J Pediatr Surg 1985;20:406.
3. Duhamel B. Embryology of exomphalos and allied malformations. Arch Dis Child 1963;38:142.
4. Cantrell JR, Haller JA Jr, Ravitch MM. A syndrome of congenital defects involving the abdominal wall, sternum, diaphragm, pericardium, and heart. Surg Gynecol Obstet 1958;107:602.
5. Allen RG. Omphalocele and gastroschisis. In: Holder TM, Ashcraft KW, eds. Pediatric surgery. Philadelphia, WB Saunders, 1980:572.
6. Bethal AL, Seashore JH, Touloukian RJ. Cesarean section does not improve outcome in gastroschisis. J Pediatr Surg 1989;24:1.
7. Fitzsimmons J, Nyberg DA, Cyr DR, Hatch E. Perinatal management of gastroschisis. Obstet Gynecol 1988;71:910.
8. Wesley JR, Drongowski R, Coran AG. Intragastric pressure measurement: a guide for reduction and closure of the Silastic chimney in omphalocele and gastroschisis. J Pediatr Surg 1981;16:264.
9. Farrell MK, Balistreri WF. Parenteral nutrition and hepatobiliary dysfunction. Clin Perinatol 1986;13:197.
10. Blane CE, Wesley JR, DiPietro MA, White SJ, Coran AG. Gastrointestinal complications of gastroschisis. AJR 1985; 144:589.
11. Evans A. The comparative incidence of umbilical hernias in colored and white infants. J Natl Med Assoc 1941;33:158.
12. Vohr BR, Rosenfield AG, Oh W. Umbilical hernia in the low-birth-weight infant (less than 1,500 gm). J Pediatr 1977; 90:807.
13. Shaw A. Disorders of the umbilicus. In: Welch KJ, Randolph JG, Ravitch MM, O'Neill JA, Rowe M, eds. Pediatric surgery. Chicago, Year Book Medical, 1986:731.
14. Rowe MI, Lloyd DA. Inguinal hernia. In: Welch KJ, Randolph JG, Ravitch MM, O'Neill JA, Rowe MI, eds. Pediatric surgery. Chicago, Year Book Medical, 1986:779.
15. Snyder WH Jr, Greanly EM Jr. Inguinal hernia. In: Benson CD, Mustard WT, Ravitch MM, Snyder WH Jr, Welch KJ, eds. Pediatric surgery. Chicago, Year Book Medical, 1962:573.
16. Rowe MI, Copelson LW, Clatworthy HW. The patient processes vaginalis and the inguinal hernia. J Pediatr Surg 1969;4:102.

17. Grosfeld JL, Cooney DR. Inguinal hernia after ventriculoperitoneal shunt for hydrocephalus. J Pediatr Surg 1974;9:311.

18. Rowe MI, Clatworthy HW. Incarcerated and strangulated hernias in children: a statistical study of high-risk factors. Arch Surg 1970;101:136.

19. Gilbert M, Clatworthy HW. Bilateral operations for inguinal hernia and hydrocele in infancy and childhood. Am J Surg 1959;97:255.

20. Holcomb GW, ed. Pediatric endoscopic surgery. Norwalk, CT, Appleton & Lange, 1994.

21. Holder TM, Ashcraft KW. Groin hernias and hydroceles. In: Holder TM, Ashcraft KW, eds. Textbook of pediatric surgery. Philadelphia, WB Saunders, 1980:594.

22. Gray SW, Skandalakis JE. Embryology for surgeons: the embryological basis for the treatment of congenital defects. Philadelphia, WB Saunders, 1972.

23. Touloukian RJ. Intestinal atresia and stenosis. In: Holder TM, Ashcraft KW, eds. Pediatric surgery. Philadelphia, WB Saunders, 1980:331.

24. Louw JH, Barnard CN. Congenital intestinal atresia: observations on its origin. Lancet 1955;2:1065.

25. Welch KJ, Randolph JG, Ravitch MM, O'Neill JA Jr, Rowe MI, eds. Pediatric surgery, ed 4. Chicago, Year Book Medical Pub, 1986.

26. Webb CH, Wangensteen OH. Congenital intestinal atresia. Am J Dis Child 1931;41:262.

27. Wilmore DW. Factors correlating with a successful outcome following extensive intestinal resection in the newborn infant. J Pediatr 1972;80:88.

28. Stauffer UG. Duodenoduodenostomy. In: Spitz L, Nixon HH, eds. Rob and Smith's operative surgery: paediatric surgery, ed 4. London, Butterworth, 1983:273.

29. Kimura K, Mukohara N, Nishijima E, et al. Diamond-shaped anastomosis for duodenal atresia: an experience with 44 patients over 15 years. J Pediatr Surg 1990;25:977.

30. Irving IM. Duodenal atresia and stenosis: annular pancreas. In: Lister J, Irving IM, eds. Neonatal surgery, ed 3. London, Butterworth, 1990:424.

31. Peña A. Atlas of surgical management of anorectal malformations. New York, Springer-Verlag, 1990.

32. Stephens FD, Smith ED. Classification, identification, and assessment of surgical treatment of anorectal anomalies. Pediatr Surg Int 1986;1:200.

33. Templeton JM, O'Neill JA. Anorectal malformations. In: Welch KJ, Randolph JG, Ravitch MM, O'Neill JA Jr, Rowe MI, eds. Pediatric surgery, ed 4. Chicago, Year Book Medical Pub, 1986:1022.

34. Ong NT, Beasley SW. Long-term continence in patients with high and intermediate anorectal anomalies treated by sacroperineal (Stephens) rectoplasty. J Pediatr Surg 1991;26:44.

35. Rehbien F. Imperforate anus: experiences with abdomino-perineal and abdomino-sacro-perineal pull-through procedures. J Pediatr Surg 1967;2:99.

36. Mollard P, Marechal JM, de Beaujeu MJ. Surgical treatment of high imperforate anus with definition of the pubo-rectalis sling by an anterior perineal approach. J Pediatr Surg 1978;13:499.

37. Hassink EA, Rieu PN, Severijnen RS, Staak FH, Feston C. Are adults content or continent after repair for high anal atresia? Ann Surg 1993;218:196.

38. Sehgal S, Ewing C, Waring P, Findlay R, Bean X, Taeusch HW. Morbidity of low-birthweight infants with intrauterine cocaine exposure. J Natl Med Assoc 1993;85:20.

39. Major CA, Lewis DF, Harding JA, Porto MA, Garite TJ. Tocolysis with indomethacin increases the incidence of necrotizing enterocolitis in the low-birth-weight neonate. Am J Obstet Gynecol 1994;170:102.

40. Parks DA, Bulkley GB, Granger DN. Role of oxygen-derived free radicals in digestive tract diseases. Surgery 1983;94:415.

41. Rubaltelli FF, Benini F, Sala M. Prevention of necrotizing enterocolitis in neonates at risk by oral administration of monomeric IgG. Dev Pharmacol Ther 1991;17:138.

42. Rowe MI. Necrotizing enterocolitis. In: Welch KJ, Randolph JG, Ravitch MM, O'Neill JA Jr, Rowe MI, eds. Pediatric surgery, ed 4. Chicago, Year Book Medical Pub, 1986:944.

43. Kliegman RM, Fanaroff AA. Neonatal necrotizing enterocolitis: a nine-year experience. Am J Dis Child 1981;135:608.

44. Ryder RW, Shelton JD, Guinan ME. Necrotizing enterocolitis: a prospective multicenter investigation. Am J Epidemiol 1980;112:1130.

45. Uauy RD, Fanaroff AA, Korones SB, Phillips EA, Phillips JB, Wright LL. Necrotizing enterocolitis in very low birth weight infants: biodemographic and clinical correlates. National Institute of Child Health and Human Development Neonatal Research Network. J Pediatr 1992;119:630.

46. Haase GM, Sfakianakis GN, Lobe TE, et al. Prospective evaluation of radionuclide scanning in detection of intestinal necrosis in neonatal necrotizing enterocolitis. J Pediatr Surg 1981;16:241.

47. Bell MJ, Kosloske A, Benton C, et al. Neonatal necrotizing enterocolitis in infancy: prevention of perforation. J Pediatr Surg 1973;8:6013.

48. Morgan LJ, Shocat SJ, Hartman GE. Peritoneal drainage as primary management of perforated NEC in the very low birth weight infant. J Pediatr Surg 1994;29:30.

49. Rowe MI, O'Neill JA, Grosfeld JL. Essentials of pediatric surgery. St Louis, CV Mosby, 1995:526.

50. Ricketts RR, Jeries ML. Neonatal necrotizing enterocolitis: experience with 100 consecutive surgical patients. World J Surg 1990;14:600.

51. Grosfeld JL, Cheu H, Schlatter M, West KW, Rescorla FJ. Changing trends in necrotizing enterocolitis: experience with 302 cases in two decades. Ann Surg 1991;214:300.

52. Statement from the National Institutes of Health workshop on population screening for the cystic fibrosis gene. N Engl J Med 1990;323:70.

53. Riordan JR, Rommens JM, Kerem B, et al. Identification of the cystic fibrosis gene: cloning and characterization of complementary DNA. Science 1989;245:1066.

54. Kerem B, Rommens JM, Buchanan JA, et al. Identification of the cystic fibrosis gene: genetic analysis. Science 1989;245:1073.

55. Drumm M, Pope H, Cliff W, et al. Correction of the cystic fibrosis defect in vitro by retrovirus-mediated gene transfer. Cell 1990;62:1227.

56. Quinton PM. Cystic fibrosis: a disease in electrolyte transport. FASEB J 1990;4:2709.

57. Quinton PM, Bijman J. Higher bioelectric potentials due to decreased chloride absorption in the sweat glands of patients with cystic fibrosis. N Engl J Med 1983;308:1185.

58. MacManus LE, Rongaus VA, Klein RL. Meconium ileus with cystic fibrosis. J Am Osteopath Assoc 1982;81:6162.

59. Rescorla FJ, Grosfeld JL. Contemporary management of meconium ileus. World J Surg 1993;17:318.

60. del Pin CA, Czyrko C, Ziegler MM, Scanlin TG, Bishop HC. Management and survival of meconium ileus: a 30-year review. Ann Surg 1992;215:179.

61. Andrassy RJ, Mahour GH. Malrotation of the midgut in infants and children. Arch Surg 1981;116:158.

62. Ladd WE, Gross RE. Abdominal surgery of infancy and childhood. Philadelphia, WB Saunders, 1941.

63. Fujimoto T, Hata J, Yokoyama S, Mitomi T. A study of the extracellular matrix protein as the migration pathway of neural crest cells in the gut: analysis in human embryos with special reference to the pathogenesis of Hirschsprung's disease. J Pediatr Surg 1989;24:550.

64. Kleinhaus S, Boley SJ, Sheran M, Sieber WK. Hirschsprung's disease: a survey of the members of the surgical section of the American Academy of Pediatrics. J Pediatr Surg 1979;14:588.

65. Burnstock G, Costa M. Inhibitory innervation of the gut. Gastroenterology 1973;64:141.

66. Frigo GM, DelTacco J, Lecchini S, et al. Some observations on the intrinsic nervous mechanism in Hirschsprung's disease. Gut 1973;14:35.

67. Larsson LT, Malmfors G, Wahlestedt C, Leander S, Hakanson R. Hirschsprung's disease: a comparison of the nervous control of ganglionic and aganglionic smooth muscle in vitro. J Pediatr Surg 1987;22:431.

68. Tomita R, Munakata K, Kurosu Y, Tanjoh K. A role of nitric oxide in Hirschsprung's disease. J Pediatr Surg 1995;30:437.

69. O'Kelly TJ, Davies JR, Tam PK, Brading AF, Mortensen NJ.

Abnormalities of nitric-oxide-producing neurons in Hirschsprung's disease: morphology and implications. J Pediatr Surg 1994;29:294.

70. Schärli AF, Meier-Ruge W. Localized and disseminated forms of neuronal intestinal dysplasia mimicking Hirschsprung's disease. J Pediatr Surg 1981;16:164.

71. Martucciello G, Caffarena PE, Lerone M, et al. Neuronal intestinal dysplasia: clinical experience in Italian patients. Eur J Pediatr Surg 1994;4:287.

72. Meier-Ruge W, Schmidt PC, Stoss F. Intestinal neuronal dysplasia and its morphometric evidences. Pediatr Surg Int 1995;10:447.

73. Puffenberger EG, Kauffman ER, Bolk S, et al. Identity-by-descent and association mapping of a recessive gene for Hirschprung disease on human chromosome. Hum Mol Genet 1994;3:1217.

74. Mulligan LM, Eng C, Attie T, et al. Diverse phenotypes associated with exon 10 mutations of the RET proto-oncogene. Hum Mol Genet 1994;3:2163.

75. Ikeda K, Goto S. Diagnosis and treatment of Hirschsprung's disease in Japan. Ann Surg 1983;199:400.

76. Thomas DFM, Malone M, Fernie DS, et al. Association between *Clostridium difficile* and enterocolitis in Hirschsprung's disease. Lancet 1982;1:78.

77. Polley TZ Jr, Coran AG, Heidelberger KP, Wesley JR. Suction rectal biopsy in the diagnosis of Hirschsprung's disease and chronic constipation. Pediatr Surg Int 1986;1:84.

78. Cilley RE, Statter MB, Hirschl RB, Coran AG. Definitive treatment of Hirschprung's disease in the newborn with a one-stage procedure. Surgery 1994;115:551.

79. Georgeson KE, Fuenfer MM, Hardin WD. Primary laparoscopic pull-through for Hirschprung's disease in infants and children. J Pediatr Surg 1995;30:1017.

80. Sieber WK. Hirschsprung's disease: current problems in surgery. Chicago, Year Book Medical Pub, 1978.

81. Vanderwinden JM, Mailleux P, Schiffmann SN, Vanderhaeghen JJ, de Laet MH. Nitric oxide synthase activity in infantile hypertrophic pyloric stenosis. N Engl J Med 1992;327:511.

82. Benson CD. Infantile pyloric stenosis. Prog Pediatr Surg 1969;1:63.

83. Lobe TE. Evolving laparoscopic and thoracoscopic procedures in infants and children. Laparoscopic Surg 1993;1:184.

84. Rumack BH, Rumack CM. Disk battery ingestion. JAMA 1983;249:2509.

85. Oldham KT, Lobe TE. Gastrointestinal hemorrhage in children. Pediatr Clin North Am 1985;32:1247.

86. McDougal WS, Izant RJ Jr, Zollinger RM Jr. Primary peritonitis in infancy and childhood. Ann Surg 1975;181:310.

87. Dehner LP. Hepatic tumors in the pediatric age group: a distinctive clinicopathologic spectrum. In: Rosenberg HS, Bolande RP. Perspectives in pediatric pathology. Chicago, Year Book Medical Pub, 1978.

88. Dehner LP, Ishak KG. Vascular tumors of the liver in infants and children: a study of thirty cases and review of the literature. Arch Pathol 1971;92:101.

89. Ezekowitz RAB, Mulliken JB, Folkman J. Interferon alfa-2a therapy for life-threatening hemangiomas of infancy. 1992;326:1456.

90. Dehner LP, Parker ME, Franciosi RA, et al. Focal nodular hyperplasia and adenoma of the liver: a pediatric experience. Am J Pediatr Hematol Oncol 1979;1:85.

91. Ein SH, Stephens CA. Benign liver tumors and cysts in childhood. J Pediatr Surg 1974;9:847.

92. Exelby PR, Filler RM, Grosfeld JL. Liver tumors in children in particular reference to hepatoblastoma and hepatocellular carcinoma: American Academy of Pediatrics surgical section survey (1974). J Pediatr Surg 1975;10:329.

93. Mahour GH, Wogu GU, Seigel SE, et al. Improved survival in infants and children with primary malignant liver tumors. Am J Surg 1983;146:236.

94. Price JB, Schullinger JN, Santuli TV. Major hepatic resections for neoplasia in children. Arch Surg 1982;117:11.

95. Randolph JG, Altman RP, Arensman RM, et al. Liver resection in children with hepatic neoplasms. Ann Surg 1978;187:599.

96. Larsen LR, Raffensperger J. Liver abscess. J Pediatr Surg 1979;14:329.

97. McCarty E, Pathmanand C, Sunakorn P, et al. Amebic abscess in childhood. Am J Dis Child 1973;126:67.

98. Gray SW, Skandalakis JE. The liver. In: Embryology for surgeons: the embryological basis for the treatment of congenital defects. Philadelphia, WB Saunders, 1972:217.

99. Lilly JR. Biliary atresia: the jaundiced infant. In: Welch KJ, Randolph JG, Ravitch MM, O'Neill JA Jr, Rowe MI, eds. Pediatric surgery, ed 4. Chicago, Year Book Medical Pub, 1986:1047.

100. Ohya T, Fujimoto T, Shimomura H, Miyano T. Degeneration of intrahepatic bile duct with lymphocyte infiltration into biliary epithelial cells in biliary atresia. J Pediatr Surg 1995;30:515.

101. Chandra RS, Altman RP. Ductal remnants in extrahepatic biliary atresia: a histopathologic study with clinical correlation. J Pediatr 1978;93:196.

102. Tan CE, Davenport M, Driver M, Howard ER: Does the morphology of the extrahepatic biliary remnants in biliary atresia influence survival? A review of 205 cases. J Pediatr Surg 1994;29:1459.

103. Morecki R, Glaser JH, Horwitz MS. Etiology of biliary atresia: the role of reo 3 virus. In: Daum F, Fisher SE, eds. Extrahepatic biliary atresia. New York, Marcel Dekker, 1983:1.

104. A-Kader HH, Nowicki MJ, Kuramoto KI, Baroudy B, Zeldis JB, Balistreri WF. Evaluation of the role of hepatitis C virus in biliary atresia. Pediatr Infect Dis J 1994;13:657.

105. Riepenhoff-Talty M, Schaekel K, Clark HF, et al. Group A retroviruses produce extrahepatic biliary obstruction in orally inoculated newborn mice. Pediatr Res 1993;33:394.

106. Schmeling DJ, Oldham KT, Guice KS, Kunkel RG, Johnson KJ. Experimental obliterative cholangitis: a model for the study of biliary atresia. Ann Surg 1991;213:350.

107. Majd M. Radionuclide studies in the evaluation of neonatal jaundice. In: Daum F, Fisher SE, eds. Extrahepatic biliary atresia. New York, Marcel Dekker, 1983:23.

108. Adelman S. Prognosis of uncorrected biliary atresia: an update. J Pediatr Surg 1978;4:389.

109. Busuttil RW, Colonna JO II, Hiatt JR, et al. The first 100 liver transplants at UCLA. Ann Surg 1987;206:387.

110. Starzl TE, Demetris AJ. Liver transplantation: a 31-year perspective. Chicago, Year Book Medical Pub, 1990.

111. Whitington PF, Emond JC, Whitington SH, et al. Small bowel length and the dose of cyclosporine in children after liver transplantation. N Engl J Med 1990;322:733.

112. Burnweit CA, Coln D. Influence of diversion on the development of cholangitis after hepatoportoenterostomy for biliary atresia. J Pediatr Surg 1986;21:1143.

113. Kasai M. Hepatic portoenterostomy for the so-called "noncorrectable" type of biliary atresia. In: Daum F, Fisher SE, eds. Extrahepatic biliary atresia. New York, Marcel Dekker, 1983:79.

114. Luketic VA, Sanyal AJ. The current status of ursodeoxycholate in the treatment of chronic cholestatic liver disease. (Review) Gastroenterologist 1994;2:74.

115. Grosfeld JL, Rescorla FJ, Skinner MA, West KW, Scherer LR. The spectrum of biliary tract disorders in infants and children: experience with 300 cases. Arch Surg 1994;129:513.

116. Ryckman F, Fischer R, Pedersen S, et al. Improved survival in biliary atresia patients in the present era of liver transplantation. J Pediatr Surg 1993;28:382.

117. Otte JB, de Ville de Goyet J, Reding R, et al. Sequential treatment of biliary atresia with Kasai portoenterostomy and liver transplantation: a review. Hepatology 1994;20:41S.

118. Dunn SP, Weintraub W, Vinocur CD, Billmire DF, Falkenstein K. Is age less than 1 year a high-risk category for orthotopic liver transplantation? J Pediatr Surg 1993;28:1048.

119. Broelsch CE, Emond JC, Thistlethwaite JR, et al. Liver transplantation, including the concept of reduced-size liver transplants in children. Ann Surg 1988;208:410.

120. Todani T, Narusue M, Watanabe Y, et al. Management of congenital choledochal cyst with intrahepatic involvement. Ann Surg 1978;187:272.

121. Todani T, Tabuchi K, Watanabe Y, et al. Carcinoma arising in the wall of congenital bile duct cysts. Cancer 1979;44:1134.

122. Flanigan DP. Biliary cysts. Ann Surg 1975;182:635.

123. O'Neill JA Jr. Choledochal cyst. In: Welch KJ, Randolph JG, Ravitch MM, O'Neill JA Jr, Rowe MI, eds. Pediatric surgery, ed 4. Chicago, Year Book Medical Pub, 1986:1056.

124. Lipsett PA, Pitt HA, Colombani PM, Boitnott JK, Cameron JL. Choledochal cyst disease: a changing pattern of presentation. Ann Surg 1994;220:644.

125. Coran AG. Pancreatic problems in infants and children. In: Zuidema GD, Turcotte JG, eds. Surgery of the alimentary tract: pancreas, biliary tract, liver, and spleen, ed 3. Philadelphia, WB Saunders, 1990:121.

126. Warshaw AL, Richter J, Schapiro RH. The cause and treatment of pancreatitis associated with pancreas divisum. Ann Surg 1983;198:443.

127. Van Camp JM, Polley TZ, Coran AG. Pancreatitis in children: diagnosis and etiology in 57 patients. Pediatr Surg Int 1994;9:492.

128. Adzick NS, Shamberger RC, Winter HS, Hendren WH. Surgical treatment of pancreas divisum causing pancreatitis in children. J Pediatr Surg 1989;24:54.

129. Warshaw AL, Simeone J, Schapiro RH, et al. Objective evaluation of ampullary stenosis with ultrasonography and pancreatic stimulation. Am J Surg 1985;149:65.

130. Keith RG, Shapiro TF, Saibil FG. Treatment of pancreatitis associated with pancreas divisum by dorsal duct sphincterotomy alone. Can J Surg 1982;25:622.

131. Cooney DR, Grosfeld JL. Operative management of pancreatic pseudocysts in infants and children: a review of 75 cases. Ann Surg 1975;182:590.

132. Grosfeld JL, Vane DW, Rescorla FJ, et al. Pancreatic tumors in childhood: anomalies of 13 cases. J Pediatr Surg 1990;25:1057.

133. Grosfeld J. Surgical management of islet cell adenoma in infancy. Surgery 1978;84:519.

134. Aynsley-Green A, Pollak JM, Bloom SR, et al. Nesidioblastosis of the pancreas: definition of the syndrome and the management of severe neonatal hyperinsulinemic hypoglycemia. Arch Dis Child 1981;56:496.

135. Schiller M, Krausz M, Meyer S, et al. Neonatal hyperinsulinism: surgical and pathologic considerations. J Pediatr Surg 1980;15:16.

136. Al-Rabeeah A, Al-Ashwal A, Al-Herbish A, Al-Jurayyan N, Sakati N, Abobakr A. Persistent hyperinsulinemic hypoglycemia of infancy: experiences with 28 cases. J Pediatr Surg 1995;30:1119.

SURGERY: SCIENTIFIC PRINCIPLES AND PRACTICE, Second Edition, edited by Lazar J. Greenfield, Michael W. Mulholland, Keith T. Oldham, Gerald B. Zelenock, and Keith D. Lillemoe. Lippincott–Raven Publishers, Philadelphia, © 1997.

CHAPTER 104
PEDIATRIC GENITOURINARY SYSTEM

DAVID A. BLOOM, MICHAEL L. RITCHEY, AND ARNOLD G. CORAN

Urinary and Testicular Anomalies

DAVID A. BLOOM, AND MICHAEL L. RITCHEY

KIDNEY

Three discrete stages occur during kidney organogenesis. The initial structure, the pronephros, undergoes complete regression, whereas elements of the second structure, the mesonephros, persist into adulthood. The mesonephric duct extends caudally to communicate with the anterior cloaca by the fifth gestational week, forming a ureteral bud near the distal end of the mesonephric duct. The cranial end of the ureter ascends to meet the mesodermal nephrogenic cord and branches into the differentiating metanephrogenic cap. Ascent of the kidney from the fourth lumbar segment to the first lumbar vertebra occurs partly from true migration and also from somatic growth of the lumbar portion of the body. The kidney also undergoes a 135-degree medial rotation before assuming its final position.

Renal Agenesis

Renal agenesis results from failure of induction of the metanephric blastema by the ureteral bud. The unilateral incidence of this is about 1 in 1100 autopsies. Contralateral renal anomalies, usually malrotation or ectopia, occur in 15% of patients with unilateral renal agenesis. Genital anomalies are present in 30% to 60% of females with renal agenesis and in 10% to 20% of males. In the female, these anomalies often assume greater clinical importance, thus leading to earlier evaluation and discovery of the absent kidney. Malformations of the lower spine, rectum, and anus occur in both sexes, suggesting that regional maldevelopment involving the posterior cloaca and adjacent mesonephric duct may be responsible.

Unilateral renal agenesis (a solitary kidney) is often detected in the first few years of life during evaluation of children with multiple-organ system anomalies. The prognosis for children with a solitary kidney was once assumed to be normal, but recent data suggest that a reduction in the number of nephrons in experimental animals with this condition adversely affects the remaining renal function because hyperfiltration of residual nephrons is associated with progressive sclerosis of the glomeruli.[1] Reports of focal glomerulosclerosis in humans with congenital solitary kidneys support this concept.

Bilateral renal agenesis, with the concomitant facial dysmorphia, pulmonary hypoplasia, and orthopedic abnormalities known as Potter syndrome, occurs in about 1 in 4000 births. These infants generally are stillborn or rapidly succumb to respiratory or renal failure.

Renal Ectopy

Renal ectopy describes a kidney that lies outside the renal fossa but remains in the ipsilateral retroperitoneal space. Failure of complete ascent is one relevant event that can be due to a number of factors, including ureteral bud or metanephric blastema deficiency, genetic abnormalities, teratogenic causes, or anomalous vasculature. Renal ectopy occurs in about 1 in 1100 people. The most common position of the ectopic kidney is in the pelvis (pelvic or sacral kidney), opposite the sacrum or below the aortic bifurcation. An intrathoracic kidney, as the name suggests, occurs when a portion or all of a kidney extends above the ipsilateral diaphragm. This unusual type of ectopy may result either from accelerated ascent before diaphragmatic closure or from delayed closure of the diaphragm allowing continued ascent.[2]

Ectopic kidneys can be difficult to visualize and are easily overlooked on excretory urography because they frequently overlie the bony structures. Oblique plain radiographs may help to establish this diagnosis. An ectopic kidney can be readily identified using ultrasound or computed tomography as well. Most patients are asymptomatic, and the incidence of ectopic kidney is routinely higher in autopsy series than in clinical studies. Many patients are detected during evaluation of problems unrelated to the ectopia. The most common surgical problem associated with renal ectopia is congenital ureteropelvic junction (UPJ) obstruction. This may be due to the renal malrotation and a high ureteral insertion or to an anomalous vessel that partially obstructs the collecting system. Treatment should be individualized, but most patients require surgical correction in the form of a dismembered pyeloplasty. Renal stones may develop in these ectopic kidneys. Screening studies are routine. Open surgical removal, often necessary in the past, has been largely replaced by extracorporeal shock-wave lithotripsy or endourologic techniques. Because the contralateral kidney may also be abnormal, every effort is made to preserve an ectopic kidney. Inadvertent removal of a solitary ectopic kidney is a potential disaster and has occurred when such kidneys were mistaken for some other pelvic mass.

Horseshoe Kidney

Unusual radiographic images result from the fusion of two or more kidney masses (Fig. 104-1). Horseshoe kidney is the most common renal fusion anomaly, with an incidence of about 1 in 750 otherwise normal people. The two renal masses join at the midline, usually at the lower poles. Horseshoe kidney is readily diagnosed by excretory urography. The isthmus that connects the two kidneys consists of renal parenchyma or fibrous tissue, and the horseshoe kidney is usually positioned low in the abdomen, with an isthmus below the junction of the inferior mesenteric artery and aorta. Although it usually passes anterior to the great vessels, the isthmus may lie posterior to the aorta or inferior vena cava. The blood supply to the isthmus is variable, frequently supplied by an arterial vessel directly from the aorta, common iliac, or inferior mesenteric arteries. The functional capacity of the isthmus parenchyma can be assessed by radionuclide imaging.

Horseshoe kidney does not adversely affect survival, and

nearly one third remain undiagnosed. Clinical problems tend to be secondary to hydronephrosis, urinary tract infection (UTI), or urolithiasis. More than 100 instances of primary renal malignancy have been reported in patients with horseshoe kidney. After adenocarcinoma, Wilms tumor is the second most common tumor associated with horseshoe kidney. A review of National Wilms Tumor Study patients found a seven-fold increase in the risk of Wilms tumor among patients with horseshoe kidney.[3] The diagnosis of horseshoe kidney was often missed preoperatively when a distorted pyelogram was presumed secondary to the renal mass.

Correction of UPJ obstruction is the most frequent surgical intervention required for patients with horseshoe kidney. In the past, dividing the isthmus was recommended to prevent ureteral obstruction at that site, but this is rarely necessary. Horseshoe kidney and other fusion anomalies may be discovered unexpectedly during retroperitoneal procedures, such as resection of abdominal aortic aneurysm.

Cystic Disease

Renal cystic disease may be congenital or acquired. Cases diagnosed at birth usually present with an abdominal mass. Cystic kidneys are among the common causes of neonatal abdominal mass. Numerous classifications categorize the different cystic disorders of the kidney based on both clinical and radiologic features, pathologic studies, and genetic associations.

Multicystic dysplastic kidney, the most common form of renal cystic disease in infants, occurs in 1 in 4000 births and is usually unilateral. Cysts vary in size and do not communicate. Ultrasound evaluation is usually diagnostic. The important differential diagnosis is obstructive hydronephrosis. Isotope renal scans reveal absent function in multicystic dysplastic kidney, but imaging the remainder of the urinary tract is important to exclude contralateral renal abnormalities and vesicoureteral reflux (VUR) because these occur in at least 20% of the solitary functioning contralateral kidneys. Surgical removal of multicystic dysplastic kidney is controversial. Long-term sequelae of these dysplastic kidneys are uncommon but include hypertension, pain, hematuria, calcification, infection, and neoplasm formation. Operative morbidity and mortality, however, are minimal. Multicystic nephrectomy in the first 2

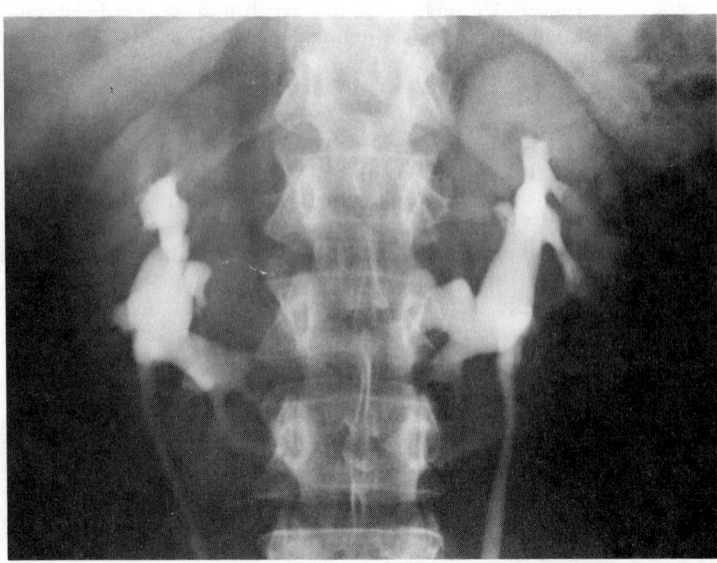

Figure 104-1. Intravenous urogram of horseshoe kidney. Abnormal rotation of kidneys, medial lower calyces, and lateral deviation of ureters are present.

years of life can be performed with 24-hour hospitalization. With modern imaging techniques, exploratory surgery is rarely indicated to establish the diagnosis, and many multicystic dysplastic kidneys completely regress within the first year of life if serially examined with ultrasound. A national registry of the American Academy of Pediatrics Section on Urology monitors retained multicystic dysplastic kidneys. The current recommendation for neonatal multicystic dysplastic kidney is ultrasonographic surveillance, reserving nephrectomy for those who fail to regress or for rare instances of symptomatic lesion.

Infantile polycystic kidney disease is better described as autosomal recessive polycystic kidney disease. This congenital disorder affects both kidneys and can become evident clinically at birth or later in childhood. All patients have some form of liver disease, ranging from biliary ectasia to congenital hepatic fibrosis. The usual neonatal presentation consists of bilateral, massive flank masses that fail to transilluminate. Renal ultrasound reveals uniformly increased echogenicity, and intravenous urography demonstrates the classic sun-ray pattern caused by streaking of contrast-filled collecting tubules. Most children develop progressive renal failure. Those who present later in childhood are more likely to develop concurrent congenital hepatic fibrosis.

Autosomal dominant polycystic kidney disease, one of the most common genetic diseases, is usually diagnosed in the third and fourth decades of life. It may also present in childhood when the initial course may be deceptively benign. The diagnosis of even a single renal cyst in childhood in a family with autosomal dominant polycystic kidney disease is suggestive of the disease.

Ureteropelvic Junction Obstruction

The most common cause of neonatal hydronephrosis is UPJ obstruction. The pathogenesis of this disorder is variable. Failure of recanalization of the fetal ureter causes some obstructions. Microscopic derangement of the muscle bundles and increased intramural collagen deposition may lead to failure of peristaltic wave propagation. Extrinsic causes of obstruction include aberrant vessels, kinks in the proximal ureter, and adherent bands. In many patients, asymptomatic UPJ obstruction is suggested in the antenatal period by ultrasonographic evidence of hydronephrosis. Signs and symptoms of UPJ obstruction later in life include

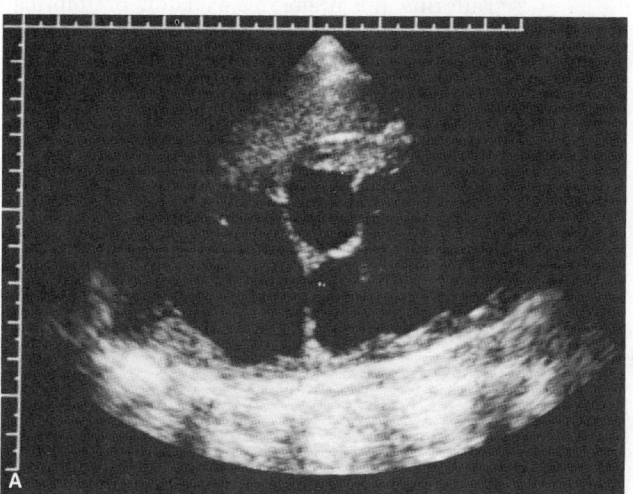

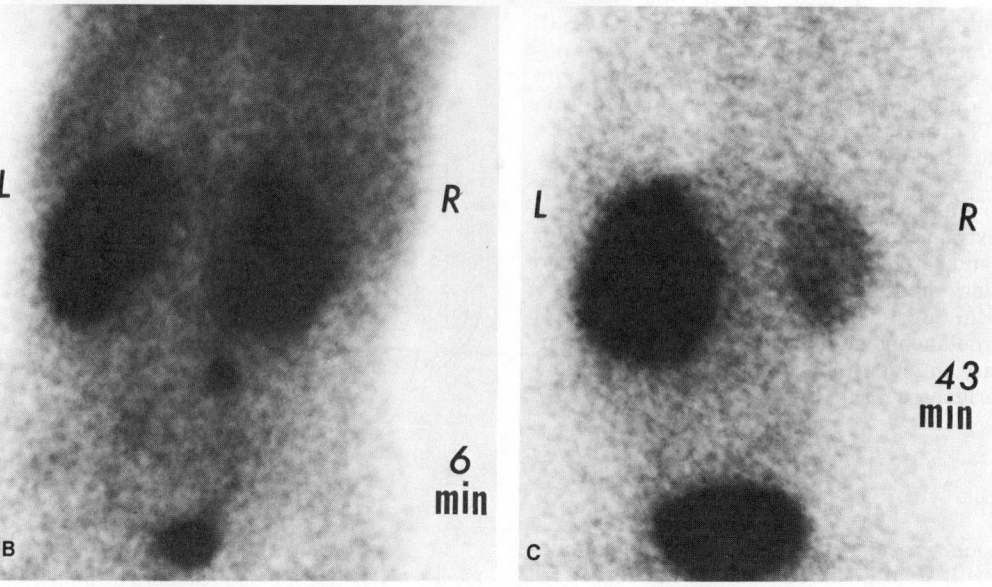

Figure 104-2. Ureteropelvic junction obstruction at the left kidney. (*A*) Ultrasound scan (dilated calyces, thin parenchyma). (*B*) Diuretic renal scan (6-minute ^{99m}Tc DTPA study, symmetric kidneys, but only the right ureter is visible). (*C*) Diuretic renal scan (43-minute study). Furosemide was given at 25 minutes. There is good washout of the right kidney but persistence of DTPA on the left.

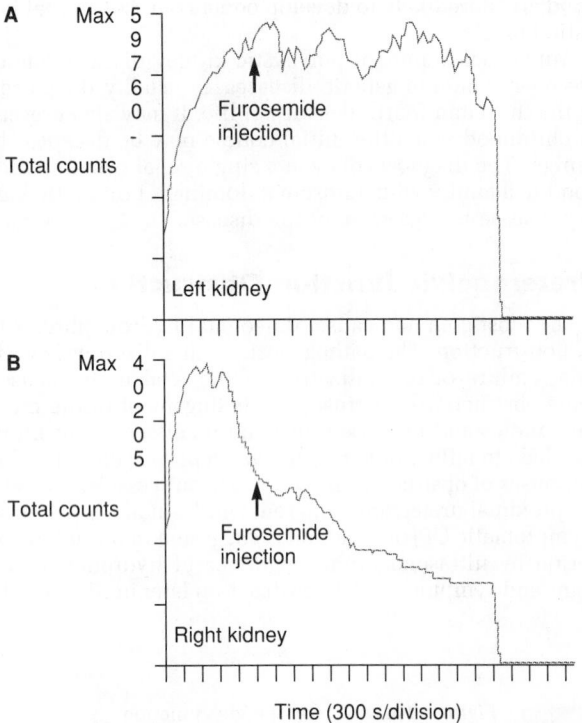

Figure 104-3. Diuretic renal scan computer analysis of washout curves. The left kidney (*A*) accumulated DTPA after diuretic with virtually no washout, whereas the right kidney (*B*) has precipitous washout after furosemide administration. This study shows an obstructed left kidney and normal right kidney.

abdominal mass, pain, hematuria, infection, or renal stones. Occasionally, UPJ obstruction is diagnosed by gross hematuria after blunt trauma because a hydronephrotic kidney is more susceptible to injury than a normal kidney.

Evaluation in children generally begins with abdominal ultrasonography (Fig. 104-2). Occasionally, excretory urography is necessary to define the renal anatomy. In some cases, it may be difficult to distinguish between true obstruction and nonobstructive dilatation. Diuretic renography or antegrade perfusion measurement (the Whitaker test) more accurately assesses obstruction[4] (Fig. 104-3). Doppler measurement of the renal resistive index is a potential tool for evaluating obstruction, although it is more dependable in adults than children. It is important to rule out bilateral UPJ obstruction.

The goal of surgical management is dependent drainage of the renal pelvis, and this is usually accomplished by dismembered pyeloplasty with resection of the obstructing segment. An extraperitoneal approach is satisfactory for most patients, and careful tissue handling is mandatory to avoid devascularizing the ureter with an ischemic stricture. A successful outcome is expected in more than 90% of patients. Percutaneous endopyelotomy has been advocated for primary and recurrent UPJ obstruction, but there is limited experience with its use in children.

URETER

Megaureter

The term *megaureter* refers to a large dilated ureter. Megaureters can result from distal ureteral obstruction or reflux, either of which may be congenital or acquired, or megaureters can be nonrefluxing and nonobstructed. *Ob-*

structed megaureters are blocked at a narrow segment of ureter, proximal to the ureterovesical junction. Histologically, the narrowed segment has increased collagen deposition, muscular deficiency, or a thickened circular band of muscle. These abnormalities impair propagation of peristalsis and cause distention of the proximal ureter. Peristalsis becomes defective in the dilated proximal ureter because of the inability of the wall to coapt. A *nonrefluxing, nonobstructed megaureter* is radiographically similar to this, with a narrowed distal ureteral segment. There is variable dilatation of the proximal ureter, and its distal aspect is generally the most dilated. This condition may be the result of prior obstruction or prior reflux that resolved spontaneously. Diuretic renography helps distinguish this entity from an obstructed megaureter.

The common manifestations of megaureters are urinary infection, hematuria, and abdominal pain. As with most congenital renal anomalies, antenatal ultrasound usually provides the first clue. Asymptomatic patients with megaureter may not require aggressive treatment. Intervention in some patients, however, prevents future functional deterioration. Conversely, some untreated patients have radiographic improvement over time without functional impairment.[5]

Surgical management consists of reimplanting the ureter into the bladder after excising the obstructing segment. Tailoring the ureter by excision or imbrication usually achieves a satisfactory antireflux mechanism.[6]

Ureteral Duplication

Complete duplication of the ureter is attributed to the embryonic formation of two ureteral buds on the mesonephric duct (Fig. 104-4). This is the most common urinary tract anomaly, and it occurs in 2% to 4% of patients evaluated with excretory urography. In completely *duplex systems*, two ipsilateral ureteral orifices enter the bladder. In *bifid systems*, the duplication is incomplete, and two

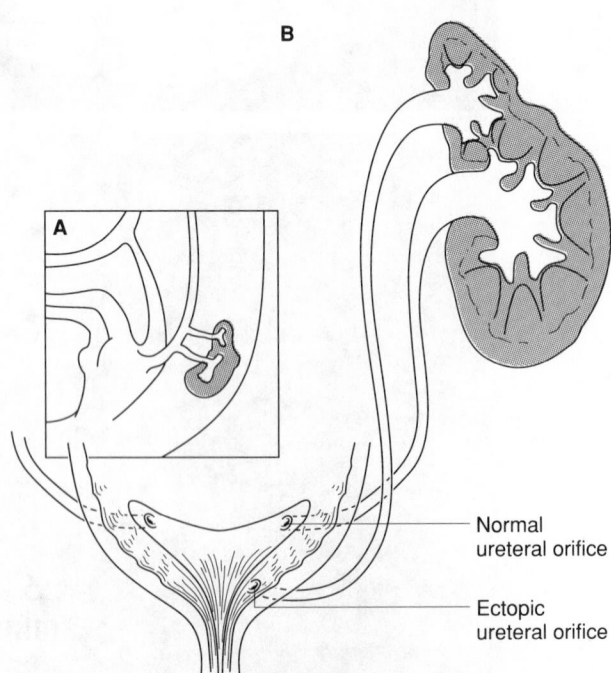

Figure 104-4. Ureteral duplication. The proposed embryology of two ureteral buds (*A*) and complete duplication with abnormal upper pole and ectopic ureteral orifice (*B*) are shown.

proximal ureters unite so that only one distal ureter enters the bladder. The most likely disorder associated with complete ureteral duplication is VUR, which occurs more frequently into the ureter from the lower renal moiety. The upper ureter is more likely to be associated with obstruction. These disorders can be explained by the embryologic development of the duplex system. The lower-pole ureter is incorporated into the bladder earlier than usual, leading to a lateral orifice position with a deficient intramural ureteral tunnel and thus an incompetent vesicoureteral valve. The upper ureter remains attached to the wolffian segment for a longer period, and entry into the bladder is delayed, leaving the ureteral orifices closer to the bladder neck or in the urethra where they are vulnerable to obstruction.

UTI is the most likely clinical presentation for patients with ectopic ureters and duplications. Urinary incontinence may occur in the female because of termination of an ectopic ureter distal to the external urinary sphincter. The ureteral orifice may be found in the uterus, cervix, or vagina, and vaginal discharge is another presenting complaint. Some patients do not become symptomatic until adult life. The surgical management of ureteral duplication follows the same principles for correcting VUR and megaureter. Many upper renal segments with ectopic ureter or ureterocele have poor function and are best managed by partial nephrectomy.

Ureterocele

Ureterocele is a congenital cystic dilation of the distal ureter. This anomaly may result from distal obstruction of the fetal ureter by persistence of Chwalla membrane, normally a transient process during organogenesis. Ureterocele may occur either in association with ureteral duplication or in a single system. In the latter circumstance, it is called *simple ureterocele* and may be an asymptomatic incidental finding in the adult patient. Occasionally, simple ureterocele is associated with obstruction, calculi, infection, reflux, or nonfunction of the renal unit. Ectopic ureterocele is usually associated with ureteral duplication and is characterized by entry of the ureterocele into the bladder neck or urethra. The most common clinical presentation is UTI. The renal segment associated with ectopic ureterocele is likely to have decreased or absent function because of dysplasia, obstruction, and infection. Obstruction of the lower renal segment can occur from compression by either the dilated upper-pole ureter or the ureterocele. Reflux is likely in the lower ureter. The bladder outlet may also be obstructed by a ureterocele, which can prolapse into the urethra. Decompression of the ureterocele from above (pyelopyelostomy or upper-pole nephrectomy) or from below (by transurethral incision) is the initial therapeutic step. One third of patients may need subsequent correction of reflux or excision of an upper-pole ureteral stump.

Vesicoureteral Reflux

Primary VUR is a congenital abnormality of the ureterovesical junction. Lateral ectopia of the ureteral orifice is attributed to an excessively caudal origin of the ureteral bud on the mesonephric duct. The ureteral bud is incorporated into the bladder prematurely and has more time to migrate cephalad and laterally. This results in a short intravesical ureter, a critical factor in the pathogenesis of VUR. Other factors that contribute to normal ureteral function include support from the detrusor muscle, ability of trigonal muscle to maintain length, closure of ureteral ostia, and peristaltic activity of the ureter. The low pressure normally present in the bladder (8 to 15 mmHg) is suffi-cient to compress the roof of the intravesical ureter against the underlying detrusor if the intravesical tunnel is long enough.

The significance of VUR was not appreciated until the 1960s. Serial radiologic studies demonstrated that renal scars in children with UTI occurred almost invariably in association with VUR.[7] Reflux of infected urine causes renal cortical damage, and the greatest vulnerability to scarring occurs in the first 5 years of life (the big bang phenomenon). Reflux of sterile urine is probably not harmful in the presence of normal bladder pressures. *Reflux nephropathy* is the term used for a scarred kidney associated with reflux. Children with even a single UTI should be evaluated by voiding cystography, which reveals VUR in about one third of patients. The long-term sequelae of reflux nephropathy include a 10% to 25% risk of hypertension. Reflux nephropathy is the cause of end-stage renal disease in 5% of transplantation patients and is the second most common cause of renal failure in children.

Most children with VUR are treated nonoperatively. The case for medical management of VUR is based on the observation that reflux tends to resolve with time, particularly in children with low-grade VUR.[8] Reflux is graded on a scale of 1 to 5, with 5 being the most severe degree. The goal of nonoperative management is to prevent urinary infection during the months or years it may take to outgrow the reflux.

When medical therapy fails or if the child does not outgrow reflux, several approaches are available for correcting reflux. Their goal is to create a long subepithelial tunnel in the bladder wall with good muscular backing (Fig. 104-5). The ureter can be approached intravesically or extravesically. Surgical cure rates exceed 95%.[9] If a ureter is dilated, its diameter must be reduced to achieve an acceptable ureteral width/length ratio of 1 to 4. This can be done by excision of the redundant portion or by a variety of imbrication techniques. Endoscopic correction of reflux offers another means of therapy.[10] This consists of subureteral injection of collagen, polytef paste, or other materials to buttress the ureterovesical junction.[11] Subtrigonal injection therapy of reflux is not as successful as surgical reconstruction, but it is less invasive and more palatable,

BLADDER

The cloaca is separated into two compartments by the urorectal septum. By the seventh week of gestation, the ventral portion is the urogenital sinus and the dorsal compartment is the rectum. Simultaneously, the genital tubercle separates from the umbilical cord by mesodermal growth of the lower abdominal wall. The mesonephric ducts enter into the urogenital sinus, with progressive absorption of the ducts distal to the ureteral bud. This results in separate terminations for the ureter and mesonephric duct. These openings migrate so that the ureteral bud moves upward and laterally and the mesonephric duct moves downward and medially. The urogenital sinus consists of two portions at the point where the müllerian ducts join the dorsal wall of the urogenital sinus. The ventral portion forms the bladder, part of the prostatic urethra in the male, and the entire female urethra. The caudal portion gives rise to the vaginal vestibule and lower third of the vagina in the female. In the male, it produces a portion of the prostatic urethra and the membranous urethra.

Urachal Abnormalities

The urachus extends from the umbilicus to the anterior bladder wall and lies in the space of Retzius. This represents the apical attachment of the cloaca to the allantois.

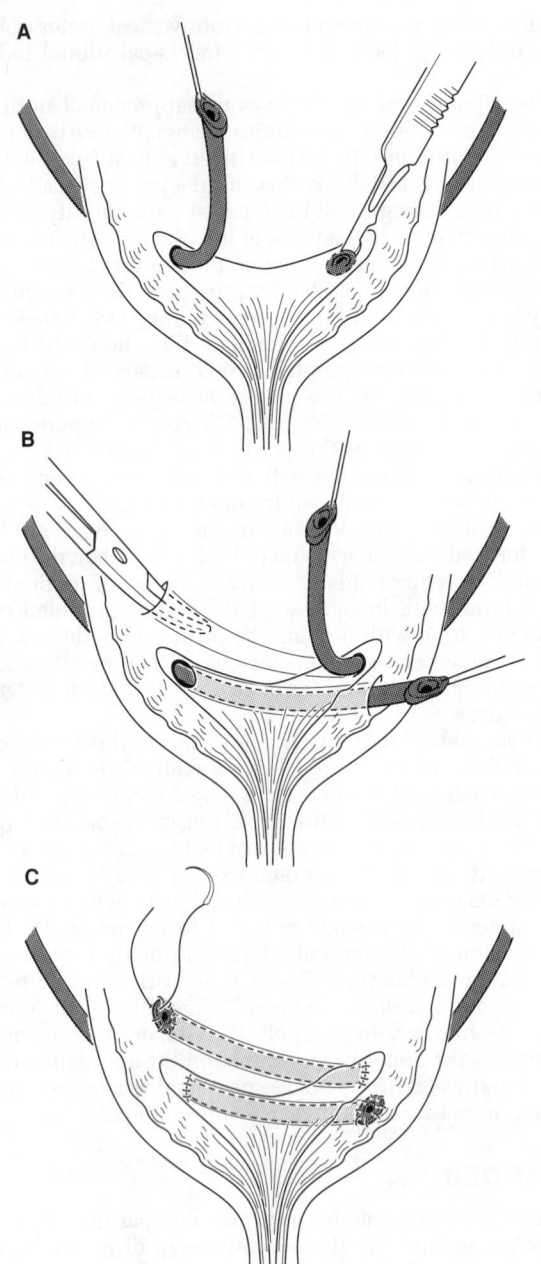

Figure 104-5. Ureteroneocystostomy (cross-trigonal reimplant).

The urachus becomes a solid cord during the fifth month of gestation, but a potential space may remain and become occluded by desquamated epithelium. Failure of involution after birth leads to several malformations. Failure of closure results in a patent urachus with a communication between the bladder and umbilicus. This is frequently seen in patients with bladder outlet obstruction and results in a wet umbilicus. The diagnosis can be confirmed radiographically. Although spontaneous closure is possible, excision of the tract and surgical closure of the bladder are usually necessary. Cysts along the course of the urachus are caused by epithelial degeneration and desquamation. These often become symptomatic in late childhood or adulthood. Patients have suprapubic pain, tenderness, and a palpable mass. Ultrasound is ideal for imaging these lesions. Treatment consists of incision and drainage followed by excision after the infection has resolved. A urachal sinus results when a urachal cyst dissects into the umbilicus causing periumbilical inflammation and drainage. Therapy consists of surgical resection of the cyst and sinus with formal surgical closure of the bladder.

Neurogenic Bladder

Spinal dysraphism, the most common cause of neurogenic bladder in children, encompasses anomalies ranging from occult dermal sinus and cord lipoma to a visible myelomeningocele (MMC). Complications of neurogenic vesical dysfunction (infection, hydronephrosis, renal failure) were a major cause of morbidity and mortality in these patients in the past, but these sequelae are largely preventable with modern urologic care. One of the great contributions to the treatment of these children was Lapides' introduction of clean intermittent catheterization.[12] Within a few years, it became widely accepted and rendered urinary diversion for neurogenic bladder nearly obsolete. Clean intermittent catheterization was a practical and effective solution for many of the problems associated with MMC. The next major advance was the concept that the leakpoint pressure was a reliable predictor of risk for renal deterioration.[13] The primary goal for children with MMC is to maintain safe intravesical pressures. There is nothing sophisticated or magical in the urodynamics necessary to do this. The pressure–volume characteristics of a normal bladder consist of a flat filling curve, ended by a (voluntary) bladder contraction with simultaneous relaxation of the bladder neck and external sphincters. In MMC, however, the pressure–volume relation is distorted, and the filling curve is hypertonic; each increment in volume results in an increase in pressure. Spontaneous voiding in these patients is unusual, and they are often incontinent. Thus, bladder storage is inadequate, and outlet resistance is inappropriate.

Evaluation in the newborn period identifies children at risk for renal damage. Children with leakage at low intravesical pressures require appropriate care before the urinary tract is damaged. The initial treatment of these children consists of intermittent catheterization and pharmacologic therapy. If bladder storage capability cannot be improved by anticholinergic therapy, surgical procedures are necessary to achieve safe urine storage and continence. Bowel and gastric segments, dilated ureters, and detrusor excision can augment bladder capacity. Sequelae of enterocystoplasty include electrolyte abnormalities, mucus production, stone formation, spontaneous perforation, and tumor formation. Bladder outlet resistance can be improved by bladder neck reconstruction, artificial urinary sphincter, pubovesical sling, urethral suspension, and injection of collagen.

PENIS AND URETHRA

The external genitalia are morphologically identical in both sexes until the 50-mm crown-to-rump stage, which occurs at about the ninth fetal week. After this, morphogenesis diverges according to sex, and the penis becomes distinct from the clitoris. The genital tubercle appears in the fifth week of fetal life. On the ventral aspect, a urethral groove is bordered by the urogenital folds. These folds unite over the urethral plate to form the urethra. The most distal portion of the penile urethra results from epithelial invagination in the glans penis. The glanular urethra then joins the terminal penile urethra. Failure of complete fusion of the urethral folds between the 5th and 12th gestational weeks results in a urethral meatus proximal to the distal tip of the glans penis. At the 12th week of gestation, the prepuce is an epithelial fold. By birth, the fold sur-

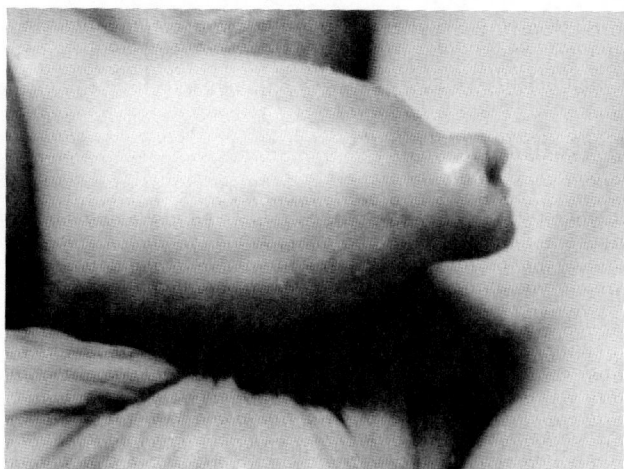

Figure 104-6. Normal nonretractile prepuce of infancy.

rounds the glans, and the inner surface fuses to the glans penis and obscures the glans and meatus.

Prepuce

The foreskin can be fully retracted in only a minority of infants (Fig. 104-6). During the first five years of life, the natural processes of intermittent erections and the progressive accumulation of desquamated residue gradually separate the inner epithelial surface of prepuce from glans. Even by 6 years of age, nearly two thirds of boys still have isolated adherent areas, particularly around the coronal margin.[14] Keratin pearls that accumulate between the glans and inner prepuce are normal in infancy and early childhood. They help make the foreskin retractable and are not to be confused with smegma that occurs in adult men. In fact, keratin pearls are sterile. They are best left alone or gently wiped away when they come to the surface. Forcible retraction of the foreskin, either by the family at home or by the physician in the office, is a common but inadvisable practice.

The American Academy of Pediatrics has published guidelines on the indications for circumcision.[15] Circumcision should be encouraged in infants with a history of urinary infection or VUR to decrease the chances of ascending infection. On the contrary, in infants with hypospadias, chordee, significant penoscrotal webbing, or other congenital problems, circumcision should be discouraged to preserve the foreskin for use in later reconstruction. Hypospadias can be associated with an intact foreskin; therefore, a glans exposed during circumcision must be inspected before the foreskin is removed. In normal infants, circumcision is completely a matter of family choice and not an important issue for medical debate.

In infants under 2 to 3 months of age, circumcision is done with a clamp or bell. In older patients, free-hand excision is done using a dorsal slit or sleeve resection under general anesthesia. Neonates are circumcised using local anesthesia and papoose-board restraint. Once the anesthetic has taken effect, adhesions between inner prepuce and glans are disrupted by clamp or probe. A small dorsal slit may be necessary to expose glans, and the entire coronal margin should be free of adhesions. Normal meatal configuration and position are confirmed, and a clamp (Gomco or Mogen) is applied. The clamp is left in place for 10 minutes, and the excess skin is excised (but never with electrocautery when a metallic clamp is adjacent to

glans). Postoperative instructions include using petroleum jelly on the meatus at each diaper change to guard against meatal stenosis. Proper neonatal circumcision has a complication rate of 0.2%, and the problems are usually minor.[16]

Phimosis is a fibrotic contraction of the preputial aperture so that retraction is impossible (Fig. 104-7). This is distinguished from the normal inability to retract the fused prepuce in the infant. Iatrogenic injury forcibly retracting the infant's prepuce is a common cause of phimosis. Preputial injury leads to cicatrix formation, which narrows the preputial aperture. Normal erections or manual retraction of the foreskin may crack or tear the narrow aperture, leading to further scarring or infection. Severe instances of phimosis can impede urinary flow. Circumcision or dorsal slit are the most effective solutions to phimosis.

Paraphimosis is the entrapment of a phimotic prepuce proximal to the coronal margin (Fig. 104-8). This initially causes lymphatic congestion, but venous congestion and arterial compromise may follow. Careful and persistent manual decompression usually solves the problem, but in unusual instances, emergency circumcision is necessary.

Hypospadias and Epispadias

Hypospadias occurs in 0.8% of all male births (Fig. 104-9). Classification of hypospadias is based on the position of the urethral meatus. This may be glanular, coronal,

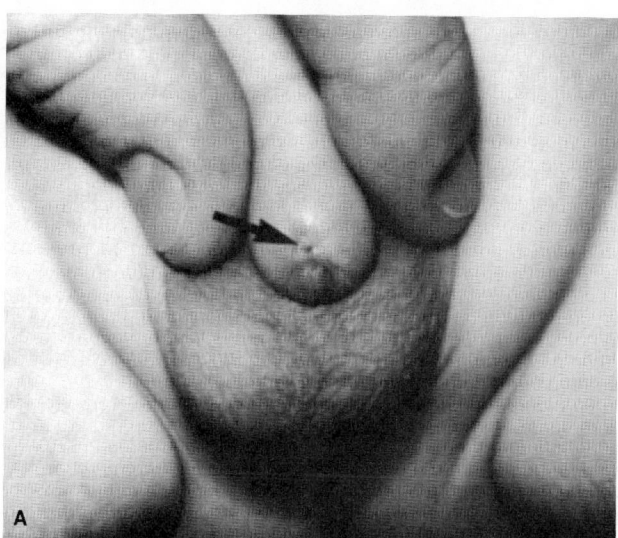

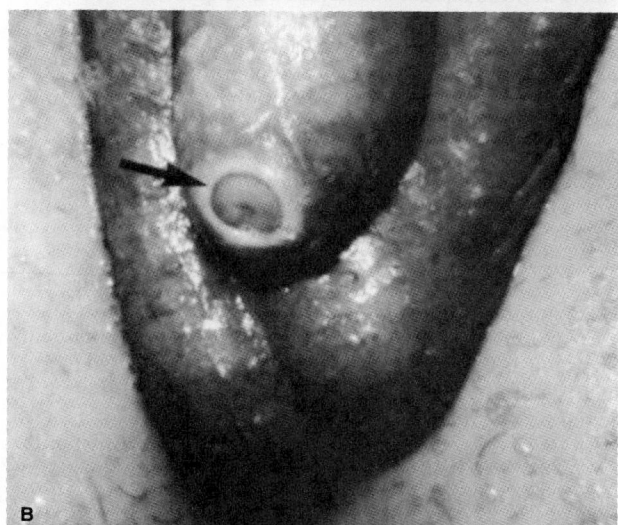

Figure 104-7. True phimosis in a child (*A*) and an adolescent (*B*).

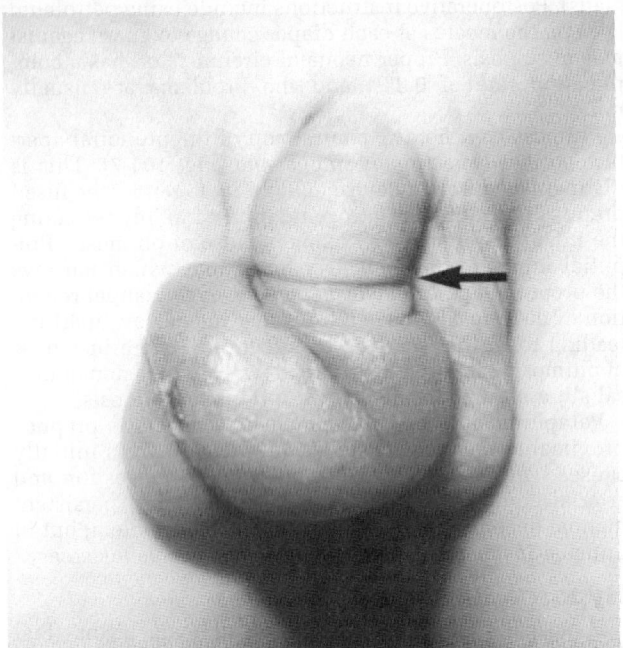

Figure 104-8. Paraphimosis (*arrow*), with distal edema.

midshaft, penoscrotal, scrotal, or perineal. Usually, the shortfall is a matter of less than 1 cm, and a mild degree of ventral penile curvature (chordee) may coexist. The distal forms of hypospadias represent over 85% of cases. More proximal variants are usually associated with severe degrees of chordee. The specific cause of hypospadias is unclear, but hormonal and genetic factors are implicated. The incidence of hypospadias is higher in brothers and fathers of a child with hypospadias. Cryptorchidism is present in 10% of boys with hypospadias. A child with severe hypospadias and an undescended testicle must be evaluated for intersex disorders. Prostatic utricle enlargement occurs in up to half of patients with perineal hypospadias. Renal abnormalities are less frequent.

More than 200 operations have been described for surgical correction of hypospadias. Principles of hypospadias repair include the correction of associated anomalies, such as chordee, careful surgical technique with optical magnification, and delicate tissue handling. Repair is undertaken after 6 months of age, usually on an outpatient basis. Most hypospadias can be corrected with a one-stage procedure. A vascularized pedicle flap is useful if skin flaps are necessary for urethral reconstruction. Severe hypospadias, particularly if associated with penoscrotal transposition, may be managed with staged reconstruction. If sufficient penile skin is not available, free grafts, such as skin, oral mucosal or bladder epithelium, are useful for urethral reconstruction. The most frequent complications after reconstructive surgery are urethrocutaneous fistula and stenosis or stricture of the neourethra. With artificial erection to assess chordee intraoperatively, persistent penile curvature is a less common problem.

Epispadias is a rare anomaly of completely different embryogenesis than hypospadias. Epispadias is related to persistence of the cloacal plate and delayed medial migration of the adjacent mesenchyme. It is seen more often with bladder exstrophy than as an isolated defect. Epispadias consists of a dorsally placed meatus proximal to the glanular tip. The degree of bending, or reverse chordee, is related to the severity of epispadias. Bladder neck insufficiency and urinary incontinence occur in severe cases. Surgical

correction of epispadias, its dorsal chordee, and bladder neck incompetence offer some of the greatest challenges in reconstructive genitourinary surgery.

Posterior Urethral Valves

Posterior urethral valves are a major cause of neonatal urinary obstruction. They occur only in males, with an incidence of 1 in 5000 births. The obstructing lesion is a membrane or valvular leaflet in the distal prostatic urethra. Different theories regarding the embryologic development of these valves have been proposed, including exaggerated development of the urethrovaginal folds, persistence of the most distal portion of the wolffian duct, and persistence of the urogenital diaphragm. A broad range of severity and radiographic appearance is related to the age and mode of presentation. Neonatal presentation typically includes a flank mass, urinary retention, urinary ascites, sepsis, azotemia, and a dysmorphic urinary tract. Older children present with hematuria, obstructive voiding symptoms, enuresis, or infection. In the neonate with hydronephrosis, evaluation includes blood chemistries, ultrasonography,

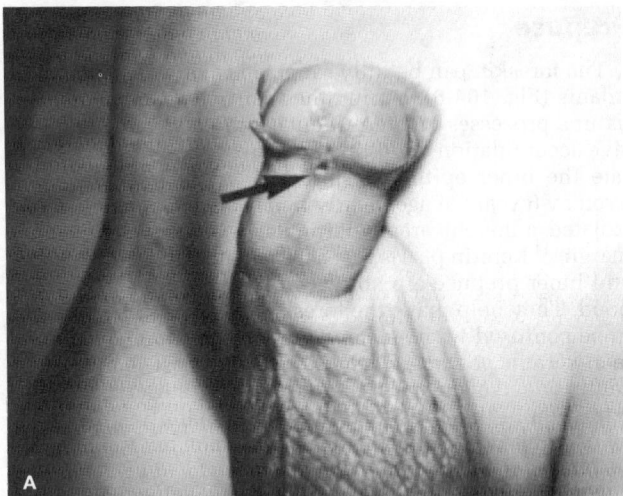

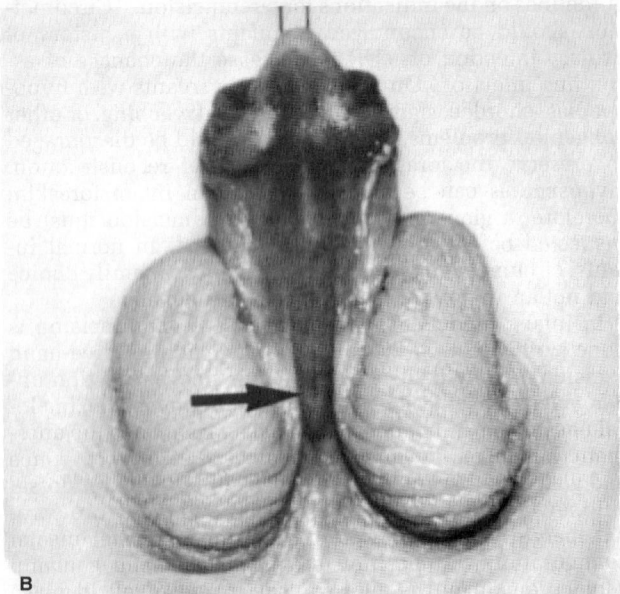

Figure 104-9. Subcoronal (*A*) and scrotal (*B*) hypospadias. The ureteral meatus is indicated by the arrow.

and voiding cystourethrography. The latter test defines the level of obstruction and identifies the 40% to 50% of children with VUR.

Management of posterior urethral valves begins with restoring electrolyte imbalances and acidosis. Initial decompression of the urinary tract is best accomplished with catheter drainage, possibly in the prenatal period. This is followed by primary endoscopic valve ablation. Advances in urologic instrumentation have decreased the likelihood of urethral damage. Cutaneous vesicostomy is useful in occasional circumstances and permits a subsequent antegrade approach for valve ablation. High urinary diversion and renal biopsy are necessary for persistent renal insufficiency, which may be due to renal dysplasia.

TESTIS

Before the sixth gestational week, the urogenital tracts of all embryos are identical, consisting of a genital tubercle, the urogenital sinus, two mesonephric (wolffian) ducts, and two paramesonephric (müllerian) ducts. Testicular embryology begins with the migration of primitive germ cells from the yolk sac endoderm along dorsal gut mesentery, reaching the genital ridge by the fifth week of gestation. Sertoli cells are recognizable at the seventh week and Leydig cells by the eighth week. Sertoli cells are the source of müllerian-inhibiting substance, which causes the müllerian ducts to regress in the ninth week. This is one of the key endocrine events in the male fetus. Leydig cells produce testosterone, which elongates the genital tubercle and encourages migration and fusion of genital folds to form the scrotum and urethra. Canalization of the sex cords creates the seminiferous tubules, and Leydig cells proliferate from the 14th through the 18th weeks.

Mesenchymal condensation at the caudal mesonephros during the fifth gestational week forms the presumptive gubernaculum. This becomes a band that joins the mesonephric duct and abdominal wall. By the eighth week, this portion of mesonephric duct becomes the caudal epididymis. A peritoneal dimple at this site, the processus vaginalis, is present at the 10th week. By the 12th week, a recognizable testis has migrated or has been pulled to that location, the future internal inguinal ring. There is little further change in testicular position until the seventh month, when the gubernaculum swells, and the processus vaginalis extends into the scrotum.

Undescended Testis

Undescended testis occurs in 30% of premature boys, 3.4% of full-term boys, 0.8% of 1-year-olds, and 0.8% of adults. If testicular descent has not occurred by 1 year of age, it is unlikely to occur subsequently. The scrotum serves an important thermoregulatory function by keeping the testes 2° to 3°C cooler than the rest of the body, to permit normal pubertal maturation and functional semen. Testes that remain undescended during childhood have a significant reduction in the number of germ cells. An undescended testis has an enhanced likelihood of malignant change. This predisposition is probably unaltered by surgical relocation in the scrotum (orchiopexy), but a scrotal position renders the testis amenable to self-examination. Undescended testes are blighted gonads, and if orchiopexy is performed, lifelong surveillance and self-examination skills must be ensured.

An undescended testis must be distinguished from a retractile testis. The latter appears to reside above the scrotum on initial examination, but gentle and persistent technique brings the testis into the scrotum, where it stays if the patient is relaxed. Some ectopic undescended testes can be maneuvered into the scrotum by the examiner, but once released, they ascend. Most undescended testes are ectopic. They have descended through the internal ring, inguinal canal, and external ring but have become trapped in a pocket known as the *superficial pouch of Denis Brown*, which is located between the Scarpa fascia and external oblique fascia. Less often, the undescended testis is in the inguinal canal.

Orchiopexy is performed at any time after 1 year of age. The testis is located and mobilized, and the spermatic cord is followed cephalad to the internal inguinal ring. A patent processus vaginalis must be dissected from the spermatic cord to adequately mobilize the testis. Further dissection in the retroperitoneum provides additional length. A subcutaneous scrotal pouch is created, and the testis is anchored within it. The epididymal configuration is often abnormal in boys with undescended testes (Fig. 104-10). Mild dysmorphism may be of no consequence, but exceedingly abnormal or unattached genital ducts make fertility from that testis unlikely. These features should be noted at the time of operation, mentioned to the family, and described in the operative note.

Hormonal treatment with either human chorionic gonadotropin or luteinizing hormone-releasing hormone has been advocated to induce testicular descent. Because most undescended testes are fixed in the superficial inguinal pouch and must be literally cut free during orchiopexy, it is difficult to understand how hormonal treatment can accomplish this, and careful randomized studies have failed to support this nonoperative approach.

An undescended testis is nonpalpable in some patients. Before this diagnosis is invoked, however, several examination techniques are necessary to rule out false nonpalpability. The genital examination of children must be patient and gentle. Application of water-soluble lubricating jelly reduces tactile friction and may permit identification of a

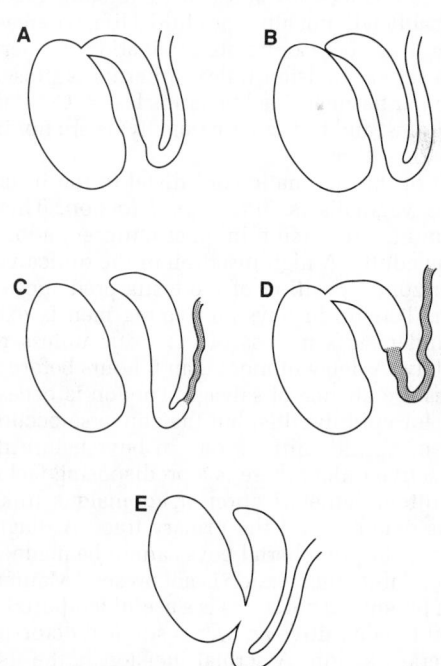

Figure 104-10. Epididymal anomalies in undescended testes. (*A*) Tenuous attachment of head of epididymis to the testis. (*B*) Complete separation of the epididymis from the testis. (*C*) Detached epididymis and atretic vas deferens. (*D*) Tenuous attachment of head. Atretic body and vasal atresia. (*E*) Section of head but partial attachment of body of epididymis tail.

testis. Reexamination of the child in a crossed-leg sitting posture may also reveal the gonad. If the testis is truly nonpalpable, the inguinal canal is explored, but if the testis is not found or its absence is proved by identifying blind-ending spermatic vessels, the search should be expanded into the peritoneal cavity. An alternative approach is laparoscopy to identify an abdominal testis or to prove its absence by revealing blind-ending spermatic vessels. Laparoscopy further allows the use of endoscopic techniques to manage abdominal testes surgically.[17]

Management of undescended testes in adults is controversial. Some have recommended they be removed in men up to 50 years of age, whereas others suggest they be ignored in men older than 32 years.[18] These recommendations are based on a greater theoretic risk of death from surgical intervention compared with risk of death from tumor at those ages. Undescended testes are usually devoid of germ cells, and therefore their removal should not alter fertility. Additionally, if these testes are nonpalpable, the risk for malignancy is obviated.

Torsion

The most common pediatric scrotal emergency is torsion, and this can occur in one of three forms. In newborns, spermatic cord torsion occurs high on the cord. The loose connection of tunica vaginalis to the scrotum permits the entire scrotal contents to twist; this is *extravaginal torsion.* The event may occur before birth or in the immediate perinatal period and seems to be completely asymptomatic. A scrotal mass resulting from perinatal torsion is often misconstrued as a tumor. Extravaginal torsion may be bilateral. Surgical salvage by immediate exploration and untwisting is possible but is a long shot at this age. Usually, the twisted testis is completely necrotic. Because the torsion occurs high on the cord, an inguinal incision is advantageous. The main advantage to prompt exploration is the opportunity to anchor the contralateral testis and thereby decrease its chances for subsequent torsion. Losing one testis probably will not alter the child's life, whereas losing both is a tragedy. Contralateral fixation is performed through a scrotal incision unless a hernia is present, and paratesticular tissue is fixed to dartos fascia. Genital ducts, parietal tunics, and testicular parenchyma are not invaded by needle or suture.

Torsion of the spermatic cord distal to the insertion of the tunica vaginalis is *intravaginal torsion.* This is the usual form of cord torsion in older children, adolescents, and young adults. A high insertion of the tunica vaginalis and a horizontal position of the testis predispose to this condition. Torsion in boys and young men is extremely painful and results in loss of the testis unless relieved immediately. A delay of more than 6 hours before surgery minimizes the chance of salvage. Torsion is occasionally mistaken for epididymitis, but the converse occurs much more often. Epididymitis is rare in boys before they are sexually active unless there is a predisposing factor, such as intermittent catheterization or anomalous linkage between vas deferens and the urinary tract. A diagnosis of epididymitis in prepubertal boys cannot be made without absolute certainty that torsion is not present. Manual detorsion with parenteral narcotics is a useful temporizing technique, but the definitive answer is surgical detorsion with contralateral fixation. A scrotal incision is the usual approach, but an inguinal approach is used when there is concern about coexisting hernia, when the twisted testis is undescended, or when there is uncertainty about the diagnosis. A frankly necrotic testis is removed, and an ischemic testis may be untwisted and observed for viability. Sympathetic orchiopathy (contralateral damage from

immunologic response to the damaged testis) is a theoretical possibility, but definitive evidence of this is lacking in the literature. It is therefore best to try to preserve a twisted testis if there is evidence of viability. Some boys experience transient or intermittent torsion. They may have acute scrotal pain, perhaps with swelling and erythema, but resolution occurs within minutes or a few hours. Some young men with definitive torsion and a completely ischemic testis have a history of previous intermittent scrotal pain. This pattern of *torsion and detorsion* is a good reason for elective bilateral orchiopexy.

Torsion of a gonadal appendage may cause as much pain as primary testicular torsion. The testicular appendix, a müllerian duct remnant, is the usual affected structure, but epididymal appendages also are susceptible to torsion. Careful examination may reveal a tender focal subcutaneous induration or a visible blue dot near the upper pole of the testis. If torsion of an appendix can be recognized at examination, no surgical course is necessary, but if confident diagnosis cannot be made, exploration is necessary to exclude torsion of the spermatic cord.

Ultrasonography is useful in instances of trauma to ascertain integrity of the tunica albuginea or to identify an underlying testicular mass. Nuclear scans are occasionally useful in the management of intrascrotal problems. In situations of scrotal pain and swelling in boys, torsion must be excluded. Astute history-taking and physical examination usually are sufficient to determine if surgical exploration is necessary. If a diagnosis other than torsion is made, it must be made with absolute confidence.

Prepubertal Testis Tumors

Prepubertal testis tumors make up only 1% of all testis tumors. The usual lesion is a yolk sac tumor, which is a variant of embryonal-cell carcinoma. The tumors present with painless enlargement of a testis. The typical age of discovery is 2 years, and orchiectomy with removal of the spermatic cord is usually curative. Nonetheless, metastatic spread can occur, and the roles of retroperitoneal node dissection and adjuvant chemotherapy still prompt debate. These tumors usually generate high levels of serum alpha-fetoprotein, which allow monitoring of patients for relapse.

OTHER GENITOURINARY DISORDERS
Antenatal Hydronephrosis

Antenatal hydronephrosis, recognized from ultrasonography during pregnancy, has created a new aspect of medical practice. Antenatal hydronephrosis has certainly existed throughout history but, most likely, only the occasional instance created a clinical postnatal problem. In some cases, the clinical problem may take decades to declare itself. Although there is no evidence that most fetuses with hydronephrosis come to harm later in their lives, the recognition of upper urinary tract dilation in the fetus has led to tremendous interest in antenatal intervention. In most situations, only a single kidney is involved, and the degree of hydronephrosis is unlikely to cause a problem with vaginal delivery. Giant hydronephrosis, larger than 10 cm, may present an argument for cesarean section delivery. Patients with bilateral hydronephrosis and normal amniotic fluid volume should be allowed to come to term, but if oligohydramnios is present, the prognosis is poor. Antenatal upper-tract decompression by means of fetal ureterostomy or placement of a percutaneous catheter is technically possible, but concomitant pulmonary dysplasia may predetermine the outcome for these fetuses.[19]

Antenatal hydronephrosis is evaluated postpartum by ultrasonography at 3 days of life; this is followed by a voiding cystogram and diuretic renal scan at 1 month. The usual conditions that cause antenatal hydronephrosis are VUR, obstruction at the ureteropelvic or ureterovesical junction, prune-belly syndrome, ureterocele, and duplication. In some cases, initial evaluation fails to demonstrate any explanation for the hydronephrosis. These patients should be followed with serial ultrasonography during childhood.

Prune-Belly Syndrome

Prune-belly syndrome, also known as Eagle-Barrett syndrome, consists of abdominal-wall muscular deficiency, dilated upper urinary tracts, and undescended testes that reside in the abdominal cavity. Incomplete syndromes and variants in females have been described. A similar pattern of dysmorphism has been created in a fetal sheep model by means of urethral ligation, thereby suggesting that prune-belly syndrome is the result of transient fetal obstructive uropathy. Three main clinical groups have been identified: (1) stillborn fetuses with severe pulmonary and renal dysplasia, (2) children with unilateral or mild bilateral renal dysplasia, and (3) children with normal renal function. Patent urachus, megalourethra, or urethral atresia sometimes occur in prune-belly syndrome. Orthopedic anomalies include clubbed feet and congenital hip dislocation. Dimpling of the outer knee or elbow is common. Other associated anomalies include intestinal malrotation, gastroschisis, Hirschsprung disease, imperforate anus, cardiac septal defects, and tetralogy of Fallot. Urinary tract reconstruction is not always necessary, but orchiopexy and abdominal wall reconstruction are usually worthwhile.[20]

Intersex, Vaginal, and Uterine Anomalies

ARNOLD G. CORAN

INTERSEX ANOMALIES

Although intersex abnormalities are uncommon, physicians involved with infants and children should have an understanding of these problems. Proper gender assignment to a neonate born with ambiguous genitalia is a social emergency that must be resolved in the newborn period.[21] Once appropriate sex assignment has been made, the next critical step is reconstruction, if necessary. Deviation from

this approach can result in severe emotional disability for the child and family.

Embryology

Normal sexual development during gestation requires the correct chromosome complement and composition, proper migration of germ cells from the yolk sac to the urogenital ridge for initial induction of the gonad, appropriate hormonal production by the gonad, and proper response by the target organs to the secreted hormones. A defect in any one of these steps can result in ambiguous genitalia.

As detailed in the first part of this chapter, the Y chromosome and other genetic instructions initiate differentiation of the primitive gonad into a testis. The first evidence of sexual dimorphism in the testis is the Sertoli cell. A factor produced by the testis leads to the differentiation of the medullary cords of the primitive gonad into seminiferous tubules. Sertoli cells in the seminiferous tubules begin to produce müllerian-inhibiting substance after the seventh fetal week. Leydig cells differentiate from interstitial cells in the testis and begin to produce testosterone at 8 to 9 weeks. Testosterone stimulates the development of the wolffian duct system to form the vas deferens, the seminal vesicles, and the epididymis. In addition, testosterone is reduced at the end-organ target sites to dihydrotestosterone, which regulates the development of the external genitalia into the penis and scrotum.

In the absence of the Y chromosome, a primitive gonad differentiates into an ovary. Female development of the müllerian duct system and external genitalia is also an autonomous process. The normal female is not exposed to müllerian-inhibiting substance; therefore, the müllerian ducts form fallopian tubes, uterus, cervix, and upper portion of the vagina. Simultaneously, in the absence of testosterone, the wolffian ducts regress. The genital tubercle, genital folds, genital swellings, and urogenital sinus develop into clitoris, labia minora, labia majora, and lower vagina, respectively, when 5-α-dihydrotestosterone is not present.

Diagnostic Evaluation

Abnormalities that result in ambiguous genitalia can be grouped into four categories—female pseudohermaphroditism, male pseudohermaphroditism, true hermaphroditism, and mixed gonadal dysgenesis.[22] During the initial evaluation of an infant with ambiguous genitalia, the symmetry of the gonads and the presence or absence of Barr bodies on buccal smear (the chromatin mass indicative of a second X chromosome) allow the differentiation among these four entities with a high degree of accuracy (Table 104-1). A chromatin-positive neonate with symmetric gonads usually is a female pseudohermaphrodite, whereas a

Table 104-1. DIFFERENTIATION OF FOUR MAJOR INTERSEX ABNORMALITIES

	Female Pseudohermaphroditism	True Hermaphroditism	Male Pseudohermaphroditism	Mixed Gonadal Dysgenesis
Buccal smear (Barr bodies)	Positive	Positive	Negative	Negative
Karyotype	XX	XX	XY	XO/XY
Urinary steroids	Positive	Negative	Negative	Negative
Gonads	Normal ovaries	Testis, ovary, ovatestis	Testes	Dysgenetic and streak ovaries

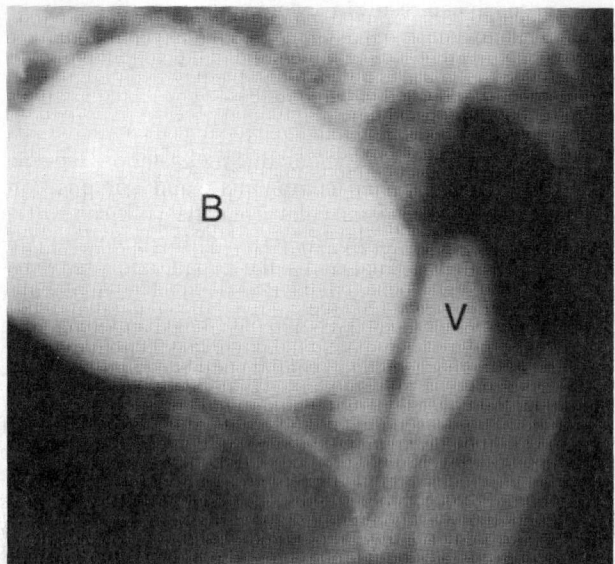

Figure 104-11. Retrograde genitogram in a patient with congenital adrenal hyperplasia. This procedure is performed with a Foley catheter inserted just inside the perineal opening with the ballon inflated. Note the low insertion of the vagina into the urogenital sinus. V, vagina; B, bladder.

chromatin-positive neonate with asymmetric gonads usually is a true hermaphrodite. A chromatin-negative neonate with symmetric gonads usually is a male pseudohermaphrodite, and a chromatin-negative neonate with asymmetric gonads usually has mixed gonadal dysgenesis.

Complete evaluation of the infant with ambiguous genitalia, in addition to a thorough physical examination (including rectal examination to check for a uterus, vaginal examination, and consideration of phallus size and shape) should include the following:

- Complete family history to determine if other family members have a similar problem (undiscovered congenital adrenal hyperplasia is suggested if female relatives died in infancy)
- Detailed evaluation of drug ingestion during pregnancy (especially androgenic agents such as progesterone)
- Karyotype
- Urinary steroid measurements
- Serum electrolytes
- Retrograde genitogram to demonstrate the location of the vaginal entrance into the urogenital sinus

Occasionally, laparotomy or laparoscopy is required for definitive sex identification, especially with true hermaphrodites.[23]

Most infants with ambiguous genitalia are assigned the female gender because the relevant surgical reconstruction is far more practical. Regardless of genotype, it is uniformly agreed that an inadequate phallus cannot be surgically corrected and that a patient fares much better in the female gender role. The exception to this is the genetic male with severe penoscrotal hypospadias and bilateral undescended testes but a functional phallus, who is always reared as a male.

Female Pseudohermaphroditism– Adrenogenital Syndrome (Congenital Adrenal Hyperplasia)

Infants with congenital adrenal hyperplasia have a 46,XX karyotype but have been exposed to excessive levels of endogenous androgens in utero. Three important enzy-

matic deficiencies are associated with this syndrome—21-hydroxylase, 11-hydroxylase, and 3-β-hydroxysteroid dehydrogenase (see Chap. 58). Each of these enzyme deficiencies results in overproduction of intermediary steroid hormones with androgenic properties that masculinize the external genitalia of the XX fetus. The phenotypic picture varies from mild clitoral enlargement alone to complete masculinization of the urethra with a normal-appearing male phallus and the urethral meatus at the glans penis. The latter clinical picture is usually associated with complete fusion of the labia.

Because of the proximal defect in glucocorticoid synthesis, these patients require cortisol replacement. In addition, those with mineralocorticoid deficiency (representing the salt-losing form of the adrenogenital syndrome) require mineralocorticoid replacement. All these children are reared as females, and they should have normal fertility because the internal genitalia are normal. Surgical therapy is designed to correct the cosmetic and functional deformities of the external genitalia, particularly the hypertrophy of the clitoris and the malformation of the vaginal introitus. The ideal surgical management is a cut-back or posterior flap vaginoplasty with a clitoral reduction or recession, usually performed when the patient is 3 to 6 months of age. (Figs. 104-11 to 104-15). If the child has the rare form of congenital adrenal hyperplasia in which the vaginal insertion into the urethra is proximal to the external sphincter, then vaginoplasty is delayed until the patient is at least 2 years of age, and a formal pull-through of the vagina to the perineum is required.[24,25]

Mixed Gonadal Dysgenesis

The syndrome of mixed gonadal dysgenesis is associated with dysgenic gonads and retained müllerian structures (Fig. 104-16). Usually, a mosaicism of the karyotype (typically 45,XO/46,XY) is present. There is a high incidence (50%) of malignant tumor development in the dysgenic gonads. Gonadoblastoma is the most common tumor; how-

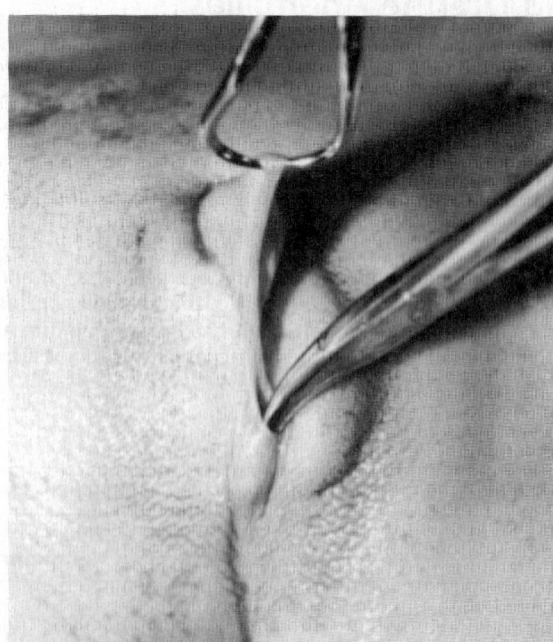

Figure 104-12. Female pseudohermaphrodite with congenital adrenal hyperplasia, moderate clitoral hypertrophy (towel clip), and urogenital sinus (hemostat).

ever, seminoma and dysgerminoma can occur, especially in the streak gonads. Because of this, bilateral gonadectomy is recommended after the first decade of life in all patients with mixed gonadal dysgenesis. Surgical reconstruction is the same as for patients with congenital adrenal hyperplasia in that all these patients are reared as females. Appropriate reconstruction of the external genitalia is required, but because of the absence of functional gonads, all these patients are infertile.

Male Pseudohermaphroditism–Testicular Feminization Syndrome

Male pseudohermaphroditism occurs in infants with an XY karyotype but deficient masculinization of their external genitalia. Male pseudohermaphroditism can result from several deficiencies, including inadequate testosterone production due to deficiencies of the enzymes necessary for its biosynthesis; inability of the external target organs to convert testosterone to dihydrotestosterone due to 5-alpha-reductase deficiency; and deficiencies in androgen receptors. Each rare form is specifically named, but the most common and well-known example is the testicular feminization syndrome, which results from an androgen receptor deficiency inherited as an X-linked recessive trait. Regardless of enzymatic defect, these patients are best raised as females since the phallus is inadequate for the male gender role. In a few cases, the diagnosis is made during routine inguinal herniorrhaphy in a phenotypic female, at which time testes are found. Because of the high risk for malignancy in the intraabdominal gonads, removal is required. Generally, this is best done at the time of discovery, but given the social issues attendant to this surprise finding, some have delayed this procedure until puberty. Occasionally, a patient may present after puberty

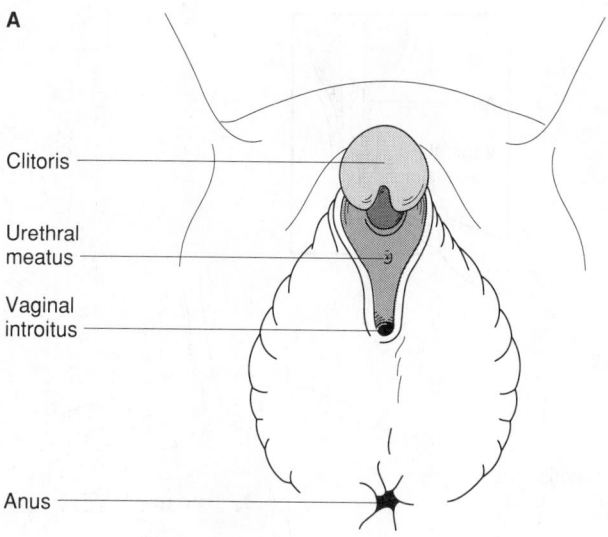

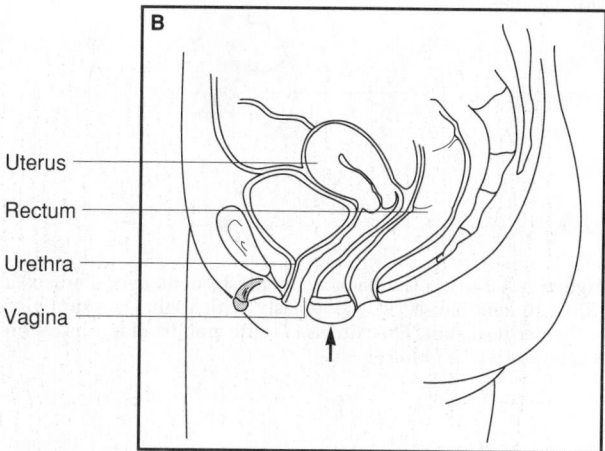

Figure 104-14. (*A*) Clitoral hypertrophy and urogenital sinus. (*B*) Low insertion of the vagina into the urogenital sinus.

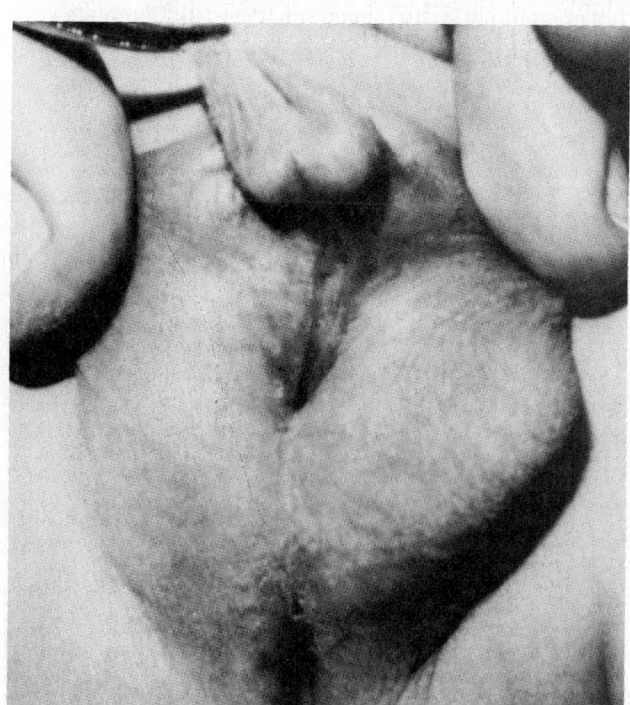

Figure 104-13. Female pseudohermaphrodite with congenital adrenal hyperplasia and severe clitoral hypertrophy, urogenital sinus, and fusion of the labia to form a scrotum. A high insertion of the vagina into the urethra was seen on genitogram and at surgery.

with amenorrhea. In this situation, bilateral gonadectomy and vaginal reconstruction, if necessary, should be done when the diagnosis is confirmed. Bilateral orchiectomy should be carried out just before puberty to prevent masculinization during puberty. These patients have a short vaginal vault; however, most can be treated with vaginal dilatation and will have a functionally adequate vaginal cavity. A few of these patients, however, require a vaginal replacement. This has been accomplished using skin grafts or pulled-through intestine, particularly the colon.[26] Occasionally, a child with this abnormality has significant clitoral hypertrophy and requires a clitoral recession. Obviously, these patients are infertile.

True Hermaphroditism

True hermaphrodites represent the rarest type of ambiguous genitalia. By definition, these patients have both normal male and normal female gonadal tissue, with an ovary on one side and a testis on the other or with an ovotestis on one or both sides (Fig. 104-17). Eighty percent of these patients have a 46,XX karyotype. Most hermaphrodites have an inadequate phallus and should be raised as females. In these patients, the testis and the testicular portion of the ovotestis should be removed, leaving the ovarian tissue in place. The surgical goals of reconstruction

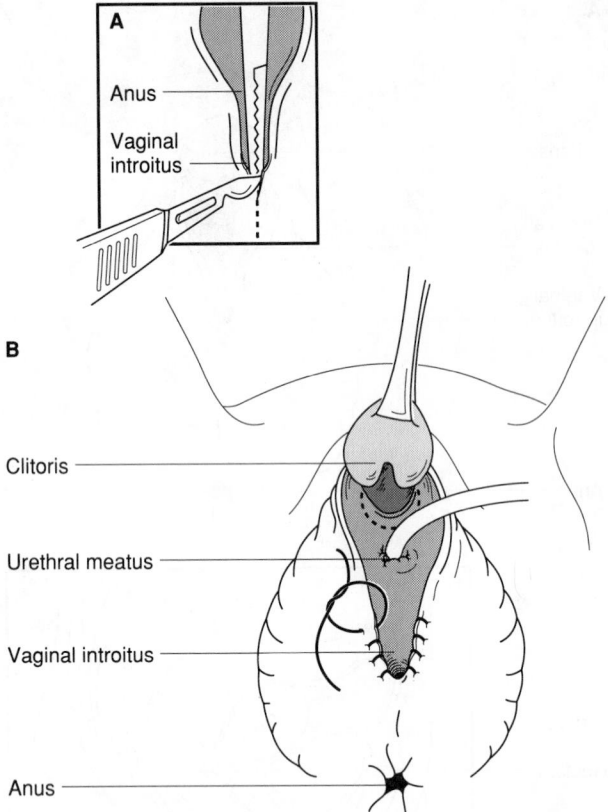

Figure 104-15. (*A*) Cut-back vaginoplasty done over a hemostat. (*B*) Completed cut-back vaginoplasty with vagina marsupialized to the perineal skin. The clitoris is being mobilized for the clitoral recession (*dashed circle*).

are similar to those for the child with congenital adrenal hyperplasia and mixed gonadal dysgenesis. Most are reared as females. Occasionally, the phallus is adequate for the male gender role, in which case all ovarian and müllerian structures are removed and hypospadias reconstruction is performed. Just after puberty, testicular prostheses may be inserted.

Surgical Considerations

The timing of the reconstructive surgical procedure represents a balance between the psychological advantages of early surgery and the technical limitations imposed by the small size of the structures. The trend is clearly toward earlier reconstruction.[27,28] The importance of the clitoris for orgasm and normal sexual function and the need to preserve all or part of it with its nerve supply has been emphasized by several investigators. Surgical options include an operation in which all of the clitoris is recessed beneath the pubic symphysis. This procedure produces an excellent cosmetic result; however, the long-term functional results are not yet known, since most of the patients who have undergone this procedure have not yet reached full sexual maturity. A small series of patients who underwent clitoral recession had good functional results.[29] An alternate approach to clitoral recession preserves the glans with its neurovascular bundle and resects the corpora. This procedure allows the clitoris to be recessed beneath the pubic symphysis without the need to accommodate the bulk of the corpora. Theoretically, the advantage of this type of recession is the elimination of dyspareunia, but no

evidence indicates that dyspareunia is a significant complication of clitoral recession without corporal resection. In addition, there is a potential for damage to the neurovascular bundle when the corpora are resected. Despite surgical preferences, no compelling data favor one procedure over the other. Surgical resection of the clitoris is inappropriate.

VAGINAL ANOMALIES

Most vaginal anomalies occur in conjunction with intersex disorders; however, isolated vaginal anomalies and vaginal anomalies in association with cloacal or urogenital abnormalities are also seen. Female urogenital embryogenesis is the result of pairing, fusion, and canalization of the müllerian ducts, which were medial to the wolffian ducts and grew caudally to join the cloaca at the müllerian tubercle. Distal fusion creates a uterovaginal canal, but the proximal nonfused Müllerian ducts become the fallopian tubes. The demarcation between the lower vagina, which arises from the urogenital sinus, and the upper vagina, which is of müllerian duct origin, is not clear; however, most studies suggest that the upper two thirds of the vagina are of müllerian origin and the lower third of cloacal or urogenital origin. The genital tubercle becomes the clitoris, and the genital swellings become the labia majora.

Urogenital sinus and cloacal anomalies are classified among the caudal regression syndromes, which present with a wide variety of vaginal, bladder, kidney, and rectal abnormalities. If the müllerian ducts do not fuse to form the müllerian tubercle, the vaginal plate does not form and join with the distal vagina. This results in the formation of a urogenital sinus.

Vaginal Atresia

Vaginal atresia can be complete, proximal, or distal. None of these should be confused with the common finding of an imperforate hymen (Fig. 104-18). Complete vagi-

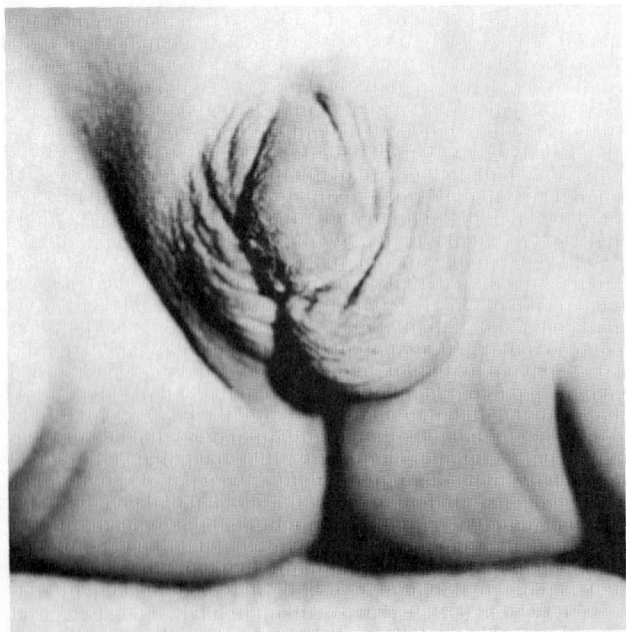

Figure 104-16. Child with mixed gonadal dysgenesis (46,XO/XY). Significant clitoral hypertrophy and a gonad in the left labioscrotal fold can be seen.

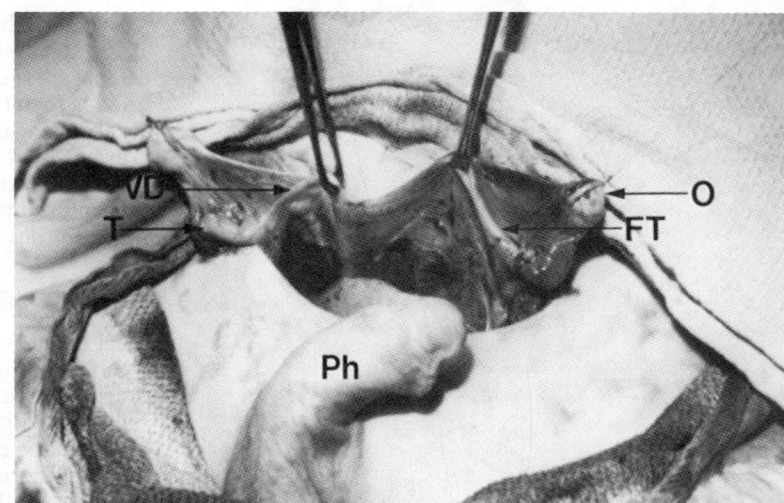

Figure 104-17. Child with true hermaphroditism. On the right side of the picture (the patient's left) are a fallopian tube (FT) and ovary (O). On the other side, a vas deferens (VD) and a testis (T) are visible. Note the large phallus (Ph). This patient was given a male gender assignment.

nal atresia results from failure of the müllerian ducts to reach the urogenital sinus. This is frequently associated with urologic anomalies, such as renal agenesis or fusion, and with duplication anomalies. In this situation, the fallopian tubes are normal, but the uterus is bicornuate and rudimentary. The ovaries are always normal. If the sino-vaginal bulbs, which originate from the urogenital sinus to form the vaginal plate, do not proliferate, then distal vaginal atresia results, and the cervix, uterus, and fallopian tubes are normal (Fig. 104-19). Proximal vaginal atresia is a result of failure of the müllerian duct to fuse to form the müllerian tubercle (Fig. 104-20). In this case, the fallopian tubes and uterus are normal, but the cervix is abnormal.

Hydrocolpos or hydrometrocolpos may present in infancy if the vagina or the vagina and uterus fill with mucus

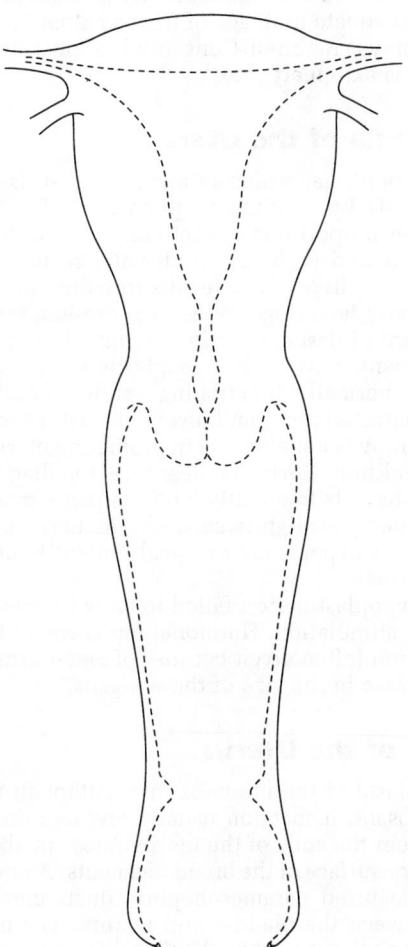

Figure 104-18. Imperforate hymen.

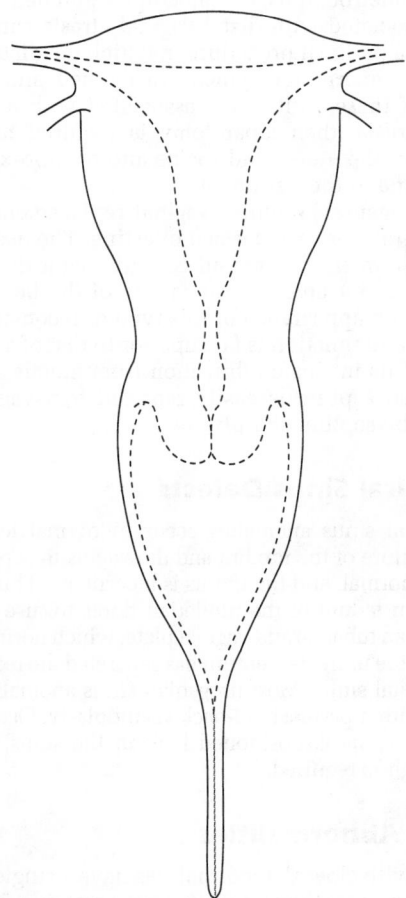

Figure 104-19. Distal vaginal atresia.

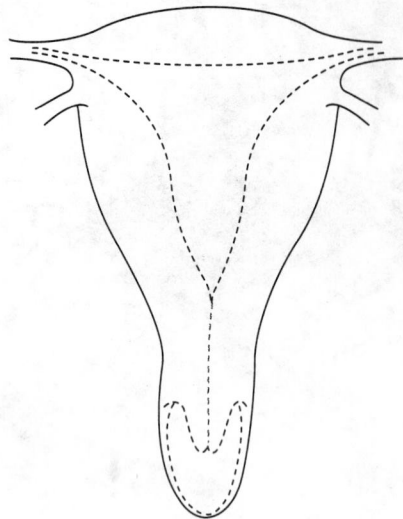

Figure 104-20. Proximal vaginal atresia with associated cervical atresia.

because of maternal estrogen stimulation of the uterine and vaginal glands. At menarche, hematocolpos or hematometrocolpos occur when the obstructed vagina fills with menstrual blood. In either situation, the patient may have a large abdominal mass. In distal vaginal atresia, the proximal vagina and uterus are normal, and episodic abdominal pain occurs at menarche. Amenorrhea is also common. In the case of proximal vaginal atresia, vaginal and uterine agenesis preclude this type of cyclical pain. Hydrocolpos, hydrometrocolpos, hematocolpos, and hematometrocolpos associated with distal vaginal atresia can be managed with a perineal procedure in which the distal vaginal atresia or imperforate hymen are opened and properly drained. If these entities are associated with a proximal vaginal atresia, then laparotomy is required to provide drainage for the uterus and vagina and to approximate the distal vagina to the perineum.

Vaginal agenesis requires vaginal replacement with either skin grafts or vascularized intestine. The use of a vascularized segment of sigmoid colon brought down to the labia minora for anastomosis is one of the best options. The cosmetic appearance of this type of reconstruction is excellent, and function is far superior to that of a skin graft because of its intrinsic lubrication from mucus secretion.

A vaginal septum is easily repaired transvaginally by dividing the septum sharply.

Urogenital Sinus Defects

Urogenital sinus anomalies occur in normal females because of failure of the urethra and the vagina to separate. The rectum is normal, and the uterus is bicornuate. This anomaly results from failure of the müllerian ducts to fuse and form the müllerian tubercle and vaginal plate, which normally takes place after the urorectal septum has separated the rectum from the urogenital sinus. Most urogenital sinus anomalies can be repaired with a perineal cut-back vaginoplasty. Occasionally, when the vagina is positioned high in the sinus, a vaginal pull-through is required.

Cloacal Abnormalities

Infants with cloacal abnormalities have a single opening on the perineum; there is no separate opening for the vagina or the rectum. The labia are often flat, and the phallus

is small. These infants can be genotypic males or females, and the assigned sex depends on the size of the phallus. Most are reared as females. Various forms of vaginal atresia are associated with cloacal abnormalities, and their surgical management depends on whether there is a vaginal agenesis, a proximal vaginal atresia, or a distal vaginal atresia. In recent years, the posterior sagittal approach has been used to repair both the rectal and vaginal abnormalities in these children.

UTERINE ANOMALIES

Fusion anomalies of the müllerian ducts result in genital tract duplication, such as duplicate vagina, uterus, and cervix (uterus didelphys). Partial fusion creates a single vagina with uterocervical duplication (uterus duplex bicollis) or a single vagina with a single cervix and two uteruses (bicornuate uterus or uterus duplex unicollis). Uterine anomalies rarely cause symptoms during childhood, and relatively few patients are symptomatic during adolescence. Most of the problems uterine anomolies create are related to infertility or are complications of pregnancy and labor.

Atresia of the Cervix

Atresia of the cervix is due to failure of the cervical portion of the fused paramesonephric ducts to develop and canalize. The condition is rare. The atretic cervix forms a solid cord of tissue between the uterine corpus above and the vagina below. When menstruation begins, a hematometra forms above it. Treatment usually consists of dilatation to obtain adequate drainage of the hematometra. Rarely, a hysterectomy is required. Congenital cervical stenosis may occur but is extremely rare.

Hypoplasia of the Uterus

True hypoplasia, which is most unusual, is characterized not only by a failure to attain normal size but also by a greater proportionate length and development of the cervix compared with the shorter and relatively smaller corpus. Severe hypoplasia results in failure of growth beyond an early fetal stage. When it is present, the uterus is a small cord of tissue, usually without a cavity.

Few patients have truly hypoplastic uteri and amenorrhea with normally functioning ovaries, normal female sexual characteristics, and cyclic breast changes. Hormonal therapy is not effective in promoting uterine growth in this condition. During adolescence, the diagnosis of an infantile uterus is frequently but incorrectly made when a patient's uterus is slightly smaller than normal. A patient with either a hypoplastic or a truly infantile uterus does not menstruate.

Some hypoplastic uteri failed to grow because of a lack of ovarian stimulation. Hormonal replacement therapy in this situation (often given because of amenorrhea) results in an increase in the size of these organs.

Aplasia of the Uterus

True aplasia of the uterus is rare. Although the uterus appears absent, inspection usually reveals thin cords extending from the ends of the uterine tubes medially along the superior surface of the broad ligaments. A midline remnant of the fused paramesonephric ducts creates a firm strand between the bladder and rectum. The ovaries are usually normal but may be displaced laterally toward the pelvic brim. In most instances, aplasia of the uterus is accompanied by poorly developed or aplastic uterine tubes. Vaginal agenesis is always present if there is a true agenesis of the uterus. Frequently, there are associated anomalies of the lower urogenital tract.

A uterus unicornis results when there is aplasia of part or all of one paramesonephric duct; the accompanying tube is usually absent or rudimentary.

Uterine Duplication

Partial or complete duplication of the uterus is caused by imperfect fusion of the paramesonephric ducts (Fig. 104-21). The genital folds fail to unite normally. The result is either a complete bicornuate uterus (ie, two cervices) or simple duplication of the uterine body.

Anomalies of the Fallopian Tubes

Anomalies of the fallopian tubes are without significance in childhood or adolescence. These malformations appear to play some role in problems of sterility and pregnancy. Small supernumerary or accessory tubes attached to the fimbriated ends or communicating with the isthmic or ampullar portions of the tubes are relatively common and may be seen when a child is operated on for some other pelvic condition. Accessory tubes of this type cause no problems and need not be disturbed.

Introital problems

Synechiae vulvae, or labial fusion, is a common condition in infancy and early childhood. The midline adherence of the labia minora is usually asymptomatic, incomplete, and flimsy such that time or mild lateral tension normalize the opening. A short course of weak topical es-

trogens usually produce enough maturation of the squamous surfaces to prevent readherence. Occasionally, however, the fusion is high grade and dense enough to interfere with micturition and precludes easy separation. In these instances, incision and suture of the skin edges is humane and reliable. A short course of topical estrogens prevents readhesion.

Girls may sometimes have urethral prolapse in which a distended inflamed urethral meatus appears for no obvious reason. Usually, these are minimally symptomatic and voiding is not compromised. These lesions usually regress with time and topical agents, although excision is sometimes necessary, particularly for symptomatic cases. Differential diagnosis includes trauma, sexual abuse, urethral caruncle, and prolapsed ureterocele.

Sexual abuse is much more prevalent than expected, and it may have consequences in terms of genitourinary function and structure.[30] A careful perineal and introital examination may reveal important clues, such as a widened introitus or asymmetry of the hymenal margin.[31]

REFERENCES

1. Shimamura T, Morrison AB. A progressive glomerulosclerosis occurring in partial five-sixths nephrectomized rats. Am J Pathol 1975;79:95.
2. N'Guessan G, Stephens FD. Congenital superior ectopic (thoracic) kidney. Urology 1984;24:219.
3. Mesrobian HJ, Kelalis PP, Hrabovsky E, et al. Wilms' tumor in horseshoe kidneys: a report from the National Wilms' Tumor Study. J Urol 1985;133:1002.
4. O'Reilly PH, Lawson RS, Shields RA, et al. Idiopathic hydronephrosis—the diuresis renogram: a new non-invasive method of assessing equivocal pelvicoureteral junction obstruction. J Urol 1979;121:153.
5. Keating MA, Escola J, McSnyder HM III, et al. Changing concepts in management of primary obstructive megaureter. J Urol 1989;142:636.
6. Kalicinski H, Kansy J, Kotarbinska B, et al. Surgery of megaureters: modification of Hendren's operation. J Pediatr Surg 1977;12:183.
7. Hodson CJ, Edwards D. Chronic pyelonephritis and vesicoureteral reflux. Clin Radiol 1960;11:219.
8. Bloom DA, Bennett CJ. Nonoperative management of vesicoureteral reflux. Semin Urol 1986;4:74.
9. Kennelly MJ, Bloom DA, Ritchey ML, et al: Outcome analysis of bilateral Cohen cross-trigonal ureteroneocystostomy. Urology 1995;46:393.
10. O'Donnell B, Puri P. Endoscopic correction of primary vesicoureteral reflux. Br J Urol 1986;58:601.
11. Leonard MP, Canning DA, Epstein JI, et al. Local tissue reaction to the subureteral injection of glutaraldehyde cross-linked bovine collagen in humans. J Urol 1990;143:1209.
12. Bloom, DA, McGuire EJ, Lapides J. A brief history of urethral catheterization. J Urol 1994;151:317.
13. Bloom DA, Knechtel JM, McGuire EJ. Urethral dilation improves bladder compliance in children with myelomeningocele and high leak point pressures. J Urol 1990;144:430.
14. Oster J. Further fate of the foreskin. Arch Dis Child 1968; 43:200.
15. American Academy of Pediatrics. Newborns: care of the uncircumcised penis. Elk Grove Village, IL, American Academy of Pediatrics, 1986.
16. Wiswell TE, Geschke DW. Risks from circumcision during the first month of life compared with those for uncircumcised boys. Pediatrics 1989;83:1011.
17. Bloom DA, Ritchey ML, Manzoni G. Laparoscopy for the nonpalpable testis. In: Holcomb GW III, ed. Pediatric endoscopic surgery. Norwalk, CT, Appelton & Lange, 1994:41.
18. Farrer JH, Walker AH, Rajfer J. Management of the postpubertal cryptorchid testis: a statistical review. J Urol 1985; 134:1071.
19. Glick PL, Harrison MR, Golbus MS, et al. Management of the fetus with congenital hydronephrosis. II. Prognostic criteria and selection for treatment. J Pediatr Surg 1985;20:376.

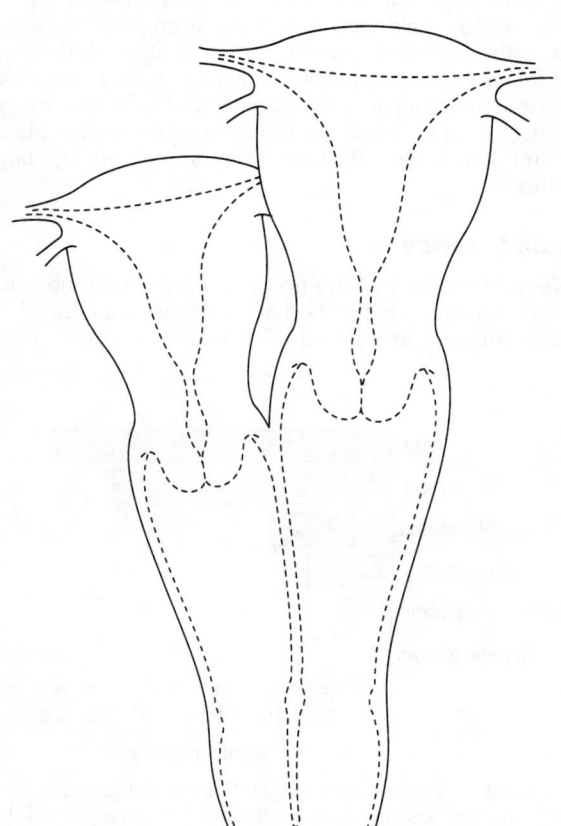

Figure 104-21. Duplication of the vagina and uterus.

20. Ehrlich RM, Lesavoy MA, Fine RN. Total abdominal wall reconstruction in the prune belly syndrome. J Urol 1986; 136:282.

21. Canty TG. The child with ambiguous genitalia: a neonatal surgical emergency. Ann Surg 1977;186:272.

22. Donahoe PK, Hendren WH. Perineal reconstruction of ambiguous genitalia in infants raised as females. Ann Surg 1984;200:363.

23. Coran AG, Polley TZ Jr. Surgical management of ambiguous genitalia in the infant and child. J Pediatr Surg 1991;26:812.

24. Hendren WH, Donahoe PK. Correction of congenital abnormalities of the vagina and perineum. J Pediatr Surg 1980; 15:751.

25. Sharp RJ, Holder TM, Campbell PH, et al. Neonatal genital reconstruction. J Pediatr Surg 1987;22:168.

26. Wesley JR, Coran AG. Intestinal vaginoplasty for congenital absence of the vagina. J Pediatr Surg 1992;27:985.

27. Donahue PK, Gustafson ML. Early one-stage surgical reconstruction of high vaginal atresia. J Pediatr Surg 1994;29:352.

28. Donahue PK, Powell DM, Lee MM. Clinical management of intersex abnormalities. Curr Probl Surg 1991;27:15.

29. Randolph JG, Wellington H, Rathlev MC. Clitoroplasty for females born with ambiguous genitalia: a long-term study of 37 patients. J Pediatr Surg 1981;16:882.

30. Bloom DA. Editorial: sexual abuse and voiding dysfunction. J Urol 1995; 153:777.

31. Bloom DA, Sanvordenker JK. Genitourinary manifestations of sexual abuse in children. Adv Urol 1993;6:1.

SURGERY: SCIENTIFIC PRINCIPLES AND PRACTICE, Second Edition, edited by Lazar J. Greenfield, Michael W. Mulholland, Keith T. Oldham, Gerald B. Zelenock, and Keith D. Lillemoe. Lippincott–Raven Publishers, Philadelphia, © 1997.

CHAPTER 105

CHILDHOOD TUMORS

MICHAEL P. LAQUAGLIA

The focus of this chapter is malignant solid tumors of infancy, childhood, and adolescence. Fortunately, these are rare conditions, especially when compared with the incidence of major adult malignancies like breast and lung cancer. This rarity, however, poses special problems to the clinical and basic science cancer researcher. For the clinician studying the effectiveness of a particular drug or surgical technique, the number of patients available for randomized trials is drastically reduced. Similarly, the basic scientist wishing to analyze the effect of a particular genetic mutation on the development or virulence of a tumor is limited in the material available for study. The solution to this problem has been the establishment of cooperative groups for the clinical and basic scientific study of pediatric malignancies. These include the Children's Cancer Group (CCG; formerly Children's Cancer Study Group, or CCSG) and the Pediatric Oncology Group (POG) in the United States, and the Societé Internacionale Oncologique Pediatrique in Europe. These agencies were originally focused on the study of hematologic malignancies. Later, collaboration was extended to the study of pediatric solid tumors, and cooperation between groups allowed prospective protocols to be done on some rare tumors. The Intergroup Rhabdomyosarcoma Study was established as a collaborative effort between POG and CCG to address the special problems posed by childhood sarcomas, most importantly rhabdomyosarcoma. The National Wilms' Tumor Study (NWTS) enrolls most Wilms tumors diagnosed in the United States. This organization has made significant progress in increasing the cure rate from Wilms tumors and

in developing therapies with minimal early and late toxicity. This and other cooperative studies, combined with pioneering single-institutional efforts, have resulting in a 40% increase in the overall survival rate for pediatric cancer since the 1970s. Overall 5-year survival rates for all stages are about 85% for Wilms tumor, 70% for hepatoblastoma, and 50% for rhabdomyosarcoma. In comparison, the survival rate was less than 20%, and closer to zero, respectively, for these malignancies before the advent of multidisciplinary therapy. Despite this progress, only 20% to 40% of children with neuroblastomas and less than 10% of children with hepatocellular carcinomas survive more than 5 years after diagnosis. As in the past, the pediatric surgical oncologist will be instrumental to future progress.

INCIDENCE OF SOLID TUMORS IN CHILDHOOD

The incidence of various pediatric solid tumors of interest to pediatric surgeons is compared in Figure 105-1 to the incidence of acute lymphoblastic leukemia and accumulated central nervous system tumors.[1,2] Neuroblastoma is the most common extracranial solid tumor, followed in incidence by Wilms tumors. Rhabdomyosarcomas have about half the incidence of the previous two, while hepatic tumors are fortunately extremely rare.

NEUROBLASTOMA
Epidemiology and Associated Conditions

Neuroblastoma is the most common extracranial solid tumor and the most common abdominal malignancy of childhood. The incidence is 10.5 per million white children and 8.8 per million black children younger than 15 years of age in the United States. This results in about 500 new cases reported each year.[3] The male/female ratio is 1.2:1, and the incidence is uniform throughout the world. The median age at diagnosis is about 2 years, and 80% of children are younger than 4 years of age at diagnosis.[4] Case reports associating neuroblastoma with fetal exposures, including the fetal alcohol syndrome, or hydantoin or phenobarbital exposure have not been supported by larger studies.[5,6]

Basic Science

Neuroblastoma was the first tumor in which molecular biologic advances in the field of oncogenes were translated into a clinically useful tool. The N-myc oncogene, whose

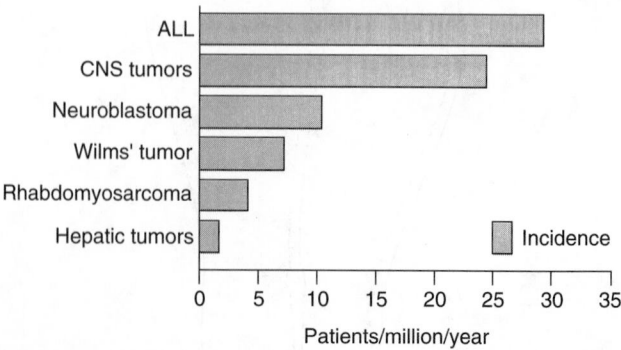

Figure 105-1. The incidence of childhood malignancies. Brain (CNS) tumors are the most common solid tumor in children. Neuroblastoma is the most common solid tumor treated by general pediatric surgeons. All, acute lymphocytic leukemia.

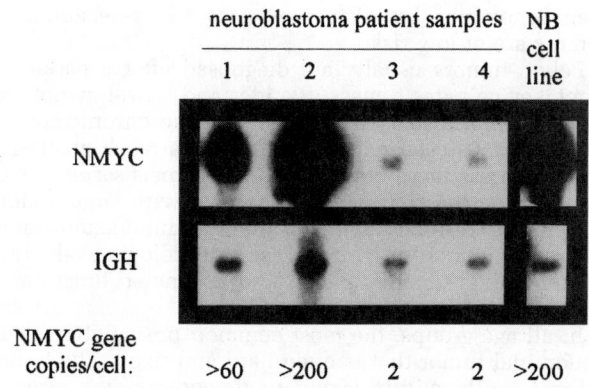

neuroblastoma patient samples | NB cell line

NMYC

IGH

NMYC gene copies/cell: >60   >200   2   2   >200

Figure 105-2. Example of N–myc amplification analysis by Southern blotting in neuroblastoma samples from four patients. The Southern blot hybridization signal obtained with the N–myc probe is normalized to that obtained on the same blot with a control probe for a gene not subject to amplification, such as the immunoglobulin heavy chain gene (IGH). The signals are then normalized to a negative control (placental DNA, not illustrated). A neuroblastoma cell line with N–myc amplification is used as a positive control. The IGH signals show that similar amounts of DNA are present in each lane, but the N–myc signals are grossly different from each other, indicating amplification in cases 1 and 2 and in the control cell line. Samples 1 and 2 show high-level N–myc amplification, exceeding 60 and 200 copies of N–myc per cell, respectively, which corresponds to greater than 30-fold and 100-fold amplification. Samples 3 and 4 contain two copies of N–myc per cell, as expected in diploid cells without amplification. (Courtesy of Marc Ladanyi, M.D., Department of Pathology, Memorial Sloan-Kettering Cancer Center)

function and mechanism of action remain the subject of investigation, was empirically shown to be a useful predictor of survival and risk. It was found that patients with an increased number of copies of the N-myc gene had a much worse prognosis.[7–9] Most authorities consider a copy number of more than 10 to be significant. It has also been shown that when N-myc is amplified in the primary tumor, the same is true for metastatic deposits or recurrent tumors.[10] Rapid assessment of the N-myc copy number can be done using the process of in situ fluorescent hybridization, while the traditional method using Southern blotting takes longer. An example of tumor analysis from a patient is presented in Figure 105-2. The mechanism of N-myc

amplification in neuroblastoma remains unknown. N-myc is a DNA-binding protein. It thus exerts control over other genes and may help to keep the cell in G_1 phase.[11]

Since the identification of the Rb gene and identification of its role as a tumor-suppressor gene, much work has been devoted to finding tumor suppressors in other systems. The usual starting point for this type of analysis is determination of a consistent cytogenetic deletion. The most common cytogenetic abnormality in neuroblastoma is deletion of a portion of the short arm of the first chromosome at 1p36.[12] The presence of a 1p deletion correlates with worse outcome in neuroblastoma and has been used as a prognostic factor. It has been shown using cell fusion that replacement of this deleted segment is associated with a marked reduction in tumorigenicity.[13] A number of laboratories are trying to identify the neuroblastoma tumor-suppressor gene 1p36.

Another active area of neuroblastoma research is the relation of nerve growth factor receptors to differentiation and clinical risk. The low-affinity nerve growth factor receptor LNGFR and the TRK protooncogene, which is a component of the high-affinity nerve growth factor receptor, are expressed in human neuroblastoma tissue. A number of authors have shown that LNGFR and TRK (TRK-A) expression are inversely correlated with N-myc amplification and are associated with lower stage at diagnosis and improved prognosis.[14–16]

Pathology

Neuroblastoma cells are derived from the primitive neural crest, as are melanocytes; Schwann cells; neuroendocrine cells (APUD cells); C cells of the thyroid gland, the autonomic nervous system, and adrenal gland; and mesenchymal cells of the midface. Neuroblastoma cells are thought to arise from primitive sympathoblasts (neuroblasts).[17] Under certain circumstances, these pluripotential cells demonstrate an ability to differentiate along a separate neural crest lineage. For instance, pure ganglioneuroma is thought to arise from complete differentiation of primitive neuroblasts into ganglion cells. Schwann cell differentiation is also clearly and frequently observed in these tumors. It is also possible to identify melanocytic differentiation in certain rare but well-reported neuroblastomas. Finally, because the sympathetic nervous system extends along the entire neuraxis, neuroblastoma can

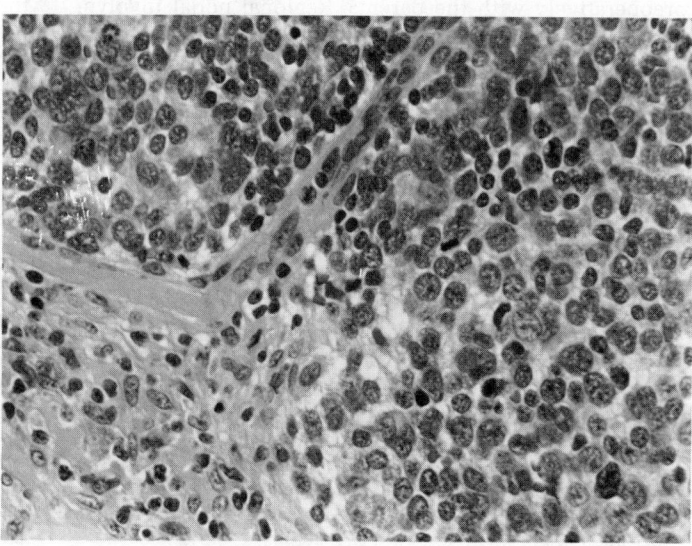

Figure 105-3. Typical neuroblastoma with monotonous cellular patterns. Note the mitotic figure (*center*; ×450).

arise from cervical, thoracic, abdominal (retroperitoneal), and pelvic primary sites.

Neuroblastoma falls into the category of a small, round, blue cell tumor of childhood characterized by sheets of cells staining with hematoxylin. Other tumors that fall into this category include primitive neuroectodermal tumors (PNET) and Ewing sarcoma, non-Hodgkin lymphomas, and undifferentiated sarcomas (certain rhabdomyosarcomas). Light microscopic diagnosis depends on the identification of Homer-Wright pseudorosettes, ganglion cells, neuropil and neuritic processes, and schwannian stroma (Fig. 105-3). Homer-Wright pseudorosettes consist of rings of dark-staining neuroblasts surrounding an eosinophilic core of neuropil. The diagnosis can be aided by immunohistochemical staining that is positive for neurofilament proteins (S-100), synaptophysin, and neuron-specific enolase. PNETs may express neuron-specific enolase but not the other neural markers.[18]

At presentation, most neuroblastomas are highly cellular and have a uniform appearance. After chemotherapy, the tumor often appears to have rests of neuroblasts contained in a schwannian stroma. This histologic appearance is called *ganglioneuroblastoma*, and although more differentiated in appearance, there is no impact on clinical risk, which is determined by the findings at initial diagnosis. It is also possible for tumors to contain significant amounts of stroma at diagnosis, and this finding is associated with improved outcome. This observation is the basis of the Shimada grading system, which is summarized in Table 105-1.[19] Because it may help predict risk, all neuroblastomas should undergo Shimada classification at diagnosis.

Neuroblastoma metastasizes to both regional lymph nodes and distant sites, most frequently bone marrow and cortical bone. The liver and rarely lungs can also be the site of metastatic spread. Cortical bone involvement as manifested by a positive bone scan is a particularly poor prognostic indicator.

Presentation, Workup, and Staging

Clinical presentation is dependent on site of origin, age at diagnosis, and the biologic aggressiveness of the tumor. The proportion of patients with cervical or pelvic tumors is increased in patients younger than 1 year when compared with older children. Cervical tumors present as a lateral neck mass, and airway compromise is not usually observed. Because they arise from cervical sympathetic ganglia, there may be associated Horner syndrome, which is often permanent after resection and should be discussed preoperatively with the parents. Regional nodal involve-

ment is common, but distant metastases are rare, and most tumors are of low risk.

Pelvic tumors usually are diagnosed after a parent or caretaker palpates a mass. Bladder and bowel symptoms like recurrent urinary tract infections and chronic constipation can be seen when pelvic tumors reach great size and compress these organs. Hydronephrosis secondary to ureteral compression is often observed with large tumors and usually resolves after resection. Epidural extension to the sacrum can also be noted, and neurologic evaluation documenting somatic motor and sphincter function is mandatory.

In all age groups, the most common presentation is an abdominal tumor that is often hard and fixed. The tumor arises from the midline sympathetic nerves or the adrenal. Often, regional nodal echelons are involved along the aorta. These involved nodes can be bulky and may extend distally to the aortic bifurcation and proximally into the mediastinum, overshadowing the primary tumor. Patients with metastatic or large bulky tumors, especially if older than 1 year of age, may appear generally ill or anemic.

Several syndromes are particularly associated with neuroblastoma: periorbital ecchymoses (raccoon eyes), opsoclonus–myoclonus syndrome, and the secretory diarrhea syndrome. Periorbital ecchymoses are caused by orbital metastases with subsequent obstruction and rupture of veins in the periorbital skin. The optic nerve and vision are not usually threatened, and the ecchymoses often take months to resolve even after the orbital tumors have regressed. Opsoclonus–myoclonus is a paraneoplastic syndrome thought to be autoimmune in nature; it is caused by development of antibodies against the tumor that cross-react with Purkinje cells in the cerebellum. Unfortunately, the symptoms may not regress after resection of the neuroblastoma, and the condition can result in devastating neurologic injury. Secretory diarrhea in this condition is caused by release of vasoactive intestinal peptide by the tumor. The watery diarrhea may require intravenous support but usually resolves with treatment. This condition is an indication of tumor differentiation and is associated with low-risk lesions.

The workup is directed toward delineation of tumor extent in the primary site and identification of metastatic deposits. The primary site is usually evaluated by computed tomography (CT) or magnetic resonance imaging (MRI); no reported analyses compare the two in neuroblastoma. If CT scans are used, they should be performed with both gastrointestinal and intravenous contrast. This is true even for cervical and thoracic primaries so that the position and course of the pharynx and esophagus are precisely determined. The volume scanned should include not only the primary tumor but also the regional lymphatics. The lower chest should be included in scans of cervical primaries, the upper abdomen and lower neck in thoracic tumors, and the entire abdomen, pelvis, and lower chest for abdominal primaries. Because of the high incidence of cortical bone involvement, especially in children older than 1 year, bone scans or radiographic series should also be performed routinely. The bone marrow is assessed by bone marrow aspiration at four iliac crest sites and bone biopsy at two. If CT or MRI scans include the liver, appropriate windows can be used to identify hepatic metastases. Ultrasound can also be used in this regard, and plain chest films are used to identify pulmonary metastases. If pulmonary metastases are present, Doppler ultrasonography can be used to identify intracaval tumor extension. It is also useful to perform a [131]I (or ^{123}I) metaiodobenzylguanidine scan to assess metastatic sites and as a baseline for evaluation of therapeutic response in the primary site. Finally, a 24-hour urine collection for measurement of meta-

---

Table 105-1. SHIMADA HISTOPATHOLOGIC CLASSIFICATION OF NEUROBLASTOMA

FAVORABLE

Stroma rich, all ages, no nodular pattern
Stroma poor, age 1.5–5 y, MKI <100
Stroma poor, age <1.5 y, MKI <200

UNFAVORABLE

Stroma rich, all ages, nodular pattern
Stroma poor, age >5 y
Stroma poor, age 1.5–5 y, undifferentiated
Stroma poor, age 1.5–5 y, differentiated, MKI >100
Stroma poor, age >1 y, MKI >200

MKI, mitosis–karyorrhexis index (number of mitoses and karyorrhexis per 5000 cells).

Table 105-2. INTERNATIONAL STAGING CRITERIA FOR NEUROBLASTOMA

Stage	Criteria	3-Year Survival Rate (%) Overall	Relapse free
1	Localized tumor confined to site of origin; complete gross resection with or without microscopic margin; all identifiable regional nodes negative, including contralateral	97	88
2A	Unilateral tumor with incomplete gross excision; nodes negative	87	72
2B	Unilateral tumor with incomplete or complete gross excision with positive ipsilateral but negative contralateral nodes	86	63
3	Infiltration across the midline with or without regional nodal involvement; unilateral tumor with positive contralateral nodes; midline tumor with bilateral nodal involvement	62	58
4	Distant metastases to lymph nodes (4N), bone, bone marrow, liver, or other organs	<40	<40
4S	Localized primary tumor as described for stage 1 or 2 with distant metastases limited to liver, skin, and bone marrow (<10% involvement)	~75	~75

nephrine, dopamine, and vanillymandelic acid may help diagnostically and as a tumor marker to assess therapeutic response.

The diagnosis of neuroblastoma requires histologic confirmation either by direct tumor biopsy or by demonstration of malignant cells in bone marrow samples. Because of the wide range of molecular biologic studies that have prognostic importance, many groups attempt to obtain enough tissue at diagnosis to allow full molecular biologic and cytogenetic analysis in addition to histologic diagnosis. When possible, several grams of tumor tissue should be obtained, and a portion should be snap frozen. Given the seriousness of this tumor, this is a reasonable objective. If the tumor is not initially resectable, a small incision or minimally invasive procedure usually is adequate exposure to obtain enough tissue for diagnostic and specialized studies.

The most widely used staging system for neuroblastoma is based on the international system, which is listed in Table 105-2. This was evolved from previous systems developed by Evans and colleagues and the POG.[4] Tumor size and location with regard to the midline remain important determinants of stage.

Risk Groups

As a result of insights gained through cooperative group studies, as well as the work done by several single institutions, it is possible to categorize neuroblastoma patients into high-, intermediate-, and low-risk groups at diagnosis. This assessment is based on age, stage, Shimada classification, and the results of specialized studies, including flow cytometry, analysis for N-myc amplification, cytogenetics, and TRK gene expression. Ancillary criteria include serum ferritin, lactic dehydrogenase, and neuron-specific enolase determinations at diagnosis and before blood transfusion. Table 105-3 lists criteria for high- and low-risk patients. Risk assignment is important because it strongly determines therapy.

Treatment

Neuroblastoma treatment depends on degree of risk, as noted earlier. In general, low-risk tumors do not require chemotherapy or radiation. Resection of the primary lesion to obtain the diagnosis and biologic markers is followed by observation. Serial imaging studies of the primary and possible metastatic sites in low-risk patients are performed. Urinary catecholamines should fall to normal levels and remain there.

High-risk neuroblastoma remains one of the central problems in pediatric oncology, with overall survival rates in the 10% to 30% range despite multidisciplinary therapy and the use of multiagent chemotherapy. Initial surgery should be confined to acquisition of diagnostic tissue, staging, and placement of a vascular access device. It has been noted that surgical complications are higher with initial attempts at complete resection without impact on survival. After a course of chemotherapy, usual four or five cycles, second-look surgery is performed (Fig. 105-4). Although controversy surrounds the issue of resectional surgery in high-risk patients, most authorities agree that complete gross resection should be the goal of second-look proce-

Table 105-3. RISK STATUS DETERMINANTS IN NEUROBLASTOMA

Parameters	Low Risk	High Risk
Age	<1 y (especially <6 mo)	>1 y at diagnosis
Stage	1, 2A, 2B, 4S	3, 4
Shimada classification	Favorable	Unfavorable
N-myc amplification	<3 copies	>3 Copies
Expression of TRK	trk Expressed	No trk expression
Flow cytometry	Hyperdiploid, triploid	Diploid
Cytogenetics	No 1p abnormality	1p Deletion
Ferritin at diagnosis	<142 ng/mL	≥142 ng/mL
Lactic dehydrogenase	≤1500 U/mL	>1500 U/mL
Neuron-specific enolase	≤100 ng/mL	>100 ng/mL

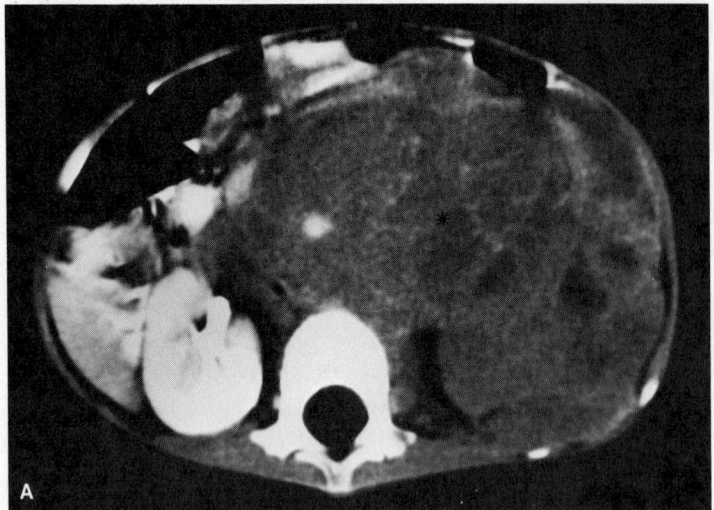

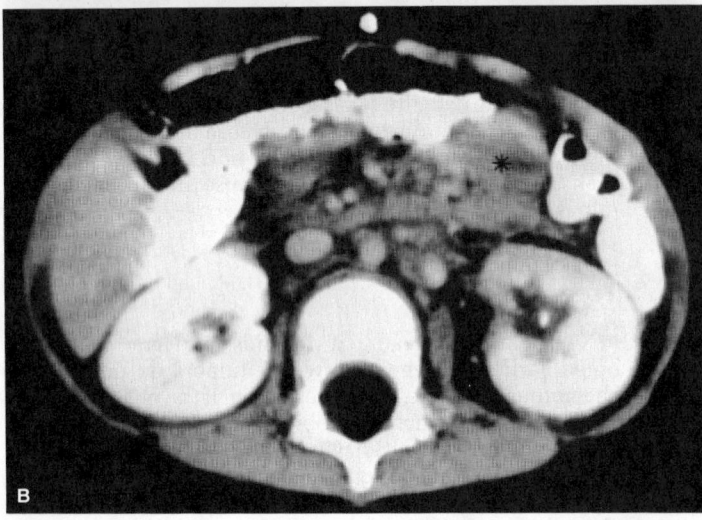

Figure 105-4. (*A*) Initial CT scan of a child with stage 4 neuroblastoma. (*B*) CT scan of the same child after incisional biopsy and cytoreductive chemotherapy. Residual tumor is present despite dramatic reduction in overall tumor size.

dures. The approach is dictated by the particular properties of the primary tumor. For upper abdominal lesions, especially those involving major midline branches of the abdominal aorta or the vena cava, thoracoabdominal exposure is helpful and well tolerated. The goal of resection is a complete vascular dissection and should encompass not only the primary but all involved regional nodal echelons.

The evolution in chemotherapy for neuroblastoma has moved toward higher dose intensities of multiple agents. *Dose intensity* is defined as the drug dose usually normalized to surface area divided by the time interval over which it is administered. In one metaanalysis, increased dose intensity correlated with improved overall and disease-free survival. In another report, primary tumor resectability correlated with increased chemotherapy intensity. There is no widely accepted regimen, and the major cooperative groups, as well as larger single institutions, have differing protocols. The CCG is planning to base part of its high-risk neuroblastoma regimen on a protocol developed at Memorial Sloan-Kettering Cancer Center. This protocol includes: cyclophosphamide, 70 mg/kg/d for 2 days, doxorubicin, 75 mg/m^2 over 72 hours, and vincristine, 2 mg/m^2 over 72 hours, given as cycles 1, 2, 4, and 6. These cycles alternate with cisplatin, 50 mg/m^2/d for 4 days, and etoposide, 200 mg/m^2/d for 3 days, for cycles 3, 5, and 7. Second-look surgery is performed after cycle 4. This regimen has resulted in a 45% disease-free survival rate at 2 years from diagnosis in high-risk stage 4 patients.[20]

Future Directions

The role of bone marrow ablation and autologous bone marrow rescue in high-risk neuroblastoma patients is being evaluated in randomized trials. Also, peripheral stem cell harvests, which may have certain advantages over autologous bone marrow, are being used to support hematopoietic function after myeloablative therapy. Similarly, the cytokine, granulocyte-colony stimulating factor, is routinely used to lessen the duration and severity of granulocytopenia after chemotherapy. Treatment with radiolabeled or cold monoclonal antibodies is also undergoing trial. Finally, various tumor vaccination strategies using gene-transfer technology are planned. This approach entails transfection of cytokines into autologous tumor cells, which are then lethally irradiated ex vivo and reinfused as a vaccine to stimulate native immunity.

WILMS TUMOR

Epidemiology and Associated Conditions

The overall incidence of Wilms tumor or nephroblastoma is 7 per 1 million children (1 per 10,000) younger than the age of 16 years, which translates into about 460 new cases in the United States and Canada per year.[21,22]

The incidence is highest for African Americans and lowest for patients of East Asian descent. Whites have an intermediate incidence. The gender ratio is about 1:1, and the peak incidence occurs between 2 and 3 years of age.[23] Median ages reported from the National Wilms' Tumor Study were 36 months for boys and 43 months for girls with unilateral disease, while boys and girls with bilateral disease presented at a median age of 23 and 30 months, respectively.[24]

Table 105-4 lists conditions associated with the development of Wilms tumor along with the associated increase in relative risk. In general, the presence of any of these conditions or syndromes should initiate a workup to rule out the presence of Wilms tumor.

Basic Science

The successful identification of the Rb gene as the tumor suppressor in retinoblastoma has led to similar investigations regarding the other pediatric solid tumors. In general, researchers attempt to find a consistent chromosomal deletion that indicates the possible site of a tumor-suppressor gene. Molecular biologic techniques are then used to identify and clone the gene. In the case of Wilms tumor, cytogenetic abnormalities have been identified on chromosomes 11p13, 1p, and 16q.[25–27] A gene called WT1 was cloned from the site on the 11th chromosome and has been shown to bind to DNA, suggesting that it functions to control gene expression. Furthermore, WT1 has been shown to be linked to the gene locus associated with aniridia but was not linked to the occurrence of Wilms tumor in three separate, multiple-case kindred.[28,29] This suggests that the Wilms tumor suppressor is probably not WT1 but may reside on a locus at 1p or especially 16q. Interestingly, NWTS-5, which is being initiated, will be directed to determining which genetic locus is associated with the development of Wilms tumor and is the most likely candidate for the Wilms tumor-suppressor gene.

Pathology

The study of Wilms tumor has benefited greatly from a central pathology review performed at the NWTS Pathology Center. Much progress in defining Wilms tumor risk categories has ensued. This underscores the need for accurate and adequate histologic analysis of all Wilms tumor specimens.

It is hypothesized that Wilms tumor arises from primitive metanephric blastema, and individual tumors often contain not only primitive metanephric cells but also cartilage, skeletal muscle, and squamous epithelium. Most tumors arise unifocally within the kidney, but about 7% of unilateral Wilms tumors are multicentric.[23] The proportion of synchronous bilateral tumors among all nephroblastoma patients ranges from 4.4% to 7%, while that of metachronous tumors is 1.% to 1.9%.[29] Wilms tumors are equally distributed with regard to the left and right side and may occur with no apparent connection to the kidneys. Usually, extrarenal Wilms tumor occurs in the retroperitoneal area, but other reported sites include pelvis, scrotum, and inguinal region.

Grossly, the tumors are globular or spherical and have a uniform pale-gray or tan color on sectioning. Calcification is not usually apparent, but "egg-shell" calcification can be observed in tumors that have undergone significant spontaneous hemorrhage. This is different from the stippled calcifications associated with neuroblastoma. Cysts may be present, and in infants, polypoid extension into the pelvicalyceal system may cause confusion with botryoid rhabdomyosarcoma.[30] Also, there is often a pseudocapsule of compressed renal parenchyma. Most tumors, unless composed of a large proportion of stromal elements, are friable and easily ruptured. This is of great significance to the operating surgeon, who must determine whether preoperative rupture has occurred and must avoid intraoperative spillage. The consequence of either of these events is upstaging of the lesion and the need for whole abdominal radiotherapy with its attendant morbidity.

Microscopically, these tumors demonstrate a triphasic pattern of blastemic, stromal, and epithelial cells. Biphasic tumors with blastemic and stromal cells are common, and some specimens consist of only a single type (Fig. 105-5). A major parameter predictive of tumor aggressiveness and patient survival is the histologic finding of anaplasia. This finding is defined by the presence of hyperdiploid mitotic figures, three-fold or greater nuclear enlargement, and hyperchromasia of enlarged nuclei. The effect of anaplasia on prognosis is so marked that tumors with these findings are designated "unfavorable histology" by the NWTS. Anaplastic tumors, which comprise about 5% of all Wilms tumors, are rare in the first 2 years of life, but their incidence increases to 13% of patients diagnosed at 5 years of age or older.

Presentation, Workup, and Staging

Most Wilms tumors are first diagnosed after appreciation of an asymptomatic abdominal mass, which can attain great size. This usually occurs during routine pediatric

Table 105-4. WILMS TUMOR–ASSOCIATED SYNDROMES AND CONDITIONS

Syndrome	Syndrome Components	Wilms Tumor Risk
Beckwith-Wiedemann	Macroglossia, somatic gigantism, visceromegaly, hypoglycemia, abdominal wall defects	About 5% (500-fold increase)
WAGR	Wilms tumor, aniridia, ambiguous genitalia, mental retardation, WT1 deletion	40%–50% (40,000-fold to 50,000-fold increase)
Neurofibromatosis	Cafe-au-lait spots, plexiform neurofibromas, predisposition to multiple tumors	About 0.26% (26-fold increase)
Denys-Drash	Pseudohermaphroditism, glomerulopathy, gonadal tumors or dysgenesis	About 60%–70% (60,000-fold to 70,000-fold increase)
Perlman familial nephroblastomatosis	Bilateral renal hamartomas, macrosomia, islet cell hypertrophy, unusual facies, mental retardation	About 60%*
Genital anomalies	Cryptorchidism, hypospadias, gonadal dysgenesis, pseudohermaphroditism	Increased

There is an increased risk of nephroblastoma in patients with the Denys-Drash and Perlman syndromes, but these are very rare, with less than 10 cases of Perlman syndrome reported. The incidence of Wilms tumor in the general population is 1 in 10000; therefore, the incidence of Wilms tumor in Beckwith-Wiedemann syndrome is 5/100 ÷ 1/10000, which is a 500-fold increase.

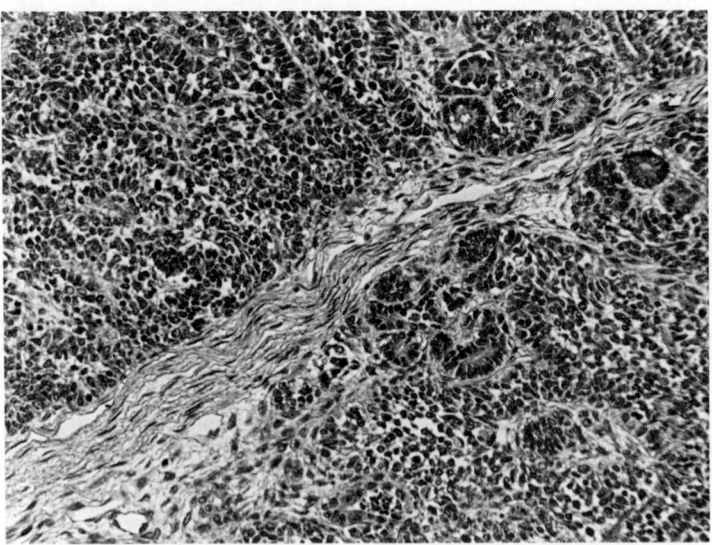

Figure 105-5. Wilms tumor. The background is blastemic cells, and some areas are suggestive of tubule formation (×140).

examination or while the children are being attended by a relative. Parents are usually surprised and feel guilty that such a mass could have gone unnoticed and need reassurance. A subset of patients develop rapid abdominal enlargement associated with pain, fever, and gross hematuria. This is attributed to intratumoral hemorrhage and may be associated with spontaneous rupture.

The NWTS recommends the following workup for suspected nephroblastoma patients. A excretory urogram is obtained to identify the tumor site; demonstrate pelvicalyceal distortion, thus localizing the process to the kidney; and assess the function of the contralateral kidney. It is acceptable to substitute CT scanning of the abdomen with intravenous and oral contrast for excretory urography (Fig. 105-6). Indeed, almost every center performs this study routinely. An abdominal, real-time Doppler ultrasound is performed to identify intracaval tumor extension, liver metastases, or enlarged retroperitoneal lymph nodes. Finally, good posteroanterior and oblique plain films of the chest are done to identify pulmonary metastases. All data concerning stage IV patients in the NWTS studies is based on the diagnosis being made by plain chest radiographs. Several studies have been performed that support the va-

lidity of this approach. In particular, patients with pulmonary metastases diagnosed by CT but not by plain chest films did as well as patients with nonmetastatic disease when staged and treated on the basis of their abdominal tumor alone. It is recommended that patients with pulmonary nodules identified by CT scan but not plain chest radiographs undergo biopsy to verify the diagnosis. This has obvious cost of care and quality of life implications. Some effort to resolve this controversy is needed given the prevalence of CT scanning.

In the United States, this initial workup is followed by surgical resection of the tumor, if possible (Fig. 105-7). This then allows surgical and histologic parameters to be included in staging. The surgeon must pay strict attention to the local tumor extent or tumor rupture and status of the regional periaortic, interaortocaval, paracaval, and perirenal lymph nodes. Direct visualization and bimanual palpation of the contralateral kidney is mandatory in all cases, even when CT scans do not indicate involvement. Preoperative assessment of the contralateral kidney is inaccurate in one third of cases. Finally, the liver should be carefully palpated and the peritoneal and diaphragmatic surfaces inspected for metastases.

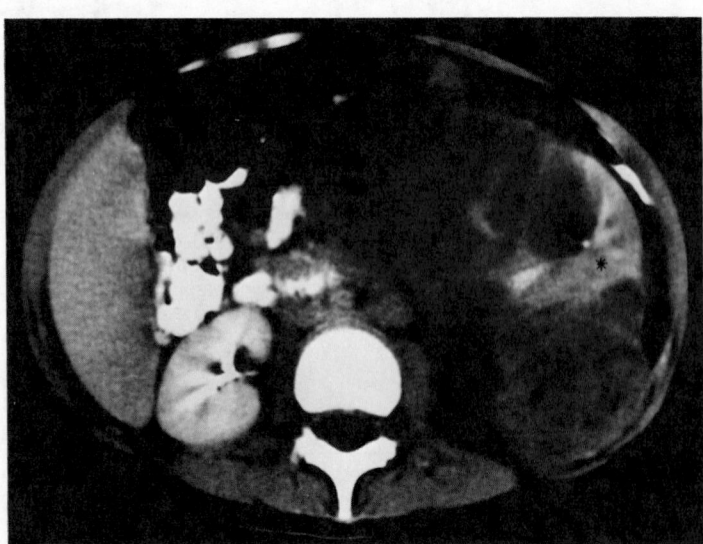

Figure 105-6. Initial CT scan of a child with a left-sided Wilms tumor. The distortion of the calyceal system is characteristic of intrinsic renal tumor. A kidney (*asterisk*) is identifiable.

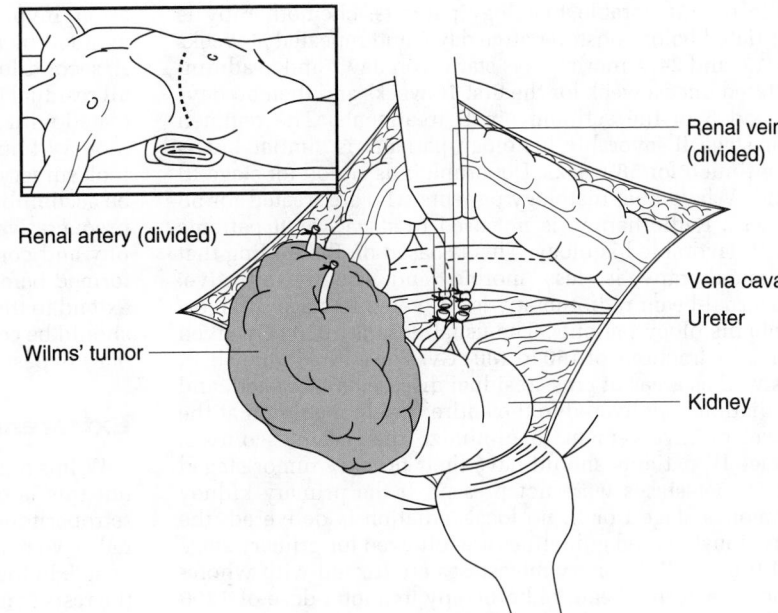

Renal vein (divided)

Renal artery (divided)

Vena cava

Ureter

Wilms' tumor

Kidney

Figure 105-7. Operative approach to resection of a right renal Wilms tumor.

Once the imaging and surgical and pathologic data are acquired, a tumor stage is assigned; the present NWTS staging schema is listed in Table 105-5. Stage is basically an assessment of risk group and has been validated by previous NWTS studies. Its importance lies in defining the least morbid treatment that results in long-term remission or cure.

Treatment

The standard of care in the United States is initial surgical resection. Exceptions to this rule include extensive intracaval tumors that require cardiopulmonary bypass for extraction, obviously unresectable tumors with documented invasion of contiguous structures, and possibly bilateral tumors, especially if it is unclear which side is most heavily involved. These special cases are discussed again later. For most patients, exploration and resection should be performed through a wide transverse incision that allows comfortable inspection and palpation of the contralateral kidney. As noted earlier, complete sampling of regional nodal echelons is mandatory, as is careful assessment of the tumor margins and possible areas of metastases. Most authors recommend early ligation of the renal vein, but most surgeons admit to not performing this maneuver because it is often difficult or unsafe, owing to the size of the tumor. The available data indicate that later ligation of the renal vein after tumor mobilization does not adversely affect prognosis. After the kidney and accompanying Gerota fascia is mobilized, the renal artery is most easily identified by posterior dissection. Radical ureterectomy does not impact outcome, but the ureter should be divided well distal to the calyceal system to make sure any polypoid pelvicalyceal extensions are encompassed.

All resectable Wilms tumor patients receive postoperative chemotherapy. There may be one exception to this rule, as reported by the Dana Farber Group. This consists of stage I favorable histology patients who are younger than 24 months of age at diagnosis and have tumors less than 250 g in weight at resection.[31,32] Beckwith suggested a further refinement of histologic criteria to identify low-risk stage I patients: no vascular invasion beyond the renal hilar plane and absence of capsular invasion.

A major effort by NWTS was the development of chemotherapy protocols for Wilms tumor that minimize toxicity while maintaining efficacy. Data accumulated from these studies has shown that in stage I or II favorable histology patients, survival is improved when combination chemotherapy using vincristine and actinomycin D is used. Stage I unfavorable histology patients have equivalent survival to stage I favorable histology patients and can be treated with the same adjuvant regimen. This emphasizes the importance of accurate surgical and pathologic staging. In stage III and IV favorable histology patients, outcome was improved for those receiving doxorubicin in addition to vincristine and actinomycin D. Recommendations for chemotherapy include intravenous actinomycin D, 75 μg/kg/course, and vincristine, 1.5 mg/m^2/dose. For stage I favor-

Table 105-5. STAGING CRITERIA FOR WILMS TUMOR

Wilms Tumor Staging System*		4-Year Survival Rate (%)
Stage 1	Tumor limited to kidney and completely excised; surface intact with no evidence of rupture	97
Stage 2	Tumor extends beyond kidney but completely excised; infiltration through the renal capsule, or extension into vessels outside the kidney substance, or local open biopsy or spillage confined to the flank; no residual tumor	95
Stage 3	Residual nonhematogenous tumor	91
Stage 4	Hematogenous metastases to lung, liver, bone, brain, etc.	78
Stage 5	Bilateral renal involvement at diagnosis	Same as for highest stage unilateral

* Survival based on outcome for favorable histology patients in the National Wilms' Tumor Study-3.

able or unfavorable histology patients, chemotherapy is initiated before postoperative day 6 and repeated at weeks 5, 13, and 24. Vincristine is started on day 7 and is administered once a week for the first 10 weeks and then on days 1 and 5 of the actinomycin D treatments. The regimen for stage II favorable histology patients is similar but is continued for 58 weeks. Doxorubicin is added for stage III and IV favorable histology patients who are treated for 58 weeks. Radiotherapy is *not* used in stage I or II patients with favorable histology. This is based on the finding that chemotherapy is less morbid and equally effective. External-beam radiotherapy is delivered to stage III favorable histology patients. The usual dose is 1080 cGy given in daily fractions of 150 to 180 cGy. The entire kidney bed, as well as areas of gross residual disease, are targeted, and radiation is delivered to the entire vertebral column at the level of involvement to minimize the risk of scoliosis. Stage IV patients should have their primary tumor staged as if metastases were not present. If the primary kidney tumor is stage I or II, no local radiation is delivered; the previously noted guidelines are followed for primary stage III tumors. Pulmonary metastases are treated with whole-thorax external-beam radiotherapy to a total dose of 1200 cGy given in 150-cGy fractions. The mediastinum is not shielded to prevent recurrence in central lymphatics or the lung margins. Nonresectable liver metastases are treated to a total of 1980 cGy. Localized liver lesions may receive focal radiation, but diffuse hepatic metastases require treatment of the entire hepatic volume. Supplemental boosts to localized areas of 500 to 1000 cGy may also be used. Bulky nodal, brain, and skeletal metastases receive 3060 cGy and supplemental focal boosts as necessary.

All unfavorable histology patients in stages II through IV are treated with actinomycin D, vincristine, and doxorubicin as well as external-beam radiation using the stage III favorable histology guidelines noted earlier.

Bilateral Wilms Tumor

The overall survival rate of patients who have bilateral Wilms tumor is 87%.[33] The survival rate for this disease is high because 90% of cases are of favorable histology, most kidneys are stage I when considered individually and advances have made treatment more successful. Because of the danger of debilitating loss of renal function, it is acceptable to administer preoperative chemotherapy based on the results of an initial exploration and biopsy. After tumor shrinkage, a second-look procedure and nephron-sparing renal resection can be performed. Using this strategy, survival rates have been achieved that are equivalent to the more traditional approach. The latter involves an initial nephrectomy of the most heavily involved kidney, followed by chemotherapy, and then reexploration.[34]

Renal Vein and Inferior Vena Caval Involvement

A study reported from NWTS-3 included 164 patients with gross and 47 patients with microscopic involvement of the renal vein beyond the kidney (11.3%). Two-year survival rates were 90%, 79%, and 72%, respectively, for patients with stages I, II, and III disease. Important predictors of outcome were histologic pattern and stage. The authors suggested that complete en bloc of the primary tumor and the renal vein extension constituted the most effective initial management.[35]

The survival rates of patients with intracaval tumor extension do not differ from those of Wilms tumor patients as a whole.[36] It has been suggested that a complicated oper-

ation involving cardiopulmonary bypass can be safely avoided by administration of preoperative chemotherapy. A second-look procedure should then be performed and all residual tumor resected. Because chemotherapy is associated with significant tumor shrinkage, and because pulmonary tumor embolus has not been a problem, second-look surgery is usually less complicated, and resection can be accomplished using conventional means. Nevertheless, preoperative workup that includes Doppler ultrasonography and contrast vena cavography should always be performed before operation. If tumor thrombus continues to extend to the proximal vena cava or right atrium, resection should be coordinated and performed under cardiopulmonary bypass.

Extrarenal Wilms Tumor

Wilms tumors can arise from areas other than the kidney, but this is extremely rare. The most common site is the retroperitoneum, followed by the pelvis and inguinal canal. Two mechanisms for this phenomenon have been proposed. In the first theory, the tumor is thought to arise from the rests of metanephric tissue. The second theory suggests that Wilms tumor develops from germinal tissue present in a teratoma. It is possible that both mechanisms are operative. Stage for stage, extrarenal Wilms tumors have a prognosis similar to renal primary tumors, and therapy should be guided by principles developed by NWTS.[37–39]

Adult and Neonatal Wilms Tumor

Wilms tumors that occur at both ends of the age spectrum are rare.[40,41] In the report by Hrabovsky and colleagues,[41] 27 of 3340 (0.8%) patients with renal tumors were younger than 30 days at presentation. Eighteen of these 27 patients had mesoblastic nephroma, 1 had a malignant rhabdoid tumor, and 4 had nonneoplastic lesions. The remaining 4 patients had Wilms tumor, and all had favorable histology. Also, none of the Wilms tumor patients had metastases at diagnosis, and all have survived. Adult Wilms tumors are associated with worse outcome, even in patients with favorable histology. A 3-year overall survival rate has been reported by NWTS and supports the use of aggressive therapy in all adult Wilms tumor patients.[42–44]

Future Directions

NWTS-5 will not ask a clinical question but rather will focus on the predictive effect on outcome of cytogenetic abnormalities at chromosomes 1, 16, and 11. This is testimony to the progress achieved by previous NWTS studies. Other areas of investigation include the role of autologous bone marrow transplantation in relapsed favorable and unfavorable histology patients, and attempts to improve outcome in the non–Wilms renal tumors that occur in childhood. In this regard, sarcoma-like protocols, using agents such as cisplatin, ifosfamide, and etoposide, are being evaluated.

NON–WILMS RENAL TUMORS OF CHILDHOOD AND ADOLESCENCE

Clear Cell Sarcoma

Clear cell sarcoma of the kidney is considered a distinct histopathologic and clinical entity from Wilms tumor.[45,46] It has a similar age distribution as that observed in Wilms tumor but a markedly worse prognosis. This tumor is characterized by a proclivity to metastasize to bones and has been called the *bone-metastasizing renal tumor of childhood* by British workers. Relapse and death occur in 75% of patients, with more than half dying within 1 year of diagnosis. Histopathologically, the tumor consists of cords and nests of pale-stained tumor cells separated by vascular structures. Confusion with classic Wilms tumor is possible, however, and central pathologic review is recommended. Clear cell sarcoma can metastasize not only to bone but also to brain. Bony metastases are usually polyostotic, but the skull is almost invariably involved. A CT scan of the abdomen or intravenous urogram, chest radiograph, MRI of the brain, and bone scan are recommended as part of the workup. The staging system is similar to that for Wilms tumor, but high rates of tumor relapse are associated with even stage I tumors, supporting the use of aggressive systemic chemotherapy in all stages. The addition of doxorubicin to the treatment regimen for these children has resulted in significant survival improvement.[47] Treatment recommendations include radical resection of the primary tumor when possible, followed by a postoperative chemotherapy regimen that includes doxorubicin, actinomycin D, and vincristine. Postoperative radiotherapy to the tumor bed is recommended regardless of stage. Usually, 1080 cGy of postoperative flank irradiation is administered. Patients should be followed with serial chest radiographs and 6-monthly brain MRI scans and bone scans for at least 3 years after treatment.

Rhabdoid Tumor

Rhabdoid tumors are rare malignancies that most commonly involve the kidney in childhood; they also can occur primarily in the mediastinum or brain.[48,49] Outcome is particularly poor, and there is no proven chemotherapy regimen. The tumor is characterized histopathologically by a rhabdomyosarcomatoid or myoblastic appearance, but the tumors do not express muscle markers and are not myoblastic in origin. Rhabdoid tumors of the kidney occur in infancy, with a median age at presentation of 13 months (range, 2 months to 5 years). Some rhabdoid tumors may be associated with the coincident development of PNETs of the brain. Extrarenal rhabdoid tumors occur in older patients. The survival rate is almost zero, and even stage I patients fare poorly. Therefore, aggressive therapy is warranted that includes surgical resection, local radiotherapy, and systemic chemotherapy. Because these tumors have been refractory to historical protocols, use of experimental dose-intense chemotherapy regimens or new chemotherapeutic agents is warranted.

Congenital Mesoblastic Nephroma

Congenital mesoblastic nephroma was first described by Bolande and colleagues[50] in 1969 and differentiated from Wilms tumor. This tumor usually occurs in infants and typically follows a benign course; however, well-documented cases have resulted in metastases and death. Histologically, the tumor consists of bundles of spindle cells, tubules of basophilic cells, and invasion into the renal parenchyma or perinephric soft tissue. The cells resemble fibroblasts or smooth muscle. Congenital mesoblastic nephroma is usually curable by radical nephrectomy alone. Tumors with high cellularity on light microscopic examination, however, and those with evident metastases require more aggressive treatment. In particular, older patients with densely cellular lesions or high mitotic indices should be considered for systemic chemotherapy.

Renal Cell Carcinoma

There are several reported series as well as scattered case reports of renal cell carcinoma occurring in childhood, adolescence, and young adults. In one study,[51] the median age was 15.5 years (range, 3 to 21 years). Histologically, the tumor is an adenocarcinoma similar to that seen in older patients. Most reported cases are of the clear cell variant of renal adenocarcinoma. There is no predilection for the right or left side, and the tumors are equally distributed between upper and lower poles and mid-kidney. Sites of metastases include lung (64%), liver (57%), bone (42%), and pleura or brain (7%). Staging is based on the adult staging system (see Chap. 109) and survival is stage dependent. Unfortunately, many of these patients present with stage IV disease. Outcome analysis has shown a correlation of survival with complete resection, although resectability was also associated with adverse prognostic factors like lymph node involvement or distant metastases. Recommended therapy is complete resection by radical nephrectomy if feasible. The role of chemotherapy is undefined, but given the poor outcome associated with higher-stage disease, it is reasonable to administer postoperative chemotherapy as an experimental protocol. This should probably be performed as part of a national cooperative study.

RHABDOMYOSARCOMA

Epidemiology and Associated Conditions

The incidence of rhabdomyosarcoma in the United States is 4 cases per 1 million white children younger than 15 years and about half that rate for black children. This translates into about 250 new cases in the pediatric population per year.[52] The male/female ratio is 1.4:1, and 80% of patients are white, 12% black, and 8% other categories.

Rhabdomyosarcoma has been observed in patients with neurofibromatosis and in patients with the Beckwith-Wiedemann syndrome. The Li-Fraumeni cancer family syndrome involves the occurrence of sarcoma, in particular rhabdomyosarcoma, along with breast, bone, or brain cancer; lung and laryngeal cancer; and adrenocortical neoplasia. In this syndrome, children with rhabdomyosarcoma have first-degree relatives afflicted with the other malignancies. In an autopsy study from the Intergroup Rhabdomyosarcoma Study, 32% of patients with rhabdomyosarcoma had congenital anomalies that included (inorder of frequency): genitourinary, central nervous system, and cardiovascular malformations.[53] Also, basal cell carcinoma has been observed in conjunction with rhabdomyosarcoma.

Basic Science

Myogenic cell differentiation can be arbitrarily divided into three broad stages: (1) commitment of a multipotent stem cell to a monopotent myoblast, (2) differentiation of a monopotent myoblast into a multinucleated myofiber expressing muscle-specific genes, and (3) maturation during which the expression of specific cellular proteins progresses through embryonic, fetal, neonatal, and adult patterns. Genetic determinants of the first stage of myogenic cell differentiation were identified first. It was initially observed that fibroblasts briefly exposed to 5-azacytidine developed a myoblastic phenotype manifested by the presence of myotubes. Genomic DNA transfection experiments verified that myoblast but not fibroblast DNA could convert

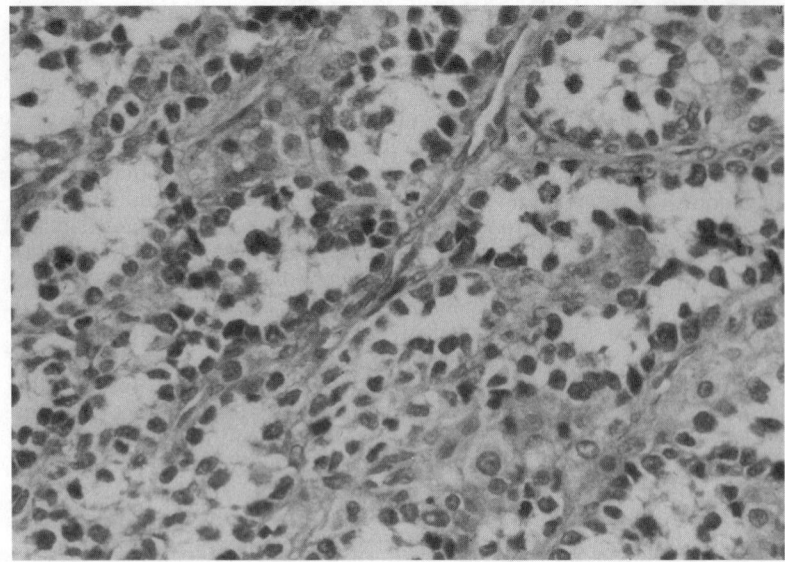

Figure 105-8. Photomicrograph illustrating the typical lunglike appearance of an alveolar rhabdomyosarcoma.

fibroblasts into stably determined myoblasts, and the frequency of conversion was consistent with a single genetic locus. This allowed the first identification of a myogenic determination gene, MyoD1.[54] MyoD is expressed exclusively in skeletal muscle as well as myoblasts derived from 5-azacytidine–treated fibroblasts. When this gene is transfected, under the control of a viral promoter, into a variety of cell types (ie, fibroblast, melanoma cells, neuroblastoma, hepatic cells, and adipocytes), expression of the MyoD cDNA induces myogenesis with expression of muscle-specific structural genes.

Pathology

Rhabdomyosarcomas are malignant tumors that arise from the ubiquitously distributed primitive mesenchyme found in the fetus. These tumors display characteristics of striated muscle, including immunohistochemical expression of skeletal muscle myosin and actin, desmin, myoglobin, and Z-band protein. Electron microscopy may show actin–myosin bundles or Z-band material. Expression of the DNA-binding protein, MyoD1, has been shown to be a lineage marker for rhabdomyosarcoma.[55]

Based on classic pathology, rhabdomyosarcoma has been divided into four main histopathologic subtypes: embryonal, alveolar, botryoid, and pleomorphic. The most common type in children is embryonal. Botryoid tumors are really of the embryonal subtype but growing into a hollow space (ie, vagina, bladder) so that they assume a characteristic grapelike appearance. Alveolar tumors are so named because of a resemblance to the microscopic structure of the lung (Fig. 105-8). Rhabdomyosarcomas are identified as alveolar if any alveolar elements are found in the tumor. Pleomorphic tumors usually occur in adults. For all histology types, sites of occurrence include (1) head and neck (orbit, infratemporal fossa), (2) genitourinary tract, including perineum and perianal area, (3) extremities, (4) trunk (chest wall, paraspinal area), (5) retroperitoneum, and (6) biliary tract.

Table 105-6. DIAGNOSTIC EVALUATION FOR SUSPECTED RHABDOMYOSARCOMA*

Examination or Test	Rationale
History and physical examination	Search for lymph nodes, size of primary mass, general condition, underlying conditions
Complete blood count	Bone marrow replacement associated with anemia or thrombocytopenia; bone marrow toxicity is the major side effect of chemotherapy
Electrolytes, renal and hepatic function tests, creatinine clearance	Renal toxicity associated with cisplatin and other alkylators; genitourinary tumors may obstruct ureters; hepatic toxicity with dactinomycin
Four-site bone marrow aspirations, two-site bone biopsies	Bone marrow metastases reported in up to 6% of patients at diagnosis (29% of stage 4 patients have marrow involvement); bone marrow assessment before chemotherapy
Bone scan	Possibility of bone and bone marrow metastases
CT of the primary site	Evaluation of tumor size, invasiveness, enlargement of regional nodes, and complicating ureteral, biliary, bowel, or airway patency
CT of possible metastatic sites	CT scanning of the lungs and liver should be done to rule out parenchymal metastases. CT scanning is superior to MR imaging in assessing the degree of bone destruction in paraspinal, extremity, and head and neck (base of skull) lesions.
MR imaging	MR imaging is done for the same rationale as CT scanning. It may give more detailed information regarding the extent of viable tumor (T2-weighted imaging) and the presence of hepatic metastases. It is also the most useful tool for evaluation of the epidural space in paraspinal or base of skull primaries.
Gallium scanning	Both the primary tumor and metastatic deposits may be identified by gallium scanning

* The same work-up is applicable to other high-grade sarcomas.

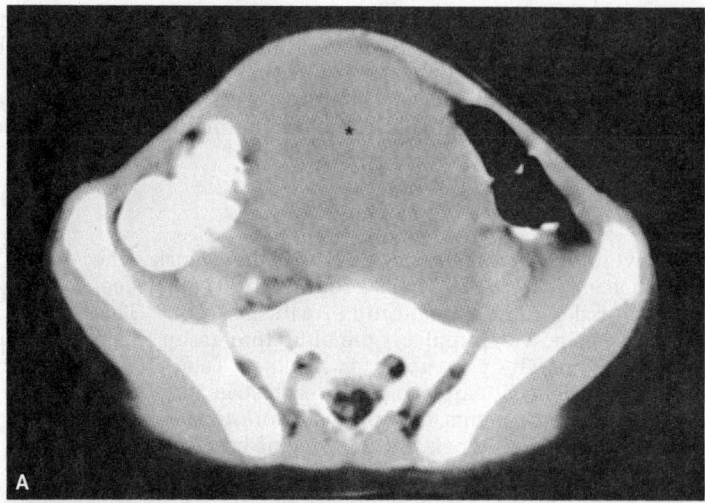

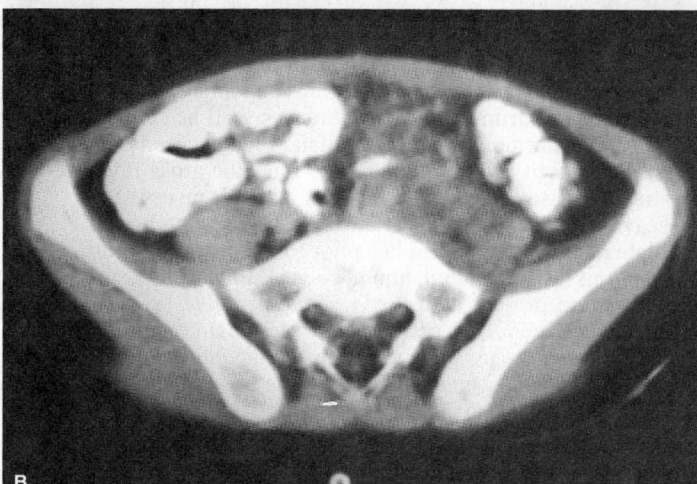

Figure 105-9. (*A*) Initial CT scan of a child with a large pelvic rhabdomyosarcoma. (*B*) CT scan of the same child after biopsy and cytoreductive chemotherapy. No tumor was demonstrable by diagnostic imaging.

Presentation and Workup

The incidence of rhabdomyosarcoma is biphasic, with one peak in infancy followed by a second in the adolescent years. Presentation is site dependent. Head and neck lesions can cause facial or cervical swelling and associated pain or skin discoloration. Sinusitis or middle ear infections can occur because the tumor blocks the normal drainage from these sites (ie, sinusal ostia, eustachian tubes). Epistaxis, proptosis, or cranial nerve palsies may also be evident in head and neck lesions. Genitourinary tumors can present with gross or microscopic hematuria, a suprapubic mass, and urinary tract infection or obstruction. Vaginal and cervical primary tumors often prolapse through the vaginal orifice as a friable polypoid mass and

may hemorrhage. Paratesticular lesions are most often observed in adolescence, and a hard mass above and separable by physical examination from the testis is observed. Extremity tumors present as a painless or painful expanding mass, and there may be an associated limp or overlying skin change. Local bony invasion may result in pathologic fractures.

Rational management depends on a thorough pretreatment workup that defines completely local tumor extent as well as evaluating regional and distant sites of metastases. Table 105-6 lists the standard workup for pediatric sarcoma patients. An extensive history, including a family history of breast cancer or other forms of sarcoma, and a thorough physical examination are elementary. Radiographic staging has been markedly facilitated by modern

Table 105-7. TNM STAGING SYSTEM FOR RHABDOMYOSARCOMA

Clinical Stage	Invasiveness	Size	Status of Nodes	Distant Metastases
I	T1	a or b	N0	M0
II	T2	a or b	N0	M0
III	T1 or T2	a or b	N1	M0
IV	T1 or T2	a or b	N0 or N1	M1

T1, noninvasive; T2, invasive; Ta, ≤5 cm; Tb, >5 cm; N0, regional nodes negative; N1, nodes positive; M0, no distant metastases at diagnosis; M1, metastases present.

imaging methods. Even greater progress in this area is promised by present efforts in the field of positron emission scanning, which allows determination of the metabolic activity of a tumor mass. Figure 105-9 is a CT scan of a large pelvic rhabdomyosarcoma originating from the bladder.

Staging

An evolution in sarcoma staging has occurred during the past 10 years, with most groups adopting the TNM system defined by the International Union Against Cancer.[56] This staging system, which replaces the older Intergroup Rhabdomyosarcoma study grouping, is listed in Table 105-7. The TNM schema attempts to divide each stage into definable clinical components. It is applied before any therapeutic interventions (although a second staging based on histologic findings of the primary tumor and regional lymph nodes after resection can also be performed).

Local tumor invasiveness is the result of cellular and molecular phenotypic properties, which are rapidly being defined by molecular analyses. The ability of cells to invade surrounding basement membranes depends on manufacture of a spectrum of lytic enzymes as well as cellular motility. Furthermore, regional or distant metastasis is not possible without initial cellular invasion. The gross invasiveness assessed for TNM staging is a rough measure of these cellular events. In this sense, the TNM system begins to relate macroscopic tumor behavior to the properties and interactions of individual tumor cells. Future directions include more precise definitions of the invasive process. Assays of collagenolytic activity and assessment of growth and invasion in nude mice are intermediate steps in this regard. Eventually, genetic determinants of invasion and metastases that are the final determinants of prognosis will be identified.

Using the TNM system, the reported overall percentage of patients with tumors greater than 5 cm ranges from 50% to 68%. The proportions of other staging variables include invasive tumors, 37% to 71%; regional nodal involvement, 7% to 28%; and distant metastases at diagnosis, 20% to 23%.

A sarcoma is adequately staged when the following criteria are met: (1) the primary tumor pathology and histopathologic subtype have been determined by biopsy, and (2) all components in the TNM staging system are known with reasonable certainty. It is preferable to biopsy metastatic regional lymph nodes, but extensive nodal dissections are not indicated. In the special case of paratesticular rhabdomyosarcoma, a limited dissection of ipsilateral, periaortic nodes is used as a determinant of the need for nodal radiation. The use of prechemotherapy nodal sampling in paratesticular rhabdomyosarcoma is controversial because many European groups favor chemotherapy along with radical orchiectomy as sole primary treatment. Most North American groups favor lymph node biopsy with consequent periaortic nodal radiation if N1 status is proved. Laparoscopic biopsy may prove a useful alternative in this regard.

Small, accessible primary lesions should undergo excisional biopsy. If this is done, the surgeon should attempt to obtain a clear microscopic margin. Larger infiltrating lesions and those whose removal would cause debilitation or deformity (ie, amputation or cystectomy) should undergo limited incisional or endoscopic biopsy. It is acceptable to perform transperineal needle core biopsies for bladder neck or perineal primary tumors. Enough biopsy material for light and electron microscopic analysis, immunohistochemistry, and cytogenetics should be obtained. It is preferable to freeze extra tissue to facilitate further specialized studies. Even though such investigations do not have direct short-term benefit for the patient, they are crucial in expanding knowledge concerning rhabdomyosarcoma. Tissue should be frozen in liquid nitrogen as soon as possible after biopsy.

Treatment

The modern treatment of rhabdomyosarcoma is multidisciplinary and includes multiagent chemotherapy, judicious resection, and radiotherapy. The intensity of therapy should be tailored to the risk of subsequent relapse, which is a function of TNM stage. In general, agents are combined to limit drug resistance while attaining a synergistic antitumor effect. A major surgical responsibility during chemotherapy is maintenance of adequate vascular access both for administration of medications as well as blood drawing. An external or implanted vascular access device usually can be inserted at the time of diagnostic biopsy.

Surgical resection of the primary tumor was the mainstay of treatment 30 years ago but only resulted in overall survival rates in the range of 20%. This rate improved to 50% with the addition of chemotherapy and resulted in uncertainty regarding the role of tumor resection in rhabdomyosarcoma. It is difficult to prove that surgical removal of the primary tumor impacts survival. One reason is that a significant proportion of patients present with distant metastases, which so profoundly influences survival that the effect of other variables is obscured. Also, most tumors that can be readily removed without serious disfigurement or disability are resected. Thus, the effect of leaving a tumor in situ cannot readily be evaluated. With present survival rates, it would be unethical to randomize patients with nonmetastatic, resectable tumors to a nonsurgical arm. Complete resection of primary tumors should be undertaken either before chemotherapy for small noninvasive lesions or after documented response with more formidable primary tumors. An example of the operative approach for a lower extremity rhabdomyosarcoma involving anterior thigh muscles is depicted in Figure 105-10. In certain situations in which chemotherapy results in complete or very good tumor regression, external-beam irradiation may be employed as a primary means of local control. Even in these circumstances, it is important to obtain biopsy specimens to document complete tumor eradication. Debilitating or disfiguring surgery should only be performed if residual tumor is present after both chemotherapy and

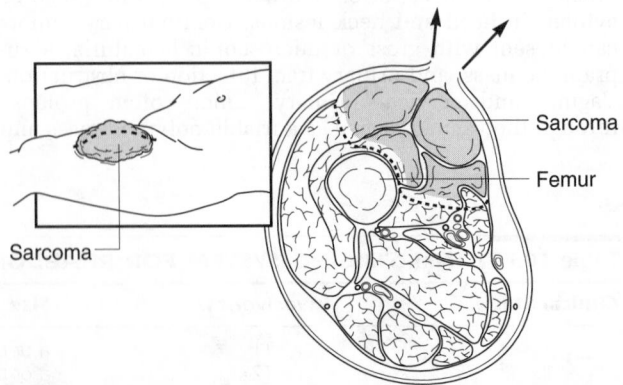

Figure 105-10. Technique for resection of a proximal lower-extremity rhabdomyosarcoma. Longitudinal incisions are always used. It is important to excise the tumor completely, with a surrounding 1- to 2-cm margin if feasible.

therapeutic irradiation. Amputation of extremity rhabdomyosarcomas does not enhance cure and should be performed only when lesions are bulky, invade bone or neurovascular structures, or are recurrent. Similarly, radical cystectomy is reserved for situations in which complete tumor eradication has not been accomplished by chemotherapy and external-beam irradiation. The guiding principle of rhabdomyosarcoma surgery is complete tumor resection, but removal of large amounts of normal tissue (ie, muscle group resection, amputation) alone does not affect outcome.

External-beam radiotherapy of the primary site or involved regional nodal echelons has contributed to locoregional control. Clinical data suggest that control of microscopic rhabdomyosarcoma can be accomplished with doses of 4000 cGy, and gross deposits require in excess of 5400 cGy for sterilization.[57]

Outcome

Table 105-8 lists the results of studies analyzing the effects of various prognostic factors on outcome in rhabdomyosarcoma.[58–64] As expected, the presence of distant parenchymal metastases at diagnosis has an overwhelming adverse effect on survival. Because of this, some groups have analyzed the effect of prognostic parameters in nonmetastatic subsets. Site and invasiveness of the primary tumor have also been independent predictors of outcome in some studies. Regarding site, most authors agree that orbital, paratesticular, and vaginal primary tumors are associated with improved outcome, while extremity, parameningeal, and truncal and retroperitoneal sites carry a worse prognosis. Survival is stage dependent. If all cases (both high and low risk) are included, the overall survival rate from rhabdomyosarcoma is about 50%.

Most studies conclude that overall and disease-free survival rates in rhabdomyosarcoma are equivalent. In the case of rhabdomyosarcoma, this means that salvage after initial relapse is negligible, making primary therapy crucial for long-term survival. This suggests that, after risk assessment by staging, therapy should be as intense as possible to eradicate the tumor. This may mean use of myeloablative therapy with autologous or peripheral stem cell rescue for high-risk patients. The effects of this intense therapy on survival remain indeterminate.

Future Directions

The results of myeloablative regimens with bone marrow or peripheral stem cell rescue are being analyzed. In addition, work is being done to refine the use of surgery and radiotherapy to maximize individual efficacy while diminishing toxicity. Interstitial brachytherapy and intraoperative radiotherapy are two areas of collaboration between the surgeon and radiation oncologist that are undergoing evaluation. Biologic or immunologic therapy for rhabdomyosarcoma is not available. It has been shown, however, that retinoid tumors have a differentiating influence on rhabdomyosarcoma cells in culture. These agents have been used clinically for certain forms of leukemia and neuroblastoma, so it is possible that they have some therapeutic effect on muscle tumors. Also, since insulin-like growth factor 2 is required for growth of rhabdomyosarcoma cells, strategies to inhibit this stimulus (suramin) may prove fruitful. These are areas of ongoing clinical and laboratory research.

NONRHABDOMYOMATOUS SOFT TISSUE SARCOMAS

Fibrosarcoma

Epidemiology

Fibrosarcomas, although rare, are the most common nonrhabdomyomatous sarcomas of infancy, childhood, and adolescence. A biphasic age incidence similar to that observed with rhabdomyosarcoma is characteristic, with one peak under 5 years of age and the second in the 10- to 15-year age group. They are most frequently encountered on extremities, with 70% of congenital fibrosarcomas occurring distally. Cases are equally distributed between the genders. Most reports suggest that prognosis is better in younger children.[65]

Pathology

Fibrosarcomas are spindle cell tumors characterized by a herringbone or interweaving pattern of tumors cells with a large amount of stromal collagen putatively arising from a fibroblastic lineage. Fibrosarcomas can be difficult, if not impossible, to distinguish from desmoid tumors or aggressive fibromatoses. For practical purposes, desmoids, fibromatoses, and low-grade fibrosarcomas can be thought of as a spectrum of similar and related neoplasms. Important characteristics of malignancy include nuclear pleomorphism, mitotic index, and basophilia. The tumor must be distinguished from undifferentiated rhabdomyosarcomas, neurofibrosarcoma, nodular fasciitis, myositis ossificans, and inflammatory pseudotumor.

Presentation and Diagnostic Evaluation

Congenital fibrosarcomas and those diagnosed in early childhood are usually located on the distal upper or lower extremity. The trunk is a secondary site. A hard, often infiltrating mass is appreciated, and there may be skin or deep fixation. Fibrosarcomas in the head and neck associ-

---

Table 105-8. COLLECTED INDICATORS OF OUTCOMES FOR RHABDOMYOSARCOMA

Institution	Year	Patients	Predictors of Outcome
Memorial Sloan-Kettering Cancer Center[58]	1994	290	Age at diagnosis, invasion, metastases, histology, regional lymph nodes
Italian Cooperative Group[59]	1991	145	Site, size, alveolar histology, clinical group
International Rhabdomyosarcoma Workshop[60]	1991	951	Invasiveness, site, interaction between invasiveness and site
Cooperative Soft Tissue Sarcoma Study (CWS-81)[61]	1991	131	Site, degree of tumor regression after 7 weeks of four-drug chemotherapy
Societé Internacionale Oncologique Pediatrique (SIOP)[62]	1988	253	Site, stage, sex
Second Intergroup Rhabdomyosarcome Study (IRS-2)[63]	1993	1115	Site, stage, alveolar histology
IRS-3[64]	1995	1062	Site, stage

ated with swallowing and airway problems are also occasionally observed and may require life-saving tracheostomy. High-grade lesions may invade bony or neural structures and metastasize to lung or liver. Multifocal lesions with multiple primary tumors affecting an extremity are sometimes seen. Bone marrow metastases do not develop. Workup is similar to that for rhabdomyosarcoma except that bone marrow aspiration and biopsy are not required.

Staging

The TNM schema is used, although lymph node metastases from fibrosarcoma are uncommon except with high-grade lesions. An adequate incisional or excisional biopsy, depending on the extent and invasiveness of the primary lesion, should be performed.

Treatment

The primary treatment of fibrosarcoma is surgical resection with negative microscopic margins if this can be done without significant debilitation or deformity. Occasionally, patients present with rapidly progressive or extensive lesions. Under these circumstances, an initial trial of systemic chemotherapy may result in gratifying tumor regression. In very young children (usually less than 5 years of age), these tumors can be indolent and may regress spontaneously. In cases in which complete resection requires mutilating surgery like amputation or laryngectomy, a plan of simple observation may be best. Often, the tumor mass is dormant for years, allowing growth of the affected part and the possibility of a less debilitating or deforming resection later. Heroic resections should only be performed if the tumor is progressive or otherwise causing severe symptoms.

There is no defined role for systemic chemotherapy. Occasionally, high-grade lesions, especially in very young children, respond to a variety of agents. Chemotherapy may be tried for unresectable, symptomatic, and progressive lesions.[66] Effective chemotherapeutic agents include doxorubicin, actinomycin D, vincristine, and cyclophosphamide, in various combinations. The combination of ifosfamide and etoposide has been shown effective in the treatment of metastatic fibrosarcoma. In summary, systemic chemotherapy may be useful for extensive or progressive lesions. A common initial regimen includes actinomycin D and vincristine, which are less toxic than alkylating agents.

In the only prospective randomized trial,[66a] use of external-beam radiotherapy was associated with a lower local recurrence rate for margin-positive low-grade sarcomas, including fibrosarcoma. Interstitial brachytherapy has been shown to lower local recurrence rates with margin-positive or negative high-grade lesions. Despite this, most patients should initially be treated by wide surgical excision.

Outcome

The survival rate for low-grade nonmetastatic fibrosarcomas occurring in infancy is more than 90%. Patients with metastatic disease have a guarded prognosis and require multidisciplinary therapy.

Tendosynovial Sarcoma

Epidemiology

Tendosynovial sarcoma is the third most common malignant pediatric soft tissue tumor. In large combined adult and pediatric series, tendosynovial sarcomas constitute about 8% of all soft tissue sarcomas. In a report of nonrhabdomyomatous soft tissue sarcomas, this histology was identified in 29% of patients.[67] The male/female distribution is 1:1.2 to 1.6. Most patients present in the early teenage years, but there is also a small incidence spike centered on 5 years of age, giving the familiar bimodal age distribution observed with other sarcomas.

Pathology

Tendosynovial sarcomas arise from the synovial tissue, which is ubiquitous in the body and helps compose tendons, joint membranes, and bursae. Synonyms include *synovioma* or *tendosynovioma, pseudoglandular synovial sarcoma, clear cell sarcoma,* and *chordoid sarcoma.* The lower extremity is the most common site of origin, with an equal distribution between the thigh, foot, and posterior knee. The shoulder and forearm are also relatively common areas of involvement. Tendosynovial sarcomas close to bone may incite a periosteal reaction. Other possible primary sites include the abdominal wall and trunk, and the head and neck, with the tongue and retropharyngeal or hypopharyngeal areas being the most common.

The most common metastatic sites are lung and pleura. Tendosynovial sarcomas are known to relapse in lung even decades after resection of the primary tumor. Metastases to regional lymph nodes and subcutaneous sites has been described but is rare. Terminally, metastases to multiple organs is possible.

Microscopically, tendosynovial sarcoma is divided into two subtypes: monophasic and diphasic. In the diphasic form, epithelioid cells and stromal spindle cells are observed. The epithelioid component is arranged in glandlike structures resembling true epithelial cells but devoid of basement membrane. The diphasic subtype has been associated with a better prognosis, but some studies have not verified this finding. The monophasic variant is the most common and consists of sheets and parallel cords of spindle-shaped cells with little cytoplasm and cigar-shaped nuclei. Prognosis has been reported to be worse with monophasic histology.

Presentation and Diagnostic Evaluation

Most patients present with an enlarging extremity mass. Pain may be prominent if bony or neural invasion is present. Regional lymph node metastases occur in 3% and distant metastases (lung) in 6% of patients at diagnosis. A workup similar to that described for rhabdomyosarcoma is appropriate. Adequate radiographic imaging of the primary site is crucial because of the impact of complete resection on outcome.

Treatment

Chemotherapy has historically been ineffective, and the primary treatment of tendosynovial sarcoma is surgical. The goal is clear microscopic margins, and every effort should be made to accomplish this, including use of amputation. Limb-sparing procedures are acceptable if complete resection is accomplished. Incomplete removal results in a high rate of local recurrence.

Rosen and colleagues[68] have reported on the use of high-dose ifosfamide in the treatment of metastases from tendosynovial sarcoma. All 13 patients treated in this study had objective responses. Chemotherapy is reserved for patients who present with metastatic disease or in whom complete resection with clear microscopic margins cannot be accomplished.

Outcome

Overall survival rates are in the range of 43% to 75%. Important prognostic indicators are large primary tumor size and high nuclear grade with extensive tumor necrosis (high grade), as well as the presence of metastases at diagnosis. Worse survival rates are correlated with tumors greater than 10 cm in diameter at diagnosis, compared with those less than 5 cm: 86% versus 22% 5-year survival. Studies have shown no effect of monophasic versus biphasic histology on outcome.[69]

Peripheral Primitive Neuroectodermal Tumor

Epidemiology, Pathology, and Clinical Presentation

Peripheral PNET (peripheral neuroepithelioma, Askin tumor, peripheral neuroblastoma) is a small, round blue cell malignancy only distinguished from Ewing sarcoma by ultrastructural and immunocytochemical features. This tumor shares the t(11;22)(q24;q12) translocation with Ewing sarcoma and esthesioneuroblastoma. The incidence is low, with 54 patients treated during a 20-year period reported from a major cancer center. About two thirds of patients are 19 years of age or younger at diagnosis, and 57% are male. The disease affects predominantly white patients, and 82% of tumors are localized at diagnosis. Common sites of involvement include chest wall (33%), pelvis (22%), paraspinal areas (13%), retroperitoneum (11%), limbs (9%), and abdomen (7%). In one study, epidural extension from the primary tumor was noted in 24% of patients at diagnosis, and 18% had distant metastases.[70] None of the patients in this series that had chest wall primary tumors had distant metastases at diagnosis. All primary tumors were greater than 5 cm in diameter in at least one dimension. Urinary catecholamines are not elevated in peripheral PNET. There is no familial or gender predilection.

Light microscopic criteria include fairly uniform, poorly differentiated round cells arranged in cords, nests, or clusters; no spindle cells with fine reticular or collagenous processes; no ganglionic or schwannian differentiation; and positive immunostaining for neuron-specific enolase. Ultrastructurally, neurosecretory-like granules and tapering ("neuritic") cytoplasmic processes are evident.

Treatment

The outcome of PNET has been historically poor, while survival rates for Ewing sarcoma, which is a related neoplasm sharing the typical (11;22) translocation, have approached 60% to 65% in patients presenting without distant metastases. There may be underlying differences in fundamental biology, but the data also suggest that the uniform, multidisciplinary approach used for Ewing sarcoma and including multiagent chemotherapy may have utility in the treatment of PNET. The diagnosis should be established by incisional biopsy and the patient quickly started on an intensive multiagent chemotherapy regimen. A dose–response effect of cyclophosphamide has been observed. Occasionally, the tumor can be completely resected before chemotherapy, and this should be done if feasible without an extensive procedure or the requirement for complicated reconstruction techniques. In most cases, definitive resection should be deferred until after administration of several cycles of systemic treatment. In general, surgery is required because complete responses to chemotherapy do not occur. External-beam radiotherapy using 4500 to 6000 cGy can shrink but not cure macroscopic tumors. Radiation may be effective in improving local control after resection, especially if margins are microscopically positive.

Outcome

In patients with localized PNET at diagnosis, complete resection of all gross disease within 3 months resulted in improved progression-free survival ($P = .0003$).[70] The ef-

fect of myeloablative therapy with autologous bone marrow rescue is being evaluated.

Desmoplastic Small Round Cell Tumor

The desmoplastic small round cell tumor a distinctive malignant neoplasm with a predilection for young males. Eighty percent of patients present before the age of 30 years, and about half are 5 to 20 years old at diagnosis.[71] There is a striking male predominance (male/female ratio, 4.1:1), and most of the patients are white. A striking feature is the frequent occurrence of divergent, multilineage differentiation with expression of epithelial, neural, and myogenic immunophenotypes.

Common presenting complaints include abdominal or back pain, abdominal distention or mass, acute abdomen, and bowel, biliary, or ureteral obstruction. Small nodules found in hernia sacs during repair have been the first indication the tumor. CT of the chest and abdomen using both gastrointestinal and vascular contrast is the most useful diagnostic procedure. Initial laparoscopic biopsy is adequate to establish the diagnosis and assess the extent of abdominal disease. Small serosal nodules not detected by imaging studies can be identified using laparoscopic magnification. A careful pelvic and serosal inspection should be carried out. Adequate tissue for immunohistochemistry, electron microscopy, and molecular biologic studies should be obtained.

Because desmoplastic small round cell tumor is a diffuse serosal malignancy, systemic chemotherapy using a dose-intense sarcoma regimen is the initial treatment. Serial abdominal CT scans can be followed to judge response, remembering that small mucosal implants may escape detection with imaging studies. After 4 to 7 cycles, exploratory laparotomy with resection of all gross disease is attempted. Consolidation chemotherapy and external-beam radiotherapy to the primary site are then employed. If diffuse peritoneal seeding is identified either at diagnostic or second-look laparotomy or laparoscopy, total abdominal irradiation is required. Myeloablative chemotherapy with autologous marrow reconstitution may also be necessary.

Of 19 reported patients with adequate follow-up, only 2 were disease-free 2 and 3.5 years after diagnosis. The other 17 died from progressive disease within 6 months to 4 years after presentation. A recent report, however, suggests that outlook may be improved using a dose-intensive multiagent chemotherapy regimen including cyclophosphamide, ifosfamide, etoposide, and doxorubicin. This justifies aggressive treatment for these patients, including extensive surgical debulking.

Neurofibrosarcoma

Neurofibrosarcomas (neurogenic sarcomas, malignant schwannomas, malignant nerve sheath tumor, malignant neurilemoma) constitute 5% to 10% of nonrhabdomyomatous soft tissue sarcomas in childhood. About 20% of all patients (children and adults) with neurofibrosarcoma have von Recklinghausen disease (neurofibromatosis type I, NF1) and 5% to 16% of patients with NF1 develop a neurofibrosarcoma. The incidence of NF1 in children with neurofibrosarcomas is as high as 66%.[72] Neurofibrosarcomas have been reported as secondary tumors after external-beam radiotherapy.

The most common sites in children are: extremity (42%), retroperitoneum (25%), and trunk. Less than 10% of patients present with metastatic disease. Microscopically, the tumor resembles fibrosarcoma but is differentiated by the presence of schwannian elements. Whorly, storiform, and tactile body–like formations are observed, and the S-100 stain is positive in about 60% of cases. Ultrastructural findings are important distinguishing criteria, and in all suspected cases, a specimen should be sent for electron microscopy. Electron microscopic findings include the presence of schwannian differentiation with cytoplasmic concavities lacking neurites. Primary neurofibrosarcoma of skin and subcutaneous tissues has also been described.

Two thirds of patients have associated neurofibromatosis type I, and aggressive diagnostic procedures, including biopsy, are warranted when enlarging extremity or truncal masses are observed. Pain may be prominent depending on location. Radicular or sciatic pain is reported with paraspinal or retroperitoneal tumors causing sciatic pressure. Spontaneous hemothorax has been reported with chest wall primary tumors. Pelvic tumors may present as a perineal or perianal mass. The primary treatment of neurofibrosarcoma is wide local excision. In one series of 20 patients (14 with neurofibromatosis), local recurrence developed in 8 of 12 patients undergoing local tumor excision plus radiation or chemotherapy but in only 1 of 6 patients treated with radical excision as well as chemotherapy or irradiation.[72] Unfortunately, a significant proportion developed distant metastases despite local control. Patients with intermediate or high-grade neurofibrosarcomas should undergo radical local excision followed by chemotherapy and irradiation.

Leiomyosarcoma

Leiomyosarcoma accounts for 7% of soft tissue sarcomas in adults but less than 2% of childhood sarcomas. The gastrointestinal (oropharynx to anus) or genitourinary tract, retroperitoneum, lungs, pulmonary artery, vascular wall (ie, middle third of the inferior vena cava, saphenous or femoral vein), popliteal artery, sinonasal area, and peripheral soft tissues (ie, extremities) are reported sites of involvement.[73] Most cases are gastrointestinal in origin. The lungs are the most common site for metastases. Regional lymph node involvement occurs in 14% of gastric (perigastric nodes) and 5% of small intestinal leiomyosarcomas at diagnosis. Dissemination to liver and brain has also been reported. Also, tumors arising from gastrointestinal structures can disseminate throughout the peritoneal cavity. Leiomyosarcoma has been reported in patients with von Recklinghausen disease and coincident with the occurrence of neurofibrosarcoma.

True leiomyosarcomas are derived from smooth muscle and are often pseudoencapsulated. Cytologically, they demonstrate uniform elongated cells with cigar-shaped nuclei. An epithelioid variant with more aggressive behavior is reported to arise in up to 40% of cases. Bone marrow metastases are not reported.

The usual presentation is pain (up to 80%) or gastrointestinal bleeding (60%). There are also reports of presentation with intussusception and perforation of a Meckel diverticulum. Congenital leiomyosarcoma associated with hydrops fetalis has also been reported. Double-contrast CT scans, gastrointestinal contrast studies, and endoscopy may aid in diagnosis.

The most effective treatment of leiomyosarcoma is complete surgical resection. This should be accomplished even when resection requires amputation or results in other disability because chemotherapy and radiation are ineffective. Reports have been made of long-term survival with resection in cases with hepatic and cerebral metastases. For gastrointestinal tumors, a 10-cm margin of bowel should be obtained along with a wide mesenteric resection. For gastric primary tumors, omentectomy is advised as well.

Overall, about half of gastrointestinal primary tumors can be resected for cure at diagnosis; in these patients, survival rates are 50% at 5 years and 35% at 10 years. In a series of gastrointestinal leiomyosarcomas reported by Ng and associates,[74] overall survival was stage dependent; survival rates were 75% for stage I disease, 52% for stage II, 28% for stage III, and 7% to 12% for stage IV. Important determinants of disease-free survival in multivariate analysis included tumor rupture ($P = .002$), contiguous organ invasion ($P = .02$), and high tumor grade ($P = .02$). Size (greater than 5 cm) and location have been found to predict outcome in other analyses. Pediatric colorectal leiomyosarcomas, although extremely rare, are reported to have a relatively favorable prognosis.

Liposarcoma and Alveolar Soft Parts Sarcoma

Liposarcomas are one of the most common type of soft tissue sarcomas in adults but are extremely rare in childhood. The peak incidence is in the second decade of life, and there is equal distribution between the genders. Most childhood tumors are of the myxoid histopathologic subtype and are low grade. The most common sites are, in order, the lower extremity, upper extremity, and retroperitoneum. The usual presenting complaint is a mass, which is often painless. Metastases are uncommon, with the lung being the most common site. Lymph node metastases are possible but extremely rare. The treatment of choice is complete surgical excision with negative microscopic margins.

Alveolar soft parts sarcoma is a rare tumor; only 102 cases were reported during a 50-year period. The tumor is associated with skeletal muscle and fascial planes, and the thigh and buttocks are the most common sites of occurrence (39.5%), followed by abdominal and chest walls. About one third of patients have metastases at diagnosis, with the most common sites being lung, bone, and brain, in that order.

The primary treatment is surgical, and the roles of chemotherapy and radiotherapy remain undefined. Unfortunately, most patients develop relapse in distant sites and die from progressive disease, although this may take 20 years or longer.

HEPATIC TUMORS

Hepatoblastoma Versus Hepatocellular Carcinoma

From 1960 to the early 1970s, there were sporadic reports of survival from hepatoblastoma after successful surgical resection. The risks of major hepatic surgery were great, however, with operative and early postoperative mortality rates approaching 25%. About two thirds of patients with hepatoblastoma had potentially resectable tumors, and complete surgical removal was associated with a 60% long-term survival rate. Systemic relapse was the most frequent cause of failure, and patients with locally unresectable disease or systemic spread at the outset were essentially incurable.

In 1975, the first consistent reports of success with doxorubicin appeared.[75] Before this, many agents had been tested with only sporadic responses. Since then, major advances have occurred in both adjuvant chemotherapy for patients with resectable disease and cytoreductive therapy for unresectable disease. In 1982, the CCSG and Southwest Oncology Group reported a significant reduction in relapse rates after complete resections of hepatoblastoma using combination chemotherapy with vincristine, cyclophosphamide, doxorubicin, and 5-fluorouracil.[76] The long-term relapse-free survival rate in stage I patients was reported at 94%.

Shortly thereafter, reports appeared of dramatic tumor necrosis and cure in patients with unresectable tumors and metastatic disease using doxorubicin and cisplatin as single or combined agents, with delayed resection.[77] Prospective trials with combinations of doxorubicin and cisplatin have confirmed these results, and patients with initially unresectable hepatoblastoma can now achieve long-term survival rates in the range of 60% to 70%.[78]

Despite this period of progress in the treatment of hepatoblastoma, the treatment of children with hepatocellular carcinoma remains problematic and their outcome poor. A complete resection is initially possible in only 10% to 20% of patients, and the problems of local and systemic relapse remain. Despite response to chemotherapy in some instances, children with unresectable disease usually remain unresectable or relapse after resection. Early diagnosis by screening of patients with genetic defects and families with hepatitis B is unlikely to have a major impact in Western nations. Research with different drug combinations, the use of new agents, and increasing the accessibility to transplantation programs may provide some hope. Developments in monoclonal antibody technology have produced exciting results with other tumors, but their use in hepatocellular carcinoma is still experimental.

Epidemiology

In Europe and North America, primary liver tumors constitute about 1.1% of childhood malignant neoplasms (1.4 cases per 1 million children in the United States).[79] The ratio of hepatoblastoma to hepatocellular carcinoma is variously reported from 1.3:1 to 6.5:1, but in areas endemic for hepatitis B, the ratio may be reversed and as low as 0.2:1. No geographic clustering of cases of hepatoblastoma has been noted. A male predominance is generally reported for both tumors, the ratio ranging from 1.5:1 to 3.1:1 for hepatoblastoma and from 1.3:1 to 3.2:1 for hepatocellular carcinoma.

Hepatoblastoma has been reported to occur sporadically in adults, but the tumor usually presents in the first 3 years of life. Congenital presentation and antenatal diagnosis have also been reported.[80] Hepatocellular carcinoma, on the other hand, is rare in infancy. In one large series of children and adults with hepatic tumors, no cases of hepatocellular carcinoma occurred in patients aged 4 years or younger in a cohort of 2286 patients. Historical series without pathologic review may report a higher rate of infantile hepatoma due to misdiagnosis of some early hepatoblastomas.

Clinical Presentation

Children with hepatoblastoma most commonly present with abdominal mass or diffuse abdominal swelling. Not infrequently, the child is in good health, and the lesion may be discovered by an observant parent or clinician on routine examination. Accompanying symptoms, such as pain, irritability, minor gastrointestinal disturbances, fevers, and pallor, occur in smaller numbers of patients. Significant weight loss is unusual, although patients may fail to thrive.

In contrast, although children and adolescents with hepatocellular carcinoma frequently present with palpable abdominal masses, these are rarely incidental. Pain is a frequent accompaniment and can occur in the absence of an obvious mass. Constitutional disturbances, such as anorexia, malaise, nausea and vomiting, and significant weight loss, occur with greater frequency. Jaundice is an uncommon feature of either disease.

In most series of hepatoblastoma and hepatocellular carcinoma, small numbers of patients present acutely with tumor rupture. Hepatoblastoma can present with sexual precocity from androgen synthesis, although this is rare.

Laboratory Studies

Mild anemia is common in both conditions, and thrombocytosis is most often seen in patients with hepatoblastoma but this has also been reported in occasional patients with hepatocellular carcinoma.[81] The cause for this is unknown but may be related to release of tumor-derived cytokines.

Liver function tests are usually nonspecifically deranged in both conditions. A high serum cholesterol level is present in 50% to 60% of cases, and there is evidence to suggest that higher elevations may correlate with a poorer prognosis. The most useful tumor marker is the serum α-fetoprotein (AFP). Elevation, often extreme, occurs in about 84% to 91% of cases of hepatoblastoma. Fewer patients with hepatocellular carcinoma have elevated AFP levels, and the elevation tends to be less marked. Although nonspecific for epithelial liver tumors, the AFP marker is used extensively to monitor both disease reduction in patients undergoing nonoperative therapy and disease recurrence in treated patients. Some reports concluded that a rise in AFP above normal in a patient with quiescent disease is more sensitive than radiology or surgical exploration at detecting recurrence.

Imaging Studies

Abdominal CT scanning is the investigation of choice both for diagnostic discrimination and to assess operability. The chest should be included to identify pulmonary metastases. The typical appearance of hepatoblastoma is that of a solitary mass with lower attenuation values than normal liver (Fig. 105-11). Dramatic contrast enhancement (as in benign vascular neoplasms), invasion of the portal vein, and lymph node involvement are unusual. Hepatocellular carcinomas have a similar appearance but are more likely to be multifocal, invade the portal vein, and metastasize to draining lymph nodes. Distinction between the two lesions cannot be definite because the pattern of disease may be atypical in either instance.

The diagnostic ability of MRI is similar to that of CT. The particular features of both hepatoblastoma and hepatocellular carcinoma on MRI are low signal intensity on T1-weighted images and high intensity on T2-weighted images. The two lesions cannot be distinguished by appearance alone.

Plain radiographs and liver–spleen scans usually indicate abnormalities but do not often contribute to diagnosis or assist in planning therapy. Angiography is indicated if embolization or infusion chemotherapy is contemplated, but this test is invasive, technically difficult in childhood, and not universally available. Similar information is available from dynamic CT scan or MRI such that these are considered adequate in most instances.

An abdominal ultrasound, in view of the low cost and ready accessibility, is probably the most useful screening investigation for children with large livers. This allows distinction between space-occupying lesions and diffuse hepatomegaly. Anatomic detail of the tumor margin is not usually sufficiently well delineated to assess resectability. Doppler ultrasound is also useful to evaluate patency of the inferior vena cava and hepatic veins, but

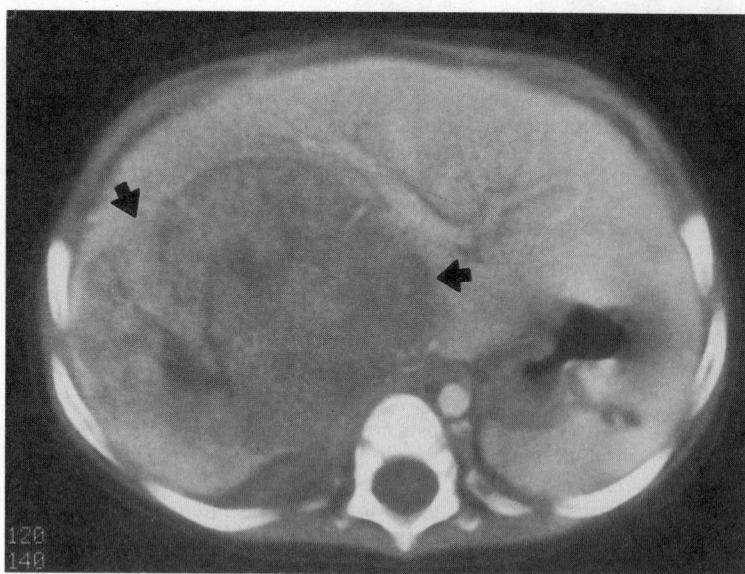

Figure 105-11. CT scan of a 2-year-old child with a large right lobar hepatoblastoma (*arrows*). Despite the large size, these lesions can often be completely resected before chemotherapy. Hepatocellular carcinoma, in contrast, often involves multiple hepatic segments, and there is a significant incidence of extrahepatic extension.

extreme compression of these vessels may prevent useful interpretation.

The ability of imaging studies to predict resectability is questionable. Resectable lesions must usually be confined to the right lobe, right lobe plus medial left lobe, or the left lobe; in addition, the hepatic veins, inferior vena cava, and portal vein must be free of disease. On occasion, the distinction between compression versus invasion of liver adjacent to the lesion cannot be made, nor can the patency of vessels be established with certainty. In rare instances, it may be obvious that metastases in the remaining liver, portal or periaortic nodes, or other intraabdominal organs preclude complete resection.

The available data do not establish any superiority of MRI or CT scan for evaluating the resectability of hepatic malignancies in children. In view of the possible advantage of primary resection, a more reliable option is to judge resectability at formal laparotomy.

Staging

A staging system was derived by the CCG and the Southwest Oncology Group to compare prognosis and outcome in various intergroup study protocols. Modifications have occurred, and the system in most frequent use is shown in Table 105-9. Stage is best determined operatively in most instances. Alternatively, a TNM (tumor, node, metastasis) classification has been proposed by the International Union Against Cancer and the American Joint Committee on Cancer, and another by the Japanese Society for Pediatric Surgery.

Pathology

Hepatoblastoma usually presents as a single, pseudoencapsulated lesion, often reaching large proportions before becoming clinically apparent. The tumor grows in an expansive fashion such that the umbilical fissure is not generally breached. Thus, despite a 30% to 40% incidence of bilobar disease, successful extended resection may still be possible. Multicentricity or massive diffuse disease within the liver occurs in less than 20% of patients, and cirrhosis of the surrounding liver is unusual.

In contrast, hepatocellular carcinoma usually lacks a distinct capsule. The tumor spreads diffusely through the liver in as many as 70% of patients, often with satellite nodules well separated from the main tumor mass. Bilobar involvement occurs in 50% to 70% of cases, and the umbilical fissure does not constitute a barrier to spread. As a result, hepatocellular carcinoma is usually unresectable. Finally, because of the association of hepatocellular carcinoma with hepatitis B infection, cirrhosis may be present in the surrounding nonneoplastic liver. This may preclude complete tumor resection if the volume of liver to be removed is likely to compromise liver function further.

The epithelial element of hepatoblastoma can display a range of differentiation from a frankly anaplastic form (indistinguishable on light microscopy from other small cell neoplasms of childhood) to embryonal differentiation (cellular arrangement resembles early ducts of embryonal liver) or fetal differentiation (cells resemble normal but small hepatocytes). In addition to the epithelial element,

Table 105-9. RELATION OF STAGING TO PROGNOSIS FOR HEPATOBLASTOMA

Clinical Group	Criteria	Relative Risk for Death of Disease
I	Complete resection of tumor as initial treatment, irrespective of resectional technique	0.16
IIA	Complete resection after irradiation or chemotherapy	0.57*
IIB	Residual disease confined to one lobe	—
III	Disease involving both hepatic lobes	2.87
IIIB	Regional nodal involvement	—
IV	Distant metastases, irrespective of the extent of the hepatic tumor	3.51

* Relative risk was assessed for stage II and III patients collectively. The relative risk is compared with other stages.

hepatoblastoma may contain varying amounts of immature stromal tissue, often containing osteoid.

A pure fetal pattern is said to be favorable and the presence of embryonal or undifferentiated histology unfavorable. Pure fetal histology has been associated with improved resectability and better long-term survival. One analysis[82] showed that resected patients with pure fetal histology have a 2-year survival rate of 92%, which is significantly better than patients with embryonal or anaplastic tumor components (63% and 0% 2-year survival rates, respectively). In contrast, anaplastic histology is unfavorable and may not be chemoresponsive. A comparison of the relative risks of death for subtypes is listed in Table 105-10.

The fibrolamellar subtype of hepatocellular carcinoma is characterized by broad fibrous septa that separate the cellular component into nodules and is most commonly seen in late childhood and adolescence. It is associated with a better prognosis and a higher resection rate. This difference, however, may not be independent of stage. Ten to 20% of hepatoblastoma patients present with distant metastases. The locations of metastases at autopsy in 46 patients in one report[83] were the lungs in 46%, portal and periaortic nodes in 11%, brain in 7%, and peritoneum and diaphragm in 4% each. The incidence of metastases is reportedly higher in patients with embryonal and anaplastic histology (80% and 100%, respectively) as opposed to fetal differentiation (29%).

Hepatocellular carcinoma presents with metastatic disease in 30% to 50% of patients. The location of metastases at autopsy was reported by the Liver Cancer Study Group of Japan.[84] The lungs were involved in 48% of patients, lymph nodes in 37%, intraperitoneal organs in 16%, peritoneum in 15%, adrenal in 11%, bone in 10%, brain in 2%, and skin in 1%. Tumor emboli were detected in the portal vein in 59.7% and in the hepatic vein in 26.6% of patients. The higher incidence of lymphatic and intraabdominal spread in hepatocellular carcinoma is relevant to local resectability and recurrence. Nodal disease in the porta hepatis and periaortic region is not readily resectable, and recurrence is inevitable if present.

Treatment

Hepatoblastoma

Complete surgical resection remains the major objective of therapy for hepatoblastoma. At presentation, about 60% of patients with hepatoblastoma have resectable tumors, and one review reported no survivors among children who underwent biopsy only or incomplete resection. More recently, sporadic patients who received nonoperative treatments have achieved complete response,[85,86] and chemo-

therapy and radiotherapy have been able to salvage some patients who tumors were incompletely resected at the primary site.

A nonanatomic resection, wedging out the tumor with a satisfactory margin, may be feasible in the uncommon instance of a small peripheral or pedunculated lesion. More often, a major anatomic resection is required, depending on tumor location and extent. As much as 85% of hepatic substance may be removed, with subsequent full and rapid regeneration despite the administration of postoperative chemotherapy.[87] The principles of safe hepatic resection are now well developed, and a considerable reduction in operative mortality has been possible in the last three decades. In two historical series, mortality was reported to be about 22%, but in more recent series, it was as low as 0% to 3%.[88,89] Invasive monitoring during anesthesia allows the precise control of central venous and arterial blood pressure to the advantage of minimizing blood loss. Clotting factors and platelets are more readily available. Postoperative measures, such as respiratory and hemodynamic support, antibiotics, and total parenteral nutrition, have all made significant contributions to overall patient care.

The surgical principles include wide exposure using a generous bilateral subcostal incision and dissection at the liver hilum with isolation of vascular and ductal structures of the segment or lobe to be resected. After hepatic arterial and portal venous inflow to the relevant area is ligated, a color demarcation acts a guide to the correct plane of division of liver substance and allows this to proceed with minimal blood loss. Technologic advances such as the Cavitron ultrasonic aspirator and metallic clip applicators have made this step less hazardous in terms of hemorrhage, although finger-fracture technique with individual vessel and duct suture-ligation remains an acceptable alternative. Hemostasis of the transected surface can be completed with use of the argon beam coagulator or electrocautery and topical agents such as thrombin and Gelfoam. A trend to eliminate use of abdominal drains in uncomplicated cases has emerged.

About 40% of hepatoblastoma patients have inoperable tumors at presentation. Bilaterality, diffuse multicentricity and metastatic lesions may all preclude resection. Various techniques have been used to increase the resectability rates. These include preoperative chemotherapy, profound hypothermia with circulatory arrest, and total hepatic vascular occlusion. These maneuvers are a useful part of the surgical armamentarium in selected instances. For truly unresectable disease, aside from transplantation, chemotherapy is the major treatment option available. During the past decade, it has become evident that some of these tumors may be rendered resectable by preoperative therapy. A randomized trial performed through an intergroup collaboration of the CCG and POG showed that survival was equivalent when either doxorubicin plus cisplatin or a combination of vincristine, cisplatin, and 5-fluorouracil was administered. In contrast, toxic side effects were significantly increased in patients receiving the former regimen. It is recommended that all hepatoblastoma patients undergo initial treatment with vincristine, cisplatin, and 5-fluorouracil.

The role of radiotherapy is not clearly defined. In treating patients with bulky disease, the tolerance of normal liver is not compatible with the doses that would be required for tumor ablation, although temporary stability may be achieved. Hepatic toxicity has been described at doses to the whole liver of greater than 25 Gy. Focal radiation up to 45 Gy can be administered with safety. There may be a place for radiation in a dose range of 25 to 45 Gy combined with chemotherapy in inoperable hepatoblastoma and in patients with postresectional residual disease.

Table 105-10. COMPARISON OF RELATIVE RISK OF DEATH FOR HISTOLOGIC SUBTYPES OF HEPATOBLASTOMA

Histopathologic Subtype	Relative Risk for Death of Disease*
Fetal	1.07
Embryonal	1.74
Mixed	0.53
Macrotrabecular pattern	1.20
Small cell undifferentiated	3.71

* Risk of death adjusted for age, sex, and stage compared with other histologic subtypes

In one report, eight patients were treated after incomplete resections (four with gross and four with microscopic residual disease) with combined irradiation and chemotherapy; six of these patients were free of disease at 4 to 83 months follow-up.[86]

Other treatments with encouraging results are in developmental phases. Intraarterial infusion chemotherapy and orthotopic liver transplantation may extend the definition of resectability as clear indications emerge. The intraarterial route allows the administration of agents directly to the tumor with the theoretic advantage of less systemic toxicity. Some agents with a high hepatic extraction (eg, doxorubicin, cisplatin, and fluorodeoxyuridine) have been shown to be useful in hepatoblastoma. Several anecdotal reports exist of dramatic responses in unresectable disease, allowing subsequent resection. Yokomori and colleagues[90] reported on the treatment of a 4-month-old infant with fetal hepatoblastoma using intraarterial therapy consisting of 5-fluorouracil, vincristine, doxorubicin, and cisplatin for 18 months. Total tumor regression occurred, and the child remained well at 6 years' follow-up. The technique, although promising, is not without hazards, such as catheter infection, thrombosis, and displacement. It is technically difficult in children. In a large review[91] of recurrence and survival rates in 597 patients who received liver transplants, a recurrence rate of 40% was found in hepatoblastoma patients, with 2- and 5-year survival rates of only 32% and 7%, respectively. Until prospective studies of arterial infusion, including chemoembolization, or hepatic transplantation are available, these modalities should be considered investigational.

With improving management of the primary lesion, mortality is increasingly the result of metastatic relapse in the lungs. If metastases demonstrate progression or relapse on therapy, surgical resection is an option. Cure of pulmonary metastatic disease has not been demonstrated with radiotherapy. One series[91] reported the operative treatment of five cases of pulmonary metastatic disease that developed after successful management of the primary tumor. All lesions developed during or soon after chemotherapy. Four patients were free of disease at 8 to 83 months' follow-up, despite having multiple lesions and requiring more than one resection in two cases. No patients with hepatoblastoma with metastases to sites other than lung or regional nodes have been reported cured.

Hepatocellular Carcinoma

Analogous to hepatoblastoma, complete surgical resection is a prerequisite for cure in hepatocellular carcinoma of childhood. Patients with incompletely resected tumors do not survive. Although patients undergoing resection survive longer than those that do not, the gain is small owing to the high local and systemic relapse rates. The Japanese Liver Cancer Study Group reported a 40% 1-year survival rate for resectable disease and 10% for unresectable lesions.

Stage for stage, the prognosis of hepatocellular carcinoma is said to be no worse than that for hepatoblastoma. Many more patients present with advanced hepatocellular carcinoma, however, owing to the prevalence of bilobar and multicentric tumors, rendering them unresectable. Nodal and systemic metastatic disease is more common at the outset. The liver may be cirrhotic in some instances, precluding an extensive resection short of transplantation.

Most series report the percentage of children with resectable hepatocellular carcinoma to be around 10% to 20%. Patients with fibrolamellar histology may be an exception, with a resection rate of 48% to 60%. Relapse after resection is common. A POG and CCG intergroup study showed no impact of either cisplatin plus doxorubicin or cisplatin, vincristine, and 5-fluorouracil on outcome in patients with hepatocellular carcinoma. Overall survival in the pediatric age group for hepatocellular carcinoma is rarely reported to exceed 20%. A role for external-beam radiotherapy has not been established. Only temporary stability of bulky disease has been demonstrated, and radiation has also failed to decrease the relapse rate in patients with minimal disease after surgical resection.

In view of poor results for conventional therapy, there may be a place for liver transplantation. In one report, treatment of nine patients who had hepatocellular carcinoma by transplantation resulted in four survivors with a median follow up of 2.3 years. Longer follow-up will be necessary to recognize the true recurrence rate and intercurrent mortality.

Outcome

After a successful complete surgical resection and without further treatment, long-term survival can be expected in about 60% to 80% of patients with hepatoblastoma. Local relapse is unusual, and the most frequent cause of failure in the remaining 20% to 40% is systemic relapse. The overall cure rate with surgery alone is about 35%, and all patients should receive preoperative or postoperative systemic chemotherapy.

REFERENCES

1. Miller RW, Dalager NA. U.S. childhood cancer deaths by cell type. J Pediatr 1974;85:664.
2. Kramer S, Meadows AT, Jarrett P, Evans A. Incidence of childhood cancer: experience of a decade in a population-based registry. JNCI 1983;70:49.
3. Young JLJ, Ries LG, Silverberg E, Horm JW, Miller RW. Cancer incidence, survival and mortality for children younger than 15 years. Cancer 1986;58(Suppl 2):598.
4. Brodeur GM, Castleberry RP. Neuroblastoma. In: Pizzo PA, Poplack DG, eds. Principles and practice of pediatric oncology. Philadelphia, JB Lippincott, 1993:739.
5. Allen RW, Ogden B, Bentley FL, Jung AL. Fetal hydantoin syndrome neuroblastoma and hemorrhagic disease in a neonate. JAMA 1980;244:1464.
6. Kinney H, Faix R, Brazy J. The fetal alcohol syndrome and neuroblastoma. Pediatrics 1980;66:130.
7. Brodeur GM, Seeger RC, Schwab M, Varmus HE, Bishop JM. Amplification of N-*myc* in untreated human neuroblastomas correlates with advanced disease stage. Science 1984;224: 1121.
8. Seeger RC, Brodeur GM, Sather H, et al. Association of multiple copies of the N-*myc* oncogene with rapid progression of neuroblastomas. N Engl J Med 1985;313:1111.
9. Grady-Leopardi EF, Schwab M, Ablin AR, Rosenau W. Detection of N-*myc* oncogene expression in human neuroblastoma by *in situ hybridization* and blot analysis: relationship to clinical outcome. Cancer Res 1986;46:3196.
10. Brodeur GM, Hayes FA, Green AA, et al. Consistent N-*myc* copy number in simultaneous or consecutive neuroblastoma samples from sixty individual patients. Cancer Res 1987; 47:4248.
11. Marui N, Sakai T, Hosokawa N, et al. N-myc suppression and cell cycle arrest at G1 phase by prostaglandins. FEBS Lett 1990;270:15.
12. Caron H. Allelic loss of chromosome 1 and additional chromosome 17 material are both unfavorable prognostic markers in neuroblastoma. Med Pediatr Oncol 1995;24:215.
13. Bader SA, Fasching C, Brodeur GM, Stanbridge EJ. Dissociation of suppression of tumorigenicity and differentiation in vitro effected by transfer of single human chromosomes into human neuroblastoma cells. Cell Growth Differ 1991; 2:245.
14. Nakagawara A, Arima M, Azar CG, Scavarda NJ, Brodeur GM. Inverse relationship between TRK expression and N-myc amplification in human neuroblastomas. Cancer Res 1992; 52:1364.

15. Nakagawara A, Arima-Nakagawara M, Scavarda NJ, et al. Association between high levels of expression of the TRK gene and favorable outcome in human neuroblastoma. N Engl J Med 1993;328:847.

16. Kogner P, Barbany G, Dominici C, et al. Coexpression of the messenger RNA for TRK protooncogene and low affinity nerve growth factor receptor in neuroblastoma with favorable prognosis. Cancer Res 1993;53:2044.

17. Le Douarin N. The neural crest. New York, Cambridge University Press, 1984.

18. Triche TJ, Askin FB, Kissane JM. Neuroblastoma, Ewing's sarcoma, and the differential diagnosis of small-, round-, blue-cell tumors. In: Finegold M, ed. Pathology of neoplasia in children and adolescents. Philadelphia, WB Saunders, 1986.

19. Shimada H, Chatten J, Newton WA Jr, et al. Histopathologic prognostic factors in neuroblastic tumors: definition of subtypes of ganglioneuroblastoma and an age-linked classification of neuroblastomas. JNCI 1984;73:405.

20. Kushner BH, La Quaglia MP, Bonilla MA, et al. Highly effective induction therapy for stage 4 neuroblastoma in children over 1 year of age. J Clin Oncol 1994;12:2607.

21. D'Angio GJ, Beckwith JB, Bishop HC, et al. The National Wilms' Tumor Study: a progress report. Proceedings of the National Cancer Conference 1972;7:627.

22. Crist WM, Kun LE. Common solid tumors of childhood. N Engl J Med 1991;324:461.

23. Breslow N, Beckwith JB, Ciol M, Sharples K. Age distribution of Wilms' tumor. Cancer Res 1988;48:1653.

24. Breslow NE, Beckwith JB. Epidemiological features of Wilms' tumor: results of the national Wilms' tumor study. JNCI 1982;68:429.

25. Rose EA, Glaser T, Jones C, et al. Complete physical map of the WAGR region of 11p13 localizes a candidate Wilms' tumor gene. Cell 1990;60:495.

26. Francke U, Holmes LB, Atkins L, et al. Aniridia-Wilms' tumor association: evidence for specific deletion of 11p13. Cytogenet Cell Genet 1979;24:185.

27. Maw MA, Grundy PE, Millow LJ, et al. A third Wilms' tumor locus on chromosome 16q. Cancer Res 1992;52:3094.

28. Grundy P, Koufos A, Morgan K, et al. Familial predisposition to Wilms' tumor does not map to short arm of chromosome 11. Nature 1988;336:374.

29. Green DM, D'Angio GJ, Beckwith JB, et al. Wilms' tumor (nephroblastoma, renal embryoma). In: Pizzo PA, Poplack DG. Principles and practice of pediatric oncology. Philadelphia, JB Lippincott, 1993:725.

30. Mahoney JP Saffos RO. Fetal rhabdomyomatous nephroblastoma with a renal pelvic mass simulating sarcoma botryoides. Am J Pathol 1981;5:297.

31. Larson E, Perez-Atayde AR, Green DM, et al. Surgery only for the treatment of patients with stage I (Cassidy) Wilms' tumor. Cancer 1990;66:264.

32. Green DM, Breslow M, Beckwith JB, et al. Treatment outcomes in patients less than two years of age with small stage I favorable histology Wilms' tumor: a National Wilms' Tumor study. J Clin Oncol 1993;11:91.

33. Malcom AW, Jaffe N, Folkman MJ, Cassady JR. Bilateral Wilms' tumor. Int J Radiat Oncol Biol Phys 1980;6:167.

34. Montgomery BT, Kelalis PP, Blute ML, et al. Extended follow up of bilateral Wilms' tumor study: results of National Wilms' Tumor Study. J Urol 1991;146:514.

35. Ritchey ML, Othersen HB Jr, de Lorimier AA, et al. Renal vein involvement with nephroblastoma: a report of the National Wilms' Tumor Study-3. Eur Urol 1990;17:139.

36. Ritchey ML, Kelalis PP, Breslow NB, et al. Surgical complications after nephrectomy for Wilms' tumor: a report from the National Wilms' Tumor Study-3. Surg Gynecol Obstet 1992;175:507.

37. Ward SP, Dehner LP. Sacrococcygeal teratoma with nephroblastoma (Wilms' tumor): a variant of extragonadal teratoma in childhood. A histologic and ultrastructural study. Cancer 1974;33:1355.

38. Luchtrath H, de Leon F, Giesen H, Gok Y. Inguinal nephroblastoma. Virchows Arch A 1984;405:113.

39. Naito K, Yokoyama O, Yamuguchi K, et al. Extrarenal nephroblastoma: report of a case and review of the literature. Hinyokika Kiyo 1985;31:1773.

40. Wexler H, Poole C, Fojaco R. Metastatic neonatal Wilms' tumor, a case report with review of the literature. Pediatr Radiol 1975;3:179.

41. Hrabovsky EE, Othersen HB Jr, deLorimier A, et al. Wilms' tumor in the neonate: a report from the National Wilms' Tumor Study. J Pediatr Surg 1986;21:385.

42. Babaian RJ, Skinner DG, Waisman J. Wilms' tumor in the adult patient: diagnosis, management, and review of the world medical literature. Cancer 1980;45:1713.

43. Byrd RL, Evans AE, D' Angio GJ. Adult Wilms' tumor: effects of combined therapy on survival. J Urol 1982;127:648.

44. Hupperets PS, Havenith MG, Blijham GH. Recurrent adult nephroblastoma: long-term remission after surgery plus adjuvant high-dose chemotherapy, radiation therapy, and allogeneic bone marrow transplantation. Cancer 1992;69:2990.

45. Marsden HB, Lawler W, Kumar PM. Bone metastasizing renal tumour of childhood: morphological and clinical features, and differences from Wilms' tumor. Cancer 1978;42:1922.

46. Beckwith JB. Wilms' tumor and other renal tumors of childhood: a selective review from the National Wilms' Tumor Study Pathology Center. Hum Pathol 1983;14:481.

47. Green DM, Moksness J, Breslow NE, Beckwith JB, D' Angio GJ. The treatment of children with clear cell sarcoma of the kidney (CCSK): a report from the National Wilms' Tumor Study (NWTS). (Abstract) Proceedings of the Annual Meeting of the American Association for Cancer Research 1994;35:A1428.

48. Beckwith JB, Palmer NF. Histopathology and prognosis of Wilms' tumor: results from the National Wilms' Tumor Study. Cancer 1978;41:1937.

49. Eftekhari F, Erly WK, Jaffe N. Malignant rhabdoid tumor of the kidney: imaging features in two cases. Pediatr Radiol 1990;21:39.

50. Bolande RP, Brough AJ, Izant RJ. Congenital mesoblastic nephroma of infancy. Pediatrics 1967;40:272.

51. Aronson DC, Medary I, Finlay JL, Herr HW, Exelby PR, La Quaglia MP. Renal cell carcinoma in childhood and adolescence: a retrospective survey for prognostic factors in 22 cases. J Pediatr Surg 1996;31:183.

52. Young JL, Miller RW. Incidence of malignant tumors in U.S. children. J Pediatr 1975;86:254.

53. Ruymann FB, Maddux HR, Ragab A, et al. Congenital anomalies associated with rhabdomyosarcoma: an autopsy study of 115 cases. A report from the Intergroup Rhabdomyosarcoma Study committee. Med Pediatr Oncol 1988;16:33.

54. Davis RL, Weintrub H, Lassar AB. Expression of a single transfected cDNA converts fibroblasts to myoblasts. Cell 1987;51:987.

55. Dias P, Parham DM, Shapiro DN, Webber BL, Houghton PJ. Myogenic regulatory protein (MyoD1) expression in childhood solid tumors: diagnostic utility in rhabdomyosarcoma. Am J Pathol 1990;137:1283.

56. Harmer MH, ed. TNM classification of pediatric tumors. Geneva, International Union Against Cancer, 1982:23.

57. Mandell L, Ghavimi F, Peretz T, et al. Radiocurability of microscopic disease in childhood rhabdomyosarcoma with radiation doses less than 4000 cGy. J Clin Oncol 1990;8:1536.

58. La Quaglia MP, Heller G, Ghavimi F, Casper ES, Vlamis V, Hajdu S, Brennan MF. The effect of age at diagnosis on outcome in rhabdomyosarcoma. Cancer 1994;73:109.

59. Carli M, Guglielmi M, Sotti G, et al. Prognostic factors in children with rhabdomyosarcoma (RMS), results of the Italian cooperative study RMS-79. (Meeting Abstract) Med Pediatr Oncol 1991;19:398.

60. Rodary C, Gehan EA, Flamant F, et al. Prognostic factors in 951 children with non-metastatic rhabdomyosarcoma: a report from the International Rhabdomyosarcoma Workshop. Med Pediatr Oncol 1991;19:89.

61. Suder J, Stienen U, Kaatsch P, et al. Analysis of prognostic factors in rhabdomyosarcoma: preliminary univariate and multivariate results of the Soft Tissue Sarcoma Study (CWS-81). Klin Padiatr 1986;198:218.

62. Rodary C, Rey A, Rezvani A, Flamant F. Prognostic factors in rhabdomyosarcomas in childhood: study carried out with 253 children registered by the International Society of Pediatric Oncology. Bull Cancer 1988;75:213.

63. Maurer HM, Gehan EA, Beltangady M, et al. The Intergroup Rhabdomyosarcoma Study-II. Cancer 1993;71:1904.

64. Crist W, Gehan EA, Ragab AH, et al. The Third Intergroup Rhabdomyosarcoma Study. J Clin Oncol 1995;13:610.

65. Soule EH, Pritchard DJ. Fibrosarcoma of infants and children: a review of 110 cases. Cancer 1977;40:1711.

66. Ninane J, Gosseye S, Pantion E, et al. Congenital fibrosarcoma. Cancer 1986;58:1400.

66a. Pisters PN, Harrison CB, Woodruff JM, et al. A prospective randomized trial of adjuvant brachytherapy in the mangement of low-grade soft tissue sarcomas of the extremity and superficial trunk. J Clin Oncol 1994;12:115.

67. Horowitz ME, Pratt CB, Webber BL, et al. Therapy of childhood soft-tissue sarcomas other than rhabdomyosarcoma: a review of 62 cases treated at a single institution. J Clin Oncol 1986;4:559.

68. Rosen G, Forscher C, Lowenbraun S, et al. Synovial sarcoma: uniform response of metastases to high dose ifosfamide. Cancer 1994;73:2506.

69. Brodsky JT, Burt ME, Hajdu SI, Casper ES, Brennan MF. Tendosynovial sarcoma: clinicopathologic features, treatment and prognosis. Cancer 1992;70:484.

70. Kushner BH, Hajdu SI, Gulati SC, Erlandson RA, Exelby PR, Lieberman PH. Extracranial primitive neuroectodermal tumor. Cancer 1991;67:1825.

71. Gerald WL, Rosai J. Desmoplastic small round cell tumor with multi-phenotypic differentiation. Zentrabl Pathol 1993;139:141.

72. Riccardi VM, Powell PP. Neurofibrosarcoma as a complication of von Recklinghausen neurofibromatosis. Neurofibromatosis 1989;2:152.

73. Swanson PE, Wick MR, Dehner LP. Leiomyosarcoma of the somatic soft tissues in childhood: an immunohistochemical analysis of six cases with ultrastructural correlation. Hum Pathol 1991;22:569.

74. Ng EH, Pollock RE, Munsell MF, Atkinson EN, Rosenthal MM. Prognostic factors influencing survival in gastrointestinal leiomyosarcomas: implications for surgical management and staging. Ann Surg 1992;215:68.

75. Olweny CL, Toya T, Kantongole-Mbidde E, et al. Treatment of hepatocellular carcinoma with Adriamycin. Cancer 1975;36:1250.

76. Evans AE, Land VJ, Newton WA, et al. Combination chemotherapy (vincristine, Adriamycin, cyclophosphamide and 5-fluorouracil) in the treatment of children with malignant hepatoma. Cancer 1982;50:821.

77. Quinn JJ, Altman AJ, Robinson HT, et al. Adriamycin and cisplatinum for hepatoblastoma. Cancer 1985;56:1926.

78. Ortega JA, Krailo MD, Haas JE, et al. Effective treatment of unresectable or metastatic hepatoblastoma with cisplatinum and continuous infusion doxorubicin chemotherapy: a report from the children's cancer study group. J Clin Oncol 1991;9:2167.

79. Ni Y, Chang M, Hsu H, et al. Hepatocellular carcinoma in childhood: clinical manifestations and prognosis. Cancer 1991;68:1737.

80. Weinberg AG, Finegold MJ. Primary hepatic tumors of childhood. Hum Pathol 1983;14:512.

81. Nickerson HJ, Silberman TL, McDona TP. Hepatoblastoma, thrombocytosis, and increased thrombopoietin. Cancer 1980;45:315.

82. Haas JE, Mukzynski KA, Krailo M, et al. Histopathology and prognosis in childhood hepatoblastoma and hepatocellular carcinoma. Cancer 1989;64:1082.

83. Lack EE, Neave C, Vawter GF. Hepatocellular carcinoma: review of 32 cases in childhood and adolescence. Cancer 1983;52:1510.

84. The Liver Cancer Study Group of Japan. Primary liver cancer in Japan. Cancer 1987;60:1400.

85. Weinblatt ME, Siegel SE, Siegel MM, et al. Preoperative chemotherapy for unresectable primary hepatic malignancies in children. Cancer 1982;50:1061.

86. Habrand JL, Nehme D, Kalifa C, et al. Is there a place for radiation therapy in the management of hepatoblastomas and hepatocellular carcinoma in children? Int J Radiat Oncol Biol Phys 1992;23:525.

87. Taylor PH, Filler RM, Nebesar NA, et al. Experience with hepatic resection in childhood. Am J Surg 1969;117:435.

88. Exelby PR, Filler RM, Grosfeld JL. Liver tumors in children in the particular reference to hepatoblastoma and hepatocellular carcinoma: American Academy of Pediatrics Surgical Section Survey-1974. J Pediatr Surg 1975;10:329.

89. Lee CS, Sung JL, Hwang LY, et al. Surgical treatment of 109 patients with symptomatic and asymptomatic hepatocellular carcinoma. Surgery 1986;99:481.

90. Yokomori K, Hori T, Asoh S, et al. Complete disappearance of unresectable hepatoblastoma by continuous infusion therapy through the hepatic artery. J Pediatr Surg 1991;26:830.

91. Black CT, Luck SR, Musemeche CA, et al. Aggressive excision of pulmonary metastases is warranted in the management of childhood hepatic tumors. J Pediatr Surg 1991;26:1082.

SURGERY: SCIENTIFIC PRINCIPLES AND PRACTICE, Second Edition, edited by Lazar J. Greenfield, Michael W. Mulholland, Keith T. Oldham, Gerald B. Zelenock, and Keith D. Lillemoe. Lippincott–Raven Publishers, Philadelphia, © 1997.

CHAPTER 106

ORTHOPEDIC SURGERY

LARRY S. MATTHEWS AND STEVEN A. GOLDSTEIN

Orthopedic surgery encompasses the diagnosis and treatment of abnormalities of the musculoskeletal system and is a broad and important field of interest. It is impossible to address all of the scientific and clinical issues relating to this specialty in this discussion. The general and specific diagnoses of musculoskeletal diseases and injuries are extensive, and the diverse biologic and engineering disciplines that influence the advancement of orthopedic surgery are growing rapidly. The emphasis of this chapter is on the structure–function relation in the musculoskeletal tissues and on the coupling of biologic and engineering principles. The selected topics provide a framework for extrapolating treatment strategies to the many musculoskeletal conditions that are not discussed.

SOFT TISSUES

Structure

Soft tissues are multiphase materials composed primarily of collagen, elastin, and a hydrophilic ground substance containing mucopolysaccharides, proteoglycans, glycosaminoglycans, and water. The relative amounts and three-dimensional organization of these constituents dictate the physical properties of the tissue. The vascular density and the degree of cellularity directly correlate with these tissues' potential for remodeling and repair.

Connective tissue consists of cells and an extracellular matrix, with a series of fibrillar protein structures encapsulated within the ground substance. Because the function of the connective tissues is primarily mechanical, the cells provide a low level of homeostatic activity except when faced with injury or damage. Perhaps the most important structural component of the connective tissues is collagen, by virtue of its high mechanical integrity. At least 15 separate collagen molecules have been identified, each with a specific conformation associated with a unique kinetic or mechanical property. The collagens can be categorized into two major groups—fiber-forming collagens and collagens that do not form regular fibers.

The fiber-forming collagens include types 1, 2, and 3. Type 1 collagen is the most abundant in the human body and is the dominant constituent in tendons, ligaments, bone, skin, vessel walls, and scar and granulation tissues. Type 2 collagen is found in cartilage, and type 3 collagen is found in tendon and ligament sheaths as well as in mus-

cle, skin, blood vessel walls, and scar tissue. The remaining collagens do not form regular fibers and include the basement membrane collagens, types 4 and 5, and the minor collagens. The minor collagens are not completely characterized, but it is hypothesized that they play a major role in the interactions between cellular and extracellular elements within the tissues. This coupling between cells and the extracellular fibrillar structures may provide structural integrity as well as a mechanism for the transduction of mechanical signal stimulation.

The other fibrillar protein of importance in connective tissues is elastin. As its name suggests, elastin is an easily deformable protein. In tendons and most ligaments, elastin is present in small amounts or not at all, although ligaments such as the ligamentum flava are dominated by elastin components. The remaining constituents of the tissues include large glycoproteins such as fibronectin and laminen, which may play a role in the regulation of collagen fiber formation and in the early phases of wound healing.

The final major constituent of the soft tissues, ground substance, is a mortar-like material in which the collagen matrices are embedded. It is composed primarily of water, which dominates its properties. Within the ground substance, proteoglycans and other large-chain polymers with pronounced hydrophilic properties regulate the amount of water in the tissue and the propensity for that water to flow within the tissues. The viscosity of the ground substance is primarily associated with hyaluronic acid.

Functional Morphology

Connective tissues transmit or resist the mechanical loads encountered by the musculoskeletal system. Their function depends on their inherent mechanical properties, for instance their ability to deform under conditions of mechanical loading. To understand the normal behavior of these tissues and the consequences of damage or degeneration, it is important to measure their normal mechanical properties. Their properties can be closely related to their morphologic and histologic appearance at the light-microscopic level.

Two important architectural features of soft tissues are collagen waviness and fiber orientation. Collagenous tissues are assembled as helical collagen molecules organized into fibrils, which are packed into fibers and eventually fiber bundles. The fiber bundles are evident under moderate magnified light and polarized light microscopy. The feature that becomes most apparent is a characteristic waviness or crimp pattern of fiber bundles. Tendons and ligaments have a low degree of waviness, whereas skin exhibits a larger wave pattern and mesentery tissue shows a large degree of waviness. The patterns are a function of chemical interactions of the collagen bundles within the ground substance or with adjacent collagen. When these tissues are loaded in tension, initial deformation occurs by straightening out the waviness. The larger the crimp pattern, therefore, the more deformable the tissue under low loads.

Because the constituent collagen fiber bundles are designed to resist tensile loads, their overall arrangement within soft tissues relates to their functional demand. For example, the fiber bundles in tendons and ligaments are primarily aligned in parallel along an axis subjected to pure tension. In skin, the fibers are organized biaxially in stacked layers, allowing skin to biaxially stretch over the organ or joint during function. A more complex triaxial organization is observed in articular cartilage, which must withstand the combination of significant shear stresses resulting from translation of joints during articulation and of compressive stresses resulting from the large contact loads transmitted across the joints.

The combined properties of the tissue constituents and their architectural arrangement dictate their response to load. An increase in crimp pattern and an increase in percentage of elastin both correlate to a high degree of deformability under load. Once the crimp pattern is lost or the elastic limit of the elastin fibers is reached, the tissue properties are dominated by the stiff, minimally deformable collagen fibers.

Two conditions that affect the mechanical properties of tissue are clinically important. The first is the effect of aging on collagenous tissues. With age, increased collagen cross-linking is observed in most tissues. Its effect is to decrease tissue deformability and increase brittleness. The second condition results from the fact that soft tissues demonstrate highly viscoelastic or time-dependent properties. The tissues behave differently with different rates of loading. In general, the faster soft tissues are loaded, the less deformation they exhibit for a given load and the higher the load required to cause catastrophic failure. This phenomenon depends completely on the viscoelastic properties of the tissue. It is easy to see how injuries might differ as a function of the rate of impact.

Mechanical Properties

Insight into the mechanical behavior and function of tissues can be gained by characterizing their response to controlled loading. Techniques similar to those used in testing engineering materials have been used extensively to evaluate the properties of biologic tissues. The general response of any soft tissue to mechanical load can be gleaned from a knowledge of its histologic construction.

Figure 106-1 illustrates load–deformation curves associated with three soft tissue structures. Characteristics from the response curve to a single cycle of load are correlated to histologic features of the model tissues. The initial deformation that occurs with load is referred to as the *toe-in region* and is associated with the degree of crimp pattern as well as the amount of elastin. The linear region is associated with the stiff collagen or collagen elastin composite. The *yield point* is defined as that amount of load or deformation that causes permanent damage to the tissue (repair is not considered at this point). The damage may be at a microscopic level or within only a portion of the fibers in the tissue. Catastrophic failure occurs at the point labeled *ultimate load* or ultimate strength. Because structures are found in many shapes and sizes, the load–deformation response characterizes the structural properties. In other words, the load–deformation characteristics of any structure can be altered by increasing the size or shape of that structure. To understand the inherent properties of the substance that makes up each structure, geometric considerations are necessary. The load–deformation response must be translated into a stress–strain response. *Stress* is defined as the load applied over a cross-sectional area of the structure, and strain is a nondimensional measure of deformation equal to the change in length divided by the

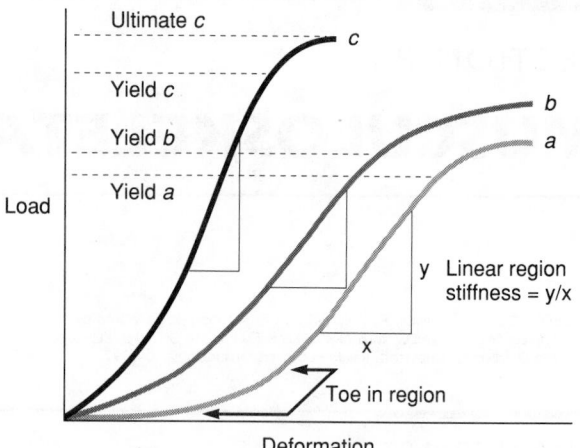

Figure 106-1. To illustrate the effect of different soft tissue constituent components on their mechanical response to load, three load-deformation curves are shown. Soft tissue response a illustrates a large toe-in region associated with a large crimp pattern and a potentially significant amount of elastin. In soft tissue response b, the toe-in region is much smaller, probably because of a smaller crimp pattern, whereas the linear portion (stiffness) is similar to tissue a and might reflect a similar composition of collagen and elastin fibers. In contrast, soft tissue response c demonstrates a small toe-in region associated with a small crimp pattern and a very steep linear portion (high stiffness), reflecting a composition that is entirely collagen. The yield and ultimate strength of these tissues would be difficult to predict from compositional information, but the cross-sectional area would contribute significantly to increased properties, since greater cross-sectional area results in greater strength.

original length. The stress–strain curve for a tendon is demonstrated in Figure 106-2. These curves are of clinical significance in understanding tissue response to load. For the tissue illustrated, damage occurs at about 10% to 12% strain with failure at nearly 20%. Translating this information into physiologic lengths can help in diagnosing injuries. For example, in testing whether the medial collateral ligament of the knee joint has been disrupted, knowledge of the biomechanical properties would suggest that a 3-inch ligament would have had to be elongated by a little less than 0.5 inch to sustain damage and by about 0.75 inch to be completely torn.

The viscoelastic properties of the tissue also provide important clinical information. For example, ligaments fail at higher loads with increased loading rate. Ligaments subjected to high-speed dramatic load tend to fail in their midsubstance, whereas at lower speeds they fail at the bone ligament insertion. Time-dependent properties are also important with respect to repeated loading. If a viscoelastic material is cyclically loaded without providing enough recovery time between each cycle, an accumulation of deformation or strain can occur with each repeated cycle. This accumulation of strain, even at low loads, has been cited as a possible causative factor in cumulative trauma disorders such as tenosynovitis and bursitis. Epidemiologic studies have shown that reducing the number of cycles or increasing the time between loading cycles can assist in preventing the onset of these chronic conditions.

Soft Tissue Repair

Soft tissues heal in stages, each of which can be correlated to recovery of mechanical properties. The first stage involves a granulation tissue, in which the collagen fibers

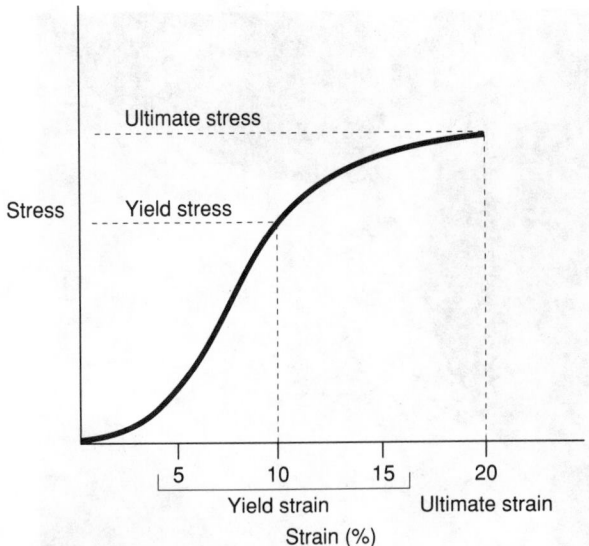

Figure 106-2. A typical stress–strain curve for a tendon is shown. By both accounting for the cross-sectional area and normalizing the deformation, this curve reflects the inherent properties of the tissue that make up the tendon. Yield occurs at about 10% and failure at greater than 20%.

are oriented in a random pattern and the degree of waviness is likewise random. This tissue is not as functional as the more optimal normal structure. In fact, some healing ligaments have been shown to acquire only 70% of their intact strength after 6 months. In time, the soft tissues remodel to produce an architecture more nearly that of the normal intact tissue. Factors associated with beneficial effects on healing include early immobilization, regulated physical stimuli, and good vascular supply. Remodeling or adaptation of soft tissues has also been shown to occur under normal physiologic loading conditions. There are reports of training effects increasing the properties of tissues and of metabolically active cells incorporated within the matrix.[1]

BONE

As for soft tissues, an understanding of the function and properties of bone tissue can be gained from examining its histologic construction. This section presents several principles that aid in the diagnosis or treatments of bone-related disorders in orthopedic practice.

There are four major functions of bone—protection of vital organs, mechanical support and locomotion, mineral homeostasis, and hematopoiesis. The architecture of bone has evolved into a form capable of supporting all four of these functions simultaneously. The mechanical and protective functions of bone are easily recognized. In addition, the hollow intramedullary canals of the appendicular skeleton, as well as the trabecular bone from metaphyseal regions, support the production of red blood cells. Bone is also the primary warehouse of calcium and phosphorus and, through a recurring process of turnover, provides a basis for mineral homeostasis in the body.

Two major types of bone are found in the human body—trabecular and cortical (Fig. 106-3). Although the chemical, molecular, and cellular components of both types are similar, the organization of these components at the ultrastructural and microstructural level leads to significant differences in their mechanical and metabolic activities. The microstructural organization of bone can be classified into

three types—primary bone, secondary bone, and woven bone. The most important characteristic of primary bone is that it must be formed on existing surfaces. The surface can be cartilaginous or preexisting bone. Primary bone is arranged in lamellar sheets, longitudinally oriented in primary lamellae and concentrically arranged surrounding a blood vessel in primary osteons. This bone is highly organized and exhibits excellent mechanical properties. Secondary osteonal bone is the primary constituent of adult cortices. Through a cellularly directed process of resorption and formation, primary bone is remodeled to form the osteons (Fig. 106-4). The formation of osteons in cortical bone is probably driven by the need to provide nutrients to the interstitial bone and to increase resistance to fracture crack propagation and possibly failure under cyclic loading. In contrast, trabecular bone is composed of longitudinal lamellae, and remodeling occurs from surfaces in discrete regions designated as trabecular packets. The spongelike structure of trabecular bone, which is found near joint surfaces in the vertebral bodies and other regions, provides a large surface/volume ratio. The significantly increased surface of bone exposed to marrow contents provides greater potential for exchange of minerals through the process of remodeling. In addition, its cancellated architecture provides an efficient energy-absorbing structure to attenuate the large loads transmitted across the joints. The final microstructural type of bone is woven bone. Although the collagen matrices in lamellar and osteonal bone are precisely organized, providing maximal mechanical properties with minimal material, woven bone is composed of disorganized yet highly mineralized tissue and is expressed in the course of fracture or damage repair. It has the advantage of being quickly deposited but the disadvantage of significantly reduced mechanical properties when compared with the highly ordered primary and secondary bone.[2]

Bone Development

The two basic mechanisms of bone development are endochondral and intramembranous bone formation. Most of the skeleton and in particular the long bones develop

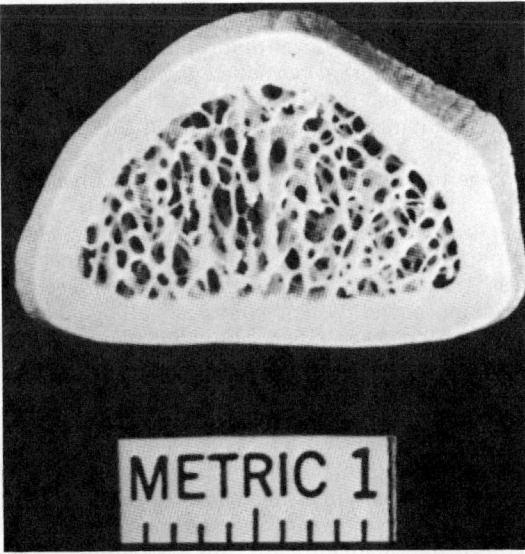

Figure 106-3. A cross-section of human long bone demonstrates the gross differences between the outer cortical or compact bony shell and the inner sponge-like trabecular bone architecture.

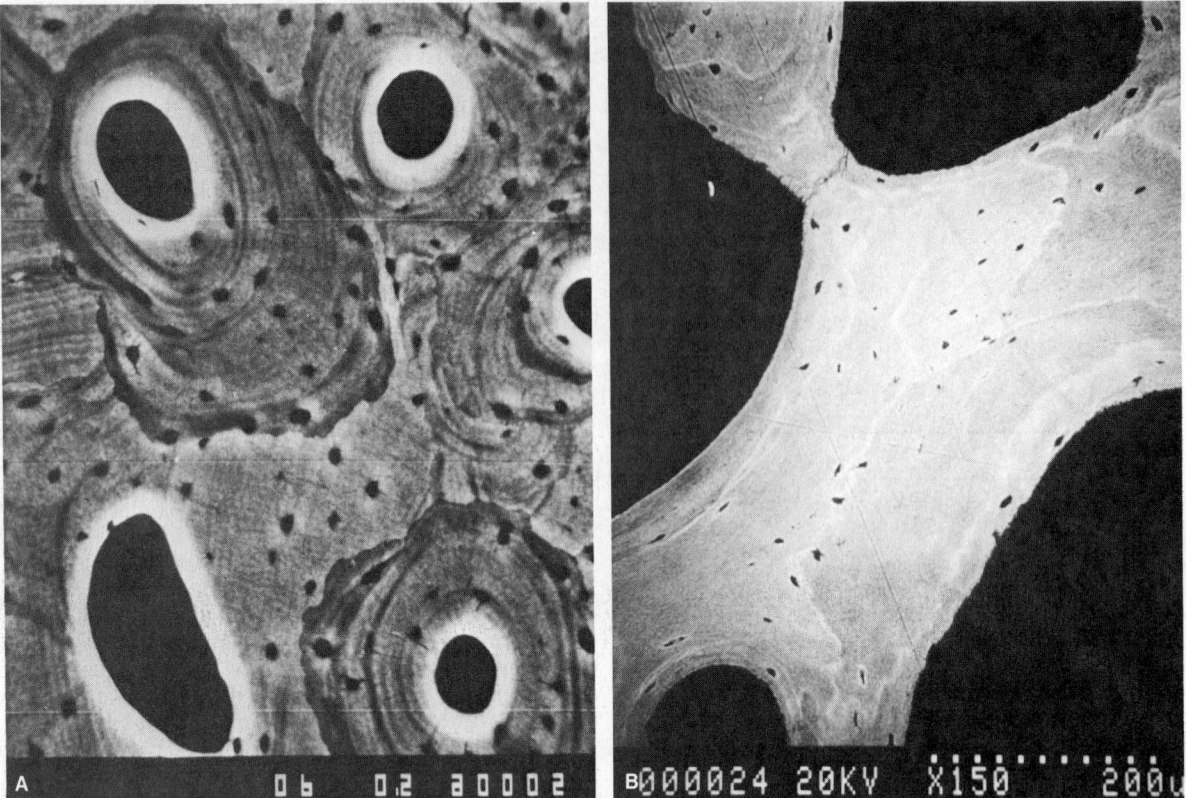

Figure 106-4. Although early anatomists considered trabecular bone an extension of porous cortical bone, the microscopic features of the two bone types are significantly different. Whereas adult cortical bone (*A*) is arranged in concentric lamellae that form osteons around a central vascular canal; individual trabeculi (*B*) are composed of irregularly shaped packets that contain nearly parallel lamellae. These microscopic features reflect the differences in remodeling mechanisms within these types of bone.

by the endochondral process, whereas several bones in the facial region and the ribs are formed by intramembranous mechanisms. An understanding of these processes is important because they continue throughout adulthood during fracture healing and, under certain circumstances, during remodeling.

Long bones begin during embryonic development as cartilaginous anlages. After an appropriate signal, cartilage cells within the central portion of the anlage become hypertrophic and the matrix that surrounds them begins to calcify. Simultaneously, progenitor cells differentiate into osteoblasts (bone-forming cells) around the periphery of the anlage to form a bone collar. Vascular invasion then proceeds into the center of the segment and appears to initiate the formation of a primary ossification center, fully initiating the endochondral bone formation process. This process is carried out through a maturation or degeneration of the chondrocytes, which express a cartilage matrix that eventually becomes calcified. The calcified cartilage serves as a template for the deposition of bone matrix, which then is mineralized. Resorption of the calcified cartilage as well as remodeling of the primary bone completes the process. Simultaneously, appositional growth continues on the periphery by the continual deposition of bone on the surface. The surface deposition is analogous to intramembranous bone formation, which is defined as bone formed without a cartilage intermediate step. This development process continues with a migration of the ossification front and an expansion of the periphery followed by initiation of the secondary ossification sites. These sites form the bound-

aries of the growth plates of the long bones. The continued growth and development of the bone occurs at the growth plates, which contribute to longitudinal growth through the endochondral process.

The cartilage of the growth plate is divided into three major zones relating to both the morphology and function of the tissue. The reserve zone is composed of what seems to be resting chondrocytes. In the proliferative zone, the cells align in a regular columnar arrangement, undergo mitosis, and begin to imbibe water and other constituents as they move into the hypertrophic zone (Fig. 106-5). At the limit of the hypertrophic zone, the matrix expressed by the chondrocytes is calcified and serves as a scaffold where bone matrix is deposited (provisional calcification zone). Factors that influence the rate of growth include vascular supply, age, hormonal effects, and mechanical stresses. The relation between mechanical stresses and growth has been defined by the Heuter-Volkman principle, which suggests that growth is inhibited by high compressive stresses and stimulated by tensile stresses. Therefore, treatment strategies for disturbed or injured growth patterns often involve the application of mechanical stresses to accelerate or decelerate growth differentially in regions of the growth plate. The exact mechanisms that control this process are unknown and remain a fertile area for research.

The growth plate's mechanical stability or resistance to damage lies in the properties of the matrix, its columnar architecture, and the surrounding tissues (eg, the perichondral ring or groove of Ranvier). Fractures of the growth

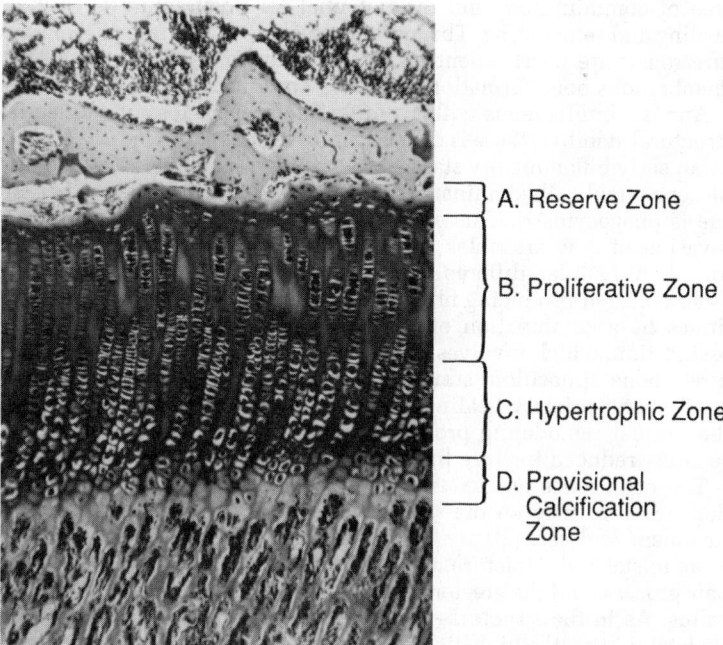

A. Reserve Zone

B. Proliferative Zone

C. Hypertrophic Zone

D. Provisional Calcification Zone

Figure 106-5. Histologic cross-section of a growth plate. The cartilaginous tissue is divided into zones that reflect the cellular activity within each.

plate are not common, but they can have severe effects on continued growth. Any treatment strategy must be designed to reduce the fracture to preserve growth-plate dynamics. Injuries leading to growth inhomogeneities often require surgical procedures to correct deformities or limb-length discrepancies.

Bone Remodeling

After the initial development and deposition of bone, it is remodeled to produce a more optimally aligned and constructed structure. This process involves resorption by osteoclasts followed by deposition of nonmineralized matrix (osteoid) by osteoblasts. During mineralization, the osteoblasts become trapped in their matrix, thereby serving as the resulting bone cells (osteocytes). Osteocytes are interconnected through a series of canaliculi to each other and to a blood vessel or marrow surface. This remodeling process can occur on the surface of trabeculi, on the surface of cortical bone, and intercortically. It proceeds as a method of normal turnover, providing access to minerals needed for normal homeostasis.[3] Under normal circumstances, the process takes about 120 days in an adult. It is through this carefully orchestrated process of remodeling that the secondary structures of cortical bone, the osteons, are formed and the geometry and directionality of the trabeculi are influenced.[2]

In addition to the requirement for continual bone turnover, the remodeling process is significantly influenced by the functional loads to which the bone is subjected. It is well established that the architecture and orientation of bone follow directly from its function, a phenomenon known as Wolff's law. Although the principle that form follows function has influenced the internal and external architecture of our bone in an evolutionary sense, it also remains active throughout adulthood. As a consequence, significant alteration in mechanical condition in a region of bone elicits an adaptation. For example, a region of bone becomes demineralized during disuse, whereas bony tissue hypertrophies with repeated and increased use. This process occurs both globally and at local levels. Perhaps

the most important expressions of bone adaptation occur at the interface between bone and an implant. As a consequence, orthopedic procedures that alter the mechanical environment elicit an adaptation response. Although the mechanisms that stimulate this response are not known, the magnitude, frequency, rate, and direction of load application significantly influence bone adaptation. Trabecular bone remodeling occurs 5 to 10 times faster than that of cortical bone remodeling, probably because of its porosity and greater surface/volume ratio.

It is important to differentiate bone remodeling from bone modeling. Bone remodeling involves the resorption of existing bone followed by formation within the resorption cavity. Modeling describes the phenomenon of bone formation without resorption. This modeling can only occur through the deposition of woven bone. It occurs during fracture healing and possibly as a result of microdamage associated with surgical procedures or severe interface conditions with prosthetic components.

Fracture Healing

The process of fracture healing follows the same principles as described for endochondral bone formation and intramembranous bone formation. In general, the repair occurs in four stages once the impact or damage has occurred—inflammation, creation of soft callus, mineralization of the callus, and remodeling of the initial mineralized tissue (see later discussion).

ORTHOPEDIC DISORDERS
Fractures

The treatment of fractures is based on an understanding of the normal healing processes and on specific geometric and functional objectives. Many factors affect the progression of healing, including patient age, nutritional status, associated soft tissue trauma, and mechanical stability. Long-term clinical success depends on location of the fracture (diaphyseal, metaphyseal, or intraarticular), the degree of comminution, and the potential for postfracture healing and remodeling. The biologic mechanisms of fracture repair are nearly identical to the endochondral and membranous bone formation processes described earlier.[4]

Almost simultaneous with a simple fracture and loss of structural stability, there is bleeding into the area followed by an early inflammatory stage and a proliferation of cells. Mesenchymal cells dominate the region, and necrotic tissue is phagocytosed. This early phase is followed by the invasion of new arterioles and capillaries, which is followed by cellular differentiation into fibrocartilage and other collagen-producing fibroblasts. The repair then continues by a combination of mechanisms—endochondral ossification, which involves a cartilage intermediate stage; direct bone apposition, similar to membranous bone formation; and primary healing involving an acceleration of the normal remodeling process directed across a stable, securely reduced fracture line.[5]

The occurrence and distribution of these mechanisms depends primarily on the stability of the fracture during treatment and secondarily on the fracture location. The more unstable the fracture, the more endochondral the repair process, and the greater the cross-sectional area of the callus. As in the structure–function relation in musculoskeletal tissues, the biologic process seems to be driven by the need to establish mechanical integrity as quickly as possible. For example, the first material formed by the osteoblasts at the fracture site is woven bone. Although woven bone has inferior mechanical properties when compared with lamellar bone (it is more brittle and less able to withstand repeated loading), it can be laid down rapidly at high density. The laws of mechanics dictate that an increase in the cross-sectional area, as produced by the surrounding callus, greatly increases the resistance of the structure to bending or torsional loads. In fact, an increase in unit diameter of the cross-section raises the strength of the structure by the fourth power of the diameter change. Therefore, even if the callus is made of inferior material, the cross-sectional attributes more than compensate for the inferior substance. Once the fracture is stabilized by the initial woven bone proliferation, secondary remodeling occurs under principles similar to the Wolff law.

The treatment of fractures has benefited greatly from advances in the biology of wound care. Application of engineering and surgical principles has helped to rapidly reestablish the accurate geometric reassembly of the parts. Stable maintenance of this geometry is important while healing takes place. Classification of open fractures has allowed estimation of the extent of soft tissue damage. Soft tissue transfer, local transposition of muscle tissue, and even free tissue transfer have allowed fracture-site coverage with viable tissue. In multiple trauma, stable fixation, early bone grafting, and skin coverage in association with systemic support and antibiotic prophylaxis have improved fracture treatment.[6]

The most significant surgical advances in the treatment of long-bone fractures are attributed to improvement in orthopedic fracture fixation implants and materials based on biomechanical principles. The first modern, well-organized, and scientifically based advance in the surgical treatment of long-bone fractures resulted from the Davos group's research on fracture healing.[7,8] They demonstrated that stable, secure, and accurate fixation of long-bone fractures with minimal surgical damage to soft tissues can result in reliable and rapid fracture healing. Application of these principles depended on the development of superior implants and surgical techniques that promoted accurate reduction of fracture fragments and sustained compression across the fracture site, enabling a higher proportion of primary healing to occur. A large array of plates, screws, and related devices are available to reconstruct unstable fractures. Again, the most important principles are to reduce the fractures accurately and to stabilize them mechanically. Unwanted motion at the fracture site may lead to malunion or nonunion (Fig. 106-6). Where possible, the plate should be affixed to the tensile side of the bone. Minimal disruption of periosteal or vascular tissues is recommended.

An appreciation of the long-term effects of device implantation is crucial to the treatment of fractures with open

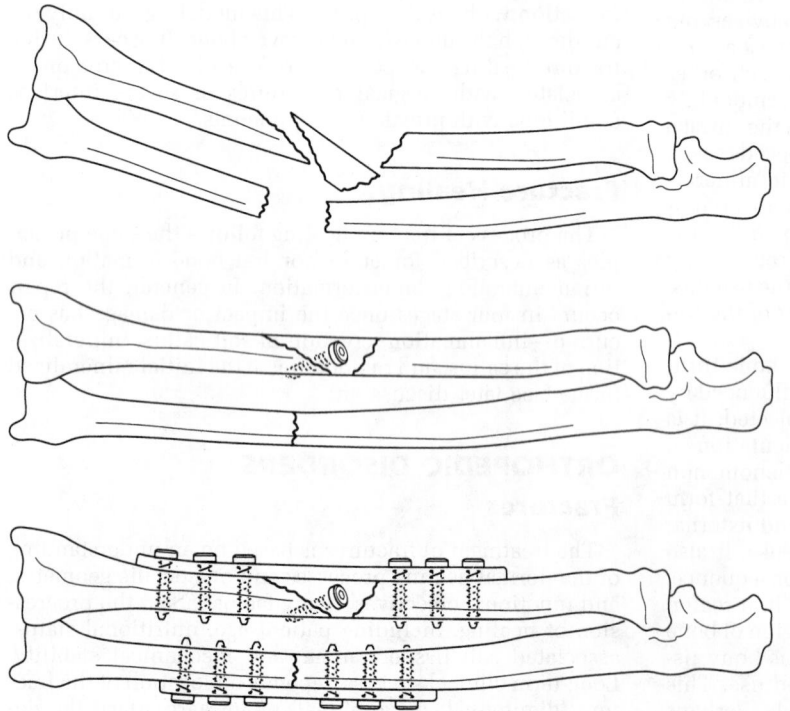

Figure 106-6. Internal fixation for a comminuted fracture of both bones of the forearm. The fractures were reduced with a combination on interfragmentary screws and compression plates and screws.

reduction and internal fixation. From a mechanical point of view, a bone and affixed implant are considered as a single composite structure. Because the fracture fixation plate is rigid stainless steel, the combined structure is significantly resistant to deformation. As a result, the bone is shielded from a proportion of the load that is normally transmitted through it during function. According to Wolff's law, bone tends to demineralize in the region beneath the plate. This phenomenon has led some surgeons to remove the devices after fracture healing in younger and more active patients. Consequently, the holes remaining after removal of the screws are themselves significant weakening defects in the bone, which may lead to refracture at a distance away from the original fracture site. This dilemma, together with the frequency of inaccurate application of the techniques, the occurrence of osteomyelitis, and the required disruption of the blood-rich periosteal tissue and initial hematoma, have limited the use of these devices to the forearm and hand and to metaphyseal fractures.

Treatment for diaphyseal fractures (particularly tibial, femoral, and humeral fractures) uses intramedullary fracture-fixation devices.[9] Previously, many of these fractures were treated with 6 weeks of traction followed by cast immobilization for 6 months to 1 year, at which time healing could be determined radiographically. The use of intramedullary rods allows early weight bearing and requires minimal immobilization of the joints above and below the fracture. Little long-term remodeling (loss of bone) has been documented. Rehabilitation is rapid, and blood loss is minimized. For simple transverse or oblique closed fractures, the infection rate is nearly zero. The introduction of intramedullary nails with provisions for proximal and distal fixation of the fracture fragments has extended the indications for this technique. Fractures close to the metaphyseal and diaphyseal junctions can be treated in this manner without compromising rotational stability. When used to treat segmented or comminuted fractures or other unstable fractures with proximal and distal bone loss, interlocking allows for a surgical reestablishment of the bone compartment and therefore limb length (Fig. 106-7). The device can maintain length until the fracture is healed. Although this technique is the optimal treatment for most fractures of the femoral shaft, applying these same principles to the tibia has not resulted in such dependable results. The blood supply for the tibia is less redundant, and the tibia is covered with less vascular soft tissue. For the femur, considerable intramedullar reaming before nail insertion ensures that a large, strong nail can be used to maximize fixation stability while preserving an adequate residual vascular supply for good healing (because of the redundant supply and massive vascular-rich tissue cuff). Reaming of the tibia results in an increased incidence of infection and nonunion and is not recommended if the fracture was open and contaminated.

Fractures Involving Joint Surfaces

For joints to last a lifetime without developing degenerative arthritis or posttraumatic arthritis, the natural precise joint surface geometrics must be preserved. These geometries work in concert with the ligaments and surrounding capsule to provide physiologic contact stresses at any functional joint position. The precision of normal anatomy provides a harmonious incongruity of the joint surfaces and maximizes physiologic nutrition and lubrication.

Any fracture that enters the joint and displaces the fracture fragments grossly disturbs this relation. Minimal displacements of articular surfaces relative to each other have profound effects on maximal contact stresses and on the nature of the contact stress distributions during joint artic-

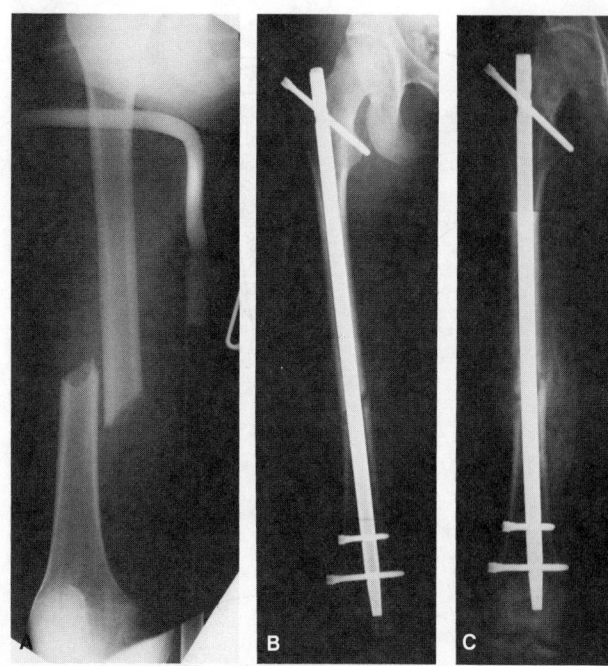

Figure 106-7. (*A*) Radiograph of a femoral shaft fracture with significant comminution. (*B*) The fracture was reduced with traction during surgery and was stabilized with an interlocking intermedullary nail. (*C*) The fracture healed rapidly, and both length and anatomic position were preserved.

ulation. Because the overwhelming importance of perfect joint geometry has been recognized in the last decade, major changes have occurred in the treatment of fractures that extend into joints. For more than two decades, displaced fractures of the malleoli of the ankle have been treated by open anatomic reduction and internal fixation. Excellent results with these fractures have supported efforts to apply the same treatment philosophy to fractures involving the tibial plateau. Elevating punched-down portions of the tibial plateau is expected to greatly improve long-term results (Fig. 106-8). There is a similar tendency to perform open reduction and internal fixation of fractures of the radius in the wrist of younger patients.

Owing to the success of aggressive surgical approach to fractures of other joints in the last decade, large operations are properly and routinely performed to restore the normal anatomy of the acetabulum for many fractures and fracture dislocations. The rationale is that restoring normal acetabular geometry allows the opposing articular cartilages to bear loads and slide past each other normally. Similarly, restoring the fracture fragments frequently leads to normal ligamentous geometry and thus to normal joint kinematics. Open surgical anatomic reduction, restoration of normal joint geometry, and strong effective internal fixation have greatly improved the functional expectations for the young person with a displaced fracture extending into the joint.[10] Although reduction and internal fixation of acetabulum fractures may not be able to indefinitely delay posttraumatic arthritis of the hip, the healed, reduced, and nearly anatomic bony pelvis around the hip socket provides a satisfactory base for future implantation of total hip replacement acetabular components.

Fracture Fixation Objectives

In summary, the major orthopedic objectives of fracture management are anatomic reduction and fixation stability. Because of the propensity for children's fractures to heal

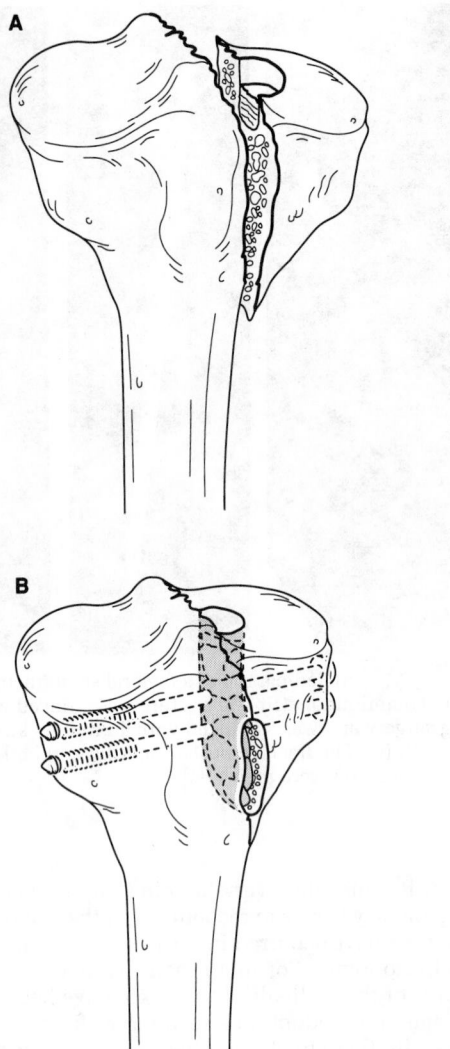

Figure 106-8. (*A*) Fracture of the lateral tibial plateau with significant inferior and lateral displacement and a punched-down region. (*B*) Accurate reduction, elevation of the punched-down region, support of the bone graft through a cortical window, and secure fixation should improve the chances for long-term joint function.

rapidly, the bulk of the discussion has been related to treating fractures in adults. Most fractures in children are treated with cast immobilization, thus avoiding the potential hazards of surgical intervention. In addition, both fracture repair and extensive remodeling occur rapidly in children because of the systemic effects of biochemical factors related to the accelerated bone formation associated with growth. Similarly, simple fractures in adults are treated with cast immobilization, particularly those involving the upper extremities.

When open reduction and internal fixation treatment are chosen, the following principles should be considered:

- Maximal maintenance of periosteal and vascular tissues without compromising stability
- Anatomic reduction and fixation stability
- The use of high-strength biocompatible implants
- The creation of fixation constructs that minimize load shielding of the underlying bone
- Maintenance of maximal soft tissue coverage and interposition between the device and skin surface

Limb-Length Discrepancy

One of the most problematic musculoskeletal conditions addressed by orthopedic surgeons is limb-length discrepancy. Whether due to polio, childhood trauma, genetic defect, or other causes, any growth-plate dysfunction leading to a limb-length discrepancy of more than 2 cm results in emotional and social losses for the individual. Efforts to lengthen limbs have been marked by serious complications and poor success rates. Osteotomy and large-gauge pin placement with subsequent elongation have been associated with unexplained hypertension, pin tract infections, and a high rate of nonunion.

Ilizarov Wire and Frame Treatment

A new and effective technique for limb-lengthening has been developed by Professor Ilizarov of Kurgan, Commonwealth of Independent States, who used firm, stable fixation of proximal and distal portions of a bone.[11,12] An encircling metal hoop with multiple small-diameter pins is mechanically placed under strong tension. Two or more pins may be placed through the bone at almost any location.

Pin placement is performed closed under image-intensifier control. A metaphyseal corticotomy is then performed through one or more small incisions, with minimal damage to the periostium and metaphyseal trabecular bone. After careful selective cortical weakening, the bone is broken in a controlled, careful manner so that the planes of the fracture are minimally separated. The periosteal and medullary blood supply are maximally preserved. Both the proximal and distal fragments are firmly maintained in position by the multiple small pins attached under tension to the strong rings that encircle the limb (Fig. 106-9).

After a short delay, the threaded extension mechanism is used to distract the segments of the bone proximal and distal to the corticotomy. The usual rate of distraction is four evenly spaced 0.25-mm adjustments per day. As the fracture separates with time, a striated density of immature bone is evident by radiography. The rate of distraction is adjusted to maintain lengthening progress while continuing to produce new bone between the bone segments. Continued weight bearing leads to a maturation of the new bone. When sufficient strength of the new bone is achieved, the frame is removed. Systematic complications, nonunion, or infections have been few. Rarely is supplementary bone grafting required.

This method has most often been applied to the femur or tibia to treat limb-length discrepancy and angular deformities, although many other sites can be treated using this modality. In segmental bone loss, this method is the treatment of choice, used in transporting a segment to fill a gap.

Mechanically Damaged Joints

Total Joint Replacement Arthroplasty

Many diseases, posttraumatic states, and conditions damage major joints and lead to pain and disability. Among these are osteoarthritis or degenerative joint disease, rheumatoid arthritis, osteonecrosis, posttraumatic arthritis, and a host of other serious abnormalities. There are many orthopedic approaches to these problems, but total joint replacement arthroplasty has earned a dominant role. The significant pain and functional limitations associated with mechanical disruption of the anatomy, loss of articular cartilage, widespread development of osteophytes, and progressive cyst formation can be relieved for many years by total joint replacement.

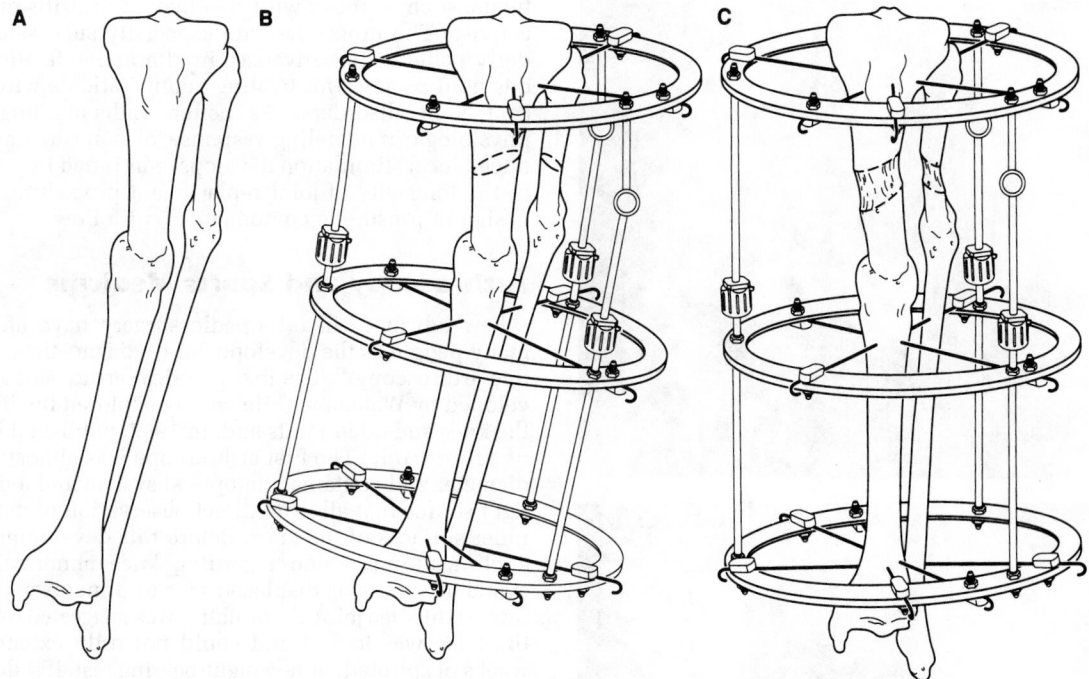

Figure 106-9. (*A*) Schematic depiction of fractures of the tibia and fibula with unacceptable shortening and a varus deformity. (*B*) The use of the Ilizarov technique, proximal corticotomies, and appropriate positioning of external fixator rings with the transfixation pins allow slow distraction for limb length and angular correction. (*C*) The angular deformity and length discrepancy were both corrected, allowing complete healing of the histogenesis site.

More than 25 years ago, Charnley[13] defined the scientific principles on which successful total joint arthroplasty depends. He emphasized low-friction bearing surfaces, the use of biocompatible materials, and intimate interfacing of the implants with bone using methylmethacrylate bone cement (Fig. 106-10). Although the principles were focused on the design and use of total hip arthroplasties, they proved applicable to developing other joint implants. Significant technological advancements in both the biomaterials and the manufacturing processes have led to dramatic improvements in total joint replacement surgery during the past 20 years. These advances include the following:

- Use of high-fatigue–strength biocompatible metallic alloys (titanium vanadium aluminum alloy and chrome cobalt molybdenum alloy)
- Low-friction articulating surfaces made from polished metal alloys opposed to a high-molecular-weight polyethylene-matched surface
- Articular surface designs that provide nearly normal ranges of motion while minimizing constraints that might subject the interface surfaces to high mechanical stresses
- Smooth geometric shapes that better match the anatomic regions in which they will be implanted
- Use of precise surgical instrumentation to create more consistent alignment and fit of the components in the recipient bones
- Improved bone surface preparation (removal of debris, reduction in bleeding) to improve penetration and interdigitation of the cement for more durable fixation

These advancements have significantly improved the longevity of artificial joints, particularly hip and knee prostheses, which are by far the most common (Fig. 106-11). Despite these advances, the procedure is still considered primarily for elderly patients. Total knee and hip prostheses have a fixation life expectancy of about 15 years or more in many patients.[14,15] Because revision total joint replacement is much less successful, total joint procedures are most frequently appropriate for patients 60 years and older. Although there are more than 200,000 implantations performed each year in the United States, many young patients with traumatic arthritis, osteonecrosis, and other conditions are unable to be treated because of the limited life expectancy of the implants.

The major failure of total joint arthroplasties is aseptic mechanical loosening at the interface between the bone, cement, and implant. Factors that contribute to loosening include excess weight, high activity level, component misalignment, and breakdown of the cement interface. A major scientific endeavor during the past 15 years has been to improve the fixation of implants by replacing the bone cement, which is known to be an inferior structural material. The most important potential advance, and one that has demonstrated some clinical success already, is the use of porous surface coated prostheses that promote biologic tissue ingrowth and fixation of the implants.[16,17] This has been made possible by manufacturing techniques that microweld small spheric beads, woven titanium wires, or sputtered metal fragments onto the surface of an implant. The sizes and shapes of the particles are selected to coat the surface with pore spaces between 100 and 500 μm in diameter, the optimal size as determined by in vivo experiments (Fig. 106-12). The implants are designed to be inserted surgically into carefully prepared bone under conditions of interference fit (tight intimate contact). It is proposed that significant bone tissue infiltration into the porous surface will begin within 8 to 12 weeks, and that after an appropriate amount of time (perhaps 1 year) long-term equilibrium bone remodeling will result in a well-fixed bone ingrowth interface that lasts for years.

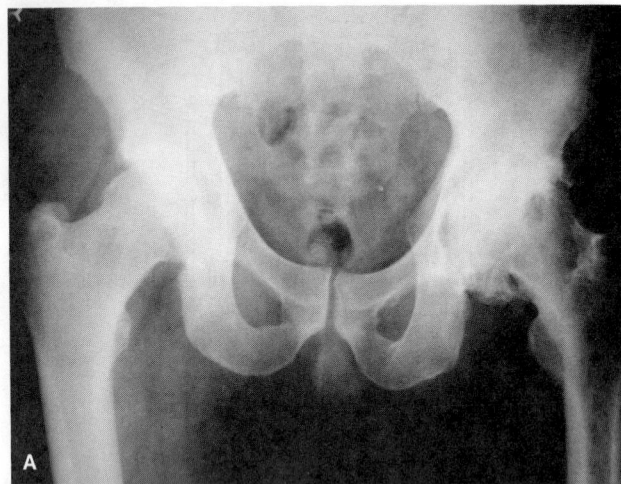

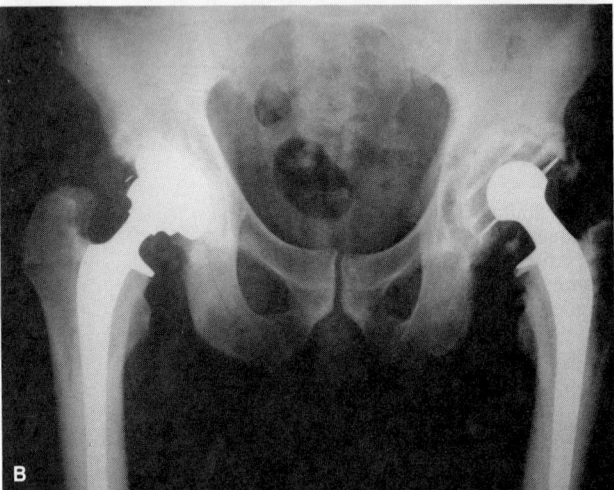

Figure 106-10. (*A*) Radiograph of patient with severe degenerative arthritis of the hip. (*B*) Cemented total hip arthroplasty is expected to provide this patient with pain-free, nearly normal hip function for more than 10 years.

Clinical data have been inconsistent. Although many acetabular components and femoral knee components have demonstrated secure ingrowth, femoral components of hips and tibial trays have been less successful. Two factors are important to secure fixation. First, the implant must be fixed rigidly within the bone during the initial ingrowth period. If micromotion occurs at the interface (probably greater than 150 μm), fibrous tissue fills the pores instead of bone, and the implant is likely to become loose and painful. Second, the local mechanical environment must promote a positive remodeling response of the supporting trabecular bone. If the local mechanical environment stimulates maintenance or hypertrophy of the supporting bone (as dictated by Wolff's law), long-term fixation may be realized. To be universally successful and to benefit the younger patient population, the implants must be significantly better than cemented devices. Because cemented implants may already last 10 to 20 years, it is difficult to evaluate the efficacy of alternative fixation techniques.

In summary, total joint replacement is one of the most significant advances for treating painful, degenerative joints. Hip and knee joint replacements have been more successful than shoulder, elbow, and other joint devices, although these are still viable treatments for selected pa-

tients, such as those with rheumatoid arthritis or limited activity. The procedures are especially successful for elderly patients, but advances in alternative fixation methods hold promise for treating young patients with significant joint disorders. As better understanding of the physiologic remodeling response of bone to implant-induced local stimulation develops, continued improvement in the longevity of joint replacement procedures and the design of prosthetic components will follow.

Arthroscopy and Sports Medicine

Few advances in orthopedic surgery have affected as many people as the development of diagnostic and operative arthroscopy.[18] The first practical arthroscope was developed by Watanabe.[19] He widely explored the interior of the knee and other joints and, in 1957, published his *Atlas of Arthroscopy*. The first arthroscope was almost 5 mm in diameter and contained an optical system and a fiberoptic light source that allowed direct observation of most of the inner surfaces of the knee. Before this development, only a clinical impression regarding knee abnormality was available. A major displaced tear of a meniscus or other important knee joint abnormality was suggested only when the knee was locked and could not fully extend after 3 weeks of splinted, non–weight-bearing rest, if it developed recurrent effusions, or if the response to flexing, maximal internal rotation, or maximal external rotation sustained with extension caused a palpable or audible clunk and severe knee joint pain. A diagnosis of internal derangement of the knee leads to a decision for exploratory arthrotomy. Unfortunately, tears of lesser severity and other knee joint abnormalities produced less severe symptoms, and often an anatomic diagnosis was not possible. Patients were sometimes treated conservatively for months before a surgical exploration provided the necessary information to surgically correct the problem. With the advent of arthrog-

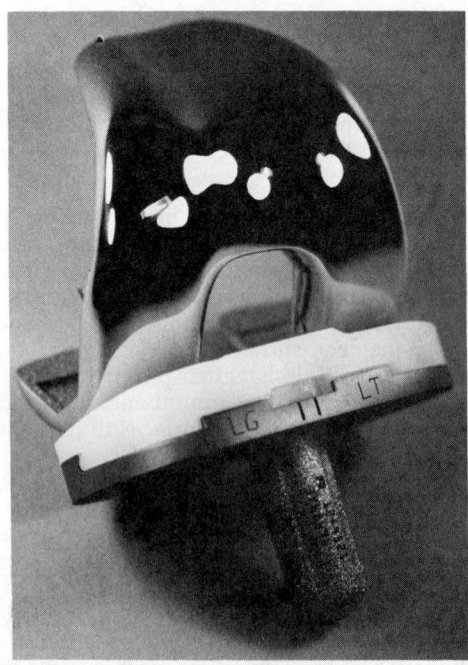

Figure 106-11. Example of a typical total knee joint arthroplasty. Similar to many available devices, the implant demonstrates a highly polished chrome cobalt molybdenum alloy femoral component that articulates against a high-molecular-weight polyethylene insert on the tibial component.

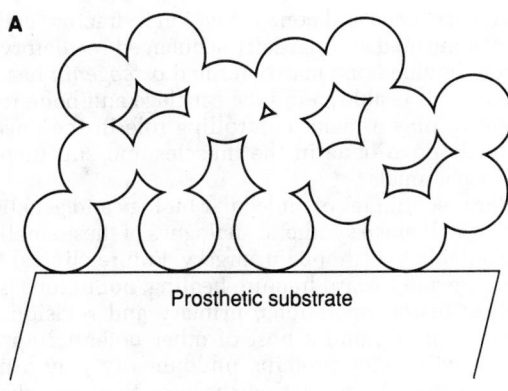

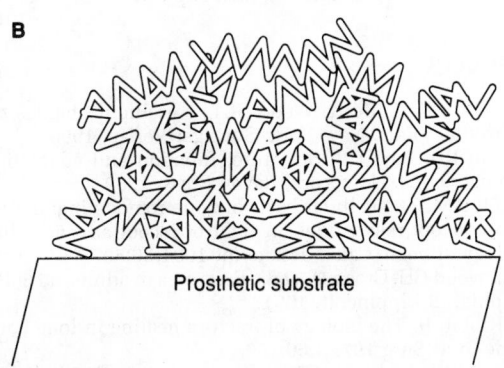

Figure 106-12. An alternative method of fixation of artificial joint components involves the use of porous surface coatings, promoting bony ingrowth for biologic fixation. Two examples of surfaces that are manufactured to produce a porous surface are microwelding of small beads (*A*) and cold diffusion of titanium wire mesh (*B*). The dimensions of the surface provide pore spaces of 100 to 500 μm.

raphy, the introduction of air and a radiographic contrast medium frequently documented a previously undiagnosed abnormality by fluoroscopy or confirming radiographs. In addition, a negative arthrogram prevented many unnecessary exploratory knee arthrotomies.

The value of arthrography depends on the skill, interest, and persistence of the radiologist. Routine arthrograms often were indeterminate, and clinical correlation was necessary since a tear or other injury could not be ruled out. If the symptoms and disability were severe enough to warrant anesthesia or to produce a small risk of infection and other infrequent surgical complications, then arthroscopy by a skilled surgeon could make a definitive anatomic diagnosis in more than 90% of cases. A correct structural or biologic diagnosis would then guide the physician to a rational treatment. It became apparent that smaller arthroscopes could allow access to other previously unapproachable joints. Arthroscopy as pioneered for the knee could also be applied to the shoulder, ankle, hip, wrist, and even the joints of the hand. Arthroscopes with diameters of less than 2 mm were made. Their small size and many angles of view made it possible to clearly visualize the posterior attachments of the knee's menisci and to examine smaller joints more completely.

Operative Arthroscopy

Surgical tools and techniques were developed quickly. Using the arthroscope, one additional portal into the knee joint, and newly developed small instruments, complete or partial meniscectomies could be done readily with little damage to the remainder of the knee structures. Treatment of meniscal injuries is best done arthroscopically. Similarly, loose bodies that had previously required open arthrotomy for removal are more easily treated with arthroscopic instrumentation. If they are too large for removal using the standard small, delicate arthroscopy instrumentation, a small, directed arthrotomy can be performed and arthroscopically directed open loose-body removal easily accomplished.

The value of the intact meniscus as a load-sharing structure was recognized almost at the same time it could be dependably visualized and excised. The menisci were demonstrated to be load-bearing structures that could distribute the loads to broad areas of the tibial plateau throughout the knee's range of flexion–extension or axial tibial and internal or external rotation. Thus, they prevented potentially damaging high-contact stresses during athletic and other activities. Some surgeons felt it was inappropriate to remove these structures and began to consider repairing torn menisci. Although much has been written about the complications and successes with repair of torn joint semilunar cartilages, indications, techniques, and outcomes need to be more fully defined before recommendations can be made.[20]

Early diagnostic and therapeutic successes have stimulated orthopedic arthroscopists to approach other more difficult abnormalities. The loose osteochondral fragment of osteochondritis dissecans can easily be observed, evaluated, and either removed or replaced into its previous location. The recipient cavity can be curetted and drilled to encourage more vascular ingrowth or otherwise prepared for return and fixation of the fragment. Anatomic fragment fixation with pegs, pins, or screws has repeatedly been accomplished with arthroscopic visualization. Arthroscopy is unquestionably the most effective method for diagnosing and treating knee ligament injuries. Previously, there was no certainty that there was a torn ligament, or how many, or whether the tears were complete. With arthroscopy, ligament injuries can be diagnosed with certainty on the day of the injury or shortly thereafter and reparative surgical treatment initiated. With better instruments and extensive experience, surgeons can definitively repair many severely injured knees using arthroscopic techniques.

Complete tears of the anterior cruciate ligament of the knees are devastating injuries. The resulting anteroposterior instability greatly increases the stress on other knee structures, particularly under fully loaded, flexed, and rotational motions. Often, there is a secondary tear of the medial or lateral meniscus, increased instability, and the early development of posttraumatic degenerative arthritis. The arthroscope allows immediate and certain diagnosis of anterior cruciate ligament tears and is a valuable tool in operative reconstruction of function. Using small external incisions, special drilling guides, and the arthroscope, strong bone-ligament-bone grafts may be placed in an anatomic location. These ligament grafts may be obtained from the patient's own patellar tendon or from autologous sources. Considerable increased stability is often achieved, allowing patients to return to high-level sports activities.

The small size of the incision, the clear visualization of the interior of the joint, and the ability to perform definitive surgical corrections with minimal damage to other structures often allow almost immediate rehabilitation. Muscular atrophy due to extensive immobilization and lack of weight bearing is prevented. The neuromuscular coordination and skills so important to the athlete are not forgotten. These advantages are crucial to the varsity and professional athlete, but they are of nearly equal importance to the laborer or the community athlete. Increased experience and further technical advances are likely to bring the same successes to the treatment of injuries and disease of other joints such as the shoulder and wrist.

Growth Factors and Other Small-Protein Cytokines

No effort to describe the scientific foundations of modern orthopedic surgery would be complete without discussing the potential effects of a family of small proteins on bone formation. These proteins are loosely referred to as *growth factors* or *cytokines*. Bone formation in vivo results from migration of bone progenitor mesenchymal cells to the area of interest. A poorly understood chemotactic mechanism is active in directing this migration. These mesenchymal stem cells then undergo rapid mitosis, forming the undifferentiated cell mass that becomes bone. Finally, under the influence of one or more of these controlling natural proteins, differentiation to cartilage and then to bone matrix occurs. Mineralization and remodeling complete this important natural process.

In many circumstances, it would be desirable to artificially initiate and manipulate this process. Control of this scheme could hasten fracture healing and potentially eliminate nonunions. Attempts at arthrodesis, particularly spine fusions, could be nearly assured of success. Proximal focal femoral deficiency or congenital pseudarthrosis of the tibia might be effectively treated. Similarly, conditions in which excess bone is formed in nonphysiologic regions could be controlled (eg, the heterotopic bone formation of spastic paraplegia or burns or a similar condition after revision total joint arthroplasty).

Orthopedists have long recognized that bone grafting greatly improves the chances of success in the treatment of nonunions. Fresh autologous trabecular bone has the greatest success, whereas fresh, freeze-dried, or irradiated allogenic bone graft material is less beneficial. A scientific explanation for the benefits of bone grafting has been slow to evolve and only recently has the identification, isolation, purification, and characterization of a family of growth factors expanded our understanding of these processes and provided an opportunity for therapeutic control.

Urist and coworkers[21] were among the first to work successfully in this field. They defined the problem and isolated a protein called *bone morphogenetic protein*, from masses of bovine bones. The extraction, separation, and purification processes are difficult, and only small amounts of the mostly purified material have been available. Yet this small protein (18.5 kd) has been demonstrated to induce cartilage and bone formation in muscle-derived mesenchymal cells. In vivo experiments have been successful in inducing bone when control animals develop none.

Similar proteins have been demonstrated to directly or indirectly influence bone induction. Platelet-derived growth factor has been derived from platelets and macrophages. It has been shown to induce migration and mitosis of mesenchymal cells in wounds and to enhance cartilage and bone formation in adult rats. Fibroblast growth factor is a mitogenic and angiogenic protein that favors new bone formation, particularly if neovascularization is required. Transforming growth factor β is secreted from bone cell cultures. This 25,000 molecular weight protein can be isolated and appears to be naturally released from platelets at the time of a fracture. It stimulates proliferation of osteoblasts and increases their production of collagen. Transforming growth factor β may be responsible for partial reg-

ulation of cartilage and bone formation in fracture callus.[22] Finally, a purified and partially sequenced regulatory protein from bovine bone matrix termed *osteogenin* has been isolated.[23,24] It is able to induce cartilage and bone formation and to play a major controlling role in the development of de novo bone in the muscles and subcutaneous tissue of mammals.

Modern techniques of molecular biology and genetic engineering will make synthetic analogues of these small proteins available to orthopedic surgery. Future clinical trials will be directed toward fracture healing, nonunions, spine and other fusion operations, primary and revision total joint arthroplasty, and a host of other potential applications. Growth factor proteins undoubtedly play a major controlling role in regulating the growth plate, shaping the developing condylar articular surfaces, wound healing, and other normal, abnormal, and reparative processes.

REFERENCES

1. Mow VC, Ratcliffe A, Wood SLY, eds. Biomechanics of diarthrodial joints. New York, Springer-Verlag, 1990.
2. Martin RB, Burr DB. Structure, function and adaptation of compact bone. New York, Raven Press, 1989.
3. Parfitt AM. The cellular basis of bone remodeling: the quantum concept reexamined in light of recent advances in cell biology of bone. Calcif Tissue Int 1984;36:537.
4. Rockwood CH, Green DP, eds. Fractures in adults, ed 3. Philadelphia, JB Lippincott, 1991.
5. McKibbin B. The biology of fracture healing in long bones. J Bone Joint Surg 1978B;60:150.
6. Gustilo RB, Anderson JT. Prevention of infection in the treatment of one thousand and twenty-five open fractures of long bones: retrospective and prospective analyses. J Bone Joint Surg 1976A;58:453.
7. Perren SM, Huggler A, Russenberger M, Straumann F, Muller ME, Allgower M. A method of measuring the change in compression applied to living cortical bone. Acta Orthop Scand 1969;125(Suppl):7.
8. Perren SM, Huggler A, Russenberger M, Straumann F, Muller ME, Allgower M. The reaction of cortical bone to compression. Acta Orthop Scand 1969;125(Suppl):19.
9. Winquist RA, Hansen ST Jr., Clawson DK. Closed intramedullary nailing of femoral fractures: a report of five hundred and twenty cases. J Bone Joint Surg 1984A;66:529.
10. Letournel E. Acetabular fractures: classification and management. Clin Orthop 1980;151:81.
11. Ilizarov GA. The tension–stress effect of the genesis and growth of tissues. I: the influence of stability of fixation and soft-tissue preservation. Clin Orthop 1989;238:249.
12. Ilizarov GA. The tension–stress effect on the genesis and growth of tissues. II: the influence of the rate and frequency of distraction. Clin Orthop 1989;239:263.
13. Charnley J, Capii Z. The nine and ten year results of the low friction arthroplasty of the hip. Clin Orthop 1973;95:9.
14. Scuderi GR, Insall JN, Windsor RE, Moran MC. Survivorship of cemented knee replacements. J Bone Joint Surg 1989B;71:798.
15. Rand JA, Dorr CA, eds. Total arthroplasty of the knee: proceedings of the knee society 1985–1986. Rockville, MA, Aspen Systems, 1986.
16. Hungerford DS, Krackow KA, Kenna RV. Cementless total knee replacement in patients 50 years old and under. Orthop Clin North Am 1989;20:131.
17. Fitzgerald RH. Non-cemented total hip arthroplasty. New York, Raven Press, 1988.
18. Johnson LL. Creating the proper environment for arthroscopic surgery. Orthop Clin North Am 1982;13:283.
19. Watanabe M. Arthroscopy: the present state. Orthop Clin North Am 1979;10:505.
20. Graf B, Docter T, Clancy W Jr. Arthroscopic meniscal repair. Clin Sports Med 1987;6:525.
21. Urist MR, De Lange RJ, Finerman GAM. Bone cell differentiation and growth factors. Science 1983;220:680.
22. Joyce ME, Terek RM, Jingushi S, Bolander ME. Role of trans-

forming growth factor β in fracture repair. Ann NY Acad Sci 1990;593:107.

23. Reddi AH, Weintraub S, Muthukumanan N. Biologic principles of bone induction. Orthop Clin North Am 1987;18:207.

24. Reddi AH, Shushan MA, Cunningham NS. Induction and maintenance of new bone formation by growth and differentiation. Ann Chir Gynaecol 1988;77:189.

SURGERY: SCIENTIFIC PRINCIPLES AND PRACTICE, Second Edition, edited by Lazar J. Greenfield, Michael W. Mulholland, Keith T. Oldham, Gerald B. Zelenock, and Keith D. Lillemoe. Lippincott–Raven Publishers, Philadelphia, © 1997.

CHAPTER 107

SURGERY OF THE HAND

BRIAN J. SENNETT AND FELIX H. SAVOIE

Hand injuries are common occurrences, reflecting the constant use of the hands in the home and workplace. To treat these injuries and pathologic conditions, a surgeon must understand not only the pathology but also the inherent function of the hand, which allows it to perform its varied tasks.

The primary functions of the hand are sensation and grasp. Sensation is critical to the hand's performance; without it, pinching, picking up objects, and holding them are difficult. Grasping is accomplished through a combination of strength and mobility. Any deficit results in disability. It is only through a thorough understanding of function and pathology that the involved hand can be adequately addressed.

FUNCTIONAL ANATOMY

Understanding the anatomy of the hand is the key to managing pathologic conditions. The nomenclature used to refer to the hand includes the terms *ulnar* and *radial* (not medial and lateral) and *volar* and *dorsal* (not anterior and posterior).

The bones of the hand form its foundation and consist of 8 carpal bones (4 in the proximal row, 4 in the distal row), 5 metacarpals, and 14 phalanges (3 in each finger, 2 in the thumb). These bones are oriented to form longitudinal and transverse arches in the hand which are architectural prerequisites to gripping, pinching, and cupping. These motions are controlled by the musculature of the upper extremities, which exert force upon the bones by tendinous insertions.

The extrinsic flexor tendons that exert these forces are encompassed by fibrous sheaths to prevent bowstringing and to improve mechanical function. Thickening of these sheaths results in pulleys that resist the tendency for tendons to bowstring in the most vulnerable regions. These flexor tendons pass across the volar side of the wrist within the carpal tunnel, a confined space formed by the carpal bones and the transverse carpal ligament. Through this tunnel pass nine flexor tendons and the median nerve. The median nerve provides sensation to the radial three and one half digits of the hand while the ulnar nerve provides sensation to the ulnar one and one half digits of the hand. The ulnar nerve enters the hand through the Guyon canal and provides innervation to 15 of the 20 intrinsic hand

muscles; the remainder of the intrinsic muscles are supplied by the median nerve (Fig. 107-1).

Examination of the dorsum of the hand reveals the extensor tendons, which are divided into six compartments as they cross the wrist (Fig. 107-2). These tendons insert distally to provide extension of the digits. The innervation of the dorsum of the hand is via the dorsal radial sensory nerve radially and the dorsal sensory branch of the ulnar nerve ulnarly.

Each of the fingers has four joints. These include the distal interphalangeal (DIP) joint, proximal interphalangeal (PIP) joint, metacarpophalangeal (MCP) joint, and carpometacarpal (CMC) joint.

The thumb only has three joints (CMC, MCP, and interphalangeal joint). Knowing the optimal position at which joints are immobilized is important when treating injuries to prevent contractures and to allow the recovery of an optimal range of motion. This position places the wrist in 30 degrees of extension, the MCP joints in 70 degrees of flexion, and the IP joints in extension.

The blood supply of the hand is via the radial and ulnar arteries. In the hand, they form a superficial and deep palmar arch from which the digital vessels arise (Fig. 107-3). Occluding both arteries and then releasing one allows the surgeon to evaluate the continuity of the arches (Allen test).

EVALUATION OF HAND INJURIES

An evaluation of the hand should be conducted in a fashion similar to that of an examination of any other area of the body. A thorough history is first obtained including the presenting complaint, evolution of the problem, and aggravating and relieving factors. In addition, one should ascertain the individual's age, gender, hand dominance, and occupation. Medical history and any preexisting conditions are often also helpful.

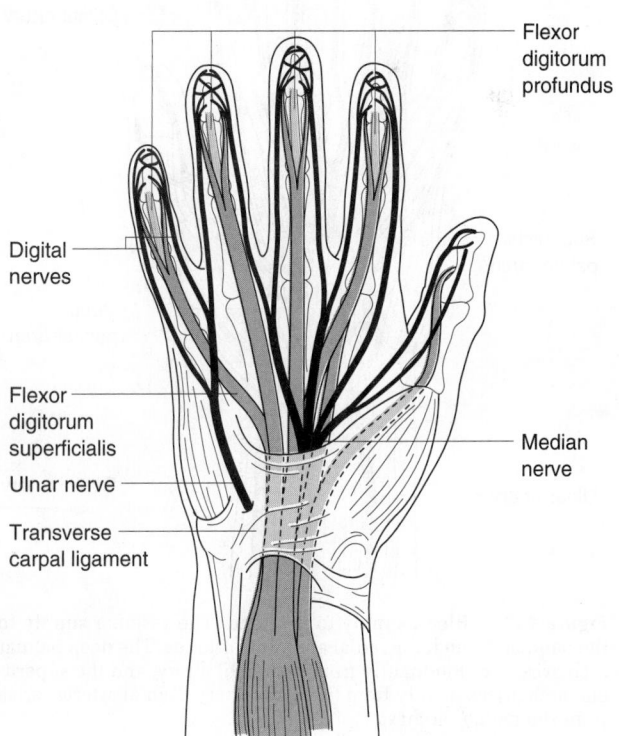

Figure 107-1. Volar anatomy of the hand and wrist.

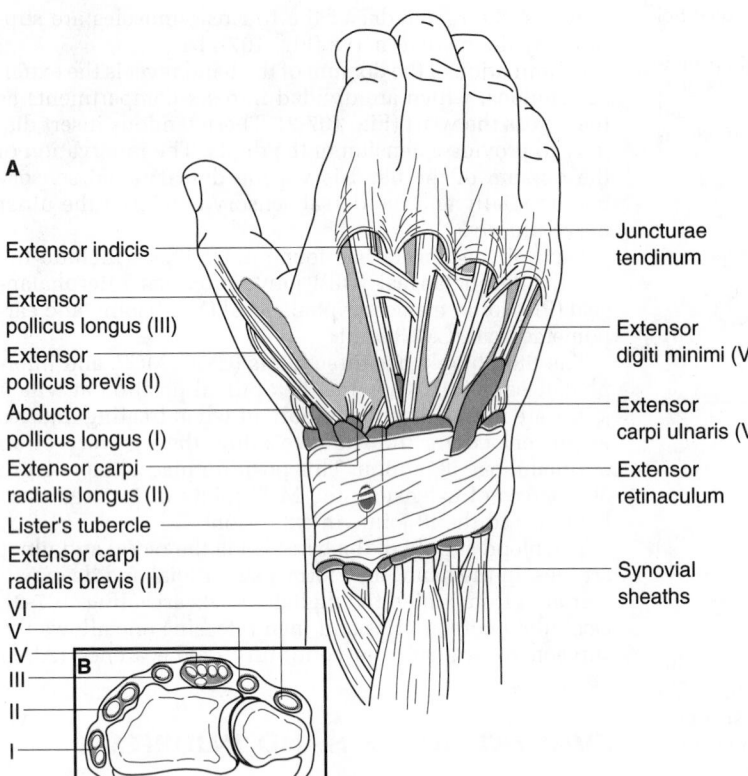

A

Extensor indicis

Extensor
pollicus longus (III)

Extensor
pollicus brevis (I)

Abductor
pollicus longus (I)

Extensor carpi
radialis longus (II)

Lister's tubercle

Extensor carpi
radialis brevis (II)

VI
V
IV
III
II
I

B

Juncturae
tendinum

Extensor
digiti minimi (V)

Extensor
carpi ulnaris (VI)

Extensor
retinaculum

Synovial
sheaths

Figure 107-2. Dorsal anatomy of the wrist. (*A*) The extensor tendons are divided into six compartments by the extensor retinaculum as they course across the dorsum of the wrist. (*B*) Cross-sectional view illustrates the compartmentalization and the relation to the radius and ulna.

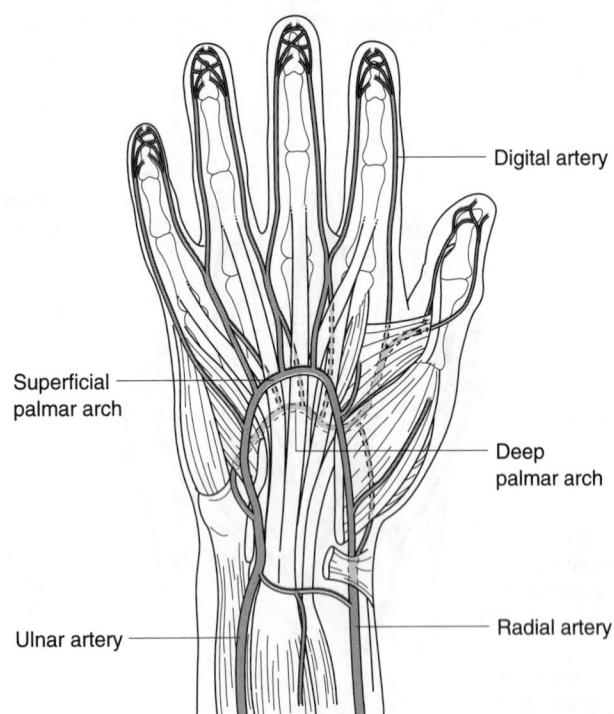

Digital artery

Superficial
palmar arch

Deep
palmar arch

Ulnar artery

Radial artery

Figure 107-3. Blood supply to the hand. The vascular supply to the hand is through the radial and ulnar arteries. The deep palmar arch arises predominantly from the radial artery, and the superficial arch arises mainly from the ulnar artery. Digital arteries arise from the palmar arches.

Physical examination should follow an orderly routine. This should include the evaluation of a patient's neck, shoulder, and elbow in addition to their forearm, wrist, and hand. Range of motion, strength, overall body habitus, muscle wasting, hypertrophy, deformities, skin changes, and areas of tenderness should all be documented. Capillary refill in the presence or absence of normal sweating patterns should be evaluated as well as the sensibility of the digits.

Radiographic examination should be considered essential and is performed on all injured extremities, regardless of the presenting complaint. More advanced testing such as electromyograms, nerve conduction studies, technetium bone scanning, computerized tomography, or magnetic resonance imaging can also be useful in evaluating the painful wrist and hand. Selective injections may also prove beneficial in determining the true etiology of a patient's pain.

NERVE INJURY AND DISEASE

Any nerve injury affecting the hand can be devastating because all nerves that supply the hand provide both sensory and motor innervation. Injuries of these nerves are generally confined to contusions, lacerations, and compressive syndromes and must be thoroughly examined to determine the cause and extent of the injury.

In evaluating nerve injuries, the examiner should first begin with a careful history of the injury. The mechanism of injury is often predictive of the structures involved and influences the prognosis. As an example, knife injuries usually lacerate every structure in their path while glass injuries can occasionally spare superficial structures and lacerate deeper ones. In contrast, crush injuries and gunshot wounds often result in significant initial neurologic findings, but recover with time.

Physical examination should include sensory evaluation of the entire hand, functional motor testing, and the presence of sweat. The absence of sweat indicates damage to the nerve innervating the involved area. Once the diagnosis of a possible nerve injury is made, the initial treatment is based on good wound care. This involves thorough irrigation, débridement of the wound edges, and closure of the wound if clean. Dressings and splints are then applied to protect the injured area.

The treatment of choice for a nerve laceration is early repair within 1 to 2 weeks with material at least as small as 8-0 nylon sutures. Lengthy delays in repairing a lacerated nerve can result in retraction of the nerve ends and result in the need for nerve grafting. Loupe magnification aids in nerve repair and is recommended. Immobilization is generally used for about 3 weeks, and axonal growth beyond the anastomosis site usually begins about 1 month postoperatively. Once axonal growth commences, it progresses at the rate of about 1 mm per day until full regeneration has occurred.

Sunderland has defined three degrees of nerve injuries—neurapraxia, axonotmesis, and neurotmesis. *Neurapraxia* is a first-degree injury in which there is a loss in axon conductivity without discontinuity. *Axonotmesis* is a second-degree injury in which axonal damage occurs but the endoneurium and perineurium remain intact. *Neurotmesis*, a third-degree injury, occurs when the nerve is completely disrupted. Contusions often result in neuropraxias whereas lacerations commonly involve disruption of the entire nerve (neurotmesis). In contrast, compressive syndromes can result in any of the three degrees of injury.

Median Nerve

The median nerve at the level of the wrist comprises about 90% sensory fascicles and 10% motor fascicles. Therefore, lacerations at this level result in a loss of sensation over the volar surface of the thumb, index, long, and radial half of the ring finger and loss of innervation of the thenar musculature. Following repair, recovery of sensation is usually adequate, but recovery of thenar muscle function is often suboptimal and requires tendon transfers to restore power and motion.

Carpal Tunnel Syndrome

Compression of the median nerve at the level of the wrist is commonly known as *carpal tunnel syndrome*. The carpal tunnel is formed by the unyielding carpal bones radi-

ally, ulnarly, and dorsally and the transverse carpal ligament volarly. The median nerve and nine flexor tendons pass through this tunnel at the level of the wrist. Any pathologic conditions that increase the pressure within the carpal tunnel results in compression of the median nerve. These conditions include nonspecific tenosynovitis, rheumatoid tenosynovitis, gout, amyloidosis, posttraumatic conditions such as Colles fractures and systemic conditions such as hypothyroidism, diabetes, obesity, pregnancy, and acromegaly.

Classic symptoms in carpal tunnel syndrome involve pain, numbness, and tingling in the median nerve distribution and occasionally weakness of the thenar musculature with symptoms often being worse at night. Physical examination often reveals decreased sensation in the median nerve distribution, a positive Tinel test over the carpal tunnel, and a positive Phalen test (increased symptoms with the wrist held in a palmar flexed position for 1 minute), and occasionally decreased thenar muscle strength. Electromyography (EMG) is often useful in establishing the diagnosis.

Conservative treatment includes the use of splints in a functional position, nonsteroidal antiinflammatory medications, and steroid injections into the carpal tunnel. All of these are directed at decreasing inflammation within the canal. If conservative management is unsuccessful, surgical decompression is necessary.

The two most common methods of carpal tunnel release include open and endoscopic techniques that release the transverse carpal ligament (Fig. 107-4). Open techniques involve a longitudinal or a transverse incision near the wrist crease. Orthopaedic surgeons favor a small longitudinal incision because it allows better definition of the entire course of the nerve and less chance of damage to the multiplicity of sensory branches to the skin of the palm. The transverse incision is more cosmetic when placed in the wrist crease, but does not allow for complete visualization of the transverse carpal ligament. Once an adequate skin incision is made, the median nerve is identified beneath the fascia of the volar forearm. A small dissector is used to free the nerve from any adhesions to the transverse carpal ligament and then kept in place while the ligament is released using a scalpel blade to protect the nerve. The nerve should be released along its ulnar border to avoid injuring the branch to the thenar musculature. The nerve should be released from the forearm through and including its branch points to the digits.

Endoscopic carpal tunnel release involves placing a slot-

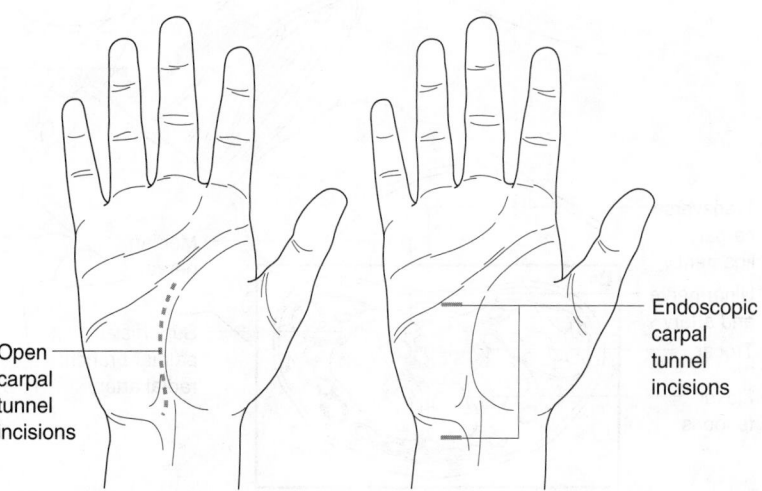

Open carpal tunnel incisions

Endoscopic carpal tunnel incisions

Figure 107-4. Carpal tunnel release incisions.

ted sheath and trocar within the carpal tunnel using one or two small incisions, replacing the trocar with a videoscope, visualizing the undersurface of the transverse carpal ligament through the slotted sheath, and releasing the ligament using specially designed cutting instruments (Fig. 107-5).

Both techniques result in excellent decompression of the median nerve. The benefits of the endoscopic technique include decreased initial palmar pain and a quicker return to activities and work. However, there is a slight increase in major nerve, artery, and tendon injuries compared with open techniques. Increased complication rates, when present, are often related to inexperience and poor training. As a result, the need for proper training in this technique can not be underestimated. The results of the two techniques at 3, 6, and 12 months are equivalent with overall excellent results.

Ulnar Nerve

The ulnar nerve also can be easily lacerated at the wrist because of its superficial location. Anesthesia usually results over the volar aspect of the small and ulnar half of the ring finger, whereas motor involvement affects the adductor pollicis, interossei muscles, and ulnar two lumbricals. This often result in a clawlike deformity of the hand due to the loss in intrinsic hand motor function. Like the median nerve, return of sensation to the ulnar nerve is often more successful than return of intrinsic hand function following repair of lacerations. As a result, tendon transfers are often required.

Compression of the ulnar nerve can occur at the Guyon canal in the wrist but is more commonly due to entrapment in the cubital tunnel at the elbow. When it occurs at the wrist, it can affect sensory only, motor only, or a combination of both. EMG is extremely helpful in pinpointing the location of compression since it is often unclear whether the lesion is occurring at the elbow or wrist. The most common cause of compression at the wrist are ganglions. Decompression of the ulnar nerve at the wrist is usually successful when a clear diagnosis has been made.

Radial Nerve

At the level of the wrist, injuries to the radial nerve affect its dorsal sensory branch, which provides sensation to the dorsum of the thumb and index finger. This nerve crosses the wrist radially in the region of the radial styloid and can often be lacerated and contused. Both can result in painful neuroma formation and decreased sensation and sometimes are unpredictable in their recovery. As a result, contusions are generally managed conservatively with exploration only being necessary in persistent cases.

Digital Nerves

Lacerations or displaced fractures can sometimes involve digital nerves. The key to managing these injuries is early diagnosis since they often do very well with early repair. The digit requires about 3 weeks of immobilization postoperatively. Axonal growth proceeds at a rate of 1 mm per day beginning about a month after repair. When there is a segmental loss of the digital nerve, a digital nerve graft can be used. The antebrachialcutaneous nerve, the sural nerve, or the terminal portion of the posterior interosseous nerve are useful for this purpose.

TENDON INJURY AND DISEASE

Tendon disorders are most likely due to lacerations, trauma, inflammatory conditions, and degenerative processes. They can affect the flexor or extensor tendons and can involve individual or multiple tendons.

Initial care of tendinous injuries involves a careful examination to determine the tendons affected. Repeated testing, the observation of the habitus of the joints, and specific tendon testing are crucial in identifying the exact pathology. The integrity of the wound dictates whether a primary or secondary tenorrhaphy will be performed. For open clean wounds, thorough irrigation, wound closure, immobilization, and prophylactic antibiotics should be instituted, followed by tendon repair within the next 7 to 10 days. For contaminated wounds, repair is delayed until the tendon bed is clean and the initial inflammatory stage has regressed.

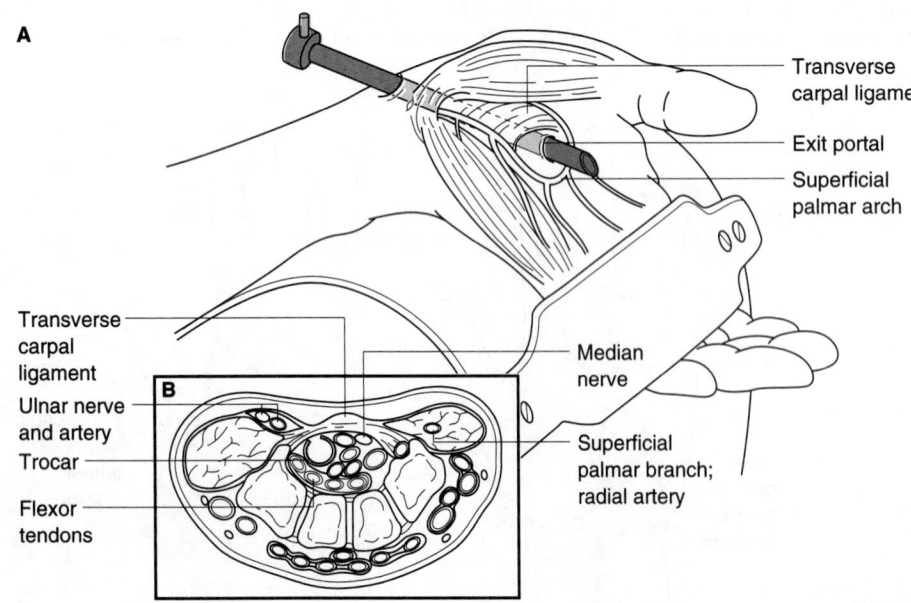

Figure 107-5. Endoscopic carpal tunnel release. (*A*) The endoscopic carpal tunnel sheath enters the wrist proximally through a small incision and exits the hand proximal to the superficial palmar arch. (*B*) Cross-sectional view demonstrates the relation between the trocar, transverse carpal ligament, and median nerve.

Adhesions are invaluable in the healing process but must be controlled to improve gliding while still providing vascularity to the healing tendon. Passive excursion of the tendons over a distance of 5 mm has been shown to have a beneficial effect on decreasing adhesion formation while not producing undue tension on the tendon repairs. Following the initial healing process (6 weeks), aggressive therapy is instituted to help remodel the scar tissue that has formed to allow the maximal range of motion to be regained.

Flexor Tendons

Flexor tendons of the fingers and thumb are divided into five different zones: zone 1 involves the area distal to the superficialis insertion; zone 2 (no man's land) includes the area between the MCP joint and the superficialis insertion; zone 3 involves the portion of the flexor tendons between the transverse carpal ligament and the MCP joint; zone 4 is the region of the carpal tunnel; and zone 5 is the area proximal to the transverse carpal ligament (Fig. 107-6).

Surgical repair of the flexor tendons is performed through Brunner zig-zag incisions to provide excellent exposure. The lacerated tendon ends are reapproximated and sutured together. A variety of repairs are described, but they are all similar in that they provide excellent purchase, minimize strangulation, avoid the dorsal blood supply of the tendon, and result in an extremely strong repair. Core sutures are generally 4-0 in diameter and are reinforced with a 6-0 epitendinous suture. Postoperatively, the repair is protected by splinting in flexion, while gentle limited passive motion decreases adhesion formation. Immobilization continues for about 4 weeks, followed by a controlled therapy program to regain motion and strength.

Flexor tendon repairs in zones 1, 3, 4, and 5 often are good, but the functional results involving zone 2 injuries are much less predictable because of tendon adhesions.

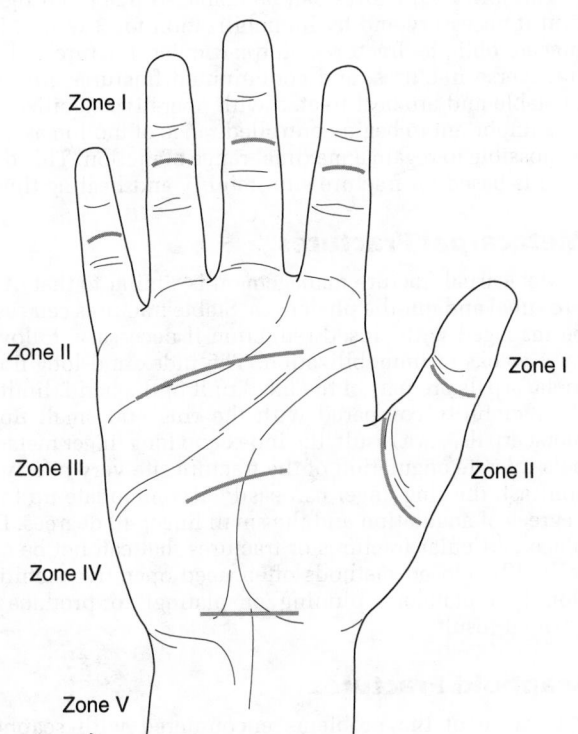

Figure 107-6. Zones of the flexor tendons.

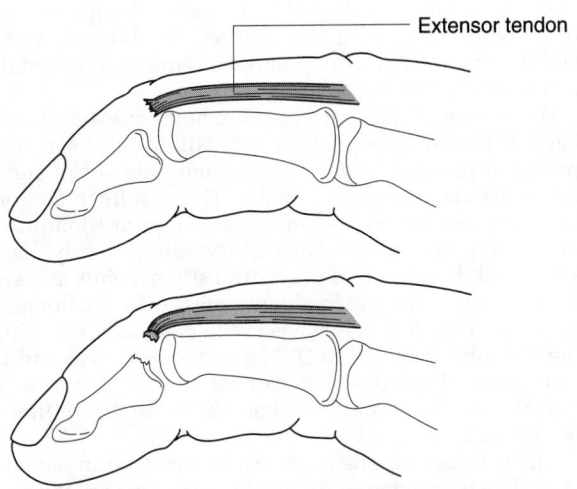

Figure 107-7. Mallet finger. Injury to the extensor tendon insertion can be caused by a rupture of the tendon (*top*) or an avulsion fracture (*bottom*) that results in a flexion deformity of the distal interphalangeal joint and the inability to actively extend the joint.

Due to these adhesion formations, it is not unlikely that a tenolysis may need to be performed to aid in mobilizing the digit.

Trigger Finger

The flexor tendons can also be involved in tenosynovitis. The most common area of involvement is located at the region of the MCP joint where the flexor tendons pass beneath the A1 pulley. Tenosynovitis in this area may result in thickening of the tendon or sheath. This thickening may result in pain, popping, or catching in this area that may prevent the finger from extending once it is fully flexed. This is the so-called triggering phenomenon as the thickening passes or attempts to pass beneath the A1 pulley. Trigger finger can often be managed conservatively using splints, local modalities, and occasional injections of the tendon sheath while avoiding the tendon itself. A 0.5- to 1-mL dose of betamethasone (Celestone) is most often used in the injection to decrease the local inflammation. In cases in which conservative management fails, surgical release of the A1 pulley through a small incision under local or regional anesthesia provides excellent relief of symptoms with rapid return of normal function.

Extensor Tendons

Extensor tendons can be affected by lacerations, closed injuries, and constrictive scenarios. Lacerations of the extensor tendons are managed similar to flexor tendons as described earlier and generally have superior results when the surgeon adheres to the principles of wound care, early repair, immobilization, and controlled therapy. Closed injuries of the extensor tendons commonly affect the PIP and DIP interphalangeal joints.

"Mallet" finger is caused by an injury of the extensor mechanism at the level of the DIP joint. This is due to an attenuation of the terminal insertion, rupture of the insertion, or an avulsion fracture of the distal phalanx often caused by sudden forceful flexion of the DIP joint (Fig. 107-7). The diagnosis is made when the DIP joint can be extended passively but not actively. These injuries can be managed with extension splinting of the DIP joint continuously for 6 weeks followed by 6 weeks of night splinting in the absence of joint subluxation. If subluxation of the DIP joint is present, closed or open reduction with stabilization of the DIP joint is necessary.

Disruption of the central tendon at its insertion into the base of the middle phalanx may allow the head of the proximal phalanx to protrude through this defect and the lateral bands to migrate laterally. This results in flexion of the PIP joint and extension of the DIP joint (Boutonniere deformity). Treatment of this injury relies on early diagnosis. Initial disruption of the central slip presents as a swollen PIP joint with maximal tenderness over the dorsum of the joint. This can be managed with extension splinting of the PIP joint leaving the DIP joint free for active and passive range of motion exercises for at least 4 weeks (Fig. 107-8). Late diagnosis necessitates sequential splinting and occasionally surgical correction.

The extensor tendons can also be involved in tenosynovitis. The most commonly involved tendons are the extensor pollicis brevis and the abductor pollicis longus (DeQuervain stenosing tenosynovitis). The tendons and overlying synovium often become thickened as they pass through the first extensor compartment located directly over the radial styloid resulting in a constrictive condition. Pain and tenderness are usually present over the radial styloid and aggravated by flexion and ulnar deviation of thumb and hand respectively (Finkelstein test). A thumb abduction splint and injection of the tendon sheaths overlying the radial styloid with 0.5 to 1 mL of betamethasone relieve the symptoms in about 75% of patients. In persistent cases, surgical release of the first extensor compartment provides excellent results. Tenosynovitis of the wrist extensors at the level of the wrist almost universally responds to splinting and conservative management.

FRACTURES

Fractures of the hands and wrist are common because of their high exposure to injury. In evaluating hand fractures, the pathomechanics of the fracture, the extent of soft

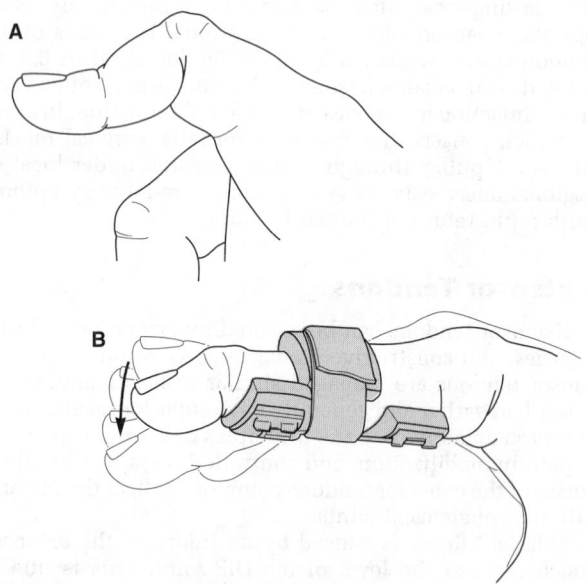

Figure 107-8. Boutonniere deformity. (*A*) Injury to the extensor tendon at the level of the proximal interphalangeal joint (central slip) results in a flexion deformity at the proximal interphalangeal joint and hyperextension of the distal interphalangeal joint. (*B*) Treatment includes dynamic extension splinting and distal interphalangeal exercises.

tissue damage, and the fracture stability must be addressed to obtain an accurate initial diagnosis and to plan a treatment course. Successful management of hand fractures results not only in bony union but also return of a full range of motion.

Distal Phalangeal Fractures

Fractures of the distal phalanx account for more than half of all hand fractures. The fractures generally occur at the tuft, shaft, or base and are generally due to crush injuries. Subungual hematomas may accompany these fractures and can be decompressed by drilling with a 19-caliber hypodermic needle or by burning a hole in the nail with an electrocautery unit. If the hematoma occupies more than half of the nail, then there is often an associated nail bed injury. Treating this injury requires removing the nail and repairing the nail bed with a fine absorbable suture and replacement of the nail to act as an external splint.

Extraarticular fractures are often quite stable and require immobilization for about 3 weeks. However, intraarticular fractures need to be assessed for joint incongruity and the presence of tendon involvement. In both scenarios, articular incongruity should be obtained to provide a functional fingertip.

Proximal and Middle Phalangeal Fractures

Shortening, angulation, and rotational forces act on the proximal and middle phalanges when fractured. These deformities can result in significant disabilities due to restriction of motion and overlap of the digits with flexion. Rotational forces can be neutralized by taping the fractured digit to the adjacent finger once an adequate reduction has been obtained. Palmar and dorsal angulation is caused by an imbalance between the intrinsic and extrinsic tendons of the hand. These effects can be minimized by immobilizing the digit and wrist in the position of function (wrist in 30 degrees of extension, MCP joint in 70 degrees of flexion). Most fractures can be managed by closed reduction if necessary and by immobilization for 3 weeks. Displaced oblique fractures, intraarticular fractures, distal transverse fractures, and comminuted fractures are often unstable and are best treated with operative stabilization. It is important to begin controlled range of motion as early as possible to regain a maximal range of motion. This decision is based on fracture site stability and healing time.

Metacarpal Fractures

Metacarpal fracture management is similar to that of the proximal and middle phalanges. Stable fractures can easily be managed with closed reduction if necessary, followed by 4 weeks of immobilization. The index and long finger metacarpals are part of the fixed unit of the hand, limiting their mobility compared with the ring and small finger metacarpals. As a result, the index and long finger metacarpals tolerate angulation of the fracture site very poorly. In contrast, the ring finger can easily accommodate up to 20 degrees of angulation and the small finger 40 degrees. Displaced articular fractures or fractures that can not be controlled by closed methods often need operative stabilization (percutaneous pinning or plating) to produce an optimal result.

Scaphoid Fractures

Because of the problems encountered with scaphoid fractures, they deserve special emphasis. It is the most commonly fractured carpal bone and can often be complicated by nonunion and avascular necrosis due to its distally based blood supply.

Diagnosis of this fracture should be suspected in any individual who has fallen on the outstretched hand and presents with pain localized to the radial aspect of the wrist. Initial radiographs are often negative, and management of a suspected scaphoid fracture should include the placement of a long arm thumb spica cast. Repeated radiographs are made at 2 weeks to confirm or dispute the presence of the fracture. If the second radiograph is also normal, the injury can be confidently managed as a sprain. This cautious approach to scaphoid fractures ensures that the diagnosis is not missed and decreases the incidence of nonunions and complications. Stable scaphoid fractures can be managed successfully with cast immobilization, whereas displaced or unstable fractures require internal fixation with pins or a Herbert screw. The arthroscope can aid in reduction and Herbert screw fixation since it minimizes the surgical exposure and decreases the length of immobilization. This has been extremely useful in managing scaphoid fractures in athletes (Fig. 107-9).

THUMB INJURIES

The thumb is clearly the most important digit of the hand since it is vital to almost all activities of the hand. Two specific injuries that require special attention include the game keeper's thumb and the Bennett fracture.

Game keeper's, also known as skier's thumb, results from an abduction injury to the MCP joint of the thumb that injures the ulnar collateral ligament. Lack of treatment results in thumb instability and difficulty with pinching and grasping activities. Partial tears can be immobilized for 4 to 6 weeks, whereas complete lesions require surgical repair followed by immobilization.

The Bennett intraarticular fracture of the base of the thumb metacarpal is often due to an impaction of the thumb. The fracture is generally unstable because of the adduction deformity of the thumb intrinsic muscles and the longitudinal pull of the abductor pollicis longus tendon. The ideal treatment includes closed reduction and percutaneous pinning of the fracture. If the articular realignment is not satisfactory, open reduction should be performed.

JOINT INJURY AND DISEASE

Dislocations

Dislocations of the finger joints, most often the PIP, are quite common. Physical examination usually reveals a painful deformed joint and the diagnosis is confirmed radiographically. Closed reduction is obtained by simultaneously applying longitudinal traction and accentuating the position that produced the deformity. Postreduction radiographs should always be obtained.

The most common dislocation involving the digits is dorsal displacement of the distal segment on the proximal one. Dorsal dislocations should be managed with closed reduction and immobilization of the joint for 7 to 10 days followed by protected mobilization. Volar dislocation of the PIP joint results in an injury to the central slip insertion of the extensor tendon and should be managed with 6 weeks of immobilization with the PIP joint in extension and the DIP joint free.

MCP dislocations are also common and are described as simple or complex. Simple dislocations are easily reduced with gentle manipulation without longitudinal traction since they can be converted into a complex dislocation.

Complex dislocations are irreducible and require surgical reduction.

Arthritides

Degenerative and rheumatoid arthritis often affects the joints of the hand and can be extremely disabling. Degenerative changes usually result in osteophyte and cyst formation in the PIP and DIP joints and are referred to as the Bouchard and Heberden nodes, respectively. Osteoarthritis also commonly involves the basal thumb CMC joint. These can often be managed conservatively with splints and medication but occasionally require surgical intervention (fusion or joint replacement).

Rheumatoid arthritis often involves the MCP and PIP joints and begins as synovial proliferation (Fig. 107-10). The synovitis results in joint destruction, tendon drift resulting in ulnar deviation of the digits, tenosynovitis, and in some cases, tendon rupture. The course is usually progressive, and treatment in the early stages is aimed at controlling the systemic disease. Useful local modalities include splinting, judicious steroid injections, and isometric exercises. Surgical treatment of deformities are based on reconstructing function. These include synovectomies, joint replacements, tendon realignment and repair, and occasionally joint fusions.

SKIN INJURY AND DISEASE

Due to its inherent exposure, the skin of the hand and its immediate underlying tissues can be affected by injuries and pathologic processes.

Thermal Burns

Burns often affect the hands because of their high exposure and lack of protective wear. Burns are often classified by depth. First-degree burns are superficial, erythematous, and hyperaesthetic. Second-degree burns are partial thickness injuries, blister, and are hyperaesthetic. Third-degree burns involve the full thickness of the skin, are dry and white in appearance, and are anaesthetic.

The urgent objective of treatment is to restore mobility with the following: (1) control of swelling with elevation, fasciotomies, and escharotomy; (2) control of pain; (3) prevention of infection; and (4) prompt débridement and skin grafting when appropriate. First-degree and mild second-degree injuries can often be managed with elevation, local ointments (Silvadene), a nonadherent dressing, and splinting. Healing usually occurs in 10 to 15 days. More severe second- and third-degree burns require extensive management including skin grafting and should be referred to a burn center.

Frostbite

Frostbite can also result in extensive soft tissue injuries. With frostbite, the hand becomes cold and numb and is graded similar to thermal burns. Initial treatment includes rapid rewarming by immersion in water at 40 to 44C until there is flushing of the digital skin. Analgesics may be required since rewarming can often be quite painful. Surgical treatment is limited to circumferential escharotomies. Generally, the involved digits are more cold sensitive after injury than before, and the patient should be informed of this.

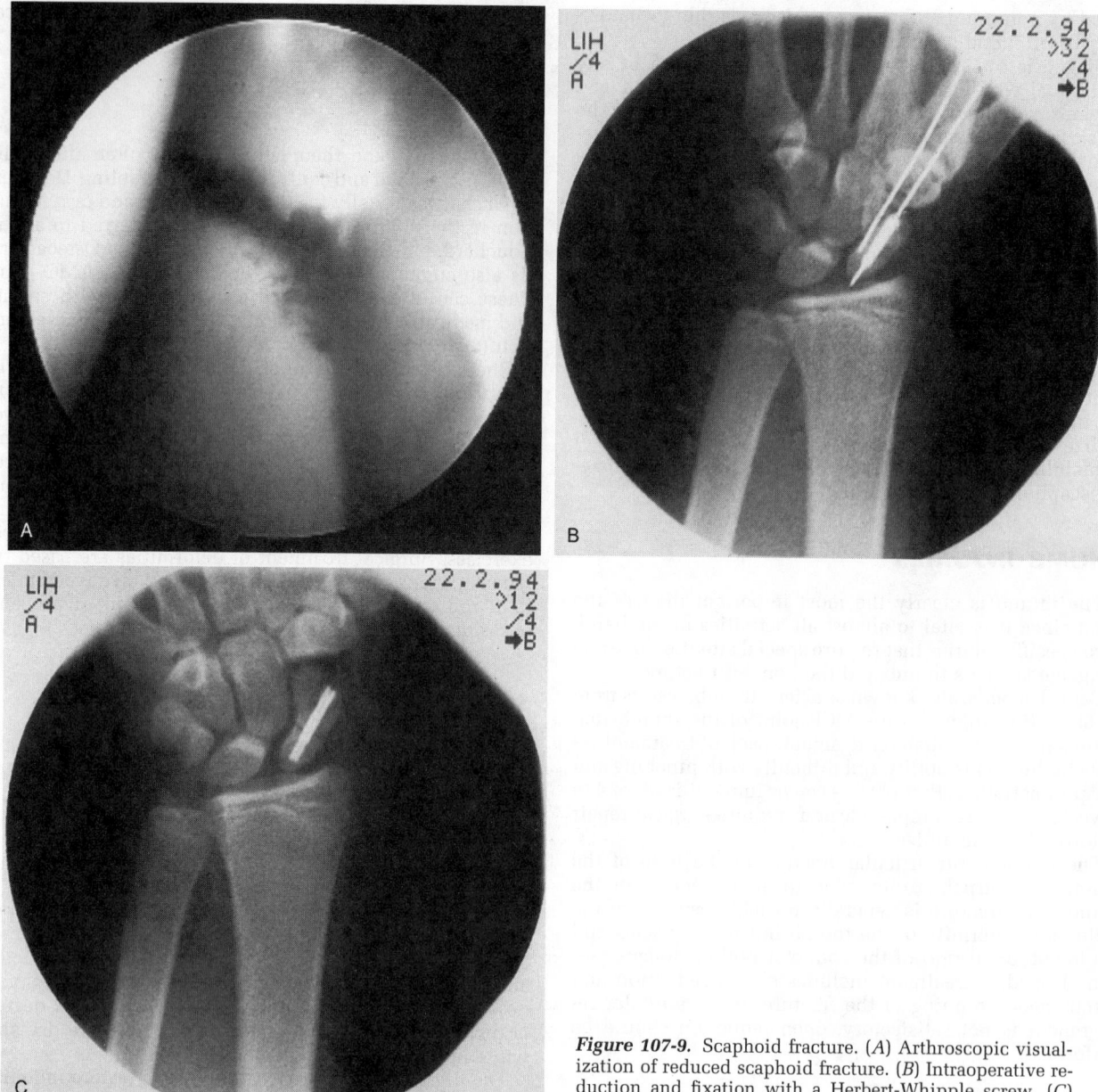

Figure 107-9. Scaphoid fracture. (*A*) Arthroscopic visualization of reduced scaphoid fracture. (*B*) Intraoperative reduction and fixation with a Herbert-Whipple screw. (*C*) Postoperative image of arthroscopic screw fixation.

Injection Injuries

Toxic substances such as paint, lubricants, sealants, and plastics can be accidentally injected into the hand under extremely high pressures. The initial injury is often deceptively small and does not represent the entire extent of damage. Because of the high pressure, the material may be injected far proximally and requires immediate, extensive débridement. Results are usually poor because of adhesion formation and loss of motion, sometimes requiring amputation.

Dupuytren Contractures

Dupuytren contractures of the hand are common and often affect middle-aged individuals. This condition is most common in men, individuals of northern European descent, and people with a positive family history. It is also associated with alcoholism and diabetes mellitus. The process involves a proliferation of the palmar fascia re-

sulting in contractures of this tissue and most commonly affects the ring and small fingers. The only effective treatment is surgical excision of the involved fascia. However, surgery is usually limited to contractures affecting the PIP joint and those causing at least a 30-degree contracture of the MCP joint of the hand.

INFECTIONS

Infections of the hand are common and are classified according to the tissue involved. Initial treatment relies on early diagnosis, débridement, elevation, splinting, antibiotics, and decompression if necessary.

Pyogenic Infections

Pyogenic infections often develop initially as a cellulitis surrounding a neglected laceration. Swelling, erythema, and tenderness are often present early and, if left un-

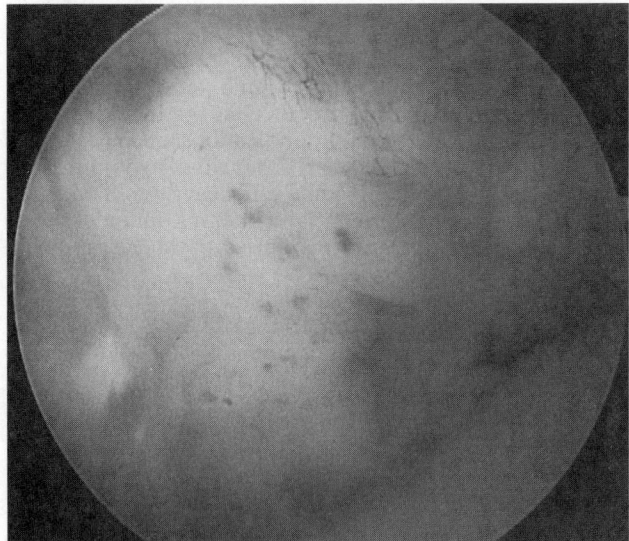

Figure 107-10. Arthroscopic visualization of rheumatoid arthritis of the wrist.

treated, result in lymphangitis and adenitis. These infections are often due to staphylococci or beta-hemolytic streptococci and are managed well with elevation, immobilization, and antibiotics. Incision and drainage is only performed when there is an actual collection of purulent material.

Pyoderma

Pyoderma is a subepithelial abscess that develops within the skin in a hair follicle, infected blister, or callus. Treatment includes incision and débridement with the application of moist dressings. If untreated, this condition can develop into a collar-button abscess.

Paronychia

The tissue surrounding the fingernail can often become traumatized and secondarily infected. A paronychia usually initially develops as a cellulitis bordering the nail and, if untreated, can involve the base of the nail. Initial treatment includes warm soaks, elevation, immobilization, and antibiotics. If an abscess forms, it generally occurs at the base corner of the nail and can be painlessly drained by incising it with a needlepoint scalpel (Fig. 107-11). Occasionally, a portion of the nail must be excised if involved.

Felon

A pyogenic infection in the terminal pulp space is called a *felon*. It requires prompt decompression to prevent necrosis of fat, skin, and bone. The incision should be placed so as to easily decompress the infection while preserving as much of the tip as possible (Fig. 107-12). Division of all the septa as described earlier deprives the pad of the tethering necessary for pinch and should be avoided. Antibiotics should also be administered.

Suppurative Tenosynovitis

Infections that spread into the flexor tendon sheaths are termed *suppurative tenosynovitis*. The four classic signs of Kanavel, which indicate this infection, are as follows:

- Tenderness along the tendon sheath
- Pain with passive motion
- Swelling along the tendon sheath
- Semiflexed posture of the involved digit

Once the diagnosis is suspected, elevation, splinting, and antibiotics are instituted. If prompt improvement does not occur, then incision and drainage should be performed by a midaxial incision or catheter irrigation (5F catheter, lidocaine, and antibiotic solution). Complications include the extension to deep spaces as proximal as the forearm and can be extremely disabling. Despite early diagnosis and aggressive treatment, significant morbidity and hand stiffness may result.

Bite Wounds

Bite wounds can be inflicted by animals or other humans. The inoculum of bacteria can often lead to infection and must be treated aggressively. Initial treatment includes thorough irrigation of the wound, antibiotics, elevation, and immobilization. These wounds should be left open. Antibiotics should include both a cephalosporin and penicillin because *Eikenella corrodens* (human bites) and *Pasturella multocida* (dog and cat bites) are only susceptible to penicillins.

TUMORS
Ganglions

Ganglion cysts are the most common tumor of the hand and result from the protrusion of a joint capsule or tendon sheath that fills with a jelly-like fluid. Most ganglions arise from the dorsal wrist joint in the region of the scapholunate interosseous ligament. Management of the ganglion can be conservative with simple observation, aspiration with

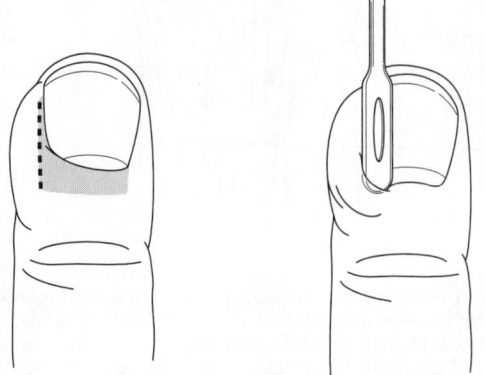

Figure 107-11. Paronychia and example of drainage.

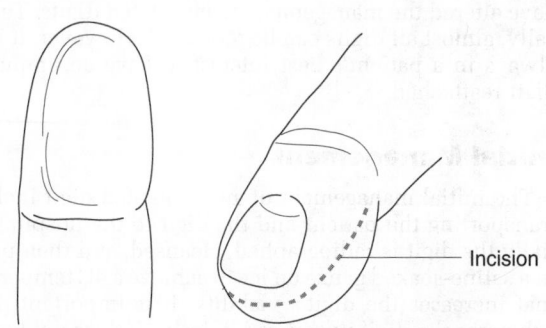

Figure 107-12. Felon involving the volar pad of the finger and recommended incision to decompress the infection.

injection of local steroids, or excision. This excision can be performed either through a small open incision or under direct arthroscopic visualization. In either case, the root of the stalk where it arises from the scapholunate interosseous ligament must be débrided to prevent recurrence.

Volar ganglions deserve evaluation of the arterial supply of the hand to ensure good digital circulation in the case of injury to the radial artery during excision of the ganglion. Volar ganglions arise most commonly from the scaphotrapeziotrapezoid joint's volar capsule.

Inclusion Cyst

When viable cells are carried deep to the dermis by injury, they can develop into a ball or cyst. This mass of keratinized cells (inclusion cyst) can compress adjacent tissue including bone. The cyst appears as a pearl and does not recur if removed completely.

Xanthoma

This tumor is also referred to as giant cell tumor of soft tissue and is an insidiously growing, painless, hard, multinodular growth that arises from the collateral ligaments or flexor sheath of the digits. The only treatment is surgical excision, and this tumor recurs unless it is entirely removed.

Neurofibroma and Schwannoma

These tumors consist of thickened nerve sheath elements and, when multiple, are part of Recklinghausen disease. The usual indication for resection is cosmetic since it is not usually symptomatic. Magnification should be used while excising the tumor to protect the nerve. If rapid growth is noted, excision should be performed since there is a rare tendency towards malignant degeneration.

Actinic Keratosis

These lesions are usually located on the dorsum of the hands and are hyperkeratotic in nature. They are common in individuals who are chronically exposed to the sun and can be treated with fluoracil or excision.

Glomus Tumor

This rare tumor is composed of blood vessels and unmyelinated nerves and may cause severe pain. It is most common in the terminal aspect of the digit and surgical excision is required to treat this tumor.

AMPUTATIONS

The technical advances in microsurgical techniques have altered the management of amputated digits. Technically, almost all digits can be replanted. However, it is not always in a patient's best interest to have an amputated digit reattached.

Initial Management

The initial management of an amputated digit includes transporting the patient and the digit to the hospital. Initially the digit is radiographed, cleansed, and then placed in a saline-soaked gauze on ice to achieve a 4C temperature that increases the digit's viability. It is important not to submerge the digit uncovered in ice so it does not become frostbitten. The cared-for digit and patient should then be transported to a hospital capable of replantation.

Indications for Replantation

Indications for replantation include injuries to multiple digits, amputations of the thumb, amputations in children, and clean amputations at the level of the hand, wrist, or distal forearm. Relative contraindications are amputations due to crush or avulsion injuries, single-digit amputations between the MCP and PIP joints, and heavily contaminated amputations. Absolute contraindications include severe medical problems, multilevel injuries, psychosis, and noncompliant patients.

Technically successful replantation occurs in about 80% of attempts. However, digital range of motion is always decreased as is sensation, and there is greater cold sensitivity. Two-point discrimination averages 13 mm in the replanted digit.

ARTHROSCOPY

Wrist arthroscopy is a recent addition to the hand surgeon's armamentarium. The arthroscope is a valuable adjunct in the diagnosis and management of wrist disorders. It allows direct visualization of numerous structures that may be difficult to assess clinically or radiographically (Fig. 107-13).

Pathologic conditions that can be addressed arthroscopically include reduction and fixation of distal radius and scaphoid fractures, repair or débridement of triangular fibrocartilage complex lesions, arthroscopic reduction and pinning of acute carpal instability patterns, wafer resections of the distal ulna in ulnar impaction syndrome, synovectomy, removal of loose bodies, and excision of the ra-

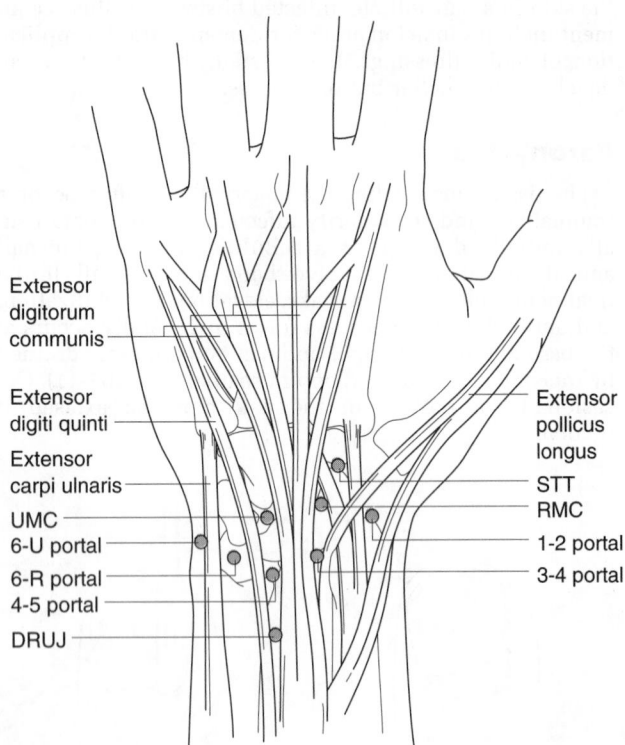

Figure 107-13. Wrist arthroscopy portals and their relation to the extensor tendons and joint. Using the multiple portals, the wrist can be well visualized while avoiding the extensor tendons. Only several of the multiple portals are used in each arthroscopic case. STT, scaphotrapeziotrapezoid; RMC, radial midcarpal; UMC, ulnar midcarpal ; DRUJ, distal radioulnar joint.

dial border of the distal ulna for distal radioulnar degenerative arthritis.

The results of these pioneering efforts in wrist arthroscopy have been extremely encouraging, resulting in the further development and increased use of the arthroscope in wrist disorders. Arthroscopic procedures of the wrist have resulted in reduced morbidity and faster recuperations, allowing rapid return to work and athletics.

Despite the advantages of direct visualization, arthroscopy of the wrist should neither preempt conservative management nor be used as a substitute for an adequate clinical examination. It should be used to facilitate the diagnosis and to aid in treatment, not to circumvent careful physical examination and basic management.

BIBLIOGRAPHY

Barron JN, Saad MN. The hand. In: Operative plastic and reconstructive surgery. Vol. 3. New York, Churchill Livingstone, 1980.

Beasley RW. Hand injuries. Philadelphia, WB Saunders, 1981.

Brand P: Clinical mechanics of the hand. St Louis, CV Mosby, 1985.

Conolly WD, Kilgore ES. Hand injuries and infections. Chicago, Mosby Year Book, 1979.

Eaton RG. Joint injuries of the hand. Springfield, IL, Charles C Thomas, 1971.

Fess EE, Gettle KS, Strickland JW. Hand splinting: principles and methods. St Louis, CV Mosby, 1981.

Flatt AE. Care of the arthritic hand. St Louis, CV Mosby, 1983.

Flatt AE. The care of minor hand injuries, ed 4. St Louis, CV Mosby, 1979.

Flynn JE. Hand surgery, ed 3. Baltimore, Williams & Wilkins, 1981.

Grabb WC, Smith JW. Hand and upper extremity plastic surgery. In: Plastic surgery: a concise guide to clinical practice, ed 3. Boston, Little, Brown, 1980, Part IV.

Green DP, ed. Operative hand surgery. New York, Churchill Livingstone, 1993.

Hopperfeld S. Surgical exposures in orthopaedics: the anatomic approach. Philadelphia, JB Lippincott, 1984.

Hunter JM, Mackin EJ, Callahan AD, et al. Rehabilitation of the hand, ed 2. St Louis, CV Mosby, 1984.

Kilgore ES Jr, Graham WP III. The hand: surgical and nonsurgical management. Philadelphia, Lea & Febiger, 1977.

Lamb DW. The practice of hand surgery. London, Blackwell Scientific, 1981.

Lister G. The hand: diagnosis and indications. New York, Churchill Livingstone, 1977.

Milford L. The hand, ed 2. St Louis, CV Mosby, 1982.

Newmeyer WL. Primary care of hand injuries. Philadelphia, Lea & Febiger, 1979.

Omer GE Jr, Spinner M. Management of peripheral nerve problems. Philadelphia, WB Saunders, 1980.

Poehling GG. Arthroscopy of the wrist and elbow. New York, Raven Press, 1994.

Schlenker JD, Kleinert HE, Tsai T. Methods and results of replantation following traumatic amputation of the thumb in sixty-four patients. J Hand Surg 1980; 5:63.

Spinner M. Injuries to the major branches of the peripheral nerves of the forearm, ed 2. Philadelphia, WB Saunders, 1978.

Strickland JW, Rettig AC. Hand injuries in athletics. Philadelphia, WB Saunders, 1992.

Tubiana R. The hand. Philadelphia, WB Saunders, 1981.

Whipple TL. Arthroscopic surgery: the wrist. Philadelphia, JB Lippincott, 1992.

Wynn-Parry CB. Rehabilitation of the hand, ed 4. London, Butterworths, 1981.

SURGERY: SCIENTIFIC PRINCIPLES AND PRACTICE, Second Edition, edited by
Lazar J. Greenfield, Michael W. Mulholland, Keith T. Oldham, Gerald B. Zelenock,
and Keith D. Lillemoe. Lippincott–Raven Publishers, Philadelphia, © 1997.

CHAPTER 108

CENTRAL NERVOUS SYSTEM

JULIAN T. HOFF AND MICHAEL F. BOLAND

A detailed history and physical examination is the foundation of neurosurgical diagnosis. Headache, altered consciousness, memory impairment, speech difficulty, visual disturbance, weakness, paresthesia, and incoordination are symptoms suggestive of central nervous system (CNS) disease. The examination should include assessment of mental status, thorough cranial nerve testing, optic funduscopy, and motor, sensory, and reflex testing.

The historical details suggest an etiology (eg, traumatic, neoplastic, vascular, infectious, degenerative, or metabolic), whereas neurologic examination permits anatomic localization of the lesion. For patients with nervous system disorders, an accurate history need be taken only once, but the examination must be repeated and recorded often to gauge the course of the illness and to judge the urgency of other diagnostic steps necessary before treatment can be given.

DIAGNOSTIC STUDIES

Once a differential diagnosis is formulated with the information gathered from the history and examination, it is necessary to confirm the principal diagnosis by use of diagnostic aids. Studies helpful in the practice of neurosurgery include plain film radiography and tomography, myelography, arteriography, computed tomography (CT), magnetic resonance imaging (MRI), ultrasonography, electromyography (EMG) and nerve conduction velocity testing, evoked potentials (visual, auditory, and somatosensory), positron emission tomography, and electroencephalography.

Plain films, especially of the spine, are useful in trauma and degenerative disorders. Myelography, both with and without CT, is useful for the evaluation of radiculopathies and, when MRI is not available, myelopathies due to trauma, tumor, and degenerative spine disease. CT and MRI provide detailed imaging of both cranial and spinal contents. They are useful in combination for visualization of bone and soft tissues, respectively. Arteriography provides detailed information about aneurysms, vascular malformations, and atherosclerotic disease. It is an essential tool in the evaluation of cerebral hemorrhage and embolic and thrombotic stroke, and in preoperative planning for tumor surgery. Ultrasound is an important adjunct in the operating room, providing visualization of tumors, cysts, vascular malformations, and congenital anomalies lying beneath the exposed surface. Ultrasound is also extensively used in brain and spinal cord imaging in the newborn.

EMG and nerve conduction velocity testing are helpful in evaluating peripheral nerve and nerve root lesions. They are also used to monitor brachial plexus and peripheral nerve recovery after traumatic injury. Visual-evoked and auditory-evoked potentials can be used in comatose patients to monitor the severity of head injury. Auditory potentials are useful in surgical excision of tumors of the eighth cranial nerve. Somatosensory-evoked potentials continually monitor spinal cord (dorsal column) function during surgical manipulation of spinal fractures and tumors. Positron emission tomography scans play an important role in epilepsy surgery, in preembolization assessment of skull-based tumors involving the cavernous sinus and surgically untreatable vascular anomalies, and in brain tumor follow-up. Electroencephalography helps delineate structural and metabolic disorders and can be used during cerebrovascular surgery as a guard against irreversible ischemia. Transcranial Doppler sonography allows noninvasive evaluation of blood flow velocity within intracranial arteries, which is useful in monitoring patients with cerebral ischemia caused by vascular spasm.

TRAUMA

Trauma is the single most common cause of death in children, adolescents, and young adults. Most accidents involving motor vehicles and falls include injury to the brain and spinal cord and their surrounding structures.[1]

Scalp Injury

Scalp injury can cause serious hemorrhage and subsequent shock if not promptly treated. Bleeding can usually be controlled with a simple pressure dressing, by firm finger pressure, or by hemostats applied to the galea, the aponeurosis of the scalp. Scalp wounds should be closed as soon as possible. Lacerations that overlie a depressed fracture or a penetrating wound of the skull require débridement in the operating room.

Simple scalp lacerations should be débrided of foreign matter, copiously irrigated, and closed primarily, taking care to approximate both the galea and skin. A good galeal closure provides excellent hemostasis. Scalp avulsions typically include all layers of the scalp, with sparing of the underlying periosteum. It the avulsion is small, closure can often be accomplished primarily. Replantation with the use of microsurgical technique is the preferred method of repair for large scalp avulsions, provided the avulsed scalp has been preserved and surgery is not delayed.

If the injured scalp is not viable but the periosteum is intact, split-thickness skin grafts can be used to close the defect. Care must be taken to keep the periosteum moist before surgery. When the periosteum is absent or desiccated, closure is more difficult, because it is through the periosteal layer that the outer skull table receives its blood supply. In this instance, closure can be accomplished with vascular flaps of greater omentum or muscle. Other methods include perforation of the outer skull to expose the diploë, which can serve as a source of granulation tissue that can then be skin grafted.

Skull Fracture

Skull fractures are classified according to whether the skin overlying the fracture is intact (closed) or disrupted (open or compound), whether there is a single fracture line (linear), several fractures radiating from a central point (stellate), or fragmentation of bone (comminuted), and whether the edges of the fracture line have been driven below the level of the surrounding bone (depressed) or not (nondepressed).

Simple skull fractures (linear, stellate, or comminuted nondepressed) require no specific treatment. They are potentially serious, however, and can be fatal if they cross major vascular channels in the skull, such as the groove of the middle meningeal artery or the dural venous sinuses. If these structures are torn, epidural or subdural hematomas, or both, can form. A simple skull fracture that extends into the accessory nasal sinuses or the mastoid air cells is considered open because it communicates with an external body surface.

Depressed skull fractures often require surgery to elevate the depressed bone fragments (Fig. 108-1). If there are no adverse neurologic signs and the fracture is closed, repair can be done electively. Intraoperatively, the dura should be inspected and repaired as described below.

Open skull fractures also require surgical intervention. Linear or stellate, nondepressed open fractures can be treated by simple closure of the scalp after thorough cleansing. Open fractures with severe comminution of underlying bone should be treated in the operating room when proper débridement can be carried out. The dura

should be inspected to ensure that a laceration has not been overlooked. If found, dural tears should be closed either primarily or with a fascial patch graft to reduce the risk of infection. Depressed, open skull fractures should be débrided, elevated, and closed in the operating room after preparations have been made for craniotomy, in case broader exposure of underlying injured dura and brain is necessary.

Basal skull fractures involve the floor of the calvarium. Bruising can occur about the eye (raccoon sign) or behind the ear (Battle sign), suggesting a fracture involving the anterior or middle fossa, respectively. Isolated cranial nerve deficits are associated with this fracture type. The facial nerve is frequently affected, with injury due to laceration (acute deficit) or swelling (delayed deficit). Almost all facial nerve deficits resolve spontaneously, especially with incomplete or delayed lesions. No specific therapy is warranted. On the other hand, complete lesions should be explored, although the timing of exploration remains a matter of debate.

Any associated cerebrospinal fluid (CSF) rhinorrhea or otorrhea should be treated expectantly. Traumatic CSF leaks typically stop within the first 7 to 10 days. Should a leak persist, lumbar CSF drainage can be implemented to seal the leak by lowering CSF volume and intracranial pressure (ICP). If this therapy fails, surgical exploration and oversewing of the defect with a fascial patch graft are indicated. Less than 5% of patients actually require surgical repair. Prophylactic antibiotics are no longer used because prospective studies have failed to demonstrate any significant benefit from their use.

Brain Injury

Injury to the brain is caused by the rapid deceleration, acceleration, and rotation associated with a blow to the head.[2] The initial impact can produce neuronal and axonal disruption, which constitutes the primary injury. Any sub-

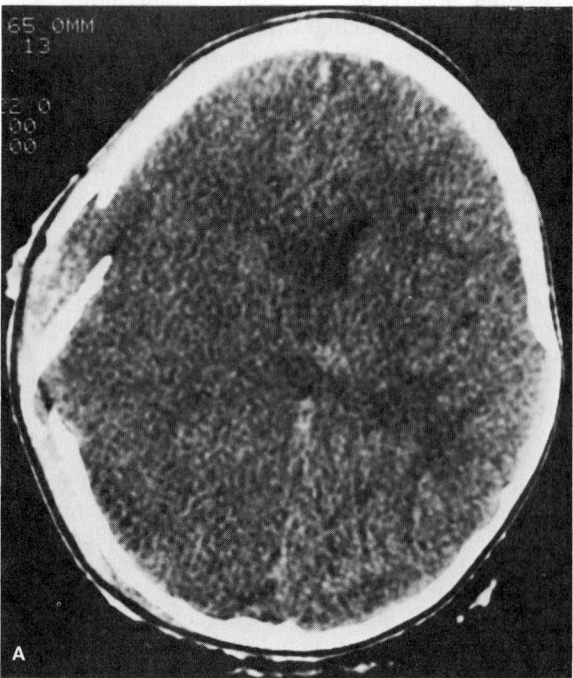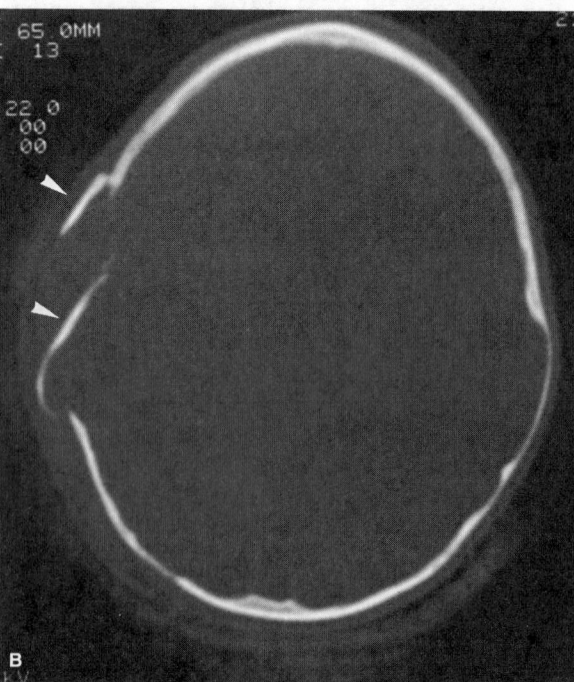

Figure 108-1. A compound, comminuted, depressed skull fracture imaged by noncontrast CT with the use of soft tissue (*A*) and bone windows (*B*). Multiple fracture fragments are visible (*arrowheads*). The overlying scalp was lacerated, and cerebrospinal fluid was leaking from the wound.

sequent complication, such as an intracranial hematoma, cerebral edema, hypoxia, hypotension, hydrocephalus, or endocrine disturbance, characterizes secondary injury and always compounds the initial insult.

Mild head injury is usually not associated with significant primary brain injury, and neurologic deficits are limited to temporary loss of consciousness (concussion). Moderate to severe head injury, on the other hand, is typically associated with deficits that may or may not be reversible. Moreover, this degree of injury is usually accompanied by secondary injury.

Distortional forces causing the primary injury can be great enough to tear intraparenchymal capillaries, superficial subdural bridging veins, or epidural vessels, thus producing uncontained blood. Vasogenic cerebral edema occurs in response to vasodilation and disruption of the blood–brain barrier. Ischemia from hypotension or hypoxia can produce cell death and consequent cytotoxic edema. Disruption of CSF absorption pathways by uncontained subarachnoid blood can lead to hydrocephalus. Inappropriate secretion of the antidiuretic hormone or the development of diabetes insipidus can aggravate cerebral edema by altering fluid and electrolyte balance. These changes, either in part or in combination, result in an elevation of ICP.

Elevated ICP contributes to secondary brain injury by reducing cerebral perfusion pressure, which, by definition, is the difference between the mean arterial blood pressure and the cerebral venous pressure. For all clinically relevant purposes, the cerebral venous pressure is identical to ICP. Thus, when ICP increases and mean arterial blood pressure remains stable, cerebral perfusion pressure decreases. When the cerebral perfusion pressure falls below 70 mmHg, cerebral blood flow is compromised, producing cerebral ischemia and compounding the primary brain injury with secondary insult.

In studies of head injury mortality, intracranial hypertension appears to be one of the most important factors affecting outcome. For this reason, aggressive management to circumvent cerebral blood flow reduction and secondary injury is imperative. Early resuscitative therapy should be initiated in the accident field with airway control and hyperventilation. In the absence of hypotension, osmotherapy can also be used.

Rapid clinical assessment is essential. Although extensive neurologic testing is limited in uncooperative or unresponsive patients, certain features of the examination are crucial. The Glasgow Coma Scale score, established in 1974, uses a numerical score to evaluate eye opening and verbal and motor behavior, both spontaneously and in response to stimulation (Table 108-1). This scale is useful for determining the patient's neurologic status and provides information regarding the ultimate outcome of the head-injured patient.

The initial neurologic examination determines whether diagnostic testing is indicated. Patients without headache, lethargy, or a focal neurologic deficit are not likely to suffer a secondary complication from their injury, and imaging studies generally are not indicated. Conversely, symptomatic patients with or without a focal deficit should undergo a CT scan of the head, using windows for soft tissue and bone detail. Should CT fail to disclose a lesion despite high clinical suspicion, carotid and cerebral angiography can help delineate a vascular abnormality that cannot be appreciated with CT.

After emergent surgical removal of any traumatic cerebral mass lesion, the goals of medical management are normalization of cerebral perfusion pressure and prevention of secondary injury to the already damaged brain. ICP monitoring may be indicated, especially in patients with

Table 108-1. GLASGOW COMA SCALE*

Parameter	Score
EYE OPENING	
Spontaneously	4
To voice stimulus	3
To pain	2
No eye opening	1
MOTOR RESPONSE	
Follows commands	6
Localizes a pain stimulus	5
Withdraws from pain	4
Flexor posturing to pain	3
Extensor posturing to pain	2
No response to pain	1
VERBAL RESPONSE	
Oriented	5
Confused	4
Inappropriate words	3
Incomprehensible sounds	2
No sounds	1

* The Glasgow Coma Scale assigns a numeric value to the responses in each of three categories with the score equal to the sum of the three responses.

marked depression or deterioration in neurologic function. Comatose patients who require emergent surgery (eg, abdominal, thoracic, orthopedic) should also be monitored, because frequent neurologic examination is not possible during general anesthesia. A ventriculostomy to measure ICP allows drainage of CSF, which significantly lowers the pressure in most instances. When the ventricular system is collapsed, intraparenchymal monitoring should be established.

Head elevation in the neutral position facilitates venous drainage. Sedation reduces posturing and reflexively combative activity, both of which worsen ICP. Moderate hyperventilation with $PaCO_2$ levels between 30 and 35 mmHg lowers cerebral blood volume and ICP without provoking cerebral ischemia. Prophylactic use of anticonvulsants prevents cerebral injury from seizures. Mild dehydration with judicious sodium replacement and prompt treatment of SIADH (syndrome of inappropriate antidiuretic hormone secretion) protect the brain from insult secondary to fluid overload. Prevention of hypotension reduces the extension of ischemic injury, whereas aggressive treatment of hypertensive episodes reduces cerebral blood volume and further disruption of the blood–brain barrier. Treatment of hyperthermia avoids an increase in the brain's metabolic demands.

If ICP remains elevated despite these measures, mannitol, 0.5 to 1 g/kg, and furosemide, 0.1 mg/kg, can be used to reduce cerebral edema. Deep sedation with narcotics and even the use of paralyzing agents such as pancuronium or atracurium can be helpful. Barbiturate coma, once commonly used for otherwise refractory ICP elevation, does not significantly change the ultimate outcome. Corticosteroids are occasionally used but have no proven benefit.

The outcome in head injury depends on many factors, including increasing age and preexisting illness, both of which are significant contributors to prognosis. Penetrating injuries, particularly gunshot wounds, have a poorer outcome compared with blunt trauma. The presence of an intracranial hemorrhage also indicates a less favorable outcome. Concomitant subdural hematoma has a poorer prognosis than epidural hematoma. Combined subdural and intracerebral hemorrhage has the worst prognosis of all. Other important factors include delay in treatment, multiple trauma, and systemic insults such as acidosis, hypoxia, and hypotension. Predictors of poor prognosis include evidence of brain-stem dysfunction on initial examination and refractory intracranial hypertension.

Epidural Hematoma

Hemorrhage between the inner table of the skull and the dura mater most commonly arises from a tear of the middle meningeal artery or one of its branches (Fig. 108-2). Arterial bleeding strips the dura from the undersurface of the bone and produces still more bleeding because the small bridging veins from the dura to the skull are torn. The hematoma rapidly increases in size and compresses the cerebral cortex.

An epidural hematoma can also arise from torn venous channels in the bone at a point of fracture or from lacerated major dural venous sinuses. Because venous pressure is low, epidural venous hematomas usually form only when a depressed skull fracture has stripped the dura from the bone and left a space in which the hematoma can develop.

Epidural hematoma classically follows a blow to the head that causes a brief period of unconsciousness. After the patient regains consciousness, there may be a lucid interval during which there are no abnormal neurologic symptoms or signs. As the hematoma enlarges, hemispheric compression occurs. With time, the medial portion of the temporal lobe is forced over the edge of the tentorium, causing compression of the oculomotor nerve and subsequent dilation of the ipsilateral pupil. Similarly, compression of the ipsilateral cerebral peduncle causes contralateral hemiparesis, which can progress to decerebrate posturing. Coma, fixed and dilated pupils, and decerebration is the classic triad suggestive of transtentorial herniation.

Epidural hematomas are curable lesions, but the mortality rate remains high because the severity of injury is often not recognized early. A patient may be seen during the lucid interval and discharged. Later, the patient can become unconscious because of progressive brain compression by the expanding hematoma.

Because of the danger of misdiagnosis, any patient with a history of a blow to the head leading to a period of unconsciousness should have a CT scan. If an epidural hematoma is found, emergent craniotomy is indicated. If the CT is normal and the patient's examination is nonfocal, the patient can be discharged, although a reliable person should be instructed to awaken the patient frequently during the next 24 hours to be certain that he or she remains arousable. Any deterioration should prompt quick return for repeat evaluation.

Subdural Hematoma

When veins bridging from the cortex to the dura or venous sinuses are torn or when an intracerebral hematoma extends into the subdural space, subdural hematomas can develop. They can be large, even though the bleeding is of venous (low pressure) origin.

Acute subdural hematomas are associated with severe head injury and arise from a combination of torn bridging veins, disruption of cortical arteries, and laceration of the cortex. The hematoma is best imaged with CT (Fig. 108-3). Evacuation of the clot can result in significant improvement, but often a major neurologic deficit remains because of the accompanying widespread neuronal and axonal injury.

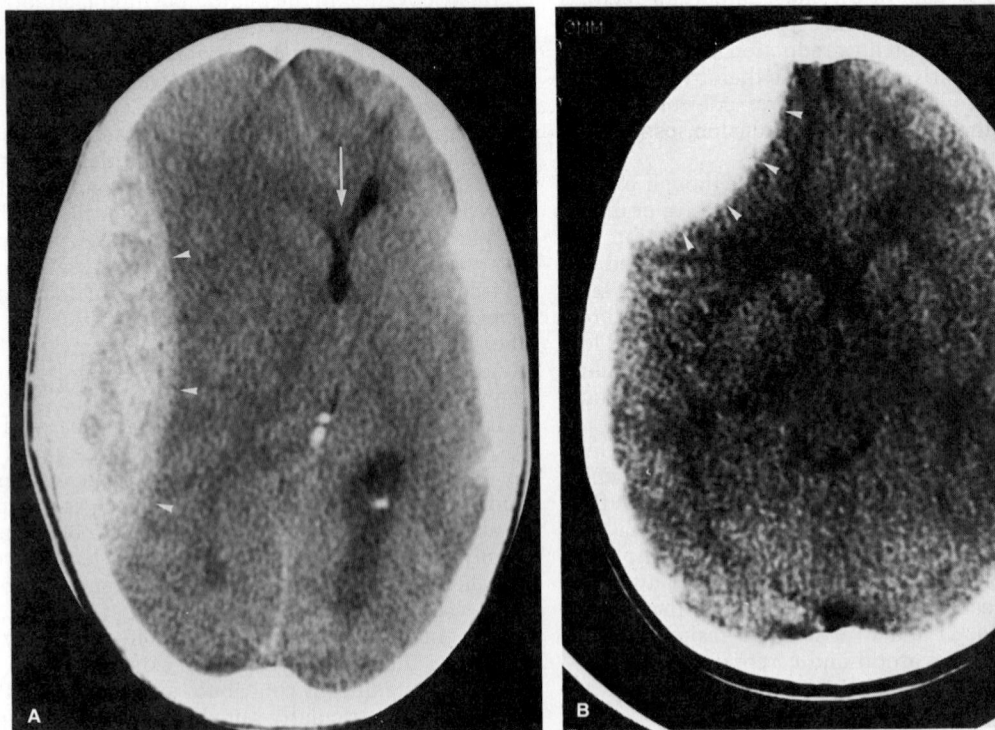

Figure 108-2. Two examples of acute epidural hematoma imaged by noncontrast CT. The increased attenuation of the lenticular-shaped mass (*arrowheads*) indicates that it is an acute lesion within the epidural space. There is a marked midline shift in *A* (*arrow*) compared with *B*. The patient in *A* was comatose and had little brain-stem function on examination. The patient in *B* was awake and conversant.

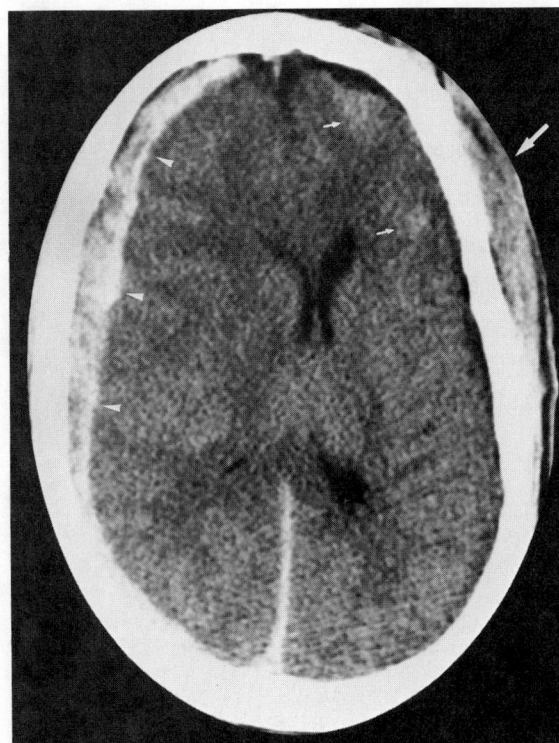

Figure 108-3. Acute subdural hematoma imaged by noncontrast CT. The high-attenuation, crescent-shaped lesion (*arrowheads*) indicates acute hemorrhage within the subdural space. Scalp swelling is visible on the contralateral side (*large arrow*), suggesting that the hematoma is due to a contrecoup injury. There are small hemorrhagic contusions in the contralateral frontal lobe as well (*small arrows*). These often accompany subdural hematomas in head trauma and signify severe injury. Midline shift is apparent.

Subacute subdural hematomas become apparent several days after injury and are associated with progressive lethargy, confusion, hemiparesis, or other hemispheric deficits. Removal of the hematoma usually produces striking improvement.

Chronic subdural hematomas arise from tears in bridging veins, often after a minor head injury. Initially, the hematoma is small. Later, it becomes encased in a fibrous membrane, liquefies, then gradually enlarges. These lesions are more common in infants and the elderly. Typical presentation includes progressive mental status changes, with or without focal signs such as hemiparesis or aphasia. Papilledema may be present. The diagnosis is confirmed by CT scanning. Treatment consists of bur hole drainage, and craniotomy may be necessary if the fluid reaccumulates.

Subdural hygromas are collections of clear or xanthochromic fluid in the subdural space. They develop when CSF escapes into the potential subdural space through a tear in the arachnoid, becomes trapped, and cannot be absorbed. The resulting fluid mass can cause the same signs and symptoms as chronic subdural hematomas. Like their hematoma counterparts, hygromas are treated by bur hole drainage. Infants may require an internalized shunt to drain the hygroma into the peritoneal space to keep it from reaccumulating.

Spinal Cord Injury

Traumatic injury of the spinal cord can result from vertebral fracture, fracture or subluxation, hyperextension of the cervical spine in the presence of a narrow spinal canal,

herniation of intervertebral disc material into the canal, and penetrating injuries such as gunshots or stabbings.[3] Neurologic involvement ranges from mild and transient to severe and permanent. Spine fracture and cord injury should be suspected in head-injured patients with or without coma and in those with multiple injuries. It is best to assume that the spine is unstable and to immobilize the patient on a backboard with a hard cervical collar until proper examination and diagnostic testing rule out injury.

Clinical findings can include spinal tenderness, extremity weakness, numbness or paresthesia, respiratory embarrassment, and hypotension. Spinal root involvement produces a radiculopathy characterized by motor and sensory impairment in the corresponding myotome and dermatome. Spinal cord involvement produces a myelopathy of variable manifestations.

Complete lesions, signifying total loss of function below the level of injury, are often referred to as *transections of the cord.* Acute transections are characterized by arreflexia, flaccidity, anesthesia, and autonomic paralysis below the level of the lesion. Arterial hypotension is invariably present when the transection is above T-5 because of the loss of sympathetic vascular tone.

Incomplete lesions can result in the Brown-Séquard syndrome, which is manifested by ipsilateral loss of motor function and position–vibratory sensation with contralateral loss of pain and temperature sensation below the level of injury. Anatomically, this presentation is explained by hemisection of the cord (Fig. 108-4*A*). The central cord syndrome is characterized by bilateral loss of motor function and pain and by loss of temperature sensation in the upper extremities, with relative preservation of these functions in the lower extremities. Typically, the distal upper extremities are more severely affected because the most medial portions of the corticospinal and spinothalamic tracts subserve these areas (see Fig. 108-4*B*). This deficit can be seen after a hyperextension injury of the cervical spine, with or without fracture. The anterior spinal artery syndrome involves the bilateral loss of motor function, pain, and temperature sensation below the level of the lesion, with sparing of position–vibratory and light touch sensation. This incomplete lesion develops when the anterior spinal artery is occluded. This renders the cord ischemic within the anterior spinal artery distribution, affecting the anterior and lateral columns bilaterally (see Fig. 108-4*C*). One common cause is an acutely ruptured cervical disc (Fig. 108-5).

Trauma to the lumbar spine can produce signs and symptoms of cauda equina compression. Presentation consists of multiple lumbosacral radiculopathies of variable severity. Lower extremity motor, sensory, and reflex functions can be affected, producing variable degrees of weakness, sensory loss (all modalities in the specific distribution of the roots involved), and diminution or absence of reflexes. Bladder distention from detrusor muscle paralysis, flaccidity of the anal sphincter, and loss of perineal sensation are common in severe injuries.

In addition to the neurologic deficit, acute spinal cord injury is accompanied by many systemic responses. If the spinal cord is damaged above C-3, respiratory efforts cease, accounting for this injury's high mortality at the scene of the accident. Although spontaneous ventilatory efforts can be initiated with injuries involving C-4 to C-6, tidal volumes are often insufficient, accounting for progressive hypoxia and carbon dioxide retention. Airway obstruction, atelectasis, and pneumonia are common complications. Assisted ventilation may be indicated, especially early after injury.

Ileus with gastric distention is common, necessitating nasogastric drainage. Similarly, bladder distention occurs

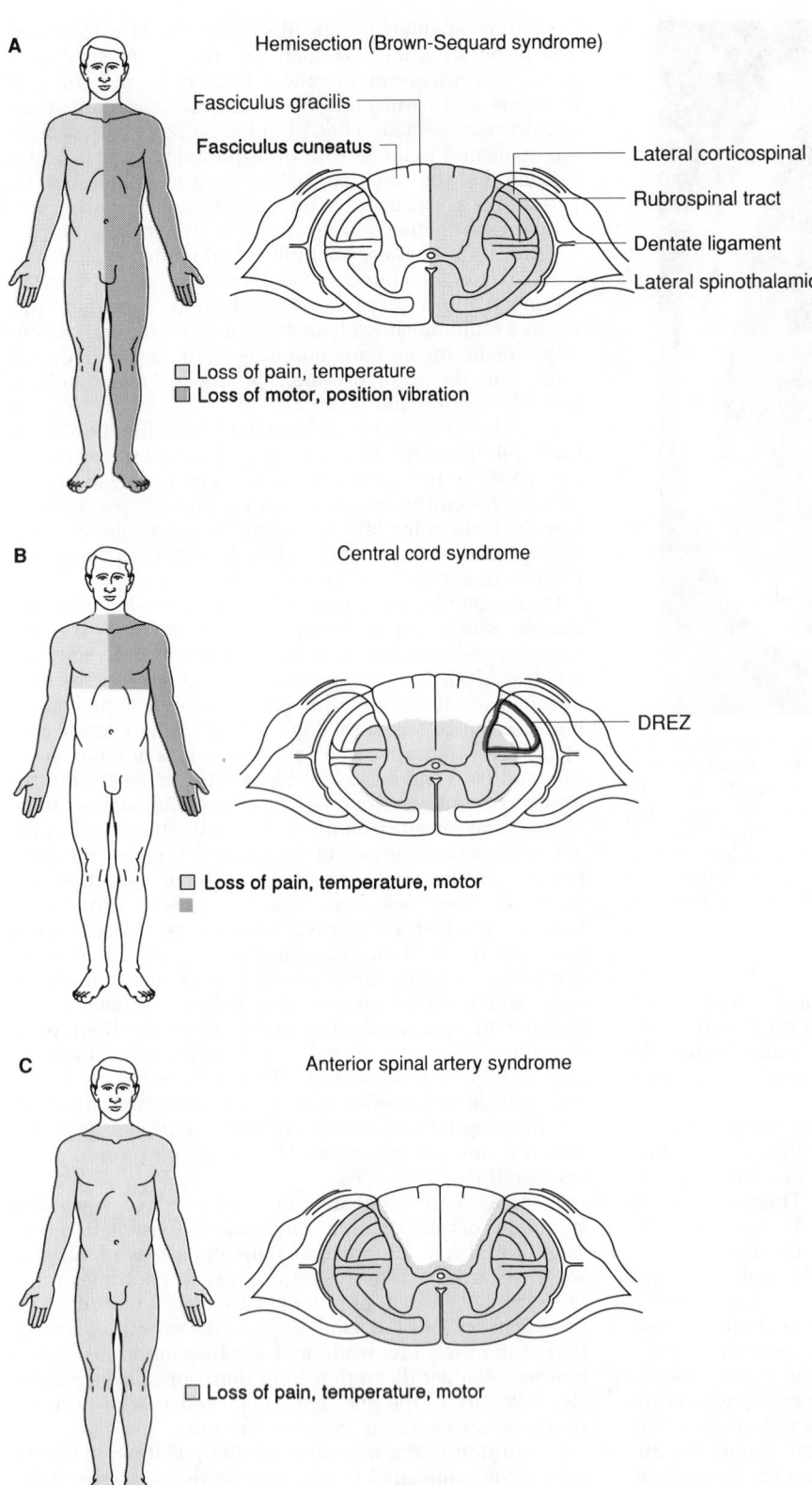

A. Hemisection (Brown-Sequard syndrome)

Fasciculus gracilis
Fasciculus cuneatus
Lateral corticospinal tract
Rubrospinal tract
Dentate ligament
Lateral spinothalamic tract

☐ Loss of pain, temperature
▨ Loss of motor, position vibration

B. Central cord syndrome

DREZ

☐ Loss of pain, temperature, motor
▨

C. Anterior spinal artery syndrome

☐ Loss of pain, temperature, motor

Figure 108-4. Schematic cross sections of the spinal cord, showing hemisection (*A*), central cord syndrome lesion (*B*), and anterior spinal artery syndrome lesion (*C*). The figure diagrams demonstrate the neurologic deficits. DREZ, dorsal route entry zone.

because the bladder and pelvic floor muscles are flaccid. Bladder drainage prevents overdistention, which can be severe enough to cause compression of the inferior vena cava and pelvic veins, impairing venous return to the heart and contributing to systemic hypotension.

Blood pressure is usually low if the cord injury is above the T-5 level. This effectively denervates the sympathetic nervous system, which leads to increased venous capacitance and decreased venous return. The resulting hypotension is controlled by the administration of intravenous fluids. Colloid is preferred to reduce the threat of vascular overload and iatrogenic pulmonary edema. Postural

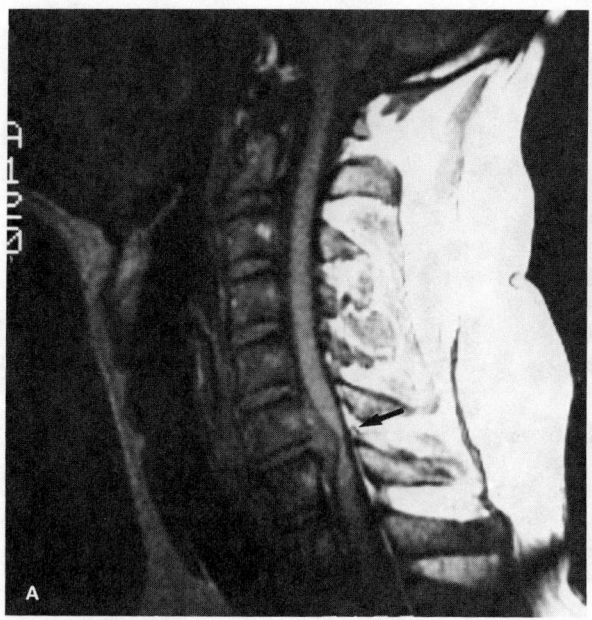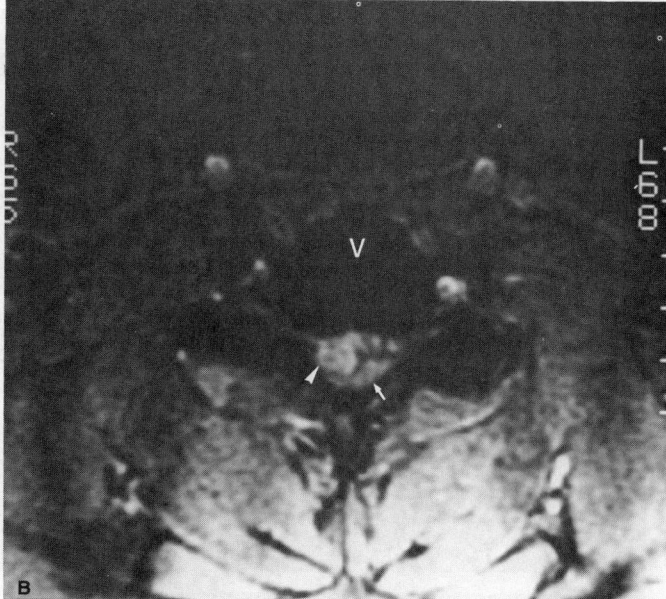

Figure 108-5. This patient developed severe neck pain and quadriparesis when he stood from a squatting position. (*A*) Sagittal cervical spine MRI scan reveals an acute herniated disc with marked cord compression (*arrow*). (*B*) Axial MRI scan shows the compressed cord (*arrow*) at the level of the herniation (*arrowhead*). V, vertebral body.

changes that will drop the blood pressure precipitously should be avoided.

Tachycardia is a common compensatory response to hypotension, but bradycardia is the rule when the cervical cord is damaged and the sympathetic input to the heart is lost. This bradycardia does not require treatment unless the patient is symptomatic or at risk for myocardial infarction or stroke because of age or other debilitating illness. If necessary, treatment with atropine and fluids is effective.

Once the patient is hemodynamically stable, spine radiographs are essential, but only while the patient remains immobilized on a backboard with a hard cervical collar firmly secured. Standard views are obtained, ensuring good visualization of the cervicothoracic junction (Fig. 108-6*A*). Comatose and severely injured patients with multiple trauma should have good plain film imaging of the complete spine. Fractured areas are further studied with CT, using both axial and sagittal views (see Fig. 108-6*B* and *C*). If no abnormality is found despite a neurologic deficit that localizes to the spinal cord level, MRI or myelography followed by CT must be used to look for traumatic intervertebral disc rupture or spinal epidural hematoma (see Fig. 108-5).

The goals of treatment are to correct spinal alignment, to protect undamaged neural tissue, to restore function to reversibly damaged neural tissue, and ultimately to achieve permanent spinal stability. Reduction and immobilization of any fracture or dislocation must receive top priority to meet these objectives. The routine administration of systemic corticosteroids (dexamethasone) is helpful in spinal cord injury.

Cervical spine malalignment can almost always be reduced by skeletal traction. Traction can be applied with skull tongs or halo apparatus. Both are seated percutaneously through the outer table of the skull while the patient is kept supine and immobilized. The patient is then transferred to a special bed and placed in cervical traction, usually in the neutral position. Frequent lateral view radiographs are obtained to ensure good reduction and to pre-

vent overdistraction, which can lead to further cord injury. Once the spinal injury is reduced, traction should be maintained. Frequent follow-up films should be taken to confirm correct alignment. Sometimes a cervical fracture cannot be reduced by traction alone without jeopardizing spinal cord function. Open reduction, usually through a posterior approach, combined with a fusion procedure may be necessary in those instances. This especially pertains to unilaterally or bilaterally locked facets.

Patients with thoracic and lumbar spine fractures are also treated with immobilization initially. Immobilization is less strict than it is with cervical fractures, but the principles remain the same. Patients are kept flat in bed without traction, and flexion, extension, lateral bending, and rotational movements are avoided. Typically, fewer systemic complications are associated with these neurologic injuries, but vigilance is required to prevent neurologic deterioration and to provide the best chance for neurologic recovery.

Indications for early operation on patients with spinal cord injury include the inability to reduce the fracture or dislocation satisfactorily by closed methods, neurologic deterioration in a patient with an initially incomplete cord lesion, severe compression of the spinal cord by an intraspinal mass shown by myelography or MRI, and a penetrating injury with or without a CSF leak. Open wounds, such as stab and gunshot wounds, should be débrided and closed whether the cord injury is complete or incomplete. Early operation to stabilize the spine is warranted, because this translates into early mobilization and rehabilitation. Either the anterior or posterior approach can be used, depending on the nature of the spine injury and the degree of instability.

If closed reduction is successful and the fracture is stable, external immobilization is necessary for a minimum of 3 months to ensure proper healing. If surgical reduction and fixation are necessary, external immobilization is still indicated. For the cervical spine, this involves a halo vest. Exceptions include anterior and posterior metal plating procedures, for which a hard cervical collar may suffice.

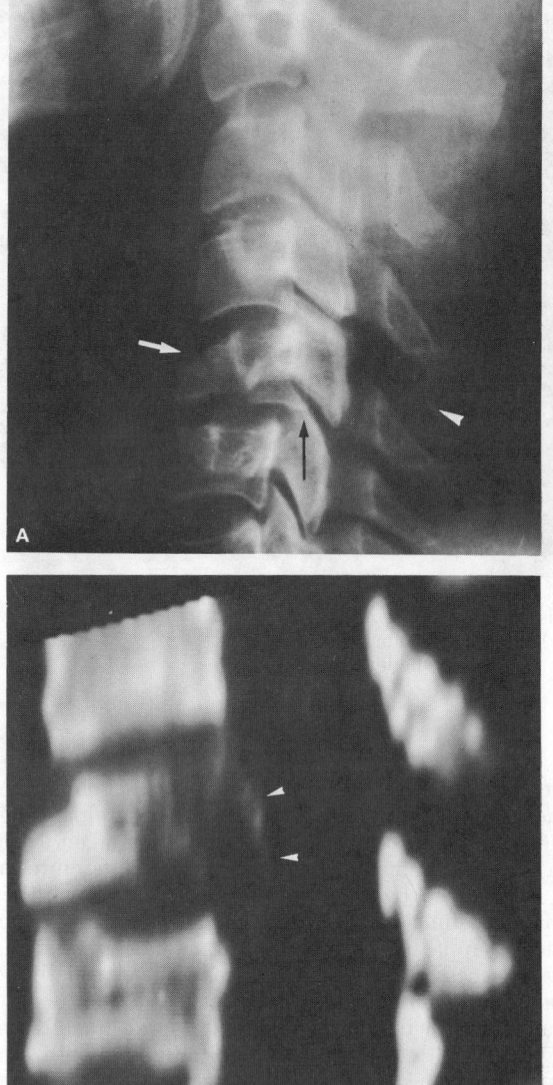

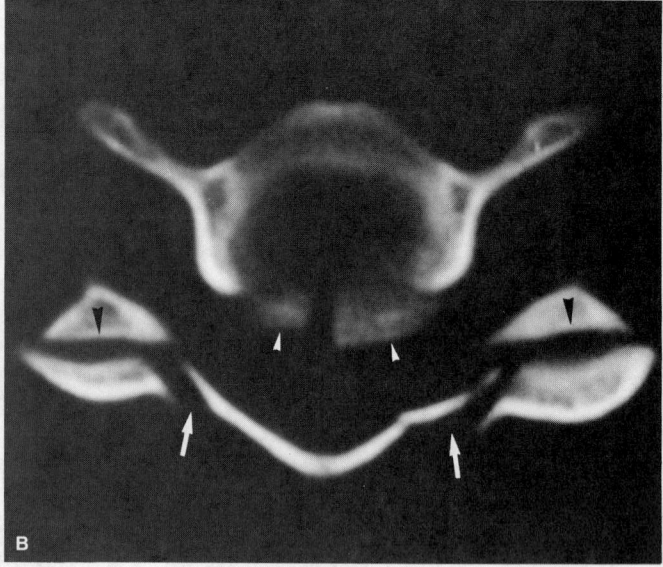

Figure 108-6. (*A*) Lateral cervical spine radiograph showing a C-5 fracture in a patient who was an unrestrained passenger in a motor vehicle accident. C-5 vertebral body compression (*white arrow*), retropulsion of a fracture fragment into the spinal canal (*black arrow*), and posterior interspinous widening (*arrowhead*) are visible. These findings are consistent with a hyperflexion injury. (*B*) Axial CT scan through the C-5 level reveals fractures of the vertebral body (white arrowheads indicate the retropulsed fragments) and the laminae (*arrows*) as well as disruption of both facet joints (*black arrowheads*). (*C*) Sagittal CT scan offers another view of the compromised spinal canal by the retropulsed fragments (*arrowheads*).

The thoracic and lumbar spines usually require a plastic body jacket or plaster cast for a minimum of 3 months. Plain films are used to monitor spinal alignment and extent of fusion after immobilization during the recovery period.

If any cord function is preserved immediately after injury, additional function usually returns if the cord and spine are protected from secondary injury. Sometimes the patient with an incomplete cord injury will walk again if early care is protective and rehabilitation is aggressive and well planned. Patients with complete injuries rarely recover function below the level of the lesion. Rehabilitation for them is directed toward self-care and vocational readjustment. Most persons with these handicaps can eventually achieve independence. Life expectancy is shortened slightly in paraplegics and significantly in quadriplegics. Long-term problems associated with skin care and recurrent urinary tract infections account for the early mortality.

Peripheral Nerve Injury

Peripheral nerve injuries can be categorized functionally. Neuropraxia is a temporary loss of function without axonal injury, and structural damage does not occur. The foot that goes to sleep after crossing the legs is an example of functional loss without abnormal change. Axonotmesis is a disruption of the axon with preservation of the axon sheath. Wallerian degeneration of the distal axon fragment occurs. Stretch or prolonged compression causes this functional and structural loss. Regeneration of the proximal axon occurs, but functional recovery depends on associated injuries, the amount of healthy proximal axon remaining after injury, and the age of the patient. Neurotmesis is disruption of both the axon and axon sheath with corresponding loss of function and is caused by transection of a nerve. Regeneration occurs, but function rarely returns to normal.

Clinically, sensory and motor changes correspond to the peripheral nerve involved. A detailed history and a precise neurologic examination can localize the site of injury with accuracy. Sensory findings are usually accurate early and remain so until regeneration is nearly complete. Compensatory motor function, often seen in the hand months after injury, is rarely seen acutely. A crude but clinically helpful sign of sensory regeneration is the Tinel sign. Percussion of the skin overlying the length of the injured nerve elicits paresthesias at the site where regeneration is occurring.

Radiographs of the injury site help find fractures or foreign bodies. EMG is not useful within the first 3 weeks of injury but is highly effective for monitoring the status of the degeneration and regeneration process that occurs later. Management decisions are often made based on EMG findings weeks to months after trauma.

Treatment of a lacerated nerve consists of primary repair when the wound is clean and uncomplicated, as in stab wounds, lacerations from glass, and surgical incisions. Secondary or delayed repair is indicated when the wound is dirty or complicated. Such wounds include gunshots and avulsions that disrupt tissue severely, making primary repair less successful. Secondary repair is best accomplished a few weeks after injury, when tissue viability is obvious, the likelihood of infection is reduced, and dissection planes are distinct. If end-to-end anastomosis is not possible because of tissue loss, nerve grafting with autologous sural nerve can be done. Intraoperative factors such as axial orientation of fascicles, proper coaptation, suture material, hemostasis, and suture line tension determine the outcome.

Nerve injuries in continuity (ie, resulting from contusion or compression without laceration) are often explored if they do not improve within 6 weeks of injury whether loss of function is complete or incomplete. Intraneural and extraneural scar tissue at the site of the lesion can prevent axonal regrowth by its constricting effect. Neurolysis releases the regenerating nerve fibers from the impinging scar and can improve functional recovery.

Prompt institution of physical therapy is also indicated for improvement of muscle function and maintenance of joint motion. It is the best means of minimizing the complications of denervation. The denervated portion of the limb is subject to muscle atrophy and fibrosis, joint stiffness, motor end-plate atrophy, and trophic skin changes. The longer the denervation persists, the less likely it is that good function will result.

Regeneration in a peripheral nerve occurs at 1 mm/d (roughly 1 inch each month), so improvement may not be obvious for many months. Factors that adversely affect the return of function include advanced age of the patient, proximal nerve injury, extensive nerve tissue loss, associated soft tissue injury, and mixed sensorimotor function. Unfortunately, incomplete neurologic recovery is often the rule. The use of tendon transfers should be considered to improve functional outcome if neurologic function is inadequate after recovery has ceased. Patients must understand that their role in treatment is an active one, and their motivation to recover must be encouraged.

NEOPLASMS

Nervous system tumors represent almost 10% of all neoplasms. Of these, 15% to 20% occur in children. Nearly 70% of adult tumors are found above the tentorium (supratentorial), whereas 70% of childhood tumors are found below (infratentorial). CNS tumors are the most common solid tumors in children. Of pediatric cancers, they are second only to leukemia in prevalence.

The incidence of nervous system neoplasia decreases in late adolescence and begins to peak again by middle age. By then, only 25% of intracranial tumors are benign. This percentage rises to 50% in the older patient, because of the increasing incidence of meningiomas and schwannomas. Overall, there is a slightly greater prevalence of tumors in men (55%), but schwannomas and meningiomas are more common in women. Of all CNS neoplasms, spinal tumors constitute about 15%.

Intracranial Tumors

Intracranial tumors exert both local and generalized effects by their presence within a closed bony structure, either arising from within or on the surface of a noncompliant brain.[4] A tumor's local influence consists of either irritative or destructive effects. Focal seizures occur because of irritation of adjacent cortex, whereas a focal neurologic deficit develops because of compressive forces on nearby functional brain.[4] More generalized effects consist of raised ICP due to the presence of the abnormal mass. This may be in the form of obstructive hydrocephalus, tumor hemorrhage, or cerebral edema, or it may simply be the result of the added volume imparted by the tumor in the closed bony compartment of the skull. The effects can be manifested as headache, occasional nausea and vomiting, decreased level of consciousness, and slowed cognitive function. Table 108-2 lists the World Health Organization's classification of intracranial tumors. The more common tumors are discussed below.

Astrocytoma

Astrocytes are glial (stromal or supporting) cells of the brain. Tumors arising from these cells make up over 60% of all intracranial tumors. Low-grade astrocytomas (grades I and II) constitute 12% of all intracranial tumors (25% of gliomas). When they involve the cerebral hemispheres, they typically arise during the fourth decade. They present with a 1- to 2-year history, producing signs and symptoms that include headaches, seizures, vomiting, mental status changes, papilledema, and focal neurologic deficits relevant to the hemisphere involved. On CT, they appear as low-attenuation lesions with minimal to mild contrast enhancement. These tumors are infiltrative and rarely can be totally excised. Surgery is generally performed for diagnosis and debulking and is usually followed by radiation therapy. The 5-year survival rate with surgery and subsequent radiation is 35% to 50%. Some low-grade astrocytomas can become anaplastic and, as such, become high-grade gliomas (see later).

Low-grade astrocytomas of the cerebellum typically occur in the pediatric population as a subtype of astrocytoma known as the *pilocytic astrocytoma*. They are often cystic with hamartomatous features, characteristics that carry a favorable prognosis. These tumors are often totally resectable. Radiation therapy is reserved for incomplete resections when follow-up has demonstrated continued tumor growth. The 10-year survival rate is over 80%.

Brain-stem gliomas are also posterior fossa tumors that occur most often in childhood. Most are benign astrocytomas. Patients may present with cranial nerve palsies, hemiparesis, and headache, often attributable to hydrocephalus. These tumors cannot be removed surgically because of significant risk of neurologic injury to the brain stem. They are treated with radiation therapy once a diagnosis is established through either open or closed biopsy. Unfortunately, prognosis is a function of their location, and 5-year survival rates are 15% to 30%.

Optic nerve gliomas are astrocytomas involving the optic pathways anterior to the optic tracts. They occur in the chiasm in 75% of cases. Two thirds of chiasmal tumors also invade the hypothalamus. The peak age of occurrence is 3 to 7 years, but their growth pattern is variable. Some remain stable for years, but others are relentlessly progressive. Those occurring strictly within one optic nerve can be excised, but the more extensive tumors are generally irradiated. The value of radiation therapy remains controversial.

High-grade astrocytomas (grades III and IV) are the most common primary intracranial tumor, constituting 25% of all

Table 108-2. WORLD HEALTH ORGANIZATION BRAIN TUMOR CLASSIFICATION (ABRIDGED)

TUMORS OF NEUROEPITHELIAL TISSUE

Astrocytic tumor
  Astrocytoma
  Pilocytic astrocytoma
  Subependymal giant cell astrocytoma
  Astroblastoma
Oligodendroglial tumor
  Oligodendroglioma
  Mixed oligoastrocytoma
Ependymal and choroid plexus tumor
  Ependymoma
    Myxopapillary ependymoma
    Subependymoma
  Choroid plexus papilloma
Pineal cell tumor
  Pineocytoma
  Pineoblastoma
Neuronal tumor
  Gangliocytoma
  Ganglioglioma
  Ganglioneuroblastoma
  Neuroblastoma
Poorly differentiated and embryonic tumor
  Glioblastoma
  Medulloblastoma
  Gliomatosis cerebri

NERVE SHEATH TUMORS

Neurilemmoma
Neurofibroma

TUMORS OF MENINGEAL AND RELATED TISSUES

Meningioma
Meningeal sarcoma
Xanthomatous tumor

PRIMARY LYMPHOMA AND BLOOD VESSEL TUMORS

Hemangioblastoma

GERM CELL TUMORS

Germinoma
Embryonal cell carcinoma
Teratoma

OTHER TUMORS AND TUMOR-LIKE LESION

Craniopharyngioma
Rathke cleft cyst
Epidermoid
Dermoid
Colloid cyst
Lipoma
Choristoma
Vascular malformations
  Capillary telangiectasia
  Cavernous hemangioma
  Arteriovenous malformation
  Venous malformation

TUMORS OF THE ANTERIOR PITUITARY

Pituitary adenoma
Pituitary adenocarcinoma

LOCAL EXTENSION FROM REGIONAL TUMORS

Glomus jugulare tumor
Chordoma
Chondroma
Chondrosarcoma
Adenoid cystic carcinoma

METASTATIC TUMORS

UNCLASSIFIED TUMORS

---

intracranial tumors and 50% of all gliomas. Age at discovery ranges from 45 to 65 years. The frontal and temporal regions are most commonly involved. Because of their infiltrative nature, many of these high-grade neoplasms involve both cerebral hemispheres by invading across the corpus callosum and are called *butterfly gliomas*. Histologically, these malignant lesions are composed of sheets of anaplastic cells with bizarre nuclei, numerous mitoses, endothelial proliferation, and abundant necrosis. Patients present with a short history of headache, focal neurologic deficit, mental status changes, or seizures (typically weeks in duration). The tumors are readily seen on CT scanning as low-attenuation lesions with marked peritumoral edema and mass effect (Fig. 108-7). Ninety percent show enhancement with intravenous contrast. Despite aggressive surgery, radiation therapy, and chemotherapy, these tumors are uniformly fatal. Although younger patients tend to do better, the average survival with surgery plus adjuvant therapy is about 12 months.

Chemotherapy is often used when tumor recurs, when the brain can no longer be irradiated, or when the tumor is not radiosensitive. It can be delivered intravenously, intraarterially, and intrathecally. Most drugs are directed at the tumor cells, whereas others indirectly attack the cells by sensitizing them to subsequent radiation. Although still in the early stages of development, immunotoxins toward tumor cells use antibodies to tumor antigens, thus using the host immune system as a means of destroying the cancerous tissue.

Meningioma

For the most part, meningiomas are benign tumors that arise from the arachnoid layer of the meninges, occurring in the fourth through sixth decades of life. They affect women in 65% of cases and arise in many typical locations. The locations of these tumors and their relative frequencies are as follows: parasagittal (falcine) 29%, sphenoid ridge 18%, convexity 13%, posterior fossa 10%, tuberculum sellae 9%, olfactory groove 5%, middle fossa 4%, and foramen magnum 2%. One percent or less occur in the orbit, gasserian ganglion, tentorium, and ventricular system. Together, meningiomas constitute about 17% of intracranial tumors.

Parasagittal (falcine) and convexity (hemispheric surface) meningiomas tend to present with seizures, focal neurologic deficits, and signs of intracranial hypertension. Sphenoid ridge tumors, classified as medial, middle, or lateral, can present with proptosis, decreased visual acuity, cranial nerve (III, IV, V, VI) palsies, seizures, or the more generalized effects of increased ICP. Posterior fossa tumors present with cerebellar signs, hydrocephalus, lower cranial nerve palsies, or long tract signs. Tuberculum sellae tumors are often accompanied by decreasing vision. Olfactory groove meningiomas can present with the classic Foster Kennedy syndrome of ipsilateral optic nerve atrophy and central scotoma with contralateral papilledema and bilateral loss of smell. Foramen magnum tumors can be difficult to recognize and are often diagnosed as multiple sclerosis, syringomyelia, or cervical spondylosis. Patients complain of neck pain, clumsiness, sensory disturbances in the upper extremities, and gait difficulties.

Either CT or MRI is the principal means of diagnosis (Fig. 108-8). Homogeneous pathologic contrast enhancement is characteristic of these neoplasms. Plain skull radiographs are abnormal 50% to 75% of the time, showing

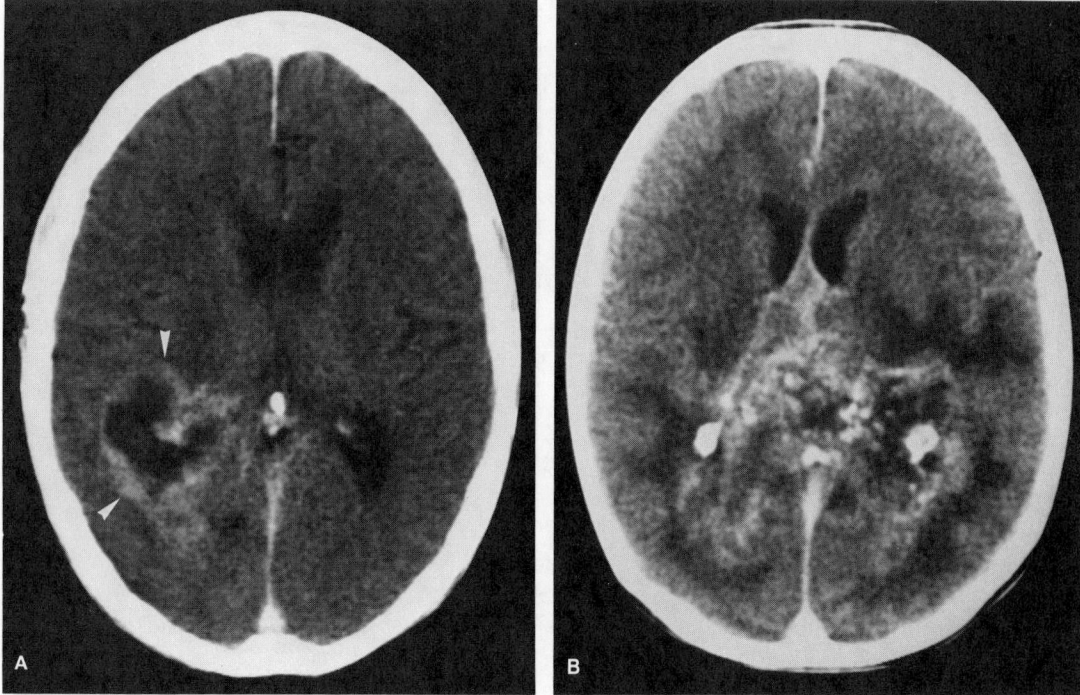

Figure 108-7. Glioblastoma multiforme (astrocytoma grade IV) discovered on contrast CT. (*A*) Typical appearance is that of a low-attenuation lesion with peripheral enhancement (*arrowheads*). (*B*) A more complex lesion demonstrating invasion across the corpus callosum.

tumor calcification, hyperostosis, increased vascular channels, or bone erosion. Angiography classically shows a blush in the late arterial phase.

The treatment for meningiomas is surgical. The techniques and goals are individualized for each tumor location, taking into account the patient's age and symptoms. In general, the goal is total excision, including the dura at the site of the tumor's attachment. If the meningeal origin cannot be excised, it is usually cauterized generously. Some meningiomas, such as those along the sphenoid ridge, may be en plaque tumors (ie, flat and tending to spread along the inner table of the skull). This feature often precludes total resection.

The recurrence rate of meningiomas after surgery depends primarily on the degree of excision and the presence of malignant histologic features. If the tumor is totally removed, including its dural attachment, the recurrence rate is about 10%. If the dural attachment can only be cauterized, the recurrence rate increases to 20%. With subtotal resection, the recurrence rate is about 40%. Nonmalignant and malignant meningiomas offer 15-year survival rates of 68% and 34%, respectively. Radiation therapy is generally reserved for malignant meningiomas, although it has also been used for incompletely removed nonmalignant meningiomas. The efficacy of this latter form of therapy remains debatable but is believed to provide prolonged survival.

Medulloblastoma

Medulloblastomas are part of the primitive neuroectodermal classification of brain tumors. They are thought to arise from primitive cells of the cerebellum, most likely the external granular layer. They constitute 8% of all gliomas and one third of all fourth ventricular region tumors. Two thirds of medulloblastomas occur in children, with an average age of onset of 14 years. In children, these tumors are more likely to occur in the midline, usually within the fourth ventricle, whereas adult tumors are fre-

quently positioned more laterally. They commonly metastasize throughout the subarachnoid space by way of the CSF and are rarely found outside the CNS.

Children with medulloblastomas commonly present with elevated ICP secondary to hydrocephalus. Cerebellar signs may be prominent with truncal ataxia and nystagmus. Some can present initially with symptoms related to spinal metastases. The diagnosis is generally made by seeing an enhancing mass on CT. Once again, MRI provides the best images of this common posterior fossa tumor. Cytologic examination of the CSF is often positive for neoplastic cells.

Treatment involves aggressive surgical removal of the tumor, followed by radiation of the brain. If CSF cytology is positive or if staging spinal myelography or MRI is positive, the spinal axis is included in the radiated field. Chemotherapy is commonly used as well. The 5-year survival rate depends on the extent of tumor resection and the efficacy of radiation therapy. Some centers report rates of 75% in patients who have had gross total tumor resections.

Schwannoma

Schwannomas are benign tumors and arise from the Schwann cells that surround axons as they leave the CNS by way of cranial nerves. Schwannomas constitute 8% of all intracranial tumors and are almost twice as common in females as males. They occur usually in the middle decades of life. If associated with von Recklinghausen disease, they can be multiple.

Schwannomas usually occur on sensory cranial nerves. The vestibular portion of the acoustic nerve is by far the most common site (acoustic neuroma). Depending on their size, these tumors usually produce hearing loss. As they enlarge, they can create facial numbness by compression of the trigeminal nerve and loss of coordination by compression of the adjacent cerebellar hemisphere. Only very late in their course do they cause facial weakness. Symp-

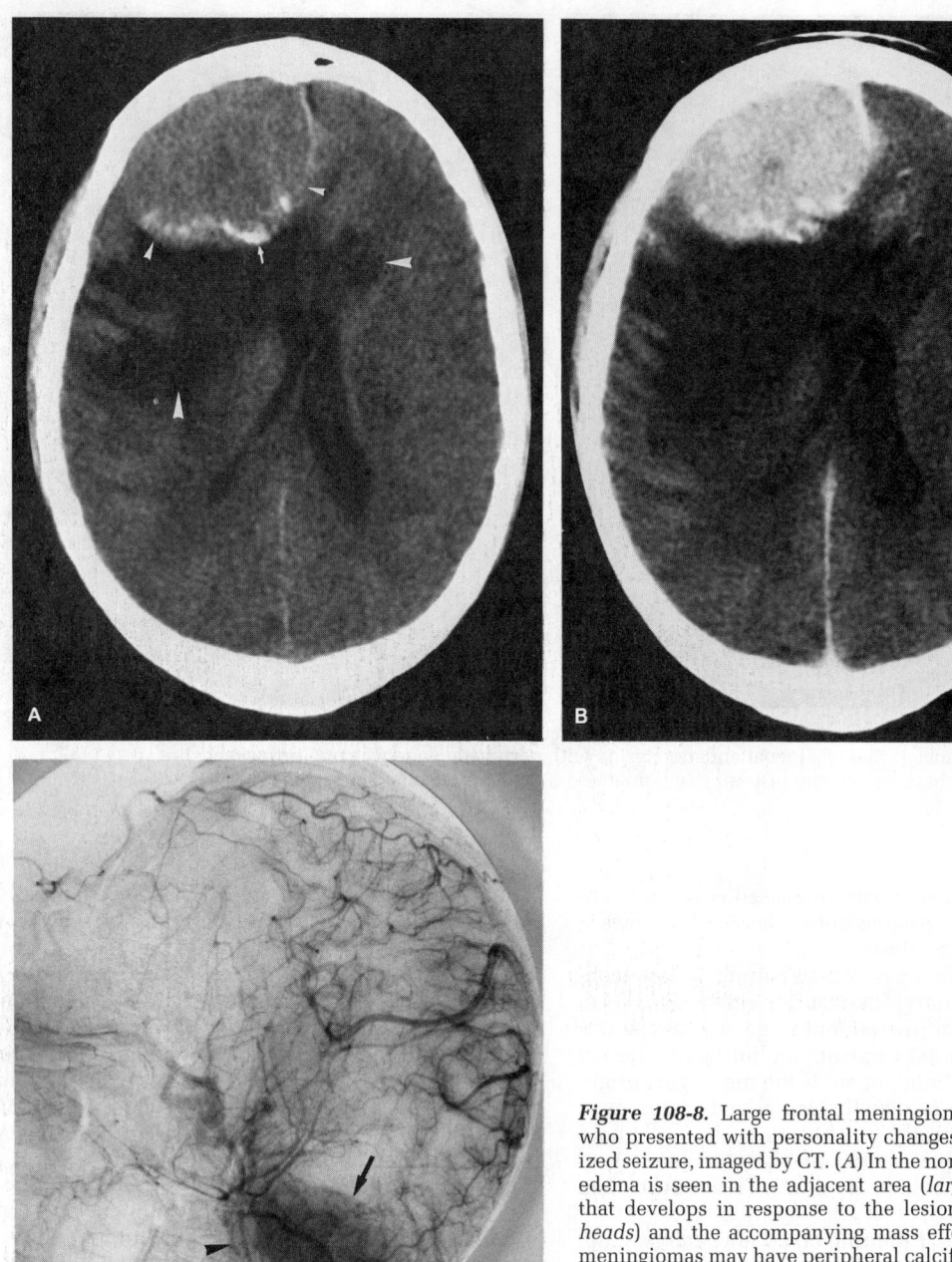

Figure 108-8. Large frontal meningioma in a patient who presented with personality changes and a generalized seizure, imaged by CT. (*A*) In the noncontrast study, edema is seen in the adjacent area (*large arrowheads*) that develops in response to the lesion (*small arrowheads*) and the accompanying mass effect. Some large meningiomas may have peripheral calcification (*arrow*). (*B*) With contrast, the lesion enhances homogeneously. (*C*) The angiogram demonstrates the classic late arterial phase blush (*arrow*). The arrowhead marks the floor of the anterior fossa (orbital roof).

toms of increased ICP due to obstructive hydrocephalus can also present late.

Much less commonly, schwannomas arise from the trigeminal nerve, presenting as a mass in the middle fossa that is associated with facial numbness. Some patients complain of lancinating, burning, and episodic pain similar to trigeminal neuralgia. Only rarely do other cranial nerves serve as the primary site of origin for schwannomas. These less common sites are more apt to be involved in cases of neurofibromatosis. Schwannomas occurring in patients with neurofibromatosis are often associated with other intracranial tumors such as meningiomas, astrocytomas, and ependymomas.

The treatment of schwannomas is surgical, and total resection is curative. Microsurgical techniques have reduced the risks of surgery and have allowed preservation of cra-

nial nerve function. Acoustic neuromas can be resected by means of the suboccipital or translabyrinthine approach, with a 95% probability of preservation of facial nerve function with small tumors. Even with the largest tumors, preservation is predictable in 50% to 70% of cases. The translabyrinthine approach is reserved for those patients who have complete hearing loss due to the presence of the mass. If this loss is incomplete, the suboccipital approach is preferred, allowing for maximal hearing preservation by leaving the middle and inner ear structures intact. Once again, preservation is directly related to tumor size. Seventy-three percent of patients with small tumors measuring 0.5 cm or less in diameter retain useful hearing. This drops to 11% for tumors measuring 2.5 cm or more. The mortality rate is a function of tumor size as well, with most deaths occurring in patients with tumors greater than 4 cm in size.

Pituitary Adenoma

Tumors arising from the pituitary gland are generally benign histologically and constitute about 8% of intracranial tumors (see Chap. 56). Focused beam radiation therapy (stereotactic radiosurgery) is an alternative method of treatment.

Ependymoma

Ependymomas originate in the ependyma, the glial cells that line the ventricular system, and constitute 5% of gliomas. Their incidence peaks at age 5 and again at 34 years of age. They arise below the tentorium, usually within the fourth ventricle, in two thirds of cases. When they occur above the tentorium, 50% are intraventricular. Infratentorial ependymomas are far more common in children. They make up about one fourth of all fourth ventricular region tumors.

The presenting symptoms are related to the tumor location. Typically, children harboring fourth ventricular tumors present with headache and vomiting related to the associated obstructive hydrocephalus. They also tend to have ataxia secondary to cerebellar compression. Patients with supratentorial tumors present with signs of raised ICP as well, but this is usually because of brain edema. Focal neurologic deficits are common. These tumors are usually well circumscribed on CT scans as enhancing masses. MRI is the study of choice when the tumor involves the posterior fossa because MRI far surpasses the imaging capabilities of CT in this region (Fig. 108-9).

Treatment involves aggressive surgical excision. Unfortunately, fourth ventricular tumors can rarely be totally removed because of invasion of the fourth ventricular floor. They are radiosensitive, so this modality clearly prolongs survival. The average 5-year survival rate with surgery and irradiation for both children and adults is in the range of 50%, with children faring less well overall. Chemotherapy is reserved for the higher grade neoplasms. All ependymomas have a propensity to recur despite aggressive management.

Oligodendroglioma

Tumors arising from the oligodendroglial cells (the supporting cells that are the source of myelin in the CNS) make up 4% of gliomas and usually occur in the cerebral hemispheres. Half of all hemispheric lesions occur in the frontal lobes. Up to one third are mixed tumors containing populations of astrocytes or ependymal cells in addition to oligodendrocytes. They are considered slow-growing with benign histologic features, but as many as 25% may show some degree of anaplasia.

Patients present with a history measured in years; 80% have a history of seizures. Patients commonly have findings of focal neurologic deficits and papilledema. These tumors are unique in their tendency to calcify, attesting to their benign nature. On CT scan, a high percentage show calcification, and most have contrast enhancement (Fig. 108-10).

Treatment involves maximum surgical resection. Radiation therapy is reserved for those tumors displaying malignant histologic features or in cases of subtotal excision. The average 5-year survival rate is 50% to 80%. There are well-documented long-term survivors, with a reported 20-year survival rate of 6%.

Craniopharyngioma

Histologically benign, craniopharyngiomas arise from nests of squamous cells within the pituitary gland. They can be found in intrasellar or suprasellar locations but are always along the craniopharyngeal canal. They are com-

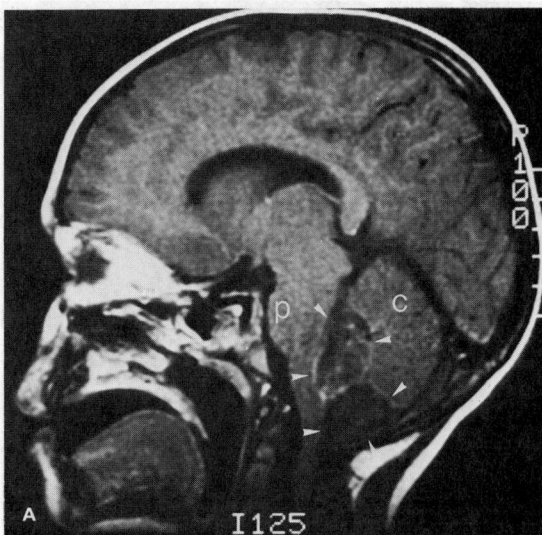

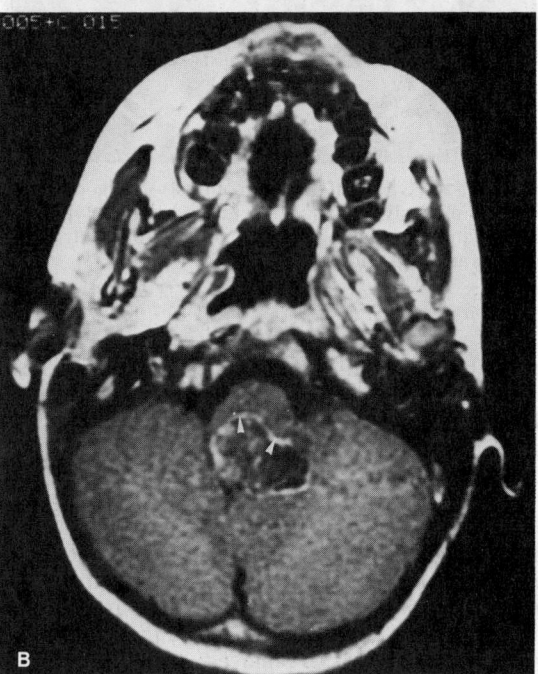

Figure 108-9. Fourth ventricular ependymoma imaged by gadolinium-enhanced MRI. (*A*) The sagittal view demonstrates the tumor (*arrowheads*) completely occupying and expanding the fourth ventricle. Note its relation to the brain stem and cerebellum (c). p, pons. (*B*) The axial view reveals marked brain-stem compression (*arrowheads*).

mon supratentorial tumors in children and constitute 3% of all intracranial tumors. More than half occur in the first two decades of life. They are largely cystic in children, containing a much larger solid component in adults. The cysts are filled with a thick fluid (sometimes described as motor oil–like) that contains cholesterol crystals. Microscopically, they are cystic epithelial tumors with both squamous and columnar elements. Tumor calcification is common and is of considerable radiologic diagnostic importance.

Patients generally present with visual difficulties, hypopituitarism, and elevated ICP. Visual problems include papilledema, visual field loss, and decreased acuity. The endocrinopathy includes diabetes insipidus, obesity, short

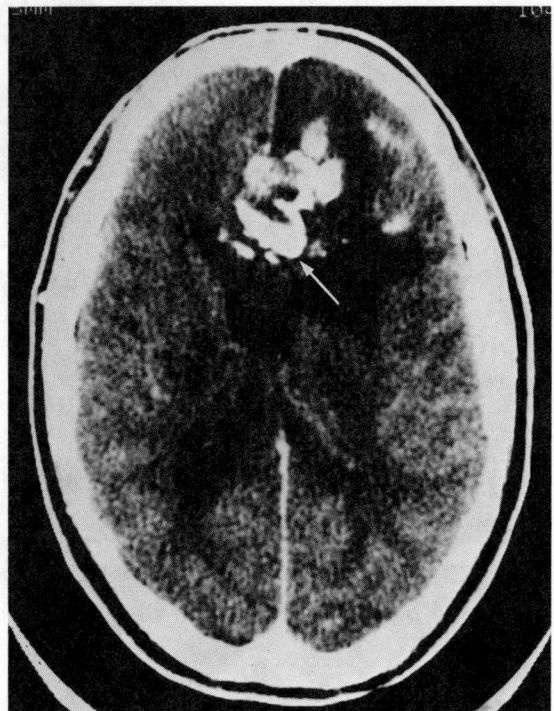

Figure 108-10. CT scan without contrast of oligodendroglioma shows the extensive calcification (*arrow*) that is typical of this lesion. Bilateral frontal lobe involvement is apparent, with tumor extending across the midline.

stature, hypothyroidism, and impaired sexual development. Elevated ICP is usually secondary to hydrocephalus.

These tumors are usually well imaged with high-resolution CT and MRI (Fig. 108-11). Treatment is usually surgical, often in combination with radiation therapy. Total surgical extirpation is possible more often in children. Recurrences are common after subtotal removals. Irradiation can be given externally or by stereotaxic placement of radioactive substances within the cystic portion. Although craniopharyngiomas can be cured with surgical removal, or controlled with radiation, many of these histologically benign tumors cannot be removed safely.

Germinoma

Germinomas occur most commonly in the region of the pineal gland and thus have been misnamed *pinealomas* in the past. The suprasellar region involving the hypothalamus is the second most common location. They are much more common in males and tend to occur in the second and third decades. They are composed of two cell populations (tumor cells and lymphocytes) and are histologically indistinguishable from testicular seminomas and ovarian dysgerminomas.

Germinomas in the pineal region tend to produce obstructive hydrocephalus and Parinaud syndrome, a midbrain syndrome characterized by upward gaze paresis, loss of convergence, and small, unreactive pupils. Those in the hypothalamic region may be associated with diabetes insipidus and emaciation (diencephalic syndrome). Germinomas are radiosensitive and do not require aggressive surgical resection, but biopsy is recommended before irradiation. The 5-year survival rate approaches 75% after radiation therapy.

Other related germ cell tumors include teratomas, embryonal cell tumors, endodermal sinus tumors, and choriocarcinomas. These tend to arise in the same locations as

germinomas. The germ cell tumors often produce compounds that serve as tumor markers. These markers are frequently identified with immunoassays of the CSF or with immunoperoxidase stains of the tissue under light microscopy. All choriocarcinomas and 10% of germinomas secrete β-human chorionic gonadotropin (HCG). Endodermal sinus tumors produce α-fetoprotein (AFP). Embryonal cell tumors typically synthesize both β-HCG and AFP. Teratomas secrete neither marker. These markers are useful for confirming the diagnoses and for measuring responses to treatment.

Epidermoid, Dermoid, and Teratoma

Epidermoids and dermoids arise from benign inclusions of epithelial elements within the CNS during closure of the embryonic neural groove. Epidermoids contain only stratified squamous epithelium. Dermoids contain skin appendages such as hair follicles, sebaceous glands, and sweat glands in addition to the squamous epithelium. Epidermoids tend to arise off the midline in locations such as the cerebellopontine angle, the parasellar region, and the diploë of the skull. Dermoids, on the other hand, usually arise in midline structures such as the cerebellar vermis or fourth ventricle. They are often accompanied by overlying bone and skin defects. Both tumor types are easily identified on CT and MRI scans. Surgical removal is the preferred treatment. Recurrences are usually managed with further surgery.

Teratomas are more common in children. By definition, they are composed of tumor cells representing all three embryonic germ cell layers. The more differentiated teratomas often contain cartilage and bone. If these elements are primitive, they are considered malignant. Like dermoids, they tend to occur in the midline in such locations as the pineal region, third ventricle, and posterior fossa. Treatment is surgical excision, along with irradiation in certain malignant types.

Hemangioblastoma

These benign tumors are vascular and usually occur in the cerebellum. They are uncommon and constitute only 1% to 2% of intracranial tumors. Typical presentation is in the fourth decade. Fifteen percent of patients have von Hippel–Lindau disease, an autosomal dominant disorder consisting of CNS hemangioblastomas, retinal angiomatosis, renal and pancreatic cysts, and renal cell carcinoma. Irrespective of this syndrome, many patients have polycythemia. Sizable neoplastic cysts are present in 60% of cases, often with only a small mural nodule of tumor. Total surgical removal is curative. Radiation therapy is used when resection is not possible. Reoperation is recommended for recurrences. Long-term survival rates are excellent, with up to 80% of patients alive at 10 years.

Metastatic Tumor

The percentage of intracranial tumors representing metastases approaches 25%. Malignant cells invade the CNS hematogenously and tend to lodge at the gray and white matter junction. Metastatic tumors occur singly or multiply and can involve virtually any portion of the brain or, less commonly, spinal cord. Although any malignancy has the potential to metastasize, the most common primary sites are the lung, breast, kidney, testis, colon, and skin. The presenting symptoms are determined by the site or sites of the metastases. The symptoms commonly include headache, mental status changes, seizures, and hemiparesis.

Metastatic lesions are best imaged with high-resolution CT scanning but can mimic other lesions such as meningiomas, abscesses, primary brain tumors, and even aneurysms. MRI is helpful in narrowing the differential diagno-

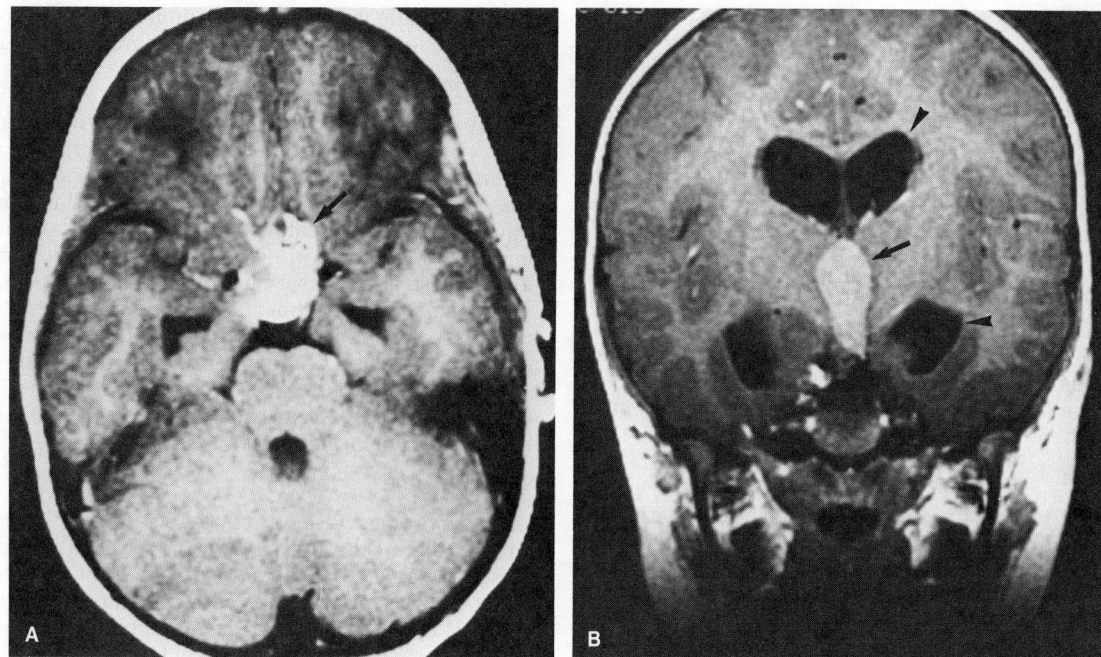

Figure 108-11. This 5-year-old child presented with decline in visual acuity and papilledema. (*A*) Axial MRI scan with gadolinium reveals an enhancing mass (*arrow*) in the region of the sella turcica. (*B*) A coronal view shows a large cyst (*arrow*) extending up into the third ventricle. There is hydrocephalus (*arrowheads*). At surgery, a craniopharyngioma was removed.

sis. If a metastasis is suspected, an extensive workup to find the primary source is recommended. If the primary site is not identified, an excisional biopsy is indicated.

In general, a symptomatic, solitary lesion that is surgically accessible should be removed. Surgery should not be undertaken for multiple lesions or in patients who are severely afflicted by their primary disease. Treatment should also include preoperative dexamethasone, as in any brain or spinal cord tumor, to reduce adjacent brain edema. Whole-brain irradiation is almost always indicated. Prognosis depends on tumor type, with median survival ranging from 1 to 2 years. Long-term survivors have been reported with surgical removal of solitary brain metastases. Quality of life is almost always improved. There is little evidence that chemotherapy plays a significant treatment role. Again, stereotaxic radiosurgery can play an increasing role in the treatment of metastatic tumors.

Tumor metastasis to the leptomeninges (meningeal carcinomatosis) is also common, particularly in the childhood leukemias and in adults with lymphoma, breast and lung cancer, and melanoma. Patients can present with cranial nerve palsies, radiculopathies, or obstructive hydrocephalus. They often have signs and symptoms suggestive of meningitis. Analysis of the CSF is usually critical, often revealing an increased opening pressure, elevated white cell count and protein levels, and a decreased glucose. There may or may not be identifiable malignant cells, but cytologic examination should always be performed.

Treatment of meningeal carcinomatosis usually involves radiation therapy and intraventricular chemotherapy. Methotrexate is a common chemotherapeutic agent. The outlook for patients with leptomeningeal tumor spread is generally poor, but a few long-term survivors emerge.

Spinal Tumors

Spinal tumors constitute about 20% of all CNS tumors. They are classified as intradural or extradural. Of the intradural type, 84% are outside the spinal cord (extramedul-lary) and 16% are within (intramedullary). Intradural tumors are almost always primary CNS tumors, whereas most extradural tumors are either metastatic or primary bone tumors of the spine. Most intradural spinal neoplasms are benign and can often be totally excised surgically. Tumors occurring within the cord (intradural, intramedullary) tend to produce weakness, increased tone usually in the form of spasticity, and sensory loss. Extramedullary lesions present with radicular pain from nerve root (lower motor neuron) compression as well as long tract (upper motor neuron) signs from cord compression. Patients with spinal tumors involving the conus region may have early loss of bladder and bowel function; those with tumors in the cauda equina present primarily with leg pain and only later develop sphincter disturbances.

The definitive study for spinal tumors is MRI, although abnormal plain films and myelograms can be diagnostic. Plain films may show widening of the interpeduncular distance, bony erosion, enlargement of the neural foramina, or a paraspinous mass. Myelography helps determine the tumor's relation to the spinal cord and dura. Postmyelogram CT can further define that relation. MRI allows refinement of the differential diagnosis.

Neurilemmoma and Neurofibroma

Typically benign, neurilemmomas and neurofibromas are the most common spinal cord tumors, making up almost 30% of the total. They are usually extramedullary intradural tumors. Of these, 13% have extradural extension through an adjacent foramen, producing the classic dumbbell shape of the neurofibroma. Fourteen percent are totally extradural. The extradural component tends to enlarge the involved foramen. Treatment is surgical removal. Adjacent or involved spinal nerve roots (usually the dorsal ones) may need to be sacrificed to obtain total excision. Multiple neurofibromas are associated with von Recklinghausen disease. In those instances, only the symptomatic tumors are removed.

Meningioma

Meningiomas constitute 26% of spinal tumors, are benign, and are usually extramedullary intradural tumors. Fifteen percent occur extradurally. Two thirds arise in the thoracic spine, affecting women in their fourth through sixth decades in 80% of cases. Surgical excision is the treatment of choice.

Ependymoma

Arising from the ependymal cells of the CNS, ependymomas are intramedullary tumors and constitute 13% of all spinal tumors. They occur more frequently in males. Nearly 60% are found in the conus region. Ependymomas should be surgically excised, and their distinct borders often allow complete resection. Radiation therapy is usually used when total removal is not possible.

Astrocytoma

These glial tumors are derived from astrocytes and are often intramedullary. Their incidence is about equal to that of spinal ependymomas. Total excision is rarely possible because of their infiltrative nature. Low-grade astrocytomas, if recurrent, are usually reoperated. Radiation therapy is reserved for malignant astrocytomas but is usually only palliative. Although the growth rate of spinal cord astrocytomas is slow, prognosis is generally poor.

Hemangioblastoma

Hemangioblastomas are rare tumors and are intramedullary 60% of the time. One third are associated with von Hippel–Lindau disease. They are benign, are well encapsulated, and should be surgically excised.

Lipoma

Lipomas constitute 10% of spinal tumors and are often associated with spina bifida and a subcutaneous lipoma. Although benign, they tend to invade the cord through a congenital dural defect and are usually only subtotally excised. These tumors do not require radiation, and mortality is low.

Dermoid

Dermoids are congenital lesions usually found in the lumbosacral area. They often have an associated sinus tract to the skin surface and can present with infection. The treatment is surgical resection, including the sinus tract. The resection of the portion entering the spinal cord is usually incomplete. The long-term prognosis is good.

Metastatic Tumor

Up to 25% of all spinal neoplasms are metastatic in origin, and most appear in an extradural location. Common primary sites include the breast, lung, prostate, and kidney. Treatment is surgical decompression with biopsy if the primary site is not known or if the neurologic decline is rapid. Otherwise, local radiation therapy is the treatment of choice. Other extradural malignant tumors include lymphoma, myeloma, plasmacytoma, chordoma, and osteogenic sarcoma. When significant bone destruction or surgical decompression renders the spine unstable, surgical stabilization through an anterior or posterior route is necessary.

Peripheral Nerve Tumors

The peripheral nervous system includes the peripheral and cranial nerves, spinal roots, and autonomic nervous system. Tumors can arise from any of these elements. The more common tumors are discussed later. More unusual tumors include gangliogliomas, neuroblastomas, paragangliomas, chemodectomas, and pheochromocytomas.

Schwannoma

Schwannomas arise from the peripheral nerve Schwann cells, which provide the myelin sheaths for axons. Schwannomas tend to displace the nerve of origin and thus usually present as a painless mass. With continued growth, they can create pain in the distribution of the nerve. As they enlarge, nerve function deteriorates. They tend to arise from sensory nerves but can also be found on motor nerves. The treatment is surgical excision. The nerve of origin can usually be preserved. At times, total excision may mean division of the parent nerve. If the nerve serves a significant function, it is preferable to leave a portion of the tumor to spare the nerve. This is possible because malignant transformation is rare.

Neurofibroma

Neurofibromas differ from schwannomas in that they actually engulf the nerve of origin within the tumor, because they arise from the nerve itself. They are often cutaneous, making it difficult to identify one specific nerve of origin. When associated with von Recklinghausen disease, they are usually multiple. When found alone, treatment is resection. When multiple tumors are present, only the symptomatic ones need to be resected. Removal requires sacrifice of the nerve, should that nerve be expendable. If the function of the nerve of origin is critical, a portion of tumor should be left attached to the nerve. Unlike patients with schwannomas, patients with neurofibromas should be followed closely, because these tumors have a higher incidence of malignant transformation.

Malignant Nerve Sheath Tumor

These tumors typically occur beyond the third decade. The treatment of choice is radical wide resection. If there is evidence of muscle or soft tissue invasion, amputation of the involved extremity is recommended. These tumors are generally resistant to radiation therapy.

CEREBROVASCULAR DISEASE

Cerebrovascular disease is the third most common cause of death in the United States and is an equally significant cause of chronic disability.[5] Death and disability are due either to ischemia causing focal or diffuse infarction or to hemorrhage causing compressive mass lesions. Cerebrovascular problems producing infarction can become hemorrhagic, and hemorrhagic lesions can lead to infarction.

Ischemic Vascular Disease (Stroke)

Ischemia and subsequent infarction of the brain can occur in the distribution of any of the cerebral vessels. Thus, any portion of the cerebrum, brain stem, or cerebellum can be affected. Because the carotid circulation provides the greatest blood supply to the brain, ischemia and infarction are most common within its distribution. Ischemia can be the result of diminished flow secondary to stenosis or occlusion of major arteries or can be due to transient or permanent occlusion of smaller arterioles from intravascular emboli.

The most common cause of stenosis or occlusion of large vessels is atherosclerosis. This often occurs extracranially at the origin of the internal carotid artery in the neck but can occur in the carotid siphon (that portion of the artery within the cavernous sinus), the distal internal carotid, or even the proximal middle cerebral artery.

Arterial emboli usually originate either from atherosclerotic ulceration in the region of the carotid bifurcation or from sources within the heart. The heart commonly becomes a source of emboli when a mural thrombus forms after a myocardial infarction or as a result of atrial fibrillation. Other risk factors for cerebral ischemia include hypertension, diabetes, hypercholesterolemia, obesity, smoking, and a family history of stroke.

Because there is no effective medical or surgical therapy for a completed stroke, the goal of surgical intervention is to identify stroke-prone patients and reduce their risk of cerebral ischemia. These high-risk patients are best identified by a history of transient ischemic attacks (TIAs). TIAs take the form of either transient cerebral ischemia or amaurosis fugax. Transient cerebral ischemia in the carotid circulation usually consists of temporary hemianesthesia, hemiparesis, or aphasia. Amaurosis fugax is transient loss of vision in one eye, usually in the form of an ascending or descending shade effect. Ischemia in the vertebrobasilar system can consist of transient diplopia, dizziness, dysarthria, dysphagia, weakness, numbness, loss of vision, or even loss of memory.

Most ischemic episodes last seconds to minutes; rarely do they last longer than 30 minutes. As long as the neurologic deficit resolves within 24 hours, the episode is a TIA. In contrast, a reversible ischemic neurologic deficit can last 24 hours to 3 weeks. Ischemic deficits lasting longer than this are considered completed strokes. Careful questioning of individuals with completed strokes reveals that of the 60% who had a history of TIAs, 20% had strokes that presented in a slow, stepwise fashion, and only 20% had strokes that were sudden in onset.

Patients with TIAs and even those with slow-onset strokes are potential candidates for preventive surgical intervention. Surgical procedures to prevent stroke are directed at either removing a source of emboli or providing increased blood flow to the brain. These consist mainly of carotid endarterectomy or a microvascular bypass procedure. Potential candidates generally undergo a CT or MRI scan of the brain to evaluate any degree of cerebral infarction and to rule out other diagnoses such as tumor, subdural hematoma, or subarachnoid hemorrhage. Patients then undergo careful angiography including the aortic arch, carotid, vertebral, and cerebral arteries. Noninvasive studies of the carotid circulation remain less accurate, although they are useful as screening procedures.

Carotid endarterectomy is indicated when ipsilateral symptoms of cerebral ischemia or amaurosis fugax exist and angiography demonstrates either significant stenosis (usually over 75%) or ulceration in the accessible portions of the common and proximal internal carotid arteries. The procedure consists of opening the affected portion of the carotid artery under systemic heparinization and removing the atherosclerotic plaque. Blood flow during the procedure may or may not be continued to the distal internal carotid artery by an internal shunt system. The mortality rate from carotid endarterectomy is about 1%, and the neurologic morbidity rate is 1% to 5% in experienced hands.

A number of patients present with cerebral ischemia ipsilateral to an occluded internal carotid artery or with stenosis of the internal carotid or middle cerebral artery that is not surgically accessible. For these patients with inadequate collateral cerebral circulation, a microvascular bypass procedure is sometimes indicated. The most common of these is the superficial temporal artery to middle cerebral artery anastomosis.

Intracranial Aneurysms

Intracranial aneurysms are diseased dilations of the cerebral arteries, their walls consisting of ballooned-out intima, media, and adventitia with a variable degree of intraluminal or mural thrombus. Most are congenital, evolving and developing during life. They can become atherosclerotic. Aneurysms typically are found at the bifurcation of the major vessels of the circle of Willis (Fig. 108-12). Up to 20% of patients with aneurysms have multiple aneurysms,

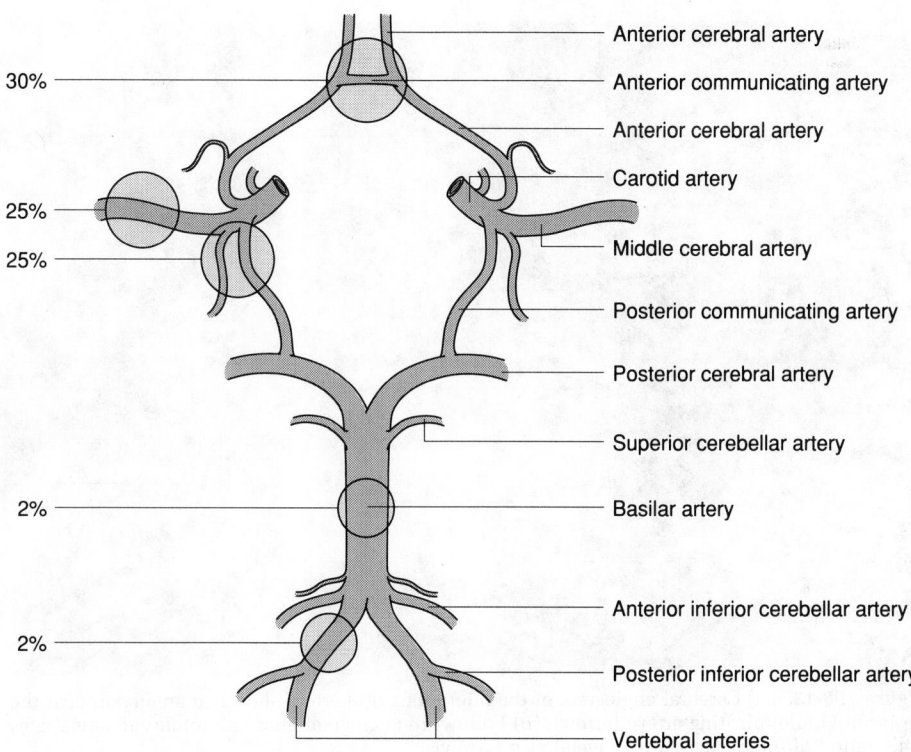

Figure 108-12. Locations of aneurysms of the circle of Willis and their relative occurrence.

- Anterior cerebral artery
- Anterior communicating artery
- Anterior cerebral artery
- Carotid artery
- Middle cerebral artery
- Posterior communicating artery
- Posterior cerebral artery
- Superior cerebellar artery
- Basilar artery
- Anterior inferior cerebellar artery
- Posterior inferior cerebellar artery
- Vertebral arteries

30%
25%
25%
2%
2%

and 1% demonstrate an associated arteriovenous malformation (AVM). If aneurysms are found more peripherally in the cerebrovasculature, a secondary cause such as trauma or infection must be considered.

Over 85% of cerebral aneurysms occur in the carotid or anterior circulation. About 30% arise from the intracranial portion of the internal carotid artery, usually at or near the origin of the posterior communicating artery (Fig. 108-13). Another 30% occur in the region of the anterior communicating artery. About 25% arise from the middle cerebral artery, usually at its first major branch point, which is commonly a trifurcation. Aneurysms of the vertebrobasilar or posterior circulation are most frequently found at the tip of the basilar artery but can occur more proximally along its trunk. The origin of the posteroinferior cerebellar artery is the next most common location.

Patients with intracranial aneurysms most commonly present with signs and symptoms of subarachnoid hemorrhage (SAH). In fact, 80% of nontraumatic subarachnoid hemorrhages are caused by aneurysm rupture. The victim reports a sudden severe headache commonly followed by neck stiffness and photophobia due to associated meningeal irritation caused by the subarachnoid blood. Transient loss of consciousness can occur. Some patients develop a focal neurologic deficit or become comatose because of the acute rise in ICP. The severity of the SAH can be graded on the Hunt and Hess criteria, as shown here. In general, the lower the grade, the better the outcome.

Grade I—No symptoms or minimal headache and slight nuchal rigidity

Grade II—Moderate to severe headache and nuchal rigidity; no neurologic deficit other than a cranial nerve palsy

Grade III—Lethargy, confusion, and mild focal neurologic deficit

Grade IV—Stupor, moderate to severe hemiparesis, possible early decerebrate posturing, and vegetative disturbances

Grade V—Deep coma, decerebrate posturing, and moribund appearance

Not all patients with aneurysms present with symptoms related to rupture. Through mass effect, an internal carotid artery aneurysm can compress the third cranial nerve, producing a palsy characterized by diplopia, ptosis, and dilated pupil. An internal carotid artery aneurysm within the cavernous sinus can compress the sixth cranial nerve and create diplopia. A giant aneurysm (more than 25 mm in diameter) of the basilar tip can block the cerebral aqueduct and create hydrocephalus. Rarely, an aneurysm can be large enough to be mistaken for a tumor.

The diagnosis of SAH is usually made clinically and confirmed either by noting blood within the subarachnoid spaces on CT or by finding bloody CSF with xanthochromia on a lumbar puncture (Fig. 108-14). The CT scan should be obtained first because it usually spares the patient a lumbar puncture and also eliminates the potential risk of brain-stem compression from herniation if an unsuspected mass lesion is present. Complete cerebral angiography is then used to identify and delineate the aneurysm and, at the same time, rule out multiple aneurysms or an associated AVM.

Once the diagnosis of aneurysmal rupture is confirmed, the patient is placed on a medical regimen to reduce the risk of rebleeding. This includes strict bed rest with the head elevated. Stimulation is kept to a minimum. Blood pressure is tightly controlled below 150 mmHg systolic. Careful observation is necessary to watch for signs of raised ICP, which may be attributable to delayed hydrocephalus. Anticonvulsants are started for seizure prophylaxis. Calcium-channel blockers are used to reduce the risk of vasospasm.

The ultimate treatment of aneurysms is microsurgical dissection and obliteration, usually by placement of a metallic clip on the aneurysm's neck by way of a craniotomy (see Fig. 108-13*B*). The timing of surgery depends on the clinical grade of the patient. Patients with a good grade (I

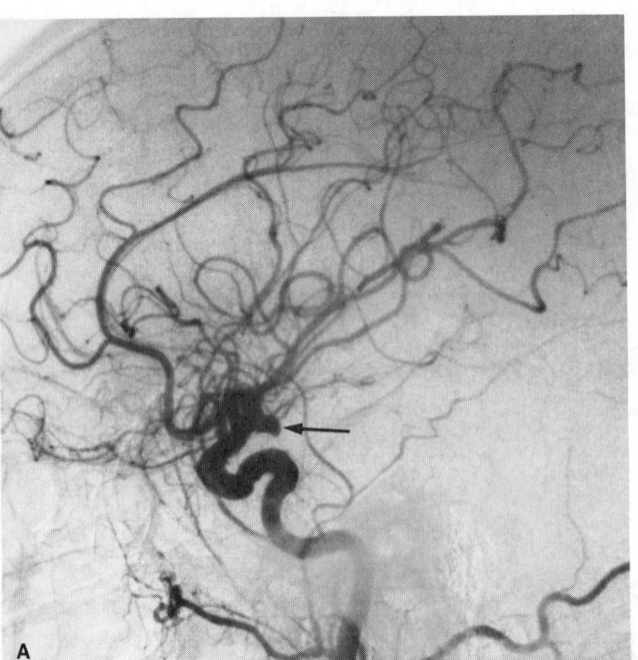
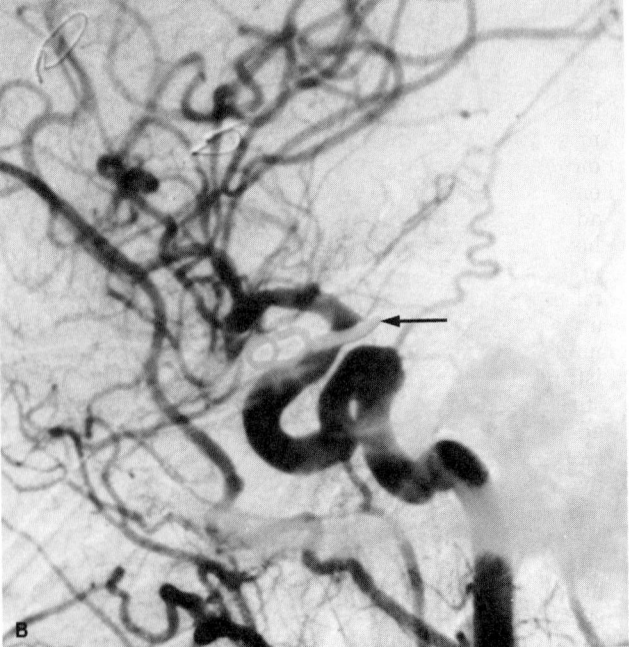

Figure 108-13. (*A*) Cerebral angiogram of the internal carotid artery shows an aneurysm near the posterior communicating artery (*arrow*). (*B*) Follow-up angiogram after craniotomy demonstrates obliteration of the aneurysm by a metal clip (*arrow*).

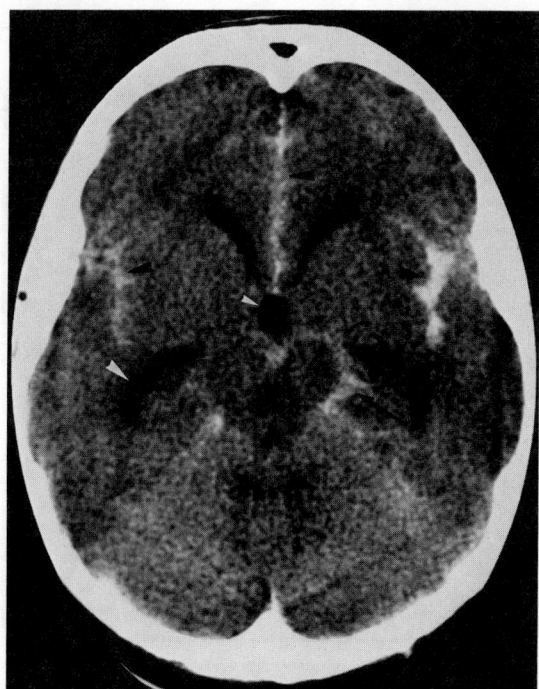

Figure 108-14. This patient presented with severe headache, nausea, and lethargy of acute onset. A noncontrast CT scan reveals diffuse subarachnoid hemorrhage with blood in the interhemispheric and bilateral sylvian fissures (*black arrowheads*) and in the subarachnoid spaces around the brain stem (*arrow*). Early hydrocephalus is evidenced by the rounding of the third ventricle (*small white arrowhead*) and visualization of the temporal horns (*large white arrowhead*).

and II) should undergo operation within 72 hours of rupture. Those with a poor grade (III and IV) should continue intensive medical management until they improve to a lower grade because mortality is higher with higher grades. Surgically accessible unruptured aneurysms should be operated on electively to prevent rupture. Some inaccessible aneurysms can be effectively obliterated by balloon embolization with interventional neuroradiologic techniques.

Complications of aneurysmal rupture include a 30% rebleeding rate within the first 8 weeks if the lesion remains unrepaired, hydrocephalus from obstruction of the arachnoid villi by subarachnoid clot, vasospasm, intracerebral hematomas, raised ICP, and seizures. The most significant and least understood of these is cerebral vasospasm. This phenomenon occurs most frequently within 4 to 7 days of the hemorrhage and results in narrowing of adjacent cerebral arteries. Vasospasm may be seen on angiography without any untoward clinical effects, or it may produce profound and life-threatening cerebral ischemia in the distribution of the involved vessels.

Because there is no effective way to reverse vasospasm and the calcium-channel blockers may not prevent its development, the best treatment is to increase cerebral blood flow to overcome the spasm. This is accomplished by increasing systemic blood pressure, often through inotropic support and intravascular volume expansion, usually by colloid and red cell transfusion. Cardiovascular status is monitored with a Swan-Ganz catheter.

Patients who undergo elective clipping of unruptured aneurysms do better than those with ruptured aneurysms because the brain has not been injured by the subarachnoid hemorrhage. In addition, aneurysms of the internal carotid artery carry less risk than those of the vertebrobasilar sys-

tem, with the exception of complex anterior communicating artery aneurysms. In general, if the aneurysm can be clipped and vasospasm avoided or effectively overcome, most patients do well.

Arteriovenous Malformations

Arteriovenous malformations occur within the CNS as congenital abnormalities in which blood is directly shunted from arteries to veins. AVMs can be small with only a single feeding artery, or they can encompass several lobes of the brain, incorporating arterial feeders from multiple sources. They can occur in almost any portion of the brain, including the cerebellum and brain stem. In the cerebral parenchyma, where they are most commonly located, they take on a conical shape with the apex deep, often reaching the lateral ventricle. Rarely, AVMs occur within the spinal cord, or they can exclusively involve the dura.

Patients with AVMs tend to present before age 30. Typical presentation is with hemorrhage (50% of cases and 10% of all intracerebral hemorrhages, second only to aneurysms). Bleeding usually occurs within the brain substance but can occur within the ventricular system or subarachnoid space. The patient experiences a sudden headache often associated with loss of consciousness and a neurologic deficit. The next most common presenting symptom is a seizure. In a few cases, seizures are frequent and refractory to medical therapy. AVMs can present with the insidious onset of a focal neurologic deficit as a result of mass effect, increased venous pressure, or vascular steal phenomenon. Occasionally, young patients with severe unrelenting headaches are found harboring an AVM.

From the time of discovery of an unruptured AVM, the risk of hemorrhage is about 1% per year cumulatively. Once an AVM has bled, the risk of rebleeding is increased to 5% per year. With each hemorrhage, the risk of death is about 10%; morbidity is at least 15%. Smaller AVMs are more likely to bleed than larger ones. Most AVMs remain stable in size, but some enlarge with time. Up to 10% have an associated aneurysm on a feeding artery. In these cases, hemorrhage is usually due to rupture of the aneurysm.

An AVM can be identified on contrast-enhanced CT scanning as a hyperdense mass, part of which has a serpentine configuration related to the presence of large draining veins. Their configuration and extent is more easily delineated with MRI (Fig. 108-15A). After hemorrhage, an unenhanced CT scan usually demonstrates intracerebral or subarachnoid blood. AVMs may be too small to be seen on CT, so careful angiography may be necessary to identify the source of hemorrhage. Lumbar puncture may be necessary if subarachnoid hemorrhage is suspected clinically but not verified by the CT scan.

In all cases of suspected or proven AVM, complete cerebral angiography must be undertaken to carefully define the extent of the malformation (see Fig. 108-15B and C). All feeding arteries, including any from the external carotid system, as well as the draining veins, must be evaluated. A treatment decision can be reached only with angiography. Should angiography fail to delineate a lesion despite suspicion, MRI can identify the angiographically occult abnormality.

The treatment of AVMs depends on the size and location of the lesion, the presenting symptoms, and the age and condition of the patient. Because of the risk of rebleeding, an AVM that has bled should be surgically excised if possible. In the patient who presents with seizures, the treatment decision is more difficult. In general, if the patient is young and the malformation is readily accessible, surgical

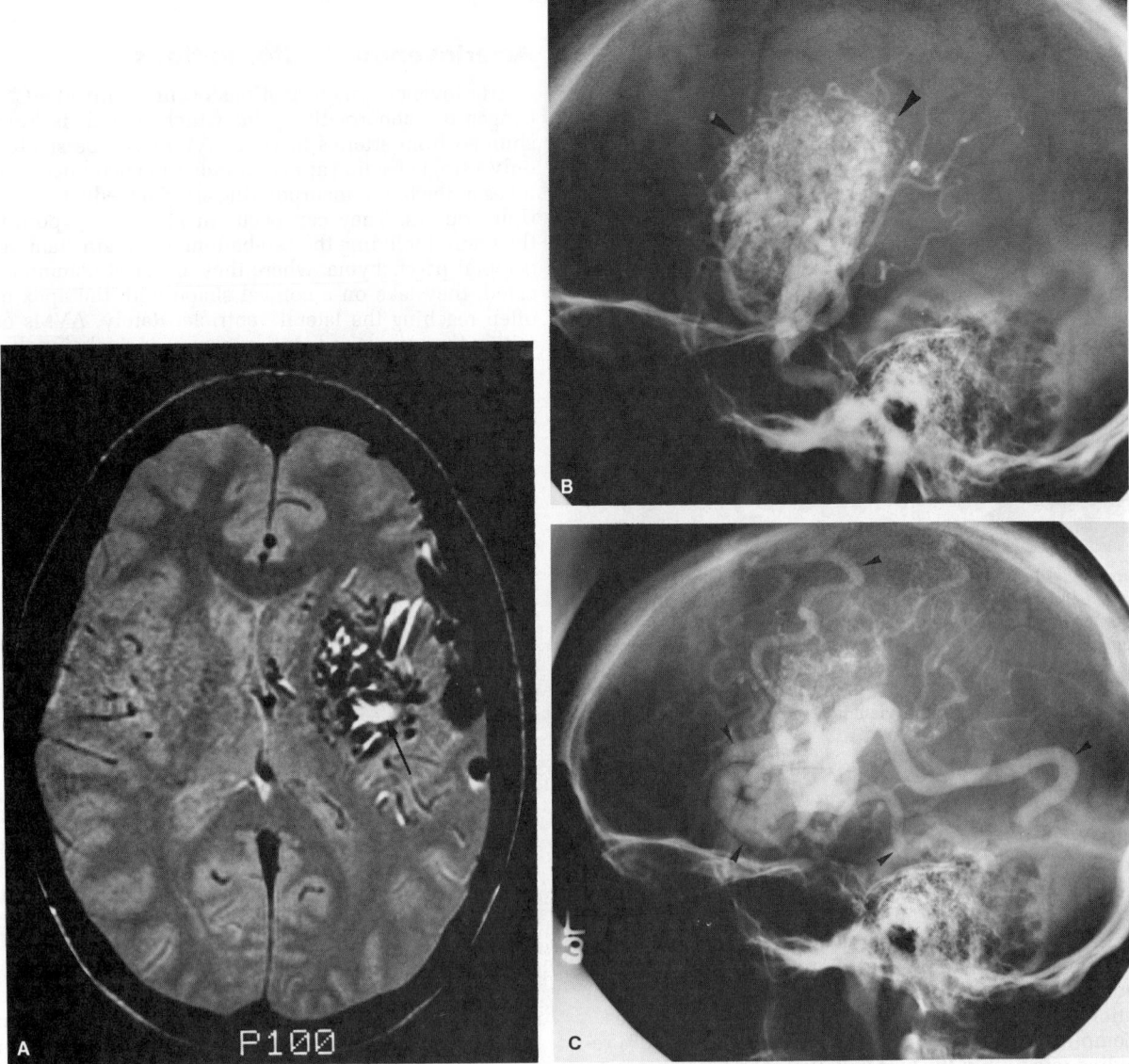

Figure 108-15. This young woman presented with a history of right arm clumsiness and seizures. (*A*) MRI scan without gadolinium shows a complex collection of tortuous blood vessels within the basal ganglia and temporal lobe consistent with an arteriovenous malformation (AVM). The bright signals within the lesion suggest previous hemorrhage (*arrow*). (*B*) Cerebral angiography (*lateral view*) on the same patient demonstrates a large AVM in the middle cerebral artery distribution (*arrowheads*). (*C*) Later phase of the angiogram reveals multiple draining veins (*arrowheads*).

resection is recommended, especially when the seizures are medically refractory. Surgery involves the microsurgical dissection and resection of the entire malformation, rather than simple ligation of feeding arteries. The results of surgery are related to the size and location of the malformation. Overall, the operative mortality rate is less than 5% and the morbidity rate is less than 10%.

Alternate or adjunctive methods of treatment include intraarterial embolization and radiation therapy. With the use of interventional neuroradiologic techniques, particulate matter or glues can be introduced into AVMs by way of feeding vessels in an attempt to occlude the arteriovenous shunt. It is rarely possible to completely obliterate these lesions with this method. This technique can reduce flow through the AVM before direct surgical intervention.

Ionizing radiation, on the other hand, can completely obliterate selected small to medium AVMs. Focused gamma or proton beam irradiation has demonstrated the best results, but an occasional success with conventional irradiation has been reported. Ionizing radiation causes endothelial proliferation and can take 6 months to 2 years to obliterate the lesion. Focused irradiation is recommended for deep, surgically inaccessible AVMs.

Brain Hemorrhage

Spontaneous hemorrhage is most commonly associated with systemic hypertension and occurs in predictable locations, including the putamen, thalamus, cerebellum, and pons. Hemorrhage can also occur within the various lobes of the brain. Nonhypertensive causes of brain hemorrhage were discussed earlier, such as rupture of AVMs and aneurysms, and hemorrhage into areas of ischemia. Additional causes include induced or endogenous coagulopathies, primary or metastatic brain tumors, and rare conditions such as amyloid angiopathy.

Chronic hypertension results in lipohyalinosis of the vessel wall, which sets the stage for either vascular occlusion or rupture. Occlusion results in infarction, whereas rupture produces an intracerebral hemorrhage. The shorter penetrating arteries of the brain appear to be the most vulnerable. The lenticulostriate and thalamoperforating vessels are involved in putamenal and thalamic hemorrhages, and affected basilar perforating branches contribute to pontine hemorrhage.

Although brain hemorrhage is often devastating, it can be surprisingly well tolerated. The hematoma tends to dissect along axonal planes, separating rather than destroying vital structures. If the resultant mass is tolerated by the patient, the blood is slowly resorbed by macrophages along the periphery, leaving only a hemosiderin-stained slit in the brain. Patients can worsen clinically after the initial hemorrhage because of associated edema formation.

Hemorrhage into the putamen accounts for most hypertensive bleeds. Presentation is characterized by lack of headache and the gradual development of hemiparesis progressing to hemiplegia. This can be associated with a hemisensory loss, aphasia, hemianopia, or ipsilateral deviation of the eyes, depending on the size of the hematoma and its direction of dissection. The patient can, of course, progress into a coma if the lesion is large. Similarly, thalamic hemorrhage presents initially with a hemisensory loss and a hemiparesis. Localizing features include downward eye deviation with limitation of vertical gaze and small sluggish pupils due to involvement of the nearby mesencephalon. Headache is uncommon.

Cerebellar hemorrhage is sudden in onset and presents with headache. Vomiting, ataxia, and dizziness are accompanying features. This hemorrhage is extremely dangerous in that it can cause coma and ultimately death due to brainstem compression and acute hydrocephalus. Brain-stem hemorrhage (usually pontine) is the most devastating and often presents with quadriparesis, decerebrate posturing, pinpoint pupils, and coma. Most patients do not survive if the hematoma is larger than 1 cm. Those who do survive have a high degree of morbidity. Lobar hemorrhage is less likely to be associated with hypertension and, in general, is better tolerated by the patient. The symptoms depend on the area of brain involved.

CT scanning has become an invaluable tool in diagnosing and defining brain hemorrhage (Fig. 108-16). CT not only delineates the hemorrhage but also assesses the ventricular size and the presence of edema, and often suggests the cause of the hemorrhage (eg, AVM, tumor, aneurysm). The hematoma appears hyperdense in the acute phase. With time, as the blood breaks down, the clot progresses to a hypodense lesion. After days or weeks, the hematoma may demonstrate an enhancing ring. If a vascular lesion is suspected, careful angiography is indicated. In all cases, appropriate coagulation studies should be obtained.

The treatment of brain hemorrhage can be medical or surgical depending on the size of the lesion, its location, and the condition of the patient. In general, if a hematoma is more than 3 cm in diameter, surgical resection is strongly considered. Surgical resection is recommended if the patient is deteriorating neurologically, no matter what the size of the hematoma. Cerebellar hematomas are particularly important to remove, because a small change in surrounding reactive edema can result in life-threatening brain-stem compression or hydrocephalus, or both.

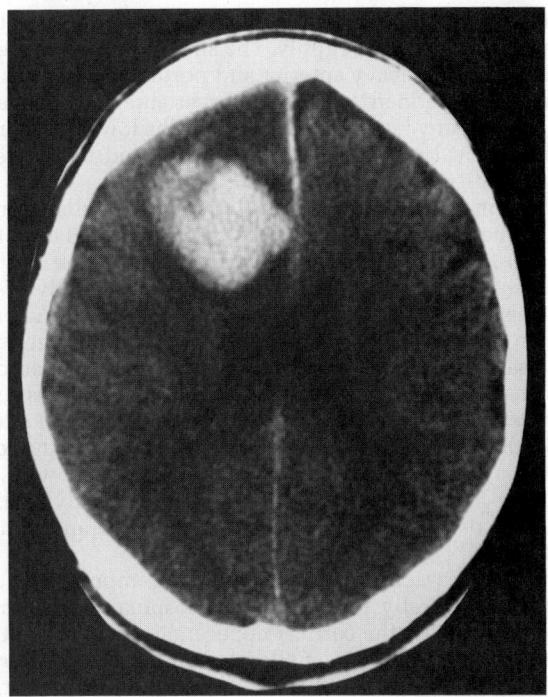

Figure 108-16. This noncontrast CT scan shows a spontaneous frontal lobe hemorrhage in a patient who was alert and complaining of headache. Examination revealed a contralateral horizontal gaze palsy secondary to involvement of the ipsilateral frontal eye field.

Because hematomas are mass lesions, medical management is directed at keeping the ICP under control. If the hemorrhage renders the patient unconscious, hyperventilation and hyperosmolar agents may be required to meet this goal. ICP monitoring can be a helpful adjunct to direct treatment. Steroids are useful in controlling brain edema if the patient bled into a tumor. Blood pressure needs close observation and tight control. Coagulopathies should be corrected. Despite medical and surgical therapy, mortality and morbidity remain high for all types of brain hemorrhage.

DEGENERATIVE SPINE DISEASE
Anatomy

The spinal column is composed of 33 vertebrae divided into the cervical (7), thoracic (12), lumbar (5), sacral (5 fused), and coccygeal (4 fused) regions. Each vertebra consists of a body, which bears weight, and the posterior elements (pedicles, laminae, spinous and transverse processes), which provide the flexibility and stability of the vertebral column. For the most part, the spinal canal has an ovoid shape in the horizontal plane, assuming a more triangular shape in the lumbar region. Most spine movement occurs in the cervical and lumbar regions. Flexion and extension are greatest in the lower cervical and lumbar segments, whereas maximal rotation occurs predominantly in the upper cervical and lumbar segments.

The intervertebral disc consists of two parts. The circumferential annulus making up the outer portion is composed of dense fibrous tissue of great strength. The central nucleus consists of fibrocartilage with little tensile strength but substantial elasticity. The nucleus is about 80% water at birth but gradually dehydrates with age, a process that leads to loss of elasticity. The fibrocartilage can then fragment acutely or degenerate gradually. It heals poorly because of limited blood supply. The annulus heals well and is buttressed by heavy anterior and posterior longitudinal ligaments for added strength. Intervertebral disc disease can occur at any level from C-1 to S-1. The lower segments of the cervical and lumbar areas are affected most often. Thoracic disc disease is rare.

The spinal cord extends from the cervicomedullary junction at the base of the skull to the conus or spinal cord tip at the L-1 to L-2 level. Within the spinal canal, the cord is centrally placed and can move rostrally and caudally a few millimeters during spinal flexion and extension. Lateral motion is restricted by the tethering of the intradural dentate ligaments. The blood supply is provided by the radicular arteries, which arise from the vertebral arteries and thyrocervical trunks in the neck, from the intercostal arteries in the thorax, and from the lumbar arteries in the low back. An arterial confluens, the artery of Adamkiewicz, is typically found in the T-10 to L-2 region, usually on the left side. It supplies the lower thoracic cord and conus medullaris.

Three fiber tracts of the spinal cord are important clinically. The laterally positioned corticospinal tracts carry motor fibers from the cortical upper motor neurons to the spinal lower motor neurons located in the ventral horns of the spinal cord. These tracts cross the midline at the pyramidal decussation in the lower medulla. The spinothalamic tract, also positioned laterally, transmits pain and temperature sensation from the contralateral side of the body. Within two or three segments of each dorsal root entry zone, the axons cross through the anterior commissure of the cord and ascend to the ipsilateral thalamus through this tract. The dorsal columns carry sensory fibers conveying position and vibratory and light touch sensation from the dorsal roots to the opposite cerebral cortex through a decussation in the brain stem.

Dorsal and ventral nerve roots emerge from the spinal cord separately, pass to their respective intervertebral foramina, and exit from the spinal canal. The roots join to form a spinal nerve within the neural foramen. In the cervical spine, the roots exit above the corresponding vertebrae. For instance, the C-5 root exits above the C-5 pedicle. Because there are eight cervical roots, C-7 exits above the C-7 pedicle, and C-8 exits above the T-1 pedicle. Consequently, all roots below C-8 exit below the pedicle of the corresponding vertebrae.

Below the conus, the lumbar and sacral roots form the cauda equina, which surrounds the filum terminale, the pial-arachnoid structure that anchors the distal cord to the caudal end of the spinal canal. The sacral roots are more centrally located adjacent to the filum. Because a lumbar root (eg, L-4) passes laterally toward the neural foramen as it descends within the spinal canal, it crosses the adjacent intervertebral disc (eg, L-4 to L-5) at its extreme lateral edge, hugging the pedicle of the vertebra laterally (Fig. 108-17). The nerve root then descends to the next lowest foramen (eg, L-5) and passes across the disc space (eg, L-4 to L-5) more medially, making that root more vulnerable to disease involving that disc.

Pathology

If the nucleus of an intervertebral disc extrudes (herniates) through the annulus, adjacent neural structures may be compressed. In the cervical and thoracic spine, compression of the spinal cord can result in paraparesis or quadriparesis, depending on the spinal segment involved. At all levels, compression of a spinal root can cause weakness and sensory loss in structures innervated by that root. The severity of the clinical syndrome depends on the site

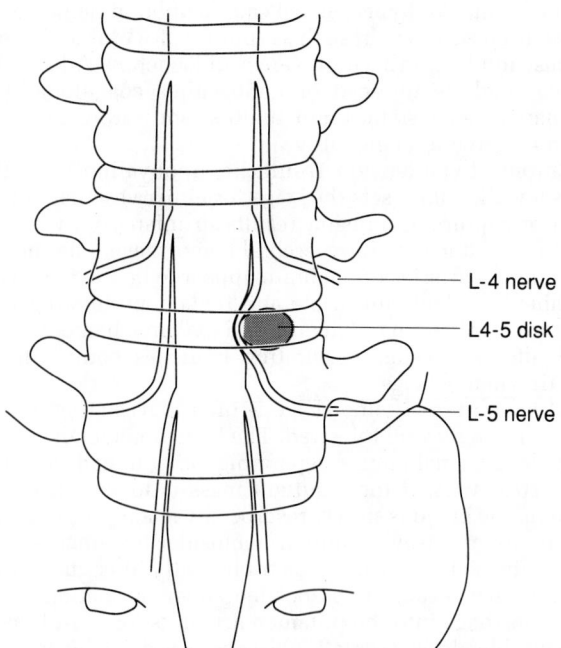

Figure 108-17. Relation between lumbar disc and nerve root exiting foramen.

L-4 nerve
L4-5 disk
L-5 nerve

and severity of compression by the displaced disc fragment. At times, the annulus and adjacent ligament hold, preventing complete extrusion of the fragmented disc. The annulus may only stretch sufficiently to allow the disc to bulge into the spinal canal or foramina.

Often the nucleus does not extrude but simply fragments in response to the forces exerted on the spinal column. This is intensified by the concomitant dehydration of the disc with loss of elasticity as it ages. The disc space gradually narrows, the joint becomes loose, and the cartilaginous end plates of the adjacent vertebral bodies abut and wear more quickly. Bony spurs (osteophytes) develop at the joint in reaction to the increased mobility and decreased elasticity.

Formation of osteophytes around the joints of vertebrae is termed *spondylosis,* a common disorder that is considered by some investigators to represent the normal process of aging. If an osteophyte forms in a neural foramen, the nerve root passing through can be chronically irritated and compressed. If the osteophyte develops within the cervical or lumbar canal, the cord or cauda equina can be compromised. Thoracic spine osteophytes causing neurologic dysfunction are rare, because their development is limited by the inherent reduced mobility of that part of the spinal column.

Cervical Spine

Clinical Presentation

The onset of symptoms and signs of an extruded disc fragment can be acute or chronic. Acute symptoms may or may not be related to trauma. In the cervical spine, neck and radicular discomfort occur simultaneously. Spinal cord symptoms are rare. There is usually limitation of neck motion, with loss of the normal cervical lordosis. With foraminal osteophytes, episodes of cervical discomfort recur over many months or years before radicular symptoms appear. Interscapular aching, suboccipital headaches, and even chest pain are common complaints.

Nerve root compression produces a radiculopathy often characterized by pain and hypoesthesia in the distribution of the involved root. Associated deep tendon reflex loss with or without weakness may be seen on examination. Cervical cord compression causes myelopathy characterized by progressive spastic paraparesis, mild to moderate sensory changes in the lower extremities and trunk, with cervical dermatomal sensory loss, weak upper extremity musculature, hyperreflexia, and plantar extensor responses.

Diagnosis

Cervical disc disease must be differentiated from other ailments, including inflammatory diseases of the soft tissues and joints of the arm and shoulder, nerve entrapment syndromes, and neoplasms. The pain must be distinguished from the pain that accompanies cardiac disease. Spinal infections, congenital lesions, and posttraumatic disorders are other important considerations.

Plain radiographs typically demonstrate loss of the lor-dotic curve of the cervical spine with narrowing of one or more disc spaces. Osteophyte formation may be seen. In cervical spondylosis, there is usually radiologic evidence of osteophytes and disc space narrowing at multiple levels. In most cases, the anteroposterior diameter of the cervical spinal canal is narrowed. Myelography with CT is useful in the diagnostic workup of a radiculopathy. The use of intrathecal contrast enhances the power of CT to delineate the lesion (Fig. 108-18). MRI is suitable for investigating myelopathies. In addition to defining the compressive lesion, MRI often shows intrinsic cord abnormalities related to the compression, consistent with edema or myelomalacia, a finding of clinical relevance. EMG can confirm the diagnosis and localize the lesion more specifically, particularly when myelographic defects are multiple.

Treatment

Painful cervical disc disease can be treated medically as long as there is no evidence of a progressive neurologic deficit (motor loss and bowel and bladder dysfunction be-

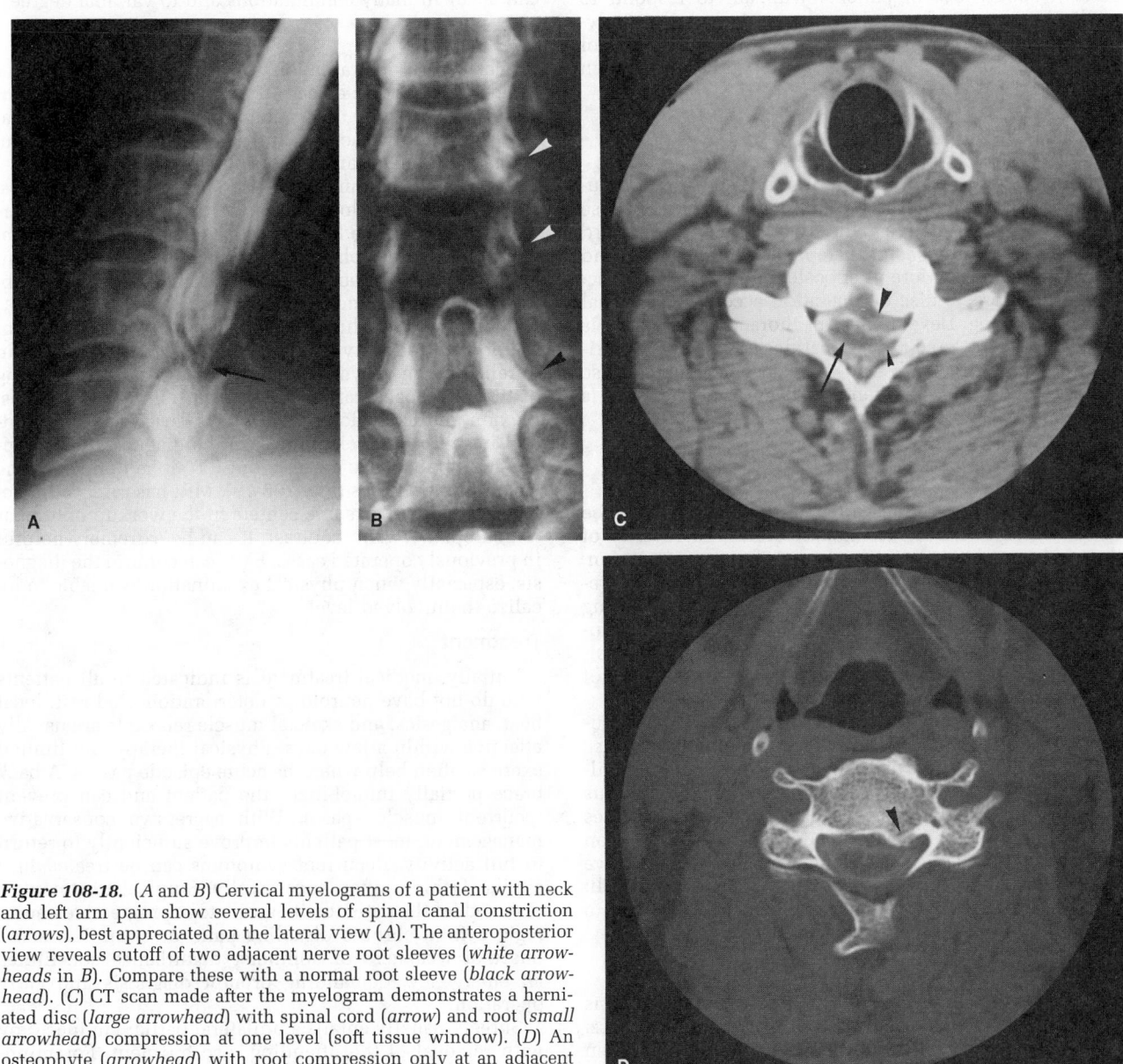

Figure 108-18. (*A* and *B*) Cervical myelograms of a patient with neck and left arm pain show several levels of spinal canal constriction (*arrows*), best appreciated on the lateral view (*A*). The anteroposterior view reveals cutoff of two adjacent nerve root sleeves (*white arrowheads* in *B*). Compare these with a normal root sleeve (*black arrowhead*). (*C*) CT scan made after the myelogram demonstrates a herniated disc (*large arrowhead*) with spinal cord (*arrow*) and root (*small arrowhead*) compression at one level (soft tissue window). (*D*) An osteophyte (*arrowhead*) with root compression only at an adjacent level (bone window).

ing most important). Adequate medical therapy includes immobilization of the neck with a soft or hard cervical collar, analgesics, muscle relaxants, and local heat. These methods, in association with a good physical therapy program, provide relief under most circumstances.

Up to 75% of patients with cervical disc disease improve after an adequate trial (10 to 14 days) of medical therapy. Some have recurrence of radicular symptoms on return to full activity. In many cases, these patients can be managed for years with intervals of cervical traction and a cervical collar, but some require surgical therapy. For the 25% who do not respond to conservative means, operation is often helpful.

There are essentially two approaches for the surgical treatment of cervical disc disease. Anteriorly, nerve roots, spinal cord, or both can be decompressed through discectomy with or without bone graft fusion. The other approach is posteriorly through a laminectomy or foraminotomy, or both. The choice of operative direction should be based on a particular patient's anatomic lesion. It is occasionally necessary to use both an anterior and a posterior approach. Regardless of approach, improvement follows operative treatment of symptomatic cervical disc disease in about 80% of patients who fail to respond to medical treatment. Surgical treatment of cervical spondylotic myelopathy results in improvement in about 60% of cases. Arrest of the progressive myelopathic deficit often occurs.

Thoracic Spine

In the thoracic spine, forceful trauma can cause the nucleus of a disc to extrude into the spinal canal. Because the canal is small relative to the spinal cord within it, cord compression readily occurs. Paraplegia is often abrupt and can be permanent. More often, osteophyte formation secondary to thoracic disc degeneration accounts for spinal canal narrowing. Development of thoracic myelopathy is more gradual. Isolated radiculopathies can also occur. Primary treatment for both acute and chronic thoracic disc disease is surgical. The offending disc fragment or spur is best removed by an anterior or lateral approach.

Lumbar Spine

Herniated lumbar intervertebral discs often produce some degree of nerve root compression. The severity of the syndrome depends on the degree of root compression. Occasionally, the entire cauda equina is involved, resulting in loss of motor and sensory function, including bowel and bladder sphincter control. Sometimes disc rupture can occur in the midline, compressing centrally positioned sacral roots preferentially, without involvement of laterally placed lumbar roots.

Fragmentation of a lumbar disc can occur without extrusion of the nucleus, as described earlier for cervical disc disease. Because of loss of elasticity within the disc, mobility of the intervertebral joint is increased. The annulus may simply bulge without tearing. With time, osteophytes can form around the degenerated disc and encroach on the spinal canal and neural foramina. This degenerative hypertrophy involves the ligamentous structures as well. Stenosis of the lumbar spinal canal is the end result, a spondylotic condition common in the elderly.

Clinical Presentation

In the lumbar spine, more than 90% of clinical problems arise from the L-4 to L-5 and L-5 to S-1 intervertebral discs. Pain is usually chronic, but its onset can be acute when associated with frank herniation. There may be back pain,

leg pain, or both. The radiation of low back pain into the buttock, posterior thigh, and calf is usually the same with disease at the L-4 to L-5 and L-5 to S-1 levels. This radiating pain can be exacerbated by coughing, sneezing, or straining. Bending and sitting accentuate the discomfort, whereas lying down characteristically relieves it. The pain is typically described as aching but frequently has a sharp or shooting element and is limited to one lower extremity. With lumbar stenosis, patients are unable to extend their spine without developing pain, numbness, or weakness, usually in both lower extremities. With upright posture, either standing or walking, the cauda equina becomes ischemic, producing neurogenic claudication. Relief is obtained by sitting or flexing forward.

Palpation usually reveals tenderness over the sciatic notch, popliteal fossa, or both. Paravertebral muscles can be in spasm. With true nerve root compression, straight leg raising produces leg pain that is accentuated by dorsiflexion of the foot. Ipsilateral leg pain produced by contralateral straight leg raising is highly suggestive of lumbar disc herniation. Other signs include the lower motor neuron findings associated with the specific root or roots involved. Sensory loss, weakness, and loss of tendon jerks can occur in many combinations and to variable degrees.

Diagnosis

Back pain with radiation to the leg has many causes besides lumbar disc disease. The differential diagnosis includes the following: bony abnormalities such as subluxation, degenerative facet fracture, and osteophyte formation; primary and metastatic tumors of the cauda equina, spine, and pelvis; inflammatory disorders, including abscess, arachnoiditis, ankylosing spondylitis, and rheumatoid arthritis; degenerative lesions of the spinal cord; peripheral neuropathies; peripheral vascular occlusive disease including abdominal aortic aneurysm; and gynecologic problems such as endometriosis.

Plain films of the lumbosacral spine can identify congenital or acquired bony changes. Disc space narrowing is an unreliable sign of symptomatic disease because narrowing of the disc space can occur without clinical symptoms. Flexion and extension lateral views reveal any concomitant instability. Myelography can be diagnostic in symptomatic lumbar disc disease, but CT alone delineates the lesion in most cases (Fig. 108-19). MRI has replaced myelography and CT at some centers in the workup of lumbar radiculopathy. With contrast, it can be extremely helpful in previously operated cases. EMG can confirm the diagnosis, especially when physical examination is unable to localize the involved level.

Treatment

Initially, medical treatment is indicated in all patients who do not have neurologic deterioration. Bed rest, local heat, analgesics, and skeletal muscle relaxants are usually effective within a few days. Physical therapy and limited exercise often help when the acute episode passes. A back brace partially immobilizes the patient and can prevent recurrent muscle spasm. With aggressive conservative management, most patients improve sufficiently to return to full activity. Recurrent symptoms can be treated in a similar fashion, often successfully. Surgical treatment is reserved for the patient with an acute or progressive neurologic deficit, chronic disabling pain, or both. The acute onset of weakness or sphincter disturbance constitutes an emergency, demanding prompt diagnosis and early operation.

Surgery usually entails a unilateral partial laminectomy with removal of the offending disc fragment. Foraminotomy may be necessary in the presence of osteophyte for-

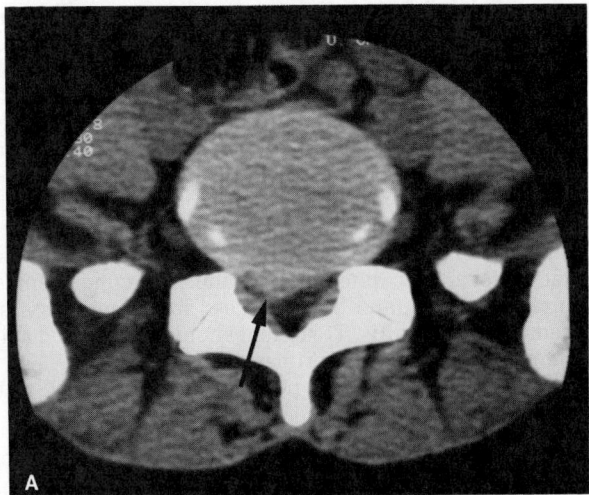
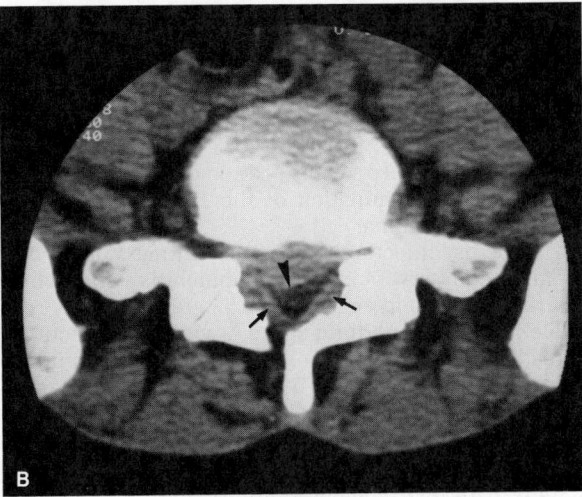

Figure 108-19. Noncontrast axial CT scan of a patient presenting with acute low back and right lower extremity pain. The slices are taken through the L-5 to S-1 disc (*A*) and 3 mm below the level of the disc (*B*). There is right paramedian herniation (*long arrow*) into the spinal canal with marked compression of the cauda equina (*arrowhead*) within the thecal sac. The short arrows identify the ligamenta flava.

mation. With lumbar stenosis, multilevel laminectomy is curative. Should plain films demonstrate any instability preoperatively, combining the laminectomy with posterior fusion, either with or without instrumentation, is generally indicated. If the imaging studies demonstrate an extruded disc fragment that accounts for the clinical signs and symptoms, 85% to 90% of patients recover with surgical treatment. If the syndrome is atypical, the myelogram equivocal, or the patient poorly motivated, operation is less effective.

INFECTIONS

The CNS can be infected by viruses, bacteria, fungi, and parasites.[6] Development of infection depends on the host's resistance (ie, immune defenses) and on the infecting agent's virulence. Bone, brain, spinal cord, meninges, and CSF can be involved separately or in combination. The routes of infection include hematogenous dissemination, local extension from a neighboring source, and direct contamination through an open wound. The infection can be diffuse, as in meningitis, or focal, as in brain abscess.

The clinical spectrum of signs and symptoms of CNS infection varies from nonspecific, such as fever, confusion, and lethargy, to highly specific, such as jacksonian epilepsy and focal neurologic deficits. Consequently, CNS infections present difficult diagnostic and therapeutic problems. Early diagnosis and treatment are crucial to a successful outcome.

Bacterial Infections

Subgaleal Abscess

Localized infection between the galea of the scalp and the pericranium constitutes subgaleal abscess. Usually, the process is initiated by contamination of an open scalp wound by staphylococci, streptococci, or anaerobic cocci. Localized scalp tenderness, warmth, and swelling are signs of abscess formation. Osteomyelitis of the skull can occur secondarily. Subgaleal infections rarely extend intracranially, unless the skull has been penetrated. Treat-

ment includes open drainage, débridement, and systemic antibiotics.

Osteomyelitis

Osteomyelitis can develop from extension of a localized infection, such as sinusitis or mastoiditis, from direct contamination at operation or after trauma, or, rarely, by hematogenous spread from a distant source such as the respiratory or urinary tract. An established skull or spine infection can extend to the epidural space and produce a localized abscess. The usual osteomyelitis pathogens are staphylococci and anaerobic streptococci. Occasionally, gram-negative organisms and fungi are responsible. Treatment consists of drainage, débridement of infected bone, and appropriate antibiotics for a prolonged period, usually 6 weeks.

Epidural Abscess

Spinal epidural abscess is much more common than intracranial epidural abscess. It is characterized by fever, local spinal tenderness, and rapid progression of neurologic deficits, often constituting a medical and surgical emergency. Radicular pain and impairment of cord function, with early motor and sensory deficits including sphincter disturbances, occur within a few days. Most epidural abscesses are caused by local extension of osteomyelitis or by hematogenous spread from a distant suppurative focus. The diagnosis is suggested by the clinical presentation. The CSF often has a markedly elevated protein level with mild pleocytosis. An MRI defines the extent of the epidural mass. If the dura is intact, infection rarely extends across it.

The most common causative organisms are *Staphylococcus aureus* and *Streptococcus* sp. Treatment should be immediate, beginning with broad antibiotic coverage until the offending agent is identified. Specific antibiotic therapy must be continued for a prolonged period of time, often up to 6 weeks. Surgical drainage is necessary when neurologic deficits progress despite aggressive medical therapy. Decadron in the perioperative period is beneficial in reducing localized edema, although prolonged use can reduce the host immune response to the infection. Recovery of neurologic function is directly related to the duration and severity of impairment before treatment.

Subdural Empyema

Subdural empyema is a purulent infection of the subdural space. It accounts for about 25% of all intracranial infections and is usually a complication of sinusitis, meningitis, or open contamination of the subdural space at operation or after trauma.

With sinusitis, infection can spread intracranially by transcranial emissary vein thrombophlebitis. Staphylococci, streptococci, and anaerobic cocci are commonly responsible. Once the subdural space is violated, infection can spread over the convexity of the brain. The accumulation of purulent material may be sufficient to produce an intracranial mass, provoking adjacent brain swelling. The clinical result is rapid neurologic deterioration, often with lateralizing signs, coma, and death. Treatment includes craniotomy with débridement, drainage, and intravenous antibiotics. The source of the infection must be treated aggressively. A sinus or mastoid drainage procedure is often required if this is the source. The mortality rate from acute fulminant subdural empyema from a paranasal source remains about 25%.

The diagnosis of intracranial subdural empyema is made readily by CT scan but can be difficult to distinguish from subacute or chronic subdural hematoma. The mass itself may be isodense, necessitating the administration of intravenous contrast. Including the sinuses on the CT scan can demonstrate the source of infection. Spinal fluid analysis is rarely diagnostic, often showing nonspecific inflammatory changes. As mentioned before, CT should be performed first, especially in a patient suspected of harboring an intracranial mass.

Spinal subdural empyema is rare. It usually develops from local extension transdurally or through the arachnoid in the presence of meningitis. Spinal cord compression and transverse myelitis can develop. Treatment is emergent, consisting of surgical drainage and prolonged antibiotic administration.

Meningitis

Bacterial meningitis is an acute, purulent infection of the leptomeninges. It is manifested by fever, lethargy, headache, nausea, vomiting, and nuchal rigidity. Seizures occur in about 20% of patients and cranial nerve palsies in about 5%. Coma can develop in up to 10% of patients with missed diagnoses, heralding a poor prognosis. Untreated bacterial meningitis is almost always fatal.

A CSF Gram stain demonstrates the offending organism in 75% of cases. Cultures provide a diagnosis 90% of the time. When CSF cultures are negative despite high clinical suspicion, as in a mild case or in an incompletely treated case of meningitis, latex agglutination studies are helpful. These immunologic studies are specifically directed at *Streptococcus pneumoniae, Haemophilus influenzae,* and *Neisseria meningitidis* and are highly sensitive when an organism is present, even with negative cultures. Blood cultures may be positive and therefore helpful in the diagnosis, particularly with infections caused by *S pneumoniae* and *N meningitidis.* CSF pleocytosis with a preponderance of polymorphonuclear cells is typical of untreated bacterial meningitis. CSF glucose is almost always reduced, whereas the protein content is typically increased.

Meningitis that develops after a penetrating wound or a neurosurgical procedure is usually caused by staphylococcal, streptococcal, or gram-negative organisms. Meningitis occurring after closed head trauma with either a skull fracture or CSF rhinorrhea is most often caused by *S pneumoniae.* Ventricular shunt and reservoir infections leading to meningitis are more likely due to *Staphylococcus epidermidis* or *S aureus.*

The treatment for acute bacterial meningitis depends on the causative organism, its antibiotic sensitivity, and the primary source of infection from which the meninges were contaminated. The presumed diagnosis is made clinically, a sample of CSF is obtained by lumbar puncture, and broad-spectrum intravenous antibiotics are immediately started. Once culture results are available, the choice of antibiotics is changed to an appropriate single agent. Bacterial endocarditis, pneumonia, sinusitis, concurrent subdural empyema, and brain abscess are sometimes associated with meningitis. Treatment should be directed at both the meningitis and the primary source.

The extent of antibiotic penetration into the CNS varies, depending on the degree of meningeal inflammation. Intrathecal administration of those antibiotics that do not readily cross the blood–CSF barrier may be necessary (the commonly used intrathecal preparations are gentamicin and vancomycin). This is especially true when an artificial substance, such as a ventricular shunt, is present. The artificial material can make eradication of the infection extremely difficult. Shunt removal is often necessary despite intravenous and intrathecal antibiotic administration. Rarely, therapy can also include the use of steroids and osmotic diuretics if ICP is elevated as a result of cerebral edema or localized brain abscess.

Complications of bacterial meningitis include communicating hydrocephalus, brain abscess, subdural empyema, and subdural effusions, particularly after *H influenzae* meningitis in infants. The risk of complications is significantly reduced by prompt, early treatment.

Brain Abscess

Brain abscess is a purulent lesion of brain tissue, beginning as a focal infection, usually in the white matter, surrounded by a typical inflammatory response. The blood–brain barrier becomes disrupted. Necrosis and liquefaction follow the acute inflammatory stage. Eventually, either the process is encapsulated by fibrous granulation tissue or the infection spreads through the parenchyma to the subarachnoid spaces and the ventricular system.

Brain abscess is usually secondary to focal infection elsewhere (Table 108-3). Abscesses that develop by direct intracranial extension are usually solitary and are typically found in the frontal and temporal lobes. Multiple brain

Table 108-3. COMMON CAUSES, TYPICAL LOCATIONS, AND MOST LIKELY ORGANISMS INVOLVED IN THE DEVELOPMENT OF BRAIN ABSCESS

Predisposing Condition	Usual Location	Common Organism
Otitis Mastoiditis	Temporal lobe Subdural abscess	*Streptococcus Bacteroides Haemophilus influenzae* Gram-negative organisms
Sinusitis	Frontal lobe Subdural abscess	*Streptococcus Staphylococcus*
Pneumonia, endocarditis, diverticulitis	Multiple brain abscesses	Various organisms (depends on source)
Penetrating wound	Site of trauma	*Staphylococcus*
Neurosurgical postoperative infection	Operative site	*Staphylococcus*

abscesses that develop in the septic patient are often related to bacterial endocarditis, pneumonia, and diverticulitis. Cyanotic congenital heart disease with concurrent infection is a frequent source. Direct contamination of the brain through a penetrating wound, especially when accompanied by in-driven bone fragments, is another cause of abscess. Abscess formation is frequent among patients with compromised immunity either from an underlying illness or during pharmacologic immunosuppression (ie, during organ transplantation).

Signs and symptoms of brain abscess are related to its mass effect. Headache, focal and neurologic deficits, and impaired mentation are often observed. There may be little or no evidence of systemic infection and the patient may be afebrile. Conversely, the patient can be deathly ill from bacteremia with fever, hypotension, and a markedly elevated white blood cell count. Seizures can occur. Progressive mass effect leads to brain shifts followed by coma.

Contrast CT and MRI are highly accurate in detecting brain abscess and should be done before the CSF is sampled. The CSF of patients with brain abscess may be entirely normal, but usually some pleocytosis is present. The causative organism can be identified and cultured from the abscess itself in 60% to 80% of cases, provided cultures are processed carefully for both aerobic and anaerobic organisms. Blood cultures are also helpful, particularly if the abscess is secondary to systemic infection.

In cases of early abscess formation or high surgical risk, medical therapy alone with the appropriate parenteral antibiotic may be sufficient. The most effective therapy is drainage of the purulent material with simultaneous administration of appropriate intravenous antibiotics. Although needle aspiration can be successful, craniotomy with evacuation and removal of the abscess wall may be necessary. Surgical drainage reduces the mass effect, thereby reducing the most critical and dangerous aspect of the infection. It also allows accurate bacteriologic analysis.

Results of treatment for brain abscess depend on the patient's neurologic status on presentation, the efficacy of the antibiotic used, the extent to which the intracranial mass is controlled by surgery, and the effective treatment of the primary source of the abscess. Despite aggressive surgical and medical management, mortality rates associated with brain abscess approach 40%, especially in the malnourished, chronically debilitated, or immunosuppressed patient.

Postoperative Infection

Any or all of the pyogenic infections described earlier can develop after operation. Once identified, characterized, and treated with appropriate antibiotics, the infection almost always subsides. Commonly isolated organisms include *S aureus* and *S epidermidis*. If a foreign body such as prosthetic material or a ventricular shunt is involved, eradicating the infection becomes more difficult, often requiring a combination of intravenous and intrathecal antibiotics with removal of the artificial material. Infrequently, infections can be satisfactorily treated in the presence of retained foreign bodies, such as a shunt, provided the infection is indolent.

Fungal Infections

As a rule, fungi are opportunistic organisms. They can become pathogenic because of depression of the host immune system, prolonged systemic antibiotic therapy, or severe systemic illness. When the CNS becomes infected, it is usually associated with pulmonary fungal infection and depressed host resistance. The CNS involvement can be a diffuse meningitis or a focal abscess. At times, multiple abscesses are present. Treatment requires long-term, systemic antifungal chemotherapy. Surgical intervention is reserved for drainage of abscesses and resection of symptomatic mass lesions. Hydrocephalus, a potential late complication, is treated with a ventricular shunt.

Parasitic Infestations

Although uncommon in North America and western Europe, parasitic diseases of the CNS are a major cause of neurologic disability and death worldwide. Control of these diseases remains a public health problem. A major emphasis is placed on their prevention, because once the CNS is infested, therapeutic options are limited. Treatment, both medical and surgical, is usually ineffective or palliative at best.

Cysticercosis

Taenia solium, the pork tapeworm, infests the human CNS by transmission of its larvae through the blood after ingestion. It is most prevalent in eastern Europe, Latin America, China, Pakistan, and India. Its presence can take one or all of four forms. Meningeal cysticercosis is characterized by parasitic vesicles throughout the basal cisterns and CSF pathways, usually with resultant hydrocephalus. Parenchymal cysticercosis diffusely involves the brain, sometimes forming large cysts. Seizures and focal deficits are common. The ventricular type resembles the meningeal form. Obstructive hydrocephalus is commonplace. Spinal cysticercosis can be intramedullary or extramedullary, producing either a transverse myelitis or a compressive myelopathy.

The diagnosis rests on serologic and radiologic testing. The presence of intracranial cysts and calcifications within skeletal muscle is often presumptive of the diagnosis. Newer anthelmintic agents can be effective, but often treatment is palliative. Anticonvulsants, CSF shunting, and occasional removal of symptomatic cysts are additional treatment options. Long-term prognosis is poor.

Echinococcosis

Hydatid disease is caused by *Echinococcus granulosus,* the dog tapeworm. It is prevalent in southern South America, northern and eastern Europe, Australia, Africa, China, and the Middle East. Humans can serve as intermediate hosts by ingesting the larvae. The liver and lungs are preferentially involved through hematogenous dissemination with subsequent formation of hydatid cysts. When the CNS is involved, cysts are usually solitary, large, and confined to white matter. There is a negligible inflammatory response.

Most cysts produce signs and symptoms related to their mass effect. Diagnosis of the infection is made serologically. CT and MRI of the brain and ultrasonography of the liver and spleen can be definitive. Chest radiographs often show calcified pulmonary cysts. Treatment consists of isolating the patient from the source and surgical removal of symptomatic cysts. Care must be taken to remove the intact cyst to avoid seeding with viable larvae. Hydatid disease of the CNS is disabling but rarely fatal if the cysts are removed when they become symptomatic.

CONGENITAL AND DEVELOPMENTAL ABNORMALITIES

About 2% of newborns possess some type of congenital abnormality.[7] Sixty percent of these involve the CNS, and over half of those are related to defective development or closure of the dorsal midline structures. Many have associated hydrocephalus. The commonly encountered neurologic malformations include the following:

- Arnold-Chiari malformation
- Dandy-Walker malformation
- Spinal dysraphism
    Meningocele
    Myelomeningocele
    Lipomyelomeningocele
    Diastematomyelia
    Dermal sinus
    Myeloschisis

Spinal Dysraphism

Between 18 and 28 days of embryonic development, the neural groove closes posteriorly in the midline to form the neural tube. This tube becomes encircled by bone derived from adjacent somites and is covered superficially by skin derived from ectoderm. Abnormal closure of the neural groove, failure of fusion of the adjacent bone, or maldevelopment of the overlying ectoderm can lead to many spinal dysraphic states. Thus, dysraphism implies an abnormal fusion of normally united parts.

Failure of the bony structures to close with normal closure of the neural groove is called spina bifida occulta. These patients have normal spinal cords and normal cord function. The abnormality usually goes unnoticed unless seen on plain radiographs. Should the meninges fail to close, a meningocele develops, producing an obvious cutaneous abnormality. The underlying neural structures develop normally, so there is no compromise of neurologic function.

Failure of the underlying neural tissue to fuse has been called spina bifida cystica or, more recently, spina bifida aperta. Myelomeningocele, the more common form, involves incomplete closure of the neural groove, usually in the lumbar region, with the abnormal, unfused neural tissue on the dorsal surface exposed through an associated defect in the spinal column. This can be partially or totally covered with epithelium. The accompanying neurologic deficit usually consists of complete absence of motor and sensory function below the level of spinal cord involvement.

The most severe form of spinal dysraphism is myeloschisis, which is much less common than myelomeningocele. The spinal cord is unfused and presents directly on the surface of the back without overlying meninges or epithelium. It usually occurs at the thoracolumbar region and is virtually always associated with paraplegia and absence of bladder function.

Both myelomeningocele and myeloschisis are associated with hydrocephalus. The hydrocephalus is caused by a developmental abnormality of the hindbrain called *Arnold-Chiari malformation,* which is associated with the more severe forms of spinal dysraphism (Fig. 108-20). This malformation is composed of caudal displacement of the cerebellar tonsils, vermis, inferior fourth ventricle, and medulla. There is a dorsal kink in the cervicomedullary junction and beaking of the quadrigeminal plate. Associated features include agenesis of the corpus callosum and obstructive hydrocephalus.

The treatment of spinal dysraphism is surgical. Meningoceles are excised and the skin is closed primarily after watertight closure of the posterior meningeal defect. Myelomeningoceles and myeloschises are closed as early as possible to reduce the risk of superficial infection and subsequent meningitis. Surgical repair is generally undertaken within 36 hours. The goal is to preserve as much neural tissue as possible, to untether the spinal cord from sur-

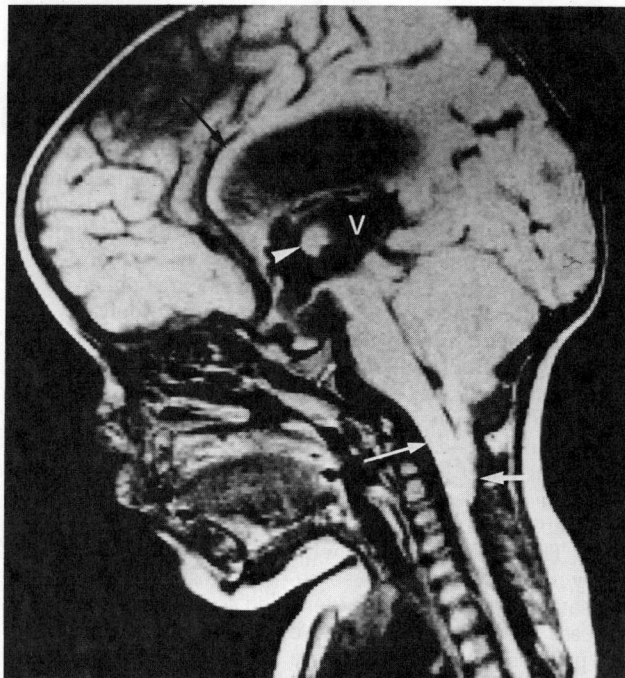

Figure 108-20. Sagittal MRI scan of the brain and upper cervical spine demonstrates some of the features of the Arnold-Chiari type II malformation. Note the herniation of the cerebellum through the foramen magnum to the level of C-4 (*short arrow*), the downward displacement of the medulla and fourth ventricle (*long arrow*), the absence of the corpus callosum, the hydrocephalus with enlargement of the third ventricle (V), and the enlarged massa intermedia (*arrowhead*).

rounding soft tissue, and to fashion a dural closure to prevent CSF leakage. Accompanying hydrocephalus is treated with shunting (see later discussion).

Survival of infants with these dysraphic states continues to improve. Despite a devastating neurologic deficit, they generally do well. Newborns with lower level lesions do better overall than do those with higher level lesions. The more severe the dysraphic state, the higher the morbidity and mortality rates. Risk of sepsis from bladder infection is reduced with intermittent catheterization when indicated. Timely revision of failed shunts placed for hydrocephalus preserves the potential for intellectual development.

Cranial Dysraphism

Cranial dysraphic states are one tenth as common as their spinal counterparts. Encephaloceles, although rare, are most commonly seen. They consist of a midline skull defect through which a small portion of brain protrudes. Most encephaloceles are covered with skin, and only about 35% have associated hydrocephalus. Once thought to arise from defects in the closure of the primitive neural tube, they probably develop because of an overlying mesodermal abnormality with subsequent perturbation of underlying cerebral tissue. In North America and Europe, 70% of encephaloceles occur in the posterior cranial vault; the remainder are found in the anterior cranial vault. In Southeast Asia, this distribution is reversed for unknown reasons.

The surgical repair involves early resection of malformed and devitalized brain with dural closure. The mortality of patients with encephaloceles varies greatly. Prognostic factors include the size and location of the anomaly, the extent of brain protrusion, and the presence of associated hydrocephalus, seizure disorder, or cerebral dysgenesis. The smaller and more anterior defects generally have a better outcome. Of those who survive, only 35% achieve normal intelligence.

Hydrocephalus

The term *hydrocephalus* implies an increase in the amount of CSF within the ventricular system. This is almost always due to a decrease in the absorption of fluid, although there are rare cases of choroid plexus papillomas causing hydrocephalus by an increase in CSF production. Hydrocephalus is traditionally referred to as *communicating* or *noncommunicating*. In the former, the ventricular system continues to communicate with the subarachnoid spaces outside the brain through the fourth ventricular foramina of Luschka and Magendie. In the noncommunicating type, often termed *obstructive,* it does not. The common causes of hydrocephalus vary with age and are listed here:

Congenital
- Arnold-Chiari malformation
- Dandy-Walker malformation
- Aqueductal atresia or stenosis
- Developmental cyst
- Encephalocele
- Neoplasm

Acquired
- Infectious meningitis
- Infectious ventriculitis
- Late-onset aqueductal stenosis
- Intraventricular hemorrhage
- Subarachnoid hemorrhage
- Neoplasm

Infantile Hydrocephalus

Hydrocephalus occurs most frequently between birth and 2 years of age and is most commonly due to congenital abnormalities of the brain. These abnormalities typically produce noncommunicating hydrocephalus. Stenosis of the cerebral aqueduct is one such common congenital anomaly. Another is the Arnold-Chiari malformation. The Dandy-Walker malformation produces a markedly enlarged fourth ventricle as a result of congenital obstruction of CSF outflow from the fourth ventricle, with resultant hydrocephalus. Other less common congenital lesions include arachnoid cysts, vascular anomalies, and congenital tumors.

Acquired hydrocephalus in the infant is often the result of meningitis or intracranial hemorrhage, both potentially causing obstruction of either the CSF absorptive mechanism or the intraventricular pathways (Fig. 108-21). Aqueductal stenosis can develop well after birth because of infection or hemorrhage and thus is termed *acquired.* Tumors can also obstruct the outflow of CSF, resulting in noncommunicating hydrocephalus.

Infants with hydrocephalus usually but not invariably present with an enlarging head circumference. They often have a tense, bulging anterior fontanelle with distended scalp veins and split cranial sutures. They may appear to have so-called sun setting of the eyes with only the tops of the irises visible (Parinaud syndrome). The head may transilluminate because of lack of cerebral substance. Neurologically, the hydrocephalus usually does not cause deficits initially because of the open cranial sutures that allow for cranial vault expansion (assuming absence of any underlying brain dysgenesis). In the more chronic forms,

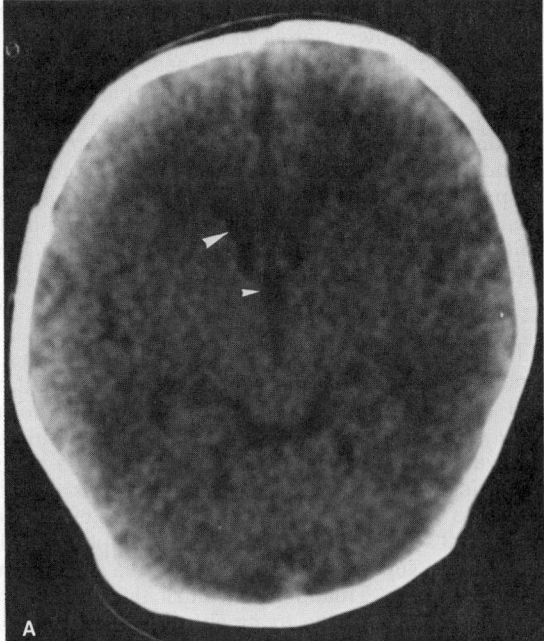

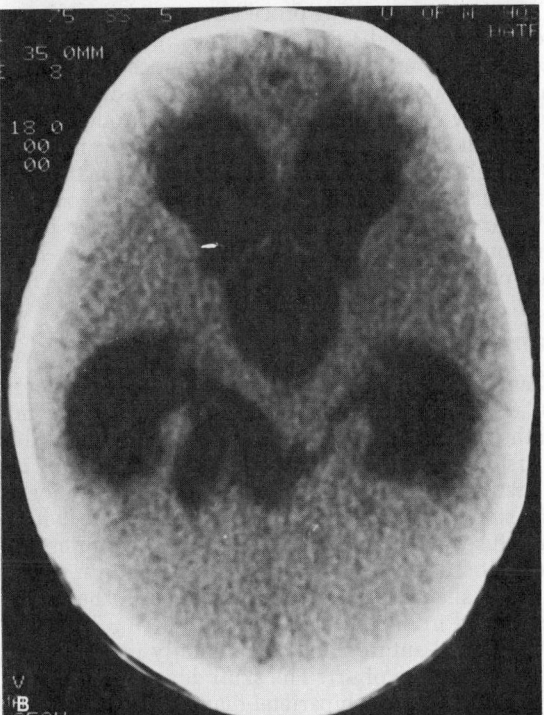

Figure 108-21. This patient suffered neonatal sepsis and subsequently developed meningitis. (*A*) Noncontrast CT scan during the first week of life shows relatively normal third (*small arrow*) and lateral (*large arrow*) ventricles. (*B*) Well after the meningitis was cured, accelerating head growth prompted another CT scan, which demonstrates marked hydrocephalus.

or in older infants with closed sutures, optic atrophy and sixth nerve palsies may be seen.

Childhood Hydrocephalus

Hydrocephalus in children older than 2 years of age can have a more acute presentation because of the decreased ability of the more mature brain and skull to accommodate the increase in CSF. Consequently, the raised ICP can acutely cause headache, nausea, vomiting, lethargy, coma, and even death. Slower onset can result in decreased mentation, behavioral changes, diminished performance in school, sixth nerve palsies, optic atrophy, paralysis of upward gaze, spastic leg weakness, and endocrine (hypothalamic) disorders. Causes of hydrocephalus in this age group include tumors, meningitis, intracranial hemorrhage (both spontaneous and traumatic), and aqueductal stenosis. Ventricular shunt malfunction can cause acute hydrocephalus in the shunt-dependent patient, regardless of the patient's age or the underlying cause.

Adult Hydrocephalus

Hydrocephalus in adults can also result from obstructive tumors, meningitis, and intracranial hemorrhage but can also be more insidious in onset. An entity called *normal pressure hydrocephalus* occurs in the older population and involves a communicating hydrocephalus with a normal intraventricular pressure. The cause remains unknown but is thought to be due to subclinical hemorrhage or infection in the patient's remote past. The classic symptom triad of ataxia, urinary incontinence, and cognitive decline suggests the diagnosis. Treatment is ventricular shunting.

Regardless of cause, the treatment of hydrocephalus is essentially the same. Either the cause must be removed (eg, tumor) or a shunting procedure must be performed to divert accumulated CSF. Sometimes, both measures are necessary. The most commonly used procedure is a lateral ventricle to peritoneal shunt with a one-way pressure-regulating valve in the system. If the peritoneal cavity is not suitable for shunting, the distal catheter can be placed in the right atrium of the heart or, rarely, in the pleural cavity. In selected cases of communicating hydrocephalus, a lumbar subarachnoid to peritoneal shunt can be used. Common complications of indwelling shunts include shunt obstruction and infection.

Craniosynostosis

Craniosynostosis is the premature closure of one or more cranial sutures typically manifested within the first 6 months of life. Because the brain doubles in size during the first 6 months of life and grows another 50% by age 2, the cranial sutures must remain open to allow for skull expansion to accommodate this growth. Usually, when one suture fuses prematurely, the brain is not compressed to a deleterious degree, but the skull develops in a distinctly abnormal shape. If more sutures are fused, the brain can be damaged from restricted growth.

The sagittal suture is most commonly involved, with a male/female ratio of 4:1. The skull develops an elongated shape with a narrow biparietal diameter, often referred to as *scaphocephaly*. The supraorbital ridge may be square shaped as a result of overexpansion of the open metopic suture. Associated congenital anomalies are rare.

The next most common suture involved is the coronal, which can close prematurely on one or both sides. Unilateral involvement produces an asymmetrically shaped forehead with flattening on the affected side and compensatory enlargement on the opposite side. This is called *plagiocephaly* and is not usually associated with other abnormalities. Bilateral coronal synostosis produces a more severe foreshortening of the entire anterior fossa and is often manifested by shallow orbits with exophthalmos and hypertelorism. This entity is often associated with inherited congenital disorders such as Crouzon disease and Apert and Carpenter syndromes.

Less common forms of craniosynostosis include premature closure of the lambdoid suture or the metopic suture. With unilateral synostosis of the lambdoid suture, the skull appears flattened in the affected occipital area, which can be confused with birth molding. With premature closure of the metopic suture, the forehead takes on a triangular shape (trigonocephaly). Neither of these forms is associated with other congenital anomalies.

The treatment of craniosynostosis is surgical and generally involves opening the affected suture along its entire length. This should be carried out as soon as possible after the diagnosis is made, because early surgical intervention provides the best cosmetic result. In cases of multiple suture involvement, prompt treatment provides early skull expansion to accommodate brain growth.

NEUROSURGICAL MANAGEMENT OF PAIN

Most neurosurgical patients have pain either as their primary complaint or as a secondary manifestation of their disease process.[2] These painful conditions can be categorized as acute processes, such as arm pain from a herniated cervical disc, or chronic processes, such as extremity pain from an invasive neoplasm. For most acute pain states, the cause can be identified and treated, but for chronic pain there is often no ready solution. The more common neurosurgical procedures available to manage chronic pain are described here.

At one time, the perception of pain was thought to involve a simple system of pathways extending from the peripheral receptors to the brain. It has subsequently been shown that this system is a complex network of pathways, with a considerable amount of modification at multiple synaptic levels. Impulses from pain receptors reach the spinal cord by way of the dorsal root ganglion and can receive significant modification in the various laminae of the dorsal horn. This information is then relayed to the thalamus but again can undergo considerable modification in the area of the brain-stem reticular formation. This sensory input is subsequently relayed to the cortex for conscious interpretation. Modifiers in this complex system include the recently identified endogenous substances labeled *endorphins, enkephalins,* and *substance P.* In addition, the psychological state of the patient influences the perception of painful stimuli.

Traditionally, neurosurgical procedures for chronic pain have been ablative or destructive, but many neuromodulating or stimulating procedures have been developed. These procedures are generally reserved for those chronic pain conditions that medical therapy has failed to alleviate.

Cerebrum

In general, few painful states warrant procedures involving the cerebral hemispheres or deep brain nuclei. Bilateral rostral cingulotomies have been performed for treatment of intractable pain. This procedure disrupts the cingulum, a large fasciculus running deep to the cingulate gyrus. It has proved useful for affective disorders involving pain when performed bilaterally. Ablative hypophysectomy can be used in the management of debilitating pain related to endocrine-dependent cancer. This is most effective when the primary malignancy is breast carcinoma, but encouraging results have also been reported with prostate cancer and, to a lesser degree, choriocarcinomas and renal cell and thyroid carcinomas.

As the primary relay station for pain impulses, the thalamus has been the target for stereotaxic ablative procedures. Thalamotomies are performed with considerable accuracy and have been used for thalamic pain disorders, phantom limb pain, and pain from invasive tumors. More recently, deep brain electrodes have been placed for stimulation rather than ablation of these structures. Permanent electrodes are positioned in the somatosensory area of the thalamus if a patient fails to experience some pain relief with an intravenous morphine trial preoperatively, or in the periaqueductal gray region of the brain stem if the patient did respond. In general, thalamic stimulation has proved useful in patients suffering from deafferentation pain, pain that typically does not respond to opiates. Conversely, brain-stem stimulation is successful in chronic painful states that are responsive to opiates. Long-term success (control of pain for a minimum of 2 years) is reported to be about 60% and 80% for the respective groups.

Cranial Nerves

Trigeminal neuralgia (tic douloureux) is one of the more commonly occurring neuropathic painful conditions. It presents as an intermittent, shocklike pain in one or more divisions of one trigeminal nerve. It most commonly involves the second (maxillary) or third (mandibular) divisions of the nerve, or both, and rarely is bilateral. The pain usually lasts for seconds, is severe, and can be incapacitating. It is often triggered by touching the face, talking, or chewing. The pain can be present for weeks or months and then spontaneously disappear, only to return with increased severity. Most patients can be initially controlled with phenytoin or carbamazepine, but eventually many require surgical intervention. A small percentage of patients can have a posterior fossa tumor causing the pain, so evaluation should include a CT or MRI scan before therapy.

In the past, surgical treatment involved ablation of the involved branches of the trigeminal nerve. This was accomplished peripherally by surgical section or alcohol ablation of the supraorbital, infraorbital, or inferior alveolar nerves. Pain control through these neurectomies was usually short-lived. Experience found that preganglionic lesions must be made for more permanent relief. Retrogasserian rhizotomy can be carried out by open surgical approaches subtemporally or through the posterior fossa, or percutaneously by placing a radiofrequency electrode through the foramen ovale. Percutaneous rhizolysis is safe, effective, and widely used. If performed properly, it has the advantage of destroying pain fibers only, leaving a variable amount of touch sensation intact.

A popular nonablative approach involves microvascular decompression of the trigeminal nerve in the posterior fossa. The theory behind this approach is that trigeminal neuralgia is caused by external pressure on the nerve by vascular structures (an artery or vein) near its entry into the brain stem. With use of the operating microscope, the offending artery can be moved or the vein ablated, thus decompressing the nerve. This procedure has a high success rate but carries more risk than the percutaneous method. An advantage is that the nerve's function remains intact.

Glossopharyngeal neuralgia is similar to trigeminal neuralgia, but much less common. Symptoms consist of lancinating, paroxysmal pain most commonly in the throat and at the base of the tongue, with occasional extension to the ear and the deep regions of the mandible and neck. Pain can be triggered by swallowing, chewing, or talking. Medical therapy is the same as that for trigeminal neuralgia. Should this fail, surgical intervention is warranted. The classic approach involves sectioning the intracranial portion of the glossopharyngeal nerve and the two superior bundles of the vagus nerve by use of a suboccipital craniectomy. Microvascular decompression has also been used with success.

Brain Stem

Trigeminal tractotomy has occasionally been used for patients with unrelenting head and neck pain secondary to invasive malignancies. This involves open surgical section of the descending trigeminal tract just inferior to the level of the obex (the opening of the fourth ventricle into the spinal canal). This technique is often combined with the division of cranial nerves IX and X, transection of the nervus intermedius of VII, and dorsal rhizotomy of C-2 through C-3. A nearly complete sensory denervation of the affected side of the head and neck is accomplished.

Spinal Cord

As with other surgical procedures for chronic pain, those involving the spinal cord have traditionally been ablative. Cordotomy, designed to obliterate the spinothalamic tract, can be performed openly or percutaneously. If the upper extremity is involved, the open technique can be achieved posteriorly through a cervical laminectomy or anteriorly through a discectomy. After gentle rotation of the spinal cord, the anterior quadrant containing the spinothalamic tract is sectioned. If the upper extremity is not involved, spinothalamic tractotomy is performed through a thoracic laminectomy. A reliable percutaneous method is available and reduces the operative risk in these often very ill patients. This method creates a functional cordotomy at the C-1 to C-2 level with a radiofrequency lesion generator. Anterolateral cordotomy can provide excellent temporary relief of pain for patients with terminal malignancies, but it is rarely effective for chronic benign conditions such as low back, postherpetic, or phantom limb pain.

For selected cases of severe pain of peripheral nerve origin, such as brachial plexus injury, postherpetic neuralgia, traumatic limb amputation, and root avulsion, ablative lesions can be made at the dorsal root entry zones of the spinal cord (Fig. 108-22). These lesions are made with a radiofrequency lesion generator or laser through an open exposure of the cord by use of a laminectomy. Several levels are usually included. About 50% of patients obtain good relief from their pain.

Chronic pain that develops in chest, flank, or abdominal incisions may warrant a surgical ablative procedure. Because these regions do not contain critical sensory areas, unilateral dorsal nerve roots can be sectioned to deprive the involved area of sensation. It is necessary to ablate at least three adjacent levels to denervate one dermatome adequately. Dorsal rhizotomy can be carried out openly through a laminectomy or percutaneously through radiofrequency thermocoagulation. Another open method, similar to rhizotomy, uses dorsal root ganglionectomy. Although pain relief from rhizotomy has been variably reported in 28% to 69% of cases, ganglionectomy offers 90% immediate relief and nearly 80% short-term relief.

Intrathecal morphine can also be given temporarily or permanently by infusion of minute but effective doses. This newer method of pain control is particularly effective in debilitated patients with terminal illnesses. The procedure involves the subcutaneous implantation of a constant infusion pump that can be recharged periodically. Morphine is delivered by this device into the CSF in small amounts sufficient to control severe pain.

In chronic painful states of nonmalignant spinal origin, such as low back and leg pain, a nonablative neuromodulation technique can play a role in therapy. This involves transcutaneous stimulation that blocks nerve conduction of pain impulses. It is simple, safe, and inexpensive. Electrodes are taped to the skin, usually over the region of the pain or directly over the affected major nerve, and then

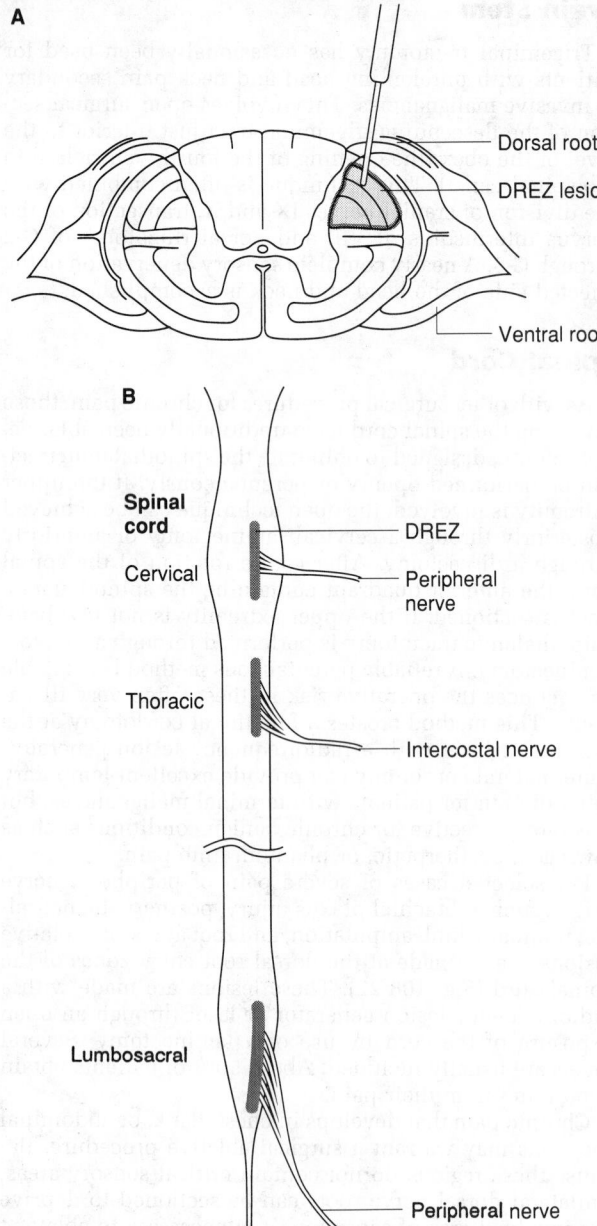

Figure 108-22. Location of dorsal root entry zone for placement of dorsal root entry zone (DREZ) lesion.

connected to a small portable stimulating device. The device has a variable pulse width, frequency, and amplitude, which can be adjusted by patients to achieve maximum pain relief. Use of this device for a brief time often provides long-lasting relief with no untoward side effects.

Peripheral Nerve

Many chronic painful states can arise from peripheral nerve or major plexus injuries. Fortunately, these painful conditions are rare, but when they do occur, they can be persistent and disabling. Pain from a partial or complete nerve injury usually involves the sensory distribution of the nerve but can include the whole extremity. Chronic pain developing after an amputation can be present in the remaining portion of the limb at the site of the amputation (stump pain) or in the nonexistent amputated portion

(phantom pain). The cause of the pain can be related to the sensory component of the nerve or to its associated sympathetic nerve supply.

With partial or complete peripheral nerve transection, a painful neuroma can form. A neuroma is a mass of misdirected axons that can develop from an injured nerve's attempt to regenerate. These axons can become sensitive to external stimuli or they can generate spontaneous pain. The usual treatment is excision of the neuroma, with prevention of recurrent formation by burying the nerve end in bone or muscle or by wrapping it in tantalum or Silastic. Neuromodulation techniques can also be applied in cases of painful neuromas. These include transcutaneous stimulation, as described earlier, and implanted devices that directly stimulate the proximal nerve.

Treatment of stump pain has included resection of neuromas, regional sympathectomy, cordotomy, and the neuromodulation techniques of transcutaneous and direct nerve stimulation. The treatment of phantom pain is more difficult but has included the treatments mentioned earlier for stump pain. In extreme cases, deep brain stimulation has been used. Dorsal root entry zone lesions have also provided relief for these chronic painful states.

Chronic pain resulting from peripheral nerve injury can be significantly altered by interruption of the sympathetic nerve supply to the affected extremity. The classic example of this dysautonomic state is major causalgia. This term implies a partial injury to a major nerve in an extremity. Minor causalgia is reserved for an injury to a more distal minor sensory nerve, which can also become a source of significant pain. It is also well recognized that a dysautonomic state can be created by major or minor trauma to an extremity that does not involve a peripheral nerve. These have been labeled *major* and *minor traumatic dystrophies*. The entire collection of causalgias and traumatic dystrophies makes up a syndrome termed *reflex sympathetic dystrophy*.

Major causalgia is most commonly related to partial injury of the sciatic or median nerves. Typically, symptoms begin in the affected nerve's distribution but can progress to involve the whole extremity. The extremity first becomes swollen, warm, erythematous, and sensitive to touch. With time, it becomes cool and pale. Hyperhidrosis (excessive sweating) can follow. Because of the lack of joint motion, the normal flexion and extension creases disappear and the skin becomes smooth and flat. Plain radiographs may demonstrate osteoporosis. Eventually, the extremity can become completely useless. A constant, burning pain develops and persists throughout these various stages. It can be exacerbated by touching or moving the extremity. Temperature changes and emotional stress can trigger worsening of the pain. Minor causalgia and the traumatic dystrophies can be accompanied by similar but less severe symptoms.

The treatment of these dysautonomic states is complex. They can be helped by disruption of the sympathetic nerve supply to the extremity. This can be accomplished temporarily with a chemical sympathectomy by use of a local anesthetic, or permanently by a surgical sympathectomy. Usually, numerous local blocks are performed initially. If these are successful, a surgical sympathectomy is performed. Sympatholytic drugs such as phenoxybenzamine can be tried, but they are rarely useful for chronic relief. Transcutaneous stimulation can be helpful but is rarely curative. Sympathetic denervation can be rewarding in major causalgia but less so in minor causalgia and the traumatic dystrophies.

Less severe and more easily treated pain can arise from chronic compression of selected peripheral nerves. The most common are compression of the median nerve at the wrist (carpal tunnel syndrome) and compression of the ulnar nerve at the elbow. Chronic compression can result in pain, paresthesias, numbness, and eventually weakness and atrophy of muscles in the distribution of the affected nerve. These compression syndromes are diagnosed clinically and confirmed by finding denervation and slowed nerve conduction on EMG and nerve conduction velocity testing. Treatment is surgical decompression of the involved nerve, with prompt and long-lasting relief in most cases.

REFERENCES

1. Apuzzo MLJ. Brain injury: complications, avoidance and management. New York, Churchill Livingstone, 1993:2365.
2. Youmans JR, ed. Neurological surgery: a comprehensive reference guide to the diagnosis and management of neurosurgical problems, ed 3. Philadelphia, WB Saunders, 1990.
3. Errico TJ, Bauer RD, Waugh T, eds. Spinal trauma. Philadelphia, JB Lippincott, 1991.
4. Russell DS, Rubinstein LJ. Pathology of tumors of the nervous system, ed 5. Baltimore, Williams & Wilkins, 1989.
5. Ojemann RG, Heros RC, Crowell RM, eds. Surgical management of cerebrovascular disease, ed 2. Baltimore, Williams & Wilkins, 1988.
6. Crockard A, Hayward R, Hoff JT, eds. Neurosurgery: the scientific basis of clinical practice, ed 2. Boston, Blackwell Scientific, 1992.
7. McLaurin RL, Venes JL, Schut L, Epstein F, eds. Pediatric neurosurgery: surgery of the developing nervous system, ed 2. Philadelphia, WB Saunders, 1989.

SURGERY: SCIENTIFIC PRINCIPLES AND PRACTICE, Second Edition, edited by
Lazar J. Greenfield, Michael W. Mulholland, Keith T. Oldham, Gerald B. Zelenock,
and Keith D. Lillemoe. Lippincott–Raven Publishers, Philadelphia, © 1997.

CHAPTER 109

MALE ANATOMY AND PHYSIOLOGY

H. BARTON GROSSMAN, WILLIAM D. BELVILLE,
GARY J. FAERBER, JOHN W. KONNAK, AND DANA A. OHL

BLADDER AND URETHRAL PHYSIOLOGY

The lower urinary tract, which includes the bladder, sphincters, and urethra, is associated with a variety of pathophysiologic processes and symptoms. The bladder is a composite of complex muscular fascicles that can both relax (and thereby accommodate urine) as well as contract to expel its contents. At the base of the bladder lies the trigone, with its specialized smooth muscle, where the ureters terminate. Most of the urinary tract lining is transitional epithelium.

The two basic functions of this unit are to store and to empty the urine it has collected, normally at low pressure. Should the bladder lose its low-pressure storage ability, it may adversely affect the ureters in the delivery of their peristaltic load. If high pressure is sustained (higher than 40 cm H_2O), ureteral dysfunction occurs, and the deleterious changes of hydroureteronephrosis may ensue.

Bladder and sphincter control are the result of a complex interaction between the central and peripheral nervous systems. During normal filling, the bladder relaxes and the smooth muscle sphincters contract. During a normal bladder contraction at voiding, both striated and smooth muscle sphincter activity cease. The initial event that triggers a normal voiding cycle is relaxation of the striated (voluntary) sphincter.[1]

Anatomic Obstructive Uropathy

Until recently, benign prostatic hypertrophy (BPH) was considered the prototype of anatomic obstructive uropathy. Work over the last decade, however, has changed much of that dogma.[2] We now know that prostatic size has little relationship to obstruction and that it can not be consistently estimated without sophisticated imaging, such as computed tomography (CT) or magnetic resonance (MR) imaging.[3]

When the bladder outlet is obstructed by some mechanism (eg, stricture, BPH, foreign body, stone), the bladder pressure usually increases with a concurrent fall in flow rate. During an extended period, this obstruction may produce bladder changes that adversely affect its storage function as well as its ability to empty completely. These clinical observations about obstruction (high bladder pressure and low flow) have been well documented.[4] Recent experience suggests that fiberoptic microtransducers may provide a less invasive, more clinically acceptable method for demonstrating these findings.[5] The increasing use of symptom scoring despite known drawbacks, however, seems to be the wave of the future for "objectively" quantifying the variable symptoms associated with lower urinary tract problems.[6]

Progressive high bladder pressure may produce no symptoms (silent prostatism) and, if sustained over 40 cm H_2O, may induce failure of ureteral emptying and thus transmit high pressure to the kidney. The end result is compromised renal function, which may occur without any noticeable reduction in urine output.

In contrast to the recent past, there is currently a variety of options, both medical and surgical, for managing BPH. Lasers, microwave, cryotherapy, and radiowave treatments are in various clinical and research stages of development. α_1-Blockers and 5α-reductase inhibitors are both approved by the Food and Drug Administration for treating BPH. Unfortunately, none of the aforementioned treatments has matched standard simple prostatectomy or intermittent catheterization in maintaining bladder compliance and standing the test of time.

Neurogenic Obstructive Uropathy

The basic problem in neurogenic obstructive uropathy begins as a failure to empty, either because of an areflexic bladder or a bladder contracting against a (dyssynergic) contracting sphincter. In neurologic injury, the fine balance between the pelvic peripheral nerves and the central nervous system is lost. If untreated, this obstruction leads to progressive loss of bladder compliance and the ensuing complications of obstruction, including reflux, stasis, stone, infection, and renal failure.

If the bladder is managed with intermittent catheterization, sphincterotomy, vesicostomy, or suprapubic or foley catheterization, these sequelae can be mostly prevented in the short term. Long-term tube management, however, is associated with frequent severe complications including malignant degeneration. While it may seem acceptable to use indwelling tubes because of convenience and the initial perception of improved continence, long-term catheterization can lead to catastrophic complications including total urethral destruction, fistulas, and squamous cell carcinoma of the bladder.

Urinary Incontinence

Urinary incontinence, excluding rare congenital anomalies and fistulas, is due to bladder or urethral dysfunction, alone or in combination. The most common form of incontinence occurs in the postpartum or overweight female and is due to loss of urethral support, which is easily corrected by a suspension procedure.

As the population ages, however, and the number of antiincontinence procedures proliferates, the number of cases involving incontinence due to inadequate closure of the vesical neck and proximal urethra is increasing. This type of incontinence, known as intrinsic sphincter dysfunction or type III stress urinary incontinence, is also seen following injury to the hypogastric nerves due to extensive pelvic trauma, radical hysterectomy, abdominal perineal resection, and other causes.[7] New advances in urodynamics have allowed easier identification of this previously difficult cohort, and new injectable therapies have proved to be an enormous breakthrough for these individuals.[8-11]

The bladder may be the primary cause of incontinence due to hyperreflexia (common) or inadequate storage ability, either volitional or idiopathic. Detrusor instability (hyperreflexia) may occur early in prostatic obstruction or result from an underlying, often subclinical neurologic cause. Fortunately, a strict regimen of anticholinergic medication (imipramine or oxybutynin) along with a regular voiding schedule often achieves social continence and dramatically improves the quality of life for these individuals.

IMPOTENCE

Erectile dysfunction is a common condition, which affects 10 million American men. The incidence increases with age, and by 55 years of age, about 8% of men are affected. By the age of 80 years, the incidence is 75%.

Mechanism of Erection

The erectile bodies of the penis are the paired corpora cavernosa surrounded by a thick fibrous investing sheath of tunica albuginea. The cavernosal tissue is spongelike and consists of lacunar spaces lined by vascular endothelium and supported by trabeculae composed of smooth muscle and fibroelastic tissue. The spaces are richly supplied with blood from the cavernosal or central arteries of the penis, which are branches of the internal pudendal arteries. Within the corpora, they give off branches called the helicine arteries, which supply the lacunar spaces. Beneath the tunica albuginea lie the subtunical venules, which drain the corpora. These join to form emissary veins, which pierce the tunica and drain into the deep dorsal vein distally and the crural veins proximally. The corpora are surrounded by a dense fibrous sheath of tunica albuginea. The penis, including the corporal bodies are richly supplied with nerves. Somatic innervation is by means of the pudendal nerves, which supply the skin and striated muscles, while autonomic innervation consists of sympathetic nerves from T-11 to L-2 and parasympathetic nerves from S-2, S-3, and S-4. Reflex or psychogenic stimulation causes dilatation of the penile arteries and the lacunar spaces with a marked increase in penile blood flow and engorgement of the corporal bodies.[12,13] The cavernous tissue expands and is compressed by the tunica. Intercavernous pressure increases, causing compression of the subtunical venules. This limits venous outflow and further increases the intercavernous pressure until a rigid erection occurs. The process is reversed in detumescence through activation of the sympathetic nerves. At the blood vessels and cavernous smooth muscle, the action of the autonomic nerves is mediated by a variety of neurotransmitters, of which some are known and others are postulated. Sympathetic innervation is mediated by norepinephrine acting on receptors in the smooth muscle. Parasympathetic postganglionic innervation may be mediated by a nonadrenergic noncholinergic neurotransmitter, likely to be nitric oxide. In addition, substances released by the vascular endothelium, chemically similar to nitric oxide, are thought to influence smooth muscle tone.

Pathogenesis

Impotence ensues from interference with the normal vascular, neurologic, psychological, endothelial, and hormonal mechanisms of erection. In many cases, the causes are multifactorial. Psychologic factors can inhibit as well as stimulate erection and account for less than half the cases of impotence. Anxiety, sexual inhibitions, and a variety of other factors can decrease potency. Organic causes are especially prevalent in older men. Although a number of systemic diseases can cause impotence, diabetes is the most common. Diabetic neuropathy and vascular disease may result in loss of potency. Other causes of impotence include debilitating diseases (renal failure, cirrhosis of the liver), drugs (alcohol, cimetidine, atenolol, clonidine, diazepam), arteriosclerotic disease, and trauma.[14] In addition to arterial disease, failure of the venous occlusive mechanism may cause venous leaking into the penile veins or into the glans or spongiosum, resulting in impotence. Impotence may also result from systemic neurologic disease such as multiple sclerosis. Spinal cord injury usually results in impotence, although reflex erections are often retained. Direct trauma to the pelvic nerves by pelvic fractures or radical pelvic surgery (radical prostatectomy) can be associated with impotence.

Hormonal disorders, such as primary hypogonadism and intersex problems, are relatively uncommon causes of impotence. An age-related fall in serum testosterone level is associated with impotence in some men and can be corrected by testosterone supplementation. Castration is usually associated with impotence, but the effect is often delayed, and some castrated men continue to be potent.

Diagnosis

A detailed sexual history can give important insight into the cause of impotence. Sudden onset or intermittent impotence may indicate a psychogenic cause. This is especially true if the patient has normal morning erections or adequate erections with masturbation. Organic impotence is usually gradual in onset and progression, and the patient is often unable to achieve a normal erection under any circumstance. A history of diabetes, hypertension, arteriosclerotic disease, or neurologic problems may indicate the cause. A list of the patient's medications should be obtained, and drug and alcohol use determined. The physical examination should include an evaluation of the general body habitus as well as detailed examination of the genitalia. A neurologic examination should be done, and peripheral pulses evaluated. Initial laboratory studies should include serum levels of testosterone, prolactin, serum lipids, and a screening test for diabetes, such as a 2-hour postprandial blood sugar. Depending on the results of the initial evaluation, additional special studies may be indicated.

Nocturnal Penile Tumescence Testing

Normal men get nocturnal erections during the rapid eye movement stage of sleep. Patients with psychogenic impotence often have a normal pattern of nocturnal erections, whereas men with organic impotence have an abnormal or absent response. A simple screening test uses a snap gauge consisting of a Velcro cuff connected to a series of bands that break if the penis expands. This can indicate whether nocturnal erections occur but does not give the pattern or duration of erection and is a poor guide to quality. Formal tumescence testing may be performed in a sleep laboratory or at home with a portable testing device. Current devices give a graphic record of frequency, duration, and quality of erection. Because this testing is cumbersome and is sometimes difficult to interpret, it is not used routinely.

Vascular Testing

A rough estimate of penile blood flow can be made through Doppler determination of penile systolic blood pressure using a penile cuff or penile plethysmography. While a normal study does not entirely rule out vasculogenic impotence, consistently low values can indicate this as a cause. This test is done in the flaccid state and does not reflect the increase in blood flow possible to cause an erection. Direct corporal injection with papaverine, a smooth muscle relaxant, or with prostaglandin E1 bypasses psychogenic and neurologic factors and produces an erection if the blood flow to the penis is normal. A poor or absent response can indicate vasculogenic impotence due to either arterial insufficiency or venous leak, although anxiety can interfere with the test. Quantitative increase in the diameter of the central arteries can be documented using duplex ultrasonography.[15] If arterial disease is suspected based on a poor response, superselective pelvic arteriography with injection of vasoactive agents is necessary to document the extent and nature of the disease. Venous leak may manifest increased diastolic flow on duplex ultrasonography. If a venous leak is suspected, cavernosometry and cavernosography should be performed.[16] This test involves perfusing the penis with saline solution after papaverine injection and measuring intracorporal pressures at various flows. Erection normally occurs at flows under 120 mL/min, with pressures approaching or exceeding blood pressure. Erection can be maintained with flows under 60 mL/min. The rate of pressure decay can also be determined. In venous leak, very high flows are necessary to initiate and maintain erection, and the pressure decay is rapid. Radiographic contrast injection is then performed to document the leak. In normal men, few if any veins are visualized during erection. With a positive test for leak, multiple veins are visualized, and leaking may be seen between the cavernosa into the spongiosum of the glans or urethra.

Hormonal Studies

Low serum testosterone may indicate hypogonadism. Elevated prolactin can indicate a pituitary neoplasm, and appropriate cerebral studies should be done.

Treatment

Nonsurgical Therapy

The treatment of impotence depends both on the etiology and the patient's willingness to pursue various therapeutic approaches. Psychogenic and mild organic impotence respond to nonspecific measures, such as the use of yohimbine and reassurance, in up to 60% of cases.[17] Sexual counseling produces excellent results in 80% of cases of psychogenic impotence if the patient and his sexual partner are willing to undergo treatment. Intracorporal papaverine or prostaglandin E1 injection can also be used as primary therapy in these patients or to help reassure them that the erectile mechanism is normal.[18] Patients with neurogenic impotence often have a dramatic effect with papaverine injection. Patients with mild vasculogenic impotence, diabetes, or nonspecific impotence are also candidates for injection therapy. Side effects of papaverine injections include priapism and fibrous plaques at the injection site. Liver toxicity has also been associated with papaverine injection. Some of these side effects can be avoided with the use of prostaglandin E1. Combi-

nations of papaverine, prostaglandin E1, and phentolamine can be formulated to maximize the beneficial effects of the individual agents and minimize the side effects of full doses of any one drug.[19] About half of all patients with decreased serum testosterone levels respond to Depo-Testosterone injections. Oral testosterone preparations should not be used because of liver toxicity and unpredictable serum levels. Recently, transdermal testosterone preparations have become available, and these should be as effective as intramuscular preparations with few side effects. Vacuum devices are also available for treating impotence. They consist of a cylinder that fits around the penis and seals at the pubic skin. A pump is used to produce a vacuum within the cylinder, which sucks blood into the penis producing an erection. An elastic band is placed tightly around the base of the penis to maintain the erection. The vacuum is then released and the cylinder is removed. Complications include penile numbness and pain, failure of ejaculation, and petechiae.

Surgical Therapy

Penile implants can be used to treat any type of intractable impotence, but they are usually reserved for patients with diabetes or vascular or neurologic dysfunction who do not respond to conservative measures. These devices are made of nonreactive materials and have cylinders that are surgically implanted into the corpora cavernosa. The device may be rigid, semirigid, or inflatable. The rigid devices produce a permanent erection, while the inflatable devices produce erection only when activated by pumping fluid into the cylinders. Two types of inflatable devices are manufactured. One is self-contained, with the pump and deflate mechanisms incorporated into the cylinders, and the other has a pump in the scrotum with a reservoir of fluid either stored in the pump or implanted suprapubically. With either type, the patient activates or deactivates the device by manual pressure through the scrotal skin or through the shaft of the penis. Complications include infection or erosion of the device in 1% to 10% of patients. Occasionally, failed parts may require replacement. In selected patients with arteriogenic vascular impotence, penile revascularization may be considered.[20] These patients are usually younger and have a localized vascular lesion. Patients with diffuse small vessel disease are not good operative candidates. The inferior epigastric artery is usually employed, and revascularization is accomplished into the dorsal penile artery if there is sufficient collateral connection to the central vessels. Occasionally, the central artery itself can be used, although this is technically more difficult. Revascularization by connecting the inferior epigastric to the deep venous system after isolating the vein to the shaft of the penis is also performed with a reported success rate of 60%. Venous leak has been treated by ligating the penile veins or occluding them by radiographic techniques. Although success rates of up to 73% have been reported, the results are generally disappointing with improvement in less than 50% of cases.[13]

MALE INFERTILITY

Infertility can be defined as the inability to conceive a pregnancy within 1 year of unprotected intercourse. About 15% of couples in the United States are affected, and in about half of them, the male contributes to the problem. The incidence of male and couple infertility may be increasing.

The structures important to male fertility include the testes, with seminiferous tubule and Leydig cell components; the excurrent duct system of the testis, consisting of the epididymis, vas deferens, and ejaculatory ducts; accessory glands, including the prostate and seminal vesicles; and the sympathetic nervous system, which supplies the majority of innervation to the other structures mentioned.

Beginning at puberty, pulsatile release of hypothalamic gonadotropin-releasing hormone (GnRH) causes release of the pituitary gonadotropins, follicle-stimulating hormone (FSH), and luteinizing hormone (LH). LH stimulates secretion of testosterone from the Leydig cells, which induces development of male secondary sex characteristics. FSH, via the Sertoli cells lining the seminiferous tubules, initiates sperm production. High intratubular levels of testosterone are also necessary, and once initiated, testosterone alone can maintain sperm production. Circulating testosterone causes negative feedback of GnRH and LH secretion. Testosterone and inhibin, a peptide hormone secreted by the Sertoli cell during active sperm production, produce negative feedback on pituitary FSH secretion.

Spermatogenesis is the process of sperm production in the seminiferous tubules and consists of three major stages[21]:

Spermatocytogenesis—mitotic division of the spermatogonia (the most immature type of male germ cell)

Meiosis—a 2N spermatogonium undergoes two cell and nuclear divisions but only one chromosomal division, resulting in four haploid spermatids. During the meiotic phase, several stages of spermatocytes are encountered.

Spermiogenesis—the morphologic conversion of round spermatids into spermatozoa with tails

Although spermiogenesis produces morphologically mature sperm, further biochemical and subtle morphologic changes to the spermatozoa occur in transit through the epididymis. Only on completing normal passage through the epididymis are spermatozoa fully functional.

The time necessary to complete spermatogenesis is about 74 days.[22] An additional 10 to 20 days is necessary for transport to the epididymal tail where sperm are stored prior to ejaculation. Thus, any factor that affects sperm production is not seen in the ejaculate for about 84 to 94 days; therefore, evaluation of treatment must be delayed until this period has elapsed.

Emission of seminal fluid in response to sexual stimulation is controlled by the sympathetic nervous system. During emission, sperm is rapidly transported from the epididymis through the vas and ejaculatory ducts into the urethra. Most of the ejaculate volume consists of fluid from the prostate and seminal vesicles, which also empty through the ejaculatory ducts. The bladder neck closes tightly to prevent retrograde ejaculation into the bladder, and rhythmic contraction of periurethral muscles causes projectile ejaculation.[23]

After ejaculation, a series of final biochemical and plasma membrane changes occur in the sperm known as *capacitation*. These changes generally take place in the female reproductive tract, but can be initiated in vitro with various media and physical maneuvers. Sperm are incapable of fertilization without undergoing capacitation. On contact with investments of the oocyte, a final change in the sperm head membrane occurs called the *acrosome reaction*, which allows penetration of the oocyte. Recent evidence has demonstrated that the binding of sperm head antigens to surface receptors of the zona pellucida is essential to the fertilization process.

Evaluation of an Infertile Man

History

A complete medical history should be performed in all patients. Special attention is directed to the history of fertility or infertility, current sexual practices, and understanding of the menstrual cycle and ovulation. Sometimes, a cursory review of such physiology and adjustment of intercourse timing is all that is needed to solve the infertility problem.

The patient is asked about congenital anomalies, systemic illness, prior surgeries (especially herniorrhaphy and bladder or scrotal surgeries), and infections or trauma of the genital and urinary tracts. Exposure to spermatogenic toxins is discerned. Some of the most common toxins encountered today are marijuana, anabolic steroids, and chemotherapeutic agents. Occasionally, pesticides and cleaning solvents may be problematic.

The urologist evaluating the male partner should also interview the woman to assess her fertility history and menstrual cycle and screen for ovulatory problems to determine proper timing of referral to a qualified gynecologist. There may be combined female and male factors in a third of infertility cases.

Physical Examination

A general physical examination is carried out in all men with attention directed to the genital organs. Body habitus and secondary sex characteristics should be typical male type. The testes should be at least 4 cm long and moderately firm in consistency. The presence or absence of the vas deferens can be determined by physical examination alone. Surgical exploration to diagnose congenital absence of the vas deferens is not needed or advisable. The epididymis should be present and not be indurated. The patient is examined standing and during valsalva maneuver to find a varicocele (dilated veins in the pampiniform plexus). Varicoceles usually occur on the left but may be bilateral and should disappear when the patient lies supine. Rectal examination is performed to assess the prostate and seminal vesicles.

Laboratory Studies

The cornerstone of male fertility evaluation is the semen analysis. The specimen should be collected at least 2 but no more than 5 days after the last ejaculation. Normal standards should be based on minimal parameters consistent with proven fertility. These parameters are shown in Table 109-1. These are not mean values but rather the "limits of adequacy," below which fertility begins to decline. Men with subnormal values may still be fertile, but with decreasing values, conception becomes statistically less likely. Because semen parameters can vary greatly between analyses in the same individual, it is important to evaluate at least three specimens before instituting therapy. *Azoospermia* is the absence of sperm in the ejaculate. *Oligospermia* refers to low sperm counts. *Asthenospermia* is low motility in the sperm sample. *Teratospermia* is defined as a high percentage of morphologically abnormal sperm.

Evidence suggests that semen abnormalities have increased during the past 50 years. Carlson and colleagues[24]

Table 109-1. NORMAL SEMEN PARAMETERS

Volume	2–5 mL
Sperm concentration	$>20 \times 10^6$/mL
Total sperm	$>60 \times 10^6$
Motility	>60%
Forward progression	>75%
Normal morphology	>60%
Fructose	Present
Agglutination	Absent
White blood cells	<5 WBCs/HPF

reviewed all publications from 1938 to 1991 that discussed semen parameters in men without a history of infertility. Data from 61 papers covering 14,947 men were included. Sperm density dropped from a mean of 113 million/mL in 1940 to 66 million/mL in 1990. Further compounding the problem was a drop in mean semen volume from 3.4 mL to 2.75 mL during the same period. These observations and an increase in incidence of testicular cancer and congenital anomalies of the testis suggest that male gonadal function and possibly male fertility may be declining.[25] That these observations may be due to environmental factors is an intriguing possibility.

Other Tests

Serum levels of FSH, LH, and testosterone are obtained on all patients with abnormal semen analysis to assess the hypothalamic pituitary–gonadal axis. Very low levels of all hormones indicate a prepubertal state or a hypothalamic or pituitary disease. A markedly elevated FSH level (more than 2.5 times the upper limit of normal) indicates irreparable testicular failure. The level is elevated because of a lack of feedback inhibition from inhibin. However, a normal FSH does not ensure spermatogenesis.

Testis biopsy and vasography are performed to investigate azoospermia. The biopsy can distinguish testicular failure from normal sperm production with obstruction of the excurrent ducts. Vasography, performed with microsurgical cannulation of the vas deferens, is used to localize the site of obstruction, so that operative therapy may be planned.

The direct immunobead test is used to detect antisperm antibodies. This is suspected in men whose sperm agglutinate or exhibit shaking motility under microscopic observation. Polyacrylamide beads coated with antihuman immunoglobulin antibodies are placed in solution with the sperm, and the percentage of sperm binding to the beads is determined. If over 20% of the sperm are bound, the direct immunobead test is positive. The presence of serum antisperm antibodies when the test is negative is insignificant.

The sperm penetration assay is a bioassay in which sperm fertilizing capability is tested in vitro against zona pellucida–free hamster eggs. Good penetration scores correlate with successful fertilization of human eggs in vitro and with prospects for pregnancy.

Sperm survival and motility in the female reproductive tract can be tested by the postcoital test. During the periovulatory period, intercourse is performed by the couple and the cervical mucus examined 2 to 6 hours later. At least five motile sperm should be found per high-power field. Abnormalities in the postcoital test may indicate hostile or inadequate cervical mucus, poor sperm survival, antisperm antibodies, or poor sperm motility.

Specific Disorders and Treatments

Complete testicular failure is diagnosed by testis biopsy showing no sperm production or by a markedly elevated FSH level. This can be congenital (germ cell aplasia) or acquired as a result of testicular toxins (chemotherapy, carbon disulfide), irradiation, trauma, infection (mumps, serious bacterial infection), or vascular insult (testicular torsion). In many cases, no cause can be found for the testicular failure. Complete testicular failure and arrest of spermatogenic maturation are not treatable conditions at the present time.

Oligospermia or oligoasthenospermia can be thought of as an incomplete testicular failure, possibly from the causes mentioned earlier. Empiric treatments such as clomiphene citrate have been used to raise gonadotropin

levels and "drive" the testes harder, but most studies involving these drugs are poorly controlled. Clomiphen treatment is probably valuable only if the serum testosterone level is less than 300 ng/mL. Intrauterine insemination and in vitro fertilization show promise since many fewer sperm are necessary to achieve conception under these circumstances.

Varicocele is found in about 15% of the general population, but in 40% of infertile men.[26] A varicocele can cause a low sperm count but more often adversely affects sperm motility and morphology. Occluding the internal spermatic system with surgery or angiographic techniques improves the semen parameters in 50% to 70% of patients and results in subsequent pregnancy rates of 25% to 50%.[27] Current surgical techniques include laparoscopic ligation and microsurgical approaches, which have both decreased operative morbidity and recovery time. The reason for the varicocele effect is not clear, but recent research points to abnormalities in testicular microcirculation. Other theories include disordered scrotal temperature regulation and retrograde flow of adrenal hormones and renal toxins.

Excurrent duct obstruction may be congenital, as in cases of absence or atresia of the epididymis, vas deferens, or ejaculatory duct. Congenital bilateral absence of the vas deferens has recently been shown to be a primary genital form of cystic fibrosis since it is believed that all such men are either homozygotes for CFTR gene mutations or compound heterozygotes with two different CFTR gene mutations.[28] This condition has been treated in recent years with microsurgical aspiration of the epididymal sperm with in vitro fertilization of partner oocytes, a technique first described by Silber and coworkers.[29]

Acquired obstruction can result from elective vasectomy, surgical injury to the epididymis (eg, hydrocele repair) or to the vas deferens (eg, herniorrhaphy) and ejaculatory duct (transurethral resection of the prostate) or from infection such as epididymitis with scarification of the epididymal tubule. Microsurgical vasovasostomy and vasoepididymostomy are performed to bypass vas deferens and epididymal obstructions, whereas transurethral resection of the ejaculatory duct orifice is done to treat that site. Technical success and pregnancy rates can be as high as 80% and 60% respectively for vasovasostomy, but only 50% and 30% respectively for the more difficult vasoepididymostomy.

Endocrine disorders are an uncommon cause of male infertility. They can be primary or secondary. Primary hypogonadotropic hypogonadism (eg, Kallman syndrome) results from a lack of hypothalamic GnRH, leading to persistence of the prepubertal hormonal status. These men can be successfully treated with exogenous gonadotropins or by pulsatile GnRH infusion pump. Secondary hypogonadotropic hypogonadism can result from mass lesions of the pituitary gland and warrants investigation with brain imaging studies.

Men with low testosterone levels and sexual dysfunction can be treated with exogenous testosterone by injection or testosterone patch (Testoderm). Unfortunately, this treatment is counterproductive in men with infertility due to low testosterone. When testosterone is given from an exogenous source, the gonadotropins decrease, leading to a lowering of the intratesticular testosterone essential for sperm production. The testosterone level must be raised by increasing endogenous production with either oral clomiphene citrate or by injection of human chorionic gonadotropin, an LH analogue.

Antisperm antibodies are found more frequently in infertile men than fertile controls.[30] They are associated with vasectomy and are postulated to occur after infection, trauma, and ischemia to the testis, which can result in alterations of the blood–testis barrier. Corticosteroids have been shown to lower sperm antibody titers, but most studies concerning pregnancy rates are poorly controlled. The potential serious side effects of corticosteroids must be considered before therapy begins. Other strategies with more potential include methods to decrease the numbers of sperm necessary to achieve pregnancy (insemination and in vitro fertilization) and development of laboratory methods to remove antibodies from the sperm.

Ejaculatory disturbances are an uncommon cause of male infertility. Premature ejaculation and idiopathic primary anejaculation (with normal nocturnal emissions) are psychogenic in origin and should be treated as such. Retrograde ejaculation can result from bladder neck surgery or neurogenic causes and is treated by retrieval of sperm from the urine, sperm washing, and artificial insemination. Complete neurogenic anejaculation can result from spinal cord injury, multiple sclerosis, diabetic neuropathy, and retroperitoneal surgery (injury to sympathetic nerve fibers). Rectal probe electrical stimulation of the ejaculatory organs with artificial insemination is the treatment of choice.[31]

Cryptorchidism results in infertility if the testes are not brought into the scrotum, probably because of higher temperatures in the abdominal cavity. To preserve future fertility, cryptorchid testes should be fixed in the scrotum early in life. Even when the surgery is performed appropriately, however, subfertility can result, suggesting a possible common cause of testicular maldescent and subtle dysgenesis of the testis.

Chromosomal abnormalities may cause male infertility. Klinefelter syndrome (47,XXY) is the most common, occurring in about 1 of every 500 male births. Patients with Klinefelter syndrome are always sterile and present with small firm testes on exam.

URINARY LITHIASIS

The advent of modern civilization changed the pattern of urinary lithiasis from a primary bladder condition to one of primary renal origin. It is estimated that 12% of the US population will develop calculus disease during their lifetime. Males have more than twice the rate of stone formation than females. Whites have between a 2 and 10 times higher incidence of renal stone disease than do blacks or Asians. There are also geographic variations in the incidence of stones. Several studies have reported that the Southeastern United States has a higher rate of lithiasis than do other parts of the nation (Fig. 109-1) In addition to geographic variations, there are also seasonal variations

Table 109-2. TYPES OF KIDNEY STONES

Stone Composition	Frequency (%)	Radiographic Appearance
Calcium oxalate ± calcium phosphate	75	Opaque
Pure calcium phosphate	7	Opaque
Magnesium ammonium phosphate (struvite)	12	Opaque
Uric acid	7	Lucent
Cystine	2	Opaque to radiolucent

with a higher incidence of lithiasis in the hot summer months than in the colder winter months. The peak incidence of lithiasis appears to be between the ages of 45 and 64 years. Those in whom a stone does form have a 50% chance of another stone's forming within 5 years.

Almost three quarters of the stones are composed of calcium oxalate in combination with calcium phosphate (Table 109-2). Magnesium ammonium phosphate (struvite) or infection stones make up about 12%, whereas pure calcium phosphate and uric acid stones each constitute 7%. Cystine stones, which constitute only 2% of all stones, develop only in patients with a rare congenital defect in the renal tubular resorption of cystine resulting in cystinuria and subsequent stone formation.[32]

Calculous Formation

The pathophysiologic basis for renal stone formation is a result of a complex interaction of many factors. Several theories of stone formation exist.[33] The nucleation theory suggests that stone formation is initiated by the presence of a crystal or foreign body, which, in supersaturated urine, promotes the growth of crystal lattice. Nucleation cannot take place in the absence of supersaturated urine, but it can take place if urine only intermittently becomes supersaturated. The intensity of nucleation is often proportional to the degree of supersaturation. An important factor in altering saturation is the urine pH, which can have a significant effect on the solubility. The matrix theory postulates that there is an organic matrix of urinary proteins that act as nidi for crystal deposition. Matrix is commonly found in the nucleus of infection stones. The inhibitor theory postulates that there are substances in the urine that prevent either crystal formation, aggregation, or both. Typical inhibitors include pyrophosphate, citrate, magnesium, glycosaminoglycans, acidic glycopeptides, and small RNA fragments.

Diagnosis

Renal stones may or may not be associated with pain, but if pain is present, it is usually dull and localizes to the flank. At times a renal stone may be associated with urinary tract infection. Ureteral stones usually present precipitously with ureteral colic (severe flank pain radiating to the groin, nausea, and vomiting). Ureteral stones that are located in the intravesical ureter also cause urgency and frequency. Urinalysis of a patient with urinary stones shows evidence of either gross or microscopic hematuria 85% to 90% of the time. In addition, pyuria may be present in up to 10% of patients presenting with stones; however, up to 5% may have completely acellular urinalysis results. For this reason, patients who present with abdominal pain should undergo both abdominal radiography and urinaly-

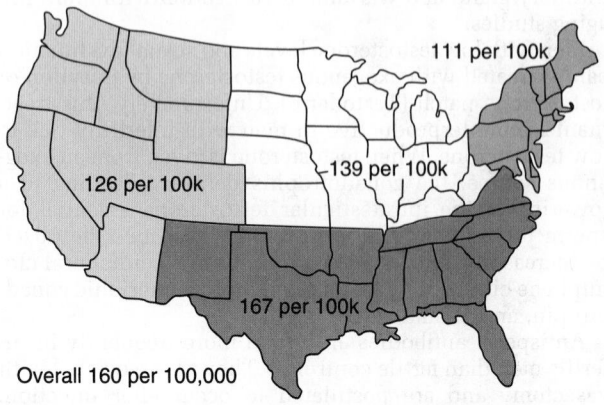

111 per 100k

139 per 100k

126 per 100k

167 per 100k

Overall 160 per 100,000

Figure 109-1. Incidence of urolithiasis in the United States.

sis in their evaluation. Between 85% and 90% of urinary stones are radiopaque and identifiable with noncontrast abdominal radiographs unless they are very small or overlie bony structures.

Treatment

Most patients pass their stones spontaneously with the aid of increased hydration and appropriate analgesics. Calculi that are less than 4 mm wide have a greater than 90% chance of passing spontaneously, whereas stones greater than 6 mm wide have less than a 10% chance of spontaneous passage. Three areas in the urinary tract system are relatively narrow and thereby impede stone passage—the ureteropelvic junction, the site where the ureter crosses over the iliac vessels, and the ureterovesical junction. These sites are also the most common sites of stone impaction.

Specific conditions known to lead to stone formation are listed in Table 109-3. In the evaluation of a patient with nephrolithiasis, it is important to query about the presence of any of these conditions. All stones passed should be retrieved for subsequent analysis. Patients passing their first stone should have serum calcium and creatinine levels and an urinalysis in addition to stone analysis. If the stone is calcium oxalate and the serum calcium level is normal, no further evaluation is necessary other than encouraging

---

Table 109-3. CONDITIONS LEADING TO URINARY LITHIASIS

INCREASED URINARY CALCIUM

Excess dietary calcium
Vitamin D toxicity
Resorptive hypercalciuria
    Prolonged immobilization
    Hyperparathyroidism
Absorptive hypercalciuria
Renal leak
Idiopathy

INCREASED SERUM CALCIUM

Hyperparathyroidism
Sarcoidosis
Vitamin D toxicity
Cushing syndrome
Milk-alkali syndrome
Thyrotoxicosis
Addison disease

INCREASED URINARY OXALATE

Excess dietary oxalate
Excess vitamin C
Gastrointestinal disorders
    Short-gut syndrome
    Gastric plication for obesity
    Small bowel resection
    Ulcerative colitis
    Regional enteritis

INCREASED URINARY URIC ACID

Excess dietary purine
Drug-induced
    Probenicid
    Sulfinpyrazone
    Salicylates
Myeloproliferative disorders
Type I glycogen storage disease
Chronic dehydration states

INCREASED URINARY CYSTINE

Autosomal recessive cystinuria

---

the patient to increase fluid intake. Any patient with stones made of uric acid, pure calcium phosphate, cystine, or struvite is at high risk for continued stone formation and should undergo more extensive metabolic evaluation. In addition, those patients with recurrent or enlarging stones, including those patients with known calcium oxalate stones should also undergo a metabolic evaluation.

Recent advances in technology have revolutionized the surgical treatment of urinary stones, virtually eliminating open surgery for renal and ureteral lithiasis. At the University of Michigan, 102 open surgeries were performed for renal and ureteral stones in 1980 alone. From 1987 to 1994, only seven open surgeries were performed. This dramatic shift away from open surgery to minimally invasive surgery was a direct result of the development of both extracorporeal shockwave lithotripsy (ESWL) and refinements in endoscopic equipment and techniques. ESWL was first developed in West Germany in the 1970s. By 1982, the Dornier HM-3 had undergone extensive clinical trials demonstrating its efficacy and reproducibility in fragmenting urinary stones, and in 1984, the first machine was installed in the United States.[34] Further, technologic developments have since led to the construction of second- and third-generation lithotripters, which now allow pain-free application of the shock wave.

The basic principles of all lithotripters include shock wave generation, focusing of the sound wave, and imaging of the stone. Within this framework differences exist, but a detailed comparison of all the different types of lithotripters is beyond the scope of this chapter. All lithotripters produce shockwaves by a spark-gap electrode or by a piezoelectric or electromagnetic element. The wave is focused via a semiellipsoid in the spark-gap machines, an acoustic lens in those employing an electromagnet to produce the shock wave, or spherical alignment in those machines using piezoceramic elements. (Fig. 109-2) Patients are either submersed in a water bath or "coupled" via a water cushion. The acoustic density of water and body tissues is essentially the same. Therefore, there is little to no impedence of the shock wave at the water–body interface. On striking the stone, which is of different acoustical density, the shock waves undergo reflection and refraction, resulting in compressive and tensile forces that fragment the stone. Localization is achieved using fluoroscopy or ultrasonography. The maximal number of shock waves delivered to the stone at one session depends on the size and composition of the stone, the energy used, and the machine type. Complications from ESWL are rare. The most common complication after ESWL is ureteral obstruction secondary to stone fragments, requiring either additional ESWL, ureteroscopic stone retrieval, or stent placement. Significant hemorrhage occurs in 0.18% to 3.8% of patients and is usually limited to those with previously unknown or inadequately corrected bleeding diathesis. Those patients with a preexisting, uncorrected coagulopathy are not candidates for ESWL therapy.

Other contraindications to ESWL are a distal anatomic obstruction precluding passage of the stone fragments, untreated urinary tract infection, pregnancy, and technical problems usually related to patient size and body habitus.

Percutaneous endoscopic renal and ureteroscopic stone removal became possible with the advent of technologic advancements in miniaturizing the endoscopic equipment required to allow atraumatic visualization of the renal collecting system and ureter. Ultrasonic, electrohydraulic, and laser probes have been developed to fragment stones under visual guidance through either rigid or flexible instruments. Percutaneous lithotripsy, alone or in combination with ESWL, results in stone-free rates of 95% for simple renal stones to 85% for complex staghorn calculi.[35]

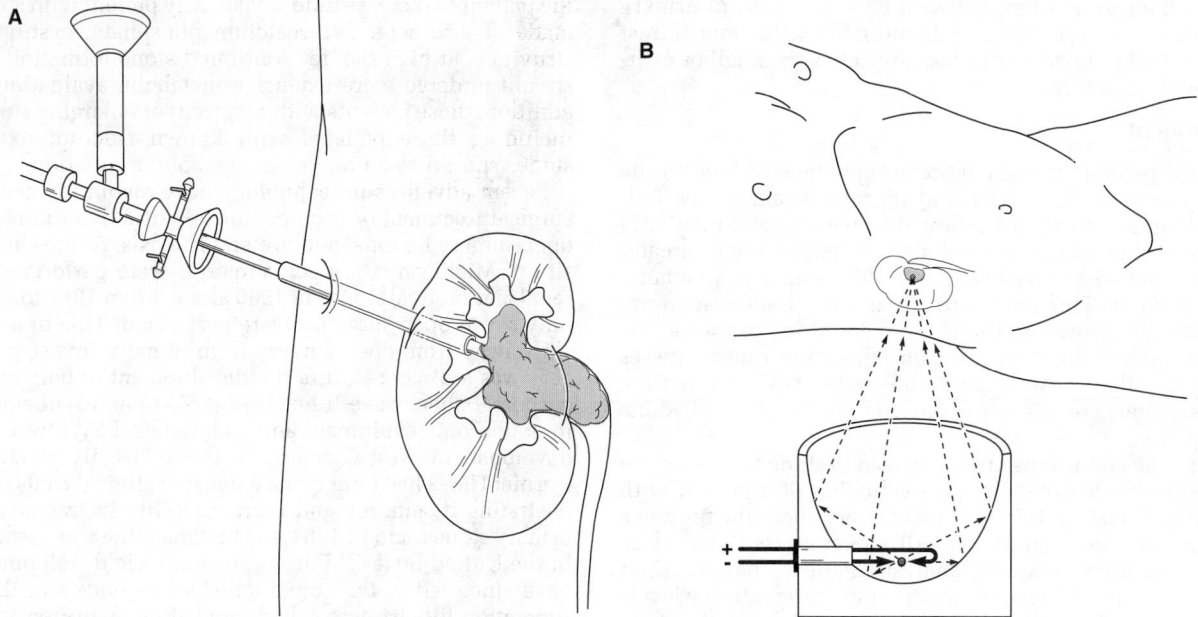

Figure 109-2. Diagram of percutaneous nephroscopy (*A*) and a lithotripsy machine (*B*).

Renal and Proximal Ureteral Stones

Extracorporeal shock-wave lithotripsy is the treatment of choice for the vast majority of renal and proximal ureteral stones, with stone-free rates ranging between 60% and 95% at 6 months.[36] Stones larger than 3 cm in diameter and branched stones such as staghorn calculi are best treated with percutaneous nephrolithotripsy alone or in combination with ESWL. ESWL monotherapy requires multiple treatments and ancillary therapies such as stent placement to prevent or treat ureteral obstruction secondary to ureteral fragments. Stone-free rates with ESWL monotherapy range between 31% and 85% with the average stone-free rate at 51%. Percutaneous nephrolithotripsy alone or in combination with ESWL results in an average stone-free rate of 84%.[37] Cystine stones are also best treated by percutaneous nephrolithotripsy because of their resistance to adequate fragmentation with ESWL.

Mid-Ureteral Stones

There are several treatment options for symptomatic mid-ureteral stones.[38] In the past, these stones were manipulated back into the kidney with guide wires, catheters, and occlusion balloons and subsequently treated with ESWL. With this approach, the reported rates of fragmentation were up to 95%. Currently, some investigators have reported treating ureteral calculi in situ with results ranging from 70% to 90% Retreatment rates were higher in the in situ group compared with the stented or manipulated group. Stone removal using either a flexible or rigid ureteroscope can also be performed.[39] Stones can be retrieved intact using a wire basket. If the calculus is too large, it can be fragmented using an electrohydraulic or ultrasonic probe or a laser fiber and subsequently removed.

Distal Ureteral Stones

Distal stones can be successfully retrieved ureteroscopically 95% to 100% of the time.[40] Although complication rates are low, they can be significant and include ureteral stricture, perforation, or avulsion.[41] To avoid some of the complications associated with ureteroscopy, ESWL of distal ureteral stones has been reported with success rates of about 85%. However, a second ESWL is required in 20% to 70% of cases for complete fragmentation.

BLADDER CANCER

A wealth of basic research and clinical data indicate that a variety of chemical carcinogens can induce bladder cancer. Occupational exposure to β-naphthylamine and para-aminodiphenyl increases the risk for bladder cancer. Epidemiologic studies have also implicated cigarette smoke as a risk factor. Bladder cancer has a strong male prevalence and is almost three times more common in men than women.

Urothelium normally expresses a transitional cell morphology but has the potential for metaplastic change to squamous or glandular epithelium. Malignant urothelium reflects these histologic alterations seen in benign disease processes. Transitional cell carcinoma accounts for about 90% of all urothelial malignancies. Squamous cell carcinomas and adenocarcinomas are much rarer. Bladder cancer is frequently multifocal and has a high incidence of recurrence.

Papillary bladder cancer and carcinoma in situ have been recognized clinically as having different presentations, appearances, and risk of progression. These clinical observations have been supported by molecular evidence that these two types of bladder cancer are fundamentally different. Superficial papillary bladder cancer is frequently associated with loss of heterozygosity (LOH) in the long arm of chromosome 9.[42] In carcinoma in situ, 9q deletions are uncommon, whereas muscle invasive tumors exhibit an intermediate level of 9q LOH.[43] This suggests that many muscle invasive tumors arise from bladder carcinoma in situ. Loss of the tumor suppressor genes *Rb* and *p53* have been implicated in progression, invasion, and metastasis of bladder cancer.

Diagnosis and Staging

The hallmark of bladder cancer is total gross painless hematuria. However, microscopic hematuria may also be the first indicator of this disease. A minority of individuals present with irritative symptoms, such as frequency and dysuria. This can be caused either by advanced local disease or carcinoma in situ. Urine cytology is effective for screening people with irritative symptoms because most people with diffuse carcinoma in situ shed neoplastic cells that are detectable by this modality as well as flow cytometry. The staging of bladder cancer is illustrated in Figure 109-3.

The usual diagnostic tests used are excretory urography and cystoscopy. The former is important because the upper tracts (renal pelves and ureters) are also at risk for the development of urothelial neoplasia. Cystoscopy is frequently not only diagnostic but also therapeutic because superficial tumors are easily excised or fulgurated (either with cautery or Nd:YAG laser) through endoscopic instruments. Patients with locally advanced tumors should undergo a metastatic evaluation usually consisting of chest radiograph and CT of the abdomen and pelvis. A bone scan can also be obtained, but the diagnostic yield from this study in asymptomatic individuals is low.

Treatment

About 70% of patients with bladder cancer present with local disease. This is associated with a 5-year age-adjusted survival rate of 88%. Close vigilance is important because the recurrence rate exceeds 50%. Between 10% and 15% of superficial tumors progress to invasive disease. Multifocal and recurrent tumors are usually treated with intravesical chemotherapy in addition to transurethral resection. Agents commonly used include thiotepa, doxorubicin, and mitomycin C. Alternatively, intravesical immunotherapy has been successfully performed with the instillation of bacillus Calmette-Guerin (BCG).[44] BCG currently appears to be the most efficacious intravesical agent for superficial bladder cancer but is associated with increased toxicity.[45]

Locally advanced tumors are usually treated with radical cystectomy (cystoprostatectomy in men and anterior exenteration in women) and urinary diversion. Radiotherapy has been used but is associated with a high rate of local recurrence. Individuals who fail on radiotherapy can often be treated with subsequent cystectomy.[46] The 5-year survival rate for patients with advanced localized disease is 20% to 50%. The development of effective systemic chemotherapy has resulted in the evaluation of several new treatments. These include cisplatin-based multidrug chemotherapy before (neoadjuvant) cystectomy, after (adjuvant) cystectomy, and with radiotherapy.

The types of urinary diversion used with radical cystectomy have changed significantly in recent years. Although ileal conduit diversion is still common, alternative methods that more closely approximate the reservoir function of the urinary bladder have gained increasing favor. In the numerous techniques that have been developed, common features include the use of intestine (large, small, or both) to create a pouch, a method to decrease the pressure in the pouch (avoiding the use of intact bowel segments), a mechanism to avoid reflux of urine into the ureters, and a mechanism to achieve continence[47,48] (Fig. 109-4). When the urinary pouch drains to the abdominal wall (eg, Kock pouch), intermittent catheterization is substituted for voiding. When the urinary pouch is anastomosed to the urethra, voiding can frequently be accomplished by abdominal straining.

Metastatic bladder cancer is usually treated with systemic chemotherapy. Cisplatin-based regimens, such as M-VAC (methotrexate, vinblastin, doxorubicin [Adriamycin], and cisplatin), has resulted in 37% complete response rates.[49] P-glycoprotein has been associated with multiple drug resistance and has been detected in bladder cancer;

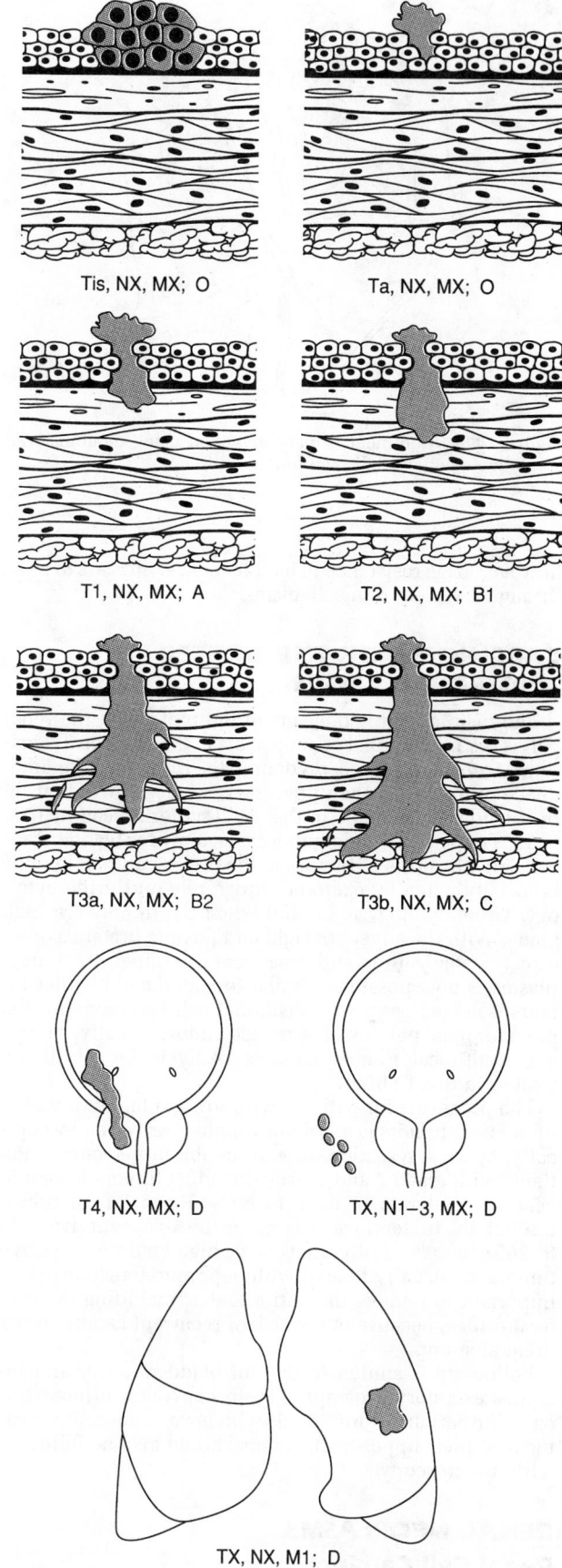

Tis, NX, MX; O

Ta, NX, MX; O

T1, NX, MX; A

T2, NX, MX; B1

T3a, NX, MX; B2

T3b, NX, MX; C

T4, NX, MX; D

TX, N1–3, MX; D

TX, NX, M1; D

Figure 109-3. Staging of bladder cancer. Both the TNM (American Joint Commission on Cancer, ed 3) and the Jewett systems are shown.

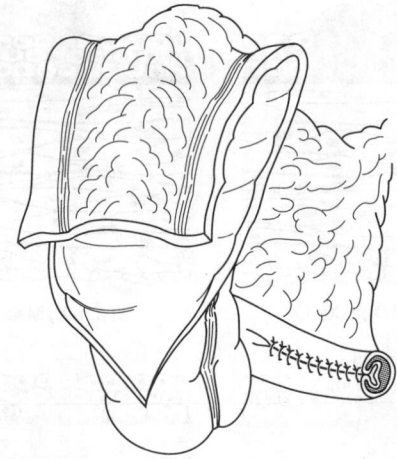

Figure 109-4. Continent urinary diversion using detubularized ascending colon and plicated terminal ilium.

however, drug resistance in bladder cancer appears to arise through a variety of mechanisms.[50]

CARCINOMA OF THE URETER AND RENAL PELVIS

The histology of neoplasms in the ureter and the renal pelvis is similar to that of neoplasms in the bladder. Transitional cell carcinomas predominate. However, the incidence of tumors in the upper tract is much lower than in the bladder. Carcinoma in the distal ureter is seen in 10% to 15% of patients undergoing cystectomy for bladder cancer. The diagnosis of tumors in the ureter and renal pelvis is usually made by excretory urography and urine cytology. Urine cytology is helpful when the tumors are high grade. With the advent of rigid and flexible ureteroscopes, direct visualization and treatment of upper tract neoplasms is now possible. Similar to superficial bladder tumors, selected cases of transitional cell carcinoma of the ureter or renal pelvis can be treated endoscopically.[51] Large and multifocal tumors are less likely to be effectively treated in this fashion.

The prognosis for patients with low-grade, noninvasive upper tract tumors is excellent whether treated endoscopically, by local resection, or with nephroureterectomy. Patients with grade 2 and muscle-invading tumors have a 5-year survival rate of 60% to 80%. Extension of tumor through the ureteral wall decreases the 5-year survival rate to 30% to 40%. Individuals with high-grade or invasive tumors are usually treated with nephroureterectomy. It is important to remove the entire ureter, including the ureteral orifice, because of the risk of recurrent cancer in the ureteral stump.

Follow-up is similar to that for bladder cancer and includes excretory urography, cystoscopy, and urine cytology. Furthermore, individuals who have endoscopic treatment of their upper-tract tumors should also be followed with ureteroscopy.

RENAL NEOPLASMS
Renal Cell Carcinoma

The most common malignant neoplasm of the renal parenchyma is the hypernephroma or renal cell carcinoma. This adenocarcinoma primarily arises from the cells of the proximal renal tubule and accounts for about 2% of all new cancers annually. It is most common after the fifth decade of life, and has a male/female ratio of about 2:1. No definite etiology has been identified, but a frequent genetic abnormality detected in renal cancer cells is the loss of heterozygosity of chromosome 3p. Multifocal bilateral tumors are associated with von Hippel–Lindau disease. The von Hippel–Lindau locus is also on the short arm of chromosome 3. The von Hippel–Lindau tumor-suppressor gene has been partially cloned and appears to play a pivotal role in the development of sporadic clear cell renal carcinoma.[52] Other possible etiologic associations include exposure to cadmium and lead, tobacco use, and renal failure.

Renal cell carcinoma is often clinically silent until late in its course. The growth rate of these tumors varies, and they may be large before symptoms or metastases occur. The classic triad consisting of flank pain, palpable mass, and hematuria is composed of late symptoms associated with advanced disease. Renal carcinomas can produce a variety of hormone or hormone-like substances (eg, erythropoietin, renin, and parathormone) and may present with a variety of symptoms including anemia, hypertension, fever, erythrocytosis, abnormalities in liver function tests, and symptoms associated with metastatic disease. Many tumors are now discovered incidentally when diagnostic studies such as intravenous urography, CT, or ultrasound are obtained for some other reason.[53] The increased detection of low-stage tumors by using these imaging modalities has resulted in an overall increase in survival.

Diagnosis and Staging

The staging of renal cell carcinoma is based on the extent of the disease. The Robson system with its TNM counterpart is shown in Figure 109-5.[54] These tumors have a predilection for growth into the renal veins with extension into the vena cava. There is not usually direct invasion of these structures, and this finding does not portend a poor prognosis. Tumor thrombi may extend superiorly into the right atrium. Perihilar and periaortic lymph nodes receive lymphatic drainage from the kidney, and nodal involvement is seen in about 30% of cases.[55] Because of ready access of tumor cells to the venous circulation, hematogenous metastases readily occur. The most common sites include lung, bone, liver, brain, adrenal gland, and the contralateral kidney. Less frequently, metastases occur in any organ, including heart, vagina, skin, and others.

Excretory urography provides a good renal image with superior detail of the collecting system. Renal masses such as benign cysts or renal cell carcinomas appear as deformities, distorting the renal outline or the collecting system. Renal cysts are far more common than renal cell carcinoma, and the main differential diagnosis of a renal mass on excretory urogaphy is between a renal cyst and a solid tumor such as renal cell carcinoma. This differentiation is sometimes obvious on excretory urography. Cysts have low-density centers with a well-defined "beak" of parenchyma surrounding them. Tumors appear dense and solid. Tomography can help make this differentiation. Renal ultrasound may be used to confirm the cystic nature of the mass. If the mass appears to be solid, CT or angiography may be used to characterize it. CT can demonstrate a solid mass, which often becomes more dense or enhances with the administration of radiographic contrast material. Hilar or periaortic lymphadenopathy or liver metastasis may be demonstrated, and the renal vein and vena cava can often be evaluated for tumor extension. Selective renal angiography shows any tumor vessels, arteriovenous fistulas, venous laking, and tumor staining characteristic of a renal cell carcinoma. Vena cavography can evaluate vena caval

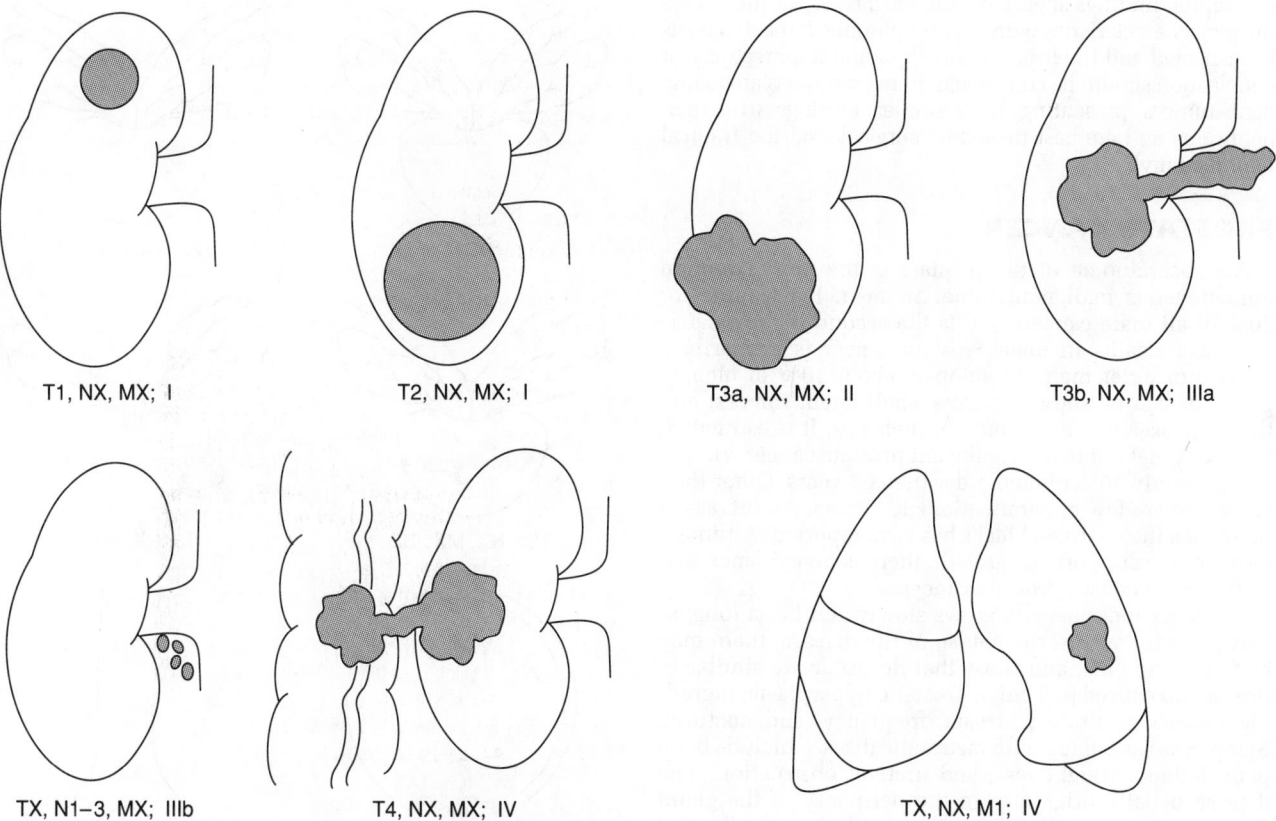

T1, NX, MX; I   T2, NX, MX; I   T3a, NX, MX; II   T3b, NX, MX; IIIa

TX, N1–3, MX; IIIb   T4, NX, MX; IV   TX, NX, M1; IV

Figure 109-5. Staging of renal cancer. Both the TNM (American Joint Commission on Cancer, ed 3) and the Robson systems are shown.

and renal vein involvement. However, MR imaging is an effective, noninvasive method for defining the extent of venous involvement. To further stage the tumor, a chest film or chest CT is used to evaluate pulmonary metastases, and a bone scan may be done to rule out osseous metastases.

Treatment

Surgical excision remains the primary mode of treatment for renal cell carcinoma. Although the need for radical nephrectomy has recently been questioned, this remains the gold standard against which less radical procedures must be judged. Radical nephrectomy is performed through an abdominal or thoracoabdominal approach and involves early control of the renal artery and vein. The tumor, together with the kidney and the perirenal fat is excised within the Gerota fascia, which is not opened. The ipsilateral adrenal gland and periaortic lymphadenectomy are often excised, although there is little evidence that this contributes to disease-free survival. Extensions of tumor into the renal vein and vena cava are also removed. If vena caval extension of tumor reaches beyond the hepatic veins or into the right atrium, cardiopulmonary bypass with hypothermia and total circulatory arrest has been used to facilitate tumor excision in a bloodless field. Preoperative angioinfarction may facilitate nephrectomy when the tumors are very large or extend into the vena cava. Resection of solitary metastases in lung, liver, bone and other organs should also be considered. The 5-year survival rate for patients with localized disease (stages 1, 2, and 3a) is 40% to 90%. The 5-year survival rate for patients with lymphatic metastases (stage 3b) is 5% to 30%. The prognosis

for patients with distant metastases (stage 4) is poor, with only 5% to 10% surviving 5 years.[56] Less radical approaches, including partial nephrectomy, have been suggested for treating smaller tumors. Results in series of highly selected patients have been comparable to the more radical technique outlined earlier, with cancer specific 5-year survival rates of over 85%.[57] This approach is especially valuable in bilateral tumors or in patients with a solitary kidney or poor overall renal function. Therapy for metastatic disease, including radiation and chemotherapy, is generally ineffective. Because of the well-documented but low incidence of spontaneous regression in renal carcinoma, a variety of immunotherapeutic approaches has been tried. Recent reports document objective remission rates of 15% to 20% using interferon, interleukin-2, and LAK cells.[58]

Other Renal Neoplasms

While less common than hypernephroma, other solid tumors involving the kidney do occur. Benign tumors include angiomyolipoma and oncocytoma, and renal sarcomas include leiomyosarcoma, liposarcoma, and hemangiopericytoma. Although angiomyolipoma does not metastasize, it can occur in multiple sites, grow large, and bleed. It is associated with tuberous sclerosis. If the tumor contains sufficient fat, it can be reliably diagnosed preoperatively with CT or MR imaging. It cannot be distinguished from hypernephroma on angiography. Small tumors may be followed if they have classic imaging characteristics. However, life-threatening hemorrhage has occurred from angiomyolipomas. Oncocytomas are also considered benign, but are difficult to differentiate from renal cell carcinoma preoperatively. Some have radiographic findings suggesting the diagnosis, but they share imaging characteristics with hypernephroma. If the diagnosis is suspected and the lesion is small, partial nephrectomy or enucleation should be considered. Renal sarcomas are malignant tumors presenting with similar findings to hypernephroma and are best treated by surgical excision (radical nephrectomy).

PROSTATE CANCER

Adenocarcinoma of the prostate is the most common noncutaneous malignant tumor in men. It accounts for 20% of all male cancers and is the second highest cause of cancer deaths in men. Prostate cancer is primarily a disease of older men. At autopsy, about 10% of men in their 50s can be shown to have small latent tumors, and this increases to 70% of men in their 80s. It is estimated, however, that clinically significant prostate cancer will develop in only 10% of men older than 65 years. Other than age, there are few apparent etiologic factors. An increased incidence in American blacks has been reported. Although testosterone supports its growth, there is no evidence that testosterone causes prostate cancer.

Prostate cancer usually grows slowly and has a long latent period. Early in the course of the disease, there may be few symptoms, and those that do occur are similar to prostatism caused by benign prostatic hyperplasia, including decreasing urinary stream, frequency, and nocturia. Symptoms associated with metastatic disease include bone pain, fatigue, weight loss, and ureteral obstruction. The disease usually originates in the periphery of the gland then progresses locally within the gland, through the capsule, and into the seminal vesicles. The primary metastatic sites are the regional lymph nodes and the osseous skeleton.

Stage and Grade

The Jewett staging system together with the TNM equivalent is shown in Figure 109-6. A histologic grading system developed by Gleason correlates with patient prognosis. In this system, the Gleason score consists of the sum of the grades of the major and minor histologic patterns of the prostatic carcinoma. Since the Gleason grade varies from 1 (well differentiated) to 5 (poorly differentiated), the Gleason score ranges from 2 to 10.[59]

Detection of Prostate Cancer

Early prostate cancer has few symptoms. Obstructive symptoms may occur, but these are also seen in benign prostatic hyperplasia. Other symptoms, such as bone pain, weight loss, and fatigue, are often signs of advanced disease. Early diagnosis requires the detection of small tumors within the prostate gland. Three modalities are used in early detection of prostate cancer—digital rectal examination, serum prostate-specific antigen (PSA), and transrectal ultrasound of the prostate. Tumors usually arise in the posterior lobe of the prostate within the sonographic peripheral zone, which surrounds the more bulky central zone of the prostate. This area is readily palpable on digital rectal examination, and early prostatic cancer presents as a small firm nodule within or at the periphery of the gland. If a 1-cm nodule is detected, it is cancer about half the time, and the differential diagnosis includes prostatic calculi, granulomas, and benign hyperplasia. Prostatic biopsy is readily performed with little morbidity and is required to confirm the diagnosis. Transrectal ultrasound of the prostate can also detect prostate cancer, which most commonly appears as a hypoechoic lesion in the peripheral zone.

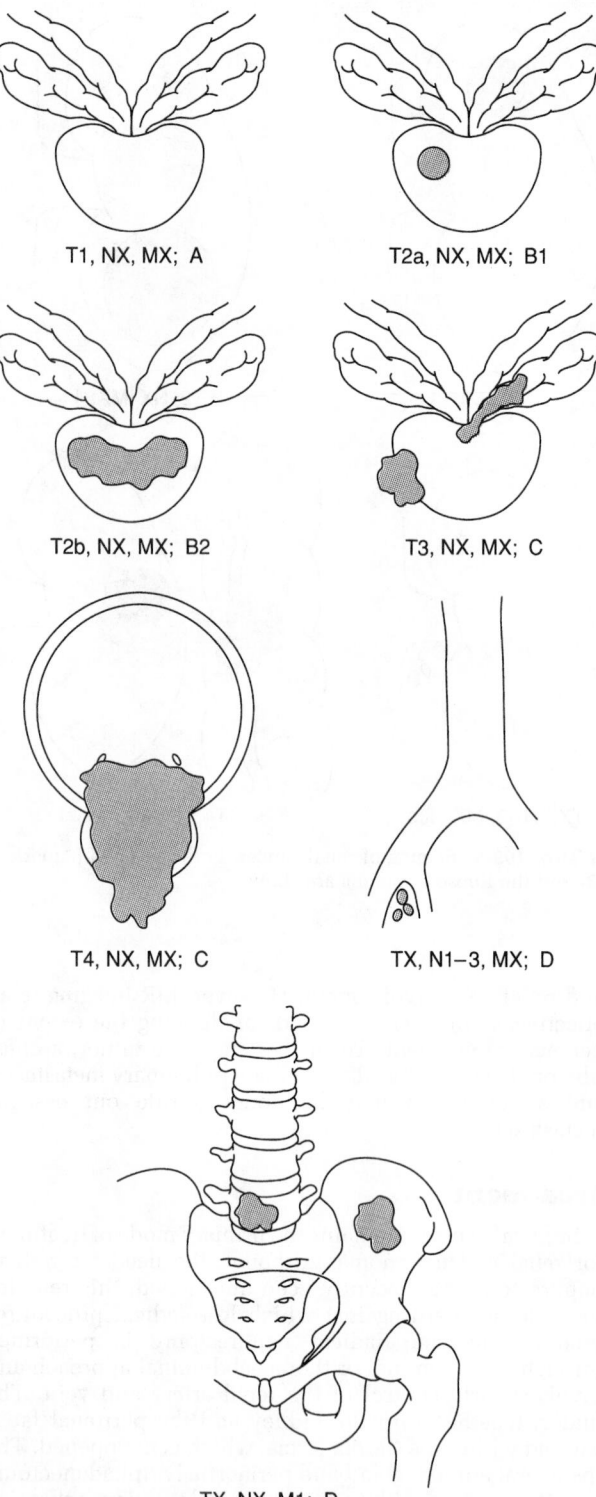

T1, NX, MX; A

T2a, NX, MX; B1

T2b, NX, MX; B2

T3, NX, MX; C

T4, NX, MX; C

TX, N1–3, MX; D

TX, NX, M1; D

Figure 109-6. Staging of prostate cancer. Both the TNM (American Joint Commission on Cancer, ed 3) and the Jewett systems are shown.

Transrectal ultrasound may detect smaller and other subtle lesions that are not easily discernible on digital rectal exam; however, digital examination discloses some carcinomas that can not be visualized with ultrasound. Ultrasonographic suspicious areas must also be confirmed with biopsy because a variety of other benign lesions can mimic the ultrasonographic appearance of prostatic cancer. When the predictive value of ultrasound and the prevalence of prostatic cancer are considered, screening for prostate cancer with transrectal ultrasonography does not appear to be an effective strategy. Serum PSA is also used to aid in the early detection of prostate cancer. PSA is elevated in 68% of men with cancer, but 33% of men with benign enlargement of the gland have an elevated PSA. Because of the specificity and sensitivity of this test, and the prevalence of prostate cancer, the use of PSA as a stand-alone screening test for prostate cancer is controversial. However, PSA testing together with digital rectal examination is widely used in early detection. The American Urological Association and the American Cancer Society currently recommend these tests for early detection of prostate cancer. In general, they should be done annually in all men older than 50 years. For men in high-risk groups, however, such as black men or those with a family history of prostate cancer, these tests should be done starting at age 40 years.

Tumor Markers

Serum prostatic acid phosphatase and serum PSA are markers for prostate cancer. Although acid phosphatase is not specific for prostate cancer, a significant elevation found on enzymatic assay usually signifies metastatic disease. However, it has largely been replaced as a tumor marker by the immunoassay for PSA. PSA is a glycoprotein specific for prostatic epithelium and is found in normal prostate tissue and in benign prostatic hyperplasia.[60] There is considerable overlap in the serum level of PSA in early prostatic carcinoma and benign prostatic hyperplasia. Attempts have been made to increase the specificity of PSA. One technique is to measure the increase in serum PSA over time. While PSA increases normally with increasing age in men,[61] it generally increases faster in men with prostate cancer.[62] This increase is called the PSA velocity, and it may be useful in detection.[63] Another technique is to measure the PSA density. This is the ratio of the serum PSA to the ultrasound-determined volume of the prostate. PSA density is often higher in patients with prostate cancer than in those with benign prostatic enlargement. In addition to its use in diagnosis, PSA is used to detect recurrences after treatment with radical prostatectomy or radiation therapy. PSA is an extremely sensitive tumor marker for recurrences after radical prostatectomy because serum levels should be undetectable if patients are tumor-free. Following radiation, the PSA level should fall and then remain stable at the lower level.

Clinical Staging

All available studies are associated with a significant staging error. Digital rectal examination is associated with a 25% staging error, largely a result of understaging. On the other hand, transrectal prostatic ultrasound frequently overstages disease confined to the prostate. Neither test can detect cancer in regional lymph nodes or at distant sites. MR imaging offers little advantage over ultrasound in assessing the primary neoplasm.[64] A bone scan is a very sensitive but relatively nonspecific method for detecting osseous metastases from prostatic cancer. Despite the incidence of positive studies from trauma and degenerative joint disease, bone scans are a valuable test for detecting distant metastases. Evaluation of the regional lymph nodes is much less satisfactory. Preoperative detection of microscopic nodal disease is virtually impossible. CT scanning and MR imaging can detect only grossly enlarged nodes. Pedal lymphangiography also has limited applicability. Surgical staging using laparoscopic techniques is more ac-

curate and may be useful before surgery or radiation in selected patients.

Treatment

Treatment of prostate cancer depends on whether the disease is localized to the prostate or advanced beyond the gland. Because prostate cancer advances slowly, the morbidity of therapy may exceed the therapeutic benefit in the elderly and debilitated. Individuals who have a limited life expectancy and low-stage disease are frequently best treated with observation only. Patients subjected to aggressive therapeutic procedures, such as radical prostatectomy, should have an estimated survival of 10 years.

If the tumor is confined within the prostatic capsule (stage A or B), treatment options include radical prostatectomy, external beam radiation therapy, and radioactive implants. Radical prostatectomy may be carried out through the perineal approach, but in recent years, the retropubic approach has been favored. Through this approach a node dissection can be done for further staging and the procedure possibly abandoned if the nodes contain tumor. In patients with a high index of suspicion for positive nodes, a laparoscopic pelvic node dissection or a dissection through an abbreviated incision can be performed to decrease postoperative morbidity. This approach may also be used in conjunction with perineal prostatectomy to evaluate the pelvic nodes. The entire prostate with its capsule and seminal vesicles is removed. A nerve-sparing approach can be used to preserve penile erection in potent patients. In this approach, the nerves involved with penile erection are excluded from the dissection. In certain cases, however, the nerves should be included in the dissection to provide a better margin of resection.

The major complications of radical prostatectomy are impotence, which drops from 100% to about 50% with the nerve-sparing approach, and incontinence, which ranges from 10% to 30%. If the disease is confined to the prostate, more than 80% of patients who do not die of other causes should be alive and disease-free at 15 years.[65] The overall disease-free survival rate is about 50%, which is the expected survival for all members of this age group. Remember that about 25% of patients are understaged clinically. A report from the Mayo Clinic indicates a similar survival with stage D1 disease (regional lymph node metastasis) if adjuvant therapy is used,[66] but most surgeons do not advocate radical prostatectomy for stage D1 disease. External beam radiation therapy has an actuarial survival rate of about 40% and 20% at 15 years for stages B and C respectively[67] and is the current treatment of choice for stage C disease. Interstitial radiation implantation is associated with fewer complications than conventional radiotherapy but has a higher local failure rate. Older patients with low-grade disease are candidates for follow-up with no treatment. Reports from Scandinavia show that the progression-free survival is good, and the cancer specific death rate at 10 years is low especially in elderly patients.[68] Several US studies support this finding.[69] All the studies have flaws, however, and there is no reliable way to tell which cancers will progress and which will remain indolent for many years. In an attempt to improve the results of therapy and decrease morbidity, a number of interesting but unproven therapeutic strategies are being explored. These include androgen ablation with luteinizing hormone-releasing hormone (LHRH) agonists and flutamide given in an attempt to downstage the disease, followed by radical surgery or radiation therapy. In addition, cryotherapy, a method for controlling prostate cancer by freezing the prostate is being reevaluated with more sophisticated equipment and ultrasound control. This method failed in the past because of excessive morbidity. Until long-term follow-up is available, these strategies must be considered investigational.

Hormonal ablation is the initial treatment of choice for advanced prostate cancer. Most prostatic cancers are androgen responsive. Androgen ablation causes improvement in 80% to 90% of patients and tumor regression in about 40%. Relapse occurs in all patients, and more than half die within 3 years. The testes are the primary source of androgen, and orchiectomy remains the gold standard and treatment of choice for advanced prostatic cancer. Estrogen produces castrate levels of testosterone, but the side effects of fluid retention and increased incidence of thromboembolic diseases such as heart attacks and strokes makes this hormone a poor choice in this high-risk age group. LHRH agonists have recently become available. These drugs produce castrate levels of testosterone by binding to receptor sites in the pituitary and blocking cyclic LH release. These drugs must be given by injection, but preparations that last 1 month are available. The need for monthly injections plus high cost are the major drawbacks to these drugs. The peripheral androgen antagonist flutamide is also available. Preliminary data suggest that this drug may improve survival when used with other methods of androgen ablation in patients with limited metastases.[70] Flutamide is also useful in preventing androgen "flare" associated with initial therapy with LHRH agonists.

Follow-Up

Prostatic carcinoma has a very slow rate of progression, and recurrences may not be manifest for many years after treatment. After treatment, patients are usually followed up every 6 months with a digital rectal examination and a PSA test. After radical prostatectomy, the PSA levels should be zero. If the level is not zero, bone scanning and other imaging studies should be done to detect metastatic disease. Local recurrences may be treated with radiation, while metastatic cancer is treated as described previously. After primary radiation therapy, the PSA levels usually fall, but the baseline may not be zero. A rise in PSA usually indicates local recurrence or metastatic disease. If local recurrence is suspected, biopsy can be performed and further follow-up, hormonal ablation, or salvage prostatectomy can be considered depending on the pathologic and clinical findings. If the PSA stabilizes at a low level, biopsy should not be considered for at least 12 months. A positive biopsy after 2 years probably indicates persistent or recurrent disease. Follow-up of patients with advanced disease includes visits every 6 months. Symptoms such as bone pain, weight loss, and fatigue are elicited, and PSA, renal function tests, and other indicated studies are performed. Relapse is usually reflected in a rise in PSA followed by symptoms of metastatic disease. Bone pain may be palliated effectively with local radiation therapy or treatment with strontium 89. After failure of hormonal therapy, changing the form or administration of androgen ablation, for instance adding flutamide, usually does not significantly alter the progression of disease. Chemotherapy has been disappointing and treatment consists mainly of palliation.

TESTIS CANCER

The gonads originate as undifferentiated abdominal structures during the fifth to sixth week of gestation. In males, the gonads differentiate into testes by 7 weeks of gestation. Descent into the scrotum occurs relatively late in fetal development. Cryptorchidism is a result of failure of normal testicular descent and is associated with an increased incidence of testicular neoplasia. The blood supply and lymphatic drainage of the adult testes reflect their intraabdominal origin in fetal life. The testicular arteries arise from the aorta below the renal arteries. The right spermatic vein enters directly into the vena cava, and the left spermatic vein joins the left renal vein. The primary lymphatic drainage of the right testis is to the interaortocaval, precaval, and preaortic lymph nodes. The lymphatic drainage of the left testis is more lateral and encompasses the paraaortic, preaortic, and interaortocaval nodes. This anatomy is important to remember in planning appropriate therapy for testis cancer.

Testis cancer is most common between the ages of 25 and 34 years and is rare in blacks. The increased risk of neoplasia associated with cryptorchid testes is not eliminated by orchidopexy. The most common malignant neoplasms of the testis arise from the germ cells and can represent a variety of histologic manifestations including choriocarcinoma, embryonal cell carcinoma, endodermal sinus tumor, seminoma, and teratoma. For therapeutic purposes, the tumors can be divided into seminomas and nonseminomas.

The usual presenting symptom is testicular enlargement that may be associated with mild discomfort. A history of scrotal trauma may be present making the correct diagnosis more difficult. Any solid testicular mass should be considered suspicious for a testis carcinoma. Scrotal ultrasound may be helpful, particularly when physical examination is difficult, for instance, in the presence of a large hydrocele. The diagnostic and therapeutic procedure for any suspected testis carcinoma is inguinal exploration with orchiectomy if the operative findings confirm the presence of a testicular mass. The inguinal approach is used to perform high ligation of the cord at the inguinal ring and to eliminate potential involvement of the inguinal lymph nodes, which are the primary area of drainage for the scrotum.

The tumor markers α-fetoprotein (AFP) and the β-subunit of human chorionic gonadotropin (β-HCG) have contributed both to the diagnosis and follow-up of testis cancer. β-HCG is measured because it is specific for this hormone. The α-subunit of HCG is similar to that of follicle-stimulating hormone, LH, and thyroid-stimulating hormone. Even with the improved specificity of the β-HCG assay, slight elevations may be seen when LH is elevated. Metastases of nonseminomatous germ cell tumors are frequently (50% to 90%) associated with elevated levels of AFP or HCG. Pure seminoma does not cause elevated AFP but can produce a moderate rise in HCG in 10% of patients. Tumor markers are helpful when obtained before and after orchiectomy to help in assessing the stage of the tumor. Furthermore, tumor markers are particularly useful for following patients with nonseminomatous germ cell tumors, aid in evaluating the response to therapy, and facilitate the early detection of tumor recurrence. The serum half-lives of AFP and HCG are 5 days and 1 day, respectively.

Radiologic evaluation of metastases is usually accomplished with CT scan of the chest, abdomen, and pelvis. Lymphangiography can also be performed. The combination of tumor markers and radiologic evaluation is accurate in determining tumor stage (Fig. 109-7). However, the sensitivity of these studies decreases as the tumor volume becomes very small. As a result, 20% to 25% of patients with stage 1 tumors have occult metastases.

Since the advent of effective chemotherapy, the prognosis for most patients is excellent. Long-term survival rate for individuals with stage 1 or 2 testis cancer exceeds 90%. The overall survival rate for patients with stage 3 disease is about 70% with prognosis related to the present extent of disease. The finding of minimum to moderate pulmonary

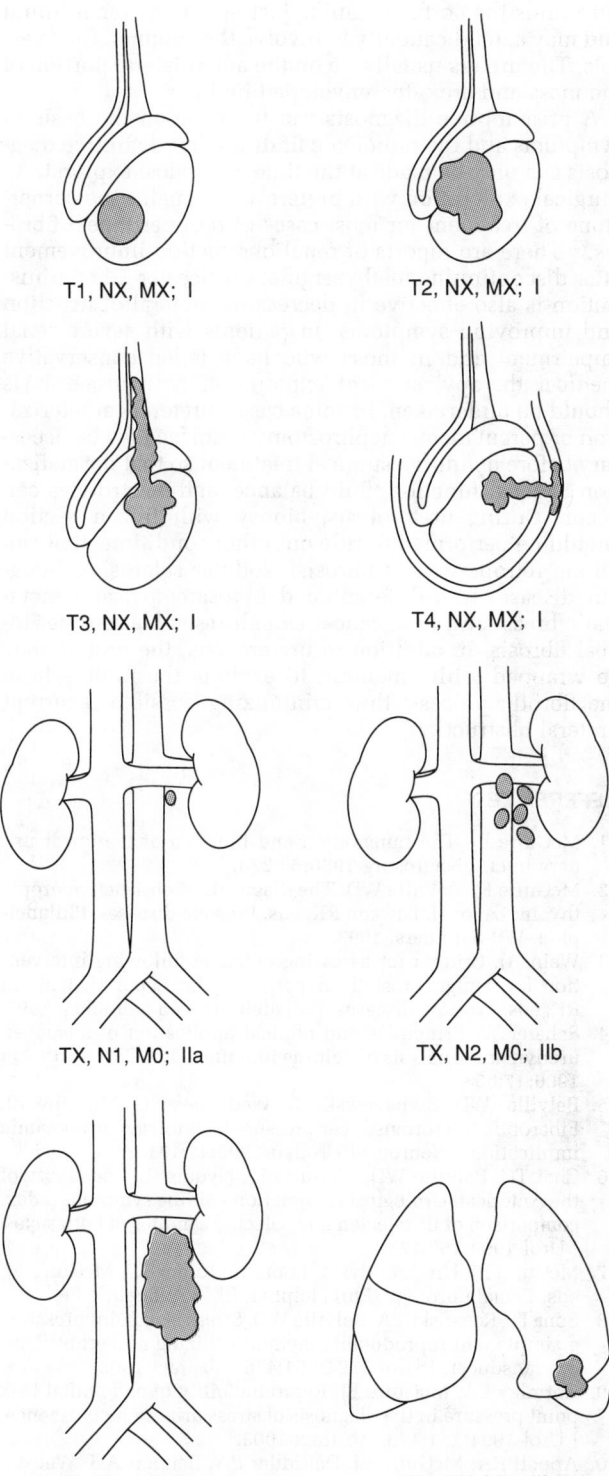

T1, NX, MX; I

T2, NX, MX; I

T3, NX, MX; I

T4, NX, MX; I

TX, N1, M0; IIa

TX, N2, M0; IIb

TX, N3, M0; IIc

TX, NX, M1; III

Figure 109-7. Staging of testis cancer. Both the TNM (American Joint Commission on Cancer, ed 3) and a commonly used descriptive system are listed.

metastases is still associated with an excellent chance for long-term survival.

Seminomas are highly responsive to radiation. Patients with minimum to moderate tumor burden (stage 1 or 2) are usually treated with radiotherapy (2500 to 3000 rad). The field of treatment encompasses the paraaortic and paracaval areas below the diaphragm and ipsilateral ingui-

nal and pelvic areas. When bulky retroperitoneal or distant metastases is present, cisplatin-based combination chemotherapy is the preferred treatment.

The treatment of nonseminomatous tumors is more controversial. Stage 1 tumors are effectively treated with retroperitoneal lymphadenectomy. Currently, nerve-sparing surgery is frequently attempted in an effort to preserve normal antegrade ejaculation. An alternative strategy is observation without any therapeutic intervention. The rationale depends on the accurate staging of tumors and the prompt administration of effective therapy at the first sign of recurrence. With aggressive follow-up and the elimination of patients with vascular invasion and invasion of the rete testis and paratesticular structures, less than 25% of patients relapse, and survival is comparable to that achieved with primary surgical therapy. Patients who elect to be treated with observation should be followed with monthly tumor markers and chest radiographs for 2 years. Furthermore, abdominal CT should be repeated at least every 3 months during this period.

Stage 2 nonseminomatous tumors smaller than 5 cm are usually managed by retroperitoneal lymphadenectomy, which not only documents the stage of disease but is therapeutic as well. Adjuvant therapy (cisplatin-based chemotherapy) is effective but may not be required. Adjuvant treatment decreases the required treatment to two cycles, while treatment at relapse usually requires four cycles of chemotherapy. Bulky stage 2 and stage 3 nonseminomatous tumors are initially treated with cisplatin-based chemotherapy, such as cisplatin, bleomycin, and etoposide. Three or four cycles of chemotherapy are administered, and restaging is performed. Evidence for residual disease with normalization of the tumor markers is usually an indication for surgical excision. The finding of residual cancer indicates the need for additional chemotherapy. A frequent pathologic finding in this circumstance is benign teratoma, which may result from the eradication of the tumor's malignant elements by chemotherapy. When benign teratoma or necrotic tumor are found, the patient need only be followed with periodic tumor markers and chest radiography.

RETROPERITONEAL TUMORS

Although primary retroperitoneal tumors are uncommon, accounting for 0.1% of all malignancies, over 85% are malignant. These tumors occur most commonly in the fifth and sixth decades of life, and typically are found to be a lymphoma or sarcoma. Congenital cystic lesions and lipomas constitute the majority of benign lesions.

Extragonadal Germ Cell Tumors

Extragonadal germ cell tumors are rare, making up only about 1% to 2% of all germ cell tumors. One of the most common sites of origin is the retroperitoneum. Two theories exist as to the origin of these neoplasms: (1) primitive germ cells fail to completely migrate into the scrotum; and (2) small rests of pluripotential cells from the morular or blastular stage persist in this location and are subject to malignant change.

When located in the retroperitoneum, these tumors generally tend to invade or envelop contiguous structures and are usually not encapsulated. Most adults who present with extragonadal tumors have advanced local disease as well as distant metastases. Accurately differentiating primary extragonadal germ cell tumors from metastatic testicular neoplasm may be difficult because primary testicular neoplasms may be small and nonpalpable. In these cases, testicular ultrasonography is helpful in making this distinction. Ultrasonography has been shown to be sensitive enough to detect primary testicular lesions as small as 2 mm. As with other retroperitoneal tumors, patients have few if any symptoms until the tumor becomes large. Again, the typical complaints are abdominal pain and nonspecific gastrointestinal symptoms. Typically, the only physical finding is an abdominal mass. Unlike sarcomas, which are more common in patients in the fourth and fifth decade of life, primary extragonadal germ cell tumors are usually seen in patients in the third decade.

Complete local excision is rarely possible because of local extension into vital adjacent organs or widespread metastatic disease. Intensive cisplatin-based chemotherapy regimens in conjunction with surgical resection of localized residual disease have achieved complete response rates ranging from 30% to 68%. Relapse rates, however, can reach 30%.

Metastatic Retroperitoneal Tumors

Retroperitoneal lymph nodes are common sites for metastases. The primary metastatic sites of testis neoplasms are the paraaortic and interaortocaval nodes. Cervical, uterine, prostate, bladder, as well as colon cancer also can metastasize to the retroperitoneal lymph nodes. Because of the proximity of the ureters, it is not uncommon for patients with significant lymphatic metastases to develop extrinsic ureteral obstruction. In addition, breast, bladder, and prostate cancer can metastasize to the ureter and cause obstruction.

Benign Retroperitoneal Conditions

Retroperitoneal fibrosis is functionally defined as any fibrotic process that involves any portion of the retroperitoneum. Although retroperitoneal fibrosis was originally considered to be a nonspecific fibrosis of unknown etiology, its association with a wide variety of autoimmune conditions, drug ingestion, and local retroperitoneal lesions suggests that it is the end result of a variety of proximate causes.[71]

Characteristically, the fibrosis envelops the aorta, iliac vessels, and ureters but rarely invades these structures. It is usually limited to the retroperitoneal space adjacent to the L-4 and L-5 vertebrae, but there are numerous reports of retroperitoneal fibrosis involving almost any major abdominal organ and blood vessel. In its early stages, biopsy specimens reveal a matrix of collagen bundles with infiltration of lymphocytes, plasma cells, and occasionally lipid-laden macrophages. In later stages, the only finding may be an acellular fibrosis. The etiology in more than two thirds of patients is unclear. In other cases, retroperitoneal fibrosis has been associated with drug use, specifically methysergide, as well as malignancies and collagen vascular diseases.

Clinically, the most common complaint is a dull, noncolicky, discomfort in the abdomen or flank, which is seen in over 90% of patients. Other patients may have clinically silent disease until they present with anuria and uremia from ureteral obstruction. Typically, retroperitoneal fibrosis affects men two to three times more often than women, with a mean age at presentation of about 50 years. Physical examination is unremarkable in most patients.

The excretory urogram usually reveals pyelocaliectasis and upper ureterectasis with medial deviation of the ureters in the lower lumber region. CT scan is the examination of choice for evaluating patients suspected of having retroperitoneal fibrosis. Typically, the fibrous plaque appears as a soft tissue mass with similar attenuation values of muscle and may enhance with contrast. The mass usually surrounds the aorta beginning just below the renal hilum and may extend caudally to involve the common iliac vessels. The ureters usually lie on the anterolateral portion of the mass and are often enveloped by it.

A presumptive diagnosis can be made on the basis of symptoms and the radiologic findings, but definitive diagnosis can only be made at the time of surgical exploration. Surgical exploration with ureterolysis remains the cornerstone of treatment for most cases of retroperitoneal fibrosis.[72] There are reports of renal obstruction improvement after discontinuing methysergide. Corticosteroid administration is also effective in decreasing ureteral obstruction and improving symptoms. In patients with severe renal impairment and in those who have failed conservative medical therapy, surgical exploration with ureterolysis should be undertaken. In some cases, ureteral catheterization or percutaneous nephrostomy drainage may be necessary before definitive surgical treatment so that normalization of renal function, fluid balance, and electrolytes can occur. During ureterolysis, biopsy with frozen section should be performed to rule out other conditions that can mimic retroperitoneal fibrosis. Nodular sclerosing Hodgkin disease, well-differentiated fibrosarcoma, and metastatic breast and lung cancer can all resemble retroperitoneal fibrosis. In addition to ureterolysis, the ureters may be wrapped with omentum to exclude the ureters from the fibrotic process, thus minimizing possible recurrent ureteral obstruction.

REFERENCES

1. McGuire EJ. The innervation and function of the lower urinary tract. J Neurosurg 1986;65:278.
2. McGuire EJ, Belville WD. The diagnosis of obstructive uropathy. In: Lepor H, Lawson RK, eds. Prostate diseases. Philadelphia, WB Saunders, 1993.
3. Wein AJ. Criteria for assessing outcome following intervention for benign prostatic hyperplasia. In: Lepor H, Lawson RK, eds. Prostate diseases. Philadelphia, WB Saunders, 1993.
4. Schafer W. Principles and clinical application of advanced urodynamic analysis of voiding function. Urol Clin North Am 1990;17:553.
5. Belville, WD, Swierzewski SJ, Wedemeyer G, McGuire EJ. Fiberoptic microtransducer pressure technology: urodynamic implications. Neurourol Urodyn 1993;12:171.
6. Chai TC, Belville WD, McGuire EJ, Nyquist L. Specificity of the American Urological Association voiding symptom index: comparison of unselected and selected samples of both sexes. J Urol 1993;150:1710.
7. McGuire EJ. Urethral dysfunction. In: Kursh ED, McGuire EJ, eds. Female urology. Philadelphia, JB Lippincott, 1994.
8. Song JT, Rozanski TA, Belville WD. Stress leak point pressure: a simple and reproducible method utilizing a fiberoptic microtransducer. J Urol 1994;151:478. Abstract 1002.
9. Gormley EA, McGuire EJ. Reproducibility of abdominal leak point pressure in the diagnosis of stress urinary incontinence. J Urol 1994;151:478. Abstract 1003.
10. Appell RA, McGuire EJ, DeRidder PA, Bennett AH, Webster GD, Badlani G. Summary of effectiveness and safety in the prospective, open, multicenter investigation of contigen implant for incontinence due to intrinsic sphincteric deficiency in females. (Abstract) J Urol 1994;151:418.
11. Goldenberg SL, Warkentin MJ. Periurethral collagen injection for patients with stress urinary incontinence. J Urol 1994;151:479. Abstract 1006.
12. Saenz de Tejada I, Goldstein I, Blanco R, Cohen RA, Krane RJ. Smooth muscle of the corpora cavernosae: role in penile erection. Surg Forum 1985;36:623.
13. Krane RJ, Goldstein I, Saenz de Tejada I. Impotence. N Engl J Med 1989;321:1648.
14. Abrahamowicz M, ed. Drugs that cause impotence. Med Lett 1987;29:65.
15. Lee B, Sikka SC, Randup ER, et al. Standardization of penile blood flow parameters in normal men using intracavernous

prostaglandin E1 and visual sexual stimulation. J Urol 1993; 149:49

16. Wespes E, Schulman C. Venous impotence: pathophysiology, diagnosis and treatment. J Urol 1993;149:1238.

17. Morales A. Nonsurgical management options in impotence. Hosp Pract 1993;28:15.

18. Padma-Nathan H, Goldstein I. The pharmacologic erection program. World J Urol 1987;5:160.

19. Bennett AH, Carpenter AJ. An improved vasoactive drug combination for a pharmacological erection program (PEP). J Urol 1991;146:1564.

20. Goldstein I. Penile revascularization. Urol Clin North Am 1987;14:805.

21. Jequier A, Crich J. Testicular function and spermatogenesis. In: Semen analysis: a practical guide. London, Blackwell Scientific Publications, 1986:8.

22. Heller GC, Clermont Y. Spermatogenesis in man: an estimate of duration. Science 1963;140:184.

23. Thomas AJ Jr. Ejaculatory dysfunction. Fertil Steril 1983; 39:445.

24. Carlson E, Gwicerman A, Kieding N, Skakkebaek N. Evidence for decreasing quality of semen during the past 50 years. BMJ 1992;305:609.

25. Gwicerman A, Carlson E, Kieding N, Skakkebaek N. Evidence for increasing incidence of abnormalities of the human testis: a review. Environ Health Perspect 1993;101(Suppl 2):65.

26. Dubin L, Amelar RD. Etiologic factors in 1294 consecutive cases of male infertility. Fertil Steril 1971;22:469.

27. Pryor JL, Howards SS. Varicocele. Urol Clin North Am 1987; 14:499.

28. Anguiano A, Oates RD, Amos JA, et al. Congenital bilateral absence of the vas deferens: a primarily genital form of cystic fibrosis. JAMA 1992;267:1794.

29. Silber SJ, Balmaceda J, Borrero C, Ord T, Asch R. Pregnancy with sperm aspiration from the proximal head of the epididymis: a new treatment for congenital absence of the vas deferens. Fertil Steril 1988;50:525.

30. Bronson R, Cooper G, Rosenfeld D. Sperm antibodies: their role in infertility. Fertil Steril 1984;42:171.

31. Ohl DA, Bennett CJ, McCabe M, Menge AC, McGuire EJ. Predictors of success in electroejaculation of spinal cord injured men. J Urol 1989;142:1483.

32. Coe FL, Parks JH, Asplin JR. The pathogenesis and treatment of kidney stones. N Engl J Med 1992;327:1142.

33. Blute ML, Segura JW, Patterson DE. Ureteroscopy. J Urol 1988;139:510.

34. Biester R, Gillenwater JY. Complications following ureteroscopy. J Urol 1986;136:380.

35. Dretler SP, Weinstein A. A modified algorithm for the treatment of ureteral calculi: 100 consecutive cases. J Urol 1988;40:732.

36. Segura JW, Patterson DE, LeRoy AJ, et al. Percutaneous removal of kidney stones: review of 1000 cases. J Urol 1985; 134:1077.

37. Lam HS, Lingeman JE, Mosbaugh PG, et al. Evolution of the technique of combination therapy for staghorn calculi: a decreasing role for extracorporeal shock wave lithotripsy. J Urol 1992;148:1058.

38. Chaussy C, Schmidt E, Jocham D, Brendel W, Forssman B, Walther V. First clinical experience with extracorporeally induced destruction of kidney stones by shock waves. J Urol 1982;127:417.

39. Drach GW, Dretler S, Fair W, et al. Report of the United States cooperative study of extracorporeal shock wave lithotripsy. J Urol 1986;135:1127.

40. Williams CM, Kaude JV, Newman RC, Peterson JC, Thomas WC. Extracorporeal shock-wave lithotripsy: long-term complications. AJR Am J Roentgenol 1988;150:311.

41. Marshall VF. Fiberoptics in urology. J Urol 1984;91:110.

42. Miyao N, Tsai YC, Lerner SP, et al. Role of chromosome 9 in human bladder cancer. Cancer Res 1993;53:4066.

43. Dalbagni G, Presti J, Reuter V, Fair WR, Cordon-Cardo C. Genetic alterations in bladder cancer. Lancet 1993;342:469.

44. Herr HW, Laudone VP, Badalament RA, et al. Bacillus Calmette-Guerin therapy alters the progression of superficial bladder cancer. J Clin Oncol 1988;6:1450.

45. Lamm DL, Blumenstein BA, Crawford ED, et al. A randomized

trial of intravesical doxorubicin and immunotherapy with Bacille Calmette-Guerin for transitional-cell carcinoma of the bladder. N Engl J Med 1991;325:1205.

46. Konnak JW, Grossman HB. Salvage cystectomy following failed definitive radiation therapy for transitional cell carcinoma of bladder. Urology 1985;26:550.

47. Hinman F Jr. Functional classification of conduits for continent diversion. J Urol 1990;144:27.

48. Carroll PR, Presti JC Jr., McAninch JW, Tanagho EA. Functional characteristics of the continent ileocecal urinary reservoir: mechanisms of urinary continence. J Urol 1989;142:1032.

49. Sternberg CA, Yagoda A, Scher HI, et al. M-VAC (methotrexate, vinblastin, doxorubicin and cisplatin) for advanced transitional cell carcinoma of the urothelium. J Urol 1988;139:461.

50. Shinohara N, Liebert M, Wedemeyer G, Chang JHC, Grossman HB. Evaluation of multiple drug resistance in human bladder cancer cell lines. J Urol 1993;150:505.

51. Grossman HB, Schwartz SL, Konnak JW. Ureteroscopic treatment of urothelial carcinoma of the ureter and renal pelvis. J Urol 1992;148:275.

52. Gnarra JR, Tory K, Weng Y, et al. Mutations of the VHL tumor suppressor gene in renal carcinoma. Nature Genet 1994;7:85.

53. Konnak J, Grossman H. Renal cell carcinoma as an incidental finding. J Urol 1985;134:1094.

54. Robson C, Churchill B, Anderson W. Radical nephrectomy for renal cell carcinoma. J Urol 1969;101:297.

55. Bennington H, Beckwith J. Atlas of tumor pathology. In: Firminger H, ed. Atlas of tumor pathology. Washington, DC, Armed Forces Institute of Pathology, 1975:93

56. Thrasher J, Paulson D. Prognostic factors in renal cell carcinoma. Urol Clin North Am 1993;0:247.

57. Morgan W, Zinke H. Progression and survival after renal conserving surgery for renal cell carcinoma: experience in 104 patients and extended follow-up. J Urol 1990;144:852.

58. Wirth M. Immunotherapy for metastatic renal cell carcinoma. Urol Clin North Am 1993;20:283.

59. Gleason D, Mellinger G. Veterans Administration Cooperative Urologic Research Group: prediction and prognosis for prostatic adenocarcinoma by combined histological grading and clinical staging. J Urol 1974;111:58.

60. Brawer M, Lang P. Prostate-specific antigen in management of prostate carcinoma. Urology 1989;33(Suppl):11.

61. Oesterling JE, Jacobsen S, Chute C, et al. Serum prostate-specific antigen in a community-based population on healthy men: establishment of age-specific reference ranges. JAMA 1993;270:860.

62. Carter H, Morell C, Pearson J, et al. Estimation of prostatic growth using serial prostate-specific antigen measurements in men with and without prostate disease. Cancer Res 1992; 52:3323.

63. Benson M, Whang I, Olsson C, McMahon D, Cooner W. The use of prostate specific antigen density to enhance the predictive value of intermediate levels of serum prostate specific antigen. J Urol 1992;147:817.

64. Waterhouse R, Resnick M. The use of transrectal ultrasound in the evaluation of patients with prostate carcinoma. J Urol 1989;141:233.

65. Lepor H, Kimball A, Walsch P. Cause-specific acturarial survival analysis: a useful method for reporting survival data in men with clinically localized carcinoma of the prostate. J Urol 1989;141:82.

66. Zinke H. Extended experience with surgical treatment of Stage D1 adenocarcinoma of the prostate: significant improvement of immediate adjuvant hormonal treatment (orchiectomy) on outcome. Urology 1989;33(Suppl 5):27.

67. Bagshaw M, Ray G. Selecting initial therapy for prostate cancer. Cancer 1987;60:521.

68. Johansson J, Adami H, Anderson S, Bergstrom R, Holmberg L, Krusemo U. High 10-year survival rate in patients with early, untreated prostate cancer. JAMA 1992;267:2191.

69. Chodak GW, Thisted RA, Gerber GS, et al. Results of conservative management of clinically localized prostate cancer. N Engl J Med 1994;330:242.

70. Crawford E, Eisenberg M, McLeod D, et al. A controlled trial of leuprolide with and without flutamide in prostatic carcinoma. N Engl J Med 1989;321:419.

71. Lepor H, Walsh PC. Idiopathic retroperitoneal fibrosis. J Urol 1979;122:1.

72. Cooksey G, Powell PH, Singh M, Yeates WK. Idiopathic retroperitoneal fibrosis: a long term review after surgical treatment. Br J Urol 1982;54:628.

SURGERY: SCIENTIFIC PRINCIPLES AND PRACTICE, Second Edition, edited by Lazar J. Greenfield, Michael W. Mulholland, Keith T. Oldham, Gerald B. Zelenock, and Keith D. Lillemoe. Lippincott–Raven Publishers, Philadelphia, © 1997.

CHAPTER 110

FEMALE GENITAL SYSTEM

W. GLENN HURT AND DAVID E. SOPER

A better understanding of gynecologic endocrinology and recent improvements in laboratory testing, imaging technology, and endoscopy have enabled gynecologists to render earlier and more accurate diagnoses of potentially serious pelvic disorders. There is no better example than what has taken place in the diagnosis and treatment of ectopic pregnancies. Quantitative serum human chorionic gonadotropin (hCG) assays and refined ultrasonography have made it possible to diagnose and treat most ectopic pregnancies, medically or endoscopically, before they rupture. Early conservative therapy minimizes damage to the tubes and ovaries and optimizes the patient's chances of having more children. It was only a few years ago that most ectopic pregnancies were not diagnosed until they had ruptured. Rupture is associated with significant morbidity and usually the loss of one tube or ovary, or both.

Improved diagnostic techniques, new antibiotic and hormone medications, the introduction of endoscopic surgery, and the recent emphasis on outpatient surgery and shortened hospitalization have revolutionized the practice of gynecologic surgery. This chapter covers the treatment of common gynecologic disorders.

EMBRYOLOGY AND SURGICAL ANATOMY

During the sixth to eighth weeks of fetal development, germ cells migrate to the genital ridges, the primitive gonads begin to descend, and sex differentiation is initiated. The fetus becomes a female if it is chromosomally determined that there is to be an ovary or if there is gonadal agenesis.

The ovaries develop from the genital ridges. The oviducts, uterus, and upper vagina develop from the paired müllerian (paramesonephric) ducts, which are invaginations of the coelomic epithelium. Failed development of the müllerian ducts causes oviduct and uterine agenesis; incomplete or failed fusion of the caudal ends of the müllerian ducts causes anomalies of the uterus and upper vagina. Developmental anomalies of the reproductive tract are often accompanied by anomalies of the urinary tract.

The upper vagina is derived from the müllerian system, which is of mesodermal origin. The lower vagina is derived from the urogenital sinus, which is of endodermal origin. Abnormal fusion of the two systems can result in the formation of a vaginal septum.

The external genitalia are derived from the genital tubercle that develops as an elevation of ectoderm on the ventral surface of the cloacal plate. By 10 to 12 weeks of fetal development, the appearance of the external genitalia permits identification of sex.

The vulva is loosely covered by skin and is affected by those pathologic processes that affect skin. Skene glands open on either side of the external urethral meatus, and the ducts of Bartholin glands open onto the fourchette. The vagina is a fibromuscular tube, 9 to 10 cm long, that is normally collapsed, with its anterior and posterior walls in apposition. The lower vagina passes from the vulva, over the perineal body, and through the levator hiatus. The middle vagina rests on the rectum and the posterior portion of the pelvic diaphragm, and the vaginal apex is suspended by the cardinal–uterosacral complex in the hollow of the sacrum. The course of the upper vagina is almost horizontal when a woman is standing erect. The urethra, trigone, and a portion of the bladder base are anterior to the vagina and are supported by the pubocervical fascia and the anterior vaginal wall. The cervix is part of the anterior vaginal wall. The vaginal apex is in direct contact with the cul-de-sac (pouch of Douglas) peritoneum at the lowest point within the peritoneal cavity. Posterior colpotomy allows access to the peritoneal cavity for pelvic surgery and drainage of abscesses. The posterior vaginal wall lies on the rectum (Fig. 110-1).

The female urethra is 4 to 5 cm long and has no anatomically dissectible sphincters. Its continence mechanism depends on its anatomic relation to the bladder, and the integrity of its mucosal, connective tissue, vascular, and muscular elements. The bladder is a highly distensible organ. It forms the posterior boundary of the retropubic space (space of Retzius). The uterine fundus is normally anteflexed in relation to the cervix and lies on the bladder anteriorly, with the intestines bearing down on its posterior wall and filling the cul-de-sac. The adnexa are composed of the oviducts, ovaries, and broad ligament structures on either side of the uterus. Anatomically, the round ligaments are anterior to the oviducts that are located anterior to the uteroovarian ligaments. Knowledge of this relation is important in performing sterilization procedures. The ovaries are attached to the uterus by the uteroovarian ligaments and to the pelvic side wall near the bifurcation of the common iliac arteries by the suspensory (infundibulopelvic) ligaments. The ureters enter the pelvis over the bifurcation of the common iliac arteries and descend retroperitoneally, parallel to the internal iliac arteries, to pass under the uterine arteries. After passing under the uterine arteries, the ureters course anteriorly through the base of the cardinal ligaments, lateral to the cervix and anterolateral to the upper vagina. The ureters then enter the ureteric tunnels, within the wall of the bladder, to open onto its trigone (Fig. 110-2).

The aorta branches on the left side of the L-4 vertebra to form the common iliac arteries. These pass over the brim

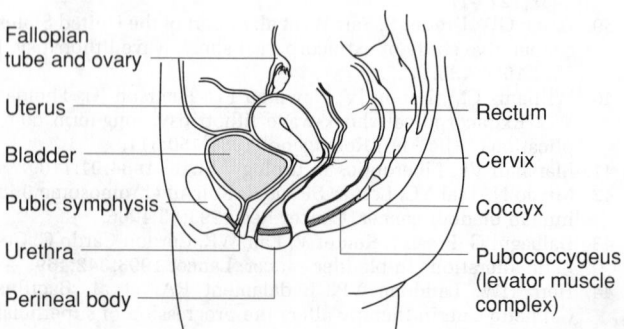

Figure 110-1. Sagittal section of female pelvis.

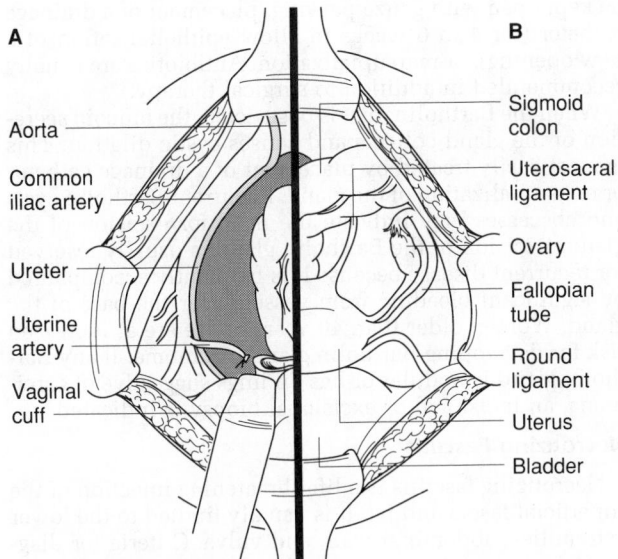

Figure 110-2. (*A*) Female pelvic cavity with uterus, fallopian tube, ovary, and peritoneum removed to show major vessels and course of ureter. (*B*) Relation of organs within pelvic cavity.

of the pelvis bilaterally and divide into the external and internal iliac arteries. The internal iliac (hypogastric) artery promptly divides into anterior and posterior branches. The posterior branch divides to form the iliolumbar, lateral sacral, and superior gluteal arteries. The anterior branch divides to form the superior, middle, and inferior vesical, middle hemorrhoidal, uterine, vaginal, obturator, internal pudendal, and inferior gluteal arteries. The blood supply to the internal genitalia is derived from the internal iliac, ovarian, and superior hemorrhoidal arteries.

The external iliac arteries are crossed at their origin by the ovarian vessels, the ureter, and the insertion of the infundibulopelvic ligament. Distally, they give off the inferior epigastric and deep iliac circumflex arteries before passing under the middle of each inguinal ligament to become the femoral arteries. The femoral artery is the primary blood supply to the lower extremity. Blood is drained from the lower extremities and pelvis by a system of veins that closely parallels the arterial supply.

An extensive collateral circulation within the pelvis permits the ligation of one, both, or all of the internal iliac and ovarian arteries or any of their branches without jeopardizing the viability of the organs. This is the reason that bilateral hypogastric artery angiographic embolization or surgical ligation can be used to lower the distal pulse pressure and permit clot formation in the control of pelvic arterial hemorrhage. It is possible for a patient to conceive and carry a pregnancy to term after these procedures. On the other hand, great care should be taken not to ligate the external iliac arteries or veins that are necessary for the viability of the lower extremities.

The lymphatics of the vulva and perineum follow the external pudendal vessels and drain to the superficial inguinal and femoral nodes. Those of the clitoris drain to the deep inguinal and external iliac nodes. The lymphatics of the upper vagina drain to the common iliac nodes, those of the middle vagina drain to the internal iliac nodes, and those of the lower vagina drain to the external iliac nodes. The lymphatics of the uterine cervix drain to the external, internal, and common iliac nodes; those of the uterine corpus drain primarily to the periaortic nodes, with some drainage to the external iliac nodes or by way of the round

ligaments to the superficial inguinal nodes. The lymphatics of the ovaries drain directly to the periaortic nodes or to the iliac nodes and then to the periaortic nodes.

The pelvic organs are supported by the pelvic and urogenital diaphragms. The endopelvic fascia that envelops the pelvic organs condenses bilaterally to form the cardinal–uterosacral ligament complexes, the perirectal fascia, and the vagina. All pelvic organs ultimately attach to and are supported by the bony pelvis. Injury to the pelvic support system can result in pelvic organ prolapse.

Potential connective tissue spaces between (retropubic or prevesical space, vesicovaginal space, rectovaginal space, retrorectal or presacral space) and alongside (paravesical spaces, pararectal spaces) the pelvic organs contribute to their independent functions. These spaces are relatively avascular and are ideal planes for anatomic dissection.

PHYSIOLOGY

The integrated function of the hypothalamus, pituitary, and ovary determines whether the normal female functions gynecologically as a child or as a reproductive or menopausal adult. Estrogen acts as a trophic hormone with respect to its action on the female breast and genitalia; estrogen deficiency causes genital atrophy. Progesterone is produced by the corpus luteum during the reproductive years and is responsible for maturation of the endometrium. Progesterone withdrawal causes shedding of the estrogen-primed endometrium.

During the reproductive years, the cyclic production of estrogen and progesterone by the ovary is responsible for orderly endometrial development and menstruation. Ovarian dysfunction can result in abnormal bleeding from an otherwise normal uterus. In most women, this abnormal bleeding is breakthrough bleeding from a proliferative or hyperplastic endometrium that is the result of unopposed estrogen stimulation due to anovulation. If the abnormal bleeding is from a secretory endometrium, it more likely has an anatomic cause, such as leiomyomas, endometrial polyps, or adenomyosis.

In the reproductive years, the ovary often contains physiologic cysts (usually less than 4 cm in diameter) as a result of follicular maturation or corpus luteum formation. Therefore, pelvic complaints associated with ovarian cysts that are detected by bimanual pelvic examination or by ultrasound, computed tomography (CT), or magnetic resonance imaging (MRI) must be correlated with knowledge of the ovarian cycle to determine their significance.

VULVA

Vulvar Intraepithelial Neoplasia

Vulvar intraepithelial neoplasia (VIN) is usually asymptomatic, but it can be a cause of vulvar pruritus. In the past, VIN was considered a disease of older women, but now half of reported cases occur in women 20 to 40 years of age. VIN often is associated with human papillomavirus (HPV) infection. It appears as white, red, or deeply pigmented lesions that can have a papular or macular configuration and can be unifocally or multifocally distributed. The application of 5% acetic acid and colposcopic examination of the vulva help to detect less obvious lesions. The location of all lesions should be documented and biopsy specimens taken. VIN should be graded histologically according to its squamous cell atypia—VIN-1 (mild dysplasia), VIN-2 (moderate dysplasia), or VIN-3 (severe dysplasia or carcinoma in situ).

VIN is best treated by local excision, by CO₂ laser vaporization (to a depth of 3 mm), or, in selected cases of extensive involvement, by a skinning vulvectomy. Systematic follow-up is necessary because of its multifocal distribution and high rate of recurrence. Older patients are at increased risk for progression of disease.

Vulvar Carcinoma

Vulvar cancer accounts for about 4% of female genital malignancies. Histologically, most vulvar cancers are squamous cell carcinoma (90%), melanoma (5%), sarcoma (2%), Bartholin gland adenocarcinoma or carcinoma, Paget disease of the vulva, or basal cell carcinoma. Except for the sarcomas, these cancers usually occur in women 55 years of age and older. Patients with HPV infection and granulomatous disease are at increased risk for developing vulvar carcinoma. Vulvar carcinoma often is surrounded by an area of VIN. Biopsy is required for a definitive diagnosis. The International Federation of Gynecology and Obstetrics (FIGO) recommends surgical staging of vulvar cancer (Table 110-1). The incidence of inguinal and pelvic node metastases with invasive squamous cell lesions less than 2 cm in diameter is 20%; with lesions larger than 2 cm, it is over 40%. Poorly differentiated lesions are more likely to metastasize than well-differentiated lesions.

Unilateral microinvasive lesions (less than 2 cm in diameter, less than 1 mm invasion, without vascular or lymphatic space involvement) can be treated by wide local excision without node dissection. Depending on location, some unilateral invasive carcinomas of the vulva can be treated by radical vulvectomy with unilateral inguinal–femoral lymphadenectomy. The remainder of cases should be treated by radical vulvectomy with bilateral inguinal–femoral lymphadenectomy. The primary complication of radical vulvectomy and lymphadenectomy is impaired wound healing. Lymphedema of the lower extremities can occur. The overall 5-year survival rate after radical vulvectomy and node dissection approximates 90% in the absence of inguinal node metastases, in contrast to 40% in the presence of inguinal node metastases and 15% in the presence of pelvic node metastases. Melanomas, sarcomas, and Bartholin gland carcinomas should be treated by radical vulvectomy and bilateral inguinofemoral lymphadenectomy. In addition, Bartholin gland carcinomas may require an abdominoperineal resection because of their pararectal and sacral lymphatic drainage. Paget disease of the vulva is a specific histologic entity that occurs in older women and may or may not be associated with an underlying adenocarcinoma. Paget disease of the vulva without an underlying adenocarcinoma is a form of intraepithelial neoplasia and is treated by wide local excision. In the presence of an underlying adenocarcinoma, radical vulvectomy and bilateral inguinofemoral lymphadenectomy is the treatment of choice. Basal cell carcinoma of the vulva is a specific histologic type of vulvar neoplasia that can be locally invasive but does not metastasize. It is most often seen in middle-aged women and should be treated by wide local excision.

Miscellaneous Disorders of the Vulva

Bartholin Gland Abscess

Bartholin gland adenitis or abscess is due to an infection that is often polymicrobial, containing bacteria similar to vaginal flora. *Neisseria gonorrhoeae* and *Chlamydia trachomatis* can also cause Bartholin gland infection. Acute adenitis can be treated by broad-spectrum antibiotics and sitz baths. Abscesses should be treated by incision and drainage near the site of the occluded duct. The site should be kept open with gauze packing, placement of a drainage catheter (for 4 to 6 weeks to allow epithelialization of a new opening), or marsupialization. Antibiotics are usually recommended in addition to surgical therapy.

When the Bartholin duct is obstructed, the mucoid secretion of the gland collects and causes cystic dilation. This is most easily treated by placement of a drainage catheter or marsupialization of the gland. Recurrent Bartholin cysts and abscesses may indicate the need for excision of the gland. Excision of the Bartholin gland is usually reserved for recurrent disease because it is frequently accompanied by significant bleeding from vessels near the base of the gland. Women older than 40 years of age are at increased risk for developing Bartholin gland carcinoma. If any Bartholin gland is nodular or has findings suggestive of carcinoma, an incisional or excisional biopsy is indicated.

Necrotizing Fasciitis

Necrotizing fasciitis is a life-threatening infection of the superficial fascia and fat. It is usually limited to the lower extremities, abdominal wall, and vulva. Criteria for diagnosis include extensive necrosis of the superficial fascia with widespread involvement of the surrounding tissues; moderate to severe systemic toxic reaction, including altered mental status; absence of major vascular occlusion; and pathologic examination of débrided tissue showing intense leukocytic infiltration, focal necrosis of fascia and surrounding tissues, and microvascular thrombosis. The condition most often affects women with diabetes (70%) or atherosclerosis. Also at risk are patients on long-term steroid or nonsteroidal antiinflammatory agent therapy and those with autoimmune diseases.

Necrotizing fasciitis can be caused by the prototype organism *Streptococcus pyogenes* (group A *Streptococcus*), with or without *Staphylococcus aureus,* or it can be of polymicrobial cause as a result of anaerobic and facultative aerobic bacteria. The infection usually starts as an insignificant skin lesion (eg, furuncle, Bartholin adenitis), in a skin abrasion, or within a surgical wound. It can remain quiescent for weeks, or it can be fulminant, with rapid extension along tissue planes. With its spread, there are changes in skin color from red to purple to blue-gray, bullae formation, skin breakdown, and frank cutaneous gangrene. The involved area becomes anesthetic as a result of thrombosis of small vessels and the destruction of superficial nerves. The patient becomes septic. Anemia can develop as a result of bacterial hemolysins and disseminated intravascular coagulation.

The clinical diagnosis is based on a constellation of symptoms and signs in association with a high index of suspicion. The hallmark of vulvar involvement is woody induration extending onto the inner thighs. If the diagnosis is suspected, an incisional biopsy with removal of at least 1 cc of subcutaneous tissue and frozen section evaluation should help differentiate necrotizing fasciitis from nonspecific ulcers, abscesses, or ischemic necrosis. If histologic evaluation of the tissue reveals necrosis of superficial fascia, polymorphonuclear infiltration of the deep dermis and fascia, fibrinoid thrombi, angiitis of vessels within the fascia, and the presence of microorganisms within the involved fascia and dermis, immediate radical débridement of all affected tissues is indicated.

Necrotizing fasciitis must be treated immediately by the correction of anemia, the restoration of fluid and electrolyte balance, the institution of broad-spectrum antibiotic therapy, and extensive surgical débridement. Skin incisions should be placed so as to remove necrotic skin but allow future reconstruction, if possible. Tunneling incisions are not advised because they are too difficult to inspect and pack. All involved subcutaneous tissue, fascia,

Table 110-1. STAGING OF GYNECOLOGIC CANCER AS RECOMMENDED BY THE INTERNATIONAL FEDERATION OF GYNECOLOGY AND OBSTETRICS

Stage	Description	Stage	Description
VULVAR CANCER		IIIA	No extension to pelvic wall
0		IIIB	Extension to pelvic wall or hydronephrosis of nonfunctioning kidney
Tis	Carcinoma in situ; intraepithelial carcinoma	IV	Carcinoma beyond true pelvis or involving mucosa of bladder or rectum
I		IVA	Spread to adjacent organs
T1, N0, M0	Tumor confined to vulva or perineum, 2 cm or less in greatest dimension. No nodal metastasis	IVB	Spread to distant organs
		UTERINE CORPUS CANCER	
II		IA	Tumor limited to endometrium
T2, N0, M0	Tumor confined to vulva or perineum, more than 2 cm in greatest dimension. No nodal metastasis	G123	
		IB	Invasion to less than half the myometrium
		G123	
III		IC	Invasion to more than half the myometrium
T3, N0, M0	Tumor of any size with:	G123	
T3, N1, M0	(1) Adjacent spread to lower urethra, vagina, anus, or	IIA	Endocervical glandular involvement only
T1, N1, M0	(2) Unilateral regional lymph node metastasis	G123	
		IIB	Cervical stromal invasion
T2, N1, M0		G123	
IVA		IIIA	Tumor invades serosa or adnexa, or presence of positive peritoneal cytology
T1, N2, M0	Tumor invades any of the following:	G123	
T2, N2, M0	Upper urethra, bladder mucosa, rectal mucosa, pelvic bone, or bilateral regional node metastasis	IIIB	Vaginal metastases
T3, N2, M0		G123	
T4, any N, M0		IIIC	Metastases to pelvic or paraaortic lymph nodes
IVB		G123	
Any T, any N, M1	Any distant metastasis including pelvic lymph nodes	IVA	Tumor invasion of bladder or bowel mucosa
Note		G123	Distant metastases including intraabdominal or inguinal lymph nodes
N (regional lymph nodes)		IVB	
N0	No lymph node metastasis	**Note**	5% or less of a nonsquamous or nonmorular solid growth pattern
N1	Unilateral regional lymph node metastasis	G1	
		G2	6%–50% of a nonsquamous or nonmorular solid growth pattern
N2	Bilateral regional lymph node metastasis		
		G3	More than 50% of a nonsquamous or nonmorular solid growth pattern
M (distant metastasis)			
M0	No clinical metastasis	**OVARIAN CANCER**	
M1	Distant metastasis (including pelvic lymph node metastasis)		Growth limited to ovaries
		I	One ovary; no tumor on external surfaces; capsule intact; no ascites present containing malignant cells
VAGINAL CANCER		IA	
0	Carcinoma in situ; intraepithelial carcinoma	IB	Both ovaries; no tumor on external surfaces; capsules intact; no ascites present containing malignant cells
I	Carcinoma limited to vaginal mucosa		
II	Carcinoma involving subvaginal tissue but not onto pelvic wall	IC	IA or IB but with tumor on surface of one or both ovaries; or with capsule ruptured; or with ascites containing malignant cells or with positive peritoneal washings
III	Carcinoma onto pelvic wall or pubic symphysis	II	Growth involving one or both ovaries with pelvic extension
			Extension or metastases to uterus or fallopian tubes
IV	Carcinoma beyond true pelvis; involvement of bladder or rectal mucosa	IIA	Extension to other pelvic tissues
		IIB	
		IIC	IIA or IIB but with tumor on surface of one or both ovaries; or with capsules ruptured; or with ascites containing malignant cells or with positive peritoneal washings
CERVICAL CANCER			
0	Carcinoma in situ; intraepithelial carcinoma	III	Tumor involving one or both ovaries with peritoneal implants outside pelvis or positive retroperitoneal or inguinal nodes; superficial liver metastases; tumor limited to pelvis but with histologically verified malignant extension to small bowel or omentum
I	Carcinoma confined to cervix		
IA	Preclinical carcinoma; diagnosed microscopically		
IA1	Minimal microscopic evidence of stromal invasion	IIIA	Tumor limited to true pelvis with negative nodes but with histologically confirmed seeding of peritoneal surfaces
IA2	Microscopic invasion from base of epithelium of 5 mm or less and lateral spread of 7 mm or less	IIIB	Tumor limited to one or both ovaries with histologically confirmed implants of peritoneal surfaces, none greater than 2 cm in diameter; nodes negative
IB	Lesions of greater dimensions than stage IA2	IIIC	Abdominal implants greater than 2 cm in diameter or positive retroperitoneal or inguinal nodes
II	Carcinoma beyond cervix but not to pelvic wall. Cancer involves vagina but not lower third	IV	Growth involving one or both ovaries with distant metastasis; pleural effusion with positive cytology; parenchymal liver metastasis
IIA	Obvious parametrial involvement	**INVASIVE GESTATIONAL TROPHOBLASTIC NEOPLASIA**	
IIB	Obvious parametrial involvement		Tumor confined to uterine corpus
III	Carcinoma to pelvic wall. No cancer-free space between tumor and pelvic wall. Tumro involves lower third of vagina. Hydronephrosis or nonfunctioning kidney not due to another cause	I	Tumor to adnexa but limited to genital structures
		II	Tumor to lungs with or without genital involvement
		III	Metastasis to other sites
		IV	

and muscle should be removed. These will appear dull gray and bloodless in comparison to the bright yellow and bloody appearance of the adjacent normal tissue. The abnormal tissue contains an exudate that resembles dishwater, and it will separate easily from the surrounding normal tissue. Frozen section biopsies may be helpful in determining tissue involvement and in establishing surgical margins. Gram stains and cultures (aerobic and anaerobic) should be performed on the resected tissue.

After adequate débridement has been performed, the wound should be packed with povidone-iodine–impregnated gauze and the patient transferred to an intensive care unit. Severe cases may require repeat surgical exploration and débridement within 24 to 36 hours to reassess the surgical margins and to facilitate wound débridement and dressing changes. When the progressive nature of the disease has been controlled, the patient can be transferred out of the intensive care unit. Antibiotics should be continued until wound induration and all systemic signs of sepsis have disappeared. The wounds can be allowed to close by secondary intention. Some may require surgical closure or skin grafting. Consultation with a plastic surgeon may be indicated to obtain optimal cosmetic and functional results.

VAGINA

Vaginal Intraepithelial Neoplasia

Vaginal intraepithelial neoplasia (VAIN) is usually asymptomatic and is detected most often by an abnormal Papanicolaou (Pap) smear. The lesion is usually located in the upper third of the vagina. VAIN tends to be multifocal and is often associated with HPV infections and neoplasia of the cervix or vulva.

Colposcopy with the application of 3% to 5% acetic acid or a Schiller test with the application of Lugol iodine solution helps identify abnormal vaginal epithelium. Epithelial abnormalities should undergo biopsy. VAIN is best treated by CO_2 laser vaporization (to a depth of 2 mm), excision of isolated lesions, or application of 5% 5-fluorouracil cream. Long-term follow-up is important because VAIN tends to recur and can be associated with other lower genital tract malignancies.

Vaginal Carcinoma

Primary vaginal cancer is rare; most cancers within the vagina are secondary to extension or metastases from cancers of the uterus or vulva. Primary vaginal cancer accounts for about 2% of female genital malignancies. The mean age at diagnosis is 65 years. It most frequently involves the upper posterior third of the vagina and is histologically a squamous cell carcinoma (90%). Adenocarcinoma (clear cell in those exposed in utero to diethylstilbestrol), sarcoma, endodermal sinus tumors, or melanoma can be found anywhere along the vaginal canal. Cytologic smears and biopsies of tissues that appear or feel abnormal are used to detect asymptomatic lesions. Abnormal vaginal discharge and painless bleeding are the most common presenting signs.

Vaginal cancer spreads primarily by direct extension and lymphatic dissemination. The location of the lesion determines paravaginal and lymph node involvement. The lymphatic drainage of the vagina is divided into thirds: the upper third drains to the common iliac, presacral, and hypogastric nodes; the middle third drains to the hypogastric nodes; and the lower third drains to the femoral and external iliac nodes. FIGO recommends clinical staging of vaginal cancer (see Table 110-1).

Surgery has a limited role in the management of vaginal cancer. Radiation therapy is recommended for most invasive squamous cell carcinomas and adenocarcinomas of the vagina. Five-year survival rates for stage I disease approximate 65%; stage II, 50%; stage III, 30%; and stage IV, 10%. Primary vaginal sarcomas, endodermal sinus tumors, and melanomas should be treated surgically. In these patients, the need for postoperative radiation therapy or chemotherapy is individualized.

Pelvic Organ Prolapse

Pelvic organ prolapse occurs as a result of weaknesses within the pelvic organ support system and the vagina.[1] Contributing factors include pregnancy and childbirth; increases in intraabdominal pressure that may be associated with chronic respiratory diseases, abdominal masses, ascites, or obesity; postmenopausal atrophy; and congenital tissue weaknesses. Additionally, iatrogenic factors, including inadequate or inappropriate surgery for correction of pelvic support defects, ventral suspensions of pelvic organs that increase the exposure of the cul-de-sac (pouch of Douglas), failure to detect and correct an enterocele, and excessive shortening of the vagina, can contribute to the development of pelvic organ prolapse. Most parous women have some evidence of pelvic organ prolapse; 10% to 15% of these women develop symptoms that require surgery.

Complaints associated with pelvic organ prolapse include pelvic pressure, a bearing-down sensation, sacral backache, coital difficulty, a protrusion from the vagina, and sometimes spotting and ulceration of the prolapsed tissues. Pelvic organ prolapse can interfere with bladder and bowel function and can cause urinary urgency and frequency, urinary incontinence, voiding difficulties or retention, and difficult defecation. The types of pelvic organ prolapse are illustrated in Figure 110-3.

The diagnosis is suggested by the history and confirmed by the pelvic examination. Contributing factors of importance are general health, sexual function, and prior attempts at surgical correction. A thorough physical examination should be performed. Special attention should be given to the evaluation of nutritional status and cardiorespiratory function. Before the patient empties her bladder, an attempt should be made to demonstrate urinary leakage by having her perform Valsalva maneuvers in the supine and erect positions. After the patient has voided, she should be catheterized to determine the urinary residual as an indicator of bladder emptying efficiency and to obtain a urine specimen for urinalysis and culture. If urinary incontinence is not demonstrated, urodynamic testing should be considered. Screening cystometry to detect an unstable bladder and stress testing to demonstrate stress incontinence can be performed by having the patient stand with a transurethral catheter in place and allowing room-temperature, sterile, normal saline to fill the bladder by gravity. The amount of saline instilled is recorded when the patient first notices an urge to void (usually after 150 to 200 mL) and when she is unable to hold any more saline (bladder capacity is usually 400 to 500 mL). The inability of the bladder to accept the sterile solution suggests detrusor instability and indicates the need for more sophisticated urodynamic testing. When the catheter is removed, at least 300 mL of fluid should remain in the bladder. Stress testing can then be performed by asking the patient to perform Valsalva maneuvers in the supine and erect positions. Squirt leakage at the acme of a sudden increase in intraabdominal pressure is suggestive of stress urinary incontinence; uncontrollable flow leakage is suggestive of an unstable bladder.

Anterior vaginal wall prolapse

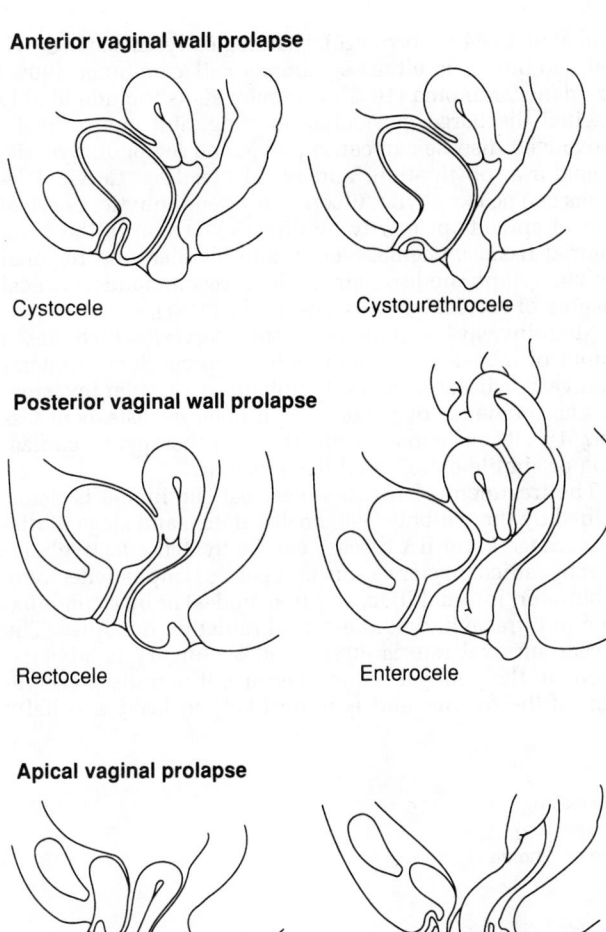

Cystocele

Cystourethrocele

Posterior vaginal wall prolapse

Rectocele

Enterocele

Apical vaginal prolapse

Uterovaginal prolapse
(with cystocele)

Vaginal vault prolapse
(with enterocele)

Figure 110-3. Types of pelvic organ prolapse.

After stress testing, the patient should be allowed to void and return to the examination table for a pelvic examination. Cytologic smears can be obtained, and the estrogenic status of the patient should be ascertained by inspection of the vaginal epithelium for rugae. A thorough pelvic examination is performed. Visualization is aided by a Sims speculum. Repeated replacement of prolapsed organs and subsequent observation of their descent during Valsalva maneuvers help determine different areas of weakness within the pelvic support system and the extent to which each of the pelvic organs is involved. The maximum degree of descent of the anterior, apical, and posterior vaginal walls should be documented. Although numerous classifications of pelvic organ prolapse have been proposed, the general trend is to classify descent as first degree if the leading point of the descending organ is to the introitus, second degree if it is within the introitus, and third degree if it extends through the introitus. The organ involved is then designated in the same manner (eg, first-, second-, or third-degree cystocele; rectocele). *Procidentia* refers to complete uterovaginal prolapse, whereby the entire uterus and vagina are outside the introitus.

A pessary can be used to reduce and support the pelvic organs of patients who are poor operative risks or who refuse surgery; definitive therapy, however, is surgical. The preferred surgical approach is transvaginal. The operation can consist of several different procedures, each aimed at correcting a specific weakness within the pelvic sup-

port system or vagina. Procedures that might be involved include vaginal hysterectomy with or without salpingo-oophorectomy, posterior culdoplasty, anterior colporrhaphy, posterior colporrhaphy, enterocele repair, and perineoplasty. Patients with stress urinary incontinence can benefit from retropubic urethropexy–colposuspension. Those with vaginal vault prolapse and inadequate cardinal–uterosacral ligaments can benefit from sacrospinous ligament fixation of the vaginal vault. Special surgical expertise is required to provide patients who have pelvic organ prolapse with a durable reconstruction of a coitally functional vagina. Colpectomy and colpocleisis are reserved for older patients who are significant surgical risks and who are not sexually active or likely to become sexually active.

Abdominal surgery for pelvic organ prolapse is usually not recommended. Abdominal colposacropexy for posthysterectomy vaginal vault prolapse is the exception. Patients with vaginal vault prolapse can be satisfactorily treated by an abdominal closure of the cul-de-sac (Moschcowitz or Halban procedure) and a colposacropexy using a fascial or synthetic strap to attach the vaginal apex to the fascia overlying the sacrum. Most of these patients benefit from a concomitant retropubic urethropexy–colposuspension because elevation of the bladder base can cause postoperative stress urinary incontinence. If the patient has a significant cystocele or rectocele, it may require anterior or posterior colporrhaphy.

UTERUS

Abnormal Cervical Cytology

Most cytology laboratories use the Bethesda system for reporting cervical–vaginal cytologic diagnoses.[2] What was known as cervical intraepithelial neoplasia is now known as a squamous intraepithelial lesion (SIL). SIL can be classified as being low grade (SIL-LG) or high grade (SIL-HG). SIL-LG includes what was formerly cervical intraepithelial neoplasia 1 or mild dysplasia; SIL-HG includes what was formerly cervical intraepithelial neoplasia 2 and 3 or moderate and severe dysplasia. The Bethesda system allows the diagnosis of atypical squamous cells of undetermined significance (ASCUS). This cytologic diagnosis reflects a degree of uncertainty as to whether or not the patient has SIL. Cytologic findings resulting in the diagnosis of ASCUS can be due to reactive or reparative changes, infection, or early neoplasia.

Squamous intraepithelial lesions (neoplasia or dysplasia) are asymptomatic conditions due to abnormal maturation of the squamous epithelium of the squamocolumnar junction of the cervix. Risk factors for the development of these squamous abnormalities include adolescent coitus, multiple sexual partners, and delivery before age 20. Cervical infection with HPV, especially types 16 and 18, is thought to play an etiologic role. Squamous intraepithelial lesions are detected by Pap smear screening and diagnosed by colposcopy, ectocervical biopsy, and endocervical curettage. Cervical conization (cold knife; loop electrosurgical excision procedure, known as LEEP; or laser) is recommended if any of the following exist:

- Significant disagreement in the grade of the lesion as determined by cytologic screening and colposcopically direct biopsy
- Endocervical curettage showing a squamous intraepithelial lesion
- Cytologic abnormality without colposcopically visible lesion
- Microinvasive carcinoma on directed biopsy

- Need to remove the neoplasia to preserve childbearing potential.

The optimal method of treatment cannot be determined until there is cytologic, colposcopic, and histologic agreement as to the grade of SIL and until the location and limits of all lesions are know. An algorithm for the management of abnormal cervical cytology is proposed in Figure 110-4.

The rate of progression of SIL-LG is considered to be minimal. A finding of SIL-HG is believed to place the patient at significant risk for developing invasive cancer if not adequately treated. Therefore, it is important to eradicate SIL-HG lesions and follow carefully all patients for persistence or recurrence to prevent the development of invasive carcinoma of the cervix.

SIL is effectively treated by cryotherapy or CO_2 laser vaporization. LEEP, CO_2 laser, or cold-knife conization can be both diagnostic and therapeutic. Hysterectomy is usually reserved for patients with SIL-HG who have completed their childbearing or those who have other gynecologic reasons for hysterectomy.

Cervical Carcinoma

Cervical carcinoma accounts for about 18% of female genital malignancies.[3,4] The mean age at diagnosis is 52 years, with a bimodal distribution (peaks at 35 to 39 years and at 60 to 64 years of age). Histologically, invasive cervical carcinoma is either squamous cell carcinoma (90%) or adenocarcinoma (10%). Common signs include bloody vaginal discharge, postcoital spotting, and metrorrhagia. Advanced disease can cause pelvic and leg pain, dysuria, hematuria, obstipation, and rectal bleeding. Cervical lesions can be exophytic, ulcerative, or endophytic. Cervical cancer spreads primarily by direct extension to the parametrial tissues, vagina, rectum and bladder, and regional pelvic lymph node chains. FIGO recommends clinical staging of cervical cancer (see Table 110-1).

Microinvasive carcinoma of the cervix, which has a depth of invasion of 3 mm or less, no confluent tongues of invasive disease, and no lymphatic or vascular invasion, has an incidence of pelvic lymph node metastasis of less than 1%. It can be treated effectively by therapeutic conization or simple extrafascial hysterectomy.

The treatment of invasive cervical carcinoma is determined by the patient's age, health status, and stage of disease. Stage I and IIA disease can be treated effectively either by radical hysterectomy and pelvic lymphadenectomy (obturator, internal iliac, and iliac nodes) or by a combination of intracavitary and external radiation therapies. The 5-year survival rate is 80% to 90%. Surgery is advantageous in the younger patient because it permits preservation of the ovaries and is more likely to leave a coitally

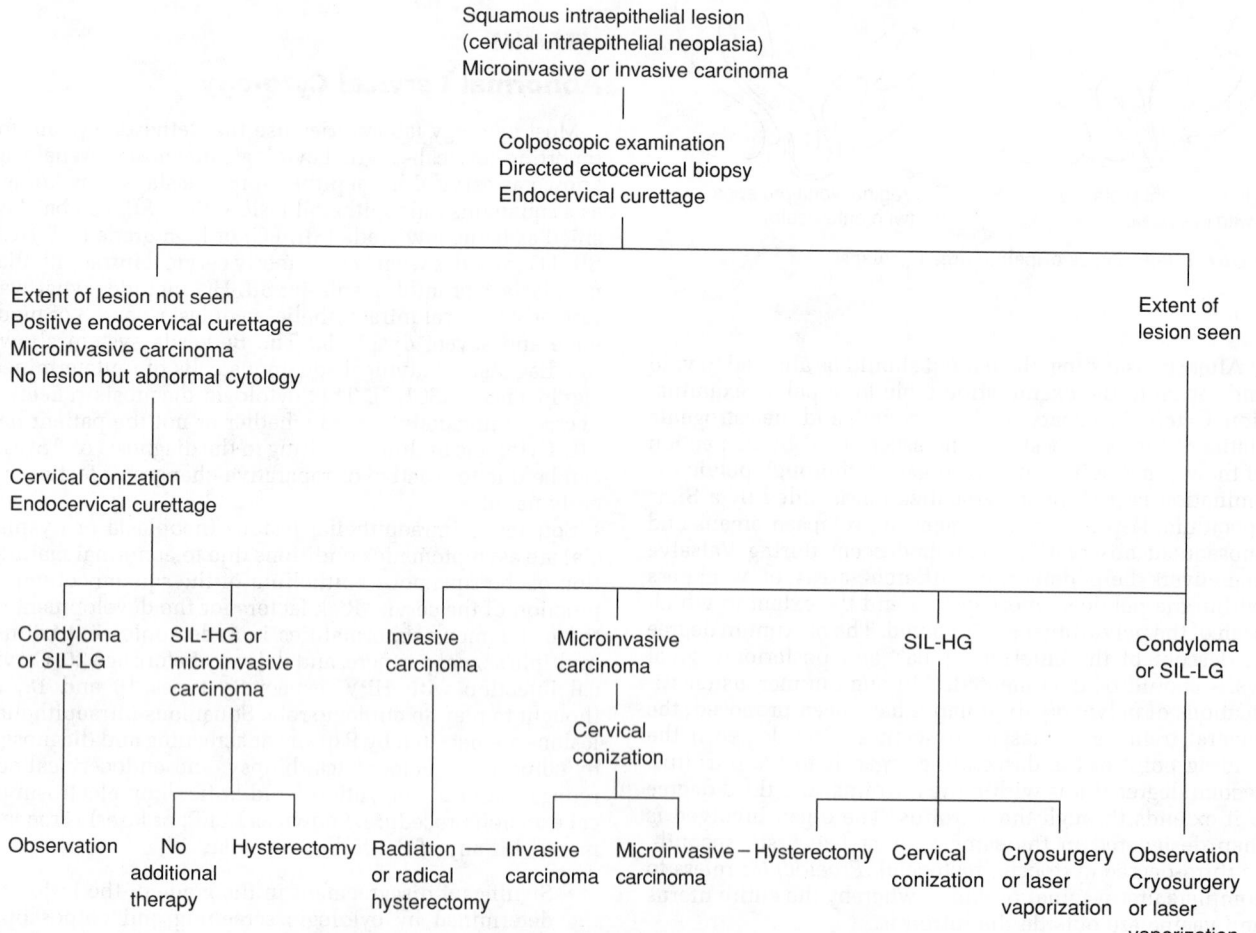

Figure 110-4. Management of abnormal cervical cytology. When the Bethesda system is used to report cervical cytology, low-grade squamous intraepithelial lesion (SIL-LG) should be considered the same as cervical intraepithelial neoplasia 1, and high grade squamous intraepithelial lesion (SIL-HG) the same as cervical epithelial neoplasia 2 and 3. Conization can be performed by cold knife (scapel), loop electrosurgical excision procedure, or laser. Frequent follow-up examinations are indicated after therapy for cervical neoplasia.

functional vagina. Stage IIB, III, and IV disease are best treated by radiotherapy. Approximate 5-year survival rates for stages III and IV are 40% and 15%, respectively. When cervical cancer is first diagnosed during pregnancy, the treatment options are essentially the same, except that the patient must decide when therapy is to be instituted based on her decision about whether to have the pregnancy terminated before or after fetal viability. Stage for stage, pregnancy does not affect 5-year survival.

Endometrial Hyperplasia

Chronic, unopposed estrogen stimulation of the endometrium due to anovulation, estrogen-producing tumors, or estrogen administration causes endometrial hyperplasia. Tamoxifen, as used in the treatment of women with breast cancer, has been reported to contribute to the development of endometrial polyps, hyperplasia, and carcinoma. Atypical adenomatous hyperplasia (complex atypical hyperplasia) is considered to be a premalignant condition when it occurs in perimenopausal women.

Adenomatous endometrial hyperplasia without atypia in premenopausal women should be treated with cyclic progestins for 6 months, either with medroxyprogesterone acetate, 20 mg/d orally for 10 days each month, or with Depo-Provera, 200 mg intramuscularly every other month for three doses, with subsequent endometrial sampling in 3 months to prove resolution of hyperplasia and subsequent periodic sampling to detect any recurrence. Perimenopausal and postmenopausal women who have adenomatous endometrial hyperplasia with atypia should be advised to undergo hysterectomy because this histologic finding is likely to be associated with endometrial cancer. Progestin therapy can be considered in the postmenopausal patient who is a poor surgical risk.

Endometrial Carcinoma

Endometrial carcinoma is the most common female genital malignancy.[3,4] The median age at diagnosis is 60 years. Histologically, it is most often an adenocarcinoma (90%). Risk factors include nulliparity, obesity, delayed menopause, chronic anovulation, and unopposed postmenopausal estrogen therapy. The most common sign is menometrorrhagia or postmenopausal bleeding. Diagnosis is made by outpatient endometrial sampling or uterine curettage. The prognosis of endometrial carcinoma is determined by histologic type, degree of cellular differentiation, extent of myometrial invasion, and presence or absence of node metastases. FIGO recommends surgical and pathologic staging of uterine corpus cancer (see Table 110-1).

The treatment of stage I endometrial carcinoma is primarily surgical. At the time of surgery, peritoneal cytology should be obtained and an extrafascial abdominal hysterectomy and bilateral salpingo-oophorectomy performed. Patients with poorly differentiated endometrial carcinomas, more than superficial myometrial invasion, or extension into the cervix should undergo selective pelvic and periaortic lymphadenectomy to determine prognosis and to aid in treatment planning (adjuvant radiation therapy). These patients may also benefit from postoperative radiotherapy. The 5-year survival rate for stage I patients is about 80%. Patients with stage II endometrial carcinoma can be treated with radical hysterectomy, bilateral salpingo-oophorectomy, and pelvic and periaortic lymphadenectomy, or with external radiotherapy and subsequent abdominal extrafascial hysterectomy and bilateral salpingo-oophorectomy. The 5-year survival rate for stage II patients is about 60%. The treatment of patients with stage III or IV disease must be individualized; treatment options

for these patients are radiotherapy or surgery, or both, and progestin therapy or chemotherapy, or both. The 5-year survival rates for patients with stage III and IV disease are about 30% and 10%, respectively.

Uterine Sarcoma

Uterine sarcomas are derived from the endometrium, myometrium, or, rarely, the vascular and connective tissues. They are usually detected in women 55 to 60 years of age. They commonly cause uterine enlargement, abnormal uterine bleeding, and pelvic pain. The primary treatment of uterine sarcomas is abdominal hysterectomy and bilateral salpingo-oophorectomy. The roles of postoperative radiation and chemotherapy are poorly defined. The 5-year survival rate for patients with stage I disease is about 50%; for stage II, III, and IV disease, the 5-year survival rate is less than 15%.

Abnormal Uterine Bleeding

The endometrium is exquisitely sensitive to circulating levels of estrogen and progesterone. Abnormal uterine bleeding during the reproductive years that is due to anovulation can be managed medically and without surgical intervention.[5] Abnormal uterine bleeding caused by anatomic lesions (eg, leiomyomas, polyps, carcinomas), however, may require surgery. The physician must determine if the cause of the abnormal bleeding is the result of endocrine or anatomic factors.

Most abnormal uterine bleeding in women younger than 40 years of age who have normal pelvic examinations is due to anovulation. Administration of medroxyprogesterone, 10 mg/d orally for 12 days beginning 14 days before the anticipated onset of the next menstrual period, usually helps correct abnormal uterine bleeding. If it does not, hysteroscopy and endometrial sampling are recommended. Diagnostic hysteroscopy can be safely performed in an outpatient setting after the oral administration of a mild analgesic, such as a nonsteroidal antiinflammatory agent. Hysteroscopy is best performed in the early proliferative phase, with CO_2 as the distending medium (45 mmHg pressure), with use of a hysteroscope and a 5-mm sheath. Visualization of the uterine cavity allows determination of whether the patient has a field abnormality or a focal lesion, such as a submucous leiomyoma, endometrial polyp, or carcinoma. Endometrial sampling allows determination of the presence or absence of endometrial hyperplasia or carcinoma within the uterus. If endometrial sampling is performed during the luteal phase, it allows documentation of ovulation.

Laser vaporization and electrical cauterization of the endometrium are used to obliterate the endometrial cavity in selected cases of menorrhagia when the patient does not respond to hormonal therapy and does not wish to have a hysterectomy, provided the possibilities of cancer or other significant anatomic abnormalities have been eliminated. Patients who have small submucous leiomyomas or polyps and whose overall uterine size does not warrant hysterectomy may be candidates for hysteroscopic resection of their lesion. Patients who wish to maintain their childbearing potential and whose abnormal bleeding is due to leiomyomas can be treated with gonadotropin-releasing hormone (GnRH) analogue therapy to shrink the leiomyomas so that hysteroscopic or laparoscopic resection or laparotomy with myomectomy can be performed more efficiently. Those who have completed childbearing and whose anatomic lesions are causing significant bleeding that does not respond to conservative therapy may be candidates for hysterectomy. When uterine, tubal, or ovarian cancer or cancer metastatic to these organs is the cause of abnormal uterine bleeding, hysterectomy is recommended.

Leiomyoma

Twenty-five percent of women in their reproductive years have uterine leiomyomas. Most are asymptomatic, but some cause abnormal bleeding, pelvic pressure, and pain. Large leiomyomas can interfere with bladder and bowel function. Rarely, leiomyomas are thought to contribute to abortion or premature labor. The risk of malignant degeneration is less than 0.5% and is not in itself an indication for surgery. Myomectomy is indicated when the patient wishes to maintain her childbearing potential and a leiomyoma is thought to be the cause of bleeding, pain, or the loss of a pregnancy. Preoperative administration of GnRH analogue therapy over a period of 2 to 3 months reduces overall uterine size and may facilitate endoscopic resection of leiomyomas or myomectomy at laparotomy. If GnRH analogue therapy is used, timing of the myomectomy is important because the uterus of a woman of reproductive age tends to escape suppression and return to its pretreatment size. Hysterectomy may be indicated for asymptomatic leiomyomas when the overall uterine size is greater than that seen at 12 to 14 weeks' gestation, or when there is rapid growth of the leiomyoma, suggesting the possibility of malignant disease. A hysterectomy may be indicated if the leiomyoma causes significant bleeding or pain despite conservative therapy.

Tubal Carcinoma

Tubal carcinoma accounts for less than 0.5% of all female genital malignancies. The average age at diagnosis is 55 years. Common complaints are a watery vaginal discharge, uterine bleeding, or pelvic pain. There may be an adnexal mass. The diagnosis is rarely made preoperatively. FIGO recommends surgical staging as if it were ovarian cancer (see Table 110-1). The treatment is surgical. Peritoneal cytology should be obtained, and abdominal hysterectomy, bilateral salpingo-oophorectomy, selective periaortic lymphadenectomy, and partial omentectomy should be performed. Postoperative radiation therapy or chemotherapy may be indicated. The 5-year survival rate for patients with stage I disease is 65%; the overall survival rate for patients with surgically treated tubal carcinoma is about 35%.

Ascending Genital Infections

Mucopurulent endocervicitis is caused by *Chlamydia trachomatis*, or *Neisseria gonorrhoeae*, or both. The clinical diagnosis is based on the finding of a yellow or green endocervical exudate on a white swab in association with cervical erythema, edema, and friability of the zone of ectopy. In pregnancy, mucopurulent cervicitis can contribute to premature delivery, postpartum endometritis, and infections in the neonate.

The pathophysiology of pelvic inflammatory disease (PID) involves the spread of microorganisms found in the endocervix through the endometrial cavity to the fallopian tubes and into the peritoneal cavity[6–8] (Fig. 110-5). Ascent of bacteria may be due to canalicular spread, spermatozoa acting as vehicles for the infecting organisms, retrograde menstruation, douching, or iatrogenic manipulation associated with endometrial biopsy, hysterosalpingograms, dilation and curettage, and insertion of an intrauterine device. The presence of bacterial vaginosis, a disorder of vaginal flora characterized by an overgrowth of anaerobic

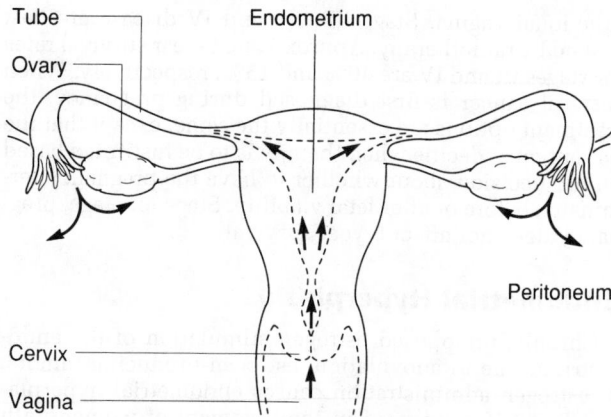

Figure 110-5. The pathophysiology of pelvic inflammatory disease involves ascending spread of microorganisms found in the endocervix.

bacteria, may facilitate the ascent of sexually transmitted and other aerobic pathogens by altering the cervical mucous barrier through enzymatic degradation by the proteolytic enzymes associated with this disorder.[9] The most common microorganisms associated with PID are *N gonorrhoeae, C trachomatis, Haemophilus influenzae,* and a variety of opportunistic aerobic and anaerobic bacteria.

Major criteria for the clinical diagnosis of PID are the following:

- A chief complaint of lower abdominal pain
- Bilateral adnexal tenderness on bimanual pelvic examination
- Vaginal leukorrhea (microscopy of a wet mount of vaginal contents revealing a marked increase in the number of inflammatory cells)

In no instance of PID will microscopy of the vaginal secretions be normal; this simple test can be used to exclude genital infection, and consequently PID, in a woman with abdominal pain.[10] Adjunctive diagnostic criteria include leukocytosis, elevated C-reactive protein or erythrocyte sedimentation rate, fever higher than 38°C, or palpable adnexal complex. Endometrial biopsy revealing plasma cell endometritis is helpful in confirming the presence of upper genital tract inflammation. Laparoscopic findings of tubal hyperemia, edema, and a sticky exudate are the gold standard for visual diagnosis. Laparoscopy is recommended for patients with a questionable diagnosis or in cases of antibiotic treatment failure. At laparoscopy, there appears to be some therapeutic benefit to the removal of free pus from the peritoneal cavity, drainage of a pyosalpinx, and lysis of adhesions.

The patient's need for hospitalization is based on the severity of the clinical illness, the likelihood of compliance with an outpatient therapeutic regimen, the suspicion of anaerobic infection, and the certainty of the diagnosis. The 1993 Centers for Disease Control and Prevention guidelines for the treatment of PID are given in Table 110-2.[11] Outpatients should be reexamined within 72 hours of the initiation of therapy to determine therapeutic response. Male sexual partners should be treated, and patients should be educated concerning the sexually transmitted nature of their disease and how to practice safe sex.

Tuboovarian abscesses are the most severe form of PID. These complexes involve loculations of pus in and about the tubes, ovaries, and bowel. Most (75%) tuboovarian abscesses can be treated with antibiotics alone. Therefore, if a patient in her reproductive years is found to have a

Table 110-2. 1993 CDC GUIDELINES FOR TREATMENT OF PID[11]

OUTPATIENT TREATMENT

Regimen A

Cefoxitin, 2 g IM, plus probenecid, 1 g PO concurrently, or ceftriaxone, 250 mg IM, or equivalent cephalosporin

plus

Doxycycline, 100 mg PO bid for 14 d

Regimen B

Ofloxacin, 400 mg PO bid for 14 d

plus

Either clindamycin, 450 mg PO qid, or metronidazole, 500 mg PO bid for 14 d

INPATIENT TREATMENT

Regimen A

Cefoxitin, 2 g IV q6h, or cefotetan,* 2 g IV q12h

plus

Doxycycline, 100 mg q12h PO or IV

Regimen B

Clindamycin, 900 mg IV q8h

plus

Gentamicin, 2 mg/kg loading dose IV or IM, followed by a 1.5-mg/kg maintenance dose q8h

NOTE

One of the above regimens is given for at least 48 hours after the patient clinically improves.

After discharge from the hospital, continue doxycycline, 100 mg PO bid for a total of 14 d, or clindamycin, 450 mg PO qid for a total of 14 d.

---

* Other cephalosporins that provide adequate gonococcal, other facultative gram-negative aerobic, and anaerobic coverage—such as ceftizoxime, cefotaxime, and ceftriaxone—may be used in appropriate doses.

---

tuboovarian abscess at laparotomy, irrigation and drainage without extirpation of the adnexa, in conjunction with broad-spectrum antibiotic therapy, should be considered as initial therapy.

Patients who fail to respond to antibiotic therapy require laparotomy and drainage of the abscess or unilateral adnexectomy. Hysterectomy with bilateral salpingo-oophorectomy is rarely necessary in the surgical management of tuboovarian abscesses and should be reserved for patients who have failed to respond to antibiotic therapy or who are septic and have bilateral disease. Laparoscopic diagnosis and drainage as well as CT-guided percutaneous drainage of tuboovarian abscesses are performed with increasing frequency and with good results.

The long-term consequences of PID include tubal factor infertility (5% to 30% after one episode of PID, depending on severity of the inflammatory process); ectopic pregnancy (sixfold increase in patients with a history of PID); and chronic pelvic pain (18%).

Toxic Shock Syndromes

Now, more than 20 years after the highly publicized epidemic of staphylococcal toxic shock syndrome, less than 300 cases are reported annually to the CDC. However, two additional microorganisms, *S pyogenes* (group A *Streptococcus*) and *Clostridium sordellii*, have been associated with toxic shock syndrome in obstetric and gynecologic patients.[7] These rare, but commonly fatal, infections challenge clinicians both diagnostically and therapeutically.

Staphylococcal Toxic Shock Syndrome

The toxic shock syndrome associated with *S aureus* is commonly associated with fever (higher than 39°C), a diffuse or palmar erythroderma progressing to subsequent peripheral desquamation, and mucous membrane hyperemia. Vomiting and diarrhea are common; multiple organ system dysfunction with rapid progression to hypotension and shock can be seen in severe cases. Menstrually related toxic shock syndrome occurs in young (ages 16 to 30) women using highly absorbent tampons. These tampons promote the production of toxic shock toxin 1, an exotoxin unique to *S aureus*, which is responsible for the clinical manifestations of this disease. Non—menstrually related cases have been associated with surgical wound infections, postpartum infections, and nonsurgical focal infections such as mastitis.

Streptococcal Toxic Shock Syndrome

The pathogenesis of streptococcal toxic shock syndrome involves the acquisition of *S pyogenes*. Mucous membranes serve as the source of this microorganism without manifesting signs of a symptomatic infection. Tissue invasion occurs, usually associated with bacterial M types 1 and 3, and if pyrogenic exotoxin A or B is expressed, shock, multiorgan failure, and tissue destruction ensue. Streptococcal toxic shock syndrome has been reported in cases of septic abortion, postpartum endomyometritis, necrotizing fasciitis, and postoperative infection. Case definition requires isolation of the group A *Streptococcus*, the presence of hypotension, and evidence of multisystem dysfunction. A rash is not a prominent presenting sign in patients with streptococcal toxic shock syndrome.

Clostridium sordellii–Associated Toxic Shock Syndrome

The toxic shock syndrome associated with *C sordellii* (CATS) is characterized by the sudden onset of weakness, nausea, and vomiting followed by progressive refractory hypotension associated with local and spreading edema. It is distinguished from staphylococcal toxic shock syndrome by the absence of *S aureus*, fever, and rash. The classic CATS has been described in patients with episiotomy infection, but it has also been associated with postpartum infections, wound infections, a vaginal foreign body, and a degenerating cervical myoma. The pathogenesis involves the production of edema-producing *Clostridium difficile*–like toxins by *C sordellii*.

All patients with toxic shock syndrome present with an evolving clinical picture resulting in shock. The management involves physiologic support, broad-spectrum antimicrobial therapy, and, in selected cases, surgical intervention. Once the diagnosis is clarified, more specific antimicrobial treatment (such as penicillin for streptococcal toxic shock syndrome or a β-lactamase–resistant antibiotic for *S aureus* toxic shock syndrome) can be initiated. Initial considerations during the physical examination include the removal of tampons, sponges, or other foreign bodies from the vagina. Culture of the mucous membranes (oropharynx, vagina), blood, focal lesions or sources (ie, endometrium), and urine should be performed to detect one of the potential pathogens. Fluid replacement to correct hypotension and physiologic monitoring in an intensive care setting are required. Recent reports suggest that intravenous immunoglobulin therapy may play an important role in the treatment of these syndromes.

OVARY

Characteristics of benign versus malignant ovarian neoplasms are listed in Table 110-3. In general, unilateral, unilocular cysts are less likely to be malignant than bilat-

Table 110-3. CHARACTERISTICS OF BENIGN VERSUS MALIGNANT OVARIAN TUMORS

Characteristic	Benign	Malignant
CLINICAL FINDINGS		
Unilateral	+++	+
Bilateral	+	+++
Cystic	+++	+
Solid	+	+++
Mobile	+++	+
Fixed	+	+++
Irregular	+	+++
Smooth	+++	+
Excrescences	–	+++
Ascites	+	+++
Cul-de-sac nodules	+	+++
Rapid growth rate	+	+++
SONOGRAPHIC FINDINGS		
Thick septa	+	+++
Internal solid parts	+	+++
Indefinite margins	+	+++
Ascites	+	+++
Matted loops of bowel	+	+++
CT FINDINGS		
Enlarged retroperitoneal nodes	–	+++
SERUM ASSAY FINDINGS		
Elevated CA-125	+	+++

(Shingleton HM, Hurt WG. Postreproductive gynecology. New York, Churchill Livingstone, 1990; modified from DiSaia PJ, Creasman WT. Clinical gynecologic oncology, ed 3. St Louis, CV Mosby, 1989)

eral, complex cysts, and solid ovarian neoplasms are suspect for malignancy at any age. When an ovarian neoplasm is associated with the acute onset of pain, nausea, and vomiting, it suggests hemorrhage, infarction, or torsion, any of which may require emergency surgery. An algorithm for the management of adnexal masses is proposed in Figure 110-6.

Benign Neoplasms of the Ovary

The size of an ovarian tumor cannot be used to predict its malignant potential. Bilateral neoplasms and those with complex or solid components are more likely malignant. Sonography, CT, or MRI can be used to determine the characteristics of ovarian neoplasms. For women in their reproductive years, it is recommended that asymptomatic unilateral, unilocular ovarian cysts smaller than 10 cm in diameter be observed for 6 to 8 weeks for resolution. In postmenopausal women, asymptomatic unilateral, unilocular ovarian cysts smaller than 5 cm in diameter are rarely (less than 2%) malignant. On the other hand, complex (septa, internal papillations, or solid components) or solid ovarian enlargements at any age are more likely to be malignant and require prompt investigation. General characteristics that help to distinguish benign from malignant ovarian tumors are presented in Table 110-3.

Follicular and corpus luteum cysts are referred to as physiologic cysts and are common in women of reproductive age. Because oral contraceptives suppress ovulation, these cysts should not develop in patients taking oral contraceptives. If unilateral, unilocular cysts develop in women of reproductive age who are not on oral contraceptive therapy, oral contraceptives can be prescribed for two or three cycles to allow time for resolution of the cysts

and to prevent the development of new cysts. Unilateral, unilocular cysts larger than 10 cm in diameter are less likely to disappear and warrant a shorter period of observation.

Theca-lutein cysts can develop during ovarian stimulation, gestational trophoblastic disease, or pregnancy. They are usually bilateral, complex, and sometimes associated with ascites. They are the only cysts fitting this description that do not require surgical exploration. They resolve with cessation of ovarian stimulation or termination of the pregnancy.

Benign cystic teratomas (dermoids) are commonly seen in women in their reproductive years. They can contain calcifications (30%) and are often bilateral (15%). Pelvic radiographs, ultrasound examinations, and CT scans are helpful in establishing a preoperative diagnosis (Fig. 110-7). Ovarian cystectomy is recommended to preserve ovarian function. If the teratoma is unilateral, the opposite ovary should be inspected, and if it is abnormal, a biopsy specimen should be taken for evaluation. Biopsy should not be performed on a perfectly normal contralateral ovary. In fact, it can cause harm to the ovary by damaging its blood supply or by contributing to adhesion formation. Perimenopausal and postmenopausal women with cystic teratomas are candidates for bilateral oophorectomy.

Serous or mucinous cystadenomas are common, benign epithelial ovarian tumors. They can be treated by cystectomy or oophorectomy. Intraoperative frozen section evaluation of these cysts is important to determine whether they contain malignant tissue. Postmenopausal women should undergo hysterectomy and bilateral salpingo-oophorectomy.

Fibromas, thecomas, and Brenner tumors of the ovary are essentially indistinguishable at surgery. Most are benign and can be treated by oophorectomy during the reproductive years or by hysterectomy and bilateral salpingo-oophorectomy during the perimenopausal and postmenopausal years. The three can be distinguished from each other by their histologic appearance.

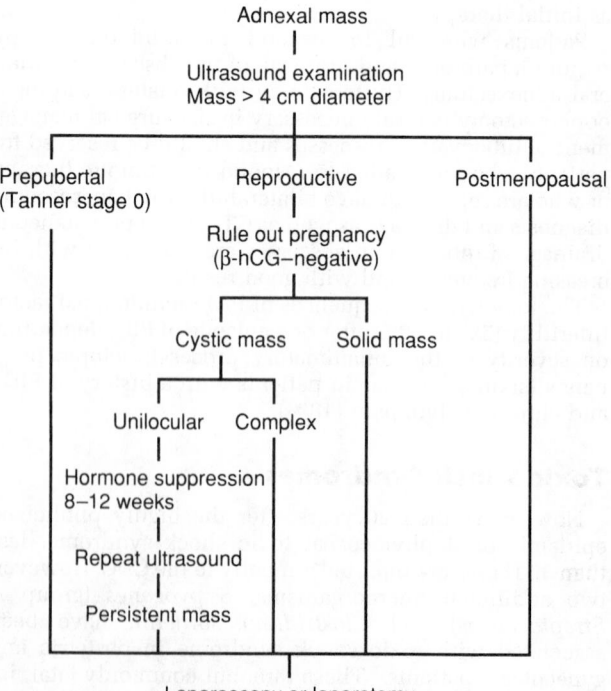

Figure 110-6. Management of adnexal mass.

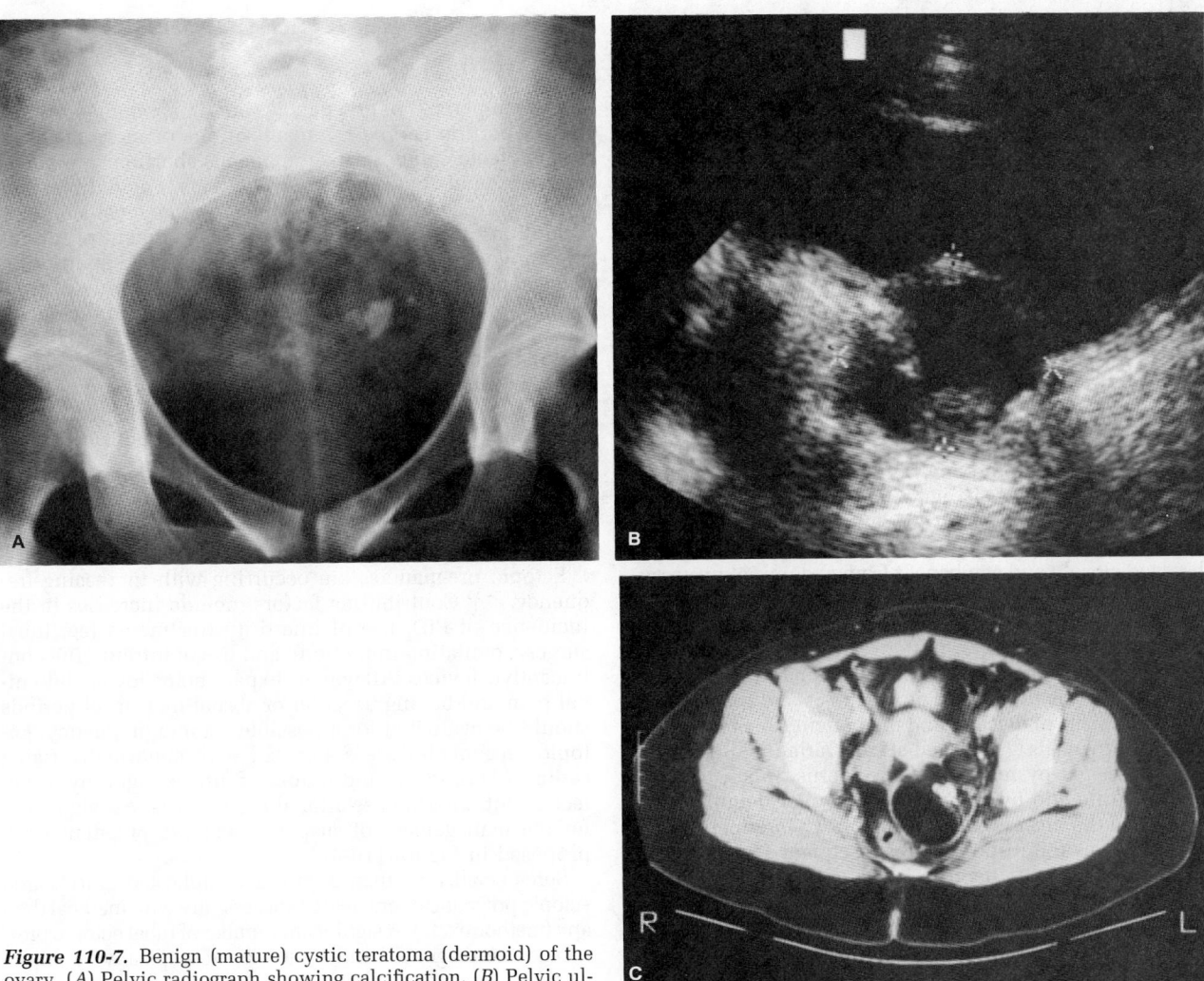

Figure 110-7. Benign (mature) cystic teratoma (dermoid) of the ovary. (*A*) Pelvic radiograph showing calcification. (*B*) Pelvic ultrasound. (*C*) Pelvic CT scan.

Endometriomas do not respond to medical therapy. Cystectomy can be performed by laparoscopy or laparotomy. Large endometriomas may require oophorectomy. Endometriosis most commonly involves the ovaries (half are bilateral); it can also involve the uterosacral ligaments, rectovaginal septum, sigmoid colon, lower genital tract, pelvic peritoneum, small intestine, bladder, and ureters. Occasionally, it implants in laparotomy or episiotomy scars or in more distant sites, such as the umbilicus, pleura, and extremities. When operating for endometriosis, every attempt should be made to remove all evidence of disease. If ovarian tissue is preserved, postoperative progesterone, danazol (Danocrine), or GnRH analogue therapy can be prescribed to suppress the growth of residual implants. In cases of extensive endometriosis, when childbearing is complete, and in perimenopausal and postmenopausal women, endometriosis is best treated by hysterectomy and bilateral salpingo-oophorectomy, with subsequent hormone replacement therapy.

Ovarian Carcinoma

Ovarian carcinoma accounts for about 25% of all female genital malignancies.[3,4] One in 70 women develops the disease. Risk factors include increased age; decreased fertility; a first-degree relative with ovarian, colon, breast, or endometrial cancer; Peutz-Jeghers syndrome; and Turner syndrome with XO/XY mosaicism. The World Health Organization's histologic classification of ovarian malignancies distinguishes them according to their derivation from coelomic epithelium, germ cells, gonadal stroma, mesenchyme, or neoplasms metastatic to the ovary. Although ovarian cancer can be seen at any age, the germ cell tumors are more common in adolescents, and the epithelial tumors are more common in postmenopausal women. The older the patient, the more likely she is to have advanced disease.

Ovarian cancer usually presents with abdominal swelling, pain, gastrointestinal symptomatology, and an adnexal mass. Evaluation of patients in whom ovarian cancer is suspected should consist of hemogram, serum chemistries, and tumor antigens, including CA-125, α-fetoprotein, and the β-subunit of hCG,[12] with selective use of abdominal CT, intravenous urogram, and radiographic evaluation of the upper and lower gastrointestinal tracts. Proctosigmoidoscopy may be indicated in patients with lower gastrointestinal symptoms. Regarding tumor-associated antigens, CA-125 is more likely to be elevated with epithelial ovarian tumors; β-hCG may be present with malignant teratomas, choriocarcinomas, and embryonal carcinomas; and

α-fetoprotein production may be associated with endodermal sinus tumors and embryonal carcinomas. In many cases, these tumor markers are more helpful in detecting persistent or recurrent disease than in establishing a preoperative diagnosis. The diagnosis of type of ovarian malignancy is dependent on histologic evaluation.

Surgical treatment of ovarian malignancies includes abdominal hysterectomy, bilateral salpingo-oophorectomy, partial omentectomy, selective periaortic and pelvic lymphadenectomy, and tumor cytoreduction. FIGO recommends surgical staging of ovarian cancer (see Table 110-1). Staging of epithelial cancers (peritoneal washings, biopsy or cytologic smear from under right hemidiaphragm, biopsy of suspicious lesions, infracolic omentectomy, biopsy of paracolic recesses and pelvic sidewalls in the absence of obvious implants, and selective lymphadenectomy of pelvic and paraaortic lymph nodes) is mandatory because it provides a basis for prognosis and appropriate postoperative chemotherapy.[3] In adolescents and women of reproductive age, it may be possible to preserve childbearing potential if the ovarian malignancy is limited to one ovary. Patients managed in this manner should be observed closely and can benefit from abdominal hysterectomy, with removal of the remaining ovary after childbearing is complete. The need for intraoperative instillations of radioactive substances, postoperative systemic chemotherapy, or radiotherapy must be individualized. Their use is determined by the histologic diagnosis and grade of the tumor, the stage of disease, and the patient's overall condition and prognosis. Advanced-stage ovarian malignancies are best treated by removal of the uterus, tubes, ovaries, and omentum and by cytoreduction (tumor debulking) of as much of the disease as is reasonable. Cytoreductive surgery improves the responses to subsequent systemic chemotherapy and radiotherapy.

The approximate 5-year survival rates for patients with epithelial ovarian cancer are 70% for stage I, 30% for stage II, 15% for stage III, and up to 5% for stage IV.

PREGNANCY-RELATED CONDITIONS

Abortion

Fifteen percent of pregnancies end in spontaneous abortion. Abortion can be the result of one or more maternal or fetal factors, but most spontaneous abortions are due to chromosomal abnormalities in the fetus. Vaginal bleeding and lower abdominal cramping are the most common symptoms associated with abortion. Treatment of uterine bleeding without cervical dilation (threatened abortion) is expectant. Quantitative β-hCG determinations and ultrasound examinations can be used to determine the subsequent course of the pregnancy. If the cervix is dilated or the patient gives a history of passage of tissue, however, an incomplete abortion probably has occurred and requires uterine suction curettage to prevent further bleeding and infection. Ultrasound imaging can help confirm the absence of a viable pregnancy in these patients.

Ectopic Pregnancy

Ectopic pregnancies are occurring with increasing frequency.[13-15] Contributing factors include increases in the incidence of PID, use of infertility treatments (eg, tubal surgery, ovulation induction), and use of intrauterine contraceptive devices. All women experiencing lower abdominal pain and having irregular or absent menstrual periods should be evaluated for a possible ectopic pregnancy. Ectopic pregnancies are associated with abnormally rising serum β-hCG levels and failure of ultrasonography to detect an intrauterine gestational sac or fetus. An algorithm for the management of suspected ectopic pregnancies is proposed in Figure 110-8.

Some small (less than 3 cm), uncomplicated, unruptured ectopic pregnancies are treated successfully with medical therapy (methotrexate). A significant number of tubal ectopic pregnancies are diagnosed and treated laparoscopically by salpin-

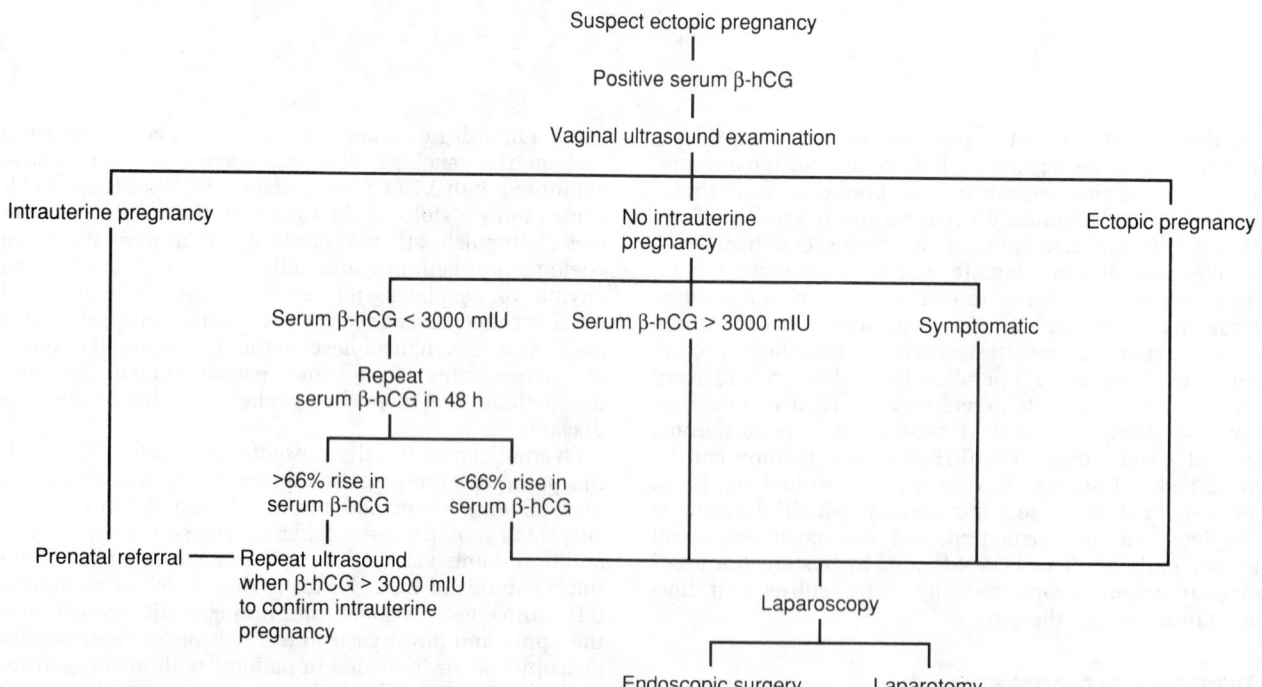

Figure 110-8. Management of suspected ectopic pregnancy. The level of serum β-hCG at which intrauterine pregnancy is detected by vaginal ultrasound examination can vary according to institution.

gostomy or salpingectomy (Fig. 110-9). Mini-laparotomy can also be used for salpingostomy or salpingectomy. Laparotomy is reserved for patients who are hemodynamically unstable, who have advanced pregnancies, or who, for some reason, require more extensive surgery.

Patients who wish to maintain their childbearing potential should undergo the most conservative procedure that allows removal of the ectopic pregnancy and preserves the integrity of their fallopian tubes. The risk of recurrent ectopic pregnancy is 15%; therefore, every effort should be made to handle tissues gently, to preserve the continuity of the tubes, and to keep adhesion formation to a minimum. The surgeon must not lose sight of the fact that specialists are able to establish and carry pregnancies to term in patients without oviducts and even without ovaries. It is therefore essential to know the patient's wishes with regard to future childbearing before taking her to the operating room.

Gestational Trophoblastic Neoplasia

Gestational trophoblastic neoplasia represents a spectrum of pregnancy-related tumors that includes hydatidiform mole, invasive mole, and choriocarcinoma. These tumors appear to be the result of abnormal fertilization. They are unique in that they are derived exclusively from fetal tissue, cytotrophoblast, and syncytiotrophoblast but have the capacity to invade maternal tissues and secrete β-hCG. Common clinical findings are irregular uterine bleeding and a uterus that is larger than estimated gestational age but contains no fetus. The preoperative evaluation should include hemogram, serum chemistries, quantitative serum β-hCG, chest radiograph, and pelvic ultrasound or abdominopelvic CT scan.

The treatment of noninvasive disease (hydatidiform mole) is suction curettage. Abdominal hysterectomy is an option only if childbearing is complete. Systematic follow-up is imperative because 15% of noninvasive disease persists or recurs. Follow-up must include weekly quantitative serum β-hCG determinations until the serum level remains within normal levels (less than 5 mIU), then monthly for 6 months. During this period of follow-up, strict contraception (use of oral contraceptives) is advised. Persistent or recurrent noninvasive disease should be treated with single-agent chemotherapy (methotrexate or actinomycin D). With close follow-up and chemotherapy, if indicated, the cure rate for noninvasive disease is 100%.

Invasive disease (invasive mole or choriocarcinoma) can follow any gestational event—hydatidiform mole, delivery of intrauterine pregnancy, abortion, or ectopic pregnancy. It can be localized to the uterus or metastasize throughout the body (lungs 90%, vagina 30%, pelvis 20%, brain 10%, liver 10%). FIGO recommends clinical staging of invasive gestational trophoblastic neoplasia (see Table 110-1). Pretreatment evaluation should include hemogram, serum chemistries, quantitative β-hCG, and imaging studies (CT of head, abdomen, and pelvis) to document metastases. Histologic diagnosis is not required when the patient has an elevated β-hCG and no evidence of gestation. Stage I disease can be treated by single-agent chemotherapy (methotrexate or actinomycin D) or by combination chemotherapy for resistant disease (etoposide, methotrexate, actinomycin D, cyclophosphamide, vincristine). Stage II, III, and IV disease should be treated with combination chemotherapy and with whole-brain radiotherapy for metastasis to the brain. Systematic follow-up should consist of weekly quantitative serum β-hCG determinations until normal for 3 consecutive weeks, then monthly determinations for 12 to 24 months. During this period of follow-up, strict contraception is advised. Patients with stage I, II, or III disease should be cured by medical therapy. Resistant disease may require combination chemotherapy and, on rare occasions, surgical resection of localized disease (uterine, pulmonary, hepatic, brain). Metastases to the brain and liver have a poor prognosis (40% to 60% survival rate). A patient cured by chemotherapy can expect to have a normal reproductive future if her uterus was not removed.

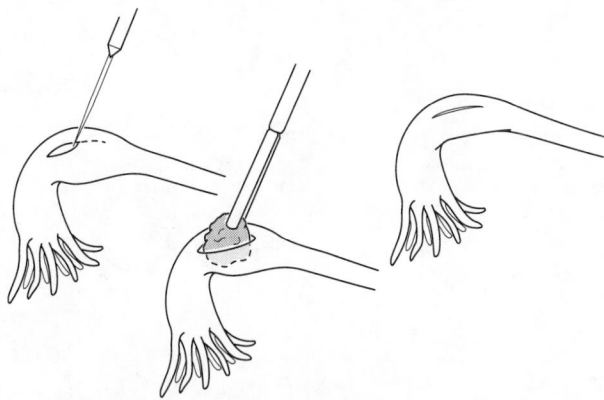

Salpingostomy using needle electrocautery

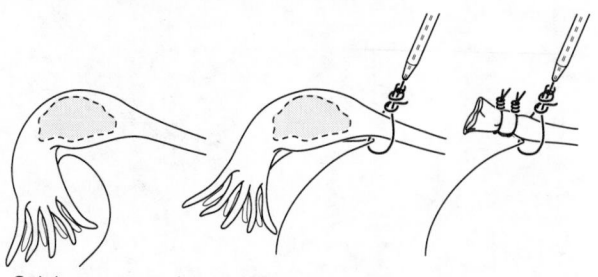

Salpingectomy using endoloop

Figure 110-9. Laparoscopic removal of ectopic pregnancy.

REFERENCES

1. Shingleton HM, Hurt WG. Postreproductive gynecology. New York, Churchill Livingstone, 1990.
2. National Cancer Institute Workshop: The 1988 Bethesda system for reporting cervical/vaginal cytologic diagnoses. JAMA 1989;262:931.
3. DiSaia PJ, Creasman WT. Clinical gynecologic oncology, ed 4. St Louis, CV Mosby, 1993.
4. Gusberg SB, Shingleton HM, Deppe G. Female genital cancer. New York, Churchill Livingstone, 1988.
5. Speroff L, Glass RH, Kase NG. Clinical gynecologic endocrinology and infertility, ed 5. Baltimore, Williams & Wilkins, 1994.
6. Holmes KK, Mardh PA, Sparling PF, et al. Sexually transmitted diseases, ed 2. New York, McGraw-Hill, 1990.
7. Pastorek JG. Obstetric and gynecologic infectious disease. New York, Raven Press, 1994.
8. Sweet RL, Gibbs RS. Infectious diseases of the female genital tract, ed 2. Baltimore, Williams & Wilkins, 1990.
9. Soper DE, Brockwell NJ, Dalton HP, Johnson D. Observations concerning the microbial etiology of acute salpingitis. Am J Obstet Gynecol 1994;170:1008.
10. Westrom L. Clinical manifestations and diagnosis of pelvic inflammatory disease. J Reprod Med 1983;38:703.
11. Centers for Disease Control. 1993 sexually transmitted diseases treatment guidelines. MMWR 1993;42:75.
12. Olt G, Berchuck A, Bast RC Jr. The role of tumor markers in gynecologic oncology. Obstet Gynecol Surv 1990;45:570.
13. Semm K, Friedrich ER. Operative manual for endoscopic abdominal surgery. Chicago, Year Book Medical, 1987.
14. Stovall TG, Ling FW, Buster JE. Outpatient chemotherapy of unruptured ectopic pregnancy. Fertil Steril 1989;51:435.
15. Weckstein LN. Current perspective on ectopic pregnancy. Obstet Gynecol Surv 1985;40:259.

SURGERY: SCIENTIFIC PRINCIPLES AND PRACTICE, Second Edition, edited by
Lazar J. Greenfield, Michael W. Mulholland, Keith T. Oldham, Gerald B. Zelenock,
and Keith D. Lillemoe. Lippincott–Raven Publishers, Philadelphia, © 1997.

CHAPTER 111

CUTANEOUS NEOPLASMS

ALFRED E. CHANG, TIMOTHY M. JOHNSON,
AND RILEY S. REES

Cutaneous neoplasms are the most commonly diagnosed malignant tumors in the United States, with an incidence of more than 900,000 annually. The most common skin cancers are the basal and squamous cell carcinomas (BCCs and SCCs). Cutaneous melanomas represent only 3% of all of skin cancers, but they account for at least 65% of skin cancer deaths. The early diagnosis and surgical treatment of these skin cancers can be curative.

MELANOMA

Epidemiology and Etiology

The incidence of melanoma in the United States is approximately 30,000 new cases per year, or 3% of all newly diagnosed cancers.[1] More important, the incidence of melanoma has increased faster than that of any other cancer. Between 1973 and 1987, the Surveillance Program of the National Cancer Institute found an 83% increase in the incidence of melanoma[2] (Fig. 111-1). Because cutaneous melanomas are readily diagnosed, this increased incidence probably is not related to improved diagnostic methods or screening. Fortunately, the mortality rates are not increasing at the same rate, primarily because patients are presenting at an earlier stage of tumor development, which allows a much higher cure rate.

The typical melanoma patient has a fair complexion and a tendency to sunburn rather than to tan, even after a relatively brief exposure to sunlight. Melanoma occurs infrequently in blacks and Asians, suggesting that skin pigment plays a protective role. Melanoma incidence is subject to large geographic and ethnic variations, mainly because of an inverse correlation with latitude and with degree of skin pigmentation.[3] Specifically, populations residing closer to the equator have a higher incidence of melanoma. In Queensland, Australia, where the predominantly fair-skinned population is perennially exposed to sunlight, one of the highest occurrences of melanoma can be found— about 28.4 per 100,000 population. Increases in incidence of melanoma at specific body sites have been reported to be consistent with changes in clothing habits over time (eg, the trunk in males, lower limbs in females, upper limbs in both sexes).[4]

The reasons for the rising incidence of melanoma are not clear but may be related to an increased exposure to ultraviolet radiation (UVR) from sunlight that reaches the earth's surface. In part, this increased UVR exposure may result from increased recreational exposure to sunlight. In addition, increased UVR exposure may be caused by decreasing levels of stratospheric ozone, which acts as a highly effective absorbing layer that prevents UVR wavelengths, especially UVB (280 to 320 nm), from reaching humans. It has been postulated that an increasing level of chlorofluorocarbons in the stratosphere has been responsible for decreased ozone levels. The causal relation between UVR and melanoma is based on indirect experimental and clinical data; the evidence for an etiologic role of UVR in the induction of nonmelanoma cancers is more compelling. In 1928, it was demonstrated that UVR can induce nonmelanoma skin cancers in experimental animals. It was later shown that this effect was restricted to wavelengths shorter than 320 nm. In patients with xeroderma pigmentosum, who are unable to repair genetic material damaged by UVR, exposure to UVR leads to the development of melanoma and nonmelanoma skin cancers, suggesting a direct causal role in the induction of these neoplasms.

Other possible mechanisms for the role of UVR in causing melanomas have been postulated. According to the classic initiation–promotion model of carcinogenesis established in experimental animal studies, the first step involves initiating factors that directly interact with the cellular DNA to induce mutations in the genome. Afterward, this process is further driven by promotional factors, which are not mutagenic by themselves but enhance the proliferation of mutated cells. In addition to the evidence that UVR is an initiating agent, it has been shown experimentally that UVR can act as a promoter of chemical carcinogens to cause cutaneous melanomas. As a promoting agent, UVR can act to influence the proliferation of an initiated (mutated) cell population or, alternatively, to influence the genetic expression of an initiated cell. Another possible mechanism by which UVR induces skin cancers may be its effect on the immune surveillance of initiated cells.[5] It has been suggested that UVR affects Langerhans cells, which are antigen-presenting cells in the epidermis and represent the most superficial sentinel of the immune system. UVR exposure has been shown to result in the development of suppressor T lymphocytes that interfere with the rejection of initiated cells. Although UVR is an etiologic agent that can cause melanoma and other skin cancers, this does not exclude other mechanisms by which these tumors can arise.

Other, nonenvironmental factors are also associated with an increased risk for melanoma. Three to 5% of patients who have had one melanoma diagnosed develop another melanoma. This risk is 10 times higher than that of the general population, in which the risk for melanoma is about 0.53%. Another group at increased risk for melanoma are those with dysplastic nevi. These patients have a 10% overall lifetime risk of developing melanoma, which is a 20-fold increase compared with the general population. Dysplastic nevi are acquired lesions of the skin that

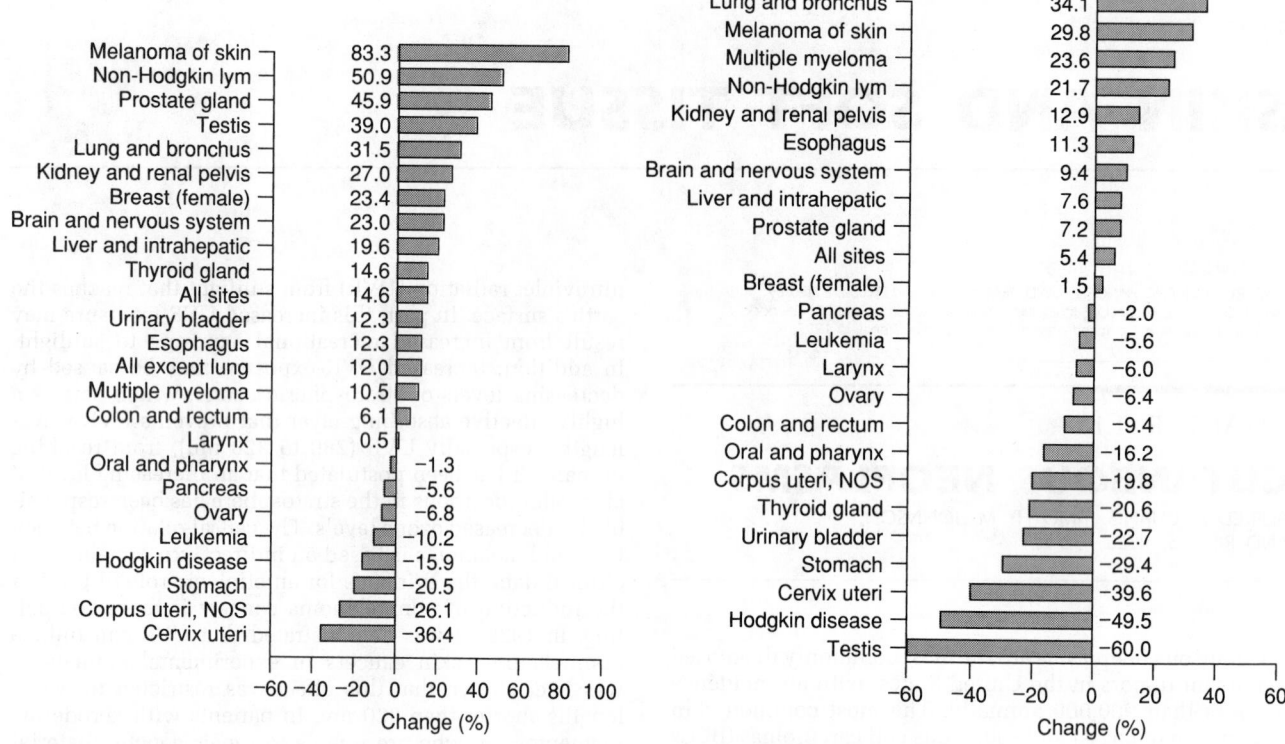

Figure 111-1. Changes in cancer incidence (*left*) and mortality (*right*) in the United States between 1973 and 1987. Data were compiled by the Surveillance Program of the National Cancer Institute. Melanoma incidence has increased faster than that of any other cancer.

have characteristics distinguishing them from common nevi. They are usually larger than common nevi, ranging from 5 to 12 mm in diameter. Anatomically, dysplastic nevi can appear anywhere on the body, and they most frequently are found on the trunk. Their concentration on covered areas, such as the buttocks, breasts, and scalp, represents a distribution different from that of most acquired nevi. Melanoma can arise within a preexisting dysplastic nevus or de novo in patients with dysplastic nevi. Dysplastic nevi can be found both in the general population (sporadic form) and in melanoma-prone families (familial form). This latter syndrome, originally known as the B-K mole syndrome, has an autosomal dominant hereditary pattern and is referred to as dysplastic nevus syndrome, familial type.[6] The lifetime risk of melanoma can approach 100% for patients with this syndrome.

Another risk factor associated with the development of melanoma is the presence of congenital nevi. A congenital nevus is a melanocytic nevus present at birth. Congenital nevi occur in 1% to 2.5% of the population. These lesions have been categorized by size into small (less than 1.5 cm diameter), medium (1.5 to 20 cm diameter), and large (more than 20 cm diameter) nevi. Ninety percent of congenital nevi are of the small type. Large congenital nevi can vary greatly in size and can occupy a major portion of the body surface. They have clinical features that include a grossly irregular surface, increased pigmentation with shades of brown, and hypertrichosis. The lifetime risk of melanoma in patients with large congenital nevi has been estimated to be between 5% and 20%. The management of large congenital nevi is complex and should be individualized to accommodate such factors as technical difficulty, cosmetic results, and perceived risk of melanoma. It is unclear to what extent melanoma develops in small

and medium congenital nevi. Data are insufficient to recommend prophylactic excision of all congenital nevi.

Genetics

Approximately 8% to 12% of cutaneous melanomas occur in persons with a familial predisposition. These individuals usually have dysplastic nevi as well. Most evidence indicates an autosomal dominant model of transmission for hereditary melanoma with variable penetrance. Some investigators propose a polygenic model of melanoma genesis involving two or more genes and inclusion of environmental factors. The theory of modulation of genetic risk by environmental factors explains the 10-fold increase in incidence of melanoma among Australian families compared with their Celtic ancestors.

The chromosomes reported to be most commonly mutated in melanoma are 1, 6, 7, 9, and 10.[7] Linkage analysis has suggested that hereditary melanoma and dysplastic nevi are associated with mutations in chromosomes 1p and 9p.[8,9] Earlier studies suggest that abnormalities in chromosome 9 may be involved in the initiating events in melanoma tumorigenesis. Abnormalities in the 1p region probably occur late in melanoma progression. A common mutation in sporadic human melanoma is deletion of the long arm of chromosome 6, which occurs in about 40% of these lesions. Correction of this genetic defect can convert a malignant melanoma cell to a normal cell phenotype, suggesting that a tumor suppressor gene may be located on chromosome 6q.[10] Abnormalities in chromosome 7 have been documented in more than half of patients with advanced melanoma. Chromosome 7 maps for the epidermal growth factor receptor, and the mutational defects on chromosome 7 appear to be correlated with overexpression of these receptors on tumor cells. Chromosome 10 translocations have been observed in DNA from melanoma tumors and from dysplastic moles, indicating that this chromosome may be involved in melanoma evolution.[11]

Clinical Diagnosis and Classification

Melanomas have a characteristic appearance (Color Fig. 111-1). Early detection by visual inspection can lead to definitive diagnosis and cure if careful attention is paid to certain features. First, color often varies: brown or black lesions may contain shades of white, red, or blue. Of all the colors, shades of blue are the most ominous. Second, an angular indentation or notching is frequently present at the perimeter of the lesion. Third, irregular elevations of the surface are characteristic. Another indication of potential malignancy is enlargement, darkening, bleeding, or ulceration of a pigmented lesion. None of these clinical signs is pathognomonic, because these features can be present in pigmented BCCs, pigmented seborrheic keratoses, Spitz nevi, dermatofibromas, or hemangiomas. Therefore, any lesion with these characteristics should be excised for biopsy.

Based on growth patterns and clinical characteristics, melanomas can be classified into four major categories: lentigo maligna melanomas, superficial spreading melanomas, nodular melanomas, and acral lentiginous melanomas.[12] Lentigo maligna melanomas constitute 10% to 15% of cutaneous melanomas and are the least aggressive of the four types. They typically occur on the sun-exposed areas of the head and neck and the dorsum of the hands. The median age at diagnosis is 70 years, and prevalence favors women. Clinically, they are large (bigger than 3 cm), flat, tan lesions with areas of dark brown or black pigmentation in some parts and areas of regression in others. Histologically, there is radial growth of abnormal melanocytes in the epidermis with minimal invasion into the papillary dermis. This radial growth process precedes vertical growth and invasion into the papillary dermis by many years. If only a radial growth component is seen, this lesion is called a *lentigo maligna,* or Hutchinson freckle, and is not a malignant melanoma (see Color Fig. 111-1*B*). The vertical growth component is associated with a focal area of elevation that may be darker or lighter than the surrounding lentigo maligna.

Superficial spreading melanomas account for about 70% of cutaneous melanomas and are of intermediate malignancy compared with the other types. These lesions usually arise in a preexisting nevus. The peak incidence is in the fifth decade of life, with an equal distribution between the sexes. There is both a radial and a vertical growth phase. The radial growth phase is characterized by the presence of melanoma tumor cells in the epidermis and papillary dermis and development of a raised, irregular surface on the skin. Vertical growth into the deeper layers of skin is associated with increasing nodularity of the lesion and a greater potential to metastasize. As is discussed later, the depth of invasion has a direct correlation with metastatic potential and prognosis. Superficial spreading melanomas are typically characterized by variation in color, irregular borders, and irregular surface.

Nodular melanomas occur in about 15% to 30% of patients with cutaneous melanoma and are the most aggressive of the four types of melanoma. The median age at diagnosis is 50 years, and these lesions occur twice as often in males as in females. They commonly arise from uninvolved skin rather than from a preexisting nevus. In general, nodular melanomas are bluish black, are more uniform in coloration than the other types, and have smooth borders. They are almost exclusively characterized by a vertical growth phase invading into the deeper layers of skin and often into the subcutis. The lack of a radial growth phase can make early diagnosis difficult.

Acral lentiginous melanoma is a distinct clinicopathologic variant of melanoma that occurs on the palms and soles and in subungual locations (see Color Fig. 111-1*G*). Acral lentiginous melanoma occurs in only 2% to 8% of whites with melanoma but in 35% to 60% of dark-pigmented people (eg, blacks, Hispanics, Asians) who have melanoma. Diagnosis usually is made in the sixth decade of life. These lesions are characterized by a radial growth phase, usually of long duration, followed by a nodular, vertical growth phase associated with metastatic potential. The radial growth phase is associated with a flat lesion with color variation. In subungual locations, this phase can present as an irregular, tan–brown streak in the nail that originates from the base of the nail bed. More than three fourths of subungual melanomas involve the great toe or thumb, and they can be confused with subungual hematoma.

Staging and Prognostic Factors

A great deal of information is available regarding various factors that correlate with the clinical outcome of patients with melanoma. Some of these prognostic factors, such as microstaging and nodal status, are of sufficient independent significance to be incorporated into staging systems with known survival rates. Other prognostic factors, such as sex, age, anatomic location of the primary melanoma, and ulceration, are of variable importance and are discussed later in this section.

Microstaging

One of the most important prognostic features of cutaneous melanoma is the stage of development of the primary tumor. Two methods have been described that assess the microstages of development. Clark and associates[12] described a system by which melanomas are classified according to depth of invasion. They described five levels of invasion related to the histologically defined layers of the skin. The levels are illustrated in Figure 111-2 and are defined as follows:

Level I: All tumor cells are confined to the epidermis with no invasion through the basement membrane (also known as melanoma in situ).

Level II: Tumor cells penetrate through the basement membrane into the papillary dermis but do not extend to the reticular dermis.

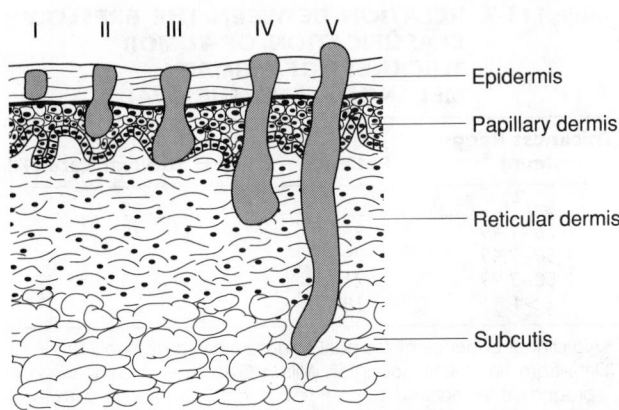

Figure 111-2. The Clark levels of invasion.

Table 111-1. RELATION BETWEEN THE CLARK CLASSIFICATION LEVEL OF INVASION OF PRIMARY MELANOMA AND SURVIVAL

Author	Patients	5-Year Survival Rate by Level (%)			
		II	III	IV	V
Clark et al[13]	208	72	47	32	12
McGovern[14]	183	82	65	49	29
Wanebo et al[15]	151	100	58	58	6
Balch et al[16]	212	85	72	57	28
Eldh et al[17]	324	100	87	72	35
TOTAL	687	$\bar{X}$ = 88	66	54	22

Level III: Tumor cells fill the papillary dermis and abut the reticular dermis but do not invade it.

Level IV: Tumor cells extend into the reticular dermis.

Level V: Tumor cells invade the subcutaneous tissues.

The correlation of the Clark level of invasion with survival is summarized in Table 111-1.[13-17] In general, patients with melanoma in situ (Clark level I) are not considered to have a malignant tumor with potential to metastasize and are adequately treated by complete excision with a 0.5-cm margin of surrounding normal skin. Patients with Clark level II, III, IV, and V tumors have 5-year survival rates of 88%, 66%, 54%, and 22%, respectively.

The other microstaging method that is used routinely was originally described by Breslow.[18] This method classifies the primary tumor according to it thickness, as measured with an ocular micrometer, from the top of the granular layer to the base of the tumor. Many investigators have documented an inverse correlation between tumor thickness and survival. A series of 1786 patients reported on by Balch and colleagues[19] is summarized in Table 111-2. In a larger series of patients, the same researchers demonstrated a continuous inverse relation between tumor thickness and 10-year mortality rate[20] (Fig. 111-3). From these data, they derived a mathematic model defining the relation between tumor thickness and survival, which was confirmed by its application to a different group of melanoma patients with localized disease.

Several studies have demonstrated that tumor thickness conveys more prognostic information than does the deter-

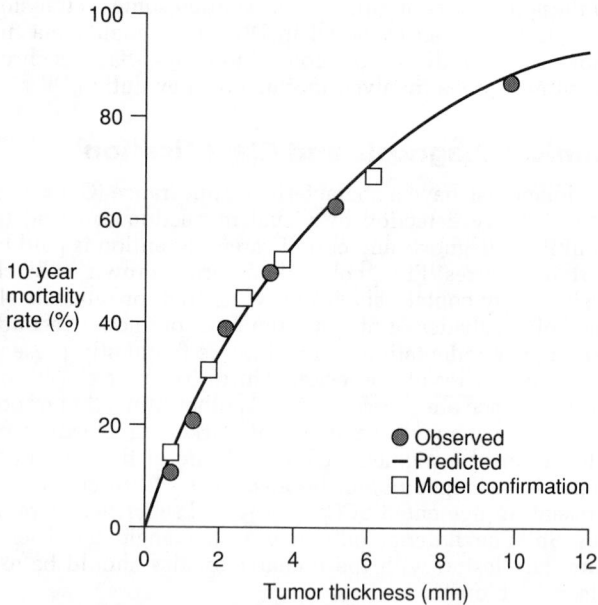

Figure 111-3. Linear relation between melanoma tumor thickness and mortality. The solid line represents mortality predicted by a mathematic model, and the closed circles demonstrate the actual mortality in 2627 patients.[20] The accuracy of the model was verified by applying it to 747 localized melanoma patients from the WHO Melanoma Group and is shown by squares.

mination of Clark level of invasion. Within a single Clark level of invasion, one can find gradations of tumor thickness that have independent prognostic significance. In addition, the measurement of tumor thickness is often more reproducible and less subjective than determination of the Clark level of invasion.

Regional Lymph Node Involvement

The presence of regional lymph node metastases is a grave sign that is associated with a poor prognosis. As in other solid malignancies, such as breast and colorectal cancer, the number of involved lymph nodes has an inverse correlation with long-term survival. The 5-year survival rate for melanoma patients with multiple involved lymph nodes is between 8% and 26%[21-24] (Table 111-3).

Table 111-2. RELATION BETWEEN THE BRESLOW CLASSIFICATION OF TUMOR THICKNESS OF PRIMARY MELANOMA AND SURVIVAL*

Thickness Range (mm)	Patients	5-Year Survival Rate (%)
≤0.75	357	89
0.76–1.49	388	75
1.50–2.49	295	58
2.50–3.99	218	46
>4	184	25

* No clinical evidence of regional or disseminated disease.
(Data from Balch CM, Soong SJ, Milton GW, et al. A comparison of prognostic factors and surgical results in 1,786 patients with localized [stage I] melanoma treated in Alabama, USA and New South Wales, Australia. Ann Surg 1982;196:677)

Table 111-3. RELATION BETWEEN POSITIVE REGIONAL LYMPH NODES AND SURVIVAL*

Investigators	Patients	Positive Lymph Nodes	Survival Rate (%)	
			5 y	10 y
Cohen et al[21]	117	1–3	55	55
		≥4	26	26
Callery et al[22]	150	1–3	45	—
		≥4	21	—
Calabro et al[23]	1001	>1	45	39
		2–4	37	28
		5–10	20	17
		>10	5	3
Bevilacqua et al[24]	176	>1	50	43
		2–3	37	37
		>3	17	8

* Patients presenting with AJC clinical stage I, II, or III.

For patients with only one or two positive lymph nodes, the range is 30% to 55%.

Clinical and Pathologic Staging

In the past, the most widely used staging system consisted of three stages: stage I for localized melanoma, stage II for regional metastases, and stage III for distant metastases. The system was simple and easy to remember, but it did not incorporate microstaging, which allows more accurate determination of prognosis in patients with localized melanoma. This is particularly relevant because it is estimated that up to 85% of newly diagnosed melanoma patients have localized disease by clinical assessment.

The American Joint Committee on Cancer (AJCC) developed a four-stage system that divides clinically localized melanomas into subgroups according to the thickness of the lesion (Table 111-4):

Stage IA—less than 0.75 mm thick
Stage IB—0.76 to 1.5 mm thick
Stage IIA—1.51 to 4 mm thick
Stage IIB—more than 4 mm thick

Stage III represents regional nodal involvement, and stage IV melanomas have evidence of disseminated metastases. Figure 111-4 shows survival rates associated with the four stages. This TNM system provides a useful classification method for clinicians involved in the treatment of melanoma patients. In general, clinically localized, thin lesions are AJCC stages IA and IB, intermediate-thickness lesions are AJCC stage IIA, and thick melanomas are classified as AJCC stage IIB.

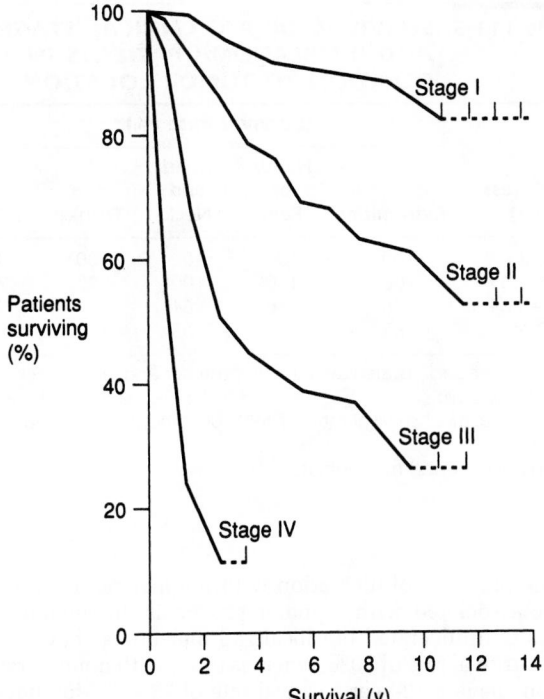

Figure 111-4. Survival according to AJC staging system. (After Balch CM, Soong S-J, Shaw HM, et al. An analysis of prognostic factors in 4000 patients with cutaneous melanoma. In: Balch CM, Milton GW, eds. Cutaneous melanoma: clinical management and treatment results worldwide. Philadelphia, JB Lippincott, 1985:321)

Table 111-4. AMERICAN JOINT COMMISSION ON CANCER MELANOMA STAGING SYSTEM, 1985

TNM DEFINITIONS

Primary Tumor

TX	Unknown, cannot be assessed
T0	Atypical melanocytic hyperplasia in situ, Clark I
T1	Clark II, 0.75 mm or smaller
T2	Clark III, 0.76–1.5 mm
T3	Clark IV, 1.51–4 mm
	Clark V, larger than 4 mm or satellites within 2 cm of
T4	primary tumor

Regional Lymph Node Involvement

NX	Unknown, cannot be assessed
N0	Negative
N1	One regional node station, nodes mobile, 5 cm in diameter or smaller, or negative nodes and fewer than five in-transit metastases
N2	More than one node station positive, nodes larger than 5 cm or fixed, more than five in-transit metastases, or any metastases with positive nodes

Distant Metastasis

MX	Unknown, cannot be assessed
M0	None
M1	Skin or subcutaneous tissue beyond the primary nodal area
M2	Visceral

STAGE GROUPING

Stage IA	T1, N0, M0
Stage IB	T2, N0, M0
Stage IIA	T3, N0, M0
Stage IIB	T4, N0, M0
Stage III	Any T, N1, M0
Stage IV	Any T, N2, M0, or any T, any N, M1–2

Other Prognostic Factors

The major prognostic factors that predict survival in melanoma patients have been accounted for in the AJCC staging system; namely, tumor microstaging, nodal status, and distant metastases. Nevertheless, because most patients with newly diagnosed melanomas have localized disease, additional prognostic information can be helpful to the patient and the clinician. Several other factors evaluated in multifactorial analyses of localized AJCC stage I and II disease are significant predictors of survival.

The anatomic location of melanomas is a significant independent prognostic indicator in patients with clinically localized disease.[25] Patients with melanomas of the extremities, excluding the hands and feet, have a better survival rate than those with lesions arising on the trunk or on the head and neck. Among patients with extremity melanomas, those with lesions on their hands and feet do significantly worse than patients with lesions on the remaining extremity sites. Certain anatomic subsites, including the upper back, posterior arm, posterior neck, and posterior scalp, appear to be associated with a poorer prognosis for intermediate-thickness melanomas (Table 111-5).

Women with melanomas have a better survival rate than men.[26] One explanation for this observation may be the different distribution sites of melanomas in men and women. In several studies, the incidence of melanomas arising in the lower extremities, a favorable anatomic location, is significantly higher in women than in men. Conversely, the incidence of truncal melanomas, which are generally associated with poorer survival, is higher in men than in women (Table 111-6). The prevalence of head, neck, and upper extremity melanomas is equal in men and women.

Table 111-5. SURVIVAL OF AJC CLINICAL STAGE I AND II MELANOMA PATIENTS IN RELATION TO TUMOR LOCATION

Thickness (mm)	Survival Rate (%)*				
	Extremities	Hands or Feet	Head and Neck	Trunk†	BANS
<0.85	100	100	100	100	98
0.85–1.69	100	100	100	97	78
1.7–3.64	86	60	64	77	58
≥3.65	83	0	65	12	33

BANS, upper back, posterolateral arm, posterior and lateral neck, and posterior scalp.

* 7.5-year acturial survival rates of 598 AJC clinical stage I and II patients.[25]

† Non-BANS truncal melanomas.

The presence of ulceration within a melanoma appears to be associated with a poorer prognosis. In general, patients with ulcerated but localized melanomas have a 10-year survival rate of 50%, whereas those with nonulcerated lesions have a 10-year survival rate of 78%.[20] Men have a higher proportion of ulcerated lesions than women (27% versus 19%), and this may be another explanation for their lower survival rate. Although ulceration appears to correlate with thickness of the melanoma, the presence of ulceration has been shown to be an independent prognostic factor.

At the cellular level, Clark and coworkers[27] further described histologic characteristics of localized melanomas that can help determine prognosis. Melanomas were described according to their particular growth phase. Lesions determined to be in the radial growth phase were nontumorigenic and were associated with an excellent prognosis. In contrast, lesions determined to have evidence of a vertical growth phase were prone to be tumorigenic. These lesions had the potential to metastasize and were associated with a poorer prognosis. The vertical growth phase was defined as the presence of larger aggregates of tumor cells within the papillary dermis, often markedly different in pigment from cells in the radial growth phase and associated with increased mitotic cells.

Genetic markers will have a more significant role as prognostic factors in the future. The presence of abnormal DNA content (DNA aneuploidy), as determined by flow cytometry, has been reported to be an unfavorable predictor of prognosis in patients with localized melanoma.[28] In patients with metastatic melanoma, structural abnormalities of chromosomes 7 or 11, as determined by cytogenetic analysis, have been reported to be associated with decreased survival.[29]

Treatment of Primary Melanoma

Biopsy

For melanoma, the tumor thickness (Breslow depth of invasion) is the single variable that most accurately determines therapy and prognosis. A full-thickness biopsy to the adipose tissue is required for any lesion suspicious for melanoma. If the melanoma is transected with a partial-thickness shave biopsy, the ability to obtain an accurate measurement of tumor thickness is lost. Therefore, a superficial shave biopsy is never recommended for a suspicious pigmented lesion. Before biopsy, a morphologic description of the lesion and a photograph can be useful for complete documentation. Also, the use of a Wood lamp can help to delineate the subclinical pigment extension, particularly with lentigo maligna melanomas on the head and neck.

Excisional biopsy with 1- to 2-mm margins is the preferred method for suspicious lesions to provide the pathologist a total specimen for histologic interpretation and microstaging. Formalin-fixed, paraffin-embedded, permanent sections should be used for biopsy diagnosis of primary cutaneous melanoma to accurately determine tumor thickness and other histopathologic prognostic variables. Frozen sections do not have a role in the microstaging of primary melanomas. If the lesion is a melanoma, the excisional biopsy represents the first stage of a two-stage procedure. The second stage is reexcision to the underlying muscle fascia with margins ranging from 0.5 to 3 cm, depending on the tumor thickness (see next section). The orientation of the biopsy is usually determined according to the ease of a potential future wide local excision and parallel orientation to the lymphatic drainage.

For suggestive lesions that are too large for complete excision and those that are located where the amount of skin is critical in terms of functional or cosmetic results, an incisional biopsy may be performed with either a scalpel or a punch tool 4 to 6 mm in diameter. Incisional biopsies for melanoma do not increase the risk of metastasis or affect patient survival. They should be performed on the most raised or most pigmented area of the lesion to maximize the obtainable diagnostic and prognostic information. The most raised area usually corresponds to the maximal thickness of the lesion. Several punch biopsies can be obtained from different areas for lesions with multiple morphologic features.

The excisional or incisional saucerization biopsy technique can also be used for melanoma. After appropriate skin preparation and establishment of local anesthesia, the scalpel blade is placed on the skin at a 45- to 60-degree angle. The skin is cut through the dermis to the adipose tissue, and the biopsy specimen is removed with pickup forceps. Homeostasis is obtained with electrocautery, chemical cautery, or fibrin foam. No sutures are used, and the wound is allowed to heal by second intention, which takes 3 to 6 weeks. Again, a shave biopsy through the dermis is never recommended for a lesion suggestive of melanoma because of the risk of transection of the lesion. One disadvantage of the saucerization biopsy technique is the risk of secondary bacterial colonization in the wound during healing. However, delay of the definitive wide local excision until complete reepithelialization has occurred is usually not necessary with the use of preoperative antibiotics.

Either incisional or excisional biopsy of skin lesions suspected to be melanoma is acceptable. Care must be taken

Table 111-6. DISTRIBUTION OF MELANOMAS WITH RESPECT TO GENDER

Location	Occurrence (%)	
	Men	Women
Scalp	7	3
Face	12	9
Neck	5	3
Arm	13	19
Front of body	16	8
Back of body	36	23
Leg	9	31
Sole of foot	2	4

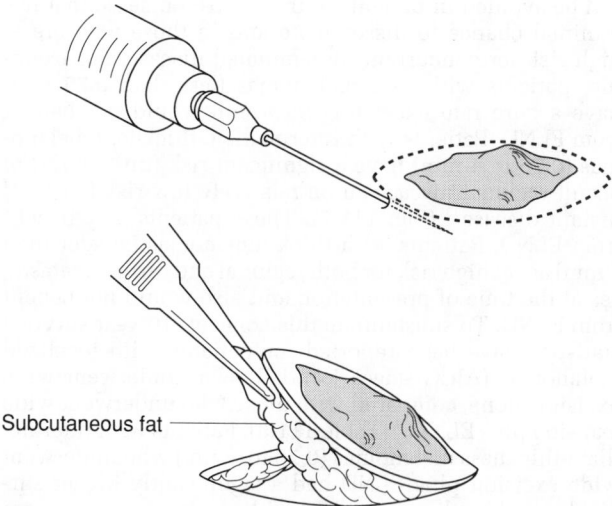

Figure 111-5. Techniques for biopsy of melanoma. (After Urist MM, Balch CM, Milton GW. Surgical management of primary melanoma. In: Balch CM, Milton GW, eds. Cutaneous melanoma. Philadelphia, JB Lippincott, 1985:74)

Subcutaneous fat

to obtain a full-thickness specimen into the subcutaneous tissue so that the pathologist can determine the microstaging of the lesion. Shave or curette biopsy is not indicated for lesions suspected to be melanoma, because microstaging cannot be ascertained from the specimen.

An excisional biopsy can easily be accomplished with lesions less than 1.5 cm in diameter. After infiltration of a local anesthetic around the lesion, but not into it, the lesion can be excised with an elliptical skin incision encompassing underlying subcutaneous tissue (Fig. 111-5). The incision should be placed so as not to compromise a subsequent wide excision. For small lesions, an excisional biopsy can be accomplished with a 6-mm punch biopsy instrument, making sure that underlying subcutaneous tissue is obtained. An incisional biopsy is performed for large lesions and for lesions of the face, hands, or feet, for which the amount of skin is critical. These biopsies can be performed with a scalpel or a 6-mm punch biopsy instrument. Care must be taken to obtain the incisional biopsy in the most raised or irregular area of the lesion.

Surgical Excision of Primary Melanoma

For melanoma in situ, excision of normal skin 0.5 cm around the lesion or previous biopsy site is acceptable for local control. For invasive cutaneous melanoma, wide excision of the primary tumor or biopsy site has been advocated for optimal local control. Limited excisions, such as excisional biopsies, are associated with local recurrence rates in the range of 30% to 60%. The optimal extent of the wide excision has been somewhat controversial. Until recently, the routine approach was to excise all primary melanomas with a 3- to 5-cm margin; this procedure often required a split-thickness skin graft for coverage. The rationale for such a generous margin was to remove clinically occult subcutaneous or intradermal satellite deposits of melanoma tumor cells. In numerous reports, wide excision of melanomas, including 3- to 5-cm margins, was associated with local recurrence rates in the range of 7% or less.

With the accumulation of more information, it has become clear that less than the traditional wide local excision is adequate for the surgical treatment of thin melanomas. The risk of local recurrence correlates more with the thickness of the melanoma than with the margin of excision.

Local recurrence after excision of melanomas less than 1 mm thick is rare regardless of the extent of the margin. The World Health Organization[30] (WHO) reported a prospective study in which patients with primary melanomas less than 2 mm thick were randomly assigned to receive excision with margins of either 1 cm (narrow) or 3 cm or more (wide). A total of 612 patients were entered into the study, 305 having narrow excisions and 307 having wide excisions. No local recurrences were seen in any patients with tumors less than 1 mm thick, regardless of the excision margin. Three local recurrences were reported in the group of patients with melanomas 1 to 2 mm thick, all of whom had undergone narrow excision. More importantly, the disease-free and overall survival rates were not significantly different between the two groups after a median follow-up of 55 months. These results clearly indicate that excision margins of 1 cm provide excellent local control for lesions less than 1 mm thick.

A prospective, randomized study evaluated the efficacy of 2-cm versus 4-cm margins for intermediate-thickness melanomas measuring 1 to 4 mm.[31] This study involved 486 patients with localized melanomas who were observed for a median of 6 years after excision. The local recurrence rate was 0.8% for patients who had 2-cm margins and 1.7% for those who had 4-cm margins; the difference was not statistically significant. As expected, the narrower margins significantly reduced the need for skin grafting and shortened the hospital stay. The results of this study demonstrated that 2-cm margins were sufficient to treat intermediate-thickness lesions. For lesions more than 4 mm thick, excision margins of at least 3 cm should be considered the standard approach. Recommended excision margins are outlined in Table 111-7.

Despite these recommendations, the site of the melanoma can affect the extent of the excision. Facial lesions usually cannot be excised with more than a 1-cm margin because of the adjacency of vital structures. Subungual melanomas should always be treated by amputation, usually at the metatarsophalangeal or metacarpophalangeal joint, so that adequate skin closure can be achieved. For plantar melanomas requiring wide excision, split-thickness skin grafts have proved simple and adequate if properly padded shoes are used.

Treatment of Regional Metastatic Melanoma

Lymphadenectomy Results and Indications

Surgical excision of metastases to regional lymph nodes is the only potentially curative therapy. The 5-year survival rate for patients who undergo lymphadenectomy for clinically positive involved nodes (AJCC stage III) ranges from 13% to 39%. In addition, for those patients not cured by lymphadenectomy, resection can avoid potential pain associated with tumor enlargement, skin breakdown, and

Table 111-7. SURGICAL MARGINS FOR MELANOMA EXCISIONS

Melanoma Thickness (mm)	Margin (cm)
In situ	0.5
<1	1
1–4	2
>4	3

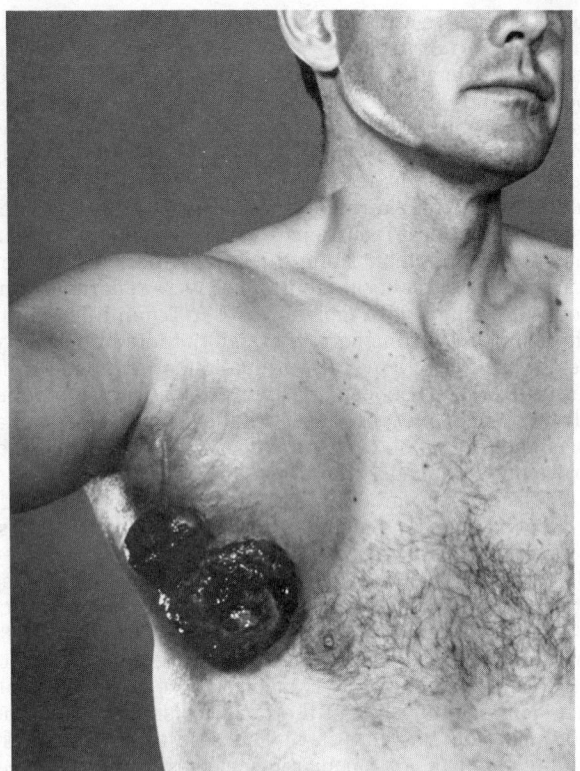

Figure 111-6. Patient with large melanoma axillary involvement with skin ulceration.

tumor necrosis (Fig. 111-6). Only 10% of patients who first present with the diagnosis of melanoma have clinical evidence of nodal metastases; about 85% have localized disease; the remaining 5% have distant metastases.[32] In less than 15% of patients, a diagnosis of melanoma is made in the absence of a definable primary lesion. If patients present with isolated nodal disease from an unknown primary site, the results of lymphadenectomy are similar to those for patients with known primary tumors.

The surgical excision of clinically positive lymph nodes is referred to as a *therapeutic lymph node dissection.* Some surgeons prefer to excise clinically normal-appearing regional lymph nodes because of the risk of occult or microscopic metastases. This procedure is known as *elective lymph node dissection* (ELND). ELND is one of the most controversial procedures in surgical oncology.

Advocates of ELND claim that resection of occult metastases in the regional nodes can prevent disseminated disease. They also argue that the results of lymph node dissections for clinically palpable disease are not as good as for nonpalpable micrometastatic disease. By contrast, advocates of delayed lymph node dissections observe all patients with clinically localized melanomas expectantly and subject them to lymphadenectomy only if there is clinical evidence of nodal spread. They reason that this "wait and watch" approach saves many patients the morbidity of unnecessary surgery without adversely affecting the survival chances of patients in whom nodal disease develops.

Several retrospective and two prospective studies have attempted to address these issues. The retrospective studies have reported conflicting data on the efficacy of ELND. The establishment of the microstaging systems has led to the hope that certain subgroups of patients can be identified who will benefit from ELND. The contention is that tumor thickness can identify those patients who may benefit from a lymphadenectomy; at the same time, dissection

can be avoided in patients with localized disease that has minimal chance to disseminate and in those who are at high risk for concurrent disseminated disease. For example, patients with thin melanomas (less than 0.75 mm) have a cure rate exceeding 95% and would not benefit from ELND. Patients with intermediate-thickness melanomas (0.76 to 4 mm) have a significant risk (up to 60%) of occult regional disease and a relatively low risk (15%) of distant disease[33] (Fig. 111-7). These patients may benefit from ELND. Patients with thick melanomas (greater than 4 mm) are at high risk for both regional and distant metastases at the time of presentation and also would not benefit from ELND. To substantiate this concept, 10-year survival statistics have been reported for patients with localized melanomas (AJCC stages I and II) who underwent wide excision alone, compared with those who underwent wide excision plus ELND[34] (Table 111-8). Patients with intermediate-thickness melanomas (0.76 to 4 mm) who underwent wide excision plus ELND had a significantly higher survival rate than those who had wide excision alone. These findings remained consistent after the analysis was stratified for tumor sites. There was no survival benefit for ELND in patients with thin (less than 0.75 mm) or thick (greater than 4 mm) lesions. Despite the results of this study, unaccounted variables may have played a role in the choice of treatment, as can occur with any retrospective analysis.[35] Therefore, the efficacy of ELND must be determined by prospective, randomized studies.

Two prospective studies have addressed ELND, and both reported no improvement in survival for patients treated by ELND. The WHO Melanoma Group conducted a study of clinically localized extremity melanoma (AJCC stages I and II) in which 267 patients were randomly assigned to receive wide excision plus ELND and 286 to have wide excision alone plus therapeutic lymphadenectomy if clinically indicated at follow-up.[36] Results from this study showed no difference in survival between the two groups (Fig. 111-8). Additional analyses by sex, tumor thickness,

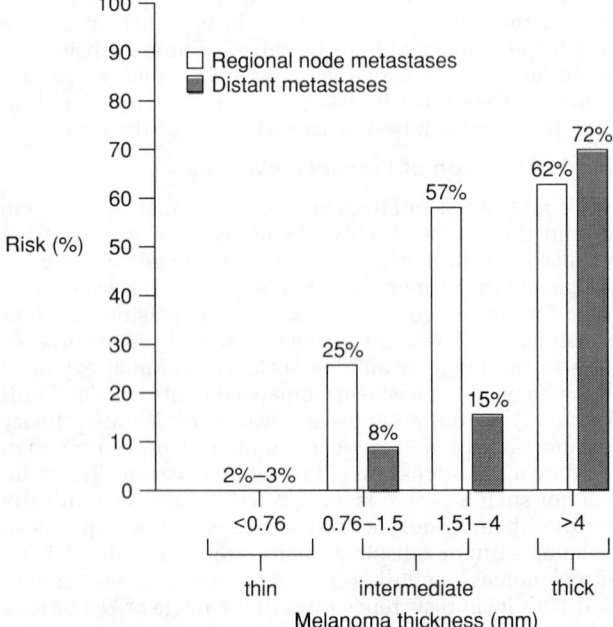

Figure 111-7. Relation of tumor thickness to risk of regional nodal and disseminated metastases. (After Balch CM. The role of elective lymph node dissection in melanoma: rationale, results, and controversies. J Clin Oncol 1988;6:163)

Table 111-8. NONRANDOMIZED EXPERIENCE WITH WIDE EXCISION VERSUS WIDE EXCISION PLUS ELECTIVE LYMPH NODE DISSECTION FOR AJC STAGES I AND II MELANOMAS*

Tumor Thickness (mm)	10-Year Survival Rate (%)			
	Extremity (N)		Trunk, Head, and Neck (N)	
	WE	WE + ELND	WE	WE + ELND
<0.76	94 (142)	100 (26)	86 (135)	83 (38)
0.76–1.49	74 (125)	92† (66)	56 (131)	80† (51)
1.5–3.99	54 (114)	80† (107)	33 (129)	64† (129)
≥4	30 (33)	44 (34)	22 (56)	26 (38)

WE, wide excision; ELND, elective lymph node dissection.

* Experience from the Sydney Melanoma Unit, Australia, and the University of Alabama, Birmingham.[34]

† Significantly different from WE alone.

level of invasion, and other variables did not identify any subgroup benefiting from ELND. About 20% of patients who underwent ELND had micrometastases in the specimens; and about 20% of patients who underwent excision alone later received therapeutic lymph node dissections. The 5-year survival rate was 50% for the subgroup of patients in whom occult micrometastases were found at ELND; this rate was not significantly different from the rate of 45% reported for patients who underwent therapeutic lymphadenectomy for clinically apparent nodal metastases.

The second prospective study was conducted by the Mayo Clinic.[37] In this study, 171 clinical AJCC stage I and II patients were randomly assigned to one of three treatment groups: 62 underwent wide excision only, 55 had ELND delayed 30 to 60 days after primary tumor excision, and 54 had concomitant ELND with excision of the primary tumor. Patients with primary lesions on the head and neck or the midline trunk were excluded. After disease-free and overall survival rates were analyzed, there were no significant differences between the groups.

Neither the WHO Melanoma Group nor the Mayo Clinic study revealed any advantage to ELND in localized extremity melanomas. A major criticism of these studies is that they included a high number of patients with thin melanomas. Clearly, from retrospective studies, ELND for thin melanomas (less than 1 mm) does not offer survival benefit, and this could have influenced the results of the prospective studies. In addition, these studies did not include patients with truncal or head and neck melanomas, which may behave differently than extremity melanomas.

Additional prospective, randomized trials are underway to evaluate ELND in high-risk melanoma patients. One study is the Intergroup Melanoma Study, which is evaluating ELND in patients with melanomas 1 to 4 mm thick and which includes extremity, truncal, and head and neck sites. A second study is being conducted by the WHO Melanoma Group and involves patients with truncal melanomas whose primary tumors measure more than 2 mm in thickness. The results of these studies may help resolve the controversy surrounding this issue.

A new technique has been developed to identify the first draining lymph node adjacent to a cutaneous melanoma, known as the "sentinel" node.[38] It has been hypothesized that melanoma involvement of a nodal basin develops in an orderly fashion and that involvement of the sentinel node is the first step of this process. By injection of a blue dye intradermally around the site of the primary mela-

noma, the sentinel node can be identified by exploration through a small incision and retrieved for histologic examination. With this blue dye technique, patients with clinically localized melanomas have been found to have tumor involvement in the sentinel node about 20% of the time.[38] Moreover, in these studies, in which a complete node dissection was performed in all patients, a negative sentinel node accurately predicted that the remaining nodes in the dissection were also uninvolved. This technique appears to be useful as a way of selecting patients, from among those who appear to have localized melanoma (AJCC stage I or II), for lymph node dissection. Whether application of this approach improves survival, compared with the wait and watch approach, remains to be evaluated in prospective studies.

Site-Specific Considerations for Regional Lymphadenectomy

The nodal drainage areas accessible for surgical excision include the ilioinguinal, axillary, cervical, and parotid regions. With truncal melanomas, or if the tumor is located in the midline, the primary nodal drainage may not be obvious. Lymphatic vessels from the upper half of the body generally drain to the axilla, and those from the lower half of the trunk drain into the inguinal region. A valid predictor of the lymphatic watershed for the groin and axillary lymph nodes is the Sappey line, which curves upward from 2 cm above the umbilicus to the level of the second and third lumbar vertebrae. Occasionally, melanomas of the upper trunk drain to the supraclavicular region.

Two contiguous, node-bearing regions exist in the ilioinguinal area. The first is composed of the superficial femoral nodes located within the femoral triangle, and the second contains the deep nodes above the inguinal ligament along the iliac and obturator vessels. Removal of the femoral nodes is referred to as a *superficial groin dissection,* and removal of the iliac and obturator nodes is called a *deep groin dissection* (Fig. 111-9).

Controversy surrounds the benefit of a deep groin dissection, which some surgeons elect to perform if there is evidence of palpable femoral lymph node involvement. In this situation, about one third of patients are likely to have

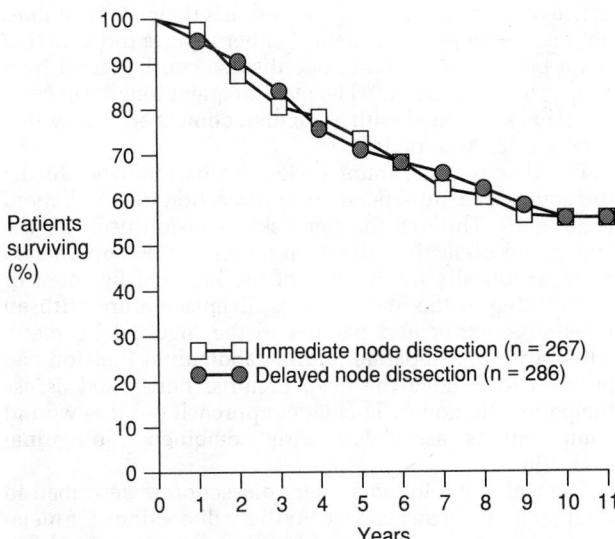

Figure 111-8. Randomized study of immediate elective lymph node dissection versus delayed therapeutic node dissection by WHO Melanoma Group. No significant difference in survival was seen between the groups.

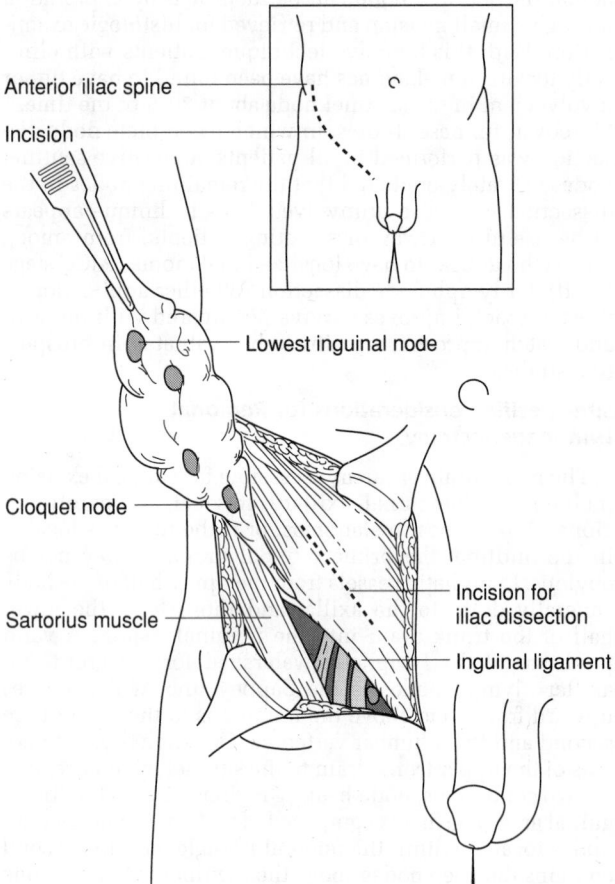

Figure 111-9. Technique of groin dissection.

tumor involvement of the deep inguinal nodes. The rarity of involvement of the deep inguinal nodes when the superficial nodes are pathologically negative or harbor only microscopic disease does not warrant a deep groin dissection in those situations. Some reports indicate that the presence of positive deep groin nodes is associated with a high incidence of disseminated disease and that their removal does not lead to long-term benefit.[39] Other reports indicate that some patients with iliac node disease can be cured by a deep groin dissection.[40] The most frequent long-term complication associated with groin dissection is edema, which occurs in 25% of patients.

The iliac and obturator nodes can be removed during the course of a superficial groin dissection by a variety of techniques. Through the same skin incision used for the superficial dissection, the deep nodes can be approached extraperitoneally by division of the inguinal ligament or by splitting of the abdominal wall musculature with an incision superior and parallel to the inguinal ligament. Alternatively, a separate midline abdominal incision can be used to remove the deep inguinal nodes and assess the paraaortic nodes. This latter approach reduces wound complications associated with combined ilioinguinal dissections.

The technique for an axillary dissection is described in Chapter 61 on breast cancer. Axillary dissections for melanoma should include removal of lymph nodes lateral, beneath, and medial to the pectoralis minor muscle (levels I to III). The axillary lymph node region is contiguous with the supraclavicular node region. Evidence of supraclavicular nodal involvement is not uncommon if bulky axillary

disease is present. There is no satisfactory procedure to remove contiguous involved axillary and supraclavicular lymph nodes. In these situations, axillary dissection is noncurative and should be considered only for palliation. Long-term complications associated with axillary dissections are infrequent; arm edema and pain occur in less than 5% of patients.

Metastases to the lymph nodes from head and neck melanomas follow predictable pathways. Melanomas arising on the scalp or face anterior to the pinna of the ear and superior to the commissure of the lip metastasize to the parotid region. Lesions inferior to the commissure of the lip spread to the cervical region. Melanomas that occur on the posterior scalp behind the pinna usually spread to occipital and posterior cervical lymph nodes. Because the parotid nodes are contiguous with the cervical nodes, a radical neck dissection to remove the cervical nodes is often performed in combination with a superficial parotid node dissection for anterior facial melanomas.

Adjuvant Therapy

Patients who undergo lymphadenectomy for AJCC stage III disease are at high risk for recurrent disease (see Fig. 111-4). These patients, as well as those who undergo surgical excision for localized deep melanomas, are in need of effective adjuvant therapy to eliminate residual micrometastatic disease. No effective adjuvant therapies are available for these patients. The WHO Melanoma Group reported on a randomized, prospective trial of 761 patients with AJCC stage IB, IIA, IIB, and III disease to evaluate chemotherapy and immunotherapy as adjuvant treatments after definitive surgical excision.[41] Patients were randomly assigned to four groups: those who received surgery alone, those who received surgery plus dacarbazine (DTIC) chemotherapy, those who received surgery plus bacille Calmette-Guérin (BCG) immunotherapy, and those patients who received surgery plus DTIC and BCG therapy. No improvement in survival was seen with any of the therapies compared with surgery alone. The identification of an effective adjuvant therapy in melanoma is an area of active investigation. Clinical trials evaluating biologic agents such as interferon-α and tumor vaccines are underway.

Treatment of Disseminated Melanoma

Evaluation for Metastatic Disease and Clinical Course

The follow-up evaluation for patients with AJCC stage I, II, or III melanoma who are rendered tumor-free by surgery should include regular histories and physical examinations. The use of extensive and frequent radiographic studies and blood work in asymptomatic, clinically disease-free patients is rarely productive. Patients with surgically excised thin (AJCC stage I) melanomas should be examined every 6 months for 5 years and yearly thereafter. Specific examination for local or regional recurrences should be performed, because surgical therapy may prove curative. In addition, a total skin examination to identify new primary melanomas should be performed. Patients with AJCC stage II or III melanomas who are clinically disease-free should be examined every 3 or 4 months for 5 years and then yearly thereafter. Yearly chest radiographs and liver function studies may be considered for evaluation of visceral disease. Lactic dehydrogenase levels have been reported to be elevated in a significant number of patients with metastatic disease. Attention should be directed to any gastrointestinal or central nervous system symptoms. Appropriate diagnostic studies can be obtained based on the clinical history and physical findings.

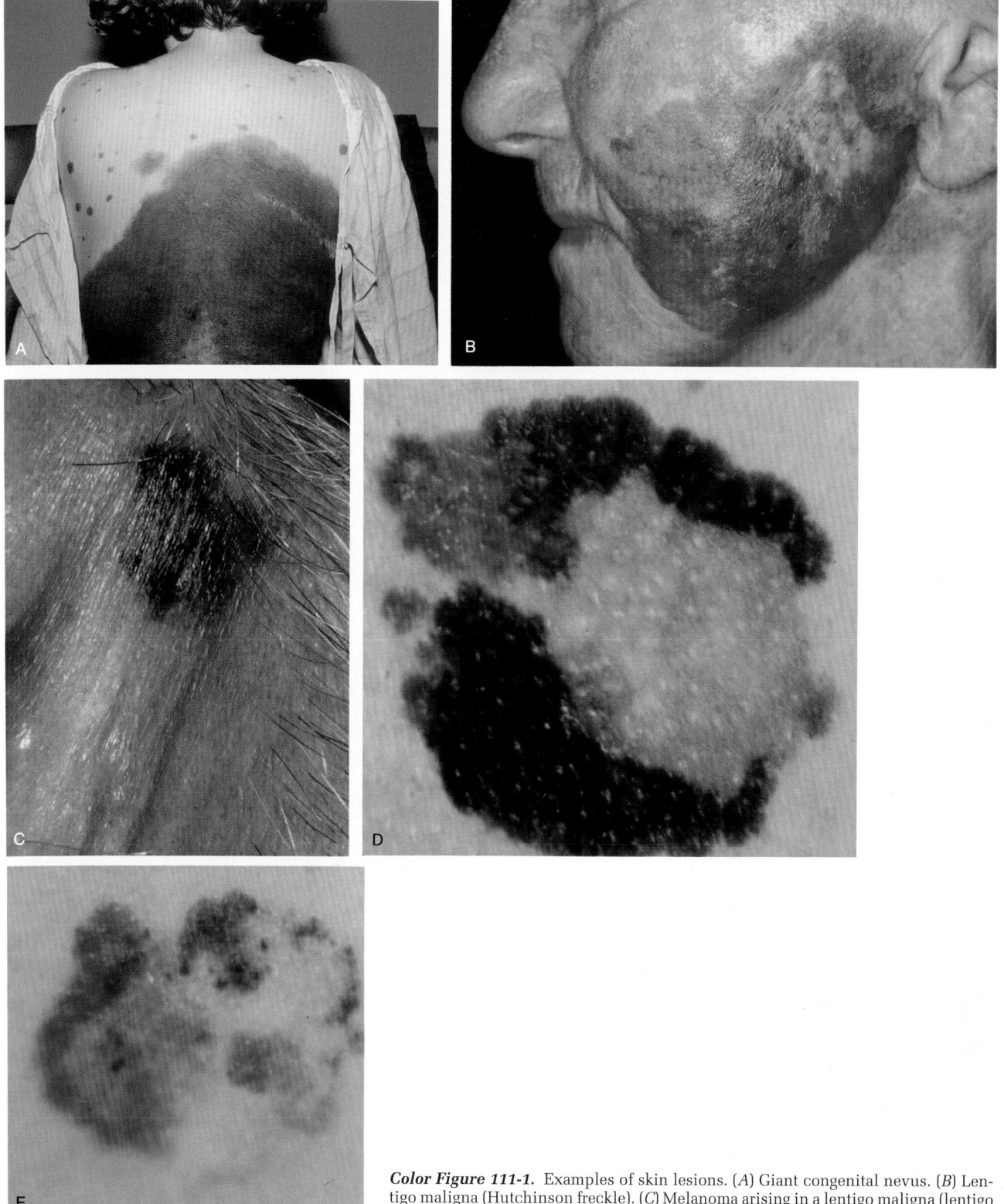

Color Figure 111-1. Examples of skin lesions. (*A*) Giant congenital nevus. (*B*) Lentigo maligna (Hutchinson freckle). (*C*) Melanoma arising in a lentigo maligna (lentigo maligna melanoma). (*D* and *E*) Superficial spreading melanoma. *(continues)*

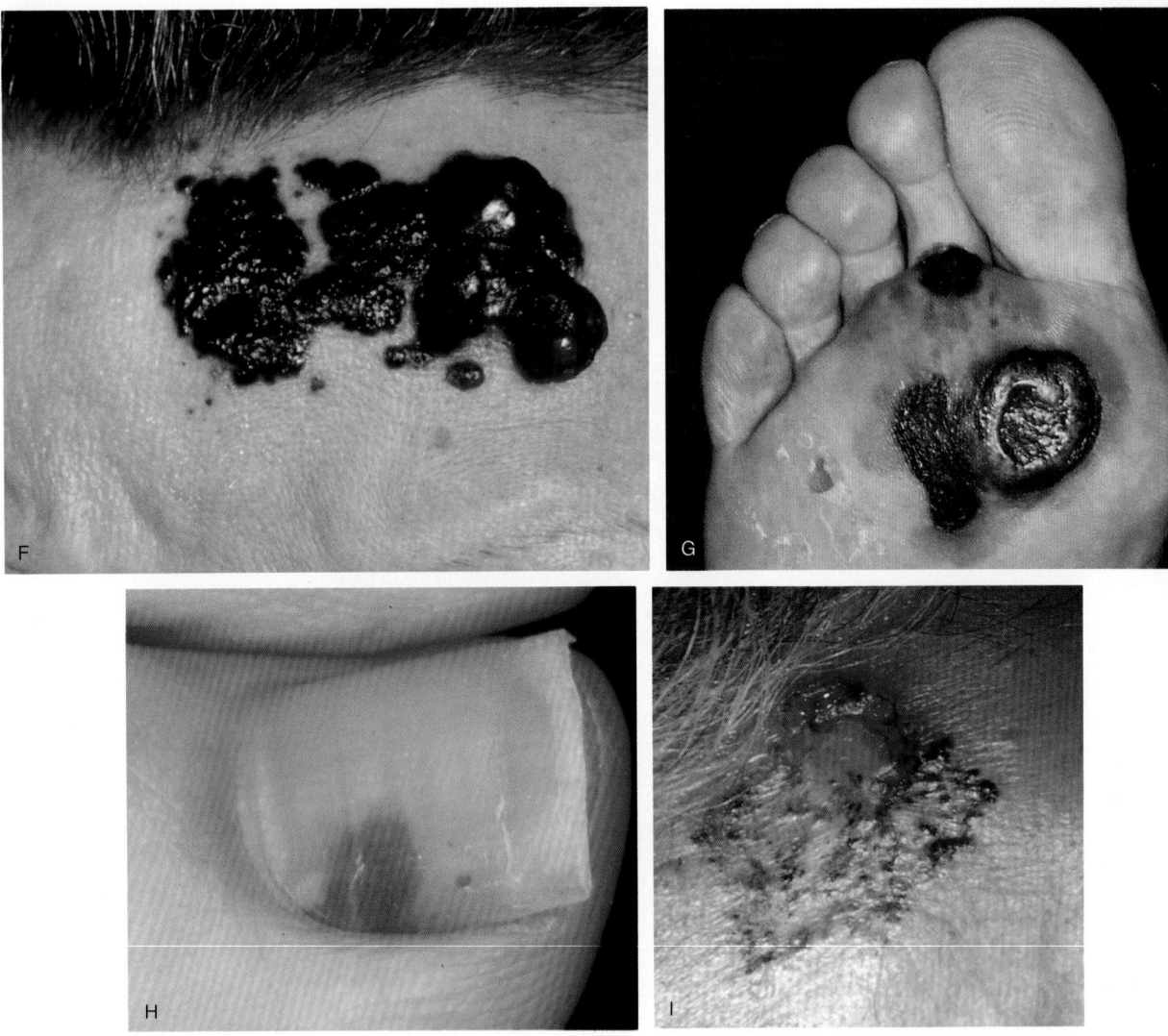

Color Figure 111-1. *(Continued)* (*F*) Nodular melanoma. (*G*) Acral lentiginous melanoma (ulcerated nodular plantar melanoma with satellite lesions). (*H*) Subungual melanoma. (*I*) Pigmented basal cell carcinoma.

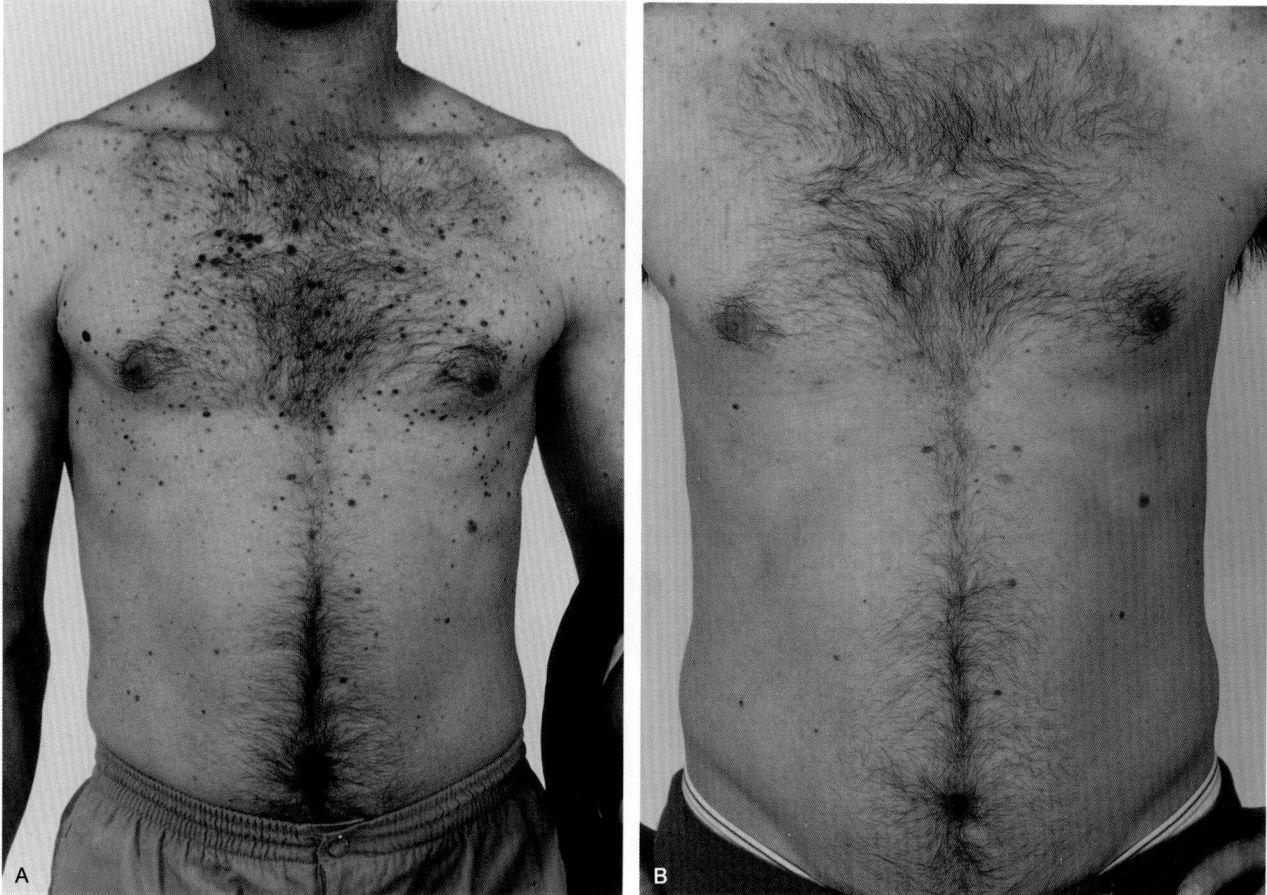

Color Figure 111-2. (*A*) Patient with disseminated melanoma metastatic to multiple cutaneous sites. (*B*) After several courses of therapy with lymphokine-activated killer cells and interleukin-2, the patient had a complete response. (Courtesy of Steven A. Rosenberg, MD, Surgery Branch, National Cancer Institute, Bethesda)

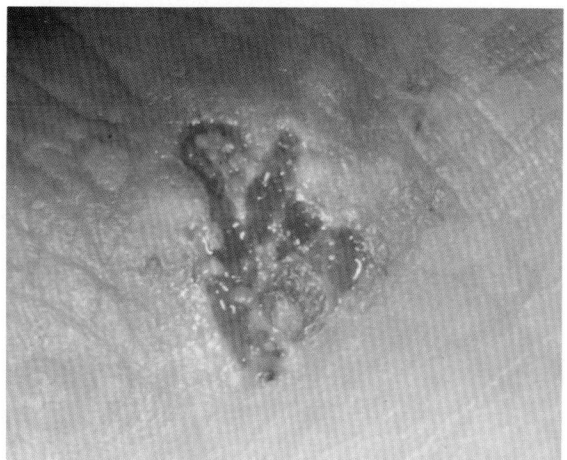

Color Figure 111-3. Squamous cell carcinoma of the hand secondary to exposure to arsenic in welding flux.

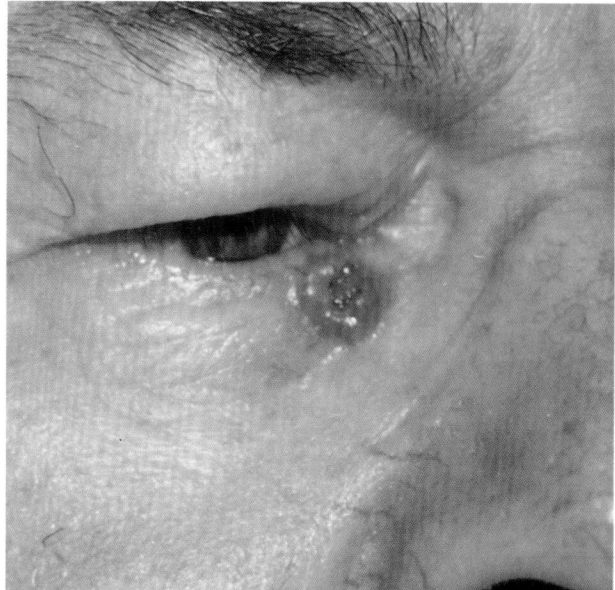

Color Figure 111-4. Basal cell carcinoma near the eye.

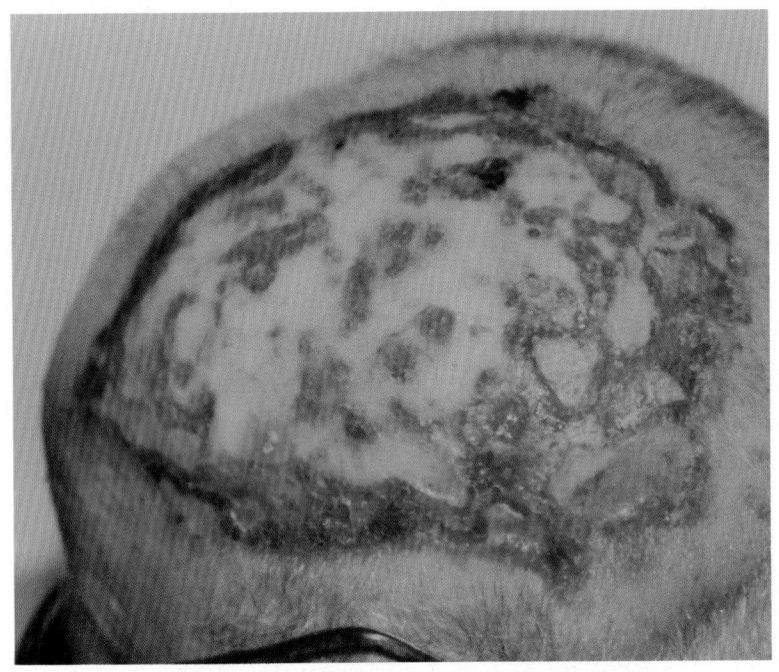

Color Figure 111-5. Morpheaform basal cell carcinoma of the scalp.

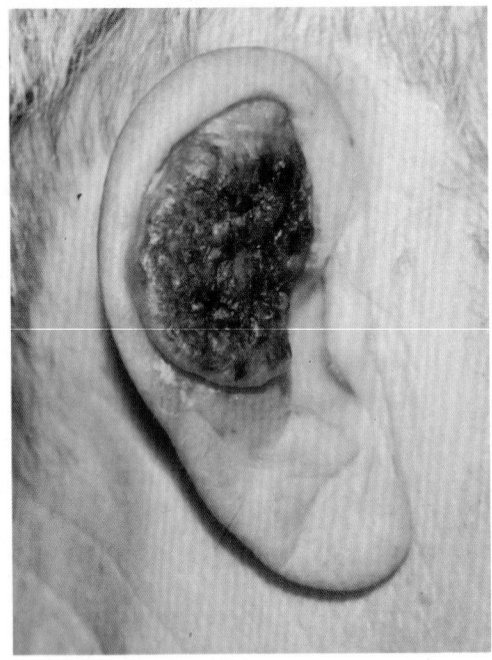

Color Figure 111-6. Ulcerative squamous cell carcinoma.

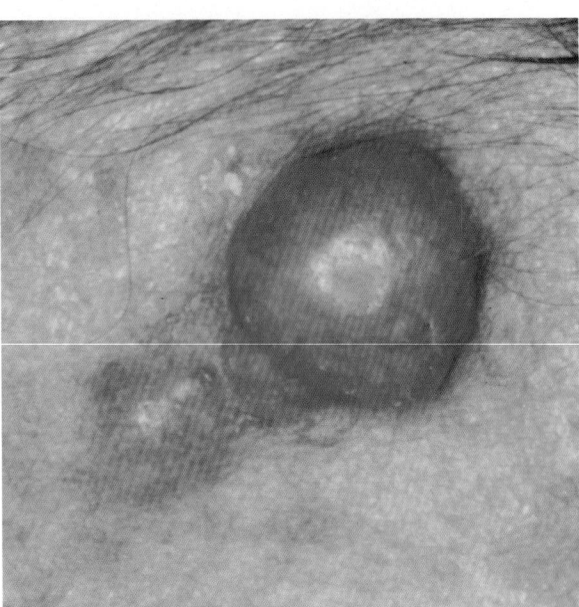

Color Figure 111-7. Merkel cell carcinoma.

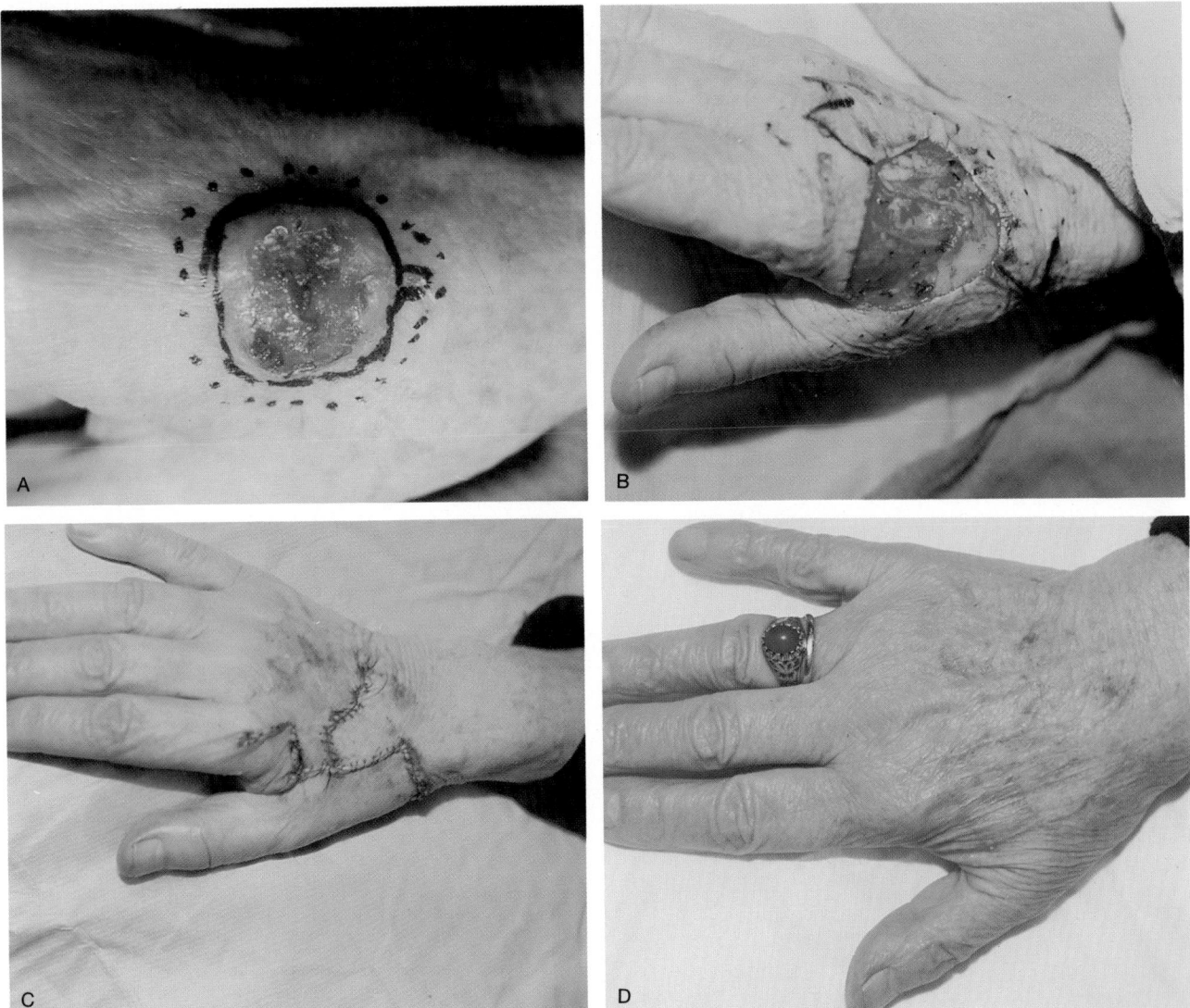

Color Figure 111-8. (*A*) Patient with a 3 × 3-cm basal cell carcinoma on the right dorsal hand with mixed nodular and aggressive growth histologic pattern. (*B*) Final Mohs surgery defect measuring 4 × 4.8 cm to the underlying tendon with preservation of tendon and nerve structures. Complete excision of the tumor required two Mohs stages (10 frozen sections). (*C*) The defect was reconstructed immediately after achievement of clear margins under local anesthesia in the Mohs Surgery Unit using birhombic flap soft tissue reconstruction. (*D*) Result 3 months after surgery.

Melanoma can disseminate to any organ. The most common sites of recurrence are skin, subcutaneous tissues, and distant lymph nodes, followed by visceral sites. Common visceral sites of metastasis, in order of decreasing occurrence, are lung, liver, brain, bone, and gastrointestinal tract. Most patients who die with disseminated disease have multiple organ involvement. Frequently, the cause of death is respiratory failure or brain complications. Patients with disseminated disease have a poor prognosis, with a mean survival of about 6 months. Cure with any treatment is rare. Selection of treatment or a decision against treatment should be based on several factors, including the patient's medical condition, the potential for palliation, and the impact of treatment on quality of life.

Surgery

Surgical excision of recurrent melanoma can be effective for palliation in patients with isolated recurrences in the skin, central nervous system, lung, or gastrointestinal tract. Surgical excision of solitary brain metastases has been shown to provide improved palliation and quality of life compared with brain irradiation. Resection of isolated pulmonary metastases or of subcutaneous recurrences is usually not considered curative but can result in significantly prolonged disease-free survival. Gastrointestinal lesions causing obstruction or bleeding should be considered for resection or bypass to relieve these symptoms.

Radiotherapy

Melanoma can respond to radiotherapy. From several reports, the best tumor responses of melanoma in the soft tissues are seen if large doses per fraction (4 to 8 Gy) are administered rather than lower conventional doses (2 to 4 Gy). Radiotherapy is commonly used for palliation of bone pain secondary to metastatic disease or brain metastasis. The average survival after brain irradiation for melanoma is about 4 months.

Chemotherapy

Melanoma is responsive to few chemotherapeutic drugs. The best single agents for treatment of melanoma are DTIC and the nitrosoureas, which have objective response rates in the range of 10% to 20%. Conventionally, objective responses have included complete disappearance of all known tumor sites (complete response) and reduction of more than half in all assessable tumor (partial response). Complete responses are rare. Responses are more frequently observed in patients with tumor in skin, subcutaneous tissue, lymph nodes, or lung. The combination regimen consisting of DTIC, carmustine (BCNU), cisplatin, and tamoxifen is being used more frequently and has been reported to have a high response rate. However, no evidence indicates that combination chemotherapy offers any better results than single-agent DTIC at this time.

Several centers have reported experience with isolated hyperthermic limb perfusion of chemotherapeutic agents to treat multiple subcutaneous (in-transit) or skin (satellitosis) metastases of the extremities. This technique requires the isolation and cannulation of the afferent and efferent vessels of the involved extremity to an extracorporeal pump. High doses of chemotherapeutic agents can be infused into the limb without systemic toxicity. Sometimes, dramatic tumor responses can be obtained. A recent European study of hyperthermic limb perfusion with a combination of melphalan, tumor necrosis factor, and interferon-γ reported 3 partial and 16 complete responses among 19 patients with melanoma lesions.[42] Tumor necrosis factor cannot be administered systemically because of its severe toxicity; the use of isolated perfusion to an extremity avoids this limitation. This approach appears to be highly effective in the small subgroup of patients with disease confined to an extremity, but confirmatory studies are needed.

Immunotherapy

The rapid evolution of recombinant DNA technology has resulted in the availability of cytokines, such as the interferons and interleukins, that can be administered to modulate a patient's immune response. In addition, hybridoma technology has allowed the development of monoclonal antibodies reactive to melanoma. These biologic agents have been used in recent immunotherapeutic trials for metastatic melanoma and demonstrate that an antitumor immune response can be generated in selected patients.

Interferon-α (IFN-α) was one of the first cytokines used in tumor therapy. IFN-α was originally produced by virus-stimulated leukocytes and is now available in recombinant form. The interferons are known to induce macrophage cytotoxicity, to enhance natural killer cell to activity, up-regulate major histocompatibility (MHC) antigens on tumors, and to up-regulate tumor-associated antigens. The objective response rates of melanoma to IFN-α administration range from 10% to 20%.

The most significant advance in melanoma immunotherapy has been associated with the use of interleukin-2 (IL-2). IL-2 is a cytokine secreted by antigen-activated helper T cells and was initially discovered because it was a T-cell growth factor. Subsequently, it was found to have many other immunologic effects, and it appears to have an important role in the enhancement of immune responses. Mulé and coworkers[43] discovered that the in vitro or in vivo exposure of lymphoid cells to high concentrations of IL-2 results in the generation of lymphokine-activated killer (LAK) cells. These cells are characterized by their ability to kill tumor cells nonspecifically in an in vitro assay. In animal studies, these researchers demonstrated that LAK cells can be administered in conjunction with IL-2 to cause tumors to regress. The use of antitumor-reactive cells as reagents to treat tumor is known as *adoptive immunotherapy*. In a clinical trial, LAK cells plus IL-2 were found to mediate regression of tumor in selected patients with disseminated melanoma[44] (Color Fig. 111-2). From these and other studies, the response rate of melanoma to LAK cells plus IL-2 has been found to be in the range of 20% to 25%. Most patients who achieved complete remission remained free of disease for prolonged periods. The evidence that antitumor-reactive cells can be used to treat established tumors has encouraged the search for more tumor-specific, and presumably more potent, cells for adoptive immunotherapy. Rosenberg and coworkers[45] showed that tumor-infiltrating lymphocytes (TIL) obtained from progressive tumors in animals are 50 to 100 times more potent in antitumor activity than LAK cells. In clinical studies, they reported that, among 86 patients with advanced melanoma treated with the combination of TIL, high-dose IL-2, and cyclophosphamide, there was a response rate of 34%.[46]

The rationale for developing T cells that are immunologically specific in their reactivity to melanoma tumors has been substantiated by the recent discovery of tumor-associated antigens expressed by melanomas. A family of melanoma antigens termed *MAGE* are expressed on tumors and act as recognition peptides for cytotoxic T cells.[47] The antigens are recognized in association with MHC HLA-A1 identity. Additional melanoma antigens have been identified by similar techniques and are restricted by HLA-A2.1 recognition.[48,49]

In addition to its use in adoptive immunotherapy, IL-2 administration alone has been associated with significant melanoma tumor regression.[50] The clinical response rate with IL-2 administration is in the range of 15% to 20% and appears to be dose related. The antitumor effects mediated by IL-2 may result from several mechanisms, including induction of LAK cells or tumor-sensitized T cells and, possibly, the secretion of other cytokines such as tumor necrosis factor and interferon-γ. Unfortunately, high doses of IL-2 can result in multiple organ system failure as the result of a leaky capillary syndrome, which is reversible on cessation of therapy. The toxicity of IL-2 is believed to be related to the induction of a variety of inflammatory mediators. New studies are being conducted that evaluate IL-2 combined with other agents such as cytokines, chemotherapeutic agents, tumor vaccines, and monoclonal antibodies.

The possibility of using a tumor vaccine derived from melanoma tumor cells or extracts of tumor cells has been studied for many years. These vaccines usually have been used as adjuvant treatment in tumor-free patients who are at high risk for recurrence in an attempt to actively produce tumor-specific immunity. To enhance the immunogenicity of these vaccine preparations, immune adjuvants, such as BCG or vaccinia virus, are sometimes included in the vaccines. In general, melanoma tumor vaccines are nontoxic and have been suggested to confer some survival benefit compared with historical controls in nonrandomized studies. Prospective, randomized trials are necessary to evaluate this approach. As indicated previously, BCG administration as a nonspecific immunostimulant has not been shown to be efficacious as an adjuvant for melanoma patients in a randomized study.[41] The recent discovery of unique melanoma tumor-associated antigens opens the door for development of highly specific reagents for tumor vaccines. These antigenic peptides will probably be used with nonspecific immunostimulants to enhance immune responsiveness.

Several monoclonal antibodies (mAb) reactive to different antigens expressed on melanoma tumor cells have been characterized. In theory, these tumor-specific reagents can be used to activate the patient's immune system to destroy tumor cells (antibody-dependent cellular cytotoxicity), or they can be conjugated with a tumoricidal agent such as a radioisotope or ricin A toxin). Objective responses have been observed in preliminary trials with mAb. One practical problem associated with the available antimelanoma mAb is that they are of mouse origin and therefore induce a human immunoglobulin G response to mouse immunoglobulin. Approaches to circumvent this problem include the construction of chimeric mAb, by fusing mouse antigen-binding sites with human immunoglobulin sequences, and development of human antimelanoma mAb. Further investigations involving therapeutic and diagnostic applications of antimelanoma mAb are required to determine the utility of this approach.

Gene Therapy

The technical feasibility of transfer of genetic material into somatic cells has established a new approach to the treatment of malignancies. Many of the gene therapy strategies for cancer have focused on modulating the host immune response by altering tumor cells to be more "immunogenic." A variety of preclinical studies have demonstrated that genetic engineering of tumor cells to secrete or express immunoregulatory peptides (ie, cytokines, costimulatory molecules, or adhesion molecules) increases the host immune response to these tumors.[51] Several clinical studies are evaluating the efficacy of genetic modification of melanoma tumor cells to secrete cytokines that can be administered to patients as tumor vaccines. A different approach, established at the University of Michigan, is genetic modification of melanoma tumors in situ by the intra-tumoral inoculation of DNA complexed with liposomes so as to induce the expression of a foreign MHC class I protein (ie, HLA-B7) by the tumor cells.[52] This procedure attempts to enhance reactivity against native tumor antigens by invoking an allogeneic immune response against a strong foreign antigen.

NONMELANOMA SKIN TUMORS

Nonmelanoma basal cell and squamous cell skin cancers are the most common type of malignancy in humans. These tumors are chiefly derived from epithelial origin. The ratio of BCC to SCC is approximately 4:1. The projected 1994 incidence of nonmelanoma (BCC and SCC) skin cancer in the United States alone is 900,000 to 1,200,000 cases. The public health burden on the US population from nonmelanoma skin cancer, for which the incidence is rapidly rising, is enormous.

Etiology

Both BCC and SCC are induced by chronic exposure to UVR, which is the most common cause of nonmelanoma skin cancer. These cancers are the predominant neoplasms on the head, neck, and hands, where sun exposure is common. Skin cancer is a significant occupational hazard for people who work outdoors, such as mail deliverers, farmers, sailors, and construction workers. The incidence of skin cancer is greater in fair-complexioned populations and is lower among darker-complexioned people. Melanin pigment in the skin appears to be the protective factor, because albino blacks have a higher incidence of skin cancer than nonalbino blacks.

Chemical carcinogens have long been implicated as etiologic agents that contribute to the formation of skin cancer. The development of scrotal carcinoma in chimney sweeps is an example: carcinogenic soot is implicated in the development of SCC. Another example is arsenic in welding flux, which is associated with carcinoma of the hand (Color Fig. 111-3). Other examples of carcinogens are coal tar, paraffin oil, creosote, and fuel oil. The mechanism may be explained by the initiation and promotion theory of skin cancer. In this scenario, initiation occurs by exposure of keratinocytes to the chemical carcinogen, and promotion occurs with repeated exposure of that area to the carcinogen.[53]

Human papillomavirus (HPV) has been implicated in the formation of SCC in humans.[54] The degeneration of a condyloma acuminata of the anus into SCC is an example of this disorder. HPV is associated with SCC in the genital, acral, and periungal regions.[55] Investigators using cDNA probes directed at herpes simplex virus have reported the presence of viral DNA in a SCC.[56] These associations strongly suggest a link between skin cancer and viruses.

The degeneration of chronic radiodermatitis into invasive SCC or BCC is well described. Typically, there is at least a 20-year latency period between radiation exposure and the development of the malignant lesion. In the past, radiotherapy was used to treat acne, facial scarring, cutaneous hemangiomas, and simple cutaneous malignancies. SCC and BCC can also develop in areas of trauma, scar, and chronic scarring disorders such as lupus erythematosus, epidermolysis bullosa acquisita, and chronic sinus tracts. Nevoid BCC syndrome and xeroderma pigmentosum are genodermatoses associated with the development of hundreds of skin cancers, usually beginning at an early age.

Basal Cell Carcinoma

Basal cell carcinoma is the most common form of skin cancer. These epithelial-derived tumors can be divided into various subtypes according to clinical appearance, histologic pattern, and biologic behavior. Although BCCs rarely metastasize, they are characterized by slow but relentless and destructive local invasion that results in high morbidity without treatment. The subclinical local invasion may be deep, extensive, and asymmetric, with finger-like extensions several centimeters beyond the clinical borders.

The most common subtype of BCC is the ulcerative, well-circumscribed nodular variety. These tumors often present as pearly papules or nodules with telangiectasias. They may be pruritic and bleed occasionally. With time, the center ulcerates to create peripheral "rolled" borders; such ulcerating BCCs are called rodent ulcers (Color Fig 111-4). Occasionally, the lesions are deeply pigmented and nodular and can be confused with melanoma. This variant has been called a *pigmented BCC* (see Color Fig. 111-1*I*). The histologic features of these tumors demonstrate isolated areas of basaloid tumor islands arising from the epidermis with peripheral palisading of nuclei and stromal retraction. In some cases, the BCC has histologic features of squamous metaplasia with keratinization. These tumors have basosquamous differentiation and can become more aggressive and develop regional lymphatic spread.

Most difficult to treat with surgical excision is the type of BCC with an aggressive growth pattern, known as morpheaform, sclerosing, or fibrosing BCC (Color Fig. 111-5). Clinically, these tumors are flat and appear to be scarlike. They have a significant incidence of recurrence because of the isolated, finger-like fronds of basal cell tumor cells that may deeply invade the surrounding structures well beyond the clinical margins of the lesion. These small, finger-like islands are often missed with standard histologic margin control.

Clinically, superficial BCCs are scaly, pink to red lesions. Frequently, they are confused with psoriasis or other eczematous, scaly dermatoses. Although these tumors are usually relatively superficial, extensive superficial subclinical involvement is common. The following risk factors are associated with extensive subclinical invasion or frequent recurrence of BCC after standard treatment, including surgical excision: recurrence after previous treatment; size greater than 2 cm; anatomic location on the central face, eyelid, or ear; aggressive growth (morpheaform, sclerosing, or fibrosing BCC); invasive histologic pattern; tumor induced by radiation; neurotropism; and incompletely excised tumor.[57-61]

Squamous Cell Carcinoma

Squamous cell carcinoma is the second most common form of skin cancer and is derived from the epithelial keratinocyte. Because these tumors can deeply invade surrounding structures or metastasize to regional lymph nodes, they must be recognized and treated aggressively. SCC causes some 2500 deaths per year in the United States. Several precursor lesions to invasive SCC exist, most commonly actinic keratoses and Bowen disease. Erythroplasia of Queyrat, another precursor lesion, represents SCC in situ on the glans penis. Clinically, SCC usually begins as an erythematous papulonodule with overlying keratotic crust or ulceration. The lesions can progress to ulceration with surrounding erythema, with or without a keratotic center. Histologically, SCC shows malignant degeneration of epithelial cells with differentiation toward keratin formation.

Ulcerative SCC is an aggressive skin malignancy that typically has a central ulceration with raised borders (Color Fig. 111-6). These tumors can arise in actinic damaged skin, solar keratoses, cutaneous horns, burn scars, or chronic wounds. These lesions infiltrate widely and can spread to regional lymphatics. In the head and neck, they commonly metastasize to the periparotid, jugular digastric, or midjugular lymph nodes. If these tumors spread to the regional lymph nodes, the prognosis is poor, with a 5-year survival rate below 50%. Tumors arising in chronic wounds or burn scars exhibit particularly aggressive behavior, and many patients present with regional lymphatic spread. In contrast, tumors that arise in actinic damaged skin demonstrate a less aggressive pattern. This is particularly true in the hand, where SCC is often indolent and grows slowly.

Accurate assessment of the higher-risk cutaneous SCCs is handicapped because of the lack of large prospective studies using multivariate analysis. Nine variables, however, have been identified as prognostic risk factors by retrospective analysis. Factors that may determine a higher risk for local recurrence, extensive subclinical invasion, and metastasis include the following[55]:

- Diameter greater than 2 cm
- Invasion to or below the reticular dermis
- Poorly differentiated histologic pattern
- Rapid growth
- Origin (scar, radiation, chronic ulcer, sinus tract)
- Anatomic site (central face, ear, lip, embryonic fusion planes)
- Host immunosuppression
- Neurotropism
- Recurrence after previous treatment

Other Tumors of Special Interest

Hundreds of cutaneous tumors exist, and their description is beyond the scope of this chapter. Three tumors that may be seen by the surgeon and are in the differential diagnosis for BCC are described here because of their potentially aggressive behavior. These are Merkel cell carcinoma, microcystic adnexal carcinoma, and sebaceous gland carcinoma.

Merkel cell carcinoma is a malignant neuroendocrine tumor with features of epithelial differentiation. Merkel cell carcinoma is biologically aggressive, with a high incidence of local recurrence and regional and systemic metastasis. The 1-, 2-, and 3-year survival rates are estimated to be 88%, 72%, and 55%, respectively. Merkel cell carcinoma typically appears as a red to purple papulonodule or indurated plaque (Color Fig. 111-7). Approximately 50% of tumors arise on the head and neck, 40% on the extremities, and 10% on the trunk. Merkel cell carcinoma is a small cell tumor with characteristic positive immunocytochemical staining for neuron-specific enolase, cytokeratin, and neurofilament protein. A chest radiograph is indicated to rule out metastatic oat cell carcinoma, which may be similar in clinical and histologic appearance. Treatment consists of wide local excision with adjuvant radiation to the primary site and the primary draining nodal groups. Careful and frequent follow-up monitoring for local, regional, or distant recurrence is warranted.[62]

Microcystic adnexal carcinoma is a rare cutaneous neoplasm with both follicular and eccrine differentiation, characterized by invasive, relentless, and destructive local growth. The incidence of neurotropism and local recurrence is very high. Microcystic adnexal carcinoma occurs primarily on the head and neck as a slowly enlarging, white to pink papuloplaque. Local invasion through the underlying muscle is common, and bony invasion occurs in up to 13% of cases. The use of standard Mohs excision (see later section) combined with permanent horizontal sectioning from the final negative Mohs stage specimens offers the highest chance of cure in most cases.[63]

Sebaceous gland carcinoma is a rare malignant tumor derived from adnexal epithelium of sebaceous glands. The tumor can arise on ocular or extraocular sites but most commonly presents as a yellowish to pink, slowly growing papulonodule on the eyelid, clinically similar to a chalazion. Local recurrence after surgical excision is relatively frequent (9% to 36%) owing to subclinical pagetoid extension and the multicentric nature of the tumor. Regional lymph node and visceral metastases occur in 14% to 25% of cases. Adjuvant radiotherapy has been shown to be beneficial in several series.[64]

Surgical Treatment of Nonmelanoma Skin Cancers

A skin biopsy for diagnosis is important before treatment of any skin cancer. Fortunately, most nonmelanoma skin cancers are small, low-risk lesions that respond with 90% to 95% cure rates to standard treatment techniques, including curettage and electrodesiccation, cryosurgery, radiotherapy, and surgical resection.[55] Many skin cancers can be removed with elliptical excisions that follow the skin tension lines. Curettage before excision is often helpful to delineate subclinical tumor extension for both BCC and SCC.[58] Margins for low-risk SCC range from 0.5 to 1 cm. Margins for low-risk BCC range from 0.3 to 0.5 cm. Mohs surgery should be considered for BCCs and SCCs that exhibit the higher-risk factors previously listed. If Mohs surgery is not available, excision with careful frozen-section control (with permanent section confirmation) is indicated.

Regional lymphadenectomy is an important component of the surgical procedure if clinically positive nodes are evident. About 80% of metastases from cutaneous SCC occur first to the primary draining regional lymph nodes. The diagnosis of metastatic SCC can easily be made with fine-needle aspiration at the time of skin biopsy. These invasive tumors have characteristic features in lymph node aspirates that allow the pathologist to secure the diagnosis. ELND for patients with SCC with clinically negative regional disease is not indicated unless the tumor extends to the parotid capsule or the lesion is large and contiguous to a draining nodal basin. BCC rarely metastasizes, and regional lymph node dissection should not be performed unless the histologic features resemble those of basosquamous cell tumors, which are more biologically aggressive lesions.

The reconstructive algorithm for the treatment of skin cancer is complex because of the variety of anatomic sites involved. Cancers of the face are treated with either full-thickness skin grafts or local skin flaps that take advantage of regional subunits of the face. This technique ensures that the involved cosmetic unit is preserved with a regional flap and that facial deformity is minimized. Full-thickness skin grafts from the preauricular area, retroauricular area, or neck are useful in nasal and eyelid reconstruction. Split-thickness grafts have little utility in the face and should be reserved for massive defects in cases in which the prognosis is poor or the patient's functional classification is poor. For very high-risk nonmelanoma skin cancers, split-thickness skin grafting may be necessary to monitor for tumor recurrence. Definitive reconstruction can then be performed at a later date. In the trunk or limbs, skin grafts or skin flaps work equally well. The exception is the hand, where preservation of tendon function requires the use of cross-finger flaps, groin flaps, reverse radial forearm flaps, or free tissue transfer.

Mohs Micrographic Surgical Treatment of Skin Cancer

Mohs surgery was developed by Dr. Frederick E. Mohs, a general surgeon from the University of Wisconsin, in the 1940s. Initially, a chemical fixative paste was applied to the skin to fix the tissue in situ; hence, the now-outdated term *Mohs chemosurgery*. The fresh tissue technique, which omitted the chemical paste, was developed and refined in the 1970s. Mohs micrographic surgery is most useful for the treatment of higher-risk nonmelanoma skin cancers. Mohs surgery is usually performed under local anesthesia in an outpatient Mohs surgical unit.[65,66] After removal of all gross tumor, the surgeon excises a thin layer of tissue, 2 to 3 mm deep and with 2- to 3-mm lateral margins. The tissue is mapped, color-coded for orientation, and sent to the technician for frozen-section processing. The specimen is flexible and flattened, with the beveled peripheral skin edge placed in the same horizontal plane with the deep margin. In this plane, both the deep and peripheral margins are examined in one horizontal cut by frozen-section analysis with total (theoretically 100%) margin control. Good-quality frozen sections may be achieved only by a skilled and experienced Mohs histotechnician. The Mohs surgeon functions as both surgeon and pathologist. After histologic interpretation of the frozen-section specimens, the precise anatomic location of any residual tumor can be identified and reexcised until all margins are tumor-free (Fig. 111-10). The Mohs surgeon's ability to microscopically track subclinical tumor extensions results in the highest cure rate with maximal preser-

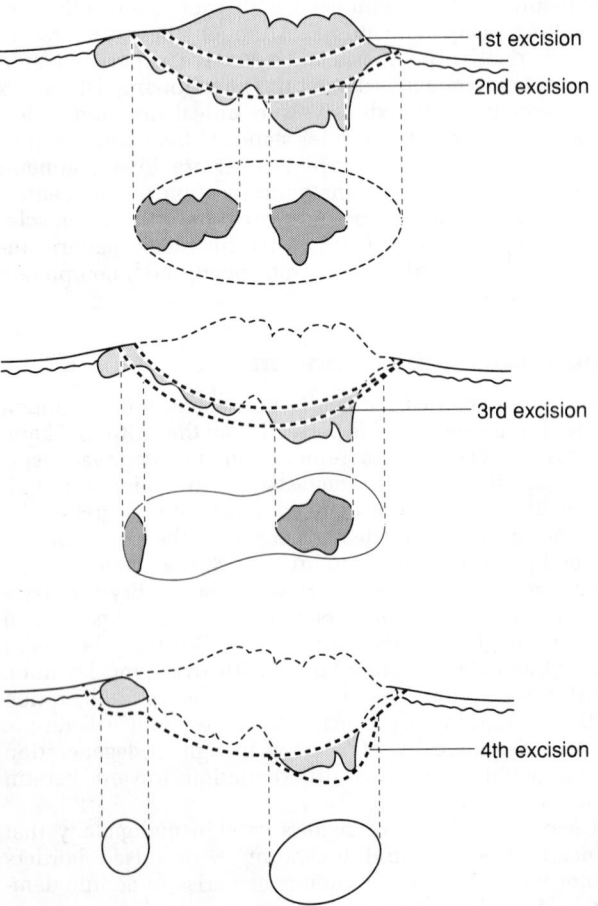

Figure 111-10. Mohs micrographic surgical technique.

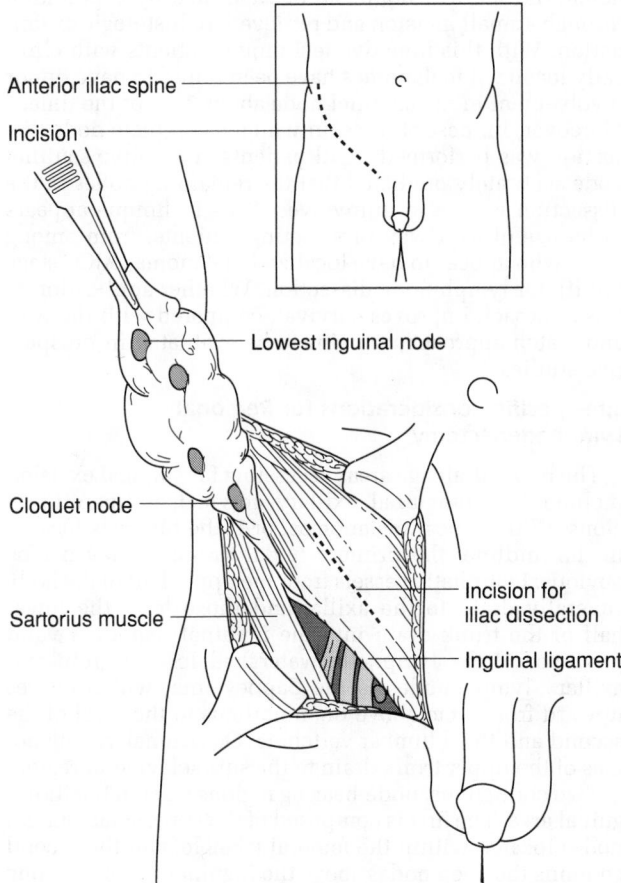

Figure 111-9. Technique of groin dissection.

tumor involvement of the deep inguinal nodes. The rarity of involvement of the deep inguinal nodes when the superficial nodes are pathologically negative or harbor only microscopic disease does not warrant a deep groin dissection in those situations. Some reports indicate that the presence of positive deep groin nodes is associated with a high incidence of disseminated disease and that their removal does not lead to long-term benefit.[39] Other reports indicate that some patients with iliac node disease can be cured by a deep groin dissection.[40] The most frequent long-term complication associated with groin dissection is edema, which occurs in 25% of patients.

The iliac and obturator nodes can be removed during the course of a superficial groin dissection by a variety of techniques. Through the same skin incision used for the superficial dissection, the deep nodes can be approached extraperitoneally by division of the inguinal ligament or by splitting of the abdominal wall musculature with an incision superior and parallel to the inguinal ligament. Alternatively, a separate midline abdominal incision can be used to remove the deep inguinal nodes and assess the paraaortic nodes. This latter approach reduces wound complications associated with combined ilioinguinal dissections.

The technique for an axillary dissection is described in Chapter 61 on breast cancer. Axillary dissections for melanoma should include removal of lymph nodes lateral, beneath, and medial to the pectoralis minor muscle (levels I to III). The axillary lymph node region is contiguous with the supraclavicular node region. Evidence of supraclavicular nodal involvement is not uncommon if bulky axillary

disease is present. There is no satisfactory procedure to remove contiguous involved axillary and supraclavicular lymph nodes. In these situations, axillary dissection is noncurative and should be considered only for palliation. Long-term complications associated with axillary dissections are infrequent; arm edema and pain occur in less than 5% of patients.

Metastases to the lymph nodes from head and neck melanomas follow predictable pathways. Melanomas arising on the scalp or face anterior to the pinna of the ear and superior to the commissure of the lip metastasize to the parotid region. Lesions inferior to the commissure of the lip spread to the cervical region. Melanomas that occur on the posterior scalp behind the pinna usually spread to occipital and posterior cervical lymph nodes. Because the parotid nodes are contiguous with the cervical nodes, a radical neck dissection to remove the cervical nodes is often performed in combination with a superficial parotid node dissection for anterior facial melanomas.

Adjuvant Therapy

Patients who undergo lymphadenectomy for AJCC stage III disease are at high risk for recurrent disease (see Fig. 111-4). These patients, as well as those who undergo surgical excision for localized deep melanomas, are in need of effective adjuvant therapy to eliminate residual micrometastatic disease. No effective adjuvant therapies are available for these patients. The WHO Melanoma Group reported on a randomized, prospective trial of 761 patients with AJCC stage IB, IIA, IIB, and III disease to evaluate chemotherapy and immunotherapy as adjuvant treatments after definitive surgical excision.[41] Patients were randomly assigned to four groups: those who received surgery alone, those who received surgery plus dacarbazine (DTIC) chemotherapy, those who received surgery plus bacille Calmette-Guérin (BCG) immunotherapy, and those patients who received surgery plus DTIC and BCG therapy. No improvement in survival was seen with any of the therapies compared with surgery alone. The identification of an effective adjuvant therapy in melanoma is an area of active investigation. Clinical trials evaluating biologic agents such as interferon-α and tumor vaccines are underway.

Treatment of Disseminated Melanoma

Evaluation for Metastatic Disease and Clinical Course

The follow-up evaluation for patients with AJCC stage I, II, or III melanoma who are rendered tumor-free by surgery should include regular histories and physical examinations. The use of extensive and frequent radiographic studies and blood work in asymptomatic, clinically disease-free patients is rarely productive. Patients with surgically excised thin (AJCC stage I) melanomas should be examined every 6 months for 5 years and yearly thereafter. Specific examination for local or regional recurrences should be performed, because surgical therapy may prove curative. In addition, a total skin examination to identify new primary melanomas should be performed. Patients with AJCC stage II or III melanomas who are clinically disease-free should be examined every 3 or 4 months for 5 years and then yearly thereafter. Yearly chest radiographs and liver function studies may be considered for evaluation of visceral disease. Lactic dehydrogenase levels have been reported to be elevated in a significant number of patients with metastatic disease. Attention should be directed to any gastrointestinal or central nervous system symptoms. Appropriate diagnostic studies can be obtained based on the clinical history and physical findings.

Table 111-8. NONRANDOMIZED EXPERIENCE WITH WIDE EXCISION VERSUS WIDE EXCISION PLUS ELECTIVE LYMPH NODE DISSECTION FOR AJC STAGES I AND II MELANOMAS*

| Tumor Thickness (mm) | 10-Year Survival Rate (%) | | | |
| | Extremity (N) | | Trunk, Head, and Neck (N) | |
	WE	WE + ELND	WE	WE + ELND
<0.76	94 (142)	100 (26)	86 (135)	83 (38)
0.76–1.49	74 (125)	92† (66)	56 (131)	80† (51)
1.5–3.99	54 (114)	80† (107)	33 (129)	64† (129)
≥4	30 (33)	44 (34)	22 (56)	26 (38)

WE, wide excision; ELND, elective lymph node dissection.
* Experience from the Sydney Melanoma Unit, Australia, and the University of Alabama, Birmingham.[34]
† Significantly different from WE alone.

level of invasion, and other variables did not identify any subgroup benefiting from ELND. About 20% of patients who underwent ELND had micrometastases in the specimens; and about 20% of patients who underwent excision alone later received therapeutic lymph node dissections. The 5-year survival rate was 50% for the subgroup of patients in whom occult micrometastases were found at ELND; this rate was not significantly different from the rate of 45% reported for patients who underwent therapeutic lymphadenectomy for clinically apparent nodal metastases.

The second prospective study was conducted by the Mayo Clinic.[37] In this study, 171 clinical AJCC stage I and II patients were randomly assigned to one of three treatment groups: 62 underwent wide excision only, 55 had ELND delayed 30 to 60 days after primary tumor excision, and 54 had concomitant ELND with excision of the primary tumor. Patients with primary lesions on the head and neck or the midline trunk were excluded. After disease-free and overall survival rates were analyzed, there were no significant differences between the groups.

Neither the WHO Melanoma Group nor the Mayo Clinic study revealed any advantage to ELND in localized extremity melanomas. A major criticism of these studies is that they included a high number of patients with thin melanomas. Clearly, from retrospective studies, ELND for thin melanomas (less than 1 mm) does not offer survival benefit, and this could have influenced the results of the prospective studies. In addition, these studies did not include patients with truncal or head and neck melanomas, which may behave differently than extremity melanomas.

Additional prospective, randomized trials are underway to evaluate ELND in high-risk melanoma patients. One study is the Intergroup Melanoma Study, which is evaluating ELND in patients with melanomas 1 to 4 mm thick and which includes extremity, truncal, and head and neck sites. A second study is being conducted by the WHO Melanoma Group and involves patients with truncal melanomas whose primary tumors measure more than 2 mm in thickness. The results of these studies may help resolve the controversy surrounding this issue.

A new technique has been developed to identify the first draining lymph node adjacent to a cutaneous melanoma, known as the "sentinel" node.[38] It has been hypothesized that melanoma involvement of a nodal basin develops in an orderly fashion and that involvement of the sentinel node is the first step of this process. By injection of a blue dye intradermally around the site of the primary mela-

noma, the sentinel node can be identified by exploration through a small incision and retrieved for histologic examination. With this blue dye technique, patients with clinically localized melanomas have been found to have tumor involvement in the sentinel node about 20% of the time.[38] Moreover, in these studies, in which a complete node dissection was performed in all patients, a negative sentinel node accurately predicted that the remaining nodes in the dissection were also uninvolved. This technique appears to be useful as a way of selecting patients, from among those who appear to have localized melanoma (AJCC stage I or II), for lymph node dissection. Whether application of this approach improves survival, compared with the wait and watch approach, remains to be evaluated in prospective studies.

Site-Specific Considerations for Regional Lymphadenectomy

The nodal drainage areas accessible for surgical excision include the ilioinguinal, axillary, cervical, and parotid regions. With truncal melanomas, or if the tumor is located in the midline, the primary nodal drainage may not be obvious. Lymphatic vessels from the upper half of the body generally drain to the axilla, and those from the lower half of the trunk drain into the inguinal region. A valid predictor of the lymphatic watershed for the groin and axillary lymph nodes is the Sappey line, which curves upward from 2 cm above the umbilicus to the level of the second and third lumbar vertebrae. Occasionally, melanomas of the upper trunk drain to the supraclavicular region.

Two contiguous, node-bearing regions exist in the ilioinguinal area. The first is composed of the superficial femoral nodes located within the femoral triangle, and the second contains the deep nodes above the inguinal ligament along the iliac and obturator vessels. Removal of the femoral nodes is referred to as a *superficial groin dissection,* and removal of the iliac and obturator nodes is called a *deep groin dissection* (Fig. 111-9).

Controversy surrounds the benefit of a deep groin dissection, which some surgeons elect to perform if there is evidence of palpable femoral lymph node involvement. In this situation, about one third of patients are likely to have

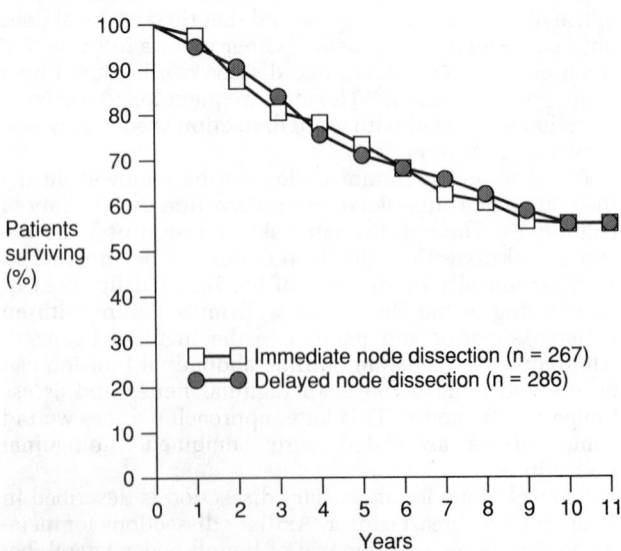

Figure 111-8. Randomized study of immediate elective lymph node dissection versus delayed therapeutic node dissection by WHO Melanoma Group. No significant difference in survival was seen between the groups.

vation of normal tissue. Soft tissue reconstruction can then be performed on the same day, after completion of Mohs surgical excision of the tumor (Color Fig. 111-8). A multidisciplinary approach involving Mohs, plastic, head and neck, and oculoplastic surgeons and radiation oncologists may be needed for extensive tumors.

Based on a review of all studies from all disciplines since 1950, the 5-year cure rate for treatment of primary (previously untreated) BCC by Mohs surgery is 99%, versus 90% to 93% for all non-Mohs modalities, including standard surgical excision.[67] For recurrent (previously treated) BCC, the 5-year cure rates are 94% for Mohs versus 60% to 84% for non-Mohs modalities.[68] In general, Mohs surgery should be considered for nonmelanoma tumors that are associated with a higher risk of recurrence after standard treatment and for tumors for which conservation of normal tissue is important. Risk factors for recurrence after standard treatment include the following:

- Recurrent tumor
- Size greater than 2 cm
- Location in the central face, eyelid, or ear
- Aggressive histologic growth pattern of BCC
- Poorly differentiated SCC
- Microcystic adnexal carcinoma
- Dermatofibroma sarcoma protuberans
- Tumor with poorly defined clinical margins
- Neurotropism
- Immunosuppressed patient with SCC
- Tumor in site of radiation
- Incompletely excised tumor

Tumors for which maximal conservation of tissue may be important include tumors on the eyelid, nose, ear, lip, digit, or genitalia and tumors in young patients. For small, low-risk lesions, Mohs surgery does not result in higher cure rates than standard techniques, but its use should be considered for all nonmelanoma skin cancers with the higher-risk factors described.

Adjuvant Radiotherapy

Radiotherapy may be useful for primary treatment of small, low-risk nonmelanoma skin cancers. For cutaneous SCC with many high-risk factors and for those with extensive neurotropism, adjuvant prophylactic radiotherapy to the primary site and the primary draining lymph nodes may decrease the risks of local recurrence and regional nodal metastasis. Prophylactic adjuvant radiotherapy should also be considered for highly aggressive, deeply invasive BCCs that exhibit extensive neurotropism.

REFERENCES

1. Boring CC, Squires TS, Tong T, et al. Cancer statistics. CA Cancer J Clin 1994;44:7.
2. NCI Division of Cancer Prevention and Control. Cancer statistics review, 1973–1987. Bethesda, US Dept of Health and Human Services, National Cancer Institute (NIH Publication 89-2789), May 1989.
3. Elwood JM, Lee JAH, Walters SD, et al. Relationship of melanoma and other skin cancer mortality to latitude and ultraviolet radiation in the United States and Canada. Int J Epidemiol 1974;3:325.
4. Magnus K. Incidence of malignant melanoma of the skin in Norway 1955–1970: variation in time and space and solar radiation. Cancer 1973;32:1275.
5. Kripke ML. Immunology and photocarcinogenesis. J Am Acad Dermatol 1986;14:149.
6. Greene MH, Clark WH, Tucker MA, et al. High risk of malignant melanoma in melanoma-prone families with dysplastic nevi. Ann Intern Med 1985;102:458.
7. Hieken TJ, Rauth S, Ronan SG, et al. Hereditary melanoma. Surg Oncol Clin North Am 1994;3:563.
8. Bale SJ, Dracopoli NC, Tucker MA, et al. Mapping the gene for hereditary cutaneous malignant melanoma–dysplastic nevus to chromosome 1p. N Engl J Med 1989;320:1367.
9. Cannon-Albright LA, Goldgar DE, Meyer LJ, et al. Assignment of a locus for familial melanoma, MLM, to chromosome 9p13–p22. Science 1992;258:1148.
10. Trent JM, Stanbridge EJ, Heyoung LM, et al. Tumorigenicity in human melanoma cell lines controlled by introduction of human chromosome 6. Science 1990;247:568.
11. Fountain JW, Bale SJ, Housman DE, et al. Genetics of melanoma. Cancer Surv 1990;9:645.
12. Clark WH Jr, Ainsworth AM, Bernardino EA, et al. The developmental biology of primary human malignant melanomas. Semin Oncol 1975;2:83.
13. Clark WH Jr, From L, Bernardino EA, et al. The histogenesis and biologic behavior of primary human malignant melanoma of the skin. Cancer Res 1969;29:705.
14. McGovern VJ. The classification of melanoma and its relationship with prognosis. Pathology 1970;2:85.
15. Wanebo HJ, Woodruff J, Fortner JG. Malignant melanoma of the extremities: a clinicopathologic study using levels of invasion (microstage). Cancer 1975;35:666.
16. Balch CM, Murad TM, Soong SJ, et al. A multifactorial analysis of melanoma: prognostic histopathologic features comparing Clark's and Breslow's staging methods. Ann Surg 1978;118:732.
17. Eldh J, Boeryd B, Peterson LE. Prognostic factors in cutaneous malignant melanoma in stage I: a clinical, morphological, and multivariate analysis. Scand J Plast Reconstr Surg 1978;12:243.
18. Breslow A. Thickness, cross-sectional area and depth of invasion in prognosis of cutaneous melanoma. Ann Surg 1970;172:902.
19. Balch CM, Soong SJ, Milton GW, et al. A comparison of prognostic factors and surgical results in 1,786 patients with localized (stage I) melanoma treated in Alabama, USA and New South Wales, Australia. Ann Surg 1982;196:677.
20. Balch CM, Soong S-J, Shaw HM, et al. An analysis of prognostic factors in 4000 patients with cutaneous melanoma. In: Balch CM, Milton GW, eds. Cutaneous melanoma: clinical management and treatment results worldwide. Philadelphia, JB Lippincott, 1985:321.
21. Cohen MH, Ketcham AS, Felix EL, et al. Prognostic factors in patients undergoing lymphadenectomy for malignant melanoma. Ann Surg 1977;186:635.
22. Callery C, Cochran AJ, Roe DJ, et al. Factors prognostic for survival in patients with malignant melanoma spread to the regional lymph nodes. Ann Surg 1982;196:69.
23. Calabro A, Singletary SE, Balch CM. Patterns of relapse in 1001 consecutive patients with melanoma nodal metastases. Arch Surg 1989;124:1051.
24. Bevilacqua RG, Coit DG, Rogatko A, et al. Axillary dissection in melanoma: prognostic variables in node-positive patients. Ann Surg 1990;212:125.
25. Day CL, Mihm MC, Lew RA, et al. Cutaneous malignant melanoma: prognostic guidelines for physicians and patients. CA Cancer J Clin 1982;32:113.
26. Mastrangelo MJ, Baker AR, Katz HR. Cutaneous melanoma. In: DeVita VT, Hellman S, Rosenberg SA, eds. Cancer: principles and practice of oncology, ed 2. Philadelphia, JB Lippincott, 1985.
27. Clark WH, Elder DE, Guerry D, et al. Model predicting survival in stage I melanoma based on tumor progression. J Natl Cancer Inst 1989;81:1893.
28. Kheir SM, Bines SD, Vonroenn JH, et al. Prognostic significance of DNA aneuploidy in stage I cutaneous melanoma. Ann Surg 1988;207:455.
29. Trent JM, Meyskens FL, Salmon SE, et al. Relation of cytogenetic abnormalities and clinical outcome in metastatic melanoma. N Engl J Med 1990;322:1508.
30. Veronesi U, Cascinelli N, Adamus J, et al. Thin stage I primary cutaneous malignant melanoma: comparison of excision with margins of 1 or 3 cm. N Engl J Med 1988;318:1159.
31. Balch CM, Urist MM, Karakousis CP, et al. Efficacy of 2 cm surgical margins for intermediate thickness melanomas (1 to

4 mm): results of a multi-institutional randomized surgical trial. Ann Surg 1993;218:262.

32. Balch CM, Karakousis C, Natarajan N, et al. Management of cutaneous melanoma in the United States. Surg Gynecol Obstet 1984;158:311.

33. Balch CM. The role of elective lymph node dissection in melanoma: rationale, results, and controversies. J Clin Oncol 1988;6:163.

34. Balch CM, Cascinelli N, Milton GW, et al. Elective node dissection: pros and cons. In: Balch CM, Milton GW, eds. Cutaneous melanoma: clinical management and treatment results worldwide. Philadelphia, JB Lippincott, 1985:131.

35. Cady B. "Prophylactic" lymph node dissection in melanoma: does it help? J Clin Oncol 1988;6:2.

36. Veronesi U, Adams J, Bandiera DC, et al. Delayed regional lymph node dissection in stage I melanoma of the skin of the lower extremities. Cancer 1982;49:2420.

37. Sim FH, Taylor WF, Pritchard DJ, et al. Lymphadenectomy in the management of stage I malignant melanoma: a prospective randomized study. Mayo Clin Proc 1986;61:697.

38. Morton DL, Wen D-R, Wong JH, et al. Technical details of intraoperative lymphatic mapping for early stage melanoma. Arch Surg 1992;127:392.

39. Coit DG, Brennan MF. Extent of lymph node dissection in melanoma of the trunk or lower extremity. Arch Surg 1989;124:162.

40. Karakousis CP, Lawrence JE, Rao UR. Groin dissection in malignant melanoma. Am J Surg 1986;152:491.

41. Veronesi U, Adamus J, Aubert C, et al. A randomized trial of adjuvant chemotherapy and immunotherapy in cutaneous melanoma. N Engl J Med 1982;307:913.

42. Lienard D, Ewalenko P, Delmotte J-J, et al. High-dose recombinant tumor necrosis factor alpha in combination with interferon gamma and melphalan in isolation perfusion of the limbs for melanoma and sarcoma. J Clin Oncol 1992;10:52.

43. Mulé JJ, Shu S, Schwartz SL, Rosenberg SA. Adoptive immunotherapy of established pulmonary metastases with LAK cells and recombinant interleukin-2. Science 1984;225:1487.

44. Rosenberg SA, Lotze MT, Muul LM, et al. A progress report on the treatment of 157 patients with advanced cancer using lymphokine-activated killer cells and interleukin-2 or high-dose interleukin-2 alone. N Engl J Med 1987;316:889.

45. Rosenberg SA, Spiess P, Lafreniere R. A new approach to the adoptive immunotherapy of cancer with tumor-infiltrating lymphocytes. Science 1986;233:1318.

46. Rosenberg SA, Yannelli JR, Yang JC, et al. Treatment of patients with metastatic melanoma with autologous tumor-infiltrating lymphocytes and interleukin 2. J Natl Cancer Inst 1994;86:1159.

47. van der Bruggen P, Traversari C, Chomez P, et al. A gene encoding an antigen recognized by cytolytic T lymphocytes on a human melanoma. Science 1991;254:1643.

48. Kawakami Y, Zakut R, Topalian SL, et al. Shared human melanoma antigens: recognition by tumor-infiltrating lymphocytes in HLA-A2.1 transfected melanomas. J Immunol 1992; 148:638.

49. Cox AL, Skipper J, Chen Y, et al. Identification of a peptide recognized by five melanoma-specific human cytotoxic T cell lines. Science 1994;264:716.

50. Chang AE, Rosenberg SA. Overview of interleukin-2 as an immunotherapeutic agent. Semin Surg Oncol 1989;5:385.

51. Miller AR, McBride WH, Hunt K, et al. Cytokine-mediated gene therapy for cancer. Ann Surg Oncol 1994;1:436.

52. Nabel GJ, Nabel EG, Yang Z-Y, et al. Direct gene transfer with DNA–liposome complexes in melanoma: expression, biological activity, and lack of toxicity in humans. Proc Natl Acad Sci U S A 1993;90:11307–11311.

53. Yupsa SH, Hennings H, Saffiotti U. Cutaneous chemical carcinogenesis: past, present, and future. J Invest Dermatol 1976; 67:199.

54. Obalek S, Jablonski S, Orth G. HPV associated intraepithelial neoplasia of external genitalia. Clin Dermatol 1985;3:104.

55. Johnson TM, Rowe DE, Nelson BR, et al. Squamous cell carcinoma of the skin (excluding lip and oral mucosa). J Am Acad Dermatol 1992;26:467.

56. Claudy AL, Chignol MC, Chardonnet Y. Detection of herpes simplex virus DNA in a cutaneous squamous cell carcinoma by in situ hybridization. Arch Dermatol Res 1989;281:333.

57. Swanson NA. Mohs surgery: technique, indications, applications, and the future. Arch Dermatol 1983;119:761.

58. Johnson TM, Tromovich TA, Swanson NA. Combined curettage and excision: a treatment for primary basal cell carcinoma. J Am Acad Dermatol 1991;24:613.

59. Salasche SJ, Amonette RA. Morpheaform basal-cell epitheliomas: a study of subclinical extensions in a series of 51 cases. J Dermatol Surg Oncol 1981;7:387.

60. Smith SP, Foley EH, Grande PJ. Use of Mohs surgery to establish quantitative proof of heightened tumor spread in basal cell carcinoma recurrent following radiotherapy. J Dermatol Surg Oncol 1990;16:1012.

61. Birkby CS, Whitaker DC. Management consideration for cutaneous neurophilic tumors. J Dermatol Surg Oncol 1988; 14:731.

62. Ratner D, Nelson BR, Brown MD, et al. Merkel cell carcinoma. J Am Acad Dermatol 1993;29:143.

63. Sebastien TS, Nelson BR, Lowe L, et al. Microcystic adnexal carcinoma. J Am Acad Dermatol 1993;29:840.

64. Nelson BR, Hamlet KR, Gillard M, et al. Sebaceous carcinoma. J Am Acad Dermatol 1995;33:1.

65. Lang PG. Mohs micrographic surgery: fresh tissue technique. Dermatol Clin 1989;7:613.

66. Zitelli JA. Mohs micrographic surgery for skin cancer. Princ Pract Oncol 1992;6:1.

67. Rowe DE, Carroll RJ, Day CL Jr. Long-term recurrence rates in previously untreated (primary) basal cell carcinoma: implications for patient follow-up. J Dermatol Surg Oncol 1989; 15:315.

68. Rowe DE, Carroll RJ, Day CL Jr. Mohs surgery is the treatment of choice for recurrent (previously treated) basal cell carcinoma. J Dermatol Surg Oncol 1989;15:424.

SURGERY: SCIENTIFIC PRINCIPLES AND PRACTICE, Second Edition, edited by Lazar J. Greenfield, Michael W. Mulholland, Keith T. Oldham, Gerald B. Zelenock, and Keith D. Lillemoe. Lippincott–Raven Publishers, Philadelphia, © 1997.

CHAPTER 112

SARCOMAS OF BONE AND SOFT TISSUE

VERNON K. SONDAK

Sarcomas are a heterogeneous group of cancers that arise from mesoderm-derived elements, including bone, cartilage, connective tissue, fat, and muscle. The soft tissues and bony structures constitute almost two thirds of the mass of the human body; despite this, sarcomas are not common. The relative rarity of sarcomas has made it difficult for any but a few specialized centers to gain wide experience with treating them. Still, sarcomas are sufficiently prevalent that a practicing surgeon can expect to encounter them at some point and must therefore be able to recognize them. In fact, an estimated 8900 new soft tissue and bone sarcomas occurred in 1995, making them more common than testicular cancer or Hodgkin disease. Soft tissue sarcomas, which account for 75% of all sarcomas, are responsible for the deaths of more patients each year than testicular cancer, Hodgkin disease, and thyroid cancer combined.[1]

The behavior of carcinomas, which arise from the ectoderm-derived tissues, varies dramatically depending on their site of origin within the body. In contrast, sarcomas typically behave in a similar fashion wherever they arise. The site of origin of a sarcoma does affect treatment, however, and hence outcome. Extremity sarcomas can usually be resected with a wide margin, although sometimes amputation is required. Because local control can be achieved in most patients with extremity lesions, emphasis is placed on preserving a functional limb. By contrast, sarcomas arising in the retroperitoneum are almost invariably situated near major organs and blood vessels. Even extensive resections often cannot include a wide margin of normal tissue around the tumor, and local recurrence is frequent. When a sarcoma arises in the head, neck, or trunk, an intermediate situation exists. Depending on the size and precise location of the tumor, wide resection may or may not be feasible, and local recurrence rates are somewhere between those of extremity and retroperitoneal sarcomas. Sarcomas arising in bone and those occurring in childhood are more sensitive to cytotoxic drugs than most adult soft tissue sarcomas. Hence, the management of these tumors is more likely to involve aggressive systemic chemotherapy. Thus, although the basic biologic and clinical behavior of all sarcomas is similar, each type requires a somewhat different management approach. Individual treatments are addressed later in this chapter.

Because of the paucity of symptoms associated with sarcomas, patients often present with locally advanced (or even metastatic) tumors. Nonetheless, surgical resection is the mainstay of treatment for patients with sarcoma, including some with metastatic disease. Surgery alone, however, is no longer the treatment of choice for most sarcoma patients. A multimodality approach that combines surgery, radiation, and in some cases, chemotherapy is the rule. In some of the more chemotherapy-responsive sarcomas (eg, Ewing sarcoma, embryonal rhabdomyosarcoma, and most types of osteogenic sarcoma), surgery has taken a secondary role to aggressive chemotherapy and is best regarded as a local adjuvant to curative systemic treatment. The surgeon must be well versed in the merits of all available therapeutic modalities to treat patients with sarcoma successfully.

EPIDEMIOLOGY

Sarcomas occur in all age groups, and they are among the most common cancers to afflict children, adolescents, and young adults. Specific sarcomas may have characteristic age distributions, but virtually any type of sarcoma can be encountered at any age. Males and females generally are equally affected, and there does not seem to be a strong tendency for sarcomas to occur in any particular ethnic or racial groups.

Most sarcomas occur in patients who have no identifiable predisposing factors—genetic or environmental. Although a history of trauma is often recalled by patients presenting with soft tissue sarcomas, traumatic injury does not seem to predispose to sarcoma development. More likely, a patient notices a soft tissue or bony lesion after an unrelated minor trauma and associates the two. Nonetheless, all patients presenting with soft tissue or bony tumors should be questioned about prior trauma because of the need to differentiate malignancy from a variety of benign posttraumatic lesions, such as myositis ossificans.

A few agents are known to cause sarcomas; these account for less than 10% of all cases.[2] Radiation exposure is clearly linked to the development of sarcomas. Sarcomas occurring in irradiated tissues are most commonly osteosarcomas or malignant fibrous histiocytomas, and they generally arise after a latency period of 7 to 20 years (Fig. 112-1). Among factory workers who were exposed to radium-226 while coating watch dials with luminous paint, several developed osteosarcomas. Radium is incor-

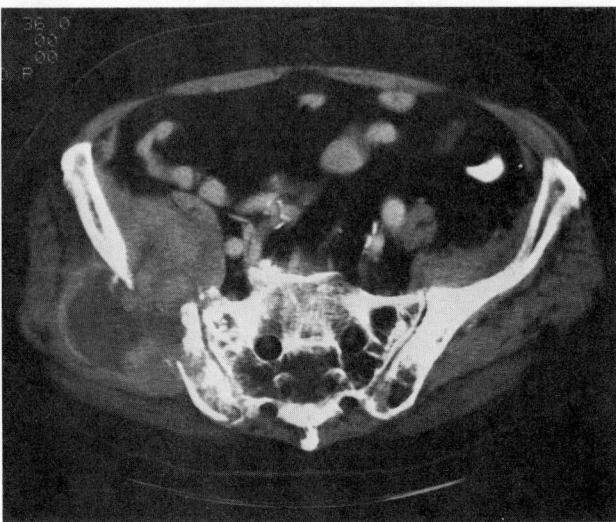

Figure 112-1. Osteosarcoma of the iliac bone that occurred 7 years after radiation therapy for cancer of the prostate and 30 years after radiation therapy for testicular cancer. The lesion was unresectable and associated with severe pain and lower extremity edema. The patient received significant palliation from two courses of intraarterial doxorubicin, after which the blood supply to the tumor was occluded by transcatheter embolization.

porated into bone in a manner analogous to calcium, and these workers were ingesting it when they used their tongues to wet the tips of their brushes. Once this practice was stopped, the epidemic ceased. The radioactive substance thorium dioxide (Thorotrast) was widely used as a contrast agent for radiologic procedures in the 1940s and 1950s. This agent predominantly accumulates in the liver where, with its half-life of over 400 years and extremely low rate of excretion, it can deliver as much as 15,000 cGy (1 cGy = 1 rad) to the hepatic parenchyma. Hepatic angiosarcomas occur with an extremely high frequency in patients who have received thorium dioxide, after a latency period of 18 to 36 years.

Certain chemicals that are not radioactive have also been implicated as causing sarcomas. These include arsenic and vinyl chloride, both of which are associated with hepatic angiosarcomas in exposed individuals. Some herbicides (phenoxyacetic acid compounds) have been linked to soft tissue sarcoma development. The highly toxic chemical dioxin is used in manufacturing these herbicides, and soft tissue sarcoma cases have been reported among workers who were exposed to dioxin and other chemicals in an industrial accident.[3] Dioxin (as well as some phenoxyherbicides) is present in small quantities in the defoliant Agent Orange, widely used during the Vietnam War. The Department of Veteran's Affairs ruled that Vietnam veterans who develop soft tissue sarcomas are entitled to compensation for their treatment, although the epidemiologic data linking Agent Orange exposure with sarcoma development remains inconclusive.[4]

In animals, infections with viruses such as the Moloney sarcoma virus can lead to sarcoma formation. In humans, infection with the human immunodeficiency virus (HIV-1) is associated with a markedly increased incidence of Kaposi sarcoma, an otherwise extraordinarily rare lesion. It is unclear whether the predilection to develop these sarcomas is due to a specific carcinogenic effect of the virus or to the underlying immunodeficiency caused by HIV infection. Because Kaposi sarcoma tends to occur only in certain subgroups of HIV-infected patients, other factors may be instrumental in its development.

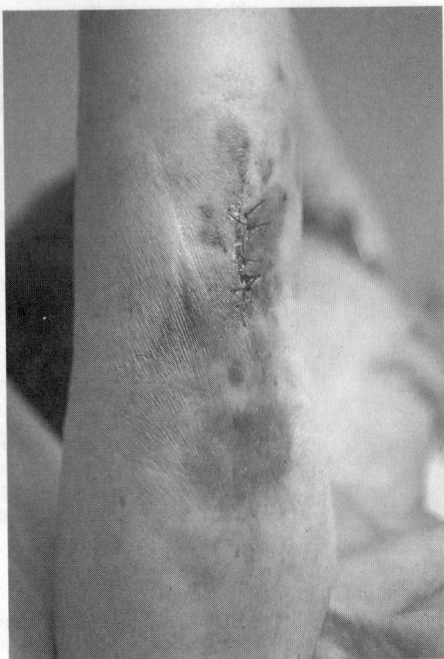

Figure 112-2. Lymphangiosarcoma of the right upper extremity occurring 21 years after a radical mastectomy and postoperative chest wall irradiation for breast cancer. At presentation, pulmonary metastases were already evident. The diffuse discoloration is more suggestive of ecchymosis than tumor. Although most instances of postmastectomy lymphangiosarcoma are associated with severe lymphedema, the extremity was relatively normal in this case.

Long-standing lymphedema of an extremity predisposes to the development of lymphangiosarcomas. Originally described in patients with arm edema after radical mastectomy and postoperative radiation (Fig. 112-2), lymphangiosarcomas have been seen in patients with severe edema from other causes as well.

Neurofibromatosis type 1 (von Recklinghausen disease) represents a condition with a genetic predisposition to sarcoma development (Fig. 112-3). An estimated 5% of neurofibromatosis patients develop a sarcoma during their lifetime. These tumors are virtually all neurofibrosarcomas (sometimes called malignant schwannomas or malignant peripheral nerve tumors) and generally arise within preexisting neurofibromas. All patients presenting with a neurofibrosarcoma should be closely examined, and a thorough family history should be obtained for evidence of neurofibromatosis. Conversely, any rapidly enlarging or newly symptomatic lesion in a patient with neurofibromatosis should be suspected of malignancy.

A genetic predisposition to sarcomas also exists in patients with retinoblastoma. Originally, a high incidence of osteosarcomas was noted in the orbit after radiation therapy for primary retinoblastoma, and these lesions were attributed to the radiation. It is now clear that the incidence of all types of sarcomas is markedly increased in these patients, even in nonirradiated areas. This increased incidence is more commonly associated with the familial than the sporadic form of retinoblastoma. The precise genetic defect responsible is now understood: mutation in one copy of the RB1 gene.

Another inherited condition is associated with childhood soft tissue sarcomas and breast cancer, as well as several other types of cancer. This condition, termed the *Li-Fraumeni syndrome*, is due to an inherited mutation in the p53 gene (also referred to as TP53), which increases affected family members' susceptibility to cancer.[5] Like the genetic defect in familial retinoblastoma, the gene involved with Li-Fraumeni syndrome is also important in sporadic sarcoma development (both of these conditions are discussed later).

With the exception of patients with these syndromes, other forms of cancer are not more common in patients with sarcomas or their relatives.

PATHOLOGIC CLASSIFICATION

Sarcomas are classified by the type of tissue formed by the tumor (histogenic classification) rather than by the type of tissue in which the tumor arises. Thus, a malignant tumor arising within a skeletal muscle but composed of malignant smooth muscle cells is termed a leiomyosarcoma, not a rhabdomyosarcoma. Bone tumors are not termed osteosarcomas unless the malignant cells clearly produce osteoid. Some bone tumors produce cartilage (chondrosarcomas); a few are fibrosarcomas or other histologic types. Occasionally, soft tissue neoplasms produce bone or cartilage; these are termed extraosseous osteosarcomas or chondrosarcomas, as appropriate. The various

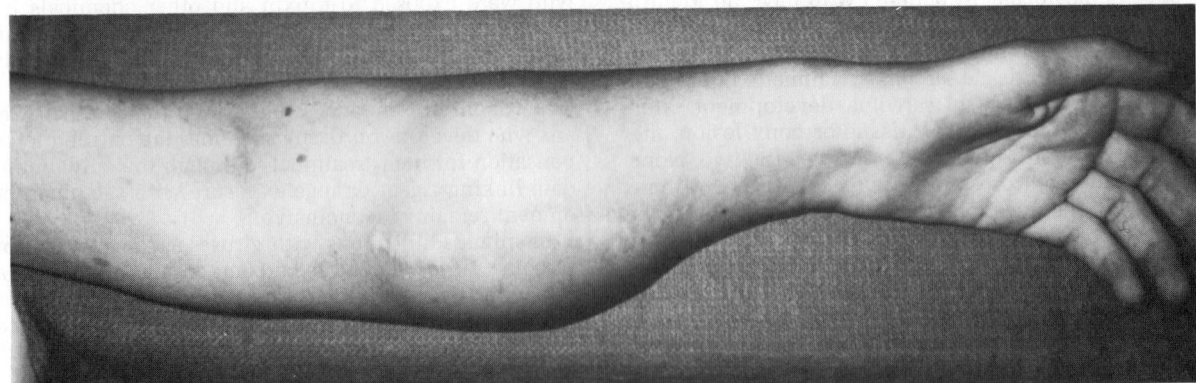

Figure 112-3. Large neurofibrosarcoma arising from the median nerve in a 17-year-old patient with neurofibromatosis. The incision is from a biopsy of the lesion 18 months before the diagnosis of malignancy. Since the earlier biopsy (which revealed only benign neurofibroma), the mass progressively enlarged and became painful, and the patient lost sensory and motor function in the median nerve distribution. There is wasting of the thenar eminence.

Table 112-1. HISTOGENIC CLASSIFICATION SCHEME FOR BENIGN AND MALIGNANT SOFT TISSUE TUMORS

Tissue Formed (Histogenesis)	Benign Soft Tissue Tumor	Malignant Soft Tissue Tumor
Fat	Lipoma	Liposarcoma
Fibrous tissue	Fibroma	Fibrosarcoma
Skeletal muscle	Rhabdomyoma	Rhabdomyosarcoma
Smooth muscle	Leiomyoma	Leiomyosarcoma
Bone	Osteoma	Osteosarcoma
Cartilage	Chondroma	Chondrosarcoma
Synovium	Synovioma	Synovial sarcoma
Blood vessel	Hemangioma	Angiosarcoma; malignant hemangiopericytoma
Lymphatics	Lymphangioma	Lymphangiosarcoma
Nerve	Neurofibroma	Neurifibrosarcoma
Mesothelium	Benign mesothelioma	Malignant mesothelioma
Tissue histiocyte	Benign fibrous histiocytoma	Malignant fibrous histiocytoma
Pluripotent	None recognized	Malignant mesenchymoma
Uncertain	None recognized	Ewing sarcoma; alveolar soft parts sarcoma; epithelioid sarcoma

types of benign and malignant soft tissue tumors are noted in Table 112-1, and the relative frequency of the different sarcomas is listed in Table 112-2.

The development of specialized markers for identifying individual types of sarcoma has led to greater precision in their classification. Available immunohistochemical stains include S-100, a marker for neural crest origin (positive in neurofibrosarcomas); factor VIII, which identifies cells of endothelial origin (positive in angiosarcomas); and myoglobin, which is found only in rhabdomyosarcomas. Although these stains are often helpful, they are not positive in every tumor of the appropriate type. Electron microscopy may reveal ultrastructural elements that are pathognomonic for a specific cell type, but in most cases sarcomas are classified by their light microscopic appearance. In a small percentage of tumors (about 10% in most series), the tumor cells are so poorly differentiated that no specific histogenesis can be determined, even using the supportive diagnostic tools mentioned.

Although the exact histologic type is an important piece of data in the evaluation of the sarcoma patient, it is not as influential in terms of prognosis and therapy as histologic grade. Histologic grade is assessed based on the degree of cellular atypia, the frequency of mitotic figures, and the presence or absence of spontaneous tumor necrosis (Fig. 112-4). Low-grade tumors have relatively little cellular atypia, few mitoses, and no tumor necrosis. Intermediate-grade tumors have more atypia and numerous mitoses, but little or no tumor necrosis. High-grade tumors show a significant degree of necrosis in addition to atypia and frequent mitotic figures.

A consistently applied grading system discriminates between tumors with good prognosis (low-grade) and those with poorer prognosis (intermediate- and high-grade). Most studies also show an important distinction between intermediate- and high-grade lesions (Fig. 112-5); thus, two-grade staging systems have largely been replaced. The pathologist should assign a histologic grade to every sarcoma biopsy specimen. For lesions in which disparate areas exist, the highest grade encountered is used to categorize the tumor.

MOLECULAR BIOLOGY

The light microscopic assessment of histologic grade is the most important single element in assessing the prognosis of sarcomas. With advances in molecular biology, however, new tools for analyzing histologic type, prognosis, and cause of these tumors have become available. Cytogenetic aberrations have been recognized in a number of soft tissue sarcomas, and some of these may be specific for certain histologic types. Alveolar rhabdomyosarcomas, myxoid liposarcomas, and synovial sarcomas have each been found to have characteristic chromosomal translocations that potentially could assist in the differentiation of these tumors from other sarcomas.[6] Flow cytometric analysis of DNA from osteosarcomas has been shown to have prognostic importance, and similar analysis of soft tissue sarcomas suggests a correlation between histologic grade and ploidy status, with most high-grade lesions being aneuploid rather than diploid. Large, prospective trials of flow cytometry and cytogenetic analysis are needed to ascertain the importance of these studies in diagnosing and treating sarcomas.

The finding of a link between familial retinoblastoma and sarcoma led researchers to search for specific genetic changes responsible for the observed susceptibility to sarcoma development. Retinoblastoma, the most common childhood malignant tumor of the eye, has been associated with a genetic defect in the retinoblastoma gene (RB1) on the long arm of chromosome 13. RB1 is a recessive oncogene

Table 112-2. RELATIVE FREQUENCY OF HISTOLOGIC TYPES OF SOFT TISSUE SARCOMAS IN ADULTS (ALL SITES)

Histologic Type	Percentage
Malignant fibrous histiocytoma	25.9
Liposarcoma	17.7
Leiomyosarcoma	14.8
Fibrosarcoma	6.6
Neurofibrosarcoma	4.0
Synovial sarcoma	3.6
Rhabdomyosarcoma	3.6
Angiosarcoma	2.9
Extraskeletal chondrosarcoma	1.2
Malignant mesenchymoma	1.0
Extraskeletal osteosarcoma	0.6
Unclassified	5.4
Other	12.7

(Modified from Lawrence W Jr., Donegan WL, Natarajan A, et al. Adult soft tissue sarcomas: a pattern of care survey of the American College of Surgeons. Ann Surg 1987;205:349)

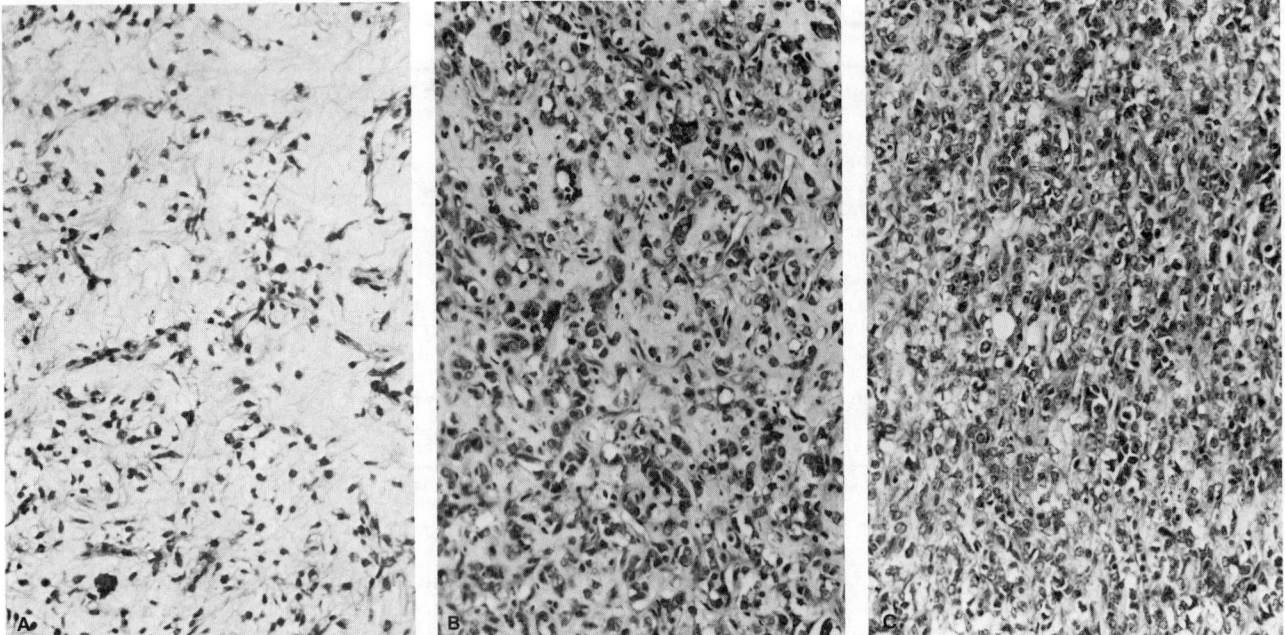

Figure 112-4. Photomicrographs of three fibrosarcomas illustrating the differing appearance of different grades of the same tumor type. The low-grade fibrosarcoma (*A*) shows relatively little cellular atypia, few mitoses, and no tumor necrosis, whereas the intermediate-grade tumor (*B*) has more atypia, numerous mitoses, and scant tumor necrosis. The high-grade tumor (*C*) shows a significant degree of necrosis in addition to atypia and frequent mitotic figures. (Courtesy of Sharon Weiss, MD, Department of Pathology, University of Michigan, Ann Arbor)

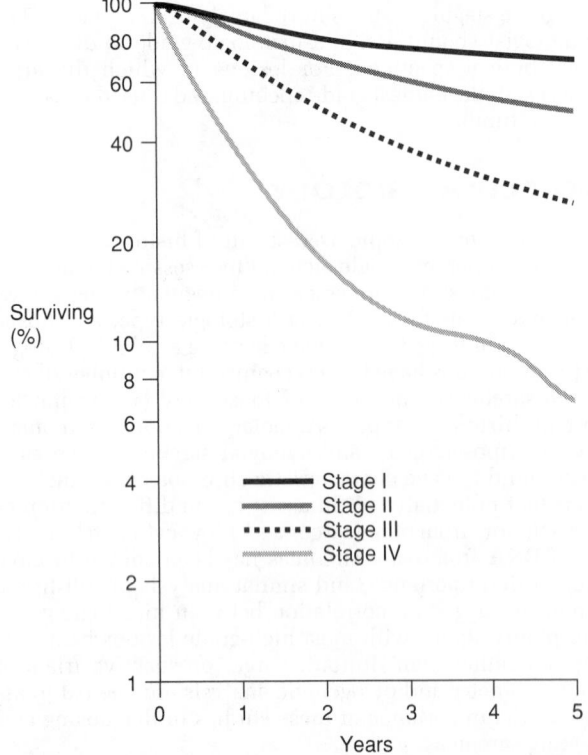

Figure 112-5. Survival of patients with sarcoma classified by AJCC stage, where stage I corresponds to low-grade, stage II to intermediate-grade, and stage III to high-grade tumors. Stage IV includes all patients with regional or distant metastases, regardless of grade of the primary tumor.

or "tumor suppressor gene," which means that both alleles must be inactivated before malignant transformation can occur. The normal product of this gene is involved in regulating cell division. Losing both normal copies of the gene predisposes to tumor formation by removing this growth control. Patients with familial retinoblastoma inherit one inactivated RB1 gene. For these individuals to develop retinoblastoma, they must undergo only one additional genetic mutation inactivating the normal gene, compared with two mutations (involving both normal RB1 genes) necessary for someone without the inherited defect. By virtue of the increased susceptibility, individuals inheriting one defective RB1 gene develop multiple, bilateral retinoblastomas at an early age (often in the first year of life).

The RB1 gene appears to affect more than retinoblastoma development. The susceptibility to sarcoma formation in familial retinoblastoma patients relates to the genetic defect in RB1 as well.[6] RB1 may also play a role in the pathogenesis of certain types of nonfamilial soft tissue sarcomas. In a study of soft tissue sarcomas in nonretinoblastoma patients, 3 of 69 cases had homozygous deletions of the RB1 gene.[7] Another 5 cases had evidence of heterozygous deletion. This illustrates an important principle of the genetics of cancer formation: it is frequently the case that the same gene involved in a familial cancer syndrome (where one inherited copy of the gene is defective and the other is presumably lost later) is also important in the spontaneous development of the relevant tumor type (where both normal copies of the gene must be lost to mutations or genetic deletions).

This principle is illustrated again with the p53 gene, associated with the Li-Fraumeni syndrome. This familial cancer syndrome involves early-onset breast cancer, sarcomas (often in childhood), and a variety of other malignancies (notably brain tumors, adrenal cortical cancers, and leukemias). Patients with Li-Fraumeni syndrome inherit a defective copy of the p53 gene, another key growth regulatory gene. Inactivation of the second, normal copy of the gene leaves the cell without the ability to regulate gene transcription, particularly after DNA damage.[8] Abnormalities of the p53 gene are also common in sporadic cases of sarcoma. One study found p53 abnormalities in about 60% of osteosarcomas and malignant fibrous histiocytomas, as well as approximately 33% of other sarcomas.[9] Interestingly, some sarcomas that do not show evidence of any p53 gene abnormalities have been found to possess amplifications of a gene called MDM2, which codes for a protein that inactivates the function of normal p53 protein.[10]

One other important genetic change in some sarcomas is the presence of the MDR1 (multidrug-resistance) gene, which is found in greater numbers of untreated sarcomas than most other tumor types.[11] The presence of this gene has been correlated in vitro with resistance to a number of cytotoxic drugs, many of which are routinely used in sarcoma chemotherapy. Experimental studies have shown the importance of MDR1 gene activation in the resistance of sarcoma cells to doxorubicin, probably the most commonly used drug for sarcoma treatment.[12] While other genetic abnormalities are likely to prove important in sarcoma development and treatment, these carefully studied genes vividly demonstrate the rapidly evolving link between the research laboratory and the clinic as well as the extent to which the practicing physician must be aware of developments in molecular biology.

DIAGNOSIS AND STAGING OF SOFT TISSUE SARCOMAS

Benign soft tissue tumors far outnumber their malignant counterparts. Because of this, prolonged delays before definitive treatment begins are common in sarcoma patients. In a survey of more than 5800 sarcoma patients, roughly half waited 4 or more months before seeking medical treatment, and 20% waited at least 6 months after seeing a physician before a correct diagnosis was made.[13] Many sarcoma patients undergo prolonged treatment for chronic hematomas or pulled muscles. Nonathletic adults rarely develop persistent soft tissue masses from either of these causes in the absence of a history of unusually strenuous activity. Only in a setting of clearcut local trauma should these diagnoses be entertained. If a soft tissue mass arises in a patient with no history of trauma or persists more than 6 weeks after local trauma, biopsy should be performed.

Soft tissue sarcomas of the extremity, trunk, head, and neck commonly present as a painless mass. Retroperitoneal sarcomas most often present as a palpable mass in association with abdominal fullness, early satiety, or vague abdominal pain. While evaluating any soft tissue mass, the physician must always remain cognizant of the possibility of malignancy. Biopsy should be done for virtually all soft tissue masses larger than 5 cm as well as for any new, enlarging, or symptomatic lesions. Small, subcutaneous lesions that have not changed for many years may be safely observed.

Biopsy

Properly performed, a timely surgical biopsy is the critical first step in a multimodality treatment approach. Improperly done, it can markedly complicate the care of the sarcoma patient and occasionally even eliminate treatment options. Excisional biopsy should be reserved for small soft tissue masses (less than 3 to 5 cm in greatest diameter), for which the chance of malignancy is low and for which

complete excision would not jeopardize subsequent treatment in the event a sarcoma was found. For all other soft tissue masses, incisional biopsy is indicated.

Several important technical factors must be considered when performing an incisional biopsy. For extremity lesions, the incision should be oriented along the long axis of the extremity. For truncal or retroperitoneal lesions, the biopsy incision should be situated so that it can be readily excised along with the tumor if a diagnosis of sarcoma is made. Any biopsy site should be placed directly over the tumor, at the point where the lesion is closest to the surface, and there should be no raising of flaps or disturbance of tissue planes superficial to the tumor (Fig. 112-6).

Many sarcomas appear to be relatively well encapsulated at the time of open biopsy. Most often, however, these tumors possess a pseudocapsule, and removing the tumor in this apparent plane leaves gross or microscopic cancer behind in most cases.[14] Soft tissue sarcomas should not be enucleated within the pseudocapsule to make a diagnosis; incisional biopsy leaving the bulk of the lesion undisturbed is preferable. Frozen-section pathologic analysis should be used to determine whether diagnostic tissue has been obtained, not to provide a definite diagnosis. Before wound closure, hemostasis should be achieved to avoid a hematoma that could disseminate tumor cells through normal tissue planes. Drains are not used routinely; in the uncommon case when a drain is required, it should exit either through or near the biopsy incision. If malignancy is diagnosed, the drain tract must be excised in continuity with the tumor mass.

Fine-needle aspiration cytology has a role in the diagnosis of some soft tissue lesions. Computed tomography (CT)–guided fine-needle aspiration has proved to be helpful in diagnosing intraabdominal and retroperitoneal tumors but is rarely needed for extremity sarcomas. Fine-needle aspiration has the advantage of minimizing the potential for tumor spillage in the peritoneal cavity that can accompany open surgical biopsy of a retroperitoneal sarcoma. Even experienced cytologists, however, often are unable to discern the grade and histologic type of a sarcoma from an aspirate.

A core needle biopsy retrieves a thin sliver of tissue (approximately 1×10 mm). As with fine-needle aspiration, the small sample size may make it difficult for a pathologist to accurately diagnose and grade the tumor, or the tissue obtained may not represent an adequate sample of the entire tumor, leading to an underestimate of the grade. Sufficient tissue to perform special stains or electron microscopy may not be available with this technique. Fears that core needle biopsies would result in a significant number of hematomas, resulting in dissemination of tumor cells, appear to be groundless. Recent series comparing core needle and open biopsies of soft tissue tumors have documented that both the histologic type and grade of a sarcoma could be correctly determined by core needle biopsy in more than 90% of cases.[15] These results have encouraged wider use of this technique, including CT-guided core needle biopsies.

Staging and Metastatic Work-Up

Once the diagnosis of sarcoma is made, the extent of the primary tumor must be assessed and the presence or absence of metastatic disease determined. Because of the prognostic importance of histologic grade, the staging of the primary tumor is based on both clinical and histologic information. The usual TNM classification is modified accordingly to a GTNM system (Table 112-3). In the absence of regional or distant metastatic disease, low-grade (G1) tumors are classified as stage I, intermediate-grade tumors as stage II, and high-grade tumors as stage III. Any tumor

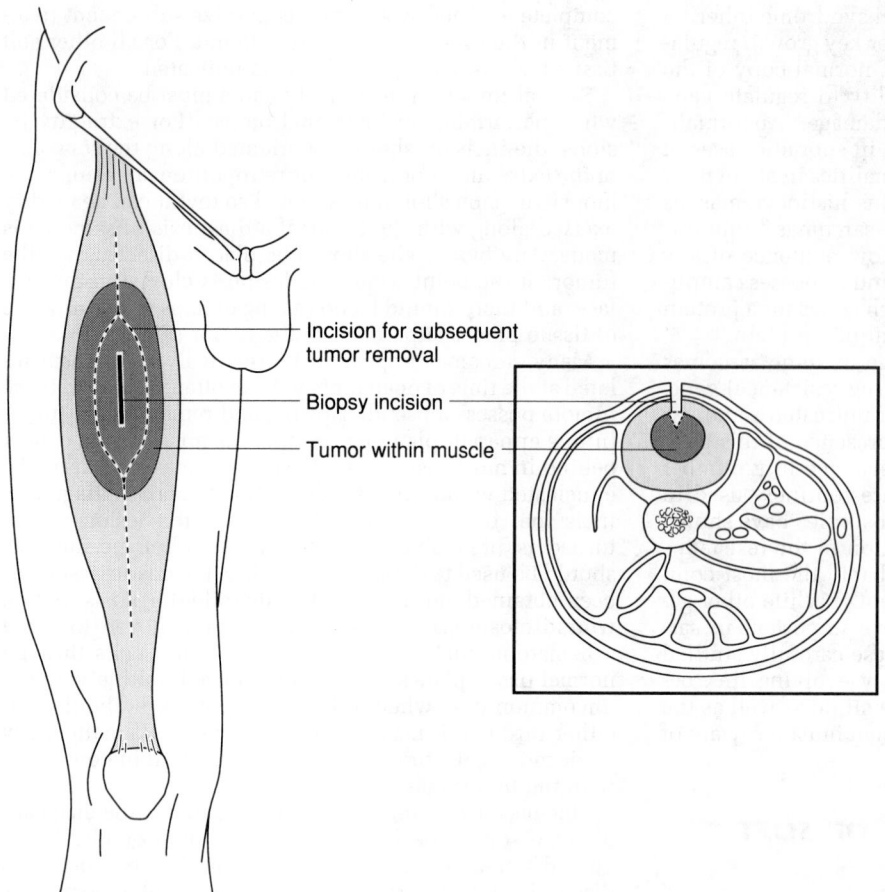

Incision for subsequent tumor removal

Biopsy incision

Tumor within muscle

Figure 112-6. Technique for biopsy of an extremity soft tissue mass suspected of being a sarcoma. The incision should be oriented along the long axis of the extremity, at the point where the lesion is closest to the surface, and situated so that it can be readily excised along with the tumor if a diagnosis of sarcoma is made. There should be no raising of flaps or disturbance of tissue planes superficial to the tumor. The mass should not be enucleated within the pseudo-capsule; rather, incisional biopsy leaving the bulk of the lesion undisturbed should be carried out. Before wound closure, hemostasis should be achieved to avoid a hematoma, which could disseminate tumor cells through normal tissue planes. Drains are not used routinely.

with regional or distant metastatic disease, regardless of the grade of the primary tumor, is classified as stage IV. This staging system is clinically useful because it separates patients into groups with clearly differing prognoses (see Fig. 112-5).

Following tumor grade, tumor size is next in prognostic importance. The larger the primary sarcoma, the greater the risk of metastatic disease and, ultimately, of death. In the GTNM system, T1 tumors are equal to or smaller than 5 cm in diameter, and T2 tumors exceed 5 cm. Each stage is subdivided into an A and B category, with T1 tumors assigned an A and T2 tumors a B. Thus, an intermediate-grade sarcoma, 8 cm in diameter without regional or distant spread (G2,T2,N0,M0) would be classed as stage IIB. Although the GTNM size cutoff is 5 cm, tumors larger than 10 cm have an even worse prognosis.

It is also recognized that superficially located tumors (ie, those situated entirely above the deep or muscular fascia of the body) have a more favorable prognosis. The AJCC system does not currently address this factor, but an alternative staging system developed at Memorial-Sloan Kettering does. In this system, size greater than or equal to 5 cm, location deep to the fascia, and high histologic grade are considered unfavorable factors, and the stage is assigned based on the number of these unfavorable factors.[16] Hence, a small, superficial, low-grade tumor (with zero unfavorable factors) would be considered stage 0, whereas a large, deep, high-grade tumor (having three unfavorable factors) would be classified as stage III. Although this system has some attractive aspects, it remains to be independently confirmed, and as yet has not been shown superior to the AJCC system.

Problematic aspects include the lack of an intermediate grade as accepted by most pathologists, as well as uncertainty as to whether a small, superficial high-grade sarcoma truly has an equivalent prognosis to either a small, deep, low-grade or a large, superficial low-grade tumor, even though all have one unfavorable factor and hence are classified as stage I. (Obviously, the same case can be made for tumors classified as stage II in this system.) Nonetheless, further investigation of the independent contribution of tumor location relative to the muscular fascia as a prognostic factor is clearly warranted.

In addition to assessing prognosis, the initial evaluation must provide information about the precise extent of the primary tumor. CT scanning and magnetic resonance imaging (MRI) are the most important studies for assessing the extent and resectability of soft tissue sarcomas, regardless of the site of origin.[17] These studies permit definition of the primary tumor in relation to bone, muscle, neurovascular structures, and adjacent organs; this is critical information when planning treatment. Both CT and MRI can provide this information, and in most cases, either study is sufficient. The choice between them is based on availability, cost, and the experience of the radiologist. Each study has advantages and disadvantages, however, and these should be considered on a case-by-case basis.

CT scans are widely available, and both the primary site and the lungs (the major site of sarcoma metastasis) can be imaged at the same sitting. Furthermore, most radiologists have more experience with CT than MRI. Tumor involvement of bone is often more clearly visible on CT scan, although bone marrow invasion may be better defined by

Table 112-3. AMERICAN JOINT COMMISSION ON CANCER GTNM CLASSIFICATION AND STAGE GROUPING OF SOFT TISSUE SARCOMAS

Stage	Description
TUMOR GRADE	
G1	Well differentiated
G2	Moderately well differentiated
G3	Poorly differentiated
G4	Undifferentiated
PRIMARY TUMOR	
T1	Tumor ≤ 5 cm in greatest diameter
T2	Tumor > 5 cm in greatest diameter
REGIONAL LYMPH NODE INVOLVEMENT	
N0	No known metastases to lymph nodes
N1	Verified metastases to lymph nodes
DISTANT METASTASIS	
M0	No known distant metastasis
M1	Known distant metastasis
STAGE GROUPING	
Stage IA	G1, T1, N0, M0
Stage IB	G1, T2, N0, M0
Stage IIA	G2, T1, N0, M0
Stage IIB	G2, T2, N0, M0
Stage IIIA	G3–4, T1, N0, M0
Stage IIIB	G3–4, T2, N0, M0
Stage IVA	Any G, any T, N1, M0
Stage IVB	Any G, any T, any N, M1

(Modified from Beahrs OH, Henson DE, Hutter RVP, Kennedy BJ. Manual for staging of cancer, ed 4. Philadelphia, JB Lippincott, 1992:132)

MRI. Disadvantages of CT scanning include the ionizing radiation and the need for intravenous iodinated contrast administration.

MRI has several advantages in evaluating sarcomas. The plane of imaging is not limited to the transverse (axial) plane of CT scans. Coronal, sagittal, and even oblique planes may be imaged with MRI. Comparative studies have also suggested that MRI better defines the relationship between tumor and normal vascular structures.[17] Because of the strong magnetic fields required for imaging, patients with implanted metallic objects, such as pacemakers, artificial joints, and some vena caval filters, may not be able to undergo MRI. Occasionally, the information obtained from CT and MRI may be complementary, but for most sarcoma patients, either study is sufficient.

Plain radiographs and radionuclide bone scans occasionally provide useful information regarding invasion of bone by tumor (Fig. 112-7), but these studies usually do not play a major role in evaluating a primary soft tissue sarcoma. Sarcomas have a characteristic arteriographic appearance, with prominent neovascularity and displacement of normal vessels. Angiography is rarely necessary for extremity lesions, although it may useful for retroperitoneal tumors. Even these, magnetic resonance angiography represents an attractive alternative (Fig. 112-8).

Regional lymph node involvement is decidedly uncommon in soft tissue sarcomas; less than 4% of cases have nodal metastases at presentation. When node involvement occurs, it conveys essentially the same prognosis as distant metastatic disease and therefore is classified as stage IV (stage IVA if only nodal metastases are present; stage IVB if both regional and distant metastases are present). Nearly all patients who ever manifest nodal involvement had high-grade primary sarcomas (Fig. 112-9). Distant metastatic disease is present in

as many as 25% of soft tissue sarcoma patients at the time of presentation. By far the most common site of metastases is the lungs. In sarcoma patients who develop metastases, the lungs are involved more than 75% of the time. About half of all sarcoma patients who die of metastatic disease have lung metastases as their only site of distant spread. Liver involvement is rare except in intraabdominal and retroperitoneal sarcomas, where it represents the second most common site of distant spread. Occasional patients develop bone or central nervous system metastases; these sites of disease are uncommon in patients who do not already have lung metastases.

For all patients with newly diagnosed soft tissue sarcomas, a chest radiograph and chest CT scan are appropriate to search for pulmonary metastases. For intraabdominal or retroperitoneal tumors, a CT scan that includes the liver should be done. Other studies, such as radionuclide bone scans, CT scanning, or MRI of the head, are not indicated in the absence of symptoms that suggest metastatic involvement.

Two new imaging modalities are being explored as adjuncts to sarcoma staging. Both studies provide functional information about tumor metabolism as opposed to the anatomic information provided by most standard imaging techniques. Phosphorus-31 MRI spectroscopy allows quantification of the amount of inorganic phosphate (P_i) relative to organic phosphate compounds, such as phosphocreatine (PC) and nucleoside triphosphates (ATP and GTP).[18] The inorganic/organic phosphate and PC/ATP ratios provide noninvasive measures of the metabolic status of a tumor, which may be correlated with tumor grade. Positron emission tomography (PET) scanning using fluoro-13-deoxyglucose also offers the potential for noninvasive analysis of tumor metabolism and has been shown to correlate with both tumor grade and response to treatment.[19]

MANAGEMENT OF EXTREMITY SOFT TISSUE SARCOMAS

The most common site of origin for sarcomas is the lower extremity (Table 112-4). Soft tissue sarcomas are most often found in the muscle groups of the thigh. The proximal upper extremity is also a common location. The distal extremities are less frequent sites of origin. Over time, there have been significant changes in the surgical approach to extremity sarcomas. Initially, attempts at limited excisions of extremity sarcomas were uniformly associated with local recurrence. These "shell-out" resections enucleated the tumor from within its pseudocapsule, invariably leaving viable tumor behind. Once this was recognized, the surgical approach to these tumors changed to one favoring radical amputation. With the advent of multimodality approaches, limb-sparing resections now can be performed in more than 90% of patients, and local recurrence rates of 10% or less are reported.

Surgery

Radical amputation is amputation at least one joint space above the most proximal extent of tumor (Fig. 112-10). For a distal thigh tumor, a radical amputation would be a hip disarticulation; for a high thigh lesion, a hemipelvectomy is required. At one time, over half of all soft tissue sarcomas of the extremity were treated with radical amputations. Even with such extensive and mutilating procedures, however, local recurrence rates of up to 20% were seen.

Radical amputation was compared with wide local excision plus postoperative radiation in a prospective, ran-

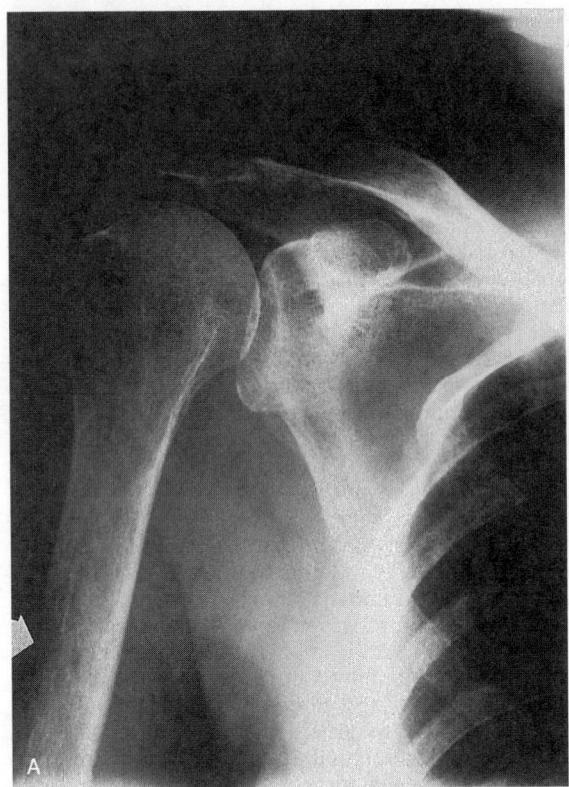

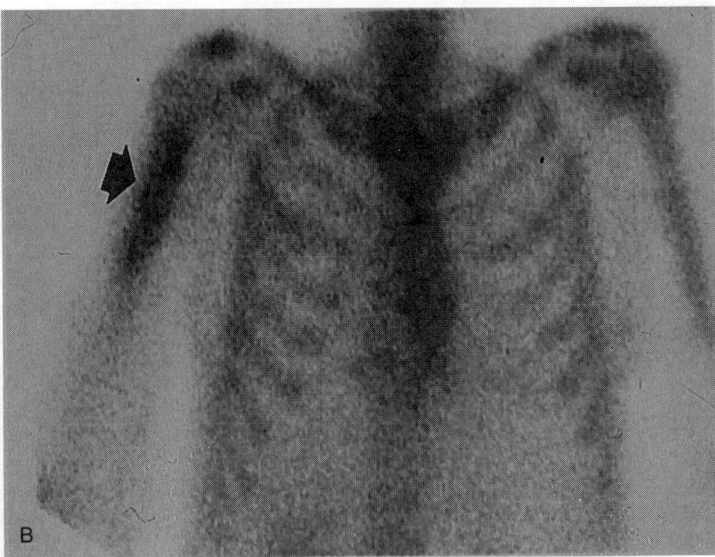

Figure 112-7. (*A*) Plain radiograph of the proximal humerus and shoulder joint, showing bony destruction (*arrow*) secondary to a large, high-grade soft tissue sarcoma adjacent to the humerus. (*B*) Radionuclide bone scan in the same patient reveals a much greater degree of involvement (*arrow*).

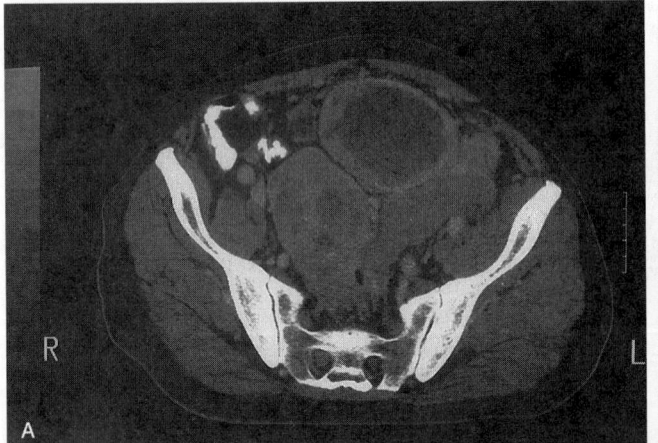

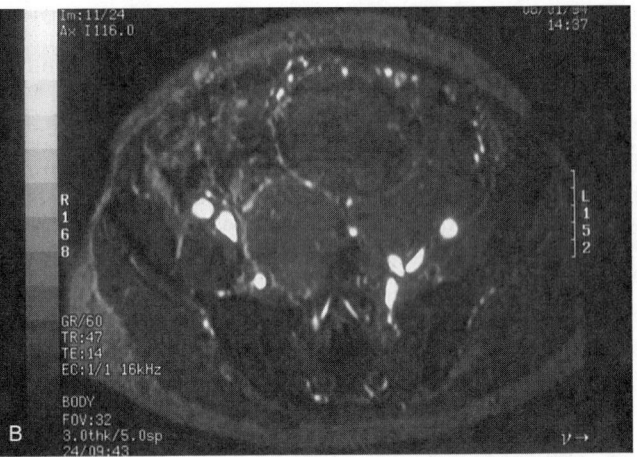

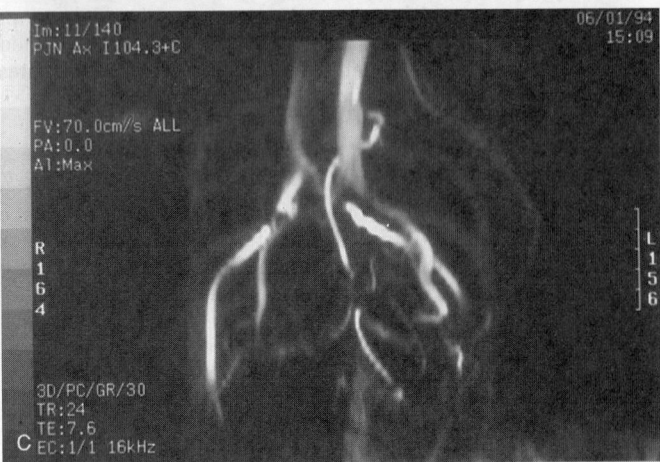

Figure 112-8. (*A*) CT scan of a large, high-grade pelvic sarcoma. There are multiple lobulations of tumor, with areas of spontaneous necrosis and a fluid–fluid level. The iliac vessels cannot be clearly distinguished as separate from the tumor mass. (*B*) MR angiogram of the same region revealing the iliac arteries and veins as prominent white spots against the dark background of tumor. (*C*) Planar reconstruction demonstrating the distal aorta and vena cava and the iliac arteries and veins. The MR angiogram suggested the vessels were free of involvement, as indeed was the case at the time of resection.

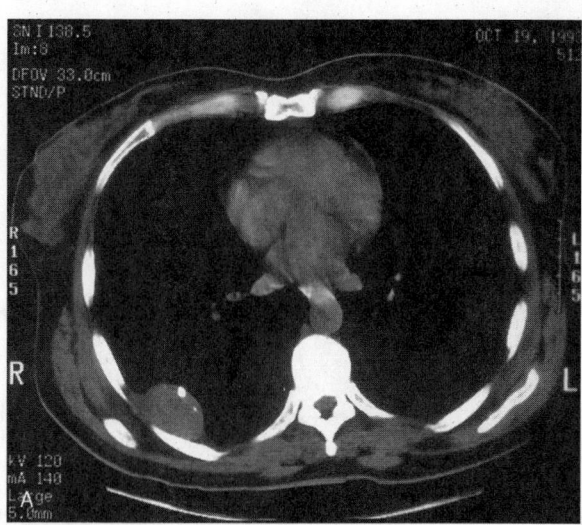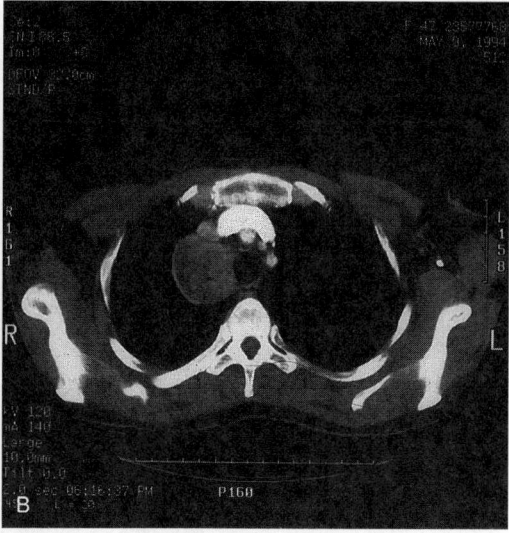

Figure 112-9. (*A*) High-grade malignant fibrous histiocytoma of the pleura. This tumor was treated with chest wall resection and postoperative radiation. (*B*) A follow-up CT scan 7 months later revealed mediastinal adenopathy, which was subsequently confirmed to represent nodal metastasis from sarcoma.

domized trial; patients who underwent limb-sparing surgery had a survival rate identical to those undergoing amputation, despite a higher local recurrence rate (19% versus 6%, difference not statistically significant).[20] This study demonstrated the merit of limb-sparing approaches to treating extremity sarcomas. Radical amputation now is reserved for patients who are not suitable candidates for limb-sparing approaches, usually because of bony invasion or large tumor size (Fig. 112-11), or for recurrence after previous limb-sparing surgery.

One of the earliest limb-sparing operations to be advocated was compartment excision. In this technique, the entire muscle group in which the sarcoma arises is removed from origin to insertion (Fig. 112-12). The belief that sarcomas spread diffusely throughout one muscular compartment but are prevented by fascial boundaries from lateral spread provided the rationale for this procedure. Unfortunately, most sarcomas are not confined within a single muscular compartment, and those that are do not usually involve the muscles for more than 2 to 3 cm beyond the grossly visible boundaries. Long, origin-to-insertion skin incisions often cross one or even two joints, making postoperative radiation and rehabilitation more difficult. Hence, compartment excision is used only in selected cases when the tumor is large but remains confined to one compartment.

Most limb-sparing protocols include a wide local excision as the definitive surgical procedure. Wide local excision involves gross total removal of the tumor with a wide margin of normal tissue, but no attempt is made to resect an entire muscle compartment (Fig. 112-13). Rather, a margin of 3 to 5 cm of normal tissue is obtained proximally and distally. On the lateral and deep margins, at least one grossly uninvolved fascial plane is resected en bloc with the tumor whenever possible. For large or deep-seated tumors, resection of uninvolved periosteum or adventitia may represent the deep margin. If necessary, major vascular structures can be resected and reconstructed with autologous or other graft material (Fig. 112-14*A*). On occasion, major nerves, such as the sciatic nerve, are sacrificed to preserve a functional, albeit neurologically compromised, extremity. When low-grade lesions are resected, because of their less aggressive nature, major vessels or nerves are not removed along with the tumor (Fig. 112-14*B*).

Radiation Therapy

For patients with small, low-grade tumors, wide local excision alone is associated with a low rate of local recurrence. Most other patients undergoing surgical excision, however, receive additional therapy to improve the chances for local control. This additional therapy usually includes radiation. Radiation also has some effectiveness as primary therapy for extremity sarcomas in patients who refuse or cannot tolerate surgery.[21] Although the results do not match the local control rates achieved with radical surgery alone, they do provide a firm basis for including radiation therapy in multimodality treatment approaches.

Postoperative Radiation

Postoperative radiation therapy after wide surgical excision provides excellent local control for primary extremity sarcomas up to 10 cm in size. The randomized trial of amputation versus wide local excision previously cited validated the concept of limb-sparing surgery combined with postoperative radiation. Generally, a dose of 6000 cGy or greater is required to ensure local control. At this dosage, the entire circumference of the extremity must not

Table 112-4. SITE OF ORIGIN OF SOFT TISSUE SARCOMAS IN ADULTS

Anatomic Site	Percentage
Lower extremity	46.4
Trunk	17.9
Upper extremity	13.1
Retroperitoneum	12.5
Head and neck	8.9
Mediastinum	1.3

(Lawrence W Jr., Donegan WL, Natarajan A, et al. Adult soft tissue sarcomas: a pattern of care survey of the American College of Surgeons. Ann Surg 1987;205:349)

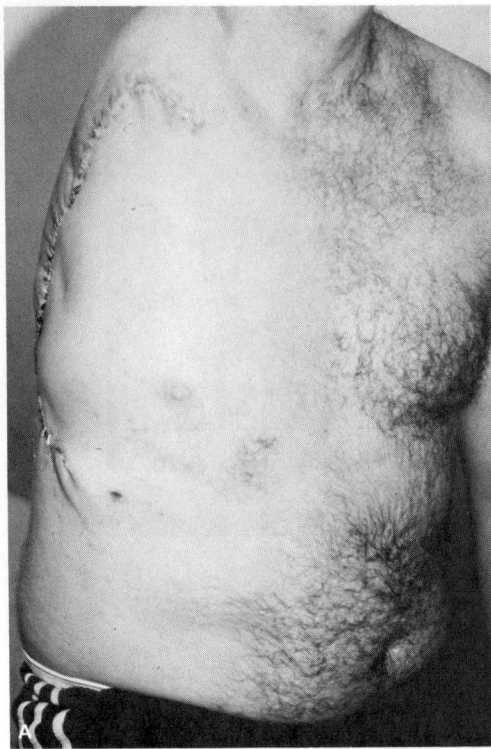
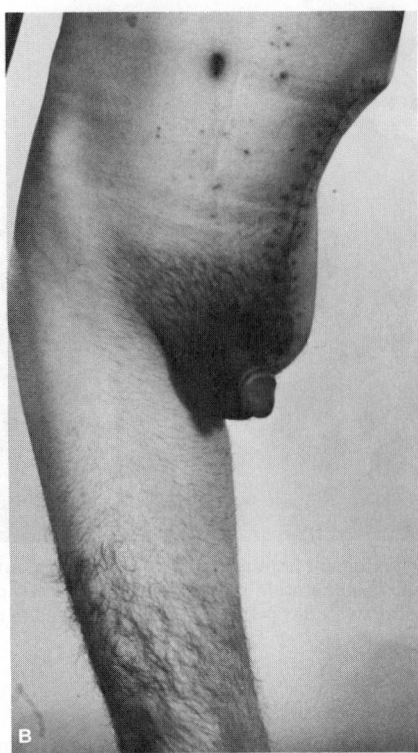

Figure 112-10. Radical amputations for extremity sarcomas include one joint above the most proximal extent of tumor. (*A*) In the upper extremity, the standard radical amputation for an upper arm tumor is a forequarter (interscapulothoracic) amputation. (*B*) In the lower extremity, the standard amputation for most tumors of the proximal thigh or buttock is a hemipelvectomy. Less-extensive amputations are possible for more distal tumors.

be irradiated, or massive lymphedema results. Generally, a strip of skin and subcutaneous tissue away from the tumor is excluded from the treatment field to prevent this complication.

Postoperative radiation can also be delivered to the tumor bed by means of implanted radioactive sources, a technique referred to as *brachytherapy*. Although this approach has the advantage of a much shorter time to completion of therapy (usually less than 1 week, compared with 6 to 7 weeks for external beam radiation), it is technically complex and requires an experienced radiation oncologist in the operating room. A randomized trial demonstrated a significant decrease in local recurrences

for high-grade sarcomas after combined surgery and postoperative brachytherapy compared with surgery alone.[22] Patients with low-grade sarcomas did not benefit from adjuvant brachytherapy, although a recent retrospective review suggested that external beam radiation is effective in decreasing local recurrence in these tumors.[23] Otherwise, from a therapeutic standpoint, brachytherapy and external beam radiation appear to be equivalent when properly administered. The data from the randomized study provide strong support for the routine inclusion of radiation therapy (by some technique) in all patients with high-grade extremity sarcomas undergoing limb-sparing surgery.

Preoperative Radiation

Experience with postoperative radiation therapy for large extremity sarcomas (10 cm or more) was more disappointing, with a high incidence of local failure. Subsequently, extensive investigations suggested that preoperative radiation offered significant advantages in this group of patients. Local control rates were considerably higher when large tumors were treated preoperatively, and in some cases, tumors initially considered unresectable without amputation shrank sufficiently to permit limb-sparing resection.[21] Although these investigations were not randomized, the prospect of preoperative treatment for large extremity sarcomas broadened the spectrum of patients for whom limb-sparing surgery could be considered.

In an effort to further extend these findings, patients with intermediate and high-grade extremity sarcomas have been treated with preoperative radiation therapy combined with regional chemotherapy. Three days of intraarterial chemotherapy with doxorubicin (Adriamycin), followed by large-fraction radiation (3500 cGy in 10 days) and wide local excision, was successful in achieving local control and in preserving a functional extremity. Significant degrees of necrosis were commonly seen in the resected tumor specimen. Local complications were frequent, however, and proved to be the most common reason for

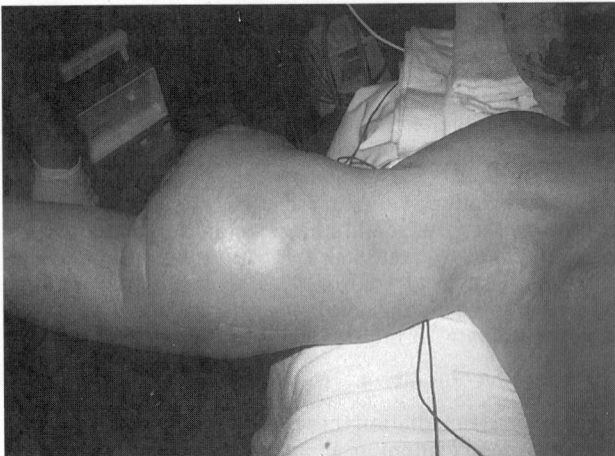

Figure 112-11. Enormous high-grade malignant fibrous histiocytoma circumferentially involving the upper arm just above the elbow. This tumor was treated with a radical amputation (shoulder disarticulation). Aggressive local or systemic treatment to shrink the tumor and avoid amputation was not used because of the patient's advanced age.

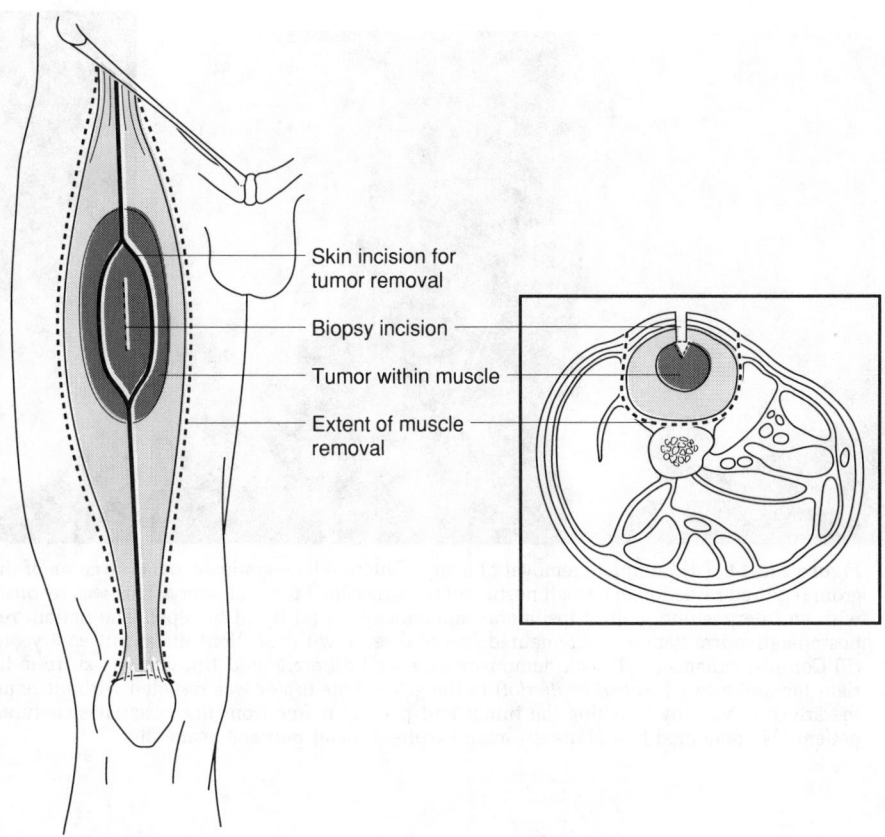

Skin incision for
tumor removal

Biopsy incision

Tumor within muscle

Extent of muscle
removal

Figure 112-12. Compartment excision
involves removal of the entire muscle
group in which the tumor arises from
origin to insertion. The skin incision
frequently crosses one or even two joint
spaces. Many large soft tissue sarcomas
are not confined to a single muscular
compartment.

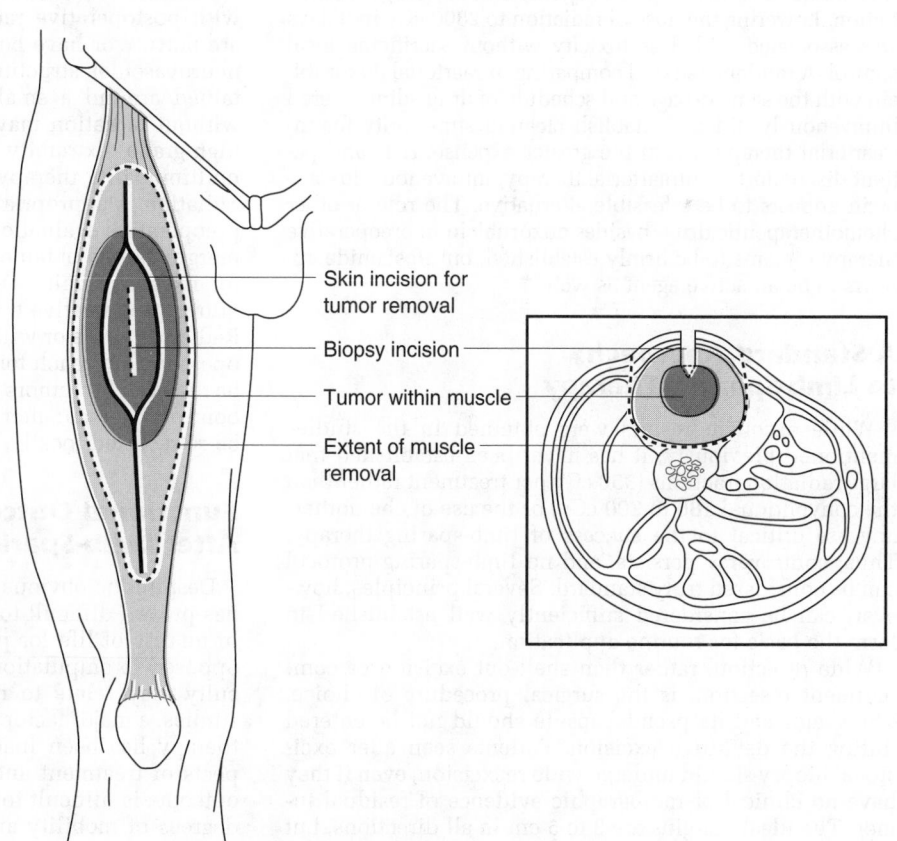

Skin incision for
tumor removal

Biopsy incision

Tumor within muscle

Extent of muscle
removal

Figure 112-13. Wide local excision involves removal of the tumor with a margin of normal tissue: 3 to 5 cm is obtained proximally and distally, and on
the lateral and deep margins, at least
one grossly uninvolved fascial plane is
resected en bloc with the tumor. No attempt is made to resect an entire muscle
compartment. If necessary, major vascular structures or nerves may be
resected.

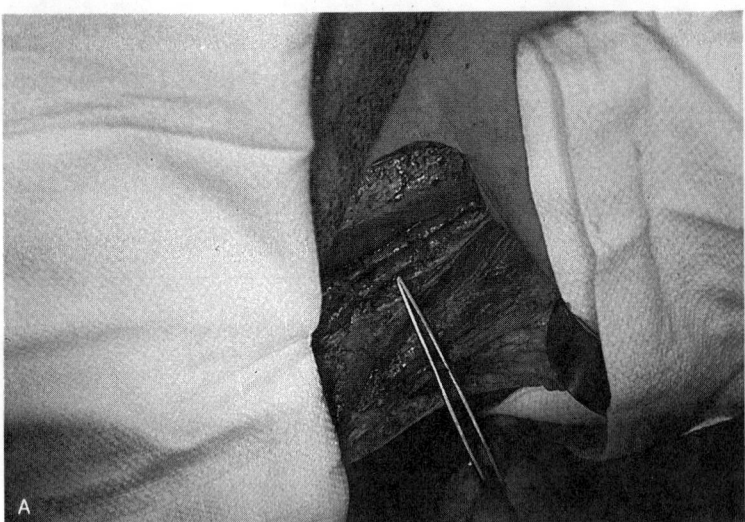
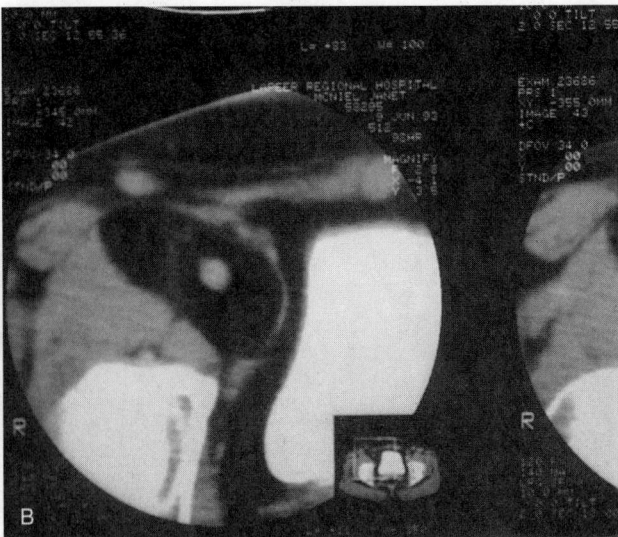

Figure 112-14. (*A*) Complete removal of a large, intermediate-grade synovial sarcoma of the right groin required resection of a small portion of the superficial femoral artery. This was reconstructed with an interposition graft of ipsilateral saphenous vein (at tip of forceps). The patient received postoperative irradiation and remained free of disease with excellent distal pulses 3 years later. (*B*) Contrast-enhanced CT scan demonstrates a well-differentiated liposarcoma surrounding the right femoral artery (*central white dot*) in the groin. This tumor was resected without removal of the artery or vein by bisecting the tumor and peeling it free from the vascular structures. This patient also remained free of disease with excellent distal pulses 3 years later.

subsequent amputation of the treated limb, which was necessary in about 5% of cases.[24]

In a series of subsequent studies, this preoperative protocol was modified to decrease toxicity and simplify drug administration. Lowering the dose of radiation to 2800 cGy in 8 days was associated with less toxicity without sacrificing local control. A randomized trial comparing intraarterial doxorubicin with the same dosage and schedule of drug administered intravenously did not establish clearcut superiority for intraarterial therapy. Given the greater expense, risk, and patient discomfort of intraarterial therapy, intravenous doxorubicin appears to be a feasible alternative. The role of other chemotherapeutic drugs besides doxorubicin in preoperative therapy remains to be firmly established, but ifosfamide appears to be an active agent as well.[24]

A Standard Approach to Limb-Sparing Therapy

While excellent results were obtained in the studies mentioned previously, it has never been established that large radiation fractions (350 cGy per treatment rather than the conventional 180 to 200 cGy) or the use of chemotherapy are critical to the success of limb-sparing therapy. Thus, controversy persists, and no limb-sparing protocol can be considered truly standard. Several principles, however, can be considered sufficiently well established to form the basis for routine application.

Wide resection, rather than shell-out excision or compartment resection, is the surgical procedure of choice. The tumor and its pseudocapsule should not be entered during the definitive excision. Patients seen after excisional biopsy should undergo wide reexcision, even if they have no clinical or radiographic evidence of residual tumor. The ideal margins are 3 to 5 cm in all directions, but at least one uninvolved fascial plane should be taken when this ideal is not achievable. If necessary, major nerves or vascular structures can be taken to achieve wide excision

of high-grade lesions. Low-grade sarcomas in close proximity to major nerves and vessels usually can be dissected safely off these structures.

Resected low-grade sarcomas of the extremity are treated with postoperative radiation if the margins of resection are narrow or have been compromised to preserve major neurovascular structures. If a wide margin has been obtained around a small, low-grade sarcoma, observation without radiation may be appropriate. Intermediate- and high-grade extremity sarcomas almost always receive multimodality therapy. Wide excision plus postoperative radiation is appropriate for tumors smaller than 10 cm if preoperative evaluation reveals that a satisfactory surgical margin can be obtained. For tumors larger than 10 cm, or for fixed extremity sarcomas, limb-sparing treatment requires preoperative treatment of the tumor in most cases. Radiation alone or with chemotherapy is a reasonable preoperative approach for these patients. Amputation should be reserved for tumors that extensively surround or involve bone or that recur after a limb-sparing approach and cannot be re-resected locally.

Functional Outcome After Limb-Sparing Surgery

Despite the obvious desirability of limb preservation, it has proved difficult to document an overall improvement in quality of life for patients undergoing limb-sparing as opposed to amputation surgeries. While part of this difficulty may relate to methodologic problems in existing studies, a major factor limiting the success of limb-sparing therapy has been inadequate attention to functional aspects of treatment and patient rehabilitation. Functional outcome is difficult to define and measure. It includes the degrees of mobility and strength achieved, the ability to return to gainful employment, and the amount of residual pain, as well as the cosmetic and body image effects. An analysis of 88 patients with extremity sarcomas who underwent multimodality limb-sparing treatment showed that performance of daily activities was not significantly impaired at either 6 or 12 months after therapy. Nevertheless, a third of the patients reported a decline in their employment status over this period. Specific treatments could not be definitively linked with changes in functional outcome or quality of life, although there were more serious wound complications and joint contractures among patients undergoing combined postoperative chemotherapy and radiation when compared with those undergoing postoperative chemotherapy alone. Quality of life in these patients was determined to be the same or better than pretreatment in 72% of patients at 6 months and in 80% at 12 months.[25] This study suggests that functional outcome and quality of life are very acceptable and may improve over time after multimodality treatment.

The functional outcome and quality of life after limb-sparing therapy can be enhanced by integrating rehabilitation specialists into the multidisciplinary treatment team. Rehabilitation efforts are best initiated before beginning therapy rather than after treatment has been completed. A dedicated team of rehabilitation specialists can assist the sarcoma treatment team in a number of ways, including treating preexisting functional deficits, counseling regarding the functional implications of limb-sparing as opposed to amputative surgeries, designing therapy programs to minimize treatment-related functional loss, and recommending adaptive techniques and equipment to compensate for the unavoidable loss of function.[26]

Chemotherapy

Chemotherapy used before surgical resection is referred to as *neoadjuvant chemotherapy*. As noted, both intraarterial and intravenous infusions of doxorubicin have been used preoperatively in extremity sarcomas. Combination chemotherapy with doxorubicin-containing regimens also has been administered preoperatively. Alternatively, some groups have used isolated limb perfusion, particularly for large or recurrent sarcomas. Isolated limb perfusion is performed by cannulating the iliac or subclavian artery and vein and directing all the blood flow for the extremity through a cardiopulmonary bypass pump. The temperature of the perfusate can be tightly regulated, and hyperthermic perfusion is generally employed. Initially, isolated limb perfusion was carried out with standard cytotoxic agents such as melphalan. Recently, the addition of tumor necrosis factor and γ-interferon to melphalan hyperthermic perfusion has been reported to have dramatically increased tumor response rates.[27] Neoadjuvant systemic chemotherapy has been validated as part of the management of osteosarcomas, but not as yet for soft tissue tumors. Hence, the precise role of preoperative chemotherapy—whether by intravenous or intraarterial infusion or hyperthermic perfusion—remains to be defined.

Adjuvant Chemotherapy

The main cause of death in soft tissue sarcoma patients is distant metastatic disease, particularly for those patients with high-grade tumors or extremity lesions.[28] As local control rates have improved, emphasis has been placed on eradicating metastatic disease with postoperative adjuvant systemic chemotherapy. Doxorubicin has undergone extensive evaluation as single-agent adjuvant chemotherapy for soft tissue sarcomas. Randomized trials, however, demonstrate that adjuvant doxorubicin does not improve overall survival compared with surgery alone.[29] A randomized, controlled trial of multiagent chemotherapy (doxorubicin, cyclophosphamide, and methotrexate) after surgery showed improved disease-free survival for patients with high-grade extremity (but not

trunk or retroperitoneal) sarcomas.[30] Toxicity of this regimen proved substantial. Symptomatic cardiac toxicity developed in 14% of patients, and many asymptomatic patients demonstrated decreased cardiac function on noninvasive testing. A subsequent study comparing this regimen to one with a lower doxorubicin dose to limit cardiotoxicity suggested that the less toxic program is equivalent to the higher-dose regimen.[31]

Despite the favorable findings from these two trials, other studies of adjuvant multidrug chemotherapy in soft tissue sarcomas have failed to demonstrate any improvement in overall survival. A recent meta-analysis of existing randomized trials pooled the available data to minimize the limitations imposed by the small sample sizes in all these studies. After combining the data from the different trials, it did appear that the likelihood of death and disease recurrence decreased in patients with high-grade extremity sarcomas.[32] Whether the magnitude of this benefit is sufficient to justify the significant toxicity of adjuvant chemotherapy remains to be determined. Patients with high-grade extremity sarcomas should be evaluated for possible adjuvant chemotherapy. Whenever possible, such patients should be enrolled in an established clinical trial so that the value of adjuvant chemotherapy can be more fully determined.

MANAGEMENT OF RETROPERITONEAL SARCOMAS

Retroperitoneal sarcomas account for about 15% of all sarcomas and about 55% of all retroperitoneal tumors. The significant advances in multimodality therapy of extremity sarcomas have not been matched by similar progress in the management of retroperitoneal tumors. Most patients with retroperitoneal sarcomas die of their disease, frequently with locally recurrent tumor as the major or sole site of failure. Unlike the situation with extremity sarcomas, even patients with low-grade retroperitoneal sarcomas usually die from progressive tumor (Fig. 112-15).

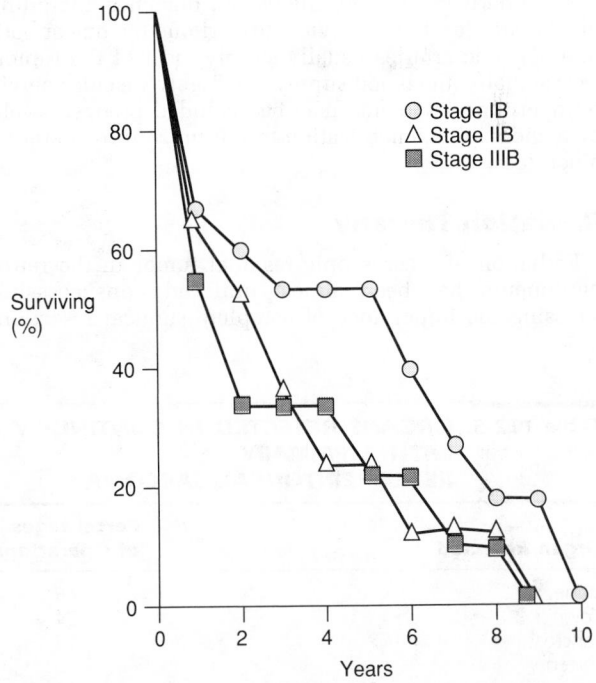

Figure 112-15. Survival of patients with retroperitoneal sarcoma classified by AJCC stage. All patients had tumors larger than 5 cm in this series. (After Storm FK, Eilber FR, Mirra J, et al. Retroperitoneal sarcomas: a reappraisal of treatment. J Surg Oncol 1980;17:1)

The poor outcome of retroperitoneal sarcomas is in part related to the inability to diagnose these tumors at an early stage. Retroperitoneal tumors rarely cause significant symptoms until they achieve large size, and even then, symptoms are generally vague and nonspecific. Abdominal pain, weight loss, early satiety, and nausea and vomiting are the most common complaints. An abdominal mass can be felt in about 80% of patients at the time of presentation. In less than 1% of cases, patients with a retroperitoneal sarcoma present with hypoglycemia simulating an insulinoma. A high index of suspicion must be maintained when evaluating patients with vague abdominal complaints if the diagnosis of a retroperitoneal sarcoma is to be made expeditiously.

Surgery

The wide margins of resection routinely obtained for extremity sarcomas are difficult to achieve in the retroperitoneum. Complete excision of all gross tumor is essential for long-term disease-free survival, but this is achievable in only about 50% of cases.[33] To remove all gross tumor, concomitant resection of adjacent organs is required more than 75% of the time (Table 112-5). Partial excisions or debulking procedures do not improve survival compared with biopsy alone (Fig. 112-16).

When a retroperitoneal sarcoma is encountered unexpectedly at laparotomy, a careful incisional biopsy with minimal disruption of surrounding tissue planes should be performed. The area of the biopsy should be isolated to prevent tumor spillage into the peritoneal cavity. When the diagnosis is confirmed, a wide excision can be carried out once the patient and surgeon are properly prepared.

A transperitoneal approach is much more likely to allow complete resection than a flank approach. Either a vertical midline or transverse incision may be used, depending on the location of the tumor. The transperitoneal approach permits resection of adjacent organs and allows for early control of the vascular supply to the tumor. In the upper retroperitoneum, the blood supply to the tumor is frequently derived from multiple small branches, including lumbar arteries. In the pelvic retroperitoneum, one or both internal iliac arteries usually supply most of the tumor. Occasionally, the blood supply to a highly vascular pelvic retroperitoneal sarcoma may be occluded preoperatively by angiographic embolization to minimize intraoperative blood loss.

Radiation Therapy

Radiation of macroscopic residual tumor in the retroperitoneum has been almost uniformly unsuccessful, stressing the importance of complete surgical resection.

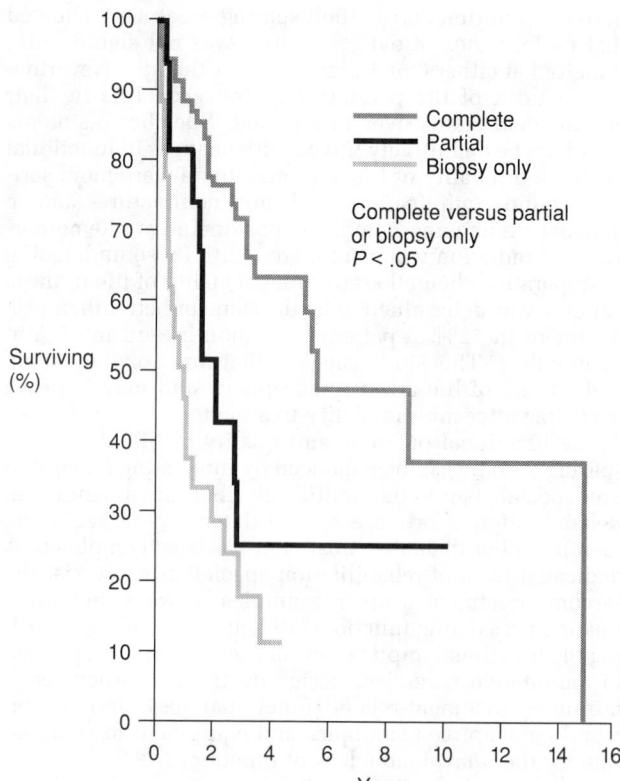

Figure 112-16. Survival of patients with retroperitoneal sarcoma classified by type of operation. Patients undergoing partial excision of their tumors had no improvement in survival compared with those deemed unresectable. (After Jacques DP, Coit DG, Hajdu SI, Brennan MF. Management of primary and recurrent soft-tissue sarcoma of the retroperitoneum. Ann Surg 1990;212:51)

Because of the difficulty in achieving wide resection margins, however, radiation is frequently used as a postoperative adjuvant. Unfortunately, the excellent local control rates obtained with postoperative radiation in extremity lesions have not been matched in the retroperitoneum.

Normal tissue tolerance to radiation is much lower in the abdomen and retroperitoneum than in the extremities. Extremity tumors can frequently be treated with 6000 cGy or more in conventional dose fractions. In contrast, the small bowel can tolerate only 4500 to 5000 cGy, and the liver and kidney even less. In an attempt to limit normal tissue toxicity, intraoperative radiotherapy has been used. This approach offers the advantage of allowing the bowel and other sensitive structures to be moved out of the field while a single high dose of radiation is administered directly to the tumor bed. Intraoperative radiotherapy is costly, logistically difficult, and associated with complications of its own, such as neurotoxicity. A randomized trial did not demonstrate any significant advantage for intraoperative radiation compared with conventional external beam radiation in retroperitoneal sarcomas.[34]

Chemotherapy

Aggressive systemic chemotherapy is poorly tolerated in patients who have just undergone a major intraabdominal procedure with resection of multiple organs. Several trials of postoperative adjuvant chemotherapy do not show any benefit for retroperitoneal sarcoma patients, and in one study, treated patients fared worse than those not receiving chemotherapy.[35] Preoperative intraarterial chemotherapy

Table 112-5. ORGANS RESECTED IN CONTINUITY WITH A PRIMARY RETROPERITONEAL SARCOMA

Organ Resected	Percentages of Operations
Kidney	46
Colon	24
Pancreas	15
Spleen	10
Major vessels (vena cava, iliac artery, or vein)	10

(Jacques DP, Coit DG, Hajdu SI, Brennan MF. *Management of primary and recurrent soft-tissue sarcoma of the retroperitoneum. Ann Surg 1990;212:51*)

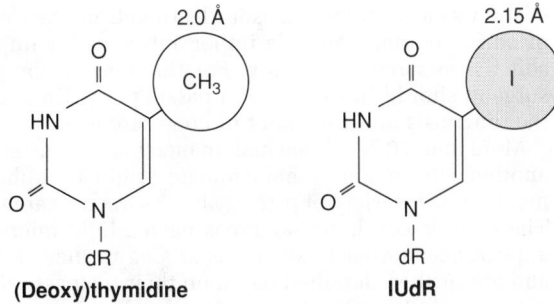

Figure 112-17. Chemical structure of the radiosensitizer iododeoxyuridine (IUdR) and the nucleotide thymidine. IUdR contains an iodine atom in place of the 5′-methyl group of thymidine. Because the atomic radii of the two are similar, IUdR is incorporated into DNA in place of thymidine. Because of iodine's greater atomic weight, cells containing IUdR in their DNA are more susceptible to damage by radiation.

is limited by the absence of a single feeder vessel in most retroperitoneal tumors. Nonetheless, a nonrandomized study suggested that preoperative doxorubicin (given intravenously in those patients without a single feeding artery) and external beam radiation followed by aggressive surgical resection led to longer survival and lower local recurrence rates than those found in a historical cohort treated with surgery with or without postoperative radiation.[36]

Radiation Sensitizers

Radiation sensitizers are being investigated as a means to improve the effectiveness of external beam radiation, particularly in the retroperitoneum, where normal tissue tolerance limits the dose that can be delivered to the tumor. Iododeoxyuridine (IUdR) and similar radiosensitizing agents are incorporated into DNA in place of thymidine (Fig. 112-17); cells containing this altered DNA are more susceptible to radiation damage. The drug IUdR is 100 times more effective than doxorubicin as a radiation sensitizer in vitro, although it does not have doxorubicin's direct cytotoxic effect. Studies of IUdR and external beam radiation in unresectable soft tissue sarcomas document impressively high rates of local control without surgery.[37]

Preoperative treatment with IUdR and radiation allows complete excision of all gross tumor for most patients with retroperitoneal sarcomas, and toxicity of this protocol has been acceptable.[38] Significant regressions have been seen, with extensive posttreatment tumor necrosis and even complete disappearance of gross tumor encountered in some cases (Fig. 112-18). It is too early to tell if this approach will alter mortality rates for patients with these difficult tumors. Unfortunately, no matter how much local control rates can be improved with aggressive local/regional therapy of retroperitoneal sarcomas, the large size of these tumors at presentation makes it likely that many will ultimately succumb to distant metastases unless better systemic treatments can be developed.

DIAGNOSIS AND MANAGEMENT OF DESMOID TUMORS

Desmoid tumors are unusual soft tissue lesions with unique characteristics but definite similarities to low-grade soft tissue sarcomas. Although clinical reports of low-grade soft tissue sarcomas often include desmoid tumors,[23] in fact desmoids virtually never metastasize even after multiple local recurrences.[39] Desmoids have also been referred to as "aggressive fibromatosis," reflecting the uncertainty that exists about their malignant potential. But whatever name is chosen, some facts are clear. Desmoid tumors present in a fashion identical to soft tissue sarcomas, as an enlarging, often painless, soft tissue mass. Clinically and radiographically, except for the special settings described later, there is nothing to distinguish a desmoid tumor from a soft tissue sarcoma. As with low-grade sarcomas, wide excision is the mainstay of treatment, but local recurrence after surgical treatment is very common. Deaths due to desmoids are infrequent since the tumors do not metastasize but can occur due to local recurrence in a critical area such as the neck.

Little is known about the etiology of desmoid tumors. There are two specific clinical settings in which desmoids arise, which have provided insights into both the cause and the therapy of these lesions. The first is during or just after pregnancy. Desmoid tumors are more common in women than men and frequently present within 1 to 2 years of delivery,

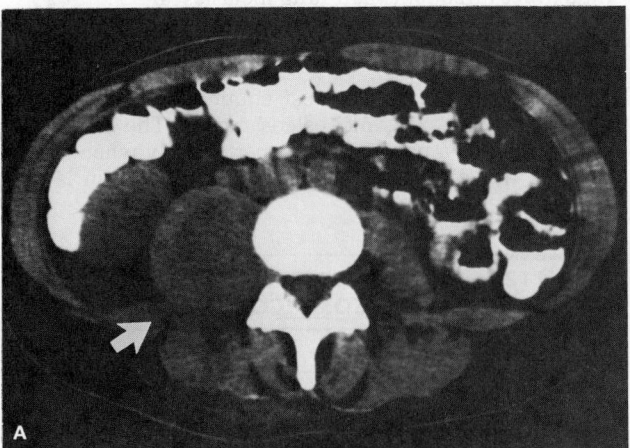
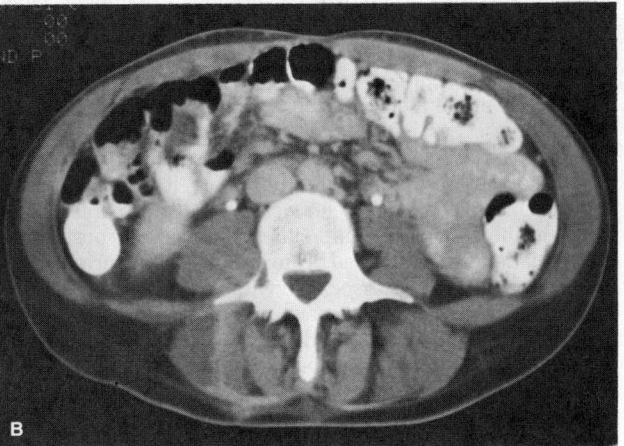

Figure 112-18. (A) Pretreatment CT scan of patient with a high-grade undifferentiated sarcoma in the paravertebral retroperitoneum. (B) After treatment with IUdR and radiation, a second CT scan shows the tumor to be significantly smaller. At surgery, only scar tissue without grossly obvious tumor was encountered. Pathologic analysis revealed three microscopic foci of viable sarcoma within the psoas muscle; no gross tumor was found.

occasionally arising in the vicinity of a cesarian section scar. These facts, combined with isolated reports of spontaneous regression of desmoids at menopause and the demonstration of estrogen receptors on some tumors, suggest a hormonal component to their development. Based on this, hormonal therapy with a variety of agents, most notably tamoxifen, has been used with occasional success. We and others have seen either complete disappearance, marked shrinkage, or stabilization of tumor growth combined with marked symptomatic improvement after treatment with tamoxifen alone or in combination with other agents (see later discussion).[39,40]

Desmoid tumors occur with greatly increased frequency in patients with familial adenomatous polyposis. The link of familial polyposis with desmoids and other soft tissue tumors was originally given the eponym *Gardner syndrome*. It is now known, however, that all patients with familial polyposis are at risk for developing desmoids and that the genetic defect in polyposis patients with and without desmoids is identical. Hence, the term *Gardner syndrome* has fallen into disuse. The desmoid tumors in polyposis patients tend to occur in the abdomen, often in the colonic mesentery after total proctocolectomy has been performed to prevent the development of adenocarcinoma of the colon. Patients with familial polyposis are born with one defective copy of the apc gene, a tumor suppressor gene. As with the RB1 and p53 genes, the second, normal copy must be lost for a tumor (either an adenomatous polyp or a desmoid) to develop. It is likely that, in a predisposed individual, surgical trauma and the resultant stimulation of fibroblast growth increases the chance that a desmoid tumor will actually develop. This may explain both the predilection for mesenteric tumors in polyposis patients and abdominal wall tumors in some women after cesarian section.

Another nonsurgical therapy for desmoids, nonsteroidal antiinflammatory drugs, was suggested by studies in familial polyposis patients. Of the available drugs, the little used arthritis medication sulindac (Clinoril) appears to be the most active. This drug has a relatively unique enterohepatic circulation, and at least some patients with familial polyposis have experienced significant reduction in the number of colonic polyps after treatment with oral sulindac. In the course of such treatment, anecdotal regressions of coexisting desmoid tumors have been seen. Alone or in combination with tamoxifen, objective regression of as many as 50% of polyposis-associated desmoid tumors has been reported.[40] Sporadic desmoids, not associated with familial polyposis, also occasionally respond to this combination. Other therapeutic modalities have been used to treat desmoid tumors. Radiotherapy has been used both as primary treatment and as postoperative adjuvant therapy.[23] Cytotoxic chemotherapy regimens have been employed, with some successes reported using relatively nontoxic regimens.[40]

The surgical approach to resectable sporadic desmoid tumors has been similar to that used for low-grade soft tissue sarcomas: resect with a histologically negative margin if possible, but do not sacrifice major neurovascular structures or adjacent organs unless absolutely necessary. If pathologic analysis of the resected specimen reveals close approximation of tumor to the surgical margin, either reexcision or postoperative radiation are employed. Unresectable or recurrent desmoids, as well as those associated with familial polyposis, are treated first with the combination of tamoxifen and sulindac. Resection or radiation are used for failures of this therapy or to eliminate residual disease after partial responses. Chemotherapy is reserved as a last resort in patients who have failed all other therapies and are severely symptomatic or in danger of dying because of compression of vital structures by tumor.

DIAGNOSIS AND MANAGEMENT OF PRIMARY BONE SARCOMAS

Primary sarcomas of bone pose certain unique challenges, but in many ways, their behavior is similar to that of soft tissue sarcomas. Lessons learned from the treatment of bone sarcomas provide important leads for improving soft tissue sarcoma therapy. For this reason, the general surgeon should have at least a passing acquaintance with the diagnosis and treatment of bone sarcomas.

More than 70% of bone malignancies are metastatic from another site or are of hematologic origin (lymphoma or myeloma). A variety of primary bone sarcomas are known. The spindle-cell bone sarcomas have a light microscopic appearance similar to sarcomas arising in the soft tissues and are further classified based on their histogenesis. This group includes osteosarcomas, chondrosarcomas, fibrosarcomas, and malignant fibrous histiocytomas arising in bone. The small round cell sarcomas include osseous Ewing sarcomas and primitive neuroectodermal tumor of bone. Osteosarcomas are by far the most common primary bone sarcomas and have been best studied in terms of therapy. They are the primary focus of this section.

Osteosarcomas occur most commonly around the knee, either in the distal femur or proximal tibia, but they can be encountered in any bone (Table 112-6). Osteosarcomas originate in the metaphyseal ends of the involved bone. Most osteosarcomas occur in childhood and adolescence; roughly 80% of patients are younger than 20 years, but there is a second peak beginning after age 60 years. This latter peak corresponds to osteosarcomas arising in bones affected with Paget disease, the most common condition predisposing to osteosarcoma development. Osteosarcomas arise in as many as 10% of patients with long-standing Paget disease. Other etiologic factors for bone sarcomas, such as exposure to radiation, have been discussed previously.

Like soft tissue sarcomas, osteosarcomas are graded using a three-part system. Most osteosarcomas are high-grade (grade III), but low-grade variants exist. These less aggressive tumors are usually parosteal or periosteal in location, in contrast to the intramedullary origin of classic osteosarcoma. As with soft tissue sarcomas, a GTNM staging system is employed. The stage groupings, however, are somewhat different than for soft tissue tumors (Table 112-7). Most osteosarcomas are stage IIB (high-grade, tumor invasion beyond cortex, no nodal or distant metastases). Involvement of regional lymph nodes is rare at the time of presentation (less than 3%). Pulmonary metastases are the most common site of distant spread and may be discovered in as many as 25% of patients at the time of presentation. Bone metastases are not uncommon in osteosarcoma, although less frequent than lung metastases.

Clinical Evaluation

A painful mass is the most common presenting complaint with an extremity osteosarcoma. The tumor may also present as a painless mass, particularly when it originates in the axial skeleton. Limitation of motion is often

Table 112-6. SITE OF ORIGIN OF OSTEOSARCOMAS

Anatomic Site	Percentage
Lower extremity	77.6
Upper extremity	12.9
Pelvis	6.0
Shoulder	2.6
Vertebrae	0.8

(Modified from Eilber F, et al. Management of stage IIB osteogenic sarcoma: experience at the University of California, Los Angeles. Cancer Treat Symp 1985;3:118)

Table 112-7. AMERICAN JOINT COMMISSION ON CANCER GTNM CLASSIFICATION AND STAGE GROUPING OF OSTEOSARCOMAS

Stage	Description
TUMOR GRADE	
GX	Grade cannot be assessed
G1	Well differentiated
G2	Moderately well differentiated
G3	Poorly differentiated
G4	Undifferentiated
PRIMARY TUMOR	
TX	Primary tumor cannot be assessed
T0	No evidence of primary tumor
T1	Tumor confined within the cortex
T2	Tumor invades beyond the cortex
LYMPH NODE INVOLVEMENT	
NX	Regional lymph nodes cannot be assessed
N0	No regional lymph node metastasis
N1	Regional lymph node metastasis
DISTANT METASTASIS	
MX	Presence of distant metastasis cannot be assessed
M0	No distant metastasis
M1	Distant metastasis
STAGE GROUPING	
Stage IA	G1, T1, N0, M0
	G2, T1, N0, M0
Stage IB	G1, T2, N0, M0
	G2, T2, N0, M0
Stage IIA	G3, T1, N0, M0
	G4, T1, N0, M0
Stage IIB	G3, T2, N0, M0
	G4, T2, N0, M0
Stage III	Not defined
Stage IVA	Any G, any T, N1, M0
Stage IVB	Any G, any T, any N, M1

(Modified from Beahrs OH, Henson DE, Hutter RVP, et al. Manual for Staging of Cancer, ed 4. Philadelphia, JB Lippincott, 1992)

present when the tumor arises near or involves a joint. A history of trauma is not uncommon, but traumatic injury has never been linked with sarcoma development. Patients occasionally present with pathologic fracture of the involved bone.

Plain radiographs of the affected bone are the first step in evaluating a suspected osteosarcoma. High-grade osteosarcomas lead to rapid destruction of bone with new bone formation and periosteal reaction. These changes are manifest radiographically by an extensive, poorly defined destructive bony lesion, often with an extraosseous component (Fig. 112-19). Codman triangles, indicative of periosteal reaction, are characteristic but not pathognomonic of osteosarcoma. If the radiographic picture suggests an osteosarcoma, further radiologic evaluation should be done before proceeding with biopsy. This allows the full anatomic extent of tumor to be defined without postsurgical artifact. More important, the radiologic evaluation allows the biopsy incision to be planned with an understanding of subsequent limb-sparing surgical options.

Radionuclide bone scanning using technetium-99m pyrophosphate can identify distant metastases to other bones as well as define skip areas of involvement within the bone of origin. Gallium-67 and thallium-201 scans may be useful for assessing the response of a primary osteosarcoma to preoperative chemotherapy. More recently, PET scanning and MRI spectroscopy have been used in this role.[18,19]

CT scanning is the most important modality in evaluating a bone sarcoma. It is excellent for assessing the degree of bony destruction, the extent of soft tissue involvement, and the relation of the tumor to adjacent neurovascular structures. The entire affected bone, including the complete joint above and below the tumor, should be visualized on the scan. A chest CT can provide evidence of pulmonary metastases too small to be seen on chest radiograph.

MRI is an important adjunct to CT scans in some patients, particularly those who are being considered for limb-sparing surgery. The excellent definition of marrow involvement by tumor allows for accurate planning of the proximal extent of the tumor resection. Angiography, while accurate in defining the relation of tumor to vessels, is rarely necessary unless intraarterial chemotherapy is used.

Biopsy

After the radiologic evaluation establishes the extent of the bony lesion, an incisional biopsy should be performed. The biopsy incision should be carefully planned so as not to jeopardize subsequent efforts at limb sparing. A vertical incision, oriented along the long axis of the extremity, is always used for arm or leg tumors. For tumors situated close to the knee, the incision is placed medially or laterally because a posterior incision can compromise the functional result of subsequent surgery. When the primary tumor is located in the pelvis or shoulder girdle, the biopsy should be performed in a location that allows its ready inclusion in the subsequent definitive operation incision.

Subject to the above constraints, the biopsy incision is generally placed over the most superficial portion of the

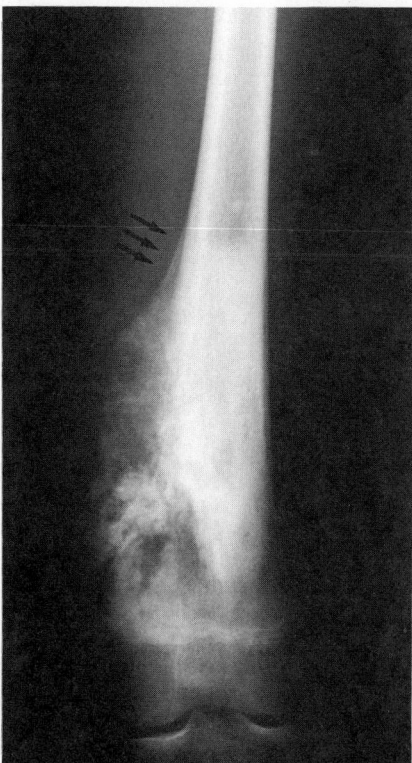

Figure 112-19. Plain radiograph of the femur showing a high-grade osteosarcoma. The tumor is an ill-defined destructive lesion with an extensive soft tissue component. Codman triangles are present (*arrows*).

tumor, and dissection is kept to a minimum. Any tissue planes entered during the biopsy are considered contaminated by tumor and must be excised in the subsequent definitive resection. If an adequate amount of tissue can be obtained by sampling the extraosseous component, this is preferable to biopsy of the bone itself. If the cortex of bone is entered, a plug of methylmethacrylate can be used to seal the bone and prevent hemorrhage or tumor spillage. Hemostasis should be achieved before closure; a drain should almost never be necessary. After the biopsy, weight-bearing on the affected limb should be restricted to minimize the chance of pathologic fracture.

Preoperative Chemotherapy

Unlike the situation for soft tissue sarcomas, preoperative (neoadjuvant) chemotherapy is sufficiently well established to be considered standard treatment for osteosarcoma patients. Historically, patients with clinically localized osteosarcoma treated by surgery alone had about a 20% 5-year survival rate. Adjuvant systemic chemotherapy after surgery improved that figure to 55% to 70% in randomized trials (Fig. 112-20). Contemporary protocols that incorporate preoperative chemotherapy into the regimen have been associated with 5-year survival rates in excess of 80%, and most of these long-term survivors have been cured of their cancer.[41]

Several significant advantages of preoperative chemotherapy for osteosarcomas have emerged. The preoperative therapy makes limb-sparing surgery more successful by decreasing the extent of soft tissue involvement and allowing time for the creation of a custom-made bone replacement. Furthermore, the tumor's response to the preoperative chemotherapy may identify those patients who require more intensive postoperative chemotherapy.

Preoperative response to chemotherapy is monitored in several ways. Many patients with osteosarcomas have an elevated serum alkaline phosphatase level, which should decline if therapy is effective. Serial scans, such as thallium-201 scans, can be used to document decreasing

tumor uptake. Failure of serum markers or scans to improve during preoperative therapy may be an indication to switch to more intensive therapy even before surgery. At the time of tumor resection, assessing the viability of the excised tumor provides the best measure of tumor response. A good response is defined as either complete absence of viable tumor cells or presence of only microscopic foci of viable cells, without any confluent areas of viable tumor. Attempts at scoring the percentage of necrosis have been less consistent, but at least 95% necrosis is necessary before a response can be considered good. Indeed, the histologic definition of a good response outlined above correlates more nearly with 98% to 99% necrosis. Patients who achieve a good response require only a short course of postoperative chemotherapy; those who do not are treated with a longer postoperative regimen that includes doxorubicin and cisplatin.

Surgery

Extremity osteosarcomas may be treated surgically either by radical amputation (amputation at least one joint above the most proximal extent of tumor) or by en bloc resection with limb sparing. Limb-sparing approaches can be considered for most patients with extremity sarcomas and no evidence of neurovascular involvement. Patients presenting initially with pathologic fractures are at higher risk for local recurrence and are less suitable candidates for limb sparing. Virtually all limb-sparing protocols for osteosarcoma incorporate some form of preoperative chemotherapy.

Essential to any limb-sparing operation is complete removal of the affected bone and soft tissues. The old biopsy site is taken in continuity with the tumor, and the adjacent joint is also resected. Generally, a proximal bone margin of 6 to 7 cm is taken beyond the highest area of abnormality on preoperative, pretherapy scans. Even if pretreatment induces some degree of tumor shrinkage, the operation should remove all areas where disease was noted at initial presentation. The marrow at the level of bony transection is curetted out and sent for frozen-section analysis to verify the adequacy of the proximal bone margin. For extensive lesions of the femur, resections of the entire femur with limb sparing can be performed.

A variety of reconstructive techniques are available after resection of an extremity osteosarcoma. Autografts (such as vascularized or nonvascularized fibular grafts), cadaver allografts, and simple arthrodeses have all been used (Fig. 112-21). Custom-made titanium endoprostheses are often used (Fig. 112-22), but their use is limited by the following: the size of bone that can accommodate them (the distal tibia is often too small to accept the prosthesis and still have adequate strength to bear weight after proximal tibial resection); the fact that many osteosarcoma patients are children who continue to grow on the unoperated side; and the long-term stresses that an active young adult puts on a prosthetic bone and joint. Technologic advances are addressing some of these issues. A new modular distal femoral prosthesis has been developed that can be periodically expanded, progressively lengthening the limb as the other leg grows. Newer materials and cementless prostheses that promote bony ingrowth rather than rely on fixative cements may provide better long-term functional results.

Some pelvic osteosarcomas can also be resected with limb sparing. Small or low-grade tumors of the bony pelvis can be removed by internal hemipelvectomy.[42] Virtually the entire hemipelvis and hip joint can be resected, leaving the neurovascular supply to the leg intact (Fig. 112-23A). Although the leg on that side is significantly shortened, weight bearing is eventually possible secondary to fibrous

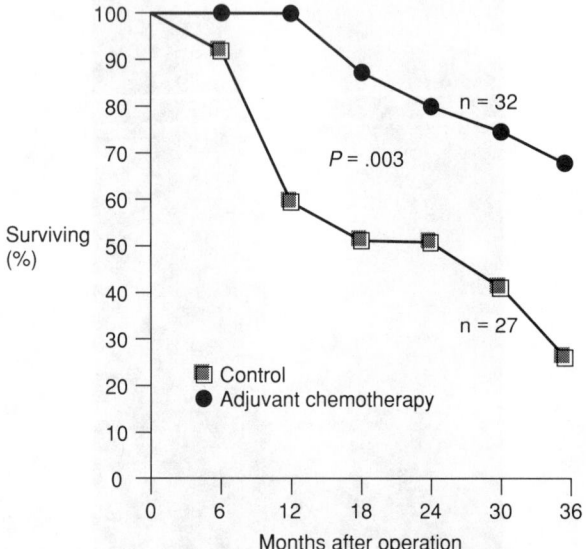

Figure 112-20. Survival of patients with surgically resected osteosarcoma treated with or without postoperative adjuvant chemotherapy in a randomized, controlled clinical trial. (After Eilber F, Giuliano A, Eckardt J, et al. Adjuvant chemotherapy for osteosarcoma: a randomized prospective trial. J Clin Oncol 1987;5:21)

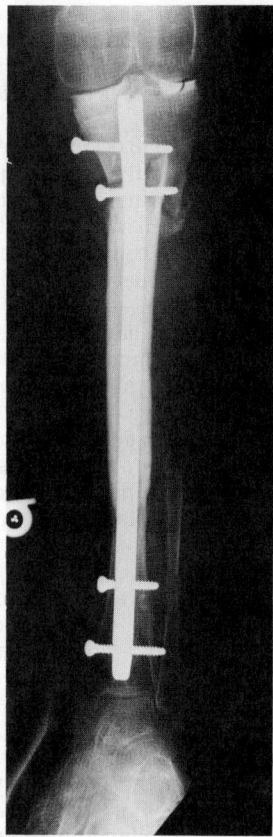

Figure 112-21. Allograft reconstruction after resection of an osteosarcoma of the proximal tibia.

adhesion of the femur to the resection site (see Fig. 112-23*B*). Alternatively, allograft reconstruction of the hemipelvis can be done to shorten the length of time until full weight bearing is possible.

Postoperative Chemotherapy

Adjuvant postoperative chemotherapy has been proved to increase survival of osteosarcoma patients after amputation or limb-sparing surgery.[43] As previously discussed, most limb-sparing regimens now incorporate preoperative chemotherapy as well. This does not replace postoperative treatment, but may influence the duration and type of postoperative chemotherapy given. The so-called T12 regimen (Fig. 112-24) is an example: patients with total or near-total tumor necrosis receive a short course of the same chemotherapy postoperatively (total duration of preoperative and postoperative treatment is 15 weeks). Those with lesser degrees of necrosis are switched to a more intensive regimen of doxorubicin and cisplatin lasting 27 weeks. Overall results of this regimen have been as good as those in which all patients receive more toxic chemotherapy. It remains to be determined, however, if the more aggressive chemotherapy is in fact improving the outcome for patients with poor initial tumor necrosis.[44] Although the optimal regimen for adjuvant chemotherapy of osteosarcoma has yet to be defined, combined preoperative and postoperative chemotherapy regimens, in which the postoperative therapy is tailored to the initial histologic response, are state of the art, particularly for patients undergoing limb-sparing surgery.

MANAGEMENT OF CHILDHOOD SOFT TISSUE SARCOMAS

Osteosarcomas occurring in the pediatric population are managed in a fashion similar to those in adults with similar results expected. Soft tissue sarcomas, however, may re-

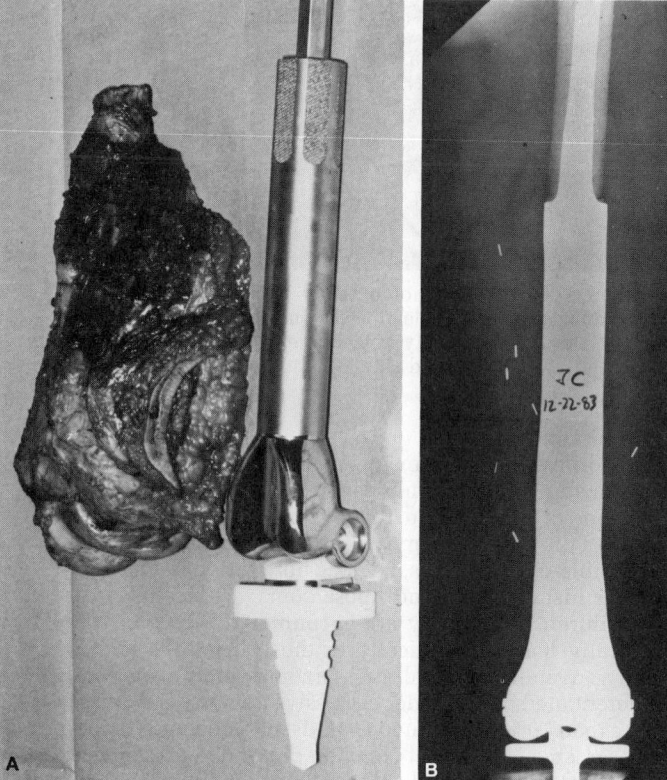

Figure 112-22. (*A*) Custom-made titanium prosthesis for replacement of the distal femur and knee joint. (*B*) Postoperative radiograph showing the prosthesis in place.

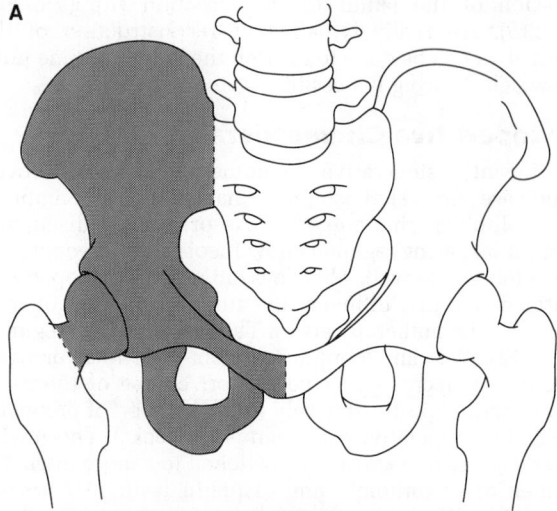

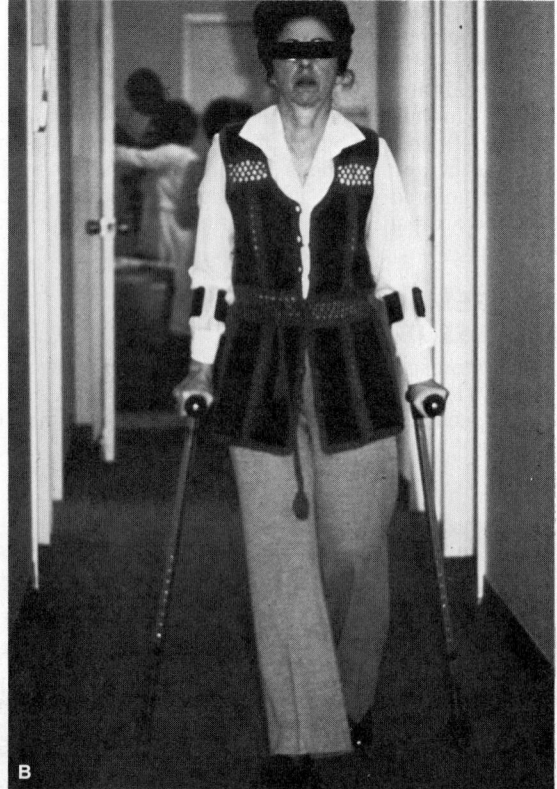

Figure 112-23. (*A*) Depiction of the bony structures removed in the conduct of an internal hemipelvectomy. (*B*) Postoperative photograph showing the ability of the patient to bear weight on the noticeably shorter operated side.

quire different management in children and adolescents than in adults. This is only partly due to differences in the behavior of sarcomas in these groups and is largely the result of the differing tumor types encountered in children.

Spindle-cell sarcomas, such as fibrosarcoma, malignant fibrous histiocytoma, and liposarcoma, are relatively rare in children. When they are encountered, however, they generally behave identically to those in adults and are managed similarly. Small-cell sarcomas, which are poorly differentiated, high-grade, aggressive tumors, account for more than 70% of childhood soft tissue sarcomas. Rhabdomyosarcoma is the most common childhood sarcoma and is the prototypical small-cell sarcoma. Extraosseous Ewing

sarcoma and primitive neuroectodermal tumor account for most of the remaining cases. Small-cell sarcomas are more sensitive to chemotherapy than most spindle-cell sarcomas; hence, chemotherapy plays a prominent role in their management.

Rhabdomyosarcomas tend to occur in three anatomic sites: the head and neck, including the orbit and paranasal sinuses (most common); the genitourinary tract; and the extremities. Most patients are younger than 5 years, although there is a second peak in adolescence composed mainly of boys with pelvic and paratesticular primary tumors. Three subtypes of rhabdomyosarcoma are seen—embryonal (most common), alveolar, and botryoid. Many adult sarcomas once classified as pleomorphic rhabdomyosarcomas are now considered to be malignant fibrous histiocytomas and are treated as any other adult soft tissue sarcoma.

In addition to their chemosensitivity, childhood rhabdomyosarcomas differ from adult sarcomas in other ways. Lymph node metastases are more common than in adult sarcomas and may be encountered in 20% to 40% of cases. The primary tumors are often locally extensive and invasive, and they often lack the pseudocapsule seen with spindle-cell sarcomas. Head and neck primaries can invade into the base of the skull or even into the brain; such extension is associated with a poor prognosis.

The locally aggressive nature of rhabdomyosarcomas, combined with their propensity to arise in sites where radical excision conveys great morbidity, has limited the role of surgery for these tumors. The initial surgical procedure should be a careful incisional biopsy, placing the incision in a way that does not complicate a subsequent excision. For most patients, chemotherapy and local irradiation play the primary roles in management. This is particularly true for rhabdomyosarcomas arising in the head and neck or pelvis. Before the routine use of adjuvant chemotherapy, 80% of children with rhabdomyosarcoma died of their disease. Now more than half are cured, and in patients presenting with limited disease amenable to complete resection after multimodality therapy, survival rates of 80% or more can be anticipated.[45]

MANAGEMENT OF RECURRENT AND METASTATIC SARCOMAS

Many adult and pediatric patients with locally recurrent or even metastatic sarcomas can be cured by aggressive surgery, often combined with radiation and chemotherapy. For this reason, all sarcoma patients should be observed carefully for recurrence. For high-grade lesions, follow-up should be directed toward detecting both local recurrence and metastases and should include periodic physical examination and chest radiograph plus CT scans of the primary site and lungs at least annually for the first 5 years. Low-grade lesions rarely metastasize in the absence of local recurrence, and follow-up should focus on the original tumor site. Low-grade sarcoma can recur up to 20 years after original resection, however, so follow-up must be maintained long-term.

Local Recurrence

Despite aggressive multimodality therapy, local recurrence remains a major mode of failure in sarcoma patients. The risk of local recurrence after surgical treatment of soft tissue sarcomas varies based on a number of factors. The most significant of these is the site of origin of the tumor, with lesions of the head and neck, trunk, and retroperitoneum all associated with a higher risk of local recurrence than lesions of the extremities. Local and regional failure

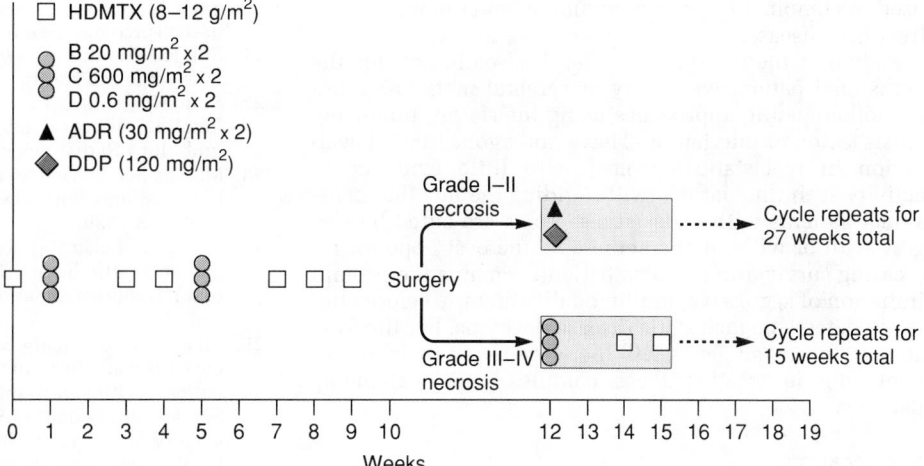

Figure 112-24. The T12 protocol employed by Rosen and colleagues for resectable osteosarcoma of the extremity. HDMTX, high-dose methotrexate; B, bleomycin; C, cyclophosphamide; D, dacarbazine; ADR, doxorubicin (Adriamycin); DDP, cisplatin (*cis*-diammine-dichloroplatinum). (After Rosen G. Preoperative [neoadjuvant] chemotherapy for osteogenic sarcoma: a 10-year experience. Orthopaedics 1985;8:659)

is the site of first recurrence after definitive resection in 50% of head, neck, and truncal sarcomas and in 75% of retroperitoneal tumors, but only 15% of extremity lesions.[46] Other factors influencing recurrence rates include the size and histologic grade of the primary tumor, deep as opposed to superficial location, and local failure of prior surgery.

Limb-sparing approaches can control and even cure local recurrence in the absence of distant metastases. For patients who were initially treated with surgery alone and who failed locally, multimodality treatment with repeat resection, radiation, and sometimes chemotherapy is associated with survival rates close to those of previously untreated patients[47] (Fig. 112-25). Patients with recurrence after surgery and radiation are more likely to require radical amputation to control recurrence in an extremity but are still candidates for salvage surgery. Locally recurrent retroperitoneal sarcomas, particularly low-grade tumors, can sometimes be resected on multiple occasions with long-term survival, but few of these patients are cured.[48]

Distant Metastases

The lungs are the most frequent site of distant spread for sarcomas and are often the only site of metastasis.[13,28] Aggressive resection of solitary or multiple lung metastases is associated with cure in about 25% to 35% of soft tissue and osteogenic sarcoma patients.[49] Even patients with bilateral metastases are candidates for surgery. This can be done either as staged thoracotomies or, preferably, as one procedure using a median sternotomy. Patients with three or fewer metastases, a long doubling time of the metastatic tumors, and unilateral disease have the best prognosis after surgical resection,[50] although patients lacking one or all of these favorable factors are still candidates for curative resection. It has been suggested that preoperative or postoperative adjuvant chemotherapy can improve the outcomes for patients undergoing complete resection of pulmonary metastases, especially from osteosarcomas.[51]

Patients with unresectable pulmonary metastases or with extrapulmonary metastases are usually treated with cytotoxic chemotherapy. Active agents include doxorubicin, ifosfamide, dacarbazine, high-dose methotrexate, and cisplatin.[52] Doxorubicin is the most active single agent for treating metastatic sarcoma. Ifosfamide is an alkylating agent closely related to cyclophosphamide and, like cyclophosphamide, is associated with severe hemorrhagic cystitis. The uroprotective agent 2-mercaptoethane sulfonate

sodium (mesna), when coadministered with ifosfamide, protects the bladder and largely eliminates hemorrhagic cystitis. Trials of ifosfamide and mesna show activity comparable to that of doxorubicin.[53] A regimen combining mesna, ifosfamide, dacarbazine, and doxorubicin (MAID regimen) has been described that showed a 49% objective response rate in previously untreated soft tissue sarcoma patients.[54] Cisplatin and high-dose methotrexate have significant activity in metastatic osteosarcoma and are often

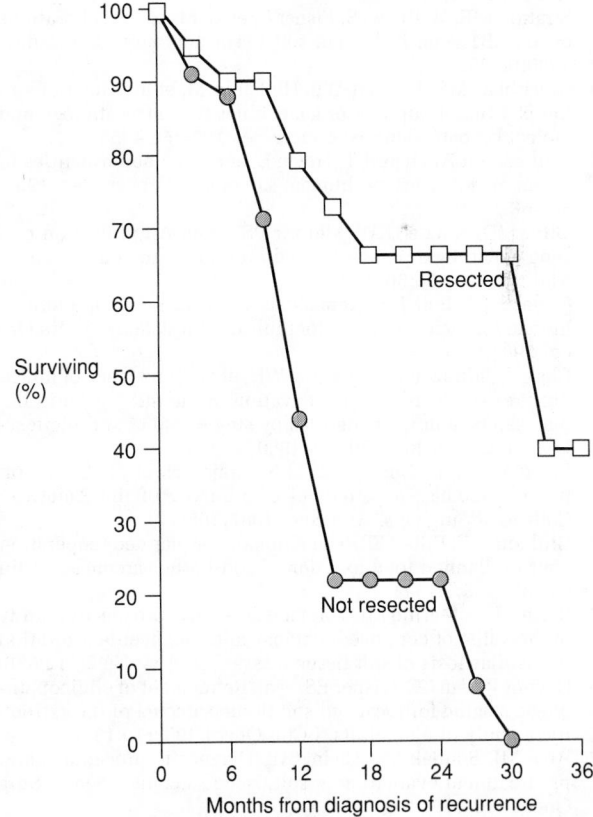

Figure 112-25. Survival of patients after resection of isolated local recurrence of an extremity soft tissue sarcoma. (After Huth J, Eilber FR. Patterns of metastatic spread following resection of extremity soft-tissue sarcomas and strategies for treatment. Semin Surg Oncol 1988;4:20)

used in combination with doxorubicin and other agents to treat this disease.

Radiation therapy may be useful as palliation for the occasional patient with bony or cerebral metastases. Immunotherapeutic approaches using interferon, tumor necrosis factor, or interleukin-2 have undergone limited evaluation in metastatic sarcoma, with little evidence of activity seen thus far. Notwithstanding the fact that occasional patients with metastatic sarcoma are cured by surgery with or without chemotherapy, the best hope for increasing survival in sarcoma patients remains the prompt initiation of aggressive, multimodality therapy before clinically detectable metastatic disease develops. For the foreseeable future, surgeons will therefore retain their prominent role in treating these complex and challenging patients.

REFERENCES

1. Parker SL, Tong T, Bolden S, et al. Cancer statistics, 1996. CA 1996;46:5.
2. McClay EF. Epidemiology of bone and soft tissue sarcomas. Semin Oncol 1989;16:264.
3. Collins JJ, Strauss ME, Levinskas GJ, et al. The mortality experience of workers exposed to 2,3,7,8-tetrachlorodibenzo-p-dioxin in a trichlorophenol process accident. Epidemiology 1993;4:7.
4. Wolfe WH, Michalek JE, Miner JC, et al. Health status of Air Force veterans occupationally exposed to herbicides in Vietnam. I: physical health. JAMA 1990;264:1824.
5. Malkin D, Li FP, Strong LC, et al. Germ line p53 mutations in a familial syndrome of breast cancer, sarcomas, and other neoplasms. Science 1990;250:1233.
6. McGuire SM, McGuire AL, McGuire MH. The genetic risk factors for bone and soft tissue tumors. Surg Oncol Clin North Am 1994;3:599.
7. Stratton MR, Williams S, Fisher C, et al. Structural alterations of the RB1 gene in human soft tissue tumours. Br J Cancer 1989;60:202.
8. Greenblatt MS, Bennett WP, Hollstein M, et al. Mutations in the *p53* tumor suppressor gene: clues to cancer etiology and molecular pathogenesis. Cancer Res 1994;54:4855.
9. Andreassen Å, Øyjord T, Hovig E, et al. *p53* abnormalities in different subtypes of human sarcomas. Cancer Res 1993;53:468.
10. Ollner JD, Kinzler KW, Meltzer PS, et al. Amplification of a gene encoding a p53-associated protein in human sarcomas. Nature 1992;358:80.
11. Gerlach JH, Bell DR, Karakousis C, et al. P-glycoprotein in human sarcoma: evidence for multidrug resistance. J Clin Oncol 1987;5:1452.
12. Chen G, Jaffrézou J-P, Fleming WH, et al. Prevalence of multidrug resistance related to activation of the *mdr*1 gene in human sarcoma mutants derived by single-step doxorubicin selection. Cancer Res 1994;54:4980.
13. Lawrence W Jr, Donegan WL, Natarajan N, et al. Adult soft tissue sarcomas: a pattern of care survey of the American College of Surgeons. Ann Surg 1987;205:349.
14. Giuliano AE, Eilber FR. The rationale for planned reoperation after unplanned total excision of soft-tissue sarcomas. J Clin Oncol 1985;3:1344.
15. Barth RJ Jr., Merino MJ, Solomon D, et al. A prospective study of the value of core needle biopsy and fine needle aspiration in the diagnosis of soft tissue masses. Surgery 1992;112:536.
16. Gaynor JJ, Tan CC, Casper ES, et al. Refinement of clinicopathologic staging for localized soft tissue sarcoma of the extremity: a study of 423 adults. J Clin Oncol 1992;10:1317.
17. Arca MJ, Sondak VK, Chang AE. Diagnostic procedures and pre-treatment evaluation of soft tissue sarcomas. Semin Surg Oncol 1994;10:323.
18. Daly PF, Cohen JS. Magnetic resonance spectroscopy of tumors and potential in vivo clinical applications: a review. Cancer Res 1989;49:770.
19. Jones DN, Brizel DM, Charles HC, et al. Monitoring of response to neoadjuvant therapy of soft tissue and musculoskeletal sarcomas using F18-FDG PET. J Nucl Med 1994;35:38P.
20. Yang JC, Rosenberg SA. Surgery for adult patients with soft tissue sarcomas. Semin Oncol 1989;16:289.
21. Suit HD, Mankin HJ, Wood WC, et al. Treatment of the patient with stage M0 soft tissue sarcoma. J Clin Oncol 1988;6:854.
22. Shiu MH, Hilaris BS, Harrison LB, et al. Brachytherapy and function-saving resection of soft tissue sarcoma arising in the limb. Int J Radiat Oncol Biol Phys 1991;21:1485.
23. Marcus SG, Merino MJ, Glatstein E, et al. Long-term outcome in 87 patients with low-grade soft tissue sarcoma. Arch Surg 1993;128:1336.
24. Eilber FR, Eckardt JJ, Rosen G, et al. Neoadjuvant chemotherapy and radiotherapy in the multidisciplinary management of soft tissue sarcomas of the extremity. Surg Oncol Clin North Am 1993;2:611.
25. Chang AE, Steinberg SM, Culnane M, et al. Functional and psychosocial effects of multimodality limb-sparing therapy in patients with soft tissue sarcomas. J Clin Oncol 1989;7:1217.
26. Sondak VK, Leonard JA Jr, Robertson JM, et al. Limb-sparing surgery for extremity soft tissue sarcomas: functional and rehabilitation considerations. Surg Oncol Clin North Am 1993;2:657.
27. Lienard D, Ewalenko P, Delmotte JJ, et al. High-dose recombinant tumor necrosis factor alpha in combination with interferon gamma and melphalan in isolation perfusion of the limbs for melanoma and sarcoma. J Clin Oncol 1992;10:52.
28. Huth JF, Eilber FR. Patterns of metastatic spread following resection of extremity soft-tissue sarcomas and strategies for treatment. Semin Surg Oncol 1988;4:20.
29. Elias AD, Antmann KH. Adjuvant chemotherapy for soft-tissue sarcoma: a critical appraisal. Semin Surg Oncol 1988;4:59.
30. Rosenberg SA, Tepper J, Glatstein E, et al. Prospective randomized evaluation of adjuvant chemotherapy in adults with soft tissue sarcomas of the extremities. Cancer 1983;52:424.
31. Chang AE, Kinsella T, Glatstein E, et al. Adjuvant chemotherapy for patients with high-grade soft-tissue sarcomas of the extremity. J Clin Oncol 1988;6:1491.
32. Tierney JF, on behalf of the Sarcoma Meta–analysis Collaboration (SMAC). A meta–analysis using individaul patient data for randomized clinical trials (RCTs) of adjuvant chemotherapy for soft tissue sarcomas (STSs). (Abstract) Proc Am Soc Clin Oncol 1996;15.
33. Storm FK, Mahvi DM. Diagnosis and management of retroperitoneal soft-tissue sarcoma. Ann Surg 1991;214:2.
34. Sindelar WF, Kinsella TJ, Chen PW, et al. Intraoperative radiotherapy in retroperitoneal sarcomas: final results of a prospective, randomized clinical trial. Arch Surg 1993;128:402.
35. Glenn J, Sindelar WF, Kinsella T, et al. Results of multimodality therapy of resectable soft-tissue sarcomas of the retroperitoneum. Surgery 1985;97:316.
36. Storm FK, Eilber FR, Mirra J, et al. Retroperitoneal sarcomas: a reappraisal of treatment. J Surg Oncol 1981;17:1.
37. Goffman T, Tochner Z, Glatstein E. Primary treatment of large and massive adult sarcomas with iododeoxyuridine and aggressive hyperfractionated irradiation. Cancer 1991;67:572.
38. Robertson JM, Sondak VK, Weiss SA, et al. Preoperative radiation therapy and iododeoxyuridine for large retroperitoneal sarcomas. Int J Radiat Oncol Biol Phys 1995;31:87.
39. Häyry P, Scheinin TM. The desmoid (Reitamo) syndrome: etiology, manifestations, pathogenesis, and treatment. Curr Probl Surg 1988;25:225.
40. Church JM. Desmoid tumors in familial adenomatous polyposis. Surg Oncol Clin North Am 1994;3:435.
41. Baker L, Crowley J, Ryan J, et al. Long term followup in the cure of osteogenic sarcoma. Proc Am Soc Clin Oncol 1989;8:320.
42. Eilber FR, Grant TT, Sakai D, et al. Internal hemipelvectomy: excision of the hemipelvis with limb preservation. Cancer 1979;43:806.
43. Eilber F, Giuliano A, Eckardt J, et al. Adjuvant chemotherapy for osteosarcoma: a randomized prospective trial. J Clin Oncol 1987;5:21.
44. Meyers PA, Heller G, Healey J, et al. Chemotherapy for nonmetastatic osteogenic sarcoma: the Memorial Sloan-Kettering experience. J Clin Oncol 1992;10:5.
45. Wexler LH, Helman LJ. Pediatric soft tissue tumors. CA Cancer J Clin 1994;44:211.

46. Potter DA, Glenn J, Kinsella T, et al. Patterns of recurrence in patients with high-grade soft-tissue sarcomas. J Clin Oncol 1985;3:353.

47. Giuliano AE, Eilber FR, Morton DL. The management of locally recurrent soft-tissue sarcoma. Ann Surg 1982;196:87.

48. Pinson CW, ReMine SG, Fletcher WS, et al. Long-term results with primary retroperitoneal tumors. Arch Surg 1989;124:1168.

49. Putnam JB, Roth JA. Resection of sarcomatous pulmonary metastases. Surg Oncol Clin North Am 1993;2:673.

50. Casson AG, Putnam JB, Natarajan G, et al. Five-year survival after pulmonary metastasectomy for adult soft tissue sarcoma. Cancer 1992;69:662.

51. Skinner KA, Eilber FR, Holmes EC, et al. Surgical treatment and chemotherapy for pulmonary metastases from osteosarcoma. Arch Surg 1992;127:1065.

52. Antmann KH, Elias AD. Chemotherapy of advanced soft-tissue sarcomas. Semin Surg Oncol 1988;4:53.

53. Antmann KH, Ryan L, Elias A, et al. Response to ifosfamide and mesna: 124 previously treated patients with metastatic or unresectable sarcoma. J Clin Oncol 1989;7:126.

54. Elias A, Ryan L, Sulkes A, et al. Response to mesna, doxorubicin, ifosfamide, and dacarbazine in 108 patients with metastatic or unresectable sarcoma and no prior chemotherapy. J Clin Oncol 1989;7:1208.

SURGERY: SCIENTIFIC PRINCIPLES AND PRACTICE, Second Edition, edited by Lazar J. Greenfield, Michael W. Mulholland, Keith T. Oldham, Gerald B. Zelenock, and Keith D. Lillemoe. Lippincott–Raven Publishers, Philadelphia, © 1997.

CHAPTER 113

AESTHETIC SURGERY

THOMAS RAY STEVENSON

BIOLOGY OF AGING SKIN

The deleterious effects of aging are produced through numerous processes, some independent and others interrelated. The major events occur in cells that are genetically directed to retard their own proliferation. Once proliferation has ceased, events within the cell transpire, including accumulation of waste product pigments, increase in the proportion of inactive enzymes, and loss of important genes. Failure of those genes that code for messenger RNA is particularly damaging.

Skin changes occur with advancing age. These changes result from the generalized aging process as well as from the effect of sun exposure.[1] Of the two, sun exposure appears more detrimental than chronologic aging alone.

Sunlight can cause redness, tanning, and cancer in human skin. Photodamaged skin in time becomes wrinkled, yellow, and leathery and displays multiple telangiectasia. Various benign, premalignant, and malignant neoplasms eventually appear. Histologically, photodamaged skin shows increased quantities of thick, altered elastic fibers. The quantity of mature collagen is diminished, and the amount of ground substance is increased. Fibroblasts are more numerous after chronic sun exposure as opposed to chronologic aging, when a decrease in the number of cellular elements is common. Sun exposure results in microvascular changes with dilatation and tortuous arteries and veins.

Ultraviolet (UV) radiation is the major offending agent in sunlight. It appears to be responsible for the observed skin changes. UVA (320 to 400 nm) makes up the major ultraviolet component in the sun's spectrum. UVB (280 to 320 nm) causes DNA damage and skin cancer and produces pyrimidine dimers in the DNA of human skin. UVA seems to play a less significant role than UVB.

REGIONAL OPERATIVE PROCEDURES

Blepharoplasty

Excess skin and fat of the upper and lower eyelids produce an aged, tired look. Fine wrinkling of eyelid skin worsens this appearance. These changes can be ameliorated by upper and lower lid blepharoplasty and fat excision.

The patient seeking blepharoplasty is evaluated preoperatively for visual acuity, ptosis of the upper eyelids, and symptoms of dry eye. In addition, a careful examination of the lower eyelids is performed, assessing the extent of lower lid laxity. If significant laxity exists and is unappreciated, an ectropion of one or both lower lids can occur postoperatively.

Blepharoplasty can be performed under local or general anesthesia.[2] Elliptical skin excisions are designed on both upper eyelids before infiltration of local anesthesia. The upper and lower eyelids are infiltrated with a solution of local anesthetic and epinephrine. The skin is removed with a strip of underlying orbicularis oculi muscle. Openings are made in the orbital septum, and excess fat is removed. The lower eyelid blepharoplasty usually involves elevation of the lower eyelid skin and underlying orbicularis oculi muscle as a composite flap. Any excess fat is removed from the inferior aspects of the orbital septum. Careful judgment is exercised when removing excess skin and muscle of the lower lid. Overly aggressive skin excision can result in lower lid ectropion. The skin wounds are closed with 6-0 silk sutures in the skin or buried 6-0 Prolene sutures.

Some patients will require no skin excision but may benefit from removal of fatty deposits of the lower lid. This can be performed under local anesthesia through an incision on the inner aspect of the lower lid (transconjunctival incision).[3] This hidden incision usually heals uneventfully. Blepharoplasty through a transconjunctival approach results in ectropion less frequently than does blepharoplasty through a transcutaneous approach.

Postoperatively, the patient is asked to rest with the head elevated to a 45-degree angle. Moist, cool compresses are applied for the first 24 hours. Artificial tears and a lubricant are used to diminish the likelihood of corneal abrasion. The patient is cautioned to return immediately if significant pain occurs or any changes in visual acuity are noted. If the procedure is done in an outpatient setting, the patient usually returns the day after the operation for evaluation. The examiner looks for evidence of hematoma or wound breakdown.

Preliminary postoperative results are apparent about 3 weeks after the operation (Fig. 113-1). By this time, much of the swelling and discoloration has resolved. Fine wrinkling of the skin can persist, but the improvement due to removal of excess skin fat should be visible. If a lower eyelid ectropion does occur, it is treated by massage and taping. Rarely, reoperation and placement of a skin graft are required to correct the ectropion.

Rhytidectomy

Age, gravity, and sun exposure combine to change facial appearance over time. Wrinkles develop in the forehead, nasolabial region, cheeks, and submental area. Skin laxity becomes apparent in the submental region, and jowls occur. An overall tired, listless expression is assumed. Ac-

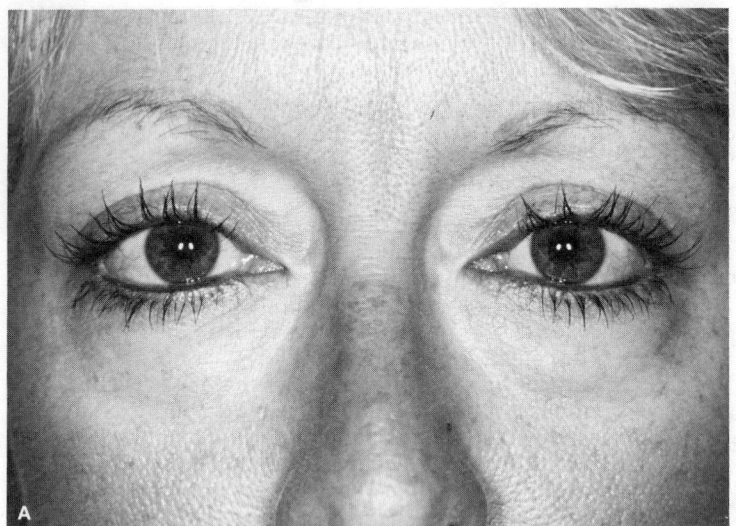

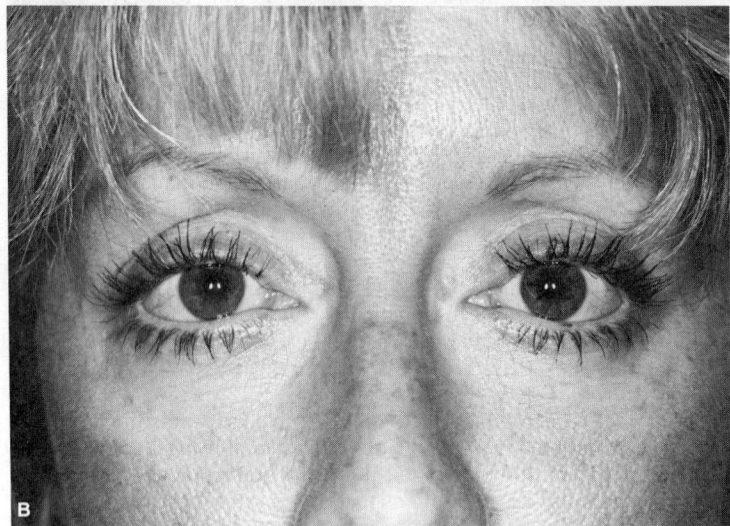

Figure 113-1. Blepharoplasty—preoperatively (*A*) and postoperatively (*B*). The patient's excess lower lid fat and upper lid skin were removed.

companying these physical changes in some people is a loss of self-esteem. Patients, both male and female, seek a more youthful appearance to improve self-image and compete successfully in business and social arenas. Preoperatively, the surgeon questions each patient regarding factors that might affect the outcome of surgery. Smokers are at an increased risk for skin necrosis after rhytidectomy. A patient with hypertension is more likely to develop a hematoma postoperatively. The use of anticoagulants or aspirin likewise increases the risk of postoperative bleeding. Preexisting surgical scars that might compromise the operative procedure are identified.

Rhytidectomy can be performed under local or general anesthesia.[4] An incision is made in the hair-bearing region of the temple about 6 cm above and slightly anterior to the root of the helix. This incision is carried to the point of attachment between the ear and scalp skin. It then passes just anterior to the ear, curves behind the earlobe, proceeds in the retroauricular sulcus to the level of the tragus, and continues posteriorly across the hairline horizontally into the scalp. The skin of the face is elevated, leaving some subcutaneous fat on its deep surface to prevent excess thinning and vascular compromise. Dissection is carried anteriorly to the nasolabial fold, and undermining progresses into the submental region. The skin flap is lifted from the sternocleidomastoid muscle and mastoid fascia. Care is

taken to maintain this plane above the parotid gland where trauma to the facial nerve might occur. Once the dissection is completed on one side of the face, the opposite side is approached and an identical procedure performed. Many plastic surgeons then isolate a portion of the superficial musculoaponeurotic system. This dissection allows identification and separation of a firm tissue plane that can be tightened, improving the effects of ultimate skin excision and reducing the amount of tension needed to close the skin incisions. Based on the surgeon's judgment, a portion of the excess skin is excised. Sutures are placed in the skin above the ear and in the retroauricular region, where tension is highest. The remaining skin is closed after hemostasis is ensured. Suction drains are often used. A compressive head dressing is applied.

Alternatively, skin redraping can be accomplished through the minimal incision technique of endoscopic surgery.[5] For both brow lift and rhytidectomy, small incisions in the hairline permit access for direct video-assisted dissection.

Postoperatively, the patient is asked to remain in a sitting position at about a 45-degree angle. Wounds are examined in the first few hours after operation and again at 24 hours for evidence of hematoma. After 24 hours, the head dressing is changed and replaced with a light dressing. Three to five days after the operation, the preauricular sutures are removed. Retroauricular and temple sutures are removed after 7 to 10 days.

Bruising that occurs as a result of the surgical procedure is usually gone after 3 weeks. Much of the facial swelling is diminished by that time; however, gradual continual reduction in swelling and relaxation of the tightened skin occur for several more months. In general, a stable postoperative result is achieved by 6 months after the procedure (Fig. 113-2).

Complications resulting from rhytidectomy can include bleeding and hematoma (Table 113-1). If a sizable hematoma occurs, it must be evacuated to prevent necrosis of the overlying skin or infection. Development of a surgical

wound infection after rhytidectomy is rare. Permanent injury to the facial nerve can occur, although the incidence appears to be less than 2% in the previously unoperated patient. Nerve paresis, especially of the buccal branches, is more common and usually resolves after several months.

Chemical Peel

Fine wrinkles of the eyelids, perioral region, and cheeks can be improved by a chemical peel.[6] This process requires production of a superficial burn with use of a solution whose active ingredient is usually phenol. Phenol has been associated with cardiac arrhythmias that are usually tran-

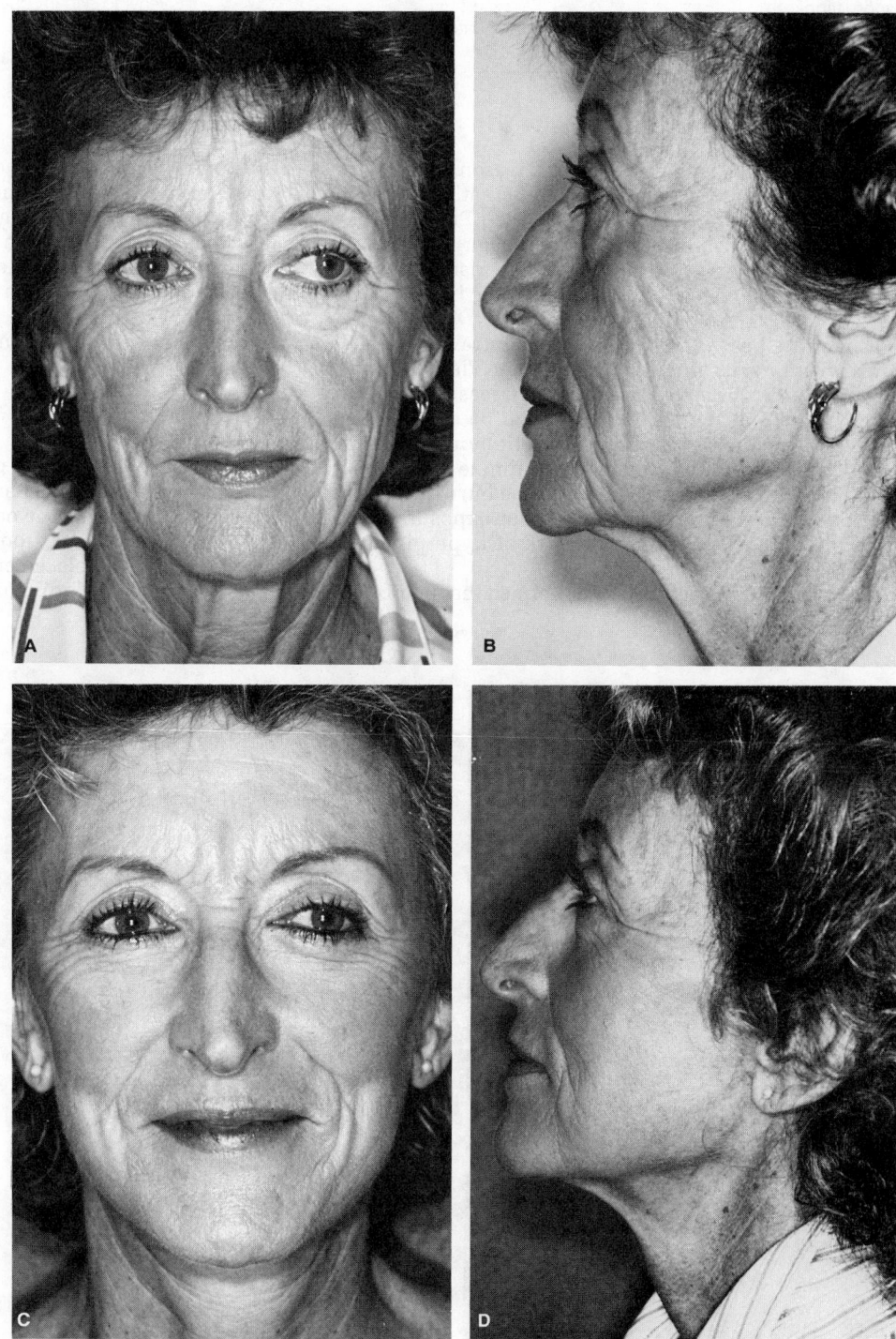

Figure 113-2. Facelift—preoperatively (*A* and *B*) and postoperatively (*C* and *D*). The excess skin of the cheeks and submental region was reduced with little visible scarring.

Table 113-1. AESTHETIC SURGERY: INDICATIONS AND COMPLICATIONS

Procedure	Indications	Complications	Incidence
Blepharoplasty	Excess eyelid skin or fat	Ectropion of lower lid	1%–3%
		Blindness	<0.001%
Rhytidectomy	Facial aging, skin excess	Skin slough	2%–10%
		Facial nerve injury	<0.05%
Chemical peel	Facial skin wrinkling	Pigmentation changes	5%–15%
		Significant scarring	<0.5%
Otoplasty	Prominent ears	Overcorrection	2%–5%
		Recurrent or persistent deformity	1%–5%
Augmentation mammaplasty	Inadequate breast size	Capsular contracture	2%–10%
Reduction mammaplasty	Breast hypertrophy	Skin breakdown	1%–10%
		Nipple loss	<1%
Brachioplasty	Skin and fat excess	Delayed healing	<5%
Abdominoplasty	Skin and fat excess	Marginal wound breakdown,	1%–5%
Liposuction	Fat excess	Overlying skin irregularities	1%–10%
Tissue expansion	Inadequate local skin	Infection	1%–5%
		Implant extrusion	1%–20%

sient but can be significant. For this reason, some physicians use trichloroacetic acid as an alternative to phenol, which results in a more superficial peel. Preoperatively, the patient must understand that although improvement in the wrinkling will occur, there is a risk of scarring, hypopigmentation, or hyperpigmentation in the treated areas.

Chemical peel is performed with intravenous sedation with or without local anesthesia. The solution is applied uniformly to the involved areas. If a deeper peel is desired, the treated areas can be covered with adhesive tape for 24 hours. Antibiotic powder or ointment is used postoperatively to minimize crusting and control superficial infection. Once the burn has healed, the patient is instructed to avoid sun exposure and to wear a sunblock to reduce the risk of hyperpigmentation (Fig. 113-3).

Superficial skin peels can be performed that improve the epidermal component of the skin, in part by removing the dead layers of keratin. Although the effects of these peels are temporary, their minimal risks make them amenable to a home skin care program and to frequent touch-up peels to maintain a fresher skin texture. Agents such as glycolic acid are applied to the skin at weekly intervals in increasing strengths. Application is followed by a moisturizing regimen and sun protection.

Rhinoplasty

Rhinoplasty is a surgical procedure whereby the contour of the external nose is changed. As a result of trauma or congenital deformity, the nose may have an unsatisfactory contour. It can appear crooked in the anterior projection, resulting from displacement or asymmetry of the nasal bones or cartilage. Individual patients can request reduc-

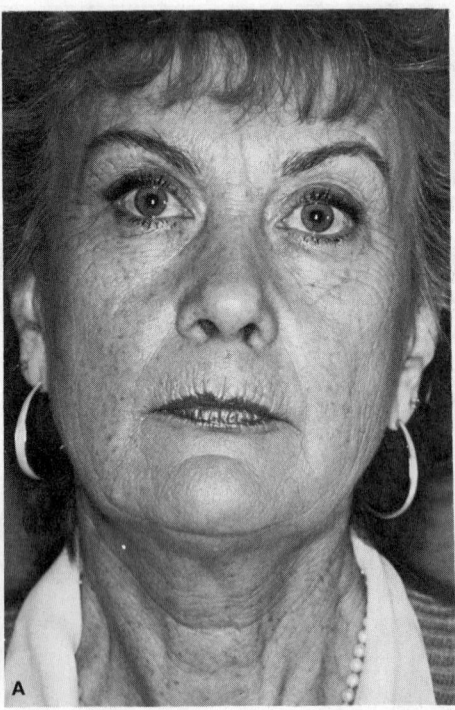 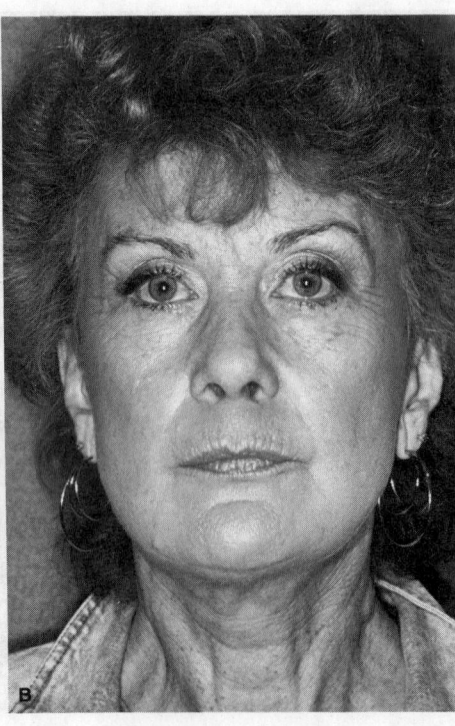

Figure 113-3. Chemical peel—preoperatively (A) and postoperatively (B). This patient has also undergone facelift and upper and lower lid blepharoplasties.

tion of a dorsal hump, refinement of a nasal tip, or correction of a drooping tip. Aesthetic rhinoplasty is directed toward the correction of these abnormalities. In those patients who suffer obstructed breathing in association with an external deformity, a simultaneous procedure on the nasal septum to improve air flow can be performed.

Photographic documentation of the external deformity is made preoperatively. Planning the operative procedure is facilitated by analysis of the preoperative photographs. It is crucial that the patient understand the goals for rhinoplasty, including proposed functional and aesthetic improvements.

Rhinoplasty can be performed under local or general anesthesia. Hemostasis is facilitated by the use of intrana-

sal vasoconstrictors as well as epinephrine-containing anesthetic solutions injected into the nose itself. Access to the bones and cartilages composing the nasal dorsum can be obtained through intranasal or external incision. Open rhinoplasty can be performed by making a small incision across the columella and extending it into intranasal incisions, permitting extensive exposure of the nasal structures. More frequently, surgical goals can be accomplished through incisions concealed inside the nose. Cartilage of the nasal tip is remodeled to improve contour if necessary. The bony and cartilaginous nasal dorsum is lowered when required through the use of a rasp, scalpel, or chisel. Nasal bones can be repositioned either to improve symmetry or to close an open deformity of the dorsum after hump re-

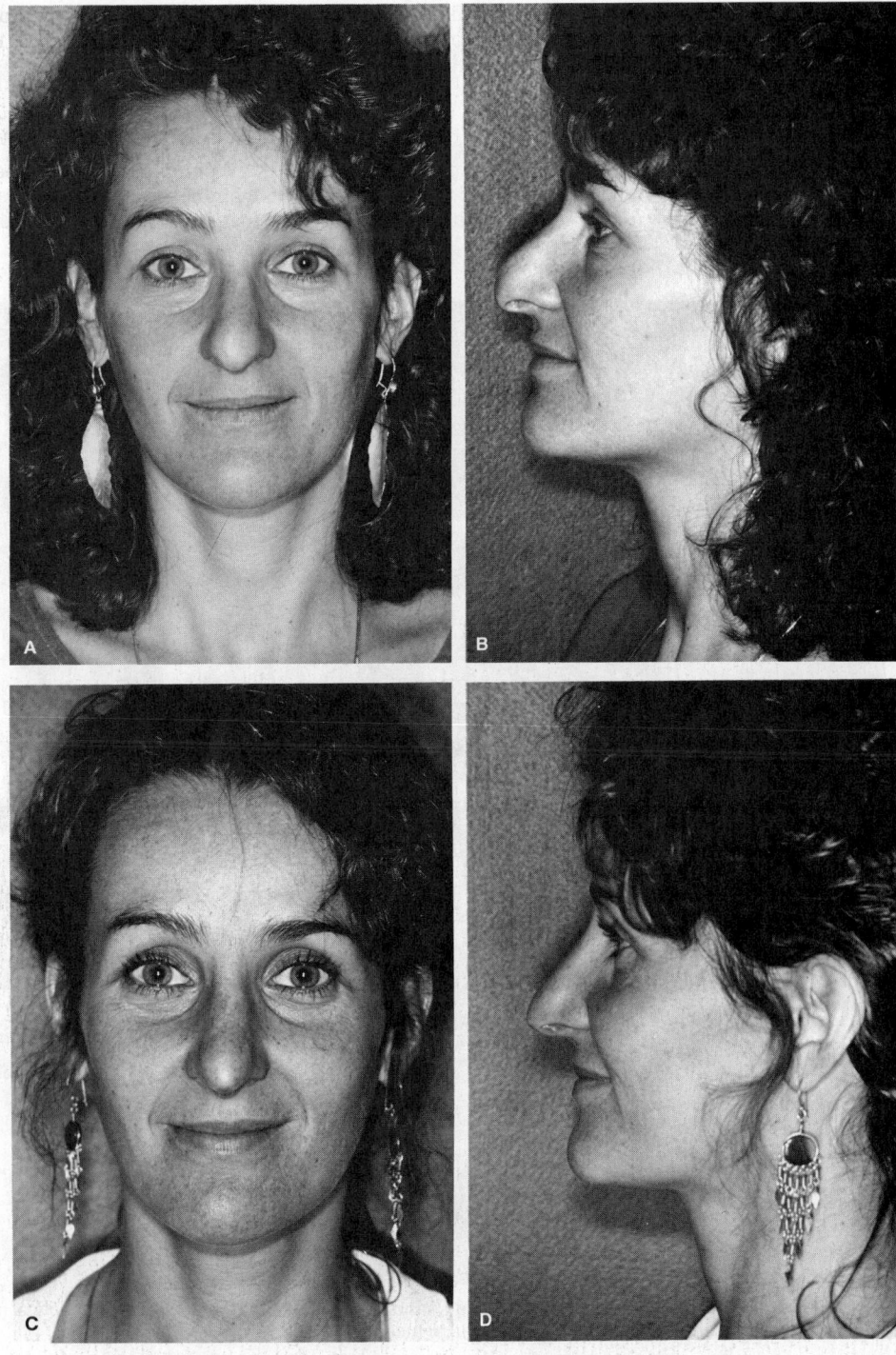

Figure 113-4. Rhinoplasty—preoperatively (*A* and *B*) and postoperatively (*C* and *D*).

moval. Bony repositioning requires osteotomies to separate the nasal bones from the maxilla.

Cartilage grafting to improve nasal contour is being used with increasing frequency. If drooping of the nasal tip is to be corrected, support for the tip is provided by a cartilage graft. This graft can be placed between the medial crura of the alar cartilages or subcutaneously in the columella.

Mild ecchymosis of the nose and eyes, as well as nasal swelling, is expected after rhinoplasty. Ice packs can minimize swelling, and oral analgesics are usually sufficient to control pain. The cartilage and bone of the nose are supported for 10 to 14 days with tape and an external splint.

Much of the swelling resolves by 3 weeks after operation. It takes several months, however, for the final result to declare itself. Because of some persistent nasal swelling, the results of a rhinoplasty may not be fully appreciated until 1 year after the procedure. During this time, repositioned bone and cartilage assume a more permanent contour (Fig. 113-4). Revision rhinoplasty is delayed for 1 year after the original procedure.

Otoplasty

Prominent ears result from an increase in conchal bowl dimensions with or without effacement of the antehelical fold. This deformity is rarely associated with hearing loss.

Otoplasty is usually performed during childhood and is done to eliminate ridicule from peers (Fig. 113-5).

Most otoplasties in children are performed under general anesthesia.[7] A lenticular segment of skin is removed from the postauricular sulcus. The conchal bowl is reduced in size and softened by judicious cartilage shaving. An antehelical fold is created through placement of horizontal mattress sutures driven through the auricular cartilage. The lobule can be repositioned by manipulation of the involved cartilage and postauricular skin. The operating surgeon must avoid overcorrection of the deformity.

Postoperative care consists of patient observation, the use of a headband at night, and the administration of analgesics. Hematoma can occur, usually heralded by increasing pain. If a hematoma occurs, it is drained immediately.

The results of otoplasty are apparent as soon as the dressings are removed. Most of the residual swelling clears by 3 to 6 weeks after operation. Occasionally, a suture is extruded months or years after the procedure. This rarely compromises the result.

Augmentation Mammaplasty

Women give many reasons for seeking augmentation mammaplasty. Some wish to restore the breast contour lost after pregnancy, breast engorgement, and subsequent

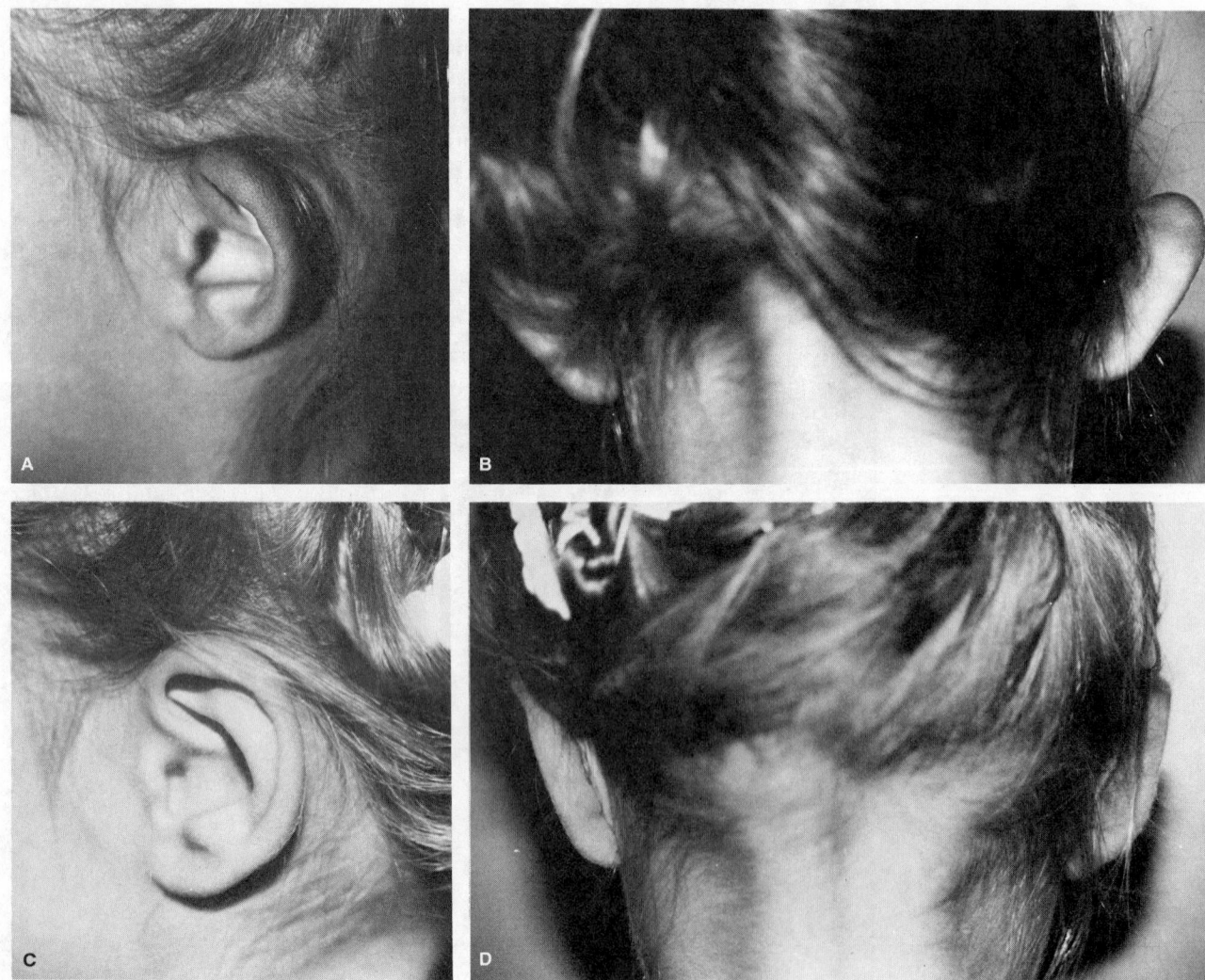

Figure 113-5. Otoplasty—preoperatively (*A* and *B*) and postoperatively (*C* and *D*). The antehelical fold was restored and the prominence of the ear reduced.

involution. Others believe that larger breasts make them more sexually attractive. Still others express a wish to improve clothing fit or overall self-esteem (Fig. 113-6).

Counseling a woman seeking breast augmentation requires careful explanation of the proposed benefits as well as potential risks of the procedure. Improved breast contour is sought through placement of a prosthesis. The prosthesis is not totally inert, and each patient must be informed regarding the effects of its placement. Evidence suggests that implants are neither carcinogenic nor likely to induce systemic illness.[8-10] The implants do cause the body to form a scar capsule. In some patients, this capsule can contract and result in uncomfortable breast hardness or a visual distortion of breast contour. Presence of an implant can complicate mammography, and the patient should be made aware of this fact (see Table 113-1). Implants vary in structure and content. The shell of most implants is composed of silicone rubber. This shell can be smooth or textured. The textured surface implant seems to be associated with a lower rate of capsular contracture and breast firmness. Most implants placed since 1991 have been saline filled. Prior to that time, silicone gel–filled implants were in common use. Concerns were raised regarding the possible association between silicone gel and autoimmune disease, resulting in FDA recommendations for marked restriction in the use of this material for breast implants.

Local or general anesthesia can be used during augmentation mammaplasty. An incision is made in either the inframammary fold, axilla, or periareolar region. A pocket is developed beneath the breast itself or beneath the pectoralis major muscle. This is performed under direct vision or endoscopically. After insertion of the prosthesis, positioning of the implant is carefully assessed to ensure symmetry.

Postoperatively, antibiotics are given for at least 24 hours, and pain medication is administered as needed. If a hematoma occurs, it is heralded by pain and swelling usually within the first 24 hours. An elastic wrap or brassiere provides breast support. Breast massage can be instituted during the first week postoperatively. This massage is believed to reduce the incidence of capsular contracture. If a capsular contracture does occur, it is usually apparent within the first 6 months. Patients who request treatment of a capsular contracture often undergo removal of the implant (with or without excision of the scar capsule) and either repositioning of the existing implant or insertion of an implant with a different composition.

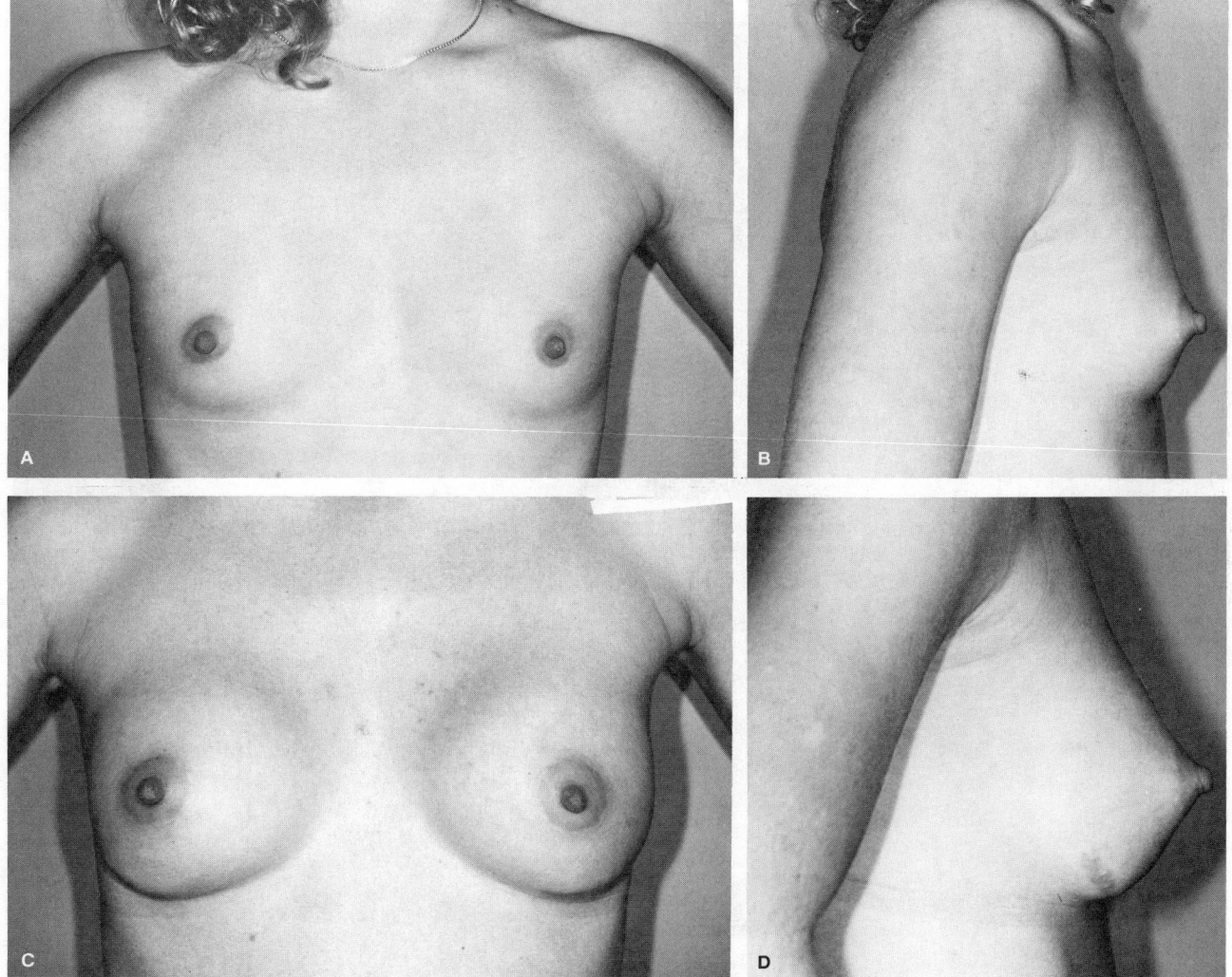

Figure 113-6. Augmentation mammaplasty—preoperatively (*A* and *B*) and postoperatively (*C* and *D*). Breast projection and distance from the center of the nipple to the inframammary fold have increased.

Mastopexy and Reduction Mammaplasty

Obesity, pregnancy, and aging contribute to drooping of the breasts that is both functionally impairing and aesthetically displeasing. The deformity can result solely from an excess of skin. More often, skin excess is accompanied by nipple enlargement, displacement of the nipple inferiorly on the breast, and an excess of breast tissue and fat. Isolated skin excess is treated by mastopexy. When other elements of breast enlargement are present, reduction mammaplasty is indicated (Fig. 113-7).

Mastopexy and breast reduction share the feature of a reduction in size of the skin brassiere. Similarly, both operations sustain nipple viability through maintenance of underlying or adjacent vascular tissue.[11] Only rarely in the massively enlarged breast is it necessary to transfer the nipple as a free nipple graft. Once the proposed skin incisions are marked and the patient is under general anesthesia, incisions are made and excess skin removed. In reduction mammaplasty, the nipple is commonly left attached to an inferiorly based pedicle of dermis, breast tissue, associated sensory nerves, and nutrient vessels. An appropriate amount of breast tissue and fat is removed, final skin trimming performed, and the incisions closed. Although mastopexy may leave only a circumareolar scar and a vertical scar below the nipple, reduction mammaplasty adds to these a scar of varying length in the inframammary fold.

Breast support is provided postoperatively by an elastic wrap or brassiere. Sutures are generally removed within the first 10 to 14 days. Hematoma, infection, and wound breakdown are rare occurrences. Some marginal skin loss or dehiscence can occur in the central portion of the inframammary wound, although this rarely requires revision. A small percentage of women experience temporary or permanent reduction in nipple sensibility, and a very small group lose the nipple entirely. Breastfeeding may or may not be possible after breast reduction.

Brachioplasty

Excess skin of the arm is often perceived by the patient as unattractive and can make it difficult to find clothing that fits appropriately. The patient who elects to undergo brachioplasty to reduce this skin and fat excess must understand that he or she is exchanging an improved contour for a scar located along the entire medial aspect of the arm (Fig. 113-8).

This procedure can be performed under local or general

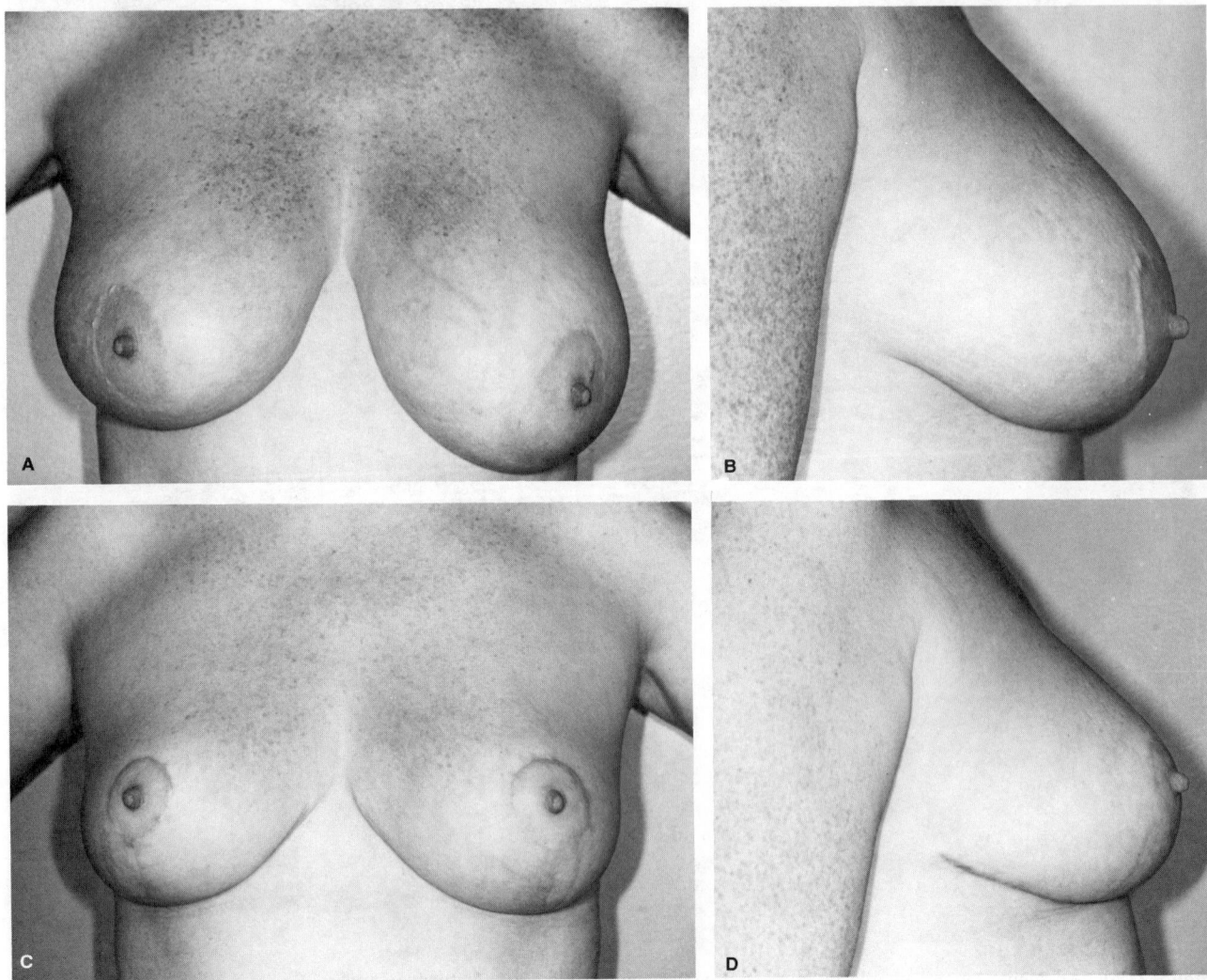

Figure 113-7. Reduction mammaplasty—preoperatively (*A* and *B*) and postoperatively (*C* and *D*). The inframammary scar is concealed beneath the breast.

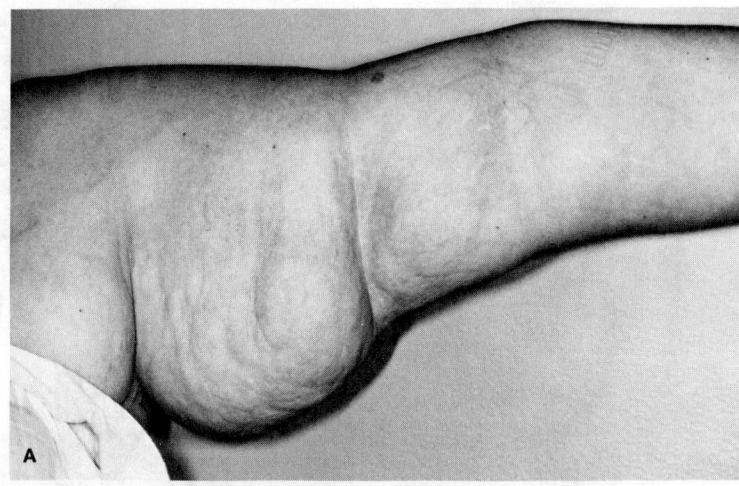

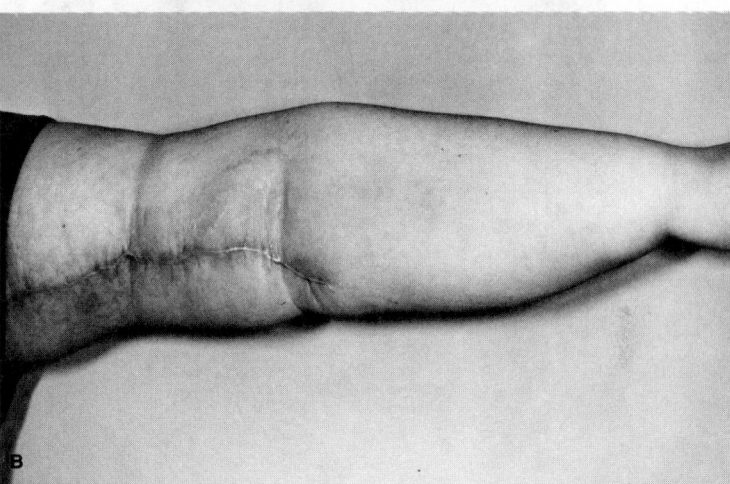

Figure 113-8. Brachioplasty—preoperatively (*A*) and postoperatively (*B*). Improved contour is accompanied by a visible scar.

anesthesia.[12] An outline for proposed skin excision is drawn on the medial arm, sometimes with a Z-plasty extension into the axilla. After skin excision, a suction drain is inserted, and the wound is closed.

Postoperative care includes close observation and the placement of a compressive dressing. Results are assessed after 3 to 6 months.

Abdominoplasty

Excess abdominal skin and fat can persist after pregnancy or can be associated with obesity. Laxity of the abdominal wall, with the separation of the rectus abdominis muscles in the midline (diastasis recti), can also be present. Indications for abdominoplasty to correct these deformities include desire for improved aesthetic appearance, better hygiene, and better clothing fit.

Markings are made preoperatively with the patient standing. A diamond-shaped excision is designed with a modification in the pubic region to permit maintenance of a normal hair pattern.[13] Once anesthesia is established, the umbilicus is circumscribed and left attached to the abdominal wall. The excess skin and fat are removed as a single unit. Remaining abdominal skin is separated from the underlying abdominal wall cephalad to facilitate wound closure. Tightening of the abdominal wall musculature is accomplished through plication of the rectus abdominis or oblique muscles, or both. Further refinement of the abdominal contour can be achieved by liposuctioning the subcutaneous fatty layers at the margins of the flaps

and along the midline. The patient is flexed at the waist, and wound closure is commenced. An opening is made in the skin to permit insertion of the umbilicus. Suction drains are placed before the completion of wound closure.

Postoperatively, it is necessary for the patient to remain in a flexed position. Prophylaxis against venous thrombosis and pulmonary embolism is maintained in the postoperative period. Over a 1- to 2-week interval, the skin stretches, and the patient is able to resume an erect posture. The resultant scar is located in the lower abdominal and suprapubic regions with a circular scar around the umbilicus (Fig. 113-9).

Liposuction

Suction-assisted lipectomy (liposuction) is a technique that permits removal of localized fat deposits from many parts of the body.[14] These include the trochanteric region, buttocks, flank, abdomen, breasts, face, thighs, knees, and ankles. The ideal patient is a young person with good skin tone who has localized fat deposits. Skin tone is important because the skin must contract and assume an improved contour once the underlying fat is removed.

The basic equipment required for liposuction includes a metal cannula with one or more holes in the tip. This cannula is connected by vacuum tubing to a suction device. The area to be treated is first infiltrated with a relatively large volume of a dilute anesthetic solution containing epinephrine.[15] A small incision is made in an adjacent area and the cannula introduced. Once the region

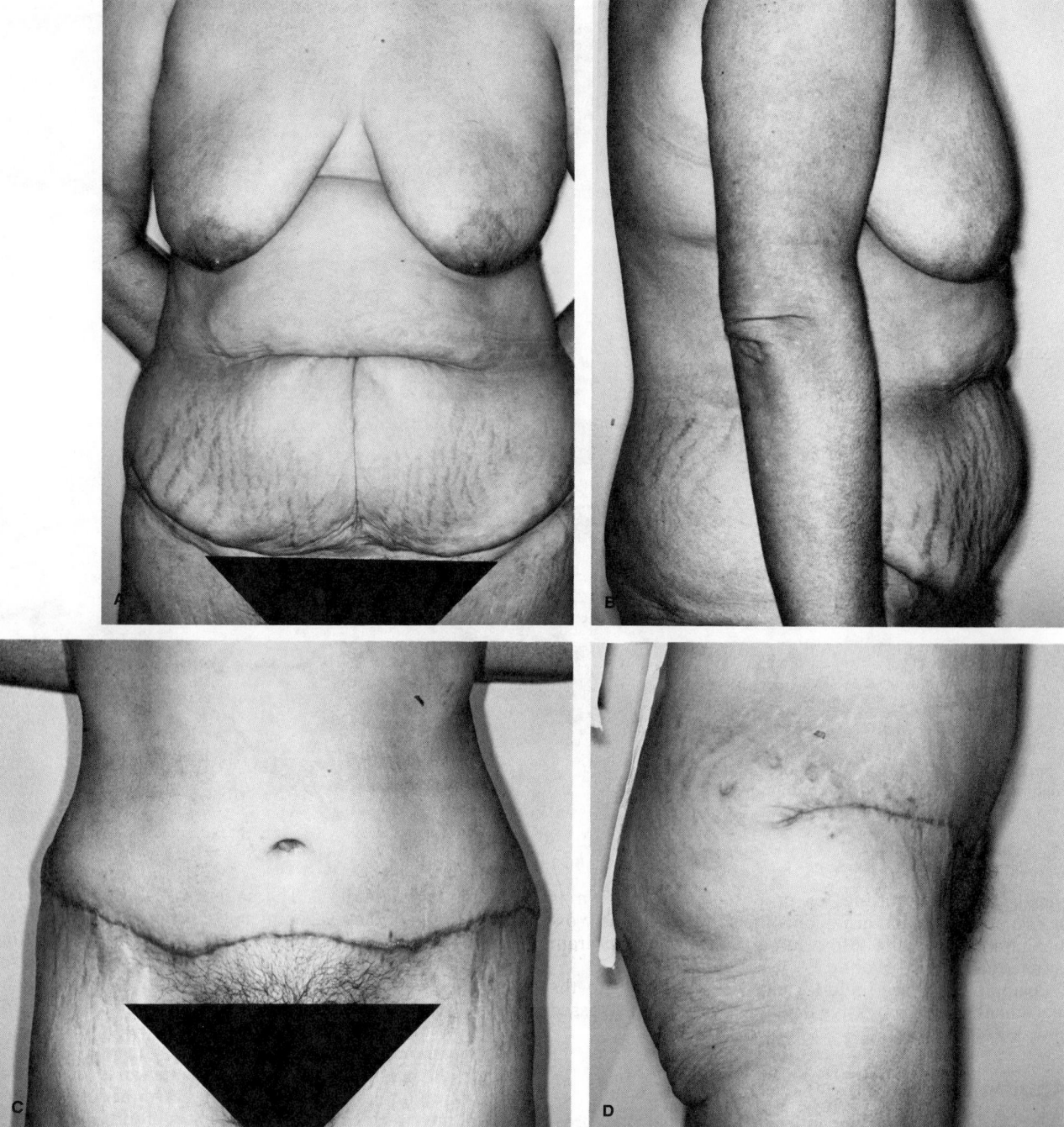

Figure 113-9. Abdominoplasty—preoperatively (*A* and *B*) and postoperatively (*C* and *D*).

to be reduced is entered with the cannula tip, suction is applied, and the cannula is passed back and forth vigorously. Individual particles of fatty tissue are drawn into the cannula, cut off by vigorous movement of the tip, and sucked through the vacuum tubing into the attached reservoir. Usually, 1500 to 1800 mL of tissue, fluid, and blood can be removed before blood transfusion is necessary.

After suction lipectomy is performed, a compressive dressing is applied. This is worn for 7 to 14 days in an attempt to reduce the likelihood of hematoma formation and to encourage uniform attachment of the skin to the underlying structures. Several weeks or months may be required to assess the final appearance (Fig. 113-10). Rippling and irregularities of the overlying skin can occur

if skin laxity was present preoperatively or if adequate shrinkage of the skin does not take place.

Tissue Expansion

Occasionally, the plastic surgeon is faced with the problem of inadequate local skin available to meet the patient's aesthetic or reconstructive needs. This skin deficiency can be seen in processes such as alopecia, localized scar formation, and the postmastectomy wound. Additional local skin can sometimes be obtained through the process of tissue expansion. A collapsed, expandable plastic shell is inserted adjacent to the area of skin deficit, usually through

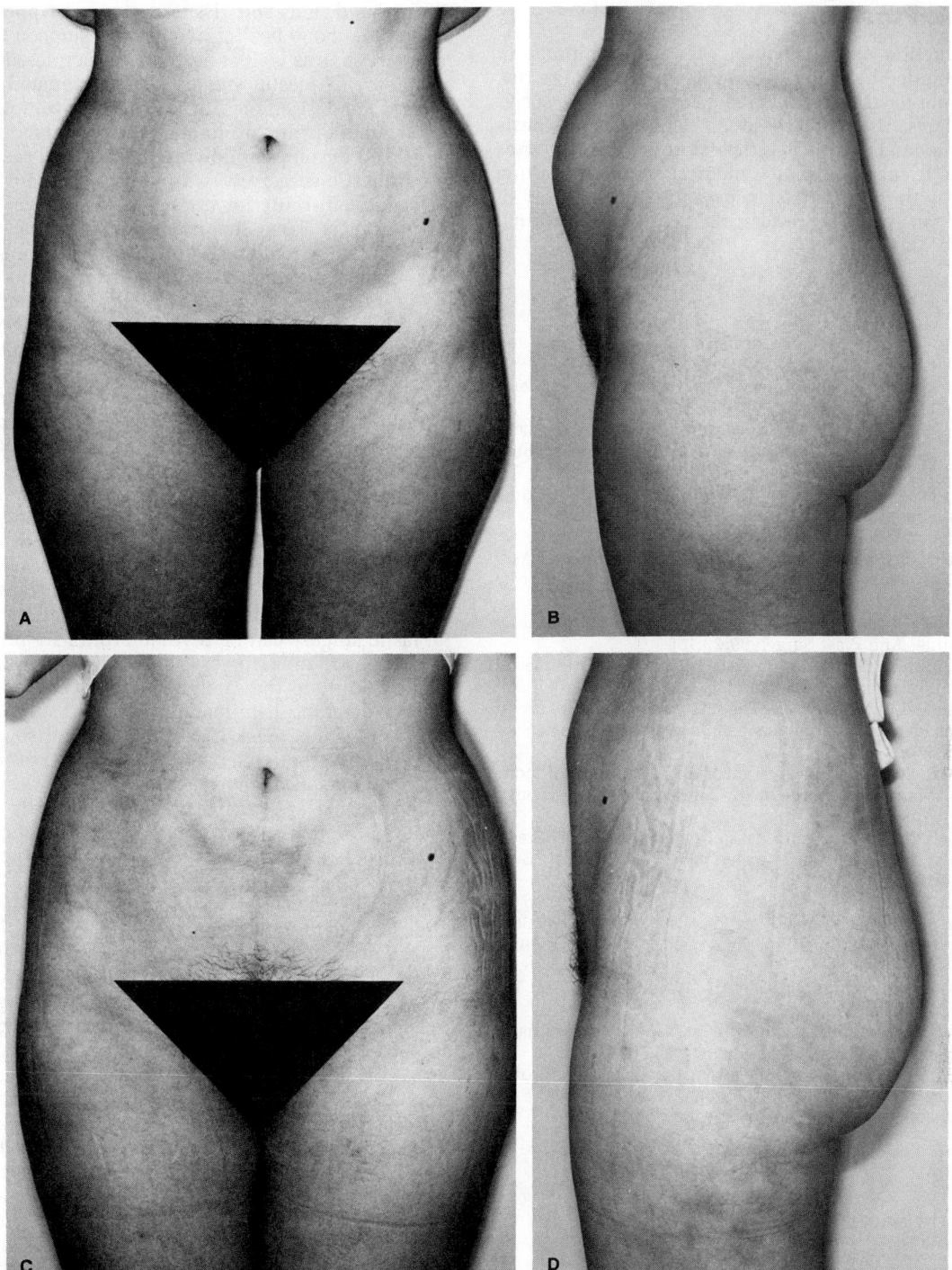

Figure 113-10. Lateral thigh and abdominal liposuction—preoperatively (*A* and *B*) and postoperatively (*C* and *D*).

an incision distant from the defect. After 1 to 3 weeks, saline is injected percutaneously into the implant through a self-sealing port. As the expander enlarges, the overlying skin begins to stretch. Recruitment of adjacent skin and production of skin cells in the involved area appear to contribute to the increase in total new surface area. The process is comparable to the abdominal skin enlargement that accompanies pregnancy. Once a sufficient amount of extra skin has been produced, the expander is removed and the new skin advanced into the required site.

Tissue expansion is not always free of complications

(see Table 113-1). During the process, rupture or leakage of the expander may require its removal and immediate replacement with an intact unit. When infection occurs, the expander is removed and a new one reinserted after the infection has cleared. Occasionally, the expander becomes exposed through wound dehiscence. This usually necessitates removal of the unit and delayed replacement. Tissue expander insertion distal to the elbow or knee is associated with a higher risk of complications, as is the use of this technique in the presence of an adjacent nonhealing or infected wound.

Aesthetic Prostheses

Reconstruction of a disfiguring wound or amputation can be precluded by patient age, systemic illness, the risk of local tumor recurrence, or inadequacy of available surgical techniques. Under these circumstances, a prosthesis can be fashioned that conceals the deformity or substitutes for missing tissue. The skilled medical sculptor working in concert with the plastic surgeon and using an array of polymers can provide restoration of a more normal appearance.

REFERENCES

1. Kligman LH. Photoaging: manifestations, prevention, and treatment. Dermatol Clin 1986;4:517.
2. Courtiss EH. Selection of alternatives in esthetic blepharoplasty. Clin Plast Surg 1981;8:739.
3. Zarem HA, Resnick JI. Expanded applications for transconjunctival lower lid blepharoplasty. Plast Reconstr Surg 1991;88:215.
4. Connell BF. Neck contour deformities. The art, engineering, anatomic diagnosis, architectural planning, and aesthetics of surgical correction. Clin Plast Surg 1987;14:683.
5. Vasconez LO, Core GB, Gamboa-Bobadilla M, Guzman G, Askren C, Yamamoto Y. Endoscopic techniques in coronal brow lifting. Plast Reconstr Surg 1994;94:788.
6. Sturzin JM, Baker TJ, Gordon HL. Chemical peel: a change in the routine. Ann Plast Surg 1989;23:166.
7. Wood-Smith D. Otoplasty. In: Rees TD, ed. Aesthetic plastic surgery. Philadelphia, WB Saunders, 1980:833.
8. McGrath MH, Burkhardt MD. The safety and efficacy of breast implants for augmentation mammaplasty. Plast Reconstr Surg 1984;74:550.
9. Cohen SB, Rohrich RJ. Evaluation of the patient with silicone gel breast implants and rheumatic complaints. Plast Reconstr Surg 1994;94:120.
10. Duffy MJ, Woods JE. Health risks of failed silicone gel breast implants: a 30-year clinical experience. Plast Reconstr Surg 1995;94:195.
11. Courtiss EH, Goldwyn RM. Reduction mammaplasty by the inferior pedicle technique. Plast Reconstr Surg 1977;59:500.
12. Guerrero-Santos J. Brachioplasty. Aesthet Plast Surg 1979; 3:1.
13. Regnault P. Abdominoplasty by the W technique. Plast Reconstr Surg 1975;55:265.
14. Courtiss EH. Suction lipectomy: a retrospective analysis of 100 patients. Plast Reconstr Surg 1984;73:780.
15. Klein JA. Tumescent technique for local anesthesia improves safety in large-volume liposuction. Plast Reconstr Surg 1993;92:1085.

SURGERY: SCIENTIFIC PRINCIPLES AND PRACTICE, Second Edition, edited by Lazar J. Greenfield, Michael W. Mulholland, Keith T. Oldham, Gerald B. Zelenock, and Keith D. Lillemoe. Lippincott–Raven Publishers, Philadelphia, © 1997.

CHAPTER 114

RECONSTRUCTIVE PLASTIC SURGERY

L. SCOTT LEVIN

Plastic surgery is the specialized branch of surgery that is concerned with repairing deformities and correcting functional deficits. Form as well as function is important in plastic surgery. Reanimation of the paralyzed face following tumor extirpation for trauma, restoration of the mu-

tilated hand, and soft tissue coverage of open fractures to facilitate bone healing require the surgeon to consider reconstructive as well as aesthetic principles. The modern principles of plastic surgery were originated by Harold Gillis. Foremost among these is the concept of replacing "like with like," the principle that allowed modern plastic surgery to develop. Following the first and second World Wars, plastic surgery was limited to the transfer of local tissues to substitute for traumatic or ablative defects following cancer. This often involved "marching" tubed random skin flaps from one part of the body to another. Little was understood about vascular territories and blood supply to different skin and muscle flaps. Anatomic research in the last three decades modernized flap surgery, resulting in a myriad of reconstructive options for complex wounds. Ideally, new tissues of adequate vascularity and dimension are transferred to areas of deficiency. One example is the use of the pectoralis major myocutaneous flap to substitute for tissue loss following radical neck dissection. This is local or regional tissue that is capped on its vascular pedicle (thoracoachromial vessels), which supply the muscle and overlying skin. If rearrangement of surrounding tissue or regional tissue is not possible, then free tissue transfer is used. With this approach, autologous tissue, including muscle, skin, bone, fascia, and others, is transplanted to substitute for tissue that has been removed.

Plastic surgery can be divided arbitrarily into aesthetic and reconstructive surgery; however, the two terms frequently apply to the same operation. For example, a patient undergoing hemimandibulectomy, oral floor resection, and radical neck dissection for oral squamous cell carcinoma has both the need for functional restoration (for mastication, speech, and feeding) and the desire for a restored normal appearance. Aesthetic surgery takes what is normal and tries to improve on appearance, whereas reconstructive surgery tries to recreate what is normal after injury, congenital deformity, or ablation.

One principle of plastic surgery is that delicate tissue handling leads to improved wound healing and diminished scar formation and distortion. Mastering atraumatic technique is therefore important. Respect and understanding of the blood supply to all tissues is paramount in plastic surgery. Tissue ischemia causes cell death, with necrosis resulting in fibrosis and possibly infection of the wound and compromised healing. Pathologic conditions of wound healing such as hypertrophic scars, or keloids, can result if soft tissue handling principles are violated. Wounds that are closed under excess tension widen and often thicken. A scar that thickens but does not go beyond the borders of the original scar is considered hypertrophic, whereas keloids are proliferative. Treatment for hypertrophic scarring requires excision of the scar and closure of the wound under circumstances different than the original closure. These scars are replaced under less tension with finer sutures to avoid recurrence of deformity. In contrast, resection and repair of the keloid scar is often complicated by recurrence and adjunctive modalities such as radiation may be needed to prevent recurrence[1].

The tools of the plastic surgeon are designed to prevent tissue injury. Fine, sharp skin hooks are traditionally used to hold flaps and retract tissue, rather than self-retaining retractors which can cause ischemia.[2] Microsurgical instruments for small vessel and nerve anastomosis and for neurorrhaphy have been developed in conjunction with very fine sutures, such as 10-0 or 11-0 suture for replantation and free tissue transfer. The dermatome is fundamental for skin grafting and is used frequently in the reconstructive plastic surgery of burns and other soft tissue defects. Recently, lasers have been developed for a variety of uses.

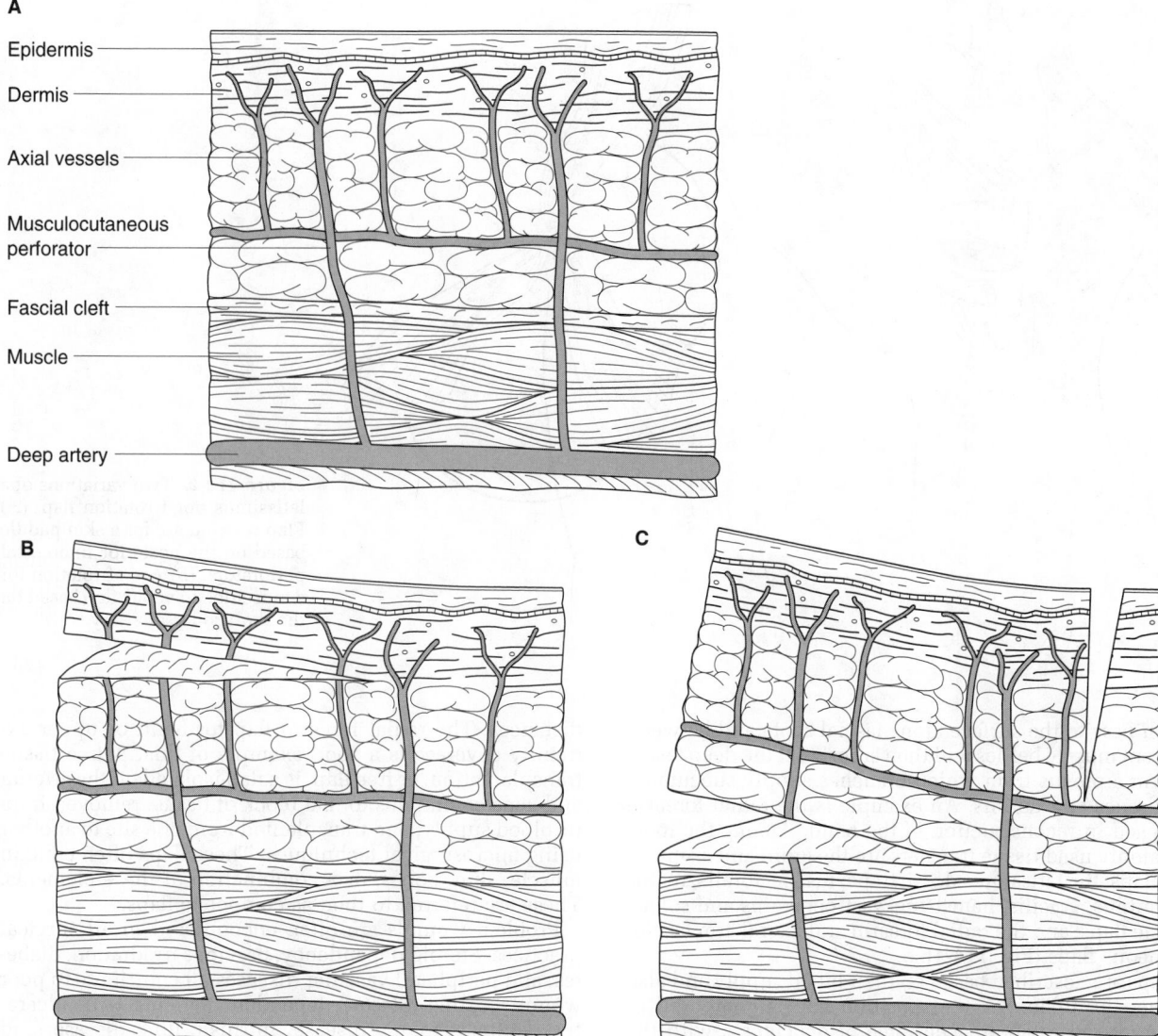

A
- Epidermis
- Dermis
- Axial vessels
- Musculocutaneous perforator
- Fascial cleft
- Muscle
- Deep artery

B

C

Figure 114-1. Flaps are classified by their vascular supply. (*A*) Normal blood supply to the skin. (*B*) Rotation or transposition flap. (*C*) Island flap with its blood supply.

PRINCIPLES OF THE FLAP

In the 1960s, the use of the deltopectoral flap was introduced for reconstruction about the head and neck.[3] This development emphasized the vascular basis of flap survival and established that axial pattern flaps could be used. This obviated the need for conventional random tube flaps that were created and advanced from one place to another in a series of operations to deliver tissue to areas of deficiency.

One example of this earlier technique involved the creation of a tube flap on the abdomen, attachment to the forearm, then division from the abdomen leaving the tube of skin attached to the forearm. The forearm graft was then attached to the face and ultimately detached from the forearm, banking or placing soft tissue in the area of necessity. These techniques are now considered obsolete.

In recent years, study of regional vascular anatomy has delineated vascular territories of the body called *angiosomes*.[4] These are territories of vascular supply based on perforating vessels from major arterial trunks. Angiosomes and venosomes of the body are consistent and provide the basis for flap design and execution. Definitive anatomic work has been done, elucidating the vascular supply to the skin.[5]

Flaps are classified according to the their vascular supply (Fig. 114-1). Skin territories can be fed either by direct cutaneous arteries, by septal perforators, or indirectly via arterioles from subadjacent muscles and skin.

An example of direct cutaneous blood supply is the deltopectoral flap, fed by the second, third, or fourth intercostal perforators from the internal mammary artery. A musculocutaneous flap has skin perforators from the underlying muscle which is supplied in turn by a named vascular pedicle. An example of this is the latissimus dorsi flap (Fig. 114-2). In this case, the skin is supplied by perforating vessels from the latissimus dorsi muscle, while the latissimus dorsi muscle itself is supplied by the thoracodorsal artery and vena commitans.

Muscle flaps are categorized in the following manner: type I flaps have a single major vascular pedicle; type II flaps have one major vascular pedicle and one minor pedicle; type III flaps have a dominant vascular pedicle and smaller segmental pedicle; type IV flaps have multiple pedicles; and type V flaps have one major and several small minor pedicles[6] (Fig. 114-3).

A fasciocutaneous flap has skin supplied by perforators

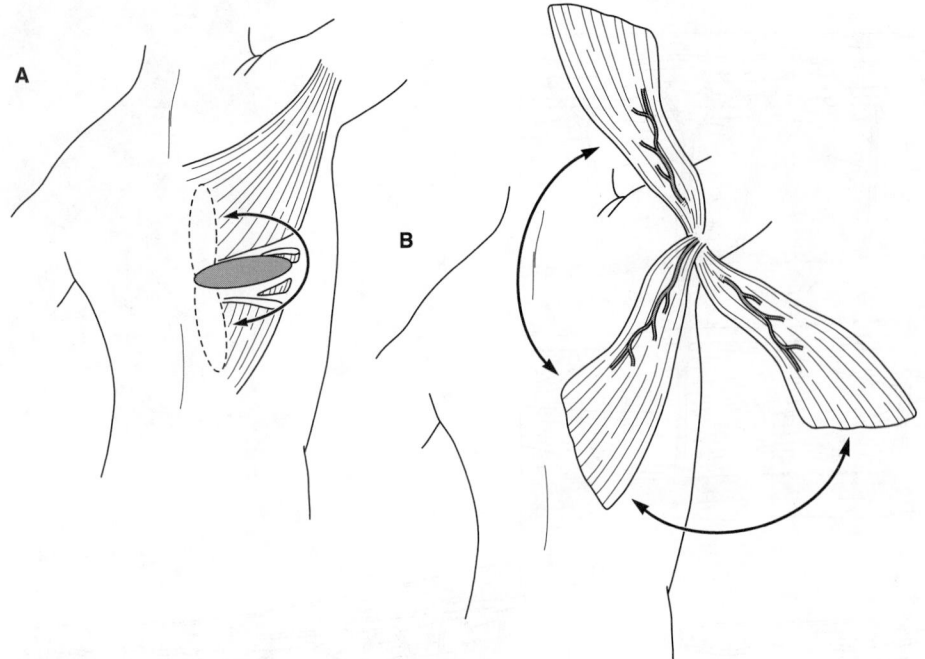

Figure 114-2. Two variations of a latissimus dorsi rotation flap. (*A*) Flap rotation arc for a skin paddle based on the posterior intercostal perforators. (*B*) Arc of rotation for a musculocutaneous flap based on the thoracodorsal artery.

which pass to the surface along fascial septa and between adjacent muscle bellies and then arborize at the deep fascia to form a plexus from which branches supply subcutaneous tissues and dermis. An example is the radial forearm flap used in reconstruction of the hand. Among the most commonly used tissue transfers are the groin and scapular skin flaps; the latissimus dorsi, trapezius, pectoralis, rectus abdominus, gracilis, hamstring, gastrocnemius and soleus muscle flaps; and the radial forearm and lateral arm fasciocutaneous flaps (Fig. 114-4).

Flaps are described based on their blood supply and also on their excursion. A transposition flap is composed of tissue moved to an adjacent area of deficiency, with the resulting defect then covered using either a skin graft or local rearrangement of adjacent tissues (Fig. 114-5).

An advancement flap is lifted on its blood supply and advanced into an adjacent defect. A notable example is the V/Y flap used for ischial pressure sores. Island pedicle flaps are created when a block of tissue is raised on an artery and vena commitans and transposed over longer

distances. The radial forearm flap for hand or upper extremity coverage is a good example of this. A free tissue transplantation, or free flap, is a flap isolated on the arterial and vena commitans to that block of tissue, removed from its blood supply, and transplanted from one site to another using microsurgical techniques. These flaps often contain muscle, skin, bones, or a combination of these elements. These are referred to then as composite flaps.

Problem wounds are often encountered in all surgical practices. Steroid dependency, previous irradiation, diabetes, and peripheral vascular diseases all contribute to poor wound healing. Steroid-dependent patients with ulcerative colitis, Crohn's disease, intrinsic lung disease, and rheumatoid arthritis are among these. These patients often have additional medical problems, and nutritional deficiencies may be among them.

Vitamin A has been shown to counteract the catabolic effects of steroids and to improve wound healing. It should be given routinely as a supplement in the perioperative period to patients on steroids. Oncology, transplant, and

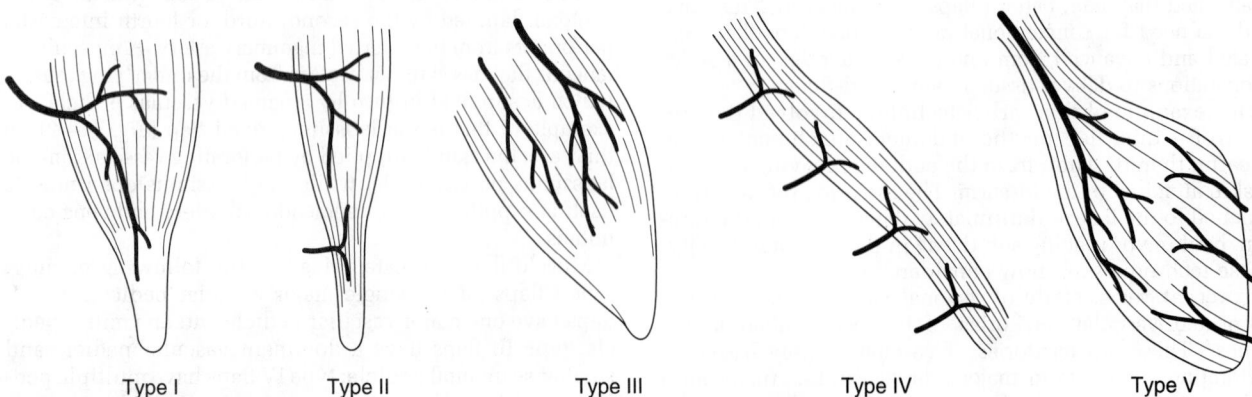

| Type I | Type II | Type III | Type IV | Type V |

Figure 114-3. Muscle vascular anatomy (flap types I to V). (After Mathes SA, Nahai F. Clinical application for muscle and musculo–cutaneous flaps. St Louis, CV Mosby, 1992:3)

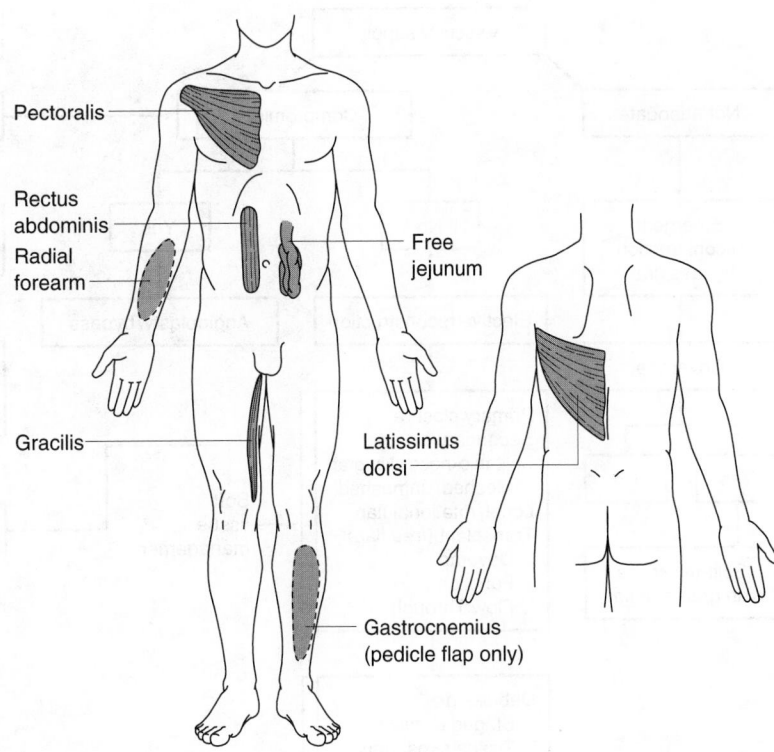

Figure 114-4. Locations of commonly used flaps.

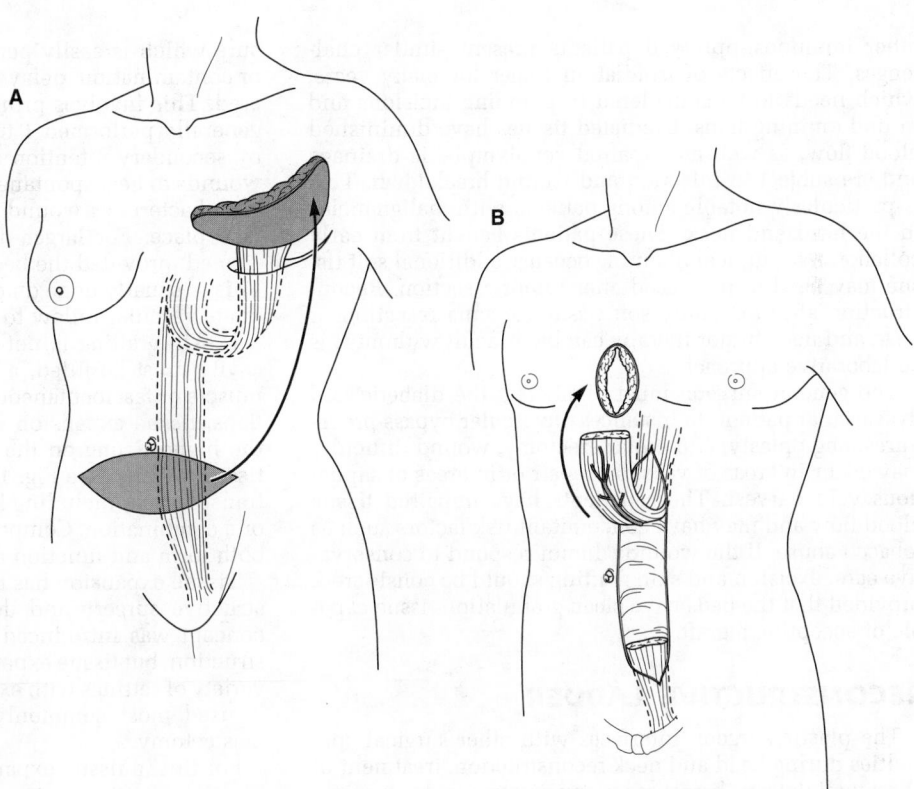

Figure 114-5. Examples of tissue transposition. (*A*) Rectus abdominis muscle flap with skin island. (*B*) Rectus abdominis muscle transposition used to close a local deficiency.

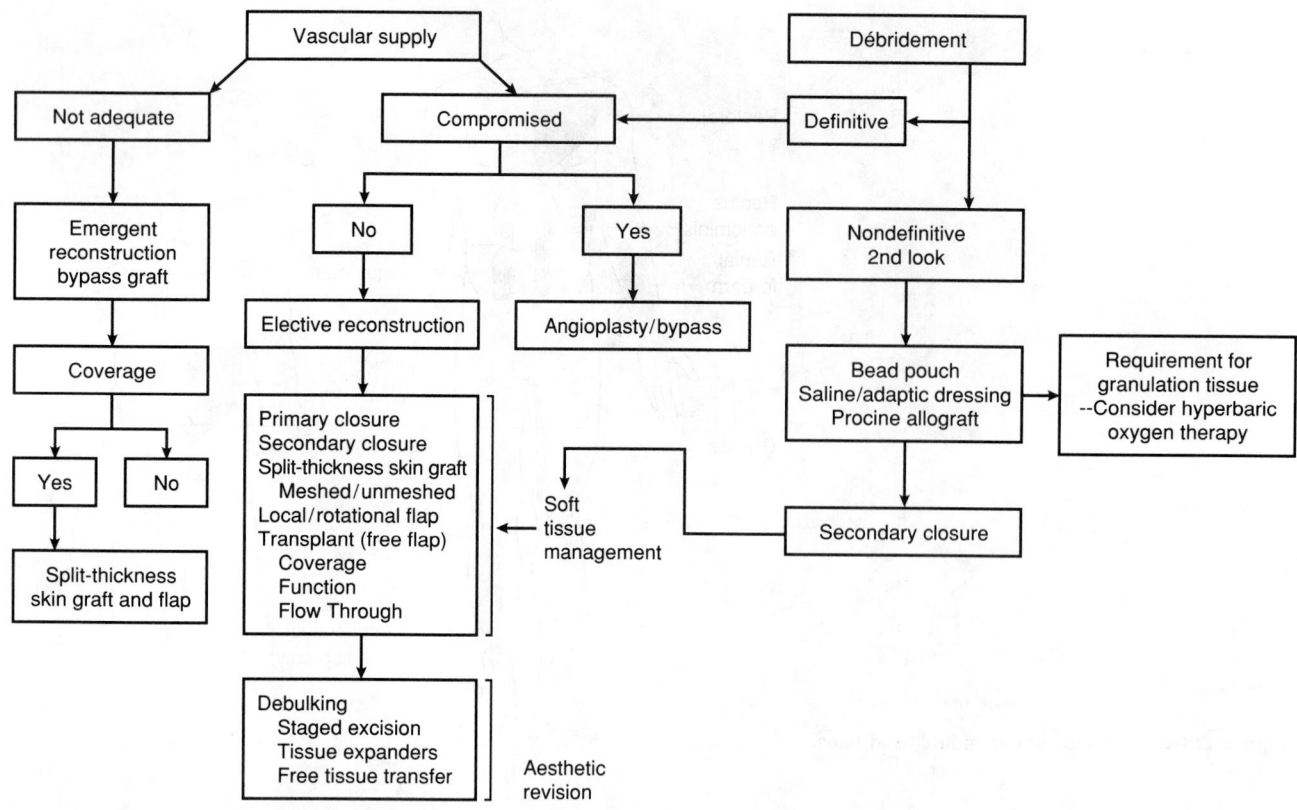

Figure 114-6. Reconstruction ladder for soft tissue defects. (After Levin LS. The reconstructive ladder: soft tissue principles for orthopaedic surgeons. Tech Orthop 1995;10:88)

other immunosuppressed patients present similar challenges. The effects of irradiation linger for many years, which needs to be considered in planning incisions and in undermining flaps. Irradiated tissues have diminished blood flow, as well as impaired venolymphatic drainage and are subject to infection and wound breakdown. This is particularly notable among patients with malignancies in the head and neck. These patients benefit from early collaborative surgical planning because additional soft tissue may need to be placed after tumor resection. Reconstruction after extremity soft tissue sarcoma resection or head and neck tumor therapy can be difficult without this collaborative approach.[7]

The general surgeon must often treat the diabetic and dysvascular patient. In instances of vascular bypass procedures, angioplasty, and endarterectomy, wound difficulty may occur in areas of vascular repair or in areas of saphenous vein harvest. These patients have impaired tissue blood flow and may have concomitant risk factors such as tobacco abuse. If the wounds do not respond to conservative care, excision and skin grafting should be considered, provided that the beds have clean granulation tissue capable of accepting a graft.

RECONSTRUCTIVE LADDER

The plastic surgeon interfaces with other surgical specialties during head and neck reconstruction, treatment of chest wall defects, breast reconstruction, vascular surgery, abdominal wall problems, and problems of the extremities. The reconstructive ladder is a classic algorithm for the plastic surgeon that summarizes the rational progression of wound closure techniques.(Fig. 114-6).

For most problems, wounds are closed by primary clo-

sure which is easily performed. In instances of infection or contamination, delayed primary closure may be considered. This involves primary wound approximation but is generally performed 1 to 5 days after wounding. Healing by secondary intention allows small open areas or small wounds to heal spontaneously. This approach avoids trapping bacteria as wound contraction and epithelialization take place. For larger defects, skin grafting can be performed, provided the bed is appropriate to receive a graft. This is usually done on clean granulation tissue with adequate vascular inflow to inosculate the graft.

If skin grafting is not satisfactory, or in cases where a cavity must be filled, a local rotation procedure using a muscle or fasciocutaneous flap is used. In addition to local flaps, tissue expansion is an option in this situation. At the highest rung on the reconstructive ladder is the free tissue transfer (see Fig. 114-6). Virtually any tissue can be transplanted, including bowel, muscle, skin, bone, fascia, or a combination. Composite flaps can provide and restore both form and function as has been described.

Tissue expansion has taken a prominent place in reconstructive surgery and deserves specific discussion. The concept was introduced in the late 1950s for ear reconstruction, but tissue expanders are currently used in a wide variety of settings with excellent results.[8] Tissue expansion is used most commonly for breast reconstruction after mastectomy.[9]

For this, a tissue expander is placed in the subpectoral position after mastectomy and the skin is closed. Because the skin envelope contracts, the tissue expander is inflated over time to maintain an appropriate configuration and is subsequently removed for placement of a permanent implant of gel silicone or saline mammary prosthesis. In general, expanders are placed in a subcutaneous pocket of

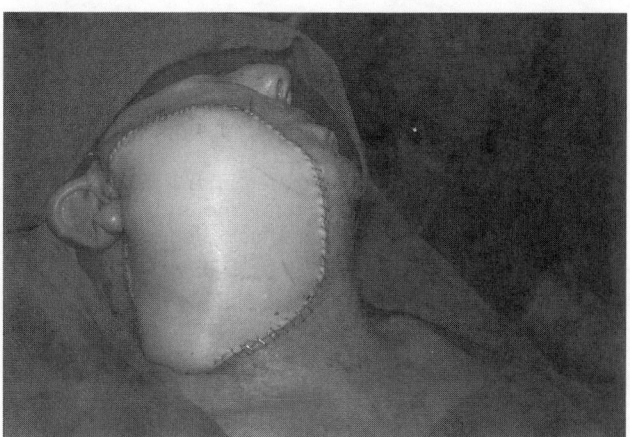

Figure 114-7. This patient underwent radical neck resection for head and neck cancer. The defect was covered with a free scapular flap.

are useful to fabricate free tissue transplants such as an expanded latissimus dorsi or scapular flap for recontouring an extremity or for reconstructing the head and neck.

HEAD AND NECK

Squamous cell carcinoma and basal cell carcinoma are often localized skin tumors on the lip, ear, and face. Definitive treatment requires complete excision, and regional lymph node dissection should be considered based on preoperative work-up and staging. Several other head and neck cancers require complex extirpative procedures which involve closure of larger defects.

Reconstruction after head and neck cancer incorporates many of the techniques noted previously. The pectoralis major myocutaneous flap is commonly used for covering radical neck dissection defects. Reconstruction after resections of oral tumors is now done in some cases with free tissue transplantation[10] (Fig. 114-7). Flaps such as the osteocutaneous fibular transplant, radial forearm flap, or scapular flap have been used effectively in head and neck and oral reconstruction as well. In certain reconstructions, particularly dental cases, osseointegrated implants are placed in revascularized bone graft, and dentures can be mounted to allow mastication and to improve function.

Microsurgical reconstruction using free flaps has become standard in certain oral cancers. The radial forearm flap is often routine in intraoral resection involving retromolar trigone, tongue, and anterior floor of the mouth where the mandible is spared. This flap has a particularly long pedicle, is pliable, can be innervated, and contours well to the inside of the mouth. More recently, free tissue transfer of

an extremity—either head, neck, or trunk. Through a portal either in the expander itself or through a remote portal, saline is sequentially injected, expanding the device and stretching the adjacent tissues including the overlying skin. A capsule forms around the expander, augmenting the vascularity of the expanded tissue. In addition, there is epidermal thickening and actual cellular recruitment during the process of tissue expansion. Once expansion is completed, the expander is removed and the stretched tissue is placed in an adjacent area of need. Tissue expanders

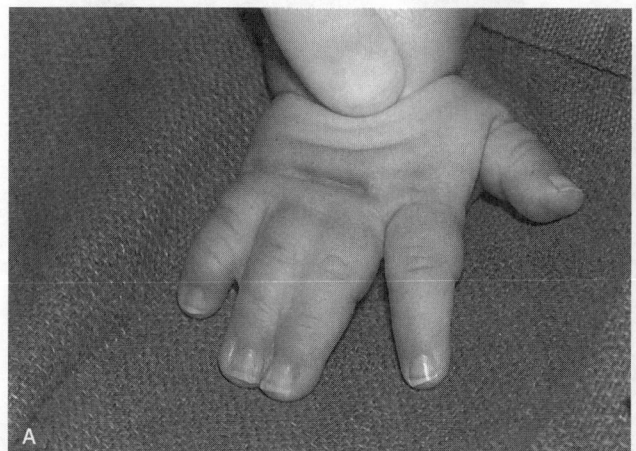

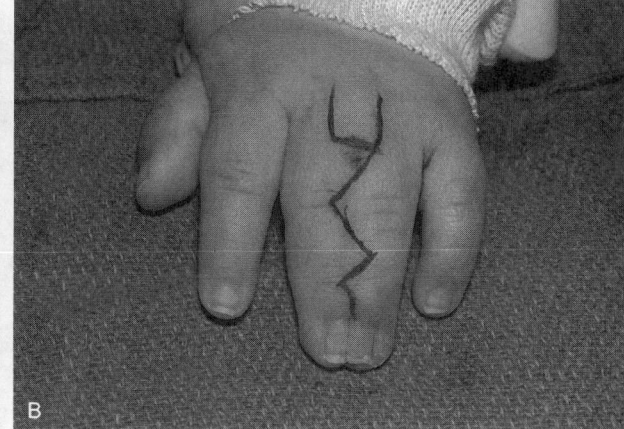

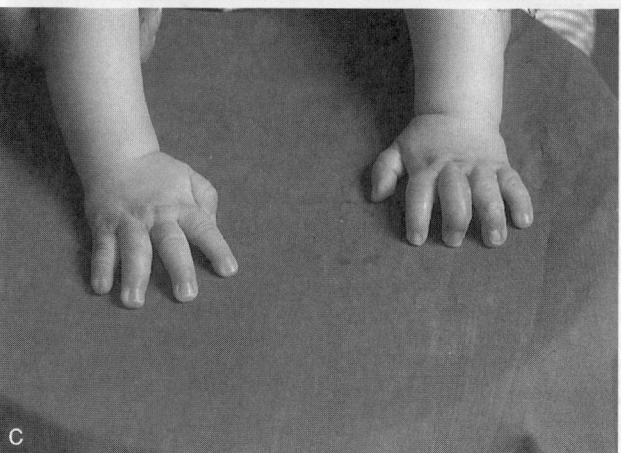

Figure 114-8. Simple syndactyly with surgical release and skin grafting.

the colon has been combined here to provide secretory capability of the intraoral lining, however this is more controversial.[11]

Similarly, the radial forearm flap and other skin flaps such as lateral arm flap or scapular flap can be used for large head and neck defects. If intraoral as well as extraoral resurfacing are required, the radial forearm flap can be divided into two separate skin paddles. A variety of skin flaps can be taken with bone but the scapular flap and the radial forearm flap are most commonly used for tongue, jaw, and neck reconstruction. The osteoseptocutaneous fibular flap is useful to recreate the bony contour of the mandible and is also useful to provide skin coverage for intraoral and extraoral defects.[12] Head and neck reconstruction commonly requires that all vascularized tissue be imported from outside the region. The pectoralis major flap, the trapezius flap, and the latissimus dorsi island pedicle flap are useful for lower neck reconstructions.

In all head and neck cancer patients, negative surgical margins should be obtained before reconstruction. This is usually done with either frozen sections, or a wound can be packed or dressed for 24 to 48 hours until the final pathology becomes available. In certain instances, tissues

such as the free jejunum or a tubed radial forearm flap can provide a conduit from the oropharynx to the esophagus. The recipient vessels for head and neck reconstruction are the external carotid, facial, and thyroid arteries. These should be preserved whenever possible during the extirpative surgery. Venous outflow is achieved with anastomosis to the anterior jugular, external jugular, internal jugular, or facial veins. Planned tracheostomy should be considered, particularly in instances of major mandibular and intraoral reconstructions because of the massive swelling that occurs during these procedures.

CONGENITAL DEFORMITIES

Craniofacial and other congenital defects such as cleft lip and palate are in the domain of plastic surgery, although these anomalies are best treated with a multidisciplinary approach that integrates otolaryngology, audiology, orthodontics, speech pathology, and others. In these children, failure of fusion of mesodermal segments during gestation results in a facial cleft that involves the palate, the lip, or both. Cleft lip and palate repair is done with one of a variety of techniques popularized by Millard (rotational advancement

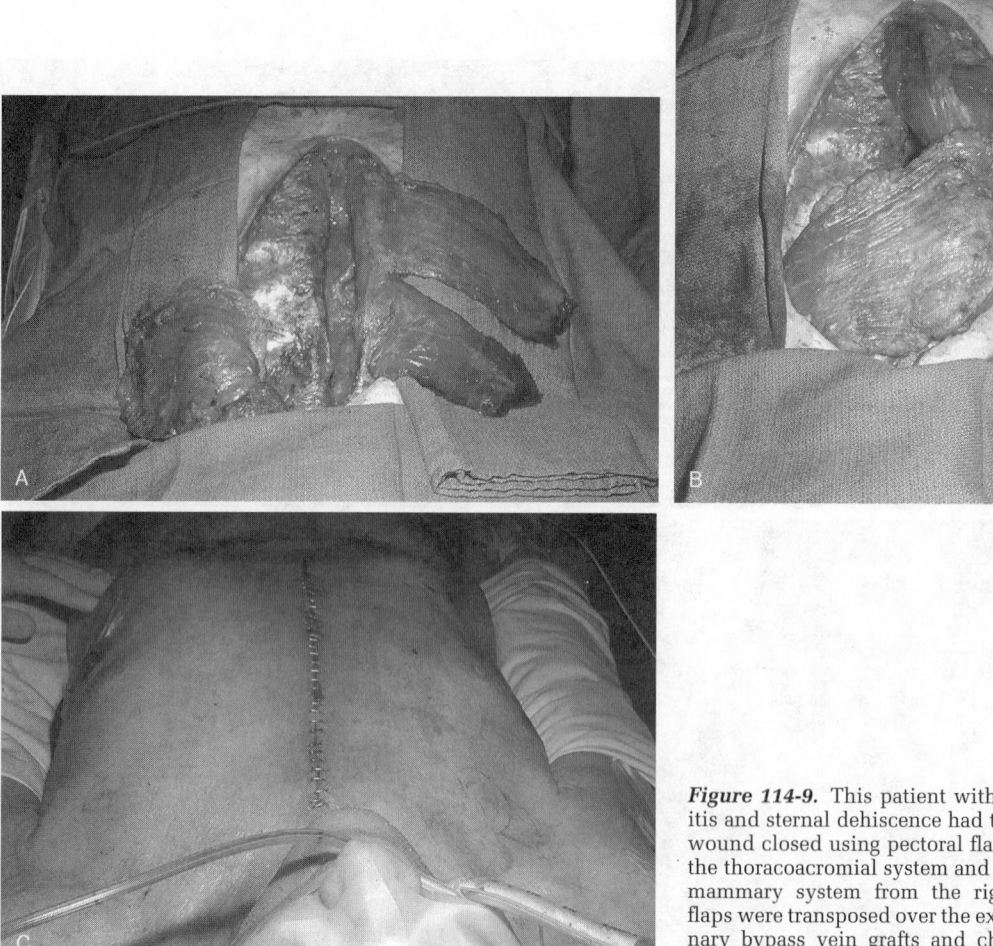

Figure 114-9. This patient with mediastinitis and sternal dehiscence had the complex wound closed using pectoral flaps based on the thoracoacromial system and the internal mammary system from the right. Muscle flaps were transposed over the exposed coronary bypass vein grafts and chest closure was successful.

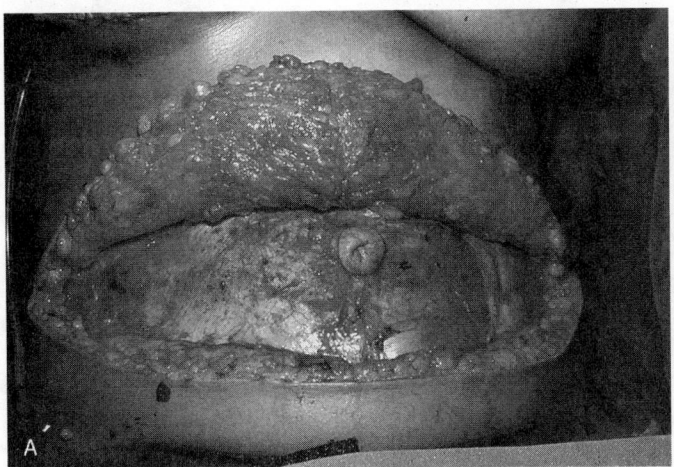 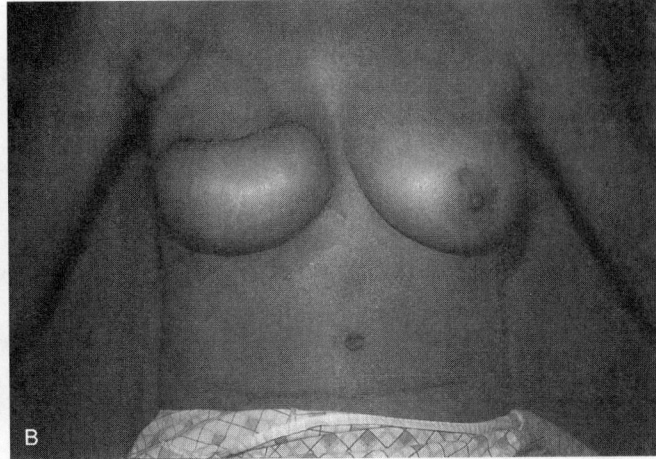

Figure 114-10. Transverse abdominal flap used for right breast reconstruction after mastectomy.

flap for lateral and bilateral lip defects).[13] Generally, lip repair is followed by palate repair, later correction of velopharyngeal incompetence, alveolar bone grafting for dental arch formation, and in adolescence, cleft lip/nasal reconstruction (rhinoplasty). Craniofacial deformities, such as those associated with Crouzon and Apert syndromes, are best treated by multidisciplinary craniofacial teams, but this is beyond the scope of this review.

Common congenital anomalies of the hand include syndactyly, polydactyly, and radial clubhand. Syndactyly can be either simple or complex (Fig. 114-8). Complex syndactyly involves the sharing of bony elements of the hand skeleton in addition to soft tissue. Simple anomalies involve only the soft tissues. Syndactyly release is performed before the first year of age if possible. The trend is to perform releases earlier to take advantage of the aspects of infant wound healing which allow wounds to heal with less scar.[14]

TRUNK AND CHEST RECONSTRUCTION

Reconstructing the trunk and chest wall may be necessary for a variety of needs after tumor resection, trauma, chronic postoperative dehiscence, or other problems. In the chest wall, flaps such as the latissimus dorsi or pectoralis major flaps are used to provide coverage in the anterior and posterior thoracic region (Fig. 114-9). The transverse rectus abdominus muscle (TRAM) flap based on the superior epigastric artery, a branch of the internal mammary artery, provides skin and subcutaneous tissue as well as muscle for postmastectomy reconstruction if expanders and saline-filled implants are not desirable[15] (Fig. 114-10). This can provide excellent results. Recently, experience with free tissue transfer in the postmastectomy patient has been excellent as well. Free transfer of the TRAM superior gluteal or lateral thigh flap can be used to provide tissue for breast reconstruction when a pedicle TRAM flap cannot be performed. The free TRAM flap is based on the deep inferior epigastric artery and usually anastomosed to the axillary artery or a branch of the thoracodorsal artery. Breast reconstruction is completed with cosmetic tatooing or surgical creation of a nipple areolar complex. Contralateral breast augmentation or reduction may be required, depending on the nature of the breast cancer and the patient's desires.

In cases in which an abdominal wall defect must be closed, the thoracoepigastric flap (an island pedicle flap based on the deep inferior epigastric artery) is quite useful (Fig. 114-11). This is particularly effective for perineal or vaginal reconstruction and is versatile for covering groin and proximal thigh wounds. For these latter defects, the rectus abdominus muscle can also be "turned down" on the inferior epigastric artery with or without skin to close groin defects. Free tissue transfers are useful for these defects as well.

PERINEAL AND GENITAL RECONSTRUCTION

The subject of genital reconstruction involves complex and individualized procedures that are largely beyond the scope of this discussion. One notable advance in genitouri-

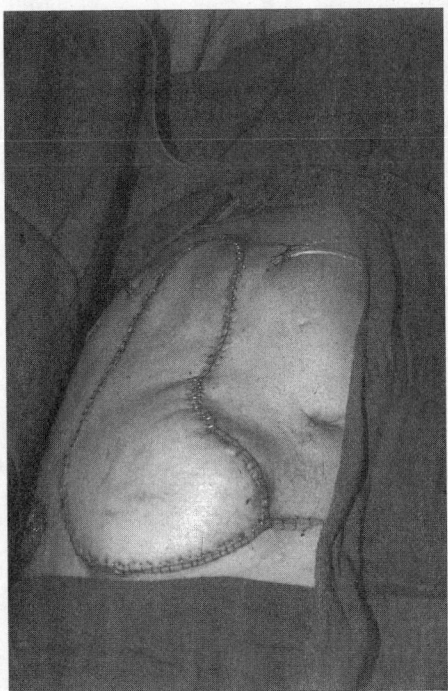

Figure 114-11. This patient had a perforated duodenal ulcer with necrotizing fasciitis of the abdominal wall, resulting in a complex defect. The patient was treated with a tensor fascia lata muscle free flap to reconstruct the abdominal wall.

Table 114-1. RECONSTRUCTION OPTIONS FOR THE LOWER EXTREMITY

FEMUR AND GROIN

Split-thickness skin graft
Tensor fascia lata
    Superior half
    Gluteus maximus
    Thoracoepigastric flap
Free flap

LEG

Tibia
    Proximal one third—gastrocnemius muscle
    Middle one third—soleus
    Distal one third—free flap

FOOT

Split-thickness skin graft
Full-thickness skin graft
Abductor hallucis muscle
Flexor hallucis brevis muscle
Plantar fascia flap
Free flap (muscle and skin—innervated?)

(Levin LS. The reconstructive ladder: soft tissue principles for orthopaedic surgeons. Tech Orthop 1995;10:88)

nary reconstruction is the development of the radial forearm flap for phallus reconstruction. This flap can be innervated and also can be used to create a urethra in instances of penile ablation due to cancer or trauma.

After tumor resection, the perineum can be reconstructed with thoracoepigastric or gracilis flaps.

DYSVASCULAR AND DIABETIC EXTREMITIES

Patients with diabetic or dysvascular feet or limbs are often best treated with arterial reconstructive procedures to revascularize complex or refractory wounds.[16] These wounds can then be closed with skin grafting. Even in these difficult situations, current techniques, especially fasciocutaneous flaps, have allowed limb salvage when amputation has previously been necessary (Table 114-1). Vascular inflow procedures and free flaps are done either sequentially or simultaneously depending on individual circumstances; however, the inflow procedure must always be done first because the flap is dependent on this blood supply. This collaboration between plastic and vascular surgeons is an important requirement for contemporary treatment of these patients.

EXTREMITY SARCOMAS

Resection of soft tissue sarcomas has often resulted in complex wounds in irradiated tissues for which primary closure attempts fail. For these patients, it is important to

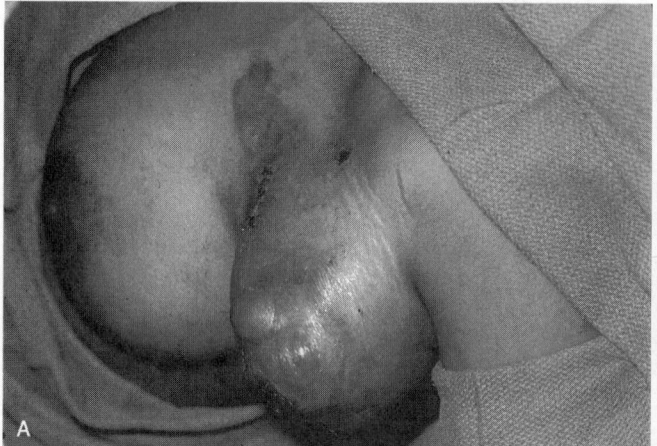
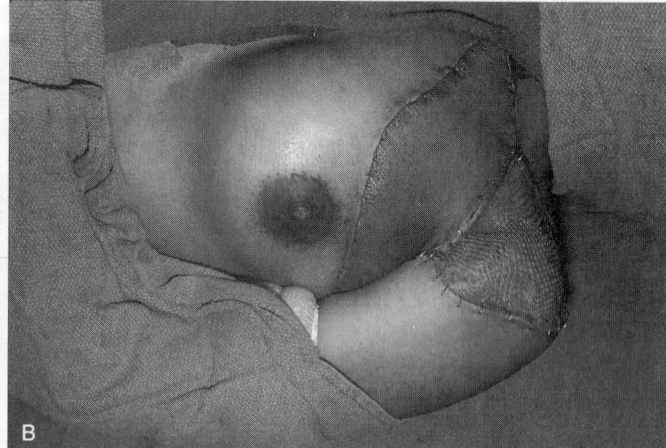
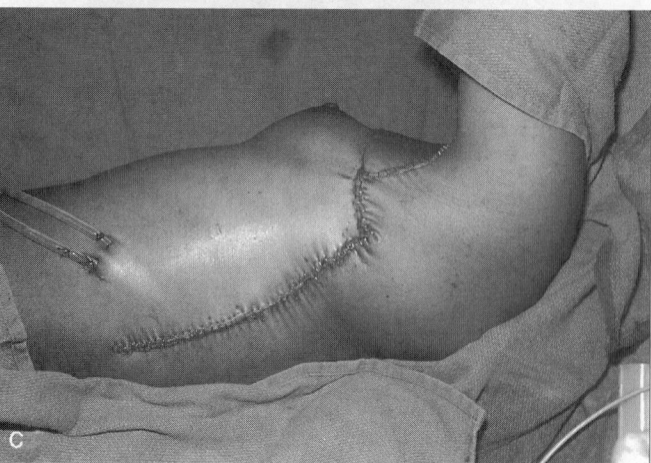

Figure 114-12. This adolescent had a malignant dermatofibrosarcoma involving the left axilla and breast. After resection, an island latissimus dorsi flap with a split-thickness skin graft was used for coverage.

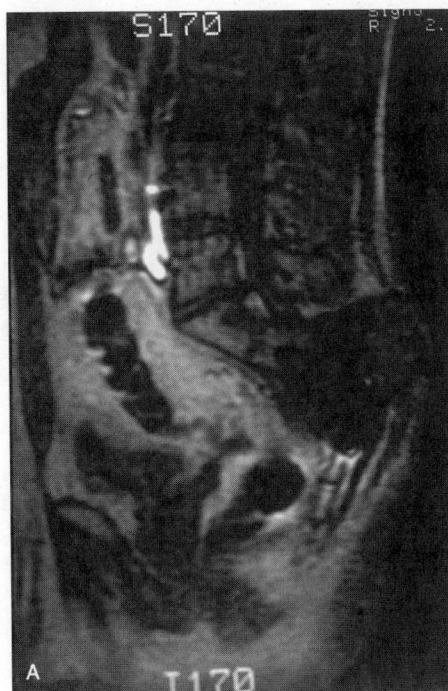
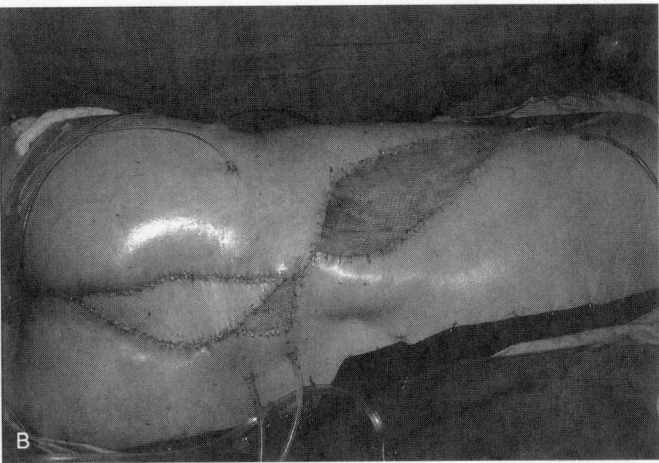

Figure 114-13. (*A*) MR image of a large angiosarcoma of the pelvis and sacrum. (*B*) Resection was followed by myocutaneous latissimus dorsi flap reconstruction. The flap was anastomosed to the thoracocostal artery and vein, using 36-cm vein grafts for both artery and vein.

consider using a well-vascularized tissue transfer at the time of tumor extirpation (Figs. 114-12 and 114-13). This approach may result in fewer wound complications, diminished morbidity, and a higher limb salvage rate.

VENOLYMPHATIC INSUFFICIENCY

Contemporary techniques in the field of reconstructive microsurgery have been used for patients with lymphedema of both upper and lower extremities.[17] Although the experience is limited and less than perfect, microscopic or venolymphatic bypass offers help where none was previously available.

O'Brien[17] reported the results of more than 100 patients with chronic lymphedema treated with microlymphaticovenous anastomosis. Objective assessment was done by limb volume and circumferential measurements. Lymphangiography was obtained initially, but this was discontinued because it resulted in injury and sclerosis of the lymphatic drainage system. Nearly 75% of the patients showed some clinical improvement with microlymphaticovenous anastomosis. Demonstrable limb volume reduction occurred in only 42%, however. Some patients were able to discontinue standard measures such as support stockings, and the incidence of cellulitis was reduced as well. It also appeared that good results correlate with earlier operations in contrast with patients operated late in their disease.

Reconstructive microsurgical techniques can also be applied for the patient with venous stasis ulcers. Resection of these chronic ulcers with coverage using well-vascularized flaps has been shown to be superior to conventional nonoperative therapy in certain patients.

REFERENCES

1. Rockwell WB, Cohen IK, Ehrlick HP. Keloids and hypertrophic scars: a comprehensive review. Plast Reconstr Surg 1989;84:827.
2. LeVan TA, Levin LS. Principles of soft tissue handling. Tech Orthop 1995;10:94.
3. Bakamjian VY. A two stage method for pharyngoesophageal reconstruction with primary pectoral skin flap. Br J Plast Surg 1970; 23:133.
4. Taylor GI, Minabe T. The angiosomes of the mammals and other vertebrates. Plast Reconstr Surg 1992;89:181.
5. Gilbert A, Macquelet AC, Heatz V. Pedicle flap of the upper limb. Boston, Little, Brown, 1992.
6. Mathes SH, Nahai F. Clinical application for muscle and musculo-cutaneous flaps. St Louis, CV Mosby, 1992:3.
7. Barwick WJ, Goldberg JA, Scully SP, Harrelson JM. Vascularized tissue transfer for closure of irradiated wounds after soft tissue sarcoma resection. Ann Surg 1992;216:591.
8. Argenta LC, Marks MW. Tissue expansion. In: Georgiade GS, Georgiade NG, Barwick WJ, et al, eds. Textbook of plastic, maxillofacial and reconstructive surgery, ed 2. Baltimore, Williams & Wilkins, 1992:103.
9. Georgiade GS, Georgiade NG. Breast reconstruction after mastectomy. In: Georgiade GS, Georgiade NG, Barwick WJ, et al, eds. Textbook of plastic, maxillofacial and reconstructive surgery, ed 2. Baltimore, Williams & Wilkins, 1992:843.
10. Shestak KC, Myers EN, Ramasastry SS, Jones NF, Johnson JT. Vascularized free tissue transfer in head and neck surgery. Am J Otolaryngol 1993;14:148.
11. Jones TR, Lee G, Emami B, Strasberg S. Free colon transfer for resurfacing large oral cavity defects. Plast Reconstr Surg 1995;96:1092.
12. Hidalgo DA. Fibula free flap: a new method of mandible reconstruction. Plast Reconstr Surg 1989:79.
13. Bauer BS, Vicari FA. Cleft palate. In: Georgiade GS, Georgiade NG, Barwick WJ, et al, eds. Textbook of plastic, maxilloficial and reconstructive surgery, ed 2. Baltimore, Williams & Wilkins 1992:299.
14. Dobysn JH, Wood WE, Bayne LG. Congenital hand deformities. In: Green DP, ed. Operative hand surgery, vol 1. New York, Churchill Livingstone 1988:255.
15. Hartrampf CR, Anton MA, Bried JT. Breast reconstruction with the transverse abdominal island (TRAM) flap. In: Georgiade GS, Georgiade NG, Barwick WJ, et al, eds. Textbook of plastic, maxillofacial and reconstructive surgery, ed 2. Baltimore, Williams & Wilkins 1992:851.
16. Oishi SN, Levin LS, Pederson WC. Microsurgical management of extremity wounds in diabetics with peripheral vascular disease. J Plast Reconstr Surg 1993;92:485.
17. O'Brien BM. Long term results after microlymphaticovenous anastomoses for the treatment of obstructive lymphadema. Plast Reconstr Surg 1990;85:562.

INDEX

Note: Page numbers followed by *f* indicate figures; those followed by *t* indicate tabular material; CF indicates color figures.

A

Abbreviated Injury Scale (AIS), 276–277, 277t
Abdomen. *See also specific organs and disorders*
  abdominoplasty and, 2272t, 2277, 2278f
  acute. *See* Acute abdomen
  anatomic divisions of, 331, 332f, 333
  in secondary survey of trauma patients, 284–285
  viscera of, vascular occlusive disease of. *See* Visceral occlusive disease
Abdominal aortic aneurysms (AAAs), 1840–1846, 1881–1891. *See also* Thoracoabdominal aortic aneurysms (TAAAs)
  arterial structure and, 1841f, 1842, 1842f
  biochemistry of, 1842–1844
    plasmin and, 1844
    protease inhibitors and, 1844
    proteases and, 1843–1844
    proteins and, 1842–1843
  cardiac risk and, assessment of, 1887–1888
  classification of, 1881–1882, 1882f
  clinical manifestations of, 1883
  diagnostic methods for, 1883–1885
    aortography, 1885, 1886f, 1886t
    imaging modalities, 1883–1885, 1884f, 1885f
  experimental, 1844
  genetics of, 1845–1846, 1846f
  iliac artery aneurysms associated with, 1891
  incidence of, 1840
  inflammation and, 1844–1845
  infrarenal, 1882, 1882f
  interventional approaches for, 1846
  juxtarenal, 1882, 1882f
  late survival and, 1887
  mycotic, 1890–1891
  pararenal, 1882, 1882f
  pathogenesis of, 1882–1883
  repair of, 1888–1890
    complications of, 1889–1890
    indications for, 1888
    operative technique for, 1888–1889
    surgical treatment risks of, 1887
  rupture of, 1883
    late survival and, 1887
    risk of, 1885–1886
  suprarenal, 1882, 1882f

Abdominal exploration, in gastric injuries, 341
Abdominal injuries, 331–353, 399–400. *See also specific injuries*
  anatomy and, 331, 332f, 333
  blunt, 333, 333t
  diagnosis of, 333–337
    abdominal paracentesis and diagnostic peritoneal lavage in, 335t, 335–336, 336f
    history in, 334
    laboratory studies in, 334
    physical examination in, 334
    radiographic examination in, 334–335
  in elderly people, 389
  indications for surgery and, 336–337
  operative approach for, 337
  pancreatitis and, 880–881
  pediatric, 382–384, 383f, 383t, 384f
  penetrating, 333, 333t
  prehospital care for, 333
  renal artery aneurysms caused by, 1906, 1907–1908
  vascular, 368–370, 370f–372f
Abdominal pain, 1246–1248, 1247f, 1248t. *See also* Acute abdomen
  in Crohn's disease, 834–835
    treatment of, 838
  in pancreatic cancer, palliative treatment for, 915
  pediatric, differential diagnosis of, 1250, 1250t
  referred, 1246, 1248
  somatic, 1246, 1247–1248
  visceral, 1246, 1247–1248
Abdominal paracentesis, in abdominal injuries, 335
Abdominal wall, 1235–1237
  anterior, anatomy of, 1207, 1208f, 1209, 1209f
  defects of, pediatric, 2028–2034
  neoplastic disease of, 1236–1237
  posterolateral (lumbar), anatomy of, 1209–1210, 1210f
  rectus sheath hematomas of, 1236
Abdominal wall defects, pediatric. *See also specific defects*
  hydroceles, 2034
Abdominoperineal resection
  for anal cancer, 1149
  for colorectal cancer, 1138, 1140f
Abdominoplasty, 2272t, 2277, 2278f
Abiomed BVS 5000 ventricular assist device, 1556, 1557f

Abiomed/THI total artificial heart, 1561f, 1561–1563
ABO compatibility, for hepatic transplantation, 596
Abruptio placentae, traumatic injuries and, 393
Abscesses
  amebic
    hepatic, 959, 960f
      pediatric, 2082
    neurologic, 2191
  anorectal, 1196–1197
    clinical manifestations of, 1197
    management of, 1197
    pathogenesis of, 1196–1197, 1198f
  of Bartholin gland, 2218
  of brain, 2190t, 2190–2191
  of breast, 1377
  in Crohn's disease, 837
    surgical treatment of, 841–842
  epidural, 2189–2190
  hepatic. *See* Hepatic abscesses
  of lung, 1478–1479
    pathogenesis of, 1478
    presentation of, 1478, 1479f
    treatment of, 1478–1479
  pancreatic, 887–888
  parapharyngeal, 636–637
  peritonsillar, 636
  retroperitoneal, 1242
  subgaleal, 2189
  tuboovarian, 2224–2225
Absorption. *See also* Malabsorption
  in colon, 1089, 1089f
  in gallbladder, 1031f, 1031t, 1031–1032, 1032f
    altered, gallstone formation and, 1039
  malabsorption and, in chronic pancreatitis, 891
    treatment of, 898t, 898–899
  in small intestine. *See* Small intestine, digestion and absorption in
Absorptive powders and pastes, 81t
Abuse, of children, 385
  sexual, introital problems related to, 2117
Access, to trauma care, 278
Accidental Death and Disability: The Neglected Disease of Modern Society, 268
Acetylsalicylic acid, See Aspirin (acetylsalicylic acid; ASA)

Acid(s)
  administration of, decreased body
      bicarbonate content due to, 261
  ingestion of, esophageal injury due to,
      712–718
    clinical features of, 713–714
    immediate diagnosis and treatment
        of, 714–715
    management of, 715–718, 718f, 718t
  organic, increased production of,
      decreased body bicarbonate
      content due to, 261
Acid-base balance, 259–266
  anion gap and, 260
  buffer systems and, 260
  definitions and, 259–260
  disturbances of, 260–266, 261t
    metabolic, 261–265. *See also specific
        disturbances*
    mixed, 266, 266f
    respiratory, 265–266. *See also
        specific disturbances*
Acidosis
  lactic, decreased body bicarbonate
      content due to, 261, 262
  metabolic. *See* Metabolic acidosis
  organic, decreased body bicarbonate
      content due to, 261–262
  pediatric, 1989
  respiratory, 261t, 265–266
    clinical features of, 265
    compensatory mechanisms in, 265
    treatment of, 265–266
  in sepsis, 56
Acid reflux test, 668
Acinar cell carcinomas
  pancreatic, 917
  of salivary glands, 641
Acinus, 863, 866f
Acoustic nerve
  neuromas of, 2175
  schwannomas of, 2175–2176
Acquired immunodeficiency syndrome
    (AIDS), 178f, 178–179. *See also*
    Human immunodeficiency virus
    (HIV) infections
  anorectal diseases in, 1204–1205
  appendicitis in, 1259
  hepatic infections associated with,
      970–971
  pericarditis in, 1576
  transmission of, by blood transfusions,
      105
  treatment of, 179
Acral lentiginous melanomas, 2233, CF
    111–1
Acromegaly
  diagnosis of, 1352, 1353f
  treatment of, 1356
Acrosome reaction, 2202
ACTHomas, 927
Actin filaments, 6–7, 7f
Actinic keratosis, of hands, 2162
Actinomycin D, 502t
  for Wilms tumor, 2125
Activated partial thromboplastin time
    (aPTT), 104
Activated protein C (APC), resistance to,
    1615
Active transport, 15–16, 16f
Acute abdomen, 1246–1251
  gynecologic causes of, 1249, 1249t
  pain and, 1246–1249, 1247f, 1248t

acute, 1248–1249
  in specific conditions, 1250t, 1250–
      1251, 1251t
  urologic causes of, 1249–1250
Acute lung injury (ALI), in shock, 190
Acute-phase proteins, 115, 116, 116t
  synthesis of, cytokine-induced, 51
Acute-phase response, 132
  mediators of, 132, 133t, 134f
  serum proteins altered during, 132,
      132t
Acute renal failure (ARF), in critically ill
    patients, 234–239, 235t
  acute tubular necrosis and, 234–235
  management of, 236–239
    general care in, 236f, 236–237
    nutrition and, 237
    renal replacement therapy in, 237–
        239, 238t
  nephrotoxic agents and, 235–236
  pigment nephropathy and, 235
  prognosis of, 239
Acute tubular necrosis (ATN)
  in critically ill patients, 234–235
  myoglobin-induced, gross pigmenturia
      and, 430, CF 12–10
  in shock, 191
Acyclovir, for herpes simplex proctitis,
    1204
Acylated plasminogen-streptokinase
    (APSAC), 99, 100, 100f, 100t
Addisonian crisis, treatment of, 204–205
Addressins, vascular, 152
Adeno-associated viruses (AAVs), as gene
    therapy vector, 521
Adenocarcinoids, of appendix, 1260
Adenocarcinomas
  of anal canal, 1148
  of appendix, 1260
  of biliary tract, pediatric, with
      choledochal cysts, 2091–2092
  colorectal. *See* Colorectal cancer
  esophageal, 700, 701f
  of gallbladder, 1058
  gastric. *See* Gastric cancer,
      adenocarcinomas
  pancreatic. *See* Pancreatic
      adenocarcinomas
  of salivary glands, 641–642
  small intestinal. *See* Small intestinal
      disorders, neoplastic disease
Adenoid cystic carcinomas
  bronchial, 1433, 1433f
  esophageal, 701
  of salivary glands, 641
Adenomas
  of bile ducts, 1013, 1056
  bronchial. *See* Bronchial adenomas
  colorectal. *See* Colorectal cancer,
      adenomas
  fibroadenomas, of breast, 1374–1375,
      1375f
    giant, 1375–1376
  of gallbladder, 1056
  hepatic
    hepatocellular, 1011–1012, 1012f
    pediatric, 2080
  hyperaldosteronism due to, treatment
      of, 1345
  of nipples, 1378
  papillary. *See* Papillomas
  pituitary. *See* Pituitary adenomas
  small intestinal, 846

Adenomatous endometrial hyperplasia,
    2223
Adenomatous polyp(s), colorectal. *See*
    Colorectal polyps
Adenomatous polyposis coli (APC),
    familial, 1110
Adenomatous polyposis coli (APC) gene
  in colorectal cancer, 1130
  in familial adenomatous polyposis,
      1120–1121, 1123, 1123f
Adenomyomas, of gallbladder, 1056
Adenosine deaminase (ADA) deficiency,
    gene therapy for, 512–513
Adenosis, sclerosing, 1376, 1376f
Adenoviruses
  recombinant, for respiratory disorders,
      513, 514f
  tumor induction by, 464
Adherens junctions, 9–10
Adhesion(s), postoperative, intestinal
    obstruction and, 824f, 824–825
Adhesion molecules
  endothelial, 116–118
    leukocytes and, 117f, 117–118, 151f,
        152
    wound repair and, 118, 118f
  in shock, 195
Adhesion receptors, antigen recognition
    and, 537–538, 538t
Adnexal carcinomas, microcystic, 2243
Adnexectomy, for tuboovarian abscesses,
    2225
Adolescents. *See also* Pediatric patients
  breast cancer in, 1383, 1383f
Adoptive cellular therapy, 504
Adoptive immunotherapy, 2241
Adrenal arteries, 1331
Adrenal disorders
  functioning tumors. *See also specific
      tumors*
    outcomes with, 1346
  nonfunctioning tumors, treatment of,
      1346
  pheochromocytomas, 1469
Adrenalectomy, 1344–1345
Adrenal glands, 1331–1346. *See also
    specific disorders*
  anatomy of, 1331, 1332f, 1333f
  cortex, 1331, 1333f
    hormone secretion by, 1331–1333,
        1334f, 1335f
  disorders of. *See also specific disorders*
    burns and, 435t
    functional assessment of, 1339–1342
      of catecholamine levels, 1341–1342
      in hyperaldosteronism, 1341, 1342t
      in hypercortisolism, 1339–1340
    localization studies of, 1342–1343
      invasive, 1343
      nonscintigraphic, 1342–1343, 1343f,
          1344f
      scintigraphic, 1343
  medulla, 1331
    hormone secretion by, 1333–1334,
        1336f
    steroidogenic enzymatic defects and,
        1334–1339
Adrenal hyperplasia, congenital, 1337,
    1337f, 1341, 2112, 2112f–2114f
Adrenal insufficiency, hypoadrenal shock
    and, 183, 204–205
  neurogenic, physiologic characteristics
      of, 197t

Adrenergic receptors, of arterioles, 186
Adrenocorticotropic hormone (ACTH)
    ectopic production of, determining
        cause of, 1340, 1340f
    in hypercortisolism, 1352
    intravenous, for ulcerative colitis, 1098
    secretion of, 1331, 1332
    in shock, 187–188
Adrenogenital syndrome, 2112, 2112f–
        2114f
Adult respiratory distress syndrome
        (ARDS), in shock, 190
Advanced trauma life support (ATLS)
    protocols for, 279
        training in, 280
    shock classification of, 286–287, 287t
Advancement flaps, 2282
Adventitia, vascular, 1585
Adventitial cystic disease, 1601–1602,
        1602f
    of popliteal artery, 1640, 1641f
Aesthetic surgery, 2269–2280. See also
        Reconstructive surgery
    abdominoplasty, 2272t, 2277, 2278f
    biology of aging skin and, 2269
    blepharoplasty, 2269, 2270f, 2272t
    brachioplasty, 2272t, 2276–2277, 2277f
    chemical peel, 2271–2272, 2272f,
        2272t
    liposuction, 2272t, 2277–2279, 2279f
    mammaplasty
        augmentation, 2272t, 2274–2275,
            2275f
        reduction, 2272t, 2276, 2276f
    mastopexy, 2276
    otoplasty, 2272t, 2274, 2274f
    prostheses for, 2280
    rhinoplasty, 2272–2274, 2273f
    rhytidectomy, 2269–2271, 2271f, 2272t
    tissue expansion, 2272t, 2278–2279,
        2284–2285
Aflatoxin B1, hepatocellular carcinoma
        associated with, 1016
Aganglionosis, congenital. See
        Hirschsprung disease
Age. See also Aging; specific age groups
    cholelithiasis and, 1034, 1035t
    hospital mortality rates related to, 445,
        445t
    of organ donors, 559, 560f
    surgical stress response and, 49–50
Agent Orange, soft tissue sarcomas and,
        2247
Aging. See also Elderly patients; Geriatric
        trauma
    atherosclerosis and, 1536
    of collagenous tissues, 2142
    of skin, biology of, 2269
    wound healing and, 79
Agkistrodon. See Bites and stings
AIDS-related complex, treatment of, 179
Air bag injuries, 271–272
Airway
    anastomotic healing of, following
        pulmonary transplantation, 613
    edema of, inhalation injury and, 433
    obstruction of, in pediatric patients,
        1994–1995
        acquired, 1995
        congenital, 1994–1995
    resistance of, pulmonary, 1984
    traumatic injuries and
        of neck, 309–310

    pediatric, 379–380, 380t
    prehospital assessment of, 280
    reassessment during resuscitation
        phase, 282
    upper
        hemorrhage of, 637
        obstruction of, 637
Alanine, loss following injury, 54
Albendazole, for hydatid disease of liver,
        960
Albumin
    during acute-phase reaction, 132, 132t
    for fluid loss, pediatric, 1989
    for shock, 288
Albumin microspheres, technetium-
        labeled, in arteriovenous fistulas,
        1921
Alcohol consumption
    liver disease due to
        cirrhosis, 974, 975, 975t
            natural history of, 976f, 976–977
        hepatic transplantation for, 583
    pancreatitis due to
        acute, 880
        chronic, 889
Aldosterone, 1331, 1337–1338
    excess of
        primary hyperaldosteronism and,
            1338, 1338f, 1338t
        screening for, 1341, 1342t
        treatment of, 1345
    normal effects of, 1337–1338
    renovascular hypertension and, 1782
    secretion of, control of, 1332–1333,
        1335f
    surgical stress response and, 53
    volume control mediation by, 247
Alfentanil, 441t
Alkali, ingestion of, esophageal injury
        due to, 712–718
    clinical features of, 713–714
    immediate diagnosis and treatment of,
        714–715
    management of, 715–718, 718f, 718t
Alkaline reflux gastritis, following
        gastrectomy, 772f, 773
Alkalosis
    metabolic. See Metabolic alkalosis
    respiratory
        clinical features of, 265
        compensatory mechanisms in, 265
        treatment of, 265
Alkylating agents, 501t
Allelic exclusion, 528
Alloimmune hemolytic anemia, 1987
Alloreactivity, 533, 533f
Alveolar collapse, in respiratory failure,
        221–222
Alveolar soft parts sarcomas, pediatric,
        2134
Alveolus(i), of breast, 1360
Amaurosis fugax, 1751
Amebic abscesses
    hepatic, 959, 960f
        pediatric, 2082–2083
    neurologic, 2191
American College of Surgeons
    Advanced Trauma Life Support course
        of, 268
    Committee on trauma of, 268
American Society of Anesthesiologists
        (ASA)

    physical status classification of, 446,
        446t
    postanesthesia care standards of, 449t,
        451
Amine precursor uptake and
        decarboxylation (APUD) cells,
        807, 918
Amino acids
    hepatic transport and storage of, 952–
        953, 953f
    metabolism of, 43, 45f–47f, 46t, 46–47
    mobilization of, cytokine-induced, 51
    signal sequences (peptides), 26
Aminoacyl tRNA synthetase, 24
9-Aminocamptothecin, 502t
Aminoglutethimide, 502t
Aminoglycosides, spectrum of activity of,
        169t
Ammonia
    amino acid metabolism and, 46
    hepatic encephalopathy and, 982
    metabolism of, in small intestine, 816–
        817
Amnesics, 442, 442t
Amnioceles. See Omphaloceles
Amniotic fluid embolism, traumatic
        injuries and, 394
Amoxicillin
    for duodenal ulcers, 765
    for gonococcal proctitis, 1203
    prophylactic, for endocarditis, 1532t
Amphotericin B
    for fungal infections, 176–177
    for monilial esophagitis, 724
Ampicillin
    for gonococcal proctitis, 1203
    prophylactic, for endocarditis, 1532t
    spectrum of activity of, 169t
Amputations
    of hands, traumatic, 2162
        indications for replantation and,
            2162
        initial management of, 2162
    lower extremity. See Lower
        extremities, amputation of
    neurosurgical pain management and,
        2196
    radical
        for osteosarcomas, 2264
        for sarcomas, 2253, 2255, 2256f
Amrinone
    for congestive heart failure, 1517
    for shock, 205–206
Amsacrine, 502t
Amylase
    pancreatic secretion of, 866
    in pancreatitis, 883–884
Amylin, 870
Amylopectin, 815
Amylose, 815
Anal canal, 1146
    anatomy of, 1180–1181, 1181f, 1182f
    cancer of. See Anal cancer
    nerve supply of, 1186
Anal cancer, 1146–1151
    of anal canal, 1148–1150
        adenocarcinomas, 1148
        epidermoid carcinomas, 1148–1150
            basaloid (cloacogenic) carcinomas,
                1149, 1150f
            mucoepidermoid carcinomas, 1149
            squamous cell carcinomas, 1149
            treatment of, 1149–1150

Anal cancer (*continued*)
of anal margin, 1147–1148
basal cell carcinomas, 1147
Bowen disease, 1147, 1148f
Paget disease, 1147–1148, 1149f
squamous cell carcinomas, 1147, 1147f
in HIV-positive patients, 1204–1205
malignant melanoma, 1150–1151
transitional (cloacogenic) zone and, 1146
Anal fissures, 1192–1196
clinical manifestations of, 1193
definition of, 1192
diagnosis of, 1193–1194
management of, 1194–1195, 1196f, 1197f
pathophysiology of, 1192–1193
secondary, 1195–1196
Anal fistulas. *See* Fistula-in-ano
Analgesics. *See* Pain management; *specific drugs*
Anal margin, 1146
cancer of. *See* Anal cancer
Anal sphincter, external, 2041
Anaphylatoxins, 133
Anaphylaxis
antivenins and, 405
Hymenoptera stings and, 407–408
Anaplastic thyroid carcinomas, 1301, 1306
Anastomotic failure, following pancreatic transplantation, 624
Anatomic dead space, 1984
Ancrod, 99
Androgens, 1336–1337
excess of, 1337, 1337f
testing for, 1341
normal effects of, 1336–1337
testosterone
for impotence, 2201
low level of, male infertility and, 2203
for male infertility, 2203
Anemias, 1266t, 1266–1269
acquired, 1268–1269
aplastic, 1268–1269
autoimmune hemolytic, 1268
congenital, 1266–1268
erythrocyte metabolism abnormalities and, 1267–1268
erythrocyte structure abnormalities and, 1266–1267
hemoglobinopathies and, 1268
in critically ill patients, management of, 237
Anesthesia, 438–453
amnesics and anxiolytics for, 442, 442t
delayed emergence from, 452t, 452–453
for facial fracture repair, 406
for hepatic transplantation, 584
for hernia repair, 1221
inhalation agents for, 439, 439t
intravenous, 441t, 441–442
local anesthetics for, 442t, 442–443
for maxillofacial repairs, 304
muscle relaxants for, 439–441, 440t
patient monitoring and, 448–451
of circulation, 450–451
of oxygenation, 448
of ventilation, 448–450
postanesthesia care standards and, 449t, 451

postoperative problems and, 449t, 450f, 450t, 451f, 451–453, 452t
in pregnancy, 393–394
preoperative evaluation for, 445–446, 446t, 447t, 448
risks associated with, 443–445
Aneurysm(s), 1840–1932
angiography in, 1693f–1695f, 1694–1695
aortic. *See* Abdominal aortic aneurysms (AAAs); Thoracic aortic aneurysms; Thoracoabdominal aortic aneurysms (TAAAs)
arterial hemodynamics and, 1665, 1667, 1667f
atherosclerotic, 1840
axillosubclavian, 1854–1857
anatomy and, 1849, 1850f
clinical manifestations of, 1855–1856
definition and etiology of, 1849
diagnosis of, 1856
etiology of, 1854–1855
incidence of, 1849, 1854
pathophysiology of, 1849
therapeutic objectives for, 1849
treatment options for, 1856f, 1856–1857
treatment results with, 1857
unresolved problems and future trends and, 1857f, 1858
of carotid artery, 1748–1749
extracranial, 1849–1852
anatomy and, 1849, 1850f
clinical manifestations of, 1851, 1852t
definition and etiology of, 1849
diagnosis of, 1851
etiology of, 1851
incidence of, 1849, 1851, 1851t
indications for intervention and, 1851–1852
pathophysiology of, 1849
therapeutic objectives for, 1849
treatment options for, 1852, 1853f–1855f
treatment results with, 1852
unresolved problems and future trends and, 1857f, 1858
of celiac artery, 1893t, 1898, 1898f
of colic artery, 1893t, 1899f, 1899–1900
diagnostic techniques for, 1677
of femoral artery, 1909–1913
arteriosclerotic, 1909–1911
clinical manifestations of, 1910
diagnosis of, 1910, 1910f
incidence of, 1909
natural history of of, 1910
treatment of, 1910–1911
mycotic, 1912–1913
clinical manifestations of, 1913
diagnosis of, 1913, 1913f
pathogenesis of, 1912–1913
treatment of, 1913
pathogenesis of, 1909
of gastric artery, 1893t, 1898f, 1898–1899
of gastroduodenal artery, 1893t, 1899f, 1900, 1900f
of gastroepiploic artery, 1893t, 1898f, 1898–1899

of hepatic artery, 1893t, 1895–1897, 1896f, 1897f
of ileal artery, 1893t, 1899f, 1899–1900
of iliac artery, with abdominal aortic aneurysms, 1891
of innominate artery, 1857–1858
anatomy and, 1849, 1850f
clinical manifestations of, 1857
definition and etiology of, 1849
diagnosis of, 1858
etiology of, 1857
incidence of, 1849, 1857
pathophysiology of, 1849
therapeutic objectives for, 1849
treatment options for, 1858
treatment results with, 1858
unresolved problems and future trends and, 1857f, 1858
intracranial, 2181f–2183f, 2181–2183
rupture of, 2182, 2183, 2183f
treatment of, 2182–2183
of jejunal artery, 1893t, 1899f, 1899–1900
mycotic, 1721
of abdominal aorta, 1890–1891
of femoral artery, 1912–1913
of thoracic aorta, 1873
of pancreatic artery, 1893t, 1899f, 1900, 1900f
of pancreaticoduodenal artery, 1893t, 1899f, 1900, 1900f
parasellar, 1355
peripheral arterial embolism and, 1622
of popliteal artery
clinical manifestations of, 1914
diagnosis of, 1914, 1914f
incidence of, 1909, 1913
natural history of, 1914
pathogenesis of, 1909
treatment of, 1914–1915
pseudoaneurysms. *See* Pseudoaneurysms
of renal artery, 1901–1908
dissecting, 1902t, 1906–1908, 1907f, 1908f
kidney preservation and, 1908
pseudoaneurysms caused by, 1906–1907, 1908f
traumatic, 1906, 1907–1908
true, 1901–1906, 1902f–1907f, 1902t
aneurysmectomy for, 1906, 1907f
nephrectomy for, 1906
rupture of, 1903–1905
of splanchnic artery, 1893t, 1893–1895, 1894f–1896f
of superior mesenteric artery, 1887–1898, 1893t, 1897f
syphilitic, 1840
ventricular, peripheral arterial embolism and, 1622
Aneurysmectomy, for renal artery aneurysms, 1906, 1907f
Aneurysm-infiltrating lymphocytes (AIL cells), 1844
Aneurysm-infiltrating macrophages (AIM cells), 1844
Aneurysmorrhaphy, for extracranial carotid aneurysms, 1852
Angiitis, hypersensitivity, 1604–1605, 1605f
Angina, visceral, 1775–1776, 1776f–1779f
Angina pectoris

in coronary artery disease, 1538, 1538f
postinfarction, as surgical indication, 1541
Prinzmetal (variant), 1538
unstable, 1538
Angiodysplasia
of right colon, 1153
of stomach and intestine, 1170
Angiogenesis
cytokines and, 120–121, 122f
in metastasis, 485–486
Angiography
diagnostic, 1678–1709
of aorta
abdominal, 1683–1684, 1684f
thoracic, 1683
in cerebrovascular disease, 1752
in chest injuries, 318
complications of, 1680, 1683
computed tomography, helical, 1679, 1680f
in congenital cystic disease of lung, 2008, 2008f
contraindications to, 1683
contrast media for, 1680, 1682f
digital, 1678–1679
future of, 1683
indications and findings on, 1688–1706
aneurysms, 1693f–1695f, 1694–1695
arterial dissections, 1695f, 1695–1697, 1696f
arterial fibrodysplasia, 1696f, 1697f, 1697–1699
arteritis, 1699
hemangiomas and vascular malformations, 1699f, 1700, 1700f
macroembolism, 1690, 1691f, 1692f
neoplasms, 1700f, 1700–1702
nonaneurysmal atherosclerosis, 1690–1694, 1692f, 1693f
peripheral venous disease, 1701f, 1702, 1705–1706
postsurgical follow-up, 1701f, 1702
pulmonary embolism, 1702f, 1706
traumatic injuries, 1697f–1699f, 1699–1700
in intracranial arteriovenous malformations, 2183, 2184f
of lower extremity arteries, 1687–1688
magnetic resonance, 1679–1680, 1681f–1682f
in abdominal aortic aneurysms, 1885
mesenteric, selective, in vascular ectasia, 1169, 1169f
normal variations simulating disease on, 1688, 1688f–1690f
outpatient, 1683
of pelvic arteries, 1684–1685
of pituitary gland and paraseltar region, 1350
radionuclide, in valvular heart disease, 1515–1516
in sarcomas, 2253, 2254f
technique for, 1678, 1679f
of upper extremity arteries, 1687
in vascular infections, 1726f, 1726–1727, 1727f

visceral
of arteries, 1685f, 1685–1686, 1686f
selective, in gastrointestinal hemorrhage, 1161, 1161f
urgent, 1771, 1774f
of veins, 1686–1687, 1687f
interventional, 1706–1709
angioplasty and, 1702f–1704f, 1706–1707
catheter fragment retrieval and, 1708f, 1709
caval interruption and, 1708f, 1708–1709
embolotherapy and, 1705f–1707f, 1708
for stress gastritis, 777–778
thrombolytic therapy and, 1705f, 1707
transjugular intrahepatic portosystemic shunts and, 1709
vascular access device placement and, 1709
Angiomatosis, encephalotrigeminal, 1930
Angiomyolipomas, renal, 2209
Angioplasty
angioscopic monitoring of, 1742, 1742f
balloon, for atherosclerosis, 1735
subclavian flap, for coarctation of aorta, 1498
transluminal, percutaneous. See Percutaneous transluminal angioplasty (PTA); Percutaneous transluminal coronary angioplasty (PCTA)
Angiosarcomas
cardiac, 1502
of spleen, 1273
Angioscopy, 1740–1742
equipment for, 1740
in-situ vein bypasses using, 1741, 1742f
for monitoring of angioplasty procedures, 1742, 1742f
technique for, 1740
thrombectomy using, 1740–1741
Angiosomes, 2281
Angiotensin-converting enzyme (ACE)
renovascular hypertension and, 1782
for vascular gene therapy, 520t
Angiotensin I, renovascular hypertension and, 1782
Angiotensinogen, 1782
Anifostine (WR-2721), for hypercalcemia, 1316
Animal bites, hand infections due to, 2161
Anion exchange-binding resins, for Clostridium difficile colitis, 1178
Anion gap, 260
Anisotropic structure, of arterial walls, 1656
Ankle-brachial index (ABI), 1669, 1671, 1671f
in infrainguinal occlusive disease, 1813
Annuloplasty, tricuspid valve, 1519, 1519f
Anoplasty, for anal fissures, 1195, 1197f
Anorectal abscesses, 1196–1197
clinical manifestations of, 1197
management of, 1197
pathogenesis of, 1196–1197, 1198f

Anorectal disorders. See also specific disorders
imperforate anus, 2041–2046
anatomy and classification of, 2041–2043, 2042f–2044f, 2043t
anomalies associated with, 2043
clinical presentation of, 2043
diagnosis of, 2043–2045
embryology of, 2041, 2041f
treatment of, 2045–2046
results and complications of, 2045–2046
in patients with acquired immunodeficiency syndrome and HIV-positivity, 1204–1205
sexually transmitted, 1202–1204
in ulcerative colitis, 1099
Anorectal flap technique, for rectovaginal fistulas, 1201, 1202f
Anorectal manometry, in Hirschsprung disease, 2059
Anorectal ulcers, in HIV-positive patients, 1205
Anorectoplasty, sagittal, posterior, 2045
Anorectum, 1180–1205. See also Anorectal entries; Anus; Rectum; specific disorders
anal continence mechanisms and, 1187
arterial supply of, 1183–1184, 1184f
defecation and, 1187–1188
lymphatic drainage of, 1184, 1186f
sensation of, 1186
venous drainage of, 1184, 1185f
Anoscopy
in fistula-in-ano, 1199
in hemorrhoids, 1188
in rectovaginal fistulas, 1200
Antacids
for duodenal ulcers, 765
for gastric ulcers, 784
prophylactic, for stress gastritis, 778
for stress gastritis, 1165
Anterior cruciate ligament tears, arthroscopic surgery for, 2151–2152
Anterior spinal artery syndrome, 2169, 2170f
Anterolateral cordotomy, for pain management, 2195
Antiarrhythmic drugs, 1567–1568. See also specific drugs
Antibiotic-associated colitis, 176, 1172–1179
Clostridium difficile, 1172
clinical diagnosis of, 1174–1176, 1175t, 1176f
clinical manifestations of, 1174, 1174f, 1175f
laboratory diagnosis of, 1176–1177
pathogenesis and prevention of, 1173t, 1173–1174
pathology of, 1172–1173
treatment of, 1177–1179
drug therapy for, 1177–1179
with relapse or recurrence, 1179
surgical, 1179
Antibiotic drugs, 167–170. See also specific drugs and drug types
for animal and human bites, of hands, 2161
antineoplastic, 502t
for appendicitis, 1258
classes of, 167–168, 168f, 169f

Antibiotic drugs (*continued*)
  for *Clostridium difficile* colitis, 1177–
      1178
  for Crohn's disease, 840–841
  directed therapy using, 169–170
  for duodenal ulcers, 765–766
  empiric therapy using, 168–169
  for gram-negative bacterial sepsis, 175–
      176
  for intraabdominal infections, 172
  for lung abscesses, 1478
  for monilial esophagitis, 724
  for pancreatitis, 885
  prophylactic, 168
    in abdominal injuries, 336–337
    in chest injuries, 319
    for endocarditis, 1531, 1532t
    for hepatic transplantation, 598
    in maxillofacial injuries, 304
  for soft tissue infections, necrotizing,
      173
  spectrum of activity of, 169t
  topical, for burns, 430–431, 431t
  for wound care, 81–82
Antibodies, 161, 162f, 163. *See also*
      Immunoglobulin(s)
  antiphospholipid, 1616–1617
  antisperm, 2203–2204
Antibody dependent cellular cytotoxicity
      (ADCC), 541
Anticholinergic drugs. *See also specific*
      drugs
  for duodenal ulcers, 763–764
  for gastric ulcers, 784
Anticoagulation. *See also* Hemostasis;
      specific anticoagulant drugs
  acute abdomen and, 1251
  for deep venous thrombosis, 1948,
      1949
  drugs for, 1619
  for pancreatic transplantation, 621–622
  for pulmonary thromboembolism,
      1953, 1954t
  in valvular heart disease, 1529t, 1529–
      1531
    complications of, 1530
    contraindications to, 1530–1531
    indications for, 1529–1530
Antidiarrheal agents, for *Clostridium*
      difficile colitis, 1178
Antidiuretic hormone (ADH)
  excess, 1348–1349
  surgical stress response and, 53
  therapeutic uses of. *See* Vasopressin
Antigen(s), 161
  class I and II, structure and function of,
      530t
  presentation of, 533
  processing of, 531–532, 532f
  recognition of, 527–530
    adhesion receptors and, 537–538,
        538t
    of altered self, 533, 533f
    anatomic organization of immune
        response and, 534
    antigen-presenting cells and, 537
    antigen recognition sites and, 534–535
    B cells and, 536–537, 537f
    cytokines and cytokine receptors
        and, 538, 539t, 540f, 540–541
    direct, 533, 533f
      by immunoglobulins, 527f, 527–
          529, 528f, 528t

homing and trafficking and, 534–
    535, 535f
  indirect, 533, 533f
  by T-cell receptors, 529–530, 529–
      531f, 530t
  T cells and, 535f, 535–536, 536f,
      536t
Antigenic modulation, 550t, 551
Antigen-presenting cells (APCs), 533, 537
Antihypertensive drugs. *See also specific*
      drugs
  for renal hypertension, 1790
Antilymphocyte globulin (ALG)
  for immunosuppression, 548, 550t, 551
  for pulmonary transplantation, 612
Antimetabolites, 501t
  for immunosuppression, 548
Antimicrobial drugs. *See* Antibiotic
      drugs; *specific drugs and drug*
      types
Antioncogenes, 471, 472t, 478, 480f
Antiphospholipid antibodies, 1616–1617
Antiplatelet agents, 98–99, 1619–1620.
      See also specific drugs
  for infrainguinal occlusive disease,
      1819
Antireflux surgery, 684–692
  Belsey Mark IV repair, 691f, 691–692
  Collis gastroplasty, 692
  failed, 693–694
  indications for, 685f, 685–686
  intraoperative complications of, 692
  Nissen fundoplication, 687, 687f–690f,
      689–690
  open Nissen fundoplication, 690
  postoperative management and, 692
  results of, 692–693, 693f
  tailored antireflux operation, 686–687,
      687f
Antisperm antibodies, 2203–2204
Antithrombin III
  deficiency of, 1615
  definition of, 89–90
  thrombosis and, 1613–1614
Antithymocyte globulin (ATG)
  for hepatic transplantation, 598
  for immunosuppression, 548, 550t, 551
Antithyroid drugs, 1291
  for Graves disease, 1295–1296
α_1-Antitrypsin (α_1AT) deficiency
  in biliary atresia, 2087
  gene therapy for, 519
Antivenin
  for snake bites, 405
  for spider bites, 407
Antral glands, 749, 749f
Antrectomy, for gastric ulcers, 786, 787f
Antroduodenal motility assessment, 666–
      670
Ant stings, 407–408
Anuria, management of, in critically ill
      patients, 236
Anus. *See also* Anal *entries*; Anorectal
      entries; Anorectum; *specific*
      disorders
  anatomy of, 2041, 2042f
Anxiolytics, 442, 442t
Aorta
  abdominal
    anatomy of, 1683–1684, 1684f
    aneurysms of. *See* Abdominal aortic
        aneurysms (AAAs)
  thoracic

anatomy of, 1683
  aneurysms of. *See* Thoracic aortic
      aneurysms; Thoracoabdominal
      aortic aneurysms (TAAAs)
  transection of, 284
Aortic arch reconstruction, direct, 1757
Aortic disorders. *See also specific*
      disorders
  hypoplastic, 1799
  infectious, management of, 1728–1730,
      1729f, 1730t
  rupture, angiography in, 1697f, 1698f,
      1699–1700
  traumatic injuries, 366–368, 367f–370f
  treatment of, 327f, 327–328
Aortic dissections. *See* Thoracic aortic
      aneurysms, dissections
Aortic insufficiency (AI), 1505, 1505t
  diagnosis of, 1512
  medical management of, 1517
  pathophysiology of, 1511
Aortic reconstruction, for aortoiliac
      disease, 1804–1805
  aortobifemoral bypass grafts for, 1804,
      1806f, 1807f
  aortoiliac endarterectomy for, 1804,
      1805f
  iliofemoral grafts for, 1804–1805, 1807f
  results of, 1809–1810
Aortic stenosis, 1487f, 1487–1488
  medical management of, 1517
  pathophysiology of, 1510–1511
  subaortic, 1488
  supravalvular, 1488
Aortic valve
  anatomy of, 1503, 1504f
  bicuspid, 1505
  replacement of, technique for, 1524f,
      1525
  stenosis of, 1503, 1504t
Aortobifemoral bypass grafts, 1804,
      1806f, 1807f
Aortoenteric fistulas, bleeding and,
      1170–1171
Aortography
  in abdominal aortic aneurysms, 1885,
      1886f, 1886t
  in arteriovenous fistulas, 1923
  in thoracoabdominal aortic aneurysms,
      1876, 1876f
  in traumatic injuries, in elderly people,
      388
  in visceral angina, 1775, 1777f
Aortoiliac occlusive disease, 1796–1810
  anatomy and, 1796–1797, 1797f–1799f
  diagnosis and evaluation of, 1800–
      1801, 1803
    arteriography in, 1801
    pressure measurements in, 1803,
        1803f
  pathophysiology of, 1797–1798, 1800f,
      1801f
  patterns and clinical manifestations of,
      1798–1800, 1802
  treatment of, 1803–1809
    direct aortic reconstruction for,
        1804–1805, 1805f–1807f
      results of, 1809–1810
    graft patency following, 1810
    indications for operation and, 1803–
        1804
    indirect revascularization methods

for, 1805, 1808f–1809f, 1808–1809
results of, 1810
procedure selection for, 1804
Aortorenal bypass, for renal hypertension, 1791f, 1791–1792
Apert syndrome, 2194
Aplastic anemia, 1268–1269
Aponeurotic flaps, for hernia repair, 1220
Apoptosis, 545
in inflammation, 153, 153t
Appendectomy
historical background of, 1251–1252
incidental, 1259–1260
interval, 1258
Appendicitis, 1253–1260
in acquired immunodeficiency syndrome, 1259
chronic versus recurrent, 1258
diagnosis of, 1254–1256
in elderly patients, 1259
pathophysiology of, 1253f, 1253–1254, 1254t
pediatric, 1258–1259
congenital abnormalities and, 1258–1259
pelvic inflammatory disease differentiated from, 1249, 1249t
during pregnancy, 1259, 1259f
treatment of, 1256–1258
antibiotics in, 1258
interval appendectomy for, 1258
laparoscopic, 1256–1257
laparotomy for, 1257
nonoperative, 1257–1258
Appendix, 1251–1260
anatomy of, 1252f, 1252–1253
neoplastic disease of, 1260
Apple-core defect, in colorectal cancer, 1132, 1133f
Aprotinin, 99
Arginine test, intravenous, 872–873
Argon laser, for endovascular surgery, 1736
Arnold-Chiari syndrome, 2192, 2192f, 2193
Arterial blood flow, evaluation of, 1673, 1674f
Arterial blood gases, in pulmonary thromboembolism, 1952
Arterial catheterization, of pediatric patients, 1981
Arterial compression syndromes, 1635–1643. *See also* Compartment syndromes
of popliteal artery, 1639–1640, 1640f, 1641f
thoracic outlet syndromes, 1635–1638, 1636f–1638f, 1761, 1763f
of vertebral artery, 1638–1639, 1639f
Arterial dilation, for renal hypertension, 1792
Arterial disorders, 1596–1607. *See also specific disorders*
affecting media, 1599–1601
peripheral, thrombolytic therapy for, 101–102
radiation-induced, 1602–1603
Arterial dissections
angiography in, 1695f, 1695–1697, 1696f
spontaneous, of carotid artery, 1748–1749

Arterial embolism, peripheral, 1621–1634
in atherosclerosis. *See* Atheroembolism
clinical manifestations of, 1625–1627, 1626f
differential diagnosis of, 1626t, 1627, 1627f, 1628f
distribution of, 1624, 1624f
pathophysiology of, 1624–1625
source and etiology of, 1621f, 1621–1624, 1623f
thromboembolectomy for, 1627–1630, 1629t
results with, 1629f, 1629–1630
Arterial embolization
arteriographic, in pelvic fractures, 356
transcatheter, for stress gastritis, 1165
Arterial fibrodysplasia
angiography in, 1696f, 1697f, 1697–1699
of renal artery, 1784, 1786
intimal, 1784, 1785f
medial, 1784, 1785f, 1786, 1786f
operative treatment of, 1793, 1794t
perimedial, 1786, 1787f
Arterial obstruction
acute, diagnostic techniques for, 1676
peripheral, of lower extremities, diagnostic techniques for, 1674–1676, 1675f
stenotic, hemodynamics and. *See* Hemodynamics, arterial
visceral, diagnostic techniques for, 1676
Arterial switch procedure, for transposition of the great arteries, 1491, 1493, 1493f
Arteria magna syndrome, 1601, 1601f
Arteries, 1585–1592. *See also specific arteries and arterial disorders*
of abdominal viscera, 1765–1768, 1766f–1771f, 1772t
baroreceptors in, 247
compliance of, 1656–1657, 1657f
function of, 1656f, 1656–1657, 1657f
hemodynamics of. *See* Hemodynamics, arterial
regulation of anticoagulated state and, 1591–1592
regulation of luminal area of, 1586–1587, 1587f
regulation of medial and luminal thickening of, 1587–1589, 1588f, 1589f
regulation of smooth muscle growth and, 1589–1591
structure of, 1585–1586, 1586f, 1656
aneurysm formation and, 1841f, 1842, 1842f
Arterio dolicho et magna, 1601, 1601f
Arteriography
in aortoiliac disease, 1801
in arteriovenous fistulas, 1921–1922, 1922f
in congenital vascular malformations, 1927, 1930f
in coronary artery disease, 1539
in dissecting renal artery aneurysms, 1907
embolization and, in pelvic fractures, 356
in infrainguinal occlusive disease, 1821
in liver masses, 1010, 1011f

lower extremity venography
ascending, 1701f, 1705
closed-system, 1705–1706
descending, 1705
magnetic resonance, in renovascular hypertension, 1787
in renovascular hypertension, 1787, 1789f
selective, in thoracoabdominal aortic aneurysms, 1876
in vascular injuries, 363
in vascular occlusive disease, of upper extremities, 1760–1761, 1762f, 1763f
Arterioles
adrenergic receptors of, 186
anatomy of, 183, 184f
Arteriomegaly, 1601, 1601f
Arteriosclerosis, femoral artery aneurysms in. *See* Aneurysm(s), of femoral artery
Arteriovenous fistulas (AVFs), 1916f, 1916–1924, 1917f
carotid cavernous sinus, 1921
congenital, 1924, 1924f
diagnosis of, 1921–1922, 1922f
for hemodialysis, 1923–1924
hemodynamic alterations and, 1917–1920
local, 1918f, 1918–1919, 1919f
systemic, 1919–1920, 1920f
hepatic artery-portal venous, 1921, 1923
signs and symptoms of, 1920–1921
treatment of, 1922–1924, 1924f
vertebral, 1921
Arteriovenous malformations (AVMs), 1916
angiography in, 1699f, 1700
hypoactive, 1929
intracranial, 2183–2184, 2184f
pulmonary, 1434
Arteritis
angiography in, 1699
immune, 1602–1606
Behçet disease, 1604
Cogan syndrome, 1604
giant cell arteritis group, 1605–1606
Takayasu arteritis, 1606, 1607f, 1748, 1761
temporal arteritis, 1605–1606, 1606f, 1748
hypersensitivity angiitis group, 1604–1605, 1605f
Kawasaki disease, 1603f, 1603–1604
polyarteritis nodosa, 1603, 1603f
of upper extremities, 1761
Arthritis
degenerative
of hand, 2159
in morbid obesity, 790
in morbid obesity, 790
rheumatoid, of hand, 2159, 2161f
Arthroplasty, total joint replacement, 2148–2150, 2150f, 2151f
Arthroscopy, 2150–2152
diagnostic, 2150–2151
operative, 2151–2152
of wrist, 2162f, 2162–2163
Articular disorders. *See* Joints; *specific disorders*

Artificial hepatic support systems. *See also specific systems*
  arteriovenous fistulas for, 1923–1924
  for fulminant hepatic failure, 979, 979t
Asbestos, tumors caused by, 462
Ascites, 986–990
  chylous, 1242–1243, 1969
  cirrhotic, 987–988, 988f
  clinical and laboratory features of, 987–988, 988f, 988t
  complications of, 988t, 988–989, 989t
  pathophysiology of, 986–987
  pediatric, 2077t, 2077–2078
  treatment of, 989–990
    diuretics in, 989
    paracentesis in, 989
    sodium and fluid restriction in, 989
    surgical, 989–990, 990f
Ascorbic acid
  pediatric requirement for, 1976t
  requirements in surgical patients, 62t
  wound healing and, 78
A Scoring Characterization of Trauma (ASCOT), 277
Asialoglycoprotein, 946t
A-sites, 24
Aspergillus infections, 177
Asphyxia, traumatic, pediatric, 381
Aspirin (acetylsalicylic acid; ASA)
  as antiplatelet agent, 98, 1620
  for claudication, 1717–1718
  gastric ulcers and, 782
  for infrainguinal occlusive disease, 1819
  metabolic acidosis due to, 262
Assist-controlled ventilation, 1986
Asthenospermia, 2202
Astler-Coller staging system, modified, for colorectal cancer, 1134, 1134f, 1135f, 1135t, 1136t
Astrocytomas
  intracranial, 2173–2174, 2175f
    high-grade, 2173–2174
    low-grade, 2173
  pilocystic, 2173
  spinal, 2180
Atherectomy, 1735–1736
Atheroembolism, 1622, 1623f, 1630f, 1630–1634, 1631t, 1798, 1801f
  arterial catheter-related, 1632
  coronary, 1633
  diffuse, 1634
  gastrointestinal, 1633
  lower extremity, 1632f, 1632–1633
  pathophysiology of, 1631, 1631f
  renal, 1633–1634
Atheromas, 1593
Atherosclerosis, 1710–1718
  aneurysms in, 1840
  aortic aneurysms in, of thoracic aorta, 1860f, 1860–1863
    operative management of, 1860, 1861f–1863f, 1862–1863
  arterial embolism in. *See* Atheroembolism
  of cardiac grafts, 605
  cerebrovascular disease and. *See* Cerebrovascular disease, ischemic
  coronary, 1536–1538
    lesions in, 1536, 1537f
    prevention of, 1537–1538
    risk factors for, 1536–1537

endovascular surgery in. *See* Endosurgery, vascular
gene therapy for, 519–520
immunosuppression and, 553
infrainguinal. *See* Infrainguinal occlusive disease
nonaneurysmal, angiography in, 1690–1694, 1692f, 1693f
nonoperative treatment of claudication in, 1715–1718
  exercise training, 1715–1716, 1716t
  pharmacologic, 1716–1718
plaques in, 1593
  Hollenhorst, 1751
  rupture of, 1631, 1631f
  soft, 1750
regression of, 1718, 1718t
renal artery aneurysms and, 1902, 1904f
renal artery occlusion and, 1783–1784, 1784f
risk factors for, 1710–1715
  diabetes mellitus, 1714t, 1714–1715, 1715t
    treatment results and, 1714–1715
  homocysteine, 1715
  hyperlipidemia, 1710–1712
    lipid-lowering therapy and, 1711–1712
    lipoproteins and, 1710–1711
  hypertension, 1714
  smoking, 1712–1714, 1713f
  following splenectomy, 1280
  theories of, 1592f, 1592–1594, 1594f
  thoracoabdominal aortic aneurysms in, 1874
tissue ischemia and, 1654–1655
upper extremity occlusive disease due to, 1761
Atracurium, 440t
Atrial natriuretic peptide (ANP), in sodium and volume control, 247
Atrial septal defect (ASD), 1483–1484, 1484f
Atrioventricular canal-type defects, 1485
Atrioventricular fistulas, coronary, 1495
Atrioventricular (AV) node, 1565
Atrioventricular septal defect (AVSD), 1483, 1496–1497
Atropine, 440t
Auerbach plexus, 1085–1086, 1087
Autocrine stimulation, 540
Autografting, for burns, 431
Automatic implantable cardioverter-defibrillator (AICD), for ventricular arrhythmias, 1570
Automaticity, 1566
Autoregulation
  to change oxygen consumption, 216f, 216–217
  to change oxygen delivery, 217, 217f
  to maintain oxygen delivery, 216
Avascular necrosis, of femoral head, 375
Axial flow pumps, 1555, 1556f
Axial spine, fractures of, 373
Axillary artery, aneurysms of. *See* Aneurysm(s), axillosubclavian
Axillary lymph node dissection (ALND), 1389, 1394
  in metastatic melanomas, 2240
  therapeutic, 1389
Axonemes, 9
Axonotmesis, 2155, 2172

Azathioprine (Imuran), 549t
  for cardiac transplantation, 602, 602t
  for Crohn's disease, 841
  for pulmonary transplantation, 612
Azithromycin, for chlamydial proctitis, 1204
Azoospermia, 2202
Azotemia, differential diagnosis in liver disease, 981, 981t

B

Bacitracin, for *Clostridium difficile* colitis, 1178
Bacteria, opsonization of, inflammation and, 134–135, 136f
Bacterial clearance, 171
Bacterial infections. *See also specific infections*
  gram-negative, sepsis caused by, 174–176, 175f
  meningitis caused by, 2190
  neurologic, 2189–2191
  peritonitis caused by, spontaneous, in ascites, 988t, 988–989, 989t
Bacterial translocation, 180
Ball-in-cage heart valves, 1525f, 1525–1526, 1530
Balloon angioplasty, for atherosclerosis, 1735
Balloon dilation
  for atherosclerosis, 1735
  for bile duct strictures, 1074–1075, 1076f, 1077t
    endoscopic, 1075, 1077t
    surgical treatment versus, 1075, 1077, 1077t
  for esophageal achalasia, 675
Balloon tamponade, for gastroesophageal varices, 994, 994f, 1166–1167
  endoscopic sclerotherapy versus, 995
Balloon valvuloplasty, 1518
  aortic, percutaneous, 1518
Barium contrast studies
  enema
    in appendicitis, 1256, 1257f
    in colorectal adenomas, 1115
    in colorectal cancer, 1132, 1133f
    in Hirschsprung disease, 2059, 2060f
    in meconium ileus, 2051, 2052f
    in ulcerative colitis, 1097
  esophageal, 658, 659f
    in congenital cystic disease of lung, 2007–2008
    in esophageal cancer, 702–703, 703f
    in gastric adenocarcinomas, 797, 798f
Baroreceptors, fluid volume and, 246–247
Barotrauma, with mechanical ventilation, 1986
Barrett's esophagus, 704
  in gastroesophageal reflux disease, 683–684
Barrett's mucosa, 700, 701f
Barrier defenses, 160
Bartholin gland
  abscesses of, 2218
  carcinomas of, 2218
Bartter syndrome, 1338
Basal body, 9
Basal cell carcinomas (BCCs)
  of anal margin, 1147
  of skin, 2242–2243, CF 111–1, CF 111–4–5

etiology of, 2242
pigmented, 2243, CF 111–1
surgical treatment of, 2244
vulvar, 2218
Basal energy expenditure (BEE), 227
Basal metabolic rate (BMR), 227
injury response and, 54
Basaloid carcinomas, of anal canal, 1149, 1150f
Basal skull fractures, 2166
Base deficit, in shock, 286, 287f
Basophils, inflammation and, 147–148
Bassini repair, for inguinal and femoral hernias, 1222, 1223f
Battle sign, 296, 2166
B cells
in antigen recognition, 536–537
T-dependent and T-independent responses and, 536, 537f
pancreatic, 869–870
receptor driven stimulation of, 545–547, 546f
BCNU (carmustine), 501t
Bed sores, healing of, 80
Bee stings, 407–408
Behçet disease, 1604
Belsey artery, 655
Belsey Mark IV repair, 691f, 691–692
Benign prostatic hypertrophy (BPH), 2199
Bennett intraarticular fracture, of base of thumb, 2159
Benzodiazepines, 442, 442t
Bernard-Soulier syndrome, 95
Bernoulli equation, modified, 1534
Bernstein test, 668
Berry, ligament of, 1284, 1284f
Beta-adrenergic blocking agents, for coronary artery disease, 1539
Betamethasone (Celestone), for trigger finger, 2157
Bicarbonate
excretion of, in hyperparathyroidism, 1321
gastric production of, 756f, 756–757
gastric secretion of, 775
mechanisms resulting in decreased body content of, 261–262
nonrenal loss of, 261
pancreatic secretion of, 865, 868f
therapeutic. See Sodium bicarbonate
Bile, 954–956
composition of, 954–955, 1036
gallbladder, hepatic bile versus, 1031t
hepatic, gallbladder bile versus, 1031t
secretion of, 954–955
Bile acid(s), metabolism of, 955, 955f
Bile acid-binding resins. See also specific drugs
for hypercholesterolemia, 1711
Bile duct(s)
adenomas of, 1013
calculous disease of. See Choledocholithiasis
extrahepatic, 1026–1028
common bile duct, 1026–1027
common hepatic duct, 1026, 1028f
cystic duct, 1026, 1029f
histology and ultrastructure of, 1029
vessels and nerves of, 1027–1028
hamartomas of, 1013
Bile duct cancer, 1060–1066
adjuvant therapy for, 1066

clinical findings in, 1061
diagnosis of, 1061f, 1061–1062
incidence of, 1060
palliative stenting for, 1065f, 1066, 1066t
staging of, 1060–1061, 1061f
surgical treatment of, 1062–1065
determination of resectability and, 1065
for hilar tumors, 1062, 1062f–1063f, 1065
for middle- and lower-third bile duct tumors, 1062
of unresectable tumors, 1064f, 1065–1066
Bile duct strictures, 1067–1081
anastomotic, 1068–1079
in cholangiohepatitis, 1080f, 1080–1081
in choledocholithiasis, 1080
in cholelithiasis, 1080
in chronic pancreatitis, 1078–1080, 1079f
clinical presentation of, 1069, 1070f
intrahepatic arterial 5-fluorouracil infusion causing, 1081
laboratory studies in, 1069–1070
in Mirizzi syndrome, 1080
nonoperative management of, 1073–1075
endoscopic balloon dilation for, 1075, 1077t
percutaneous balloon dilatation for, 1074–1075, 1076f, 1077t
surgical management versus, 1075, 1077, 1077f
pathogenesis of, 1067–1069, 1068f, 1069f
preoperative management of, 1070, 1072
in primary sclerosing cholangitis, 1077t, 1077–1078, 1078f, 1079f
hepatic transplantation for, 582–583
radiographic examination in, 1070, 1071f, 1072f
surgical management of, 1072–1073
elective repair of established strictures, 1072–1073, 1074f
immediate repair of intraoperative bile duct injury, 1072
morbidity and mortality associated with, 1073
nonoperative management versus, 1075, 1077, 1077f
Bile micelles, 816
Bile probes
esophageal, 669, 669f
gastric, 666–670
Bile salts, absorption of, from small intestine, 816
Biliary atresia, 2083–2090
anatomy of, 2084f, 2083–2084
microscopic, 2083–2084, 2085f
clinical presentation and diagnosis of, 2085–2087, 2086t
correctable and uncorrectable, 2083
hepatic transplantation for, 583
pathophysiology of, 2084–2085
treatment of, 2087–2090
hepatic transplantation for, 2089–2090

portoenterostomy for, 2087–2089, 2088f, 2089f
results and complications of, 2088–2089
Biliary colic, in cholelithiasis, 1043, 1043f
Biliary disorders. See also specific disorders
calculous. See Choledocholithiasis; Cholelithiasis
in chronic pancreatitis, treatment of, 898f, 899f, 899–900
neoplastic, 1056–1066
benign, 1056–1057
clinical findings in, 1057
diagnosis and treatment of, 1057
pathology of, 1056
malignant. See Bile duct cancer; Gallbladder cancer
obstructive
cirrhosis due to, 975–976
following hepatic transplantation, 592
sphincter of Oddi dysfunction, 1031
in ulcerative colitis, 1096
Biliary diversion, colonic motor dysfunction following, 1092
Biliary leakage, following hepatic transplantation, 592–593, 596f
Biliary reconstruction, in hepatic transplantation, 588, 591f, 592f
Biliary sludge, 1040
Biliary tract, 1023–1081. See also Bile duct(s); Gallbladder
anatomy of, 1023–1028
extrahepatic biliary ducts, 1026–1028
vessels, nerves, and lymphatics, 1023–1024, 1026, 1026f, 1027f
embryology of, 1023, 1024f
histology and ultrastructure of, 1029
lecithin and cholesterol secretion by, 955
motor function of, 1029–1030, 1030f
neurohormonal regulation of, 1030–1031
pediatric, 2083–2093. See also specific disorders
embryology of, 2083, 2083f
proteins of, 955–956
sphincter of Oddi and, 1028f, 1030
dysfunction of, 1031
Biliopancreatic diversion, partial, for morbid obesity, 792–793
Bilirubin, excess of
conjugated hyperbilirubinemia, 2086
pediatric, 1990–1991
Bilirubin uridine diphosphoglucuronate glucuronyl transferase deficiency, gene therapy for, 518–519
Billroth I operation, for gastric ulcers, 785, 785f
Billroth II operation, for gastric ulcers, 785–786
Bimolecular layer, of plasma membrane, selectivity and energy conversion and, 12–13, 13f
Biobrane, for burns, 431
Biochemical markers
in colorectal cancer, 1138
recurrent, 1144, 1144t
in germinomas, 2178

Biochemical markers (*continued*)
  for melanomas, 2236
  for pancreatitis, 883–884
  in prostate cancer, 2211
  in testis cancer, 2212
Biofeedback, for anal incontinence, 1201
Biologic therapy. *See* Immunotherapy
Bio-Medicus Bio-Pump, 1555
Bioprosthetic heart valves, 1525, 1525f
  complications of, 1526, 1526f
Biopsies. *See specific sites and techniques*
Biotin
  pediatric requirement for, 1976t
  requirements in surgical patients, 62t
Biphosphonates, for hypercalcemia, 1315
Birth
  premature, 1973
    thermoregulation and, 1979–1980
    transitional circulation at, 1980–1981
Bismuth subsalicylate (Pepto-Bismol), for
      duodenal ulcers, 765
Bites and stings, 402–408
  human and animal bites, hand
      infections due to, 2161
  Hymenoptera stings, 407–408
  lizard bites, 406
  scorpion stings, 408
  snake bites, 402t, 402–403, 403f
    clinical evaluation of, 404
    signs and symptoms of, 404
    treatment of, 405–406
    venom and, 403–404, 404t
  spider bites, 406f, 406–407, 407f
Björk-Shiley valve, 1526, 1526f
Black widow spider bites, 406, 407, 407f
Black widow syndrome, 1845
Bladder
  cancer of, 490, 2206–2208
    diagnosis and staging of, 2206–2207,
      2207f
    metastatic, 2207–2208
    treatment of, 2207–2208, 2208f
  neurogenic, pediatric, 2106
  pediatric, 2105–2106
  physiology of, 2199
  traumatic injuries of, 358, 359f
    pediatric, 384
Blalock-Hanlon septectomy, for
      transposition of the great
      arteries, 1491
Blalock-Taussig shunt
  for tetralogy of Fallot, 1490
  for univentricular heart, 1499
Blastomas, pulmonary, in pediatric
      patients, 2010
Bleeding. *See also* Hemorrhage
  uterine, abnormal, 2223–2224
Bleeding disorders, 92–95
  coagulation factor deficiency, 92–94,
      93f, 94f
    gene therapy for, 519
  fibrinolytic abnormalities, 95
  with fibrinolytic agents, 100–101
  platelet disorders, 94–95, 95f
Bleeding time assays, 103
Bleomycin, 502t
Blepharoplasty, 2269, 2270f, 2272t
Bloating, in gastroesophageal reflux
      disease, 681
Blood
  ABO compatibility of, for hepatic
      transplantation, 596

viscosity of, arterial flow and energy
      loss and, 1660–1662, 1661f
Blood dyscrasias, upper extremity
      occlusive disease and, 1762–
      1763
Blood flow
  arterial. *See* Hemodynamics, arterial
  cerebral, intracranial pressure and,
      292–293, 293f
  coronary, 1535–1536
    metabolic regulation of, 1536
    physical regulation of, 1536
  in critically ill patients
    regional, 226–227
    systemic, 226–227
  gastric, 757, 775
  hepatic, 948
    blood cleansing function and, 948
    control of, 948, 948f
  intestinal, mechanical bowel
      obstruction and, 820
  laminar, arterial flow and energy loss
      and, 1660–1661, 1661f
  as mechanism protecting against
      thrombosis, 1610f, 1618–1619
  nonlaminar, 1610f, 1618–1619
  renal, pediatric, 1987
  turbulent, local effects of, 1662, 1663f
  venous, 1937–1938
Blood gases
  arterial, in pulmonary
      thromboembolism, 1952
  correction of, in hypothermia, 409–410
Blood pressure. *See also* Hypertension;
      Hypotension
  central venous
    in pulmonary thromboembolism,
      1952
    in shock, 286, 288
  direct measurement of, 1672
  femoral, in aortoiliac disease, 1803,
      1803f
  hypothermia and, 410
  indirect measurement of, 1669–1672,
      1670f
    ankle pressure, 1669, 1671, 1671f
    segmental leg pressures, 1671
    toe pressure, 1671, 1671f
    upper extremity pressures, 1671–
      1672, 1672f
Blood transfusions
  for gastrointestinal hemorrhage, 1159
  massive, complications of, 105
  nonhemolytic reactions to, 104–105
  risks of, 104–105
  in shock, 289, 289t
    autotransfusion for, 289
    encapsulated hemoglobin for, 290
    stroma-free hemoglobin for, 290
    type O, Rh-negative blood for, 289
    type-specific blood for, 289
Blood volume
  arteriovenous fistulas and, 1920
  cardiac function and filling pressure
      and, 226
  in portal hypertension, 985–986
  stress response and, 48
Blow-out fractures, management of, 305–
      306
Blunt injuries. *See* Traumatic injuries
B lymphocytes. *See* B cells
Bochdalek hernias, 2020, 2022–2027

anatomy and physiology and, 2020,
      2022f, 2022–2024, 2023f
  fetal circulation and, 2022–2024,
      2024f
  anomalies associated with, 2025
  diagnosis of, 2024, 2024f
  extracorporeal membrane oxygenation
      for, 2026
  high-frequency ventilation for, 2026
  liquid ventilation for, 2026–2027
  medical management of, 2025
  operative management of, 2025f, 2025–
      2026
    pulmonary transplantation, 2026
    results of, 2026
    in utero, 2026
Body cavity lavage, for rewarming, 412
Body composition, 42–43, 43f, 43t
  surgical stress response and, 49
Body fluids. *See also* Extracellular fluid
      (ECF); Intracellular fluid (ICF)
  acid-base balance of. *See* Acid-base
      balance
  atrial and renal natriuretic peptides
      and, 247–248
  compartments and, 242t, 242–243
    pediatric, 1987–1988
  composition of, 243t, 243–247
    changes in, 255–259. *See also*
      specific electrolytes and
      electrolyte imbalances
    concentration and, 243
    effective circulating volume and,
      245–246
    osmotic activity and, 243–245, 244f
    volume control and. *See* Fluid
      volume
  concentration of, 243. *See also specific*
      electrolyte imbalances
    changes in, 253f, 253–255
  fluid and electrolyte therapy and. *See*
      Fluid and electrolyte therapy
  monitoring of fluid status and, 252
  normal salt exchange and, 249
  normal water exchange and, 248–249,
      249t
  total body water and, 242t, 242–243
    pediatric, 1987
Bone(s), 2143f, 2143–2145, 2144f. *See*
      also Fractures; *specific fractures*
      and sites
  development of, 2143–2145, 2145f
  formation of, growth factors and other
      small-protein cytokines and,
      2152
  functions of, 2143
  grafting of, 2152
  of hand, 2153
  hyperparathyroidism and, 1320f, 1320–
      1321
  long, development of, 2144
  primary, secondary, and woven, 2143
  remodeling of, 2145
    pediatric, 384
  sarcomas of. *See* Osteosarcomas
  trabecular and cortical, 2143, 2143f
Bone marrow suppression, wound
      healing and, 79
Bone-metastasizing renal tumor of
      childhood, 2127
Bone morphogenetic protein, 2152
Boundary layer separation, 1662, 1663f
Boutonniere deformity, 2158, 2158f

Bowel. *See* Intestinal *entries;* Intestine(s); *specific regions of bowel*
Bowen disease, of anal margin, 1147, 1148f
Brachial artery
catheter injuries of, 1763
traumatic injuries of, 370, 372f
Brachioplasty, 2272t, 2276–2277, 2277f
Brachytherapy, 491–492
adjuvant, with head and neck surgery, 650–651
intraoperative, 490
Bradykinin
lysyl, production in tissue, 136
production in plasma, 135–136
Brain
electrodes in, for pain management, 2195
irradiation of
for gestational trophoblastic neoplasia, 2229, 2229f
for metastatic intracranial tumors, 2179
Brain death, 561–562
definition of, 561–562
etiology of, 562
pathophysiology of, 562
Brain disorders. *See also specific disorders*
abscesses, 2190t, 2190–2191
hemorrhagic, 2184–2185, 2185f
traumatic injuries, 2166–2168, 2167t. *See also* Head injuries
Brain-stem gliomas, 2173
Branchial cleft remnants, 1995–1998
anatomy and embryology of, 1995, 1995f, 1996f
clinical issues in, 1996
operative considerations and outcome of, 1996–1998, 1997f, 1998f
Branham sign, 1926
BRCA-1 gene, breast cancer and, 1381
BRCA-2 gene, breast cancer and, 1381
Breast(s), 1357–1412
anatomy of, 1358–1361
adult, 1358–1359, 1360f
histology and functional architecture, 1360, 1361f
lymphatic drainage, 1359–1360, 1360f
in males, 1360–1361
cell regulation and, 1361
embryology and development of, 1358, 1359f
examination of, 1363–1366
imaging in, 1364t, 1364–1366, 1365f, 1366f
patient history and, 1363
physical examination, 1363, 1364f
lactation and. *See* Breast feeding; Lactation
male
anatomy of, 1360
diseases of, 1410–1412
cancer, 1411t, 1411–1412
gynecomastia, 1410–1411
mammaplasty and
augmentation, 2272t, 2274–2275, 2275f
reduction, 2272t, 2276
mastopexy and, 2276
menopause and, 1363
menstruation and, 1361–1362, 1362f

postlactational involution of, 1362
during pregnancy, 1362
radial scars of, 1376f, 1376–1377
Breast biopsies, 1366, 1367f, 1368t, 1368–1370, 1389
core-needle, 1369
fine-needle aspiration, 1368t, 1368–1369, 1369f
incisional and excisional, 1369, 1369f
wire localization, 1369–1370, 1370f
Breast cancer, 1379–1410
adenoid cystic carcinomas, 1384
adjuvant systemic therapy for, 1396–1399
cytotoxic chemotherapy, 1397–1399
hormonal, 1397
rationale for, 1396t, 1396–1397, 1397f
apocrine carcinomas, 1384
biology of, 1384–1386
of cancer dissemination, 1385–1386, 1386f
cellular and molecular, 1384–1385
in children and adolescents, 1383, 1383f
counseling and support for, 1399
ductal carcinoma in situ, 1403t, 1403–1404
clinical presentation of, 1403
management of, 1403–1404, 1404t
pathology of, 1403, 1404f
prognosis of, 1403
ductal carcinomas, 1382, 1383f
variants of, 1382–1383, 1383f
epidemiology and risk factors for, 1379f, 1379t, 1379–1380, 1380f
familial, 460
follow-up procedures for, 1399, 1399t
grave signs in, 1386
historical background of, 1358, 1358t
hyperplasia and, 458–459, 460f
inflammatory, 1387, 1387f
inherited syndromes and, 1381
intraductal papillomas, 1378
invasive carcinomas, 1382–1384
ductal, 1382, 1383f
variants of, 1382–1383, 1383f
lobular, 1383–1384
lobular carcinoma in situ, 1383–1384, 1403t, 1404–1405
clinical presentation of, 1405
management of, 1405
pathology of, 1405
prognosis of, 1405, 1405t
locally advanced, 1386
management of, 1399–1400
in males, 1411t, 1411–1412
mastectomy for. *See* Mastectomy
medullary carcinomas, 1382–1383
atypical, 1382–1383
metaplastic carcinomas, 1384
metastases from
management of, 1401t, 1401–1402
chemotherapy for, 1402
hormonal therapy for, 1402
mastectomy for, 1402
radiotherapy for, 1402
occult cancer presenting as, 1409–1410
mucinous (colloid) carcinomas, 1383
noninvasive. *See* Breast cancer, ductal carcinoma in situ; Breast cancer, lobular carcinoma in situ

occult, presenting as axillary metastases, 1409–1410
operable
radiotherapy for, 1395–1396
after lumpectomy, 1395, 1396f
after mastectomy, 1395–1396
surgery for, 1391–1395
axillary lymph node dissection, 1394
breast-conserving procedures, 1392, 1392t
breast reconstruction, 1394f, 1394–1395
mastectomy, 1392–1394, 1393f
Paget disease of nipple, 1409, 1409f
pathology of, 1381–1384, 1382f
precursor lesions and, 1385
during pregnancy and lactation, 1409
prophylaxis of
mastectomy for, 1405–1407
nonsurgical, 1407
recurrent, management of, 1400–1401
after breast-conserving surgery, 1401
after mastectomy, 1400f, 1400–1401
regional nodal, 1401
sarcomas, 1407–1409
arising after treatment of breast cancer, 1407–1409, 1408f
cystosarcoma phyllodes, 1407, 1408f
stromal (monomorphic), 1407, 1408f
scirrhous carcinomas, 1382, 1383f
secretory (juvenile) carcinomas, 1383, 1383f
squamous carcinomas, 1384
staging of, 1386–1389
clinical, 1386–1387, 1387f, 1387t
diagnostic imaging and clinical laboratory adjuncts for, 1389, 1389t
pathologic, 1388t, 1388–1389
surgeon's role in, 1387–1388
TNM, 1386, 1387t
treatment planning for, 1389–1391
locoregional approaches and, 1390t, 1390–1391, 1391t
adjuvant therapy for, 1391
function and cosmesis and, 1391
local control and, 1390–1391
regional control and, 1391
process of, 1391
terminology and, 1389–1390
tubular carcinomas, 1383
Breast conservation, 1389, 1391–1392, 1392t
Breast disorders. *See also specific disorders*
abscesses, 1377
cancer. *See* Breast cancer
cellulitis, 1377
of extramammary origin, 1410
fat necrosis, 1377
fibroadenomas, 1374–1376, 1375f
fibrocystic disease, 1370, 1372–1374
breast cancer risk and, 1380
clinical evaluation of, 1370, 1372–1374
epidemiology and risk factors for, 1370
galactoceles, 1377, 1378f
infectious, 1377
in males, 1410–1412
cancer, 1411t, 1411–1412
gynecomastia, 1410–1411

Breast disorders (*continued*)
  masses, 1373
    cysts, 1373
    dominant, 1367f
    evaluation of. *See* Breast biopsies
    fibrocystic changes in, 1373
    malignant. *See* Breast cancer
    thickenings, 1367f
  mastodynia (mastalgia), 1372t, 1372–1373
  Mondor disease, 1377–1378
  of nipple disorders. *See* Nipples
  periductal mastitis (mammary duct ectasia; plasma cell mastitis), 1377
  sclerosing adenosis, 1376, 1376f
Breast feeding. *See also* Lactation
  hyperbilirubinemia and, 1991
  maternal transfer of humoral immunity during, 1991
  nutrition and, 1978
Breast reconstruction, 1390, 1394f, 1394–1395
  following prophylactic mastectomy, 1406–1407
Breast self-examination (BSE), 1363
Breathing, traumatic injuries and
  pediatric, 379–380, 380t
  prehospital care and, 280–281
  during resuscitation phase, 282
Brenner tumors, ovarian, 2226
Bromocriptine, for acromegaly, 1356
Bronchial adenomas, 1432–1433
  adenoid cystic carcinomas, 1433, 1433f
  mucoepidermoid, 1433
  mucous gland, 1433
  in pediatric patients, 2009
Bronchial cancer, 490
Bronchial injuries, 284
  pediatric, 381
  treatment of, 326–327, 327f
Bronchiectasis, 1479–1480
  cylindric, 1479
  diagnosis of, 1480, 1480f
  pathogenesis of, 1479–1480
  saccular (cystic), 1480
  treatment of, 1480
  varicose, 1480
Bronchiolitis, obliterative, following pulmonary transplantation, 613–614
Bronchogenic carcinomas, in pediatric patients, 2009–2010
Bronchogenic cysts, 1471, 1471f
  congenital, 2006, 2007f
Bronchopleural fistulas, posttraumatic, 398
Bronchoscopy, in tracheal stenosis1473
  in esophageal cancer, 703
  in lung abscesses, 1478–1479
Brown recluse spider bites, 406f, 406–407
Brown-Séquard syndrome, 2169, 2170f
Brunner glands, 807
Brunner zig-zag incisions, for hand surgery, 2157
Buccal mucosa, cancer of, 638
Budd-Chiari syndrome, 976, 991, 991t, 1958
  clinical course of, 991
  hepatic transplantation for, 583
  portal hypertension associated with, 993
  treatment of, 991, 992f

Buerger's disease, 1597–1599, 1599f, 1762
Buffer systems, 260
Burhenne technique, 1052f, 1053, 1054, 1054t
Burkitt lymphoma, Epstein-Barr virus and, 464
Burns, 422–437
  carbon monoxide and cyanide exposure and, 433–434
  chemical, 428, CF 12–7
  child abuse and, 428–429, 429t, CF 12–9
  complications of, 434, 435t–436t, 436
  definitive wound closure for, 431–433
    for face, ocular adnexae, and ears, 431–432, 432f, CF 12–11
    for genitals, 432–433
    for hands and feet, 432, CF 12–12
  in elderly people, 387
  electrical, 428, CF 12–5
  epidemiology of, 423, CF 12–1
  fluid resuscitation for, 429–430, 430t, CF 12–10
  future management of, 437
  of hands, 2159
  inhalation injury and respiratory failure and, 433, 433t
  initial evaluation of, 424–429
    of chemical injuries, 428, CF 12–7
    of electrical injuries, 428, CF 12–5, CF 12–6
    of injuries of abuse, 428–429, 429t, CF 12–9
    systemic, 424, 424f, 425t–426t, 426–428, 427f, 428f, 428t, CF 12–2–12–4
    of tar injuries, 428, CF 12–8
  initial wound excision and biologic closure for, 430–431
    estimation of burn depth and, 430
    excision techniques for, 431
    temporary wound closure alternatives for, 431
    topical antimicrobials for, 430–431, 431t
  management philosophy for, 422–423
  natural history of, 423f, 423–424
    local response to injury and, 423
    systemic response to injury and, 423–424
  nutritional support for, 434
  in pregnancy, 393, 393t
  rehabilitation and reconstruction for, 436–437
    hypertrophic scarring and, 436–437, CF 12–13
  stress gastritis and, 777
  tar, 428, CF 12–8
  total parenteral nutrition and, 59–60
  vascular access techniques for, 434
Buschke-Löwenstein tumor, 1203
Bushmaster bites. *See* Bites and stings
Busulfan, 501t
Butterfly gliomas, 2174, 2175f

C

Cabrol modification, 1865f, 1866
Cachectin. *See* Tumor necrosis factor (TNF)
Calcification, of heart valves, 1504–1505

Calciphylactic arteriopathy, 1763
Calcitonin
  calcium and phosphate metabolism and, 1313
  for hypercalcemia, 1315
Calcitonin gene-related peptide (CGRP), vasodilation induced by, 757
Calcitoninomas, 927
Calcitriol, for hypocalcemia, 1317
Calcium, 257–259. *See also* Hypercalcemia; Hypocalcemia
  biliary, gallstone formation and, 1038–1039
  homeostasis of, 257, 258f
  metabolism of, parathyroid gland and, 1310
    regulation of, 1312t, 1312–1313
  pediatric requirements for, 1977, 1988–1989
Calcium carbonate, for hypocalcemia, 1317
Calcium-channel blocking agents. *See also specific drugs*
  for coronary artery disease, 1539
Calcium gluconate
  for hyperkalemia, pediatric, 1989
  for hypocalcemia, 1317
  for spider bites, 407
Calcium homeostasis, abnormalities of, in shock, 187
Calcium ions
  as intracellular messengers, 40f, 40–41, 41f
  organ preservation injury and, 557
Calf claudication, 1639
Calories, 44
  requirements for, 44, 44t, 45t, 54
Camptothecins, 502t
Cancer, 455–505. *See also specific cancers and sites*
  causes of, 459–464
    chemical carcinogenesis, 462–463
    familial and ethnic influences, 459–461
    immunodeficiency, 459
    physical carcinogenesis, 461–462
    viral, 463–464, 464f
  chemotherapy for. *See* Cancer chemotherapy
  clinical research in, 491
  congenital patterns of expression of, 478–481, 480f–482f
  as contraindication to organ donation, 560–561
  epidemiology of, 455–457
    geographic patterns and, 455, 456f, 456t, 457f
    statistics and, 455–457, 457f–459f, 457t
  gene therapy for. *See* Gene therapy, for cancer
  of head and neck. *See* Head and neck cancer; *specific sites and cancers*
  hypercalcemia and, 1314–1315
  hypersplenism and, 1271
  immunosuppression and, 552–553
  immunotherapy for. *See* Immunotherapy
  metastasis of. *See* metastatic disease
  neurosurgical pain management techniques for, 2194, 2195–2196
  nutritional support and, 57–59
    enteral, 58

patient selection for, 57–58, 58f
total parenteral nutrition, 58–59
oncogenesis and. *See* Oncogene(s);
    Oncogenesis
palliative care and, 491
peripheral arterial embolism and, 1623,
    1623f
radiotherapy for. *See* Radiotherapy
reduction of surgical mortality,
    morbidity, and cost and, 490–
    491
rehabilitation and, 491
spectrum of neoplasia and, 458–459,
    460f, 461f
surgeon's role and, 489–490
thrombosis associated with, 1617–1618
Cancer chemotherapy, 494, 496–500,
    497f
  adjuvant, 499
    for bile duct cancer, 1066
    for colorectal cancer, 1142–1144,
      1143f
    with head and neck surgery, 650
    for osteosarcomas, 2265, 2267f
    for sarcomas, 2259
    surgery with, for pancreatic cancer,
      913, 913f
  administration of, 499–500
  for anal cancer, 1150
  for bladder cancer, metastatic, 2207–
    2208
  for breast cancer, 1397–1399
    duration, dose intensity, and
      coordination with other
      modalities, 1398–1399
    metastases from, 1402
    neoadjuvant, 1398
    in node-negative patients, 1398
    in postmenopausal, node-positive
      patients, 1398
    in premenopausal, node-positive
      patients, 1397–1398, 1398ft
  for desmoid tumors, of abdominal wall,
    1237
  for desmoplastic small round cell
    tumors, pediatric, 2133
  dose intensity and, 498–499, 2122
  enteritis due to, total parenteral
    nutrition for, 60
  for gallbladder cancer, 1060
  for gastric adenocarcinomas, 802
  for gastrinomas, 925
  for gestational trophoblastic neoplasia,
    2229, 2229f
  for hepatoblastomas, pediatric, 2137
  induction (first-line), 499
  intraarterial, 499
    gastric ulcers and, 783
  for intracranial astrocytomas, 2174
  for liver cancer, primary, 1019
  for lung cancer, non-small cell
    stage I and II, 1427
    stage IIIa, 1428–1431, 1429t, 1430t
  malignant cell resistance to, 497f, 497–
    498, 498f, 498t
  for metastatic disease
    in head and neck cancer, 650t, 651,
      651t
    intracranial, 2179
    melanomas, 2240
    metastatic, 2241
  neoadjuvant (primary), 499
    for osteosarcomas, 2264, 2264f

neoadjuvant, for sarcomas, 2259
  for neuroblastomas, pediatric, 2122
  for neurofibrosarcomas, pediatric, 2134
  for pancreatic cancer, palliative, 915
  for peripheral primitive
    neuroectodermal tumors,
    pediatric, 2133
  postoperative, 489–490
  preoperative, 489
  regimens for, 496t
  regional, 499–500
  salvage regimens, 499
  sanctuary sites and, 499
  for sarcomas, 2256, 2259
    metastatic, 2267–2268
    retroperitoneal, 2260–2261
  for small intestinal cancer, 848, 850,
    851, 855
  for tenosynovial sarcomas, pediatric,
    2132
  for testis cancer, 2213
  therapeutic responses and toxicity of,
    500, 501t–503t
  for Wilms tumor, 2125–2126
  wound healing and, 79
Candidal infections, 176–177
  esophagitis due to, 724, 725f
Cantrell, pentalogy of, 2030
Capacitation, 2202
Capacitive model, 41
Capillaries, anatomy of, 183, 184f, 185,
  185f
Capnography, in persistent pulmonary
    hypertension of newborn, 1985
Captopril, for shock, 206
Carbapenems, spectrum of activity of,
  169t
Carbohydrates. *See also specific*
    carbohydrates
  digestion and absorption of, in small
    intestine, 814–815, 815f
  as energy source, 229, 230t
  metabolism of, hepatic. *See* Liver,
    carbohydrate metabolism in
  pediatric requirements for, 1975
Carbon dioxide
  insufflation with, for laparoscopic
    surgery, 736, 738, 738t
  optimizing removal of, in respiratory
    failure, 224
  transfer in lung, 220, 220f
  ventilation and metabolism of, 218,
    218f, 219f
Carbon dioxide laser, for endovascular
    surgery, 1736
Carbon monoxide, inhalation of, burns
    and, 433–434
Carboplatin, 501t
Carboxypenicillins, spectrum of activity
    of, 169t
Carcinoembryonic antigen (CEA) assay,
    in colorectal cancer, 1138
  recurrent, 1144, 1144t
Carcinogenesis. *See* Cancer
Carcinoid tumors
  of appendix, 1260
  colorectal, 1145
  gastric, 803–804
  of lung, 1431, 1432f
  pulmonary, in pediatric patients, 2009,
    2009f, 2010f
  rectal, 1119–1120
  small intestinal, 852–855

carcinoid syndrome and, 854–855
  origin of, 852, 853f
  presentation and diagnosis of, 852–
    854, 853f, 854f
  prognosis and survival and, 855
  treatment of, 854, 855
Carcinomas. *See specific sites and*
    carcinomas
Carcinomatosis, meningeal, 2179
Carcinosarcomas, esophageal, 701
Cardiac arrhythmias, 1565–1574
  catheter technique for management of,
    1569
  conduction system anatomy and, 1565,
    1565f
  drug therapy for, 1567–1568
  electrophysiologic testing in, 1567,
    1567f
  physiology of, 1565–1567, 1566f
  postoperative, 1568
  reentrant, 1566f, 1566–1567
  spinal cord injuries and, 2171
  surgical management of, 1569–1574
    implantable devices for, 1570
    for supraventricular arrhythmias,
      1570–1574, 1571f–1573f, 1571t,
      1573t
  sustained and nonsustained, 1567
  ventricular, 1568t, 1568–1574
Cardiac catheterization
  arteriovenous fistulas due to, 1923
  in valvular heart disease, 1514t, 1514–
    1515, 1515f
Cardiac conduction system, anatomy of,
    1565, 1565f
Cardiac contraction, in shock, 188, 189f
Cardiac death, sudden, ventricular
    arrhythmias and, 1568, 1568t
Cardiac disorders. *See also*
    Cardiovascular disorders;
    specific disorders
  in morbid obesity, 788–789
  sepsis and, 57
Cardiac failure, posttraumatic, 399
Cardiac function, in critically ill patients,
    225–226, 226f
  blood volume and filling pressure and,
    226
Cardiac glands, 748
Cardiac output
  arteriovenous fistulas and, 1919–1920
  hypothermia and, 410
  low, following coronary artery bypass
    grafting, 1546
  in pediatric patients, 1982
Cardiac surgery
  abdominal complications of, 1250
  cardiac tamponade related to, 1578–
    1579
  intraaortic balloon pump during, 1552
Cardiac tamponade, 1577–1579
  causes and diagnosis of, 1577–1578,
    1578f
  clinical findings in, 201
  following coronary artery bypass
    grafting, 1546–1547
  following surgery, 1578–1579
  treatment of, 328–330, 329f
Cardiac transplantation, 599–606
  coronary artery bypass grafting versus,
    1549
  graft atherosclerosis and, 605

Cardiac transplantation (*continued*)
  graft rejection and, 602–604, 603f–
    605f
  historical background of, 599
  for hyperplastic left heart syndrome,
    1500
  immunosuppression for, 602, 602t
  indications for, 599
  operative technique for, 600–602
    for heterotopic transplantation, 602
    for orthotopic transplantation, 600–
      602, 601f
  pediatric, 604–605
  postoperative care for, 602
  preoperative evaluation and selection
    criteria for, 600, 600t
  research and future concerns in, 605–
    606
  results and survival following, 605
Cardiogenic shock, 182–183, 199–201
  compressive, 201
  intrinsic, 199–201
  after myocardial infarction, as surgical
    indication, 1541–1542
  physiologic characteristics of, 197t
Cardiomegaly, arteriovenous fistulas and,
    1920, 1920f
Cardiomyopathy, ischemic, 1538
Cardioplegia solutions, 1544
Cardiopulmonary bypass
  for aortic stenosis, 1488
  for atrial septal defect, 1484
  for coronary artery bypass grafting,
    1544, 1545
  postoperative care and, 1527
  for rewarming, 412
  for thoracic aortic aneurysms, 1860,
    1869
  for valvular heart disease, technique
    for, 1520, 1520f
  for ventricular septal defects, 1486
Cardiovascular disorders. *See also*
    specific disorders
  anesthesia and, 443–445, 452
  brain death and, 562
  burns and, 435t
  in chronic liver disease, 979–980
  hypothermia and, 408
  posttraumatic, 399
Cardiovascular system. *See also specific*
    organs
  age-related changes in, 387
  normal pressures for, 196t
  pediatric. *See* Pediatric patients,
    cardiovascular physiology of
  in shock, 188–189
    cardiac dynamics and, 188, 189f
    peripheral vascular response and, 189
    venous system and, 188–189
CardioWest C-70 total artificial heart,
    1558, 1559f
Carmustine (BCNU), 501t
L-Carnitine (levocarnitine), for
    claudication, 1716
Carotid artery
  aneurysms of. *See* Aneurysm(s), of
    carotid artery
  common, left, traumatic injuries of,
    367, 368f
  infections of, management of, 1730
  occlusive disease of. *See*
    Cerebrovascular disease;
    ischemic

  traumatic injuries of, management of,
    313t, 313–314
Carotid bruits, in cerebrovascular disease,
    1752
Carotid cavernous sinus fistulas, 1921
Carotid endarterectomy, 1753–1757
  for cerebrovascular disease, 1745, 2181
  complications of, 1754–1756
    neurologic, 1754–1755
    nonneurologic, 1755f, 1755–1756
  efficacy for prevention of stroke, 1756t,
    1756–1757
  external, 1757, 1757f
  for extracranial carotid aneurysms,
    1849
  technique for, 1753–1754, 1754f
Carotid siphon, 1746–1747
Carotid stenosis, recurrent, carotid
    endarterectomy and, 1755f,
    1755–1756
Carpal tunnel, 2196–2197
Carpal tunnel syndrome, 2155f, 2155–
    2156, 2156f
Carpenter syndrome, 2194
Carrier proteins, 13, 14f, 18, 20f–22f, 20–
    21
Cartilage, of growth plates, 2144, 2145f
Catabolism, surgical stress response and,
    53
Catalase, hydrogen peroxide removal by,
    154
Catalytic receptors, cell surface, 37, 37f
Catecholamines, 1338–1339
  excess of, 1339, 1339t
  measurement of, 1341–1342
  normal effects of, 1338–1339
Catenins, colorectal polyps and, 1110
Cathepsin D, in breast cancer, 1389
Catheter(s). *See* Nutritional support;
    Vascular catheters/
    catheterization; *specific types of*
    catheters
Catheter ablation, for ventricular
    arrhythmias, 1569, 1573–1574
Catheter fragments, retrieval of,
    angiography and, 1708f, 1709
Catheter sepsis, 176, 401
Cationic peptides, in inflammation, 155f,
    156
Cattell maneuver, 343, 344f
Causalgia, major and minor, 2196
Caustic ingestions, esophageal injury due
    to, 712–718
  clinical features of, 713–714
  immediate diagnosis and treatment of,
    714–715
  management of, 715–718, 718f, 718t
Cavitation, traumatic injuries and, 269
C-cell hyperplasia, 1327–1328
CCF/Nimbus total artificial heart, 1561,
    1562, 1562f, 1563
CCNU (lomustine), 501t
Cecum
  diverticulitis of, 1156–1157
  perforation of, 1093
Cefotetan, for pelvic inflammatory
    disease, 2225t
Cefoxitin, for pelvic inflammatory
    disease, 2225t
Ceftriaxone
  for gonococcal proctitis, 1203
  for pelvic inflammatory disease, 2225t

Celestone (betamethasone), for trigger
    finger, 2157
Celiac artery
  anatomy of, 1685, 1685f
  aneurysms of, 1893t, 1898, 1898f
Cell(s), 3–42
  of breast, regulation of, 1361
  composition of, determination of, 12,
    12f
  cytoskeleton of, 6–9
    actin-based filaments of, 6–7, 7f
    intermediate filaments of, 7–8, 8f
    microtubules of, 8f, 8–9, 9f
  diversity of, metastasis and, 487–489,
    488f
  endoplasmic reticulum of, 5, 5f, 6f
  energy of, organ preservation injury
    and, 557–558, 558f
  Golgi complex of, 5
  lysosomes of, 6
  membrane transport and. *See*
    Membrane transport
  mitochondria of, 5, 5f
  neoplastic transformation of. *See*
    Oncogene(s); Oncogenesis
  nucleus of, 4f, 4–5
  plasma membrane of, 3–4, 4f. *See also*
    Plasma membrane
  programmed death of, 545
  regulation of function, 34f, 34–42
    intracellular messengers, 39–42
    intracellular receptors and gene
      expression, 35f, 35–36, 36f
    transduction by cell surface
      receptors, 36–39, 37f–39f
  structure of, 3f, 3–9
  tumor
    death or loss of, 469
    heterogeneity of, in breast cancer, 1385
    tumor cell cycle and, 469, 469f, 470t
    vaccines and, 503
      for metastatic melanoma, 2242
  volume regulation and, 21–22, 23f
Cell-cell interactions, 9–11
  cell junctions and, 9–10, 10f
  cell-matrix adhesion and, 10–11
Cell culture, in *Clostridium difficile*
    colitis, 1176
Cell injury and death, in inflammation,
    152–158
  cationic peptides and proteins and,
    155f, 156
  general characteristics of, 152–153,
    153f, 153t
  oxidants and, 154t, 154–155
  proteinases and, 155–156
Cell junctions, 9–10, 10f
Cell-surface receptors, hepatic, 945, 946f,
    946t, 947, 947f
Cellular defenses, 163
Cellulitis
  of breast, 1377
  of hands, 2160–2161
  in lymphedema, 1970
Cell web, 7
Celosomia. *See* Omphaloceles
Centimorgans, 506
Central cord syndrome, 2169, 2170f
Central splenorenal shunt, 1000f
Central venous catheters
  for monitoring fluid status, 252
  in pediatric patients, 1981
  placement technique for, 65–66, 1709

Central venous pressure (CVP)
  in pulmonary thromboembolism, 1952
  in shock, 286, 288
Centrifugal pumps, 1555, 1555f
Cephalosporins, spectrum of activity of,
    169t
c-*erb*-A oncogene, 477
Cerebellar hemorrhage, 2185
Cerebral blood flow (CBF), intracranial
    pressure and, 292–293, 293f
Cerebral contusions, in head injuries,
    296–297, 297f
Cerebral edema
  in fulminant hepatic failure, 978
  head injuries and, 293
Cerebral ischemia, in low-flow states. *See*
    Cerebrovascular disease,
    ischemic
Cerebral perfusion pressure (CPP),
    intracranial pressure and, 292–
    293, 293f
Cerebrospinal fluid (CSF)
  in bacterial meningitis, 2190
  hydrocephalus and. *See*
    Hydrocephalus
  rhinorrhea and otorrhea and, 2166
Cerebrovascular disease, 2180–2185
  aneurysms, 2181f–2183f, 2181–2183
  arteriovenous malformations, 2183–
    2184, 2184f
  brain hemorrhage, 2184–2185, 2185f
  diagnostic techniques for, 1676
  ischemic, 1745–1757, 2180–2181
    anatomy and, 1746–1747, 1747f,
      1748f
    clinical presentation of, 1751
    following coronary artery bypass
      grafting, 1547
    diagnosis of, 1751–1752
    epidemiology of, 1745–1746, 1746f,
      1746t
    in low-flow states, 1750–1751
    management of, 1753–1757
      medical therapy for, 1753
      surgical therapy for, 1753–1757,
        2181
    natural history of, 1752–1753
      in asymptomatic disease, 1752–
        1753
      in symptomatic disease, 1752
    during or after carotid
      endarterectomy, mechanisms of,
      1754–1755
    pathophysiology of, 1747–1751,
      1749t, 1750f
    transient ischemic attacks, 1751,
      2181
  lacunar, 1751
Ceruloplasmin, hepatic copper
    metabolism and, 957
Cervical atresia, 2116
Cervical carcinomas, 2222–2223
  immunosuppression and, 553
Cervical lymph node biopsy, 643, 645f
Cervical spine
  degenerative disease of, 2186–2188
    clinical presentation of, 2186–2187
    diagnosis of, 2187, 2187f
    treatment of, 2187–2188
  traumatic injuries of, 301, 2171
    with neck injuries, 310
Cesarean section, postmortem, 394
c-fos oncogene, 477

Chaperones, 26
Chelating agents, for hypercalcemia, 1315
Chemical carcinogenesis, 462–463
  soft tissue sarcomas and, 2247
Chemical injuries
  burns, 428, CF 12–7
  cirrhosis and, 975
  esophageal, 712–718
    clinical features of, 713–714
    immediate diagnosis and treatment
      of, 714–715
    management of, 715–718, 718f, 718t
Chemical peels, 2271–2272, 2272f, 2272t
Chemoattractants, neutrophil stimulation
    by, 143–144
Chemotactic factors, leukocyte-
    endothelial cell interactions and,
    118–119, 119t
Chemotherapy, antineoplastic. *See*
    Cancer chemotherapy
Chenodeoxycholic acid (CDCA), for
    cholelithiasis, 1047
Chest
  flail, treatment of, 321–322, 322f
  in secondary survey of trauma patients,
    284
Chest injuries, 317–331
  adjunctive diagnostic modalities for,
    318
  anatomy and, 317
  evaluation of, 317–318
  treatment of, 319–331
    general conduct of surgery for, 319f,
      319–320, 320f
    general considerations in, 319
    indications for surgery and, 319
    for mediastinal injuries, 326–331
    for parenchymal injuries, 325–326
    for pleural space injuries, 323–325
    for thoracic cage injuries, 320–323
Chest pain, noncardiac
  diagnosis of, 665
  in gastroesophageal reflux disease, 681
Chest radiography. *See also* Radiographic
    examination
  in chest injuries, 318
  in esophageal cancer, 703
  in persistent pulmonary hypertension
    of newborn, 1985
  in pulmonary thromboembolism,
    1951–1952
Chest tubes
  in chest injuries, 319
  for thoracic empyema, 1457, 1458f
  in trauma patients, 280–281
Chest wall. *See also* Rib(s); Sternum
  anatomy of. *See* Thoracic anatomy
  deformities of, in pediatric patients,
    2001–2003
    embryology of, 2001
    pectus carinatum, 2003, 2003f
    pectus excavatum, 2002, 2002f
    Poland syndrome, 2003
    sternal clefts, 2001f, 2001–2002
  injuries of, indications for surgery and,
    319
  reconstruction of, 2286f, 2287, 2287f
  tumors of, 1444–1451
    chest wall reconstruction and, 1449–
      1451
      muscle flaps for, 1450–1451,
        1452f–1454f

techniques for, 1449–1450, 1450f,
  1451f
    chest wall resection for, 1449
    clavicular, 1448
    diagnosis of, 1445–1446
    preoperative evaluation of, 1445
    presentation of, 1445
    soft tissue sarcomas, 1448
Chief cells, in hyperparathyroidism,
    1318f, 1319
Chilblain, 412
Child abuse, 385
  burns caused by, 428–429, 429t, CF
    12–9
  sexual, introital problems related to,
    2117
Children. *See* Pediatric patients
Child-Turcotte risk classification method,
    for gastroesophageal varices,
    993, 993t
Chlamydial proctitis, 1203–1204
Chlorambucil, 501t
Chloramphenicol, spectrum of activity of,
    169t
Chloride ions, in cystic fibrosis, 2050
2-Chloroprocaine, 442t
Cholangiocarcinomas, 1018
Cholangiography. *See also* Endoscopic
    retrograde cholangiography
    (ERC)
  intraoperative, during cholecystectomy,
    1047
  transhepatic, percutaneous
    in bile duct cancer, 1061, 1061f
    in bile duct strictures, 1070, 1071f
    in choledocholithiasis, 1052
Cholangiohepatitis, bile duct strictures
    due to, 1080f, 1080–1081
Cholangiohepatocellular carcinoma, 1018
Cholangiopancreatography. *See*
    Endoscopic retrograde
    cholangiopancreatography
    (ERCP)
Cholangitis, primary sclerosing, 1077t,
    1077–1078, 1078f, 1079f
  hepatic transplantation for, 582–583
Cholecystectomy, 1044–1047
  bile duct injury during, 1067, 1068f,
    1069f
    immediate repair of, 1072
  delayed versus early, 1045–1047
  extended, for gallbladder cancer, 1059
  intraoperative cholangiography in,
    1047
  laparoscopic, 1045, 1045f, 1045t, 1046f
    for gallbladder cancer, 1060
  management of common bile duct
    stones found during, 1052f,
    1052–1054
  open, 1044t, 1044–1045, 1045t
  radical, for gallbladder cancer, 1059
Cholecystitis
  acute, 1043f, 1043–1044
    bacteriology of, 1044
    pathogenesis of, 1043–1044
    pathology of, 1044
  complications of, 1050–1051
  emphysematous, 1050
Cholecystocholedochal fistulas, 1051
Cholecystoenteric fistulas, 1050
Cholecystography
  cholecystokinin, in cholelithiasis, 1042
  oral, in cholelithiasis, 1041, 1041f

Cholecystokinin (CCK)
  biliary tract regulation by, 1030–1031
  small intestinal, 807
Cholecystokinin cholecystography, in
    cholelithiasis, 1042
Cholecystolitholysis, transhepatic,
    percutaneous, for cholelithiasis,
    1047–1048, 1048f
Choledochal cysts, 2090–2093
  anatomy of, 2090, 2090f, 2091f
  clinical presentation and diagnosis of,
    2092f, 2092–2093
  embryogenesis of, 2083
  treatment of, 2093, 2093f
    complications and results of, 2093,
    2093t
Choledochoceles, 2090
Choledochoduodenostomy
  for bile duct strictures, 1079–1080
  for choledocholithiasis, 1055
Choledochojejunostomy
  for bile duct cancer, 1062
  Roux-en-Y
    for bile duct strictures, 1079
    for choledocholithiasis, 1055
Choledocholithiasis, 1051–1055
  bile duct strictures due to, 1080
  clinical evaluation and diagnosis of,
    1051–1052
  in elderly patients, 1049
  incidence of, 1051
  management of
    recurrent stones and, 1055
    retained stones and, 1052f–1054f,
      1054t, 1054–1055
    stones found during cholecystectomy
      and, 1052f, 1052–1054
  natural history of, 1051
  in pancreatitis, 879–880, 881f
  pathogenesis and morphology of, 1051
Choledochoscopy, in choledocholithiasis,
    1053
Cholelithiasis, 1033–1055
  acalculous, 1048–1049
  asymptomatic, 1040–1041
  bile duct strictures due to, 1080
  biliary sludge and, 1040
  cancer associated with, 1057f, 1057–
    1058, 1058f
  cholesterol gallstones and, 1036–1039
    altered gallbladder absorption and,
      1039
    biliary calcium and, 1038–1039
    biliary prostaglandins and, 1039,
      1039f
    cholesterol saturation and, 1037,
      1037f
    cholesterol solubilization and, 1036f,
      1036–1037, 1037f
    gallbladder stasis and, 1038, 1039f
    normal bile composition and, 1036
    nucleation and mucus secretion and,
      1037–1038, 1038f
  in cirrhosis, 1049
  clinical features of, 1042–1044
    acute cholecystitis, 1043f, 1043–
      1044
    biliary colic, 1043, 1043f
    nonspecific symptoms, 1042–1043
  in diabetes mellitus, 1049
  diagnosis of, 1041–1042
  in elderly patients, 1049
  epidemiology of, 1034–1036

gallstone classification and, 1033–
    1034, 1034f
  following gastric surgery for morbid
    obesity, 793
  incidence of, 1034
  management of, 1044–1048
    biliary lithotripsy for, 1048
    cholangiography in, 1047
    cholecystectomy for. See
      Cholecystectomy
    contact dissolution for, 1047–1048,
      1048f
    medical dissolution for, 1047
    unresolved issues concerning, 1048
  pigment gallstones and, 1039–1040
    classification of, 1039–1040
    pathogenesis of, 1040
  total parenteral nutrition-induced,
    1049–1050
Cholescintigraphy, 666–670
Cholestasis, nonspecific, following
    hepatic transplantation, 591–592
Cholesterol
  atheroemboli and, 1630
  bile saturation with, 1037, 1037f
  biliary secretion of, 955
  metabolism of, hepatic, 951–952, 953f
  nucleation of, 1037–1038, 1038f
  solubilization of, 1036f, 1036–1037,
    1037f
Cholesterol gallstones. See Cholelithiasis
Cholesterolosis, 1056
Cholesterol polyps, 1056
Cholestyramine
  for Clostridium difficile colitis, 1178
  for hypercholesterolemia, 1711, 1712
Chondromas, of ribs, 1446
Chondrosarcomas, of ribs, 1447, 1447f
Chordoid sarcomas. See Sarcomas,
    tenosynovial
Choriocarcinomas, 2229, 2229f
Christmas factor deficiency, 93, 93f
  gene therapy for, 519
Chromaffin tumors. See
    Pheochromocytomas
Chromium, requirements in surgical
    patients, 62t
Chromocell system, adrenomedullary,
    1331
Chromosome 18q, allelic loss of, in
    colorectal cancer, 1130
Chronic lymphocytic leukemia (CLL),
    1275, 1276f
Chronic myelogenous leukemia (CML),
    1275
Chronic venous insufficiency (CVI),
    1939–1943, 1958–1965
  diagnosis of, 1960–1962
    invasive studies for, 1960–1962,
      1963f
    noninvasive studies for, 1960, 1961f,
      1962f
  management of, 1940–1941, 1941f,
      1942f, 1943, 1962–1965
    for primary venous incompetence,
      1962–1963, 1963f, 1964f, 1965
    for venous obstruction, 1965, 1965f
    for venous ulceration, 1965
  pathophysiology of, 1958–1960, 1959f,
      1960f
Chylomicron(s), atherosclerosis and, 1711
Chylomicron remnants, 946t
Chylothorax, 1461–1463, 1462f, 1462t

Chylous ascites, 1242–1243, 1969
Chyluria, 1969
Chymotrypsinogen, pancreatic secretion
    of, 866, 867
Cigarette smoking. See Smoking
Cimetidine, 764f
  for duodenal ulcers, 762, 763t, 764f
Cinefluoroscopy, 1739–1740
Circulation
  collateral. See Collateral circulation
  fetal, 1980, 1980f, 2022–2024, 2024f.
      See also Persistent pulmonary
      hypertension of the newborn
      (PPHN)
  monitoring, postoperative, 450–451
  in shock. See Shock, microcirculatory
      response to
  transitional, at birth, 1980–1981
  traumatic injuries and
    in elderly people, 388
    pediatric, 380t, 380–381
    prehospital care and, 281
    during resuscitation phase, 282
Circulatory support. See Intraaortic
    balloon pumps (IABPs);
    Mechanical circulatory support;
    Ventricular assist devices (VADs)
Circumcision, indications for, 2107
Cirrhosis, 972t, 972–977
  alcoholic, 974, 975
    hepatic transplantation for, 583
    natural history of, 976f, 976–977ic
  ascites in, 987–988, 988f
  biliary, 974
    primary, 975–976
  cardiac, 976
  cholelithiasis and, 1035, 1049
  clinical features of, 977, 977t
  etiology of, 974–976
    biliary duct obstruction in, 975–976
    chemical injury in, 975, 975f
    microbiologic injury in, 975
    venous outflow obstruction in, 976
  hepatocellular carcinoma associated
      with, 1015–1016
  histologic classification of, 973f, 973–
      974
  macronodular, 972–973, 973
  micronodular, 972
  morphologic classification of, 972–973,
      973f
  natural history of, 976f, 976–977
  pathogenesis of, 974, 974f
  portal hypertension and, 986
  portosystemic shunt surgery in, 1003
  postnecrotic, 974
  primary biliary, hepatic transplantation
      for, 582
  septal (trabecular), 973
  varices in. See Varices,
      gastroesophageal
  venoocclusive, 974
Cisplatin, 501t
c-jun oncogene, 477
Claudication
  in atherosclerosis, nonoperative
      treatment of, 1715–1718
    exercise training, 1715–1716, 1716t
    pharmacologic, 1716–1718
  calf, 1639
  intermittent, in infrainguinal occlusive
      disease, 1811–1812, 1812t, 1813
    evaluation of, 1814

Clavicle, tumors of, 1448
Clear cell sarcomas. *See also* Sarcomas,
    tenosynovial
  renal, pediatric, 2126–2127
Cleft lip and palate, plastic surgery for,
    2286–2287
Clindamycin
  for pelvic inflammatory disease, 2225t
  spectrum of activity of, 169t
Clinical research, in cancer, 491
Clinoril (sulindac)
  for desmoid tumors, 2262
  for familial adenomatous polyposis,
    1124
Cloacal abnormalities, 2116
Cloacogenic carcinomas, of anal canal,
    1149, 1150f
Clofibrate, for hypercholesterolemia, 1712
Clonal abortion, 547
Clonal anergy, 547
Clonal deletion, 547
Clonality, 464, 464f
Closing capacity, 1983
Clostridium difficile, colitis and. *See*
    Antibiotic-associated colitis
Clostridium sordellii-associated toxic
    shock syndrome (CATS), 2225
Clotrimazole, for monilial esophagitis,
    724
Cluster determinants (CDs), 529
Coagulation. *See also* Hemostasis
  disorders of. *See also specific disorders*
    in pancreatitis, 885
  extrinsic pathway of, 83–84, 84f, 85,
    85f
  hypothermia and, 411
  intrinsic pathway of, 84
  mechanisms of, 1613
Coagulation factors, deficiencies of, 92–
    94, 93f, 94f
Coagulation tests, 104
Coagulopathy
  intraoperative management of, for
    hepatic transplantation, 584–
    585, 585f
  in shock, 291
Coarctation of the aorta (COA), 1497–
    1498
Coccidioides immitis infections, 177
Codman triangles, in osteosarcomas, 2263
Codons, 22
Cogan syndrome, 1604
Cold-immersion foot, 412
Cold injury, 412–414
  treatment of, 413–414
Cold stress, infants and, 1979
Colectomy
  segmental, for diverticulitis, 1154–
    1155
  subtotal, for ulcerative colitis, 1100f,
    1100–1101
  transverse, right, 1138
Colestipol
  for *Clostridium difficile* colitis, 1178
  for hypercholesterolemia, 1711
Colic, biliary, in cholelithiasis, 1043,
    1043f
Colic artery, aneurysms of, 1893t, 1899f,
    1899–1900
Colitis
  antibiotic-associated. *See* Antibiotic-
    associated colitis
  indeterminate, 834

ulcerative. *See* Inflammatory bowel
    disease; Ulcerative colitis
Colitis cystica profunda, 1119
Collagen(s)
  abdominal aortic aneurysms and, 1882
  aneurysm formation and, 1843
  arterial compliance and, 1656
  mutation of, aneurysm formation and,
    1845
  in soft tissues, 2141–2142
  types of, 69, 71t
  wound healing and
    proliferative phase of, 68–69, 71f
    remodeling phase of, 70–71, 72f
Collagenases
  aneurysm formation and, 1843
  metastasis and, 483, 484t
  for wound care, 82
Collateral circulation
  arterial hemodynamics and, 1665
  in Buerger's disease, 1598, 1599f
  infrainguinal, 1811, 1812f
  pelvic, 2217
  portosystemic, in portal hypertension,
    985, 985f
  visceral, 1767, 1769f–1770f
Collis gastroplasty, 692
Colloid(s), in shock, 288–289
Colloid oncotic pressure, 244
Coloanal anastomosis, for colorectal
    cancer, 1138, 1141, 1141f, 1142f
Colon. *See also* Colorectal *entries*
  anatomy of, 1083–1086
    epithelium and, 1083, 1085
    general considerations in, 1083,
      1084f–1086f
    muscular structure of colonic wall
      and, 1085
    neural components and, 1085–1086
  defecation and, 1089–1090
  epithelial transport in, 1089, 1089f
  free tissue transfer of, 2285–2286
  motor function of
    contractile electrical complex and,
      1087
    dysfunction of, 1090t, 1090–1091.
      See also Constipation; Diarrhea
    postoperative, 1092
    electric control activity and, 1087
    giant migrating contractions and,
      1087
    individual phasic contractions and,
      1087
    neurohumeral control of, 1087–1088
    physiology of, 1086–1087
      alterations in, 1088–1089
Colon bypass, for esophageal cancer, 706
Colonic disorders. *See also specific
    disorders*
  angiodysplasia of right colon, 1153
  cancer. *See* Colorectal cancer
  diverticulitis of ascending colon,
    1156–1157
  diverticulosis, 1091, 1091f
    hemorrhage in, 1167, 1168
  giant colonic diverticulum, 1157, 1157f
  irritable colon syndrome, 1091–1092
  perforation, in ulcerative colitis, 1099
  pseudoobstruction, 829, 1092f, 1092–
    1093
  traumatic injuries, 351–352
  vascular ectasia, hemorrhage in, 1167,
    1168–1170, 1169f

Colonic inertia, 1090
Colonization resistance, 160
Colonoscopy
  in *Clostridium difficile* colitis, 1176
  in colorectal adenomas, 1115–1116
  in colorectal cancer, 1133
  in gastrointestinal hemorrhage, 1160–
    1161
  in ulcerative colitis, 1096
  in vascular ectasia, 1169
Colorectal cancer, 1128–1145
  adenocarcinomas
    clinical risk factors for, 1131–1132
      familial, 1131, 1131t
      inflammatory bowel disease, 1131
      polyps, 1131–1132, 1132f, 1132t
    diagnosis of, 1132–1134
      screening and, 1133–1134
      symptoms and, 1132
      tests in, 1132–1133, 1133f
    epidemiology of, 1128, 1128f
    etiology of, 1128–1131
      dietary factors in, 1128–1129,
        1129f
      molecular genetics and, 1129–
        1131, 1130f
      mutagenesis in, 1129
    metastatic, to liver, 1019–1020,
      1020f, 1021t
    primary, treatment of, 1137–1144
      adjuvant chemotherapy for, 1142–
        1144, 1143f
      adjuvant immunotherapy for, 1144
      adjuvant radiotherapy for, 1141–
        1142
      of intraperitoneal colon and upper
        third of rectum, 1138, 1140f
      invasive cancers, 1137–1141,
        1139f
      of middle and lower third of
        rectum, 1138, 1140, 1140f–
        1142f, 1141
      neoplastic polyps and, 1137
    recurrent, treatment of, 1144t, 1144–
      1145
      disseminated disease and, 1145
      hepatic metastases and, 1144,
        1145f
      local recurrence and, 1144
      pulmonary metastases and, 1144
    staging of, 1134–1137
      Dukes classification for, 1134,
        1134f, 1136t
      modified Astler-Coller staging
        system for, 1134, 1134f, 1135f,
        1135t, 1136t
      natural history and, 1135–1137,
        1137f
      pathology and, 1134
      prognostic factors and, 1135, 1136t
      TNM classification for, 1135, 1136t
  adenomas, 1114–1117
    diagnosis of, 1115
    management of, 1115–1116
    primary prevention of recurrence of,
      1116–1117
    serrated, 1118
  carcinoid tumors, 1119–1120, 1145
  genetics of, 461, 481, 482f
  hereditary nonpolyposis. *See*
    Hereditary nonpolyposis
    colorectal cancer (HNPCC)
  lymphomas, 1145

Colorectal cancer (*continued*)
  perforated, diverticulitis versus, 1153
  in Peutz-Jeghers syndrome, 1126
  polyps and. *See* Colorectal polyps,
    mucosal, neoplastic
  sarcomas, 1145
  in ulcerative colitis, prophylaxis of,
    1099
Colorectal polyps, 1109–1127
  classification of, 1109t, 1109–1110
  mucosal, neoplastic, 1110–1117, 1131–
    1132, 1132f, 1132t
    adenomas associated with, 1114–
      1117, 1132, 1132t
      diagnosis of, 1115
      management of, 1114–1115
      primary prevention of recurrence
        of, 1116–1117
    clinical features of, 1114
    epidemiology of, 1111–1114
      anatomic distribution and, 1111
      associated disease states and, 1114
      heredity and, 1111–1112
      natural history and, 1112–1114
      prevalence and, 1111
    histopathology and malignant
      potential of, 1111, 1112f–1114f
    management of, 1116, 1117f, 1137
    pathogenesis of, 1110–1111
      abnormal proliferation and, 1111
      molecular biology of, 1110f, 1110–
        1111
  mucosal, nonneoplastic, 1117–1118
    hyperplastic, 1117–1118, 1118f
    inflammatory, 1118, 1119f
    juvenile (retention), 1118
  pedunculated, 1109
  polyposis syndromes and, 1120–1127,
    1131, 1131t. *See also specific*
    syndromes
  sessile, 1109
  submucosal, 1118–1120, 1119f
Colostomy
  for colonic and rectal injuries, 352
  diverting, for anorectal malformations,
    2045
  for soft tissue infections, necrotizing, 174
Colovaginal fistulas, in diverticular
    disease, diagnosis and treatment
    of, 1156
Colovesical fistulas, in diverticular
    disease, diagnosis and treatment
    of, 1156
Colposacropexy, for vaginal vault
    prolapse, 2221
Colposcopy, for vaginal intraepithelial
    neoplasia, 2220
Colubridae. *See* Bites and stings
Combined segment disease, aortoiliac,
    1799
Comminuted skull fractures, 2166
Commissurotomy, mitral, 1519
Common bile duct
  anatomy of, 1026–1027
  stones in. *See* Choledocholithiasis
Common hepatic duct, anatomy of, 1026,
    1028f
Communicating hydrocephalus, 2193
Compartment excision, for sarcomas,
    2255, 2257f
Compartment syndromes, 1640–1642,
    1642f
  abdominal, in shock, 208

following burns, 427
intraabdominal, posttraumatic, 400
in lower extremities, 1642
orthopedic injuries and, 375
posttraumatic, 401
following snake bites, 404
in upper extremities, 1642
following vascular injuries, 365, 365f
Compensatory mechanisms
  loss of, in shock, 286
  in metabolic acidosis, 263
  in metabolic alkalosis, 264, 264t
  in respiratory acidosis, 265
  in respiratory alkalosis, 265
Competitive inhibitors, 439
Complement
  humoral defenses and, 163
  inflammation and, 132–135, 135f
    alternative complement pathway
      and, 134
    C3 and bacterial opsonization and,
      134–135, 136f
    classic complement pathway and,
      134
  in shock, 193
Compliance, of lungs, 1984
Computed tomography (CT)
  in abdominal aortic aneurysms, 1884,
    1885f
  in abdominal injuries, 335
    pediatric, 382, 383t
  in adrenal disorders, 1342–1343, 1343f
  in appendicitis, 1255f, 1255–1256,
    1256f
  in arteriovenous fistulas, 1922
  in brain hemorrhage, 2185, 2185f
  in bronchiectasis, 1480, 1480f
  in cerebrovascular disease, 1752
  in chronic pancreatitis, 892, 893f
  in congenital cystic disease of lung,
    2007, 2008f
  in degenerative spine disease
    cervical, 2187, 2187f
    lumbar, 2188, 2189f
  in duodenal injuries, 345
  esophageal, 658, 660f, 661f
    in esophageal cancer, 703
  in gastric adenocarcinomas, 797–798,
    799f
  in hernias, 1217
  in hyperparathyroidism, 1322
  in intestinal obstruction, 822–823
  in intracranial arteriovenous
    malformations, contrast-
    enhanced, 2183, 2184f
  of liver, 935, 937
    in hepatoblastomas, pediatric, 2135,
      2136f
    in hepatocellular carcinomas,
      pediatric, 2135, 2136f
    in liver masses, 1009, 1010f
  in maxillofacial injuries, 302, 304f
  in osteosarcomas, 2263
  in pancreatic cancer, 906t, 906–907,
    907f
  in pancreatic injuries, 350
  in pancreatic neoplastic disease, 918–
    919, 919f, 920f
  in pancreatitis, 883
  in pericardial disease, 1575
  of pituitary gland and parasellar
    region, 1350
  in renal injuries, 357, 357f

in sarcomas, 2252–2253
in small intestinal injuries, 351
in thoracoabdominal aortic aneurysms,
  1876, 1876f
of thyroid gland, 1294
tracheal, 1473, 1474f
in traumatic injuries, in pregnancy, 393
in vascular disorders, 1669, 1670f
in vascular infections, 1725, 1725f
in Wilms tumor, 2124, 2124f
Computed tomography angiography,
  helical, 1679, 1680f
Computed tomography angioportography
  (CTAP), in liver masses, 1009
Condensing vacuoles, 31
Conduction, heat transfer by, 1979
Condylomata acuminata, anal, 1202–
  1203
Congenital adrenal hyperplasia, 1337,
  1337f, 1341, 2112, 2112f–2114f
Congenital heart disease, 1483–1500
  aortic stenosis, 1487f, 1487–1488
  atrial septal defects, 1483–1484, 1484f
  atrioventricular septal defect, 1483,
    1496–1497
  coarctation of aorta, 1497–1498
  coronary artery anomalies, 1495–1496
  double-outlet right ventricle, 1493–
    1494
  hyperplastic left heart syndrome, 1500,
    1501f
  patent ductus arteriosus, 1496
  tetralogy of Fallot, 1488–1490, 1489f
  transposition of the great arteries,
    1490f–1493f, 1490–1491, 1493
  truncus arteriosus, 1494f, 1494–1495
  univentricular heart, 1498–1499, 1499f
  ventricular septal defects, 1485f, 1485–
    1487
Congenital hypertrophy of retinal
    pigmented epithelium (CHRPE),
    in familial adenomatous
    polyposis, 1120
Congenital malformations. *See specific*
    organs and malformations
Congenital nevi, melanomas and, 2232
Congenital vascular malformations
    (CVMs), 1924–1932
  etiology of, 1925
  signs and symptoms of, 1925–1928,
    1929f–1932f
    cutaneous, 1925–1926, 1926f–1928f
  treatment of, 1928–1930, 1932, 1932f
Congestive heart failure (CHF), 1505–
    1509
  anesthesia and, 443, 444, 444t
  backward, 1507
  forward, 1507
  medical management of, 1516–1517
  myocardial failure in, 1507f, 1507–
    1509, 1508f
    peripheral manifestations of, 1508–
      1509
Conjoined area, 1211
Conjoined tendons, 1211
Connective tissue(s), 2141. *See also*
    specific tissues
  functional morphology of, 2141–2142
Connective tissue disease, pericarditis in,
    1577
Connexins, 10
Connexons, 10
Consent, for organ donation, 562–563

Constipation, 1090, 1090t
  idiopathic, chronic, 1090
  slow transit, 1090
Contact dissolution, for cholelithiasis, 1047–1048, 1048f
Continence, anal, mechanism of, 1187
Continuous arteriovenous hemofiltration (CAVH), for critically ill patients, 238t, 238–239
Continuous arteriovenous rewarming, 412
Continuous positive airway pressure (CPAP), 1986
Contraceptives, oral, thrombosis associated with, 1618
Contractile electrical complex, colonic, 1087
Contractions, colonic. See Colon, motor function of
Contractures
  Dupuytren, 2160
  following lower extremity amputation, 1836
Contrast media
  for angiography, 1680, 1682f
  nephrotoxicity of, 235–236
Controlled ventilation, 1986
Convection, heat transfer by, 1979
Convexity meningiomas, 2174
Cooley anemia, 1268
Cooper ligaments, 1211, 1360
  repair of, for inguinal and femoral hernias, 1222, 1224f
Copper
  hepatic metabolism of, 957
  requirements in surgical patients, 62t
  wound healing and, 78
Copperhead bites. See Bites and stings
COPs, 29
Coral snake bites. See Bites and stings
Cordotomy, for pain management, 2195
Core needle biopsies
  of breast masses, 1369
  of sarcomas, 2251
Corkscrew collaterals, 1598, 1599f
Corkscrew esophagus, 679, 679f
Coronary artery bypass grafting (CABG), 1543–1548
  cardiac transplantation versus, 1549
  cooperative studies of, 1548–1549
  indications for, 1543t, 1543–1544
  long-term outcomes of, 1548
  postoperative management and, 1545–1547
    bleeding and, 1546
    infection and, 1547
    low cardiac output and, 1546
    postpericardiotomy syndrome and, 1547
    stroke and, 1547
    tamponade and, 1546–1547
  reoperative, 1548
  risk factors for operative mortality and, 1547t, 1547–1548
  surgical technique for, 1544–1545, 1545f, 1546f
  for ventricular arrhythmias, 1569
Coronary artery disease (CAD), 1534–1549
  with abdominal aortic aneurysms, evaluation for, 1887–1888
  acute myocardial infarction and. See Myocardial infarction (MI), acute

anesthesia and, 443–444, 444t
atherosclerosis and, Aee Atherosclerosis
blood flow and, 1535–1536
  metabolic regulation of, 1536
  physical regulation of, 1536
cardiac transplantation for, coronary artery bypass grafting versus, 1549
clinical presentation of, 1538f, 1538–1539
coronary artery bypass grafting for. See Coronary artery bypass grafting (CABG)
coronary veins and, 1535
diagnosis of, 1539
medical management of, 1539
percutaneous transluminal coronary angioplasty for. See Percutaneous transluminal coronary angioplasty (PCTA)
Coronary artery disorders, 1534–1535, 1535f. See also specific disorders
anomalies of, 1495–1496
atheroembolism of, 1633
Coronary Artery Surgery Study, 1549
Coronary blood flow, 1535–1536
  metabolic regulation of, 1536
  physical regulation of, 1536
Coronary veins, 1535
Corpus luteum cysts, 2226
Corticospinal tracts, 2186
Corticosteroids, 1331. See also specific drugs
  for Crohn's disease, 839–840, 840f
  for infections, 180
Corticotropin-releasing hormone (CRH), 1331–1332
  determining cause of hypercortisolism and, 1340
Cortisol, 1335–1336
  excess of. See Hypercortisolism
  normal effects of, 1335–1336
  secretion of, control of, 1331–1332, 1334f
  in shock, 187–188
  surgical stress response and, 52–53
Cortisone acetate, for hypercortisolism, 1344
Cottonmouth bites. See Bites and stings
Counseling, for breast cancer patients, 1399
Countertransporter, 15–16, 16f
Cowden syndrome, 1127
Cranial dysraphism, 2192–2193
Cranial nerves. See also specific nerves
  injuries of, carotid endarterectomy and, 1755
  neurosurgical pain management and, 2195
Cranial sutures, premature closure of, 2194
Craniopharyngiomas, 2177–2178, 2179f
Craniosynostosis, 2194
C-reactive protein, during acute-phase reaction, 132, 132t
Creatine kinase, in myocardial infarction, 1540
Cricothyroidotomy, 1476–1478, 1479f
  in traumatic injuries, pediatric, 380
Critical care, 215–240. See also Traumatic injuries; specific injuries

acute renal failure and, 234–239, 235t
blood volume and hemodynamics and, 225–227
metabolism and nutrition and, 227, 229–234
multiple organ failure and, 239t, 239–240
oxygen kinetics in, 215–218
for pregnant patients, 394
respiratory physiology and pathology and, 218–225
for traumatic injuries
  in elderly people, 389
  pediatric, 385
Critical Reynolds number, 1662
Crohn's disease, 831–843. See also Inflammatory bowel disease
anal fissures in, 1195–1196
anal fistulas in, 1199
colorectal cancer and, 1131
complications of, 836t, 836–837, 837f
definition of, 831
diagnosis of, 837–838
differential diagnosis of, 838, 839t
in elderly patients, 843
epidemiology of, 831
immunogenetic causes of, 832f, 832–833, 833f
infectious causes of, 832
intestinal obstruction and, 826–827
medical management of, 838–843
  for abdominal pain, 838
  for diarrhea, 838
  drug therapy in, 839–840, 840f
  nutritional therapy in, 838–839
pathology of, 833–836
  clinical features, 834–836, 835t, 836t
  macroscopic appearance, 833–834, 834f
  microscopic features, 834, 834f, 835t
pediatric, 843
in pregnancy, 843
surgical treatment of, 841–843
  in colonic disease, 842
  fistulas and abscesses and, 841–842
  in perianal disease, 842–843
  preoperative preparation for, 841
  recurrence and, 842
  strictures and, 842
  technical aspects of, 841
ulcerative colitis versus, 1096, 1097t
Cronkhite-Canada syndrome, 1127, 1127f
Crossmatching, for organ transplantation, 554, 554f
  positive crossmatch and, 542
Crotalidae. See Bites and stings
Crotalus. See Bites and stings
Croton oil, tumors caused by, 462
Crouzon disease, 2194
Cryotherapy, for prostate cancer, 2211–2212
Cryptococcus neoformans infections, 177
Cryptorchidism, 2204
Crypts of Lieberkühn, 807
Crystalloids, in shock, 288, 289
Cultures
  in Clostridium difficile colitis, 1176
  for human immunodeficiency virus detection, 178t
  microbiological, culture and sensitivity determinations and, 166t, 166–167

Cultures (*continued*)
  mixed lymphocyte, for organ
      transplantation, 554
  techniques for, 166
Cushing syndrome. *See* Hypercortisolism
Cushing ulcers, 777
Cutaneous neoplasms, 2231–2245. *See
      also specific neoplasms*
C-X-C chemokines
  angiogenesis and, 121, 122f
  leukocyte-endothelial cell interactions
      and, 119, 119t
Cyanide, inhalation of, burns and, 433–
      434
Cyanosis
  in tetralogy of Fallot, 1489
  in transposition of the great arteries,
      1490
Cyclic adenosine monophosphate
      (cAMP), as intracellular
      messenger, 39f, 39–40, 40f
Cyclooxygenase, in inflammation, 138
Cyclophosphamide, 501t
  for neuroblastomas, pediatric, 2122
  for peripheral primitive
      neuroectodermal tumors,
      pediatric, 2133
Cyclosporine (CsA; Sandimmune), 548,
      549t
  for cardiac transplantation, 602, 602t
  for Crohn's disease, 841
  for hepatic transplantation, 598
  for pulmonary transplantation, 612
  for renal transplantation, 577
  for ulcerative colitis, 1098
Cylindromas, of salivary glands, 641
Cyst(s)
  adventitial, 1601–1602, 1602f
      of popliteal artery, 1640, 1641f
  branchial cleft remnant-derived, 1995–
      1998
      anatomy and embryology of, 1995,
          1995f, 1996f
      clinical issues in, 1996
      operative considerations and
          outcome of, 1996–1998, 1997f,
          1998f
  of breast, 1373
  bronchogenic, 1471, 1471f
      congenital, 2006, 2007f
  choledochal. *See* Choledochal cysts
  corpus luteum, 2226
  enteric (duplication; enterogenous),
      1471, 1471f, 2074–2075, 2075f
      in pediatric patients, 2009
  esophageal, 698, 699f
  follicular, 2226
  ganglion, 2161–2162
  hepatic. *See* Hepatic cysts
  inclusion, of hands, 2162
  of lung, congenital. *See* Pulmonary
      disorders, congenital cystic
      disease
  lymphocysts, 1969
  mesenteric, 1240–1241, 2075–2076,
      2076f
  of nipples, 1378
  omental, 1241, 2075–2076, 2076f
  pancreatic pseudocysts, 886f, 886–887,
      887f
      following pancreatic injuries, 349
      pediatric, 2096–2097
  pericardial, 1471
      in pediatric patients, 2009

pleural, 1463
Rathke, 1355
renal, pediatric, 2102–2103
  multicystic, 2102–2103
  polycystic, 2103
retention, pancreatic, pediatric, 2097
splenic, 1275–1276, 1276f
theca-lutein, 2226
thymic, in pediatric patients, 2008–
    2009
thyroglossal duct, 1283, 1998–1999
  anatomy and embryology of, 1998,
      1998f
  clinical issues in, 1998
  operative considerations and
      outcome of, 1998–1999
Cystadenocarcinomas
  of appendix, 1260
  pancreatic, 916, 916f
Cystadenomas
  mucinous
      of appendix, 1260
      pancreatic, 916
  ovarian, 2226
  serous, pancreatic, 915–916, 916f
Cystathionine synthase deficiency, 1606–
    1607, 1616
Cystectomy, radical, for bladder cancer,
    2207
Cystic adenomatoid malformations
    (CAMs), congenital, 2005, 2005f
Cystic duct
  anatomy of, 1026, 1029f
  histology and ultrastructure of, 1029
  stones in, 1050–1051
Cysticercosis, neurologic, 2191
Cystic fibrosis
  diagnosis of, 2050
  gene therapy for, 514–515, 516f, 522
  meconium ileus and, 2049–2050
  pathophysiology of, 2050, 2050f
Cystic fibrosis transmembrane
    conductance regulator (CFTR)
    gene, 514–515, 516f
Cystic hygromas, 1966
  of head and neck, 1999
      anatomy and embryology of, 1999,
          1999f
      clinical issues in, 1999
      operative considerations and
          outcome of, 1999
  mediastinal, 2009
Cystic medial necrosis, 1599–1600
Cystic teratomas
  ovarian, 2226, 2227f
  in pediatric patients, 2009
Cystometry, screening, for vaginal
    prolapse, 2220
Cystoprostatectomy, for bladder cancer,
    2207
Cystoreduction, abdominal, 2228
Cystosarcoma phyllodes, 1407
  clinical presentation of, 1407
  management of, 1407
  pathology of, 1407, 1408f
Cytochromes P-450
  hepatic biotransformation and, 956
  pediatric, 1990
Cytokines, 108–126, 109f, 110f, 110t. *See
    also specific cytokines*
  antigen recognition and, 538, 539t,
      540f, 540–541
  bone formation and, 2152

host defenses and, 163–165, 164f
inflammation and, 109–119, 110f, 111f,
    132, 133t
multiple organ system failure and, 110t
organ preservation injury and, 559
priming of neutrophil function by, 147,
    148f
production of, 109
receptors for, antigen recognition and,
    538, 539t, 540f, 540–541
recombinant, for cancer, 503–504,
    510t, 510–511, 511f
surgical stress response and, 50–52,
    51f
ulcerative colitis and, 1094–1095
wound healing and, 119–126, 120f,
    121f, 121t. *See also specific
    cytokines*
  angiogenesis and, 120–121, 122f
  fibroblasts and. *See* Fibroblast(s),
      cytokines and
Cytokine syndrome, 550t, 551
Cytomegalovirus (CMV) infections, 177–
    178
  anorectal, in HIV-positive patients,
      1204
  immunosuppression and, 552
  following pulmonary transplantation,
      613
  transmission of, by blood transfusions,
      105
Cytoplasm, 5
Cytosine arabinoside, 501t
Cytoskeleton, 6–9
  actin-based filaments of, 6–7, 7f
  intermediate filaments of, 7–8, 8f
  microtubules of, 8f, 8–9, 9f
Cytosol, composition of, 11, 11f
Cytoxan, 549t

D

Dacarbazine, 501t
Damus-Kaye-Stanzel operation
  for double-outlet right ventricle, 1494
  modified, for univentricular heart, 1499
Danazol, for mastodynia, 1372–1373
Dandy-Walker malformation, 2193
Dapsone, for spider bites, 407
Daunorubicin, 502t
Dead-space ventilation, 1984
Death. *See* Mortality
Débriding agents, 82
Declamping hypotension, following
      abdominal aortic aneurysm
      repair, 1889
Decompression, surgical, for acute
      epidural or subdural hematomas,
      297–298, 298f
Decompressive procedures, for peripheral
      nerve compression, 2197
Decortication, for thoracic empyema,
      1457–1458
Decubitus ulcers, healing of, 80
Deep brain electrodes, for pain
      management, 2195
Deep groin dissection, 2239–2240, 2240f
Deep postanal space, anatomy of, 1182,
      1183f
Deep venous thrombosis (DVT), 1944–
      1951
  diagnosis of, 1946–1948

Duplex studies for, 1947, 1947f, 1948f
fibrin and fibrinogen product assays for, 1948
impedance plethysmography for, 1947–1948
radionuclide scanning for, 1948
venography for, 1946f, 1946–1947
etiology and pathogenesis of, 1944–1946, 1945f
following lower extremity amputation, 1837
posttraumatic, 399
in elderly people, 389
prophylaxis of, 1948–1949
mechanical measures for, 103
thrombolytic therapy for, indications for, 101
treatment of, 1949–1950
anticoagulation for, 1949
fibrinolysis for, 1949–1950
surgical, 1950f, 1950–1951
Defecation
anorectum and, 87088
colon and, 1089–1090
Degenerative aneurysms, 1863f, 1863–1866
operative management of, 1864, 1864f, 1865f, 1866
Degenerative joint disease
of hand, 2159
in morbid obesity, 790
Degenerative spinal disease. See Spine, degenerative disease of
Dehydration
hypertonic, 253, 253f
hypotonic, 253, 253f
isotonic, 253, 253f
Delorme procedure, modified, for rectal prolapse, 1191, 1195f
Delphian lymph nodes, 1284
Deltopectoral flaps, 2281
Denis Brown, superficial pouch of, 2109
Depressed skull fractures, 2166, 2166f
De Quervain stenosing tenosynovitis, 2158
De Quervain thyroiditis, 1298–1299
Dermal analogues, for burns, 437
Dermoid tumors
intracranial, 2178
ovarian, 2226, 2227f
spinal, 2180
Desmoid tumors
of abdominal wall, 1237
in familial adenomatous polyposis, 1120
mesenteric, 1240
treatment of, 2261–2262
Desmoplastic small round cell tumors, pediatric, 2133
Desmopressin acetate, 99
Desmosomes, 10
Devascularization, procedures, for varices, 1005
Dexamethasone test, high-dose, for hypercortisolism, 1340, 1340f
Dextran, 102–103
in shock, 288
Diabetes insipidus, pediatric, 1989
Diabetes mellitus, 615–617
atherosclerosis and, 1536, 1714t, 1714–1715, 1715t
treatment results and, 1714–1715

cholelithiasis and, 1035, 1049
extremity reconstruction in, 2288, 2288t
foot ulcers in, healing of, 80
gene therapy for, 521–522
infections in, lower extremity amputations and, 1824–1825
insulin-dependent (type I), 615–616
islet transplantation for, 625f, 626f, 626–627
late complications of, 616
in morbid obesity, 790
pancreatic transplantation for. See Pancreatic transplantation
pathogenesis of, 616, 616f
prevalence and incidence of, 616
secondary complications of, pathogenesis of, 616–617
wound healing in, 79
of foot ulcers, 80
Diabetic ketoacidosis (DKA), treatment of, 263–264
Diacylglycerol, as intracellular messenger, 41f, 41–42
Diagnostic peritoneal lavage (DPL), 284, 335t, 335–336, 336f
pediatric, 382, 383t
in pelvic fractures, 353, 355f
in pregnancy, 393
in small intestinal injuries, 350, 351
Dialysis
hemodialysis
arteriovenous fistulas for, 1923–1924
for critically ill patients, 237–238, 238t
peritoneal, for critically ill patients, 238, 238t
Diapedesis, transalveolar, myocardial failure and, 1509
Diaphragm
congenital abnormalities of, 2019–2027
anatomy and, 2020, 2021f
Bochdalek hernias. See Bochdalek hernias
embryology of, 2019f, 2019–2020, 2020f
eventration, 2027
Morgagni hernias, 2027
pelvic, 1213, 1215, 1215f
rupture of, transection of, 284
traumatic injuries of, 337, 337f
pediatric, 381
Diarrhea
in Crohn's disease, 835
treatment of, 838
mechanisms causing, 1090–1091
ulcerative colitis and. See Ulcerative colitis
Diazepam (Valium), 442t
Diazoxide, for nesidioblastosis, pediatric, 2098
Diet. See also Nutrition
colorectal cancer and, 1128–1129, 1129f
for gastric ulcers, 785
for morbid obesity, 790
Diet-induced thermogenesis, 1974
Dieulafoy vascular malformations, 1170
Diffuse esophageal spasm (DES), 677, 679, 679f
Diffusion, 1984
Difluorodeoxycytidine, 501t
Digestion, in small intestine. See Small

intestine, digestion and absorption in
Digital angiography, 1678–1679
Digitalis glycosides, for congestive heart failure, 1517
Digital nerves, disorders of, 2156
Dilaudid, for patient-controlled analgesia, 454t
D-Dimer fragment, 85–86
Dimethadione (DMO) test, 871–872
Dionosil Oily, for thoracic empyema, 1457
Dioxin, soft tissue sarcomas and, 2247
Dipyridamole (Persantine), as antiplatelet agent, 98
Direct immunobead test, in male infertility, 2203
Disc disease, spinal. See Spine, degenerative disease of
Discectomy, for cervical spine disease, 2188
Discomfort, cytokine-induced, 52
Disintegrins, 99
Dislocations
of hand, 2159
with potential for neurovascular compromise, 375
Disodium etidronate, for hypercalcemia, 1315
Dissecting aneurysms, of renal artery. See Aneurysm(s), of renal artery
Dissections, arterial
angiography in, 1695f, 1695–1697, 1696f
aortic. See Thoracic aortic aneurysms, dissections
Disseminated intravascular coagulation (DIC), 92
Diuretics. See also specific drugs
for ascites, 989
thiazide, hypercalcemia and, 1315
Diversity (D) regions, 528
Diverticular disease, 1151–1157
of cecum, 1156–1157
clinical presentation and differential diagnosis of, 1152–1153
in diverticulitis, 1152–1153
in diverticulosis, 1152, 1153f
hemorrhage and, 1153, 1154f
obstruction and, 1153
colonic, 1091, 1091f, 1156–1157
diverticulosis, hemorrhage in, 1167, 1168
perforated colon cancer versus, 1153
diagnosis and therapy of, 1153–1156
for diverticulitis, 1154–1155, 1155f
for diverticulosis, 1153
for fistulas, 1156
for obstruction, 1155–1156
diverticulitis, 1151, 1156–1157
in Meckel's diverticulum, 2070–2071
diverticulosis, 1091, 1091f, 1151
esophageal. See Esophageal diverticula; Zenker diverticula
giant colonic diverticulum, 1157, 1157f
giant diverticulum, 2074–2075, 2075f
Meckel's diverticulum. See Meckel's diverticulum
pathologic anatomy of, 1152, 1152f
pathophysiology of, 1152
peridiverticulitis, 1151
small intestinal, 1171

DNA
  recombinant. *See* Gene therapy
  structure of, 22, 23f
  synthesis of, 22–23, 24f
  transcription of, 23, 24f
DNA amplification, 471, 472f, 472t
DNA footprinting, 35
DNA ploidy, in papillary thyroid
    carcinomas, 1302–1303
DNA-protein complexes, for hepatic
    disorders, 516
DNA tumor viruses, 470
Dobutamine
  for congestive heart failure, 1517
  for shock, 205
Docetaxel (Taxotere), 502t
Docking proteins, 26–27
Dolicho et mega-artere, 1601, 1601f
Dopamine
  for congestive heart failure, 1517
  for shock, 205
Doppler effect, 1751–1752
Doppler studies, 1668, 1668f, 1673
  in chronic venous insufficiency, 1960,
      1962f
  color-coded flow mapping, 1673
  in congenital vascular malformations,
      1926–1927
  laser, 1673
  in valvular heart disease, 1514
  in vascular injuries, 362
  in vascular occlusive disease
    cerebrovascular, 1752
    of upper extremities, 1759–1760
Dorsal nerve roots, 2186
Dorsal root entry zone (DREZ) lesions, for
    pain management, 2195, 2196f
Double-outlet right ventricle (DORV),
    1493–1494
Down-regulation, 1338
  of receptors, 33–34
Doxacurium, 440t
Doxorubicin, 502t
  for neuroblastomas, pediatric, 2122
  for sarcomas, 2259
  for Wilms tumor, 2126
Doxycycline
  for chlamydial proctitis, 1203
  for gonococcal proctitis, 1203
  for pelvic inflammatory disease, 2225t
Drainage. *See also* Chest tubes
  for lung abscesses, 1479
  for maxillofacial repairs, 305
  pancreatic, following traumatic
      injuries, 347–348, 349f
  pericardial, 1582
  of pilonidal sinuses, 1199
  thoracoscopic, for chylothorax, 1463
  of tuboovarian abscesses, 2225
Dressings
  occlusive, for chronic venous
      insufficiency, 1940
  for open wounds, 77–78
  types of, 80–81, 81t
Dressler syndrome, 1576
Drop attacks, 1751
Drug(s). *See also specific drugs and drug
      types*
  metabolic acidosis due to, 262
  nephrotoxic, 235–236
  pancreatitis and, 881
  during pregnancy, 394
  radiation sensitizing, 493, 493f

Duct(s) of Luschka, 1029
Ductography, of breasts, 1365, 1366f
Ductus diverticulum, aneurysms of, 1873
Duhamel procedure, Martin modification
    of, 2061, 2062f
Dukes classification, for colorectal
    cancer, 1134, 1134f, 1136t
Dumbbell neurogenic tumors,
    mediastinal, 1468f, 1468–1469
Dumping syndrome, following
    gastrectomy, 772
Duodenal drainage studies, in
    cholelithiasis, 1042
Duodenal ulcers, 759–773
  bleeding from, 1162
  diagnosis of, 761
  drug treatment of, 761–766, 762f, 763f,
      763t
    antacids in, 765
    antibiotics in, 765–766
    anticholinergic drugs in, 763–764
    histamine-receptor antagonists in,
        761–763, 764f
    prostaglandin analogues in, 765, 765f
    proton-pump blockers in, 764
    sucralfate in, 764–765
  epidemiology of, 759
  hemorrhage and, 769–770
  intractable, 769, 769t
  obstruction due to, 770–771, 771f
  operative treatment of, 766–769
    goals of, 766
    operative procedures for, 766f–768f,
        766–768
    physiologic consequences of, 768t,
        768–769
  pathophysiology of, 759t, 759–761
    acid secretory status and, 760
    environmental factors and, 759–760
    Helicobacter pylori and, 760
    mucosal defense against peptic
        injury and, 760–761
  perforation of, 770, 771f
  postgastrectomy syndromes and, 771–
      773
    alkaline reflux gastritis, 772f, 773
    dumping, 772
Duodenoduodenostomy, for duodenal
    atresia/stenosis, 2040f, 2040–
    2041
Duodenogastric reflux, gastric ulcers and,
    782–783
Duodenum. *See also specific disorders*
  gross anatomy of, 805–806, 806f
  mucosal defenses of, 760–761
  obstruction of
    neonatal. *See* Intestinal atresia/
        stenosis, duodenal
    in pancreatic cancer, palliative
        treatment for, 914
    pancreatitis and, 882
  traumatic injuries of, 343–346
    blunt, 345–346
    penetrating, 343f–346f, 343–345
Duplex scanning, 1668
  in arteriovenous fistulas, 1922
  in cerebrovascular disease, 1752
  in chronic venous insufficiency, 1960,
      1962f
  in deep venous thrombosis, 1947,
      1947f, 1948f
  in vascular injuries, 362–363
Duplication(s)

gastrointestinal, 1471, 1471f, 2074–
    2075
  cystic, 2074–2075, 2075f
  in pediatric patients, 2009
  tubular, 2075, 2075f
  ureteral, 2104f, 2104–2105
  uterine, 2117, 2117f
Dupuytren contractures, 2160
Dust, tumors caused by, 462
Dye injection, for lymphatic
    visualization, 1967–1968
Dynamic compliance, 1984
Dysfibrinogenemia, 1616
Dysphagia
  in esophageal cancer, 702
  in gastroesophageal reflux disease, 681
  nonobstructive, diagnosis of, 665
  sideropenic, 705, 705f
Dysplasia, 459
  colorectal polyps and, 1111, 1114f
  fibromuscular, 1597, 1597f, 1598f, 1748
  fibrous, of ribs, 1446, 1446f
Dysplastic nevi
  genetic factors in, 460–461
  melanomas and, 2231–2232
Dyspnea, myocardial failure and, 1508
Dysvascular extremities, reconstruction
    of, 2288, 2288t

E

Eagle-Barrett syndrome, 2111
Ears
  burns of, management of, 431–432
  otoplasty and, 2272t, 2274
Eastern Cooperative Oncology Group
    Performance Status Scale, 503t
E-cadherin, 9–10
Ecchymoses, periorbital, neuroblastomas
    and, 2120
Echinococcosis
  hepatic, 960
  neurologic, 2191
Echocardiography
  Doppler. *See* Doppler studies
  in pericardial disease, 1575
  in valvular heart disease, 1513–1514
Ectopia cordis, 2030, 2030f
Ectopic pregnancy, 2228f, 2228–2229,
    2229f
  acute abdomen and, 1249
Eczema
  of nipples, 1378
  venous, 1959
Edema
  cerebral
    in fulminant hepatic failure, 978
    head injuries and, 293
  wound healing and, 77, 79
Edrophonium, 440t
Edrophonium test, 668–669
Effective circulating volume, 245–246
Effective refractory period, 1565–1566
Effort thrombosis, 1635
Ehlers-Danlos syndrome, 1599, 1600,
    1600f
Eicosanoids. *See also specific eicosanoids*
  inflammation and, 136–140, 137t,
      138f–140f
    cyclooxygenase products and, 138
    lipoxygenase pathways and, 138–140
  in shock, 193f, 193–194

Ejaculatory disturbances, 2204
Elapidae. *See* Bites and stings
Elastase, aneurysm formation and, 1843
Elastin
    aneurysm formation and, 1842–1843
    mutation of, aneurysm formation and,
        1845
    in soft tissues, 2141
    thoracoabdominal aortic aneurysms
        and, 1874
Elderly people
    appendicitis in, 1259
    cholelithiasis in, 1049
    coronary artery bypass grafting in, 1547
    Crohn's disease in, 843
    traumatic injuries of. *See* Geriatric
        trauma
Elective lymph node dissection (ELND),
    2238f, 2238–2239, 2239f, 2239t
Electrical burns, 428, CF 12–5
Electric control activity (ECA), colonic,
    1087
Electrocardiography (ECG)
    in coronary artery disease, 1539
    in myocardial infarction, 1540, 1540f
    in pulmonary thromboembolism, 1951
    in trauma patients, 284
    in valvular heart disease, 1513
Electrocauterization, for abnormal uterine
    bleeding, 2223
Electrochemical potential gradient, 14, 15f
Electrocoagulation, for peptic ulcers,
    1163
Electrohydraulic shock wave lithotripsy
    (ESWL)
    in choledocholithiasis, 1048
    in cholelithiasis, 1048
    complications of, 2205
    for urinary lithiasis, 2205, 2206
Electrolytes. *See also* Fluid and
        electrolyte therapy; *specific
        electrolytes*
    abnormalities of. *See also specific
        electrolyte abnormalities*
        in critically ill patients, management
            of, 236–237
    absorption of, from small intestine,
        813f, 813–814, 814f
    body fluid concentrations of. *See* Body
        fluids; *specific electrolytes and
        electrolyte imbalances*
    in parenteral solutions, 249t, 249–250
Electrophysiologic testing, in cardiac
        arrhythmias, 1567, 1567f
Elliptocytosis, hereditary, 1267
Embolectomy, pulmonary
    catheter, transvenous, for pulmonary
        thromboembolism, 1955, 1957f
    for pulmonary thromboembolism,
        1954–1955, 1955f, 1956f
Embolism
    following abdominal aortic aneurysm
        repair, 1890
    amniotic fluid, traumatic injuries and,
        394
    arterial. *See* Arterial embolism;
        Atheroembolism
    atheromatous, 1798, 1801f
    cerebrovascular disease and, 1751
    macroembolism, angiography in, 1690,
        1691f, 1692f
    mesenteric, 1768–1769, 1773f
    paradoxical, 1483

Embolization
    angiographic, 1705f–1707f, 1708
        in pelvic fractures, 356
    for arteriovenous fistulas, 1923
    complications of, 1923
    for intracranial arteriovenous
        malformations, 2184
    transcatheter, for stress gastritis, 1165
Embolus(i)
    cerebrovascular disease and, 2180–
        2181
    paradoxical, 1623–1624
Emergency Medical Service Act of 1973,
    268
Emphysema, mediastinal
        (pneumomediastinum), 1471–
        1472
Empty-sella syndrome, 1355
Empyema
    in cholecystitis, 1050
    contamination by gastric contents and,
        341, 342f, 343
    pleural (thoracic), 1456t, 1456–1458,
        1457f–1459f
    posttraumatic, 398
    subdural, 2190
Encapsulated hemoglobin, in shock,
    290
Encephaloceles, 2192–2193
Encephalopathy
    hepatic. *See* Hepatic encephalopathy
    in pancreatitis, 885
Encephalotrigeminal angiomatosis, 1930
Encrustation hypothesis, of
        atherosclerosis, 1593
Endarterectomy
    aortoiliac, 1804, 1805f
    carotid. *See* Carotid endarterectomy
    for renal hypertension, 1792–1793,
        1793f
    for visceral angina, 1776, 1779f
Endocardial resection, for ventricular
        tachycardia, 1570
Endocarditis, 1505, 1531–1532
    management of, 1531–1532, 1532f,
        1532t
    pathology of, 1531
    presentation of, 1531
Endocervicitis, mucopurulent, 2224
Endocrine insufficiency, in chronic
        pancreatitis, 891t, 891–892
Endocrine pancreas. *See* Pancreas,
        endocrine
Endocytosis, 32–34, 33f
    receptor-mediated, 32–33
Endoesophageal intubation, for
        esophageal cancer, 705–706,
        706f
Endometrial carcinomas, 2223
Endometrial hyperplasia, 2223
Endometriomas, ovarian, 2227
Endometriosis, small intestinal, 847
Endopelvic fascia, 2217
Endoplasmic reticulum, 5, 5f, 6f
    hepatic, 947
Endorectal dissection, Rehbein, for
        anorectal malformations, 2045
Endorectal pull-through, laparoscopically
        assisted, for Hirschsprung
        disease, 2062, 2065f
Endorphins, 2194
Endoscopic retrograde cholangiography

(ERC), in bile duct strictures,
        1070, 1072f
Endoscopic retrograde
        cholangiopancreatography
        (ERCP)
    in bile duct cancer, 1061
    in bile duct strictures, 1079
    in choledocholithiasis, 1052, 1055
    in pancreas divisum, 2095, 2095f
    in pancreatic cancer, 907–908, 908f
    in pancreatic injuries, 347, 350
    in pancreatitis
        acute, 883
        chronic, 892, 893f, 894f
    pancreatitis following, 880
Endoscopic therapy
    balloon dilation, for bile duct
        strictures, 1075, 1077t
    for carpal tunnel syndrome, 2155f,
        2155–2156
    for gastroesophageal varices, 1166,
        1166f
    for gastrointestinal hemorrhage, 1162–
        1164, 1164f, 1164t
    for pain in chronic pancreatitis, 893
    percutaneous urinary stone removal,
        2205–2206
    polypectomy, in colorectal polyps,
        1116, 1117f
    sclerotherapy, for gastroesophageal
        varices, 994–996
        complications of, 995
        injection techniques for, 994, 995f
        long-term survival following, 996
        sclerosant choice for, 994–995
        surgery versus, 995–996, 996t
        type of scope for, 994
        vasopressin and balloon tamponade
            versus, 995
    sphincterotomy, 1051
        for choledocholithiasis, 1054, 1054f,
            1054t, 1055
        for pancreatitis, 885–886
    for stress gastritis, 777, 1165
    variceal ligation, 996f, 997f, 998–1000
Endoscopy
    diagnostic
        in Crohn's disease, 837, 838t
        esophageal, 657–658, 658f, 658t
        in gastric adenocarcinomas, 797,
            798f
        in gastric ulcers, 779
        in gastrointestinal hemorrhage,
            1159–1161
        in ulcerative colitis, 1097
    ultrasonography directed by
        in gastric adenocarcinomas, 798–799
        in pancreatic cancer, 908, 908f
Endosomes, hepatic, 947
Endosurgery, 735–743. *See also*
        Laparoscopic therapy;
        Thoracoscopic surgery
    vascular, 1733–1745
        atherectomy, 1735–1736
        atherosclerotic lesion distribution
            and, 1733f–1735f, 1733–1734
        endoluminal grafts, 1738–1739,
            1739f
        future of, 1744t, 1745
        intraluminal access techniques for,
            1734–1735
        intraluminal imaging techniques and,
            1739–1745

Endosurgery (*continued*)
    angioscopy. *See* Angioscopy
    cinefluoroscopy, 1739–1740
    ultrasonography, 1742–1745,
        1743f, 1744f
    intravascular stenting, 1738
    laser therapy, 1736–1737
        recanalization devices for, 1737
    thrombolytic therapy and, 1737–
        1738
    transluminal dilation, 1735
Endothelial cells
    leukocyte interactions with, 116–119
        adhesion molecules and, 117f, 117–
          118, 118f
        chemotactic factors and, 118–119, 119t
        wound repair and, 118, 118f
    vascular. *See* Vascular endothelium
Endothelial growth factor (EGF),
        vascular, for vascular gene
        therapy, 520t
Endothelial-leukocyte adhesion molecule-
        1 (E-LAM 1), 152
Endothelins, volume control and, 248
Endothelium-derived relaxing factor
        (EDRF)
    arterial luminal area and, 1587
    inflammation and, 152
    nitric acid produced by, 1610, 1611
Endothoracic fascia, 1441
Endotracheal intubation
    tracheal stenosis due to, 1473, 1473f
    tracheoinnominate artery fistulas
        caused by, 1474–1475
    in traumatic injuries, 280
        complications of, 398
        indications for, 397, 397t
        pediatric, 379–380, 380t
Endovascular surgery. *See* Endosurgery,
        vascular
Energetics
    of active transport, 15–16, 16f
    of membrane transport, 13–14, 15f
    of water flow, 14–15, 15f
Energy
    arterial hemodynamics and. *See*
        Hemodynamics, arterial
    balance of, in critically ill patients,
        231–232
    cellular, organ preservation injury and,
        557–558, 558f
    conversion of
        energy-converting membrane
          transport and, 11–12, 12f
        membrane composition and, 12–13,
          13f
    metabolism of, 43–45, 44t, 45t
        in critically ill patients, 227, 229f
    requirements for
        of critically ill patients, estimating
          and measuring, 227, 229
        lower extremity amputation levels
          and, 1826, 1826t
        pediatric, 1974–1975
        in surgical patients, 44t, 44–45, 45t
    sources of, 43–44, 229–230, 230t. *See*
        also Carbohydrates; Fat(s);
        Protein(s)
        endogenous, 230–231
    tissue ischemia and, 1646–1649, 1648f
    transfer of, traumatic injuries and, 269
Enflurane, 439t
Enkephalins, 2194

Entamoeba histolytica, hepatic abscesses
        due to, 959, 960f
    pediatric, 2082
Enteral feeding, 63
    for cancer patients, 58
    for critically ill patients, 232–233, 233t
    for infants, 1976t, 1978
    for multiple organ failure syndrome,
        210
    in pancreatitis, 885
Enteric cysts, 1471, 1471f, 2074–2075,
        2075f
Enteric disorders, burns and, 435t
Enteritis
    chemotherapy-induced, total parenteral
        nutrition for, 60
    radiation-induced
        intestinal obstruction and, 827
        total parenteral nutrition for, 60
Enterocolitis, necrotizing. *See*
        Necrotizing enterocolitis (NE)
Enterocutaneous fistulas, total parenteral
        nutrition for, 59
Enterogenous cysts, 1471, 1471f, 2074–
        2075, 2075f
    in pediatric patients, 2009
Enteroglucagon, small intestinal, 808
Enteroinsular axis, 869
Enteroscopy, intraoperative, in
        gastrointestinal hemorrhage,
        1161
Envenomation injuries. *See* Bites and
        stings
Enzyme(s)
    hepatic biotransformation and, 956
    pancreatic secretion of, 865–867, 869f
    replacement of, for pain in chronic
        pancreatitis, 892–893, 894f
Enzyme-linked immunosorbent assay
        (ELISA), 167
    in *Clostridium difficile* colitis, 1176–
        1177
    for human immunodeficiency virus
        detection, 178, 178f
Eosinophils, inflammation and, 147
Ependymomas, 2177, 2177f
    intracranial, pediatric, 2177
    spinal, 2180
Epidermal analogues, for burns, 437
Epidermal growth factor (EGF)
    for burns, 437
    gastric, 752
    hepatic, 946t
    lung cancer and, 1419
    for wound care, 82, 82t
Epidermoid tumors
    carcinomas, of anal canal. *See* Anal
        cancer
    intracranial, 2178
Epididymal obstructions, 2203
Epidural abscesses, 2189–2190
Epidural analgesia, opiate, 454, 454t
Epidural hematomas, 2168, 2168f
    in head injuries, 296, 297f
    treatment of, 297–298, 298f
Epigastric artery, inferior, 1212
Epigastric hernias, 1227–1228, 1228f
Epigastric pain
    in chronic pancreatitis, 890f, 890–891
        treatment of, 892–898
    in gastroesophageal reflux disease, 681
Epiglottitis, acute, in pediatric patients,
        1995

Epinephrine
    normal effects of, 1338–1339
    in shock, 187, 205
Epiphrenic diverticula, 728–729, 729f
Epipodophylotoxins, 502t
Epispadias, 2108
Epistaxis, 301
Epithelial cells, polarized secretion of, 32
Epithelial growth factor (EGF), fibroblasts
        and, wound healing and, 123–
        124
Epithelialization, 72–74, 73f–74f, 75, 76,
        76f
Epithelium
    colonic, 1083, 1085
        transport and, 1089, 1089f
    gastric. *See* Gastric epithelium
Epstein-Barr virus (EBV) infections, 178
    Burkitt lymphoma and, 464
Equilibrium, membrane transport, 13–14,
        15f
Erectile dysfunction. *See* Impotence
Ergocalciferol. *See* Vitamin(s), vitamin D
        (ergocalciferol)
Erythroblastosis fetalis, 1987
Erythrocytes
    inflammation and, 151, 151f
    metabolic abnormalities of, 1267–1268
    splenic maintenance of, 1265
    structural abnormalities of, 1266–1267
Erythromycin
    for chlamydial proctitis, 1203
    for gonococcal proctitis, 1203
    prophylactic, for endocarditis, 1532t
    spectrum of activity of, 169t
Escharotomies, for burns, 426, 427f
E-selectin, in shock, 195
Esophageal achalasia, 704–705
Esophageal atresia, 2011–2016
    anomalies associated with, 2012, 2014t
    classification of, 2011, 2012f–2013f
    diagnosis of, 2012, 2014f
    embryology of, 2011
    incidence of, 2011
    pathophysiology of, 2011–2012
    preoperative treatment of, 2012
    surgical treatment of, 2012–2016,
        2015f
        complications of, 2014–2015, 2015t
        operative technique for, 2013–2014
        results of, 2015–2016, 2016f
Esophageal body, manometric assessment
        of, 666, 667f
Esophageal cancer, 490, 698–712
    adenocarcinomas, 700, 701f
    anatomic and physiologic
        considerations in, 694–695
    cervicothoracic, 711–712, 712f–716f
    diagnosis of, 702–704
        esophagoscopy in, 703–704
        history and physical examination in,
          702
        radiographic examination in, 702–
          703, 703f
    pathophysiology of, 701–702
        local effects and, 701–702
        systemic effects and, 702
    premalignant lesions and, 704–705,
        705f
    squamous cell carcinomas, 698–700
    tracheoesophageal fistulas and, 732,
        732f, 733f, 734
    treatment of, 705–711

bypass in, 706
intubation in, 705–706, 706f
laser fulguration in, 706
multimodality, 710–711
radiotherapy in, 705
resection in, 706–710
radical, 709–710, 712t
transhiatal, 708f–711f, 708–709, 712t
transthoracic, 706–708, 707f
Esophageal disorders. *See also specific disorders*
caustic injuries, 712–718, 717f
clinical features of, 713–714
immediate diagnosis and treatment of, 714–715
management of, 715–718, 718f, 718t
in dermatologic disorders, 730
of esophageal body, 674–680
foreign bodies, 2071, 2072f
functional, 665–670
ambulatory esophageal manometry in, 669
dual esophageal pH monitoring in, 668
esophageal bile probe in, 669, 669f
provocative testing in, 668–669
stationary esophageal manometry in, 665–666
24-hour pH monitoring in, 666–667
gastroesophageal reflux disease. *See* Gastroesophageal reflux disease (GERD)
pharyngoesophageal, 670–674
investigation of, 672, 672f
pathophysiology of, 670, 671f, 672
treatment of, 672–674, 673f
premalignant, 704–705, 705f
primary esophageal body disorders
achalasia, 674–677, 675f, 676f
diffuse esophageal spasm, 677, 679, 679f
hypertensive lower esophageal sphincter, 679–680
nonspecific, 680
nutcracker esophagus, 679
rare, 730f–732f, 730–731
secondary motor disorders, 680
structural abnormalities, 657–658
barium studies in, 658, 659f
computed tomography in, 658, 660f, 661f
endoscopy in, 657–658, 658f, 658t
traumatic injuries, management of, 316, 330f, 330–331, 331f
tumors, 694–711
anatomic and physiologic considerations in, 694–695
cysts, 698, 699f
granular cell myoblastomas, 698
hemangiomas, 697
heterotopic, 698
leiomyomas, 695–696, 696f, 697f
malignant. *See* Esophageal cancer
papillomas, 698
polyps, 696–697, 697f, 698f
varices. *See* Varices, gastroesophageal
Esophageal diverticula, 725–729
epiphrenic, 728–729, 729f
mid-esophageal, traction, 728, 728f
pharyngoesophageal (Zenker), 670–674, 726f, 726–728, 727f
investigation of, 672, 672f

pathophysiology of, 670, 671f, 672
treatment of, 672–674, 673f
true and false, 725
Esophageal duplications, 2016
Esophageal fistulas, 731–734
malignant, 732, 732f, 733f, 734
nonmalignant, 731–732
Esophageal manometry
stationary, 665–666
of esophageal body, 666, 667f
for lower esophageal sphincter assessment, 665, 665f, 666f
for upper esophageal sphincter assessment, 666
24-hour, 669
Esophageal perforation, 718–724, 719t
clinical features of, 718
diagnosis of, 719
management of, 719–724
nonoperative, 719
operative, 719–724
for cervical and upper thoracic perforations, 719–720, 720f
for late perforations, 722, 724
for perforations associated with intrinsic disease, 721–722, 723f
for thoracoesophageal perforations, 720–721, 721f, 722f
Esophageal stenosis, congenital, 2016
Esophageal strictures
after chemical burns, 716–718, 718f
in gastroesophageal reflux disease, 683
Esophageal transection, for varices, 1004f, 1005, 1005f
Esophageal ulceration, in gastroesophageal reflux disease, 683
Esophageal webs, distal, 729, 730f
Esophagitis, 658, 658t
Barrett's, 704
in gastroesophageal reflux disease, 683–684
in gastroesophageal reflux disease, 681, 682–684
infectious, 724–725
monilial, 724, 725f
reflux, 704
Esophagoesophagostomy, for esophageal atresia and tracheoesophageal fistulas, 2012–2016, 2015f
complications of, 2014–2015, 2015t
operative technique for, 2013–2014
results of, 2015–2016, 2016f
Esophagogastrojejunostomy, Roux-en-Y, for gastric ulcers, 786
Esophagogastroscopy, in gastrointestinal hemorrhage, 1159–1160
Esophagography, 330, 330f
barium, 658, 659f
Esophagoscopy
basic principles and anatomic relations and, 703–704
in esophageal cancer, 703–704
vital staining and ultrasonography and, 704
Esophagus
abdominal, 654, 654f
blood supply and venous drainage of, 654–655, 655f, 656f
cervical, 653
embryology of, 653
gastric function testing and, 669–670
innervation of, 656

lymphatics of, 655–656, 657f
physiology of, 658–665, 661f
antireflux barrier and, 664f, 664–665
of esophageal body, 661–662, 663f, 664
of lower esophageal sphincter, 654
of pharyngoesophageal segment, 660–661, 662f
Schatzki ring of, 729, 730f
thoracic, 653–654
Estrogens, 1336–1337, 2217
antineoplastic, 502t
breast cancer and, 1379–1380, 1385
breast cell regulation by, 1361
excess of, 1337, 1337f
normal effects of, 1336–1337
Ethanol. *See* Alcohol consumption
Ethylenediaminetetraacetic acid (EDTA), for snake bites, 405
Ethylene glycol, metabolic acidosis due to, 262
Etoposide (VP-16), 502t
for neuroblastomas, pediatric, 2122
European Coronary Surgery Study, 1549
Evaporation, heat transfer by, 1979
Ewing sarcomas, of ribs, 1447
Excisional biopsies
of breast masses, 1369
in melanomas, 2236–2237, 2237f
Excretory ducts, of breast, 1360
Excretory sinuses, of breast, 1360
Excretory urography, in renal cell carcinomas, 2208
Exenteration, anterior, for bladder cancer, 2207
Exercise, for infrainguinal occlusive disease, 1815t, 1815–1816
Exercise testing, 1673–1674
Exocrine pancreas. *See* Pancreas, exocrine
Exocytosis, 30–32, 32f
polarized secretion in epithelial cells and, 32
Exomphalos. *See* Omphaloceles
Exons, 23
Expiratory reserve volume, 1983
Extraanatomic bypass, for traumatic injuries, 365
Extracellular fluid (ECF). *See also* Body fluids
composition of, 11, 11f
effective circulating volume of, 245–246
volume of, 242–243
Extracellular matrix
cell-matrix adhesion and, 10–11
proteins of, aneurysm formation and, 1842–1843
Extracorporeal circulation, for rewarming, 411–412
Extracorporeal membrane oxygenation (ECMO), 1553
for diaphragmatic hernias, 2026
Extrasphincteric fistulas, 1198
Extravaginal torsion, 2110
Extremities. *See also* Lower extremities; Upper extremities
limb-length discrepancy and, 2148
Ilizarov wire and frame treatment for, 2148, 2149f
limb-sparing operations and
for osteosarcomas, 2264–2265, 2266f

Extremities (*continued*)
for sarcomas, 2255, 2257f, 2258f, 2258–2259
functional outcome following, 2258–2259
mangled, 376–377
osteosarcomas of. *See* Osteosarcomas
reconstructive surgery of
for dysvascular and diabetic extremities, 2288, 2288t
following resection for sarcomas, 2288f, 2289, 2289f
for venolymphatic insufficiency, 2289
traumatic injuries of
pediatric, 385
in secondary survey, 285
Extrinsic pathway inhibitor, 85
Exudates, wound healing and, 77
Eye(s)
burns and, 435t
pupils of, in head injuries, 294, 294f
Eyelids, blepharoplasty and, 2269, 2270f, 2272t

F

Face
burns of, management of, 431, 432f
injuries of. *See* Maxillofacial injuries
Facial fractures, management of, 305–308, 306f–308f
Facial nerve, 300
lacerations of, repair of, 305, 305f
Factor deficiency, 94
Factor IX
deficiency of. *See* Hemophilia B
for vascular gene therapy, 520t
Factor V deficiency, 94
Factor VII
deficiency of, 94
elevation of, thrombosis associated with, 1618
Factor X deficiency, 94
Factor XI deficiency, 93
Factor XIII deficiency, 95
Fallopian tubes
anomalies of, 2117
carcinomas of, 2224
Falls, 272, 272f
in children, 377
in elderly people, 386, 386f
Familial adenomatous polyposis (FAP), 1110, 1120–1124, 1121f
desmoid tumors in, 1120
diagnosis of, 1123–1124
extraintestinal features of, 1120, 1122f–1123f
gastrointestinal features of, 1120
genetic basis of, 1120–1121, 1123, 1123f
management of, 1127
variants of, 1127
Familial hypercholesterolemia (FH), gene therapy for, 517–518, 518f
Familial hypocalciuric hypercalcemic hyperparathyroidism, 1315
Famotidine, 764f
for duodenal ulcers, 762, 763, 763t, 764f
Fasciitis, necrotizing, 173
Fasciocutaneous flaps, 2281–2282, 2283f
Fasciotomy, for compartment syndromes, 1642

Fasts, monitored, in insulinomas, 921–922
Fat(s). *See also* Lipid(s); *specific lipids*
digestion and absorption of, in small intestine, 816
as energy source, 229–230, 230t
metabolism of
injury response and, 54
sepsis and, 56
Fat embolism syndrome, orthopedic injuries and, 376
Fat necrosis, of breast, 1377
Fatty acid(s)
free, metabolism of, 44
long-chain, absorption from small intestine, 816
metabolism of, 43
hepatic, 951–952, 952f
cholesterol and, 951–952, 953f
phospholipids and, 952
in infants, 1975
pediatric requirements for, 1975
wound healing and, 78
Fatty acid-binding protein, 816
Fatty acid CoA esters, 951, 952
Fatty streak, 1749
in atherosclerosis, 1536, 1537f, 1592f, 1592–1593
Fc receptors (FCRs), 541
Fear, stress response and, 49
Fecal fat test, 871
Fecal leukocyte test, in *Clostridium difficile* colitis, 1174–1175, 1176f
Fecal occult blood tests, in colorectal cancer, 1133
adenomas, 1115
Feeding catheter jejunostomy, 65
Feet, burns of, management of, 432
Felons, 2161, 2161f
Felty syndrome, hypersplenism and, 1271
Female genitourinary system, 2216–2229. *See also* Pregnancy; *specific organs and disorders*
embryology and surgical anatomy of, 2216f, 2216–2217, 2217f
physiology of, 2217
Femoral artery
anatomy of, 1687, 1810–1811, 1811f
aneurysms of. *See* Aneurysm(s), of femoral artery
catheterization of, arteriovenous fistulas due to, 1923
common, cannulation of, 1734
pressure in, in aortoiliac disease, 1803, 1803f
superficial, traumatic injuries of, 370, 372f
thrombectomy of, angioplastic, 1741
Femoral head, avascular necrosis of, 375
Femoral hernias, 1221–1226, 1222f–1226f
diagnosis of, 1217
Femoral sheath, 1211
Femoral vein
deep, 1935
thrombectomy of, angioplastic, 1741
Femoropopliteal artery, infections of, management of, 1730, 1731f
Femoropopliteal occlusive disease. *See* Infrainguinal occlusive disease
Fentanyl, 441t

Ferritin, hepatic iron metabolism and, 957
Fetal heart rate, in traumatic injuries, 392
α-Fetoprotein (AFP)
in hepatocellular carcinoma, 1017–1018
in testis cancer, 2212
Fetus. *See also* Pregnancy
assessment of, in traumatic injuries, 392
circulation of, 1980, 1980f, 2022–2024, 2024f. *See also* Persistent pulmonary hypertension of the newborn (PPHN)
fluid spaces of, 1987–1988
growth and maturation of, 1973
hepatic system of, 1990
hydronephrosis in, 2110–2111
intrauterine growth retardation of, 1973
fluid spaces and, 1987–1988
nutrient requirements of, for water, 1974
surgery of, for diaphragmatic hernia repair, 2026
thermoregulation in, 1979
wound healing in, 83
Fever
cytokine-induced, 51–52
intraabdominal infections and, 172
Fiber, digestion and absorption of, in small intestine, 815
Fibric acid derivatives, for hypercholesterolemia, 1712
Fibrillin, aneurysm formation and, 1843
Fibrin, 85
assays of, in deep venous thrombosis, 1948
thrombosis and, 1614
Fibrin degradation products, thrombosis and, 1614
Fibrinogen, 86
deficiency of, 94
elevation of, thrombosis associated with, 1618
Fibrinogen products, assays of, in deep venous thrombosis, 1948
Fibrinolysis, 85–86, 86f–88f
abnormalities in, 95
congenital disorders of, 1616
defective, 91–92
tests of, 104
thrombosis and, 1614
Fibrinolytic therapy. *See* Thrombolytic therapy
Fibrin-stabilizing factor deficiency, 95
Fibroadenomas, of breast, 1374–1375, 1375f
giant, 1375–1376
Fibroblast(s), cytokines and, 121–126, 124t
epithelial growth factor, 123–124
interleukin-1, tissue remodeling and, 122, 123f
platelet-derived growth factor, 125
transforming growth factor-β, 124–125, 125f
tumor necrosis factor and interleukin-6, 122–123, 124f
Fibroblast growth factor (FGF)
arterial smooth muscle growth and, 1590
bone formation and, 2152
for vascular gene therapy, 520t
for wound care, 82, 82t

Fibrocystic disease, of breasts, 1370, 1372–1374
  breast cancer risk and, 1380
  clinical evaluation of, 1370, 1372–1374
  epidemiology and risk factors for, 1370
Fibrodysplasia, arterial. *See* Arterial fibrodysplasia
Fibrogenesis, in cirrhosis, 974
Fibromas, ovarian, 2226
Fibromuscular dysplasia (FMD), 1597, 1597f, 1598f, 1748
Fibrosarcomas
  neurofibrosarcomas, pediatric, 2133–2134
  pediatric, 2131–2132, 2266
    epidemiology of, 2131
    outcome of, 2132
    pathology of, 2131
    presentation and diagnosis of, 2131–2132
    staging of, 2132
    treatment of, 2132
Fibrosis, 125
  retroperitoneal, 1243–1244, 2214
Fibrous caps, 1749
Fibrous dysplasia, of ribs, 1446, 1446f
Fibrous histiocytomas, malignant
  of chest wall, 1448
  pediatric, 2266
Fick equation, modified, 1534
Filling pressure, in critically ill patients, cardiac function and blood volume and, 226
Films, 81t
Filters, vena caval
  for deep venous thrombosis, 1950f, 1950–1951
    percutaneous insertion of, 1950f, 1951
  for thrombophlebitis, 1957, 1958
Fine-needle aspiration (FNA)
  of breast masses, 1368t, 1368–1369, 1369f
  of liver masses, 1010, 1011f
  of sarcomas, 2251
  of solitary thyroid nodules, 1300
  in thyroid cancer, 1304
Finkelstein test, 2158
Fire ant stings, 407–408
Firearm injuries. *See* Traumatic injuries
Fissurectomy, for anal fissures, 1195, 1197f
Fistula(s)
  aortoenteric, bleeding and, 1170–1171
  arteriovenous. *See* Arteriovenous fistulas (AVFs)
  atrioventricular, coronary, 1495
  branchial cleft remnant-derived, 1995–1998
    anatomy and embryology of, 1995, 1995f, 1996f
    clinical issues in, 1996
    operative considerations and outcome of, 1996–1998, 1997f, 1998f
  bronchopleural, posttraumatic, 398
  cholecystocholedochal, 1051
  cholecystoenteric, 1050
  colovaginal, in diverticular disease, diagnosis and treatment of, 1156
  colovesical, in diverticular disease, diagnosis and treatment of, 1156

  in Crohn's disease, 836t, 836–837
    surgical treatment of, 841–842
  enterocutaneous, total parenteral nutrition for, 59
  horseshoe, 1199
  pancreatic, following pancreatic injuries, 347–349
  rectovaginal, 1200f, 1200–1201, 1202f
  thyroglossal duct, 1283
  tracheoesophageal. *See* Tracheoesophageal fistulas
  tracheoinnominate artery, 1474–1475, 1475f
Fistula-in-ano, 1197–1199
  classification of, 1198, 1198f
  clinical manifestations of, 1198–1199
  in Crohn's disease, 1199
  management of, 1199
Fistulotomy, for fistula-in-ano, 1199
FK 506 (Prograf; tacrolimus), 548, 549t
Flail chest, treatment of, 321–322, 322f
Flaps, for reconstructive surgery, 2281–2282, 2282f–2283f, 2284
Flora. *See* Microorganisms
Flow cytometry (FCM)
  in breast cancer, 1389
  neoplastic cell growth and proliferation and, 466, 467f, 468, 468f
Floxuridine, 501t
Fluconazole, for monilial esophagitis, 724
Fludarabine, 501t
Fluid and electrolyte therapy, 249–252. *See also* Fluid therapy
  goals of, 250
  intraoperative, 252
  maintenance, 251, 251t
  parenteral solutions for, 249t, 249–250, 250t
  pediatric, 1988t, 1988–1989
    for correction of existing deficits or excesses, 1989
    maintenance requirements for, 1988, 1988t
    for replacement of ongoing losses, 1989, 1990t
  postoperative, 252
  for replacement of ongoing fluid losses, 251–252, 252t
  for volume deficits, 250–251
  for volume excesses, 251
Fluid restriction, in ascites, 989
Fluid sequestration, after shock, 187
Fluid spaces, 242t, 242–243
  pediatric, 1987–1988
Fluid therapy. *See also* Fluid and electrolyte therapy
  for burns, 429–430, 430t
    in children, 429
  for gastrointestinal hemorrhage, 1158–1159
  in head injuries, 294–295
  for hypercalcemia, 1315
  for pancreatitis, 884
  pediatric, 1988t, 1988–1989
    for correction of existing deficits or excesses, 1989
    maintenance requirements for, 1988, 1988t
    for replacement of ongoing losses, 1989, 1990t
  in shock, 288–290
    colloids for, 288–289

  crystalloids for, 288
  experimental fluids for, 289–290
  in traumatic injuries
    in elderly people, 388
    pediatric, 380
Fluid volume
  control of, 246–247
    baroreceptor function and, 246–247
    baroreceptor modulation of, 246
    hormonal mediators of, 247
    hypervolemia and, fluid and electrolyte therapy for, 251
    hypovolemia and, pediatric, physiologic response to, 378
    reduced. *See* Hypovolemia
Flumazenil (Romazicon), 442t
5-Fluorouracil (5-FU), 501t
  for anal cancer, 1150
  intrahepatic arterial infusion of, bile duct strictures due to, 1081
  for pancreatic cancer, 915
Flutamide, for prostate cancer, 2211
Foam(s), 81t
Foam cells, 1592, 1592f
Focal nodular hyperplasia (FNH), 1012–1013
  hepatic, pediatric, 2080
Folate, pediatric requirement for, 1976t
Folic acid, requirements in surgical patients, 62t
Follicle-stimulating hormone (FSH), in males, 2202, 2203
Follicular cysts, 2226
Fontan procedure
  for hyperplastic left heart syndrome, 1500
  for univentricular heart, 1499
Foot. *See* Lower extremities
Foramen of Winslow hernias, 1235
Foramen ovale, 1483
Foraminectomy, for cervical spine disease, 2188
Foraminotomy, for lumbar spine disease, 2188–2189
Foreign bodies, 2071–2072
  in distal gastrointestinal tract, 2071–2072
  esophageal, 2071, 2072f
  tracheobronchial, in pediatric patients, 2017–2019
    clinical picture in, 2017f, 2018, 2018f, 2018t
    management of, 2018–2019, 2019f
    pathophysiology of, 2017
Foreign-body tumors, 461–462
Fossa ovalis defects, 1483
Foster Kennedy syndrome, 2174
Fournier gangrene, 174
Fractionation, 494, 495f
Fractures, 2145–2148, 2146f, 2147f. *See also specific fractures and sites*
  diaphyseal, treatment of, 2147, 2147f
  fixation of, 376
    device implantation for, 2146f, 2146–2147, 2147f
    objectives of, 2147–2148
  Gustilo classification of, 375, 375t
  healing of, 2145
  involving joint surfaces, 2147, 2148f
  open, 375, 375t, 401
Frank-Starling relation, 1506, 1507f
  pediatric patients and, 1982
Free fatty acids, metabolism of, 44

Freehand variceal injection, 994, 995f
Free radicals, cell injury and, 154, 154t
Free T$_4$, 1292
Free T$_4$ index, 1292
Free wall rupture, after myocardial
    infarction, as surgical indication,
    1542
Friderichsen-Waterhouse syndrome, 1270
Frontal bone, anatomy of, 299
Frontal sinus fractures, management of,
    305, 306f
Frostbite, 412–414
    of hands, 2159
    treatment of, 413–414
Frostnip, 412
Functional residual capacity (FRC), 1983
    diseases decreasing, in pediatric
        patients, 1983–1984
Fungal infections, 176–177. *See also*
        specific infections
    aneurysmic
        of abdominal aorta, 1890–1891
        of femoral artery, 1912–1913
        of thoracic aorta, 1873
    aneurysms and, 1721
    neurologic, 2191
    treatment of, 176, 177
Furosemide, for intracranial
        hypertension, 2167

G

Gag reflex, in fulminant hepatic failure,
    978
Galactoceles, 1377, 1378f
Galactorrhea, 1373
Gallbladder
    absorption in, 1031f, 1031t, 1031–
        1032, 1032f
        altered, gallstone formation and,
            1039
    anatomy of, 1023, 1025f, 1026f
    embryology of, 1023, 1024f
    histology and ultrastructure of, 1028–
        1029
    secretion by, 1032
Gallbladder cancer, 1057–1060
    diagnosis of, 1059
    incidence of, 1057f, 1057–1058, 1058f
    pathology of, 1058f, 1058–1059, 1059t
    prognosis of, 1060
    treatment of, 1059–1060, 1060f
Gallbladder disorders. *See also specific*
            disorders
    dyskinesia, 1031
    neoplastic disease
        benign, 1056–1057
            clinical findings in, 1057
            diagnosis and treatment of, 1057
            pathology of, 1056
        malignant. *See* Gallbladder cancer
    perforation, in cholecystitis, 1050–
        1051
Gallbladder stasis, 1038, 1039f
Gallium nitrate, for hypercalcemia,
        1315–1316
Gallstone ileus, 1050
    intestinal obstruction and, 825f, 825–
        826
Gallstones. *See* Choledocholithiasis;
            Cholelithiasis
Game keeper's thumb, 2159

Gamma-aminobutyric acid (GABA),
        hepatic encephalopathy and,
        982f, 982–983
Ganglion cysts, 2161–2162
Ganglioneuroblastomas, pediatric, 2120
Ganglioneuromas, mediastinal, 1467–
        1468
    in pediatric patients, 2011
Ganglioside GM$_1$, for spinal cord injury,
        374
Gangrene, Fournier, 174
Gap junctions, 10
Gardner syndrome, 2262
Gas exchange
    in critically ill patients,
            pathophysiology of, 218–221,
            219f
        carbon dioxide transfer in lung and,
            220, 220f
        pulmonary mechanics and, 220–221,
            221f
        persistent pulmonary hypertension of
            newborn and, 1984
Gastrectomy
    distal, for gastric ulcers, 785, 785f, 786
    for gastric lymphomas, 803
    postgastrectomy syndromes and, 771–
        773
        alkaline reflux gastritis, 772f, 773
        dumping, 772
    total, for gastrinomas, 924
Gastric acid, secretion of, 752–755
    cellular events and, 752, 753f, 754,
        754f
    duodenal ulcers and, 760
    gastric secretory studies and, 784
    gastric ulcers and, 780–781
    hypersecretion, gastroesophageal reflux
        and, 665
    regulation of, 754–755, 755f
    stress gastritis and, 776–777
Gastric acid analysis, 666–670
Gastric angiodysplasia, 1170
Gastric artery, aneurysms of, 1893t,
        1898f, 1898–1899
Gastric bypass
    for esophageal cancer, 706
    for morbid obesity, 791–792, 792f
        gastroplasty versus, 792, 792f
Gastric cancer, 795–804
    adenocarcinomas, 795–802
        chemotherapy for, 802
        clinical features of, 797, 797f, 797t
        curative treatment for, 800, 801f,
            802, 802f
        diagnosis and screening for, 797–
            799, 798f, 799f
        epidemiology of, 795, 795f, 796f
        palliative treatment for, 802
        pathology of, 799–800, 800f, 800t
        premalignant lesions and, 795–796
    carcinoids, 803–804
    lymphomas, 802–803
        clinical features of, 802–803
        diagnosis of, 803
        treatment of, 803, 803f
    sarcomas, 804
Gastric contents, contamination by,
        empyema and, 341, 342f, 343
Gastric dilatation, in abdominal injuries,
        pediatric, 383
Gastric dilation, gastroesophageal reflux
        and, 664

Gastric emptying, assessment of, 669
Gastric epithelium, restitution of, 774–
        776
    endogenous prostanoids and, 775
    mucosal blood blow and, 775
    mucus and bicarbonate secretion and,
        775
    trophic peptides and, 776
Gastric function tests, 669–670
Gastric inhibitory peptide (GIP), small
        intestinal, 808
Gastric injuries, traumatic, 341, 342f, 343
Gastric leakage, following gastric surgery
        for morbid obesity, 793
Gastric motility, 757–758
    coordination of contraction and, 758
    gastric ulcers and, 781
    smooth muscle and, 757–758, 758f
Gastric outlet obstruction, duodenal
        ulcers and, 770–771, 771f
Gastric peptides, 749–752. *See also*
        specific peptides
Gastric reservoir, gastroesophageal reflux
        and, 664–665
Gastric surgery, previous,
        adenocarcinomas and, 796
Gastric tonometry, in shock, 196
Gastric transection, for varices, 1005
Gastric ulcers, 779–787
    acid and pepsin secretion and, 780–
        781
    acid secretory studies in, 784
    bleeding from, 1162
    definition of lesions and, 779, 779f
    diagnosis of, 784
    dietary restrictions for, 785
    duodenogastric reflux and, 782–783
    endoscopic identification of, 779
    environmental factors and, 781–782
    gastric motility and, 781
    following gastric surgery for morbid
        obesity, 793
    gastritis and, 782
    giant, 787
    histologic appearance of, 779
    incidence of, 780, 782t
    infection and, 783
    Helicobacter pylori, treatment of, 785
    intraarterial chemotherapy and, 783
    location of, 779–780, 780f–782f
    medical therapy for, 784–785
    natural history of, 783
    nonsteroidal antiinflammatory drug-
        induced, treatment of, 785
    presentation of, 784
    surgical treatment of, 785–787
        for complications, 787
        indications for, 785
        for type I ulcers, 785f, 785–786, 786f
        for type II ulcers, 786, 787f
        for type III ulcers, 786
        for type IV ulcers, 786
        for type V ulcers, 786
Gastrin, 749–751, 750f, 751f
    glycine-extended, 750
Gastrinomas, 919t, 923t, 923–925, 924f
    in multiple endocrine neoplasia, 1326–
        1327
    pediatric, 2097
Gastrinoma triangle, 924, 924f
Gastritis
    adenocarcinomas and, 796
    gastric ulcers and, 782

reflux, alkaline, following gastrectomy, 772f, 773
stress. *See* Stress gastritis
Gastrocolic reflex, 1088
Gastroduodenal artery
anatomy of, 1766
aneurysms of, 1893t, 1899f, 1900, 1900f
Gastroenterostomy, for duodenal obstruction, in pancreatic cancer, 914
Gastroepiploic artery, aneurysms of, 1893t, 1898f, 1898–1899
Gastroesophageal reflux disease (GERD), 680–694
antireflux barrier and, 664f, 664–665
clinical features of, 680–681
complications of, 681–684, 682f, 682t, 683f
diagnosis of, 665
in morbid obesity, 790
pathophysiology of, 680
surgical treatment of. *See* Antireflux surgery
Gastrointestinal disorders. *See also specific disorders*
following abdominal aortic aneurysm repair, 1890
duplications, 2074–2075
cystic, 2074–2075, 2075f
tubular, 2075, 2075f
foreign bodies, 2071–2072
distal, 2071–2072
esophageal, 2071, 2072f
hyperparathyroidism and, 1321
microembolism, 1633
sepsis and, 57
in systemic inflammatory response syndrome, 210
varices. *See* Varices, gastroesophageal
Gastrointestinal hemorrhage, 1158t, 1158–1171
in angiodysplasia of stomach and intestine, 1170
aortoenteric fistulas and, 1170–1171
clinical presentation of, 1158–1162
diagnostic procedures for, 1159–1162, 1160f
in Dieulafoy vascular malformation, 1170
hematemesis and, 1158
hematochezia and, 1158
in inflammatory bowel disease, 1171
initial evaluation and resuscitation for, 1158–1159
lower gastrointestinal, 1167–1170
in colonic diverticulosis, 1168
in colonic vascular ectasia, 1168–1170, 1169f
in Mallory-Weiss syndrome, 1167
in Meckel's diverticulum, 1171
melena and, 1158
pediatric, 2072–2074, 2073t, 2074t
diagnosis of, 2073–2074
in infants, 2073
neonatal, 2072–2073
in older children, 2073
in young children, 2073
in peptic ulcer disease, 1162–1164
endoscopic treatment for, 1164f, 1164t, 62064
in small intestinal diverticulum, 1171
in stress gastritis, 1164–1165
variceal. *See* Varices, gastroesophageal

Gastrointestinal polyposis syndromes, 1120–1127. *See also specific syndromes*
Gastrointestinal tract. *See also specific organs*
immunoresponsiveness of, 810–811
microbial flora of, 160
nutritional support of. *See* Nutritional support, for critically ill patients
in pregnancy, 391
total parenteral nutrition effects on, 61–62
Gastrojejunostomy, for gastric ulcers, 785–786, 786, 787
Gastroplasty
Collis, 692
for morbid obesity, 791, 791f, 792f
gastric bypass versus, 792, 792f
Gastroschisis, 2028–2029
anatomy, embryology, and pathophysiology of, 2028–2029, 2029f
clinical issues in, 2030
operative considerations, subsequent management, and outcome of, 2031f, 2031–2032
Gastrostomy, placement technique for, 65
Gating, of ion channels, 17f, 17–18
modulation of, 18, 19f, 20f
Gaucher disease, hypersplenism and, 1270–1271
Gemcitabine, 501t
Gemfibrozil, for hypercholesterolemia, 1712
Gender
cholelithiasis and, 1035
coronary artery bypass grafting and, 1547
melanomas and, 2235, 2236t
surgical stress response and, 50
Gene(s). *See also* Oncogene(s); *specific genes*
expression of, regulation of, 35f, 35–36, 36f
mutant, gene therapy directed toward, 511–512, 512f, 512t, 513f
structure of, 22–24, 23f, 24f
transcription of, 23, 24f
General anesthetics. *See* Anesthesia
Gene therapy, 506–522, 507f, 555
for cancer, 504t, 505, 510–513
adenosine deaminase deficiency and, 512–513
cytokine gene transfer and, 510t, 510–511, 511f
gene mutation-directed, 511–512, 512f, 512t, 513f
metastatic melanoma, 2242
suicide drug therapy strategy for, 512
ex vivo, 507
general approaches to, 507, 507t
gene transfer strategies in hematopoietic system and, 509f, 510
for hepatic disorders, 515–519, 516t
α_1-antitrypsin deficiency, 519
bilirubin UDP deficiency, 518–519
DNA-protein complexes for, 516
ex vivo, 516–517
familial hypercholesterolemia, 517–518, 518f
hemophilia B, 519

ornithine transcarbamylase deficiency, 518
Human Genome Project and, 506–507
muscle cells as delivery vehicles for secreted proteins and, 520
for muscular dystrophy, 520
for neurologic disorders, 521
Parkinson disease, 521
viral vectors for, 521
for pancreatic disorders, 521–522
cystic fibrosis and, 522
diabetes mellitus, 521–522
islets of Langerhans and, 522
islet transplantation and, 522
recombinant retroviruses in, 507–508, 508f, 510
for respiratory disorders, 513–515
adenoviruses for, 513, 514f
cystic fibrosis, 514–515, 516f
liposomes for, 514, 514f, 515f
for vascular disorders, 519–520, 520t
preclinical models for, 520
in vivo, 507
Genetic factors
aneurysm formation and, 1845–1846, 1846f
in cancer, 459–461
of breast, 1381, 1385
colorectal, 1129–1131, 1130f
melanomas, 2232–2233
sarcomas, 2248
in cholelithiasis, 1034–1035
in colorectal polyps, 1110
in Crohn's disease, 832
in familial adenomatous polyposis, 1120–1121, 1123, 1123f
in hyperparathyroidism, 1318
in pancreatitis, chronic, 889
in ulcerative colitis, 1095
Genetic markers. *See also* Biochemical markers
for melanomas, 2236
Genitourinary disorders. *See also specific disorders*
burns, 435t
management of, 432–433
genital reconstruction and, 2287–2288
injuries, pediatric, 384
intersex anomalies. *See* Intersex anomalies
Genitourinary system. *See also specific organs*
female, 2216–2229
embryology and surgical anatomy of, 2216f, 2216–2217, 2217f
physiology of, 2217
male, 2199–2214
pediatric, 2101–2117
Gentamicin
for pelvic inflammatory disease, 2225t
prophylactic, for endocarditis, 1532t
Geriatric trauma, 386–390
abdominal, 389
anatomic and physiologic characteristics of aging and, 387, 387t
head injuries, 389
initial evaluation and resuscitation of or, 388
intensive care considerations in, 389
mechanisms of injury and, 386–387
outcome prediction and, 389–390, 390t
prevention of, 390
thoracic, 388

Germ cell tumors, extragonadal, 2213–2214

Germinomas, intracranial, 2178

Gestational trophoblastic neoplasia, 2229

Giant cell arteritis, 1605–1606
systemic, 1605–1606, 1606f
Takayasu arteritis, 1606, 1607f, 1748, 1761
temporal arteritis, 1605–1606, 1606f, 1748

Giant colonic diverticulum, 1157, 1157f

Giant migrating contractions, colonic, 1087

Gila monster bites, 406

Gingiva, cancer of, 638

Glanzmann thrombasthenia, 95

Glasgow Coma Scale (GCS), 282, 283t
brain injuries and, 293–294, 294f, 2167, 2167t
in elderly people, 389

Glenn procedure, for hyperplastic left heart syndrome, 1500

Gliomas
brain-stem, 2173
butterfly, 2174, 2175f
of optic nerve, 2173

Glomerular filtration rate (GFR)
elevation of, in diabetes mellitus, 617
pediatric, 1987
in shock, 191

Glomerulosclerosis, in diabetes mellitus, 617

Glomerulus, enlargement of, in diabetes mellitus, 617

Glomus jugulare tumors, of head and neck, 643

Glomus tumor, 2162

Glossopharyngeal neuralgia, neurosurgical pain management for, 2195

Glucagon
pancreatic synthesis, secretion, and action of, 868–869
in shock, 188
small intestinal, 808

Glucagonomas, 919t, 926, 926t

Glucocorticoid(s). See also specific drugs
for hypercalcemia, 1315
for immunosuppression, 548, 549t
wound healing and, 79

Glucocorticoid response elements, 35

Gluconeogenesis, 949–950, 951

Glucose. See also Hypoglycemia
homeostasis of, in chronic liver disease, 981
for hyperkalemia, pediatric, 1989
metabolism of, 43
injury response and, 54
sepsis and, 55–56

Glucose intolerance, in chronic liver disease, 981

Glucose-6-phosphate dehydrogenase (G6PD) deficiency, 1267

Glucose tolerance tests
intravenous, 872
oral, 872, 873t

Glucose transporters, 867, 870f

Glucuronidation, hepatic biotransformation and, 956

Glutamine
loss following injury, 54
metabolism of

sepsis and, 56, 56f
in small intestine, 816–817, 817f

Glutathione S-transferases, hepatic biotransformation and, 956

Glycine-extended gastrin, 750

Glycogenesis, 949, 949f

Glycogenolysis, 949, 949f

Glycolysis, 949, 950f

Glycopyrrolate, 440t

Goiters, 1470
multinodular, toxic, 1297–1298
tracheal compression due to, 1473

Goldie-Coldman hypothesis, 1396

Golgi complex, 5, 947

Gonadal appendages, torsion of, 2110

Gonadal dysgenesis, mixed, 2112–2113

Gonadotropin-releasing hormone (GnRH), in males, 2202

Gonococcal proctitis, 1203

Gorlin equation, 1534

G protein(s)
oncogenes and, 474–475, 475f, 476f
in signal transduction, 144f, 144t, 144–147, 145f
activation of NADPH oxidase and, 145, 147f
alternative signal pathways and, 145, 147
coupling to phospholipase C and subsequent events in neutrophils and, 145, 146f

G-protein-linked receptors, 37–39, 38f, 39f

Gracilis muscle transposition, for anal incontinence, 1201–1202

Grafts
bone, 2152
free, nonviable, for hernia repair, 1220
infections of, following abdominal aortic aneurysm repair, 1890
organ, rejection of. See Antigen(s), recognition of; Transplantation; Transplantation immunology; specific organs
skin
for burns
autografts, 431
porcine xenograft, 431
split-thickness, for scalp injuries, 2165–2166
thrombosis of, following pancreatic transplantation, 623
vascular. See Vascular grafts

Graft-versus-host disease (GVHD), 553

Granular cell(s), 1780

Granular cell myoblastomas, esophageal, 697–698

Granulation tissue, 119–120

Granulocyte(s). See Polymorphonuclear leukocytes (PMNs); specific polymorphonuclear leukocytes

Granulocyte colony-stimulating factor, acute-phase response mediation by, 133t

Granulocyte-monophage colony-stimulating factor, acute-phase response mediation by, 133t

Granulomatous diseases. See also specific granulomatous diseases
hypercalcemia and, 1315

Granulomatous thyroiditis, 1298–1299

Graves disease, 1295–1297
clinical manifestations of, 1295

diagnosis of, 1295
medical treatment of, 1295–1296
surgical treatment of, 1296–1297

Great vessels
transposition of, 1490f–1493f, 1490–1491, 1493
traumatic injuries of, 366–368, 367f–370f

Greenfield filter, 103
for deep venous thrombosis, 1950f, 1950–1951
for thrombophlebitis, 1957, 1958

GRFomas, 927

Ground substance, in soft tissues, 2141

Growth factors. See also specific growth factors
bone formation and, 2152
breast cell regulation by, 1361
inflammation and, 142
lung cancer and, 1419
neuroblastomas and, 2119
oncogenes and, 472–474, 473f–475f
promoting intestinal mucosal growth, 63–64
for wound care, 82, 82t

Growth hormone (GH)
in acromegaly, 1352, 1353f
for burns, 437
glucose homeostasis and, in chronic liver disease, 981
hepatic, 946t
for wound care, 82

Growth plates
cartilage of, 2144, 2145f
mechanical stability of, 2144–2145

Guide wires, for intraluminal vascular access, 1734–1735

Gunshot wounds. See Traumatic injuries

Gut decontamination, for infections, 180

Gut mucosal barrier, dysfunction of, stress response mediation by, 52

Gynecologic disorders, acute abdomen and, 1249, 1249t

Gynecomastia, 1410–1411

H

Hairy cell leukemia, 1274, 1276f

Halothane, 439t

Hamartomas
of bile ducts, 1013
mesenchymal, pediatric, 2079
of pituitary gland, 1355
pulmonary, 1433–1434
of spleen, 1273

Hands, 2153–2163
amputation of, 2162
indications for replantation and, 2162
initial management of, 2162
arthroscopy of, 2162f, 2162–2163
burns of, management of, 432, CF 12–12
cold-immersion, 412
fractures of, 2158–2159
distal phalangeal, 2158
metacarpal, 2158
proximal and middle phalangeal, 2158
scaphoid, 2158–2159, 2160f
of thumb, 2159
functional anatomy of, 2153, 2153f, 2154f

infections of, 2160–2161
  bites causing, 2161
  felons, 2161, 2161f
  paronychia, 2161, 2161f
  pyoderma, 2161
  pyogenic, 2160–2161
  suppurative tenosynovitis, 2161
joint injury and disease of, 2159
  arthritides, 2159, 2161f
  dislocations, 2159
nerve injury and disease of, 2154–2156
  of digital nerves, 2156
  of median nerve, 2155–2156
  of radial nerve, 2156
  of ulnar nerve, 2156
skin injury and disease of, 2159–2160
  Dupuytren contractures, 2160
  frostbite, 2159
  injection injuries, 2160
  thermal burns, 2159
tendon injury and disease of, 2156–
    2158
  of extensor tendons, 2157f, 2157–
    2158, 2158f
  of flexor tendons, 2157, 2157f
  trigger finger, 2157
traumatic injuries of, evaluation of,
    2153–2154
tumors of, 2161–2162
Hashimoto disease, 1298
Hasselbalch triangle, 1212, 1212f
Head and neck, 639–651. See also
    Cervical spine; Neck
benign lesions of, 635–637
diagnostic approach to, 635
malignant lesions of. See Head and
    neck cancer; specific cancers
in secondary survey of trauma patients,
    283–284
surgical treatment of. See Head and
    neck surgery; specific sites and
    procedures
Head and neck cancer, 637–651. See also
    specific sites and cancers
metastatic, 642, 642f, 642t, 650t, 651,
    651t
molecular biology of, 637
mucosal, 638, 640–641
staging of, 638, 639t, 640t
surgical treatment of. See Head and
    neck surgery; specific sites and
    procedures
Head and neck disorders, pediatric,
    1994–2000
airway obstruction and, 1994–1995
  acquired, 1995
  congenital, 1994–1995
branchial cleft remnants and, 1995–
    1998
  anatomy and embryology of, 1995,
    1995f, 1996f
  clinical issues in, 1996
  operative considerations and
    outcome of, 1996–1998, 1997f,
    1998f
hemangiomas and, 2000
  clinical issues in, 2000, 2000f
  treatment and outcome of, 2000
lymphadenopathy and, 1999–2000
  operative considerations and
    outcome of, 2000
lymphangioma and cystic hygroma
    and, 1999

anatomy and embryology of, 1999,
    1999f
  clinical issues in, 1999
  operative considerations and
    outcome of, 1999
thyroglossal duct cysts and, 1998–1999
  anatomy and embryology of, 1998,
    1998f
  clinical issues in, 1998
  operative considerations and
    outcome of, 1998–1999
Head and neck surgery, 643–650. See
    also specific sites and
    procedures
adjuvant treatment with, 650–651
cervical lymph node biopsy, 643, 645f
radical neck dissection, 644, 646, 648f,
    649f
reconstructive, 649f, 649–650, 2285f,
    2285–2286
rehabilitation following, 650
Head injuries, 291–298, 2165–2169
brain injury and, 2166–2168, 2167t
clinical assessment of, 293–294
definitive management of, 297–298
in elderly people, 389
epidemiology of, 291
epidural hematomas and, 2168, 2168f
initial treatment of, 294–297
  in absence of clinical signs of
    herniation, 295
  in presence of clinical signs of
    herniation, 295
  radiographic priorities in, 295–297
organ donation and, 399
pathophysiology of, 291–293
  cerebral edema and osmolar therapy
    and, 293
  intracranial pressure and, 292–293,
    293f
  primary injury and, 291–292
  secondary injury and, 292
pediatric, 384
of scalp, 2165–2166
skull fractures, 2166, 2166f
subdural hematomas and, 2168–2169,
    2169f
Healing. See also Wound healing
of fractures, 2145
of soft tissues, 2142–2143
Health care reform, nutritional support
    and, 66, 66t
Heart. See also Cardiac entries;
    Cardiovascular entries;
    Myocardial entries; Pericardial
    entries; Pericardium
artificial, 1558
  permanent, 1561f, 1561–1563, 1562f
  temporary, 1558, 1559f
conduction system of, anatomy of,
    1565, 1565f
congenital vascular malformations and,
    1927
neoplastic disease of, primary, 1500,
    1502
preservation of, 569
suitability for donation, 561
univentricular, 1498–1499, 1499f
Heartburn, in gastroesophageal reflux
    disease, 680–681
Heart disease
congenital. See Congenital heart
    disease

ischemic. See Coronary artery disease
    (CAD)
rheumatic, 1503–1504, 1504t
valvular. See Valvular heart disease
HeartMate 1000 IP ventricular assist
    device, 1556, 1557f, 1558
HeartMate VE ventricular assist devices,
    1559
Heat clamp, 1979
Heineke-Mikulicz pyloroplasty, for
    duodenal ulcers, 767
Helicobacter pylori infections
  adenocarcinomas and, 796
  duodenal ulcers and, 760
  gastric ulcers and, 783
  treatment of, 785
Heller myotomy, for esophageal
    achalasia, 675, 676–677, 677f,
    678f
Heloderma horridum bites, 406
Heloderma suspectum bites, 406
Hemangioblast(s), 1585
Hemangioblastomas
  intracranial, 2178
  spinal, 2180
Hemangioendotheliomas, hepatic,
    pediatric, 2079
Hemangiomas
  angiography in, 1699f, 1700, 1700f
  cardiac, 1502
  cavernous, hepatic, 1013, 1014f
  esophageal, 697
  hepatic, pediatric, 2078–2079
  in pediatric patients, 2000
    clinical issues in, 2000, 2000f
    treatment and outcome of, 2000
  small intestinal, 847
  of spleen, 1273
Hematemesis, 1158
  in esophageal cancer, 702
Hematochezia, 1158
Hematocolpos, in infancy, 2116
Hematogenous metastasis, 483, 485
Hematologic disorders
  burns and, 435t
  following snake bites, 404
Hematomas
  epidural, 2168, 2168f
    in head injuries, 296, 297f
    treatment of, 297–298, 298f
  intramural, duodenal, 345–346
  pulmonary, treatment of, 325–326,
    326f
  rectus sheath, 1236
  retroperitoneal, 352f, 352–353
  subdural. See Subdural hematomas
  submucosal, pediatric, 383
Hematometrocolpos, in infancy, 2116
Hematopoietic system, gene transfer
    strategies in, 509f, 510
Hematuria, renal injuries and, 356
Heme, metabolism of, 956, 957
Hemicolectomy
  left, for colorectal cancer, 1138, 1139f,
    1140f
  right, for colorectal cancer, 1138, 1139f
Hemifontan procedure
  for hyperplastic left heart syndrome,
    1500
  for univentricular heart, 1499
Hemifundoplication, for esophageal
    achalasia, 675

Hemodialysis
  arteriovenous fistulas for, 1923–1924
  for critically ill patients, 237–238, 238t
Hemodynamic disorders. *See also*
        specific disorders
  in pancreatitis, 885
  in systemic inflammatory response
        syndrome, 210
Hemodynamic monitoring
  in gastrointestinal hemorrhage, 1159
  normal parameters for, 196t
  of pediatric patients, 1981–1982, 1982f
  in shock, 195–196, 196t, 197t
Hemodynamics
  arterial, 1656–1667
    aneurysms and, 1665, 1667, 1667f
    arterial structure and function and,
        1656f, 1656–1657, 1657f
    blood flow and energy loss and,
        1659–1662
      inertial energy loss, 1662
      local effects of turbulent flow and,
        1662, 1663f
      measurement of, 1659–1660
      viscosity and laminar blood flow
        and, 1660–1661, 1661f
      viscous energy loss, 1661–1662
    blood flow control and, 1657–1658
      flow-related, 1658
      humoral, local, 1658
      local, 1657
      neurologic, 1657–1658
    evaluation of, 1673, 1674f
    pressure and energy and, 1658–
        1659, 1660f
      determinants of arterial pressure
        curve and, 1658–1659
      energy in ideal system and, 1659,
        1660f
    stenosis and, 1662–1665
      collateral circulation and, 1665
      critical, 1663
      energy loss and, 1662–1663, 1664f
      multiple stenoses and, 1665, 1666f
      subcritical, 1663–1665, 1664f
  arteriovenous fistulas and, 1917–1920
    local effects and, 1918f, 1918–1919,
        1919f
    systemic effects and, 1919–1920, 1920f
  in critically ill patients, algorithm for,
        227, 228f
  of pediatric patients, 1981t, 1981–1982
  in pregnancy, 390–391
  following valvular heart surgery, 1529
Hemodynamic stability, of organ donors,
        560
Hemoglobinopathies, 1268
Hemolysis, prosthetic heart valves and,
        1527
Hemolytic anemia
  alloimmune, 1987
  autoimmune, 1268
Hemolytic uremic syndrome, 1270
Hemophilia A, 92–93, 93f
Hemophilia B, 93, 93f
  gene therapy for, 519
Hemorrhage. *See also specific sites;*
        specific sites and disorders
  during antireflux operations, 692
  in brain, 2184–2185, 2185f
  congenital vascular malformations and,
        1928
  control of, in shock, 288

following coronary artery bypass
        grafting, 1546
  in diverticular disease, 1153, 1154f
  duodenal ulcers and, 769–770
  from facial injuries, 301
  fluid shift after, 186t
  fracture-related, 374
  in fulminant hepatic failure, 978
  following hepatic transplantation, 593
  intraabdominal, posttraumatic, 400
  massive, during splenectomy, 1279–
        1280
  in Meckel's diverticulum, 2070
  from ovarian cysts, acute abdomen
        and, 1249
  following pancreatic transplantation,
        624
  pelvic fractures and, 353–354, 355f,
        356, 356f
  subarachnoid, 2182, 2183f
  in traumatic injuries, in pregnancy, 395
  in ulcerative colitis, 1099
  of upper airway, 637
  variceal. *See* Varices, gastroesophageal
  vascular injuries and, 362
Hemorrheologic drugs, for infrainguinal
        occlusive disease, 1815t, 1817
Hemorrhoid(s), 1188–1190
  classification of, 1188
  clinical manifestations of, 1188
  examination of, 1188
  treatment of, 1188–1190
    in inflammatory bowel disease, 1190
    in portal hypertension, 1190
    for postpartum hemorrhoids, 1190
    for strangulated hemorrhoids, 1190
    for thrombosed external
        hemorrhoids, 1189–1190
Hemorrhoidectomy, 1189, 1189f
Hemostasis, 83–105. *See also*
        Anticoagulation; Coagulation
  antiplatelet agents for, 98–99
  basic considerations in, 83–84, 84f, 85f
  bleeding disorders and. *See* Bleeding
        disorders; *specific disorders*
  blood transfusion risks and, 104–105
  dextran for, 102–103
  fibrinolysis and, 85–86, 86f–88f
  fibrinolytic agents for, 99–102, 100f,
        100t, 102t
  heparin for, 95–97
  laboratory monitoring of, 103–104
    coagulation tests for, 104
    fibrinolytic tests for, 104
    platelet function tests for, 103–104
  for maxillofacial repairs, 304
  mechanical measures for, 103
  natural anticoagulant mechanisms and,
        84–85, 85f, 86f
  new agents for, 99
  procoagulant states and. *See*
        Hypercoagulable states
  thrombosis and inflammation and, 87,
        88f, 89
  warfarin for, 97f, 97–98, 98f
Hemothorax
  caked or clotted, treatment of, 324f,
        324–325, 325f
  chest injuries and, 318, 319
  in trauma patients, 284
  treatment of, 324, 324f
Heparin, 95–97, 1619

  for deep venous thrombosis, 1948,
        1949
  low-dose, 96
  low-molecular-weight, 96
  reversal of anticoagulation with, 96–97
  thrombocytopenia associated with, 89,
        1617
  thrombosis induced by, 1617
Hepatic abscesses
  amebic, 959, 960f
    pediatric, 2082
  pyogenic, 958–959
    pediatric, 2081–2082
Hepatic arteries
  anatomy of, 935, 935t, 936f, 1766
  aneurysms of, 1893f, 1895–1897,
        1896f, 1897f
  thrombosis of, following hepatic
        transplantation, 593–595
Hepatic artery-portal vein fistulas, 1921,
        1923
Hepatic cysts, 1013–1015
  acquired, 1015
  congenital
    polycystic disease and, 1014–1015
    solitary, 1013–1014, 1015f
  pediatric, 2080
Hepatic disorders. *See also specific*
        disorders
  chronic, 979–984
    cardiorespiratory manifestations of,
        979–980
    glucose homeostasis disorders and,
        981
    pulmonary manifestations of, 980,
        980t
    renal manifestations of, 980–981
    systemic manifestations of, 979
  gene therapy for. *See* Gene therapy, for
        hepatic disorders
  hydatid, 960
  portal hypertension associated with,
        992
  schistosomal, 960–961
  in ulcerative colitis, 1096
Hepatic duct, common, anatomy of, 1026,
        1028f
Hepatic encephalopathy, 981–984
  clinical features of, 983
  in fulminant hepatic failure, 978
  course o, 967, 968t
  management of, 983t, 983–984
  pathogenesis of, 982f, 982–983
Hepatic failure
  acute (fulminant), 967–970, 968t, 977–
        979
    clinical features of, 978
    encephalopathy course in, 967, 968t
    etiologic factors and pathogenesis of,
        977–978, 978t
    hepatic transplantation for, 583
    intracranial hypertension in, 969–
        970
    management of, 968–970, 978–979
    predicting outcome in, 968, 969t,
        970f
  in multiple organ failure syndrome,
        240
  sepsis and, 57
  total parenteral nutrition for, 59
Hepatic lobectomy, for bile duct cancer,
        1062–1063, 1065f

Hepatic necrosis, subacute, predicting
    outcome in, 968, 969t, 970f
Hepatic reserve, preoperative evaluation
    of, 937, 939
    correlation of computed tomography
        with segmental anatomy and,
        937f, 939
    oncologic considerations in hepatic
        resection and, 939
Hepatic resistance, in portal
    hypertension, 985–986
Hepatic system. *See also* Liver
    pediatric, 1990–1991
        bilirubin metabolism and, 1990–
            1991
        enzyme function and
            pharmacokinetics and, 1990
Hepatic transplantation, 581–599
    anesthetic management for, 584
    for biliary atresia, 2089–2090
    elective, preoperative assessment and
        management for, 584
    for hepatoblastomas, pediatric, 2138
    immunosuppression for, 598
    indications for, 581–583, 582t
    intraoperative management of
        coagulopathy for, 584–585, 585f
    postoperative complications of, 590–
        596
        biliary leak or obstruction, 592–593,
            596f
        hemorrhage, 593
        intraabdominal sepsis, 595–596
        neurologic, 596
        nonspecific cholestasis, 591–592
        primary nonfunction, 590–591
        thrombotic, 593–595
    rejection and, 596–598
        acute, treatment of, 598
        antibody-mediated, 596
        cell-mediated, 596–597, 597f, 597t,
            598f
        chronic, 597–598
    results with, 598–599
    surgical technique for, 585–590
        for anhepatic phase and implantation
            of donor liver, 587–588, 589f–
            591f
        for auxiliary liver transplantation,
            589–590, 594f–595f
        for dissection of recipient liver, 585–
            587, 586f–588f
        for postrevascularization phase and
            biliary reconstruction, 588, 591f,
            592f
        for reduced-size transplantation,
            588–589, 593f
    urgent, preoperative assessment and
        management for, 584
Hepatic veins
    anatomy of, 933–934, 934f, 1686
    outflow obstruction of. *See* Budd-
        Chiari syndrome
    thrombophlebitis of. *See* Budd-Chiari
        syndrome
Hepatitis, 961t, 961–967
    hepatitis A, 179, 961–962, 962f
        prophylaxis of, 962
    hepatitis B, 179, 962–965, 963f–965f
        hepatic transplantation for, 583
        hepatitis D coinfection and
            superinfection in, 966–967, 967f

hepatocellular carcinoma associated
        with, 1015, 1016
    precore mutant virus in, 962
    prophylaxis of, 964–965
    hepatitis C, 179, 965–966, 966f
    hepatitis D, 179, 966–967, 967f, 968f
        coinfection and superinfection in
            hepatitis B and, 966–967, 967f
        tests for, 967
    hepatitis E, 967
    non-A, non-B
        acute hepatic failure due to, 977
        hepatic transplantation for, 583
Hepatoblastomas, pediatric, 2080f, 2080–
    2081, 2081f, 2134–2138
    clinical presentation of, 2135
    epidemiology of, 2135
    hepatocellular carcinoma versus,
        2134–2135
    imaging in, 2135–2136, 2136f
    laboratory studies in, 2135
    outcome of, 2138
    pathology of, 2136–2137, 2137t
    staging of, 2136, 2136t
    treatment of, 2137–2138
Hepatocellular adenomas, 1011–1012,
    1012f
Hepatocellular carcinomas (HCCs),
    pediatric, 2081, 2134–2138
    clinical presentation of, 2135
    epidemiology of, 2135
    hepatoblastomas versus, 2134–2135
    imaging in, 2135–2136, 2136f
    laboratory studies in, 2135
    outcome of, 2138
    pathology of, 2136–2137, 2137t
    treatment of, 2138
Hepatocytes
    allogenic, for hepatic disorders, 516–
        517
    heterogeneity of, 943
    plasma membrane of, 943, 944f, 945,
        945f
Hepatorenal syndrome, 980–981, 981t
Hereditary nonpolyposis colorectal
    cancer (HNPCC), 461, 1110, 1131
    adenomas in, 1114–1117
        diagnosis of, 1115
        management of, 1115–1116
        primary prevention of recurrence of,
            1116–1117
    genetic factors in, 461, 1131
Hermaphroditism
    pseudohermaphroditism
        female, 2112, 2112f–2114f
        male, 2113
    true, 2113–2114, 2115f
Hernias, 1215–1235
    clinical manifestations of, 1217–1219
        complications and, 1218–1219
        of uncomplicated hernias, 1217–
            1218
    diagnosis of, 1217
    diaphragmatic
        Bochdalek. *See* Bochdalek hernias
        compressive cardiogenic shock due
            to, 201
        Morgagni, 2027
    epidemiology of, 1215–1216
    epigastric, 1227–1228, 1228f
    femoral, 1221–1226, 1222f–1226f
        diagnosis of, 1217
    incarcerated, 1218

incisional, 1215, 1235, 1235f
inguinal, 1215, 1221–1226, 1222f–
        1226f, 2032–2034
    anatomy, embryology, and
        pathophysiology of, 2032, 2033f
    clinical issues in, 2033
    diagnosis of, 1217
    differential diagnosis of, 1217
    direct, 2032
    femoral, 2032
    indirect, 2032
    operative considerations and
        outcome of, 2033–2034
internal, 1233–1235
    foramen of Winslow, 1235
    mesenteric, 1234–1235
    paraduodenal, 1234
interparietal, 1229
intestinal obstruction caused by, 825,
    1218
lumbar, 1230–1231, 1231f
mesocolic, 2054–2055
    treatment of, 2056–2057
obturator, 1231–1232
paraumbilical, 1215–1216, 1217,
    1226–1227, 1227f
pathobiology of, 1216–1217
    biochemical and metabolic
        alterations and, 1216
    chronic injury and, 1216
    congenital anatomic variants and,
        1216–1217
    physiologic alterations and, 1216
perineal, 1233, 1234f
recurrence of, 1221
Richter, 1218, 1218f
sciatic, 1232f, 1232–1233, 1233f
sliding, treatment of, 1219, 1219f
Spigelian, 1228, 1228f, 1229f
strangulated, 1218f, 1218–1219
supravesical, 1229–1230, 1230f
treatment of, 1219–1221
    anesthesia for, 1221
    complications of, 1220–1221
    for inguinal hernias, 2032, 2033–
        2034
    for massive hernias, 1221
    preoperative and postoperative care
        and, 1221
    principles of, 1219f, 1219–1220,
        1220f
umbilical, 1215–1216, 1217, 1226–
        1227, 1227f, 2032
    anatomy and embryology of, 2032
    clinical issues with, 2032
    operative considerations and
        outcome of, 2032
    of umbilical cord. *See* Omphaloceles
ventral, diagnosis of, 1217
Herpes simplex virus (HSV), as gene
    therapy vector, 521
Herpes simplex virus (HSV) infections,
    178
    proctitis due to, 1204
Herpes simplex virus (HSV) thymidine
    kinase, for vascular gene
    therapy, 520t
Herpesviruses. *See also specific viruses*
    infections caused by, 177–178, 177–
        179. *See also specific infections*
    tumor induction by, 464
Hespan (hetastarch; hydroxyethyl starch),
    in shock, 288–289

Hetastarch (Hespan; hydroxyethyl starch), in shock, 288–289

Hiatal hernia, in gastroesophageal reflux disease, 681–682

High-density lipoproteins (HDLs), atherosclerosis and, 1711

High-dose dexamethasone test, for hypercortisolism, 1340, 1340t

High endothelial venules, 152

High-frequency ventilation, 1986
for diaphragmatic hernias, 2026
jet, 1986
oscillatory, 1986

High linear energy transfer (LET) radiation, 494, 496f

Hirschsprung disease, 2057–2066
anatomy of, 2057–2058
clinical features of, 2058–2059
incidence and associations, 2058
presentation, 2058–2059
diagnosis of, 2059, 2060f, 2061f
embryology of, 2057
pathophysiology of, 2058
treatment of, 2059–2066
Duhamel procedure for, 2061, 2062f
laparoscopically assisted endorectal pull-through for, 2062, 2065f
rectal myectomy for, 2062, 2064
results of, 2064, 2066
Soave procedure for, 2061–2062, 2063f
Swenson procedure for, 2062, 2064f
for total colorectal aganglionosis, 2064

Hirudin, 99

Histamine, 764f

Histamine receptor(s), gastric acid secretion and, 752, 753f

Histamine-receptor antagonists
for duodenal ulcers, 761–763, 764f, 765–766
for gastric ulcers, 784, 784t
prophylactic, for stress gastritis, 778
for stress gastritis, 1165

Histiocytomas, fibrous, malignant
of chest wall, 1448
pediatric, 2266

Histiocytosis X, of ribs, 1446–1447

Histones
hepatic, 947
nuclear, 5

Histoplasma capsulatum infections, 177

HLA matching, for organ transplantation, 553–554

Hoarseness, in esophageal cancer, 702

Hodgkin disease
of head and neck, 643
spleen and, 1273–1274, 1274t, 1275f

Hodgkin lymphoma, in pediatric patients, 2010

Hollenhorst plaques, 1751

Homer-Wright pseudorosettes, 2119f, 2120

Homocysteine, plasma, atherosclerosis and, 1654–1655

Homocysteinemia, 1606–1607

Homocystinuria, 1606–1607, 1616
atherosclerosis and, 1715

Hormonal ablation, for prostate cancer, 2211, 2212

Hormonal failure, brain death and, 562

Hormonal studies, in impotence, 2201

Hormone(s). *See also specific glands and hormones*
biliary tract regulation by, 1030–1031
breast cell regulation by, 1361
cholelithiasis and, 1035
counterregulatory, surgical stress response and, 50
small intestinal, 807–808
volume control mediation by, 247

Hormone receptors, gene expression control and, 35f, 35–36, 36f

Hormone-sensitive lipase, 44

Hormone therapy
for breast cancer
adjuvant, 1397
metastases from, 1402
for desmoid tumors, 2262
for gastrinomas, 925
for mastodynia, 1372–1373
for menopausal symptoms, breast cancer risk and, 1379–1380
postoperative, 489–490
for undescended testes, 2109

Horner syndrome, in pediatric patients, 2011

Hornet stings, 407–408

Horseshoe fistulas, 1199

Horseshoe kidney, 2102, 2102f

Hospital care, for traumatic injuries, 278

Host defenses, 160–165
barriers, 160
cellular, 163
cytokines, 163–165, 164f
humoral, 161, 162f, 163
interactions among components of, 165, 165f
microbial flora, 160–161, 161f
modulation of, therapeutic, 180–181
therapeutic modulation of, 180–181

Host factors
metastasis and, 486
surgical stress and. *See* Stress response, surgical stress and

Human bites, hand infections due to, 2161

β-Human chorionic gonadotropin (β-HCG), in testis cancer, 2212

Human Genome Project, 506–507

Human immunodeficiency virus (HIV) infections. *See also* Acquired immunodeficiency syndrome (AIDS)
anorectal diseases in, 1204–1205
detection of, 178f, 178–179
hepatic infections associated with, 970–971
placental transmission of, 1992
transmission of, 179

Human papillomavirus (HPV)
condylomata acuminata and, 1202–1203
squamous cell carcinomas of skin and, 2242

Humoral defenses, 161, 162f, 163

Humoral hypercalcemia of malignancy (HHM), 1314–1315

Hürthle cell carcinomas, 1301, 1305–1306

Husni bypass, for venous obstruction, 1965

Hutchinson freckle, 2233, CF 111–1

Hydatid disease
of liver, 960
neurologic, 2191

Hydatidiform moles, 2229, 2229f

Hydroceles, 2034
acute, 2034
communicating, 2034

Hydrocephalus, 2193–2194
adult, 2194
childhood, 2193–2194
communicating and noncommunicating, 2193
infantile, 2193, 2193f
normal pressure, 2194
in spinal dysraphism, 2192, 2192f

Hydrocolloid dressings, 80–81, 81t

Hydrocolpos, in infancy, 2115–2116

Hydrocortisone, for addisonian crisis, 204–205

Hydrocytosis, hereditary, 1267

Hydrogel dressings, 81t

Hydrogen ions, organ preservation injury and, 556–557, 557f

Hydrogen peroxide, cell injury and, 154, 154t

Hydrometrocolpos, in infancy, 2115–2116

Hydronephromas, 2208–2209
diagnosis and staging of, 2208–2209, 2209f
treatment of, 2209

Hydronephrosis
antenatal, 2110–2111
ureteropelvic junction obstruction and, 2103f, 2103–2104, 2104f

Hydrophyidae. *See* Bites and stings

Hydrops, in cholecystitis, 1050

Hydrops fetalis, 1987–1988

18-Hydroxycorticosterone, in hyperaldosteronism, 1341, 1342t

Hydroxyethyl starch (Hespan; hetastarch), in shock, 288–289

Hydroxyl radical, cell injury and, 154t, 154–155

Hygromas
cystic. *See* Cystic hygromas
subdural, 2169

Hymen, imperforate, 2114, 2115f

Hymenoptera stings, 407–408

Hyperaldosteronism
primary, 1338, 1338f, 1338t
screening for, 1341, 1342t
treatment of, 1345

Hyperbaric oxygen therapy, for soft tissue infections, necrotizing, 174

Hyperbilirubinemia
conjugated, 2086
pediatric, 1990–1991

Hypercalcemia, 257–258, 1314–1316
causes of, 257
clinical manifestations of, 257–258, 1314, 1314t
differential diagnosis of, 1314–1315
in hyperparathyroidism, 1321
hypercalcemic crisis and, 1325
medical treatment of, 1315–1316, 1316t
metabolic alkalosis due to, 264
treatment of, 258

Hypercholesterolemia
familial, gene therapy for, 517–518, 518f
treatment of, 1711–1712

Hypercoagulable states, 89–92, 1614–1618

acquired, 1616–1618
antithrombin III deficiency, 89–90
congenital, 1614, 1615–1616
deep venous thrombosis and, 1945
defective fibrinolytic activity, 91–92
disseminated intravascular coagulation, 92
heparin-associated thrombocytopenia, 89
lupus anticoagulant-antiphospholipid syndrome, 91
platelet aggregation abnormalities, 92
protein C and S deficiencies, 90, 90f
resistance to activated protein C, 90–91
Hypercortisolism, 1336, 1337t
determining cause of, 1340, 1340f, 1340t
diagnosis of, 1352, 1353f
screening for, 1339–1340
treatment of, 1343–1345, 1355–1356
nonoperative, 1343–1344
operative, 1344–1345
Hyperdynamic state, in portal hypertension, 984
Hyperemia, reactive, 1673–1674
Hypergastrinemia, disease states associated with, 923, 923t
Hyperglycemia, injury response and, 54
Hyperinsulinemia
fetal, 1973
pediatric, 2096f, 2098
Hyperkalemia, 255–256
causes of, 255–256
clinical features of, 256
in critically ill patients, management of, 236–237
pediatric, 1989
treatment of, 256
Hyperlipidemia, atherosclerosis and, 1537, 1710–1712
lipid-lowering therapy and, 1711–1712
lipoproteins and, 1710–1711
Hyperlipoproteinemia, pancreatitis and, 881
Hypermagnesemia, 259
causes of, 259
clinical features of, 259
treatment of, 259
Hypermetabolism
burns and, 424
future management of, 437
nutritional support and, 434
in critically ill patients, mediators of, 230
injury response and, 54
sepsis and, 55
Hypernatremia, 254–255
causes of, 254
clinical features of, 254
pediatric, 1989
treatment of, 254–255
Hyperosmolar nonketotic acidosis, treatment of, 264
Hyperparathyroidism, 1317–1326
carcinomas and, 1326
definitions of, 1317
diagnosis of, 1321
etiology of, 1318
hypercalcemic, 1314
hypercalcemic crisis and, 1325
hypocalciuric, familial, 1315
incidence of, 1317–1318, 1318t

localization of, 1321–1322
neonatal, 1325
pancreatitis and
acute, 881, 881f
chronic, 889
pathology of, 1318–1319
carcinomas and, 1319
single- versus multiple-gland disease and, 1318f, 1318–1319, 1319f, 1319t
persistent or recurrent, 1324–1325, 1325f
in pregnancy, 1325
primary, 1317
secondary, 1317, 1325–1326
systemic effects of, 1319–1321, 1320t
tertiary, 1317
treatment of, 1322–1324
of asymptomatic disease, 1322–1323
extend of resection and, 1324
indications for surgery and, 1322
parathyroid autotransplantation techniques for, 1324
surgical principles for, 1323f, 1323–1324
Hyperplasia, 458–459, 460f
adrenal, congenital, 1337, 1337f, 1341, 2112, 2112f–2114f
breast cancer and, 458–459, 460f
C-cell, 1327–1328
endometrial, 2223
focal nodular, hepatic, pediatric, 2080
Hyperplastic left heart syndrome (HLHS), 1500
Hyperprolactinemia, diagnosis of, 1352, 1354, 1354f, 1354t
Hypersensitivity angiitis group, 1604–1605, 1605f
Hypersplenism, 1271–1273
Hypertensinogen, 1782
Hypertension
anesthesia and, 443
atherosclerosis and, 1536, 1714
intracranial. See Intracranial hypertension
portal. See Portal hypertension; Varices
pregnancy-induced, 394
pulmonary. See Persistent pulmonary hypertension of the newborn (PPHN)
renovascular. See Renovascular hypertension
venous, chronic venous insufficiency and, 1959
Hypertensive urography, in renovascular hypertension, 1788–1789
Hyperthyroidism, 1295–1298. See also Graves disease
hypercalcemia and, 1315
solitary toxic nodule and, 1298
toxic multinodular goiter and, 1297–1298
Hypertonic saline solutions, 249t, 250
in shock, 289–290
Hypertrophic scars, 83
burns and, 436–437, CF 12–13
Hyperviscosity syndrome, 1607
Hypervolemia, fluid and electrolyte therapy for, 251
Hypoadrenal shock, 183, 204–205
neurogenic, physiologic characteristics of, 197t
Hypocalcemia, 258–259, 1316–1317

causes of, 258
clinical features of, 259, 1316, 1316t
differential diagnosis of, 1316–1317
medical treatment of, 1317
in pancreatitis, 885
treatment of, 259
Hypochlorous acid, cell injury and, 154t, 155
Hypoferremia, cytokine-induced, 51
Hypoglycemia
in fulminant hepatic failure, 978
pediatric, 2096f, 2097f, 2097–2098
Hypogonadism, hypogonadotropic, primary and secondary, 2203
Hypogonadotropic hypogonadism, primary and secondary, 2203
Hypoinsulinemia, fetal, 1973–1974
Hypokalemia, 256–257
causes of, 256
clinical features of, 256
metabolic alkalosis due to, 264
pediatric, 1989
treatment of, 256–257
Hypomagnesemia, 259
causes of, 259
clinical features of, 259
in hyperparathyroidism, 1321
hypocalcemia and, 1317
treatment of, 259
Hyponatremia, 249, 253–254
causes of, 253
clinical features of, 253–254
diagnosis of, 254
pediatric, 1989
treatment of, 254
Hypoparathyroidism
idiopathic, hypocalcemia and, 1316–1317
postoperative, hypocalcemia and, 1316
Hypoperfusion
in critically ill patients, management of, 227, 228f, 229
distal, vascular injuries and, 362
stress response and, 48
Hypopharynx, cancer of, 640
Hypophysectomy, ablative, for pain management, 2194
Hypoplasia, uterine, 2116
Hypoplastic aorta syndrome, 1799
Hypospadias, 2107–2108, 2108f
Hyposplenism, 1273
Hypotension
in critically ill patients, management of, 227, 228f, 229
declamping, following abdominal aortic aneurysm repair, 1889
orthopedic injuries and, 373–374
in shock, 187
spinal cord injuries and, 2170–2171
Hypothenar hammer syndrome, 1763, 1764f
Hypothermia, 408t, 408–412, 409f
prevention of, in organ donors, 563
in shock, 291
rewarming and, 207
in trauma patients, 410–411
in traumatic injuries, in elderly people, 389
treatment of, 411–412
Hypovolemia
fluid and electrolyte therapy for, 250–251

Hypovolemia (*continued*)
   microvascular and cellular response to,
      186t, 186–187
   pediatric, 1989
      physiologic response to, 378
   in shock, 188, 189f
Hypovolemic shock, 182, 196–199, 198t
   diagnosis of, 197–198
   physiologic characteristics of, 197t
   treatment of, 198–199
Hypoxemia, pulmonary
      thromboembolism and, 1953
Hypoxia, respiratory alkalosis and, 265
Hysterectomy
   abdominal
      extrafascial, for endometrial
         carcinomas, 2223
      for ovarian carcinomas, 2228
      for tubal carcinomas, 2224
      for uterine sarcomas, 2223
   for abnormal uterine bleeding, 2223–
      2224
   radical, for cervical carcinomas, 2222
   for uterine leiomyomas, 2224
Hysteroscopy, diagnostic, for abnormal
      uterine bleeding, 2223

I

Iatrogenic complications, posttraumatic,
      396
ICAM-1, 1611
Idarubicin, 502t
Ifosfamide, 501t
   for tenosynovial sarcomas, pediatric,
      2132
Ileal artery, aneurysms of, 1893t, 1899f,
      1899–1900
Ileal pouch dysfunction, following
      ileoanal anastomosis, 1104–1106
Ileoanal anastomosis
   continent, 1101–1106, 1102f–1107f
   for familial adenomatous polyposis,
      1124
Ileorectal anastomosis, for ulcerative
      colitis, 1100, 1100f
Ileostomy
   abdominal, for ulcerative colitis, 1100,
      1100f
   continent, for ulcerative colitis, 1101,
      1101f
Ileum, gross anatomy of, 806, 807f
Ileum duplex, 2074–2075, 2075f
Ileus, 827–829
   diagnosis of, 828f, 828–829
   etiology of, 827–828, 829t
   gallstone, 1050
      intestinal obstruction and, 825f,
         825–826
   management of, 829
   meconium. *See* Meconium ileus
   postoperative
      with laparoscopic surgery, 738–739
      total parenteral nutrition for, 60
Iliac arteries. *See also* Aortoiliac
      occlusive disease
   aneurysms of, with abdominal aortic
      aneurysms, 1891
   common, 2216–2217
   external, 2217
   internal (hypogastric), 2217
Iliac lymph nodes, dissection of, in
      metastatic melanomas, 2240

Iliac veins
   common, 1936, 1938f
   external, 1935–1936
   internal, 1936
   thrombectomy of, angioplastic, 1741
Iliococcygeal muscle, anatomy of, 1181,
      1182f
Iliofemoral bypass grafts, 1804–1805,
      1807f
Iliohypogastric nerve, 1212
Ilioinguinal nerve, 1212
Iliopubic tract, 1211
Imaging. *See also* Radiographic
      examination; *specific modalities,
      sites, and disorders*
   of breasts, 1364t, 1364–1366, 1365f,
      1366f
   in pulmonary thromboembolism, 1952,
      1952f
   in valvular heart disease. *See* Valvular
      heart disease
Immobilization
   hypercalcemia and, 1315
   for spinal fractures, 2171–2172
   systemic impact of, 375–376
Immune arteritis. *See* Arteritis, immune
Immune function
   age-related changes in, 387
   alterations in, posttraumatic, 395–396,
      396t
   ontogeny of immune system and, 1991
   splenic, 1265–1266
Immune thrombocytopenic purpura
      (ITP), 1269t, 1269–1270
Immunocompetence, preservation of,
      with laparoscopic surgery, 739
Immunocompromised patients
   acute abdomen in, 1250, 1251t
   hepatic infections in, 970–971
Immunodeficiency, cancer and, 459
Immunoglobulin(s). *See also*
      Antibody(ies)
   antigen recognition by, 527f, 527–529,
      528f, 528t
   immunoglobulin A (IgA)
      hepatic, 946t
      secretory, 161
      structural properties of, 528t
   immunoglobulin D (IgD), 161, 163
      structural properties of, 528t
   immunoglobulin E (IgE), 161, 163
      structural properties of, 528t
   immunoglobulin G (IgG), 161
      maternal transfer of, 1991
      structural properties of, 528t
   immunoglobulin M (IgM), 161
      structural properties of, 528t
Immunoglobulin supergene family
   antigen recognition and, 538, 538t
   leukocytes and, 117–118
Immunology
   of carcinogen-induced tumors, 462f,
      463, 463f
   of Crohn's disease, 832f, 832–833, 833f
   developmental. *See* Pediatric patients,
      immunology and infection in
   of pancreatitis, 882
   small intestinal. *See* Small intestine,
      immunology of
Immunometric assays (IMAs), 1292, 1293
Immunomodulation, posttraumatic, 396
Immunoradioassays (IRAs), 1292
Immunostimulants, 181

Immunosuppression
   for cardiac transplantation, 1500
   clinical, 548, 549t, 550t, 551
   complications of, 552f, 552–553
   drug toxicity and, 553
   for hepatic transplantation, 598
   for pancreatic transplantation, 621–622
   for pulmonary transplantation, 612
   for renal transplantation, 576f, 577
      sequential therapy and, 577
   in shock, 208–209
   for ulcerative colitis, 1098
Immunotherapy
   adjuvant
      for colorectal cancer, 1144
      with head and neck surgery, 650
   adoptive, 2241
   for cancer, 500–505
      biologic, 503–505
         adoptive, 504
         multiagent, 504
         new approaches to delivery of,
            504–505
         recombinant cytokines for, 503–504
         tumor cell vaccines for, 503
      gene therapy, 504t, 505
      host immune response and, 500–
         501, 503
   for metastatic melanomas, 2240, 2241–
      2242, CF 111–2
Impedance plethysmography, in deep
      venous thrombosis, 1947–1948
Imperforate anus. *See* Anorectal
      disorders, imperforate anus
Imperforate hymen, 2114, 2115f
Impotence, 2200–2201
   diagnosis of, 2200–2201
   mechanism of erection and, 2200
   pathogenesis of, 2200
   treatment of, 2201
Impregnated dressings, 81t
Imuran (azathioprine), 549t
   for cardiac transplantation, 602, 602t
   for Crohn's disease, 841
   for pulmonary transplantation, 612
Incarcerated hernias, 1218
Incision(s)
   for abdominal aortic aneurysm repair,
      1888
   Brunner zig-zag incisions, for hand
      surgery, 2157
   healing of, 77
   relaxing, for hernia repair, 1220, 1222–
      1223, 1224f
   subxiphoid pericardial window, 329,
      329f
   for vulvar necrotizing fasciitis, 2218
Incisional biopsies
   of breast masses, 1369, 1369f
   of melanomas, 2236
   of osteosarcomas, 2263–2264
   of sarcomas, 2251, 2252f
Incisional hernias, 1215, 1235, 1235f
Incisura pancreatis, 859
Inclusion cysts, of hands, 2162
Incontinence
   anal, 1201–1202
      in rectal prolapse, 1191–1192
      treatment of, 1201–1202, 1203f
   urinary, 2199–2200
Indomethacin
   as antiplatelet agent, 98
   for patent ductus arteriosus, 1496

Infants. *See also* Pediatric patients
  breast feeding of, 1978. *See also*
        Lactation
    hyperbilirubinemia and, 1991
    maternal transfer of humoral
        immunity during, 1991
    nutrition and, 1978
  formulas for, 1976t, 1978
  growth and development of, 1973–
        1974
  hydrocephalus in, 2193, 2193f
  infections in, 1991–1992
  intestinal obstruction in, 2034–2066,
        2035t. *See also specific
        conditions causing obstruction*
  liver resection in, 2081
  mechanical ventilation in, 1986
  persistent pulmonary hypertension of
        newborn and. *See Persistent
        pulmonary hypertension of the
        newborn (PPHN)*
  premature, 1973
    thermoregulation and, 1979–1980
  thermoregulation in, 1979–1980
  Wilms tumor in, 2126
Infection(s), 159–181. *See also
        Abscesses; Sepsis; specific
        infections*
  following abdominal aortic aneurysm
        repair, 1890
  branchial cleft remnant-derived, 1995–
        1998
    anatomy and embryology of, 1995,
        1995f, 1996f
    clinical issues in, 1996
    operative considerations and
        outcome of, 1996–1998, 1997f,
        1998f
  of catheters, 176, 401
  cirrhosis due to, 975
  clinical manifestations of, 170
  as contraindication to organ donation,
        560
  following coronary artery bypass
        grafting, 1547
  Crohn's disease and, 832
  fever with, 172
  fungal, 176–177. *See also specific
        infections*
  gram-negative bacterial sepsis, 174–
        176, 175f
  of hands, 2160–2161
  of head and neck, 635–637, 636f
  hepatic, in immunocompromised hosts,
        970–971
  host defenses against. *See Host
        defenses*
  hypersplenism and, 1271
  immunosuppression and, 552, 552f
  intraabdominal, 170–173, 171f, 172f
    posttraumatic, 400
  invasive, stress response and, 49
  following lower extremity amputation,
        1835–1836
  lower extremity amputations and,
        1824–1825
  mastitis and breast abscesses and, 1377
  microbiological diagnostic techniques
        for, 166–167
    culture and sensitivity
        determinations, 166t, 166–167
    newer, 167
    staining, 166

  in multiple organ failure syndrome,
        210
  multiple organ system failure and. *See
        Multiple organ failure syndrome
        (MOFS)*
  necrotizing enterocolitis due to, 2046
  neonatal, 1991–1992
  neurologic, 2189–2191
    bacterial, 2189–2191
    fungal, 2191
    parasitic, 2191
  nosocomial, pneumonia, 176
  pancreatitis and, 881–882, 882t
  parasitic, 180
  pericarditis associated with, 1576
  of prosthetic devices, 176
  protozoan, 180
  following pulmonary transplantation,
        612, 613
  pyogenic, of hands, 2160–2161
  soft tissue, necrotizing, 173–174
  transmission of, by blood transfusions,
        105
  treatment of, 180–181
    antibiotic drugs in. *See Antibiotic
        drugs*
    gut decontamination in, 180
    immunostimulants in, 181
    lipopolysaccharide neutralization in,
        180–181
  ulcerative colitis and, 1094
  urinary, 176
    in ureteral duplication, 2105
  of urinary tract, 176
  vascular. *See Vascular disorders,
        infections*
  viral. *See Viral infections; specific viral
        infections*
  of wounds, 170
    following lower extremity
        amputation, 1835–1836
    posttraumatic, 400–401
Inferior vena cava (IVC), 1936
  bypass of, for venous obstruction,
        1965
  thrombophlebitis of, 1957
  Wilms tumor and, 2126
Infertility, male, 2201–2204
  evaluation of, 2202–2203
  specific disorders and treatments for,
        2203–2204
Inflammation, 130–158
  acute-phase response and, 132
    mediators of, 132, 133t, 134f
    serum proteins altered during, 132,
        132t
  anatomy and cell development and,
        130–132, 131f
  aneurysm formation and, 1844–1845
  cellular components of, 142–152
    erythrocytes, 151, 151f
    granulocytes, 142–148. *See also
        Polymorphonuclear leukocytes
        (PMNs); specific
        polymorphonuclear leukocytes*
    lymphocytes, 149
    mast cells, 148
    mononuclear phagocytes, 148–149,
        149f
    platelets, 149–151, 150t
    vascular endothelium, 151–152
  cellular injury in. *See Cell injury and
        death, in inflammation*

  humoral components of, 132–142
    complement, 132–135, 135f
    cytokines, 109–119, 110f, 111t, 132,
        133t, 141–142. *See also specific
        cytokines*
      localization of inflammation and,
        51
    eicosanoids, 136–140, 137t, 138f–
        140f
    growth factors, 142
    kinins, 135–136, 137f
    platelet-activating factor, 140–141,
        141f, 142f
  localization of, cytokine-induced, 51
  mastitis and breast abscesses and, 1377
  in shock. *See Shock,
        immunoinflammatory responses
        to*
  thrombosis associated with, 87, 88f, 89,
        1618
  tissue ischemia and, 1651–1652, 1652f
Inflammatory bowel disease. *See also
        Crohn's disease; Ulcerative
        colitis*
  bleeding in, 1171
  colorectal cancer and, 1131
  hemorrhoids in, treatment of, 1190
Inflammatory phase, of wound healing,
        67–68, 68t, 69f–70f
Inflammatory polyps, of gallbladder, 1056
Inflammatory response, alterations in,
        posttraumatic, 396
Infrainguinal occlusive disease, 1810–
        1823
  anatomy and, 1810–1811, 1811f
  atherosclerosis and, natural history of,
        1813f, 1813t, 1813–1814
  collateral circulation and, 1811, 1812f
  nonoperative treatment of, 1815–1819
    exercise for, 1815t, 1815–1816
    pharmacologic, 1815t, 1817, 1819
    smoking cessation and, 1816–1817
  operative treatment of, 1819–1823
    arteriography and, 1821
    indications for, 1820
    primary amputation, 1816f, 1821
    prosthetic bypass grafting, 1823
    vein bypass grafting, 1817f–1821f,
        1821–1823
      complications of, 1821f, 1822t,
        1822–1823
  pathophysiology of, 1811–1813, 1812t
  patient evaluation in, 1813f, 1815,
        1816f
Infrapiriform foramen, 1213, 1215f
Infrapopliteal occlusive disease. *See
        Infrainguinal occlusive disease*
Infundibular ventricular septal defects,
        1485
Inguinal anatomy, 1207–1213
  of anterior abdominal wall, 1207,
        1208f, 1209, 1209f
  of inguinal region, 1210–1213, 1211f–
        1213f
  of posterior abdominal wall, 1209–
        1210, 1210f
Inguinal canal, 1211–1212
Inguinal hernias, 1215, 1221–1226,
        1222f–1226f
  diagnosis of, 1217
  differential diagnosis of, 1217
Inguinal ligament, 1211, 1211f

Inguinal lymph nodes
  deep, dissection of, in metastatic
      melanomas, 2240
  dissection of, for anal cancer, 1150
Inhalation injury, 433, 433t
Initiation factors, 23
Injection injuries, of hands, 2160
Injury response, 48, 48t, 54–55
  ebb phase of, 54
  flow phase of, 54
  nutritional support and, 54–55
  time course of, 54
Injury Severity Score (ISS), 277
Innominate artery
  aneurysms of. *See* Aneurysm(s), of
      innominate artery
  traumatic injuries of, 366–368, 367f–
      370f
Inorganic carcinogens, 463
Inotropic agents. *See also specific drugs*
  for congestive heart failure, 1517
  for hypoperfusion, in critically ill
      patients, 227, 229f
  for organ donors, 563
  for shock, 205–206
      cardiogenic, 200–201
Insensible water loss, 248, 249, 249t
  pediatric, 1988
Inspiratory capacity, 1983
Inspiratory reserve volume, 1983
Insulin
  fetal and postnatal growth and
      development and, 1973–1974
  glucose homeostasis and, in chronic
      liver disease, 981
  hepatic, 946t
  for hyperkalemia, pediatric, 1989
  for pituitary evaluation, 1351–1352
  in shock, 188
  synthesis, secretion, and action of,
      867–868, 869f, 870f
Insulin-like growth factor 1 (IGF-1)
  hepatic, 946t
  for wound care, 82, 82t
Insulinomas, 919t, 921t, 921–923, 922f
  malignant, 922–923
  in multiple endocrine neoplasia, 1327,
      1327f
Insuloacinar portal system, 864
Integrins, 124
  antigen recognition and, 538, 538t
  cell-matrix adhesion and, 10–11
  leukocytes and, 117
Intensive care unit (ICU). *See* Critical
      care
Intercostal space, 1441, 1442f
Interdigestive myoelectric complex, 812
Interferon(s), recombinant, for cancer,
      503–505
Interferon-α (IFN-α), for metastatic
      melanomas, 2241
Interferon-*gamma (IFN-*gamma)
  acute-phase response mediation by, 133t
  recombinant, for cancer, 510, 510t
  surgical stress response and, 51
Interleukin(s)
  1 (IL-1)
      acute-phase response mediation by,
          132, 133t
      fibroblasts and, tissue remodeling
          and, 122, 123f, 124t
      gram-negative bacterial sepsis and,
          175

inflammation and, 114f, 114–115
      metabolic and inflammatory effects
          of interleukin-1 and, 114f, 114–
          115, 115t, 116t
      in shock, 194–195
      surgical stress response and, 50–51
      for wound care, 82, 82t
  2 (IL-2)
      acute-phase response mediation by,
          133t
      for metastatic melanomas, 2241–
          2242
      recombinant, for cancer, 504, 510,
          510t, 511f
  4 (IL-4)
      acute-phase response mediation by,
          133t
      recombinant, for cancer, 510, 510t
  6 (IL-6)
      acute-phase response mediation by,
          133t
      fibroblasts and, wound healing and,
          123
      gram-negative bacterial sepsis and,
          175
      inflammation and, 115–116, 116f
      surgical stress response and, 51
  8 (IL-8)
      acute-phase response mediation by,
          133t
      in shock, 195
  3 (IL-3), acute-phase response
      mediation by, 133t
  5 (IL-5), acute-phase response
      mediation by, 133t
  7 (IL-7), acute-phase response
      mediation by, 133t
  9–13 (IL-9–13), acute-phase response
      mediation by, 133t
  ulcerative colitis and, 1094–1095
Intermaxillary fixation (IMF), 307–308,
      308f
Intermediate-density lipoproteins (IDLs),
      atherosclerosis and, 1711
Intermediate filaments, 7–8, 8f
Intermittent claudication, in infrainguinal
      occlusive disease, 1811–1812,
      1812t, 1813
  evaluation of, 1814
Intermittent mandatory ventilation, 1986
Internal mammary artery (IMA) grafts,
      1544
International Classification of Diseases,
      277
Interparietal hernias, 1229
Interposition grafts, for coarctation of
      aorta, 1498
Intersex anomalies, 2111–2114
  diagnosis of, 2111t, 2111–2112
  embryology of, 2111
  female pseudohermaphroditism, 2112,
      2112f–2114f
  male pseudohermaphroditism, 2113
  mixed gonadal dysgenesis, 2112–2113
  surgical considerations in, 2114
  true hermaphroditism, 2113–2114,
      2115f
Intersphincteric abscesses, 1197
Intersphincteric fistulas, 1198
Intersphincteric space, anatomy of, 1182,
      1183f
Interstitial radiation implantation, for
      prostate cancer, 2211

Interstitial space, treatment of, in
      respiratory failure, 225
Intervertebral disc disease. *See* Spine,
      degenerative disease of
Intestinal atresia/stenosis, 2035–2038
  anatomy and embryology of, 2036,
      2036f
  clinical presentation of, 2036–2037
  diagnosis of, 2037
  duodenal, 2038–2041
      anatomy and embryology of, 2038,
          2038f, 2039f
      clinical presentation of, 2038, 2040
      diagnosis of, 2040, 2040f
      treatment of, 2040f, 2040–2041
          results and complications of, 2041
  treatment of, 2037f, 2037–2038, 2040f,
      2040–2041
      results and complications of, 2038
Intestinal cancer. *See also specific sites*
  intestinal obstruction and, 827, 827f
Intestinal fluid, mechanical bowel
      obstruction and, 820
Intestinal gas, mechanical bowel
      obstruction and, 819
Intestinal ischemia, following abdominal
      aortic aneurysm repair, 1890
Intestinal malrotation, 2053–2057
  anatomy of, 2054–2055
      mesocolic hernias and, 2054–2055
      mixed or incomplete rotation and,
          2054, 2055f
      nonrotation and, 2054, 2054f
  clinical presentation of, 2055
  diagnosis of, 2055, 2056f
  embryology of, 2053f, 2053–2054,
      2054f
  treatment of, 2055–2057, 2057f
      results and complications of, 2057
Intestinal obstruction, 817–827
  colonic pseudoobstruction, 829, 1092f,
      1092–1093
  in diverticular disease in diverticular
      disease, clinical presentation and
      diagnosis of, 1153
  hernias and, 825, 1218
  large intestinal, in diverticular disease,
      diagnosis and treatment of,
      1155–1156
  mechanical, 818–827
      adhesions and, 824f, 824–825
      in cholecystitis. *See* Gallstone ileus
      classification of, 818f, 818–819, 819t,
          820f
      clinical presentation and diagnosis
          of, 821
      closed-loop, 819, 820f
          complications of, 820–821
      complete, 818
      complications of, 820–821
      in Crohn's disease, 826–827
      gallstone ileus and, 825f, 825–826
      hernias and, 825
      incomplete, 818
      intussusception and, 826, 826f
      malignant, 827, 827f
      management of, 823–824
          laparoscopic surgery for, 827
      neurogenic (functional), 818
      open-loop, 819, 820f
          closed-loop, 821
      pathophysiology of, 819–820
      radiation enteritis and, 827

radiographs and imaging in, 821–823
simple, 818, 818f
strangulation, 818
terminology for, 818
volvulus and, 827
in Meckel's diverticulum, 2070
neonatal, 2034–2066, 2035t. *See also specific conditions causing obstruction*
in ulcerative colitis, 1099
Intestine(s). *See also specific regions and disorders*
angiodysplasia of, 1170
blood flow of, mechanical bowel obstruction and, 820
motility of. *See also* Ileus
mechanical bowel obstruction and, 820
traumatic injuries of, pediatric, 383
viability of, recognition of, 1774, 1776t
second-look procedures for, 1774
Intima, vascular, 1585
Intimal cell mass hypothesis, of atherosclerosis, 1594
Intraabdominal infections, 170–173, 171f, 172f
Intraaortic balloon counterpulsation (IABC), for shock, cardiogenic, 201
Intraaortic balloon pumps (IABPs), 1550–1553, 1551f, 1552f
complications of, 1553
indications for, 1551–1552
insertion technique for, 1552–1553
operation for, 1553
Intracellular fluid (ICF). *See also* Body fluids
composition of, 11, 11f
Intracellular receptors, activation of, 35
Intracerebral hemorrhage, in head injuries, 296–297, 297f
Intracranial hypertension
brain injuries and, 2167–2168
in fulminant hepatic failure, 969–970
in head injuries, computed tomography evaluation of, 296, 296f
head injuries and, 292–293, 293f
after head injury, pediatric, 384
posttraumatic, 399
Intracranial pressure (ICP), 292
elevation of. *See* Intracranial hypertension
monitoring of
in brain hemorrhage, 2185
in head injuries, 298
Intragastric pressure, gastroesophageal reflux and, 664
Intraluminal shunts, for traumatic injuries, 364–365
Intramural hematomas, duodenal, 345–346
Intrauterine growth retardation (IUGR), 1973
fluid spaces and, 1987–1988
Intravaginal torsion, 2110
Intravenous pyelography (IVP)
in renal injuries, 356
in ureteral injuries, 359
Intrinsic factor, 756
vitamin B_{12} absorption and, 816
Introns, 22
Intussusception, 826, 826f, 2067–2069

anatomy and pathophysiology of, 2067f, 2067–2068, 2068t
clinical presentation of, 2068
diagnosis of, 2068, 2069f
treatment of, 2068–2069
results of, 2069
Intussuscipiens, 2067
Intussusciptum, 2067
In utero surgery, for diaphragmatic hernia repair, 2026
Invariant chains, 532
Invasive moles, 2229, 2229f
Iodine-131
for Graves disease, 1296
for thyroid cancer, 1306–1307
Iodine, thyroid gland and, 1288
Iodine-123 imaging, of thyroid gland, 1294
Iodine-131 scans, of thyroid gland, 1306
Iododeoxyuridine (IUdR), for sarcomas, retroperitoneal, 2261, 2261f
Ion channels, 16–18
blockade of, 18
gating of, 17f, 17–18
modulation of, 18, 19f, 20f
ligand-gated, 18, 20f
receptors of, 36, 37f
Ionizing radiation. *See* Radiation
Irnotecan (CPT-II), 502t
Iron
hepatic metabolism of, 956–957
requirements in surgical patients, 62t
Irritable colon syndrome, 1091–1092
Ischemia
following abdominal aortic aneurysm repair, 1890
cerebrovascular. *See* Cerebrovascular disease, ischemic
in coronary artery disease. *See* Coronary artery disease (CAD)
inflammation and, 156, 158
lower extremity, angiography in, 1693–1694
mesenteric
angiography in, 1693, 1693f
nonocclusive, low-flow, 1772–1773, 1774f
posttraumatic, 395
severe, of lower extremities, diagnostic techniques for, 1674–1675, 1675f
in shock, 208
tissue injury and. *See* Tissue ischemia
following vascular injury, 362
visceral. *See* Visceral occlusive disease
wound healing and, 79, 79t
Ischemic penumbra, 1664, 1666f
Ischemic rest pain, in infrainguinal occlusive disease, 1812
Ischemic therapy, for liver cancer, primary, 1019
Ischemic ulcers, 1940
in infrainguinal occlusive disease, 1812
Ischioanal abscesses, 1197
Ischioanal space, anatomy of, 1182, 1183f
Islet cell tumors, nonfunctional, 927
Islets of Langerhans, 863, 867f
gene transfer in, 522
transplantation of, 625f, 626f, 626–627
for diabetes mellitus, 522
Isoflurane, 439t
Isoproterenol, for shock, 205
Isotonic saline solution, 249t, 250

Isotopic renography, in renovascular hypertension, 1789
Isthmectomy
for carcinomas, 1303
for solitary thyroid nodule, 1301
Ivalon sponge wrap operation, for rectal prolapse, 1191

J

Jaundice
in pancreatic cancer, palliative treatment for, 914, 914f
physiologic, neonatal, 2086
Jejunal artery, aneurysms of, 1893t, 1899f, 1899–1900
Jejunoileal bypass, for morbid obesity, 790–791, 791f
Jejunostomy
feeding catheter, 65
Witzel, 65
Jejunum, gross anatomy of, 806, 807f
Jewett staging system, for prostate cancer, 2210, 2210f
Joining (J) regions, 528
Joints. *See also specific joints*
degenerative disease of
of hand, 2159
in morbid obesity, 790
fractures involving surfaces of, 2147, 2148f
of hand, 2153, 2154f, 2159
arthritides of, 2159, 2161f
dislocations of, 2159
total joint replacement arthroplasty and, 2148–2150, 2150f, 2151f
in ulcerative colitis, 1096
Juvenile polyposis, 1126f, 1126–1127

K

Kallidin, production in tissue, 136
Kallikrein, inhibition of, 99
Kaposi sarcoma, 2247
anorectal, in HIV-positive patients, 1204
immunosuppression and, 553
Karnofsky Performance Status Scale, 503t
Kasabach-Merritt syndrome, 1925
Kawasaki disease, 1603f, 1603–1604
Keloids, 82
Keratosis, actinic, of hands, 2162
Kernicterus, 1990
Ketamine, 441t, 441–442
Ketoacidosis
decreased body bicarbonate content due to, 261–262
diabetic, treatment of, 263–264
Ketoconazole, for monilial esophagitis, 724
17-Ketosteroids, 1331
Kidney(s). *See also* Renal *entries*
atheroembolism of, 1633–1634
baroreceptors in, 246–247
enlargement of, in diabetes mellitus, 617
horseshoe, 2102, 2102f
pediatric, 2101–2104. *See also specific disorders*
traumatic injuries of, 384
preservation of, 568–569, 573t

Kidney(s), preservation of (*continued*)
  in dissecting renal artery aneurysms, 1908
  suitability for donation, 561
  traumatic injuries of, 356–358, 357f
    pediatric, 384
Kidney plasminogen activator, 1738
Kinin(s), inflammation and, 135–136, 137f
  bradykinin production in plasma and, 135–136
  cellular kininogenase activity and, 136
  kinin production in tissue and, 136
Kininogenase, cellular activity of, 136
Klatzkin tumors, 1061
Klinefelter syndrome, 2204
Klippel-Trenaunay syndrome, 1926, 1927–1928, 1929f, 1930, 1930f, 1932f
  lymphatics in, 1967
  port wine stains in, 1930, 1932
Knees
  arthroscopic meniscectomy and, 2151
  total joint replacement and, 2149, 2150f
Kocher maneuver, 343, 343f, 347
Kock ileostomy, continent, 1101, 1101f
K-*ras* point mutations, lung cancer and, 1419
K value, 872

L

Labor, hemorrhoids following, 1190
Laboratory studies. *See also specific tests and disorders*
  in abdominal injuries, 334
  of adrenal gland. *See* Adrenal gland
  in bile duct strictures, 1069–1070
  in chronic pancreatitis, 892
  in hyperparathyroidism, 1321
  for male infertility, 2202t, 2202–2203
  in pancreatic cancer, 905–906
  of pancreatic function, 870–873
    endocrine, 872–873, 873t
    exocrine, 870–872, 872t
  in pregnancy, 391–392
  of thyroid function, 1291–1293
  in vascular occlusive disease, of upper extremities, 1760
Lacis cells, 1780
Lacrimal duct injuries, repair of, 305
Lactated Ringer solution, 249t, 249–250
Lactation, 1362. *See also* Breast feeding
  breast cancer during, 1409
  breast involution following, 1362
Lactation mastitis, 1377
Ladd procedure, for malrotation, 2055–2057, 2057f
Lambl excrescence, 1502
Lamellae, aneurysm formation and, 1842–1843
Laminectomy
  for cervical spine disease, 2188
  for lumbar spine disease, 2188, 2189
Laminograms, tracheal, 1473, 1474f
Langerhans, islets of, 863, 867f
  gene transfer in, 522
  transplantation of, 625f, 626f, 626–627
    for diabetes mellitus, 522
Laparoscopic therapy, 736–740
  access for, 736, 737f, 738f
  advantages and disadvantages of, 739

for appendicitis, 1256–1257
cholecystectomy, 1045, 1045f, 1045t, 1046f
  cholangiography during, 1047
  for gallbladder cancer, 1060
complications of, 740, 740t
current status of, 739–740
future of, 740
gasless, 736, 738
for hernia repair, of inguinal and femoral hernias, 1225, 1226f
insufflation for, 736, 738, 738t
for intestinal obstruction, 827
Nissen fundoplication, 687, 687f–690f, 689–690
physiology and, 736, 738t, 738–739
splenectomy, 1280
Laparoscopy, diagnostic
  in abdominal injuries, 335
  in cancer, 490
Laparoscopy therapy, endorectal pull-through, for Hirschsprung disease, 2062, 2065f
Laparotomy
  in abdominal injuries, 336–337
  in pelvic fractures, 353–354
  in pregnancy, 394
  in renal injuries, 357–358
  in splenic injuries, 338
    pediatric, 383
  staging, in Hodgkin's disease, 1274, 1274t, 1275f
  therapeutic, in appendicitis, 1257
  for tuboovarian abscesses, 2225
Lap belt injuries, 271
Laplace law, 1506, 1534
Laryngeal nerve
  recurrent. *See* Recurrent laryngeal nerve (RLN)
  superior, 1286
Laryngectomy, 647, 649
Laryngotracheoesophageal cleft, 2016
Larynx
  cancer of, 640–641
  traumatic injuries of, management of, 314–316, 316f
Laser-induced fluorescence, 1736
Laser therapy
  for abnormal uterine bleeding, 2223
  for cancer, 490
  continuous wave versus pulsed lasers for, 1736
  endovascular, 1736–1737
  fulguration, for esophageal cancer, 706
  for peptic ulcers, 1162–1163
Latissimus dorsi flaps, 2281, 2282f
Latissimus dorsi island pedicle flaps, 2286
Latissimus dorsi muscle, 1443f, 1444
Latissimus dorsi muscle flaps, for chest wall reconstruction, 1450, 1452f
Latrodectus mactans bites, 406, 407, 407f
Lecithin, biliary secretion of, 955
LeFort fractures, 299f, 299–300
  repair of, 307
Left anterior descending (LAD) artery, 1534
Leg. *See* Lower extremities
Leiomyomas
  esophageal, 695–696, 696f, 697f
  small intestinal, 846
  uterine, 2224
Leiomyosarcomas

gastric, 804
pediatric, 2134
small intestinal, 849–850
  origin of, 849
  presentation and diagnosis of, 849, 849f
  prognosis and survival and, 850
  treatment of, 849–850
Lentigo maligna, 2233, CF 111–1
Leptomeninges, metastases to, 2179
Leukemia
  hairy cell, 1274, 1276f
  lymphocytic, chronic, 1275, 1276f
  myelogenous, chronic, 1275
  treatment of, 1275
Leukocytes, endothelial cell interactions with, 116–119
  adhesion molecules and, 117f, 117–118, 118f, 151f, 152
  chemotactic factors and, 118–119, 119t
  high endothelial venules and, 152
  wound repair and, 118, 118f
Leukocytosis
  cytokine-induced, 51
  peripheral, in spontaneous bacterial peritonitis, 988
Leukotrienes
  in inflammation, 137t
  in shock, 193f, 193–194
Levator ani muscle, 2041
  anatomy of, 1181, 1182f
LeVeen peritoneovenous shunt, for ascites, 990f
Levocarnitine (L-carnitine), for claudication, 1716
Lidocaine, 442t
Lieberkühn crypts, 807
Li-Fraumeni syndrome, 1381, 2248, 2250–2251
Ligament of Berry, 1284, 1284f
Ligand-gated ion channels, 18, 20f
Ligandins, hepatic biotransformation and, 956
Ligand-receptor interaction, in endocytosis, 33–34
Ligation
  for extracranial carotid aneurysms, 1852
  of perforating veins, 1941, 1941f, 1943
  of varicose veins, 1939
Limb-length discrepancy, 2148
  Ilizarov wire and frame treatment for, 2148, 2149f
Limbs. *See* Extremities; Lower extremities; Upper extremities
Limb-sparing operations
  for osteosarcomas, 2264–2265, 2266f
  for sarcomas, 2255, 2257f, 2258f, 2258–2259
    functional outcome following, 2258–2259
Linear skull fractures, 2166
Lip(s), cleft, plastic surgery for, 2286–2287
Lipases, 44
  pancreatic secretion of, 866
  in pancreatitis, 884
Lipid(s). *See also specific lipids*
  metabolism of, hepatic. *See* Liver, lipid metabolism in
  pediatric requirements for, 1975
  plasma membrane, selectivity and

energy conversion and, 12–13, 13f
priming of neutrophil function by, 147, 148f
in total parenteral nutrition, 60–61
Lipid bilayer, solubility-diffusion and, 15, 15f
Lipid insudation hypothesis, of atherosclerosis, 1593
Lipodermatosclerosis, 1959
Lipodystrophy, isolated, 1238–1239
Lipogranulomas, of mesentery, 1238–1239
Lipogranulomatosis, sclerosing, 1238–1239
Lipomas
of abdominal wall, 1236
colorectal, 1118
small intestinal, 846
spinal, 2180
Lipomatous tumors, mesenteric, 1240
Lipopolysaccharides (LPSs), neutralization of, 180–181
Lipoprotein(s)
atherosclerosis and, 1710–1711
metabolism of, 44
Lipoprotein(a), 1616
atherosclerosis and, 1711
Lipoprotein-associated coagulation inhibitor, 85
Lipoprotein lipase, 44
endothelial-bound, atherosclerosis and, 1711
Liposarcomas, pediatric, 2134, 2266
Liposomes, for respiratory disorders, 514, 514f, 515f
Liposuction, 2272t, 2277–2279, 2279f
Lipoxins, in inflammation, 137t
Lipoxygenase pathways, inflammation and, 138–140
Liquid ventilation, for diaphragmatic hernia repair, 2026–2027
Lithiasis
biliary. *See* Choledocholithiasis; Cholelithiasis
urinary. *See* Urinary lithiasis
Lithostathine, 890
Lithotripsy
basic principles of, 2205, 2206f
biliary
in choledocholithiasis, 1048
in cholelithiasis, 1048
contraindications to, 2205
for urinary lithiasis, 2205, 2206
Livedo reticularis, 1632, 1632f
Liver. *See also* Hepatic *entries*
anatomy of, 931–943
morphologic and functional, 932–935, 933f
of hepatic arteries, 935, 935t, 936f
of hepatic veins, 933–934, 934f
of portal veins, 934–935, 935f
topographic, relations to perihepatic structures and, 931f, 931–932, 932f
artificial hepatic support systems for, 979, 979t
bile and. *See* Bile *entries;* Biliary *entries*
biotransformation in, 956
blood flow in, 948
blood cleansing function and, 948
control of, 948, 948f

carbohydrate metabolism in, 948–950
gluconeogenesis and, 949–950, 951f
glycogenesis and glycogenolysis and, 949, 949f
glycogen storage and metabolism and, 949
glycolysis and, 949, 950f
phosphogluconate pathway and, 949, 951f
heme and porphyrin metabolism in, 956, 957f
histologic organization of, 943, 944f
imaging of, 935–937
computed tomographic, 935, 937
magnetic resonance imaging for, 937
positron emission tomography scanning for, 937
ultrasonographic, 935, 936f
intraoperative assessment of, 938f–940f, 939, 941
lipid metabolism in, 950–953
fatty acids and, 951–952, 952f
cholesterol and, 951–952, 953f
phospholipids and, 952
lipid transport into liver and, 950–951
lobes of, 932–933, 933f
major lobectomy of, 941
metabolism of, 953–954, 954f
metal metabolism in, 956–957
neoplastic disease of, 1008–1022
benign, 1010–1015
cystic, 1013–1015
solid tumors, 1011–1013
vascular lesions, 1013
diagnostic evaluation of, 1008–1010, 1009f–1011f, 1009t
malignant. *See* Liver cancer
parenchymal cell ultrastructure of, 943–947
pediatric, 2078–2082
embryology of, 2083, 2083f
neoplastic disease of, 2078–2081, 2079t
benign, 2079–2080
liver resection for, 2081, 2082f
malignant, 2080–2081
preoperative evaluation of hepatic reserve and, 937, 939
correlation of computed tomography with segmental anatomy and, 937f, 939
oncologic considerations in hepatic resection and, 949
preservation of, 568–569, 573t, 574f
protein metabolism in, 952–953
amino acid transport and storage and, 952–953, 953f
formation of plasma protein formation and, 953, 954t
protein uptake and degradation and, 953
segmental resections of, 940f–942f, 941, 943
suitability for donation, 561
traumatic injuries of, 338–341, 339f, 340f
pediatric, 382, 383, 383f, 384f
ultrastructure of
cell-surface receptors and, 945, 946f, 946t, 947, 947f
endoplasmic reticulum and Golgi complex and, 947

endosomes, multivesicular bodies, and lysosomes and, 947
mitochondria and, 947
nucleus and, 947
plasma membrane and, 943, 944f, 945, 945f
vitamin metabolism in, 957
Liver biopsies
in biliary atresia, 2086–2087
in liver masses, 1010, 1011f
Liver cancer, 1015–1022
cholangiocarcinomas, 1018
hepatic transplantation for, 583
hepatocellular carcinoma (primary), 1015–1018
clinical presentation of, 1016–1017
diagnosis of, 1017–1018
epidemiology, etiology, and pathogenesis of, 1015–1016
natural history of, 1018
pathology of, 1016, 1016f, 1017f
screening for, 1018, 1018t
metastatic, 1019–1022
biology of, 1019
from colorectal cancer, 1136
treatment of, 1144, 1145f
from colorectal primaries, natural history of, 1019–1020, 1020f, 1021t
evaluation of, 1020, 1021t, 1022f
treatment of, 1020–1022
for extrahepatic disease, 1020
intrahepatic distribution and, 1021
margin of resection for, 1020–1021
number of metastases and, 1021
size of metastases and, 1021
surgical options for, 1021–1022
primary, treatment of
curative therapy for, 1018–1019
liver transplantation for, 1019
palliative therapy for, 1019
sarcomas (primary), 1018
Liver resection, in infants and children, 2081
Liver transplantation
for hepatocellular carcinoma, 1019
orthotopic
for Budd-Chiari syndrome, 991, 992f
for fulminant hepatic failure, 979, 979f
Lizards, venomous, 406
Loading, of soft tissues, 2142, 2142f, 2143f
Lobar overinflation, congenital, 2005, 2006f
Lobectomy, for, 2008
Lobules, of breast, 1360
Local anesthetics, 442t, 442–443
Lomustine (CCNU), 501t
Long terminal repeats, 508
Lorazepam (Ativan), 442t
Lovastatin, for hypercholesterolemia, 1712
Low-density lipoproteins (LDLs)
atherosclerosis and, 1711
hepatic, 946t
Lower esophageal sphincter
hypertensive, 679–680
manometric assessment of, 665, 665f, 666f
physiology of, 664
Lower extremities
amputation of, 1823t, 1823–1838

Lower extremities (*continued*)
above-knee, 1826f, 1832–1833, 1836t
rehabilitation and prosthetic management for, 1838
below-knee, 1826f, 1830–1832, 1834t, 1835f
rehabilitation and prosthetic management for, 1838
complications of, 1834–1837
additional limb loss, 1837
deep venous thrombosis, 1837
mortality, 1834–1835
of stumps, 1835–1837
digital and ray, 1826f, 1828, 1828t, 1829f
rehabilitation and prosthetic management for, 1837
hip disarticulation, 1826f, 1834
indications for, 1823–1824, 1824t
operative management of, 1827–1834
above-knee amputations, 1826f, 1832–1833, 1836t
below-knee amputations, 1826f, 1830–1832, 1834t, 1835f
digital and ray amputations, 1826f, 1828, 1828t, 1829f
general considerations in, 1827–1828
hip disarticulation, 1826f, 1834
Syme amputations, 1826f, 1829–1830, 1832f–1833f
transmetatarsal amputations, 1826f, 1828–1829, 1830t, 1831f
postoperative care and, 1834
preoperative management for, 1824–1827
of infectious problems, 1824–1825
medical evaluation and, 1824, 1824t
multidisciplinary evaluation for, 1827
potential for revascularization and, 1825
selection of amputation level and, 1825–1827, 1826f, 1826t
timing of operative intervention and, 1827
primary, for infrainguinal occlusive disease, 1816f, 1821
rehabilitation and prosthetic management and, 1837–1838
general considerations in, 1837, 1837t
specific levels and, 1837–1838
Syme, 1826f, 1829–1830, 1832f–1833f
rehabilitation and prosthetic management for, 1838
transmetatarsal, 1826f, 1828–1829, 1830t, 1831f
rehabilitation and prosthetic management for, 1837
arteries of, anatomy of, 1687–1688
atheroembolism of, 1632f, 1632–1633
blood pressure measurement in, 1669, 1670f, 1671, 1671f
calf claudication of, 1639
compartment syndromes in, 1642
diabetic foot ulcers and, healing of, 80
fractures of, fixation of, 376
ischemia of
following abdominal aortic aneurysm repair, 1890
angiography in, 1693–1694

leg ulcers and, healing of, 80
peripheral arterial obstruction of, diagnostic techniques for, 1674–1676, 1675f
sarcomas of, 2253, 2253t
trench (cold-immersion) foot and, 412
vascular trauma to, 370, 373f
veins of, 1935–1937, 1936f–1938f
pressure in, 1937
venous disease of, angiography in, 1701f, 1705
Loxosceles reclusa bites, 406f, 406–407
Lumbar hernias, 1230–1231, 1231f
Lumbar nerve roots, 2186, 2186f
Lumbar spine
degenerative disease of, 2188–2189
clinical presentation of, 2188
diagnosis of, 2188, 2189f
treatment of, 2188–2189
traumatic injuries of, 2169, 2171
Lumpectomy, 1389, 1390–1391, 1392, 1392t
for ductal breast cancer, 1403–1404, 1404f
local recurrence following, management of, 1401
radiotherapy after, 1395, 1396f
reexcision, 1389
Lundh test, 872
Lung(s). *See also* Pulmonary *entries;* Respiratory *entries*
acute injury of, in shock, 190
biochemical maturation of, 1983
carbon dioxide transfer in, in critically ill patients, 220, 220f
collapse of, in chest injuries, 319
compliance of, 1984
preservation of, 569
Lung cancer, 1417–1433, 1434–1438
adenomas, 1432–1433
adenoid cystic carcinomas, 1433, 1433f
mucoepidermoid, 1433
mucous gland, 1433
biology of, 1418–1420
carcinoid tumors, 1431, 1432f
in pediatric patients, 2009, 2009f, 2010f
incidence and epidemiology of, 1417
large cell neuroendocrine tumors, 1431
metastatic, 1434–1438
clinical presentation and diagnosis of, 1435, 1435f, 1436f
from colorectal cancer, treatment of, 1144
of head and neck cancer, 651
historical background of, 1434–1435
from sarcomas, management of, 2267
surgical resection for. *See* Pulmonary resection
non-small cell, 1417, 1420t, 1420–1431
clinical presentation and diagnosis of, 1421, 1421f, 1422f
selection of treatment for, 1421–1423, 1422f, 1423f
surgical resection for. *See* Pulmonary resection
treatment of
for stage I and II disease, 1423–1427, 1424f–1426f
for stage IIIa disease, 1427–1431
pathologic classification of, 1417–1418, 1418t

in pediatric patients, 2009f, 2009–2010, 2010f
small cell, 1417, 1418, 1431–1432
squamous cell, 1417
Lung capacities, 1983
Lung scans, in pulmonary thromboembolism, 1952
Lung volumes, 1983
Lupus anticoagulant, 1616–1617
Lupus anticoagulant-antiphospholipid syndrome, 91
Luschka, ducts of, 1029
Luteinizing hormone (LH), in males, 2202
Luteinizing hormone-releasing hormone (LHRH), for prostate cancer, 2211
Lymph, analysis of, 1968
Lymphadenectomy
axillary, 1389, 1394
for metastatic melanomas, 2240
delayed, total mastectomy with, 1390
elective, 2238f, 2238–2239, 2239f, 2239t
of iliac nodes, for metastatic melanomas, 2240
of inguinal nodes
for anal cancer, 1150
for metastatic melanomas, 2240
inguinofemoral, for vulvar carcinomas, 2218
for metastatic melanomas, 2237–2240
results and indications for, 2237–2239, 2238f, 2239f, 2239t
site-specific considerations for, 2239–2240, 2240f
of obturator nodes, for metastatic melanomas, 2240
pelvic
abdominal, 2228
for uterine carcinomas, 2222
periaortic
abdominal, 2228
for tubal carcinomas, 2224
regional, for skin cancer, 2244
retroperitoneal, for testis cancer, 2213
Lymphadenitis
mesenteric, acute, 1238
suppurative, acute, in pediatric patients, 1999
Lymphadenopathy
benign, of head and neck, 639
in pediatric patients, 1999–2000
operative considerations and outcome of, 2000
Lymphangiomas
cystic, mesenteric, 1239
in pediatric patients, 1999
anatomy and embryology of, 1999, 1999f
clinical issues in, 1999
operative considerations and outcome of, 1999
of spleen, 1273
Lymphangiosarcomas, 1966, 1968f
etiology of, 2248, 2248f
Lymphangitis, 1970
Lymphatic metastasis, 483–484
Lymphaticovenous anastomoses, 1970
Lymphatic system. *See also specific disorders*
anatomy of, 1966, 1967f

lymph node dissection and. *See* Lymphadenectomy

nodes of
   barrier function of, 484–485
   biopsies of, cervical, 643, 645f
   Delphian, 1284
   in melanomas, 2234t, 2234–2235

Lymphedema, 1966–1968
   classification of, 1969
   diagnosis of, 1966–1968
     lymphatic visualization for, 1967–1968, 1968f
     tissue fluid analysis for, 1968
   management of, 1969–1970
     conservative, 1969–1970
     operative treatment for, 1970
   pathophysiology of, 1966, 1968f
   primary, 1969
   reconstructive surgery for, 2289
   secondary, 1969, 1970

Lymphocysts, 1969

Lymphocytes
   development of, 544–545, 545f
   inflammation and, 149

Lymphocytotoxic antibodies, hepatic transplantation and, 596

Lymphography, radiographic, 1968, 1968f

Lymphoid nodules, isolated, colorectal, 1118–1119

Lymphoid tissue, small intestinal
   aggregated, 809–810, 810f
   nonaggregated, 809, 809f

Lymphokine-activated killer (LAK) cells, interleukin-2 and, 2241

Lymphokines, 163

Lymphomas
   anorectal, in HIV-positive patients, 1204
   of appendix, 1260
   Burkitt, Epstein-Barr virus and, 464
   colorectal, 1145
   gastric, 802–803
     clinical features of, 802–803
     diagnosis of, 803
     treatment of, 803, 803f
   Hodgkin, in pediatric patients, 2010
   immunosuppression and, 553
   mediastinal, 1470
   pancreatic, 916–917, 917f
   small intestinal, 850–852
     Mediterranean, 852
     origin of, 850, 850t
     presentation and diagnosis of, 850–851, 851f
     prognosis and survival and, 851–852
     treatment of, 851

Lymphoreticular system, 130–131, 131f

Lynch syndrome. *See* Hereditary nonpolyposis colorectal cancer (HNPCC)

Lysosomes, 6
   hepatic, 947

Lysyl bradykinin, production in tissue, 136

Lytic therapy. *See* Thrombolytic therapy; *specific agents*

M

Machinery murmurs, 1921

Macroembolism, angiography in, 1690, 1691f, 1692f

Macrophage colony-stimulating factor, acute-phase response mediation by, 133t

Macrophages, inflammation and, 148–149, 149f

Macula densa, 1780

Magnesium, 259. *See also* Hypermagnesemia; Hypomagnesemia
   pediatric requirement for, 1977

Magnetic resonance angiography, 1679–1680, 1681f–1682f
   in abdominal aortic aneurysms, 1885

Magnetic resonance arteriography, in renovascular hypertension, 1787

Magnetic resonance imaging (MRI)
   in abdominal aortic aneurysms, 1884–1885
   in adrenal disorders, 1343, 1344f
   in arteriovenous fistulas, 1922
   of breasts, 1366
   in cerebrovascular disease, 1752
   in congenital vascular malformations, 1927, 1931f
   of liver, 937
     in liver masses, 1009
   in osteosarcomas, 2263
   of pituitary gland and parasellar region, 1350, 1351f
   in sarcomas, 2253
   in thoracoabdominal aortic aneurysms, 1876, 1877f
   of thyroid gland, 1294
   in vascular disorders, 1669, 1670f
     infections, 1725, 1725f

Major histocompatibility complex (MHC), antigen recognition by T-cell receptors and, 529f–530f, 529–530, 530t

Malabsorption, in chronic pancreatitis, 891
   treatment of, 898t, 898–899

Malar complex fractures, repair of, 307

Male genitourinary system, 2199–2214. *See also specific organs and disorders*

Male infertility, 2201–2204
   evaluation of, 2202–2203
   specific disorders and treatments for, 2203–2204

Malignant fibrous histiocytomas
   of chest wall, 1448
   pediatric, 2266

Malignant melanomas. *See* Melanomas

Mallet finger, 2157f, 2157–2158

Mallory bodies, cirrhosis and, 973f, 973–974

Mallory-Weiss syndrome, bleeding in, 1167

Mall's space, 948, 948f

Malnutrition
   in Crohn's disease, 835
   stress response and, 49
   in trauma patients, consequences of, 55

Malrotation, intestinal. *See* Intestinal malrotation

Mammaplasty
   augmentation, 2272t, 2274–2275, 2275f
   reduction, 2272t, 2276, 2276f

Mammary duct ectasia, 1377

Mammography, 1364t, 1364–1365, 1365f

Mandible
   anatomy of, 300, 300f
   fractures of, repair of, 307–308, 308f

Manganese, requirements in surgical patients, 62t

Mannitol
   for cerebral edema, 293
   for intracranial hypertension, 2167

Manometry
   anorectal, in Hirschsprung disease, 2059
   esophageal. *See* Esophageal manometry

MAP kinase, activation of, 37, 38f

Marfan syndrome, 1599–1600, 1600f
   aortic aneurysms in, 1864
     operative management of, 1864, 1864f, 1865f, 1866

Marion-Clatworthy cavomesal shunt, 1000f

Marlex methyl methacrylate sandwich, for chest wall reconstruction, 1449, 1450f

Maryland Institute of Emergency Medicine, 268

Masaoka staging system, for thymomas, 1470, 1470t

Mastalgia, 1372t, 1372–1373

Mast cells, inflammation and, 148

Mastectomy, 1392–1394
   cancer dissemination and, 1385–1386, 1386f
   for ductal breast cancer, 1403–1404, 1404t
   for lobular breast cancer, 1405
   local recurrence following, management of, 1400f, 1400–1401
   lymphedema following, 1966, 1968f
   for metastic breast cancer, 1402
   prophylactic, 1405–1407
     choice of operation for, 1406
     indications for, 1406, 1406t
     reconstruction following, 1406–1407
   radical, 1389
     modified, 1389–1390, 1390, 1391t, 1392–1394, 1393f
   radiotherapy after, 1395–1396
   subcutaneous, 1389
   toilet, 1402
   total, 1389, 1390–1391
     with delayed lymph node dissection, 1390

Mastitis
   lactation, 1377
   periductal (mammary duct ectasia; plasma cell mastitis), 1377

Mastodynia, 1372t, 1372–1373

Mastopexy, 2276

Matrix, of growth plates, 2144–2145

Maxilla
   anatomy of, 299
   fractures of, repair of, 307f, 307–308, 308f

Maxillofacial injuries, 298–308
   anatomy and, 299f, 299–300, 300f
   definitive care for, 302, 304–308
     bony injury management in, 305–308, 306f–308f
     infection prophylaxis in, 304
     soft tissue injury management in, 304–305, 305f
     timing of repair and, 302, 304
   early considerations in, 300–301
   evaluation of, 301–302

Maxillofacial injuries, evaluation of (*continued*)
    physical examination in, 301–302, 302f, 303f
    radiographic, 302, 303f, 304f
Maximal voluntary ventilation, 231
Maze procedure, 1574
MDR1 gene, sarcomas and, 2251
Mechanical circulatory support, 1550–1563. *See also* Intraaortic balloon pumps (IABPs); Ventricular assist devices (VADs)
    extracorporeal membrane oxygenation for, 1553
    permanent, future of, 1563
    temporary, CardioWest C-70, 1558, 1559f
    total artificial hearts, 1558
      permanent, 1561f, 1561–1563, 1562f
Mechanical heart valves, 1525f, 1525–1526
    complications of, 1526–1527
Mechanical ventilation
    in cardiogenic shock, 200
    complications of, 397t, 397–398
    for diaphragmatic hernias, 2026
    for multiple organ failure syndrome, 210
    for pediatric patients. *See* Ventilatory support, pediatric
    for respiratory failure, 224–225, 225f
    ventilatory modes for, 1985–1986
Mechlorethamine, 501t
Meckel's diverticulum, 1171, 2069–2071
    anatomy and embryology of, 2069f, 2069–2070, 2070f
    anomalies associated with, 2071
    clinical presentation of, 2070t, 2070–2071
    as incidental finding, 2071
    treatment of, 2071
Meconium ileus, 2049–2052
    clinical presentation of, 2050–2051
    cystic fibrosis and, 2049–2050
    diagnosis of, 2051, 2051f
    meconium plug syndrome and, 2052
    treatment of, 2051–2052
      nonoperative, 2051
      operative, 2051–2052
        postoperative care and results of, 2052
Meconium plug syndrome, 2052
Media, vascular, 1585, 1656
Medial necrosis, cystic, 1599–1600
Median arcuate ligament syndrome, 1778, 1789f
Median nerve, 2153, 2153f
    disorders of, 2155–2156
      carpal tunnel syndrome, 2155f, 2155–2156, 2156f, 2196–2197
Mediastinal injuries, indications for surgery and, 319
Mediastinitis, 1465–1467
    acute, 1465–1466
    following coronary artery bypass grafting, 1547
    granulomatous, chronic, 1466–1467
    necrotizing, descending, 1466
    following valvular heart surgery, 1528
Mediastinum, 1465f, 1465–1472, 1466f.
    See also specific disorders
    anatomy of. *See* Thoracic anatomy
    cysts of, 1471, 1471f
      neurogenic, 1467–1469, 1468f
      in pediatric patients, 2008–2009

emphysema of, 1471–1472
infections of, 1465–1467
neoplastic disease of, 1467–1471
    neurogenic, 1467–1469, 1468f
    in pediatric patients, 2010–2011
Medroxyprogesterone, for abnormal uterine bleeding, 2223
Medullary carcinomas of thyroid (MCTs), 1301, 1304–1305
    in multiple endocrine neoplasia, 1327–1328, 1328f
Medulloblastomas
    in familial adenomatous polyposis, 1120
    intracranial, 2175
      pediatric, 2175
Megamitochondria, in cirrhosis, 974
Megaureters, 2104
    nonrefluxing, nonobstructed, 2104
    obstructed, 2104
Megestrol acetate (Megace), for breast cancer, metastases from, 1402
Meiosis, spermatogenesis and, 2202
Meissner plexus, 1085, 1087
Melanomas, 2231–2242
    acral lentiginous, 2233, CF 111–1
    anal, 1150–1151
    clinical diagnosis and classification of, 2233, CF 111–1
    epidemiology and etiology of, 2231–2232, 2232f
    esophageal, 701
    genetics of, 2232–2233
    of head and neck, 643
    lentigo maligna, 2233, CF 111–1
    metastatic, disseminated, treatment of, 2240–2242
      chemotherapy for, 2241
      evaluation for, 2240–2241
      gene therapy for, 2242
      immunotherapy for, 2241–2242, CF 111–2
      radiotherapy for, 2241
      surgical, 2241
    metastatic, regional, lymphadenectomy for, 2237–2240
      adjuvant therapy and, 2240
      indications and results of, 2237–2239, 2238f, 2239f, 2239t
      site-specific considerations for, 2239–2240, 2240f
    nodular, 2233
    primary, treatment of, 2236–2237
      biopsy and, 2236–2237, 2237f
      surgical excision for, 2237, 2237t
    staging and prognostic factors for, 2233–2236, 2236t
      clinical and pathologic staging, 2235, 2235f, 2235t
      microstaging and, 2233f, 2233–2234, 2234f, 2234t
      regional lymph node involvement and, 2234t, 2234–2235
    superficial spreading, 2233
    ulceration within, 2236
    vulvar, 2218
Melena, 1158
Melphalan, 501t
Membrane anchor sequences, 27
Membrane transport, 11f, 11–22
    active, 15–16, 16f
    carrier proteins and, 18, 20f–22f, 20–21

energetics and mechanism of, 13–14, 15f
energy-converting, 11–12, 12f
    membrane composition and, 12–13, 13f
ion channels and, 16–18
    blockade of, 18
    gating of, 17f, 17–18
      modulation of, 18, 19f, 20f
macromolecule synthesis, transport, and organization and. *See* DNA; Protein(s); RNA
mechanisms of, 16, 16f, 17f
membrane composition and, 12–13, 13f
membrane proteins and, 13, 14f
selectivity and its modulation and, 11
    membrane composition and, 12–13, 13f
volume regulation and, 21–22, 23f
water channels and, 18
water flow and, 14–15, 15f
Meningeal carcinomatosis, 2179
Meningiomas
    intracranial, 2174–2175, 2176f
      parasagittal and convexity, 2174
      recurrence of, 2175
    of pituitary gland, 1354–1355
    spinal, 2180
Meningitis, bacterial, 2190
Meniscectomy, arthroscopic, 2151
Menopause, breasts and, 1363
Menstruation, 2217
    breasts and, 1361–1362, 1362f
Meperidine, 441t
    for patient-controlled analgesia, 454t
6-Mercaptopurine, 501t
    for Crohn's disease, 841
Merkel cell carcinomas, of skin, 2243, CF 111–7
Mesenchymomas, malignant, pediatric, 2081
Mesenteric arteries
    inferior, anatomy of, 1766, 1768f
    superior
      anatomy of, 1685f, 1685–1686, 1686f, 1766, 1767f, 1797
      aneurysms of, 1887–1898, 1893t, 1897f
      angiography of, 1693, 1693f
Mesenteric cysts, 2075–2076, 2076f
Mesenteric embolism, 1768–1769, 1773f
Mesenteric hernias, 1234–1235
Mesenteric ischemia, nonocclusive, low-flow, 1772–1773, 1774f
Mesenteric thrombosis, 1769, 1771–1772, 1774f
Mesenteritis, retractile, 1238–1239
Mesentery, 1237–1241. *See also specific disorders*
    anatomy of, 1237–1238
    cysts of, 1240–1241
    inflammatory diseases of, 1238–1239
    neoplastic disease of, 1239–1240
Mesoblastic nephromas, congenital, 2127
Mesocolic hernias, 2054–2055
    treatment of, 2056–2057
Mesonephros, 1987
Mesothelial cysts, 1240–1241
Mesotheliomas
    mesenteric, 1239–1240
    pleural, 1463–1465
      benign, localized, 1463–1464

malignant
diffuse, 1464t, 1464–1465
localized, 1464
Messenger RNA (mRNA), 23–24
Metabolic acidosis, 261t, 261–264
clinical features of, 263
compensatory mechanisms in, 263
extrarenal, 261
for hyperosmolar nonketotic acidosis, 264
mechanisms resulting in decreased body bicarbonate content and, 261–262
renal, 261, 262–263
in shock, 290–291
treatment of
for acute acidosis, 263
for chronic acidosis, 263
for diabetic ketoacidosis, 263–264
Metabolic alkalosis, 264–265
causes of, 264
clinical features of, 264–265
respiratory compensation in, 264, 264t
treatment of, 265
Metabolic control, following pancreatic transplantation, 624
Metabolic disorders. See also specific disorders
of erythrocyte metabolism, 1267–1268
hernias and, 1216
inherited, hepatic transplantation for, 583
in pancreatitis, 885
in shock, 191, 192f
following valvular heart surgery, 1527–1528
Metabolic rate, 44, 44t, 45t
basal, injury response and, 54
Metabolic support, for multiple organ failure syndrome, 211, 211t
Metabolism. See also Hypermetabolism
age-related changes in, 387
of amino acids, 45f–47f, 46t, 46–47
of bile acids, 955, 955f
of calcium, parathyroid glands and, 1310
regulation of, 1312t, 1312–1313
of carbohydrates, hepatic. See Liver, carbohydrate metabolism in
of carbon dioxide, in critically ill patients, ventilation and, 218, 218f, 219f
of energy, 43–45, 44t, 45t
in critically ill patients, 227, 229f
of fat
injury response and, 54
sepsis and, 56
of fatty acids
hepatic, 951–952, 952f
cholesterol and, 951–952, 953f
phospholipids and, 952
in infants, 1975
of glucose
injury response and, 54
sepsis and, 55–56
of heme, 956, 957
hepatic, 953–954, 954f
interleukin-1 effects on, 114f, 114–115, 115t, 116t
of lipids, hepatic. See Liver, lipid metabolism in
of metals, hepatic, 956–957

of phosphate, parathyroid glands and, 1310, 1312
regulation of, 1312t, 1312–1313
of porphyrin, 956
of proteins. See Liver, protein metabolism in; Protein(s), metabolism of
stress response and. See Injury response; Sepsis, metabolic response to; Stress response
thermoregulation and, 47
of trace minerals, sepsis and, 57
tumor necrosis factor effects on, 113
of vitamins, hepatic, 957
Metabolism-enhancing drugs, for infrainguinal occlusive disease, 1817, 1819
Metacarpal fractures, 2158
Metal(s), hepatic metabolism of, 956–957
Metalloproteinases, aneurysm formation and, 1843–1844
Metanephros, 1987
Metaplasia, 459, 461f
Metastatic disease, 482–489
from breast cancer. See Breast cancer, metastases from
esophageal, 731, 732f
of head and neck, 642, 642f, 642t, 650t, 651, 651t
hepatic. See Liver cancer, metastatic
heterogeneity of, 486
intracranial, 2178–2179
invasion and, 482–486, 484t
angiogenesis and, 485–486
barrier function of lymph nodes and, 484–485
hematogenous spread and, 483, 485
host factors and, 486
lymphatic spread and, 483–484
metastatic cascade and, 485, 485f
origin of cellular diversity and, 487–489, 488f
pancreatic ductal adenocarcinomas and, 903t, 903–904, 904f
pericarditis due to, 1576
pleural, 1465
primary tumors and, 486–487
pulmonary. See Lung cancer; Pulmonary resection
retroperitoneal, 2214
sarcomas and, 2253, 2255f
management of, 2267–2268
skip metastases and, 484
small intestinal, 855
spinal, 2180
Methanol, metabolic acidosis due to, 262
Methemalbumin, in pancreatitis, 884
Methimazole, 1291
Methotrexate, 501t
for Crohn's disease, 841
Methylprednisolone
for acute hepatic graft rejection, 598
for cardiac transplantation, 602, 602t
for spinal cord injury, 374
Methyl tert-butyl ether (MTBE), for cholelithiasis, 1047–1048
Methylxanthines, as antiplatelet agents, 98
Metronidazole
for amebic hepatic abscesses, 959
for Clostridium difficile colitis, 1178, 1179
for duodenal ulcers, 765

for pelvic inflammatory disease, 2225t
spectrum of activity of, 169t
Mexican beaded lizard bites, 406
Microangiopathy, diabetic, 616–617
Microbiologic diagnostic techniques, 166–167
in vascular infections, 1728
Microcirculation, in shock. See Shock, microcirculatory response to
Microcystic adnexal carcinomas, 2243
Microembolism, following abdominal aortic aneurysm repair, 1890
Microlymphatic bypass, for secondary lymphedema, 1970
Microorganisms. See also specific microorganisms and infections
commensal, 160–161, 161f
intestinal, mechanical bowel obstruction and, 819–820
vascular infections and, 1724, 1724t
Microprostol, for duodenal ulcers, 763t
Microsurgery
for intracranial aneurysms, 2182–2183
reconstructive, 2285–2286
for venolymphatic insufficiency, 2289
Microtubule(s), 8f, 8–9, 9f
Microtubule-associated proteins (MAPs), 9
Microtubule-organizing center, 8
Microvascular decompression, of cranial nerves, for pain management, 2195
Microvilli, 7
Midazolam (Versed), 442t
Migrating motor complex (MCC), 812
Milk-alkali syndrome, hypercalcemia and, 1315
Milk leg, 1946
Milk line, 1358, 1359f
Minerals, 230
homeostasis of, parathyroid gland and, 1313–1314, 1314f
pediatric requirements for, 1977
requirements in surgical patients, 62t
wound healing and, 78–79
Minimal inhibitory concentration (MIC), 166
Minimyosin, 6–7
Minithoracotomy, transaxillary, for spontaneous pneumothorax, 1461, 1461f
Mirizzi syndrome, 1080
Misoprostol, for duodenal ulcers, 765
Mithramycin, for hypercalcemia, 1315
Mitochondria, 5, 5f
hepatic, 947
protein targeting and, 27–29, 28f
Mitomycin C, 501t
for anal cancer, 1150
Mitotane, 502t
for hypercortisolism, 1344
Mitoxantrone, 502t
Mitral annular calcification, 1504
Mitral commissurotomy, 1519
Mitral insufficiency, 1505, 1505t
Mitral regurgitation (MR), 1505t, 1505–1506
diagnosis of, 1512–1513, 1513t
medical management of, 1517
after myocardial infarction, as surgical indication, 1542
pathophysiology of, 1511–1512

Mitral stenosis
  diagnosis of, 1513
  echocardiography in, 1514
  medical management of, 1517
  pathophysiology of, 1509f, 1509–1510, 1510t
Mitral valve
  anatomy of, 1503, 1504f
  endocarditis and, 1531
  repair of, technique for, 1520–1521, 1521f, 1522f
  replacement of, technique for, 1521, 1523, 1523f, 1525
Mivacurium, 440t
Mixed acid-base disorders, 266, 266f
Mixed gonadal dysgenesis, 2112–2113
Mixed lymphocyte culture, for organ transplantation, 554
Mixed tumors, malignant, of salivary glands, 641–642
Mohs micrographic surgical treatment, for skin cancer, 2244f, 2244–2245, CF 111–8
Mondor disease, 1377–1378
Monilial esophagitis, 724, 725f
Monitored fasts, in insulinomas, 921–922
Monobactams, spectrum of activity of, 169t
Monoclonal antibodies (mAbs), for metastatic melanoma, 2242
Monoclonal hypothesis, of atherosclerosis, 1593–1594
Monocytes, inflammation and, 148–149, 149f
Monokines, 163
Mononuclear phagocytes, inflammation and, 148–149, 149f
Monosaccharides, digestion and absorption of, in small intestine, 815
Morbid obesity, 788–794, 789f, 789t
  cardiac dysfunction and, 788–789
  central versus peripheral obesity and, 788
  degenerative joint disease and, 790
  diabetes mellitus and, 790
  dietary management of, 790
  pulmonary dysfunction and, 789–790
  surgical management of, 790–794, 793f, 794f
    complications of, 793
    failure of, 793–794
    gastric procedures for, 791–794
    jejunoileal bypass for, 790–791, 791f
    venous stasis disease and, 790
Morgagni diaphragmatic hernias, 2027
Morphine, 441t
  intrathecal, 2195
  for patient-controlled analgesia, 454t
Mortality
  following abdominal aortic aneurysm repair, 1890
  age, preoperative disease, and surgery related to, 445, 445t
  coronary artery bypass grafting and, risk factors for, 1547t, 1547–1548
  following lower extremity amputation, 1834–1835
  lower extremity ischemia and, 1813f, 1813t, 1814
  sudden cardiac death, ventricular arrhythmias and, 1568, 1568t

in systemic inflammatory response syndrome, 210
  after traumatic injury, peaks of, 267f, 267–268
  following valvular heart surgery, 1528–1529, 1529f
Motilin, small intestinal, 808
Motorcycle accidents, 272
Motor function
  of biliary tract, 1029–1030, 1030f
    disorders of, 1031
  colonic. See Colon, motor function of
  examination of, in head injuries, 294
Motor vehicle collisions. See Traumatic injuries, motor vehicle collisions as cause of
Mouth. See also Oral cavity
  floor of, cancer of, 638
Mucocutaneous lymph node syndrome, 1603f, 1603–1604
Mucoepidermoid carcinomas
  of anal canal, 1149
  bronchial, 1433
  of parotid gland, 641
Mucor infections, 177
Mucosa, oral, cancer of, 638
Mucosal defenses
  duodenal, against peptic injury, 760–761
  gastric, against peptic injury, 773–774, 774f
Mucous gland adenomas, bronchial, 1433
Mucus
  gallbladder secretion of, cholesterol gallstone formation and, 1038
  gastric, 775
Multidrug resistance, 498
Multiple endocrine neoplasia (MEN), 1326–1330
  genetic factors in, 461
  hyperparathyroidism and, 1318
  medullary thyroid carcinomas in, 1304, 1305
  MEN I, 1326–1327
    gastrinomas associated with, 925
    pancreatic tumors in, 1326–1327, 1327f
    parathyroid disease in, 1326
    pituitary adenomas in, 1327
  MEN II, 1327–1330
    medullary thyroid carcinomas in, 1327–1329, 1328f
    nonendocrine manifestations of, 1329f, 1330
    parathyroid disease in, 1330
    pheochromocytomas in, 1329–1330
  pathogenesis of, 1326
Multiple organ failure syndrome (MOFS), 182, 195, 209–211, 211t, 239–240. See also Systemic inflammatory response syndrome (SIRS)
  burns and, 434, 435t–436t, 436
  criteria for, 239t
  cytokines and, 110t
  management of, 240
  phases of, 240
  traumatic injuries and, in elderly people, 389
Multivesicular bodies, hepatic, 947
Murmurs, arteriovenous fistulas and, 1921
Muscle(s). See also Musculoskeletal

disorders; Musculoskeletal system; *specific muscles*
  of colonic wall, 1085
  inguinal, 1211, 1211f
  myoblasts as delivery vehicles for secreted proteins and, 521
  papillary, 1506
  pelvic, 1213, 1214f, 1215, 1215f
  of pelvic floor, anatomy of, 1181–1182, 1182f
  skeletal, actin filaments of, 6, 7f
  smooth
    arterial, 1588f, 1588–1589
      regulation of growth of, 1589–1591
    gastric, 757–758, 758f
    thoracic, 1442, 1443f, 1444
Muscle flaps, for chest wall reconstruction, 1450–1451, 1452f–1454f
Muscle relaxants, 439–441, 440t
  competitive inhibitors, 439
  nondepolarizing, 440t, 440–441
  reversal of, 439
Muscular dystrophy, gene therapy for, 520–521
Musculoaponeurotic flaps, for hernia repair, 1220
Musculoskeletal disorders, 2145–2163
  arthroscopy for, 2150–2152
    diagnostic, 2150–2151
    operative, 2151–2152
  burns and, 436t
  dislocations
    of hand, 2159
    with potential for neurovascular compromise, 375
  growth factors and other small-protein cytokines and, 2152
  of hands. See Hands
  limb-length discrepancy, 2148
    Ilizarov wire and frame treatment for, 2148, 2149f
  posttraumatic, 373–377, 401. See also Fractures; *specific injuries and sites*
    compartment syndromes and. See Compartment syndromes
    considered in primary survey, 373–374
    emergencies, 374–375
    strategy and timing for management of, 377
    systemic impact of, 375–376
  total joint replacement arthroplasty for, 2148–2150, 2150f, 2151f
Musculoskeletal system, 2141–2163. See also Bone(s); Muscle(s); *specific muscles*
  orthopedic surgery and, 2145–2163. See also *specific disorders*
  in pregnancy, 391
  soft tissues of. See Soft tissue(s); *specific tissues*
Mustard operation, for transposition of the great arteries, 1491, 1491f, 1493
Mutagenesis, colorectal cancer and, 1129
Myasthenia gravis, thymus gland and, 1469
myc oncogene family, 477
Mycotic aneurysms
  of abdominal aorta, 1890–1891
  of femoral artery, 1912–1913
  of thoracic aorta, 1873

Myectomy, rectal, for Hirschsprung disease, 2062, 2064
Myelofibrosis, with myeloid metaplasia, hypersplenism and, 1272–1273
Myeloid metaplasia, myelofibrosis with, hypersplenism and, 1272–1273
Myelomeningoceles (MMCs), 2192
  hydrocephalus associated with, 2192, 2192f
  neurogenic bladder and, 2106
Myeloproliferative disorders, 1617
Myeloschisis, 2192
  hydrocephalus associated with, 2192, 2192f
Myocardial contusions
  in elderly people, 388
  treatment of, 328
Myocardial dysfunction, in septic shock, 202–203
Myocardial failure, 1507f, 1507–1509, 1508f
  peripheral manifestations of, 1508–1509
Myocardial infarction (MI)
  acute, 1539–1552, 1540f
    diagnosis of, 1540, 1540f
    early evolving, 1540–1541
    management of, 1540–1542
      mechanical intervention for, 1541
      surgical indications and, 1541–1542
    presentation of, 1540
  anesthesia and, 444, 444t
  intraaortic balloon pump in, 1551–1552
  pericarditis associated with, 1576
  peripheral arterial embolism and, 1622
  thrombolytic therapy for, 102
Myocardial ischemia, anesthesia and, 452
Myoepitheloid cells, 1780
Myosin I, 6–7
Myxomas, cardiac, 1500

N

NADPH oxidase, activation of, 145, 147f
Na$^+$-K$^+$-ATPase, 11–12, 21, 22f
  organ preservation injury and, 556
Narcotic antagonists, for infections, 180
Narcotics
  as anesthetics, 441, 441t
  intrathecal, 2195
  for postoperative pain control, 453t, 453–454, 454t
Nasal bones, anatomy of, 299
Nasoduodenal feeding catheters, 64
Nasoethmoid fractures, management of, 305, 306f
Nasogastric intubation
  feeding catheters and, 64, 65f
  for gastrointestinal hemorrhage, 1159
Nasopharynx, cancer of, 640
Nausea
  anesthesia and, 451f, 452
  in gastroesophageal reflux disease, 681
Nd:YAG laser, for endovascular surgery, 1736
Neck. *See also* Cervical spine; Head and neck; Head and neck cancer; Head and neck surgery
  exploration of

    in hyperparathyroidism, 1323f, 1323–1324
    in traumatic injuries, 312, 313f
  injuries of, 309–317
    anatomy and, 309, 309f, 310f
    initial management of, 309–311, 311t
    neurologic, management of, 317
    operative exploration of, 312, 313f
    pharyngeal and esophageal, management of, 316
    selective versus mandatory exploration of, 311t, 311–312
    tracheal and laryngeal, management of, 314–316, 316f
    vascular, management of, 312–313
Neck dissection, radical, 644, 646, 648f, 649f
Necrosis
  avascular, of femoral head, 375
  fat, of breast, 1377
  hepatic, subacute, predicting outcome in, 968, 969t, 970f
  in inflammation, 152–153, 153f
  medial, cystic, 1599–1600
  of skin, after rhytidectomy, 2270
  wound healing and, 77
Necrotizing enterocolitis (NE), 2046–2049
  clinical presentation of, 2047
  diagnosis of, 2047–2048, 2048f
  pathophysiology of, 2046, 2047f
  treatment of, 2048–2049
    nonoperative, 2048t, 2048–2049
    operative, 2049
    results and complications of, 2049
Necrotizing fasciitis, 173
  vulvar, 2218, 2220
Needle aspiration. *See also* Fine-needle aspiration (FNA)
  ultrasound-guided, in pancreatitis, 883
Needle biopsy, in solitary thyroid nodule, 1300
Nelson syndrome, 1354–1355
  differential diagnosis of, 1354t, 1354–1355
Neonates, hyperparathyroidism in, 1325
Neoplastic cysts, hepatic, 1015
Neoplastic disease, 458–459, 460f, 461f. *See also* Cancer; Oncogene(s); Oncogenesis; *specific neoplasms*
  angiography in, 1700f, 1700–1702
  of appendix, 1260
  mesenteric, 1239–1240
  omental, 1241–1242
  pancreatic, pediatric, 2097
  pericardial, 1575
  retroperitoneal, 1244
Neostigmine, 440t
  muscle relaxant reversal by, 439
Nephrectomy
  for renal artery aneurysms, 1906
  for renal hypertension, 1793
Nephroblastomas. *See* Wilms tumor
Nephrogenesis, 1987
Nephromas, mesoblastic, congenital, 2127
Nephropathy
  diabetic, 617
    following pancreatic transplantation, 625
  pigment, in critically ill patients, 235
  reflux, 2105

Nephrotic syndrome, thrombosis associated with, 1618
Nephrotoxic agents, 235–236
Nerve blocks
  for abdominal pain, in pancreatic cancer, 915
  for postoperative pain control, 452f, 453
Nerve growth factors, neuroblastomas and, 2119
Nerve regeneration, 2172, 2173
Nerve roots, spinal, 2186
Nerve sheath tumors, malignant
  pediatric, 2133–2134
  of peripheral nerves, 2180
    etiology of, 2248, 2248f
Nesidioblastosis, pediatric, 2096f, 2097f, 2098
Neurapraxia, 2155
Neurilemmomas
  malignant, pediatric, 2133–2134
  spinal, 2179
Neuroblastomas, pediatric, 2118–2122
  associated conditions and epidemiology of, 2118
  basic science of, 2118–2119, 2119f
  future directions for, 2122
  mediastinal, 1468, 2011
  pathology of, 2119f, 2119–2120, 2120t
  presentation, workup, and staging of, 2120–2121, 2121t
  risk groups for, 2121, 2121t
  treatment of, 2121–2122, 2122f
Neuroectodermal tumors, primitive, peripheral, pediatric, 2133
  outcome of, 2133
  treatment of, 2133
Neuroendocrine system. *See also specific glands and hormones*
  in shock, 187–188
Neurofibromas
  etiology of, 2248, 2248f
  mediastinal, 1467
    in pediatric patients, 2011
  mesenteric, 1240
  of peripheral nerves, 2180
    of hands, 2162
  spinal, 2179
Neurofibrosarcomas
  etiology of, 2248, 2248f
  pediatric, 2133–2134
Neurogenic bladder, pediatric, 2106
Neurogenic sarcomas, pediatric, 2133–2134
Neurogenic shock, 183, 203–204
  physiologic characteristics of, 197t
Neurogenic tumors, mediastinal, 1467–1469, 1468f
Neurologic disorders, 2165–2197. *See also specific disorders*
  of brain. *See* Brain disorders; Head injuries; *specific disorders*
  burns and, 435t
  cerebrovascular. *See* Cerebrovascular disease
  following hepatic transplantation, 596
  hypothermia and, 410
  infections, 2189–2191
    bacterial, 2189–2191
    fungal, 2191
    parasitic, 2191
  injuries
    of brain. *See* Head injuries

Neurologic disorders, injuries (*continued*)
of cranial nerves. *See also specific nerves*
carotic endarterectomy and, 1755
degrees of, 2155, 2172
of neck, management of, 317
of peripheral nerves, 2172–2173
of hands. *See* Hands
spinal. *See* Spinal cord injuries
neoplastic, 2173–2180. *See also specific neoplasms*
intracranial, 2173–2179, 2174t
of peripheral nerves, 2180
spinal, 2179–2180
of peripheral nerves
of hands. *See* Hands
injuries, 2172–2173
neoplastic, 2180
neurosurgical pain management and, 2196–2197
posttraumatic, 399
following snake bites, 404
spinal. *See* Spinal cord injuries; Spine; *specific disorders; specific spinal regions*
following valvular heart surgery, 1527
Neurologic examination
brain injuries and, 2167
in burns, 426
of trauma patients, 282, 283t
Neuromas
acoustic, 2175
following lower extremity amputation, 1836–1837
neurosurgical pain management and, 2196
Neuromodulation technique, nonablative, for pain management, 2195–2196
Neuromuscular blocking agents, 439–441, 440t
competitive inhibitors, 439
nondepolarizing, 440t, 440–441
reversal of, 439
Neuromuscular system, hyperparathyroidism and, 1321
Neuronal system, adrenomedullary, 1331
Neuropathy, diabetic, 617
following pancreatic transplantation, 625
Neuropraxia, 2172
Neurosurgery, for pain management. *See* Pain management, neurosurgical
Neurotensin, small intestinal, 808
Neurotmesis, 2155, 2172
Neurotransmitters
false, hepatic encephalopathy and, 982f, 982–983
small intestinal, 808
Neurotrophic ulcers, 1940
Neutrophils
inflammation and, 142–147, 143t
cytokine and lipid priming of neutrophil function and, 147, 148f
G proteins in signal transduction and, 144f, 144t, 144–147, 145f
inhibitory pathways and, 147
signal transduction to neutrophils and, 143
stimulation by chemoattractants and, 143–144
recruitment of, 119
in shock, 195
wound healing and, 119
Nevus(i)

congenital, melanomas and, 2232
dysplastic
genetic factors in, 460–461
melanomas and, 2231–2232
Niacin
for hypercholesterolemia, 1711–1712
pediatric requirement for, 1976t
requirements in surgical patients, 62t
Nipples
discharge from, 1373–1374, 1374f
Paget disease of, 1409, 1409f
skin lesions of, 1378
tumors of, 1378
Nissen fundoplication
laparoscopic, 687, 687f–690f, 689–690
open, 690
transabdominal, 686–687, 687f
Nitric oxide (NO)
organ preservation injury and, 559
produced by endothelium-derived relaxing factor, 1610, 1611
in shock, 195
volume control and, 248
Nitric oxide synthase (NOS), inflammation and, 152
Nitrogen balance, 46
Nitrogen losses, 45f, 45–46, 46f
injury response and, 54
Nitroglycerin
for acute myocardial infarction, 1541
for coronary artery disease, 1539
for shock, 206
Nitroprusside, for shock, 206
Nitrosoureas, 501t
Nitrous oxide, as anesthetic, 439t
Nocturnal penile tumescence testing, 2200–2201
Nodular melanomas, 2233
Non-A, non-B hepatitis, hepatic transplantation for, 583
Nonadrenergic noncholinergic (NANC) neurons, colonic, 1087–1088
Nonanatomic vascular bypasses, 1757
for renal hypertension, 1792
Noncommunicating hydrocephalus, 2193
Noncoronary cusp, 1534
Nonrotation, intestinal, 2054, 2054f
Nonsteroidal antiinflammatory drugs (NSAIDs). *See also specific drugs*
for desmoid tumors, 2262
duodenal ulcers and, 759–760
gastric ulcers and, 782
treatment of, 785
peptic ulcers and, 1162
prophylactic, for colorectal adenomas, 1117
Nonviable free grafts, for hernia repair, 1220
Norepinephrine
normal effects of, 1338–1339
in shock, 187, 205
Normal pressure hydrocephalus, 2194
Nose, rhinoplasty and, 2272–2274, 2273f
Nosebleeds, 301
Novacor N100 ventricular assist device, 1558, 1558f, 1559–1560
Nuclear oncogenes, 477, 477f, 477t, 478f
Nuclear pores, 5
Nuclear proteins, targeting of, 27
Nucleation, of cholesterol, 1037–1038, 1038f
Nucleus

of hepatic cells, 947
structure of, 4f, 4–5
Nutcracker esophagus, 679
Nutrition. *See also* Diet
age-related changes in, 387
biochemistry of, 42–47. *See also* Metabolism
body composition and, 42–43, 43f, 43t
deficits of
in Crohn's disease, 835
stress response and, 49
in trauma patients, consequences of, 55
of pediatric patients. *See* Pediatric patients, growth and maturation of
wound healing and, 78–79
Nutritional status
assessment of
in critically ill patients, 234, 234f, 235f
in surgical patients, 53
surgical stress response and, 49
Nutritional support
for burn patients, 434
for cancer patients, 57–59
enteral, 58
patient selection for, 57–58, 58f
total parenteral nutrition, 58–59
central venous catheters for, 65–66
for children, 385
for critically ill patients, 232–234
in acute renal failure, 237
energy and protein for, 232
enteral, 232–233, 233t
of gut, 62–64
alternatives to, 64
enteral, 63
growth factors for, 63–64
gut-specific nutrients for, 63
nutritional assessment and, 234, 234f, 235f
parenteral, 233t, 233–234
for Crohn's disease, 838–839
enteral. *See* Enteral feeding
feeding catheter jejunostomy for, 65
gastrostomy placement for, 65
health care reform and, 66, 66t
for pancreatitis, 885
parenteral. *See* Parenteral feeding; Total parenteral nutrition (TPN)
perioperative, 60
peripheral intravenous feedings for, 65
requirements for, determination of, 53
routes for, 53
for sepsis, 57
for surgical patients, 53, 59–64. *See also* Total parenteral nutrition (TPN), for surgical patients
transnasal feeding catheters for, 64, 65f
for trauma patients, 54–55
goals of, 55
Witzel jejunostomy, 65
Nystatin, for monilial esophagitis, 724

O

Obesity
anesthesia and, 445, 445t
central versus peripheral, 788
cholelithiasis and, 1035

morbid. *See* Morbid obesity
Obesity hypoventilation syndrome, 789
Oblique muscles
  external, 1211
  internal, 1211
Obstructive sleep apnea syndrome, in
  morbid obesity, 789–790
Obstructive uropathy, 2199
Obturator canal, 1213, 1214f
Obturator hernias, 1231–1232
Obturator internus muscle, 1213, 1214f
Obturator lymph nodes, dissection of, in
  metastatic melanomas, 2240
Obtuse marginal branches, 1534
Ocular adnexae, burns of, management
  of, 431, CF 12–11
Oddi, sphincter of, 1028, 1030f
  dysfunction of, 1031
Ofloxacin
  for chlamydial proctitis, 1204
  for pelvic inflammatory disease, 2225t
Ogilvie syndrome, 829, 1092f, 1092–1093
OKT3, 550t, 551
Oligoasthenospermia, 2203
Oligodendromas, intracranial, 2177,
  2178f
Oligospermia, 2202, 2203
Oliguria, management of, in critically ill
  patients, 236
Omental cysts, 2075–2076, 2076f
Omentectomy, partial
  abdominal, 2228
  for tubal carcinomas, 2224
Omentum, 1241–1242
  anatomy of, 1241
  cysts of, 1241
  neoplastic disease of, 1241–1242
  torsion of, 1241
Omeprazole
  for duodenal ulcers, 763t, 764, 765–766
  for gastric ulcers, 784
Omphaloceles, 2029–2030
  anatomy, embryology, and
    pathophysiology of, 2029f,
    2029–2030, 2030f, 2030t
  clinical issues in, 2030–2031
  operative considerations, subsequent
    management, and outcome of,
    2031–2032
  upper celosomia, 2030, 2030f
Omphalomesenteric duct. *See* Meckel's
  diverticulum
Oncocytomas, renal, 2209–2210
Oncogene(s), 469–472, 471f–482f, 472t,
  473t, 477t
  activation of, 470–471, 472f, 472t, 475,
    476f, 478, 479f
  antioncogenes and, 471, 472t, 478, 480f
  c-*erb*-A, 477
  c-fos, 477
  c-jun, 477
  congenital patterns of malignancy
    expression and, 478–481, 480f–482f
  DNA amplification and, 471, 472f, 472t
  G proteins and, 474–475, 475f, 476f
  mutation of, 478
  myc, 477
  nuclear, 477, 477f, 477t, 478f
  peptide growth factors and, 472–474,
    473f–475f
  protooncogenes, 469, 470

signal transduction and, 474
  tumor viruses, 469–470
Oncogenesis, 464–469
  characteristics of transformed cells
    and, 464–465, 465f, 4564f
  growth and proliferation of neoplastic
    cells and, 465–468
  parameters affecting tissue growth and,
    468–469
Oophorectomy, for breast cancer, 1397
  metastases from, 1402
Open skull fractures, 2166
Ophthalmic disorders, burns and, 435t
Opioid(s)
  as anesthetics, 441, 441t
  intrathecal, 2195
  for postoperative pain control, 453t,
    453–454, 454t
Opioid antagonists, for infections, 180
Opsoclonus-myoclonus, neuroblastomas
  and, 2120
Optic nerve gliomas, 2173
*Optimal Hospital Resources for the Care
  of the Seriously Injured*, 268
Oral cavity
  cancer of, 638
  surgery of, 646–647
  in ulcerative colitis, 1096
Oral contraceptives, thrombosis
  associated with, 1618
Orbit, anatomy of, 299
Orbital apex fractures, management of,
  306, 306f
Orbital blow-out fractures, management
  of, 305–306
Orchiopexy, 2109, 2109f
Organ donors, 399
  cadaveric, 559–563
    brain death and, 561–562
      definition of, 561–562
      etiology of, 562
      pathophysiology of, 562
    determination of suitability for
      donation and, 559–561
      age and, 559, 560f
      contraindications and, 560–561
      general considerations in, 559
      hemodynamic stability and, 560
      overall premorbid health and,
        559–560
      specific organ dysfunction and,
        561
    for kidneys, 574–575, 576f
    maintenance of, 563
    non-heartbeating, 563
    request for permission from next of
      kin and, 562–563
  living, for kidneys, 573–574, 575f
  for pancreatic transplantation,
    assessment of, 619
  for pulmonary transplantation, 608–
    609, 609f
Organelles, transport in cytoplasm, 9, 9f
Organic carcinogens, 462
Organ preservation, 556–563, 568–571
  donor maintenance and, 563
  of heart, 569
  of kidneys, 568–569, 573t, 574f, 575–577
  of liver, 568–569, 573t, 574f
  of lungs, 569, 609–610
  for pancreas, 568–569, 573t, 574f

of pancreas, 568–569, 573t, 574f, 619–620
  pathophysiology of organ preservation
    injury and, 556–559
    cellular energy and, 557–558, 558f
    cytokine-mediated effects and, 559
    ionic composition and, 556–557,
      557f
    nitric oxide-mediated effects and,
      559
    oxygen free radical-mediated effects
      and, 558, 558f
    reperfusion injury and, 558
    structural integrity and, 556
  for small intestine, 569, 571
Organ procurement, 563–568
  surgical technique for, 564–566, 565f–572f, 568
  United Network for Organ Sharing and
    team coordination for, 563–564,
    564f
Organ procurement organizations (OPOs),
  563–564
Organ transplantation. *See* Antigen(s),
  recognition of; Transplantation;
  Transplantation immunology
Ornithine transcarbamylase (OTC)
  deficiency, gene therapy for, 518
Oropharynx
  cancer of, 640
  microbial flora of, 160
Orthopedic surgery, 2145–2163. *See also*
  Musculoskeletal disorders;
  specific disorders
Orthopnea, myocardial failure and, 1508
Osmoregulation, 245, 245f, 246f
Osmotic activity, of body fluids, 243–245, 244f
  colloid oncotic pressure and, 244
  osmoregulation and, 245, 245f, 246f
  sodium concentration and water
    balance and, 245, 246f
Osteochondritis dissecans, arthroscopic
  surgery for, 2151
Osteochondromas, of ribs, 1446, 1446f
Osteogenic sarcomas, of ribs, 1447
Osteogenin, 2152
Osteomyelitis, 2189
Osteons, 2143
Osteophytes, in spondylosis, 2186
Osteosarcomas, 2262t, 2262–2265, 2263t
  biopsy of, 2263–2264
  clinical evaluation of, 2262–2263,
    2263f
  postoperative chemotherapy for, 2265,
    2267f
  preoperative chemotherapy for, 2264,
    2264f
  of ribs, 1447
  surgical treatment of, 2264–2265,
    2265f, 2266f
Osteoseptocutaneous fibular flaps, 2286
Ostium primum, 1483
Ostium secundum defects, 1483
Otologic disorders, burns and, 435t
Otoplasty, 2272t, 2274, 2274f
Ovaries
  cysts of, hemorrhage from, acute
    abdomen and, 1249
  development and anatomy of, 2216
  irradiation of, for breast cancer, 1397
  neoplastic disease of, 2225–2228,
    2226f

Ovaries, neoplastic disease of (*continued*)
  benign, 2226t, 2226–2227, 2227f
  carcinomas, 2227–2228
Oxidants
  cell injury and, 154t, 154–155
  in inflammation, peroxidase synergism
      with, 155–156
Oximetry
  pulse, in persistent pulmonary
      hypertension of newborn, 1985
  venous, in pediatric patients, 1982
Oxygen
  consumption of
    in critically ill patients, 215–216
      autoregulation to change, 216f,
          216–217
      hypothermia and, 410
  delivery of
    in critically ill patients, 216, 216f
      autoregulation to change, 217, 217f
      autoregulation to maintain, 216
      optimizing, in respiratory failure,
          223–224
    supranormal, for shock, 207–208
  transport of, calculations for, 197t
  wound healing and, 76–77
Oxygenation
  extracorporeal membrane oxygenation
      and, 1553
    for diaphragmatic hernias, 2026
  monitoring, postoperative, 448
  of organ donors, 563
Oxygen free radicals, organ preservation
    injury and, 558, 558f
Oxygen tension, measurement of, 1673
Oxygen therapy, hyperbaric, for soft tissue
    infections, necrotizing, 174
Oxyntic glands, 748, 749

P

Paclitaxel (Taxol), 502t
Paget disease
  of anal margin, 1147–1148, 1149f
  of nipples, 1409, 1409f
  vulvar, 2218
Pain
  in chronic pancreatitis. *See*
      Pancreatitis, chronic
  in claudication. *See* Claudication
  in esophageal cancer, 702
  ischemic rest pain, in infrainguinal
      occlusive disease, 1812
  noncardiac, in chest
    diagnosis of, 665
    in gastroesophageal reflux disease,
        681
  orthopedic assessment and, 374
  in peripheral arterial embolism, 1625
  phantom, following lower extremity
      amputation, 1837
  stress response and, 49
Pain management. *See also* Anesthesia
  after chest injury, 399
  in chronic pancreatitis, 893–894
  neurosurgical, 2194–2197
    brain stem and, 2195
    cerebrum and, 2194–2195
    cranial nerves and, 2195
    peripheral nerves and, 2196–2197
    spinal cord and, 2195–2196, 2196f
  postoperative, 452f, 452t–454t, 453–
      454

Palate
  cleft, plastic surgery for, 2286, 2287
  hard, cancer of, 638
Palliative care, for cancer, 491
Pancreas, 857–927
  anatomy of, 857f, 857–863
    embryology, 857, 858f, 859f
    surgical, 857, 859–863
      of arterial supply, 860, 861f
      of innervation, 862–863, 864f, 865f
      of lymphatic drainage, 862, 863f
      of pancreatic ducts, 859–860, 861f
      relations to other structures and,
          857, 859, 860f
      of venous drainage, 860, 862, 862f
  endocrine
    function of, 867–870
      amylin secretion and action and,
          870
      glucagon synthesis, secretion, and
          action and, 868–869
      insulin synthesis, secretion, and
          action and, 867–868, 869f, 870f
      intraislet regulation of hormone
          secretion and, 870, 871f
      pancreastatin secretion and action
          and, 870
      pancreatic polypeptide synthesis,
          secretion, and action and, 870
      somatostatin synthesis, secretion,
          and action and, 869–870
      tests of, 872–873, 873t
    following pancreatic transplantation,
        621–622
    structure of, 863, 867f
    surgical stress response and, 53
  exocrine
    function of, 864–867
      bicarbonate secretion and, 865,
          868f
      enzyme groups and, 866–867
      enzyme secretion and, 865–866,
          869f
      tests of, 870–872, 871t, 872t, 892
    following pancreatic transplantation,
        621–622
    structure of, 863, 866f
  intravascular pattern of, 864, 868f
  pediatric, 2093–2094. *See also specific
      disorders*
    embryology of, 2093–2094, 2095f
    neoplastic disease of, 2097
    preservation of, 568–569, 573t
    suitability for donation, 561
Pancreas divisum, 2095f, 2095–2096
Pancreastatin, 870
Pancreatectomy
  distal, 348
    for VIPomas, 926
  for nesidioblastosis, pediatric, 2096f,
      2097f, 2098
  radical, extended, for pancreatic
      cancer, 912f, 912–913
  total, for pancreatic cancer, 912
Pancreatic abscesses, 887–888
Pancreatic adenocarcinomas, ductal,
    901–915
  curative treatment of, 908–913
    surgery alone for, 908–913
    surgery with adjuvant chemotherapy
        for, 913, 913f
    surgery with intraoperative
        radiotherapy for, 913

diagnosis of, 905–908
  clinical signs and symptoms and,
      905, 905t
  laboratory studies and, 905–906
  radiographic examination and, 906t,
      906–908, 907f, 908f
epidemiology and etiology of, 901f,
    901–902
palliative treatment of, 913–915
  antineoplastic, 915
  for symptoms, 914–915
pathology of, 902t, 902–905, 903f
  location and, 902–903
  precursor and precancerous lesions
      and, 902
  sites and frequency of local
      extension and, 903
  sites and frequency of metastatic
      disease and, 903t, 903–904, 904f
  staging and, 904t, 904–905
Pancreatic artery, aneurysms of, 1893t,
    1899f, 1900, 1900f
Pancreatic disorders. *See also specific
    disorders*
  gene therapy for, 521–522
  neoplastic disease. *See also specific
      neoplasms*
    of endocrine pancreas, 918–927,
        919t
      localization and staging of, 918–
          920, 919f–921f
      surgical exploration of, 920–921
    of exocrine pancreas, 901–917
    in multiple endocrine neoplasia,
        1326–1327, 1327f
  traumatic injuries, 346–350
    blunt, 349–350
    pediatric, 383–384
    penetrating, 346–349, 347f, 349f
Pancreatic ducts
  adenocarcinoma of. *See* Pancreatic
      adenocarcinomas
  anatomy of, 859–860, 861f
  obstruction of, pancreatitis and
    acute, 882
    chronic, 890
Pancreatic fistulas, following pancreatic
    injuries, 347–349
Pancreaticoblastomas, pediatric, 2097
Pancreaticoduodenal arteries, 805
  aneurysms of, 1893t, 1899f, 1900,
      1900f
Pancreaticoduodenectomy
  blind, for gastrinomas, 924–925
  for pancreatic cancer, 908–912, 909f–
      910f
    postoperative course after, 911
    results of, 911t, 911–912
Pancreaticojejunostomy, for chronic
    pancreatitis, 894–895, 895f–897f
Pancreatic polypeptides, synthesis,
    secretion, and action of, 870
Pancreatic pseudocysts, 886f, 886–887,
    887f
  following pancreatic injuries, 349
  pediatric, 2096–2097
Pancreatic resection, for chronic
    pancreatitis, 897f, 897–898, 898f
Pancreatic stone protein, 890
Pancreatic transplantation, 556
  anticoagulation for, 622
  for diabetes mellitus, 617–626
    indications for, 618–619

donor organs for, 619–620
  donor assessment and, 619
  no-touch dissection technique and, 619
  preservation of, 619–620
  vascular anatomic considerations in, 619, 620f
endocrine function and, 622
exocrine function and, 622
immunosuppression for, 621–622
late complications of, 624–626
metabolic control following, 624
operative technique for, 620–621
  anatomic and physiologic bases for, 620–621
  with segmental grafts, 621
  with whole-organ, composite pancreaticoduodenal grafts, 621, 621f
pancreatic transplantation alone, 619
postoperative complications of, 622t, 622–624
  immunologic, 622–623
  nonimmunologic, 623–624
results with, 623f, 624f, 625t, 626
simultaneous renal-pancreatic transplantation, 618
Pancreatitis
acute, 874–888
  abdominal trauma and, 880–881
  biliary tract stone disease and, 879–880, 881f
  diagnosis of, 883–884
  drugs and, 881
  duodenal or pancreatic duct obstruction and, 882
  ethanol and, 880
  etiology and clinical associations of, 879, 880t
  hyperlipoproteinemia and, 881
  hyperparathyroidism and, 881
  immunologic factors in, 882
  incidence and demographics of, 877, 879, 879t
  infections and, 881–882, 882t
  management of, 884–886
    medical therapy in, 884–886
    surgical treatment in, 885–886
  pancreatic abscesses and, 887–888
  pancreatic pseudocysts and, 886f, 886–887, 887t
  pathology of, 874, 875f
  pathophysiology of, 874–877, 876f–879f
  pediatric, 2094–2095
  postprocedural, 880
  pregnancy and, 882
  presentation of, 882t, 882–883
  vascular disease and, 882
chronic, 889–900
  bile duct strictures secondary to, 1078–1080, 1079f
  biliary complications of, treatment for, 898f, 899f, 899–900
  causes of, 889–890
  classification of, 889, 889f
  diagnosis of, 892
  endocrine insufficiency in, 891t, 891–892
  incidence of, 889
  malabsorption and weight loss in, 891
    treatment for, 898t, 898–899

obstructive, 890
pain in, 890f, 890–891, 892–898
  abstinence for, 892
  analgesics for, 893–894
  endoscopic therapy for, 893
  enzyme replacement for, 892–893, 894f
  surgical treatment for, 894–898
pathogenesis of, 890
prognosis of, 900, 900f
senile, 890
tropical, 889
following pancreatic transplantation, 623–624
posttraumatic, 349
pediatric, 383–384
Pancreatoblastomas, 917
Pancreatography, transduodenal, intraoperative, 347
Pancuronium, 440t
Panel reactive antibody (PRA), for organ transplantation, 554
Panniculitis, mesenteric, 1238–1239
Pantothenic acid
  pediatric requirement for, 1976t
  requirements in surgical patients, 62t
Papaverine injections, for impotence, 2201
Papillary-cystic neoplasms, of pancreas, 915
Papillary muscles, 1506
Papillomas
  of bile ducts, 1056
  of breast, intraductal, 1378
  esophageal, 698
  of gallbladder, 1056
Papillomatosis, of gallbladder, 1056
Papovaviruses, tumor induction by, 464
Paraaminobenzoic acid (PABA) test, 872
Paracentesis
  abdominal, in abdominal injuries, 335
  diagnostic, in ascites, 987
  therapeutic, for ascites, 989
Paracrine substances, small intestinal, 808
Paradoxical embolism, 1483, 1623–1624
Paraduodenal hernias, 1234
Paragangliomas, vagal, 643
Parapharyngeal abscesses, 636–637
Paranasal sinuses, cancer of, 641
Parapharyngeal abscesses, 636–637
Paraphimosis, 2107, 2108f
Paraplegia
  following abdominal aortic aneurysm repair, 1890
  following thoracic aortic aneurysm repair, 1872–1873, 1873f
Parasagittal meningiomas, 2174
Parasellar region, imaging of, 1350, 1351f
Parasitic infections, 180. See also specific infections
  neurologic, 2191
  pericarditis associated with, 1576
Parathryoid glands, carcinoma of, 1319
Parathyrinomas, 927
Parathyroid glands, 1286–1287, 1308–1330. See also Hyperparathyroidism
  anatomy of, 1308–1309, 1309f–1311f
  autotransplantation of, for hyperparathyroidism, 1324
  calcium metabolism and, 1310. See also Hypercalcemia; Hypocalcemia
    regulation of, 1312t, 1312–1313

carcinomas of, 1326
mineral homeostasis and, 1313–1314, 1314f
mineral metabolism and, 1310, 1311f
multiple endocrine neoplasia and. See Multiple endocrine neoplasia (MEN)
phosphate metabolism and, 1310, 1312
  regulation of, 1312t, 1312–1313
resection of, for hyperparathyroidism, 1324
Parathyroid hormone (PTH). See also Hyperparathyroidism
  assays of, in hyperparathyroidism, 1321, 1322f
  calcium and phosphate metabolism and, 1312f, 1312–1313
  deficiency of, metabolic alkalosis due to, 264
Parenchymal cells, ischemic injury of, 1649f, 1649–1650, 1650f
Parenteral feeding, for critically ill patients, 233t, 233–234
Parenteral nutrition. See also Total parenteral nutrition (TPN)
  in pancreatitis, 885
Parietal cell(s), 748f, 748–749
  activation of, 752, 754
Parietal cell proton pump, 752, 754
Parinaud syndrome, 2178, 2193
Parkinson disease, gene therapy for, 521
Paronychia, 2161, 2161f
Parotid duct injuries, repair of, 305
Parotid gland
  cancer of, 641, 642t
  surgery of, 643–644, 646f–647f
Parotitis, 176
Paroxysmal nocturnal dyspnea, myocardial failure and, 1508
Partial thromboplastin time (PTT), 104
Patent ductus arteriosus (PDA), 1496, 2023, 2024f
Patent processus vaginalis, 2032
Paterson-Kelly syndrome, 705, 705f
Patient-controlled analgesia (PCA), 453t, 454, 454t
Peau d'orange, 1387, 1387f
Pectineal ligament, 1211
Pectoralis major muscle, 1442, 1443f
Pectoralis major muscle flaps, 2286
  for chest wall reconstruction, 1450–1451, 1453f
Pectoralis minor muscle, 1442, 1443f
Pectus carinatum, 2003, 2003f
Pectus excavatum, 2002, 2002f
Pedestrian injuries, 272
  of elderly people, 386–387
Pediatric patients, 1973–2138. See also specific disorders
  abdominal pain in, differential diagnosis of, 1250, 1250t
  appendicitis in, 1258–1259
    congenital abnormalities and, 1258–1259
  biliary tract of, 2083–2093
    embryology of, 2083, 2083f
  breast cancer in, 1383, 1383f
  cardiac transplantation in, 604–605
  cardiovascular physiology of, 1980–1986
    fetal circulation and, 1980, 1980f
    monitoring and hemodynamic

Pediatric patients, cardiovascular physiology of (*continued*)
    assessment and, 1981t, 1981–1982, 1982f
    persistent pulmonary hypertension of the newborn and, 1982–1985
        evaluation of respiratory function and, 1985
        respiratory mechanics and gas exchange in, 1983f, 1983–1984
        surfactant and, 1984–1985
    transitional circulation and, 1980–1981
  chest wall deformities in. *See* Chest wall, deformities of
  child abuse and, 385
    burns caused by, 428–429, 429t, CF 12–9
    sexual, introital problems related to, 2117
  colorectal polyposis in, 1126f, 1126–1127
  congenital cystic disease of lung in. *See* Pulmonary disorders, congenital cystic disease
  congenital esophageal stenosis in, 2016
  congenital heart disease in. *See* Congenital heart disease
  congenital malformations in. *See* *specific organs and malformations*
  congenital tracheal stenosis in, 2017
  Crohn's disease in, 843
  esophageal duplications in, 2016
  fluid therapy in, for burns, 429
  gastrointestinal disorders in, 2034–2078. *See also specific disorders*
  genitourinary system of, 2101–2117. *See also specific disorders*
  growth and maturation of, 1973–1979
    nutrition requirements for, 1974–1977
        for energy, 1974–1975
        enteral feeding and, 1967t, 1978
        parenteral feeding and, 1977t–1979t, 1978–1979
        for protein, 1975, 1977
        for trace elements and minerals, 1977
        for vitamins, 1976t, 1977
        for water, 1974
    postnatal, 1973–1974
    prenatal, 1973
  head and neck of. *See* Head and neck disorders, pediatric
  hepatic physiology of, 1990–1991
    bilirubin metabolism and, 1990–1991
    enzyme function and pharmacokinetics and, 1990
  hydrocephalus in, 2193f, 2193–2194
  immunology and infection in, 1991–1992
    immune system ontogeny and, 1991
    maternal transfer of humoral immunity and, 1991
    neonatal sepsis and, 1991–1992
    viral sepsis and, 1992
  laryngotracheoesophageal cleft in, 2016
  liver of. *See* Liver, pediatric
  liver resection in, 2081
  mediastinal cysts in, 2008–2009
  medulloblastomas in, 2175
  neoplastic disease in, 2118–2138. *See also specific tumors*

    solid tumor incidence and, 2118, 2118f
  neuroblastomas in, mediastinal, 1468
  pancreas of, 2094–2098
    embryology of, 2094, 2095f
    neoplastic disease of, 2097
  pedestrian injuries of, 272
  portal hypertension in, 1005–1006
  renal physiology of, 1986–1989
    fluid and electrolyte management and, 1988t, 1988–1989
    fluid spaces and, 1987–1988
    renal function and, 1986–1987
  renovascular hypertension in, operative treatment of, 1793, 1794t
  sarcomas in, soft tissue, management of, 2265–2266
  thermoregulation in, 1979–1980
  thoracic tumors in, 2009–2011
    of lung, 2009–2010
        metastatic, 2010
        primary, 2009f, 2009–2010, 2010f
    mediastinal, 2010–2011
  tracheobronchial foreign bodies in, 2017–2019
    clinical picture in, 2017f, 2018, 2018f, 2018t
    management of, 2018–2019, 2019f
    pathophysiology of, 2017
  traumatic injuries of, 377–386
    abdominal, 382–384, 383f, 383t, 384f
    anatomic and physiologic considerations in, 378, 379f
    child abuse and, 385
    genitourinary, 384
    initial evaluation and resuscitation for, 378–381
        airway and breathing in, 378–380, 380t
        circulation in, 380t, 380–381
    intensive care considerations in, 385
    mechanisms of injury and, 377f, 377–378
    neurologic, 384
    pelvic fractures and extremity trauma, 384–385
    prevention of, 385–386
    quality assurance and, 385
    resuscitation algorithm for, 381, 381f
    thoracic, 381–382
    triage and prehospital care for, 378, 379t
  umbilical hernias in, 1226–1227, 1227f
  vascular rings in, 2016–2017
    complete, 2016–2017
    incomplete, 2017
  ventilatory support for. *See* Ventilatory support, pediatric
Pediatric Trauma Score, 378, 379t
Pelvic anatomy, 1213, 1214f, 1215, 1215f
Pelvic arteries, anatomy of, 1684–1685
Pelvic floor muscles, anatomy of, 1181–1182, 1182f
Pelvic fractures, 353–354, 354f–356f, 356, 374
  pediatric, 384–385
Pelvic inflammatory disease (PID), 2224f, 2224–2225, 2225t
  acute abdomen and, 1249
  appendicitis differentiated from, 1249, 1249t
Pelvic organ prolapse, 2220–2221, 2221f
Pelvic plexus, 1185

Pelvis
  osteosarcomas of, limb-sparing therapy for, 2264–2265, 2266f
  in secondary survey of trauma patients, 285
Penetrating injuries. *See* Traumatic injuries
Penicillins
  penicillin G
    for gonococcal proctitis, 1203
    spectrum of activity of, 169t
  penicillin V, prophylactic, for endocarditis, 1532t
  prophylactic, for endocarditis, 1532t
  spectrum of activity of, 169t
Penile implants, for impotence, 2201
Penile tumescence testing, nocturnal, 2200–2201
Penis
  disorders of. *See specific disorders*
  pediatric, 2106–2109. *See also specific disorders*
  prepuce of, 2107, 2107f, 2108f
Penn State total artificial heart, 1558, 1559f
Penn State ventricular assist device, 1560f, 1560–1561
Pentalogy of Cantrell, 2030
Pentostatin, 501t
Pentoxifylline
  for claudication, 1716, 1717t
  for infrainguinal occlusive disease, 1815t, 1817
Pepsin, 755–756
  secretion of, gastric ulcers and, 780–781
Peptic ulcers
  duodenal. *See* Duodenal ulcers
  gastric. *See* Gastric ulcers
  hemorrhage in, 1162–1164
    endoscopic treatment of, 1162–1164, 1164f, 1164t
  stress. *See* Stress gastritis
Peptides
  colonic motor activity and, 1088
  gastric, 749–752. *See also specific peptides*
  trophic, gastric, 776
Peptide YY (PYY), small intestinal, 808
Percutaneous aortic balloon valvuloplasty, 1518
Percutaneous biopsy, of liver masses, 1010
Percutaneous endoscopic urinary stone removal, 2205–2206
Percutaneous transhepatic cholangiography (PTC)
  in bile duct cancer, 1061, 1061f
  in bile duct strictures, 1070, 1071f
  in choledocholithiasis, 1052
Percutaneous transhepatic cholecystolitholysis, for cholelithiasis, 1047–1048, 1048f
Percutaneous transluminal angioplasty (PTA), 1702f–1704f, 1706–1707
  renal, for renal hypertension, 1790–1791
Percutaneous transluminal coronary angioplasty (PCTA)
  cooperative studies of, 1548–1549
  intraaortic balloon pump during, 1552
  for ischemic heart disease, 1542–1543
    complications of, 1543

indications for, 1542–1543
results with, 1543
Perfluorocarbons, in shock, 290
Perforating veins, 1936
ligation of, 1941, 1941f, 1943
Perianal abscesses, 1197
Perianal space, anatomy of, 1182, 1183f
Pericardial cysts, 1471
in pediatric patients, 2009
Pericardial effusions, 1577
Pericardial tamponade. *See* Cardiac
tamponade
Pericardiectomy, 1580f, 1581f, 1582
Pericardiocentesis, 1579f, 1580–1582
Pericardiotomy, postpericardiotomy
syndrome and, 1547
Pericarditis, 1575–1577
causes of, 1576–1577
in connective tissue disease, 1577
constrictive, 1579–1580
diagnosis of, 1579–1580
pathophysiology of, 1578f, 1579
treatment of, 1580
iatrogenic, 1576–1577
idiopathic (nonspecific), 1576
infectious, 1576
myocardial infarction and, 1576
treatment of, 1577
uremic, 1576
Pericardium, 1574–1582
anatomy and embryology of, 1574
biopsy of, 1580f, 1582
cardiac tamponade and. *See* Cardiac
tamponade
congenital abnormalities of, 1575
diagnostic studies of, 1575
drainage of, 1582
neoplastic disease of, 1500, 1502
congenital abnormalities of, 1575
physiology of, 1574–1575
Peridiverticulitis, 1151
Periductal mastitis, 1377
Perimembranous ventricular septal
defects, 1485
Perineal hernias, 1233, 1234f
Perineum
development and anatomy of, 2217
reconstruction of, 2287–2288
Peripheral intravenous feedings, 65
Peripheral nerve disorders. *See*
Neurologic disorders, of
peripheral nerves
Peripheral primitive neuroectodermal
tumors (PNETs), pediatric, 2133
outcome of, 2133
treatment of, 2133
Peripheral resistance, arteriovenous
fistulas and, 1919
Peripheral resistance units, 1661
Perirectal spaces, anatomy, 1182–1183,
1183f
Peritoneal dialysis, for critically ill
patients, 238, 238t
Peritoneal lavage
diagnostic. *See* Diagnostic peritoneal
lavage (DPL)
for pancreatitis, 886
Peritoneovenous shunts, for ascites, 989–
990, 990f
Peritonitis
bacterial, spontaneous, in ascites, 988t,
988–989, 989t

following colonic and rectal injuries,
352
in Crohn's disease, 837
following gastric surgery for morbid
obesity, 793
primary, pediatric, 2076–2077
tertiary (persistent), 170–171
Peritonsillar abscesses, 636
Pernio, 412
Peroneal artery, anatomy of, 1687–1688
Peroneal veins, 1935, 1938f
Peroxynitrite, cell injury and, 154t, 155
Persistent pulmonary hypertension of the
newborn (PPHN), 1982–1985,
2023–2024
evaluation of respiratory function and,
1985
pharmacologic management of, 2023–
2024
respiratory mechanics and gas
exchange in, 1983f, 1983–1984
surfactant and, 1984–1985
Pessaries, for vaginal prolapse, 2221
Peutz-Jeghers syndrome, 846–847, 1124,
1126
complications of, 1126
gastrointestinal features of, 1125f, 1126
management of, 1126
skin lesions in, 1126
Peyer patches, 807
in intussusception, 2068
p53 gene
in colorectal cancer, 1130
lung cancer and, 1419
sarcomas and, 2248, 2250–2251
Phagocytosis, 34
Phalangeal fractures, 2158
Phantom extremity pain, following lower
extremity amputation, 1837
Pharyngoesophageal diverticula, 670–
674, 726f, 726–728, 727f
enker diverticula, pathophysiology of,
670, 671f, 672
investigation of, 672, 672f
treatment of, 672–674, 673f
Pharynx
bleeding from, 301
cancer of, 638, 640
surgery of, 649, 649f
traumatic injuries of, management of, 316
Pheochromocytomas
catecholamine excess and, 1339, 1339t
catecholamine measurement in, 1341–
1342
mediastinal, 1469, 1469f
in multiple endocrine neoplasia, 1329–
1330
nonfunctioning, 1339
treatment of, 1345–1346
nonoperative, 1345
operative, 1346
Phimosis, 2107, 2107f
Phlebography, ascending, in chronic
venous insufficiency, 1941
Phlegmasia alba dolens, 1946
Phlegmasia cerulea dolens, 1946
pH monitoring
esophageal
dual, 668
24-hour, 666–667
indications for, 666–667
interpretation of, 667, 668f, 668t
technique for, 667

gastric, 24-hour, 666–670
Phosphate(s)
for hypercalcemia, 1315
in hyperparathyroidism, 1321
metabolism of, parathyroid glands and,
1310, 1312
regulation of, 1312t, 1312–1313
Phosphatidylinositides, 752
Phosphogluconate pathway, 949, 951f
Phospholipase C, G-protein binding to,
145, 146f
Phospholipids
metabolism of, hepatic, 952
in surfactant, 1985
Phosphorus, pediatric requirement for,
1977
Phosphorus-31 magnetic resonance
imaging spectroscopy, in
sarcomas, 2253, 2255f
Phosphorylation, tyrosine kinase
regulation by, 474
Photocoagulation
infrared, for hemorrhoids, 1189
laser, for peptic ulcers, 1163
Photoplethysmography (PPG), in chronic
venous insufficiency, 1940,
1960, 1961f
Phrenic nerve, course in diaphragm, 341,
342f
Phylloquinone, requirements for
pediatric, 1977
in surgical patients, 62t
Physical therapy, for peripheral nerve
injuries, 2173
Physiologic dead space, 1984
Pickwickian syndrome, 789
Pierce-Donachy ventricular assist device,
1556, 1556f
Pigment gallstones, 1039–1040
classification of, 1039–1040
pathogenesis of, 1040
Pigment nephropathy, in critically ill
patients, 235
Pigmenturia, acute tubular necrosis and,
myoglobin-induced, 430, CF 12–
10
Pilonidal sinuses, 1199–1200
clinical manifestations of, 1199
complicated by carcinoma, 1200
diagnosis of, 1199
postoperative care and, 1200
treatment of, 1199–1200
Pinealomas, 2178
Pipecuronium, 440t
Pituitary adenomas
acromegaly and, 1352, 1353f
cell analysis methods for, 1349–1350,
1350f, 1350t
Cushing disease and, 1352, 1353f
hyperprolactinemia and, 1352, 1354,
1354f, 1354t
in multiple endocrine neoplasia, 1327,
1327f
Nelson syndrome and, 1354t, 1354–
1355
treatment of, 1355–1357
for acromegaly, 1356
for Cushing disease, 1355–1356
for nonfunctioning adenomas, 1355
for prolactinomas, 1356–1357
macroadenomas, 1356–1357
microadenomas, 1357

Pituitary apoplexy, 1355
Pituitary gland, 1347–1357
  adenohypophysis, 1347, 1348f
  adenomas of. See Pituitary adenomas
  clinical evaluation of, 1351
  embryology, anatomy, and physiology
    of, 1347f–1349f, 1347–1349
  endocrine evaluation of, 1351–1352
  imaging of, 1350, 1351f
  neurohypophysis, 1347, 1348f, 1348–
    1349
Pit viper bites. See Bites and stings
Plant alkaloids, 502t
Plaques, atherosclerotic, 1593
  Hollenhorst, 1751
  rupture of, 1631, 1631f
  soft, 1750
Plasma cell mastitis, 1377
Plasmacytomas, of ribs, 1448, 1448f
Plasma expanders, 250, 250t
Plasma membranes, 3–4, 4f
  composition of, implications for
    selectivity and energy
    conversion, 12–13, 13f
  of hepatocytes, 943, 944f, 945, 945f
  membrane transport and. See
    Membrane transport
Plasma osmolality, 244
Plasmin, 85
  aneurysm formation and, 1844
  thrombosis and, 1614
Plasminogen, activation of, 86. See also
    Thrombolytic therapy; specific
    fibrinolytic agents
Plastic meshes/sheets, for hernia repair,
    1220
Plastic surgery. See Aesthetic surgery;
    Reconstructive surgery
Platelet(s)
  activation of, 94–95, 95f
    factors derived from activated
      platelets and, 150, 150t
  adhesion of, 1612, 1612f
  aggregation of, 1612f, 1612–1613
    abnormal, 92
    stimulation of, 1612–1613
    testing for, 103–104
  disorders of, 94–95, 95f
    in critically ill patients, management
      of, 237
  function of, hypothermia and, 411
    tests of, 103–104
  inflammation and, 149–151, 150t
  secretion of, 1612, 1612f
Platelet-activating factor (PAF)
  inflammation and, 140–141, 141f, 142f
  in shock, 194
Platelet coagulant activity, 1612, 1612f,
    1613
Platelet count, 103
Platelet-derived growth factor (PDGF)
  acute-phase response mediation by,
    133t
  arterial smooth muscle growth and,
    1590
  bone formation and, 2152
  fibroblasts and, wound healing and,
    125
  for vascular gene therapy, 520t
  for wound care, 82, 82t
Platelet release reaction, 1612–1613
Pleiotropic drug resistance, 498

Pleomorphic adenomas, of salivary
    glands, 641, 641t
Plethysmography, 1669, 1672f, 1672–
    1673
  air, in chronic venous insufficiency,
    1940–1941, 1941f
  in chronic venous insufficiency, 1940–
    1941
  digital, 1672–1673
  impedance, in deep venous
    thrombosis, 1947–1948
  outflow, in chronic venous
    insufficiency, 1960
  photoplethysmography, in chronic
    venous insufficiency, 1960,
    1961f
  segmental, 1672, 1673f
  in vascular occlusive disease, of upper
    extremities, 1760
Pleura, 1451–1465. See also specific
    disorders
  anatomy of, 1444, 1445f, 1451–1452
  cysts of, 1463
  tumors of, 1463–1465
    benign, 1463–1464
    malignant, 1464t, 1464–1465
    metastatic, 1465
Pleural effusions, 1452–1456
  ascites and, 987
  exudates, 1452–1453
  malignant, treatment of, 1455–1456
  physical and chemical characteristics
    of, 1453–1455
  subpulmonic, 1453
  transudates, 1452–1454
Pleural empyema, 1456t, 1456–1458,
    1457f–1459f
Pleural space injuries, indications for
    surgery and, 319
Pleurectomy, for pleural effusions, 1455–
    1456
Pleurodesis, chemical, for pleural
    effusions, 1455
Plummer-Vinson syndrome, 705, 705f
Pneumatic antishock garment (PASG)
  in pelvic fractures, 354
  for shock, 206–207
  for trauma patients, 281
Pneumatoceles, treatment of, 326, 326f
Pneumatosis cystoides intestinalis, 1119
Pneumatosis intestinalis, ion necrotizing
    enterocolitis, 2047, 2048f
Pneumocystis carinii infections, 180
Pneumomediastinum, 1471–1472
Pneumonia, nosocomial, 176
  posttraumatic, 398t, 398–399
Pneumonitis, with esophageal atresia and
    tracheoesophageal fistulas, 2012
Pneumoperitoneum
  carbon dioxide, for laparoscopic
    surgery, 736, 738, 738t
  progressive, for massive hernia repair,
    1221
Pneumothorax
  during antireflux operations, 692
  chest injuries and, 318, 319
  open, treatment of, 323
  simple, treatment of, 323, 323f
  spontaneous, 1458–1461, 1460f, 1461f
  tension
    pediatric, 381
    treatment of, 323, 324f

Poiseuille's equation, 185, 1509, 1534,
    1661–1662
Poland syndrome, 1358, 2003
Polyarteritis nodosa (PAN), 1603, 1603f
Polycystic kidney disease, pediatric, 2103
Polycythemia vera, hypersplenism and,
    1273
Polyhydramnios
  duodenal obstruction and, 2040
  esophageal atresia and
    tracheoesophageal fistulas and,
    2012
Polymerase chain reaction (PCR), 167
  for human immunodeficiency virus
    detection, 178f, 178–179
Polymorphonuclear leukocytes (PMNs).
    See also specific
    polymorphonuclear leukocytes
  inflammation and, 142–152
Polyneuropathy, following gastric surgery
    for morbid obesity, 793
Polyp(s)
  cholesterol, 1056
  colorectal. See Colorectal polyps;
    specific syndromes
  esophageal, 696–697, 697f, 698f
  gastric, 795–796
  inflammatory, of gallbladder, 1056
  of nipples, 1378
  pseudopolyps, in ulcerative colitis,
    1097
Polypectomy
  endoscopic, in colorectal polyps, 1116,
    1117f
  index, in colorectal adenomas, 1115–
    1116, 1116f
Polyposis syndromes, 1120–1127. See
    also specific syndromes
Polypropylene mesh repair, for inguinal
    and femoral hernias, 1223, 1225f
Polyribosomes, 25
Popliteal artery
  adventitial cystic disease of, 1640,
    1641f
  anatomy of, 1810–1811, 1811f
  aneurysms of. See Aneurysm(s), of
    popliteal artery
Popliteal artery entrapment syndrome,
    1639–1640, 1640f, 1641f
Popliteal vein, 1935
Porcine xenograft, for burns, 431
Pores, nuclear, 5
Porphyrin, metabolism of, 956
Portal decompression, for Budd-Chiari
    syndrome, 991
Portal hypertension, 984–986
  differential diagnosis of, 991–993, 992t
  hemorrhoids in, treatment of, 1190
  hypersplenism and, 1270
  idiopathic, 992–993
  pediatric, 1005–1006
  physiology of, 984–986
    blood volume and hepatic resistance
      and, 985–986
    portosystemic collaterals and
      hyperdynamic state and, 984,
      985f
    variceal hemorrhage and. See Varices,
      gastroesophageal
Portal vein(s)
  anatomy of, 934–935, 935f, 1686
  thrombophlebitis of, 1958
  thrombosis of

allogenic hepatocytes and, 517
following hepatic transplantation, 595
traumatic injuries of, 369–370
Portal vein-hepatic artery fistulas, 1921, 1923
Portoenterostomy, for biliary atresia, 2087–2089, 2089f
results and complications of, 2088–2089
Portosystemic collaterals, in portal hypertension, 985, 985f
Portosystemic shunts
for ascites, intrahepatic, transjugular, 990
for gastroesophageal varices, 998f–1000f, 1000, 1002–1005
end-to-side, 998f, 1002
intrahepatic, transjugular, 997f, 998–1000, 1167
lateral, 999f, 1000f, 1002
mesocaval, interposition, 1002–1003
preoperative and postoperative care and, 1002t, 1003
results with, 1002t, 1003f, 1003–1005
selective, 1002
Port wine stains, in Klippel-Trenaunay syndrome, 1930, 1932
Positive crossmatch, 542
Positron emission tomography scanning (PET)
of breasts, 1365–1366
of liver, 937
in sarcomas, 2253, 2255f
Postcoital test, 2203
Posterior descending artery (PDA), 1534–1535
Posterior urethral valves, 2108–2109
Posterior wall fractures, management of, 305, 306f
Postgastrectomy syndromes, 771–773
alkaline reflux gastritis, 772f, 773
dumping, 772
Postoperative fluid therapy, 252
Postpericardiotomy syndrome, 1547
Postphlebitic syndrome. See Chronic venous insufficiency (CVI)
Postsplenectomy sepsis (PSS), 1270–1271
prophylaxis of, 1280
Postthrombotic syndrome. See Chronic venous insufficiency (CVI)
Posttransplantation lymphoproliferative disease (PTLD), 845, 852
Potassium, 255–257. See also Hyperkalemia; Hypokalemia
in hyperaldosteronism, 1341, 1342t
pediatric requirements for, 1988
Potassium balance, normal, 249
Pouchitis, following ileoanal anastomosis, 1104–1106
Precursor lesions, breast cancer and, 1385
Prednisone
for cardiac transplantation, 602, 602t
for hepatic transplantation, 598
for ulcerative colitis, 1098
Preeclampsia, 394
Pregnancy, 2228–2229
abortion and, 2228
anesthesia in, 393–394
anticoagulation in, 1530–1531

appendicitis during, 1259, 1259f
breasts during, 1362
cancer and, 1409
Crohn's disease in, 843
ectopic, 2228f, 2228–2229, 2229f
acute abdomen and, 1249
gestational trophoblastic neoplasia and, 2229
hemorrhoids following labor and, 1190
high-risk, 1973
hyperparathyroidism during, 1325
intrauterine growth retardation and, 1973
fluid spaces and, 1987–1988
maternal transfer of humoral immunity during, 1991
pancreatitis and, 882
polyhydramnios during
duodenal obstruction and, 2040
esophageal atresia and tracheoesophageal fistulas and, 2012
thrombosis associated with, 1618
traumatic injuries during, 390–395
anatomy and physiology and, 390–392, 391t
gastrointestinal changes and, 391
hemodynamic changes and, 390–391
laboratory studies and, 391–392
musculoskeletal system and, 391
pulmonary changes and, 391
renal system and, 391
initial assessment and management of, 392–393
diagnostic modalities for, 392–393, 393t
fetal assessment and monitoring in, 392
history and physical examination in, 392
management of, 393–395
amniotic fluid embolism and, 394
for blunt trauma, 393
for burns, 393, 393t
critical care and, 394
hemorrhage and, 395
medications in, 394
for minor trauma, 395
operative, 393–394
thromboembolism and, 394
toxemia and preeclampsia and, 394
Prehospital care, for traumatic injuries. See Traumatic injuries, prehospital care for
Prekallikrien, inhibition of, 99
Premature birth, 1973
thermoregulation and, 1979–1980
Premorbid health, of organ donors, 559–560
Prenatal period. See Fetus; Pregnancy
Prenzepine, for duodenal ulcers, 763t
Preoperative evaluation, for anesthesia, 445–446, 446t, 447t, 448
Pressure assist ventilation, 1986
Pressure control ventilation, 1986
Pressure-regulated volume control ventilation, 1986
Pressure sores, healing of, 80
Pressure support ventilation, 1986
Primary survey, of trauma patients, 282–283, 283t

Pringle maneuver, 339, 339f
Prinzmetal angina, 1538
Proaccelerin deficiency, 94
Probenecid
for gonococcal proctitis, 1203
for pelvic inflammatory disease, 2225t
Procarbazine, 501t
Procidentia, 2221
Proconvertin deficiency, 94
Proctitis
chlamydial, 1203–1204
gonococcal, 1203
herpes simplex, 1204
Proctocolectomy, total
for familial adenomatous polyposis, 1124
for ulcerative colitis, 1100
Proctoscopy, in hemorrhoids, 1188
Proctosigmoidoscopy, in colorectal cancer, 1132–1133
Progastrin, 749–750
Progesterone, 1331, 2217
deficiency of, 1341
Prolactinomas, treatment of, 1356–1357
for macroadenomas, 1356–1357
for microadenomas, 1357
Proliferative phase, of wound healing, 68–69, 71f, 71t
Promoter regions, 23
Pronephros, 1987
Propofol, 441, 441t
Propranolol
for gastroesophageal varices, 994
for Graves disease, 1296–1297
prophylactic, for aortic aneurysms, 1846
Propylthiouracil (PTU), 1291
Prostacyclins, gastric, 775
Prostaglandin(s)
biliary, gallstone formation and, 1039, 1039f
gastric, 775
for gastric ulcers, 785
in inflammation, 137t
prophylactic, for stress gastritis, 778–779
prostaglandin E1, for impotence, 2201
renal, volume control and, 248
in shock, 193, 193f
Prostaglandin analogues, for duodenal ulcers, 765, 765f
Prostaglandin synthetase, for hypercalcemia, 1315
Prostate cancer, 2210–2212
clinical staging of, 2211
detection of, 2210–2211
follow-up for, 2212
stage and grade of, 2210, 2210f
treatment of, 2211–2212
tumor markers in, 2211
Prostatectomy, radical, for cancer, 2211
Prostate-specific antigen (PSA), in prostate cancer, 2211, 2212
Prosthetic devices
aesthetic, 2280
infections associated with, 176
following lower extremity amputation, 1837–1838
general considerations in, 1837
specific levels and, 1837–1838
surfaces of, anticoagulation and, 99
Prosthetic heart valves, 1525f, 1525–1527, 1526f

Prosthetic heart valves (*continued*)
  bioprosthetic, 1525, 1525f
    complications of, 1526, 1526f
  complications of, 1526f, 1526–1527
  endocarditis and, 1531
  hemodynamics and, 1526, 1526t
  mechanical, 1525f, 1525–1526
    complications of, 1526–1527
  peripheral arterial embolism and, 1622
Protamine sulfate, for reversal of heparin
    anticoagulation, 96–97
Protease(s), aneurysm formation and,
    1843–1844
Protease inhibitors, aneurysm formation
    and, 1844
τ protein, 9
Protein(s). *See also specific proteins*
  aneurysm formation and, 1842–1843
  biliary, 955–956
  carrier, 13, 14f, 18, 20f–22f, 20–21
  digestion and absorption of, in small
    intestine, 815–816
  as energy source, 229, 230t
  metabolism of, 45f–47f, 45–47, 46t
    in critically ill patients, 227, 229f,
      230
      mediators of, 230
    hepatic. *See* Liver, protein
      metabolism in
    injury response and, 54
    sepsis and, 56, 56f
  pediatric requirements for, 1975, 1977
  plasma, hepatic formation of, 953, 954t
  plasma membrane, transport pathways
    for, 13, 14f
  requirements for, in critically ill
    patients, estimating and
    measuring, 230
  secretory pathway and, 29f–31f, 29–30
  sources of, 230
    endogenous, 230–231
  synthesis of, 24–25, 25f
  targeting of, 26–29
    nuclear and mitochondrial, 27–29,
      28f
    secretory pathway, 26f–28f, 26–27
Proteinase(s), in inflammation, 155–156
α₁-Proteinase inhibitor (α₁-PI), during
    acute-phase reaction, 132, 132t
Protein C
  activated, resistance to, 90–91, 1615
  deficiency of, 1615
  definition of, 90, 90f
  thrombosis and, 1614
Protein kinase C, activation of, 475, 476f,
    478, 479f
Protein S
  deficiency of, 1615–1616
  definition of, 90, 90f
Protein-sparing effect, 229
Proteoglycans, wound healing and,
    remodeling phase of, 71
Prothrombic states. *See* Hypercoagulable
    states
Prothrombin time (PT), 104
Proton-pump blockers, for duodenal
    ulcers, 764
Protooncogenes, 469, 470
Protozoan infections, 180
Pro-urokinase (pro-UK), 1738
Prune-belly syndrome, 2111
Pseudoaneurysms
  of aortic isthmus or proximal arch
    vessels, 368, 369f, 370f

dissecting renal artery aneurysms as
    cause of, 1906–1907, 1908f
  of femoral artery
    anastomotic, 1911–1912
      clinical manifestations of, 1911
      diagnosis of, 1911, 1911f
      incidence of, 1911
      pathogenesis of, 1911
      treatment of, 1911–1912
    catheter-induced, 1912
Pseudoappendicitis syndrome, 1238
Pseudocysts, pancreatic, 886f, 886–887,
    887f
  following pancreatic injuries, 349
  pediatric, 2096–2097
Pseudodiverticulosis, 679, 679f
Pseudoglandular synovial sarcomas. *See*
    Sarcomas, tenosynovial
Pseudohermaphroditism
  female, 2112, 2112f–2114f
  male, 2113
Pseudohyponatremia, 253
Pseudohypoparathyroidism,
    hypocalcemia and, 1317
Pseudomembranous colitis (PMC). *See*
    Antibiotic-associated colitis
Pseudoobstruction, with gastroschisis or
    omphalocele, 2032
Pseudopolyps, in ulcerative colitis, 1097
Pseudotumor(s), of gallbladder
    (strawberry gallbladder), 1056
Pseudotumor cerebri, in morbid obesity,
    790
Pseudoxanthoma elasticum, 1600–1601
P-sites, 24
Psoriasis, cytokines and, 121
PSU/Sarns total artificial heart, 1562,
    1562f, 1563
Psychologic disorders,
    hyperparathyroidism and, 1321
Pubococcygeal muscle, anatomy of, 1182,
    1182f
Puborectalis muscle, 2041
Pull-through procedure, for anorectal
    malformations, 2045
Pulmonary artery, coronary artery
    originating from, 1495–1496
Pulmonary artery catheters
  in pediatric patients, 1981–1982
  in shock, 195–196, 196t, 197t
Pulmonary blastomas, in pediatric
    patients, 2010
Pulmonary contusions
  pediatric, 381
  in trauma patients, 284
  treatment of, 325
Pulmonary disorders. *See also specific
    disorders*
  abscesses, 1478–1479
    pathogenesis of, 1478
    presentation of, 1478, 1479f
    treatment of, 1478–1479
  anesthesia and, 444–445
  bronchiectasis, 1479–1480
    diagnosis of, 1480, 1480f
    pathogenesis of, 1479–1480
    treatment of, 1480
  burns and, 435t
  in chronic liver disease, 980, 980t
  congenital cystic disease, 2003–2008
    bronchogenic cysts and, 2006, 2007f
    cystic adenomatoid malformations
      and, 2005, 2005f

diagnosis of, 2006–2008, 2007f
  embryology of, 2003
  lobar overinflation and, 2005, 2006f
  pulmonary sequestrations in, 2003–
    2005, 2004f
  treatment of, 2008
cystic disease, congenital. *See*
    Pulmonary disorders, congenital
    cystic disease
in fulminant hepatic failure, 978
in morbid obesity, 789–790
neoplastic disease
  benign, 1433–1434, 1434t
    arteriovenous malformations, 1434
    hamartomas, 1433–1434
  malignant. *See* Lung cancer
in pancreatitis, 884
posttraumatic, 396–399, 397t, 398t
following valvular heart surgery, 1527
Pulmonary edema, in respiratory failure,
    222
Pulmonary embolectomy
  catheter, 103
  open, 103
Pulmonary embolism
  angiography in, 1702f, 1706
  orthopedic injuries and, 376
  posttraumatic, 399
  thrombolytic therapy for, 101
Pulmonary hematomas, treatment of,
    325–326, 326f
Pulmonary hypertension
  persistent, of newborn. *See* Persistent
    pulmonary hypertension of the
    newborn (PPHN)
  in pulmonary thromboembolism, 1954,
    1955–1956
Pulmonary infarction, pulmonary
    thromboembolism and, 1953
Pulmonary lacerations, treatment of, 325
Pulmonary mechanics, in critically ill
    patients, 220–221, 221f
Pulmonary resection
  for non-small cell lung cancer, 1423–
    1431
    stage I and II, 1423–1427, 1424f–
      1426f
      adjuvant therapy and, 1425, 1427
      patterns of recurrence and, 1425
      survival and, 1424–1425, 1427t
    stage IIIa, 1427–1428, 1428t, 1429–
      1431
  of pulmonary metastases, 1434–1438
    criteria for, 1435–1437, 1436t, 1437t
    historical background of, 1434–1435
    preoperative evaluation for, 1437
    results with, 1437t, 1438, 1438t
    surgical technique for, 1437–1438
  for small cell lung cancer, 1431–1432
Pulmonary sequestrations, congenital,
    2003–2005, 2004f
Pulmonary system. *See also* Lung(s)
  in pregnancy, 391
  in shock, 189–190
Pulmonary thromboembolism, 1951–
    1956
  anticoagulation for, 1953, 1954t
  chronic, 1955–1956
  clinical presentation of, 1951, 1951t
  diagnosis of, 1951–1952
  embolectomy for, 1954–1955
    catheter, transvenous, 1955, 1957f
    pulmonary, 1954–1955, 1955f, 1956f

pathophysiology of, 1952–1953
pulmonary hypertension and, 1954, 1955–1956
surgical approaches for, 103
thrombolytic therapy for, 1953–1954
Pulmonary transplantation, 606–615
complications of, 612–614, 613t
for diaphragmatic hernia repair, 2026
donor considerations for, 608–609, 609f
future of, 615
indications for, 606–608, 607f, 608t
lung preservation for, 609–610
operative technique for, 610–612
for double-lung transplantation, 611f, 611–612
for single-lung transplantation, 610, 611f
posttransplantation physiology and, 614f, 614t, 614–615
results with, 612, 612t
Pulmonary valve, anatomy of, 1503, 1504f
Pulse oximetry
in persistent pulmonary hypertension of newborn, 1985
postoperative, 448
Pulse volume recordings, 1672, 1673f
Pulsus paradoxus, in cardiac tamponade, 1577
Pulsus parvus et tardus, in valvular heart disease, 1512
Pupils, in head injuries, 294, 294f
Purpura fulminans, 90
diagnosis of, 429t
Putamen, hemorrhage into, 2185
Pyelonephritis, acute abdomen and, 1250
Pyloric exclusion, 344–345, 346f
Pyloric stenosis, hypertrophic, infantile, 2066–2067
anatomy and pathophysiology of, 2066
clinical presentation of, 2066
diagnosis of, 2066f, 2066–2067
treatment of, 2067, 2067f
Pyloroplasty
for duodenal ulcers, 766f–767f, 767
for gastric ulcers, 786, 787
Pyoderma, 2161
Pyogenic hepatic abscesses, 958–959
Pyridostigmine, 440t
Pyridoxine
pediatric requirement for, 1976t
requirements in surgical patients, 62t
Pyropoikilocytosis, hereditary, 1267
Pyruvate kinase deficiency, 1267–1268

Q

Quality assurance, pediatric trauma care and, 385
Quinolones, spectrum of activity of, 169t

R

Race, cholelithiasis and, 1034–1035
Radial artery
anatomy of, 1687
catheter injuries of, 1763
Radial forearm flaps, 2285, 2286
Radial nerve, disorders of, 2156

Radial scars (sclerosing lesions), of breast, 1376f, 1376–1377
Radiation
heat transfer by, 1979
ionizing
biology of, 492
principles of, 491, 492f
soft tissue sarcomas and, 2247, 2247f
tumors caused by, 462
ultraviolet. See Ultraviolet radiation (UVR)
Radiation injury
arterial, 1602, 1602f
enteritis and
intestinal obstruction and, 827
total parenteral nutrition for, 60
risk of, in pregnancy, 393, 393t
wound healing and, 79
Radiation sensitizers, for sarcomas, retroperitoneal, 2261, 2261f
Radiodermatitis
basal cell carcinomas of skin and, 2242
squamous cell carcinomas of skin and, 2242
Radiographic contrast agents
for angiography, 1680, 1682f
nephrotoxicity of, 235–236
Radiographic examination. See also specific modalities
in abdominal injuries, 334–335
in bile duct strictures, 1070, 1071f, 1072f
in chest injuries, 318
in cholelithiasis, 1041
in chronic pancreatitis, 892, 893f, 894f
in Clostridium difficile colitis, 1176
in Crohn's disease, 837–838, 838t, 839f
in duodenal injuries, 345
of hand, 2154
in head injuries, 295–297
in Hirschsprung disease, 2059
in intestinal obstruction, 821–822, 821–823, 822f
of liver. See Liver, imaging of
in maxillofacial injuries, 302, 303f, 304f
in meconium ileus, 2051, 2051f
in necrotizing enterocolitis, 2047–2048, 2048f
in osteosarcomas, 2263, 2263f
in pancreatic cancer, 906t, 906–908, 907f, 908f
in pancreatitis, 883
of pituitary gland and parasellar region, 1350
in pleural effusions, 1453
in sarcomas, 2253, 2254f
in spinal cord injuries, 2171, 2172f
in thoracic empyema, 1456, 1457f
in traumatic injuries
in elderly people, 388
in pregnancy, 393, 393t
in ulcerative colitis, 1097, 1097f
in valvular heart disease, 1513
in vascular occlusive disease, of upper extremities, 1760f–1762f, 1760–1761
Radioimmunoassays (RIAs), 1292
Radionuclide scanning
in adrenal disorders, 1343
in biliary atresia, 2086, 2087f
of bone, in osteosarcomas, 2263
in deep venous thrombosis, 1948

in gastrointestinal hemorrhage, 1161–1162
ion necrotizing enterocolitis, 2048
in liver masses, 1009–1010
of lymphatic clearance, 1968
of thyroid gland, 1294, 1306
in solitary thyroid nodule, 1299–1300
in vascular infections, 1727
Radiosensitivity, 492f, 492–493, 493f
Radiotherapy, 491–494
for acromegaly, 1356
adverse effects and biology of normal tissue and, 492f, 492–493, 493f
for anal cancer, 1150
for bile duct cancer, adjuvant, 1066
for bladder cancer, 2207
brachytherapy, 491–492
adjuvant, with head and neck surgery, 650–651
intraoperative, 490
for breast cancer, 1390, 1391, 1395–1396
after lumpectomy, 1395, 1396f
after mastectomy, 1395–1396
metastases from, 1402
sarcomas induced by, 1407–1409, 1408f
for colorectal cancer, adjuvant, 1141–1142
for desmoid tumors, of abdominal wall, 1237
for desmoplastic small round cell tumors, pediatric, 2133
for esophageal cancer, 705, 705f
external-beam, for pancreatic cancer, 915
for fibrosarcomas, pediatric, 2132
for gallbladder cancer, adjuvant, 1060
with head and neck surgery, adjuvant, 650–651
for hepatoblastomas, pediatric, 2137–2138
intraoperative, 490
for pancreatic cancer, 913, 915
ionizing radiation and, 491, 492f
for liver cancer, primary, 1019
for lung cancer, non-small cell
stage I and II, 1425, 1427
stage IIIa, 1428, 1430t, 1430–1431
for metastatic intracranial tumors, 2179
whole-brain irradiation, 2179
gestational trophoblastic neoplasia and, 2229, 2229f
for metastatic melanomas, 2241
for neurofibrosarcomas, pediatric, 2134
for pancreatic cancer, intraoperative, 913, 915
pharmacologic modification of, 493, 493f
during pregnancy, contraindication to, 1409
radiation biology and, 492
for rhabdomyosarcomas, pediatric, 2131
for sarcomas, 2255–2256, 2258
postoperative, 2256, 2258
preoperative, 2255–2256
retroperitoneal, 2260
for skin cancer, adjuvant, 2245
for small intestinal cancer, 848, 850, 851, 855
with surgery, 494

Radiotherapy (*continued*)
teletherapy, 492
for testis cancer, 2213
tumor biology and, 493f, 493–494
fractionation and, 494, 495f
high linear energy transfer radiation and, 494, 496f
for uterine carcinomas, 2222–2223
whole-brain irradiation, for metastatic intracranial tumors, 2179
gestational trophoblastic neoplasia and, 2229, 2229f
for Wilms tumor, 2126
Ranitidine, 764f
for duodenal ulcers, 762, 763t, 764f
Rapamycin, 548
Rathke cysts, 1355
Rathke pouch, 1347, 1347f
Rattlesnake bites. *See* Bites and stings
Raynaud phenomenon, 1758–1759
Raynaud syndrome, 1759
Rb gene, neuroblastomas and, 2119
RB1 gene, sarcomas and, 2249–2250
Reaction-to-injury hypothesis, of atherosclerosis, 1589, 1593
Reactive hyperemia, 1673–1674
Recanalization, for acute myocardial infarction, 1541
Receptor(s). *See also* Ligand-receptor interaction; *specific receptors*
cell surface, transduction of, 36–39, 37f–39f
intracellular, gene expression control and, 35f, 35–36, 36f
Receptor down-regulation, 33–34
Receptor-mediated endocytosis, 32–33
Recombinant DNA. *See* Gene therapy
Reconstructive surgery, 2280–2289
aortic. *See* Aortic reconstruction
of breast, 1390, 1394f, 1394–1395
for burns, 436–437, CF 12–13
of chest wall, 1449–1451
muscle flaps for, 1450–1451, 1452f–1454f
techniques for, 1449–1450, 1450f, 1451f
for congenital deformities, 2285f, 2286–2287
for extracranial carotid aneurysms, 1852, 1853f–1855f
of extremities
dysvascular and diabetic, 2288, 2288t
following resection for sarcomas, 2288f, 2289, 2289f
for venolymphatic insufficiency, 2289
flap principles for, 2281f–2283f, 2281–2282, 2284
of head and neck, 649f, 649–650, 2285f, 2285–2286
perineal and genital, 2287–2288
reconstructive ladder for, 2284f, 2284–2285
of renal artery, for renal hypertension, 1792
following resection of extremity osteosarcomas, 2264, 2265f
following skin cancer, 2244
of trunk and chest, 2286f, 2287, 2287f
venous, direct, 1943
Rectal biopsy, in Hirschsprung disease, 2059, 2061f

Rectal myectomy, for Hirschsprung disease, 2062, 2064
Rectal prolapse, 1190–1192
anatomic abnormalities and, 1190
classification of, 1190
clinical manifestations of, 1190–1191
complications of, 1191
diagnosis of, 1191
evaluation of, 1191
incontinence in, 1191–1192
pathophysiology of, 1190
pediatric, 2078, 2078f
treatment of, 1191, 1192f–1195f
Rectal sling operation, 1191, 1192f
Rectoanal reflex, 1187
Rectopexy, for rectal prolapse, 1191, 1193f
Rectosigmoidectomy, perineal, for rectal prolapse, 1191, 1194f
Rectosigmoid resection, transabdominal, for rectal prolapse, 1191, 1193f
Rectovaginal fistulas, 1200f, 1200–1201, 1202f
Rectum. *See also* Anorectal *entries;* Anorectum; Colorectal *entries; specific disorders*
anatomy of, 2041, 2042f
cancer of, 490
nerve supply of, 1184–1186, 1187f
traumatic injuries of, 351–352
Rectus abdominis muscle flaps, for chest wall reconstruction, 1451, 1454f
Rectus sheath hematomas, 1236
Recurrent laryngeal nerve (RLN), 656, 1284, 1284f, 1285f–1287f, 1285–1286
traumatic injuries of, management of, 317
Reduplication, 2074–2075, 2075f
Referred pain, abdominal, 1246, 1248
Reflex sympathetic dystrophy, 2196
Reflux
duodenogastric, gastric ulcers and, 782–783
gastric. *See* Gastroesophageal reflux disease (GERD)
Reflux nephropathy, 2105
Regurgitation, in esophageal cancer, 702
Rehabilitation
for burns, 436
for cancer, 491
following head and neck surgery, 650
following lower extremity amputation, 1837–1838
general considerations in, 1837, 1837t
specific levels and, 1837–1838
for traumatic injuries, 278
Relaxing incision, for hernia repair, 1220, 1222–1223, 1224f
Release factors, protein synthesis and, 25
Remodeling, of bone, 2145
pediatric, 384
Remodeling phase, of wound healing, 70–71, 72f
Renal acidosis. *See* Metabolic acidosis
Renal agenesis, 2101
Renal artery
aneurysms of. *See* Aneurysm(s), of renal artery
occlusive disease of. *See* Renal hypertension

reconstruction of, ex vivo, for renal hypertension, 1792
stenosis of, developmental, 1786, 1788f
Renal blood flow, pediatric, 1987
Renal cell carcinomas, 2208–2209
diagnosis and staging of, 2208–2209, 2209f
pediatric, 2127
treatment of, 2209
Renal compensation, in metabolic acidosis, 263
Renal cystic disease, pediatric, 2102–2103
multicystic, 2102–2103
polycystic, 2103
Renal disorders. *See also specific disorders*
burns and, 435t
in chronic liver disease, 980–981
neoplastic, pediatric, 2122–2127. *See also* Wilms tumor
in pancreatitis, 884–885
in systemic inflammatory response syndrome, 210
following valvular heart surgery, 1527
Renal ectopy, 2101–2102
Renal failure
following abdominal aortic aneurysm repair, 1889–1890
acute. *See* Acute renal failure (ARF)
in diabetes mellitus, 617
posttraumatic, 401–402
sepsis and, 57
in shock, 190–191
Renal function, pediatric, 1986–1987
Renal hypertension, 1780–1794
clinical features of, 1786–1787, 1789f
diagnosis of, 1787–1790, 1790f, 1791f
pathology of, 1783–1786
arterial fibrodysplasia and, 1784, 1785f–1787f, 1786
atherosclerosis and, 1783–1784, 1784f
developmental renal artery disease and, 1786, 1788f
pathophysiology of, 1780–1783, 1781f–1783f
treatment of, 1790–1794
bypass procedures for, 1791f–1793f, 1791–1793
percutaneous transluminal renal angioplasty for, 1790–1791
pharmacologic, 1790
renal revascularization for, 1791
results of operative therapy and, 1793t, 1793–1794, 1794t
Renal natriuretic peptide, in sodium and volume control, 247
Renal pelvis, carcinomas of, 2208
Renal replacement therapy. *See also specific modalities*
for critically ill patients, 237–239, 238t
Renal revascularization, for renal hypertension, 1791
Renal system. *See also* Kidney(s)
age-related changes in, 387
hyperparathyroidism and, 1320, 1320f
pediatric, 1986–1989
fluid and electrolyte therapy and, 1988t, 1988–1989
fluid spaces and, 1987–1988
renal function and, 1986–1987
in pregnancy, 391
transalveolar, 1509

Renal transplantation, 571–581
  cadaveric, 574–575, 576f
  complications of, 581
  high-risk groups and, 577f–579f, 577–578
  immunosuppression for, 576f, 577
  indications for, 571–572, 574t
  living donors for, 573–574, 575f
  organ preservation for, 575–577
  outcome of, 578–580, 579f, 580t
    phase 1, 579, 580f
    phase 2, 579–580, 580f, 580t, 581f
    phase 3, 580
    phase 4, 580
  procedure for, 572–573
Renal tubular acidosis (RTA). See Metabolic acidosis
Renal vein(s)
  anatomy of, 1687
  Wilms tumor and, 2126
Renal vein renin ratio (RVRR), in renovascular hypertension, 1788, 1790f
Renin
  activity in peripheral and renal venous blood, in renovascular hypertension, 1788
  renovascular hypertension and, 1780–1783, 1781f–1783f
  secretion of, 1332
  in shock, 188
  for vascular gene therapy, 520t
Renin-angiotensin system
  renovascular hypertension and, 1781–1783, 1782f
  volume control mediation by, 247
Renin-systemic renin index (RSRI), in renovascular hypertension, 1788, 1791f
Renography
  diuretic, in ureteropelvic junction obstruction, 2104, 2104f
  isotopic, in renovascular hypertension, 1789
Renovascular hypertension, pediatric, operative treatment of, 1793, 1794t
Renovascular occlusive disease, angiography in, 1692f, 1692–1693
Reperfusion
  tissue ischemia and, 1652, 1653t
  of visceral circulation, 1771–1772
Reperfusion injury
  of donor organs, 558
  posttraumatic, 395
  in shock, 208
Replantation, of amputated hand, indications for, 2162
Residual lung volume, 1983
Resistance vessels, 1588
Resources for the Optimal Care of the Injured Patient, 279
Respiration
  anatomy of, 1440
  mechanics of, persistent pulmonary hypertension of newborn and, 1983f, 1983–1984
  neonatal, assessment of, 1985
Respiratory acidosis, 261t, 265–266
  clinical features of, 265
  compensatory mechanisms in, 265
  treatment of, 265–266

Respiratory alkalosis, 261t, 265
  clinical features of, 265
  compensatory mechanisms in, 265
  treatment of, 265
Respiratory compensation
  in metabolic acidosis, 263
  in metabolic alkalosis, 264, 264t
Respiratory depression
  in fulminant hepatic failure, 978
  hypothermia and, 408–410
Respiratory disorders. *See also specific disorders*
  in chronic liver disease, 979–980
  in esophageal cancer, 702
  in gastroesophageal reflux disease, 681
  gene therapy for, 513–515
    adenoviruses for, 513, 514f
    in cystic fibrosis, 514–515, 516f
    liposomes for, 514, 514f, 515f
Respiratory distress
  diaphragmatic hernias and, 2024, 2024f, 2025
  in shock, 190
Respiratory failure
  in critically ill patients, 221–225
    management of, 222–225, 223f
      mechanical ventilation in, 224–225, 225f
      treatment of interstitial space in, 225
    pathophysiology of, 221–222
      alveolar collapse and, 221–222
      pulmonary edema and, 222
    inhalation injury and, 433, 433t
Respiratory insufficiency
  in morbid obesity, 789
  sepsis and, 57
Respiratory quotient (RQ), 44–45, 231–232
Respiratory system. *See also* Pulmonary *entries; specific organs*
  age-related changes in, 387
Response elements, 35
Resting energy expenditure, 227
Restraint device injuries, 271–272
Retention cysts, pancreatic, pediatric, 2097
Retinoblastoma(s)
  congenital pattern of expression of, 478–480, 480f, 481f
  familial, sarcomas associated with, 2249–2250
Retinoblastoma protein, for vascular gene therapy, 520t
Retinol. *See* Vitamin(s), vitamin A (retinol)
Retinopathy, diabetic, following pancreatic transplantation, 625–626
Retrogasserian rhizotomy, 2195
Retroperitoneal disorders. *See also specific disorders*
  abscesses, 1242
  chylous ascites, 1242–1243
  fibrosis, 1243–1244
  neoplastic disease, 1244, 2213–2214
    benign, 2214
    germ cell, 2213–2214
    metastatic, 2214
    soft tissue sarcomas, management of, 2259f, 2259–2261
      chemotherapy for, 2260–2261

radiation sensitizers for, 2261, 2261f
  surgical, 2260, 2260f, 2260t
  traumatic injuries, 353–361. *See also specific injuries*
    hematomas and, 352f, 352–353
Retroperitoneum, 1242–1244
  anatomy of, 352f, 352–353, 1242
Retroviruses
  recombinant, for gene therapy, 507–508, 508f, 510
  tumor induction by, 470, 471f
Revascularization. *See also* Endosurgery, vascular
  for aortoiliac disease, indirect, 1805, 1808f–1809f, 1808–1809
  evaluation of potential for, prior to amputation, 1825
  percutaneous transluminal coronary angioplasty for. *See* Percutaneous transluminal coronary angioplasty (PCTA)
  renal, for renal hypertension, 1791
  for ventricular arrhythmias, 1569
  for visceral angina, 1776, 1778f, 1779f
Revised Trauma Score (RTS), 275t, 275–276, 276f
  pediatric patients and, 378, 379t
Rewarming
  active, 411–412
  for frostbite, 413
  for hypothermia, 411–412
  passive, 411
  for shock, 207
Reynold equation, 1534
Rhabdoid tumors, pediatric, 2127
Rhabdomyomas, cardiac, 1500, 1502
Rhabdomyosarcomas
  of chest wall, 1448
  pediatric, 2127–2131, 2266
    associated conditions and epidemiology of, 2127
    basic science of, 2127–2128
    future directions for, 2131
    outcome of, 2131, 2131t
    pathology of of, 2128, 2128f
    presentation and workup of, 2128t, 2129f, 2129–2130
    staging of, 2129t, 2130
    treatment of, 2130f, 2130–2131
Rheumatic heart disease, 1503–1504, 1504t
Rheumatoid arthritis, of hand, 2159, 2161f
Rhinoplasty, 2272–2274, 2273f
Rhizopus infections, 177
Rhizotomy, retrogasserian, 2195
Rhytidectomy, 2269–2271, 2271f, 2272t
Rib(s), 1440–1441, 1441f
  chondromas of, 1446
  chondrosarcomas of, 1447, 1447f
  fibrous dysplasia of, 1446, 1446f
  fractures of
    in elderly people, 388
    treatment of, 320–321, 321f
  histiocytosis X and, 1446–1447
  osteochondromas of, 1446, 1446f
  plasmacytomas of, 1448, 1448f
  sarcomas of
    Ewing sarcomas, 1447
    osteogenic, 1447
Riboflavin
  pediatric requirement for, 1976t
  requirements in surgical patients, 62t

Richter hernias, 1218, 1218f
Riedel struma, 1299
Rifampin, for *Clostridium difficile* colitis, 1178
RNA
  messenger, 23–24
  synthesis of, 23–24
  transfer, 24–25, 25f
RNA polymerase II, 23
RNM classification, for colorectal cancer, 1135, 1136t
Rocuronium, 440t
Rokitansky-Aschoff sinuses, 1028–1029
Roller-head pumps, 1554–1555
Rollover accidents, 271
Rotamase inhibitors, 548
Rotational advancement flaps, 2286–2287
Rubber band ligation, for hemorrhoids, 1188–1189, 1189f

S

Sacral nerve roots, 2186
Sacral plexus, 1186
St. Jude heart valve, 1526, 1526f
Saline solutions, 249t, 250
  in shock, 289–290
Salivary glands
  benign tumors of, 641, 641t
  cancer of, 641–642, 642t
  infections of, 637
  surgery of, 643–644, 646f–647f
Salpingectomy, for ectopic pregnancy, 2229, 2229f
Salpingo-oophorectomy, bilateral abdominal, 2228
  for endometrial carcinomas, 2223
  for tubal carcinomas, 2224
  for uterine sarcomas, 2223
Salpingostomy, for ectopic pregnancy, 2228–2229, 2229f
Salt exchange, normal, 249
Sandimmune, See Cyclosporine (C$_S$A; Sandimmune)
Sandwich technique, for hernia repair, 1220, 1220f
Saphenous vein, greater, 1935, 1936f
Saphenous vein bypass, for infrainguinal occlusive disease, 1817f–1821f, 1821–1823
  complications of, 1821f, 1822t, 1822–1823
Saphenous vein grafts
  crossover, for venous obstruction, 1965, 1965f
  for traumatic injuries, 364
Sarcoidosis
  hypercalcemia and, 1315
  hypersplenism and, 1271
Sarcomas. *See also specific sarcomas*
  alveolar soft parts, pediatric, 2134
  of bone. *See Osteosarcomas*
  of breast, 1407–1409, 1408f
    arising after treatment of breast cancer, 1407–1409, 1408f
    cystosarcoma phyllodes, 1407, 1408f
    stromal (monomorphic), 1407, 1408f
  clear cell, renal, pediatric, 2126–2127
  colorectal, 1145
  Ewing, of ribs, 1447
  familial retinoblastomas associated with, 2249–2250

gastric, 804
hepatic, 1018
  pediatric, 2081
Kaposi, 2247
  anorectal, in HIV-positive patients, 1204
  immunosuppression and, 553
  metastatic, 2253, 2255f
  neurogenic, pediatric, 2133–2134
  renal, 2210
  soft tissue, 2246–2262. *See also* Leiomyosarcomas
    biopsy of, 2251, 2252f
    of chest wall, 1448
    desmoid. *See Desmoid tumors*
    epidemiology of, 2247f, 2247–2248, 2248f
    of extremities, management of, 2253, 2254t, 2255–2259
      chemotherapy for, 2259
      functional outcome after limb-sparing surgery and, 2258–2259
      radiotherapy for, 2255–2256, 2258
      reconstructive surgery following resection and, 2288f, 2289, 2289f
      standard approach to limb-sparing therapy for, 2258
      surgical, 2253, 2255, 2256f–2258f
    of head and neck, 642–643
    metastatic, management of, 2267–2268
    molecular biology of, 2249–2251
    pathologic classification of, 2248–2249, 2249t, 2250f
    pediatric, management of, 2265–2266
    recurrent, management of, 2266–2267, 2267f
    retroperitoneal. *See Retroperitoneal disorders, neoplastic disease*
    staging and metastatic work-up for, 2251–2253, 2253t, 2254f, 2255f
  spindle-cell, pediatric, 2266
  tenosynovial, pediatric, 2132–2133
    epidemiology of, 2132
    outcome of, 2132–2133
    pathology of, 2132
    presentation and diagnosis of, 2132
    treatment of, 2132
  uterine, 2223
  vulvar, 2218
Sarfeh shunt, 1001f, 1002
Sarns centrifugal pump, 1555, 1555f
Saucerization biopsy technique, in melanomas, 2236
Scalp injuries, 2165–2166
Scaphocephaly, 2194
Scaphoid fractures, 2158–2159, 2160f
Scars, 73–74, 82–83
  facial, 305
  hypertrophic, 83
    burns and, 436–437, CF 12–13
  keloids, 82
  radial (radial sclerosing lesions), of breast, 1376f, 1376–1377
  unsightly, 83
Schatzki ring, 729, 730f
Schistosomiasis, hepatic, 960–961
Schwannomas
  of hands, 2162
  intracranial, 2175–2176
  malignant
    etiology of, 2248, 2248f
    pediatric, 2133–2134

of peripheral nerves, 2180
Sciatic hernias, 1232f, 1232–1233, 1233f
Scimitar syndrome, 1483
Scintigraphy, hepatobiliary, in cholelithiasis, 1041–1042
Scissurae, hepatic, 932
Sclerosing adenosis, 1376, 1376f
Sclerotherapy
  complications of, 1167
  endoscopic. *See Endoscopic therapy, sclerotherapy*
  for gastroesophageal varices, 1167
  for peptic ulcers, 1163
  for varicose veins, 1939
Scorpion stings, 408
Screening
  for colorectal cancer, 1133–1134
  for hypercortisolism, 1339–1340
Scrotal torsion, 2110
Sebaceous gland carcinomas, 2244
Secondary survey, of trauma patients, 283–285
Second-hit phenomenon, 182
Secretin, small intestinal, 807
Secretin test, 870–871, 871t
Secretory proteins
  targeting, 26f–28f, 26–27
  vesicular transport of, 29f–31f, 29–30
Segmental pressures
  lower extremity, 1671
    in infrainguinal occlusive disease, 1813f, 1815
  upper extremity, 1759–1760
Seldinger technique
  for arteriography, in vascular injuries, 363
  for intraaortic balloon pump insertion, 1552–1553
Selectins
  antigen recognition and, 538, 538t
  leukocytes and, 117, 118
Selective arterial secretin stimulation test, in pancreatic neoplastic disease, 919–920, 921f
Selective mesenteric angiography, in vascular ectasia, 1169, 1169f
Selective visceral angiography, in gastrointestinal hemorrhage, 1161, 1161f
Selectivity, of plasma membrane, 11
  membrane composition and, 12–13, 13f
Semilunar valves, anatomy of, 1503, 1504f
Seminomas, 2212–2213, 2213f
Sengstaken-Blakemore tubes, for gastroesophageal varices, 994, 994f
Sensitivity determinations, 166t, 166–167
Sepsis
  bacterial, gram-negative, 174–176, 175f
  as contraindication to organ donation, 560
  intraabdominal, following hepatic transplantation, 595–596
  metabolic response to, 55–57
    nutritional requirements and feeding problems and, 57
    time course of, 55
  neonatal, 1991–1992
  nutritional support for, 57

following pancreatic transplantation, 624

postsplenectomy, 1270–1271

shock and. *See* Septic shock

traumatic injuries and, in elderly people, 389

Sepsis syndrome, effective circulating volume and, 246

Septectomy, Blalock-Hanlon, for transposition of the great arteries, 1491

Septicemia, pneumococcal, postsplenectomy, 338

Septic shock, 183, 201–203

hyperdynamic, 183

physiologic characteristics of, 197t

hyperdynamic response in, 202

hypodynamic, 183

physiologic characteristics of, 197t

hypodynamic response in, 202

intraaortic balloon pump in, 1552

myocardial dysfunction in, 202–203

treatment of, 203, 204f

Serine protease inhibitors, 1613–1614

Serratus anterior muscle, 1442, 1443f

Serum sickness, antivenins and, 405

Serum total T₃, 1292

Serum TSH, 1292–1293

Sex steroids, 1336–1337. *See also specific hormones*

excess of, 1337, 1337f

testing for, 1341

normal effects of, 1336–1337

Sexually transmitted diseases. *See also specific disorders*

anorectal, 1202–1204

Shear strain injuries, 270

Shock, 182–211

cardiogenic, 182–183, 199–201

compressive, 201

intrinsic, 199–201

physiologic characteristics of, 197t

cardiovascular response to, 188–189

cardiac dynamics and, 188, 189f

peripheral, 189

venous, 188–189

classification of, 182–183

complications of, 208–211

abdominal compartment syndrome, 208

immunosuppression, 208–209

ischemia-reperfusion injury, 208

multiple organ failure syndrome, 209–211, 211t

decompensated, 187

gastric tonometry in, 196

hemodynamic monitoring in, 195–196, 196t, 197t

hemorrhagic, traumatic injuries and, 282

hypoadrenal, 183, 204–205

neurogenic, physiologic characteristics of, 197t

hypothermia in, 411

hypovolemic, 182, 196–199, 198t

diagnosis of, 197–198

physiologic characteristics of, 197t

treatment of, 198–199

immunoinflammatory responses to, 191–195

adhesion molecules and, 195

complement and, 193

eicosanoids and, 193f, 193–194

interleukin-1 and, 194–195

interleukin-8 and, 195

nitric oxide and, 195

platelet-activating factor and, 194

tumor necrosis factor and, 194

metabolic abnormalities in, 191, 192f

microcirculatory response to, 183–187, 186t

anatomy and, 183, 184f, 185, 185f

physiology and, 185–186

neuroendocrine response to, 187–188

neurogenic, 183, 203–204

physiologic characteristics of, 197t

posttraumatic, 395

pulmonary response to, 189–190

renal response to, 190–191

septic. *See* Septic shock

following snake bites, 404

in trauma patients, 285–291

classification of, 286–287, 287t

complications of, 290–291

evaluation of, 286, 287f

pathophysiology of, 285–286

loss of compensation and, 286

rapid response and, 285

sustained response and, 285–286

treatment of, 287–290

traumatic, 182, 199

physiologic characteristics of, 197t

treatment of, 205–208

for hypovolemic shock, 198–199

inotropic agents in, 205–206

pneumatic antishock garment for, 206–207

rewarming in, 207

for septic shock, 203, 204f

supranormal resuscitation in, 207–208

Trendelenburg position for, 206

vasodilators in, 206

Shock lung, 209

Short-bowel syndrome, total parenteral nutrition for, 59

Short esophagus, in gastroesophageal reflux disease, 684, 684f

Shunts

peritoneovenous, for ascites, 989–990, 990f

portosystemic. *See* Portosystemic shunts

Sickle cell disease, 1268

Sigmoidoscopy

in colorectal adenomas, 1115

flexible

in *Clostridium difficile* colitis, 1176, 1176f

in ulcerative colitis, 1096, CF 45-1–3

rigid, in colorectal cancer, 1132

Signal peptidase, 26

Signal recognition particles (SRPs), 26–27

Signal sequences (peptides), 26

Signal transduction

hepatic cell-surface receptors and, 947, 947f

in neutrophils, 143

G proteins and. *See* G protein(s), in signal transduction

oncogenes and, 474

Simple skull fractures, 2166

Single-chain urokinase-type plasminogen

activator (SCU-PA), 99, 100, 100f, 100t

Sinoatrial (SA) node, 1565

Sinuses

branchial cleft remnant-derived, 1995–1998

anatomy and embryology of, 1995, 1995f, 1996f

clinical issues in, 1996

operative considerations and outcome of, 1996–1998, 1997f, 1998f

pilonidal. *See* Pilonidal sinuses

Sinusitis, 176, 635–636, 636f

posttraumatic, 401

Sinusoids, in portal hypertension, capillarization of, 986

Sistrurus. See Bites and stings

Skeletal muscle, actin filaments of, 6, 7f

Skeletal traction, for cervical spine malalignment, 2171

Skier's thumb, 2159

Skin, aging of, biology of, 2269

Skin biopsies, in melanomas, 2236–2237, 2237f

Skin disorders. *See also specific disorders*

of hands. *See* Hands, skin injury and disease of

necrosis, after rhytidectomy, 2270

neoplastic diseases, 2231–2245. *See also specific neoplasms*

surgical treatment of, 2244–2245

Mohs micrographic, 2244f, 2244–2245, CF 111–8

of nipples, 1378

in ulcerative colitis, 1096

Skin grafts

for burns

autografts, 431

porcine xenograft, 431

split-thickness, for scalp injuries, 2165–2166

Skip metastases, 484

Skull fractures, 2166

basilar, 296

depressed, 295–296

linear, 295, 296f

open, 296

Skull radiographs, in head injuries, 295–296, 296f

Sleep apnea. *See* Obstructive sleep apnea syndrome

Sliding hernias, treatment of, 1219, 1219f

Slow-reacting substance of anaphylaxis, in shock, 194

Small cell (oat cell) carcinomas, esophageal, 700–701

Small intestinal disorders. *See also specific disorders*

Crohn's disease. *See* Crohn's disease

diverticula, 1171

neoplastic disease, 844–855

adenocarcinomas, 847–849

origin of, 847, 848f

presentation and diagnosis of, 847–848, 848f

prognosis and survival and, 849

treatment of, 848, 849f

adenomas, 846

benign, 846t, 846–847

clinical presentation of, 845, 845t

conditions mimicking, 847

Small intestinal disorders, neoplastic
    disease (*continued*)
    diagnosis of, 845–846
    epidemiology of, 844
    etiopathogenesis of, 844–845
    incidental masses and, 855
    malignant, 847–855
        in Peutz-Jeghers syndrome, 1126
    posttransplantation lymphoproliferative
        disease, 845, 852
    strictures, in Crohn's disease, surgical
        treatment of, 842
    traumatic injuries, 350–351
Small intestine, 805–855. *See also*
        Duodenum; Ileum; Jejunum
    digestion and absorption in, 812–816
        bile salt absorption, 816
        of carbohydrates, 814–815, 815f
        electrolyte absorption, 813f, 813–
            814, 814f
        of fats, 816
        of proteins, 815–816
        vitamin absorption, 816
        water absorption, 812–813
    glutamine and ammonia metabolism
        in, 816–817, 817f
    gross anatomy of, 805–806
    histology of, 806–807, 808f
    hormones, neurotransmitters, and
        paracrine substances of, 807–808
    immunology of, 808–811
        aggregated lymphoid tissue and,
            809–810, 810f
        migratory pathways and
            gastrointestinal
            immunoresponsiveness and,
            810–811
        nonaggregated lymphoid tissue and,
            809, 809f
        secretory immune system and, 810
    microbial flora of, 160–161
    motility of, 811–812
        interdigestive pattern of, 812
        intrinsic electrical activity and, 811f,
            811–812
    preservation of, 569, 571
Smoking
    abdominal aortic aneurysms and, 1883
    atherosclerosis and, 1537, 1712–1714,
        1713f
    cessation of
        atherosclerosis and, 1713–1714
        in infrainguinal occlusive disease,
            1816–1817
    gastric ulcers and, 782
    skin necrosis after rhytidectomy and,
        2270
    wound healing and, 79
Smooth muscle
    arterial, 1588f, 1588–1589
        regulation of growth of, 1589–1591
    gastric, 757–758, 758f
Snake bites. *See* Bites and stings
SNAREs, 30, 30f
Soave procedure, 2061–2062, 2063f
Sodium. *See also* Hypernatremia;
        Hyponatremia
    pediatric requirements for, 1988
    water balance and, 245, 246f
Sodium balance, normal, 249
Sodium bicarbonate
    for hyperkalemia, pediatric, 1989
    for hypocalcemia, 1317

Sodium handling, in chronic liver
        disease, 980
Sodium restriction, in ascites, 989
Sodium tripolyphosphate, ingestion of.
        See Caustic ingestions
Soft tissue(s), 2141–2143. *See also*
        specific tissues
    functional morphology of, 2141–2142
    healing of, 2142–2143
    mechanical properties of, 2142, 2142f,
        2143f
    structure of, 2141
    viscoelastic properties of, 2142
Soft tissue disorders. *See also specific*
        soft tissue disorders
    burns and, 436t
    necrotizing infections, 173–174
    posttraumatic, 401
    sarcomas. *See* Leiomyosarcomas;
        Sarcomas, soft tissue
Solid and cystic tumors, of pancreas, 915
Solubility-diffusion, membrane transport
        and, 15, 15f, 16, 16f, 17f
Somatic pain, abdominal, 1246, 47048
Somatomedin C (Sm-C), for wound care,
        82, 82t
Somatostatin
    gastric, 751f, 751–752
    for gastroesophageal varices, 994
    pancreatic synthesis, secretion, and
        action of, 869–870
    small intestinal, 807–808
Somatostatin analogues, for acromegaly,
        1356
Somatostatinomas, 919t, 926, 926t
Somatostatin receptor staging, in
        pancreatic neoplastic disease,
        919
Space of Mall, 948, 948f
Spectinomycin, for gonococcal proctitis,
        1203
Spermatic cord, 1212
Spermatocytogenesis, 2202
Spermatogenesis, 2202
Sperm formation, 2202
    disorders of, 2202–2204
Spermiogenesis, 2202
Sperm penetration assay, 2203
Spherocytosis, hereditary, 1266–1267
Sphincterectomy, internal, lateral, for
        anal fissures, 1194–1195, 1196f
Sphincter of Oddi, 1028, 1030f
    dysfunction of, 1031
Sphincteroplasty
    for anal incontinence, 1201, 1203f
    transduodenal, for choledocholithiasis,
        1055
Sphincterotomy, endoscopic, 1051
    for choledocholithiasis, 1054, 1054f,
        1054t, 1055
    for pancreatitis, 885–886
Sphincters
    anal, external, 2041
    extrasphincteric fistulas and, 1198
    intersphincteric abscesses and, 1197
    intersphincteric fistulas and, 1198
    intersphincteric space and, anatomy of,
        1182, 1183f
    lower esophageal
        hypertensive, 679–680
        manometric assessment of, 665, 665f,
            666f
        physiology of, 664
    of Oddi, 1028, 1030f

dysfunction of, 1031
    suprasphincteric fistulas and, 1198
    transsphincteric fistulas and, 1198
    upper esophageal, manometric
        assessment of, 666
Sphincter-saving surgery, for colorectal
        cancer, 1138, 1141, 1141f,
        1142f
Spider bites, 406f, 406–407, 407f
Spigelian hernias, 1228, 1228f, 1229f
Spina bifida aperta, 2192
    neurogenic bladder and, 2106
Spina bifida occulta, 2192
Spinal cord injuries, 374–375, 2169–
        2172, 2170f–2172f
    cervical, 2171
    complete lesions, 2169
    fracture reduction for, 2171–2172
    hypotension and, 2170–2171
    incomplete lesions, 2169, 2170f
    lumbar, 2169, 2171
    paraplegia and
        following abdominal aortic aneurysm
            repair, 1890
        following thoracic aortic aneurysm
            repair, 1872–1873, 1873f
    pediatric, 384
    radiographic examination in, 2171,
        2172f
    tachycardia and, 2171
    thoracic, 2171
Spinal dysraphism, 2192, 2192f
    neurogenic bladder and, 2106
Spinal epidural abscesses, 2189–2190
Spinal nerve roots, 2186
Spinal stabilization, 374–375
Spindle-cell sarcomas, pediatric, 2266
Spine. *See also specific regions*
    degenerative disease of, 2185–2189
        anatomy and, 2185–2186, 2186f
        cervical, 2186–2188
            clinical presentation of, 2186–
                2187
            diagnosis of, 2187, 2187f
            treatment of, 2187–2188
        lumbar, 2188–2189
            diagnosis of, 2188, 2189f
            treatment of, 2188–2189
        pathology of, 2186
        thoracic, 2188
    immobilization of, 374
    neoplastic disease of, 2179–2180
        metastatic, 2180
Spinothalamic tract, 2186
Spinothalamic tractotomy, 2195
Spironolactone, for ascites, 989
Splanchnic artery, aneurysms of, 1893t,
        1893–1895, 1894f–1896f
Spleen, 1262–1280
    anatomy of, 1262–1265
        blood supply, 1262, 1264f
        embryology, 1262, 1263f, 1264f
        histology, 1262, 1264–1265, 1265f
    erythrocyte maintenance and, 1265
    immune function of, 1265–1266
    transplantation of allogenic
        hepatocytes into, 517
    vascular capacity of, 1266
Splenectomy, 338, 1276–1280
    for autoimmune hemolytic anemia,
        1268
    complications of, 338, 1280

for glucose-6-phosphate dehydrogenase deficiency, 1267
for hypersplenism, 1271–1273
for immune thrombocytopenic purpura, 1269
laparoscopic, 1280
massive bleeding during, 1279–1280
partial, 1277, 1279f, 1280
postsplenectomy sepsis and, 1270–1271
postsplenectomy sepsis following, prophylaxis of, 1280
techniques for, 1277, 1277f–1279f, 1279–1280
Splenic artery, anatomy of, 1765
Splenic autotransplantation, 1270
Splenic biopsies, 1274, 1275f
Splenic disorders. *See also specific disorders*
cystic, 1275–1276, 1276f
neoplastic disease, 1273–1275
Hodgkin's disease, 1273–1274, 1274t, 1275f
leukemia, 1274–1275, 1276f
non-Hodgkin's lymphoma, 1274
primary tumors, 1273
surgical injury, during antireflux operations, 692
traumatic injuries, 337–338, 338t
pediatric, 382–383
Splenic salvage techniques, 1277
Splenic vein thrombosis, hypersplenism and, 1270
Splenomegaly, 1276
Splenorrhaphy, 1279f, 1280
Splicing, 22
Split renal function studies, in renovascular hypertension, 1789–1790
Split tolerance, 547
Spondylosis, 2186
Spontaneous bacterial peritonitis (SBP), in ascites, 988t, 988–989, 989t
Sports medicine, arthroscopy in, 2150–2152
diagnostic, 2150–2151
operative, 2151–2152
Squamous cell carcinomas (SCCs)
of anal canal, 1149
of anal margin, 1147, 1147f
esophageal, 698–700
immunosuppression and, 552
in pilonidal sinuses, 1200
of skin, 2242, 2243, 2244
etiology of, 2242, CF 111–3
Squamous intraepithelial carcinomas (SILs), 2221–2222, 2222f
SRP receptors, 26–27
Stab wounds. *See* Traumatic injuries
Staining techniques, 166
Standing waves, 1688, 1689f
Staphylococcal scalded skin syndrome, diagnosis of, 429t
Staphylococcal toxic shock syndrome, 2225
Starch
digestion and absorption of, in small intestine, 815
structure of, 815, 815f
Starling's law, 185
Starr-Edwards heart valve, 1525f, 1525–1526, 1530
Starvation adaptation, 229

Static compliance, 1984
Steam inhalation, injury caused by, 433
Stein-Leventhal syndrome, in morbid obesity, 790
Stellate skull fractures, 2166
Stents
for arteriovenous fistulas, 1923
for bile duct cancer, 1065f, 1066, 1066t
for jaundice, in pancreatic cancer, 914, 914f
transanastomotic, for bile duct strictures, 1073, 1074f
transhepatic, for primary sclerosing cholangitis, 1078, 1079f
for varices, 997f, 998–1000
vascular, 1738
Sternal clefts, 2001f, 2001–2002
Sternal dehiscence, following coronary artery bypass grafting, 1547
Sternal fractures, treatment of, 321, 322f
Sternocleidomastoid muscle, 1442, 1443f
Sternotomy
median, 320, 320f
for great vessel injuries, 367, 367f
for thymomas, 1470, 1470f
Sternum, 1440
tumors of, 1448
Steroids. *See also specific steroids*
sex, 1336–1337. *See also specific hormones*
excess of, 1337, 1337f
testing for, 1341
normal effects of, 1336–1337
for ulcerative colitis, 1098
for upper extremity occlusive disease, 1764
Stimulus-secreting coupling, 31–32
Stings. *See* Bites and stings
Stomach. *See also* Gastric *entries*
anatomy of
gross, 745–747, 746f–748f
microscopic, 748f, 748–749, 749f
bicarbonate production by, 756f, 756–757
blood flow of, 757, 775
mucosal defenses of, 773–774, 774f
mucus of, 775
Stop codons, 22
Stop transfer sequences, 27
Strangulated hernias, 1218f, 1218–1219
Strawberry gallbladder, 1056
Streptococcal toxic shock syndrome, 2225
Streptokinase, 99, 100, 100f, 100t, 1737, 1738
allergic reactions to, 1949
complications of, 1953–1954
for deep venous thrombosis, 101
for pulmonary thromboembolism, 1953–1954
Streptozocin, 501t
Stress gastritis, 776–779
angiographic therapy for, 777–778
bleeding in, 1164–1165
definition of lesions in, 776
endoscopic therapy for, 777
luminal acid secretion and, 776–777
medical treatment of, 777
predisposing factors for, 776, 776t, 777
presentation and diagnosis of, 777
prophylaxis of, 778t, 778–779
surgical therapy for, 778

Stress proteins, in inflammation, 153t, 154
Stress response, 47–57
components of, 48–49
infection, 49
malnutrition and its consequences, 49
pain and fear, 49
tissue damage, 48
volume loss and tissue underperfusion, 48
mediators of, 49–52
age, 49–50
body composition, 49
counterregulatory hormones, 50
cytokines, 50–52, 51f
gender, 50
gut mucosal barrier dysfunction, 52
nutritional status, 49
surgical stress and, 48, 48t, 52–53
mediators of, 49–50
nutritional support and, 53
physiologic responses and, 52f, 52–53
traumatic injuries and. *See* Injury response
Stress ulceration, posttraumatic, 400
Stretch marks, 74
Stretch receptors, fluid volume and, 246–247
Strokes. *See* Cerebrovascular disease, ischemic
Stroke volume, arteriovenous fistulas and, 1920
Stroma-free hemoglobin, in shock, 290
Stromal tumors, mesenteric, 1240
Struma lymphomatosa, 1298
Stuart-Power factor deficiency, 94
Stumps
complications of, following lower extremity amputation, 1835–1837
neurosurgical pain management and, 2196
Sturge-Weber syndrome, 1930
Subarachnoid hemorrhage (SAH), 2182, 2183f
in head injuries, 297
Subarterial ventricular septal defects, 1485
Subclavian artery
aneurysms of. *See* Aneurysm(s), axillosubclavian
right, traumatic injuries of, 366–368, 367f–370f
Subclavian catheters, insertion of, 61f
Subclavian flap angioplasty, for coarctation of aorta, 1498
Subclavian vein, thrombophlebitis of, 1957
Subdural empyema, 2190
Subdural hematomas, 2168–2169, 2169f
in elderly people, 388
in head injuries, 296, 297f
acute, 2168–2169, 2169f
chronic, 2169
treatment of, 297–298, 298f
Subdural hygromas, 2169
Subgaleal abscesses, 2189
Submandibular gland, surgery of, 644, 648f
Submucosal hematomas, pediatric, 383

Substance abuse, as contraindication to organ donation, 561

Substance P, 2194

Succinylcholine, 440t

Sucralfate
  for duodenal ulcers, 763t, 764–765
  for gastric ulcers, 784–785
  prophylactic, for stress gastritis, 778

Sudden cardiac death (SCD), ventricular arrhythmias and, 1568, 1568t

Sufentanil, 441t

Suicide drug therapy, 512

Sulfasalazine
  for Crohn's disease, 840
  for ulcerative colitis, 1097–1098

Sulfotransferases, hepatic biotransformation and, 956

Sulindac (Clinoril)
  for desmoid tumors, 2262
  for familial adenomatous polyposis, 1124

Summit lesions, in *Clostridium difficile* colitis, 1176

Sump syndrome, 1055

Superficial groin dissection, 2239

Superficial pouch of Denis Brown, 2109

Superficial spreading melanomas, 2233

Superior vena cava syndrome, 1472

Superoxide anion, cell injury and, 154, 154t

Support, for breast cancer patients, 1399

Suppression, leukocytes and, 547

Supracristal ventricular septal defects, 1485

Supralevator abscesses, 1197

Supralevator spaces, anatomy of, 1182–1183, 1183f

Supranormal resuscitation, for shock, 207–208

Suprapiriform foramen, 1213, 1215f

Suprasphincteric fistulas, 1198

Supravesical hernias, 1229–1230, 1230f

Surfactant, persistent pulmonary hypertension of newborn and, 1984–1985

Surgeons
  role in breast cancer staging, 1387–1388
  role in cancer treatment, 489, 490
  role in trauma system, 278–279

Surgical decompression, for acute epidural or subdural hematomas, 297–298, 298f

Surgical patients
  energy requirements of, 44t, 44–45, 45t
  nutritional support for, 53
  vitamin requirements of, 62t

Surgical procedures. *See also* Intraoperative *entries*; Postoperative *entries*; specific *procedures and disorders*
  hospital mortality rates related to, 445, 445t

Suspensory ligaments of Cooper, 1360

Suturing
  for hernia repair, 1220, 1220f
  for maxillofacial repairs, 304–305

Swan-Ganz catheters, in shock, 195–196, 196t, 197t

Swenson procedure, 2062, 2064f

Sympathectomy
  chemical, 2196
  total, 442–443

Synchronized intermittent mandatory ventilation, 1986

Syndactyly, plastic surgery for, 2285f, 2287

Syndrome of inappropriate antidiuretic hormone (SIADH), 1348–1349

Synoviomas. *See* Sarcomas, tenosynovial

Syphilis
  aneurysms in, 1840
  esophagitis in, 725

Systemic inflammatory response syndrome (SIRS), 182. *See also* Multiple organ failure syndrome (MOFS)

Systemic lupus erythematosus (SLE), hypersplenism and, 1271

T

Takayasu arteritis, 1606, 1607f, 1748, 1761

Tamoxifen, 502t
  for breast cancer, metastases from, 1402
  for desmoid tumors, 2262

Tandem disease, aortoiliac, 1799

Tapeworms
  hepatic infections caused by, 959, 960f
  neurologic infections caused by, 2191

Tar, burns caused by, 428, CF 12–8

T_4 assay, 1292

Taxanes, 502t

Taxol (paclitaxel), 502t

T cell(s)
  in antigen recognition, 535f, 535–536, 536f, 536t
  in neonates, 1991
  receptor driven stimulation of, 545–547, 546f

T-cell receptors (TCRs), antigen recognition by, 529f–530f, 529–530, 530t

Technetium-labeled albumin microspheres, in arteriovenous fistulas, 1921

Technetium-99m-iminodiacetic acid ($_{99m}$Tc-IDA), in biliary atresia, 2086, 2088f

Technetium-99m methylene diphosphonate bone scanning, in frostbite, 414

Technetium-99m scanning, of thyroid gland, 1294
  in solitary thyroid nodule, 1300

Teletherapy, 492

Temporal arteritis, 1605–1606, 1606f, 1748

Tendons, of hands, 2153, 2153f, 2154f
  disorders of, 2156–2158
    of extensor tendons, 2157f, 2157–2158, 2158f
    of flexor tendons, 2157, 2157f
    trigger finger, 2157
  infections of, 2161

Teniposide (VM-26), 502t

Tenosynoviomas. *See* Sarcomas, tenosynovial

Tenosynovitis
  of extensor tendons of hand, 2158
  of flexor tendons of hand, 2157
  stenosing, De Quervain, 2158
  suppurative, of hands, 2161

Tensile strain injuries, 270

Tension-time index (TTI), 1550

Teratomas
  cardiac, 1502
  cystic
    ovarian, 2226, 2227f
    pediatric, 2009
  hepatic, pediatric, 2080
  intracranial, 2178
    pediatric, 2178
  mediastinal, 1469
    pediatric, 2011

Teratospermia, 2202

Testes
  biopsy of, in male infertility, 2203
  cancer of, 2212–2213, 2213f
  inguinal hernias and. *See* Hernias
  pediatric, 2109–2110. *See also specific disorders*
  prepubertal tumors of, 2110
  retractile, 2109
  undescended, 2109f, 2109–2110

Testicular failure, 2203

Testicular feminization syndrome, 2113

Testicular torsion, acute abdomen and, 1250

Test-meal PP response, 872, 872t

Testosterone
  for impotence, 2201
  low level of, male infertility and, 2203
  for male infertility, 2203

Tetanus prophylaxis
  in abdominal injuries, 337
  for snake bites, 405

Tetracaine, 442t

Tetracycline(s)
  for chlamydial proctitis, 1203
  for duodenal ulcers, 765
  for gonococcal proctitis, 1203
  spectrum of activity of, 169t

Tetralogy of Fallot, 1488–1490, 1489f

Tetrodotoxin, ion channel blockade by, 18

Thalamotomy, for pain management, 2194

Thalassemia, 1268

Theca-lutein cysts, 2226

Thecomas, ovarian, 2226

Therapeutic lymph node dissection. *See* Lymphadenectomy

Thermal coagulation, for peptic ulcers, 1163

Thermogenesis, diet-induced, 1974

Thermoregulation, 47
  in pediatric patients, 1979–1980
  thermoregulatory drive and, 410

Thiamine
  deficiency of, following gastric surgery for morbid obesity, 793
  pediatric requirement for, 1976t
  requirements in surgical patients, 62t

Thiazide diuretics, hypercalcemia and, 1315

Thick filaments, 6

Thionamide, for Graves disease, 1296

Third-space loss, pediatric, 1989

Thoracentesis, for pleural effusions, 1455

Thoracic anatomy, 1440–1444
  anatomic landmarks, 1444
  blood supply, venous drainage, and lymphatics, 1442
  musculature, 1442, 1443f, 1444
  pleura, 1444, 1445f

respiration and, 1440
skeletal support, 1440–1441, 1441f, 1442f
Thoracic aortic aneurysms, 1859–1873
  atherosclerotic, 1860f, 1860–1863
    operative management of, 1860, 1861f–1863f, 1862–1863
  degenerative, 1863f, 1863–1866
    operative management of, 1864, 1864f, 1865f, 1866
  dissections, 1867–1869
    classification of, 1866f, 1867
    diagnosis of, 1867, 1867f, 1869
    operative management of, 1868f, 1869, 1870f–1871f
    surgical results with, 1871f, 1872f, 1879
  of ductus diverticulum, 1873
  mycotic, 1873
  paraplegia following surgery for, 1872–1873, 1873f
  traumatic, 1869–1872
Thoracic duct
  ligation of, transabdominal, for chylothorax, 1463
  traumatic injuries of, 1969
Thoracic empyema, 1456t, 1456–1458, 1457f–1459f
Thoracic injuries. *See also specific injuries*
  in elderly people, 388
  pediatric, 381–382
Thoracic outlet syndromes (TOSs), 1635–1638, 1636f–1638f, 1761, 1763f
Thoracic spine
  degenerative disease of, 2188
  traumatic injuries of, 2171
Thoracoabdominal aortic aneurysms (TAAAs), 1873–1881
  classification of, 1874, 1875f
  clinical manifestations of, 1874–1875
  diagnosis of, 1875–1876, 1877f
  diseases associated with, 1875
  epidemiology of, 1873–1874
  etiology of, 1874
  management of, 1876–1881
    patient selection and, 1876–1877
    risk factor assessment and, 1877, 1878t
    surgical, 1877–1881
      operative technique for, 1878–1880, 1879f, 1880f
      postoperative management and, 1880
      preoperative preparation for, 1878
      results of, 1880–1881
  natural history of, 1874
  pathophysiology of, 1874
Thoracoepigastric flaps, 2287, 2287f
Thoracoscopic surgery, 741–743
  advantages and disadvantages of, 742
  anesthesia for, 741
  chylothorax drainage, 1463
  current status of, 742, 742t, 743t
  future of, 742–743
  for spontaneous pneumothorax, 1460f, 1460–1461
  technical aspects of, 741f, 741–742
Thoracoscopy, in chest injuries, 318
Thoracotomy
  anterolateral, 329
  emergency, 319–320, 320f
  in trauma patients, 282–283

in traumatic injuries, pediatric, 380–381
Thrombectomy
  angioscopic, 1740–1741
  for deep venous thrombosis, 1950, 1950f
  for traumatic injuries, 364
Thrombin, 85
  platelet aggregation and, 1612–1613
Thrombin clotting time, 104
Thromboangiitis obliterans, 1597–1599, 1599f, 1762
Thrombocytopenia
  heparin-associated, 89, 1617
  immune thrombocytopenic purpura, 1269t, 1269–1270
  thrombotic thrombocytopenic purpura, 1270
Thrombocytosis, 103
  following splenectomy, 1280
Thromboembolectomy
  femoropopliteotibial, angioscopic, 1741
  of iliac artery, transfemoral, angioscopic, 1741
  for peripheral arterial embolism, 1627–1630, 1629t
    results with, 1629f, 1629–1630
Thromboembolism. *See also* Deep venous thrombosis (DVT); Embolism; Thrombosis
  in mitral rheumatic disease, 1529–1530
  mural, mitral stenosis and, 1510, 1510t
  pulmonary. *See* Pulmonary thromboembolism
  traumatic injuries and
    in elderly people, 389
    in pregnancy, 394
Thrombolytic therapy
  for acute myocardial infarction, 1541
  agents for, 99–102, 100f, 100t, 102t, 1620. *See also specific agents*
  angiography and, 1705f, 1707
  angioscopic, 1737–1738
  complications of, 1541
  contraindications to, 102, 102t
  for deep venous thrombosis, 1949–1950
  intraoperative, 102
  for pulmonary thromboembolism, 1953–1954
Thrombomodulin, tumor necrosis factor regulation of expression of, 87
Thrombophlebitis, 1956–1958
  of breast veins, 1377–1378
  of hepatic veins. *See* Budd-Chiari syndrome
  of inferior vena cava, 1957
  migrans, 1956–1957
  of portal vein, 1958
  of subclavian vein, 1957
  suppurative, management of, 1730
Thrombosis, 1608–1620
  effort, 1635
  heparin-induced, 1617
  following hepatic transplantation, 593–595
  inflammation related to, 87, 88f, 89
  location and histologic composition of thrombi and, 1609
  mechanisms protecting against, 1609–1619

blood flow and thrombosis, 1618–1619, 1619f
  circulating inhibitory proteins and fibrinolytic system, 1613–1618
    fibrinolytic system, 1614
    hypercoagulable syndromes and, 1614–1618
    serine protease inhibitors, 1613–1614
  endothelium and vessel wall reactions, 1609–1613
    coagulation reactions, 1613
    endothelial physiology and, 1609–1610, 1610f
    platelet reactions, 1612f, 1612–1613
    vessel wall damage and, 1610–1612, 1611f
  mesenteric, 1769, 1771–1772, 1774f
  mural, mitral stenosis and, 1510, 1510t
  following pancreatic transplantation, 623
  of splenic vein, hypersplenism and, 1270
  therapeutic implications of, 1619–1620
  following vascular injuries, 362, 366
  venous. *See* Deep venous thrombosis (DVT); Pulmonary thromboembolism; Thrombophlebitis; Venous thrombosis
Thrombotic thrombocytopenic purpura (TTP), 1270
Thromboxane A_2
  plate aggregation and, 1613
  tissue ischemia and, 1652, 1654
Thromboxane synthase inhibitors, as antiplatelet agents, 98–99
Thumb
  joints of, 2153
  traumatic injuries of, 2159
Thymectomy, 1469
Thymic cysts, in pediatric patients, 2008–2009
Thymidine-labeling index, in breast cancer, 1388–1389
Thymomas
  mediastinal, 1469–1470, 1470f, 1470t
  in pediatric patients, 2011
Thyroglobulin, serum, 1293
Thyroglossal duct cysts, 1283, 1998–1999
  anatomy and embryology of, 1998, 1998f
  clinical issues in, 1998
  operative considerations and outcome of, 1998–1999
Thyroglossal duct fistulas, 1283
Thyroid antibodies, serum, 1293
Thyroid cancer, 1301–1307
  anaplastic, 1301, 1306
  follicular, 1301, 1303–1304
  Hürthle cell, 1301, 1305–1306
  iodine-131 treatment for, 1306–1307
  medullary, 1301, 1304–1305
    in multiple endocrine neoplasia, 1327–1328, 1328f
  papillary, 1301–1303
Thyroid disorders. *See also specific disorders*
  cancer. *See* Thyroid cancer
  ectopic thyroid tissue, 1283
  functional, 1295–1299

Thyroid disorders (*continued*)
solitary nodules, 1299–1300
diagnosis of, 1299–1300
operative treatment of, 1301
Thyroidectomy
for carcinomas, 1303–1304
for Graves disease, 1296, 1297
for toxic multinodular goiter, 1297–1298
Thyroid gland, 1283–1307
anatomy of, 1283–1288
anatomic relations, 1283–1288, 1284f–1291f
embryology, 1283
imaging of, 1293–1295
approach to, 1294–1295
lingual, 1283
physiology of, 1288–1293
laboratory tests of thyroid function and, 1291–1293
pharmacologic factors and, 1291
surgical approach to, 1287–1288, 1289f–1291f
Thyroid hormone(s), 1288–1293
assays for, 1292–1293
fetal and postnatal growth and development and, 1974
thyroid-stimulating hormone suppression by, in solitary thyroid nodule, 1300–1301
Thyroid hormone response elements, 35
Thyroiditis, 1298–1299
chronic lymphocytic (Hashimoto disease), 1298
Riedel struma and, 1299
subacute (de Quervain; granulomatous), 1298–1299
Thyroid lobectomy
for carcinomas, 1303
for solitary thyroid nodule, 1301
Thyroid sheath, 1284
Thyroid-stimulating hormone (TSH), 1289–1290
serum, 1292–1293
suppression of, in solitary thyroid nodule, 1300–1301
Thyrotoxicosis. *See* Graves disease; Hyperthyroidism
Thyrotropin-releasing hormone (TRH), TRH test and, 1293
Thyroxine (T_4), 1288–1289
free T_4 and, 1292
free T_4 index and, 1292
T_4 assay and, 1292
Tibial artery, anatomy of, 1687
Tibial vein, posterior, 1935, 1937f
Tic doloreux, neurosurgical pain management for, 2195
Ticlopidine, 1620
as antiplatelet agent, 99
for infrainguinal occlusive disease, 1819
Tidal volume, 1983
Tilting-disk heart valves, 1526, 1526f
Tinel sing, 2172
Tissue damage, stress response and, 48
Tissue expansion, 2272t, 2278–2279, 2284–2285
Tissue factor pathway inhibitor, 85
Tissue ischemia, 1643f, 1643–1655
activation of secondary cascades and, 1652
cellular and molecular aspects of, 1654–1655

endothelial injury and, 1650, 1651f
energy failure and, 1646–1649, 1648f
inflammatory systems and, 1651–1652, 1652f
parenchymal cell injury and, 1649f, 1649–1650, 1650f
remote or systemic effects of, 1652, 1654
reperfusion effects and, 1652, 1653t
tolerance and, 1644f–1648f, 1644–1646, 1647t
Tissue perfusion
following burns, 426–427
in organ donors, 563
reduced
in critically ill patients, management of, 227, 228f, 229
distal, vascular injuries and, 362
stress response and, 48
Tissue plasminogen activator (tPA), 85, 99, 100, 100f, 100t, 1738
for deep venous thrombosis, 101
for pulmonary thromboembolism, 1954
thrombolytic therapy for, 101
for vascular gene therapy, 520t
Tissue transfer, 2284, 2284f
of colon, 2285–2286
T lymphocytes
in antigen recognition, 535f, 535–536, 536f, 536t
in neonates, 1991
receptor driven stimulation of, 545–547, 546f
receptors for, antigen recognition by, 529f–530f, 529–530, 530t
TNM staging
for bile duct cancer, 1061
for breast cancer, 1386, 1387t, 1388, 1388t
for esophageal cancer, 700
postsurgical, 709, 712t
for gallbladder cancer, 1059, 1059t
for head and neck cancer, 638, 639t
for liver cancer, 1018, 1018t
for mesotheliomas, 1464t, 1464–1465
for pancreatic cancer, 904t, 904–905
for prostate cancer, 2210, 2210f
for renal cell carcinomas, 2208, 2209f
for rhabdomyosarcomas, 2129t, 2130
for sarcomas, 2251, 2253t
Tobacco use. *See* Smoking
Tocopherol
pediatric requirement for, 1976t, 1977
requirements in surgical patients, 62t
wound healing and, 78
Toe-in region, 2142
Toe pressure, 1671, 1671f
Tolbutamide response test, 873
Tolerance
to ischemic injury, 1644f–1648f, 1644–1645, 1647t
organ transplantation and, 547
Tongue, cancer of, 638
Topotecan, 502t
TORCH complex, 1992
Torsion
omental, 1241
scrotal, 2110
testicular, acute abdomen and, 1250
Total artificial hearts (TAHs), 1558
permanent, 1561f, 1561–1563, 1562f
temporary, 1558, 1559f
Total body water (TBW), 242t, 242–243
pediatric, 1987

Total dead space, 1984
Total joint replacement arthroplasty, 2148–2150, 2150f, 2151f
Total lung capacity, 1983
Total parenteral nutrition (TPN)
for cancer patients, 58–59
cholelithiasis induced by, 1035–1036, 1036t, 1049–1050
in Crohn's disease, 839
for multiple organ failure syndrome, 210
for pediatric patients, 1977t–1979t, 1978–1979
with gastroschisis or omphalocele, 2031–2032
for surgical patients
complications of, 61, 63t, 64f
effects on gastrointestinal tract, 61–62
formulas for, 60–61, 61f, 61t, 62t
as primary therapy, 59–60
as secondary therapy, 60
Total sympathectomy, 442–443
Tourniquets, for snake bites, 405
Toxemia, of pregnancy, 394
Toxic epidermal necrolysis, diagnosis of, 429t
Toxic injuries, of hands, 2160
Toxic megacolon (toxic dilation)
in Crohn's disease, 837, 837f
in ulcerative colitis, 1097, 1097f, 1099–1100
Toxic multinodular goiter, 1297–1298
Toxic shock syndromes, 2225
Toxins, metabolic acidosis due to, 262
Toxoplasma gondii infections, 180
Trace elements
metabolism of, sepsis and, 57
pediatric requirements for, 1977
requirements in surgical patients, 62t
wound healing and, 78
Trachea, 1472–1478. *See also specific disorders*
diagnosis of pathology of, 1473, 1474f
displacement of, in pediatric patients, 2011
fistulas of, 1474–1476
obstructing lesions of, treatment of, 1473–1474
stenosis of, inflammatory, 1473, 1473f
surgery to, 1476–1478. *See also specific procedures*
traumatic injuries of, management of, 315–316
tumors of, 1472–1473
extrinsic compression and, 1473
primary, 1472
secondary, 1472–1473
treatment of, 1473–1474
Tracheal stenosis, 1473, 1473f
pediatric patients, 2017
Tracheal strictures, 1473
Tracheobronchial foreign bodies, in pediatric patients, 2017–2019
clinical picture in, 2017f, 2018, 2018f, 2018t
management of, 2018–2019, 2019f
pathophysiology of, 2017
Tracheobronchial injuries, treatment of, 326–327, 327f
Tracheoesophageal fistulas, 731–734, 1475–1476, 1477f

malignant, 732, 732f, 733f, 734
nonmalignant, 731–732
in pediatric patients, 2011–2016
anomalies associated with, 2012, 2014t
classification of, 2011, 2012f–2013f
diagnosis of, 2012, 2014f
embryology of, 2011
incidence of, 2011
pathophysiology of, 2011–2012
preoperative treatment of, 2012
surgical treatment of, 2012–2016, 2015f
complications of, 2014–2015, 2015t
operative technique for, 2013–2014
results of, 2015–2016, 2016f
Tracheoinnominate artery fistulas, 1474–1475, 1475f
Tracheostomy, 643, 644f, 1476, 1478f
tracheoinnominate artery fistulas caused by, 1474–1475
in traumatic injuries, pediatric, 380
Tractotomy, trigeminal, 2195
Transamination, 47
Transblot techniques, 167
for human immunodeficiency virus detection, 178f, 178–179
Transcapillary refill, shock and, 286
Transcobalamins, 816
Transcription factors, 23
Transcutaneous stimulation, for pain management, 2196
Transduodenal intraoperative pancreatography, 347
Transferrin, hepatic, 946t
iron metabolism and, 956–957
Transfer RNA (tRNA), 24–25, 25f
Transforming growth factors
breast cancer and, 1385
transforming growth factor-α (TGF-α)
lung cancer and, 1419
for wound care, 82, 82t
transforming growth factor-β (TGF-β)
acute-phase response mediation by, 133t
bone formation and, 2152
fibroblasts and, wound healing and, 124–125, 125f
for wound care, 82, 82t
Transfusion therapy. See Blood transfusions
Trans-Golgi network, 30
Transient ischemic attacks (TIAs), 1751, 2181
Transitional elements, 29
Transjugular intrahepatic portosystemic shunts (TIPs)
angiography and, 1709
for ascites, 990
for varices, 997f, 998–1000, 1167
Transluminal dilation, 1735
Translymphatic absorption, 171
Transnasal feeding catheters, 64, 65f
Transplantation. See also specific organs
cellular, 556
gene therapy and, 555
graft rejection and, 541–544. See also specific organs
acute, 542, 543f, 544f
chronic, 542–544
hyperacute, 541–542, 542f

immunology of. See Antigen(s), recognition of; Transplantation immunology
organ donors for. See Organ donors
organ preservation for. See Organ preservation
organ procurement for, 563–568
surgical technique for, 564–566, 565f–572f, 568
United Network for Organ Sharing and team coordination for, 563–564, 564f
Transplantation immunology, 527–554
cellular transplants and, 556
effector mechanisms of immune response and, 541–544
cellular, 541
clinical syndromes related to, 541–544, 542f–544f
soluble, 541
immune response initiation and, 527–541
alloreactivity and, 533, 533f
antigenicity and, 533–534
antigen presentation and antigen-presenting cells and, 533
antigen processing and, 531–532, 532f
antigen recognition and. See Antigen(s), recognition of
immune response regulation and, 544–554
antigenicity and immunity aspects important for clinical transplantation and, 553–554, 554f
clinical immunosuppression and, 55t, 548, 549t, 551
complications of immunosuppression and, 552f, 552–553
loci for inducing nonresponsiveness and, 547–548
lymphocyte development and, 544–545, 545f
receptor driven stimulation of T and B responses and, 545–547, 546f
tolerance and, 547
xenotransplantation and, 555
Transposition of the great arteries (TGA), 1490f–1493f, 1490–1491, 1493
Transpulmonary shunting, 219
Transsphincteric fistulas, 1198
Transverse rectus abdominis myocutaneous (TRAM) flaps, 2287, 2287f
for breast reconstruction, 1395
Transverse scissura, hepatic, 932
Transversus abdominis muscle, 1211
Trapezius flaps, 2286
Trapezius muscles, 1442, 1443f, 1444
Trauma team, composition of, 281–282
Traumatic cysts, hepatic, 1015
Traumatic dystrophies, major and minor, 2196
Traumatic injuries, 267–414. See also specific injuries
assessment of, 274–278
Abbreviated Injury Scale and, 276–277, 277t
Injury Severity Score and, 277
Revised Trauma Score and, 275t, 275–276, 276f
TRISS methodology and, 277–278

biomechanics of, 269–272
of blunt trauma, 269–272
cavitation and, 269
energy transfer and, 269
of penetrating injuries, 273f, 273–274
bites. See Bites and stings
blunt
anatomic considerations in, 272–273, 273t
biomechanics of, 269–272
burns. See Burns
cold-induced, 412–414
treatment of, 413–414
complications following, 395–402
abdominal, 399–400
alterations in immune and inflammatory response and, 395–396, 396t
cardiovascular, 399
immunomodulation and, 396
infections, 400–401
neurologic, 399
orthopedic, 401
provider-related, 396
pulmonary, 396–399, 397t, 398t
renal failure, 401–402
shock, ischemia, and reperfusion injury and, 395
soft tissue, 401
in elderly people. See Geriatric trauma
epidemiology of, 269
historical development of trauma care and, 268t, 268–269
hypothermia following, 410–411
injury response in. See Injury response
local effects of tissue injury and, 395
lower extremity amputations and, 1824
of lymphatic system, 1969
mortality peaks after, 267f, 267–268
motor vehicle collisions as cause of, 270–272
in children, 378
in elderly people, 386
frontal and rear impact and, 270, 271f
lateral impact, rotational impact, and rollover and, 270–271
motorcycles and, 272
pedestrians and, 272
restraint device injury and, 271–272
nitrogen loss following, 54
nutritional support for, 54–55
goals of, 55
pediatric. See Pediatric patients, traumatic injuries of
penetrating
anatomic considerations in, 274, 275f
biomechanics of, 273f, 273–274
peripheral arterial embolism and, 1622–1623
in pregnancy. See Pregnancy, traumatic injuries during
prehospital care for, 278, 279–281
airway assessment in, 280
breathing and, 280–281
circulation and, 281
personnel for, 280
resuscitation care for, 281–285
primary survey and, 282–283, 283t
secondary survey and, 283–285
team composition and, 281–282
shear strain injuries, 270

Traumatic injuries (*continued*)
 shock in. *See* Shock
 stings. *See* Bites and stings
 tensile strain injuries, 270
 thermal. *See* Burns
 thoracic aortic aneurysms due to,
  1869–1872
 trauma systems for, 278–279
  components of, 278
  development of, 279
  primary role of surgeons in, 278–279
 vascular, angiography in, 1697f–1699f,
  1699–1700
Traumatic shock, 182, 199
 physiologic characteristics of, 197t
T12 regimen, for osteosarcomas, 2265,
  2267f
Trench foot, 412
Trendelenburg position, for shock, 206
Trephination, in head injuries, 298, 298f
T$_3$ resin uptake test, 1292
TRH test, 1293
Triangle of auscultation, 1444
Tricuspid regurgitation, 1506, 1506t
 diagnosis of, 1513
 medical management of, 1517
Tricuspid stenosis
 diagnosis of, 1513
 medical management of, 1517
 pathophysiology of, 1512
Tricuspid valve, anatomy of, 1503, 1504f
Tricuspid valve annuloplasty, 1519,
  1519f
Trigeminal nerve, schwannomas of, 2175
Trigeminal neuralgia, neurosurgical pain
  management for, 2195
Trigeminal tractotomy, 2195
Trigger finger, 2157
Triglycerides, metabolism of, 44
Trigonocephaly, 2194
Triiodotyrosine (T$_3$), 1288
 serum total, 1292
 T$_3$ resin uptake test and, 1292
Trimethoprim-sulfamethoxazole,
  spectrum of activity of, 169t
Triolein breath test, 872
Tripod fractures, repair of, 307
Triskelion, 32
TRISS methodology, 277–278
 children and, 385
Truncus arteriosus, 1494f, 1494–1495
Trunk reconstruction, 2286f, 2287, 2287f
Trypsinogen, pancreatic secretion of,
  866–867
Tubercle of Zuckerandl, 1286, 1286f
Tuberculosis
 esophagitis in, 724–725
 pericarditis associated with, 1576
Tuboovarian abscesses, 2224–2225
Tubular duplications, 2075, 2075f
Tubular function, pediatric, 1987
Tubulin, 8
Tumor(s). *See* Cancer; Neoplastic disease;
  Oncogene(s); Oncogenesis;
  specific tumors and sites
Tumor cell(s)
 death or loss of, 469
 heterogeneity of, in breast cancer, 1385
Tumor cell cycle, 469, 469f, 470t
Tumor cell vaccines, 503
 for metastatic melanoma, 2242
Tumor growth fraction, 469, 469t
Tumor markers. *See* Biochemical markers
Tumor necrosis factor (TNF)

acute-phase response mediation by,
  132, 133t
 fibroblasts and, wound healing and,
  122–123, 124f
 gram-negative bacterial sepsis and, 175
 host defense and, 164–165
 inflammation and, 110–114, 111f
  mechanisms of injury and, 111–113,
   112f, 112t, 113f
  metabolic effects of tumor necrosis
   factor and, 113
  pathologic changes induced by
   tumor necrosis factor and, 111
  tumor necrosis factor kinetics and
   tolerance and, 113–114
 recombinant, for cancer, 510, 510t
 in shock, 194
 surgical stress response and, 50
 thrombomodulin expression regulation
  by, 87
Tumor-specific transplantation antigens
  (TSTAs), 462f, 463
Tumor-suppressor genes, 471, 472t, 478,
  480f
Tumor volume doubling time, 466, 466f,
  467f
Turcot syndrome, 1115, 1120
Two-pillow orthopnea, 1508

U

Ulcer(s)
 anorectal, in HIV-positive patients,
  1205
 Cushing, 777
 decubitus, healing of, 80
 esophageal, in gastroesophageal reflux
  disease, 683
 of foot, healing of, 80
 ischemic, 1940
  in infrainguinal occlusive disease,
   1812
 of leg, healing of, 80
 in melanomas, 2236
 neurotrophic, 1940
 peptic
  gastric. *See* Gastric ulcers
  stress. *See* Stress gastritis
 of stump, following lower extremity
  amputation, 1836
 venous, 1940
  in chronic venous insufficiency,
   management of, 1965
Ulcerative colitis, 1093–1108. *See also*
  Inflammatory bowel disease
 causes of, 1094–1095
 clinical features of, 1096
 Crohn's disease versus, 1096, 1097t
 diagnosis of, 1096–1097, 1097f, 1097t
 epidemiology of, 1093–1094
 medical management of, 1097–1098
 pathology of, 1095t, 1095–1096
 surgical management of, 1098–1106
  approaches for, 1100–1106
  indications for, 1098–1100
   extracolonic disease as, 1098–1099
   intractable disease as, 1098
   prophylactic, for cancer, 1099
   surgical emergencies and, 1099–
    1100
Ulnar artery, anatomy of, 1687
Ulnar nerve, 2153, 2153f
 disorders of, 2156, 2197

Ultimate load, 2142
Ultrasonography
 abdominal
  in cholelithiasis, 1041, 1042f
  in hepatocellular carcinomas,
   pediatric, 2135–2136
 in appendicitis, 1254–1255, 1255f
 for atherosclerotic plaque ablation,
  1737
 in bile duct cancer, 1061, 1061f
 in biliary atresia, 2086
 of breasts, 1365, 1366f
 in chronic pancreatitis, 892
 Doppler. *See* Doppler studies
 duplex. *See* Duplex scanning
 endoscopic
  in gastric adenocarcinomas, 798–799
  in pancreatic cancer, 908, 908f
  in esophageal cancer, 704
 hydrocolonic, in colorectal adenomas,
  1115
 intraoperative
  in cancer, 490
  real-time, in insulinomas, 922, 922f
 intravascular, 1742–1745, 1743f, 1744f
 of liver, 935, 936f
 in pancreatitis, 883
 real-time B-mode
  in insulinomas, 922, 922f
  in vascular disorders, 1668, 1669f
   abdominal aortic aneurysms,
    1883–1884, 1884f
 of renal artery, in renovascular
  hypertension, 1787–1788
 in solitary thyroid nodule, 1300
 of thyroid gland, 1294
 transabdominal, in liver masses, 1009,
  1010f
 transcutaneous, in pancreatic cancer,
  906
 transrectal, in prostate cancer, 2210–
  2211
 in traumatic injuries, in pregnancy,
  392
 in ureteropelvic junction obstruction,
  2103f, 2104
 in vascular infections, 1724–1725
Ultraviolet radiation (UVR)
 aging of skin and, 2269
 basal cell carcinomas of skin and, 2242
 melanomas and, 2231
 squamous cell carcinomas of skin and,
  2242
Umbilical anomalies, with Meckel's
  diverticulum, 2071
Umbilical cord, hernias of. *See*
  Omphaloceles
Umbilical hernias, 1215–1216, 1217,
  1226–1227, 1227f, 2032
 anatomy and embryology of, 2032
 clinical issues with, 2032
 operative considerations and outcome
  of, 2032
 pediatric, 1226–1227, 1227f
Undernutrition. *See* Nutrition, deficits of
Uniform Anatomical Gift Act, 562–563
United Network for Organ Sharing
  (UNOS), 563, 564f
Univentricular heart, 1498–1499, 1499f
Universal precautions, 179
Unna boots, for chronic venous
  insufficiency, 1940
Unstable angina, 1538

Upper esophageal sphincter (UES), manometric assessment of, 666
Upper extremities
arteries of, anatomy of, 1687
blood pressure measurement in, 1671–1672, 1672f
brachioplasty and, 2272t, 2276–2277, 2277f
compartment syndromes in, 1642
fractures of, fixation of, 376
hands. *See* Hands
vascular occlusive disease of, 1758–1764
clinical examination for, 1759
diagnosis of, 1761–1763
of distal arterial lesions, 1762–1763, 1763f, 1764f
of proximal arterial lesions, 1761–1762, 1763f
history taking in, 1758–1761, 1759t
laboratory examination for, 1760
noninvasive examination for, 1759–1760
radiographic examination for, 1760f–1762f, 1760–1761
symptoms of, 1758–1759
treatment of, 1764
vascular trauma to, 370, 372f
Upper gastrointestinal series, in duodenal injuries, 345
Up-regulation, 1338–1339
Urachal abnormalities, 2105–2106
Urea, synthesis of, 46–47
Ureidopenicillins, spectrum of activity of, 169t
Uremia
pericarditis in, 1576
platelet disorders in, 95
Uremic acidosis. *See* Metabolic acidosis
Ureter(s)
carcinomas of, 2208
duplication of, 2104f, 2104–2105
megaureters and, 2104
traumatic injuries of, 350f, 358–359
ureteroceles and, 2105
vesicoureteral reflux and, 2105, 2106f
Ureteroceles, 2105
Ureteropelvic junction (UPJ) obstruction, 2103f, 2103–2104, 2104f
Ureteroscopic stone removal, 2205–2206
Urethra. *See also specific disorders*
female, development and anatomy of, 2216
male, physiology of, 2199
pediatric, 2106–2109
posterior valves and, 2108–2109
Urethral injuries, 358, 359–361, 361f
pediatric, 384
Uridine diphosphoglucuronate glucuronyl (UDP) transferases
bilirubin, deficiency of, gene therapy for, 518–519
hepatic biotransformation and, 956
Urinary bladder. *See* Bladder
Urinary diversion, for bladder cancer, 2207, 2208f
Urinary incontinence, 2199–2200
Urinary lithiasis, 2204f, 2204t, 2204–2206
calculus formation in, 2204
diagnosis of, 2204–2205
treatment of, 2205t, 2205–2206, 2206f
for distal ureteral stones, 2206

for mid-ureteral stones, 2206
for renal and proximal ureteral stones, 2206
Urinary tract. *See* Genitourinary system; *specific organs*
Urinary tract infections (UTIs), 176
in ureteral duplication, 2105
Urodilatin, 247
Urogenital organs, nerve supply of, 1184–1186, 1187f
Urogenital sinus defects, 2116
Urography
excretory, in renal cell carcinomas, 2208
hypertensive, in renovascular hypertension, 1788–1789
Urokinase, 99–100, 100f, 100t, 1707, 1737–1738
for deep venous thrombosis, 101
Urologic disorders, acute abdomen and, 1249–1250
Ursodeoxycholic acid (UDCA), for cholelithiasis, 1047
Utah total artificial heart, 1561
Uterine disorders. *See also specific disorders*
abnormal bleeding, 2223–2224
abnormal cervical cytology and, 2221–2222, 2222f
aplasia, 2116–2117
ascending genital infections, 2224f, 2224–2225, 2225t
carcinomas, 2222–2223, 2224
cervical atresia, 2116
endometrial hyperplasia, 2223
fallopian tube anomalies and, 2117
hypoplasia, 2116
introital, 2117
leiomyomas, 2224
rupture, 393
sarcomas, 2223
toxic shock syndromes, 2225
Uterus, 2116–2117, 2221–2225. *See also* Pregnancy
activity of, in traumatic injuries, in pregnancy, 392
development and anatomy of, 2216, 2217
duplication of, 2117, 2117f
Uvomorulin, 9–10

V

Vaccines, tumor cell, 503
Vagal nerves, 746–747, 747f
Vagina, 2114–2115, 2220–2221
atresia of, 2114–2115, 2115f, 2116f
carcinomas of, 2220
cloacal abnormalities of, 2116
development and anatomy of, 2216
intraepithelial neoplasia of, 2220
prolapse of, 2220–2221, 2221f
urogenital sinus defects of, 2116
Vaginal intraepithelial neoplasia (VAIN), 2220
Vagotomy
cholelithiasis and, 1035

for duodenal ulcers, 766f, 766–767
gastric, proximal
for duodenal ulcers, 767–768
for gastric ulcers, 786, 786f, 787
physiologic consequences of, 768
parietal cell, for gastrinomas, 924
truncal
for duodenal ulcers, 767, 768f
for gastric ulcers, 786, 787f
physiologic consequences of, 768t, 768–769
Valvular heart disease, 1503–1532
anatomy and pathology and, 1503f, 1503–1506, 1504f, 1504t–1506t
anticoagulation for, 1529t, 1529–1531
complications of, 1530
contraindications to, 1530–1531
indications for, 1529–1530
congestive heart failure and, 1506–1509
diagnosis of, 1512–1513
electrocardiography in, 1513
physical examination in, 1512t, 1512–1513
endocarditis and, 1531–1532
management of, 1531–1532, 1532f, 1532t
pathology of, 1531
presentation of, 1531
imaging in, 1513–1516
cardiac catheterization, 1514t, 1514–1515, 1515f
chest roentgenography, 1513
echocardiography, 1513–1515
radionuclide angiography, 1515–1516
medical management of, 1516fm 1516t, 1516–1517
for congestive heart failure, 1516–1517
myocardial failure and, 1507f, 1507–1509, 1508f
peripheral manifestations of, 1508–1509
pathophysiology of, 1506, 1507f, 1509–1512
of aortic insufficiency, 1511
of aortic stenosis, 1510–1511
of mitral regurgitation, 1511–1512
of mitral stenosis, 1509f, 1509–1510, 1510t
of multivalvular disease, 1512
of tricuspid stenosis, 1512
surgical management of, 1518–1529
indications for, 1518, 1519f
options for, 1518–1519, 1519f
postoperative care and, 1527–1528, 1528f
preoperative care and, 1519
prosthetic valves and, 1525f, 1525–1527, 1526f
complications of, 1526f, 1526–1527
hemodynamics and, 1526, 1526t
results with, 1528–1529
functional, 1529
hemodynamic, 1529
mortality and, 1528–1529, 1529f
surgical technique for, 1519–1525
for cardiopulmonary bypass, 1520, 1520f
for mitral valve repair, 1520–1521, 1521f, 1522f

Valvular heart disease, surgical technique
for (continued)
for valve replacement, 1521, 1523,
1523f, 1524f, 1525
Valvuloplasty, balloon, 1518
aortic, percutaneous, 1518
Vancomycin
for Clostridium difficile colitis, 1177–
1178
prophylactic, for endocarditis, 1532t
spectrum of activity of, 169t
Van't Hoff equation, 244
Variant angina, 1538
Varicella-zoster virus (VZV) infections, 178
Varices, gastroesophageal, 1165–1167,
1166f
in portal hypertension, 986
local factors and, 986
portal and variceal pressure and, 986
variceal size and appearance and,
986, 986t
treatment of, 993–1005
choice of therapy for, 993, 993t
devascularization and transection
procedures for, 1004f, 1005,
1005f
endoscopic ligation for, 996f, 997f,
998–1000
endoscopic sclerotherapy for. See
Endoscopic therapy,
sclerotherapy
medical, 993–994
portosystemic shunts for. See
Portosystemic shunts
prophylactic, 996–998
Varicoceles, 2203
Varicose veins, 1938–1939
in congenital vascular malformations,
1925–1926, 1926f–1928f
primary and secondary, 1938
treatment of, 1938–1939
Vascular access. See also Vascular
catheters/catheterization
in burn patients, 434
for endovascular surgery, 1734–1735
for interventional angiography, 1709
for laparoscopic therapy, 736, 737f,
738f
Vascular addressins, 152
Vascular bypass procedures
aortobifemoral, 1804, 1806f, 1807f
aortorenal, for renal hypertension,
1791f, 1791–1792
for axillosubclavian aneurysms, 1856f,
1856–1857
direct, for aortoiliac disease. See Aortic
reconstruction
iliofemoral, 1804–1805, 1807f
indirect, for aortoiliac disease, 1805,
1808f–1809f, 1808–1809
results of, 1810
nonanatomic, 1537
for renal hypertension, 1792
prosthetic, for infrainguinal occlusive
disease, 1823
saphenous vein, for infrainguinal
occlusive disease, 1817f–1821f,
1821–1823
complications of, 1821f, 1822t,
1822–1823
for thoracic aortic aneurysms, 1860,
1861f–1863f, 1862–1863
heparin-bonded shunts for, 1862–
1863

for thoracoabdominal aortic aneurysms.
See Thoracoabdominal aortic
aneurysms (TAAAs)
for upper extremity occlusive disease,
1764
venous, in-situ, angioscopy-assisted,
1741, 1742f
for venous obstruction, 1942f, 1943,
1965, 1965f
Vascular catheters/catheterization
arterial
atheroembolism associated with, 1632
in pediatric patients, 1981
cardiac catheterization
arteriovenous fistulas due to, 1923
in valvular heart disease, 1514t,
1514–1515, 1515f
catheter ablation and, for ventricular
arrhythmias, 1569, 1573–1574
central venous catheters
for monitoring fluid status, 252
in pediatric patients, 1981
placement technique for, 65–66,
1709
complications of
arteriovenous fistulas, 1923
atheroembolism, 1632
brachial artery injuries, 1763
femoral artery pseudoaneurysms,
1912
fragment retrieval, angiography and,
1708f, 1709
infectious, 176, 401
radial artery injuries, 1763
renal artery aneurysms, 1906
pulmonary artery
in pediatric patients, 1981–1982
in shock, 195–196, 196t, 197t
Vascular disorders. See also specific
disorders
diagnostic techniques for, 1668–1677.
See also specific techniques
clinical applications of, 1674–1677
methods and instruments for, 1668–
1669
physiologic and anatomic basis of,
1668
physiologic measurements and,
1669–1674
hernia repair and, 1220–1221
infections, 1720–1732
anatomic distribution of, 1721,
1722f, 1723t
classification of, 1721
clinical manifestations of, 1721, 1722
diagnosis of, 1724–1728
anatomic imaging techniques in,
1724–1727, 1725f–1727f
functional imaging techniques in,
1727
microbiologic testing and, 1728
management of, 1728f, 1728–1732,
1729t
for aortic infections, 1728–1730,
1729f, 1730t
for carotid artery infections, 1730
for femoropopliteal arterial
segment infections, 1730, 1731f
results and late outcome and,
1730, 1732
for suppurative thrombophlebitis,
1730
for visceral artery infections, 1730

pathophysiology of, 1722–1724
bacteriology and, 1724, 1724t
predisposing factors and, 1723–
1724
following vascular injuries, 366
injuries, 361–373
abdominal, 368–370, 370f–372f
complications of, 366
diagnosis of, 362–363, 363t
of extremities, 370, 372f, 373f
of neck, management of, 312–314
nonoperative management of, 363
operative management of, 363–366,
364t, 365f
outcome in, 370–371, 373
pathophysiology of, 362
pediatric, 385
of thoracic great vessels, 366–368,
367f–370f
malformations
congenital. See Congenital vascular
malformations (CVMs); specific
specific malformations
Dieulafoy, 1170
mesenteric tumors, 1240
occlusive. See Cerebrovascular
disease;Renal hypertension;
Upper extremities, vascular
occlusive disease of; Visceral
occlusive disease
pancreatitis and, 882
in shock. See Shock, microcirculatory
response to
venous
occlusive, hepatic, 991
peripheral, angiography in, 1701,
1702, 1705–1706
Vascular ectasia, colonic, hemorrhage in,
1167, 1168–1170, 1169f
Vascular endothelium, 1585
cell injury and, in inflammation, 156f,
157f, 158
inflammation and, 151–152
high endothelial venules and
lymphocytes and, 152
leukocyte adhesion to endothelial
cells and, 151f, 152
ischemic injury of, 1650, 1651f
as nonthrombogenic surface, 86, 87f
physiology of, 1609–1610, 1610f
tumor necrosis factor-induced injury
of, 111–113, 112f, 112t, 113f
Vascular grafts. See also Coronary artery
bypass grafting (CABG)
angioplastic thrombectomy for, 1741
aortobifemoral, 1804, 1806f, 1807f
in aortoiliac occlusive disease, patency
of, 1810
endoluminal, 1738–1739, 1739f
iliofemoral, 1804–1805, 1807f
infections of, 1721–1722
for infrainguinal occlusive disease. See
Infrainguinal occlusive disease,
operative treatment of
internal mammary artery, 1544
interposition, for coarctation of aorta,
1498
saphenous vein
crossover, for venous obstruction,
1965, 1965f
for traumatic injuries, 364
for traumatic injuries, 364

Vascular reservoir, as splenic function, 1266
Vascular rings
  esophageal, 730–731
  in pediatric patients, 2016–2017
    complete, 2016–2017
    incomplete, 2017
Vascular surgery. *See also* Endosurgery, vascular
  reconstructive, for traumatic injuries, 364–366, 365f
Vascular testing, in impotence, 2201
Vasculitis. *See* Arteritis
Vas deferens obstructions, 2203
Vasoactive intestinal polypeptide (VIP), biliary tract regulation by, 1031
Vasoconstriction
  in shock, 189
  shock and, 185–186
Vasodilation
  gastric, 757
  neurogenic shock and, 183
  shock and, 185–186
Vasodilators. *See also specific drugs*
  for shock, 206
Vasography, in male infertility, 2203
Vasopressin
  for gastroesophageal varices, 993–994, 1166
    endoscopic sclerotherapy versus, 995
  for stress gastritis, 1165
Vasospastic disease, diagnostic techniques for, 1676
VATER (VACTERL) associations, with anorectal malformations, 2043
Vecuronium, 440t
Vein(s). *See also specific veins and venous disorders*
  blood flow in, 1937–1938
  deep, disorders of, 1939–1943. *See also specific disorders*
  insufficiency of. *See* Chronic venous insufficiency (CVI)
  of lower extremities, 1935–1937, 1936f–1938f
    pressure in, 1937
  perforating, 1936
    ligation of, 1941, 1941f, 1943
  physiology of, 1937–1938, 1939f
  structure of, 1585–1586, 1586f
  superficial, disorders of, 1938–1939
    treatment of, 1938–1939
  valves of, 1936–1937
    absence of. *See* Chronic venous insufficiency (CVI)
    incompetence of, 1939–1940
    surgery of, 1942f, 1943
  varicose, 1938–1939
    in congenital vascular malformations, 1925–1926, 1926f–1928f
    primary and secondary, 1938
    treatment of, 1938–1939
  vessel wall damage and, deep venous thrombosis and, 1945–1946
Vena cava. *See also* Inferior vena cava (IVC)
  superior vena cava syndrome and, 1472
  thrombosis of, following hepatic transplantation, 595
  traumatic injuries of, 369–370

Vena caval interruption
  for deep venous thrombosis, 1950f, 1950–1951
  for venous thromboembolism, 103
Venoconstriction, in shock, 188–189
Venodilation, neurogenic shock and, 183
Venography
  contrast, in chronic venous insufficiency, 1960–1962, 1963f
  in deep venous thrombosis, 1946f, 1946–1947
Venolymphatic insufficiency, reconstructive surgery for, 2289
Venous admixture, 219
Venous disorders. *See also specific disorders*
  occlusive, hepatic, 991
  peripheral, angiography in, 1701, 1702, 1705–1706
Venous eczema, 1959
Venous lakes, 1935
Venous obstruction, in chronic venous insufficiency, management of, 1965, 1965f
Venous oxygen saturation monitoring. *See* Oximetry, venous
Venous pressure, ambulatory, in chronic venous insufficiency, 1962
Venous saturation monitoring, in critically ill patients, 217–218, 218f
Venous stasis
  deep venous thrombosis and, 1944–1945, 1945f
  in morbid obesity, 790
Venous thrombosis. *See also* Deep venous thrombosis (DVT); Pulmonary thromboembolism; Thrombophlebitis
  mesenteric, 1776, 1778
  peripheral arterial embolism arising from, 1623–1624
  prophylaxis of, heparin for, 96
Venous ulcers, 1940
  in chronic venous insufficiency, management of, 1965
Ventilation
  carbon dioxide metabolism and, 218, 218f, 219f
  dead-space, 1984
  mechanical. *See* Mechanical ventilation
  monitoring, postoperative, 448–450
  of organ donors, 563
Ventilation/perfusion matching, 1984
Ventilatory support. *See also* Mechanical ventilation
  pediatric, 1985–1986
    classification of positive-pressure ventilators for, 1985, 1985f
    complications of, 1986
    in neonates, 1986
    pediatric, 1986
    ventilatory modes for, 1985–1986
Ventral hernias, diagnosis of, 1217
Ventral nerve roots, 2186
Ventricular assist devices (VADs), 1554t, 1554–1558
  nonpulsatile, 1554–1555
    axial flow pumps, 1555, 1556f
    centrifugal, 1555, 1555f
    roller-head pumps, 1554–1555

  permanent, 1559–1561
    HeartMate VE, 1559
    Novacor N100, 1559–1560
    Penn State, 1560f, 1560–1561
  pulsatile, 1555–1558
    Abiomed BVS 5000, 1556, 1557f
    HeartMate 1000 IP, 1556, 1557f, 1558
    Novacor N1000, 1558, 1558f
    Pierce-Donachy, 1556, 1556f
Ventricular function
  coronary artery bypass grafting and, 1547
  in pediatric patients, 1982
Ventricular septal defect (VSD), 1485f, 1485–1487
  atrioventricular canal-type defects, 1485
  in double-outlet right ventricle, 1493–1494
  after myocardial infarction, as surgical indication, 1542
  perimembranous, 1485
  supracristal (infundibular; subarterial), 1485
  in tetralogy of Fallot, 1489
Ventricular septation procedures, for univentricular heart, 1499
Venules, anatomy of, 183, 184f, 185
Verner-Morrison syndrome, 919t, 925t, 925–926
Vertebral artery
  compression of, 1638–1639, 1639f
  traumatic injuries of, management of, 314, 314f, 315f
Vertebral artery reconstruction, 1757
Vertebrobasilar insufficiency, 1751
Very low-density lipoproteins (VLDLs), 816
  atherosclerosis and, 1711
Vesicoureteral reflux (VUR), 2105, 2106f
  ureteral duplication and, 2104–2105
Veterans Administration Cooperative Study, 1548–1549
Vibration syndrome, upper extremity occlusive disease and, 1763
Vinblastine, 502t
Vinca alkaloids, 502t
Vincristine, 502t
  for neuroblastomas, pediatric, 2122
  for Wilms tumor, 2125, 2126
Viperidae. *See* Bites and stings
VIPomas, 919t, 925t, 925–926
Viral infections, 177–179. *See also specific infections*
  as contraindication to organ donation, 560
  neonatal, 1992
Virchow triad, 1944–1945
Viruses
  as gene therapy vectors, 504t
  tumor induction by, 463–464, 464f, 469–470
Visceral arteries
  anatomy of, 1685f, 1685–1686, 1686f
  infections of, management of, 1730
Visceral occlusive disease, 1764–1778, 1765f
  acute, 1768–1769, 1771–1774
  anatomy and, 1765–1768, 1766f–1771f, 1772t
  causes of, 1773–1774, 1776t
    iatrogenic, 1773, 1775f
  chronic, 1775–1780

Visceral occlusive disease (*continued*)
   pathophysiology of ischemic injury
      and, 1768
   recognition of intestinal viability and,
      1774, 1776t
      second-look procedures for, 1774
Visceral pain, abdominal, 1246, 47048
Visceral veins, anatomy of, 1686–1687,
   1687f
Viscoelastic properties, of soft tissues,
   2142
Vital capacity, 1983
   myocardial failure and, 1508
Vital signs, lack of, after chest trauma, in
   elderly people, 388
Vitamin(s)
   absorption of, from small intestine, 816
   for critically ill patients, 230
   hepatic metabolism of, 957
   pediatric requirements for, 1976t, 1977
   requirements in surgical patients, 62t
   vitamin A (retinol)
      intoxication by, hypercalcemia and,
         1315
      pediatric requirement for, 1976t,
         1977
      requirements in surgical patients, 62t
      wound healing and, 78, 2282
   vitamin B (thiamine)
      deficiency of, following gastric
         surgery for morbid obesity, 793
      pediatric requirement for, 1976t
      requirements in surgical patients, 62t
   vitamin B_2 (riboflavin)
      pediatric requirement for, 1976t
      requirements in surgical patients, 62t
   vitamin B_6 (pyridoxine)
      pediatric requirement for, 1976t
      requirements in surgical patients, 62t
   vitamin B_{12}
      absorption from small intestine, 816
      pediatric requirement for, 1976t
      requirements in surgical patients, 62t
   vitamin C (ascorbic acid)
      pediatric requirement for, 1976t
      requirements in surgical patients, 62t
      wound healing and, 78
   vitamin D (ergocalciferol)
      calcium and phosphate metabolism
         and, 1313, 1313f
      deficiency of, hypocalcemia and,
         1317
      intoxication by, hypercalcemia and,
         1315
      pediatric requirement for, 1976t,
         1977
      requirements in surgical patients, 62t
   vitamin E (tocopherol)
      pediatric requirement for, 1976t, 1977
      requirements in surgical patients, 62t
      wound healing and, 78
   vitamin K (phylloquinone)
      pediatric requirement for, 1977
      requirements in surgical patients, 62t
      wound healing and, 78–79
Vitelline duct. *See* Meckel's diverticulum
Volcano lesions, in *Clostridium difficile*
   colitis, 1176
Volume assist ventilation, 1986
Volume control ventilation, 1986
Volume resuscitation. *See also* Fluid and
      electrolyte therapy; Fluid
      therapy

for shock
   hypovolemic, 198
   neurogenic, 204
   septic, 203
Volvulus, 827
   midgut, 2055
Vomiting
   anesthesia and, 451f, 452
   in pancreatic cancer, palliative
      treatment for, 914
Von Hippel-Lindau disease, 2178, 2208
Von Recklinghausen disease. *See*
   Neurofibromas
Von Willebrand factor (vWF), deficiency
   of, 93, 94f
VP-16 (etoposide), 502t
   for neuroblastomas, pediatric, 2122
Vulva, 2217–2220
   Bartholin gland abscesses of, 2218
   carcinomas of, 2218, 2219t
   development and anatomy of, 2217
   intraepithelial neoplasia and, 2217–
      2218
   necrotizing fasciitis of, 2218, 2220
Vulvar intraepithelial neoplasia (VIN),
   2217–2218
Vulvectomy, radical, for carcinomas,
   2218

W

Wangensteen-Rice invertogram, 2044f,
   2044–2045
Warfarin, 97f, 97–98, 98f, 1619
   for deep venous thrombosis, 1949
Warren shunt, 1001f, 1002
Warthin tumors, of salivary glands, 641,
   641t
Wasp stings, 407–408
Water
   absorption of, from small intestine,
      812–813
   balance of, sodium concentration and,
      245, 246f
   flow across cell membranes, 14–15, 15f
   losses of
      insensible, 248, 249, 249t
         pediatric, 1988
      normal, 248–249, 249t
   pediatric requirements for, 1974, 1988,
      1988t
   renal handling of, in chronic liver
      disease, 980
Water channels, 18
Water intoxication, pediatric, 1989
Water moccasin bites. *See* Bites and
   stings
Weight loss
   in chronic pancreatitis, 891
   in esophageal cancer, 702
Western immunotransblot, for human
      immunodeficiency virus
      detection, 178f, 178–179
Whipple procedure, for bile duct cancer,
   1062
Whipple triad, 921, 921t, 2098
Whole-brain irradiation
   for gestational trophoblastic neoplasia,
      2229, 2229f
   for metastatic intracranial tumors, 2179
Wilms tumor, 2122–2126
   adult and neonatal, 2126

associated conditions and
      epidemiology of, 2122–2123,
      2123t
   basic science of, 2123
   bilateral, 2126
   extrarenal, 2126
   future directions for, 2126
   pathology of, 2123, 2124f
   presentation, workup, and staging of,
      2123–2125, 2124f, 2125f, 2125t
   renal vein and inferior vena cava
      involvement with, 2126
   treatment of, 2125–2126
Wire localization biopsy, of breast
   masses, 1369–1370, 1371f
Witzel jejunostomy, 65
Wolff-Parkinson-White (WPW) syndrome,
   1567, 1567f
   surgical management of, 1571, 1571f,
      1571t, 1573t, 1573–1574
Wound(s)
   burn. *See* Burns
   localization of, cytokine-induced, 51
Wound healing, 67–83, 68f
   of acute wounds, 75–77
      clinical features of, 76f, 76–77
      wound contraction and, 75–76
   of chronic wounds, 77
   clinical implications of, 74–75
   cytokines and, 119–126, 120f, 121f,
         121t. *See also specific cytokines*
      angiogenesis and, 120–121, 122f
      fibroblasts and. *See* Fibroblast(s)
   epithelialization and, 72–74, 73f–74f,
         75, 76, 76f
   of fetal wounds, 83
   granulation tissue and, 119–120
   inflammatory phase of, 67–68, 68t,
         69f–70f
   moist conditions for, 76, 76f
   proliferative phase of, 68–69, 71f, 71t
   remodeling phase of, 70–71, 72f
   scarring and. *See* Scars
   vitamin A and, 2282
Wound infections, 170
   following lower extremity amputation,
         1835–1836
   posttraumatic, 400–401
Wound management, 77–82
   antibiotic drugs for, 81–82
   for burn wounds. *See* Burns
   for chronic wounds, 79–80
   débriding agents for, 82
   dressings for, 80–81, 81t
      for open wounds, 77–78
   in maxillofacial injuries, 304
   pharmacologic agents for, 82, 82t
   of surgical incisions, 77
   sutures in, 75
   systemic factors affecting, 78–79
   in vascular injuries, 365–366
Wrist, arthroscopy of, 2162f, 2162–2163

X

Xanthogranulomas, retroperitoneal,
   1238–1239
Xanthomas, of hands, 2162
Xenotransplantation, 555
Xerocytosis, hereditary, 1267

Y

Y chromosomes, 2111
Years of productive life lost (YPLL),
    269
Yield point, 2142

Z

Zenker diverticula, 670–674, 726f, 726–
    728, 727f
  investigation of, 672, 672f

pathophysiology of, 670, 671f, 672
  treatment of, 672–674, 673f
Zinc
  hepatic metabolism of, 957
  requirements in surgical patients, 62t
  wound healing and, 78
Zollinger-Ellison syndrome, 919t, 923t,
    923–925, 924f
  in multiple endocrine neoplasia, 1326–
    1327
  pediatric, 2097

Zona fasciculata, 1331, 1333f
Zona glomerulosa, 1331, 1333f
Zona reticularis, 1331, 1333f
Z-plasty, for pilonidal sinuses, 1199–
    1200
Zuckerandl, tubercle of, 1286, 1286f
Zygoma, anatomy of, 299
Zygomatic arch fractures, repair of,
    307